CEREBROSPINAL FLUID NORMAL VALUES

Bilirubin	0
Cells	0-5/mm^3, all lymphocytes
Chloride	110-129 mEq/L
Glucose	48-86 mg/dl or ≥60% of serum glucose
pH	7.34-7.43
Pressure	7-20 cm water
Protein, lumbar	15-45 mg/dl
Albumin	58%
α_1-globulins	9%
α_2-globulins	8%
β-globulins	10%
γ-globulins	10 (5-12)%
Protein, cisternal	15-25 mg/dl
Protein, ventricular	5-15 mg/dl

ENDOCRINOLOGIC NORMAL VALUES

Hormone and Metabolite Normal Values

Adrenocorticotropin (ACTH), serum	15-100 pg/ml
Aldosterone (mean ± standard deviation)	
Serum	
210 mEq/day sodium diet	
Supine	48 ± 29 pg/ml
Upright (2 hr)	65 ± 23 pg/ml
110 mEq/day sodium diet	
Supine	107 ± 45 pg/ml
Upright (2 hr)	532 ± 228 pg/ml
Urine	5-19 µg/24 hr
Calcitonin, serum	
Basal	0.15-0.35 ng/ml
Stimulated	<0.6 ng/ml
Catecholamines, free urinary	<110 µg/24 hr
Chorionic gonadotropin, serum	
Pregnancy	
First month	10-10,000 mIU/ml
Second and third months	10,000-100,000 mIU/ml
Second trimester	10,000-30,000 mIU/ml
Third trimester	5000–15,000 mIU/ml
Nonpregnant	<3 mIU/ml
Cortisol	
Serum	
8 AM	5-25 µg/dl
8 PM	<10 µg/dl
Cosyntropin stimulation (30-90 min after 0.25 mg cosyntropin intramuscularly or intravenously)	>10 µg/dl rise over baseline
Overnight suppression (8 AM serum cortisol after 1 mg dexamethasone orally at 11 PM)	≤5 µg/dl
Urine	20-70 µg/24 hr
C-peptide, serum	0.28-0.63 pmol/ml
11-Deoxycortisol, serum	
Basal	0-1.4 µg/dl
Metyrapone stimulation (30 mg/kg orally 8 hr prior to level)	>7.5 µg/dl
Epinephrine, plasma	<35 pg/ml
Estradiol, serum	
Male	20-50 pg/ml
Female	25-200 pg/ml

Estrogens, urine (increased during pregnancy; decreased after menopause)	*Male*	*Female*
Total	4-25 µg/24 hr	5-100 µg/24 hr
Estriol	1-11 µg/24 hr	0-65 µg/24 hr
Estradiol	0-6 µg/24 hr	0-14 µg/24 hr
Estrone	3-8 µg/24 hr	4-31 µg/24 hr

Etiocholanolone, serum	<1.2 µg/dl
Follicle-stimulating hormone, serum	
Male	2-18 mIU/ml
Female	
Follicular phase	5-20 mIU/ml
Peak midcycle	30-50 mIU/ml
Luteal phase	5-15 mIU/ml
Postmenopausal	>50 mIU/ml
Free thyroxine index, serum	1-4 ng/dl
Gastrin, serum (fasting)	30-200 pg/ml
Growth hormone, serum	
Adult, fasting	<5 ng/ml
Glucose load (100 g orally)	<5 ng/ml
Levodopa stimulation (500 mg orally in a fasting state)	>5 ng/ml rise over baseline within 2 hr
17-Hydroxycorticosteroids, urine	
Male	2-12 mg/24 hr
Female	2-8 mg/24 hr
5′-Hydroxyindoleacetic acid (5′-HIAA), urine	2-9 mg/24 hr
Insulin, plasma	
Fasting	6-20 µU/ml
Hypoglycemia (serum glucose <50 mg/dl)	<5 µU/ml
17-Ketosteroids, urine	
Under 8 years old	0-2 mg/24 hr
Adolescent	0-18 mg/24 hr
Adult	
Male	8-18 mg/24 hr
Female	5-15 mg/24 hr
Luteinizing hormone, serum	
Male adult	2-18 mIU/ml
Female adult	
Basal	5-22 mIU/ml
Ovulation	30-250 mIU/ml
Postmenopausal	>30 mIU/ml
Metanephrines, urine	<1.3 mg/24 hr
Norepinephrine	
Plasma	150-450 pg/ml
Urine	<100 µg/24 hr
Parathyroid hormone, serum	
C-terminal	150-350 pg/ml
N-terminal	230-630 pg/ml
Pregnanediol, urine	
Female	
Follicular phase	<1.5 mg/24 hr
Luteal phase	2.0-4.2 mg/24 hr
Postmenopausal	0.2-1.0 mg/24 hr
Male	<1.5 mg/24 hr
Progesterone, serum	
Female	
Follicular phase	0.02-0.9 ng/ml
Luteal phase	6-30 ng/ml
Male	<2 ng/ml
Prolactin, serum	
Nonpregnant	
Day	5-25 ng/ml
Night	20-40 ng/ml
Pregnant	150-200 ng/ml
Radioactive iodine (^{131}I) uptake (RAIU)	5%-25% at 24 hr (varies with iodine intake)
Renin activity, plasma (mean ± standard deviation)	
Normal diet	
Supine	1.1 ± 0.8 ng/ml/hr
Upright	1.9 ± 1.7 ng/ml/hr
Low-sodium diet	
Supine	2.7 ± 1.8 ng/ml/hr
Upright	6.6 ± 2.5 ng/ml/hr
Diuretics and low-sodium diet	10.0 ± 3.7 ng/ml/hr
Testosterone, total plasma	
Bound	
Adolescent male	<100 ng/dl
Adult male	300-1100 ng/dl
Female	25-90 ng/dl
Unbound	
Adult male	3-24 ng/dl
Female	0.09-1.30 ng/dl
Thyroid-stimulating hormone, serum	<10 µU/ml
Thyroxine (T_4), serum	
Total	4-11 µg/dl
Free	0.8-2.4 ng/dl
Thyroxine-binding globulin capacity, serum	15-25 µg T_4/dl
Thyroxine index, free	1-4 ng/dl
Tri-iodothyronine (T_3), serum	70-190 ng/dl
T_3 resin uptake	25%-45%
Vanillylmandelic acid (VMA), urine	1-8 mg/24 hr

Endocrine Function Tests

Adrenal gland	
Glucocorticoid suppression: overnight dexamethasone suppression test (8 AM serum cortisol after 1 mg dexamethasone orally at 11 PM)	≤5 μg/dl
Glucocorticoid stimulation: cosyntropin stimulation test (serum cortisol 30-90 min after 0.25 mg cosyntropin intramuscularly or intravenously)	>10 μg/ml more than baseline serum cortisol
Metyrapone test, single dose (8 AM serum deoxycortisol after 30 mg/kg metyrapone orally at midnight)	>7.5 μg/dl
Aldosterone suppression: sodium depletion test (urine aldosterone collected on day 3 of 200 mEq day/sodium diet)	<20 μg/24 hr
Pancreas	
Glucose tolerance test* serum glucose after 100 g glucose orally)	
60 min after ingestion	<180 mg/dl
90 min after ingestion	<160 mg/dl
120 min after ingestion	<125 mg/dl
Pituitary gland	
Adrenocorticotropic hormone (ACTH) stimulation. See Adrenal gland, Metyrapone test	
Growth hormone stimulation: insulin tolerance test (serum growth hormone after 0.1 U/kg regular insulin intravenously after an overnight fast to induce a 50% fall in serum glucose concentration or symptomatic hypoglycemia)	>5 ng/ml rise over baseline
Levodopa test (serum growth hormone after 0.5 g levodopa orally while fasting)	>5 ng/ml rise over baseline within 2 hr
Growth hormone suppression: glucose tolerance test (serum growth hormone after 100 g glucose orally after 8 hr fast)	<5 ng/ml within 2 hr
Luteinizing hormone (LH) stimulation: gonadotropin-releasing hormone (GnRH) test (serum LH after 100 μg GnRH intravenously or intramuscularly)	4- to 6-fold rise over baseline
Thyroid-stimulating hormone (TSH) stimulation: thyrotropin-releasing hormone (TRH) stimulation test (serum TSH after 400 μg TRH intraveneously)	>2-fold rise over baseline within 2 hr
Thyroid gland	
Radioactive iodine uptake (RAIU) suppression test (RAIU on day 7 after 25 μg tri-iodothyronine orally 4 times daily)	<10% to <50% baseline
Thyrotropin-releasing hormone (TRH) stimulation test. See Pituitary gland, Thyroid-stimulating hormone (TSH) stimulation	

*Add 10 mg/dl for each decade over 50 years of age.

HEMATOLOGIC NORMAL VALUES

Table 2. Differential cell count of bone marrow

Myeloid cells	
Neutrophilic series	
Myeloblasts	0.3%-5.0%
Promyelocytes	1%-8%
Myelocytes	5%-19%
Metamyelocytes	9%-24%
Bands	9%-15%
Segmented cells	7%-30%
Eosinophil precursors	0.5%-3.0%
Eosinophils	0.5%-4.0%
Basophilic series	0.2%-0.7%
Erythroid cells	
Pronormoblasts	1%-8%
Basophilic normoblasts	
Polychromatophilic normoblasts	7%-32%
Orthochromatic normoblasts	
Megakaryocytes	0.1%
Lymphoreticular cells	
Lymphocytes	3%-17%
Plasma cells	0%-2%
Reticulum cells	0.1%-2.0%
Monocytes	0.5%-5.0%
Myeloid/erythroid ratio	0.6-2.7

FOURTH EDITION

INTERNAL MEDICINE

Editor-in-Chief

JAY H. STEIN, MD

Section Editors

JOHN J. HUTTON, MD PETER O. KOHLER, MD
ROBERT A. O'ROURKE, MD HERBERT Y. REYNOLDS, MD
MARTIN A. SAMUELS, MD MERLE A. SANDE, MD
JERRY S. TRIER, MD NATHAN J. ZVAIFLER, MD

with 1185 illustrations

Mosby

St. Louis Baltimore Boston Chicago London Madrid Philadelphia Sydney Toronto

Mosby
Dedicated to Publishing Excellence

Publisher: George Stamathis
Acquisition Editor: Stephanie Manning
Developmental Editor: Kathryn H. Falk
Assistant Editor: Ellen Baker Geisel
Project Manager: Gayle May Morris
Production Editors: Sheila Walker, Lisa Nomura
Manufacturing Supervisor: Theresa Fuchs
Book and Cover Designer: Susan Lane
Logo Calligraphy: Charles Mullen

NOTE: The indications for and dosages of medications recommended conform to practices at the present time. References to specific products are incorporated to serve only as guidelines; they are not meant to exclude a practitioner's choice of other, comparable drugs. Many oral medications may be given with more scheduling flexibility than implied by the specific time intervals noted. Individual drug sensitivity and allergies must be considered in drug selection. Adult doses are provided as a gauge of the maximum dose commonly used.

Every attempt has been made to ensure accuracy and appropriateness. New investigations and broader experience may alter present dosages schedules, and it is recommended that the package insert of each drug be consulted before administration. Often there is limited experience with established drugs for neonates and young children. Furthermore, new drugs may be introduced, and indications for use may change. This rapid evolution is particularly noticeable in the use of antibiotics and cardiopulmonary resuscitation. The clinician is encouraged to maintain expertise concerning appropriate medications for specific conditions.

FOURTH EDITION

Printed in the United States of America
Composition by the Clarinda Company
Printing/binding by Rand McNally

Mosby-Year Book, Inc.
11830 Westline Industrial Drive
St. Louis, Missouri 63146

Library of Congress Cataloging in Publication Data

Internal medicine / editor-in-chief, Jay H. Stein ; section editors,
John J. Hutton . . . [et al.]. —4th ed.
p. cm.
Includes bibliographical references and index.
ISBN 0-8016-6911-1
1. Internal medicine. I. Stein, Jay H.
[DNLM: 1. Internal Medicine. WB 115 I605 1994]
RC46.I475 1994
616—dc20
DNLM/DLC
for Library of Congress 93-22168
CIP

93 94 95 96 97 / 9 8 7 6 5 4 3 2 1

Editors

Editor-in-Chief

JAY H. STEIN, M.D.
Professor of Medicine
Senior Vice President and Provost
University of Oklahoma Health Sciences Center
Oklahoma City, Oklahoma
Renal and Electrolyte Disorders
Special Topics in Internal Medicine

Section Editors

JOHN J. HUTTON, M.D.
Professor of Pediatrics and Medicine
Dean of College of Medicine
University of Cincinnati
Cincinnati, Ohio
Hematology and Oncology

PETER O. KOHLER, M.D.
President, Oregon Health Sciences University
Portland, Oregon
Endocrinology, Metabolism, and Genetics

ROBERT A. O'ROURKE, M.D.
Charles Conrad Brown Distinguished Professor
in Cardiovascular Disease
Director, Division of Cardiology
University of Texas Health Science Center, San Antonio
San Antonio, Texas
Diseases of the Heart and Blood Vessels

HERBERT Y. REYNOLDS, M.D.
J. Lloyd Huck Professor of Medicine
Chairman, Department of Medicine
Milton S. Hershey Medical Center
Pennsylvania State University
College of Medicine
Hershey, Pennsylvania
Pulmonary and Critical Care Medicine

MARTIN A. SAMUELS, M.D.
Professor of Neurology
Harvard Medical School
Chief of NeurologyBrigham and Women's Hospital
Boston, Massachusetts
Neurologic Disorders

MERLE A. SANDE, M.D.
Professor and Vice Chairman of Medicine
University of California, San Francisco
School of Medicine
Chief, Medical Service
San Francisco General Hospital
San Francisco, California
Infectious Diseases

JERRY S. TRIER, M.D.
Professor of Medicine
Harvard Medical School
Division of Gastroenterology
Senior Physician
Division of Gastroenterology
Brigham and Women's Hospital
Boston, Massachusetts
Alimentary Tract, Liver, Biliary Tree, and Pancreas

NATHAN J. ZVAIFLER, M.D.
Professor of Medicine
University of California, San Diego
Medical Center
San Diego, California
Clinical Immunology, Rheumatology, and Dermatology

To

Dr. Robert G. Petersdorf

the ombudsman of academic medicine

with the greatest fondness

Contributors

Richard S. Abrams, M.D.
Associate Clinical Professor of Medicine and Obstetrics and Gynecology, University of Colorado Health Sciences Center School of Medicine; Staff Physician, Rose Medical Center, Denver, Colorado

Shelley Albert, M.D.
Research Associate/Visiting Scientist, Renal-Electrolyte Division, University of Pennsylvania, Department of Medicine, Hospital of the University of Pennsylvania, Philadelphia, Pennsylvania

Joseph S. Alpert, M.D.
Professor of Medicine and Head, Department of Medicine, University of Arizona Health Science Center, Tucson, Arizona

Grant J. Anhalt, M.D.
Associate Professor, Department of Dermatology, Director, Immunodermatology Division, Johns Hopkins University School of Medicine, Baltimore, Maryland

Aśok C. Antony, M.D., F.A.C.P.
Professor of Medicine, Division of Hematology-Oncology, Department of Medicine, Indiana University School of Medicine, Indianapolis, Indiana

Frederick R. Appelbaum, M.D.
Professor of Medicine, University of Washington School of Medicine, Member, Fred Hutchinson Cancer Research Center, Seattle, Washington

Jane Appleby, M.D.
Assistant Professor, Department of Medicine, Medical Center Hospital, Audie L. Murphy Memorial Veterans Hospital; Co-Director, Medical Consultation Service, University of Texas Health Science Center, San Antonio, Texas

Michael D. Apstein, M.D.
Chief, Gastroenterology Section, Department of Medicine, Brockton/West Roxbury V.A. Medical Center, West Roxbury, Massachusetts; Associate Physician, Brigham and Women's Hospital, Assistant Professor of Medicine, Harvard Medical School, Boston, Massachusetts

Tomás Aragón, M.D., M.P.H.
Fellow, Infectious Diseases, University of California, San Francisco, School of Medicine, San Francisco, California

Gordon L. Archer, M.D.
Professor of Medicine and Microbiology/Immunology, Department of Medicine and Microbiology/Immunology, Medical College of Virginia; Chairman, Division of Infectious Diseases, Department of Medicine, Medical College of Virginia, Virginia Commonwealth University, Richmond, Virginia

John P. Atkinson, M.D.
Busch Professor and Chairman, Department of Medicine, Professor of Medicine and Molecular Microbiology, Washington University School of Medicine, St. Louis, Missouri

Vicki V. Baker, M.D.
Associate Professor and Director, Division of Gynecologic Oncology, University of Texas Medical School, Houston, Texas

George L. Bakris, M.D.
Director, Clinical Research, Hypertension Fellowship Program; Assistant Professor, Departments of Internal and Preventive Medicine, Rush-Presbyterian–St. Luke's Medical Center, Chicago, Illinois

Stanley P. Balcerzak, M.D.
Professor of Internal Medicine, Director, Division of Hematology and Oncology, Department of Internal Medicine, The James Cancer Hospital, Columbus, Ohio

H. Verdain Barnes, M.D.
Professor and Chairman, Department of Medicine, Wright State University School of Medicine, Dayton, Ohio

Richard J. Barohn, M.D.
Internal Medicine (Neurology), University of Texas Health Science Center at San Antonio, Medical Center Hospital, San Antonio, Texas

Françoise Basset, M.D.
Directeur de recherche INSERM, INSERM U82, Faculte Xavier Bichat, Paris, France

Richard L. Bauer, M.D., M.Sc.
Associate Professor, Department of Medicine, Audie L. Murphy Memorial Veterans Administration Hospital; Associate Chief of Staff for Ambulatory Care, San Antonio, Texas

Sabrina G. Beacham, R.EEG/EPT.
Lab Manager, Division of Electrodiagnostics, Thomas Jefferson University Hospital, Department of Neurology, Jefferson Medical College, Philadelphia, Pennsylvania
106 Electroencephalography and Evoked Responses

Lisa A. Beck, B.A., M.D.
Clinical Instructor of Dermatology, Johns Hopkins University, Baltimore, Maryland
327 Psoriasis
334 Dermatologic Manifestations of Gastrointestinal Disease

William S. Beckett, M.D., M.P.H.
Associate Professor of Medicine, Yale University School of Medicine, Attending Physician, Department of Internal Medicine, Yale-New Haven Hospital, New Haven, Connecticut
211 Occupational Lung Diseases

Norman H. Bell, M.D.
Professor of Medicine and Pharmacology, Medical University of South Carolina; Staff Physician, Ralph Johnson Veterans Affairs Medical Center, Charleston, South Carolina
182 Osteomalacia and Disorders of Vitamin D Metabolism

Rodney D. Bell, M.D.
Associate Professor of Neurology, Jefferson Medical College of Thomas Jefferson University; Attending Neurologist, Thomas Jefferson University Hospital, Philadelphia, Pennsylvania
106 Electroencephalography and Evoked Responses

George A. Beller, M.D.
Professor of Medicine, University of Virginia Health Sciences Center, Charlottesville, Virginia
5 Cardiac Noninvasive Techniques

Gordon R. Bernard, M.D.
Associate Professor of Medicine, Chief, Medical Intensive Care, Department of Internal Medicine, Vanderbilt University Hospital, Vanderbilt University Medical School, Nashville, Tennessee
202 Pulmonary Edema

Roger D. Bies, M.D.
Section of Cardiology, Baylor College of Medicine, Houston, Texas
2 Molecular Biology of Cardiovascular System

Timothy D. Bigby, M.D.
Assistant Professor, Department of Medicine, University of California, San Diego; Staff Physician, Department of Veterans Affairs Medical Center, San Diego, California
300 Asthma

John P. Bilezikian, M.D.
Attending Physician, Department of Medicine, Columbia-Presbyterian Medical Center; Professor of Medicine and Pharmacology, Chief, Division of Endocrinology, College of Physicians and Surgeons, Columbia University, New York, New York
177 Hypercalcemia
178 Hypocalcemia
187 Primary Hyperparathyroidism

Peter McL. Black, M.D., Ph.D.
Franc D. Ingraham Professor of Neurosurgery, Harvard Medical School; Neurosurgeon in Chief, Brigham and Women's Hospital and Children's Hospital, Boston, Massachusetts
131 Head Trauma

Joseph R. Bloomer, M.D.
Professor of Medicine, Director of Division of Gastroenterology, Hepatology, and Nutrition, Department of Medicine, University of Minnesota Hospital and Clinic, Minneapolis, Minnesota
176 Disorders of Porphyrin Metabolism

Harry G. Bluestein, M.D.
Professor of Medicine, University of California, San Diego, School of Medicine, La Jolla, California; Attending Physician, University of California, San Diego Medical Center, San Diego, California
297 Immunodeficiencies
302 Periarticular Rheumatic Complaints

David H. Boldt, M.D.
Professor of Medicine, Chief, Division of Hematology, University of Texas Health Science Center, San Antonio, Texas
81 Abnormal Nucleated Blood Cell Counts
82 Lymphadenopathy and Splenomegaly
92 Abnormalities of Phagocytes, Eosinophils, and Basophils

Kenneth D. Brandt, M.D.
Professor of Medicine, Head, Rheumatology Division, Indiana University School of Medicine, Indianapolis, Indiana
318 Osteoarthritis

Glenn D. Braunstein, M.D.
Professor of Medicine, University of California, Los Angeles, School of Medicine; Chairman, Department of Medicine, Cedars-Sinai Medical Center, Los Angeles, California
160 Disorders of the Hypothalamus and Anterior Pituitary

Debra L. Breneman, M.D.
Associate Professor, Department of Dermatology, University of Cincinnati College of Medicine, Cincinnati, Ohio
96 Melanoma, Kaposi's Sarcoma, and Mycosis Fungoides

Kenneth L. Brigham, M.D.
Professor of Medicine and Director, Center for Lung Research, Vanderbilt University School of Medicine, Nashville, Tennessee
202 Pulmonary Edema

Roy G. Brower, M.D.
Associate Professor of Medicine, Johns Hopkins University School of Medicine; Director, Medical Intensive Care Unit, Johns Hopkins Hospital, Baltimore, Maryland
192 Pulmonary Blood Flow

Adam P. Brown, M.D.
Department of Neurological Surgery, Washington University School of Medicine, St. Louis, Missouri
234 Brain Abscess and Perimeningeal Infections

Robert H. Brown, Jr., M.D., Ph.D.
Assistant Professor, Harvard Medical School; Associate Neurologist, Massachusetts General Hospital, Boston, Massachusetts
125 Muscle Disease

Richard E. Bryant, M.D.
Professor of Medicine, Director, Division of Infectious Diseases, Oregon Health Sciences University, Portland, Oregon
235 Skin and Subcutaneous Infections

Jean-Paul Butzler, M.D., Ph.D.
Professor and Chairman, Director World Health Organization Collab., Centre for Enteric Campylobacter, Department of Clinical Microbiology, St. Pierre University Hospital, Free University of Brussels, Belgium
266 Infections Caused by *Campylobacter* and *Helicobacter* Species

T. Edward Bynum, M.D.
Associate Professor, Department of Medicine, Harvard Medical School, Boston, Massachusetts
36 Abdominal Pain
44 Intestinal Obstruction and Peritonitis
46 Vascular Diseases of the Intestine

Grant L. Campbell, M.D.
Epidemiologist, Bacterial Zoonoses, Branch, Division of Vector-Borne Infectious Diseases, National Center for Infectious Diseases, Centers for Disease Control and Prevention, Fort Collins, Colorado
275 Infections Caused by *Borrelia* (Relapsing Fever and Lyme Disease)

Robert L. Capizzi, M.D.
Executive Vice President, Worldwide Research and Development, U.S. Bioscience, West Conshohocken, Pennsylvania
72 Principles of Treatment of Cancer

Louis R. Caplan, M.D.
Neurologist-in-Chief, Department of Neurology, New England Medical Center; Professor and Chairman, Neurology, Professor of Medicine, Tufts University School of Medicine, Boston, Massachusetts
120 Cerebrovascular Disease (Stroke)

Martin C. Carey, M.D., D.Sc.
Senior Physician, Department of Medicine, Brigham and Women's Hospital; Professor of Medicine, Department of Medicine, Harvard University Medical School, Boston, Massachusetts
51 Bile Production and Secretion
65 Biliary Tract Stones and Associated Diseases

Dennis A. Carson, M.D.
Professor of Medicine, Department of Medicine; Director, Sam And Rose Stein Institute for Research on Aging, University of California, San Diego, California
294 Rheumatoid Factors

John E. Carter, M.D.
Associate Professor, Departments of Medicine (Neurology) and Ophthalmology, University of Texas Health Science Center, San Antonio, Texas
134 Ocular Manifestations of Neurologic Disorders

Henry F. Chambers III, M.D.
Associate Professor of Medicine, Department of Medicine, University of California San Francisco School of Medicine; Head, Division of Infectious Diseases, San Francisco General Hospital, San Francisco, California
241 Fevers and Infections in Travelers

Charles K. Chan, M.D.
Assistant Professor of Medicine, University of Toronto Faculty of Medicine; Consultant in Respiratory and Critical Care Medicine, Wellesley and Princess Margaret Hospitals, Toronto, Canada
217 Pulmonary Thromboembolism

Kanu Chatterjee, M.B., F.R.C.P.
Professor of Medicine, Lucie Stern Professor of Cardiology, Associate Chief, Division of Cardiology, Department of Medicine, Moffitt/Long Hospitals; Director, Coronary Care Unit, Department of Medicine, University of California, San Francisco, California
13 Ischemic Heart Disease

Melvin D. Cheitlin, M.D.
Chief, Cardiology Division, San Francisco General Hospital; Professor of Medicine, University of California, San Francisco, California
24 Cardiac Tumors; Cardiac Manifestations of Endocrine, Collagen Vascular, and HIV Disease; and Traumatic Injury of the Heart

Neil S. Cherniack, M.D.
Professor of Medicine and of Physiology and Biophysics, Vice President for Academic Affairs; Dean, School of Medicine, Case Western Reserve University School of Medicine, Cleveland, Ohio
190 Abnormalities of the Control of Breathing

Sanjiv Chopra, M.D.
Associate Professor of Medicine, Harvard Medical School; Physician and Director, Clinical Hepatology, Beth Israel Hospital, Boston, Massachusetts
62 Liver Abscesses and Cysts
63 Hepatic Tumors
68 Diseases of the Peritoneum, Mesentery, and Omentum

Anthony W. Chow, M.D., F.R.C.P.(C)
Professor and Head, Division of Infectious Diseases, Department of Medicine, Vancouver General Hospital; Professor and Head, Division of Infectious Diseases, Department of Medicine, University of British Columbia, Vancouver, British Columbia, Canada
270 Infections Caused by *Bacteroides* and Other Mixed, Nonsporulating Anaerobes

Steven L. Chuck, M.D.
Assistant Research Physician, Department of Microbiology and Immunology, Department of Medicine, University of California, San Francisco, California
247 Rabies

Philip J. Clements, M.D.
Professor of Medicine, Division of Rheumatology, University of California, Los Angeles, School of Medicine, Los Angeles, California
317 Antirheumatic Drugs

William E. Clutter, M.D.
Associate Physician, Department of Medicine, Barnes Hospital; Associate Professor of Medicine, Department of Medicine, Washington University School of Medicine, St. Louis, Missouri
169 Hypoglycemia

C. Glenn Cobbs, M.D.
Chief, Medical Service, Veterans Affairs Medical Center; Professor and Vice Chairman for V.A. Affairs, University of Alabama, Birmingham, Alabama
239 Gram-Negative Bacteremia and the Sepsis Syndrome

Dewey J. Conces, Jr., M.D.
Associate Professor of Radiology, Indiana University School of Medicine, Indianapolis, Indiana
197 Pulmonary Diagnostic Imaging

J. Allen Cooper, Jr., M.D.
Associate Professor of Medicine, University of Alabama at Birmingham, School of Medicine; Chief, Pulmonary Section, Veterans Affairs Medical Center, Birmingham, Alabama
212 Adverse Pulmonary Reactions to Drugs and Other Therapeutic Modalities

Robert B. Couch, M.D.
Professor and Chairman, Department of Microbiology and Immunology, Baylor College of Medicine, Houston, Texas
245 Orthomyxovirus Infections (Influenza)

William G. Couser, M.D.
Head, Division of Nephrology, Professor of Medicine, Department of Medicine, University of Washington School of Medicine, Seattle, Washington
354 Glomerular Diseases

William F. Crowley, Jr., M.D.
Chief of Reproductive Endocrine Unit, Massachusetts General Hospital; Professor of Medicine, Department of Medicine, Harvard Medical School, Boston, Massachusetts
156 Amenorrhea
165 Disorders of the Ovary

Philip E. Cryer, M.D.
Physician, Department of Medicine, Barnes Hospital; Professor of Medicine, Department of Medicine, Washington University School of Medicine, St. Louis, Missouri
169 Hypoglycemia

Ralph G. Dacey, Jr., M.D.
Professor and Chairman, Department of Neurological Surgery, Washington University School of Medicine, St. Louis, Missouri
234 Brain Abscess and Perimeningeal Infections

James A. Dalen, M.D.
Professor of Medicine and Dean, College of Medicine, University of Arizona Health Science Center, Tucson, Arizona
20 Pulmonary Hypertensive Heart Disease

Walter J. Daly, M.D.
James O. Ritchey Professor of Medicine, Dean, Indiana University School of Medicine, Indianapolis, Indiana
189 Respiratory Pathophysiology

James H. Dauber, M.D.
Division of Pulmonary, Allergy, and Critical Medicine, Department of Medicine, University of Pittsburgh; Pulmonary Service, Veterans Administration Medical Center, Pittsburgh, Pennsylvania
220 Pulmonary Transplantation

John Davenport, M.D., C.M.
Assistant Chief, Neurology Service, Director, Clinical Neurophysiology Laboratory, Veterans Affairs Medical Center; Assistant Professor, Department of Neurology, University of Minnesota, Minneapolis, Minnesota
117 Epilepsy

David M. Dawson, M.D.
Chief, Neurology Service, Department of Neurology, Brockton/West Roxbury V.A. Hospital; Professor of Neurology, Harvard University, Boston, Massachusetts
121 Demyelinating Diseases

John L. Decker, M.D.
Scientist Emeritus, National Institutes of Health, Bethesda, Maryland
306 Systemic Lupus Erythematosus

Louis J. Dell'Italia, M.D.
Associate Professor of Medicine, Division of Cardiology, University of Alabama at Birmingham, Department of Medicine, Birmingham, Alabama
7 Chest Pain

David T. Dennis, M.D.
Chief, Bacterial Zoonoses, Branch, Division of Vector-Borne Infectious Diseases, National Center for Infectious Diseases, Centers for Disease Control and Prevention, Fort Collins, Colorado
275 Infections Caused by *Borrelia* (Relapsing Fever and Lyme Disease)

Peter Densen, M.D.
Professor, Department of Internal Medicine, The University of Iowa, Iowa City, Iowa
222 Basic Principals of Infectious Diseases
223 Host Defense Against Infection: The Roles of Antibody, Complement, and Phagocytic Cells

Colin Derdeyn, M.D.
Professor of Surgery and Radiology, Departments of Neurological Abscess, and Mallinckrodt Institute of Radiology, Washington University School of Medicine, St. Louis, Missouri
234 Brain Abscess and Perimeningeal Infections

Emmanuel N. Dessypris, M.D.
Professor of Medicine, Medical College of Virginia; Chief, Section of Hematology, Oncology, Department of Veterans Affairs, H.H. McGuire Medical Center, Richmond, Virginia
80 Abnormal Hematocrit

Gerald F. DiBona, M.D.
Professor and Vice Chairman, Department of Internal Medicine, University of Iowa College of Medicine; Chief, Medical Service, Veterans Affairs Medical Center, Iowa City, Iowa
359 Glomerular and Interstitial Hereditary Nephropathies

Renuka Diwan, M.D.
Director of Dermatologic Surgery, Assistant Professor, Departments of Dermatology and Otolaryngology/Head and Neck Surgery, Johns Hopkins Hospital, Baltimore, Maryland
326 Cutaneous Malignancies

Jeremiah P. Donovan, M.D.
Assistant Professor of Medicine, Department of Internal Medicine, University of Nebraska Medical Center, Omaha, Nebraska
64 Liver Transplantation

R. Gordon Douglas, Jr., M.D.
President, Merck Vaccine Division, Merck and Company, Inc., Whitehouse Station, New Jersey; Clinical Professor, Department of Medicine, Cornell University Medical College, New York, New York
244 Picornavirus Infections (Enterovirus and Rhinovirus)

Ian R.G. Dowdeswell, M.D.
Associate Professor, Indiana University School of Medicine; Chief, Pulmonary Section, Assistant Chief, Medical Service, Veterans Administration Medical Center, Indianapolis, Indiana
218 Pleural Diseases
219 Diseases of the Mediastinum

Thomas A. Drake, M.D.
Associate Professor of Pathology and Laboratory Medicine, University of California, Los Angeles, School of Medicine; Chief, Outpatient Laboratory, University of California, Los Angeles Medical Center, Los Angeles, California
226 Use of Laboratory Tests in Infectious Diseases

Frank W. Drislane, M.D.
Associate in Neurology, Beth Israel Hospital; Instructor, Department of Neurology, Harvard Medical School, Boston, Massachusetts
142 Neuropulmonology

Herbert L. DuPont, M.D.
Mary W. Kelsey Professor and Director, Center for Infectious Diseases, The University of Texas Medical School/School of Public Health, Hermann Hospital and Lyndon B. Johnson General Hospital, University of Texas Health Science Center, Houston, Texas
236 Gastrointestinal Infections

David T. Durack, M.B., D.Phil.
Professor, Departments of Medicine and Microbiology, Chief, Division of Infectious Diseases and International Health, Duke University Medical Center, Durham, North Carolina
256 Rickettsial Infections
265 Infections Caused by *Haemophilus* Species

Frances M. Dyro, M.D.
Assistant Professor of Neurology, Harvard Medical School, Boston, Massachusetts; Chief, Neuro-urology Laboratory, Brighton Medical Center, Portland, Maine
135 Neurology of the Lower Urinary Tract

J. Donald Easton, M.D.
Professor and Chairman, Department of Clinical Neurosciences, Brown University School of Medicine; Neurologist-in-Chief, Rhode Island Hospital, Providence, Rhode Island
105 Spinal Fluid Examination
111 Coma and Related Disorders
112 Faintness and Syncope

Gregory L. Eastwood, M.D.
President, State University of New York Health Science Center, Syracuse, New York
34 Gastrointestinal Bleeding
39 Gastritis and Other Gastric Diseases

John Edmeads, M.D.
Professor of Medicine (Neurology), University of Toronto; Head, Division of Neurology, Sunnybrook Health Science Center, Toronto, Ontario, Canada
113 Headache and Facial Pain

John E. Edwards, Jr., M.D.
Chief, Division of Infectious Diseases, Harbor/University of California, Los Angeles; Professor of Medicine, University of California Los Angeles Medical Center, Los Angeles, California
278 Infections Caused by *Candida, Actinomyces, and Nocardia* Species

M. Joycelyn Elders, M.D.
Professor of Pediatric Endocrinology, University of Arkansas College of Medicine; Attending Pediatrician and Director of Pediatric Endocrinology, Arkansas Children's Hospital, Little Rock, Arkansas
172 Lipodystrophies

George M. Eliopoulos, M.D.
Associate Professor of Medicine, Harvard Medical School; Assistant Chairman, Department of Medicine, New England Deaconess Hospital, Boston, Massachusetts
224 Principles of Anti-Infective Therapy

Murray Epstein, M.D.
Professor of Medicine, Department of Medicine, V.A. Medical Center and Jackson Memorial Medical Center; Professor of Medicine, Department of Medicine, University of Miami School of Medicine, Miami, Florida
351 Disorders of Sodium Balance

Marie-Claude Faugere, M.D.
Associate Research Professor, Division of Nephrology, Bone and Mineral Metabolism, Department of Internal Medicine, University of Kentucky Medical Center, Lexington, Kentucky
186 Renal Bone Disease

Mark Feldman, M.D.
Chief, Medical Service, Veterans Affairs Medical Center; Southland Distinguished Chair and Vice Chairman, Department of Internal Medicine, University of Texas Southwestern Medical Center, Dallas, Texas
27 Gastric Secretion
37 Nausea, Vomiting, and Anorexia

Steven R. Feldman, M.D., Ph.D.
Assistant Professor, Departments of Dermatology and Pathology, Bowman Gray School of Medicine, Wake Forest University, Winston-Salem, North Carolina
336 Cutaneous Manifestations of Sarcoidosis

Robert B. Fick, Jr., M.D.
Associate Director, Pulmonary, Genentech, Inc., South San Francisco, California; Clinical Associate Professor of Medicine, Stanford University School of Medicine, Stanford, California
213 Cystic Fibrosis and Bronchiectasis

William F. Finn, M.D.
Professor of Medicine, Department of Medicine, University of North Carolina, Chapel Hill, North Carolina
347 Acute Renal Failure
357 Toxic Nephropathy

Charles Fisch, M.D.
Distinguished Professor of Medicine, Indiana University School of Medicine, Indianapolis, Indiana
9 Cardiac Arrhythmias

Suzanne W. Fletcher, M.D.
Editor, Annals of Internal Medicine, Adjunct Professor of Medicine, University of Pennsylvania; Adjunct Professor of Medicine, Jefferson Medical College, Philadelphia, Pennsylvania
372 The Periodic Health Examination

Barry S. Fogel, M.D.
Professor, Department of Psychiatry and Human Behavior, Associate Director, Center for Gerontology and Health Care Research, Brown University, Providence, Rhode Island
127 Anxiety
128 Mood Disorders
129 Personality Disorders, Maladaptive Illness Behavior, and Somatization
130 Thought Disorders

Marvin Forland, M.D.
Professor of Medicine, Associate Dean for Clinical Affairs, Attending Physician, Medical Center Hospital, Audie L. Murphy Memorial Veterans Hospital, Medical School, University of Texas Health Science Center, San Antonio, Texas
339 Urinalysis
344 Dysuria

George R. Fournier, Jr., M.D.
Assistant Professor of Urology, University of California, San Francisco School of Medicine; Staff Physician, Urology Service, San Francisco Veterans Administration Medical Center, San Francisco, California
240 Urinary Tract Infections

Robert I. Fox, M.D., Ph.D.
Associate Member, Department of Rheumatology, Scripps Clinic and Research Foundation, La Jolla, California
305 Sjögren's Syndrome

Gregory L. Freeman, M.D.
Associate Professor of Medicine, Division of Cardiology, University of Texas Health Science Center, San Antonio, Texas
1 Cardiovascular Physiology

Roy Freeman, M.B., Ch.B.
Assistant Professor of Neurology, Division of Neurology, New England Deaconess Hospital, Boston, Massachusetts
109 Autonomic Nervous System
126 Behavioral Neurology

Marvin J. Fritzler, M.D., Ph.D.
Professor and Head, Division of Rheumatology, Clinical Immunology and Dermatology, Department of Medicine, Foothills Hospital, University of Calgary, Calgary, Alberta, Canada
293 Autoantibodies

Jack D. Fulmer, M.D., F.A.C.P., F.C.C.P.
Ben V. Branscomb Professor of Medicine in Respiratory Diseases, Department of Medicine, Division of Pulmonary and Critical Care Medicine, University of Alabama, Birmingham, Alabama
206 Interstitial Lung Disease

William H. Gaasch, M.D.
Professor of Medicine, University of Massachusetts Medical School; Chief of Cardiology, The Medical Center of Central Massachusetts, Worcester, Massachusetts
6 Cardiac Catheterization and Angiography

Hasan Garan, M.D.
Associate Professor of Medicine, Harvard Medical School; Co-Director, Cardiac Arrhythmia Service, Massachusetts General Hospital, Boston, Massachusetts
12 Sudden Death

Alan J. Garber, M.D., Ph.D.
Professor of Medicine, Biochemistry and Cell Biology, Baylor College of Medicine; Chief of Endocrinology, Diabetes and Metabolism, The Methodist Hospital, Houston, Texas
168 Diabetes Mellitus
170 Heritable Disorders of Carbohydrate Metabolism
174 Lysosomal Storage Diseases

J. Bernard L. Gee, M.D.
Professor of Medicine, Department of Internal Medicine, Yale University School of Medicine, New Haven, Connecticut
211 Occupational Lung Diseases

Thomas D. Gelehrter, M.D.
Professor and Chairman, Department of Human Genetics, Professor of Internal Medicine, University of Michigan Medical School; Attending Physician, Division of Molecular Medicine and Genetics, Department of Internal Medicine, University of Michigan Hospital, Ann Arbor, Michigan
175 Phakomatoses

James N. George, M.D.
Professor of Medicine, Chief, Hematology-Oncology Section, University of Oklahoma Health Sciences Center; Attending Physician, Oklahoma Memorial Hospital, Oklahoma Veterans Administration Medical Center, Oklahoma City, Oklahoma
70 Hemostasis and Fibrinolysis
76 Evaluation of Hemostasis and Thrombosis
83 Excessive Bleeding and Clotting

Thomas D. Geppert, M.D.
Associate Professor, Department of Internal Medicine—Rheumatology, University of Texas Southwest Medical Center, Dallas, Texas
286 Cellular Immunity
291 Evaluation of Cellular Immune Function

Julie Louise Gerberding, M.D., M.P.H.
Assistant Professor of Medicine, University of California, San Francisco, School of Medicine; Physician Specialist and Director, Center for Hospital Epidemiology and Infection Prevention, San Francisco General Hospital, San Francisco, California
242 Acquired Immunodeficiency Syndrome

Meghan B. Gerety, M.D.
Associate Professor, Division of Geriatrics and Gerontology, Department of Medicine, University of Texas Health Science Center at San Antonio; Associate Director for Clinical Activities, Geriatric Research, Education and Clinical Center, Audie L. Murphy Memorial Veterans Hospital, San Antonio, Texas
370 Gerontology and Geriatric Medicine

Bernard J. Gersh, M.B., Ch.B., D.Phil.
Consultant, Division of Cardiovascular Diseases and Internal Medicine, Mayo Clinic and Mayo Foundation; Professor of Medicine, Mayo Medical School, Rochester, Minnesota
14 Acute Myocardial Infarction

Abraham A. Ghiatas, M.D.
Associate Professor, Department of Radiology, University of Texas Health Science Center, San Antonio, Texas
341 Imaging of Renal Disorders

David N. Gilbert, M.D.
Director, Medical Education and Earle A. Chiles Research Institute, Providence Medical Center; Professor of Medicine, Department of Medicine, Oregon Health Sciences University, Portland, Oregon
262 Clostridial Infections

George G. Glenner, M.D.
Attending Physician, Department of Pathology, University of California, San Diego Medical Center; Research Pathologist, Department of Pathology, University of California, San Diego School of Medicine, La Jolla, California
322 The Amyloidoses

Vay Liang W. Go, M.D.
Professor of Medicine, Department of Medicine, School of Medicine, University of California, Los Angeles, California
52 Pancreatic Secretion
54 Evaluation of Pancreatic Diseases
67 Pancreatic Diseases

Stanley Goldfarb, M.D.
Clinical Professor of Medicine, University of Pennsylvania; Vice President for Patient Care, Education and Research, Graduate Health System, Graduate Hospital, Philadelphia, Pennsylvania
179 Disorders of Phosphate Homeostasis
180 Disorders of Magnesium Homeostasis
355 Diabetic Nephropathy
360 Disorders of Renal Tubular Transport

Alan Goldfien, M.D.
Professor of Medicine, Emeritus, Departments of Medicine, Obstetrics and Gynecology and Reproductive Sciences, and The Cardiovascular Research Institute, School of Medicine, University of California, San Francisco, California
164 Disorders of the Adrenal Medulla

Fred H. Goldner, M.D.
Clinical Associate Professor of Medicine, University of Texas Health Science Center at San Antonio; Chief, Department of Medicine, Brooke Army Medical Center, San Antonio, Texas
43 Idiopathic Inflammatory Bowel Disease

Markus Goldschmiedt, M.D.
Assistant Professor of Internal Medicine, Department of Gastroenterology, Parkland Memorial Hospital, Dallas V.A. Medical Center, University of Texas Southwestern Medical Center, Dallas, Texas
27 Gastric Secretion

Daniel M. Goodenberger, M.D.
Director, Pulmonary Consultation Service, Barnes Hospital; Assistant Professor of Medicine, Respiratory and Critical Care Division, Washington University School of Medicine, St. Louis, Missouri
204 Pulmonary Rehabilitation

Peter D. Gorevic, M.D.
Professor of Medicine and Pathology, Department of Medicine, University Hospital; Head, Division of Allergy, Rheumatology and Clinical Immunology, Department of Medicine, State University of New York, Stony Brook, New York
314 Cryoglobulinemia

Leonard J. Gorkun, M.D.
Director, Section of Occupational and Environmental Health Services; Clinical Assistant Professor of Medicine, Department of Medicine, UMDNJ-New Jersey Medical School, Newark, New Jersey
365 Occupational and Environmental Health

Raj K. Goyal, M.D.
Chief, Gastroenterology Division, Beth Israel Hospital; Charlotte F. and Irving W. Rabb Professor of Medicine, Harvard Medical School, Boston, Massachusetts
26 Alimentary Tract Motor Function

Christopher J. Grace, M.D.
Assistant Professor, Division of Infectious Disease, Department of Medicine, University of Vermont, College of Medicine, Burlington, Vermont
272 Infections Caused by Legionellae

Jared J. Grantham, M.D.
Professor, Department of Medicine, Kansas University Medical Center, Kansas City, Kansas
358 Cystic Diseases of the Kidney

John R. Graybill, M.D.
Professor of Internal Medicine, Chief, Division of Infectious Diseases, University of Texas Health Science Center at San Antonio, Audie L. Murphy Memorial Veterans Hospital, San Antonio, Texas
277 Infections Caused by Fungi

F. Anthony Greco, M.D.
Director, Sarah Cannon Cancer Center, Centennial Medical Center; Professor of Medicine, Department of Medicine (Oncology), Vanderbilt University Hospital, Nashville, Tennessee
102 Carcinoma of Unknown Primary Site

Thomas M. Grogan, M.D.
Professor of Pathology, Department of Pathology, University of Arizona, Tucson, Arizona
94 Hodgkin's Disease and Non-Hodgkin's Lymphoma

Allen B. Gruber, M.D.
Neurologist, Santa Rosa Northwest Hospital, San Antonio, Texas
107 Electromyography

Scott M. Grundy, M.D., Ph.D.
Professor of Internal Medicine and Biochemistry, Center for Human Nutrition, University of Texas Southwestern Medical School, Dallas, Texas
171 Disorders of Lipids and Lipoproteins

Richard L. Guerrant, M.D.
Thomas M. Hunter Professor of International Medicine, Head, Division of Geographic Medicine, University of Virginia School of Medicine; Attending Physician, University of Virginia Health Sciences Center, Charlottesville, Virginia
267 Infections Caused by *Vibrio* Species

Paul A. Gutierrez, M.D.
Spinal Cord Injury Service, Long Beach V.A. Medical Center, Department of Neurology, University of California, Irvine, Irvine, California
132 Spinal Cord Injury

Jack M. Gwaltney, Jr., M.D.
Wade Hampton Frost Professor of Medicine, Head Division of Epidemiology and Virology, Department of Internal Medicine, University of Virginia Health Sciences Center, Charlottesville, Virginia
230 Upper Respiratory Infections (Colds, Pharyngitis, Sinusitis)

John D. Hainsworth, M.D.
Associate Director, Sarah Cannon Cancer Center, Centennial Medical Center; Associate Professor, Department of Medicine, Vanderbilt University Hospital, Nashville, Tennessee
102 Carcinoma of Unknown Primary Site

Allan J. Hance, M.D.
Directeur de recherche INSERM, INSERM U82, Faculte de Medicine Xavier Bichat, Paris, France
209 Langerhans' Cell Granulomatosis (Histiocytosis X, Eosinophilic Granuloma)

Stephen C. Hauser, M.D.
Assistant Professor, Department of Medicine, Harvard Medical School; Physician and Director of Gastroenterology Clinics, Gastroenterology Division, Brigham and Women's Hospital, Boston, Massachusetts
61 Hepatic Veno-Occlusive Diseases
66 Other Diseases of the Gallbladder and Biliary Tree

Frederick G. Hayden, M.D.
Stuart S. Richardson Professor of Clinical Virology, Department of Internal Medicine, University of Virginia School of Medicine; Associate Director, Clinical Microbiology Laboratory, Department of Pathology, University of Virginia Health Sciences Center, Charlottesville, Virginia
246 Paramyxovirus, (Measles, Parainfluenza, Mumps, and Respiratory Syncytial Virus), Rubella Virus, and Coronavirus Infections

Gregory F. Hayden, M.D.
Professor of Pediatrics, Department of Pediatrics, University of Virginia School of Medicine, Charlottesville, Virginia
246 Paramyxovirus (Measles, Parainfluenza, Mumps, and Respiratory Syncytial Virus), Rubella Virus, and Coronavirus Infections

J. Owen Hendley, M.D.
Professor of Pediatrics, Head, Division of Pediatric Infectious Diseases, Department of Pediatrics, University of Virginia Health Sciences Center, Charlottesville, Virginia
271 *Bordetella pertussis* Infection (Whooping cough)

Nancy K. Henry, Ph.D., M.D.
Assistant Professor of Pediatrics, Mayo Medical School, Rochester, Minnesota
269 Infections Caused by *Brucella, Francisella tularensis, Pasteurella,* and *Yersinia* Species

Daniel B. Hier, M.D.
Chief, Neurology Service, University of Illinois Hospital; Professor and Head, Department of Neurology, University of Illinois, Chicago, Illinois
116 Disorders of Speech and Language

John L. Ho, M.D.
Assistant Professor of Medicine, Cornell University Medical College; Assistant Attending Physician, New York Hospital, New York, New York
261 Gram-Positive Aerobic Bacillary Infections: *Corynebacterium* and *Listeria*

Ronald Hoffman, M.D.
Bruce Kenneth Wiseman Professor of Medicine and Pathology, Hematology-Oncology Section, Department of Medicine, Indiana University School of Medicine, Indianapolis, Indiana
69 Molecular and Cellular Biology of Hematopoiesis

Antoinette F. Hood, M.D.
Professor, Department of Pathology and Dermatology, Indiana University School of Medicine, Indianapolis, Indiana
332 Cutaneous Manifestations of Drug Reactions

Edward W. Hook III, M.D.
Professor of Medicine, University of Alabama School of Medicine; Director, Sexually Transmitted Disease Control Program, Jefferson County Department of Health, Birmingham, Alabama
264 *Neisseria gonorrhoeae* Infections

Philip C. Hopewell, M.D.
Chief, Division of Pulmonary and Critical Care Medicine, San Francisco General Hospital; Professor of Medicine, Department of Medicine, University of California, San Francisco, California
276 Tuberculosis and Nontuberculous Mycobacterial Infections

Thomas D. Horn, M.D.
Assistant Professor of Dermatology and Pathology, Department of Dermatology, Johns Hopkins Hospital, Baltimore, Maryland
337 Cutaneous Features of the Human Immunodeficiency Virus Infection

Edward S. Horton, M.D.
Medical Director, Joslin Diabetes Center, Boston, Massachusetts
153 Obesity

Anastacio M. Hoyumpa, M.D.
Professor of Medicine, Department of Medicine/Gastroenterology and Nutrition, University of Texas Health Science Center, San Antonio, Texas
56 Principal Complications of Liver Failure

Jerome F. Hruska, M.D., Ph.D.
Associate Professor of Medicine, Department of Internal Medicine, University of Nevada School of Medicine, Las Vegas, Nevada
249 Bunyavirus and Togavirus Infections (Viral Encephalitis and Dengue and Yellow Fever)

Leonard D. Hudson, M.D.
Professor of Medicine and Head, Division of Pulmonary and Critical Care Medicine, Department of Medicine, University of Washington School of Medicine, Seattle, Washington
200 Acute Respiratory Failure

Russell D. Hull, M.B., M.Sc.
Professor, Department of Medicine, Foothille Hospital; Professor, Department of Medicine, University of Calgary, Calgary, Alberta, Canada
86 Thrombosis and Anticoagulation

Gene G. Hunder, M.D.
Professor of Medicine, Mayo Medical School, Department of Internal Medicine; Chairman, Division of Rheumatology, Mayo Medical Center, Rochester, Minnesota
307 Vasculitic Syndromes

Gary W. Hunninghake, M.D.
Professor and Director, Department of Internal Medicine, Pulmonary Diseases Division, University of Iowa College of Medicine, Iowa City, Iowa
207 Sarcoidosis

Debra K. Hunt, M.D., M.P.H.
Assistant Professor, Division of General Medicine, Department of Medicine, University of Texas Health Science Center, San Antonio, Texas
367 Substance Abuse

John J. Hutton, M.D.
Professor of Pediatrics and Medicine, Dean, College of Medicine, University of Cincinnati, Cincinnati, Ohio
93 The Leukemias and Polycythemia Vera

Steven E. Hyman, M.D.
Associate Professor of Psychiatry and Neuroscience, Harvard Medical School; Director of Research, Department of Psychiatry, Massachusetts General Hospital, Boston, Massachusetts
137 Neuroendocrinology

Michael C. Iannuzzi, M.D.
Assistant Professor of Internal Medicine, Division of Pulmonary and Critical Care Medicine, University of Michigan Medical School, Ann Arbor, Michigan
214 Neoplasms of the Lung

David H. Ingbar, M.D.
Associate Professor of Medicine, Departments of Pulmonary Medicine and Critical Care, University of Minnesota School of Medicine; Co-Director, Medical Intensive Care Unit, University of Minnesota Hospital and Clinics, Minneapolis, Minnesota
203 Respiratory Therapy and Monitoring

Richard S. Irwin, M.D.
Professor of Medicine, University of Massachusetts Medical School; Director, Pulmonary and Critical Care Medicine, University of Massachusetts Medical Center, Worcester, Massachusetts
20 Pulmonary Hypertensive Heart Disease

Lisa J. Istorico-Sanders
Assistant Professor, Division of Infectious Diseases, University of South Florida, Tampa, Florida
239 Gram-Negative Bacteremia and the Sepsis Syndrome

Waldemar G. Johanson, M.D., M.P.H.
Professor and Chairman, Department of Medicine, UMDNJ-New Jersey Medical School, Newark, New Jersey
365 Occupational and Environmental Health

Warren D. Johnson, Jr., M.D.
Professor of Medicine and Chief, Division of International Medicine, Cornell University Medical College; Attending Physician, New York Hospital, New York, New York
261 Gram-Positive Aerobic Bacillary Infections: *Corynebacterium* and *Listeria*
268 Infections Caused by *Salmonella* and *Shigella* Species

M. Colin Jordan, M.D.
Director, Division of Infectious Diseases, Department of Medicine, University of Minnesota Hospital; Professor of Medicine and Microbiology, University of Minnesota, Minneapolis, Minnesota
251 Herpesvirus Infections (Herpes Simplex Virus, Varicella-Zoster Virus, Cytomegalovirus, Epstein-Barr Virus)

Richard M. Jordan, M.D.
Professor of Medicine, Chief, Division of Endocrinology, East Tennessee State University, Quillen-Dishner College of Medicine, Johnson City, Tennessee; Chief, Medical Service, Veterans Administration Medical Center, Mountain Home, Tennessee
147 Principles of Endocrine Physiology
150 Laboratory Diagnosis in Endocrinology
152 Weight Loss

Rafael Jurado, M.D.
Assistant Professor, Department of Medicine, Emory School of Medicine; Assistant Chief, Veterans Administration Medical Center, Atlanta, Georgia
243 Fever in the Hospitalized Patient

Abdulhay A. Kadri, M.D.
Assistant Professor of Medicine, University of Texas Health Science Center, San Antonio, Texas
367 Substance Abuse

Martin F. Kagnoff, M.D.
Professor of Medicine, Director, Laboratory of Mucosal Immunology, Department of Medicine, University of California, San Diego School of Medicine, La Jolla, California
29 Intestinal Immunity

Gary C. Kanel, M.D.
Associate Pathologist, Department of Pathology, Rancho Los Amigos Medical Center; Associate Professor of Pathology, Department of Pathology, USC School of Medicine, Los Angeles, California
59 Alcoholic Liver Disease

Ashwani Kapila, M.D.
Associate Clinical Professor of Radiology, University of Texas Health Science Center at San Antonio; Attending Radiologist, Santa Rosa Hospital and Humana Metropolitan Hospital, San Antonio, Texas
108 Neuroradiologic Studies

Marshall M. Kaplan, M.D.
Professor of Medicine, Tufts University School of Medicine; Chief, Gastroenterology Division, New England Medical Center, Boston, Massachusetts
53 Evaluation of Hepatobiliary Diseases
60 Primary Biliary Cirrhosis, Wilson's Disease, Hemochromatosis, and Other Metabolic and Fibrotic Liver Diseases

Norman M. Kaplan, M.D.
Professor, Department of Internal Medicine, University of Texas Southwestern Medical Center, Dallas, Texas
23 Arterial Hypertension

Adolf W. Karchmer, M.D.
Chief, Division of Infectious Diseases, Department of Medicine, New England Deaconess Hospital; Associate Professor of Medicine, Harvard Medical School, Boston, Massachusetts
315 Infections of the Joints

B.S. Kasinath, M.D.
Associate Professor, Department of Medicine, University of Texas Health Science Center; Chief, Renal Division, Audie L. Murphy V.A. Medical Center, San Antonio, Texas
342 Hematuria
343 Proteinuria
345 Acute Nephritic Syndrome

Michael S. Katz, M.D.
Professor and Chief, Division of Geriatrics and Gerontology, Department of Medicine, University of Texas Health Science Center at San Antonio; Director, Geriatric Research, Education and Clinical Center, Associate Chief of Staff for Extended Care, Audie L. Murphy Memorial Veterans Hospital, San Antonio, Texas
370 Gerontology and Geriatric Medicine

David A. Katzenstein, M.D.
Assistant Clinical Professor of Medicine, Stanford University Medical Center; Associate Medical Director, AIDS Clinical Trials Unit, Stanford University Medical Center, Stanford, California
251 Herpesvirus Infections (Herpes Simplex Virus, Varicella-Zoster Virus, Cytomegalovirus, Epstein-Barr Virus)

Arnold F. Kaufmann, D.V.M., M.S.
Acting Chief, Mycotic Diseases Branch, Division of Bacterial Disease, National Center for Infectious Diseases, Centers for Disease Control and Prevention, Atlanta, Georgia
274 Infections Caused by Leptospires (Leptospirosis)

Sanjiv Kaul, M.D.
Professor of Medicine, University of Virginia Health Sciences Center, Charlottesville, Virginia
5 Cardiac Noninvasive Techniques

Donald Kaye, M.D.
Klinghoffer Professor and Chairman, Department of Medicine, Medical College of Pennsylvania, Philadelphia, Pennsylvania
240 Urinary Tract Infections

John Kendall, M.D.
Department of Medicine, Oregon Health Sciences University and Portland V.A. Medical Center, Portland, Oregon
163 Disorders of the Adrenal Cortex

L. Lyndon Key, Jr., M.D.
Associate Professor of Pediatrics, Department of Pediatrics, Medical University of South Carolina, Charleston, South Carolina
182 Osteomalacia and Disorders of Vitamin D Metabolism

A. Daniel King, M.D.
Postdoctoral Fellow, Department of Dermatology, University of Cincinnati College of Medicine, Cincinnati, Ohio
96 Melanoma, Kaposi's Sarcoma, and Mycosis Fungoides

Barbara J. Kircher, M.D.
Assistant Professor of Medicine, Division of Cardiology, University of Florida Medical Center, Jacksonville, Florida
216 Pulmonary Hypertension: Primary and Secondary Causes

Saulo Klahr, M.D.
Physician-in-Chief, Department of Medicine, Jewish Hospital of St. Louis; Simon Professor and Co-Chairman, Department of Medicine, Washington University School of Medicine, St. Louis, Missouri
361 Obstructive Uropathy

Irwin Klein, M.D.
Professor of Medicine & Cell Biology, Chief, Division of Endocrinology, North Shore University Hospital, Cornell University Medical College, New York, New York
162 Disorders of the Thyroid

John H. Klippel, M.D.
Clinical Director, National Institute of Arthritis and Musculoskeletal and Skin Disease, Clinical Center, National Institutes of Health, Bethesda, Maryland
306 Systemic Lupus Erythematosus

Sidney Kobrin
Renal Electrolyte Division, Hospital of the University of Pennsylvania, University of Pennsylvania, School of Medicine, Philadelphia, Pennsylvania
180 Disorders of Magnesium Homeostasis
360 Disorders of Renal Tubular Transport

Peter O. Kohler, M.D.
President, Oregon Health Sciences, University School of Medicine, Portland, Oregon
147 Principles of Endocrine Physiology
150 Laboratory Diagnosis in Endocrinology
152 Weight Loss

Michael A. Kolodziej, M.D.
Assistant Professor of Medicine, Hematology-Oncology Section, Department of Medicine, University of Oklahoma Health Sciences Center; Attending Physician, Oklahoma Memorial Hospital, Oklahoma Veterans Administration Medical Center, Oklahoma City, Oklahoma
70 Hemostasis and Fibrinolysis
76 Evaluation of Hemostasis and Thrombosis
83 Excessive Bleeding and Clotting

Donald P. Kotler, M.D.
Gastrointestinal Division, Department of Medicine, St. Luke's Roosevelt Hospital Center, College of Physicians and Surgeons, Columbia University, New York, New York
48 Gastrointestinal Manifestations of HIV Infection and AIDS

Sumner C. Kraft, M.D.
Professor of Medicine and Committee on Immunology, University of Chicago Pritzker School of Medicine; Attending Physician, University of Chicago Hospital and Clinics, Chicago, Illinois
43 Idiopathic Inflammatory Bowel Disease

Stephen M. Krane, M.D.
Persis, Cyrus and Marlowe B. Harrison Professor of Medicine, Harvard Medical School; Physician and Chief, Arthritis Unit, Massachusetts General Hospital, Boston, Massachusetts
323 Heritable and Developmental Disorders of Connective Tissue

Eric H. Kraut, M.D.
Professor of Internal Medicine, Division of Hematology/Oncology, Chief of Staff, Arthur James Cancer Hospital and Research Institute, Columbus, Ohio
79 Complications of Cancer and Cancer Therapy

G. Gopal Krishna, M.D.
Attending Physician, Department of Medicine, Hospital of University of Pennsylvania; Associate Professor, Department of Medicine, University of Pennsylvania, Philadelphia, Pennsylvania
350 Disorders of Water Balance

Theodore G. Krontiris, M.D., Ph.D.
Physician, Department of Medicine, New England Medical Center Hospitals; Associate Professor, Departments of Medicine, Molecular Biology and Microbiology, Tufts University School of Medicine, Boston, Massachusetts
71 Molecular and Cellular Biology of Cancer

Satish Kumar, M.D.
Assistant Professor of Medicine, University of Oklahoma Health Sciences Center, Oklahoma City, Oklahoma
347 Acute Renal Failure

Robert C. Kurtz, M.D.
Director, Gastrointestinal Endoscopy Unit, Attending Physician and Member, Gastroenterology and Nutrition Service, Memorial Sloan-Kettering Cancer Center, New York, New York
40 Tumors of the Stomach

Neil A. Kurtzman, M.D.
Chairman and Arnett Professor, Department of Internal Medicine, Texas Tech University Health Sciences Center, Lubbock, Texas
353 Disorders of Acid-Base Balance

Robert A. Kyle, M.D.
Consultant, Division of Hematology and Internal Medicine, Mayo Clinic and Mayo Foundation; Professor of Medicine and Laboratory Medicine, Mayo Medical School, Rochester, Minnesota
75 Evaluation of Monoclonal Proteins in Serum and Urine
95 Multiple Myeloma and the Disproteinemias

Douglas R. LaBrecque, M.D.
Professor of Medicine, Director, Liver Service, Internal Medicine, University of Iowa Hospitals and Clinics; Chief, GI/Hepatology, Medicine, V.A. Medical Center, Iowa City, Iowa
57 Acute and Chronic Hepatitis

Melvin E. Laski, M.D.
Associate Professor, Internal Medicine and Physiology, Texas Tech University Health Sciences Center, Lubbock, Texas
353 Disorders of Acid-Base Balance

Valerie Ann Lawrence, M.D.
Associate Professor, Department of Medicine, Medical Center Hospital, Audie L. Murphy Memorial Veterans Hospital; Director, Medical Consultation Service, University of Texas Health Science Center, San Antonio, Texas
373 Preoperative Medical Evaluation

Makau Lee, M.D., Ph.D.
Fellow in Gastroenterology, Department of Internal Medicine, University of Texas Southwestern Medical Center, Dallas, Texas
37 Nausea, Vomiting, and Anorexia

James H. Leech, M.D.
Associate Professor, Department of Medicine, University of California, San Francisco; Attending Physician, Department of Medicine and Division of Infectious Diseases, San Francisco General Hospital, San Francisco, California
280 Infections Caused by Protozoa

Jacob Lemann, Jr., M.D.
Professor of Medicine, Chief, Nephrology Division, Medical College of Wisconsin, Froedtert Memorial Lutheran Hospital, Milwaukee, Wisconsin
349 Nephrolithiasis

Gerald S. Levey, M.D.
Senior Vice President, Department of Medical and Scientific Affairs, Merck and Company, Inc., Whitehouse Station, New Jersey
162 Disorders of the Thyroid

Matthew E. Levison, M.D.
Chief, Division of Infectious Diseases, Professor of Medicine, Department of Medicine, Medical College of Pennsylvania, Philadelphia, Pennsylvania
232 Intra-Abdominal Infections

Jay A. Levy, M.D.
Professor, Department of Medicine, Research Associate, Cancer Research Institute, School of Medicine, University of California, San Francisco, California
252 Human Retrovirus Infections

Michael J. Lichtenstein, M.D.
Associate Professor, Division of Geriatrics and Gerontology, Department of Medicine, University of Texas Health Science Center; Staff Physician, Geriatric Research, Education and Clinical Center, Audie L. Murphy Memorial Veterans Hospital, San Antonio, Texas
70 Gerontology and Geriatric Medicine

J.T. Lie, M.D.
Professor and Director of Anatomic Pathology, Department of Pathology, University of California Davis Medical Center, Sacramento, California
307 Vasculitic Syndromes

Charles J. Lightdale, M.D.
Director of Clinical Gastroenterology, Columbia-Presbyterian Medical Center; Professor of Clinical Medicine, Columbia University College of Physicians and Surgeons, New York, New York
45 Tumors of the Small and Large Intestines

David A. Lipschitz, M.D., Ph.D.
Director, Geriatric Research, Education and Clinical Center, John L. McClellan Memorial Veterans Hospital; Professor of Medicine, Physiology, and Biophysics, Director, Division of Aging, Department of Medicine, University of Arkansas for Medical Sciences, Little Rock, Arkansas
87 Iron Deficiency Anemia, the Anemia of Chronic Disease, Sideroblastic Anemia, and Iron Overload

Peter E. Lipsky, M.D.
Professor of Internal Medicine and Microbiology, Director, Rheumatic Diseases Division, Director, Harold C. Simmons Arthritis Research Center, Department of Internal Medicine, University of Texas Southwestern Medical Center, Dallas, Texas
286 Cellular Immunity
291 Evaluation of Cellular Immune Function

M. Kathryn Liszewski, B.S.
Lab Manager, Department of Rheumatology, Washington University School of Medicine, St. Louis, Missouri
287 Complement System and Immune Complex Diseases
290 Complement Measurements
298 Inherited Complement Deficiencies

Francisco Llach, M.D.
Chief of Nephrology, Professor of Medicine, University of California, Los Angeles, California
346 Nephrotic Syndrome

Eric L. Logigian, M.D.
Assistant Professor of Neurology, Harvard University School of Medicine; Physician, Brigham and Women's Hospital, Boston, Massachusetts
123 Diseases of Peripheral Nerve and Motor Neurons

Jacob S.O. Loke, M.D.
Attending Physician, Department of Internal Medicine, Yale New Haven Hospital; Clinical Professor of Medicine, Department of Internal Medicine, Yale University School of Medicine, New Haven, Connecticut
189 Respiratory Pathophysiology
195 Pulmonary Function Testing

D. Lynn Loriaux, M.D., Ph.D.
Clinical Director, National Institute for Child Health and Human Development, National Institutes of Health, Bethesda, Maryland
155 Hirsutism
163 Disorders of the Adrenal Cortex

Robert G. Luke, M.D.
Taylor Professor of Medicine, Director, Department of Internal Medicine, University of Cincinnati Medical Center; Physician-in-Chief, University Hospital, University of Cincinnati College of Medicine, Cincinnati, Ohio
348 Chronic Renal Failure

Jamson S. Lwebuga-Mukasa, M.D., Ph.D.
Associate Professor of Medicine, Director, Pulmonary and Critical Care Division, Department of Internal Medicine, State University of New York, Buffalo General Hospital, Buffalo, New York
194 Mechanisms of Lung Injury and Repair

John S. MacGregor, M.D., Ph.D.
Director, Cardiac Catheterization Laboratory, San Francisco General Hospital; Assistant Professor of Medicine, University of California, San Francisco, San Francisco, California
24 Cardiac Tumors; Cardiac Manifestations of Endocrine, Collagen Vascular, and HIV Disease; and Traumatic Injury of the Heart

Jon T. Mader, M.D.
Professor, Division of Infectious Diseases, Department of Internal Medicine, University of Texas Medical Branch, Galveston, Texas
237 Osteomyelitis

R. Ellen Magenis, M.D.
Professor, Department of Molecular and Medical Genetics, University Hospital and CCD, Oregon Health Sciences University, Portland, Oregon
149 Principles of Genetic Disorders

Barry J. Make, M.D.
Associate Professor of Medicine, University of Colorado Health Science Center; Director, Pulmonary Rehabilitation, National Jewish Center for Immunology and Respiratory Medicine, Denver, Colorado
204 Pulmonary Rehabilitation

Hartmut H. Malluche, M.D.
Professor and Director, Division of Nephrology, Bone and Mineral Metabolism, Department of Medicine, University of Kentucky Medical Center, Lexington, Kentucky
186 Renal Bone Disease

Gerald L. Mandell, M.D.
Professor of Medicine, Owen R. Chatham Professor of Sciences, University of Virginia School of Medicine; Head, Division of Infectious Diseases, University of Virginia Health Sciences Center, Charlottesville, Virginia
223 Host Defense Against Infection: The Roles of Antibody, Complement, and Phagocytic Cells

Theodore W. Marcy, M.D.
Associate Professor of Medicine, Pulmonary Division, University of Vermont School of Medicine, Burlington, Vermont
203 Respiratory Therapy and Monitoring

Diana L. Marquardt, M.D.
Associate Professor of Medicine, Department of Medicine, University of California, San Diego Medical Center, San Diego, California
301 Anaphylaxis

John C. Marshall, M.D., Ph.D.
Professor and Chair, Department of Medicine, University of Virginia Health Sciences Center, Charlottesville, Virginia
157 Impotence and Altered Libido
158 Gynecomastia

Liam Martin, M.B., M.R.C.P.I, F.R.C.P.(C)
Assistant Professor of Medicine, Department of Medicine, Foothills Hospital; Assistant Professor of Medicine, Department of Medicine, Division of Rheumatology, Clinical Immunology and Dermatology, University of Calgary, Calgary, Alberta, Canada
293 Autoantibodies

R. Michael Massanari, M.D., M.S.
Director, Hospital Epidemiology, Associate Director, Professional Practice Review Group, Department of Internal Medicine, Henry Ford Hospital; Adjunct Professor, Department of Epidemiology, School of Public Health, University of Michigan, Detroit, Michigan
225 Hospital Infection Control

Jean K. Matheson, M.D.
Co-Director, Sleep Disorders Center, Department of Neurology, Beth Israel Hospital; Instructor, Department of Neurology, Harvard Medical School, Boston, Massachusetts
110 Sleep and Its Disorders

Suzanne M. Matsui, M.D.
Assistant Professor of Medicine, Department of Medicine (Gastroenterology), Stanford University School of Medicine, Stanford, California, Veterans Administration Medical Center, Palo Alto, California
250 Rotavirus and Norwalk-Like Virus Infections

Richard A. Matthay, M.D.
Professor and Associate Chairman, Department of Internal Medicine, Yale University School of Medicine, New Haven, Connecticut
217 Pulmonary Thromboembolism

John H. McAnulty, M.D.
Professor of Medicine, Department of Medicine, Division of Cardiology, Oregon Health Sciences University, Portland, Oregon
4 Electrocardiography

David McCall, M.D., Ph.D.
Director, Coronary Intensive Care Unit, Medical Center Hospital; Professor, Department of Medicine, University of Texas Health Science Center, San Antonio, Texas
10 Congestive Heart Failure
11 Hypotension and Cardiogenic Shock

Daniel J. McCarty, M.D.
Will and Cava Ross Professor of Medicine, Director, Arthritis Institute, Department of Medicine, Medical College of Wisconsin, Milwaukee, Wisconsin
320 Arthritis Associated with Calcium-Containing Crystals

Brian McGovern, M.D.
Assistant Professor of Medicine, Harvard Medical School; Co-Director, Cardiac Arrhythmias Service, Massachusetts General Hospital, Boston, Massachusetts
12 Sudden Death

John E. McGowan, Jr., M.D.
Professor of Pathology and Laboratory Medicine, and Medicine (Infectious Diseases), Emory University, School of Medicine, Grady Memorial Hospital, Atlanta, Georgia
243 Fever in the Hospitalized Patient

T. Dwight McKinney, M.D.
Professor of Medicine, Department of Medicine, Indiana University School of Medicine; Clinical Research Physician, Eli Lilly and Company, Indianapolis, Indiana
340 Renal Function Tests
364 Renal Cell Carcinoma

Thomas A. Medsger, Jr., M.D.
Professor of Medicine, Chief, Division of Rheumatology and Clinical Immunology, Department of Medicine, University of Pittsburgh School of Medicine, Presbyterian University Hospital, Montefiore University Hospital, Pittsburgh, Pennsylvania
309 Systemic Sclerosis (Scleroderma)

Schlomo Melmed, M.D.
Professor of Medicine, University of California, Los Angeles, School of Medicine; Director, Division of Endocrinology and Metabolism, Cedars-Sinai Medical Center, Los Angeles, California
160 Disorders of the Hypothalamus and Anterior Pituitary

Jay E. Menitove, M.D.
Deputy Director, Medical Services, Hoxworth Blood Center; Professor, Department of Internal Medicine, University of Cincinnati College of Medicine, Cincinnati, Ohio
77 Blood Transfusion

Thomas P. Miller, M.D.
Professor of Medicine, Arizona Cancer Center, University of Arizona, Tucson, Arizona
94 Hodgkin's Disease and Non-Hodgkin's Lymphoma

John Mills, M.D.
Scientific Director, MacFarlane Burnet Centre; Consultant, Fairfield Infectious Diseases Hospital, Melbourne, Australia
253 Adenovirus Infections
255 Mycoplasmal Infections

Charlotte E. Modly, M.D.
Clinical Assistant Professor, Department of Dermatology, University of Maryland School of Medicine, Baltimore, Maryland
329 Acne

Robert C. Moellering, Jr., M.D.
Shields Warren-Mallinckrodt Professor of Medical Research, Harvard Medical School; Physician-in-Chief, New England Deaconess Hospital, Boston, Massachusetts
224 Principles of Anti-Infective Therapy

Warwick L. Morison, M.D.
Associate Professor, Department of Dermatology, Johns Hopkins Hospital, Baltimore, Maryland
327 Psoriasis
330 Photodermatoses

John F. Morrissey, M.D.
Emeritus Professor of Medicine, Section of Gastroenterology, University of Wisconsin Medical School, Madison, Wisconsin
30 Gastrointestinal Endoscopy

Robb E. Moses, M.D.
Professor and Chairman, Department of Molecular and Medical Genetics, Oregon Health Sciences University, Portland, Oregon
149 Principles of Genetic Disorders

Gregory R. Mundy, M.D.
Professor and Head, Department of Medicine, Division of Endocrinology and Metabolism, University of Texas Health Science Center, San Antonio, Texas
148 Physiology of Bone and Mineral Homeostasis
151 Diagnostic Approach to Bone and Mineral Disorders
184 Osteopetrosis
185 Fibrous Dysplasia
188 Malignant Disease and the Skeleton

Joseph P. Murgo, M.D.
Clinical Professor of Medicine, Louisiana State University School of Medicine in New Orleans; Section Head, Cardiology, Oschner Medical Institutions, New Orleans, Louisiana
6 Cardiac Catheterization and Angiography

Jock Murray, O.C., M.D., F.R.C.P.(C), F.A.C.P., L.L.D., D.Sc.
Professor of Medical Humanities, Director, Dalhousie Multiple Sclerosis Research Unit, Department of Medicine, Dalhousie Medical School, Halifax, Nova Scotia, Canada
103 Neurologic History and Examination

Diya F. Mutasim, M.D.
Assistant Professor, Department of Dermatology, University of Cincinnati, Cincinnati, Ohio
325 Bullous Diseases

Kenneth K. Nakano, M.D., M.P.H.
Medical Director, Straub Foundation, Department of Neurology, Straub Clinic and Hospital, Honolulu, Hawaii
114 Neck and Back Pain
141 Neurorheumatology

Robert G. Narins, M.D.
Head, Division of Nephrology and Hypertension, Department of Internal Medicine, Henry Ford Hospital, Detroit, Michigan
350 Disorders of Water Balance
352 Disorders of Potassium Balance

Eric G. Neilson, M.D.
Chief, Renal-Electrolyte Division, Professor of Medicine, University of Pennsylvania, Department of Medicine, Hospital of the University of Pennsylvania, Philadelphia, Pennsylvania
362 Tubulointerstitial Diseases

James R. Nethercott, M.D.
Attending Physician, Department of Dermatology, Johns Hopkins Hospital; Professor, Department of Dermatology, Johns Hopkins University, Baltimore, Maryland
328 Dermatitis

Harold C. Neu, M.D.
Professor of Medicine and Pharmacology, Chief, Division of Infectious Diseases, College of Physicians and Surgeons, Columbia University, Columbia Presbyterian Medical Center, New York, New York
231 Pneumonia

James J. Nordlund, M.D.
Professor and Chairman, Department of Dermatology, University of Cincinnati, Cincinnati, Ohio
96 Melanoma, Kaposi's Sarcoma, and Mycosis Fungoides

Kathryn A. O'Connell, M.D., Ph.D.
Research Associate, Department of Dermatology, Johns Hopkins School of Medicine, Baltimore, Maryland
337 Cutaneous Features of the Human Immunodeficiency Virus Infection

G. Richard Olds, M.D.
Director, Division of Geographic Medicine and Clinical Immunology, Department of Medicine, Miriam Hospital, Professor of Medicine; Director, International Health Institute, Brown University, Providence, Rhode Island
282 Infections Causes by Helminths

Robert A. O'Rourke, M.D.
Charles Conrad Brown Distinguished Professor in Cardiovascular Disease, Director of Cardiology, University of Texas Health Science Center, San Antonio, Texas
1 Cardiovascular Physiology
8 Palpitations
11 Hypotension and Cardiogenic Shock
21 Diseases of the Aorta
112 Faintness and Syncope

C. Kent Osborne, M.D.
Professor, Department of Medicine/Oncology, University of Texas Health Science Center at San Antonio, Attending Physician, Medical Center Hospital, San Antonio, Texas
97 Breast Cancer
99 Cancer of the Testis and Prostate

J. Donald Ostrow, M.D., M.Sc.
Medical Investigator, Research Service, D.V.A. Lakeside Medical Center; Professor, Department of Medicine, Northwestern University Medical School, Chicago, Illinois
55 Jaundice and Disorders of Bilirubin Metabolism

Ann Ouyang, M.B.
Professor of Medicine, University of Pennsylvania School of Medicine; Chief, Division of Gastroenterology, Milton S. Hershey Medical Center, Pennsylvania State University, Hershey, Pennsylvania
41 Diarrhea, Constipation, and Irritable Bowel Syndrome

David L. Page, M.D.
Professor of Pathology, Director of Anatomic Pathology, Department of Pathology, Vanderbilt University Medical Center, Nashville, Tennessee
167 Benign Disorders of the Breast

Jean William Pape, M.D.
Associate Professor, Department of Medicine, State University Hospital of Haiti, Hatian National Institute for Laboratory and Research, Haiti; Associate Professor, Department of Medicine, Cornell University Medical College, New York, New York
268 Infections Caused by *Salmonella* and *Shigella* Species

Irvin L. Paradis, M.D.
Division of Pulmonary, Allergy, and Critical Care Medicine, Department of Medicine, University of Pittsburgh, Pittsburgh, Pennsylvania
220 Pulmonary Transplantation

Stephen W. Parker, M.D.
Assistant Professor in Neurology, Harvard Medical School; Director, Otoneurology, Department of Neurology and Otolaryngology, Massachusetts General Hospital, Boston, Massachusetts
115 Otoneurology

Harold E. Paulus, M.D.
Professor of Medicine, Division of Rheumatology, University of California, Los Angeles, School of Medicine, Los Angeles, California
317 Antirheumatic Drugs

Nancy J. Pelc, M.D.
Postdoctoral Fellow, Department of Dermatology, University of Cincinnati College of Medicine, Cincinnati, Ohio
96 Melanoma, Kaposi's Sarcoma, and Mycosis Fungoides

John R. Perfect, M.D.
Assistant Professor of Medicine, Duke University School of Medicine, Division of Infectious Disease, Department of Medicine, Duke University Hospital, Durham, North Carolina
265 Infections Caused by *Haemophilus* Species

Henry S. Perkins, M.D.
Associate Professor of Medicine, Department of Medicine, The University of Texas Health Science Center, San Antonio, Texas
374 The Fiduciary Concept: A Basis for an Ethics of Patient Care

Roger M. Perlmutter, M.D., Ph.D.
Professor and Chairman, Department of Immunology, Professor of Medicine (Medical Genetics) and Biochemistry, University of Washington; Investigator, Howard Hughes Medical Institute, Seattle, Washington
285 Antibodies: Structure and Genetics

Joseph K. Perloff, M.D.
Streisand/American Heart Association, Professor of Medicine and Pediatrics, Departments of Medicine and Pediatrics, University of California, Los Angeles, Center for Health Science, Los Angeles, California
3 Physical Examination of Cardiovascular System

Carolyn Petersen, M.D.
Assistant Professor, Department of Medicine, University of California, San Francisco; Attending Physician, Department of Medicine and Division of Infectious Diseases, San Francisco General Hospital, San Francisco, California
280 Infections Caused by Protozoa

Walter L. Peterson, M.D.
Professor of Medicine, University of Texas Southwestern Medical School, Dallas, Texas
32 Evaluation of Gastroduodenal Diseases
38 Peptic Ulcer Disease

Robert V. Pierre, M.D.
Professor of Pathology, Department of Pathology, University of Southern California, Los Angeles, California
73 Evaluation of Cells in the Peripheral Blood and Bone Marrow
74 Molecular Diagnostics

Graham F. Pineo, M.D., F.R.C.P.(C), F.A.C.P.
Professor of Medicine, Department of Medicine, Calgary General Hospital; Professor of Medicine, Department of Medicine, University of Calgary, Calgary, Alberta, Canada
86 Thrombosis and Anticoagulation

Paul H. Plotz, M.D.
Chief, Connective Tissue Diseases Section, Arthritis and Rheumatism Branch, National Institute of Arthritis and Musculoskeletal and Skin Diseases, National Institutes of Health, Bethesda, Maryland
311 Inflammatory Myopathies

Frisso A. Potts, M.D.
Instructor in Neurology, Harvard Medical School, Chief, Neurophysiology, Brockton/West Roxbury, Veterans Administration Medical Center; Visiting Physician, Division of Neurology, Brigham & Women's Hospital, Boston, Massachusetts
122 Myelopathies

Sumanth D. Prabhu, M.D.
Assistant Professor of Medicine, Division of Cardiology, University of Texas Health Science Center, San Antonio, Texas
1 Cardiovascular Physiology

Thomas T. Provost, M.D.
Noxell Professor and Chairman of Dermatology, Johns Hopkins University School of Medicine, Baltimore, Maryland
Co-Editor of Dermatology section
324 Cutaneous Manifestations of Connective Tissue Diseases

Amy A. Pruitt, M.D.
Assistant Professor of Neurology, Department of Neurology, Hospital of the University of Pennsylvania, Philadelphia, Pennsylvania
136 Neuro-Oncology

William E.M. Pryse-Phillips, M.D., F.R.C.P., F.R.C.P.(C)
Division of Neurology, Department of Medicine, Health Sciences Centre, Professor of Medicine, Neurology, Faculty of Medicine, Memorial University of Newfoundland, St. John's, Newfoundland, Canada
104 Psychologic Testing

Robert J. Pueringer, M.D.
Assistant Professor, Department of Internal Medicine, Pulmonary Diseases Division, The University of Iowa College of Medicine, Iowa City, Iowa
207 Sarcoidosis

Michael D. Rader, M.D., Ph.D.
Resident in Dermatology, Department of Dermatology, Johns Hopkins Hospital, Baltimore, Maryland
324 Cutaneous Manifestations of Connective Tissue Diseases

Shahbudin H. Rahimtoola, M.B., F.R.C.P.
George C. Griffith Professor of Cardiology, Chairman, Griffith Center; Professor of Medicine, University of Southern California, Los Angeles County and University of Southern California Medical Center, Los Angeles, California
16 Valvular Heart Disease

Lawrence G. Raisz, M.D.
Professor of Medicine, Department of Medicine, Head, Division of Endocrinology and Metabolism, John Dempsey Hospital; Attending Physician, University of Connecticut School of Medicine, Farmington, Connecticut
181 Osteoporosis

John A. Rankin, M.D.
Associate Professor of Medicine, Yale University School of Medicine, Departments of Pulmonary and Critical Care/Internal Medicine, Yale New Haven Hospital and West Haven Veterans Hospital, West Haven, Connecticut
196 Invasive Diagnostic Techniques

Gary E. Raskob, M.D.
Assistant Professor, Department of Biostatistics and Epidemiology, University of Oklahoma, Oklahoma City, Oklahoma
86 Thrombosis and Anticoagulation

Charles A. Reasner II, M.D.
Assistant Professor, Department of Medicine, Division of Endocrinology and Metabolism, University of Texas Health Science Center, San Antonio, Texas
148 Physiology of Bone and Mineral Homeostasis
151 Diagnostic Approach to Bone and Mineral Disorders
184 Osteopetrosis
188 Malignant Disease and the Skeleton

Guy S. Reeder, M.D.
Consultant, Division of Cardiovascular Diseases and Internal Medicine, Mayo Clinic and Mayo Foundation; Associate Professor of Medicine, Mayo Medical School, Rochester, Minnesota
14 Acute Myocardial Infarction

Patrick T. Regan, M.D.
Chairman, Department of Medicine, Columbia Hospital; Associate Clinical Professor, Department of Medicine, Medical College of Wisconsin, Milwaukee, Wisconsin
67 Pancreatic Disease

Mark Reichelderfer, M.D.
Director of Gastrointestinal Endoscopy, Associate Professor of Medicine (CHS), Department of Medicine, University of Wisconsin Hospital and Clinics, Madison, Wisconsin
30 Gastrointestinal Endoscopy

Michael F. Rein, M.D.
Attending Physician, Department of Internal Medicine, University of Virginia Health Sciences Center; Professor of Internal Medicine (Infectious Diseases), Department of Internal Medicine, University of Virginia, Charlottesville, Virginia
238 Sexually Transmitted Diseases (Urethritis, Vaginitis, Cervicitis, Proctitis, Genital Lesions)
273 Infections Caused by *Treponema* Species (Syphilis, Yaws, Pinta, Bejel)

James A. Reinarz, M.D.
Professor, Department of Internal Medicine/Infectious Diseases, University of Texas Medical Branch, Galveston, Texas
263 *Neisseria meningitidis* Infections

Donald Resnick, M.D.
Professor of Radiology, Department of Radiology, University of California, San Diego Medical Center; Chief, Osteoradiology Section, Department of Radiology, V.A. Medical Center, San Diego, California
296 Imaging Evaluation of Patients with Arthritis

Ellen B. Rest, M.S., M.D.
Assistant Professor, Department of Dermatology, University of Minnesota, Minneapolis, Minnesota
333 Cutaneous Manifestations of Internal Malignancy

Herbert Y. Reynolds, M.D.
J. Lloyd Huck Professor of Medicine, Chairman, Department of Medicine, Milton S. Hershey Medical Center, Pennsylvania State University College of Medicine, Hershey, Pennsylvania
193 Host Defense Mechanisms in the Respiratory Tract
199 Approach to Patient with Respiratory Disease: History, Physical Examination, and Assessment of Major Symptoms
208 Hypersensitivity Pneumonitis

Telfer B. Reynolds, M.D.
Clayton G. Loosli Professor of Medicine, Department of Medicine, Division of Gastrointestinal and Liver Diseases, University of Southern California School of Medicine, Los Angeles, California
59 Alcoholic Liver Disease

Robert R. Rich, M.D.
Professor and Head, Immunology Section, Vice President and Dean of Research, Baylor College of Medicine, Department of Microbiology and Immunology and Medicine, Baylor College of Medicine, Houston, Texas
283 Human Immune Response

Charles T. Richardson, M.D.
Clinical Professor of Internal Medicine, University of Texas Southwestern Medical Center at Dallas; Attending Physician, Baylor University Medical Center, Dallas, Texas
38 Peptic Ulcer Disease

Lee W. Riley, M.D.
Assistant Professor, Division of International Medicine, Cornell University Medical College; Attending Physician, New York Hospital, New York, New York
268 Infections Caused by *Salmonella* and *Shigella* Species

Jean E. Rinaldo, M.D.
Professor of Medicine, Division of Pulmonary Medicine, Vanderbilt University, Nashville, Tennessee
201 Multiple Organ Dysfunction Syndrome (MODS) in the Context of ARDS

Robert Roberts, M.D.
Chief of Cardiology, Section of Cardiology, Methodist Hospital, Professor of Medicine and Cell Biology, Section of Cardiology, Baylor College of Medicine, Houston, Texas
2 Molecular Biology of Cardiovascular System

Gary L. Robertson, M.D.
Professor of Neurology and Medicine, Department of Neuroendocrinology, Northwestern Memorial Hospital; Director, Clinical Research Center, Northwestern University Medical School, Chicago, Illinois
161 Disorders of the Posterior Pituitary

Sander J. Robins, M.D.
Director, Section of Lipid Metabolism and Atherosclerosis Prevention, Department of Medicine, Boston V.A. Medical Center; Associate Professor of Medicine, Department of Medicine, Boston University School of Medicine, Boston, Massachusetts
51 Bile Production and Secretion

Dudley F. Rochester, M.D.
E. Cato Drash Professor of Medicine, Department of Internal Medicine, University of Virginia Health Sciences Center; Head, Departments of Pulmonary and Critical Care Medicine, University of Virginia Health Sciences Center, Charlottesville, Virginia
191 Respiratory Muscles and Respiratory Muscle Failure

G. David Roodman, M.D.
Chief, Hematology Section, Audie Murphy V.A. Hospital; Professor, Department of Medicine, University of Texas Health Science Center, San Antonio, Texas
90 Hemolytic Anemia

Allan H. Ropper, M.D.
Chief of Neurology, St. Elizabeth's Hospital; Professor of Neurology, Tufts University School of Medicine, Boston, Massachusetts
139 Principles of Neurologic Emergencies and Intensive Care

Robin D. Rothstein, M.D.
Assistant Professor of Medicine, University of Pennsylvania School of Medicine, Department of Medicine, Division of Gastroenterology, Philadelphia, Pennsylvania
41 Diarrhea, Constipation, and Irritable Bowel Syndrome

Lewis J. Rubin, M.D.
Professor of Medicine and Physiology, University of Maryland School of Medicine; Head, Division of Pulmonary and Critical Care Medicine, University of Maryland Medical System, Baltimore, Maryland
216 Pulmonary Hypertension: Primary and Secondary Causes

Jeremy N. Ruskin, M.D.
Associate Professor of Medicine, Harvard Medical School; Director, Cardiac Arrhythmia Service, Division of Cardiology, Massachusetts Hospital, Boston, Massachusetts
12 Sudden Death

Michael S. Saag, M.D.
Associate Professor of Medicine, Department of Medicine, Division of Infectious Diseases, University of Alabama, Birmingham, Alabama
279 *Cryptococcus neoformans* Infections

Seymour M. Sabesin, M.D.
Josephine Dyrenforth Professor of Medicine, Rush Medical College; Director, Digestive Diseases, Rush-Presbyterian—St. Luke's Medical Center, Chicago, Illinois
50 Hepatic Metabolism

Sharon Safrin, M.D.
Attending Physician, Medical and Infectious Diseases Services, San Francisco General Hospital; Assistant Clinical Professor, Departments of Medicine, Epidemiology and Biostatistics, University of California, San Francisco, California
281 *Pneumocystis carinii* Infection

Stephen M. Sagar, M.D.
Assistant Chief of Neurology, Neurology Service, Veterans Affairs Medical Center, San Francisco; Professor, Department of Neurology, University of California, San Francisco, California
138 Metabolic and Toxic Disorders

Martin A. Samuels, M.D.
Professor of Neurology, Harvard Medical School; Chief of Neurology, Brigham and Women's Hospital, Boston, Massachusetts
140 Neurocardiology
142 Neuropulmonology
143 Neurogastroenterology
144 Neurohepatology
145 Neurohematology
146 Neuronephrology

Merle A. Sande, M.D.
Professor and Vice Chairman, Department of Medicine, University of California, San Francisco School of Medicine; Chief, Medical Service, San Francisco General Hospital, San Francisco, California
15 Infective Endocarditis
222 Basic Principles of Infectious Diseases
228 Fever and Rash
242 Acquired Immunodeficiency Syndrome

Richard J. Santen, M.D.
Evan Pugh Professor of Medicine, Pennsylvania State University College of Medicine; Vice Chairman, Department of Medicine, Chief, Division of Endocrinology, Diabetes, and Metabolism, Milton S. Hershey Medical Center, Hershey, Pennsylvania
166 Disorders of the Testis

David J. Sartoris, M.D.
Chief, Quantitative Bone Density, Department of Radiology, University of California, San Diego, Medical Center; Associate Professor of Radiology, Musculoskeletal Imaging Section, Department of Radiology, University of California, San Diego, California
296 Imaging Evaluation of Patients with Arthritis

Julius Schachter, Ph.D.
Professor of Epidemiology, Department of Laboratory Medicine, University of California, San Francisco; Director, World Health Organization Collaborating Center for Reference and Research on Chlamydia, San Francisco, California
254 Chlamydial Infections

Andrew I. Schafer, M.D.
Chief, Medical Service, Houston Veterans Affairs Medical Center, W.A. and Deborah Moncrief Professor and Vice Chairman, Department of Medicine, Baylor College of Medicine, Houston, Texas
84 Thrombocytopenia and Disorders of Platelet Function

Michael Schatz, M.D.
Associate Clinical Professor, Department of Medicine, University of California, San Diego; Staff Allergist, Department of Allergy, Kaiser Permanente Medical Center, San Diego, California
299 Rhinitis

W. Michael Scheld, M.D.
Professor of Medicine and Neurosurgery, Associate Chair for Residency Programs, University of Virginia School of Medicine, Charlottesville, Virginia
233 Acute Meninigitis

Steven Schenker, M.D.
Professor of Medicine and Pharmacology, Division Chief, Department of Medicine/Gastroenterology and Nutrition, University of Texas Health Science Center at San Antonio; Staff Physician, Audie L. Murphy Memorial Veterans Hospital, San Antonio, Texas
56 Principal Complications of Liver Failure
371 Drug Interactions

Robert C. Schlant, M.D.
Professor of Medicine (Cardiology), Chief of Cardiology, Grady Memorial Hospital, Department of Cardiology, Emory University School of Medicine, Atlanta, Georgia
19 Congenital Heart Disease

Charles J. Schleupner, M.D.
Professor of Internal Medicine, University of Virginia School of Medicine; Chief, Medical Service, Veterans Affairs Medical Center, Salem, Virginia
248 Arenavirus Infections (Lymphocytic Choriomeningitis, Lassa Fever, Hemorrhagic Fevers), Colorado Tick Fever, and Parvovirus Infection

George P. Schmid, M.D.
Chief, Clinical Research Branch, Division of STD/HIV Prevention, National Center for Prevention Services, Centers for Disease Control and Prevention, Atlanta, Georgia
275 Infections Caused by Borrelia (Relapsing Fever and Lyme Disease)

Konrad S. Schulze-Delrieu, M.D., F.R.C.P.C.C.
Professor, Department of Internal Medicine, University of Iowa College of Medicine, Veterans Administration Medical Center, Iowa City, Iowa
31 Evaluation of Esophageal Disease
35 Esophageal Diseases

Benjamin D. Schwartz, M.D., Ph.D.
Director, Department of Immunology, Monsanto Corporate Research; Research Professor, Department of Medicine (Rheumatology), Washington University School of Medicine; Physician, Department of Medicine (Rheumatology), Jewish Hospital, St. Louis, Missouri
284 Human Leukocyte Antigen Complex

J. Edwin Seegmiller, M.D.
Professor of Medicine, Associate Director, Sam and Rose Stein Institute for Research on Aging, University of California, San Diego, School of Medicine, San Diego, California
321 Ochronosis and Alkaptonuria

Marjorie E. Seybold, M.D., M.P.I.A.
Neuro-Ophthalmologist, Department of Ophthalmology, Scripps Clinic, La Jolla, California; Staff Neurologist, V.A. Medical Center; Adjunct Professor, Department of Neurosciences, University of California, San Diego, California
124 Diseases of the Neuromuscular Junction

Ralph Shabetai, M.D.
Professor of Medicine, University of California, San Diego, School of Medicine; Chief of Cardiology, Veterans Administration Hospital, La Jolla, California
18 Pericardial Disease and Pericardial Heart Disease

Pravin M. Shah, M.D.
Professor of Medicine, Attending Cardiologist, Director of Academic Program, Cardiology Section, Loma Linda University Medical Center, Loma Linda, California
17 Cardiomyopathies

Bhagwan T. Shahani, M.D., D.Phil.
Professor and Head, Department of Physical Medicine and Rehabilitation; Professor, Department of Neurology, University of Illinois at Chicago, College of Medicine, Chicago, Illinois
133 Principles of Neurorehabilitation

John N. Sheagren, M.D.
Chairman, Department of Internal Medicine, Illinois Masonic Medical Center; Professor of Medicine, University of Illinois College of Medicine, Chicago, Illinois
257 *Staphylococcus aureus* Infections

Duane Sigmund, M.D.
Assistant Professor, Department of Internal Medicine, University of Cincinnati College of Medicine, Cincinnati, Ohio
101 Lung Cancer

Richard M. Silver, M.D.
Associate Professor, Department of Internal Medicine, Medical University of South Carolina, Charleston, South Carolina
308 Raynaud's Phenomenon
310 Diffuse Fasciitis with Eosinophilia

Eva Simmons-O'Brien, M.D.
Resident in Dermatology, Department of Dermatology, Johns Hopkins Hospital, Baltimore, Maryland
324 Cutaneous Manifestations of Connective Tissue Diseases
334 Dermatologic Manifestations of Gastrointestinal Disease

Frederick R. Singer, M.D.
Medical Director, Osteoporosis/Metabolic Bone Disease Program, Saint John's Hospital and Health Center; Director, Skeletal Biology Laboratory, John Wayne Cancer Institute, Santa Monica, California
183 Paget's Disease of Bone

Richard M. Slataper, M.D.
Consultant, Department of Medicine, Ochsner Clinic, New Orleans, Louisiana
363 Renovascular Diseases

Peter M. Small, M.D.
Howard Hughes Medical Institute, Stanford University, Palo Alto, California
276 Tuberculosis and Nontuberculous Mycobacterial Infections

Peter Smolens, M.D.
Professor of Medicine, University of Texas Health Science Center at San Antonio; Clinical Associate, Medical Center Hospital, Audie L. Murphy Memorial Veterans Hospital, San Antonio, Texas
356 Renal Manifestations of Dysproteinemias

Gordon L. Snider, M.D.
Chief, Medical Service, Department of Medicine, Boston V.A. Medical Center; Maurice B. Strauss Professor of Medicine, Boston and Tufts University Schools of Medicine, Boston, Massachusetts
205 Chronic Obstructive Pulmonary Disease

Michael F. Sorrell, M.D.
Robert L. Grissom Professor of Medicine, Department of Internal Medicine, University of Nebraska Medical Center, Omaha, Nebraska
64 Liver Transplantation

K. Vincent Speeg, Jr., M.D., Ph.D.
Professor of Medicine, Division of Gastroenterology and Nutrition, Department of Medicine, University of Texas Health Science Center, San Antonio, Texas
371 Drug Interactions

John A. Spittell, Jr., M.D.
Professor of Medicine, Mayo Medical School; Consultant, Cardiovascular Disease, Mayo Clinic, Rochester, Minnesota
22 Diseases of the Peripheral Arteries and Veins

Peter C. Spittell, M.D.
Senior Associate Consultant, Division of Cardiovascular Diseases, Mayo Clinic and Mayo Foundation, Rochester, Minnesota
22 Diseases of the Peripheral Arteries and Veins

Jay H. Stein, M.D.
Professor of Medicine Senior Vice President and Provost, University of Oklahoma Health Sciences Center, Oklahoma City, Oklahoma
338 Principles of Renal Physiology
347 Acute Renal Failure
356 Renal Manifestations of Dysproteinemias

Alfred D. Steinberg, M.D.
Principal Scientist, The MITRE Corporation, McLean, Virginia
289 Tolerance and Autoimmunity

Martin H. Steinberg, M.D.
Associate Chief of Staff for Research, V.A. Medical Center; Professor of Medicine, University of Mississippi, School of Medicine, Jackson, Mississippi
89 Hemoglobinopathies and Thalassemias

Richard H. Sterns, M.D.
Associate Professor of Medicine, Department of Medicine, University of Rochester School of Medicine, Rochester General Hospital, Rochester, New York
352 Disorders of Potassium Balance

Dennis L. Stevens, Ph.D., M.D.
Chief, Infectious Diseases, Department of Medicine, Veterans Affairs Medical Center, Boise, Idaho; Professor of Medicine, Department of Medicine, University of Washington, Seattle, Washington
259 *Streptococcus pyogenes* Infections

Lynne Warner Stevenson, M.D.
Assistant Professor of Medicine, Director, Ahmanson-UCLA Cardiomyopathy Center, Department of Medicine, University of California, Los Angeles Medical Center, Los Angeles, California
25 Cardiac Transplantation

James G. Straka, Ph.D.
Research Associate in Medicine, University of Minnesota, Minneapolis, Minnesota
176 Disorders of Porphyrin Metabolism

Larry J. Strausbaugh, M.D.
Hospital Epidemiologist and Staff Physician, Medical Service, Portland Veterans Affairs Medical Center; Professor, Department of Internal Medicine, School of Medicine, Oregon Health Sciences University, Portland, Oregon
260 Enterococcal and Other Non-Group A Streptococcal Infections

Terry B. Strom, M.D.
Professor of Medicine, Harvard Medical School; Physician and Director of Clinical Immunology, Beth Israel Hospital, Boston, Massachusetts
348 Chronic Renal Failure

Lewis R. Sudarsky, M.D.
Assistant Professor of Neurology, Harvard Medical School, Boston, Massachusetts; Assistant Chief, Neurology Service, Brockton/West Roxbury Veterans Administration Medical Center, West Roxbury, Massachusetts
119 Parkinsonism and Movement Disorders

Stephen B. Sulavik, M.D.
Professor and Head, Division of Pulmonary Medicine, University of Connecticut School of Medicine, Farmington, Connecticut; Clinical Professor of Medicine, Yale University School of Medicine, New Haven, Connecticut
210 Primary Granulomatous Pulmonary Vasculitis

Thomas Y. Sullivan, M.D.
Medical Director, Pulmonary Function, Exercise, and Sleep Laboratories, Methodist Hospital; Associate Clinical Professor, Department of Internal Medicine, Indiana University School of Medicine, Indianapolis, Indiana
215 Solitary Pulmonary Tumor

Robert W. Summers, B.S., M.D.
Medical Director, Diagnostic and Therapeutic Unit, James A. Clifton Center for Digestive Diseases, University of Iowa Hospitals and Clinics; Professor, Division of Gastroenterology-Hepatology, Department of Internal Medicine, University of Iowa College of Medicine, Veterans Administration Medical Center, Iowa City, Iowa
31 Evaluation of Esophageal Disease
35 Esophageal Diseases

J. T. Sylvester, M.D.
David Marine Professor of Medicine, Department of Medicine, Johns Hopkins Hospital; Director, Division of Pulmonary and Critical Care Medicine, Department of Medicine, Johns Hopkins University School of Medicine, Baltimore, Maryland
192 Pulmonary Blood Flow

Randy Taplitz, M.D.
Fellow, Infectious Diseases, Division of Infectious Diseases, Department of Medicine, University of California, San Francisco School of Medicine, San Francisco, California
228 Fever and Rash

Angelo Taranta, M.D.
Professor of Medicine, New York Medical College; Director, Department of Medicine, Cabrini Medical Center, New York, New York
316 Rheumatic Fever

Robert D. Tarver, M.D.
Associate Professor, Department of Radiology, Indiana University School of Medicine, Indianapolis, Indiana
197 Pulmonary Diagnostic Imaging

Martin G. Täuber, M.D.
Attending Physician, Medical Service, San Francisco General Hospital; Assistant Professor, Department of Medicine and Infectious Diseases, University of California, San Francisco, California
227 Fever of Unknown Origin

Robert A. Terkeltaub, M.D.
Chief, Rheumatology Section, Department of Medicine, San Diego Veterans Affairs Medical Center; Associate Professor of Medicine in Residence, Department of Medicine, University of California, San Diego, California
319 Gout and Hyperuricemia

Jess G. Thoene, M.D.
Professor of Pediatrics, Director of Biochemical Genetics and Metabolism, Department of Pediatrics, University of Michigan, C.S. Mott Children's Hospital, Ann Arbor, Michigan
173 Disorders of Amino Acid Metabolism

Knox H. Todd, M.D.
Research Fellow, Division of Emergency Medicine, Department of Medicine, University of California, Los Angeles School of Medicine, Center for the Health Sciences, Los Angeles, California
368 Environmental Emergencies, Bites, and Stings

Galen B. Toews, M.D.
Professor and Chief of Pulmonary and Critical Care Medicine, Department of Internal Medicine, University of Michigan Medical Center, Ann Arbor, Michigan
214 Neoplasms of the Lung

Jerry S. Trier, M.D.
Professor of Medicine, Harvard Medical School, Division of Gastroenterology; Senior Physician, Division of Gastroenterology, Brigham and Women's Hospital, Boston, Massachusetts
28 Intestinal Absorption
33 Evaluation of Intestinal Diseases
42 Diseases of Intestinal Absorption

Allan R. Tunkel, M.D., Ph.D.
Assistant Professor of Medicine, Department of Internal Medicine (Infectious Diseases), Medical College of Pennsylvania, Philadelphia, Pennsylvania
233 Acute Meningitis
240 Urinary Tract Infections

Manjeri A. Venkatachalam, M.B., B.S.
Professor of Pathology and Medicine, Department of Pathology, University of Texas Health Science Center, San Antonio, Texas
343 Proteinuria

David L. Vesely, M.D., Ph.D.
Professor of Internal Medicine, Physiology, and Biophysics, University of South Florida Medical School; Attending Physician, Department of Internal Medicine, James A. Haley Veterans Hospital and Tampa General Hospital; Director of the Atrial Natriuretic Peptides Research Laboratories, Tampa, Florida
154 Weakness

Vernon A. Vix, M.D.
Professor, Department of Radiology and Department of Medicine, Indiana University School of Medicine, Indianapolis, Indiana
197 Pulmonary Diagnostic Imaging

Daniel D. Von Hoff, M.D.
Professor of Medicine, Head, Section of Drug Development, University of Texas Health Science Center, San Antonio, Texas
100 Head and Neck Cancer

Michael Vulpe, M.D.
Spinal Cord Injury Service, Long Beach V.A. Medical Center, Department of Neurology, University of California, Irvine, California
132 Spinal Cord Injury

David H. Walker, M.D.
Professor and Chairman, Department of Pathology, University of Texas Medical Branch, Galveston, Texas
256 Rickettsial Infections

Robert E. Wall, M.D.
Chairman, Department of Obstetrics and Gynecology, Rose Medical Center; Associate Clinical Professor, Department of Obstetrics and Gynecology, University of Colorado School of Medicine, Denver, Colorado
369 Medical Disorders During Pregnancy

Richard A. Walsh, M.D.
Director of Cardiology, University of Cincinnati College of Medicine, Cincinnati, Ohio
8 Palpitations
112 Faintness and Syncope

Thomas M. Walshe III, M.D.
Assistant Professor of Neurology, Harvard Medical School; Associate Chief of Neurology, Brockton-West Roxbury V.A. Medical Center, Brockton, Massachusetts
118 Cognitive Failure Dementia

Stephen I. Wasserman, M.D.
H.M. Ranney Professor and Chairman, Department of Medicine, University of California, San Diego, California
288 Immediate Hypersensitivity
292 Laboratory Methods in Immediate Hypersensitivity
300 Asthma

Rosemarie M. Watson, M.D.
Associate Professor of Dermatology, Johns Hopkins University School of Medicine; Clinical Director, Dermatology Ambulatory Care Unit, Johns Hopkins Hospital, Baltimore, Maryland
335 Cutaneous Manifestations of Endocrine Disorders

William A. Watson, Pharm.D.
Clinical Associate Professor, Diplomat, American Board of Applied Toxicology, Department of Emergency Medicine, Truman Medical Center; Clinical Associate Professor, Emergency Medicine and Pharmacy Practice, Schools of Medicine and Pharmacy, University of Missouri-Kansas City, Kansas City, Missouri
366 Clinical Toxicology

David L. Weinbaum, M.D.
Clinical Assistant Professor of Medicine, University of Pittsburgh School of Medicine; Chief, Division of Infectious Diseases, Western Pennsylvania Hospital, Pittsburgh, Pennsylvania
223 Host Defense Against Infection: The Roles of Antibody, Complement, and Phagocytic Cells

Michael H. Weisman, M.D.
Professor of Medicine, University of California, San Diego, School of Medicine, LaJolla, California; Attending Physician, University of California, San Diego, Medical Center, San Diego, California
312 Spondyloarthropathies
315 Infections of the Joints

Jay D. Wenger, M.D.
Acting Chief, Meningitis and Special Pathogens Branch, Division of Bacterial and Myotic Diseases, National Center for Infectious Diseases, Centers for Disease Control and Prevention, Atlanta, Georgia
274 Infections Caused by Leptospires (Leptospirosis)

Richard P. Wenzel, M.D., M.Sc.
Professor, Department of Internal Medicine, University of Iowa College of Medicine; Director, Division of Clinical Epidemiology, University of Iowa Hospitals and Clinics, Iowa City, Iowa
225 Hospital Infection Control

Elliot Weser, M.D.
Professor and Deputy Chairman, University of Texas Health Science Center at San Antonio; Chief, Medical Service, Audie L. Murphy Memorial Veterans Hospital, San Antonio, Texas
49 Nutrition and Internal Medicine

Gilbert C. White II, M.D.
Professor of Medicine, University of North Carolina at Chapel Hill, School of Medicine; Attending Physician, North Carolina Memorial Hospital, Chapel Hill, North Carolina
85 Disorders of Blood Coagulation

S. Elizabeth Whitmore, M.D.
Assistant Professor of Dermatology, Department of Dermatology, Johns Hopkins Hospital Medical Institutions, Baltimore, Maryland
328 Dermatitis

Herbert P. Wiedemann, M.D.
Chairman, Department of Pulmonary and Critical Care Medicine, Cleveland Clinic Foundation, Cleveland, Ohio
198 Intensive Care Monitoring and Mechanical Ventilation

Laurel Wiegand, M.D.
Associate Professor of Medicine, Division of Pulmonary and Critical Care Medicine, Department of Medicine, Milton S. Hershey Medical Center, Pennsylvania State University, Hershey, Pennsylvania
221 Sleep-Related Respiratory Disorders

David A. Williams, M.D.
Associate Professor Pediatrics and Medical and Molecular Genetics and Kipp Investigator of Pediatrics, Herman B. Wells Center for Pediatric Research; Associate Investigator, Howard Hughes Medical Institute, Indiana University School of Medicine, Indianapolis, Indiana
69 Molecular and Cellular Biology of Hematopoiesis

Eric S. Williams, M.D.
Professor of Medicine, Indiana University School of Medicine, Indianapolis, Indiana
9 Cardiac Arrhythmias

Penny Williams, M.D.
Division of Infectious Disease, Department of Medicine and Department of Surgery, University of Pittsburgh, Pittsburgh, Pennsylvania
220 Pulmonary Transplantation

Barbara Braunstein Wilson, M.D.
Associate Professor, Department of Dermatology, University of Virginia Health Sciences Center, Charlottesville, Virginia
331 Superficial Fungal Infections

Mary E. Wilson, M.D.
Associate Professor of Internal Medicine, Department of Internal Medicine, University of Iowa College of Medicine, Iowa City, Iowa
267 Infections Caused by *Vibrio* Species

Walter R. Wilson, M.D.
Professor of Medicine, Mayo Medical School, Rochester, Minnesota
269 Infections Caused by *Brucella, Francisella tularensis, Pasteurella,* and *Yersinia* Species

Washington C. Winn, Jr., M.D.
Director, Clinical Microbiology Laboratory, Department of Pathology, Medical Center Hospital of Vermont; Professor of Pathology, Department of Pathology, University of Vermont College of Medicine, Burlington, Vermont
272 Infections Caused by Legionellae

Birgit Winther, M.D.
Assistant Professor, Otolaryngology and Head and Neck Surgery, and Pediatrics, University of Virginia Health Sciences Center, Charlottesville, Virginia
230 Upper Respiratory Infections (Colds, Pharyngitis, Sinusitis)

Victor A. Yanchick, M.D.
Dean, College of Pharmacy, Professor of Pharmacy, University of Oklahoma Health Sciences Center, Oklahoma City, Oklahoma
371 Drug Interactions

Eleanor A. Young, Ph.D., RD/LD
Professor, Department of Medicine, University of Texas Health Science Center, San Antonio, Texas
49 Nutrition and Internal Medicine

Lowell S. Young, M.D.
Director, Kuzell Institute for Arthritis and Infectious Diseases, Department of Medicine, California Pacific Medical Center; Clinical Professor, Department of Medicine, University of California, San Francisco, California
229 Fever in the Compromised Host

Robert R. Young, M.D.
Professor and Vice Chair, Department of Neurology, University of California, Irvine, California; Chief, Neurology Service, Long Beach V.A. Medical Center, Long Beach, California
132 Spinal Cord Injury

Miguel Zabalgoitia, M.D.
Director, Non-Invasive Laboratories, Audie L. Murphy Memorial Veterans Hospital and Medical Center Hospital; Assistant Professor of Medicine, Department of Medicine/Cardiology, University of Texas Health Science Center, San Antonio, Texas
21 Diseases of the Aorta

Robert S. Zeiger, M.D., Ph.D.
Clinical Professor of Pediatrics, Department of Pediatrics, University of California, San Diego; Chief of Allergy, Department of Allergy, Kaiser Permanente Medical Center, San Diego, California
299 Rhinitis

Hyman J. Zimmerman, M.D.
Professor of Medicine, Emeritus, George Washington University School of Medicine; Distinguished Physician, Emeritus, Armed Forces Institute of Pathology, Hepatic Department, Washington, D.C.
58 Drug- and Toxin-Induced Liver Disease

Fuad N. Ziyadeh, M.D.
Assistant Professor of Medicine, Department of Medicine, Hospital of the University of Pennsylvania, Renal-Electrolyte Division, University of Pennsylvania, Philadelphia, Pennsylvania
179 Disorders of Phosphate Homeostasis
355 Diabetic Nephropathy

Nathan J. Zvaifler, M.D.
Professor of Medicine, University of California, San Diego Medical Center, San Diego, California
295 Synovial Fluid Analysis
303 Evaluation of Joint Complaints
304 Rheumatoid Arthritis
313 Uncommon Arthropathies

Preface

We are very excited about the fourth edition of *Internal Medicine*. Our editorial group continues to believe that the basic format is appropriate for students, house officers, and practicing physicians. Each part, except for one on special topics, is divided into three primary sections: an introductory section on basic principles of a given organ system, a section on laboratory tests, including review of the differential diagnosis, and a detailed section on various disease entities.

Although the basic format has remained constant, the text has changed dramatically. From the outset, we made a commitment to change at least one third of the authors and chapters with each edition to ensure that the book is as current as possible. In addition, many new chapters have been added and several have either been deleted or combined. For example, there are new chapters on molecular biology of the cardiovascular system, cardiac transplantation, gastrointestinal manifestations of HIV infection and AIDS, faintness and syncope, principles of neurorehabilitation, spinal cord injury, multiple organ dysfunction syndrome in the context of ARDS, pulmonary transplantation, sleep-related respiratory disorders, fever in the hospitalized patient, infections caused by the *Candida, Actinomyces,* and *Nocardia* species, periarticular rheumatic complaints, and Raynaud's phenomenon.

Internal medicine and medicine in general are changing rapidly. What our practice will look like in 10 years is far from clear. I would like to think that, even in this age of information explosion and curriculum and health care reform, we are able to create, in a single volume, a work that is both readable and encyclopedic, and ultimately of great value to the busy clinician.

Acknowledgements

We would once again like to thank our secretaries for their long hours of patience in this endeavor. George Stamathis and Stephanie Manning at Mosby have been fantastic. I would especially like to thank Kathy Falk, who has overseen the development of the manuscript. She certainly has the greatest patience with such a low-key group of editors.

JAY H. STEIN

Contents

PART TWO

Alimentary Tract, Liver, Biliary Tree, and Pancreas

ALIMENTARY TRACT

I Physiologic, Biochemical, and Immunologic Principles

II Diagnostic Procedures and Tests

III Clinical Syndromes and Specific Disease Entities

LIVER, BILIARY TREE, AND PANCREAS

I PHYSIOLOGIC, BIOCHEMICAL, AND IMMUNOLOGIC PRINCIPLES

II DIAGNOSTIC PROCEDURES AND TESTS

III CLINICAL SYNDROMES AND SPECIFIC DISEASE ENTITIES

PART THREE

Hematology and Oncology

BASIC PRINCIPLES I

LABORATORY TESTS II

II Clinical Syndromes

III Neurologic Diseases

The Neurology of Behavior IV

Neurology in General Medicine and Surgery V

III Clinical Syndromes and Therapeutic Modalities

IV Specific Disease Entities

PART SEVEN

Infectious Diseases

Basic Principles I

II Laboratory Tests

III Clinical Syndromes

Organisms Infective to Humans IV

Viral Diseases

PART EIGHT

Clinical Immunology, Rheumatology, and Dermatology

I Principles of Immunology

II Laboratory and Diagnostic Tests

Clinical Immunology III

Atopic Diseases and Related Syndromes IV

Rheumatic Disorders V

III Basic Clinical Syndromes

IV Disorders of Electrolyte and Acid-Base Balance

PART TEN

Special Topics in Internal Medicine

APPENDIX

Color Plates

Plate I

1. Color flow velocities in diastole.
2. Color flow velocities in systole.
3. Color Doppler image—aortic regurgitation.
4. Color Doppler image—mitral regurgitation.

Plate II

1. Reflux esophagitis.
2. Lower esophageal ring.
3. Esophageal varices actively bleeding.
4. Carcinoma of stomach.
5. Benign gastric ulcer.
6. Duodenal ulcer that has recently bled.
7. Cholangiocarcinoma with common bile duct obstruction bypassed with an endoscopically placed expandable stent.
8. Benign colon polyp.
9. Carcinoma of sigmoid colon.
10. Severe Crohn's colitis.
11. Diverticulum of colon.
12. Pseudomembranous colitis caused by *Clostridium difficile*.
13. Perivenular fibrosis closing off terminal hepatic vein (alcoholic hepatitis).
14. Hepatocyte containing alcoholic hyalin (alcoholic hepatitis).
15. Hypertrophic liver (alcoholic cirrhosis).
16. Uniform micronodules (alcoholic cirrhosis).
17. Primary biliary cirrhosis, stage I.
18. Primary biliary cirrhosis, stage II.
19. Left-sided heart failure.
20. Alpha-1 antitrypsin deficiency.
21. Schistosomiasis.
22. Mulberry-shaped solitary cholesterol gallstone.
23. Close-packed faceted cholesterol gallstones.
24. Round solitary cholesterol gallstone.
25. Black polymer pigment gallstones.
26. Polarized light microscopy of bile-rich duodenal fluid.

Plate III

1. Normal bone marrow.
2. Colony forming unit grown from human bone marrow.
3. Maturing erythroid precursors in bone marrow.
4. Erythrocyte morphology in peripheral blood.
5. Lymphocyte morphology in peripheral blood.
6. Granulocyte morphology in peripheral blood.
7. Iron in normal bone marrow.
8. Ringed sideroblasts in sideroblastic anemia.
9. Plasma cells in multiple myeloma.
10. Cutaneous manifestations of acute graft-versus-host disease.
11. Bone marrow in polycythemia vera.
12. Petechiae and hemorrhagic bullae in acute idiopathic thrombocytopenic purpura.
13. Megaloblastic bone marrow.
14. Malignant melanoma.
15. Mycosis fungoides.

Plate IV

1. Background diabetic retinopathy.
2. Exudative diabetic retinopathy.
3. Proliferative diabetic retinopathy.
4. Osteomalacia with tetracycline labeling.
5. Predominant hyperparathyroid bone disease.
6. Mixed uremic osteodystrophy.
7. Low turnover osteomalacia.

Plate V

1. Mature oocyst of *Isospora belli* in unstained fecal smear.
2. *Treponema pallidum* by dark field microscopy.
3. Quellung reaction with pneumococcal omni serum.
4. Staphylococci.
5. *Haemophilus influenzae*.
6. Gram-negative rods in *Klebsiella* pneumoniae or others caused by enterobacteriaceae or pseudomonas.
7. Gram-stained expectorated sputum or transtracheal aspirate in aspiration anaerobic pneumonia.
8. Gram stain of centrifuged cerebrospinal fluid in *Haemophilus influenzae* type B meningitis.
9. Gram stain of centrifuged cerebrospinal fluid in meningococcal meningitis.
10. Giemsa stain of bronchial washings demonstrating *Pneumocystis carinii* cysts.
11. Giemsa stain of conjunctiva scraping showing typical cytoplasmic inclusion of *Chlamydia trachomatis*.
12. *Leishmania* amastigotes in cutaneous leishmaniasis.
13. Photomicrographic scraping from base of herpes blister demonstrating multinuclear giant cells.
14. Giemsa-stained blood smear in *Plasmodium falciparum* malaria.
15. Giemsa-stained blood smear in *Plasmodium vivax* malaria.
16. Trypomastigotes of *Trypanosoma brucei rhodesiense* in Giemsa-stained thick blood smear.
17. Trypomastigote of *Trypanosoma cruzi* in Giemsa-stained blood smear.
18. Petechial and purpuric skin lesions in severe case of Rocky Mountain spotted fever.

Plate V *continued*

19. Rocky Mountain spotted fever.
20. Cutaneous lesions in meningococcemia (close-up).
21. Cutaneous lesions in meningococcemia.
22. Cutaneous lesion in disseminated gonococcal infection.
23. Cutaneous lesion in leukemic patient with overwhelming *Pseudomonas aeruginosa* septicemia.
24. Desquamation following toxic shock syndrome.
25. Cutaneous sporotrichosis.
26. Specificity in diagnosing pneumococcal pneumonia.
27. Erysipelas.
28. Periorbital *H. influenzae* cellulitis.
29. Hot tub folliculitis.
30. Staphylococcal scalded skin syndrome.
31. Acute gangrene of arm.
32. Elephantiasis nostras.
33. *Mycobacterium marinum.*
34. Modified Kinyoun stain of stool specimen demonstrating *Cryptosporidium.*
35. Oocysts of *Cryptosporidium.*
36. Chancre of penis.
37. Hematoxylin and eosin preparation from peripheral lymph node.
38. Acid-fast stain of lymph node biopsy.
39. Transbronchial biopsy specimen in cytomegalovirus pneumonitis.
40. Cutaneous Kaposi's sarcoma lesions.
41. Kaposi's sarcoma lesion in colonic mucosa.
42. Typical lesion of bacillary angiomatosis.
43. Retinochoroiditis due to cytomegalovirus infection.
44. Oral hairy leukoplakia.
45. Typical maculopapular rash of measles.
46. Petechial rash of atypical measles.
47. "Strawberry tongue" exanthem.
48. Negri bodies in human rabies.
49. Typical focus of rickettsial vasculitis in an arteriole.
50. Small intradermal hemorrhage at a focus of vasculitis.
51. Secondary syphilis.
52. Palmar lesions of secondary syphilis.
53. Blastomycosis.
54. Sporotrichosis.
55. Actinomycosis.
56. *Entamoeba histolytica* in fecal specimen.
57. *Giardia lamblia* trophozoite and cyst.

Plate VI

1. Crystals in synovial fluids as viewed with compensated polarized light.
2. Reiter's disease.
3. Lupus erythematosus.
4. Dermatomyositis (Gottron's papules).
5. Dermatitis herpetiformis.
6. Psoriasis.
7. Porphyria cutanea tarda.
8. Stevens-Johnson syndrome.
9. Erythema nodosum.
10. Exanthematous eruption developing after the administration of trimethoprim-sulfamethoxazole.
11. Cutaneous leukocytoclastic vasculitis.
12. Toxic epidermal necrolysis.
13. Metastatic carcinoma.
14. Neurofibromatosis.
15. Pyoderma gangrenosum.
16. Addison's disease: hyperpigmentation of skin and palmar and digital creases.
17. Addison's disease: hyperpigmentation of gums along dentate margins.
18. Vitiligo.
19. Necrobiosis lipoidica diabeticorum.
20. Acanthosis nigricans.
21. Papular lesions of sarcoidosis.
22. Lesions of lupus pernio.
23. Noncaseating granulomas of sarcoidosis.
24. Kaposi's sarcoma.

INTERNAL MEDICINE

Color Plates

I-VI

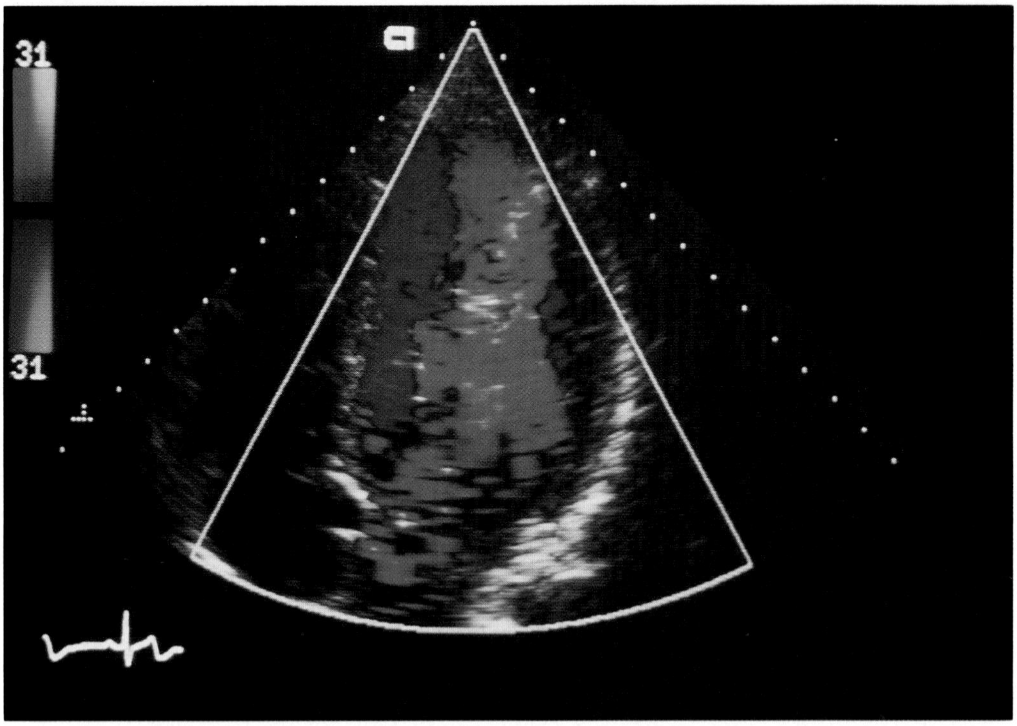

Plate I-1. Flow velocities in diastole coming towards the transducer (which is located over the apex) and depicted in red.

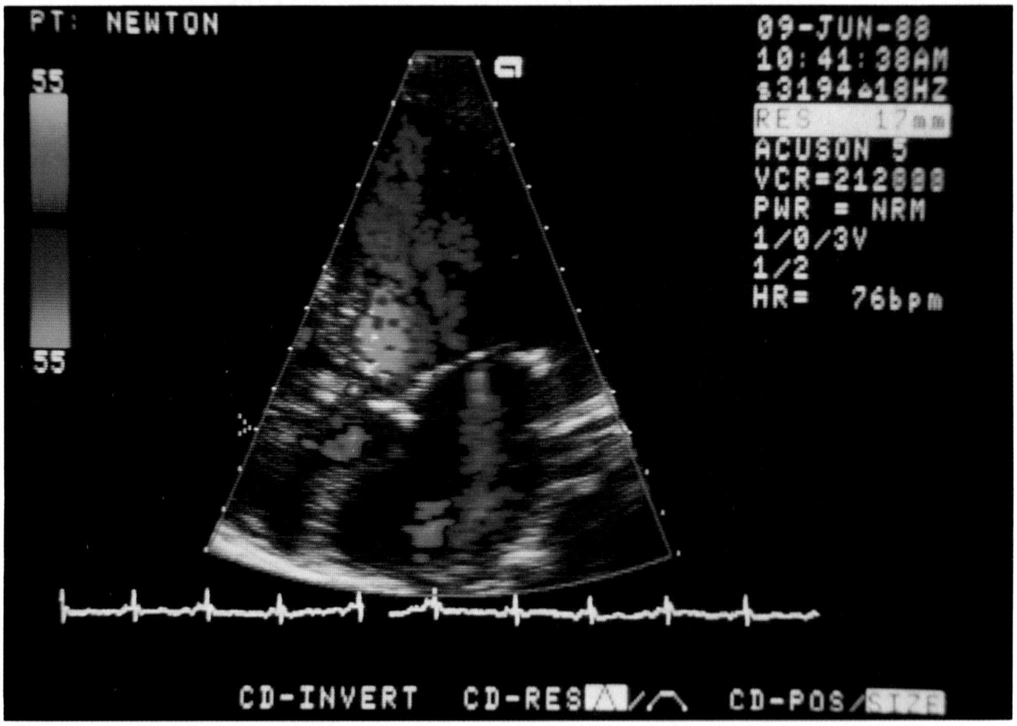

Plate I-2. Flow velocities in systole moving away from the transducer (which is located over the apex) and depicted in blue.

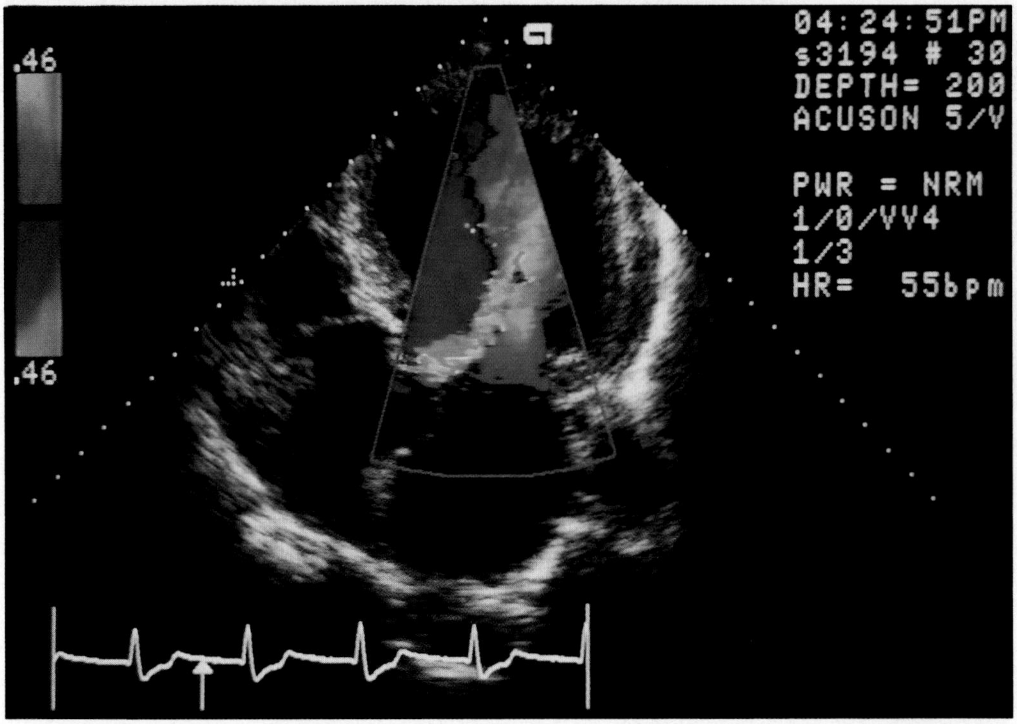

Plate I-3. Doppler image from a patient with aortic regurgitation. This diastolic image showing the aortic regurgitant jet directed into the left ventricular cavity was acquired using transthoracic echocardiography.

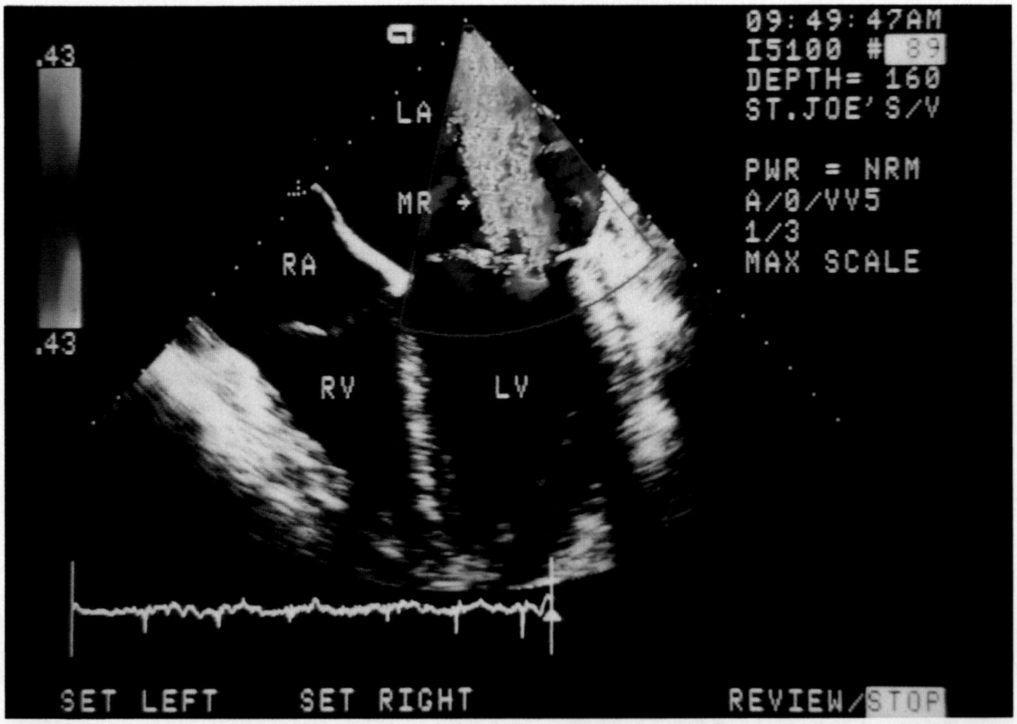

Plate I-4. Doppler image from a patient with mitral regurgitation. This systolic image showing the mitral regurgitant jet directed into the left atrium was acquired using transesophageal echocardiography.

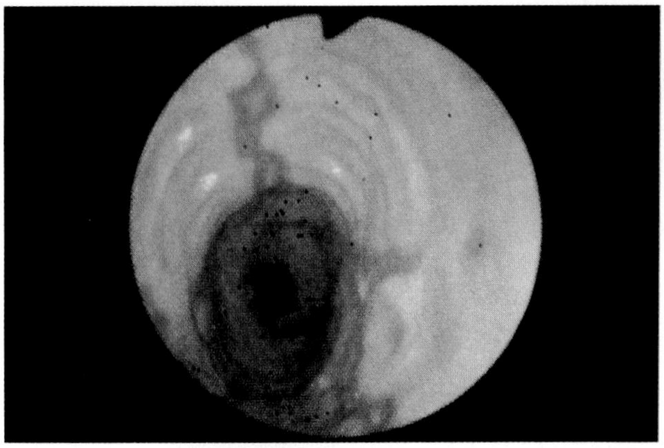

Plate II-1. Reflux esophagitis.

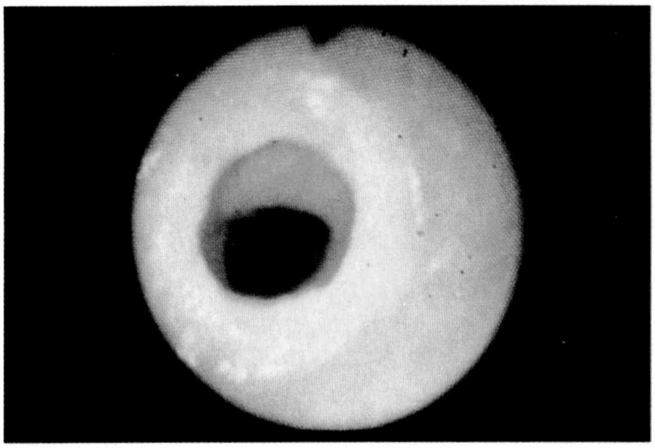

Plate II-2. Lower esophageal ring.

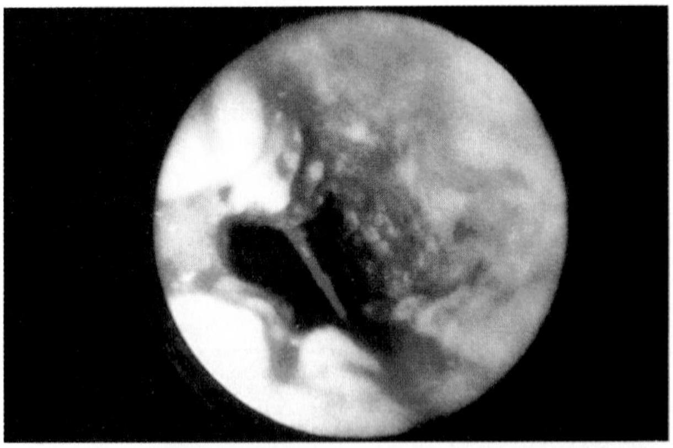

Plate II-3. Esophageal varices actively bleeding.

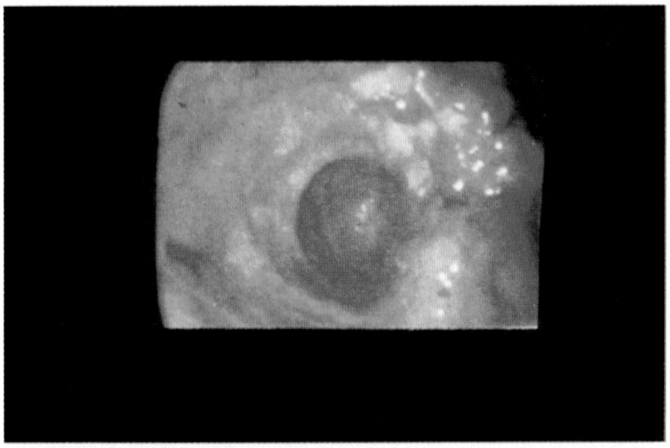

Plate II-4. Carcinoma of stomach.

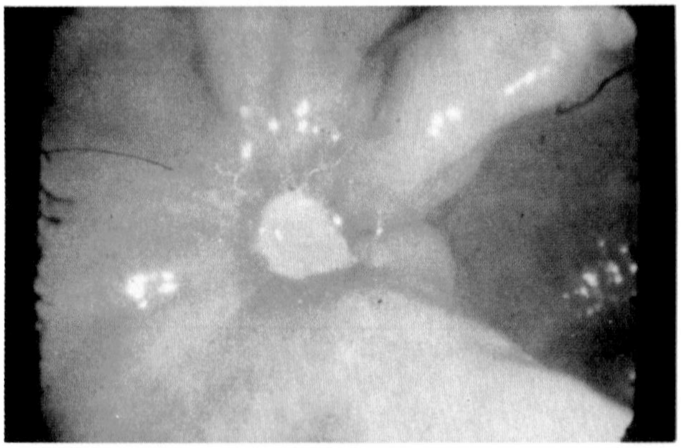

Plate II-5. Benign gastric ulcer. (Photographed with the intragastric camera of a gastrocamera fiberscope.)

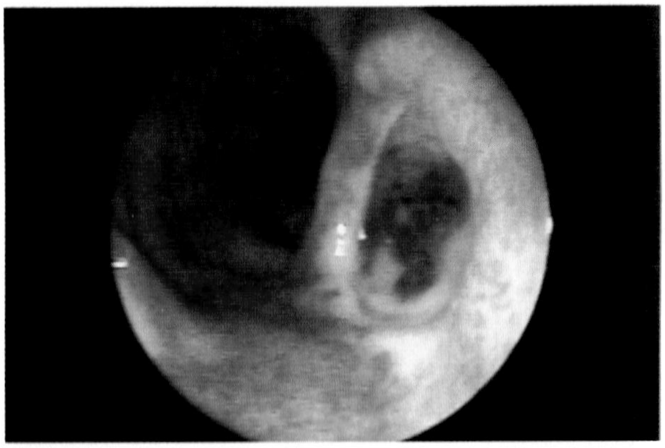

Plate II-6. Duodenal ulcer that has recently bled; there is a visible vessel in the ulcer base.

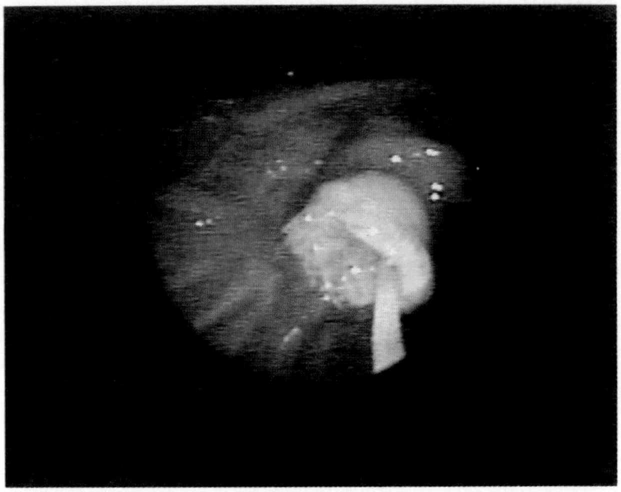

Plate II-7. Cholangiocarcinoma with common bile duct obstruction, bypassed with an endoscopically placed expandable stent. A 2 mm ERCP catheter has been passed through the stent.

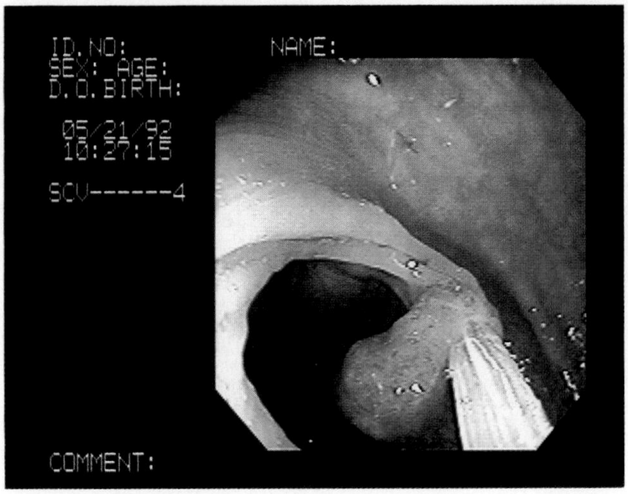

Plate II-8. Benign colon polyp snared before electrosurgical removal. (Photographed with a videoendoscope.)

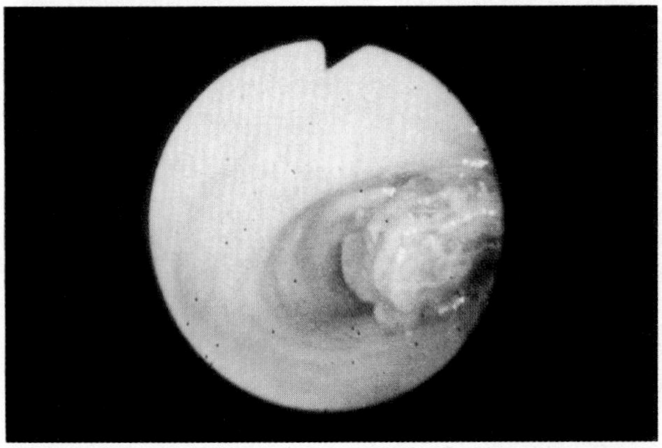

Plate II-9. Carcinoma of sigmoid colon.

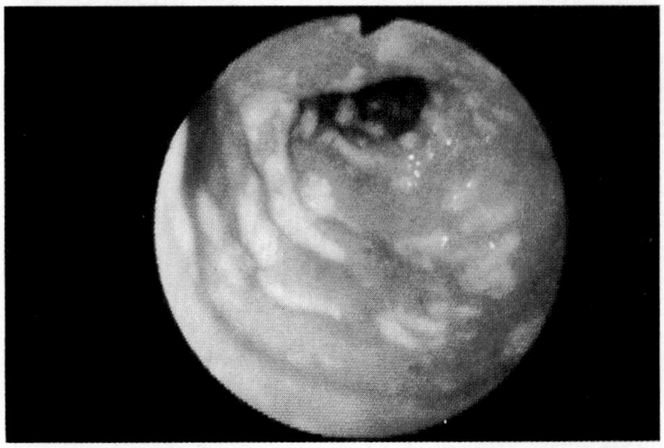

Plate II-10. Severe Crohn's colitis.

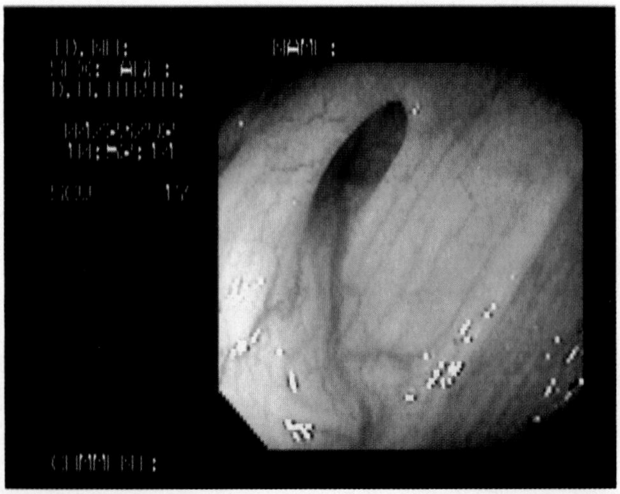

Plate II-11. Diverticulum of colon showing its relation to perforating blood vessels. (Photographed with a videoendoscope.)

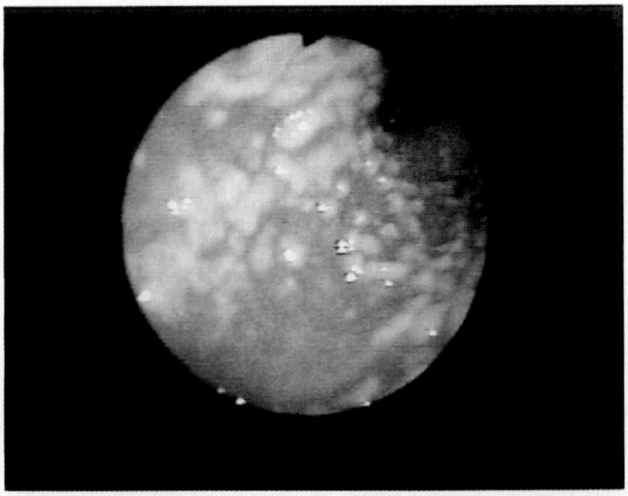

Plate II-12. Pseudomembranous colitis caused by *Clostridium difficile*, following antibiotic therapy.

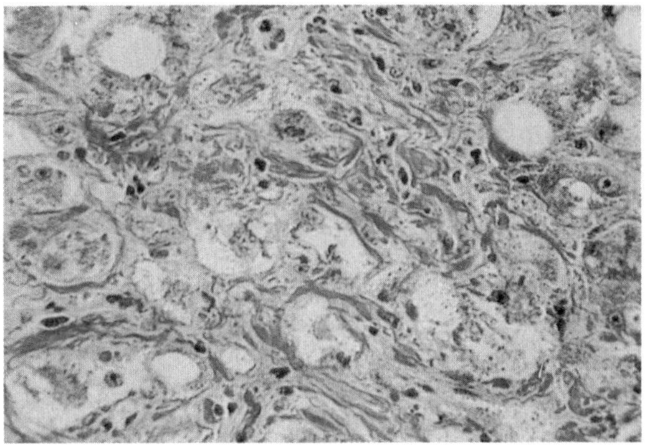

Plate II-13. Perivenular fibrosis closing off the terminal hepatic vein (alcoholic hepatitis.)

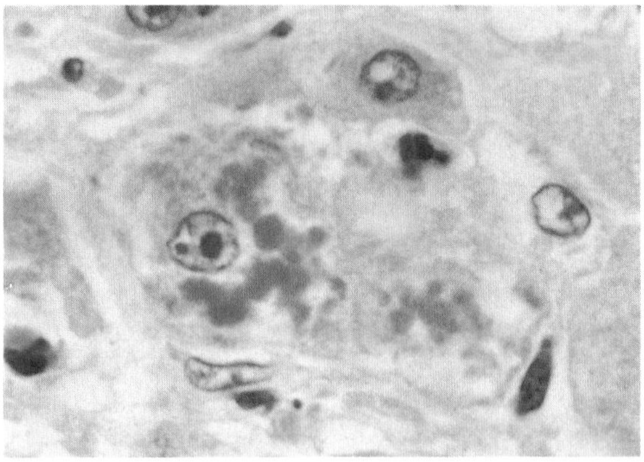

Plate II-14. Hepatocyte containing alcoholic hyalin (alcoholic hepatitis).

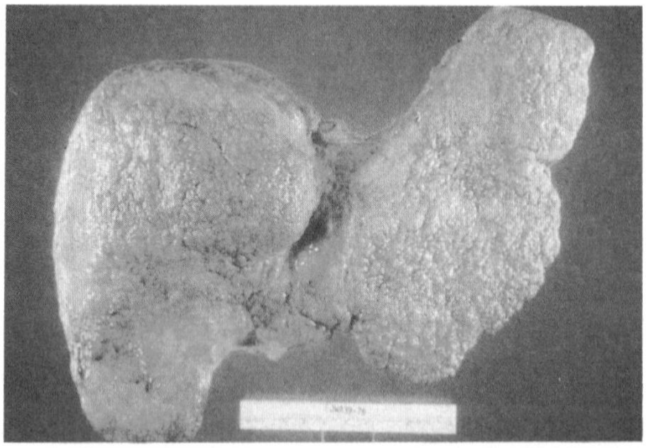

Plate II-15. Hypertrophic liver (alcoholic cirrhosis).

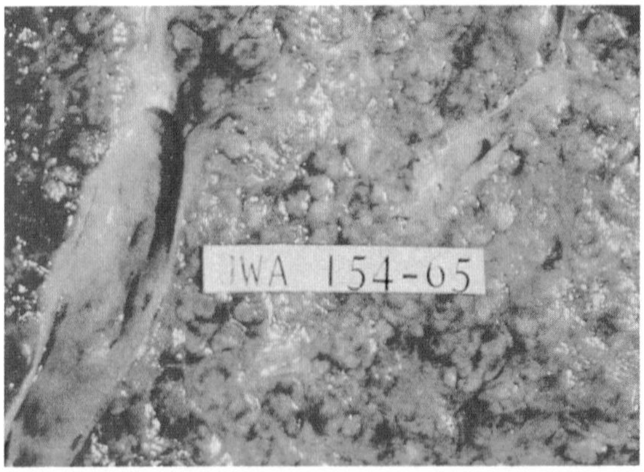

Plate II-16. Uniform micronodules (alcoholic cirrhosis).

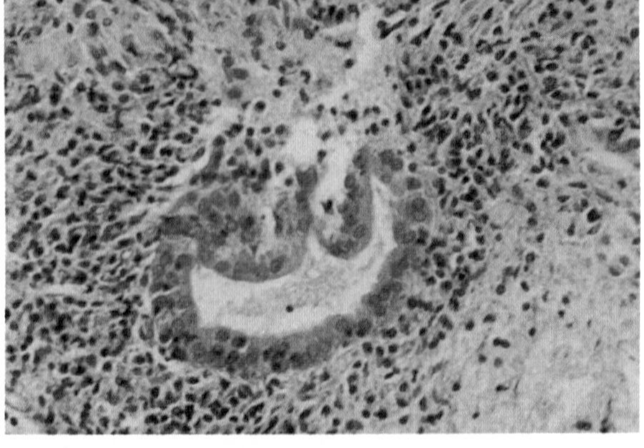

Plate II-17. Primary biliary cirrhosis, stage I. Interlobular bile duct is eccentrically damaged and about to rupture. It is surrounded by lymphocytes and plasma cells. Percutaneous needle biopsy, fixed in Carnoy's solution. Masson trichrome. × 67.5.

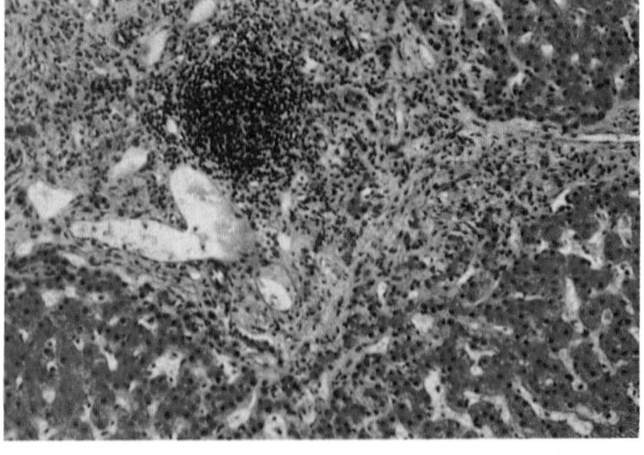

Plate II-18. Primary biliary cirrhosis, stage II. Enlarged portal triad containing atypical ductules and a small lymphoid follicle. Percutaneous needle biopsy, fixed in Carnoy's solution. Masson trichrome. × 31.

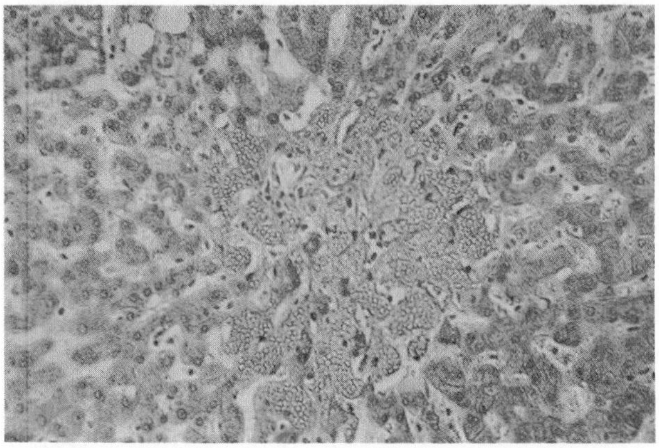

Plate II-19. Left-sided heart failure. Pericentral hepatocytes within hepatic plates have been replaced by red blood cells. There is no sinusoidal dilatation. Percutaneous needle biopsy, fixed in Carnoy's solution. Masson trichrome. × 31.

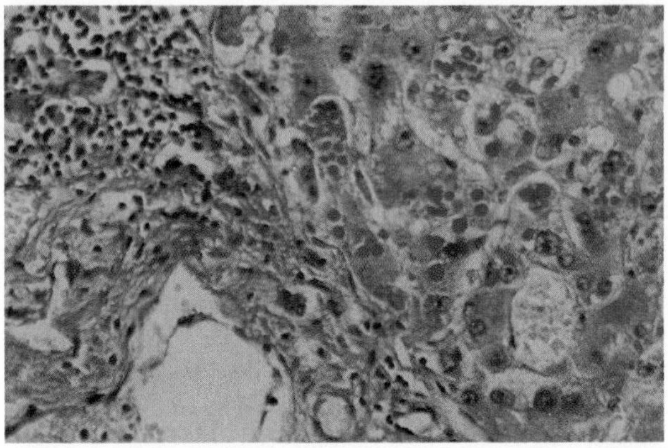

Plate II-20. Alpha-1 antitrypsin deficiency. Periportal hepatocytes demonstrating numerous PAS-positive globules of varying size. Autopsy, formalin fixation. PAS. × 67.5.

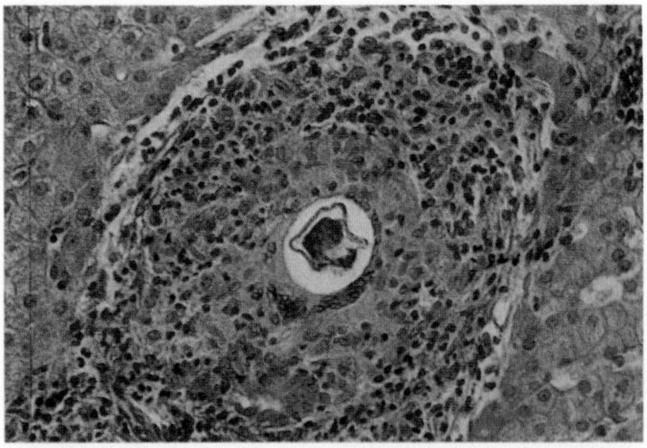

Plate II-21. Schistosomiasis. *Schistosoma mansoni* egg, surrounded by a giant cell, is at the center of a noncaseating granuloma. Percutaneous needle biopsy, fixed in Carnoy's solution. Masson trichrome. × 67.5.

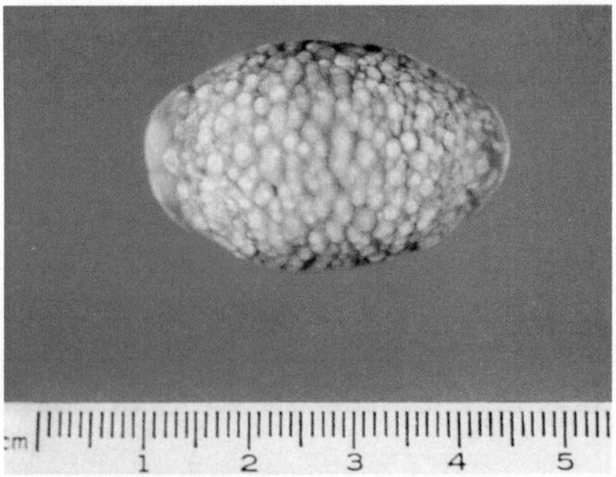

Plate II-22. Mulberry-shaped solitary cholesterol gallstone (3.5 cm × 2.0 cm). (Courtesy of David E. Cohen, Boston.)

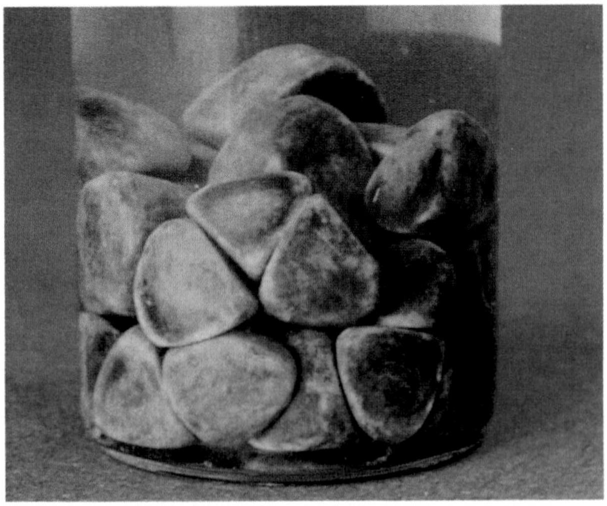

Plate II-23. Close-packed faceted cholesterol gallstones conforming to the shape of a cylindric vessel.

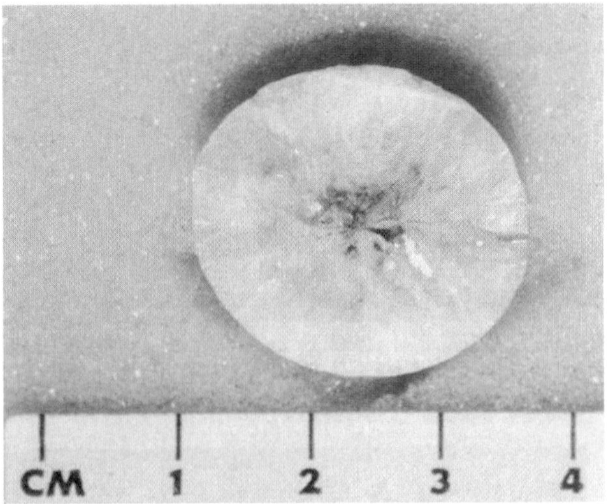

Plate II-24. Round solitary cholesterol gallstone with cut surface displaying a pigmented nucleus composed of the acid salt of calcium bilirubinate.

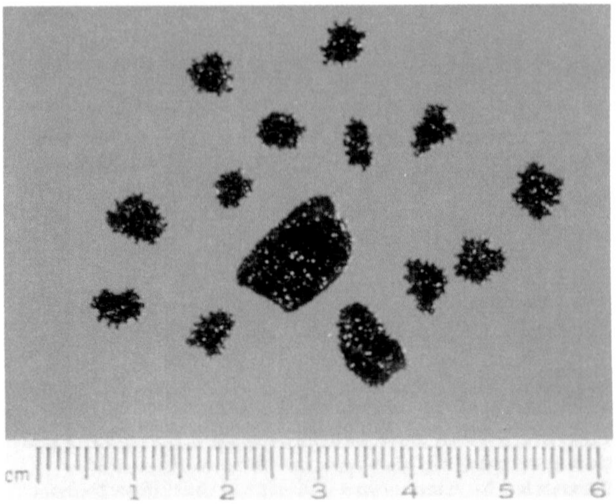

Plate II-25. Black polymer pigment gallstones formed in a gallbladder. Most are small and spiculated; one is large and flat.

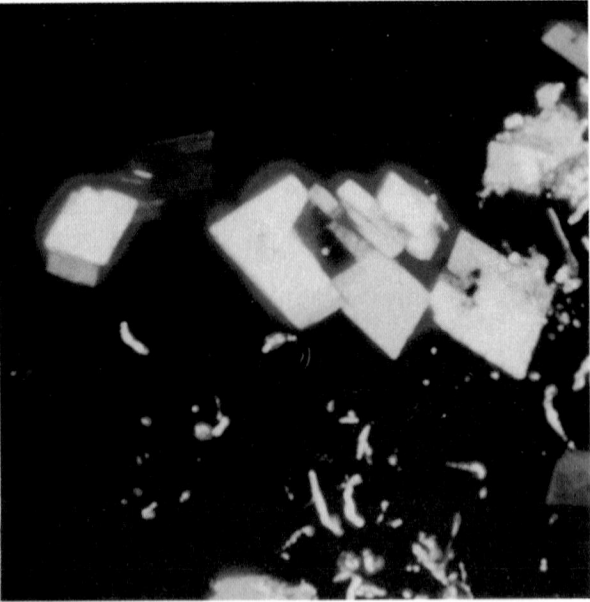

Plate II-26. Polarized light microscopy of bile-rich duodenal fluid showing rhombohedral cholesterol monohydrate crystals and amorphous golden-yellow bilirubin precipitates. × 40.

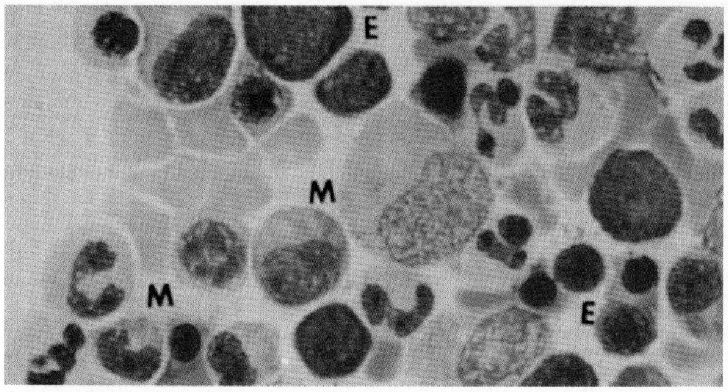

Plate III-1. Normal bone marrow. *M*, myeloid precursor, *E*, erythroid precursor. × 600.

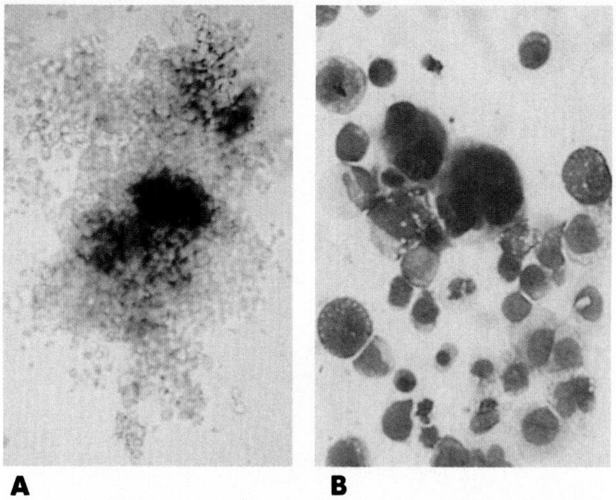

Plate III-2. Colony-forming unit grown from human bone marrow. **A,** CFU-GEMM colony derived from a pluripotent stem cell grown in methycellulose. The colony contains granulocytes, erythrocytes, macrophages, and megakaryocytes. **B,** A Wright-stained smear of a single colony (CFU-GEMM) containing granulocytes, erythrocytes, macrophages, and megakaryocytes.
(Courtesy of H. A. Messner.)

Plate III-3. Maturing erythroid precursors in bone marrow. **A,** Pronormoblast. **B,** Basophilic normoblasts. **C,** Polychromatophilic and orthochromatophilic normoblasts with a megaloblastic appearance.

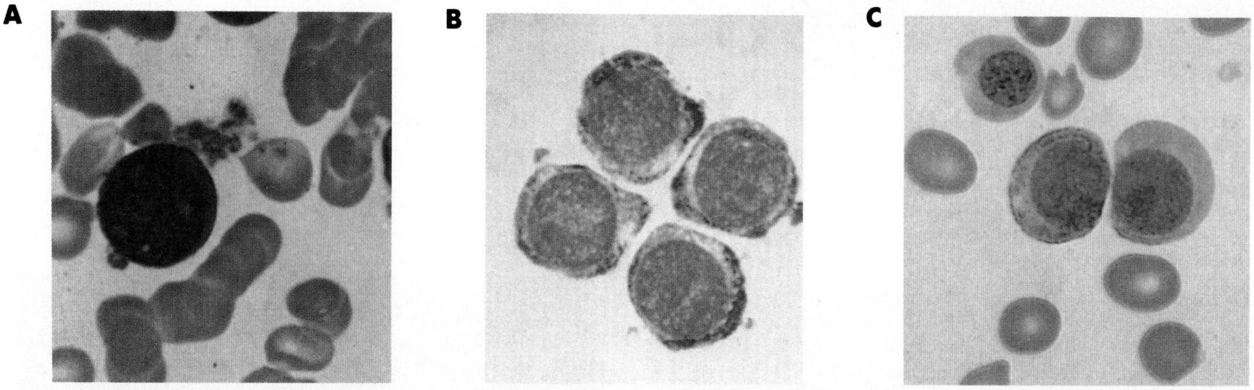

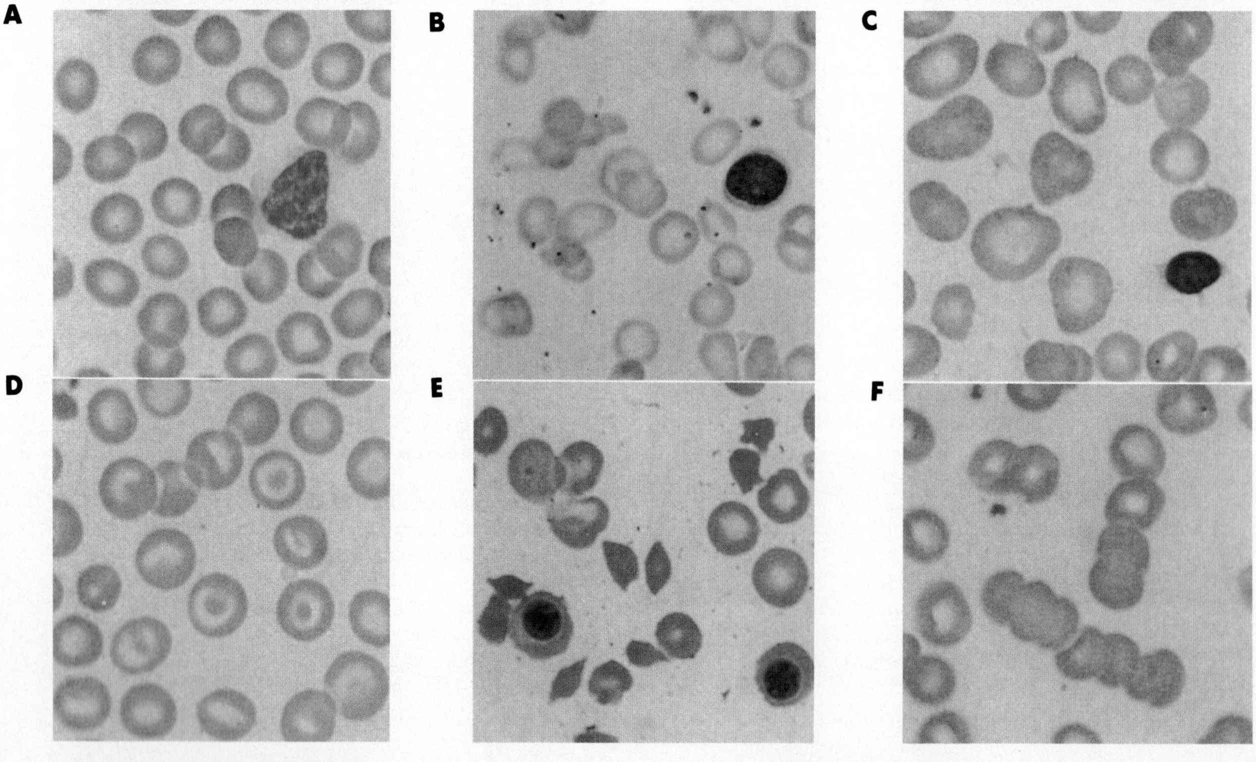

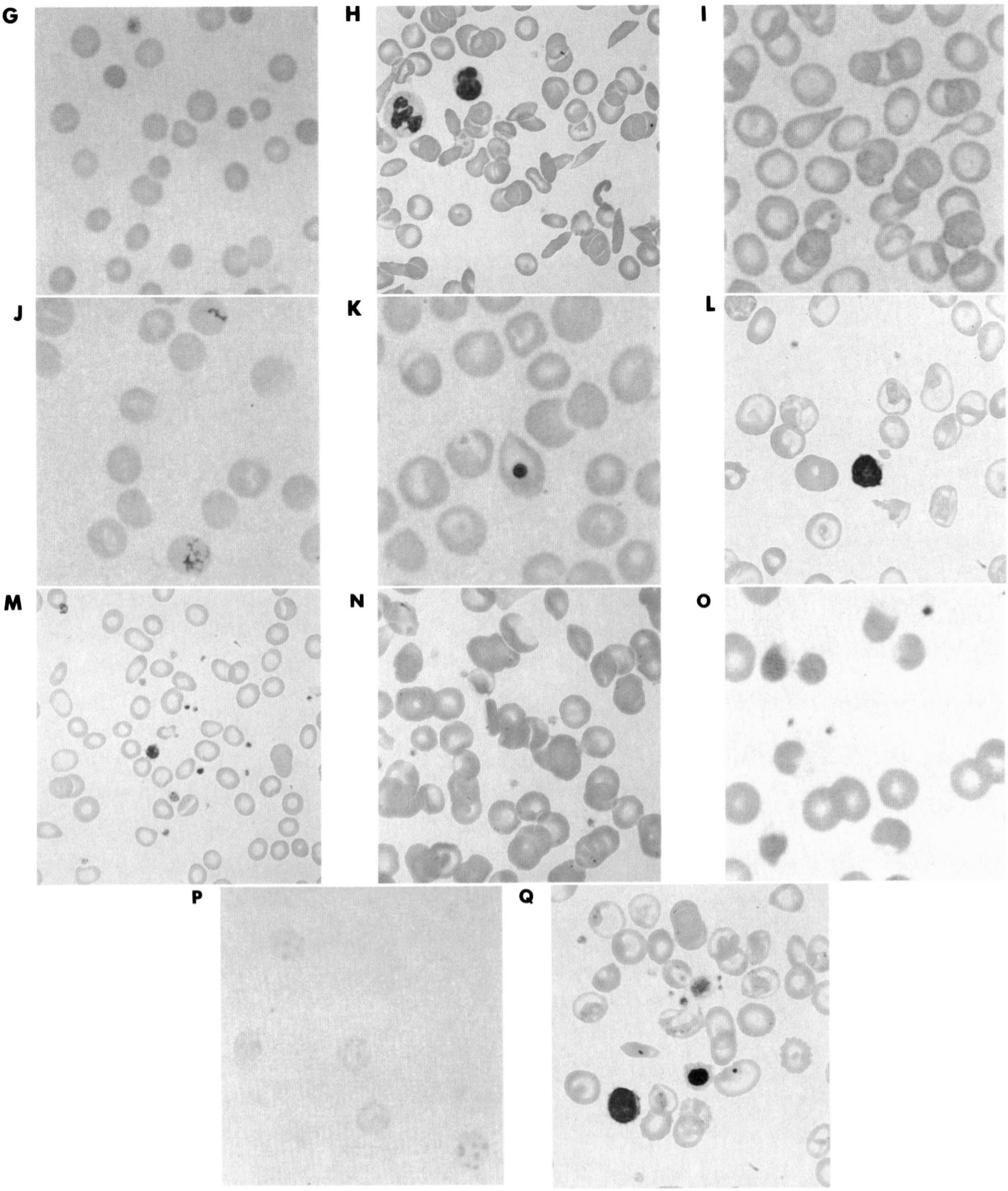

Plate III-4. Erythrocyte morphology in peripheral blood. Wright's stain. × 1000. **A,** Normal red cells. **B,** Microcytic hypochromic cells typical of iron deficiency. **C,** Macrocytosis typically seen in megaloblastic anemia. **D,** Target cells. **E,** Schistocytes and nucleated red cells. **F,** Rouleau formation. **G,** Normal red cells and microspherocytes in hereditary spherocytosis. **H,** Sickle cell anemia, showing sickled cells, a Howell-Jolly body, and polychromatophilia. **I,** Teardrop poikilocytes. **J,** Reticulocytes (special stain). **K,** Howell-Jolly body (nuclear remnant). **L,** Homozygous beta-thalassemia, showing microcytic and hypochromic erythrocytes, anisocytosis and poikilocytosis, basophilic stippling, a Howell-Jolly body, target cells, and polychromatophilia. **M,** Heterozygous beta-thalassemia, showing hypochromia and microcytosis. **N,** Hemoglobin sickle cell disease, showing an HbC crystal, target cells, a folded taco-shaped cell, polychromatophilia, and Pappenheimer bodies. **O,** Eccentrocytes (blister cells) with a lop-sided distribution of hemoglobin. Typically seen during a hemolytic episode in G6PD deficiency. **P,** Heinz bodies (supravital stain). **Q,** HbS-beta^{0}-thalassemia, showing a nucleated erythrocyte, Howell-Jolly and Pappenheimer bodies, a sickle cell, target cells, polychromatophilia, hypochromia, and microcytosis.

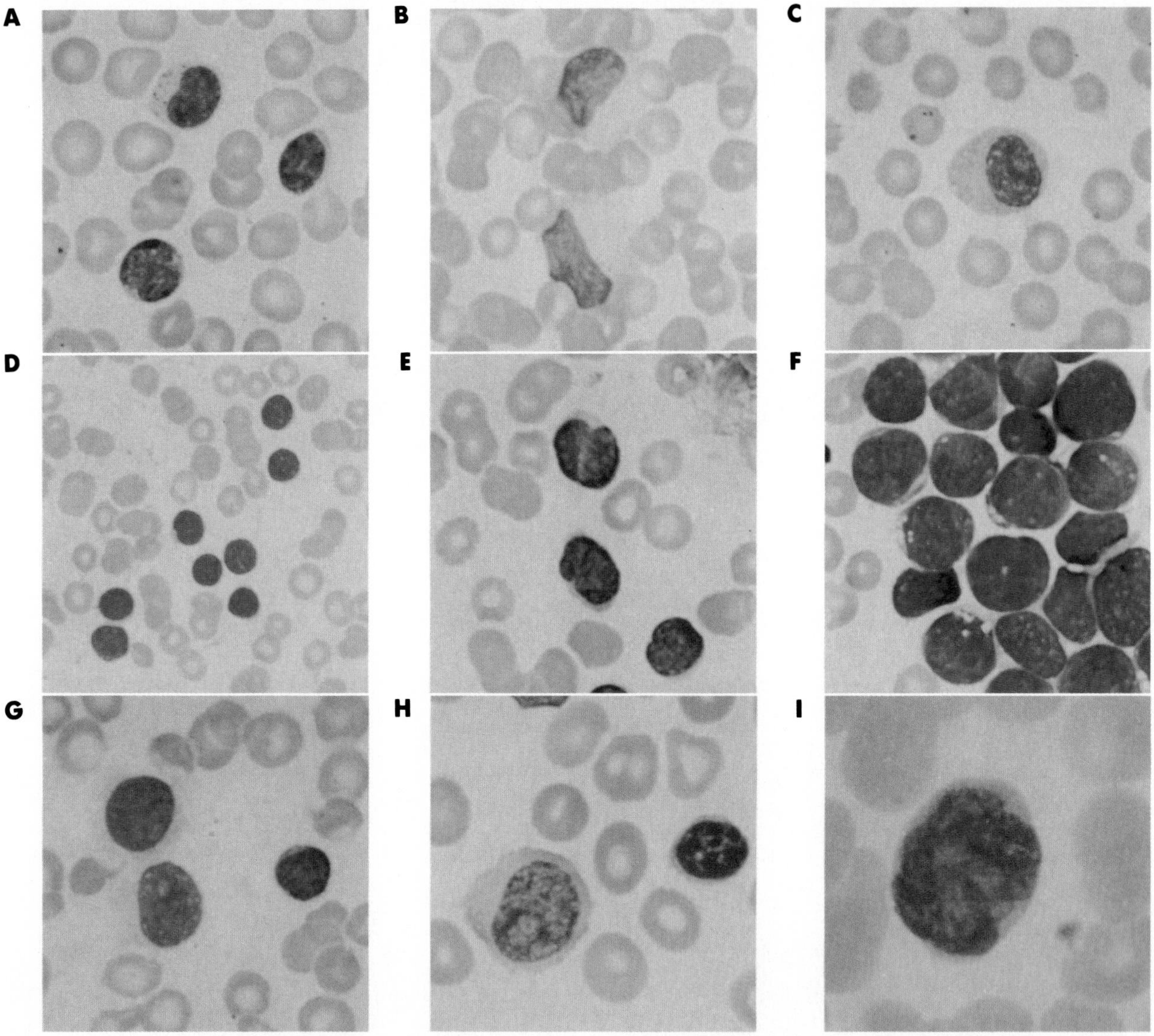

Plate III-5. Lymphocyte morphology in peripheral blood. Wright's stain. × 1000. **A,** Normal lymphocytes. **B,** Atypical lymphocytes (infectious mononucleosis). **C,** Plasmacytoid lymphocyte. **D,** Chronic lymphocytic leukemia. ×600. **E,** Lymphosarcoma "buttock" cells. **F,** Acute lymphoblastic leukemia. **G,** Hairy cells. **H,** The large cell is a prolymphocyte, the small cell is a normal, mature lymphocyte. **I,** Sézary cell with a lobulated, convoluted nucleus. × 2000.

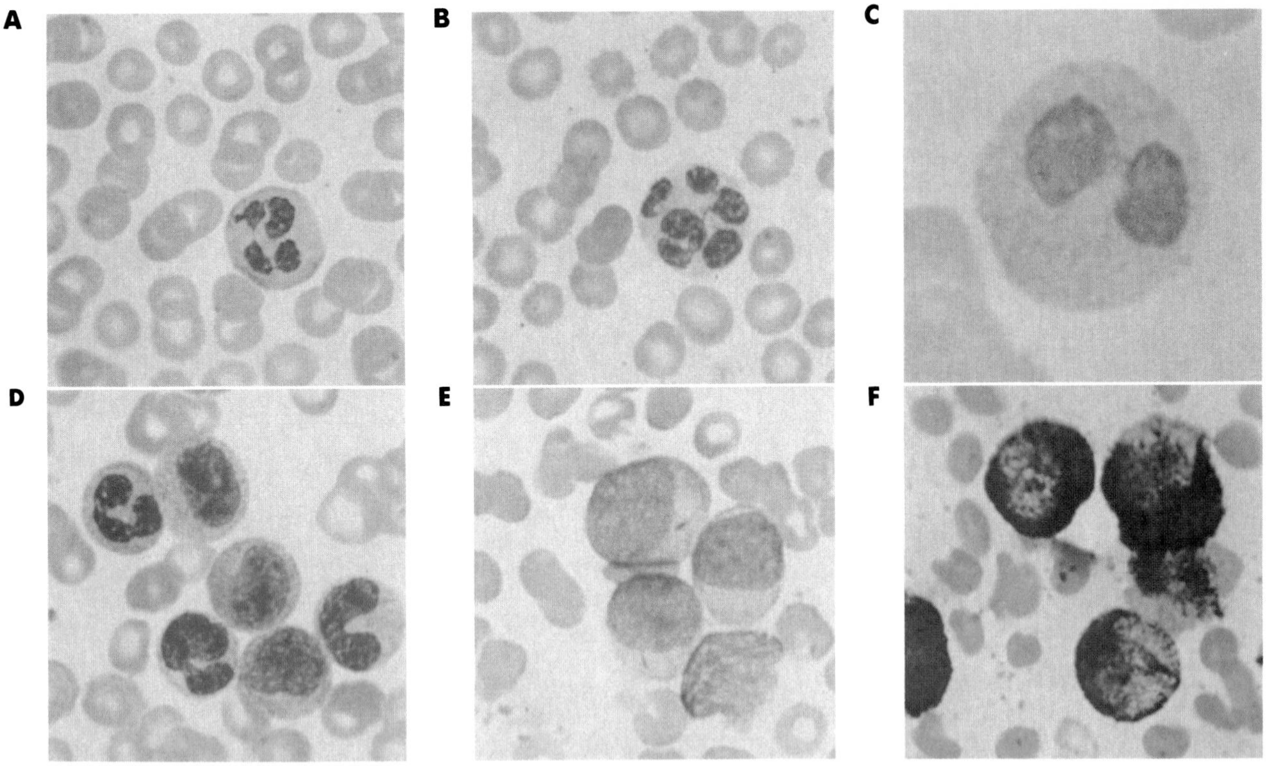

Plate III-6. Granulocyte morphology in peripheral blood. Wright's stain. × 1000. **A,** Normal neutrophil. **B,** Hypersegmented neutrophil. **C,** Pelger-Huët anomaly (bilobed neutrophil, magnified). **D,** Chronic myelogenous leukemia showing granulocytes at several stages of differentiation. **E,** Leukemic myeloblasts with Auer rods in the cytoplasm. **F,** Leukemic blasts that stain with Sudan black B.

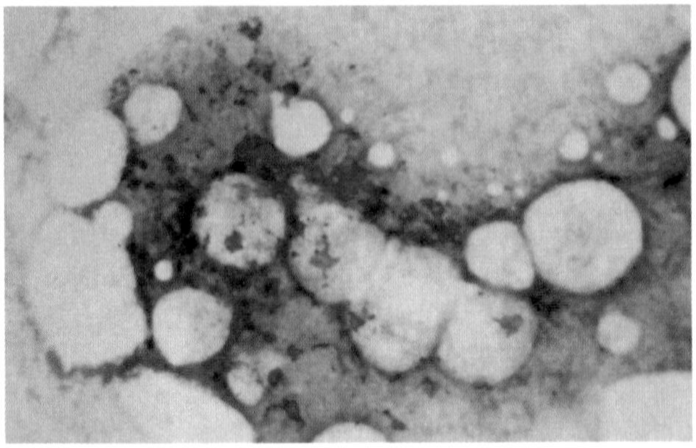

Plate III-7. Iron in normal bone marrow stained with Prussian blue. × 100.

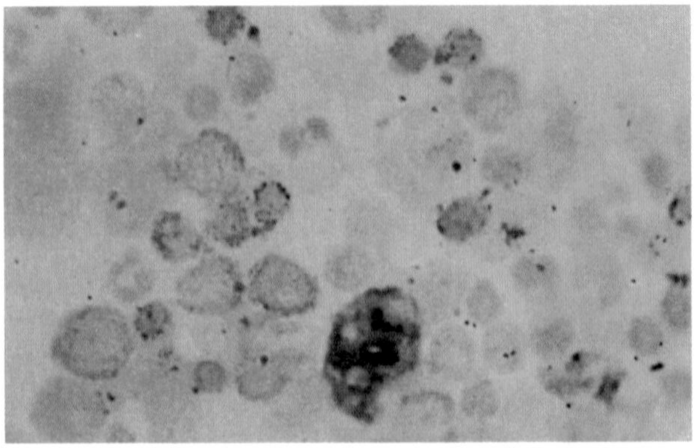

Plate III-8. Ringed sideroblasts in the bone marrow from a patient with sideroblastic anemia. Prussian blue stain. × 1000.

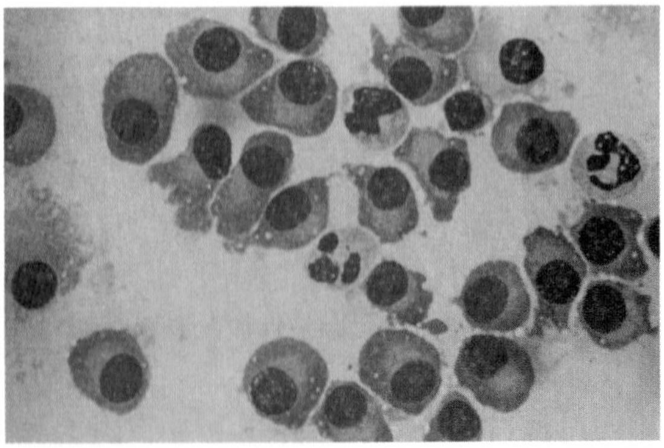

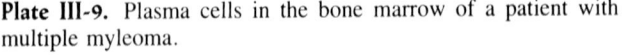

Plate III-9. Plasma cells in the bone marrow of a patient with multiple myleoma.

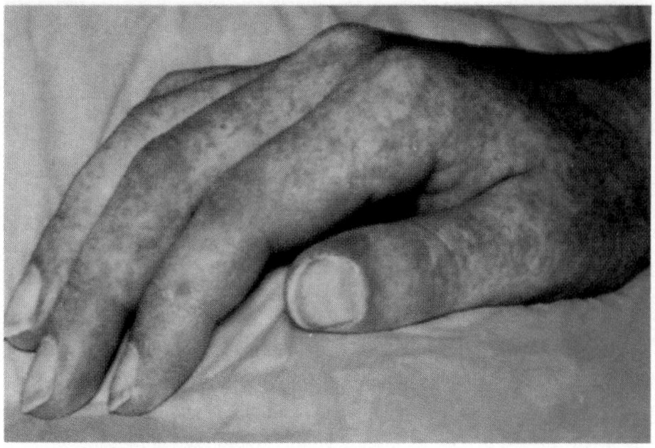

Plate III-10. Cutaneous manifestations of acute graft-versus-host disease seen on the hands of a patient 18 days after bone marrow transplantation.

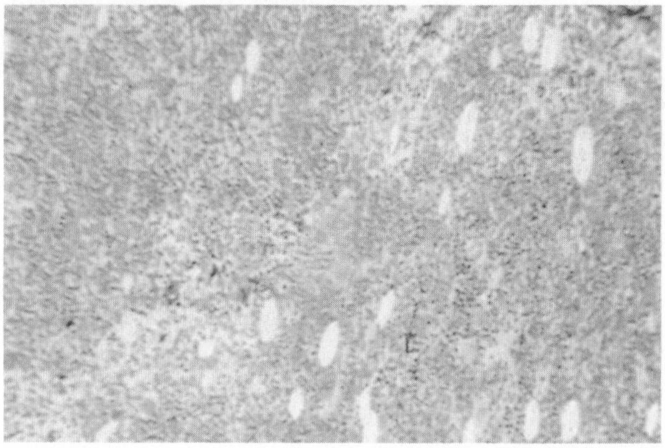

Plate III-11. Bone marrow in polycythemia vera. Increased cellularity, prominent erythropoiesis, and cluster of megakaryocytes are characteristic features. × 100.

A **B**

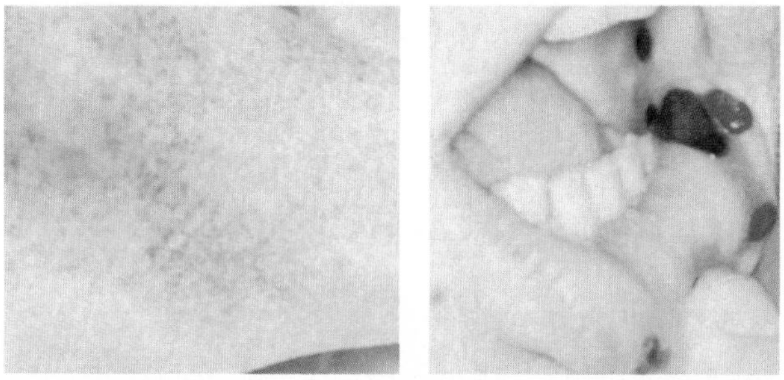

Plate III-12. Petechiae and hemorrhagic bullae in a patient with acute idiopathic thrombocytopenic purpura. These photographs were taken on the first day of illness in a previously healthy 25-year-old man. **A,** Petechiae over the lateral surface, right ankle, and foot. **B,** Hemorrhagic bullae in his oral mucous membranes.

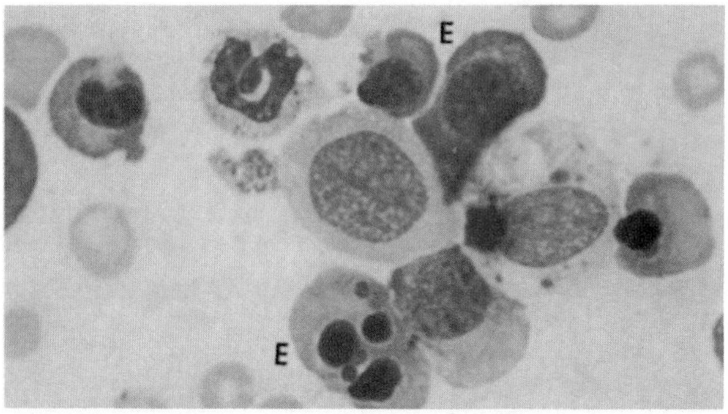

Plate III-13. Megaloblastic bone marrow. *E,* the large megaloblastic erythroid precursors containing abnormal nuclei and multiple nuclear fragments are characteristic. × 1000.

A **B**

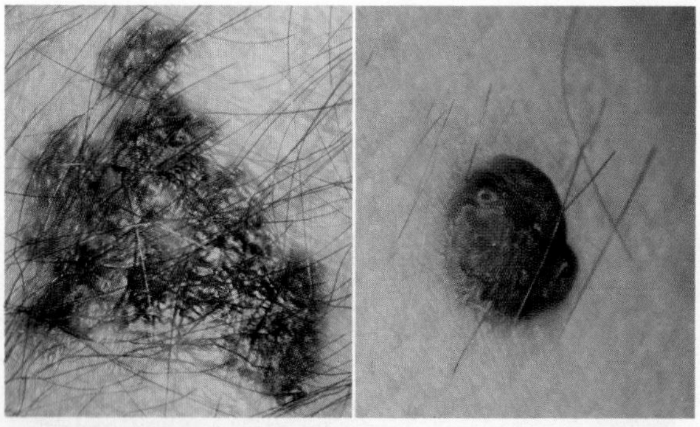

Plate III-14. Malignant melanoma. **A,** Superficial spreading melanoma. **B,** Nodular melanoma.

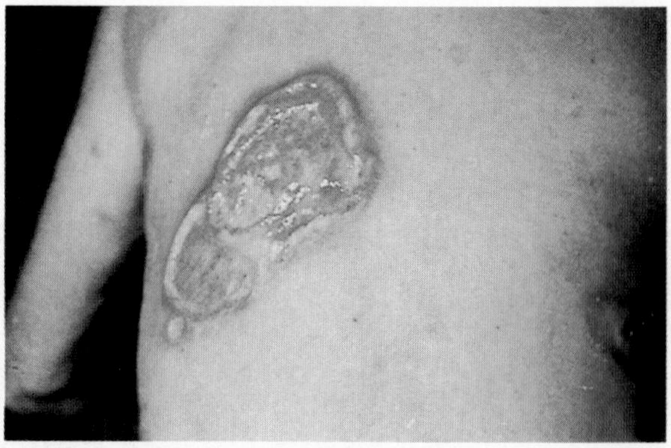

Plate III-15. Mycosis fungoides.

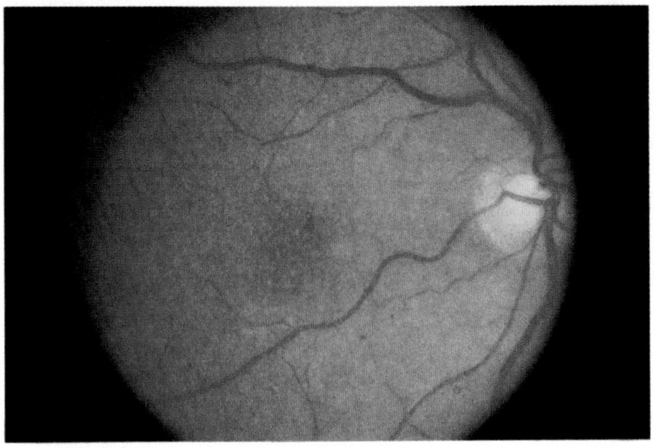

Plate IV-1. Nonproliferative or background diabetic retinopathy. The characteristic features of nonproliferative retinopathy include microaneurysms, dot hemorrhages, slightly larger and irregular blot hemorrhages, and occasionally cotton-wool patches. Flame-shaped hemorrhages in the nerve fiber layer of the retina may also occur.

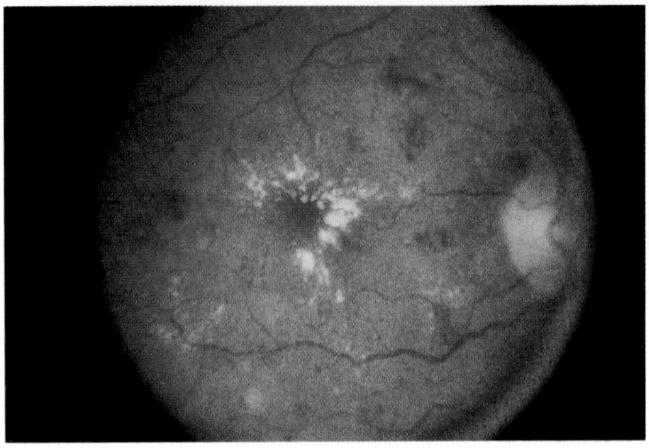

Plate IV-2. Exudative diabetic retinopathy. Hard exudates, composed of lipid, carbohydrate, and protein, which are left in the retina after long-standing capillary endothelial leakage of serum, may take a variety of shapes. Rings of exudates suggest that microangiopathy in the center of the ring is leaking. Almost always, other evidence of nonproliferative retinopathy is present.

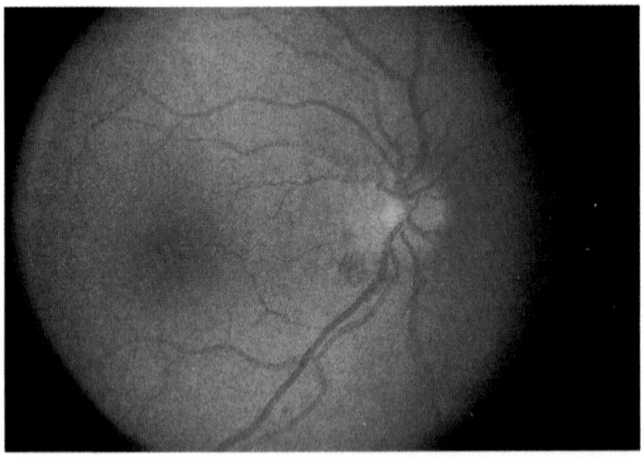

Plate IV-3. Proliferative diabetic retinopathy. At a more advanced stage of diabetic retinopathy, new blood vessels form and grow from previously existing normal vessels. Their larger-than-normal caliber, their unusual lacelike arrangement following no anatomic patterns, and their elevation above the retinal plane as they evolve distinguish them from other alterations of preexisting normal retinal vessels.

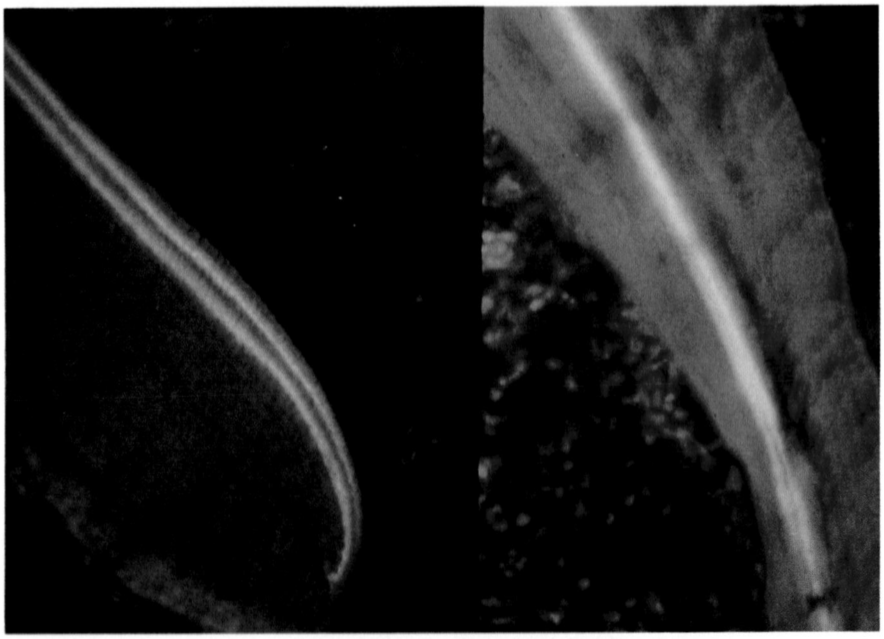

Plate IV-4. Biopsies of iliac crest showing tetracycline labeling at the mineralization front in a normal subject *(left)* and a patient with osteomalacia *(right)*. Note the two separate bands of fluorescence in the normal subject and the coalescence of the two bands in the patient. (Dr. Robert Weinstein.)

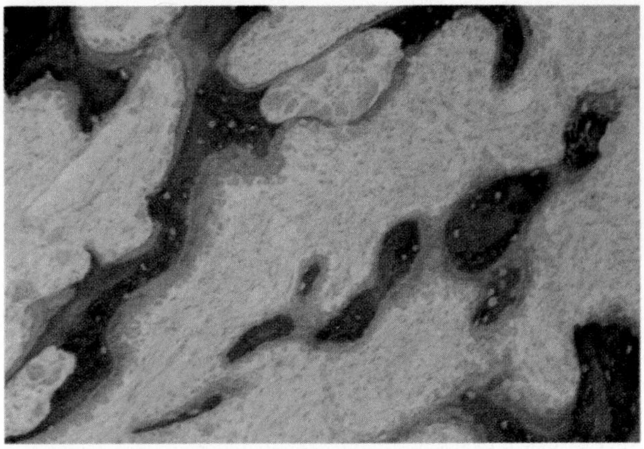

Plate IV-5. Predominant hyperparathyroid bone disease. Undercalcified 3-μm thick section of anterior iliac bone from chronically dialyzed patient. Abundance of osteoclasts, osteoblasts, and osteocytes. Marrow fibrosis. Irregular trabecular surface and tunneling resorption of mineralized bone underneath osteoid. Modified Masson-Goldner stain. Original magnification ×8. (Reprinted with permission from Malluche HH and Faugere MC: Atlas of mineralized bone histology. New York, 1986, Karger.)

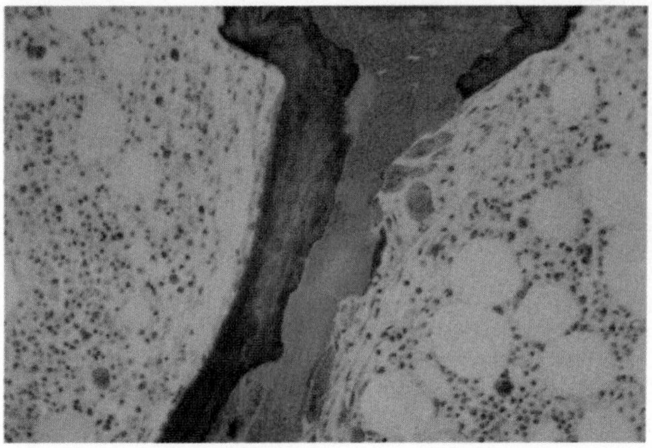

Plate IV-6. Mixed uremic osteodystrophy. Undecalcified 3-μm thick section of anterior iliac bone from chronically dialyzed patient. Presence of multinucleated osteoclasts resorbing bone and new bone apposition at the opposite side of the trabeculum. Increased osteoid seam thickness. Mild peritrabecular fibrosis. Modified Masson-Goldner stain. Original magnification × 20. (Reprinted with permission from Malluche HH and Faugere MC: Atlas of mineralized bone histology. New York, 1986, Karger.)

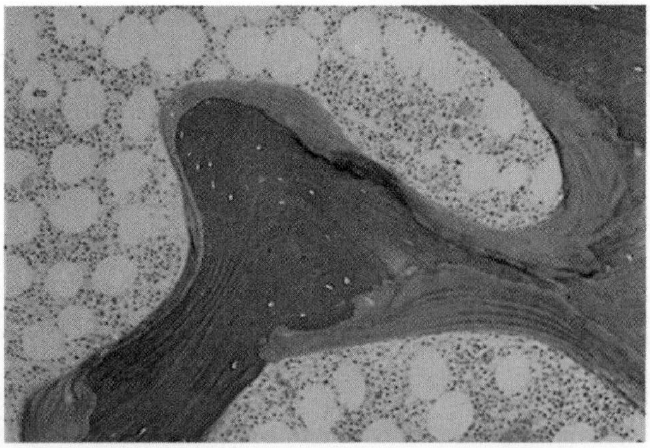

Plate IV-7. Low turnover osteomalacia. Undecalcified 3-μm thick section of anterior iliac bone from chronically dialyzed patient. High osteoid volume caused by increased fraction of trabecular surface covered by osteoid seams and increased osteoid seam width. Irregular interface between osteoid and mineralized bone, reflecting previously enhanced resorptive activity. Absence of peritrabecular and marrow fibrosis. Paucity of bone-forming and bone-resorbing cells. Modified Masson-Goldner stain. Original magnification ×12.5 (Reprinted with permission from Malluche HH and Faugere MC: Atlas of mineralized bone histology. New York, 1986, Karger.)

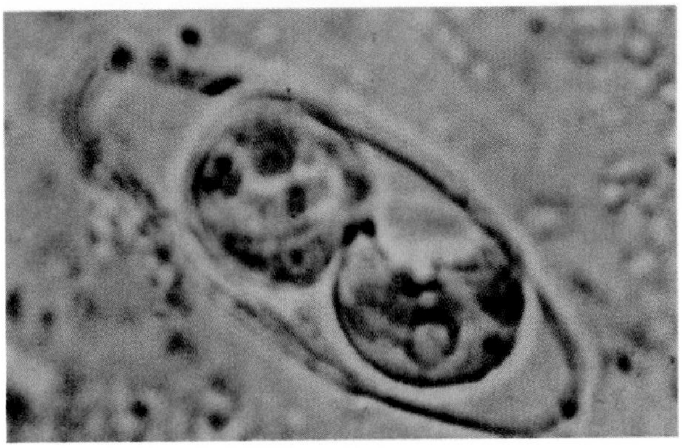

Plate V-1. Mature oocyst of *Isospora belli* in unstained fecal smear. The oocyst is typically elongated, measures 20 to 33 μm by 10 to 19 μm, and has a wall consisting of two layers. Two sporocysts may be seen within the oocyst. × 2000. (Courtesy of Dr. Keith Hadley, San Francisco General Hospital.)

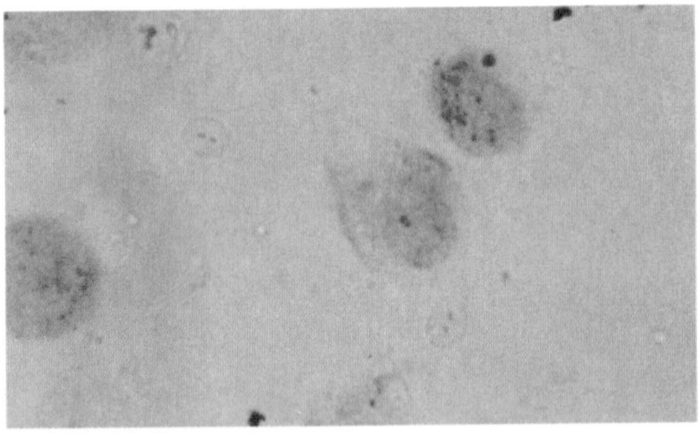

Plate V-3. Inspection for a quellung reaction with pneumococcal omni serum improves the correlation of the Gram stain with the culture of nearly 90%, chiefly by reducing the number of false-positive smears caused by the otherwise indistinguishable oral alpha-hemolytic streptococcus.

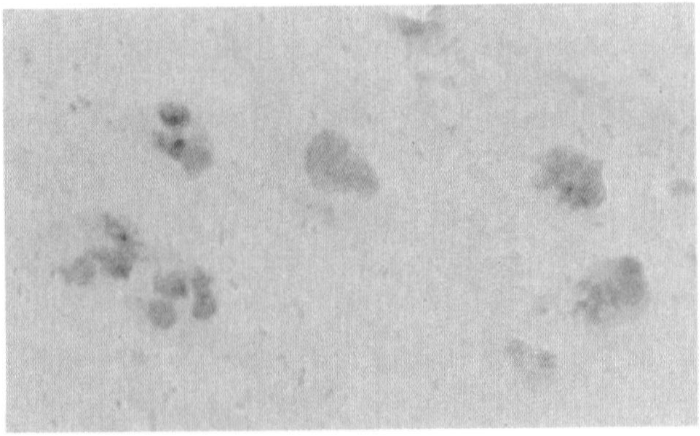

Plate V-5. *Haemophilus influenzae* is often difficult to see because the gram-negative coccobacillary forms may be poorly stained and may blend with the red background.

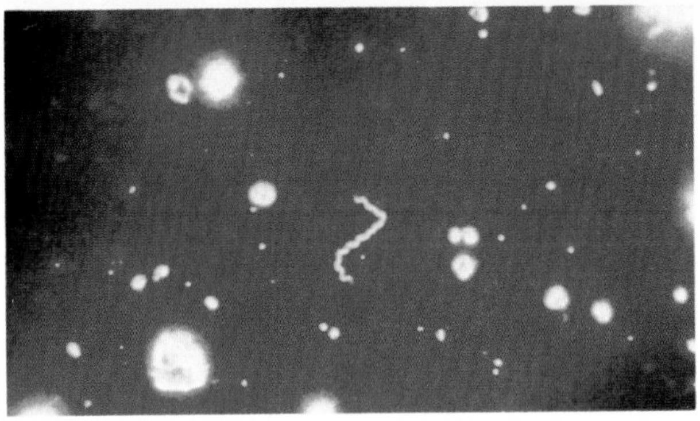

Plate V-2. *Treponema pallidum* by dark field microscopy. × 1000. Note the distinct spirals and characteristic bending. (Courtesy of Centers for Disease Control.)

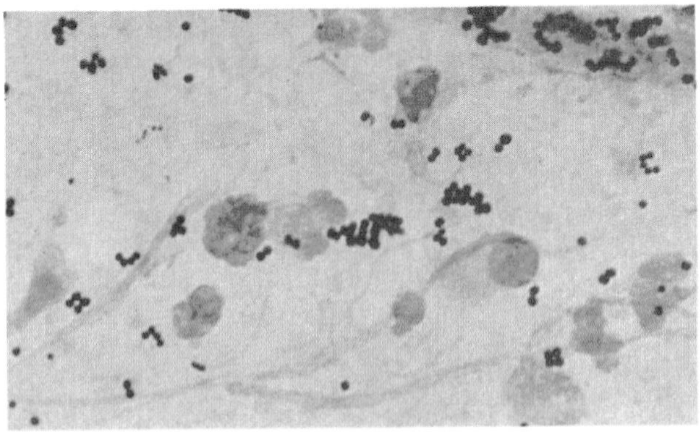

Plate V-4. Staphylococci can be identified by the typical clustering (like grapes on a stem) of gram-positive cocci.

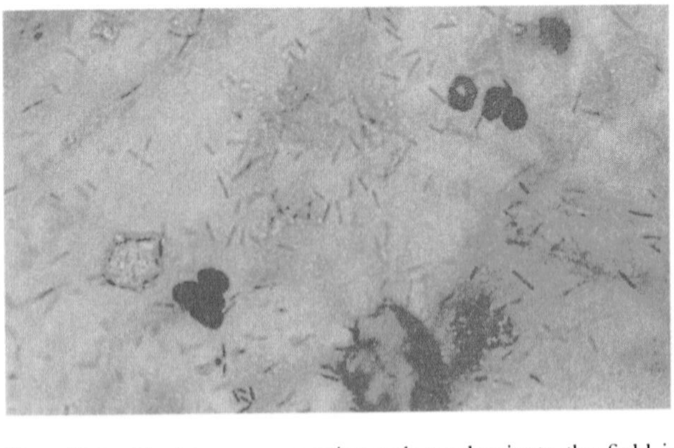

Plate V-6. The big gram-negative rods predominate the field in *Klebsiella pneumoniae* or others caused by the enterobacteriaceae or pseudomonas.

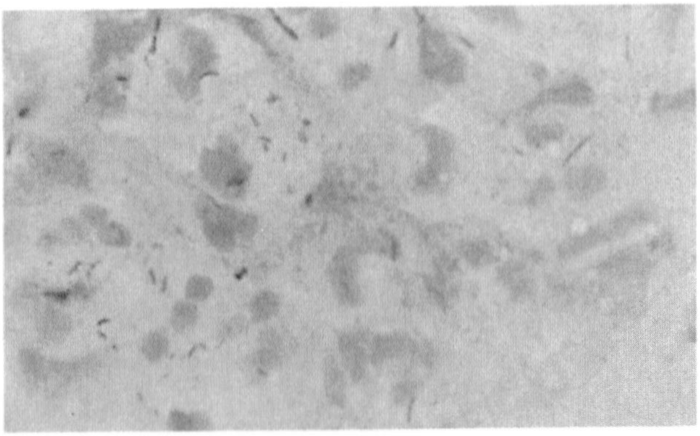

Plate V-7. Gram-stained expectorated sputum or transtracheal aspirate from patients with aspiration anaerobic pneumonia typically shows a mixture of gram-positive cocci rods with bizarre morphologic forms.

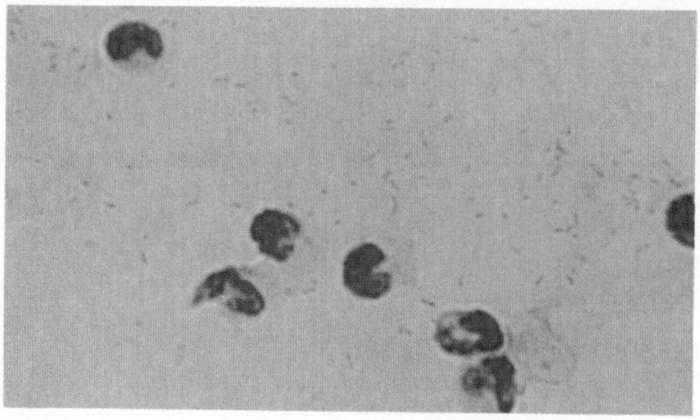

Plate V-8. Gram stain of spun cerebrospinal fluid from a patient with *Haemophilus influenzae* type B meningitis. Note presence of coccobacillary organisms in conjunction with polymorphonuclear leukocytes.

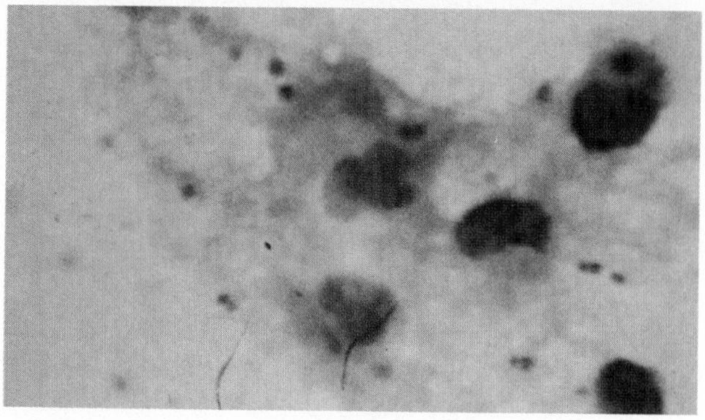

Plate V-9. Gram stain of centrifuged cerebrospinal fluid from a patient with meningococcal meningitis. Note presence of gram-negative cocci in pairs associated with polymorphonuclear leukocytes.

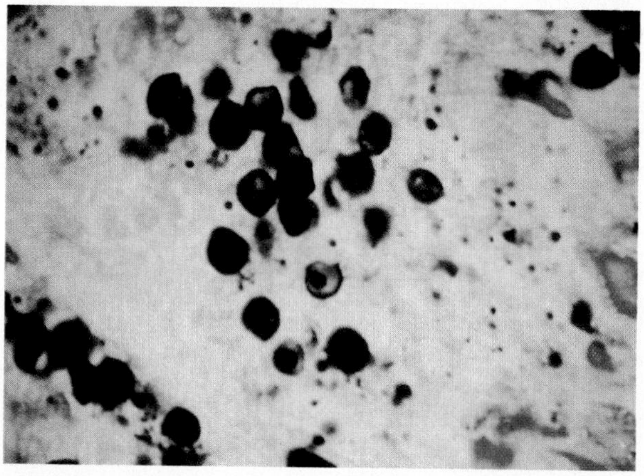

Plate V-10. Giemsa stain of bronchial washings demonstrating *Pneumocystis carinii* cysts.

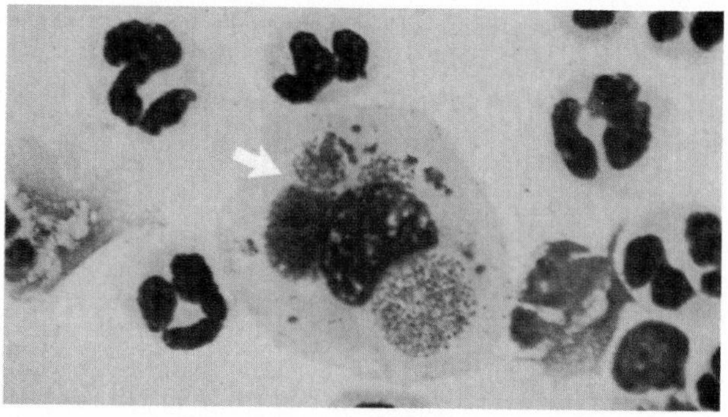

Plate V-11. Giemsa stain of conjunctiva scraping showing typical cytoplasmic inclusion of *Chlamydia trachomatis*.

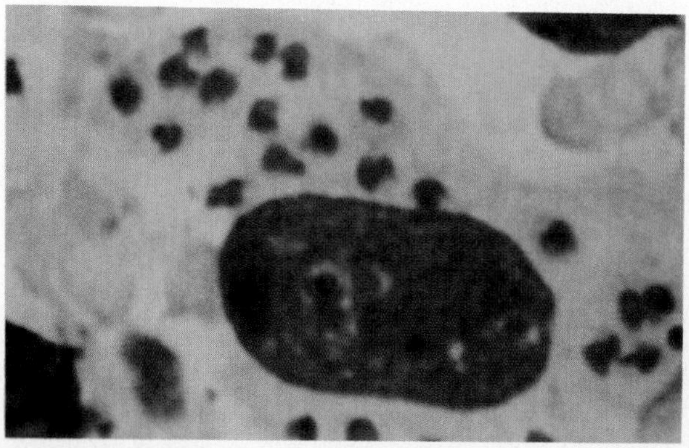

Plate V-12. *Leishmania* amastigotes within an impression smear in cutaneous leishmaniasis. Giemsa stain. ×2000. (Courtesy of Dr. Keith Hadley, San Francisco General Hospital.)

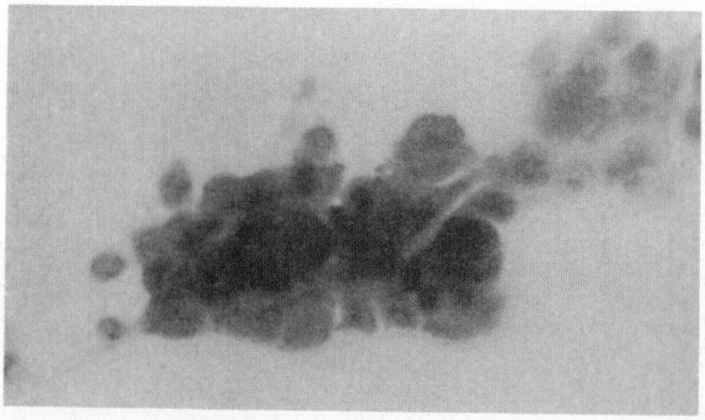

Plate V-13. Photomicrographic scraping from base of herpes blister demonstrating multinuclear giant cells.

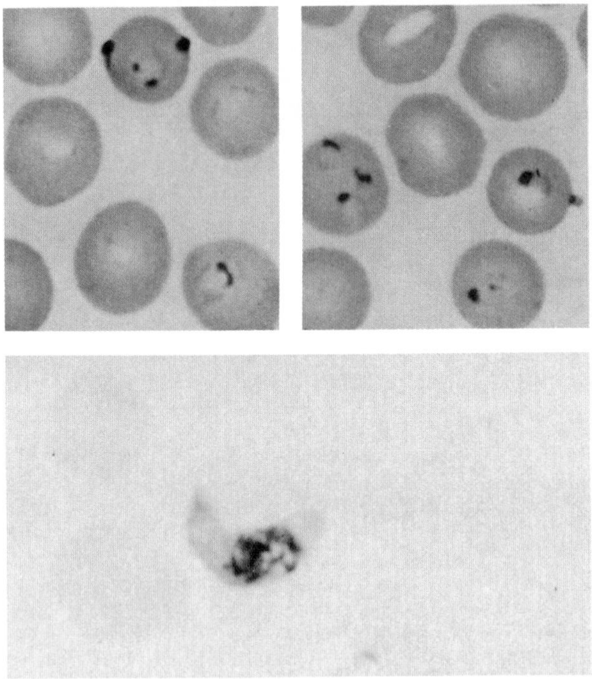

Plate V-14. Giemsa-stained blood smear in *Plasmodium falciparum* malaria. Asexual parasites (top *left* and *right*): note that ring forms predominate, some erythrocytes contain multiple parasites, and some parasites contain double nuclei. ×2000. Gametocyte *(bottom)* has pathognomonic crescent shape. ×2000.

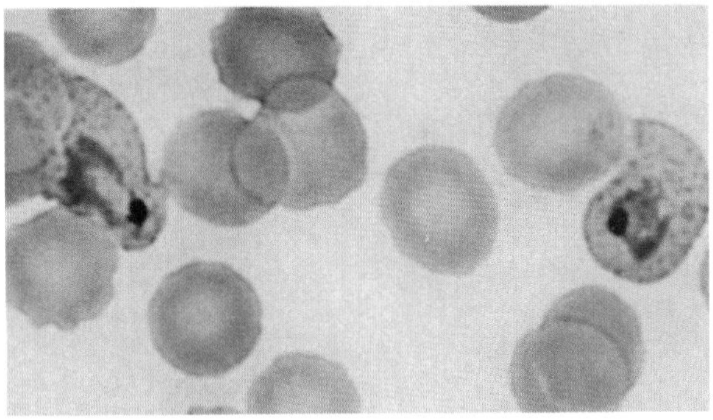

Plate V-15. Giemsa-stained blood smear in *Plasmodium vivax* malaria. Asexual parasites. Note that the parasites are large and ameboid, the infected erythrocytes are the largest cells in the field (because they are reticulocytes), and the erythrocytes contain numerous pink dots (Shüffner's dots). ×2000.

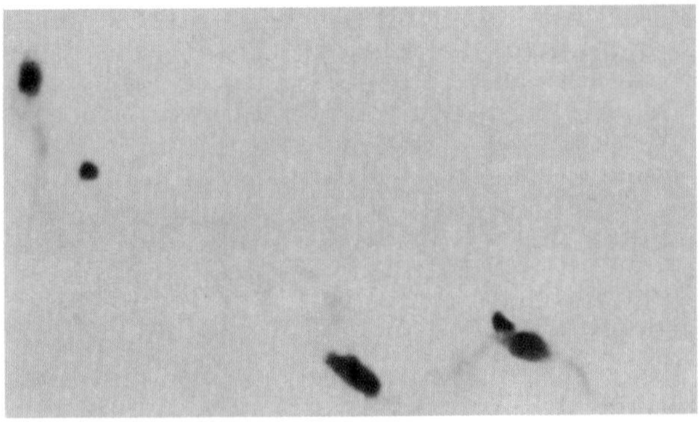

Plate V-16. Trypomastigotes of *Trypanosoma brucei rhodesiense* in a Giemsa-stained thick blood smear. There is a central reddish nucleus, and the kinetoplast cannot be distinguished. ×2000 (Courtesy of Dr. Keith Hadley, San Francisco General Hospital.)

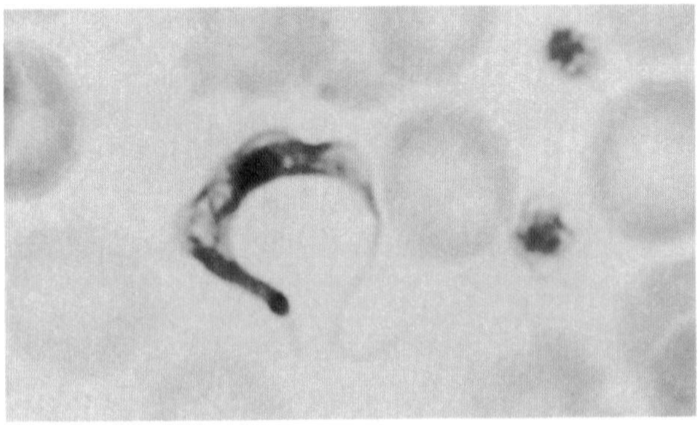

Plate V-17. Trypomastigote of *Trypanosoma cruzi* in a Giemsa-stained blood smear. A central nucleus, flagellum, and posterior kinetoplast can be seen. ×2000. (Courtesy of Dr. Keith Hadley, San Francisco General Hospital.)

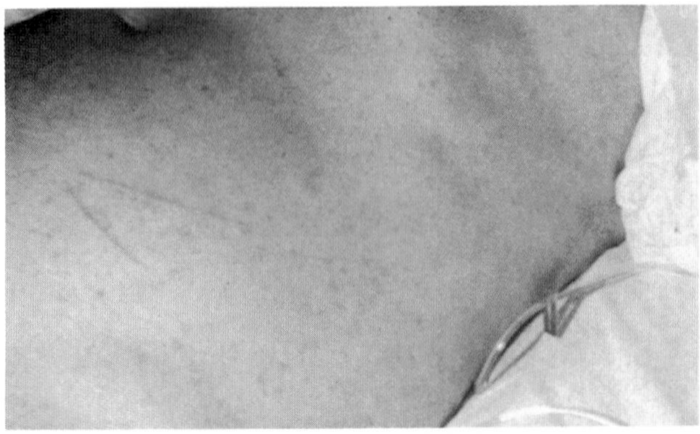

Plate V-18. Petechial and purpuric skin lesions in a severe case of Rocky Mountain spotted fever, 7 days after onset of symptoms.

Plate V-19. In Rocky Mountain spotted fever, the rickettsia invade the vasculature of the integument as well as other organs and can be demonstrated in vessel walls by immunofluorescence.

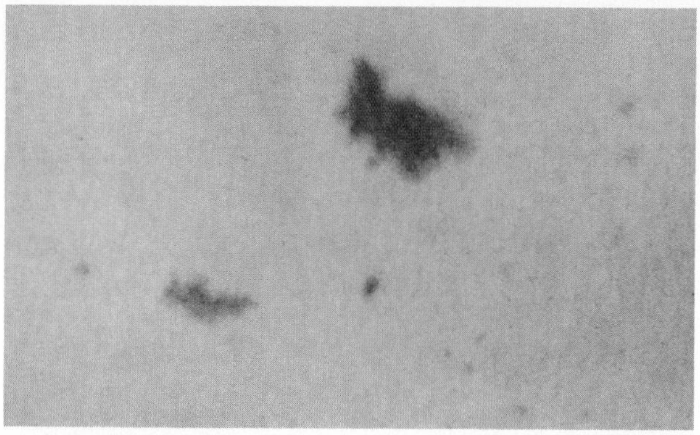

Plate V-20. Cutaneous lesions in a patient with meningococcemia (close-up).

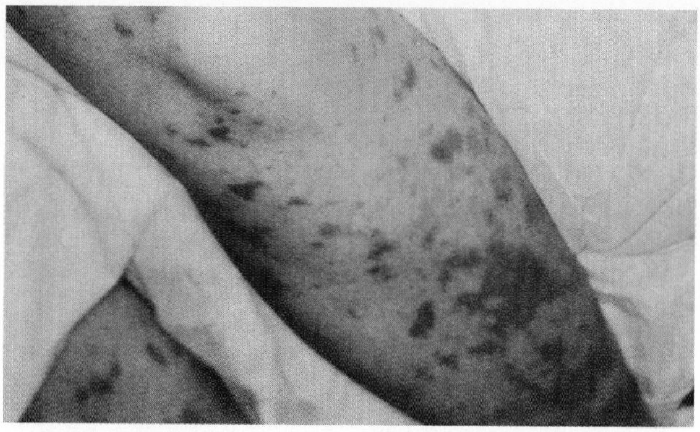

Plate V-21. Cutaneous lesions in a patient with meningococcemia.

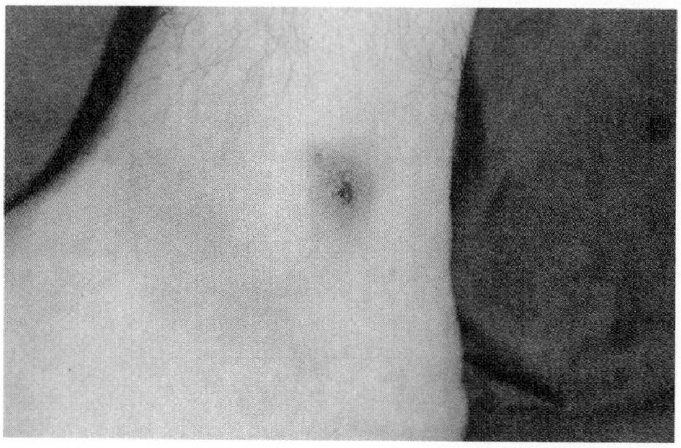

Plate V-22. Cutaneous lesion from a patient with disseminated gonococcal infection. Note the characteristic appearance of the gray necrotic ulcer on an erythematous base in the typical location on the ankles.

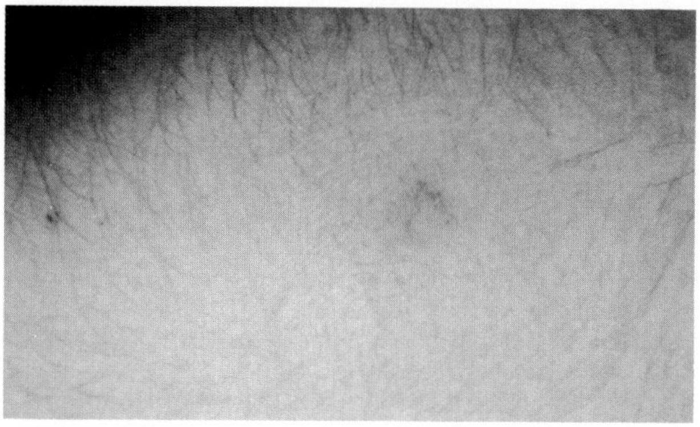

Plate V-23. Cutaneous lesion in a leukemic patient with overwhelming *Pseudomonas aeruginosa* septicemia. Lesion is called *ecthyma gangrenosum*. Note the characteristics of the bluish central discoloration.

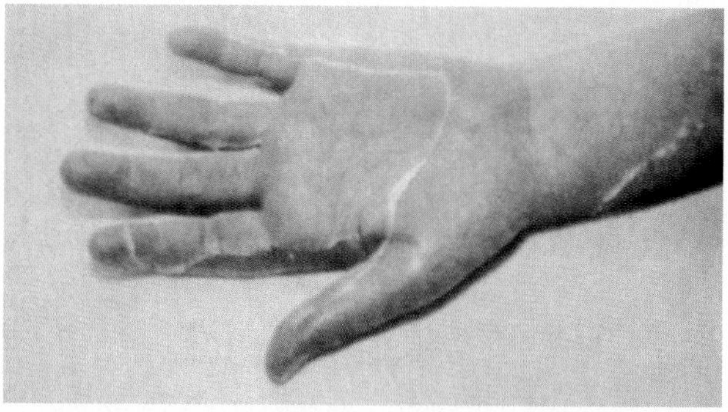

Plate V-24. Desquamation following toxic shock syndrome.

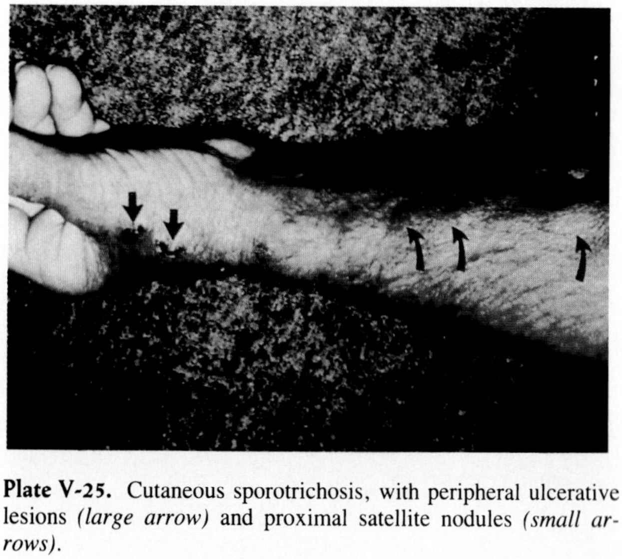

Plate V-25. Cutaneous sporotrichosis, with peripheral ulcerative lesions *(large arrow)* and proximal satellite nodules *(small arrows)*.

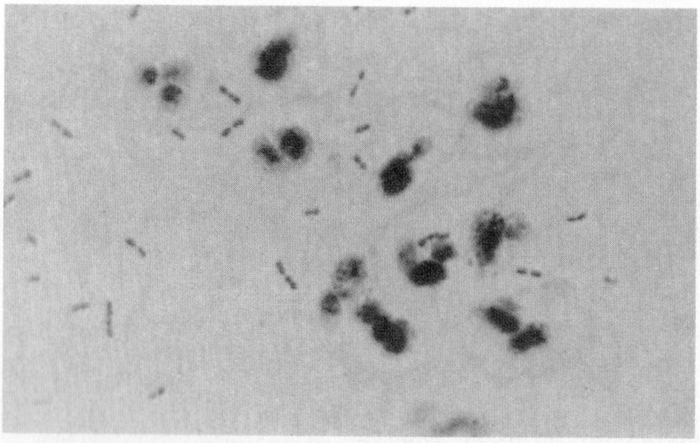

Plate V-26. If more than 10 gram-positive diplococci appear in a high-power (×1000) field, the specificity of diagnosing pneumococcal pneumonia is 85% with a sensitivity of 62%.

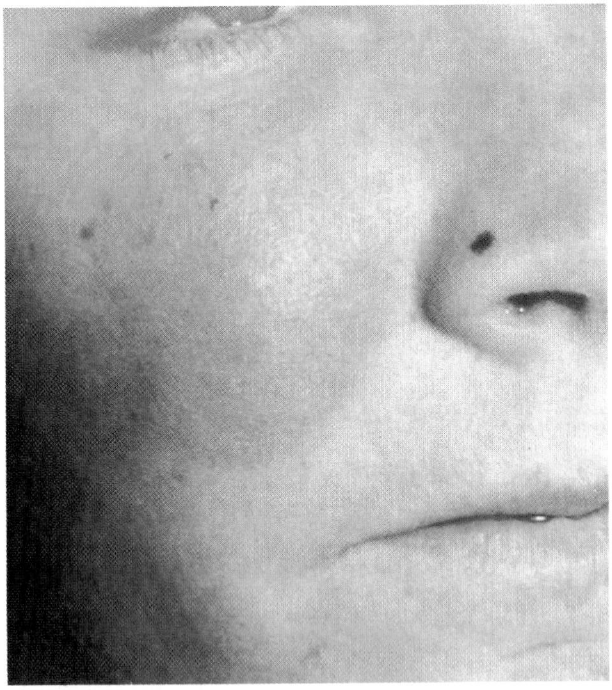

Plate V-27. Erysipelas.

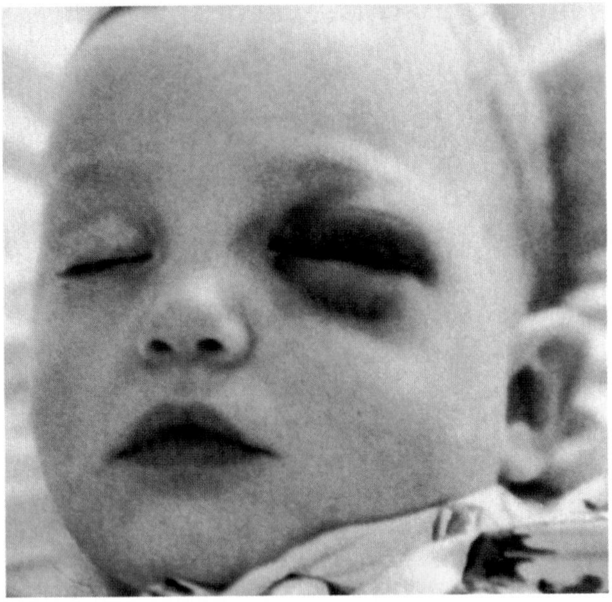

Plate V-28. Periorbital *H. influenzae* cellulitis.

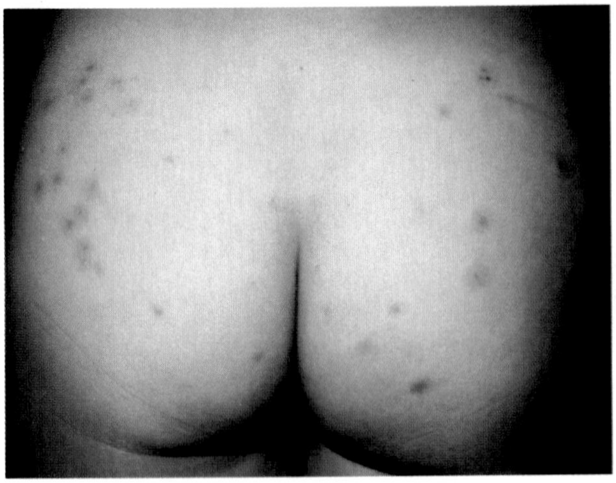

Plate V-29. Hot tub folliculitis.

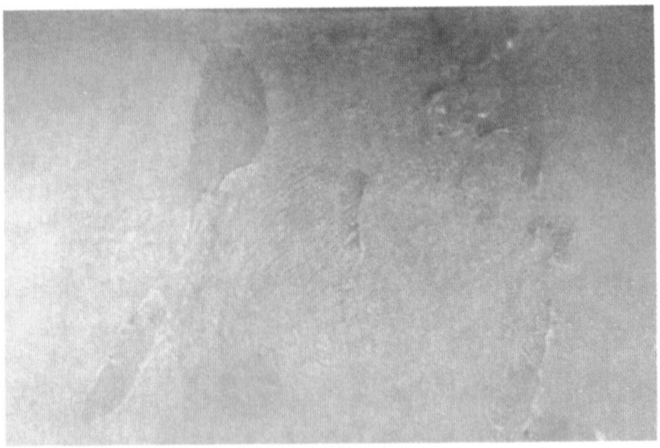

Plate V-30. Staphylococcal scalded skin syndrome.

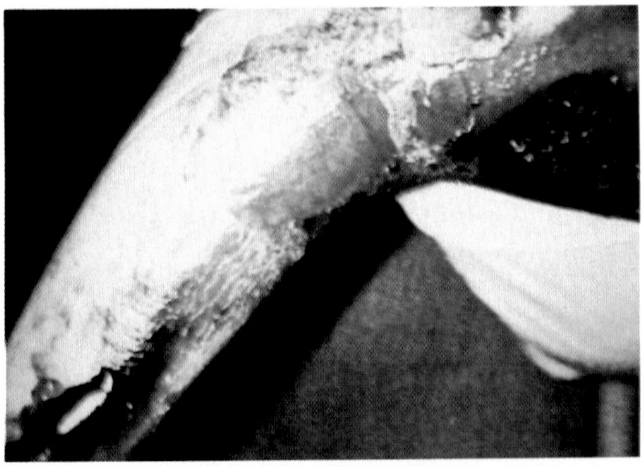

Plate V-31. Acute gangrene of the arm caused by *Streptococcus pyogenes*, group A, type 12. (From Arch Intern Med 112:937, 1963, American Medical Association. With permission.)

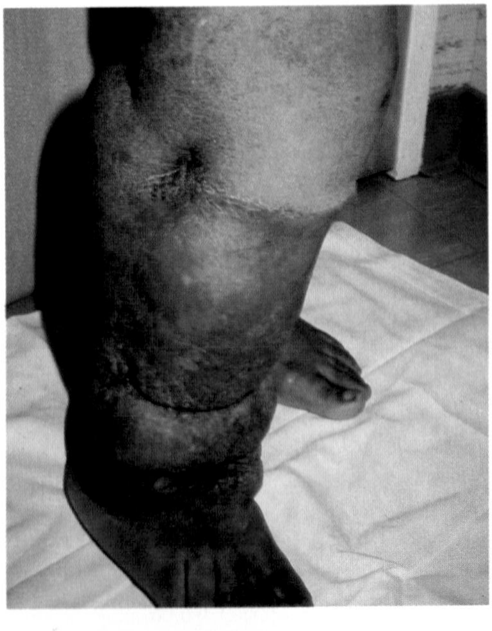

Plate V-32. Elephantiasis nostras.

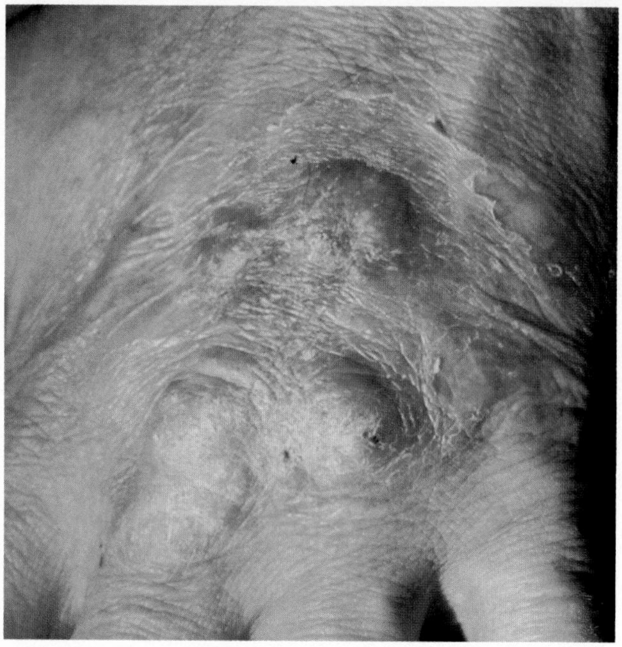

Plate V-33. *Mycobacterium marinum.*

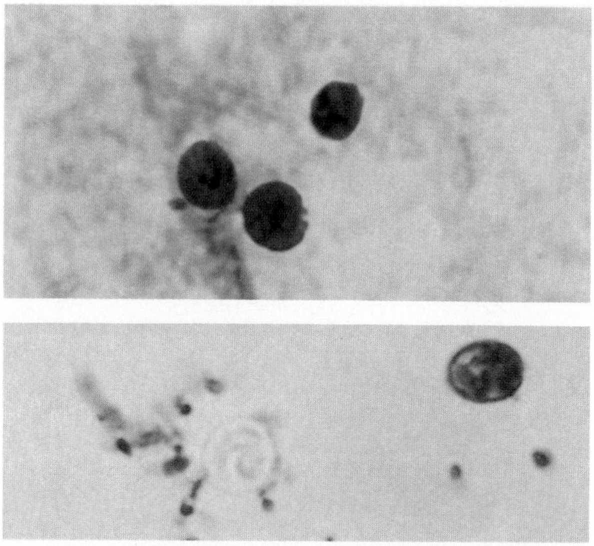

Plate V-35. Oocysts of *Cryptosporidium*. Oocysts are acid-fast and can be stained with modified Kinyoun stain or Ziehl-Neelsen stain *(top)* (×2000). Periodic acid Schiff (PAS) stain can assist in differentiating *Cryptosporidium* from yeast *(bottom)*. Yeast stains with PAS; *Cryptosporidium* does not. ×2000. (Courtesy of Dr. Keith Hadley, San Francisco General Hospital.)

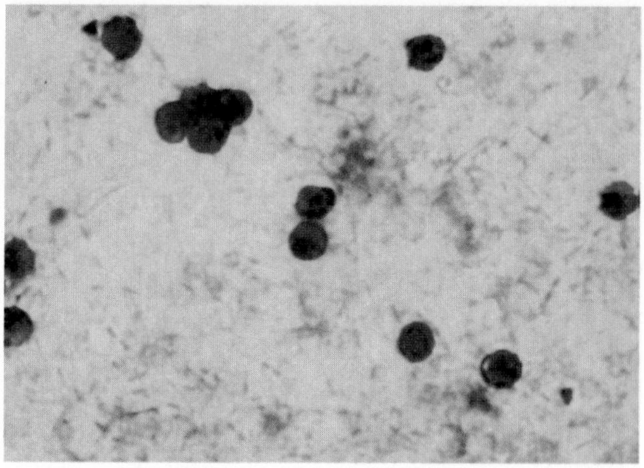

Plate V-34. Modified Kinyoun stain of stool specimen demonstrating the numerous oval, red cryptosporidia.

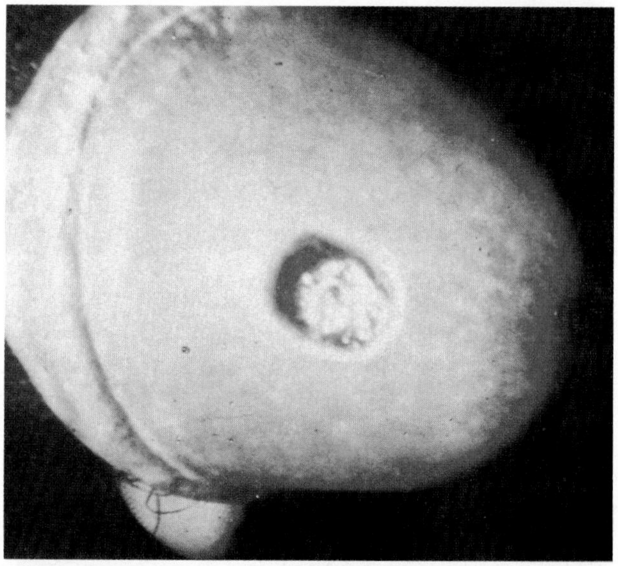

Plate V-36. Chancre of the penis in primary syphilis. (Courtesy of Centers for Disease Control.)

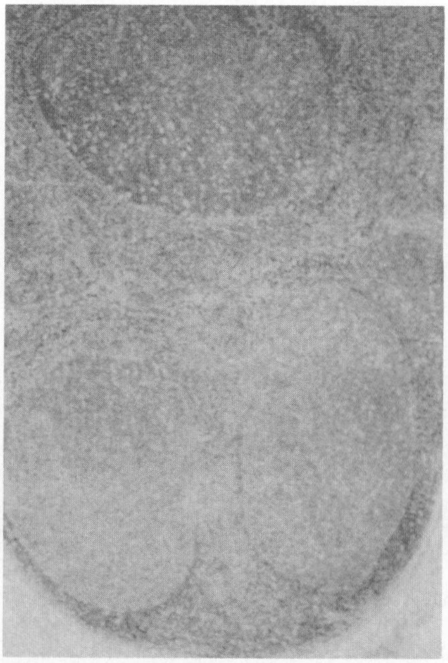

Plate V-37. Hematoxylin and eosin preparation of biopsy specimen from peripheral lymph node demonstrating reactive hyperplasia.

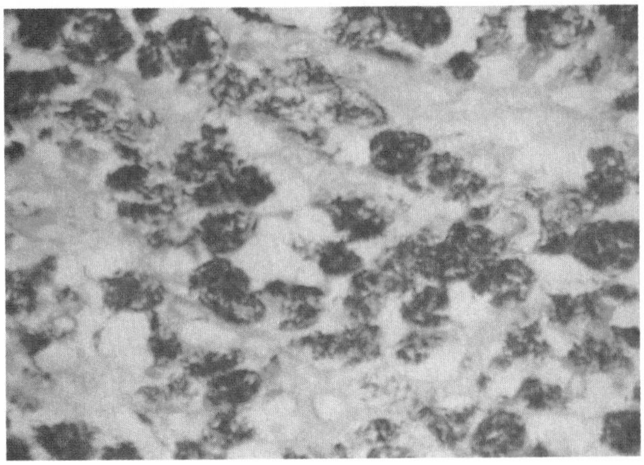

Plate V-38. Acid-fast stain of lymph node biopsy demonstrating macrophages filled with numerous red-staining *Mycobacterium avium* organisms.

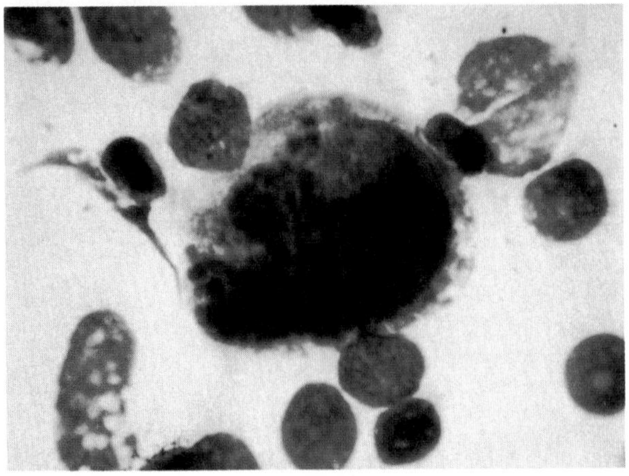

Plate V-39. Transbronchial biopsy specimen from a patient with cytomegalovirus pneumonitis demonstrating a multinucleated cell with intranuclear and cytoplasmic inclusions.

A

B

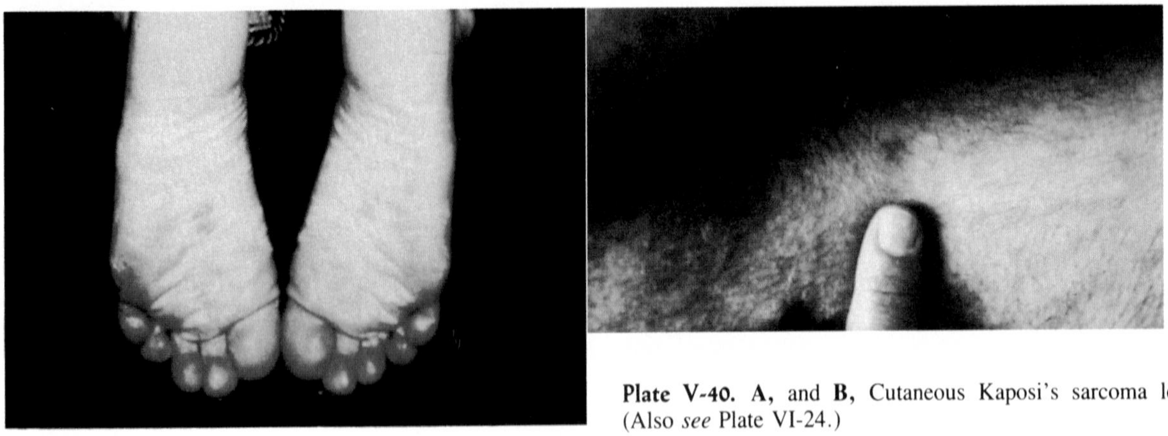

Plate V-40. A, and **B,** Cutaneous Kaposi's sarcoma lesions. (Also *see* Plate VI-24.)

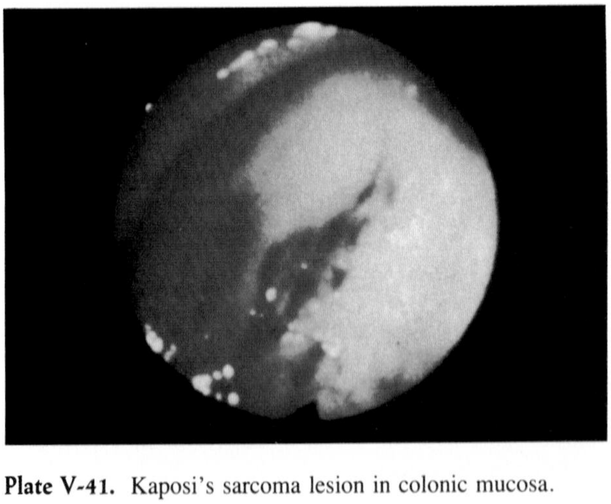

Plate V-41. Kaposi's sarcoma lesion in colonic mucosa.

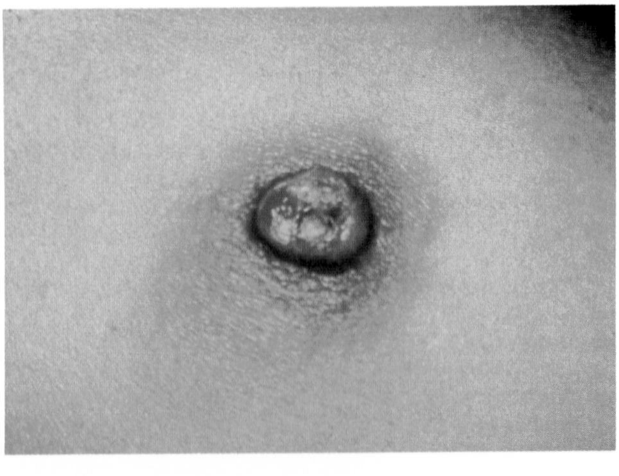

Plate V-42. Typical lesion of bacillary angiomatosis.

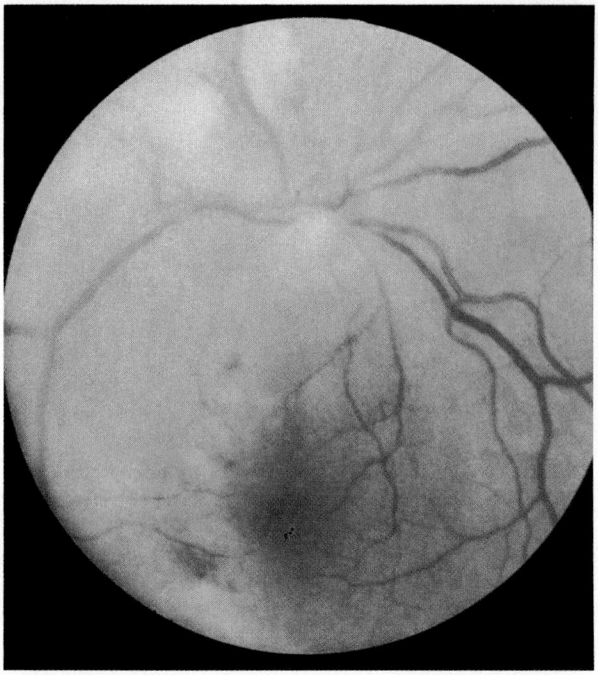

Plate V-43. Retinochoroiditis caused by cytomegalovirus infection.

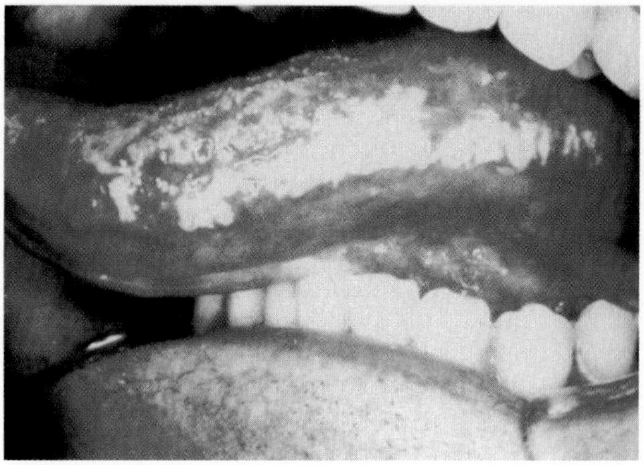

Plate V-44. Oral hairy leukoplakia.

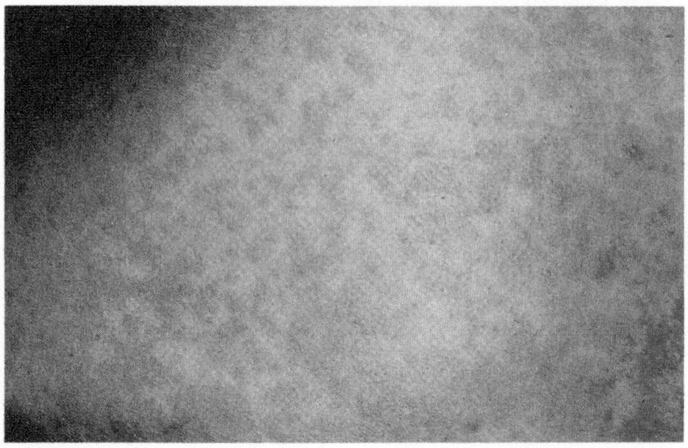

Plate V-45. Typical maculopapular rash of measles.

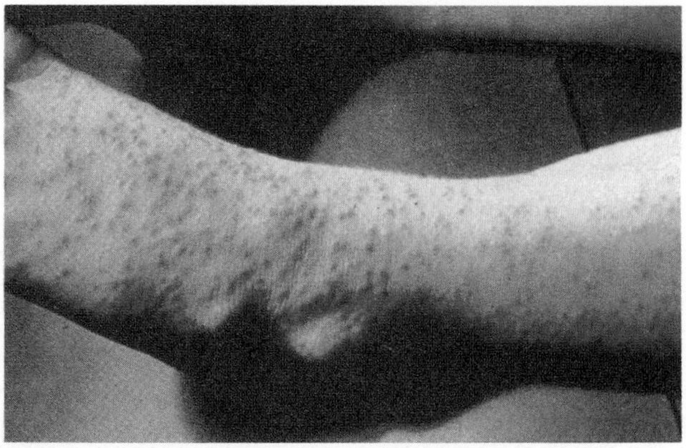

Plate V-46. Petechial rash of atypical measles.

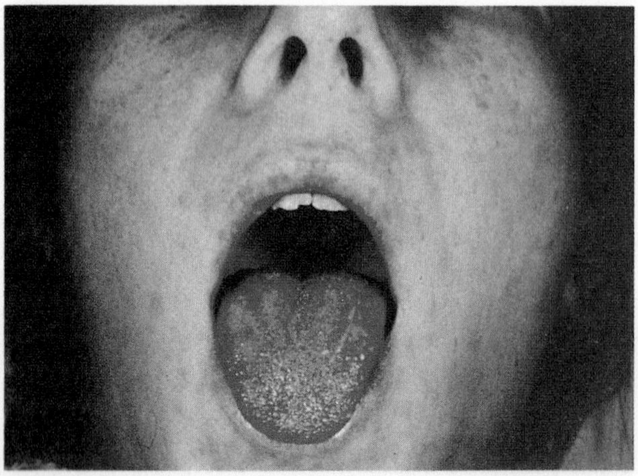

Plate V-47. "Strawberry tongue" exanthem seen in association with the erythematous maculopapular exanthem of atypical measles.

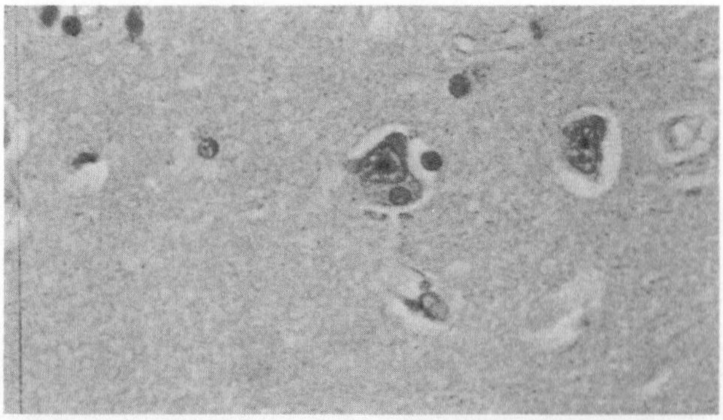

Plate V-48. Negri bodies in human rabies. In the center is a well-defined cell with a nucleus and a cytoplasmic Negri body. Hematoxylin-eosin stain. ×200. (Courtesy of Dr. Jerry Winkler, Centers for Disease Control.)

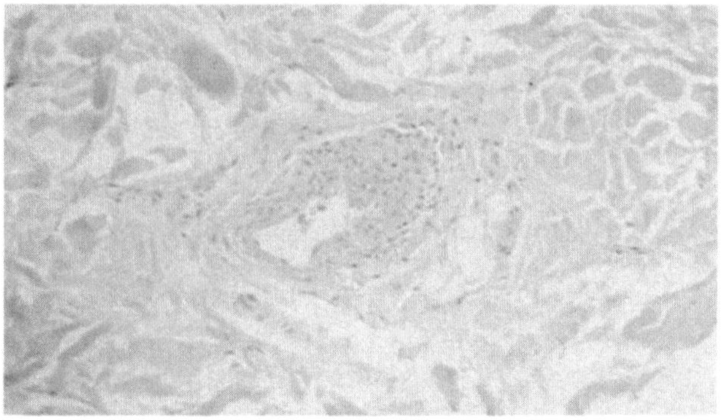

Plate V-49. Typical focus of rickettsial vasculitis in an arteriole, with mononuclear inflammatory infiltrate and a small, nonocclusive thrombus.

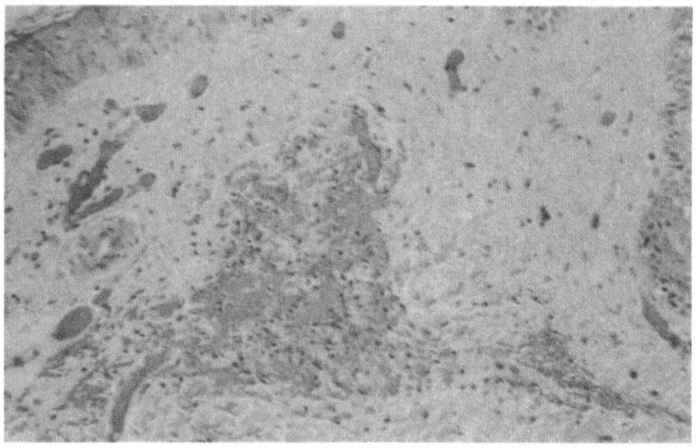

Plate V-50. Small intradermal hemorrhage at a focus of vasculitis. This causes the palpable, petechial rash that does not blanch on pressure.

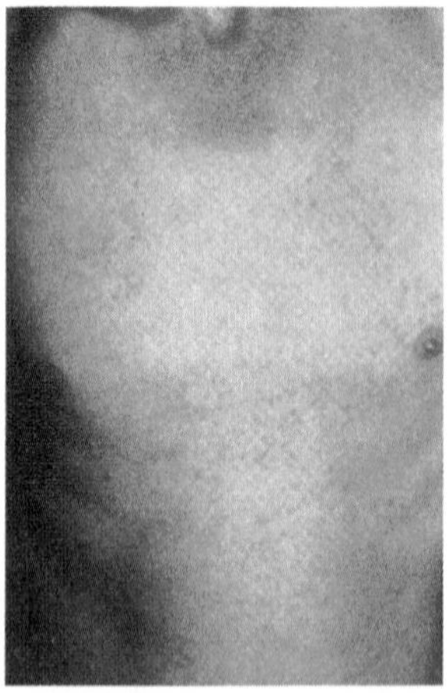

Plate V-51. Secondary syphilis. (Courtesy of Dr. Charles J. Schleupner.)

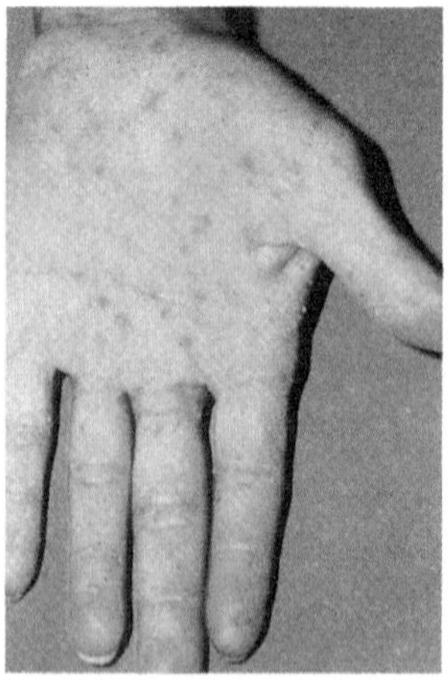

Plate V-52. Palmar lesions of secondary syphilis. (Courtesy of Dr. Charles J. Schleupner.)

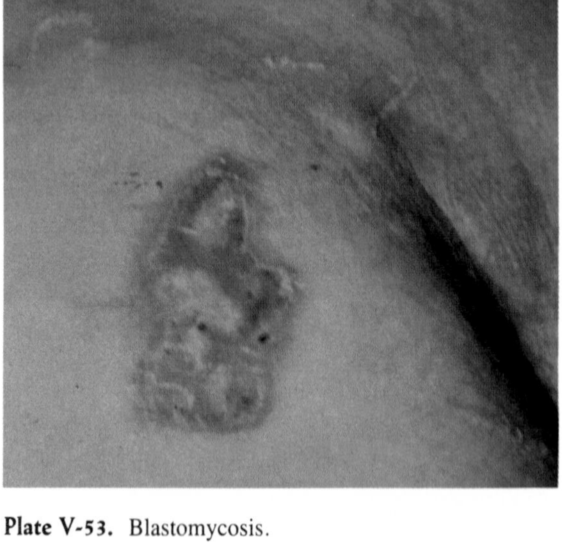

Plate V-53. Blastomycosis.

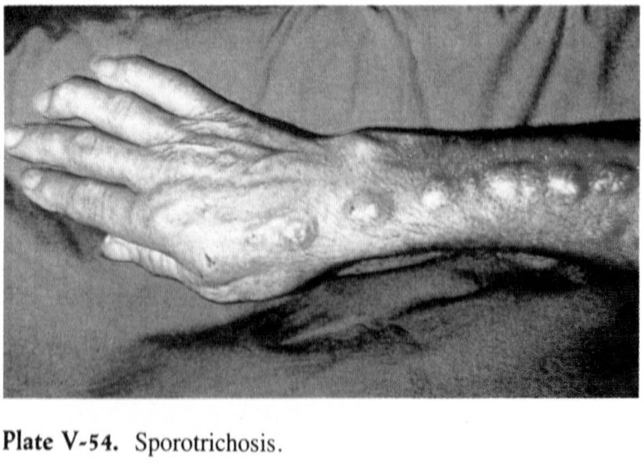

Plate V-54. Sporotrichosis.

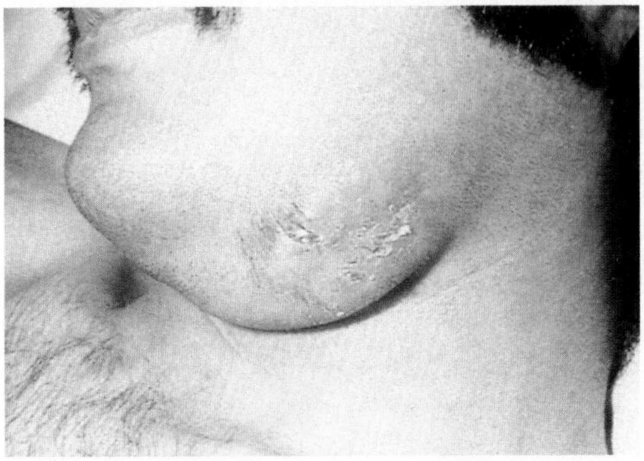

Plate V-55. Actinomycosis.

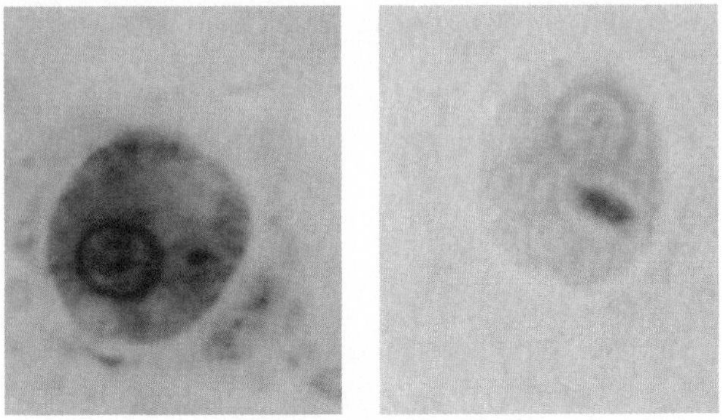

Plate V-56. *Entamoeba histolytica* in fecal specimen (trichrome stain). On the left is a trophozoite or a very early cyst. Trophozoites measure 10 to 60 μm in diameter and may contain phagocytized erythrocytes. On the right is a cyst containing a chromatoidal bar and a single nucleus. Mature cysts are 10 to 20 μm in diameter and most often contain four nuclei. ×2000. (Courtesy of Dr. Keith Hadley, San Francisco General Hospital.)

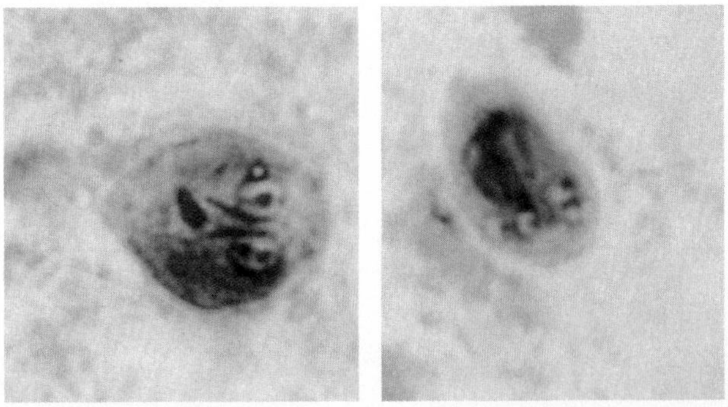

Plate V-57. *Giardia lamblia* trophozoite *(left)* and cyst *(right)*. The trophozoite contains two nuclei and a flagellum. The cyst contains four nuclei. ×2000. (Courtesy of Dr. Keith Hadley, San Francisco General Hospital.)

A

B

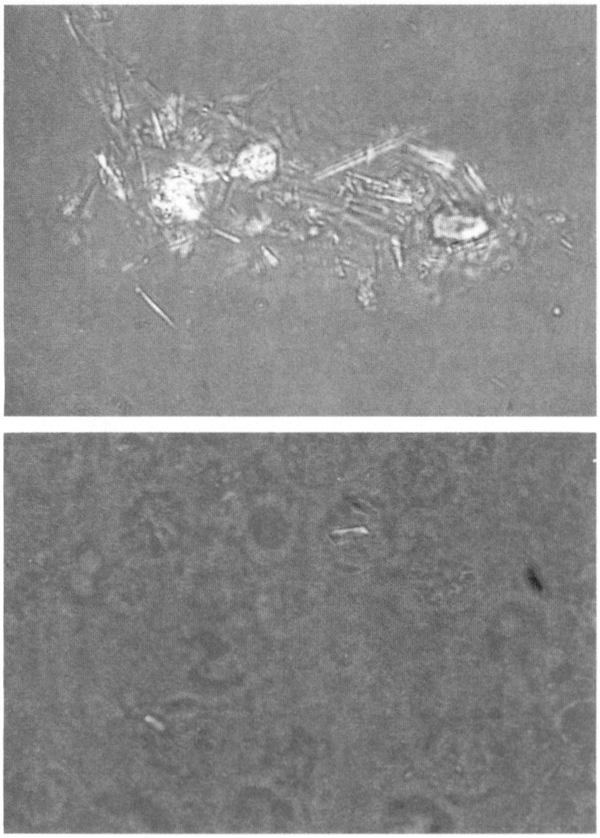

Plate VI-1. The appearance of crystals in synovial fluids as viewed with compensated polarized light. **A,** Intracellular and extracellular negatively birefringent, needle-shaped monosodium urate crystals. **B,** Faint, positively birefringent rhomboid crystals of calcium pyrophosphate dihydrate (CPPD).

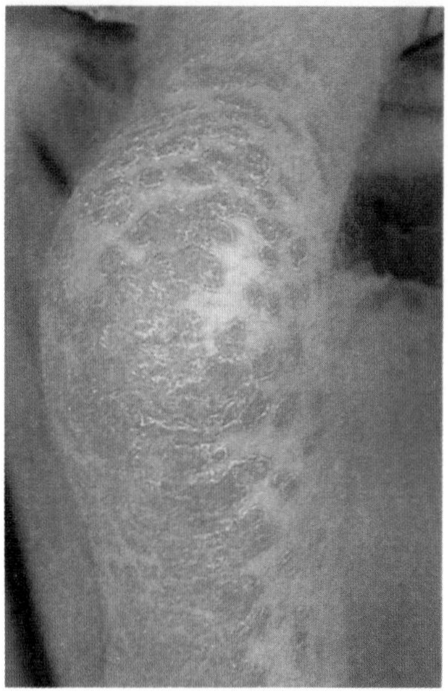

Plate VI-2. Reiter's disease.

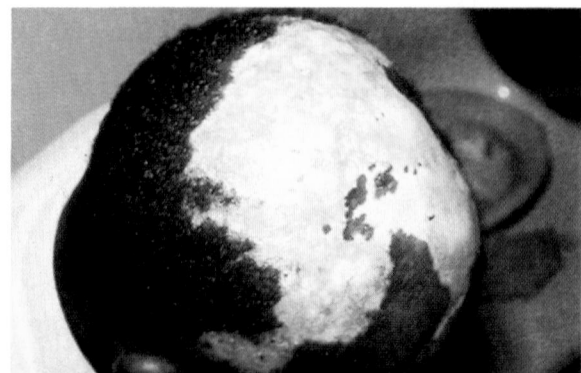

Plate VI-3. Lupus erythematosus.

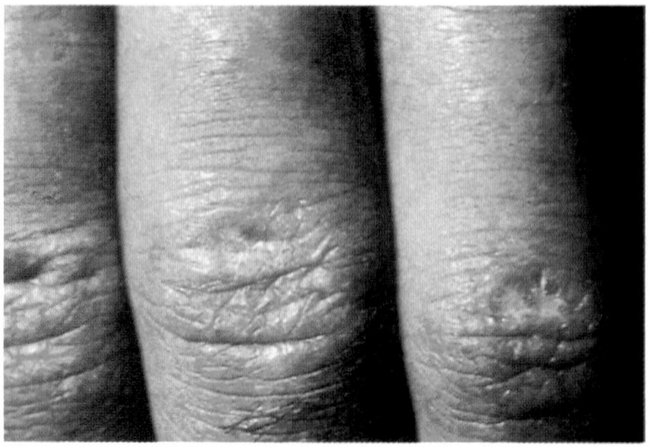

Plate VI-4. Dermatomyositis (Gottron's papules.)

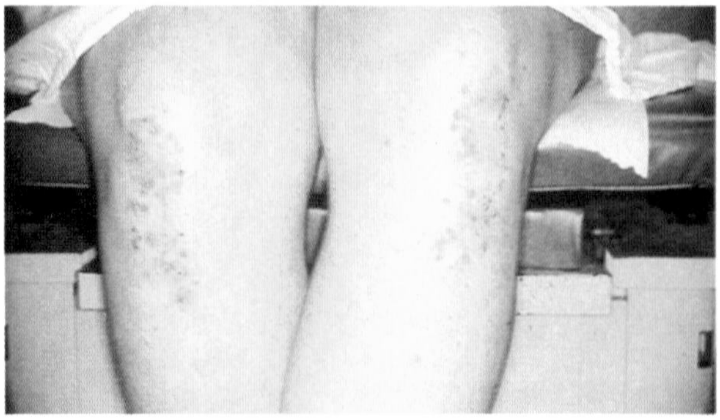

Plate VI-5. Dermatitis herpetiformis.

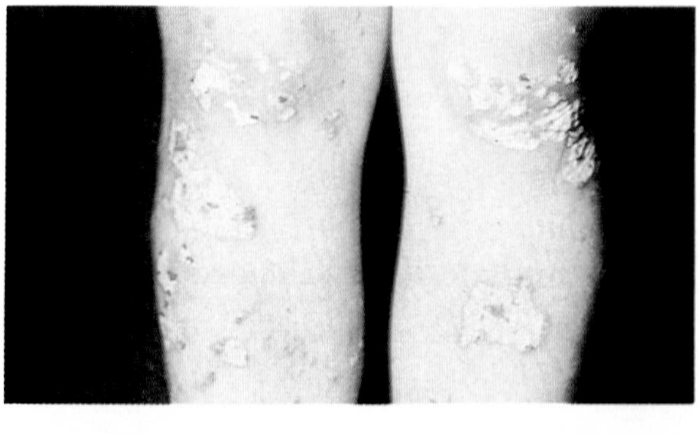

Plate VI-6. Psoriasis.

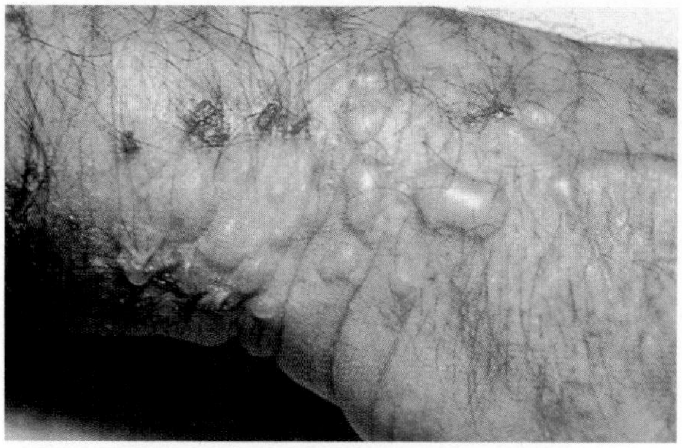

Plate VI-7. Porphyria cutanea tarda.

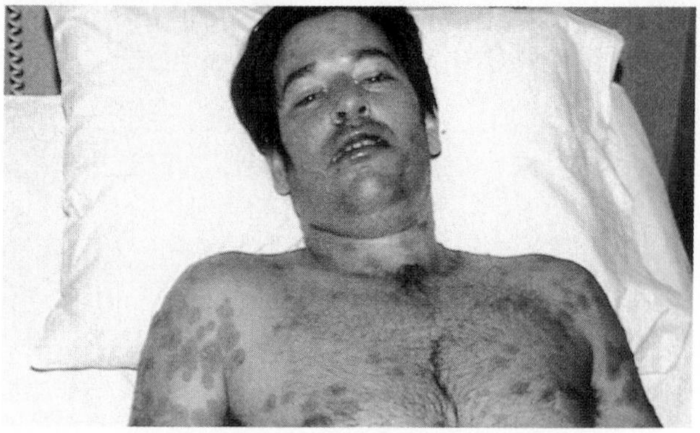

Plate VI-8. Stevens-Johnson syndrome.

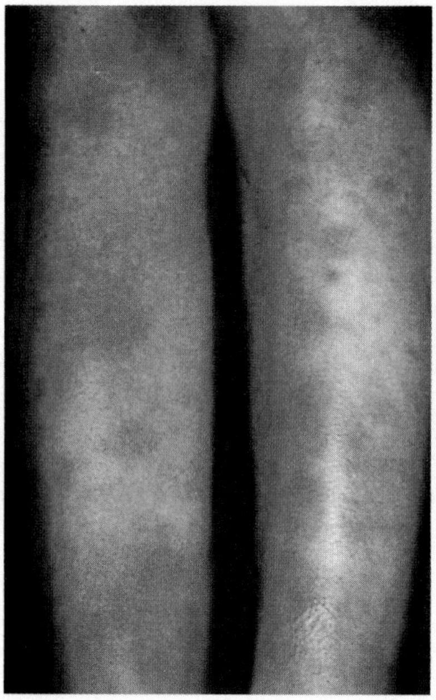

Plate VI-9. Erythema nodosum.

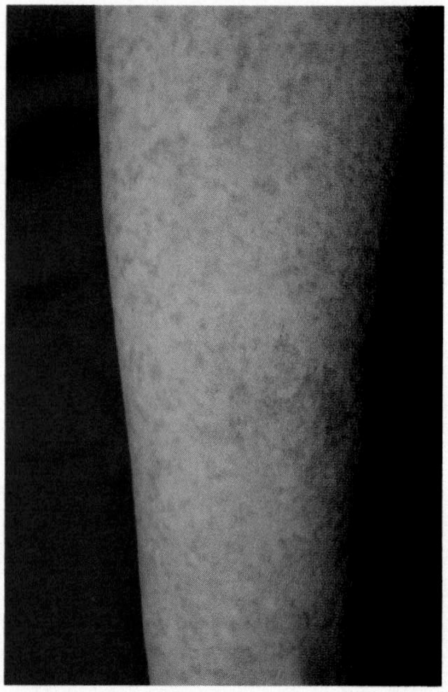

Plate VI-10. Exanthematous eruption developing after the administration of trimethoprim-sulfamethoxazole.

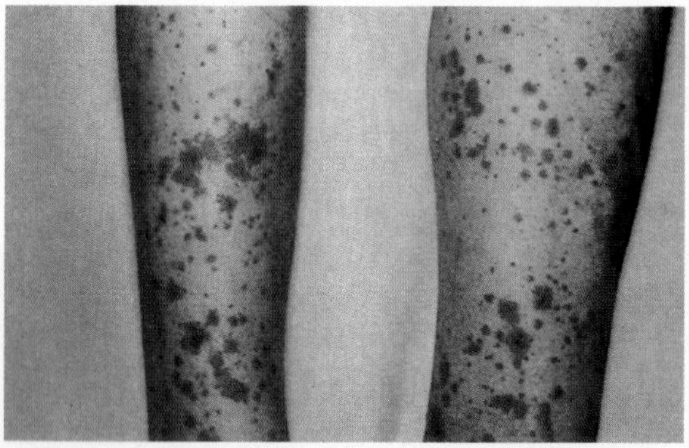

Plate VI-11. Cutaneous leukocytoclastic vasculitis.

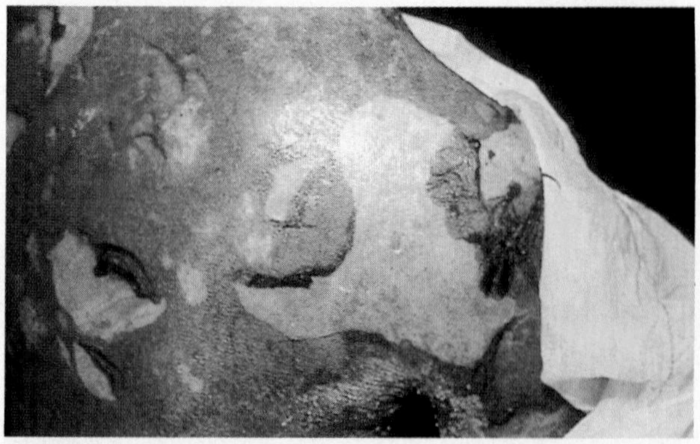

Plate VI-12. Toxic epidermal necrolysis.

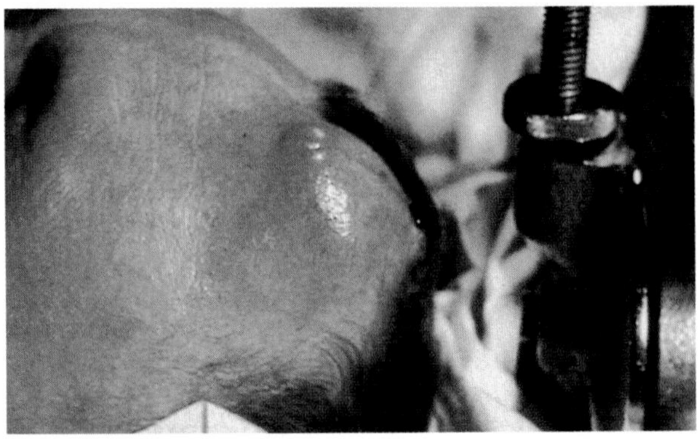

Plate VI-13. Metastatic carcinoma.

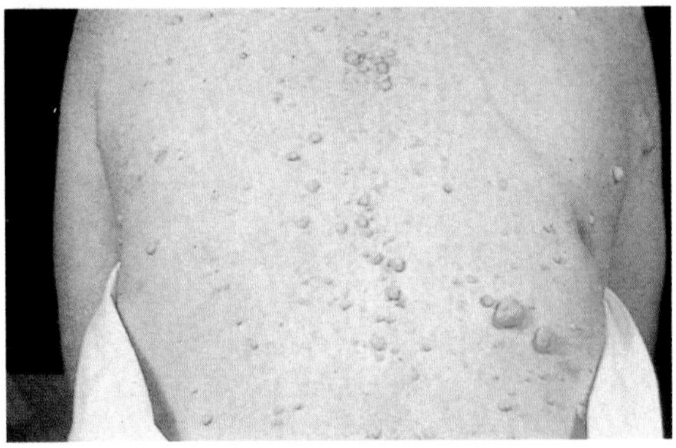

Plate VI-14. Neurofibromatosis.

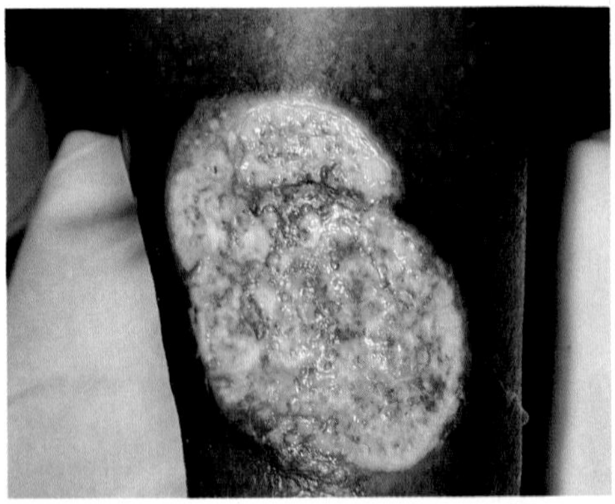

Plate VI-15. Pyoderma gangrenosum.

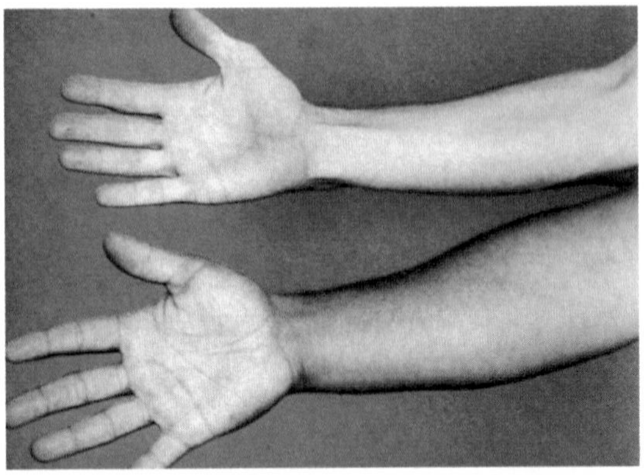

Plate VI-16. Addison's disease: hyperpigmentation of skin and palmar and digital creases.

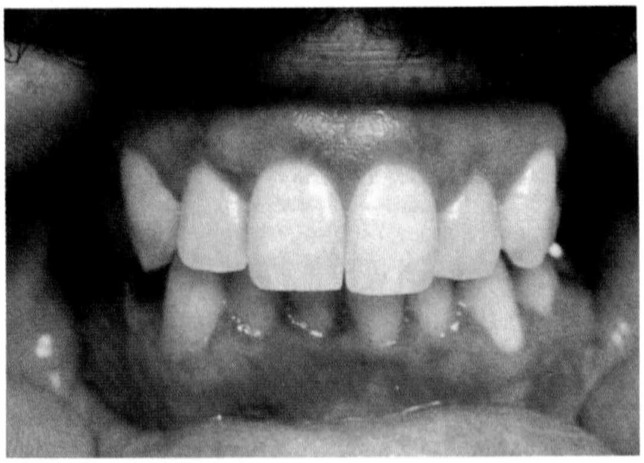

Plate VI-17. Addison's disease: hyperpigmentation of gums along dentate margins.

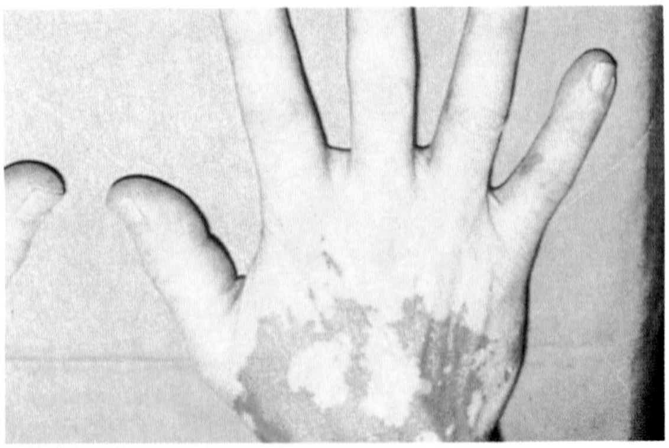

Plate VI-18. Vitiligo.

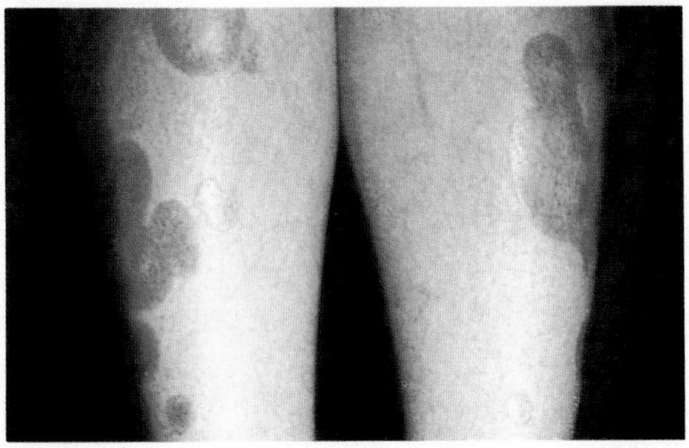

Plate VI-19. Necrobiosis lipoidica diabeticorum.

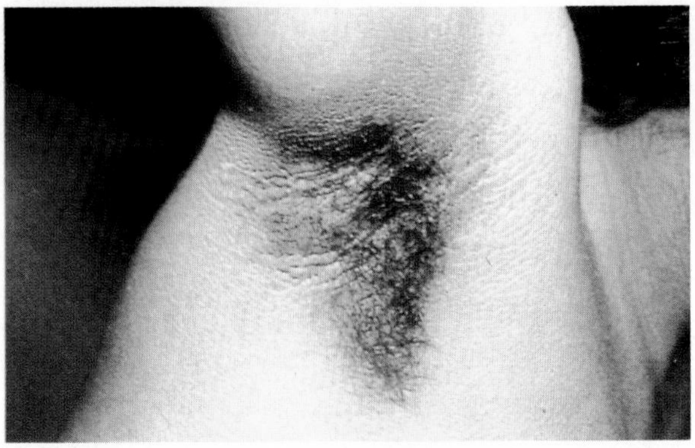

Plate VI-20. Acanthosis nigricans.

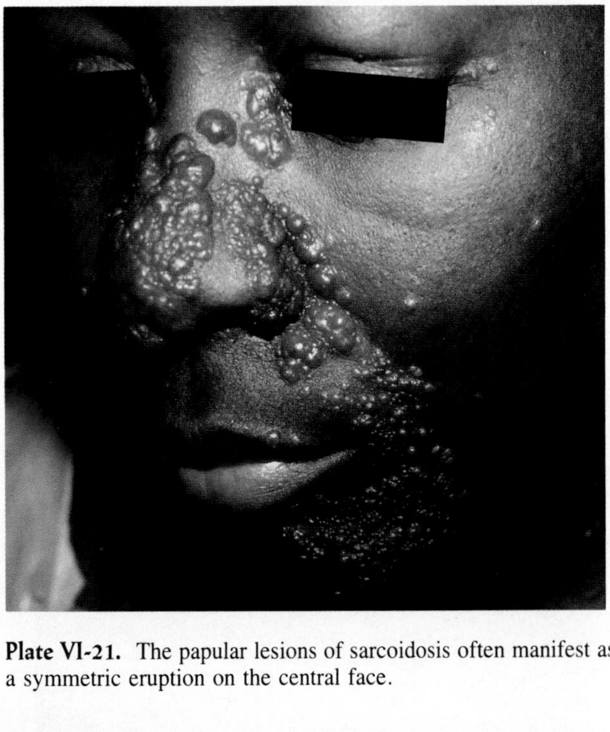

Plate VI-21. The papular lesions of sarcoidosis often manifest as a symmetric eruption on the central face.

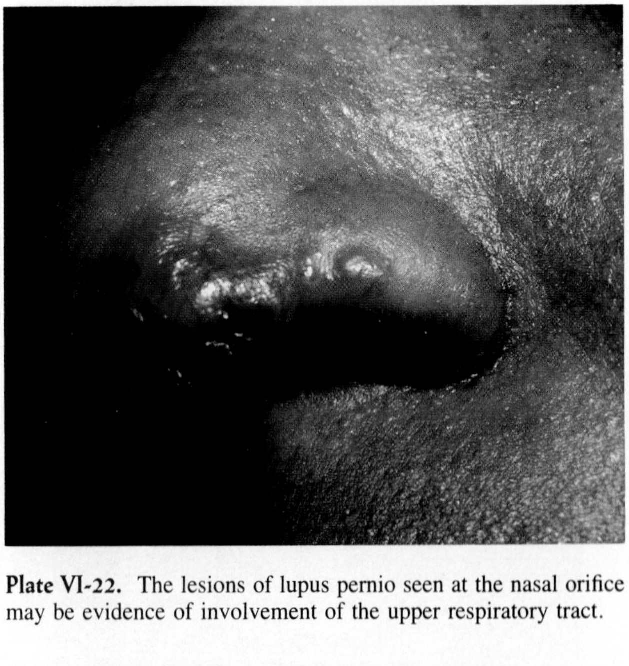

Plate VI-22. The lesions of lupus pernio seen at the nasal orifice may be evidence of involvement of the upper respiratory tract.

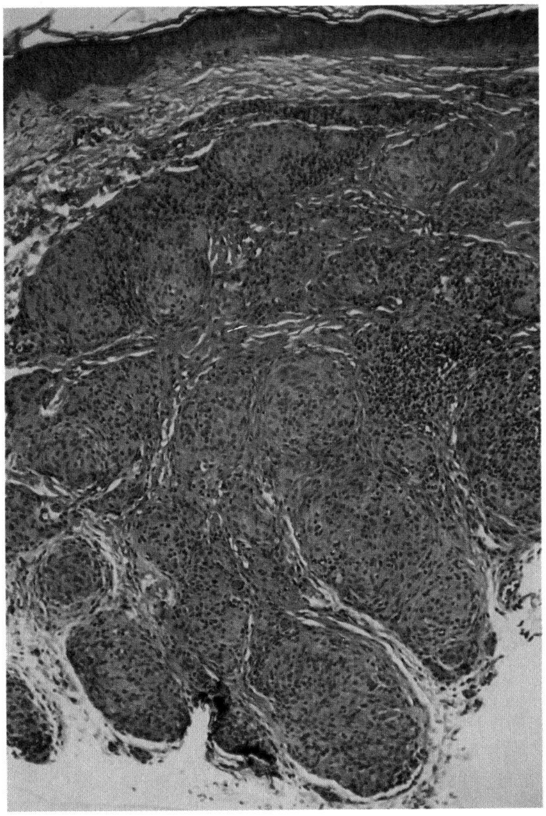

Plate VI-23. The noncaseating granulomas of sarcoidosis may extend deep into the dermis. There is a relative paucity of small lymphocytes.

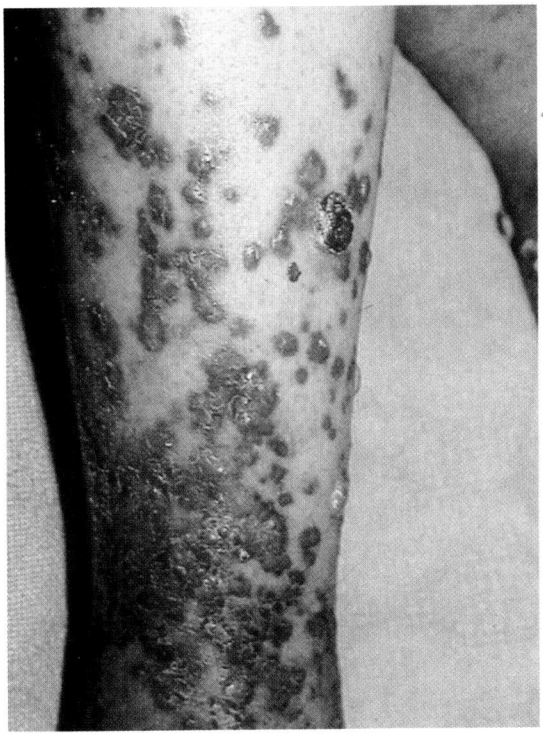

Plate VI-24. Kaposi's sarcoma. (Also see Plate V-40, **A** and **B**.)

PART ONE

Diseases of the Heart and Blood Vessels

I BASIC PHYSIOLOGY

CHAPTER

1 Cardiovascular Physiology

Gregory L. Freeman
Sumanth D. Prabhu
Robert A. O'Rourke

*Webster's Dictionary** defines the heart as "a muscular organ which is the propelling agent of blood in the body. . . . By its alternate dilatation and contraction the circulation is carried on." In physiologic terms this is an amazingly accurate description of the heart. It is composed of fully differentiated, postmitotic muscle cells, which are activated by electrical depolarization. Its rhythmic properties permit efficient pumping by cyclic filling and emptying, and it moves the blood through the vasculature so that oxygen and nutrients are supplied to the metabolizing tissues and waste products are removed.

Although this description is simple, it belies the extreme complexity and sophistication of the heart and the vascular system to which it is coupled. The intrinsic cardiac regulatory mechanisms, as well as the control provided by the autonomic nervous system, allow the heart to maintain appropriate systemic blood flow under a remarkably wide range of conditions. This chapter outlines the basic functional properties of the cardiovascular system, providing the knowledge of normal cardiac function necessary for properly interpreting the cardiovascular physical examination. Moreover, a basic knowledge of normal physiology is necessary for recognizing and understanding the manifestations and significance of pathologic conditions affecting the cardiovascular system.

Fig. 1-1 provides a schematic map of how the parts of the cardiovascular system interact to produce cardiac output. Because much basic and clinical literature is available on each of these specific topics, one can easily focus narrowly and thus lose sight of how these systems function together. From a conceptual viewpoint, emphasis must be given to the heart's primary function: to provide blood flow to the body. By keeping this in mind, one can see how each component participates in providing that flow and can predict how a malfunction of any component would interfere with it.

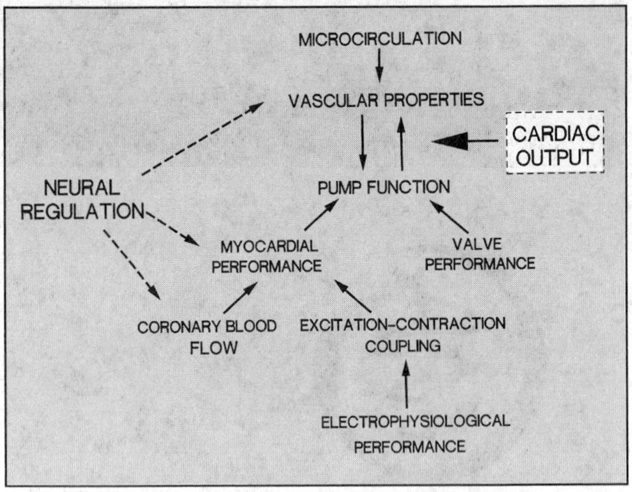

Fig. 1-1. Schematic drawing of the basic components of the cardiovascular system. Cardiac output is measured as forward flow out of the heart into the systemic circulation; it is affected by both the heart and the vasculature. Dotted lines indicate neural regulatory mechanisms.

BASIC ELECTROPHYSIOLOGY

Resting potential

Under resting conditions, differences in ionic concentrations across the sarcolemma of cardiac cells produce a difference of electrical potential such that the cells are polarized. For ventricular and atrial myocytes the resting potential is about −90 mV, with the cell's inside negative to its outside; for the sinus node the resting potential is about −65 mV. In the extracellular fluid the concentrations of sodium and chloride are high, about 145 and 120 mM, respectively; the concentration of potassium is low, about 4 mM. In the intracellular space, by contrast, the concentration of potassium is high, about 150 mM; sodium and chloride are present in low concentrations of about 15 and 6 mM, respectively.

The maintenance of these ionic gradients depends on several mechanisms. The first is a membrane pump, which exchanges intracellular sodium for extracellular potassium in a ratio of 3:2. To transport the ions against their concentration gradients and to maintain the sarcolemma in a polarized state, the sodium-potassium pump requires the hydrolysis of the high-energy phosphate, adenosine triphosphate (ATP), which occurs as a result of the action of a membrane-bound ATPase. This mechanism is clinically important because it is the site of action of the digitalis glycosides.

The second important mechanism active in maintaining the resting potential is sodium-calcium exchange. This does not directly depend on ATP hydrolysis but is linked to the movement of sodium resulting from the sodium-potassium pump. Sodium-calcium exchange moves calcium ions out of the cell in exchange for an increase in intracellular sodium. Thus, under resting conditions, a countertransport of sodium ions occurs: sodium ions removed from the cell by the sodium-potassium pump move back into the cell, whereas calcium ions are removed to the extracellular space. Recent observations suggest that the sodium-calcium exchange mechanism is sensitive to transmembrane potential and also plays a role in ion currents during the repolarization phase of the action potential.

*Webster's new twentieth century dictionary of the English language, unabridged, ed 2. New York, 1979, Simon & Schuster.

Action potential

The cyclic nature of the heart's mechanical behavior depends on rhythmic depolarization of the myocytes, which leads to contraction. Fig. 1-2 demonstrates the action potentials of a ventricular myocyte and a sinus node cell. The fully polarized, diastolic portion of the action potential is termed *phase 4*. In myocytes this potential is constant; in specialized conduction tissue, phase 4 of the action potential has a positive slope, and membrane potential approaches the depolarization threshold. When threshold is reached, rapid depolarization of the membrane (phase 0) ensues, and depolarization spreads to the rest of the heart by means of the specialized conduction tissue. The mechanism for phase 0 depolarization is the movement of sodium ions along their electrochemical gradient into the cell. This results by means of "fast" sodium channels that are open very briefly; their inactivation is both time and voltage dependent and occurs within a few milliseconds (ms). Phase 1 represents early, rapid depolarization and likely results from inactivation of sodium channels and a transient, outward potassium current.

The second inward current that plays a major role in cardiac depolarization results from calcium entry via channels that have extremely different kinetics from the sodium channels. The behavior of these "slow" calcium channels is reflected by the action potential of the sinus node cell shown in Fig. 1-2. The threshold of these channels is higher than that of the sodium channels, and the rate of voltage increase caused by this inward calcium current is slower. These channels play the dominant role in the electrophysiology of the sinus and atrioventricular (A-V) nodes but are present in all myocardial cells. Stimulation of the heart by catecholamines increases the amount of current carried via these channels by inducing the presence of more channels in the membrane and possibly by prolonging the time they are open.

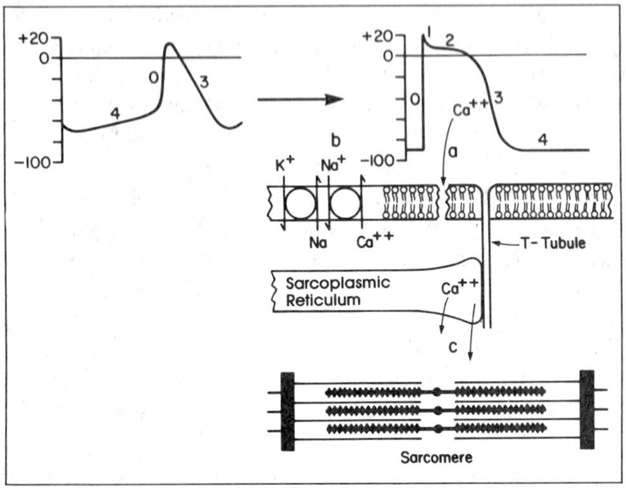

Fig. 1-2. Schematic drawing of a myocardial cell showing the principal movements of calcium. *a,* Entry of calcium into the cell by means of a slow channel; *b,* sodium-calcium exchange; *c,* release of calcium from the sarcoplasmic reticulum. Action potentials from a sinus node cell *(upper left)* and from myocardium *(upper right)* are shown.

Unlike skeletal muscle, cardiac tissue remains depolarized for a prolonged period, about 100 ms. During phase 2 of the action potential, only a small net voltage change occurs. The transition to phase 3, or more rapid repolarization, results from inactivation of the slow inward (calcium channel) current, the onset of an outward potassium current, and possibly extrusion of calcium via the sodium-calcium exchange mechanism.

EXCITATION-CONTRACTION COUPLING

The interaction of actin and myosin, which leads to sarcomere shortening, depends on the presence of free intracellular calcium. Calcium entry into the myoplasm is facilitated by the T tubules, which radially invaginate the cell's interior. The amount of calcium entering the myocyte during the action potential is not sufficient to activate contraction but leads to the release of large amounts of calcium from intracellular stores, which are probably located in the sarcoplasmic reticulum. This "calcium-triggered calcium release" is likely the key mechanism in excitation-contraction coupling in the heart. The amount of calcium released from the sarcoplasmic reticulum depends on the amount of calcium entering the cell by the slow channels; therefore the contractility of cardiac muscle responds to interventions that influence these channels' behavior. Such interventions include the administration of catecholamines, as well as drugs such as diltiazem, nifedipine, or verapamil, which specifically block the channels.

MYOCARDIAL PERFORMANCE

The myocyte's basic contractile unit is the sarcomere, which consists of an array of actin and myosin filaments (Fig. 1-3). Under resting conditions the filaments are prevented from interacting by the regulatory proteins troponin and tropomyosin. When calcium ions are present in the myoplasm, they bind to a portion of the troponin molecule (troponin C), causing a stearic change in the molecule, which allows the interaction of actin and myosin. Sarcomere shortening results from cross-bridge cycling, a process that requires hydrolysis of ATP and that leads to tension generation and/or shortening of the muscle. As shown in Fig. 1-3, the overlap of the actin and myosin filaments present at the onset of contraction depends on the precontractile sarcomere length, which is maximal at about 2.2 μ. Thus the force that can be generated depends on the resting sarcomere length, a relationship that underlies the well-known Frank-Starling mechanism of the heart.

Papillary muscle studies

The myocardium's mechanical behavior has been extensively explored through studies on isolated papillary muscle. The apparatus used in such studies is shown in Fig. 1-4. The muscle is placed between a tension transducer, which measures the force or load that it carries, and a lever used to control that load. The muscle is stretched to its

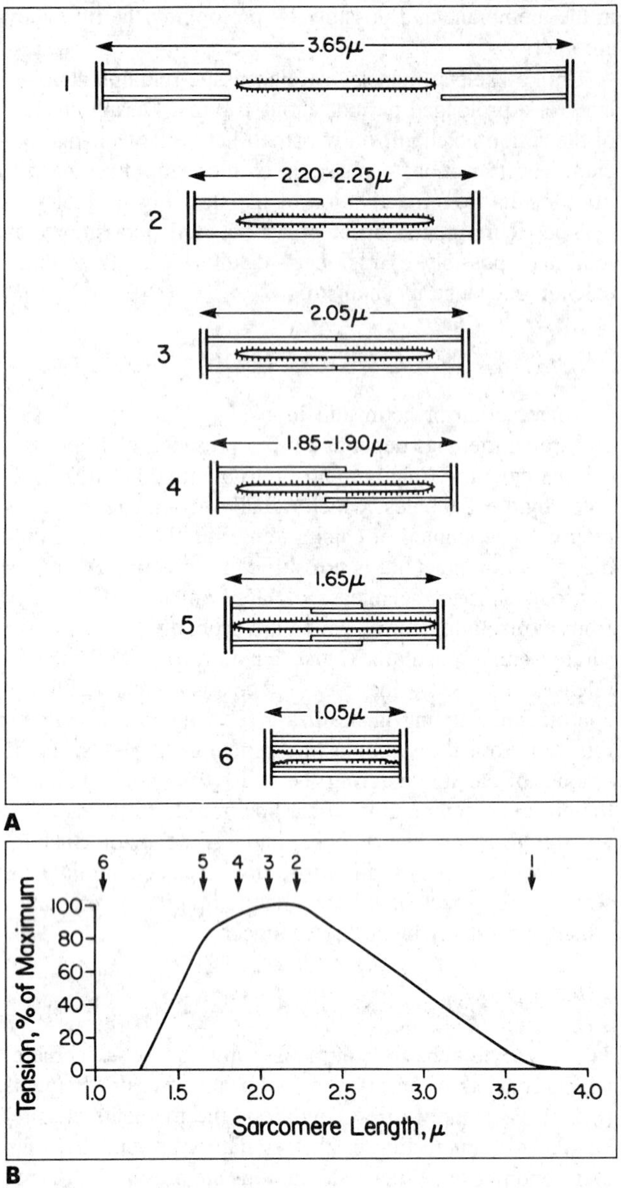

Fig. 1-3. A, Amount of overlap between the actin and myosin filaments varies with precontractile sarcomere length. **B,** Tension development at each sarcomere length (*1* to *6*). (Modified from Braunwald E, Ross J Jr, and Sonnenblick EH, editors: Mechanisms of contraction of the normal and failing heart. Boston, 1976, Little, Brown.)

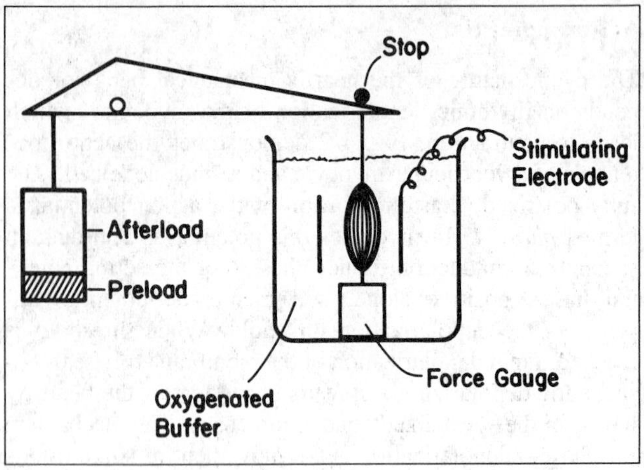

Fig. 1-4. Apparatus used for papillary muscle experimentation.

precontractile length by a load that is added to the lever while the muscle is quiescent; this weight constitutes the *preload*. Further lengthening is prevented by a stop placed above the lever, after which additional weight is added to the lever. Under resting conditions this additional weight is not supported by the muscle, but after the muscle has been stimulated and contraction begins, overall shortening of the muscle cannot take place until the force generated by the muscle is sufficient to overcome both the preload and the additional weight, termed the *afterload*. Once this amount of force has been generated, shortening occurs.

In Fig. 1-5, *A*, the results of an experiment in which no shortening was allowed (isometric contraction) are shown, with muscle length on the abscissa and force (tension) on the ordinate. The bottom curves show the passive-elastic properties of the myocardium, which demonstrate the resting tissue's response to increased preload. The amount of elongation that occurs in response to an increment in preload clearly depends on the muscle's initial length. When the initial length is low, the muscle is easily stretched; substantial elongation results from a small increment of preload. However, when the initial length is longer, further elongation requires a substantial increase in tension.

The upper curves in Fig. 1-5, *A*, show tension generated by the muscle after stimulation, both before (open circles) and after (closed circles) inotropic stimulation with calcium. Under either inotropic state, tension developed depends on the muscle's initial length, increasing as the muscle is stretched. The relationship of tension generation to initial muscle length is a fundamental property of the myocardium and is termed the *Frank-Starling mechanism*. With calcium added, the amount of tension produced from any given resting length is increased, reflecting an increase in the muscle's contractility. Although increased contractility alters the muscle's active, tension-generating properties, reflected by a shift of the isometric length-tension relation, its passive-elastic behavior is unchanged.

The results of an experiment in which shortening is allowed to occur are shown in Fig. 1-5, *B*. Two contractions are plotted, both starting from the same initial length. In contraction 1 the afterload is lower than in contraction 2, and the muscle shortens more against this lower load. The inotropic state, or muscle contractility, is the same in the two contractions shown in Fig. 1-5, *B*, and the difference in shortening results from the difference in afterload. The dashed line represents the isotonic length-tension relation, which is similar to the isometric length-tension relation just discussed. For any combination of preload and afterload, this relation defines how much muscle shortening will occur.

Another important observation is that the rate of shortening depends on the load against which the muscle short-

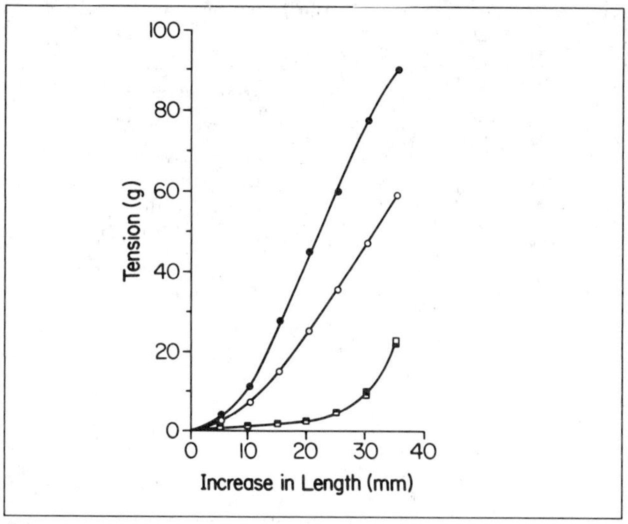

A

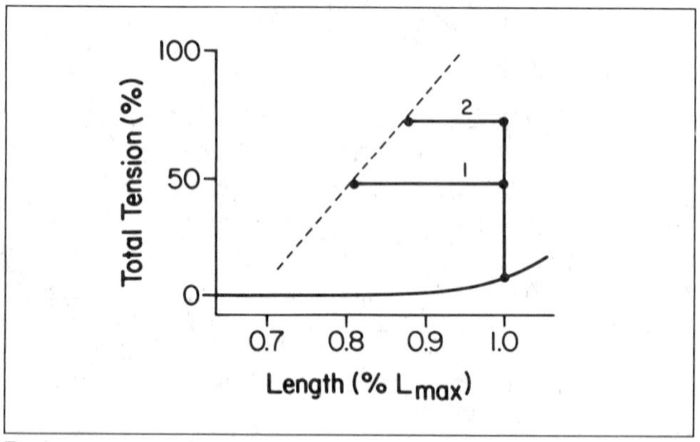

B

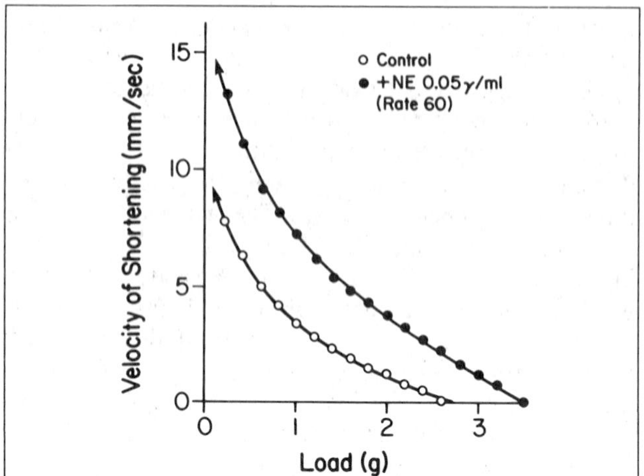

C

Fig. 1-5. A, Isometric length-tension relation. The squares show passive behavior of the tissue, and the circles show tension generated after stimulation. Open symbols show control conditions, and closed symbols are conditions after inotropic stimulation with calcium. **B,** The dashed line shows isotonic length-tension relation. The shortening that occurs depends on the afterload against which the muscle must work. **C,** The force-velocity relation, before *(open circles)* and after *(closed circles)* inotropic stimulation with norepinephrine *(NE)*. (Modified from Braunwald E, Ross J Jr, and Sonnenblick EH, editors: Mechanisms of contraction of the normal and failing heart. Boston, 1976, Little, Brown.)

ens. This force-velocity relation is shown in Fig. 1-5, *C*, under control conditions (open circles) and after inotropic stimulation with norepinephrine (closed circles). The x intercept represents isometric contraction, where force is maximal, but no shortening occurs. As the load against which the muscle contracts is reduced, the speed at which it shortens increases. The maximum rate at which shortening could occur, termed V_{max}, is represented by this plot's y intercept. This value must be extrapolated because one cannot perform an experiment with totally unloaded shortening. The addition of norepinephrine increases the velocity of shortening against any given afterload and increases V_{max}. For this reason, V_{max} has been considered an index of the myocardium's contractile state.

Thus the myocardium's overall performance is controlled by three key determinants. The first is *preload,* a measure of the initial sarcomere length at the onset of contraction. The second is *afterload,* the force that the muscle must generate before shortening can occur. The third is *contractility,* the muscle's inotropic state. These three determinants of myocardial performance also control the intact heart's performance.

MECHANICS OF INTACT HEART: PUMP FUNCTION

Cardiac cycle

To understand the heart's mechanical performance, one must know the events that occur during the cardiac cycle in both the atria and the ventricles. These events are illustrated in Fig. 1-6. During diastole, when the pressure in the ventricles falls below that in the atria, the A-V valves open, allowing rapid emptying of the atrial chambers. This rapid emptying is followed by a period of slow filling, since atrial and ventricular pressures are almost equal, and further filling depends on continued venous return to the heart. After the sinus node depolarizes, the atria contract, again producing a pressure gradient between the atria and ventricles and additional ventricular filling. Importantly, the atrial contraction accounts for about 20% to 25% of ventricular filling, an effect that is not present during atrial fibrillation.

With the onset of ventricular depolarization, the pressure in the ventricles rises, and the A-V valves close. For a brief period, termed *isovolumic systole,* no change in intraventricular volume occurs because the A-V valves are closed and the pressure in the ventricles is not yet high enough to open the semilunar valves. When ventricular pressures rise above those in the aorta and pulmonary artery, ejection begins. When ejection is complete, the pressure in the ventricle begins to fall. When it has fallen below the pressure in the aorta and pulmonary arteries, the semilunar valves close. Again, for a brief period, termed *isovolumic diastole* (or isovolumic relaxation), no change in ventricular volume can occur because the semilunar valves are closed, and the pressure in the ventricles is still higher than the pressure in the atria. When the ventricular pressure falls below the pressure in the atria, the A-V valves open, and the cycle begins again.

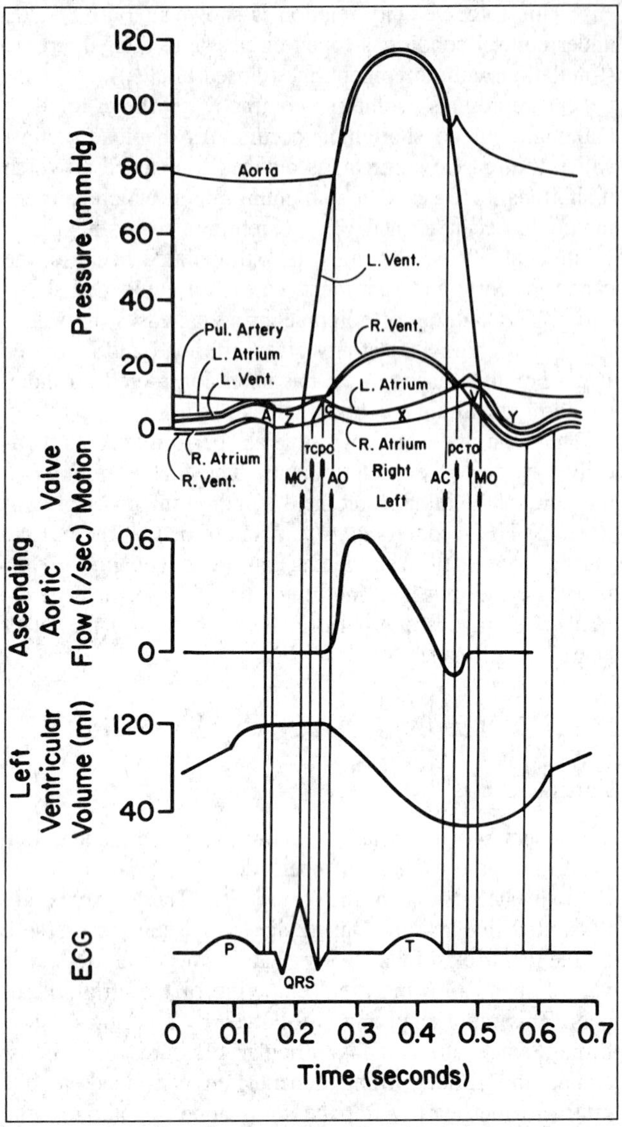

Fig. 1-6. Electrical and mechanical events during the cardiac cycle. *MC* and *TC*, Mitral and tricuspid closure; *PO* and *AO*, pulmonic and aortic valve opening; *AC* and *PC*, aortic and pulmonic valve closure; *TO* and *MO*, tricuspid and mitral valve opening; *L*, left; *R*, right; *Vent*, ventricle; *Pul*, pulmonary. (Modified from Hurst JW, editor: The heart, ed 5. New York, 1982, McGraw-Hill.)

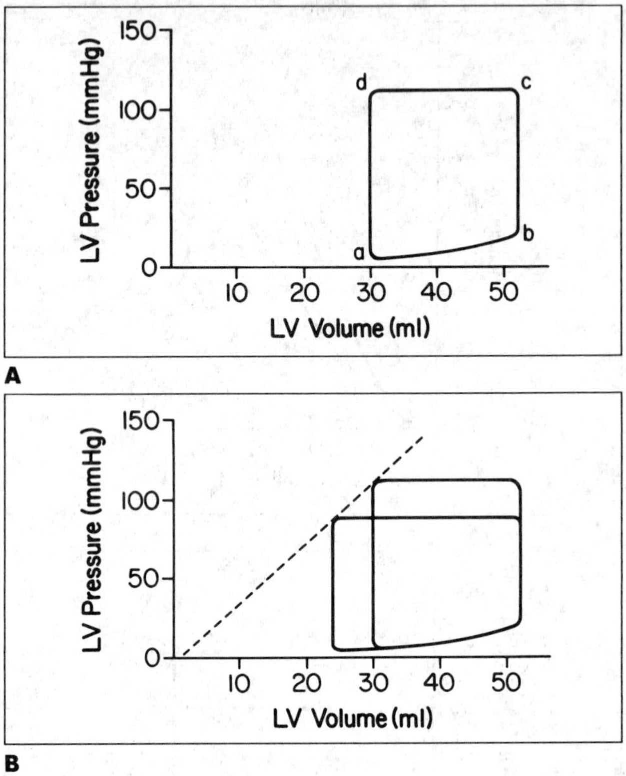

Fig. 1-7. A, One pressure-volume loop from the left ventricle (*LV*). **B,** Two pressure-volume loops, beginning from the same end-diastolic volume. As in Fig. 1-5, *B*, the shortening that occurs depends on the afterload against which the muscle must work.

Ventricular performance during systole

The simplest way to apply the concepts of myocardial mechanics just discussed to the intact heart is to consider the left ventricle's behavior during the cardiac cycle. A pressure-volume loop for a single cardiac cycle of the left ventricle is shown in Fig. 1-7, *A*. Ventricular filling (*a* to *b*) is followed by isovolumic systole (*b* to *c*), ejection (*c* to *d*), and isovolumic relaxation (*d* to *a*). In Fig. 1-7, *B*, two loops are shown in a manner similar to Fig. 1-5, *B*. It is evident that from any preload and for any contractile state, the ejection that occurs depends on the afterload; that is, when the afterload is higher, less ejection occurs.

The intact ventricle's performance, as with that of the isolated myocardium, depends on the determinants of preload, afterload, and contractility. Although these factors can be manipulated independently in experimental preparations, their interaction in patients makes assessment of ventricular performance more difficult. Although several indexes have been proposed to quantify myocardial contractility, none is without limitations. The maximum rate of rise of ventricular pressure (dP/dt_{max}) can be easily measured in a catheterization laboratory and is related to contractility. Unfortunately this parameter depends on preload and varies from patient to patient, to the extent that it does not provide a reliable way of comparing patients or for following a single patient over time. A second index, the velocity of circumferential fiber shortening (V_{cf}), can be determined from angiographic or echocardiographic studies of the ejecting heart and reflects the force-velocity relation discussed earlier. However, V_{cf} also depends on loading conditions and varies from patient to patient. Therefore its measurement also does not allow definitive identification of abnormal contractility or comparison of groups of patients. A third approach to evaluating left ventricular (LV) performance, which has received much attention in the recent past, is the end-systolic pressure-volume relation (Fig. 1-7), since the slope of this relation is thought to reflect contractility. This relation can be determined in patients by generating pressure-volume loops, using angiography or echocardiography to image the heart at three or more different afterloads. The technical difficulty of defining the relation, as well as the substantial range of values that occur in normal hearts, reduce the clinical utility of this index as a means of defining cardiac contractility.

Thus, even though each index provides insight into how the heart functions as a pump, none is ideal for quantifying the myocardium's contractile state. How to best describe systolic performance in patients remains a challenge. One simple measure of ventricular performance is the *ejection fraction* (EF), which represents the fraction of the ventricular volume present at end-diastole that is ejected during systole. This measurement can be made by contrast cineventriculography, two-dimensional (2D) echocardiography, or radioventriculography. The EF is influenced by afterload, as shown in Fig. 1-7, and any heart will fail if the afterload is raised high enough. This is illustrated by the clinical picture in hypertensive crisis, in which a patient with a normally functioning left ventricle may develop signs of heart failure. In this instance a mismatch occurs between the ventricle's functional capacity and the load that it confronts. This phenomenon has been termed *afterload mismatch.* When the arterial pressure is returned to the normal range, the ventricle's systolic performance, as reflected by the EF, is normal.

The EF's usefulness lies in the ease with which it can be quantified. When the LV preload is adequate and arterial pressure is in the normal range, the LVEF should be in the range of 50% to 65%. If the EF is reduced to 40% or less, the likelihood of LV dysfunction must be considered. This occurs both in patients with global cardiac dysfunction, such as primary cardiomyopathy, and in those with regional LV dysfunction resulting from atherosclerotic coronary artery disease. Moreover, numerous studies have shown that a reduced EF is associated with substantially increased morbidity and mortality in patients with cardiac disease, verifying that this is a clinically useful index of systolic ventricular performance.

Ventricular performance during diastole

During diastole, two distinct phenomena occur. The first is the process of *relaxation,* when the tension generated by the sarcomeres dissipates, and pressure in the ventricle falls to a level where filling can occur. The second is *passive filling,* by which the sarcomeres are stretched to their precontractile length, setting the stage for the next systole. The governing mechanisms for these processes are different, and each of them may be affected by disease processes, leading to diastolic cardiac dysfunction.

At the cellular level, cardiac relaxation likely results from removal of calcium ions from the myoplasm. This process, caused by reuptake of calcium by the sarcoplasmic reticulum, requires the hydrolysis of ATP by a membrane-bound enzyme present in this structure. Some evidence also indicates that calcium is transported out of the cell during this time by the sodium-calcium exchange mechanism. Since intraventricular volume does not change during isovolumic relaxation, the rate at which pressure falls during this period probably reflects the kinetics of the active reuptake of calcium in the cell. Numerous studies have shown that during isovolumic relaxation the decay of intraventricular pressure is exponential, allowing it to be quantified by a time constant of relaxation. This index of relaxation, usually termed *T* or *tau,* has undergone intense study. Although *T* is affected by several factors, including the heart rate and the afterload at which it is evaluated, experimental evidence suggests that in both cardiac ischemia and cardiac hypertrophy, myocardial relaxation occurs more slowly than it does under normal conditions. The degree to which this alteration in relaxation is manifested clinically remains unclear, but the data suggest that abnormalities in diastolic physiology contribute to the elevated end-diastolic pressure often seen in patients with these conditions.

Unlike relaxation, which is an active process in the heart, cardiac filling is primarily a passive process, depending on the diastolic pressure gradient between the atrium and the ventricle and on the ventricular chamber's elastic properties. Fig. 1-8 shows the LV diastolic pressure-volume relation, which is similar to the passive length-tension curves shown in Fig. 1-5, *A.* Two important observations can be made. First, when intraventricular volume is low, additional filling (ΔV) does not cause much increase in pressure (ΔP). This applies to clinical situations in which the arterial blood pressure is low because of hypovolemia, such as with hemorrhage or dehydration. In this setting, volume infusion improves systolic performance by the Starling mechanism without greatly raising LV end-diastolic pressure. By contrast, when intraventricular volume is high, additional filling (ΔV) causes a substantial increase in pressure (ΔP), and further recruitment of systolic performance by the Starling mechanism can only occur at the expense of an elevated LV end-diastolic pressure, which may result in pulmonary venous congestion.

The second important observation from Fig. 1-8 is that under certain conditions the entire diastolic pressure-

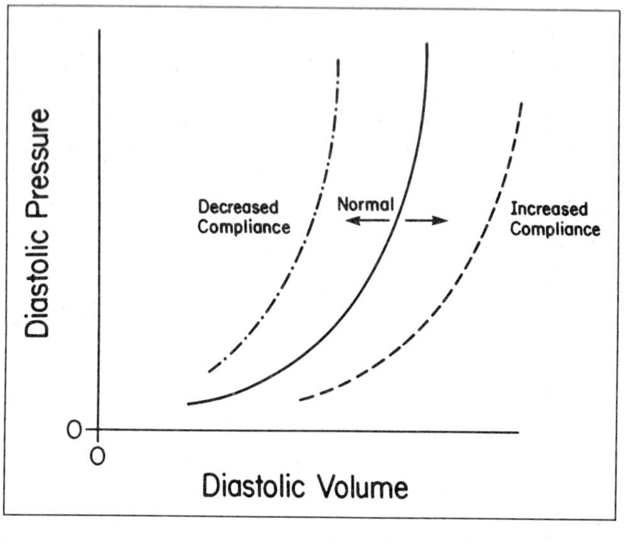

Fig. 1-8. The relation of pressure and volume during passive filling of the left ventricle. The relation is altered when compliance of the chamber is changed.

volume curve is shifted. When the curve is shifted upward (or leftward), more intraventricular pressure is required to distend the heart to any given volume, and the compliance of the chamber ($\Delta V/\Delta P$) is reduced. The most common cause of reduced compliance of the LV chamber is *pressure overload hypertrophy,* as occurs in many patients with chronic arterial hypertension. If the LV compliance is greatly reduced, adequate filling can only occur if the end-diastolic pressure is elevated. Thus, although systolic cardiac function is normal, patients may have pulmonary congestion as a result of diastolic ventricular dysfunction.

When the diastolic pressure-volume curve is shifted downward (or rightward), less intraventricular pressure is required to distend the heart to any given volume, and the chamber's compliance is increased. This may occur in conditions of chronic *volume overload hypertrophy*. In this case, LV end-diastolic pressure may be low, despite a large end-diastolic volume.

Concept of wall stress

In studies of isolated muscle segments the relation of mechanical performance to sarcomere dynamics is relatively straightforward, since the fibers are all oriented in a single direction. In the intact ventricle, where the orientation of myofibers varies greatly at different depths in the heart wall, the actual load on specific myofibers cannot be measured. The force present in the intact heart's wall can be estimated through the calculation of wall stress, which is a measure of force per cross-sectional area of the myocardium. Fig. 1-9 shows the factors that determine the wall stress. The most frequently used formula for calculating wall stress is based on the law of Laplace, which assumes that the heart is a thin-walled sphere. Wall stress is directly proportional to intraventricular pressure and to the chamber's radius, which reflects intraventricular volume, and is inversely related to the ventricular wall thickness.

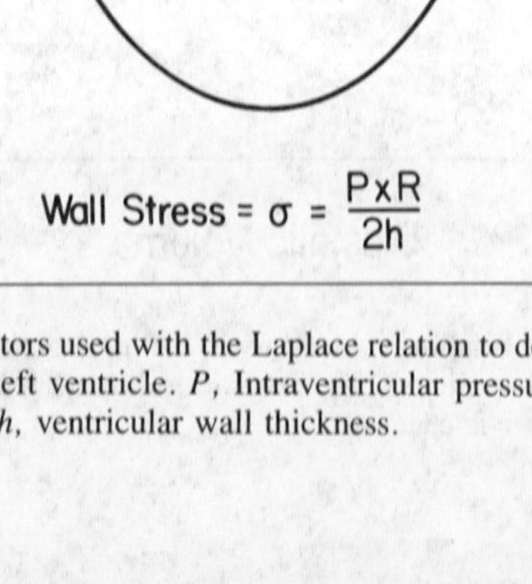

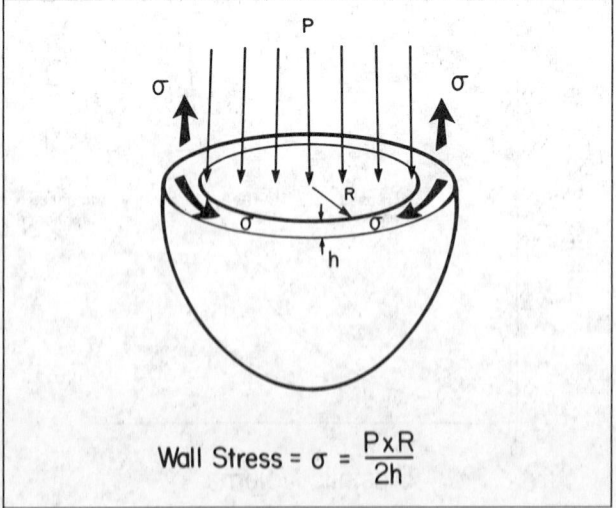

$$\text{Wall Stress} = \sigma = \frac{P \times R}{2h}$$

Fig. 1-9. Factors used with the Laplace relation to determine wall stress in the left ventricle. *P*, Intraventricular pressure; *R*, chamber's radius; *h*, ventricular wall thickness.

The left ventricle is not spheric throughout the cardiac cycle, and the wall thickness is not uniform at all points in the left ventricle. Thus the actual stress exerted across the chamber's wall can only be estimated. Although the absolute measurement of stress is most important in experimental studies on cardiac mechanics, an understanding of this concept has practical importance, since wall stress has been shown to be an important determinant of myocardial oxygen (O_2) demand. This is not surprising, since the amount of force exerted by a myofiber, an energy-dependent process, should be related to O_2 consumption. To understand properly the impact of pharmacologic therapy on the patient with myocardial ischemia, the effects on ventricular volume, pressure, and wall thickness, as factors determining wall stress and thus affecting myocardial O_2 consumption, must be considered. In the patient with congestive heart failure resulting from symptomatic coronary artery disease who is receiving diuretics, a reduction in intracardiac volume will reduce wall stress through a reduction of chamber radius, a reduction of intraventricular pressure, and an increase in wall thickness. Each of these effects leads to a reduction in myocardial O_2 demand, a beneficial effect in the patient with ischemic heart disease.

FACTORS CONTROLLING CARDIAC OUTPUT

Under normal conditions, cardiac output is about 5 L/min, which is sufficient for the metabolic needs of body tissues. If the body's metabolic needs increase, such as with exercise, cardiac output must rise. Various mechanisms are involved in the control of cardiac output, some of which influence the heart's pumping function and some of which influence the peripheral circulation. In Fig. 1-10 the interrelations of the various factors that control cardiac output are illustrated in a flow chart.

The relation of cardiac output to ventricular filling, Starling's law of the heart, is shown in Fig. 1-11 as a cardiac function curve. From this relation, for a specific contractile state, the key determinant of cardiac output clearly is the heart's end-diastolic volume, which results from venous return from the periphery. Thus, for cardiac output to increase, either the contractile state of the heart or the venous return to the heart must increase.

The box on p. 9 lists factors that play a role in altering these determinants of cardiac output. Cardiac filling is influenced by several determinants. Of primary importance is the amount of blood available for return to the heart by the venous system. Venous return is not only altered when a change occurs in total blood volume, but also when a change occurs in the amount of blood pooled in the capacitance vessels of the venous system. The simplest example of the latter effect occurs when a person who is standing up lies down. During the upright position, a substantial increase in the gradient to venous return results from gravity, and venous pooling occurs in the lower extremities. This gradient is removed when the person assumes the supine position. Thus, although the total intravascular volume is not changed, more blood is returned to the heart. This

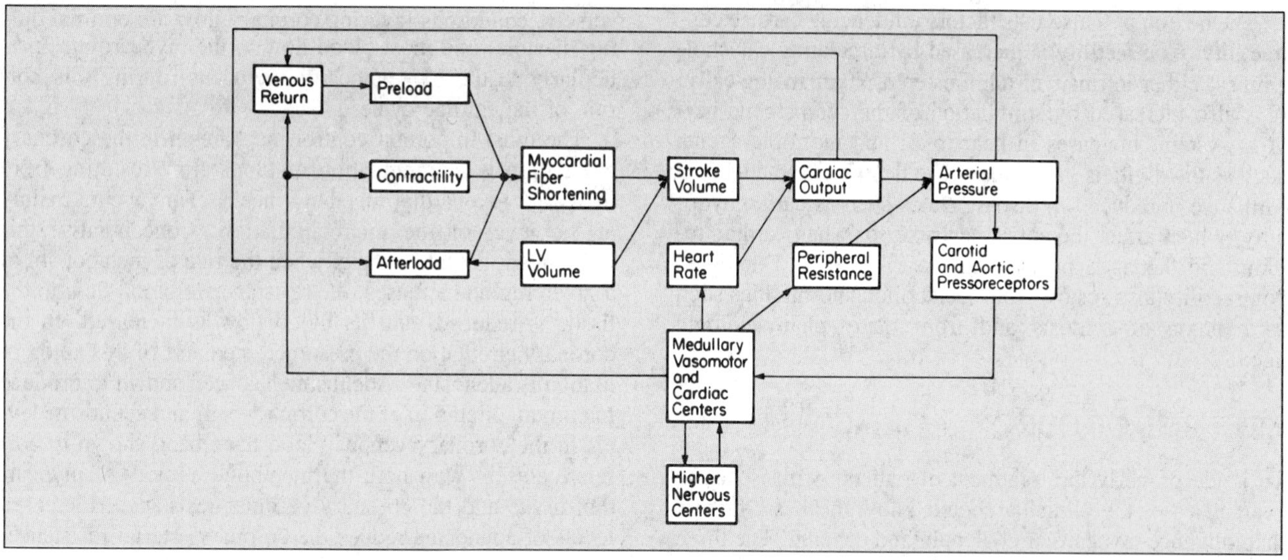

Fig. 1-10. Flow diagram of mechanisms governing the cardiovascular system. *LV,* Left ventricular.

method of increasing venous return is used when patients are placed in the Trendelenburg position. Similarly, sympathetically mediated increases in venous tone and increases in lower extremity muscular activity both tend to increase venous return to the heart. The relation of venous capacitance to cardiac filling is relevant in the management of patients receiving vasodilator therapy, which may directly reduce cardiac preload by this mechanism.

Various physical factors can affect venous return to the heart by limiting or augmenting cardiac filling. Increases in the pressure surrounding the heart, such as increased intrapericardial pressure caused by cardiac tamponade, will reduce the gradient for venous return. A similar influence occurs in patients on ventilators requiring positive end-expiratory pressure, in whom the pressure in the intrathoracic fossa surrounding the heart is increased. Another important physical factor in cardiac filling is a properly timed atrial contraction. As discussed previously, atrial systole contributes a substantial amount to end-diastolic filling of the ventricle. In patients with atrial fibrillation, cardiac filling is reduced, even when the other factors promoting venous return are unchanged.

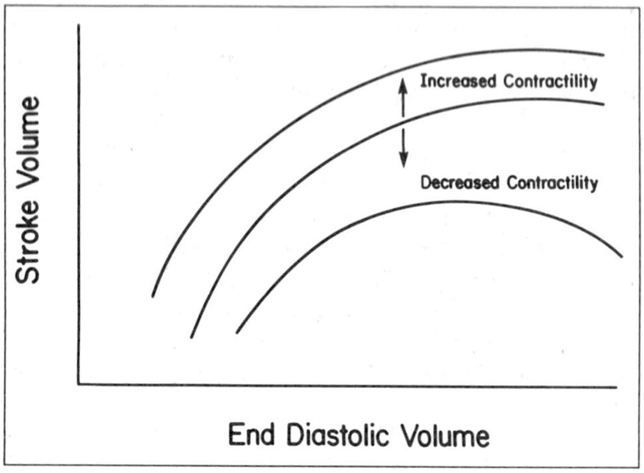

Fig. 1-11. Cardiac function curves showing the relation of stroke volume to end-diastolic volume. The curve is shifted upward by increased contractility and downward by decreased contractility.

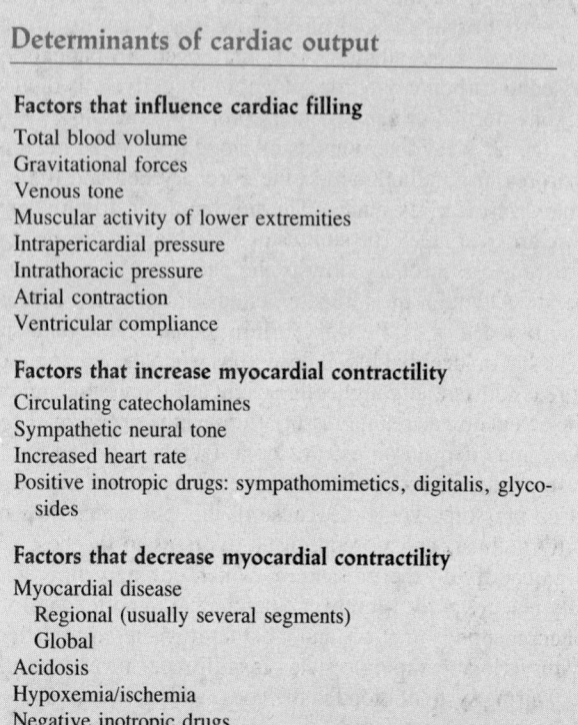

Determinants of cardiac output

Factors that influence cardiac filling

Total blood volume
Gravitational forces
Venous tone
Muscular activity of lower extremities
Intrapericardial pressure
Intrathoracic pressure
Atrial contraction
Ventricular compliance

Factors that increase myocardial contractility

Circulating catecholamines
Sympathetic neural tone
Increased heart rate
Positive inotropic drugs: sympathomimetics, digitalis, glycosides

Factors that decrease myocardial contractility

Myocardial disease
- Regional (usually several segments)
- Global

Acidosis
Hypoxemia/ischemia
Negative inotropic drugs

The box on p. 9 also lists factors influencing cardiac contractility. Contractility is increased by circulating catecholamines, either intrinsic or administered pharmacologically. It is also increased by stimulation of the sympathetic nervous system, increases in heart rate, and inotropic agents such as the digitalis glycosides. The heart's contractile performance is reduced in disease states such as cardiomyopathy, which affect the entire ventricle, or when cardiac regions are damaged by ischemic heart disease. Depressed contractility also results from metabolic abnormalities such as hypoxia or acidosis and from many pharmacologic agents.

CONTROL OF CORONARY CIRCULATION

To guide properly the treatment of patients with ischemic heart disease, the clinician should know the basic factors that influence myocardial O_2 supply and demand. The three key determinants of myocardial O_2 demand are the wall stress, which reflects the mechanical load on the myocyte; the heart rate; and the contractile state. The myocardium's O_2 demand varies directly with these factors. Because near maximum O_2 extraction from the blood occurs at all times in the coronary bed, increased myocardial O_2 needs are met by increased delivery of blood to the myocardium, or O_2 deficit will result.

The distinction between myocardial ischemia caused by inadequate blood flow through the tissue bed and hypoxemia caused by inadequate O_2 delivery *alone* should be made. Under conditions of ischemia not only is O_2 delivery decreased, but flow is insufficient to wash out metabolic by-products that accumulate in the tissue bed, leading to reduced pH and increased carbon dioxide (CO_2). In hypoxemia, on the other hand, the only abnormality is a decreased tissue O_2 and blood flow is adequate to prevent by-product accumulation. This may occur in patients exposed to carbon monoxide, in whom O_2 delivery is reduced despite normal or supranormal coronary blood flow.

The physical determinants of blood flow to the heart are the pressure gradient across the coronary bed and the coronary vascular resistance. The upstream, or driving, pressure arises at the aortic sinuses of Valsalva; the downstream pressure for coronary flow is the subject of some controversy. Although the ultimate venous drainage for myocardial blood flow is the right atrium, considerable data suggest that myocardial blood flow stops when the driving pressure is substantially higher than right atrial pressure and that the actual downstream pressure (termed the *pressure at zero flow*) may depend on extravascular factors that lead to closure of the microcirculation at pressures greater than right atrial pressure. The exact cause of this phenomenon is not fully defined, and no consensus exists as to the best way for quantifying the pressure at which coronary flow actually reaches zero. Moreover, the clinical importance of this phenomenon is unclear, and whether it is altered in patients with various pathologic states is still under investigation.

During systole, blood in the aortic root moves away from the coronary ostia, and the tension in the myocardium is high. As a result, little myocardial blood flow occurs. Conversely, conditions favoring coronary flow are optimal during diastole, and most blood flow to the myocardium, particularly to the LV endocardium, occurs during this portion of the cardiac cycle.

The most important control mechanism in the coronary circulation is autoregulation of blood flow resulting from increased myocardial metabolic needs. This occurs mainly at the level of the microcirculation. Conceptually, this mechanism is quite simple: when the rate of metabolism of a given region increases, the resistance to blood flow to the tissue is reduced, and its blood flow is increased. In the coronary circulation the presumed mediator of this autoregulation is adenosine. Adenosine has been shown to produce maximum dilatation of the coronary bed, and adenosine levels in the coronary venous blood have been shown to correlate closely with both the metabolic activity of myocardial tissue and the coronary vascular resistance. Increased levels of adenosine reduce the coronary arterial resistance, with a subsequent increase in local blood flow.

Under normal conditions the myocardial blood flow can increase by up to 400%, allowing normal O_2 and nutrient delivery during exercise or other conditions producing cardiovascular stress. The difference between resting coronary flow and the highest flow that can be achieved is the *coronary flow reserve,* which represents the maximum increase in flow that can occur before nutrient and O_2 delivery limit myocardial performance. When the coronary circulation is normal, the flow reserve is great enough that an individual's overall exercise capacity generally depends on the performance of the skeletal muscles; peripheral exhaustion precedes cardiac exhaustion, and cardiac function does not limit exercise performance. However, the situation is different when severe coronary artery stenoses are present. In this case the driving pressure for flow to the microcirculation is no longer the pressure measured in the aortic root but rather the pressure *distal* to the coronary artery occlusion. Thus significant lesions reduce the driving pressure for flow to the myocardium, and autoregulation must occur to maintain adequate flow under resting conditions. When such partial vasodilatation is present at rest, the coronary flow reserve is reduced. If such a patient exercises, myocardial O_2 demand may exceed supply, and regional ischemia, often with angina pectoris, may ensue.

NEURAL CONTROL OF CIRCULATION

Regulatory mechanisms mediated by the autonomic nervous system play a key role in the control of cardiovascular function. The integrated action of the sympathetic and parasympathetic nervous systems allows the heart to maintain adequate tissue perfusion under a wide range of conditions, both by direct cardiac effects and by effects on the peripheral circulation.

Relative to central cardiovascular control, the complex interactions of medullary pressor and depressor regions and how they affect arterial pressure, resting autonomic tone to the circulation, and cardiac reflexes have been the subject of intensive research. A few points merit specific consideration. First, central inhibitory and excitatory stimuli interact in ways that are at times antagonistic and at times synergistic to modulate the cardiovascular system's behavior. Under resting conditions, neural input to the circulation results from the balance of these factors. Second, the central regions that influence cardiovascular control are in the brainstem and are active even when higher cortical function is absent. As such, discrete loss of central cardiovascular control is very rare clinically. Although bilateral ablation of the nucleus tractus solitarius may lead to hypertension in an otherwise normal laboratory animal, a tumor or cerebrovascular accident (stroke) damaging these regions in a patient would be accompanied by major loss of higher function. Finally, some degree of cardiovascular control is exerted by the spinal cord. The observation that blood pressure not only gradually returns to control levels but that cardiovascular reflexes also can be elicited in patients with spinal cord transection underscores the spinal cord's role in integration and expression of central cardiovascular control.

Cardiac innervation

The heart is innervated by postsynaptic sympathetic and parasympathetic efferents, which have generally opposite effects, and cardiac autonomic tone depends on the balance between them. Cardiac sympathetic nerves arise from paravertebral ganglia and are distributed to the coronary vasculature, to the atrial and ventricular myocytes, and to the sinus and A-V nodes. Although the coronary vasculature likely is supplied by alpha-adrenergic nerves, the bulk of the sympathetic innervation to the heart is composed of beta-adrenergic fibers, and the postsynaptic receptors are of the $beta_1$ subtype. Cardiac sympathetic stimulation, mediated either by norepinephrine released from nerve terminals or by circulating epinephrine, leads to three major physiologic effects. The first is an increase in heart rate (positive chronotropic effect), resulting from innervation of the sinus node. The second is improved A-V conduction (positive dromotropic effect). The third is improved contractility (positive inotropic effect), resulting from direct myocardial innervation. Under situations of stress, or during exercise when sympathetic tone is enhanced, all these mechanisms are elicited. The importance of these mechanisms is also apparent in patients treated with beta-blocking drugs because the side-effect profile of these agents includes sinus bradycardia, impaired A-V nodal conduction, and depressed cardiac contractility.

Cardiac parasympathetic innervation is mediated by the vagus nerves. These nerves richly supply the sinus and A-V nodes, and they are also distributed to the atrial and ventricular myocytes, particularly those of the inferoposterior left ventricle. Cardiac parasympathetic stimulation, mediated by the neurotransmitter acetylcholine, leads to reduced chronotropic and dromotropic effects and to mildly negative inotropic effects. The bradycardia and hypertension seen more often with inferior than anterior myocardial infarction may reflect this differential distribution of parasympathetic innervation.

Cardiac reflexes

Cardiac reflexes occur as a result of specific receptors in the heart or vascular system. The best known cardiac reflex results from stimulation of baroreceptors located in the carotid sinuses and the aortic arch. These receptors are sensitive to arterial pressure, and as pressure is elevated, they fire with increased frequency. The afferent impulses from these baroreceptors travel to the brain, producing a dual effect: sympathetic tone to the peripheral vasculature is reduced, and vagal tone to the heart is increased. Both a reduction of arterial pressure and a slowing of heart rate result. If arterial pressure is reduced below normal levels, the opposite effect occurs: sympathetic tone and heart rate are both increased. Thus this reflex modulates arterial pressure, buffering acute changes in this variable. Clinically this reflex is used to slow the heart rate during carotid sinus massage (Chapter 9). The carotid baroreflex also is important in patients in whom the reflex is abnormally augmented. In these patients, torsion or compression on the carotid artery can lead to excessive baroreceptor activity and marked bradycardia with syncope.

A second type of reflex is mediated by chemical stimuli: hypoxia, reduced pH, and hypercapnea. Chemoreceptors sensitive to these stimuli are also located in the aortic arch and in the carotid bodies, which are near the carotid sinus baroreceptors. When arterial O_2 content is low, during acidosis, or when arterial CO_2 content is high, these receptors trigger an increase in heart rate and hyperventilation.

Another reflex mediated by chemical stimuli is the *Bezold-Jarisch phenomenon*. In experimental animals the administration of veratradine to the atria or into the coronary arteries leads to bradycardia and a reduction of arterial pressure. This cardiodepressor response, which is reversed by atropine, is thought to be the mechanism that underlies the bradycardia and the hypotension that sometimes occur during coronary arteriography in patients with normal coronary arteries.

Autonomic control of peripheral circulation

Several facts regarding autonomic control of the circulation should be emphasized. Little or no parasympathetic innervation to the peripheral vessels occurs. The influence of vagal tone and reflexes is mainly limited to direct effects on the heart. On the other hand, direct sympathetic innervation of almost the entire circulation occurs, with a distribution to both arterial and venous beds. Under normal conditions, resting sympathetic tone contributes to the maintenance of arterial and venous pressure. These efferents are important under stressful circumstances, when general sympathetic circulatory stimulation can occur. In this case (the fight-or-flight reaction), stimulation to the arterial circulation increases blood pressure, and sympathetic vasodilatation of the skeletal muscles increases flow to these tissues. Stimulation to the venous circulation increases venous return to the heart, leading to an increase in cardiac output, and stimulation of the heart elicits the inotropic, chronotropic, and dromotropic responses discussed earlier. This acute neural response brings the cardiovascular system to a state of readiness for maximum response to the stressful stimulus.

MICROCIRCULATORY CONTROL

The microvasculature comprises arterioles, capillaries, venules, and arteriovenous anastomoses, as shown in Fig. 1-12. Regulation of peripheral vascular resistance is provided by the microcirculation, predominantly at the level of the precapillary sphincter. Using dynamic regulatory mechanisms, the microcirculation determines the level and distribution of blood flow and thereby controls the delivery of nutritive substances to the various tissue beds.

Autoregulation

This mechanism of microcirculatory control refers to the maintenance of steady-state blood flow in response to changes in perfusion pressure, as well as the redistribution of blood flow in response to the metabolic needs of the local tissue bed. The primary mechanism underlying autoregulation concerns the production of tissue metabolic factors. Vasodilator metabolites accumulate in tissue regions that are hypoperfused or have increased metabolic rates. A principal metabolite is adenosine, a degradation product of adenine nucleotide metabolism, produced when ATP utilization exceeds the resynthesis of high-energy phosphate compounds. Accumulation of adenosine leads to vasodilatation, presumably at the level of the precapillary sphincter (Fig. 1-12), decreasing vascular resistance and increasing local blood flow. In addition to adenosine, other metabolic factors have been implicated as mediators of autoregulation, including prostaglandins and kinins. Tissue hypoxia also produces direct vasodilatation of precapillary sphincters in many vascular beds. Other mechanisms involved in autoregulation include myogenic factors (stretch-induced contraction of vascular smooth muscle) and endothelial regulation of vascular tone.

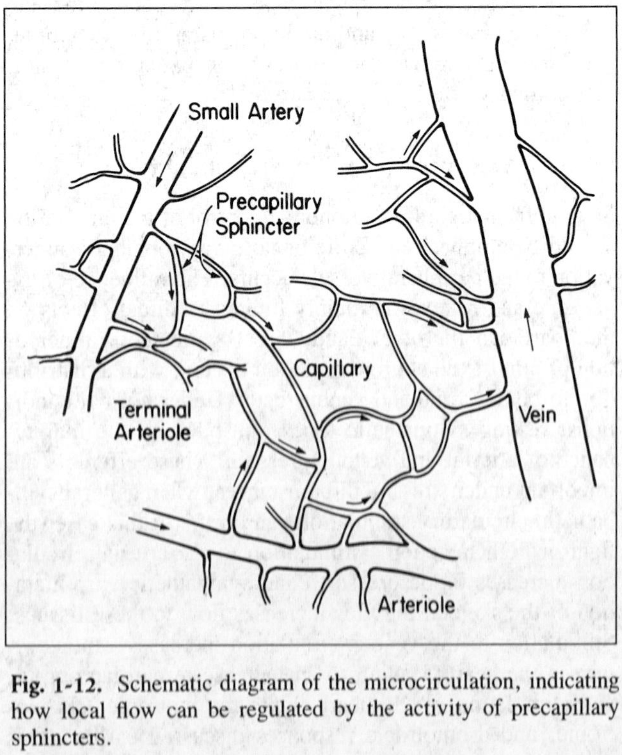

Fig. 1-12. Schematic diagram of the microcirculation, indicating how local flow can be regulated by the activity of precapillary sphincters.

Functions of vascular endothelium

The endothelium lines the lumen of the entire vascular tree as a cellular monolayer. Endothelial cells perform several specialized and complex functions and are important mediators of vascular tone. The endothelial layer forms a continuous nonthrombogenic surface between blood and the vessel wall and serves as a selective permeability barrier controlling the transport of ions, water, and macromolecules in both directions (away from and into the lumen) by the process of endocytosis. The endothelium is responsible for the uptake of certain circulating hormones (e.g., norepinephrine) and for certain metabolic functions (e.g., conversion of angiotensin I to angiotensin II). The endothelium also produces a variety of vasoactive substances that directly or indirectly modulate vascular tone. Additionally, these cells produce anticoagulant and antiplatelet substances such as prostacyclin (PGI_2), fibrinolytic substances such as plasminogen activator, procoagulants such as von Willebrand factor, and connective tissue macromolecules.

Endothelium-derived relaxing factor (EDRF) and PGI_2 are two principal vasorelaxing and platelet-inhibiting agents produced by the endothelium (Fig. 1-13). PGI_2 is a metabolite of arachidonic acid and is produced in response to a variety of stimuli, including hemodynamic stress, tissue hypoxia, and ATP. PGI_2 serves to relax vascular smooth muscle (VSM) and inhibit platelet aggregation by increas-

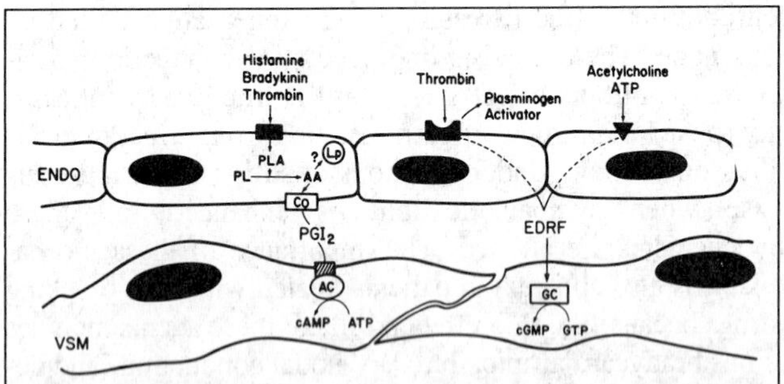

Fig. 1-13. Endothelium-dependent mechanisms of vasodilatation. Stimulation of endothelial cell *(ENDO)* surface receptors by various vasoactive substances results in activation of "second messenger" systems in the vascular smooth muscle *(VSM)* in the blood vessel wall. These systems may be activated by various eicosanoids (e.g., prostacyclin, or PGI_2) or endothelium-derived relaxing factor *(EDRF)*. *AA*, Arachidonic acid; *AC*, adenylate cyclase; *ATP*, adenosine triphosphate; *cAMP*, adenosine 3′,5′-cyclic monophosphate; *CO*, cyclo-oxygenase; *GC*, guanylate cyclase; *GTP*, guanosine triphosphate; *cGMP*, guanosine 3′,5′-cyclic monophosphate; *Lp*, lipoxygenase; *PL*, phospholipid; *PLA*, phospholipase.

ing intracellular levels of the second messenger, cyclic adenosine monophosphate (cAMP). EDRF is a thiolated form of nitric oxide (NO) and also relaxes VSM and inhibits platelet aggregation. EDRF is secreted in response to a variety of substances acting through specific cell surface receptors. These include acetylcholine, thrombin, histamine, bradykinin, adenosine nucleotides, and catecholamines (acting through $alpha_2$ adrenoreceptors). EDRF is also generated in response to serotonin and thromboxane A_2, expressed by aggregating platelets. Thus these substances require an intact endothelium to exert their vasorelaxant effects. In this manner the endothelium serves to produce and/or enhance the actions of vasodilators such as acetylcholine, histamine, and adenosine nucleotides, as well as oppose the vasoconstrictor effects of serotonin, thromboxane, and catecholamines. Acting in concert, EDRF, PGI_2, and plasminogen activator are important counterregulators of thrombotic and vasoconstrictor stimuli. In the presence of dysfunctional endothelium (e.g., atherosclerosis), this capacity is lost (Chapter 171).

EDRF acts by increasing intracellular concentrations of a different second messenger, cyclic guanosine monophosphate (cGMP). EDRF-induced increases in cGMP lead to the inhibition of calcium ion (Ca^{2+}) release from VSM sarcoplasmic reticulum (SR), resulting in relaxation. Pharmacologic agents such as nitroglycerin and nitroprusside also act in this manner by generating NO. Unlike the endogenous vasodilator substances previously listed, however, these drugs do not require an intact endothelium to produce vasorelaxation (see box below). Thus nitroglycerin produces vasodilatation even in the presence of dysfunctional endothelium and is of benefit to patients with coronary artery disease (Chapter 13).

Vascular smooth muscle

The resting potential of VSM is smaller than that of cardiac muscle, approximately −40 to −55 mV. VSM cell membranes lack fast sodium channels and are less permeable to potassium. In response to depolarization by stretch, neurotransmitters, or electrical stimulation, voltage-dependent Ca^{2+} channels carry an inward Ca^{2+} current. This can then lead to Ca^{2+}-induced Ca^{2+} release similar to that seen in cardiac muscle, producing excitation-contraction coupling.

Dependence of vasoactive substances on intact endothelium

Endothelium dependent	Endothelium independent
Acetylcholine	Nitrates
Bradykinin	Sodium nitroprusside
Thrombin	Ca^{2+} blockers
Histamine	Beta-adrenergic blockers
Adenine nucleotides	Atrial natriuretic factor
	Minoxidil

Contraction of VSM occurs through the interaction of actin and myosin. Phosphorylation of one of the myosin light chains (LC_{20}) by Ca^{2+}, calmodulin, and the enzyme myosin light chain kinase (MLCK) initiates cross-bridge cycling and VSM contraction. Unlike cardiac muscle, VSM can maintain contraction for long periods without fatigue, a necessity for the maintenance of vascular tone. This may be related to the so-called latch state of VSM, in which tension is maintained despite significantly lower intracellular Ca^{2+} and significantly slower cross-bridge cycling.

VSM contraction can also be induced by various hormones and drugs without membrane depolarization (Fig. 1-14). Such pharmacologic and hormonal signal transduction is achieved by membrane-bound G (guanosine nucleotide–binding) proteins and the production of intracellular second messengers from the phosphoinositide (phosphatidylinositol) pathway. In response to such compounds as $alpha_2$-adrenoreceptor agonists, receptor-coupled G proteins stimulate phospholipase C, which hydrolyzes phosphatidylinositol diphosphate to inositol-1,4,5-triphosphate (IP_3) and diacylglycerol (DAG). IP_3 subsequently stimulates SR Ca^{2+} release, increasing intracellular Ca^{2+} and stimulating contraction. DAG produces the activation and membrane translocation of protein kinase C (PK_C). Proposed mechanisms by which PK_C may stimulate VSM contraction include increased sodium-hydrogen and consequent sodium-calcium exchange, increased open time of sarcolemmal slow Ca^{2+} channels, and sensitization of the contractile apparatus to Ca^{2+}. These events are summarized in Fig. 1-14. This mode of VSM contraction is important in hormonally mediated increased vascular tone, such as that produced by catecholamines or angiotensin II.

EXERCISE PHYSIOLOGY

During isotonic exercise the heart must provide a greater output to support the needs of the working muscles. Cardiovascular adaptation in exercise involves the peripheral circulation, the heart, and the sympathetic nervous system, allowing the cardiac output to rise to levels four to five times that present at rest. This is useful clinically because assessment of cardiovascular performance during exercise tolerance testing is a useful tool for diagnosis of cardiac disease, assessment of functional capacity, and assessment of the effectiveness of therapy in patients with cardiac disease.

Dynamic exercise leads to microvascular autoregulation of working muscles, which promotes blood flow to these beds. This vasodilatation facilitates the increased cardiac output while not causing excessive afterload to the left ventricle. A second peripheral vascular response to exercise is venoconstriction, which directly leads to an increased gradient for venous return to the heart. In addition to the impact of venoconstriction, venous return is augmented by increased lower extremity muscle activity and by contraction of abdominal muscles, which increases abdominal venous return.

During exercise a complex interplay occurs between the factors that control cardiac performance. Despite substan-

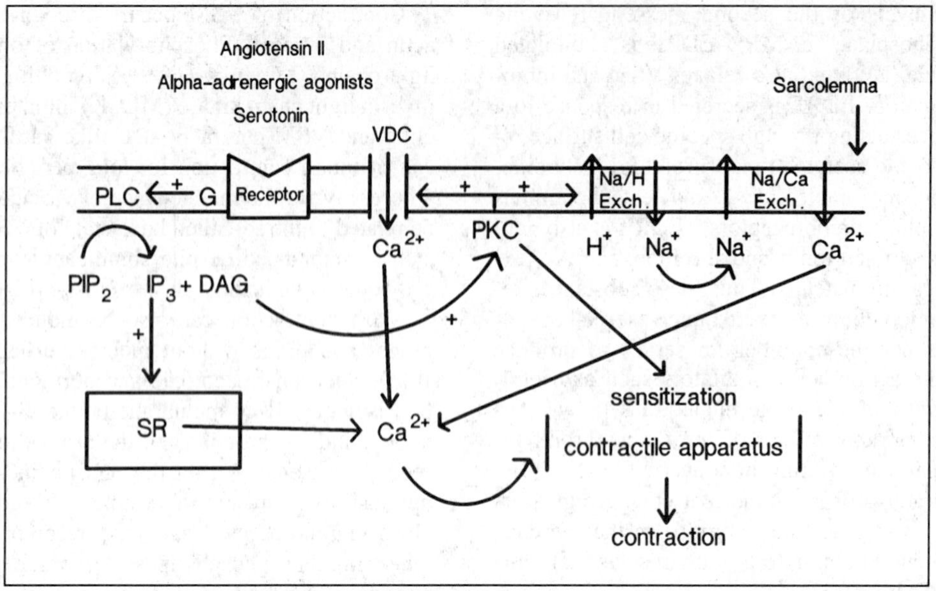

Fig. 1-14. Schematic diagram of cellular events leading to contraction in vascular smooth muscle as a result of hormonal stimulation. Receptor-coupled, membrane-bound G proteins *(G)* stimulate phospholipase C *(PLC)*, which in turn hydrolyzes phosphatidylinositol diphosphate *(PIP_2)* to form inositol-1,4,5-triphosphate *(IP_3)* and diacylglycerol *(DAG)*. These second messengers activate a variety of cellular processes (see text), ultimately leading to increased intracellular calcium, contractile apparatus sensitization, and contraction. *VDC*, Voltage-dependent Ca^{2+} channel; *PKC*, protein kinase C.

tial increases in cardiac output, arterial blood pressure (afterload) is only moderately elevated. Left ventricular volume (preload) is not greatly altered when the level of exertion is moderate but may increase during heavy exertion. Contractility, on the other hand, is substantially increased during dynamic exercise, as a function of both the sympathetic stimulation and the concordant increase in heart rate. Thus the increase in cardiac output is accompanied by an increase in stroke volume, primarily because of a decrease in end-systolic LV chamber size.

The sympathetic nervous system plays an important role during exercise. Sympathetic stimulation leads to systemic venoconstriction, which improves venous return, and also leads to vasoconstriction of vascular beds not participating in exercise. This vasoconstriction serves to limit flow to these beds to the amount needed for their baseline function; if vasoconstriction did not occur, flow to these beds would increase as a result of the increase in cardiac output. Sympathetic stimulation and parasympathetic withdrawal also lead to increases in heart rate and contractility that underlie the increase in cardiac output.

The cardiovascular changes just discussed occur during isotonic exercise. Isometric exercise, such as the hand-grip maneuver, leads to somewhat different changes. In this circumstance the arterial pressure (afterload) is substantially elevated, such that the ejection fraction is not increased to the extent that it is in dynamic exercise. Also, since isometric exercise generally involves a smaller increase in overall metabolic demand than isotonic exercise, the changes in cardiac output and heart rate are less pronounced.

REFERENCES

Abboud FM and Thames MD: Interaction of cardiovascular reflexes in circulatory control. In Berne R and Sperelakis N, editors: Handbook of physiology: the cardiovascular system, vol 3. Bethesda, Md, 1983, American Physiological Society.

Braunwald E and Sobel BE: Coronary blood flow and myocardial ischemia. In Braunwald E, editor: Heart disease: a textbook of cardiovascular medicine, ed 4. Philadelphia, 1992, Saunders.

Braunwald E, Ross J Jr, and Sonnenblick EH, editors: Mechanisms of contraction of the normal and failing heart. Boston, 1976, Little, Brown.

Brown AM: Cardiac reflexes. In Berne R and Sperelakis N, editors: Handbook of physiology, vol 1. Bethesda, Md, 1983, American Physiological Society.

Feigl EO: Coronary physiology. Physiol Rev 63:1, 1983.

Guyton AC: The circulation. In Guyton AC, editor: Textbook of medical physiology, ed 7. Philadelphia, 1986, Saunders.

Hathaway DR et al: Vascular smooth muscle: a review of the molecular basis of contractility. Circulation 83:382, 1991.

Jaffe EA, editor: Biology of endothelial cells. Boston, 1984, Nijhoff.

Nathan RD, editor: Cardiac muscle: the regulation of excitation and contraction. New York, 1986, Academic.

Peach MJ, Singer HA, and Loeb AL: Mechanisms of endothelium dependent vascular smooth muscle relaxation. Biochem Pharmacol 34:1867, 1985.

Randall W, editor: Nervous control of cardiovascular function. New York, 1984, Oxford University.

Sperelakis N, editor: Physiology and pathophysiology of the heart. Boston, 1984, Nijhoff.

CHAPTER

2 Molecular Biology of Cardiovascular System

Roger D. Bies
Robert Roberts

The study of the mechanisms controlling cardiovascular function has recently undergone a dramatic evolution from the traditional physiologic and anatomic paradigms that have dominated the field for many years to an intense interest in the cascade of molecular interactions responsible for cardiac and vascular development, growth, hypertrophy, adaptation to physiologic stress, cholesterol metabolism, thrombosis, and hormonal and autonomic effects in the myocardium. Molecular biology offers a unique technology that allows one to study the molecular diversity within the heart. Rare molecules difficult to detect at the protein level because of their low concentrations can now be analyzed. The specific gene product as well as the regulatory mechanisms that control when a protein is expressed and in what cell or tissue to perform a programmed biologic function can now be explored. This can be accomplished either in isolated cells or in the intact organism using recombinant deoxyribonucleic acid (DNA) technology, such as in a transgenic animal. Unique molecular control and expression of genes to generate specific proteins are important in the development of the myocardium, the valvular apparatus, the conduction system, and the vascular system. Recombinant DNA technology promises to provide not only an understanding of the basic mechanisms of cardiovascular science but also a therapeutic benefit. This chapter is an introduction to basic molecular biology, common molecular laboratory technology, and the recent advances made in molecular cardiology and cardiovascular genetics.

THE DNA CODE

The human chromosome, the largest molecule in the human body, comprises a long double-stranded helical molecule of DNA associated with different nuclear proteins. Each strand consists of a chain of deoxyribose sugars missing a hydroxyl group on the second carbon atom of the sugar ring. The deoxyribose sugar chain is linked by phosphodiester bonds between the fifth (5′) carbon atom on one sugar to the third (3′) carbon in the ring on the preceding sugar molecule. The first carbon of the sugar ring is linked to one of the four nucleotide bases found in all DNA molecules. Thus, by convention, DNA is arranged in a 5′ to 3′ direction through its phosphodiester linkages. *Genes* are discrete regions of DNA arranged sequentially along the molecule. Each gene contains a specific DNA code that directs the synthesis of a unique messenger ribonucleic acid (mRNA), a mirror image of the code contained on the DNA. The mRNA is processed and transported from the nucleus to the cellular cytoplasm. In the cytoplasm the genetic code is "read" by a large molecule called a *ribosome*. It translates the code into amino acid sequence and synthesizes a unique protein from the mRNA to perform a specific cell function. Some genes, the so-called housekeeping genes, are turned on in all cells and provide the common proteins for cell structure, cellular organelles, and metabolic enzymes that perform basic cell function. In the heart and vascular system, some genes are specifically turned on or off to give a group of cells their tissue-specific characteristic to perform the unique function typical of that organ system.

The specificity of the DNA code is spelled out by a simple four-letter code designated by the nucleotide bases. These letters A, C, G, and T refer to adenine, cytosine, guanine, and thymine, respectively. The variation in the linear sequence of these four letters contains the specificity of the DNA code and is a sequence unique for each specific gene. The two DNA strands are held together by hydrogen bonds between exclusive nucleotide base pairs such that each strand has a complementary strand that perfectly matches its mate (Fig. 2-1). Adenine only binds to thymine with two hydrogen bonds (A=T), and guanine only binds to cytosine with three hydrogen bonds (G≡C). The uniqueness of any particular stretch of nucleotide base sequence and the highly specific complementary nature of hy-

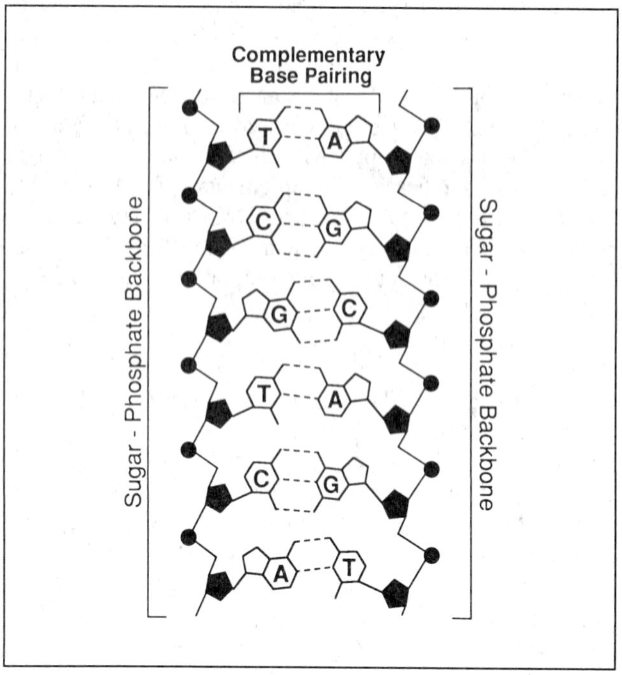

Fig. 2-1. Specificity of deoxyribonucleic acid (DNA) base pairing. The two strands of DNA are bound together by hydrogen bonds between the nucleotide bases on each strand. The bonds are formed by strict pairing between two complementary bases, A—T or C—G, such that each strand reflects the exact sequence of the opposite strand. *A*, Adenine, T, thymine; G, guanine; C, cytosine. The sugar *(dark pentamer)* and phosphate *(dark circle)* linkages form the backbone of the DNA strand. (From Roberts R et al: A primer of molecular biology. New York, 1992, Elsevier.)

drogen bond base pairing between A and T or G and C account for the specificity of the DNA code and serve as a basis for the sensitive techniques of detection currently used in molecular biology.

Although chromosomal DNA is only found within the cell's nucleus, a small amount of nonchromosomal DNA is found within mitochondria and serves as a template to encode for a few enzymes used in mitochondrial oxidative metabolism. mRNA is also present initially in the nucleus, where it is synthesized as a mirror image from the DNA template of a particular active gene. The mRNA found in a particular cell represents the activity of only those specific genes required for that particular cell's function. mRNA is a single-stranded molecule very similar to DNA in that it is composed of a long chain of ribose sugars, each linked to a nucleotide base. The mRNA code is identical to the DNA code from which is made, except that the nucleotide base, thymine, is not found in RNA and is replaced by the nucleotide base, uracil (U); as with thymine, uracil only associates with adenine. mRNA is a processed form of nuclear RNA that is transported to the cell's cytoplasm, where the unique coding sequence is translated into a protein. A group of three nucleotide bases is called a *codon,* and a unique combination of the A, U, G, and C bases encodes for each of the 20 common amino acids found in protein molecules.

The amino acid content and sequence for a particular protein are encoded from a unique mRNA molecule, which is synthesized from a chromosomal gene. Therefore the isolation and identification of the sequence of an individual mRNA molecule reveal much information. One drawback to the study of mRNA is that it is an easily degraded, single-stranded molecule. One "trick" used in molecular biology to produce a stable copy of the information contained in mRNA is to synthesize a complementary DNA molecule (cDNA) from the RNA template. cDNA is a stable copy of the mRNA that can then be manipulated for cloning, sequencing, or producing recombinant proteins in vivo.

GENE REGULATION

Normal and abnormal molecular responses to biologic or pharmacologic stress include changes in contractile protein isoforms in cardiac hypertrophy and failure, activation of endogenous injury and repair mechanisms in myocardial necrosis, changes in sodium channel properties during prolonged therapy with antiarrhythmic drugs, or regulation of cardiac beta-receptor density with cardiac beta-blocker therapy. Regulation of these processes occurs at multiple levels, from the gene in the cardiac cell to modification or phosphorylation of the resultant protein.

Gene transcription is the process of activation of a particular gene and the synthesis of that gene's specific RNA message. The regulation and selectivity of gene expression by a particular cell is the basis for cell differentiation and is what makes cardiac muscle different from skeletal muscle or smooth muscle. Before transcription can occur, the DNA at the site of the gene of interest must unravel and expose its sequence to an enzyme that can synthesize an RNA copy of the gene. DNA is normally compacted around a class of well-characterized proteins called *histones,* which may act to regulate the availability of a particular segment of DNA for gene activity. Histones bind with the DNA, and changes in histone DNA binding may allow a confirmational configuration in the DNA helix such that RNA polymerase can bind and begin synthesis of an RNA molecule. At the start site of a particular gene, the presence or absence of methyl (CH_3) groups in the dinucleotide sequence, —C—G—, has also been shown to be an important factor as to whether or not the gene is active in a particular cell. Gene activation involves the binding of RNA polymerase to a specific segment of the gene called the *promoter.* Once this binding occurs, RNA polymerase moves down the DNA molecule, reading and synthesizing an RNA copy of the gene until the end of the gene is reached and the RNA polymerase falls off. Several complex factors regulate the rate and frequency of RNA polymerase binding. Other unique elements at the start site of a gene include *enhancer* sequences, which interact with the promoter and regulate RNA polymerase binding, whereas other elements inhibit transcription and are referred to as *silencers* (Fig. 2-2).

Transcription factors are an identified heterogeneous group of proteins that bind to promoter, enhancer, and silencer sequences and further modulate RNA polymerase binding. They are nuclear proteins that can regulate the tissue-specific and physiologic activation of certain genes.

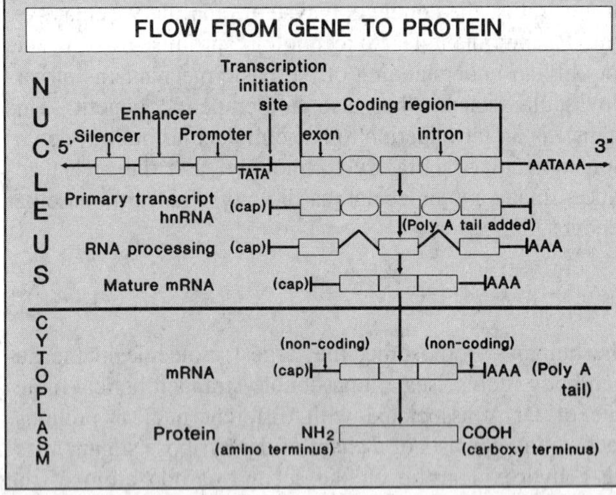

Fig. 2-2. Regulation of gene activation. Schematic diagram of the components of gene structure that contribute to gene activation and protein synthesis. Ribonucleic acid (RNA) polymerase binds to a site at the beginning of a gene (promoter region), which often contains a TATA box. Other gene elements (enhancers) may regulate this process. A heteronuclear RNA copy of the gene (hnRNA) is produced, which contains protein-coding (exons) and noncoding (introns) sequences. The noncoding introns are spliced out, and the RNA is "capped" at the 5′ end and polyadenylated at the 3′ end (Poly A tail) to form a mature messenger RNA (mRNA). The mRNA is used to synthesize the protein encoded for by this gene in the cell cytoplasm. (From Roberts R et al: A primer of molecular biology. New York, 1992, Elsevier.)

One familiar group of transcription factors are the glucocorticoid and thyroid receptor proteins. These proteins represent a distinct class of specific DNA binding proteins that contain what is termed *zinc finger* motif, where a finger-like loop is stabilized at the base by a single zinc ion to form a common DNA binding structure. Thyroid hormone, which binds to its cell surface receptor on cardiac myocytes, is transported as a receptor complex to the nucleus, where it is shown to be a prominent regulator of myosin heavy chain (MHC) gene expression. *Oncogene proteins* form a second category of transcription factors that regulate cardiac gene expression. Two well-studied oncogene proteins in the heart include c-*jun* and c-*fos*. These oncogene proteins generally form dimers held together by the interaction of four or five leucine residues, spaced seven residues apart in the sequence of each protein. These leucine residues can interdigitate, forming a zipperlike dimer and resulting in the term *leucine zipper* motif, which is used to describe this class of transcription factor proteins. The promoter region of some genes involved in cardiac hypertrophy contain a conserved DNA sequence (e.g., the AP1 site) that binds leucine zipper–type proteins. Pressure and volume overload of cardiac tissue have been shown to induce the expression of oncogene proteins, which may then regulate the genes involved in compensatory hypertrophy or structural remodeling of the ventricular wall.

Some transcription factors are able to activate the genes that determine the tissue characteristics of a specific cell. For example, a transcription factor protein called myo-D is capable of turning on the gene programs that create a normal skeletal muscle cell. This protein's influence is so strong that if the myo-D protein is introduced into a nonmuscle cell such as a fibroblast, it can transform that cell into a skeletal muscle by imposing its regulatory properties. Myo-D is a nuclear protein in the class of molecules called *helix-loop-helix* proteins, which describe a common structural conformation for this class of transcription factor proteins.

The next step in the regulation of gene expression is the process of *posttranscriptional regulation,* the cell's ability to modify or process the RNA transcript once it has been produced. One important mechanism of posttranscriptional regulation is the process of alternative mRNA splicing. This occurs in the nucleus before export of the mature RNA into the cytoplasm. Alternative splicing is a mechanism whereby a single RNA code from a single gene can be "edited" by the cell by splicing out or inserting some of the coding sequences, which ultimately results in a change in a portion of the protein's peptide sequence produced by that gene. In this way, multiple *isoforms* of a protein can be produced from a single gene. It has been demonstrated that various cardiac proteins, including the contractile elements, troponin T and tropomyosin, and dystrophin, a cytoskeletal protein in the heart, are expressed as tissue-specific and developmentally specific isoforms that may confer variations in molecular function tailored for the cell's specific needs.

Further regulatory steps that modulate the ultimate quantity and activity of a particular protein product from an activated gene occur in the cell cytoplasm. For example, the quantity of protein produced can be regulated at the level of the ribosome. Modifications of a protein's activity can occur after translation and include proteolysis, which can cleave off a peptide fragment to form an active molecule, glycosylation, phosphorylation, the formation of sulfhydryl bonds, or the coupling of fatty acids, which may affect the protein's destination within the cell. All these steps are potential targets for pharmacologic or genetic therapies.

ISOLATION AND DIGESTION OF DNA

Molecular techniques using DNA have proved useful in the development of diagnostic tools to analyze cardiovascular diseases and have provided a unique approach to structure/function analysis of molecular interactions in the heart. DNA can be isolated from any human tissue, including blood. The white cells provide an easily accessible source of DNA and can be extracted manually or with an automatic DNA extraction device. About 200 μg of DNA can be obtained from 10 to 20 ml of blood, which can be stored almost indefinitely at subzero temperatures. The lymphocytes can be transformed with Epstein-Barr virus to propagate indefinitely in cell culture as immortal cell lines to provide a renewable source of DNA. In performing molecular genetic studies, researchers routinely use lymphocytes, since a renewable source of DNA precludes the necessity of obtaining further blood from the family.

DNA is present in extremely large molecules because each chromosome is essentially a single, long DNA molecule. The smallest chromosome (chromosome 21) has about 50 million base pairs (bp), whereas the largest chromosome (chromosome 1) has more than 250 million bp. The techniques for identification and analysis of DNA became feasible and readily accessible with the discovery of restriction endonuclease enzymes found in bacteria. These particular enzymes made it possible to cut DNA into smaller fragments of specific sizes, a process usually referred to as digestion. They have specific recognition sites that vary from 2 to 8 bp in length. These enzymes only cut at these specific recognition sites, and thus the number of fragments generated for a particular DNA molecule remain consistent with the number of recognition sites and provide predictable patterns after separation by electrophoresis.

SEPARATION AND IDENTIFICATION OF DNA BY ELECTROPHORESIS

Separation of the DNA fragments after digestion is simplified by exploiting the observation that DNA is negatively charged. The phosphate groups have a net negative charge; thus the universally employed technique for separation of DNA fragments is electrophoresis, in which the fragments migrate in the gel in proportion to their length. The longer fragments migrate slower relative to the shorter fragments and give rise to a particular pattern of size-separated DNA. The electrophoresis is usually performed using either agarose or polyacrylamide gel, after which the fragments are stained with ethidium bromide and visualized in ultraviolet light as "bands" on the gel. Electrophoresis is used universally and routinely in the separation and detection of DNA fragments. The use of ethidium bromide staining provides for visualization of all DNA fragments but does not always give the desired resolution. However, resolution is improved by the use of a radiolabeled probe, which specifically hybridizes only with the fragment of interest. After hybridization the gel is exposed to x-ray film, and only the fragments of interest emit radioactivity and are visualized on the autoradiograph. A further modification of this technique is the transferral of the DNA fragments by diffusion from the gel to a nylon filter developed by E.M. Southern and discussed in the next section.

The size of the fragments of double-stranded DNA is indicated by their length in base pairs (nucleotides). For example, a 200 bp fragment is a piece of double-stranded DNA, with each complementary strand being 200 nucleotide bases in length. A 1000 bp fragment is 1 kilobase (kb) in length, and a 1 million bp fragment is 1 megabase (Mb) in length. Many DNA endonucleases are now commercially available, each of which is specific for a particular DNA sequence. Each enzyme has only one recognition site, which may be a 4, 5, 6, or 8 bp sequence and will only cut a section of DNA that contains that particular sequence.

SOUTHERN, NORTHERN, AND WESTERN BLOTTING

The analysis of a few hundred bp of DNA in the region of interest may be difficult when the DNA from all the human chromosomes (which amounts to 3 billion nucleotide bp) are cut and separated on the same gel. This dilemma is resolved by using a DNA probe tagged with an easily recognizable marker such as a radionuclide. The technique has been further modified, with the DNA fragments transferred by osmotic diffusion from the gel to a solid support consisting of either nitrocellulose or nylon.

The method developed by E.M. Southern involves digestion of DNA and separation by electrophoresis, as described previously. Smaller fragments of DNA move more rapidly in the gel, whereas larger fragments move more slowly, each fragment moving a characteristic distance proportional to its size. The DNA is then transferred to a "hard copy" nitrocellulose or nylon membrane. The pattern of DNA separated and transferred onto the membrane is identical to the pattern of DNA separated on the agarose gel. This membrane can then be dried and used to detect DNA fragments of interest. To do this, a DNA probe is used. A probe is a fragment of DNA that contains a nucleotide sequence specific for the gene or chromosomal region near the region of interest. The detection method requires that the probe be labeled with some identifiable tag, usually radioactive phosphorus-32 (^{32}P), and then denatured into a single DNA strand. The DNA on the membrane must also be denatured into single strands such that the radioactive strand added in a solution to the membrane can bind to the specific complementary fragments on the membrane. The binding of a DNA probe to fragments containing complementary sequences is called *hybridization*. The membrane can then be washed and exposed to an x-ray film in a process called *autoradiography*. Only those fragments that have bound to the probe and contain the DNA of interest will be exposed on the film, and their sizes and pattern can be determined (Fig. 2-3).

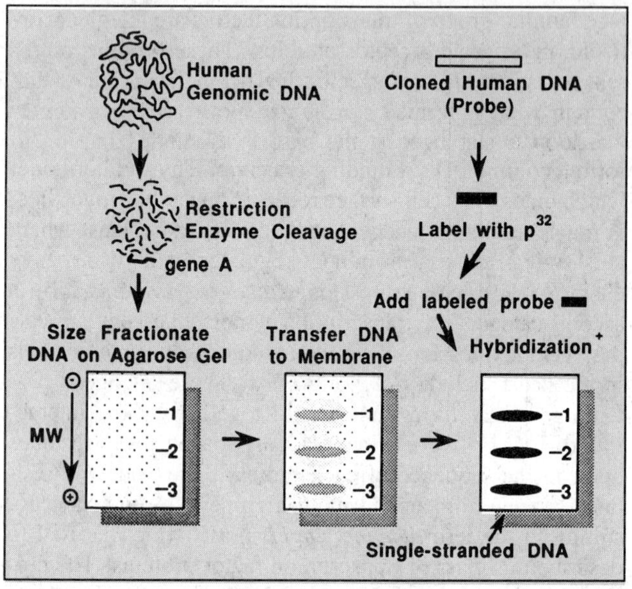

Fig. 2-3. Southern blotting technique. Human DNA is isolated and digested with a restriction enzyme, creating small fragments that are then size separated on an agarose gel using electrophoresis. In this case, gene *A* is analyzed and is found to contain restriction enzymes sites cleaving it into three different-sized fragments labeled *1*, *2*, and *3*. The largest fragment, *1*, moves most slowly through the gel, and *3*, the smallest fragment, moves farthest in the electric field. The complex DNA mixture is denatured into single-stranded molecules and then transferred to a solid-support nylon membrane for further manipulation and detection. Detection is accomplished by labeling a cloned complementary DNA probe containing the transcribed sequences from gene *A* with radioactive phosphorus-32. The labeled probe is then capable of binding to (hybridizing) the complementary sequences of DNA that have been size separated. The filter is washed and exposed to x-ray film, and only fragments *1*, *2*, and *3*, which have hybridized with the probe, are detected at the size position they have migrated to from the gel. Different individuals may vary by containing a different number of restriction enzyme sites within a particular gene, leading to different fragment patterns on the Southern blot autoradiogram. (From Roberts R et al: A primer of molecular biology. New York, 1992, Elsevier.)

If the material being isolated and identified is DNA, the procedure is referred to as Southern blotting, whereas if the material is RNA, it is called Northern blotting. Correspondingly, the separation and membrane transfer of protein for detection is referred to as Western blotting. The probe used for Southern or Northern blotting is usually a radionuclide-labeled DNA fragment, whereas Western blotting usually employs a chemically tagged antibody.

DNA CLONING

DNA cloning is a method of isolating and producing multiple copies of a DNA fragment of interest. These cloned fragments can then be used as DNA probes or sequenced to analyze the specific sequences of the cloned fragment. Cloned fragments representing a complete gene can be used for pharmaceutical purposes by producing vast amounts of a purified (recombinant) protein such as rtPA, now used daily in the treatment of myocardial infarction (Chapter 14). Cloned genes can also be used to express a particular protein in vivo in a transgenic animal. This type of experiment is very useful in studying the physiologic function of a particular molecule and how it interacts with other proteins in the cell.

DNA cloning techniques are fundamentally similar in that they all involve inserting a segment of the DNA of interest into a second piece of DNA that can replicate the desired fragment, called *vector* DNA. Vector DNA is DNA recognized by a host cell system and can be replicated many times, resulting in amplification of a single fragment of DNA of interest. Vector DNA and the DNA to be cloned are first both cut with a restriction enzyme. The DNA to be cloned is then inserted into vector DNA, and an enzyme called DNA ligase is used to link the DNA fragments together to assemble the vector into a functioning piece of DNA. The vector DNA plus the desired cloned DNA insert are then incorporated into a host cell system that recognizes vector sequences and propagates them within the cell as if it were its own native DNA. Four general classes of cloning systems are currently in use. The choice of sys-

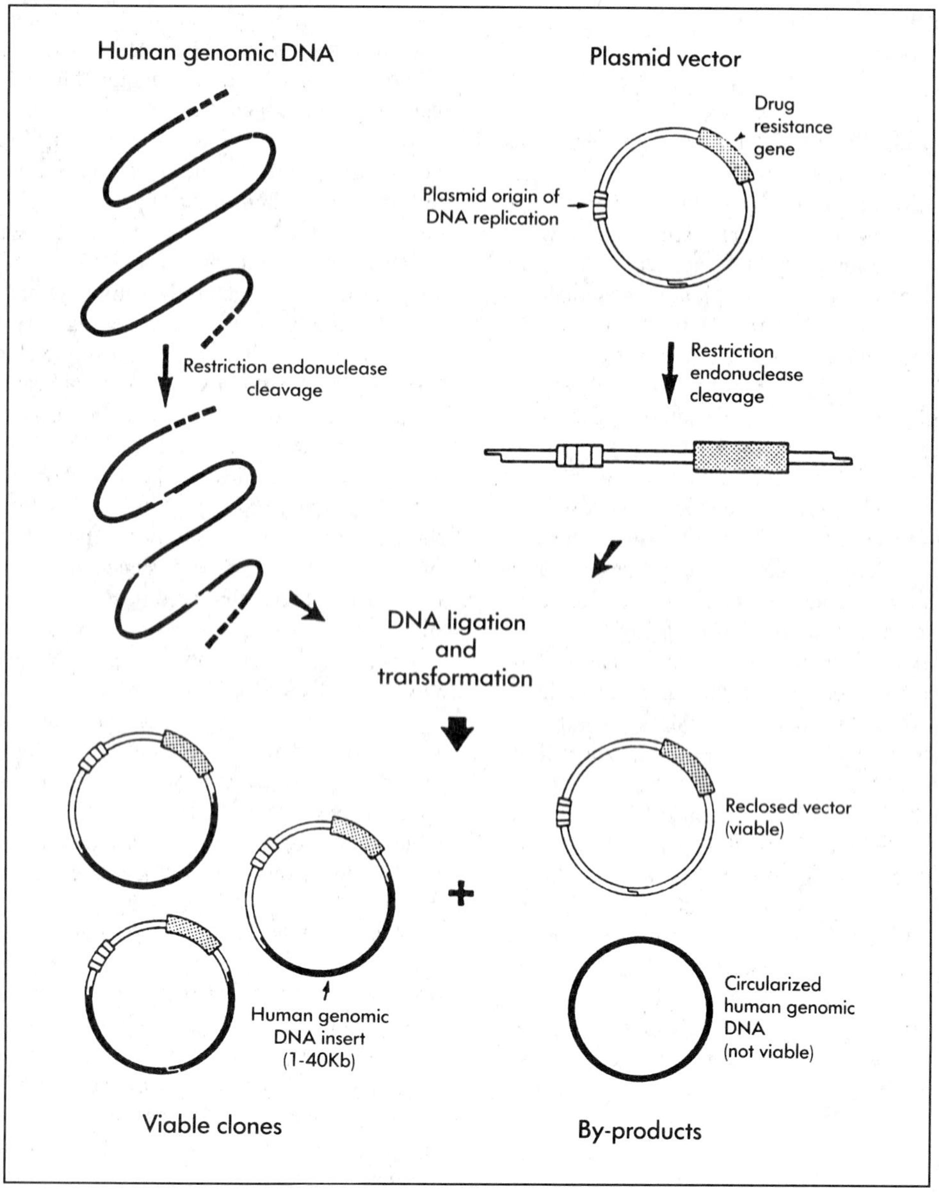

Fig. 2-4. Cloning of a DNA fragment using a plasmid as the vector. Initially the human genomic DNA is cleaved with a restriction enzyme and then inserted into the plasmid vector that contains a means of replication and a selectable marker, such as a drug-resistance gene. Various by-products of the procedure (i.e., closed vector, circularized human DNA) are also represented. (From Roberts R et al: A primer of molecular biology. New York, 1992, Elsevier.)

tem depends on the DNA fragment's size and the purpose of using a particular cloning technique:

1. Small DNA fragments 5 to 15 kb in size are generally cloned into a piece of circular DNA vector called a *plasmid,* which is incorporated into bacterial cells and replicated many times. Plasmids contain an origin of DNA replication and also often contain sequences for a drug-resistance gene (Fig. 2-4).
2. *Phage* cloning systems can handle DNA pieces up to 20 kb in size, which are incorporated into a bacteriophage that invades and multiplies in a bacterial host.
3. A combination vector system called a *cosmid* can clone DNA pieces up to 50 kb in size.
4. A new system using yeast rather than bacteria have allowed insertions of 1 Mb (1 million bp) of human DNA fragments into *yeast* DNA.

RNA ANALYSIS

Only about 5% of chromosomal DNA actually represents genes that encode for proteins. Therefore routine analysis of DNA is complicated by many noncoding sequences, the significance of which is still under investigation. mRNA, on the other hand, represents only DNA sequences that have been transcribed to perform a cell function; these sequences encode for the 50,000 to 100,000 proteins formed in the different cells. Although the DNA content of different cells is the same, mRNA isolated from cardiac tissue varies significantly from mRNA isolated from another organ, such as the liver. The translated proteins from the mRNA in these two organs are very different and perform quite different functions. Therefore the mRNA sequences provide unique information about tissue-specific proteins produced in a particular organ and can define tissue-specific protein isoforms that may differentially regulate function in these different tissues. mRNA can directly predict the amino acid sequence of proteins that have not yet been discovered. The mRNA sequence can also be used as a probe to analyze DNA fragments and find the gene that produces a particular protein. Northern blotting, one method of analyzing RNA, is performed similar to the Southern blot technique described earlier except that instead of using DNA, RNA is used and separated electrophoretically, then blotted onto a membrane and probed with a radioactive probe.

Because full-length mRNA transcripts can directly encode for a desired protein, it is often desired to clone the mRNA sequence into an "expression vector" to allow one to make the recombinant protein and study its function. mRNA is single stranded and a relatively unstable molecule that is often converted in the laboratory to a more stable cDNA copy of the sequence.

DNA LIBRARIES

The terms *DNA libraries* and *cDNA libraries* refer to cloned fragments of DNA from two very different sources. A DNA library is derived from genomic DNA (chromosomal) that has been digested with a restriction enzyme and cloned into one of the cloning systems described previously. Such a library contains multiple fragments of different sizes of DNA that may have exons from genes, introns from noncoding regions within genes, and very large portion of noncoding genomic DNA existing between genes that performs structural and regulatory functions for the DNA. To access the library, one must have a probe to *screen* all the clones present to find those that contain complementary sequences found in the probe.

In contrast, a cDNA library is derived from RNA, which does not contain these upstream, nontranscribed sequences; thus they would not be found in a cDNA library. However, by using cDNA probe, one can select a clone from the genomic DNA library that contains both transcribed and nontranscribed regulatory sequences upstream from the gene's coding region. Analysis of these sequences have been useful in demonstrating the various factors that regulate an important gene's activity. Promoters and enhancers that are active in cardiac tissues can be isolated in this way. Although DNA libraries contain information important in gene regulation and gene coding, cDNA libraries (from RNA) are useful in the study of gene function. cDNA libraries allow one to focus on the unique transcripts produced in individual organ types and thus allow a more focused selection of gene activity in the heart.

The screening methods for DNA and cDNA libraries are very similar. In a bacterial cloning system the bacteria cells are diluted and spread out on an agarose plate such that a single bacterial cell containing a single cloned fragment can grow as a single colony. These colonies grow as small dots on top of the culture plate. A nylon membrane is laid on top, and the colonies are then "lifted" onto a membrane. The bacterial colonies are then lysed on the membrane, and the DNA content of each clone is denatured and adheres to the membrane at the location of the "lifted" colony. These membranes can then be screened with a radioactive probe to identify which lifted colony contains the cloned fragment of interest. This colony can then be selected and grown to make a large preparation of a single cloned fragment of DNA or cDNA.

The expression, regulation, and function of a particular gene and its protein can now be studied by manipulating and piecing together different cloned fragments of DNA from different sources. For example, cloned promoters and enhancers, which initiate gene function, can be ligated to a cDNA clone encoding for a particular protein. Recombinant human proteins such as rtPA are produced by ligating the human cDNA clone to the gene regulatory sequences active in bacteria. In this way a human protein can be artificially produced in a bacterial system in large quantities. The properties that control regulation of promoter and enhancer sequences in a human cardiac gene can be studied by ligating the regulating sequences to what is called a *reporter* gene. Reporter genes synthesize a product not normally found in human tissues, and easily quantifiable as a measure of gene activity.

SEQUENCING

DNA sequencing is an essential aspect of molecular biology. The DNA, cDNA, or RNA sequence information is used to derive the amino acid sequence of a protein, find a particular endonuclease restriction enzyme site for molecular analysis, or detect mutations in a gene that produce human disease through deletions, insertions, or substitutions within the genetic code.

The Sanger technique involves the use of DNA polymerase to copy a cloned piece of DNA. Four separate reactions are performed for each of the four nucleotides, A, T, C, and G. The DNA synthesis reaction mixture for each base contains a contaminating source of nucleotide base–specific terminating molecules. These are dideoxy nucleotides that lack the 3′ sugar hydroxy group required for the next phosphodiester linkage. As a result, each reaction mixture contains different copy fragment lengths of the original DNA that are terminated at the site of the terminating base used in that reaction. For example, the thymine reaction contains copies of the sequence terminated each time a thymine dideoxy base is added. The four reactions, each specific for A, T, G, or C, are then run side by side on a polyacrylamide gel in four lanes. Resolution is such that a single bp difference in size can be separated on a gel. The DNA sequence is read so that the nucleotide base gel lane that contains the next longest strand determines the base next in the sequence. Standard sequencing gels can sequence approximately 250 bp/gel, so sequencing of a few thousand bp of DNA or cDNA is still a relatively time-consuming undertaking. The development of new automated sequencers have greatly enhanced the output.

RESTRICTION FRAGMENT LENGTH POLYMORPHISM

The DNA sequence is highly conserved, so when a particular segment of DNA from a variety of different individuals is compared, the size of DNA fragments generated by a particular enzyme generally is similar. Thus the number and size of DNA fragments produced when a region of DNA is cut with a particular enzyme form a recognizable pattern that can be analyzed after separation by electrophoresis. Small variations in the sequence between unrelated individuals may cause a restriction enzyme recognition site to be lost or added to a particular region of the DNA, which would produce different-sized DNA fragments, resulting in a different pattern from that expected. This difference is referred to as *polymorphic*. The restriction fragment pattern from maternal and paternal DNA is passed on to the offspring such that a restriction fragment length polymorphism (RFLP) is distinguishable from each parental chromosome. When the RFLP pattern is analyzed in the region of a particular gene, the inheritance of that gene from each parent can be determined (Fig. 2-5). If one parent is a carrier of a genetic disease, such as hypertrophic cardiomyopathy (HCM), the likelihood of an offspring inheriting that disease can be determined from the offspring's RFLP pattern by a comparison with the RFLP pattern from the affected parent. If the RFLP from the disease-carrying region of the affected parent's DNA matches the son's or daughter's pattern, the likelihood of inheriting the disease is significant. With HCM, various families have been identified who have inherited mutations in the beta-MHC gene, which appear to cause the disease.

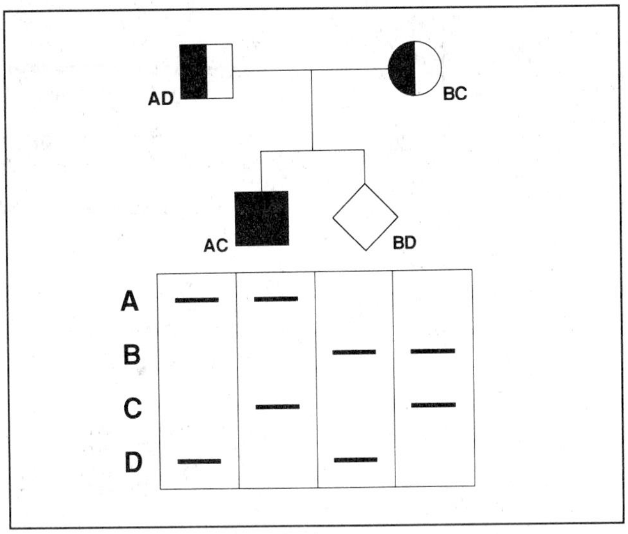

Fig. 2-5. Restriction fragment length polymorphism (RFLP) detection of autosomal recessive disease transmission. Restriction fragment bands *A, B, C,* and *D* detected on Southern blot using a disease-linked probe. A small family pedigree is shown above. On the basis of the affected child's inheritance *(solid square below),* the father's diseased allele cosegregates with band *A,* and the mother's diseased allele cosegregates with band *C.* The normal offspring *(open diamond)* inherited the father's *B* and the mother's *D* bands, both of which are linked to the normal gene. A child containing only one diseased allele from either parent *(not shown)* would be a carrier for the disease. (From Roberts R et al: A primer of molecular biology. New York, 1992, Elsevier.)

POLYMERASE CHAIN REACTION

The polymerase chain reaction (PCR) technique provides for rapid isolation and purification of a desired fragment of DNA by selective logarithmic amplification. The desired piece of DNA can be amplified from a complex mixture of very diluted DNA or a single copy of the target fragment within a few hours without the need for cloning and purification. The technique requires some knowledge of the DNA sequences in the region to be amplified. First, small specific oligonucleotide molecules approximately 25 bases in length must be synthesized to act as "primers" for the reaction. The DNA to be copied is denatured with heat such that the strands separate and then cool so the small, short, sequence-specific oligonucleotide primers can bind to the desired region of the DNA. The heat-stable *Taq* polymerase enzyme is used to initiate synthesis at the precise region of DNA bound by primer. This process is called *primer extension*. By selecting oligonucleotide primers flanking the region of interest and oriented inward toward each other, the intermediate sequence is amplified by doubling the amount of DNA copy in that particular region with each cycle. The DNA is repeatedly denatured and copied in this one region. Repeated cycles can synthesize approximately 1 million copies of the piece of DNA of interest in about 3 hours (Fig. 2-6). The PCR method is most efficient for pieces of DNA less than 1000 bp in size, although fragments up to 5000 to 7000 bp have been produced. The technique is so rapid and simple that it has quickly gained wide popularity in both diagnostic and research laboratories.

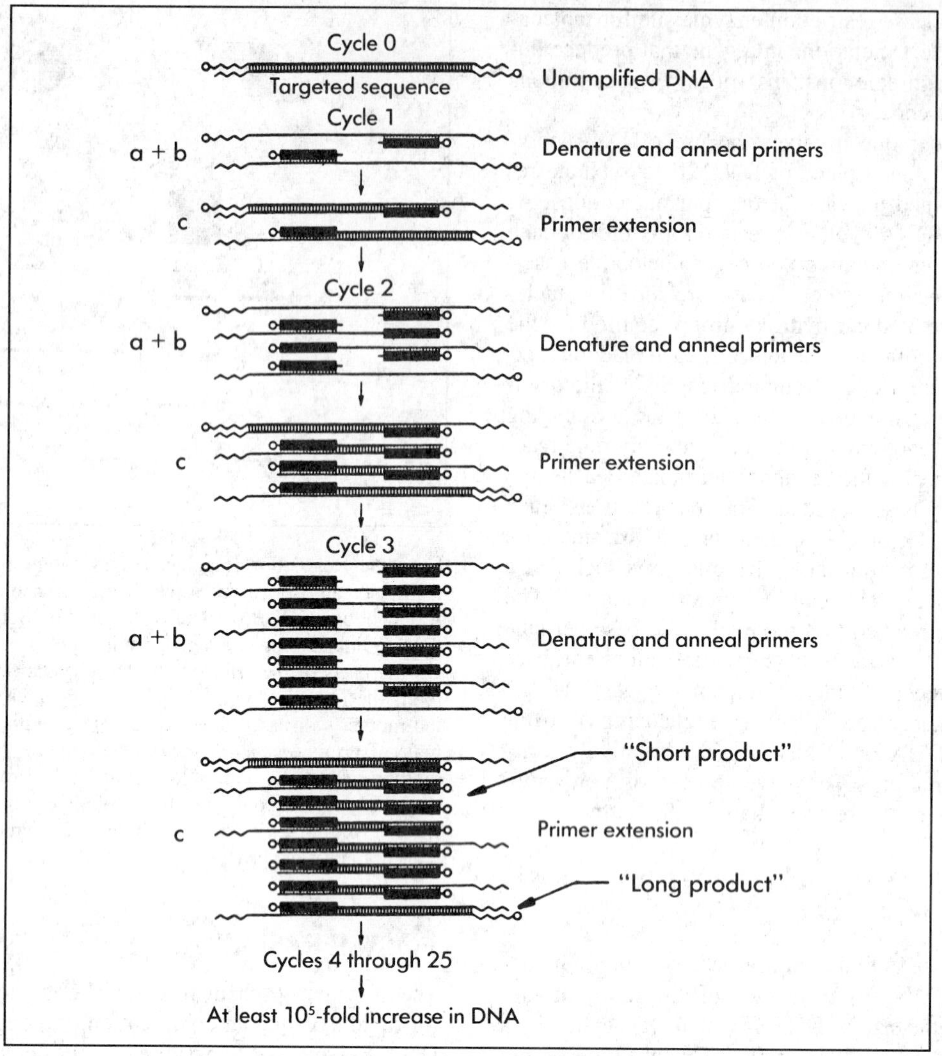

Fig. 2-6. Polymerase chain reaction (PCR). Amplification of a selected region is accomplished by separating the two strands of DNA with heat denaturation and subsequent annealing of short oligonucleotide primers complementary to and flanking the region to be amplified (steps *a* and *b*). In step *c* the enzyme *Taq* polymerase is used to extend synthesis from the primer, creating double-stranded DNA in the selected region for amplification. A second cycle of denaturation and annealing of primers followed by primer extension again doubles the amount of double-stranded DNA in the region of interest, with some copies terminating at the site of the downstream primer. These "short products" eventually dominate the reaction, creating a single-size DNA fragment selected by the separation distance of the two primers used in the reaction. The PCR product is often visualized by agarose gel electrophoresis and ethidium bromide staining of the DNA *(not shown)*. (From Roberts R et al: A primer of molecular biology. New York, 1992, Elsevier.)

GENE TRANSFER

Numerous methods have now been developed to transfer foreign DNA into mammalian cells. Each method has its own advantages and pitfalls in terms of efficacy and utility of gene transfer. Transgenic animals provide a useful source for studying the impact of gene expression or gene mutations in the intact animal. Determination of a particular protein's or enzyme's function and its effect on the pathophysiology of disease may be best accomplished by this method. A foreign DNA vector designed to express a particular protein under the control of a selected promoter and enhancer system is introduced by injection into a fertilized ovum. The genetically altered ovum is then implanted into the uterus of a surrogate maternal animal, and the offspring's phenotypic effects are studied. Recently the effect of the intracellular calcium modulator *calmodulin* on cardiac growth has been studied in transgenic mice. Calmodulin was expressed specifically in the heart under the control of the promoter for atrial natriuretic factor. This expression vector overexpressed calmodulin in the atria of the offspring mouse hearts, causing myocyte growth and hypertrophy and often early death (C. Grurer, personal communication).

Gene transfer in the cardiovascular system is a relatively new field, but several interesting test systems have already been developed. Using tissue culture, one can now induce cardiac myocytes, vascular smooth muscle cells, and endothelial cells to incorporate exogenous DNA into the cells by a variety of methods. Cellular uptake of exogenous DNA can be enhanced with the use of calcium phosphate, DEAE-dextran, liposomes (lipofection), electroporation, retrovirus transfection, adenovirus transfection, direct injection, or the use of DNA-coated microprojectiles in a system developed by Dupont called the "gene gun." The more difficult task has been to accomplish gene transfer and have its protein product expressed in the differentiated cells of a live animal. One successful technique is to transplant genetically modified cells from tissue culture into an intact animal.

CARDIAC GROWTH AND HYPERTROPHY

Although the human heart exhibits remarkable physiologic reserve, the nondividing cardiac myocyte is limited in its ability to preserve function in response to disease or injury. The major compensatory response to ischemia, infarction, hypertension, and/or heart failure is cellular hypertrophy and adaptations in the intracellular constituents, including contractile proteins and proteins that mediate excitation-contraction coupling. Cell division in heart tissue terminates during fetal development. However, some genes continue to show developmental differences in gene expression, such as the slow cardiac calcium adenosine triphosphatase (Ca-ATPase), which is dramatically increased in the adult human ventricle. In contrast, atrial natiuretic factor, which is expressed in the embryonic ventricle, is turned off as the heart matures into the adult stage. Differences in the cardiac myocyte's ability to divide or express different proteins or protein isoforms are regulated by transcription factors that determine cardiac gene expression during development and disease. Various physiologic stressors (e.g., pressure overload) can cause induction and re-expression of fetal genes, which may provide insight into the adaptative cellular response seen in patients with cardiac hypertrophy. For example, in patients with cardiac failure the atrial natiuretic gene is re-expressed in the diseased ventricular muscle, whereas in persons with healthy ventricles this gene is quiescent.

The signaling mechanisms that induce changes in the cascade of proteins affecting differential function in cardiac hypertrophy and failure have broad potential in the treatment of heart disease (Fig. 2-7). Several initiating signals

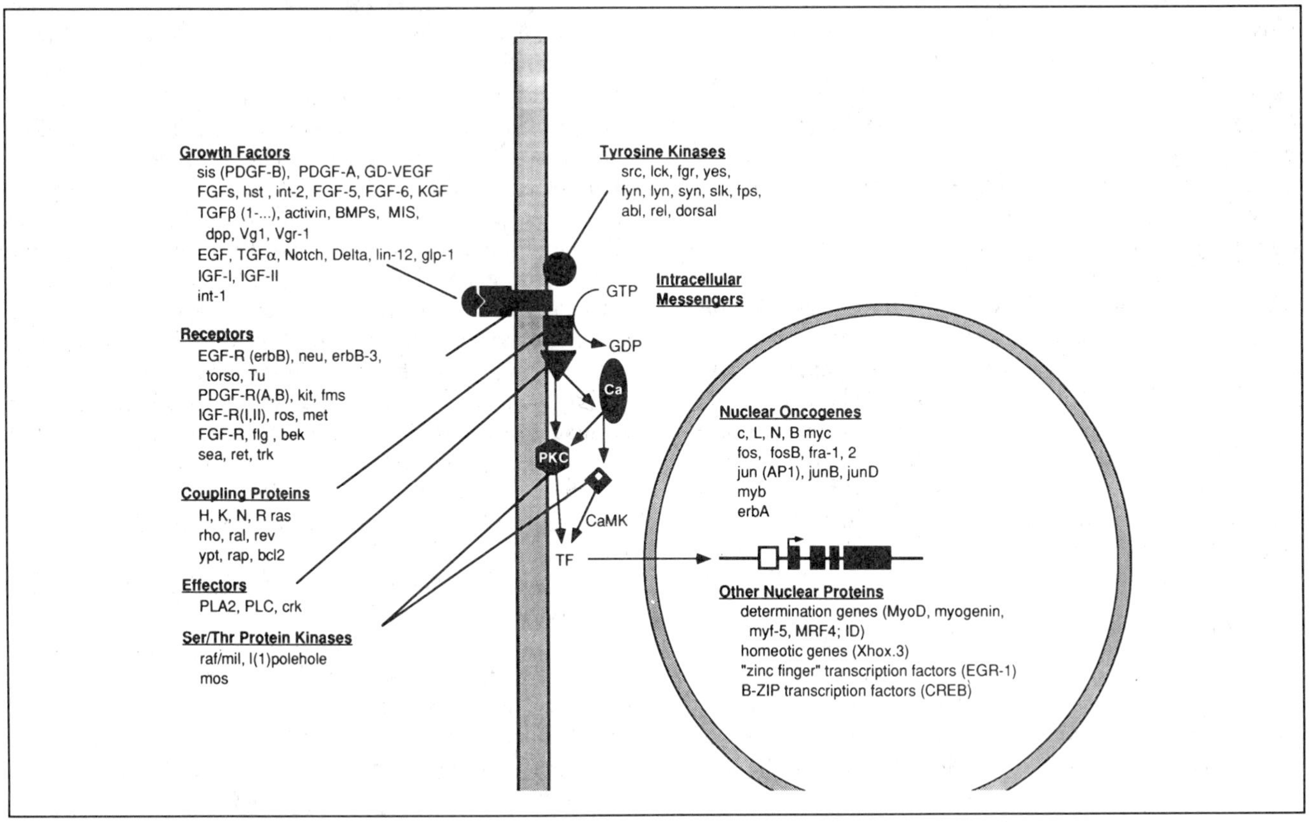

Fig. 2-7. Oncogene proteins and cardiac growth and hypertrophy. Cellular oncogenes encode several proteins that may be involved in cardiac growth. The stimulus for cardiac gene regulation involves extracellular forces (i.e., pressure), neurotransmitters, hormones, or growth factors that stimulate membrane receptors and regulate cardiac gene transcription through various coupling proteins, tyrosine kinases, and intracellular messengers. These cellular mechanisms appear to regulate production of nuclear oncogenes, which encode transcription factors, leading to cardiac gene regulation.

have been identified that alter cardiac gene expression. Norepinephrine has been shown to alter beta-MHC gene expression and skeletal alpha-actin expression in cultured cardiac cells. Mechanical stretch of isolated ventricular myocytes on distensible membranes has also been shown to induce RNA synthesis, beta-MHC expression, and expression of the skeletal alpha actin and atrial myosin light chain. The observation that crude extracts from hypertrophied hearts could provoke hypertrophy when infused in vivo provides evidence that locally produced trophic substances are important as initiating signals for hypertrophy and alterations in cardiac gene expression. The acidic and basic fibroblast growth factors and transforming growth factor beta (TGF-β) are the peptide growth factors that have been studied most extensively. These growth factors have been shown to recapitulate partially the fetal cardiac phenotype by increasing production of atrial natiuretic factor and decreasing production of calcium ATPase in ventricular myocardium. Although these growth factors have been identified in myocardial cells, some have suggested that fibroblasts may play the major role in the production of distinct trophic substances during injury or stress. Release of these growth factors has been demonstrated in ischemic myocardium and in the surviving myocardium surrounding infarcted cardiac muscle.

The nuclear oncogene proteins c-*myc,* c-*fos,* and c-*jun* have received considerable attention in the context of cardiac growth and hypertrophy. In the normal adult ventricle, relatively little expression of c-*myc* and c-*fos* occurs. However, during physiologic stress, these proteins increase dramatically in the cell nucleus. As previously discussed, these proteins are transcription factors that bind to the regulatory regions of genes and direct their activity. For example, a *fos/jun* heterodimer binds to the regulatory regions of the atrial natiuretic gene, which is activated in ventricular muscle during pressure overload hypertrophy. Serum growth factors and norepinephrine have both been shown to induce c-*myc* expression in cultured ventricular cells. C-*fos* is induced by both acidic and basic fibroblast growth factors and by passive stretch, angiotensin, and endothelin. Depending on the initiating signal, a variety of receptors, coupling proteins, and signaling proteins transmit the extracellular stress to the nucleus, where nuclear transcription factors act to alter cell function.

ADRENERGIC RECEPTORS AND G PROTEINS

Autonomic tone plays a pivotal role in the regulation of cardiac contractile function, heart rate, and conduction through the atrioventricular node. Muscarinic receptors in the heart interact with the neurotransmitter *acetylcholine,* which is released by the parasympathetic division of the autonomic nervous system via the vagus nerve. Alpha and beta receptors in the heart interact with the neurotransmitter *norepinephrine,* released from sympathetic nerve terminals, and *epinephrine,* released from the adrenal cortex. Pharmacologic stimulation or inhibition of these receptors has proved useful in cardiovascular therapies for patients with congestive heart failure, hypertension, acute myocardial infarction, and bradyarrhythmias. Maladaptive responses to chronic stimulation of these receptors also occur, such as the induction of tachyarrhythmias and the alteration in gene expression and cellular proteins demonstrated in congestive heart failure. Several isoforms of each receptor class have now been purified and cloned, allowing their study in both in vitro and in vivo experimental systems. Currently, three subtypes of the $alpha_1$-adrenergic receptor ($alpha_{1a}$, $alpha_{1b}$, $alpha_{1c}$), three subtypes of the $alpha_2$-adrenergic receptor ($alpha_{2a}$, $alpha_{2b}$, $alpha_{2c}$), and three subtypes of the beta-adrenergic receptor ($beta_1$, $beta_2$, $beta_3$) have been identified. Five different muscarinic receptors have also been cloned (M_1, M_2, M_3, M_4, M_5). These receptors are all membrane proteins that share general features, including up to seven stretches of hydrophobic amino acids, each long enough to span the lipid bilayer. The amino terminus of the receptor proteins is usually outside the cell, and the carboxy terminus is in the cytoplasm. Each receptor contains glycosylation sites as well as amino acids that serve as substrates for protein kinases. Protein kinases can phosphorylate the receptor and influence its activity.

The general mechanism for signal transduction for these receptor proteins involves *G proteins*. G proteins are so named because of their ability to bind guanosine triphosphate (GTP). This high-energy phosphate complex activates adenyl cyclase, which catalyzes the conversion of adenosine triphosphate (ATP) to adenosine 3′,5′-cyclic monophosphate (cAMP). The $beta_1$, $beta_2$, and $beta_3$ receptors are coupled to a G protein called G_s, which stimulates adenyl cyclase. The $alpha_{2a}$ and $alpha_{2b}$ receptors and the M_2 and M_4 receptors are coupled to a G protein called G_i, which inhibits adenyl cyclase. With the M_2 receptor the G-protein coupling may also directly activate the cardiac potassium channel. Not all these receptors work through adenyl cyclase. The $alpha_1$ receptor and M_1, M_3, and M_5 receptors appear to couple to an unknown G protein that activates phospholipase C. Both cAMP and phospholipase C can modulate a variety of cellular processes, including cardiac growth metabolism and ion channel activity. cAMP positively regulates the activity of protein kinase A (PK_A), which can have several effects. Cardiac calcium channels are regulated by PK_A-mediated phosphorylation of the channel protein. Overstimulation of the beta receptors appear to cause PK_A-modulated desensitization of beta-receptor activity. The decrease in the capacity of the beta receptor to activate the G_s protein results from a feedback loop in which PK_A phosphorylates the $beta_2$ receptor. The promoter region of the $beta_2$ receptor has also been sequenced and analyzed. PK_A mediates active removal of the receptors from the membrane by downregulation and has also been shown to decrease synthesis of new receptors by influencing $beta_2$-receptor mRNA stability. PK_A appears to cause destruction of the $beta_2$-receptor mRNA in the cell's cytoplasm.

The activation of phospholipase C through the $alpha_1$-adrenergic receptor and several muscarinic receptors stimulates two separate pathways of cell regulation. Phospholipase C cleaves membrane phospholipids to produce both inositol phosphates and diacylglycerol. Diacylglycerol activates protein kinase C (PK_C), whereas inositol phosphates regulate intracellular calcium. Although PK_C cannot be stimulated by activation of the beta receptor, several sites for PK_C phosphorylation exist on the $beta_2$ receptor. Therefore stimulation of alpha and muscarinic receptors may affect beta-receptor function.

G proteins consist of a three-subunit G protein complex that associates with a signal-transducing cell surface receptor. Alpha, beta, and gamma (α, β, γ) subunits and isoforms of each have been identified. Initially, all three subunits are in contact with the receptor. When the receptor is stimulated by hormone (i.e., epinephrine), the alpha subunit releases bound guanosine diphosphate (GDP), and the receptor undergoes a structural change, increasing its affinity for hormone. The empty alpha subunit can then bind GTP, which causes a release of the alpha subunit from the receptor (beta/gamma subunit) complex. The GTP-activated alpha subunit binds to and activates adenyl cyclase, converting ATP to cAMP (Fig. 2-8). Some G proteins, such as G_k (activated by a muscarinic receptor), can directly modify the activity of the cardiac potassium channel without acting through a protein kinase. Molecular techniques have allowed modifications of cDNAs that express these various receptors and G proteins in an in vitro system in which the receptor's mutation has allowed identification of ligand binding sites and sequences that interact with the G proteins.

An important beta-receptor regulator called *beta-adrenergic receptor kinase* (BARK) has been cloned and purified and shown to be capable of phosphorylating the beta receptor, but only in the presence of an agonist. The action of BARK is mediated by a second protein called beta arrestin. The sequence of receptor deactivation requires binding of an agonist to the receptor, followed by the receptor's phosphorylation by BARK near the G protein binding site. This phosphorylated site is recognized by beta arrestin, which binds to the receptor and prevents its binding to the G_s protein. Because receptor occupancy is required for BARK activity, BARK probably plays a physiologic role when receptors are exposed to high concentrations of agonists, such as in synaptic clefts. BARK may also play a role in beta-receptor desensitization in patients with high catecholamine states, such as end-stage congestive heart failure. BARK-mediated beta-receptor desensitization contrasts greatly with the model for desensitization mediated by PK_A.

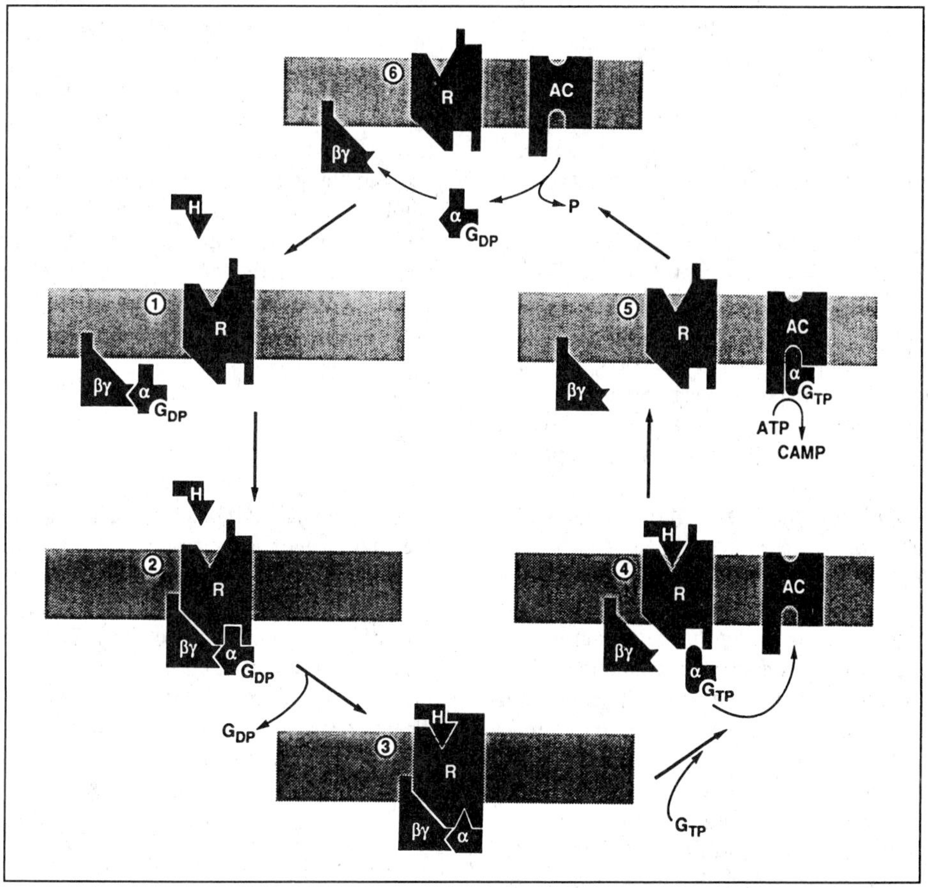

Fig. 2-8. Outline of a cycle of signal transduction for the $beta_2$-adrenergic receptor. The components include the hormone *(H)* epinephrine, the $beta_2$ receptor *(R),* the subunits of G_s *(alpha, beta/gamma),* and adenyl cyclase *(AC).* See text for discussion.

ION CHANNELS

Membrane depolarization and excitation-contraction coupling are mediated by an important class of transmembrane proteins known as ion channels. These proteins are important pharmacologic targets that regulate the flow of sodium, calcium, and potassium currents across the cardiac myocyte plasma membrane and sarcoplasmic reticulum. The gating of ion channels generally fall into two categories: voltage dependent and receptor mediated. Many voltage-dependent channels are highly regulated by receptor-mediated modulation of voltage sensitivity.

Calcium channels

Three cation pump enzymes catalyze the movement of calcium against its concentration gradient: (1) the ryanodine receptor, the calcium ATPase of the sarcoplasmic reticulum (SRCA); (2) the dihydropyridine receptor, the calcium ATPase of the plasma membrane (PMCA); and (3) the sodium/calcium exchanger powered by the sodium gradient created by the sodium/potassium ATPase (NKA), which secondarily moves calcium out of the cell. NKA has an alpha-catalytic subunit, which is stabilized by a beta subunit that can be glycosylated. Both PMCA and SRCA contain an alpha-catalytic subunit, which can act as the functional unit. ATP hydrolysis converts the catalytic subunit into a high-affinity protein conformation to activate the channel.

PMCA, SRCA, and NKA are each encoded by tissue-specific, developmentally regulated gene families. Many of these mRNA gene products are alternatively spliced for multiple isoforms of the channel, encoded by a single gene. These isoforms' functional significance is currently under investigation.

Alternate mechanisms for inducing cardiac hypertrophy clearly cause differential effects on expression of SRCA. For example, in cardiac hypertrophy induced by hyperthyroidism, thyroid hormone receptor appears to bind to the promoter region of SRCA to enhance expression and enzymatic activity. In contrast, pressure overload hypertrophy induces up to a 50% decrease in SRCA levels. Expression of NKA is also enhanced by both thyroid hormone and glucocorticoid induction.

SRCA is modulated by other intracellular proteins, including phospholamban, which reduces the enzyme's affinity for calcium. Phospholamban can be dissociated from the SRCA by phosphorylation through cAMP-dependent protein kinase and calmodulin-dependent protein kinase, both of which can be activated by cell surface receptors. PMCA is also activated by intracellular proteins, with calmodulin-dependent protein kinase and direct activation by calmodulin being the most important.

SRCA has been extensively studied as a recombinant molecule expressed in tissue culture cell systems. Site-directed mutagenesis of various regions of the protein has identified the ion binding sites and the ATP binding site for the protein. These homologous regions contained within both PMCA and NKA suggest that these sequences are partially conserved motifs.

Beta-adrenergic stimulation causes a fivefold increase in calcium currents through G protein stimulation of adenyl cyclase and PK_A. Acetylcholine decreases cardiac calcium currents only after they have been stimulated by beta-adrenergic agonists, a process mediated by an inhibitory G protein mechanism. PK_C phosphorylation has a biphasic effect, with initial calcium current stimulation followed by inhibition.

Sodium channels

The voltage-dependent cardiac sodium channel has been cloned and studied electrophysiologically in the cell system of the *Xenopus* frog oocyte. Initial rapid membrane depolarization is achieved via fast changes in sodium permeability through a voltage-activated gate. Cardiac sodium channel activation has a fast phase opening and closing, followed by a slow component characterized by "burst" openings that last several milliseconds. This burst component of the cardiac channel characterizes the late sodium current plateau typical of cardiac sodium channels.

The cardiac sodium channel is susceptible to gating modification by beta-adrenergic stimulation. The G_s protein appears to be responsible for modulating cardiac sodium currents through cAMP-dependent phosphorylation or direct interaction of G_s with the channel. Adrenergic stimulation depresses the sodium current and slows conduction, which may produce a substrate for re-entrant arrhythmias or ventricular fibrillation. A decrease in action potential threshold may also be mediated by angiotensin II, which stimulates PK_C-mediated modulation of the cardiac sodium channel. Angiotensin-converting enzyme inhibitor drugs may have an antiarrhythmic effect by blocking cardiac angiotensin II effects on sodium currents. Antiarrhythmic agents such as lidocaine exert their effect through binding to open depolarized inactivated sodium channels, which slows their recovery from inactivation (Chapter 9). The effect is to prevent impulse generation from the damaged depolarized tissue.

Potassium channels

Cardiac potassium channels have been studied less than the sodium and calcium channels. Acetylcholine stimulation of the muscarinic M_2 receptor appears to cause an unidentified G protein to interact directly with the cardiac potassium channel. The possibility of comediated PK_C activation of the channel has not been excluded. Another pathway for G protein–mediated modulation of the cardiac potassium channel may be via the cardiac adenosine receptor. These receptors may be particularly important for activating potassium channels in ischemic cardiac muscle.

CONTRACTILE AND CYTOSKELETAL PROTEINS

The observation that the contractile and cytoskeletal proteins undergo isoform transitions both in cardiac hypertrophy and in cardiomyopathy has led to an intense investigation regarding the pathophysiology of these diseases and the fundamental cellular defects. The cardiac sarcomere is composed of thick and thin filaments (Chapter 1). Thick filaments are composed of two myosin heavy chains (MHCs) together with two pairs of myosin light chains (MLCs). MHCs are encoded by both an alpha-MHC gene and a beta-MHC gene, which allow the formation of three possible MHC combinations: alpha/alpha, alpha/beta, or beta/beta. Alpha/alpha-MHC has a fourfold to fivefold greater ATPase activity than the beta/beta-MHC combination. The predominant form in the adult ventricle is beta-MHC, whereas the alpha form appears to be present primarily in the adult atrium. In patients with cardiac hypertrophy, beta-MHC expression increases. Mutations in beta-MHC have been described in families with the inherited form of hypertrophic cardiomyopathy.

Changes in MLC expression have also been described, and several MLC isoforms exist. Absent or significantly reduced MLC 2 (the regulatory MLC, which can be phosphorylated) has been found in patients with idiopathic dilated cardiomyopathy. Dramatically reduced or absent MLC 2 may alter ATPase activity and result in generalized destabilization of the sarcomere's lattice geometry.

Each thick filament of myosin is associated with six thin-filament protein complexes. The thin filament contains two chains of globular actin associated with the dimeric superhelix tropomyosin molecule and three different troponin molecules. Troponin C binds calcium, troponin I binds actin, and troponin T stabilizes the complex and binds it to tropomyosin. Both troponin T and I can also be phosphorylated and may induce changes in the activity of these molecules during contraction. Phosphorylation of troponin I appears to decrease the sensitivity for calcium and may account for the lusitropic effect of beta-adrenergic agonists on cardiac relaxation. The tropomyosin genes encode both alpha and beta subunits and are capable of alternative splicing to produce a variety of tropomyosin isoform proteins. Similarly, the alpha-actin protein is present in three different isoforms produced by separate genes: the skeletal, cardiac, and smooth muscle alpha actins. Although the smooth muscle alpha actin has been found in embryonic myocardium, only the skeletal and cardiac alpha actins are present in the adult ventricle. No consistent differences in alpha actin have yet been observed in human cardiac disease.

Several intermediate and accessory proteins are associated with the contractile proteins and are involved in their assembly, stability, and organization. *Desmin* is an intermediate filament found in muscle cells that appears to tie the edges of the Z disks (lines) together. Intermediate filament assembly is controlled through phosphorylation by protein kinases. Interestingly, alterations in desmin and other cytoskeletal proteins have been described in patients with cardiomyopathy. Thick filaments of myosin are linked to the Z disk via a large 2500 kd (kilodalton) protein called *titin,* whereas actin filaments within the sarcomere are linked to the Z disk via an elongated 600 kd protein called *nebulin. Alpha actinin* is another Z disk–associated protein, which acts within the sarcomere to bundle actin molecules and link these filaments together near their attachment to the Z disk. Spectrin is a 280 kd protein localized to the cytoplasmic surface of the cardiocyte membrane. Spectrin forms a complex with the protein ankyrin and binds to a number of important molecules, including the voltage-dependent sodium channel, sodium ATPase, and the acetylcholine receptor. In cardiac pressure overload, volume overload, hypercontractile states, and failure, the forces exerted on the heart's cytoskeletal contractile elements may cause pathophysiologic responses in the organization and relative content of these various filaments.

Various mutations in the gene that encodes the cytoskeletal protein *dystrophin* cause the skeletal and cardiac disease seen in Duchenne and Becker muscular dystrophies. Dystrophin is localized to the cell membrane's cytoplasmic surface, where it is associated with a large transmembrane, glycoprotein complex. Skeletal muscle and cardiac cells deficient in dystrophin display elevated intracellular calcium levels and increased calcium leakage across the cell membrane. These data have led to speculation that dystrophin is associated with molecules that modify calcium activity at the cell membrane. Dystrophin is alternatively spliced at the carboxy terminus, producing multiple isoforms, some of which are specific for cardiac tissue. The cardiomyopathy and conduction defects seen in Duchenne and Becker muscular dystrophies are directly related to the defective expression of dystrophin in the heart.

LIPOPROTEINS, APOLIPOPROTEINS, AND ATHEROSCLEROSIS

Atherosclerosis and accelerated atherogenesis remain the most recognized and most treatable forms of cardiac disease (Chapter 171). Diagnosis and treatment of the major dyslipoproteinemias have been mainly advanced by molecular techniques that have elucidated the various mechanisms for this heterogeneous group of disorders. Premature cardiovascular disease is caused either by defects in lipoprotein receptors or by the associated apolipoproteins that modulate their metabolism. Elevated levels of low-density lipoprotein (LDL), beta–very-low-density lipoprotein (beta-VLDL), and lipoprotein a (LPa) and diminished levels of high-density lipoprotein (HDL) all increase the risk of early atherosclerotic ischemic heart disease (Chapter 171).

Plasma lipids are important substrates for energy metabolism, membrane integrity, and steroid synthesis. They are transported as lipoproteins and are separated into five major classes by the content of triglycerides, cholesterol, cholesterol esters, phospholipids, and apolipoproteins. Intestinally absorbed lipids are transported to the liver as large, hydrated lipoproteins called *chylomicrons.* The intestines, liver, and capillary endothelium modify these particles by the addition of lipoproteins and by interactions with the enzyme hepatic lipase. Lecithin-cholesterol acetyltransferase (LCAT) also catalyzes the esterification of plasma cholesterol to cholesterol esters in the liver and is active in lipoprotein lipase in the capillary endothelium. Triglyceride-rich VLDL secreted by the liver is converted to the cholesterol-rich LDL by the combined action of these lipolipases (Chapter 171).

The pathologic mechanisms for the accumulation of plasma lipids within macrophages with subsequent foam cell formation and the formation of an occlusive atherosclerogenic plaque are now largely understood (Chapter 171). The dyslipoproteinemias result in increased transport and transudation of lipoproteins into the intima of the coronary vessels, where blood-derived macrophages also migrate. Oxidative modification of LDL enhances uptake by macrophages and foam cell formation. Cytokinins liberated by macrophages stimulate additional migration of blood-borne macrophages and migration and proliferation of smooth muscle cells into the intima, which ultimately progress into a complex atherosclerotic lesion.

The structural similarity of LPa to plasminogen has led to a proposal that this lipoprotein particle may enhance thrombosis formation by binding tissue plasminogen activator and deactivating it, resulting in diminished steady-state thrombolysis and enhanced thrombogenesis. HDLs have been proposed to play a pivotal role in retarding foam cell formation by removing excess cholesterol from peripheral cells and transporting the cholesterol back to the liver, where it is secreted as free cholesterol or bile acids. Diminished HDL levels alter the equilibrium of cholesterol deposition by reducing cholesterol removal and transport back to the liver, which promotes lipid accumulation in peripheral cells.

The apolipoproteins associated with these various lipid particles are responsible for their receptor recognition, enzyme activation, secretion, and cellular uptake. For example, apolipoprotein B100 and E interact with the LDL receptor to initiate endocytosis and cellular uptake of LDL. Apolipoprotein A1 on HDL is believed to interact with an HDL receptor to facilitate the removal of cholesterol from peripheral cells.

Genetic diseases that alter expression of the LDL receptor or one of the apolipoprotein molecules can severely affect cholesterol metabolism. The LDL receptor gene is located on chromosome 19, where the genes for apolipoproteins E, C2, and C1 are also located. The genes for apolipoproteins A1, C3, and A4 are found on chromosome 11. The apolipoprotein B isoproteins are synthesized from a single gene on chromosome 2, and LPa is a polymorphic apolipoprotein with multiple genetic alleles present at a single locus on chromosome 6.

Familial hypercholesterolemia established the importance of LDL levels in atherogenesis and has now been characterized by four classes of mutations in the LDL receptor gene. Patients who are heterozygous for the disease have LDL cholesterol levels of 250 to 500 mg/dl, and homozygous patients have concentrations of 600 to more than 1200 mg/dl. The dramatic coronary disease in these patients may appear as early as age 2 years to as late as the mid-20s. Class I mutations result from failure of LDL receptor biosynthesis. Class II mutations are characterized by an LDL receptor that cannot be transported to the cell surface from the endoplasmic reticulum. Class III mutations produce an LDL receptor that is present at the cell surface but cannot bind LDL normally. Class IV mutations lead to receptors that bind LDL at the cell membrane but that cannot be normally internalized and metabolized by the cell. Triple drug therapy is often required to treat patients with familial hypercholesterolemia. Liver transplantation is the most effective, although the most costly, treatment. Gene therapy using recombinant LDL receptor has shown promise in the LDL-deficient Watanabe rabbit.

Type III lipoproteinemia (dys-beta-lipoproteinemia) is characterized by a structural or functional defect in apolipoprotein E. The genetic defects in this disease cause either an apolipoprotein E deficiency or the production of a functionally defective apolipoprotein E. The altered E variants have a decreased affinity for the LDL receptor, producing delayed catabolism and accumulation of remnant lipoprotein particles. Although these patients develop premature cardiovascular disease, in contrast to those with LDL receptor disorders, they respond well to diet and medical therapy (Chapter 171).

Patients with low HDL levels have been characterized by several genetic defects in apolipoprotein A1. Several families have been described who have increased catabolism of A1, whereas other families have an A1 deficiency from structural mutations in the gene. Patients with combined deficiency of A1, C3, and A4 often have reduced levels of HDL and VLDL, with relatively normal LDL levels.

Increased LPa levels have also been shown to increase fivefold the relative risk of premature vascular disease. The genetic mechanism for increased plasma levels of LPa has not yet been defined. Elevated LPa levels are not effectively reduced by diet, and the only medication shown to reduce LPa levels consistently is niacin (Chapter 171).

The disorder designated *familial combined hyperlipidemia* (FCH) is probably a heterogeneous disease and is the most common of all the dyslipoproteinemias. The gene frequency of this codominantly inherited disease has been estimated as 1 in 300 in the U.S. population. The lipid and lipoprotein profile of these patients varies, and elevations in cholesterol, triglycerides, or both may be observed in the plasma. Patients with FCH often have an abnormal cholesterol/apolipoprotein B ratio, and plasma HDL levels are frequently reduced. They generally respond to diet and medical therapy for control of their hyperlipidemia.

APPLICATION OF MEDICAL GENETICS TO CARDIOMYOPATHIES

Major advances have been made in uncovering the molecular basis for cardiomyopathy in patients who have inherited genetic diseases that influence their cardiac function. This group of diseases dramatically illustrates the important interplay of many different cellular elements and how defects in many different aspects of cellular physiology can produce a cardiomyopathic phenotype. Defects in contractile proteins, such as mutations in the beta-MHC, have been implicated in hypertrophic cardiomyopathy. Defective expression of the cytoskeletal protein dystrophin is responsible for the cardiomyopathy and conduction defect seen in patients with Duchenne and Becker muscular dystrophies. The cardiomyopathy seen in those with myotonic dystrophy is probably caused by the altered expression of a protein kinase in cardiac tissues. Maternally inherited mitochondrial defects have also been described in patients with cardiomyopathy, in whom impaired oxidative phosphorylation may cause both conduction defects and congestive heart failure.

Congenital long Q-T syndrome has recently been mapped to the short arm of chromosome 11; X-linked cardiomyopathy, to the short arm of the X chromosome; and a form of complete atrial standstill and muscle weakness called Emery-Dreifuss muscular dystrophy, to the distal long arm of the X chromosome. Several families with idiopathic dilated cardiomyopathy have been described, suggesting an as yet unknown gene mutation that may account for some patients with this disease.

To identify the gene and gene product responsible for an inherited disease, an approach called *positional cloning* is employed. This strategy refers to identifying and cloning the region of a chromosome that is consistently inherited with the disease. Thousands of markers are now available that identify the individual chromosomes as well as subregions of each chromosome. When a particular marker is consistently coinherited with the disease, that marked region of a particular chromosome is said to be genetically linked to the disease. The use of RFLP patterns described previously has proved to be a powerful technique in mapping disease inheritance using these linked markers. Once a chromosomal region has been identified, the arduous process of cloning overlapping segments of DNA in this region and searching for candidate genes that may be responsible for the disease begins. The identification of the causal gene depends on finding a gene expressed in cardiac tissue exhibiting the disease, then demonstrating a causal relationship between the mutation and the defective protein's effect on tissue function.

Familial hypertrophic cardiomyopathy

Familial hypertrophic cardiomyopathy (FHCM) has long been an interesting disease for the cardiologist, since its clinical, hemodynamic, and morphologic profile may be used as a paradigm for many other cardiac diseases (Chapter 17). The disease is known to have an autosomal dominant pattern of inheritance and was the first primary cardiac disorder for which the causative gene was isolated. Although FHCM may be genetically heterogeneous, it has now been shown in several North American families that a major locus is on the long arm of chromosome 14 and that the gene is beta-MHC. About nine different mutations have now been identified in the beta-MHC gene and been shown to cosegregate with the disease. Most of these mutations have been missense mutations located in the portion of the gene that gives rise to the globular head of the myosin protein. The most common missense mutation appears to be in exon 13, where the nucleotide adenine substitutes for guanine, resulting in the amino acid arginine substituting for the amino acid glutamine in the beta-MHC protein.

The linkage data from several families with FHCM showing the locus on chromosome 14q are compelling, and the mutations recognized in the beta-MHC gene in these families suggest that they are the cause of the disease. However, it requires several years of study to prove that the mutations in that particular gene do cause the disease, as has been the case for Duchenne muscular dystrophy and cystic fibrosis. Nevertheless, considerable progress has been made, and recently it was documented that the missense mutation in exon 13 is translated into the mRNA isolated from myocardium of a patient with FHCM. Furthermore, the mutation was expressed in the beta-MHC mRNA of this patient's skeletal muscle. Despite many families having the disease as a result of beta-MHC mutations on chromosome 14q, several families clearly are not linked to beta-MHC, and studies are being undertaken to determine alternate chromosomal loci for FHCM.

Cardiomyopathy of Duchenne and Becker muscular dystrophy

Duchenne and Becker muscular dystrophies are allelic X-linked recessive disorders caused by mutations in the gene encoding the cytoskeletal protein dystrophin. These diseases affect approximately 1 in 3500 newborn males and are the most common and devastating of the human muscular dystrophies. Phenotypic effects of dystrophin gene mutations are primarily manifested in limb skeletal muscle, although patients usually die from respiratory failure, congestive heart failure, or cardiac conduction abnormalities. Dystrophin is also expressed in brain tissue, and one third of all patients have some degree of mental retardation. Patients who have a milder form of Becker dystrophy often express detectable amounts of a truncated form of dystrophin because of intragenic deletions that presumably occur in noncritical regions of the molecule. In contrast, patients with Duchenne dystrophy have been characterized by low levels or complete absence of dystrophin caused by mutations and presumably resulting in premature chain termination, message instability, protein degradation, or inability of the altered protein to localize to the cell membrane. Dystrophin is a cytoskeletal protein localized to the sarcolemma, although it appears to lack a transmembrane domain. Dystrophin is associated with an integral membrane glycoprotein complex that links the cytoskeleton to the extracellular molecule laminin. When dystrophin is absent from dystrophic muscle, the integral membrane glycoproteins are also lost. The dystrophin-glycoprotein complex may be involved in the regulation of intracellular calcium. Biochemical studies have shown increased calcium leakage in dystrophic muscle and elevated intracellular calcium levels.

Molecular correlations between gene mutation and disease severity have implicated the dystrophin's carboxy terminus as an important domain for dystrophin function. It has been demonstrated that carboxy terminal mutations, particularly those occurring within the cysteine-rich domain, confer a severe disease phenotype, even when mutant dystrophin protein can be shown to be correctly localized at the dystrophic muscle sarcolemma.

Heart block in myotonic muscular dystrophy

Myotonic muscular dystrophy (Steinert disease) is a systemic disease that has many nonmyopathic features, including frontal baldness, cataracts, and muscle atrophy with a characteristic long face and slightly nasal voice (Chapter 125). As many as 80% of patients have interventricular conduction defects, which may culminate in fatal Stokes-Adams episodes unless anticipated and treated by pacemaker insertion. The gene responsible for this disease has been localized to the long arm of chromosome 19, and sequence homology has shown that the gene appears to be a protein kinase.

The unusual pattern of inheritance with a more severe phenotype in the offspring has been termed *anticipation*. The genetics of this type of disease mutation involves the progressive expansion of a repetitive sequence of DNA within the disease gene. In myotonic dystrophy, amplification of a repeating triplet (GCT) occurs in the noncoding 3′ region of the DNA transcript and presumably causes altered expression of the encoded protein kinase in diseased tissues. This novel protein kinase, termed *myotonin,* is alternatively spliced, encoding for isoforms of the protein, and qualitative differences in these isoforms may affect the varied tissue manifestations of the disease.

Mitochondrial cardiomyopathies

Several reports have described abnormalities in mitochondrial morphology and mitochondrial gene deletions in patients either with isolated cardiomyopathy or with multisystem diseases who primarily manifest cardiac conduction defects. The mitochondrial defects in these patients probably represent a heterogeneous group of diseases that affect mitochondrial function. One family with an apparent X-linked recessive inheritance pattern for disease was characterized by the deaths of four related male infants from dilated cardiomyopathy and heart failure. Morphologic studies revealed mitochondria that were greatly enlarged with irregular shape and increased crista and that contained unidentified dense granules. The incidence of these mitochondrial changes were noted four times more frequently in cardiac tissues than in skeletal muscle and the diaphragm at autopsy. Electron microscopy of a biopsy sample from a mother of the proband revealed no abnormalities. The genetic defect in this disorder has not yet been identified but illustrates the potential importance of mitochondrial dysfunction in a subgroup of patients with cardiomyopathy.

Kearns-Sayre syndrome is a well-described myopathy characterized by external ophthalmoplegia pigmentary retinopathy, and heart block. The morphologic changes in skeletal muscle observed using a trichrome strain involve the identification of so-called ragged red fibers. Cardiac involvement appears almost exclusively to affect the specialized conduction system rather than the myocardium. Patients with this disorder have been shown to have deletions in the genes encoded by the mitochondrial genome. Kearns-Sayre syndrome is transmitted by maternal inheritance because all the mitochondria in the ovum during the zygote's formation are from the mother. As a result, the affected mother passes the disease to all children, but only her daughters can transmit the mitochondrial abnormality to subsequent generations. The relative proportion of mitochondrial genomes affected varies from 30% to 85% in different patients. Biochemical analysis of the mitochondrial enzymes from muscle extracts shows widely scattered values. However, most patients have reduced activity of four enzymes in the respiratory chain: cytochrome *c* oxidase, cytochrome *c* oxoreductase, rotenone-sensitive NADH–cytochrome *c* reductase, and NADH dehydrogenase (cytochrome *c* reductase).

Congenital long Q-T syndrome

Several disorders have been shown to target the cardiac conduction system through unknown mechanisms that prolong the Q-T interval (Chapter 9). These patients have a high incidence of sudden death from episodic ventricular arrhythmias and also have Stokes-Adams attacks, characterized by fainting spells and usually precipitated by exertion or emotional stress. Antiarrhythmic drugs that modulate the activity of ion channels can prolong the Q-T interval, prompting speculation that these disorders involve gene defects in proteins involved in membrane repolarization.

The *Romano-Ward syndrome* is predominantly a childhood illness, usually with onset before age 3 years, although some patients do not show clinical signs until age 30. Affected individuals are generally healthy except for episodes of palpitations, chest pain, and sudden loss of consciousness or sudden death. Romano-Ward syndrome is inherited as an autosomal dominant trait, and linkage analysis has mapped the disease to the distal portion of the short arm of chromosome 11. The genetic probe used to show linkage to this region of the chromosome is the gene encoding the Harvey-*ras* oncogene (H-*ras*-1). The genetic odds favoring linkage of the disease near or at the H-*ras*-1 gene are greater than 10^{16} to 1. Although still under investigation, no mutations have yet been identified in the coding sequence of the H-*ras*-1 gene in patients with long Q-T syndrome, and therefore this gene cannot yet be implicated as a causative gene in the disease.

Jervell and Lange-Nielsen syndrome is an autosomal recessive inherited disease associated with a cardiac abnormality similar to that seen in Romano-Ward syndrome; however, these patients also have bilateral high-tone perceptive deafness. The incidence is about 1 in 300,000 persons in the general population and about 1 in 100 among all deaf children. Histologic abnormalities in the artery to the sinus and atrioventricular nodes have been demonstrated, and the administration of digitalis can reduce the Q-T interval and diminish the frequency of syncopal attacks. The chromosomal location and molecular defect in these individuals remain undefined.

Familial cardiomyopathies

Idiopathic dilated cardiomyopathy (IDC) represents a heterogeneous group of entities, some of which have a genetic basis, most likely caused by a single gene defect (Chapter 17). Clinical evaluation of these patients requires exclusion of numerous metabolic, toxic, or inflammatory processes that may be the primary cause for cardiac failure. As many as 26% of patients with IDC have specific autoantibodies to the heart circulating in their blood. It has been suggested that some of these patients develop autoimmune heart disease. Cardiac-specific anti-alpha-MHC and anti-beta-MHC isoform antibodies have been found in as many as 86% of patients. Specific biochemical defects have also been described, including absence of or significant reduction in the amount of regulatory MLC 2, which may affect both ATPase activity and filament assembly in the myopathic hearts. This effect results from increased activity in a specific but as yet uncharacterized protease that cleaves MLC 2 and inactivates it in these patients.

Electron micrographs of hearts from patients with IDC demonstrate cellular hypertrophy with a dramatic lack of myofibrils in many cellular areas. Cytoskeletal proteins, including the intermediate filament protein desmin, are increased in the diseased myocardium and irregularly distributed within the cells beyond their normal presence at the Z disks (lines). Increased amounts of tubulin and vinculin have also been described, indicating abnormal cytoskeletal reorganization. As expected, increased expression of vimentin, a protein found in connective tissue cells, was found in the interstitial spaces.

Several pedigrees have demonstrated an autosomal dominant pattern of inheritance in patients with IDC. These patients experience cardiomegaly, congestive heart failure, arrhythmias, syncope, and sudden death. Prognosis is highly variable, with some affected individuals remaining asymptomatic for several years. Others die of heart failure and arrhythmias as young adults. Histologically, the affected hearts typically show diffuse fibrosis with severe hypertrophy of the remaining muscle fibers, as demonstrated in sporadic cases of IDC already described. The clinical identification of families and referral for linkage analysis and molecular studies clearly offer the only hope of progress in determining a specific mechanism(s) causing IDC.

An *X-linked cardiomyopathy* was reported in 1987. In this 63-member pedigree the males tend to develop heart failure in their late teens or early 20s with relatively few skeletal muscle manifestations. The females manifest the disease much later in the fifth or sixth decade of life and typically have a very mild form of cardiomyopathy. Linkage analysis has shown that the disease in this pedigree appears to be linked to the proximal (5′) region of the dystrophin gene, the gene responsible for Duchenne and Becker muscular dystrophies. Although no definite abnormalities and dystrophin have been demonstrated, a defect in the dystrophin locus may result in a cardiomyopathy without clinical evidence of skeletal muscle disease.

REFERENCES

Bean BP, Cohne CJ, and Tsien RW: Lidocaine block of cardiac sodium channels. J Gen Physiol 81:613, 1983.

Berko BA and Swift M: X-linked dilated cardiomopathy. N Engl J Med 316:1186, 1987.

Bies RD et al: Expression and localization of dystrophin in human cardiac Purkinje fibers. Circulation 86:147, 1992.

Caforio ALP et al: Identification of α- and β-cardiac myosin heavy chain isoforms as major autoantigens in dilated cardiomyopathy. Circulation 85:1734, 1992.

Darnell J, Lodish H, and Baltimore D, editors: Molecular cell biology, ed 1. New York, 1990, Freeman.

Fu Y-H et al: An unstable triplet repeat in a gene related to myotonic muscular dystrophy. Science 255:1256, 1992.

Keating M et al: Linkage of a cardiac arrhythmia, the long QT syndrome, and the Harvey *ras*-1 gene. Science 252:704, 1991.

Lim CS et al: Direct in vivo gene transfer into the coronary and peripheral vasculatures of the intact dog. Circulation 83:2007, 1991.

Mares A et al: Molecular biology for the cardiologist. Curr Probl Cardiol 17:1, 1992.

Margossian SS et al: Light chain 2 profile and activity of human ventricular myosin during dilated cardiomyopathy: identification of a causal agent for impaired myocardial function. Circulation 85:1720, 1992.

Ozawa T et al: Multiple mitochondrial DNA deletions exist in cardiomyocytes of patients with hypertrophic or dilated cardiomyopathy. Biochem Biophys Rev Commun 170:830, 1990.

Parker TG and Schneider MD: Growth factors, proto-oncogenes, and plasticity of the cardiac phenotype. Annu Rev Physiol 53:173, 1991.

Perryman MB et al: Expression of a missense mutation in the mRNA for B-myosin heavy chain in myocardial tissue in hypertrophic cardiomyopathy. J Clin Invest 90:271, 1990.

Russell DW, Esser V, and Hobbs HH: Molecular basis of familial hypercholesterolemia. Arteriosclerosis 9(suppl I):1, 1989.

Schaper J et al: Impairment of the myocardial ultrastructure and changes of the cytoskeleton in dilated cardiomyopathy. Circulation 83:504, 1991.

Schneider MD and Parker TG: Molecular mechanisms of cardiac growth and hypertrophy: myocardial growth factors and proto-oncogenes in development and disease. In Roberts R, editor: Molecular basis of cardiology, Cambridge, Mass, 1991, Blackwell.

Tanigawa G et al: A molecular basis for familial hypertrophic cardiomyopathy: an α/β cardiac myosin heavy chain hybrid gene. Cell 62:991, 1990.

Towbin JA et al: X-linked cardiomyopathy: molecular genetic evidence of linked to the Duchenne muscular dystrophy locus. Pediatr Res 27:25A, 1990.

Vybiral T et al: Human cardiac and skeletal muscle spectrins: differential expression and localization. Cell Motil Cytoskeleton 21:291, 1992.

II LABORATORY TESTS AND DIAGNOSTIC METHODS

CHAPTER

3 Physical Examination of Cardiovascular System

Joseph K. Perloff

An accurate diagnosis of the nature and extent of a patient's cardiovascular disease often can be obtained by performing a physical examination of the heart and the circulation, including the chest, abdomen, and retina and by recognizing signs of noncardiac diseases that modify or explain the cardiovascular findings. Assessment of the heart and circulation includes five areas: physical appearance, the arterial pulses, the jugular pulse and peripheral veins, the heart's movements (observation, palpation, and percussion of the precordium), and auscultation. The chest (thorax, lungs, pleura), abdomen, and optic fundi typically reflect changes secondary to or associated with cardiac and vascular disorders. The infant, child, or young adult with a cardiac abnormality is likely to be otherwise healthy. With advancing age, however, coexisting noncardiac diseases frequently develop, and their physical signs cannot be ignored if one puts the cardiovascular examination in proper perspective. Not only is systematic identification of physical signs required, but also a synthesis of information based on these signs. No organ system lends itself better than the heart and circulation to a close association among physical signs, structure, and function. Laboratory characterization of cardiovascular anatomy and physiology has validated the accompanying physical signs and in turn has permitted remarkably precise pathophysiologic inferences to be drawn from them. Excitement, satisfaction, and a feeling of confidence and security are generated when an abundance of accurate, practical information is assembled with the unaided senses apart from a stethoscope, a sphygmomanometer, an ophthalmoscope, and a pocket flashlight.

PHYSICAL APPEARANCE

Attention should focus first on the patient's general physical appearance and then on details. Certain distinctive appearances permit accurate prediction of specific coexisting cardiac diseases. The general appearance of patients manifesting the catabolic effects of chronic congestive heart failure is familiar: edematous legs, protruding ascitic abdomen, and muscle wasting of the pectorals, shoulder girdle, and arms. Conversely, acute pulmonary edema is dramatically reflected in the struggling, frightened, diaphoretic patient with dyspnea and tachypnea while sitting bolt upright. The general appearance of the patient with suspected coronary artery disease may be useful, such as a short, balding, mesomorphic, middle-aged, overweight male with nicotine-stained fingers, an ashtray filled with cigarette butts, and bulging briefcases nearby, symbols of deadlines he feels driven to meet.

The physical appearance of the patient with marked obesity is familiar, but obesity with hypersomnolence (Pickwickian syndrome) is associated with *pulmonary* hypertension. Obesity that is principally truncal, with abdominal striae and relatively thin extremities (Cushing syndrome), is accompanied by *systemic* hypertension. The general appearance of the patient with Marfan syndrome (dislocated lenses and hyperextensible joints noted as details) predicts aortic root disease, myxomatous abnormality of the mitral valve, and an ectatic mitral annulus. Cyanosis and clubbing are well recognized but should be characterized not only by their presence and degree but also by their distribution. Cyanosis and clubbing of the toes with sparing of the fingers mean reversed shunt through a patent ductus arteriosus that joins the aorta distal to the left subclavian artery. Down syndrome is readily recognized and predicts the presence of an endocardial cushion defect. In the female with short stature, webbing of the neck, sexual infantilism (absent or scanty pubic and axillary hair), wide-set nipples, low hairline, small chin, and wide-carrying angle of the arms (Turner syndrome), bicuspid aortic valve and coarctation of the aorta are often present.

Gestures and *gait* may be important features of physical appearance. A clenched fist pressed against the sternum is a time-honored gesticulation used to describe the oppressive pain of myocardial infarction. The importance of gait was emphasized by James Mackenzie (Perloff JK, 1990), who wrote, "When the patient presents . . . for examination, the physician naturally scrutinizes him and makes a mental note of his gait . . . and how he deports himself generally." Today, however, physicians (except neurologists) seldom pointedly observe their patients' walk, even though an abnormal gait may be the first evidence of a systemic neuromuscular disease with cardiac involvement. The child with classic Duchenne muscular dystrophy has a characteristic clumsy, waddling walk caricatured by the exaggerated lumbar lordosis and protuberant abdomen; myocardial dystrophy (predictably posterobasal left ventricular wall) is frequently present. An ataxic gait accompanied by pes cavus and hammer toe is typical of Friedreich's ataxia, in which cardiac involvement takes the form of hypertrophic cardiomyopathy or less often, dilated cardiomyopathy.

Detailed physical appearance can be of equal diagnostic importance. Coronary artery disease is suspected from certain minor details (e.g., corneal arcus and ear lobe creases) and certain major details (e.g., cutaneous and tendon xanthomas). Some xanthomas (dorsum of the hand) are not recognizable unless the fingers are gently flexed, imparting subcutaneous motion to the dorsal tendons. The diagnosis of infective endocarditis benefits from identification of such details as petechiae, Osler's nodes, and Janeway lesions. In patients with pulmonary arteriovenous fistulas, the most distinctive detailed appearance is coexisting mucocutaneous telangiectasia (tiny ruby lesions on the face, nasal and oral mucous membranes, tongue, lips, skin, and nailbeds). Ulnar deviation of the fingers and thick interphalangeal joints identifies rheumatoid arthritis and warrants careful auscultation for the soft, diastolic murmur of mild aortic regurgitation. In Jaccoud arthritis, patients' hands superficially resemble those of patients with rheumatoid arthritis, but the fingers can easily be moved into correct alignment (correction of the ulnar deviation); no thickening of the interphalangeal joints occurs, and accompanying rheumatic mitral and aortic regurgitation is likely. Vitiligo, especially if symmetric, sometimes occurs with hyperthyroidism and may prove diagnostically useful in older patients with apathetic Graves disease, atrial fibrillation, and heart failure.

Examination of the eye's internal appearance requires an ophthalmoscope. Skilled use of this instrument is therefore a necessary part of the cardiac and vascular physical examination. The optic fundi provide unique access to the appearance of small arteries, arterioles, veins, venules, and capillaries. The appearance of patients with hypertensive retinopathy includes increased light reflex, copper wire appearance, arteriovenous nicking, increased tortuosity, and irregular caliber of the arterioles (permanent or relatively permanent changes), accompanied at times by hemorrhages, exudates, "cotton-wool" patches, and papilledema (changes that tend to disappear with control of blood pressure). Less well known is the distinctive appearance of retinal arteries when hypertension results from coarctation of the aorta: tortuous, frequent "U turns" but not the aforementioned changes of hypertensive retinopathy. In patients with cyanotic congenital heart disease, retinal veins are large in caliber, even toward the periphery, a pattern related to the increase in red cell mass. The occasional papilledema and retinal edema are responses to the decrease in arterial oxygen saturation.

Retinal arterial emboli sometimes have distinctive appearances that reflect their origins. Calcific emboli tend to be dull, white, and close to the disc margin. Lipid emboli are yellowish and are seen peripherally, especially at bifurcations. Cholesterol emboli (Hollenhorst plaques) are highly refractile. Fibrin-platelet emboli appear as whitish plugs that are sometimes seen moving through the retinal arteries.

In the retina of patients with infective endocarditis, boat-shaped hemorrhages should be distinguished from Roth spots, which have a cotton-wool appearance (perivascular collections of lymphocytes in the retina's nerve layer) surrounded by hemorrhage. However, these distinctive retinal signs now occur relatively infrequently.

ARTERIAL PULSES

Examination

The ancient art of feeling the pulse can be applied in contemporary context to considerable diagnostic advantage. The radial, brachial, carotid, femoral, dorsalis pedis, and posterior tibial pulses are all accessible and should be palpated routinely. Technique is important. For the radials, brachials, carotids, and femorals, tactile impression is heightened by palpation with a single digit, preferably the thumb. When two pulses are compared (right and left or upper and lower extremity), both arteries should be palpated at the same time or in rapid succession. The alternating method is appropriate for the carotids, which should not be compressed simultaneously.

In assessing the pulse's quality, the brachials and carotids are preferred because their waveform is more likely to reflect the central aortic pulse. Sitting comfortably at the patient's right side, the examiner can support the subject's relaxed elbow with the right hand, freeing that thumb to explore the antecubital fossa for the brachial pulse (Fig. 3-1). The elbow's optimum position can be determined by gently raising the patient's forearm while simultaneously palpating the brachial pulse. Similarly, the examiner can place the right thumb comfortably on the patient's left carotid artery, a position that also permits subsequent timing of the contralateral jugular venous pulse (Fig. 3-2). Once the thumb is in place, the degree of pressure applied to the artery should be varied until the maximum pulsation is elicited.

Digital pulses can be conveniently assessed when the examiner's fingertips gently grip the patient's fingertips. This technique is sufficiently sensitive to identify occasionally even normal digital pulses. Assessment of digital pulsations is enhanced by transilluminating a fingertip with a small flashlight in a dark room while inspecting the nailbed for cyclic blanching synchronous with the pulse.

Nonpalpable but otherwise normal dorsalis pedis and posterior tibial pulses can sometimes be identified after the vasodilator effect of sublingual nitroglycerin. When feeling or assessing radial pulses is difficult, Allen's test is useful. Radial and ulnar arteries are simultaneously compressed by the examiner's two thumbs while the patient vigorously opens and closes the fist to induce blanching of the palm. Selective arterial refilling is judged by the rate of

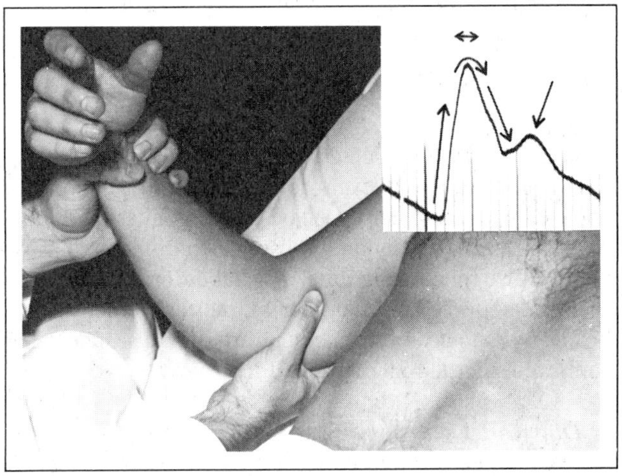

Fig. 3-1. Technique for palpating the right brachial arterial pulse with the examiner's right thumb. The patient's arm is in a relaxed position. The insert shows a normal brachial arterial pulse, with attention to ascending limb, crest, and descending limb. The dicrotic wave *(last arrow)* is not normally felt.

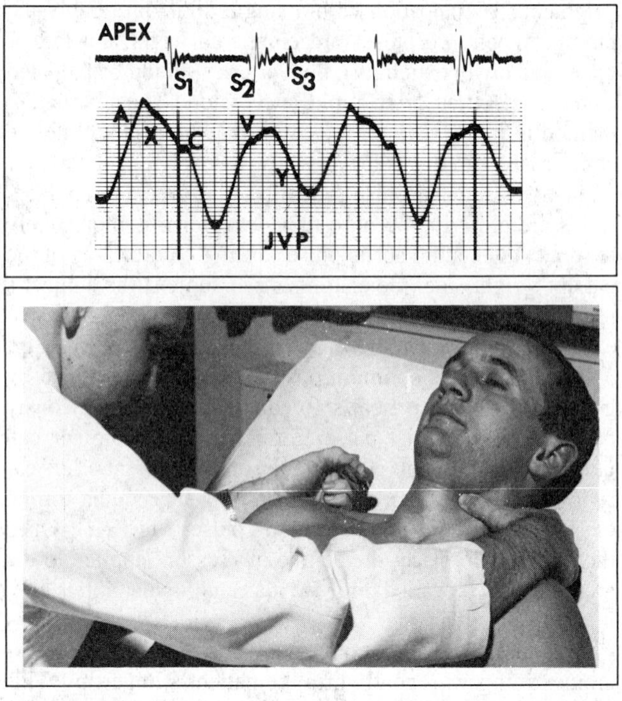

Fig. 3-2. Upper tracing shows simultaneous phonocardiogram and normal jugular venous pulse *(JVP)*. The jugular pulse is characterized by an *A* wave and *X* descent and a *V* wave and *Y* descent. The *C* wave is the movement imparted by the carotid pulse. S_1, S_2, and S_3 are the first, second, and third heart sounds, respectively. The photograph shows a recommended technique for observing the JVP. The examiner's right thumb gently palpates the patient's left carotid artery for timing purposes. The examiner's left hand holds a pocket flashlight, the beam of which is directed obliquely across the patient's right neck, throwing the undulations of the JVP into bolder relief. The patient's trunk is adjusted from the horizontal to provide maximum excursion of the deep jugular vein.

color return to the opened, but not hyperextended, palm as pressure is sequentially released from the radial and ulnar arteries.

Information

Rate and rhythm. Impressions of rate and rhythm of arterial pulses are useful even though that information can be obtained by more precise methods. An irregular rhythm increases interest in subsequent observation of the jugular venous pulse, anticipating atrial fibrillation or multiple ventricular ectopic beats. Occasionally, pulsus alternans is sufficiently pronounced to halve the arterial pulse rate when compared with the rate at the cardiac apex.

Differential pulsations. The most frequent cause of selective diminution or absence of an arterial pulse, especially in carotids and femorals, is occlusive atherosclerotic vascular disease. In this context, attention should be directed to pulses not routinely palpated, the subclavians (above the clavicle) and the popliteals. Assessment of lower extremity (distal) blood flow in patients with peripheral vascular disease benefits from observing the rate of arterial refilling in each foot by raising the legs (blanching) with the patient lying supine, then lowering the legs over the bedside while the differential rates of refilling are observed in the feet and toes. The presence and degree of dependent rubor is another indication of the adequacy or inadequacy of distal lower extremity arterial blood flow.

Comparative palpation of two pulses (paired upper extremity pulses or upper and lower extremity pulses) can yield important diagnostic information. To detect coarctation of the aorta, simultaneous palpation of brachial and femoral arteries is advised. In patients with mild coarctation the femoral arteries may be readily perceived and initially considered normal until simultaneous comparison with the brachial pulse reveals a diagnostic difference in timing and pulse pressure. If coarctation involves the left subclavian artery, the left brachial pulse is conspicuously smaller than the right, and unilateral notching of the right ribs can be anticipated on the chest radiograph. Isolated diminution of the left brachial pulse arouses suspicion of a subclavian "steal" and requires palpation of the subclavian artery on the same side. In the presence of aortic stenosis, conspicuous asymmetry of the carotid and brachial pulses (right greater than left) implies that the obstruction is supravalvular.

For routine indirect determination of blood pressure at the bedside, the sphygmomanometer compression cuff, the hand-operated rubber bulb for inflation, and the adjustable valve for cuff deflation should be in perfect working order. The inflatable rubber bag must be contained completely within a sealed inelastic cuff that permits secure application and that exerts an even pressure over the area to which it is applied. The width of the compression cuff within its inelastic covering should be about 20% greater than the limb's diameter or about half the limb's circumference (American Heart Association standards). The manometer can be either mercury or aneroid.

Brachial arterial pressure is routinely determined with the patient lying comfortably in the supine position and the arm at approximately the level of the heart. Blood pressure should be taken in both arms because the systolic tends to be higher in the right arm (as much as 15 mm Hg in adults). It is useful to palpate the brachial artery while inflating the cuff 20 to 30 mm Hg above the pressure required to obliterate the pulse. The adjustable screw valve is then used for controlled deflation, with the peak systolic pressure identified by the appearance of clear Korotkoff sounds for two or more consecutive beats. Continued deflation of the cuff determines the diastolic pressure, which can be considered as either the level of abrupt muffling of Korotkoff sounds or the level at which these sounds vanish. The disappearance point is recommended because it is more reproducible when sequential observations by the same examiner are compared, when one observer's findings are compared with another's, or when results are compared with intra-arterial diastolic pressure. When the pulse pressure is wide, however, the point of muffling is closer to the intra-arterial diastolic pressure. If the difference between muffling and disappearance of Korotkoff sounds is considerable, both pressures should be recorded in addition to the systolic.

If cuff deflation is too slow, venous congestion serves to elevate diastolic pressure and decrease the intensity of Korotkoff sounds so that systolic pressure is underestimated and diastolic pressure overestimated. The cuff should be deflated rapidly after the diastolic blood pressure is determined, and at least 1 minute should pass before blood pressure determinations are repeated in the same limb.

If Korotkoff sounds are difficult to hear in the brachial artery, audibility is improved by having the patient open and close the fist vigorously six times. A silence occasionally separates the initial appearance of Korotkoff sounds from reappearance at a lower level. This silence is called the *auscultatory gap*. The clinical importance of the auscultatory gap lies in misjudging systolic pressure when the sphygmomanometer cuff is inflated to a level within the gap itself. This error is avoided by inflating the cuff to 20 or 30 mm Hg above the level necessary to obliterate the brachial pulse (see earlier discussion).

A prevailing misconception concerns the accuracy of sphygmomanometer determinations of brachial arterial pressure in patients with obese arms. Error is unlikely or minimal, however, when the compression cuff is the appropriate size, as noted earlier, and exerts an even pressure over the enclosed area. Errors arise when an inflatable bag fails to enclose the arm or bulges through its inelastic cover. These faulty or poorly fitting cuffs result in spuriously high arterial pressure readings.

If the only available cuff does not adequately encircle the arm, the cuff can be applied to the forearm while the stethoscope is applied to the radial artery for the detection of Korotkoff sounds. This technique is appropriate for a forearm of relatively uniform circumference (cylindrical) but not when a conical forearm prevents uniform cuff application. Properly determined forearm blood pressure is a reasonable estimate of brachial arterial blood pressure.

In adults, especially those beyond middle age, brachial arterial pressure should be recorded both supine and standing. When a normal person assumes an upright position, at most a transient decline in systolic pressure of 5 to 15 mm Hg occurs, whereas diastolic pressure tends to rise. These changes are accompanied by slight reflex tachycardia.

The seemingly outmoded technique of palpation for estimating arterial pressure occasionally serves a useful purpose in modern bedside monitoring. Palpation prevents the examiner from being misled by the auscultatory gap. Systolic and diastolic pressures can be estimated by palpation when Korotkoff sounds are indistinct or inaudible. The cuff should first be inflated in the standard manner 20 to 30 mm Hg above the level required to obliterate the brachial pulse. When the cuff is slowly deflated, the approximate peak systolic pressure is that level at which a palpable brachial pulse first consistently reappears. The diastolic pressure is then estimated by detecting the distinctive snapping quality of the palpable pulse as the cuff is deflated further.

It is sometimes useful to determine blood pressure in the legs. Interestingly, when *intra-arterial* brachial and femoral pressures are compared in normal subjects, there is no significant difference in systolic, diastolic, or mean pressure, but the *auscultatory systolic* femoral pressure is about 10 mm Hg higher than the intra-arterial measurement. Upper extremity blood pressure is routinely taken in the supine position, but lower extremity blood pressure using the popliteal artery is recorded with the patient prone. A cuff of appropriate size and fit is applied to the thigh. Slow inflation is important to avoid discomfort, if not pain, induced by rapid compression of the thigh. Systolic and diastolic pressures are then estimated by auscultation of Korotkoff sounds in the popliteal fossa, as described for the brachial artery. Only systolic popliteal Korotkoff sounds may be clearly delineated. If this technique proves unsatisfactory, the patient can be returned to the supine position and a cuff of appropriate size (often an arm cuff) applied to the calf's lower half. Korotkoff sounds can then be sought by applying the stethoscope's bell to the dorsalis pedis or posterior tibial artery first identified by palpation.

Arterial thrills. The neck should be examined for thrills. Palpation must be selective over the carotid and subclavian arteries and in the suprasternal notch. Brachiocephalic arterial thrills originate from three sources. The most frequent, and perhaps the most important, source is atherosclerotic obstruction. The second is transmitted murmurs within the thorax, especially the murmur of valvular aortic stenosis. The third source is at the origins of the brachiocephalic arteries of perfectly normal, healthy children and young adults with loud, innocent supraclavicular systolic murmurs that attenuate or vanish with hyperextension of the shoulders.

Waveform. Analysis of waveform is one of the most important uses of the arterial pulse. For this purpose the brachials and carotids are, with few exceptions, the most useful because they reflect the central aortic pulse more closely than do peripheral pulses, which are damped and distorted. A clear appreciation of the tactile impression of a normal arterial pulse requires experience based on repeated assessments in healthy patients of all ages under varying conditions of relaxation and tension. Specific attention should be paid to the ascending limb, the peak, and the descending limb (see Fig. 3-1). Normally, the examiner appreciates a smooth, uninterrupted, but not abrupt upstroke, a single unsustained peak, and a discernible but not abrupt downstroke; the dicrotic wave is not normally felt.

To detect pulsus alternans, the femoral and radial pulses have the advantage of peripheral amplification that is not compromised by waveform distortion. Each beat should be compared with the next during quiet respiration to detect the cyclic differences characteristic of pulsus alternans. What the examiner feels is a variation in the rate of rise rather than a definable difference in pulse pressure. Alternation may affect every other beat or, more often, is variable from beat to beat. Pulsus alternans is often precipitated or augmented by an ectopic ventricular beat, which the examiner should deliberately anticipate in order to take advantage of analysis of the next beats.

Detection of pulsus paradoxus requires comparison of quality and amplitude during quiet respiration to identify the inspiratory decline in pulse pressure. Deep inspiration in some normal people causes a perceptible fall in systemic pulse pressure, but the slight inspiratory fall during quiet respiration is not detected in patients with normal hearts. Casual inspiration in a healthy person results in no more than a 3 to 4 mm Hg decline in systolic pressure; even relatively deep inspiration causes a decline not exceeding 10 mm Hg. The term *pulsus paradoxus* applies when the inspiratory decrease *exceeds* 10 mm Hg.

In patients with cardiac disease, the paradoxical pulse occurs most frequently with pericardial tamponade and less often with chronic constrictive pericarditis. In both of these disorders, inspiration is accompanied by abnormal decreases in systolic *and* diastolic pressures, reflecting an exaggerated inspiratory decline in left ventricular volume. The most common noncardiac cause of pulsus paradoxus is pulmonary emphysema. The decrease in lung compliance (stiff lungs) exaggerates the normal inspiratory fall in left ventricular volume and in systolic and diastolic arterial pressures. When airway obstruction (bronchospasm) coexists, the respiratory effects on the pulse are even greater because inspiration continues to cause an exaggerated fall in systolic and diastolic pressures, whereas exhalation is accompanied by an exaggerated *rise* in systolic pressure *above* normal, as in phase II of the Valsalva maneuver.

To elicit a paradoxical pulse, the patient should be positioned comfortably with the trunk raised to a level that minimizes the amplitude of respiratory excursions. Specific instructions should be given to breathe as regularly and quietly as comfort permits. The examiner's thumb should be applied to the brachial arterial pulse with enough compression to elicit the maximum systolic impact. Compression is gradually released while the examiner observes the patient's respiratory movements by glancing at the chest or abdomen. As pressure on the brachial artery decreases in a gradual stepwise manner, a level is reached at which the pulse diminishes or even vanishes during inspiration. The paradoxical pulse can often be elicited with a sphygmomanometer whether or not an abnormal decrease is detected by palpation. In fact, the paradox is even more readily detected with a sphygmomanometer. The cuff is inflated above systolic pressure. Korotkoff sounds are sought over the brachial artery while the cuff is deflated at a rate of approximately 2 to 3 mm Hg per heartbeat. The peak systolic pressure during expiration should first be identified and reconfirmed. The cuff is then deflated very slowly to establish the pressure at which Korotkoff sounds become audible during *both* inspiration and expiration. When the difference between these two observed levels reaches or exceeds 10 mm Hg during quiet respiration, a paradoxical pulse is present.

A small arterial pulse implies a decrease in pulse pressure. If the peak is unsustained, the low pulse pressure is likely to reflect the reduced ventricular stroke volume of heart failure. If the rate of rise is slow, the peak sustained, and the downstroke imperceptible, the likely cause is valvular aortic stenosis. On the other hand, a normal pulse pressure with a brisk rate of rise is a feature of pure mitral regurgitation, ventricular septal defect, or some forms of hypertrophic cardiomyopathy. The term *small water-hammer pulse* has been associated with the latter conditions. The more frequent use of the term *water-hammer pulse* applies to an abnormally abrupt upstroke, an unsustained peak, and a rapid collapse with a wide pulse pressure characteristic of aortic regurgitation. Corrigan's pulse (free aortic regurgitation) often imparts a to-and-fro ballistic movement to the head. The large water-hammer pulse is readily visible, especially in the neck, as Corrigan originally described.

The normal arterial pulse has a single systolic crest. The most common cause of twin peaking is the pulsus bisferiens of moderate to marked aortic regurgitation. Twin peaking also occurs in hypertrophic obstructive cardiomyopathy but with a normal pulse pressure. A third type of twin peaking, the least common, results from a single systolic crest followed by a palpable dicrotic wave (the dicrotic pulse).

JUGULAR PULSE AND PERIPHERAL VEINS

Method of examining jugular venous pulse

Information derived from examination of the jugular veins includes (1) waveform and pressure, (2) anatomic-physiologic inferences, and (3) arrhythmias and conduction defects. The deep (internal) and superficial (external) jugular veins provide convenient, accurate, reproducible means of assessing right atrial pressure and waveform. Since the jugular veins normally are passively distended in the supine position, the patient's trunk must be elevated to the level at which excursions of the *deep* jugular veins are maximal, generally about 35 to 45 degrees above the horizontal (see Fig. 3-2). The patient's head can then be adjusted upward or to either side by gently moving the chin, but the head should not be tilted too far upward or turned too sharply, because these maneuvers tense the sternocleidomastoid muscle and compress or obliterate the underlying deep jugular vein. An oblique light source should be directed across the area under examination to highlight the venous waves. It is convenient for the examiner to place the right thumb on the patient's left carotid artery while inspecting the venous pulsations on the opposite side (see Fig. 3-2). The free left hand can adjust the beam of a pocket flashlight. The superficial jugular vein is readily recognized because it distends as a column when the vessel is compressed just above the clavicle. When compression is released, the crest of the distended column falls to a level approximating the mean right atrial pressure. This procedure is not needed when the venous pressure is elevated.

Deep jugular venous pulsations must be distinguished from the carotid pulse. Pulsations asynchronous with the carotid cannot be arterial and therefore must be venous. The carotid pulse is palpable, but the venous pulse is not. Carotid pressure remains the same or falls slightly with inspiration, whereas the jugular venous A wave and X descent become more prominent, despite the fall in mean right atrial pressure. Venous pulsations cease if the deep jugular vein is compressed at the root of the neck; the pressure required does not affect the carotid pulsation. Abdominal compression with the palm may transiently augment venous but not arterial pulsations. The compression need not be in the right upper quadrant (hepatojugular reflux). Technique is important because sudden abdominal compression provokes a Valsalva response, which abruptly elevates the central venous pressure. Compression should be firm but gradual.

Jugular venous waveform

The deep jugular vein pulsates in response to phasic changes in right atrial pressure. Individual components of the venous pulse can be identified by timing with readily accessible clinical references, especially the carotid pulse (see Fig. 3-2) but also the heart sounds. It is more practical to time the venous pulse initially with the carotid so that the physical examination is not interrupted for auscultatory orientation. During subsequent auscultation the venous pulse can be reassessed if necessary to confirm or identify specific features that remain unresolved using the carotid reference alone.

Two positive venous waves (crests) and two descents (troughs) occur in each normal cardiac cycle (see Fig. 3-2). The first positive wave is the A wave of atrial contraction immediately preceding the carotid pulse. The first trough—the X descent, or descending limb of the A wave—is interrupted by the carotid pulse with which it coincides. The second positive wave, the V wave of passive atrial filling, follows the carotid pulse by a perceptible interval. The second trough, the Y descent, is clearly diastolic and represents the descending limb of the V wave. The Y descent begins early in diastole as the tricuspid valve opens and right atrial pressure falls passively.

Timing of the jugular pulse with heart sound references requires selection of a precordial site where the first and second sounds are easily heard. The examiner holds the stethoscope in place with the right hand while a source of oblique light is adjusted with the left hand. The A wave coincides with or immediately precedes the first heart sound. The Y descent begins just after the second sound, when the tricuspid valve opens.

Jugular venous pressure

The vertical levels (crests) of the A wave, V wave, and superficial jugular vein are determined after the patient's trunk has been elevated above the horizontal to an angle coinciding with the maximum excursion of the deep jugular vein. The sternal angle of Louis is the most suitable reference for quantifying the crests of the waves. A centimeter ruler serves as a measure and should be placed vertically at the sternal angle with a tongue blade crossing perpendicularly at the level of the wave crest under study. Height in centimeters above the sternal angle is then read. Although the superficial jugular vein usually reliably reflects mean right atrial pressure, venoconstriction occasionally collapses the vessel despite an elevated venous pressure. If the measured heights of the waveforms are normal or borderline, additional information can be gained by observing the response to gradual sustained abdominal compression—abdominojugular reflux. Compression is maintained for at least 30 seconds (at most 60 seconds) while the external and internal jugular veins are scrutinized. Normally, in response to augmented venous return, prominence of the external jugular vein and the crests and troughs of the internal jugular transiently increase (for a few beats) (see previous discussion). This initial increase is followed promptly by a fall to control levels as abdominal compression continues. In patients with right ventricular failure, the initial rise in jugular venous pressure is *not* followed by a prompt fall but instead is maintained during the entire 30 to 60 seconds of compression.

Abnormal jugular venous waveforms

Conduction defects and arrhythmias are sometimes diagnosed from the jugular pulse with surprising precision. In sinus rhythm, an A wave precedes each carotid pulse. Prolongation of the A wave to carotid (C) interval reflects prolongation of the P-R interval. Progressive prolongation of the A-C interval ending in an A wave without a palpable carotid pulse reflects the progressive P-R interval prolongation and nonconducted beat of Wenckebach second-degree atrioventricular block. The A wave disappears in atrial fibrillation, occurs twice as often as the carotid pulse in 2:1 heart block, and amplifies synchronously with the carotid pulse in junctional rhythms. In complete heart block, A waves bear no constant relationship to the carotid pulse, but when right atrial contraction fortuitously coincides with a closed tricuspid valve (synchronous with ventricular contraction), the A wave amplifies, producing intermittent "cannon" waves.

Anatomic and physiologic inferences can be drawn from the jugular venous pulse and represent some of the most important insights gained from it. A giant A wave means that a hypertrophied right atrium is contracting against an increased resistance, either within the right atrium (myxoma), at the tricuspid valve (tricuspid stenosis), or in the thick-walled, hypertrophied right ventricle of pulmonary hypertension or isolated pulmonic stenosis. In the normal right atrial pulse the A wave is slightly dominant, whereas in the normal left atrium, A and V crests are equal. When the two atria are in common communication (large ostium secundum atrial septal defect), the right atrial pressure pulse resembles the left; that is, the A and V crests are equal. In patients with right ventricular failure, the mean right atrial pressure rises, and the crests of the A and V waves rise with it. The X and Y descents become brisker. This waveform reaches its ultimate expression in constrictive pericarditis, in which A waves and V waves are so high that their crests are not clearly delineated, whereas the brisk X and Y descents dominate the venous pulse. In either case—severe right ventricular failure or constrictive pericarditis—examination benefits from observation of the jugular pulse with the patient sitting upright or even standing. In tricuspid regurgitation with sinus rhythm, the X descent is first decreased, then obliterated as the V wave increases and the Y descent becomes brisker. With severe tricuspid regurgitation the venous pulse is represented by a large systolic venous (V) wave and a collapsing Y descent. A tall V wave with gradual Y descent implies obstruction to right atrial flow, as in patients who have tricuspid stenosis with atrial fibrillation.

Peripheral veins

Examination of peripheral veins generally focuses on the lower extremities, but the axillary veins should not be ignored. Much information can be gathered from inspection alone. Asymmetric leg edema can be seen and confirmed by simple digital pressure to elicit pitting. Assessment of superficial veins for distention (varices) is incomplete unless the veins are examined with the patient standing. In chronic venous stasis, the overlying skin tends to have a reddish, cyanotic hue or may be discolored by brownish pigmentation; stasis ulcers appear over the malleoli. In patients with acute superficial thrombophlebitis, a red subcutaneous chord is sometimes visible. Palpation provides further information. The skin is usually warm, and overlying muscle may be indurated, especially the calf. The phlebitic vein is generally tender to touch, or deep compression may reveal tenderness. In applying pressure, care must be taken to avoid squeezing the calf; instead, pressure should be applied with the fingers against the calves and in Hunter's canal. The visible red chord is usually palpable as tender induration along the course of the subcutaneous vein. Homans sign (calf pain elicited by forced dorsiflexion of the foot) is unreliable because of the frequency of both false-positive and false-negative responses.

PRECORDIAL PALPATION AND MOVEMENTS

Most of the important movements transmitted by the heart can be palpated or seen. Information so obtained includes (1) systolic movements caused by the ventricles, (2) vibrations or movements caused by heart sounds, and (3) transmitted vibrations of murmurs (i.e., thrills). Percussion usually supplies little additional information, but before beginning methodic palpation, it is important to percuss briefly to identify visceral situs: left thoracic heart, left stomach, and right liver (situs solitus); right thoracic heart, right stomach, and left liver (situs inversus); or right thoracic heart, left stomach, and right liver (situs inversus with dextrocardia).

Palpation should be conducted systematically and is preceded by careful observation of precordial movements, which are sometimes more readily seen than felt. An oblique light serves to emphasize the movements, which can be brought into further relief by putting an ink mark (X) on the skin at the site under observation (Fig. 3-3, *A*). The visualized movements can then be timed with the carotid pulse or the heart sounds. With experience, the examiner can determine not only whether an impulse is systolic or diastolic but whether the impulse occurs in middiastole, presystole, early systole, or late systole. For observation and palpation, each of the following sites should be interrogated, although not necessarily routinely: apex, left and right sternal borders (interspace by interspace from first to fifth), subxiphoid, suprasternal notch, right sternoclavicular junction, and ectopic sites, especially above the cardiac apex. Each movement should be sought first with the flat portion of the fingers, then with the fingertips, and finally as precisely as possible with the tip of the first or second finger. Parasternal impulses (right ventricle, pulmonary trunk, ascending aorta) are appreciated better during exhalation and are best analyzed with the patient supine. How-

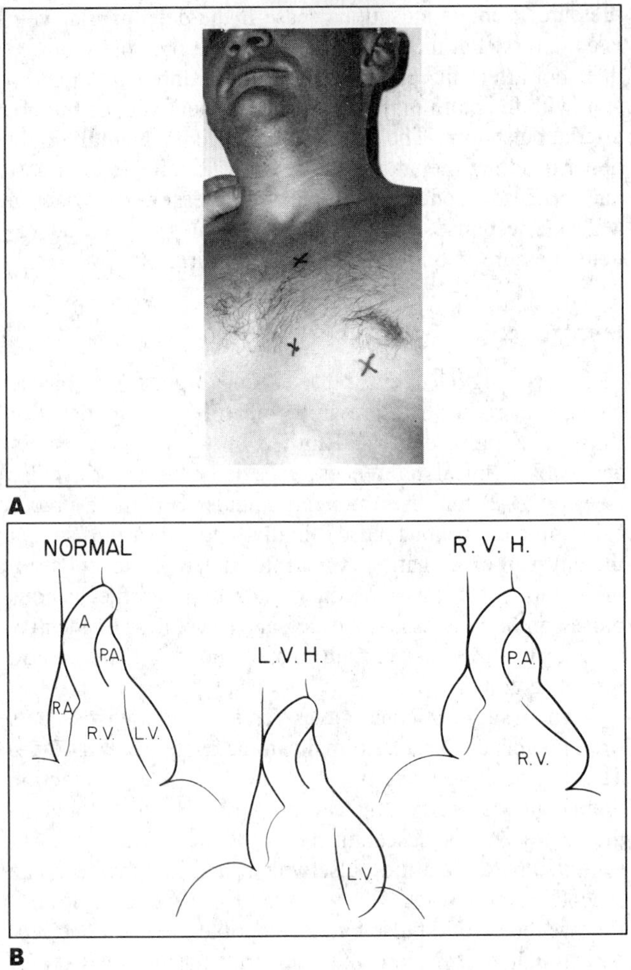

Fig. 3-3. A, Photograph showing how the sites of left ventricular, right ventricular, and pulmonary arterial impulses can be marked and timed. The examiner's thumb is on the patient's right carotid pulse for timing purposes. **B,** Topographic anatomy of the normal heart and of hypertrophy of the left *(LV)* and right *(RV)* ventricles. Normally the LV occupies the apex, yielding a gentle, unsustained anterior systolic movement with medial retraction (interventricular sulcus dividing RV from LV, as illustrated). With LV hypertrophy *(LVH)* the LV occupies the apex but yields a more sustained (pressure overload) or dynamic (volume overload) impulse with medial retraction. With RV hypertrophy *(RVH)* the RV may occupy the apex, yielding a left sternal edge systolic impulse with apical retraction. A dilated main pulmonary artery *(PA)* is sometimes palpated. *RA,* Right atrium.

ever, apical movements are best defined with the patient in a partial left lateral decubitus position.

Systolic movements of ventricles

Identification, localization, and characterization of ventricular movements should replace the imprecise term *point of maximum impulse;* recognition of left and right ventricular impulses is essential (Fig. 3-3, *B*).

When the *left* ventricle forms the apex, a positive systolic movement with medial retraction identifies the plane of the ventricular septum (interventricular sulcus) and confirms that the lateral impulse is left ventricular (LV). Although the quality of the LV impulse is more accurately assessed with the patient in the left lateral decubitus position, LV size is best estimated by returning the patient to the supine position while keeping a finger over the ventricle. Normally the LV impulse is a gentle, localized tap; excitement or exercise increases its prominence but not its duration. As stroke volume and ejection rate increase, the impulse becomes appropriately quick, abrupt, and dynamic; as resistance to LV ejection increases, the impulse becomes sustained and heaving.

Right ventricular (RV) movement is assessed at the left sternal border (third through fifth interspaces) and subxiphoid. The infundibulum underlies the third left interspace, and the RV body underlies the fourth and fifth interspaces. If the examining hand is placed beneath the xiphoid and directed upward toward the left hemidiaphragm, the right ventricle imparts an impulse to the fingertips. A brief, tapping RV impulse is normal at birth and is occasionally found in normal children and young adults with thin chest walls.

In patients with small, linear hearts the LV impulse is close to the sternal edge and may be difficult to distinguish from a RV impulse until the patient is turned into the left lateral position. The heart then moves away from the midline, so the left ventricle can be identified as such by observing medial retraction not apparent with the patient supine. As the right ventricle enlarges, normal left sternal border retraction is replaced by a positive systolic impulse with *lateral* retraction (Fig. 3-3, *B*). A pure RV impulse causes positive movement at the left sternal edge, with retraction at the apex. A pure LV impulse causes positive movement at the apex with medial retraction. With combined ventricular impulses, the positive movements at the apex and left sternal edge are separated by an area of retraction in the region of the interventricular sulcus.

Impulses of aorta, pulmonary trunk, and dilated atria

A dilated aortic root may cause a distinct impulse in the second or third right interspace (aortic aneurysm), and a right aortic arch may cause subtle right sternoclavicular systolic movement. Systolic distention of an enlarged pulmonary trunk transmits an impulse to the second left interspace (Fig. 3-3, *B*).

Systolic expansion of dilated atria, especially in patients with mitral or tricuspid regurgitation, may impart distinctive movements to the chest wall. The left atrium is a posterior chamber, so systolic expansion moves the heart forward; the rigid vertebral column serves as an immobile fulcrum, limiting posterior displacement. The movement may be mistaken for an intrinsic RV impulse, but left atrial expansion occurs perceptibly later than impulses imparted by either ventricle. This subtle difference in timing can sometimes be detected by simultaneously timing the first heart sound with the stethoscope. Systolic expansion of an enlarged right atrium with systolic movement of a large right hepatic lobe causes dramatic late systolic movement of the entire right lower chest in patients with gross tricuspid regurgitation.

Palpable heart sounds and murmurs

Heart sounds may be palpable because of their vibrations' intensity or their discrete precordial movements. The loud first heart sound (S_1) of mitral stenosis is generally felt over the LV impulse. Pulmonic ejection sounds are palpated in the second left interspace and may increase with exhalation and decrease with inhalation. The impact of the pulmonic component of the second heart sound (P_2) (pulmonary hypertension) is characteristically identified in the second left interspace, although this sound may be palpated as a tap in some normal children and thin young adults. An augmented atrial contribution to ventricular filling is characterized by presystolic distention of either the left or the right ventricle and may be more readily detected by palpation than by the auscultatory counterpart (fourth heart sound, S_4). Rapid ventricular filling is sometimes associated with LV middiastolic distention, corresponding to an abnormal third heart sound (S_3). A physiologic or normal S_3 is rarely palpable or visible.

A palpable murmur is defined as a *thrill*. It is therefore redundant to use the term *palpable thrill*. Murmurs that reach grade IV (of VI) usually transmit their vibrations through the chest wall. A thrill is best characterized according to its site of maximum intensity, the direction of its radiation, and its duration. Thrills should be sought at precordial sites and in the neck (suprasternal notch, subclavians; see earlier discussion). Thrills are often better appreciated with the heads of the metacarpal bones than with the fingertips, but the hand should not be arched when the metacarpals are applied because this decreases cutaneous sensitivity.

AUSCULTATION

Accurate cardiac auscultation requires a quiet room, a comfortable patient, and a good stethoscope equipped with bell, diaphragm, and well-fitting earpieces. Auscultation should be conducted in the supine, sitting, and left lateral positions and should be performed during appropriate physical and respiratory maneuvers.

S_1 and S_2 establish the framework within which murmurs and additional sounds can be placed. If the stethoscope is applied to the chest with the right hand, the thumb

Systolic Sounds

1. Early systolic
   a. Ejection sounds (aortic/pulmonic)
   b. Aortic prosthetic valve sounds
2. Mid/late systolic
   a. Mitral clicks
   b. "Remnants of rubs"

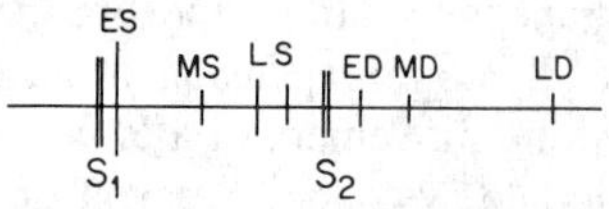

Diastolic Sounds

1. Early diastolic
   a. Opening sounds (snaps)
   b. Early S_3 (EDS of constrictive pericarditis, ventricular knock of mitral regurgitation)
   c. Mitral prosthetic valve opening
   d. "Tumor plop"
2. Middiastolic
   a. Third heart sounds
   b. Summation sounds (S_3 + S_4)
3. Late diastolic (presystolic)
   a. Fourth heart sounds
   b. Pacemaker sounds

Fig. 3-4. The first *(S_1)* and second *(S_2)* heart sounds form the auscultatory framework within which additional sounds can be placed. *ES,* Early systolic; *MS,* midsystolic; *LS,* late systolic; *ED (EDS),* early diastolic (sounds); *MD,* middiastolic; *LD,* late diastolic.

of the left hand is free to palpate the carotid pulse, which times the first sound, even at rapid heart rates. Alternatively, S_1 and S_2 can be identified at the heart's base, where cadence and comparative intensities often make recognition easier. The stethoscope is then moved stepwise toward the sternal edge and apex, so that the timing established at the base is not lost.

Once the framework of the cardiac cycle has been fixed, auscultatory events should be analyzed sequentially: S_1, early systole, midsystole, late systole, S_2, early diastole, middiastole, and presystole (Figs. 3-4 and 3-5). The topographic sequence of auscultation is best related to the normal direction of blood flow, that is, the inflow valves (apex and lower left sternal edge), followed by the outflow valves (left and right bases). Consistent use of the same sequence minimizes the chance of oversight. Attention should also be directed to nonprecordial sites, including the axilla, back, neck, and abdomen.

Heart sounds

Heart sounds are relatively brief, discrete auditory vibrations of varying intensity (loudness), frequency (pitch), and quality (timbre). S_1 identifies the onset of ventricular systole, and S_2 signals the onset of diastole. The basic heart sounds are S_1, S_2, S_3, and S_4. Each can be normal or abnormal. Other heart sounds are, more often than not, abnormal; still others are iatrogenic (e.g., prosthetic sounds, pacemaker sounds). Heart sounds within the auscultatory framework formed by S_1 and S_2 are designated as *early systolic, midsystolic, late systolic, early diastolic, middiastolic,* and *late diastolic* (Fig. 3-4).

An early systolic sound can be an ejection sound (aortic or pulmonic) or an aortic prosthetic sound. Midsystolic and late systolic sounds are generally mitral clicks (prolapse). Early diastolic sounds are usually opening snaps but may be S_3 (early diastolic sounds of constrictive pericarditis, ventricular knock of mitral regurgitation), a prosthetic sound, or a "tumor plop." Middiastolic sounds are typically S_3 and occasionally summation sounds (synchronous S_3 and S_4), whereas late diastolic sounds are almost always S_4; rarely, they are pacemaker sounds.

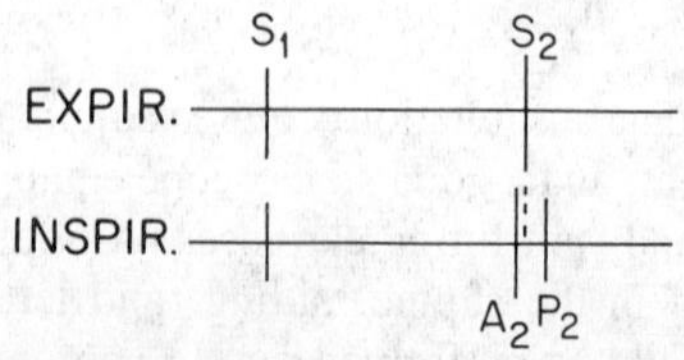

Fig. 3-5. Normal splitting of second heart sound *(S_2)*. During inspiration, S_2 splits into aortic *(A_2)* and pulmonic *(P_2)* components. The splitting results mainly from later occurrence of P_2. *S_1*, First heart sound.

First heart sound. The initial major component of S_1 is most prominent at the cardiac apex (when the apex is occupied by the left ventricle). A second component is sometimes heard at the lower left sternal edge, occasionally at the apex, but seldom at the base. In addition to the presence and degree of splitting, S_1 should be characterized by its quality and intensity. The qualities (pitch) of the two components are similar and are best appreciated with the stethoscope's diaphragm or firm pressure of the bell. When S_1 is split, the first component is normally the louder, with a softer second component confined to the lower left sternal edge or apex.

Second heart sound. S_2 has two components, the first designated the *aortic component* (A_2) and the second, the *pulmonic component* (P_2). S_2 normally splits into its two components during inspiration and is single during expiration. Splitting is best identified in the second left intercostal space because the softer P_2 is normally confined to that area, whereas the louder A_2 is heard at the base, sternal edge, and apex. Each component of S_2 coincides with the dicrotic incisura of the relevant great arterial pressure pulse and represents sequential closure of the aortic and pulmonic valves (Fig. 3-5).

Splitting of S_2 deviates from normal in several important respects. S_2 can remain single throughout the respiratory cycle because of either the absence of one component or synchronous occurrence of the two components. Paradoxical splitting, a reversed sequence of semilunar valve closure, results in expiratory splitting with inspiratory fusion, as in complete left bundle branch block. *Persistent* splitting means that the two components are audible during *both* phases of respiration, with appropriate inspiratory and expiratory directional changes, as in complete right bundle branch block. Persistent splitting sometimes occurs when healthy young patients are examined supine, especially during shallow breathing. In these patients an erroneous impression of abnormally wide splitting can be avoided by reexamining the patient in the sitting position. A persistent split becomes *fixed* when the degree of splitting remains unchanged during respiration, as in uncomplicated ostium secundum atrial septal defect.

The normal inspiratory increase in the A_2-P_2 interval mainly results from a delay in the P_2 and less from earlier occurrence of the A_2. Interpretation of the relative intensities of the two components of S_2 requires comparison when the sounds are heard simultaneously. The statement that "A_2 is greater than P_2" correctly applies only when both components of the S_2 are heard simultaneously. A_2 and P_2 do *not* refer to a comparison of a single S_2 at the right and left bases. An accentuated P_2 can be transmitted to the cardiac apex or right base. Increased intensity of P_2 in the second left interspace may prevent identification of a closely preceding A_2. In that event, auscultation at the lower left sternal edge or apex permits identification of the transmitted but attenuated P_2, allowing ready detection of splitting.

Third and fourth heart sounds. Two diastolic filling periods occur in each cardiac cycle in sinus rhythm, one passive and relatively early in diastole, the other active and in late diastole or presystole (after atrial contraction) (see Fig. 3-2). The sounds that accompany these two filling periods are S_3 and S_4. These sounds may be normal (physiologic) or abnormal (pathologic). The presence of the sounds, individually or together, may produce a cadence called *gallop rhythm*. Accordingly, gallop rhythm can be caused by S_3, S_4, or the presence of both S_3 and S_4. When diastole is short or the P-R interval long, atrial contraction is synchronous with the passive filling phase, and S_3 and S_4 coincide to form a summation sound or a summation gallop rhythm. The presence of these filling sounds is more important than the rhythm they create. For example, when S_3 or S_4 sounds coexist with murmurs or other sounds, it is more appropriate to refer to the presence of S_3 and S_4 as such, rather than to say that gallop sounds exist without gallop rhythm. *Third and fourth heart sounds* are terms that apply to specific events in the cardiac cycle, not to the total number of sounds at any given time. When S_1 and S_2 are accompanied by S_3 or S_4, a *triple* rhythm is created. When S_1 and S_2 are accompanied by S_3 and S_4, a *quadruple* rhythm is established. Gallop rhythm is a pathologic designation that should be avoided unless one is certain that the additional sound is abnormal. Children and young adults often have normal S_3 but not normal S_4 sounds. The converse is the case in older adults.

How can normal and abnormal S_3 or S_4 be distinguished? This can be done generally by the "company they keep" rather than by distinctive auscultatory properties of the sounds themselves. The abnormal heart sounds that cause the gallop rhythms are not merely exaggerations of normal S_3 and S_4 at relatively rapid rates but instead result from the inappropriate presence of these sounds. Because two diastolic filling periods are features of the cardiac cycle on *both* sides of the heart, it follows that S_3 and S_4 can originate in either the left or the right ventricle. It also follows that the atrial contribution to ventricular filling requires active atrial transport; thus this filling phase and the accompanying S_4 disappear when coordinated atrial contraction ceases, as in atrial fibrillation.

S_3 and S_4 are relatively low-frequency events that are often soft and require special stethoscopic techniques for detection. Soft low-frequency sounds are most readily heard in a quiet room, when the stethoscope's bell is placed on the skin just lightly enough to form an air seal. S_3 and S_4 originate within the cavity of the left ventricle and are best heard over the LV impulse, especially when that impulse is brought closer to the chest wall by turning the patient into the left lateral decubitus position. *Right* ventricular S_3 and S_4 are best heard along the lower left sternal edge or in the subxiphoid region. The latter site is especially useful in older patients with emphysema. Exercise, by increasing venous return and accelerating atrioventricular flow, augments third and fourth sounds. A few sit-ups usually suffice. Occasionally, ventricular filling sounds appear or are augmented when venous return is increased by raising a recumbent patient's legs or by transiently increasing the heart rate by having the patient cough. Respiration has a selective effect on augmenting a *right* ventricular S_3 and S_4. During inspiration, venous return to the right side of the heart increases; thus RV filling sounds tend to become louder. The converse is true with LV filling sounds. When the heart rate is fast, atrial contraction coincides with the passive filling phase, making it impossible to determine whether an accompanying filling sound is S_3, S_4, or a summation sound. Carotid sinus pressure transiently slows the heart rate and separates the two diastolic filling periods; auscultation can then discriminate where in diastole a given sound occurs.

Additional heart sounds. The most common *early systolic sound* is an ejection sound, either aortic or pulmonic. Ejection sounds typically coincide with movement of the relevant semilunar valve to its maximum open position. The sounds are of relatively high frequency ("clicking"). However, the term *ejection sound* is preferred to *ejection click* to distinguish a great artery ejection sound from a click of mitral valve origin (see later discussion) and to avoid the awkward term *nonejection click*. Aortic ejection sounds are best heard at the cardiac apex and right base, whereas pulmonic ejection sounds are best heard at the left base and often selectively and distinctively decrease in intensity during inspiration. An early systolic sound accompanies a ball-

and-cage aortic prosthesis (Starr-Edwards), is less apparent with a tilting-disk aortic valve, and is absent with a tissue prosthesis. The caged ball sometimes produces a trill of sounds as it "seats" in the apex of its cage.

The most common *midsystolic to late systolic sounds* are clicks associated with mitral valve prolapse (Chapter 16). Variability epitomizes systolic click(s), which at any given time may be absent, single, or multiple, and may be midsystolic or late systolic. A patient with an isolated midsystolic click on one examination may on reexamination exhibit one or more midsystolic or late systolic clicks or a burst of discrete clicks or crackles.

The most familiar *early diastolic sound* is the opening sound (opening snap) of the mitral valve. Opening sounds or snaps originate in mitral (most frequently) or tricuspid (infrequently) valves, usually because of atrioventricular valve stenosis but occasionally because of augmented flow rates across anatomically normal valves. The opening snap of mitral stenosis is best heard with the stethoscopic diaphragm at the lower left sternal edge; when loud, however, it is readily heard at the cardiac apex and base. Transmission to the left base invites a mistaken interpretation of wide splitting of S_2. Careful auscultation avoids this error by detecting two sounds on exhalation (synchronous aortic and pulmonic components followed by the opening snap) and three sounds on inspiration (A_2 and P_2 followed by the opening snap).

Early diastolic sounds occur in constrictive pericarditis and mitral regurgitation and have been designated *early diastolic sounds* and *ventricular knocks,* respectively. These are merely rapid filling sounds that occur early and are usually loud, because a high atrial pressure decompresses rapidly across an unobstructed valve into a recipient ventricle with decreased compliance. An early diastolic sound caused by a rigid prosthesis in the mitral location coincides with the opening of the prosthesis. Early diastolic sounds are also caused by atrial myxoma, either left or right. The chief requirement for generation of these "tumor plops" is a highly mobile tumor attached to the atrial septum by a long stalk. The sound results from abrupt diastolic seating of the mobile mass within its atrioventricular orifice (Chapter 24).

Middiastolic sounds are for all practical purposes normal or abnormal S_3 or summation sounds (see earlier discussion).

The most common *late diastolic (presystolic) sound* is S_4, discussed earlier. Rarely an RV pacemaker produces a presystolic *pacemaker sound,* which occurs immediately after the onset of the pacing stimulus. The sound precedes S_1 and is characteristically high pitched and clicking, unlike a low-frequency S_4. The pacemaker sound is believed to originate from contraction of chest wall muscle, but this does not necessarily imply RV perforation.

Heart murmurs

It is now appropriate to discuss systolic, diastolic, and continuous murmurs. A cardiovascular murmur is a relatively prolonged series of auditory vibrations characterized according to intensity (loudness), frequency (pitch), configuration (shape), quality, duration, direction of radiation, and timing in the cardiac cycle. Correct assessment of these features sets the stage for diagnostic conclusions that can be drawn from a murmur of a given description.

The intensity, or loudness, of murmurs is graded from I to VI. A grade I murmur is so faint that it is heard only with special effort. A grade II murmur is faint but readily recognized. A grade III murmur is prominent but not loud; a grade IV murmur, loud; and a grade V murmur, very loud. A grade VI murmur is loud enough to be heard with the stethoscope just removed from contact with the chest. Frequency (pitch) varies from high to low. A murmur's configuration, or shape, may be crescendo, decrescendo, crescendo-decrescendo (diamond shaped), plateau (sustained), or uneven (variable). A murmur's quality is best characterized by descriptive terms such as *harsh, rough, rumbling, scratchy, buzzing, grunting, blowing, musical, squeaking,* or *whooping.* A murmur's duration can be long or short, with all gradations in between. Long murmurs occupy all or almost all of systole or diastole. A loud murmur generally radiates from its site of maximum intensity, and the direction of radiation sometimes provides information on the murmur's origin.

The three basic categories of murmurs are systolic, diastolic (Fig. 3-6), and continuous (Fig. 3-7). A systolic murmur begins with or after S_1 and ends at or before S_2 on its side of origin. A diastolic murmur begins with or after S_2 on its side of origin and ends at or before S_1. A continuous murmur begins in systole and continues without interruption through the timing of S_2 into all or part of diastole.

Systolic murmurs are descriptively classified according to their time of onset and termination as midsystolic, holosystolic, early systolic, or late systolic (Fig. 3-6). A midsystolic murmur begins after S_1 and ends before the S_2 on its side of origin. Midsystolic murmurs originating in the left side of the heart end before A_2; midsystolic murmurs originating in the right side of the heart end before P_2. A holosystolic murmur begins with S_1, occupies all of systole, and ends with S_2 on its side of origin.

Diastolic murmurs are descriptively classified according to their time of onset as early diastolic, middiastolic, or late diastolic (presystolic) (Fig. 3-6). An early diastolic murmur begins with either A_2 or P_2. A middiastolic murmur begins at a clear interval after S_2. A late diastolic or presystolic murmur begins immediately before S_1.

Systolic murmurs. The chief settings in which *midsystolic murmurs* occur are:

1. Obstruction to ventricular outflow
2. Dilatation of the aortic root or pulmonary trunk
3. An increased rate of flow into the great arteries
4. Morphologic changes in the semilunar valves or their lines of attachment without obstruction
5. Some forms of mitral regurgitation

It should be emphasized that midsystolic murmurs are not synonymous with "ejection." A case in point is the mitral midsystolic murmur of papillary muscle dysfunction.

Holosystolic murmurs are generated by flow from a chamber or vessel whose pressure throughout systole is

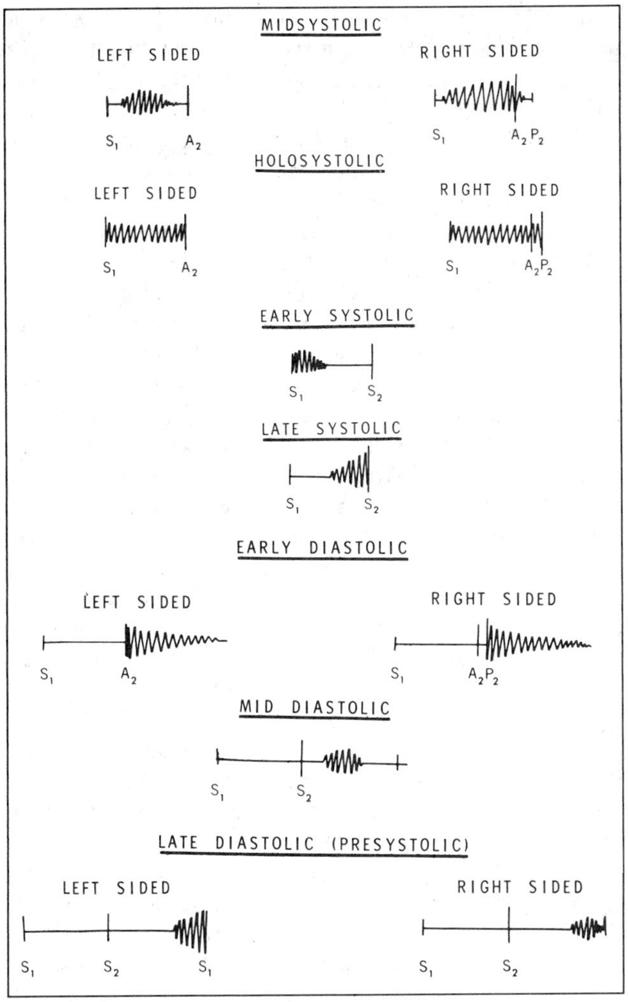

Fig. 3-6. Sketch illustrates murmurs: midsystolic (left and right sided), holosystolic (left and right sided), early systolic, late systolic, early diastolic (left and right sided), middiastolic, and late diastolic or presystolic (left and right sided). A_2, Aortic component; P_2, pulmonic component; S_1, S_2, first, second heart sounds.

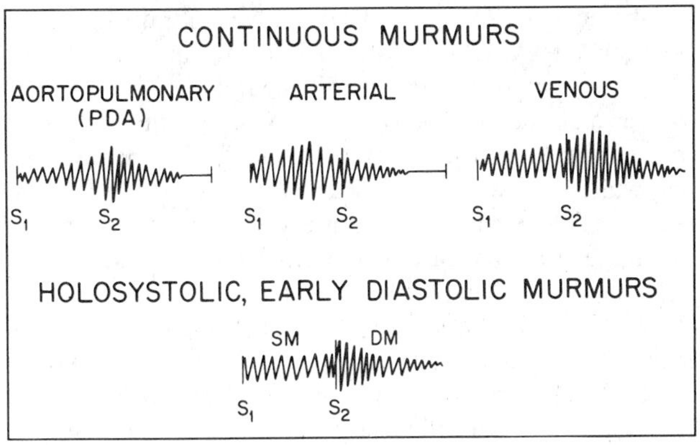

Fig. 3-7. Continuous murmurs begin in systole and *continue without interruption* through the timing of the second heart sound *(S_2)* into all or part of the diastole. These murmurs are aortopulmonary, as in patent ductus arteriosus *(PDA);* arterial, as in an obstructed carotid artery; or venous, as in a venous hum. Holosystolic *(SM)* plus early diastolic *(DM)* murmurs may occupy all the cardiac cycle, but they are two separate murmurs rather than a continuous murmur. S_1, First heart sound.

higher than the pressure in the recipient chamber or vessel. Such murmurs accompany mitral or tricuspid regurgitation, ventricular septal defect, and, under certain circumstances, aortopulmonary connections. The murmur of mitral regurgitation caused by papillary muscle dysfunction can be holosystolic, early systolic, late systolic, or midsystolic, whereas the murmur of acute severe mitral regurgitation is typically early systolic.

Early systolic murmurs begin with S_1, are decrescendo, and end before subsequent S_2 sometimes at or just after midsystole. Such murmurs are associated with certain types of ventricular septal defects, mitral regurgitation, or tricuspid regurgitation. For example, a soft, high-frequency early systolic decrescendo murmur is typical of a tiny ventricular septal defect in which the shunt is confined to early systole. Acute, severe mitral regurgitation into a small, unprepared left atrium tends to produce a large V wave that approaches LV pressure in later systole. The regurgitant flow is maximal in early systole and minimal in later systole, and the murmur mirrors this pattern. A similar systolic murmur is a feature of tricuspid regurgitation without RV hypertension. This is in contrast to the high-frequency holosystolic murmur of tricuspid regurgitation with *elevated* RV systolic pressure.

A *late systolic murmur,* especially when preceded by one or more midsystolic to late systolic clicks, is the auscultatory hallmark of mitral valve prolapse. If no murmur is heard with the patient in the supine position, a murmur can sometimes be provoked by physical maneuvers, such as the left lateral decubitus position, sitting, leaning forward, or standing, especially standing rapidly from a squatting position. In a small proportion of patients with mitral prolapse, a striking systolic honk or whoop is intermittently heard either spontaneously or with physical maneuvers.

Systolic arterial murmurs (extracardiac systolic murmurs) originate in systemic or pulmonary arteries. Detection underscores the value of auscultation at nonprecordial sites. Such murmurs are caused by anatomic abnormalities in an artery, such as tortuosity or luminal narrowing, or by increased flow through normal arteries. The rise and decline of pulsatile systolic flow imparts to the murmur a crescendo-decrescendo shape. The most frequent cause of systolic arterial murmurs is atherosclerotic obstruction of the carotid, subclavian, or iliofemoral arteries. Innocent or normal supraclavicular systolic murmurs are heard in normal children and adolescents. These latter murmurs originate within normal brachiocephalic arteries, probably near their origins, and decrease or vanish with hyperextension of the shoulders, that is, bringing the elbows behind the back so that the shoulder girdle muscles are taut.

Diastolic murmurs. *Early diastolic murmurs* are epitomized by chronic aortic regurgitation. The murmur begins with A_2 and is generally decrescendo, reflecting the progressive decline in volume and rate of regurgitant flow during the course of diastole. The high velocity of regurgitation generates a high-frequency, blowing murmur. Faint, high-frequency murmurs of aortic regurgitation are difficult to hear and must be specifically sought by firmly pressing the stethoscopic diaphragm at the middle left sternal border while the patient sits, leans forward, and holds the breath in full exhalation. Soft or equivocal murmurs of aortic regurgitation increase in intensity when squatting or isometric exercise (handgrip) transiently raises systemic resistance. The early diastolic murmur of pulmonary hypertension (Graham Steell murmur) may be difficult or impossible to distinguish from mild aortic regurgitation when the murmur is soft and the systemic arterial pulse normal.

With the notable exception of the murmur of pulmonary valve regurgitation not caused by pulmonary hypertension (i.e., congenital, endocarditis), *middiastolic murmurs* typically occur across atrioventricular (A-V) valves during the rapid filling phase. Such murmurs originate at the mitral or tricuspid orifice because of A-V valve obstruction or abnormal patterns of A-V flow. The middiastolic murmur of mitral stenosis should be sought by placing the stethoscope's bell lightly against the skin at the site of the LV impulse, best localized with the patient in the left lateral decubitus position. In addition, middiastolic murmurs occur at normal A-V valves in the presence of augmented volume and velocity of flow across the mitral valve in ventricular septal defect or pure mitral regurgitation, and across the tricuspid valve in atrial septal defect or tricuspid regurgitation. These middiastolic murmurs are short and medium pitched, tend to occur with large shunts or appreciable A-V valve regurgitation, and are often preceded by S_3 sounds. The Austin Flint murmur may be middiastolic or presystolic and results from antegrade flow across a mitral valve that is closing rapidly because of simultaneous LV filling from aortic regurgitation.

Late diastolic or *presystolic murmurs* occur during the period of late (active) ventricular filling in response to atrial contraction. At normal cardiac rates, these murmurs imply sinus rhythm. As with middiastolic murmurs, presystolic murmurs originate at either the mitral or the tricuspid orifice, usually because of obstruction, but occasionally because of abnormal patterns of presystolic A-V flow. An example of the latter is the presystolic Austin Flint murmur. The presystolic murmur of mitral stenosis occurs when the left ventricle begins to contract in the face of appreciable flow across the mitral orifice in response to atrial contraction. In tricuspid stenosis with sinus rhythm, the presystolic murmur typically occurs with absent or trivial middiastolic vibrations and selectively increases with inspiration.

Continuous murmurs. The term *continuous* is best applied to murmurs that begin in systole and continue without interruption through S_2 into all or part of diastole; the presence of a murmur during all phases of the cardiac cycle is not a requirement. Accordingly, a systolic murmur that extends beyond S_2 into diastole is continuous, even if the murmur finishes before subsequent S_1. Continuous murmurs generally occur as blood flows from a higher-pressure to a lower-pressure zone without interruption from systole to diastole. Such murmurs result mainly from aortopulmonary connections, arteriovenous connections, disturbances of flow patterns in arteries and disturbances of flow patterns in veins (Fig. 3-7).

The continuous murmur of patent ductus arteriosus with low pulmonary vascular resistance is representative of murmurs generated by aortopulmonary connections. Continuous murmurs caused by arteriovenous connections are illustrated by congenital or acquired disorders, such as systemic arteriovenous fistulas, coronary arterial fistulas, and communication from a sinus of Valsalva to the right side of the heart. Continuous murmurs occasionally result from disturbances of flow patterns in constricted systemic or pulmonary arteries provided a constant difference exists in pressure on the two sides of the narrowed segment. Critical atherosclerotic obstruction of a large brachiocephalic or femoral artery may result in such a continuous murmur. The examiner should remember that arterial continuous murmurs, especially in constricted arteries, are typically louder in systole. Disturbances of flow patterns in nonconstricted arteries sometimes produce continuous murmurs, as illustrated by systemic to pulmonary arterial collaterals in certain types of cyanotic congenital heart disease (e.g., pulmonary atresia with ventricular septal defect). The "mammary souffle" is an innocent murmur heard during late pregnancy and early postpartum; the souffle may be systolic or continuous. These murmurs are believed to be arterial in origin and, when continuous, are louder in systole.

The venous hum is an example of a continuous murmur caused by altered flow patterns in normal veins. To elicit the hum, the patient should be examined in the sitting position; a stethoscopic bell is applied to the medial aspect of the right supraclavicular fossa while the examiner's left hand grasps the patient's chin from behind and pulls it tautly to the left and upward. The hum is characteristically louder in diastole and is instantaneously abolished by digital pressure on the ipsilateral deep jugular vein. Radiation of a loud venous hum below the clavicles invites the mistaken diagnosis of an intrathoracic continuous murmur. Pressure applied to the appropriate jugular vein obliterates the hum and avoids this error.

Pericardial rubs are occasionally mistaken for intracardiac murmurs because rubs occur in systole (generally in midsystole), middiastole, and late diastole (presystole). Rubs are best heard at the lower left sternal edge and often increase in intensity (or appear) with firm pressure of the stethoscopic diaphragm, during inspiration, and when the precordium is examined with the patient supported on elbows and knees. The rub's systolic component is the most consistent, followed by the presystolic component. Diagnosis of a rub is most difficult (often impossible) when only the systolic phase remains.

CHEST AND ABDOMEN

Examination of the chest begins with observation of respiratory patterns and appearance, the latter to detect scoliosis, kyphosis, pectus carinatum or excavatum, or simple loss of thoracic kyphosis, all of which can alter cardiac physical signs. Auscultation and percussion of the thorax may identify isolated *left* lower lobe rales or effusion, suggesting pulmonary embolism rather than cardiac failure. Crepitant inspiratory rales are features of pulmonary edema in the adult, but in infants pulmonary edema is largely interstitial, so rales are absent. Auscultation generally focuses on breath sounds and rales, but examination in the axillae and back is necessary to detect the peripheral systolic murmurs of pulmonary artery stenosis, the lower lobe systolic murmur of pulmonary arteriovenous fistula (which may be heard only during deeply held inspiration or Müller's maneuver), or the continuous murmur of systemic arterial collaterals in pulmonary atresia with ventricular septal defect.

Assessment of the abdomen includes appearance, palpation, percussion, and auscultation. Examination begins with inspection, which may detect the bulging flanks of ascites. Palpation is important to identify the hepatic enlargement of congestive hepatomegaly, the tender spleen tip of infective endocarditis, the normal aorta above the umbilicus, or an aortic aneurysm below the umbilicus. Auscultation serves to detect the systolic murmurs of iliofemoral or abdominal aortic obstruction or of renal arterial stenosis.

EYEGROUNDS

Examination of the retina provides direct access to small arteries and veins. Systemic hypertension may be accompanied by subtle changes in arterioles (narrowing, straightening, increased light reflex, loss of small arteriolar branches, early compression of underlying veins) or, at the other end of the spectrum, the obvious changes of the retinopathy in malignant hypertension. Diabetic retinopathy begins with subtle microaneurysms that can be overlooked unless meticulously sought. Roth spots indicating infective endocarditis should also be sought.

REFERENCES

Basta LL and Bettinger JJ: The cardiac impulse: a new look at an old art. Am Heart J 97:96, 1979.

Benchimol A and Tippit HC: The clinical value of the jugular and hepatic pulses. Prog Cardiovasc Dis 10:159, 1967.

Cogan DG: Ophthalmic manifestations of systemic vascular disease. Philadelphia, 1974, Saunders.

Fisher J: Jugular venous values and physical signs. Chest 85:685, 1984.

Ishimitsu T et al: Origin of the third heart sound: comparison of ventricular wall dynamics in hyperdynamic and hypodynamic types. J Am Coll Cardiol 5:268, 1985.

Kirkendall WM et al: AHA committee report: recommendations of human blood pressure determined by sphygmomanometers. Circulation 62:1146, 1983.

Linfors EW and Neelson FA: The case for bedside rounds. N Engl J Med 303:1230, 1980.

Manning DM, Kurchirka C, and Kaminski J: Miscuffing: inapprorpate blood pressure cuff application. Circulation 68:763, 1983.

Maxwell MH et al: Error in blood-pressure measurement due to incorrect cuff size in obese patients. Lancet 2:33, 1982.

Perloff JK: The clinical recognition of congenital heart disease, ed 3. Philadelphia, 1987, Saunders.

Perloff JK: Physical examination of the heart and circulation, ed 2. Philadelphia, 1990, Saunders.

Perloff JK: Heart sounds and murmurs: physiological mechanisms. In Braunwald E, editor: Heart disease, ed 4. Philadelphia, 1992, Saunders.

Perloff JK: Neurological disorders and heart disease. In Braunwald E, editor: Heart disease, ed 4. Philadelphia, 1992, Saunders.

Silverman ME: Causes of valve disease: visual clues. J Cardiovasc Dis 8:340, 1983.

CHAPTER

4 Electrocardiography

John H. McAnulty

The electrocardiogram (ECG), which assesses the heart's electrical activity, has become an invaluable part of clinical care. Normal electrical patterns have been established, and the electrical changes caused by anatomic abnormalities, drugs, metabolic changes, and heart disease have been defined. In the 8 decades since Einthoven and his colleagues first introduced electrocardiography, many investigators and teachers have contributed to what we know and are currently learning. Criteria for diagnosis are still being created, and different methods for recording the heart's electrical activity are being developed. Currently available equipment and criteria have made the ECG particularly useful for two purposes: the definition of structural and disease changes and the evaluation of rhythm abnormalities. Rhythms are discussed in other chapters. This chapter focuses on the interpretation of the ECG and its contributions to the diagnosis of many disease states.

ELECTRICAL ACTIVITY IN HEART AND ECG

The cardiac rhythm and conduction system has two properties: *automaticity* and *conductivity*. The first is unique. Under normal circumstances, some cardiac cells have the ability to activate or "depolarize" spontaneously and then return to electrical neutrality or "repolarize." With modification by the autonomic nervous system and humoral agents, this cycle continually repeats itself. The other property of the rhythm system, conductivity, allows the rapid spread of this electrical activity to other regions of the heart that ordinarily do not have automaticity. The ECG allows assessment of each of these properties.

All forms of electrocardiography are based on the concept of measurement of change in electrical vectors. A *vector* is a force (in this case electrical, which is measured as voltage) with magnitude and direction. The changes in the vectors (both direction and magnitude) are the direct result of the automaticity and the conduction characteristics of the heart. As electrical current flows through the heart, the magnitude and direction of the electrical potential between various regions of the heart continually change. This creates a continually changing sequence of electrical vectors until depolarization and then repolarization of all cells have occurred. This sequence repeats itself with each normal c diac cycle. This spread of electrical activity is initiated by cells with automaticity that stimulate the cells next to them, which in turn activate adjacent cells. This process occurs more rapidly within the heart's conduction system, but cell-to-cell spread occurs in myocardial tissue as well.

To understand this flow of change in vectors, consideration of a row of cells and measurement of their electrical activity may be helpful (Fig. 4-1). In their deactivated state, no potential difference exists between the cells at one end compared with the other. In each of the cells, the membrane surface is relatively positive compared with the intracellular potential (the result of ion transfer that is both passive and active). Electrodes recording electrical activity from this group of cells would show no electrical activity. If the cell at one end of the row were stimulated, for example, by the conduction system next to the cell, its membrane surface would become relatively more negative compared with those next to it. This cell's activation would in turn stimulate the cell next to it, and by this process the electrical current would pass down the row of cells.

An electrode (Fig. 4-1, electrode *C*) recording this electrical activity from the end where the cells are relatively positive would, if attached to a penwriter, cause an upward deflection (by convention). It would continue to do so until all the cells were activated and the cells closest to the lead were no longer more positive than those next to it. An electrode (Fig. 4-1, electrode *A*) recording exactly the same electrical activity from the other end of the row of cells would sense the cells on its end as relatively more negative compared with the other cells, and this negative charge would be recorded as a downward deflection by a penwriter. An electrode positioned at the center (Fig. 4-1, electrode *B*) would initially sense the cells at its position being more positive than those at the negative end and would record a

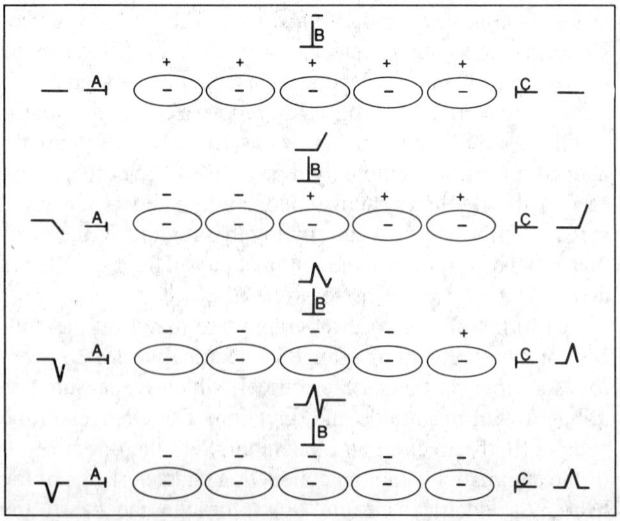

Fig. 4-1. Schematic presentation of a row of cells undergoing activation. Electrode *A* is at the end where the cells are relatively negative, electrode *C* at the end where the cells are relatively positive, and electrode *B* at the center where the flow of change of charges produces a positive followed by a negative deflection.

positive deflection. When the flow of change of charges reached electrode *B*, no potential difference would exist. As flow proceeded past the electrode, it would record a relative negative charge, and there would be a downward deflection of the pen. By convention, this flow of current, or change in relative vectors, is said to flow from negative to positive. Depending on the cells' orientation and the degree of charge difference among the cells, the electrical potential would have magnitude and direction.

At any one instant, the change in electrical vectors proceeds in multiple directions because the heart is a three-dimensional structure. Any external lead, however, can only interpret the electrical activity as a summation of the overall electrical events and thus records an overall vector at any instant in time. Thus, although some forces may be going away from a lead, an even larger number of the forces may be going relatively toward it, resulting in a positive deflection at that time. At another time during the cardiac cycle, some electrical forces may be going toward a lead, but most may be going away from it, resulting in a negative deflection.

Several different forms of electrocardiography exist, although each records a sequential change of electrical vectors. Although the heart's electrical activity can be recorded from leads placed directly on or within it, this is not a practical approach in most patients. In 1913 Einthoven and his colleagues first described recording of electrical activity from the heart using an *external lead system*. They in turn created the first set of standard leads, the bipolar "limb" leads labeled I, II, and III. Interpretation of the recordings made from these leads is based on various assumptions that are not completely accurate but have become applicable. The first assumption is that the body is a homogeneous, uniform volume conductor and that any pair of bipolar leads placed on the body will record the same electrical activity. The second assumption is that the heart is at any given instant in time a single *dipole*, that is, a pair of spatially separated regions with one region having a positive charge compared with another. According to the Einthoven theory, this dipole is located in the center of an equilateral triangle, and an electrode on the right arm and one on the left arm form the top of the triangle. Recording between these two electrodes can then be assumed to be viewing the heart horizontally; this has been labeled *lead I* (Fig. 4-2). Electrodes on the right arm and left leg form another side of the triangle, and the recording made from this bipolar electrode has been labeled *lead II* and views the heart at an angle of 60 degrees below the view seen by lead I. *Lead III* is recorded between the left arm and left leg and views the heart from an angle of 120 degrees away from lead I. Three additional frontal plane leads have been established. These are unipolar leads using any single electrode to record from, with the remaining leads being converted to a common ground. Altering resistances of these leads has led to the creation of the augmented limb leads, *aVR*, *aVL*, and *aVF*, which view the heart from the angles shown in Fig. 4-2. The six limb leads view the heart from a single frontal plane.

Subsequently, another set of unipolar leads was stan-

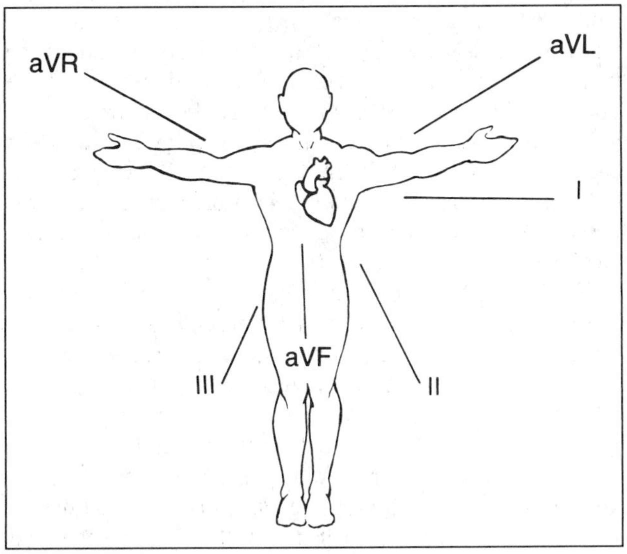

Fig. 4-2. The torso with the six limb leads in a single frontal plane.

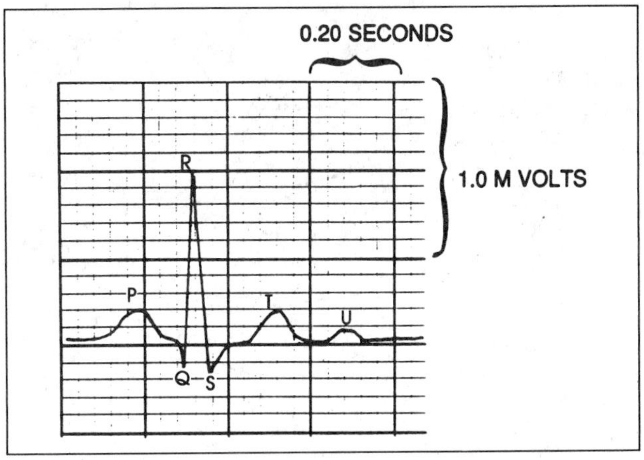

Fig. 4-4. Schematic representation of the various components of the scalar ECG P-QRS-T wave complex (see text) and the strip chart paper on which it is recorded.

dardized, the precordial leads labeled V_1 to V_6 (Fig. 4-3). These are positioned across the front and left lateral chest, and being unipolar, they provide a signal that views the heart from their geographic position on the chest. Even though it would theoretically be feasible to create any number of lead systems, these 12 leads have become the convention for the *scalar* ECG. They allow evaluation of the direction, magnitude, duration, and frequency of the electrical events occurring in the heart.

The arrangement of the leads allows evaluation of the electrical events from different directions. Leads V_1 and aVR, being somewhat to the right of the heart, are considered right-sided leads. Leads aVL, I, II, and $V_{5,6}$ are left-sided leads. Leads II, III, and aVF are inferior leads, and leads V_1 to V_4 view the heart from the anterior wall and are anterior leads (Figs. 4-2 and 4-3).

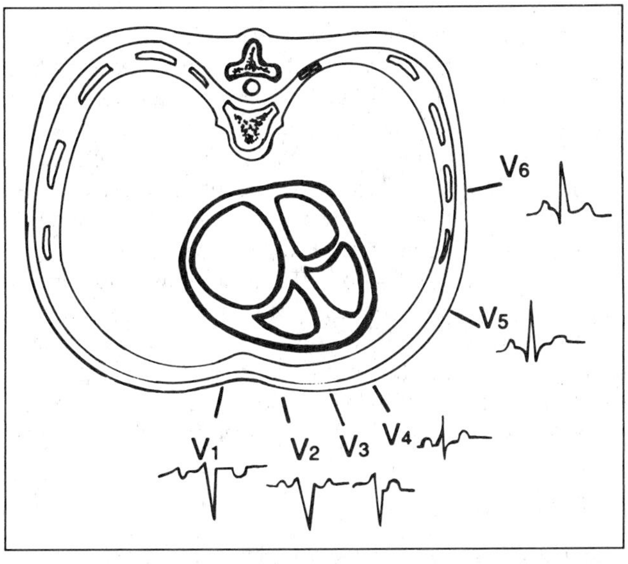

Fig. 4-3. Cross section of the upper torso with the position of the six (V_1 to V_6) unipolar precordial leads.

The machines used to record the ECGs have evolved into reliable and relatively easy-to-use instruments. The paper used on the strip chart recorder is designed to make interpretation easy (Fig. 4-4). By convention it runs at 25 mm/sec, and the paper is divided by lines that are separated by 1 mm, and given the speed of the paper, a small box on the tracing inscribes a period of 0.04 second. On each machine a calibration switch provides a 1 mV signal. By convention, the standard calibration is 1 mV for each 10 mm deflection on the paper, but if the voltage recorded is too large for the recording paper, this standardization can be changed.

NORMAL ELECTRICAL ACTIVITY AND NORMAL ECG

P wave

The electrical activity (Fig. 4-4) in the heart begins at the sinus node, which is located at the junction of the right atrium and superior vena cava. Although the sinus node's electrical activity is insufficient to be recorded by surface leads, it initiates the spread of electrical activity through the atria. As the atrial cells are depolarized, a large enough force is created to cause a recognizable electrical event: the P wave on the ECG. Because of its location in the right atrium, the sinus node activates that chamber first. As right atrial activation is occurring, it blends into activation of the left atrium. Leads II and V_1 are most important for evaluation of the P waves (Figs. 4-4 and 4-5).

Lead II looks at the heart from the left and from an angle 60 degrees below the horizontal. In a normal heart the P waves in this lead are always positive because electrical activity in both atria proceeds toward the left. Two other features of the normal P wave have been recognized. First, in the normal person, atrial activity takes less than 0.12 second to be completed, and thus the normal P wave is less

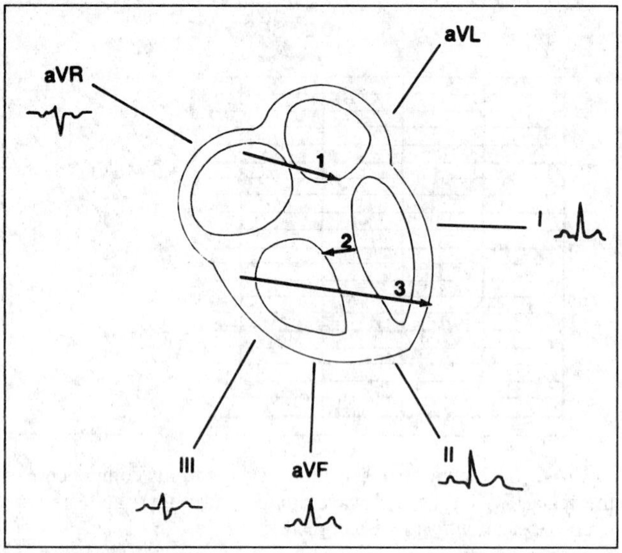

Fig. 4-5. Normal activation sequence in the heart. Atrial activation *(arrow 1)* results in a P wave that is positive in lead II. The first portion of ventricular activation occurs in the intraventricular septum *(arrow 2)*. Since it proceeds from left to right, the initial portion of the QRS complex is negative in the left-sided leads (i.e., a narrow Q wave is often seen at these levels). Although continued ventricular activation occurs to the left and the right (also anteriorly and posteriorly), the preponderance of forces are to the left *(arrow 3)*, resulting in that latter portion of the QRS complex being positive in the left-sided leads (i.e., an R wave) and negative in the right-sided leads (i.e., an S wave).

than 0.12 second in length in lead II. Additionally, the voltage of the P wave in lead II in a normal population is less than 0.25 mV (i.e., less than 2.5 small boxes tall with normal standardization).

The normal P wave in V_1 is somewhat more variable. In most persons, it is a biphasic wave, with the initial portion of the P wave being positive as the right atrium is activated toward the front and with the second portion being negative as the left atrium is activated posteriorly. Although it is standard to position V_1 in the fourth intercostal space just to the right of the sternum, anatomic positional variation can result in some patients having a completely positive P wave in lead V_1.

P-R segment

As the electrical activity leaves the atrium and passes through the atrioventricular (A-V) node, the His bundle, and the bundle branches, its magnitude is insufficient to be recorded on the surface ECG. Thus the recordings return to baseline in all the leads.

QRS complex

The bundle branches and the Purkinje fibers rapidly spread electrical activity throughout the ventricle. Ventricular depolarization results in the QRS complex on the ECG. Although the term *QRS complex* relates to activation of the ventricle, in some leads there may be no Q wave, or no R wave, or no S wave. By definition in a given lead, if the first electrical activity causes a negative deflection of the initial portion of the QRS, that negative deflection is called a *Q wave*. Any electrical activity seen coming toward a lead causing a positive deflection results in an *R wave*. Electrical activity going away from a lead after an R wave has already been inscribed results in a negative deflection called an *S wave*.

The ventricle's earliest depolarization occurs on the left side of the septum and results from activation by the left bundle branch. The activation spreads from the septum's left side toward the right, and thus the earliest forces in the QRS complex go from left to right. This results in a Q wave in many of the left-sided leads (particularly lead V_6) and an initial R wave in the right-sided leads, aVR and V_1 (Figs. 4-4 and 4-5). Two important features of this initial deflection have been recognized. First, in the normal heart, this portion of the QRS complex is usually completed in less than 0.04 second (one small box at a paper speed of 25 mm/sec). Second, the magnitude of this initial force is generally less than 25% of the overall QRS height in any one lead. Alterations in these observations suggest specific abnormalities, as discussed later.

While the septum is being activated, electrical activity continues to spread rapidly through the bundle branches and into the ventricles. Right ventricular and left ventricular activation occur at approximately the same time and immediately follow the septal activity. Since the left ventricle is 5 to 10 times as thick as the right ventricle, the forces going toward the left predominate. Because of this, the remainder of the QRS complex is positive in the left-sided leads and negative in the right-sided leads. Occasionally the final portion of the ventricular activation may be directed toward the right, causing an S wave in the left-sided leads and a terminal positive wave (an R′) in the right-sided leads.

Certain features of the QRS complex have been recognized as normal. First, the duration of the QRS is less than or equal to 0.10 second. This remarkably rapid activation results from the conduction capabilities of the bundle branches. Second, normal voltage or magnitude criteria have been determined (this is reviewed when abnormal voltage situations are described under ventricular hypertrophies). Third, normal values for the overall electrical direction of ventricular activation, the mean QRS axis, have been established. A significant deviation of the mean electrical axis can indicate heart disease. The normal mean QRS axis ranges from a position 30 degrees above the horizontal (arbitrarily called −30 degrees) to +110 degrees away from the horizontal (Fig. 4-6). Inclusion of axes as abnormal that are either less negative or less positive than this may make the use of axis deviation a somewhat more sensitive marker for heart disease, but specificity would be lost.

S-T segment

After depolarization of the ventricles, a plateau phase of electrical activity occurs with no significant changes in the vectors. The inscribing pen on the ECG returns to the base-

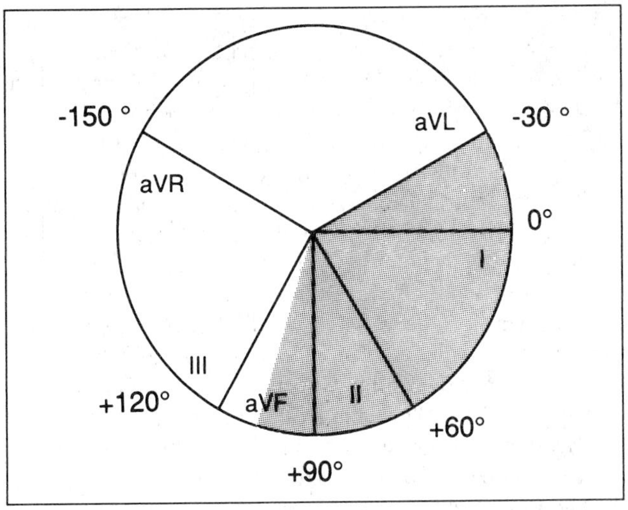

Fig. 4-6. Positions of the six limb leads and their extent of positivity or negativity (in degrees), with the gray area indicating the normal limits of the mean QRS axis in the frontal plane.

line. This region is called the S-T segment. It extends from the end of the QRS complex (called the J point) to the beginning of the T wave. When interpreting an ECG, the S-T segment should be evaluated for three features: *position* (elevated or depressed); *configuration* (convexity downward, which has been called "scooping," convexity upward, which has been called "coving," or straight noncurving segments); and *location* (i.e., are S-T segment changes diffuse or localized).

Ordinarily the S-T segment is positioned along the baseline, although slight elevation may occur. Additionally, the normal S-T segment is straight or has a slight convexity, downward configuration (i.e., is scooped).

T wave

The T wave is formed by repolarization of the ventricle. Depolarization occurs from endocardium to epicardium; repolarization begins in the epicardium and moves to the endocardium. Generally the T wave goes in the same direction as the QRS complex, but exceptions exist. In lead III the QRS is often positive and the T wave is negative (or vice versa), and in leads V_1 and V_2 the T wave may be positive and the QRS complexes negative. In the limb leads the overall mean axis of the T wave should be within 60 degrees of the mean QRS axis. Separation in axis beyond this degree raises the concern of a myocardial abnormality. There are no rules about the height or width of a T wave. Hyperacute ischemia and hyperkalemia are known to cause tall and peaked T waves, but tall T waves are common in normal patients, and thus the findings have to be interpreted carefully.

U wave

The exact origin of the U wave is still debated, but some supportive evidence suggests that it is caused by repolarization of the His-Purkinje system. A normal U wave has the same polarity as the T wave, although the U wave has less voltage. It is more prominent with slower heart rates. When a U wave exceeds or equals the T wave's height or when it appears to be inverted (this is difficult to assess), a cardiac abnormality is likely. Syndromes causing these changes are discussed later.

APPROACH TO ECG

All ECGs should be evaluated systematically for the following:

1. P wave rate and regularity
2. QRS complex rate and regularity
3. Interval measurement: P-R, QRS, and Q-T
4. Duration, magnitude, and configuration of the P waves, QRS complexes, S-T segments, T waves, and U waves

Failure to be systematic may allow recognition of one problem but may neglect equally important findings. Most normal values for intervals were established by using the limb lead system only, a reason that the precordial leads (which frequently detect a longer QRS complex) are not used for these measurements. The P-R interval extends from the beginning of the P wave to the beginning of the QRS complex (normal is 0.12 to 0.20 second). An argument could be made for using the shortest P-R interval because, occasionally in individuals with pre-excitation, the early ventricular activation wave (delta wave) may be seen in some leads but not in others. Still, in the absence of pre-excitation, it is standard to measure the longest. The QRS interval measurement should be made from the beginning to the end of the QRS complex, where it is best seen to be the longest (normal is less than or equal to 0.10 second). The Q-T interval measurement should be made from the beginning of the QRS complex to the end of the T wave. Normalcy of the Q-T interval is related to heart rate. Charts are available for interpretation. The importance of measuring the Q-T interval and correcting it for the heart rate (using available charts or the formula, $\text{Q-Tc} = \frac{\text{Q-T interval}}{\sqrt{\text{R-R interval}}}$ is worth emphasizing because a prolonged value is associated with sudden death syndromes.

ECG ABNORMALITIES

Intraventricular conduction abnormalities

Bundle branch block. At least four reasons exist to be able to interpret bundle branch block (BBB) on the ECG. Because of the following fourth reason, students of electrocardiography should be able to recognize this abnormality before considering any others.

1. BBB occurs quite often, and because it is found in 1% to 2% of the population, anyone interpreting ECGs will frequently encounter this finding.
2. BBB is an indication of heart disease. The exceptions to this are so unlikely that the general rule is applicable.
3. BBB is an indication of conduction system disease

and suggests that a patient is at increased risk of bradycardias as well as tachycardias.

4. BBB precludes some other interpretations, so the diagnosis should be made before considering other abnormalities on the tracing.

The unifying rule and requirement for BBB is a QRS complex that is 0.12 second or longer.

Right bundle branch block. In normal conduction, as ventricular activation begins, the first fibers activating the septum come off the left bundle and result in a left-to-right septal activation. This results in a small Q wave in the left-sided leads (less than 0.04 second in duration and less than one fourth of the overall QRS height) and a small R wave in the right-sided leads. Right BBB (Fig. 4-7) does not alter this initial activation of the ventricle. Normally, as septal activation is being completed, activation spreads rapidly through both the left and the right bundles. The external leads, however, sense an overwhelming dominant force going toward the left because of left ventricular (LV) size, and this results in a large R wave in the left-sided leads and a large S wave in the right-sided leads. Right BBB does not change the normal activation toward the left, so this portion of the QRS complex is also unchanged. In the normal heart, by the time the LV activation is complete, so is that of the right. However, in the person with right BBB, because the right ventricle was not activated through the rapid bundle branch conduction mechanism, electrical activity moves through the myocardium toward the right at a much slower pace, presumably on a cell-to-cell basis. After LV activation is completed, electrical activation is still moving toward the right to activate the right ventricle. Although the electrical forces are no greater than normal, at this time they are unopposed by left-sided forces, and they are seen as an electrical potential moving toward the right, causing a secondary R wave (an R′) in the right-sided leads and an S wave in the left-sided leads. Because the conduction is not by the rapid conduction pathway, this takes longer than usual, resulting in the QRS complex of 0.12 second or greater. This abnormal depolarization causes repolarization changes best seen in the right-sided leads: S-T segment depression and T wave inversion. This adds up to the abnormalities required for making the diagnosis of right BBB:

1. QRS complex of 0.12 second or longer
2. Delayed right ventricular (RV) forces, resulting in the terminal R waves in the right-sided leads and S wave in the left-sided leads
3. Right-sided S-T segment depression and T wave inversion

Right BBB on the ECG makes the diagnosis of RV hypertrophy (see later criteria) unreliable. Additionally, it is inappropriate to assume that right-sided ST-T changes could result from causes other than the BBB (although they might be).

Some controversy exists as to the best way to determine the mean QRS axis in individuals with right BBB. Some have suggested that the terminal portion of the QRS complex (final 0.04 second) should not be included because it is not part of normal conduction. However, most of the clinical studies evaluating the significance of right BBB have used the entire QRS complex for determination of axis. Because of this, it is recommended that axis determination in patients with right BBB be determined in this way.

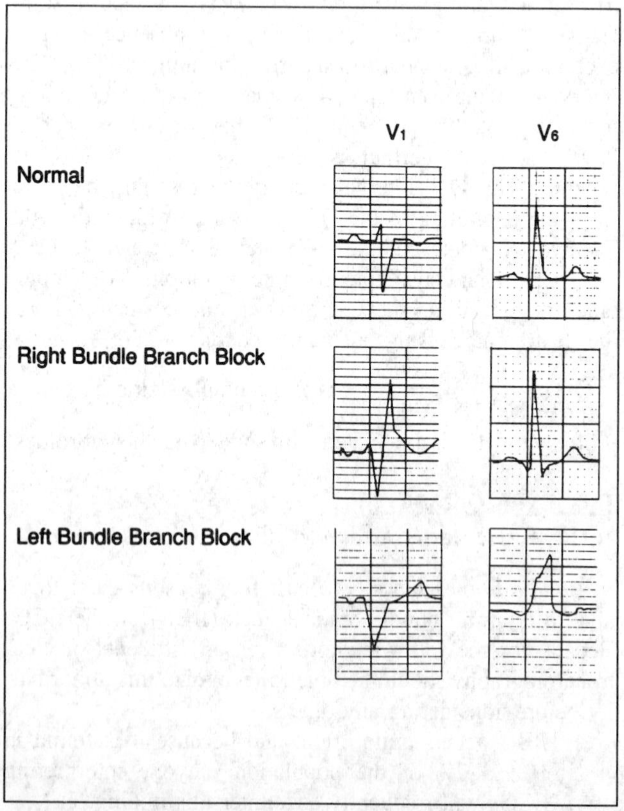

Fig. 4-7. V_1 and V_6 ECG complexes when no conduction abnormality exists and when right or left bundle branch block is present (see text).

Left bundle branch block. Normally the initial activation of the septum comes from the left bundle, resulting in initial left-to-right electrical activity. With left BBB (Fig. 4-7), the septum is not activated by the left bundle but rather by distal right bundle fibers, and septal activation proceeds from right to left. Thus left BBB results in a change in the early portion of the QRS complex with loss of the normal small Q waves seen in the left-sided leads and the small R waves seen in the right-sided leads. Electrical activation continues rapidly through the right bundle toward the right ventricle. Because the left ventricle is not activated by the left bundle, spread through the left ventricle begins on a cell-to-cell or segment-to-segment basis. Despite its slow activation, again LV dominance results in enough electrical forces going toward the left that often the rapid activity toward the right is not seen. Electrical activity continues to spread toward the left, resulting in a long, broad R wave in the left-sided leads until LV activation is completed. This abnormal depolarization results in abnormal repolarization with left-sided ST-T wave changes. The criteria for reading left BBB are:

1. QRS complex greater than or equal to 0.12 second
2. Delayed LV activation
3. Loss of the normal "septal Q wave" in the left-sided leads
4. Left-sided S-T segment depression and T wave inversion

Left BBB interferes with interpretation of other abnormalities. Although a myocardial infarction may be the cause of a left BBB, it is best not to try to interpret this finding on the ECG. Patients with left BBB may have ST-T abnormalities from other causes, but they should not be evaluated when this conduction abnormality is present. The same is true for those with LV hypertrophy. If striking day-to-day changes occur in the QRS or ST-T segments in a patient with left BBB, the examiner could assume that some event is the cause but should take care in using the ECG alone as the diagnostic tool.

Intraventricular conduction delays. Occasionally the QRS complex is wide and does not meet the criteria for the BBBs. This is generally associated with ST-T abnormalities. The significance of this finding is not always clear clinically, but its presence makes a cardiac abnormality likely.

Fascicular block. Block of individual fascicles of the left bundle can be suggested by ECG changes. The rules required for left anterior fascicular block are a mean QRS axis less than or equal to -30 degrees; initial R waves in leads II, III, and aVF; and Q waves in leads I and aVF.

Left posterior fascicular block is suggested by a mean right axis deviation (i.e., $\geq +110$ degrees) with Q waves in II, III, and aVF and initial R waves in leads I and aVF. This diagnosis is uncertain until right ventricular hypertrophy has been excluded as a cause of these changes.

Ischemic heart disease

The ECG is particularly useful in the diagnosis of ischemic heart disease, but the changes caused by this process are complex and variable. Because the coronary blood vessels reach the epicardial surface first and then divide into smaller branches as they penetrate the myocardium, the endocardium is most vulnerable to limitations in myocardial blood flow and oxygen supply. Ischemia, injury, and necrosis of the endocardium cause different ECG changes than they do with epicardial involvement. The ECG can demonstrate the presence of the myocardial ischemic process, can depict endocardial versus epicardial involvement, can localize the process as anterior, inferior, or lateral, and, with serial tracings, can define the timing of the process.

Changes caused by limitation of blood flow from coronary artery disease tend to be localized, tend to be associated with reciprocal abnormalities, and can have a typical evolutionary pattern. As a general rule, myocardial ischemia results in T wave changes, injury causes S-T abnormalities, and damage or necrosis and scarring result in changes in the QRS complex. These rules are not rigid, and a person can have full-thickness myocardial damage without QRS changes.

In the typical full-wall-thickness infarction, an evolutionary pattern of changes can be observed in the leads closest to, or looking most directly at, the process. For example, leads II, III, and aVF would reflect these changes with an inferior myocardial infarction. As shown in Fig. 4-8, with initial occlusion of the coronary blood vessel, ischemia occurs first and may result in T wave changes. Briefly, a tall peaked T wave can develop and persist for seconds, minutes, or hours. With continued occlusion of the blood

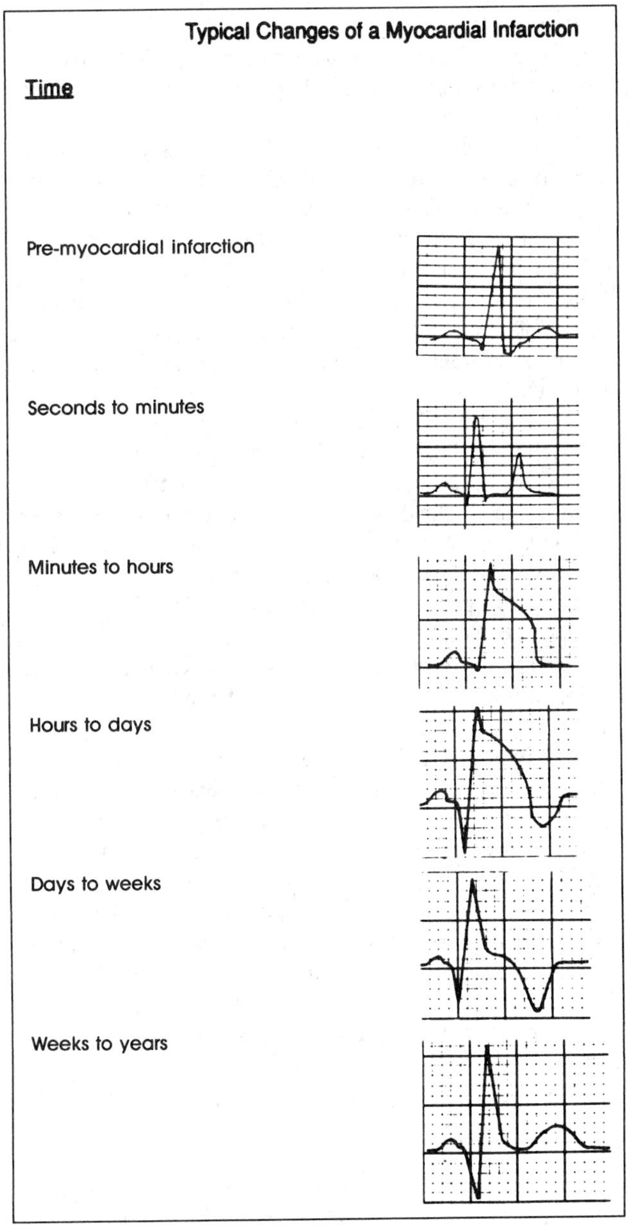

Fig. 4-8. Normal preinfarction ECG complex followed from above downward by the evolutionary ECG changes of acute Q wave (transmural) myocardial infarction (see text).

vessel, ischemia persists and myocardial injury occurs. This results in S-T segment elevation with a coved (convexity upward) configuration. At about the same time the T waves become inverted. Within a matter of minutes to hours to days, if the process continues and myocardial necrosis occurs, the QRS changes may occur. Typically, this results in the development of a pathologic Q wave, that is, a Q wave that is 0.04 second or greater in duration, which usually contributes to greater than 25% of the overall QRS height.

In approximately 1 week, the S-T segments return to baseline. Persistent elevation of the S-T segment has been correlated to some degree with the development of an LV aneurysm at the infarction site. The T wave inversion is unpredictable. In some patients it remains inverted; in others it returns to normal. Once the abnormal Q wave develops, it persists indefinitely in approximately 90% of patients with anterior infarction and 80% of those with inferior myocardial infarction.

These typical evolutionary changes may not occur, even in patients with a full-thickness infarction. Conversely, they may be observed in patients eventually shown to have a partial-wall-thickness infarction. When endocardial changes alone occur, the leads looking most directly at the involved region typically depict S-T segment depression. This is the pattern most often observed with exercise testing when transient subendocardial ischemia and injury are provoked.

The abnormal Q wave is the ECG finding most specific for a myocardial infarction. However, other syndromes may cause Q waves, which by themselves would meet the criteria for making the diagnosis of infarction. Potential causes for this so-called pseudoinfarction pattern are listed in the box above. One in particular is worth discussing: the "poor R wave progression." Normally a recording from the precordial leads will reveal an R wave that gradually increases in size from leads V_1 to V_6. The R wave exceeds the magnitude of the S wave in V_3 or in V_4. Failure of the R wave to become larger than the S wave can result from several causes. Probably more frequently than warranted, it has been attributed to an anterior myocardial infarction. Individuals with an anterior myocardial infarction sometimes may not develop true Q waves in these leads but rather only have smaller R waves. However, this is unusual, and this pattern of poor R wave progression occurs so often that it is inappropriate to be definitive about the diagnosis of an infarction. Perhaps the most common explanation for this ECG pattern is the presence of associated chronic obstructive pulmonary disease.

Syndromes and ECG patterns suggesting myocardial infarction when one has not occurred

Syndromes

Left ventricular hypertrophy
Right ventricular hypertrophy
Hypertrophic cardiomyopathy
Dilated and restrictive cardiomyopathies
Myocardial trauma
Myocardial tumor
Pulmonary embolism
Wolff-Parkinson-White syndrome
Metabolic abnormalities (e.g., hyperkalemia)
Congenital heart disease

ECG patterns

Left bundle branch block
Left anterior fascicular block
Normal repolarization pattern
Poor R wave progression
ECG lead misplacement

Atrial and ventricular enlargement and hypertrophy

Atrial enlargement. The ECG is not the ideal procedure for diagnosing atrial enlargement, but ECG features suggest its presence (Fig. 4-9). Left atrial enlargement affects the latter half of the P wave, causing an atrial conduction delay as well as voltage changes best seen in leads II and V_1. Criteria for left atrial enlargement are a P wave of 0.12 second (three small boxes) or greater in lead II or the presence of a negative component of the biphasic P wave that exceeds 0.04 second and 0.1 mV (one small box at a normal standardization) in depth in lead V_1.

With right atrial enlargement the P wave in lead II can

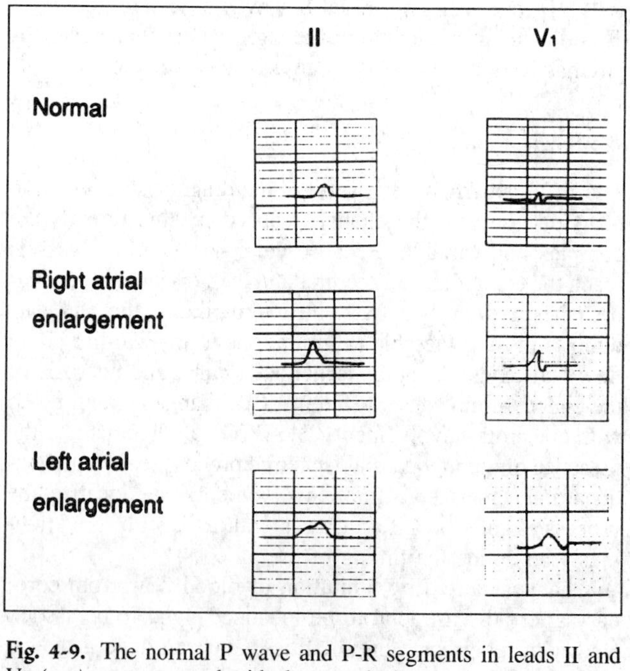

Fig. 4-9. The normal P wave and P-R segments in leads II and V_1 *(top)* are contrasted with those typically seen with right atrial *(middle)* and left atrial enlargement *(bottom)*.

exceed 0.25 mV (2.5 boxes tall or greater) and usually has a vertical axis. Often the initial positive vector is particularly prominent in leads V_1 to V_3. The large-magnitude P wave in lead II can occasionally be found in normal people, particularly those with faster heart rates.

Left ventricular hypertrophy. Multiple criteria exist for the diagnosis of LV hypertrophy (Fig. 4-10). Each has problems with sensitivity and specificity. Voltage criteria and repolarization abnormalities are required for the diagnosis.

Voltage measurement is affected by tissue around the heart, lung tissue, adipose tissue, breast tissue, and body position. Additionally, voltage may vary from day to day. Even measurement with one machine may not be equivalent to that measured by another (because of differences in frequency response). Thus it is difficult to define criteria that apply to all people. A conservative recommendation is that the diagnosis of LV hypertrophy should not be made until the combination of the S wave in V_1 and the R wave in V_5 or the S wave in V_2 and the R wave in V_6 equals or exceeds 3.5 mV (35 small boxes) or until the R wave in lead aVL exceeds 1.1 mV (11 small boxes). Using voltage criteria alone, 5% to 10% of the population would be erroneously given the diagnosis of LV hypertrophy. Therefore associated ST-T abnormalities are required to make the diagnosis more specific. Typically, they occur in the left-sided leads and include S-T segment depression with a convexity upward configuration and T wave inversion. This has been called the *strain pattern* (Fig. 4-10). When present without voltage criteria, these ST-T abnormalities could be the result of LV hypertrophy, but they are not a specific finding.

Associated left axis deviation, left atrial enlargement, and intraventricular conduction often occur but are not necessary for the diagnosis.

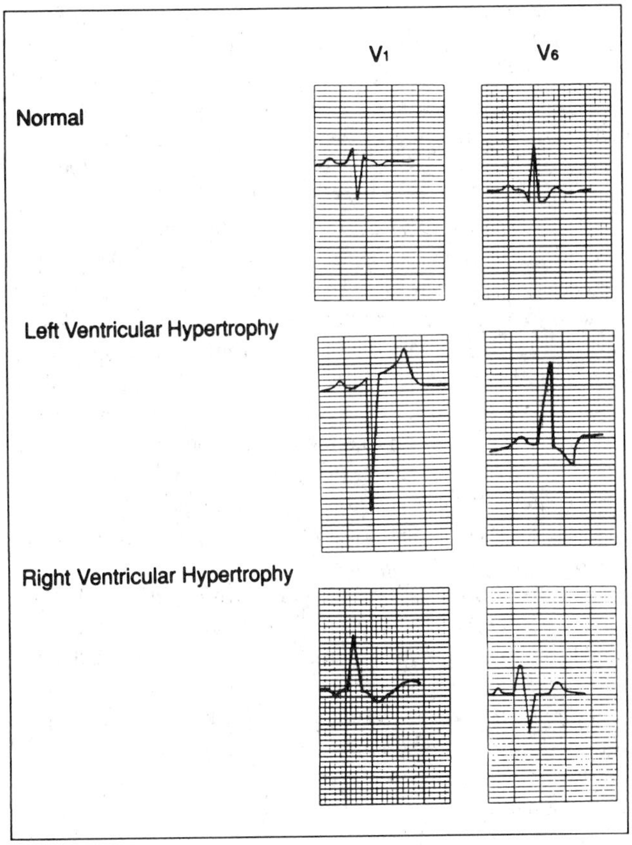

Fig. 4-10. The ECG complex in V_1 and V_6 in the normal subject *(top)* is contrasted with that frequently seen in patients with left ventricular hypertrophy *(middle)* and right ventricular hypertrophy *(bottom)*.

Right ventricular hypertrophy. Hypertrophy of the right ventricle (Fig. 4-10) causes electrical forces that can equal or exceed those seen in the left ventricle. This results in the criteria for RV hypertrophy, which is an R wave in lead V_1 that is at least as great or greater in magnitude than the S wave in that lead. ST-T changes similar to those described for LV hypertrophy occur in the right-sided leads. Right atrial enlargement and a vertical mean QRS access frequently accompany RV hypertrophy.

Syndromes that alter S-T and T waves

Inconsistency in interpretation of ST-T changes often occurs, but these changes occasionally are useful in clinical diagnosis. Some syndromes for which ST-T analysis is important (BBB, ventricular hypertrophy, coronary artery disease) have already been discussed (Fig. 4-11). In others, changes in the ST-T segments are the major manifestation on the ECG.

"Two almost-always-right rules." Although making any rigid recommendations about interpreting the S-T segments is probably unwise, I have found "two almost-always-right rules" helpful. The first states that although S-T segment elevation may be a normal variation, S-T segment depression is never normal. The second suggests that even though S-T segment scooping (convexity downward) may be normal, coving (convexity upward) of the S-T segment is not acceptable as normal.

These rules require some discussion. The first is the stronger of the two. The one exception is J point depression with rapid rise of the S-T segment to the baseline. This is a common finding in normal persons during exertion. The difficulty in knowing whether the J point is depressed versus the whole S-T segment is that no absolute rules exist about how rapidly the S-T segment must rise to reach the baseline to be considered normal. Some criteria have been established for exercise testing. If the S-T segment remains 1 mm below the baseline (as defined by the P-R segment) at 0.08 second (two small boxes) after the J point, a cardiac abnormality is likely. The criteria for a resting ECG have not been established. However, as a general rule, if S-T segment depression does not quickly return to the baseline, the examiner should recognize that it correlates highly with cardiovascular abnormalities.

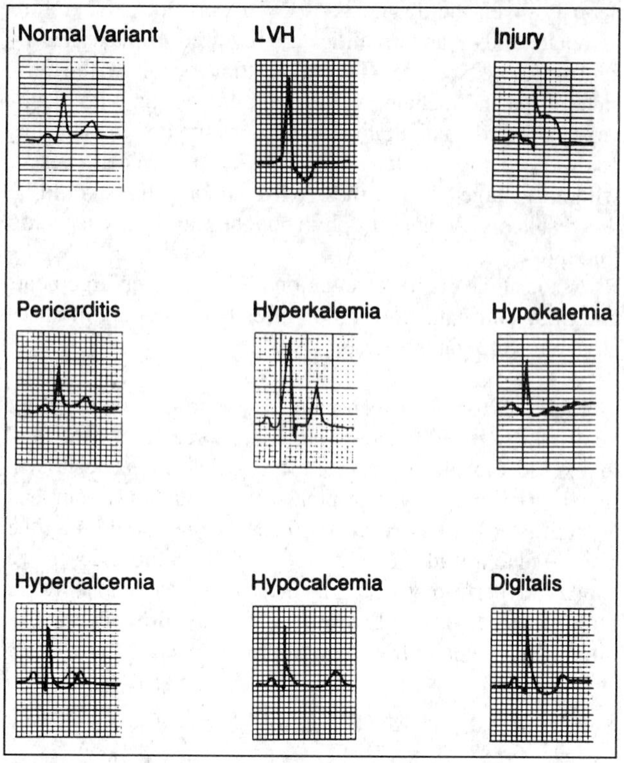

Fig. 4-11. Changes involving primarily the ST-T wave complex, which may be normal, result from hypertrophy or can be caused by injury or pericarditis and are contrasted with those caused by electrolyte abnormalities or drug therapy (see text). *LVH,* Left ventricular hypertrophy.

The second rule is somewhat less helpful. True coving can be difficult to define because in order for the S-T segment to enter a negative T wave (which is a normal finding in the right-sided leads), a convexity upward or a coved appearance may be present. If this is found in more than one lead, however, it also should raise the concern that the individual has heart disease.

Pericarditis. A patient may have pericarditis (Fig. 4-11) and have no ECG changes. When the changes do occur, however, they can strongly support the diagnosis. Diffuse S-T segment elevation characterizes the disease, which makes some sense because the pericardium surrounds the heart. Only leads V_1 and aVR have S-T segment depression, which also makes some sense because they view the heart from above and not through the pericardium as do the other leads. These elevated S-T segments have a convex downward or scooped appearance, often with some blunting of T wave height. No reciprocal changes occur, as are often seen with coronary artery disease changes. The P-R segments may appear depressed. The configuration and diffuse presence of the S-T segment changes differentiate them from the changes of ischemic heart disease. The evolution of S-T changes seen with pericarditis also differs from that occurring with coronary artery disease. Classically, before any T wave changes occur, the S-T segments of pericarditis return to normal, and then the T waves may become inverted. Coronary artery disease results in T wave inversion while the S-T segments are still elevated.

If a person develops pericardial fluid along with the pericarditis, QRS voltage can be reduced. With very large effusions, the heart can swing in the fluid. This may cause the QRS complex in any one lead to alternate from positive to negative on a beat-to-beat basis, a phenomenon called *electrical alternans.*

Since S-T segment elevation with a downward convexity can be a normal variant, it can be difficult to make the diagnosis of pericarditis from the ECG. The more diffuse the S-T changes, the more likely pericarditis is present. Additionally, blunting of the T waves (difficult to quantitate) also favors pericarditis.

Metabolic abnormalities. Any metabolic abnormalities can alter the ECG. Changes in levels of sodium, magnesium, pH, and other minor elements can cause ST-T abnormalities, but not predictably. Extreme excess or depletion of potassium or calcium, however, can result in recognizable patterns on the ECG.

Hypokalemia. An increase in ventricular ectopy is one manifestation of hypokalemia, but changes in the ST-T waves can be more diagnostic (Fig. 4-11). Typically the S-T segment is depressed, the T wave is flattened, and the U wave exceeds the height of the T wave. Occasionally the U wave can be confused with a T wave, suggesting a prolonged Q-T interval. Actually, with hypokalemia, this can be true, but it is difficult to measure the Q-T interval because of the presence of the U wave. These changes generally occur with a serum potassium level of less than 3.0 mEq/L.

Hyperkalemia. The changes from hyperkalemia can be evolutionary as the potassium level increases. As the potassium exceeds 6.0 mEq/L, T waves can become tall and peaked (changes similar to those seen with hyperacute ischemia) (Fig. 4-11). As the potassium level increases, intraventricular conduction is affected, causing widening of the QRS interval and the P-R interval. In the extremes the P-R interval can be so long that the P wave blends with the previous T wave; this, along with increasing QRS width, can give a sine wave appearance. These changes are readily reversible with administration of calcium chloride or bicarbonate.

Calcium abnormalities. Hypercalcemia (Fig. 4-11) results in a short Q-T interval. This is occasionally associated with S-T segment depression. Extreme hypercalcemia can cause sinus arrest and A-V conduction blocks.

Perhaps not surprisingly, hypocalcemia results in a prolonged Q-T interval. This is often associated with some broadening of the T wave and, generally, with a normal S-T segment.

Drug effects. Any medication can potentially affect the heart and thus the ECG. Some can cause predictable changes.

The phenothiazine drugs can cause ventricular ectopy and repolarization changes: S-T segment depression, T wave flattening, and abnormal U waves (changes indistinguishable from those caused by hypokalemia). The tricyclic antidepressant agents also can cause increased ventricular and atrial ectopy and at extreme levels can cause heart block.

Digitalis causes typical ECG changes (Fig. 4-11). The ST-T changes are not a reason to stop the drug. Typically, digitalis causes Q-T shortening (similar to hypercalcemia) as well as S-T segment depression with a convexity downward configuration. Digitalis can increase ventricular ectopy and with increased levels can cause A-V block.

The class IA antiarrhythmic drugs can also cause typical ST-T changes. These changes also are indistinguishable from those described for hypokalemia: S-T segment depression, T wave flattening, and a prominent U wave.

Changes from pacemakers

Implantable electronic pacemakers and evaluation for malfunction are discussed in Chapter 9. Those interpreting ECGs should be aware of several pacemaker features. An abrupt, absolutely vertical deflection on the ECG is not characteristic of any cardiac electrical activity and should suggest the presence of electronic pacemaker activity. If the pacemaker stimulus precedes each P wave, the pacemaker wire is pacing the atrium. When this is true, the QRS complex, the S-T segments, and the T waves can be interpreted normally. If the stimulus precedes each QRS complex, the pacemaker is stimulating the ventricle. When this is true, further interpretation of QRS, S-T, and T is inappropriate. Some patients have dual-chamber pacemakers, and both atrial and ventricular pacing may be detected on the ECG.

Pre-excitation syndromes

The significance and management of the pre-excitation syndromes are also discussed elsewhere (Chapter 9). Their presence, however, also can alter interpretation of the ECG. Each of these syndromes is associated with a short P-R interval. If the P-R interval is short but the QRS complex is narrow ($\leq$ 0.10 second), the pre-excitation is likely to result from rapid A-V node conduction or an A-V node bypass tract that inserts proximal to the bundle branches, since a narrow QRS can only be the result of conduction through the bundle branches. Patients with this finding may have recurrent re-entry supraventricular tachycardia and thus have the Lown-Ganong-Levine syndrome. Normal interpretation of the QRS complex, S-T segments, and T waves is appropriate with this syndrome.

If the short P-R interval is associated with a wide QRS complex and ST-T abnormalities, the pre-excitation is most likely caused by an accessory A-V bypass tract (Kent bundle). This also predisposes individuals to recurrent arrhythmias: the Wolff-Parkinson-White syndrome. When this form of pre-excitation is present on the ECG, further interpretation of QRS, S-T, and T may be misleading. Wolff-Parkinson-White syndrome is one cause of the pseudoinfarction patterns, and the usual rules for ST-T evaluation of hypertrophy may not be applicable.

REFERENCES

Algra A et al: QTc prolongation measured by standard 12-lead electrocardiography is an independent risk factor for sudden death due to cardiac arrest. Circulation 83:1888, 1991.

Devereaux RB et al: Electrocardiographic detection of left ventricular hypertrophy using echocardiographic determination of left ventricular mass as the reference standard. J Am Coll Cardiol 3:82, 1984.

Ginzton LE and Laks MM: The differential diagnosis of acute pericarditis from the normal variant: new electrocardiographic criteria. Circulation 56:1004, 1982.

Goldberger AL and O'Konski M: Utility of the routine electrocardiogram before surgery and on general hospital admission: critical review and new guidelines. Ann Intern Med 105:552, 1986.

Hurd HP et al: Comparative accuracy of ECG and vector criteria for inferior wall myocardial infarction. Circulation 63:1025, 1981.

Lee YC et al: ECG lead reversals: a common source of misinterpretation. Prim Cardiol 18:64, 1992.

Murphy ML et al: Descriptive characteristics of the electrocardiogram from autopsied men free of cardiopulmonary disease. Am J Cardiol 52:1275, 1983.

Sridharan MR and Flowers NC: Computerized electrocardiographic analysis. Mod Concepts Cardiovasc Dis 53:37, 1984.

Willems JL et al: The diagnostic performance of computer programs for the interpretation of electrocardiograms. N Engl J Med 325:1767, 1991.

CHAPTER

5 Cardiac Noninvasive Techniques

George A. Beller
Sanjiv Kaul

Cardiac noninvasive techniques refer to those diagnostic procedures that do not necessitate the placement of intravascular or intracardiac catheters. This chapter includes information on all frequently used noninvasive cardiac diagnostic methods except standard electrocardiography (Chapter 4). In ordering noninvasive tests, the physician should reflect on the quality of the available laboratory for performing the test(s), the accuracy and cost of the test(s) compared with alternative diagnostic methods, and the influence of test results on subsequent clinical decision making.

CHEST RADIOGRAPH

Before the advent of echocardiography, the chest radiograph was the only means of estimating cardiac size and status of the pulmonary vasculature. The radiograph is still useful in determining associated pulmonary pathology in patients with cardiac disorders and in determining the presence of pulmonary edema, particularly when other pulmonary conditions (e.g., pneumonia) coexist. Mediastinal widening on the chest radiograph may be the first indication of aortic pathology (e.g., dissection, aneurysm).

Fig. 5-1 illustrates the cardiac structures that can be seen in different views on the chest radiograph. Because

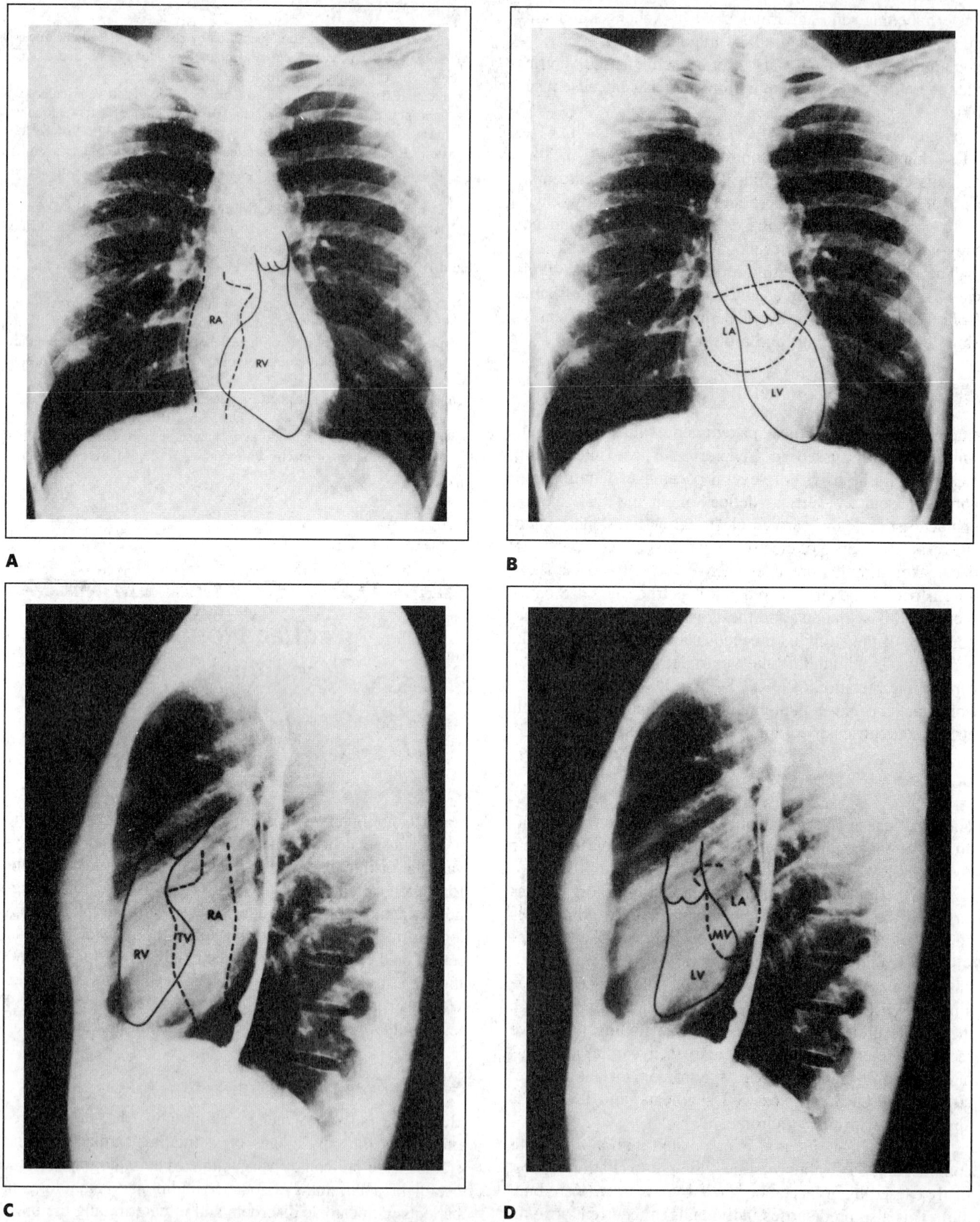

Fig. 5-1. Posterior anterior and lateral views of the normal heart showing major structures, including cardiac chambers. **A** and **C,** Right-sided heart chambers; **B** and **D,** left-sided heart chambers. *RA,* Right atrium; *RV,* right ventricle; *TV,* tricuspid valve; *LA,* left atrium; *LV,* left ventricle; *MV,* mitral valve. (From Dinsmore RE: Chest roentgenography. In Pohost GM and O'Rourke RA, editors: Principles and practice of cardiovascular imaging. 1991, Boston, Little, Brown. With permission.)

the cardiac silhouette represents a "summation" planar image, it is difficult to determine the exact cause of increased heart size, which can occur from enlargement of any chamber or the presence of pericardial effusion. Images from different views (Fig. 5-1, *A* to *D*) sometimes can assist in this purpose. Certain characteristic features on the cardiac silhouette and pulmonary vasculature are noted in specific cardiac conditions such as mitral stenosis (Chapter 16) and left-to-right cardiac shunts (Chapter 19). A rough estimate of these conditions' severity can be derived from the chest radiograph. However, echocardiography (with Doppler) provides accurate assessments of these conditions and generally has replaced the radiograph for this purpose.

The findings of pulmonary venous congestion, such as prominent superior pulmonary veins, interstitial or alveolar edema, Kerley B lines, and the presence of fluid in the interlobar fissures, are usually noted with left atrial pressures greater than 20 mm Hg (Chapter 10). When these findings are present on the radiograph, they are usually also evident on physical examination. Sometimes, however, coexisting pulmonary disease may make it difficult to separate these from other findings.

Calcification of the aorta or coronary arteries indicates atherosclerosis of these structures. Calcification may also be noted in the mitral annulus, mitral valve, aortic valve, left ventricular (LV) mural thrombus, LV aneurysm, or left atrial or LV tumors. The presence and type of prosthetic valve can also be seen and correct placement of a pacemaker lead confirmed on the chest radiograph.

The presence of dextrocardia, with or without situs inversus, may assist in the echocardiographic examination, particularly in the identification of abnormally placed structures. Classic radiographic patterns, such as "a boot-shaped heart" (Chapter 19), are usually associated with tetralogy of Fallot and may narrow the differential diagnosis in a child with central cyanosis. An anomalous pulmonary vein draining into the inferior vena cava may lead to the "scimitar" sign. Similarly, increased pulmonary vasculature may indicate the presence of undetected left-to-right cardiac shunts, and lack of pulmonary vasculature may indicate pulmonic or subpulmonic stenosis (Chapter 17).

In summary, the chest radiograph has had an important historic role in the evaluation of patients with cardiac disorders and is still useful, particularly in determining coexisting pulmonary pathology.

EXERCISE ELECTROCARDIOGRAPHIC TESTING

Electrocardiographic (ECG) stress testing is a clinically valuable technique that provides important diagnostic and prognostic information in patients with suspected or known coronary artery disease. The two major types of muscular exercise that can be used to stress the cardiovascular system are isometric (static) and isotonic (dynamic). Exercise is considered *isometric* when sustained muscular contraction occurs without motion (e.g., with handgrip), whereas isotonic exercise is defined as muscular contraction that results in some motion (e.g., running). Isometric exercise, which presents primarily a pressure load to the left ventricle, is rarely used for diagnostic ECG stress testing but can be employed as an adjunct to pharmacologic stress, as with intravenous dipyridamole or adenosine infusion. *Isotonic* exercise, which imposes a volume load to the left ventricle, is the preferred mode of exercise used for stress testing, and the cardiovascular response to isotonic exercise is proportional to the exercise's intensity.

Physiology

When a subject maximally exercises, the cardiac output may increase from 5 to 25 L/min, which results in increased systemic arterial pressure despite vasodilatation in the skeletal muscles, which assists the increase in flow. The increase in stroke volume during exercise varies and depends on the intensity of exercise and the posture in which exercise is performed. Although stroke volume usually increases, the primary mechanism for the rise in cardiac output is by an augmented heart rate. The increase in heart rate with exercise is attributed to a diminished vagal tone, followed by an increase in sympathetic neural outflow to the heart and blood vessels. Maximum heart rate decreases with age; this usually can be calculated by 220 minus the subject's age.

When isotonic exercise commences at a certain intensity, oxygen (O_2) uptake by the lung increases, then remains stable at a steady state after 2 minutes. At this steady state, heart rate, cardiac output, arterial blood pressure, and pulmonary ventilation are maintained at relatively constant levels. The *maximum oxygen uptake* ($\dot{V}O_{2max}$) is the maximum O_2 a person consumes when performing isotonic exercise. For exercise stress testing, the *metabolic equivalent* (MET) is used as a surrogate for $\dot{V}O_2$ and is expressed in multiples of resting requirements. One MET is equal to 3.5 ml O_2/kg of body weight/min. A person walking on a level surface at 4 miles/hr would exercise at a workload of 4 METs. $\dot{V}O_{2max}$ is also equal to the maximum cardiac output times the maximum arteriovenous O_2 difference. Because cardiac output is equal to the product of stroke volume and heart rate, $\dot{V}O_2$ is directly proportional to heart rate.

Myocardial $\dot{V}O_2$ is the product of heart rate and systolic blood pressure, often referred to as the *double product* or *rate-pressure product*. The major determinants of myocardial $\dot{V}O_2$ include myocardial wall tension, myocardial contractility, and heart rate (Chapter 1). The increase in myocardial O_2 demand during exercise is met by an increase in myocardial blood flow. Regional myocardial ischemia develops during exercise when a patient with a coronary artery stenosis cannot produce enough blood flow to supply the myocardium's increased metabolic needs (Chapter 13). In a patient with symptomatic coronary artery disease, angina pectoris usually occurs at the same double product regardless of the activity.

Procedures

Exercise testing should be conducted solely by well-trained personnel with basic knowledge of exercise physiology and who are trained to provide cardiopulmonary resuscitation (CPR). Testing should be performed under the supervision of a physician familiar with general indications and contraindications to the test and familiar with normal and abnormal responses. Competency standards for performance of exercise testing have been defined by a joint statement from the American College of Physicians, American College of Cardiology, and American Heart Association Task Force on Clinical Privileges in Cardiology. The physician or physician's assistant responsible for supervising an exercise test must first ask pertinent questions about the patient's medical history, should perform a brief physical examination, and must review a standard 12-lead ECG acquired immediately before testing.

General contraindications to exercise testing for myocardial ischemia include very recent acute myocardial infarction (less than 5 days); active unstable angina with rest pain; potentially life-threatening arrhythmias; acute pericarditis; severe aortic stenosis; marked elevation of arterial blood pressure (>200 mm Hg systolic or 120 mm Hg diastolic); severe symptomatic LV dysfunction; acute pulmonary embolus or infarction; acute or serious noncardiac disorder; acute thrombophlebitis or deep venous thrombosis; neurologic, musculoskeletal, or arthritic condition precluding adequate exercise; and inability or lack of motivation to perform the test.

Technical aspects

The ECG recording electrodes are placed on the trunk and should mimic the standard 12-lead conventional system. A recorder designed to capture high-quality ECG data during exercise is mandatory, and microprocessors are useful for generating average waveforms and for making certain ECG measurements. The exercise test can be performed on a treadmill or a mechanically or electrically braked cycle. A treadmill should have both variable-speed and variable-grade capability and must be accurately calibrated. The treadmill should have front and siderails for patients to steady themselves; patients should not tightly grasp siderails because this decreases $\dot{V}O_2$, increases exercise time, and enhances muscle artifact. Bicycle ergometers are most often used to evaluate the functional capacity and response to therapy with cardiovascular drugs in patients with coronary artery disease or heart failure.

Before commencing the exercise test protocol, a 12-lead ECG tracing should be obtained in the standing position when performing treadmill exercise and after voluntary hyperventilation. The latter may induce ST-T wave changes that must be taken into account when interpreting exercise-induced alterations. Clinical testing consists of an initial warm-up load, progressive uninterrupted exercise with an adequate duration at each level, and a recovery period. The 12-lead ECG is recorded each minute, with frequent three-lead recordings taken according to clinical circumstances. Blood pressure determinations are made frequently, and the patient is observed closely for limiting end-points or complications. The exercise workload is usually changed every 3 minutes, and testing for detection of coronary artery disease is conducted to symptom-limited end-points. The Bruce protocol is the most popular one used in the United States, and its advantages include a seventh or final stage that cannot be completed by most individuals. The optimum protocol should last 6 to 12 minutes and should be individualized to the patient. Submaximum testing is most often conducted during the predischarge phase after recovery from an uncomplicated acute myocardial infarction.

Indications for terminating an exercise test include a drop in systolic blood pressure to below baseline levels despite an increase in exercise workload, new-onset or increasing anginal chest pain, central nervous system symptoms, signs of poor peripheral perfusion, high-grade ventricular arrhythmias, and the patient's request to cease. Frequently a test is terminated when marked (>4.0 mm) ischemic S-T segment depression is observed or new S-T segment elevation appears in leads without Q waves. This latter finding reflects transmural ischemia, which may result from exercise-induced vasospasm or rarely from sudden occlusion of a coronary vessel. Similarly, a less serious arrhythmia (e.g., supraventricular tachycardia) may result in premature termination of the test.

Since abnormal responses may occur only during recovery after exercise, patients should be continuously monitored in the supine position during the postexercise periods for at least 5 minutes.

Clinical applications

The main indication for exercise testing is to assist in the diagnosis of coronary artery disease in patients with chest pain (Chapter 13). A second major indication is to evaluate functional capacity and aid in assessing the prognosis of patients with known coronary artery disease. When exercise stress is sufficient to produce a mismatch between myocardial O_2 supply and demand, myocardial ischemia will develop and often is identified by certain alterations in the ECG's S-T segment. Although anginal chest pain induced by the test is strongly predictive of coronary artery disease, 1.0 mm of horizontal or downsloping S-T segment depression is considered a positive end-point for ischemia (Chapter 4). The S-T depression must persist for 80 milliseconds (ms) or longer and must be recognized in at least three consecutive beats with a steady ECG baseline. Increasing S-T segment elevation can often be seen in leads demonstrating pathologic Q waves at rest in patients with prior myocardial infarction. These changes are predominantly observed in patients with a depressed ejection fraction and severe regional myocardial asynergy.

A review of published studies shows that the sensitivity of exercise ECG stress tests averaged 68%, with average specificity of 77% for detection of coronary artery disease. The extent of coronary artery disease may affect the test's sensitivity. An ischemic ECG response occurs in 85% or more of patients with three-vessel disease but in only 45%

to 50% of patients with single-vessel disease. The administration of antianginal drugs may influence exercise stress test results. Beta-adrenergic blockers, calcium antagonists, and nitrates may prevent the appearance of abnormal S-T segment changes. Beta blockers may prevent the patient from attaining the desired heart rate–blood pressure product at which ischemic S-T segment depression would appear.

An ECG stress test is considered to be "diagnostic" when 85% or more of the maximum predicted heart rate adjusted for age is attained. Sensitivity is reduced if the test is terminated at suboptimum heart rates in the absence of limiting symptoms.

In certain situations, horizontal or downsloping S-T segment depression can appear in the absence of significant coronary artery disease. Causes of false-positive S-T segment responses include ST-T wave abnormalities on the resting ECG caused by digitalis administration, LV hypertrophy, mitral valve prolapse syndrome, hyperventilation, electrolyte abnormalities such as hypokalemia, bundle branch block, Wolff-Parkinson-White syndrome, pericardial disease, systemic hypertension, and noncardiac disorders such as nonischemic cardiomyopathy.

Although sensitivity and specificity values define a test's essential accuracy, the interpretation of any patient's test results depends on the pretest likelihood of coronary artery disease in that individual or in the overall population being tested. Bayes' theorem expresses the posttest likelihood of disease as a function of the test's sensitivity and specificity and the disease's prevalence in the population being tested. A diagnostic test such as exercise electrocardiography is of greatest value with an intermediate probability of disease in the range of 50%, where uncertainty is greatest. In a population with a high prevalence of coronary artery disease, a positive test merely confirms the presence of disease, but a negative test does not exclude disease. In a low-prevalence population, a negative test merely confirms the absence of disease, but a positive test result does not establish disease presence because such a response may represent a false-positive test result.

Conversely, although ECG exercise testing does not add substantially to the diagnosis of coronary artery disease in male patients with typical angina pectoris, the test may be useful for prognostication. Several high-risk exercise test variables are associated with an increased cardiac event rate and a high incidence of left main or three-vessel coronary artery disease (see box, above right). Patients with 2.0 mm or more of S-T segment depression, particularly when manifested at a low exercise heart rate or workload, have a higher incidence of high-risk anatomic disease compared with patients with lesser degrees of S-T segment depression. Patients failing to progress farther than stage 1 of the Bruce protocol or to achieve a workload of at least 4 METs are at higher risk for subsequent ischemic cardiac events compared with patients with better exercise capacity. Peak heart rate alone on exercise testing is related to survival. Patients achieving a heart rate of only 120 beats/min or less on exercise testing have a significantly worse survival compared with patients whose heart rate exceeds 120 beats/min.

Exercise ECG and thallium-201 (^{201}Tl) imaging variables associated with high-risk coronary artery disease

Exercise ECG stress testing

- Impairment of exercise tolerance
- Ischemic S-T segment depression and/or angina at 4 METs or less
- 2 mm or more of horizontal or downsloping S-T depression
- Ischemic S-T depression lasting longer than 5 minutes into recovery period
- S-T depression observed in five or more ECG leads
- Decrease in systolic blood pressure of 10 mm Hg or greater with exercise

Exercise ^{201}Tl scintigraphy

- Multiple perfusion defects, particularly of the redistribution type, in more than one coronary supply region
- Increased lung ^{201}Tl uptake
- Transient left ventricular cavity dilatation observed on exercise images

Patients who attain exercise heart rates greater than 160 beats/min have a much lower subsequent cardiac event rate even with S-T segment depression. Normally the systolic blood pressure increases with exercise because of the increased cardiac output with maintenance of stroke volume. Exercise-induced mechanical dysfunction resulting in impaired systolic contraction from ischemia often causes a failure to increase the systolic blood pressure by 10 mm Hg or more or may result in exercise-induced hypotension. A decrease in systolic blood pressure of 10 mm Hg or more during exercise has been shown to predict left main or three-vessel coronary artery disease. Finally, the demonstration of complex ventricular ectopy at peak exercise is associated with increased risk of an adverse outcome.

CONTINUOUS AMBULATORY ELECTROCARDIOGRAPHIC RECORDING

The initial objective of ambulatory electrocardiography was to detect arrhythmias in ambulatory patients with symptoms such as dizziness, palpitations, and syncope, and this still remains its major role. Three or four ECG leads are placed on the chest wall and connected to a small tape recorder, which the patient clips to a belt. Usually the ECG is continuously recorded on tape for 24 hours. However, the recordings may last up to 72 hours. A diary is usually provided so the patient can record symptoms and the time when these occurred. In some patients an *event monitor* is used. This unit is attached to the patient for up to a month at a time, and several seconds to minutes of the most recent ECG recordings are retained within the device's computer memory. When patients experience a symptom, they can trigger the device and play back the recordings to an analysis system via the telephone.

The data on the recording devices are played back on an

automated analysis system that scans the data extremely rapidly. Abnormalities are detected and printed out with the time at which they occurred. Such data as slowest and fastest heart rates, total premature atrial and ventricular beats, and abnormal pauses are all noted. The physician then can correlate these with the patient's symptoms.

Another use of ambulatory ECGs is the detection of S-T segment elevation when symptoms are or are not present. The entity of *silent myocardial-ischemia* (Chapter 13) was first described when painless S-T elevation was first documented on the ambulatory ECG in patients with coronary artery disease. However, spontaneous and painless S-T elevation may occur without ischemia, such as during meals or hyperventilation. Exercise testing with cardiac imaging (radionuclide, echocardiographic) is more accurate for detecting myocardial ischemia and provides more prognostic information than ambulatory electrocardiography.

Patients with variant angina (Chapter 13) are more likely to show ECG ST-T wave changes during normal activity than during exercise testing. Ambulatory electrocardiography may be useful in such patients, particularly for monitoring the results of therapy. The results of therapy can also be assessed by this technique in patients with arrhythmias (Chapter 9).

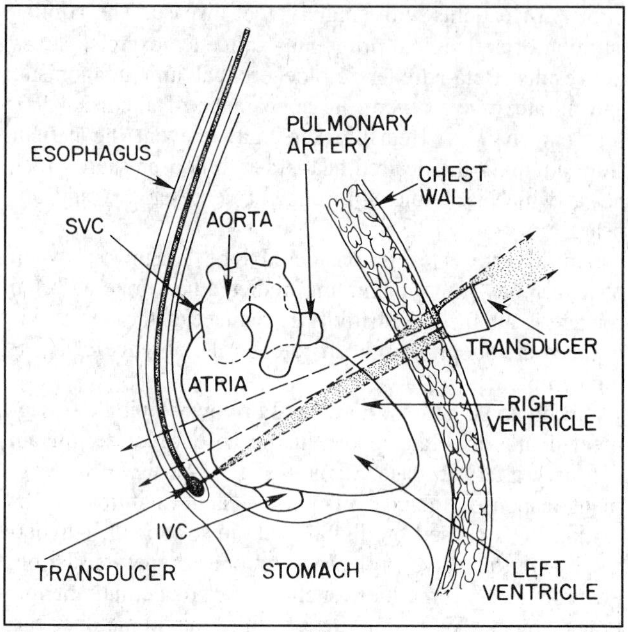

Fig. 5-2. Methods of acquiring images of the heart using echocardiography. The transducer placed on the chest wall can be used to acquire most images. Because of its proximity to these structures, however, the transducer placed in the esophagus can be used to acquire better images of the posterior cardiac structures and the great vessels.

ECHOCARDIOGRAPHY

Echocardiography is used to image cardiac structures and function and also flow direction and velocities within cardiac chambers and vessels. Usually these images are obtained from several positions on the chest wall and abdomen using a hand-held transducer (Fig. 5-2); this technique is referred to as *transthoracic* echocardiography. In some circumstances a specially designed transducer is inserted into the esophagus and stomach to obtain images from behind the heart; this technique is referred to as *transesophageal* echocardiography (Fig. 5-2). Although traditionally considered "noninvasive," echocardiography is now often used in the operating room, where either transesophageal echocardiography is used or the transducer is hand-held directly over the heart's surface. In the cardiac catheterization laboratory, miniature transducer-tipped catheters are inserted directly into coronary arteries to obtain cross-sectional images of the arterial lumen and wall or into the cardiac chambers to visualize cardiac structures.

Imaging cardiac structures and function

Echocardiography uses ultrasound to image the heart. Ultrasound is emitted by piezoelectric crystals housed within a transducer. When these crystals' shape is changed electronically, they emit ultrasound waves that travel within tissue at 1540 cm/sec and are reflected back from tissues and tissue-blood interfaces. The returning sound waves distort the piezoelectric crystals within the transducer, and the energy is transformed into an electric signal, which is converted to a video signal for display on a screen. The video signal's intensity is proportional to that of the reflected sound wave, and the signal's location on the screen indicates the time for the sound wave to return from the tissue. Because the time for the sound wave to return from a structure within the heart is inversely related to the structure's distance from the transducer, cardiac structures are displayed on the video screen in their true anatomic orientation.

When a beam created by a single crystal is directed through the heart, it interrogates the heart as an "ice pick." This method is called *M-mode* echocardiography and provides excellent axial and temporal resolution. Fig. 5-3 depicts an M-mode image through the heart at the mitral valve level in a normal subject and in a patient with dilated cardiomyopathy. Because the tracing represents an ice pick view, cardiac structures are not represented in a tomographic format, and only a very limited view of the cardiac chambers is provided.

To image more of the heart at the same time, several individual beams can be emitted from several piezoelectric crystals housed within the same transducer, creating a wide beam capable of imaging the heart in an entire plane. This beam can be created either mechanically, in which the crystals are moved within the transducer using a motor, or electronically, in which the crystals are stimulated one after the other to produce a wide-angled beam. The beam can be of any size and contains several imaging lines produced by individual sound waves. Because the speed of sound in tissue is constant, the rate at which each sector is created depends on the number of lines to be formed and their length. For a 90-degree sector with a depth of 20 cm, the frame rate is 30/sec.

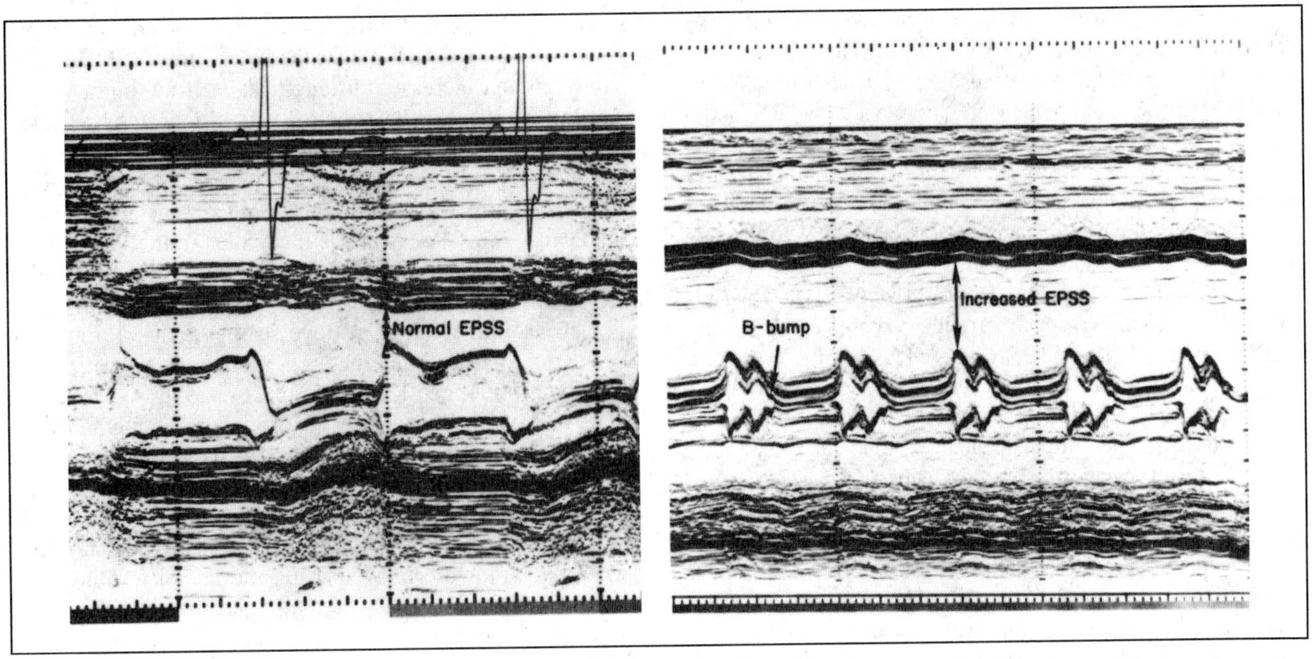

Fig. 5-3. M-mode echocardiogram through the left ventricle at the mitral valve level in a normal subject *(left)* and in a subject with dilated ischemic cardiomyopathy *(right)*. *EPSS,* E-point septal separation, indicating the distance between the anterior mitral leaflet and the interventricular septum in diastole.

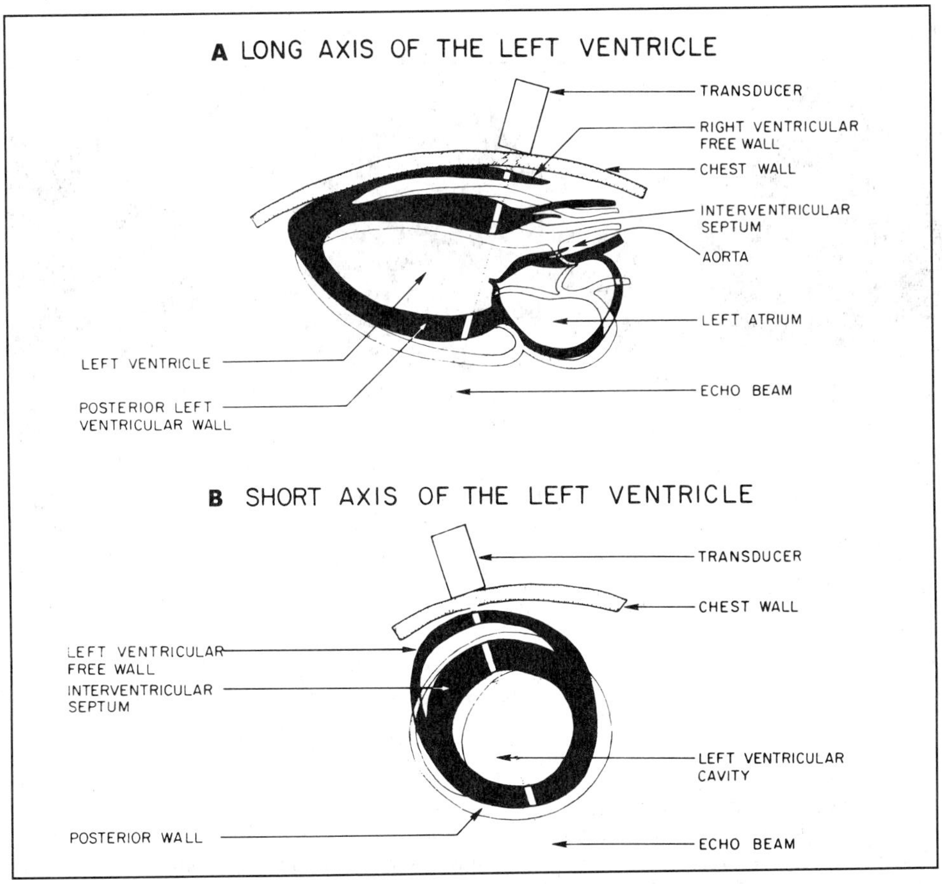

Fig. 5-4. Diagrammatic representation of parasternal long-axis **(A)** and short axis **(B)** views on two-dimensional (2D) echocardiography obtained in end-diastole *(white)* and end-systole *(black)*. The M-mode beam can be guided using the 2D image. (From Kaul S: Am Heart J 112:568, 1986. Reproduced with permission.)

This imaging method is termed *two-dimensional* (2D) echocardiography and is the standard format used for imaging the heart. The same transducer can also be used to obtain M-mode data, which are more valuable when the M-mode beam is guided from the 2D image, because the exact orientation of the beam is known (Fig. 5-4). Using the transthoracic approach, 2D images are acquired from three standard locations: parasternal, apical, and subcostal. The parasternal approach provides long-axis and short-axis images of the LV (Fig. 5-4) and right ventricular (RV) inflow. The apical approach provides two-chamber, four-chamber (Fig. 5-5), and long-axis views of the LV. The subcostal approach often is not needed if the parasternal and apical images are adequate; however, in some patients in whom these images are inadequate, subcostal views provide useful information. Also, the subcostal four-chamber view provides the best approach for imaging the interatrial septum.

By using several planes, the heart can be imaged comprehensively in real time using 2D echocardiography. Cardiac chamber dimensions and wall thickness can be measured and valve structure and motion assessed. In addition, proximal portions of the great vessels can be imaged and any echo-free space within the pericardial cavity noted. Classic patterns can be used to define disease entities, as shown in Fig. 5-3, which compares images from a normal subject and a patient with dilated cardiomyopathy. Compared with the normal image, the other shows a dilated LV cavity and an increased distance between the mitral valve and the interventricular septum, which indicates low ejection fraction. A "B bump" is also noted on the anterior mitral leaflet, which indicates a high LV end-diastolic pressure. The end-systolic four-chamber view of the same patient (Fig. 5-5, *C*) also shows incomplete mitral leaflet closure, indicating mitral regurgitation and a thrombus in the LV apex.

Because the echo beam traverses tissue and is reflected back from intervening structures, it becomes weaker when it reaches structures located farthest away from the transducer. The echo beam can be artificially strengthened at greater depth, a technique called *time-gain compensation*. However, despite this modification, structures located farthest from the transducer may not be imaged as clearly as those nearest to the transducer. This is particularly true when structures are imaged using the lateral resolution of ultrasound. For instance, structures such as the left atrial appendage, the pulmonary veins, and the aorta are not imaged well using the transthoracic approach.

Since the esophagus is close to both the atria and the great vessels, a transducer positioned in it (see Fig. 5-2) provides significantly better detail of these structures. Fig. 5-6 is an example of dissection of the thoracic aorta noted

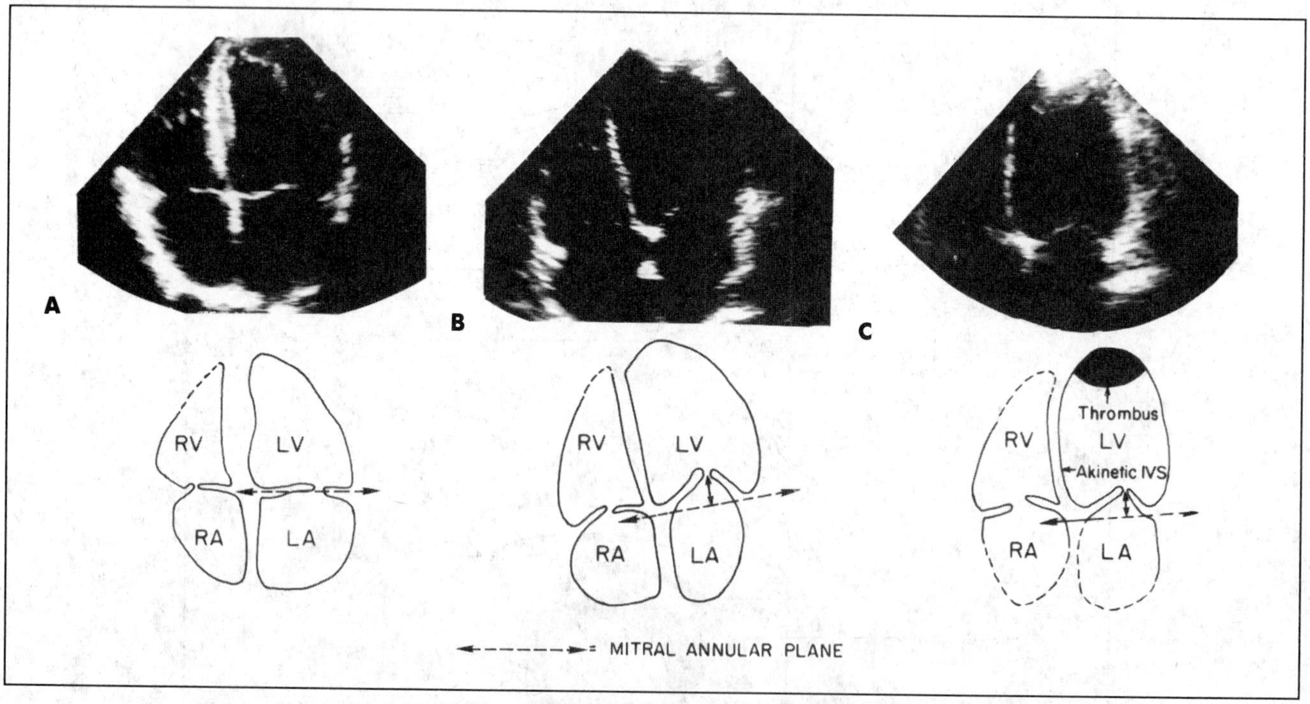

Fig. 5-5. Four-chamber views from three different subjects. **A,** Normal subject with normal left ventricular size and normal end-systolic position of the mitral leaflets in relation to the mitral annulus. **B,** Patient with dilated cardiomyopathy and *incomplete mitral leaflet closure,* in which the leaflets hang up in the left ventricle in end-systole and result in mitral regurgitation. **C,** Patient with dilated cardiomyopathy similar to one in **B,** with the additional finding of a thrombus in the left ventricular apex. The interventricular septum *(IVS)* is also akinetic. This patient's M-mode echocardiogram is depicted in the right panel in Fig. 5-3. (From Kaul S: Am Heart J 118:963, 1989. Reproduced with permission.)

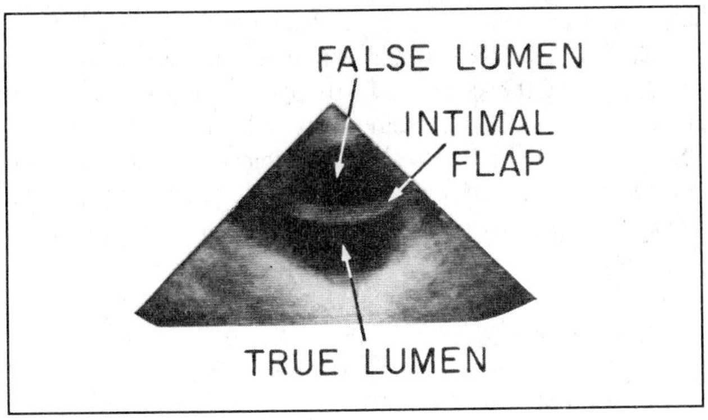

Fig. 5-6. Dissection of the thoracic aorta noted on transesophageal echocardiography.

on transesophageal echocardiography. Fig. 5-7 illustrates a thrombus in a mechanical prosthetic mitral valve that could not be visualized from the transthoracic approach because of "shadowing" created by the prosthesis. However, the thrombus was clearly seen on transesophageal echocardiography (Fig. 5-7, *A*), and its position was confirmed when the prosthetic valve was surgically removed (Fig. 5-7, *B*). Moreover, since there is no intervening lung and the imaging depth from the transesophageal approach is less, requiring less tissue penetration, higher-frequency transducers can be used, resulting in even better resolution.

Despite the definitely superior image quality obtained with transesophageal echocardiography, the procedure is uncomfortable for the awake patient, who requires sedation and a local anesthetic to the pharynx. The procedure is also more time and resource consuming: a nurse is required to assist, and a trained physician is required to perform it. This differs from transthoracic echocardiography, which can be performed by a trained sonographer. Therefore the transesophageal procedure should only be performed when the information required cannot be obtained by other less involved methods.

Imaging flow velocities and direction

When a moving source of light is interrogated from a stationary object, the frequency of light emitted from the moving source changes, becoming higher as it moves toward the stationary object (white to red) and lower as it moves away (white to blue). The direction of shift in frequency therefore indicates the moving source's direction of motion and has been termed the *Doppler effect* after the Austrian physicist who described this phenomenon. This same phenomenon is noted when ultrasound is emitted from a stationary transducer and the reflected waves from the red blood cells (RBCs) within cardiac chambers and great vessels are received by the same or another stationary transducer. The direction of shift in ultrasound frequency is used to determine the direction of flow of the RBCs in relation to the transducer. This direction of flow can be displayed as a spectral velocity profile, with the profile oriented toward the transducer for blood coming toward it or oriented away from the transducer for blood flowing away.

Fig. 5-8 illustrates the spectral display of signals from the LV outflow tract using a continuous-wave Doppler transducer positioned at the heart's apex, with the ultrasound beam directed from the LV apex to the aortic root. The flow signals directed upward are oriented toward the transducer, and those directed downward are oriented away from the transducer. These signals indicate that the patient has aortic regurgitation because in diastole, flow is directed toward the transducer (toward the LV apex). The flow directed downward indicates the maximum peak velocity in systole is along the line of interrogation. This is normal (almost 1 m/sec), indicating the absence of any obstruction in the LV outflow tract.

The direction of flow can also be depicted by using color coding of velocity shifts within the cardiac chambers. Red depicts blood directed toward the transducer (see Color Plate I-1), and blue depicts blood moving away from the transducer (see Color Plate I-2). Not only can the direction of RBC flow be assessed, but the RBC cell velocity can be

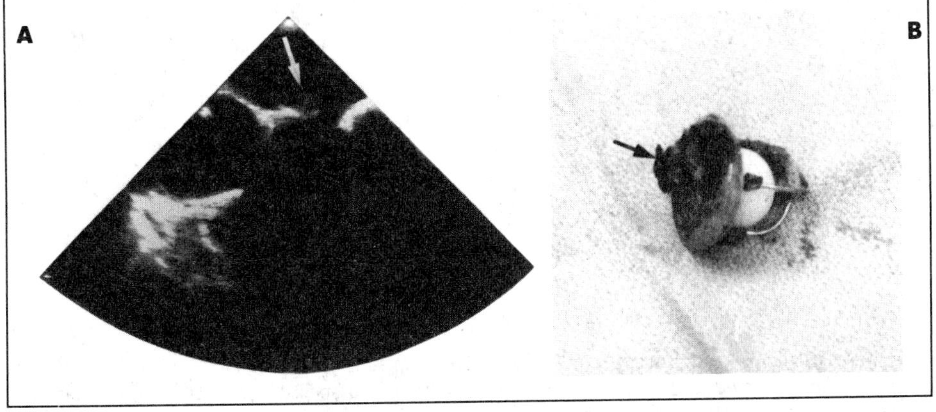

Fig. 5-7. A, Thrombus on the left atrial aspect of the prosthetic mitral valve noted on transesophageal echocardiography. **B,** Presence of the thrombus was confirmed with inspection of the valve after it was surgically removed.

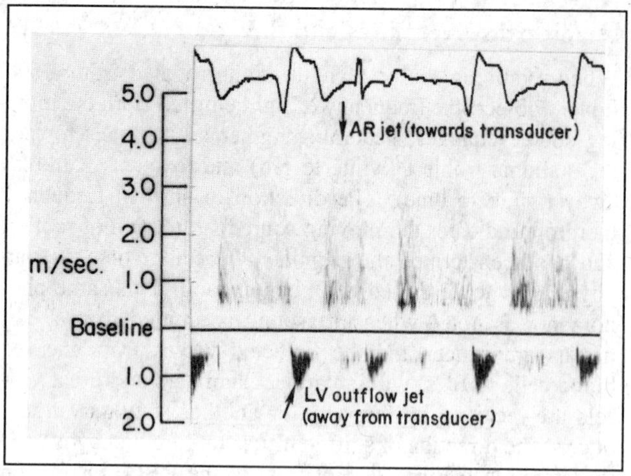

Fig. 5-8. Continuous-wave Doppler recordings obtained from a line of interrogation extending from the left ventricular *(LV)* apex to the LV outflow tract. It depicts abnormal diastolic flow oriented toward the transducer, indicating aortic regurgitation *(AR),* and normal systolic velocity, indicating absence of any obstruction in the entire outflow tract.

measured as well. Unlike imaging cardiac structures, in which the best resolution is obtained when the structure is imaged with the echo beam perpendicular to it, accurate measurement of RBC velocity is obtained by having the beam as parallel to the cells as possible. The degree of shift in the frequency of ultrasound after it strikes the RBCs reflects the velocity at which the RBCs are moving. The faster they move, the greater is the frequency shift. As long as the RBCs are sampled along their direction of flow (±15 degrees), the Doppler shift produced by them provides an accurate assessment of RBC velocity.

This velocity information can be used to quantify flow and to measure pressures within cardiac chambers. Because flow equals velocity times area, if the aortic root area (2D imaging of the heart) and the flow velocity across the aortic valve are known, the stroke volume can be calculated. When multiplied by heart rate, the stroke volume can provide the cardiac output. The same principle can be used to measure valve area, using the continuity equation, which is based on energy proximal to a stenosis being the same as distal to it. Since velocity times area equals flow, this

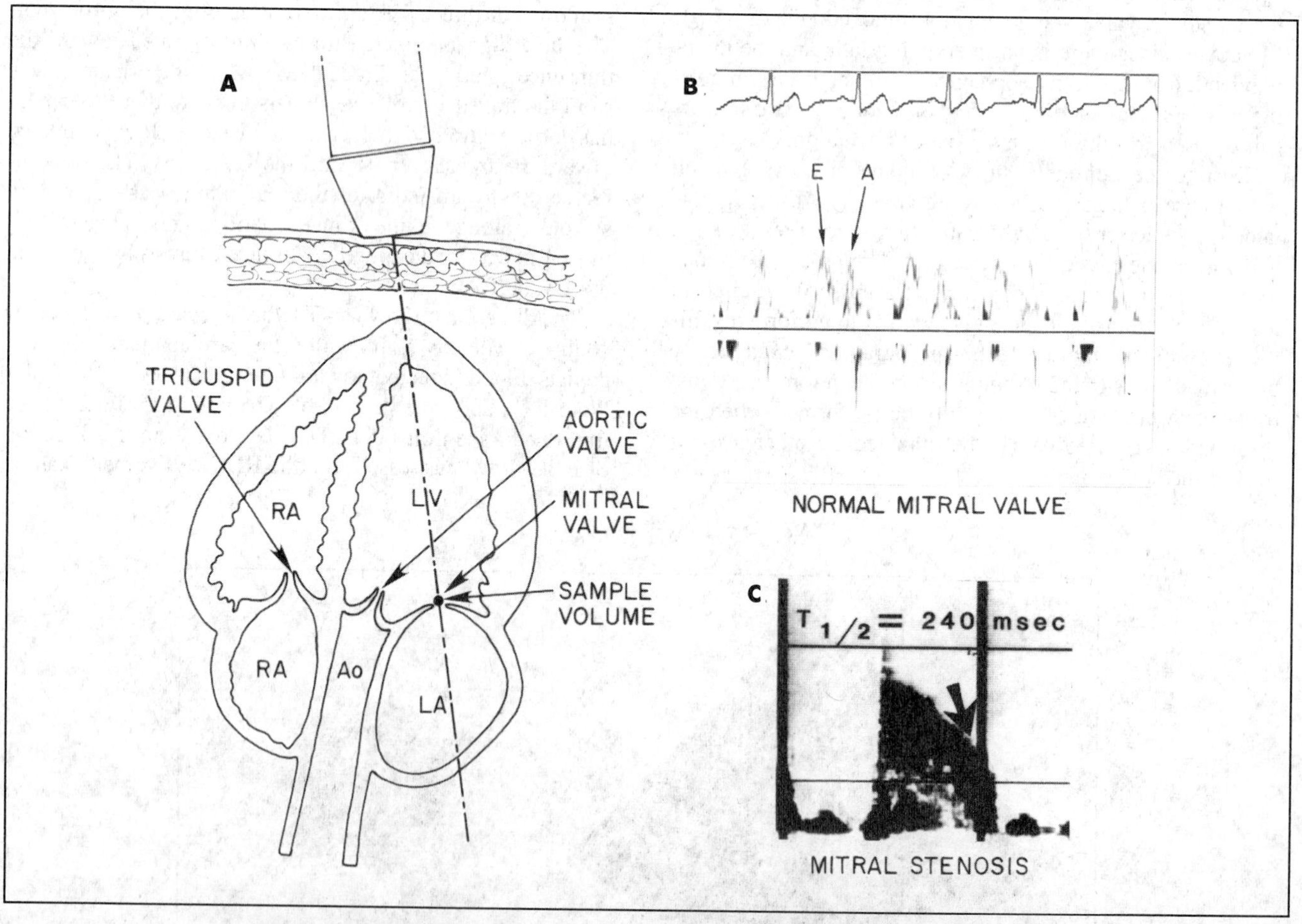

Fig. 5-9. Method of acquiring spectral velocity profiles using the pulsed-Doppler method. **A,** Sample volume is located at the mitral valve tips, resulting in a spectral velocity profile oriented toward the transducer (**B** and **C**). **B,** Normal mitral velocity profile in which the E wave results from early LV filling and the A wave from LV filling caused by left atrial contraction. **C,** Velocity profile from a patient with severe mitral stenosis in which the pressure half-time is 240 ms. No A wave exists because the patient is in atrial fibrillation.

flow should be the same downstream as upstream from a stenosed aortic valve. If the aortic root area just proximal to the valve (from 2D imaging) and the mean velocity at this plane are known, aortic valve area can be calculated by dividing the product of these two by the velocity across the stenotic aortic valve.

In practice, measurement of velocities is performed using either the *pulsed-Doppler* or the *continuous-wave Doppler* technique. For the pulsed technique a sample volume is placed over a region where the velocity has to be measured, such as at the mitral leaflet tips (Fig. 5-9, *A*). As the ultrasound signals return from the heart, all except those returning from this sample volume will be rejected. The signals from the sample volume are then depicted as a spectral display, with time on the x axis. Fig. 5-9, *B*, illustrates pulsed-Doppler signals from a normal mitral valve, whereas *C* illustrates those from a patient with mitral stenosis. This technique is excellent for quantification of velocities at a discrete site; however, it is limited by the maximum velocity it can measure and is not used for the quantification of velocities greater than 2 m/sec.

Unlike pulsed Doppler, in which the transducer emits ultrasound and then goes into the "receive mode" to acquire the returning waves, continuous-wave Doppler uses two transducers: one to emit ultrasound and the other to receive it. Although this technique cannot localize the exact region within the beam length producing the greatest Doppler shift, it can measure very high velocities, such as those created by valvular stenosis and regurgitation and intracardiac shunts.

Using the modified Bernoulli equation ($P = 4V^2$), the peak instantaneous velocity across a region (V) can be converted to the peak instantaneous pressure gradient (P) across it. For instance, if V across a stenotic aortic valve is 5 m/sec, P across it is 100 mm Hg. V can be converted to mean gradient by integrating the velocity profile. Similarly, as shown in Fig. 5-10, if V measured from a regurgitant jet across the tricuspid valve during systole is 4.8 m/sec, the gradient across the tricuspid valve in systole is 92 mm Hg. If, based on the jugular venous pressure, the mean right atrial pressure is estimated to be 10 mm Hg, the peak ventricular systolic (and hence the pulmonary artery systolic pressure, unless pulmonic stenosis is present) pressure is 102 mm Hg. Pulmonic valve motion on M-mode images in the patient whose Doppler signal is depicted in Fig. 5-10, *A*, also shows the classic "flying W" pattern for pulmonary hypertension, as depicted in *B*.

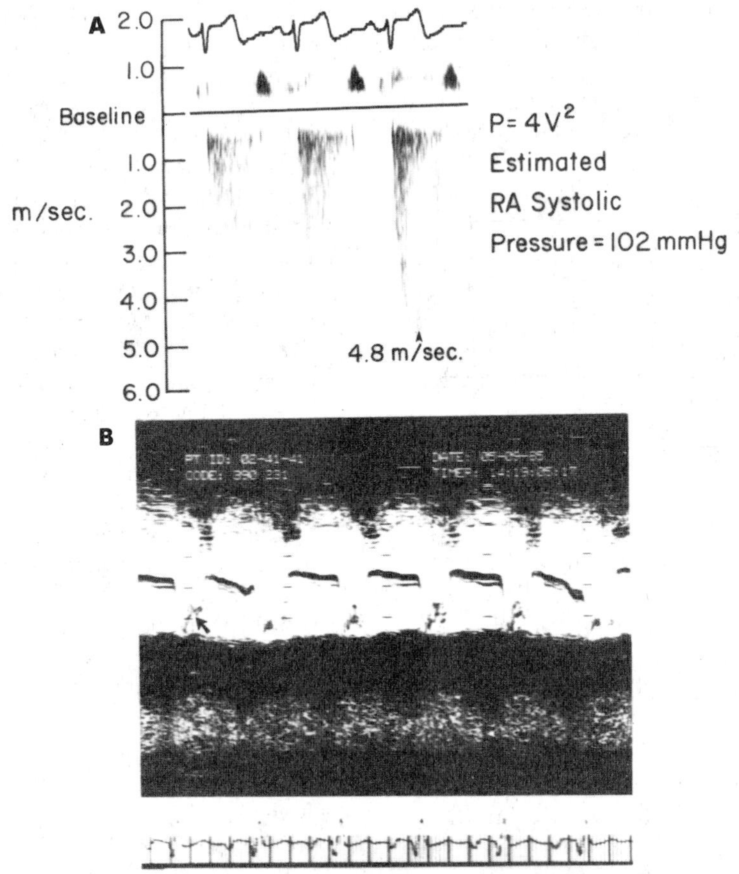

Fig. 5-10. Continuous-wave Doppler (**A**) and M-mode tracings (**B**) from a patient with pulmonary hypertension (see text for details).

The rate of pressure gradient decline across a stenotic mitral valve provides an estimate of the severity of stenosis. The time required during diastole to go from peak pressure gradient to half that value provides a direct assessment of mitral stenosis; the longer this interval, the more severe is the mitral stenosis. The simultaneous left atrial and LV pressure recordings in a patient with mitral stenosis (Fig. 5-11) indicate a 260 ms interval (normal, 20 to 60 ms) for the maximum pressure gradient to reach half its original value and severe mitral stenosis. Fig. 5-9, *C,* illustrates a Doppler signal from the same patient. The pressure half-time of 240 ms derived from pulsed Doppler was very close to the 260 ms obtained at cardiac catheterization.

The information available from pulsed-Doppler echocardiography in terms of mean velocities and turbulent flow can also be obtained by simultaneously color-coding velocities in different regions of the cardiac cavities and great vessels. Differently colored maps can be used, and higher velocities of blood are coded brighter. When turbulence is present, the range of velocities within a region is large. The variance from the mean velocity therefore is great compared with the situation when flow is laminar. This variance is color-coded as a mosaic pattern. For instance, aortic regurgitation causes a mosaic pattern in the LV outflow tract in diastole on a transthoracic image (see Color Plate I-3), and a mosaic pattern is noted in the mitral regurgitant jet in the left atrium in systole on a transesophageal image (see Color Plate I-4). Although providing similar information as pulsed Doppler, color Doppler has the added advantage of depicting images of normal and abnormal flow and direction of flow superimposed on routine 2D images. Whereas color Doppler improves the ease with which the heart can be examined for flow patterns, spectral Doppler displays are needed for a quantification of peak and mean velocities when assessing pressure gradients across valves. Similarly, color Doppler, as with pulsed Doppler, provides only a semiquantitative assessment of the severity of regurgitation.

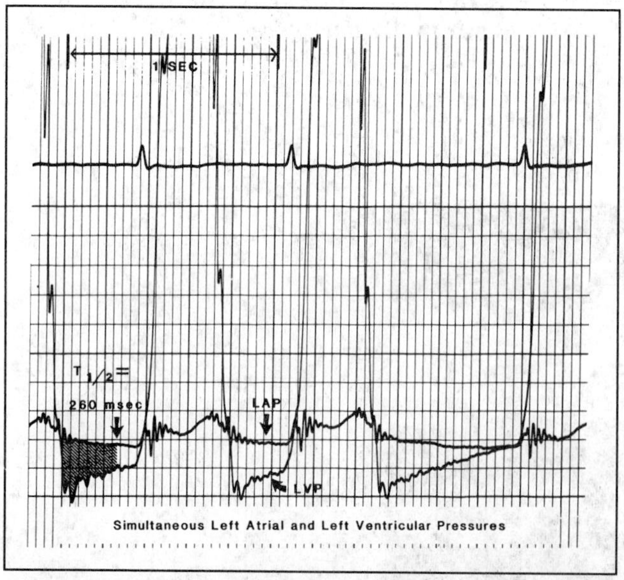

Fig. 5-11. Simultaneous left atrial and left ventricular pressure tracings from a patient with mitral stenosis to illustrate the principle of *pressure half-time*. It takes 260 ms for the maximum pressure gradient between the left atrium *(LAP)* and left ventricle *(LVP)* in diastole to reach half that value. This patient had a pressure half-time of 240 ms with the pulsed-Doppler method.

Clinical indications

Since most heart diseases involve the cardiac structures, echocardiography is useful for the evaluation of almost all cardiovascular diseases. Being portable, echocardiography equipment can be brought to the patient's bedside and can provide an immediate diagnosis and the hemodynamic status of critically ill patients. The causes of hypotension, pulmonary edema, or both can be determined (Chapters 10 and 11). When the causes are noncardiac, cardiac function and structures are usually normal. When the causes are cardiac, they can be easily diagnosed on echocardiography.

Echocardiography can be used for the assessment of patients with acute and chronic forms of coronary artery disease (Chapters 13 and 14). In these patients, it can be used for the early detection of acute myocardial infarction, determination of in-hospital prognosis and complications after infarction (infarct expansion, ventricular remodeling), demonstration of myocardial "stunning," diagnosis of RV infarction, detection of LV thrombus, and assessment of viable myocardium using pharmacologic stress testing. In patients with chronic coronary artery disease, echocardiography can be used for detection of disease using either exercise or pharmacologic stress and for assessment of long-term effects of infarction, such as global LV dysfunction, ischemic mitral regurgitation, and aneurysm formation.

Echocardiography is excellent for evaluating patients with primary myocardial disorders such as ventricular hypertrophy (obstructive or nonobstructive) and restrictive and dilated cardiomyopathies (Chapter 17). In the former, it can serve to define the distribution of hypertrophy and estimate the severity of outflow tract obstruction and mitral regurgitation; in the latter, it can be used to examine LV function and may provide characteristic diagnostic findings.

As can be noted in the previous examples, echocardiography is very useful in assessing the cause of valvular disease (e.g., rheumatic, degenerative) and the hemodynamic assessment of the severity of valvular disease (Chapter 16). This technique has revolutionized the diagnosis of congenital heart disease in children and continues to be important in the assessment of the common and uncommon congenital disorders in adults (Chapter 19). Echocardiography also has become important in the postoperative management of patients with congenital heart disease.

Although it cannot be used to determine the degree of pericardial thickening or the presence of pericardial inflammation, echocardiography is the "gold standard" for the diagnosis of pericardial effusion and can be used to evaluate cardiac tamponade and discriminate constrictive pericarditis from restrictive cardiomyopathy (Chapter 18). Echocardiography is extremely useful for the diagnosis of cardiac masses and for the diagnosis of diseases affecting the great vessels (Chapter 24).

Indications for transesophageal echocardiography

Aortic pathology
Aortic dissection
Aortic root abscess
Aortic valve endocarditis (native/prosthetic)
Aortic atheromatous debris

Mitral valve pathology
Mitral valve endocarditis (native/prosthetic)
Mitral regurgitation (unclear etiology)

Atrial pathology
Atrial thrombus/tumor
Patent foramen ovale
Small atrial septal defect

Transesophageal echocardiography is also the gold standard for the diagnosis of left atrial thrombus and prosthetic mitral valve dysfunction. It is also very useful for the diagnosis of aortic pathology, such as aortic dissection, aortic abscess, and atheromatous debris in the aorta. Transesophageal echocardiography can also detect a thrombus in the main or left or right pulmonary artery in patients with pulmonary embolus and can visualize the proximal portions of the coronary arteries. The indications for transesophageal echocardiography are listed in the box above.

Newer developments

Echocardiography is being used with increasing frequency in the operating room, especially in evaluating the success of valve repair and replacement. Transesophageal echocardiography is also being used for the on-line intraoperative monitoring of patients undergoing noncardiac surgery, especially those at risk for ischemic events during aortic cross-clamping. In the future, intracardiac catheters likely will have transducers capable of imaging the heart, which can be placed in the right side of the heart and will allow continuous on-line cardiac imaging of the left and right ventricles of critically ill patients.

Echocardiography is now frequently used in the cardiac catheterization laboratory as an adjunct to coronary angiography. Doppler techniques are used to measure coronary blood flow. Microbubbles of air are injected into the coronary arteries to assess myocardial perfusion. This technique has the potential for the assessment of collateral blood flow and myocardial viability. It also has potential for assessing myocardial perfusion after intravenous (IV) injection of bubbles capable of transpulmonary transit. Catheter-tipped transducers are introduced into coronary arteries to obtain cross-sectional images, particularly after intervention procedures, and have the potential for quantification of residual atheroma and the detection of thrombus.

Finally, new technology, such as three-dimensional (3D) imaging, is being developed to both acquire and depict cardiac data in three dimensions using ultrasound.

NUCLEAR CARDIOLOGY TECHNIQUES

Considerable progress has been made in the ability to image the heart with radionuclide techniques. After the IV administration of various radiolabeled agents, either the myocardium or the cardiac blood pools and great vessels can be imaged with the patient at rest or during exercise by employing a scintillation or positron camera and appropriate computer processing. Many diagnostic and prognostic applications of nuclear cardiology techniques are based on the principle that physiologic and functional information, rather than just structural or anatomic information, is the ultimate value of this noninvasive methodology. Myocardial perfusion imaging or radionuclide angiography performed in conjunction with exercise electrocardiography can provide clinically relevant data regarding presence and extent of ischemia. Prognostically, this may be more important than the mere classification of the number of diseased vessels by angiography.

With the emergence of coronary angioplasty and thrombolytic therapy as highly effective interventions for patients with acute ischemic syndromes, nuclear cardiology tests have been used frequently for the noninvasive determination of the efficacy of revascularization or reperfusion with these therapeutic approaches. Finally, significant advances have been made in the application of nuclear cardiology techniques for assessing myocardial viability in patients with LV dysfunction. Infarct-avid imaging with radiolabeled antimyosin antibody and positron emission tomographic imaging of myocardial blood flow and metabolism are gaining increased attention as noninvasive approaches for evaluating patients with ischemic heart disease or acute myocardial infarction.

Myocardial perfusion imaging

Myocardial perfusion imaging usually is performed with exercise ECG testing for detecting coronary artery disease and determining prognosis. Thallium-201 (^{201}Tl) is the perfusion agent most often employed, but a new agent, technetium-99m (^{99m}Tc) sestamibi (Cardiolite), is gaining increased clinical use, particularly with single-photon emission computed tomographic (SPECT) imaging.

Thallium-201 imaging. Thallium, a metallic element in group IIIA of the periodic table, is transported intracellularly by both passive and active mechanisms. Early myocardial uptake of IV ^{201}Tl is directly proportional to regional myocardial blood flow and the extraction fraction of ^{201}Tl by the myocardium. After the initial phase of myocardial uptake, there is continuous exchange of myocardial ^{201}Tl and ^{201}Tl from the extracardiac compartments. ^{201}Tl is continually washing out of normally perfused myocardium and replaced by recirculating ^{201}Tl from residual activity in the blood pool compartment. This process of continuous exchange forms the basis of the phenomenon of *^{201}Tl redis-*

tribution that is observed when the tracer is administered during transient underperfusion of the myocardium, as induced by exercise in patients with significant coronary artery disease. In clinical imaging studies, ^{201}Tl redistribution is defined as the total or partial resolution of initial postexercise defects when assessed by repeat imaging 2½ to 4 hours after tracer administration. The ^{201}Tl perfusion scan is most often performed with conventional treadmill exercise testing. A dose of 2.5 to 3.0 mCi of ^{201}Tl is administered through a freely flowing IV cannula during symptom-limited end-points such as angina pectoris, shortness of breath, fatigue, lower extremity claudication, or hypotension. The patient then exercises for another 30 to 45 seconds to ensure that the initial myocardial uptake phase will reflect the perfusion pattern present at peak exercise. Within 5 minutes after cessation of exercise, the patient is positioned under the collimator of a gamma camera to obtain anterior and multiple oblique projection images for the planar approach and for multiple-angle images acquired using the SPECT technique, with rotation of the camera around the patient.

Areas of diminished ^{201}Tl uptake on the immediate images after exercise represent either zones of stress-induced transient ischemia or myocardial scar. To differentiate the two, delayed images are obtained to look for redistribution. Redistribution or reversible defects imply stress-induced ischemia, whereas persistent or fixed defects on serial images suggest myocardial scar. Approximately 30% of persistent defects actually represent severe ischemia rather than scar. Recently, reinjection of a second dose of ^{201}Tl, with the patient at rest after acquisition of the redistribution images, has shown further reversibility in approximately 40% of defects that appear fixed at 2½ to 4 hours. In addition, some have advocated late redistribution imaging at 24 hours to identify further defect reversibility that is not evident on 4-hour delayed images. Approximately 20% to 25% of the defects that remain persistent on 4-hour delayed images show additional defect reversibility on 24-hour images.

Planar or SPECT ^{201}Tl scintigraphy performed with symptom-limited exercise stress testing has enhanced both sensitivity and specificity of detecting coronary artery disease. Sensitivity and specificity of qualitative visual ^{201}Tl scintigraphy using planar imaging technology are reported to be about 84% and 87%, respectively. When early and delayed ^{201}Tl scintigrams are assessed quantitatively by computer-assisted analysis, both sensitivity and specificity increase to about 90%. SPECT ^{201}Tl imaging further improves sensitivity for detection of coronary artery disease compared with planar imaging, although at a somewhat reduced specificity (more false-positive results). The SPECT technique permits more of a 3D delineation of in vivo ^{201}Tl uptake. Compared with planar imaging, SPECT has some distinct advantages. Images are free of background, and lesion contrast is higher. Localization of defects is more precise and more readily appreciated. The extent and size of defects are better defined by tomographically reconstructed views.

Several factors increase or decrease sensitivity of ^{201}Tl scintigraphy for detecting coronary artery disease. With both planar and SPECT imaging, it is more difficult to resolve lesions of the left circumflex coronary artery. Also, branch stenoses of the major coronary arteries are more difficult to resolve than when more proximal narrowings are present. As with exercise ECG testing, sensitivity for detecting single-vessel disease is less than that for detecting two- or three-vessel disease. The level of exercise achieved during stress testing influences the exercise ECG more than the ^{201}Tl scintigram. Throughout the range of exercise workloads or peak heart rates achieved, the frequency of ^{201}Tl scan abnormalities is more prevalent than exercise S-T segment depression. Similarly, antianginal drugs have little influence on results of myocardial perfusion imaging compared with exercise ECG stress testing.

Exercise ^{201}Tl imaging is useful for the noninvasive assessment of prognosis in patients with chest pain syndromes or known coronary artery disease. The box on p. 59 summarizes the high-risk ^{201}Tl scan variables. On initial postexercise images, high-risk scan findings include multiple ^{201}Tl defects and/or washout abnormalities in one or more coronary supply regions, increased ^{201}Tl uptake in the lung that can be quantitated using the lung/heart ratio, and exercise-induced transient LV cavity dilatation. Presence of redistribution compared with solely persistent defects indicates a higher risk for subsequent cardiac events. The extent of stress-induced hypoperfusion, as reflected by the total number of defects identified, is one of the best prognostic predictors of subsequent death and reinfarction in patients with coronary artery disease. This is particularly true when extensive hypoperfusion is observed at low exercise heart rates and workloads and is accompanied by ischemic S-T segment depression. Patients with chest pain and completely normal myocardial ^{201}Tl perfusion scans have been shown to have an excellent prognosis, with less than a 1% per year death or infarction rate. Increased lung uptake of ^{201}Tl reflects ischemia-induced LV diastolic dysfunction with development of pulmonary edema. A portion of the ^{201}Tl dose equilibrates with this pulmonary interstitial edema fluid, giving the appearance of increased ^{201}Tl activity in the lung on the anterior view. Some observers have reported that an increased lung/heart ^{201}Tl ratio is even a better predictor of prognosis than the number of perfusion defects identified. Fig. 5-12 shows serial postexercise images in a patient with inferior and anteroseptal defects reflecting multivessel coronary artery disease.

^{201}Tl imaging can be performed solely in the resting state to identify residual myocardial viability in regions of severe wall motion abnormalities. Patients with chronic coronary artery disease and LV dysfunction caused by "hibernation" demonstrate preservation of ^{201}Tl uptake at rest (Chapter 13). With this technique, IV ^{201}Tl is administered, and initial and delayed rest images are acquired at 20 minutes and 4 hours after tracer injection. Areas of resting hypoperfusion will demonstrate initial defects that show a late filling or redistribution. Zones of myocardial asynergy showing preserved ^{201}Tl uptake exhibit improved regional systolic function after revascularization. This technique is

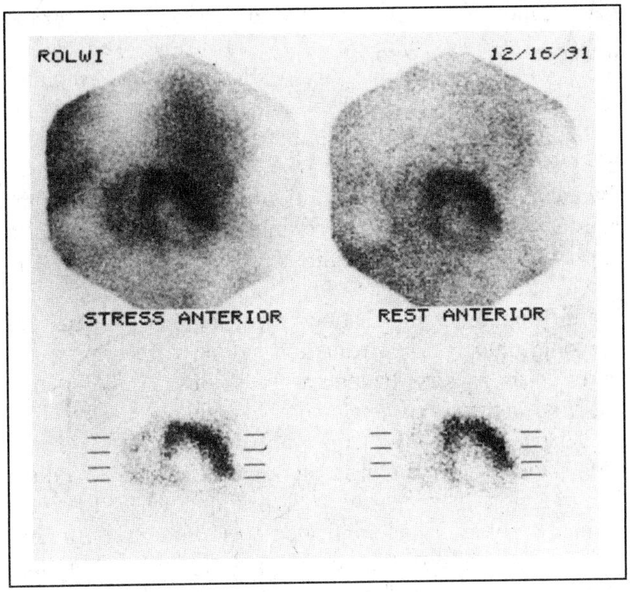

A

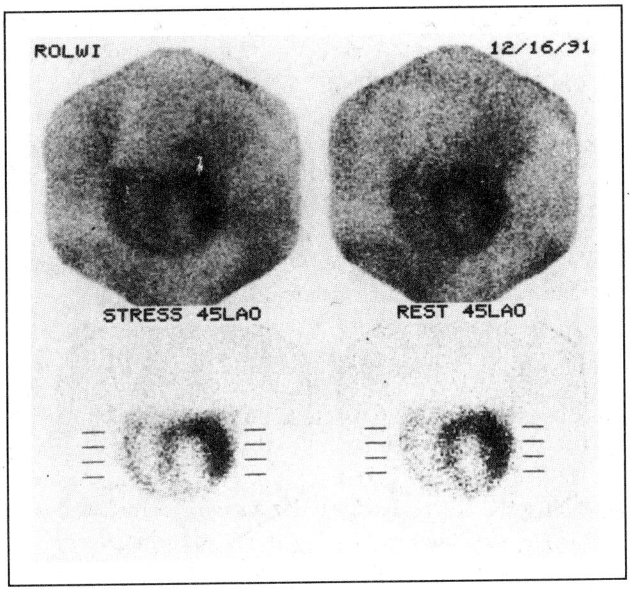

B

Fig. 5-12. A, Postexercise and delayed (after rest) anterior view, planar, thallium-201 (^{201}Tl) images obtained 10 minutes and 2½ hours after ^{201}Tl injection, respectively. Note increased ^{201}Tl uptake in the lung and an extensive inferior wall defect that is predominantly persistent. The background-subtracted images are shown below the processed images. **B,** Postexercise and delayed 45-degree left anterior oblique (LAO) images in the same patient showing an anteroseptal defect with partial delayed redistribution.

now used clinically to assist in the selection of patients with coronary artery disease and severely depressed LV ejection function who will benefit most from revascularization.

^{201}Tl imaging has some significant limitations. Visual interpretation of ^{201}Tl images may be difficult if one is not knowledgeable regarding attenuation artifacts and variants of normal. Breast tissue interposed between the camera head and the chest wall may produce the appearance of perfusion defects in women because of the absorption effect and the resulting ^{201}Tl attenuation. A large RV blood pool overlying the inferior wall on the anterior projection image may also cause an attenuation artifact. A high left hemidiaphragm overlying the posterior wall will cause an attenuation artifact, seen most evidently on the 70-degree left anterior oblique (LAO) or lateral projection image. With SPECT imaging, relatively less ^{201}Tl activity is observed in the inferobasilar segments on the short-axis images because of attenuation of ^{201}Tl activity. This may result in false-positive scan interpretations.

Technetium-99m sestamibi imaging. ^{99m}Tc sestamibi is a lipophilic cationic ^{99m}Tc complex that, as with ^{201}Tl, is taken up in myocardial tissue in proportion to regional myocardial blood flow. The 140 keV photon energy peak of ^{99m}Tc is ideal for gamma camera imaging and can produce higher-quality images than those produced by ^{201}Tl. The relatively short half-life (6 hours) of ^{99m}Tc provides favorable patient dosimetry and permits administration of 10 to 15 times larger doses than with ^{201}Tl, yielding better images in a shorter period.

Since ^{99m}Tc sestamibi does not redistribute over time after IV administration, separate injections of the radionuclide must be administered during stress and resting states to differentiate between transient ischemia and myocardial scar. Perhaps the most direct protocol using this radionuclide is to perform the exercise and resting studies 24 hours apart. Each imaging procedure employs 20 to 30 mCi of ^{99m}Tc sestamibi. Images are acquired 30 to 45 minutes after ^{99m}Tc sestamibi administration, permitting clearance of activity from the lungs and splanchnic organs. In clinical practice a protocol involving separate rest and stress injections separated by 24 hours may not be very practical. To overcome this limitation, an abbreviated same-day protocol has been proposed.

Sensitivity and specificity for detection of coronary artery disease with ^{99m}Tc sestamibi are comparable to those cited for ^{201}Tl and are reported to be in the 85% to 90% range. The higher photon energy and enhanced count rate with somewhat decreased attenuation and scatter make ^{99m}Tc sestamibi a better radionuclide for SPECT imaging compared with ^{201}Tl. Specificity is therefore enhanced because of superior image quality and fewer image artifacts. Some have reported that more individually stenosed arteries are detected by ^{99m}Tc sestamibi SPECT than by ^{201}Tl SPECT. Two other potential advantages of ^{99m}Tc sestamibi imaging exist: the ability to gate the perfusion images with the ECG in order to assess regional wall thickening. Assessment of regional systolic function and perfusion simultaneously may assist in the noninvasive detection of viability. Finally, first-pass radionuclide ventriculography can be undertaken with the IV bolus injection of ^{99m}Tc sestamibi before acquisition of myocardial perfusion scans. The LV ejection fraction (LVEF) can be measured both at rest and during exercise. The ability to measure LVEF and regional myocardial perfusion simultaneously with a single IV injection of ^{99m}Tc sestamibi may significantly enhance this agent's prognostic value.

Some limitations to ^{99m}Tc sestamibi imaging deserve mention. First, because the agent does not redistribute over time, it may not be as useful for assessing myocardial viability in the resting state in patients with coronary artery disease and LV dysfunction. ^{99m}Tc sestamibi uptake in the lung has not been validated as a prognostic variable and thus may somewhat diminish the agent's prognostic usefulness.

Technetium-99m teboroxime imaging. ^{99m}Tc teboroxime is a boronic acid adduct of technetium dioxime (BATO) compound that is a neutral lipophilic agent with high initial myocardial extraction and rapid myocardial clearance. Because of its rapid myocardial clearance, all imaging protocols must be performed rapidly; ideally, no more than 1 minute should pass between ^{99m}Tc teboroxime injection and the onset of imaging. SPECT acquisition is difficult using this radionuclide perfusion agent because of the short imaging time needed to acquire high-quality scintigrams. Another drawback of this agent is the substantially high level of liver activity that is seen in some patients, causing difficulty in assessing the heart's inferior wall. Nevertheless, despite these limitations, sensitivity and specificity of exercise ^{99m}Tc teboroxime imaging have been shown to be in the 85% to 90% range.

Pharmacologic stress imaging. Pharmacologic stress is an appropriate substitute for exercise stress imaging for detecting significant coronary artery stenoses and separating high-risk and low-risk subgroups of patients with coronary artery disease. When either IV dipyridamole or adenosine is administered in the patient with a critical coronary stenosis, flow reserve is impaired in the stenotic region. Also, the degree of vasodilatation is significantly less relative to the increase in flow in response to these vasodilators in normally perfused zones. When ^{201}Tl is administered during dipyridamole's or adenosine's peak effect in the patient with significant coronary narrowing, diminished uptake and delayed clearance of the radionuclide occur in the stenosis zone, producing an initial defect and delayed redistribution.

The sensitivity and specificity of dipyridamole or adenosine ^{201}Tl imaging for detection of coronary artery disease are comparable to those of exercise scintigraphy. Dipyridamole ^{201}Tl stress scintigraphy is performed in the following manner. First, no caffeinated beverages are permitted for 12 hours before imaging. Patients receiving theophylline compounds are not eligible for testing unless these drugs have been discontinued. After baseline hemodynamic values are obtained, 0.56 mg/kg of dipyridamole is infused over 4 minutes. A dose of 2.0 to 3.0 mCi of ^{201}Tl is injected at 9 minutes, and initial images are obtained 5 minutes later. As with exercise scintigraphy, delayed images are obtained 2½ to 4 hours later. Vital signs and serial 12-lead ECGs are obtained every minute during dipyridamole infusion and for at least 5 minutes thereafter. Aminophylline (50 to 100 mg IV) can be administered to reverse dipyridamole-associated side effects, such as systemic hypertension, chest pain, and nausea. The adenosine protocol involves infusion of IV adenosine (140 μg/kg/min), which is maintained for 6 minutes. After 3 minutes at this infusion rate, a 2.0 to 3.0 mCi dose of ^{201}Tl is injected in a contralateral vein and flushed with normal saline. The adenosine infusion is maintained for 3 additional minutes after ^{201}Tl administration. Early and delayed images are acquired in a manner similar to that after exercise stress or dipyridamole imaging.

Dipyridamole or adenosine ^{201}Tl imaging can provide useful prognostic information, particularly in patients undergoing preoperative evaluation before peripheral vascular or aortic surgery. Patients who demonstrate ^{201}Tl redistribution defects preoperatively experience a sevenfold higher perioperative ischemic cardiac event rate compared with patients not demonstrating such scan abnormalities. Dipyridamole or adenosine ^{201}Tl scintigraphy can be performed early after uncomplicated acute myocardial infarction for separation of high-risk and low-risk subgroups. Pharmacologic stress imaging is safe when performed as early as 4 days after onset of infarction in patients who remain asymptomatic after the early acute phase of hospitalization. Patients with recurrent angina at rest should not be considered for pharmacologic stress imaging.

Side effects of either dipyridamole or adenosine imaging are predominantly minor, with chest pain and S-T segment depression occurring more frequently after adenosine infusion than after dipyridamole administration. Chest pain occurs even in the absence of underlying coronary artery disease. S-T segment depression after infusion of dipyridamole occurs in approximately 10% to 15% of patients.

Radionuclide angiography

Imaging of ventricular function differs significantly from myocardial perfusion imaging in that the radioactive tracer remains in the blood pool during scintigraphy, and cardiac dynamics are assessed in a similar manner as employed with contrast ventriculography. An in vivo labeling technique with ^{99m}Tc radiopharmaceuticals is the approach most often used. With this technique, unlabeled IV stannous pyrophosphate reconstituted in normal saline is injected 15 to 20 minutes before injection of 15 to 30 mCi of ^{99m}Tc. Radionuclide angiography implies the dynamic imaging of the LV and RV blood pools employing ECG gating. Two approaches to gated radionuclide angiography have emerged: the first-pass and the equilibrium methods.

The *equilibrium radionuclide method* is also referred to as a *MUGA* nuclear scan study because of *mu*ltiple-*g*ated *a*cquisition with repetitive sampling of blood pool counts from equal subdivisions of the cardiac cycle's R-R interval. Generally a framing interval of 30 to 50 ms is used for the resting state and 20 to 30 ms for exercise. Imaging is performed for as many as 200 successive cardiac cycles, with the R wave of the ECG used as the marker to initiate acquisition of count data with each cycle. From these "resultant" images, both regional wall motion and global ventricular function are evaluated. The equilibrium-gated radionuclide angiogram is then displayed in an endless-loop format in which frames are displayed in a cine (movie) mode. This averaged cardiac cycle is displayed over and over again and simulates the beating heart compared with that observed in contrast ventriculography. Chamber size and segmental wall motion are assessed visually, and ventricular EF and end-systolic and end-diastolic volumes can be measured by computer-assisted quantitation techniques.

Changes in radioactivity that occur within the left and right ventricles during the cardiac cycle can be digitized and displayed in the form of a relative volume curve (Fig. 5-13). This curve is based on the principle that a change in radioactivity is proportional to the change in blood volume. When corrections for background have been performed, the LV time-activity curve represents the average change in blood volume when all the cardiac cycles have been integrated to form a composite cycle.

To assess regional ventricular function, multiple imaging views are obtained. They include the anterior, 45-degree LAO, and steep 70-degree LAO projections.

Perhaps the most useful parameter derived from the radionuclide angiogram is the LVEF. The method for calculation of the LVEF is called the *area-counts technique*. The supposition for this technique is that proportionality exists between ^{99m}Tc counts and the LV blood pool and actual blood volume. The end-diastolic counts are proportional to the end-diastolic volume, and the end-systolic counts are proportional to the end-systolic volume. The change in radioactivity in the LV blood pool between end-diastole and end-systole is proportional to stroke volume, and this change is referred to as *stroke counts*. The EF is computed as the end-diastolic counts minus the end-systolic counts divided by the end-diastolic counts after adjusting for background radioactivity. The area-counts technique for calculation of EF correlates well with EF assessed from contrast ventriculography (Fig. 5-13).

Other indices that can be obtained from the radionuclide angiogram include peak systolic ejection rate, ejection time, RVEF, regurgitant fraction, and diastolic filling time. Left-to-right intracardiac shunts can also be quantitated using radionuclide angiographic methods. A semiquantitative assessment of valvular regurgitation can be assessed by measuring the ratio of the LV stroke volume to the RV stroke volume.

With the *first-pass radionuclide method*, a single bolus of ^{99m} Tc is injected rapidly through the IV route, and analysis is limited to the initial transit of radioactivity through the central circulation. A multicrystal scintillation camera is preferable to the single-crystal Anger camera for first-pass radionuclide angiography, since high count rates of up to 400,000 counts/sec are obtained with the multicrystal device.

Clinical uses. In most patients the etiology of congestive heart failure can be ascertained by the history, physical findings, chest radiographic manifestations, and ECG patterns (Chapter 10). However, in certain patients the cause of heart failure is not evident. In such patients a gated radionuclide angiogram at rest may be useful in distinguishing between ischemic cardiomyopathy and primary idiopathic dilated cardiomyopathy. Patients with ischemic cardiomyopathy have multiple segmental wall motion abnormalities, whereas patients with primary myocardial disease usually have diffuse hypokinesis.

Resting radionuclide angiography can be very valuable in the evaluation of patients with chronic ischemic heart disease and those with recent myocardial infarction. The LVEF is one of the most useful prognostic variables that can be obtained. As with echocardiography, radionuclide angiography can be used for assessing myocardial viability. Preservation of systolic wall motion after infarction or in patients with chronic coronary artery disease and heart failure implies residual viability. Such patients may benefit

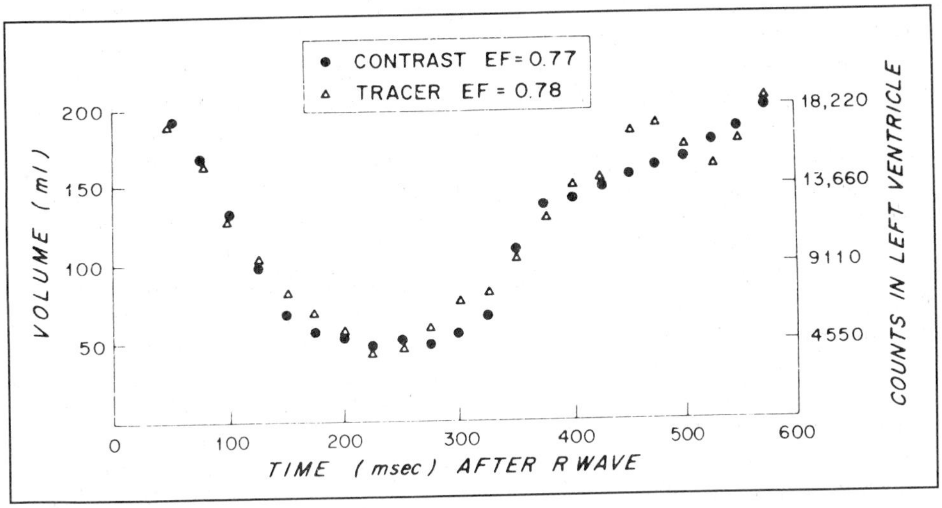

Fig. 5-13. Technetium-99m (^{99m}Tc) activity represented by "counts" in the LV region of interest versus time curve and the LV volume from contrast angiography versus time curve plotted on the same axes. The ejection fraction *(EF)* is almost identical for the two techniques. (From Burow RD et al: Circulation 56:1024, 1977. With permission.)

from revascularization, with improvement in function coincident with amelioration of symptoms. The resting radionuclide angiogram is also well suited for recognition of aneurysmal LV dilatation, which can be distinguished from pseudoaneurysms and thinned myocardial segments that are unsuitable for surgery.

Radionuclide angiography has been successfully employed in cancer patients to evaluate cardiotoxicity of doxorubicin by serial assessment of LVEF. Imaging RV size and contraction pattern is particularly useful in the evaluation of patients who have inferior wall infarction and signs of low cardiac output. Patients with hemodynamically significant RV infarction show a depressed RVEF and RV dilatation, although the LVEF may be normal or only mildly reduced. RV dynamics can also be evaluated in patients with chronic obstructive pulmonary disease. Radionuclide angiography can be performed with supine bicycle exercise to detect coronary artery disease and determine prognosis (Chapters 13 and 14). Coronary artery disease is detected by demonstrating an exercise-induced decrease or a failure to increase LVEF from rest to exercise. Inducible ischemia with exercise stress is manifested by a new regional wall motion abnormality when compared with the resting assessment.

The patient with regurgitant valvular disease may experience irreversible myocardial dysfunction before the appearance of clinical symptoms (Chapter 16). A substantial number of patients with asymptomatic aortic regurgitation have an abnormal EF response during exercise. However, most observers have not found the assessment of the exercise EF very useful in patients with aortic regurgitation in regard to timing of valvular surgery. Certainly a change in the *resting* EF over serial observations is a more compelling indication for intervening with valvular surgery.

Myocardial infarction imaging

The principle of techniques for imaging acute myocardial infarction is that the radiopharmaceutical is preferentially sequestered in necrotic myocardial tissue, yielding a "hot spot" of radioactivity that can be imaged with a gamma scintillation camera (Chapter 14). The first agent used for this imaging approach was ^{99m}Tc pyrophosphate, which concentrates in myocardial zones of irreversible cellular injury. ^{99m}Tc pyrophosphate deposition presumably occurs in necrotic areas of calcium overload. Myocardial ^{99m}Tc pyrophosphate scintigrams become abnormal 12 to 24 hours after myocardial infarction; thus this technique is not very useful for the acute detection of infarction in patients with chest pain. The optimum images are acquired 24 hours after the onset of necrosis, and scans may remain positive for 1 week or longer.

More recently, interest has focused on the use of indium-111 (^{111}In) antimyosin antibodies as an infarct-avid imaging agent. Myosin molecules remain as insoluble myofibrils after irreversible ischemic injury, and the myosin heavy chains do not clear from damaged myocardium. Myosin-specific antibodies bind to their antigens only in necrotic myocardial tissue, whereas normal myocardial cell membranes prevent the antibodies' intracellular entry.

For clinical imaging, Fab fragments of antimyosin antibodies labeled with ^{111}In are employed. Images of Fab antimyosin uptake are obtained 24 hours after tracer administration. Antimyosin antibody uptake is maximal in the central region of necrosis, whereas ^{99m}Tc pyrophosphate uptake is maximal at the periphery of the infarct region, where there is more residual blood flow.

Clinical uses. Myocardial infarct imaging is rarely required in clinical practice because the diagnosis of acute myocardial infarction can readily be made by clinical history, typical ECG changes, and measurement of creatine kinase and its MB fraction (Chapter 14). However, some patients may have an equivocal history, a nondiagnostic ECG, and enzyme levels that do not show a typical rise-and-fall pattern characteristic of acute infarction. Some patients seen 2 days or longer after the presumed onset of infarction may have normal creatine kinase levels but demonstrate an abnormal ^{99m}Tc pyrophosphate or ^{111}In antimyosin antibody scan.

^{111}In antimyosin antibody imaging has also been found to be clinically useful in establishing the diagnosis of acute myocarditis and detecting acute and chronic allograft rejection in patients with heart transplants.

Positron emission tomography

Positron emission tomography (PET) provides the capability for quantitative noninvasive imaging of regional concentration of positron-emitting radioisotopes. PET is undertaken after the IV administration of short-lived positron emitters such as carbon-11 (^{11}C), nitrogen-13 (^{13}N), oxygen-15 (^{15}O), fluorine-18 (^{18}F), and rubidium-82 (^{82}Rb). ^{82}Rb is generator produced and has a half-life of 75 seconds. The myocardial uptake of ^{82}Rb is proportional to regional blood flow, and this agent is given during peak vasodilator stress after dipyridamole or adenosine administration. Sensitivity and specificity for detection of coronary artery disease with ^{82}Rb PET are about 90%. Clinical imaging studies employ approximately 20 mCi of ^{13}N ammonia. ^{15}O-labeled water, another positron-emitting flow tracer, has a first-pass extraction fraction approaching 100% and an ultrashort half-life of 2 minutes, which requires administration of high doses of tracer activity.

Perhaps the most interesting and potentially useful application of PET is the noninvasive assessment of myocardial metabolism. ^{18}F, 2-fluoro-2-deoxyglucose (FDG), is a glucose analog employed with PET imaging to assess regional glucose metabolism in the myocardium. The magnitude of FDG activity reflects the magnitude of glucose consumption. Under conditions of severe ischemia, increased FDG uptake reflects substrate utilization in the glycolytic pathway. Increased FDG activity on PET images in areas of diminished perfusion is characteristic of "hibernating myocardium" and reflects preservation of myocardial viability. Areas showing FDG/blood flow mismatch usually

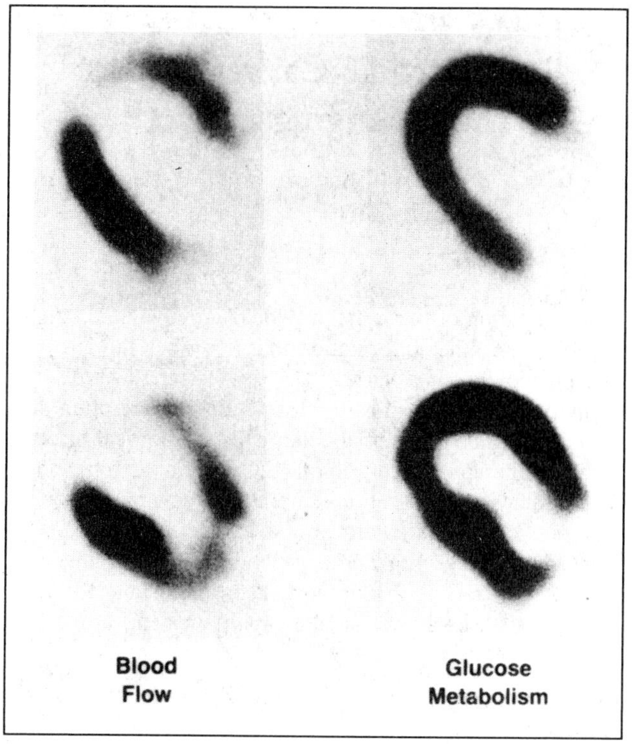

Fig. 5-14. Positron emission tomographic (PET) images of blood flow *(left)* and glucose metabolism *(right)* obtained at two levels of the heart's midportion. Note that the perfusion abnormalities on the nitrogen-13 (^{13}N) ammonia PET images of blood flow correspond to increased FDG uptake on the glucose metabolism images indicative of a mismatch pattern characteristic of preserved viability. (From Brunken R: J Am Coll Card 10(3):563, 1987.)

demonstrate improved regional function after coronary revascularization. Regions of myocardium that show both diminished perfusion and diminished FDG uptake rarely demonstrate improved systolic function after bypass surgery or angioplasty. Fig. 5-14 is an example of diminished myocardial perfusion, as evaluated by ^{13}N ammonia imaging, and increased FDG uptake indicative of viable myocardium in this region.

COMPUTED TOMOGRAPHY OF CARDIOVASCULAR SYSTEM

Ultrafast scanning

Ultrafast computed tomographic (CT) scanning can acquire images faster and at multiple levels without scanner or patient movement when compared with conventional CT scanning. The resolution of most ultrafast CT devices is in the range of 0.7 to 1.5 mm, and the slice thickness can be varied from 3 to 10 mm. The scanner is operable in either a cine mode, a flow mode, or a volume mode. Contrast enhancement is mandatory in order for CT to distinguish the blood pool from the myocardium. Clinical applications include the detection of coronary calcification in the proximal coronary vessels; quantitation of LV mass; measurement of LVEF and end-diastolic, end-systolic, and stroke volumes; evaluation of regional myocardial systolic contraction; and evaluation of myocardial perfusion after bolus injection of contrast medium.

Conventional scanning

Perhaps the most frequently used clinical application of conventional CT for cardiovascular imaging is the evaluation of the thoracic aorta for presence of an aneurysm (Chapter 24). Conventional CT with contrast medium allows for a highly sensitive diagnosis of an aneurysm and can accurately measure its diameter and determine the presence or absence of intraluminal thrombus. Although aortography provides the most definitive diagnostic study for a dissecting aortic aneurysm, conventional CT demonstrates clearly the segment of aortic dissection, showing an intimal flap between the true and false lumina. Contrast medium is also injected for detection and localization of aortic dissection. Pericardial disease can also be well evaluated using conventional CT. Pericardial cysts, neoplastic pericardial infiltration, effusions, and constrictive pericarditis are well delineated by conventional CT.

MAGNETIC RESONANCE IMAGING

Magnetic resonance imaging (MRI) has revolutionized imaging of the brain and other body structures. It is a true 3D imaging modality because it acquires data from an entire volume of tissue, which can then be depicted in tomographic slices. MRI involves placing the body region to be imaged within a large-bore superconducting magnet, which for most imaging requires a field strength of 1 to 2 Tesla. Because the heart moves as a result of both cardiac contraction and respiration, the best-quality images are obtained by ECG and respiratory gating.

The theory of MRI and physics of image construction are beyond the scope of this chapter. In brief, however, MRI depends on the absorption and re-emission of radiofrequency (RF) energy from certain nuclei when these are placed within a magnetic field. To create cardiac images, the hydrogen nuclei are used most often because these are abundant in the body. When placed in a magnetic field, these nuclei align themselves parallel to the field. If the proper RF pulse is then applied, the alignment of the nuclei changes in relation to the magnetic field, and this change depends on the RF signal's strength and duration. The signal generated by the movement of the nuclei away from their aligned positions within the magnetic field can be detected by a receiver coil placed within the magnet.

After the RF pulse stops, the nuclei begin to realign themselves again parallel to the magnetic field of the external magnet, which can be measured by T1 and T2 relaxation times. These values vary for different tissues and are used to provide contrast in the images. The signals detected within the tissue are subjected to fast-Fourier transform, and the number of times the nuclei have to be perturbed to produce an image depends on the resolution required. This, coupled with the number of images required during the cardiac cycle and the heart and respiratory rates, will determine how long the patient needs to be within the magnet. Different pulse-generating sequences used to create different types of images also affect the imaging time.

The images produced by MRI are of excellent resolution, and because the data are acquired in three dimensions, measurements of cardiac mass and volume can be very precise. In addition, by using certain imaging sequences, flow through cardiac chambers can be measured. Newer imaging sequences allow for fast acquisition with greater temporal resolution, so images can be viewed in a cine loop similar to radionuclide cineangiography. MRI contrast agents provide the potential for measuring myocardial blood flow. MR spectroscopy offers the capability for studying myocardial metabolism.

MR images are particularly useful in the diagnosis of aortic disease (e.g., dissection, aneurysm), constrictive pericarditis, anomalous pulmonary venous connections, and systolic pulmonary arterial shunts. MRI also is being used with increased frequency for detecting intracardiac masses, defining complex congenital heart disease, assessing myocardial infarction and viability, and determining coronary artery bypass graft patency. However, MRI's clinical usefulness compared with other available noninvasive techniques (e.g., transthoracic and transesophageal echocardiography, nuclear imaging techniques, CT) remains to be clarified.

REFERENCES

Bansal RC and Shah PM: Transesophageal echocardiography. Curr Probl Cardiol 15:47, 1990.

Bateman TM: X-ray computed tomography. In Pohost GM and O'Rourke RA, editors: Principles and practice of cardiovascular imaging. Boston, 1991, Little, Brown.

Beller GA: Current status of nuclear cardiology techniques. Curr Probl Cardiol 15:447, 1991.

Dinsmore RE: Chest roentgenography. In Pohost GM and O'Rourke RA, editors: Principles and practice of cardiovascular imaging. Boston, 1991, Little, Brown.

Eagle KA et al: Combining clinical and thallium data optimizes preoperative assessment of cardiac risk before major vascular surgery. Ann Intern Med 110:859, 1989.

Feigenbaum H: Echocardiography, ed 4. Philadelphia, 1985, Lea & Febiger.

Fletcher GF et al: Exercise standards: a statement for health professionals from the American Heart Association. Circulation 82:2286, 1990.

Gibbons RJ: The use of radionuclide techniques for identification of severe coronary disease. Curr Probl Cardiol 15:307, 1990.

Kaul S: Echocardiography in coronary artery disease. Curr Probl Cardiol 15:235, 1990.

Kaul S et al: Prognostic utility of the exercise thallium-201 test in ambulatory patients with chest pain: comparison with cardiac catheterization. Circulation 77:745, 1988.

Matle L and Angelsen B: Doppler ultrasound in cardiology: physical principles and clinical applications, ed 2. Philadelphia, 1993, Lea & Febiger (in press).

Rehr R: Cardiovascular nuclear magnetic resonance imaging and spectroscopy. Curr Probl Cardiol 16:127, 1991.

Schelbert HR: Current status and prospects of new radionuclides and radiopharmaceuticals for cardiovascular nuclear medicine. Semin Nucl Med 17:145, 1987.

Weyman AE, editor: Principles and practice of echocardiography. Philadelphia, 1993, Lea & Febiger (in press).

CHAPTER

6 Cardiac Catheterization and Angiography

William H. Gaasch
Joseph P. Murgo

Catheterization of the heart provides hemodynamic, angiographic, and other information that describes the anatomy and physiology of a variety of disease states. These data include valuable prognostic information and are often necessary to evaluate potential candidates for surgical or other forms of therapy. In addition to this diagnostic function of the cardiac catheterization laboratory, several important therapeutic procedures are now available for the management of patients with coronary, valvular, and congenital heart disease. Thus it is important to understand the indications and risks as well as the capabilities and limitations of the procedure.

INDICATIONS

Patients with known or suspected coronary artery disease may require cardiac catheterization to assess the presence or extent of disease. Fixed atherosclerotic lesions, intimal disruption, thrombus, and coronary artery spasm may be visualized and ventricular function assessed.

The severity of valvular disease may be evaluated at rest and during exercise or other hemodynamic stress. Ventricular function is assessed, and associated conditions such as coronary artery disease and pulmonary hypertension are evaluated.

Hemodynamic and angiographic studies are necessary to define the type and complexity of congenital heart disease and assess the possibility of associated coronary or other abnormalities.

Diseases of the pericardium, myocardium, or endocardium require extensive diagnostic evaluation that often includes catheterization. It is particularly important to identify patients with treatable disorders, especially pericardial disease.

In patients with congestive heart failure, catheterization is used to assess and evaluate ventricular function and to rule out intracardiac shunts and valvular, coronary, and other associated abnormalities.

Postoperative catheterization may provide diagnostic information in patients who have undergone coronary bypass surgery, valve replacement, repair of congenital defects, or other surgical procedures.

Pulmonary hypertension and its severity can be assessed, and the potential causes (e.g., intracardiac shunts, pulmonary embolic disease, pulmonary venous hypertension) can be identified.

The authors gratefully acknowledge Stephen H. Humphrey's and William E. Craig's contributions to this revised chapter.

Right heart catheterization, generally performed with a balloon flotation catheter in the intensive care unit, provides diagnostic information and allows an assessment of the response to therapy. Although complete right and left heart catheterization with angiography may eventually be necessary, an early right heart catheterization can be invaluable in patients with heart failure and in those with acute coronary syndromes, especially those with the mechanical complications of myocardial infarction (i.e., mitral regurgitation and ventricular septal defect).

An endomyocardial biopsy can provide diagnostic information in patients with heart failure. It is typically used to identify rejection after cardiac transplantation, but it can also be useful in patients with myocardial dysfunction of unknown cause. Electrophysiologic studies can provide a specific diagnosis as well as an evaluation of therapeutic interventions (Chapter 9).

Percutaneous transluminal coronary angioplasty is the most common therapeutic procedure performed in the cardiac catheterization laboratory, but coronary atherectomy and coronary stints are increasingly used (Chapter 13). Balloon catheter valvotomy of stenotic mitral or aortic valves also can be effective in selected patients with valvular heart disease (Chapter 16). Therapeutic procedures (e.g., balloon septostomy or dilatation of aortic coarctation) may be especially valuable in children with congenital heart disease.

RISKS

The mortality associated with diagnostic cardiac catheterization is approximately 0.1%, but the frequency of nonfatal complications is greater. These complications include myocardial infarction, perforation of the heart or great vessels, ventricular fibrillation, induction of atrial arrhythmias or atrioventricular block, thromboembolic complications such as cerebrovascular accident (stroke) or peripheral embolization, bleeding, infection, and hypersensitivity reactions to angiographic contrast materials.

The complications of therapeutic procedures such as coronary angioplasty or balloon valvuloplasty are considerably greater than those of diagnostic cardiac catheterization. For example, abrupt closure occurs in 1% to 3% of patients undergoing coronary angioplasty; some of these patients require urgent bypass surgery. These are relatively new procedures, and the complication rate will undoubtedly decline as experience grows and the techniques evolve.

The risks of cardiac catheterization can be minimized if relative contraindications are considered. These include uncontrolled arrhythmias as well as hypokalemia and digitalis intoxication, uncontrolled hypertension or heart failure, allergy to radiographic contrast agents, and intercurrent febrile or other illness. Heparin is usually substituted for oral anticoagulants before catheterization. Special arrangements must be made for patients with severe renal insufficiency.

TECHNIQUES

Many techniques allow specially designed catheters to be introduced into peripheral blood vessels and (with fluoroscopic and/or pressure monitoring) selectively advanced into the various chambers or great vessels. Once in place, catheters are used for a variety of purposes, such as pressure and flow measurements, angiography, blood sampling, indicator injection and sampling, recording of electrophysiologic data, biopsy, and therapeutic procedures.

Right heart catheterization has classically been performed with the patient under local anesthesia by direct exposure of an antecubital vein; the catheter is introduced through a small venotomy and is guided into the heart. A percutaneous approach through the femoral, jugular, or subclavian veins may also be used; this technique involves cannulation of the vessel with a needle through which a guidewire is introduced. When the wire is satisfactorily positioned, the needle is removed, and the catheter is guided over the wire into the vessel. The wire is then removed, and the catheter is advanced into the heart. Alternatively, a vein dilator with sheath may be advanced over the wire. The wire is then removed, and a catheter is inserted through the sheath. As the catheter is advanced through the right side of the heart, pressure measurements are made, blood samples are obtained for blood gas analysis, and cardiac output can be measured.

A balloon flotation catheter may be introduced directly into an exposed vein or through a sheath. The catheter is advanced while monitoring pressure, and when it approaches the right atrium, the balloon is inflated. Blood flow through the right side of the heart usually carries the balloon catheter through the right ventricle, into the pulmonary artery, and finally to the "pulmonary artery wedge" position, where pulmonary venous pressure is measured. This technique may be used without fluoroscopic assistance, but it is essential to monitor pressure continuously and to avoid excessive balloon inflations.

Left heart catheterization may be performed by introducing the catheter into an exposed artery by a percutaneous approach similar to that just described. The use of vascular sheaths for catheter insertion and exchange has greatly reduced the potential for trauma to the artery. The catheter is advanced under fluoroscopic guidance from the brachial or femoral arteries to the ascending aorta and then retrograde across the aortic valve into the left ventricle. Pressures are measured, blood samples are obtained for blood gas analysis, and angiography is performed. It is difficult to enter the left atrium using the retrograde approach, and thus the pulmonary artery wedge pressure is used as a close approximation of left atrial pressure.

The transseptal approach to the left atrium and left ventricle may be used. This method is especially useful in the presence of severe aortic stenosis or a prosthetic aortic valve. The technique employs a unique catheter through which a specially designed needle and stylet can be advanced from the femoral vein and inferior vena cava through the interatrial septum into the left atrium.

Coronary arteriography is performed with specially designed catheters, inserted via brachial or femoral arteries, that allow selective injection of contrast material in the right and left coronary arteries (Fig. 6-1). *Transluminal coronary angioplasty* requires initial placement of a guiding catheter

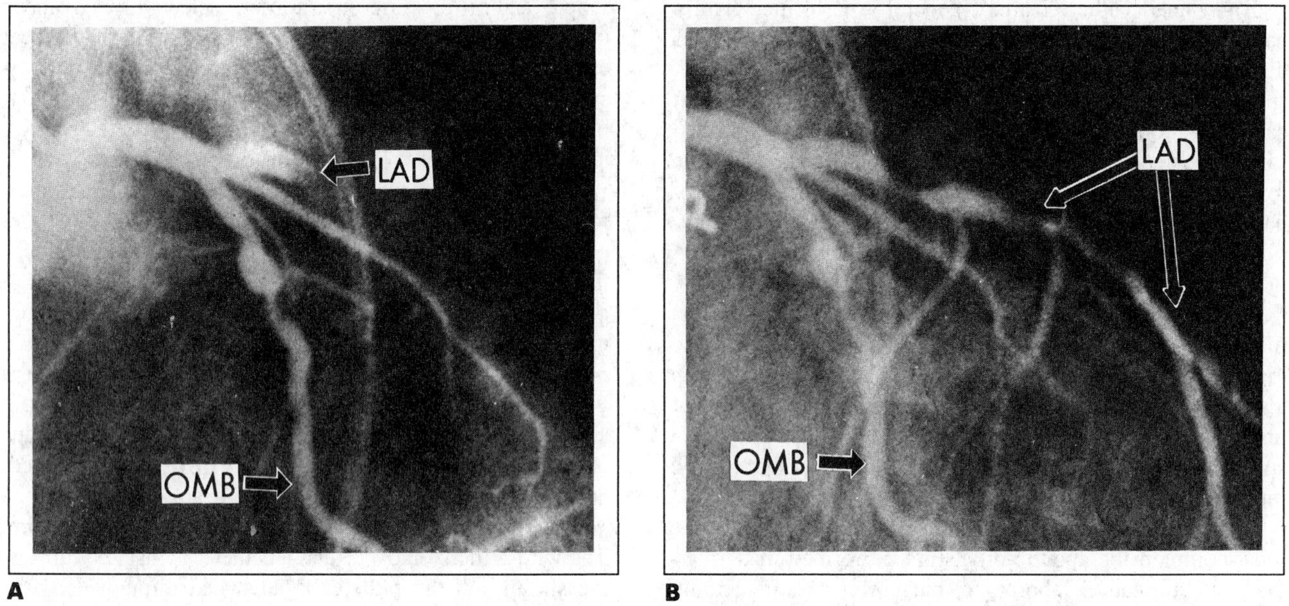

Fig. 6-1. **A,** Arteriogram of left coronary artery (right anterior oblique projection) in a patient 2 hours after onset of myocardial infarction. The arrow indicates site of total occlusion of left anterior descending artery *(LAD)*. **B,** Same coronary artery after 60 minutes of intracoronary streptokinase administration; antegrade flow in the LAD has been restored. *OMB,* Obtuse marginal branch.

at the ostium of the coronary artery to be dilated. After selective coronary arteriography is performed to confirm significant obstruction, the balloon dilatation catheter and guidewire are introduced into the guiding catheter and advanced into the coronary artery. When appropriately positioned across the obstructing lesion, the balloon is inflated and the obstructing lesion compressed (Fig. 6-2). Arteriography is then repeated to confirm a successful dilatation. Coronary stents can be used to maintain vessel patency. Administration of intracoronary thrombolytic agents for acute myocardial infarction requires selective cannulation of the thrombosed coronary artery. This procedure may be accompanied by transluminal angioplasty.

PRESSURE MEASUREMENT

Cardiovascular pressures are measured with specially designed catheters and transducers. These instruments allow

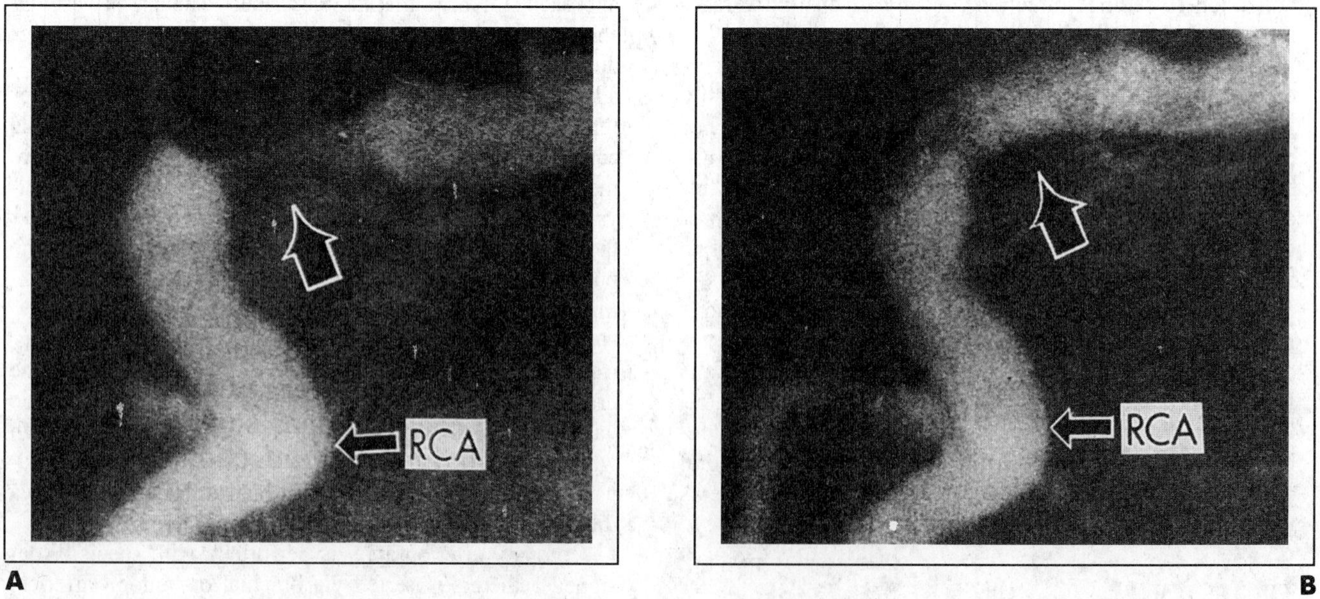

Fig. 6-2. **A,** Arteriogram of proximal right coronary artery *(RCA)* in the 60-degree left anterior oblique projection showing a segment of high-grade obstruction before angioplasty. **B,** Same RCA moments later after successful balloon dilatation.

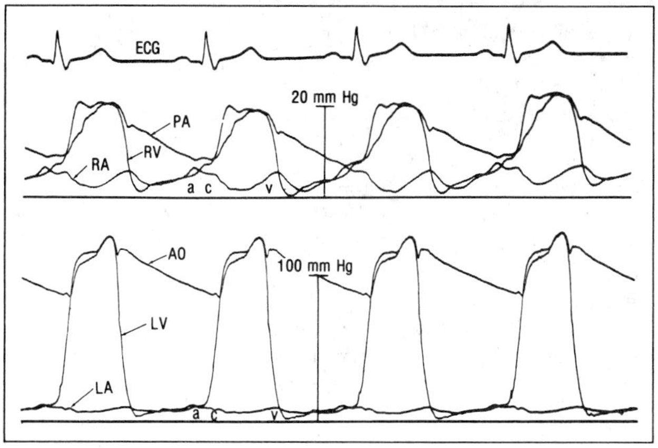

Fig. 6-3. Normal pressure recordings from the great arteries and cardiac chambers. Simultaneous high-fidelity tracings were obtained with special catheters on which multiple micromanometers were mounted. *ECG,* electrocardiogram; *PA,* pulmonary artery; *RV,* right ventricle; *RA,* right atrium; *AO,* aorta; *LV,* left ventricle; *LA,* left atrium. The *a, c,* and *v* refer to right and left atrial pressure waveform.

the pressure pulse to displace or deform a mechanical device such as a membrane or diaphragm; mechanical displacement is transformed into an electrical signal by *pressure transducers.* The electrical signals produced by the transducers are subsequently amplified and displayed or recorded. By convention, cardiovascular pressures are measured relative to middle right atrial position and atmospheric pressure.

The fidelity with which a transducer electrically represents a pulsatile pressure wave depends on the frequency response of the catheter and transducer system. Conventional fluid-filled catheter transducer systems provide a limited frequency response. Therefore proper care is necessary to eliminate or minimize the factors that limit frequency response (e.g., excessively long tubing, presence of air bubbles). For more accurate measurements, miniaturized transducers have been mounted on cardiac catheters so that pressure signals are converted to electrical signals at the site of interest in the cardiovascular system.

The normal pressure relationships of the chambers of the human heart and great vessels are shown in Fig. 6-3. Small physiologic flow-related pressure gradients between the ventricle and great vessels persist until midsystole; the flow of blood continues until the arterial dicrotic notch (incisura). Normal pressure values are listed in Table 6-1.

CARDIAC OUTPUT

During catheterization the cardiac output can be measured by methods based on the Fick principle, indicator-dilution techniques, or angiography. The *Fick principle* states that the uptake or release of a substance by an organ equals the product of blood flowing through the organ and the arteriovenous (A-V) difference of the substance. By measuring the oxygen (O_2) content of pulmonary arterial (mixed-venous) and pulmonary venous (or systemic arterial) blood, the pulmonary blood flow is measured. In the absence of intracardiac shunts (see following discussion), the pulmonary blood flow is assumed to be equal to the systemic blood flow. The formula for measurement of cardiac output (CO, L/min) by the Fick principle for O_2 is as follows:

(EQ.1)

$$CO = \frac{\dot{V}O_2}{\text{Arterial } O_2 \text{ content} - \text{Mixed-venous } O_2 \text{ content}}$$

where $\dot{V}O_2$ is oxygen uptake (ml/min), arterial O_2 content is systemic arterial oxygen content (ml/L), and mixed-venous O_2 content is pulmonary arterial oxygen content (ml/L).

O_2 consumption has been classically determined by spirometry and chemical analysis of the expired gas. In the resting subject, $\dot{V}O_2$ is approximately 3.5 ml O_2/kg/min, or in a 70 kg man, approximately 245 ml O_2/min. Because about 25% of the O_2 bound to hemoglobin is removed during each passage of blood through the systemic circulation, the normal A-VO_2 difference is 3 to 4 ml O_2/dl (assuming fully oxygenated blood with normal hemoglobin concentration, the arterial O_2 content is 20 ml O_2/dl blood). Therefore the cardiac output of this 70 kg man is 245 ml/min divided by 3.5 ml/dl, or 7 L/min. Normal flow data are shown in Table 6-1.

A second technique for measuring cardiac output is the *indicator-dilution method,* based on the principle that the volume of fluid in a system can be determined if a known amount of an indicator (e.g., indocyanine green) is added to the system and if the resultant concentration of the indicator can be measured:

(EQ.2)

$$\text{Vol} = \frac{\text{Amount of indicator}}{\text{Resultant concentration of indicator}}$$

where vol is volume (ml), amount of indicator is indocyanine green (mg) added to the venous system, and resultant concentration is concentration (mg/ml) in the arterial blood. This concentration is determined by sampling arterial blood and measuring the concentration with a densitometer over time and thus measuring volume as a function of time or cardiac output in milliliters per minute. Assumptions about mixing and sampling are necessary, but the indocyanine green method is acceptable for determining the cardiac output. The *thermodilution* (i.e., cold saline) *method* is somewhat easier to use because no arterial puncture is required and no blood need be withdrawn. Use of a cold fluid as the indicator employs the same principle, but the site of injection must be close to the site of observation. Special adaption of the balloon-tipped, flow-directed catheter allows the indicator (5 to 10 ml of cold saline) to be injected rapidly in the right atrium and sensed by a thermistor located 25 to 30 cm away (at the catheter tip in the main pulmonary artery). Substituting temperature for concentration of indicator in equation 2, a bedside computer determines the cardiac output. Properly performed, the indicator-dilution methods have an error of only 5% to 10%. They are most

Table 6-1. Hemodynamic data in normal humans at rest (±1 SD)

Pressure data			
Right atrium		Pulmonary capillary wedge	
A wave	5 ± 3 mm Hg	A wave	8 ± 3 mm Hg
V wave	4 ± 3 mm Hg	V wave	8 ± 3 mm Hg
Mean	4 ± 2 mm Hg	Mean	7 ± 2 mm Hg
Right ventricle		Left ventricle	
Systolic	21 ± 3 mm Hg	Systolic	115 ± 11 mm Hg
End diastolic	6 ± 2 mm Hg	End diastolic	8 ± 3 mm Hg
		dP/dt_{max}	1600 ± 360 mm Hg/sec
Pulmonary artery		Aorta	
Systolic	19 ± 2 mm Hg	Systolic	115 ± 11 mm Hg
Diastolic	8 ± 2 mm Hg	Diastolic	74 ± 8 mm Hg
Mean	12 ± 2 mm Hg	Mean	93 ± 8 mm Hg
Flow data			
Hemoglobin (Hb) oxygen-carrying capacity			1.36 ml/g Hb
Oxygen consumption			126 ± 24 ml/min/m^2
Arteriovenous oxygen difference			3.6 ± 0.5 vol/dl
Cardiac index			3.6 ± 0.5 L/min/m^2
Stroke index			48.0 ± 9 ml/beat/m^2
Stroke work index			0.54 ± 0.12 joules/m^2
Systemic and pulmonary vascular resistance			
Total pulmonary resistance			144 ± 33 dynes-cm-sec^{-5}
Pulmonary arteriolar resistance			62 ± 29 dynes-cm-sec^{-5}
Systemic vascular resistance			1086 ± 270 dynes-cm-sec^{-5}

dP/dt_{max}, Maximum rate of rise of ventricular pressure.

accurate in normal or high cardiac output states and are much less accurate in the presence of valvular regurgitation or low output states, when Fick cardiac outputs are more reliable.

Stroke volume (ml/beat) is the cardiac output (ml/min) divided by the heart rate (beats/min). The cardiac index (L/min/m^2) is the cardiac output (L/min) divided by the body surface area (m^2).

CIRCULATORY SHUNTS AND RESISTANCES

A special use of blood flow measurements is to detect and quantitate intracardiac shunts. Left-to-right shunts mix fully oxygenated blood from the left side of the heart with the desaturated blood in the right side of the heart. For example, a left-to-right shunt will occur in the patient with an atrial septal defect when right ventricular diastolic stiffness is lower than left ventricular diastolic stiffness. The shunt may be detected and an increase or "step up" in blood O_2 content noted as blood is sampled in the right heart chambers. A left-to-right shunt may be quantitated by using the Fick principle. First, flow through the pulmonary circuit is calculated by using equation 1. Next, systemic blood flow (SBF, L/min) is calculated as follows:

(EQ.3)

$$SBF = \frac{\dot{V}O_2}{\text{Arterial } O_2 \text{ content} - \text{Mixed-venous } O_2 \text{ content}}$$

where $\dot{V}O_2$ is oxygen uptake, arterial O_2 content is systemic arterial oxygen content, and mixed-venous O_2 content is venae cavae content. The calculation of the A-VO_2 difference for the systemic circuit requires a sample of mixed-venous blood from the venae cavae (proximal to the shunt); the calculation for the pulmonary circuit requires blood from the pulmonary artery (distal to the shunt). Thus the magnitude of a left-to-right intracardiac shunt (L/min) is calculated as follows:

(EQ.4)

$$\text{Shunt} = \text{PBF} - \text{SBF}$$

where PBF is pulmonary blood flow (L/min) and SBF is systemic blood flow (L/min). In the case of an atrial septal defect, a pulmonary/systemic flow ratio exceeding 1.5 indicates a significant shunt. Smaller shunts cannot be detected reliably with the oxymetry method.

Right-to-left intracardiac shunts cause a mixture of desaturated blood from the right side of the heart with oxygenated blood returning from the pulmonary circuit. Detection and localization of the shunt are accomplished by noting a decrease in O_2 content as blood is sampled in the left heart chambers and aorta. Application of the methods outlined earlier permits quantitation of a right-to-left shunt. Bidirectional shunting also may occur, but a discussion of methods for estimating the severity of complex intracardiac shunts is beyond the scope of this chapter.

Indicators other than O_2, such as indocyanine green dye or ascorbic acid, are often used in the detection of intracardiac shunts. Other agents, such as hydrogen or krypton-85, may be introduced at the pulmonary capillary level by inhalation and detected in the right side of the heart by special techniques that permit the detection of even very small left-to-right shunts. Angiographic methods also permit detection and precise localization of intracardiac shunts. Flow data are summarized in Table 6-1.

The principle for calculating systemic and pulmonary vascular resistances is that resistance is directly proportional to the pressure drop across the vascular bed and inversely proportional to the flow through the bed. Thus systemic vascular resistance (SVR, Wood units) is calculated as follows:

$$\text{SVR} = \frac{\text{AOP} - \text{RAP}}{\text{SBF}} \quad \text{(EQ.5)}$$

where AOP is mean aortic pressure (mm Hg), RAP is mean right atrial pressure (mm Hg), and SBF is systemic blood flow (L/min). Similarly, pulmonary arteriolar resistance (PAR, Wood units) is calculated as follows:

$$\text{PAR} = \frac{\text{PAP} - \text{LAP}}{\text{PBF}} \quad \text{(EQ.6)}$$

where PAP is mean pulmonary artery pressure (mm Hg), LAP is mean left atrial (or pulmonary artery wedge) pressure (mm Hg), and PBF is pulmonary blood flow (L/min). These formulas give resistances in arbitrary (Wood) units; multiplication of these units by a factor of 80 produces metric units of dynes-cm-sec^{-5}.

An increase in flow results in an increase in pressure if downstream vascular resistance remains constant; if vasoconstriction produces an increase in resistance, maintenance of normal flow requires a ventricle to generate increased pressure. These principles partly form the basis for vasodilator therapy in patients with congestive heart failure (Chapter 10).

VALVE ORIFICE SIZE

A special case of resistance to blood flow is that produced by stenotic valves. As valve orifice area decreases, an exponential increase in the pressure gradient across the stenotic valve is generated for any given flow. Conversely, a minor increase in flow, as occurs during exercise, is associated with large increases in the pressure gradient. These predictions are based on the hydraulic orifice-area formulas developed by Gorlin and Gorlin. The effective orifice areas (cm^2) of stenotic, aortic, and mitral valves may be calculated as follows:

$$\text{Aortic valve area} = \frac{\text{Flow/SEP}}{44.5\sqrt{\Delta P}} \quad \text{(EQ.7)}$$

$$\text{Mitral valve area} = \frac{\text{Flow/DFP}}{38\sqrt{\Delta P}} \quad \text{(EQ.8)}$$

where flow is flow across the orifice (ml/beat), SEP is systolic ejection period (sec/beat), DFP is diastolic filling period (sec/beat), and ΔP is the mean pressure gradient across the orifice. Thus the pressure gradient across a stenotic orifice provides a reasonable estimate of the orifice area when the cardiac output is normal but not when heart failure is present. These orifice equations are not valid in the presence of significant valvular regurgitation if systemic blood flow (Fick or indicator dilution) is used in the equations; because only forward stroke volume is considered by this method, the orifice size will be underestimated. If, however, the total stroke volume is determined, the orifice formulas may be used in patients with mixed stenotic and regurgitant lesions.

ANGIOGRAPHY

Angiography permits assessment of cardiac volume and morphology and allows analysis of cardiac motion. To create and record a visual image of cardiovascular structures, a radiopaque material is injected into the chamber or vessel of interest. Various x-ray techniques then record the silhouette created by the contrast material. Most often, recording is done on 35 mm film at imaging speeds of 30 to 60 frames/sec, producing a cineangiogram that allows study of the chamber or vessel in real-time, slow-motion, and single-frame modes.

With the newer technique of digital angiography, the x-ray image is detected by a high-resolution television camera rather than on film. The analog signal output from the camera is digitized and sent to a central processing unit for storage, display, and processing. Subsequent computer processing of the images obtained by digital angiography allows better quantitative assessment of parameters such as coronary stenosis and ventricular volumes. Computerized assessment and quantification of video densitometry from coronary arteriography may provide estimates of myocardial perfusion and coronary blood flow. Most importantly, the increased contrast enhancement allows for a significant reduction in the amount of contrast material required for injection.

Angiography of the *right side of the heart* is useful in

evaluating congenital abnormalities as well as acquired disorders such as tricuspid regurgitation or constrictive pericarditis. Injection of radiopaque material in the pulmonary arteries provides images for detecting pulmonary thromboemboli and congenital abnormalities of the pulmonary vasculature and, after passage through the lungs, for determining left heart size and morphology.

Angiography of the *left side of the heart* is used to assess mitral and aortic valves and the size and function of the left heart chambers and the ascending aorta. Selective left ventriculography may be employed to diagnose and assess the severity of mitral regurgitation and to define abnormalities of the mitral leaflets and subvalvular structures. Ventriculography is also used to assess the ventricular outflow tract, the presence of mural thrombi, the aortic valve, and left-to-right shunts at the ventricular level.

Global and regional function of the left ventricle can be assessed by analyzing the ventriculogram, most often using the right arterior oblique projection alone. However, the accuracy is improved substantially if a left arterior oblique projection is also obtained. Thus it is possible to detect and

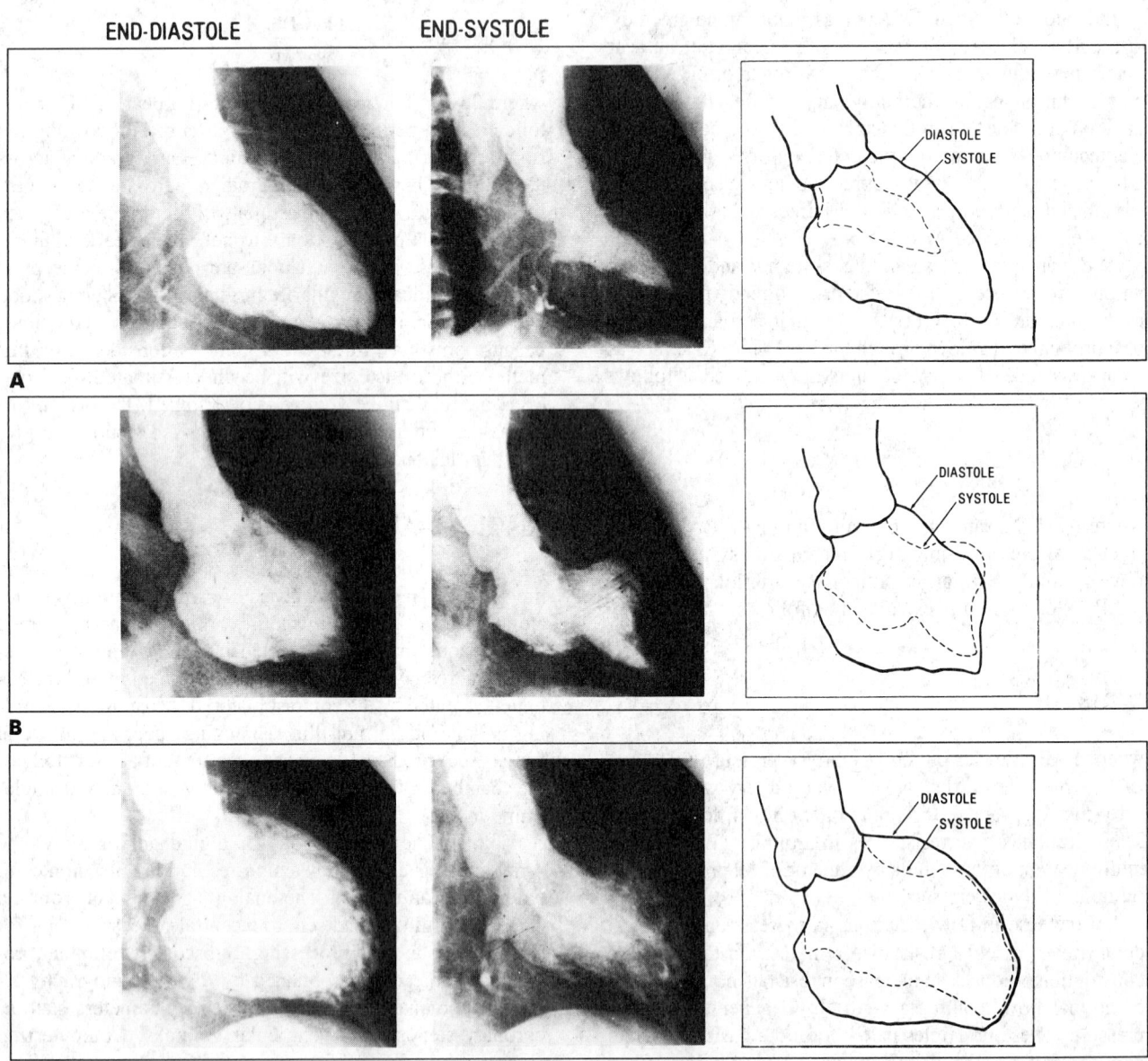

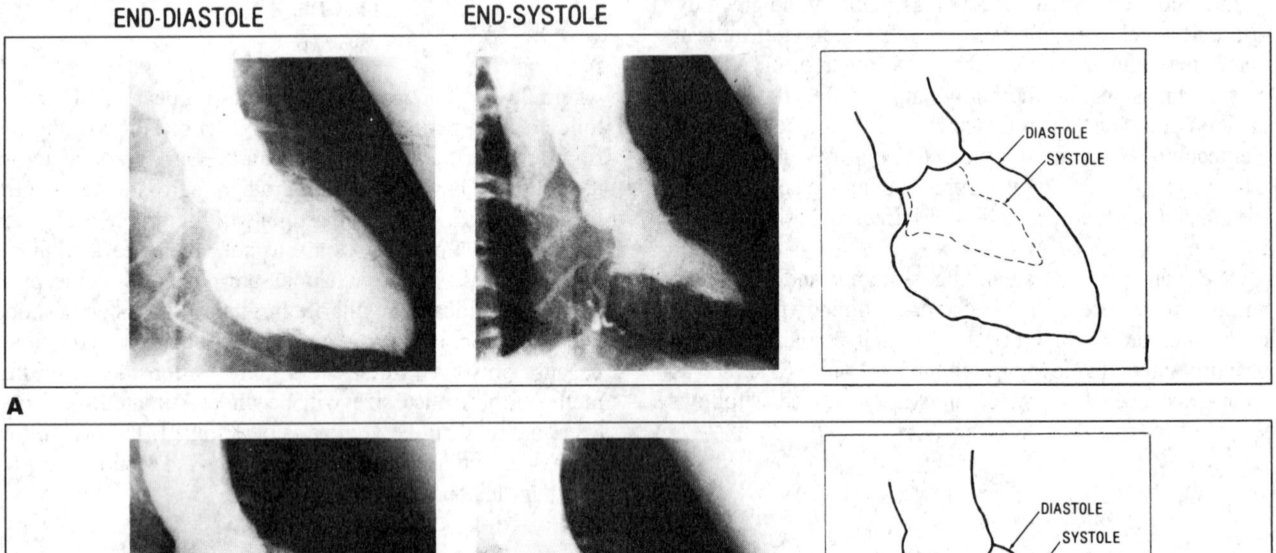

Fig. 6-4. End-diastolic and end-systolic frames from the left ventricular cineangiograms (right anterior oblique projection) of three different patients. Superimposed silhouette outlines are shown in the panels on the right. **A,** Normal left ventriculogram showing symmetric left ventricular contraction. **B,** Ventriculogram from a patient who had multiple myocardial infarctions, showing dyskinesis of the anterior ventricular wall and hypokinesis of the inferior wall. **C,** Ventriculogram from a patient with extensive anterior infarction; akinesis of the anterior and apical portions of the left ventricle is demonstrated.

assess quantitatively wall motion abnormalities (ventricular asynergy). Fig. 6-4 shows examples of regional wall motion abnormalities: reduced motion (hypokinesis), absent motion (akinesis), and paradoxical systolic expansion (dyskinesis).

By modeling the left ventricle as an ellipsoid and determining a radiographic magnification factor, its end-diastolic and end-systolic volumes can be calculated. Thus total stroke volume can be determined. If the effective stroke volume (Fick or indicator-dilution technique) is known, the regurgitant volume can be measured in patients with mitral or aortic regurgitation.

Angiography of the ascending aorta is performed to assess the severity of aortic regurgitation and to define aortic root anatomy of congenital or acquired disorders, including aortic dissection.

Selective coronary arteriography provides detailed visualization of the coronary arteries. Atherosclerotic and congenital lesions and collateral vessels can be assessed, coronary spasm or thrombus diagnosed, and coronary bypass graft patency confirmed. Finally, coronary arteriography is an essential ingredient in therapeutic procedures such as transluminal angioplasty and during or after the administration of thrombolytic agents.

LEFT VENTRICULAR FUNCTION

The evaluation of left ventricular (LV) function and myocardial contractility has been extensively investigated. Various indices derived from the pre-ejection and ejection phases of the cardiac cycle have been devised to assess and evaluate systolic function. Similarly, diastolic function (i.e., heart's ability to fill without a compensatory increase in diastolic pressure) has been studied by measuring relaxation and filling parameters as well as the myocardium's passive elastic properties. Systolic and diastolic dysfunction often coexist, but it is well established that elevated filling pressures (diastolic dysfunction) may be present in the absence of systolic failure.

Of the pre-ejection or isovolumic indices of contractility, the first derivative of LV pressure with respect to time, the rate of rise of ventricular pressure (*dP/dt,* mm Hg/sec), is the simplest to obtain and interpret. If LV end-diastolic pressure and volume remain relatively constant, changes in the maximum rate of rise of pressure (dP/dt_{max}) reflect changes in contractility. Calculations of contractile element velocity and other derived indices can reflect acute changes in contractility, but they are of very limited use in the assessment of basal contractile state in diseased hearts (Chapter 1).

The ejection phase indices of contractility or systolic function can be derived from an analysis of the LV cineangiogram. The *ejection fraction* (EF, %), defined as the ratio of stroke volume to end-diastolic volume, is calculated as follows:

(EQ.9)

$$EF = \frac{\text{Stroke volume}}{\text{End-diastolic volume}}$$

where the stroke volume is end-diastolic volume minus end-systolic volume. A major advantage of this parameter is that absolute ventricular volume calculations are not necessary. Moreover, because the EF is a normalized parameter, interpatient comparisons may be made without considering body size. Since cineangiographic techniques permit description of the time course of volume change, special techniques may be applied to calculate the rate of change of ventricular dimensions or volume. When coupled with pressure measurements, ventriculographic dimension and wall thickness data may be used to calculate LV wall tension or stress and thus to construct LV stress–dimension-shortening plots, which may be used to assess ventricular function and contractility. These analyses are based on the well-known inverse relation between afterload (systolic stress) and shortening (Chapter 1).

The stroke work (SW, joules) performed by the left ventricle may be calculated as follows:

(EQ.10)

$$SW = (LVSP - LVEDP) \cdot SV \cdot 0.136$$

where LVSP is LV systolic pressure (mm Hg), LVEDP is end-diastolic pressure (mm Hg), SV is stroke volume (ml), and 0.136 is a conversion factor of mm Hg to metric units (joules). Comparing values for SW among patients of different size requires normalization of the SV for body surface area. By plotting the SW index (joules/m^2) against LVEDP in different physiologic states (e.g., rest, exercise, drug administration), a modified "Starling" ventricular function curve can be generated (Chapter 1).

Diastolic pressure-volume and stress-strain data are used to assess LV passive elastic stiffness. Stiffness may be increased in hypertrophied and fibrotic hearts, in the presence of infiltrative disease, and in chronic constrictive pericarditis.

Abnormalities of LV diastolic relaxation may be assessed by measuring the rate of isovolumetric pressure decline and/or the rate and timing of ventricular filling. These relaxation parameters, which are determined in part by active energy-requiring processes, may be abnormal in chronic disease states (e.g., hypertrophy, cardiomyopathy) and during acute or transient disorders (e.g., angina pectoris). Relaxation abnormalities often precede impaired systolic function (Chapters 1 and 10).

CATHETERIZATION DATA IN VARIOUS DISEASES

Ischemic heart disease

An imbalance between myocardial blood supply and demand underlies the manifestations of ischemic heart disease. Coronary arteriography is used to determine the cause of inadequate myocardial blood supply and its severity; the technique allows identification of fixed coronary obstruction caused by atherosclerosis, obstructions caused by coronary artery spasm or thrombus, and congenital or traumatic coronary abnormalities.

An abnormal left coronary arteriogram is shown in Fig.

6-1. The left anterior descending artery is completely occluded, and there is moderate disease in the obtuse marginal branch. After the administration of intracoronary streptokinase, flow is restored, but a severe fixed obstruction persists. An example of a successful coronary angioplasty procedure is shown in Fig. 6-2. Complete coronary arteriography requires multiple contrast injections and filming in multiple radiographic projections. Such information is important in planning myocardial revascularization and provides valuable prognostic information.

Coronary artery spasm causes or contributes to myocardial ischemia in Prinzmetal's variant angina and in a variety of other ischemic syndromes (Chapter 13). The intravenous (IV) administration of ergonovine maleate during coronary arteriography may permit the detection of coronary artery spasm in patients with atypical clinical presentations. The angiographic demonstration of coronary spasm provides the clinician with important information about the cause of the myocardial ischemia and aids in planning therapy.

The evaluation of ventricular function in the patient with coronary artery disease is very important. Of the many variables by which ventricular function may be assessed, measurement of ventricular filling pressure and cardiac output and angiographic determination of LV size, wall motion, and EF are the most frequently used.

Examples of information obtained from left ventriculography in patients with coronary artery disease are shown in Fig. 6-4. Three ventriculograms are presented. Drawings of the end-diastolic and end-systolic silhouettes are also provided to aid in the interpretation of the systolic contraction pattern. Fig. 6-4, *A,* depicts a normal left ventricle, and Fig. 6-4, *B,* illustrates a ventricle damaged by infarction. During systole the anterior wall of the damaged ventricle bulges outward (i.e., dyskinesis). The remainder of the ventricular silhouette is irregular in the systolic frame. The apex of the chamber demonstrates decreased inward motion (i.e., hypokinesis). Fig. 6-4, *C,* demonstrates akinesis. The anterior and apical portions of this patient's left ventricle show absent motion during systole. The end-diastolic ventricular dimension is enlarged because of the ventricle's diminished pumping capacity.

By combining angiographic and hemodynamic data, cardiac catheterization should provide information regarding the cause of myocardial ischemia, a description of the heart's functional state, and a determination of the damage already produced by the disease.

Aortic stenosis

As aortic stenosis develops, an abnormal pressure difference or gradient is generated across the valve. This results in an increase in LV pressure and high flow velocities in the narrowed orifice. The resultant turbulent flow is associated with the characteristic murmur of aortic stenosis (Chapter 16). Catheterization data in aortic stenosis are illustrated in Fig. 6-5, *A.* Simultaneous LV and aortic pressure curves illustrate the high LV pressure and the pressure gradient across the stenotic valve.

Fig. 6-5, *B,* is a representative aortic root angiogram in a patient with significant aortic stenosis. A prominent bulge in the aortic root is the site of poststenotic dilatation of the vessel, an abnormality that arises in response to the turbulent blood flow across the narrowed, thickened, and irregular aortic valve. The left ventriculogram, shown in Fig. 6-5, *F,* demonstrates the greatly thickened aortic valve that is prevented from opening fully during systole. The valve appears domelike, and the narrowed orifice is easily seen. The LV systolic dimensions are small as a result of concentric hypertrophy.

Aortic regurgitation

Examples of the different pressure waveforms obtained from patients with acute and chronic aortic regurgitation are shown in Fig. 6-5, *C* and *E.* A major difference between acute and chronic aortic regurgitation is the relatively normal LV chamber size and high diastolic pressures in the

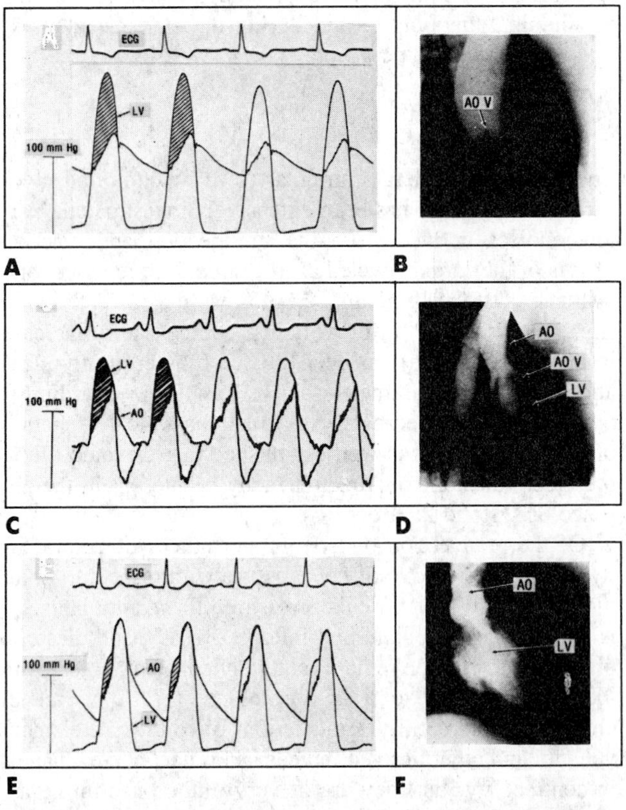

Fig. 6-5. Pressure and angiographic data from patients with aortic valve disease. **A,** Simultaneous micromanometer recordings of left ventricular *(LV)* and aortic *(AO)* pressure from a patient with severe aortic stenosis showing a pressure gradient *(shaded area)* between the left ventricle and the aorta. **B** and **F,** Aortic root and LV angiograms, respectively, showing thickening and doming of the aortic valve *(AO V),* poststenotic dilatation of the aortic root, and concentric hypertrophy of the left ventricle. **C** and **E,** LV and AO pressure tracings from patients with acute and chronic aortic regurgitation, respectively. **D,** Aortic root angiogram from a patient with aortic regurgitation reveals reflux of radiopaque material across the aortic valve into the left ventricle.

acute form in contrast to ventricular dilatation and increased chamber compliance in the chronic form.

In acute aortic regurgitation a substantial elevation in LV diastolic pressure may be seen; in some patients it may increase to such an extent that equilibration with aortic pressure occurs before the end of diastole (Fig. 6-5, *C*). A considerable systolic pressure gradient may be observed between the left ventricle and the aorta. Such gradients may result from ejection dynamics of increased blood flow associated with a large volume load and do not necessarily imply associated valvular stenosis.

LV and aortic pressure tracings from a patient with chronic aortic regurgitation are shown in Fig. 6-5, *E*. This ventricle is compliant and accepts the large diastolic volume without major changes in diastolic pressure. The physical characteristics of the ascending aorta also change with chronic aortic regurgitation so that flow-related systolic gradients are generated across the aortic valve but are extremely different in magnitude and duration when compared with the hemodynamics of acute aortic regurgitation.

An aortic root angiogram performed in a patient with aortic regurgitation is shown in Fig. 6-5, *D*. The early diastolic frame reveals regurgitation of opacified blood across the aortic valve into the left ventricle.

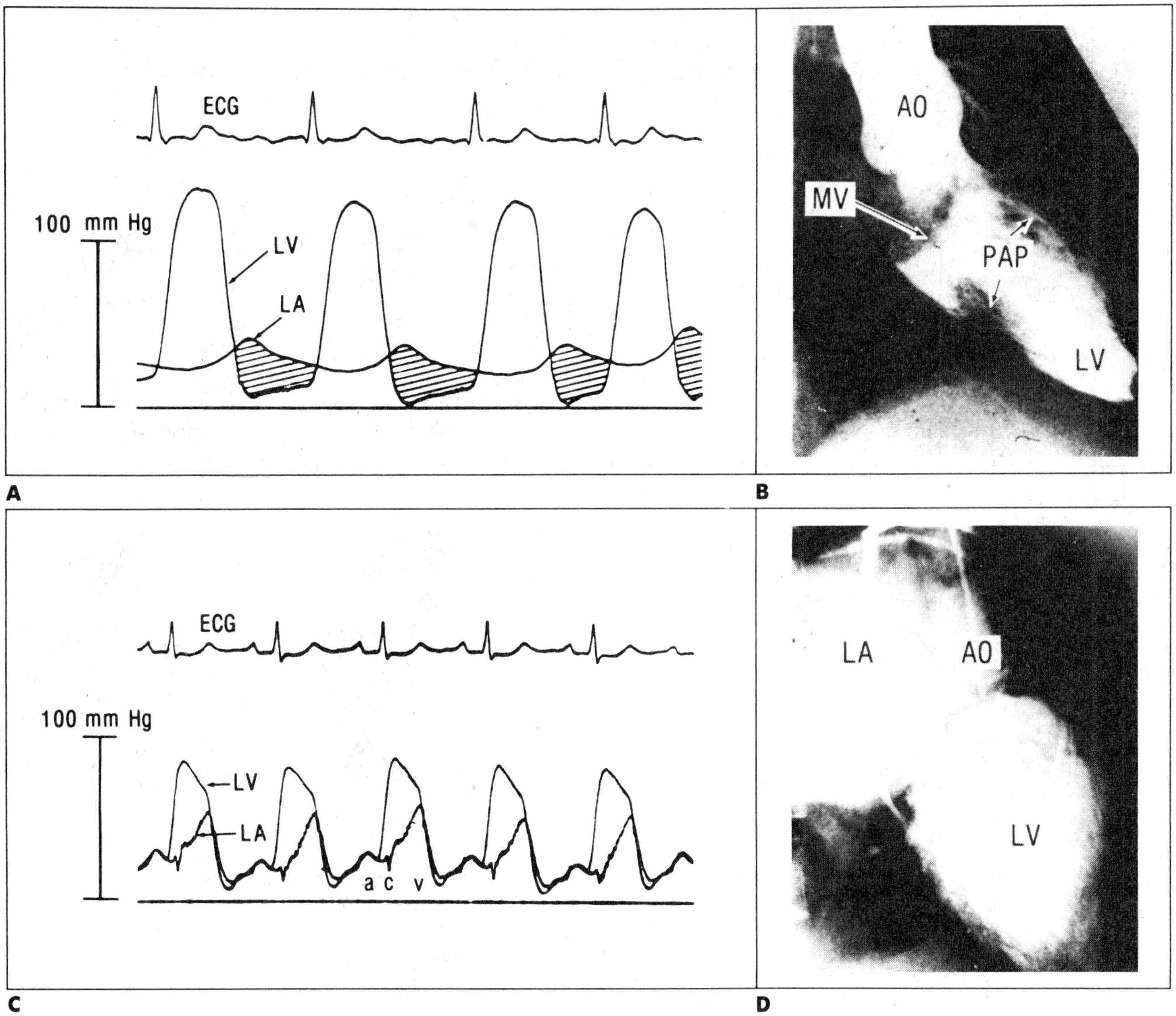

Fig. 6-6. Pressure and angiographic data from patients with mitral valve disease. **A,** Simultaneous left ventricular *(LV)* and left atrial *(LA)* pressure recordings from a patient with mitral stenosis. The "left atrial" pressure was recorded indirectly through the pulmonary wedge position. This example illustrates a pandiastolic pressure gradient *(shaded area)* across the mitral valve. **B,** LV angiogram from the same patient shows a thickened mitral valve *(MV)*, prominent papillary muscle *(PAP)*, and a small LV cavity. *AO*, Aorta. **C,** LV and LA pressure tracings from a patient with acute mitral regurgitation showing a prominent regurgitant wave *(v)* in the left atrium. The *a* and *c* also refer to LA pressure waves. **D,** Left ventriculogram from a patient with chronic mitral regurgitation showing an enlarged LV cavity and a massively enlarged left atrium.

Mitral stenosis

As mitral stenosis develops, a progressive rise in left atrial (LA) pressure is required to maintain adequate flow across the valve. As shown in Fig. 6-6, *A,* the elevated LA pressure and the diastolic pressure gradient across the mitral valve are present throughout diastole, but the presence of atrial fibrillation causes a beat-to-beat variation in the diastolic pressure gradient. When the diastolic filling period is shortest, the end-diastolic LA pressure (and the pressure gradient) is highest.

In patients whose heart rates are well controlled, long diastolic filling periods may allow adequate decompression of the left atrium, resulting in surprisingly low filling pressures during rest or when cardiac output demands are at a minimum. Thus an adequate evaluation of the severity of mitral stenosis is achieved by increasing heart rate and cardiac output by exercise. If the valve orifice area is significantly decreased, substantial increases in pressure will occur in the left atrium, pulmonary capillary bed, and the pulmonary artery. Pressure information and valve gradient measurements alone do not provide an adequate characterization of the degree of stenosis. Blood flow rates and a calculation of valve orifice area should be a part of the evaluation of all stenotic valves.

The typical angiographic appearance of the mitral valve and left ventricle in a patient with rheumatic mitral stenosis is shown in Fig. 6-6, *B*. A diastolic frame is shown. The limited excursion of the thickened mitral valve produces a sharp line of demarcation between the nonopacified blood in the left atrium and the contrast medium in the small left ventricle. Since the rheumatic process involves the entire mitral apparatus, the angiographic appearance of the ventricle also reveals prominent papillary muscles, with

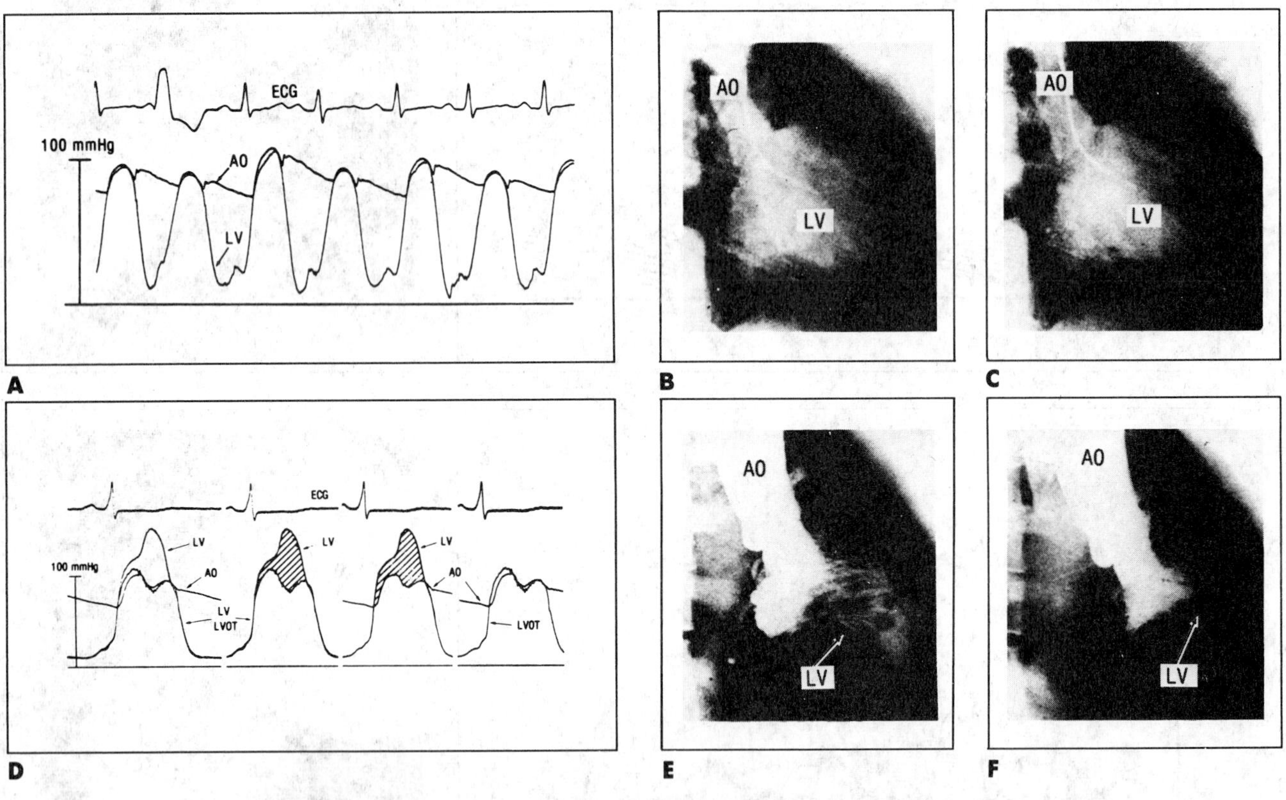

Fig. 6-7. Pressure and angiographic data from patients with cardiomyopathy. **A,** Left ventricular *(LV)* and aortic *(AO)* pressure tracings from a patient with congestive (dilated) cardiomyopathy demonstrating elevated LV diastolic pressure and LV alternans after a ventricular ectopic beat. **B** and **C,** End-diastolic and end-systolic frames from the left ventriculogram of a patient with congestive cardiomyopathy. The left ventricle is dilated and the ejection fraction is greatly reduced. **D,** Simultaneous high-fidelity pressure tracings from a patient with hypertrophic obstructive cardiomyopathy demonstrating the characteristic pressure gradient *(shaded area)* between the LV body and outflow tract *(LVOT)*. In the first cardiac cycle, pressures are recorded in the LV cavity, LVOT, and ascending aorta by three micromanometers mounted on a single catheter. In the second cycle the ascending aortic pressure tracing has been eliminated, revealing a systolic pressure gradient between the LV body and LVOT. In the third cycle the LVOT pressure has been eliminated, revealing a pressure gradient between the LV body and the aorta. In the fourth cycle the pressure tracing from the LV body has been removed; no abnormal pressure gradient exists across the aortic valve. **E** and **F,** End-diastolic and end-systolic frames, respectively, from the LV cineangiogram of the same patient shown in **D.** The LV cavity is small in diastole and almost obliterated in systole.

their tips positioned close to the mitral annulus as a result of chordal fusion and shortening.

Mitral regurgitation

As with aortic regurgitation, substantial hemodynamic differences exist between acute and chronic mitral regurgitation (Chapter 16). In patients with acute mitral regurgitation the left atrium remains small and noncompliant, and a sudden regurgitant volume into a small left atrium produces a marked rise in LA pressure, with a large regurgitant v wave in the LA pressure pulse (Fig. 6-6, *C*). In chronic mitral regurgitation, progressive LA dilatation with an associated increase in LA compliance allows large regurgitant volumes of blood without significant increases in LA pressure. The left ventriculogram in Fig. 6-6, *D*, demonstrates the marked LA dilatation that accompanies significant chronic mitral regurgitation. Because progressive, insidious damage to LV myocardium may occur in the disease's more advanced stages, an accurate evaluation of LV function is especially important in these patients.

Cardiomyopathies

Although cardiomyopathy is complex and diverse, the clinical examples chosen illustrate the two most common disorders of cardiac muscle: congestive (dilated) and hypertrophic cardiomyopathies (Chapter 17).

Congestive cardiomyopathies are primarily characterized by the heart's reduced ability to eject blood. The end-diastolic and end-systolic frames from an LV cineangiogram are shown in Fig. 6-7, *B* and *C*. There is diffuse hypokinesis of the left ventricle, a reduced EF, and a low cardiac output. The LV and aortic pressure tracings are shown in Fig. 6-7, *A*. In addition to the elevated LV end-diastolic pressure, LV alternans is present in the beats after a premature ventricular contraction. In patients with congestive cardiomyopathy the purposes of cardiac catheterization are to identify the cause when possible, determine the degree of functional impairment, and assess responses to pharmacologic interventions, such as afterload reduction or inotropic agents.

Hypertrophic cardiomyopathies are characterized by an asymmetric myocardial hypertrophy, small LV cavities, and hypercontractile systolic function (Chapter 17). Abnormalities of diastolic function, often caused by the extraordinary hypertrophy that accompanies this disorder, result in marked reductions of LV diastolic compliance.

The typical angiographic appearance of the left ventricle in a patient with hypertrophic cardiomyopathy is shown in Fig. 6-7, *E* and *F*. In the diastolic frame (Fig. 6-7, *E*), a distorted, highly trabeculated ventricular chamber is illustrated. The left ventricle's hypercontractile quality is illustrated in Fig. 6-7, *F*, which shows that the chamber's apical portions are virtually obliterated during systole.

In some patients, systolic anterior movement of the mitral valve may be associated with the presence of intraventricular pressure gradients (Fig. 6-7, *D*). Not all patients

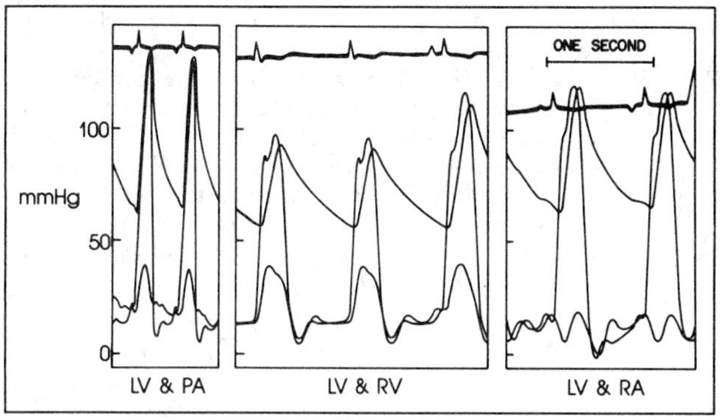

Fig. 6-8. Simultaneous micromanometer recordings of right and left ventricular pressure from a patient with chronic constrictive pericarditis. Diastolic pressures in the left ventricle *(LV)*, pulmonary artery *(PA)*, right ventricle *(RV)*, and right atrium *(RA)* are equal. The contribution of atrial systole to end-diastolic and developed systolic pressures in this noncompliant heart is illustrated by the transition from junctional to atrial rhythm *(middle panel)*.

with hypertrophic cardiomyopathy demonstrate such gradients, and various interventions, such as the production of a premature ventricular contraction, inhalation of amyl nitrite, or an infusion of isoproterenol, may be employed to produce such gradients during cardiac catheterization. Some investigators interpret the presence of such a gradient as indicating an obstruction to LV outflow. Others, who believe that ejection is not impeded, interpret a gradient as the result of combined hyperdynamic ejection and geometric factors. The interpretation and significance of these intraventricular gradients remain controversial.

Chronic constrictive pericarditis

When scarring and fibrosis affect the pericardium, diastolic filling is impaired, whereas systolic function is preserved. The insidious progression of chronic constrictive pericarditis eventually results in systemic and pulmonary venous hypertension and the signs and symptoms of congestive heart failure (Fig. 6-8). Thus the diagnosis of constrictive pericarditis should be considered in all patients with heart failure. Complete right-sided and left-sided heart catheterization is performed to exclude the diagnosis of restrictive cardiomyopathy, confirm the diagnosis of pericardial constriction, and evaluate the presence of other disease.

REFERENCES

Abrams HL, editor: Abrams angiography: vascular and interventional radiology, ed 3. Boston, 1983, Little, Brown.

Cannon SR, Richards KL, and Crawford M: Hydraulic estimation of stenotic orifice area: a correction of the Gorlin formula. Circulation 71:1170, 1985.

Grossman W: Cardiac catheterization and angiography, ed 4. Philadelphia, 1991, Lea & Febiger.

Kennedy JW: Complications associated with cardiac catheterization and angiography. Cathet Cardiovasc Diagn 8:5, 1982.

King SB and Douglas JS: Coronary arteriography and angioplasty. New York, 1985, McGraw-Hill.

Kruger RA and Riederer SJ: Basic concepts of digital subtraction angiography. Boston, 1984, GK Hall.

Levine HJ and Gaasch WH, editors: The ventricle: basic and clinical aspects. Boston, 1985, Martinus Nijhoff.

Reiber JH et al: Assessment of short-, medium-, and long-term variations in arterial dimensions for computer-assisted quantitation of coronary arteriograms. Circulation 71:280, 1985.

Vas R et al: Digital quantification eliminates intraobserver and interobserver variability in the evaluation of coronary artery stenoses. Am J Cardiol 57:718, 1985.

Yang SS et al: From cardiac catheterization data to hemodynamic parameters, ed 3. Philadelphia, 1988, Davis.

III Clinical Syndromes

CHAPTER

7 Chest Pain

Louis J. Dell'Italia

Chest pain, often described as "chest discomfort," is a common symptom of patients seeking medical evaluation. An accurate assessment of the cause and significance of the various types of chest discomfort is important and in some instances lifesaving. Etiologies of chest pain can be separated into two major categories, cardiac and noncardiac (see the box on the right).

Differential diagnosis of chest pain

Cardiovascular

Ischemic in origin
- Coronary atherosclerosis
- Aortic stenosis
- Hypertrophic cardiomyopathy
- Severe systemic hypertension
- Severe right ventricular hypertension
- Aortic regurgitation
- Severe anemia/hypoxia

Nonischemic in origin
- Aortic dissection
- Pericarditis
- Mitral valve prolapse/autonomic dysfunction

Gastrointestinal

Esophageal reflux
Esophageal spasm
Esophageal rupture

Pulmonary

Pulmonary embolus
Pneumothorax
Pneumonia

Neuromusculoskeletal

Thoracic outlet syndrome
Degenerative joint disease of cervical/thoracic spine
Costochondritis (Tietze's syndrome)
Herpes zoster

Psychogenic

Anxiety
Depression
Cardiac psychosis
Self-gain

CARDIAC CAUSES OF CHEST PAIN

Ischemic causes

Although no uniform presenting symptom exists for ischemic heart disease, chest pain or discomfort represents the most common reason for seeing a physician. William Heberden is credited with the original description of his own angina in 1768:

> But there is a disorder of the breast marked with strong and peculiar symptoms, considerable for the kind of danger belonging to it, and not extremely rare, which deserves to be mentioned more at length. The seat of it and sense of strangling and anxiety with it is attended, make it not improperly called angina pectoris.
>
> They who are afflicted with it are seized while they are walking (more especially if it be up a hill and soon after eating) with a painful and most disagreeable sensation in the breast, which seems as if it would extinguish life if it were to increase or to continue; but the moment they stand still, all this uneasiness vanishes.

Angina pectoris is defined as chest pain or discomfort of cardiac origin that results from a temporary imbalance between myocardial oxygen (O_2) supply and demand (Chapter 13). A patient's description of ischemic chest pain may take many forms, including burning, viselike tightness, squeezing, choking, heaviness, knifelike, and suffocating. This variety of descriptions may be further modified by the patient's intelligence, education, and sociocultural background. However, the patient is usually able to describe a deep rather than a superficial origin of the pain. Although the etiology of the various forms of discomfort is complex and not fully understood, an adequate anatomic explanation exists for the many patterns of referred pain that can be manifested in the neck, jaw, left shoulder, and left arm. It is thought that nonmedullated, small sympathetic nerve fibers that parallel the coronary arteries provide the afferent sensory pathway for angina and enter the spinal cord in the lowest cervical and upper thoracic segments (C8-T4). Here these sympathetic afferent impulses converge with impulses from somatic thoracic structures onto the same ascending spinal neurons. Thus impulses reaching visceral afferent neurons may stimulate nearby intermediate neurons that are receptors for somatic impulses and subsequently may produce a sensation of discomfort in the various referred areas in the chest, neck, or arms. Because the quality or character of the chest discomfort can be difficult to interpret, the location, radiation, duration, precipitating factors, and means of relief are very important in the systematic assessment of the patient with chest pain (see the box on p. 89).

Localization of the site of discomfort may help in determining its cause. Although the deep, visceral character of ischemic chest pain often defies localization, anginal pain usually begins in the midsternum or slightly to the left of the midline. Pain localized to a discrete area of the chest by pointing a finger to the inframammary region or cardiac apex usually is not angina pectoris. However, one or two clenched fists held by the patient over the sternum (Levine's sign) when describing the discomfort strongly suggests angina. Pain that originates entirely outside the thorax or epigastrium and subsequently radiates to the chest is not caused by myocardial ischemia. However, ischemic pain may only be felt in the arm or may start in the arm and radiate to the chest. As discussed, the patterns of *radiation* can vary because of the convergence of visceral and somatic impulses. In general, however, angina does not radiate to the upper jaw, the lower back, or below the umbilicus.

The assessment of chest pain is not complete without an evaluation of *precipitating factors* that elicit chest discomfort. This information is not only of diagnostic value but also provides an index of the severity of narrowing in the coronary vessel(s). Chest discomfort usually is induced by exercise, cold environment, or emotion or after eating a large meal. All these activities increase the O_2 demand of cardiac muscle by increasing heart rate, blood pressure, and myocardial contractility mediated through sympathetic stimulation. Increased O_2 demand must be balanced by an augmentation in coronary blood flow because the coronary circulation is not capable of increasing its O_2 extraction, since oxygen extraction is near maximal at baseline. The *double product* (heart rate times blood pressure) has been used as a bedside index of the heart's myocardial O_2 demand. Although it does not include contractility, the double product demonstrates a high correlation with directly measured O_2 consumption in the normal left ventricle. An increase in heart rate decreases diastolic filling time when most blood flow to left ventricular (LV) endocardium occurs. An augmentation in pressure increases the tension developed in the ventricular wall (Laplace's law = Pressure × Radius/Wall thickness), and in the normal ventricle a higher pressure indicates greater contractility. However, one can appreciate how larger increments in myocardial O_2 demand can occur for a comparatively lower heart rate times pressure product in the dilated ventricle as opposed to the normal-sized ventricle because of differences in wall stress. Nevertheless, myocardial O_2 supply depends greatly on the ability to increase coronary blood flow. Therefore the extent of physical activity (double product) that precipitates angina is related to the degree of fixed coronary artery stenosis but is not necessarily related to the number of coronary arteries with obstructive lesions. However, many episodes of angina, especially variant and unstable angina, are probably caused by coronary vasoconstriction or thrombosis without an increase in myocardial O_2 demand.

Typical angina pectoris usually comes on gradually and reaches its maximum intensity over 2 to 3 minutes. If pain is related to exertion, *relief* should occur within 2 to 3 minutes after cessation of exercise or with administration of sublingual nitroglycerin (Chapter 13). Nitroglycerin dilates the coronary vessels, thereby increasing blood flow and O_2 delivery through the diseased vessel and by way of collateral vessels. Nitroglycerin also decreases both preload and afterload through its venous and arterial vasodilating properties, thereby decreasing both diastolic and systolic wall stress. However, nitroglycerin's effect on arterial vasodilatation may not be apparent by a simple cuff sphygmomanometer pressure recording. Recent data have demonstrated that nitroglycerin's effect on arterial afterload reduction is accomplished by decreasing wave reflection in the arterial circulation (Fig. 7-1). Delayed relief at 10 to 15 minutes after nitroglycerin administration is not compatible with ischemic chest pain and may be caused by a placebo effect. Pain that occurs after exercise or at the end of a stressful day is not consistent with ischemic chest pain. Occasionally, patients experience dissipation of angina during continuation of exercise (walk-through phenomenon) or absence of chest pain during a subsequent exercise effort (warm-up phenomenon) that previously elicited angina. These phenomena have been attributed to opening of important collaterals during the initial episode of ischemia.

Other precipitating factors unrelated to physical activity can increase myocardial O_2 demand (double product) through reflex discharge of catecholamines. When the patient is carefully questioned, the physician may find that episodes of *chest pain at rest* may be associated with emotional lability such as occurs during anger, fright, or uncomfortable situations. Exposure to cold air causes an increase in systemic arterial pressure and heart rate, whereas extreme heat results in an augmented cardiac output from vasodilatation. Use of tobacco may elicit chest pain at rest or at a lower level of physical activity by two mechanisms. Carbon monoxide, which is a combustion product in ciga-

The Canadian Cardiovascular Society's classification of angina pectoris

1. Ordinary physical activity, such as walking and climbing stairs, does not cause angina. Angina with strenuous or rapid or prolonged exertion at work or recreation.
2. Slight limitations of ordinary activity. Walking or climbing stairs rapidly, walking uphill, walking or stair climbing after meals, or in cold, or in wind, or under emotional stress, or only during the few hours after awakening. Walking more than two blocks on the level and climbing more than one flight of ordinary stairs at a normal pace and in normal conditions.
3. Marked limitation of ordinary physical activity. Walking one to two blocks on the level and climbing one flight of stairs in normal conditions and at normal pace.
4. Inability to carry on any physical activity without discomfort—anginal syndrome may be present at rest.

From Campeau L: Letter to the editor. Circulation 54:522, 1976. Reproduced with permission of the American Heart Association and the author.

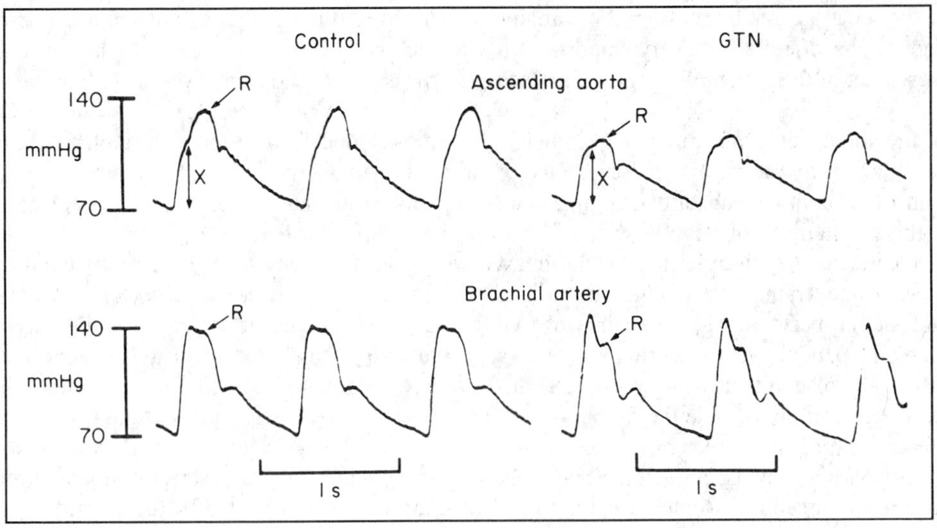

Fig. 7-1. High-fidelity pressure waveforms in the same patient from the brachial artery and ascending aorta at control valves and after nitroglycerin glyceryl trinitrate *(GTN),* administration. Reduction in amplitude of the reflected wave *(R)* by GTN is responsible for a change in contour of ascending aortic and brachial arterial waveforms. Because R constitutes a large part of the aortic pressure waveform, GTN produces a fall in the central systolic pressure. (From Kelly RP et al: Eur Heart J 11:138, 1990. Reproduced by permission of the European Society of Cardiology.)

rette smoke, may combine with hemoglobin and shift the hemoglobin-oxygen dissociation curve to the left, thereby reducing tissue O_2 delivery. The absorption of nicotine through the lungs increases myocardial O_2 demand by increasing heart rate, systolic arterial pressure, and contractility through the release of endogenous catecholamines.

Some patients with exertional angina pectoris experience *angina at rest* as a result of progression of disease severity or as an isolated clinical event. Coronary vasomotor tone is an important determinant of coronary blood flow and is influenced by several factors, including autonomic activity, metabolic products, and circulatory neurohumoral substances (Chapter 13). One or a combination of these factors is presumably responsible for an acute decrease in myocardial O_2 supply in patients with fixed coronary disease and in those with otherwise normal coronary arteries. This added feature may produce variable clinical manifestations of angina, ranging from angina at rest on certain days to pain that can only be elicited with maximum physical exertion at other times. Another cause of an acute decrease in myocardial O_2 supply includes coronary thrombosis superimposed on coronary atherosclerosis with spontaneous thrombolysis or coronary artery embolism. Angina at rest may also be caused by intermittent tachyarrhythmias that increase myocardial O_2 demand while decreasing diastolic filling time for coronary perfusion. Alternatively, labile hypertension acutely increases myocardial wall stress, resulting in rest angina. Another mechanism of rest angina may occur just before sleep, soon after the patient reclines. This results from an increase in LV wall stress caused by the increased LV volume resulting from an augmentation in venous return in the supine position. However, angina that occurs in the early morning hours usually results from increased coronary vasomotor tone, which has been demonstrated to be common during this time of the day.

From the previous discussion it is apparent that many potential causes of ischemic rest pain are unrelated to the number of diseased coronary vessels. Therefore, despite the more malignant natural history observed in many patients with angina at rest, the predictive value of the history alone is not as accurate as with exertional angina, which can be related to O_2 demand by the double product. However, the number of diseased vessels and the amount of myocardium at risk are directly related to prognosis, and the likely severity often can be estimated from a careful history. A classification of the functional severity of angina pectoris is detailed in the box on p. 87. Episodes of angina pectoris can be *associated with symptoms* that result from ischemic LV dysfunction or life-threatening arrhythmias. Severe ischemia may produce an increase in diastolic filling pressures or papillary muscle dysfunction, resulting in pulmonary venous congestion and symptoms of shortness of breath. This may also be the only manifestation of ischemia, or "anginal equivalent," in the absence of chest discomfort, particularly in diabetic patients. Low cardiac output may produce other associated symptoms of fatigue, weakness, or dizziness resulting from arrhythmias or ischemic LV dysfunction. Prolonged, severe pain associated with shortness of breath results from elevated LV diastolic pressures caused by ischemia involving a large amount of myocardium. These patients are clearly at increased risk. In addition, prolonged, severe pain at rest associated with nausea, vomiting, and diaphoresis suggests myocardial infarction. Furthermore, myocardial infarction is more frequently associated with signs of LV dysfunction (dyspnea, orthopnea) and autonomic nervous system hyperactivity

Characteristics of angina pectoris

Quality

Pressure of heavy weight on the chest
Burning
Tightness
Constriction about the throat
Visceral quality (deep, heavy, squeezing, aching)
Gradual increase in intensity followed by gradual fading

Location

Over sternum or very near to it
Anywhere between epigastrium and pharynx
Occasionally limited to left shoulder and left arm
Rarely limited to right arm
Limited to lower jaw
Lower cervical or upper thoracic spine
Left interscapular or suprascapular area

Radiation

Medial aspect of left arm
Left shoulder
Jaw
Occasionally right arm

Duration

30 seconds to 30 minutes

Precipitating factors

Relationship to exercise
Effort that involves use of arms above the head
Cold environment
Walking against the wind
Walking after a large meal
Emotional factors involved with physical exercise
Fright, anger, anxiety
Coitus

Nitroglycerin relief

Relief of pain occurring within 45 seconds to 5 minutes after taking nitroglycerin

Associated symptoms

Shortness of breath
Dizziness, lightheadedness, syncope
Palpitations
Weakness

(tachycardia, diaphoresis, bradycardia). However, up to 25% of patients may have no pain or may have atypical symptoms, particularly elderly and diabetic patients.

An evaluation of the patient who complains of chest pain is not complete without an assessment of the risk factors for coronary artery disease. Increased age, hypertension, diabetes, hypercholesterolemia, and cigarette smoking are established independent risk factors for coronary artery disease. Other important risk factors include a family history of premature coronary artery disease, obesity, sedentary lifestyle, type A personality, hypertriglyceridemia, and hyperuricemia. This information, coupled with a detailed history of the chest pain (see the box at left), should permit the physician to categorize the patient as being at low, intermediate, or high risk for coronary artery disease. This interview process is extremely important not only in determining whether an exercise test is necessary, but also in interpreting exercise test results to rule out the diagnosis of coronary artery disease, especially in the patient with a low pretest likelihood of disease. More importantly, a careful history may alert the physician to an unstable pattern. For example, an older patient with multiple risk factors complaining of frequent painful episodes relieved by two or three nitroglycerin tablets, recent onset of rest angina, angina with minimum exertion, or angina with associated symptoms may be at increased risk for exercise. In this particular patient it may be more appropriate to proceed directly to cardiac catheterization. These examples underscore the importance of a physician-patient interaction that results in a comprehensive chest pain history based on the known physiology of the coronary circulation and the bedside hemodynamic determinants (double product) of myocardial O_2 demand. Taken in this manner, this history stratifies the patient into low risk versus high risk and stable versus unstable, thereby providing important supplemental information to noninvasive and invasive testing (Chapter 13).

It is important at this point to emphasize that angina is a symptom and not solely a manifestation of coronary atherosclerosis. For example, classic symptoms of exertional angina may occur in the patient with *aortic stenosis* (Chapter 16), in whom increased resistance to LV ejection occurs with each heartbeat. This imbalance in myocardial O_2 demand results from increased systolic tension, a prolonged ejection period relative to the diastolic filling period (when most coronary flow occurs), and decreased coronary perfusion to the subendocardium caused by a thicker muscle mass and high diastolic filling pressures. Chronic elevation of afterload produces a similar physiologic mechanism for exertional angina in patients with *systemic hypertension* and *pulmonary hypertension* resulting from primary or secondary causes. In contrast, the patient with hypertrophic cardiomyopathy has an increased muscle mass that is not induced by an afterload stimulus. In this patient, hypercontractility and impaired coronary perfusion create an imbalance of myocardial O_2 supply and demand, especially at high heart rates. Severe *anemia* or *hypoxia* increases the heart's workload at a time when O_2 delivery is compromised, resulting in symptoms of angina at rest or angina with minimum exertion, even in the patient with normal coronary anatomy.

Severe *aortic regurgitation* (Chapter 16) may produce nocturnal angina during sleep when vagally induced bradycardia results in a longer diastole, more regurgitation, and greatly decreased coronary perfusion pressure caused by equilibration of aortic diastolic and LV diastolic filling pressures. Several reports have described certain patients with typical exertional chest pain and angiographically normal coronary arteries. Although these patients have been classified as having microvascular angina, metabolic and functional evidence of inducible ischemia has been demonstrated in only a small subset of patients having limited flow responses to pharmacologic or metabolic stress. These patients include a higher percentage of females, have a decreased number of coronary risk factors, and are less likely to have relief of pain after taking sublingual nitroglycerin or other antianginal drugs that are usually effective in patients with myocardial ischemia caused by obstructive coronary artery disease. At this time, the underlying cause of this chest pain syndrome is highly speculative; however, these patients' life expectancy appears no different from that of an age-matched and sex-matched population without chest discomfort.

Nonischemic causes

Pericarditis is a common cause of nonischemic cardiac pain (Chapter 18). The chest pain of pericarditis is usually sharp and penetrating. In contrast to ischemic cardiac chest pain, this pain comes on suddenly and lasts for hours to days. In addition, pericardial pain is worsened by deep inspiration and by lying in a flat, recumbent position. The pain is relieved by nonsteroidal anti-inflammatory agents and by sitting upright and leaning forward. Radiation of the discomfort may involve the shoulders, upper back, and neck. This pattern of radiation can be explained by the innervation of the pericardium. The visceral pericardium is virtually insensitive to pain, whereas pain fibers originating in the parietal pericardium innervate only the diaphragmatic surface. Consequently, radiation of the discomfort of pericarditis may involve the shoulders, upper back, and neck because of irritation of the diaphragmatic pleura, which is innervated through the phrenic nerve by fibers originating in the cervical sympathetic ganglia (C3 to C5). Occasionally the pain of acute pericarditis may mimic that observed in acute myocardial infarction, possibly because of periadventitial coronary artery nerve stimulation. In addition, because the pain is sharp, it must be differentiated from that of acute aortic dissection.

As mentioned earlier, the pain of *acute aortic dissection* must be differentiated from that of acute myocardial infarction and acute pericarditis (Chapter 21). The pain of aortic dissection is sudden in onset, in contrast to the pain of acute myocardial infarction, which increases in intensity with time. The pain is usually sharp and may radiate into the neck, back, flanks, and legs. The pattern of radiation depends on the location of the arterial dissection. Patients frequently characterize the pain as "tearing" in quality and the most excruciating pain that they have ever experienced. Manifestations of arterial occlusion may occur, including syncope and other neurologic symptoms when dissection involves the carotid and cerebral arteries and vascular insufficiency of the limbs when dissection extends to the subclavian and femoral arteries. In general, most patients have a longstanding history of systemic arterial hypertension, except patients with Marfan syndrome or idiopathic cystic medial necrosis.

Chest pain is a frequent complaint of patients with *mitral valve prolapse* (Chapter 16). The pain may be substernal but is more often perceived in the left anterior thorax. The pain is described in many ways, including a sharp or sticking pain or less frequently a dull ache. In addition, the pain's duration is highly variable, often being characterized as momentary or lancinating, but it may also last several minutes to several hours. In contrast to ischemic chest pain, the chest pain of mitral valve prolapse is usually nonradiating. In addition, the pain is usually not related to exercise and tends to occur in clusters, particularly during periods of emotional stress. The pain is not relieved by sublingual nitroglycerin and has no consistent relieving factors. In some patients the chest discomfort actually represents palpitations from premature ventricular contractions. Many patients complain that their heart is "jumping out of their chest." Many studies have demonstrated that mitral valve prolapse and panic disorder may frequently exist. Again, chest pain is the symptom in both these conditions that most often brings the patient to medical attention.

NONCARDIAC CAUSES OF CHEST PAIN

Gastrointestinal causes

The clinical history of pain originating in the gastrointestinal tract, particularly that of esophageal origin, frequently cannot be differentiated from ischemic cardiac pain. Recent studies of *reflux esophagitis* with prolonged esophageal pH and pressure monitoring demonstrate that the chest pain seems to be related primarily to an acid-sensitive mucosa, whereas motility disorders occur much less frequently than previously suggested by conventional laboratory tests. Gastroesophageal reflux disease and heart disease increase in prevalence as the population grows older. In addition, drugs used to treat coronary artery disease, such as nitrates, beta blockers, and calcium entry blockers, may decrease lower esophageal sphincter pressure and contraction amplitude, thereby aggravating or predisposing to gastroesophageal reflux. Therefore reflux-induced chest pain occurs frequently in patients with obstructive coronary artery disease.

Gastroesophageal reflux pain is usually burning and is located in the epigastric or retrosternal area. The pain is frequently precipitated by the recumbent position or by bending over. However, gastroesophageal reflux pain may be triggered by exercise. Symptoms suggesting an esophageal origin of chest pain include pain that continues for hours, retrosternal pain without lateral radiation, pain that occurs after meals or interrupts sleep, and pain that is relieved with antacids. Other esophageal symptoms can often be elicited, including regurgitation, dysphagia, and odynophagia.

Esophageal spasm results from a neuromuscular disorder of the esophagus that produces pain frequently confused with ischemic chest pain. This condition may occur in any age group but most often affects those between ages 50 and 60 years. As with ischemic chest pain, pain from esophageal spasm is located in the retrosternal area and often radiates to the back, arms, and jaw. The pain may be described as a burning, squeezing, or aching sensation. Features that may distinguish it from ischemic chest pain include associated symptoms of dysphagia, regurgitation of gastric contents, and pain during or after ingestion of extremely hot or cold drinks. Patients may have pain precipitated by exercise; this pain can be relieved with sublingual nitroglycerin, which relaxes esophageal smooth muscle. The definitive diagnosis is made by demonstrating abnormal esophageal motility on cine-esophagrams or by performing esophageal manometry.

Acute esophageal rupture may occur after a prolonged bout of vomiting or retching or after esophageal instrumentation. The event is characterized by severe retrosternal pain resulting from the chemical mediastinitis produced by acidic gastric contents. The pain of peptic ulcer disease and biliary colic may be confused with ischemic chest pain because both conditions may be associated with a burning sensation in the epigastrium.

Pulmonary causes

The acute substernal chest pain of *pulmonary embolus* (Chapter 20) often occurs in a specifical clinical setting, such as during the postoperative period, during long trips, in patients with congestive heart failure, and in patients with deep vein thrombophlebitis. The chest pain is usually sharp and may be located in the right or left thorax, depending on the location of the embolus. Frequently the chest pain is also aggravated by inspiration. Although the clinical findings of acute pulmonary embolus may be quite variable, massive embolus is often associated with dyspnea, tachypnea, and cyanosis. The physical examination may also reveal an elevated jugular venous pressure, tricuspid regurgitation, and other signs of acute right-sided heart failure.

Acute spontaneous pneumothorax may also be associated with chest pain. However, this condition may be readily differentiated from ischemic chest pain because it usually occurs in young, otherwise healthy males in the third and fourth decades of life. The clinical presentation is typically marked by the sudden onset of agonizing, unilateral, pleuritic chest pain accompanied by severe shortness of breath. The plain or expiratory chest radiograph provides the definitive diagnosis. The chest pain of *pneumonia* results from pleural irritation, which manifests as a sharp, pleuritic pain frequently accompanied by decreased inspiratory efforts. This condition is usually associated with fever, chills, and increased sputum production.

Neuromusculoskeletal causes

The various *thoracic outlet syndromes* may produce symptoms that are sometimes confused with cardiac chest pain. Compression of the neurovascular bundle by a cervical rib or the scalenus anterior muscle may cause discomfort radiating to the chest, neck, and ulnar surface of either arm. The prominence of associated paresthesias, the lack of clear relation of the pain to physical exercise, and its aggravation by certain body positions are helpful differential features.

Tietze's syndrome, or *idiopathic costochondritis,* is an occasional cause of anterior chest wall pain that is aggravated by movement and deep breathing. The reproduction of the chest pain syndrome by direct pressure over the involved costochondral junction and the relief of pain after local infiltration with lidocaine are helpful diagnostic maneuvers. Degenerative arthritis of the cervical and thoracic vertebrae may cause bandlike pain confined to the chest, neck, or back, which often radiates to the arms. Radiologic evidence of degenerative changes involving the cervical and thoracic vertebrae is often found in asymptomatic elderly patients. The production or exacerbation of pain by various postures, movement, sneezing, or coughing is more useful in the diagnosis of chest discomfort caused by vertebral disease.

The prevesicular phase of *herpes zoster* may be characterized by bandlike chest pain in a dermatomal distribution. The patient's advanced age, the presence of hyperesthesia on physical examination, and the eventual eruption of typical lesions 3 or 4 days after the onset of symptoms resolve any diagnostic difficulties.

Psychogenic causes

Chest pain of emotional origin may be difficult to distinguish from chest pain resulting from angina pectoris because both may be precipitated by anxiety. However, a careful history (see the box on p. 89) will document that chest pain of emotional origin is frequently sharp, left inframammary in location, and usually very well circumscribed. Psychogenic chest pain may be described as stabbing or lightninglike episodes of pain lasting less than 1 minute and not precipitated by any activity. Alternatively, the patient may complain of a substernal ache that lasts for hours or days and is unrelieved by nitroglycerin. Although these symptoms of chest discomfort may be associated with other symptoms, they are very dissimilar from those resulting from myocardial ischemia. Patients may complain of atypical symptoms such as air hunger, palpitations, giddiness, circumoral paresthesias, and other multiple somatic complaints that may suggest a neurasthenic personality. The patient often admits to having mild episodes of discomfort during the history and physical examination. During this time, nonverbal communication, such as a flat or worried facial expression, retarded motor activity, and hand wringing, may indicate underlying depression. As stated previously, many studies have demonstrated that mitral valve prolapse and psychogenic chest pain may frequently coexist. Recent studies of patients with mitral valve prolapse syndrome have demonstrated that faulty autonomic regulation can easily lead to inappropriate tachycardia or bradycardia, orthostatic hypotension, dyspnea, reduced effort tolerance and fatigability, chest pain, and rhythm disturbances. The similarity between these symptoms and the somatic expressions of anxiety just described may be related to autonomic dysfunction rather than a collection of neurotic complaints. Therefore appropriate tests of the autonomic nervous system may be indicated in some patients.

LIMITATIONS OF CHEST PAIN HISTORY

Although a complete history as outlined earlier provides a framework for further diagnostic workup in the patient with chest pain, the history may be misleading because of several factors. The physician's inability to interview the patient systematically results in incomplete data. This may result from different physicians' variable skill in obtaining a correct history or from the patient's inability to describe accurately the symptom complex because of sociocultural or educational reasons. Furthermore, many patients may withhold symptoms from the physician to maintain job security. In contrast, other patients may fabricate symptoms to obtain disability.

Finally, it must be emphasized that a typical history of angina pectoris does not necessarily coincide with the extent of coronary atherosclerosis. In addition, the physician must be alert to the existence of obstructive coronary artery disease in the absence of chest pain, especially in the diabetic patient. In these situations a high index of suspicion should lead the physician to appropriate diagnostic tests to rule out the presence of significant obstructive coronary artery disease.

REFERENCES

Alpert MA et al: Mitral valve prolapse, panic disorder and chest pain. Med Clin North Am 75:1119, 1991.

Berman DS, Rozanski A, and Knowbel SB: The detection of silent ischemia: cautions and precautions. Circulation 75:101, 1987.

Cannon RO: Microvascular angina: cardiovascular investigations regarding pathophysiology and management. Med Clin North Am 75:1097, 1991.

Coghlan HC: Autonomic dysfunction in the mitral valve prolapse syndrome: the brain-heart connection and interaction. In Boudoulas H and Wooly CF, editors: Mitral valve prolapse and mitral valve prolapse syndrome. Mount Kisco, NY, 1988, Futura.

Dell'Italia LJ and O'Rourke RA: Evaluation of the patient with signs and symptoms of ischemic heart disease. In Chatterjee K and Parmley WW, editors: Cardiology. Philadelphia, 1991, Lippincott.

Richter JE: Gastroesophageal reflux disease as a cause of chest pain. Med Clin North Am 75:1065, 1991.

Samson JJ and Cheitlen M: Pathophysiology and differential diagnosis of cardiac pain. Prog Cardiovasc Dis 13:507, 1971.

Uhl GS and Froelicher V: Screening for asymptomatic coronary artery disease. J Am Coll Cardiol 1:946, 1983.

Weiner DA et al: Correlations among history of angina, ST-segment response, and prevalence of coronary artery disease in the coronary artery surgery study (CASS). N Engl J Med 301:230, 1979.

CHAPTER

8 Palpitations

Robert A. O'Rourke
Richard A. Walsh

Patients use the term *palpitation* to denote an unpleasant awareness of the heartbeat that may result from an alteration in cardiac rate, rhythm, stroke volume, and/or contractility. This symptom is frequently encountered, is nonspecific, and often reflects a functional rather than an organic problem. Although some patients with definite heart disease may be unaware of severe arrhythmias, other patients with various anxiety states may describe palpitations resulting from normal heart action. The latter are particularly noted during introspective moments and at night, just before sleep, rather than during periods of marked physical activity. Such individuals may be convinced that palpitations result from underlying heart disease and indicate impending death. These concerns cause apprehension, increase autonomic nervous system activity, and often eventuate in a vicious cycle that results in complete emotional disability and cardiac neurosis. Frequently, palpitations may be the initial or only manifestation of important cardiac arrhythmias. Thus, whether palpitations are a manifestation of incapacitating anxiety requiring empathy and reassurance or a result of arrhythmias necessitating further diagnostic testing and treatment, they deserve careful assessment.

PATHOGENESIS

A patient's awareness of normal or abnormal heart action may result from several mechanisms. Anxiety may sensitize individuals to normal cardiac motion within the thoracic cavity. Normal persons exposed to stressful situations experience forceful sensations of cardiac motion as a consequence of increased circulating catecholamines and resultant augmented heart rate and contractility. Stressful pathologic states, such as fever, hyperthyroidism, anemia, and pheochromocytoma, may cause palpitations on a similar basis.

Forceful, regular palpitations may be described by patients with abnormally increased stroke volume, such as occurs with aortic and mitral regurgitation or ventricular septal defect and a variety of hyperkinetic circulatory states (e.g., anemia, thyrotoxicosis, arteriovenous fistula). These patients frequently complain of palpitations at night while lying on the left side, when the heart most closely approximates the chest wall.

Intermittent tachyarrhythmias, bradyarrhythmias, or isolated premature contractions may cause palpitations by sporadic, irregular alterations in heart motion. Palpitations are most often perceived during the onset or at the termination of the arrhythmia. Patients may describe the ectopic beat and/or the enhanced ventricular contraction after the postectopic pause.

CAUSES OF PALPITATION

Acute or chronic anxiety reaction

The symptom of palpitation is most often described by patients with an acute or chronic anxiety reaction. Many of these patients are distressed by the awareness of normal heart action during daily exercise, such as walking up stairs or doing housework. A history of the gradual onset and offset of this sensation corresponding to a period before and after intense physical activity usually suggests sinus tachycardia as the underlying mechanism. In addition to increased awareness of normal heart action, anxious patients may be more sensitive to the presence of premature beats.

Both atrial and ventricular premature depolarizations have been documented frequently by ambulatory electrocardiographic (ECG) recordings in otherwise healthy adults, particularly during periods of emotional stress and fatigue. Finally, anxious patients often describe palpitations in the absence of any objective evidence of cardiac arrhythmia.

Palpitations may be part of a chronic anxiety neurosis that is manifested by protracted autonomic nervous system overactivity. This condition has been variously termed *neurocirculatory asthenia, soldier's heart, DaCosta's syndrome, cardiac neurosis,* and *functional cardiovascular disease*. These patients often have physical findings of a hyperkinetic circulatory state manifested by resting sinus tachycardia, excessive perspiration, widened arterial pulse pressure, and a functional systolic murmur in the absence of other physical findings or laboratory data that suggest hyperthyroidism (Chapter 162). The common association of nonspecific ST-T wave changes on the ECG with the patient at rest, together with the frequent complaints of chest pain (Chapter 7), may lead to the mistaken diagnosis of coronary artery disease. Diagnostic error may be compounded by stress ECG testing because hyperventilation alone may provoke S-T segment depression in some patients.

A subgroup of patients with the mitral valve prolapse syndrome has been recognized as having a psychologic profile and signs of autonomic dysfunction similar to patients with neurocirculatory asthenia (Chapter 16). These observations, when combined with atrial or ventricular arrhythmias and/or false-positive ECG exercise test results, often complicate evaluation of the patient with mitral prolapse who has anxiety, atypical chest pain, and palpitations. Symptoms suggestive of hyperventilation (giddiness, circumoral/distal paresthesias) associated with transient or extremely prolonged and well-circumscribed "stabbing" chest pain in the region of the cardiac apex suggests a functional etiology rather than organic heart disease.

Successful treatment of palpitations resulting from a chronic anxiety state may simply require reassurance or, in patients with more severe symptoms, long-term counseling and psychotherapy, along with appropriate use of sedatives and tranquilizers. Beta blockade with propranolol in doses ranging from 80 to 320 mg/day may be useful in treating difficult patients with palpitations associated with sinus tachycardia or some patients with the mitral valve prolapse syndrome.

Premature ventricular depolarizations

Usually the diagnosis of premature ventricular beats is suspected from the patient's history. The premature and the postectopic beats are often described as "flip-flops"or "a skipped beat." The postectopic pause may be perceived as an actual cessation of heartbeat ("my heart stopped"), in contrast to the complete lack of awareness of similar pauses during atrial fibrillation. When premature beats are frequent, clinical differentiation from atrial fibrillation may be aided by physical exercise. Exercise-induced sinus tachycardia may abolish premature beats, whereas ventricular contractions remain irregular in atrial fibrillation.

Table 8-1. Value of the history in detecting the cause of palpitations

Description of palpitations	Defining likely cause
Occasional "flip-flops," "skipped beats"	Premature beats
Sudden onset, rapid, regular	Supraventricular tachycardia
Sudden onset, rapid, irregular	Paroxysmal atrial fibrillation
Gradual onset, regular with exercise	Sinus tachycardia
Associated with drugs	Tobacco, coffee, tea, catecholamines, xanthines, thyroid hormone
Associated with atypical chest pain and hyperventilation symptoms	Anxiety state, mitral valve prolapse syndrome

Tachyarrhythmias and bradyarrhythmias

Observant patients may describe the sudden onset of rapid, regular palpitations not associated with exercise or other forms of environmental stress, suggesting the diagnosis of supraventricular tachycardia. Some patients have taken their pulse during the palpitations or have had a companion do so. A rate of 100 to 140 beats/min suggests sinus tachycardia, a regular rate of 150 beats/min suggests atrial flutter, and a regular rate exceeding 160 beats/min suggests paroxysmal supraventricular tachycardia (Chapter 9). By contrast, the gradual onset and cessation of palpitations associated with stress or exercise suggest sinus tachycardia. Ventricular tachycardia is not usually associated with palpitations, perhaps because of the reduced cardiac output. However, prominent cerebral symptoms often occur. Episodic second- or third-degree atrioventricular block may be accompanied by slow, forceful palpitations, often associated with varying degrees of lightheadedness or frank syncope. If the patient is seen between attacks, the initial diagnostic possibilities depend greatly on the history (Table 8-1). However, the precise characterization of the basis for palpitations depends on the correlation of symptoms with ECG evidence of arrhythmias.

Ambulatory ECG recording often fails to disclose irregularities of heart rhythm in patients complaining of palpitations. In patients with infrequent episodes, long-term ambulatory ECG recordings may have to be performed on multiple occasions to detect the rhythm during symptoms (Chapters 5 and 9). An alternative approach is ECG telephone transmission during symptoms or the use of a patient-activated recording system with a 30-second memory loop.

REFERENCES

Braunwald EB, editor: Heart disease: a textbook of cardiovascular medicine, ed 4. Philadelphia, 1992, Saunders.

Hurst JW, editor: The heart, ed 7. New York, 1990, McGraw-Hill.

Knudson MP: The natural history of palpitations in a family practice. J Fam Pract 24:357, 1989.

Ruddy R, Roman-Smith P, and Barbey JT: Palpitations: evaluation and management. Prog Cardiol 1/2:231, 1988.

CHAPTER

9 Cardiac Arrhythmias

Eric S. Williams
Charles Fisch

Arrhythmia denotes an alteration of the normal site or rate of electrical impulse generation within the heart or an alteration of the impulse's orderly spread through the cardiac conducting system.

Cardiac arrhythmias are very common and can occur in the presence or absence of heart disease. Occasionally they are the first clinical manifestation of underlying cardiac pathology. Arrhythmias vary greatly in their clinical significance. They may be undetected by patients or result in symptoms that range from merely bothersome to incapacitating. Some arrhythmias, despite their potential to produce symptoms, do not adversely affect the patient's long-term outlook. Other arrhythmias, whether associated with symptoms or not, can sometimes be independent risk factors for subsequent death.

The correct identification of an arrhythmia is thus important for both prognostic and therapeutic reasons. However, the assessment does not end with recognition of the specific arrhythmia. The physician must, to the degree possible, also understand (1) the underlying cause of the arrhythmia (particularly whether or not there is underlying heart disease and its severity), (2) the clinical situation in which the arrhythmia occurs, and (3) the arrhythmia's effect on the patient's quality of life and on the heart's hemodynamic performance. It is important that an arrhythmia be considered within the context of a complete cardiac diagnosis because the prognosis and the choice of therapy depend largely on the factors just listed. Moreover, such an approach will permit the physician to avoid exposing the patient who does not require aggressive therapy to the risks and expense of antiarrhythmic drugs.

This chapter is divided into two sections. The first deals with general principles governing arrhythmias and the second with specific arrhythmias.

GENERAL PRINCIPLES

Anatomy and physiology of specialized conduction system

Many arrhythmias originate within the specialized conduction system; less often, and only in presence of a significant myocardial disorder, they arise in the myocardial contractile fibers. The specialized conduction system includes the sinoatrial (SA) node located at the entrance of the superior vena cava and the right atrium, the atrioventricular (A-V) node, the bundle of His, right and left bundle branches (the latter with anterior and posterior divisions), and the Purkinje fibers. Specialized pathways connect the SA and A-V nodes, but their functional significance is controversial. Occasionally, discrete myocardial fibers provide a pathway for electrical activity between the atria and ventricles. These accessory connections provide a means for an electrical impulse to bypass the A-V node, resulting in ventricular pre-excitation (see later discussion). The SA and AV nodes are richly innervated by sympathetic and parasympathetic fibers, and their function is influenced to a great extent by this autonomic innervation.

The blood supply to the SA node is through the SA nodal artery, which arises from the right coronary artery in approximately 60% and from the circumflex artery in about 40% of individuals. Primary blood supply to the A-V nodal area is via the A-V nodal artery, which originates from the right coronary artery in 90% and from the left circumflex artery in 10% of persons. The bundle branches obtain much of their blood supply from the left anterior descending vessel. Not surprisingly, therefore, A-V conduction block during inferior infarction (from right coronary obstruction) is usually at the level of the A-V node, whereas heart block complicating extensive anterior infarction can be the result of the interruption of conduction more distally in the bundle branches.

The normal cardiac impulse originates in the SA node and activates the atria, and this activation is registered on the electrocardiogram (ECG) as a P wave. The impulse is physiologically delayed in the A-V node, resulting in the P-R interval. The impulse then traverses the bundle of His, the two bundle branches, and the Purkinje system to activate the ventricular myocardium. The current generated by activation of the ventricular myocardium is responsible for the QRS complex. Normally the activation of the ventricle occurs rapidly and in an orderly sequence, yielding a narrow (<0.10 second in duration) complex with a characteristic contour. An interruption of this orderly sequence (e.g., with right or left bundle branch block) results in a wide QRS complex with an aberrant contour. A wide QRS also results when ventricular activation arises from the ventricle (e.g., premature ventricular contraction). It is important to recognize that although an arrhythmia is often a manifestation of disordered function of the specialized conduction system, its activity is not directly reflected in the ECG waveform. Rather, the P wave and the QRS complex reflect the activation of the "working" myocardium. Consequently an ECG diagnosis of an arrhythmia may have to be based on deductive analysis, with the abnormal behavior of the specialized conduction tissue deduced from the electrical behavior of the atrial and ventricular myocardium. This may make an ECG diagnosis of some arrhythmias difficult.

The electrophysiologic mechanisms underlying most arrhythmias result from altered automaticity or conduction or both, concepts that may be best understood in light of an isolated cell's behavior, as described next. It must be emphasized, however, that the electrophysiologic mechanism of a specific arrhythmia in humans is often impossible to identify at the bedside.

The resting transmembrane voltage estimated with an intracellular microelectrode is negative; the magnitude of the negativity depends on the cell studied (Fig. 9-1). For example, the resting transmembrane voltage is approximately

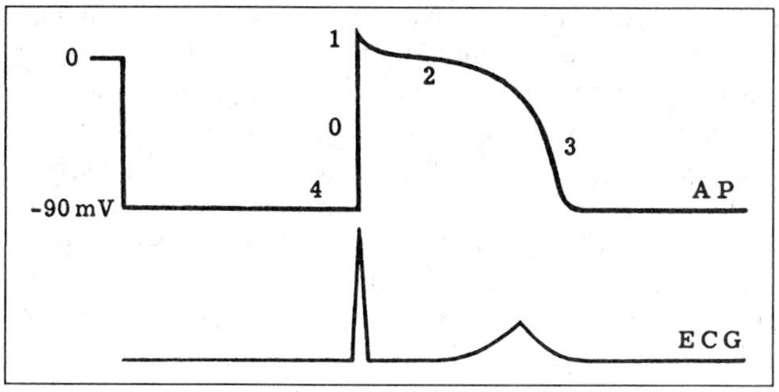

Fig. 9-1. Correlation of the transmembrane action potential *(AP)* with the surface electrocardiogram *(ECG)*. (From Heger JJ and Fisch C: Cardiac arrhythmias. In Spittel JA Jr, editor: Clinical medicine, vol 6. Philadelphia, 1982, Lippincott. Reproduced with permission.)

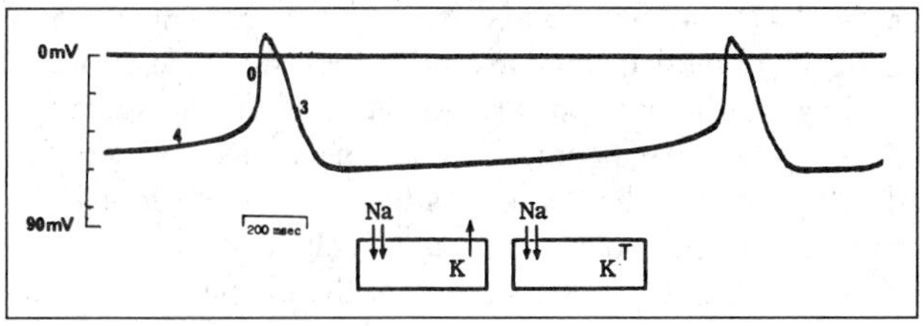

Fig. 9-2. Automatic sinoatrial node fiber showing gradual spontaneous loss of phase 4 transmembrane voltage. When the declining transmembrane voltage reaches the threshold level, a propagated transmembrane action potential is generated.

−60 mV in a SA nodal cell and −90 mV in a Purkinje fiber. The intracellular negativity is potassium dependent, the result of an efflux of the potassium cation (K^+) during the resting phase, or phase 4, of the transmembrane action potential (TAP). Activation of the cells is associated with a sudden influx of positively charged sodium (Na^+), reversing the intracellular negativity to a positive voltage of about 10 to 20 mV, the so-called overshoot. The sudden reversal of the intracellular negativity is phase 0, and the positive overshoot is phase 1 of the TAP. The ECG reflection of phases 0 and 1 is the QRS complex. Phase 2 follows and is characterized by a relatively stable voltage. Changes in phase 2 voltage are caused largely by slow calcium channel movement. The cells in which slow-channel calcium-dependent voltage plays a significant role in generation of the TAP include those of the SA and A-V nodes. Phase 2 of the TAP is reflected in the ECG by the S-T segment. Phase 3 of TAP, the T wave of an ECG, results from an efflux of K^+, which restores the intracellular negativity. At this point in the cycle the cell contains an excess of Na^+ and a deficit of K^+; the restitution of the normal ionic concentrations occurs during phase 4, the isoelectric baseline of the ECG. This process is energy consuming and is accomplished by the sodium, potassium, and calcium adenosine triphosphatase (ATPase) pumps. In the normal cell, complete restitution of the intracellular ionic concentration and transmembrane negativity precedes the subsequent cardiac activation.

The SA node, or more specifically a cell of the SA node, acts as the normal primary pacemaker (Fig. 9-2). During phase 4 there is a gradual influx of Na^+ or diminished efflux of K^+ or both, resulting in a gradual spontaneous loss of phase 4 negativity. When the phase 4 transmembrane voltage is reduced to the level of the threshold potential, a TAP is generated. The spontaneous loss of transmembrane negativity during phase 4 of a TAP defines automaticity. Acceleration or deceleration of the heart rate results from an accelerated or decelerated loss of phase 4 negativity, respectively. Normally the gradual loss of phase 4 voltage, or automaticity, is the property of the primary pacemaker, the SA node, with the remainder of the specialized conduction system having the property of latent automaticity. Automaticity of myocardial fibers is rare, occurring only in the patient with significant pathology.

The automatically generated TAP acts as a stimulus to the adjoining cells, which in turn stimulate adjacent cells, leading to propagation of the impulse. Activation of the contiguous cells by the TAP is caused by a reduction of their respective transmembrane resting potentials to threshold potential. The voltage difference between phase 4 and threshold potentials defines excitability. The narrower the difference, the more excitable is the cell, because a stimulus of lesser strength is required to reduce phase 4 potential to threshold potential. The speed of conduction does not necessarily parallel the excitability. In fact, an increase in excitability may result in reduced speed of conduction. This paradox results from the dependence of the speed of conduction on the integrity of the stimulus, namely, the TAP (Fig. 9-3). The integrity of TAP as a stimulus depends

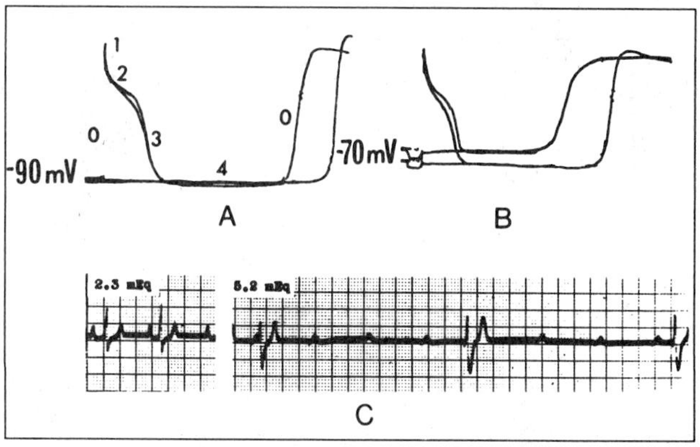

Fig. 9-3. ECG (**C**) demonstrates atrioventricular block caused by K^+ in a digitalis-intoxicated dog and the electrophysiologic mechanism responsible for the block. The two control action potentials recorded at the left in **A** are about 1 mm apart. The phase 0 is shown blown up on the right. After infusion of KCl (**B**) the phase 4 potential is reduced from −90 to −70 mV; the *dV/dt* (the rate of change of voltage) of phase 0 is reduced: the amplitude of the action potential is reduced, and the conduction between the two microelectrodes is greatly delayed, as indicated by an increase in the distance between the two action potentials (**B,** *right*). (From Fisch C: Relation of electrolyte disturbances to cardiac arrhythmias. Circulation 47:408, 1973. Reproduced with permission of the American Heart Association.)

on the TAP's amplitude and the speed of phase 0 voltage rise. Both of these depend in turn on the magnitude of phase 4 voltage at the moment of TAP generation, the so-called takeoff potential. In other words, the more negative the takeoff potential, the "better" is the resultant TAP and the more rapid is the conduction. Conversely, a reduced, or less negative, transmembrane voltage at the moment of activation results in a reduced speed of phase 0 voltage rise and reduced magnitude of the TAP. The altered TAP may fail to stimulate the adjoining cells adequately, and as a result the rate of propagation may be depressed or blocked.

The two mechanisms responsible for most ectopic arrhythmias are *automaticity* and *re-entry* (Fig. 9-4). (It is not clear whether "triggered" automaticity—a separate and specific mechanism of arrhythmias described at the cellular level—is responsible for clinical arrhythmias.) Re-entry is the result of unequal, or more specifically regional, unidirectional block of conduction. It can be illustrated by assuming that an impulse proceeds normally along one limb of a Y-shaped Purkinje fiber but is blocked in the other limb. The normally conducted impulse participates in the heart's activation. It also re-enters the blocked fiber in a retrograde direction and exits through the normally conducting branch. The second activation of the heart is registered as an ectopic impulse. The impulse is able to re-enter the fiber's blocked branch because the block is unidirectional, that is, in the antegrade direction only. Perpetuation of the re-entrant conduction results in a re-entrant tachycardia.

Diagnosis

Clinical diagnosis. Arrhythmias can often be detected, or at least suspected, by the symptoms and physical findings

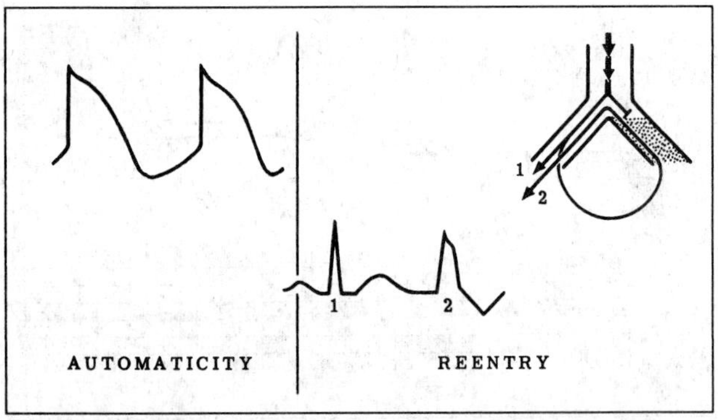

Fig. 9-4. Mechanisms responsible for most ectopic arrhythmias. Automaticity is manifested by a gradual loss of resting membrane potential (phase 4), which on reaching the threshold potential generates a propagated action potential. In re-entry an impulse arrives at an area of unequal conduction. It is conducted normally along one pathway and takes part in ventricular activation, which gives rise to the normal QRS. Re-entry can result from localized unidirectional block *(far right),* which means that forward conduction is blocked. After cardiac excitation the impulse enters the blocked area in a retrograde direction and re-enters the tissue via the normally conducting pathway, giving rise to the second, or re-entrant, or ectopic, QRS complex. (From Fisch C: Electrophysiological basis of clinical arrhythmias. Heart Lung 3:51, 1974. Reproduced with permission.)

they produce. The most common symptom is palpitation, which denotes an awareness of the heartbeat. Palpitation can be the result of alterations in heart rate, rhythm, or force of contraction (Chapter 8). Individuals vary remarkably in the degree to which they are aware of such alterations. Some seem to feel every premature beat, whereas others are unaware of grossly irregular rhythms or even runs of ventricular tachycardia. In evaluating a patient with palpitations, it is important to inquire about the nature of the palpitation (e.g., rapid, regular or irregular) and whether any associated symptoms are present. It can be helpful to have patients "tap out" with the hand their recollection of an arrhythmia to help identify its rate and regularity.

Patients may complain of a "skipped beat" or that "the heart stops." This usually results from the pause and subsequent forceful systole after a premature contraction. Premature heartbeats are occasionally accompanied by a momentary sharp or stabbing sensation at the cardiac apex. Paroxysms of rapid arrhythmias may be felt as a fluttering, pounding, or racing of the heart or a beating in the throat. Arrhythmias that are sufficiently fast or slow can limit cardiac output and cerebral perfusion, leading to weakness, lightheadedness, or syncope. In patients with ischemic heart disease, rapid arrhythmias can provoke angina pectoris. Arrhythmias can also precipitate or exacerbate congestive heart failure. It is important to recognize that arrhythmias can result in these associated symptoms (lightheadedness, syncope, chest pain, dyspnea) in the absence of any sensation of palpitation. Also, some patients with palpitations do not have arrhythmia. Other factors, including elevated blood pressure or anxiety, can contribute to awareness of the heartbeat. The medical history should include inquiry about the circumstances associated with the palpitations and the factors that seem to precipitate them. For example, at what age did they begin and how frequently do they occur, is there a history of underlying heart disease, do they occur with exertion or without obvious provocation, after meals or caffeine or ethanol ingestion, or during periods of emotional stress? The manner of onset and termination of palpitation can be helpful (Chapter 8). Re-entrant A-V nodal tachycardia, for example, is typically abrupt in onset and termination, whereas sinus tachycardia associated with anxiety typically resolves more slowly. In some elderly patients, marked bradycardia with syncope can follow stimulation of a hypersensitive carotid sinus on turning the head abruptly, shaving, or buttoning a tight collar.

Arrhythmias can be a side effect or toxic effect of certain medications (e.g., digitalis, antiarrhythmic drugs) and can be precipitated by hypokalemia or perhaps hypomagnesemia caused by diuretic therapy. Thus careful inquiry into the medication history is an important part of the evaluation of the patient with suspected arrhythmias.

As indicated previously, a careful search for any historic or physical examination evidence of underlying heart disease and assessment of its severity are essential parts of the evaluation. The effects of an arrhythmia are influenced by the intrinsic cardiac function, and some cardiac disorders predispose patients to certain arrhythmias. Moreover, signs of extracardiac disease should be sought because some such disorders can cause or contribute to arrhythmia. Examples include thyrotoxicosis and acute or advanced pulmonary disease.

In evaluating the patient with ongoing arrhythmia, the first goal of the bedside evaluation is assessment of the effects of the arrhythmia on cardiac pumping function (e.g., blood pressure, sensorium). This serves to identify the urgency with which treatment is instituted. Compromised blood flow may be manifested to varying degrees by diminished blood pressure (often with narrowed pulse pressure), diminished mentation, and cool skin. In some patients, particularly those with underlying heart disease, pulmonary rales from congestive heart failure may be evident.

Physical examination during a rhythm disturbance may also help identify the specific arrhythmia. The rate, regularity, and the pattern of any irregularity of the heartbeat should be noted. The presence of grossly irregular ("irregularly irregular") rhythm, for example, suggests the presence of atrial fibrillation. In some patients a pulse deficit may be present: simultaneous palpation of the radial pulse and auscultation over the precordium reveals beats that do not generate enough cardiac output to result in a peripheral pulse beat. In patients with a regular rhythm, intermittent changes in the amplitude of the pulse or the systolic blood pressure may be the result of A-V dissociation (independent atrial and ventricular activation) as the cardiac output is enhanced in those beats when atrial systole occurs by chance just before ventricular systole. The examination should include careful analysis of the jugular venous pulse with particular attention to signs of A-V dissociation. During A-V dissociation the magnitude of the jugular A wave characteristically varies, based on its occurrence relative to the independent ventricular systole. When atrial and ventricular systole fortuitously occur simultaneously, large or cannon A waves result as atrial contraction against the closed tricuspid valve propels blood in a retrograde manner. Ventricular tachycardia (VT), for example, frequently results in A-V dissociation and intermittent cannon A waves. Signs of A-V dissociation in a patient with a slow heart rate (e.g., less than 40/min) raise suspicion that heart block, another cause of A-V dissociation, is present. In some arrhythmias, large A waves occur with each heartbeat because of near-simultaneous activation of atria and ventricles (Chapter 3). Examples include A-V nodal re-entrant tachycardia and junctional or ventricular tachycardia in which the atria are activated in a retrograde manner. Since A waves are the result of effective atrial contraction, they are not present during atrial fibrillation.

Examination during certain maneuvers can also provide important diagnostic information. Vagal stimulation by means of carotid sinus massage or Valsalva maneuver in a patient with suspected atrial flutter, for example, characteristically reduces the ventricular rate abruptly from an initial 150 to 75/min. Atrial flutter is not terminated; the slower rate is the result of a vagally mediated reduction of A-V node conduction of the flutter waves to the ventricle (from 2:1 to 4:1). After termination of the maneuver the 150/min rate typically returns. Supraventricular tachycardias that require the A-V node for their genesis (e.g., A-V nodal re-entrant tachycardia, A-V re-entrant tachycardia associated with Wolff-Parkinson-White [WPW] syndrome) typically respond in an all-or-none manner to vagal stimulation. That is, the tachycardia is terminated abruptly by the vagal stimulation or is unaffected by it. Vagal stimulation also affects sinus node discharge. The typical response of sinus tachycardia is gradual slowing during vagal stimulation.

Laboratory diagnosis: electrocardiogram. Although specific arrhythmias may be suggested by the history and physical findings, the ECG remains the "gold standard" for diagnosis and permits documentation of the arrhythmia in the medical record. As with any laboratory procedure, the ECG does have limitations. An important example is the occasional wide QRS tachycardia in which the distinction cannot be made between VT and supraventricular tachycardia with aberrant conduction.

Ambulatory ECG recordings (Holter or event monitoring). This technique is frequently used in patients with unexplained episodic palpitations, dizziness, or syncope. The goal is both to document the suspected arrhythmia and, importantly, to define the temporal relationship of the recorded arrhythmia with the patient's symptoms. Absence of such a temporal relationship may spare the patient potentially hazardous antiarrhythmic therapy or permanent pacing and stimulate the search for alternative etiologies such as neurologic disorders. Ambulatory monitoring is sometimes performed in asymptomatic patients thought to be at high risk for serious arrhythmias and in some patients to assess effectiveness of antiarrhythmic therapy.

Ambulatory ECG monitoring is limited by many serious arrhythmias and symptoms being episodic; neither may occur during the monitoring period. It is important to emphasize also that certain types of arrhythmias may be recorded by ambulatory monitoring in individuals without symptoms or heart disease and may be of little or unknown clinical significance. In analyzing the results of ambulatory ECG monitoring, the physician must consider not only the specific arrhythmias detected but also the characteristics of the patient and the clinical situation in which they occur.

Intracardiac ECG. In most patients with arrhythmias the information from the clinical findings and ECG recordings permits the physician to make the correct diagnosis and decisions about the need for and form of therapy. In selected patients, however, additional useful diagnostic information can be obtained by intracardiac ECG recordings (Fig. 9-5). It can be helpful, for example, in the differentiation of VT from aberration when the distinction cannot be made from ECG and physical examination. The technique can also aid in the diagnosis and localization of accessory A-V bypass tracts. This is particularly important for patients with WPW syndrome for whom ablation therapy is contemplated.

Intracardiac catheterization techniques have also been used in some clinical situations to help in the selection of patients for antiarrhythmic therapy and in the prediction of effectiveness of various antiarrhythmic drugs.

Therapy

The first and most important decision regarding antiarrhythmic therapy is not which treatment to use but rather which

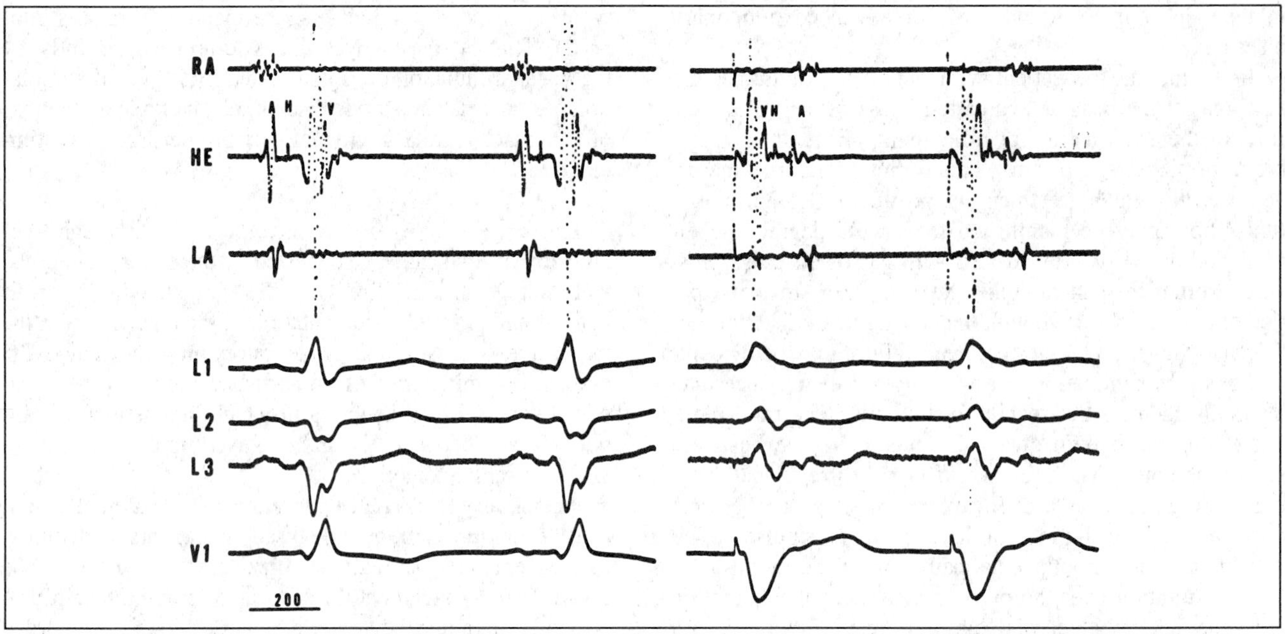

Fig. 9-5. Intracardiac electrocardiogram. The normal, spontaneous sequence of activation begins in the right atrium *(RA)*. The His bundle tracing *(HE)* records atrial activity *(A)*, His bundle activity *(H)*, and excitation of the ventricles *(V)*. When the impulse originates in the ventricles *(right panel)*, the ventricular complex *(V)* precedes the His potential *(H)*, and in this example retrograde conduction reaches the right and left atria *(LA)* and atrial potential *(A)* is recorded. (From Fisch C: Diagnosis and management of cardiac arrhythmias. Curr Probl Cardiol 1(12):1, 1977. Reproduced with permission.)

patients to treat. This decision is often made more difficult and important by the limited effectiveness and the side effects of many of the available therapeutic agents. Therapeutic intervention is generally indicated when (1) symptoms caused by the arrhythmia interfere unacceptably with the patient's quality to life or (2) the arrhythmia compromises the patient's hemodynamic status (Fig. 9-6). Depending on the specific arrhythmia, the decision may also be influenced by the rate and duration of the arrhythmia (e.g., sustained versus nonsustained) and by its frequency and likelihood of recurrence and progression. The presence or absence of underlying heart disease is important, as is the clinical situation in which the arrhythmia occurs.

Before considering specific forms of antiarrhythmic therapy, it is important to emphasize again that whenever possible, the treatment should include measures to improve or remove the underlying or precipitating causes of the arrhythmia. This includes both cardiac etiologies and extracardiac factors such as hypoxemia, hypokalemia, and toxicity or side effects of medications.

A variety of pharmacologic and nonpharmacologic measures are used in the treatment of patients with arrhythmias. For different arrhythmias, therapy may involve maneuvers or drugs to change vagal tone directly or indirectly, drugs to alter automaticity or conduction, cardiac pacing, or electric shock for cardioversion or defibrillation. In recent years, techniques have been developed to remove or destroy focal areas in the heart necessary for the genesis or perpetuation of certain arrhythmias. Some of these techniques are

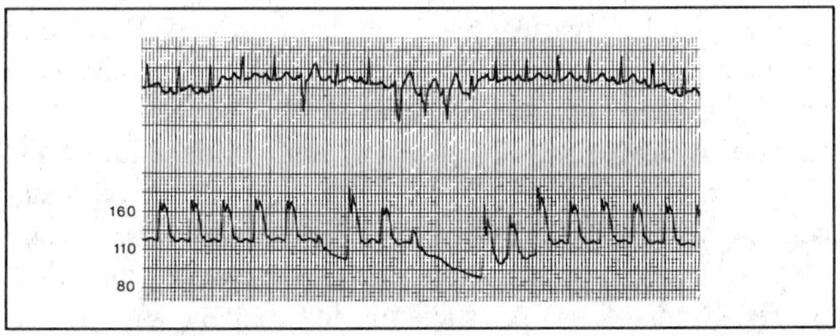

Fig. 9-6. Hemodynamic deterioration caused by ventricular arrhythmias. The depression is not only a function of accelerated rate because it is also present following a single premature ventricular complex occurring late in diastole *(top row)*. The deterioration in arterial pressure (measured in mm Hg, *lower panel*) probably is related to loss of atrial contribution and abnormal intraventricular conduction. (From Fisch C: Diagnosis and management of cardiac arrhythmias. Curr Probl Cardiol 1(12):1, 1977. Reproduced with permission.)

performed in the surgical suite, whereas others (e.g., radiofrequency catheter ablation) are performed in the electrophysiology laboratory. Furthermore, implantable devices with the potential to detect and to defibrillate or cardiovert patients with advanced refractory ventricular arrhythmias have been developed.

If antiarrhythmic drug therapy is indicated, the selection of the specific agent is based on the type of arrhythmia and an estimation of the relative risk/benefit ratio of treatment with the available drugs in the patient under consideration.

Therapy is often influenced by the underlying heart disease and ventricular function and by coexistent hepatic, renal, or pulmonary disease, since these may alter the drug's metabolism or place the patient at enhanced risk for one or more of its potential side effects. The patient's age may be similarly important, as well as his or her ability to comply with the necessary regimen. Important drug interactions can also occur between certain antiarrhythmic drugs and other medications (e.g., enhanced or reduced quinidine clearance by phenytoin or cimetidine, respectively) and can influence the choice or dose of antiarrhythmic drug. These points emphasize the importance of full understanding of the actions, pharmacokinetics, toxicity, and side effects of antiarrhythmic drugs before prescribing them.

For some antiarrhythmic drugs, selection of the appropriate dosage and dosing interval can be aided by the determination of the drug's blood levels. The blood level must be obtained at the appropriate time (e.g., trough level before next planned dose) and after the patient has been taking the agent long enough to approach a steady-state condition. Moreover, the physician must understand the limitations of blood levels of individual drugs and the considerable variability of individual patient response. Determination of blood levels can be helpful also in monitoring patient compliance, in patients with suspected drug toxicity or drug interaction, or when altered drug metabolism occurs, such as with impaired hepatic or renal function. Nonetheless, it is important to recognize that toxicity can occur in some patients despite "therapeutic" levels of antiarrhythmic drugs. For some drugs the issue is further complicated by the presence of drug metabolites that can exert or interfere with antiarrhythmic actions or contribute to side effects or toxicity.

Evaluation of an antiarrhythmic drug's efficacy in preventing arrhythmia recurrence can be difficult, particularly when an arrhythmia is episodic and infrequent. Also, spontaneous variability of an arrhythmia can simulate a beneficial response to the antiarrhythmic agent. These problems can be particularly vexing when treating patients with ventricular arrhythmias. For these reasons, some have proposed that the inducibility of ventricular arrhythmias by premature stimulation during invasive intracardiac electrophysiologic study serve as a guide to drug selection, particularly in high-risk patients.

For most arrhythmias, selection of an antiarrhythmic drug is largely a function of clinical judgment, and the effectiveness of therapy is assessed by the clinical response and by the rhythm monitoring (e.g., Holter monitoring studies).

Particularly when treating patients with ventricular arrhythmias, the assessment of drug effectiveness must also take into account the potential for most antiarrhythmic agents occasionally to induce or worsen arrhythmias. This "proarrhythmic" effect can lead to incessant and life-threatening ventricular arrhythmias. An example of proarrhythmia is torsade de pointes, a polymorphous VT associated with drug-induced prolongation of the Q-T interval. Reduced left ventricular function as well as diuretic-induced hypokalemia may increase the risk of serious proarrhythmia. Treatment with antiarrhythmic drugs with the potential for proarrhythmia should generally be initiated in the hospital with close patient monitoring. This is particularly important when significant underlying heart disease is present.

Unfortunately, it is now clear from the Cardiac Arrhythmia Suppression Trial (CAST) that the risk of serious proarrhythmia, at least with some drugs and in some situations, is not consistently predicted by the patient's early response to the drug. In this trial, survivors of acute myocardial infarction with complex nonsustained ventricular arrhythmias who were deemed to be at enhanced risk for late sudden death were treated with antiarrhythmic drugs or placebo. Although treated patients responded to the therapy and tolerated it in the hospital, the subsequent mortality was greater in those treated with encainide or flecainide than in those treated with placebo. The relationship of this finding to other drugs and clinical situations is not yet clear. Troubling observations about long-term mortality risk have also emerged from meta-analyses of chronic antiarrhythmic therapy in patients with supraventricular arrhythmias (i.e., quinidine for atrial fibrillation). These experiences and observations emphasize the importance of restricting treatment with drugs that have proarrhythmia potential to patients with a clear indication and of careful in-hospital institution and follow-up. The patient should also be aware of the risks of therapy.

Much is known about the cellular actions of antiarrhythmic drugs, and this information forms the basis of classification systems, as outlined next. However, these systems are limited. Many drugs, for example, exert several cellular effects, and drugs in the same class may share some common actions but differ in others. The relationship of any one or all of these cellular actions, as defined in the research laboratory, with its antiarrhythmic actions in humans is often unclear.

Class I drugs characteristically block the fast sodium channel. Based on variable actions, they are subclassified into class IA (quinidine, procainamide, disopyramide), class IB (tocainide, mexiletine, phenytoin), and class IC (flecainide, propafenone). Class II drugs (propranolol, metoprolol, atenolol, others) block beta-adrenergic receptors. Class III drugs (bretylium, amiodarone, sotalol, *N*-acetylprocainamide [NAPA]) block potassium channels and prolong repolarization. Class IV drugs (verapamil, diltiazem) block the slow calcium channel, primarily affecting SA and A-V nodal cells.

Beyond their electrophysiologic actions, antiarrhythmic drugs can variably affect the heart's contractile function. Prominent examples include disopyramide and flecainide, the negative inotropic actions of which can precipitate cardiac failure when administered to patients with significant left ventricular dysfunction. Some antiarrhythmic drugs also alter peripheral vascular tone and can worsen, for example, orthostatic hypotension.

Selected antiarrhythmic drugs are described briefly in the following paragraphs. Physicians using these drugs should consult additional sources and have a full understanding of the drugs' actions, pharmacokinetics, drug interactions, and

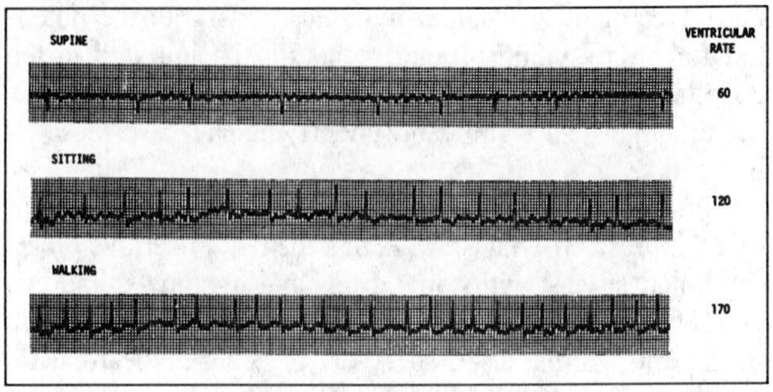

Fig. 9-7. Vagal effect of digitalis on atrioventricular (A-V) conduction and ventricular rate in atrial fibrillation. The slow ventricular response in the supine position is overcome promptly by change to a sitting position and with walking. The vagal effect depressed A-V conduction, prolonged A-V nodal refractoriness, enhanced concealment, and resulted in a slow ventricular response. However, this was not the optimum desired effect of digitalis. To control the ventricular rate during usual daily activities and with exertion, the extravagal effect of digitalis is required. In this instance, additional digitalis had to be administered despite the supine, resting ventricular rate of 60/min. (From Fisch C, Zipes DP, and Noble RJ: Digitalis toxicity: Mechanisms and recognition. Prog Cardiol 4:37, 1975. Reproduced with permission.)

toxicity. The specific use of some of the drugs is included with the later discussion of individual arrhythmias.

Digitalis. Digitalis is not included in the previous classification but is frequently used in patients with certain rapid supraventricular arrhythmias, particularly atrial fibrillation, in whom the primary goal is to limit the ventricular rate. This effect results from digitalis' vagal and direct actions to slow A-V conduction. The clinical importance of this dual action of digitalis on the A-V node is illustrated in Fig. 9-7. The degree to which digitalis can promote the return of sinus rhythm or prevent recurrences of atrial fibrillation is controversial. Digitalis is also used to slow the ventricular response to atrial flutter and can be used in the treatment and prevention of A-V nodal re-entrant tachycardia.

Familiarity with digitalis pharmacokinetics is essential for proper use of the drug and avoidance of toxicity. This includes understanding the effects of extracardiac disorders

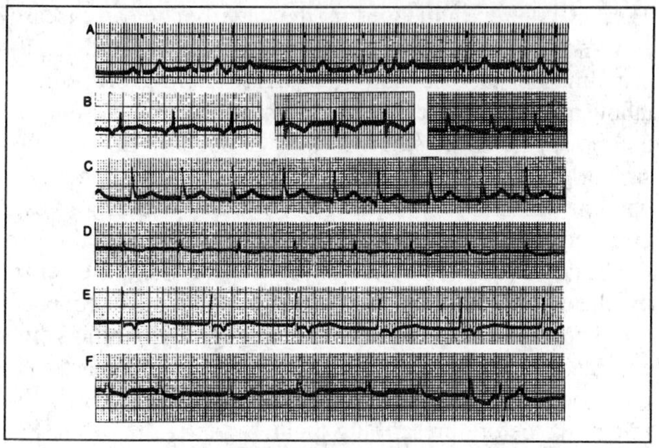

Fig. 9-9. **A,** Junctional premature beats with negative (retrograde) P waves in lead II. **B,** Junctional (A-V nodal) tachycardia with retrograde P wave preceding, superimposed on, and following the QRS complex. **C,** Nonparoxysmal junctional tachycardia (NPJT) interrupted by conducted sinus P waves. **D,** Atrial fibrillation with a regular ventricular rhythm at a rate of 75 beats/min, characteristic of NPJT. **E,** Junctional rhythm with retrograde P waves after the QRS. **F,** Junctional escape rhythm and A-V dissociation caused by slowing of the sinus rate. As soon as the sinoatrial node accelerates, it assumes control of the cardiac rhythm.

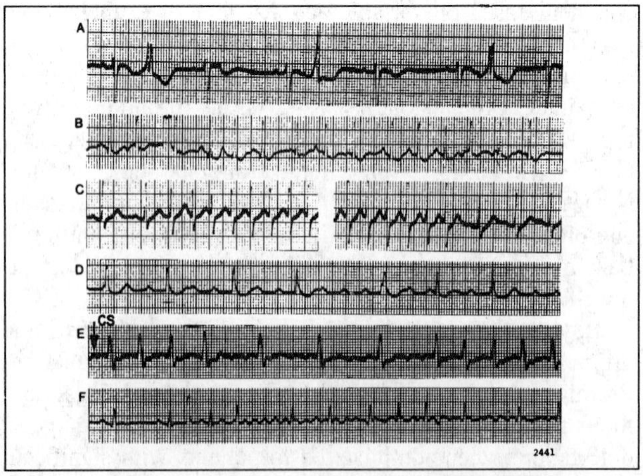

Fig. 9-8. **A,** Atrial bigeminy with nonconducted (blocked) and aberrantly conducted atrial premature complex (APC). The latter may be confused with ventricular premature complex. **B,** Multifocal, multiform ("chaotic") APC. **C,** Paroxysmal supraventricular tachycardia showing an abrupt onset and termination. **D,** Atrial tachycardia with block. **E,** Effect of carotid stimulation (CS) on atrial flutter. **F,** Onset of atrial fibrillation.

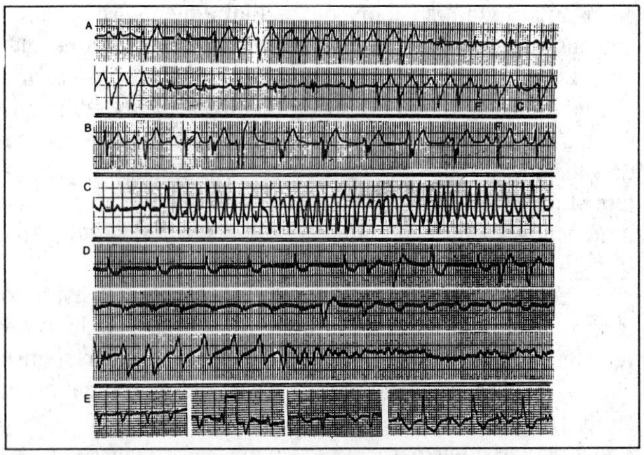

Fig. 9-10. **A,** Premature ventricular complex (PVC) with a full compensatory pause followed by ventricular tachycardia (VT) with fusions *(F)* and captures *(C)*. **B,** Accelerated idioventricular rhythm with a fusion complex *(F)*. **C,** VT with rotation of direction of QRS. When associated with a prolonged Q-T interval, it is termed *torsade de pointes*. **D,** Atrial fibrillation with PVC in first tracing, followed by VT from two different foci in middle tracing terminating in ventricular fibrillation from digitalis intoxication *(third tracing)*. **E,** Bidirectional VT caused by digitalis intoxication.

and other medications on the metabolism of digitalis. Digoxin, the primary preparation used clinically, is cleared by the kidney; its dosage must be reduced as renal function declines. Although digitalis toxicity may affect nearly every system of the body, the potentially lethal manifestations result from cardiotoxicity. The diagnosis of cardiotoxicity is often difficult and requires a careful correlation of the ECG with other clinical and laboratory findings. One of the reasons that digitalis toxicity can be difficult to diagnose is that arrhythmias identical to those induced by digitalis toxicity can be caused by the underlying heart disease or other medications. For example, although premature ventricular complexes (PVCs) are likely the most common cardiac manifestation of digitalis intoxication, they are also the least specific. Arrhythmias that are highly suggestive of digitalis intoxication include atrial tachycardia (AT) with block (Fig. 9-8), nonparoxysmal junctional tachycardia (NPJT) (Fig. 9-9, *C* and *D*), "bidirectional" VT (Fig. 9-10, *E*), ectopic rhythms arising from multiple sites of the specialized conduction tissue (Fig. 9-10, *D*), depression of the SA pacemaker (Fig. 9-11, *D*), significant depression of the A-V conduction (i.e., second- or third-degree A-V block) (Fig. 9-12, *B* and *E*), exit block (Fig. 9-11, *E*), ectopic rhythms with simultaneous depression of conduction, and A-V dissociation caused by an acceleration of a subsidiary pacemaker (Fig. 9-9, *B*). The approach to selected digitalis-induced arrhythmias (including the importance of withholding the digitalis and ensuring normal blood potassium levels) is described later in this chapter. In the patient with life-threatening digoxin intoxication, cardiac glycoside–specific Fab fragments have been beneficial in the reversal of arrhythmias.

Quinidine. Quinidine can be effective in the suppression or conversion of several supraventricular and ventricular arrhythmias. Because of its action to prolong the accessory pathway's refractory period in patients with WPW syndrome, quinidine also has the potential to reduce the ventricular rate in these patients during atrial flutter or fibrillation. Quinidine exerts a vagolytic effect and can enhance A-V nodal conduction. When given to patients with atrial flutter or fibrillation (in the absence of WPW syndrome) who are not taking digitalis, the ventricular rate can rise precipitously (Fig. 9-13). Quinidine also has alpha-adrenergic blocking action and can cause peripheral vasodilatation and hypotension. Quinidine's effectiveness is tempered by a significant incidence of undesirable side effects, most often gastrointestinal symptoms such as diarrhea, anorexia, and nausea. Central nervous system symptoms (cinchonism) may also occur. Idiosyncratic or allergic reactions include fever, rash, thrombocytopenia, and hemolytic anemia. As with all class I drugs, quinidine oc-

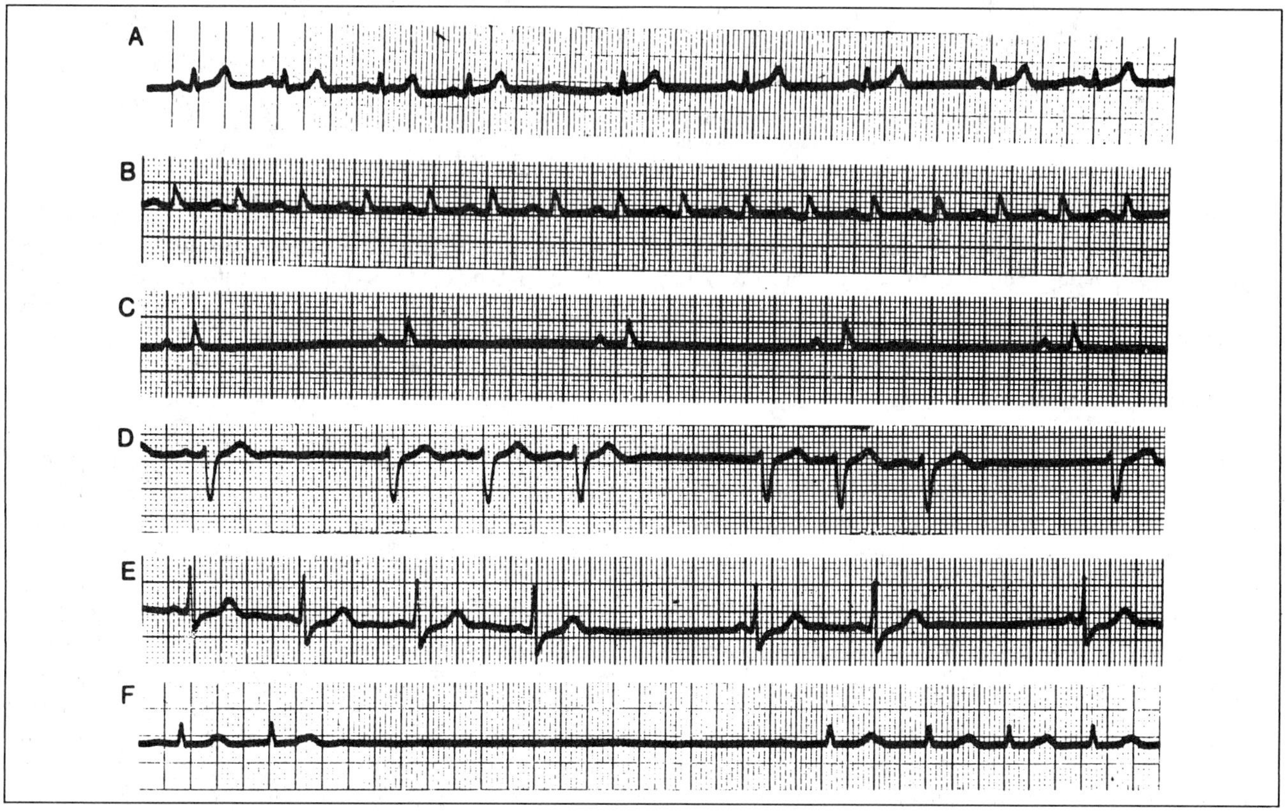

Fig. 9-11. A, Sinus arrhythmia. **B,** Sinus tachycardia. **C,** Sinus bradycardia. **D,** Sinus arrest with pauses terminated by junctional escape. **E,** 2:1 sinoatrial block. The longer pause is twice the length of the basic sinus cycle length. **F,** Atrial tachycardia with long periods of atrial arrest (tachycardia-bradycardia syndrome).

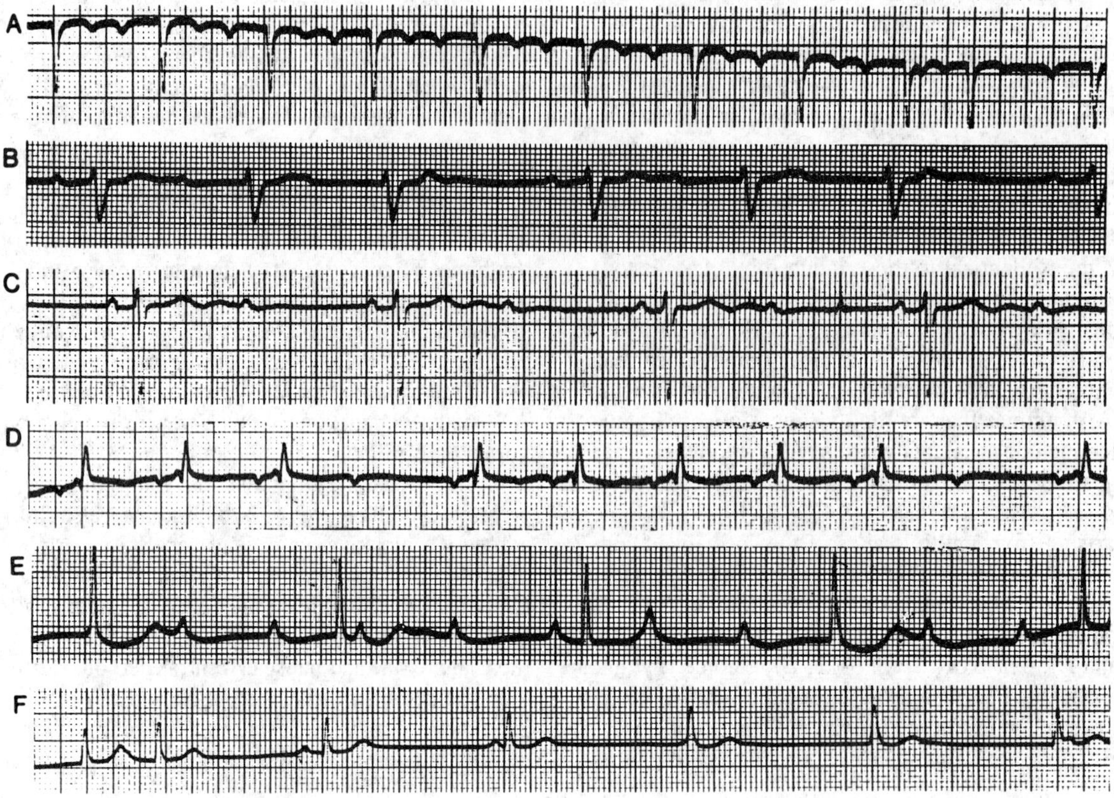

Fig. 9-12. A, First-degree A-V block with a P-R interval of 0.30 second. The third QRS from the right is followed by an early P wave, which in turn activated the ventricles earlier than expected, indicating presence of a *re-entrant impulse,* an *echo,* or *reciprocation* (these terms are interchangeable). **B,** Mobitz type I, or Wenckebach, A-V block. **C,** 2:1 A-V block. **D,** Mobitz type II A-V block. **E,** Complete A-V block. **F,** A-V dissociation caused by slowing of the sinus rhythm, with the P waves "marching" through the QRS.

casionally worsens ventricular arrhythmias and can underlie torsades de pointes (Fig. 9-10, *C*), producing, for example, syncope. Quinidine syncope is not directly related to the drug's plasma concentrations. Syncope may be more likely in patients with pronounced prolongation of the Q-T interval (some prolongation of Q-T interval is expected with quinidine therapy). Quinidine toxicity can impair conduction, leading to prolongation of QRS duration and PR interval. Both hepatic and renal clearance of quinidine are important. Quinidine interacts with several other medications. Its administration to patients taking digoxin can significantly raise the blood level of digoxin. Various quinidine preparations, including sustained release, are available. The usual dose of quinidine sulfate, for example, is 300 to 600 mg four times a day.

Procainamide. The therapeutic uses of procainamide are similar to those of quinidine. Procainamide is safer than quinidine when intravenous (IV) administration is required, although careful blood pressure and ECG monitoring is still necessary. It is also less likely to cause gastrointestinal symptoms during chronic therapy. Procainamide use can be complicated by immune-mediated reactions, including fever and agranulocytosis. Many patients develop antinuclear antibodies. A clinically important lupuslike syndrome can also occur and appears to be more likely in patients whose metabolism is characterized by slow hepatic acetylation. Several regimens have been used when emergent IV administration of procainamide is required. One approach includes 25 to 50 mg over 1 to 2 minutes, repeated every 5 minutes until the arrhythmia is controlled, the blood pressure declines, the QRS complex is prolonged more than 50%, or the upper dose limit is reached. Therapy can be maintained with a constant IV infusion at 2 to 6 mg/min. Procainamide has a relatively short half-life, and its oral use can be facilitated by a prolonged-release preparation, which often can be given every 6 hours. Typically the total daily dose is 2 to 4 g. In the patient with impaired metabolism or excretion, the dosage or dosing interval may be reduced. Procainamide is acetylated to *N*-acetylprocainamide (NAPA), which exerts its own electrophysiologic and toxic effects. NAPA is excreted by the kidney. In the patient with renal failure, NAPA (and procainamide) levels rise and must be monitored.

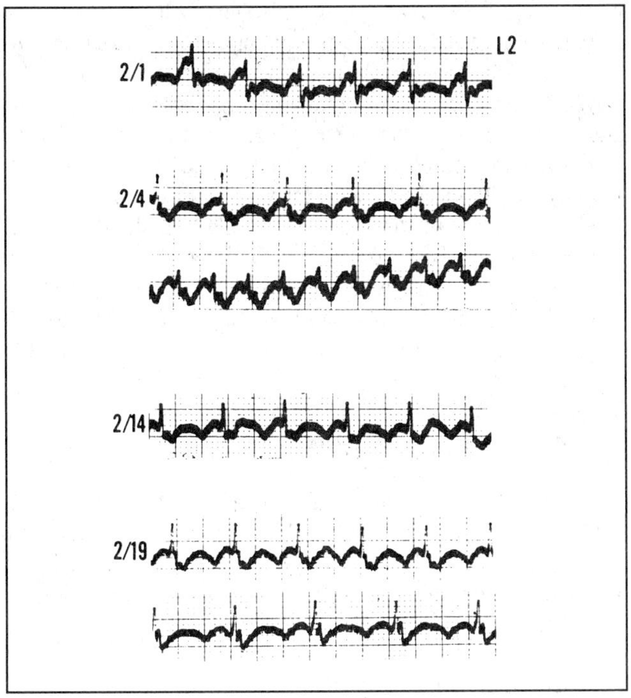

Fig. 9-13. Effect of quinidine and digitalis on the ventricular rate in atrial flutter over 19 days. After administration of quinidine and digitoxin, a 2 : 1 atrial flutter *(2/1)* converted to a 1 : 1 flutter *(2/4)* with prompt hemodynamic deterioration. Because of the 1 : 1 response after administration of quinidine, additional digitalis was administered over the next 15 days, followed by quinidine on 2/19. Despite a significant slowing of the atrial rate caused by quinidine, a 2 : 1 A-V conduction was maintained because of suppression of A-V nodal conduction by digitalis. (From Fisch C: Diagnosis and management of cardiac arrhythmias. Curr Probl Cardiol 1(12):1, 1977. Reproduced with permission.)

Disopyramide. Disopyramide is similar to quinidine and procainamide in its antiarrhythmic actions and efficacy. It cannot be used in patients with significant left ventricular dysfunction because of its more pronounced negative inotropic effect. Common side effects include dry mouth, constipation, and blurred vision because of the drug's anticholinergic action. The risk of urinary tract obstruction limits its use in middle-age and elderly men. As with the other class I drugs, disopyramide can occasionally precipitate or worsen ventricular arrhythmias. Unlike quinidine (but similar to procainamide), disopyramide does not significantly alter digitalis levels. Dosage of disopyramide is usually 100 to 200 mg about every 6 hours.

Lidocaine. Lidocaine, administered intravenously, is often the treatment of choice for acute ventricular arrhythmias. Lidocaine is generally not effective for treatment of supraventricular arrhythmias. Lidocaine is metabolized by the liver, and the dosage must be reduced in the patient with hepatic dysfunction or reduced hepatic blood flow, as may occur with cardiac failure or shock. Adverse effects include central nervous system symptoms such as confusion, delirium, lethargy, and seizures. These can usually be avoided by careful attention to dosage and blood levels of the drug. Lidocaine can also depress sinus node function. Several lidocaine loading regimens have been used, with attention to avoiding a drop in its blood level 20 minutes or longer after an initial bolus. For example, an initial bolus dose of 1 to 2 mg/kg body weight (20 to 50 mg/min) can be followed about 30 minutes later by a second bolus of 0.5 mg/kg. Throughout this period and thereafter, a continuous infusion of 1 to 4 mg/min is employed, with careful clinical monitoring and subsequent determination of blood levels of the drug.

Tocainide and *mexiletine* are orally administered drugs developed to exert antiarrhythmic actions similar to lidocaine. Their adverse effects include central nervous system symptoms and nausea. These effects may be reduced by administering the drugs with meals, which limits the rate of absorption and the peak blood level.

Flecainide and encainide. Flecainide and encainide are more recently developed antiarrhythmic agents. These drugs are effective in suppressing arrhythmias in many patients and perhaps less likely than other drugs to result in "nuisance" symptoms (e.g., gastrointestinal intolerance). However, they were shown in the CAST of nonsustained ventricular arrhythmias in survivors of myocardial infarction to result in enhanced mortality when compared with placebo treatment. In light of these data and the concern about proarrhythmia, the drugs should be limited to patients with life-threatening sustained ventricular arrhythmias who have not responded to other agents. Encainide has been withdrawn from the market. Flecainide also exerts negative inotropic effects and cannot be used in patients with significant left ventricular dysfunction.

Beta-adrenergic blocking drugs. The properties and actions of beta blockers, including their roles in patients with cardiac ischemia or hypertension, are described in detail elsewhere in this book. Their effects on cardiac arrhythmias stem from their action to block adrenergic stimulation of cardiac beta ($beta_1$) receptors. Several beta-adrenergic blocking drugs are available, including oral and IV preparations, and some differ in their relative specificity for the $beta_1$ receptor, their duration of action, and their side-effect profile—factors that can affect the selection of a specific drug in individual patients. They slow SA nodal discharge rate and thus can be effective in patients with a hyperdynamic sinus rate. They may also help in the control of other arrhythmias precipitated by emotional stress or physical exertion. They can prolong A-V node refractoriness, thus decreasing A-V conduction. Because of this, they can be effective against arrhythmias originating in or using the A-V junction as their site of origin or perpetuation (e.g., A-V nodal re-entrant tachycardia). They slow the ventricular response to atrial fibrillation and flutter.

It is established that some beta-adrenergic blocking drugs, (e.g., propranolol, timolol, metoprolol, atenolol) reduce mortality in survivors of acute myocardial infarction.

This effect has not been established for beta-adrenergic blocking drugs with intrinsic sympathomimetic activity (ISA). For other indications, beta blockers with ISA may offer an advantage if concern exists about a relatively slow resting heart rate. Adverse effects include excessive slowing of heart rate or A-V conduction and hypotension. The drugs exert negative inotropic effects that can precipitate or exacerbate congestive heart failure in patients with significantly impaired ventricular systolic function. Because of their effect on $beta_2$ receptors, the drugs can precipitate bronchospasm in patients with asthma or chronic obstructive lung disease. They have the potential to worsen claudication in patients with peripheral vascular disease. Beta-adrenergic blocking drugs may increase hypoglycemia risk in insulin-dependent diabetic patients and can adversely affect serum lipid levels. In patients with coronary heart disease the abrupt withdrawal of beta blockers can lead to exacerbation of cardiac ischemia and arrhythmias.

Amiodarone. Amiodarone can be effective in the control of several supraventricular arrhythmias, including those associated with the WPW syndrome, as well as ventricular arrhythmias. Its FDA approval, however, is restricted to life-threatening ventricular arrhythmias unresponsive to more conventional drugs. This stems from the numerous side effects, some of which (e.g., pulmonary dysfunction, pneumonitis) are dangerous. Other undesirable effects include gastrointestinal symptoms, disturbances of thyroid function, photosensitivity and skin discoloration, cerebellar dysfunction, and depression of ventricular function. Because many toxic effects are dose related, the smallest effective dose must be used. Periodic monitoring of various laboratory parameters is necessary.

Amiodarone can also lead to proarrhythmia and can interact with several other drugs, including digoxin, the dosage of which must be reduced. Administration must include consideration of the unusual pharmacokinetic properties of amiodarone, which binds extensively in body tissues and has a very long half-life. Considerable delay occurs before steady state is reached and the drug's full action becomes evident. Similarly, a prolonged period of elimination follows withdrawal of therapy. Because of these factors, amiodarone is reserved for patients with incapacitating or life-threatening arrhythmias who are unresponsive to conventional agents.

Verapamil and diltiazem. Verapamil and diltiazem block the calcium-dependent slow-channel transmembrane current. Because the action potentials of the SA and A-V nodal cells are influenced to a greater extent by this current, these cells are most affected by electrophysiologic actions of verapamil and diltiazem. IV verapamil is very effective in terminating A-V nodal re-entrant tachycardia that has not responded to vagal maneuvers or adenosine (see next discussion). The usual dose is 10 mg administered over 1 to 2 minutes while blood pressure and cardiac rhythm are monitored. If necessary, a second dose can be given 30 minutes later. Verapamil and diltiazem can also transiently reduce the ventricular response in patients with atrial flutter or fibrillation. IV verapamil can also terminate narrow-QRS A-V re-entrant tachycardia in patients with the WPW syndrome, since one limb of the re-entrant cycle typically traverses the A-V node. Verapamil may indirectly accelerate conduction over the bypass tract in patients with WPW syndrome and therefore should not be used in these patients if atrial fibrillation is present. IV verapamil is generally not effective against ventricular tachycardia and should not be given to patients with this or wide-QRS tachycardia because it can result in hemodynamic collapse. Oral verapamil or diltiazem may be effective in preventing recurrence of A-V nodal re-entrant tachycardia and controlling the ventricular rate in patients with atrial flutter or fibrillation (in the absence of a bypass tract).

Adverse effects of verapamil and diltiazem include A-V block, excessive sinus node suppression, and a negative inotropic effect in patients with underlying left ventricular dysfunction. The drugs should be avoided in patients who are hemodynamically unstable or at enhanced risk for these adverse effects. Verapamil can also reduce the excretion of digoxin.

Adenosine. Adenosine is an endogenous nucleoside (not included in the previously described classification system) used in the treatment of supraventricular arrhythmias. It initially slows sinus node discharge and depresses conduction in the A-V node, often with transient A-V block. Rapid IV injection (6 to 12 mg) results in termination of most cases of re-entrant A-V nodal tachycardia. It is better tolerated than verapamil in patients with impaired ventricular function or hypotension, and therefore some believe adenosine is the drug of choice for patients with re-entrant A-V nodal or A-V tachycardias. Side effects include flushing and chest pressure sensation, which is typically transient. Adenosine is competitively inhibited by methylxanthines; with therapeutic levels of theophylline, adenosine's effects may be blocked. Conversely, dipyridamole blocks the uptake of adenosine and can enhance its actions. In this situation, smaller doses of adenosine should be used.

Pacing. Permanent artificial pacemakers are most often used in patients with symptomatic bradycardia (Fig. 9-14), either intermittent or persistent, when the underlying cause of the bradycardia cannot be reversed. The bradycardia may be the result of A-V block (Fig. 9-15) or sinus node dysfunction, such as marked sinus bradycardia, SA block, or SA nodal arrest. In some patients the sinus dysfunction is a component of the bradycardia-tachycardia syndrome, in which case a pacemaker may be required because of the intrinsic bradycardia and to allow treatment of the tachycardia component with medications that have the potential to worsen the bradycardia component. The indications for permanent pacemaker placement in patients who have yet to experience but are thought to be at significant risk for symptoms (e.g., syncope, sudden death) are more controversial. Pacing is generally recommended for such patients with type II A-V block or acquired complete heart block. The use of temporary pacemakers in patients with acute myocardial infarction and selected conduction abnormali-

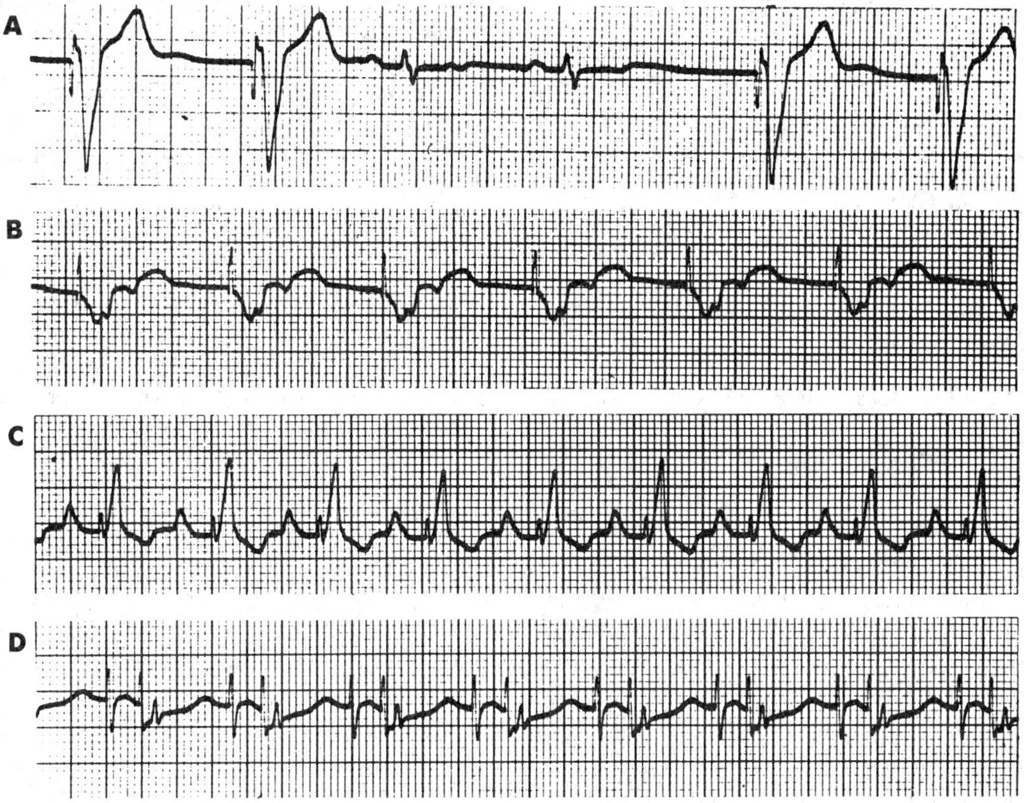

Fig. 9-14. **A,** Tracing from a single-chamber, ventricular-inhibited sensing pacemaker. **B,** Rhythm strip showing ventricular pacing with retrograde atrial conduction. **C,** Ventricular pacing in synchrony with sensed atrial activity. **D,** Tracing showing pacing of both atrial and ventricular chambers in synchrony.

ties is described in Chapter 14. Temporary pacemaker therapy is also required in some patients in the early postoperative period after cardiac surgery. It can also be effective in some patients with ventricular arrhythmias by means of overdrive suppression. Temporary pacing can help some patients in the control of ventricular arrhythmias associated with a long Q-T interval. Atrial pacing techniques can be used to terminate certain supraventricular arrhythmias, such as re-entrant A-V nodal tachycardia and atrial flutter. Atrial pacing is not effective in termination of atrial fibrillation.

A variety of permanent pacemakers is available. They are programmable (see Fig. 9-14), permitting subsequent adjustment of sensing and pacing functions, including the rate of pacing, in a noninvasive manner. The different pacemakers vary in their mode of action and their pacing sites, such as single or dual chamber. The latter is designed to preserve or enhance cardiac output by maintaining effective atrial contribution when possible. A similar goal underlies the rate-responsive ventricular pacemaker. Although single chamber in function, it is designed to increase the paced rate during physical activity.

A five-component classification scheme and code has been used for permanent pacemakers. The typically used first three components include, in order, the cardiac chamber paced, the chamber sensed by the pacemaker, and the pacemaker's response to a sensed beat (i.e., the pacemaker is inhibited or triggered by it). In this scheme, *V* and *A* denote ventricle and atrium, respectively. Dual *(D)* indicates both atrium and ventricle; *O* denotes none. *I* and *T* indicate inhibited or triggered, respectively. Thus a standard VVI pacemaker both senses in and paces the ventricle, and it is inhibited by a sensed impulse. A DDI pacemaker has the ability to sense and to pace either the atrium or ventricle or both.

Selection of the appropriate pacemaker requires consideration of the underlying rhythm/conduction abnormality and the patient's clinical characteristics, including age. Pacemakers depend on their power source, which must be replaced when signs of impending exhaustion become evident. Periodic surveillance is required to replace the power source before overt pacemaker failure. This may include ECG assessment (obtained telephonically or at the bedside) of the intrinsic pacing rate, which is designed to slow as the battery power declines. The rate of pacing during placement of a magnet over the pacemaker can also be determined. More sophisticated measurements of pacemaker function and power expenditure, requirements, and reserve can be performed at the bedside with the pacemaker programmer. Pacemakers can also malfunction and at times can precipitate arrhythmias. Because of the complexity of

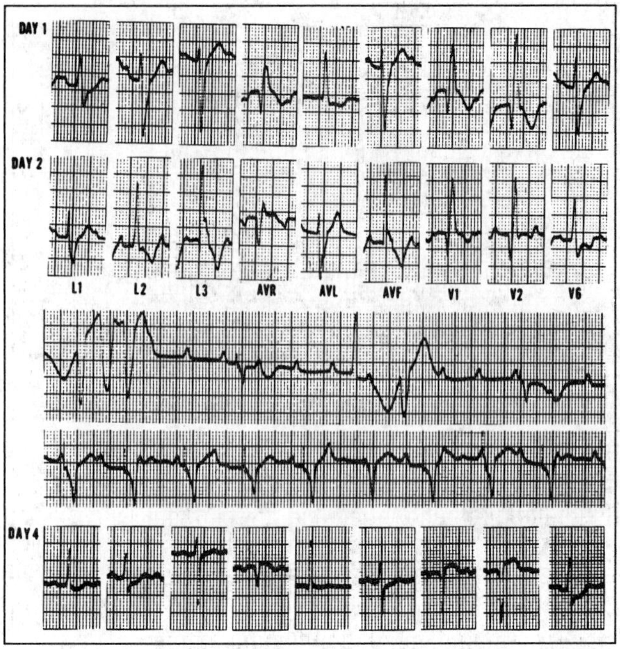

Fig. 9-15. Acute anterior mycardial infarction complicated by right bundle branch block (RBBB) and left anterior fascicular block *(day 1)* and by RBBB and left posterior fascicular block *(day 2)*. Complete A-V block followed *(third tracing)*. The patient was treated with a transvenous pacemaker *(fourth tracing)*. On day 4 the intraventricular conduction normalized. (From Fisch C: Diagnosis and management of cardiac arrhythmias. Curr Probl Cardiol 1(12):1, 1977. Reproduced with permission.)

modern permanent pacemaker therapy, selection of the type of pacemaker, its mode of action, follow-up surveillance, and recognition of malfunction are best left to those with expertise in this area.

In recent years, pacemakers with the capacity to recognize ventricular fibrillation and the ability to accomplish internal defibrillation have been developed. They have been used in certain high-risk patients, such as survivors of sudden cardiac death, and those whose advanced ventricular arrhythmias are refractory to conventional medical therapy. Pacemakers designed to detect and electrically cardiovert ventricular tachycardia have also been developed.

For details regarding the indications for and the selection of appropriate permanent pacemakers, the reader is referred to the guidelines compiled by a joint task force of the American College of Cardiology and the American Heart Association.

Ablation and surgical therapy. As indicated previously, some arrhythmias may be terminated or prevented or their effects mitigated through the use of catheter-delivered ablation therapy in the electrophysiology laboratory. In this treatment, energy (e.g., radiofrequency energy) is used to destroy small amounts of myocardium necessary for the genesis, perpetuation, or conduction of arrhythmias. A prominent example is the ablation of the accessory pathway in patients with WPW syndrome. The technique has also been used in selected patients with re-entrant A-V nodal tachycardia; in these patients, therapy can be complicated infrequently by the development of complete heart block. Other complications include injury to the coronary circulation and embolic events. In unusual cases of refractory atrial flutter or fibrillation in which the ventricular rate cannot be medically controlled, catheter ablation can be used to produce complete heart block intentionally; this carries the requirement for permanent pacemaker therapy.

Surgical techniques or cryoablation during cardiac surgery can also be used for selected supraventricular arrhythmias. Surgical therapy has also been employed in some patients with refractory life-threatening ventricular arrhythmias, usually those with advanced coronary heart disease and left ventricular dysfunction. The procedure may be combined, as indicated, with coronary revascularization and ventricular aneurysm resection.

SPECIFIC ARRHYTHMIAS

Accelerated rhythms

Sinus tachycardia. Sinus tachycardia (see Fig. 9-11, *B*) is nearly always a response to some stimulus rather than an independent rhythm disturbance. The stimulus is often physiologic, such as exercise or anxiety. In individuals with hyperkinetic circulatory states the heart rate response to stimuli is exaggerated in degree. Sinus tachycardia is an expected finding in patients with many cardiac disorders, such as heart failure and pericarditis, and in patients with extracardiac disorders, such as hypovolemia or hyperthyroidism. Sinus tachycardia is often asymptomatic but may result in palpitations. Moreover, it can precipitate angina pectoris in patients with underlying coronary artery disease.

The ECG features of sinus tachycardia include a heart rate greater than 100 but uncommonly above 180 beats/min, with P waves of normal morphology preceding each QRS complex. With very rapid rates, the P wave may be difficult to identify because of its superimposition on the preceding T wave. In the absence of an associated intraventricular conduction disturbance, the QRS complex is normal, measuring less than 0.10 second in duration. Sinus tachycardia typically shows some variability in rate over time, and the characteristic response to vagal maneuvers is a gradual slowing followed by a gradual resumption of the rate after termination of the maneuver. If the stimulus responsible for the sinus tachycardia is intense, the heart rate may be unaffected by vagal maneuvers.

The treatment of sinus tachycardia focuses on alleviation of the underlying cause, which should always be sought when unexplained or persistent sinus tachycardia is detected.

Atrial premature complexes. Atrial premature complexes (APCs) (see Fig. 9-8, *A*) arise from ectopic atrial foci. By definition, the impulse occurs before the next expected sinus discharge. Usually, APCs are conducted through the A-V node to activate the ventricles. However, very premature APCs may not reach the ventricles because the A-V node is still refractory from the preceding depolarization. APCs occur in normal individuals and in some may be exaggerated by caffeine, alcohol, and other stimulants. APCs may also be a manifestation of cardiac disease and at times are precursors of more advanced arrhythmias, including atrial fibrillation. APCs, although most often asymptomatic, may give rise to palpitations.

Frequent, multiform, "chaotic" APCs can occur in older persons and in patients with lung disease, and these may be mistaken for atrial fibrillation (see Fig. 9-8, *B*).

The ECG features of APCs include a premature P wave that differs from sinus P waves in morphology. Often the ectopic P wave occurs during the preceding T wave and alters its contour. Because the P wave is premature, its conduction through the A-V node may be depressed, producing a prolonged P-R interval. If sufficiently premature, the atrial impulse is blocked and fails to reach the ventricle. The pause that results from suppression of the SA node by an APC is characteristically less than the full compensatory pause associated with a premature ventricular complex. That is, the sinus P-P interval encompassing the APC is less than twice the P-P interval of the normal sinus rhythm. However, if the APC occurs early and fails to enter the SA node, or if the SA node is inordinately suppressed by the APC, the pause can be fortuitously near or fully compensatory. An APC may also activate the His-Purkinje system while it is still partly refractory, producing a wide QRS complex because of aberrant conduction.

APCs usually require no specific therapy. Rarely, patients with frequent and symptomatic APCs require treatment. This can be accomplished with digitalis, which may suppress the APCs or decrease the likelihood of conduction to the ventricle, or with beta-adrenergic blocking drugs. In patients with APCs caused by heart disease, the approach should always include treatment of the underlying disorder.

Paroxysmal supraventricular tachycardia. Paroxysmal supraventricular tachycardia (PSVT), previously termed *paroxysmal atrial tachycardia* or *paroxysmal junctional tachycardia,* (see Fig. 9-8, *C*) is frequently found in individuals without evidence of cardiac disease, including healthy young individuals. PSVT may also complicate the course of patients with valvular, myocardial, and coronary heart diseases.

PSVT is typically abrupt in onset and termination. It can be associated with a wide range of symptoms, which depend in part on the heart rate, the presence or absence of underlying heart disease, and the patient's age. Palpitations are the sole manifestation in some individuals, whereas lightheadedness, shortness of breath, and weakness occur in others. At times, the paroxysms are accompanied by polyuria. The pulse rate is usually regular at 180 to 220/min but may be irregular early after the onset of the arrhythmia. The jugular venous A wave may be prominent. This is noted when the atria and ventricles are depolarized at approximately the same time, resulting in atrial contraction against a closed tricuspid valve. The first heart sound is typically monotonous in quality.

Intracardiac electrophysiologic studies have confirmed that PSVT is actually a group of arrhythmias with different mechanisms. These include re-entry within the SA or A-V node or re-entry using both the A-V node and an accessory pathway. Most often, PSVT results from sustained re-entry within the A-V node. In this case, there appear to be functionally or anatomically distinct pathways for conduction within the A-V node, and they differ in refractory periods and conduction speeds. Thus an APC can block, for example, in the fast pathway and conduct to the ventricle via the slow pathway. This impulse may then conduct retrogradely over the fast pathway to the atrium and thereby begin a reciprocating tachycardia. The retrograde P wave is often not evident on the ECG because it typically occurs during the QRS complex. If P waves are evident during A-V nodal re-entrant tachycardia, they usually occur just after the QRS complex. The QRS complex during A-V nodal re-entrant tachycardia is normal in duration unless there is an associated intraventricular conduction defect or functional aberration.

The treatment of patients with PSVT caused by A-V node re-entry involves interventions that alter the critical relationship of conduction and refractoriness in the A-V node. The most frequently used measures interrupt the re-entry cycle by producing a further slowing of conduction. Carotid sinus pressure and the Valsalva maneuver accomplish this by increasing vagal tone. These maneuvers are useful from both diagnostic and therapeutic standpoints and are usually the first measures used. In patients with infrequent and only mildly symptomatic PSVT, they may be the only therapy required. Carotid sinus pressure can be dangerous in patients with carotid occlusive vascular disease; in its presence, this maneuver should not be used. The characteristic response of re-entrant PSVT to vagal stimulation is "all or none"; that is, the maneuver typically terminates the tachycardia or has no substantial effect on its rate. Although vagal stimulation may slow the tachycardia rate slightly, it does not induce transient block at the A-V node level. This result is understandable in light of the re-entrant nature of arrhythmia within the A-V node. If a block develops, the re-entry cycle is interrupted and the arrhythmia stops. When atrial tachycardia is associated with A-V block, the mechanism of the rapid rhythm most likely is not from A-V node re-entry but is presumed to be automatic (or re-entry within the atrium).

If simple vagal stimulation maneuvers do not terminate A-V nodal re-entrant tachycardia in a hemodynamically stable patient, the treatment of choice is IV adenosine or verapamil. If arrhythmia persists, a short-acting beta-adrenergic blocking drug or IV digitalis can be administered. Other forms of therapy include the anticholinesterase drug edrophonium, now largely supplanted by adenosine and verapamil.

If immediate termination of arrhythmia is required because of the patient's hemodynamic state, external synchronized electrical countershock should be employed. Often a low energy level (e.g., 25 to 50 joules) is successful. Atrial pacing can also be employed in selected patients to restore sinus rhythm. Capture of the atria by the paced premature impulse terminates the tachycardia by interrupting the re-entry pathway.

As indicated earlier, when deciding whether to prescribe chronic drug therapy to reduce the likelihood of recurrence of re-entrant A-V nodal tachycardia, one must consider the frequency and severity of the episodes. For some patients, avoidance of caffeine, alcohol, and other stimulants seems to reduce the likelihood of recurrence. If prophylactic drug treatment is required, digitalis is usually the drug of choice provided the WPW syndrome is not present (see next paragraphs). Digitalis may be preferred largely because it can be administered in a single daily dose. Alternative (or additional) therapy may include beta-adrenergic or calcium blocking drugs. Antiarrhythmic drugs, such as the class IA agents, can also be effective. For patients with refractory symptomatic A-V nodal re-entrant tachycardia despite medical therapy, surgical and catheter techniques are available.

PSVT in patients with WPW syndrome (tachyarrhythmias resulting from ventricular pre-excitation) requires special consideration. Ventricular pre-excitation refers to activation of a portion of the ventricle via A-V connections that bypass the usual decremental conduction of the A-V node. The most common accessory pathway, which is composed of myocardial fibers, is termed *Kent's bundle*. In patients with ventricular pre-excitation, the typical QRS complex during sinus rhythm represents a fusion between the premature ventricular activation and that occurring via the A-V node. The resultant P-R interval is short (<120 ms) and the QRS complex in some leads demonstrates a delta wave (slurred upstroke). The QRS complex is prolonged (>120 ms), and secondary ST-T wave changes occur.

Patients with WPW syndrome can experience PSVT because of re-entry that involves both the A-V node and an accessory pathway (A-V re-entrant tachycardia). Although the accessory pathway generally conducts more rapidly than the A-V node, its refractory period is longer. Thus an APC may block in the accessory pathway and conduct to the ventricle via the A-V node. If the accessory pathway cells have then regained their excitability, the impulse can retrogradely activate the atrium and initiate reciprocating tachycardia. Since the re-entrant pathway typically is antegrade through the A-V node and retrograde over the accessory pathway, the QRS complex during tachycardia is usually narrow and normal in appearance; this is also termed *orthodromic conduction*. Less often the tachycardia can travel antegrade over the accessory pathway, in which case the QRS is wide. Interestingly, in some patients with an accessory pathway the impulse is capable only of retrograde conduction. In these patients the QRS morphology is normal during sinus rhythm as well as during tachycardia.

The presence of WPW syndrome alters the medical approach to PSVT. If the QRS during tachycardia is narrow (orthodromic tachycardia), the initial approach is similar to A-V nodal re-entrant tachycardia (e.g., vagal maneuvers, IV adenosine or verapamil). If additional therapy is required, a drug that prolongs the refractory period of the accessory pathway (e.g., procainamide) can be used, or electric cardioversion employed, based on the clinical situation. Digitalis can shorten the accessory pathway refractory period and has been reported to speed conduction over it, leading to life-threatening rapid ventricular rates if atrial fibrillation develops. Thus digitalis should generally not be given to WPW patients and certainly not in the absence of concomitant treatment with a drug that slows conduction over the accessory pathway. Although atrial fibrillation and flutter are considered later in this chapter, it is necessary to include here some special considerations about them in patients with WPW syndrome. Atrial fibrillation and flutter can be particularly dangerous in WPW patients because of very rapid ventricular rates that can result from conduction over the accessory pathway, which does not exhibit the decremental conduction of the A-V node. In this case the resultant QRS is wide and very fast. Prompt electric cardioversion is often required. Drug therapy may require a combination of agents that acts to slow conduction over both the accessory pathway (e.g., procainamide) and the A-V node (e.g., beta-adrenergic blocking agent). As noted previously, IV verapamil should not be administered to patients with wide-QRS tachycardias.

Establishment of an effective oral regimen to prevent PSVT in patients with WPW syndrome can be complex and difficult. It generally involves drugs (e.g., class IA or IC agents) that slow the accessory pathway conduction, at times in conjunction with agents (e.g., beta-adrenergic blocking drugs) that affect the A-V node. For symptomatic WPW patients with recurrent arrhythmias, ablative therapy has been employed increasingly and earlier. This is because of the complexity of treatment that may otherwise be required and the potential side effects of the antiarrhythmic drugs, particularly since the patients are often young and face long-term treatment.

Atrial tachycardia with block. Unlike re-entrant A-V nodal tachycardia, atrial tachycardia (AT) with block (see Fig. 9-8, *D*) rarely occurs in patients without significant cardiac disease or digitalis intoxication. The physical findings during the AT depend on the atrial rate and on the degree of the associated A-V block. Regularly occurring atrial A waves may be detected in the jugular venous pulse, and their amplitude depends on their relation to the ventricular contraction. Variable A-V block results also in an irregular pulse and changing intensity of the first heart sound.

The atrial rate is usually 150 to 200/min, with P waves that differ in contour from those of sinus origin; however, the difference may be quite subtle. The ventricular rate depends on the degree of associated A-V block, which is typically 2:1, occasionally greater, and at times variable. Wenckebach periodicity is often present. Vagal maneuvers typically reduce the ventricular rate by increasing the degree of A-V block, but unlike with re-entrant A-V nodal tachycardia, they do not terminate the arrhythmia. These maneuvers should not be performed when digitalis excess is a potential cause of the AT because the maneuver may occasionally initiate a ventricular arrhythmia or result in excessive A-V block.

The treatment of AT with block depends both on the resultant hemodynamic effects and on the cause of the arrhythmia. When caused by digitalis excess, the approach is to discontinue the drug and to maintain a normal serum potassium level. Because the ventricular rate in such patients is often not excessive, this may be all that is necessary. If additional treatment is required, a beta-adrenergic blocking drug or phenytoin may be tried. When not caused by digitalis intoxication, AT with block can be treated with digitalis or a beta blocker (if no other contraindication exists) to slow the ventricular rate while measures are undertaken to treat the underlying cardiac disease. If AT with block persists, other antiarrhythmic agents (e.g., class IA drugs) may be effective.

Atrial flutter. Atrial flutter (see Figs. 9-8, *E*, and 9-13) occurs in patients with a variety of cardiac and some extracardiac disorders. It is found only rarely in normal individuals. Common causes include ischemic heart disease, particularly acute myocardial infarction; valvular heart disease; and chronic or acute pulmonary disease, including acute pulmonary embolus.

The degree to which atrial flutter contributes to symptoms and findings of cardiac failure, lightheadedness, or angina pectoris depends both on the ventricular heart rate and on the severity of the underlying cardiac disease. Similarly, the prognosis depends in large part on the precipitating and underlying causes of the arrhythmia. Atrial flutter typically is an unstable rhythm, usually converting either to atrial fibrillation or to sinus rhythm. Chronic atrial flutter, although infrequent, does occur. The risk of systemic embolization during atrial flutter is less than that during atrial fibrillation, presumably because of the flutter's organized atrial activity.

During atrial flutter the atrial rate is usually about 300/min. The A-V node is unable to conduct at such rapid rates. Usually, every other flutter wave is conducted to the ventricles, resulting in a pulse rate of approximately 150/min. In fact, atrial flutter should always be considered in patients who have a regular pulse rate of 150/min. Occasionally, rapid and regular "flutter waves" can be observed in the jugular venous pulse.

The ECG features include regular saw-tooth-like flutter waves most prominent in leads II, III, aVF, and V_1. Although the flutter waves typically occur at a frequency of about 300/min, the rate may range from 250 to 350/min. In untreated patients the QRS complexes characteristically occur at a rate one-half that of the atria. Slower ventricular rates may be observed, particularly if coexistent A-V nodal disease is present or if the patient has been treated with drugs such as digitalis or verapamil, which slow conduction through the A-V node. In these patients the usual 2:1 A-V conduction may be decreased to 4:1 or less. Less often, varying A-V block results in an irregular ventricular response. At times the characteristic saw-tooth ECG pattern of atrial flutter is difficult to discern. Vagal maneuvers or IV verapamil can aid in diagnosis by abruptly decreasing the ventricular response, thereby exposing the flutter waves (see Fig. 9-8, *E*).

Various therapeutic approaches are available for management of atrial flutter. The choice and timing of specific therapy is based on two factors: (1) the degree of hemodynamic compromise caused by the rapid heart rate and (2) the nature and reversibility of the cause of the arrhythmia. For patients whose hemodynamic status is compromised, direct current (DC) cardioversion is the treatment of choice. Usually, a low level of energy, such as 20 to 50 joules, is successful in converting atrial flutter to sinus rhythm or, less frequently, to atrial fibrillation. In the latter case, cardioversion with higher energy levels can be employed in an attempt to restore sinus rhythm, or digitalis can be given to control the ventricular rate; the choice depends on the clinical situation. Considering the success of electrical cardioversion of sustained atrial flutter and the difficulty that can occur with the medical control of ventricular rate, cardioversion is often chosen as the initial treatment even for patients who are only mildly or moderately compromised by the arrhythmia. This approach presumes, however, that additional measures to prevent a prompt recurrence of the flutter are likely to be successful. This presumption often requires effective treatment of the underlying cause. Rapid atrial pacing can also be used to restore sinus rhythm or induce atrial fibrillation. Because this procedure uses very low-level energy, it may be particularly advantageous in the occasional patient for whom conventional DC cardioversion might carry enhanced risks, such as in the patient who has received large amounts of digitalis.

For patients in whom electrical cardioversion is not chosen as initial therapy, an IV infusion of a calcium channel blocker or beta blocker (e.g., the ultra-short-acting esmolol) may slow the ventricular rate. Digitalis also can be administered to slow the ventricular rate. Unfortunately, control of the ventricular response to atrial flutter with digitalis is not as effective or predictable as in patients with atrial fibrillation. At times, manifestations of digitalis intoxication become evident before the rate of ventricular response to atrial flutter is reduced. Moreover, administration of large doses of digitalis may render the subsequent use of DC cardioversion dangerous. If the ventricular response to atrial flutter does not respond to "adequate" amounts of digitalis, and if no contraindications exist to the use of beta-adrenergic blocking drugs, the latter can be added to the regimen. Although the beta blocker acts to reduce the conduction of atrial impulses to the ventricle, it does not appear to affect the underlying atrial arrhythmia.

In patients who fail to respond to the preceding measures or who have recurrences of flutter, other antiarrhythmic drugs (e.g., class IA or IC agents) may act to restore or maintain sinus rhythm. Because some of these agents exert a vagolytic effect as well as slow the flutter rate, their administration may result in 1:1 A-V conduction with rapid hemodynamic deterioration. Therefore such drugs should not be administered until the patient has received sufficient amounts of digitalis (or beta blocker or calcium channel blocker) to delay A-V conduction and thus prevent 1:1 ventricular response (see Fig. 9-13). Consideration of these type I drugs must be accompanied by concern about their potential for proarrhythmia and other side effects, as outlined previously. They should not be selected for long-term use unless their benefits are thought to outweigh these risks in the individual patient.

Atrial fibrillation. Atrial fibrillation (see Figs. 9-7; 9-8, *F;* 9-9, *D;* and 9-10, *D*) can complicate the course of patients with a variety of heart and systemic diseases and occasionally occurs in individuals without clinically evident heart disease. Hypertensive cardiovascular disease, ischemic heart disease, and mitral valve disease are disorders frequently associated with atrial fibrillation. Presumably, an important underlying mechanism in these conditions is elevation of left atrial pressure. Atrial injury, such as can occur with pericarditis or heart trauma, can result in atrial fibrillation, as can the metabolic insult of excessive alcohol or thyroid hormone stimulation. Atrial septal defect is often complicated by supraventricular arrhythmias, including atrial flutter and fibrillation.

Regardless of the etiology, atrial fibrillation results in loss of effective atrial contraction and a rapid, irregular ventricular response. Atrial fibrillation carries the additional risk of systemic embolization. The risk of embolization during atrial fibrillation is most pronounced when associated with mitral stenosis and an enlarged left atrium.

Atrial fibrillation may be paroxysmal or chronic. Its onset is often recognized because of irregular, rapid palpitations. The occurrence of other manifestations, including symptoms of cardiac failure and angina pectoris, depends on the rate of the ventricular response and the severity of the underlying cardiac disease. The hemodynamic consequences of atrial fibrillation are most profound with coexistent mitral stenosis or a noncompliant left ventricle, such as accompanies left ventricular hypertrophy caused by hypertension, aortic stenosis, or hypertrophic cardiomyopathy. In these conditions the atrial contribution to ventricular filling and cardiac output is most important, and its loss with onset of atrial fibrillation is most likely to compromise the patient's hemodynamic status.

Atrial fibrillation is diagnosed at the bedside by the "irregularly irregular" pulse rate, a pulse deficit, and a varying arterial pulse amplitude. These physical findings are caused by varying diastolic filling periods with resultant differing stroke volumes. The stroke volume during the more rapid beats may be insufficient to generate a palpable pulse. Similarly, the first heart sound typically varies in intensity, being louder after a shorter cycle length. The jugular pulse contour occasionally exhibits irregular fibrillatory undulations. Frequently the jugular venous findings are confined to loss of the A wave resulting from the absence of organized atrial activity.

The ECG features of atrial fibrillation include the absence of P waves, which are replaced by irregular fibrillatory waves at rates varying from 350 to 500/min. The fibrillatory waves may be coarse or fine; thus the designation of *coarse* or *fine* atrial fibrillation. The distribution of QRS complexes appears random. The ventricular rate in untreated patients without concomitant A-V nodal disease as a rule varies from 150 to 200/min. In the absence of an intraventricular conduction defect, the QRS complexes are normal in duration and contour. It is important to recognize, however, that aberrant conduction frequently occurs in patients with atrial fibrillation because of Ashman's phenomenon. This form of aberrant intraventricular conduction occurs when a relatively long R-R interval is followed by a relatively short R-R interval. It results from the direct relationship of the refractory period of the intraventricular conduction system, especially of the right bundle, with the length of the preceding R-R cycle. The aberrant complex that follows the short cycle typically has a right bundle branch configuration. Moreover, the aberrant conduction can at times be perpetuated for several cycles, simulating VT. Occasionally it may not be possible definitely to distinguish perpetuation of aberration from VT. Although aberration from Ashman's phenomenon can occur with any supraventricular arrhythmia, it is most frequently encountered during atrial fibrillation because of the irregular cycle lengths.

As with the other supraventricular arrhythmias, atrial fibrillation of recent onset that seriously compromises the patient's hemodynamic status should be terminated promptly with DC cardioversion; higher energy levels are usually required for atrial fibrillation than for atrial flutter. For most patients, however, the initial treatment of atrial fibrillation focuses on control of the ventricular heart rate (e.g., with digitalis) while efforts are undertaken to identify and remove the precipitating cause of the arrhythmia. The apical heart rate is used as a guide to the digitalis therapy. Digitalis blood levels do not permit precise identification of the optimum dose for control of the ventricular response and can be misleading in some patients. The goal of digitalis therapy usually is to reduce the resting apical heart rate to about 70 to 80 beats/min and, importantly, to ensure that the rate does not rise excessively (i.e., >110/min) with mild exertion (see Fig. 9-7). It must be emphasized, however, that the expectation for control of heart rate must be tempered by the patient's overall clinical condition. In patients with thyrotoxicosis, myocarditis, severe heart failure, infection, pulmonary embolus, lung disease, or other conditions that evoke physiologic increases in heart rate, it may not be possible or desirable to lower the ventricular rate 70 to 80/min. Attempting to do so with large amounts of digitalis may evoke toxicity.

Because additional or alternative drugs to slow the ventricular rate are available, it is not necessary to "push" digitalis to near toxic doses. Beta-adrenergic or calcium blocking drugs can be cautiously added or used in place of digitalis. In some patients, usually elderly ones, the ventricular response to atrial fibrillation is intrinsically slow because of concomitant A-V node disease. In such patients, treatment may not be necessary.

An additional goal in the treatment of many patients with atrial fibrillation is restoration of effective atrial contraction through conversion to sinus rhythm. However, the decision to employ drugs or electric shock to meet this goal must include a careful assessment of the likelihood that sinus rhythm will be maintained. This likelihood in turn depends on several factors, including the duration of the atrial fibrillation, the size of the left atrium, and the underlying cardiac disease. Evidence suggests that less than half of patients successfully cardioverted remain in sinus rhythm at the end of 1 year. The probability of success is greatest when the atrial fibrillation is of brief duration, perhaps less than 12 months, and when the left atrium (estimated by echocardiography) is not greatly enlarged. Cardioversion can be attempted with usual doses of quinidine, after the ventricular rate has been controlled with digitalis. In most patients, however, the method of choice for cardioversion is external electric shock.

Quinidine is often administered before the elective DC cardioversion of atrial fibrillation in hopes of enhancing the likelihood of restoring and maintaining sinus rhythm. In fact, the quinidine may restore sinus rhythm in approximately 10% of patients, obviating the need for the planned electrical cardioversion. Cardioversion should be avoided in patients with digitalis intoxication because of the risk of ventricular fibrillation. Class 1A drugs (e.g., quinidine) may help maintain sinus rhythm but carry the risk of proarrhythmia and other side effects. As indicated previously, concern has been raised about these risks on long-term outcome. Amiodarone, which also carries proarrhythmia potential as well as other important possible side effects, can be helpful in selected patients.

The emergence of a regular heart rate during treatment of chronic atrial fibrillation with digitalis rarely indicates restoration of sinus rhythm. Regularization of the heart rate should raise the suspicion of high-degree heart block when the rate is slow or of junctional or ventricular tachycardia when the rate is rapid. Recognition of these arrhythmias is critical because they usually indicate severe digitalis intoxication.

As indicated previously, atrial fibrillation carries the risk of systemic embolization. Because of this, anticoagulation has traditionally been used in selected patients with chronic atrial fibrillation, particularly those with associated mitral stenosis, prior embolic episode, or a mechanical valve prosthesis. Although the guidelines for anticoagulant therapy and the optimum regimen are still evolving, recent studies have emphasized the embolic risk in patients with atrial fibrillation and nonvalvular heart disease, as well as the value of anticoagulant therapy in decreasing this risk. Aspirin appears to confer some protection in patients less than 75 years of age. Most physicians, however, subscribe to data indicating the superiority of warfarin in preventing cerebrovascular accident (stroke). The decision to use warfarin must also take into account the patient's age, clinical situation, and risk of bleeding. In individuals at high risk for trauma, falls, or bleeding, warfarin is not used prophylactically. It is also generally recommended that patients with atrial fibrillation receive warfarin for 2 to 3 weeks (if no contraindication exists) before elective cardioversion and for several weeks after restoration of sinus rhythm.

Nonparoxysmal junctional tachycardia. The intrinsic rate of spontaneous discharge of A-V junctional tissue in a normal individual is 40 to 60 beats/min. When the sinus rate falls below this level, the junctional tissue becomes the dominant pacemaker, activating the ventricles as an "escape" rhythm. By contrast, several pathologic states can lead to accelerated junctional rhythms, with rates in excess of the physiologic escape rate. An example is nonparoxysmal junctional tachycardia (NPJT), in which the rate usually ranges from 70 to 130/min (see Fig. 9-9, *C* and *D*). The mechanism of NPJT is presumed to be enhanced automaticity of junctional tissue. It occurs as a manifestation of digitalis intoxication, after open heart surgery, during acute myocardial infarction, and in myocarditis. Infrequently, NPJT is present in individuals without overt cardiac disease.

The ECG recognition of NPJT is most straightforward when identifiable independent atrial rhythm and normal intraventricular conduction exist (see Fig. 9-9, *C* and *D*). If atrial depolarization results from retrograde conduction from the junctional focus, as illustrated by the junctional tachycardia in Fig. 9-9, *B*, the resultant P waves are negative in leads II, III, and aVF. Antegrade conduction from the junction to the ventricles may be irregular because of second-degree, often type I, antegrade A-V block.

Because the rate of NPJT is not excessive, it may not impair ventricular function except for the loss of effective atrial contraction. Specific antiarrhythmic therapy is usually not required. The treatment focuses on the underlying cause. This focus is particularly important when the cause is digitalis intoxication, since NPJT denotes a severe degree of drug poisoning. If suppression of NPJT is necessary, potassium, lidocaine, phenytoin, or a beta blocker may be tried. If digitalis is not responsible, the treatment of the underlying cause coupled with careful patient monitoring may suffice. In a patient who has not taken digitalis, control of the arrhythmia may be achieved by cautious administration of the glycoside.

Premature ventricular complexes. PVCs (see Fig. 9-10, *A*, *B*, and *D*) can occur in normal individuals, and their frequency may increase with advancing age, emotional stress, and excessive use of alcohol, tobacco, or caffeine. The prevalence and frequency of PVCs increase with underlying cardiac disease. Toxicity from a variety of drugs, such as digitalis glycosides, theophylline compounds, and sympathomimetic drugs, may also be manifested by PVCs. Marked bradycardia can be associated with PVCs as well.

Patients vary greatly in their sensitivity to PVCs. Some with frequent PVCs are asymptomatic; others are incapacitated by palpitations from similar degrees of arrhythmia. If the PVCs are very premature and frequent, as with ventricular bigeminy, in which every sinus beat is followed by a PVC, the arrhythmia may result in reduction of the cardiac output and consequent fatigue.

In addition to prematurity of the pulse and subsequent compensatory pause, the physical findings associated with PVCs depend on the temporal relationship of the atrial and ventricular contractions. If both occur simultaneously, large, jugular cannon A waves are produced. The simultaneous atrial and ventricular contractions responsible for the cannon A waves may be a result either of fortuitous timing of independent atrial and ventricular contractions or of retrograde activation of the atria by the ventricular impulse.

Because PVCs arise below the bundle of His, the ventricle's activation is anomalous and results in a bizarre, prolonged QRS complex. The T wave is usually opposite in polarity to the QRS complex. By definition, the PVC occurs before the next expected sinus beat. Although the ventricular impulse may not fully traverse the A-V node in the retrograde direction, it typically blocks the conduction of the subsequent sinus P wave. A full compensatory pause follows. A full compensatory pause is thus present when the R-R interval encompassing the PVC is twice the length of the basic R-R interval (see Fig. 9-10, *A*). A less-than-compensatory (noncompensatory) pause may result when the PVC reaches and depolarizes the atrium, "resetting" the SA node in a manner analogous to an APC. When a PVC occurs during slow sinus rates, the A-V node may have time to recover after the PVC, allowing activation of the ventricles by the next sinus impulse. No compensatory pause occurs, and the PVC is termed an *interpolated* PVC. The fortuitous appearance of a PVC just after an antegrade atrial impulse reaches the ventricle results in ventricular activation by both the PVC and the supraventricular impulse. This interrelationship results in a *fusion complex,* with QRS morphology intermediate between that of the normal sinus impulse and that of the PVC (see Fig. 9-10, *A* and *B*). Fusion complexes are diagnostic of arrhythmias originating in the ventricles. PVCs may be classified by several ECG criteria, including their relationship to the dominant rhythm (e.g., bigeminy, trigeminy, quadrigeminy), and by their morphology (i.e., uniform or multiform). The decision to employ antiarrhythmic therapy for patients with PVC is usually based on associated symptoms.

Ventricular tachycardia. VT (see Fig. 9-10) is defined as three or more consecutive complexes originating below the bifurcation of the bundle of His at a rate greater than 100/min. Generally the rate of VT is 150 to 180/min and the rhythm regular. However, the rates may be faster or slower and the rhythm irregular. VT can also be classified as sustained or nonsustained in duration. Atrial activity and ventricular activity are most often independent during VT, resulting in A-V dissociation. Occasionally the atria are depolarized in a retrograde direction by the ventricle. Ventricular rhythm at a rate less than 100/min but greater than the normal passive ventricular escape rate of 20 to 40/min is termed *accelerated idioventricular rhythm* (see Fig. 9-10, *B*).

VT may complicate most forms of heart disease and, as with PVC, may result from drug toxicity, hypoxia, and electrolyte imbalance. Although occurring infrequently in the normal individual, VT occasionally occurs in the absence of detectable cardiovascular disease or other precipitating factors.

The presence and severity of symptoms depend on rate and duration of the tachycardia and on severity of the underlying heart disease. The stroke volume may be reduced because of the very rapid rates, the loss of effective atrial contraction, and the ventricles' asynchronous contraction. The resultant reduction of cerebral perfusion can lead to lightheadedness and syncope. VT may exacerbate heart failure and precipitate angina pectoris in patients with coronary artery disease. When VT is associated with A-V dissociation, cannon A waves can be detected in the jugular venous pulse. With 1:1 retrograde conduction to the atria, each ventricular contraction may be accompanied by a jugular A wave.

The ECG diagnosis of VT is usually based on wide, bizarre QRS complexes; A-V dissociation; and the previously described fusion complexes. Furthermore, a P wave occurring when the A-V node and ventricle are not refractory may activate or "capture" the ventricle, thereby interrupting the course of VT. In this circumstance the normal QRS morphology of the "capture" complex after a cycle length shorter than that of the tachycardia proves that the wide QRS complexes are ventricular in origin and not supraventricular with aberrant intraventricular conduction (see Fig. 9-10, *A*).

Despite these useful criteria, the diagnosis of VT and its differentiation from supraventricular tachycardia with aberration is often difficult and occasionally impossible. This is particularly true when atrial activity cannot be identified during wide-QRS tachycardia. The pattern of the wide QRS on the scalar ECG can at times suggest that its origin is ventricular or supraventricular with aberrancy (see the box below). In selected patients, intracardiac electrocardiography is required to determine the tachycardia's origin (see *A* in Fig. 9-5).

The acute treatment of patients with VT depends on the clinical situation. If VT results in hemodynamic compromise, electrical cardioversion is the treatment of choice, unless digitalis intoxication is present. If the VT is satisfactorily tolerated, IV lidocaine can be administered. If this is not effective, IV procainamide can be tried. The decision to employ chronic antiarrhythmic therapy for recurrent VT usually includes a consideration of the presence or absence of symptoms and underlying heart disease. The VT's rate and duration may also influence the decision. Class I drugs are usually used, but other drugs (described previously) or combinations of drugs may be required. Enthusiasm for antiarrhythmic therapy must be tempered by the risks (some-

ECG features that can support ventricular tachycardia as rhythm underlying wide-QRS tachycardia

Fusion beats
"Capture" beats
A-V dissociation

Marked left axis
QRS complex of 0.14 second or longer
If right bundle branch block morphology: monophasic R, biphasic qR, QR, or RS complex in lead V_1
If left bundle branch block morphology: R wave in V_1 greater than 30 ms or onset of R wave to nadir of S wave ≥70 msec; any Q wave in V_5 or V_6
Similar QRS appearance across precordium (concordance)

times including life-threatening proarrhythmia) and limited effectiveness of the drugs and the lack of proof that they reduce the risk of progression to sudden death (besides beta blockers in postinfarction patients). In selected patients the treatment of recurrent life-threatening VT may require surgical or ablative therapy.

The morphology of the QRS complexes may vary during VT. An interesting and clinically important example is the polymorphic VT, in which the QRS complexes change direction, appearing to twist about the isoelectric line (see Fig. 9-10, *C*). This type of arrhythmia occurs most often in association with a prolonged Q-T interval, in which case it is termed *torsades de pointes*. This form of ventricular arrhythmia may be congenital in origin or may result from administration of drugs that prolong the Q-T interval. The treatment may include temporary pacing to increase the underlying heart rate and thereby shorten the Q-T interval. When torsade results from drugs, immediate discontinuation of the offending agent is obviously important. IV magnesium has been reported to be beneficial.

More rare examples of VT include *bidirectional* VT (see Fig. 9-10, *E*), characterized by shifting of the QRS axis in the frontal plane, and *multifocal* VT (see Fig. 9-10, *D*), most often the result of digitalis intoxication.

The approach and treatment of the patient with ventricular fibrillation, including electric defibrillation and cardiopulmonary resuscitation, is described elsewhere in this text.

Accelerated idioventricular rhythm. Accelerated idioventricular rhythm (AIVR) (see Fig. 9-10, *B*) occurs most often in patients with acute myocardial infarction. Occasionally, AIVR may be associated with other cardiac disorders or may result from digitalis intoxication. Because the rates of AIVR, usually 70 to 100/min, are in the range of sinus rhythm, the two rhythms typically alternate in their control of the heart, with the short runs of AIVR frequently beginning and ending with fusion beats. Because the rate of AIVR is not excessive, it is usually well tolerated by patients unless the loss of the atrial contribution to cardiac output proves to be critical.

AIVR is often a benign, short-lived arrhythmia and may not require specific antiarrhythmic therapy. Careful observation of the patient is required. AIVR can occasionally represent underlying VT with a 2:1 exit block from the ventricular focus. Sudden disappearance of the exit block can lead to rapid VT and clinical decompensation. Treatment of AIVR is indicated when the loss of atrial contraction contributes to cardiac failure. Antiarrhythmic therapy may also be considered when more rapid ventricular arrhythmias accompany AIVR. If treatment is required, lidocaine is usually the antiarrhythmic drug of choice. By accelerating the sinus rate, atropine can suppress AIVR but, by increasing the heart rate, may also contribute to myocardial ischemia.

Bradycardias

Sinus bradycardia. Sinus bradycardia (see Fig. 9-11, *C*), defined as a sinus rate of less than 60/min, can result from physiologic influences or intrinsic disease of the SA node. Sinus bradycardia is a common finding in young and well-conditioned individuals. It may be exaggerated during sleep, when heart rates of 40/min or slower are not rare. It may be associated with intracranial hemorrhage, carotid stimulation, inferior myocardial infarction, hypothyroidism, and drugs such as beta-adrenergic blocking agents, clonidine, verapamil, and infrequently, digitalis.

The ECG recorded during sinus bradycardia displays P waves of normal morphology at a rate less than 60/min. Although the rhythm is often regular, sinus bradycardia frequently is associated with sinus arrhythmia. Sinus arrhythmia can be respiratory, in which case the changes in sinus discharge rate are coincident with vagal tone alterations caused by respiration, or can be independent of respiration. The former is usually a physiologic response; the latter is most often an abnormal finding.

In most individuals, sinus bradycardia produces no symptoms, does not adversely affect prognosis, and requires no therapy. In fact, sinus bradycardia is often beneficial because of the attendant reduction in cardiac work and oxygen demand. Excessive bradycardia should prompt a careful review of the patient's medications and general medical condition to identify a possible extracardiac contribution to the slow heart rate. If the sinus bradycardia leads to symptoms or findings requiring prompt therapy, atropine is the drug of choice. In patients with persistent symptomatic sinus bradycardia, transvenous pacing may be indicated.

Sinus arrest and sinoatrial exit block. Sinus arrest (see Fig. 9-11, *D*) is manifested by an unexpected and abrupt cessation of atrial electrical activity because of arrest of the spontaneous depolarization of the SA nodal pacemaker cells. A sudden pause in atrial activity may be a manifestation also of SA exit block (see Fig. 9-11, *E*), during which normal SA nodal depolarization continues, but the electrical activity generated by the SA node fails to activate the atria. In either case the presence and severity of associated symptoms depend on the pause's duration. Often the pause is terminated by a junctional escape complex (see Fig. 9-11, *D*) or rhythm at a rate of 40 to 60/min, and no serious symptoms result. In the absence of an appropriate escape rhythm, prolonged sinus arrest may lead to lightheadedness and syncope.

Electrocardiographically, sinus arrest is characterized by unexpected absence of P waves. When vagal influences contribute to sinus arrest, the SA rate may gradually slow before the prolonged pause. If the mechanism of the sudden pause is SA exit block, the pause's duration is typically a multiple of the basic P-P interval. However, the degree of the exit block can vary and rarely may exhibit Wenckebach periodicity. The latter makes the distinction of SA exit block from sinus arrest difficult if not impossible. If symptomatic sinus pauses persist despite attempts to remove the underlying cause, permanent transvenous pacing may be required.

Tachycardia-bradycardia syndrome. Abnormalities of SA node function, including inappropriate sinus bradycardia,

SA block, or sinus arrest, are occasionally accompanied by intermittent ectopic supraventricular tachycardias (see Fig. 9-11, *F*). In this case the bouts of tachycardia characteristically result in exaggerated suppression of the sinus node. Consequently the tachycardia is followed by longer than expected pauses before the resumption of atrial or junctional activity. Some patients have an associated intraventricular conduction defect. Taken together, these findings suggest that the tachycardia-bradycardia syndrome can indicate diffuse involvement of the specialized cardiac conduction system.

The management of patients with the tachycardia-bradycardia syndrome depends on the specific manifestations and the symptoms' severity. For many symptomatic patients the treatment includes permanent pacing to control excessive bradycardia and digitalis to control the supraventricular tachycardia.

Atrioventricular nodal (junctional) rhythm. A-V nodal rhythm (see Fig. 9-9, *E*) is generally a passive rhythm assuming control of the ventricle in the presence of marked sinus bradycardia, sinus or atrial standstill, or A-V block at the A-V nodal level. The A-V nodal rhythm is typically regular, and the rate is usually about 40 to 60/min. In the absence of pre-existing abnormal intraventricular conduction, the QRS complexes are normal in duration. The atria may be activated in a retrograde direction.

Atrioventricular conduction disturbances. Abnormalities of A-V conduction are generally classified by degree and by the site of the conduction disturbance. First-degree A-V block (see Fig. 9-12, *A*) indicates slowing of conduction but with each impulse successfully traversing the A-V junction to activate the ventricles. Second-degree block (see Fig. 9-12, *B* to *D*) is characterized by failure of some of the atrial impulses to activate the ventricles. In third-degree block (see Fig. 9-12, *E*), or complete heart block, none of the atrial impulses reaches the ventricles. Heart block can result from a proximal conduction disturbance in the A-V nodal area or in the distal conducting system below the bundle of His. The site of the block is often suggested by the type of block and the ECG morphology of the QRS complex.

First-degree A-V block. First degree A-V block (see Fig. 9-12, *A*) is almost always the result of slowed conduction within the A-V node. Because each atrial impulse activates the ventricles, first-degree block does not produce symptoms. The ECG feature is a P-R interval greater than 0.22 second, with each of the P waves followed by a QRS complex.

Second-degree A-V block. Second-degree A-V block may produce symptoms if it results in significant bradycardia. Second-degree A-V block is further classified as Mobitz type I (see Fig. 9-12, *B*) and type II (see Fig. 9-12, *D*). Mobitz type I, or Wenckebach, A-V block is characterized by progressive slowing of A-V conduction of successive atrial impulses, culminating in a nonconducted atrial impulse. Mobitz type II A-V block exists when a sudden unexpected failure of atrial conduction occurs without the progressive prolongation of A-V conduction in preceding complexes. The site of the type I block typically is the A-V nodal area. Type I block can result from heightened vagal tone and can occur in young, normal individuals during sleep. It is a frequent complication in acute inferior myocardial infarction and can also result from a variety of drugs. The ECG manifestations of type I second-degree A-V block include progressive lengthening of the P-R interval, culminating in a nonconducted P wave. The increment of slowing of A-V nodal conduction decreases with each successive P wave of the Wenckebach cycle. Thus the R-R intervals typically, but not invariably, shorten as the P-R interval lengthens (see Fig. 9-12, *B*).

Usually, type I second-degree A-V block requires no therapy other than measures to correct the underlying disturbance. If type I block progresses to complete heart block, it is usually accompanied by an acceptable junctional escape rhythm. If prompt treatment of type I block is necessary, atropine often improves the A-V conduction. Persistent, symptomatic type I second-degree A-V block may require pacemaker insertion.

Type II second-degree A-V block is almost always a manifestation of organic heart disease and less often of serious drug toxicity. It has the potential to progress to high-degree or complete heart block. Moreover, because the site of the block is typically distal to the bundle of His, the escape rhythm, should complete heart block develop, is ventricular in origin, usually at rates slower than 40/min that are not tolerated by the patient. Electrocardiographically, type II A-V block is characterized by the abrupt failure of a P wave to be conducted to the ventricle, without progressive lengthening of the antecedent P-R intervals. The intraventricular conduction of the conducted beats is usually abnormal, exhibiting a bundle branch block configuration. Type II second-degree A-V block usually requires pacing, particularly in the patient with acute myocardial infarction. The long-term prognosis of patients with type II A-V block, however, is usually related to the underlying cardiac disease.

Distinction of type I from type II block is not possible in the presence of 2:1 A-V block (see Fig. 9-12, *C*). Statistically, however, 2:1 A-V block in the presence of a normal QRS morphology is nearly always type I. With wide QRS complexes, 2:1 block may represent proximal or distal block.

Third-degree A-V block. Third-degree A-V block (complete heart block) (see Fig. 9-12, *E*) is characterized by failure of all atrial impulses to be conducted to the ventricles. As with second-degree A-V block, the site of the complete block may be the A-V node, bundle of His, or distally in the bundle branches. Block at the A-V node area is usually associated with a junctional escape rhythm with a narrow QRS complex, if the intraventricular conduction is normal. Block below the bundle of His results in a ventricular escape rhythm with bizarre QRS complexes.

Complete A-V block at the A-V node area complicates acute inferior infarction. As such, the block is often transient and the junctional escape rate stable. If prompt treatment is required, atropine may be administered but temporary pacing is generally recommended. Complete A-V block at the A-V node area may also result from chronic fibrosis within the septum and rarely from digitalis intoxication. The site of congenital complete heart block is also most often above the bifurcation of the bundle of His. In this case the junctional escape rate is faster than that associated with acquired supra-His block. Moreover, the junctional rhythm associated with congenital heart block often accelerates in response to exertion. Pacemaker therapy is generally not required in supra-His congenital heart block unless associated symptoms are present.

Complete heart block distal to the A-V node may result from idiopathic fibrosis of the conduction system or fibrocalcific degeneration of the cardiac skeleton, conditions that can occur in elderly persons. Other causes include myocarditis, cardiomyopathy, sarcoidosis, calcific valvular heart disease, and extensive acute myocardial infarction, usually anterior in location. Patients with distal-His complete A-V block are usually symptomatic; they characteristically do not respond well to atropine. In acutely symptomatic patients, isoproterenol can be used emergently to increase heart rate until temporary pacing can be instituted. However, this drug must be used with caution in patients with ischemic heart disease because of the potential to increase myocardial oxygen demand. Permanent pacing is indicated for most patients with distal-His complete A-V heart block.

Atrioventricular dissociation. The term *atrioventricular dissociation* indicates the presence of independent atrial and ventricular rhythms. It can be the result of complete heart block, as just described. Alternatively, A-V dissociation can result from physiologic interference, in which the A-V conduction system is rendered refractory to the sinus impulse because of earlier depolarization by another impulse (see Fig. 9-12, *F*). A-V dissociation can occur from slowing of the sinus rate with escape of a lower focus or from an inappropriate acceleration of a junctional or ventricular focus. The resultant A-V dissociation leads to the P wave "marching through" the QRS-T complex. When a sinus P wave is sufficiently removed from the preceding QRS-T and outside of the A-V nodal refractory period, the sinus impulse is conducted to the ventricles.

Intraventricular conduction abnormalities

Interruption of the normal orderly sequence of ventricular activation, resulting either from slowing or block of conduction in a portion of the intraventricular conduction system, leads to prolonged and bizarre QRS complexes. Characteristic QRS patterns on the scalar ECG permit localization of the conduction abnormality when the site is in the right or left bundle branches or in the anterior or posterior divisions (fascicles) of the left bundle. Nonspecific intraventricular conduction defects are presumed to be the result of more diffuse conduction abnormalities, distal to the conducting system's major branches.

Intraventricular conduction abnormalities such as right or left bundle branch block (RBBB, LBBB) can at times be intermittent and/or dependent on heart rate. *Acceleration* (or tachycardia-dependent) block is much more common than *deceleration* (or bradycardia-dependent) block. As described earlier, functional conduction block (primarily right bundle branch pattern) can occur via Ashman's phenomenon.

Left anterior fascicular block. Conduction block in the anterior fascicle (see Fig. 9-15) of the left bundle occurs frequently. It is associated with a variety of cardiac disorders, including ischemic heart disease, systemic hypertension, aortic valve disease, and cardiomyopathy. Moreover, left anterior fascicular block occurs in some individuals with no clinical evidence of cardiovascular disease. The ECG features of left anterior fascicular block (including QRS axis from −45 degrees to −90 degrees) are detailed in Chapter 4.

Left posterior fascicular block. Conduction block isolated to the posterior fascicle of the left bundle rarely occurs (see Fig. 9-15). When present, it is usually accompanied by evidence of significant cardiac disease and often by conduction delay in the right bundle branch. The ECG features of left posterior fascicular block are listed in Chapter 4. Diagnosis usually requires not only the presence of the characteristic ECG pattern but also documentation of change from an earlier normal tracing.

Left bundle branch block. LBBB may result from conduction block in the proximal left bundle or from simultaneous block in the anterior and posterior fascicles. Most patients with LBBB have underlying cardiovascular disease, usually caused by hypertension, coronary artery disease, or cardiomyopathy. The conduction disturbance can occasionally precede other signs of the heart disease. The prognosis of patients with LBBB generally depends on the etiology and severity of the underlying condition.

The left ventricle's delayed electrical activation from LBBB results in a delay of left ventricular contraction and thus the reversed or paradoxical splitting of the second heart sound.

The ECG criteria of LBBB are included in Chapter 4. It is important to recognize the limitation that LBBB imposes on the recognition of myocardial infarction patterns. Because the septal activation proceeds from right to left, the intraventricular cavity is initially positive. Q waves of infarction are no longer reliably recorded. Consequently, with LBBB, the diagnosis of myocardial infarction in most patients must be made without the aid of the ECG.

Right bundle branch block. Slowing or block of conduction in the right bundle branch (see Figs. 9-12, *D*, and 9-15) can result from various cardiac disorders. Occasionally, however, RBBB may be recorded in individuals without clinical evidence of cardiovascular disease. RBBB in young individuals without signs of underlying disease is associated with a good prognosis. The prognosis of the RBBB in patients with heart disease is primarily that of the underlying disorder. RBBB delays the right ventricular contraction and pulmonic valve closure, producing wide splitting of the second heart sound. Respiratory variation of the second sound is usually maintained. The ECG features of RBBB are described in Chapter 4.

Right bundle branch block and fascicular blocks. A relatively common form of bifascicular block is the combination of RBBB and left anterior fascicular block (see Fig. 9-15). This pattern is recognized by the abnormal left axis of the QRS complex in the limb leads and by the simultaneous RBBB pattern in the right precordial leads. Interestingly, this form of bifascicular block is occasionally recorded in patients without clinical evidence of heart disease. Unless the patient has recently had acute myocardial infarction, this type of bifascicular block seldom progresses to complete block, and prophylactic pacing is not required.

Other combinations of bundle branch and fascicular blocks (see Fig. 9-15) rarely occur and usually are overshadowed by the associated heart disease.

REFERENCES

Braunwald E: Heart disease: a textbook of cardiovascular medicine, ed 4. Philadelphia, 1992, Saunders.

Cardiac Arrhythmia Suppression Trial (CAST) investigators: Preliminary report: effect of encainide and flecainide on mortality in a randomized trial of arrhythmia suppression after myocardial infarction. N Engl J Med 321:406, 1989.

Fisch C: William Withering: an account of the foxglove and some of its medical uses, 1785-1985. J Am Coll Cardiol 5:1A, 1985.

Fisch C: Electrocardiography of arrhythmias. Philadelphia, 1990, Lea & Febiger.

Guidelines for permanent cardiac pacemaker implantation: a report of the Joint American College of Cardiology/American Heart Association Task Force on Assessment of Cardiovascular Procedures. J Am Coll Cardiol 14:1827, 1989.

Kindwall K, Brown J, and Josephson ME: Electrocardiographic criteria for ventricular tachycardia with wide complex left bundle branch block. Am J Cardiol 61:1279, 1988.

Minardo J et al: Clinical characteristics of patients with ventricular fibrillation during antiarrhythmic drug therapy. N Engl J Med 319:257, 1988.

Wellens JHH, Bar FW, and Lie KI: The value of the electrocardiogram in the differential diagnosis of a tachycardia with a widened QRS complex. Am J Med 64:247, 1978.

CHAPTER

10 Congestive Heart Failure

David McCall

Despite the declining mortality from cardiovascular disease and cerebrovascular accident (stroke) in the United States, congestive heart failure (CHF) continues to be a major cause of morbidity. In fact, the incidence of CHF appears to be increasing: hospitalizations for CHF quadrupled between 1970 and 1985. Several factors could account for this. Heart failure increases with increasing age, and the U.S. population is an aging one. Better pharmacologic approaches and advanced interventions now enable health care professionals to keep more people alive than in the 1960s and 1970s. In patients over age 65, CHF is the most common hospital discharge diagnosis, and in all age groups it represents the fourth most common diagnosis. Clearly, CHF remains a major public health problem. Annually, approximately 500,000 men and women in the United States develop heart failure, and the overall prevalence is 2.3 to 2.5 million.

Heart failure, the end-stage of many cardiovascular diseases, including coronary artery disease, hypertensive heart disease, valvular disease, and the cardiomyopathies, remains one of the most challenging clinical dilemmas facing the physician. *Heart failure* may be defined as a pathophysiologic state in which cardiac output is not adequate to meet the body's metabolic needs. This definition, however, could potentially be ambiguous. It could denote either primary cardiac pump dysfunction in the presence of normal peripheral requirements or, conversely, increased tissue demands that cannot be met by a normal or augmented cardiac output. A more simple operating definition would be to consider heart failure as *a state in which cardiac dysfunction results in a diminished functional capacity and thus an impaired quality of life*. This not only defines the clinical syndrome but also sets the stage for at least two therapeutic objectives. Another major concern is that, despite recent therapeutic advances, the mortality for patients with CHF from any etiology remains high. For all functional classes the 5-year mortality is approximately 50%, and for patients in New York Heart Association (NYHA) Functional Class IV the 1-year mortality is 60%. Therefore a third therapeutic objective is to improve survival.

The syndrome of heart failure is extremely complex; a variety of primary cardiovascular disorders blend with varying compensatory mechanisms and adaptive responses, resulting in a wide spectrum of clinical symptoms and signs. Although the compensatory mechanisms initially tend to offset the circulatory failure, many ultimately have a deleterious effect and contribute to the continued deterioration in cardiac performance. In view of the high mortality, each patient with CHF should undergo a diligent search for any primary and precipitating causes so that such factors may be satisfactorily corrected. Failure to identify and correct underlying and precipitating factors is the most common reason for treatment failure. Despite a better understanding of heart failure and changing options for therapy, only in recent years have specific interventions been shown to improve survival.

This chapter focuses on the common pathophysiologic mechanisms that underlie CHF regardless of its etiology. The chapter also discusses traditional and recent therapeutic approaches designed to improve systolic function, improve the patient's functional capacity and quality of life, and prolong survival through a direct approach to the pathophysiologic processes.

CLASSIFICATION

Although CHF never occurs in the absence of some specific cardiac abnormality, one must remember that CHF per se is not a specific disease. Rather, it is a pathophysiologic condition that results from the interplay between the primary cardiac disorder and the compensatory mechanisms, some of which eventually adversely affect the cardiovascular system. Therefore a diagnosis of CHF must *never* be accepted and is *never* complete until the underlying cardiac disorder has been identified.

Heart failure occurs because of a mechanical abnormality, a cardiac muscle disease, and/or an arrhythmia (see the box below). Mechanical abnormalities may affect systolic performance, diastolic performance, or both. The systolic group includes conditions causing ventricular pressure overload (e.g., hypertension, aortic stenosis) and volume overload (valvular regurgitation, intracardiac or extracardiac shunts). The diastolic group comprises disorders of the pericardium (e.g., constrictive pericarditis), restrictive myocardial disease (e.g., cardiac amyloidosis), and mitral or tricuspid stenosis. Although these conditions may selectively involve the left or right ventricle, a disorder affecting one pumping chamber of two pumps in series must invariably affect the other, although the chronologic sequence of this involvement is variable.

Classification of cardiac failure

I. Mechanical abnormalities
  A. Increased resistance to forward outflow (pressure overload)
  B. Increased ventricular inflow (volume overload): valvular regurgitation, shunts, increased blood volume
    1. Primary
    2. Secondary (valvular regurgitation from ventricular dilatation)
  C. Pericardial disease (constriction and tamponade)
  D. Restrictive heart disease (endocardial or myocardial)
  E. Ventricular aneurysm
II. Myocardial failure
  A. Primary
    1. Cardiomyopathy
    2. Myocarditis
    3. Metabolically induced muscle dysfunction (hypothyroidism)
    4. Reduction in muscle mass (myocardial infarction)
  B. Secondary
    1. Dysdynamic heart failure (longstanding volume or pressure overload)
    2. Drug induced
    3. Cardiac involvement in systemic disease
III. Electrical disorders
  A. Asystole
  B. Ventricular fibrillation
  C. Heart block
  D. Ventricular tachycardia

Disease of cardiac muscle may be either primary, as with myocarditis leading to cardiomyopathy and heart failure, or secondary, when a longstanding overload state results in dysfunction of cardiac muscle. The latter condition, known as *dysdynamic heart failure,* may occur in longstanding, severe valvular regurgitation. CHF associated with the localized loss of muscle mass (e.g., acute myocardial infarction, infiltration of myocardium with tumor) is also classified as myocardial dysfunction.

Arrhythmias may precipitate a severe reduction in cardiac output, aggravating pre-existing heart failure or initiating overt clinical heart failure when only subclinical cardiac dysfunction was present previously.

It is important to distinguish CHF from *circulatory congestion,* which may develop from impaired sodium and water balance in the absence of cardiac disease. Thus renal failure may cause salt and water retention and clinical symptoms and signs of heart failure when cardiac performance is normal.

PATHOGENESIS

The initial pathophysiologic event in CHF is a decrease in cardiac output at any given ventricular end-diastolic pressure or atrial pressure (Fig. 10-1). This can result from (1) excessive afterload, which shifts the ventricular function curve downward and to the right; (2) depressed contractility, which also shifts the curve downward and to the right; (3) valvular regurgitation or intracardiac shunting, which reduces the "effective" forward stroke volume for any end-diastolic pressure; or (4) reductions in total cardiac compliance, which shift the diastolic pressure-volume curve upward and to the left. The fourth alteration, as discussed in Chapter 1, also results in a depression of the ventricular function curve downward and to the right. In a sense, this is also the primary pathophysiologic problem in mitral or tricuspid stenosis, since the inability to fill the ventricles at

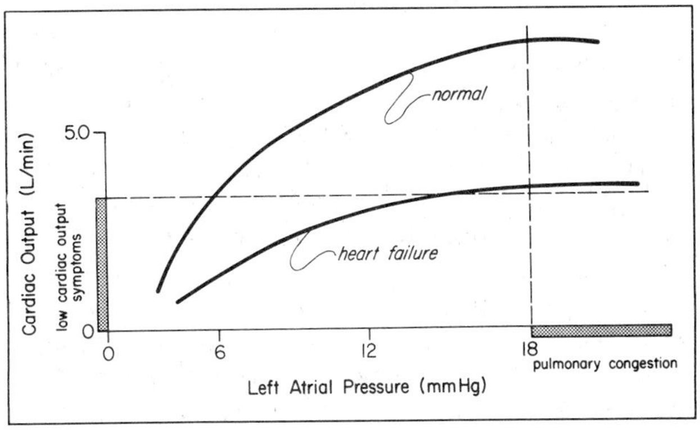

Fig. 10-1. Ventricular function curve in congestive heart failure (CHF) compared with normal curve. At any level of left atrial pressure, cardiac output is decreased in the failing heart. Dotted areas indicate levels of cardiac output and filling pressure at which symptoms develop. (Modified from Mason DT, editor: Congestive heart failure. New York, 1976, Yorke Medical Books.)

a normal atrial pressure results in a downward shift of the Frank-Starling relation when cardiac output is plotted against atrial pressure.

The time course involved in the downward displacement of the cardiac output–filling pressure curve varies greatly. An acute hypertensive crisis may rapidly depress the curve downward and produce immediate symptoms, whereas chronic, progressive increases in afterload (e.g., aortic stenosis) may require years to produce that same downward displacement. In part, this is caused by the development of compensatory mechanisms, such as hypertrophy and dilatation (see later discussion on acute and chronic compensatory adjustments), which may greatly modify the Frank-Starling relationship.

The downward shift of the ventricular function curve in the presence of a normal venous return curve results in a new intersection of the two curves at a lower cardiac output and higher atrial pressure (Chapter 1). If the output is sufficiently low (generally less than 2.2 L/min/m^2), there will be symptoms of low cardiac output; if atrial pressure is sufficiently high (more than 18 mm Hg on the left side), there will be symptoms of pulmonary or systemic congestion resulting from transudation of fluid into the interstitial spaces.

Myocardial failure

The depression of the ventricular function curve from an intrinsic decrease in myocardial contractility is one of the mechanisms of CHF, called *myocardial failure,* or *myocardial dysfunction.* It is a particularly important form of heart failure because it may complicate existing forms of cardiac disease (chronic pressure, volume loading) and is generally not reversible once present.

The basic defect in myocardial failure is the heart muscle's inability to generate sufficient force despite adequate ventricular filling. Many indices have been developed, both clinically and in experimental animals, in an attempt to document or quantify myocardial contractility. These include simple ejection phase indices, such as ejection fraction, peak velocity of circumferential fiber shortening (V_{cf}), fractional shortening, and stroke volume (Chapter 1). These indices may be useful in assessing baseline levels of contractility, but one must remember that all these ejection phase indices are extremely affected by afterload. From a practical standpoint, however, it is probably most convenient to use the ejection fraction, although the limitations of this must be considered.

Other indices have examined the isovolumetric phase of ventricular systole to assess contractility and changes in contractility. Of these, dP/dt_{max}, the maximum rate of rise of ventricular pressure, has had the greatest popularity. Other indices include V_{max}, the extrapolated shortening velocity at zero load. This seems to have little advantage over the more simply derived dP/dt_{max}. Finally, from ventricular pressure-volume loops, it is possible to derive E_{max} as probably the most load-independent index of myocardial contractility (Chapter 1). However, many of these are very difficult to derive in the clinical setting and therefore have very limited usefulness.

In the whole heart the reduction in *muscle* contractile performance results in a depression of *ventricular* contractile performance, characterized by a displacement downward and to the left of the stroke volume–wall tension curve at constant preload, or a displacement downward and to the right of the stroke volume–end-diastolic volume relationship at constant afterload (Chapter 1). Frequently, these contractility changes are associated with increases in muscle stiffness, which means that the diastolic pressure-volume curve is displaced upward and to the left (see Fig. 1-8). When these relationships are combined to form the classic ventricular function curve (i.e., stroke volume or cardiac output plotted against end-diastolic ventricular or atrial pressure), marked downward displacement of this relationship occurs in patients with myocardial failure compared with control subjects.

Various cellular abnormalities have been described in the myocardium, both from patients and from experimental animals with heart failure. Among the earliest was the demonstration that cardiac norepinephrine stores were depleted in patients with severe heart failure, a finding that appears to be specific for the failing myocardium. A more interesting and a consistent biochemical change in the failing myocardium is a decrease in myosin adenosine triphosphatase (ATPase) activity. This change appears to be caused by a change in the individual isoenzymes of myosin, resulting in a preponderance of the slow over the fast component. Diminished myosin ATPase activity results in a decrease in cross-bridge interaction between actin and myosin, which in turn results in a reduced velocity of muscle shortening. Although this observation represents an interesting correlation between biochemistry and muscle mechanics, its significance is unclear. As with many other biochemical changes in the myocardium, this may represent an adaptive response designed as an energy-sparing process to minimize ATP utilization. Our better understanding of molecular biology (Chapter 2) is making it increasingly clear that this, similar to other adaptive responses, represents an alteration in gene-specific expression.

Other studies have demonstrated a decrease in calcium (Ca) transport by the sarcoplasmic reticulum (SR). This finding, together with ATP depletion, could influence diastolic as well as systolic parameters of myocardial function. It has been clearly demonstrated in experimental animals and in tissue obtained from human hearts at biopsy that a decrease occurs in the activity of the Ca ATPase system responsible for SR Ca transport. Most recently, samples from human biopsies have shown a decrease in the expression of messenger ribonucleic acid (mRNA) for the Ca ATPase of the SR. Other studies have demonstrated abnormalities of mitochondrial function and a decrease in high-energy phosphate production. Nevertheless, a causal relationship between decreased ATP levels and diminished contractile activity of the failing myocardium has not been established.

Despite these observations of significant biochemical

dysfunction, the relationship between these biochemical changes and the contractile properties of the failing myocardium has yet to be established. They may well represent a secondary phenomenon but equally well may represent primary and basic underlying abnormalities that could precipitate, or at least perpetuate, the CHF state.

High output failure

High output failure is a form of CHF in which cardiac output is elevated compared with values for the normal resting state in man. However, many symptoms and physical findings are identical to those of low output failure. The primary physiologic abnormality in high output failure is either circulatory shunting or greatly increased peripheral demands for blood. Examples of high output failure include arteriovenous (AV) fistula, anemia, thyrotoxicosis, Paget's disease (multiple AV fistulas in bone), and beriberi. Although actual cardiac output is high (> 3.6 L/min/m^2), the "effective" cardiac output arriving at the peripheral tissues is low for any given atrial pressure. This is true in an absolute sense with AV shunting and in a relative sense with anemia. The effective cardiac output versus atrial pressure curve is depressed downward and to the right. In high output states, however, myocardial performance may remain normal or even augmented. Thus absolute cardiac output for any given end-diastolic *volume* may be normal or increased. Consequently, treatment in these conditions should be directed primarily toward relieving the defect that renders stroke volume inadequate rather than toward improving myocardial performance.

Acute and chronic compensatory adjustments in heart failure

The downward displacement of the ventricular function curve in CHF stimulates several acute and chronic adjustments that tend to restore the curve toward normal. Improved cardiac function results from the positive inotropic effect of augmented activity of the sympathetic nervous system. Early in heart failure, increased contractility is modulated by locally released norepinephrine from cardiac sympathetic fibers. Later, however, the failing heart appears to be supported by elevated circulating catecholamines. Heightened sympathetic influences may also redistribute peripheral flow and provide adequate perfusion to muscle during exercise, despite an inadequate global cardiac output. The role of increased catecholamines in supporting the failing heart is clear from observations that beta-adrenergic blockade in patients with borderline CHF may cause overt decompensation.

Although generalized sympathetic enhancement may be beneficial, a net increase in total peripheral resistance can feed back negatively on the compromised ventricle through the inverse relationship between stroke volume and afterload (Chapter 1). A deleterious increase in systemic vascular resistance forms the rationale for the vasodilator therapy of CHF.

An increase in blood volume through sodium and water retention by the kidneys, as well as a decrease in venous capacitance through augmented sympathetic tone, increases ventricular filling and end-diastolic volume, promoting an enhanced stroke volume via the Frank-Starling relationship. Increases in end-diastolic volume, however, produce increases in end-diastolic pressure, depending on the stiffness of the ventricular chamber. Furthermore, at high end-diastolic volumes, the augmentation in cardiac output for a given increment in heart size is reduced, whereas the increment in *diastolic pressure* for the same increase in heart size is greater. The net effect is that substantial increments in end-diastolic pressure produce relatively little increase in cardiac output at high end-diastolic pressures (i.e., there is a prominent plateau to the ventricular function curve). Thus the Frank-Starling mechanism may be relatively ineffectual in CHF; small increases in venous return create large increases in ventricular diastolic pressure and pulmonary congestion but only slight augmentation of forward output. Of equal importance for therapy, however, is that only a slight drop in cardiac output may accompany considerable reduction in filling pressure when end-diastolic pressure is greater than 20 mm Hg.

A third, equally important cardiac adaptation to the presence of chronic heart failure is a change in ventricular size and geometry. *Stroke volume* is the change in ventricular volume during systole, and, as such, it varies with the radius squared or radius cubed, depending on the model chosen to represent ventricular shape during the cardiac cycle. Thus, for a given percentage change in ventricular circumference, stroke volume will be greater at a larger ventricular diameter. Consequently, cardiac *dilatation* alone is capable of effecting a greater stroke volume for a given degree of initial fiber stretch when afterload is held constant. However, when dilatation occurs without an increase in ventricular mass, wall thickness must decrease; thus afterload (i.e., wall stress) must increase by the Laplace relationship:

$$\sigma = \frac{P \times r}{2h}$$

where σ is wall stress, P is chamber pressure, r is chamber radius, and h is chamber thickness (Chapter 1). Thus, in a nonhypertrophied heart, the geometric advantages of dilatation are largely offset by the enhanced afterload, and stroke volume does not improve. Under such circumstances, a low-to-normal stroke volume and an elevated end-diastolic volume result in a reduced ejection fraction, consistent with impaired cardiac performance. However, if increases in wall thickness occur simultaneously with enlargement in chamber size, leading to an increase in ventricular mass (i.e., *eccentric hypertrophy*), substantial augmentation in stroke volume can result. In patients with eccentric hypertrophy, considerable increases in cardiac output can be maintained for years without the signs or symptoms of CHF. However, dilatation and/or eccentric hypertrophy may cause enlargement of the atrioventricular

(A-V) valve rings and distortion of the supporting apparatus of the mitral and/or tricuspid valves (papillary muscles, chordae tendineae). Such altered geometry may lead to valvular regurgitation, which may further compromise forward stroke volume for any level of filling pressure. The reduction in heart size that accompanies the therapy of CHF may result in marked diminution of such secondary valvular incompetence.

A slightly different form of geometric adaptation accompanies chronic pressure overload. An increase in chamber pressure results in an increase in wall stress. As previously discussed, this tends to depress the ventricular function curve downward and to the right. However, increases in wall thickness without changes in internal chamber dimension develop, tending to return wall stress toward normal values. Such "afterload reduction" accomplished by *concentric hypertrophy* elevates the ventricular function curve toward pre-existing levels, although typically, hypertrophy also induces an increase in chamber stiffness. Consequently, an elevation in the filling pressure may be necessary to achieve a given end-diastolic volume and thus a given stroke volume. Frequently, symptoms of patients with pressure overload and concentric hypertrophy derive primarily from elevated filling pressures and not from low cardiac output.

Myocardial oxygen requirements in heart failure

Myocardial oxygen (O_2) demands in CHF may be elevated, normal, or low. However, since coexistent coronary artery disease often compromises the coronary circulation in patients with CHF, and since ischemia may further aggravate depressed myocardial performance, it is important to identify factors that tend to augment myocardial oxygen demand ($M\dot{V}O_2$). This may occur with increased peak ventricular pressure, as in valvular disease or hypertension, or with ventricular enlargement (i.e., dilatation without adequate eccentric hypertrophy). Finally, $M\dot{V}O_2$ may be increased through enhanced fiber shortening accompanying valvular regurgitation or high output states. The ultimate interaction of these factors in determining O_2 consumption is complex. For example, in patients with CHF, ventricular dilatation, and symptoms of ischemic heart disease, administration of a positive inotropic agent such as digitalis may actually decrease myocardial O_2 consumption and improve ischemic symptoms if heart rate and size are reduced.

PERIPHERAL SEQUELAE

Alterations in kidney function

See Chapter 352.

Alterations in peripheral blood flow

The increased sympathetic tone during CHF results in alterations in the normal distribution of regional vascular resistance that are most marked during exercise. In addition, local factors increase arteriolar stiffness at rest and contribute to the observed resistance changes. Such factors may be related to the increased sodium content of vessels in heart failure or to increased tissue pressure caused by excess extracellular fluid. In either case the impedance of the arterial tree is altered considerably, often resulting in extreme changes in the character of central and peripheral arterial pressure pulses.

These resistance changes mediate a redistribution of blood flow away from the skin and other less metabolically active tissues. In profound CHF, resting flow to the limbs and the kidneys and other abdominal viscera may be reduced to provide more adequate perfusion of such organs as the heart and brain. Even in mild CHF, the stress of exercise produces marked declines in visceral and renal blood flow to supply the increased O_2 demands of muscle. Despite these adjustments, however, limb blood flow is still often reduced during exercise as compared with normal. During moderate exertion, O_2 demands are partially satisfied by increased O_2 extraction from the blood, but during strenuous exercise, O_2 supply is still inadequate, and a significant shift to anaerobic metabolism results. Many of these changes in peripheral blood flow, O_2 extraction, and lactate production account for the symptoms of fatigue and inability to exercise in patients with CHF.

Vascular congestion

The increases in venous return in patients with CHF result in a rise in atrial pressure. Whether an increase occurs in left or right atrial pressure or in both depends on whether the left or right ventricular function curve is displaced downward. These elevations of filling pressure are reflected back into the pulmonary and/or systemic veins.

Fluid accumulation in the tissue interstitium is governed by Starling's law of capillary-interstitial fluid exchange:

$$\text{Fluid accumulation} = K[(P_c + \pi_i) - (P_i + \pi_c)] - \text{Lymph flow}$$

where K is permeability coefficient, P_c is mean intracapillary pressure, π_i is oncotic pressure of interstitial fluid, P_i is mean interstitial fluid pressure, and π_c is oncotic pressure of intracapillary fluid.

When P_c rises because of an elevation in venous pressure, fluid tends to leave the capillary and enter the interstitium. Normally, increases in lymph flow can accommodate the transudation of fluid, but with marked increases in capillary pressure, obstruction of lymphatics, or disruption of capillary membranes (altering the permeability coefficient), fluid can accumulate, leading to pulmonary or peripheral edema.

In the lungs, initial accumulation of fluid is confined to the interstitial spaces, resulting in decreased pulmonary compliance. Consequently, ventilatory effort is increased, and the Hering-Breuer reflex is activated, causing tachypnea with decreased tidal volume. Further net gain of interstitial fluid results in deterioration of gas exchange, manifested by a fall in arterial O_2 tension and the appearance of fluid in the interlobular septa. Since intracapillary pressures are higher in dependent portions of the lung, usually the bases, pathophysiologic events are often most evident there. Thus local decreases in O_2 tension at the base may produce vasoconstriction and redistribute pulmonary blood flow to the apices, although reflex mechanisms and increased resting vessel stiffness may also play a role. Eventually, further elevations in pulmonary venous pressure cause disruption of the junctions between alveolar cells, and fluid moves into alveolar spaces and small airways, terminating gas exchange (pulmonary edema). The progressive hypoxemia induced by these events may further depress ventricular function, leading to a cycle of increasing cardiac failure, more pulmonary edema, and eventually death.

Increases in right atrial pressure are reflected back into the systemic venules and capillaries, leading to peripheral edema, particularly in dependent portions of the body, where intracapillary pressures are the highest. Venous engorgement of the abdominal viscera can greatly enlarge these organs (e.g., liver, spleen) and may interfere with their metabolic functions. Thus chronic congestion of the liver in patients with CHF can impair metabolism of drugs and endogenous hormones (e.g., aldosterone); congestion of the gastrointestinal tract can reduce absorption of orally administered therapeutic agents. The latter is also associated with a protein-losing enteropathy, which further aggravates extracellular fluid retention by decreasing capillary oncotic pressure.

Venous congestion may also result in the accumulation of free fluid in body cavities, such as the peritoneal and pleural spaces, producing ascites and/or hydrothorax. Because the pleural veins drain into both pulmonary and systemic veins, pleural effusion may be present in predominantly right-sided heart or left-sided heart failure alone. Large amounts of ascitic and pleural fluid can further compromise pulmonary gas exchange, further accelerating the total pathophysiologic deterioration.

CLINICAL MANIFESTATIONS

Symptoms

Disturbances of respiration. The rise in left atrial pressure in patients with CHF causes pulmonary venous congestion, which results in *dyspnea,* a sensation of difficult or impaired respiration. Dyspnea is partly caused by increased afferent nerve activity from respiratory muscles performing augmented work in the presence of insufficient blood flow. This symptom is usually interpreted by the patient as an inability to obtain sufficient air or "shortness of breath." In mild failure, dyspnea frequently occurs only on exertion, with the increased venous return producing an elevation in left atrial pressure (i.e., dyspnea on exertion). In more severe failure, dyspnea may occur at rest, particularly in the presence of frank pulmonary edema. Two specific characteristics of this breathlessness are often present. In *orthopnea,* shortness of breath is more pronounced on assuming a recumbent position, so that the patient prefers an upright or sitting posture. In *paroxysmal nocturnal dyspnea,* the patient awakes from sleep with breathlessness and sits on the side of the bed or by an open window for 5 to 10 minutes for relief. These symptoms presumably arise from the positional dependence of pulmonary interstitial fluid accumulation and perhaps the reabsorption of peripheral edema fluid into the central circulation during sleep. Other disturbances of respiration include (1) Cheyne-Stokes respiration; (2) cough, which is usually nonproductive and may occur only at night; and (3) wheezing, or cardiac asthma, which results from bronchospasm precipitated by high left atrial pressures.

The ultimate disturbance of respiration caused by CHF is acute *pulmonary edema,* with frank, rapid transudation of fluid into the alveolar spaces (Chapter 202). Pulmonary edema is manifested by extreme shortness of breath, frequently accompanied by wheezing and "rattling" sounds emanating from the trachea. The patient may expectorate frothy fluid that is occasionally blood tinged (hemoptysis). If significant arterial desaturation exists, cyanosis may also be present. Acute pulmonary edema is a medical emergency, and prompt, appropriate therapy may be lifesaving.

Disturbances of forward cardiac output. *Weakness, easy fatigability,* and *lassitude* are common symptoms in patients with CHF, generally relating to inadequate cardiac output. Such symptoms are frequently precipitated by exertion, when the demands of exercising muscle cannot be met by compensatory increases in peripheral blood flow. Elderly patients with low cardiac output may have disturbances of mentation, characterized by confusion, disorientation, and somnolence, which are most profound in the presence of cerebrovascular disease or psychoactive agents. Reductions in renal blood flow accompanying CHF may be manifested by daytime *oliguria* (decreased frequency and volume of urination), since renovascular resistance is greatly augmented during activity. However, during bed rest, renal resistance may return to normal levels, resulting in a nocturnal diuresis, or *nocturia* (increased frequency and volume of urination at night). In severe failure, persistently inadequate O_2 delivery to peripheral tissues results in generalized catabolism, loss of body mass, and the development of *cardiac cachexia.* However, because of substantial fluid retention, net body weight may remain unchanged when serial measurements are taken.

Symptoms resulting from systemic congestion. Elevation in systemic venous pressure results in transudation of fluid into the dependent portions of the body, leading to *edema* in the pretibial region and ankles in ambulatory patients and the presacral area in patients on bed rest. Fluid may also accumulate in the peritoneal cavity, causing *ascites,* manifested by increasing abdominal girth. Enlargement of the abdominal viscera, particularly the liver, may precipitate right upper quadrant pain, abdominal fullness, anorexia, nausea, and vomiting. Rarely, hepatic dysfunction related to CHF may produce clinical jaundice. Some patients with prominent venous pressure waves accompanying elevations of mean venous pressure (i.e., tricuspid regurgitation or constrictive pericarditis) may note abnormal pulsations in the supraclavicular area.

Physical findings

Arterial system. The *blood pressure* may be high, low, or normal in patients with CHF, depending on the primary cardiac and/or peripheral arterial disease. Characteristically, in severe heart failure caused by myocardial dysfunction, mean arterial pressure is low to normal and pulse pressure is attenuated, reflecting the low ventricular stroke volume and the high systemic vascular resistance. With hypertensive heart disease or significant salt and water retention, however, mean pressure may be elevated despite advanced myocardial disease. The peripheral pulse may be normal but usually is of low amplitude, reflecting the reduced pulse pressure. Occasionally, the arterial pulse is distorted by the primary cardiac pathology (e.g., aortic valve disease; Chapter 3) or by abnormalities of the peripheral circulation (e.g., AV fistulas). In severe low output states, two distinct arterial pulse disturbances may be present. The *dicrotic pulse,* characterized by palpable systolic and diastolic pressure waves, results from a reduced stroke volume in the presence of marked peripheral vasoconstriction. *Pulsus alternans* is manifested by alternating high-amplitude and low-amplitude peak systolic pressure waves. The mechanism of pulsus alternans is incompletely understood, but alternating end-diastolic volumes with alternating Frank-Starling effects and/or alternating excitation-contraction coupling in local myocardial segments may play some role (Chapter 3).

Venous system. Inspection of the jugular venous system in patients with CHF may reveal abnormalities, depending on the right ventricle's mechanical status. If right ventricular function is normal, *venous pressure* may be normal, even in the presence of severe left ventricular decompensation (e.g., acute myocardial infarction). Usually, however, right ventricular diastolic pressure is elevated and is reflected back into the right atrium and jugular system. Abnormalities in the waveforms can be detected, depending on the nature of the disease affecting the right side of the heart (Chapter 3). Thus, in tricuspid regurgitation, the V wave will occur earlier and be accentuated; in severe right ventricular hypertrophy, right ventricular compliance will be reduced, and a prominent A wave will be present. The increase in right ventricular stiffness that often occurs with right-sided heart failure may induce a marked rise in venous pressure when venous return is enhanced. This may lead to *Kussmaul's sign,* a paradoxical increase in venous pressure with inspiration, or *hepatojugular reflux,* the appearance of jugular venous distention when sustained pressure (>30 seconds) is applied to the right upper abdominal quadrant.

A chronic elevation in right atrial pressure, as previously noted, can cause engorgement of abdominal organs and edema. Consequently, hepatomegaly, rarely splenomegaly, ascites, and presacral and/or ankle edema may be detected in patients with CHF. It must be stressed that peripheral edema is probably the least specific sign of CHF and that the diagnosis should never be made on this basis alone.

Pulmonary findings. The patient with CHF may have either rapid, shallow breathing or Cheyne-Stokes respirations. On percussion, evidence of bilateral or unilateral *pleural effusion* may be present; unilateral effusions have a predilection for the right side. When elevations in pulmonary venous pressure are only moderate and transudation of fluid is confined to the interstitium, the auscultatory findings are often normal. Occasionally, pulmonary interstitial edema may irritate small airways and produce bronchospasm, resulting in audible wheezes. However, when pulmonary capillary pressure reaches levels sufficient to cause alveolar fluid accumulation, moist inspiratory *rales,* initially confined to the lung's dependent portions, are heard. Rales are not specific for CHF and may be heard in primary lung disease as well, posing a difficult diagnostic dilemma. In acute pulmonary edema, rales and rhonchi are usually evident throughout the lung fields and may become very coarse and sibilant.

Cardiac findings. The *apical impulse* frequently is laterally displaced in patients with CHF, resulting from the compensatory development of dilatation and/or hypertrophy. However, if the heart failure is of rapid onset (e.g., acute myocardial infarction) or related to disorders of diastolic filling (e.g., restrictive heart disease or mitral stenosis), the left ventricle may be normal in size, and the cardiac apex will not be displaced. In conditions in which concentric hypertrophy has developed (e.g., hypertension, aortic stenosis), the apical impulse is frequently normally located but increased in amplitude and duration. Right ventricular involvement, either with dilatation or hypertrophy, may be indicated by a palpable impulse to the left of the sternum or beneath the xiphoid process.

On auscultation, the findings may be dominated by the primary disease process, such as a harsh systolic outflow murmur in aortic stenosis. In general, however, several auscultatory events accompany CHF of any cause. These include (1) a third heart sound, coincident with rapid ventricular filling and thought to arise from reduced ventricular compliance or increased early diastolic flow across the A-V valves, and (2) a presystolic fourth heart sound, resulting from atrial ejection of blood into a poorly compliant ventricle (Chapter 3).

In CHF from myocardial disease, the first heart sound may be decreased in intensity because the rate of rise of left ventricular pressure is reduced. Reversed splitting of the second heart sound may be present, accompanying either electrocardiographically (ECG) manifested left bundle branch block or marked mechanical delay of left ventricular ejection (Chapter 3). Finally, dilatation of either ventricular chamber may distort the supporting apparatus of the A-V valves, and the systolic murmurs of mitral and tricuspid regurgitation may be audible.

Electrocardiogram

No specific ECG alterations are associated with CHF, although arrhythmias precipitating or aggravating heart failure may be present. There may be evidence of specific chamber enlargement, either as a compensatory mechanism (e.g., left ventricular hypertrophy) or as a reflection of the basic primary disease (e.g., left atrial enlargement in mitral stenosis). In CHF associated with coronary artery disease, the ECG may identify an acute or healed myocardial infarction as the cause of the cardiac decompensation. Frequently, electrolyte abnormalities or drug effects (e.g., digitalis) that are of therapeutic importance may be detected on the ECG.

Chest radiograph

The chest radiograph may reveal enlargement of specific cardiac chambers or abnormalities of the pulmonary vasculature, which may be helpful in establishing the diagnosis of CHF or in identifying underlying cardiac disease. Frequently the cardiac silhouette in the posteroanterior projection is greater than half the total thoracic diameter, reflecting compensatory ventricular dilatation (Fig. 10-2). This may result from right, or left, or biventricular enlargement, and a lateral projection may help to identify the specific chamber responsible (Fig. 10-2). Frequently, the elevation in left atrial pressure accompanying CHF results in left atrial enlargement (Chapter 5).

Elevation of pulmonary venous pressure often results in characteristic radiographic changes. When only moderate interstitial edema fluid is present, the upper pulmonary lobe vessels may be more prominent than those to the lower lobes. Edema in the wall of the bronchioles may thicken these structures when viewed in cross section (i.e., peribronchiolar cuffing). Fluid in the interlobular septa near the periphery of the lungs may be visible as Kerley B lines, which are horizontal 1 cm markings at the edge of the lung fields. More marked accumulation of interstitial fluid results in prominence of the interstitial central lung markings and haziness of the central arterial and venous shadows. Ultimately, with frank alveolar fluid, confluent infiltrates occur, particularly in the perihilar areas, creating a "butterfly" appearance (Fig. 10-2, *A*). The presence of pleural effusion in CHF is suggested by the obscuring of the costophrenic and costovertebral angles.

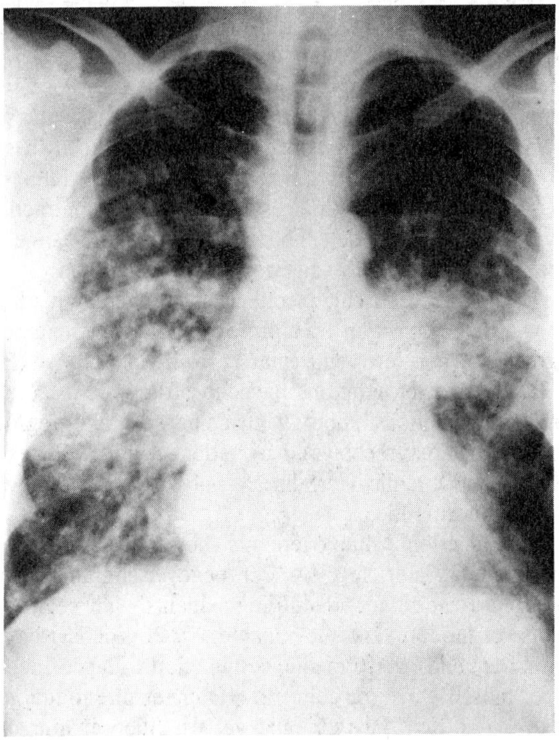

A

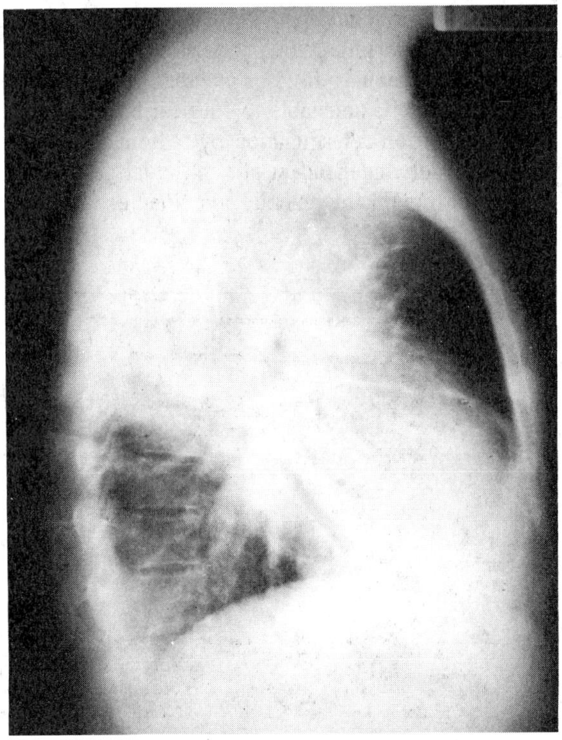

B

Fig. 10-2. Posteroanterior (**A**) and lateral (**B**) chest radiographs of patient in heart failure. There is cardiac enlargement, which is seen on the lateral projection as primarily left ventricular. Lung fields demonstrate the typical "butterfly" pattern of pulmonary edema.

Noninvasive studies

The development of noninvasive techniques has aided the evaluation of patients with CHF (Chapter 5). M-mode echocardiography has been particularly useful in characterizing valvular abnormalities (primarily mitral stenosis) and identifying right ventricular, left atrial, and left ventricular chamber enlargement (Fig. 10-3). The diagnosis of pericardial effusion as a cause of increased heart size has been greatly facilitated by two-dimensional (2D) and M-mode echocardiography.

Before the advent of echocardiography and radionuclide angiography, it was difficult by noninvasive methods to separate patients with myocardial disease from those with low "effective" cardiac outputs but normal contractility.

Now, both techniques provide reasonable estimates of the left ventricular ejection fraction, a measure of myocardial performance. Patients with depressed function generally have low ejection fractions (<50%), whereas those with normal contractility have normal or supernormal values.

M-mode echocardiography may also be used to assess the mean V_{cf}, percentage of minor dimension shortening (% ΔD), and other clinical indices of myocardial contractility (Fig. 10-3). In M-mode echocardiography the distance between the E point of the anterior mitral leaflet and the left side of the interventricular septum varies inversely with the left ventricular ejection fraction. Septal E point separation is greatest when left ventricular performance is low (Fig. 10-3). Such determinations by echocardiography requires certain assumptions about ventricular size and regional function that may be invalid in patients with CHF, especially when ischemic heart disease may cause regional wall motion abnormalities.

This objection can be overcome, however, by the use of high-quality, multiple-view 2D echocardiograms. Such studies are useful for identifying patients with segmental disease of the left ventricle (Chapter 5). 2D echocardiography is frequently performed in conjunction with continuous-wave, pulsed-wave, or color flow Doppler interrogation of the A-V, aortic, and pulmonic valves. Such examination allows not only an evaluation of overall ventricular performance but also the accurate detection and semiquantitation of stenotic and/or regurgitant valvular disease. This approach is therefore important in identifying patients with CHF caused by valvular diseases or other structural abnormalities that may be amenable to surgical intervention.

Ejection fraction determination by radionuclide angiography is relatively independent of ventricular geometry and regional wall motion. In general, combined echocardiography and radionuclide angiography yield extensive, valuable information about the causes and compensatory mechanisms of CHF. However, the cost of these studies is considerable, and their appropriate application to patients must be determined individually.

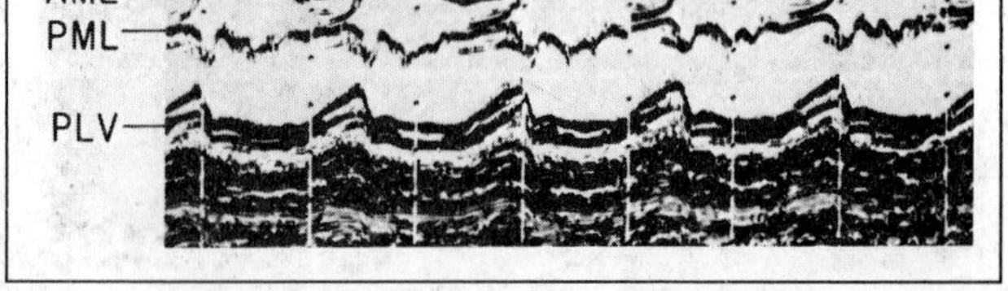

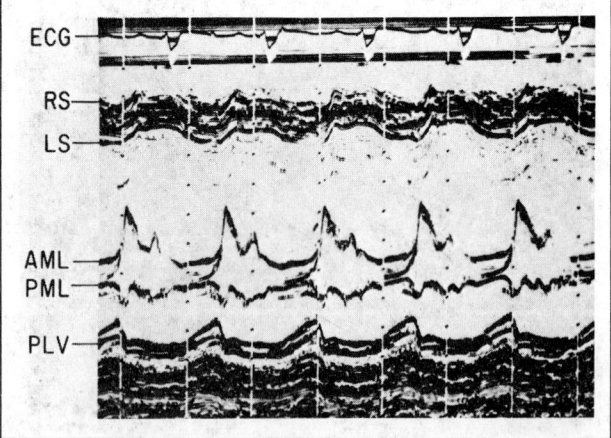

Fig. 10-3. M-mode echocardiogram at the level of the left ventricle and mitral valve in a patient with CHF. Marked left ventricular dilatation and reduced systolic shortening are present. There is also increased separation between the side of the septum and the anterior mitral leaflet. *RS,* Right septum; *LS,* left septum; *AML,* anterior mitral leaflet; *PML,* posterior mitral leaflet; *PLV,* posterior left ventricular wall. Distance between the two ventricle dots is 1 cm.

Cardiac catheterization

The ultimate diagnostic tool for establishing the cause and pathophysiologic features of CHF is cardiac catheterization (Chapter 6). Although the findings at catheterization may be dominated by the primary cardiac disease (e.g., a left ventricle to aorta pressure gradient in aortic stenosis), several features are typical of heart failure in general. First, intracardiac diastolic pressures are elevated. If mitral or tricuspid stenosis is present, this elevation is at the level of the atrium, whereas in the absence of A-V valve obstruction, both end-diastolic ventricular pressure and mean atrial pressure are increased. Depending on the relative involvement of the ventricles, either right or left, or both, ventricular diastolic pressures may be elevated. Second, pulmonary artery pressures are usually increased because of elevated left-sided filling pressures, primary disease in the pulmonary vasculature, or hypoxemia. Cardiac output at rest may be low, normal, or high, as may the AV O_2 content difference in an inverse manner. In the presence of normal or high cardiac outputs, exercise during catheterization often reveals impaired cardiac reserve. Normally during exercise, cardiac output should increase 6 dl/min for each deciliter increase in O_2 consumption (i.e., the normal exercise factor), and filling pressures should remain constant. In patients with CHF the exercise factor may be reduced, and filling pressures may rise during adequate exertion.

Angiographic data may be used to determine chamber size, detect the presence of valvular regurgitation, and assess global and regional shortening characteristics of the ventricle (e.g., ejection fraction). In CHF with compensatory dilatation and/or hypertrophy, ventricular volumes may be increased, and mitral or tricuspid regurgitation can be detected even in the absence of characteristic hemodynamic changes. If either local or global myocardial disease is present, the ejection fraction may be reduced (to <50%). Finally, coronary arteriography may be performed to assess the potential role of myocardial ischemia in the pathophysiology of CHF in a given patient.

TREATMENT

Treatment of the patient with CHF should be directed toward specific therapeutic goals. The first is to improve ventricular performance either by inotropic stimulation or by manipulation of both preload and afterload to obtain an effective ejection fraction. The second objective is to decrease the cardiac filling pressures, thereby improving the patient's functional capacity and quality of life. The third therapeutic goal, which is now being attained through some of the newer treatment modalities, is to improve survival. The exact approach to therapy for an individual patient largely depends on the specific cause and pathophysiologic features.

In every patient the search for primary and precipitating causes of CHF should be undertaken to ensure maximum success of long-term therapy.

Reduction in peripheral demands

Significant reductions in peripheral demands for cardiac output accompany bed rest, an often neglected therapeutic modality. Physical and emotional rest decreases skeletal muscle needs for blood flow and provides for redistribution of cardiac output to the kidneys, promoting diuresis. Bed rest should be maintained until heart failure has stabilized; the increased risk of thromboembolism may be ameliorated by anticoagulants, footboards, and elastic stockings. In the patient with chronic heart failure, daily activity should be limited, with periodic rest sessions. Smoking should be discontinued because nicotine increases peripheral and myocardial O_2 requirements and may elevate systemic vascular resistance, further compromising ventricular function. Alcohol consumption should be kept to a minimum because its ingestion may impair ventricular performance transiently or chronically.

Dietary management, especially sodium restriction, has traditionally played a significant role in the treatment of patients with CHF. The average American diet contains 3 to 6 g of sodium, which is sufficient to aggravate the tendency to salt and water retention seen in heart failure. Therefore mildly symptomatic patients (NYHA Functional Class II) should be discouraged from adding salt at the table and should eliminate highly salted foods, such as potato chips, pretzels, and soups. These simple measures should reduce the dietary sodium to 1.5 to 3.0 g/day. More symptomatic patients (NYHA Functional Class III and Class IV) should reduce dietary sodium intake to 1.0 to 1.5 g/day by eliminating salt from cooking. Diets enforcing an even more stringent reduction of sodium are not only expensive but are extremely unpalatable and are unlikely to be adhered to by any patient, no matter how conscientious. Other dietary measures, such as attainment and maintenance of ideal body weight, should be advised in an attempt to improve functional capacity. Heavy meals impose unnecessary circulatory demands through the digestive process, and patients should be advised of the relative benefits of frequent small meals.

Other associated diseases that augment peripheral needs for blood should be identified and treated. These include (1) infections, (2) anemia, (3) hyperthyroidism, and (4) thiamine deficiency (beriberi), which impairs ATP production and simulates cellular anoxia.

Enhancement of ventricular function curve

Displacement of the ventricular function curve upward and to the left results in an increased cardiac output and a reduced atrial pressure for any given venous return curve (Fig. 10-4). This may be accomplished by increasing the inotropic state of the ventricle or reducing the afterload. A further possibility in patients with certain cardiac arrhythmias is the restoration of normal sinus rhythm. In patients

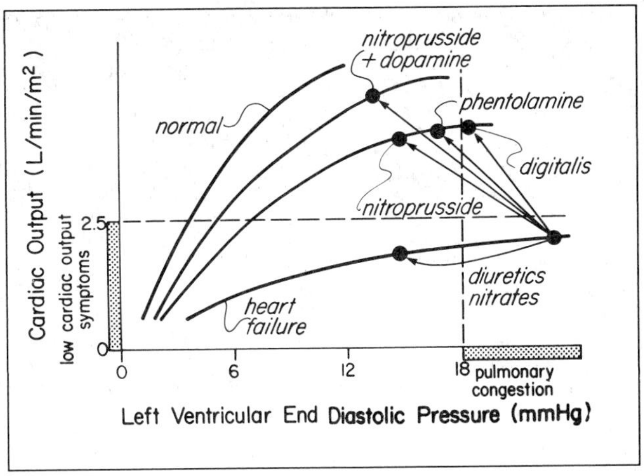

Fig. 10-4. Effects of various therapeutic interventions on the ventricular function curve in patients with CHF. Afterload reduction and/or positive inotropic agents displace the relationship upward, whereas diuretics and nitrates reduce filling pressure without displacing the curve. Dotted areas indicate levels at which symptoms of low cardiac output or pulmonary congestion occur. (Modified from Mason DT, editor: Congestive heart failure. New York, 1976, Yorke Medical Books.)

with atrial fibrillation the restoration of atrial contraction may increase cardiac output by up to 30%, particularly in those with left ventricular pressure overload and/or diminished left ventricular compliance.

Increase in inotropic state. Enhanced contractility is accomplished primarily by the administration of positive inotropic drugs. Currently, digitalis is the only such therapeutic agent available for long-term oral use. The mechanism in the enhanced contractility mediated by digitalis is still unknown, but the glycoside may act by indirectly increasing intracellular calcium through its inhibitory effects on the (Na^+, K^+)-ATPase pump. Digitalis is particularly effective in low cardiac output states caused by depressed ventricular function and in CHF accompanied by supraventricular tachyarrhythmias, in which digitalis reduces A-V nodal conduction. In high output states, when myocardial function is normal or supranormal, digitalis is of questionable therapeutic benefit. In hypertrophic cardiomyopathy, it may be contraindicated (Chapter 17).

In addition to its positive inotropic properties, digitalis has recently been shown to modulate neurohumoral compensatory mechanisms in patients with CHF. The acute administration of a cardiac glycoside to these patients results in decreases in muscle sympathetic nerve activity, in circulating norepinephrine levels, and in circulating plasma renin levels. These neurohormonal changes are accompanied by peripheral vasodilatation and increased forearm blood flow. How important are these neuroendocrine effects? This remains unanswered, but they may contribute to the beneficial effects of digitalis in CHF.

The administration of the glycoside depends on the preparation and how rapidly a clinical effect is desired. Both therapeutic and toxic effects are related somewhat to the

Table 10-1. Cardiac glycoside preparations

Agent	Gastrointestinal (GI) absorption	Onset of action (min)*	Peak effect (hr)	Average half-life	Principal excretory pathway	Average digitalizing dose (mg) Oral	Average digitalizing dose (mg) Intravenous	Usual daily oral maintenance dose (mg)
Ouabain	Unreliable	5-10	½-2	21 hr	Renal; some GI excretion		0.3-0.5	
Digoxin	60%-85%†	15-30	1½-5	36-42 hr	Renal; some GI excretion	1.25-1.5	0.75-1.0	0.25-0.5
Digitoxin	90%-100%	25-120	4-12	4-6 days	Hepatic‡; renal excretion of metabolites	0.7-1.2	1.0	0.10-0.15

*For intravenous dose.
†For tablet form of administration (may be less in malabsorption syndromes and in formulations with poor bioavailability).
‡Enterohepatic cycle exists.

serum level achieved. In patients with severe CHF, a loading dose optimizes the early effects of digitalis therapy. In patients with mild CHF, digoxin therapy can be initiated with a maintenance dose.

The pharmacokinetic properties of the frequently used digitalis preparations are summarized in Table 10-1. Maintenance doses must be adjusted when major excretory pathways are compromised (i.e., glomerular filtration with digoxin, hepatic function with digitoxin). Also, the maintenance dose of digoxin must often be reduced in patients receiving concomitant quinidine therapy. Except for the ventricular response to atrial fibrillation, therapeutic efficacy and borderline toxicity are difficult to judge. The availability of serum drug level determinations has been a significant advance in glycoside therapy.

Sympathomimetic amines, which enhance contractility by stimulation of cardiac beta receptors, are another class of agents that provide inotropic support. The typically used drugs are isoproterenol, dopamine, and dobutamine, all of which must be given by constant intravenous (IV) infusion. Their positive inotropic effects are powerful, and short-term administration in an intensive care unit (ICU) setting may be particularly beneficial in patients with severe or refractory CHF and/or cardiogenic shock (Chapter 11).

Dopamine, in addition to its beta-agonist properties, can enhance renal blood flow and facilitate a diuresis by stimulation of a dopaminergic receptor in the renal vasculature. However, at doses greater than 10 μg/kg/min, the drug also acts on alpha receptors, increasing peripheral vascular resistance, blood pressure, and therefore ventricular afterload. This may reverse its otherwise beneficial properties. Dobutamine, on the other hand, has little alpha-adrenergic activity and, despite its beta-stimulating properties, has relatively little effect on heart rate. Dobutamine does not primarily increase renal blood flow, as does dopamine, but may effect an indirect diuresis by increasing cardiac output. In addition to its short-term use for the acutely decompensated patient, dobutamine has been given on to support patients awaiting cardiac transplantation. These patients are given an infusion of dobutamine, 5 μ/kg/min for 8 hours, on an outpatient basis, and this may be repeated weekly.

Several new inotropic agents appear to improve cardiac function by mechanisms different from those of the cardiac glycosides. With some of these agents the positive inotropic effect appears to be catecholamine-mediated action secondary to beta-adrenoreceptor stimulation, whereas with others the effect is independent of catecholamines.

Beta-adrenoreceptor agonists can be divided into two groups, those that directly activate myocardial $beta_2$ receptors (prenalterol) and those whose primary action is to improve cardiovascular performance through $beta_1$-receptor-mediated systemic vasodilatation (pirbuterol, albuterol, terbutaline). Although it is tempting to group these agents in this way pharmacologically, the distinction probably is lost in clinical doses, and both types of beta adrenoreceptors most likely are activated by both groups of drugs. When these drugs are administered acutely to patients with severe CHF, significant increases in cardiac output and decreases in left ventricular end-diastolic pressure result. These changes, together with a diminished systemic vascular resistance, are present both at rest and during exercise. However, with long-term administration of these agents, the hemodynamic improvement is progressively lost, probably because of a "downregulation" of beta adrenoreceptors, that is, fewer beta receptors to be stimulated. Moreover, the improvement in cardiac function with beta-receptor agonists is accompanied by significant increases in heart rate and myocardial O_2 consumption and renders their use in patients with coronary artery disease inadvisable, since these drugs tend to exacerbate angina pectoris. Other serious potential adverse effects of these agents are ventricular and supraventricular tachyarrhythmias. Therefore, despite the demonstrated hemodynamic benefits of beta-receptor agonists when given acutely, it is unlikely that they constitute a major therapeutic modality in the management of CHF.

Both positive inotropic actions and peripheral vasodilator effects can be ascribed to noncardiac glycoside, noncatecholamine inotropic agents such as amrinone, milrinone, enoximone, and piroximone. Although these compounds' exact mechanisms of action are unknown, it has been shown that all inhibit myocardial phosphodiesterase activity and therefore presumably improve cardiac contractility through an increase in calcium availability mediated by cyclic adenosine monophosphate (cAMP). Of this group of agents, the most clinical experience has been gained with the bipyridine compound amrinone. Studies have shown both acute and sustained hemodynamic improvement in patients with severe CHF when given IV or oral amrinone. Only the IV form has received Food and Drug Administration (FDA) approval and is available for short-term use in the ICU setting.

Preliminary studies with milrinone, enoximone, and piroximone suggested that the drugs produced sustained hemodynamic improvement both at rest and with exercise. Subsequent long-term follow-up, however, indicated that patients taking these drugs had a significantly higher mortality than those taking the placebo. Therefore it is unlikely that any of these agents will be recommended as long-term, positive inotropic, oral agents for the treatment of CHF. IV milrinone recently has been approved for the treatment of severe CHF. It is more potent than amrinone but has similar vasodilator and positive inotropic effects. Milrinone has been particularly beneficial in patients with severe pulmonary hypertension and diminished cardiac output.

The precise role of all the new inotropic agents in the long-term management of chronic heart failure remains undefined. Although conceptually an agent conferring both inotropic and vasodilatory benefits would appear ideal, many unresolved issues remain at this time, including drug tolerance with chronic administration. Many of these compounds are undergoing extensive clinical trials, but only the IV forms of amrinone and milrinone have been released for general use.

Afterload reduction. As discussed previously, a sympathetically mediated net increase in total peripheral vascular resistance typically occurs in CHF. The increased peripheral resistance increases ventricular afterload, thereby further impairing cardiac output from an already compromised ventricle because of the inverse relationship between stroke volume and afterload (Chapter 1). For this reason, arterial vasodilators have been increasingly used to decrease peripheral vascular resistance, and thus afterload, in patients with CHF in an attempt to improve forward cardiac output and decrease ventricular filling pressures. Although the rationale for the use of arterial vasodilators in heart failure is based on sound principles, two limitations of this approach must be stressed.

First, the ability of vasodilator therapy to increase cardiac output depends on the adequacy of venous return. Many agents currently employed clinically for afterload reduction have venodilating properties that increase venous capacitance, decrease mean circulatory pressure, and shift the venous return curve downward and to the left (Chapter 1). Depending on the new intersection of the enhanced ventricular function curve and the altered venous return curve, cardiac output may be increased, decreased, or unchanged. Patients whose plasma volume is normal or reduced may have no improvement or a reduction in cardiac output.

Second, depending on the ultimate level of cardiac output achieved, arterial pressure may remain relatively unchanged or fall. Because coronary flow largely depends on aortic pressure in diastole, a fall in diastolic pressure below 60 mm Hg may be associated with myocardial ischemia, particularly in the patient with coronary artery disease. Ischemia will aggravate myocardial dysfunction, and the net effect may be diastrous. At present, it is difficult on clinical grounds alone to identify clearly patients who will benefit from afterload reduction. Therefore the most judicious use of these agents requires invasive hemodynamic monitoring with actual measurement of filling pressures and cardiac output.

Vasodilator therapy appears particularly useful in patients with pulmonary edema, severe mitral regurgitation, and refractory CHF from myocardial disease. In the acute setting, nitroprusside (arterial and venous dilatation), by continuous IV infusion, is the most widely used agent. It has a rapid onset, brief duration of action, and minimum toxicity during short-term administration. However, cyanide is liberated by the combination of nitroprusside with sulfhydryl groups in red cells and tissue; cyanide is converted by the liver to thiocyanate, which is excreted by the kidney. In the patient with impaired renal or hepatic function, cyanide and/or thiocyanate can accumulate, causing metabolic acidosis, confusion, and seizures. With low infusion rates, lasting less than 72 hours, toxicity is almost never observed. In infusions of greater duration, thiocyanate levels may serve as a guide to potential toxicity in that levels less than 10 mg/dl are generally well tolerated. Signs and symptoms of cyanide or thiocyanate poisoning usually resolve quickly with discontinuation of the drug.

For oral afterload reduction, hydralazine (arterial dilatation) and prazosin (arterial and venous dilatation) are the agents most widely employed. However, the long-term use of prazosin, an alpha-adrenergic antagonist, is controversial, and some studies have demonstrated tachyphylaxis to its initially favorable hemodynamic effects. On the other hand, sustained hemodynamic benefit has been shown after long-term oral administration of hydralazine. However, the precise role of long-term oral vasodilators in the management of patients with CHF requires further clarification. Nevertheless, prazosin, hydralazine, and hydralazine plus long-acting nitrates (venous dilatation) are being used for long-term therapy in many patients with congestive cardiomyopathy (Chapter 17).

Recognition of the role of the renin-angiotensin system as an important contributor to the increased systemic vascular resistance in chronic heart failure has lead to clinical trials of angiotensin-converting enzyme (ACE) inhibitors as adjuvant or even primary vasodilator therapy. The orally active ACE inhibitor captopril has produced impressive hemodynamic improvement in many patients with CHF. This drug, and its more recent analog, enalapril, blocks the conversion of angiotensin I to angiotensin II. The latter is the vasoactive form, which causes arteriolar vasoconstriction. Administration of an ACE inhibitor often results in marked hemodynamic improvement both at rest and with exercise. Long-term treatment is accompanied by sustained improvement in cardiac output and reduced filling pressures, thus ameliorating symptoms and improving functional capacity. Several controlled clinical trials have shown that captopril in doses of 25 to 50 mg three times daily can result in long-term (up to 2 years) hemodynamic improvement in as many as 70% of patients treated for CHF. Hemodynamic tolerance is rare with ACE inhibitors, and adverse reactions occur infrequently. Symptomatic hypotension may occur, especially within the first 24 hours of treatment and especially in patients who have received large doses of an IV diuretic or who have severe hyponatremia. A maculopapular skin rash occurs in 8% to 10% of patients taking captopril, and an elevation of blood urea nitrogen has been reported in about 20% of such patients. The latter effect, which usually responds to a reduction in diuretic therapy, most frequently occurs in patients in whom the left ventricular filling pressure and cardiac output are both reduced. Proteinuria and neutropenia reported with high-dose captopril therapy are rarely seen with the lower dosage currently used in the management of chronic heart failure. The incidence of enalapril-induced side effects is approximately half that seen with captopril, although the spectrum of side effects with both drugs is similar. Overall experience indicates that most patients with severe chronic CHF respond favorably to therapy with an ACE inhibitor and that adverse reactions to the drugs are rarely sufficient to discontinue therapy.

During the past several years, it has clearly been established that vasodilator therapy results in significant hemodynamic improvement in patients with CHF. Cardiac output is increased, and filling pressures are reduced. The patients are less symptomatic, and because of the reduced filling pressures, their exercise tolerance is increased, and their overall quality of life is greatly improved. Only recently, however, has it been shown that vasodilator therapy has additional benefits in patients with CHF. Large multicenter clinical trials have demonstrated that both hydralazine, in combination with a long-acting nitrate, and the ACE inhibitor enalapril effect a significant improvement in longevity in heart failure patients, in addition to providing symptomatic relief (Fig. 10-5). Given the overall hemodynamic benefits, therefore, in conjunction with the salutary effect on longevity, it now seems reasonable that vasodilator therapy should be attempted in all patients with NYHA functional class III and class IV heart failure and should be seriously considered even for those who are less symptomatic (NYHA functional class II).

This latter point is particularly strengthened by two recently published clinical trials, in which an ACE inhibitor was given to patients who had depressed left ventricular function but who had not developed overt clinical CHF. In one study the number of patients developing CHF over the course of the study significantly decreased. In the other study, involving patients with depressed left ventricular function after a Q wave, anterior wall myocardial infarction, the administration of an ACE inhibitor resulted in an improved survival and a decrease in left ventricular dysfunction. In view of this, serious consideration must now be given to administering ACE inhibitors as early as possible during the course of CHF in an attempt to prevent progression of the disease.

Reduction in cardiac filling pressures

As previously mentioned, elevation of pulmonary and systemic venous pressures is responsible for many of the symp-

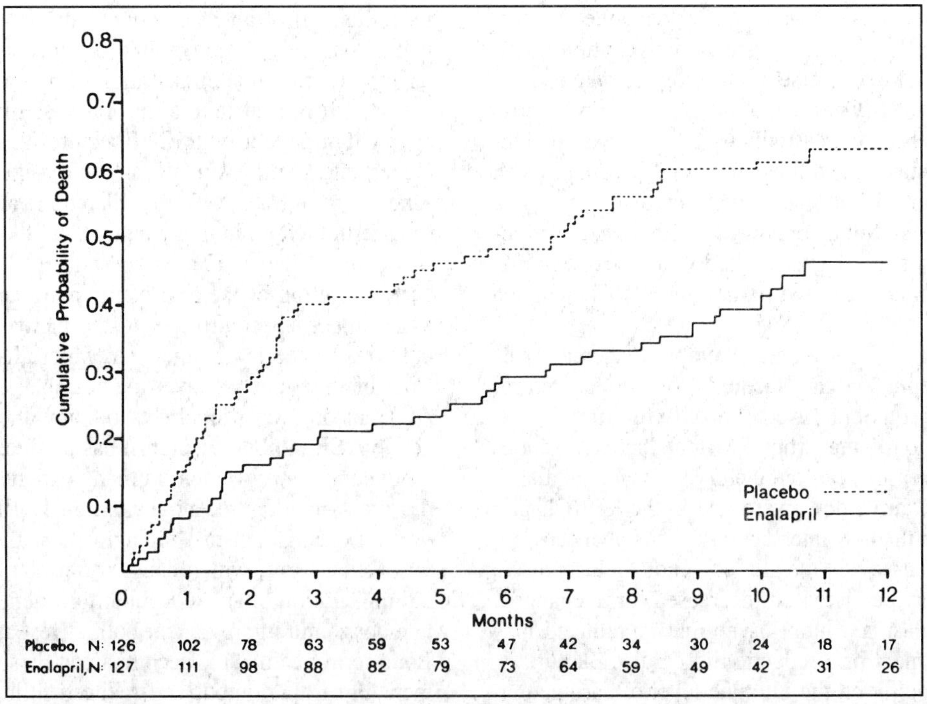

Fig. 10-5. Cumulative probability of death in patients with NYHA functional class IV heart failure randomized to either placebo or enalapril. Therapy was adjunctive to conventional treatment. Difference at 1 year is statistically significant ($P < 0.007$). (From CONSENSUS Trial Study Group: N Engl J Med 316:1429, 1987. Reprinted by permission.)

toms of CHF. Therefore one of the main objectives of treatment is to decrease atrial pressure below levels at which congestive symptoms arise. This is partly accomplished by the therapeutic interventions previously described, but additional benefit is often derived from primary reductions in venous return. Atrial pressure, as discussed in Chapter 1, is determined by the intersection of the venous return curve with the ventricular function curve. Consequently, a displacement of the venous return curve downward and to the left, accomplished by either a reduction in blood volume or an increase in venous capacitance, results in a lower atrial pressure. A decrease in plasma volume is facilitated by diuretics, which enhance salt and water excretion by the kidney; increases in venous capacitance may follow venodilator administration. However, a downward displacement of the venous return curve reduces cardiac output, as well as atrial pressure. Thus venodilator or diuretic therapy in a patient with low cardiac output may aggravate CHF, although patients with predominantly congestive symptoms and relatively "adequate" cardiac outputs because of compensatory mechanisms may benefit significantly. Furthermore, because ventricular size is a major determinant of wall stress, a reduction in atrial pressure may decrease afterload and even improve the ventricular function curve, resulting in no net change in cardiac output.

A variety of diuretic agents are available to increase sodium and water excretion by the kidney. The choice of a specific drug depends partly on the condition's severity and the patient's electrolyte status. For mild CHF, the thiazide diuretics are effective by preventing reabsorption of sodium in the distal tubule. Thiazides may also act indirectly by depleting sodium from vessel walls, thereby decreasing the resting stiffness component of arterioles and thus reducing total peripheral resistance. For more severe fluid retention, furosemide or ethacrynic acid is appropriate. These potent agents inhibit active sodium chloride reabsorption in the ascending loop of Henle. This leads to a decrease in the urinary concentrating action, often increasing urine flow to as much as one third of glomerular filtration. However, furosemide, ethacrynic acid, and the thiazides enhance potassium excretion by stimulating the Na^+-K^+ exchange mechanism in the distal tubule and may also interfere with free water excretion. Consequently, profound hypokalemia, which may predispose to digitalis toxicity, and dilutional hyponatremia may complicate long-term administration. The hypokalemia may in part be attenuated by concomitant therapy with spironolactone or triamterene, drugs that inhibit the Na^+-K^+ exchange mechanism in the distal tubule. Although by themselves these agents are relatively weak diuretics, with the thiazides or furosemide or in patients with secondary hyperaldosteronism, they can potentiate the resultant diuresis. However, with severe renal compromise, either primary or secondary to advanced CHF, spironolactone or triamterene may precipitate fatal hyperkalemia. This is particularly true if these agents are used with an ACE inhibitor. In fact, it is not recommended that a potassium-sparing diuretic be given in conjunction with any ACE inhibitors.

The principal venodilators are the nitrates, although, as mentioned, some arterial vasodilators (prazosin, nitroprusside, phentolamine) also have considerable action on the venous bed. Sublingual nitroglycerin, although effective, is generally too short acting to have great clinical utility as a venodilator in CHF. Therefore the principal agents are nitroglycerin ointment and isosorbide dinitrate. These drugs are most effective in patients with symptoms of pulmonary congestion but relatively adequate cardiac output, since administration usually reduces filling pressure and stroke volume. In patients with ischemic heart disease, myocardial function may improve with the decline in myocardial O_2 demands that follows the decrease in wall tension mediated by these agents.

• • •

Most patients first seek medical advice for heart failure while their symptoms are still moderate (NYHA functional class II). It is imperative at this stage to identify and, if possible, treat the underlying cause of the pathophysiologic state. Therapy at this time should include the general measures previously discussed: physical and emotional rest, moderate restriction of dietary sodium, and institution of digitalis and diuretic therapy. In view of recent studies, serious consideration should also be given to the administration of an ACE inhibitor. The patient's failure to respond to these measures requires more aggressive afterload reduction, increased diuretic dosage, or a more potent diuretic; further symptomatic improvement may result from the administration of a venodilator such as isosorbide dinitrate.

The various therapeutic modalities and their effects on the ventricular function curve are summarized in Fig. 10-4. Frequently the combination of a positive inotropic drug and a vasodilator can considerably enhance the cardiac output obtainable at any level of atrial pressure.

TREATMENT OF ACUTE PULMONARY EDEMA

As mentioned earlier, elevations in left atrial pressure that result in the rapid accumulation of alveolar fluid constitute a medical emergency. Since cardiac output and arterial pressure in this situation are generally adequate, therapy must be directed toward prompt lowering of left atrial pressure. In addition to the measures already discussed (positive inotropic agents, rapidly acting diuretics, vasodilators), the following measures should be instituted.

1. *Oxygen, 100%.* Fluid in alveolar spaces impairs gas exchange in the lung, resulting in arterial hypoxemia and often in retention of carbon dioxide. This further increases peripheral demands for cardiac output and may primarily depress myocardial performance, further elevating filling pressure. If hypoxemia cannot be corrected with O_2 inhalation by mask, intubation with positive end-expiratory pressure may be required.

2. *Morphine sulfate.* Parenteral morphine is a venodilator and will decrease venous return. Also, through its sedative properties, morphine may reduce the intense alpha-adrenergic stimulation that accompanies anxiety, thereby decreasing both preload and afterload. However, respira-

tory depression from overdosage must be monitored; if necessary, a morphine antagonist (naloxone) can be administered.

3. *Aminophylline*. Bronchospasm frequently complicates acute pulmonary edema, and aminophylline is useful for reversing airway constriction. In addition, the drug has a positive inotropic action, which may be related to its inhibition of phosphodiesterase, the enzyme that catalyzes the breakdown of cAMP. Aminophylline also may dilate smooth muscle in the vasculature, increase renal blood flow, and enhance sodium excretion—actions that contribute to its salutary effects. However, ventricular arrhythmias and, rarely, hypotension may be encountered. Therefore aminophylline must be administered slowly (over 20 minutes) in a dilute form, avoiding doses greater than 300 mg.

PITFALLS IN DIAGNOSIS AND TREATMENT

Heart failure is a complex pathophysiologic state; its understanding in a given patient requires a synthesis of physical findings, laboratory tests, and principles of cardiovascular physiology and pathology. Several common errors in evaluation and treatment follow.

1. *Failure to interpret mean venous pressure properly*. Inability to evaluate right atrial pressure makes differentiation of CHF from other edematous states (e.g., cirrhosis, venous obstruction) difficult.

2. *Failure to identify cardiac and pulmonary components of dyspnea*. As mentioned in Chapter 1, both elevation of left atrial pressure and primary lung disease may cause dyspnea and identical pulmonary physical findings. The presence of cardiomegaly, left-sided diastolic gallop sounds, and reduced left ventricular performance on noninvasive studies favor a cardiac origin, whereas reduced performance on pulmonary function tests suggests lung disease. Frequently, precise differentiation cannot be made on clinical grounds alone, and cardiac catheterization is required to clarify the pathophysiology.

3. *Failure to identify aggravating and precipitating causes of CHF*. Cardiac disease is frequently exacerbated by the development of secondary processes that further impair a compromised myocardium or increase peripheral demands for cardiac output. Failure to recognize and treat these aggravating factors often results in an unsatisfactory response to therapy. Therefore all patients with CHF should be examined for the following complicating conditions:

a. Recent myocardial infarction (which may be silent) or other evidence of increasing myocardial ischemia
b. Pulmonary embolism
c. Infection, including bacterial endocarditis
d. Anemia, pregnancy, and thyrotoxicosis, which increase peripheral flow demands
e. Systemic hypertension
f. Cardiac arrhythmias

Frequently, physicians attribute increasing chronic heart failure to excessive dietary intake of salt and water or noncompliance with a pharmacologic regimen, ignoring one of these more important mechanisms.

4. *Failure to identify surgically remediable causes of CHF*. With the advent of modern cardiovascular surgery, CHF caused by valvular lesions and other mechanical abnormalities (e.g., intracardiac shunts, ventricular aneurysms, constrictive pericarditis) is primarily correctable. Therefore the hemodynamic significance of valvular abnormalities and ventricular function should be assessed by physical examination and noninvasive studies. Ultimately, cardiac catheterization may be required for definitive evaluation and diagnosis.

5. *Failure to identify systemic illness associated with CHF*. Systemic diseases, including collagen vascular, metabolic, and endocrine, congenital, and neuromuscular disorders, have varying degrees of cardiac involvement and may present with heart failure. Since specialized forms of therapy may be required to treat the primary pathologic entity, an awareness of these associations is vital to management of the patient.

6. *Failure to use cardiac glycosides properly*. Digitalis is an agent with a narrow therapeutic index. Inadequate dosage often results in a suboptimum positive inotropic effect, whereas overdosage often precipitates toxicity. Therefore a proper understanding of glycoside pharmacology is imperative for maintaining an appropriate drug level. For digoxin, a level of 1 to 2 ng/ml of serum is generally considered therapeutic, although the reliability of such values in a given laboratory must be established. Factors that decrease absorption (e.g., intestinal edema from severe right-sided heart failure) and decrease excretion (e.g., fall in glomerular filtration rate) must be considered in adjusting maintenance doses. In patients with atrial fibrillation, the ventricular response to atrial fibrillation, not the serum level, is the best measure of adequate digitalization.

7. *Overdiuresis of patients with moderate-to-severe CHF*. As previously mentioned, diuretics alone generally do not improve cardiac output; they are most effective for relieving symptoms of circulatory congestion by promoting excretion of salt and water. In patients with low cardiac output the Frank-Starling mechanism may be vital for maintaining stroke volume, and overdiuresis can therefore aggravate the condition, primarily by decreasing further renal blood flow. In such patients, cardiac output must be improved. In patients without frank pulmonary congestion, this can be accomplished by rehydration; in those with extremely elevated left-sided pressures, parenteral inotropic agents and/or vasodilator therapy may be required. Also, electrolyte disturbances often accompany overzealous diuretic use, and hypokalemic, hypochloremic alkalosis should be corrected by the administration of potassium chloride.

REFERENCES

Captopril Multicenter Research Group: A placebo-controlled trial of captopril in refractory chronic congestive heart failure. J Am Coll Cardiol 2:755, 1984.

Cohn JN et al: Effect of vasodilator therapy on mortality in congestive heart failure: results of a Veterans Administration Cooperative Study (V-HeFT). N Engl J Med 314:1547, 1986.

Cohn JN et al: A comparison of enalapril with hydralazine–isosorbide dinitrate in the treatment of chronic congestive heart failure. N Engl J Med 325:303, 1991.
CONSENSUS Trial Study Group: Effects of enalapril on mortality in severe congestive heart failure: results of the Cooperative North Scandinavian Enalapril Survival Study (CONSENSUS), N Engl J Med 316:1429, 1987.
Ferguson DW et al: Sympathoinhibitory responses to digitalis glycosides in heart failure patients: direct evidence from sympathetic neural recordings. Circulation 80:65, 1989.
Franciosa JA, Dunkman WB, and Leddy CL: Hemodynamic effects of vasodilators and long term response in heart failure. J Am Coll Cardiol 3:1521, 1984.
Francis GS et al: The neurohumoral axis in congestive heart failure. Ann Intern Med 101:370, 1984.
McCall D and O'Rourke RA: Congestive heart failure. I. Biochemistry, pathophysiology, and neurohumoral mechanisms. Mod Concepts Cardiovasc Dis 54:55, 1985.
McCall D and O'Rourke RA: Congestive heart failure. II. Therapeutic options, old and new. Mod Concepts Cardiovasc Dis 54:61, 1985.
Packer M: Vasodilator and inotropic therapy for severe chronic heart failure: passion and skepticism. J Am Coll Cardiol 2:841, 1983.
Packer M, editor: Physiologic determinants of survival in congestive heart failure. Circulation 75(suppl 4):1, 1987.
Pfeffer MA et al: Effect of captopril on progressive ventricular dilatation after anterior myocardial infarction. N Engl J Med 319:80, 1988.
Scholz H: Inotropic drugs and their mechanism of action. J Am Coll Cardiol 4:389, 1984.
The SOLVD Investigators: Effect of enalapril on survival in patients with reduced left ventricular ejection fractions and congestive heart failure. N Engl J Med 325:293, 1991.

CHAPTER

11 Hypotension and Cardiogenic Shock

Robert A. O'Rourke
David McCall

Circulatory shock remains one of the few true medical emergencies. It represents the most severe complication of a variety of primary diseases, and the complex clinical picture results from an amalgam of the primary process and various cardiac and vascular compensatory mechanisms. The emergent nature of the syndrome of circulatory shock is such that it is frequently a harbinger of death. However, with prompt diagnosis, careful clinical and hemodynamic evaluation, and appropriate monitored therapy, complete survival is possible for many patients. Although the etiologies of hypotension and ultimately shock are diverse, the secondary pathophysiologic processes, many of which are responsible for the clinical picture and the ultimate downhill course, are common to all patients. These processes, which at the outset are compensatory and may lead to stabilization, frequently are progressive and, unless their vicious cycle is interrupted, can lead to steady deterioration of cardiovascular function. When progressive, the compensatory vasoconstriction may lead to ischemic failure of vital organs and to secondary metabolic changes (e.g., systemic acidosis) that will have a further deleterious effect on cardiovascular function. Knowledge of these pathophysiologic mechanisms is fundamental to the understanding of the syndrome of circulatory shock and is essential in devising appropriate therapeutic interventions. These interventions depend on an understanding of organ physiology, regulation of blood pressure, and the importance of tissue perfusion in the maintenance of organ homeostasis. The fundamental role played by maintenance of intravascular volume and the mechanisms of pharmacologic interventions, both vasoactive and inotropic, must be understood. Disturbances of both intravascular volume and myocardial performance are common to most types of circulatory shock. Therefore this discussion focuses primarily on hypovolemic shock and cardiogenic shock; the latter continues to be an important cause of death despite advances in the management of acute myocardial infarction.

DEFINITION AND ETIOLOGIC CLASSIFICATION OF SHOCK

Hypotension and shock are not synonymous. Simple lowering of the arterial blood pressure will result in hypotension, but without activation of the multiple compensatory operational cardiovascular reflexes, the clinical picture of shock is not present. Hypotension, however, is an obligatory component of shock. The term *shock* is reserved for a situation when an initial hypotension results in a general disorder of blood flow in which tissue perfusion and oxygen (O_2) delivery are reduced to levels below those required to meet metabolic demands. This decrease in flow and tissue perfusion, rather than the decrease in pressure, causes the rapid course of untreated shock with progressive circulatory failure, impaired tissue and cellular metabolism, and ultimately death.

Therefore the cardinal feature of circulatory shock is inadequate tissue perfusion and blood flow, and its differentiation from simple hypotension has important physiologic significance. Blood flow depends not only on perfusion pressure but also on vascular resistance. Flow can fall below the critical level required for cellular viability, and yet arterial blood pressure may be maintained by a compensatory increase in total systemic vascular resistance. Thus circulatory shock can occur without severe hypotension; in fact, hypotension is a relatively late sign in the course of shock and usually indicates a failure of compensatory mechanisms.

The distinction between shock and hypotension is also important therapeutically. In treating shock, the clinician must remember that flow is more important than pressure, and the immediate goal in treatment should be to restore adequate nutrient blood flow rapidly. If arterial pressure is simply raised by increasing vascular resistance, including to that of vital organs, nutrient flow may actually diminish, resulting in further ischemia and organ dysfunction.

The shock syndrome is better understood when the various initiating factors are classified according to several basic pathophysiologic mechanisms. For this purpose, it is helpful to view the circulatory system as composed of three fundamental components: the *cardiac pump,* the *circulating blood volume,* and the *vascular system,* comprising the arteries, veins, and microcirculation, which includes the arterioles, capillaries, and venules. A critical reduction in nutrient blood flow may result from a derangement in any one or several of these components. Based on the specific primary hemodynamic abnormality involved, circulatory shock can be classified into four major categories: (1) impairment of cardiac pump function *(cardiogenic shock),* (2) reduction in effective circulating blood volume *(hypovolemic shock),* (3) mechanical obstruction to central blood flow, and (4) vasomotor and microcirculatory dysfunction *(distributive shock).*

An acute reduction in cardiac output caused by hypovolemia or myocardial infarction is the most common cause of shock. Cardiogenic shock may result from mechanical dysfunction (decreased contractility) or electrical dysfunction (arrhythmias). Hypovolemic shock results from a decrease in intravascular volume that leads to a decrease in systemic filling pressure and venous return. Mechanical obstruction to blood flow can occur at any site along the circulatory system. For example, a massive pulmonary embolus can obstruct blood flow through the pulmonary arteries, whereas a pericardial effusion with cardiac tamponade may reduce blood flow into the right and left ventricles. Vascular dysfunction may result from a decrease in overall vasomotor tone or from failure of the microcirculation to supply adequate nutrient flow. A reduction in vasomotor tone leads to an increase in vascular capacity and a relative hypovolemia ("venous pooling" effect), which is seen in various forms of neurogenic shock (e.g., spinal cord injury). Microcirculatory failure may result from arteriovenous shunting, excessive arteriolar or precapillary sphincter constriction, or increased capillary permeability. These microvascular mechanisms play major roles in septic and anaphylactic shock.

An etiologic classification of shock and common precipitating factors are given in the box at right. Often, more than one mechanism contributes to progressive cardiovascular deterioration, particularly in the late stages of shock.

Etiologic factors in shock

I. Inadequate circulating blood volume (hypovolemic shock)
  A. Acute hemorrhage (e.g., trauma, gastrointestinal bleeding, retroperitoneal bleeding, hemoptysis, hemothorax, ruptured aortic aneurysm)
  B. Plasma volume loss
    1. Intestinal obstruction
    2. Peritonitis, pancreatitis, rapid accumulation of ascites
    3. Splanchnic ischemia
    4. Extensive burns or exudative skin disease
    5. Increased capillary permeability (prolonged hypoxia and ischemia, extensive tissue injury, anaphylaxis, sepsis)
  C. Excessive water and electrolyte losses
    1. Inadequate fluid and salt intake
    2. Excessive sweating
    3. Severe vomiting or diarrhea
    4. Excessive urinary losses (diabetes mellitus, diabetes insipidus, nephrotic syndrome, salt-losing nephropathy, postobstructive uropathy, diuretic phase of acute renal failure, excessive diuretic use)
    5. Acute adrenocortical insufficiency
II. Impairment of cardiac pump function (cardiogenic shock)
  A. Acute myocardial infarction
  B. Acute valvular regurgitation
  C. Cardiac rupture
  D. Severe congestive heart failure from any cause (ischemic, hypertensive, or valvular heart disease; cardiomyopathy; myocarditis)
III. Mechanical obstruction to central blood flow
  A. Obstruction to venous return or left ventricular filling
    1. Vena cava obstruction
    2. Cardiac tamponade
    3. Tension pneumothorax
    4. Prosthetic mitral valve thrombus
    5. Atrial myxoma
  B. Obstruction to left ventricular output
    1. Dissecting aortic aneurysm
    2. Prosthetic aortic valve thrombus
    3. Severe aortic stenosis
IV. Vasomotor and microvascular dysfunction
  A. Loss of vasomotor tone (neurogenic shock)
    1. Deep general anesthesia, spinal anesthesia
    2. Spinal cord or brain damage (vasomotor center)
    3. Drugs (adrenergic- and ganglionic-blocking agents, barbiturate and other drug overdoses)
    4. Anaphylaxis
  B. Microvascular failure
    1. Infection (septic shock)
      a. Gram-negative sepsis
      b. Other severe bacterial infections
    2. Anaphylaxis
    3. Prolonged shock from any cause

REGULATION OF TISSUE BLOOD FLOW AND OXYGEN DELIVERY

Since the essential feature of shock, regardless of etiology, is a critical reduction of nutrient flow, an understanding of pathophysiology requires a basic knowledge of the determinants of tissue blood flow and O_2 delivery (Fig. 11-1). Blood flow to any organ is determined by perfusion pressure and regional vascular resistance. The perfusion pressure is the driving force for flow and is the difference between arterial and venous pressure. Regional arterial pressure may be less than central aortic pressure because of changes in vessel size and arterial disease. This is especially important in the coronary vascular bed, where segmental atherosclerotic narrowing may create a substantial resistance to flow, with a fall in arterial pressure distal to the stenosis. Systemic arterial pressure is determined by cardiac output and total vascular resistance, which is the sum of all parallel and series resistances of the entire vascular tree. Cardiac output is controlled predominantly by factors that regulate heart rate, ventricular end-diastolic volume, and myocardial contractility. Regional vascular resistance is largely a function of the caliber of the arterioles (Poi-

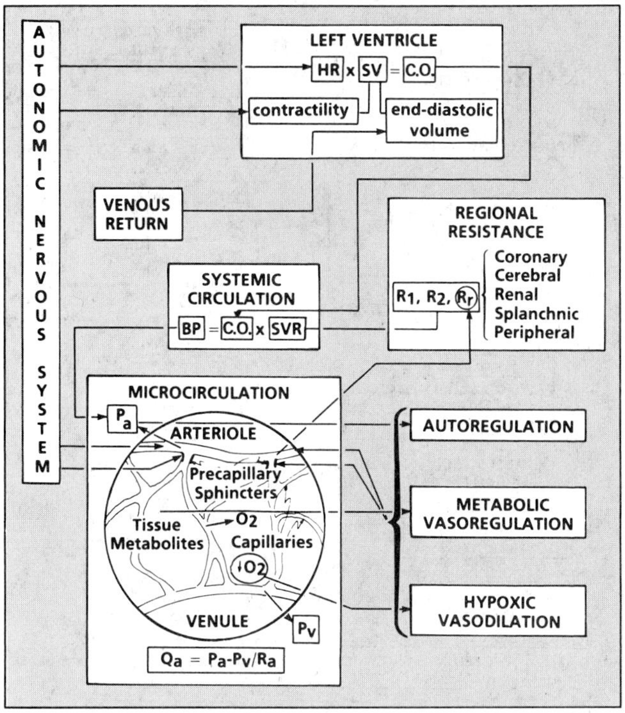

Fig. 11-1. Hemodynamic determinants and regulation of tissue flow and oxygen delivery. *HR,* Heart rate; *SV,* stroke volume; *C.O.*, cardiac output; *BP,* arterial blood pressure; *SVR,* systemic vascular resistance; R_1, R_2, R_r, regional organ resistances; P_a, arteriolar pressure; P_v, venular pressure; Q_a, arteriolar flow; R_a, arteriolar resistance.

seuille's law). Thus blood flow to any organ or tissue depends on systemic hemodynamics for generation of perfusion pressure and on regional vascular resistance.

Because perfusion pressure is relatively constant and the major resistance to blood flow occurs at the arterioles, these vessels are the primary site for blood flow regulation. The distribution of arterial flow through the capillary network for blood-tissue metabolic exchange is controlled by a precapillary sphincter, which by controlling the number of perfused capillaries, regulates the surface area available for diffusion and capillary-to-cell diffusion distances. These in turn determine the efficiency of O_2 delivery and metabolic exchange in the tissue.

In addition to transcapillary O_2 and metabolic exchange, the microcirculation also participates in the regulation of intravascular volume. The net movement of fluid across the capillary wall is determined by the balance between transmural capillary hydrostatic pressure and transmural oncotic pressure, by the permeability of the capillary membrane to water, small solutes, and proteins, and by the capillary surface area. The capillary hydrostatic pressure is related to the level of the arterial and venous pressures and also depends on the relationship of precapillary to postcapillary resistance. An increase in this resistance ratio will decrease capillary pressure and favor movement of fluid from the interstitial to the intravascular space, whereas a decrease in this ratio will increase capillary pressure and favor movement of fluid out of the intravascular space.

Regulation of tissue blood flow and O_2 delivery occurs largely at the microcirculatory level and results from changes in vascular smooth muscle tone that determine arteriolar resistance and transcapillary exchange. Vascular muscle tone is primarily influenced by the autonomic nervous system, circulating vasoactive neurohumoral agents, and local metabolic and myogenic factors (Fig. 11-1). The autonomic nervous system regulates resistance and blood pressure primarily through baroreceptor reflexes (Chapter 1). Sympathetic and parasympathetic efferent activity modulates vasomotor tone and also regulates cardiac output by influencing heart rate, contractility, and end-diastolic volume. In addition to baroreceptors, peripheral chemoreceptors, which are activated by hypoxia, may also enhance sympathoadrenal activity. Several hormonal systems involved in blood pressure homeostasis are also under autonomic control, including the adrenal medullary secretion of catecholamines and adrencorticotropic hormone (ACTH), the renin-angiotensin-aldosterone system, and antidiuretic hormone (ADH) release by the pituitary.

In addition to neurohumoral control of regional resistance and capillary exchange, several local control mechanisms also are important in regulating tissue blood flow and O_2 delivery. These mechanisms are independent of the autonomic nervous system and include metabolic vasoregulation, hypoxic vasodilatation, and autoregulation (Chapter 1). *Metabolic vasoregulation* refers to the control mechanism that matches O_2-substrate supply to metabolic demands. *Hypoxic vasodilatation* refers to the increase in blood flow that accompanies a reduction in arterial O_2 content. *Autoregulation,* the control mechanism by which blood flow is maintained relatively constant despite changes in perfusion pressure, is most pronounced in the coronary, cerebral, and renal vascular beds.

PATHOPHYSIOLOGY OF SHOCK

Despite the many etiologies of circulatory shock, the pathophysiologic mechanisms involved share many features (Figs. 11-2 and 11-3).

Hemodynamic abnormalities

In most shock states the initial hemodynamic alteration involves a reduction in cardiac output. The two mechanisms responsible for inadequate cardiac output are reduction in circulatory blood volume and impairment of cardiac pump function (Fig. 11-2). A reduction in circulating blood volume diminishes systemic venous pressure and cardiac filling, resulting in a decrease in end-diastolic volume, with a subsequent reduction in stroke volume and cardiac output. Cardiac function may be impaired by a decrease in myocardial contractility, by mechanical defects such as mitral regurgitation or ventricular aneurysm, or by an arrhythmia that reduces cardiac output by affecting heart rate and cardiac filling. Ventricular arrhythmias and conduction disturbances also may alter contractile function. Although most patients in shock demonstrate a low cardiac output, this is not always the case. For example, shock may develop in a patient with an abnormally high cardiac output caused by

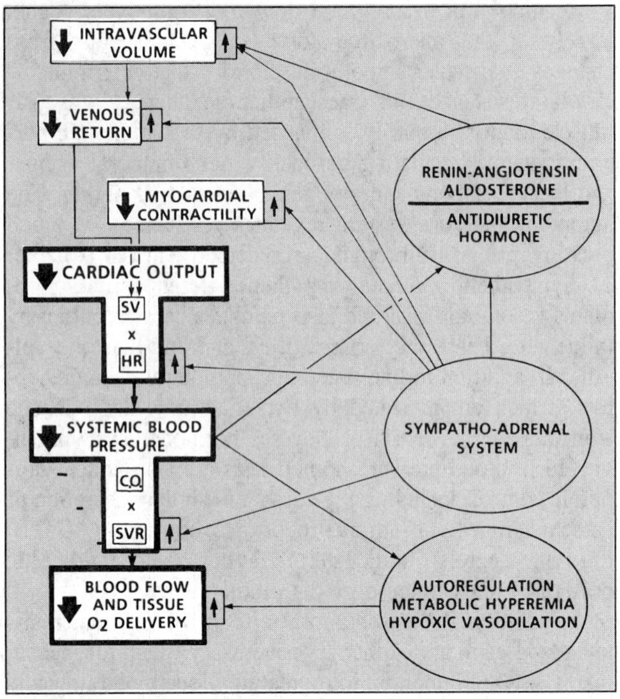

Fig. 11-2. Pathophysiology of the shock syndrome: compensatory mechanisms in early shock. In the early stages of shock, compensatory *negative feedback mechanisms* operate to restore perfusion pressure and blood flow to vital organs. The compensatory adjustments are mediated by the sympathetic nervous system, by release of humoral agents in response to decreases in perfusion pressure, and by release of local vasodilator metabolites in response to tissue ischemia. *SV,* Stroke volume; *HR,* heart rate; *C.O.,* cardiac output; *SVR,* systemic vascular resistance.

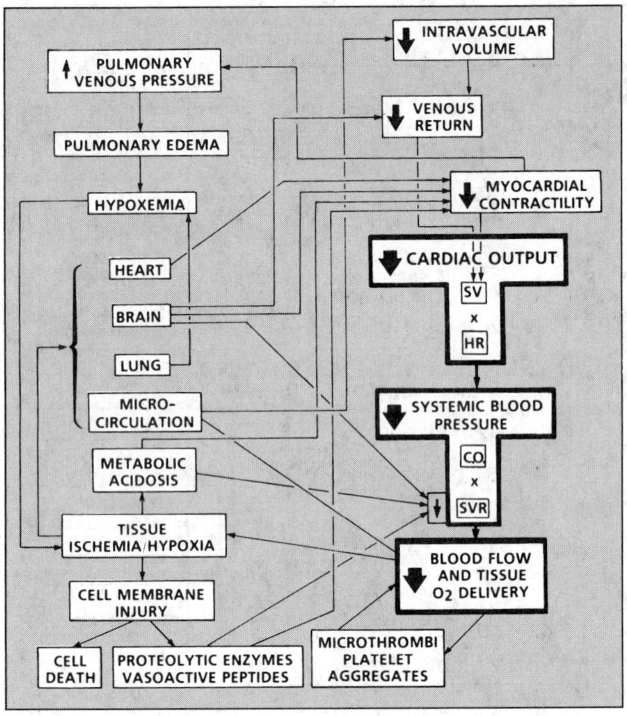

Fig. 11-3. Pathophysiology of the shock syndrome: progressive shock. If adequate blood flow is not restored after an acute reduction in perfusion pressure, *positive feedback mechanisms* eventually lead to progressive shock and irreversible cellular damage. *SV,* Stroke volume; *HR,* heart rate; *C.O.,* cardiac output; *SVR,* systemic vascular resistance.

anemia, thyrotoxicosis, or liver disease when the cardiac output falls to normal, which may then be inadequate to meet tissue metabolic demands.

Since systemic pressure is determined by cardiac output and total vascular resistance, any reduction in cardiac output without a compensatory increase in vascular resistance will result in hypotension. Because tissue blood flow is a function of perfusion pressure and regional vascular resistance, a fall in pressure will result in decreased tissue flow unless vascular resistance also decreases. If blood flow and O_2 delivery fall below a critical level, cellular ischemia occurs. Severe cellular ischemia results in inhibition of mitochondrial electron transport function, with subsequent depletion of high-energy phosphate compounds required for normal cellular metabolic function and membrane integrity. The final outcome, if the condition is left untreated, is irreversible cellular damage, vital organ deterioration, and eventually death.

Compensatory mechanisms

Fortunately, several compensatory negative feedback mechanisms operate to restore blood flow to vital organs following a reduction in cardiac output and blood pressure (Fig. 11-2). These compensatory adjustments are mediated through the sympathetic nervous system, release of endogenous neurohumoral substances, and local vasoregulatory mechanisms. A reduction in mean arterial pressure, pulse pressure, or rate of pressure rise will inhibit baroreceptor activity, resulting in enhancement of sympathetic tone and reduction in vagal tone. In addition, a decrease in left ventricular size during hypovolemia further augments sympathoadrenal efferent activity by inhibiting cardiac sensory afferent stretch receptors. This integrated cardiovascular response augments cardiac output by increasing heart rate, myocardial contractility, and venous tone and maintains systemic pressure through arterial vasoconstriction. In addition, increased sympathetic activity increases adrenal medullary synthesis and release of catecholamines. If blood pressure falls to extremely low levels, resulting in tissue ischemia, a chemoreceptor reflex is activated that further augments sympathoadrenal activity. It is important to realize that sympathoadrenal-mediated arteriolar constriction, although widespread, is not a homogeneous response. Vasoconstriction is most pronounced in skeletal muscle and splanchnic and cutaneous vascular beds; the coronary and cerebral circulations are least affected. This allows a reduced cardiac output to be redistributed to organs essential for immediate survival.

In addition to maintaining blood pressure and cardiac output, the sympathoadrenal system also influences intravascular volume regulation. Sympathetic-mediated vasoconstriction results in an increase in the ratio of precapillary-to-postcapillary resistance and a fall in capillary hydrostatic pressure, thus facilitating the osmotic movement of interstitial fluid into the vascular compartment to restore blood volume. The sympathoadrenal mechanism is capable of completely compensating for an acute blood loss of as much as 10% of the intravascular volume in a previously healthy person. With a volume deficit of 15% to 25% or more, however, cardiac output and blood pressure can no longer be maintained, and tissue blood flow is reduced. When pump failure caused by acute myocardial infarction is the initiating mechanism in shock, sympathetic baroreflexes may be impaired. Activation of cardiac sensory afferent receptors resulting from dyskinesia of the infarcted ventricle may inhibit sympathoadrenal activity, causing hypotension and bradycardia. Inability to maintain coronary perfusion pressure in this setting often leads to further myocardial ischemia and necrosis and progressive cardiovascular deterioration.

The renin-angiotensin-aldosterone system also contributes to the maintenance of blood pressure and intravascular volume (Chapter 23). The reduction in renal perfusion pressure and sympathetic stimulation of renal nerves result in the secretion of renin from the juxtaglomerular apparatus. Renin converts the circulating globulin angiotensinogen to angiotensin I, the latter being enzymatically transformed to angiotensin II by converting enzyme. Angiotensin II is the most potent endogenous vasoconstrictor and also stimulates the release of aldosterone by the adrenal cortex. Aldosterone in turn stimulates sodium and water reabsorption by the renal tubules, which helps to maintain intravascular volume. Another hormonal system that plays a role in volume regulation during shock is vasopressin (ADH), which is released from the posterior pituitary after activation of baroreceptor reflexes in response to hypotension. Vasopressin increases the permeability of the renal tubular cells in response to changes in osmolality and activation of baroreceptor reflexes following hypotension. The result is an increase in water reabsorption.

Several local vasoregulatory mechanisms also act to maintain tissue blood flow during circulatory shock. Tissue ischemia leads to an accumulation of vasoactive metabolites (e.g., adenosine), which act on arterioles and precapillary sphincters to cause vasodilatation. The reduction in arteriolar resistance increases regional blood flow (metabolic hyperemia). The decrease in precapillary sphincter tone increases total capillary surface area, facilitating blood-tissue exchange. Hypoxia also relaxes arteriolar smooth muscle and increases blood flow. Experimental data support the possible involvement of several local mechanisms in addition to the direct effect of low tissue O_2 tension on the vasculature. Autoregulation is a third local vascular response, with changes in perfusion pressure altering vascular smooth muscle tone independently of neurogenic or neurohumoral factors. In shock states the lowered perfusion pressure elicits a vasodilatory response, resulting in increased flow. Since the coronary, cerebral, and renal circulations demonstrate strong autoregulation, whereas skeletal muscle and skin exhibit weak autoregulation, relative differences in regional autoregulation favor redistribution of blood flow to the vital organs.

The shock syndrome may develop rapidly or gradually, depending on the severity of the initial insult and the adequacy of compensatory mechanisms. If the negative feedback mechanisms can maintain adequate pressure and cardiac output, a compensated "preshock" state may exist. If compensatory mechanisms are insufficient to restore effective perfusion to vital organs, either because of the severity of the initial insult or its prolonged duration, clinical evidence of reduced organ perfusion or shock will be apparent. If aggressive therapy is instituted at this point, the shock syndrome may still be reversible. However, if severe reductions in tissue perfusion continue, irreversible cellular changes eventually occur, and death will ensue.

Progressive shock

A critical point occurs in the course of shock in which dysfunction of vital organs, through positive feedback mechanisms, leads to further reductions in blood pressure and cardiac output and progressive cardiovascular deterioration (see Fig. 11-3). One of the more deleterious mechanisms involves progressive myocardial ischemia and pump failure. When systemic pressure falls below 60 mm Hg, coronary perfusion is impaired, and if coronary blood flow is reduced below levels required to meet myocardial metabolic needs, ischemia results. This causes a decrease in contractility; a further reduction in cardiac output, blood pressure, and coronary blood flow; and more impairment of cardiac function. This vicious cycle is particularly likely to occur in patients with atherosclerotic coronary artery disease, in whom distal coronary pressure may be considerably less than systemic pressure.

The accumulation of metabolic acids and toxic humoral factors produced by severely ischemic tissue may further depress cardiac function in shock. Metabolic acidosis results from excess lactate production associated with anaerobic metabolism and also from impaired renal excretion of organic acids.

Acidosis has a direct adverse effect on myocardial systolic and diastolic performance. Increased hydrogen ion concentrations impair calcium (Ca) entry through the slow Ca channel and decrease Ca release from the sarcoplasmic reticulum, thus exerting a negative inotropic effect. Intracellular acidosis also impairs Ca reuptake by the sarcoplasmic reticulum; diastolic relaxation is prolonged, which contributes to a progressive elevation in left ventricular end-diastolic pressure. In addition to perpetuating shock directly by decreasing cardiac output, progressive left ventricular dysfunction also results in increased pulmonary venous congestion and hypoxemia, which further decrease the available tissue O_2 supply.

The vasodilator effect of ischemia is more pronounced in the precapillary resistance vessels, and thus the ratio of precapillary-to-postcapillary resistance may actually decrease in the course of shock. The resulting increase in capillary hydrostatic pressure leads to movement of fluid out of the intravascular compartment, which reduces cardiac output. Loss of intravascular fluid and protein may also result from ischemic endothelial injury, which increases capillary permeability. The decrease in intravascular volume further reduces blood pressure and cardiac output, which reflexly increases sympathetic activity, causing more severe vasoconstriction and thus perpetuating the shock state.

Other deleterious circulatory effects may be initiated by ischemic damage to the central nervous system, lungs, gastrointestinal tract, kidney, and reticuloendothelial system. When arterial pressure falls to below 40 to 50 mm Hg, the cerebral ischemia produced results in intense central sympathetic activity. If the ischemia is prolonged, however, vasomotor function is impaired, resulting in a loss of compensatory baroreflexes and a further reduction in blood pressure and cardiac output.

Damage to the pulmonary capillary endothelial cell increases capillary permeability and interstitial and alveolar edema, and hemorrhage and impaired gas exchange may occur (shock lung). The resulting hypoxemia and respiratory acidosis will further decrease tissue O_2 delivery and vital organ function. Ischemia of the intestinal mucosa also increases permeability, allowing bacteria and their toxins to enter the bloodstream, causing sepsis and circulatory dysfunction. Renal ischemia may result in acute tubular necrosis with its consequent fluid, electrolyte, and metabolic disturbances. Ischemic dysfunction of the reticuloendothelial system may impair the patient's ability to withstand infection, which could further increase tissue demands.

Ischemic injury to the microvascular system frequently results in both functional and structural impairment that can perpetuate the shock state. Prolonged hypoxia, acidosis, and the accumulation of vasodilator metabolites may offset the sympathetic vasoconstriction, resulting in further hypotension and further decreases in blood flow to vital organs. Venodilatation of the capacitance vessels decreases venous return and cardiac filling, and hypoxic and metabolic vasodilatation may open up anatomic arteriovenous channels, leading to a decrease in capillary or nutrient flow. This is most pronounced in the mesenteric circulation in shock.

Finally, in severe shock, intravascular clotting from the formation of microthrombi and platelet aggregates may occur. This is likely precipitated by a low cardiac output with stasis, capillary endothelial damage with fibrin deposition, and catecholamine-induced platelet aggregation. The net result of intravascular clotting in arterioles and capillaries is to further reduce nutrient blood flow.

CLINICAL ASSESSMENT OF SHOCK

The clinical diagnosis of well-advanced circulatory shock is usually evident. The criteria used to diagnose shock are based on evidence of cardiovascular dysfunction resulting in inadequate tissue blood flow and impairment of vital organ function. The classic signs of shock include:

1. Hypotension (auscultatory systolic pressure <90 mm Hg or 30 mm Hg below previous basal levels)
2. Cool, clammy skin
3. Altered mentation
4. Reduced urine output (<20 ml/hr)
5. Metabolic acidosis

Hypotension and clinical signs of ischemic organ failure occur late in the course of fully developed, progressive shock and are associated with a very high mortality despite aggressive medical therapy. Thus the importance of recognizing early cardiovascular dysfunction is evident, and prompt treatment at this early stage greatly improves the patient's chances of survival.

The initial assessment of the cardiovascular system in the patient with suspected shock states involves careful evaluation of several important clinical variables that reflect adequate blood flow.

Heart rate and blood pressure

The earliest hemodynamic signs of a reduced cardiac output, which may occur before any significant reduction in blood pressure, include tachycardia and a decrease in the arterial pulse pressure. A relatively small reduction in cardiac output and blood pressure will stimulate reflexly the sympathoadrenal system, tending to restore systemic pressure by increasing heart rate, contractility, and systemic resistance. This results in a tachycardia and an increase in diastolic pressure. The systolic pressure may be slightly decreased or unchanged, depending on whether or not stroke volume is maintained. A reduction in cardiac output may be suspected by a decrease in pulse pressure before systolic pressure is significantly reduced. With more severe reductions in cardiac output, blood pressure will fall despite compensatory mechanisms.

Peripheral and central pulses

Gauging the pulsations felt over an artery depends on the ability to detect differences in vessel caliber during systole and diastole. This depends not only on intra-arterial pressure but also on extremity blood flow and the vessel's distensibility. Weak, thready, or even absent pulses during shock are often caused by a reduced arterial pressure but also may result from high peripheral resistance with decreased flow and reduced vessel distensibility despite normal intravascular pressure. When the skin is warm, reduced pulses usually reflect hypotension in the absence of peripheral vascular disease. The carotid and femoral pulses will provide better information about central pressure than more peripheral pulses, since there is greater flow in, and less constriction of, these larger vessels.

Skin temperature

The skin temperature in the absence of fever is an indicator of the adequacy of cutaneous blood flow. Warm skin indicates adequate cutaneous flow; cool, clammy skin indicates reduced flow. In shock, reflex sympathetic vasoconstriction frequently reduces cutaneous flow. Thus the skin temperature reflects the intensity of the sympathoadrenal discharge in shock. However, not all patients in shock demonstrate cutaneous vasoconstriction. For example, warm skin can occur in early septic shock or after myocardial infarction, despite inadequate cardiac output. In sepsis this may result from circulating vasodilator agents; in myocardial infarction, pathologic reflexes from the ischemic myocardium have been implicated.

Sensorium

A reduction in cerebral perfusion pressure and blood flow is reflected by altered mentation. In the early stages of shock this is manifested by restlessness, agitation, and confusion. With further reduction in cerebral perfusion, lethargy and obtundation occur.

Urine output

The urine output during shock, in the absence of diuretic therapy, correlates well with renal blood flow, which depends on cardiac output. A urine flow of less than 20 ml/hr in the absence of obstruction indicates inadequate renal flow and decreased cardiac output. Urinary sodium concentration and osmolality can provide earlier indications of reduced renal perfusion in shock before oliguria develops. A decrease in glomerular filtration and activation of the renin-angiotensin-aldosterone system cause an increase in sodium and water reabsorption. As a result, urinary sodium concentration will be low (<20 mEq/L), and osmolality will be high (urine/serum osmolality ratio >1.2:1.0).

HEMODYNAMIC MONITORING IN SHOCK

Hemodynamic monitoring of the patient in shock is invaluable not only in establishing the pathophysiologic mechanisms causing or perpetuating the shock syndrome but also in quickly evaluating the adequacy of therapy.

Heart rate and cardiac rhythm

Continuous monitoring of heart rate and rhythm is useful for early detection of changes in the patient's cardiopulmonary status and reflex autonomic function. A gradual increase in heart rate may alert the physician to the possibility of worsening cardiac performance or decreasing intravascular volume. Electrocardiographic (ECG) monitoring instantly detects any ventricular premature beats, which, if left untreated, may precipitate more serious ventricular arrhythmias. Other arrhythmias, as well as conduction disturbances, can be promptly identified and appropriate treatment instituted.

Blood pressure

Accurate measurement of the blood pressure in the patient in shock is critical, since the level of systemic pressure greatly influences the adequacy of tissue blood flow as well as myocardial O_2 demands. It is important to recognize that the auscultatory blood pressure measured with a sphygmomanometer in the patient in shock may be grossly inaccurate, especially when reflex vasoconstriction is prominent. In the presence of reflex sympathetic vasoconstriction, the forearm resistance may be high enough to prevent adequate blood flow despite a normal or even high intra-arterial pressure. In this setting, cuff pressure may be low or unobtainable, whereas intra-arterial pressure may actually be normal or even high. Intra-arterial pressure can be measured by cannulating the radial, brachial, or femoral arteries; cannulation of the radial artery has a lower potential for causing ischemic damage to the extremity. An 18-gauge cannula can be quickly inserted percutaneously if a pulse is palpable or by cutdown when no pulse can be felt. The arterial cannula also allows frequent determination of blood gases and pH.

Cardiac filling pressures and ventricular function

Once the diagnosis of shock has been established and the patient's condition initially stabilized, the next goal is to determine the precise etiologic and pathophysiologic mechanism(s) responsible for the shock state. Measurement of cardiac filling pressures and left ventricular function enables the physician to determine if the primary hemodynamic abnormality responsible for inadequate tissue perfusion is reduced blood volume, impaired cardiac pump function, or a combination of both.

Central venous pressure. Central venous pressure (CVP), the pressure in the thoracic vena cava, reflects mean right atrial and right ventricular end-diastolic pressures in the absence of mechanical obstruction to flow. Because venous pressure is determined not only by blood volume but also by venomotor tone and right ventricular compliance, an increase or decrease in CVP may result from changes in venous resistance or right ventricular function, as well as changes in absolute intravascular volume. CVP is measured with a catheter inserted into the superior vena cava from the antecubital, external or internal jugular, or subclavian vein. The clinical usefulness of monitoring CVP as an index of intravascular volume in certain shock states is based not on a single value but rather on the patient's response to volume loading. If a 1 to 2 dl fluid challenge over 10 minutes produces an improvement in blood pressure and tissue perfusion with little or no change in CVP (<3 mm Hg), hypovolemia is playing a role in the shock state, and further volume replacement is indicated. If, however, the fluid challenge results in a rapid rise in CVP (>5 mm Hg), with no hemodynamic improvement or actual deterioration, underlying myocardial dysfunction is more likely.

The usefulness of CVP as an index of left ventricular filling pressure is limited to patients in whom ventricular function and pulmonary vascular resistance are both normal. For example, in patients with pneumonia, pulmonary embolism, or predominant right ventricular infarction, CVP may be high and left ventricular filling pressure low, and fluid replacement may be required. On the other hand, in patients with acute myocardial infarction, left ventricular end-diastolic pressure is usually higher than CVP, which may be normal or even low. Fluid administration in these patients could result in pulmonary edema and critically worsen cardiac performance.

Pulmonary capillary wedge pressure. Measurement of left ventricular diastolic pressure during shock provides two important pieces of hemodynamic information. First, filling pressure is an indirect index of left ventricular function; second, it reflects the level of pulmonary capillary hydrostatic pressure, a factor related to the propensity for the development of pulmonary edema. This information provides a rational basis for planning specific therapy and assessing the adequacy of that therapy. Left ventricular filling pressure can be indirectly determined safely at the bedside by measuring pulmonary capillary wedge pressure (PCWP) using a flow-directed, balloon-tipped catheter (Chapter 6). The pressure measured at the catheter tip with the balloon inflated in the pulmonary artery is the PCWP and reflects left atrial pressure, which is transmitted retrogradely through the pulmonary veins. In patients with diminished ventricular compliance, atrial systole can substantially augment left ventricular end-diastolic pressure without altering mean PCWP, which then underestimates the ventricular filling pressure. On the other hand, increased mean PCWP in patients with mitral stenosis or regurgitation may overestimate left ventricular filling pressure. Despite these limitations, PCWP usually is a very reliable and useful index of left ventricular filling pressure in the critically ill patient in shock. The measured PCWP is influenced not only by intravascular volume and myocardial contractility but also by left ventricular and venous compliance and the diastolic filling period.

When PCWP cannot be obtained, the pulmonary artery end-diastolic pressure may be used as an index of left ventricular filling. There are several limitations to using the latter to assess left ventricular function. When pulmonary vascular resistance is elevated, pulmonary artery end-diastolic pressure may greatly exceed mean PCWP and left ventricular end-diastolic pressure. In the patient with reduced ventricular compliance, the atrial contribution to left ventricular end-diastolic pressure may not be totally transmitted across the pulmonary bed, so pulmonary artery end-diastolic pressure would be lower than left ventricular end-diastolic pressure.

Cardiac output. Although cardiac filling pressures are extremely useful in the diagnosis and management of shock, they do not provide a direct index of blood flow, and no single optimum cardiac filling pressure exists for every patient in shock. For example, during fluid administration to a patient in hypovolemic or septic shock who has normal ventricular function, increasing PCWP to 12 mm Hg or less generally results in optimum cardiac performance. Further elevation of PCWP in this patient is not associated with significant increases in cardiac output, mean arterial pressure, or left ventricular stroke work index. However, in patients with acute myocardial infarction and reduced left ventricular compliance, a PCWP of 14 to 20 mm Hg may be required to improve cardiac performance. Simultaneous measurement of PCWP and cardiac output can be used to construct left ventricular function curves at the bedside (Chapter 10). In this way the PCWP that maximizes cardiac output without causing pulmonary edema can be determined. Serial measurement of cardiac output can be quickly and reproducibly done with a flow-directed thermodilution catheter. A thermistor at the end of the catheter records changes in pulmonary arterial blood temperature produced by a right atrial bolus injection of cold 5% glucose. Cardiac output is calculated from a "negative-heat" dilution curve.

Within certain limitations the arteriovenous (AV) O_2 difference may be used as a rough index of cardiac output. The AV O_2 difference is determined from simultaneous blood samples drawn from a systemic artery and the pulmonary artery. Because O_2 consumption shows such wide variation in the critically ill patient in shock, absolute values have less meaning than overall trends. In general, an AV O_2 content greater than 5.2 cc/dl is associated with a reduced cardiac output. The AV O_2 difference may overestimate cardiac output when AV shunting is prominent, as in septic shock.

Blood gases

Because acidosis and hypoxia are typical consequences of shock states and result in further cardiovascular deterioration and tissue ischemia, their prompt recognition and correction are essential in preventing progressive shock. This requires frequent evaluation of arterial blood gases and pH. Plasma lactate levels and the lactate/pyruvate ratio may provide a more accurate assessment of inadequate tissue perfusion, but these measurements are not routinely available. Although the classic acid-base abnormality in the patient with established shock is metabolic acidosis, respiratory alkalosis is frequently present in the early stages. The hyperventilation probably represents a nonspecific response to stress and increased sympathetic activity mediated through baroreceptor reflexes.

MANAGEMENT OF SHOCK

The primary goal in treating the patient in circulatory shock is to restore adequate tissue blood flow rapidly in order to meet existing metabolic requirements. The management of the patient in shock can be divided into three stages: (1) initial resuscitation and general supportive measures; (2) specific pharmacologic therapy to maintain adequate blood volume, systemic pressure, cardiac output, and vital organ blood flow; and (3) identification of the underlying factor(s) responsible for the shock and institution of definitive therapy (see the box on p. 139). Mechanical circulatory assist for the patient in cardiogenic shock may constitute another stage.

Resuscitation and general measures

In any critically ill patient the first priority in resuscitation is establishing an adequate airway and effective ventilation. If respiratory function is seriously compromised, endotracheal intubation and mechanical ventilation are required. Since marked reduction of central pulses and profound hypotension may cause rapid, irreversible cerebral and myocardial damage, immediate therapy to restore perfusion pressure is indicated. The patient should be placed in the horizontal position with the legs slightly elevated to increase venous return and supplemental O_2 administered to maintain an O_2 tension of at least 70 mm Hg. In the pres-

Management of shock

I. Initial resuscitation and supportive measures
   A. Establish effective ventilation and adequate oxygenation (O_2 tension >70 mm Hg).
   B. Restore viable central pulses with dopamine or norepinephrine.
   C. If hypovolemia is suspected, begin rapid volume replacement.
   D. Treat pain, arrhythmias, and acid-base abnormalities.
II. Pharmacologic therapy
   A. Initiate volume replacement to optimize cardiac filling pressures and cardiac output.
   B. Administer vasoactive-inotropic drugs (dopamine, norepinephrine) to maintain mean arterial pressure at 65 to 70 mm Hg and improve cardiac output.
   C. Administer vasodilator drugs (nitroprusside, phentolamine) to improve tissue perfusion in the patient with excessive vasoconstriction. Do not use these drugs unless hypovolemia is corrected and systolic blood pressure is ≥80 mm Hg.
   D. Administer diuretics (furosemide, ethacrynic acid) to reduce elevated cardiac filling pressures, reduce pulmonary edema, and increase urine flow.
III. Mechanical circulatory assist (cardiogenic shock): use in conjunction with pharmacologic therapy to improve coronary perfusion and cardiac performance.
IV. Definitive therapy: establish underlying cause(s) and institute specific therapy.

ence of obvious circulatory collapse, inotropic vasoconstrictor drugs such as dopamine (200 to 2000 μg/min) or norepinephrine (2 to 20 μg/min) should be given intravenously (IV) while the patient is being clinically evaluated and arterial and venous catheters are being inserted. These drugs will rapidly raise systemic vascular resistance, augment myocardial contractility, and increase central perfusion pressure. Infusion of the minimum dose required to establish a viable pulse is the immediate goal. If hypovolemic shock is suspected, immediate, rapid volume replacement is instituted simultaneously. ECG monitoring is also begun for the detection of rhythm or conduction disturbances. Blood samples are sent for determination of hematocrit, blood gases, pH, and electrolytes.

Maintenance of adequate oxygenation and correction of acid-base disturbances and arrhythmias are essential in the early resuscitative stage of treatment. Pain should be relieved with morphine sulfate (2 to 5 mg IV) or meperidine (50 to 100 mg IV), starting with small doses, which can be repeated if needed.

Specific pharmacologic therapy

Intravascular volume in shock. Because the two major mechanisms for reduced tissue perfusion in shock are inadequate cardiac filling and impaired myocardial performance, the first step is to decide which of these two mechanisms is responsible. This is readily accomplished by measuring cardiac filling pressures. If the patient is clearly volume depleted (e.g., by blood loss) and has no known or apparent cardiopulmonary disease, CVP monitoring can be used as a guide to fluid replacement. If, on the other hand, the patient has had an acute myocardial infarction or the cause of shock is uncertain, a balloon catheter should be inserted to measure PCWP. The pressure should be raised to a level that restores blood pressure and tissue perfusion, as assessed by mental status, urine output, skin temperature, cardiac output, and blood pH. In general, raising CVP in the patient with volume-responsive shock to 10 to 15 mm Hg should restore adequate circulation unless left ventricular dysfunction or other etiologic factors are playing a role. In cardiogenic shock a PCWP of 14 to 18 mm Hg or a pulmonary artery diastolic pressure of 20 to 24 mm Hg is frequently required to achieve adequate ventricular filling and cardiac output. Raising left ventricular filling pressure is not without risk and can precipitate pulmonary edema. It should be re-emphasized that pulmonary edema may occur during fluid therapy in the presence of a normal CVP or even a normal PCWP. The lung's ability to resist pulmonary edema formation at a given capillary hydrostatic pressure depends on the tissue pressure, plasma and interstitial fluid oncotic pressure, capillary permeability, and lymph flow rate. Various studies in experimental animals and in humans have demonstrated that the plasma oncotic pressure is of major importance in preventing the movement of fluid into the tissues because of increased capillary hydrostatic pressure. For example, if the difference between oncotic pressure and PCWP remains greater than 8 mm Hg, the risk of pulmonary edema is small. If, however, PCWP approaches or exceeds the level of oncotic pressure, pulmonary edema usually develops. Also, the oncotic pressure of protein exerted across the capillary depends on the permeability of the capillary membrane to protein. If capillary permeability is increased (e.g., shock lung, endotoxic shock), plasma oncotic pressure becomes ineffective in preventing pulmonary edema.

The type and amount of fluid used in treating shock depend on the specific clinical situation. For example, when blood loss is apparent or the hematocrit is less than 30, whole blood or packed cells are the most effective agents for restoring pressure and tissue perfusion.

Acellular fluids used in the treatment of shock include crystalloids and colloids. Dextrose solutions are not efficient volume expanders. Crystalloids include isotonic saline solutions (normal saline, Ringer's lactate) and are distributed in the extracellular space, of which 25% is plasma volume. In critically ill patients with increased capillary permeability and reduced oncotic pressure, less than 25% of an infused volume of saline will remain in the intravascular space.

For better distribution and restriction of fluid therapy into the intravascular space, colloids of large molecular weight (MW) may be used. These include human serum albumin, plasma substitutes, and glucose polymers (dextrans, hydroxyethyl starch). Human serum albumin (5 g/dl) is an excellent volume expander, particularly in the edematous hypovolemic patient with low serum albumin. Because of its high cost, it should not be used indiscriminately. The use of plasma to increase blood volume carries the risk of transmitting hepatitis. Purified plasma protein derivatives do not transmit hepatitis, but they contain vasoactive contaminants that can cause hypotensive reactions. Dextrans are glucose polymers produced by streptococci. A 6% solution of dextran-70 (MW, 70,000) expands blood volume by 130% of injected volume. Dextran-70 remains intravascular for longer periods than do crystalloid solutions (70% remaining at 3 hours and 30% percent after 24 hours). The ability of dextran-40 (MW, 40,000) to expand the intravascular volume is similar to that of dextran-70, but the hemodynamic effects of dextran-40 are dissipated within 90 minutes. Dextrans also facilitate blood flow through the microcirculation by altering red blood cell aggregation, in part by reducing blood viscosity. Toxic side effects of the dextrans include anaphylactic reactions and bleeding caused by interference with platelet function and coagulation. The dextrans should be avoided in patients with active bleeding, coagulation disorders, or thrombocytopenia and should be used cautiously in patients receiving heparin. Dextran-40 may cause renal failure by increasing urine viscosity. Dextran administration should probably be discontinued if unexplained renal failure develops or urine output does not increase appropriately. Hydroxyethyl starch is another polysaccharide colloid that is similar to dextran-70 in its capacity to augment blood volume but has several other advantages. It is relatively nonallergenic, causes much less bleeding (in doses less than 1500 ml), and does not cause renal failure. Nevertheless, close monitoring of coagulation factors and platelets is recommended, particularly if used in large volumes or in combination with other volume expanders. Because amylase complexes with hydroxyethyl starch, serum amylase will usually be elevated for up to 4 days after discontinuation of therapy and should not be used as evidence of pancreatic or biliary tract disease.

Initial volume therapy should consist of 1 to 2 dl of fluid rapidly infused over 5 to 10 minutes, with continuous hemodynamic monitoring and observation of signs of increased tissue perfusion. If beneficial effects are observed without evidence of pulmonary edema, further fluids are given, with careful hemodynamic monitoring. If volume expansion increases filling pressures without increasing cardiac output and vital organ flow, further volume expansion is unlikely to be helpful and only increases the risk of precipitating pulmonary edema.

Controversy surrounds the safest, most effective form of volume replacement in the treatment of circulatory shock. It seems likely that both crystalloids and colloids have a place in the treatment of shock. Daily fluid and electrolyte losses, including additional losses from fever, vomiting, diarrhea, or nasogastric suction, require replacement with balanced salt solutions. In patients with mild-to-moderate blood loss, crystalloids can be used to replace interstitial fluid losses. Whole blood or packed red cells restore tissue O_2 delivery in patients with excessive bleeding. Once the hemoglobin is adequate (>10 g/dl), one third to one half of additional volume deficits can be administered as colloid with the remainder as crystalloid. In nonbleeding hypovolemic patients who require volume replacement, a combination of colloid and crystalloid (1:2 ratio) will restore interstitial fluid losses and also will be effective in expanding intravascular volume. In severely hypoproteinemic patients, albumin is appropriate. If the serum albumin is normal, dextrans or hydroxyethyl starch can be used. Hydroxyethyl starch is safer in patients with underlying bleeding disorders.

Diuretics. The most effective means of establishing an adequate urine output in the patient in shock is by correcting reduced intravascular volume and restoring renal perfusion pressure. Treatment of the hypovolemic, hypotensive patient with potent diuretics is dangerous and will only worsen tissue perfusion. Diuretics are useful in the patient in shock with high PCWP and pulmonary venous congestion, although in certain patients, vasodilator therapy may be even more advantageous. If diuretics are used, the smallest effective dose should be employed to maintain a urine output of at least 40 to 50 ml/hr, with careful monitoring of blood pressure and cardiac filling pressure.

Vasoconstrictor and inotropic drug therapy. If blood flow is not restored after adequate volume expansion, drugs that alter systemic vascular resistance and augment myocardial contractility will be necessary to support the circulation. However, vasoconstrictor drugs are a temporary form of therapy and should not be used for long periods to maintain blood pressure. Extensive and unnecessary vasoconstriction will increase central blood pressure but at the expense of decreasing tissue perfusion and increasing myocardial O_2 demands.

The most frequently used cardiovascular drugs in the treatment of patients in shock are the sympathomimetic amines, the effects of which are mediated through action on alpha- and beta-adrenergic receptors. Stimulation of alpha receptors causes vasoconstriction, whereas stimulation of beta receptors causes vasodilatation. Activation of myocardial beta receptors increases heart rate and contractility. The various adrenergic drugs differ in their relative alpha and beta effects. In addition, the cardiovascular effects of any single drug depend on the dose and the specific vascular bed on which it acts.

The rationale for using drugs with positive inotropic and vasoconstrictor properties for patients in shock is to increase cardiac output by augmenting myocardial contractility and to improve blood flow to vital organs by increasing perfusion pressure. A necessary hemodynamic consequence of increasing perfusion pressure by elevating total vascular resistance is that blood flow is reduced through some vascular beds. Ideally, selective vasoconstriction to nonvital structures would increase systemic resistance and provide the elevated pressure needed to improve perfusion to more vital organs. Unfortunately, most sympathomimetic amines are relatively nonspecific with respect to their vasoconstrictor action. Several drugs, most notably dopamine, do have selective constrictor and dilator activity, which results in a favorable redistribution of blood flow to the heart, brain, kidneys, and sphlanchnic organs.

Norepinephrine increases myocardial contractility by

stimulating $beta_1$ receptors and causes arteriolar and venous constriction by stimulating alpha receptors. The actual effect on cardiac output depends on the dose. In small doses the beta effect predominates, and cardiac output and blood pressure are increased. In very high doses, however, extensive vasoconstriction causes a marked increase in systemic resistance and a fall in cardiac output despite the positive inotropic effect. The vasoconstrictor effects of norepinephrine are most prominent in the cutaneous, skeletal muscle, and splanchnic beds. In the heart the relative beta effect results in coronary artery dilatation. Thus norepinephrine may exert beneficial effects in shock by increasing cardiac output and redistributing blood flow to the heart and brain. The average dose of norepinephrine bitartrate is 4 to 12 μg/min. Norepinephrine is best administered through an indwelling catheter in a large vein, since extravasation can result in severe subcutaneous tissue necrosis.

Dopamine, the naturally occurring precursor of norepinephrine, is one of the most widely used drugs in the treatment of shock, particularly cardiogenic shock. Dopamine possesses several unique properties that offer major hemodynamic advantages (Chapter 10). In low doses (2 to 5 μg/kg/min), it produces nonadrenergic vasodilatation of renal and mesenteric vascular beds. In very large doses (20 μg/kg/min), generalized alpha-mediated vasoconstriction predominates, which opposes the selective beneficial vasodilatation seen at lower doses.

The vasoactive drugs of choice in shock are norepinephrine and dopamine because of their favorable redistribution of blood flow away from the skin and muscle and toward the heart and brain. Dopamine has the added advantage of redistributing blood to the kidney and splanchnic beds. Other sympathomimetic amines are also used in the treatment of shock, but most of them are hemodynamically less advantageous than dopamine and norepinephrine.

Epinephrine is a potent beta inotropic and chronotropic catecholamine that causes vasodilatation of skeletal muscle beds and vasoconstriction of splanchnic and renal beds. Although epinephrine increases cardiac output, the effects on regional resistance do not favor redistribution of blood flow to the vital organs. However, epinephrine is indicated in anaphylactic shock, in which temporary alpha constriction is beneficial.

Dobutamine is a relatively selective $beta_1$-adrenergic synthetic sympathomimetic amine with minimum $beta_2$- and alpha-adrenergic effects. In patients with heart failure and elevated left ventricular filling pressure, dobutamine (2.5 to 20 μg/kg/min IV) increases myocardial contractility, augmenting stroke volume and cardiac output, and decreases ventricular diastolic pressure (Chapter 10). The decrease in heart size reduces wall tension and myocardial O_2 demands. In contrast to dopamine, dobutamine has little direct effect on heart rate or systemic vascular resistance. Modest increases in systolic blood pressure with dobutamine are mediated by changes in cardiac output, and decreases in systemic vascular resistance are mainly caused by withdrawal of sympathetic tone. Dobutamine has proved beneficial in cardiogenic shock in selected patients, particularly in those with low cardiac output and high filling pressures and without severe hypotension. Because dobutamine fails to increase systemic pressure substantially, it should not be used alone in patients with severe hypotension. Dobutamine has been used in combination with nitroprusside when systemic vascular resistance is elevated and also in combination with dopamine in patients with mild-to-moderate hypotension.

Pure alpha-adrenergic agents, such as phenylephrine and methoxamine, have no place in the treatment of circulatory shock because they have no inotropic properties and increase resistance without favorably redistributing blood flow to vital organs.

Extreme caution is required when drugs with potent vasoconstrictor properties are used in the treatment of patients in shock because excessive or prolonged vasoconstriction is potentially harmful. This is especially true if vasoconstrictor drugs are given to maintain blood pressure in hypovolemic patients. In addition, excessive elevation of systemic resistance and pressure increases myocardial O_2 demands and may reduce cardiac output. Unfortunately, no optimum blood pressure exists for all patients in shock because the extent of atherosclerotic narrowing of various vascular beds, which influences regional perfusion pressure, is unknown, as are the relative effects of changing afterload on myocardial O_2 supply and demand. As a general guide, however, a mean arterial pressure of 65 to 70 mm Hg is required to perfuse the brain adequately, and a diastolic pressure of 60 mm Hg is required to perfuse the heart. Therefore the dosage of the drug employed should be titrated to maintain a systolic pressure of at least 80 to 90 mm Hg and a diastolic pressure of 60 to 70 mm Hg.

Digitalis has very limited use in the treatment of patients in acute shock states associated with severe myocardial failure. As an inotropic agent in this clinical setting, digitalis is relatively weak compared with the more potent sympathomimetic amines. In addition, the hypoxia, acidosis, and impaired renal function common in shock states predispose patients to potentially dangerous digitalis-induced arrhythmias. However, digitalis may be useful in the treatment of refractory supraventricular tachyarrhythmias and mild-to-moderate pump failure when the patient is being weaned from more potent inotropic agents.

Vasodilator therapy. Some patients in shock show evidence of excessive vasoconstriction and poor tissue perfusion despite volume replacement and normal or perhaps even high systemic pressures. These patients may also be receiving vasoconstrictor drugs to maintain adequate perfusion pressure. Vasodilator therapy may be beneficial to these patients. Although generalized sympathetic vasoconstriction is a useful compensatory mechanism for maintaining systemic pressure, excessive arteriolar and precapillary constriction can reduce tissue blood flow despite adequate or even high perfusion pressure. In addition, progressively increasing postcapillary resistance will result in an increase in capillary hydrostatic pressure and loss of intravascular volume, which reduces cardiac output and reflexly increases sympathetic activity even further.

The rationale for using vasodilator therapy for patients in shock is to break the deleterious positive feedback cycle in which widespread vasoconstriction causes a decrease in cardiac output and blood pressure, resulting in further sympathetic-induced vasoconstriction. The beneficial effects of vasodilators include (1) dilatation of arterioles, precapillary sphincters, and venules, which improves capillary flow; (2) reduction in capillary hydrostatic pressure caused by a greater decrease in postcapillary resistance, which favors movement of fluid into the intravascular space; and (3) reduction in myocardial O_2 demands by decreasing both preload and afterload. The vasodilator drugs have no direct inotropic action on the heart. Their effects in increasing cardiac output are entirely mediated by changes in preload and afterload. The major drawback of vasodilator therapy is that the reduction in systemic resistance and decrease in preload may be excessive and could cause a severe decrease in systemic pressure despite an increase in cardiac output. This may be prevented by adequate volume replacement and careful monitoring of filling pressure before and during vasodilator therapy and by titrating the dose so that systemic pressure does not fall more than 10 mm Hg or below 80 to 90 mm Hg systolic. Severe hypotension is a contraindication to using vasodilator drugs.

The vasodilator agents most often used for patients in shock states are nitroprusside and phentolamine. Nitroprusside is administered IV, beginning with a dose of 0.5 μg/kg/min, with gradual increments depending on the hemodynamic response. Additional volume replacement may be required if filling pressure falls excessively (Chapter 10). Phentolamine is an alpha-adrenergic blocking agent with no depressant effects on myocardial contractility, and it inhibits venoconstriction relatively more than arteriolar constriction. This action can cause a rapid decrease in cardiac filling pressure, so adequate volume replacement is essential before starting therapy. Phentolamine is given IV in a dose of 0.3 to 1.0 μg/kg/min.

Corticosteroids. The use of pharmacologic doses of corticosteroids for patients in shock remains controversial. Their beneficial effects in animal models appear to be primarily related to their stabilizing effects on capillary and lysosomal membranes. Large doses of steroids (methylprednisolone, 30 mg/kg) may improve chances of survival if given early in the course of gram-negative septic shock. Steroids cannot be recommended for patients in cardiogenic shock because they may impair the inflammatory and healing processes, predisposing to the development of ventricular aneurysm and rupture.

Mechanical circulatory assist in cardiogenic shock

Despite advances in the management of patients with acute myocardial infarction, such as thrombolytic therapy and emergent percutaneous transluminal coronary angioplasty, (PTCA), the incidence of cardiogenic shock apparently has not declined over the last decade. Recent studies would indicate that cardiogenic shock complicates acute myocardial infarction in about 5% to 15% of patients, regardless of the application of recent therapeutic interventions (Chapter 14). This reflects extensive myocardial necrosis occurring in a set percentage of patients with acute myocardial infarction, and those developing cardiogenic shock usually have involvement of more than 40% of the left ventricular muscle mass. Cardiogenic shock most frequently complicates a large anterior myocardial infarction initiated by a proximal thrombotic occlusion of the left anterior descending coronary artery. Mortality from cardiogenic shock also has not declined over the past decade. Once cardiogenic shock develops, the mortality remains 70% to 80% unless some very specific interventions, such as revascularization with coronary artery bypass grafting, is undertaken. Therefore attempts have been made to provide mechanical circulatory assist in patients with cardiogenic shock.

The most frequently used device is the intra-aortic balloon counterpulsation that supports left ventricular function. In this technique a catheter with a distal balloon is advanced to the descending thoracic aorta after percutaneous insertion into the femoral artery. Using the ECG for synchronization, the 30 to 40 cc balloon is inflated during diastole and immediately deflated just before left ventricular ejection.

The rationale behind counterpulsation is to increase coronary blood flow by augmenting diastolic perfusion pressure (balloon inflation) and to decrease myocardial O_2 demands and improve cardiac output by reducing afterload (balloon deflation). The hemodynamic effects of aortic balloon counterpulsation in patients with cardiogenic shock include an augmentation of diastolic pressure, often with an increase in coronary blood flow; a decrease in systolic pressure and thereby left ventricular systolic wall stress; little change in mean arterial pressure; an increase in cardiac output (10% to 20%); and a reduction in left ventricular diastolic filling pressure. Contraindications for the use of balloon counterpulsation include aortic regurgitation and abdominal or thoracic aortic dissection or aneurysms. The two most frequent complications of balloon insertion are lower extremity ischemia and dissection of the aorta or iliofemoral vessels, necessitating removal of the balloon. Although balloon counterpulsation frequently results in hemodynamic and clinical improvement, the beneficial effect is often only short lived, or the patient becomes "balloon dependent" for maintenance of adequate circulation. When this occurs, cardiac catheterization is indicated to assess the possibility of definitive surgical treatment. Emergency surgery for cardiogenic shock is most beneficial in patients with infarction associated with a major mechanical impairment of ventricular performance, such as a large aneurysm, severe mitral regurgitation, or a ventricular septal defect (Chapter 14). Repair of the mechanical defect together with myocardial revascularization should not be delayed if the patient fails to show hemodynamic improvement or cannot be weaned from the balloon pump.

More recently, other peripheral circulatory assist devices have been developed. Many of these devices improve cardiac output to a greater extent than the intra-aortic balloon pump. Many limitations of the intra-aortic balloon pump are also limitations of the more powerful circulatory assist devices. In particular, many patients have persistent heart failure after their episode of cardiogenic shock and become dependent on the circulatory assist device. In addition, despite assist devices being able to produce cardiac outputs as high as 6 to 10 L/min, their use has not been associated with a significant increase in the survival rate for patients with cardiogenic shock. The survival rate has remained as low as 10% to 40% in a nationally maintained clinical registry of mechanical ventricular assist devices. The greatest use for these additional assist devices probably is to support the hemodynamic status of patients with end-stage heart failure while they are awaiting cardiac transplantation.

Prompt intervention with thrombolytic agents (streptokinase, rt-PA) to establish coronary reperfusion may be helpful, but it is unlikely that this in itself will make a major impact on either the incidence or the treatment of cardiogenic shock. For this reason, attempts have been made in recent years at several medical centers to revascularize the myocardium more aggressively with coronary artery bypass surgery or PTCA. It must be emphasized that these trials have involved only limited numbers of patients with cardiogenic shock. However, several of these studies have shown that, despite an increased morbidity in such patients, coronary artery bypass is feasible and may result in a significant improvement in mortality. The use of PTCA in patients with cardiogenic shock is even more promising; the available studies indicate that it may offer some benefit in many patients. Despite the apparent logic underlying these more aggressive approaches to re-establishing coronary perfusion and thereby eliminating the initiating ischemic insult, this mode of therapy is undergoing extensive clinical evaluation in order to define which subgroups will benefit most.

Clinical experience at several institutions has shown that mechanical ventricular assist pumps can effectively support the circulation in patients with cardiogenic shock for up to several weeks. At present, mechanical assist devices have been used primarily in selected patients with postcardiotomy cardiogenic shock who cannot be weaned from cardiopulmonary bypass despite conventional medical therapy and intra-aortic balloon counterpulsation. The use of mechanical assist devices in patients with cardiogenic shock from acute myocardial infarction who are unresponsive to medical therapy requires further evaluation.

Definitive therapy for shock

Circulatory shock is best considered a severe symptom that requires immediate supportive therapy for the patient while every attempt is made to identify the underlying disease process. If the primary cause of shock is not ultimately treated, the eventual outcome is likely to be fatal despite treatment directed at correcting secondary cardiovascular, respiratory, and metabolic derangements. In hemorrhagic shock, for example, the source of bleeding must be identified and surgically corrected. The successful treatment of septic shock requires appropriate antibiotics and identification of the source of infection, which may require surgical intervention (e.g., intra-abdominal abscess, gangrenous gallbladder). Even in cardiogenic shock, the recognition and surgical correction of reversible mechanical pump dysfunction may prove lifesaving in certain patients with intractable cardiac failure.

REFERENCES

Abboud FM et al: Reflex control of the peripheral circulation. Prog Cardiovasc Dis 18:371, 1976.

Altura BA, Lefer AM, and Schumer W, editors: Handbook of shock and trauma, vols 1 and 2. New York, 1983, Raven.

Cohn JN: Recognition and management of shock and acute pump failure. In Hurst JW, editor: The heart, ed 5. New York, 1982, McGraw-Hill.

Cowley RA and Trump BE, editors: Pathophysiology and shock, anoxia and ischemia. Baltimore, 1982, Williams & Wilkins.

Dole WP and O'Rourke RA: Pathophysiology and management of cardiogenic shock. Curr Probl Cardiol 8:1, 1983.

Drake RE and Gabel JC: Role of colloid osmotic pressure in shock resuscitation. Contemp Anesth Pract 6:101, 1983.

Goldberg RJ et al: Cardiogenic shock after a myocardial infarction: incidence and mortality from a community wide perspective, 1975 to 1988. N Engl J Med 325:1117, 1991.

Guyton RA et al: Emergency coronary bypass for cardiogenic shock. Circulation 76(suppl 5):V-22, 1987.

Lefer AM and Schumer W, editors: Progress in clinical and biological research, vol 3, Molecular and cellular aspects of shock and trauma. New York, 1982, Alan R Liss.

O'Neill WW: Management of cardiogenic shock. In Topol EJ, editor: Acute coronary intervention. New York, 1987, Alan R Liss.

Ross AD and Angaran DM: Colloids versus crystalloids—a continuing controversy. Drug Intell Clin Pharm 18(3):202, 1984.

Shoemaker WC: Diagnosis in management of shock. In Shoemaker WC et al, editors: Textbook of critical care. Philadelphia, 1984, Saunders.

CHAPTER

12 Sudden Death

Jeremy N. Ruskin
Brian McGovern
Hasan Garan

Sudden death is defined as an unexpected, nontraumatic, non-self-inflicted fatality occurring in patients with or without pre-existing disease who die within 6 hours of the onset of the terminal event. Sudden death is the leading mode of death in most industrially developed areas of the world. In the United States alone, 400,000 to 500,000 sudden deaths occur annually. More than half of these individuals succumb to *instantaneous death,* which is defined as sudden and unexpected death occurring within seconds to minutes in persons who were engaged in normal activity immediately before their collapse.

With the advent of rapid-response emergency care systems, it became apparent that most sudden deaths were cardiac in origin and that the most common terminal events were *ventricular tachycardia* (VT) and *ventricular fibrillation* (VF). Asystolic cardiac arrest appears to account for a small percentage of sudden deaths. Ambulatory electrocardiogram (ECG) recordings in sudden death victims have confirmed VT or VF preceded by VT of variable duration as the mechanism of death in a large majority of patients. Prodromal warning symptoms in these patients appear to occur infrequently.

PATHOPHYSIOLOGY

Extensive atherosclerotic coronary artery disease is by far the most common pathologic finding in patients with sudden cardiac death (SCD). Associated ventricular damage from prior myocardial infarction is also present in most SCD victims. In a study of 166 survivors of out-of-hospital cardiac arrest unassociated with acute myocardial infarction at the Massachusetts General Hospital, 125 patients (75%) had coronary artery disease. Three-vessel disease was documented in 60%, two-vessel disease in 20%, and single-vessel disease in 20% of patients. The mean left ventricular ejection fraction was 0.41 ± 0.18.

In studies from Seattle and other cities, acute coronary artery thrombosis and recent acute myocardial infarction were observed in a minority (10% to 30%) of patients with SCD. Thus the typical pathologic background for SCD in the community is severe epicardial coronary artery disease with or without previous myocardial infarction. Recent thrombotic coronary artery occlusion and fresh myocardial infarction are present in only a minority of patients. These observations support the concept that SCD is predominantly an electrical event and not a sequela of acute myocardial infarction in most patients.

Except for coronary artery disease, the presence of hypertension, cardiac enlargement, heart failure, ventricular hypertrophy, and chronic pulmonary disease have been identified as factors associated with an increased risk of sudden death. In addition, various discrete clinical entities other than atherosclerotic coronary artery disease are associated with ventricular arrhythmias and account for approximately 20% of sudden deaths in most series (see the box above). These include congestive (dilatated) cardiomyopathy, hypertrophic cardiomyopathy, aortic valve disease, mitral valve prolapse, congenital heart disease, long Q-T interval syndromes, and primary electrical heart disease. Other less common causes of sudden death include cardiac or papillary muscle rupture, massive pulmonary embolism, primary pulmonary hypertension, sickle cell anemia, and central nervous system disease.

Among the nonischemic heart diseases associated with increased risk for SCD, the cardiomyopathies are the most common (Chapter 17). Ventricular arrhythmias occur frequently in patients with both congestive and hypertrophic cardiomyopathy, and sudden death is the most frequent mode of death in both syndromes. Several studies have documented a high incidence (50% or more) of complex ventricular ectopic activity in patients with either form of cardiomyopathy. In patients with congestive cardiomyopathy, the incidence of complex ventricular arrhythmias and risk for SCD increase with the severity of ventricular enlargement and systolic dysfunction. In patients with hypertrophic cardiomyopathy, with or without a left ventricular outflow tract gradient, the occurrence of VT on ambulatory ECG recordings predicts a substantially increased risk of sudden death.

Clinical entities associated with sudden death

Coronary artery disease
Dilatated cardiomyopathy
Hypertrophic cardiomyopathy
Aortic valve disease
Mitral valve prolapse
Cyanotic congenital heart disease
Long Q-T interval syndromes
Primary electrical heart disease

Studies seeking to identify important clinical variables that would help to identify patients at high risk for SCD have focused predominantly on populations of patients with ischemic heart disease. These prospective studies, carried out primarily but not exclusively in patients who had a myocardial infarction, have identified left ventricular ejection fraction, the extent and severity of coronary artery disease, the presence of frequent and repetitive ventricular arrhythmias, and age as important predictors of risk for subsequent SCD. In patients after myocardial infarction, several nonarrhythmic risk factors are typically associated with the occurrence of complex (frequent, multiform, repetitive) ventricular ectopic activity. These include impaired ventricular function, large infarction size, left ventricular aneurysm formation, and an abnormal response to exercise testing (Chapter 14). Despite these associations, most studies have found the presence of high-grade ventricular arrhythmias, particularly VT, to be powerful independent predictors of risk for subsequent sudden death.

The Cardiac Arrhythmia Suppression Trial (CAST) examined whether or not the suppression of asymptomatic ventricular premature beats (VPBs) with antiarrhythmic drugs would reduce risk for sudden cardiac death in patients who had a myocardial infarction. In this trial, two class IC drugs, encainide and flecainide, were associated with a significant increase in sudden death and total mortality compared with placebo. Furthermore, this increase in mortality occurred despite effective suppression of ventricular ectopic activity in the drug treatment group. In the third arm of CAST, another class I antiarrhythmic drug, moricizine, was also compared with placebo. In this phase of the trial, no significant difference in sudden death or total mortality was observed between the two groups. In the subsequent CAST-II report, use of moricizine to suppress VPBs in patients after myocardial infarction was associated with excess mortality at 14 days. These data do not support the routine use of antiarrhythmic drugs in patients with asymptomatic ventricular arrhythmias after myocardial infarction.

Most sudden deaths are associated with extensive atherosclerotic coronary artery disease, and of the nonischemic causes of SCD, the most common are the cardiomyopathies. In patients with ischemic heart disease the extent and severity of coronary atherosclerosis is an important but not easily quantified determinant of risk for sudden death. However, most studies indicate that in patients with either coronary disease or cardiomyopathy, the extent of ventricular damage, as assessed by the left ventricular ejection fraction, is the most powerful independent determinant of risk for subsequent sudden death. Frequent and repetitive ventricular arrhythmias, particularly nonsustained VT, are also associated with increased risk for SCD in both populations of patients, independent of the degree of left ventricular dysfunction. Unfortunately a lethal ventricular arrhythmia may be the first symptomatic manifestation of heart disease in up to half of the patients who experience SCD. Much progress is being made, however, in identifying those patients with clinically apparent heart disease who are at high risk for life-threatening arrhythmias and sudden death. The challenge in these patients will be the identification and implementation of safe, effective prophylactic interventions for the prevention of this lethal syndrome.

PATIENT EVALUATION AND THERAPY: GENERAL CONSIDERATIONS

The evaluation and management of patients at high risk for SCD may be divided into two broad categories: the primary prevention of SCD in patients with heart disease who are at high risk and the secondary prevention of recurrent cardiac arrest and sudden death in patients who have been successfully resuscitated from an episode of cardiac arrest. Because of the limited data available on the primary prevention of SCD in patients with structural heart disease, this section focuses primarily on the evaluation and management of survivors of out-of-hospital cardiac arrest. Patients who experience cardiac arrest during the very early (acute) phase of a new transmural (Q wave) myocardial infarction are not at increased risk for late sudden death because of this event. Their evaluation and long-term management therefore do not differ from that of other patients with recent acute myocardial infarction. However, patients who experience out-of-hospital cardiac arrest unassociated with new transmural myocardial infarction are at high risk for recurrent cardiac arrest and sudden death. In this latter group of patients a detailed cardiac evaluation and individualized prophylactic therapy are indicated to reduce the risk of subsequent SCD. In most patients this requires therapy directed at the underlying heart disease as well as specific antiarrhythmic therapy.

The treatment of the patient with cardiac arrest in the community is based on the immediate initiation of cardiopulmonary resuscitation (CPR) by a bystander or trained emergency medical personnel. Neurologic recovery and long-term survival depend heavily on the speed with which CPR is initiated and the duration of time between collapse and the delivery of definitive treatment (usually defibrillation) for the underlying arrhythmia. The recent development of automatic advisory external defibrillators that can be used in the field by minimally trained medical or lay personnel constitutes an important advance toward increasing the survival rate among victims of out-of-hospital cardiac arrest.

After successful resuscitation from out-of-hospital cardiac arrest, a thorough investigation of possible precipitating causes is indicated. An attempt should be made to document clearly the arrhythmia at the time of resuscitation. Patients should be assessed for abnormalities (see the box below) that might predispose them to the occurrence of VT or VF, including acute reversible myocardial ischemia, hypoxemia, acidosis, electrolyte imbalance (particularly hypokalemia and hypomagnesemia), stimulation of the sympathetic nervous system, cardioactive drug toxicity, or substance abuse (e.g., cocaine). Acidosis, hypoxemia, drug toxicity, and electrolyte disturbances, when present, should be treated promptly to prevent recurrent arrhythmias. Other than ischemia, these reversible factors, although important, are rarely solely responsible for the occurrence of out-of-hospital cardiac arrest. Furthermore, moderate hypokalemia is frequently observed after resuscitation from cardiac arrest and is more likely the result of a transient catecholamine-induced entry of potassium into skeletal muscle than a primary causal abnormality. Nevertheless, it is prudent to monitor the serum potassium concentration closely in all patients with life-threatening ventricular arrhythmias, especially when diuretic therapy is employed, and to initiate potassium supplementation to maintain the serum potassium concentration in the range of 4.5 mEq/L. Finally, it is important to recognize the arrhythmogenic potential of a wide range of pharmacologic agents, including sympathomimetic drugs, cocaine, ethyl alcohol, methylxanthines, phenothiazines, tricyclic antidepressants, digitalis glycosides, volatile hydrocarbons, and all antiarrhythmic drugs. With the advent and widespread use of sensitive, precise monitoring and electrophysiologic testing techniques to assess cardiac arrhythmias, the high incidence of drug-induced aggravation of ventricular arrhythmias has become increasingly apparent. A drug-related cause for cardiac arrest should be considered in any patient who manifests exacerbation of an arrhythmia during therapy with an antiarrhythmic drug.

After stabilization of the cardiac rhythm and resolution of any neurologic and pulmonary complications, all patients surviving an out-of-hospital cardiac arrest unassociated with a new transmural myocardial infarction should undergo a detailed anatomic and functional cardiac evaluation. With rare exceptions, diagnostic cardiac catheterization with cor-

Precipitating causes of sudden cardiac death

Acute reversible ischemia
Hypoxemia
Electrolyte abnormalities
Increased sympathetic activity
Cardioactive drug toxicity
Substance abuse

onary angiography, left ventricular angiography, and hemodynamic assessment are indicated. In some patients with coronary artery disease, exercise or dipyridamole-thallium imaging may add useful functional information on the physiologic significance of coronary stenoses (Chapter 5). Confirmation of severe coronary artery disease, especially left main or advanced three-vessel disease, generally warrants surgical revascularization. Lesser degrees of coronary artery disease are usually managed with aggressive anti-ischemic medical therapy or percutaneous transluminal coronary angioplasty (PTCA). Limited data from uncontrolled studies suggest that coronary artery bypass surgery may reduce recurrence rate and total mortality in survivors of out-of-hospital cardiac arrest. However, no data from prospective controlled trials are available to address this important issue. In patients who undergo coronary artery bypass surgery after prehospital cardiac arrest, we recommend that intracardiac electrophysiologic studies (EPS) be performed both before and after surgical revascularization. In some patients with well-preserved left ventricular function and inducible VF at EPS, surgical revascularization may result in the elimination of inducible VF at postoperative EPS. In such patients, surgical revascularization alone is associated with a highly favorable outcome. However, in patients with inducible monomorphic VT occurring in association with one or more left ventricular wall motion abnormalities, revascularization alone is rarely sufficient to suppress either spontaneous or inducible VT. In such patients, additional therapy in the form of antiarrhythmic drugs, map-guided antiarrhythmic surgery, or implantable defibrillators is necessary (Chapter 9).

Left ventricular dysfunction and congestive heart failure are major risk factors for sudden death. The significance of the increased mortality associated with digitalis and diuretic use in patients after myocardial infarction is uncertain and may result, at least in part, from differences in baseline left ventricular function. Total body potassium depletion resulting from chronic diuretic therapy may increase susceptibility to VF, particularly during acute ischemia. Thus diuretics should be used with care, and close attention should be paid to maintaining electrolyte balance with supplemental potassium in this patient population. Afterload and preload reduction with vasodilator drugs may reduce myocardial oxygen demand and fiber stretch and thereby afford additional protection against ventricular arrhythmias and provide significant improvement in congestive symptoms in some patients. Two studies, one with hydralazine and isosorbide dinitrate and one with enalapril, have shown a reduction in total mortality in patients with congestive heart failure. In one study a favorable effect on sudden death rate was demonstrated in patients with heart failure who were treated with enalapril. Beta-adrenergic receptor blocking agents have been demonstrated to reduce substantially the risk for sudden death in patients after myocardial infarction, and this protective effect appears to be particularly prominent in patients with left ventricular dysfunction. Unfortunately the presence of congestive heart failure frequently limits the use of these agents in patients at highest risk for sudden death. The optimum treatment for ventricular dysfunction in patients with ischemic and nonischemic heart disease remains to be defined, although available data strongly support the use of angiotensin-converting enzyme (ACE) inhibitors and, when tolerated, beta blockers. Furthermore, the very early use of thrombolytic therapy and ACE inhibitors in patients with acute myocardial infarction appears to be associated with preservation of ventricular function and reduced mortality.

DETECTION AND TREATMENT OF ARRHYTHMIAS

Two main approaches to the detection and treatment of arrhythmias have been used in survivors of out-of-hospital cardiac arrest unassociated with acute myocardial infarction. These include the suppression of spontaneous high-grade ventricular arrhythmias, as detected by ambulatory ECG recording techniques, and the use of therapy guided by invasive EPS. In the former approach, baseline spontaneous ventricular ectopic activity (VEA) is graded by frequency and repetitiveness and quantitated by 24 to 48 hours of ambulatory ECG recordings in the absence of antiarrhythmic drugs. Ambulatory recordings, sometimes in conjunction with exercise stress testing, are then repeated in the presence of steady-state concentrations of an antiarrhythmic drug to assess the efficacy of the regimen in suppressing spontaneous VEA. Because of the high degree of spontaneous day-to-day variability in the frequency of VPBs within individual patients, VPB suppression rates in the range of 90% are required to attribute an observed effect to an antiarrhythmic drug with confidence. In recent years, emphasis at most centers has shifted away from the quantitative suppression of isolated VPBs toward the abolition of high-risk repetitive forms (e.g., couplets and salvos of nonsustained VT). Data from a small number of centers suggest that the elimination by an antiarrhythmic drug of repetitive forms of VEA, provided these were present with high frequency during a baseline recording, is associated with a low risk for SCD in patients with a history of life-threatening ventricular arrhythmias.

This approach has several advantages, including being noninvasive and using equipment and techniques familiar and available to most cardiologists. The addition of exercise testing adds a dynamic component to the evaluation of drug efficacy that may be of importance in selected patients. Furthermore, the testing can be conveniently repeated to assess continued drug efficacy during long-term outpatient follow-up. The principal disadvantage of ambulatory recording-guided therapy in survivors of out-of-hospital cardiac arrest is the relative lack of sensitivity and specificity of spontaneous VEA as an end-point for antiarrhythmic therapy. Less than 50% of patients at most centers manifest sufficient quantities of spontaneous VEA on ambulatory ECG recordings to allow this technique to be used as a therapeutic end-point. Furthermore, the number of patients who manifest frequent repetitive forms of VEA, a more specific therapeutic end-point, is much lower than 50%. Thus more than half the patients in most series of survivors of out-of-hospital cardiac arrest do not qualify for therapy guided by ambulatory recording techniques. Finally, the high degree of spontaneous variability of VEA frequently poses problems in the interpretation of the results of drug testing.

Electrophysiologic testing studies are widely used in the evaluation and management of arrhythmias in survivors of cardiac arrest, particularly those in whom only low levels of spontaneous VEA are observed during ambulatory ECG recordings. Most patients (70% to 80%) have an inducible ventricular arrhythmia in response to programmed electrical stimulation. In 166 survivors of cardiac arrest studied at the Massachusetts General Hospital, programmed ventricular stimulation initiated reproducible runs of presyncopal nonsustained VT in 45 patients (27%), sustained monomorphic VT in 61 patients (37%), and polymorphic VT-VF in 25 patients (15%). In 35 patients (21%), no ventricular arrhythmias were induced. The use of EPS in this patient population thus allows the physician to detect clinically significant arrhythmias not apparent during ambulatory recordings and to characterize the rate, QRS morphology, hemodynamic consequences, and ease of induction of the arrhythmia. Once the baseline arrhythmia has been defined, serial electrophysiologic studies are performed to assess the effects of one or more antiarrhythmic drugs in preventing or modifying the induction of VT and VF. In patients in whom drugs are ineffective, EPS is used to evaluate suitability for antiarrhythmic surgery or implantation of an automatic cardioverter/defibrillator. The results of EPS are highly predictive of outcome in survivors of cardiac arrest. In patients with inducible arrhythmias that are suppressed by antiarrhythmic therapy, the combined incidence of recurrent cardiac arrest and sudden death in patients who comply with medical therapy is less than 10% at 2 years. In patients with persistently inducible VT or VF despite antiarrhythmic therapy, this incidence is approximately 33% at 2 years. Recent observations from our laboratory indicate that the persistence of inducible VT or VF, the presence of impaired left ventricular function, and the absence of cardiac surgery are all strong independent predictors of outcome in this patient population. Furthermore, the relative risks associated with these predictors are multiplicative, so that patients with a left ventricular ejection fraction less than 0.30 (relative risk, 2.6) and persistently inducible VT (relative risk, 4.0) have a 10-fold increased risk of recurrent cardiac arrest compared with patients who do not have these characteristics. Patients with no inducible arrhythmia at baseline EPS compose a heterogeneous group in whom an intermediate (20%) 2-year risk of recurrent cardiac arrest and SCD has been observed. Recent data suggest that a specific subset of patients without inducible ventricular arrhythmias—those with reversible myocardial ischemia and well-preserved ventricular function—are at very low risk for recurrent cardiac arrest when treated only with anti-ischemic medical or surgical revascularization therapy. By contrast, those patients without inducible arrhythmias who have severely impaired ventricular function are at high risk for recurrent cardiac arrest and generally warrant therapy with an implantable defibrillator.

The use of EPS to guide therapy in patients with a history of sustained VT or VF is well established. However, physicians are frequently confronted with the problem of patients with structural heart disease, left ventricular dysfunction, and recurrent nonsustained VT who are known to be at increased risk for but have not yet experienced a life-threatening ventricular arrhythmia. At present, the role of EPS in such patients is controversial. Nevertheless, several recent clinical studies have provided observations suggesting that patients with recurrent nonsustained VT related to coronary artery disease who manifest inducible sustained VT at EPS are at particularly high risk for spontaneous sustained VT or sudden death over the next 1 to 2 years. Those patients without inducible sustained VT at EPS appear to have an excellent short-term prognosis without antiarrhythmic therapy. These data are preliminary, however, and large-scale prospective trials will be required to provide more definitive data on optimum approaches to the evaluation and management of these high-risk patients.

In recent years a relatively new noninvasive test known as the *signal-averaged electrocardiogram* (SAECG) has been employed to identify patients with cardiac disease at high risk for ventricular arrhythmias and SCD. The test involves the recording of large numbers of QRS complexes with standard orthogonal (X, Y, Z) leads during sinus rhythm. The recorded signals are amplified, digitalized, averaged, and filtered to eliminate artifact and then combined into a vector magnitude representing the high-frequency content from the three orthogonal leads. The resultant SAECG is then analyzed for the presence of high-frequency, low-voltage signals in the terminal portion of the QRS complex (late potentials) and for prolongation of the averaged QRS complex duration. It is hypothesized that late potentials on the SAECG represent slow conduction in diseased areas of the myocardium, reflecting an anatomic substrate for re-entrant ventricular arrhythmias. Several studies have demonstrated late potentials on SAECG to be a sensitive predictor of risk for both inducible and spontaneous VT, particularly in patients with recent myocardial infarction. As with most noninvasive tests in this population, however, the SAECG, when used alone, has poor specificity for patients at high risk for VT and sudden death. Recent observations suggest that the combined use of the SAECG, ambulatory ECG recordings, and radionuclide ventriculography may provide a much more specific means of identifying patients with myocardial infarction at high risk for life-threatening ventricular arrhythmias than the use of any single test alone. One such study found that an abnormal SAECG combined with complex VEA on ambulatory ECG monitoring or an ejection fraction of less than 0.40 identified patients with myocardial infarction at risk for a major arrhythmic event, with a sensitivity of 65% to 80% and a specificity of 89%. Thus good stratification by risk for VT and VF can be accomplished in these patients using a combination of noninvasive tests, although some problems achieving an optimum balance of sensitivity and specificity remain.

Furthermore, although the efficacy of beta-adrenergic blocking agents in reducing risk for sudden death after myocardial infarction is well established, the role of other therapeutic interventions in high-risk patients requires further study. The results of CAST demonstrate that patients with a history of myocardial infarction and asymptomatic or mildly symptomatic ventricular arrhythmias should not be treated with sodium-channel-blocking antiarrhythmic drugs. Whether these patients would benefit from other forms of antiarrhythmic therapy directed at the prevention of sudden cardiac death is unknown at present.

TREATMENT

Currently, antiarrhythmic drugs constitute the mainstay of therapy for the prevention of recurrent arrhythmias and SCD in survivors of out-of-hospital cardiac arrest. Experience with a wide range of antiarrhythmic agents from several centers has affirmed the importance of using specific, reproducible end-points to guide the selection of a safe, effective pharmacologic regimen. In many referral centers, EPS is the preferred approach, particularly in patients who fail to manifest spontaneous, repetitive ventricular arrhythmias on ambulatory ECG recordings. In patients in whom conventional antiarrhythmic agents alone and in combination fail to suppress inducible VT and VF, therapy with amiodarone or investigational agents should be considered. As with conventional drugs, the results of EPS are predictive of clinical efficacy during long-term therapy with these agents. The sequence in which antiarrhythmic drugs are tested is determined by the patient's prior drug history and ventricular function, as well as physician experience and preference. In general, drugs such as disopyramide, flecainide, encainide, and sotalol should be avoided in patients with severely impaired ventricular function (Chapter 9).

When antiarrhythmic drugs fail to suppress ventricular arrhythmias adequately in survivors of cardiac arrest, nonpharmacologic therapeutic options, including map-guided antiarrhythmic surgery and implantable cardioverter/defibrillators, should be contemplated. Map-guided ventricular resection and cryoablation are generally considered in patients with structural heart disease and drug-resistant, sustained monomorphic VT. This technique involves the use of electrical activation sequence mapping to locate and guide the resection or ablation of the putative region of VT origin. The approach is best suited to patients with VT associated with ventricular aneurysms and is generally combined with a standard aneurysmectomy. Many centers employ cryothermal ablation in addition to ventricular endocardial resection because the former technique enhances the surgeon's ability to ablate arrhythmogenic sites on the interventricular septum and at the base of papillary muscles, where excision cannot be performed safely. The operative mortality of the technique is in the range of 5% to 10% at most centers, and the procedure's efficacy in eliminating inducible VT at postoperative EPS is 60% to 80%. In patients with persistently inducible VT after surgery, antiarrhythmic drug therapy is generally effective in suppressing spontaneous VT, although implantable defibrillators are sometimes required.

The *automatic implantable cardioverter/defibrillator* (ICD) is a comparatively new, highly effective therapy for prolonging survival in patients at high risk for SCD. This device is designed to detect the presence of VT or VF and to convert these arrhythmias to sinus rhythm by delivering one or more synchronized 25- to 35-joule DC shocks. The 300 g pulse generator, which is considerably larger than a standard pacemaker, is implanted subcutaneously in a paraumbilical position. Several configurations for the sensing and shocking leads have been employed but are not reviewed here. More than 25,000 ICD devices have been implanted worldwide. The operative mortality is 1% to 3%, and approximately 50% of patients discharged are given antiarrhythmic drugs to reduce the frequency of spontaneous VT and VF and to control supraventricular arrhythmias. During the first 18 months after implantation, approximately 40% to 50% of patients experience at least one discharge from the ICD under circumstances consistent with a malignant ventricular arrhythmia. The incidence of sudden death in recipients of the ICD is 1% to 2% at 1 year and 5% at 3 years. These figures are far below the best attainable survival statistics achieved with other forms of therapy and represent a striking reduction in anticipated sudden death rates in this high-risk population. At present, implantation of the ICD is indicated in patients surviving one or more episodes of cardiac arrest or syncopal-sustained VT unassociated with acute myocardial infarction or a reversible cause in whom inducible VT or VF cannot be suppressed with aggressive medical or surgical therapy. Survivors of cardiac arrest in whom no arrhythmias are induced at baseline EPS and in whom treatable precipitants such as severe proximal coronary artery disease are not present are also candidates for implantable defibrillators.

Problems with the ICD include complications of the thoracotomy implantation procedure, infection, pocket hematomas and effusions, transient arrhythmias, lead and pulse generator malfunction, premature battery depletion, and device discharges for sinus tachycardia and supraventricular arrhythmias. Third-generation or tiered therapy devices, currently in clinical trials, are widely programmable and incorporate bradycardia and antitachycardia pacing as well as low-energy cardioversion, high-energy defibrillation functions, and advanced diagnostic capabilities. Furthermore, the use of transvenous endocardial lead electrodes in conjunction with submuscular or subcutaneous patch electrodes will eliminate the need for a thoracotomy during implantation in many patients. With these technologic advances and the survival statistics already achieved, implantable arrhythmia control devices will likely assume a major role in the management of patients at high risk for sudden death.

REFERENCES

Baum RS, Alvarez H III, and Cobb LA: Survival after resuscitation from out-of-hospital ventricular fibrillation. Circulation 50:1231, 1974.

Bigger J et al: The relationships among ventricular arrhythmias, left ventricular dysfunction and mortality in the two years after myocardial infarction. Circulation 69:250, 1984.

Brooks R et al: The automatic implatable cardiovertory defibrillator: early development, current utilization and future directions. In Braunwald E, editor: Heart disease update. Philadelphia, 1990, Saunders.

CAST-II investigators: Effects of the antiarrhythmic agent moricizine on survival after myocardial infarction. N Engl J Med 327:227, 1992.

Consensus Trial Study Group: Effects of enalapril on mortality in severe congestive heart failure: results of the Cooperative North Scandinavian Enalapril Survival Study. N Engl J Med 316:1429, 1987.
Echt DS et al: Mortality and morbidity in patients receiving encainide, flecainide or placebo: the Cardiac Arrhythmia Suppression Trial, N Engl J Med 324:781, 1991.
Garan H et al: Electrophysiologic studies before and after myocardial revascularization in patients with life-threatening ventricular arrhythmias. Am J Cardiol 51:519, 1983.
Holmes DR et al: The effect of medical and surgical treatment on subsequent sudden cardiac death in patients with coronary artery disease: a report from the Coronary Artery Surgery Study. Circulation 73:1254, 1986.
Kelly P et al: The automatic implantable cardioverter/defibrillator: efficacy, complications and survival in patients with malignant ventricular arrhythmias. J Am Coll Cardiol 11:1278, 1988.
Norwegian Multicenter Study Group: Timolol-induced reduction in mortality and reinfarction in patients surviving acute myocardial infarction. N Engl J Med 304:801, 1981.
Ruskin J et al: Antiarrhythmic drugs: a possible cause of out-of-hospital cardiac arrest. N Engl J Med 309:1302, 1983.
Swerdlow CD, Winkle RA, and Mason JW: Determinants of survival in patients with ventricular tachyarrhythmias. N Engl J Med 308:1436, 1983.
Wilber DJ et al: Out-of-hospital cardiac arrest: role of electrophysiologic testing in the prediction of long-term outcome. N Engl J Med 318:19, 1988.

IV Specific Disease Entities

CHAPTER

13 Ischemic Heart Disease

Kanu Chatterjee

The manifestations and pathophysiologic consequences of ischemic heart disease are protean. Ischemic heart disease may be totally silent or may manifest in angina, arrhythmias, and heart failure. Myocardial ischemia stems from the imbalance between myocardial oxygen (O_2) requirements and O_2 supply. Myocardial O_2 supply (arterial O_2 content times coronary blood flow) primarily depends on coronary blood flow; in most patients, arterial O_2 saturation and content are normal. An imbalance between myocardial O_2 supply and demand can occur from a primary decrease in coronary blood flow or from a disproportionate increase in myocardial O_2 requirements or their combination. In some clinical syndromes of ischemic heart disease, the capacity to increase coronary blood flow for the increment in myocardial O_2 demand is limited, and myocardial ischemia results whenever this reserve for myocardial perfusion is exceeded. Impaired myocardial perfusion, caused by primary decrease in coronary blood flow resulting from fixed or dynamic increase in the coronary arterial resistance and/or abnormalities of the coronary vascular autoregulatory mechanisms, appears to be the principal cause for myocardial ischemia in other clinical syndromes. Conceivably the mechanisms for myocardial ischemia may vary in the same individuals in different circumstances, and, as a result, the clinical manifestations may also change. Considerable advances have been made in the last few years in the understanding of the pathophysiologic mechanisms of myocardial ischemia in the different clinical syndromes of chronic ischemic heart disease.

ETIOLOGY

Obstructive coronary artery disease caused by atherosclerosis is the most common cause of chronic ischemic heart disease. In addition, manifestations of chronic and episodic myocardial ischemia can occur from nonatherosclerotic coronary artery disease and in the absence of any coronary artery disease.

Debate over the precise mechanism by which atherosclerotic lesions of the coronary arteries develop in patients with chronic ischemic heart disease continues (Chapter 171). Nevertheless, it is generally believed that the intimal layer is principally involved in atherosclerosis, and three different types of lesions can be identified: the fatty streak, the fibrous plaque, and the complicated lesion. Current evidence suggests that intimal endothelial injury is important in initiating the atherosclerotic process. Experimental studies suggest that the endothelial barrier, broken by mechanical or chemical injury, is associated with a tissue response that includes local platelet adhesion and aggregation. Various factors, including hypertension and hyperlipidemia, can injure the arterial endothelium and trigger this tissue response. The disruption of endothelium exposes the subendothelial connective tissue to platelets, as well as to circulating lipids. With repeated or continuous endothelial injury, deposition of intracellular and extracellular lipids and proliferation of arterial smooth muscle then contribute to the formation of obliterative atherosclerotic lesions. Cellular necrosis, hemorrhage, lipid deposition, and smooth muscle proliferation then lead to complicated lesions that contain newly formed connective tissue and lipids that may eventually calcify.

Alternative hypotheses have also been promulgated to explain human coronary artery atherosclerosis (Chapter 171). Cellular mechanisms for lipid deposition might be involved in the development of the atherosclerotic process. Continued, enhanced synthesis of cholesterol, deficient high-density (alpha) lipoproteins (HDLs), and a defective lysosomal lipoprotein transport mechanism have been proposed as potential contributory mechanisms in the pathogenesis of coronary artery atherosclerosis.

Precisely how well-recognized, important risk factors such as hypertension, smoking, diabetes mellitus, increased low-density lipoproteins (LDLs), and decreased HDL levels contribute to the development of atherosclerotic coronary artery lesions has not been established. Hypertension is regarded as an important contributing factor for the entrance of lipids. The ingredients of cigarette smoke that are thought to promote atherosclerosis are carbon monoxide and nicotine, but the mechanisms remain unclear. Diabetic patients have been reported to have circulating substances that promote muscle proliferation, as well as an increased propensity to bind lipoproteins.

High levels of total cholesterol and increased levels of LDL fraction, decreased total HDL, and its subfractions HDL_2 and HDL_3, particularly HDL_2, have been found important risk factors for coronary artery disease. Insulin resistance, which may be associated with impaired glucose tolerance, hyperinsulinemia, elevated plasma triglyceride levels, and decreased HDL cholesterol, has been identified as a risk factor for atherosclerotic coronary artery disease.

Hyperlipidemia may be secondary (mainly dietary) or primary (from familial defects in cellular LDL receptors). The mechanism of the "protective" effects of HDLs needs clarification. Nevertheless, recent studies suggest that modification is feasible in clinical practice and may be associated with halting the progression and even with regression of atherosclerosis. Thus modification of risk factors is important in the management of chronic ischemic heart disease.

Although atherosclerotic obstructive coronary artery disease is the most common cause of chronic myocardial ischemia, myocardial ischemia can result from nonatherosclerotic coronary artery disease, as well as appear in the absence of coronary artery lesions (see the box at right). Congenital anomalies of the coronary arteries (e.g., anomalous origin of the left coronary artery from the pulmonary artery) can precipitate myocardial ischemia and infarction. Hereditary metabolic disorders are infrequently associated with nonatherosclerotic coronary artery lesions. Systemic collagen vascular disease, irradiation, chest trauma, and extrinsic compression of the coronary arteries by tumors can infrequently be a cause of obstructive lesions and myocardial ischemia.

When myocardial ischemia occurs in the presence of normal coronary arteries, several pathologic conditions should be considered. If coronary artery spasm is demonstrated, variant angina (Prinzmetal's angina) is most likely the diagnosis. Although acute episodes of myocardial ischemia can result from coronary artery embolism, chronic myocardial ischemia is a rare sequela.

Increase in myocardial O_2 requirements and impaired myocardial perfusion may precipitate myocardial ischemia in patients with valvular heart disease and hypertrophic cardiomyopathy. In dilated nonischemic cardiomyopathy, myocardial O_2 demand may also increase disproportionately because of a marked increase in left ventricular wall stress. Decreased transmyocardial pressure gradient caused by elevated left ventricular diastolic pressure and impaired coronary vasodilatory reserve may also compromise myocardial perfusion and induce myocardial ischemia.

Causes of myocardial ischemia in presence and absence of coronary artery disease

- I. Atherosclerotic obstructive coronary artery disease
- II. Nonatherosclerotic coronary artery disease
  - A. Coronary artery spasm
  - B. Congenital coronary artery anomalies
    1. Anomalous origin of coronary artery from pulmonary artery
    2. Aberrant origin of coronary artery from aorta or another coronary artery
    3. Coronary arteriovenous fistula
    4. Coronary artery aneurysm
- III. Acquired disorders of coronary arteries
  - A. Coronary artery embolism
  - B. Dissection
    1. Surgical
    2. During percutaneous coronary angioplasty
    3. Aortic dissection
  - C. Extrinsic compression
    1. Tumors
    2. Granulomas
    3. Amyloidosis
  - D. Collagen vascular disease
    1. Polyarteritis nodosa
    2. Temporal arteritis
    3. Rheumatoid arthritis
    4. Systemic lupus erythematosus
    5. Scleroderma
  - E. Miscellaneous disorders
    1. Irradiation
    2. Trauma
    3. Kawasaki disease
  - F. Syphilis
- IV. Hereditary disorders
  - A. Pseudoxanthoma elasticum
  - B. Gargoylism
  - C. Progeria
  - D. Homocystinuria
  - E. Primary oxaluria
- V. "Functional" causes of myocardial ischemia in absence of anatomic coronary artery disease
  - A. Syndrome X
  - B. Hypertrophic cardiomyopathy
  - C. Dilated cardiomyopathy
  - D. Muscle bridge
  - E. Hypertensive heart disease
  - F. Pulmonary hypertension
  - G. Valvular heart disease; aortic stenosis, aortic regurgitation

PATHOPHYSIOLOGY

Determinants of myocardial oxygen demand

The major determinants of myocardial oxygen demand ($M\dot{V}O_2$) and perfusion are shown in the box on p. 151 (see also Chapter 1). Even under conditions of no increased stress, the myocardium extracts approximately 75% of the available O_2. This O_2 is used to provide energy by oxidative metabolism, and the rate of myocardial O_2 consumption parallels the cardiac energy requirements.

Heart rate is a major determinant of $M\dot{V}O_2$, which increases as heart rate increases. Tachycardia also produces deleterious effects on myocardial perfusion because of the decreased duration of diastole, during which left ventricu-

Major determinants of myocardial oxygen consumption and coronary blood flow

I. Myocardial oxygen consumption
  A. Heart rate
  B. Contractility
  C. Wall stress
    1. Intraventricular pressure
    2. Ventricular volume
    3. Wall thickness
II. Myocardial perfusion
  A. Perfusion pressure (arterial diastolic pressure)
  B. Epicardial coronary artery resistance, including resistance at the site of stenosis
  C. Coronary arteriolar resistance
  D. Extravascular resistance
  E. Left ventricular diastolic pressure and coronary sinus venous pressure

lar perfusion occurs. Reduction of heart rate is therefore associated with decreased $M\dot{V}O_2$ and improved left ventricular myocardial perfusion. Intraventricular systolic pressure (same as systemic arterial pressure in the absence of left ventricular outflow obstruction), ventricular volume, and wall thickness are the major determinants of left ventricular wall stress. Increased ventricular volume and/or pressure increase wall stress; increased wall thickness (hypertrophy) decreases wall stress. The rationale for reducing arterial pressure and/or left ventricular volume in order to decrease $M\dot{V}O_2$ is apparent. Enhanced contractility increases $M\dot{V}O_2$. Therefore reduction of contractility is another potential method of decreasing O_2 requirements.

In clinical practice, the most frequently used index of $M\dot{V}O_2$ is the product of peak systolic pressure and heart rate *(double product)*. This index, however, does not incorporate changes in contractility or ventricular volume. The tension-time index *(triple product)* includes the area under the systolic portion of the arterial pressure curve, left ventricular ejection time, and heart rate but excludes left ventricular volume and contractility. Little difference exists between the double product and the triple product as indices of $M\dot{V}O_2$.

Determinants of coronary blood flow and myocardial oxygen supply

Myocardial O_2 supply is a function of O_2 delivery and extraction. Arterial O_2 content cannot be significantly increased under normal atmospheric conditions, and myocardial O_2 extraction is nearly maximum at rest. Thus augmenting coronary blood flow remains the principal means of providing increased O_2 supply.

Coronary blood flow is directly related to the perfusion pressure (aortic diastolic pressure) and the duration of diastole and is inversely proportional to coronary vascular bed resistance, the latter being determined by a number of factors (Chapter 1). The degree of epicardial coronary artery stenosis is a major determinant of coronary blood flow in patients with atherosclerotic ischemic heart disease. In addition the autonomic activity, circulating neurohumoral substances, and local vasoactive components modulate the epicardial coronary arterial tone. Alpha-adrenergic stimulation is associated with decreased caliber and increased tone of the epicardial coronary arteries. The role of local and circulating vasoactive substances (prostacyclin, thromboxane, endothelial-derived relaxing factor, endothelin, serotonin, histamine, angiotensin) in the regulation of the coronary vascular tone, either in normal or in pathologic conditions, has not been clearly delineated. It has been suggested, however, that the dynamic variations in the caliber of both the normal and the stenosed coronary artery segments may occur in response to these vasoactive stimuli.

The extravascular mechanical compression of the intramyocardial coronary arteries offers resistance to coronary blood flow during systole. The resistance offered by arteriolar vessels, the site of autoregulation, modulates coronary vascular resistance and plays a major role in regulating myocardial perfusion with or without coronary artery disease. The arteriolar tone is influenced by autonomic activity, metabolic products, circulating neurohumoral substances, and various pharmacologic agents. During increased myocardial metabolic demand, such as during exercise, arteriolar resistance declines, which augments blood flow (autoregulatory reserve). With increasing severity of epicardial coronary artery stenosis, the autoregulatory reserve is progressively diminished, and with very severe coronary artery stenosis, the distal coronary vascular bed resistance may reach minimum levels. In such circumstances, myocardial perfusion primarily depends on perfusion pressure, and a reduction in arterial diastolic pressure may precipitate myocardial ischemia.

Left ventricular diastolic pressure and coronary sinus venous pressure also serve to resist myocardial perfusion, particularly to the subendocardium. A decrease in left ventricular diastolic pressure, without a concomitant reduction in arterial diastolic pressure, increases the transmyocardial pressure gradient and thereby improves subendocardial perfusion.

Angina of effort (classic angina). By far the most common cause of *exertional angina* is atherosclerotic narrowing of the large epicardial coronary arteries. The resulting intraluminal resistance is added to the autoregulatory resistance of the arterioles and contributes significantly to the total coronary arterial resistance to blood flow.

In patients with effort angina, resting coronary blood flow is adequate and proportional to $M\dot{V}O_2$ at rest, indicating that stenotic resistance and the resistance of the distal coronary vascular bed are below the critical level required to limit flow at rest. During exercise, there is a twofold to fourfold decrease in resistance of the distal coronary vascular bed mediated by local metabolites that promote coronary blood flow to meet the increased $M\dot{V}O_2$. Although such vasodilatation always increases flow to the potentially ischemic myocardial zones, the increment in flow for a given increase in demand becomes progressively curtailed as the degree of stenosis increases, resulting in relative myocardial ischemia. The principal mechanism for the increased $M\dot{V}O_2$ is increased heart rate and arterial pressure, as well as a reflex increase in contractility (Figs. 13-1 and 13-2). A relative increase in left ventricular diastolic volume and pressure and decreased diastolic perfusion time might also be contributory in some patients. The mechanism for the efficacy of pharmacologic agents that decrease $M\dot{V}O_2$ in effort angina is apparent.

Absolute reduction of coronary blood flow to the potentially ischemic myocardial zones can also occur during increased myocardial stress and during exercise. This reduction in flow may result from a decrease in the perfusion pressure distal to the stenosis associated with increased flow velocity through the stenosis and/or diversion of flow from the subendocardium toward the epicardium. Thus exertional angina may result from either an excessive increase in myocardial O_2 requirements, causing an imbalance of O_2 demand and supply, or an absolute reduction of flow, producing true myocardial ischemia. An increase in the coronary arterial tone, either at the site of stenosis or at the nonatherosclerotic segments, may occur during exercise and may contribute to decreased coronary blood flow.

Variant angina (Prinzmetal's angina). Variant angina is characterized by cyclically recurrent angina at rest, usually unrelated to effort. It is often associated with S-T segment elevation on the electrocardiogram (ECG) during angina.

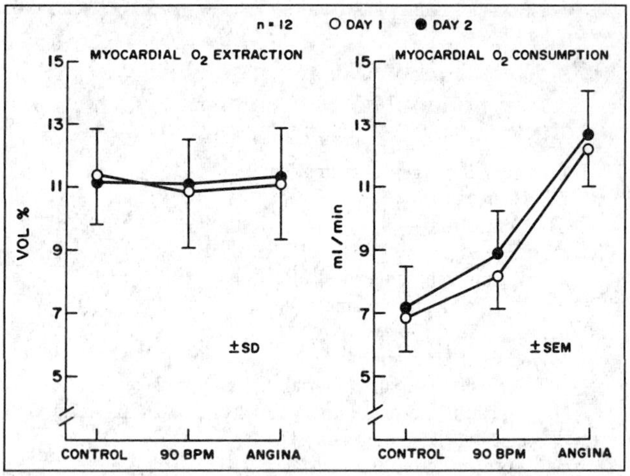

Fig. 13-2. Myocardial O_2 extraction *(left panel)* and myocardial O_2 consumption *(right panel)* during pacing-induced angina on 2 consecutive days. Myocardial O_2 extraction does not vary. $M\dot{V}O_2$ increased as pacing rate was increased but was essentially the same at the onset of angina on both days. (Published with permission from Chatterjee K et al: JAMA 252:1170, 1984.)

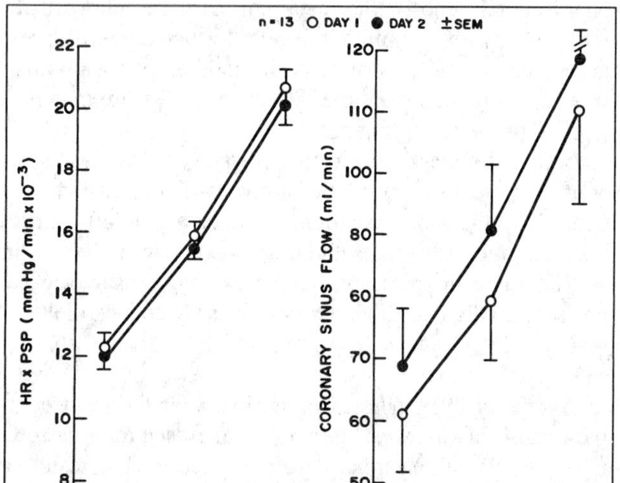

Fig. 13-1. Angina threshold and coronary reserve during pacing-induced angina. Changes in heart rate–peak systolic blood pressure product *(HR × PSP)*, an index of $M\dot{V}O_2$ *(left panel)*, at control, subangina (90 beats/min [BPM]), and angina heart rates on 2 consecutive days. The HR × PSP index at angina was the same on both days, suggesting that the angina threshold remained unaltered during pacing-induced angina. Coronary sinus blood flow *(right panel)* increased as paced heart rate increased, with only slight differences in flow level on the two days. (Published with permission from Chatterjee K et al: JAMA 252:1170, 1984.)

The primary mechanism of variant angina is a spontaneous decrease in coronary blood flow unrelated to changes in $M\dot{V}O_2$. Coronary sinus venous O_2 content tends to decrease, suggesting a decrease in coronary blood flow. Coronary blood flow frequently decreases or fails to increase even when an increase occurs in perfusion pressure, heart rate, and $M\dot{V}O_2$ during spontaneous angina. Most important, arteriographic studies have documented transient complete or incomplete, localized or diffuse narrowing of the epicardial coronary arteries (coronary artery spasm), causing interruptions of flow to the ischemic myocardium during spontaneous angina. Coronary artery spasm can also be provoked by intravenous (IV) injection of vasoconstrictors such as ergonovine or by hyperventilation. Such spasm is usually accompanied by symptoms and ECG changes similar to those associated with the patient's spontaneous angina attacks. The mechanism for the focal or diffuse spasm of the coronary arteries still remains speculative. Activation of histamine or serotonin receptors, an imbalance between the beta- and alpha-adrenoreceptor activity, an imbalance between vasodilator prostacyclin and vasoconstrictive thromboxane activity, and decreased production of endothelial-derived relaxing factors in the presence of atherosclerosis have been regarded as potential mechanisms. It must be emphasized that both the precise mechanism for coronary artery spasm and the precise triggering mechanism in individual patients remain unclear.

Most patients with variant angina also have fixed obstructive coronary artery lesions of varying severity. Only a few have completely normal coronary arteries. The sites of coronary artery spasm may vary, although they most frequently occur at, or in the vicinity of, atherosclerotic lesions. However, in the same patient, single or multiple coronary arteries, different coronary arteries, or different locations in the same artery may demonstrate coronary artery spasm during anginal attacks. This variability should be considered in the management of patients with variant angina.

Silent myocardial ischemia. Myocardial ischemia can occur in the absence of any symptoms referable to ischemia. The existence of "silent ischemia" has been documented by arteriographic, scintigraphic, metabolic, ECG, and hemodynamic studies. Reversible wall motion abnormalities during contrast ventriculography or radioisotope angiography performed during pacing or exercise-induced stress or spontaneously without angina provide good evidence for silent ischemia. Reversible myocardial thallium perfusion defects or decreased myocardial rubidium-82 uptake during exercise, cold pressor tests, or during spontaneous unprovoked S-T segment shifts in the ECG occur in the absence of angina. Abnormal myocardial lactate metabolism without angina before coronary artery bypass surgery and its normalization after surgery provides metabolic evidence for silent myocardial ischemia. Transient decline in regional ventricular relaxation and systolic wall motion, along with an increase in left ventricular end-diastolic pressure in the absence of angina, provide hemodynamic evidence for silent ischemia. ECGs during exercise testing or ambulatory ECGs frequently reveal horizontal or downsloping ischemic S-T segment depressions in the absence of angina in patients with documented coronary artery stenoses. Thus, ample evidence is available for the existence of silent myocardial ischemia in some patients with coronary artery disease.

The mechanism for silent ischemia during exercise appears to be similar to that for exercise-induced angina, that is, increased myocardial O_2 requirements producing imbalance between O_2 demand and supply. Continuous ambulatory ECG and blood pressure monitoring in patients with chronic stable angina reveals that both heart rate and blood pressure increase frequently during a few minutes preceding the onset of ischemic S-T segment changes, suggesting that increased myocardial O_2 demand may, in part, be a potential mechanism for silent ischemia in these patients. Decreased heart rate or lack of increase in heart rate with beta-adrenergic blocking agents associated with reduction in the frequency and duration of silent ischemia also provides evidence for increased $M\dot{V}O_2$ as a contributory mechanism for silent ischemia. Spontaneous episodes of silent ischemia, however, may occur without any increase in the $M\dot{V}O_2$. Heart rate preceding or during the episodes of ischemia is often lower than that during exercise-induced angina. During the episodes of unprovoked ischemic S-T segment depression without angina, decreased myocardial uptake of rubidium-82 has been demonstrated by positron emission tomography. This suggests that a primary decrease in coronary blood flow may be the principal mechanism for spontaneous episodes of silent myocardial ischemia. The mechanisms for the primary decrease or an inadequate increase in coronary blood flow when there is an increment in $M\dot{V}O_2$ may be different in the different anginal syndromes. It is likely that in patients with variant angina, the mechanisms that precipitate symptomatic myocardial ischemia also induce silent myocardial ischemia.

In patients with unstable ischemic syndromes (unstable angina, postinfarction angina), spontaneous episodes of silent ischemia probably result from formation of labile nonocclusive thrombi at the site of ruptured or fissured atheromatous plaques, causing transient interruption of blood flow. Coronary arterial vasoconstriction mediated by vasoactive substances released because of platelet and endothelial dysfunction may further decrease coronary blood flow and compromise myocardial perfusion. Increased coronary vascular tone resulting from heightened sympathetic activity and/or platelet aggregation, release of vasoactive substances such as thromboxane, and a reduced vasodilating regulatory effect of endothelial-derived relaxing factors are other potential mechanisms for spontaneous silent myocardial ischemia. Until the mechanism for silent ischemia can be determined, the therapy, when indicated, will remain empirical, with the use of nonspecific coronary vasodilators or reperfusion therapy.

Mixed angina. Patients with mixed angina are those whose clinical profiles are not typical of either classic angina or variant angina. Since the exercise threshold is variable, alterations in coronary vascular tone and spontaneous changes in coronary blood flow have been implicated as causes of ischemia. Variable responsiveness of the coronary vascular bed to adrenergic stimulation might explain the changes in coronary vasculature resistance. A simultaneous increase in $M\dot{V}O_2$ also contributes to mixed angina. Although these patients have variable exercise thresholds, the rate-pressure product at the onset of angina or S-T segment depression during exercise remains unchanged.

Postprandial angina. The mechanism of postprandial angina also needs further clarification. The hypothesis that the diversion of blood flow from the myocardium to the gastrointestinal system precipitates postprandial angina has not been substantiated. The hemodynamic changes associated with ingestion are characterized by increased heart rate and blood pressure caused by reflex sympathetic stimulation. Thus increased $M\dot{V}O_2$ provides a possible explanation, particularly when angina occurs during exercise after meals. In these patients, significant obstructive atherosclerotic lesions are likely to be present. However, it is also possible that an inappropriate increase in coronary vascular tone resulting from sympathetic stimulation causes a primary reduction in coronary blood flow, causing postprandial angina. Despite increased heart rate and blood pressure, which increase $M\dot{V}O_2$, coronary blood flow is not proportionately increased and may even fall. Thus both a "vasoactive mechanism" and increased $M\dot{V}O_2$ likely contribute to postprandial angina.

Unstable angina. The syndrome of unstable angina is clinically characterized by angina of changing character, duration, and intensity in patients with either a relatively long history of stable angina or a recent onset of angina.

Discrete, single, or multiple episodes of prolonged rest angina are important features of the clinical profile.

Patients with stable angina may become "unstable" because of the development of concurrent illness such as severe anemia, hyperthyroidism, and aortic stenosis (secondary unstable angina). However, in most patients such secondary causes are absent, and a primary change in the pathoanatomy of the coronary artery lesions appears to precipitate unstable angina syndrome. The distribution of coronary artery lesions is similar in patients with stable and unstable angina, but the type of lesions in patients with unstable angina may be different from those in patients with stable angina. In unstable angina an eccentric atheromatous plaque with irregular surface protruding into the lumen of the coronary artery (type IIb) is the most frequent type of lesion identified angiographically. In patients with stable angina, smooth concentric (type I), smooth eccentric (type IIa), or diffuse lesions (type III) are more frequent. The lesions' irregular surface probably represent fissuring or ulceration of the plaques, which may initiate platelet aggregation and adhesion and formation of labile nonocclusive thrombi at the site or vicinity of the atheromatous plaque. Although the mechanisms of plaque fissuring or ulceration remain unclear, ample evidence is available to indicate that such changes in coronary artery lesions are probably fundamental in the pathogenesis of unstable angina. Mechanical obstruction at the site of disturbed atheromatous plaque caused by recurrent platelet or fibrin thrombi formation may produce episodes of rest ischemia.

Increased platelet aggregability and increased production of vasoconstrictor thromboxane A_2 appear to occur more frequently in patients with unstable angina than in patients with stable angina or acute myocardial infarction. Furthermore, intraoperative angioscopic studies have demonstrated thrombus at the site of the atheromatous plaque, causing partial or total occlusion of the offending coronary artery. The increased serum concentrations of fibrin-related antigen, D dimer, the principal breakdown fragment of fibrin and of fibrin monomer, an intermediate product of fibrin formation, in the serum of patients with unstable angina, compared with that of control subjects and patients with chronic stable angina provides indirect evidence for the presence of an active thrombotic process in patients with unstable angina. Fibrinopeptide A concentration is also higher in patients with unstable angina. Coronary arteriographic studies have demonstrated the presence of severe, fixed atherosclerotic coronary artery lesions in most patients with unstable angina and the presence of thrombus in the artery supplying the area of ischemia. These findings form the basis for the use of antiplatelet drugs or thrombolytic agents in the management of unstable angina.

In some hemodynamic studies, an increase in heart rate and/or arterial pressure, along with elevated left ventricular diastolic pressure, has been shown to accompany rest angina, suggesting that increased myocardial O_2 requirements may precipitate myocardial ischemia in some patients. It has also been suggested that some forms of stress cause increased $M\dot{V}O_2$ and increased blood flow to the relatively nonischemic myocardium but not to regions perfused by severely obstructed coronary arteries. However, there is general agreement that rest angina in patients with unstable angina syndrome results most frequently from partial thrombotic occlusion of a coronary artery.

Nocturnal angina. The mechanism for angina that occurs after a patient has retired to bed is unlikely to be similar in all patients. Two distinct types of nocturnal angina are recognized: (1) pain that affects the patient soon after retiring or lying down, even before going to sleep, and (2) pain that wakes the patient several hours after resting, usually in the early morning.

Nocturnal angina occurring soon after going to bed is most likely caused by an increase in $M\dot{V}O_2$ associated with increased left ventricular volume and as a result of an increment in left ventricular wall tension.

Nocturnal angina occurring in the early morning hours may be related to increased coronary vascular tone, although the precise triggering mechanism remains unclear.

Syndrome X. Typical exertional or stress-induced angina occurring in the absence of angiographically documented epicardial coronary artery disease is defined as syndrome X. Secondary causes of angina in patients with normal coronary arteries, such as aortic and mitral valvular disease, pulmonary hypertension, and muscle bridge, need to be excluded before the diagnosis of syndrome X can be considered. During treadmill exercise tests, patients develop typical angina associated with ischemic changes in the stress ECG. In some patients, focal impairment of myocardial perfusion, as evident from reversible myocardial thallium defects and transient reduction of blood flow to vascular territory, may be observed. The mechanism for myocardial ischemia in syndrome X remains unclear; abnormality of vasodilatation of coronary microvasculature, regional or global, is the proposed explanation of stress-induced angina, which is also the reason for other term for syndrome X, *microvascular angina*. The prognosis of patients with this syndrome generally is excellent. Calcium channel blockers and nitrates are effective in controlling angina.

CLINICAL MANIFESTATIONS

Several syndromes resulting from ischemic heart disease are recognized clinically, although myocardial ischemia can be entirely asymptomatic. Acute myocardial infarction may be the first evidence of ischemic heart disease (Chapter 14). Infrequently, arrhythmias and congestive heart failure can be the predominant consequence of ischemic heart disease. However, angina pectoris is by far the most common clinical manifestation.

Angina

The term *angina,* first used by Dr. William Heberden in 1768, was intended to indicate a sense of strangling associated with anxiety and frequently accompanied by a sense of death (angor animi). However, this classic description of precordial discomfort is not uniformly expressed by patients with angina pectoris, whose distress can otherwise be described as "viselike," "constricting," "suffocating," "crushing," "a heaviness," "a tightening," "pressure," or even "indigestion." Some patients complain of a burning sensation in the chest; others of the chest "expanding or bursting" (Chapter 7).

The location of chest discomfort is most frequently retrosternal but can be left pectoral or epigastric. Infrequently the discomfort can be located only in the interscapular or epigastric regions.

Radiation is common and usually occurs down the medial aspect of the left arm. Radiation can also occur to both arms, throat, lower jaw, back, and epigastrium. Rarely the discomfort may start distally, in arms, elbows, and wrists, and radiate centrally toward the chest. The absence of radiation does not exclude a diagnosis of angina pectoris.

The duration of chest discomfort may vary in the different anginal syndromes. However, discomfort of a fleeting, stabbing, or shocklike nature that lasts for only 2 to 3 seconds is not caused by myocardial ischemia; similarly, discomfort that lasts for several hours or days without any remission is unlikely to be angina.

Precipitating factors should be evaluated for a diagnosis of angina. Classic angina is most frequently experienced during exercise. In patients with chronic stable angina, the level of exercise that precipitates angina is usually reproducible and predictable. The extent of physical activity that precipitates angina appears to be inversely related to the severity (but not necessarily to the extent) of coronary artery lesions.

Angina pectoris may develop after less effort than usual in the morning, in a cold environment, walking against the wind, and walking after a large meal. Emotional states (e.g., anger, anxiety), isometric exercises, and sexual intercourse can also induce angina.

Analysis of the mode of relief of chest discomfort is helpful in diagnosing angina pectoris. Typical angina dissipates gradually over a period of minutes, usually as a result of cessation of the activity that precipitated it. Angina pectoris also begins gradually and reaches its maximum intensity over a period of minutes (Chapter 7). Relief of "chest discomfort" in response to nitroglycerin is also a helpful diagnostic clue. Relief of angina typically occurs within 45 seconds to 5 minutes after the sublingual administration of nitroglycerin. However, chest pains associated with esophageal spasm are also relieved by nitroglycerin; thus response to nitroglycerin is not specific for angina pectoris. In some patients, carotid sinus massage can cause relief of angina by decreasing heart rate and blood pressure.

The character, location, and radiation of angina are similar in the different clinical syndromes. However, the duration, precipitating factors, and clinical presentations are different. In patients with classic angina the duration is usually brief, precipitated by physical activity and relieved by the cessation of activity. The intensity of the discomfort is extremely variable. Emotional stress, various forms of isometric exercise, and activity after meals may precipitate angina. When nocturnal angina is experienced by patients with classic angina, it usually occurs soon after retiring or after lying down and is usually relieved promptly by sitting up.

In patients with variant angina, repeated episodes of angina occur at rest, usually without a history of predictable effort-induced angina. The duration can be considerably longer (30 to 40 minutes), and the angina dissipates either spontaneously or in response to nitroglycerin. ECGs obtained during prolonged episodes of angina often reveal reversible S-T segment elevation, indicating transmural myocardial ischemia. Cyclic occurrence (i.e., angina recurring more or less at the same time of the day or night in the same patient) is also observed. Nocturnal angina is usually experienced long after retiring to bed, frequently in the early morning hours, and is not relieved by assuming an upright position. An increased prevalence of migraine headache and Raynaud's phenomenon has been noted in patients with variant angina, suggesting a general propensity to vasoreactivity.

The typical clinical presentation, however, may be lacking in variant angina. In addition to rest angina, some patients may experience angina during physical activity, although the level of physical activity that induces angina is unpredictable. The cyclic occurrence and nocturnal angina might be absent, and an ECG might demonstrate S-T segment depression (subendocardial ischemia) instead of S-T segment elevation.

The clinical characteristics of angina in patients with unstable angina depend on the definition used to distinguish this syndrome. Presently, *unstable angina* is most frequently defined according to criteria used in the National Institutes of Health (NIH)–sponsored National Cooperative Study. The diagnosis depends on the presence of one or more of the following history features: (1) angina pectoris of new onset (usually within 1 month and brought on by minimum exertion); (2) development of more severe, prolonged, or frequent (crescendo) angina superimposed on a pre-existing pattern of relatively stable, effort-related angina pectoris; or (3) angina pectoris at rest as well as with minimum exertion.

Because rest angina is an important criterion, variant angina is sometimes diagnosed as unstable angina; however, variant angina should be distinguished from unstable angina.

The duration of this discomfort is usually longer (up to 40 minutes), and the intensity may be more severe. Relief of angina in response to nitroglycerin is frequently incomplete. In patients with a history of stable angina, a sudden reduction in the level of physical activity that induces angina or an increase in frequency, severity, and duration of angina should be suspected of heralding the onset of unstable angina. A new site of radiation or the onset of new symptoms, such as dyspnea, palpitations, and diaphoresis, along with angina, may also suggest unstable angina.

The incidence of the unstable angina syndrome in patients with new onset of angina remains unclear. Different studies have reported that between 25% and 88% of patients with unstable angina give a history of new onset of angina.

Dyspnea

Dyspnea without associated angina is an infrequent clinical manifestation of myocardial ischemia. However, concomitant with angina, many patients with classic angina experience "a sensation of being unable to take a deep breath." In patients with variant or unstable angina, severe dyspnea may accompany prolonged episodes of angina caused by marked increase in pulmonary venous pressures. Symptoms and signs of low cardiac output may also be seen in these patients. Nocturnal dyspnea soon after retiring indicates myocardial ischemia in some patients; the dyspnea is relieved by assuming an upright posture and also by nitroglycerin.

Dizziness, palpitations, and syncope

Palpitations alone are infrequent in patients with chronic ischemic heart disease (Chapter 8) but can be experienced along with angina. They result most frequently from premature ventricular beats. Dizziness and syncope caused by ventricular tachycardia or fibrillation during myocardial ischemia rarely occur without being preceded by angina. These complications may be precipitated by physical activity (e.g., treadmill exercise). In patients with variant or unstable angina, dizziness or syncope during prolonged episodes of angina may result from ventricular tachyarrhythmias or atrioventricular conduction disturbances.

Syncope caused by hypotension is an infrequent clinical manifestation of myocardial ischemia. However, its occurrence indicates severe ischemia involving large segments of myocardium, results in severe pump failure, and carries an ominous prognosis.

Several cardiac and noncardiac disorders can cause chest discomforts that mimic angina pectoris (Chapter 7). With a careful clinical history, physical examination, and appropriate laboratory tests, these disorders can usually be distinguished from angina.

PHYSICAL EXAMINATION

The physical examination may yield entirely normal findings or may reveal manifestations of risk factors for coronary artery disease. Tendon xanthomas, xanthelasma, and corneal arcus, particularly in younger subjects, may suggest lipid abnormalities. A diagonal ear lobe crease may be more prevalent in patients with ischemic heart disease.

Cardiovascular examination should include determination of blood pressure, examination of peripheral pulses, and funduscopic examination (Chapter 3). Detection of hypertension or its manifestations and peripheral vascular disease is important because there is a higher prevalence of atherosclerotic coronary artery disease in these patients. In young patients, coarctation of the aorta and supravalvular aortic stenosis should be excluded because these conditions are associated with premature atherosclerosis.

Cardiac examination may reveal manifestations and sequelae of ischemic heart disease, as well as the causes of angina other than coronary artery disease. In patients with chronic ischemic cardiomyopathy, particularly those with overt heart failure, physical examination may reveal signs of left-sided and right-sided heart failure (Chapter 3). However, these physical findings are not specific for ischemic cardiomyopathy and are present in patients with dilated congestive cardiomyopathy of any etiology.

Certain physical findings may provide information regarding the presence and severity of ischemic heart disease. Third and fourth heart sound gallops are palpable in some patients with coronary artery disease. During hand-grip exercise, which may induce myocardial ischemia, palpable or audible gallops may appear transiently. During exercise-induced angina or spontaneous angina, these physical findings are frequently present. Fourth heart sounds are detected during auscultation in most patients with symptomatic coronary artery disease, and third heart sounds are also common, but neither is specific for ischemic heart disease (Chapter 3).

Abnormalities of the outward movement of the apical impulse can be detected in some patients. A sustained apical impulse often indicates the presence of dyskinetic myocardial segments and/or a depressed left ventricular ejection fraction. This abnormal finding is most frequently appreciated in patients with a previous myocardial infarction and chronic left ventricular aneurysms. However, it can appear transiently during either spontaneous or hand-grip exercise–induced ischemia.

Paradoxical (reversed) splitting of the second heart sound can occur transiently during an anginal attack. Transient depression of left ventricular function and a prolonged ejection time appear to be the mechanisms. The murmur of mitral regurgitation can be detected in some patients; papillary muscle dysfunction is the most frequent cause, but left ventricular dilatation may also be contributory. A relatively high-frequency diastolic murmur or a continuous murmur along the left parasternal area, associated with proximal coronary artery stenosis, usually of the left anterior descending coronary artery, occurs infrequently.

LABORATORY STUDIES

Electrocardiography

ECG evaluation is an important tool in the diagnosis of ischemic heart disease (Chapter 4). A normal resting ECG is found in 50% of patients with chronic stable angina without a history of previous myocardial infarction and does not exclude significant coronary artery disease. Q waves, diagnostic of anterior or inferior myocardial infarctions, are highly specific indicators of left ventricular wall motion abnormalities related to previous myocardial infarction and also indicate atherosclerotic obstructive coronary artery disease in a vast majority of patients. Other ECG abnormalities may be observed in patients with ischemic heart disease, but they are not specific; they are minor ST-T changes, conduction disturbances, including left bundle branch block and left anterior hemiblock, and ventricular arrhythmias.

The resting ECG, when recorded during an episode of variant or unstable angina, may reveal a variety of abnormalities indicative of myocardial ischemia (Chapter 4). Reversible S-T segment elevation suggests transmural myocardial ischemia, whereas S-T segment depressions suggest subendocardial ischemia. S-T segment alternans, occasionally seen during acute ischemic episodes, is usually associated with later development of ventricular tachyarrhythmias or advanced conduction disturbances. Transient Q waves have been observed infrequently in patients with severe myocardial ischemia without infarction. T wave inversions, the appearance of "U" waves or negative "U" waves, normalization of pre-existing T wave changes, transient prolongation of the Q-T interval, and appearance of arrhythmias may indicate myocardial ischemia; however, the predictive value of these changes for the diagnosis of myocardial ischemia remains undetermined. Nevertheless, an ECG obtained during an episode of chest pain that does not show changes in the S-T segments or T waves is strong evidence against myocardial ischemia as the cause of chest pain. When the resting ECG shows left ventricular hypertrophy or a conduction defect, the reliability of any ECG change as a predictor of myocardial ischemia is reduced. In patients with unstable or variant angina, ECG changes are transient and normalize partially or completely with relief of myocardial ischemia.

A resting ECG is useful for the diagnosis of previous myocardial infarction. In patients with variant or unstable angina, the ECG should be obtained during chest pain, both to detect myocardial ischemia and to define the likely ischemic myocardial region.

The exercise ECG is more useful than the resting ECG in detecting myocardial ischemia (Chapter 5). Downsloping S-T segments are highly specific for coronary artery disease; most patients with this response have double- or triple-vessel involvement. Horizontal or slowly upsloping S-T segments are much less specific indicators of coronary artery disease. Marked S-T segment depression (0.2 mV or more) in symptomatic patients is associated with a high incidence of multivessel coronary artery disease and left main artery disease. Earlier onset of S-T segment depression and greater persistence of S-T segment changes after the cessation of exercise strengthen the diagnosis of coronary artery disease. S-T segment changes occurring in the early stages of exercise and persisting for 8 minutes or longer after exercise are strongly associated with extensive coronary artery disease.

The value of exercise ECG findings for the diagnosis of coronary artery disease is related to the prevalence of coronary artery disease in the patient population being evaluation (Bayes theorem) (Chapter 5). An abnormal resting ECG caused by left ventricular hypertrophy, intraventricular conduction abnormalities, or electrolyte disturbances or by drug therapy (e.g., digitalis) decreases the predictive value of stress electrocardiography for the diagnosis of coronary artery disease. On the other hand, hemodynamic abnormalities observed during exercise in association with an abnormal stress ECG improve the predictive value. A fall in systolic blood pressure, the lack of significant increase in heart rate, a low heart rate–blood pressure product at the onset of S-T segment changes, and significant dyspnea during exercise all increase the probability of extensive coronary artery disease (Chapter 5).

Ambulatory ECG recordings may reveal evidence of transient myocardial ischemia (S-T segment shifts) in patients with ischemic heart disease (Chapter 5). Angina may not accompany the S-T segment changes. Ambulatory ECG recording has been recommended for the diagnosis of variant angina. The ambulatory ECG is frequently employed to detect episodes of silent myocardial ischemia. A flat or downsloping S-T segment depression of at least 1.0 mm or more below an isoelectric baseline and lasting for at least 1 minute is regarded as evidence for myocardial ischemia in patients with known coronary artery disease. Such ECG changes correlate well with other markers of myocardial ischemia, such as changes in myocardial thallium-201 or rubidium-82 uptake. Characteristic S-T depression occurs less frequently in totally asymptomatic patients without any other evidence of coronary artery disease. J point depression with upsloping S-T segments, however, occur frequently, in up to 36% of normal individuals. It needs to be emphasized that although characteristic S-T segment changes in the absence of angina often indicate silent myocardial ischemia in patients with known coronary artery disease, caution must be used in interpreting such changes in asymptomatic persons. The ECG changes must be supported by other evidence for myocardial ischemia.

Chest radiograph

Plain chest radiographs usually do not reveal any diagnostic information in patients with ischemic heart disease. Intracardiac linear calcification involving the apical portion of the cardiac silhouette may indicate chronic left ventricular aneurysm and, indirectly, the presence of ischemic heart disease, since previous myocardial infarction resulting from atherosclerotic coronary heart disease is the most frequent cause. Coronary artery calcification of more than one major coronary artery branch is frequently associated with significant coronary artery disease. However, this is an infrequent finding on standard chest films; fluoroscopy is more sensitive in detecting intracardiac calcification. Cardiac fluoroscopy, along with an exercise treadmill test, has a higher predictive value for the diagnosis of significant coronary artery disease. Computed cardiac tomography (cardiac CT) is useful to detect coronary artery calcification and can be of value for diagnosis of coronary atherosclerotic disease. When coronary artery calcification is detected in an individual with a positive exercise test, significant obstructive coronary artery disease is almost always present. In patients with prolonged episodes of chest pain, radiographic findings of pulmonary venous hypertension are strong evidence for myocardial ischemia. Unusual causes of ischemic heart disease, such as calcific aortic stenosis, coarctation of aorta, pseudo–xanthoma elasticum, and coronary artery aneurysm, occasionally are suggested by standard chest films.

Standard laboratory tests

Hyperlipidemia and carbohydrate intolerance are established risk factors for coronary artery disease. Therefore assessment of lipid profile and carbohydrate tolerance should be considered in patients with ischemic heart disease.

Among relatively young patients (i.e., under the age of 50 years) with arteriographically proved coronary artery disease, the incidence of carbohydrate intolerance or type II or I hyperlipoproteinemia may be as high as 90%.

Noninvasive imaging studies

In the diagnosis of ischemic heart disease and its severity, myocardial perfusion scintigraphy, gated blood pool scintigraphy, and echocardiography are of value in appropriate subsets of patients (Chapter 5). These studies aid in establishing the diagnosis of ischemic heart disease, as well as in localizing and quantitating the ischemic myocardial segments. The box below lists their potential clinical applications.

Myocardial perfusion scintigraphy. Thallium-201 myocardial perfusion scintigraphy is often employed in the diagnosis of ischemic heart disease. Images made at the peak of dynamic exercise, the time of maximum blood flow and therefore of isotope distribution, are compared with resting images made later (Chapter 5). Perfusion abnormalities related to reversible myocardial ischemia are transient and normalize when the ischemia is relieved. In contrast, image abnormalities caused by myocardial infarction or scar tissue are persistent. The appearance of perfusion defects during stress-induced myocardial ischemia and subsequent normalization of the defects on relief of the ischemia form the basis for stress thallium myocardial perfusion scintigraphy.

IV dipyridamole-thallium myocardial perfusion scintigraphy is an alternative technique to exercise thallium perfusion scintigraphy, and its sensitivity, specificity, and predictive value in the diagnosis of significant coronary artery disease appear to be very similar to those of exercise thallium scintigraphy (Chapter 5). Dipyridamole blocks adenosine deaminase and prevents adenosine reuptake by red blood cells, increasing local concentration of adenosine. Adenosine, being a potent coronary vasodilator, decreases coronary vascular resistance and increases coronary blood flow. However, the magnitude of reduction of coronary vascular resistance and therefore the magnitude of increase in coronary blood flow is related to the severity of coronary artery stenosis. After dipyridamole administration in patients with varying degrees of coronary artery stenosis in the different vascular territories, heterogeneity of flow distribution and thus of thallium uptake occurs, which allows the diagnosis of coronary artery disease. IV adenosine is expected to produce similar results, but its relative advantage compared with dipyridamole has not been established. Dipyridamole-thallium perfusion scintigraphy is safe and is indicated in patients who cannot perform adequate exercise (i.e., with peripheral vascular disease) or when exercise testing is contraindicated.

Many studies have demonstrated the improved sensitivity of the thallium perfusion scintigraphic technique compared with stress electrocardiography in the diagnosis of coronary artery disease, particularly in the identification of single- and double-vessel disease. Thus an exercise thallium myocardial perfusion scan is useful for excluding significant coronary artery disease in patients who have atypical chest pains, for establishing presence of high-risk coronary artery disease (left main coronary artery or triple-vessel involvement), and in patients in whom stress electrocardiography shows an equivocal response or cannot be interpreted because of baseline repolarization abnormalities, ST-T changes from drugs, left ventricular hypertrophy, or conduction disturbances. Stress thallium myocardial perfusion scintigraphy also provides information regarding the distribution and extent of myocardial ischemia.

Clinical use of radioisotopic imaging in the diagnosis of unstable and variant angina is limited by logistic problems. Diagnosis should be made primarily by the history and the ECG evidence of myocardial ischemia. Thallium scintigraphy may aid in the diagnosis of rest angina by demonstrating decreased segmental myocardial perfusion defects during prolonged episodes of chest pain (Chapter 5). The new radionuclide tracer technetium-99m ^{99m}Tc sestamibi, a lipophilic cationic compound with a short half-life, is taken

Noninvasive studies in anginal syndromes

1. Classic angina
   a. History, physical examination, and resting ECG
   b. Normal resting ECG: stress electrocardiography to detect high-risk patients or to assess response to therapy
   c. Abnormal resting ECG (uninterpretable): stress thallium myocardial perfusion scan to detect high-risk patients
   d. In patients with poor exercise tolerance: dipyridamole-thallium myocardial perfusion scan to detect severity of coronary artery disease
   e. In patients in whom concurrent assessment of left ventricular function is indicated: resting and exercise gated blood pool scintigraphy or two-dimensional (2D) echocardiography
   f. In patients with previous myocardial infarction and stable angina: stress thallium myocardial perfusion scan (in patients with adequate exercise tolerance) or dipyridamole-thallium myocardial perfusion scan or exercise ventriculography to assess the severity of coronary artery disease and to localize the new vascular territory involved with atherosclerosis
2. Atypical chest pain syndrome
   a. Normal resting ECG: stress electrocardiography
   b. Abnormal resting ECG: stress thallium myocardial perfusion scintigraphy or stress ventriculography (in the absence of other detectable heart disease)
   c. Mitral valve prolapse, chest pain, and abnormal resting ECG: echocardiography and stress thallium myocardial perfusion scintigraphy
   d. Suspected valvular heart disease: 2D echocardiography
3. Variant and unstable angina
   a. History
   b. ECG during chest pain
   c. In patients with prolonged chest pain and uninterpretable ECG: 2D echocardiography; thallium myocardial perfusion scintigraphy and/or gated blood pool scintigraphy

up by the myocardium receiving coronary blood flow without undergoing significant redistribution.

^{99m}Tc teboroxime is a neutral lipophilic complex that is rapidly taken up by the myocardium, with also rapid myocardial washout. Its relative advantages for the detection of coronary artery disease needs to be determined.

Gated blood pool scintigraphy. Global and regional myocardial wall motion may be studied by gated blood pool scintigraphy (Chapter 5). Regional wall motion abnormalities and decreased global ejection fraction are frequently observed in patients with previous myocardial infarction, ischemic cardiomyopathy, and chronic left ventricular aneurysm. Assessment of left ventricular function during exercise by gated blood pool scintigraphy is an alternative approach to thallium myocardial perfusion scintigraphy for detecting ischemic heart disease. Decreased global left ventricular ejection fraction or the appearance of new segmental wall motion abnormalities may suggest significant coronary artery disease. However, a decrease or lack of an increase in left ventricular ejection fraction can also be observed in patients without coronary artery disease (Chapter 5).

Echocardiography. Echocardiography can also be used to study global and regional cardiac wall motion, particularly reversible segmental wall motion abnormalities (Chapter 5). Exercise echocardiography to assess abnormalities of regional and global left ventricular systolic function may provide indirect evidence for the presence of obstructive coronary artery disease. Inotropic stimulation with dobutamine may induce left ventricular wall motion abnormalities in patients with obstructive coronary artery disease. Similarly, left ventricular wall motion abnormalities during dipyridamole or adenosine infusion detected by transthoracic two-dimensional echocardiography may also indicate the presence of significant coronary artery disease. The sensitivity, specificity, predictive value, and relative advantages and disadvantages of stress echocardiography in detecting coronary artery disease remain to be established, and the study should be used only in special circumstances.

Coronary arteriography

The definitive diagnosis of coronary artery disease and its anatomic extent can be made only by coronary angiography. Techniques are described in Chapter 6. This section's discussion is confined to indications for the technique and interpretation of the information gained.

Indications for coronary arteriography

1. In patients with classic angina, coronary arteriography is not required for the diagnosis of coronary artery disease.
2. In patients with stable angina in whom a stress ECG or a thallium myocardial perfusion scan suggests high-risk coronary artery disease (e.g., left main coronary artery stenosis), coronary arteriography is indicated.
3. In patients with stable angina, when revascularization surgery or angioplasty is contemplated, coronary arteriography must be performed.
4. In occasional patients with atypical chest pain (e.g., patients admitted to a coronary care unit several times to rule out myocardial infarction), when other diagnostic tests have failed to clarify the diagnosis, coronary arteriography may be required to exclude coronary artery disease.
5. In patients with angina and valvular heart disease, coronary arteriography is required to delineate the coronary anatomy and establish the mechanism of angina.
6. In most patients with unstable angina, coronary arteriography is indicated. Timing of coronary arteriography, however, is variable, largely depending on the response to medical therapy. In patients who have partial or no relief of angina with medical therapy, coronary arteriography should be done promptly.
7. In patients with variant angina who have S-T elevation or depression during angina, coronary arteriography is indicated to determine whether the coronary arteries are normal of if fixed coronary artery stenosis is present.
8. When a diagnosis of variant angina is strongly suspected but cannot be documented by noninvasive studies, coronary arteriography with ergonovine provocation is indicated.

Interpretation of arteriographic findings. In patients with stable angina the incidence of single-, double-, and triple-vessel coronary artery disease is approximately the same. Abnormalities of left ventricular wall motion can be detected by contrast ventriculography in approximately 60% of patients with chronic ischemic heart disease. Asynergy is usually caused by scar tissue and reflects previous myocardial infarction. However, abnormal segmental wall motion and decreased global ejection fraction may also result from reversible myocardial ischemia (hibernating myocardium). In the catheterization laboratory, intervention ventriculography can be performed (with nitroglycerin or post-extrasystolic potentiation) to differentiate between scar tissue and reversible ischemic myocardial segments. Reversible hypokinetic myocardial segments often demonstrate improved systolic motion after nitroglycerin or with post-extrasystolic potentiation. Contrast left ventriculogram also reveals mitral regurgitation when present.

In patients with unstable angina, single-, double-, and triple-vessel disease also occur with approximately equal frequency. However, the following exceptions or qualifications may be noted. The incidence of single-vessel disease is higher in patients with recent onset of angina. Left main coronary artery stenosis is also more frequent in patients with unstable angina. The left anterior descending coronary artery is the most frequently affected vessel. Less developed collateral circulation has been observed in patients with unstable angina than in those with chronic stable angina. In approximately 10% of patients diagnosed with unstable angina, coronary arteriography does not reveal hemodynamically significant coronary artery stenosis. Coronary artery spasm is considered to be the mechanism for rest angina in these patients. Type IIb coronary artery lesions are more frequently encountered, and in patients with an abnormal resting ECG, thrombus at the site of coronary artery stenosis is also discovered more frequently.

As described earlier, hemodynamic abnormalities are variable in patients with unstable angina. In some patients, severe depression of cardiac function may be observed during ischemic episodes, whereas the hemodynamics may be normal between episodes of angina.

In patients with variant angina, coronary arteriography reveals atherosclerotic lesions of varying severity involving at least one major coronary artery in most patients (Chapter 6), although in some patients, arteriographically detectable lesions are absent. Coronary artery spasm as the mechanism for variant angina has been well documented. In some patients with suspected variant angina, provocation of coronary artery spasm is required to confirm the diagnosis (Chapter 6). Ergonovine, methacholine, and hyperventilation have been used to provoke coronary artery spasm; IV injection of ergonovine (0.05 to 0.4 mg) appears to be the method most likely to provoke coronary artery spasm. Demonstration of coronary artery spasm alone, however, does not confirm a diagnosis of variant angina. Unless the provoked coronary artery spasm is accompanied by the patient's usual chest pain, along with ECG changes indicating myocardial ischemia, the diagnosis of variant angina is not established. In patients with severe fixed coronary artery stenosis, an ergonovine provocation test should be avoided because of the risk of precipitating a myocardial infarction.

At catheterization, atrial pacing is used occasionally to induce myocardial ischemia by increasing heart rate; however, it is considerably less sensitive and specific for diagnosing coronary artery disease than treadmill exercise testing.

MEDICAL MANAGEMENT

Management of a patient with ischemic heart disease should incorporate modification of risk factors for coronary atherosclerosis along with interventions to prevent adverse consequences of myocardial ischemia. Thus treatment of hypertension, hyperlipidemia, obesity, and diabetes and cessation of smoking should be part of the routine management of such patients.

Physical exercise has been advocated for patients with ischemic heart disease to decrease the complications of coronary artery disease. The relationship between physical activity and the development of coronary artery disease is unclear, but physical training clearly produces beneficial effects on cardiac performance. Furthermore, physical activity provides patients with a sense of well-being. Thus regular physical exercise is recommended for patients with chronic stable angina. Aggressive "lipid control" modification of other risk factors, vigorous exercise, and stress reduction have the potential to cause regression of established atherosclerotic coronary artery disease; however, such a rigid lifestyle is difficult to maintain.

The treatment of angina and other manifestations of myocardial ischemia is based on a reduction of $M\dot{V}O_2$ and an increase in coronary blood flow to the potentially ischemic myocardium. Pharmacologic agents, in general, decrease $M\dot{V}O_2$, although some agents have the potential to enhance myocardial perfusion. Revascularization surgery and transluminal coronary angioplasty, on the other hand, increase coronary blood flow and O_2 delivery to the myocardium.

Pharmacologic agents: nitroglycerin and nitrates

Nitroglycerin and nitrates are direct-acting smooth muscle relaxants and cause vasodilatation of the peripheral vascular bed. It is generally accepted that "the nitrate receptors," which contain sulfhydryl (SH) groups, are probably located on the myocytes rather than on the vascular endothelium. After receptor binding, nitrosothiols (NO) groups are formed, which stimulate guanylate cyclase to produce cyclic guanosine monophosphate (GMP) in the smooth muscles. The mechanism of cyclic GMP–mediated vasodilatation is unclear but may be related to decreased calcium entry to the cell or increased calcium uptake by the sarcoplasmic reticulum. The SH groups, required for the stimulation of guanylate cyclase, are oxidized by excess exposure to nitrates. The depletion of SH groups is the proposed mechanism for nitrate tolerance, and this hypothesis is supported by the observations that SH donor *N*-acetylcysteine at least partially reverses nitrate tolerance. It has been suggested that the augmented cyclic adenosine monophosphate (cAMP) production in response to prostaglandins contributes to nitrate-induced vasodilatation.

Nitroglycerin and nitrates produce more pronounced vasodilatation of the venous capacitance bed than the arteriolar resistance bed. The hemodynamic effects of nitroglycerin are characterized by decreased ventricular diastolic volumes associated with decreased systemic and pulmonary venous pressures. Arterial pressure tends to decrease, and heart rate and contractility may increase. Decreased arterial pressure and left ventricular volume are associated with decreased wall tension and a resulting decreased $M\dot{V}O_2$. In rare instances a paradoxical increase in $M\dot{V}O_2$ may occur because of excessive reflex tachycardia and increased contractility.

Nitroglycerin also dilates the large epicardial conductance coronary arteries. Coronary arteriolar resistance tends to decrease, although to a much lesser extent. Since collateral coronary arteries tend to respond in the same way as larger arteries, nitroglycerin can potentially increase collateral blood flow.

The potential beneficial and deleterious effects of nitroglycerin and nitrates in the treatment of angina are summarized in Table 13-1. In patients with stable angina associated with fixed obstructive coronary artery disease, nitroglycerin exerts its beneficial effects primarily by decreasing $M\dot{V}O_2$.

Relaxation of the smooth muscles of the epicardial coronary arteries and relief of coronary artery spasm are the mechanisms of beneficial effects in patients with variant angina. Increases in regional coronary blood flow and myo-

Table 13-1. Potential beneficial and deleterious effects of nitroglycerin and other nitrates in management of angina

Effects	Results
Beneficial	
Decreased ventricular volume	
Decreased arterial pressure	Decreased $M\dot{V}O_2$
Decreased ejection time	
Decreased left ventricular diastolic pressure	Improved subendocardial perfusion
Increased collateral flow	Improved perfusion to ischemic myocardium
Vasodilatation of epicardial coronary arteries	Relief of coronary artery spasm
Deleterious	
Reflex tachycardia	Increased $M\dot{V}O_2$
Reflex increase in contractility	
Decreased diastolic perfusion time because of tachycardia	Decreased myocardial perfusion

Reprinted with permission from Chatterjee K, Rouleau J-L, and Parmley WW: JAMA 252:1173, 1984.

Table 13-2. Nitrate and nitrite drugs used in treatment of angina

Drug	Dosage	Duration of action
Short acting		
Nitroglycerin, sublingual	0.15-1.2 mg	10-30 min
Isosorbide, sublingual	2.5-5.0 mg	10-60 min
Amyl nitrite, inhalant	0.18-0.3 ml	3-5 min
Long acting		
Nitroglycerin, oral sustained-action	6.5-13 mg/6-8 hr	6-8 hr 3-6 hr
Nitroglycerin, 2% ointment	½-2 inches/4 hr	3-6 hr
Nitroglycerin, slow-release buccal	1-2 mg/4 hr	1½-2 hr
Nitroglycerin, slow-release transcutaneous	10-25 mg/24 hr	24 hr or longer
Isosorbide dinitrate, sublingual	2.5-10 mg/2 hr	4-6 hr
Isosorbide dinitrate, oral	10-60 mg/4-6 hr	4-6 hr
Isosorbide dinitrate, chewable	5-10 mg/2-4 hr	2-3 hr
Pentaerythrityl tetranitrate	40 mg/6-8 hr	6-8 hr
Erythrityl tetranitrate	10-40 mg/6-8 hr	6-8 hr

Published with permission from Katzung BG and Chatterjee K: Basic and clinical pharmacology. Los Altos, Calif, 1983, Lange.

cardial perfusion are associated with the relief of angina. For maintenance therapy, long-acting nitrates or nitroglycerin administered transcutaneously are frequently effective. In general, relatively larger doses of these agents are needed compared with those used for the treatment of stable angina.

Nitroglycerin and nitrates are effective in decreasing the frequency and duration of episodes of spontaneous S-T segment shifts without angina in patients with stable angina and with vasospastic angina. Enhanced left ventricular regional wall motion provides additional evidence for its effectiveness in ameliorating silent myocardial ischemia.

Nitroglycerin and nitrates are also useful in the treatment of unstable angina, although the precise mechanism is not clear. Both decreased $M\dot{V}O_2$ and increased myocardial perfusion, associated with decreased coronary vascular tone, might be contributory. In patients with repeated episodes of rest angina, administration of nitroglycerin by the IV route is preferable because it permits easier control of angina.

Some of the forms of nitroglycerin and nitrates used in the treatment of angina are listed in Table 13-2. The onset of action of sublingual nitroglycerin is rapid (1 to 3 minutes), which is why it is the most frequently used agent for the immediate treatment of angina pectoris. Because of its shorter duration of action (not exceeding 20 to 30 minutes), it is not a suitable agent for maintenance therapy. The onset of action of IV nitroglycerin is also rapid (5 minutes), but its hemodynamic effects are quickly reversed on discontinuation of its infusion. Its clinical application is therefore restricted to the treatment of recurrent rest angina. However, tolerance to the hemodynamic effects of nitroglycerin certainly occur both in patients with angina and with heart failure. It has been suggested that an 8-hour to 12-hour nitroglycerin-free period avoids the development of tolerance. Cross-tolerance to isosorbide dinitrate has been documented; thus substitution of nitroglycerin by isosorbide dinitrate is not effective. Improvement in exercise tolerance of patients with stable angina is more apparent when given three times rather than four times daily, presumably because an 8-hour nitrate-free period is required to prevent tolerance. Buccal and oral preparations and several transdermal forms of nitroglycerin are also available. It is claimed that these formulations provide effective blood concentrations for long periods, but their effectiveness in the maintenance therapy of angina remains uncertain. Treadmill exercise tests have demonstrated that the beneficial effects of "nitroglycerin patches" do not last more than 6 to 8 hours.

The onset of action of sublingual or chewable isosorbide dinitrate, pentaerythrityl tetranitrate, and erythrityl tetranitrate is rapid (2 to 3 minutes), but their duration of action is relatively short (1½ to 3 hours). Isosorbide 5-mononitrate does not undergo liver metabolism and is fully bioavailable after oral administration. Its elimination half-life is 4 to 6 hours and duration of action about 8 hours.

The most common undesirable effect of nitrate therapy is a throbbing headache, which tends to decrease with continued therapy. Postural dizziness and weakness also occur, but frank syncope is rare. Because of the potential for withdrawal symptoms, nitrate therapy should be tapered rather than abruptly stopped.

Methemoglobinemia is virtually never seen in the clinical management of angina and has been observed only when very large (nonpharmacologic) doses of nitrates have been used. Nitrates do not worsen glaucoma, once thought to be

Table 13-3. Effects of beta-adrenergic blocking drugs, nitrates, and combined beta blocker–nitrate therapy in patients with angina pectoris

	Beta blockers	Nitrates	Combined nitrates and beta blockers
Heart rate	Decrease	Reflex increase	Decrease
Atrial pressure	Decrease	Decrease	Decrease
End-diastolic volume	Increase	Decrease	None or decrease
Contractility	Decrease	Reflex increase	None
Ejection time	Increase	Decrease	None
Diastolic perfusion time	Increase	Decrease	Increase

Published with permission from Katzung BG and Chatterjee K: Basic and clinical pharmacology. Los Altos, Calif, 1983, Lange.

a contraindication, and nitrates can be used safely in the presence of increased intraocular pressure. However, nitrates are contraindicated if intracranial pressure is elevated.

Beta-adrenergic blocking agents

The beneficial effects of beta-blocking agents are primarily related to their potential to decrease $M\dot{V}O_2$. In general, beta-blocking drugs decrease heart rate, blood pressure, and contractility, which in turn decrease $M\dot{V}O_2$. Exercise-induced increases in heart rate and blood pressure are also blunted by beta-blocker therapy. Decreased heart rate is associated with a larger left ventricular end-diastolic volume, which increases $M\dot{V}O_2$, but the net effect in most patients is reduction of $M\dot{V}O_2$.

Some beta-blocking drugs have the potential to enhance myocardial perfusion because of their differential effects on coronary vascular resistance in the relatively ischemic and nonischemic myocardial segments. Myocardial perfusion also may improve because of increased diastolic perfusion time associated with decreased heart rate. It has been suggested that beta-blocking agents may decrease platelet aggregation and also cause a rightward shift of the oxyhemoglobin dissociation curve, which increases O_2 delivery. However, decreased $M\dot{V}O_2$ seems to be the most important mechanism for the relief of myocardial ischemia.

Beta-blocker therapy enhances exercise tolerance and delays the onset of angina and S-T segment depression during exercise in patients with effort angina. The magnitude of S-T segment depression may also decrease. Although exercise tolerance improves, the heart rate–blood pressure product at the onset of myocardial ischemia remains unchanged.

The increase in end-diastolic volume that results from relative bradycardia is an undesirable effect of beta-blocking drugs. Furthermore, a significant reduction in contractile function, if it occurs, may also increase left ventricular end-systolic and end-diastolic volumes and end-diastolic pressure. These potential deleterious effects can be overcome by the concomitant use of nitrates. Beta-blocking drugs and nitrates tend to offset each other's deleterious effects of $M\dot{V}O_2$ (Table 13-3), and the net result is a decrease in $M\dot{V}O_2$. An additive effect of the two agents in improving exercise tolerance has been observed, although it may not occur in all patients with chronic stable angina. The differences in the important properties of the different beta-blocking agents are summarized in Table 13-4.

No conclusive evidence proves that any particular beta-blocking drug is superior to any other for the management of stable angina. Relatively cardioselective beta blockers are competitive antagonists to $beta_1$ receptors, and nonselective beta blockers are antagonists to both $beta_1$ and $beta_2$ receptors. Nonselective beta blockers therefore may have the potential to increase coronary vascular tone because of

Table 13-4. Properties of various beta-adrenergic blocking agents

Agent	Cardioselectivity	Intrinsic sympathetic activity	Lipid solubility	Plasma half-life (hours)	Usual dose for angina
Propranolol	−	−	+++	1-6	60-320 mg/day
Metoprolol	+	−	+	3	100-200 mg/day
Nadolol	−	−	0	16-24	80-240 mg/day
Timolol	−	−	+	4-5	15-45 mg/day
Atenolol	+	−	0	6-9	50-100 mg/day
Pindolol	−	+++	+	4	5-20 mg/day
Acebutolol	+	++	0	8-12	600-1200 mg/day
Labetolol (combined beta- or alpha-blocking effects)	−	−	+++	3-4	300-600 mg/day

unopposed alpha-adrenergic activity. Worsening leg claudication and Raynaud's phenomenon are observed more frequently with nonselective than with cardioselective beta blockers. $Beta_2$ receptor inhibition is associated with increased serum potassium levels. Correction of hypokalemia therefore is more likely to occur with nonselective beta blockers than with cardioselective beta blockers. Beta-blocking agents with intrinsic sympathetic stimulating activity attenuate the exercise-induced increase in heart rate and blood pressure without causing a significant decrease in heart rate or blood pressure. In clinical circumstances in which reduction of resting heart rate or blood pressure is not required or undesirable, beta-blocking agents with intrinsic sympathetic activity may provide some advantage.

The side effects profile of different beta-blocking drugs may differ and should be considered in the selection of a particular beta-blocking agent in the long-term management of patients with angina pectoris. Bronchospasm is more likely to occur with nonselective beta blockers. Intensification of insulin-induced hypoglycemia is more common with nonselective beta-blocking drugs. Depression of cardiac function and precipitation of overt congestive heart failure may complicate beta-blocker therapy, particularly in patients with already compromised left ventricular function. Beta-blocking agents with intrinsic sympathetic-stimulating activity theoretically are less likely to precipitate heart failure. Central nervous system side effects (e.g., fatigue, depression, lack of concentration) have been reported less frequently with beta-blocking drugs that do not substantially cross the blood-brain barrier (lipophilic beta blockers). Gastrointestinal side effects and sexual dysfunction are common with all beta-blocking agents.

The effective dose of any beta-blocking drug varies considerably from patient to patient; dose titration in individual patients against both resting and exercise heart rates is desirable, along with monitoring of changes in blood pressure and cardiac function. In patients with severe effort angina, considerable reduction in resting heart rate (50 to 60 beats/min) and maximum heart rate during exercise (100 to 120 beats/min) may be required to control angina effectively.

For maintenance therapy of stable angina, beta-blocking drugs with a relatively long half-life are preferred because of improved patient compliance. The potential disadvantage of the long-acting beta blockers, however, is the longer persistence of hemodynamic effects and untoward effects when, in certain clinical circumstances, withdrawal of beta-blocker therapy becomes necessary. It must be emphasized that sudden withdrawal of effective beta-blocker therapy in ambulatory patients may result in worsening of angina and precipitation of acute ischemic episodes, including myocardial infarction. During elective withdrawal of beta-blocker therapy, patients should be instructed to reduce their physical activity, and withdrawal should be gradual.

Despite the potential for the beta-blocking drugs to increase coronary vascular tone (unopposed alpha-adrenergic effect), in clinical practice, many patients (50% to 85%) become free of anginal attacks on a regimen of combined beta-blocker and nitrate therapy. The effectiveness of beta-blocker therapy is more satisfactory in patients with a history of effort-induced angina. For patients who have not been on beta-blocker therapy, relatively short-acting beta-blocking drugs should be administered to decrease resting heart rate to between 50 and 60 beats/min and systolic blood pressure to 100 to 110 mm Hg without precipitating heart failure or compromising organ perfusion. In some patients, therapy may be initiated with IV propranolol (0.1 to 0.2 mg/kg) or the short-acting beta blocker esmolol. In patients already receiving beta-blocker therapy, the dose of beta-blocking drugs should be increased to achieve the desired hemodynamic effects. In patients with unstable angina, beta blockers should be used in conjunction with nitrates and frequently with calcium blocking agents for those who continue to experience rest angina.

In patients with variant angina, beta blockers do not appear to be effective; coronary vasodilators remain the primary therapy. Interestingly, beta blockers can decrease the frequency and duration of silent episodes of spontaneous S-T segment depressions in patients with stable angina caused by obstructive coronary artery disease. The mechanisms for the beneficial effect, however, remain unclear.

Calcium channel blocking agents

Drugs that block the slow inward current of a propagated cardiac impulse, frequently called calcium channel blocking agents, have emerged as an important addition to the pharmacotherapy of anginal syndromes. Calcium channel blocking drugs have the potential to decrease $\dot{M}VO_2$ as well as to increase coronary blood flow.

All calcium channel blocking drugs possess a negative inotropic effect: they decrease myocardial contractile force because of decreased availability of calcium to the contractile elements. These agents also inhibit calcium entry to the smooth muscles of the peripheral vascular bed and cause peripheral vasodilatation. Arterial and intraventricular pressures decrease because of the decreased systemic vascular resistance. Heart rate may also decrease with the use of some calcium channel blocking agents. These hemodynamic effects (decreased contractility, heart rate, and arterial pressure) decrease $M\dot{V}O_2$.

Calcium channel blocking agents may increase coronary blood flow and myocardial perfusion by several mechanisms. All calcium channel blocking agents can cause dilatation of the epicardial coronary arteries and thus relieve and prevent vasospasm of the large coronary arteries. Arterial dilatation results partly from the direct effect on smooth muscles and partly from inhibition of the vasoconstrictive effect of the alpha receptors. Evidence also shows that calcium channel blocking agents have the potential to promote coronary collateral blood flow.

Other physiologic effects of calcium channel blocking agents, such as improved left ventricular diastolic function and myocardial relaxation and decreased myocardial injury in the presence of ischemia from decreased myocardial calcium overload, have been observed. However, the significance of these effects in the treatment of ischemic heart disease remains undetermined.

Several calcium channel blocking drugs are available for clinical use (Table 13-5). Tiapamil and bepridil appear to possess sodium channel blocking effects in addition to calcium channel blocking properties. Nifedipine, verapamil, and diltiazem are structurally different, and there are also differences in their cardiovascular effects. Sinoatrial and atrioventricular nodal tissues, which are mainly composed of "slow-response cells," are affected by verapamil and diltiazem but not by nifedipine. Thus verapamil and diltiazem decrease atrioventricular conduction and are effective for the treatment of supraventricular tachycardia and for decreasing ventricular responses in atrial fibrillation or flutter. In patients with a history of supraventricular tachycardia or atrial fibrillation and flutter, diltiazem or verapamil provides advantages over nifedipine. However, in patients with sinoatrial or atrioventricular nodal disease, nifedipine is preferable. All three agents decrease arterial pressure; however, nifedipine seems to be a more potent arteriolar dilator, and the hypotensive response to nifedipine is usually more pronounced. Negative inotropic effects, least likely with diltiazem, can cause a depression in left ventricular pump function. Reduction of systemic vascular resistance and a decrease in left ventricular afterload usually compensate for the potential deleterious consequences of their negative inotropic effects on cardiac performance. Thus the overall left ventricular pump function may remain unchanged. However, verapamil is not well tolerated by patients with significantly depressed left ventricular function.

Concomitant use of beta blockers should also be avoided in patients with depressed left ventricular function because of the risk of precipitating overt heart failure from the combined negative inotropic effects of both classes of agents.

It has been demonstrated that both nonspecific sympathetic antagonism and alpha-adrenergic antagonism can occur with some calcium channel blocking agents. Nonspecific sympathetic antagonism is most marked with diltiazem and much less with verapamil. Nifedipine does not seem to have this effect. Thus reflex tachycardia, in response to hypotension, occurs most intensely with nifedipine and less so with verapamil. With diltiazem, heart rate may even decrease despite a fall in arterial pressure. Consequently, in patients with bradycardia in whom further reduction in heart rate is not desired, nifedipine is preferable to verapamil or diltiazem. Conversely, when reduction in heart rate is desired, verapamil or diltiazem is more likely to produce this effect than nifedipine.

Drug interaction, such as with digitalis, is a practical clinical problem with the use of some calcium channel blocking agents. Serum digoxin levels consistently increase with verapamil, and digitalis toxicity can occur. Both decreased distribution volume and impaired clearance of digoxin appear to contribute to increased serum digoxin levels. Serum digoxin levels have rarely been found to increase after nifedipine or diltiazem therapy.

In the treatment of effort angina, all three agents increase exercise tolerance and the duration of exercise before the onset of angina or S-T segment depression. However, the heart rate–blood pressure product at the onset of myocardial ischemia usually remains unchanged. Clinical studies suggest that a reduction in $M\dot{V}O_2$ is the primary mechanism by which currently available calcium channel blocking agents produce their beneficial effects in patients with effort angina.

In the management of unstable angina, calcium channel blocking agents are useful in certain subsets of patients. Controlled studies have suggested that these agents are more likely to control angina in patients who are already taking beta blockers and/or nitrates and that the beneficial

Table 13-5. Calcium channel blocking agents potentially useful in management of angina syndromes

Agent	Usual dose	Absolute or relative contraindications
Dihydropyridines		
Nifedipine	Oral: 30-120 mg/day Sublingual: 10 mg q4-6 h	Hypotension
Nitrendipine	20-40 mg/day	Hypotension
Felodipine (potent vasodilator)	15-30 mg/day	Hypotension
Nimodipine (useful in cerebral ischemia)	0-35 mg/kg, 4 hourly	Hypotension
Nisoldipine	30-60 mg/day	Hypotension
Nicardipine	15-90 mg/day	Hypotension
Verapamil	IV bolus: 5-10 mg in 10 min IV infusion: 1 mg/min to total of 10 mg Oral: 120-480 mg/day	Sick sinus syndrome, A-V conduction defects, sinus bradycardia, digitalis toxicity, overt heart failure, hypotension
Diltiazem	IV: 0.15-0.25 mg/kg over 2 min Oral: 90-230 mg/day	As for verapamil
Mixed agents		
Tiapamil (as with verapamil, also a sodium blocker)	1500 mg/day	As for verapamil
Bepridil (mixed sodium blocker)	200-400 mg/day	Prolonged Q-T interval

effects are observed particularly in patients who develop S-T segment elevations during spontaneous rest angina. The mechanisms for the beneficial effects of calcium channel blocking agents in unstable angina have not been clarified. A reduction of myocardial O_2 requirements is likely to be contributory in certain patients; in others, improved myocardial perfusion caused by a primary decrease in coronary vascular tone must also play a role. Nifedipine used alone can enhance myocardial ischemia and increase the incidence of infarction and adverse cardiac events; thus nifedipine and probably other dihydropyridine calcium channel blocking agents alone should be avoided for management of ischemia in patients with unstable angina.

Nifedipine, verapamil, and diltiazem are all effective in preventing a recurrence of anginal episodes in patients with variant angina. In approximately 70% of patients, anginal attacks are completely abolished; in another 20% a marked reduction in frequency can be expected. The prevention of coronary artery spasm is the principal mechanism for this beneficial effect. Nifedipine, administered sublingually, can cause prompt relief of angina.

Although nitroglycerin and nitrates are also effective in the management of variant angina, the incidence of undesirable side effects with nitrates compared with calcium entry blocking agents is higher. Furthermore, beneficial effects of calcium channel blocking agents have been documented in patients refractory to nitrate therapy.

All three of the calcium channel blocking agents (diltiazem, verapamil, nifedipine) decrease the frequency and duration of the silent episodes of ischemia. A decrease in coronary vascular tone and improved myocardial perfusion are the likely mechanisms. Diltiazem has been found effective in decreasing the incidence of silent and symptomatic myocardial ischemia, as well as of acute cardiac events in patients with non–Q wave myocardial infarction.

Relative vasoselective calcium channel blocking agents (nicardipine, felodipine, isradipine) appear to possess more potent vasodilating properties and less negative inotropic effects compared with other calcium channel blocking agents. However, the relative advantages and potential complications of these agents in the management of angina have not been established. The usual dose of isradipine is 5 to 20 mg/day.

The side effects of the different calcium channel blocking agents differ to some extent. Symptoms related to hypotension (e.g., dizziness) can occur with any of these agents but are more frequent with nifedipine. Headaches, flushing, gastrointestinal symptoms (e.g., nausea, constipation), and dependent edema are common to all the agents. Nonspecific central nervous system symptoms are observed infrequently after administration of calcium channel blocking drugs. Frank psychosis (mania) has been reported after the use of diltiazem, although this complication is extremely rare. Bradyarrhythmias occur more frequently with verapamil than with diltiazem. As described earlier, overt heart failure and elevation of serum digoxin levels are more likely to occur with verapamil than with nifedipine and diltiazem.

For treatment of angina with the calcium channel blocking agents, it is necessary to administer adequate doses. The usual effective doses of the typically used agents are as follows: nifedipine (30 to 120 mg/day), verapamil (240 to 480 mg/day), and diltiazem (180 to 360 mg/day).

Other antianginal therapies

Long-term anticoagulant therapy with coumadin derivatives does not appear to have any role in the management of chronic ischemic heart disease. Aspirin decreases the incidence of acute cardiac events (infarction, sudden death, need for coronary artery bypass surgery) almost by 50% in patients with unstable angina. IV heparin has been found more effective than beta blockers and aspirin in controlling angina and decreasing the incidence of adverse cardiac events in patients with unstable angina. Thus IV heparin therapy should be considered in patients who continue to experience angina, despite aspirin and antianginal pharmacotherapy.

Ticlopidine, another antiplatelet agent, with different mechanisms of action than aspirin, is also effective in reducing the incidence of ischemia and infarction in patients with unstable angina. Ticlopidine, at a dose of 250 mg twice daily, given for 6 months may reduce the incidence of mortality and of myocardial infarction by 50%. Ticlopidine primarily inhibits the adenosine diphosphate pathway of platelet aggregation but, unlike aspirin, does not inhibit the cyclo-oxygenase pathway; it does not prevent the production of thromboxane by platelets or the production of prostacyclin by endothelial cells. Ticlopidine can be used when aspirin is contraindicated; its gastrointestinal and bleeding complications are similar to those of aspirin.

IV prostacyclin, although it increases coronary blood flow, does not improve the angina threshold in patients with effort angina. Similarly, it does not provide any advantage, compared with conventional therapy, in patients with unstable angina.

Beneficial effects were anticipated in the treatment of vasospastic angina with alpha-adrenergic blocking agents; however, controlled studies have failed to demonstrate the efficacy of alpha-blocking agents, such as prazosin, in variant angina.

Intra-aortic balloon counterpulsation is effective in controlling episodes of rest angina in patients with unstable angina. "Systolic unloading" decreases $M\dot{V}O_2$, and diastolic augmentation has the potential to enhance myocardial perfusion. Patients with preserved left ventricular function and stable hemodynamics usually do not require intra-aortic balloon counterpulsation. In patients with significantly depressed left ventricular function and unstable hemodynamics, intra-aortic balloon counterpulsation is useful for stabilization. Recurrent thrombotic occlusions at the site of fissured or ruptured atheromatous plaques are regarded as a probable mechanism for prolonged rest angina and threatened infarction in patients with unstable angina, the rationale for use of thrombolytic agents.

CORONARY ANGIOPLASTY AND MYOCARDIAL REVASCULARIZATION SURGERY

Coronary angioplasty

Percutaneous transluminal dilatation of the coronary arteries is an effective method for reducing the degree of coronary artery stenosis. The technical details of this procedure are described in Chapter 6.

Coronary angioplasty as an effective method for the treatment of angina is now well established. Many appropriately selected patients have become asymptomatic after angioplasty. In patients with effort angina, exercise tolerance invariably improves after successful angioplasty. Thallium-201 scintigraphy during exercise usually demonstrates enhanced perfusion of previously underperfused myocardial segments. Regional systolic and diastolic function also improve. Angioplasty decreases or eliminates the resistance at the site of stenosis, and thus increased perfusion is the mechanism for the beneficial effects of angioplasty.

Coronary angioplasty provides some advantages over coronary artery bypass surgery. Thoracotomy, with its complications, prolonged hospitalization for postoperative care, and protracted convalescence, can be avoided. Cost-effectiveness also favors angioplasty. The incidence of angioplasty-related myocardial infarction appears to be less than the incidence of perioperative myocardial infarction. Furthermore, the option for surgery at some future date remains available to patients who have undergone successful angioplasty.

The potential complications of angioplasty include coronary artery dissection and rupture, cardiac tamponade, and myocardial infarction. Emergency revascularization surgery is required in some patients as a result of complications from angioplasty. The most common serious complication, however, is restenosis, with a reported incidence of approximately 30%.

The success rate for angioplasty varies. It certainly depends on clinicians' skill and experience. The reported success rate in experienced hands is as high as 90%. With the advent of steerable catheters and "kissing balloon" techniques, angioplasty is being performed with greater frequency and a higher success rate. Left main coronary artery lesions, heavily calcified uncompressible lesions, long-segment stenoses, and very distal coronary artery lesions are relative contraindications for angioplasty. Initially, patients with total occlusion, calcified lesions, and multivessel and multiple stenoses were not considered to be candidates for angioplasty. However, with increasing experience and improved techniques, physicians in many specialized centers have been successfully dilating such complex lesions, which are no longer regarded as absolute contraindications for angioplasty.

Selection of patients for angioplasty remains largely empirical and depends partly on available facilities and the clinician's skill and experience. Nevertheless, successful angioplasty can cause a marked improvement in angina, and it is recommended that patients refractory to medical therapy be considered for coronary angioplasty.

Directional atherectomy, rotablator atherectomy, and laser angioplasty are newer mechanical techniques for relieving coronary artery atherosclerotic stenosis. Each technique appears to have some specific advantages; however, the overall restenosis rates (30% to 50%) with these techniques presently are similar to those after balloon angioplasty.

Coronary artery bypass surgery

Surgical creation of a bypass shunt from the aorta to a diseased coronary artery beyond the area of fixed obstruction is now an established therapy for ischemic heart disease (see the box below). Most often, a saphenous vein is used for the shunt material, although other veins may also be used. The internal mammary artery is being used with increasing frequency and in most patients is the vessel of choice for left anterior descending coronary artery lesions because of its higher long-term patency rate.

Perioperative mortality in patients with normal or slightly depressed left ventricular function is presently quite low at 1.0% to 2.5%. In patients with depressed left ventricular function, operative mortality is considerably higher, approximately 10% to 30%, and the operative risk increases with the increasing severity of depressed cardiac function. Left main coronary artery stenosis, incomplete revascularization, a combined surgical procedure (bypass grafts along with aneurysmectomy or valve replacement), and female sex appear to influence operative risk adversely.

The incidence of perioperative myocardial infarction has also declined with the availability of better myocardial protection techniques (cold cardioplegia). The incidence of clinically significant perioperative infarction is presently 5% or less.

The early graft patency rate (within 6 months) exceeds 80%. Early graft occlusion usually results from thrombosis. The saphenous vein graft patency rate after 6 to 10 months is 70% to 86%, and the graft closure rate decreases significantly after the first year. After the first year the graft attrition rate is approximately 2% per year. The patency rate of the internal mammary artery grafts is higher than that of saphenous vein grafts. Fibrous intimal, medial, and adven-

Indications for coronary artery bypass surgery in patients with stable effort angina

1. Significant left main coronary artery stenosis
2. Left main coronary artery stenosis, with significant right coronary artery stenosis and depressed left ventricular function
3. Stable angina and normal left ventricular function
   a. Refractory to medical therapy
   b. Intolerance to pharmacologic agents because of side effects
   c. Quality of life with medical therapy unacceptable
4. In patients with moderately to severely depressed left ventricular function *when angina but not heart failure* is the predominant manifestation of ischemic heart disease

tial proliferation and atherosclerotic involvement of the bypass grafts are the principal causes of late graft occlusion. The risk for late graft occlusion is significantly higher in patients with higher LDL and lower HDL cholesterol. Thus control of hyperlipidemia should be considered as an important part of management after bypass surgery. Aspirin started during the immediate preoperative period also decreases the rate of graft occlusion, which is the rationale for aspirin therapy in patients undergoing coronary artery bypass surgery.

Between 70% and 95% of patients with stable or unstable angina report either complete or marked relief of anginal symptoms. Improved exercise tolerance and improved quality of life are expected for most patients. Improvements in regional and global myocardial mechanical and metabolic function also occur (Fig. 13-3). Coronary artery bypass surgery also decreases the frequency and duration of the silent episodes of spontaneous S-T segment depression.

Improvement in survival with revascularization surgery varies with the subset of patients. In patients with significant left main coronary artery stenosis, particularly those with associated right coronary artery lesions and depressed left ventricular function, long-term survival is better with surgical therapy than with medical therapy. Recent studies also suggest that for patients with moderately to severely decreased ventricular ejection fraction (40% or less), surgical therapy offers a better long-term prognosis than does medical therapy, provided angina is the predominant symptom. This beneficial effect is observed regardless of the number of coronary vessels involved and despite the higher operative mortality. Improvement in quality of life is significantly greater after surgical therapy than with medical therapy. Thus surgical therapy should be considered when angina becomes refractory to medical therapy or when improvement in quality of life becomes a priority.

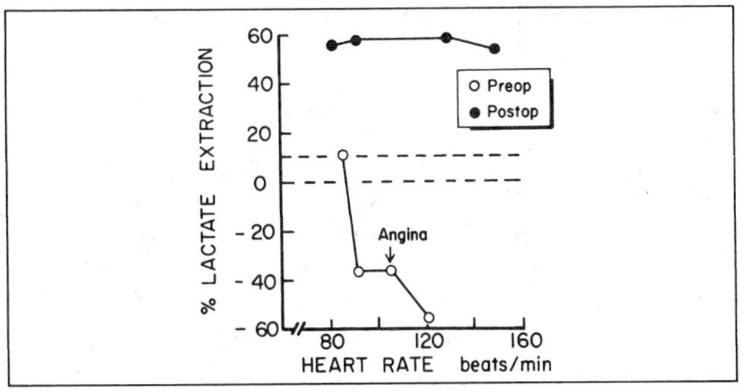

Fig. 13-3. Changes in myocardial lactate extraction during atrial pacing before and after coronary artery bypass surgery. Positive values indicate lactate extraction by the myocardium and thus adequate O_2 supply. Negative values indicate lactate production and myocardial ischemia. Preoperatively with increased heart rate and at the onset of angina, myocardial lactate production rather than extraction occurred. Postoperatively, despite a higher pacing rate, lactate extraction was normal and angina did not develop. These findings suggest that revascularization surgery can improve angina threshold and prevent myocardial ischemia. (Published with permission from Katzung BG and Chatterjee K: Basic clinical pharmacology. Los Altos, Calif, 1983, Lange.)

Indications for and timing of revascularization surgery in patients with unstable angina remain controversial (Fig. 13-4). The NIH National Cooperative Study compared medical and surgical therapy; improvement in survival following surgical therapy was not demonstrated. It appears established, however, that emergency revascularization surgery is rarely required and that most patients can be "cooled off" with aggressive medical therapy, as outlined previously. Thus coronary arteriography and the decision regarding revascularization surgery can be made electively following the cooling-off period in most patients, usually during the same hospitalization. Some patients who develop angina with limited physical activity or who continue to experience rest angina require early coronary arteriography for consideration of semiemergent reperfusion therapy. Patients who remain asymptomatic with medical therapy and tolerate medical therapy well can undertake a stress test electively. If evidence of myocardial ischemia is detected during the early stage of exercise, despite medical therapy, coronary arteriography and reperfusion therapy are recommended. If myocardial ischemia does not appear during the stress test, medical therapy can be continued and surgery deferred.

When a vasospastic mechanism for unstable angina is suspected from the clinical profile, coronary arteriography must be performed during the same hospitalization to delineate the coronary anatomy. If fixed coronary artery lesions are revealed, decisions regarding medical and surgical therapy can then be made in the same way as in pa-

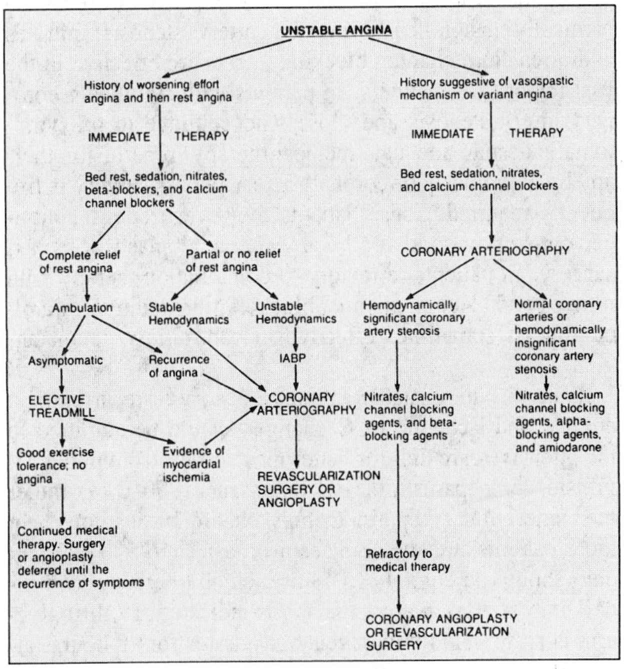

Fig. 13-4. Guidelines for the management of unstable angina. In all patients with unstable angina, aspirin therapy should be considered until it is contraindicated *(not indicated in figure)*. For patients who continue to have rest angina despite antianginal and aspirin therapy, heparin therapy should be considered *(not indicated in figure)*. A few of these patients may also benefit from thrombolytic therapy. *IABP*, Intra-aortic balloon pump.

tients with a history of effort angina. Patients with normal coronary arteries or with hemodynamically insignificant coronary artery stenosis should be regarded as having variant angina, and aggressive medical therapy should be continued.

The benefits of revascularization surgery in patients with variant angina have been unimpressive, even when significant fixed obstructive lesions are present. Episodes of coronary artery spasm may continue despite revascularization surgery. Therefore surgery is recommended only when aggressive medical therapy has failed and only in patients with associated severe fixed coronary artery stenosis. It has been suggested that cardiac sympathectomy along with coronary artery bypass surgery may provide better results than coronary artery bypass surgery alone.

SUGGESTED THERAPEUTIC APPROACHES

In patients with chronic stable angina, once the diagnosis is established, pharmacotherapy is initiated usually with nitrates, and then beta-adrenergic blocking agents and/or calcium channel blocking agents are added to control angina. Reperfusion therapy with angioplasty or coronary artery bypass surgery is considered in patients who become refractory to pharmacotherapy or cannot tolerate pharmacotherapy because of either the drug's side effects or poor acceptance of the quality of life during pharmacotherapy. Coronary artery bypass surgery should also be considered in patients with hemodynamically significant left main coronary artery stenosis or triple-vessel coronary artery disease with a large extent of myocardium at risk.

In patients with variant angina, with normal or hemodynamically insignificant coronary artery stenosis, nitrates and/or calcium channel blocking agents are effective in the vast majority of patients. In patients with significant coronary artery stenosis and those who continue to be symptomatic despite adequate medical therapy, reperfusion therapy by angioplasty or coronary artery bypass surgery is frequently required. These patients, however, require continued coronary vasodilator therapy after angioplasty or bypass surgery. In patients refractory to combination therapy with nitrates and calcium channel blockers, the addition of amiodarone is sometimes effective in controlling variant angina.

Patients with unstable angina, a history of recurrent rest angina, and ischemic ECG changes should be admitted to the intensive care unit for better monitoring. Continuous IV infusion of heparin (5000 U bolus and 1000 U/hr) rather than intermittent heparin therapy should be instituted. In those patients already taking aspirin, aspirin (75 to 325 mg/day) should be continued. Aspirin should be continued indefinitely if conservative therapy is indicated. IV nitroglycerin is preferable to nonparenteral nitrates for 48 hours, although continuous infusion of nitroglycerin may produce tolerance. IV esmolol has been shown to be effective in reducing the frequency of ischemic episodes and thus is preferable to other beta-blocking agents for initial management. For maintenance therapy, nonparenteral beta-blocking drugs are titrated according to the changes in heart rate and blood pressure. Nifedipine and probably other dihydropyridines alone should be avoided for treatment of unstable angina because of increased risk of infarction; these agents, however, can be used in combination with nitrates and beta blockers. Presently available data suggest that thrombolytic agents (e.g., rt-PA) are less effective than heparin in reducing the frequency of ischemic episodes in unstable angina; thus thrombolytic agents are only indicated in a very select group of patients. Patients refractory to aspirin, heparin, and antianginal drugs require coronary arteriography with a view to revascularization. Patients with hemodynamic instability and severely depressed left ventricular function may benefit from prophylactic intra-aortic balloon counterpulsation therapy before coronary arteriography.

Silent myocardial ischemia occurs frequently in patients who had manifestations and/or complications of coronary artery disease previously. In patients with documented prior myocardial infarction, chronic stable angina, unstable angina, and variant angina, more than half the episodes of ischemia occur without angina. The incidence of coronary artery disease in patients who never had manifestations of coronary artery disease but exhibit evidence of silent myocardial ischemia is relatively small, approximately 4%.

Frequent episodes of silent myocardial ischemia in patients with unstable angina and acute myocardial infarction appear to indicate a worse prognosis. The prognosis of patients with chronic stable angina or variant angina and episodes of "silent ischemia" has not been adequately assessed. It also remains uncertain whether pharmacotherapy or reperfusion therapy influences the ultimate prognosis. Nevertheless, until such evidence is available, it is reasonable to assess for silent myocardial ischemia in certain high-risk groups. In these specific subsets of patients, one should consider pharmacotherapy initially and later even more aggressive therapy such as angioplasty or coronary artery bypass surgery. However, in the "low-risk group" or in patients without prior evidence of coronary artery disease, any therapeutic intervention for the prevention of silent myocardial ischemia is unnecessary and unjustified.

PROGNOSIS

Manifest ischemia such as angina is associated in the United States with an annual mortality of approximately 4%. In the Framingham Study the annual mortality of those who had a nonfatal myocardial infarction was 5%. However, recurrent myocardial infarctions are associated with a higher mortality. Hypertension, cigarette smoking, an abnormal ECG, ventricular arrhythmias, and ischemic S-T segment changes during exercise all are adverse prognostic indicators in patients with ischemic heart disease.

The extent and severity of coronary artery disease and the state of left ventricular function appear to be the most important prognostic factors for all patients with ischemic heart disease. With significant stenosis of only one of the major coronary arteries, the annual mortality rate is approximately 2%. With two-vessel disease, the annual mortality rate is about 7%. In patients with significant triple-vessel disease, it is 11%. Left main coronary artery stenosis carries an ominous prognosis: the 5-year mortality has been reported to be as high as 57%.

Evidence of heart failure from left ventricular dysfunction is associated with a mortality almost three times as high as the mortality in patients without heart failure who have a similar extent of coronary artery disease. The degree of depression of left ventricular function appears to bear a direct relation to mortality. In patients with three-vessel coronary artery disease and with normal ejection fraction, the 2-year mortality is approximately 12%; with an ejection fraction less than 50%, 2-year mortality increases to 36%. In patients with diffuse left ventricular dysfunction (usually an ejection fraction of 25% or less) and with triple coronary artery disease, a 5-year mortality rate of 90% has been reported.

Current medical therapy, particularly with beta blockers, appears to influence the long-term prognosis of patients with stable angina. The Coronary Artery Surgery Study (CASS) reported an annual mortality of 1.6% in patients with mild to moderate angina and preserved left ventricular function. Even in patients with decreased ejection fraction, the prognosis is better than expected.

The prognosis for patients with unstable angina has been evaluated by both retrospective and prospective studies. Early studies had reported an early mortality ranging from 10% to 60%, with an incidence of myocardial infarction of 20% to 80%. More recent studies have suggested, however, that the early mortality rate (within 1 month of hospitalization) is 1% to 2% and that the infarction rate is approximately 10%. The NIH National Cooperative Study reported an in-hospital mortality of 3% and late mortality of 7% during follow-up (average 30 months). In patients with progressively worsening effort angina or rest angina, a very unfavorable long-term prognosis has been reported. Five-year and 10-year mortality rates of 39% and 52%, respectively, have been observed. In patients whose angina is not relieved within 48 hours of bed rest, 1-year mortality may be as high as 57%. Spontaneous S-T segment depression unaccompanied by angina, particularly lasting for 1 hour or longer per 24 hours of ECG monitoring, is also associated with worse prognosis in patients with unstable angina.

The prognosis of patients with variant angina remains undetermined. However, sudden death has been reported in approximately 15% of patients with severe variant angina, usually within 3 months of the onset of symptoms. Patients with variant angina and with normal coronary arteries appear to have a better prognosis than do those with fixed obstructive coronary artery lesions.

REFERENCES

Ambrose JA et al: Angiographic morphology and the pathogenesis of unstable angina pectoris. J Am Coll Cardiol 5:609, 1985.

Chatterjee K, Rouleau JL, and Parmley WW: Medical management of patients with angina: has first-line management changed? JAMA 252:1170, 1984.

Cohn PF: Total ischemic burden: definition, mechanisms and therapeutic implications. Am J Med 81(suppl 4A):2, 1986.

Cohn PF: Silent myocardial ischemia: present status. Mod Concepts Cardiovasc Dis 56:1, 1987.

Deanfield JE et al: Transient ST-segment depression as a marker of myocardial ischemia during daily life. Am J Cardiol 54:1195, 1984.

DeFeyter PJ et al: Emergency coronary angioplasty in refractory unstable angina. N Engl J Med 313:342, 1985.

Dell'Italia LJ and O'Rourke RA: Evaluation of the patient with signs and symptoms of ischemic heart disease. In Chatterjee K and Parmley WW, editors: Cardiology. Philadelphia, 1991, Lippincott.

Epstein SE, Quyyumi AA, and Bonow RO: Myocardial ischemia—silent or symptomatic? N Engl J Med 318:1058, 1988.

Hammermeister KE, DeRoven TA, and Dodge HT: Comparison of survival of medically and surgically treated patients in Seattle Heart Watch. Circulation 65:535, 1982.

Karliner JS: Stable angina pectoris. In Chatterjee K and Parmley WW, editors: Cardiology. Philadelphia, 1991, Lippincott.

Kirklin JW et al: ACC/AHA guidelines and indications for coronary artery bypass graft surgery. J Am Coll Cardiol Circulation 83:1125, 1991.

Lewis HD et al: Protective effects of aspirin against acute myocardial infarction and death in men with unstable angina. N Engl J Med 309:396, 1983.

Ludmer PL et al: Paradoxical acetylcholine-induced coronary artery constriction in patients with coronary artery disease. N Engl J Med 315:1045, 1986.

Maseri A, Chierchia S, and L'Abbate A: Pathogenetic mechanisms underlying the clinical events associated with atherosclerotic heart disease. Circulation 62:(suppl. 5):V, 1980.

Opie LH et al: Drugs for the heart, ed 2. New York, 1987, Harcourt Brace Jovanovich.

Ouyang P et al: Variables predictive of successful medical therapy in patients with unstable angina: selection by multivariate analysis from clinical, electrocardiographic and angiographic evaluations. Circulation 70:367, 1984.

Passamani E et al: The CASS principal investigators and their associates. A randomized trial of coronary artery bypass surgery: survival of patients with a low ejection fraction. N Engl J Med 312:1665, 1985.

Pepine CJ: Acute and chronic ischemic heart disease: unstable angina. In Chatterjee K and Parmley WW editors: Cardiology. Philadelphia, 1991, Lippincott.

Pepine CJ and Feldman RL: Dynamic coronary blood flow reduction: supply side considerations. Int J Cardiol 3:3, 1983.

Rankin JS et al: Clinical characteristics and current management of medically refractory unstable angina. Ann Surg 200:457, 1984.

Silverman KJ and Grossman NW: Angina pectoris: natural history and strategies for evaluation and management. N Engl J Med 310:1712, 1984.

Takaro T: The Veteran's Cooperative Randomized Study of Surgery for Coronary Arterial Occlusive Disease: subgroup with significant left main lesions. Circulation 54:III, 1976.

CHAPTER

14 Acute Myocardial Infarction

Guy S. Reeder
Bernard J. Gersh

INCIDENCE

Despite the approximate 40% decline in cardiovascular deaths during the last 3 decades, atherosclerotic cardiovascular disease still represents the most frequent cause of death in the United States. There are approximately

700,000 coronary artery-related deaths per year and more than 1 million myocardial infarctions (MIs), with early death in 10% to 15% and a subsequent 1-year mortality of 10% to 15%. The decreasing individual mortality from MI, possibly accounted for by earlier detection, widespread use of coronary care units, advances in drug therapy, reperfusion with thrombolytic agents or balloon angioplasty, and better methods of risk stratification, may be offset by the general aging of the population. These older patients at risk for atherosclerotic heart disease make up a group in whom the case-fatality rate for acute MI remains high.

PATHOPHYSIOLOGY

Acute MI occurs when profound and prolonged ischemia leads to irreversible myocardial cell damage and necrosis. In most patients, this results from thrombotic coronary occlusion. Infrequently, MI may occur with prolonged or severe coronary spasm in the absence of underlying coronary artery disease; this mechanism is implicated in cases related to cocaine use, ergot therapy, and severe emotional stress. Rare causes of MI include spontaneous coronary artery dissection, nitroglycerin withdrawal, serum sickness and various allergic conditions, profound hypoxemia, sickle cell crisis, carbon monoxide poisoning, and acquired hypercoagulable states. Epidemiologic studies demonstrate an increase in MI event rates in the early morning hours, probably related to circadian variation in coronary vascular tone, catecholamines, and coagulability (Fig. 14-1). This phenomenon is blunted by beta-adrenergic receptor blockade.

Recently, much investigation has centered on complex atherosclerotic plaque as a precursor of MI and unstable angina. Postmortem studies demonstrated that the nidus for intracoronary thrombus formation is usually disruption of a lipid-rich atherosclerotic plaque with exposure of thrombogenic plaque material to the bloodstream (Fig. 14-2). Serial angiographic studies demonstrated that plaque rupture and thrombosis in mild stenoses more often lead to MI than similar processes involving tight lesions, presumably as a result of better distal collateralization in the latter.

The sequence of events leading to plaque rupture is not fully understood, but it is known that lipid-rich plaques have an increased risk of rupture. Such plaques usually have an eccentrically located lipid pool separated from the vessel lumen by only a thin, fibrous cap. Plaque rupture usually occurs at the junction between the fibrous cap and the normal vessel wall, probably from increased stress at this area. Whether increased shear forces caused by the stenosis, repeated oscillatory stress resulting from contraction of the heart, or changes in coronary tone related to circulating catecholamines act singly or in concert to potentiate plaque rupture remains conjectural. Once rupture occurs, platelets adhere to the exposed collagen and lipid matrix, and the thrombotic cascade is initiated.

Totally occlusive thrombus in patients with inadequate distal collateralization most often results in Q wave MI. Transiently occluding thrombus, with spontaneous lysis, or distal collateralization may yield lesser degrees of necrosis and produce non–Q wave MI. Patients with intermittent or subtotal occlusive thrombi, adequate collateralization, or both may have the syndrome of unstable or prolonged angina in the absence of myocardial necrosis. Thus a common underlying process (i.e., plaque rupture and superimposed thrombus) is responsible for unstable angina, non–Q wave MI, Q wave MI, and probably sudden death in many patients. Extent of MI relates to the size of the territory supplied by the infarct-related vessel, the presence and adequacy of distal collateralization, and the metabolic needs of the jeopardized myocardium. In the majority of nonreperfused Q wave infarcts, most of the jeopardized myocardium becomes necrotic, whereas in non–Q wave in-

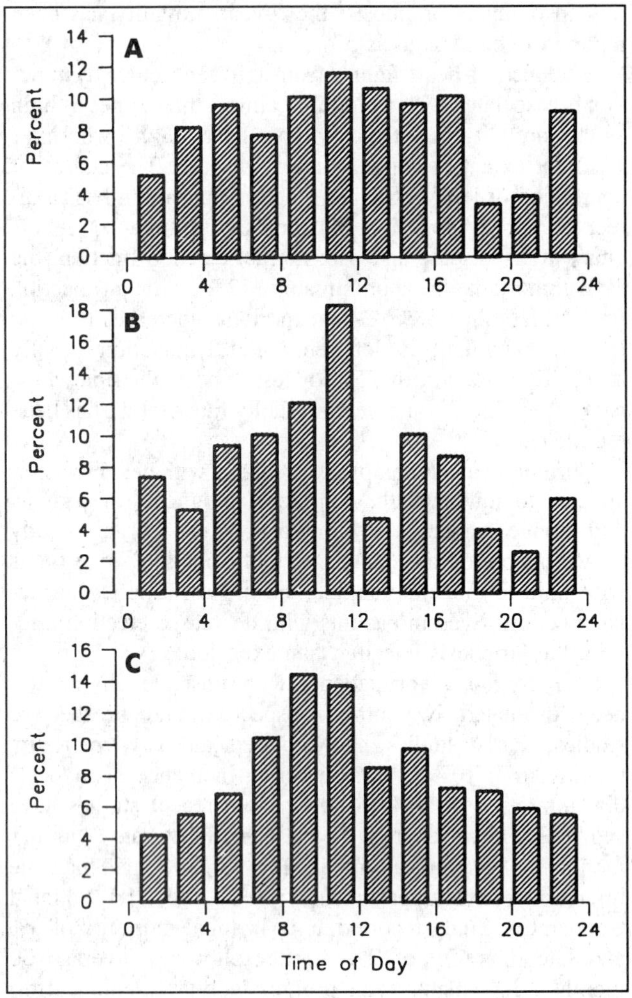

Fig. 14-1. Diurnal variation in myocardial infarction (MI). **A,** Incidence of MI in 206 patients receiving beta-adrenergic receptor blocker therapy before their MI. Morning incidence of MI did not increase. Percent of MIs per 2-hour interval is indicated on *y* axis, and time of day is indicated on *x* axis (military time). **B,** Incidence of MI in 147 patients receiving calcium antagonists before their MI. Morning incidence of MI increased ($P < 0.01$) similar to that observed in total study population. **C,** Incidence of MI in 1473 patients who did not receive beta-adrenergic receptor blocker therapy. Morning incidence of MI is increased ($P < 0.001$). (From Willich SN et al: Circulation 80:853, 1989. By permission of the American Heart Association.)

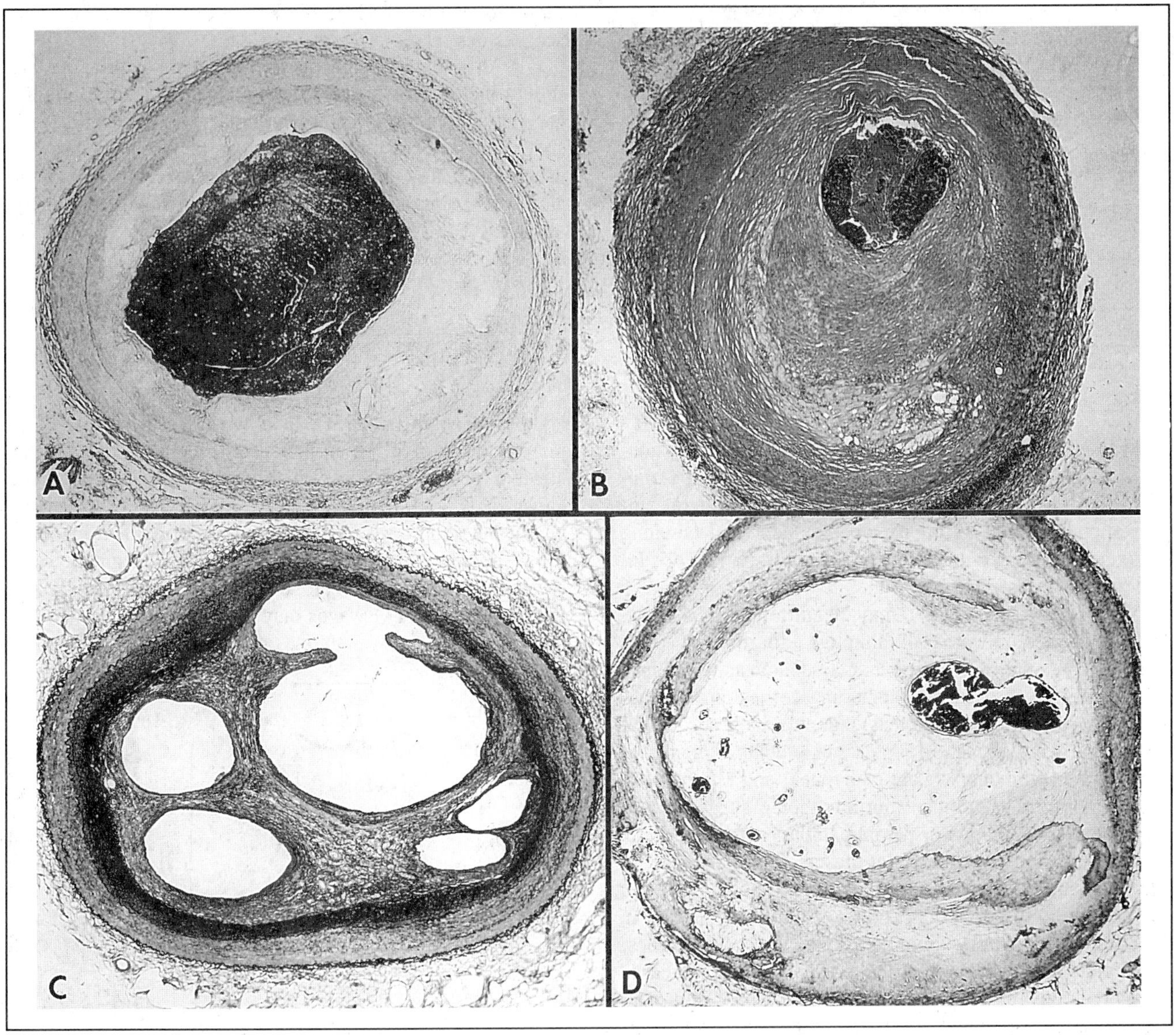

Fig. 14-2. Coronary thrombosis and its consequences. Occlusive thrombi involving grade 2 plaque **(A)** and grade 4 plaque **(B)**. Organization and fibrosis of thrombus with **(C)** and without **(D)** appreciable lysis and recanalization. (From Edwards WD: In Gersh BJ and Rahimtoola SH, editors: Current topics in cardiology: acute myocardial infarction. New York, 1991, Elsevier. By permission of Elsevier Science Publishing Company.)

farcts and unstable angina, a substantial amount of residual jeopardized (ischemic) myocardium has not yet become necrotic.

Myocardial necrosis leads to an inflammatory response with infiltration of neutrophils and monocytes. Necrotic myocardium is gradually replaced by the deposition of collagen fibers and scar tissue. This healing process is complete within 4 to 6 weeks after necrosis.

CLINICAL PRESENTATIONS

The classic symptom of acute MI is discomfort in the central area of the chest that may radiate to the neck, back, or arms. It is persistent (unrelieved by nitrates) and is frequently associated with diaphoresis, nausea, weakness, and fear of impending death. The discomfort gradually builds to maximum intensity over several minutes, and this feature may help to differentiate MI from other conditions, such as aortic dissection or perforated peptic ulcer, in which maximum pain is usually instantaneous. In patients with preexisting angina pectoris the pain of MI is usually similar but persistent.

At least one fifth of MIs are clinically unrecognized because of atypical symptoms, especially in elderly patients (Table 14-1), or absence of chest discomfort. Painless MI is known to occur in elderly persons, in patients with diabetes mellitus, and in postoperative patients, especially those receiving analgesics. If the pain of myocardial ischemia is perceived in the epigastrium, back, or in one arm only, the diagnosis may not be considered by the patient

Table 14-1. Atypical symptoms of myocardial infarction (MI) in elderly patients

	Patients (%)		
Symptoms	**65-74 years**	**75-84 years**	**≥85 years**
Chest pain	78	60	38
Dyspnea	41	44	43
Sweating	34	23	14
Syncope	3	18	18
Confusion	3	8	19
Stroke	2	7	7

Modified from Bayer AJ et al: J Am Geriatr Soc 34:263, 1986.

and sometimes not by the physician (Chapter 7). Occasionally, MI may be recognized in retrospect only by the clinical occurrence of a complication, such as peripheral embolization of mural thrombus, development or worsening of congestive heart failure, new mitral regurgitation, or syncope caused by arrhythmia.

The physical examination may be entirely normal in patients with uncomplicated MI, although a fourth heart sound is typical. A minority of patients may demonstrate findings that suggest hyperlipidemia, including corneal arcus, xanthelasma, or tendon xanthomas. Patients with substantial left ventricular dysfunction at presentation may demonstrate tachycardia, pulmonary rales, tachypnea, and a third heart sound. A mitral regurgitant murmur should suggest papillary muscle dysfunction or partial papillary muscle rupture; however, the latter is unlikely at presentation. An aortic regurgitant murmur occurs infrequently and should suggest the possibility of aortic dissection, as should asymmetry in blood pressure or pulse amplitude in the upper extremities.

In patients with right ventricular involvement, increased jugular venous pressure, Kussmaul's sign, and a right ventricular third heart sound may be present. Such patients virtually always have inferior MIs and may demonstrate exquisite blood pressure sensitivity to nitrates. In patients with massive left ventricular dysfunction, shock is indicated by hypotension, diaphoresis, cool skin and extremities, pallor, oliguria, and possible confusion. These patients have a high mortality. Some estimation of prognosis at presentation is possible with the use of the Killip classification (Table 14-2). However, more accurate stratification of risk of early mortality can be obtained by the use of hemodynamic subsets, as described later.

The differential diagnosis of the patient with acute MI should include aortic dissection, pericarditis, acute pulmonary embolism, intercostal neuralgia, costochondritis, and abdominal visceral disorders such as peptic ulcer disease, pancreatitis, and biliary colic. The physical examination alone often allows accurate differentiation of MI from many of these other disorders, as do the electrocardiogram (ECG) and other laboratory tests.

Table 14-2. Killip class and hospital mortality

Killip class		Hospital mortality (%)
I	No CHF	6
II	Mild CHF, rales, S_3 heart sound, congestion on chest radiograph	17
III	Pulmonary edema	38
IV	Cardiogenic shock	81

Modified from Killip TK III and Kimball JT: Am J Cardiol 20:457, 1967.
CHF, Congestive heart failure.

ELECTROCARDIOGRAPHIC MANIFESTATIONS

The ECG remains the most useful test for making the diagnosis of MI (Chapter 4). In Q wave MI the initial ECG manifestation involves an increase in the amplitude of the T wave (peaking) followed within minutes by S-T segment elevation (Fig. 14-3). The R wave may initially increase in height but soon decreases as Q waves form. If the jeopardized myocardium is reperfused, the S-T segment may promptly revert to normal, although T waves usually remain inverted and Q waves may or may not regress. In the

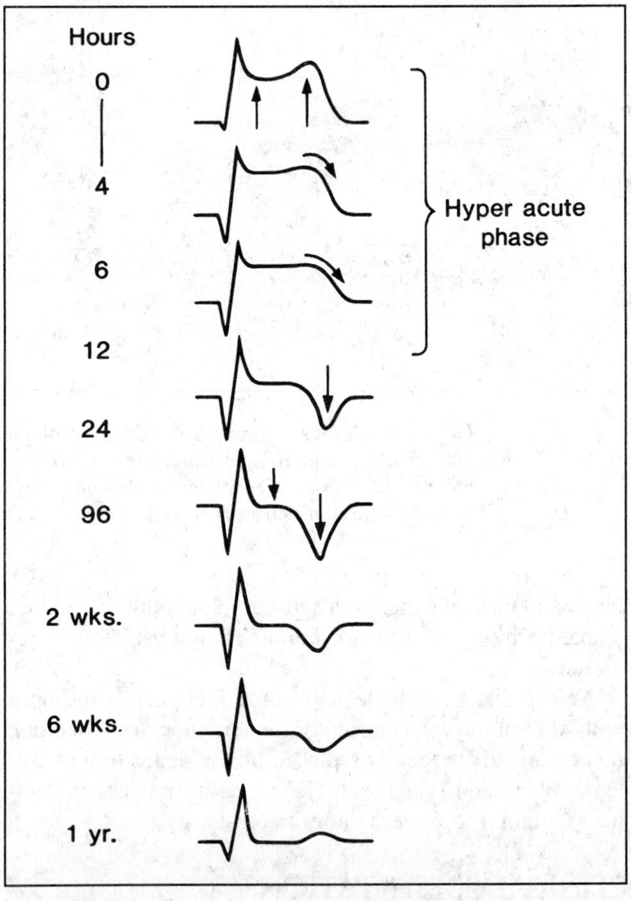

Fig. 14-3. Evolution of electrocardiographic changes in MI. Serial, morphologic, typical QRST changes with time after transmural MI are depicted. (From Gau GT: In Brandenburg RO et al: editors: Cardiology: fundamentals and practice, vol 1. Chicago, 1987, Mosby–Year Book. By permission of Mayo Foundation.)

absence of reperfusion the S-T segment gradually returns to baseline in several hours to days, and T waves are symmetrically inverted. These changes describe anterior and inferior transmural MI. Posterior transmural MI is an exception to these rules because there generally is S-T depression in leads V_1 to V_3 at presentation, and MI may therefore be mistaken for an anterior non–Q wave MI. Conduction disturbances are common with inferior MI and may include first-, second-, or third-degree atrioventricular block or, less often, sinus bradycardia (Chapter 4).

Patients with non–Q wave MI may demonstrate various nonspecific S-T segment and T wave abnormalities but most often demonstrate S-T depression with or without T wave inversion; Q waves do not evolve.

"Reciprocal" S-T segment depression may occur in leads remote from those with S-T segment elevation. The presence of reciprocal depression denotes a patient at higher risk for later complications. In some patients a large MI may produce reciprocal depression simply because of electrical phenomena. In other patients, the presence of remote depressions indicates "ischemia at a distance" and the presence of multivessel disease or compromised collateralization. Finally, S-T depression in leads V_1 to V_3 may represent posterior injury rather than anterior ischemia (Chapter 4).

OTHER LABORATORY TESTS

Measurement of the serum level of creatine kinase (CK) is useful for confirmation of MI. The MB isoenzyme of CK (CK-MB) is present in largest concentration in myocardium, although small amounts (1% to 2%) can be found in skeletal muscle, especially the tongue, small intestine, and diaphragm. CK-MB appears in serum within approximately 3 hours of MI onset, reaches peak levels at 12 to 24 hours, and has a mean duration of activity of 1 to 3 days. Because of the short time for release of this enzyme, phlebotomy for CK-MB analysis should be performed at admission, 12 to 18 hours later, at 24 to 30 hours, and possibly at 36 to 48 hours. False-positive cardiac increases in CK-MB levels can occur after cardioversion, cardiac surgery, myopericarditis, percutaneous transluminal coronary angioplasty, and occasionally after rapid tachycardia. Noncardiac causes of false-positive increases in CK-MB levels may occur with extensive skeletal muscle trauma, rhabdomyolysis, the muscular dystrophies, and some other neuromuscular disorders. Rarely, some patients may have low and constant elevations of serum levels of CK-MB for no known cause.

In patients who are first seen more than 24 hours after symptom onset, MB-CK activity may be decreasing or normal, and in selected patients it may be useful to measure serum levels of aspartate aminotransferase (AST) or lactic dehydrogenase (LDH). Although these enzymes have a longer duration of increased levels in the bloodstream, they are not specific for myocardium, and therefore their routine measurement is not justified. Moreover, in a patient with an infarct confirmed on the basis of creatine phosphokinase analyses, the AST level provides little additional information and is expensive to measure.

Occasionally the concentration of CK-MB isoenzyme may be increased in patients with normal total levels of CK enzyme. This finding usually indicates a small amount of myocardial necrosis in a patient whose baseline total CK enzyme level is at the low-normal end of the range, a not unusual finding in the elderly patient.

The chest radiograph is useful in patients with acute MI primarily for exclusion of complications, such as pulmonary edema, or other conditions in the differential diagnosis, such as pneumothorax or aortic dissection.

CARDIAC IMAGING

There are many applications of cardiac imaging in acute MI (e.g., diagnosis, prognosis, management of complications, assessment of underlying diseases) (Chapter 5) but the current focus on cost-effectiveness warrants a re-evaluation of the *incremental* information provided by the imaging technique. Presently, only selective coronary arteriography is a reliable method for assessing the coronary anatomy, and its indications in MI are presented later.

Various imaging techniques are used to visualize the cardiac chambers, cardiac valves, or both (Chapter 5). Left ventricular systolic function, as measured by the ejection fraction, is a strong prognostic indicator for survival in patients with coronary artery disease. Measurements of left ventricular function can be obtained with contrast-enhanced left ventriculography, two-dimensional (2D) echocardiography, radioisotope ventriculography, and fast computed tomography (CT) techniques. Use of perfusion imaging to indicate the extent of MI may help to determine response to reperfusion; helpful techniques include either thallium scintigraphy or, more recently, the use of sestamibi, a technetium isotope that initially distributes in a manner similar to thallium but does not undergo late redistribution. This allows demonstration of the initial perfusion defect even with delayed imaging, unlike with thallium.

When viability of tissue is in question, resting thallium imaging with 4- and 24-hour views or positron emission tomography (PET) have been used. Application of PET is limited to the few centers that have this technology.

When mechanical complications of MI are suspected, 2D echocardiography and frequently transesophageal echocardiography are the methods of choice for detecting left ventricular mural thrombus, right ventricular MI, papillary muscle and valve pathology, pericardial effusion and tamponade, and cardiac rupture. Left ventricular wall motion analysis and quantitation of valvular regurgitation can also be performed with contrast-enhanced ventriculography. In many institutions, however, patients are initially evaluated with 2D echocardiography and color flow Doppler imaging because of the low cost, absence of risk, and convenience of this technology, which can be used at the patient's bedside.

Routine application of any imaging modality in every patient with MI cannot be justified from either an intellectual or a financial standpoint. The quality and availability of each technique at an institution are crucial to the use of a particular imaging modality. Before performing any imaging technique on the patient who has had an MI, the physician must have firmly in mind the clinical question to be answered as well as the likelihood that the test results will affect clinical decision making.

APPROACH TO THE PATIENT

There are four immediate goals in the management of the patient with acute MI: (1) relief of ischemic pain, (2) stabilization of hemodynamics, (3) reduction of myocardial oxygen demand ($M\dot{V}O_2$), and (4) maintenance or increase of myocardial perfusion. As much as possible, these goals should be achieved simultaneously.

1. Pain relief is best achieved with O_2, nitroglycerin, and intravenously (IV) administered morphine sulfate.
2. Estimation of the patient's volume status and the presence of left ventricular failure can be established to some extent by the results of the physical examination. If the patient is hypertensive, the careful IV administration of nitroglycerin and beta-adrenergic receptor blockers can be beneficial. If the patient is hypotensive without pulmonary congestion or rales, cautious fluid administration can be performed, perhaps with 2D echocardiographic imaging of left and right ventricular function.
3. Reduction of $M\dot{V}O_2$ is achieved with sedation, pain relief, reduction of the heart rate (if tolerated) to 70 beats/min or less with IV administration of beta-adrenergic receptor blockers, and IV administration of nitroglycerin as long as a mean arterial pressure of 80 mm Hg is preserved. In patients in whom concern exists regarding precipitation of left ventricular failure, a short-acting beta-adrenergic receptor blocker such as esmolol is useful.
4. To maintain myocardial perfusion, aspirin (325 mg chewable) and IV administered heparin (5000 to 10,000 U boluses) are used for antiplatelet and anticoagulant effect. Although these measures provide some relief of pain and partial resolution of S-T segment deviation in many patients, the cornerstone of modern therapy for MI is early reperfusion, either with thrombolytic therapy or emergent angioplasty. Therefore patients must be assessed rapidly as candidates for one of these interventions.

Thrombolytic therapy for patients with MI

Indications

Ongoing Q wave MI longer than 30 minutes and less than 6 hours manifested by S-T segment elevation of 1 mV or greater in two or more ECG leads
Ongoing Q wave MI longer than 6 and less than 24 hours with continued ischemic pain
Chest pain and S-T depression in anterior precordial leads coupled with imaging test demonstrating posterior left ventricular wall motion abnormality
Patient consent
Absence of absolute contraindications

Contraindications

Absolute
- Active bleeding
- Recent (< 6 weeks) major surgical procedure or arterial puncture in noncompressible area or recent major trauma
- Symptomatic cerebrovascular disease or intracranial pathologic condition

Relative
- History of gastrointestinal bleeding or active ulcer disease
- Recent (6 months) administration of streptokinase or allergy to this drug (applies only to streptokinase)
- Cardiogenic shock
- History of bleeding diathesis
- Remote history of cerebrovascular disease
- Prolonged cardiopulmonary resuscitation

Thrombolytic therapy

The rationale of thrombolytic therapy is largely based on laboratory investigations of experimental acute MI. The appreciation that myocardial necrosis occurs in a progressive wave front from the endocardium to the epicardium and that this progression could be halted with prompt reperfusion led to the concept of myocardial salvage by lysis of intracoronary thrombi, using IV thrombolytic agents. General indications and contraindications for IV thrombolytic therapy are shown in the box above. Patients with evidence of Q wave MI who are not judged to be at increased risk for bleeding complications may be considered for thrombolysis. Table 14-3 illustrates features of the currently available thrombolytic agents. These vary with respect to fibrin selectivity, antigenicity, side effects, and cost. Even though fibrin-selective agents, such as tissue plasminogen activator (t-PA), have been shown conclusively to produce higher 90-minute patency rates compared with nonselective agents (i.e., streptokinase), the clinical results in terms of mortality and left ventricular function are remarkably similar.

Fig. 14-4 shows pooled mortality data from five trials involving more than 28,000 patients treated within 6 hours of symptom onset and demonstrates an average mortality reduction of approximately 27 ± 3% compared with those receiving placebo. Additionally, two large trials directly compared different thrombolytic agents with each other, as opposed to placebo. In GISSI-2 and its international arm, 20,000 patients were randomized to t-PA (100 mg) or streptokinase (1.5 million U), with a second randomization to heparin (12,500 U given subcutaneously two times a day) or placebo. All received aspirin, and 36% received beta-adrenergic receptor blocking agents. The mortality in the streptokinase arm was 8.5% and in the t-PA arm, 8.9%. In the Third International Study of Infarct Survival (ISIS-3) involving 46,000 patients randomized to streptokinase, activated plasminogen streptokinase activator complex (APSAC), or t-PA, the respective 5-week mortalities were 10.5%, 10.6%, and 10.3%, respectively (Fig. 14-5). The rate of hemorrhagic stroke was slightly higher in the t-PA (0.7%) and APSAC (0.6%) groups compared with the streptokinase group (0.3%).

Table 14-3. Features of thrombolytic agents

Agent	Fibrin selectivity	Antigenicity	Hypotension	Cost ($)*	Usual dosage
Streptokinase	−	+	+	206	1.5 million U/3 hr
Urokinase†	−	−	−	3192	3 million U/3 hr
scu-PA	+	−	−	NA	NA
t-PA	+	−	−	2244	100 mg/3 hr
APSAC	−	+	+	1665	30 Unit bolus

*Pharmacy cost at one institution in 1992 dollars.
†Not approved for this use.
scu-PA, Single-chain urokinase-type plasminogen activator; *t-PA,* tissue plasminogen activator; *APSAC,* activated plasminogen streptokinase activator complex; *NA,* not applicable.

Despite these trials, the choice of thrombolytic agent is still an area of controversy. Several ongoing trials (GUSTO, LATE) will likely resolve the issues of adjunctive heparin administration and the time of reperfusion.

The effects of thrombolytic therapy on left ventricular ejection fraction, as a surrogate of myocardial salvage, have been moderate. Pooled data from trials of thrombolytic therapy demonstrate an average change in ejection fraction of only 9% between treatment and control groups. More recent imaging techniques using technetium sestamibi, however, do document unequivocally that successful reperfusion results in significant salvage (approximately 40% to 50% of the area at risk). The substantial improvement in survival with thrombolytic therapy is probably not totally explainable by myocardial salvage alone. Repeated observations that survival is better with an open infarct-related rather than a closed infarct-related artery led to the so-called open artery hypothesis. Potential explanations for a survival benefit included improved tissue healing, less cavity dilatation, and a source for collaterals if another artery becomes jeopardized in the future. Additionally, electrical instability of the myocardium may be decreased in the presence of an open infarct-related artery.

The general acceptance of the efficacy of thrombolytic therapy in Q wave MI and the enhanced benefits of early treatment led to investigational use of prehospital administration of thrombolytic agents. Those likely to gain the most benefit from thrombolysis include patients with large MIs, continued pain at presentation, and collaterals to the infarct-related vessel and patients in whom myocardial O_2 consumption can be decreased before and during thrombolytic therapy.

At present, controversy exists about the application of thrombolytic therapy to certain patient subsets.

Elderly. There has been reluctance to apply thrombolysis to elderly patients because of an increased risk of bleeding. However, because these patients have a highly in-

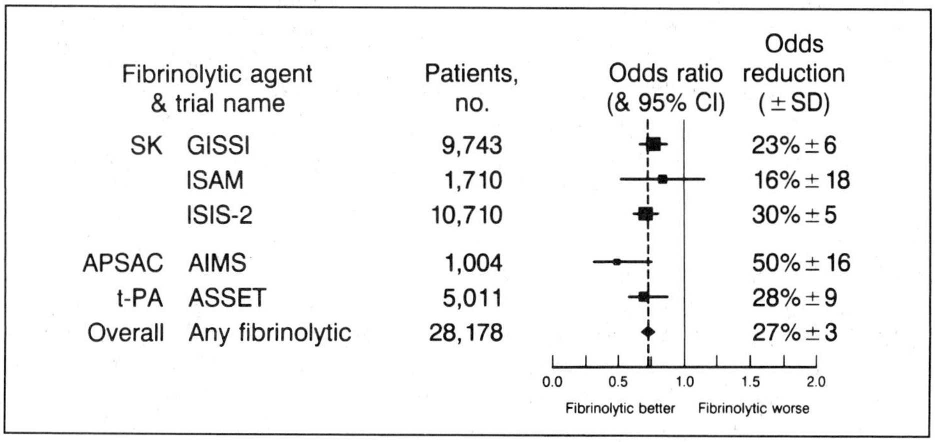

Fig. 14-4. Mortality reduction in five large randomized trials of thrombolysis versus placebo for MI. Trial size is represented by size of square; relative mortality reduction is shown by position of square in relation to vertical line; confidence limits *(CI)* are demonstrated by horizontal line. Diamond shows pooled results of trials, with an average 27% mortality reduction. *SD,* Standard deviation; *SK,* streptokinase; *t-PA,* tissue plasminogen activator. (Modified from Topol EJ, editor: Textbook of interventional cardiology. Philadelphia, 1990, Saunders.)

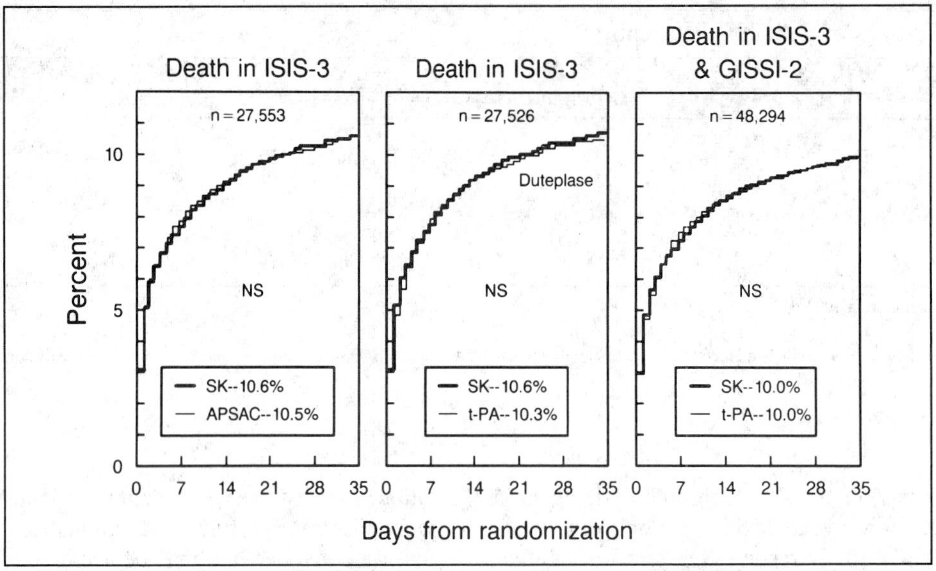

Fig. 14-5. Cumulative percent mortality in ISIS-3 and GISSI-2: comparison of thrombolytic agents. *SK,* Streptokinase; *APSAC,* activated plasminogen streptokinase activator complex; *t-PA,* single-chain tissue plasminogen activator. Survival curves are nearly identical for all agents. (From ISIS-3 [Third International Study of Infarct Survival] Collaborative Group: Lancet 339:753, 1992. By permission of the Lancet.)

creased risk of death with MI, the potential for gain is increased, and in general, thrombolytic therapy in elderly patients has been underused. No upper age limit exists for thrombolysis; however, the older the patient, the more rigorous should be the search for contraindications.

Late presentation. The use of thrombolytic therapy in patients who first appear late after the onset of symptoms (≥6 hours) is an important but unresolved issue that applies to a substantial number of patients. The benefits clearly diminish with time, as does the potential for myocardial salvage; the risk of rupture may increase with time as well. Nonetheless, there remains a sizable proportion of patients with stuttering MI, perhaps with extensive collateralization or intermittent occlusion and reopening of the infarcted vessel, who will still benefit. Pending results of ongoing trials, a rational strategy is to treat patients with persistent pain, if accompanied by S-T segment elevation, regardless of the duration of symptoms.

S-T segment depression. The bulk of evidence suggests that thrombolytic therapy has little value in patients with non–Q wave infarction. Although most of these patients have persistent chest pain and S-T segment depression, a subset of these patients (i.e., those with S-T depression in leads V_1 to V_3) may have posterior Q wave MI (in the area of the circumflex coronary artery), and such patients may benefit from thrombolytic therapy.

New left bundle branch block. The presence of new left bundle branch block is a marker for extensive MI. Although the conduction abnormality may mask the diagnosis of Q wave MI, several trials demonstrated a benefit of thrombolytic therapy in this group, and such patients should be considered candidates unless contraindications to thrombolysis exist.

Reocclusion. Reocclusion of the infarct-related vessel occurs in 15% to 20% of patients and is silent in half of these. Causes of vessel reocclusion are probably multifactorial but relate to persistence of thrombus, the underlying thrombogenic lesion, and possibly activation of the clotting system by lytic therapy itself. The timing and route of administration of adjunctive heparin therapy also remain controversial. Additionally, some physicians advocated the use of front-loaded thrombolytic drug administration with claims of higher initial patency but with uncertain results as to reocclusion.

Angioplasty

Percutaneous transluminal coronary angioplasty has assumed an important role in treatment of patients with acute MI (Fig. 14-6).

Direct angioplasty implies the use of this technique instead of thrombolytic therapy early in acute MI. Patency rates of 80% to 95% (higher than that achievable with thrombolytic therapy) are possible with reocclusion rates, and in-hospital mortality is similar to that reported in trials of thrombolysis. Advantages of this approach include the avoidance of thrombolytic therapy with its small but important risk of intracranial hemorrhage and the production of wide patency in the infarct-related vessel. However, this approach is limited by the lack of universal availability of catheterization facilities and the resultant delays for many patients located far from available centers.

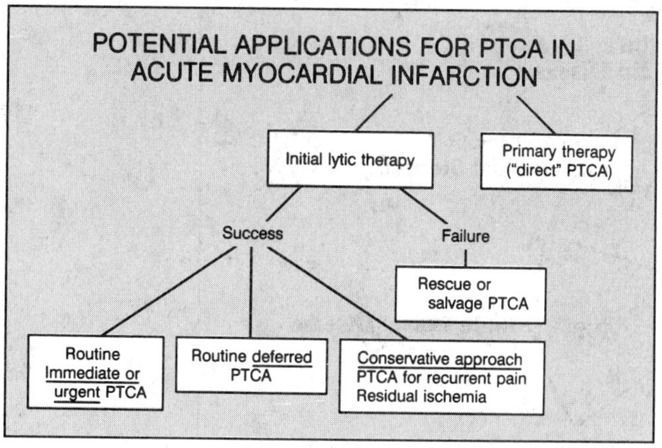

Fig. 14-6. Potential application of percutaneous transluminal coronary angioplasty *(PTCA)* during acute myocardial infarction. (From Holmes DR Jr and Gersh BJ: In Gersh BJ and Rahimtoola SH, editors: Current topics in cardiology: acute myocardial infarction. New York, 1991, Elsevier. By permission of Elsevier Science Publishing Company.)

Recently, several randomized trials comparing results of direct angioplasty to thrombolytic therapy have been reported. Results in 103 patients in one trial from the Mayo Clinic demonstrated no significant difference in myocardial salvage between these two initial treatment strategies, with approximately half of myocardium at risk salvaged in each group. Complications, overall mortality, and aggregate cost were also similar.

For most of the U.S. population, however, primary angioplasty is limited by logistic constraints, and it is reassuring to see that thrombolytic drugs are equally effective in achieving myocardial salvage. Nonetheless, an important role exists for primary angioplasty in institutions with the available resources. Furthermore, direct angioplasty should be strongly considered (1) when a contraindication to thrombolytic therapy exists or (2) when the diagnosis of MI is uncertain by ECG criteria. Also, several uncontrolled series of patients with cardiogenic shock demonstrated an apparent marked decrease in mortality compared with historical control subjects and with results of trials of thrombolysis for patients in whom little or no benefit was apparent. Therefore it is reasonable to offer direct angioplasty to patients who have cardiogenic shock for whom mortality otherwise may reach 80% to 90%.

Angioplasty performed after thrombolytic therapy can be subdivided into three clinical situations: routine, rescue, and late elective angioplasty (see Fig. 14-6). *Routine* angioplasty implies early use of the technique after thrombolytic therapy, despite the presence of an open infarct-related artery. Three large-scale randomized trials investigated this approach (TIMI, TAMI, European Cooperative Study Group). Each trial demonstrated a higher mortality, increased bleeding complications, no decrease of reocclusion, and a higher rate of emergency coronary bypass surgery in the early angioplasty group. Early routine angioplasty in asymptomatic patients after thrombolytic therapy therefore cannot be recommended and is contraindicated.

Rescue angioplasty implies the early use of angioplasty in patients whose arteries failed to recanalize after thrombolytic therapy. Success rates for angioplasty in these patients are lower than for direct angioplasty but still are 70% to 80%. Mortality rates and vessel reocclusion are higher than for patients undergoing direct angioplasty or thrombolysis. No randomized trials comparing rescue angioplasty with a control group of patients with unopened nondilated infarct-related vessels have been reported, although one trial is in progress (RESCUE trial). The current inability to assess noninvasively the patency of an infarct-related artery is a major limitation to the more widespread use of rescue angioplasty and to the conduct of a trial. Currently it is reasonable for patients who have continued pain and S-T segment elevation after thrombolytic therapy to undergo cardiac catheterization for determination of infarct vessel patency and to undergo angioplasty if the vessel remains occluded.

Late elective angioplasty implies the selective use of angioplasty in the convalescent stage of myocardial infarction. Both the TIMI-2 trial and the SWIFT trial compared a conservative strategy of angioplasty for patients with spontaneous or exercise-induced ischemia after MI versus an invasive strategy of routine catheterization and angioplasty at 18 to 48 hours. At follow-up the number of deaths and repeat infarctions and the measurements of ejection fraction were similar in the conservative and routine catheterization groups, demonstrating no definite advantage for the latter.

The findings from these large multicenter trials are consistent and emphasize that a conservative policy of watchful waiting accompanied by angiography for these patients with spontaneous or exercise-induced ischemia is not only safe but the correct and most cost-effective approach for those with a stable clinical course after thrombolytic therapy.

Whereas the role of angioplasty after thrombolytic therapy has been clarified, an issue of continued debate is the role of routine predismissal angiography in stable postthrombolytic patients, as opposed to exercise or pharmacologic stress testing.

Fig. 14-7 shows the proportion of patients in various anatomic subgroups found at angiography after thrombolytic therapy. Some patients, those with left main coronary artery disease or three-vessel disease, might be selected for early surgical revascularization on the basis of findings from routine postinfarction angioplasty. However, identification of high-risk patients is also likely from predismissal exercise testing (although the predictive value of such testing may be decreased in the postthrombolytic patient).

The major argument against routine angiography after MI is "reperfusion momentum": the temptation to intervene with angioplasty for an anatomically severe lesion that may or may not be clinically important. At present, one may recommend either routine, post-MI angiography or a more conservative approach of selective angiography on the basis of spontaneous or exercise-induced ischemia. If routine angiography is elected, subsequent revascularization must be limited to patients with high-risk coronary anatomy, demonstrable ischemia, or both.

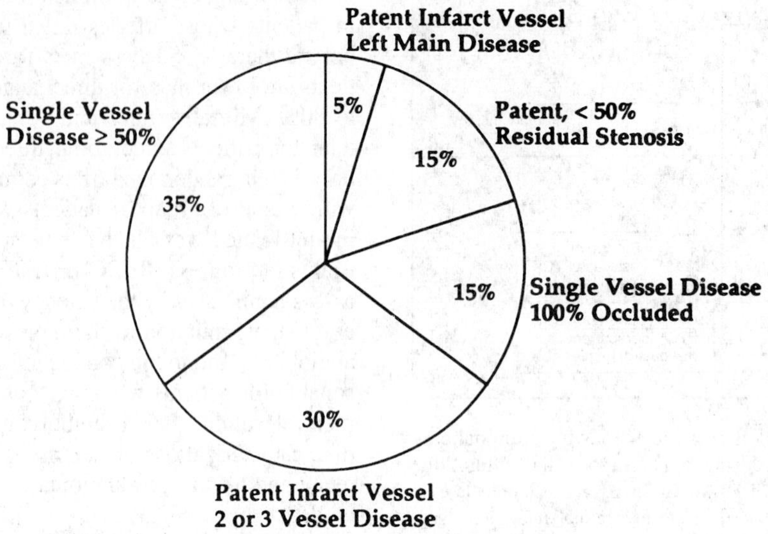

Fig. 14-7. Proportion of patients in each of five anatomic subsets distinguished after thrombolytic therapy. (From Topol EJ, Holmes DR, and Rogers WJ: Ann Intern Med 114:877, 1991. By permission of the American College of Physicians.)

ADJUNCTIVE THERAPY

Pharmacologic therapy for patients with acute MI retains an important role in patient management, with or without the use of reperfusion techniques.

Oxygen

Low-flow O_2 therapy delivered by nasal cannula should be routinely given during the first days of acute MI in most patients. Mild hypoxemia may occur, even in the absence of apparent pulmonary congestion. Additionally, some patients may have dyspnea related to acute changes in left ventricular compliance and secondarily increased pulmonary interstitial fluid.

Morphine sulfate

Morphine sulfate has traditionally been used to relieve the pain of myocardial ischemia and is best administered IV in boluses of 2 to 5 mg, to a maximum of 10 to 15 mg for a normal adult. Caution is necessary in treating patients with chronic obstructive pulmonary disease. Naloxone should be available for reversal of respiratory depression if this occurs. Additionally, the reduction in preload by morphine may exacerbate hypotension, particularly in elderly patients.

Nitrates

The cautious use of nitroglycerin is a mainstay in the early treatment of MI, particularly large Q wave anterior wall infarctions. Nitrates have several salutary effects, including dilatation of venous capacitance vessels, arterial resistance vessels, and coronary arteries, and possibly redistribution of flow to ischemic areas. Animal experiments demonstrated reduction in infarct size when nitroglycerin was administered IV within the first 4 to 6 hours after coronary occlusion, and several clinical studies in certain subgroups of patients support these findings.

IV nitroglycerin, starting at a dose of 5 to 10 μg/min, can be used in most patients early in the course of MI and is often useful as initial treatment for relief of pain. In normotensive patients the usual goal is to decrease systolic blood pressure by 10%; in hypertensive patients a 30% decrease is allowable, but adequate perfusion pressure must be maintained because infarct size can actually increase if mean blood pressure decreases below 80 mm Hg. IV nitroglycerin is usually administered for 24 to 48 hours, depending on the patient's clinical condition and the use of nitrates given orally or of other afterload-reducing agents. Approximately 10% of patients demonstrate a sensitivity to nitroglycerin manifested by a profound decrease in blood pressure after administration of even a small dose. This vagally mediated reflex is especially prominent in patients with inferior wall MI and those with substantial right ventricular involvement. Nitroglycerin therapy is best avoided in this subgroup of patients. Additionally, nitrate tolerance may occur, even within the first 24 hours of continuous IV infusion.

Beta-adrenergic receptor blockers

The use of beta-adrenergic receptor blockade in patients with acute MI is logical, and the theoretic advantages have been supported by much data from clinical trials. Nonetheless, it appears that these agents are still underused, particularly in the United States.

Mechanisms whereby beta-adrenergic receptor blockers may be beneficial include (1) a reduction in myocardial O_2 consumption, which by slowing the rate of necrosis can increase the time available for myocardial salvage and decrease the risk of recurrent ischemia; (2) antagonism of arrhythmogenic and toxic biochemical effects of catecholamines; and (3) a possible direct effect on myocardial ventricular fibrillation threshold. Also, in ISIS-1, with a trial of IV atenolol, a reduction in mortality was achieved by a highly significant decrease in the frequency of cardiac rupture compared with placebo treatment.

The results of clinical trials document an impressive decrease in early and late mortality despite minimum change in left ventricular function. In pooled data from 28 trials of beta-adrenergic receptor blockers, the average mortality decrease was 28% at 1 week, with most benefit obtained in the first 48 hours. An average 18% reduction in reinfarction and 15% reduction in cardiac arrest were also documented. The long-term effects of beta-adrenergic receptor blockade by agents without intrinsic sympathetic activity in secondary prevention of death after MI were established by large-scale randomized trials (Fig. 14-8). Although most of the benefit of beta-adrenergic receptor blockade was demonstrated within the first week of infarction and occurred in patients at increased risk, continuing benefit in terms of decreased mortality was documented up to 1 year later.

Many experts recommend the early IV administration of beta-adrenergic receptor blockers followed by beta blockers given orally for most patients with MI who do not demonstrate overt congestive heart failure or shock at admission. Major left ventricular dysfunction is not necessarily a contraindication; when concern exists regarding this, IV administration of a short-acting beta blocker, such as esmolol, can be used, with rapid termination of its effects if hypotension or increased pulmonary congestion occurs.

Calcium channel blockers

Most studies of the calcium channel blockers failed to demonstrate any definite benefit in patients with Q wave MI. In a meta-analysis of 22 trials, no improvement in mortality, reduction of infarct size, or reduction in the incidence of reinfarction was documented (Fig. 14-9). The lack of benefit probably relates to the negative inotropic action of the calcium channel blockers, with an adverse effect in patients with left ventricular failure and the potential for nifedipine reflexly to increase heart rate and myocardial O_2 consumption. In patients with non–Q wave MI, two trials (Diltiazem Reinfarction Study, Multicenter Diltiazem Postinfarction Trial) demonstrated a decreased incidence of reinfarction and post-MI angina in patients treated with diltiazem compared with placebo. Further analysis in one of these trials demonstrated that patients with left ventricular failure, manifested by pulmonary congestion, actually had

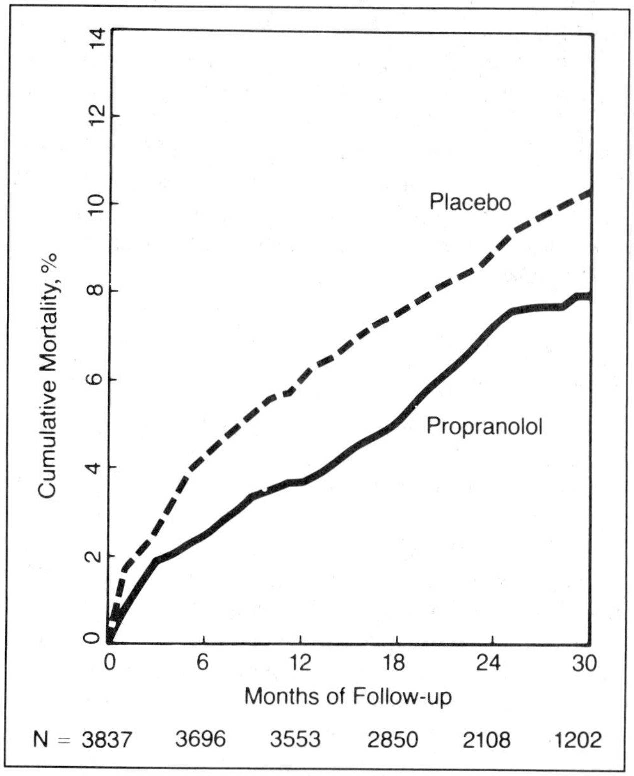

Fig. 14-8. Survival after acute MI: the BHAT trial. Life table cumulative mortality curves for propranolol hydrochloride and placebo groups. *N* denotes total number of patients followed up through each time point. (From Friedman L et al: JAMA 246:2073, 1981.)

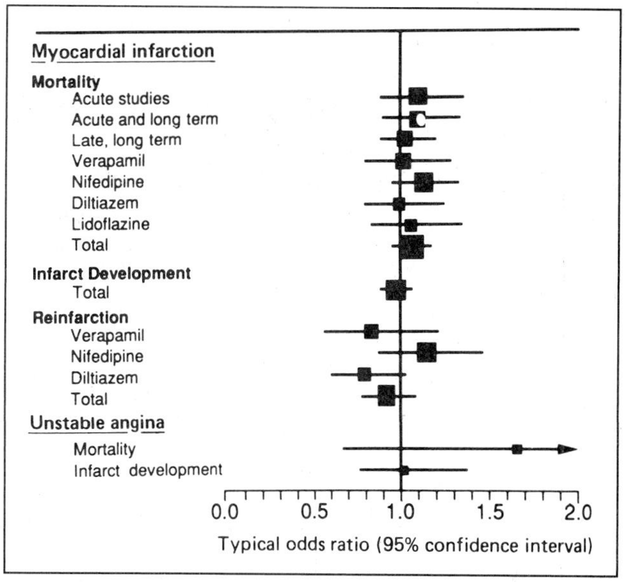

Fig. 14-9. Published studies of calcium channel blockers in patients with acute MI. Typical odds of death, infarct development, and reinfarction according to disease, types of trials, and drug used. Area of squares proportional to number of patients. Bars indicate 95% confidence intervals. Portions to left of vertical line (corresponding to odds ratio < 1) indicate reduced risk with treatment; portions to right of vertical line indicate increased risk with treatment. Upper 95% confidence limit for effect on mortality in unstable angina, 6.2. Note that treatment does not seem to reduce risk of any event. (From Held PH, Yusuf S, and Furberg CD: Br Med J 299:1187, 1989. By permission of British Medical Journal.)

an adverse response to diltiazem, with benefit limited to those without pulmonary congestion.

Although it is reasonable to treat a subgroup of patients who have non–Q wave MI with diltiazem, most such patients undergo invasive study and prompt revascularization.

Aspirin

Aspirin decreases mortality in patients with MI, undoubtedly through its antiplatelet effects. This was perhaps best illustrated in the ISIS-2 study (Fig. 14-10), in which patients were randomized to treatment with aspirin, streptokinase, or placebo, with later heparin therapy. The decrease in the death rate with aspirin and heparin was 23% compared with 25% for streptokinase and heparin and 41% for the combination of all three agents. Thus the effect of aspirin was nearly as great as that of streptokinase in this study, and the benefits of each were partially additive. Currently, 325 mg of chewable aspirin usually is administered when the patient with acute MI is first seen.

Prophylactic use of lidocaine

Prophylactic use of lidocaine can decrease the risk of primary ventricular fibrillation but also appears to increase the risk of fatal asystolic events. In a recent meta-analysis of six trials of prophylactic use of lidocaine in patients with acute MI, the mortality was slightly higher in the lidocaine group. Currently, prophylactic use of lidocaine is not recommended for patients with acute MI.

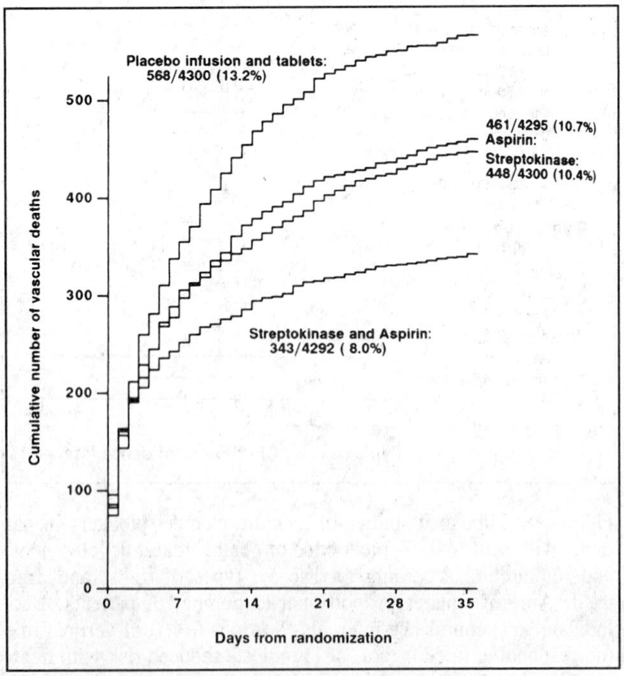

Fig. 14-10. Effect of aspirin, streptokinase, both, or neither on 35-day vascular mortality in the ISIS-2 study. (From ISIS-2 [Second International Study of Infarct Survival] Collaborative Group: Lancet 2:349, 1988. By permission of the Lancet.)

Heparin

Heparin is a key adjunctive agent for treatment of patients with acute MI. Heparin acts to inhibit the thrombotic cascade by its potentiation of antithrombin III and by a direct antithrombin effect. It has recently become clear that thrombosis occurs simultaneously with thrombolysis and may even be potentiated by thrombolytic agents such as streptokinase or t-PA. Additionally, thrombin is a strong inducer of platelet aggregation, and these factors undoubtedly account in part for the propensity toward reocclusion after successful artery recanalization.

The major benefit of heparin in patients receiving thrombolytic therapy appears to be in decreasing reocclusion rather than in enhancing initial salvage. However, controversy surrounds the timing and administration of heparin. Probably the best method for administration of heparin is bolus IV administration followed by a continuous drip with titration to an activated partial thromboplastin time of 2.0 to 2.5 times normal. Although heparin can be administered before, during, or after the conclusion of thrombolytic therapy, we elect to administer it at the onset of treatment.

Hospitalization for uncomplicated infarction

During the past 10 years, hospital stay for patients with uncomplicated MI has decreased. For patients without recurrent ischemic pain or hemodynamic or electrical instability, 48 hours of observation in an intensive care bed is usually followed by 48 hours of observation in a step-down area or monitored bed and 24 to 48 hours in a nonmonitored bed. Even shorter hospital stays (3 to 4 days) have been safely accomplished for patients after successful thrombolysis and angiographic documentation of low-risk coronary anatomy and preserved left ventricular function. The determination of the optimum length of stay must be individualized.

Management of patients with non–Q wave myocardial infarction

The differentiation between Q wave and non–Q wave MIs is useful because the management, clinical course, and late prognosis differ between the two entities. Pathologic studies of non–Q wave MIs demonstrate an incomplete MI in relation to the myocardial territory at risk. Even though the incidence of severe coronary artery disease is roughly similar in Q wave and non–Q wave MIs, patients with non–Q wave MIs are two to four times more likely to have a patent infarct-related artery at presentation, with residual severe stenosis or prominent collateralization. Because of the smaller amount of infarcted tissue, the risk of congestive heart failure and significant arrhythmia is lower than with Q wave MI, as is in-hospital mortality. However, in the 6 to 12 months after non–Q wave MI, the cumulative mortality reaches or exceeds that for patients dismissed from the hospital after Q wave MI because of a higher incidence of reinfarction.

Risk factors for further events in patients with non–Q wave MI include anterior location, persistent S-T segment depression at dismissal, occurrence or progression of S-T depression with angina, and inability to perform a low-level stress test. On the other hand, patients with non–Q wave MI who have no S-T segment depression are in a lower-risk group.

The immediate treatment of patients with non–Q wave MI should consist of aspirin, IV heparin, reduction of excess myocardial O_2 consumption, and perhaps treatment with diltiazem, depending on the presence or absence of pulmonary congestion. In general, at our institution, patients with non–Q wave MI, particularly if the extent of enzyme release is small, are treated similarly to patients with angina at rest. The initial step is stabilization of the symptoms and hemodynamics, followed by coronary angiography. Thereafter, therapy is individualized on the basis of the coronary anatomy, left ventricular function, age, and other clinical variables. An alternative approach after stabilization is for the patient to begin mobilization under observation. In the absence of recurrent symptoms, angiography may be limited to patients with documented ischemia during stress testing.

COMPLICATIONS

Because of the ubiquity of cardiac rhythm monitoring, most patients who die in the hospital from acute MI do so because of either extensive myocardial damage with pump failure or mechanical complication of MI, such as severe mitral regurgitation or cardiac rupture. The mechanical complications are potentially curable and should be in the forefront of any differential diagnosis in the patient with failure and hemodynamic deterioration.

Left ventricular failure

More than 20 years ago, Killip and Kimball (see Table 14-2) described the outcome of patients without or with various degrees of left ventricular failure occurring during hospitalization for acute MI. In patients with mild congestive heart failure characterized by rales covering less than 50% of the lung fields or an S_3 gallop, mortality was 17%, whereas those with pulmonary edema had a doubling of mortality to approximately 38%. Treatment of the patient with mild congestive heart failure during the post-MI course may require no more than usual methods, such as sodium restriction, digitalis, afterload reduction, and diuretics. Most patients with adequate peripheral perfusion and urine output do not require invasive hemodynamic monitoring.

Severe left ventricular dysfunction (pump failure) may present as florid pulmonary edema or cardiogenic shock, with hypotension, cool underperfused extremities, oliguria, and evidence of cerebral and visceral hypoperfusion (Chapters 10 and 11). These patients constitute a high-risk subset. Shock from severe left ventricular dysfunction occurs in approximately 7% of patients with MIs and carries a historical mortality of about 80%. The goals for management of these patients are twofold: (1) hemodynamic stabilization to ensure adequate oxygenation, acid-base balance, and tissue perfusion and (2) rapid investigation of any potentially reversible causes for the patient's condition. Hypovolemia may present as hypotension and decreased peripheral perfusion in the absence of pulmonary congestion (Chapter 11). Such patients should receive a cautious trial of volume expansion in the absence of overt pulmonary congestion.

In patients with more than mild pulmonary congestion, with or without hypotension, invasive hemodynamic monitoring using a balloon-tipped pulmonary artery catheter allows immediate access to valuable hemodynamic information and guides therapy. The management of such patients has been described on the basis of hemodynamic subsets related to pulmonary artery wedge pressure and cardiac output (see the box below). The basic goals of this approach include adjustment of volume status to bring pulmonary artery capillary wedge pressure to 18 to 20 mm Hg, optimization of cardiac output with inotropic agents or vasodilators, or both. In hypotensive patients, dopamine is the preferred inotropic agent because of its peripheral constricting properties with preservation of renal perfusion. Nitroglycerin is the preferred vasodilator and may be added cautiously once an acceptable systemic pressure has been obtained. Nitroprusside is less desired because of its potential coronary steal effect. For normotensive patients with low cardiac output, dobutamine, which has mixed inotropic and vasodilatory properties, may be preferable.

Severely hypotensive patients can be temporarily aided by intra-aortic balloon pumping or possibly by a ventricular assist device (Chapter 11). However, the benefits from these mechanical treatments are often temporary and may carry a significant risk of complications. Therefore, in patients with incipient cardiogenic shock, the search for a correctable condition, such as one of the mechanical complications of MI, is of the utmost importance.

Therapy by hemodynamic subset in Killip class I through IV patients (see Table 14-2)

I	No treatment other than standard (aspirin, beta-adrenergic receptor blockers, heparin)
II	Diuretic therapy to lower pulmonary artery wedge pressure to 18 mm Hg (also consider IV nitroglycerin and afterload reduction with angiotensin-converting enzyme inhibitors)
III	Volume expansion to a pulmonary artery wedge pressure of 18 mm Hg (also consider dobutamine)
IV	Afterload reduction with IV nitroglycerin, nitroprusside, or angiotensin-converting enzyme inhibitors with or without an inotrope such as dobutamine or dopamine (search for correctable complication of MI)

Modified from Forrester JH et al: N Engl J Med 295:1356, 1976.

Mechanical complications

The mechanical complications of acute MI occur infrequently but are important because they are potentially reversible. Moreover, among patients who die of mechanical complications, infarct size is considerably smaller than in patients dying of arrhythmias or primary pump failure. Thus the mechanical complication per se is the major cause of death and not left ventricular dysfunction.

The mechanical complications of MI include myocardial free wall rupture, ventricular septal defect, acute ischemic disruption of the mitral valve with severe regurgitation, and right ventricular infarction. Infarction expansion or extension and left ventricular aneurysm formation are also mechanical complications, but these do not generally result in major acute deterioration of hemodynamics.

Although use of the balloon-tipped pulmonary artery flotation catheter provides useful diagnostic information and is helpful in monitoring therapy, the most efficient method for diagnosing the mechanical complications is bedside 2D echocardiography, including the use of the transesophageal approach when necessary. With these two modalities, virtually every patient who has experienced a mechanical complication can be rapidly diagnosed and plans for corrective therapy instituted.

Acute mitral regurgitation

Although the presence of transient mitral regurgitation caused by papillary muscle dysfunction is common in patients with MI, severe mitral regurgitation from papillary muscle rupture (Fig. 14-11) is a life-threatening, eminently correctable complication. Papillary muscle rupture accounts for approximately 5% of deaths in patients with acute MI, as determined by autopsy studies. Rupture of the entire papillary muscle is rapidly fatal because of the torrential mitral regurgitation that results. Usually, survivors have had partial tearing of one or more heads of the papillary muscle, with severe regurgitation caused by a flail mitral segment. Papillary muscle rupture usually involves the posterior medial papillary muscle, presumably because its blood supply is derived only from the posterior descending artery, whereas the anterolateral papillary muscle has a dual blood supply from both left anterior descending and circumflex branches.

The clinical presentation of papillary muscle rupture is the acute onset of pulmonary edema, usually within 2 to 7 days after inferior MI. The characteristics of the murmur vary; no murmur may be audible as a result of a rapid increase of pressure in the left atrium. Therefore a high degree of suspicion, especially in the patient with inferior wall infarction, is necessary for diagnosis. 2D echocardiographic examination demonstrates the severed papillary muscle

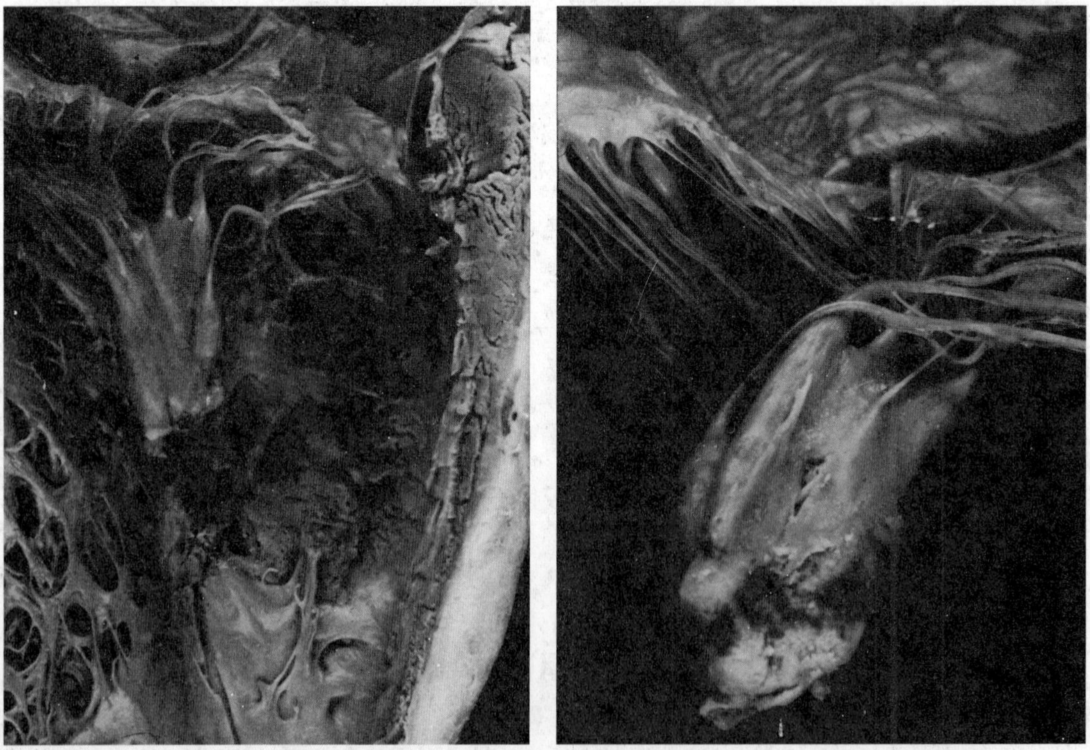

Fig. 14-11. Pathologic specimen demonstrates complete transection of papillary muscle *(left)* and close-up view *(right)* caused by MI. Severe mitral regurgitation and death resulted. (Photo courtesy of William Edwards, MD.)

head and a flail segment of the mitral valve. Left ventricular function is hyperdynamic as a result of the severe regurgitation into the low-impedance left atrium; this finding alone should suggest the diagnosis.

The cornerstone of successful therapy is prompt diagnosis and emergency surgery. Surgical correction requires mitral valve replacement in most patients; repair is possible in a minority. The current approach of emergency surgery accrues an overall operative mortality of approximately 25%, but this appears to be decreasing, and the late results of this approach are excellent.

Myocardial rupture

Rupture of the free wall of the left ventricle accounts for approximately 10% of deaths in patients with acute MI. The characteristics of patients with free wall rupture are similar to those with rupture of the papillary muscle or ventricular septum. Rupture of the free wall of the left ventricle typically occurs in small infarcts (Fig. 14-12), often in patients with single-vessel disease and poor collaterals and typically in elderly females with first MIs. Although any wall may be involved, rupture of the lateral wall probably occurs most often. Rupture occurs within the first 5 days of infarction in 50% of patients and within 14 days in 87%. The area of rupture always occurs within the MI area but usually is eccentrically located near the junction with normal myocardium.

The clinical presentation involves sudden electromechanical dissociation. The great majority of patients die even when rapid resuscitative measures, including pericardiocentesis, balloon pumping, and urgent rush to cardiac surgery, are attempted. Occasionally, rupture may be subacute, with periodic small amounts of blood leaking into the pericardial space. Persistent, severe pericardial pain may be a manifestation of this phenomenon, and the subsequent inflammatory process may wall off the area of pericardial leakage from the remaining pericardial space. In this way a false aneurysm or pseudoaneurysm of the left ventricle may form. The entity is easily and reliably detected by 2D echocardiography and mandates early surgical intervention because of the risk of further expansion of the false aneurysm or release of its contents into the remaining pericardial space, producing tamponade and death. The major impediment to surgical correction of acute free wall rupture is logistic, but among the few patients who can undergo surgery early enough, immediate surgery can be performed with gratifying results.

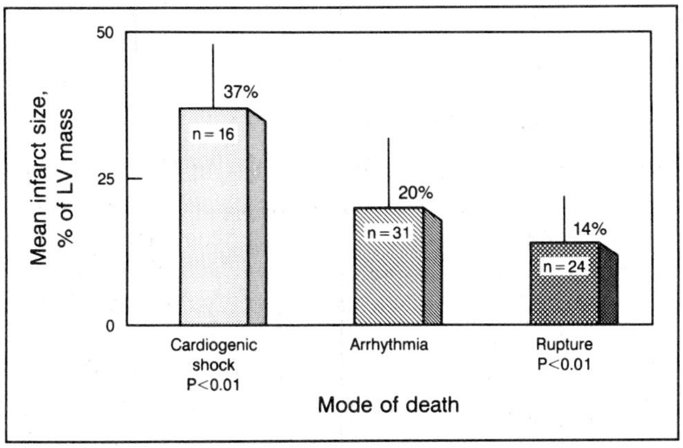

Fig. 14-12. Mean infarct size as percentage of left ventricular mass in patients dying of cardiogenic shock, arrhythmia, and cardiac free wall rupture. *LV*, Left ventricular. (Data from Saffitz JE, Fredrickson RC, and Roberts WC: Am J Cardiol 57:1249, 1986.)

Ventricular septal rupture

Rupture of the ventricular septum occurs in 1% to 3% of patients with acute MIs and causes approximately 5% of peri-infarction deaths. The substrate is quite similar to that of free wall rupture in terms of number of vessels diseased and infarct size. Typically, ventricular septal rupture associated with anterior MI is located in the apical septum, and that associated with inferior MI is located in the basal inferior septum. Involvement of anterior and inferior MIs is approximately equal, unlike papillary muscle rupture.

The diagnosis should be suspected clinically when a new pansystolic murmur is present. Once again, echocardiography, including the transesophageal approach, can diagnose this condition. Additionally, withdrawal of venous samples from the pulmonary artery catheter and an arterial line, as well as measurement of O_2 consumption, allow calculation of the percentage of shunt. As with other cardiac ruptures, aggressive and early angiography and surgical management are advocated, although the outcome in these patients is not as gratifying as in those with acute mitral regurgitation because the extent of myocardial necrosis is generally larger.

Right ventricular infarction

Involvement of the right ventricle (Fig. 14-13) is a common sequela of acute inferior MI. However, hemodynamically significant right ventricular dysfunction occurs much less often in relatively few patients with right ventricular infarction.

The diagnosis of hemodynamically significant right ventricular infarction rests on the clinical triad of hypotension, increased jugular venous pressure, and clear lung fields in a patient with acute inferior wall MI. A more sensitive finding suggestive of right ventricular involvement is a positive Kussmaul's sign. Additional diagnostic techniques that can document right ventricular involvement include ECG S-T segment elevation in right-sided chest leads (V_3R or V_4R), visualization of right ventricular wall motion abnormalities, and right ventricular dilatation on radionuclide angiography or echocardiography.

From a management standpoint, it is crucial to identify the patient in whom the abnormal hemodynamic profile is predominantly the result of right ventricular involvement, that is, dominant right ventricular infarction. Documentation that right ventricular function rapidly improves in a few days and the usually favorable response of the hemodynamic abnormality to fluid loading with or without inotropic support emphasize the importance of correctly identifying

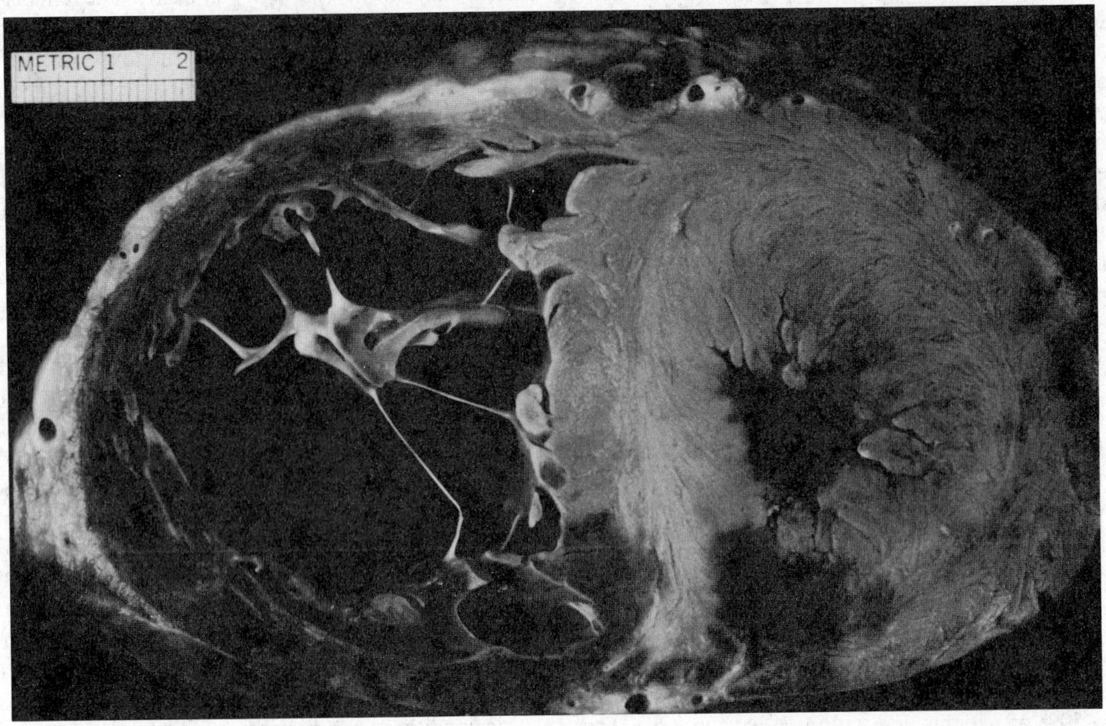

Fig. 14-13. Extensive right ventricular MI associated with inferior wall infarction. Severe right ventricular failure resulted in patient's death. (Photograph courtesy of William D. Edwards, MD.)

this problem. In patients with normal hemodynamics, the need to diagnose right ventricular infarction is debatable. If it is suspected, avoidance of preload reduction is sufficient.

Pulmonary artery balloon-tipped flotation catheter measurements in patients with significant right ventricular infarction demonstrate elevation of the right atrial pressure, usually greater than 10 mm Hg, and often show a right atrial pressure/pulmonary artery wedge pressure ratio of 0.8 or greater. However, in patients with significant left ventricular dysfunction and elevation of the wedge pressure, this ratio may be lower and does not exclude the presence of significant right ventricular involvement. The incidence of high-grade atrioventricular (A-V) block is also increased in patients with right ventricular infarction.

Treatment of patients with right ventricular infarction typically involves volume loading with normal saline to achieve a pulmonary artery wedge pressure of 18 to 20 mm Hg. In some patients, this alone is sufficient to improve cardiac output and systemic pressure. However, some patients will not respond to fluid-loading alone. Recent investigations suggest that this may be the result of marked right ventricular enlargement within a relatively noncompliant pericardium, which may result in functional left ventricular compression caused by ventricular interaction. When volume loading alone does not suffice, the use of an inotropic agent, such as dobutamine, has been advocated and has demonstrated limited success. Cautious use of agents such as nitroprusside may occasionally be warranted.

Most patients, even those with substantial right ventricular dysfunction, spontaneously improve in 48 to 72 hours after the acute event. Patients in shock may benefit from attempted angioplasty of the occluded right coronary artery or even possibly the temporary use of a right ventricular assist device; however, many of these patients have associated significant left ventricular dysfunction complicating the picture. The overall balance between the extent of right ventricular and left ventricular dysfunction is a major determinant of long-term outcome.

Infarct expansion and left ventricular aneurysm

Infarct expansion refers to thinning and dilatation of the infarct segment, usually without clinical manifestations of myocardial enzyme release. This is in contradistinction to infarct extension, in which recurrent pain and another increase in the CK-MB values are generally observed. Infarct expansion has been described primarily in sequential echocardiographic studies and is a precursor of aneurysm formation and myocardial rupture in a minority of patients.

The formation of a left ventricular true aneurysm occurs in the days and weeks after MI, probably beginning with infarct expansion, necrosis and removal of dead cellular elements, and replacement with fibrous scar tissue. Patients at increased risk for aneurysm formation include those with large infarcts, those with uncontrolled hypertension, and those receiving corticosteroids or nonsteroidal anti-inflammatory agents. The early development of apical dyskinesis or aneurysm formation predisposes to mural thrombus and embolization during the first 3 to 6 months after MI. Furthermore, it appears likely that early infarct expansion, by altering regional wall stress, predisposes to ventricular remodeling, with dilatation of the noninfarct portion of the left ventricle and ultimately late congestive heart failure and death.

Left ventricular thrombus

Left ventricular thrombus (Fig. 14-14) can be observed in 10% to 40% of anterior wall infarcts and rarely in inferior wall infarcts. Thrombus is usually located within hypokinetic or dyskinetic segments, that is, in areas of relative stasis of blood flow, usually the left ventricular apex. Large or mobile thrombi, as observed on echocardiographic examination, have a relatively high risk of embolization. We usually provide 3 to 6 months of anticoagulant therapy in patients with (1) large anterior MI, (2) congestive heart failure, (3) documented mural thrombus, or (4) large apical aneurysmal or dyskinetic segments.

The incidence of left ventricular thrombus formation probably is decreased by the early use of thrombolytic therapy because extent of MI and degree of wall motion abnormality may be decreased and because of a direct effect against thrombus formation.

Pericarditis

Pericarditis frequently occurs early in the course of transmural MI. It may manifest as a pericardial rub, pleuritic chest pain, or pericardial effusion seen on 2D echocardiography, or it may be clinically silent (Chapter 18). Late pericardial inflammation (2 weeks to 3 months after MI) has been termed *Dressler's syndrome* and is probably related to an autoimmune mechanism. It is becoming increasingly infrequent for reasons unknown. Treatment with salicylates, nonsteroidal anti-inflammatory agents, or colchicine is preferred to the use of corticosteroids because of the high frequency of relapse when corticosteroid therapy is discontinued. Echocardiography in patients with pericarditis is useful to determine the extent of effusion and to exclude the possibility of partial rupture or pseudoaneurysm.

Electrical complications

Conduction disturbances. Conduction disturbances in patients with acute MI generally result from two mechanisms: ischemic injury to the conduction system or surrounding myocardium and abnormal reflexes that are usually vagally

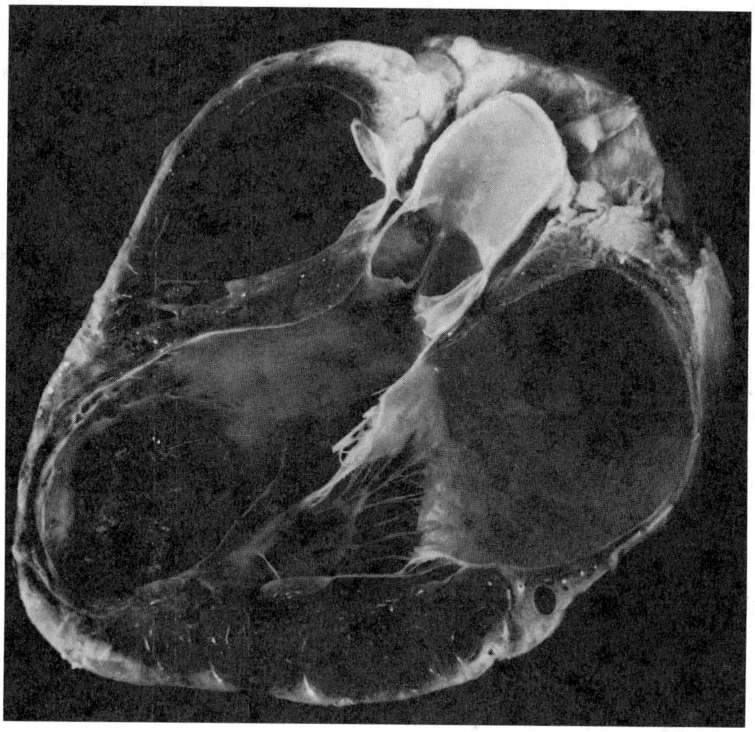

Fig. 14-14. Left ventricular thrombus. Extensive anterior and apical MI with apical thrombus. Systemic embolization occurred before death. (From Edwards WD: In Gersh BJ and Rahimtoola SH, editors: Current topics in cardiology: acute myocardial infarction. New York, 1991, Elsevier. By permission of Elsevier Science Publishing Company.)

mediated and precipitated by MI. The blood supply (Fig. 14-15) to the sinus node arises from the proximal right coronary artery in 55% of patients and from the proximal left circumflex in 45%. The blood supply to the A-V node arises from the distal branches of the right coronary artery in 90% of patients and from the distal portions of the left circumflex artery in 10%. There is usually a dual blood supply to the A-V node and bundle of His, which accounts for the lack of necrosis of these structures even with extensive MI. The right bundle branch is supplied primarily by the septal perforator vessels originating from the left anterior descending artery, as is the distal portion of the anterior left bundle branch. The main left bundle branch has a dual supply from both distal branches of the right coronary and proximal circumflex vessels, and the posterior division of the left bundle branch is supplied from branches of the circumflex coronary artery.

In general, all conduction disturbances associated with inferoposterior MI are related largely to enhanced vagal activity, tend to be more transient, are often responsive to atropine, and imply a more benign outcome than those involved in anterior MI. Conversely, major conduction disturbances associated with anterior MI usually imply extensive septal necrosis and more significant reduction in left ventricular function.

Sinus bradycardia. Sinus bradycardia and sinus pauses occurring in either anterior or inferior MI are usually benign and are generally observed unless prolonged asystole or symptoms are present. First-degree A-V block occurs in 4% to 13% of patients with MI. Observation and avoidance of any medications that might prolong A-V conduction are all that is required.

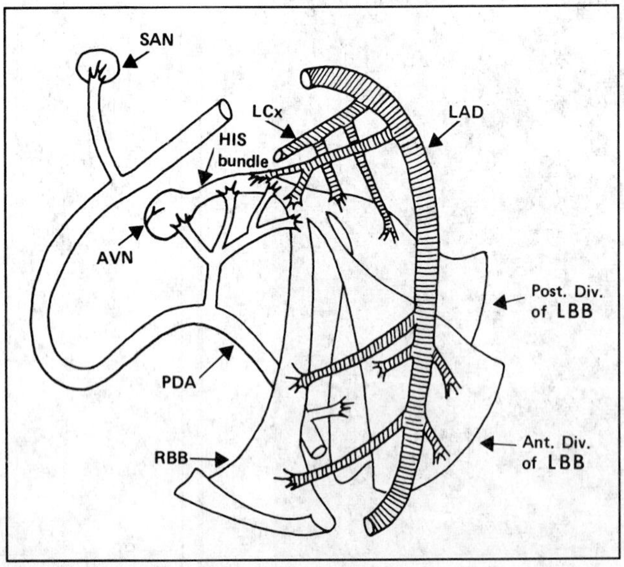

Fig. 14-15. The conduction system and its blood supply. *AVN,* Atrioventricular node; *LAD,* left anterior descending; *LCx,* left circumflex; *LBB,* left bundle branch; *PDA,* posterior descending artery; *RBB,* right bundle branch; *SAN,* sinoatrial node. (From DeGuzman M and Rahimtoola SH: Cardiovasc Clin 13:191, 1983. By permission of FA Davis Company.)

Second-degree atrioventricular block. This usually develops within the first 24 hours of MIs in 3% to 10% of individuals. With type I second-degree A-V block, progressive prolongation of the P-R interval is observed; this usually occurs with inferoposterior MI and may often respond to atropine. A narrow QRS complex is usually present, and careful observation is the rule unless the ventricular rate decreases below 45 beats/min or symptoms of ischemia or impaired perfusion develop. Type II second-degree A-V block is identified by intermittent dropped beats in the absence of progressive P-R prolongation and implies extensive infranodal conduction system injury. Often the QRS complex is wide, indicating associated bundle branch block (BBB), and progression to complete heart block occurs in approximately one third of these patients. Most patients with anterior MI and type II second-degree A-V block receive temporary transvenous pacing because of the unpredictable risk of complete heart block.

Complete heart block. This occurs in 3% to 7% of patients with acute MIs. In general, patients with inferoposterior MI progress to third-degree heart block after a period of second-degree block and again may demonstrate some responsiveness to atropine. Often a reliable junctional escape rhythm is present, and recovery tends to occur within 3 to 7 days, although occasionally it can be delayed. Many of these patients can be observed, in some with standby, temporary, transcutaneous pacing patches in place. Complete heart block in patients with anterior MI usually indicates an extensive area of myocardial necrosis, may occur unpredictably, and carries a poor prognosis. Most patients require temporary transvenous pacing, and some physicians advocate permanent transvenous pacing. Late mortality in these patients is usually caused by pump failure or ventricular fibrillation rather than persistent, high-grade A-V block.

The occurrence of any new BBB with acute MI also identifies patients with extensive infarction who are at higher risk for later complications. Unifascicular block, especially left anterior hemiblock, occurs in approximately 5% of patients and has a relatively benign prognosis. Complete right or left BBB occurs in 10% to 15% of patients and most often involves the right bundle branch. In the past, the new occurrence of left or right BBB has been a generally accepted indication for temporary transvenous pacing. However, mortality in these patients is related primarily to pump failure or ventricular fibrillation.

The indications for temporary transvenous pacing were a source of discussion and interest in the 1970s. The indications still apply, but the availability of transcutaneous pacing (if capture can be documented in advance) simplifies the management in patients with marginal indications or in whom venous access is limited.

Late postinfarction bradyarrhythmias. Permanent transvenous pacing is indicated in patients with persistent complete or high-grade A-V block or persistent, type II second-degree A-V block after MI and in patients with a new BBB and transient but resolved complete heart block during the acute course of MI. However, this indication remains controversial, and no proved benefit of pacing exists in this subgroup of patients. Occasionally, patients may require electrophysiologic study to determine the site of A-V block and to aid in the decision of whether permanent pacing is indicated. Permanent pacing may also be indicated in the rare patient with profound sinus node dysfunction.

Tachyarrhythmias. The genesis of tachyarrhythmias in patients with MI is multifactorial. Decreased blood flow leads to anaerobic metabolism, and decreased venous outflow allows accumulation of by-products of this process, resulting in acidosis, increased extracellular potassium concentration, and increased intracellular calcium concentration. In addition, there may be alterations in sympathetic and vagal tone and increased concentrations of circulating catecholamines. The electrophysiologic correlates of these cellular abnormalities include slowing of conduction and prolongation of refractoriness, and the inhomogeneous nature of the MI process produces an ideal situation for the occurrence of re-entrant arrhythmias (Chapter 9). The presence of injury currents may directly enhance phase IV depolarization of Purkinje cells, resulting in increased automaticity. Fiber stretch, resulting from increased atrial and ventricular end-diastolic pressures, is also arrhythmogenic. Finally, reperfusion, possibly from intracellular calcium overload or production of free O_2 radicals, may generate reperfusion arrhythmias, which may be either automatic or re-entrant.

Supraventricular arrhythmias. Sinus tachycardia occurs in up to 25% of patients with acute MI and often results from pain, anxiety, and sometimes hypovolemia. Persistent sinus tachycardia, related to increased circulating catecholamines, may be a marker of severe left ventricular dysfunction and is a poor prognostic sign. Whatever the cause, sinus tachycardia is undesired because of increased O_2 demand. After relief of pain and assessment for the presence of pulmonary congestion, it is desirable to decrease the heart rate below 70 beats/min by IV administration of beta-adrenergic receptor blockers. A short-acting beta-adrenergic receptor blocker, such as esmolol, may be appropriate for patients in whom the extent of left ventricular dysfunction is of particular concern.

Atrial premature beats typically occur in patients with acute MI and may represent increased left atrial pressure. They may also be a harbinger of other atrial tachyarrhythmias. However, when they occur in isolation, observation alone suffices.

Atrial fibrillation occurs in 10% to 15% of patients with acute MI. Its presence early signifies atrial ischemia; later it may also represent atrial stretch from increasing filling pressures. Immediate cardioversion is the best treatment for patients with symptomatic rapid atrial fibrillation or in whom the rapid ventricular response produces ischemia. If the ventricular response is only moderate and the patient is asymptomatic, IV diltiazem or esmolol is useful for control of heart rate, along with digoxin given orally; the latter may take 4 to 8 hours for full effect. Recurrent episodes of atrial fibrillation should be suppressed with an antiarrhythmic agent such as procainamide or quinidine. The treatment of atrial flutter is similar to that of atrial fibrillation except that drug treatment is less effective in producing an easily controlled ventricular response. Occasionally, atrial overdrive pacing may be used to terminate atrial flutter without resorting to cardioversion.

A-V nodal re-entrant tachycardia (supraventricular tachycardia) occurs infrequently in patients with acute MI, probably relates to underlying dual A-V nodal pathways, and may respond to adenosine or digitalis, among other agents. Accelerated junctional rhythm is a benign disorder that may be observed.

Ventricular tachyarrhythmias. Although many patients with MI may have ventricular premature beats, few develop more advanced arrhythmias. Conversely, ventricular fibrillation or tachycardia may develop without warning. Suppression of ventricular premature beats can be accomplished if they are symptomatic, are frequent (more than 5/min), or occur in runs of bigeminy. Otherwise, they may be observed.

The ubiquity of early ventricular ectopy and primary ventricular arrhythmias is well established in patients seen within the first few hours of MI. These rhythms remain a major indication for the prompt initiation of ECG monitoring during the treatment of acute MI, and they typically decrease in frequency during the first 24 to 36 hours of infarction. In contrast, ventricular arrhythmias occurring late after the completion of MI are usually a manifestation of underlying left ventricular dysfunction and thus have been termed *secondary* ventricular arrhythmias. Such rhythms portend a less benign prognosis, not only because of the electrical disturbance per se, but also because this indicates significant systolic dysfunction.

Accelerated idioventricular rhythm may occur in up to 40% of continuously monitored patients and may signify reperfusion in some. Although this rhythm disturbance is generally considered benign and is usually untreated, idioventricular rhythms that accelerate to 110 to 120 beats/min may then be more appropriately considered automatic ventricular tachycardias with a less benign prognosis, and these more rapid rhythms should be suppressed with lidocaine.

Ventricular tachycardia occurs in up to 15% of patients during acute MI. The ventricular rate is usually 140 to 200 beats/min, and this rhythm disturbance may degenerate to ventricular fibrillation. The rhythm disturbance usually responds to IV lidocaine. However, procainamide, bretylium, cardioversion, ventricular overdrive pacing, or amiodarone may all be required in the acute stages for resistant cases (Chapter 9). The use of lidocaine prophylactically for prevention of ventricular tachycardia remains controversial.

Ventricular fibrillation is seen in approximately 8% of patients surviving to hospitalization for acute MI. It is more frequent in large Q wave infarcts and may occur with or without warning arrhythmias. The occurrence of ventricular fibrillation within the first 24 hours of hospitalization was thought not to confer any long-term risk to patients successfully resuscitated. However, recent studies indicate poorer outcome for patients with ventricular fibrillation at any time during their hospital course. Ventricular fibrillation or tachycardia occurring late in the hospital course may result from pump failure, severe electrolyte imbalance, effects of antiarrhythmic medications, or other metabolic derangements. However, it is usually associated with decreased left ventricular systolic function and portends a poor prognosis. *Sustained monomorphic* ventricular tachycardia, occurring early or late during the hospital course, occurs infrequently but implies an arrhythmogenic substrate and a propensity for recurrence after discharge. An invasive electrophysiologic study can be justified in these patients before dismissal.

Treatment of ventricular fibrillation in the early phase of MI involves immediate cardioversion and lidocaine given IV for 24 to 36 hours as prophylaxis for a recurrent episode. Late-phase ventricular fibrillation should prompt a search for severe residual ischemia or reinfarction.

The treatment of patients with asymptomatic, late-phase, nonsustained ventricular tachycardia remains problematic and is the current focus of several randomized trials. Nonsustained ventricular tachycardia is an independent predictor of mortality and sudden death after MI. Decreased left ventricular systolic function and late potentials on signal-averaged ECGs are also independent additional predictors of mortality.

Electrophysiologic testing was proposed as a procedure to assess asymptomatic patients at increased risk for ventricular fibrillation and sudden death, but the results have been disappointing; although quite sensitive, the test is nonspecific. At present such testing remains investigational. A second problem in treatment of such patients relates to antiarrhythmic drugs (Chapter 9). The bulk of available data indicates that antiarrhythmic therapy for asymptomatic, nonsustained ventricular tachycardia in patients after MI worsens survival.

The only pharmacologic treatments that have been shown to improve survival in the patient after MI include beta-adrenergic receptor blockade, thrombolytic therapy, and aspirin, and these agents should be used whenever possible. Additionally, patients with late-phase, nonsustained ventricular tachycardia should have a thorough search for residual myocardial ischemia, which, in conjunction with left ventricular dysfunction and ventricular arrhythmias, identifies a subgroup at high risk for sudden cardiac death in whom coronary revascularization may be of benefit.

LATE MANAGEMENT

Late management of patients with MI includes risk stratification, rehabilitation, and preventive cardiology.

Risk stratification

Reasonable estimates of survival and morbidity after MI can be established by using clinical and noninvasive laboratory parameters. The history and physical examination can identify factors such as advanced age, prior MI, presence of New York Heart Association (NYHA) class II to IV congestive heart failure, postinfarction angina, mechanical complications of MI, and non–Q wave MI, all of which identify patients at higher risk for reinfarction and death in the first 6 months after MI. As stated previously, decreased ejection fraction, complex ventricular ectopy, and late potentials on the signal-averaged ECG also identify individuals at increased risk for continued problems. The absence of these clinical and noninvasively determined risk factors identifies a population at low risk for reinfarction and death in the months immediately after MI.

Exercise testing, with or without the use of radioisotopes, has also proved useful in detecting patients at relatively higher or lower risk for a poor outcome. In patients who do not manifest pump failure or severe ischemia, have negative results of a predischarge exercise test, have an ejection fraction greater than 40%, and have negative results of a symptom-limited outpatient exercise test at 6 weeks, a 1-year mortality of 5% or less can be expected.

Virtually all the studies examining prognosis after MI were performed in the prethrombolysis era. As a group, such patients might typically have a 1-year post-MI mortality of up to 30%, and these risk stratification algorithms remain useful in patients not receiving thrombolytic or reperfusion therapy. However, the increasingly aggressive use of reperfusion strategies (thrombolysis, acute angioplasty, myocardial revascularization) and the selection process for thrombolytic therapy resulted in 1-year postdischarge cumulative mortality rates of 2% to 5% in some studies. The previously established criteria for risk stratification in the prethrombolysis era may not apply to most patients treated with thrombolytic drugs or mechanical reperfusion.

Rehabilitation and preventive cardiology

The goals of cardiac rehabilitation are to enhance quality of life, facilitate return to normal activities, and provide secondary prevention to correct risk factors for further ischemic events. At our institution a four-phase program is instituted for patients after uncomplicated MI. An interdisciplinary approach involving members of the medical and nursing staff, social and vocational rehabilitation counselors, occupational therapists, dietitians, and an exercise physiologist allows an integrated strategy to patient education, modification of risk factors, vocational adjustment, and improvement in quality of life.

The phase I program begins when the patient is hemodynamically and electrically stable in the coronary care unit and continues until discharge. It begins with passive range-of-motion exercises and progresses to sitting in a chair twice daily, minimum self-care exercises, then ambulating with physical therapists, having bathroom privileges, showering in a wheelchair, and gradually increasing levels of supervised activities. Initially an upper limit heart rate of 20 beats/min above the standing rate is used, but by the end of phase I, the patient can generally walk at a pace of 1 to 2 miles/hr for up to 10 minutes three times a day. At this stage a predismissal or an early postdismissal rehabilitation treadmill exercise test is performed, usually using the Naughton protocol with a target of either symptoms or achievement of 5 metabolic equivalents (METs) of activity. A positive result on such a test or intercurrent symptoms are usually an indication for an invasive study.

Phase II begins at patient discharge and generally continues for 1 to 3 months. Objectives include continued patient education, modification of risk factors, preparation for gradual return to occupational and avocational activities, and improvement of cardiovascular fitness by aerobic exercise. In general a standard program includes three visits weekly for supervised exercise sessions as well as unsupervised and regular home exercise sessions, sometimes including telephone ECG transmission for monitoring of ischemia or arrhythmia. A symptom-limited treadmill exercise test is performed at the beginning and end of phase II to establish a safe upper-limit heart rate during exercise and to assess aerobic improvement during the program's course.

After successful completion of phase II, the phase III program is initiated with the goal of continued improvement in cardiorespiratory fitness, usually with group exercise and education sessions at a community exercise facility or a strictly home exercise program without direct supervision. Exercise to 50% to 70% of functional aerobic capacity is usually prescribed as long as no ischemia is present during treadmill testing to this level. The duration of phase III is 6 months to 1 year, and patients are released from this program when their functional capacity can be sustained at 8 METs with a stable rest and exercise ECG and without symptoms of angina or dyspnea at normal activity levels.

Finally, patients may enter a phase IV program, designed to maintain the exercise capacity achieved in phase III, and the length of this program is indefinite.

A mandatory aspect of the rehabilitation program is modification of risk factors. Smoking cessation is the most important, in addition to blood pressure control and treatment of hyperlipidemia and diabetes mellitus. Periodic reinforcement and regular follow-up are essential.

REFERENCES

ACC/AHA guidelines for the early management of patients with acute myocardial infarction (special report). Circulation 82:664, 1990.

β-Blocker Heart Attack Study Group: The β-Blocker Heart Attack Trial. JAMA 246:2073, 1981.

Cardiac Arrhythmia Suppression Trial (CAST) investigators: Preliminary report: effect of encainide and flecainide on mortality in a randomized trial of arrhythmia suppression after myocardial infarction. N Engl J Med 321:406, 1989.

Chesebro JH et al: Thrombolysis in Myocardial Infarction (TIMI) Trial, Phase I: a comparison between intravenous tissue plasminogen activator and intravenous streptokinase: clinical findings through hospital discharge. Circulation 76:142, 1987.

Cohn JN et al: Right ventricular infarction: clinical and hemodynamic features. Am J Cardiol 33:209, 1974.

DeWood MA et al: Prevalence of total coronary occlusion during the early hours of transmural myocardial infarction. N Engl J Med 303:897, 1980.

Ellis SG et al: Coronary angioplasty as primary therapy for acute myocardial infarction 6 to 48 hours after symptom onset: report of an initial experience. J Am Coll Cardiol 13:1122, 1989.

Gersh BJ and Rahimtoola SH, editors: Current topics in cardiology: acute myocardial infarction. New York, 1991, Elsevier.

Gomes JA et al: The prognostic significance of quantitative signal-averaged variables relative to clinical variables, site of myocardial infarction, ejection fraction and ventricular premature beats: a prospective study. J Am Coll Cardiol 13:377, 1989.

Gruppo Italiano per lo Studio della Sopravvivenza nell'Infarto Miocardico: GISSI-2: a factorial randomised trial of alteplase versus streptokinase and heparin versus no heparin among 12,490 patients with acute myocardial infarction. Lancet 336:65, 1990.

Held PH, Yusuf S, and Furberg CO: Calcium channel blockers in acute myocardial infarction and unstable angina: an overview. Br Med J 299:1187, 1989.

Hine LK et al: Meta-analysis of empirical long-term antiarrhythmic therapy after myocardial infarction. JAMA 262:3037, 1989.

ISIS-1 (First International Study of Infarct Survival) Collaborative Group: Mechanisms for the early mortality reduction produced by beta-blockade started early in acute myocardial infarction: ISIS-1. Lancet 1:921, 1988.

ISIS-2 (Second International Study of Infarct Survival) Collaborative Group: Randomised trial of intravenous streptokinase, oral aspirin, both, or neither among 17,187 cases of suspected acute myocardial infarction: ISIS-2. Lancet 2:349, 1988.

ISIS-3 (Third International Study of Infarct Survival) Collaborative Group: ISIS-3: a randomised comparison of streptokinase *vs* tissue plasminogen activator *vs* anistreplase and of aspirin plus heparin *vs* aspirin alone among 41,299 cases of suspected acute myocardial infarction. Lancet 339:753, 1992.

Jugdutt BI and Warnica JW: Intravenous nitroglycerin therapy to limit myocardial infarct size, expansion, and complications: effect of timing, dosage, and infarct location. Circulation 78:906, 1988.

Killip T III and Kimball JT: Treatment of myocardial infarction in a coronary care unit: a two year experience with 250 patients. Am J Cardiol 20:457, 1967.

MacMahon S et al: Effects of prophylactic lidocaine in suspected myocardial infarction: an overview of results from randomized, controlled trials. JAMA 260:1910, 1988.

MIAMI Trial Research Group: Metoprolol in acute myocardial infarction (MIAMI): a randomized placebo-controlled international trial. Eur Heart J 6:199, 1985.

TIMI Study Group: Comparison of invasive and conservative strategies after treatment with intravenous tissue plasminogen activator in acute myocardial infarction: results of the Thrombolysis in Myocardial Infarction (TIMI) Phase II Trial. N Engl J Med 320:618, 1989.

Willich SN et al: Increased morning incidence of myocardial infarction in the ISAM Study: absence with prior β-adrenergic blockade. Circulation 80:853, 1989.

CHAPTER

15 Infective Endocarditis

Tomás Aragón
Merle A. Sande

Infective endocarditis is a localized infection consisting of fibrin, platelets, and microorganisms that adhere to the cardiac valves or other endothelial surfaces. The clinical manifestations are systemic and include fever, cardiac murmurs, anemia, splenomegaly, petechiae, pyuria, and peripheral emboli. Without appropriate treatment, the mortality approaches 100%, though its pace varies from a subtle, indolent, wasting condition to fulminant, overwhelming sepsis. Endocarditis must be considered early in the differential diagnosis of a wide variety of conditions; prompt diagnosis and aggressive appropriate antibiotic therapy are critical.

Successful therapy requires close cooperation between the internist and the surgeon since emergency cardiac surgery has become a critical therapeutic intervention in some patients.

PATHOPHYSIOLOGY

Normal native cardiac valves are remarkably resistant to attachment of bacteria and subsequent infection; intravenous injection of very high titers of pyogenic bacteria into experimental animals fails to produce endocarditis. Damage to the endothelial surface either by scarring (as from rheumatic heart disease) or direct trauma (as from turbulent blood flow or jet streams produced by intracardiac shunts) renders the tissue susceptible to colonization of circulating microorganisms. The critical predisposing lesion seems to be a deposit of platelets and fibrin on the endothelium—so-called nonbacterial thrombotic endocarditis. Studies in animals have shown that these clotting elements are the receptive surface for adhesion of circulating microorganisms and subsequent infection (Fig. 15-1). Preexisting structural cardiac diseases that result in scarring or lead to turbulent blood flow can be identified in over half of all patients with endocarditis. Most of the others probably have clinically undetectable abnormalities.

Recently the epidemiology of conditions predisposing to infective endocarditis has changed, primarily for three reasons: decreasing incidence of rheumatic heart disease, increased recognition and diagnosis (because of widespread use of echocardiography) of mitral valve prolapse, and the aging of the population, which has increased the prevalence of degenerative heart disease. In previous series, rheumatic heart disease accounted for 40% to 60% of recognized preexisting diseases; in more recent series, it accounts for less than than 25% of native valve endocarditis (Table 15-1). Stenosis and/or regurgitation of the mitral (85%), aortic (50%), and tricuspid (less than 10%) valves are the predisposing valve lesions.

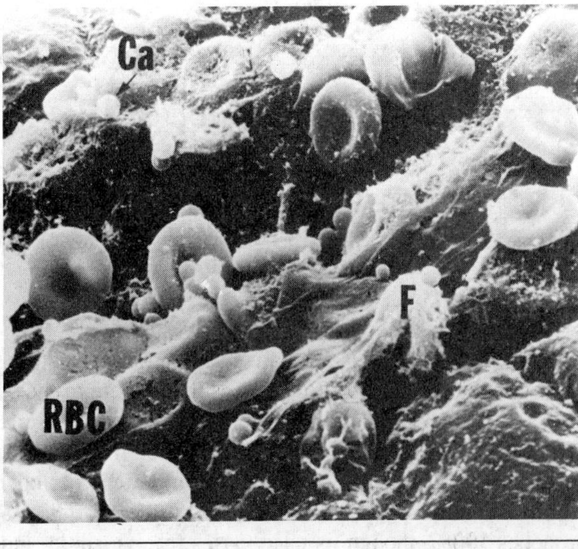

Fig. 15-1. Traumatized heart valve endothelium showing adherent erythrocyte (RBC) and fibrin (F). Note the erythrocyte covered by fibrin. Yeast cells (Ca) are also present on the developing vegetation.

In many centers mitral valve prolapse has surpassed rheumatic heart disease as the most common predisposing condition for infective endocarditis (Chapter 16). The prevalence of mitral valve prolapse is 4% in unselected populations, and the risk for infective endocarditis is three to eight times higher in persons with mitral valve prolapse than in the general population. However, this increased risk is greater in the subset of patients with mitral valve prolapse associated with a systolic murmur of mitral regurgitation. In addition, patients with mitral valve prolapse and diffusely thickened redundant leaflets on echocardiogram (with or without mitral regurgitation) have a higher risk of endocarditis than patients without this condition (Chapter 16). Although the risk of endocarditis is relatively low among persons with mitral valve prolapse, this condition is common in the general population, which accounts for the increased proportion of cases of endocarditis. In most recent series, mitral valve prolapse accounts for 20% to 25% of the cases of endocarditis. Therefore, mitral valve prolapse with mitral regurgitation and/or myxomatous proliferation (leaflet thickening and redundancy) may account for a majority of cases of endocarditis.

Congenital heart disease accounts for approximately 20% of identifiable lesions. These include all high-pressure shunts, such as ventricular septal defects, tetralogy of Fallot, and patent ductus arteriosus, as well as stenotic lesions, including coarctation of the aorta and congenital valvular and subvalvular lesions of the pulmonic and aortic valves. In hypertrophic obstructive cardiomyopathy, the infection is usually found on either the mitral or aortic valve. Endocarditis is rare in patients with isolated secundum atrial septal defects, probably because of the low-pressure shunt with little turbulence.

Degenerative heart diseases, including Marfan's syndrome, luetic aortitis, calcification of the mitral anulus, and calcific nodular lesions resulting from arteriosclerosis, account for the largest proportion of cases without demonstrable underlying valvular disease.

Many iatrogenic conditions render the host susceptible to endocarditis and endarteritis. They include arterioarterial

Table 15-1. Approximate distribution of predisposing conditions to native valve endocarditis*

Predisposing condition	Percentage
Mitral valve prolapse	20-25
Rheumatic heart disease	15-20
Congenital heart disease	20
Degenerative heart disease	20
None	20

*Distribution may vary markedly depending on geographic location, hospital, and patient population.

fistulas, hemodialysis shunts or fistulas, peritoneovenous shunts, and intracardiac pacemaker wires. Hospitalized patients who are compromised hosts and undergo invasive intravascular access procedures, including Swan-Ganz or central venous pressure monitoring and the insertion of hyperalimentation lines, are particularly susceptible. Endocarditis also complicates implanted prosthetic cardiac valves in 0.5% to 2.0% of cases. These infections frequently result from intraoperative contamination, but the presence of the foreign body and the turbulence created by the prosthesis also render these valves susceptible to colonization by circulating microorganisms. Intravenous drug abusers have a high incidence of infective endocarditis, and in two thirds of such patients there are no known predisposing cardiac lesions. Over half the patients have tricuspid valve involvement, a distribution that remains unexplained.

The infection is usually localized along the line of closure of the damaged valve leaflet on the atrial side of the atrioventricular valves and on the ventricular surface of the semilunar valves, distal to the stenosis of a coarctation of the aorta; on the low-pressure side of an intracardiac shunt; or at the jet stream impact area on the ventricular wall of a ventricular septal defect. These are the areas where fibrin-platelet thrombi are deposited and where turbulent flow and eddy currents are present, providing a receptive surface for attachment of circulating microorganisms.

Bacteria that cause endocarditis reach the heart through the bloodstream; in general, the organisms that produce disease are those that most commonly produce transient bacteremia (i.e., streptococci and staphylococci) (Table 15-2). Bacteremia is extremely common in humans and seems to occur whenever a heavily colonized mucous membrane or infected area is traumatized. Procedures in or manipulations of the oral cavity and genitourinary and gastrointestinal tracts commonly produce transient bacteremia.

The level of bacteremia (i.e., titers of circulating organisms) probably depends on the degree of trauma and the number of microorganisms colonizing or infecting the traumatized site. In one study, 10% of patients with severe gingival disease had detectable bacteremia even before undergoing any dental procedure, and in a recent study over 60% had positive blood cultures 5 minutes after simple dental cleaning. Experiments in animals with damaged cardiac valves have demonstrated that a critical level of bacteremia is required to produce endocarditis and that this level is species-specific and even strain-specific. Interestingly, the infectious dose for gram-negative rods such as *Escherichia coli* is nearly 100 times higher than for gram-positive cocci such as *Staphylococcus aureus* and viridans streptococci. This difference in median infective dose (ID_{50}) correlates with the relative frequency with which these organisms produce disease in man.

Nonpathogenic organisms that rarely produce other common infections (oral streptococci, diphtheroids, and *S. epidermidis*) are important pathogens in infective endocarditis, suggesting that classic virulence factors (such as are found in *S. aureus* and gram-negative bacilli) may be less important in the pathogenesis of this disease. The ability of bacteria to adhere firmly to fibrin and platelets, however, seems to be a critical characteristic. For example, species of viridans streptococci that produce extracellular dextran from sucrose strongly adhere to dental enamel and produce dental plaque. These same dextran-producing strains are responsible for the majority of cases of streptococcal endocarditis, even though non-dextran-producing strains are more commonly isolated from the bloodstream after dental procedures. In animal models, dextran formation by *Streptococcus sanguis* has been shown to increase its ability to produce endocarditis (lower ID_{50}). The presence of fibronectin, a glycoprotein produced by endothelial cells, also appears to markedly increase adherence of streptococci and staphylococci but not *E. coli*. Thus, as the bacteria are rapidly swept past the damaged valve, the strains that can most strongly adhere to the receptive surface of fibrin and platelets are the organisms that have the best chance of producing disease.

After adherence and multiplication of the organism, further deposition of platelets and fibrin occurs, leading to the development of the mature vegetation. This lesion consists of a friable mass of bacteria in very high titers (10^8 to 10^{10} bacteria per gram) tightly encased in the fibrin platelet mesh. Few phagocytic cells are present in the deep recesses of the vegetation; thus, the organisms appear protected from the host's major defenses. Vegetation propagation (platelet and fibrin deposition) continues until the organisms are eradicated by antimicrobial agents or surgery. In some instances, especially when disease is caused by *S. aureus*, the infection may dissect into the valve ring, producing abscesses or aneurysms of the sinus of Valsalva, and may burrow through the interventricular septum to involve the conduction system, producing arrhythmias, or out to the pericardium, producing purulent pericarditis or cardiac rupture. Cardiac valves may be quickly destroyed by the more virulent organisms (*S. aureus* and *Streptococcus pneumoniae*).

The more indolent streptococcal vegetations usually grow more slowly but may reach a large size. Involvement of the chordae tendineae or papillary muscles may lead to

Table 15-2. Approximate distribution of organisms causing endocarditis

Organism	Native valve (percentage)	Prosthetic valve* <2 mo (percentage)	Prosthetic valve* >2 mo (percentage)
Viridans and other streptococci	60	10	30
Staphylococcus aureus	25	20	15
Enterococci	10	5	10
Coagulase-negative staphylococci	<1	30	20
Gram-negatives†	5	15	10
Candida species	<1	10	5
Other	<1	10	10

*Time after valve implantation.
†HACEK organisms for native valve endocarditis and other gram-negative aerobic bacilli for prosthetic valve endocarditis.

rupture and acute valvular regurgitation or to outflow obstruction, both resulting in acute congestive heart failure. Progressive scarring of the valve after successful treatment may also eventually lead to hemodynamically significant regurgitation. Fungi *(Candida* and *Aspergillus)* tend to produce very large friable vegetations that frequently embolize, obstructing major arteries.

The extracardiac manifestations of the disease are usually the result of arterial embolization of pieces of the friable vegetation. Embolization to the vaso vasorum of major arteries or contiguous spread from a septic arterial embolus may produce a mycotic aneurysm. These commonly occur at the bifurcation of medium-sized arteries, and 50% occur in the brain; the thorax and abdomen are involved in 40% and the extremities in 10%. Embolizations to all major arteries may occur. When the coronary vessels are involved, myocardial infarction may result. Cerebral embolization may produce temporary vascular insufficiency or stroke. Metastatic abscess formation is common in the spleen, kidney, or other vital organs when the disease is caused by *S. aureus* and, occasionally, viridans streptococci (*S. anginosus,* also called *S. milleri* group). Many of the unique peripheral manifestations of the disease (Janeway lesions, cutaneous infarcts, Osler's nodes) are thought also to be the result of small-vessel embolization.

Immune-complex deposition also appears to play a role in the pathophysiology of extracardiac manifestations of endocarditis, especially those in the kidney. Abnormalities in renal architecture can be found in nearly all cases of infective endocarditis. In the preantibiotic era the incidence of glomerulonephritis was greater than 75% in subacute endocarditis but less than 40% in acute endocarditis, suggesting that infections with less virulent organisms and a more prolonged antigenic challenge produce high levels of circulating immune complexes and concomitant glomerulonephritis. Glomerulonephritis has been reported in 2% to 60% of patients treated with antibiotics for endocarditis, but the true incidence has not been established. *S. aureus* endocarditis is frequently associated with glomerulonephritis, particularly in parenteral drug abusers, regardless of the duration of the illness. Glomerular lesions may be focal or diffuse, and crescents may be present. Interstitial involvement may produce tubular damage, endarteritis, and arteriosclerosis. Embolization is common, and septic renal infarcts occur in nearly all patients with fatal *S. aureus* endocarditis. Since this disease is associated with a constant intravascular antigenic challenge, it is not surprising that high titers of antibodies of several classes are found. Circulating immune complexes can be identified in more than 90% of patients with infective endocarditis of long duration and fall with institution of appropriate antibiotic therapy. Some of the peripheral manifestations of endocarditis (Roth's spots, Osler's nodes, petechiae, and some diffuse purpuric lesions) may be due in part to immune complex deposition.

CLINICAL SYNDROME

The clinical presentation of infective endocarditis is primarily that of unexplained fever and cardiac murmur. However, the disease may present in a wide variety of ways. The symptoms and signs may be protean, and essentially any organ system can be involved. Four pathophysiologic processes contribute to the clinical picture: (1) the infectious process on the valve, (2) arterial embolization of vegetation, (3) bacteremia with metastatic infection, and (4) immunopathologic manifestations.

The clinical presentation is to a large extent determined by the nature of the infective organism. With pyogenic bacteria such as *S. aureus* and, less commonly, *Streptococcus pneumoniae* and *Neisseria gonorrhoeae,* the disease may be acute and fulminant, with high fever, multiple metastatic abscesses and peripheral embolic phenomena, rapid valve destruction, and a high mortality. About one third of patients with staphylococcal endocarditis have a history of a preceding staphylococcal infection, and symptoms generally start within 2 weeks of the initial infection. This form of acute bacterial endocarditis may involve a normal valve, in contrast to the subacute infection, which almost always occurs on a damaged valve. All age groups are involved, but mortality is particularly high in patients over 50 years of age. Narcotic abusers have a particular predilection for developing *S. aureus* endocarditis, although the disease may be less fulminant than in a nonaddicted population. Staphylococcal endocarditis may be confused with other severe acute infectious diseases, such as gram-negative sepsis with endotoxemia, meningococcemia, and occasionally with an acute vasculitis such as systemic lupus erythematosus. Of patients with staphylococcal bacteremia, 60% in older autopsy series and 10% in recent reports show evidence of endocarditis.

The subacute form of infective endocarditis accounts for approximately two thirds of cases and is usually caused by either viridans streptococci or enterococci. A history of dental procedures is found in 15% to 20% of patients with viridans streptococcal endocarditis, and about 50% of patients with enterococcal disease have had a preceding genital or urologic procedure. In the vast majority of cases, symptoms begin within the 2-week period after the procedure, but because of the protean nature of the disease, the diagnosis is usually not made for 5 weeks. Eighty percent of these patients have a previous history of cardiac disease. Symptoms usually begin insidiously with anorexia, weakness, weight loss, fatigue, feverishness with night sweats, and arthralgias. The nonspecific presentation often leads to incorrect diagnoses, such as various malignancies, collagen vascular diseases, tuberculosis, fever or anemia of unknown origin, glomerulonephritis of unknown origin, and other chronic diseases. Although the distinction between acute and subacute forms of the disease is clinically important, they represent the two extremes of a continuum, and there is considerable overlap between the clinical syndromes produced by the individual organisms. The various clinical presentations of endocarditis are listed in the box on p. 193.

The physical findings in infective endocarditis can provide important diagnostic clues. Almost all patients have fever, but elderly patients and those with renal failure, severe disability, or congestive heart failure may not. The fever is usually remittent and rarely exceeds 39.5° C (103°

Clinical presentations of endocarditis

Fever and heart murmur
Sepsis
Fever of unknown origin
Transient ischemic attacks or stroke
Meningitis
Subarachnoid hemorrhage
Peripheral arterial embolization
Myocardial infarction
Unexplained congestive heart failure
Pulmonary infarction, necrotizing pneumonia
Constitutional symptoms suggestive of
- Neoplasm
- Hematologic malignancy
- Collagen vascular disease

Musculoskeletal complaints suggestive of
- Polymyalgia rheumatica
- Acute rheumatic fever
- Rheumatoid arthritis

Anemia
Renal failure

F) except in acute endocarditis. Heart murmurs are present in over 85% of patients but may not be detected in patients with tricuspid disease. The detection of a changing murmur or appearance of a new murmur during the course of disease is an important diagnostic clue, but such a change is found in only 3% to 10% of patients.

Cutaneous manifestations are found in approximately 50% of patients. Petechiae are the most common and usually appear in the conjunctiva, palate, buccal mucosa, and extremities. They occur most frequently in patients with prolonged illness. They present as small, nonblanching lesions in crops but discolor and disappear within 2 to 3 days. Osler's nodes are small, painful nodular lesions, usually in the pads of the fingers or toes or occasionally on the thenar eminence. They range in size from 2 to 15 mm, may be multiple, and disappear in hours to days. They are most common in patients with subacute endocarditis but may also be found in systemic lupus erythematosus or marantic endocarditis, hemolytic anemias, and gonococcal infections, and in extremities with cannulated radial arteries. Janeway lesions are hemorrhagic, macular, flat, painless plaques with a predilection for the palms and the soles. They are most commonly found in patients with acute staphylococcal endocarditis and are frequently multiple. Roth's spots are pale, oval retinal lesions with a peripheral area of hemorrhage that are usually found near the optic disc. They are rare (<5% of cases) and can also be identified in patients with anemia, leukemia, or connective tissue disorders (systemic lupus erythematosus). Splinter hemorrhages are subungual, linear, reddish brown streaks found in the fingernails or toenails. They are most suggestive of endocarditis when located proximally in the nail bed. Distal splinter hemorrhages are also seen in patients with occupational trauma to the nails. Clubbing of the nail beds has been found and is especially common when the disease is of long duration.

Splenomegaly is reported in up to 60% of patients, and its incidence correlates with the duration of disease. Musculoskeletal complaints are common, occurring in as many as 44% of patients. They usually appear early in the disease, may be the only initial complaint, and include arthralgias, arthritis, low back pain, and diffuse myalgias. Neurologic manifestations occur in 30% to 40% of patients and may dominate the clinical picture, especially in staphylococcal endocarditis. A sudden neurologic event in a young person should always suggest the possibility of infectious endocarditis. Major cerebral emboli are found in 10% to 30% of patients and may produce transient or permanent neurologic defects. Mycotic aneurysms of the cerebral vessels occur in up to 10% of patients and are usually clinically silent but may present as an expanding mass lesion of the brain or, with rupture, as a subarachnoid hemorrhage, resulting in a severe headache, stiff neck, and fever. Other features include seizures, visual changes, choreoathetoid movement, mononeuropathy, cranial nerve palsies, and toxic encephalopathies.

Major embolic episodes occur in approximately one third of patients with endocarditis, often early in the disease or after therapy has been completed. The incidence appears to be highest in those with large vegetations as determined by echocardiogram. Splenic infarctions are common and may present as left upper quadrant pain radiating to the left shoulder, accompanied by a splenic or pleural friction rub and a left pleural effusion. An embolus lodging in the mesenteric artery may precipitate signs and symptoms of an acute abdominal process. Emboli to large peripheral arteries may produce acute occlusion of blood flow to a limb. Pulmonary emboli arise from right-sided (tricuspid) infection and are a common feature in narcotic-associated endocarditis. Coronary artery emboli usually arise from the aortic valve and may produce acute myocardial infarction.

Congestive heart failure may predominate in the presentation and may result from valvular dysfunction, associated myocarditis that commonly complicates endocarditis early in the course of the disease, or myocardial infarction. The signs of uremia, once a common presenting feature of bacterial endocarditis, are now rarely observed. However, 10% to 15% of patients with endocarditis may present with immune-complex glomerulonephritis, and signs of azotemia are occasionally present.

LABORATORY FINDINGS

The laboratory manifestations of endocarditis are summarized in Table 15-3. Most patients with endocarditis have the anemia characteristic of chronic disease, with normochromic, normocytic indices, low serum iron, and low iron-binding capacity. The anemia progressively worsens with the duration of the illness. Leukocytosis is found primarily in patients with the acute form, whereas leukopenia may be found in the subacute disease and is usually associated with splenomegaly. Large histiocytes (mononuclear cells) can be detected in peripheral blood. The presence of these

Table 15-3. Laboratory manifestations of endocarditis

Laboratory finding	Incidence (percentage)
Hematologic	
Anemia	70-90
Thrombocytopenia	5-15
Leukocytosis*	20-30
Leukopenia	5-15
Histiocytosis	25
Elevated ESR	90-100
Serologic	
Hypergammaglobulinemia	20-30
Rheumatoid factor	40-50
Hypocomplementemia	5-15
Immune complexes	90-100
Mixed cryoglobulins	80-95
Urine	
Proteinuria	50-65
Microscopic hematuria	30-50
RBC casts	10-12
Bacteremia	
Positive blood cultures	95
Intraleukocytic bacteria	50

*Primarily in acute endocarditis.

cells is not diagnostic of endocarditis; they may also be seen in patients with malaria, typhoid fever, and tuberculosis. The erythrocyte sedimentation rate (ESR) is nearly always elevated; however, it may be normal in patients with renal failure, congestive heart failure, or disseminated intravascular coagulation. Rheumatoid factor can be detected in the majority of patients who have had symptoms of endocarditis for at least 6 weeks.

Detection of bacteremia with blood culture is the single most important diagnostic test. Bacteremia is usually continuous and low grade (less than 100 bacteria/ml of blood) in the subacute form of the disease but may be high grade in acute staphylococcal endocarditis. In patients who eventually have positive blood cultures, 80% of the first set of blood cultures drawn are positive, as are 89% of the first two sets and 99% of the first three sets. Therefore, if subacute bacterial endocarditis is suspected, three cultures (each consisting of 5 to 10 ml of blood obtained from separate venipuncture sites) are collected over a 24-hour period and cultured with both aerobic and anaerobic techniques. In acute situations, several cultures may be drawn at approximately 20-minute intervals before starting empiric therapy.

Modern blood-culturing techniques fail to identify the etiologic agents of endocarditis in about 5% of cases. If initial cultures are negative at 48 to 72 hours, additional cultures should be obtained and all should be held for 2 to 3 weeks with periodic Gram's stains and subculturing. If gram-positive cocci are grown initially but fail to grow in subculture, a nutritionally deficient variant streptococci should be suspected, which may require broth supplemented with pyridoxal hydrochloride or cysteine. Possible etiologies of culture-negative endocarditis are extensive and include antimicrobial therapy before obtaining cultures; fastidious organisms (anaerobic bacteria, nutritionally variant streptococci, HACEK-group and other fastidious organisms, *Brucella* species); *Chlamydia psittaci* (psittacosis); *Rickettsia* such as *Coxiella burnetti* (Q fever); fungi (e.g., *Candida, Aspergillus*); chronic endocarditis; marantic endocarditis; atrial myxoma; Libman-Sacks endocarditis; and incorrect diagnosis. When endocarditis cultures are negative, a careful history should be taken and more extensive evaluation for unusual causes should be initiated. Patients with endocarditis caused by fungi frequently have negative blood cultures, but large vegetations are usually detected by echocardiogram, and embolic complications are common.

Serologic detection of antigen or antibodies is useful in diagnosing some forms of endocarditis. Serologies are becoming increasingly important in the diagnosis of candidal and aspergillus endocarditis. Serologic evidence of infection with *Chlamydia psittaci* and the causative agent of Q fever would be diagnostic of endocarditis in some clinical situations.

Echocardiography has become a valuable tool for patients suspected of having endocarditis (Chapter 5). The evaluation of endocarditis has benefited dramatically from developments in noninvasive cardiology, particularly with regard to 2D transthoracic echocardiography (TTE), Doppler echocardiography, and transesophageal echocardiography (TEE). The TEE procedure is very safe, usually lasts about 10 to 15 minutes, and is well tolerated by patients. Transesophageal echocardiography has improved visualization of the cardiac structures by taking advantage of the anatomic relationship of the esophagus to the heart; structures of 1 to 2 mm in size can be visualized. Valvular morphology and valve structures, chordae, and attachments are better defined by TEE than TTE. Major advantages of TEE over TTE include improved image quality, particularly in technically difficult studies; superior visualization of valve ring abscesses, mycotic aneurysms, prosthetic valve abnormalities, and small vegetations; improved hemodynamic assessment of prosthetic valve dysfunction; intraoperative assessment of cardiac hemodynamics and structures; and clarification of abnormal but nondiagnostic TTE studies. The disadvantages of TEE are that the procedure is more invasive and more labor-intensive and carries a potential risk of bacteremic seeding of abnormal valves. Though both TTE and TEE have high specificity, TEE is much more sensitive than TTE in detecting vegetations and abscesses involving left-sided structures of the heart, especially in the setting of prosthetic valves (Table 15-4). In endocarditis, TEE should be performed when the site, extent of infection, and effect on cardiac function have not been clearly defined by TTE, when persistent fever, bacteremia, or other evidence suggests ongoing infection and possible abscess formation, or when a prosthetic heart valve may limit the accuracy of TTE. Transesophageal echocardiography should not replace TTE, but should complement it when TTE is nondiagnostic or if additional data will influence therapy, management, or surgical approach. Doppler echo-

Table 15-4. Comparison of test characteristics of transesophageal echocardiography (TEE) and transthoracic echocardiography (TTE) in endocarditis

	TTE		TEE	
	sens (%)	spec (%)	sens (%)	spec (%)
Valvular vegetations*	60	>95	90	>95
Abscesses†	28	97	87	95

*Estimate based on various studies.
†Data from Daniel WG et al: Improvement in the diagnosis of abscesses associated with endocarditis by transesophageal echocardiography. N Engl J Med 324:795, 1991. Surgery or autopsy results used as gold standard to calculate test characteristics in a severely ill study population (n = 118).

cardiography uses sound waves to identify and quantitate flow through intracardiac and extracardiac vascular structures; it can be used to measure a variety of hemodynamic parameters. For evaluation of endocarditis, Doppler echocardiography enables the severity of valvular regurgitation to be estimated and is an integral part of TTE and TEE. In evaluating mitral valve dysfunction and mitral regurgitation, the Doppler TEE is far superior to the standard TTE approaches.

The echocardiogram provides important prognostic information as well, since patients with vegetative lesions by echocardiography have a higher incidence of congestive failure, embolization, need for surgery, and death than those lacking detectable vegetations. Large vegetations (>1 cm), multiple vegetations, left-sided vegetations, and vegetations increasing in size on antibiotic therapy indicate a particularly high-risk subpopulation. The echocardiogram can also be used to assess left ventricular function in patients with aortic regurgitation (Chapter 16).

DIFFERENTIAL DIAGNOSIS

Although the diagnosis of endocarditis may be obvious in patients with underlying cardiac valvular disease who present with fever and peripheral embolic phenomena, these classic findings are frequently absent. Up to 50% of patients do not exhibit peripheral manifestations, and the murmur may be absent or subtle; this is particularly common in intravenous drug users with right-sided endocarditis. In the elderly there may be no fever, and the patient may present with no more than confusion, wasting, anorexia, and lethargy.

The classic manifestations of endocarditis may mimic those of other diseases. Fever, petechiae, splenomegaly, microscopic hematuria, and anemia with a cardiac murmur may resemble acute rheumatic fever with carditis, collagen vascular diseases such as systemic lupus erythematosus with cardiac involvement, or neoplasms such as atrial myxomas. The clinical picture may be dominated by the manifestations of arterial embolization mimicking acute myocardial infarction, transient cerebral ischemic attacks, stroke, sudden occlusion of a major artery, or splenic or renal infarction.

SPECIAL CONSIDERATIONS

Infection in intravenous drug users

Intravenous drug users have a unique predilection for developing infective endocarditis and in some large metropolitan hospitals account for the majority of cases. The bacteremia in intravenous drug abusers occurs with injection and probably arises from bacterial colonization of their skin and nares. The disease tends to differ from conventional forms in location and microbiology. In over 70% the tricuspid valve is involved, followed in frequency by the aortic (and mitral) valves. Approximately three fourths of the cases are caused by *S. aureus*. There is an appreciable incidence of community-acquired methicillin resistance in the *S. aureus* isolated in Detroit, Michigan, but this currently appears to be a localized phenomenon. *Pseudomonas aeruginosa, P. cepacia,* and other gram-negative aerobic bacilli account for an additional 15%, *Candida albicans* and various streptococci for about 10%. The latter two organisms affect the aortic and mitral valves more commonly than the tricuspid valve. The effect of an increasing prevalence of human immunodeficiency virus (HIV) disease on the epidemiology and clinical management of endocarditis in this group remains to be seen.

A diagnosis of endocarditis must be considered in all febrile intravenous drug abusers since fever may be the only manifestation. Prospective studies of the emergency-room evaluation of such patients have shown that neither signs, symptoms, laboratory tests, nor clinical judgment can be used to accurately predict which patients have endocarditis, which provides the rationale for admitting all febrile intravenous drug users to the hospital. When the tricuspid valve is involved, the clinical presentation frequently reflects septic pulmonary involvement, including fever, chills, pleurisy, cough, and hemoptysis. Signs of tricuspid regurgitation, such as a short or pansystolic murmur that increases with inspiration (Chapter 16), may also be present. A chest x-ray may reveal several poorly defined peripheral infiltrates, which may cavitate, reflecting septic pulmonary infiltrates. Pyuria caused by either septic renal emboli or immune-mediated renal injury is frequently seen.

Therapy with appropriate antimicrobial drugs is usually successful. Traditional therapy consists of 4 weeks of intravenous antibiotics, but recent trials have shown comparable results with a 2-week combination of nafcillin and an aminoglycoside in selected drug abusers who have isolated, uncomplicated right-side *S. aureus* endocarditis. The mortality from staphylococcal endocarditis in this patient population is relatively low (up to 10%), compared with 30% to 40% in the nonaddict population. The reasons for these differences are not clear but in part reflect the high incidence of right-sided disease and the youthful population involved. Therapy of highly resistant microbes, such as *Pseudomonas cepacia,* may require surgical excision of the tricuspid valve. Once infection has occurred, these patients are highly susceptible to recurrent episodes of endocarditis.

Prosthetic valve endocarditis

Infective endocarditis is a relatively common (0.5% to 2.0% incidence) and devastating complication of prosthetic cardiac valve or tissue graft valve replacement. With the increasing use of valve replacement, the prevalence of this disease has continued to rise, and in some major hospitals accounts for up to 30% of all cases of infective endocarditis. The disease has been separated for convenience into two forms: early (within the first 2 months after surgery; one third of the patients) and late (more than 2 months after valve replacement; two thirds of the patients).

In early disease the organism is probably introduced at the time of surgery or stems from infectious complications of the procedure, such as wound infections, urinary tract infections, and intravenous catheter infections. This is reflected in the causative organisms in early prosthetic valve endocarditis. Half of the cases are caused by staphylococcal species (*S. epidermidis,* approximately 30%; *S. aureus,* 20%). *Pseudomonas* and Enterobacteriaceae account for 15% to 20% and fungi, particularly *Candida* and *Aspergillus* species, account for an additional 15%. Streptococci occur in less than 10% of cases. Early endocarditis is frequently fulminant and rapidly progressive. The aortic valve is more commonly affected than the mitral valve. Initial clinical manifestations include fever, a regurgitative murmur associated with perivalvular leak, or a systolic murmur suggestive of outflow obstruction. The opening and closing prosthetic valve sounds may be muted by vegetation invasion of the cage. Peripheral manifestations are unusual except for petechiae, which occur in about 50% of patients. However, emboli to major organs are common; large emboli can be especially common in patients with *Aspergillus* or *Candida* prosthesis infection. A traumatic (impact) hemolytic anemia may occur as a result of perivalvular leak. The incidence of early prosthetic valve endocarditis appears to have decreased in the last decade, probably because of perioperative antibiotic prophylaxis and improved surgical care. Mortality, however, remains high (approaching 80% in some series), reflecting the virulence of the etiologic agents.

Late prosthetic valve endocarditis is similar to natural valve endocarditis. Predisposing factors include oral-dental and genitourinary procedures. Streptococci account for approximately 40% of cases, *S. epidermidis* for 25%, and *S. aureus* for 15%. Gram-negative organisms, particularly fastidious organisms such as *Haemophilus aphrophilus,* other *Haemophilus* species, and *Actinobacillus,* and fungi are uncommon, occurring in less than 10% of patients. The clinical manifestations of late prosthetic valve endocarditis are similar to those found in natural valve disease and are, again, dictated by the virulence of the infecting organism. Prognosis is somewhat better with late infection, and mortality is approximately 40%. Infection in both early and late prosthetic valve endocarditis is usually at suture lines and may result in ring abscess formation with dissection, fistula formation, rarely purulent pericarditis, valve dysfunction with dehiscence leading to instability of the prosthesis, or vegetation growth with valvular outflow obstruction.

When prosthetic valve endocarditis is suspected, cinefluoroscopy may detect alterations in the rocking motion of the valve. The ECG may reveal conduction disturbances, such as those commonly occurring with a ring abscess. Because of the multiple echoes caused by the prosthesis itself, the transesophageal echocardiogram is clearly superior to the transthoracic echocardiogram for the hemodynamic assessment of prosthetic valve dysfunction and the visualization of vegetations and ring abscesses. As in native valve endocarditis, the diagnosis is established by detecting bacteremia (or fungemia) by serial blood culture techniques. All patients with bacteremia in the postoperative period do not have endocarditis. This is especially true with gram-negative rod infections, in which bacteremia may result from urinary tract infection from indwelling urinary catheters, septic phlebitis from intravenous catheters, or respirator-induced gram-negative pneumonic or sternal wound infections. However, when bacteremia persists after the local infection is eradicated or foreign bodies are removed, patients should be considered to have prosthetic valve endocarditis and treated accordingly.

The differential diagnosis of fever in the postoperative period involves considering a long list of conditions, including those that have been listed, as well as postcardiotomy syndrome, drug fever, thrombophlebitis, transfusion-induced hepatitis, cytomegalovirus infection, and mononucleosis. Repeated blood culturing is therefore critical in identifying cases of endocarditis and in instituting appropriate therapy.

Antimicrobial therapy of prosthetic endocarditis needs to be specifically tailored to the infecting organism (Table 15-5). Even with appropriate antimicrobials, surgical intervention is frequently required in patients with staphylococcal, fungal, or gram-negative infection or who develop hemodynamic compromise.

THERAPY FOR ENDOCARDITIS

Successful therapy for infective endocarditis entails administering rapidly bactericidal antimicrobial agents in high enough dosages and for long enough periods to sterilize the vegetations completely. This therapy should be coupled with aggressive surgical management of complications, including valve replacement and drainage of myocardial abscesses when clinically indicated.

Antimicrobial therapy

Infective endocarditis is unique because the focus of infection is contained within the protective environment of the valvular vegetation. Few phagocytic cells are present within this tightly woven matrix of fibrin, platelets, and very high numbers of microorganisms. Host defenses appear to be relatively ineffective in eradicating the infective organisms. Thus, the antimicrobial regimen used must be bactericidal

Table 15-5. Current recommendations for treatment of bacterial endocarditis

Antibiotics	Dosage[a]	Administration	Duration	Comments
Penicillin-susceptible viridans streptococci and *Streptococcus bovis* (MIC ≤ 0.1 μg/ml)				
1. Penicillin G	2 million units every 4 hr	IV	4 wk	Preferred in patients >65 years old and those with renal or eight cranial nerve impairment, heart failure, or CNS complications. Effective for other penicillin-susceptible nonviridans streptococci.
2. Penicillin G	2 million units every 4 hr	IV	2 wk	Uncomplicated patient: age <65; no renal or eight cranial nerve impairment; no CNS complication; no severe heart failure; not nutritionally deficient variant; viridans streptococci and *S. bovis* only.
& gentamicin[b]	1 mg/kg (not to exceed 80 mg) q8h	IV	2 wk	
3. Penicillin G	2 million units every 4 hr	IV	4 wk	Nutritionally deficient variants; relapse; complications such as shock or extracardiac focus of infection; 6 wks of penicillin for prosthetic valve infection.
& gentamicin[b]	1 mg/kg (not to exceed 80 mg) q8h	IV	2 wk	
4. Vancomycin[c]	15 mg/kg (not to exceed 1 g) q12h	IV	4 wk	Penicillin allergy.
5. Cefazolin[d]	1-2 g every 8 hr	IV	4 wk	Penicillin allergy.
6. Ceftriaxone[d]	2 g once daily	IV or IM	4 wk	Uncomplicated patient with viridans streptococci; candidate for outpatient therapy; penicillin allergy.
Strains of viridans streptococci & *S. bovis* relatively resistant to penicillin G (0.1 μg/ml < MIC < 0.5 μg/ml)				
1. Penicillin G	2 million units every 4 hr	IV	4 wk	For MIC >0.5 μg/ml, treat same as enterococcus. For prosthetic valve infection, give 6 wk of penicillin and 6 wk of gentamicin.
& gentamicin[b]	1 mg/kg (not to exceed 80 mg) q8h	IV	2 wk	
2. Vancomycin[c]	15 mg/kg (not to exceed 1 g) q12h	IV	4 wk	Penicillin allergy; avoidance of gentamicin.
3. Cefazolin[d]	1-2 g every 8 hr	IV	4 wk	Penicillin allergy; avoidance of gentamicin.
Enterococci *(E. faecalis)* (or viridans streptococci with MIC ≥0.5 μg/ml)				
1. Penicillin G	4 million units every 4 hr	IV	4-6 wk	Increase to 6-8 wks for symptoms longer than 3 months, complicated course, or prosthetic valve infection. Some would use ampicillin, but no evidence of superiority available.
& gentamicin[b]	1 mg/kg (not to exceed 80 mg) q8h	IV	4-6 wk	
2. Vancomycin[c]	15 mg/kg (not to exceed 1 g) q12h	IV	4-6 wk	Penicillin allergy.
& gentamicin[b]	1 mg/kg (not to exceed 80 mg) q8h	IV	4-6 wk	
Staphylococcus aureus				
1. Nafcillin	1.5 g every 4 hr	IV	4 wk	Methicillin-susceptible strain; increase duration to 6 wks for complicated infection; omit gentamicin for significant renal impairment. Some recommend gentamicin for 5-7 days.
& gentamicin[b]	1 mg/kg (not to exceed 80 mg) q8h	IV	3-5 days	
2. Vancomycin[c]	15 mg/kg (not to exceed 1 g) q12h	IV	4-6 wk	Penicillin allergy or methicillin-resistant strain; increase duration to 6 wks or longer for complicated infection.
3. Cefazolin[d]	2 g every 8 hr	IV	4-6 wk	Penicillin allergy; increase duration to 6 wks for complicated infection.
4. Nafcillin	1.5 g every 4 hr	IV	2 wk	Methicillin-susceptible strain; intravenous drug user, tricuspid valve infection only, no extrapulmonary infection, no renal impairment.
& gentamicin[b]	1 mg/kg (not to exceed 80 mg) q8h	IV	2 wk	
5. Nafcillin	1.5 g every 4 hr	IV	6-8 wk	Prosthetic valve infected with methicillin-susceptible strain; for methicillin-resistant strain substitute vancomycin for nafcillin.
& rifampin[e]	300 mg every 12 hr	PO or IV	6 wk	
& gentamicin[b]	1 mg/kg (not to exceed 80 mg) q8h	IV	2 wk	

[a]Dosages are for patients with normal renal function.

[b]Streptomycin 500 mg every 12 hr intramuscularly may be used instead of gentamicin. Gentamicin doses should be adjusted to achieve a peak serum concentration of 3 μg/ml, and streptomycin a peak serum concentration of 20 μg/ml.

[c]Vancomycin peak serum concentrations 1 hour after infusion should be in the range of 30 to 45 μg/ml.

[d]Cephalosporins should be avoided in patients with an immediate type hypersensitivity reaction to penicillin.

[e]This use of rifampin is not listed in the manufacturer's official directive.

[f]*Haemophilus* species, *Actinobacillus actinomycetemcomitans, Cardiobacterium hominis, Eikenella corrodens, Kingella kingii.* MIC = minimum inhibitory concentration.

Continued.

Table 15-5. Current recommendations for treatment of bacterial endocarditis—cont'd

Antibiotics	Dosage[a]	Administration	Duration	Comments
Coagulase-negative staphylococci or prosthetic valve infection				
1. Nafcillin	1.5 g every 4 hr	IV	6-8 wk	Methicillin-susceptible strain; vancomycin recommended in case of uncertain methicillin susceptibility.
& rifampin	300 mg every 12 hr	PO or IV	6-8 wk	
& gentamicin[b]	1 mg/kg (not to exceed 80 mg) q8h	IV	2 wk	
2. Vancomycin[c]	15 mg/kg (not to exceed 1 g) q12h	IV	6-8 wk	Methicillin-resistant strain; penicillin allergy.
& rifampin	300 mg every 12 hr	PO or IV	6-8 wk	
& gentamicin[b]	1 mg/kg (not to exceed 80 mg) q8h	IV	2 wk	
HACEK group#				
1. Ampicillin	2 g every 4 hr	IV	4 wk	Definitive regimen determined by in vitro susceptibilities.
& gentamicin[b]	1 mg/kg (not to exceed 80 mg) q8h	PO or IV	4 wk	
2. Ceftriaxone[d]	2 g once daily	IV or IM	6 wk	Penicillin allergy.

and given in high enough dosages to ensure adequate bactericidal activity. Bacteriostatic drugs should never be used. The antimicrobial regimen must be tailored to the infecting organism. Thus, isolation of the organism is vital to optimum management. Once the organism has been isolated and identified, its susceptibility to antimicrobial agents should be determined by serial tube dilution techniques in broth. The disk sensitivity method has little value in managing this disease.

Antibiotics should be administered parenterally and meticulous attention should be given to aminoglycoside levels to prevent toxicity. Specific recommendations are outlined in Table 15-5. There is no merit to routinely monitoring serum bactericidal levels since this test, even when performed in a standardized manner, has not been shown to provide clinically useful information in the majority of patients. Its utility in patients with infections caused by unusual organisms or who exhibit inadequate clinical responses to standard treatment regimens remains to be determined.

Highly penicillin-susceptible viridans streptococci and *S. bovis* are sensitive to penicillin and have minimum inhibitory concentrations (MICs) less than or equal to 0.1 μg/ml. A regimen of 4 weeks of penicillin G alone has been successful in nearly 99% of patients treated. The addition of an aminoglycoside increases the rate of bacterial killing in vitro and has been shown in experimental animals to increase the rate at which organisms are eradicated from the vegetations in vivo. Four weeks of penicillin alone is preferred for patients likely to have side effects with an aminoglycoside. Therapy with 2 weeks of penicillin and gentamicin is as effective as 4 weeks of penicillin alone and is appropriate for uncomplicated infections. For nutritionally deficient variant strains or complicated infections, 4 weeks of penicillin plus 2 weeks of gentamicin is recommended. For prosthetic valve infection, appropriate therapy is 6 weeks of penicillin plus 2 weeks of gentamicin. For penicillin-allergic patients with a history of a rash, vancomycin, cefazolin, and ceftriaxone are acceptable alternatives. However, ceftriaxone is reserved for patients with uncomplicated infections caused by viridans streptococci and who are candidates for outpatient therapy. Patients should be carefully evaluated and stabilized in the hospital before management as outpatients is considered. Cephalosporin antibiotics should be avoided in patients with immediate-type hypersensitivity reactions to penicillin.

Relatively penicillin-resistant viridans streptococci (and *S. bovis*) have MICs between 0.1 and 0.5 μg/ml. The recommended therapy is 4 weeks of penicillin plus 2 weeks of gentamicin. For penicillin-allergic patients with a history of a rash, 4 weeks of cefazolin is an appropriate alternative. For patients with an immediate-type hypersensitivity reaction to penicillin, 4 weeks of vancomycin is recommended. Infection caused by viridans streptococci with an MIC greater than 5 μg/ml should be treated with the same regimen used for infections caused by enterococci.

Enterococci are unique because of their relative resistance to penicillin and their universal resistance to cephalosporins. Therapy with these drugs alone is frequently ineffective; the synergistic combination of penicillin and gentamicin or streptomycin must be administered. For enterococci, or viridans streptococci with an MIC greater than 0.5 μg/ml, 4 weeks of penicillin plus 4 weeks of gentamicin is recommended. Duration of therapy should be extended to 6 weeks for prolonged disease (symptoms for 3 months or longer), a complicated course, or prosthetic valve infection. For penicillin-allergic patients, vancomycin should be substituted for penicillin. The degree of resistance to aminoglycosides is variable. Highly resistant enterococci (MIC greater than or equal to 2000 μg/ml) are not synergistically killed by an aminoglycoside combined with penicillin or vancomycin in vitro or in experimental models. Susceptibility of the enterococci should guide final selection of the appropriate aminoglycoside, but tobramycin is not recommended because *E. faecium* is highly resistant to it. Prolonged use of aminoglycosides, particularly gentamicin, in patients with renal insufficiency may be associated with auditory and vestibular toxicity; serum levels in these patients should be monitored carefully during therapy. Irreversible vestibular toxicity is reported in 20% of patients who receive streptomycin for 4 weeks. The incidence of nephrotoxicity (rise in serum creatinine of greater than 5 mg/dl) with gentamicin ranges from 20% (doses of 3 mg/kg or less) to 100% (doses greater than 3 mg/kg), although the drug-associated nephrotoxicity can be reversible. Antibiotic susceptibility, the nature of the toxicity associated with each agent, and the ease of monitoring therapy should be weighed in choosing the most appropriate antibiotic regimen.

Staphylococcal endocarditis is caused by *S. aureus* or coagulase-negative staphylococci (e.g., *S. epidermidis*). Acute *S. aureus* endocarditis continues to have a mortality of 30% to 40% (except in drug addicts). Death is usually the result of the complications of the disease, that is, valve destruction, rupture of mycotic aneurysms, or myocardial or metastic abscess formation in vital organs; only rarely is it caused by failure of antimicrobial therapy. For methicillin-susceptible *S. aureus,* 4 weeks of nafcillin plus 3 to 5 days of gentamicin is recommended. Experimental and clinical data suggest that the addition of gentamicin for the first several days increases the rate of both clinical response and clearance of the bacteremia. Recent studies have demonstrated that vancomycin may not be as effective as nafcillin for therapy of *S. aureus* endocarditis; vancomycin should be reserved only for patients infected with methicillin-resistant *S. aureus* (4 weeks of vancomycin is recommended) or for those who are penicillin-allergic (4 weeks of either vancomycin or cefazolin can be used). For complicated *S. aureus* endocarditis, therapy is extended for 6 weeks or longer. *S. aureus* prosthetic valve infection with methicillin-susceptible strains requires 6 weeks of nafcillin plus 6 weeks of rifampin plus 2 weeks of gentamicin therapy. With a methicillin-resistant strain, vancomycin is substituted for nafcillin. Unless unequivocal in vitro tests show it to be methicillin-susceptible, coagulase-negative staphylococcal native or prosthetic valve endocarditis should be treated with 6 weeks of vancomycin plus 6 weeks of rifampin plus 2 weeks of gentamicin. Fastidious gram-negative coccobacilli such as the HACEK group (*Haemophilus, Actinobacillus, Cardiobacterium, Eikenella,* and *Kingella* species) occasionally cause native valve endocarditis. In vitro they are susceptible to ampicillin, cephalosporins, aminoglycosides, and penicillin-aminoglycoside combinations. Ampicillin plus gentamicin for 4 weeks is recommended; ceftriaxone is highly active in vitro and may be a suitable alternative.

The mainstay of therapy for fungal endocarditis is surgery combined with antifungal treatment. Amphotericin B up to 1 mg/kg/day intravenously is given to a minimum total dose of 40 to 50 mg/kg (2.5 to 3.5 g). Flucytosine 150 mg/kg/day in four divided doses orally is usually added. To avoid bone marrow suppression, 2-hour postdose flucytosine levels should be between 50 to 100 μg/ml.

Antimicrobial therapy for other organisms, including anaerobes, gram-negative cocci, and gram-negative bacilli, should be tailored according to the in-vitro sensitivities of the organisms. Empiric therapy in patients suspected of having endocarditis should be instituted after appropriate blood cultures have been obtained. For acute native valve endocarditis, empiric therapy should include antibiotics that are bactericidal against streptococci, staphylococci, and enterococci. The three-drug combination of nafcillin plus penicillin plus gentamicin can be used. Nafcillin can be omitted if *S. aureus* is not suspected, such as in subacute endocarditis. For penicillin-allergic patients, vancomycin can be substituted for both nafcillin and penicillin. Empiric therapy for endocarditis in intravenous drug users must be active against *S. aureus;* for example, a nafcillin-gentamicin combination. In some communities, unusual organisms (e.g., methicillin-resistant *S. aureus* or *Pseudomonas*) may be more prevalent, and empiric therapy must be extended to cover them. In patients with prosthetic valves, agents should be active against staphylococci, both *S. aureus* and coagulase-negative and gram-negative organisms. Vancomycin, gentamicin, and rifampin are recommended. Culture-negative endocarditis should be evaluated for fastidious or slow-growing organisms and other unusual causes; empiric therapy should be directed against enterococci and viridans streptococci. Four weeks of penicillin (or vancomycin for the penicillin-allergic patient) plus gentamicin is recommended. With right-sided endocarditis, an acute clinical course, a history of intravenous drug use, or lack of response to penicillin plus aminoglycoside, *S. aureus* should be suspected and nafcillin added or vancomycin substituted for penicillin. For culture-negative prosthetic valve endocarditis, vancomycin plus rifampin plus gentamicin should be used to cover against coagulase-negative staphylococci.

The exact role of cardiac surgery in infective endocarditis is controversial, and decisions regarding surgical intervention are best made on an individual basis in consultation with an experienced surgeon. In general, surgery should be considered for patients who, despite appropriate medical therapy, develop deep-seated myocardial abscesses (frequently manifested by emerging conduction defects), persistent bacteremia, or fungal endocarditis or who have infected prosthetic valves. Aortic insufficiency resulting in shock requires emergent cardiac valve replacement. Patients with valvular insufficiency with congestive heart failure should be treated aggressively with diuretics and afterload reduction; surgery is indicated if they do not improve within 24 hours. Patients with hemodynamically stable valvular insufficiency should be treated with a full course of antibiotics before being evaluated for cardiac surgery.

ENDOCARDITIS PROPHYLAXIS

The use of chemoprophylaxis to prevent bacterial endocarditis in high-risk patients has become accepted practice. Although its value has never been proved in humans, administration of bactericidal antibiotics has been shown to prevent endocarditis in experimental animals. Current recommendations are based on these animal studies as well as on clinical, epidemiologic, and bacteriologic data. Patients at risk are those with cardiac or vascular disease known to be associated with endocarditis (see box below). Penicillin-sensitive oral streptococci (various species of viridans streptococci) are likely to be isolated from the bloodstream in patients undergoing dental, oral, or respiratory tract procedures; enterococci, which are more resistant to penicillin, are seeded in patients undergoing genitourinary or gastrointestinal procedures (see box, right). Drug selection is based on the sensitivity of the endocarditis-producing organisms likely to disseminate during a given procedure, and current recommendations are set forth in the 1990 American Heart Association guidelines (Table 15-6). The new AHA recommendations emphasize the use of oral over parenteral regimens, of amoxicillin over penicillin V as the standard oral regimen, and of prophylaxis for patients with mitral valve prolapse when mitral regurgitation is present (Chapter 16). Amoxicillin is as active as penicillin V against oral streptococci, but plasma levels and half-life are increased. The oral regimen is also recommended for high-risk patients (e.g., patients with prosthetic valves) undergoing dental, oral, or respiratory tract procedures; however, some authorities would still select the parenteral regimens provided. When used in other countries for high-risk patients, oral amoxicillin therapy has been associated with better compliance and few failures. For penicillin-allergic patients, clindamycin and erythromycin are recommended. Because patients taking oral penicillins for secondary prevention of rheumatic fever or for other purposes may harbor oral streptococci relatively resistant to the penicillins, erythromycin or clindamycin should be used for prophylaxis. The main prophylactic regimens recommended for genitourinary or gastrointestinal procedures are still parenteral for standard or high-risk patients. However, for standard-risk patients undergoing minor (low-risk) procedures, an oral amoxicillin regimen is optional. When infected tissue is manipulated, antibiotic selection should be based on the sensitivities of the most likely infecting or-

Common cardiac conditions at risk for endocarditis

Endocarditis prophylaxis recommended

Prosthetic cardiac valves
Previous bacterial endocarditis
Most congenital cardiac malformations
Rheumatic and other acquired valvular dysfunction
Hypertrophic cardiomyopathy
Mitral valve prolapse with valvular regurgitation*

Endocarditis prophylaxis not recommended

Isolated secundum atrial septal defect
Surgical repair without residua beyond 6 mo. of secundum ASD, VSD, or PDA
Previous coronary artery bypass surgery
Mitral valve prolapse without mitral regurgitation*
Physiologic, functional, or innocent heart murmurs
Previous Kawasaki disease without valvular dysfunction
Previous rheumatic fever without valvular dysfunction
Cardiac pacemakers and implanted defibrillators

Modified from Dajani AS et al: Prevention of bacterial endocarditis: recommendations by the American Heart Association. JAMA 264:2919, 1990.

*Prophylaxis is recommended for patients with MVP with a holosystolic murmur of mitral regurgitation or leaflet redundancy (myxomatous degeneration) on echocardiography. Prophylaxis is optional in patients with late systolic murmur or echocardiographic mitral regurgitation that is nonaudible on physical exam. ASD, atrial septal defect; VSD, ventricular septal defect; PDA, patent ductus arteriosis.

Dental or surgical procedures at higher risk to cause bacteremia that results in endocarditis

Endocarditis prophylaxis recommended

Dental procedures known to induce gingival or mucosal bleeding, including professional cleaning
Tonsillectomy and/or adenoidectomy
Surgical operations that involve intestinal or respiratory mucosa
Bronchoscopy with a rigid bronchoscope
Sclerotherapy for esophageal varices
Esophageal dilatation
Gallbladder surgery
Cystoscopy
Urethral dilatation
Urethral catheterization if urinary tract infection is present*
Prostatic surgery
Incision and drainage of infected tissue*
Vaginal hysterectomy
Vaginal delivery in the presence of infection*

Endocarditis prophylaxis not recommended†

Dental procedure not likely to induce gingival bleeding
Injection of local intraoral anesthesia (except intraligamentary)
Shedding of primary teeth
Tympanostomy tube insertion
Endotracheal intubation
Bronchoscopy with a flexible bronchoscope with or without biopsy
Cardiac catheterization
Gastrointestinal endoscopy with or without biopsy
Cesarean section
In the absence of infection for urethral catheterization, dilatation and curettage, uncomplicated vaginal delivery, therapeutic abortion, sterilization procedures, or insertion or removal of intrauterine devices

Modified from Dajani AS et al: Prevention of bacterial endocarditis: recommendations by the American Heart Association. JAMA, 264:2919, 1990. This table is not meant to be all-inclusive.

*In addition to the prophylactic regimen for genitourinary procedures, antibiotic therapy should be directed against the most likely bacterial pathogen.

†In patients at high risk for endocarditis (those with prosthetic valves or history of endocarditis), physicians may choose to administer prophylactic antibiotics even for low-risk procedures.

Table 15-6. Recommended prophylactic antibiotic regimens for patients at risk having dental, oral, upper respiratory tract, genitourinary, or gastrointestinal procedures

Procedure	Risk factor	Dosing regimen*	Comments
Dental, oral, or upper respiratory tract	Standard risk† with native valve	**Amoxicillin** 3 g orally 1 hr before procedure, then 1.5 g after initial dose.	Standard oral regimen
		Erythromycin 1 g orally 2 hr before procedure, then 0.5 g 6 hr after initial dose.	Amoxicillin/penicillin allergy.
		Clindamycin 300 mg orally 1 hr before procedure, then 150 mg 6 hr after initial dose.	Amoxicillin/penicillin allergy or unable to tolerate erythromycin.
		Ampicillin 2 g IV or IM 30 min before procedure, then 1 g IV or IM 6 hr after initial dose.	Unable to take oral medications.
		Clindamycin 300 mg IV 30 min before procedure, then 150 mg 6 hr after initial dose.	Unable to take oral medications; amoxicillin/ampicillin/penicillin allergy.
	High risk† (prosthetic valve or history of endocarditis)	**Ampicillin** 2 g IV or IM plus **Gentamicin** 1.5 mg/kg (not to exceed 80 mg) IV or IM 30 min before procedure, then amoxicillin 1.5 g orally 6 hr after initial dose.	Alternatively, instead of oral amoxicillin the IV regimen can be repeated 8 h after initial dose.
		Vancomycin 1 g IV starting 1 hr before procedure.	Amoxicillin/ampicillin/penicillin allergy; no repeat dose necessary.
Genitourinary or gastrointestinal	Standard or high risk	**Ampicillin** 2 g IV or IM plus **gentamicin** 1.5 mg/kg (not to exceed 80 mg) IV or IM 30 min before procedure, then amoxicillin 1.5 g orally 6 hr after initial dose.	Alternatively instead of oral amoxicillin the IV regimen can be repeated 8 hr after initial dose.
		Vancomycin 1 g IV plus **gentamicin** 1.5 mg/kg (not to exceed 80 mg) IV or IM starting 1 hr before procedure. May repeat gentamicin 8 hr after initial dose.	Amoxicillin/ampicillin/penicillin allergy; no repeat dose necessary for vancomycin.
	Low risk (minor procedures)‡	**Amoxicillin** 3 g orally 1 hr before procedure, then 1.5 g after initial dose.	Not for amoxicillin/penicillin-allergic patients.

Modified from Dajani AS et al: Prevention of bacterial endocarditis: recommendations by the American Heart Association. JAMA, 264:2919, 1990. Reader should refer to article for more detailed discussion of this topic.

*In patients with impaired renal function it may be necessary to omit second dose of gentamicin.

†Standard oral regimens can be used in higher risk patients as per AHA recommendations, however, clinicians may choose parenteral regimens.

‡Patients without prosthetic valve and no history of endocarditis and no urinary tract infection undergoing minor procedures.

ganism. Antibiotic prophylaxis should start 30 to 60 minutes before the procedure and, unless indicated clinically, should not be continued beyond the recommended postprocedure dose. Maximum protective benefit is probably derived within the first 6 to 8 hours, and prolonged antibiotic administration predictably leads to the emergence of resistant strains.

In patients with mitral valve prolapse, the AHA recommends antibiotic prophylaxis only for those with mitral regurgitation. However, exactly how mitral regurgitation should be defined in this setting (by physical examination or echocardiography) has not been clarified. In addition, a recent echocardiographic study defined a subset of patients with mitral valve prolapse with thickened mitral valve leaflets and redundancy who are at high risk for endocarditis. Based on current knowledge, prophylaxis is recommended for patients with mitral valve prolapse with a holosystolic murmur of mitral regurgitation or with leaflet thickening and redundancy (myxomatous proliferation) on echocardiography. Prophylaxis is optional in patients with a late systolic murmur or with echocardiographic mitral regurgitation that is nonaudible on physical examination (Chapter 16). Antibiotic prophylaxis is recommended perioperatively in patients undergoing open heart surgery, valve replacement, or placement of intracardiac materials. The antibiotic chosen should be directed against *S. aureus* and coagulase-negative staphylococci and tailored to the pathogens most commonly isolated in the particular institution. Prophylaxis should be given in the years after most heart or valvular surgery in patients undergoing high-risk dental, oral, respiratory tract, genitourinary, gastrointestinal, or other procedures. This is not recommended for patients who have undergone coronary artery bypass graft surgery. All patients at risk for endocarditis should establish and maintain the best possible oral health and dental hygiene to reduce potential sources of bacterial seeding, and should receive regular dental care.

REFERENCES

Bisno AL et al: Antimicrobial treatment of infective endocarditis due to viridans streptococci, enterococci, and staphylococci. JAMA 261:1471, 1989.

Chambers HF, Miller T, Newman M: Two-week therapy of *Staphylococcus aureus* right-sided endocarditis and bacteremia in intravenous drug users. Ann Intern Med 109:619, 1988.
Dajani AS et al: Prevention of bacterial endocarditis. Recommendations by the American Heart Association. JAMA 264:2919, 1990.
Daniel WG et al: Improvement in the diagnosis of abscesses associated with endocarditis by transesophageal echocardiography. N Engl J Med 324:795, 1991.
Devereux RB et al: Mitral valve prolapse: causes, clinical manifestations, and management. Ann Intern Med 111:305, 1989.
Dinubile MJ: Surgery in active endocarditis. Ann Intern Med 96:650, 1982.
Erbel R et al: Improved diagnostic value of echocardiography in patients with infective endocarditis by transesophageal approach. A prospective study. Eur Heart J 9:43, 1988.
Francioli P et al: Treatment of streptococcal endocarditis with a single daily dose of ceftriaxone sodium for 4 weeks. Efficacy and outpatient treatment feasibility. JAMA 267:264, 1992.
Freedman LR and Valone J Jr: Experimental infective endocarditis. Prog Cardiovasc Dis 23:169, 1979.
Kaye D: Prophylaxis for infective endocarditis: an update. Ann Intern Med 104:419, 1986.
Kaye D and Abrutyn E: Prevention of bacterial endocarditis: 1991. Ann Intern Med 114:803, 1991 (editorial).
Marks AR et al: Identification of high-risk and low-risk subgroups of patients with mitral-valve prolapse, N Engl J Med 320:1031, 1989.
McKinsey DW et al: Underlying cardiac lesions in adults with infective endocarditis. The changing spectrum. Am J Med 82:681, 1987.
Pelletier LL Jr and Petersdorf RG: Infective endocarditis: review of 125 cases from the University of Washington Hospitals, 1963-72. Medicine (Baltimore) 56:287, 1977.
Sande MA, Kaye D, and Root RK, editors: Endocarditis. vol 2, Contemporary issues in infectious diseases. New York, 1984, Churchill Livingstone.
Sande MA and Scheld WM: Combination antibiotic therapy of bacterial endocarditis. Ann Intern Med 92:390, 1980.
Scheld WM and Sande MA: Endocarditis and intravascular infections. In Mandell GL, Douglas RG Jr, Bennett JE, editors: Principles and practice of infectious diseases. New York, 1990, Wiley.
Shapiro SM and Bayer AS: Transesophageal and doppler echocardiography in the diagnosis and management of infective endocarditis, Chest 100:1125, 1991.
Small PM and Chambers HF: Vancomycin for *Staphylococcus aureus* endocarditis in intravenous drug users. Antimicrob Agents Chemother 34:1227, 1990.
Van Scoy RE: Culture-negative endocarditis. Mayo Clin Proc 57:149, 1982.
Wolfson JS and Swartz MN: Serum bactericidal activity as a monitor of antibiotic therapy. N Engl J Med 312:968, 1985.

CHAPTER

16 Valvular Heart Disease

Shahbudin H. Rahimtoola

The clinical assessment and management of valvular heart disease have undergone many changes in the last three decades. The incidence of acute rheumatic fever has declined, and as a result rheumatic heart disease is not the most important cause of valve disease. Prolapse of the mitral valve and congenital aortic valve disease are now the most common valvular lesions. Valve surgery has been the major therapeutic advance in treating severe valve disease; in fact, most patients with severe valve disease are now considered candidates for operation. Doppler echocardiography (Chapter 5) has an important role in the diagnosis and follow-up of these patients. Catheter balloon valvuloplasty is an exciting new intervention technique for the treatment of stenotic cardiac valves.

AORTIC STENOSIS

Etiology

Aortic stenosis is obstruction to outflow of blood from the left ventricle to the aorta. The obstruction may be at the valve, above the valve (supravalvular), or below the valve (subvalvular). Supravalvular aortic stenosis is a congenital lesion. Subvalvular aortic stenosis results either from a discrete fibromuscular obstruction, which is a congenital lesion, or from a muscular obstruction (hypertrophic cardiomyopathy).

Congenital abnormalities of the aortic valve account for more than 90% of cases of isolated aortic valve stenosis. The commonest cause of acquired aortic stenosis is rheumatic heart disease; patients with this disease usually have additional mitral valve disease. Rare disorders that produce aortic valve stenosis include rheumatoid disease and atherosclerosis associated with severe hypercholesterolemia.

Pathology

In congenital aortic valve stenosis, the valve may be unicuspid, bicuspid, or tricuspid, depending on the patient's age. In the first two decades of life, over 90% of stenotic valves are either unicuspid or bicuspid, whereas in patients 65 years of age or over, 90% of the valves are tricuspid. Unicuspid valves produce severe obstruction in infancy and are the most frequent malformation found in fatal valvular aortic stenosis in children under the age of 1 year (Chapter 19). Congenital bicuspid valves are capable of producing severe obstruction to left ventricular outflow after the first few years of life. The valvular abnormality produces turbulent flow, which traumatizes the leaflets and eventually leads to fibrosis, rigidity, and calcification of the valve. In a congenitally abnormal tricuspid aortic valve, the cusps are of unequal size and have some degree of commissural fusion; the third cusp may be diminutive. Eventually, the abnormal structure leads to changes similar to those seen in a bicuspid valve, and significant left ventricular outflow obstruction often results.

Rheumatic aortic stenosis results from adhesions and fusion of the commissures and cusps. The leaflets and the valve ring become vascularized, which leads to retraction and stiffening of the cusps. Calcification occurs, and the aortic valve orifice is reduced to a small triangular or round opening, which is frequently regurgitant as well as stenotic. Importantly, the heart exhibits other evidence of rheumatic heart disease, namely, involvement of the mitral valve and presence of Aschoff's nodules in the myocardium. Rheumatoid aortic stenosis is extremely rare and results from nodular thickening of the valve leaflets and the involvement of the proximal part of the aorta. In severe forms of hypercholesterolemia, lipid deposits occur not only in the aortic wall but also in the aortic valve and occasionally produce valvular stenosis.

The left ventricle is concentrically hypertrophied. The hypertrophied cardiac muscle cells are increased in size, with their transverse diameters ranging from 15 to 70 μm (normal, 10 to 15 μm). There is a variable amount of fibrous tissue (collagen fibrils) in the interstitial tissue. Usually, the cardiac muscle cells do not degenerate in patients with aortic valve stenosis.

Subclinical calcific emboli are commonly found if diligently sought.

Abnormal physiology

With reduction in the aortic valve area, energy is dissipated during the transport of blood from the left ventricle to the aorta. The aortic valve area has to be reduced by 50% of normal before a measurable gradient can be demonstrated in humans. When a pressure gradient develops between the left ventricle and the ascending aorta, left ventricular pressure rises; aortic pressure remains within the normal range until end-stage heart failure occurs. The relationship of the valve area to cardiac output and pressure gradient is discussed in the section on mitral stenosis. As left ventricular pressure rises, ventricular wall stress increases, which leads to impaired left ventricular function. Therefore, the heart normalizes wall stress by becoming hypertrophic (Chapter 1). Since aortic stenosis develops slowly over the years in humans, hypertrophy develops in proportion to increased intraventricular pressure, and myocardial stress remains normal. Thus, the major compensatory mechanism by which the heart copes with left ventricular outflow obstruction is ventricular hypertrophy. Left ventricular mass in patients with severe aortic stenosis undergoing valve replacement averages 229 g per square meter (normal, 105 g/m^2); at autopsy, left ventricles weighing as much as 1000 g have been reported. However, left ventricular volume is within the normal range. Therefore, there is a considerable thickening of the left ventricular wall.

The diastolic properties of the left ventricle are affected in aortic stenosis. There is a resistance to left ventricular filling, because the hypertrophied left ventricle per se offers increased resistance to filling, the stiffness of the left ventricle is increased, or both. As a result, left ventricular end diastolic pressure is elevated, but this cannot be used as a measure of left ventricular failure. Powerful atrial contraction produces the required left ventricular filling and results in an elevated left ventricular end diastolic pressure (atrial booster pump function). The necessary left ventricular filling and fiber length are achieved by atrial systole, which occupies only a small part of the cardiac cycle. Therefore, there is a transient increase in left atrial pressure due to the large A wave, but mean left atrial pressure remains in the normal range or is only minimally increased.

Left atrial contraction is therefore of considerable benefit to these patients. Loss of effective atrial contraction, either because of atrial fibrillation or because of an inappropriately timed atrial contraction (e.g., that associated with first-degree heart block or with atrioventricular [AV] dissociation), results in elevations of mean left atrial pressure, reduction of cardiac output, or both, and may precipitate heart failure.

Left ventricular systolic pump function is determined by myocardial (muscle) function and by a combination of left ventricular afterload and preload (Chapter 1). Thus, impaired left ventricular systolic pump function (as measured by ejection fraction) may be the result of impaired myocardial function, afterload-preload mismatch, or both. Left ventricular systolic pump function is normal in most patients with severe aortic stenosis. When the left ventricular hypertrophy alone is not adequate to overcome the outflow obstruction, the left ventricle uses the Frank-Starling mechanism (preload reserve) to maintain systolic pump function. When the preload reserve is no longer adequate, a reduction of left ventricular systolic pump function occurs. In aortic stenosis, use of the preload reserve is not a good compensatory mechanism. Even small increases in left ventricular volume result in major increases in left ventricular end-diastolic pressure, because the left ventricle is on the very steep portion of its diastolic pressure-volume curve, and the corresponding increase in mean left atrial pressures produces pulmonary edema. Eventually, pulmonary artery, right ventricular, and right atrial pressures are elevated. Peripheral edema results from increases in systemic venous pressure and salt and water retention.

In most patients with aortic valve stenosis, cardiac output is in the normal range and initially increases normally with exercise. Later, as the severity of aortic stenosis increases progressively, the cardiac output remains within the normal range at rest, but, on exercise, it no longer increases in proportion to the amount of exercise undertaken or does not increase at all (fixed cardiac output). With the development of congestive heart failure, there is a reduction in the resting cardiac output and a tachycardia. As a result, stroke volume may be so lowered that it results in a small gradient across the left ventricular outflow tract in spite of severe aortic stenosis.

In severe aortic stenosis, myocardial oxygen needs are increased because of an increased muscle mass (hypertrophy), elevations in ventricular pressures, and prolongation of the systolic ejection time. Blood flow to the myocardium, particularly flow to the subendocardium, is inadequate, because the abnormally elevated pressure compresses the coronary arteries as they traverse the myocardium to supply the subendocardium, and the elevated left ventricular end-diastolic pressure lowers the diastolic aortic–left ventricular pressure (coronary perfusion pressure) gradient. Associated obstructive coronary artery disease from atherosclerosis further increases the imbalance between myocardial oxygen needs and supply.

Clinical manifestations

History. Patients with congenital valve stenosis may give a history of a murmur since childhood or infancy; those with rheumatic stenosis may have a history of rheumatic fever. Most patients with valvular aortic stenosis, including a few with severe valve stenosis, are asymptomatic. The symptoms of aortic stenosis are angina pectoris, syncope, exertional presyncope, and the symptoms of heart failure. It must be emphasized that once symptoms occur in a patient with severe aortic stenosis, the life span of the patient is very short without surgical treatment. Sudden cardiac death occurs in 5% of patients with aortic stenosis. It occurs only in those with severe valve stenosis, most of whom have had some cardiac symptoms before the fatal episode. Typical angina pectoris occurs with or without associated coronary artery disease and results from an imbalance between myocardial oxygen demand and supply, as previously discussed.

Syncope is the result of reduced cerebral perfusion. Syncope occurring on effort is caused by either systemic vasodilatation in the presence of a fixed or inadequate cardiac output, an arrhythmia, or both. Syncope at rest is usually due to a transient ventricular tachyarrhythmia, from which the patient recovers spontaneously. Other possible causes of syncope include transient atrial fibrillation or transient AV block during which the ventricle is deprived of the powerful atrial booster pump function and/or the ventricular rate is slow.

Dyspnea on exertion, orthopnea, paroxysmal nocturnal dyspnea, and pulmonary edema result from varying degrees of pulmonary venous hypertension. Systemic venous congestion with enlargement of the liver and peripheral edema results from increased systemic venous pressure and salt and water retention. There is an increased incidence of gastrointestinal arteriovenous malformations. As a result, these patients are susceptible to gastrointestinal hemorrhage and anemia. Calcific systemic embolism may occur.

Physical findings. The arterial pulse rises slowly, taking a longer time than normal to reach peak pressure, and the peak is reduced; the pulse pressure may be narrowed. The anacrotic notch on the upstroke is best appreciated in the carotid arteries. The more severe the valve stenosis, the lower the anacrotic notch on the arterial pulse. A systolic thrill may be felt in the carotid arteries. The jugular venous pulse is normal unless the patient is in congestive heart failure. In the absence of heart failure, the heart size is normal. The cardiac impulse is heaving and sustained in character, and there may be a palpable fourth heart sound (S_4). An aortic systolic thrill often is present at the base of the heart. In 80% to 90% of adult patients with severe aortic stenosis, there is an S_4 gallop sound, a midsystolic ejection murmur that peaks late in systole, the second heart sound (S_2) is single, and there is a faint early diastolic murmur of minimal aortic regurgitation. In the young patient with valvular aortic stenosis, a systolic ejection sound initiates the systolic murmur but later tends to disappear as aortic stenosis becomes severe. The S_2 may be paradoxically split, and there may be no early diastolic murmur. In many patients, particularly the elderly, the systolic ejection murmur is atypical, may be soft or cooing, and may be heard only at the apex of the heart. In the presence of congestive heart failure, the jugular venous pressure often is increased, the left ventricle is dilated, there is a third heart sound, and the systolic murmur may be very soft or absent. Thus, the clinical features on physical examination resemble those of heart failure from a variety of causes such as cardiomyopathy, rather than aortic stenosis.

Severe valvular aortic stenosis is common in patients 60 years of age or older. The clinical features in many of these patients tend to be somewhat different from those typical of younger patients. Systemic hypertension is common, occurring in about 20% of the patients, half of whom have moderate or severe systolic and diastolic hypertension. A fifth of the patients first present in congestive heart failure. The male/female ratio is 2:1. Because of thickening of the arterial wall and its associated lack of distensibility, the arterial pulse rises normally or even rapidly, and the pulse pressure is wide. The S_2 is either absent or single.

Chest radiograph. The characteristic finding is a normal-sized heart with a dilated ascending aorta (Fig. 16-1). Calcium in the aortic valve can be seen on the lateral film but is best appreciated by fluoroscopy with image intensification. Calcium in the aortic valve is the hallmark of aortic stenosis in adults 40 to 45 years of age. In patients aged 45 years or above, the diagnosis of aortic valve stenosis of any severity is not tenable if calcium in the aortic valve is not present. However, the presence of calcium does not necessarily denote that the aortic stenosis is severe. In patients with heart failure, the cardiac size is increased because of dilatation of the left ventricle and left atrium; the lung fields show pulmonary edema and pulmonary venous congestion with redistribution of blood flow. In the presence of congestive heart failure, the right ventricle and the right atrium may be dilated.

Electrocardiogram. The ECG in severe aortic stenosis shows left ventricular hypertrophy with or without secondary ST-T wave changes (Chapter 4). However, it is important to recognize that in about 10% to 15% of patients with severe aortic stenosis, left ventricular hypertrophy cannot be appreciated on the ECG. In fact, the ECG may be entirely normal in some of these patients. The P wave abnormalities of left atrial enlargement and hypertrophy or conduction delay are usually present. The ECG may show left bundle branch block, right bundle branch block with left or right axis deviation, or, occasionally, isolated right bundle branch block. In some of the patients, the conduction abnormality results from aortic valve calcification extending into the specialized conducting tissue. The patients are usually in sinus rhythm. The presence of atrial fibrillation indicates the presence of either associated mitral valve disease, coronary artery disease, or heart failure secondary to aortic valve disease.

Special laboratory studies. On the echocardiogram, the aortic valve leaflets normally are barely visible in systole, and the normal range of aortic valve opening is 1.6 to 2.6 cm (Chapter 5). In the presence of a bicuspid aortic valve, eccentric valve leaflets may be seen. The aortic valve leaflets may appear to be thickened as a result of calcification and/or fibrosis; however, the older patient without valve stenosis may also have thickened cusps. The aortic valve may have a reduced opening, but this also occurs in other con-

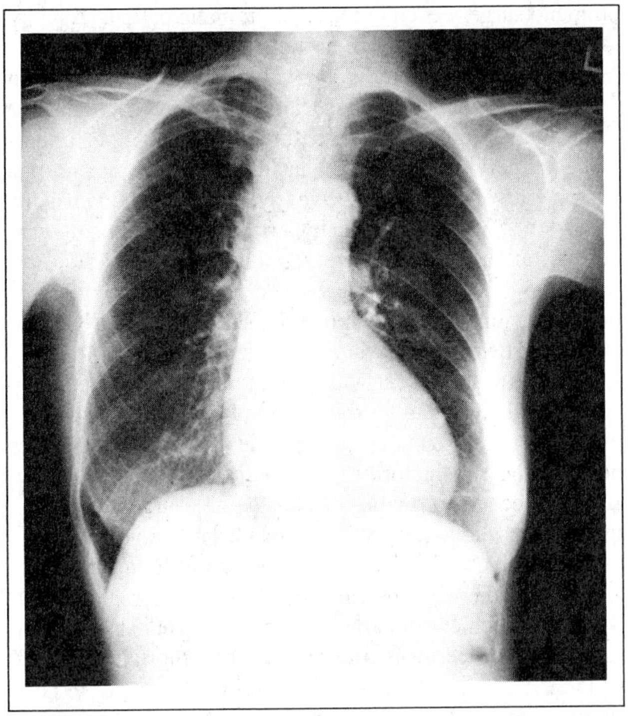

A

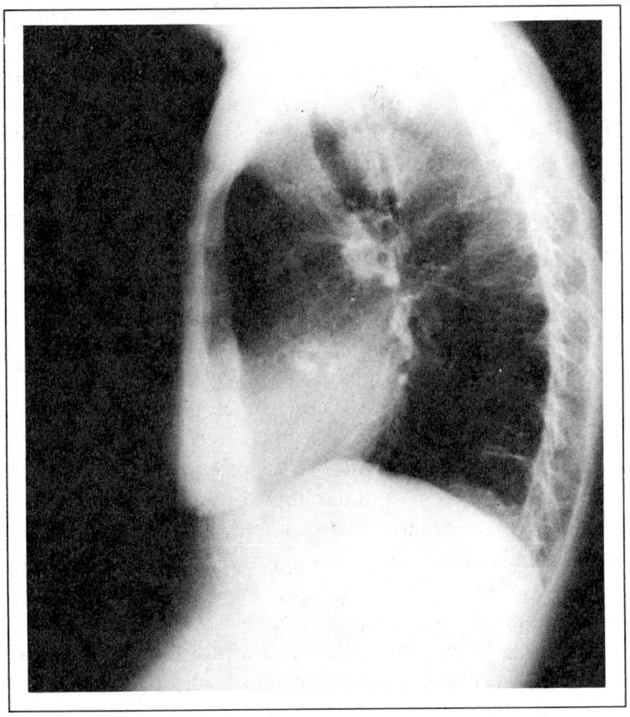

B

Fig. 16-1. Chest radiograph in the frontal **(A)** and left lateral **(B)** projection in a patient with severe aortic stenosis. The aortic valve is heavily calcified, a finding best appreciated on the lateral projection **(B)** or with fluoroscopy.

ditions in which the cardiac output is reduced. The left ventricular hypertrophy often results in thickening of both the interventricular septum and the posterior left ventricular wall. The left ventricular size is normal. All these abnormalities are better appreciated on two-dimensional (2D) echocardiography. When left ventricular function is impaired, the left ventricle and left atrium are dilatated and the percentage of dimensional shortening (Chapter 5) is reduced.

In many patients, the severity of aortic valve stenosis is incorrectly estimated by M-mode or 2D echocardiography. Neither is a completely reliable technique for assessing the severity of valvular aortic stenosis. However, the presence of normal movement of thin aortic leaflets on the echocardiogram is strong evidence against severe aortic stenosis in adults.

Doppler echocardiography, when properly applied, is useful for obtaining the valve gradient and valve area noninvasively (Chapter 5). When compared to that obtained at cardiac catheterization, the standard error of the estimate of the mean gradient in the best laboratories is 10 mm Hg. Thus, the mean gradient obtained by Doppler can be expected to be within ± 20 mm Hg of that obtained at catheterization. Similarly, the valve area will be within ± 0.3 cm^2 of that obtained at cardiac catheterization.

Cardiac catheterization remains the standard technique to confirm the diagnosis of valvular aortic stenosis and to accurately assess its severity (Chapter 6). This is done by measuring simultaneous left ventricular and systemic arterial pressure (see Fig. 6-3) and measuring cardiac output by either the Fick principle or the indicator-dilution technique. The aortic valve area can be calculated. Aortic valve stenosis can be considered to be severe when the aortic valve area index is 0.6 cm^2 per square meter or less or the valve area is 1.0 cm^2 or less. The state of left ventricular pump function can be quantitated by measuring left ventricular volumes and ejection fraction. It must be recognized that ejection fraction underestimates myocardial function in the presence of the increased afterload of aortic stenosis. The presence of coronary artery disease and its site and severity can be estimated only by selective coronary angiography, which should be performed in patients with angina, those with left ventricular systolic dysfunction, those with risk factors for coronary artery disease, and all patients 35 years of age or older being considered for aortic valve surgery. The incidence of associated coronary artery disease is related to the prevalence of coronary artery disease in the population. In general, in persons 50 years of age or older it is about 50%.

Gated blood pool radionuclide scans provide information on ventricular function similar to that provided by left ventricular cineangiography (Chapter 5). These studies are of particular value in the occasional patient in whom left ventricular cineangiography is unsuccessful.

It is recommended that exercise tests of any kind not be undertaken in patients with severe aortic stenosis unless there is a specific reason for such studies. Exercise tests in these patients may precipitate ventricular tachyarrhythmias and ventricular fibrillation. If there is doubt about the severity of aortic stenosis and concern that the patient's symptoms may not be caused by aortic stenosis, then it is usually wise to document the absence of severe aortic stenosis before performing an exercise test.

Ambulatory ECG recording may be needed in an occasional patient suspected of having an arrhythmia, since symptoms occur only during arrhythmias in some patients with mild or moderate aortic stenosis.

Natural history and prognosis

Valvular aortic stenosis is frequently a progressive disease, the severity increasing over time. The factors that control this progression and the time it takes for severe outflow obstruction to develop are unknown. In a recent study in patients with "mild" stenosis, the rate of progression to moderate or severe stenosis was 12% in 10 years and 62% in 25 years. The duration of the asymptomatic period after the development of severe aortic valve stenosis is also unknown; some recent data suggest it may be less than 2 years. The overwhelming majority of adults with severe aortic stenosis who are seen by cardiologists have symptoms. Severe disease in adults is lethal, with a prognosis that is worse than for many forms of neoplastic disease. The 3-year mortality is approximately 36% to 52%. The 5-year mortality is about 52% to 80% and the 10-year mortality is 80% to 90%. A recent study of elderly patients (average age 77 years) showed 1-year and 3-year mortalities were 44% and 75%, respectively. With the onset of severe symptoms (angina, syncope, or heart failure) the average life expectancy is 3 years. A combination of symptoms is much more ominous, a sign of a greatly reduced survival. Sudden death, like syncope, occurs in the presence of severe aortic stenosis. Its exact incidence is difficult to determine but is probably about 5%. Most, but not all, of these patients have had some cardiac symptoms before the fatal episode; at times, the only symptom has been exertional presyncope.

Management

All patients with aortic stenosis need antibiotic prophylaxis against infective endocarditis (Chapter 15). Those in whom the valve lesion is of rheumatic origin need additional rheumatic fever prophylaxis (Chapter 316). Patients with mild or moderate stenosis rarely have symptoms or complications and do not need any specific medical therapy. In mild stenosis, the patient should be encouraged to lead a normal life. Those with moderate valve stenosis should avoid moderate to severe physical exertion and competitive sports. In patients with mild or moderate disease, if atrial fibrillation should occur, it should be reverted rapidly to sinus rhythm. In severe stenosis, reversion to sinus rhythm often becomes a matter of some urgency.

Operation should be advised if the patient has severe aortic valve stenosis. In young patients, if the valve is pliable and mobile, simple commissurotomy may be feasible, and it will relieve outflow obstruction to a major degree; overly enthusiastic commissurotomy with production of significant aortic regurgitation should be avoided. This is probably a palliative procedure that puts off valve replacement for many years. Older patients and even young patients with calcified, rigid valves need valve replacement. In view of the natural history of severe aortic valve stenosis, that is, a 10-year mortality of 80% to 90%, it is reasonable to recommend surgery even to the asymptomatic patient. Asymptomatic adults with severe aortic stenosis are uncommon.

The operative mortality of valve replacement is about 5% or less. Patients with associated coronary artery disease should have coronary bypass surgery at the same time as valve surgery. Left ventricular function remains normal postoperatively if perioperative myocardial damage has not occurred. Left ventricular hypertrophy regresses toward normal; after 2 years, the regression continues at a slower rate up to 8-10 years after valve replacement. Surviving patients are functionally improved. The 10-year survival is 60% or better; 15-year survival is 45% or better.

Patients who present with heart failure should be hospitalized and treated with digitalis and diuretics and should undergo surgery as soon as possible. If heart failure does not respond satisfactorily and rapidly to medical therapy, surgery becomes a matter of considerable urgency. Catheter balloon valvuloplasty is an important bridge procedure that usually greatly improves the patients' hemodynamics and makes them better candidates for valve replacement. Valve replacement in patients with aortic stenosis and heart failure can be performed at an operative mortality of 10% or less. Although this is higher than in patients not in heart failure, the risk is justified, because late survival in those who live through the operation is excellent and is far superior to that which can be expected with medical therapy. The 7-year survival of patients who survive operation is 84%. The impaired left ventricular function improves in *all* such patients provided there has been no perioperative myocardial damage and becomes normal in two thirds of the patients. In addition, the operative survivors are functionally much improved. Left ventricular hypertrophy and dilatation (if present preoperatively) regress toward normal.

Despite the excellent results of valve replacements in patients with severe aortic stenosis who are in heart failure, it is important to recognize that surgery should *not* be delayed until heart failure develops.

The role of catheter balloon valvuloplasty in the older patient has now been clarified. In calcific aortic stenosis after catheter balloon valvuloplasty, the average increase in valve area is 0.3 cm^2 and the final aortic valve area usually averages 0.8 cm^2; thus, many patients continue to have severe aortic stenosis. The 30-day, 1-year, and 3-year mortalities average 14%, 35%, and 71%, respectively, in the older patient with calcific aortic stenosis. This technique is indicated in those who have an expected limited short life span, as a bridge procedure in those who need emergent noncardiac surgery and in those who are in heart failure, when operative risks are considered to be prohibitively high, and in those who refuse surgery.

CHRONIC AORTIC REGURGITATION

Etiology

In North America, the most common cause of isolated severe aortic regurgitation is aortic root dilatation that is presumably the result of medial disease. Other common causes include a congenital (bicuspid) valve, previous infective endocarditis, and rheumatic disease. Chronic aortic regurgitation also occurs in association with a variety of other diseases, such as

1. Congenital lesions, for example, supravalvular and discrete subvalvular aortic stenosis, ventricular septal defect, and aneurysm of the sinus of Valsalva.
2. Connective tissue diseases, for example, Marfan's syndrome, osteogenesis imperfecta, and Ehlers-Danlos syndrome.
3. Autoimmune diseases, for example, ankylosing spondylitis, rheumatoid arthritis, and systemic lupus erythematosus.
4. Various forms of aortitis and arteritis, for example, giant-cell arteritis and Takayasu's disease.
5. Syphilis.

Forty percent to 60% of the surgically removed valves from patients with isolated severe aortic regurgitation are classified as idiopathic. Half of these (or 20% to 30% of all the valves removed) showed histologic criteria of myxomatous degeneration.

Pathology

Depending on the cause, the valve cusps show thickening, shortening, commissural lesions, and calcification. Regardless of the cause, the left ventricle is dilated and hypertrophied; some of the largest ventricles have been described in association with chronic severe aortic regurgitation. Little pockets may be seen in the left ventricular outflow tract. These are pouches out of the endocardial lining formed by the regurgitant jet's striking the left ventricle.

The myocardium is hypertrophied, with replication of sarcomeres in series, elongation of fibers, and wall thickening. The wall is not as thickened as in patients with aortic stenosis. Ultrastructural changes in the myocardial cells are similar to those seen in aortic stenosis; an important difference, however, is the frequent presence of degenerated cardiac muscle cells in patients with severe aortic regurgitation. Cardiac muscle cells with mild degeneration show focal myofibrillar lysis, with preferential loss of thick myofilament and focal proliferation of tubules of the sarcoplasmic reticulum. Moderately degenerated muscle cells show a marked decrease in the number of myofibrils and T tubules and proliferation of sarcoplasmic reticulum, mitochondria, or both. Severely degenerated muscle cells usually are present in areas of marked fibrosis; they are often atrophic, have thickened basement membranes, and have lost their intercellular connections. These degenerated cardiac muscle cells may represent the ultrastructural basis for impaired left ventricular function, which is seen more commonly in severe aortic regurgitation than in severe aortic stenosis.

In patients with rheumatoid arthritis and ankylosing spondylitis, nodules on the outer surface of the anterior leaflet of the mitral valve have been described.

Abnormal physiology

The left ventricle responds to chronic aortic regurgitation by an increase in left ventricular diastolic volume, the increment in end diastolic volume being proportional to the amount of regurgitation. The left ventricle hypertrophies to normalize stress (Chapter 1). The left ventricular wall is not as thickened as in aortic stenosis; however, the total left ventricular mass is greatly increased, and the wall is usually thicker than normal.

Because of the leak of blood from the ascending aorta to the left ventricle in diastole, the aortic diastolic pressure is reduced and is frequently below 50 mm Hg. The large left ventricular stroke volume (a combination of forward stroke volume and regurgitant volume) results in elevation of the aortic systolic pressure, and thus the pulse pressure is considerably increased. The left ventricular end diastolic pressure is increased because the regurgitant volume increases ventricular end-diastolic volume. However, the relation between left ventricular end-diastolic volume and end-diastolic pressure is not linear (Chapter 1), and in any group of patients there is a considerable scatter between the two measurements. In fact, many patients have a normal ventricular end-diastolic pressure in spite of severe aortic regurgitation and large left ventricles, indicating a shift of the ventricular pressure-volume curve to the right.

The increased left ventricular end-diastolic volume is associated with a normal ejection fraction, and, as a result, left ventricular stroke volume is large. The left ventricle in aortic regurgitation is ejecting against systemic resistance, and the myocardial tension that is developed to open the aortic valve and eject the huge stroke volume is great. This contrasts with another volume-overload lesion, mitral regurgitation, in which there is a low-resistance chamber into which the left ventricle is also emptying (the left atrium). Thus, for the same degree of regurgitant volume, myocardial tension or afterload is higher in aortic regurgitation.

Left ventricular stroke volume in aortic regurgitation consists of the forward stroke volume (blood delivered to the body tissues and the heart), which, multiplied by heart rate, makes up the forward cardiac output and the regurgitant volume (the volume of blood that regurgitates back to the left ventricle). In the early stages, even in severe aortic regurgitation, the forward cardiac output and left ventricular ejection fraction are normal at rest. During exercise, end-diastolic volume is reduced and ejection fraction is increased. As in normal subjects, the systemic vascular resistance is decreased, and the heart rate is increased, which reduces the length of diastole. Both these factors reduce the regurgitant volume, and forward stroke volume and cardiac output are increased during exercise.

Progressive impairment of left ventricular function in aortic regurgitation produces the following changes: at first, left ventricular ejection fraction fails to increase normally or actually diminishes during exercise, with the resulting increment in cardiac output with exercise being inadequate. However, current data suggest that an abnormal response of the left ventricular ejection fraction (failure to increase) on exercise is also related to lack of an adequate fall in systemic vascular resistance during exercise. Thus, a decline in ejection fraction on exercise cannot be used as a specific marker of left ventricular function in these patients. However, an ejection fraction on exercise of less than 0.50 has been shown to correlate with increased left atrial pressure during exercise and an abnormal left ventricular contractile state at rest. Further impairment of left ventricular function produces demonstrable abnormalities at rest; there is a further increase in left ventricular end-diastolic volume, which helps to maintain forward stroke volume. The resting left ventricular ejection fraction is reduced, and mean left atrial pressure begins to increase. Even at this stage, the forward cardiac output may be maintained in the normal range. The increases in left atrial pressure may produce various grades of pulmonary edema. Finally, in the state of severe heart failure, ejection fraction may be low, left ventricular end-diastolic volume is large, and end-diastolic pressure is greatly increased and is associated with increases in left atrial, pulmonary, right ventricular, and right atrial pressures. Cardiac output is no longer normal. An increase in systemic venous pressure in association with salt and water retention produces engorgement of systemic organs (e.g., the liver) as well as peripheral edema.

Because of the increase in left ventricular mass, myocardial oxygen needs are increased. Coronary blood flow is inadequate with stress because of the reduction in the aortic diastolic pressure and increased diastolic ventricular pressure. The inadequate coronary blood flow jeopardizes the subendocardium, which may become ischemic. Associated obstructive coronary artery disease exacerbates the reduction in coronary blood flow.

Clinical manifestations

History. Patients with mild to moderate aortic regurgitation usually do not have symptoms that can be attributed to the heart. Even patients with severe aortic regurgitation may be asymptomatic. They may complain of pounding of the head or palpitations, which result from their awareness of the beating of a dilated left ventricle that undergoes a large volume change in systole, during either sinus beats or post-ectopic beats. The main symptoms of severe aortic regurgitation result from elevated pulmonary venous pressures and include dyspnea on exertion, orthopnea, and paroxysmal nocturnal dyspnea. When congestive heart failure occurs, patients complain of fatigue and weakness. Angina pectoris occurs in 20% of such patients and may be present even if the coronary arteries are normal. Angina associated with syphilitic aortic regurgitation may be due to associated ostial stenosis of the coronary arteries. In such patients, angina often occurs at rest and is difficult to control.

Physical findings. A variety of interesting but not very useful signs may be present in patients with chronic severe aortic regurgitation. These include de Musset's sign (bobbing of the head with each heartbeat), Traube's sign (pistol-shot sound heard over the femoral artery), Duroziez's sign (systolic murmur over the femoral artery when it is compressed proximally and diastolic murmur when it is compressed distally), and Quincke's pulse (capillary pulsations that can be detected by pressing a glass slide on the patient's lip or transmitting a light through the patient's fingertips).

The arterial pulse is very characteristic and consists of an abrupt distention with a rapid rise and a quick collapse (Corrigan's pulse). The arterial pulse may be bisferious, a double impulse during systole that signifies severe aortic regurgitation (Chapter 3). The systolic arterial pressure is increased, the diastolic pressure is reduced, and the Korotkoff's sounds persist down to 0 mm Hg. Even in such instances, however, the recorded intra-arterial pressure rarely falls below 30 mm Hg. The vasoconstriction that occurs in the presence of severe heart failure may result in some elevation of the arterial diastolic pressure. The jugular venous pressure is normal except in heart failure and in instances in which the greatly dilated ascending aorta obstructs the superior vena cava.

On inspection, the chest may rock and the cardiac impulse may be visible. The cardiac impulse is hyperdynamic. There may be a systolic thrill at the base of the heart, over the carotids, and in the suprasternal notch. This results from a large left ventricular stroke volume across a diseased aortic valve. A diastolic thrill signifies severe aortic regurgitation. The first heart sound is usually soft, because the mitral valve leaflets are close to each other at the onset of systole, or, if valve closure is premature, the valve is closed. This is exaggerated if the P–R interval is prolonged. The S_2 is usually single because the aortic valve does not close properly, or because the left ventricular ejection time is prolonged, and the P_2 may not be heard. Often, a systolic ejection murmur that is sometimes very loud is present. The sine qua non of aortic regurgitation is an early or immediate decrescendo diastolic murmur beginning after the S_2. It is best heard with the diaphragm of the stethoscope at the left sternal border, or, in difficult instances, by having the patient sit up and lean forward and by auscultating in held respiration at the end of a deep expiration. In severe aortic regurgitation, the murmur may be holodiastolic. When it is soft, its intensity can be increased by doing isometric exercise, for example, a handgrip, which increases aortic diastolic pressure. At times, this murmur is better heard along the right sternal border, which should draw attention to the possibility that the cause of the aortic regurgitation is aortic root disease. Classically, rupture of the sinus of Valsalva into the right heart chambers produces a continuous murmur.

In many patients with severe aortic regurgitation, an Austin Flint murmur is present in presystole and/or mid-diastole (Chapter 3). Two inferences can be drawn from the presence of an Austin Flint murmur: (1) It signifies that the aortic regurgitation is severe, and (2) it requires that associated mitral stenosis be excluded. The most helpful sign at the bedside is the response of the murmur to the inhalation of amyl nitrite. The vasodilatation produced by amyl nitrite increases forward flow, reduces the regurgitant volume, and results in the Austin Flint murmur becoming much softer or disappearing. On the other hand, the increased cardiac output and the tachycardia accentuate or increase the murmur of mitral stenosis. Alternatively, echocardiography can easily demonstrate the presence of organic mitral stenosis.

Chest radiograph. The left ventricle is increased in size, and this can be appreciated on the chest x-ray by an increase in the cardiothoracic ratio (Fig. 16-2). Since the upper limit of normal of the cardiothoracic ratio is 0.49, many patients with increased left ventricular size have an enlarged ventricular volume and still have a cardiothoracic ratio within the normal range. The ascending aorta is dilated, and there may be calcium in the aortic valve. There might be evidence of an enlarged left atrium and an increased left atrial and pulmonary venous pressure, which are manifested in the pulmonary vascular shadows by a redistribution of blood flow, pulmonary congestion, and pulmonary edema.

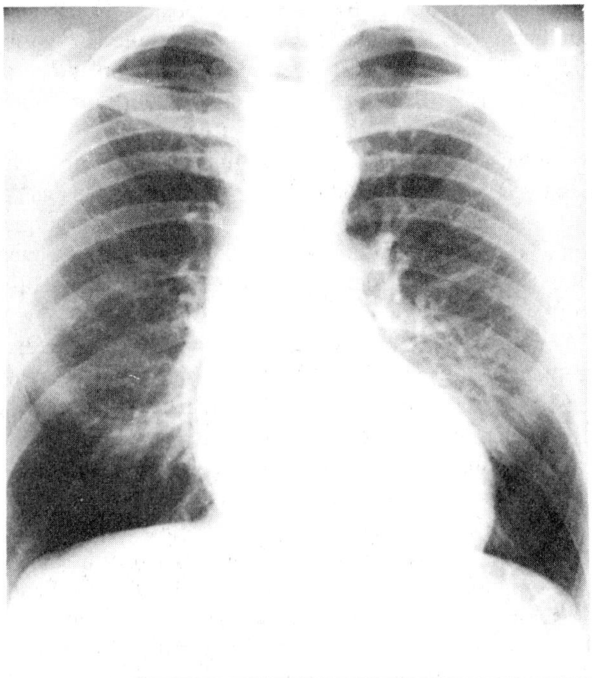

A

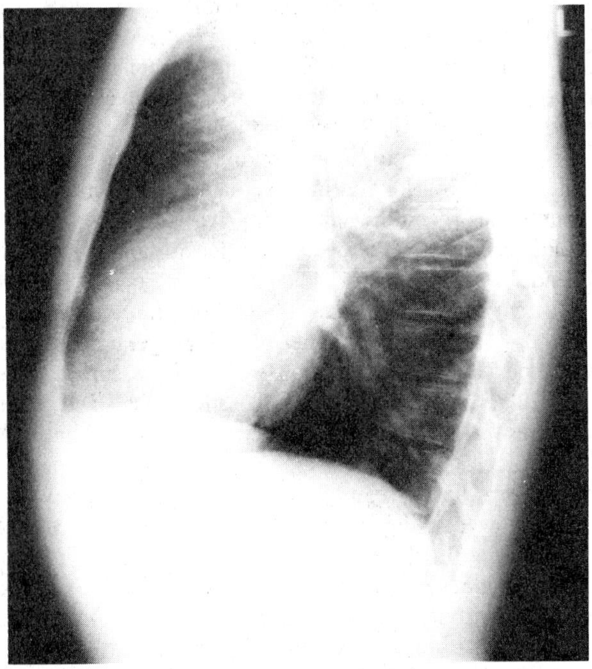

B

Fig. 16-2. Chest radiograph in the frontal (**A**) and left lateral (**B**) projection in a patient with severe aortic regurgitation. The ascending aorta and left ventricle are enlarged.

Electrocardiogram. The ECG shows left ventricular hypertrophy with or without associated secondary ST-T wave changes. In a small percentage of patients, ECG evidence of left ventricular hypertrophy is absent in spite of severe aortic regurgitation. Conduction abnormalities, such as left bundle branch block or right bundle branch block with or without axis deviation, may be present. The P–R interval may be prolonged, particularly in patients with ankylosing spondylitis. The rhythm is usually sinus. The presence of atrial fibrillation should make one suspect the presence of associated mitral valve disease or heart failure.

Special laboratory studies. The sign of aortic regurgitation on echocardiography is diastolic fluttering of the anterior leaflet of the mitral valve (Chapter 5). Echocardiography is of particular value for excluding the presence of associated mitral stenosis in patients with an Austin Flint diastolic murmur. Left ventricular dimensions are increased, and if ventricular function is normal, the percentage of dimensional shortening is normal. Because of the increase in left ventricular dimensions caused by the volume overload, there is separation between the open anterior leaflet of the mitral valve and the endocardial surface of the interventricular septum (septal–E point separation), but this does not necessarily indicate impaired left ventricular function when aortic regurgitation is present. In aortic regurgitation, as in other volume-overloaded lesions, the response in mild volume overload is an elongation of the heart. Since M mode echocardiography takes a pencil look at the short axis of the heart, left ventricular dimensions by M-mode echocardiography may appear to be normal. 2D echocardiography (Chapter 5) is much superior to the M-mode technique for assessing left ventricular volumes and systolic function in such patients. A dilated ascending aorta can be detected on echocardiography and so can an enlarged left atrium. Aortic valve vegetations suggest infective endocarditis. Some unusual conditions can easily be detected by echocardiography, for example, prolapse of the aortic leaflet into the left ventricle in diastole. Doppler echocardiography (Chapter 5) is useful for diagnosing and assessing the severity of aortic regurgitation. There is a significant incidence of false positives in the mild grade. There is also an overlap between the various grades of severity of assessment of aortic regurgitation by Doppler when compared to angiography.

Cardiac catheterization allows the measurement of intracardiac and intravascular pressures and cardiac output both at rest and on exercise and demonstrates the changes described under Abnormal Physiology, p. 207. In addition, other valvular diseases, for example mitral stenosis, aortic stenosis, and mitral regurgitation, can be excluded. Left ventricular angiography demonstrates enlarged left ventricular volumes and allows the calculation of ejection fraction. Angiography performed with injection of contrast medium in the ascending aorta demonstrates aortic regurgitation and allows a semiquantitative assessment of the degree of aortic regurgitation (Chapter 6). In addition, the angiogram demonstrates the dimension of the aortic root and the state of the ascending aorta. Selective coronary angiography allows assessment of the site, severity, and extent of associated obstructive coronary artery disease and should be performed in patients with angina, those with left ventricular systolic dysfunction, those with risk factors for coronary artery disease, and those 35 years of age or older who are being considered for surgery.

Gated blood pool radionuclide scans also allow the measurement of left ventricular volumes and ejection fraction. In addition, with this technique, it is now possible to quantify the amount of aortic regurgitation. However, these scans assess regurgitation present at both the aortic and mitral valves. Thus, if both valves are incompetent, the total amount of regurgitation present at both valves will be evaluated. This technique also allows measurement of left ventricular ejection fraction on exercise and on serial studies.

A treadmill exercise test provides an objective assessment of the degree of functional impairment and documentation of arrhythmias related to exertion.

Ambulatory ECG recording may be needed in an occasional patient suspected of having an arrhythmia.

Natural history and prognosis

Patients with mild aortic regurgitation that does not progress should have a normal life expectancy. Their major risk is the development of infective endocarditis and further valve destruction. Patients with moderate aortic regurgitation, if their disease does not progress, would be expected to have a life expectancy that is reasonably close to the normal range. However, the disease does progress, and mortality at the end of 10 years appears to be about 15%.

Patients with severe aortic regurgitation are known to have a long asymptomatic period before the condition is discovered. In asymptomatic patients with normal left ventricular function at rest, symptoms and/or left ventricular dysfunction and/or sudden death developed at the rate of less than 4% per year. The predictor of development of symptoms is left ventricular systolic dysfunction at rest. In those with normal left ventricular systolic function at rest, the predictors are an increased left ventricular size (left ventricular dimension at end-diastole of $\geq$ 70 mm, at end-systole of $\geq$ 50 mm, and left ventricular end-diastolic volume index of $\geq$ 150 ml/m^2) and abnormal left-ventricular ejection fraction on exercise of $<$ 0.50. Sudden death in asymptomatic patients appears to occur only in those with a massively dilated left ventricle (left ventricular end-diastolic dimension of $\geq$ 80 mm). It is likely that left ventricular dysfunction first appears on exercise and later also at rest; eventually, heart failure ensues. However, severe symptoms may occur even when left ventricular systolic pump function is normal at rest. The 5-year mortality of symptomatic patients with severe aortic regurgitation is about 25% and the 10-year mortality averages 50%. Once symptoms occur in patients with aortic regurgitation, it is likely that the rate of deterioration will be rapid. Most patients with angina are dead within 4 years. The 2- to 3-year mortality of those in heart failure is 50% to 70%. The overall 5-year and 10-year mortalities after appearance of mild to moderate symptoms without overt heart failure are approximately 30% and 50% respectively.

Management

All patients with aortic regurgitation need antibiotic prophylaxis to prevent infective endocarditis (Chapter 15). Patients with aortic regurgitation of a rheumatic origin need antibiotic prophylaxis to prevent recurrences of rheumatic carditis (Chapter 316). Patients with syphilitic aortic regurgitation need a course of antibiotics to treat syphilis.

Patients with mild aortic regurgitation need no specific therapy. They do not need to restrict their activities and can lead a normal life. Patients with moderate aortic regurgitation also usually need no specific therapy. However, these patients should avoid heavy physical exertion, competitive sports, and isometric exercise.

Patients with severe aortic regurgitation need medical treatment and eventually surgical treatment, which usually consists of valve replacement. Medical treatment consists of the administration of digitalis, diuretics, and vasodilators. Digitalis acts by increasing myocardial contractility, often reducing end-diastolic volume while increasing the ejection fraction and also the cardiac output if it is reduced in the resting state. Digitalis is clearly indicated in patients with symptoms. The need for and benefits of this therapy in asymptomatic patients have not been well documented. Diuretics are of value when the left atrial pressure is elevated and in the presence of congestive heart failure.

Vasodilators are either arterial, venous, or both. Vasodilators act by reducing the peripheral arterial resistance, which favors forward cardiac output and reduces regurgitant volume; initially, the total left ventricular stroke volume remains unchanged. If the left atrial pressure is elevated and left ventricular ejection fraction reduced, vasodilators frequently result in an improvement in both.

The value of long-term vasodilators in asymptomatic patients has been evaluated in two placebo-controlled randomized trials. Hydralazine produced modest reduction of end-diastolic volume and increase in ejection fraction; however, because of side effects, long-term compliance was poor. A calcium-channel blocking agent, nifedipine, produced significant reduction in blood pressure and left ventricular end-diastolic volume and mass, and major increases in left ventricular ejection fraction. Almost all patients completed the trial. All asymptomatic patients with severe aortic regurgitation should be treated with a vasodilator (calcium channel blocking agent, nifedipine) and digitalis. Long-term hydralazine therapy in symptomatic patients results in significant benefit in 20% to 35% of patients. Vasodilators are indicated in patients who refuse surgery or are not operative candidates for any reason. It is also indicated for short-term therapy in patients awaiting valve replacement to optimize their hemodynamics (reduce filling pressures and increase cardiac output) and thus reduce their operative risks.

Vasodilators are of considerable short-term benefit in patients in functional classes III and IV but ideally should be started after the institution of hemodynamic monitoring, that is, measurement of pulmonary artery wedge pressure and cardiac output with the use of balloon flotation catheters. Hemodynamic monitoring identifies patients who need the therapy, whereas clinical judgments can be wrong. It establishes whether arterial dilators alone will suffice or additional venodilators are needed. Finally, it provides information on the optimum dosage of vasodilator therapy. After the initial hemodynamic measurements are made, arterial dilators are given in progressively increasing dosage until an optimum effect on cardiac output has been obtained. If cardiac output does not show any further increase but left atrial pressure is still very high, additional venodilator therapy should be given. If the patient is very ill or the hemodynamic abnormalities are marked, intravenous therapy (for example, sodium nitroprusside) may be the vasodilator of first choice. Recent data show that small doses of hydralazine (≤50 mg) are without therapeutic effect and that larger doses (≥150 mg) need to be given only twice daily. The twice-daily regimen reduces the incidence of side effects and can be expected to improve patient compliance. Alternatively, patients can be given angiotensin-converting enzyme inhibitors.

Patients with severe chronic aortic regurgitation need valve replacement. The correct timing of surgical therapy has not been fully clarified. Valve replacement should be performed before irreversible left ventricular dysfunction occurs. However, the major problem is identifying the precise point at which left ventricular dysfunction will occur. Here, two major difficulties are encountered: (1) Patients may already have impaired left ventricular systolic pump function at rest when they first present or at the time of the first symptom; and (2) patients with severe symptoms may have normal left ventricular systolic pump function. Patients may be in functional class III (symptoms with less than ordinary activity), with a normal left ventricular ejection fraction, or they may be in functional class I (asymptomatic), with a reduced left ventricular ejection fraction. A reduced ejection fraction by 2D echocardiography and/or radionuclide ventriculography are the best noninvasive indicators of depressed systolic ventricular function (Chapter 5).

Decisions about surgery in aortic regurgitation should be based on the functional class and on the left ventricular ejection fraction at rest. Patients with chronic severe aortic regurgitation who are in functional class III or IV (symptoms at rest) need valve replacement. Benefit from valve replacement has been demonstrated even when the left ventricular ejection fraction is 0.25 or less. As opposed to aortic stenosis, in which no lower level of ejection fraction indicates inoperability, it is likely that some patients with aortic regurgitation and a low ejection fraction will become inoperable. This level has not been precisely defined but may be about 0.15 or less. Patients who are in functional class II (symptoms with ordinary activity) and those who have impaired left ventricular systolic pump function (reduced ejection fraction) at rest should be offered valve replacement. Although there is some disagreement about recommending valve replacement to patients with normal ejection fraction who are in functional class II, we would do so. Although the issue is controversial in some countries, we believe that patients who are in functional class I and have a reduced ejection fraction at rest should be offered aortic valve replacement. If the ejection fraction is normal at rest, one should consider valve replacement in class I patients if the left ventricle is huge (left ventricular end-diastolic volume ≥150 ml/m^2, left ventricular internal dimension on M-mode echocardiogram of ≥70 mm at end diastole, ≥50 mm at end systole) and/or the left ventricular ejection fraction shows a new, persistent reduction to ≤0.54 to 0.60, if the patients have reduced exercise capacity on treadmill testing, or if ambulatory ECG monitoring demonstrates ventricular tachyarrhythmias. It is suggested that such patients undergo an exercise test with right heart catheterization, and valve replacement is recommended if the pulmonary artery wedge pressure on exercise is greater than or equal to 20-24 mm Hg. Patients with associated significant coronary artery disease should have coronary bypass surgery performed at the time of valvular surgery.

Aortic valve replacement, with or without associated coronary bypass surgery for obstructive coronary disease, can be performed at many surgical centers with an operative mortality of 5% or less. If aortic valve replacement is successful and uncomplicated, left ventricular volume and hypertrophy regress but do not return to normal. Impaired left ventricular systolic pump function improves postoperatively in 50% or more of the patients; recent data show improvement is more likely to occur if left ventricular dysfunction was present preoperatively for 12-14 months or less. Even if left ventricular systolic pump function does not improve, there is a reduction in end-diastolic volume and hypertrophy; from a cardiac point of view, this is advantageous to the patient. The 5-year survival of patients undergoing aortic valve replacement in severe aortic regurgitation is 85% (includes operative and late cardiac deaths). The 5-year survival of patients with a left ventricular ejection fraction of 0.45 or greater is 87% versus 54% in patients with an ejection fraction less than 0.45. Late survival after valve replacement for chronic severe aortic regurgitation is best predicted by variables indicative of left ventricular systolic pump function.

Recently, new techniques of aortic valve repair are being developed and evaluated. Eventually, it is possible that some patients may need to have valve repair rather than valve replacement for aortic regurgitation.

ACUTE AORTIC REGURGITATION

Etiology

Infective endocarditis is the usual etiology of acute aortic regurgitation. It may also be caused by aortic dissection and trauma to the heart. Severe systemic hypertension is often associated with transient aortic regurgitation, which disappears as the blood pressure is brought under control.

Abnormal physiology

The major difference between acute and chronic severe aortic regurgitation is the extent of left ventricular enlargement. The left ventricle is large in chronic aortic regurgitation but is only somewhat dilated in patients with acute aortic regurgitation. However, there is a limit to how much the left ventricle can increase its volume acutely (probably no more than 20% to 30%) and the left ventricle often appears normal both on physical examination and on the chest x-ray. Nevertheless, the increase in left ventricular volume is inadequate for the amount of regurgitation. Since the left ventricle is only slightly increased in size, the increase in left ventricular stroke volume is limited even if the ejection fraction is increased. Most of the left ventricular stroke volume is regurgitated back into the left ventricle; as a result, the forward stroke volume to the body and the cardiac output may be severely compromised in spite of a marked compensatory sinus tachycardia. An acute increase in left ventricular end-diastolic volume results in a marked increase in left ventricular end-diastolic pressure, because the left ventricle is operating on the steep portion of the diastolic pressure-volume curve. If, in addition, the left atrial pressure is normal or mildly increased, the mitral valve may close prematurely. If the left atrial pressure rises considerably, pulmonary edema and passive pulmonary hypertension commonly occur. Compensatory tachycardia is the rule; it helps to shorten diastole, hence the time available for aortic regurgitation to occur, and attempts to maintain the cardiac output. The left ventricular and aortic systolic pressure remain normal. The aortic diastolic pressure cannot fall below the elevated left ventricular end-diastolic pressure, and thus the arterial pulse pressure may be in the normal range. It is important to recognize that left ventricular systolic pump function is frequently normal in these patients at least in the initial stages.

Clinical manifestations

The patient may have a history of trauma and exhibit the clinical features of infective endocarditis. Usually, however, the symptoms of heart failure are predominant.

On physical examination, these patients have tachycardia. The peripheral pulse shows a rapid rate of rise in arterial pressure, but the systolic pressure is normal. The diastolic pressure is normal or even reduced, and the pulse pressure is often normal. Thus, although the classic peripheral signs of chronic severe aortic regurgitation are often absent, an important diagnostic clue is the rapid rate of rise of arterial pressure. If there is frank congestive heart failure, the usual clinical manifestations of heart failure are present. The left ventricle is often hyperkinetic. The S_1 is soft; the S_2 is soft and often single. There is usually a loud diastolic gallop (S_3). An aortic systolic murmur is often present, and the classic early or immediate diastolic murmur of aortic regurgitation is present. An Austin Flint murmur may be heard.

The ECG often shows nonspecific ST-T wave changes and a sinus tachycardia. However, the ECG may be normal. The chest radiograph shows that the cardiothoracic ratio may be within the normal range. The aorta is not dilated unless aortic root disease or dissection of the aorta is the cause of the acute regurgitation. The lung fields show the signs of increased pulmonary venous pressure and of pulmonary edema.

One must be aware of the typical clinical picture of patients with gross acute aortic regurgitation in severe heart failure to recognize it. These patients are often intravenous drug abusers and have marked sinus tachycardia and pulmonary edema. However, an aortic diastolic murmur may be absent or difficult to appreciate, which often causes the diagnosis to be missed. The chest x-ray shows a "normal" heart size with pulmonary edema. The important diagnostic clues include (1) a peripheral arterial pulse that has a rapid rate of rise and fall, even though the pulse pressure is small; (2) the telltale signs of intravenous drug abuse; and (3) "normal" heart size with pulmonary edema on chest x-ray.

Echocardiography shows the diastolic flutter of the anterior leaflet of the mitral valve. In addition, the echocardiogram may show vegetations on the aortic valve, prolapse of an aortic valve leaflet into the left ventricle in diastole, and premature mitral valve closure. The mitral valve may be seen to open for only a short time because the stroke volume is limited. Occasionally, the aortic valve leaflets have been totally destroyed, and none is seen on the echocardiogram. Doppler can easily demonstrate the aortic regurgitation and provides an estimate of its severity. For detection of dissection of the aorta, transesophageal echocardiography/Doppler is overall probably the best of the noninvasive tests for most patients, however, magnetic resonance imaging has the highest specificity and should be used in stable patients if the diagnosis has not been already made. Cardiac catheterization and angiography show the abnormal physiology described, and aortography shows gross aortic regurgitation. A radionuclide gated blood pool scan may be helpful in demonstrating normal left ventricular ejection fraction and a mild increase in left ventricular volumes.

The natural history of this condition is variable. If the aortic regurgitation is mild to moderate in severity, these patients are likely to do well with medical therapy. Eventually, the changes of chronic aortic regurgitation will be seen. In patients with severe aortic regurgitation, the natural history depends on whether they have heart failure. If heart failure is present, which is common, the prognosis is very poor.

Management

The underlying cause of the regurgitation must be treated, which often is difficult. In patients with infective endocarditis, the appropriate antibiotic therapy has to be given. If the aortic regurgitation is mild, no other specific therapy may be needed. If aortic regurgitation is moderate, digitalis therapy is advisable; vasodilators may be beneficial. Aortic regurgitation caused by dissection of the aorta is an indication for surgery regardless of the degree of regurgitation.

For patients with severe aortic regurgitation, the choices

of medical therapy include digitalis, diuretics, and vasodilators. Patients with heart failure should be given digitalis, diuretics, and vasodilators. In patients with moderate or severe heart failure, despite medical therapy, aortic valve replacement is indicated. If the patient responds dramatically to digitalis, diuretics, and vasodilators, surgical therapy often can be delayed until heart failure and the infection (when caused by endocarditis) are controlled, and the patient is in a more stable condition. If the patient does not respond immediately and dramatically to therapy, valve replacement should not be delayed, even if the infection is uncontrolled or the patient has had little antibiotic therapy.

MITRAL STENOSIS

Etiology

Mitral stenosis is an obstruction to blood flow between the left atrium and the left ventricle caused by abnormal mitral valve function. Congenital mitral stenosis is uncommon. It is usually caused by a "parachute" deformity of the valve in which shortened chordae tendineae insert in a large, single papillary muscle. In virtually all adult patients, the cause of mitral stenosis is previous rheumatic carditis. However, about 60% of patients with rheumatic mitral valve disease do not give a history of rheumatic fever or chorea, and about 50% of patients with acute rheumatic carditis do not eventually have clinical valvular heart disease. Mitral stenosis, usually rheumatic, in association with atrial septal defect is called *Lutembacher's syndrome*. A rare cause of mitral stenosis is massive mitral valve anular calcification. This process occurs most frequently in elderly women and produces mitral stenosis by limiting leaflet motion. The degree of stenosis, when present, is usually mild. Other causes of obstruction to left atrial outflow include a left atrial myxoma, massive left atrial ball thrombus, and cor triatriatum, in which a congenital membrane is present in the left atrium.

Pathology

In temperate climates and developed countries, there is usually a long interval (an average of 20 years) between an episode of rheumatic carditis and the clinical presentation of symptomatic mitral stenosis. In tropical and subtropical climates and in less developed countries, the latent period is often shorter, and mitral stenosis may occur during childhood or adolescence. The pathologic hallmark of rheumatic carditis is Aschoff's nodule. The most common lesion of acute rheumatic endocarditis is mitral valvulitis. The mitral valve has vegetations along the line of closure and chordae tendineae. Mitral regurgitation may be present during the acute episode.

Mitral stenosis is usually the result of repeated episodes of carditis alternating with healing and is characterized by the deposition of fibrous tissue. Ultimately, the deformed valve is subject to nonspecific fibrosis and calcification. Lesions along the line of closure result in fusion of the commissures and contracture and thickening of the valve leaflets. The chordal lesions are manifested as shortening and fusion of these structures. The combination of commissural fusion, valve leaflet contracture, and chordae tendineae fusion results in a narrow, funnel-shaped orifice, which restricts the flow of blood from the left atrium to the left ventricle. The rapidity with which patients become symptomatic with this lesion may depend on the number and severity of repeated bouts of rheumatic valvulitis. Frequently, the rheumatic episodes are not clinically apparent.

In pure mitral stenosis, the left ventricle is usually normal, but there may be evidence of previous carditis with deposition of fibrous tissue. The left atrium is enlarged and hypertrophied as a consequence of left atrial hypertension. Mural thrombi are often found in the left atrium, particularly if atrial fibrillation has been present. Calcification of the mitral valve frequently also involves the mitral anulus.

Abnormal physiology

The pathophysiologic features of mitral stenosis all result from obstruction of the flow of blood between the left atrium and the left ventricle. With reduction in valve area, energy is lost to friction during the transport of blood from the left atrium to the left ventricle. Accordingly, a pressure gradient is present across the stenotic valve. The relationship between valve area, cardiac output, flow period, and average diastolic gradient between the left atrium and the left ventricle is defined by the formula of Gorlin and Gorlin (Chapter 6).

It is readily apparent that maintaining cardiac output when the valve area is small requires a high gradient and thus elevated left atrial pressure. Similarly, an increased demand for cardiac output, such as occurs during exercise or in pregnancy, results in an increase in gradient and high left atrial pressures. More subtle is the effect of the length of the flow period on the relationship between output and gradient. The time available for diastole is that part of the cardiac cycle not taken up by isovolumetric contraction and relaxation or by ejection. As the heart rate increases, the total amount of time spent during systole increases despite a reduction in the systolic time per beat. Thus, time available for diastole decreases as the heart rate increases. Because blood can flow through the mitral valve only during diastole, the flow rate is inversely proportional to the flow period at a constant cardiac output. Of course, a higher flow rate results in a greater loss of energy to friction and requires a larger gradient and higher left atrial pressures.

The pressure gradient between the left atrium and the left ventricle, which increases markedly with increased heart rate or cardiac output, is responsible for left atrial hypertension. The left atrium gradually enlarges and hypertrophies. Pulmonary venous pressure rises with left atrial pressure and is passively associated with an increase in pulmonary arterial pressure. In up to 20% of patients, the pulmonary vascular resistance is also elevated, which further increases pulmonary artery pressure. Pulmonary arterial hypertension results in right ventricular hypertrophy and right ventricular enlargement. The changes in right ventricular function eventually result in right atrial hypertension and enlargement and in systemic congestion.

Pulmonary venous hypertension alters lung function in several ways. Distribution of blood flow in the lung is altered, with a relative increase in flow to the upper lobes and therefore in physiologic dead space. Pulmonary compliance generally decreases with increasing pulmonary capillary pressure, adding to the work of breathing, particularly during exercise. Chronic changes in the pulmonary capillaries and pulmonary arteries include fibrosis and thickening. These changes protect the lungs from transudation of fluid into the alveoli (pulmonary edema). Indeed, it is not uncommon to find patients with severe mitral stenosis whose resting pulmonary artery wedge pressure (indirect left atrial pressure) exceeds 30 mm Hg. However, capillary and alveolar thickening further add to the abnormalities of ventilation and perfusion. Pulmonary vascular changes result in increasingly elevated pulmonary vascular resistance.

In some patients with high pulmonary vascular resistance and right ventricular dysfunction, cardiac output may be low. The body maintains oxygen consumption by extracting more oxygen from the arterial blood, and mixed venous oxygen content falls. The hemoglobin oxygen dissociation curve is shifted to the right, facilitating the unloading of oxygen from hemoglobin to the tissues. The reduced cardiac output results in surprisingly small gradients across the mitral valve despite severe stenosis. Although pulmonary congestion may be less striking in these patients, the cardiac output does not increase normally with exercise, and, typically, the patients are severely limited by fatigue.

Long-standing mitral stenosis with severe pulmonary hypertension and resultant right ventricular dysfunction may be accompanied by chronic systemic venous hypertension. Tricuspid regurgitation is frequently present, even in the absence of intrinsic disease of this valve. Functional pulmonic regurgitation may also be present. Dependent edema formation and visceral congestion directly reflect elevated venous pressure and salt and water retention. Chronic passive congestion in the liver leads to central lobular necrosis and eventually cirrhosis.

Clinical manifestations

History. An asymptomatic interval is usually present between the initiating event of acute rheumatic fever and the presentation of symptomatic mitral stenosis. During this interval, the patient feels well. Initially, there is little or no gradient at rest, but with increased cardiac output, left atrial pressure rises, and exertional dyspnea develops. As mitral valve obstruction increases, dyspnea occurs at lower work levels. The progression of disability is so subtle and so protracted that many patients adapt by circumscribing their lifestyles. It becomes imperative, then, to document what activities the patient can perform without symptoms, and at what activity level symptoms begin; failure to do this often results in an underestimation of disability.

As obstruction progresses, the patients note orthopnea and nocturnal dyspnea that apparently results from redistribution of blood to the thorax on assuming the supine position. With severe mitral stenosis and elevated pulmonary vascular resistance, fatigue rather than dyspnea may be the predominant symptom. Dependent edema, nausea, anorexia, and right upper quadrant pain reflect systemic venous congestion resulting from right heart failure.

Palpitations are a frequent complaint in mitral stenosis and may represent frequent premature atrial contractions or paroxysmal atrial fibrillation. Of patients with severe symptomatic mitral stenosis, 50% or more have chronic atrial fibrillation. Paroxysmal atrial fibrillation may produce pulmonary edema in some patients with mitral stenosis. The acute increase in left atrial pressure that produces pulmonary edema results both from a decrease in the diastolic flow period caused by increased heart rate and from a loss of atrial transport function.

Systemic embolism, a frequent complication of mitral stenosis, may result in stroke, occlusion of extremity arterial supply, occlusion of the aortic bifurcation, or visceral or myocardial infarction. Atrial fibrillation, increasing age of the patient, increasing left atrial size, and a previous history of embolism are associated with an increased incidence of systemic embolism. Hemoptysis may result from increased pulmonary venous pressure. Blood streaking of pulmonary edema fluid may result, or hemoptysis may be severe and, rarely, life-threatening. Pulmonary embolism, which is more common in patients with heart failure, also may cause hemoptysis.

Exertional chest pain, typical of angina pectoris, may be present in some patients with severe mitral stenosis but normal coronary arteries. Severe pulmonary hypertension has been postulated as a cause. Infective endocarditis is an uncommon complication of pure mitral stenosis.

Progression of symptoms in mitral stenosis is generally slow but relentless. Thus, a sudden change in symptoms rarely reflects a change in valve obstruction. Rather, there usually is a noncardiac precipitating event or paroxysmal atrial fibrillation. Fever, pregnancy, and noncardiac surgery, all of which increase cardiac output, can precipitate decompensation in patients with moderate to severe obstruction.

Physical findings. During the latent, presymptomatic interval, incidental physical findings may be normal or may provide evidence of mild mitral stenosis. Frequently, the only characteristic finding noted at rest will be a loud S_1 and a presystolic murmur. A short diastolic decrescendo rumble may be heard only with exercise. In patients with symptomatic mitral stenosis, the findings are more obvious, and careful physical examination usually leads to the correct diagnosis.

The general appearance of the patient in mitral stenosis is usually normal. The mitral stenosis facies, characterized by malar flush, is uncommon and is caused by peripheral cyanosis, which is usually associated with a low cardiac output and severe pulmonary hypertension. Tachypnea may be present if left atrial pressure is high. The jugular venous pressure may be normal or may show evidence of elevated right ventricular end diastolic pressure or tricuspid regurgitation (Chapter 3). Atrial fibrillation produces an irregular venous pulse with absent A waves. The arterial pulse is normal except for irregularity in atrial fibrillation and low volume when cardiac output is reduced. All peripheral pulses should be carefully examined because of the frequency of systemic embolism. The chest findings may be normal or may reveal signs of pulmonary congestion with rales or pleural fluid (dullness and absent breath sounds). Marked left atrial enlargement may produce egophony at the tip of the left scapula.

The precordium is usually unremarkable on inspection. On palpation, the apical impulse should feel normal. An abnormal left ventricular impulse suggests disease other than pure mitral stenosis. A diastolic thrill usually is appreciated only when the patient is examined in the left lateral decubitus position. When pulmonary hypertension is present, a sustained right ventricular lift along the left sternal border and pulmonic valve closure may be palpable. On auscultation in the supine position, the only abnormality appreciated may be the accentuated S_1. Failure to examine the patient in the left lateral decubitus position accounts for most of the misdiagnoses of symptomatic mitral stenosis. The diastolic rumble is heard best with the bell of the stethoscope applied at the apical impulse. Nevertheless, the murmur may be localized, and the region around the apical impulse also should be auscultated. The opening snap is heard best with the diaphragm and is often most easily appreciated midway between the apex and the left sternal border. In this intermediate region, the S_1, the pulmonary component of the second heart sound (P_2), and the opening snap can be identified.

The opening snap occurs after the left ventricular pressure falls below left atrial pressure in early diastole. When left atrial pressure is high, as in severe mitral stenosis, the snap occurs earlier in diastole. The converse is true with mild mitral stenosis. The interval between the A_2 and the opening snap varies from 40 to 120 ms. Although the opening snap is present in most cases of mitral stenosis, it is absent in patients with stiff, fibrotic or calcified leaflets. Thus, absence of the opening snap in severe mitral stenosis indicates that mitral valve replacement rather than commissurotomy may be necessary.

The diastolic rumble follows the opening snap. In some patients with low cardiac output or mild mitral stenosis, brief exercise, such as sit-ups or walking, is adequate to increase flow and bring out the murmur. The murmur is low pitched, rumbling, and decrescendo. In general, the more severe the mitral stenosis, the longer the murmur. Presystolic accentuation of the murmur occurs in sinus rhythm and has been reported even in atrial fibrillation. A diastolic rumble is not diagnostic of mitral stenosis (Chapter 3).

Systolic murmurs also may be heard in association with the murmur of mitral stenosis. A blowing holosystolic murmur at the apex suggests associated mitral regurgitation, whereas a systolic blowing murmur heard best at the lower left sternal border that increases with inspiration usually signifies tricuspid regurgitation. The Graham Steell murmur is a high-pitched diastolic decrescendo murmur of pulmonic regurgitation caused by pulmonary hypertension. In most patients with mitral stenosis, such a murmur usually indicates aortic regurgitation. In general, a left-sided third heart sound (S_3) is not compatible with important mitral stenosis, with the possible exception of concomitant severe aortic regurgitation and significant left ventricular systolic dysfunction. If an S_3 and a rumble are present, mitral regurgitation is usually the predominant lesion.

Chest radiograph. The posteroanterior and lateral chest films are often so typical that experienced clinicians can make the tentative diagnosis from the film before the history and physical examination are complete (Fig. 16-3). The thoracic cage is normal. The lung fields show evidence of elevated pulmonary venous pressure. Blood flow is redistributed to the upper lobes, resulting in prominence of upper lobe vascularity. Increased pulmonary venous pressure results in transudation of fluid into the interstitium. Accumulation of fluid in the interlobular septa produces linear streaks in the bases, which extend to the pleura (Kerley B lines). Interstitial fluid may also be seen as perivascular or peribronchial cuffing. With transudation of fluid into the alveolar spaces, pulmonary edema is seen. Chronic hemosiderin deposition results in an interstitial radiodensity that does not resolve after the relief of stenosis. Pulmonary hypertension results in enlargement of the main pulmonary trunk and right and left main pulmonary arteries. These changes are not specific for mitral stenosis but represent long-standing elevated left atrial pressure.

The cardiac silhouette usually does not show generalized cardiomegaly, but the left atrium is invariably enlarged. This is manifested in the posteroanterior film by a density behind the right atrial border (double atrial shadow), prominence of the left atrial appendage on the left heart border between the main pulmonary artery and left ventricular apex, and elevation of the left main bronchus. The lateral film shows the left atrium bulging posteriorly. The left ventricular silhouette is normal. The right ventricle may be enlarged if pulmonary hypertension has been present. Right ventricular enlargement is usually noted by filling of the retrosternal space but is an unreliable sign in adults. The combination of a normal-sized left ventricle, enlarged left atrium, and pulmonary congestion should immediately raise the possibility of mitral stenosis. Mitral valve calcification is occasionally seen on the plain chest film.

Electrocardiogram. The ECG is not usually as helpful as the chest x-ray. For patients in sinus rhythm, the widened P wave is caused by interatrial conduction delay and/or prolonged left atrial depolarization (Chapter 4). The P wave is broad and notched in lead II and biphasic in lead V_1, and measures 0.12 s or more. Atrial fibrillation is common. Left ventricular hypertrophy is almost never present unless there are associated lesions. Right ventricular hypertrophy may be present if pulmonary hypertension is marked.

Clinical indications of severe mitral stenosis. Some clinical features make it virtually certain that mitral stenosis is severe. These include (1) moderate to severe pulmonary hypertension as indicated by clinical and ECG evidence of right ventricular hypertrophy or pulmonary hypertension, or both, and/or (2) moderate to severe elevation of left atrial pressure as indicated by orthopnea, a short P_2-OS interval, a diastolic rumble that occupies the whole length of a long

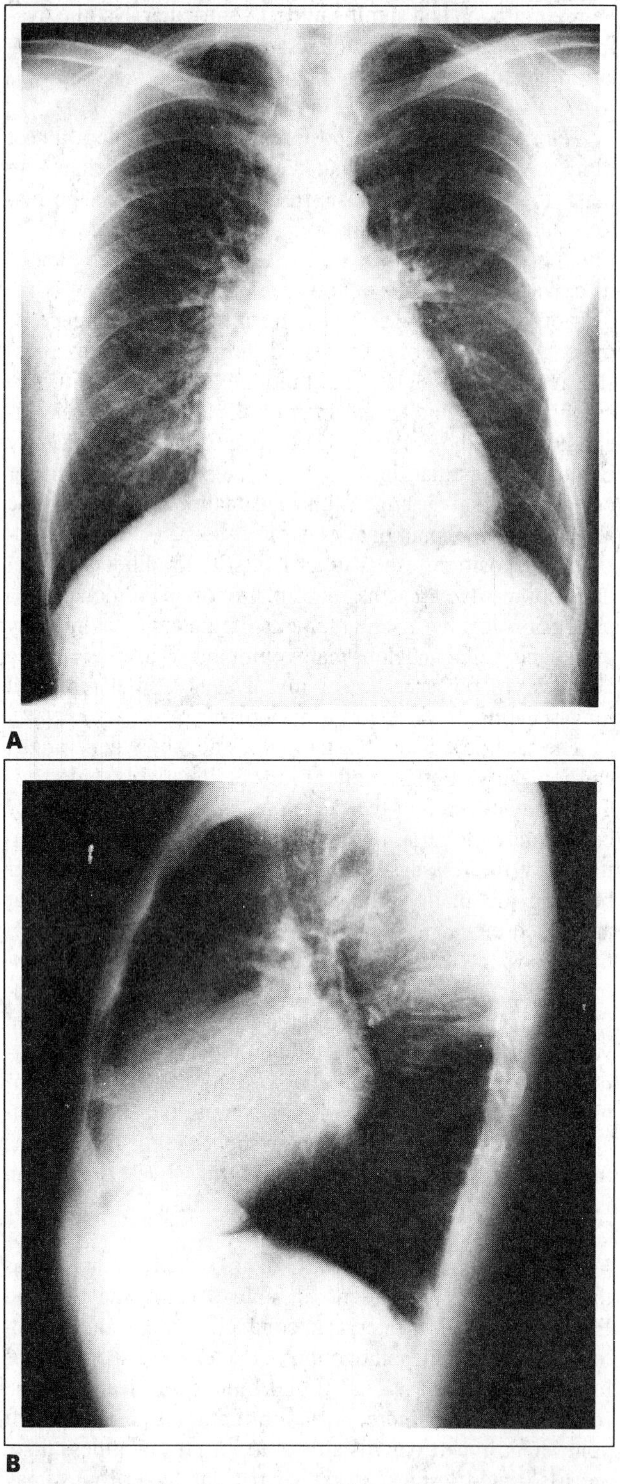

Fig. 16-3. Chest radiograph in the frontal (**A**) and left lateral (**B**) projection in a patient with severe mitral stenosis. Marked left atrial enlargement and pulmonary vascular engorgement are present in the absence of left ventricular enlargement.

diastolic interval in patients with atrial fibrillation, and pulmonary edema on the chest x-ray. In both these clinical circumstances, one must be certain that there is no other cause for the elevated left atrial pressure and that left atrial hypertension is not caused mainly by a correctable transient elevation of left ventricular diastolic pressure.

Special studies. Echocardiography has proved to be both sensitive and specific for mitral stenosis when adequate studies are done (Chapter 5). False positives and false negatives are uncommon. M-mode and 2D echocardiography do not reliably predict the severity of mitral stenosis. Doppler studies provide an estimate of mitral valve area that is within ± 0.4 cm^2 (prior to interventional therapy) of that obtained by cardiac catheterization. The echographic findings of mitral stenosis reflect the loss of normal valve function. The fusion of commissures results in movement of the anterior and posterior leaflets anteriorly in parallel during diastole. In patients in sinus rhythm, there is an absence of further opening of the valve that is normally seen with atrial contraction. Other findings include decreased E-to-F slope, decreased mitral valve leaflet excursion, and multiple echoes, indicating thickening or calcification of the valve. Left atrial enlargement is seen. Abnormal pulmonary valve motion and right ventricular enlargement may signify pulmonary hypertension.

Echocardiography is of great value in patients with equivocal signs, in patients with gross pulmonary hypertension, to differentiate mitral stenosis from an Austin Flint murmur of aortic regurgitation, and in the rare patient with "silent" mitral stenosis. It is used to assess left and right ventricular and atrial size and function, to evaluate the aortic and tricuspid valves, and to estimate pulmonary artery pressure.

In the majority of patients with disabling symptoms from presumed mitral stenosis, right and left heart catheterization should be performed as part of a preoperative assessment. Simultaneous measurement of cardiac output and the gradient between the left atrium and the left ventricle and calculation of valve area remain the "gold standard" for assessing the severity of mitral stenosis (Chapter 6). Left ventricular angiography assesses the competence of the mitral valve, an important determinant of operability for mitral commissurotomy. Quantification of left ventricular function provides a useful prognostic indicator of operative and late survival and of the expected functional result. Aortic and tricuspid valve function can be assessed when there is a question of coexisting lesions. Selective coronary arteriography establishes the site, severity, and extent of coronary artery disease and should be performed in patients with angina, in those with left ventricular systolic dysfunction, in those with risk factors for coronary artery disease, and in those 35 years of age or older who are being considered for surgery.

Natural history

The population presenting with mitral stenosis is changing because of the sharp decline in the incidence of acute rheumatic fever in the past 40 years. Native-born American citizens with symptomatic mitral stenosis are presenting at an older age. Young adults in the third and fourth decades with symptomatic mitral stenosis are more likely to come from low socioeconomic backgrounds and from the inner city or be immigrants, particularly from Latin America, Middle East, Southeast Asia, or the Orient. Therefore, the latent period between acute rheumatic fever and symptomatic mitral stenosis is variable and appears to be related to the presence of repeated streptococcal infection. Females with mitral stenosis outnumber males by almost 2:1. The most important feature of the asymptomatic interval, then, is the susceptibility to repeated bouts of both rheumatic valvulitis and streptococcal infection. The mechanism for the progression from no symptoms to mild to severe symptoms is progressive stenosis of the mitral valve.

With the onset of exertional dyspnea and fatigue, the valve area is usually reduced to one half to one third its normal size. Further small reductions in valve area markedly obstruct flow and result in symptoms with minimal exertion. The interval from initial mild symptoms to disabling symptoms may be 10 years. During this time, the patient is at little risk of death, permanent injury, or irreversible cardiac damage, except from atrial fibrillation with rapid ventricular rate resulting in pulmonary edema and from systemic embolus. Unfortunately, it is not possible to predict who is at risk of embolism. When functional class III symptoms are present, the valve area is usually 1.0 cm^2 or less, and both rest and exercise hemodynamics are deranged. Further small reductions in valve area result in symptoms at rest. The survival of patients with functional class III symptoms treated nonsurgically is markedly reduced, and fewer than 50% can be expected to survive 10 years and almost none with class IV symptoms will survive 10 years.

Management

Mitral stenosis can be prevented through two approaches. First, all streptococcal infections should be diagnosed and correctly treated. This prevents most initial episodes of acute rheumatic fever. Second, all patients with known previous acute rheumatic fever should receive appropriate antibiotic prophylaxis (Chapter 316).

Although the incidence of infective endocarditis is low, in isolated mitral stenosis, all patients exposed to bacteremia should receive appropriate prophylaxis against infective endocarditis (Chapter 15). Family and vocational planning should be considered. Women with this disease should consider bearing children before symptoms occur, since pregnancy is usually well tolerated with mild mitral stenosis. Occupations that require strenuous exertion in middle age and later should probably be avoided if possible. When patients reach the symptomatic threshold, medical treatment may be of some benefit. Digitalis offers no improvement for the patient with normal sinus rhythm and normal left ventricular function. When atrial fibrillation is present, however, digitalis plays a critical role in controlling ventricular rate. In selected patients beta-adrenergic blocking agents or diltiazem may be added to reduce exercise-induced severe tachycardia. Beta-adrenergic blocking agents should be used with great caution or not at all in patients with impaired left ventricular function or associated significant aortic stenosis. In my view, digoxin and diltiazem is probably the best combined therapy. Diuretics reduce pulmonary congestion and peripheral edema and allow most patients freedom from salt restriction. For the patient with mild symptoms, maintenance of sinus rhythm is desirable. Cardioversion of atrial fibrillation and maintenance of antiarrhythmic therapy with digitalis and quinidine should be offered to these patients. Anticoagulation is usually begun about 1-2 weeks in advance of cardioversion. Patients with chronic atrial fibrillation and those with a previous history of embolism should receive anticoagulation unless there is a specific contraindication.

Unless there is a contraindication, surgery should be recommended to a mitral stenosis patient with functional class III or IV symptoms. For younger patients with a pliable valve and without important mitral regurgitation, this means commissurotomy. Because of the low morbidity and mortality of mitral commissurotomy, surgery is also offered to these patients when functional class II symptoms are present. The results of successful commissurotomy are excellent, and surgical mortality is less than 1%. Late mortality at 10 years is less than 5%, the thromboembolism rate is 2% per year or less, and the reoperation rate ranges from 0.5 to 4.5% per year. The return of symptoms after commissurotomy usually is the result of an incomplete operation, other valvular lesions, or deterioration of myocardial function. In less-developed countries, excellent results have been reported in a very high percentage of patients for up to 25 years.

For the older patient with a stiff or calcified valve, or when moderate mitral regurgitation is present, mitral valve replacement is usually performed. Valve replacement carries a higher operative mortality than does commissurotomy (approximately 5%) and the morbidity that is associated with prostheses (see Prosthetic Valves, p. 229). Survival at 10 years after mitral valve replacement for functional class III and IV patients is better than 60% (Fig. 16-4).

Catheter balloon commissurotomy with use of the double balloon technique or the Inoue balloon produces immediate and 3-month hemodynamic and clinical results comparable to those obtained by surgical commissurotomy. The results of catheter balloon commissurotomy are greatly influenced by the characteristics of the valve and its supporting apparatus, which are best determined by 2D echocardiography. In the appropriate patient, in centers with skilled and experienced staff, catheter balloon commissurotomy is the procedure of first choice for relief of severe mitral stenosis.

MITRAL REGURGITATION

Etiology

Competent mitral valve function requires functioning of individual mitral leaflets, chordae tendineae, anulus, left atrium, papillary muscles, and supporting left ventricular segments. Disruption of the function of any of these elements can cause mitral valve regurgitation. The abnormalities causing mitral regurgitation reflect the multiple elements necessary for normal function. The valve leaflets are the most delicate components of this system, and disruption of leaflet substance invariably leads to important mitral regurgitation. For this reason, rheumatic fever, which most commonly attacks the mitral leaflets, has been a leading cause of mitral regurgitation. With the sharp decline in primary and secondary cases of rheumatic fever in this

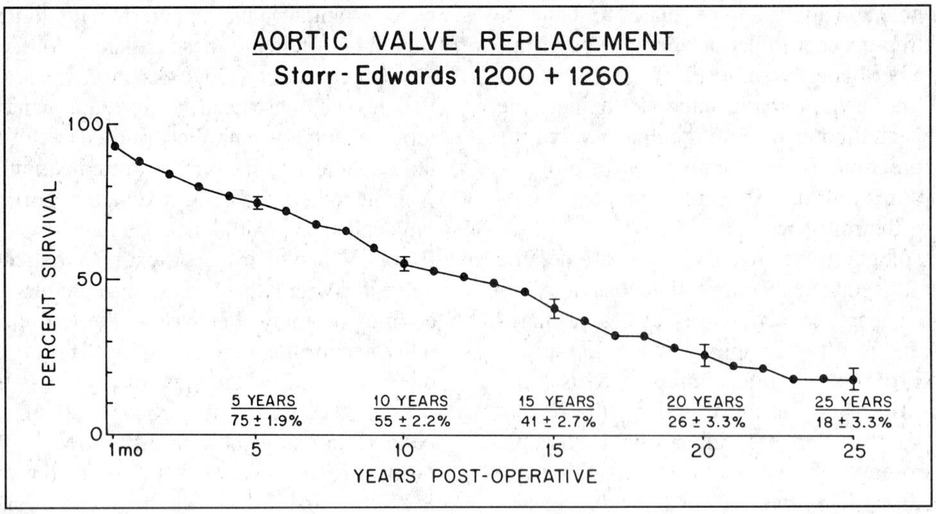

A

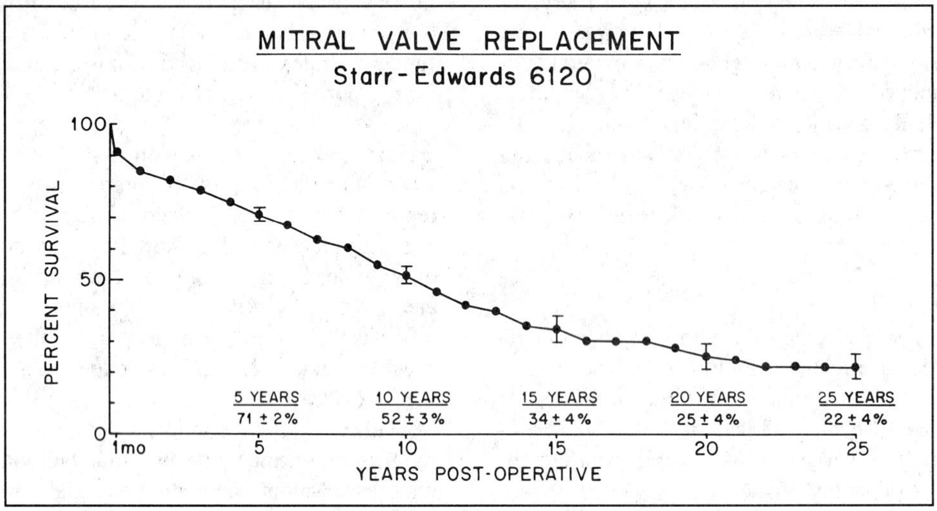

B

Fig. 16-4. Survival after aortic **(A)** or mitral **(B)** valve replacement with a non-cloth-covered, caged Silastic ball prosthesis. The numbers indicate percentages of survival with one standard error.

country, isolated mitral regurgitation caused by rheumatic disease requiring surgery is now less common.

Mitral valve prolapse (see Mitral Valve Prolapse, p. 223) is now one of the commonest causes of isolated mitral regurgitation requiring surgery. Rupture of chordae tendineae may occur in both rheumatic and prolapsing mitral valves and may result from trauma or endocarditis. In a substantial number of patients, however, the cause remains unknown. Mitral valve anular dilatation, which occurs in marked left ventricular and left atrial enlargement and in Marfan's syndrome, prevents normal coaptation of the leaflets, leading to mitral regurgitation. Idiopathic mitral anular calcification prevents the anulus from contracting normally during systole, again promoting regurgitation. There is a known association between mitral valve prolapse, anular calcification, and chordal rupture with or without Marfan's syndrome.

Left ventricular enlargement also impairs normal papillary muscle function by displacing the muscles laterally. The most common cause of papillary muscle dysfunction is coronary artery disease. Dysfunction may result from ischemia or necrosis of the muscles themselves or of the underlying left ventricular wall. Aneurysmal bulging of the left ventricle may also compromise papillary muscle function. Myocardial infarction is the usual setting in which papillary muscle rupture occurs and it results in catastrophic mitral regurgitation. Mitral regurgitation in hypertrophic cardiomyopathy is caused by the characteristic systolic anterior motion of the anterior leaflet of the mitral valve, which results in failure of adequate leaflet coaptation.

Congenital abnormalities of the mitral valve caused by abnormal development of the endocardial cushions and resultant cleft mitral valve may result in mitral regurgitation. Systemic illnesses may also affect the mitral valve leaflets. The most common of these are systemic lupus erythematosus, rheumatoid arthritis, and ankylosing spondylitis. Methysergide, a drug used to treat headaches, may cause leaflet thickening and regurgitation; the regurgitation may disappear on cessation of therapy. Infective endocarditis may also involve the valve leaflet primarily, causing leaflet perforation and mitral regurgitation.

Pathology

The pathology of mitral regurgitation is as varied as the causes. The changes caused by rheumatic fever and mitral valvulitis were reviewed in the section on mitral stenosis. The specific pathologic feature of rheumatic valvulitis that results in mitral regurgitation is loss of leaflet area through contracture. There is severe fibrosis and rigidity of the whole of the valvular apparatus. Unlike mitral stenosis, mitral regurgitation may be present from the initial episode of acute rheumatic fever. Commissural fusion is an unimportant feature of rheumatic mitral regurgitation. When it is present, mixed mitral stenosis and mitral regurgitation result. The regurgitation of blood into the left atrium during systole results in left atrial enlargement and hypertrophy. The left ventricle is also enlarged and hypertrophied to maintain the large left ventricular stroke volume.

Abnormal physiology

The fundamental abnormality of mitral regurgitation is that the left ventricle simultaneously ejects blood through two orifices, the aorta and the incompetent mitral valve. There are three direct results of this abnormality. First, the volume of blood that moves through the aortic valve, that is, the effective cardiac output, is less than the left ventricular stroke volume. This requires that the actual left ventricular end-diastolic and stroke volumes be increased to supply the normal circulatory demands. Second, the regurgitation of blood back into the left atrium during systole increases the volume, and therefore the pressure, of the left atrium. Third, the total impedance (left atrium and aorta) against which the left ventricle ejects is reduced. The reduction of impedance enhances left ventricular systolic pump function by allowing the ventricle to empty more rapidly early in systole and thereby decreases left ventricular radius and therefore wall stress. The reduction in stress permits greater shortening and, accordingly, stroke volume is increased for a given preload, aortic resistance, and myocardial contractility.

To compensate for the fraction of stroke volume lost to the left atrium, left ventricular stroke volume must be increased. As previously described, the reduction in impedance to ejection increases stroke volume. However, additional mechanisms are necessary. With acute valvular regurgitation, preload (sarcomere length) is increased. This mechanism, however, is sharply limited by the diastolic pressure-volume curve of the ventricle and pericardium. Thus, acute severe mitral regurgitation frequently results in high filling pressure and pulmonary edema. The chronic adaptation to volume overload uses increased numbers of sarcomeres in an enlarged circumference operating at their optimum length. Left ventricle volume and mass are increased, and the pressure-volume curve is shifted to the right. Long-standing, severe volume overload often leads to myocardial dysfunction, the cause of which is not understood. Continued left ventricular enlargement is used to compensate for decreased left ventricular function. Left ventricular and left atrial enlargement further impair mitral valve function, increasing mitral valve regurgitation. Left ventricular end-diastolic pressure and left atrial pressure eventually rise, whereas cardiac output falls. The ability to increase cardiac output with exercise is markedly impaired. Pulmonary and systemic congestion are present.

Regurgitation of blood into the left atrium during systole results in left atrial volume and pressure overload. The effects on pulmonary venous and arterial pressures and the significance of these changes are similar to those seen in mitral stenosis. Because of the increased volume of blood in the atrium during systole, a large V wave may be present. The size of the V wave depends on the amount of mitral regurgitation and the volume and compliance of the left atrium and pulmonary veins. Characteristically, acute severe mitral regurgitation has a high V wave because the left atrium has not had time to enlarge. The other extreme is the patient with severe mitral regurgitation and aneurysmal dilatation of the left atrium in whom the V wave is small and the mean left atrial pressure is normal. In severe mitral regurgitation, mean left atrial pressures usually are not elevated to the same extent as in severe mitral stenosis. In addition to the pulmonary artery wedge pressure tracing, the V wave may also be reflected back to the pulmonary artery and be seen in the pulmonary artery pressure waveform. In some of these patients, pulmonary venous blood can be picked up in the distal pulmonary artery, as demonstrated by an increase in oxygen saturation of blood in the distal pulmonary arteries.

The reduced impedance to ejection in mitral regurgitation may cause an overestimate of left ventricular function. This stems from the fact that ejection fraction, commonly used in determining left ventricular systolic pump function, is sensitive to changes in afterload. This becomes important in selecting patients for surgery. After mitral regurgitation is surgically stopped, the impedance to left ventricular ejection is suddenly increased. In the presence of poor left ventricular function, this increased afterload may result in cardiac decompensation and perioperative death or a poor postsurgical result.

The presence of parallel impedances to left ventricular ejection also has another implication. Factors that affect the impedance in either the aorta or the left atrium determine their relative flows. Thus, factors that increase impedance in the left atrium or decrease impedance in the aorta favor blood flow to the aorta and decrease regurgitant fraction and increase forward stroke volume.

Clinical manifestations

History. Because of the compensatory mechanisms available, mild mitral regurgitation does not produce cardiac symptoms, and patients with moderate to severe mitral regurgitation may have long asymptomatic intervals. In contrast, acute severe mitral regurgitation is usually associated with congestive heart failure.

The predominant symptoms relate to pulmonary and systemic venous congestion and impaired rest and exercise cardiac output. As a consequence, patients are most frequently limited by exertional dyspnea and fatigue. Orthopnea and paroxysmal nocturnal dyspnea may result from redistribution of blood volume in the supine position. Acute episodes of pulmonary edema are less common than with mitral stenosis unless an acute change in mitral valve function occurs with chordae tendineae or papillary muscle rupture, or valve perforation with endocarditis. Long-standing pulmonary hypertension results in tricuspid regurgitation and systemic venous congestion, manifested by peripheral edema, abdominal pain, and swelling. Systemic embolism and hemoptysis are less common than with mitral stenosis. Patients with anular calcification may have calcific systemic emboli. Chest pain typical of angina pectoris usually indicates coexisting coronary artery disease. As with many volume-overload lesions, patients frequently complain of palpitations, which often represent an awareness of the large left ventricle contracting to expel the large stroke volume. Irregular palpitations indicate ectopic beats or atrial fibrillation, which may be present in up to 75% of these patients. Infective endocarditis may occur on damaged leaflets, further compromising mitral valve function.

Physical findings. The general appearance shows no features characteristic of mitral regurgitation, but tachypnea, cyanosis, and edema may be readily apparent in patients with end-stage mitral regurgitation and severe heart failure. The jugular venous pressure is elevated when pulmonary hypertension has been long-standing. A prominent A wave reflects increased filling pressure, and a large V wave may represent tricuspid insufficiency. Only a CV wave is present in patients with atrial fibrillation. The carotid pulse is normal or shows a brisk upstroke, except with severe reduction in cardiac output, which results in a small-volume pulse. The precordium is hyperactive. The left ventricular impulse is laterally and caudally displaced and larger than usual. An apical systolic thrill is not infrequent. A right ventricular impulse and pulmonary valve closure may also be felt along the left sternal border when pulmonary hypertension is present. An impulse along the left sternal border may represent sustained left atrial filling during systole. This expansile pulsation of the left atrium may displace the right ventricle and has to be distinguished from a right ventricular heave.

The sine qua non of clinical diagnosis of mitral regurgitation is the mitral systolic murmur; therefore, careful auscultation is important. A typical murmur may be notably absent in severe prosthetic perivalvular leak and in some patients may be very localized and heard in only one spot on the precordium. When mitral regurgitation is caused by leaflet damage, such as with rheumatic heart disease or endocarditis, the murmur is holosystolic. The exception to this rule is acute severe mitral regurgitation due to chordal rupture or leaflet perforation. In this setting, the left atrium is small and noncompliant. The V wave in the left atrium may approach left ventricular pressure toward the end of systole, reducing regurgitant flow and causing the murmur to be early and midsystolic in timing. As the lesion becomes less acute, the murmur becomes holosystolic. Murmurs not caused by leaflet damage may vary in intensity and duration during systole.

The murmur of mitral regurgitation is typically high frequency and blowing in quality. It is heard best with the diaphragm of the stethoscope placed firmly over the left ventricular impulse. The murmur often radiates well to the axilla. The exception to this rule is acute chordal rupture of the posterior leaflet, which produces a loud murmur that radiates to the left sternal border. The murmur is thus frequently confused with ventricular septal defect and aortic stenosis. With anterior leaflet involvement, the murmur radiates to the back and the spine and can be conducted to the top of the head. A characteristic of mitral regurgitation murmurs caused by leaflet damage is the constancy of the murmur at different cycle lengths. This helps to differentiate this murmur from that of idiopathic hypertrophic cardiomyopathy and aortic stenosis. Thus, the careful listener can use the natural variation of cycle length in atrial fibrillation or fortuitous extrasystoles to help confirm the presence of mitral regurgitation and its cause. The S_1 is reduced in intensity and may be obscured by the murmur. An S_4 is uncommon except in acute mitral regurgitation. A third heart sound, or S_3, often is present with severe mitral regurgitation. In some patients with severe mitral regurgitation, a diastolic rumble is present because of increased diastolic flow. The pulmonary component of S_2 is increased when pulmonary arterial hypertension is present.

Chest radiograph. The thoracic cage is normal except in patients with mitral valve prolapse or Marfan's syndrome, who have a higher incidence of scoliosis, pectus excavatum, and thin chest with decreased anteroposterior diameter. The lung fields show evidence of elevated pulmonary venous pressure, and the findings are similar to, but less marked than, those seen in mitral stenosis. The pulmonary arteries are enlarged in long-standing pulmonary hypertension. The cardiac silhouette usually shows overall enlargement; left ventricular and left atrial enlargement constitutes most of this increase. The left atrium reaches larger dimensions than in any other cardiac disease in long-standing severe mitral regurgitation, and in some patients the left atrium is aneurysmal. Right ventricular and right atrial enlargement reflect elevated pulmonary pressures. Calcification of the anulus of the mitral valve may be present, but leaflet calcification is uncommon in pure mitral regurgitation. Left ventricular aneurysm may be present when coronary artery disease is the cause of mitral regurgitation.

Electrocardiogram. Atrial fibrillation is present in up to 75% of patients with chronic severe mitral regurgitation. Signs of left atrial enlargement or increased pressure or interatrial conduction delay are manifested in patients with sinus rhythm by broad-notched P waves in lead II and biphasic P waves in V_1. Signs of left ventricular hypertrophy are frequently present in chronic severe mitral regurgitation.

Biventricular hypertrophy and biatrial enlargement may also be demonstrated when pulmonary artery pressure is elevated. In acute severe mitral regurgitation, the ECG may be entirely normal.

Special studies. Unlike the echocardiogram in mitral stenosis, the echocardiogram of mitral regurgitation may not be diagnostic of mitral valve dysfunction. Occasionally, ruptured chordae tendineae, or flail leaflets, are seen with severe acute mitral regurgitation. Multiple or thick echoes on the leaflets suggest fibrosis or calcification and are typically seen with rheumatic heart disease. Vegetations may be seen on the valve in infective endocarditis. The left atrium and left ventricle are enlarged, reflecting the severity of the mitral regurgitation. More important, echocardiography can be used serially to assess left ventricular dimensions and function. Doppler echocardiography (Chapter 5) is useful for diagnosing and assessing the severity of mitral regurgitation. There is a significant incidence of false positives in the mild grade, and the lesion may be erroneously judged to be severe in the presence of significant aortic stenosis. There is also an overlap between the various grades of severity of assessment of mitral regurgitation by Doppler when compared to angiography. Transesophageal echocardiography is of considerable value in defining mitral valve morphology and assessing the severity of mitral regurgitation (Chapter 5).

Radionuclide-derived ejection fractions can be used to assess left ventricular function reliably. Comparison of simultaneous right and left ventricular stroke counts may be used to assess the severity of left-sided regurgitant lesions; this technique does not distinguish between aortic and mitral regurgitations. The effect of exercise on left ventricular systolic function can be obtained with this technique (with the limitations mentioned under Chronic Aortic Regurgitation, p. 206), as can serial evaluations.

Right and left heart catheterization remains the cornerstone of evaluation of patients with symptomatic mitral regurgitation. Left ventricular cineangiography is used to assess quantitatively left ventricular volume and function, as well as the degree of valvular regurgitation. Pulmonary vascular resistance and cardiac output are measured. The effect of exercise on hemodynamics and cardiac function can be evaluated. Coexisting lesions of the aortic and tricuspid valves are assessed. Coronary arteriography determines the presence, site, and severity of coronary arterial obstruction and should be performed in patients with angina, in those with risk factors for coronary artery disease, in those with left ventricular systolic dysfunction, and in those 35 years of age or older who are being considered for cardiac surgery.

Natural history

The course of mitral regurgitation is determined by the cause and the interplay between the severity of the regurgitation and the ability of the left ventricle to compensate. Chronic mild mitral regurgitation is rarely responsible for symptoms because of adequate compensation; the major risk in such patients is infective endocarditis. With moderate to severe mitral regurgitation, there may be a long asymptomatic interval, and, when symptoms occur, they may progress slowly. However, functional capacity with severe mitral regurgitation may decline because of deterioration of left ventricular function rather than worsening of valve function. Or worsening of function may be caused by chordal rupture. Survival of symptomatic patients with important mitral regurgitation is about 60% at 10 years, but additional studies are needed to determine the natural history of severe mitral regurgitation.

Management

As with mitral stenosis, primary or secondary rheumatic fever prophylaxis reduces the incidence of rheumatic mitral regurgitation. Prevention of myocardial infarction reduces the incidence of mitral regurgitation caused by coronary artery disease.

Infective endocarditis prophylaxis is essential for all patients with mitral regurgitation, including the patient with trivial or mild valvular regurgitation (Chapter 15). Patients with rheumatic mitral regurgitation need antibiotic prophylaxis to prevent recurrence of rheumatic carditis (Chapter 316).

The patient with mild mitral regurgitation needs no specific therapy. The symptomatic patient can be helped by medical treatment through several approaches. Symptoms of systemic and pulmonary congestion are improved with diuretics. Digitalis reduces symptoms by improving left ventricular systolic pump function and controlling ventricular rate in patients with atrial fibrillation. Reduction of aortic impedance by decreasing systemic vascular resistance also helps relieve symptoms of mitral regurgitation and improve hemodynamic abnormalities. Afterload and preload reduction are helpful, but the effect of chronic vasodilator therapy on the natural history of mitral regurgitation is unknown; preliminary results are disappointing. It is recognized that any treatment that tends to reduce left ventricular size may reduce mitral regurgitation by improving the function of the mitral apparatus. Thus, the combination of decreased activity, diuresis, digitalis, and vasodilators reduces symptoms and improves hemodynamics in most patients. Maintenance of sinus rhythm is not as important for patients with mitral regurgitation as for those with mitral stenosis. Unless there is a clear reduction in function after the onset of atrial fibrillation, most patients with severe mitral regurgitation should probably be left in atrial fibrillation, with the rate controlled by digitalis; others may need small doses of beta-blocking agents or diltiazem to control ventricular rate adequately.

The optimum timing of operation for the patient with chronic severe mitral regurgitation has not been determined. The problem of timing of valve replacement in chronic mitral regurgitation arises from the observation that disabling symptoms may be the result of irreversible left ventricular dysfunction. Thus, the best time to intervene in chronic mitral regurgitation is just before irreversible left ventricular dysfunction occurs. It is clear that this point cannot be determined from the symptoms. Furthermore, ejection phase indices commonly used to assess left ventricular function are elevated by the reduced impedance to ejection in mitral regurgitation. It is generally agreed that as the left ventricle enlarges and function decreases, a point is reached when mitral valve replacement is not beneficial. It may not be possible to determine this point prospectively in each patient. However, a recent study suggests that when the end diastolic dimension is greater than 7 cm and the fractional shortening is reduced or low normal, a reduction in left ventricular volume and mass does not occur after mitral valve replacement, and ventricular function may actually deteriorate. Clinical use of this information should be tempered by knowledge of the difficulties intrinsic to M-mode echocardiography, including reproducibility of measurements and effects of volume overload on geometry. For these reasons, our current practice is to recommend mitral valve replacement to patients with severe mitral regurgitation and evidence of borderline or reduced left ventricular function even if symptoms are mild or absent. Factors that favor the balance toward surgery include a valve that is suitable for repair, a rheumatic or prolapse etiology, potential for major hemodynamic benefit, potential for correction of a large area of myocardial ischemia, and a dramatic response to medical treatment. Patients with disabling symptoms and good left ventricular function are ideal candidates for surgery. Because of the increased operative mortality and poor postoperative results, we are reluctant to routinely recommend surgery in patients with ejection fractions of 0.30 or less. Pending new data, these patients should be treated vigorously with digitalis, diuretics, and vasodilators. If there is good improvement with this therapy, they should be reevaluated for surgery.

The expected results of mitral valve replacement for rheumatic mitral regurgitation are similar to those for mitral stenosis. In patients with mitral regurgitation caused by coronary artery disease, the results are poorer. Patients with significant associated coronary artery disease should also have coronary bypass surgery at the time of valve replacement. Patients who postoperatively have a left ventricular ejection fraction of greater than or equal to 0.50 have much better long-term survival than those with a left ventricular ejection fraction of less than 0.50. Preoperative predictors of postoperative left ventricular ejection fraction of 0.50 or more are left ventricular ejection fraction of at least 0.50, left ventricular end-systolic volume index of no more than 50 ml/m^2, and absence of pulmonary hypertension.

The current trend is to perform mitral valve repair, rather than replacement, when feasible. When successful, the results of valve repair are similar to those of valve replacement and left ventricular function may be better with valve repair. Moreover, the incidence of many of the complications of prosthetic heart valves and especially of systemic emboli is much lower with valve repair. It is uncertain whether valve repair results in better survival compared with valve replacement.

ACUTE MITRAL REGURGITATION

Etiology

Acute mitral regurgitation usually results from infective endocarditis or trauma, both of which may result in rupture or perforation of the valve leaflets and chordae tendineae. Chordal rupture also occurs in rheumatic and prolapsing mitral valves, but in many patients the cause is unknown. Spontaneous chordal rupture is more common in men and in patients with systemic hypertension, acute left ventricular dilatation from any cause, or fibrosis of the papillary muscles. Papillary muscle dysfunction from ischemia, infarction, or fibrosis of the papillary muscle, the underlying left ventricular muscle, or both often causes acute mitral regurgitation. The most common cause of papillary muscle dysfunction is coronary artery disease. Rupture of a papillary muscle from myocardial infarction or trauma usually causes acute, catastrophic mitral regurgitation, particularly when the belly rather than an apical head of a papillary muscle is affected.

Abnormal physiology

The major difference between acute and chronic severe mitral regurgitation is the extent of left ventricular and left atrial enlargement and the magnitude of left atrial (and pulmonary venous) hypertension. The left ventricle is large in chronic mitral regurgitation but is only somewhat dilated in acute mitral regurgitation. To compensate for the left ventricular stroke volume lost to the left atrium, total left ventricular stroke volume has to increase. This is achieved by an "increase" of ejection fraction and an increase of left ventricular end-diastolic volume and sarcomere length. However, this compensatory mechanism is limited by the characteristic sarcomere length-tension curve and the diastolic pressure-volume relationships of the left ventricle and the pericardium. The left ventricle can increase acutely probably by no more than 20% to 30%, which accounts for its "normal size" on both physical examination and chest x-ray. This increased size is usually inadequate to maintain forward stroke volume; the compensatory tachycardia is often inadequate to maintain a normal forward cardiac output. The regurgitant volume increases left atrial volume. However, increases of left atrial size are limited by the left atrial pressure-volume curve and, as a result, left atrial pressure rises precipitously, producing pulmonary edema. Pulmonary hypertension is common. The regurgitant volume frequently cannot be accommodated in the left atrium and is transmitted into the pulmonary veins. In the absence of myocardial infarction, left ventricular systolic pump function frequently is normal in these patients; indeed, measured indicators of left ventricular systolic function may yield increased values because of the reduced impedance to left ventricular emptying.

Clinical manifestations

The patient may have a history of trauma or myocardial infarction, and the patient may exhibit the clinical features of infective endocarditis. Usually the symptoms of heart failure are predominant.

On physical examination, these patients have tachycardia; they may also be orthopneic. The usual clinical manifestations of heart failure often are present. As opposed to patients with chronic mitral regurgitation, of whom 75% are in atrial fibrillation, patients with acute mitral regurgitation are usually in sinus rhythm. The left ventricle is hyperkinetic. The S_1 is soft, and a loud S_3 is the rule. In contrast to patients with a chronic lesion, patients with acute mitral regurgitation usually have a presystolic gallop (fourth heart sound). They have a mitral systolic murmuring that may be holosystolic, late systolic, or crescendo-decrescendo. There may be a diastolic mitral flow murmur. The P_2 is increased in intensity.

The electrocardiogram often shows nonspecific ST-T wave changes and a sinus tachycardia. However, the ECG may be normal or may demonstrate the findings of a myocardial infarct. On the chest radiograph the cardiothoracic ratio may be within the normal range. The lung fields show signs of increased pulmonary venous pressure and of pulmonary edema.

Echocardiography (M-mode, 2D, or transesophageal) may show a variety of abnormalities, which include vegetations, prolapse of the mitral valve, flail leaflets, mitral valve aneurysm, mitral anular calcification, and the changes of a myocardial infarction. Two-dimensional echocardiography is also of value in determining left ventricular size and function, left atrial size, and presence of other cardiac lesions. Doppler echocardiography (Chapter 5) may be useful in demonstrating mitral regurgitation in those rare instances when there is no characteristic murmur (also see Mitral Regurgitation, p. 217). A radionuclide gated blood pool scan may help demonstrate normal left ventricular ejection fraction and an increase in left ventricular volumes.

The natural history of this condition is variable. If the mitral regurgitation is mild to moderate in severity, patients are likely to do well with medical therapy. Eventually, the changes of chronic mitral regurgitation occur. In patients with severe mitral regurgitation, the natural history depends on whether they have heart failure, coronary artery disease, papillary muscle rupture, or a combination. If heart failure is present, which is common, the prognosis is very poor. If coronary artery disease is the cause, the prognosis is that of the coronary artery disease and its complications. If papillary muscle rupture is present, 95% or more of patients die within 48 hours.

Management

The underlying cause of regurgitation must be treated, which often is difficult. In patients with infective endocarditis, the appropriate antibiotic therapy must be given. If the mitral regurgitation is mild, no other specific therapy may be needed. If mitral regurgitation is moderate, digitalis, diuretics, and vasodilators may be advisable.

For patients with severe mitral valve regurgitation, the choices of medical therapy include digitalis, diuretics, and vasodilators. Patients with heart failure should be given digitalis, diuretics, and vasodilators. In patients with mild, moderate, or severe heart failure that persists despite medical therapy, surgery is indicated. If the patient responds dramatically to digitalis, diuretics, and vasodilators, surgical therapy often can be delayed until heart failure and the infective endocarditis are controlled so that the operation is performed when the patient is in a more stable condition. If the patient does not respond immediately and dramatically to medical therapy, surgery should not be delayed, even if the infection is uncontrolled or the patient has had little antibiotic therapy. Surgery usually involves mitral valve replacement, but if the valve is suitable for repair, valvuloplasty is the procedure of choice. Associated or causative coronary artery disease requires coronary artery bypass surgery if it is technically feasible. Valve rupture, if diagnosed, is an indication for immediate valve surgery.

MITRAL VALVE PROLAPSE

Etiology

Mitral valve prolapse occurs in the presence of redundant mitral valve leaflets, elongated chordae tendineae, enlarged mitral anulus, and abnormally contracting left ventricular wall segments. Mitral valve prolapse is associated with the physical findings of one or more systolic clicks and a late systolic murmur. Echocardiographic and angiographic studies reveal protrusion of the mitral leaflet or leaflets beyond the plane of the mitral anulus and into the left atrium, with associated mitral regurgitation. The cause of mitral valve prolapse is at present unknown. Our inability to determine the cause probably means that the clinical features have heterogeneous origins.

The syndrome has been noted in all ages but is most common (5%) in women of childbearing age. Autosomal dominant inheritance has been demonstrated both with, and in the absence of, muscular dystrophy. Many patients with Marfan's syndrome have mitral valve prolapse. Mitral valve prolapse associated with segmental wall motion abnormalities develops in some patients with coronary artery disease. Mitral valve prolapse has been demonstrated in up to 37% of patients with ostium secundum atrial septal defect. Myxomatous proliferation of the mitral leaflet tissue is often found in patients with mitral valve prolapse who require valve surgery or are studied at autopsy. The incidence of myxomatous proliferation of the mitral valve in patients with incidental findings of prolapse is unknown and may be small.

Thus, the clinical syndrome that we know as mitral valve prolapse does not have a single cause. It may occur as an autosomal dominant heritable disorder, as part of a generalized connective tissue abnormality, or sporadically in otherwise normal people. Our imprecise knowledge of the natural history, complications, and treatment of this disorder naturally follows from our inability to characterize its etiology or the significance of the click-murmur syndrome or isolated echocardiographic findings of mitral valve prolapse in individual patients. It is possible that mitral valve prolapse is being significantly overdiagnosed.

Pathology

The presumed normal life span of most patients with mitral valve prolapse has limited the pathologic examination of the heart and the mitral valve to a small subset of patients who have severe mitral regurgitation or who die suddenly or accidentally. Pathologic findings most commonly include redundant mitral leaflet tissue involving predominantly the posterior leaflet. The chordae tendineae may be elongated. In the absence of coronary artery disease, the papillary muscles underlying the left ventricular myocardium are normal. The mitral anulus of patients with mitral valve prolapse and severe mitral regurgitation may be strikingly enlarged. Histologic examination shows myxomatous infiltration of the valve leaflets, with increased acid mucopolysaccharides. The normal collagenous and elastic elements are disrupted. These changes, however, are not specific for this syndrome. There is great variability in the amount of myxomatous tissue (spongiosa portion of leaflet) present in otherwise normal valves, but in the mitral valve prolapse syndrome, the spongiosa portion of the mitral leaflet actually invades and disrupts the fibrosa portion (elastin and collagen tissue). There is an increased incidence of associated mitral anular calcification and ruptured chordae tendineae, particularly in elderly patients with mitral valve prolapse.

Abnormal physiology

Except for the mitral valve, the cardiovascular system functions normally in most persons with mitral valve prolapse. The major pathophysiologic event is mitral regurgitation. Mitral regurgitation may be absent, trivial, slowly progressive, or sudden and severe in onset, with chordae tendineae rupture. When mitral regurgitation is hemodynamically important, pathophysiologic changes of left ventricular volume overload and regurgitation into the left atrium are present and are identical to those previously discussed under Mitral Regurgitation, p. 217. The systolic click and murmur of mitral valve prolapse result from abnormal valve function. Early in systole, the valve is competent. However, as the ventricle contracts and becomes smaller, the redundant mitral leaflets and/or chordae tendineae allow the affected leaflet to fall back into the left atrium, disrupting leaflet coaptation and allowing mitral regurgitation. At the moment of maximum prolapse, the chordae tendineae and leaflets tense, producing the click or multiple clicks. Events that alter left ventricular size, contractility, and/or aortic impedance affect the timing of maximum prolapse and thus the systolic click and murmur. A reduction of ventricular volume (by standing up), an increase in myocardial contractility (exercise), or a decrease in arterial resistance (amyl nitrite) often accentuates a systolic click or murmur and causes this auscultatory finding to occur earlier in systole.

Autonomic dysfunction has been demonstrated in women with mitral valve prolapse and is characterized by decreased parasympathetic and increased alpha-adrenergic tone. Arrhythmias, including supraventricular and ventricular tachycardia, are common in patients with this syndrome (the mechanism is unknown), and the rare occurrence of sudden death is presumed to be on this arrhythmic basis. Abnormal electrophysiologic function has not otherwise been documented in mitral valve prolapse. Shortened platelet survival time has been noted in some patients with mitral valve prolapse, and there is an increased incidence of mitral valve prolapse in young persons with cerebrovascular accidents. This is probably caused by fibrin emboli from the abnormal mitral leaflet tissue, as several postmortem studies suggest.

Clinical manifestations

Most patients with mitral valve prolapse are asymptomatic and therefore are diagnosed only because the characteristic click and murmur are heard incidentally during a physical examination or on echocardiographic/Doppler study performed for some other indication. Occasionally, the patient hears a loud whoop on standing up and seeks medical help. In others, the diagnosis is actively pursued because of atypical chest pain, palpitations, cerebrovascular episodes, or history of heart murmur.

History. There is no symptom complex diagnostic of mitral valve prolapse. In the rare instances of severe mitral regurgitation, the previously described symptoms of shortness of breath, fatigue, weakness, orthopnea, and paroxysmal nocturnal dyspnea predominate. Some patients with mitral valve prolapse seek medical attention because of atypical (for angina) chest pain, unusual shortness of breath, easy fatigability, syncope, and palpitations. These complaints are not specific for mitral valve prolapse and frequently occur in patients without cardiac or other organic disease.

Chest pain in mitral valve prolapse is usually not related to exertion. It may last for hours and yet may allow continued activity. The pain responds poorly to nitroglycerin. Since both mitral valve prolapse and coronary artery disease are common, some patients with coronary artery disease also have mitral valve prolapse. Shortness of breath and fatigue may be only subjective or may be demonstrable on a graded exercise test. Palpitations are a frequent subjective complaint and may or may not correlate with arrhythmias documented by ambulatory ECG recording. Occasional patients report frank syncopal episodes in addition to lightheadedness and dizzy spells. These may or may not correlate with arrhythmias. There is an association between mitral valve prolapse and transient cerebral or retinal ischemic events or stroke.

Physical findings. The diagnosis of mitral valve prolapse is most frequently made by physical examination. Although the patient's general appearance may be normal, the incidence of thoracic skeletal abnormalities is high and warrants careful inspection. Loss of the normal dorsal thoracic kyphosis (straight back), scoliosis, pectus excavatum, and decreased anteroposterior/transverse diameter ratio are present singly or in combination in over half of the affected patients. Diseases with a high incidence of mitral valve prolapse (e.g., Marfan's syndrome, myotonic dystrophy, atrial septal defect) have their own characteristic findings.

In the absence of hemodynamically important mitral regurgitation, most are restricted to auscultation of the heart. The precordial examination may reveal a sharp midsystolic tap, coincident with the click. The auscultatory phenomena are diagnostic of mitral valve prolapse. These include a nonejection click or multiple clicks heralding a midsystolic or late systolic murmur. The clicks and murmur are best heard at the apex, and the murmur is typically soft and blowing, sometimes with radiation to the axilla, consistent with mitral regurgitation. Occasionally, a loud whoop or honk is heard. It is important to note that the click(s) and murmur are variable and may be heard only intermittently; at times, only the click or the murmur is heard. When present, the click and murmur behave in the following manner: Maneuvers that decrease left ventricular size move the click and murmur closer to or simultaneous with the S_1. With standing up from a supine position or amyl nitrite inhalation, therefore, the click moves closer to S_1 and the duration of the murmur lengthens. In some, a holosystolic murmur follows these manipulations. Maneuvers that increase left ventricular size cause the click and the onset of the murmur to occur later in systole. Squatting, passive leg lifting in the supine position, or sustained hand grip exercise thus move the click and the murmur to later in systole and may even abolish one or both. In patients with suggestive symptoms and normal auscultatory findings, the physical examination is incomplete without a provocative maneuver to bring on the click and/or murmur. In some patients, the murmur is holosystolic.

Chest radiograph. The abnormalities of the thoracic skeleton previously described are readily recognized on the chest x-ray (scoliosis, straight back, pectus excavatum). The lungs and cardiac silhouette are normal unless hemodynamically important mitral regurgitation is present; these changes are described under Mitral Regurgitation, p. 217.

Electrocardiogram. The scalar ECG may show flat or inverted T waves in the inferior leads (II, III, aVF) in about one third of patients with mitral valve prolapse. These abnormalities may fluctuate with time and may be readily confused with myocardial ischemia. The Q-T interval may be prolonged. Most often the ECG is entirely normal.

Special laboratory studies

Echocardiography. After the physical examination, the test most commonly used to diagnose mitral valve prolapse is echocardiography. The specific findings on M-mode echocardiography are abrupt late systolic or, occasionally, pansystolic movement of the closed mitral valve toward the left atrium. Caudal angulation (Chapter 5) of the transducer must be avoided because it may produce an artifact resembling pansystolic prolapse. As with auscultation, maneuvers that change left ventricular volume change the echocardiographic timing of prolapse, and the diagnostic sensitivity may be enhanced. Two-dimensional echocardiography also demonstrates prolapse and is probably the more sensitive of the two techniques. The combination of M-mode and 2D echocardiography is superior to either alone (Chapter 5). However, the absence of the classic findings of prolapse on the echocardiogram does not exclude the diagnosis of mitral valve prolapse, since false-negative results are obtained in up to 10% of patients.

Cardiac catheterization and angiography. Hemodynamic and angiographic procedures are not indicated to make the diagnosis of mitral valve prolapse. These invasive tests may be useful in evaluating the occasional patient with hemodynamically important mitral regurgitation. Coronary arteriography may be necessary in some patients with anginal pain to establish whether coronary obstructive disease is present. The left ventriculogram shows posterior displacement of the mitral leaflets across the plane of the mitral anulus and into the left atrium during systole. Both 30-degree right anterior oblique and 60-degree left anterior oblique views are necessary to assess the mitral apparatus for prolapse accurately by left ventriculography.

Radionuclide studies. Myocardial perfusion scintigraphy in association with a graded exercise test may be used successfully to differentiate patients with mitral valve prolapse and anginal pain from those with and without associated obstructive coronary artery disease. Blood pool scans are not as effective for the diagnosis of prolapse.

Exercise testing. Exercise testing may induce frequent and complex ventricular extrasystoles, particularly during the recovery period. The high incidence of false-positive S-T segment depression in patients with mitral valve prolapse during exercise testing diminishes the importance of this finding. Exercise testing also enables one to evaluate objectively the degree of functional impairment.

Ambulatory ECG recordings. Ambulatory ECG recordings reveal premature atrial contractions or premature ventricular contractions in half the patients studied. Supraventricular or ventricular tachycardias have been observed in 6% of patients who have been evaluated by ambulatory ECG recording. However, these recorded arrhythmias often do not correspond in time to symptoms such as palpitations.

Natural history

Mitral valve prolapse is found at all ages in both sexes but is most prevalent in women of childbearing age. Consequently, most of those who reach the physician's office for evaluation of a heart murmur or symptoms subsequently found to be related to mitral valve prolapse are young women. Most patients with mitral valve prolapse are asymptomatic, and the diagnosis of prolapse is usually made in these patients during routine physical examination or from an echocardiographic examination performed for some other purpose.

Complications of mitral valve prolapse are infrequent but important. Chest pain is not common and is usually atypical for angina pectoris. Since prolapse and coronary artery disease are both common disorders, it is not surprising that some patients have severe associated atherosclerotic obstructive coronary artery disease. Endocarditis may occur in patients with prolapse, even in the absence of previously documented mitral regurgitation; mitral regurgitation often is intermittent. Progressive mitral regurgitation may occur because of increasing mitral dilatation, lack of leaflet coaptation, or chordae tendineae rupture. Acute severe mitral regurgitation may follow chordal rupture involving a large segment of leaflet. There is a known association between mitral valve prolapse and mitral anular calcification. These patients are also likely to have supraventricular and ventricular tachyarrhythmias. Some patients have associated preexcitation, and in most the accessory pathway appears to be on the left side of the heart. Sudden death is rare in prolapse and is probably caused by ventricular fibrillation or tachycardia; it occurs usually in those with symptomatic ventricular tachyarrhythmias. There is a relationship between mitral valve prolapse and cerebral and retinal ischemic events. Platelet survival is known to be shortened in some patients with mitral valve prolapse. Two-dimensional echocardiography of the mitral valve and the left atrium in some patients with mitral valve prolapse, stroke, and normal cerebral angiograms has shown densities consistent with thrombus on the mitral valve or in the left atrium, in the groove between the prolapsing valve and the left atrial wall. Transesophageal echocardiography may be of particular value in demonstrating thrombus in the left atrium when it is not seen on transthoracic echocardiography. Data show that patients with mitral valve prolapse who also have a thickened mitral valve on 2D echocardiography have a higher incidence of associated cardiovascular abnormalities and of complications of mitral valve prolapse.

Management

Because of the good prognosis in most patients with prolapse, management should be supportive. For patients who are incidentally found to have mitral valve prolapse on physical examination, echocardiographic examination with a brief explanation of the problem, a recommendation for infective endocarditis prophylaxis (Chapter 15), and reassurance seem most appropriate. If the physical findings are not classic for prolapse, the echocardiogram can be used to substantiate the diagnosis. Left ventricular cineangiography is unwarranted for diagnosis alone in most patients. Patients with mitral valve prolapse (whether they have a mitral systolic murmur, midsystolic click, or both) need antibiotics to prevent infective endocarditis.

For patients who have symptoms, with chest pain, palpitations, dyspnea, or possibly cerebral or retinal emboli, a more extensive evaluation may be indicated. Echocardiography can aid in supporting the clinical diagnosis of prolapse, in evaluating left ventricular function and volume overload (if significant mitral regurgitation is present), and in showing ruptured chordae. If the patient has had cerebrovascular episodes, anticoagulant and/or antiplatelet therapy is reasonable. Patients with recurrent tachyarrhythmias or syncope or who survive sudden death should undergo electrophysiologic study with provocative stimulation to determine whether they have abnormal conduction function or an accessory pathway and to guide drug therapy. Mitral regurgitation is managed as described previously.

In the absence of coronary artery disease, hemodynamically important mitral regurgitation, or a symptomatic arrhythmia, most patients with mild symptoms can be treated with reassurance. For those with refractory chest pain or palpitations, beta-adrenergic blocking agents may be effective. These agents also may be effective for the treatment of supraventricular tachyarrhythmias or premature ventricular contractions. Except for the management of important mitral regurgitation, significant obstructive coronary artery disease, or life-threatening arrhythmias in association with an accessory pathway, surgical therapy is not recommended. In the appropriate patient, catheter ablation therapy or implantation of a cardioverter defibrillator with or without a pacemaker may be indicated.

TRICUSPID STENOSIS

Etiology

Tricuspid stenosis is almost always rheumatic in origin. It rarely occurs as an isolated lesion and is associated with mitral valve disease (often stenosis) and with aortic stenosis. Tricuspid stenosis in the cardinoid syndrome is usually accompanied by tricuspid regurgitation. Obstruction of right atrial outflow occurs with a right atrial myxoma and, rarely, with a particular form of constrictive pericarditis.

Pathology

The valvular abnormalities in tricuspid stenosis are similar to the findings in rheumatic mitral valve disease; calcification of the valve, however, is rare. The normal area of the tricuspid valve is 7 cm^2; in severe tricuspid stenosis, the area is less than 1.5 cm^2. Although tricuspid stenosis is diagnosed in 3% to 4% of patients with multivalvular disease, it has been detected at autopsy and by 2D echocardiography in 10% or more of these patients.

Abnormal physiology

Stenosis of the tricuspid valve prevents adequate filling of the right ventricle and may lower cardiac output. The right atrium is enlarged and its pressure elevated, whereas the right ventricle is of normal size. Severe tricuspid stenosis may prevent or ease the pulmonary congestion resulting from associated severe mitral stenosis. In severe tricuspid stenosis, the altered hemodynamics are similar to those in mitral stenosis with two exceptions: (1) Instead of pulmonary congestion and pulmonary edema, these patients have systemic congestion and systemic edema; and (2) since the right ventricle is much more compliant than the left, right ventricular, and therefore right atrial, pressures are lower than the left atrial pressures that are seen in mitral stenosis.

Clinical manifestations

History. The age and sex ratio are the same as in mitral stenosis. The symptoms are dominated by the left-sided valvular disease, but effort intolerance and easy fatigability may be caused in part by tricuspid stenosis. If increased jugular venous pressure and liver enlargement are present, they may be caused mainly by tricuspid stenosis. The lack of pulmonary congestion in patients with severe mitral stenosis may be caused by severe tricuspid stenosis. If there is no pulmonary venous hypertension, hemoptysis, pulmonary edema, orthopnea, and paroxysmal nocturnal dyspnea are also usually absent.

Physical findings. The arterial pulse is normal. When sinus rhythm is present, giant A waves are present in the jugular pulse (Chapter 3). In such patients, if a right ventricular heave is absent, the diagnosis of right atrial obstruction is nearly certain. In atrial fibrillation, large V waves with a *slow* Y descent are the characteristic finding in this condition. A diastolic murmur and, if the patient is in sinus rhythm, a presystolic murmur are audible at the left sternal edge. It may be difficult to distinguish these murmurs from those caused by mitral stenosis, but an increase in intensity of the murmur(s) during inspiration suggests tricuspid stenosis. An opening snap is rarely heard or is difficult to distinguish from the mitral opening snap; when it is heard, it is present after the mitral opening snap. Since tricuspid stenosis may be associated with regurgitation, a holosystolic murmur that increases during inspiration may also be heard in the same area.

Chest radiograph. The right atrium may be enlarged. Calcification of the tricuspid valve is rare. Signs of associated mitral stenosis are often present.

Electrocardiogram. If sinus rhythm is present, tall, pointed P waves indicating right atrial enlargement and/or hypertension may be identified. Atrial fibrillation is common.

Echocardiography. An echocardiogram of the tricuspid valve shows a pattern similar to that in mitral stenosis. Findings on 2D echocardiography, namely, doming of the tricuspid valve, are more specific than those of M-mode echocardiography. In patients with suspected tricuspid stenosis, careful 2D echocardiographic and Doppler study of the tricuspid valve must be performed. Evidence of mitral and aortic valve disease may be seen.

Cardiac catheterization. Simultaneous recording of right ventricular and right atrial pressures is the way to demonstrate a gradient across the tricuspid valve. The gradient is often small and can be difficult to detect, especially when atrial fibrillation or a low cardiac output is present. The gradient can be increased with exercise. Normally, there is less than a 1-mm Hg diastolic gradient across the tricuspid valve. A gradient greater than 3 mm Hg suggests moderate stenosis, whereas a gradient greater than 5 mm Hg is associated with severe stenosis. If sinus rhythm is present, tall A waves can be seen in the right atrial pressure tracing.

Natural history

Tricuspid stenosis is never a primary lesion. The mitral and aortic valvular abnormalities usually dominate and determine the clinical course. Diuretics should be used with some caution in moderate to severe tricuspid stenosis, because when venous pressure is lowered, right ventricular filling and output are reduced. As a consequence, left ventricular filling and output may be compromised. Tricuspid commissurotomy is the usual treatment if severe stenosis is present. Valve replacement may be indicated if significant regurgitation through the valve is also present.

TRICUSPID REGURGITATION

Etiology

Tricuspid regurgitation most commonly results from right ventricular dilatation caused by left ventricular failure, mitral stenosis, pulmonary hypertension, pulmonary stenosis, or atrial septal defect. It may resolve after correction of the primary abnormality, but tricuspid regurgitation associated with rheumatic disease is usually permanent. Causes not associated with right ventricular dysfunction are infective endocarditis, carcinoid, and trauma. Thus, the patients most likely to have tricuspid regurgitation are those with severe heart failure or with severe mitral valve disease and intravenous drug abusers with infective endocarditis. Prolapse of the tricuspid valve usually occurs with mitral valve prolapse. Rarely, tricuspid regurgitation has been associated with a protein-losing enteropathy, lymphocytopenia, and immunologic deficiency. Congenital lesions, such as Ebstein's anomaly and endocardial cushion defect, also cause tricuspid regurgitation (Chapter 19).

Abnormal physiology

The physiologic effects of tricuspid regurgitation are anallogous to those of mitral regurgitation, except that the right atrium is more compliant than the left atrium, and right ventricular systolic pressure is lower than that present in the left ventricle. Thus, in tricuspid regurgitation, the right ventricle is delivering blood into a more compliant atrium at a lower driving pressure than in mitral regurgitation. Forward flow may be decreased, and right ventricular volume is increased.

Clinical manifestations

History. Symptoms are usually dominated by the underlying disease. Symptoms that may be primarily related to tricuspid regurgitation are fatigue and dyspnea on exertion, a throbbing in the neck or abdomen, epigastric distention, nausea, loss of appetite, and peripheral edema.

Physical findings. Large V waves with a rapid Y descent are noted in the jugular venous pulse. The neck vein findings are often not prominent because the right atrium is very compliant. Atrial fibrillation is present in 80% of patients. The right ventricle feels hyperdynamic. A holosystolic murmur that increases with inspiration (Carvallo's sign) is heard best at the xiphoid area and adjacent to the left sternal edge.

Chest radiograph. The chest x-ray may reveal evidence of right atrial enlargement. If the tricuspid regurgitation is related to other problems, the overall heart size is usually increased.

Electrocardiogram. The rhythm is usually atrial fibrillation. Evidence of right atrial and ventricular enlargement may be present.

Echocardiogram. The M-mode echocardiogram provides only indirect evidence of tricuspid valve regurgitation. Diminished or paradoxical interventricular septal motion reflecting volume and/or pressure overload of the right ventricle may be present. Intravenous injection of indocyanine green or microscopic air bubbles allows detection of tricuspid regurgitation on 2D echocardiography. Vegetations may be seen on the tricuspid valve, as may a right-sided myxoma. Flail leaflet, Ebstein's anomaly, and endocardial cushion defects may be seen, as may tricuspid valve prolapse. Doppler studies are of particular value in diagnosing and assessing the severity of tricuspid regurgitation. However, there is an incidence of false-positive for the mild lesion.

Cardiac catheterization. It is difficult to quantitate the degree of tricuspid regurgitation by catheterization. Right ventricular angiography and indicator-dilution curves show tricuspid regurgitation and provide semiquantification, but there is a high incidence of false-positive findings as a result of technical problems, for example, a catheter across the valve or atrial fibrillation. Demonstration of a systolic murmur in the right atrium by intracardiac phonocardiography may be necessary to establish the diagnosis but is usually not clinically necessary.

Natural history and management

The hemodynamic burden of tricuspid incompetence is usually well tolerated. An exception is the acute type that results from rupture of the valve or its supporting structure.

Mild to moderate tricuspid regurgitation usually requires no specific therapy. Severe regurgitation can be treated by digitalis and diuretics. As in tricuspid stenosis, overenthusiastic use of diuretics entails some danger. In all forms of tricuspid regurgitation, therapy is directed to the primary lesion or to associated left-sided valvular lesions. If the regurgitation is secondary to another problem, and at operation for that problem the tricuspid valve appears normal, correcting the primary cause is usually sufficient. In some patients, tricuspid valvuloplasty corrects the severe regurgitation. However, valve replacement may be necessary for regurgitation that is part of multivalve rheumatic disease. Some intravenous drug abusers with severe tricuspid insufficiency and no right ventricular systolic hypertension may be treated temporarily by valve resection alone.

PULMONIC STENOSIS

Pulmonic valve stenosis is usually a congenital lesion and is considered in detail in Chapter 19. It may be produced in rare instances by carcinoid, rheumatic disease, myxoma, and myxosarcoma of the pulmonary valve. Extrinsic compression from tumors and aneurysm of the aorta or sinus of Valsalva and a particular kind of constrictive pericarditis may produce right ventricular outflow obstruction. The abnormal hemodynamics, history, and physical findings are dependent on the degree of obstruction and are similar to those seen in congenital valve stenosis. Diagnosis is usually made by cardiac catheterization and angiography. Treatment, if needed, is usually directed to the primary cause. Resection of the tumor and valve replacement may be necessary.

PULMONIC REGURGITATION

Etiology

Pulmonic regurgitation can occur as a primary or secondary lesion. Primary regurgitation associated with normal pulmonary artery pressure is caused by congenital absence or deformity of the valve, infective endocarditis, or dilatation of the pulmonary artery from any cause, including the idiopathic variety or, perhaps most commonly, pulmonary-valve surgery. However, most cases of pulmonic regurgitation are secondary and are associated with elevated pulmonary artery pressure (>80 mm Hg) caused by mitral stenosis, primary pulmonary hypertension, cor pulmonale, and other sources of pulmonary hypertension. Rare causes include rheumatic disease, carcinoid, trauma, and syphilis.

Abnormal physiology

Since there is normally only a 5 mm Hg gradient in diastole across the pulmonary valve, pulmonic regurgitation with normal pulmonary artery pressure is usually of no hemodynamic consequence. As pulmonary artery pressure and diastolic gradient increase, so does the hemodynamic significance of the lesion. Occasionally, right ventricular enlargement and failure result.

Clinical manifestations

History. In patients with normal pulmonary artery pressure, symptoms are absent. In patients with high pulmonary artery pressure, symptoms are usually related to the underlying lesion but may be aggravated by the pulmonic regurgitation.

Physical findings. Pulmonic regurgitation is usually diagnosed only by auscultation. With normal pulmonary artery pressures, the heart sounds are normal; P_2 is followed by a short pause, then by a short, rough, low-pitched decrescendo murmur that ends well before the S_1. It is best heard in the second or third left intercostal space. If pulmonary hypertension is present, the murmur occurs immediately after a P_2, which is usually louder than normal. It is a higher-pitched, blowing, decrescendo diastolic murmur (Graham Steell's murmur).

Chest radiograph and electrocardiogram. The chest x-ray and ECG are usually normal. If the pulmonic regurgitation is secondary to another lesion, both reflect the original lesion.

Cardiac catheterization. With severe pulmonic valve regurgitation, the pulmonary artery diastolic pressure approaches right ventricular diastolic pressure and its pressure tracing is similar to the right ventricular tracing. Injection of a contrast agent into the pulmonary artery demonstrates pulmonic regurgitation.

Natural history and prognosis

Although large series are not available, it appears that patients with pulmonic regurgitation without pulmonary hypertension do reasonably well for long periods of time. Surgical removal or destruction of the valve does not produce heart failure unless pulmonary hypertension is present. However, some of these patients are now presenting 10 to 20 years later with severe right ventricular dilatation and impaired cardiac performance. Thus, pulmonic regurgitation with low pulmonary artery pressure may not be totally benign. In patients with high pulmonary pressure, symptoms and complications are usually related to the primary lesion.

Management

Pulmonic regurgitation with normal pulmonary artery pressure requires no special treatment. Valve replacement can be performed if the regurgitation causes major hemodynamic and cardiac problems. When it is secondary to another lesion, treatment is directed toward the primary cause.

MULTIVALVULAR DISEASE

Multivalvular disease occurs frequently. Common forms of this disease include stenosis and regurgitation at one valve, for example, mitral stenosis and mitral regurgitation, aortic stenosis and aortic regurgitation. Also very common are various combinations of stenosis and regurgitation of the aortic, mitral, and tricuspid valves. Many combinations are possible.

The abnormal physiology, history, and physical and other findings depend on the combination of valves affected, the degree of stenosis and regurgitation, and associated factors such as pulmonary hypertension and coronary artery disease.

PROSTHETIC VALVES

Intracardiac prosthetic heart valves have been in use for 33 years. Because of the success of valve replacement in improving symptoms and offering some patients prolonged survival (Fig. 16-4), hundreds of thousands of patients now have prosthetic heart valves. These patients are not cured but still have serious heart disease. They have exchanged native valve disease for prosthetic valve disease (see box, below) and must be followed with the same care as patients with native valvular disease. The clinical course of patients with prosthetic heart valves is influenced by several factors.

Ventricular dysfunction

Despite relief of valvular obstruction or regurgitation, some patients fail to improve or even deteriorate after valve replacement because of impaired myocardial function. The cause of dysfunction may be carditis associated with rheumatic disease, myocardial degeneration and fibrosis from long-standing pressure or volume overload, ischemic damage at the time of valve replacement, coronary artery disease, or other associated diseases such as congestive (dilated) cardiomyopathy. Perioperative myocardial damage is an important cause of postoperative ventricular dysfunction. The importance of myocardial protection at the time of valve surgery is now recognized, and current operative techniques reduce myocardial oxygen consumption by hypothermic, potassium-arrest cardioplegia.

Other cardiac lesions

Cardiac diseases affecting primarily one valve often affect other valves, the conduction system, coronary arteries, and pulmonary vasculature. With the exception of pulmonary hypertension and functional tricuspid regurgitation, these

Major complications of valve replacement

1. Operative mortality
2. Perioperative myocardial infarction
3. Prosthetic endocarditis
4. Prosthetic dehiscence
5. Prosthetic dysfunction
   a. Obstruction: usually thrombotic, occasionally due to item 3, 4, or 8
   b. Regurgitation
   c. Hemolysis
   d. Structural failure
6. Thromboemboli
7. Hemorrhage with anticoagulant therapy
8. Valve prosthesis–patient mismatch
9. Prosthetic replacement often caused by item 3, 4, or 5; occasionally caused by item 6, 7, or 8
10. Late mortality, including sudden, unexplained death

disorders do not improve after isolated valve replacement. Rheumatic disease typically affects both mitral and aortic valves but not necessarily with the same severity at the same time. Therefore, patients who have mitral valve replacement may subsequently require aortic valve replacement years later, or vice versa. Calcification of the aortic and mitral valve anuli accompanying disease of these valves may extend to the conduction system. High-degree or complete atrioventricular block may occur at the time of surgery or during the late postoperative period, requiring pacemaker implantation. Coronary artery disease is very common in the age range of patients requiring valve replacement. We recommend that coronary arteriography be performed preoperatively in all patients with myocardial ischemic pain, in those with left ventricular systolic dysfunction, in those with risk factors for coronary artery disease, and in those 35 years of age or older. Coronary bypass surgery of technically suitable vessels is performed at the time of valve replacement.

Prosthesis-related problems

As stated, the patient with a heart valve prosthesis has traded native valvular disease for prosthetic valvular disease.

Operative mortality for valve replacement averages 5% (range 2% to 10%) for aortic valve replacement and averages 8% (range 5% to 12%) for mitral valve replacement. Operative mortality is related to older age of patient, functional classes III to IV, increased left ventricular size, left ventricular dysfunction, heart failure, pulmonary hypertension, low cardiac output, and presence of associated diseases such as systemic hypertension, diabetes, and renal and hepatic failure. Coronary bypass surgery performed at the same time as valve replacement increases the operative mortality modestly, but associated coronary artery disease if not bypassed increases the operative and late mortality significantly. Other very important factors include the occurrence of perioperative myocardial infarction, the duration of the operation, aortic cross-clamp time, and whether the patient needed reoperation within 1 to 2 weeks after the initial operation, and on an elective or emergency basis.

The risk of prosthetic endocarditis is about 3% in the first year and 0.5% in subsequent years. Despite therapy, infections in the early postoperative period (up to 2 to 12 months) are the result of hospital-based organisms. They are difficult to cure and have a high mortality (about 77%); early reoperation is usually recommended. Mortality from late (2 to 12 months or later) postoperative infection is approximately 40%. About half the patients can be treated successfully with medication alone. The infected valve should be replaced in patients who do not respond to medical treatment or who have evidence of heart failure, anular invasion, embolism, prosthetic dysfunction, unstable prosthesis, or gram-negative, staphylococcal, or fungal infection. The importance of adequate antibiotic prophylaxis for the prevention of endocarditis cannot be overemphasized (Chapter 15).

Prosthetic dehiscence is the result of sutures pulling out of the cardiac tissues. It may result from infection, inadequate surgical technique, or diseased cardiac tissue (e.g., edema, necrosis, calcification).

Because of the continued proliferation of new types and models of prostheses and their relatively brief history of clinical use, the natural history of prosthetic failure is incompletely determined. Although some mechanical prostheses had initial problems with component failure, the most common cause for prosthetic dysfunction today is thrombotic obstruction. The incidence of thrombotic obstruction with the Björk-Shiley spherical occluder valve is higher than that seen with the Starr-Edwards or St. Jude valves, particularly in the mitral position. Failure of tissue valves is more common than failure of mechanical prostheses because of leaflet deterioration or calcification; progressive prosthetic regurgitation is the rule. Bioprosthesis failure is greater in younger patients and in the mitral position. In patients over 50 years old, failure of mitral prosthesis usually starts at 7-8 years and of aortic prosthesis at 8-10 years. It is unlikely that the tissue valves currently in use will be able to provide the long-term performance demonstrated by the ball valve mechanical prosthesis.

Red cells are fractured by turbulence and contact with foreign surfaces. Some degree of hemolysis is present with all mechanical prostheses but not with bioprostheses. However, important hemolysis may occur with a perivalvular leak or severe prosthetic obstruction regardless of prosthesis type. Serum lactic dehydrogenase (LDH) is usually the simplest and most reliable index of hemolysis to follow in patients with prosthetic valves. A sudden increase in LDH may indicate prosthesis dysfunction, perivalvular leak, or cloth tear. Iron and folate therapy usually correct anemia. Valve re-replacement may be required for severe, refractory hemolytic anemia.

Important systemic embolization is an unfortunate complication of prosthetic valve replacement. Anticoagulation is recommended for all patients with mechanical prostheses. Despite long-term anticoagulation, patients with mechanical prostheses face a 1% to 2% or less per year embolic rate for aortic prostheses and a 3% to 4% or less per year rate for mitral prostheses. If patients experience an embolism, dipyridamole is added to the anticoagulant therapy. Tissue prostheses in the aortic position have a similar embolic rate *without* anticoagulation. Tissue mitral prostheses do not have a lower incidence of emboli than do mechanical prostheses when atrial fibrillation is present. Therefore, long-term anticoagulation is recommended in patients with this rhythm. Cessation of anticoagulation in patients with mechanical prostheses should be avoided because it carries a 20% to 25% incidence of systemic embolism in the first year. If it is necessary to discontinue anticoagulation temporarily, it is recommended that it be slowly tapered.

Long-term anticoagulant therapy is associated with bleeding episodes. The incidence of minor bleeding is about 2% to 4% per year or less. The incidence of major bleeding is about 1% to 2% per year or less, with a mortality of about 0.5% per year or less. The incidence of these complications is lower in patients who take their medications reliably and in those in whom smooth long-term anticoagulation can be achieved. When using oral anticoagulation, prothrombin times should be 1.3 to 1.7 times (average 1.5) the control time; those with mitral prostheses should have higher ratios than those with aortic prostheses. Higher degrees of anticoagulation increase the incidence of bleeding without reducing the incidence of thromboembolism.

No prosthesis currently employed has an effective orifice as large as that of the native valve, and valve prosthesis–patient mismatch may occur. All patients with prosthetic heart valves have mild to moderate stenosis. Patients with aortic valve prostheses have obstruction to left ventricular outflow (aortic stenosis), and patients with mitral valve prostheses have obstruction to left atrial emptying (mitral stenosis). This is most important with the large patient in whom a small prosthesis must be placed for technical reasons. The resulting patient-prosthesis mismatch contributes to incomplete relief of symptoms. The long-term effect of intrinsic prosthetic stenosis on survival and ventricular dysfunction is unknown. The presence of intrinsic prosthetic stenosis must be considered when advising patients with prosthetic heart valves concerning activity.

Reoperation to replace a prosthetic heart valve is a serious complication. It is usually required for moderate to severe prosthetic dysfunction and dehiscence, for prosthetic endocarditis, and occasionally for recurrent thromboembolism, severe recurrent bleeding from anticoagulant therapy, and valve prosthesis–patient mismatch.

Late cardiac death may result from ventricular dysfunction, other cardiac lesions, or prosthesis-related causes. Late, sudden death is not uncommon. It may result from a bradyarrhythmia, a tachyarrhythmia that is often associated with ventricular dysfunction, prosthetic dysfunction or mismatch, coronary artery disease, or a combination of these.

Management

All patients with prosthetic valves need appropriate antibiotics for prophylaxis against infective endocarditis (Chapter 15). Patients with rheumatic heart disease continue to need antibiotics as prophylaxis against the recurrence of rheumatic carditis. Adequate anticoagulation is needed for appropriate patients. At present, this means anticoagulation with sodium warfarin unless there is a specific contraindication to such therapy. Anticoagulation is needed in *all* patients with *any* type of mechanical prosthesis and in patients with bioprostheses who are in atrial fibrillation.

During the first 6 weeks after surgery, the physician and surgeon jointly manage the patient, directing their attention toward relieving postoperative discomfort, readjusting cardiac medications, and instituting anticoagulation if not contraindicated. A graduated plan of activity is started that, in most cases, enables the patient to return to full activity in 6 weeks.

Several syndromes are peculiar to the postoperative period. The postperfusion syndrome, which occurs in up to 5% of patients, usually appears in the third or fourth postoperative week. Characterized by fever, splenomegaly, and atypical lymphocytes, it is benign and self-limited. Another effect of surgery, the postpericardiotomy syndrome, occurs in up to 25% of the patients and is characterized by fever and pleuropericarditis. It usually develops in the second or third postoperative week but can appear as late as 1 year after surgery and sometimes recurs. Although this syndrome is usually self-limited, most patients benefit from taking anti-inflammatory drugs, such as aspirin or indomethacin, and a short course of corticosteroids is also occasionally required.

Even though the pericardium is left open at the end of surgery, cardiac tamponade has been known to occur during the first 6 weeks. The critically ill patient improves promptly with pericardial drainage, which underscores the need to consider this uncommon postoperative complication. Usually, anticoagulants have been given and the fluid is hemorrhagic.

The 6-week postoperative visit is critical, because by this time the patient's physical capabilities and expected improvement in functional capacity can usually be assessed. At this time, the physician should assemble essential records and data for the subsequent office followup, including the preoperative catheterization report, surgeon's operative report, and hospital discharge summary. The prosthesis model, serial number, and size should of course be recorded.

The work-up on this visit should include an interval or complete initial history and physical examination, ECG, chest x-ray, echocardiography/Doppler studies, complete blood count, electrolytes, LDH, and prothrombin time, if indicated. The examination's main focus is on physical signs that relate to functioning of the prosthesis or suggest the presence of a myocardial, conduction, or valvular disorder. The auscultatory sounds to expect with some normally functioning prostheses are listed in Table 16-1. Severe perivalvular mitral regurgitation may be inaudible on physical examination, a fact to remember when considering possible causes of functional deterioration in a patient.

The interval between routine follow-up visits depends on the patient's needs. Anticoagulant regulation does not require office visits.

Multiple noninvasive tests have emerged for assessing valvular and ventricular function. Fluoroscopy can reveal abnormal rocking of a dehiscing prosthesis or limitation of the occluder if the latter is opaque. Phonocardiography can detect variant poppets if "normal" sounds were previously established. Radionuclide angiography is useful to determine whether functional deterioration is the result of reduced ventricular function. M-mode echocardiography has proved unreliable in assessing ventricular and prosthetic function, but 2D echocardiography with Doppler velocity recordings yields useful information about both.

"Heart failure" after valve replacement may be the result of (1) preoperative left ventricular dysfunction that improved partially or not at all, (2) periopertive myocardial damage, (3) other valve disease that has progressed, (4) complications of prosthetic heart valves, and (5) associated

Table 16-1. Normal auscultatory findings in patients with prosthetic heart valves

Type of prosthetic valve	Auscultatory finding*	
	Aortic	Mitral
Starr-Edwards ball valve	Sharp opening sound after S_1	Sharp opening sound after S_2, 0.07-0.15 s
	Sharp closing sound at S_2	Sharp closing sound at S_1
	Ball "rattles" during systole	Ball "rattles" during diastole
	SEM	SEM
Björk-Shiley spherical occluder	Soft opening sound after S_1	Soft opening sound after S_2, 0.07-0.15 s
	Sharp closing sound at S_2	Sharp closing sound at S_1
	SEM	
Xenograft	SEM	Diastolic rumble†
		SEM

*Absence of opening or closing sounds with mechanical prostheses usually signifies severe prosthetic dysfunction.
†Indicates bioprosthetic obstruction or prosthesis-patient mismatch.
SEM, systolic ejection murmur.

heart disease, such as coronary artery disease and systemic hypertension.

Any patient with a prosthetic heart valve who does not improve after the surgery or who later shows deterioration of functional capacity should undergo appropriate testing, including cardiac catheterization and angiography to determine the cause. Such studies are also necessary for patients

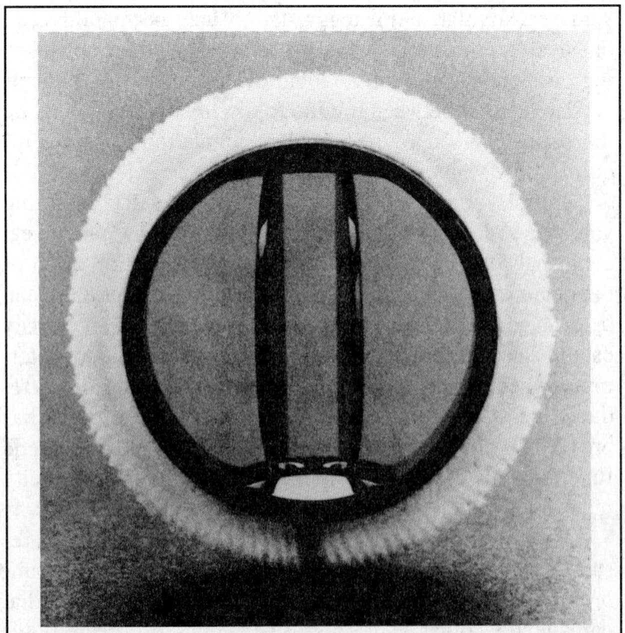

Fig. 16-5. St. Jude valve.

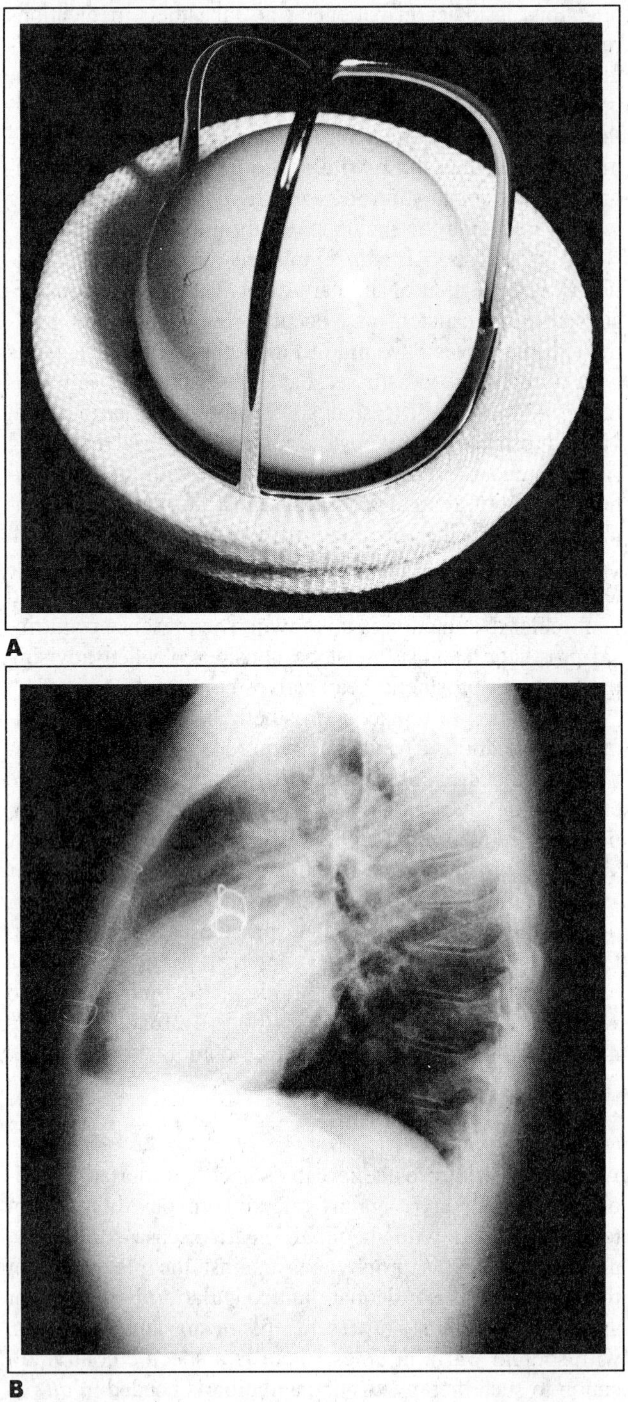

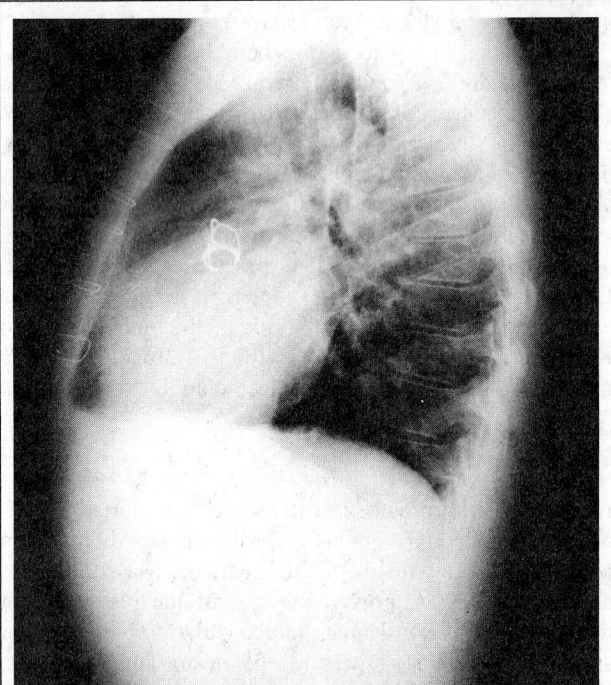

Fig. 16-6. A, Starr-Edwards model 1260 aortic prosthesis. **B,** The radiolucent Silastic poppet is not seen on the chest radiograph.

who require reoperation for endocarditis or repeated embolism, to determine the hemodynamics and anatomy for the surgeon.

The indications for reoperating on a patient with prosthetic valve endocarditis have already been discussed. The patient in stable condition, without prosthetic valve endocarditis, can probably undergo reoperation with slightly greater risk than that accompanying the initial surgery. For the patient with catastrophic dysfunction, surgery is clearly indicated and urgent. The patient without endocarditis or severe dysfunction requires careful hemodynamic evaluation, and the decision about reoperation should then be based on the hemodynamic abnormalities, the symptoms, ventricular function, and current knowledge of the natural history of the particular prosthesis.

Choice of prosthesis

In the United States, two main kinds of prosthetic heart valves are presently being implanted: mechanical prostheses and bioprostheses. The three main types of mechanical valves that are being used are a bileaflet (St. Jude) valve (Fig. 16-5), a ball and cage (Starr-Edwards) valve (Fig. 16-6), and the Medtronic Hall valve; the tilting disk valve (e.g., the Bjork-Shiley spherical occluder valve) is no longer being used in the United States. The bioprostheses are porcine heterografts (e.g., Hancock and Carpentier-Edwards) (Fig. 16-7).

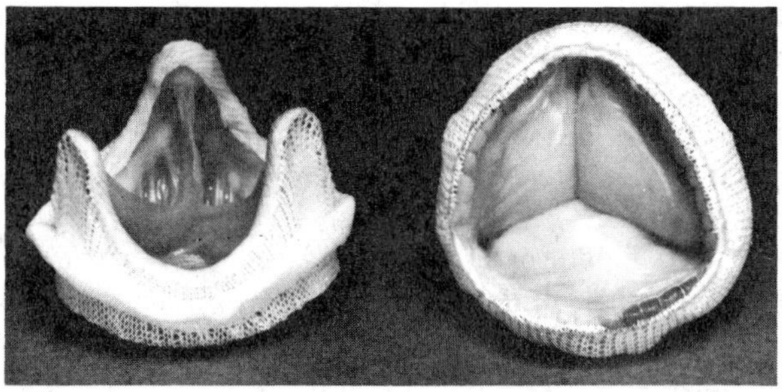

A

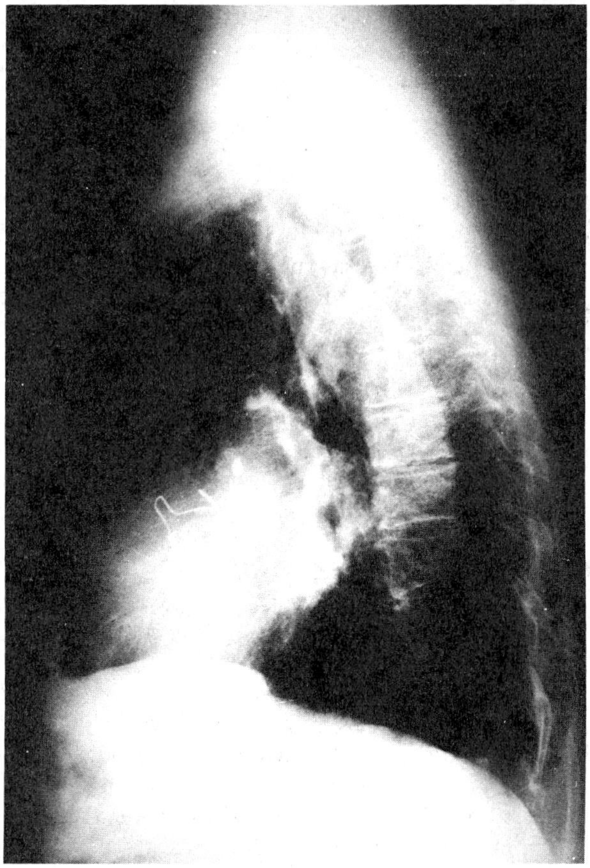

B

Fig. 16-7. **A,** Carpentier-Edwards aortic prosthesis. **B,** Only the wire stent of this bioprosthesis is visualized on the chest roentgenogram.

The main advantages of the mechanical prostheses are their *proved* durability (Starr-Edwards valves last for up to 33 years; the Björk-Shiley spherical occluder valve, for up to 10 to 15 years) and the accumulated knowledge of their complications, including rate of occurrence. The later model Björk-Shiley 60-degree convexoconcave prosthesis has a high incidence of strut fracture and is no longer available for clinical use. Follow-up on the St. Jude valve is available for 8-10 years. The main advantage of porcine heterografts is that anticoagulant therapy is not required for patients in sinus rhythm. Since mechanical valves with anticoagulation and heterografts without anticoagulation have demonstrated similar thromboembolism rates, the main disadvantage of mechanical valves is the need for anticoagulant therapy and its associated morbidity and mortality. The main disadvantage of heterografts is their limited durability. At present, heterograft valve failure (degeneration and obstruction) occurs at an average rate of less than or equal to 5% at 5 years, 10%-20% at 10 years, and 40%-65% at 15 years.

Antibiotic sterilized homograft valves have a low incidence of many complications, in particular of prosthetic endocarditis. However, they are more difficult to insert and the failure rate averages 19% at 10 years, 54% at 14 years, and 88% at 20 years. Viable cryopreserved homografts may have a very low failure rate.

The prosthetic valve should be chosen after a careful consideration of all factors. Bioprostheses are indicated for patients who should not or cannot take anticoagulants, for women of childbearing age who want to bear a child, and for patients whose life expectancy from other diseases is likely to be less than 7 to 10 years after valve replacement. Mechanical prostheses are indicated for all patients in atrial fibrillation, for patients who require valves in the smaller sizes, for patients with a long life expectancy, and for patients who want to reduce the chance of reoperation to a minimum.

REFERENCES

Bloomfield P et al: Twelve-year comparison of a Bjork-Shiley mechanical heart valve with porcine bioprosthesis. N Engl J Med 324:573, 1991.

Bonaw RO et al: Serial long-term assessment of natural history of asymptomatic patients with chronic aortic regurgitation and normal left ventricular systolic function. Circulation 84:1625, 1991.

Cheitlin MD and Byrd RC: Prolapsed mitral valve: the commonest valve disease? Curr Probl Cardiol January 8(1):1984.

Crawford M et al: Determinants of survival and left ventricular performance following mitral valve replacement. Circulation 81:1173, 1990.

Grunkemeier GL et al: Prosthetic heart valve performance: long-term follow-up. Curr Probl Cardiol 17(6): 1992.

Hammermeister KE et al: Comparison of outcome after valve replacement with a bioprosthetic versus a mechanical prosthesis. Initial five-year results of a randomized trial. J Am Coll Cardiol 10:719, 1987.

Kawanishi DT and Rahimtoola SH: Catheter balloon commissurotomy for mitral stenosis: complications and results. J Am Coll Cardiol 19:192, 1992.

Kulick DL et al: Catheter balloon valvuloplasty in adults. Curr Probl Cardiol July, August 15(7&8):1990.

O'Rourke RA and Crawford MH: Mitral valve regurgitation. Curr Probl Cardiol. May 1984.

Rahimtoola SH: Perspective on valvular heart disease. Update II. In Knoebel S, editor: Era in cardiovascular medicine. New York, 1991, Elsevier.

Rahimtoola SH: Vasodilator therapy in chronic, severe aortic regurgitation. J Am Coll Cardiol 16:430, 1990.

Rahimtoola SH: Lessons learned about the determinants of the results of valve surgery. Circulation 78:1503, 1988.

Rahimtoola SH: Valvular heart disease: a perspective. J Am Coll Cardiol 1:199, 1983.

Rahimtoola SH: The need for cardiac catheterization and angiography in valvular heart disease is not disproven. Ann Intern Med 97:433, 1982.

Rahimtoola SH: The problem of valve prosthesis—patient mismatch. Circulation 58:20, 1978.

Waller BF: Morphological aspects of valvular heart disease. Curr Probl Cardiol October and November 8(10&11):1984.

Walsh RA and O'Rourke RA: The diagnosis and management of acute left-sided valvular regurgitation. Curr Probl Cardiol December 3(12): 1979.

CHAPTER

17 Cardiomyopathies

Pravin M. Shah

MYOCARDITIS

Myocarditis is inflammation of the myocardium that is commonly caused by infectious agents, particularly viruses. It may occur in an acute, subacute, or chronic form, and the inflammation may involve the myocardial cell, interstitium, and/or vascular elements. Any infectious agent may produce cardiac inflammation by direct invasion of the myocardium, by production of a myocardial toxin, or by autoimmunity. The viral etiologies include echovirus, poliovirus, and coxsackie A and B, coxsackie B being the most frequent. Myocarditis may also be caused by pharmacologic agents, chemicals, metabolic disorders, radiation, or other physical agents. In some patients, myocarditis presents as acute congestive heart failure; in others, it results in chronic insidious congestive cardiomyopathy. In most patients with acute myocarditis, the inflammatory process is transient and subclinical, and no evidence of persistent cardiac disease exists.

The clinical manifestations are highly variable and may fall into one of the following categories: (1) Asymptomatic patients generally have focal myocarditis, diagnosed as an incidental finding at autopsy, with a reported incidence varying between 1% and 7%. (2) Symptomatic patients may have a predominantly systemic illness with few or no signs of cardiac involvement except for subtle clues such as persistent tachycardia or electrocardiographic changes. (3) Cardiac presentation includes chest pain of myopericarditis or symptoms of heart failure. (4) Uncommonly, focal myocarditis with features of acute myocardial infarction is noted. (5) Similarly, presentation with arrhythmia and occasionally with sudden death has been described. (6) Some patients may present with pulmonary or systemic emboli.

Myocarditis may result in nonspecific symptoms, including fatigue, dyspnea, palpitations, and precordial discomfort. Chest pain is usually caused by associated pericarditis but may suggest myocardial ischemia.

Physical examination commonly reveals tachycardia. The first heart sound (S_1) is often soft; third or fourth heart sounds (S_3, S_4) are frequent, and a soft apical systolic murmur (mitral regurgitation) may be present. Diastolic murmurs are rare. A friction rub is often heard in patients who have associated pericarditis.

Clinical evidence of congestive heart failure is present in the more severe cases. The heart size is usually normal in asymptomatic patients, but may be enlarged in patients with heart failure or pericardial effusion. Pulmonary and systemic embolism may occur.

The most common electrocardiogram abnormalities involve the S-T segment and the T wave, but atrial and ventricular arrhythmias and atrioventricular (AV) conduction defects may result. Pathologic Q waves are rare. Complete AV block is usually transient but occasionally results in sudden death. Chest x-rays may reveal a normal or enlarged heart, with or without signs of pulmonary venous hypertension.

The diagnosis is often based on determining the associated systemic illness and its characteristics. Methods for identifying the responsible infectious agents are described in Chapter 226. In experienced hands, transvenous endomyocardial biopsy is a safe method of establishing the diagnosis and assessing the results of therapy in severe cases of myocarditis. Although the biopsy does not usually identify the responsible infectious agent, a diagnosis of active myocarditis may be made on the basis of inflammatory infiltrate accompanied by necrosis of adjacent myocytes. When clinically indicated, repeat biopsies may be designated as "ongoing," "resolving," or "resolved" myocarditis. Although the histologic appearance of acute myocarditis is often characteristic, the criteria for diagnosis of chronic, indolent, resolving "myocarditis" are often subtle and subject to considerable interobserver variability. The more subtle changes are relevant only when earlier biopsy has demonstrated characteristic cellular response. Furthermore, the inflammatory changes may be spotty, requiring several biopsy specimens from different regions to provide diagnostic information. Noninvasive techniques, such as echocardiography and radionuclide angiography (Chapter 5), may be useful for detecting impaired left ventricular performance or pericardial effusion during the systemic illness. Continuous ambulatory ECG recordings have been used to document atrial and ventricular arrhythmias in various infectious diseases. Positive gallium scans, although not specific for myocarditis, have been reported in a subgroup of patients responsive to immunosuppressive therapy.

Treatment is often supportive and includes rest and adequate oxygenation. Congestive heart failure is treated in the usual manner with digitalis, diuretics, and vasodilators, with particular attention to the possibility of digitalis toxicity. Important arrhythmias should be treated with the usual antiarrhythmic agents. The use of corticosteroids in acute viral myocarditis is controversial; it is generally believed to be contraindicated unless severe cardiovascular compromise unresponsive to conventional modalities has occurred. In-vitro studies indicate that the use of corticosteroids during the acute viral illness may actually exacerbate the infectious process. However, some patients with myocarditis proved by endomyocardial biopsy have been shown to respond favorably to a combination of immunosuppressive drugs and corticosteroids. However, the predictive value of histologic findings remains undefined. Currently, most authorities recommend that immunosuppressive therapy in acute viral myocarditis be used only as a last resort. Some patients have been reported to respond dramatically, although spontaneous recovery may also be observed. Prolonged bed rest also has been advocated, but its benefit in preventing long-term sequelae has not been established.

CARDIOMYOPATHY: GENERAL CONSIDERATIONS

Cardiomyopathy is best defined as diffuse myocardial disorder attributable neither to pressure or volume overload nor to segmental loss of muscle function secondary to ischemic damage. This definition does not exclude the coexistence of valvular, hypertensive, or coronary artery disease; it merely requires that these be judged not responsible for the myocardial dysfunction. Hence, the diagnosis of cardiomyopathy involves identifying concomitants and excluding other causes.

The current definition used by the World Health Organization/International Society of Cardiology Task Force on Cardiomyopathies specifically describes these as "heart muscle disease or diseases of unknown cause or causes." The previous use of etiologic classification into primary and secondary types is therefore redundant. However, it is important to consider etiologies that may result in cardiac involvement simulating cardiomyopathies (box, above).

It is generally unnecessary to subject every patient to laboratory investigation for each possible cause, since clinical clues to the probable cause are often present. The potentially correctable conditions—hemochromatosis, hypophosphatemia, and, rarely, beriberi and endocrine states without other end-organ features—should be carefully considered. Similarly, it may be necessary to examine the possible role of toxic agents such as alcohol, since these may add to myocardial dysfunction even when not causing the disease.

The pathophysiologic classification (box, right) offers an excellent opportunity to characterize the underlying myocardial dysfunction and thus approach therapy more physiologically. Although there is some overlap, the dilated cardiomyopathies are characterized by abnormal systolic pump function; the hypertrophic cardiomyopathies, by disordered diastolic function from reduced distensibility; and the restrictive cardiomyopathies, by elements of both.

Conditions that may simulate cardiomyopathies

Infective (e.g., viral, rickettsial, protozoal, bacterial, Chagas' disease)
Metabolic and infiltrative (e.g., hemochromatosis, amyloidosis, glycogen storage disease)
Toxic (e.g., alcohol, anticancer agents, amphetamines, cobalt)
Radiation
Endocrine (e.g., hyperthyroidism, hypothyroidism, acromegaly, Cushing's disease)
Deficiency (e.g., beriberi, hypophosphatemia)
Ischemic (e.g., diffuse nonsegmental ischemic dysfunction)
Collagen disease (e.g., periarteritis nodosa, rheumatic fever, rheumatoid arthritis)
Immunologic (transplant rejection, peripartum)
Neuromuscular

DILATED (CONGESTIVE) CARDIOMYOPATHY

As the term implies, the most frequent underlying anatomic change in dilated (congestive) cardiomyopathy is chamber (ventricular) dilation, generally accompanied by a physiologic alteration in systolic pump function that results in the clinical syndrome of congestive heart failure. Although most patients in the past came under observation only after symptoms of heart failure developed, current noninvasive diagnostic techniques permit recognition of the disorder in the early, asymptomatic phase. The underlying disorder remains undetected before chamber dilation, unless a conduction disturbance, for example, bundle branch block, heralds the early onset of the disease.

Pathology

Postmortem examination reveals enlargement and dilatation of all four cardiac chambers. The cardiac valves are intrinsically normal, as are the coronary arteries. However, cardiomyopathy may coexist in a patient with associated val-

Pathophysiologic classification of cardiomyopathies

I. Dilated (congestive) cardiomyopathy
II. Hypertrophic cardiomyopathy
   A. Asymmetrical
      1. Dynamic outflow obstruction
      2. Absence of resting or provoked outflow obstruction
   B. Concentric: dynamic outflow obstruction is uncommon
III. Restrictive cardiomyopathy

vular or coronary artery disease. Mural thrombi are often noted in the ventricles or the atria.

Histologic examination reveals myocardial cell degeneration and areas of necrosis and fibrosis; cellular infiltration is generally not pronounced except in patients with an acute inflammatory process. It has been reported that patients with predominantly mononuclear lymphocytic infiltration respond favorably to steroid therapy. Confirmation of these observations by an ongoing multicenter study may provide an important indication for myocardial needle biopsy in patients with primary cardiomyopathies.

Needle biopsy was introduced as a technique for evaluating myocardial damage caused by specific conditions. However, the usefulness of needle biopsy has so far been limited to occasional conditions such as amyloid disease, hemochromatosis, and acute myocarditis.

Pathophysiology

Diffuse myocardial damage leading to dilated cardiomyopathy predominantly affects systolic pump function. In the early phases, the only objective evidence may be signs of circulatory insufficiency occurring with imposed stress, such as physical exercise. Progressive impairment of cardiac function subsequently develops. Chamber dilation is the result of increased residual volume caused by reduced ejection fraction, but in turn may provide a partial compensation on the basis of the Frank-Starling mechanism. Eventually, however, hypertrophy results, with an increase in muscle mass. All patients with dilated cardiomyopathy, except those with the most acutely fulminant disease (i.e., acute myocarditis), have cardiac hypertrophy (i.e., increased muscle mass), although wall thicknesses are generally normal (i.e., so-called eccentric hypertrophy).

The symptomatic phase of dilated cardiomyopathy is generally the result of elevated filling pressures and resulting venous congestion, although reduced cardiac output may contribute by decreasing glomerular filtration rate and increasing sodium reabsorption. In addition, a prominent symptom of generalized fatigue results from subnormal resting cardiac output. The symptom complex in dilated cardiomyopathy may differ from that in congestive heart failure from other causes, in which primary involvement of the left heart chambers with pulmonary congestion, edema, and pulmonary arterial hypertension precedes the development of right heart failure. Most patients with dilated cardiomyopathy have simultaneous involvement of both left and right heart chambers. Thus, the sequence of progressive symptomatology is different and involves systemic venous congestion in the early phases. Rarely, isolated left or right ventricular cardiomyopathy may be present.

Clinical and laboratory manifestations

Dyspnea is a common early symptom. The clinical and laboratory features are summarized in Table 17-1. Effort intolerance is often a rapidly progressive symptom. In advanced disease, orthopnea develops, requiring the use of two or more pillows for head elevation. Episodes of paroxysmal nocturnal dyspnea generally denote severe degrees of pulmonary venous congestion and edema. Episodic coughing with frothy expectoration may accompany dyspnea. Some patients can comfortably lie flat despite pulmonary edema, especially when it is chronic or is associated with severe right ventricular failure.

Palpitation may represent sinus tachycardia with minimum exertion or commonly occurring arrhythmias. Sustained episodes of awareness of a rapid heartbeat may be associated with supraventricular or ventricular tachycardia. Easy fatigability is often due to low cardiac output and may replace dyspnea as a prominent presenting symptom.

Dependent edema is secondary to systemic venous congestion and constitutes evidence of right ventricular failure, whereas right upper quadrant abdominal pain with tenderness indicates hepatic congestion. Generally, weight loss and anorexia are late features, although apparent weight gain from water retention may mask muscle wasting.

The physical examination may provide important diagnostic clues in the more advanced phase, but is generally not helpful in the early phase of minimum or no symptoms.

Signs of systemic venous congestion may include jugular venous distention, hepatomegaly, dependent edema, ascites, and, in advanced cases, mild jaundice and cachexia. Signs of pulmonary venous congestion include pulmonary rales and pleural effusions.

There is lateral and caudal displacement of a sustained left ventricular apical impulse, and the diastolic rapid-filling phase (S_3) and presystolic (S_4) phase of the left ventricle are often palpable. A prominent pulmonic component of S_2 is heard in patients with severe pulmonary hypertension. The presence of an apical S_3 is related to an increased left atrial (filling) pressure, dilated chamber, and reduced cardiac output. An apical S_4 is related to diminished left ventricular compliance and strong atrial contraction. The presence of both S_3 and S_4 results in a quadruple rhythm and, in the presence of tachycardia, may simulate a middiastolic rumble. When S_3 and S_4 are superimposed during tachycardia, a loud summation gallop sound may be heard. Not infrequently, the S_3 or summation gallop sound may be the loudest sound appreciated over the apex. Similar gallop sounds originating in the right heart are generally best heard over the lower left sternal edge and subxiphoid areas (Chapter 3).

An apical systolic murmur of mitral regurgitation may be heard as a high-pitched, blowing murmur of variable duration and intensity. A similar murmur at the lower left sternal edge may represent tricuspid regurgitation. A diastolic rumble suggests a more severe degree of mitral regurgitation.

Pulsus alternans is often noted as an evidence of ventricular dysfunction (Chapter 3). It is generally accentuated by upright posture and other maneuvers resulting in decreased ventricular volume.

On the chest x-ray, cardiomegaly with enlargement of all chambers is generally noted in symptomatic patients. The lung fields show signs of pulmonary venous congestion and edema.

On the ECG, sinus tachycardia, intraventricular conduction disturbances, signs of left ventricular or biventricular enlargement, signs of left or biatrial enlargement, and low voltage are noted, singly or in combination. Although first- or second-degree AV block may be observed, higher degrees of heart block are uncommon.

The M-mode echocardiogram is extremely useful to confirm diagnosis and to, as quantitatively assess ventricular function. The left ventricular internal dimension is increased, often in excess of 7 cm; its percentage of dimensional shortening is markedly reduced (Chapter 5). The ventricular septum and posterior left ventricular walls are of normal thickness. The percentage of thickening and excursions of both walls during systole are reduced. The degree of left ventricular dilatation is variable and some symptomatic patients may have a normal-sized left ventricle despite marked reduction of contractile function. A characteristic appearance of the mitral leaflets in the middle of the left ventricular cavity may draw attention to the diagnosis (Fig. 10-3). The diastole opening E point of the anterior mitral leaflet is further removed from the left side of the interventricular septum, denoted as E point–septal separation. This distance may be well in excess of 1 cm and reflects reduced ejection fraction. In advanced disease, with the ejection fraction below 25%, the E point–septal separation is often greater than 2.5 cm. A prominent beta notch in the mitral valve echo indicates elevated left ventricular end diastolic pressure. The valves are structurally normal in the absence of coexisting organic valvular heart disease. The left atrium and the right ventricle are often enlarged. The prognostic value of echocardiography was reported in a large series of patients with myocardial failure. The ratio of left ventricular dimension to wall thickness and the E point–septal separation were more predictive of long-term mortality.

Two-dimensional echocardiography permits a more accurate evaluation of chamber size and overall ventricular function. It also helps the differentiation from coronary artery disease with congestive heart failure by demonstrating local areas of asynergy when ischemic heart disease is present. Doppler echocardiography commonly demonstrates regurgitation across the mitral and tricuspid valves even in the absence of murmurs. Mitral inflow velocity pattern may show tall, peaked E wave with rapid deceleration suggesting elevated left atrial pressure. Right ventricular and pulmonary artery pressures can be estimated by the use of continuous-wave Doppler signal of tricuspid regurgitation. Cardiac output measured by Doppler methods may be useful for following the clinical course of patients, along with 2D echocardiographic estimates of ejection fraction and chamber dilatation.

Radionuclide angiography allows accurate assessment of ejection fraction, as well as semiquantitative evaluation of regional wall motion abnormalities. Radionuclide ejection fraction may be used as a noninvasive index of ventricular pump function in follow-up studies to determine the course of the disease. Quantitation of ejection fraction and segmental wall motion by echocardiography is equally reliable.

A diagnosis of dilated cardiomyopathy may be made in most patients from the clinical and noninvasive studies. Cardiac catheterization may be indicated (1) to assess the severity of coexisting valvular heart disease, (2) to assess the presence of associated coronary artery disease, and (3) to evaluate the acute effects of therapeutic interventions.

Extensive multivessel coronary artery disease may coexist without symptomatic ischemic events. This probably unfavorably alters the prognosis. The term *ischemic cardiomyopathy* is often used to describe patients with global dysfunction secondary to chronic global ischemia (hibernating myocardium) without clinically evident myocardial infarction. Those with truly ischemic cardiomyopathy may benefit from myocardial revascularization (e.g., coronary bypass surgery) with improved ejection fraction.

Management

Since the underlying cause in most cases of dilated cardiomyopathy is unknown or no longer relevant, the principles of management are largely symptomatic or supportive (Table 17-1). These may best be considered under (1) reduction in cardiac work, (2) supportive measures, (3) measures directed toward specific causes, and (4) radical therapy.

Burch has advocated prolonged complete bed rest for 6 months to 1 year based on his experience that marked reduction in heart size was observed in over 50% of patients so treated. These results are difficult to interpret, since a large number of the patients were alcoholic, and alcohol withdrawal may have been largely responsible for the improvement. This type of protracted complete bed rest resulting in muscle wasting is unacceptable to most patients. However, the current trend in management is to recommend moderate levels of activity.

The introduction of vasodilator therapy in the treatment of acute or chronic congestive failure with or without acute myocardial infarction is a major therapeutic advance (Chapter 10). Patients with dilated or congestive cardiomyopathy are often managed effectively with the use of these agents. The usefulness of vasodilators is well established in the presence of moderate or severe heart failure despite digitalis and diuretic therapy. Reductions of both preload and afterload by vasodilator therapy are desirable end points in the setting of increased filling pressures and result in decreased ventricular volume, reduced wall tension, decreased oxygen and metabolic demands, and often an increase in cardiac output. Vasodilator agents currently in use include intravenous sodium nitroprusside, sublingual and oral nitrates, intravenous and oral hydralazine, oral prazosin, and converting enzyme inhibitors such as captopril or enalapril (Chapter 10).

The arteriolar smooth muscle dilator hydralazine, in a dosage of 25 to 100 mg three or four times a day, produces an increase in cardiac output with minor effects on filling pressures, arterial pressure, or heart rate in most patients with chronic heart failure. Side effects of this drug, especially a lupuslike syndrome, may seriously limit its long-term use in large dosages.

The antihypertensive drug prazosin is a potent alpha-adrenergic blocking agent with balanced vasodilator effects on venous and arterial beds. It is effective orally and requires an initial dose of 1 mg to minimize symptomatic se-

Table 17-1. Differential features of the cardiomyopathies

Feature	Dilated or congestive	Hypertrophic	Restrictive
Symptoms	Dyspnea, fatigue, orthopnea, cough, leg edema, ascites	Dyspnea, angina, dizziness, syncope, palpitations	Dyspnea, fatigue, leg edema, ascites
Physical findings	Moderate to severe cardiomegaly, sustained apical impulse, S_3 and S_4 common, murmur of mitral or tricuspid regurgitation	Mild cardiomegaly, sustained or bifid apical impulse with prominent atrial impulse, brisk carotid upstroke, S_4 common; ejection systolic murmur along left sternal edge, longer apical systolic murmur, both often increased during Valsalva strain	Mild to moderate cardiomegaly, prominent S_3, mitral or tricuspid regurgitation common, inspiratory increase in venous pressure
Electrocardiogram	Sinus tachycardia, ventricular and atrial enlargement, arrhythmia, bundle branch block	Left ventricular hypertrophy, short P-R, abnormal Q waves, arrhythmias	Low voltage, interventricular and AV conduction defects
Echocardiogram	Dilated cavities, normal wall thicknesses, decreased fractional shortening, evidence of reduced ejection fraction, MR and TR	Normal or small left ventricular cavity, asymmetrical hypertrophy, systolic anterior motion, small left ventricular outflow, characteristic Doppler velocity profile of LVOT obstruction	Normal to mild dilatation of cavity, reduced systolic function, thick walls, pericardial effusion, mitral inflow patterns of LV diastolic dysfunction
Medical treatment			
Digitalis	Yes	No	Perhaps
Diuretics	Yes	Perhaps	Yes
Vasodilators	Yes	No	Yes
Sympathomimetic amines	Perhaps	No	Perhaps
Vasoconstrictors	No	Yes	No
Beta blockers	No	Yes	No
Calcium blockers	No	Yes	No
Ace inhibitors	Yes	No	No
Disopyramide	No	Yes	No
Surgical treatment	? Transplantation	Ventriculomyectomy	? Transplantation
Prognosis	Progressive worsening	Generally stable	Rapid worsening
Complications	Heart failure, arrhythmias, systemic or pulmonary embolism	Sudden death, arrhythmias, infective endocarditis, heart failure, systemic embolism	Heart failure, arrhythmias

Modified from Wynne J and Braunwald E: The cardiomyopathies and myocarditides, In Braunwald E, editor: Heart disease, Philadelphia 1980, Saunders.

vere hypotension, which is often seen with the first dose. The drug may be given in a twice-a-day regimen, generally in a dosage not to exceed 10 mg twice daily. This drug has been shown to increase cardiac output and decrease filling pressures (Chapter 10).

The agents captopril and enalapril inhibit conversion of angiotensin I to angiotensin II and the degradation of bradykinin. They cause a reduction in systemic vascular resistance and ventricular filling pressures, with an increase in cardiac output and no change in heart rate.

The long-term efficacy of oral vasodilators in double-blind cooperative studies shows improved survival after use of hydralazine-nitrate combination, and of enalapril. Enalapril, when administered to patients receiving digitalis and diuretics, improved survival compared to a placebo. This beneficial effect was seen in patients with mild symptoms (class II), as well as with more advanced symptoms (classes III or IV). Enalapril improved survival in a head-to-head comparison with hydralazine–isosorbide dinitrate combination, and tends to be better tolerated with fewer side effects for long-term use. Administration of prazosin was not associated with improved survival when compared to placebo.

Long-term oral administration of digitalis has long-established effectiveness in treating chronic congestive heart failure (Chapter 10). The drug is generally used before vasodilators are administered. The basic therapeutic use of digitalis in patients with dilated cardiomyopathy is similar to that for congestive heart failure from any cause. It is especially indicated in the presence of resting sinus tachycardia and supraventricular arrhythmias, including atrial fibrillation.

Among the catecholamines and other sympathomimetic amines, the agents with the most therapeutically potent beta-adrenergic effects on the myocardium are dopamine and dobutamine (Chapters 10 and 11). The role of these agents in dilated cardiomyopathy with congestive heart failure is restricted to advanced refractory heart failure. They favorably influence circulatory and metabolic balance. Intravenous infusions of either drug over 5 to 10 days may be attempted with pulmonary artery and wedge pressure monitoring using a flow-directed balloon catheter in an intensive care unit setting. Intra-arterial pressures are usually also monitored. Frequent measurements of filling pressures, cardiac output, blood gases, and urinary output are necessary as a guide to the proper dosage and to monitor the therapeutic response. These agents may be less effective and possibly detrimental in the absence of high filling pressure (wedge pressure < 15 mm Hg). Newer inotropic agents, for example amrinone and milrinone, are often beneficial when administered acutely; however, a deleterious effect on survival with their chronic use is reported (Chapter 10).

Long-term oral anticoagulant therapy may be considered in patients on prolonged bed rest, since the likelihood of venous thromboembolic disease is increased in the setting of low cardiac output. Similarly, patients with chronic or frequent atrial fibrillation, echocardiographically demonstrated intracardiac clots, or evidence of systemic or pulmonary thromboembolism are candidates for anticoagulant therapy. There are no prospective studies showing improved risk-benefit ratio to justify routine use of anticoagulents in all cases. Chronic hepatic congestion and previous alcohol-induced hepatic damage may complicate successful anticoagulant therapy.

The long-term use of beta-adrenergic blocking agents is controversial, but has been reported to produce favorable results in about half the patients, with resultant decreases in heart size and amelioration of heart failure. However, these drugs depress myocardial function and, as a rule, are contraindicated in the presence of heart failure.

Antiarrhythmic drugs may be required in patients with dilated cardiomyopathy who have documented arrhythmias. Both supraventricular and ventricular arrhythmias are frequent, and the latter probably explains many of the sudden deaths observed in these patients. It remains to be demonstrated if the use of antiarrhythmic agents improves survival in this subset of patients. Indeed, increased proarrhythmia with class I agents may produce an adverse outcome.

Cardiac transplantation (Chapter 25) may be considered for younger patients with advanced myocardial damage refractory to medical therapy who show no evidence of severe pulmonary hypertension or other organ involvement. This procedure is carried out at selected centers. The 1-year patient survival rate is in excess of 80%, which is comparable to the survival rate with cadaver kidney transplants. With improved understanding of the immunologic aspects of rejection, as well as improved availability of donor organs, transplantation may offer considerable promise for patients with advanced dilated cardiomyopathy.

A large body of evidence incriminates heavy alcohol intake in dilated cardiomyopathy. In early cases, total abstinence may produce dramatic recovery. The cardiac depressant effects of alcohol make it an undesirable substance for such patients, even when no definite causal connection appears likely.

Severe hypophosphatemia in burn patients, prolonged respiratory alkalosis, chronic phosphate-binding antacid use, and treatment of diabetic ketoacidosis resulting in serum phosphate levels below 1.0 mg per deciliter may lead to dilated cardiomyopathy and congestive heart failure. Replenishment of phosphate rapidly leads to complete recovery.

Lithium carbonate used in manic-depressive disorders may result in toxic damage to the myocardium, with cardiac dilatation, ventricular arrhythmias, and sudden death. High doses of cyclophosphamide have been associated with congestive heart failure and death from hemorrhagic myocarditis with cardiac dilatation.

Doxorubicin therapy is associated with progressive cardiomegaly and depression of cardiac function. The toxicity is dose related and is observed in about 2% of patients so treated. Ingestion of a toxic dose is fatal in over half the patients. Its occurrence may be prevented if a cumulative dose of less than 500 mg/m^2 is given. Daunorubicin shows a greater propensity than doxorubicin for cardiac toxicity in the doses used. Patients receiving these agents should be followed by periodic echocardiograms to reveal early evidence of cardiac involvement.

Beriberi heart disease, although rare in Western countries, may cause high-output congestive heart failure with cardiomegaly in nutritionally deprived parts of the world. It is rapidly reversible with replacement of thiamine.

HYPERTROPHIC CARDIOMYOPATHIES

Hypertrophic cardiomyopathy (HCM) is a form of primary myocardial disease with a characteristic clinical and pathologic expression. Several terms have been used for the disorder: *idiopathic hypertrophic subaortic stenosis* (IHSS) in the United States, *muscular subaortic stenosis* in Canada, and *hypertrophic obstructive cardiomyopathy* (HOCM) in Europe.

A term that includes "subaortic stenosis" is unfortunate, since the disorder may be expressed without left ventricular outflow obstruction, and since patients with isolated infundibular subpulmonic stenosis have been described. It is more accurate and potentially less confusing to refer to the disorder as *hypertrophic cardiomyopathy* and add the word *obstructive* if either left or right ventricular outflow obstruction can be demonstrated.

Etiology

Despite considerable progress in understanding the clinical hemodynamic, pathologic, and function aspects of HCM, the underlying cause and pathogenesis of this disease are largely unknown. The asymmetrical type of HCM is commonly a genetically transmitted disorder, but sporadic cases are also recognized. The findings of a recent study on the genetic aspect using echocardiography to identify asymmetrical septal hypertrophy suggested an autosomal dominant transmission.

An abnormal response of the myocardium to normal catecholamines has been postulated as a pathogenetic mechanism. The clinical association between HOCM and pheochromocytoma, neurofibromatosis, and lentiginosis suggests a genetic disorder of neural crest tissue. Experimental production of massive left ventricular hypertrophy with outflow obstruction after a small, sustained infusion of norepinephrine lends support to this postulate.

Disproportionate septal thickness and myofiber disarray are found in normal embryonic and fetal cardiac morphogenesis. Therefore, HCM may represent failure of regression rather than postnatal development. Increased sympathetic stimulation or increased receptor-site sensitivity may play a role in the failure of regression. Alternatively, it is possible that the manifest disorder represents a genetically determined response of hypertrophy to circulatory overload. Once the process is initiated, the abnormal arrangement of the myofibers results in systolic and diastolic malfunction, which in turn may provide a stimulus for further hypertrophy. More recent molecular-genetic studies have linked familial hypertrophic cardiomyopathy to the cardiac myosin heavy-chain genes on chromosome 14 in some but not all families, indicating genetic heterogeneity. The presence of different disease genes or different mutations within a given gene may account for differences in clinical expression of familial HCM. A recent report has identified nearly 50% of families with a beta cardiac myosin heavy-chain mutation. Additionally, knowledge of the precise mutation in an individual patient may provide prognostic information. Future research into molecular-genetic studies is expected to shed additional light on this subject.

Pathology

The pathologic findings observed at autopsy are remarkably uniform and include massive and asymmetrical hypertrophy. Thickening of the walls involves both the atria and the ventricles, although the most characteristic findings involve the left ventricle. The interventricular septum is generally much more massively hypertrophied than the free wall. This peculiar asymmetrical septal hypertrophy may provide the necessary hemodynamic conditions that produce a dynamic outflow obstruction. Localization of such hypertrophy in the midlateral wall may result in midventricular obstruction and its distribution in the right ventricular infundibulum in subpulmonic stenosis.

In a subgroup of patients defined by 2D echocardiographic, cineangiographic, and/or postmortem examination, the hypertrophy involved primarily the apical portion of the left ventricular rather than the outflow tract. This is termed asymmetric apical hypertrophy and such patients have none of the clinical features of intraventricular obstruction.

Striking pathologic features common to most patients with outflow obstruction include fibrous thickening of the anterior mitral leaflet and plaques in the upper interventricular septum constituting the left ventricular outflow tract. The former is thought to represent the result of frequent collisions of the anterior mitral leaflet against the interventricular septum. The endocardial plaques in the septum may be the result of jet lesions distal to the obstruction. The aortic valve is generally normal, and the coronary arteries are large and patent in the absence of coexisting disease.

On microscopy, a bizarre and disorderly array of muscle fibers is a striking feature and is associated with increased connective tissue that interrupts and crisscrosses muscle bundles. Myofibril disarray is not pathognomonic for this disease and is often spotty in distribution, but the disarray is quantitatively more severe in this condition than in others. Additional features include deep clefts in the septum, abnormal narrowing of small intramural coronary arteries, and sclerosis of the sinus node.

One report has emphasized the importance of the peculiar catenoid shape of the interventricular septum: it is convex to the left in the apex-to-base plane, but concave on its left ventricular surface in the cross sections. This bizarre and characteristic shape is thought to be responsible for the adynamic nature of the septum. It is hypothesized that fiber disarray and local hypertrophy could result from isometric contraction of a catenoid septum.

Pathophysiology

The functional end results of the abnormal anatomy are characteristic. They include changes in both systolic and diastolic left ventricular function, with profound effects on pressures and flow.

The integrity of overall systolic function is rather well preserved until the end stage; indeed, hypercontractility is a hallmark of the disorder. The cardiac output is generally normal or even increased; the ejection fraction is often supernormal. The rate of ejection is accelerated, so it is mostly completed in the first 60% to 80% of systole. Although global function is well preserved, regional abnormalities occur; for example, the upper interventricular septum is often hypodynamic and shows reduced thickening during systole. The free walls are generally hypercontractile.

Left ventricular outflow obstruction is dynamic and variable. The variability can be observed within the same cardiac cycle, from one beat to the next and from one physiologic state to another. When present, outflow obstruction begins after the onset of early uninterrupted ejection. Present evidence suggests that the obstruction is caused by a sharp systolic anterior motion (SAM) of the anterior mitral leaflet, which obliterates the outflow space. The actual mechanism of SAM is not clear, although it is likely to be the result of a Venturi effect from the rapid ejection of a jet of blood through an anatomically narrowed outflow space. The degree of left ventricular outflow obstruction can be accentuated by factors that reduce preload (end-diastolic volume), diminish afterload (arterial pressure), or increase contractility or heart rate. Echocardiographic recordings have demonstrated that SAM of the mitral valve is both exacerbated and prolonged by interventions that accentuate the outflow obstruction, and vice versa. Some investigators interpret intraventricular pressure gradients as not indicative of true obstruction, since left ventricular emptying is normal or exaggerated. These have been attributed to cavity obliteration. Recent echocardiographic and Doppler techniques have elucidated differences between true gradients resulting from obstruction and those caused by cavity obliteration.

Mitral regurgitation is demonstrated by color-flow Doppler echocardiography in about 90% of obstructive patients and is related to the dynamic outflow obstruction in the vast majority. Thus, when outflow obstruction is accentuated with a more persistent and prominent SAM, mitral regurgitation is more severe. The factors that decrease outflow obstruction tend to reduce the degree of mitral regurgitation.

Severe right ventricular infundibular stenosis is rare and may occur either independently or concurrently with left ventricular outflow obstruction. The mechanism of right ventricular outflow obstruction is different from that on the left side, since the infundibulum is circumferentially bound by muscle. Excessive muscle contraction in this disorder results in outflow obstruction, and the factors resulting in increased contractility tend to accentuate obstruction. The tricuspid valve does not appear to play any important role in the right-sided outflow obstruction.

Distensibility and compliance of the hypertrophied ventricles are reduced, with resulting elevation in end-diastolic pressure without an increase in volume. The abnormalities of early diastolic relaxation coupled with reduced distensibility tend to influence the pattern of diastolic filling. Thus, early, rapid, passive filling is notably impaired, necessitating a stronger atrial contraction to deliver diastolic inflow into a relatively nondistensible left ventricle. This dependence on atrial contraction to maintain efficient flow is exemplified by a sudden drop in cardiac output when atrial fibrillation supervenes. Although this abnormality of diastolic compliance has important hemodynamic consequences, namely, elevations of left atrial and pulmonary venous pressures with resultant pulmonary congestion and edema, actual obstruction to inflow is rare.

Clinical features

The clinical findings in HCM are summarized in Table 17-1. Effort dyspnea and paroxysmal nocturnal dyspnea constitute the most common symptoms and represent evidence of pulmonary congestion. Because elevations in pulmonary venous and left atrial pressures occur in the presence of a hyperdynamic, hypercontractile left ventricle, they must be attributed to increased stiffness of the hypertrophic ventricles. In some patients, especially those with volume overload, frank pulmonary edema may be noted.

Frank syncope and dizziness short of loss of consciousness (presyncope) are common. These may be effort-related, although they are not predictably so. The frequency of the episodes is highly variable. The exact mechanism is obscure; however, it is probably related to reflex vasodilatation and hypotension induced by stretching the left ventricular baroreceptors. Alternatively, arrhythmia may play a role by producing a decrease in cardiac output.

Typical effort angina simulating symptomatic coronary artery disease is frequent, although episodes of chest pain may be prolonged and may occur spontaneously at rest. Typically, sublingual nitroglycerin fails to provide prompt relief, although this is not a universal finding. In the presence of large, patent coronary arteries, ischemia is probably caused by intramyocardial compression of coronary arteries and increased myocardial tension and muscle mass, with oxygen requirements outstripping oxygen delivery.

Palpitations may merely represent awareness of forcible heartbeats, especially in the left lateral decubitus position. More commonly, atrial and ventricular arrhythmias are responsible. Tachyarrhythmias are poorly tolerated and are often associated with symptoms of low output and hypotension. Isolated or short runs of ventricular and supraventricular premature depolarizations often occur without symptoms.

The physical signs also tend to vary considerably from minimal or nonspecific to highly characteristic. The characteristic signs include evidence of left ventricular hypertrophy and obstruction of left ventricular outflow, left ventricular inflow, and right ventricular outflow.

A powerful systolic thrust of the left ventricle on palpation indicates an increase in muscle mass, and, although less frequent, the characteristic bifid apex in systole is virtually diagnostic of this condition. A prominent atrial contraction imparts a strong presystolic impulse that is palpable at the apex. A trifid impulse composed of a prominent A wave and bifid systolic peaks is sometimes palpable and often recordable on apex cardiogram. Such a finding is highly characteristic of this disease. S_4 is present in virtually every patient in sinus rhythm.

A jerky arterial pulse with sharp upstroke is typical, although not diagnostic. Occasionally, a bifid (bisferiens) pulse may be left, especially in the carotid artery (Chapter 3). A bifid arterial pulse in association with a normal pulse pressure is highly characteristic of HOCM (Fig. 17-1). The pulse contour in HOCM is influenced by the presence and severity of outflow obstruction. In the absence of resting obstruction, the arterial pulse is essentially normal.

A systolic murmur of variable intensity is present along the left sternal border and apex. It is poorly transmitted to the aortic area and neck vessels. It is medium pitched or high pitched, with onset after the S_1. The murmur resembles a long ejection murmur along the left sternal border and attains a regurgitant quality (high pitched, blowing) toward the apex. The apical murmur may be well transmitted to the axilla. The S_2 is clearly audible, and both com-

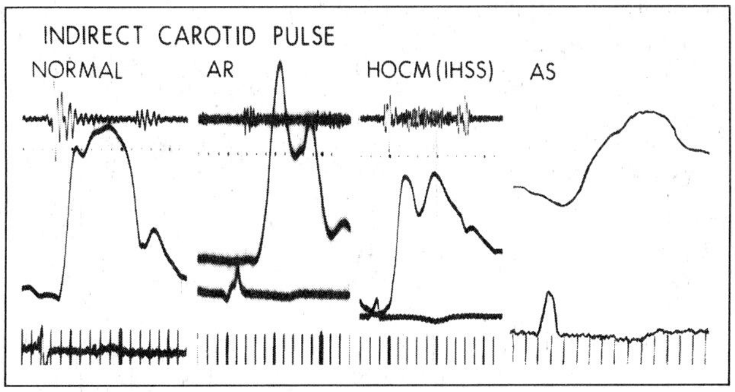

Fig. 17-1. Contour of indirect carotid pulse in hypertrophic obstructive cardiomyopathy, HOCM (IHSS), compared with normal, aortic regurgitation (AR), and aortic stenosis (AS). Note the bifid systolic pulse in AR and HOCM, although the former is associated with wide pulse pressure and the latter with normal pulse pressure.

ponents are well preserved. Reverse splitting with a delayed aortic component is diagnostic of severe outflow obstruction in the absence of left bundle branch block. The signs of outflow obstruction, including intensity of the systolic murmur, are accentuated by maneuvers that augment the severity of obstruction (Table 17-2 and Fig. 17-2).

The blowing apical murmur of mitral regurgitation also generally varies in intensity with dynamic outflow obstruction. In a few patients, associated severe mitral valve regurgitation independent of outflow obstruction may be present. The presence of independent mitral valve regurgitation can be determined by raising the blood pressure with methoxamine or angiotensin, which, while relieving outflow obstruction, do not diminish murmur intensity if the regurgitation is unrelated to obstruction. These patients may require mitral valve surgery; hence, this differentiation is clinically important.

Whereas a prominent atrial sound (S_4) is a constant feature of a noncompliant hypertrophied left ventricle, a mitral diastolic murmur simulating mitral stenosis may occasionally lead to consideration of rheumatic mitral disease. The absence of an opening snap and the presence of severe, unexplained left ventricular hypertrophy should point to a correct diagnosis.

The systolic murmur of infundibular pulmonic stenosis is similar to that noted in congenital infundibular pulmonic stenosis. The murmur is not prominent at the lower left sternal edge. The ejection sound is absent, and the pulmonary closure sound is delayed. When infundibular obstruction accompanies left ventricular outflow obstruction, the clinical signs of the latter dominate. However, isolated right ventricular outflow obstruction may be difficult to differentiate from congenital infundibular pulmonic stenosis until evidence for unexplained left ventricular hypertrophy is sought.

The common conditions to be considered in the differential diagnosis include other forms of left ventricular outflow obstruction, mitral regurgitation, and coronary artery disease.

Table 17-2. Effects of physiologic and pharmacologic maneuvers in hypertrophic obstructive cardiomyopathy

Intervention	Left ventricular outflow obstruction	Murmur
Valsalva		
Phase 2–3	Increased	Increased
Phase 4	Decreased	Decreased
Squatting	Decreased	Decreased
Upright posture	Increased	Increased
Exercise	Increased	Increased
Amyl nitrite inhalation	Increased	Increased
Methoxamine	Decreased	Decreased
Isoproterenol	Increased	Increased
Propranolol	Decreased or unchanged	Decreased or unchanged

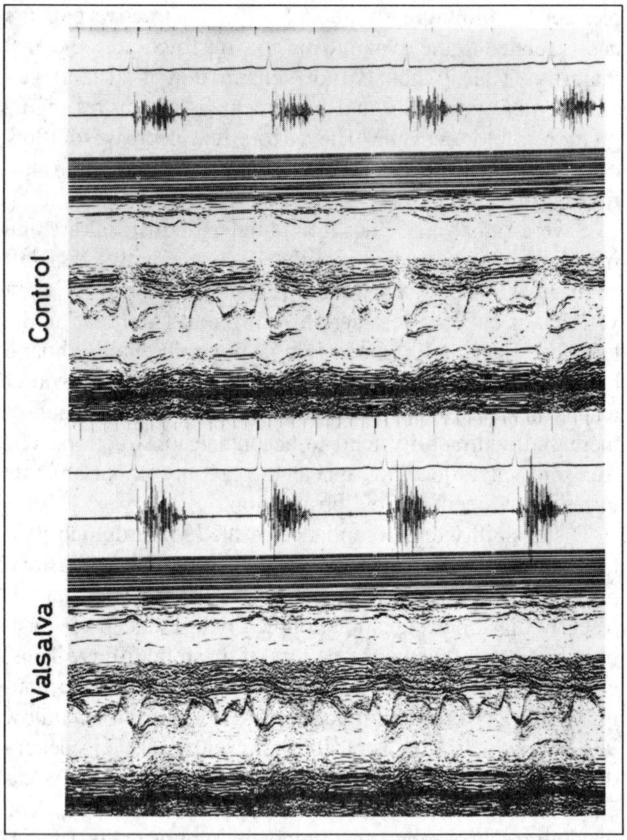

Fig. 17-2. Effects of Valsalva maneuver on the murmur intensity and SAM of the mitral valve are shown in the control *(upper panel)* and during Valsalva strain *(lower panel)*. Note the increase in amplitude of the murmur along with more prominent systolic motion.

Laboratory diagnosis

The laboratory findings in HCM are summarized in Table 17-1. A routine 12-lead ECG often discloses evidence of left ventricular hypertrophy with increased QRS voltage or ST-T wave changes in the lateral precordial leads (V_4 to V_6). All signs of left ventricular hypertrophy are absent in about 10% of patients despite the massive increase in cardiac muscle mass. Hence, a normal ECG does not exclude the diagnosis of HCM. Occasionally, large, abnormal Q waves simulating myocardial infarction are noted because of septal depolarization. These changes of pseudoinfarction are present in less than 10% of patients.

Other features include a short P-R interval, Wolff-Parkinson-White syndrome, left-axis deviation caused by left anterior hemiblock, and complete left or right bundle branch block. Atrial and ventricular premature depolarizations are common, but may be detected only with ambulatory ECG recording. Complete heart block is rare.

Posteroanterior and lateral chest x-rays are often normal. Evidence of left ventricular enlargement may be subtle, since the cavity size is not increased. Left atrial size is either normal or only slightly increased, except in a stage of advanced decompensation. Pulmonary venous engorgement may be seen, but frank pulmonary edema and signs of pulmonary arterial hypertension are infrequent.

Echocardiography (Chapter 5) is an important method of diagnosing HCM (Fig. 17-3). This technique is useful for evaluating the thickness of the interventricular septum and left ventricular posterior wall; their movements in systole; the end-diastolic and end-systolic dimensions of the left ventricular cavity along its minor axis; the left ventricular outflow size, defined as the space between the anterior mitral leaflet and interventricular septum; and the functional aspects of mitral and aortic valve motion. It also permits differentiation of concentric from asymmetrical hypertrophy. In the former, the interventricular septum/left ventricular posterior wall ratio is close to unity; in the latter, the ratio exceeds 1.3:1.0. When the ratio of 1.3:1.0 is used, some degree of overlap is observed, but a ratio greater than 1.5:1.0 is more specific for asymmetry.

Dynamic left ventricular outflow obstruction is diagnosed by analyzing the systolic motion of the mitral valve. Abnormal SAM of the anterior mitral leaflet with its apposition against the interventricular septum localizes the outflow obstruction in HOCM. The SAM begins sometime after completion of early ejection and is terminated in end-systole before the S_2.

The dynamic nature of obstruction may be interpreted from variations in the extent of SAM with different maneuvers designed to alter the dynamic obstruction. Patients without resting obstruction usually have small and incomplete SAM, whereas those with high resting gradients tend to have complete SAM consistently noted from one beat to the next. Since SAM of the anterior mitral leaflet is probably caused by a Venturi effect from rapid, early ejection across the left ventricular outflow space, its occurrence in other conditions may be predicted. It has been noted in hyperkinetic circulatory states, in aortic regurgitation, and during infusion of dopamine in a patient in shock. Echocardiographic simulation of SAM may be observed in mitral valve prolapse and in pericardial effusion, but the differentiation is generally easy. As a result of the dynamic midsystolic obstruction to outflow, the aortic valve cusps may show premature closure with late systolic reopening. Diastolic movement of the mitral valve is impaired, with a flat E to F slope (Chapter 5).

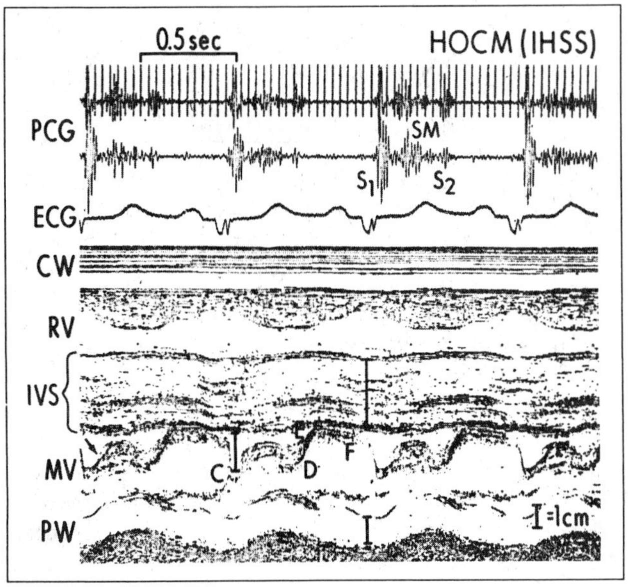

Fig. 17-3. M-mode echocardiogram in a patient with HOCM. The interventricular septum (IVS) is markedly thickened (2 cm) and is more than 1.5 times the thickness of the posterior wall (PW). The mitral valve (MV) echo shows systolic anterior motion *(arrow),* which starts after closure point C and returns to baseline before diastolic opening point D. The open valve in early diastole at point E comes in contact with the IVS, and the diastolic slope (E–F) is attenuated. PCG, phonocardiogram.

A combination of narrow left ventricular outflow space, thickened interventricular septum, and the typical SAM of the anterior mitral leaflet is virtually diagnostic of HOCM. When the interventricular septal wall/posterior wall ratio exceeds 1.5:1.0, asymmetrical hypertrophy can be diagnosed confidently. With rare exceptions, patients with HCM demonstrate asymmetrical septal hypertrophy, although the latter is not specific for HCM. Two-dimensional echocardiography may reveal the asymmetric hypertrophy to involve the lateral free wall, the apex, the distal septum, and rarely the posterioinferior wall. Additional findings include midsystolic preclosure of one or more aortic valve cusps (Fig. 17-4), a hypodynamic interventricular septum with diminished systolic motion, and reduced diastolic slope of the anterior mitral leaflet. When SAM is absent at rest and following provocative maneuvers (i.e., Valsalva maneuver or amyl nitrite inhalation), it may be inferred that HCM, if present, is of the nonobstructive type. When numerous criteria are observed, a diagnosis can be made from the echocardiographic examination alone. However, in the absence of clear evidence to support the diagnosis, further evaluation may be undertaken.

The advent of Doppler methods has demonstrated (1) mitral regurgitation, (2) localization of outflow obstruction with increased velocity, and (3) quantitation of outflow gradients using continuous-wave Doppler method. The 2D echocardiography technique (Fig. 17-5) generally permits differentiation of SAM involving the mitral leaflet from that involving the chordae tendineae. The leaflet SAM is more characteristically associated with outflow obstruction, whereas the chordal SAM may represent passive buckling of the chordae tendineae in a rapidly emptying left ventricle. With the advent of Doppler echocardiography, it is possible to obtain information on flow and pressure dynamics using pulsed- and continuous-wave modes. The pulsed-wave Doppler method can localize the site of obstruction by showing aliasing or turbulence below the aortic valve when obstruction is localized in the left ventricular outflow tract; the measurement of high velocities by the continuous-wave Doppler method can be used to estimate the pressure drop across the subvalvular obstruction. The contour of the outflow tract velocity profile mirrors the profile of the pressure drop from the left ventricular cavity to the outflow tract and assumes a characteristic dagger shape. As ventricular ejection begins, the early velocity is around 1.5 meters/second commensurate with the rapid early ejection. Subse-

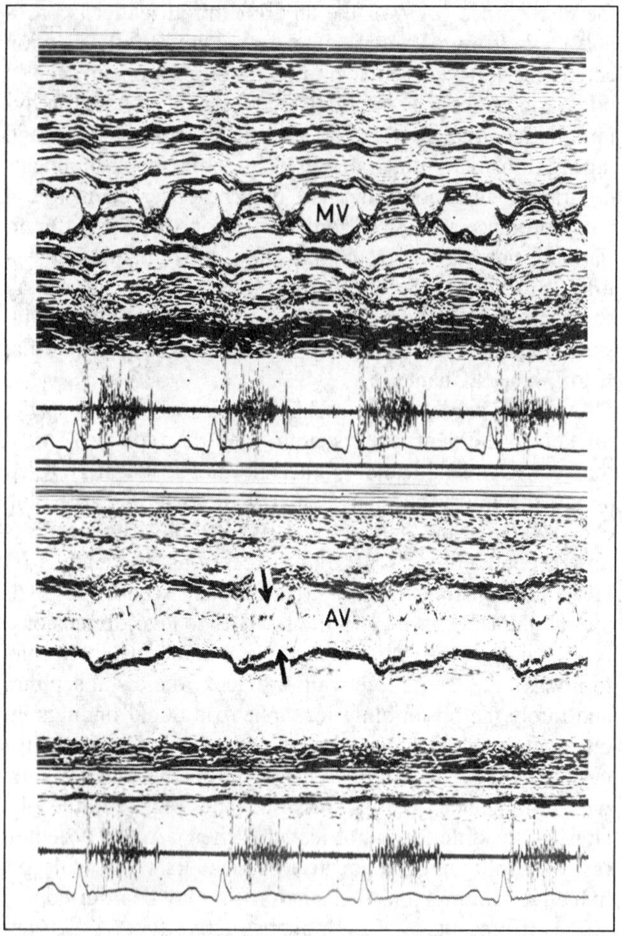

Fig. 17-4. M mode echocardiogram at the levels of the mitral valve (MV) *(upper panel),* and aortic valve (AV) *(lower panel),* in a patient with HOCM. Note the systolic anterior motion of the mitral valve and midsystolic aortic valve closure *(arrow).* Simultaneous ECG and phonocardiograms are shown in both panels. Note the phonocardiogram showing a late-onset murmur that ends before the S_2.

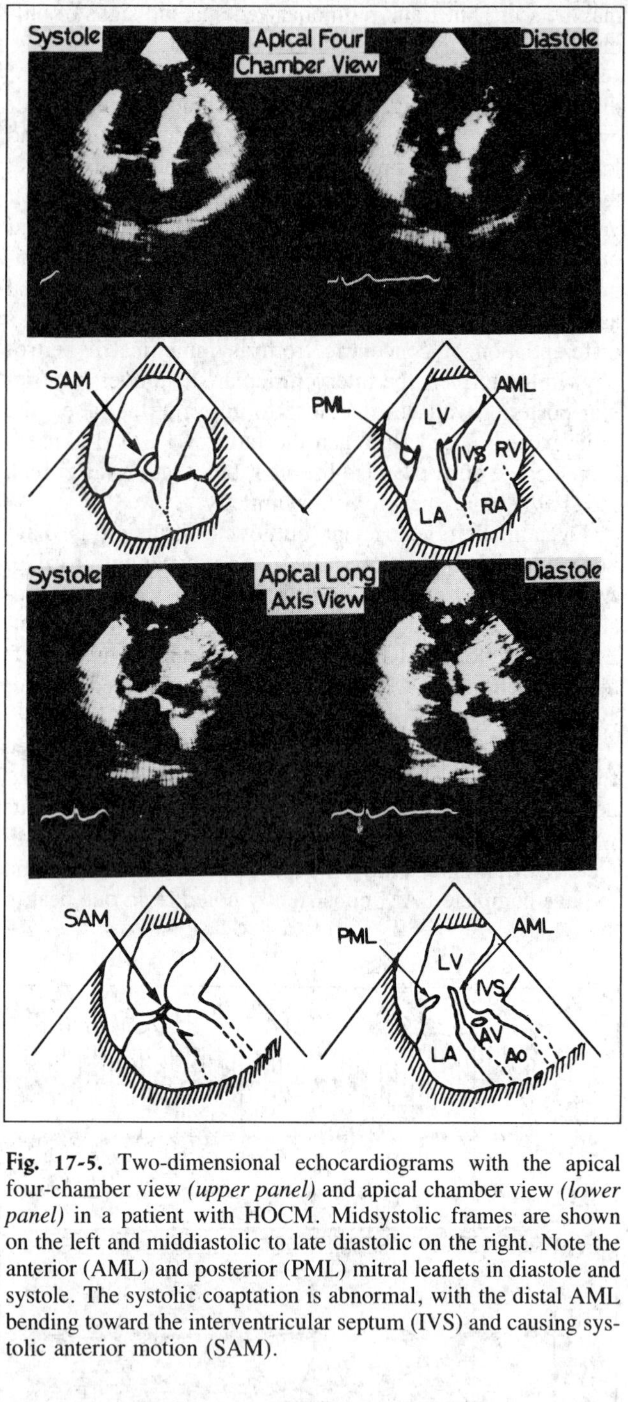

Fig. 17-5. Two-dimensional echocardiograms with the apical four-chamber view *(upper panel)* and apical chamber view *(lower panel)* in a patient with HOCM. Midsystolic frames are shown on the left and middiastolic to late diastolic on the right. Note the anterior (AML) and posterior (PML) mitral leaflets in diastole and systole. The systolic coaptation is abnormal, with the distal AML bending toward the interventricular septum (IVS) and causing systolic anterior motion (SAM).

quently, the Doppler velocity increases progressively to reach a peak in mid to late systole and returns to baseline at the end of ejection. This profile differs sharply from that seen in fixed obstruction, such as valvular aortic stenosis, where a smooth contour of increasing velocity is observed, even when it peaks in midsystole (Fig. 17-6). In addition, the presence and severity of mitral regurgitation can be assessed. A similar approach can be used to evaluate right ventricular infundibular obstruction.

Until the advent of echocardiography, final confirmation of diagnosis rested with cardiac catheterization and selective cardiac angiography (Chapter 6). A key diagnostic feature is the demonstration of dynamic left ventricular outflow obstruction. Special care must be taken, however, to avoid recording an artifactual gradient from entrapment of the catheter. Analysis of the recorded arterial pressure and pressure gradient during a postectopic beat often provides an important clue. Typically, the arterial pulse pressure is narrower in the postectopic beat than the sinus beat, in contrast to the normal and the fixed forms of left ventricular outflow obstruction (e.g., valvular aortic stenosis), when the pulse pressure is wider in the postectopic beat. Accentuation of outflow gradient with the Valsalva maneuver, amyl nitrite inhalation, or isoproterenol infusion provides added confirmation.

Selective left ventricular cineangiography demonstrates the characteristic anatomic and functional features (Chapter 6). Ventricular geometry is altered, the cavity assuming a sausage shape in the right anterior oblique projection. In a few patients, simultaneous left and right ventricular angiograms have been reported to demonstrate a massively

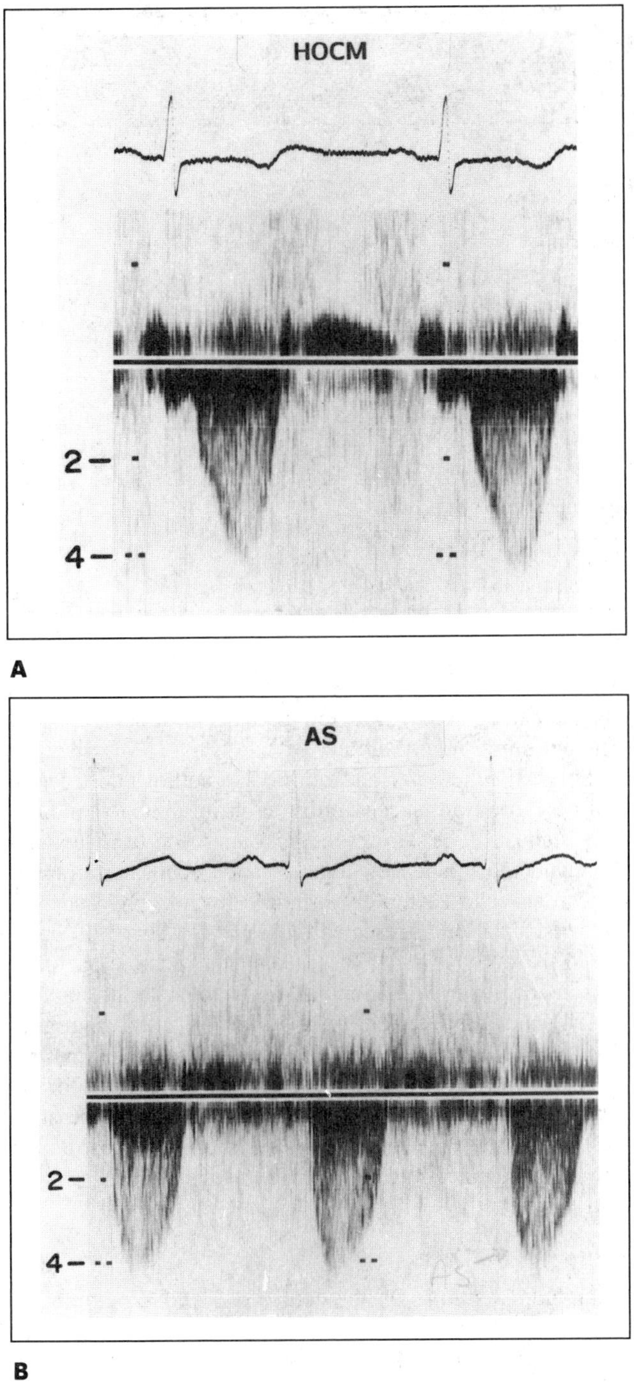

Fig. 17-6. The continuous-wave Doppler spectral display of velocity profile of outflow obstruction in hypertrophic obstructive cardiomyopathy (HOCM—**A**) shows a characteristic dagger shape. The peak velocity is reached in mid to late systole of 4.0 m/s consistent with peak systolic gradient of 64 mm Hg ($\Delta P = 4.V^2$). In contrast, the velocity profile in aortic valve stenosis (AS—**B**) shows a smooth progressive rise to a peak. The striking difference in the shapes of the velocity profiles by continuous-wave Doppler provides an important clue of dynamic (HOCM) versus fixed (AS) outflow obstruction.

thickened interventricular septum, especially in its midportion. Since echocardiography provides a reliable means of diagnosing HCM, catheterization-angiography studies are reserved for selected patients and situations and need to be carried out on rare occasions for diagnostic confirmation.

Management

Both medical and surgical management are palliative, since the cause of this bizarre cardiomyopathy is unknown. The major objectives of therapy are to improve symptoms, ameliorate outflow obstruction, improve left ventricular compliance, suppress arrhythmias, and prevent and treat major complications, that is, bacterial endocarditis and thromboembolism.

Medical management. The cardiac drugs commonly used for symptomatic relief of dyspnea or angina in other cardiac disorders are either contraindicated or must be used with caution (Tables 17-1 and 17-3). Thus digitalis must be avoided except to treat rapid atrial fibrillation when beta-adrenergic blockade and calcium channel blockers are unsuccessful or poorly tolerated. Nitrates are generally contraindicated and are often ineffective in relieving angina. Diuretics must be used with caution so as not to produce hypovolemia.

Beta-adrenergic blocking agents have been used extensively. Slowing the heart rate is generally beneficial. Although amelioration of obstruction induced by exercise and beta-adrenergic stimulation has been demonstrated, resting gradients are reduced only in some patients with labile obstruction. Symptomatic improvement is striking in some patients and may last several years, although increasing doses may be needed; others fail to experience sustained improvement. A daily dose in excess of 480 mg may be required for some patients. Recent observations of improved left ventricular compliance with beta-adrenergic blockage, if confirmed, may provide a rational explanation for symptomatic relief. These agents have not been shown to decrease the incidence of ventricular arrhythmias or sudden death. The dose of propranolol should be increased gradually and the effects monitored, especially in those without a major component of outflow obstruction.

A beneficial effect of the calcium channel–blocking drugs verapamil and long-acting nifedipine has been reported. Symptomatic amelioration is frequently observed; however, worsening of heart failure may result. In some patients with undue hypotensive effect, severe deterioration or even death may ensue. The use of these agents should be carefully monitored. Disopyramide (norpace) has been used for its negative inotropism to provide symptomatic improvement in some patients with hypertrophic obstructive cardiomyopathy.

The use of antiarrhythmic agents may become one of the most important medical interventions in HCM. Sudden cardiac death is overwhelmingly the most common mode of demise, probably from arrhythmias, although their causal role has not yet been definitely established. Atrial and ventricular arrhythmias occur in the majority of patients with

Table 17-3. Drugs used in hypertrophic cardiomyopathy

Cardiovascular drugs	Indications for use	Generally contraindicated
Propranolol and other beta blockers	Obstruction, arrhythmias, and (?) decreased left ventricular compliance	
Digitalis	Rapid, uncontrolled atrial fibrillations	Yes
Diuretics	Pulmonary and systemic congestion	With hypovolemia
Antianginal agents—nitrates and other vasodilators		Yes
Inotropic agents—isoproterenol, dopamine, epinephrine, bitartrate		Yes
Vasopressors—angiotensin, methoxamine	Hypotension	
Atropine sulfate	Extreme bradycardia	Yes
Antiarrhythmic agents—procainamide, quinidine sulfate, quinidine gluconate, amiodarone	Arrhythmias	
Oral anticoagulants	Atrial fibrillation or thromboembolism	
Calcium blockers—verapamil, nifedipine	Symptoms caused by obstruction or decreased left ventricular compliance	
Disopyramide	Symptoms caused by outflow obstruction	

HCM regardless of the symptomatic or hemodynamic state. Although supraventricular tachycardias may worsen symptoms, they have not been shown to be associated with sudden death. Ventricular tachycardia and other high-grade ventricular arrhythmias have been demonstrated in at least 30% of patients monitored by 72-hour ambulatory ECG recordings. Asymptomatic family members screened and found to have HCM also have a high incidence of asymptomatic ventricular arrhythmias. Treatment of ventricular tachycardia in all patients with HCM regardless of the presence of obstruction or symptoms is currently recommended. Unfortunately, ventricular arrhythmias generally have been found to be refractory to conventional agents alone or in combination with beta-adrenergic blockade. Amiodarone, a class III antiarrhythmic agent (Chapter 9), has been shown to suppress the majority of atrial and ventricular arrhythmias and is reported in an uncontrolled clinical trial to prevent sudden cardiac death in this disorder.

Bacterial endocarditis is a well-known complication, and the use of prophylactic antibiotics at times of risk is recommended. Thromboembolism is observed, especially in the presence of intermittent or sustained atrial fibrillation. Anticoagulation with sodium warfarin is advised in this clinical setting, particularly if an embolic episode has been diagnosed.

Surgical management. Considerable experience has been reported with transaortic ventriculomyotomy or ventriculomyectomy in patients with HOCM. Although the amount of muscle removed is small, several echocardiographic and cardiac catheterization studies have reported postoperative relief of outflow obstruction. Symptomatic improvement is often dramatic, along with reduction or abolition of the systolic murmur and other features of left ventricular outflow obstruction. The more recent surgical approach of mitral valve replacement to relieve outflow obstruction is usually not indicated, except in a few patients with severe, independent mitral regurgitation.

Surgical relief of right ventricular outflow obstruction can be carried out successfully, as in infundibular pulmonary stenosis. The current surgical approach to myectomy is considerably aided by intraoperative echocardiography. Epicardial echo accurately localizes hypertrophy and permits visualization of resected muscle in the shape of a tunnel in the outflow tract. Transesophageal echo is useful to demonstrate normalization of systolic anterior motion (SAM) and improvement or abolition of mitral regurgitation. This operation, to achieve consistent and optimal results, requires a team effort by an operating surgeon and cardiologist-echocardiographer. The present-day operative risk should not exceed 5% to 10% and relief of obstruction should be realized in over 95% of cases.

Natural history

Longitudinal studies on the course of HCM are limited in length of follow-up, but future long-term studies with additional anatomic and functional observations using echocardiography and ambulatory ECG recordings should provide useful data on its natural course.

A retrospective, multicenter study of 190 patients with verified HOCM, having a left ventricular outflow gradient either at rest or on provocation, examined the progression of the disease with an average follow-up of 5.2 years. In this study, older patients tended to have more symptoms (New York Heart Association functional class III or IV), possibly indicating a progressive course of disease. Clinical symptoms did not correlate with the severity of outflow obstruction or murmur intensity. After the follow-up period, 83% of the 141 surviving patients were either clinically improved or their condition had become stable.

Sudden cardiac death is the most common cause of death in patients with HCM regardless of symptomatic or hemodynamic states. Sudden death is statistically increased in patients who have a family history of sudden death and does not seem to be altered by treatment with beta-adrenergic blockers, calcium channel blockers, or surgical myotomy-myectomy, although patients surviving surgery are reported to have a lower incidence of sudden death in some series. Studies currently in progress suggest that ventricular tachycardia as documented by ambulatory ECG recordings is associated with sudden death, but a significant causal relationship has not yet been established. Furthermore, prevention of sudden death by the use of antiarrhythmic drugs remains to be demonstrated.

Progressive congestive heart failure with visceral congestion was rare, although this outcome may be more common during the end-stage disease with a longer follow-up. Twelve percent of patients had atrial arrhythmias, and almost half of those patients had established atrial fibrillation. Overall mortality from complications of the disease was 18% during the follow-up period, giving an attrition rate of approximately 3.4% per year.

The disorder cannot be considered benign, and the danger of sudden death exists despite clinical stability. Clinical observations suggest that in some families, without distinguishing features, there is a strong probability of sudden death in several closely related members.

Although slow progression of the disease and clinical stability are the rule in hypertrophic cardiomyopathy, sudden cardiac death may intervene at any stage of the clinical course. Identifying patients at high risk of sudden death will be the focus of continuing and future investigations on altering the mortality of this disease. As noted above, recent molecular-genetic studies offer this promise.

RESTRICTIVE CARDIOMYOPATHY

The term *restrictive cardiomyopathy* describes a characteristic syndrome of myocardial disease with features simulating constrictive pericarditis. The predominant hemodynamic abnormalities include evidence of diastolic restriction of ventricular filling. The resulting ventricular pressure pulse recording shows a rapid decline of pressure in early diastole, followed by a brisk rise to a plateau (termed the *square root sign*). The venous or atrial pressure pulses show a rapid Y descent and often a rapid X descent. Some evidence of systolic dysfunction may also be evident, especially on noninvasive testing.

Etiology

A variety of specific processes associated with infiltrative or fibrotic pathology involving the myocardium or endomyocardium may be responsible. Primary or idiopathic cases are rare. Secondary causes include amyloidosis, sarcoidosis, endomyocardial fibrosis, Loeffler's hypereosinophilic endocarditis, carcinoid, endocardial fibroelastosis, and hemochromatosis.

Pathology

The conspicuous features are infiltration and fibrosis involving to a varying degree the myocardium and endocardium. The ventricular size is often normal or mildly enlarged. The muscle is often stiff and thickened. The endocardium may be scarred and thickened. The atria may be conspicuously dilated. The valves are generally spared except in endomyocardial fibrosis, in which the AV valves are predominantly involved. The etiologic diagnosis rests on histologic identification of the specific infiltration. Needle biopsy may be especially useful in this regard and may assist in therapy in some instances, for example, hemochromatosis or sarcoidosis.

Pathophysiology

The diastolic restriction of ventricular filling common to this syndrome results in elevations of atrial and venous pressures. Sinus tachycardia is a compensatory feature and helps to maintain cardiac output, since the stroke volume may be relatively fixed by diastolic restriction. The venous congestion may be evident in both the lungs and the systemic organs, depending on the relative severity of involvement of the two ventricles. The ventricular pressure pulse shows a dip and plateau (square root sign). The resulting atrial pressure pulse finding is a rapid Y descent. In addition, the X descent may be prominent in some cases.

Clinical manifestations

The clinical features (see Table 17-1) are predominantly those of pulmonary and systemic venous congestion, as in dilated cardiomyopathy. Clinical evidence of cardiomegaly usually is conspicuous by its absence. The symptoms and signs of left and right heart failure are often present (Chapter 10).

On the chest x-ray marked atrial enlargement with mild ventricular enlargement and pulmonary venous congestion, pulmonary edema, and pleural effusions are commonly present. On the ECG, sinus tachycardia with low voltage and diffuse ST-T changes are noted. Atrial fibrillation is frequently present.

The characteristic features of the echocardiogram include thickened walls with a normal or slightly enlarged ventricular cavity and moderate to marked dilatation of the atria. The systolic function, as measured by fractional shortening, may be reduced. The echo appearance of the ventricular walls in amyloidosis shows a typical granular or sparkling appearance.

The pressure waveforms and intracardiac pressures obtained during cardiac catheterization are highly suggestive of constrictive pericarditis. However, differences in end-diastolic pressures in the two ventricles, with exercise, volume loading, or catecholamine infusion, are seen more often with restrictive cardiomyopathy. Right ventricular end-diastolic pressure is frequently more than one third of the peak systolic pressure in constrictive pericarditis, but is less commonly so in restrictive cardiomyopathy.

Differentiation from constrictive pericarditis may not be possible despite all the invasive and noninvasive testing and may require thoracotomy for confirmation. Such a radical approach may be needed, since constrictive pericarditis is a surgically remediable lesion.

Treatment

The basic principles of treatment (see Table 17-1) are similar to those in dilated or congestive cardiomyopathy, with the following differences. First, it may be neither practical nor desirable to reduce venous pressure markedly toward normal, because a sharp reduction in cardiac output and a drop in blood pressure may result. Second, moderate tachycardia is beneficial in maintaining cardiac output, since the stroke volume is limited by diastolic restriction of filling. Third, digitalis therapy may have no beneficial effect in the absence of left ventricular enlargement, and the resulting bradycardia may reduce cardiac output. Finally, a beneficial role of vasodilator drugs has not been demonstrated.

Clinical course and prognosis

Most of the conditions causing restrictive cardiomyopathy have a poor prognosis and frequently a rapidly deteriorating course. Some patients with hemochromatosis may be improved by phlebotomy, and valve replacement may be indicated in those with carcinoid heart disease. Surgical resection of fibrotic endocardium has been undertaken with some success in patients with endomyocardial fibrosis in endemic areas. Treatment of the other associated infiltrative disorders is not satisfactory.

REFERENCES

Anderson JL et al: A randomized trial of low-dose beta-blockage therapy for idiopathic dilated cardiomyopathy. Am J Cardiol 55:471, 1985.

Bonow RO et al: Verapamil induced improvement in left ventricular diastolic filling and increased exercise tolerance in patients with hypertrophic cardiomyopathy; short and long term effects. Circulation 72:853, 1985.

Cohn JN et al: Effect of vasodilator therapy on mortality in chronic congestive heart failure. N Engl J Med 314:1547, 1986.

Dec GW Jr et al: Active myocarditis in the spectrum of acute dilated cardiomyopathies. N Engl J Med 312:885, 1985.

Goodwin JF: Prospects and predictions for the cardiomyopathies. Circulation 50:210, 1974.

Holmes J et al: Arrhythmias in ischemic and nonischemic dilated cardiomyopathy: Prediction of mortality by ambulatory electrocardiography. Am J Cardiol 55:146, 151, 1985.

Kowey PR, Eisenberg R, and Engel TR: Sustained arrhythmias in hypertrophic obstructive cardiomyopathy. N Engl J Med 310:1566, 1984.

Maron BJ et al: Hypertrophic cardiomyopathy: Interrelations of clinical manifestations, pathophysiology and therapy. N Engl J Med 316:780, 844, 1987.

McKenna WJ et al: Arrhythmia in hypertrophic cardiomyopathy. I. Influence of prognosis. Br Heart J 46:168, 1981.

McKenna WJ et al: Arrhythmia in hypertrophic cardiomyopathy. II. Comparison of amiodarone and verapamil in treatment. Br Heart J 46:173, 1981.

Nippoldt TB et al: Right ventricular endomyocardial biopsy, clinicopathologic correlates in 100 consecutive patients. *Mayo Clin Proc* 57:407, 1982.

O'Connell JB: Dilated cardiomyopathy: emerging role of endomyocardial biopsy. Curr Probl Cardiol 11:450, 1986.

O'Connell JB: Immunosuppression for dilated cardiomyopathy. N Engl J Med 321:1119, 1989.

Report on the WHO/ISFC task force on the definition and classification of cardiomyopathies. Br Heart J 44:672, 1980.

Shabetai R: Cardiomyopathy: how far have we come in 25 years, how far yet to go? J Am Coll Cardiol 1:252, 1983.

Shah PM: Controversies in hypertrophic cardiomyopathy. Curr Probl Cardiol 11:567, 1986.

The SOLVD Investigators: Effect of enalapril on survival in patients with reduced left ventricular ejection fraction and congestive heart failure. N Engl J Med 325:293, 302, 1991.

Umverferth DV et al: Factors influencing the one-year mortality of dilated cardiomyopathy. Am J Cardiol 54:147, 1984.

Watkins H et al: Characteristics and prognostic implications of myosin missense mutations in familial hypertrophic cardiomyopathy. N Engl J Med 326:1108, 1992.

CHAPTER

18 Pericardial Disease and Pericardial Heart Disease

Ralph Shabetai

The term *pericarditis* designates all disorders of the pericardium. Most, however, are not infectious, and indeed many are not inflammatory. Therefore, a more suitable term is *pericardial disease*. In many cases, the clinical manifestations are cardiac rather than pericardial; for these, the preferred term is *pericardial heart disease*.

The pericardium can be involved in a variety of systemic diseases, but once involved may dominate the clinical picture. The frequency of pericardial involvement in systemic diseases is greater when postmortem rather than clinical criteria are employed. A good example is rheumatoid disease, in which clinical manifestations of pericardial involvement, although dramatic, are uncommon, whereas pathologic changes are often found at autopsy.

ETIOLOGY

The diseases that may affect the pericardium are so numerous that an encyclopedic enumeration is not useful. The box on p. 249 includes the majority of causes. Idiopathic pericardial disease heads the list, since in many cases the cause of pericardial disease is never discovered despite extensive investigation. Like any list of possible causes, the box should be regarded only as a guideline. For example, there is considerable overlap between idiopathic pericarditis and suspected but unproved viral or tuberculous pericarditis. Pericardial disease caused by immune reactions of the pericardium is the unifying mechanism of several kinds of pericardial disease listed in the box. AIDS is now one of the most common causes of pericardial effusion.

Causes of pericardial disease

- Idiopathic disease
- Connective tissue disease
  - Rheumatoid arthritis
  - Rheumatic fever
  - Scleroderma
  - Lupus erythematosus
- Neoplastic disease
  - Bronchogenic carcinoma
  - Breast cancer
  - Lymphoma
  - Primary pericardial disease
- Infectious disease
  - **AIDS**
  - Viral pericarditis
  - Tuberculous pericarditis
  - Histoplasmosis and other fungal diseases
  - Acute pyogenic pericarditis, especially in children
    - *Haemophilus influenzae*
    - *Neisseria meningitidis*
  - Infectious endocarditis
  - Reiter's syndrome
  - Protozoal pericarditis
- Trauma
  - Sharp or blunt trauma
  - Iatrogenic trauma
  - Radiation
- Metabolic disease
  - Hemodialysis
  - Uremia
  - Myxedema
  - Chylopericardium
  - Cholesterol pericarditis
- Amyloidosis
- Drug-induced and immune reaction disease
  - Procainamide
  - Hydralazine
  - Anticoagulant
  - Nicotinic acid
  - Postpericardiotomy syndrome
- Myocardial infarction
  - Acute myocardial infarction
  - Dressler's syndrome
- Rupture
  - Cardiac rupture
  - Ruptured aorta
  - Aneurysm of the ascending aorta
  - Dissecting hematoma

Neoplastic pericardial disease

Neoplasm is an important cause of pericardial disease, especially in patients over 50 years of age. The leading causes are bronchogenic carcinoma and carcinoma of the breast. Lymphoma frequently involves the mediastinum and the pericardium and is the most common cause of malignant pericardial disease in the young. Since almost any malignant tumor may metastasize to the thorax, pericardial involvement complicates a variety of neoplastic diseases. Primary pericardial neoplasm is rare, but mesothelioma is the commonest.

AIDS

Pericardial effusion and pericarditis are the most common manifestations of AIDS. In some cases but by no means all, cardiomyopathy is associated. Pericarditis is usually caused by commensal infection with organisms such as atypical tubercle bacillus.

Infectious nontuberculous pericarditis

Virtually any organism can infect the pericardium, but of especial importance are coxsackie A and B and ECHO virus. The syndrome of acute idiopathic pericarditis is often considered synonymous with viral pericarditis, but investigations of sporadic cases of acute idiopathic pericarditis seldom prove a viral cause.

Tuberculous pericarditis

Tuberculosis is an important cause of pericarditis. In tuberculous pericarditis, it is the exception to find evidence for either miliary tuberculosis or a parenchymal lung lesion. The diagnosis of tuberculous pericarditis is established when tubercle bacilli are found by stain or culture of pericardial fluid, but these techniques are diagnostic in only one third to one half of the cases. The diagnosis is often presumptive and based on indirect evidence such as contact or conversion of tuberculin skin test.

Trauma

Sharp chest injuries result in one of the several syndromes of pericardial disease when the heart or one of the great vessels has been penetrated. Blunt injury may also affect the pericardium; steering wheel contact or other physical violence, for example, often causes myocardial contusion and pericardial disease. The manifestations of pericardial disease may be early, as when significant hemorrhage into the pericardium occurs, or late, as when a secondary, probably immune reaction occurs after a small amount of blood appears in contact with injured mesothelial cells of the pericardium. Clinical presentation may be delayed for weeks, months, or years after the trauma. Early reactions include dry fibrinous pericarditis and acute tamponade. Delayed manifestations include chronic or recurrent pericardial effusion and constrictive pericarditis.

A disconcerting proportion of cases of traumatic pericardial disease are iatrogenic, caused, for example, by radiation therapy, perforation of the heart during cardiac catheterization and angiography, or insertion of a pacing electrode. Closed chest cardiac massage, complications of endoscopy, and drugs that sensitize the pericardium are other iatrogenic causes. Pericardial disease, sometimes associated with myocardial disease, may occur late after mediastinal irradiation for tumors involving the thorax, and it is often difficult to distinguish it from recurrence of the neoplastic disease.

Metabolic disorders affecting the pericardium

Pericardial disease is a common manifestation of end-stage renal failure. Pericardial disease occurring during the course of chronic hemodialysis is of greater practical importance. It may occur as a manifestation of uremic pericardial disease, but since the blood urea nitrogen and creatinine are usually maintained at levels below those associated with pericardial involvement in chronic uremia, the etiology may be different. Some consider pericardial disease to be caused by "middle molecules" that are not dialyzed or to be related to immunologic abnormalities induced by dialysis itself. Dialysis patients are unduly susceptible to infection, and thus viral or tuberculous pericarditis may develop. Pericardial disease is becoming less common in well-managed dialysis units.

Drug-induced pericardial disease

Hydralazine often induces systemic lupus erythematosus, frequently resulting in pericarditis. Several other agents, such as procainamide and isoniazid, are also capable of producing a pericardial reaction.

Pericardial involvement after myocardial infarction

A pericardial friction rub is apparent in at least 10% of patients with acute myocardial infarction. Pericardial rub in these patients is usually benign, although it has been stated that the prognosis of acute myocardial infarction is worse when a pericardial friction rub occurs. The difference in prognosis may be related to the association of pericardial involvement with larger myocardial infarctions. The occurrence of pericardial friction rubs with inferior and posterior infarctions and with anterior infarctions suggests that the pericardial involvement may not be a continuous localized patch but may be more generalized. Dressler's syndrome is characterized by fever, pericardial friction rub, pain, and, frequently, pericardial effusion. Other common features include leukocytosis, pleurisy with or without effusion, and pulmonary infiltrates. The prevalence of Dressler's syndrome is declining, perhaps as a consequence of reduced use of warfarin. There is probably a relation between Dressler's syndrome, which is now uncommon, and two other, similar syndromes, the postpericardiotomy syndrome and pericardial disease that follows blunt chest trauma. Common to these entities is the occurrence of damaged mesothelial pericardial cells and bleeding into the pericardial space. These may be the linking ingredients that initiate the pericardial reaction. Convincing evidence shows that the postpericardiotomy syndrome occurs after the combination of viral infection and the release of myocardial antibodies.

A pericardial friction rub does not contraindicate thrombolytic treatment.

PATHOLOGY

Acute pericarditis

When the pericardium is acutely inflamed, a fibrinous reaction occurs. The plentiful deposition of fibrin gives the pericardium a shaggy appearance which, together with edema, produces a slight thickening of the membrane. In addition, there may be considerable vascularity, which may partly explain the propensity for bleeding into the pericardial space in patients with pericardial disease who are receiving anticoagulants.

Pericardial effusion

Frequently, pericardial disease is accompanied by effusion. These effusions can be detected clinically by their pathophysiologic effects or by laboratory examination. On the other hand, in congestive heart failure, a considerable volume of transudate may be found in the pericardial space at autopsy, although these effusions are seldom recognized by clinical means or by echocardiography and practically never cause symptoms. The nature of the fluid varies with the cause of the pericardial disease—for example, exudates in inflammatory disease, chyle in injury or disease of the thoracic duct, cholesterol crystals in cholesterol pericarditis, or blood in a variety of conditions.

Chronic pericardial disease

Chronic disease of the pericardium may result in formation of a firm scar. The pericardium thickens and in extreme cases, especially in tuberculosis, may become calcified. In advanced cases the pericardium, normally 1 to 3 mm, may become more than 1 cm thick. The specific cause of the pericardial scar may be found by histologic examination—for example, caseation in tuberculous pericarditis, neoplastic cells in primary or secondary malignant disease of the pericardium, and amyloid. Causative organisms may be stained or cultured from the pericardium or from pericardial fluid.

CLINICAL MANIFESTATIONS

The physical and laboratory findings in pericardial disease are listed in the box at upper right.

Acute pericarditis

The major causes of acute pericarditis are viral or idiopathic, but most of the conditions listed in the box on p. 249 can cause acute pericarditis. The pathologic finding is

Syndromes of pericardial disease

- Acute pericarditis
  - Pain
  - Fever
  - Friction rub
  - ECG changes
  - May be recurrent
  - May be associated with effusion
- Pericardial effusion
  - Abnormal chest radiograph
  - Recognized by echocardiography
  - ECG changes
  - Chronic effusive pericarditis
- Cardiac tamponade
  - Raised jugular venous pressure
  - Prominent X descent, absent Y descent
  - Pulsus paradoxus
- Constrictive pericarditis
  - Raised jugular venous pressure
  - Prominent Y descent
  - Simulates right heart failure
  - Effusive constrictive pericarditis
  - Occult pericardial constriction

usually a fibrinous pericarditis, sometimes hemorrhagic, and sometimes associated with pericardial effusion in varying amounts.

The cardinal symptom of acute pericarditis is chest pain of variable severity. Pericardial pain may be similar to the pain of acute myocardial infarction or indistinguishable from pleurisy. Frequently, however, the pain suggests a pericardial origin. Thus, it may be retrosternal yet be aggravated by inspiration or coughing and relieved by sitting up. The pain may radiate in the manner of ischemic pain, but a characteristic location is the trapezius ridge. The patient usually has fever. In infectious cases, a period of general malaise may precede the onset of fever and pericardial pain.

The finding on physical examination that is pathognomonic of pericarditis is the pericardial friction rub, an extraneous sound accompanying heart sounds but not a cardiac murmur. Pericardial friction rubs are usually scratchy and "superficial" and vary in quality from fine to coarse (Chapter 3). Sometimes, a pericardial friction rub is palpable. The quality of a pericardial friction rub is similar to that of a pleural friction rub, but the timing is associated with the cardiac rather than the respiratory cycle.

The characteristic pericardial friction rub is triphasic, having one component in presystole, another in ventricular systole, and a third in diastole. When all three components are present, recognition is simple, but in nearly half the cases only two components, or sometimes only the systolic component, is present. Two component friction rubs must be distinguished from the murmurs of valvular heart disease. This distinction is usually straightforward but may become difficult when the heart sounds are muffled and the heart rate is rapid. Pericardial friction rubs confined to systole are commonly mistaken for systolic murmurs. Attention to details of timing, quality, pitch, radiation, and response to maneuvers usually obviates this error. The greatest difficulty arises when a murmur and a pericardial friction rub are both present.

The differential diagnosis includes

1. Cardiac murmurs
2. Ejection sounds and mitral or tricuspid clicks
3. Artifact caused by surgical emphysema
4. Mediastinal crunch (Hamman's sign) caused by air in the mediastinum
5. Pleural friction rub
6. Skin rubbing on the stethoscope chest piece

The intensity of a pericardial friction rub may vary with respiration, sometimes disappearing altogether during part of the respiratory cycle. When the intensity of a rub is greatly modulated by respiration, it is often termed *pleuropericardial friction rub*. Pericardial friction rubs are usually best appreciated when the diaphragm of the stethoscope is applied with firm pressure. In view of the effects of posture on pericardial friction rubs, the physician should auscultate with the patient in several positions, including supine and sitting. Pericardial friction rub may be evanescent, and it is often necessary to auscultate frequently.

The patient with acute pericarditis may appear acutely distressed and have rapid, guarded breathing. Frequently the patient is febrile and flushed, and the heart rate is rapid. The chest radiograph may be normal. If a previous chest radiography is available for comparison, it may be observed that the heart size has increased slightly. However, since pericardial effusion may be absent or its quantity small, one cannot rely on this finding. Since many causes of acute pericarditis are associated with pleurisy, pleural effusions may be present. In addition, infiltrates may be evident in the lungs.

The electrocardiogram (ECG) can be helpful in making the diagnosis (Fig. 18-1) (Chapter 4). The characteristic finding in the earliest stages is generalized S-T segment elevation. Commonly, it is present in all leads except aVR and V_1, where S-T segment depression may be found. This pattern is difficult to distinguish from the normal variant,

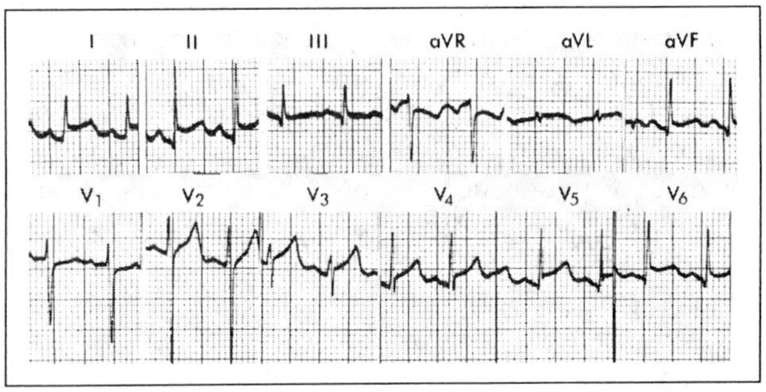

Fig. 18-1. Electrocardiogram of a patient with acute pericarditis. The S-T segment is elevated in leads I, II, III, aVF, and V_4 to V_6. Depression is seen in aVR and V_1. The P-R segment is depressed. This record is characteristic of acute pericarditis.

early repolarization. After several days, the S-T segment returns to the baseline and the ECG may appear normal. In some cases, the tracing evolves with widespread T wave inversions characteristic of chronic pericarditis. Except when chronic pericarditis supervenes, the ECG eventually becomes normal, whether or not there was a phase of T wave inversion. A less common but highly specific ECG abnormality is depression of the PR segment.

The echocardiogram is helpful when the clinician suspects acute pericarditis because in some instances it reveals a small unsuspected pericardial effusion (Chapter 5).

Modest elevation of the serum level of creatine kinase and other cardiac enzymes may be found. The cardiac isoenzymes may be present in slightly increased amounts, and gallium scans of the heart may be positive.

The natural history and prognosis of acute pericarditis depend on the cause. The idiopathic and viral forms of acute pericarditis are usually relatively brief, even when severe, and resolve without sequelae. The illness usually responds rapidly to treatment with anti-inflammatory agents, and thus an unaltered natural history is rarely observed.

In some patients with idiopathic or viral pericarditis, the troublesome syndrome of recurrent pericarditis occurs, characterized by relapses of acute pericarditis that follow either spontaneous or treatment-induced apparent cure. The relapses may be frequent and may recur over many years. They are usually associated with a return of all the features that characterized the initial episode.

Acute tuberculous pericarditis is associated with early pericardial effusion and does not improve until specific antituberculous chemotherapy is instituted. Acute pericarditis occurring in the course of rheumatoid arthritis may lead to the development of constrictive pericarditis.

Acute pericarditis may occur during the course of chronic hemodialysis. It may be manifested by fever and pericardial friction rub, and there is often an associated pericardial effusion. In some patients, cardiac tamponade occurs after recurrent bouts of pericardial inflammation; in others, constrictive pericarditis may be the end result. In patients receiving hemodialysis, the clinical presentation of pericarditis varies from a trivial illness characterized by pericardial friction rub to a serious one characterized by a large pericardial effusion and cardiac tamponade.

Acute pericarditis induced by drugs such as hydralazine or procainamide usually disappears promptly after the drug is discontinued. There is no evidence linking pericardial friction rub in the early stage of acute myocardial infarction to the subsequent appearance of Dressler's syndrome.

The management of acute pericarditis is usually straightforward; it most often responds well to simple anti-inflammatory agents. Aspirin usually suppresses the clinical manifestations of viral and idiopathic acute pericarditis within 24 hours; more commonly, indomethacin is employed in standard dosage. In fact, any of the nonsteroid anti-inflammatory agents is likely to suppress acute pericarditis. In patients in whom the syndrome cannot be ameliorated by large doses of indomethacin, and when other causes of acute pericarditis such as tuberculosis or acute bacterial infection have been ruled out, steroid therapy is required, as it also is for the more tenacious instances of recurrent pericarditis and for a few of the most recalcitrant episodes of Dressler's syndrome. For patients requiring steroid therapy, it is appropriate to begin with large doses, for example, 60 mg or more per day of prednisone. This dosage should be maintained for 2 to 3 weeks, after which the dose is slowly and gradually lowered until the minimum dose that suppresses the illness is discovered. This minimum dose is maintained for 1 to 2 months and then is tapered and finally discontinued. Colchicine, 0.6 to 1.2 mg daily, may reduce dependency on prednisone.

Patients with recurrent pericarditis usually show the same or similar manifestations with each relapse and tend to respond to the same therapeutic regimen. Every effort should be made to treat the patient completely and yet minimize the risks of long-term steroid and perhaps azathioprine therapy. Combinations of steroid and indomethacin can be used. In some patients, alternate-day therapy with these drugs is effective.

When recurrences are frequent and severe and have occurred over a period of several years in spite of potentially dangerous doses of steroids, pericardiectomy may be considered. Some recurrences may be seen even after the surgical procedure, or the primary site of the disease may shift to the pleura. However, after pericardiectomy, the disease sometimes abates more rapidly. When pericarditis is a component of myopericarditis, treatment is focused on the myocardial component and is thus directed against heart failure. The role of immunosuppressive treatment is under active investigation.

Pericardial effusion

Transudate, exudate, or blood may accumulate in the pericardial space in most of the forms of pericardial disease listed in the box on p. 251. With echocardiography, small effusions can be detected in the conditions that used to be designated "dry pericarditis." In many of these conditions, the effusion is of no importance except that it helps establish the diagnosis of pericardial involvement.

In pericardial disease of idiopathic or inflammatory origin, the pericardial fluid is usually exudative. Frank pus may be found in the worst cases of pneumococcal and staphylococcal pericarditis. In rupture of the heart or a great vessel, the pericardial fluid is blood.

The entity *chronic effusive pericarditis* is of unknown origin. Enormous volumes of pericardial fluid may be present, but the condition develops slowly, permitting the pericardium to stretch. Stretching of the pericardium allows the immense pericardial effusion to exist at pressures only slightly above normal; therefore, hemodynamics are only slightly altered.

The physician who suspects pericardial effusion should seek a history compatible with disorders that commonly affect the pericardium. A history of recent viral or flulike illness may precede acute pericarditis. Trauma victims should be questioned and examined for evidence of injury to the chest that may have induced pericardial effusion or hemorrhage. Patients receiving chronic hemodialysis are always at risk for the development of pericardial effusion, sometimes with tamponade. Contact with tuberculosis, symptoms suggestive of pulmonary tuberculosis, and conversion of a tuberculin skin test to positive may be clues leading to the diagnosis of tuberculous pericardial effusion. The patient in whom fever, precordial pain, and possibly a pericardial friction rub develop after myocardial infarction or cardiac surgery is likely to have Dressler's syndrome or postpericardiotomy syndrome.

On examination, signs of pericardial effusion are absent unless the pericardial fluid is under increased pressure when the manifestations of cardiac tamponade appear. In perhaps half the patients with pericardial effusions of appreciable volume, cardiac activity cannot be palpated at the precordium. In patients with a large pericardial effusion and a palpable apex beat, it is possible to percuss cardiac dullness beyond the apex beat. This sign is of value provided there is no disease of the left lower lobe or left pleural cavity. These limitations combine to make this physical finding of little practical use. Pericardial friction rub may be present in spite of a larger pericardial effusion.

The chest radiograph appears entirely normal in the presence of small pericardial effusion. When a larger effusion is present, there is a proportionate increase in the cardiopericardial silhouette. It then becomes necessary to distinguish between pericardial effusion and cardiac enlargement. In the absence of other clues pointing to pericardial effusion, this differentiation is rarely possible by chest radiograph, although in a minority of patients the separate edges of the left heart border and the pericardium can be seen. Pericardial effusion is suggested when the cardiopericardial silhouette is considerably enlarged yet the lung fields are clear and do not show redistribution of blood flow. Enlargement of all four chambers of the heart with tricuspid regurgitation can produce a similar chest radiogram.

The ECG may be normal, but when pericardial effusions are large, voltage may be diminished. Following pericardiocentesis, the voltage increases. Electrical alternans is a sign of cardiac tamponade but usually does not occur with pericardial effusions under low pressure.

Echocardiography is the most sensitive, most specific, and most convenient means of determining whether pericardial fluid is present and in roughly what amount. The test has replaced all other noninvasive and invasive procedures as the ideal method for making these determinations. With meticulous echocardiographic technique and awareness of the pitfalls (Chapter 5), false-positive results related to cysts, pleural effusion, and tumors should be rare. The diagnosis is seldom missed when proper use is made of the damping and gain controls to locate precisely the position of the pericardium (Chapter 5). The pericardial effusion appears as an echo-free space between the moving epicardium and the stationary pericardium (Figure 18-2). Smaller effusions are usually confined to the area behind the posterior wall of the left ventricle, whereas larger effusions are found anterior to the anterior wall of the right ventricle as well. The echo-free space usually disappears or diminishes as the beam is swept from the left ventricle to the left atrium. Two-dimensional (2D) echocardiography more precisely localizes the distribution of the pericardial fluid and is helpful in guiding pericardiocentesis. The echocardiogram shows normal size of the cardiac chambers and normal ventricular systolic function.

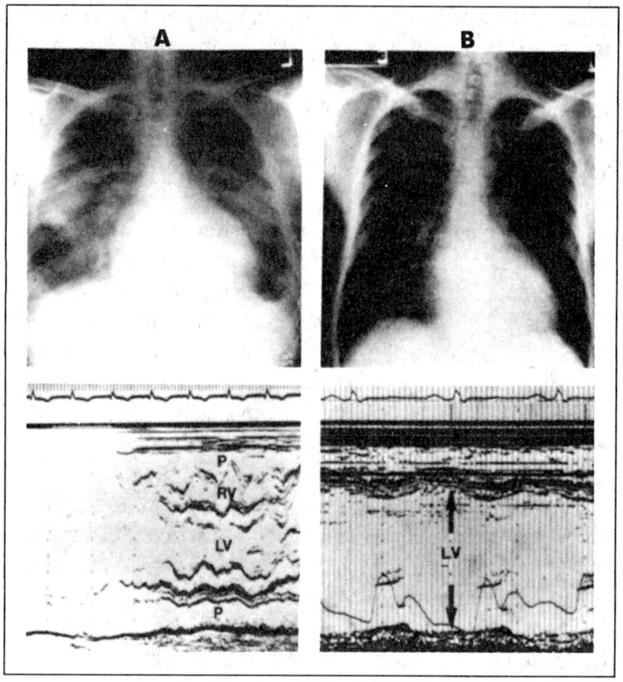

Fig. 18-2. Chest radiograph and M-mode echocardiogram in a patient with pericardial effusion **(A)** compared with a patient with cardiomyopathy **(B)**. **A** shows cardiomegaly, vascular redistribution, and bilateral pleural effusions on radiograph suggesting congestive heart failure. Diagnosis of effusive pericarditis is evident on echocardiogram. **B** demonstrates cardiomegaly on radiograph, which is defined as left ventricular enlargement on echocardiogram. *LV,* left ventricle; *P,* pericardial effusion; *RV,* right ventricle. (Reproduced by permission. From Forst D and O'Rourke RA: Cardiovascular complications of chronic renal disease. In Stein JH and Brenner BM, editors: Contemporary Issues in Nephrology, vol 7. New York, 1981, Churchill-Livingstone.)

A radionuclide blood pool scan demarcates a cold area around the heart and a separation of cardiac radioactivity from that in the liver. Radionuclide scanning is not the preferred tool but may be employed when echocardiography is not available. Furthermore, when blood pool scans are carried out for other reasons, pericardial effusion is sometimes detected as an incidental finding.

It is unnecessary to perform cardiac catheterization for the sole purpose of detecting pericardial effusion. When cardiac catheterization is being performed for other purposes or to evaluate the hemodynamics of pericardial effusion, and the catheter is manipulated within the right atrium, its tip cannot be made to engage the right edge of the cardiopericardial silhouette in the posteroanterior projection. Angiocardiography reveals a large, stationary fluid density surrounding the smaller, active, opaque density of the cardiac chambers. Frequently, the edge of the right atrium becomes straight or concave.

Physicians encountering a victim of major blunt or sharp

chest injury who has hypotension, a raised venous pressure, and possibly pulsus paradoxus may urgently explore the pericardium for blood, since the patient may have cardiac tamponade, which will prove fatal before echocardiography and other studies can be undertaken to determine if pericardial effusion and cardiac tamponade are present. In all other circumstances, it is not justifiable to explore the pericardium to diagnose pericardial effusion.

Pericardiocentesis and pericardial drainage are discussed in more detail under Cardiac Tamponade, below. Other indications besides cardiac tamponade include suspicion of pyopericardium and the need to establish the etiologic diagnosis, for example, tuberculosis, neoplastic cell type, or systemic disease. The cautious physician will recall that when both pleural and pericardial effusions are present, aspiration and biopsy of the former may provide the diagnosis. Acute pericarditis with effusion but without tamponade is not an indication for removal of pericardial fluid unless it persists after a week or more of vigorous anti-inflammatory treatment.

The natural history and prognosis of pericardial effusion are related to the cause of the effusion and the presence or absence of cardiac tamponade.

Cardiac tamponade

Cardiac tamponade is a condition in which pericardial fluid under increased pressure impedes diastolic filling and secondarily reduces cardiac output and arterial blood pressure.

The abnormal physiology resulting from cardiac tamponade explains its signs and symptoms. The normal intrapericardial pressure measured by a conventional catheter or needle is subatmospheric. During quiet respiration, intrapericardial pressure is −1 or −2 mm Hg during expiration and −5 mm Hg during inspiration. Pericardial surface pressure measured by a flat balloon is higher, approximating right atrial pressure. Which of these is the "physiologic pressure" remains to be settled, but the reader should be aware of this important new development in physiology. The pericardium is less compliant than the cardiac chambers that it snugly invests. Intrapericardial volume is slightly larger than the cardiac volume, the difference being the reserve volume of the pericardium.

When fluid is injected into the pericardium of an intact animal, there is only a slight rise in intrapericardial pressure with the first deciliter or so. Thereafter, the pressure rises steeply. This pericardial pressure–volume relationship explains why a relatively small volume of fluid appearing rapidly in the pericardial space induces cardiac tamponade. As soon as the residual volume of the pericardial space has been filled, further accumulation of fluid greatly increases the intrapericardial pressure because the noncompliant pericardium does not stretch. Thus, after perforation of the heart, severe cardiac tamponade becomes manifest after only 2 or 3 dl of blood have gathered in the pericardial sac. Removing only a small portion of the pericardial fluid causes pericardial pressure to drop steeply, with rapid clinical and hemodynamic improvement. On the other hand, in chronic effusive pericarditis, the pericardial effusion may measure more than a liter, while the conventionally measured intrapericardial pressure is only a few millimeters of mercury. Between these extremes, pericardial effusions of several deciliters that have accumulated over days, weeks, or months cause varying severity of cardiac tamponade.

Severe cardiac tamponade is associated with intrapericardial pressure of 10 to 20 mm Hg or more. (When there is pericardial effusion, liquid and surface pericardial pressures are the same.) Moderate cardiac tamponade results from pericardial pressure in the range of 10 to 15 mm Hg. Mild cardiac tamponade with intrapericardial pressure in the range of 8 to 10 mm Hg is a definite clinical entity but is more difficult to recognize.

The essential pathophysiologic abnormality in cardiac tamponade is that the increased intrapericardial pressure impedes diastolic filling. As the intrapericardial pressure increases, systemic and pulmonary pressures increase to the level required to prevent collapse caused by compression of the cardiac chambers. Thus, the right atrial, left atrial, and two ventricular diastolic pressures approach and eventually equal intrapericardial pressure.

In the normal heart, the conventionally measured intrapericardial pressure averages −2 or −3 mm Hg, the right atrial filling pressure averages 4 mm Hg, and the left atrial pressure is approximately 7 mm Hg. Thus, the transmural filling pressures using conventional techniques for the two sides of the heart average 7 and 10 mm Hg, respectively. In cardiac tamponade, since the cardiac filling pressures and the pericardial pressure are in equilibrium, the transmural filling pressures of the two sides of the heart are close to zero, whether measured conventionally or with a pericardial balloon; that is, preload or distending pressure is greatly reduced, decreasing cardiac output. The combination of high cardiac filling pressure and reduced cardiac output resembles cardiac failure, but the resemblance is only superficial because in cardiac tamponade, impaired tissue perfusion is caused not by myocardial failure but by reduced preload (Chapters 1 and 10).

In cardiac tamponade, the pericardial pressure prevents diastolic filling when cardiac volume is at a maximum. During ventricular ejection, cardiac volume shrinks, inducing a slight decline in intrapericardial pressure, which permits venous return to the heart. The mean venous pressure is greatly elevated, and the jugular venous pulse is characterized by a sharp X descent, corresponding to a surge of venous return, but there is no Y descent, reflecting the impossibility of cardiac filling when cardiac volume is maximum.

Cardiac tamponade, except when loculated or caused by clot, is caused by greatly increased intrapericardial pressure that equally affects left and right heart-filling pressures.

When pericardial fluid is present and the intrapericardial pressure is elevated, cardiac tamponade is present when the following criteria are met: (1) the right atrial pressure is elevated and equals the intrapericardial pressure; (2) pericardiocentesis lowers the intrapericardial pressure and the right atrial pressure until the right atrial pressure returns to normal and the intrapericardial pressure falls below the right atrial pressure, restoring a significant transmural right heart pressure; and (3) cardiac output and arterial blood pressure increase after pericardiocentesis.

Pulsus paradoxus is a characteristic finding in cardiac tamponade. Other conditions, notably bronchial asthma and severe obstructive airway disease, may cause pulsus paradoxus, perhaps by different mechanisms. The pathophysiology of pulsus paradoxus in cardiac tamponade is complex, no single mechanism being responsible. During inspiration, venous return to the right side of the heart increases, causing increased volume of the right heart. Since the pericardium is tense, this increased volume produces a slight increase in intrapericardial pressure, further compromising the performance of the left ventricle. In addition, expanded right ventricular volume is achieved partly by bowing of the intraventricular septum into the left ventricle, thereby decreasing its volume and its apparent compliance. Also, the inspiratory increase in right ventricular stroke volume does not appear in the aorta until expiration. The effect of respiratory variations in stroke volume is exaggerated when the cardiac output is decreased. Finally, the descent of the diaphragm during inspiration pulls on the pericardium, further increasing pericardial pressure. All these factors combine to create a major decline in arterial blood pressure during inspiration.

It is helpful to establish whether conditions predisposing to pericardial effusion and cardiac tamponade are present. A history of viral infection, tuberculosis, cancer of the lung or breast, chest trauma, previous radiation, the administration of procainamide or hydralazine, renal disease and hemodialysis, or the presence of a systemic disease may be the first clue pointing to cardiac tamponade.

If cardiac tamponade is extreme, the patient may be unable to report symptoms. In severe but less extreme circumstances, patients complain of varying degrees of dyspnea or fullness in the chest. In acute cardiac tamponade, there may be precordial pain. In mild or moderate cardiac tamponade, specific complaints are frequently lacking.

The findings on examination vary with severity. In the most severe cases, the patient may be stuporous, and the findings of shock may be present. In less severe cases, these findings may be absent. Between these two extremes, one may encounter patients in varying degrees of acute and chronic distress.

Inspection of the neck veins is the single most important part of examining a patient for cardiac tamponade (Chapter 3). Almost invariably, the venous pressure is elevated. In patients with severe tamponade, the intrapericardial pressure, and consequently the central venous pressure, may rise to 20 mm Hg or more. Elevation of the jugular venous pressure to such high levels cannot be appreciated when the patient is supine or semirecumbent, because the venous pressure is so high that the neck veins cease to pulsate. It becomes necessary, then, to alter the patient's position, sometimes until the thorax is at an angle of 90° to the horizontal plane, to appreciate the level of the venous pressure.

The jugular venous pulse is characterized by a sharp X descent, which can be recognized at the bedside as an inward movement of the jugular pulse synchronous with the pulse of the carotid artery, and an absent Y descent. The level of venous pressure usually falls slightly during inspiration.

In extreme cases, the arterial blood pressure may not be audible; in other cases, varying degrees of hypotension are found. In mild cases, the arterial blood pressure is normal. Pulsus paradoxus is appreciated as a distinct decrease in the volume of the arterial pulse during inspiration. In extreme cases the peripheral pulse disappears at the height of inspiration. With hypotension, it may not be possible to appreciate pulsus paradoxus because of the combination of rapid heart rate and small pulse volume. When pulsus paradoxus cannot be appreciated in a distal artery, it should be sought in the carotid or femoral vessels, where it may still be observed.

Pulsus paradoxus can be estimated with a sphygmomanometer. The cuff is inflated to a value exceeding the systolic pressure and then is slowly deflated. The blood pressure sounds are auscultated while respirations are observed. Initially, the first Korotkoff sound is heard only during expiration, but as the cuff pressure falls, a pressure reading is obtained at which the sounds can be heard throughout the respiratory cycle. The difference between these pressure readings in mm Hg estimates pulsus paradoxus.

In following patients for changing signs of cardiac tamponade, serial observations of the jugular venous pressure and of the estimated pulsus paradoxus are of key importance.

The precordial examination may be unremarkable. In some cases, a pericardial friction rub is audible. It may or may not be possible to elicit the signs of pericardial effusion (see Acute Pericarditis p. 250). Usually, the lungs are clear. The chest radiograph is the same as that described under Pericardial Effusion, p. 252.

The ECG may be normal, but in some cases may show low voltage. When there is extreme distress, sinus tachycardia is present. In some cases, electrical alternans is found. This is caused by swinging of the heart in the fluid-filled pericardial sac. Alternans of P, QRS, and T waves is specific for cardiac tamponade, but alternans of the QRS complex alone, although less diagnostic, is much more common.

The echocardiogram shows an echo-free space behind the posterior wall of the left ventricle and usually also in front of the anterior wall of the right ventricle. The diagnosis of cardiac tamponade is unlikely if a good-quality echocardiogram fails to confirm the presence of considerable pericardial effusion. In most cases, specific echocardiographic abnormalities of cardiac tamponade are present (Chapter 5). These include diastolic collapse of the ventricle and compression of the right atrium, an excessive shift of the septum toward the left ventricle during inspiration, a decreased E to F slope of the anterior leaflet of the mitral valve during inspiration, and occasionally pseudoprolapse of the mitral valve. The right ventricular dimensions are reduced in cardiac tamponade but not by pericardial effusion without tamponade. Echocardiography confirms the swinging motion of the heart that causes electrical alternans. Except in life-threatening emergencies, the diagnosis of cardiac tamponade is an indication to catheterize at least the right side of the heart to confirm the diagnosis, provide safe hemodynamic monitoring, and guide the course of pericardiocentesis.

Right atrial compression and right ventricular diastolic collapse are early signs of tamponade, appearing soon after pericardial and right atrial pressures equilibrate. At this state, pulsus paradoxus is absent and reductions of systemic arterial pressure and cardiac output are modest. When pericardial pressure rises to higher levels, these hemodynamic markers become severe, which defines decompensated tamponade.

The right atrial waveform is characterized by a prominent X descent but no Y descent (Fig. 18-3); the right ventricular diastolic pressure is elevated but does not display an early diastolic dip. Right ventricular and pulmonary arterial systolic pressures are elevated to approximately 40 mm Hg, and there is little difference between the pulmonary wedge, arterial diastolic, and right atrial pressures.

The arterial pressure tracing confirms pulsus paradoxus and allows accurate measurement of its degree. If the left heart is catheterized, left atrial and ventricular diastolic pressures are found equal to the corresponding pressures on the right. Cardiac output is usually reduced. When the pericardial sac is cannulated, the intrapericardial pressure is precisely equal to the right atrial pressure.

Untreated, severe cardiac tamponade is fatal. Treatment consists of removing the pericardial fluid and thus reducing intrapericardial pressure. In extreme cases, pericardiocentesis must be accomplished immediately, wherever the patient is found. In the vast majority of cases, however, the procedure is preceded by electrocardiography and the

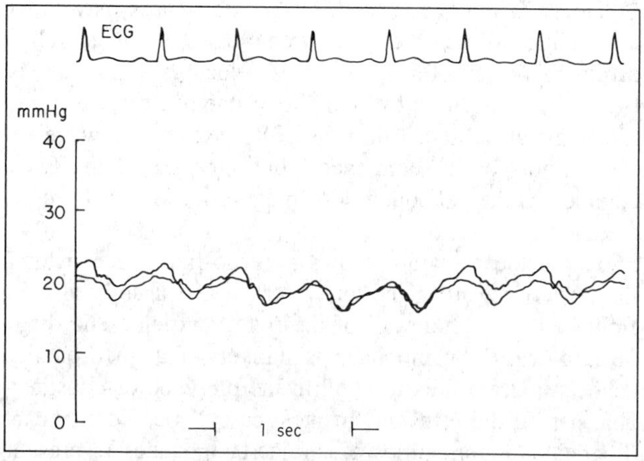

Fig. 18-3. Simultaneously recorded pressure tracings from a patient with severe cardiac tamponade (right atrium and pericardium). The venous pressure is elevated to approximately 20 mm Hg. This pressure is virtually identical to the simultaneously recorded intrapericardial pressure. Toward the middle of the tracing, a small decline in these pressures is observed because of the effect of inspiration. Note that the right atrial pressure shows an X descent but no Y descent. This waveform is characteristic of cardiac tamponade. Correspondingly, an early diastolic dip does not occur in the ventricular diastolic pressure in patients with cardiac tamponade.

pericardium is drained during an elective surgical procedure, or needle pericardiocentesis is carried out electively under controlled conditions.

The choice between open surgical drainage and pericardiocentesis varies with clinical circumstances, institutions, and physicians. Surgical drainage has the advantage that it is often more complete and allows generous biopsy of the pericardium. Surgical drainage is performed under direct vision, and the surgeon may have the opportunity to break down adhesions and free loculation of the fluid. There is also less danger of lacerating the heart or a coronary artery. A malignant pericardial effusion can be managed by balloon pericardiotomy.

Pericardiocentesis has the advantage of not requiring the services of a surgeon, an anesthesiologist, and operating room staff, and it is easier to obtain accurate intrapericardial and cardiac pressures. Thus, pericardiocentesis allows the physician to confirm the diagnosis of cardiac tamponade, estimate its severity, and judge the immediate hemodynamic effects of the removal of pericardial fluid. Finally, pericardiocentesis is of great value in diagnosing effusive constrictive pericarditis. The advent of 2D echocardiography has greatly increased the safety of pericardiocentesis.

Except in extreme emergencies, pericardiocentesis should be performed or supervised by skilled, experienced personnel in the cardiac catheterization laboratory or an equivalent facility. The patient should be placed in a semirecumbent position. Two-dimensional echocardiography, if available, should be used to locate the area of maximum pericardial effusion and the place where it is closest to the skin to determine the site of puncture. Otherwise, the subxiphoid route is preferred: after local anesthesia, the needle is directed from the subxiphoid area cephalad with a slight posterior tilt. The needle may be directed toward the left or right shoulder. An ECG monitor lead attached to the needle may be used to warn the physician when the needle has touched the heart. A pericardial tube may be left in place for several hours or up to several days. The tube may be used for continuous pericardial drainage and should obviate the need for repeated pericardiocentesis. The tube may be used to administer chemotherapeutic agents into the pericardial sac—for example, tetracycline, 5-fluorouracil, or nitrogen mustard for malignant disease; steroids for other pericardial effusions.

There is no agreement concerning the proper management of cardiac tamponade in hemodialysis patients. The signs of pericarditis and pericardial effusion are usually best managed by increasing the frequency of hemodialysis and administering indomethacin. Some regard the onset of cardiac tamponade under these circumstances as a clear indication for prompt pericardiectomy. Others, including ourselves, do not support this view, even though the operation can be performed easily and with minimum morbidity and mortality. We favor managing cardiac tamponade in patients undergoing hemodialysis by pericardiocentesis. A nonabsorbable steroid, for example, triamcinolone, may be instilled into the pericardial sac to hasten reabsorption of the effusion.

The pericardial aspirate should be carefully examined

and cultured, lest the clinician miss an unsuspected case of tuberculous or viral pericarditis in a patient undergoing hemodialysis. Recurrences of cardiac tamponade in dialysis patients are best managed by pericardiectomy.

For all but the mildest cardiac tamponade, definitive and proper treatment is removal of the pericardial fluid. When there is a delay in preparing for pericardiocentesis or pericardial drainage, the patient is supported by adjunctive pharmacologic measures. It is important first to expand the blood volume with saline, dextran, or blood; when the blood volume is expanded, blood pressure increases, and the patient responds favorably. At this point, cautious intravenous administration of nitroprusside results in greatly improved perfusion while the blood pressure is maintained. It is highly desirable to monitor the blood pressure, central venous pressure, pulmonary wedge pressure, and cardiac output during these pharmacologic interventions until the pericardial fluid is removed. If nitroprusside therapy is not appropriate, considerable hemodynamic improvement can be obtained by a combination of intravenous isoproterenol and blood volume expansion. None of these temporizing measures, however, constitutes definitive treatment of cardiac tamponade.

Constrictive pericarditis

Constrictive pericarditis is a condition in which the diastolic filling of the heart is impeded by scar in the pericardium that restricts the diastolic volume and causes a marked increase in the end-diastolic pressure of both ventricles.

Etiology. In the World War II era, tuberculosis was the commonest cause of chronic constrictive pericarditis; with improvement in the treatment of tuberculosis, it has become an uncommon cause in the United States and Western Europe, but is still a common cause in South Africa and less-developed countries. The cause of most cases of constrictive pericarditis in the United States is never discovered. Neoplasm is an important cause of constrictive pericarditis, which often is considerably less chronic that the idiopathic and tuberculous types of pericarditis. Carcinoma of the lung and breast are two extremely important causes of constrictive pericarditis. In appropriate regions of the country, histoplasmosis should be considered in the patient with clinical features suggesting tuberculosis.

Subacute constrictive pericarditis may appear after blunt chest trauma and in rheumatoid arthritis. Constrictive pericarditis may occur early after *Haemophilus influenzae* infection in children and may follow radiation of the chest for treatment of malignant disease. Constriction may occur weeks to years after the irradiation. Postoperative constrictive pericarditis complicates about 0.3% of cardiac operations.

Pathophysiology. In chronic constrictive pericarditis, the abnormal pericardium is greatly thickened. The normal pericardium is 1 to 3 mm thick. In long-standing chronic constrictive pericarditis, the pericardium may be more than 1 cm thick, literally imprisoning the heart. No reserve volume remains, and the pericardium is totally unyielding. In the more chronic cases, especially those of tuberculous or idiopathic origin, heavy calcification may be present, and the scar may intimately involve the superficial layers of the myocardium and the major coronary arteries. In subacute cases, calcification is absent, and although the pericardium is rigid, it may be only a few millimeters thick.

As in cardiac tamponade, the basic pathophysiology is impaired cardiac filling, but there are pathophysiologic differences: restriction of cardiac filling is minimal at end-systole and is total when, at the end of the first third of diastole, cardiac volume reaches the limits set by the noncompliant pericardial scar. Ventricular end-diastolic pressure is elevated (as in cardiac tamponade) because of the external impediment to both sides of the heart. When cardiac size is minimal at end-systole, venous return occurs, and the X descent of venous pressure is manifested. During the first third of ventricular diastole, cardiac filling is rapid, causing the ventricular pressure to fall sharply. Ventricular diastolic pressure then rises rapidly to an elevated level and remains there until the onset of the subsequent systole. This elevated plateau of pressure exists because the ventricles, from the end of the rapid filling phase on, are filled to the capacity permitted by the constricting epicardial scar. This pattern of ventricular diastolic pressure has been termed *dip and plateau,* or the "square root" sign, and is observed in both ventricles (Fig. 18-4). During diastole, the jugular veins and right atrium are in free communication with the right ventricle, and therefore the early diastolic dip of ventricular pressure is seen as a prominent Y descent in the venous pulse. Thus, in cardiac tamponade, the Y descent is absent, whereas in constrictive pericarditis

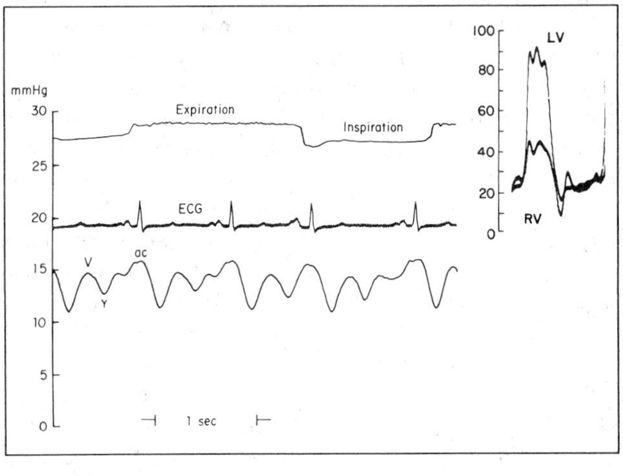

Fig. 18-4. Venous pressure tracing in a patient with constrictive pericarditis. Note the following features: the ECG demonstrates P mitrale, which is common in constrictive pericarditis. Respiratory variation is absent from the venous pressure tracing, and the waveform shows prominent X and Y descents. The inset is a recording of left *(LV)* and right *(RV)* ventricular pressure from a patient with subacute constrictive pericarditis. Note the early diastolic dip of pressure in both ventricles and the equilibration of the mid-diastolic and later diastolic plateaus of pressure in the two ventricles.

it is predominant, a further point of distinction from tamponade.

Ventricular systolic function usually remains normal. However, because the heart is deprived of the normal diastolic stretch, cardiac output is reduced.

The clinical manifestations of constrictive pericarditis mimic those of congestive heart failure and those of liver disease, from which they must be distinguished. A history of cancer of the breast or lung, tuberculosis, radiation therapy, or chest trauma may lead to studies that establish the diagnosis of constrictive pericarditis.

In addition to this relevant history, patients usually complain of weight gain, increase in abdominal girth, and swelling, which may be confined to the ankles but in severe cases is frequently generalized. They also complain of fatigue and shortness of breath. Palpitation may be noted. Some patients give a history of previous acute pericarditis.

The single most important physical finding is an abnormal jugular venous pulse. The venous pressure is elevated and displays prominent X and Y descents or a small X descent and a prominent Y descent (Chap. 3). These abnormalities of the jugular venous pulse in a patient with dyspnea, edema, hepatomegaly, and perhaps ascites virtually assure that the correct diagnosis is either severe tricuspid regurgitation or constrictive pericarditis. This final differential diagnosis can often be settled clinically or by Doppler echocardiography.

In severe cases, the arterial blood pressure and pulse pressure are reduced; this abnormality is not found in mild and moderate cases. In subacute constrictive pericarditis, especially when pericardial effusion is also present, pulsus paradoxus may be detected. This sign is uncommon in long-standing chronic constrictive pericarditis. Atrial fibrillation eventually supervenes in most patients with chronic constrictive pericarditis.

Precordial examination is often abnormal. Systolic retractions of the lower left chest may be observed or cardiac activity may be invisible and impalpable. Contrary to statements in the literature, the heart is not necessarily small. A systolic murmur is frequent, but its pathophysiology has not been explained.

A loud third heart sound, the "pericardial knock," is usually audible. This sound is related to the sudden checking or rapid ventricular filling at the onset of the plateau of ventricular filling and pressure that is to last for the final two thirds of diastole.

Fluid retention, manifested by peripheral edema, pleural effusions, and ascites, is the rule in severe chronic disease. The liver is enlarged and firm and pulsates synchronously with the jugular pulse. Signs of hepatic insufficiency secondary to long-standing severe congestion are commonly found in more severe chronic disease. Chronic reduction in cardiac output and elevation of venous pressure result in a severely wasted appearance, which contrasts startlingly with swollen extremities and distended abdomen.

When the liver is affected by long-standing chronic congestion, liver function test results become abnormal and jaundice appears. The clinical and laboratory evidence of hepatic insufficiency frequently leads to a mistaken diagnosis of cirrhosis of the liver. There is often considerable albuminuria. Plasma proteins are frequently abnormal because of a combination of chronic disease, hepatic and renal congestion, and protein-losing enteropathy.

On the chest radiograph the heart may be normal in size but is frequently enlarged. Radiographic diagnosis of a chronic calcific pericardium constitutes an easily seen abnormality, especially on the oblique projections. Subacute constrictive pericarditis and chronic pericarditis not of tuberculous origin are frequently not calcific. Occasionally calcification is found in the pericardium in the absence of constrictive pericarditis or any demonstrable pathophysiologic condition.

There are several characteristic abnormalities in the ECG. They are low voltage, especially in the limb leads, P mitrale, S-T segment abnormalities, and T wave inversions. In long-standing disease, atrial fibrillation is frequently seen. The Q waves and atrioventricular or intraventricular conduction disturbances occasionally seen have been ascribed to penetration of the superficial myocardium and epicardial coronary arteries by the scar.

The echocardiogram is less helpful than in pericardial effusion (Chapter 5). Nonetheless, it can sometimes establish that the pericardium is thickened. Restricted motion of the heart during the final two thirds of diastole has been observed in several patients with constrictive pericarditis. In subacute disease, pericardial effusion may be found in addition to the thick, immobile pericardium. Notching of the interventricular septum corresponds to the wide biphasic P wave and is associated with a transient reversal of left and right ventricular end-diastolic pressures. In patients in whom adhesions are developing, the thickened pericardium may be observed to move with the epicardium. The echocardiogram may help distinguish between constrictive pericarditis and restrictive cardiomyopathy, because of increased myocardial thickness in the latter.

Increased pericardial thickness is more reliably imaged by computed tomography or nuclear magnetic resonance imaging. Combined with the functional abnormalities shown by echocardiography, this is of great diagnostic value.

Effusive-constrictive pericarditis is a syndrome most frequently associated with malignant disease in which features of constrictive pericarditis combine with features of cardiac tamponade. In these patients, the pericardium is thickened and scarred, but pericardial effusion is present as well. Frequently, the initial presentation is more that of cardiac tamponade but, following pericardiocentesis, the venous pressure remains elevated, displays the classic Y descent, and fails to fall during inspiration. Pulsus paradoxus is not uncommon in effusive-constrictive pericarditis.

Mild constrictive pericarditis may not be clinically evident. The patients usually give a history of previous acute pericarditis and complain of fatigue, dyspnea, and chest pain. Normal hemodynamics are found by cardiac catheterization, but when studies are repeated after the rapid intravenous infusion of a large quantity of fluid, left and right heart-filling pressures equilibrate and develop the dip-and-plateau configuration.

Cardiac catheterization, often with endomyocardial biopsy, is indicated to assess the severity of constrictive pericarditis, to ascertain that restrictive cardiomyopathy is not the correct diagnosis, and to uncover myocardial, valvular, and coronary artery abnormalities masked by the dominant picture of constrictive pericarditis. As in cardiac tamponade, right and left atrial pressures, right and left ventricular diastolic pressures, and pulmonary arterial diastolic pressure are equal. However, in constrictive pericarditis, the ventricular diastolic pressures are characterized by a deep early diastolic dip, followed by an elevated plateau (see Fig. 18-4). Pulmonary hypertension is usually mild and cardiac output is frequently diminished. In severe cases, the ventricular filling pressures exceed 20 mm Hg, but frequently, in the days or weeks preceding cardiac catheterization, intensive diuretic therapy has greatly reduced the cardiac filling pressure. Filling pressures on the two sides of the heart are equal. This finding, however, is of limited value in distinguishing from restrictive cardiomyopathy in which these pressures may also be equal, although sometimes left ventricular diastolic pressure exceeds right.

The natural history of most cases is of advancing severity with increasing compression of the heart and congestion of systemic tissues. The liver is usually severely affected in chronic cases, and liver failure is the mode of death in some. Cardiac output progressively declines, and the tissues suffer from severe passive congestion and hypoperfusion. Almost inevitably, atrial fibrillation appears after two decades and heralds a sharp downward turn.

In contrast to this clinical picture is the very rapid development of significant compression in the weeks or months following *Haemophilus influenzae* infection in childhood or early signs of acute pericarditis in rheumatoid arthritis.

For the majority the treatment is pericardiectomy. The operation is usually straightforward and carries a low risk. There are, however, two important exceptions. Constrictive pericarditis with a dense scar, heavy calcification, and invasion of the epicardium is more difficult to cure surgically, increasing the risk. It may be impossible to dissect a plane, so significant cardiac damage may complicate the operation. Furthermore, cardiac failure and damage to the liver may be irreversible. The second group in which the operation may be more difficult and risky consists of those with a thin peel of epicardial scar constricting the heart. In such patients the epicardial constriction must be removed, but the heart may be lacerated during the tedious dissection. At the other end of the spectrum are patients with mild or even occult constrictive pericarditis who, in the absence of symptoms and especially when they can be followed carefully, do not require pericardiectomy.

In summary, patients with moderate to severe constrictive pericarditis enjoy dramatic improvement after pericardiectomy. For patients with occult constrictive pericarditis, the operation is premature, whereas for some patients with extreme constrictive pericarditis, it is too late for the operation to be safe and provide significant improvement. Improvement can be brought about in the late stage by diuretic therapy and, especially when atrial fibrillation has appeared, digitalis.

Even after successful pericardial resection, several months may elapse before full improvement occurs and the jugular venous pressure returns to normal.

REFERENCES

Bush CA et al: Occult constrictive pericardial disease. Diagnosis by rapid volume expansion and correction by pericardiectomy. Circulation 56:924, 1977.

Dressler W: The post-myocardial infarction syndrome: A report on 44 cases. Arch Intern Med 103:28, 1959.

Gaasch WH, Peterson KL, and Shabetai R: Left ventricular function in chronic constrictive pericarditis. Am J Cardiol 34:107, 1974.

Galve E et al: Pericardial effusion in the course of myocardial infarction: incidence, natural history and clinical relevance. Circulation 73:294, 1986.

Leimgruber PP et al: The hemodynamic derangement associated with right ventricular diastolic collapse in cardiac tamponade: an experimental echocardiographic study. Circulation 68:612, 1983.

Reddy PS et al: Cardiac tamponade: hemodynamic observations in man. Circulation 58:265, 1978.

Schoenfeld MH et al: Restrictive cardiomyopathy versus constrictive pericarditis: role of endomyocardial biopsy in avoiding unnecessary thoracotomy. Circulation 75:1012, 1987.

Shabetai R, editor: Cardiology clinics (diseases of the pericardium) vol 8, Philadelphia, 1990, WB Saunders.

Shabetai R et al: Pulsus paradoxus. J Clin Invest 44:1882, 1965.

Shabetai R, Fowler NO, and Guntheroth WG: The hemodynamics of cardiac tamponade and constrictive pericarditis. Am J Cardiol 26:480, 1970.

Shabetai R and Rostand SG: Nephrogenic pericardial disease. Contemporary Issues Nephrol 13:89, 1984.

Skhvatsabaja LV et al: Secondary malignant lesions of the heart and pericardium in neoplastic disease. Oncology 43:103, 1986.

Spodick DH: Diagnostic electrocardiographic sequences in acute pericarditis: significance of PR segment and PR vector changes. Circulation 48:575, 1973.

Tei C et al: Atrial systolic notch on the interventricular septal echogram: an echocardiographic sign of constrictive pericarditis. J Am Coll Cardiol 1:907, 1983.

Tyberg JV et al: The relationship between pericardial pressure and right atrial pressure: an intraoperative study. Circulation 73:428, 1986.

CHAPTER

19 Congenital Heart Disease

Robert C. Schlant

Congenital heart disease, present at birth, occurs in approximately 8 infants per 1000 live births when individuals with mitral valve prolapse and bicuspid aortic valve are excluded (Chapter 16).

ETIOLOGY

In most instances of congenital heart disease, the exact cause of the defect in development is not known. Only infrequently is a specific cause identified. One of the few identified causes is the intrauterine rubella syndrome, in which maternal rubella during early pregnancy may result in a variety of defects, including microcephaly, cataracts, deafness, and cardiovascular abnormalities, such as pulmonary artery branch stenosis, patent ductus arteriosus, or pulmonic stenosis. The fetal alcohol syndrome, related to excessive alcohol intake by the mother, is associated with multiple defects, including microcephaly, microophthalmia, micrognathia, poor growth and development, and often congenital heart disease, particularly septal defects. Lithium use during pregnancy has been associated with Ebstein's anomaly. The many forms of heritable or possibly heritable types of congenital heart disease that are attributed to recognized chromosomal abnormalities probably account for only 5% to 10% of congenital defects; however, there is a tendency for congenital heart disease to run in families. The Holt-Oram syndrome consists of a hypoplastic thumb or other skeletal abnormalities and is often associated with an ostium secundum defect. The Ellis–van Creveld syndrome (chondroectodermal dysplasia) is an autosomal recessive defect consisting of dwarfism, polydactyly of the hands and occasionally the feet, and a common atrium. Down's syndrome is associated with trisomy 21 and in about 20% with endocardial cushion defect. Patent ductus arteriosus is more common in infants born at high altitudes (above 1500 m) and, like ventricular septal defect, in infants born prematurely. Bicuspid aortic valve, aortic atresia, and complete transposition of the great arteries occur more commonly in male infants while ostium secundum atrial septal defect, partial endocardial cushion defects, and patent ductus arteriosus are more frequent in females.

THE FETAL CIRCULATION AND CHANGES ASSOCIATED WITH BIRTH

The fetus obtains all of its nutrition and oxygen from the placental circulation. The fetal circulation is characterized by three special vascular channels, all of which normally disappear after birth: (1) the foramen ovale in the atrial septum, through which blood passes from the right atrium to the left atrium; (2) the ductus arteriosus, through which most of the blood reaching the pulmonary artery reaches the aorta; and (3) the ductus venosus, which shunts about half of the blood returning from the placenta through the liver to the inferior vena cava, where much of it preferentially streams to the heart and across the foramen ovale and into the left atrium and systemic circulation. Blood from the superior vena cava, on the other hand, preferentially streams across the tricuspid valve into the right ventricle. Because of the right-to-left shunts through the foramen ovale and the ductus arteriosus, the output of the right ventricle is twice that of the left ventricle and relatively little blood (about 8% of the total cardiac output) reaches the uninflated lungs. Soon after birth there is an eightfold to tenfold increase in pulmonary blood flow and a marked decrease in the resistance to blood flow in the lungs; this is related to the inflation of the previously collapsed lungs and to a decrease in pulmonary arterial vasoconstriction produced by changes in pulmonary arterial oxygen tension, prostaglandin PGI_2, and leukotrienes. The increased systemic vascular resistance produced by vasoconstriction or by tying of the umbilical cord and umbilical arteries increases the systemic vascular resistance and the pressures in the left ventricle and left atrium. The increase in left atrial pressure, decrease in inferior vena cava blood return to the right heart, and decrease in right atrial pressure permit the foramen ovale to be closed by the opposition of the valve of the foramen ovale (the septum primum) against the edge of the crista terminalis. Usually, the valve becomes adherent and permanently closed in a few months, but in about 35% normal adults, a potential opening persists.

Since the pulmonary and systemic circulations are in communication before birth, the systolic pressures in the left and right ventricles, the aorta, and the pulmonary artery are all nearly equal. With the abrupt fall in pulmonary vascular resistance shortly after birth and the subsequent closure of the ductus arteriosus, the pulmonary artery pressure initially decreases rather abruptly and then more slowly until, after about 2 to 6 weeks, it reaches normal values. The decrease in pulmonary vascular resistance is associated with a marked regression of the thick medial muscle layers of the pulmonary arteries and arterioles. This normal regression of the pulmonary vasculature within the first few weeks or months after birth may permit the development of an increasing left-to-right shunt in patients born with a large ventricular septal defect or patent ductus arteriosus.

ATRIAL SEPTAL DEFECT

Except for mitral valve prolapse and bicuspid aortic valve, atrial septal defect (ASD) is the most frequent type of congenital heart disease in adolescents and adults. The most frequent defect is the ostium secundum type; it is occasionally associated with mitral valve prolapse. Many patients with associated mitral valve prolapse do not have myxomatous, floppy, or billowing mitral valve leaflets, and the prolapse is probably produced by distortion of the left ventricle and the mitral apparatus by the markedly dilated right ventricle. Defects of the sinus venosus type in the superior portion of the septum are much less frequent; they are often associated with partial anomalous pulmonary venous connection from the right upper or middle lobe to the superior vena cava or right atrium. Defects in the ostium primum involve the inferior portion of the atrial septum and are grouped as endocardial cushion defect or common atrioventricular canal defects (see Common Atrioventricular Canal Defects [Endocardial Cushion Defect]). After birth, the foramen ovale usually closes, although patency to a probe persists permanently in about 35% of adults. Very rarely, such patients may acquire a functional atrial septal defect ("blown-open foramen ovale") if the left atrial pressure increases markedly as a result of mitral valve disease, stretching the atrial septum and permitting a left-to-right shunt to develop. Conversely, if the right atrial pressure increases markedly, as in acute pulmonary embolus, a right-to-left shunt may develop or a paradoxical embolus may occur. ASD often occurs in association with other lesions. The combination of ostium secundum ASD and mitral stenosis is known as Lutembacher's syndrome.

The relative magnitude of the left-to-right (L-R) or right-to-left (R-L) shunt depends on the size of the ASD, the relative compliance of the two atria, the resistance to flow across the tricuspid and mitral valves, and especially the relative distensibility of the right and left ventricles. At birth, the two ventricles have similar diastolic filling characteristics, since they function at nearly the same systolic pressures in utero. As a result, there is little or no L-R shunting until the normal regression of the fetal pulmonary vasculature occurs and the normal growth hypertrophy of the left ventricle causes it to become less compliant than the right ventricle. With medium or large atrial septal defects, there is no significant pressure difference between the two atria, and the direction and amount of shunting are determined primarily by the relative compliance of the right and left ventricles. Some atrial defects present at birth may spontaneously close over the ensuing 5 years. Because of the tremendous reserve of the pulmonary circulation, the pressure in the pulmonary artery may not be elevated in some patients with a pulmonary flow three times greater than the systemic flow. After at least 20 years, however, a minority of patients (perhaps 15%) develop progressively more severe pulmonary vascular disease, which eventually may markedly increase pulmonary vascular resistance and, consequently, pulmonary artery and right ventricular pressure. Eventually, the stroke volume and the compliance of the hypertrophied right ventricle may decrease, causing the L-R shunt to decrease and, eventually, to reverse. When there is sufficient R-L shunt to produce significant arterial oxygen unsaturation and clinical cyanosis, the patient is said to have the Eisenmenger reaction. In general, this syndrome develops much later (usually between 20 and 40 years of age), and less often in patients with ASD than in patients with a large ventricular septal defect or a patent ductus arteriosus. Patients with the Eisenmenger reaction may have exertional syncope, hemoptysis, angina, and polycythemia. Patients who develop the Eisenmenger reaction have a high operative mortality for closure of the defect, and a high percentage of such patients do not have a decrease in the pulmonary artery or right ventricular pressure after surgery. On the other hand, children who have surgical correction at a young age may be dramatically improved and may be capable of normal physical activities.

Children with ASD tend to be thin, asthenic, and relatively gracile in habitus. ASD occurs twice as often in girls as in boys. A history of frequent upper respiratory tract infections and slight effort intolerance or dyspnea is frequently noted, but many patients reach adolescence or young adulthood with only mild or no symptoms. As these patients get older, however, they have a progressively increasing prevalence of cardiac symptoms, primarily fatigue and dyspnea on exertion. In patients over age 40, congestive heart failure may develop, often with supraventricular arrhythmias, especially atrial fibrillation.

The pathophysiology of heart failure in ASD is frequently complex and multifactorial. In patients with a medium- or large-sized ASD, the right and left atrial pressures and therefore the filling pressures of both ventricles are essentially equal. When this pressure becomes elevated, there are symptoms and signs of increased venous pressure in both the pulmonary and the systemic circulation. In many patients it is not possible to determine whether the failure was caused primarily by dysfunction of the left or the right ventricle.

In general, a decrease in left ventricular diastolic distensibility increases the left-to-right shunt and RV stroke volume, whereas a decrease in right ventricular distensibility decreases the left-to-right shunt and RV stroke volume and may even produce a right-to-left shunt across the ASD. The causes of changes in LV distensibility in patients with ASD include the following: age-related changes in LV distensibility, coronary artery disease, systemic arterial hypertension, mitral regurgitation, idiopathic myocardial dysfunction, and right ventricular dysfunction. Changes in the right ventricular distensibility may be produced by the chronic volume load from the ASD; the pressure load from pulmonary hypertension, particularly when marked; right ventricular ischemia; and left ventricular dysfunction. In patients with a chronically overloaded RV whose right ventricles remain abnormal after surgery, the right ventricle may transmit the diastolic pressure abnormalities to the left ventricle. Patients with ASD and heart failure frequently have atrial fibrillation, which may be either a contributing factor or a worsening consequence.

The physical findings vary considerably with the size of the L-R shunt and the pulmonary vascular resistance. The jugular venous pulse tends to have equal A and V waves or more prominent A waves if there is pulmonary hypertension. Since the pressures in the left and right atria are essentially equal with a large defect, the jugular venous pressure directly reflects the filling pressure of both ventricles. In patients with a significant shunt, right ventricular dilatation and hypertrophy may be manifest as a hyperdynamic right ventricular lift along the left parasternal border and a palpable pulmonary trunk and pulmonary component of the second heart sound (P_2). The first sound is usually loud and prominently split. The two components (A_2 and P_2) of the second heart sound are classically widely split, and during expiration the interval between the two sounds is fixed or does not decrease or disappear in the normal fashion (Chapter 3). A systolic murmur of grade III or less in the second or third left intercostal space is usually present, sometimes with an early ejection sound. Patients with a large L-R shunt may have a low-pitched diastolic murmur along the lower left sternal border produced by high flow across the tricuspid valve. This may disappear if the L-R shunt decreases as a result of the Eisenmenger reaction or marked RV hypertrophy. Some patients have evidence of mitral valve prolapse (Chapter 16). Mitral regurgitation caused by thickening of the anterior mitral valve leaflet, perhaps related to improper mitral leaflet coaptation produced by the dilated RV, occurs in about 15% of patients over age 50 and may increase in frequency and severity with age. Rarely, high flow in the pulmonary vessels may produce systolic murmurs that can be heard over the posterior lung fields and that may extend past the second heart sound. Rarely, a decrescendo, blowing diastolic murmur of pulmonary regurgitation from pulmonary hypertension is heard

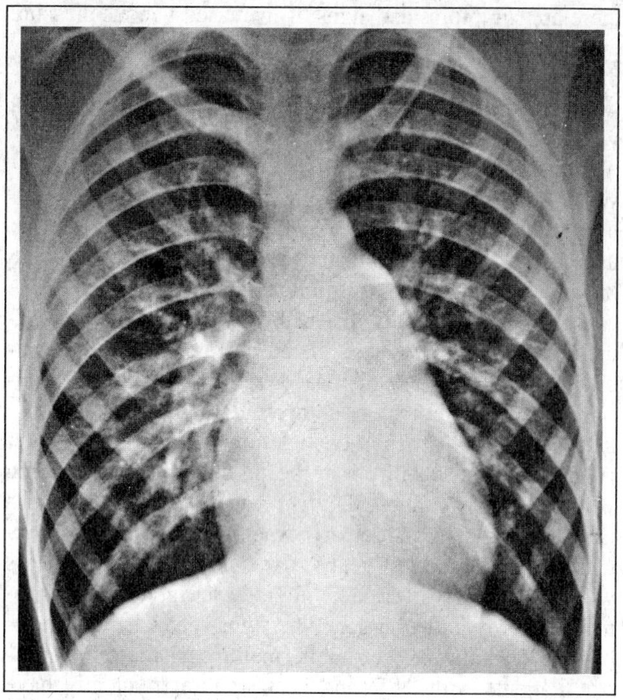

Fig. 19-1. Chest film of a 12-year-old patient with ostium secundum ASD showing mild cardiomegaly and increased pulmonary blood flow through enlarged main and peripheral pulmonary vessels. (Film provided by Dr. Wade H. Shuford, Professor of Radiology, Emory University School of Medicine.)

along the upper left sternal border. Patients with severe right ventricular hypertension and dilatation may develop tricuspid regurgitation. Cyanosis and clubbing may be present in individuals in whom the Eisenmenger reaction develops.

The chest radiograph characteristically shows slight or moderate cardiomegaly with prominence of the pulmonary outflow tract and increased pulmonary vascular markings when the pulmonary flow is at least twice as great as systemic flow (Fig. 19-1). Dilatation of the right ventricle may occasionally be evident on the lateral view; RA and RV dilatation produce marked cardiomegaly. Calcification can be seen in pulmonary vessels with severe hypertension. In patients with severe pulmonary vascular disease, the pulmonary vasculature has a "pruned-tree" appearance, with prominent central vessels but decreased small, distal vasculature. The left atrium is usually enlarged only in adults with congestive heart failure and atrial fibrillation.

The electrocardiogram (ECG) classically shows right axis deviation and incomplete right bundle branch block (Fig. 19-2). The rhythm is usually sinus until age 20, after which there is a progressive increase in supraventricular arrhythmias, including atrial fibrillation, atrial flutter, and atrial tachycardia. The development of right ventricular hypertrophy may be reflected in further widening of the QRS complex and in increased amplitude of the R′ wave in lead V_1. The P-R interval is prolonged in about 20% of patients. The P axis is usually nearly vertical in ostium secundum defects but tends to be horizontal in sinus venosus defects.

Two-dimensional (2D) or transesophageal (TEE) echocardiography may directly image the atrial septal defect, in addition to demonstrating dilatation of the right ventricle and paradoxical motion of the ventricular septum. The diagnosis is often aided by color Doppler or contrast echocardiography. Pulmonary hypertension may be reflected in abnormal motion of the pulmonic valves. Doppler echocardiography (Chapter 5) may provide evidence of the L-R shunt. Clinical and echocardiographic evidence of mitral valve prolapse is present in about 10% to 20% of patients with an ostium secundum ASD, but may disappear after surgical correction of ASD.

At cardiac catheterization the catheter may pass freely from the right to the left atrium through the defect, and blood samples demonstrate an abnormal step-up in the oxygen content of blood sampled from the superior vena cava and right atrium caused by the L-R shunt of oxygenated blood from the left atrium (Chapter 6). The quantities of L-R and R-L shunts and pulmonary and systemic blood flows can be estimated. The presence of anomalous pulmonary venous drainage may be detected. The pressures in the pulmonary artery and right ventricle can be directly measured and the pulmonary vascular resistance calculated by dividing the pulmonary pressure by the pulmonary flow. It is important to distinguish patients with a high pulmonary artery pressure in association with a high flow (and therefore normal or low pulmonary vascular resistance) from patients with high pulmonary artery pressure with a low flow (and high pulmonary vascular resistance). In the presence of a large L-R shunt, there may be a function peak pres-

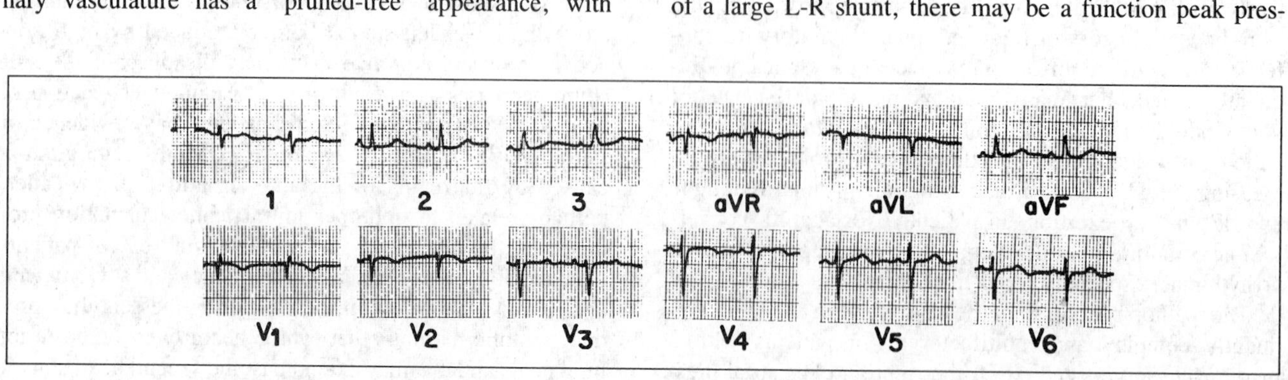

Fig. 19-2. Electrocardiogram of a patient with ostium secundum ASD with right axis deviation and incomplete right bundle branch block.

sure gradient across the pulmonary valve, which is usually only 5-20 mm Hg but can be 50-60 mm Hg.

Most individuals with ASD and a pulmonary flow more than 1.7 times systemic flow should have the defect repaired, preferably between the ages of 3 and 6 years, to prevent the subsequent development of pulmonary vascular disease and/or heart failure. Surgical repair can also be successfully performed in adults, including those over the age of 60. Individuals with pulmonary flow that is calculated to be 1.5 to 1.7 times systemic flow are in a borderline zone, although many probably should undergo surgery. Individuals with normal pressures and calculated pulmonary flow less than 1.5 times systemic flow usually do not require repair. Surgical closure is less clearly indicated in older patients, adult patients with sinus venous defects with pulmonary flow less than 1.8 times systemic flow, and patients with severe pulmonary vascular disease or mitral regurgitation. A few patients with severe pulmonary vascular disease have had transplantation of one lung, although it is probable that severe pulmonary vascular disease will eventually develop in this lung. In contrast to most other forms of congenital heart disease, patients with isolated ostium secundum ASD rarely acquire infective endocarditis. Patients with chronic atrial fibrillation should be maintained on low-dose warfarin. Closure of an ASD with a double-umbrella device introduced by a catheter is feasible if the defect is circular, is less than 2 cm in diameter, and has a well-defined rim. These necessary conditions for this investigational technique are often not present in adult patients.

After successful closure of an ASD before the age of 20, the heart size usually returns to normal and the pulmonary vasculature on chest radiograph returns to normal. The electrocardiographic evidence of incomplete right bundle branch block and the abnormal splitting of the second heart sound often persist although the splitting may vary with respiration if the conduction disturbance regresses.

After surgical repair of an atrial septal defect, a small percentage of patients may have a small residual L-R shunt of no hemodynamic consequence. Years after successful repair of an ASD, a small percentage of patients develop atrial arrhythmias such as sinus bradycardia, atrial fibrillation, or atrial flutter. Patients who have their ASD closed with a patch of synthetic material and who subsequently develop mitral regurgitation can have intravascular hemolysis from a jet of regurgitant blood striking the patch.

Most women who have had an ASD repaired tolerate pregnancy well but have a risk of about 6% of having a child with the same defect. The risk is about 1.5% if only the father has had an ASD.

PARTIAL TRANSPOSITION OF THE PULMONARY VEINS (PARTIAL ANOMALOUS PULMONARY VENOUS CONNECTION)

In this condition, one or more of the four pulmonary veins is connected to the right atrium or a systemic vein. The most frequent type is abnormal connection of the veins from the right upper and middle lobes to the superior vena cava or right atrium in patients with a sinus venosus type of ASD. The defect can readily be repaired at the time of repair of the ASD. When isolated transposition of the pulmonary veins occurs, it has the physiologic effects of an ASD with L-R shunt. Occasionally, the abnormal right pulmonary vein appears on the chest radiograph as a crescentlike shadow (scimitar syndrome) in the right lung field before it enters the inferior vena cava either just above or just below the diaphragm. There are often associated abnormalities and hypoplasia of the lung segments connected to the anomalous vein, hypoplasia of the right pulmonary artery, and a shift of the heart to the right side of the chest. Other cardiac defects are common.

COMMON ATRIOVENTRICULAR CANAL DEFECTS (ENDOCARDIAL CUSHION DEFECT)

This group of anomalies encompasses a variety of abnormalities, including ostium primum defects of the inferior atrial septum, with or without defects of the high ventricular septum, and defects or clefts in the mitral and/or tricuspid valves that result in mitral and/or tricuspid regurgitation. In some patients only one atrioventricular valve is present. Ostium primum defects are common in patients with Down's syndrome.

The combination of L-R shunt and atrioventricular valve regurgitation is usually associated with earlier and more severe disability than is ostium secundum ASD. In childhood, upper respiratory infections are common and weight gain tends to be retarded, as in patients with ostium secundum defects. If significant mitral regurgitation is present, there may be dyspnea and fatigue on exertion or even pulmonary edema. In general, elevation of pulmonary artery pressure and the development of pulmonary vascular disease tend to occur earlier than in ostium secundum defects. Adults may develop atrial fibrillation, complete heart block, and heart failure.

The findings on physical examination are similar to those of a patient with ostium secundum ASD plus possible evidence of mitral or, less frequently, tricuspid regurgitation (Chapter 16). The chest radiograph is similar to that of an ostium secundum ASD except for dilatation and hypertrophy of the left ventricle if there is significant mitral regurgitation. In contrast to patients with other types of chronic mitral regurgitation, the left atrium is only mildly enlarged, if at all.

The ECG is often the first clue to the presence of an ostium primum type of endocardial cushion defect rather than an ostium secundum ASD. The characteristic findings are the combination of incomplete right bundle branch block with an rSr′ in lead V_1 in combination with a QRS axis between 0 and −150 degrees (Fig. 19-3). If there is significant mitral regurgitation, there may also be increased R wave voltage in the left precordial leads. The P-R interval is usually prolonged.

The 2D transthoracic (TTE) or transesophageal (TEE) echocardiogram may demonstrate the low atrial septal defect as well as abnormal motion of the mitral or tricuspid

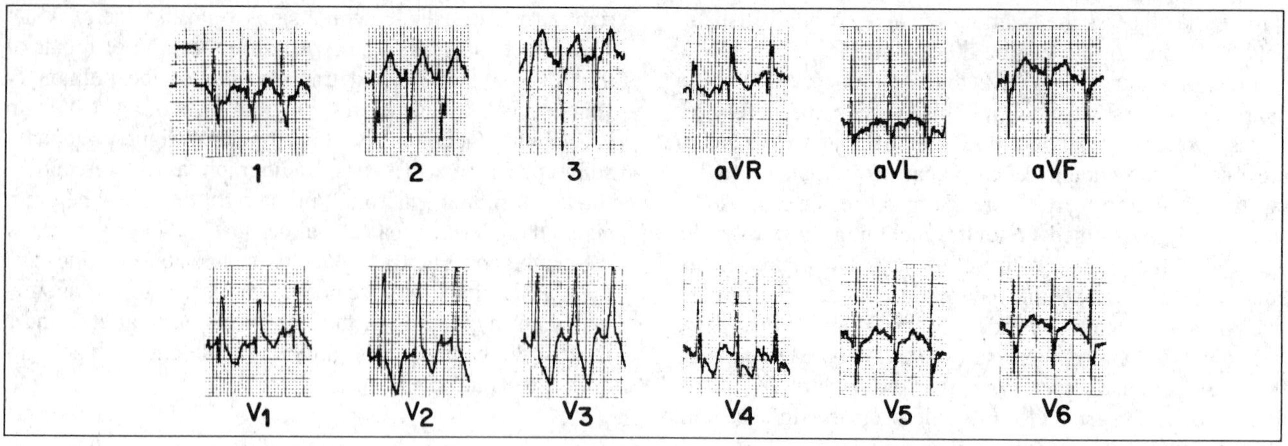

Fig. 19-3. Electrocardiogram of a patient with ostium primum ASD, showing incomplete right bundle branch block and marked left axis deviation.

valve leaflets or even complete absence of the tissues formed at the middle of the heart from the endocardial cushion. Dilatation of both ventricles may be present. Doppler echocardiography provides an estimate of the severity of the regurgitation.

Cardiac catheterization provides evidence of an ASD with an increase in oxygen content in blood samples from the right atrium compared with those in the superior vena cava. It may be possible to pass the catheter across the defect into the left atrium and ventricle. Left ventricular angiography demonstrates a characteristic "gooseneck" deformity of the left ventricular outflow tract in the presence of a cleft anterior mitral valve leaflet. It may also demonstrate the L-R shunt, at times directly from the left ventricle to the right atrium, or mitral regurgitation.

Patients with an endocardial cushion defect require antibiotic prophylaxis against endocarditis during any dental procedure or surgical procedure likely to be associated with bacteremia. When only an ostium primum defect is present, surgical repair of an endocardial cushion defect is very similar to that of an ostium secundum defect; however, clefts in the mitral or tricuspid valves are much more difficult to repair satisfactorily without residual regurgitation. Some patients require repair or pulmonary artery banding in the first year of life. Occasionally, the valve cannot be repaired and must be replaced with a prosthetic valve.

A woman with an endocardial cushion defect has about a 14% likelihood of having a child with the same defect. The risk is 1% if only the father is affected.

VENTRICULAR SEPTAL DEFECT

In infants ventricular septal defect (VSD) is the most common recognized congenital heart defect after mitral valve prolapse or bicuspid aortic valve. About 10% of adolescents and adults with congenital heart disease have an isolated VSD. It is unusual in adults over age 40. The majority of infants who are born with a VSD experience spontaneous closure of the defect. Such closure is most likely to occur in the first 10 years and with small defects, but closure can occur later, and even large defects may close. The defects may be small or large and single or multiple. Defects are located usually in the superior, membranous portion of the ventricular septum (infracristal defect) and less frequently in the subpulmonic (supracristal) area or in the inferior muscular portion.

The clinical course and natural history of VSD vary markedly with the size of the defect(s). Small defects (less than 0.5 cm^2/m^2) produce a loud holosystolic murmur and thrill along the lower left sternal edge but only a small L-R shunt of no hemodynamic consequence. Such a defect, however, predisposes the patient to infective endocarditis. This type of defect, maladie de Roger, is very likely to close spontaneously. Intermediate-size defects (0.5 to 1.0 cm^2/m^2) permit a moderate to large L-R shunt and produce mild to moderate elevation of right ventricular and pulmonary artery pressures. In patients with large defects (more than 1.0 cm^2/m^2), who usually have equal pressures in both ventricles and the hemodynamics of a single ventricle, the direction and amount of shunt between the two ventricles depend on the compliance of the two ventricles and the relative impedance to the ejection of blood out the aorta and out the pulmonary artery. Patients with a large VSD have both increased pulmonary blood flow and increased pulmonary artery pressure. Thus, they are likely to develop the Eisenmenger reaction much earlier and more severely than patients with an ostium secundum ASD.

Infants with a large VSD may have little L-R shunt at birth when the pulmonary vasculature is still markedly hypertrophied and the pulmonary vascular resistance is high. As hypertrophy of the media in the pulmonary vessels regresses over the first 3 to 12 weeks in full-term infants at sea level, the pulmonary vascular resistance decreases, allowing a much greater L-R shunt and exposing the pulmonary capillaries to relatively high pressures. Also, the increasing L-R shunt imposes a volume load on the left ventricle, which may cause an elevation of the diastolic pressures in the left ventricle, left atrium, and pulmonary veins, further contributing to the development of pulmonary edema. In many, perhaps most, children a secondary increase in the pulmonary vascular resistance begins after a few days or weeks. This increase in resistance tends to decrease the L-R shunt, to "protect" the pulmonary capillaries from the high pulmonary artery pressure, and to decrease the volume load on the left ventricle. In patients with a large VSD the pulmonary vascular resistance often increases excessively after a variable period of time, usually 3 to 20 years, with the development of severe pulmonary vascular disease and the Eisenmenger reaction. At that stage, the pulmonary vascular resistance, which is usually more than 600 dynes/sec/cm^{-5}, or about 7 units per square meter, is so high relative to the systemic vascular resistance that the L-R shunt decreases or even disappears completely, together with the murmur from the shunt across the VSD. Surgical correction is usually prohibitive when the pulmonary vascular resistance is more than 800 dynes/sec/cm^{-5}, or 11 units per square meter, in adults. Such patients often have dyspnea on exertion, chest pain, hemoptysis, and syncope. A R-L shunt may develop, together with a marked right ventricular left parasternal lift, arterial unsaturation, cyanosis, clubbing, and polycythemia. At this stage, the pulmonary vascular disease is largely irreversible; surgical repair of the defect is of limited benefit and is associated with a high operative mortality. Pregnancy and oral contraceptives are prohibited for such patients. In a few adolescents or adults with a large VSD, a marked infundibular stenosis develops, which decreases the L-R shunt and can also produce a R-L shunt and cyanosis. Therapy with combined cardiac and pulmonary transplantation is a potential form of therapy for patients with Eisenmenger's syndrome.

Patients with small VSDs usually have no symptoms. Those with medium or large defects may develop congestive heart failure at 3 to 12 weeks, which may be misdiagnosed as pneumonia. If the child survives this period, it may then be only mildly symptomatic with exertional dyspnea, failure to thrive, and fatigue but with relatively poor growth until the subsequent development of the Eisenmenger reaction, with cyanosis, clubbing, dyspnea, and weakness. Eventually, such patients may die suddenly, or may develop biventricular heart failure and/or pulmonary emboli and thrombi.

At birth there may be no murmurs, although usually a moderately loud holosystolic murmur is heard along the lower left sternal border at a few days of age. Often the murmur is accompanied by a thrill. In patients with a small defect and small L-R shunt, there is no parasternal lift or accentuated P_2, but usually there is a hyolosystolic murmur and thrill along the lower left sternal border. The murmur and L-R shunt may end in midsystole if the defect is in the muscular septum. In patients with a small VSD the ECG and chest radiograph are normal. Patients with moderate or large defects and shunts have a similar murmur, but the apical impulse may be sustained, forceful, and displaced, together with a forceful left parasternal impulse, reflecting the volume load on both ventricles. The components of the second heart sound are normally or moderately widely split, usually with a loud pulmonic component. An early diastolic, low-frequency murmur and third heart sound may be heard at the apex, reflecting the increased flow across the mitral valve into the LV.

The chest radiograph of patients with large defects shows enlargement of all four chambers and the pulmonary artery, together with pulmonary plethora. Patients with Eisenmenger's reaction may have a pruned-tree appearance with normal or decreased pulmonary blood flow (Fig. 19-4). The ECG may show biatrial and left ventricular or biventricular hypertrophy (Fig. 19-5). Patients with VSD and Eisenmenger's reaction may be inoperable when they have lost the ECG evidence of left or combined ventricular hypertrophy and have only right ventricular hypertrophy. The 2D echocardiogram or transesophageal echocardiogram may demonstrate the VSD directly in addition to dilatation of both ventricles and evidence of pulmonary hypertension. Doppler echocardiography provides evidence of the magnitude and direction of ventricular shunt.

Cardiac catheterization (Chapter 6) permits measurements of pressures in the cardiac chambers and blood sampling to estimate the direction and magnitude of intracardiac shunts and to estimate pulmonary vascular resistance. Left ventricular angiography may demonstrate the shunt to the right ventricle. Coronary arteriography is usually performed in adults, especially those with risk factors for coronary artery disease. The VSD and the size of both ventricles can also be demonstrated by nuclear magnetic resonance imaging (NMRI).

Patients with small VSDs, a small L-R shunt, and a pul-

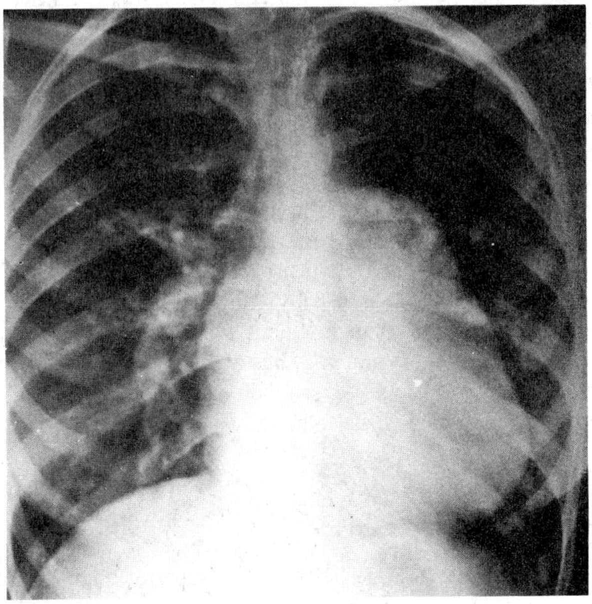

Fig. 19-4. Chest film of a patient with a large VSD and the Eisenmenger reaction. The film shows moderate cardiomegaly, enlarged main and central arteries, and a pruned-tree appearance of the distal pulmonary arteries. (Film provided by Dr. Wade H. Shuford, Professor of Radiology, Emory University School of Medicine.)

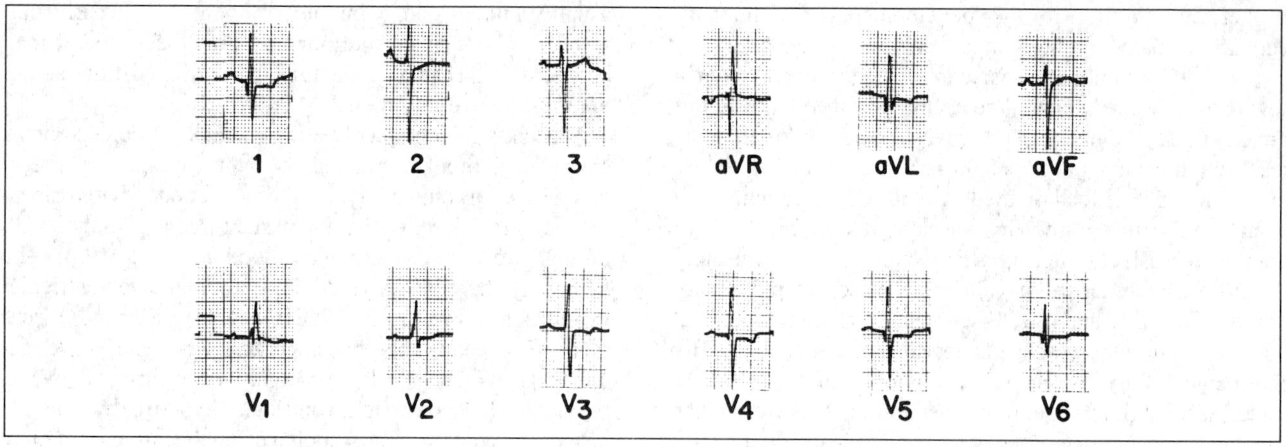

Fig. 19-5. Electrocardiogram of patient with VSD and biventricular hypertrophy. Tracing also shows incomplete right bundle branch block but no definite left atrial abnormality.

monary to systemic flow ratio less than 1.5:1.0 require only prophylaxis for bacterial endocarditis (Chapter 15). Most of these small defects close spontaneously, and those that remain open do not require surgery. If pulmonary edema develops in an infant with a large VSD and does not respond to therapy with digitalis and diuretics, the patient may require primary closure of the defect or, less frequently, pulmonary artery banding to decrease the pulmonary artery flow. Patients with a persistent large defect who survive infancy with medical therapy or with pulmonary artery banding should have complete repair when the child is about 12 to 24 months of age. In patients in whom the Eisenmenger reaction develops, there is a much higher operative mortality and only a slight chance of a significant decrease in the pulmonary vascular resistance or pressure. Patients who develop infundibular stenosis with a R-L shunt may develop secondary polycythemia. In patients with hyperviscosity symptoms the hematocrit can be lowered to below 65% by phlebotomy with fluid replacement to decrease the likelihood of thrombosis. Repeated phlebotomy may require iron therapy to avoid iron deficiency. Some of these patients can have corrective surgery with good results. In adults without severe pulmonary vascular disease, surgical correction of a VSD is usually indicated if the pulmonary blood flow is more than 1.4 times systemic flow.

A woman who has a VSD has about a 9.5% likelihood of having a child with the same defect, whereas the likelihood is only 2.5% if the father has had a VSD.

VENTRICULAR SEPTAL DEFECT WITH AORTIC REGURGITATION

There is usually a large defect in the superior, supracristal portion of the membranous ventricular septum just under the right coronary cusp of the aortic valve. In most patients the support for the aortic valve is adequate until early childhood, when the diastolic murmur of aortic regurgitation first is heard. The clinical course of such patients is usually more problematic than is that of patients with an isolated VSD. Often the aortic regurgitation becomes progressively more severe and may require valve replacement. Occasionally, the VSD closes spontaneously, leaving only moderate to severe aortic regurgitation. The aortic regurgitation may be directly demonstrated by aortography, which may also demonstrate the VSD. Echocardiography may demonstrate the VSD and may show diastolic fluttering of the anterior mitral valve leaflet produced by the aortic regurgitation. Doppler echocardiography provides an estimate of both the regurgitation and the L-R shunt.

The VSD should be repaired if there is moderate pulmonary artery hypertension with a significant L-R shunt. At times, repair of the VSD can correct the support of the aortic valve and decrease or eliminate the aortic regurgitation; more often, however, it is necessary to replace the aortic valve.

PATENT DUCTUS ARTERIOSUS

Patent ductus arteriosus (PDA) is common in infants and children but accounts for only about 2% of congenital heart defects in adults. It tends to occur with higher frequency in siblings and can result from maternal rubella in the first trimester of pregnancy. Persistence of PDA is more frequent in females, in premature infants, and in infants born at high altitudes.

The ductus arteriosus is normally patent during fetal life, when it provides a shunt from the pulmonary artery to the aorta. After birth, the ductus normally closes functionally over the first 24 to 48 hours of life and anatomically over the first 3 months; closure at a later age occurs but is infrequent. PDA may occur with many other defects, especially coarctation of the aorta and VSD.

The hemodynamic consequences and physiologic changes produced by a PDA are related to the vascular resistance through the ductus and to the pulmonary vascular resistance. In infants with high-resistance PDA, there may be only a very small L-R shunt and little hemodynamic consequence other than increased susceptibility to infective endarteritis. Infants with large, low resistance PDA and large L-R shunts may develop left ventricular failure and pulmonary edema at 3 to 12 weeks, when the fetal vasculature undergoes its normal regression of early infancy. Usually, the left ventricle is able to compensate for the increased L-R shunt by dilatation and hypertrophy and the pulmonary vasculature increases its resistance. Although the PDA closes spontaneously in many children within 3 months, a large ductus may persist and can eventually result in Eisenmenger's reaction with pulmonary vascular resistance equal to or greater than systemic resistance and a R-L shunt through the PDA with cyanosis of the lower extremities. This can occur at any age beyond 3 years.

Individuals with a small PDA may have no symptoms. Infants with a large PDA may develop pulmonary edema with severe dyspnea, cyanosis, and tachypnea at about 6 to 12 weeks of age. The heart failure and respiratory distress tend to occur in the first week in premature infants and in the second or third month in nonpremature infants. Children who survive this period may be relatively asymptomatic except for mild exertional fatigue and dyspnea. Some patients with medium or large defects and a chronic volume load on the left ventricle develop left ventricular failure after the age of 20. Right ventricular failure caused by the chronic pressure load may also occur.

The classic finding of PDA is a thrill and continuous "machinery" murmur with a late systolic accentuation that is loudest in the first to third left parasternal intercostal spaces (Chapter 3). Some patients have only a systolic murmur. The murmur is often not present immediately after birth in full-term infants. The arterial pulse pressure tends to be increased, reflecting the large diastolic runoff into the pulmonary circuit. In patients with a large L-R shunt the apical impulse is displaced leftward and sustained. Patients with a large L-R shunt through the PDA may have a mitral flow middiastolic murmur and a third heart sound at the apex. Patients who develop Eisenmenger's reaction with severe pulmonary vascular obstructive disease and a R-L shunt may have a right ventricular lift and a loud pulmonic component of the second heart sound, no ductus thrill or murmur, but differential cyanosis with cyanosis of the toes, intermediate cyanosis of the left fingers, and no cyanosis of the right fingers.

The chest radiograph may be normal in patients with a very small PDA, while patients with a large PDA may have pulmonary plethora together with enlargement of the ascending aorta and aortic knob, left ventricle and atrium, and pulmonary artery (Fig. 19-6). Patients who develop severe pulmonary vascular disease may have a normal left ventricle and atrium but a pruned-tree appearance of the peripheral pulmonary vasculature. Older patients occasionally have calcification of the PDA. The ECG in patients with a significant L-R shunt usually shows evidence of left ventricular hypertrophy and left atrial abnormality. Right ventricular hypertrophy may be present in patients with pulmonary hypertension. Echocardiography may demonstrate the ductus, dilatation and hyperfunction of the left ventricle, and occasionally left atrial enlargement. Doppler echocardiography may be used to diagnose and quantify the shunt. Cardiac catheterization permits direct measurement of cardiac pressures and estimation of any L-R or R-L shunts. Aortography demonstrates the PDA, as does NMRI.

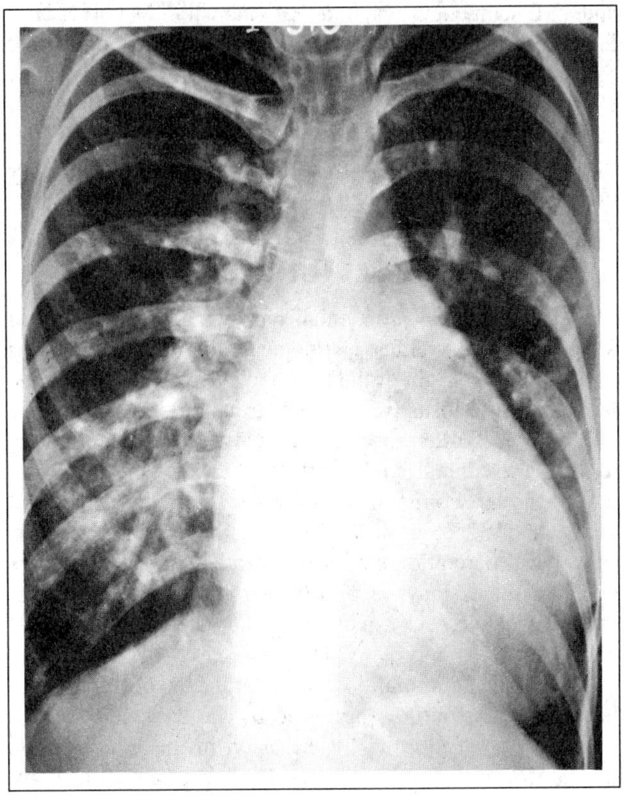

Fig. 19-6. Chest film of a patient with a PDA showing moderate cardiomegaly and very prominent peripheral pulmonary vessels. In this film the aorta is not enlarged. (Film provided by Dr. Wade H. Shuford, Professor of Radiology, Emory University School of Medicine.)

Infants with PDA in whom congestive heart failure develops may be treated with indomethacin (which inhibits synthesis of prostaglandins) in an attempt to induce closure of the ductus, but most full-term infants eventually require elective surgical closure at 1 to 2 years of age. A patent ductus in premature infants is more likely to close either spontaneously or with indomethacin, although some require surgical closure. All patients should receive prophylaxis against infective endarteritis of the ductus. In general, any child or adult discovered to have a PDA should have it surgically corrected unless the patient has already developed an Eisenmenger reaction or is elderly.

A mother who has a PDA has a 4% likelihood of having a child with the same defect. The likelihood is 2% if only the father has had a PDA.

AORTOPULMONARY SEPTAL DEFECT

This relatively rare defect consists of a communication, or "window," which is often relatively large, between the ascending aorta and the main pulmonary artery. A large aortopulmonary artery communication permits equalization of their pressures and, in most instances, a large L-R shunt until the development of severe pulmonary vascular disease and an Eisenmenger reaction. Patients with this defect clinically resemble those with a large, low-resistance PDA, and the two lesions can coexist. The distinction is usually made by passage of a catheter across the defect or by TTE or TEE, left ventricular angiography, aortography, or NMRI. Early surgical repair is necessary to prevent progressive pulmonary vascular disease.

COARCTATION OF THE AORTA

There is a discrete, congenital narrowing of all layers of the aorta, usually either just opposite the ductus arteriosus or distal to the origin of the left subclavian artery just above the ductus arteriosus (preductal coarctation). In adolescents or adults, it is often located just below the ligamentum arteriosus (postductal coarctation). Rarely, it may be proximal to the left common carotid artery or in the abdominal aorta. About 25% to 46% of patients have a bicuspid aortic valve. Coarctation may be associated with other defects and in females may be part of Turner's syndrome (short stature, webbed neck, small chin, and other skeletal abnormalities).

The basic abnormality is the significant obstruction to left ventricular outflow produced by the coarctation. As a consequence of systolic hypertension in the left ventricle and upper body, the patient may develop a number of complications. These include left ventricular failure, which may develop at any time from infancy to adulthood; cerebral hemorrhage, which may be from a berry aneurysm in the circle of Willis; aortic rupture or dissection, which usually involves either the ascending aorta or poststenotic dilatation just beyond the coarctation; and infective endocarditis or endarteritis, which usually involves a coexisting bicuspid aortic valve but can rarely involve the coarctation itself. Extensive collaterals develop between the arterial circulation proximal to the coarctation and the circulation distal to the coarctation.

Isolated coarctation occurs much more frequently in males. Symptoms and signs of right and/or left ventricular failure develop in about half of infants with coarctation, while others have no symptoms. Occasionally, there may be headache, frequent nosebleeds, or excessive fatigue or discomfort of the legs on exertion. Most adult patients have isolated coarctation without other cardiac defects.

The hallmark of aortic coarctation is an abnormal systolic pressure difference (equal to or greater than 30 mm Hg) between the right arm and the legs (Chapter 3). The pressure in the left arm may be equal to or less than that in the right arm, depending on the site of coarctation. The diastolic pressure below the coarctation is often normal or nearly normal. In some patients the pressure difference between the right arm and the legs is relatively mild at rest but increases dramatically during exercise. The carotid pulses are often very forceful while the pulses in the leg are delayed, weak, or impalpable. The legs are occasionally poorly developed relative to the chest and arms. The apical impulse is sustained, forceful, and displaced leftward and inferiorly. Patients with a bicuspid aortic valve may have a harsh midsystolic murmur and thrill along the second right intercostal space and an early systolic ejection click at the apex. In addition, there may be a blowing, decrescendo diastolic murmur of aortic regurgitation along the left sternal border. A midsystolic blowing murmur from the coarctation may often be heard faintly along the left sternal border or louder posteriorly in the left interscapular space. At times, this murmur extends into early diastole. Collateral vessels produce systolic murmurs that may continue into or throughout diastole and are commonly heard over the posterior chest wall beyond childhood. At times, these collateral intercostal vessels are palpable, particularly over the posterior chest.

The chest radiograph may show prominence of the ascending aorta and enlargement of the left ventricle and left atrium. The poststenotic dilatation of the aorta and the dilated proximal left subclavian artery and aorta may produce a "figure 3" sign along the left side of the upper descending thoracic aorta. Classically, notching on the undersurfaces of the posterior ribs bilaterally is present after the age of 7 or 8 (Fig. 19-7). If the coarctation is proximal to the origin of the left subclavian artery, however, notching may occur only on the right side, whereas patients with coarctation of the abdominal aorta may have no notching of the upper ribs.

The usual ECG findings are those of left ventricular hypertrophy and left atrial abnormality (Chapter 4). Infants may have right ventricular or combined ventricular hypertrophy, often in association with an interatrial L-R shunt.

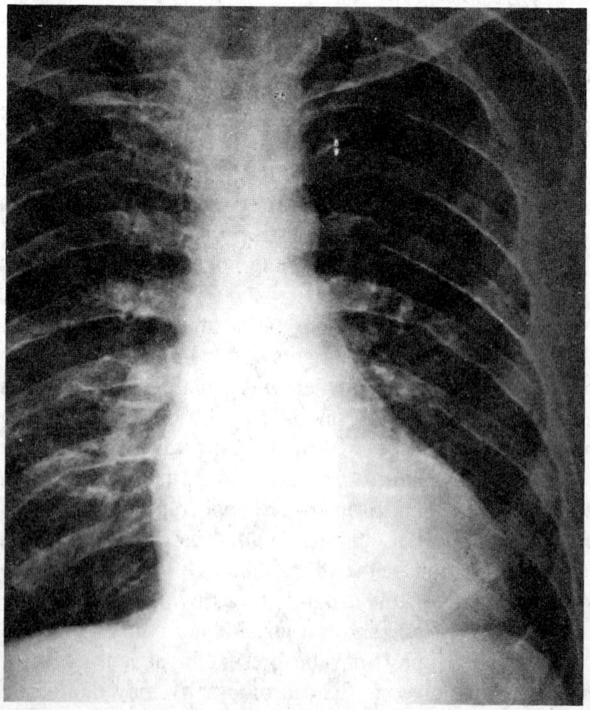

Fig. 19-7. Chest film of a patient with coarctation of the aorta showing mild cardiomegaly and notching on the undersurfaces of the posterior ribs. (Film provided by Dr. Wade H. Shuford, Professor of Radiology, Emory University School of Medicine.)

Aortography proximal to the suspected site demonstrates the character of the coarctation and the collateral vessels and may also demonstrate aortic regurgitation or a bicuspid aortic valve. Two-dimensional echocardiography, especially transesophageal, and NMRI can also demonstrate the coarctation. Upper- and lower-extremity blood pressure measurements during exercise are useful in assessing the significance of systolic pressure differences that are only mild at rest.

Most young patients with significant coarctation should undergo cardiac catheterization to assess possible associated lesions. Children with isolated coarctation should have elective surgical repair at age 4 to 6 to decrease the likelihood of heart failure, aortic dissection or rupture, and cerebral hemorrhage. Balloon dilatation has been used successfully in children and a few adults. Older children and young adults should have surgical repair as soon as feasible. In patients over age 50 without evidence of a complication, the indication for surgery is less definite. After surgical repair, some patients with coarctation have a postcoarctation syndrome of acute abdominal pain, ileus, and even a necrotizing mesenteric vasculitis soon after repair that appears to be related to suddenly exposing the abdominal vessels to a higher than usual blood pressure. This can usually be prevented or satisfactorily controlled by careful blood pressure control with sodium nitroprusside and beta blockers; very rarely, it may require emergency surgery. Patients should be followed consistently after repair of the coarctation, since many have an associated bicuspid aortic valve and many redevelop systemic hypertension for which they will require therapy. A small percentage of patients operated on in childhood develop evidence of recurrence of the stenosis at the site of coarctation. Such patients can usually be managed with balloon dilatation or pharmacologically to control their hypertension; only rarely do they require repeat surgery.

A woman with coarctation of the aorta has about a 4% chance of having a child with the same defect. The likelihood is 2.5% if only the father has had a coarctation.

CONGENITAL AORTIC STENOSIS (SEE ALSO ACQUIRED AORTIC STENOSIS, CHAPTER 16)

The obstruction may be either supravalvular, valvular, or subvalvular. Supravalvular stenosis is usually produced by a fibrous band or ring just above the aortic valve. Valvular stenosis in infants or children is usually produced by cuspal fusion of a bicuspid valve, or by a unicuspid (unicommissural) or noncommissural valve. It is four times as frequent in males. Congenital subvalvular stenosis is usually produced by a discrete fibromembranous or fibromuscular band or ring that extends from the anterior leaflet of the mitral valve to the ventricular septum just below the aortic valve. In older children or adults, subvalvular obstruction is usually produced by hypertrophic obstructive cardiomyopathy (Chapter 16).

Infants and children may die suddenly without significant symptoms. Others have symptoms of dyspnea or distress on feeding or on exertion, fatigue, exertional angina, or syncopal or near-syncopal episodes. In occasional infants, the stenosis is critical at birth or in the first 6 months and requires prompt surgical correction to prevent congestive heart failure. More often, the symptoms of congestive heart failure or of distress while eating, which are equivalent to angina pectoris in an older patient, occur after several years or during the rapid growth phase of childhood. Valvular aortic stenosis is usually associated with an ejection click, which is often loudest at the apex. Half the patients with subvalvular aortic stenosis have the murmur of aortic regurgitation caused by fibrosis and retraction of the aortic valve leaflets from the jet of blood through the subvalvular obstruction.

Some patients with supravalvular aortic stenosis have a particular elfin appearance with mental retardation, retarded growth, small chin, and malformed teeth. Peripheral pulmonary artery stenosis is frequently an associated condition. Hypercalcemia has occasionally been noted in infancy. Usually the blood pressure is higher in the right arm than in the left, and there is no ejection click. The midsystolic murmur is usually loudest in the first right intercostal space and radiates to both carotids. A fourth heart sound may be heard at the apex in this and all other types of moderate to severe aortic stenosis.

The examination of patients with valvular aortic stenosis is similar except that the murmur is usually loudest in the second right intercostal space, frequently with a systolic thrill. An ejection click is heard either in this area or at the apex, and occasionally the murmur of aortic regurgitation is heard along the left sternal border. In infants or children with valvular aortic stenosis, the carotid pulse may be normal and the aortic component of the second heart sound may be well preserved. The presence of paradoxical splitting of the second heart sound is rare and implies severe obstruction (Chapter 3). A fourth heart sound is frequently heard with moderate or severe obstruction.

The chest radiograph may show slight convexity of the left ventricle. Prominence of the ascending aorta is usual in valvular stenosis, but is unusual in supravalvular stenosis, and is only occasionally found in subvalvular stenosis. Calcification is usually seen only in valvular stenosis after age 20. Evidence of pulmonary edema may be present.

All forms of aortic stenosis usually have electrocardiographic evidence of left ventricular hypertrophy and left atrial enlargement when the obstruction is significant. Doppler echocardiography demonstrates the location and provides a good estimate of the severity of the obstruction. NMRA can also demonstrate the location of the obstruction, while cardiac catheterization and left ventricular angiography permit estimation of the effective orifice of the obstruction and evaluation of left ventricular function in addition to outlining the obstruction. Coronary arteriography is performed on all patients with angina and most adult patients. In patients with low peak or mean gradients across the aortic valve, it is important to calculate the valve area since a decreased stroke volume can result in there being only a mild pressure gradient across a severely stenotic valve. Some patients have a progressive increase in the severity of obstruction over 3 to 5 years.

Surgery is generally indicated in children or adolescents with a peak pressure difference between the left ventricle and the aorta of 75 mm Hg or greater or a valve area less than 0.5 cm^2 per square meter. Surgery may also be indicated with less severe obstruction in patients with symptoms, cardiomegaly, or ECG changes (Chapter 16).

A woman with congenital AS has about an 18% chance of having offspring with the same defect, whereas the likelihood is only 5% if the father has had congenital AS.

BICUSPID AORTIC VALVE

This lesion, which may be the most common type of congenital heart disease other than mitral valve prolapse, occurs more frequently in males, with an incidence of 1% to 2%. In most instances one leaflet is larger than the other. It often occurs in association with PDA, coarctation of the aorta, or interruption of the aortic arch.

A bicuspid aortic valve is the most frequent cause of significant valvular aortic stenosis in infancy and childhood, of congenital aortic regurgitation, and of isolated calcific stenosis before the age of 65. While some bicuspid aortic valves are fully competent at birth, the abnormal structure of the valve produces abnormal stresses on the valve that eventually result in premature fibrosis and calcification after 30 to 60 years. A minority of patients have aortic regurgitation from early life. Infective endocarditis is a constant threat to any patient with a bicuspid aortic valve. While the majority of patients with a bicuspid aortic valve eventually develop valvular fibrosis and calcification with calcific aortic stenosis (Chapter 16), a rare patient over the age of 70 is found at autopsy to have only mild fibrosis with no significant stenosis. There is a suggestion that calcification and stenosis occur earlier in patients with systemic hypertension or hypercholesterolemia.

Patients with a functionally normal bicuspid aortic valve have no symptoms. Patients who have congenitally significant stenosis or regurgitation, however, may develop symptoms of congestive heart failure, angina, or syncope in infancy or childhood (Chapter 16). The presence of a bicuspid aortic valve can be suggested in a young patient who is found to have a midsystolic murmur loudest in the second right intercostal space together with an ejection click, which is often heard loudest at the apex. An early diastolic blowing murmur of aortic regurgitation may occasionally be heard along the left sternal border. The diagnosis and management of patients with significant aortic stenosis or regurgitation are described in Chapter 16. For most of their lives, the main danger is infective endocarditis. With the development of any one of the classic triad of symptoms—congestive heart failure, angina, or syncope—patients are candidates for prompt surgery because of the high risk of sudden death without such therapy (Chapter 16).

VALVULAR PULMONIC STENOSIS WITH INTACT VENTRICULAR SEPTUM

There is usually a dome-shaped stenosis of the pulmonic valve with fused commissures, often associated with poststenotic dilatation of the main pulmonary artery. The severe obstruction is associated with marked hypertrophy of the right ventricle, which at times is associated with secondary muscular infundibular stenosis of the outflow tract. Maternal rubella may be associated with pulmonic stenosis, although patent ductus arteriosus and pulmonary artery branch stenosis are more frequent.

Many patients have no symptoms even with severe stenosis. When present, the most frequent symptoms are easy fatigability and dyspnea on exertion. Angina pectoris on exertion and syncope can also occur, especially with severe stenosis.

In patients with moderate or severe pulmonic stenosis there is usually a prominent A wave in the jugular venous pulse; a palpable, sustained right ventricular lift along the left sternal border; a widely split second heart sound with a delayed and usually faint or inaudible pulmonic component; a moderately loud and long, harsh, spindle-shaped midsystolic murmur, often with a thrill that is loudest in the second left intercostal space and tends to radiate to the left infraclavicular area and the neck; and a right-ventricular fourth heart sound along the left sternal border. In patients with mild to moderate pulmonic stenosis, a pulmonic ejection sound may be heard at the base or upper left sternal edge (Chapter 3). Patients with severe pulmonic stenosis and elevation of right atrial pressure may have arterial oxygen unsaturation and cyanosis from a R-L shunt through a patent foramen ovale.

The chest radiograph may show varying degrees of prominence of the right atrium and right ventricle, occasionally producing marked enlargement of the heart. There is often prominence of the main and/or left pulmonary artery produced by poststenotic dilatation; however, the pulmonary blood flow appears normal or diminished (Fig. 19-8, *A*). In adults, the pulmonic valve may be calcified.

There is a reasonably good correlation between the severity of stenosis and the relative ECG evidence for right ventricular hypertrophy in lead V_1. In addition, there is usually right axis deviation and right atrial enlargement. Doppler echocardiography provides a good estimate of the severity of pulmonic stenosis and of right ventricular function. Contrast echocardiography may document a R-L shunt at the atrial level. Cardiac catheterization permits direct measurements of the pressure difference across the stenotic valve and right ventricular pressures and permits calculation of the effective valve orifice. Right ventricular angiography visualizes the dome-shaped stenosis and poststenotic dilatation of the pulmonary artery (Fig. 19-8, B).

Patients with pulmonic stenosis are susceptible to infective endocarditis, for which they should receive appropriate antibiotic prophylaxis (Chapter 15). Balloon valvuloplasty (valvotomy) is the treatment of choice for most patients with isolated congenital pulmonic stenosis. In gen-

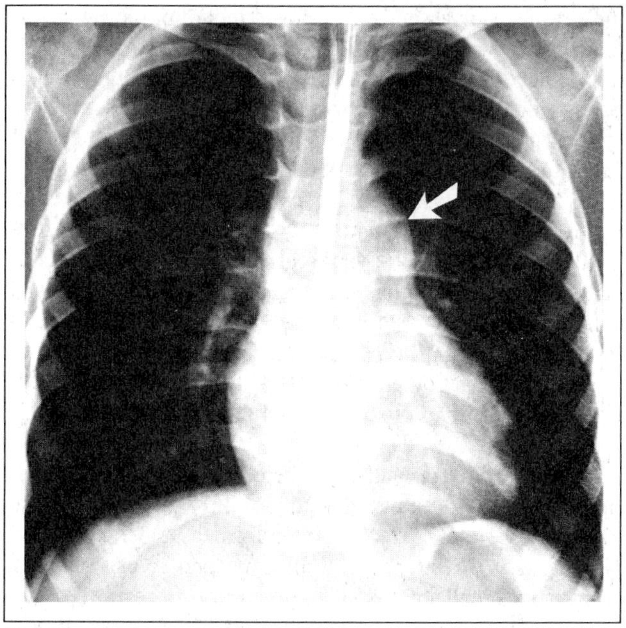

A

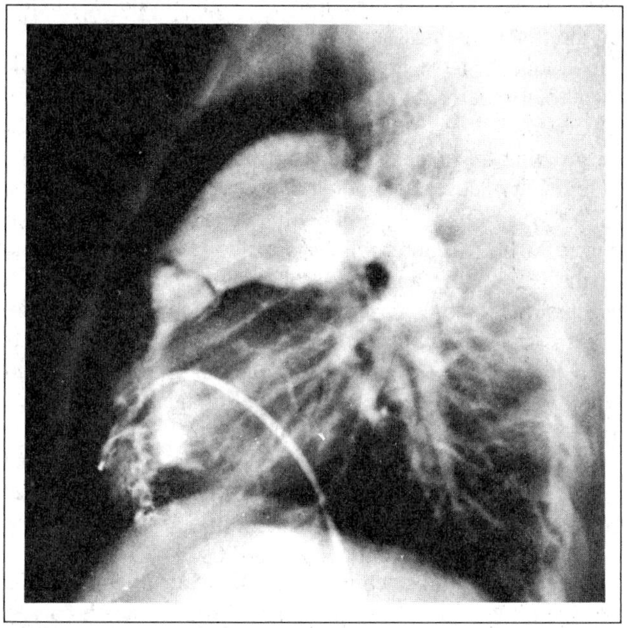

B

Fig. 19-8. Chest film **(A)** and right ventricular angiogram **(B)** in a patient with isolated pulmonic stenosis. The chest film shows a slight prominence of the main pulmonary artery *(arrow)* and diminished pulmonary blood flow. The angiogram shows dome-shaped stenosis of the pulmonary valve with poststenotic dilatation of the main pulmonary artery. (Film provided by Dr. Wade H. Shuford, Professor of Radiology, Emory University School of Medicine.)

eral, valvotomy is indicated, preferably in childhood, if the peak systolic pressure difference between the right ventricle and the pulmonary artery is 80 mm Hg or more and is indicated for many, but not all, patients with a resting pressure difference of 50 to 79 mm Hg. Occasionally, balloon valvotomy is indicated in symptomatic patients with pressure differences of 25 to 49 mm Hg at rest, but only very rarely is it indicated with lower pressure differences. If catheter balloon valvuloplasty is not successful, surgical valvotomy may be performed. Surgery should include infundibular resection if hypertrophy of this region is thought to contribute significantly to the obstruction.

In contrast to valvular aortic stenosis, patients over the age of 12 with pulmonic stenosis who have serial cardiac catheterizations usually show no increase in a pressure difference of less than 50 mm Hg across the valve. Most children and many adults do very well after balloon valvuloplasty or surgical valvotomy, whereas some adults occasionally do not, perhaps because of right ventricular fibrosis and persistent hypertrophy. Many patients have mild pulmonary regurgitation after pulmonic valvotomy; occasionally this regurgitation is severe and leads to right ventricular volume overload and tricuspid regurgitation. Rarely, pulmonic stenosis can recur after valvotomy.

A woman with pulmonary stenosis has a 6.5% chance of having a child with the same defect, whereas the likelihood is 2% if only the father is affected.

TETRALOGY OF FALLOT

Tetralogy of Fallot is the most common type of cyanotic congenital heart disease in older children and adults. The four features of the syndrome are a large VSD, pulmonic stenosis of varying severity but usually predominantly infundibular, overriding of the aorta over the VSD, and right ventricular hypertrophy. Other cardiac lesions are frequently present, including a right aortic arch in about 30% of patients. There is great variation in the pathology and pathophysiology, depending on the severity of pulmonic stenosis and the size of the VSD. Thus, some patients initially have only mild infundibular stenosis and have a L-R shunt from the large VSD. Subsequently, they may develop marked infundibular stenosis and a R-L shunt and cyanosis. The level of systemic vascular resistance also influences the amount of pulmonary blood flow and, therefore, of cyanosis.

Cyanosis is usually noted shortly after birth in patients with severe pulmonic stenosis. A systolic murmur along the left sternal border may also be noted shortly after birth if there is moderate obstruction to pulmonary flow, but the murmur may be faint or absent if there is very severe pulmonic stenosis or pulmonic atresia. Episodic loss of consciousness or hypercyanotic episodes may occur in association with severe stenosis, often after exertion or crying, and is often caused by transient worsening of infundibular stenosis. Classically, infants or children with tetralogy assume the knee-chest position or squat to obtain relief from exertional cyanosis. These maneuvers compress the femoral arteries and increase systemic resistance, producing an increase in pulmonary blood flow and increasing arterial oxygen saturation; they also increase venous return.

Growth and development often are below average. Some patients have no detectable cyanosis, while others have marked generalized cyanosis with clubbing of the fingers and toes. In most cyanotic patients there is a faint right ventricular impulse felt along the lower left sternal edge and a midsystolic murmur that is loudest in the third intercostal space near the sternum and is often associated with a thrill. In most patients with cyanosis and tetralogy of Fallot the pulmonic component of the second heart sound is not heard; only a loud, single aortic component is heard. In patients who have mild pulmonic stenosis and so-called acyanotic tetralogy or pink tetralogy, the findings are similar to those of patients with a large VSD, including a widely split second heart sound.

The classic chest film of patients with cyanosis shows a boot-shaped heart produced by right ventricular hypertrophy, small pulmonary artery, and small left ventricle, in association with relatively clear lung fields. In patients with acyanotic tetralogy of Fallot, the pulmonic stenosis is mild, and there may even be a L-R shunt across the VSD with increased pulmonary vascular markings. The aortic arch is on the right side in about 30% of patients (Fig. 19-9).

The ECG in cyanotic patients usually shows right-axis deviation, right ventricular hypertrophy, absent Q waves over the left pericardium, and often right atrial abnormality. In patients with mild pulmonic stenosis, the ECG shows Q waves and higher R waves in the left precordial leads.

Two-dimensional echocardiography or NMRI usually provides an accurate picture of the anatomy and permits a reasonable evaluation of ventricular function. Cardiac catheterization and angiography provide an accurate assessment of the severity of the pulmonic stenosis, the amount of R-L shunting, the character of the ventricular septal defect, and the presence of associated lesions, including coronary artery anomalies.

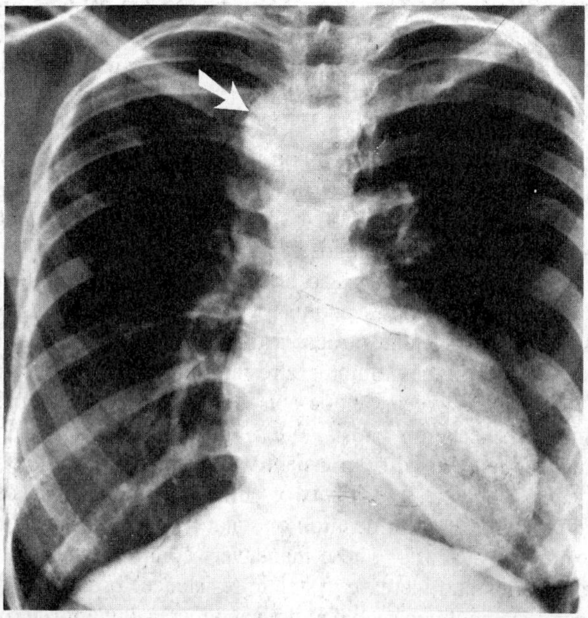

Fig. 19-9. Chest film of a patient with tetralogy of Fallot showing mild cardiomegaly, uplifting of the cardiac apex, decreased pulmonary blood flow, and a right aortic arch *(arrow)*. (Film provided by Dr. Wade H. Shuford, Professor of Radiology, Emory University S hool of Medicine.)

Medical management consists primarily of trying to prevent brain abscess, cerebrovascular accidents, and infective endocarditis. Infants and children rarely have congestive heart failure, which does occasionally occur in adult patients. In some patients, the cyanosis is associated with marked polycythemia, which can produce headaches, fullheadedness, or, rarely, cerebral venous thrombosis. Repeated phlebotomy may be necessary for hyperviscosity symptoms, which usually do not occur unless the hemotrocrit is more than 65%. Repeated phlebotomy can produce iron deficiency anemia unless iron supplementation is provided. Propranolol is often useful in preventing hypoxic spells.

Surgery should usually be offered to patients with tetralogy of Fallot who have more than mild cyanosis. Preferably, elective total correction is performed at age 4 or 5, or, if necessary, in infancy. In some instances, especially in some very small infants, it is necessary to perform a palliative shunt procedure such as a Blalock-Taussig procedure, in which a subclavian artery from the opposite side of the aortic arch is anastomosed to a pulmonary artery. Most patients have a complete right bundle branch block after total repair.

Complications of the Blalock-Taussig procedure include outgrowing the size of the anastomosis and, rarely, the development of severe pulmonary vascular obstructive disease (PVOD). PVOD is more likely to occur in adults who have had a Potts procedure, which is a side-to-side anastomosis of the descending aorta to the left pulmonary artery, or a Waterston-Cooley anastomosis, in which the ascending aorta is anastomosed to the right pulmonary artery. Patients who have had a palliative procedure in childhood should usually have total correction at an early age before they either outgrow the shunt or develop severe PVOD.

Patients with uncorrected tetralogy have an increased morbidity and mortality during pregnancy. Patients who have had a palliative procedure continue to be at risk of brain abscess and infective endocarditis.

Overall, the most common cause of death in patients with tetralogy after surgical repair is sudden death caused by ventricular arrhythmias. Patients should be followed regularly after repair to detect ventricular arrhythmias on routine ECG, as well as on periodic ambulatory ECG and/or 24-hour ambulatory ECG. Ventricular arrhythmias detected should be treated aggressively. Other causes of death include congestive heart failure related to residual ventricular defect and severe PVOD after a palliative procedure.

A woman with tetralogy of Fallot has a 2.5% chance of producing a child with the same defect. The likelihood is 1.5% if only the father is affected.

EBSTEIN'S ANOMALY OF THE TRICUSPID VALVE

In this defect there is downward displacement of the septal and posterior leaflets of the tricuspid valve, which are broadly attached to the wall of the right ventricle below the true anulus of the valve and have poorly developed papillary muscles and chordae tendineae. Usually the anterior leaflet is attached normally to the anulus. The wall of the "atrialized" portion of the right ventricle above the abnormal tricuspid valve is abnormally thin. The markedly reduced pumping ability of the small functional right ventricle is further hindered by the bulging of the anterior leaflet into the right atrium during systole. The tricuspid valve is usually regurgitant, although it can be stenotic. There is usually an ASD or a patent foramen ovale, through which a large R-L shunt develops. A significant number of patients have the Wolff-Parkinson-White (WPW) syndrome (Chapter 9) and have recurrent supraventricular tachycardias. In a few patients there is evidence that the maternal use of lithium may have been a factor in the development of Ebstein's syndrome.

A few patients are acyanotic, although there may be a history of cyanosis at birth that subsequently decreased or of chronic cyanosis together with episodes of tachycardia in association with fatigue and breathlessness. At times, chest pain occurs. Ebstein's anomaly is relatively rare beyond the fourth decade, although survival to age 85 has been reported.

Although there is usually a R-L shunt, many patients are not clinically cyanotic. There may be systolic pulsations of the jugular veins with large V waves, and an early to midsystolic murmur of tricuspid regurgitation along the left sternal border. The murmur may increase with inspiration (Càrvallo sign) and may be associated with a thrill. Occasionally, there is a low-pitched murmur of tricuspid stenosis along the left sternal border. There is usually no parasternal lift or right ventricular hypertrophy. Usually, there is wide splitting of both the first and second heart sounds, which, together with loud right ventricular third and fourth heart sounds, produces a loud cacophony of sounds.

The chest radiograph characteristically shows a large heart without enlargement of the right ventricle or main pulmonary artery. The pulmonary vasculature is normal or diminished. In about 10% of patients, the ECG shows a short P-R interval and evidence of type B WPW syndrome (Chapter 9). Other ECGs in patients with Ebstein's anomaly show prominent, right atrial P waves, a prolonged P-R interval, and complete or incomplete right bundle branch block. Right ventricular hypertrophy is absent.

Echocardiography shows that closure of the tricuspid valve occurs more than 65 ms later than mitral valve closure in association with abnormally increased motion of the tricuspid leaflet. The abnormal displacement of the tricuspid valve into the right ventricle is well shown by 2D echocardiography, and the location of the R-L shunt can be identified by contrast and Doppler echocardiography. NMRI also shows the essential anatomic features. Cardiac catheterization permits the recording of right ventricular electrocardiograms from the lower portion of the "right atrium" that is formed by the atrialized portion of the right ventricle. Cardiac catheterization and right ventricular angiography also permit estimation of the severity of tricuspid regurgitation, evaluation of right ventricular function, identification of any associated abnormalities, and localization of the site of R-L shunting.

Management varies greatly, as do the many abnormalities that may be encountered in mild to severe cases. Most patients die from either congestive heart failure or sudden death before the age of 25. In general, surgery should be considered in any patient with progressive cyanosis, heart failure, or effort intolerance. The most encouraging surgical results have been from anuloplasty with plication of the atrialized portion of the right ventricle, although the results have been only fair. Patients with recurrent supraventricular tachycardia and type B WPW syndrome can usually be controlled medically, but intracardiac mapping and surgical division of the anomalous pathway may be necessary.

TRUNCUS ARTERIOSUS (COMMON AORTOPULMONARY TRUNK)

In this condition a single large vessel leaves the base of the heart, usually above a ventricular septal defect. There is a single semilunar valve at the base of the truncus, which gives rise to the coronary arteries, the pulmonary arteries, the aorta, and all systemic arteries. There is moderate variation in the origins of the pulmonary arteries, which occasionally are partially stenotic near their origins. Such stenosis tends to decrease the pulmonary flow and to protect the pulmonary arteries from systemic arterial pressure.

Most children have mild to moderate cyanosis from birth and a large L-R shunt, develop PVOD, and die in childhood. A rare patient with stenosis near the origin of the pulmonary arteries may live to young adulthood without surgery.

Echocardiography and NMRI can usually establish the diagnosis. The complete study of the condition requires cardiac catheterization, right ventricular angiography, and aortography. Both medical and surgical management are unsatisfactory. Surgery can be attempted with construction of a conduit containing a prosthetic valve from the right ventricle to the pulmonary arteries. Both the conduit tubing and the prosthetic heart valve should be carefully monitored for dysfunction.

COMPLETE (DEXTRO-) TRANSPOSITION OF THE GREAT ARTERIES

The basic defect is the origin of the aorta from the right ventricle anterior and to the right of the pulmonary artery, which arises from the left ventricle. The ventricles are in the normal position ("D-loop"), and the atria and ventricles are normally related. To sustain life, some communication must exist between the two circulations. Most patients have a patent foramen ovale, about two thirds have a PDA, and one third have a VSD. Other defects that may be present include a rudimentary right ventricle and tricuspid atresia or stenosis. The lesion is more frequent in males and in children of diabetic mothers. It accounts for about 4% of functional cardiac malformations at birth and about 10% of all patients with cyanotic heart disease. It is the most common cyanotic congenital lesion requiring treatment in the first weeks of life and is rarely encountered in adults.

Most children have cyanosis and dyspnea from birth and exhibit growth retardation with symptoms of congestive heart failure. In infants without a communication between the two circulations, there may be marked cyanosis and distress but no murmurs. Other patients may have the continuous machinery murmur of PDA or the holosystolic murmur and thrill of a VSD.

There is a great variation in the chest film, depending on the associated lesions and the amount of pulmonary blood flow. There may be an enlarged, typical egg-shaped cardiac shadow with a narrow pedicle. There is often evidence of increased pulmonary blood flow. The ECG is normal for age with right ventricular predominance. Doppler echocardiography and NMRI can usually provide the diagnosis and define the associated defects although cardiac catheterization and angiography may be necessary.

Infants in acute distress should have emergency cardiac catheterization and balloon atrial septostomy to allow communication between the two circulations and thus survival until a more definitive procedure can be attempted. Survival depends on the associated lesions and the rate of development of PVOD.

CONGENITALLY CORRECTED TRANSPOSITION OF THE GREAT ARTERIES

The two basic defects are transposition of the aorta and the pulmonary artery and inversion of the ventricles ("L-loop"). Thus, there is functional correction with systemic venous blood passing through the morphologic right atrium to a bicuspid mitral valve into a right-sided morphologic left ventricle and into the pulmonary artery, while pulmonary venous blood passes through a morphologic left atrium and a tricuspid valve into a left-sided morphologic right ventricle and into the aorta, which is anterior to the pulmonary artery. There may be no symptoms unless there is an associated defect, for example, Ebstein's anomaly of the tricuspid valve, VSD, obstruction to outflow of the venous ventricle, mitral regurgitation, pulmonic stenosis, congenital heart block, or variations in the pattern of coronary arteries; most patients have an associated defect. There may be no abnormalities on physical examination, but one fourth of the patients have a loud single second sound that is loudest in the second left intercostal space and is produced by aortic valve closure. An apical holosystolic murmur is heard in about half the patients.

In some patients the chest film is essentially normal. The normal shadow of the main pulmonary artery may be absent, and there may be a convexity, or "shoulder," on the left middle cardiac border produced by the displaced anterior aorta. The ECG may show a prolonged P-R interval, and there may be small Q waves over the right precordium but not in the lateral chest leads. Supraventricular arrhythmias, including paroxysmal atrial tachycardia, atrial fibrillation, and atrial flutter, may occur. The abnormal location of the aorta, pulmonary artery, and atrioventricular valves can be demonstrated by echocardiography, NMRI, or cardiac catheterization and selective angiography. Palliative surgery may be necessary for associated defects.

DOUBLE-OUTLET RIGHT VENTRICLE (PARTIAL TRANSPOSITION)

In this relatively rare condition, the aorta is transposed and originates from the right ventricle, medial to the pulmonary artery, which also arises from the right ventricle. There is almost always a VSD, and pulmonic stenosis is present in more than half the cases. Depending on the size of the VSD and the presence or absence of pulmonary stenosis, the patient's symptoms and clinical findings may resemble those of patients with a large VSD or those of patients with tetralogy of Fallot. Echocardiography and NMRI both provide reasonably accurate images of the defects, while cardiac catheterization and angiography permit precise measurements of pressures, shunts, and resistances as well as excellent visualization of the major defects. Medical management is symptomatic. Patients with pulmonic stenosis can be treated with palliative arterial shunts to the pulmonary artery. In some patients more complex operative procedures are required for correction.

TOTAL ANOMALOUS PULMONARY VENOUS CONNECTION

In this syndrome, the four pulmonary veins return oxygenated blood from the lungs to the right atrium or to one of its tributaries. In the right atrium some blood is shunted to the left atrium through an atrial septal defect and produces systemic cyanosis, which may be mild or marked. Physiologically, there is a large L-R shunt and a smaller R-L shunt. Most infants have cyanosis with increased fatigue on exertion and develop congestive heart failure and die by the age of 1 year. The chest radiograph shows increased pulmonary blood flow, and the heart may have a figure-of-eight or "snowman" appearance if the pulmonary venous blood enters a vertical vein in the left upper chest and a dilated superior vena cava is in the right upper chest. The ECG usually shows evidence of right axis deviation, right ventricular hypertrophy, and right atrial enlargement. Echocardiography and NMRI can visualize the dilated right atrium and right ventricle and, in many cases, the anomalous pulmonary veins joining the right atrium or a tributary. Doppler echocardiography provides an estimate of the location, magnitude, and direction of shunts. Cardiac catheterization and selective pulmonary angiography are used for precise delineation of the anatomic defects and for confirmation of the R-L and L-R shunts.

Emergency balloon atrial septostomy may provide temporary relief if the atrial defect is too small, but most patients require complete surgical correction with connection of the pulmonary venous return to the left atrium and closure of the ASD to prevent death from congestive failure in the first year of life.

TRICUSPID ATRESIA

The rare syndrome of atresia of the tricuspid valve is always associated with an interatrial communication and often with hypoplasia of the right ventricle. The systemic blood returns to the right atrium, where it passes into the left atrium. Pulmonary blood flow, which is usually markedly decreased, is achieved by a patent ductus arteriosus or a VSD. There is usually marked cyanosis, a single first heart sound, and left axis deviation on the ECG. If the interatrial communication is inadequate in size, balloon septostomy can be utilized to increase pulmonary blood flow, along with other palliative procedures, such as the creation of a systemic arterial-pulmonary artery shunt. More nearly complete correction of the defect involves the anastomosis of the right atrium to the right ventricle or creation of a conduit between the right atrium and the pulmonary artery in combination with closure of the interatrial communication. Very few children with this defect live to adulthood.

AORTIC SINUS ANEURYSM (SINUS OF VALSALVA FISTULA)

In this condition, which is more common in males, there is a congenital defect between the anulus fibrosis of the aortic valve and the media of the aorta. Over a period of three to four decades, the aortic pressure causes progressive dilatation and aneurysm formation at the area of weakness. Eventually, the aneurysm ruptures, most often into the right ventricle, less frequently into the right atrium, and, rarely, into the left ventricle, left atrium, or pericardium. Occasionally, bacterial endocarditis is responsible for the rupture.

There are no symptoms until the aneurysm ruptures. There may be the abrupt onset of severe, tearing chest pain and symptoms of acute heart failure. There may be a wide pulse pressure with bounding arterial pulses. Classically, there is a very loud continuous precordial murmur with thrill; occasionally, the murmur can be heard from the foot of the bed.

The diagnosis of the aneurysm and the location of the fistula and the chamber into which it ruptures can be confirmed by aortography, transthoracic Doppler echocardiography, transesophageal echocardiography, or NMRI (Chapter 5). It is possible to diagnose an asymptomatic aortic sinus aneurysm before rupture if one of these procedures happens to be performed for some other reason.

Surgical repair is indicated for virtually all individuals in whom a fistula develops from an aortic sinus aneurysm. On the other hand, if an aneurysm is incidentally discovered before it ruptures to form a fistula, surgery is probably not indicated, since it is difficult to know exactly the location and extent of the congenital defect until it ruptures.

COR TRIATRIATUM

A relatively rare syndrome, cor triatriatum is produced by a congenital fibromuscular band that divides the left atrium into a superior and posterior chamber and an inferior and anterior chamber and produces obstruction to the flow of pulmonary venous blood through the left atrium into the left ventricle. The symptoms resemble those of mitral stenosis with progressive dyspnea and pulmonary congestion (Chapter 16). There may be evidence of pulmonary artery hypertension and right ventricular hypertrophy, but a loud snapping S_1, opening snap, and diastolic rumble are absent. The condition can be demonstrated by transthoracic or, preferably, transesophageal echocardiography, NMRI, or pulmonary angiography. The abnormal diaphragm can be surgically excised with excellent results.

HYPOPLASTIC LEFT HEART SYNDROME

In hypoplastic left heart syndrome the mitral valve, left ventricle, aortic valve, and ascending aorta are markedly hypoplastic, and the right ventricle provides all the blood flow to the lungs and, via a patent ductus arteriosus, to the body. Echocardiography can readily confirm the diagnosis. The condition is usually incompatible with life for more than a few days. Surgery, including cardiac transplantation, has been tried with only limited success.

ABERRANT RIGHT SUBCLAVIAN ARTERY

The aberrant right subclavian artery arises from the aorta distal to the origin of the left subclavian artery and passes behind the esophagus to the right arm. It may occur as an isolated lesion or together with other lesions, particularly right aortic arch, tetralogy of Fallot, or coarctation of the aorta. In the presence of aortic coarctation, the pressure in the right arm can be lower than that in the left arm if the aberrant artery originates distal to the coarctation. The anomaly rarely produces symptoms, although formerly it was thought to produce dysphagia. The diagnosis can usually be confirmed by barium swallow. No treatment is necessary.

MALPOSITIONS OF THE HEART

Situs inversus refers to a condition in which the arrangement of organs is the reverse of normal. In complete situs inversus the heart and cardiac apex and abdominal organs are located on the opposite side of normal (mirror-image dextrocardia), and the heart is usually normal. On the other hand, when there is situs inversus of the viscera but the heart is in the left side of the chest (isolated levocardia), a serious cardiac malformation is usually present. *Dextroversion* refers to the condition in which the viscera, atria, and aortic arch are in their normal position but the cardiac apex is on the right. Congenital heart disease is usually present, particularly corrected transposition of the great arteries, pulmonic stenosis, or VSD. In patients in whom the visceral situs is indeterminate, complex heart disease is usually present, together with asplenia or polysplenia.

CONGENITAL ABNORMALITIES OF THE CORONARY ARTERIES

The three congenital anomalies of the coronary arteries encountered most frequently in adult patients are an ectopic origin of a coronary artery from the aorta, an anomalous origin of a coronary artery from the pulmonary artery, and coronary arteriovenous fistula.

Ectopic origin of a coronary artery from the aorta is an isolated finding in approximately 0.6% of individuals undergoing coronary arteriography. Of the numerous variations, two are especially likely to produce clinical symptoms: either an ectopic left coronary artery arising from the right sinus of Valsalva or an ectopic right coronary artery arising from the left sinus of Valsalva. Both ectopic arteries may pass between the aorta and the pulmonary artery. The coronary circulation can be compromised either by hypoplasia of the coronary ostia or of the proximal coronary artery or, less frequently, by compression between the aorta and pulmonary artery or extreme angulation of the proximal coronary artery. It is likely that only a minority of patients with this condition have myocardial ischemia from the anomaly. Clinical manifestations may include angina pectoris, myocardial infarction, ventricular tachycardia, and sudden death. Symptoms may occur in adolescence or young adult life, depending on the degree of proximal narrowing, mass of muscle supplied, and collateral circulation. Echocardiography, especially transesophageal, can often provide the diagnosis, but coronary arteriography is necessary for proper definition of the abnormality.

Patients with significant objective evidence of myocardial ischemia should be treated by coronary artery bypass graft surgery. An ectopic right coronary artery incidentally discovered at coronary arteriography requires no specific therapy. Many other varieties of ectopic origin and unusual course of the coronary arteries occur; they seldom produce symptoms and are usually discovered incidentally. Knowledge of aberrant coronary arteries before surgery for congenital heart disease is important if the surgery involves ventriculotomy, in which an aberrant coronary artery might be damaged. This damage is especially likely to occur in patients with tetralogy of Fallot. Knowledge of the presence of an aberrant coronary artery is also important in patients undergoing intraoperative myocardial perfusion by coronary cannulation.

In anomalous origin of the left coronary artery from the pulmonary artery, the left main coronary artery originates from a sinus just above the pulmonic valve, whereas the right coronary artery originates from its normal aortic sinus. In utero, the pressures in the pulmonary artery and aorta are nearly equal, and myocardial perfusion is reasonably normal. After birth, however, pressure in the pulmonary artery rapidly declines and the perfusion pressure in the pulmonary artery and the left coronary artery is no longer high enough to perfuse the left ventricle, which has a much higher intramyocardial systolic pressure. As a consequence, the heart is perfused by the right coronary artery originating from the right aortic sinus, while collateral vessels carry some blood from the right coronary artery to the anomalous left coronary artery and to the pulmonary artery. The infant or child usually develops myocardial ischemia or infarction, often within the first 6 months of life. Mitral regurgitation frequently results from the myocardial infarction.

Some infants have no symptoms preceding sudden death, while others have great distress, which probably represents angina pectoris, while feeding. Most children die before the age of 12, usually from sudden death or chronic left ventricular failure from myocardial scarring and mitral regurgitation. Some patients, however, may survive until adulthood. Often, there is no clear history of chest pain, since the infarction occurs in infancy before the child can describe symptoms. There may be evidence of a left ventricular aneurysm, left ventricular hypertrophy, and an apical holosystolic murmur from mitral regurgitation. Occasionally, there is a continuous murmur produced by the intercoronary anastomoses.

The chest radiograph usually shows evidence of left ventricular hypertrophy and often pulmonary congestion. The ECG often shows evidence of an extensive anterolateral myocardial infarction. Coronary arteriography and aortic root aortography demonstrate the right coronary artery originating normally from the aorta and connecting by collaterals to the left coronary artery, which drains into the pulmonary artery. Left ventricular angiography or echocardiography can demonstrate the area of myocardial infarction and dyskinesia and may also demonstrate mitral regurgitation. Transesophageal echocardiography can also demonstrate the abnormal origin of a coronary artery.

If the extent of myocardial infarction is not excessive, the left coronary artery can be anastomosed to either the aorta or the subclavian artery. Heart transplantation should be considered in some patients. Otherwise, management is purely supportive for symptoms of myocardial ischemia and heart failure.

In congenital coronary arteriovenous fistula, the right and left coronary arteries originate normally from the aorta, but one or more branches form a fistula with a cardiac chamber or the pulmonary artery. Most fistulas originate from a branch of the right coronary artery and communicate with the right ventricle, right atrium, or coronary sinus. The fistula functions as a L-R shunt but usually does not seriously interfere with myocardial oxygenation, so angina and myocardial infarction usually do not occur. On the other hand, the shunt can be so large that it imposes a volume load on the left ventricle and whatever right-sided chambers the shunt involves.

Many patients have no symptoms. Others may have retarded growth, mild exertional fatigue, and dyspnea. The fistula can also become the site of infective endarteritis, with symptoms similar to those of infective endocarditis (Chapter 15). If the fistula enters the right atrium, right ventricle, or coronary sinus, there may be evidence of biventricular enlargement with both a parasternal impulse and a displaced and sustained apical impulse. The hallmark is a continuous murmur, which often is less loud than the murmurs of PDA and usually is located in a lower position on the chest. At times it is maximal to the right of the sternum. The systolic murmur is often loudest during systole if the fistula enters the right atrium, loudest during either systole or diastole if it enters the right ventricle, and loudest about the second heart sound if it enters the pulmonary artery.

If the fistula is large, the chest radiograph usually shows left ventricular, right ventricular, and pulmonary artery dilatation, except for the small number of cases in which the fistula enters the pulmonary artery, producing only dilatation of the left ventricle and pulmonary artery. The pulmonary vasculature is often increased because of the large L-R shunt and increased pulmonary flow. Occasionally, the cardiac border is slightly irregular as a result of the aneurysmal dilatation of the involved coronary artery.

There may be ECG evidence of left or combined ventricular hypertrophy. Coronary arteriography or aortography delineates the size and course of the involved coronary artery and the site of entry into the right heart or pulmonary artery. NMRI and echocardiography, especially transesophageal, can also delineate the involved coronary artery when it is markedly dilated. Coronary arteriovenous fistulas should usually be surgically corrected to decrease the risk of infective endarteritis, abolish the L-R shunt, and perhaps improve the coronary blood flow reserve.

CONGENITAL PERICARDIAL DEFECTS

Congenital defects may involve any portion of the parietal pericardium, although the left side is more frequent. Most patients are asymptomatic, but partial defects can rarely cause chest pain, which can resemble angina pectoris. Herniation and strangulation, particularly of the left atrial appendage through a partial pericardial defect, can occur and produce sudden death. The presence of partial left defect may be suggested on a chest film by a prominence in the area of the pulmonary artery produced by herniation of the left atrial appendage. Echocardiography, particularly transesophageal, and NMRI usually provide a proper diagnosis. Partial defects should usually be surgically corrected by closure to prevent herniation and strangulation of the left atrium or ventricle. Complete pericardial absence or large defects do not require therapy.

DISTURBANCES OF CONDUCTION

The Wolff-Parkinson-White syndrome, the Romano-Ward syndrome (prolonged QT interval with deafness), and the Jervell and Lange-Nielsen syndrome (prolonged QT interval without deafness) are discussed in Chapter 9.

REFERENCES

Adams FH, Emmanouilides GC, and Riemenschneider TA, editors: Moss' heart disease in infants, children, and adolescents, ed 4. Baltimore, 1989, Williams and Wilkins.

Dexter L: Atrial septal defect. Brit Heart J 18:209, 1956.

Engle MA and Perloff JK, editors: Congenital heart disease after surgery: benefits, residua, sequelae. New York, 1983, Yorke.

Garson A Jr et al: Prevention of sudden death after repair of tetralogy of Fallot: treatment of ventricular arrhythmias. J Am Coll Cardiol 6:221, 1985.

Giuliani ER et al: Cardiology: fundamentals and practice, ed 2. St. Louis 1991, Mosby Year Book.

Graham TP Jr: Ventricular performance in congenital heart disease. Circulation 84:2259, 1991.

McNamara DG: The adult with congenital heart disease. Curr Probl Cardiol 14:57, 1989.

Nora JJ, Berg K, and Nora AH: Cardiovascular diseases: genetics, epidemiology, and prevention. New York, 1991, Oxford University Press.

Nugent EW et al: The pathology, abnormal physiology, clinical recognition, and medical and surgical treatment of congenital heart disease. In Hurst JW et al, editors: The heart, ed 7. New York, 1990, McGraw Hill.

Parmley WW and Chatterjee K, editors: Cardiology. Vol 2: Cardiovascular disease. Philadelphia, 1988–1991, Lippincott.

Perloff JK: Congenital heart disease in adults. In Braunwald E, editor: Heart disease, ed 4. Philadelphia, 1992, Saunders.

Perloff JK and Child JS, editors: Congenital heart disease in adults. Philadelphia, 1991, Saunders.

Perloff JK et al: Adults with cyanotic congenital heart disease: hematologic management. Ann Int Med 109:406, 1988.

Roberts WC: Adult congenital heart disease. Philadelphia, 1987, FA Davis.

CHAPTER

20 Pulmonary Hypertensive Heart Disease

Joseph S. Alpert
Richard S. Irwin
James A. Dalen

The resistance to pulmonary blood flow is only one twelfth the resistance across the systemic bed in normal individuals. The mean pulmonary artery (PA) pressure is only 12 $\pm$ 2 mm Hg and the mean left atrial pressure is only 6 $\pm$ 2 mm Hg in normals. Thus the left pressure gradient across the normal pulmonary circulation is only 6 $\pm$ 2 mm Hg. A normal cardiac output of 5 to 6 liters per minute flows from the right ventricule to the left atrium with a pressure drop of only 6 mm Hg, as opposed to a pressure drop of about 90 mm Hg in the systemic circulation between the left ventricle and right atrium. The resistance of the pulmonary vascular bed is much lower than that of the systemic circulation because the media of the precapillary pulmonary arterioles are thin compared with the more muscular media of the systemic arterioles. The low resistance of the pulmonary circulation accounts for a right ventricle that is less than half as thick as the left ventricle.

Pulmonary hypertension occurs if resistance to flow across the pulmonary bed increases. Such an increase occurs as a result of a variety of diseases that affect the pulmonary circulation. Pulmonary hypertension is present when mean PA pressure exceeds 20 mm Hg, and in the vast majority of cases, it is secondary to cardiac or pulmonary diseases. Pulmonary hypertension can be subdivided into three categories based on its pathophysiology: precapillary, passive, and reactive. In precapillary pulmonary hypertension the abnormality that leads to elevated pulmonary pressures is located in the pulmonary arteries or arterioles. Individuals with passive pulmonary hypertension have diseases that lead to increased pulmonary venous pressure that, in turn, produces secondary elevations in pulmonary arterial pressure, for example, mitral stenosis. Patients with reactive pulmonary hypertension have long-standing elevated pulmonary venous pressure complicated by pulmonary arteriolar vasoconstriction (Table 20-1). The only "pure" form is the rare entity primary pulmonary hypertension. Examination of this entity will allow elucidation of the clinical manifestations of pulmonary hypertension from any cause. In most patients with secondary pulmonary hypertension, the clinical manifestations are overshadowed by the underlying cardiac or pulmonary disease. The natural history, prognosis, and management also depend on the underlying disease.

An approach to the differential diagnosis of pulmonary hypertension is shown in Table 20-1.

PRECAPILLARY PULMONARY HYPERTENSION

Pathophysiology

In patients with precapillary pulmonary hypertension, the disease involves the pulmonary circulation proximal to the pulmonary capillaries, that is, the PAs or arterioles. Pressure in the PA is increased (mean PA pressure >20 mm Hg), but wedge pressure and left atrial pressure remain normal (<12 mm Hg). As a result, the mean PA to left atrial pressure gradient is increased and exceeds 12 mm Hg.

Patients with precapillary pulmonary hypertension have dyspnea, but because their pulmonary venous pressure is normal, they do not experience orthopnea, paroxysmal nocturnal dyspnea, or pulmonary edema. On physical examination such patients are often observed to have tachypnea, but the auscultatory findings in the lungs are usually normal. The chest x-ray may show evidence of right ventricular enlargement and prominent pulmonary arteries, but the left ventricle is normal. Pulmonary venous redistribution and Kerley B lines do not occur. The electrocardiogram (ECG) usually demonstrates right ventricular hypertrophy or right axis deviation.

Table 20-1. Differential diagnosis of pulmonary hypertension

Pressure variable	Precapillary	Passive	Reactive
PA mean pressure	↑/↑↑	↑	↑↑
Left atrial pressure	Normal	↑	↑
PA left atrial pressure gradient	>12 mm Hg	<12 mm Hg	>12 mm Hg

Causes of precapillary pulmonary hypertension

The causes of precapillary pulmonary hypertension are listed in the box below.

Primary pulmonary hypertension. Primary pulmonary hypertension is the rarest cause of pulmonary hypertension, but it is described here in detail because it illustrates the clinical manifestations of pulmonary hypertension not accompanied by other cardiac or pulmonary disease.

Primary pulmonary hypertension is a disease of unknown origin, characterized by diffuse pathologic changes in the pulmonary vasculature. Patients with primary pulmonary hypertension do not have intrinsic pulmonary or cardiac disease or extrinsic causes of pulmonary vascular obstruction.

Several theories have been advanced concerning the cause of primary pulmonary hypertension. Some authorities argue that it is the result of recurrent episodes of asymptomatic pulmonary embolism. Supporting this theory is the common autopsy finding of clinically unrecognized, organizing, or recanalized pulmonary emboli in patients with primary pulmonary hypertension. An alternative explanation for the development of primary pulmonary hypertension is thrombosis in situ of small pulmonary arteries, with resultant widespread pulmonary vascular obstruction. Various abnormalities of coagulation, including abnormal platelet function and defective fibrinolysis, have been demonstrated in patients with primary pulmonary hypertension. Arrayed against recurrent pulmonary thromboembolism or in-situ arterial thrombosis as the cause are the findings of several pathologic studies that demonstrate clear morphologic differences between patients with thromboembolic or thrombotic pulmonary hypertension and those with primary pulmonary hypertension. However, veno-occlusive disease affecting the majority of small pulmonary venules has been observed in a number of patients with primary pulmonary hypertension (see Reactive Pulmonary Hypertension).

Drug hypersensitivity has also been suggested as a cause

Causes of pulmonary hypertension

- Precapillary pulmonary hypertension
  - Primary pulmonary hypertension
  - Disorders of ventilation
  - Congenital heart disease with pulmonary vascular disease
  - Pulmonary embolism
  - Schistosomiasis
- Passive pulmonary hypertension
  - Left ventricular failure
  - Mitral valve disease
  - Cor triatriatum
  - Obstruction of major pulmonary veins
- Reactive pulmonary hypertension
  - Some patients with mitral valve disease
  - Rarely, other causes of pulmonary venous hypertension, including pulmonary veno-occlusive disease

of primary pulmonary hypertension, although allergic vasculitis would be unlikely to affect only the pulmonary vasculature. Some type of immunologic process may play a role in the development of primary pulmonary hypertension, but the nature and extent of such a process remain unknown.

Increased pulmonary vascular reactivity and pulmonary vasoconstriction have been demonstrated in patients with primary pulmonary hypertension, leading to the conclusion that a marked vasospastic or vasoconstrictive tendency underlies the development of primary pulmonary hypertension in predisposed persons. Heightened autonomic nervous system activity is considered by some to be a factor in the development of primary pulmonary hypertension. Primary pulmonary hypertension is more common at high altitudes than at sea level, suggesting that hypoxic pulmonary vasoconstriction predisposes to this condition. Patients with primary pulmonary hypertension appear to have increased pulmonary vasomotor tone early during their illness. However, as the disease progresses, functional changes progress to fixed, anatomic pulmonary vascular lesions.

A number of pathologic findings are common to almost all patients with primary pulmonary hypertension: (1) intimal thickening and fibrosis in small pulmonary arteries and arterioles, producing a characteristic "onion-skin" configuration; (2) increased medial thickness of small muscular pulmonary arteries and arterioles; (3) dilated, thin-walled side branches of muscular pulmonary arteries known as *plexiform lesions;* and (4) necrotizing arteritis and fibrinoid necrosis in the walls of muscular pulmonary arteries.

Most patients with primary pulmonary hypertension come to the attention of a physician late in the course of the disease, or when symptoms of right ventricular failure develop. Women with primary pulmonary hypertension outnumber men 3:1 or 4:1. The disease occurs sporadically or with a familial pattern suggestive of autosomal dominant inheritance with variable penetrance.

Patients with primary pulmonary hypertension usually complain of exertional dyspnea without orthopnea, as well as effort syncope, anginal chest pain, and weakness. Late in the disease, dyspnea occurs at rest. Palpitations are commonly reported and may be related to the sudden death of some patients. Occasionally, patients complain of cough and/or hemoptysis.

Physical examination of patients with primary pulmonary hypertension discloses findings consistent with pulmonary hypertension and right ventricular pressure overload: a large A wave in the jugular venous pulse; left parasternal (right ventricular) heave; pulmonic ejection sound and flow murmur; prominent pulmonic component of the second heart sound; right ventricular fourth heart sound; and signs of right ventricular failure (hepatomegaly, peripheral edema, and even ascites). Patients with severe pulmonary hypertension may also have a prominent V wave in the jugular venous pulse, a right ventricular third heart sound, and murmurs of tricuspid and/or pulmonic regurgitation. The lungs are clear, but the respiratory rate is increased, even at rest.

The results of routine laboratory tests are usually normal in patients with primary pulmonary hypertension. Abnormal platelet function, defects in fibrinolysis, and other abnormalities of coagulation are occasionally noted in such patients. The ECG demonstrates right ventricular hypertrophy and right atrial enlargement (P pulmonale). Chest radiography in patients with primary pulmonary hypertension demonstrates enlargement of the main pulmonary artery and its major branches, with marked tapering of peripheral arteries (Fig. 20-1). The lung fields are strikingly lucent. The right ventricle and atrium are often enlarged.

The results of pulmonary function tests are usually normal. Arterial blood gas analysis usually reveals evidence of hyperventilation, with a low PCO_2 and elevated pH. The arterial PO_2 may be normal or reduced. Echocardiography demonstrates enlarged right ventricular dimensions, small or normal left ventricular dimensions, and a thickened interventricular septum. Right ventricular systolic and diastolic dysfunction may be present. Doppler echocardiographic examination usually demonstrates tricuspid and pulmonic regurgitation. Perfusion lung scans in patients with primary pulmonary hypertension are usually normal or demonstrate small, nonspecific defects. Lung scanning may be hazardous late in the course of the disease, because the macroaggregated albumin particles used in scanning may significantly reduce the cross-sectional area of the already critically limited pulmonary vascular bed.

The diagnosis of primary pulmonary hypertension cannot be confirmed without cardiac catheterization and pulmonary angiography to exclude other cardiac or pulmonary causes of pulmonary hypertension. Some patients are too ill for one or both these procedures, and, in such patients, the diagnosis remains tentative. Right heart catheterization reveals markedly elevated pulmonary arterial and right ventricular pressures. Right atrial pressure is increased if right ventricular failure is present. Left ventricular, left atrial, and pulmonary capillary wedge pressures are low or normal. Pulmonary angiography demonstrates large central pulmonary arteries, with marked peripheral tapering (Fig. 20-2). It should be noted that pulmonary angiography presents a potential risk of death to the patient with primary pulmonary hypertension; subselective injections are usually employed rather than injection into the main pulmonary artery.

The differential diagnosis of primary pulmonary hypertension entails ruling out many causes of secondary pulmonary hypertension. Entities that must be excluded before a clinical diagnosis of primary pulmonary hypertension can be entertained include mitral stenosis, congenital cardiac defects with Eisenmenger's reaction, recurrent pulmonary embolism, sickle cell disease, collagen vascular disease, and such rare entities as cor triatriatum and pulmonary venous obstruction.

No universally effective treatment is currently available for this condition. It has been noted that some vasodilators may transiently lower PA pressure. Long-term reduction in the level of pulmonary hypertension has been reported following chronic oral diazoxide, diltiazem, nifedipine, or hydralazine administration in a few patients. Hemodynamic and clinical worsening has also been described after vaso-

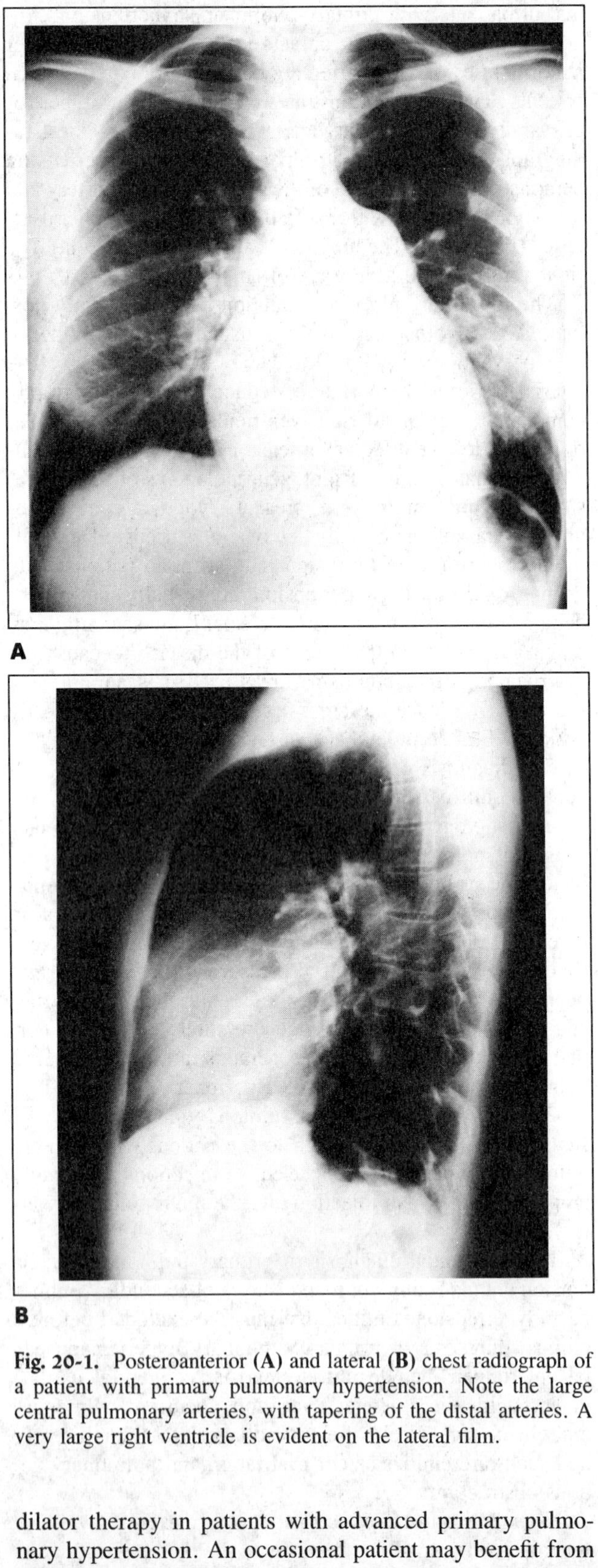

Fig. 20-1. Posteroanterior (**A**) and lateral (**B**) chest radiograph of a patient with primary pulmonary hypertension. Note the large central pulmonary arteries, with tapering of the distal arteries. A very large right ventricle is evident on the lateral film.

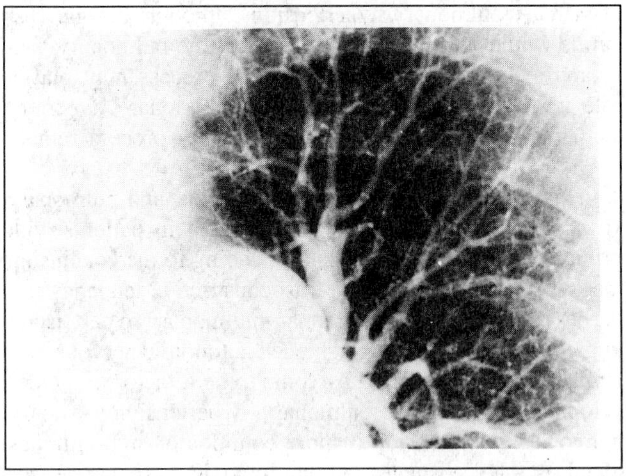

Fig. 20-2. Pulmonary angiogram in a patient with primary pulmonary hypertension (same patient as in Fig. 19-1). The contrast medium was injected into the left upper pulmonary artery. Note the large central pulmonary arteries, with marked tapering of the distal branches.

dilator therapy in patients with advanced primary pulmonary hypertension. An occasional patient may benefit from chronic sublingual administration of isoproterenol. Some patients achieve dramatic and long-lasting reduction in pulmonary arterial pressure during high-dose diltiazem or nifedipine therapy. Right ventricular hypertrophy regresses after such sustained reductions in pulmonary arterial pressure.

Anticoagulants are widely used in this condition, either because of a clinical diagnosis of recurrent pulmonary embolism or as prophylaxis against thromboembolism in patients with right ventricular failure. There is suggestive clinical evidence that anticoagulation ameliorates the clinical course of primary pulmonary hypertension. Other agents have been tried without effect. Combined heart/lung or single lung transplant is being evaluated as therapy for these patients. Rarely, the disease process seems to remit spontaneously, with return of PA pressure to normal.

The natural history of primary pulmonary hypertension is generally that of gradual decline. Sudden death occurs on occasion but refractory right ventricular failure is the usual cause of death. As noted earlier, some individuals respond dramatically to vasodilators such as diltiazem and nifedipine while others have spontaneous remissions.

Disorders of ventilation. The ventilatory respiratory diseases that can cause precapillary pulmonary hypertension include vasoconstriction of the pulmonary vascular bed, anatomic restriction of the pulmonary vascular bed, or a combination of both, as shown in the box at upper right.

Pulmonary vasoconstriction occurs in response to a number of different stimuli. The most potent, clinically important, and best documented is alveolar hypoxia. The mechanism of hypoxic vasoconstriction is not well understood. Alveolar hypoxia occurs in a number of different pulmonary diseases as a consequence of alveolar hypoventilation or ventilation-perfusion inequalities (Chapter 205). Increases in plasma hydrogen ion concentration (acidemia), particularly when produced by hypercapnia, not only cause pulmonary vasoconstriction directly but also augment the effect of alveolar hypoxia. Although these two stimulants may produce only modest increases in pressure in normal subjects at sea level, the vasoconstrictive effects may become greatly magnified and sustained in various clinical situations.

Disorders of ventilation that can cause precapillary pulmonary hypertension

I. Alveolar hypoxia (with or without acidemia)
   A. With structurally normal pulmonary parenchyma and vascular bed
      1. High-altitude pulmonary hypertension (residence at or above 3000 m)
      2. Primary central hypoventilation
      3. Peripheral, obstructive sleep apnea
      4. Obesity-hypoventilation syndrome
      5. Paralytic poliomyelitis
      6. Myasthenia gravis
   B. With pulmonary parenchymal disease
      1. Chronic bronchitis
      2. Emphysema
      3. Cystic fibrosis
II. Anatomic restriction of the pulmonary vascular bed
   A. Diffuse lung disease
      1. Sarcoidosis
      2. Progressive systemic sclerosis
      3. Idiopathic interstitial fibrosis
      4. Adult respiratory distress syndrome
   B. Extensive lung resection
   C. Extensive fibrothorax
III. Vasoconstriction plus anatomic restriction of the pulmonary vascular bed
   A. Kyphoscoliosis
   B. Chronic fibrotic tuberculosis

High-altitude pulmonary hypertension is caused by the hypoxic vasoconstrictive effects of chronic alveolar hypoxia and occurs in humans born and raised at high altitude. As long as these persons reside at altitudes above 3000 m, pulmonary hypertension is sustained because of persistent pulmonary vasoconstriction. However, it can be reversed on return to sea level, since alveolar hypoxia is no longer present.

Pulmonary hypertension may occur in a wide variety of extrapulmonary respiratory diseases solely on the basis of alveolar hypoventilation, even with a structurally normal pulmonary parenchyma and vascular bed, for example, peripheral, obstructive sleep apnea.

The main determinants of pulmonary hypertension in patients with the chronic obstructive pulmonary diseases (COPD), chronic bronchitis, and emphysema are alveolar hypoxia and acidemia (Chapter 205). Pulmonary hypertension occurs in many patients with COPD and cystic fibrosis when PaO_2 is less than 50 mm Hg and $PaCO_2$ is greater than 45 mm Hg. These degrees of hypoxemia and hypercapnia become predictable in COPD patients when the absolute value of FEV_1 is less than 1 liter. Although respiratory acidosis and other factors, such as anatomic restriction of the pulmonary vascular bed, increased cardiac output, polycythemia, and an expanded lung volume may contribute, all these influences are secondary to alveolar hypoxia in the pathogenesis of the pulmonary hypertension of COPD.

Anatomic restriction of the pulmonary vascular bed may also cause pulmonary hypertension. The cross-sectional area of the pulmonary vascular bed can be reduced in several ways. In diffuse interstitial lung diseases, parenchymal disease probably compresses and gradually obliterates the small pulmonary arteries, causing increased resistance to blood flow, with resultant pulmonary hypertension. Since hypoxic vasoconstriction does not appear to contribute significantly to the resistance to blood flow in these diseases, other pulmonary function tests can be useful in predicting the presence of pulmonary hypertension. When the vital capacity is 50% of the predicted value in sarcoidosis or idiopathic interstitial fibrosis, pulmonary hypertension may well be present at rest; when it is between 50% and 80% of predicted, pulmonary hypertension may develop with exercise. In progressive systemic sclerosis, a diffusing capacity of less than 43% of predicted is a better predictor of pulmonary hypertension than is a vital capacity of less than 50% of predicted; in this disease, diffusing capacity has a sensitivity of 67% in predicting definite pulmonary hypertension.

A combination of vasoconstriction plus anatomic restriction of the pulmonary vascular bed is involved in the pathogenesis of pulmonary hypertension in diseases such as kyphoscoliosis and long-standing fibrotic tuberculosis complicated by fibrothorax, thoracoplasty, and/or an acute respiratory infection (Chapters 230 and 231).

Although idiopathic kyphoscoliosis affects 2% to 3% of the population of the United States, a deformity of the thoracic spine severe enough to produce pulmonary hypertension is found in a relatively small number of these patients. Pulmonary hypertension at rest in this disease should not be anticipated unless the vital capacity is less than 60% of predicted.

The clinical manifestations of pulmonary hypertension fall into two categories: those resulting from the primary ventilatory disorder and those resulting from abnormal cardiac function. Against the background of the primary ventilatory clinical manifestations are the signs and symptoms of pulmonary hypertension and cor pulmonale (see Primary Pulmonary Hypertension).

In addition to the pulmonary function studies that help predict the presence of pulmonary hypertension and often determine its cause, chest radiographs frequently are useful for determining the type of pulmonary disease.

The diagnostic value of the ECG in pulmonary hypertension and cor pulmonale depends on the underlying ventilatory disorder. Although the ECG is reliable in demonstrating right ventricular hypertrophy in diseases that anatomically restrict the vascular bed, it is less reliable in vasoconstrictive diseases, since the levels of pulmonary hypertension are generally less. Perhaps because of the hyperinflated lungs, episodic hypoxemia, and respiratory acidosis that occur in COPD patients, ECG evidence of right ventricular hypertrophy is uncommon. Serial changes are the ones most likely to occur. When arterial PO_2 falls below 50 mm Hg in COPD patients with pulmonary hypertension, one or more of the following ECG changes should be seen: a rightward shift of the mean QRS axis, T wave abnormalities in right precordial leads, S-T depressions in leads II, III, and aVF, and transient right bundle branch block. With improvement in gas exchange, all these changes should subside.

Pulmonary hypertension caused by ventilatory disorders may be treated in a variety of ways. For primary central hypoventilation, a respiratory center stimulant such as progesterone may suffice. For the morbidly obese hypoventilator, weight reduction is the primary mode of therapy. For peripheral obstructive sleep apnea, nasal continuous positive airway pressure (CPAP) is often helpful and a permanent tracheostomy may be curative. While cessation of cigarette smoking and a Milwaukee brace prevent pulmonary hypertension from occurring in many patients with minimal COPD and kyphoscoliosis, respectively, continuous oxygen therapy may be helpful late in the course of both diseases (see Chapter 205). Decortication may be curative in pulmonary hypertension caused by fibrothorax, as may corticosteroids in idiopathic interstitial fibrosis and sarcoidosis. Treatment of the adult respiratory distress syndrome includes supportive as well as specific measures (see Chapter 200). Finally, since the vasoconstrictive component in combined anatomic and vasoconstrictive disorders is the only element that can be reversed, alveolar hypoxia must always be considered and treated with supplemental oxygen. Although prostaglandin E_1 and nifedipine can acutely inhibit hypoxic, pulmonary vasoconstriction, it is not known at this time what role the long-term administration of these agents or other vasodilators will play in the treatment of pulmonary hypertension caused by ventilatory disorders.

Congenital heart disease. Congenital heart disease can lead to precapillary pulmonary hypertension (Chapter 19). The most frequent congenital lesions leading to pulmonary hypertension in adults are those characterized by a left-to-right shunt: ventricular septal defect, patent ductus arteriosus, and ostium secundum atrial septal defect (ASD). As the pulmonary vascular resistance increases, the magnitude of the left-to-right shunt decreases. Late in the course, the patient may be cyanotic as a result of right-to-left shunting. The development of severe pulmonary hypertension in patients with these cardiac defects is termed the Eisenmenger reaction. The clinical findings and/or symptoms of ventricular septal defect and patent ductus arteriosus usually lead to their detection in childhood. However, the clinical manifestations of ASD are subtle, and therefore this lesion can remain undetected until adult life.

The primary symptom of ASD is decreased exercise tolerance. Such patients are not disabled but often avoid strenuous athletic activities and adjust their lifestyle to their modest limitation. On physical examination, there is a systolic pulmonic murmur and usually fixed splitting of the second heart sound (Chapter 19). The ECG usually indicates a right ventricular volume overload, and the chest radiograph often shows increased pulmonary vascular markings, an enlarged right ventricle, and a small aortic knob.

An echocardiogram usually confirms the clinical diagnosis by demonstrating right ventricular volume overload. Doppler echocardiographic examination or first-pass radionuclide angiography demonstrates the left-to-right shunt and yields an estimate of its size. Cardiac catheterization quantifies the magnitude of the left-to-right shunt and determines whether the lesion is complicated by pulmonary hypertension.

Pulmonary hypertension in patients with ASD may be modest and associated with increased pulmonary blood flow. This condition is termed *hyperkinetic pulmonary hypertension*. In this circumstance, the pulmonary hypertension is reversible if the left-to-right shunt is eliminated by closure of the ASD. However, PA pressure may reach systemic levels and be associated with a minimal left-to-right shunt or even a net right-to-left shunt. When ASD is complicated by pulmonary hypertension, patients note dyspnea; with severe pulmonary hypertension, they may experience chest pain, hemoptysis, and syncope. The ECG demonstrates right ventricular hypertrophy, and the chest x-ray shows very prominent proximal pulmonary arteries with tapered distal arteries. The outlook is poor when ASD is complicated by precapillary pulmonary hypertension. Death occurs within 10 years in at least half of such patients.

The cause of pulmonary hypertension in patients with ASD is unclear. Although some patients survive to advanced age without the development of pulmonary hypertension, it occurs in about 30% of adults with ASD. Pulmonary hypertension is a response of the pulmonary arterioles to the large pulmonary blood flow associated with ASD. The media of the arterioles hypertrophy, thereby increasing resistance to flow and increasing PA pressure. Intimal proliferation may occur, with a resultant further increase in resistance and pressure. Why this process develops in some patients with ASD and not others is unknown. The size of the defect does not determine in which patients pulmonary hypertension develops as long as the ASD is greater than 1 cm in diameter.

In patients with ASD living at sea level, pulmonary hypertension rarely occurs before age 20, but it may do so in ASD patients living at modest altitudes (>1220 m). This earlier incidence in patients with ASD living at higher altitudes has been attributed to the effects of mild alveolar hypoxia.

Serial cardiac catheterizations have demonstrated the development of pulmonary hypertension in patients with ASD whose PA pressure was normal at the first study. However, patients age 50 or older with ASD and normal pulmonary artery pressures rarely develop subsequent pulmonary hypertension.

The inability to predict which patients with ASD will develop pulmonary hypertension and the poor prognosis once severe pulmonary hypertension develops are facts favoring the surgical closure of ASD when first detected, especially in patients under age 50. The operative risk of closing an uncomplicated ASD is less than 1% (Chapter 19).

Pulmonary embolism. Pulmonary embolism is the commonest cause of acute pulmonary hypertension. There are two mechanisms by which pulmonary hypertension occurs in patients with acute pulmonary embolism: embolic obstruction of the pulmonary circulation and vasoconstriction.

The major factor causing pulmonary hypertension in pulmonary embolism is the embolic obstruction of the pulmonary vascular bed. Significant pulmonary hypertension does not occur unless more than 50% of the pulmonary bed is obstructed. It should be noted that in patients without previous heart or lung disease, pulmonary embolism, even when massive, does not cause severe pulmonary hypertension. In response to acute increases in afterload, the normal right ventricle can only generate 40 to 50 mm Hg pressure, at which point it dilates and fails.

Mild pulmonary hypertension is found in patients with minor pulmonary embolism (obstruction of less than 25% of the pulmonary circulation). Pulmonary hypertension in this case cannot be explained on a mechanical basis. It is very probably caused by pulmonary vasoconstriction, secondary to hypoxemia.

Pulmonary hypertension secondary to pulmonary embolism is reversible. As the degree of pulmonary embolic obstruction and the hypoxemia decrease, the PA pressure returns to normal levels.

Chronic pulmonary hypertension is rare when acute pulmonary embolism is treated with anticoagulation or venous interruption. Patients with chronic pulmonary hypertension secondary to pulmonary embolism usually have had multiple symptomatic episodes of pulmonary embolism that were not treated.

Pulmonary hypertension caused by repeated attacks of silent pulmonary embolism is a very rare syndrome. Clinically, it is difficult to distinguish such patients from those with the equally rare syndrome of primary pulmonary hypertension. Ventilation-perfusion lung scans and a search for deep venous thrombosis are essential to distinguish between these two entities.

Schistosomiasis. Although schistosomiasis is not endemic in the United States, it is a worldwide problem that affects 200 million people in 71 countries. It is the leading cause of chronic pulmonary hypertension in the world. The infection occurs when individuals are exposed to water infested by snails that serve as hosts for the blood flukes *Schistosoma mansoni* and *S. japonicum*. Cercariae penetrate the skin and are carried by the blood to the liver, where they mature into adult parasites (Chapter 282). If ova enter the venous circulation, they lodge in pulmonary arterioles, where they produce an inflammatory lesion and granulomas. The obstruction of pulmonary arterioles results in pulmonary hypertension. With extensive involvement of the arterioles, PA pressure reaches systemic levels. The main pulmonary arteries may become aneurysmal. Death occurs secondary to chronic pulmonary hypertension with right ventricular failure.

There is no effective treatment once pulmonary hypertension occurs. Prevention consists of avoiding wading and swimming in fresh water contaminated with the snail host.

PASSIVE PULMONARY HYPERTENSION

Pathophysiology

A variety of diseases result in elevation of pulmonary venous pressure (box, p. 278). As pulmonary venous pressure increases, PA pressure must rise if pulmonary blood flow is to continue. This mandatory increase in PA pressure in response to increased pulmonary venous pressure is termed *passive pulmonary hypertension*. The gradient across the pulmonary bed remains normal, that is, less than 12 mm Hg. Since pulmonary venous pressure is rarely sustained above 25 to 30 mm Hg, mean PA pressure in patients with passive pulmonary hypertension rarely exceeds 35 to 40 mm Hg. The increased PA pressure places a burden on the right ventricle and may eventually lead to right ventricular failure.

In evaluating patients with pulmonary hypertension, a first step is to distinguish between passive and precapillary pulmonary hypertension. The primary clue to the diagnosis of passive pulmonary hypertension is the presence of pulmonary venous hypertension, which is recognized by the following symptoms: dyspnea, orthopnea, and paroxysmal nocturnal dyspnea. Radiographic signs of pulmonary venous hypertension include prominence of the upper lobe pulmonary veins, increased density of the central lung fields, and Kerley B lines. Kerley B lines are particularly useful in detecting chronic pulmonary venous hypertension and are caused by interstitial edema or fibrosis in the interlobular septa. They appear as fine, dense, horizontal linear densities in the lateral lower lobes, just above the diaphragm (Fig. 20-3).

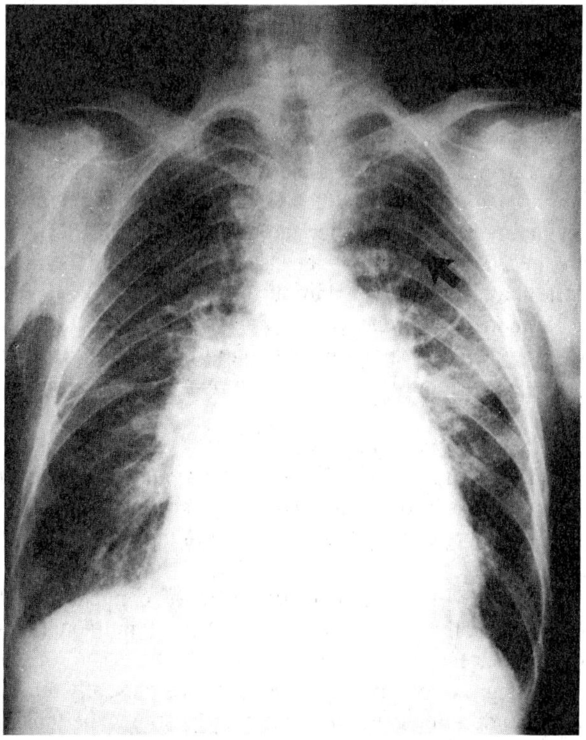

Fig. 20-3. Chest radiograph from a patient with severe mitral stenosis and pulmonary venous hypertension. Note pulmonary vascular redistribution *(arrow),* fluid in the major fissure of the left lung, and hazy infiltrates of interstitial edema bilaterally.

Causes of passive pulmonary hypertension

Any disease that causes left ventricular failure results in increased pulmonary venous pressure and thereby leads to passive pulmonary hypertension (Chapter 10). The commonest causes of left ventricular failure are systemic hypertension, congestive cardiomyopathy, and ischemic heart disease. In all of these conditions symptoms of left ventricular failure, including dyspnea, orthopnea, and paroxysmal nocturnal dyspnea, occur before signs of passive PA hypertension appear. Signs of right ventricular failure do not appear until pulmonary venous hypertension has been sufficiently sustained to lead to PA hypertension.

Aortic valve disease may lead to passive pulmonary hypertension by causing left ventricular failure and pulmonary venous hypertension. Right ventricular failure secondary to passive pulmonary hypertension in patients with aortic stenosis is particularly ominous. Without aortic valve replacement, death occurs within a year of the appearance of right ventricular failure.

Mitral valve disease, particularly mitral stenosis, may lead to pulmonary venous hypertension without left ventricular failure. That is, left atrial pressure, and thus pulmonary venous pressure, may be increased to 20 to 30 mm Hg, whereas the left ventricular filling pressure remains normal. Mitral stenosis is one of the commonest causes of prolonged pulmonary venous hypertension, hence one of the commonest causes of chronic passive pulmonary hypertension. Since mitral stenosis may be silent, it should be considered whenever one evaluates a patient with unexplained pulmonary hypertension. Echocardiography is particularly helpful in diagnosing silent mitral stenosis.

Two rare forms of congenital heart disease may lead to passive pulmonary hypertension: cor triatriatum and pulmonary vein stenosis (Chapter 19).

Cor triatriatum is characterized by the presence of a membrane that separates the left atrium into two chambers. The pulmonary veins enter the "third atrium." Blood enters the true left atrium by means of opening(s) in the membrane that separates the third atrium from the true atrium.

Pulmonary vein stenosis is most likely to occur at the junction of the pulmonary veins with the left atrium. If the lesion affects multiple veins, pulmonary hypertension occurs.

The diagnosis of these two rare causes of pulmonary hypertension is made by echocardiography and cardiac catheterization. Pulmonary artery and pulmonary wedge pressures are increased, whereas pressure in the true left atrium is normal.

Patients with these two rare forms of congenital heart disease usually present with symptoms of pulmonary venous hypertension very early in life.

The signs of passive PA hypertension are usually masked by the underlying cause of pulmonary venous hypertension. However, pulmonary hypertension should be suspected whenever the chest radiograph shows enlargement of the pulmonary arteries or right ventricle, or when the ECG shows biventricular hypertrophy in a patient expected to have left ventricular hypertrophy.

Treatment

Passive pulmonary hypertension is clearly reversible if the underlying cause of pulmonary venous hypertension is corrected. Treatment of systemic hypertension or correction of valvular disease lowers pulmonary venous pressure and thereby also relieves passive pulmonary hypertension.

REACTIVE PULMONARY HYPERTENSION

In certain patients with long-standing pulmonary venous hypertension, PA pressure may rise out of proportion to the increased pulmonary venous pressure. The pressure gradient from the PA to the left atrium increases, and PA pressure may reach systemic levels. This reaction to pulmonary venous hypertension is most likely to occur in patients with mitral valve disease, particularly mitral stenosis. It is uncommon in patients with left ventricular failure secondary to aortic valve disease, coronary heart disease, or systemic hypertension; individuals with the latter two conditions usually succumb before reactive pulmonary hypertension can develop. When the gradient is more than 12 mm Hg in patients with these diseases, one should suspect associated mitral valve disease or some superimposed cause of precapillary pulmonary hypertension, such as pulmonary embolism or chronic lung disease.

The cause of this inordinate increase in PA pressure and pulmonary vascular resistance in patients with reactive pulmonary hypertension resides in the precapillary pulmonary arterioles. These arterioles demonstrate medial hypertrophy and possibly intimal proliferation—findings similar to those noted in patients with severe precapillary pulmonary hypertension secondary to congenital heart disease.

Reactive pulmonary hypertension greatly increases the patient's disability. Right ventricular hypertrophy develops, and right ventricular failure may follow. Cardiac output and exercise tolerance decrease markedly.

The ECG shows right ventricular hypertrophy, and the chest radiograph demonstrates right ventricular enlargement with very prominent central pulmonary arteries. On physical examination, a systolic parasternal heave is present, and the pulmonic component of the second heart sound is loud. The stigmata of right ventricular failure (distended neck veins, hepatomegaly, peripheral edema) may be present.

Even though the pathologic findings are similar to those in patients with severe precapillary pulmonary hypertension secondary to congenital heart disease, reactive pulmonary hypertension is reversible if pulmonary venous pressure is returned to normal. When patients with mitral stenosis complicated by passive and reactive pulmonary hypertension have mitral valve replacement, passive pulmonary hypertension resolves immediately after surgery, although the PA to left atrial pressure gradient may persist. Follow-up catheterizations months to years after mitral valve replacement demonstrate a progressive decrease in the gradient and a return of PA pressure to near-normal levels.

An additional cause of reactive pulmonary hypertension is pulmonary veno-occlusive disease. This disease is characterized by diffuse, patchy involvement of small pulmonary veins and venules. The affected veins show fibrous narrowing or obliteration of the intima. Some observers believe that these lesions represent organized or recanalized thromboses of pulmonary veins. The disease affects children and young adults and is usually fatal within 2 years. It leads to severe pulmonary hypertension resembling that seen in primary pulmonary hypertension.

Pulmonary hypertension resulting from pulmonary veno-occlusive disease is differentiated from primary pulmonary hypertension by the presence of pulmonary venous hypertension in the former. Therefore, patients with venoocclusive disease often have orthopnea and paroxysmal nocturnal dyspnea, and their chest radiographs usually show Kerley B lines.

It is difficult to measure wedge pressure accurately in this disease. It may be elevated, normal, or "zero." Left atrial pressure is normal. The cause of veno-occlusive disease is unknown, and no treatment is available except for combined heart/lung or single lung transplantation.

REFERENCES

D'Alonzo GE et al: Survival in patients with primary pulmonary hypertension—results from a National Prospective Registry. Ann Int Med 115:343, 1991.
Fuster V et al: Primary pulmonary hypertension: natural history and the importance of thrombosis. Circulation 70:580, 1984.
Harvey RM, Enson Y, and Ferrer MI: A reconsideration of the origins of pulmonary hypertension. Chest 59:82, 1971.
Kawakami Y et al: Relation of oxygen delivery, mixed venous oxygenation and pulmonary hemodynamics to prognosis in chronic obstructive pulmonary disease. N Engl J Med 308:1045, 1983.
Packer M, Medina N, and Yushak M: Adverse hemodynamic and clinical effects of calcium channel blockade in pulmonary hypertension secondary to obliterative pulmonary vascular disease. J Am Coll Cardiol 4:890, 1984.
Pietra GG et al: Histopathology of primary pulmonary hypertension—a qualitative and quantitative study of pulmonary blood vessels from 58 patients in the National Heart, Lung, and Blood Institute Primary Pulmonary Hypertension Registry. Circulation 80:1198, 1989.
Rich S and Brundage BH: High-dose calcium channel-blocking therapy for primary pulmonary hypertension: evidence for long-term reduction in pulmonary arterial pressure and regression of right ventricular hypertrophy. Circulation 76:135, 1987.
Round S and Hill NS: Pulmonary hypertensive diseases. Chest 85:397, 1984.
Thadani U et al: Pulmonary veno-occlusive disease. Q J Med 44:133, 1975.
Voelkel NF: Mechanisms of hypoxic pulmonary vasoconstriction. Am Rev Respir Dis 133:1186, 1986.
Wagenvoort CA, and Wagenvoort N: Pathology of pulmonary hypertension, ed 2. New York, 1977, Wiley.
Walcott G, Burchell HB, and Brown AL: Primary pulmonary hypertension. Am J Med 49:70, 1970.

CHAPTER

21 Diseases of the Aorta

Miguel Zabalgoitia
Robert A. O'Rourke

Anatomically, the aorta is divided into the ascending aorta, aortic arch, descending thoracic aorta, and abdominal aorta. In the normal adult, the ascending aorta extends from the base of the heart up to 5 to 6 cm cephalad. It continues as the aortic arch, from which the three brachiocephalic arteries (innominate, left common carotid, and left subclavian) take off. The descending thoracic aorta is the continuation of the aorta beyond the arch. It courses in front of the spine and behind the esophagus, measures approximately 20 cm in length, and ends at the level of the diaphragm. The aortic isthmus is the junction between the arch and the descending thoracic aorta where coarctations of the aorta are usually located. The abdominal aorta is the continuation of the thoracic aorta below the diaphragm. It gives off the splanchnic vessels, measures about 15 cm in length, and ends at the point of its bifurcation into the common iliac arteries.

The aortic wall is composed of a thin intima layer lined by endothelium, a thick media layer containing elastic tissue arranged in a spiral, and a thin adventitia layer, composed mainly of collagen, that contains the vasa vasorum and lymphatics. The great tensile strength of the aorta lies in its elastic medium, which serves as an expansible reservoir and accommodates each stroke volume ejected by the left ventricle during early systole. It then recoils during late systole and diastole, propelling the column of blood distal to the arterial bed. This converts the pulsatile inflow into a continuous outflow.

In addition to the conductance and pumping functions, the aorta plays a role in the control of systemic vascular resistance and heart rate. Baroreceptors analogous to those in the carotid sinus lie in the ascending aorta and the aortic arch and send afferent signals to the vasomotor center in the brain stem by way of the vagus nerves (Chapter 1). Raising the aortic pressure causes reflex bradycardia and reduction of systemic vascular resistance, whereas lowering the blood pressure increases the heart rate and systemic resistance.

The systolic aortic pressure is a function of the *volume* of blood ejected, the *compliance* of the aorta, and the *resistance* to blood flow (Chapter 1). The aorta and its branches tend to stiffen with age, which accounts for the increase in systolic blood pressure with advancing age. Specific disease entities that affect the aorta deserve a brief description.

Atherosclerosis

Atherosclerosis is the most common cause of aortic aneurysms in adults over 50 years of age. Atherosclerosis starts during early adult life in the abdominal aorta, and from there extends in both cephalad and caudal directions. On pathologic examination, the atherosclerotic process is frequently seen to extend from the intima into the media, where the elastic and muscular supports of the aorta are destroyed. A combination of atherosclerotic plaque and thrombus is common in atherosclerotic aneurysms. Distal arterial embolization of cholesterol crystals and small thrombi may produce catastrophic consequences.

Marfan syndrome (cystic medial necrosis)

Histologically, cystic medial necrosis consists of multiple clefts of mucoid material within the aortic media. The nature of the process responsible for the degeneration of elastic and collagen fibers is unknown, but the development of the lesion seems to be accelerated by hypertension and pregnancy. The typical lesion is a fusiform aneurysm affecting the ascending aorta and the sinuses of Valsalva. Aortic regurgitation may be present as a result of dilatation of the aortic ring. This condition is particularly prevalent in patients with Marfan syndrome. However, careful examination of patients with annuloaortic ectasia and cystic medial necrosis reveals that about 25% to 50% of these patients may have some, but not all, of the clinical features of the Marfan syndrome, indicating that many patients represent a forme fruste of this disorder.

The physical examination in patients with Marfan syndrome may reveal abnormal pulsation of the dilated ascending aorta over the second and third right intercostal spaces. As with other cases of aortic regurgitation secondary to dilatation of the ascending aorta, the intensity of the diastolic murmur is greater to the right of the sternum; in patients with aortic regurgitation secondary to primary valvular abnormality, on the other hand, the murmur is best heard along the left sternal border (Chapter 3).

The chest radiograph shows a markedly dilated ascending aorta and left ventricular dilatation proportional to the severity of aortic regurgitation. Calcification of the ascending aorta and aortic valve is uncommon. Conventional transthoracic echocardiography demonstrates an abnormally widened aortic root, aneurysmal dilatation of the sinuses of Valsalva, and incomplete coaptation of the aortic cusps during diastole (Chapter 5).

Complications of aneurysms of the ascending aorta account for more than 90% of deaths from Marfan syndrome. Elective composite-graft repair of the aorta is recommended when the aortic root diameter reaches 6.0 cm, even if the patient is asymptomatic. Surgical correction is also advised when aortic regurgitation is severe, causing symptoms of congestive heart failure. The risks of failure of aortic valve replacement and aneurysm resection in this group of patients are between 10% and 15%. Recently, a 90% postsurgical survival at 8 years has been reported for ascending aortic aneurysms in patients with Marfan syndrome.

Mycotic aneurysms

The so-called mycotic aneurysms of the aorta are of bacterial, not fungal, origin. Since the intact endothelium is quite resistant to bacterial invasion, a previously damaged area almost always provides the site for infection. Bacterial endocarditis is the usual setting in which mycotic aneurysms occur, but they may also develop during sepsis or by direct spread of infection from surrounding tissues. Direct invasion of the wall of the aorta adjacent to an aortic valve endocarditis may result in a valve ring abscess or in sinus of Valsalva rupture. Mycotic aneurysms tend to be saccular in appearance. Staphylococci, streptococci, and salmonellae are the usual infectious agents. Treatment includes parental antibiotics followed by surgical excision.

Diseases of the aorta are primarily the result of degenerative changes in the aortic wall. Among the factors that lead to this degeneration are aging and hypertension. Diseases of the aorta can be classified into the following categories (box below).

AORTIC ANEURYSMS

An aneurysm of the aorta is a pathologic dilatation of any of its anatomic segments. A *true aneurysm* includes all three layers of the wall, as opposed to a *pseudoaneurysm,* in which disruption of the intima and media layers has occurred and the wall is composed of the adventitia and thrombus. According to their gross appearance, aneurysms may be described as *fusiform,* when the entire circumfer-

Classification of diseases of the aorta

- Aneurysm
  - Thoracic
    - Ascending
    - Arch
    - Descending
  - Abdominal
    - Suprarenal
    - Infrarenal
- Dissection
  - Type I } Type A
  - Type II } Type A
  - Type III }Type B
- Aortitis
  - Syphilitic
  - Rheumatic diseases
    - Rheumatoid arthritis
    - Ankylosing spondylitis
    - Psoriatic arthritis
    - Reiter's syndrome
    - Relapsing polychondritis
    - Enteropathic arthropathies
  - Takayasu's arteritis
  - Giant-cell arteritis
- Arterial obstruction
  - Atherosclerotic
  - Thrombotic
  - Embolic
- Trauma
- Coarctation (Chapter 19)

ence is affected resulting in a diffusely dilated lesion, or *saccular,* when only a portion of the circumference is affected resulting in a diverticular formation.

Regardless of the cause and location of an aneurysm, it has a tendency to expand. The Laplace relation describes the reason for such expansion:

$$T = R \cdot P$$

where *T* is the wall tension of a hollow organ, *R* is the radius of the organ, and *P* is the pressure being supported by the wall. As the radius increases, the wall tension increases and rupture becomes more likely. Pseudoaneurysms are more prone to rupture than true aneurysms because of the relative weakness of the wall formed by thrombus and connective tissue.

Aortic aneurysms are frequently asymptomatic. However, when symptoms occur, they may be caused by (1) pain at the site of aneurysm expansion; (2) compression of adjacent structures; (3) embolism of a mural thrombus; and (4) rupture into pleural, peritoneal, or retroperitoneal spaces. The most common cause of death in patients with thoracic or abdominal aneurysms is rupture with resultant exsanguination. Thoracic aneurysms tend to rupture into the left pleural space, whereas abdominal aneurysms tend to rupture into the retroperitoneal space.

Thoracic aortic aneurysms

In the normal adult, the ascending aorta measures 3.5 cm or less, the aortic arch between 2.8 and 3.5 cm, and the thoracic descending aorta between 2.2 and 3.0 cm in diameter. The signs and symptoms of a thoracic aortic aneurysm depend on its size and location. Many thoracic aneurysms are asymptomatic, being recognized on routine chest radiograph as a mediastinal widening. Thus, an aortic aneurysm should be considered in the differential diagnosis of any mediastinal mass. Further investigation should include noninvasive methods such as computed tomography scanning, magnetic resonance imaging, or transesophageal echocardiography. If surgical repair is indicated, contrast aortography may be needed. Since progressive layering of thrombus may occur within the aneurysmal sac and because an arteriogram shows only the intraluminal dimensions, the true size of the aneurysm may be underestimated. The exact dimensions of the aneurysm, including the thickness of the thrombus, can be better measured by computed tomography, magnetic resonance imaging, or transesophageal echocardiography.

Chronic chest pain, arising from compression of adjacent structures, may radiate into the neck, shoulders, or back. Severe chest pain in patients with a thoracic aneurysm may represent sudden expansion, rupture, or dissection. Compression of the left main-stem bronchus or the trachea may produce respiratory symptoms. Compression of the left recurrent laryngeal nerve may produce hoarseness, and esophageal compression may result in dysphagia. Aortic regurgitation is unusual in arteriosclerotic ascending aortic aneurysms but common with annuloaortic ectasia or dissections. Thrombus formation along the inner wall of the aneurysm can develop, and distal emboli may produce a cerebrovascular event.

Management depends on the size and location of the aneurysm, the clinical presentation, and the relative risks of rupture versus operation. Rupture is the most serious complication of an aneurysm. It has an exceedingly high mortality rate, whereas elective repair in a low-risk patient can be performed safely with less than 10% mortality. A direct relationship exists between aneurysmal size and risk of rupture. Aneurysms larger than 6 cm in patients with low operative risk should be considered for elective repair. In other patients, computed tomography scanning, magnetic resonance imaging, or transesophageal echocardiography should be obtained at 6- or 12-month intervals to assess aneurysmal growth. These include asymptomatic patients with stable aneurysms less than 6 cm in diameter, asymptomatic patients with Marfan syndrome and an aneurysm less than 5 cm in diameter, and high-risk patients with large thoracic aneurysms. In the presence of signs and symptoms of expansion suggesting impending rupture (pain, compression of adjacent structures, new diastolic murmur, and objective evidence of aneurysmal growth), urgent surgical intervention is needed.

Aneurysms are repaired by replacing the dilated segment of the aorta with a Dacron graft. If the aortic valve and the fibrous ring are involved, resulting in aortic regurgitation, replacement of the aortic valve with reimplantation of the coronary arteries is required. Serious complications after repair include myocardial infarction, stroke, and respiratory and renal failure. Therefore, complete preoperative assessment is mandatory to establish the operative risk on an individual basis.

Abdominal aortic aneurysms

Since atherosclerosis is most common in the descending abdominal aorta, 75% of atherosclerotic aneurysms are found in the distal abdominal aorta below the renal arteries. An abdominal aneurysm commonly produces no symptoms and is usually detected on routine examination as a palpable, pulsatile, and nontender mass or as an incidental finding on abdominal radiograph or abdominal ultrasound obtained for other reasons. Some patients may complain of pulsations in the abdomen, others of low back pain. During periods of rapid expansion, abdominal aneurysms produce pain in the low back, abdomen, or groin; the pulsatile mass frequently becomes tender and appears more fixed than in the asymptomatic patient. Acute pain and hypotension occur with rupture of the aneurysm, requiring an emergent operation.

An abdominal aneurysm should be suspected when physical examination reveals a pulsatile, expansible, and occasionally tender mass between the xiphoid process and the umbilicus. The diagnosis is confirmed by abdominal ultrasound, which delineates the size, location, and tissue characteristics of the aneurysmal sac contents. A mural thrombus is present in almost all cases. In addition, serial abdominal ultrasound studies are extremely useful for documenting aneurysm expansion. Computed tomography and magnetic resonance imaging have also been used for this purpose. Contrast aortography is essential in the preoperative evaluation to document the extent of atherosclerosis in adjacent vascular territories. However, aortography may underestimate the diameter of the aneurysm since the presence of mural thrombus reduces the intraluminal size.

The risk of rupture for abdominal aneurysms also increases with its size. The mortality of patients with abdominal aneurysms exceeding 6 cm in diameter is approximately 50% in 1 year, 75% in 2 years, and 90% in 3 years; in those with lesions between 4 and 6 cm, it is 25% in 1 year, 28% in 2 years, and 30% in 3 years. Thus, operative resection of the aneurysm is indicated in symptomatic patients, in those with evidence of rapidly expanding aneurysms regardless of their size, and in patients with aneurysms larger than 5 cm in diameter, regardless of their symptoms. For aneurysms less than 5 cm in diameter, serial follow-up with abdominal ultrasound is recommended.

The prognosis depends upon the extent, location, and severity of atherosclerosis in vessels supplying vital organs. Frequently, the severity of accompanying coronary artery and cerebrovascular disease determines the long-term prognosis. Thus, careful preoperative cardiac and general medical evaluation are essential in all surgical candidates. Operative mortality ranges between 1% and 5% in most centers. However, after acute rupture, the mortality of an emergent operation is generally more than 50%.

DISSECTION OF THE AORTA

Aortic dissection is usually initiated by an intimal tear that allows blood driven by arterial pressure to dissect through the aortic media, separating the intima from the adventitia and creating a double-lumen vessel. Since most dissections occur in the outer half of the medial layer of the aorta, the false lumen wall is exceedingly thin and prone to rupture. Occasionally, the false lumen reenters the true lumen in a more distal location through a spontaneous fenestration of the intimal flap.

Most aortic dissections occur in patients ages 40 to 60, and in men more than in women by a ratio of 3:1. Predisposing factors to aortic dissection include systemic hypertension, coarctation of the aorta, atherosclerosis, pregnancy, cystic medial necrosis, and trauma. The elevated incidence noted in patients with systemic hypertension and coarctation of the aorta is probably related to abnormally high wall stress. In elderly patients with extensive atherosclerosis, dissection may originate from perforation of an atheromatous plaque. The increased incidence of dissection in females in the third trimester of pregnancy may be a result of changes in connective tissue that occur late in pregnancy.

The two widely accepted classifications of aortic dissections are those of DeBakey and Stanford. DeBakey classifies dissections into type I, which originates in the ascending aorta and extends into the descending aorta; this form accounts for 60% to 70% of cases. Type II affects only the ascending aorta; this form is most commonly noted in patients with annuloaortic ectasia and accounts for 10% of cases. Type III originates from the upper descending aorta and extends distally; this form accounts for 20% to 30% of cases. Stanford's classification separates dissections into Type A, which involves the ascending aorta, and type B, which is limited to the descending aorta.

Severe chest pain occurs in more than 90% of patients. It is frequently described as a sudden, tearing pain associated with diaphoresis. The pain of aortic dissection is so severe it tends to persist despite the use of narcotics. The location of the pain may be useful in localizing the site and extent of the dissection. As a general rule, pain in the chest, neck, and jaw suggests dissection involving the ascending aorta, whereas pain in the back suggests involvement of the descending aorta. The presence of pain implies activity of the dissection; movement of the pain from chest to back or from upper to lower back suggests extension of the dissection.

Other clinical features of acute onset of aortic dissection are manifestations of its four major complications: (1) compression of adjacent structures such as superior cervical ganglia (Horner's syndrome), superior vena cava (superior vena cava syndrome), left laryngeal nerve (hoarseness), bronchus (dyspnea), and esophagus (dysphagia); (2) occlusion of major branch vessels; (3) retrograde extension into the aortic valve; and (4) rupture into a body space. Myocardial ischemia or infarction may occur as a result of coronary artery involvement. Since most type A dissections extend along the greater aortic curvature, the right coronary artery is more commonly affected than the left. Neurologic ischemic symptoms may occur as a result of occlusion of cerebral or spinal arteries. Ischemic signs and symptoms affecting the upper and lower extremities may result from involvement of the subclavian or iliac arteries. Splanchnic vascular occlusion can result in bowel infarction and renal failure. Severe hypertension in a patient with a type B dissection should suggest renal artery involvement. Hemopericardium and cardiac tamponade may complicate a type A lesion with retrograde dissection.

Although half of the patients with aortic dissection present with hypertension, others present with normal or low blood pressure. If significant hypotension is present, aortic rupture into the left pleural cavity or into the pericardial space (with resultant cardiac tamponade) should be suspected. Examination of the jugular veins is helpful in distinguishing between cardiac tamponade and hypovolemia (Chapter 18). An emergent echocardiogram is mandatory to confirm this diagnosis.

Physical examination reveals an acutely distressed patient. Neurologic deficit or a pulse discrepancy between the arms may indicate compromise of the aortic arch vessels. Similarly, acute abdominal pain or diminished femoral pulses may suggest splanchnic or iliofemoral vessel involvement. Aortic regurgitation in a patient with aortic dissection strongly suggests that the dissecting process has extended into the aortic root or the aortic ring, particularly if signs and symptoms of severe heart failure are present.

The electrocardiogram usually excludes acute myocardial ischemia unless there is coronary artery involvement. As seen in Fig. 21-1, the chest radiograph may be helpful in suggesting the presence of aortic dissection. The unusually widened mediastinum may be present in either type A

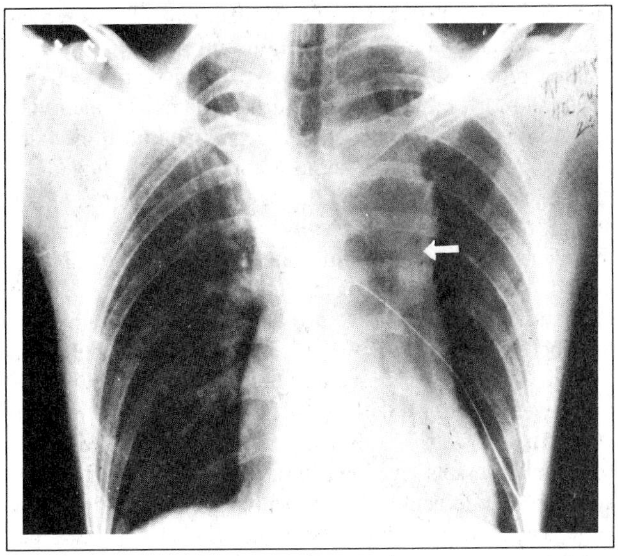

Fig. 21-1. Posteroanterior chest radiograph of a patient with acute aortic dissection caused by anuloaortic ectasia associated with Marfan syndrome. Note the wide mediastinal shadow. (Reprinted with permission from Walsh RA and O'Rourke RA: The diagnosis and management of acute left-sided valvular regurgitation. Curr Probl Cardiol 4(9):1-34, December 1979.)

or type B dissection. Although a nonspecific finding, a widened mediastinum should lead to more specific diagnostic procedures. Conventional transthoracic echocardiography can reveal dilatation and double-lumen of the aortic root in type A dissections, although false-positive and false-negative results are frequent.

The method of choice for diagnosing aortic dissection is transesophageal echocardiography (Chapter 5). Other imaging modalities such as magnetic resonance imaging and computed tomography with contrast have also been shown to be highly accurate in detecting aortic dissection. However, transesophageal echocardiography has the following advantages over magnetic resonance imaging and computed tomography scanning: (1) it can be performed as a bedside procedure in the emergency room or in the intensive care area, (2) it requires less than 20 minutes, (3) it does not require contrast media. Fig. 21-2 illustrates a patient with type I aortic dissection. The separation between the true lumen and the false lumen by the intimal flap is clearly identified. A moderate amount of anterior pericardial effusion is also evident. Contrast aortography may be needed to determine the status of the coronary and aortic arch arteries (Fig. 21-3).

The prognosis for survival in untreated patients with aor-

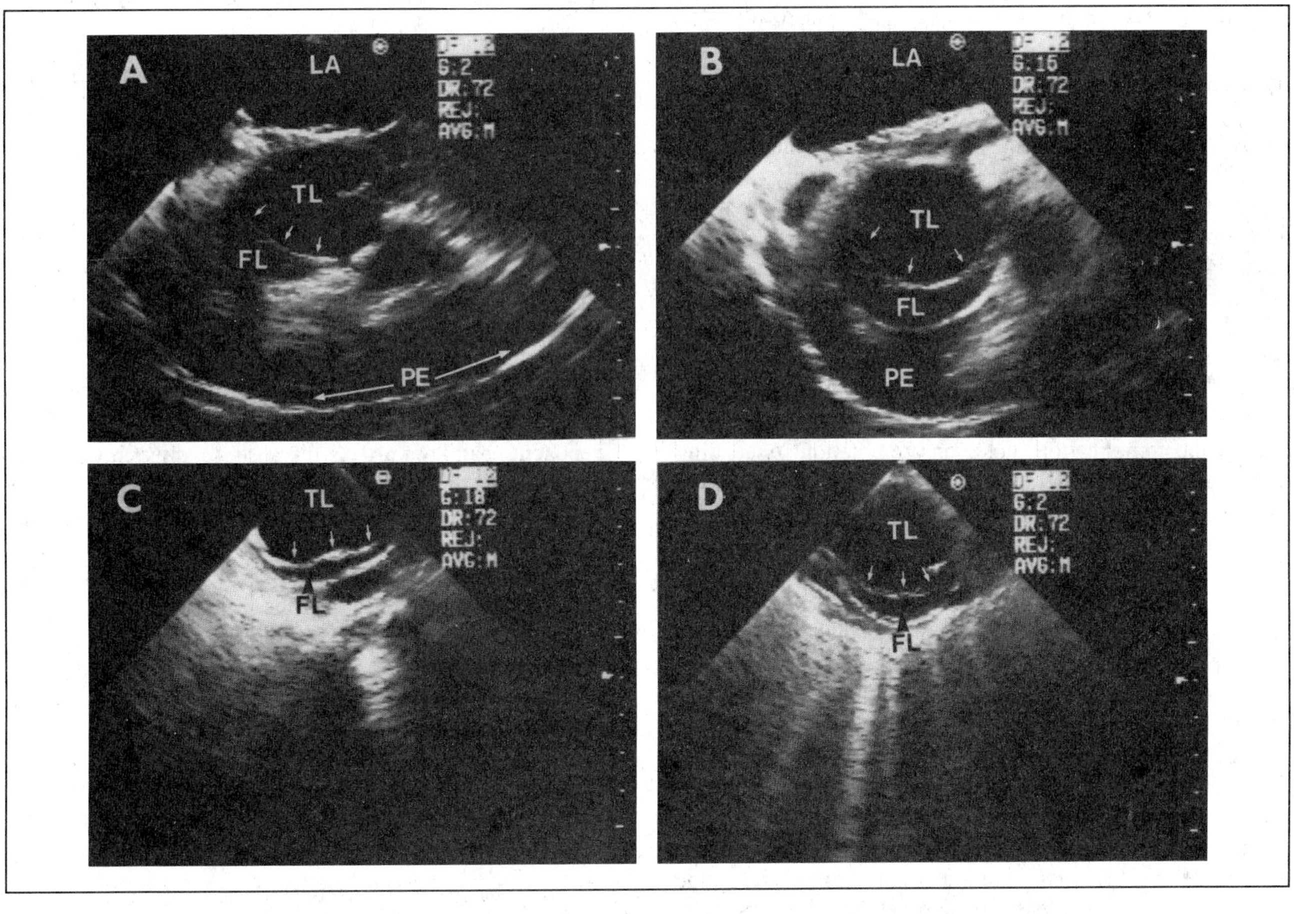

Fig. 21-2. Transesophageal echocardiography in a patient with type I acute aortic dissection. The true lumen *(TL)* and the false lumen *(FL)* are clearly separated by an intimal flap *(arrows)*. A moderate amount of anterior pericardial effusion *(PE)* is also noted. **(A),** Image at the level of the aortic valve and aortic root. **(B),** Image at the level of the ascending aorta. **(C),** Image at the level of the aortic arch. **(D),** Image at the level of the middescending thoracic aorta.

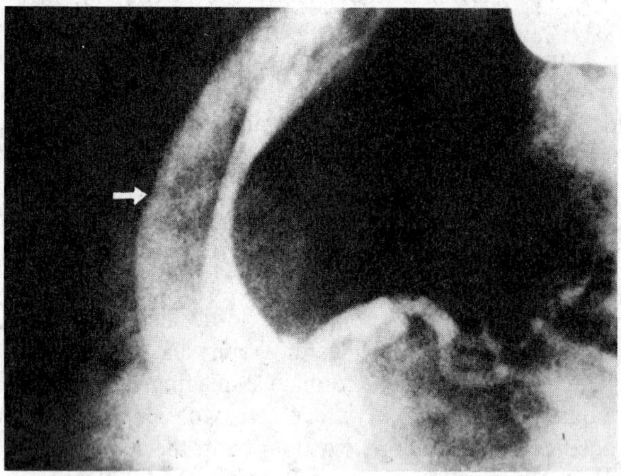

Fig. 21-3. Angiogram of a patient with acute aortic dissection of the ascending aorta. Contrast material fills the true lumen; the false lumen is to the left. (Reprinted with permission from Walsh RA and O'Rourke RA: The diagnosis and management of acute left-sided valvular regurgitation. Curr Probl Cardiol 4(9):1-34, December 1979.)

tic dissection is extremely poor. In one series of 505 patients, one third died within 48 hours of presentation; three fourths were dead within 2 weeks; and nine out of ten did not survive 1 year. Thus, transesophageal echocardiography should be performed as soon as possible in all patients in whom aortic dissection is suspected.

Medical therapy should be initiated as soon as the diagnosis is suspected. Unless hypotension is present, therapy should be aimed at reducing cardiac contractility and systemic arterial pressure, and thereby shear stress. Systolic blood pressure should be maintained between 100 and 120 mm Hg. A beta-adrenergic blocker should be immediately administered simultaneously with sodium nitroprusside infusion. Direct vasodilators, such as diazoxide and hydralazine, are contraindicated since these agents can increase hydraulic shear and may propagate dissection.

Definitive therapy is dictated by the type of dissection and by the complications noted on presentation. Ascending aortic dissections (type A) are unstable and pose the threat of retrograde dissection, rupture, acute severe aortic regurgitation, or fatal pericardial tamponade; thus surgical intervention is the preferred treatment. The goals of surgery are to correct complications and to limit the dissecting process. The intimal tear is either excised or oversewn; the false lumen is obliterated by oversewing the aorta. Restoration of the vascular integrity of aortic branches frequently requires use of Dacron grafts if the aortic arch is involved. In the presence of aortic regurgitation, the leaflets may be resuspended, rendering the valve competent. The distal dissection plane, which may extend into the descending thoracic or abdominal aorta, often becomes obliterated. The major causes of perioperative mortality and morbidity include myocardial infarction, paraplegia, renal failure, tamponade, hemorrhage, and sepsis.

For patients with descending aorta dissection (type B) who are stable without vascular complications, medical therapy is the preferred mode of treatment. Transesophageal echocardiography may be useful in the decision-making process in patients with type B dissections. If the upper and lower margins of the dissection can be identified and are limited to the thoracic descending aorta, if the false lumen is completely or almost completely occupied by thrombus, and if active circulation between the true lumen and the false lumen is not evident by color-flow Doppler, the decision for medical management alone is well supported. However, if the distal end of the dissection cannot be identified because it extends beyond the diaphragm into the abdominal aorta, if the false lumen is not obliterated by thrombus, and if there is evidence of blood-flow activity between the true and the false lumens, emergent thoraco-abdominal contrast aortography is recommended to detect splanchnic vessels and lower limb involvement. The decision for an emergent operation should be based upon these angiographic results. Fig. 21-4 illustrates serial transesophageal echocardiographic images in a patient with type B dissection.

Long-term management of patients with aortic dissection treated either medically or surgically should include careful control of blood pressure with the use of long-acting beta-adrenergic blockers and serial noninvasive follow-up by means of computed tomography scanning, magnetic resonance imaging, or transesophageal echocardiography.

AORTITIS

Though the causes of aortitis are diverse, the pathologic consequences are similar: aneurysm formation or stenosis of aortic branch vessels. Syphilis, ankylosing spondylitis, and rheumatoid arthritis result in inflammation, scarring, and weakening of the aortic media. Involvement of the aortic ring and cusps often results in aortic regurgitation. In contrast, Takayasu's arteritis and giant-cell arteritis produce obstruction of aortic branches and ischemic symptoms.

Syphilis (Chapter 273)

Treponema pallidum affects the aorta by direct invasion of the adventitia layer. The spirochetes spread through the lymphatics into the aortic media and produce an obliterative endarteritis of the vasa vasorum. Inflammation leads to destruction of elastic tissue and eventually to scar formation and calcification within the media along the ascending aorta. The characteristic radiographic appearance of dilatation and calcification of the ascending aorta (not the aortic knob) should suggest syphilitic aortitis. Other clinically important manifestations of tertiary syphilis of the aorta include aortic regurgitation and coronary ostial stenosis. Positive serologic tests support the diagnosis. Penicillin therapy as recommended for tertiary syphilis is necessary.

Chronic rheumatoid diseases

Aortitis involving predominantly the ascending aorta has been documented in patients with rheumatoid arthritis (Chapter 304), ankylosing spondylitis (Chapter 312), psor-

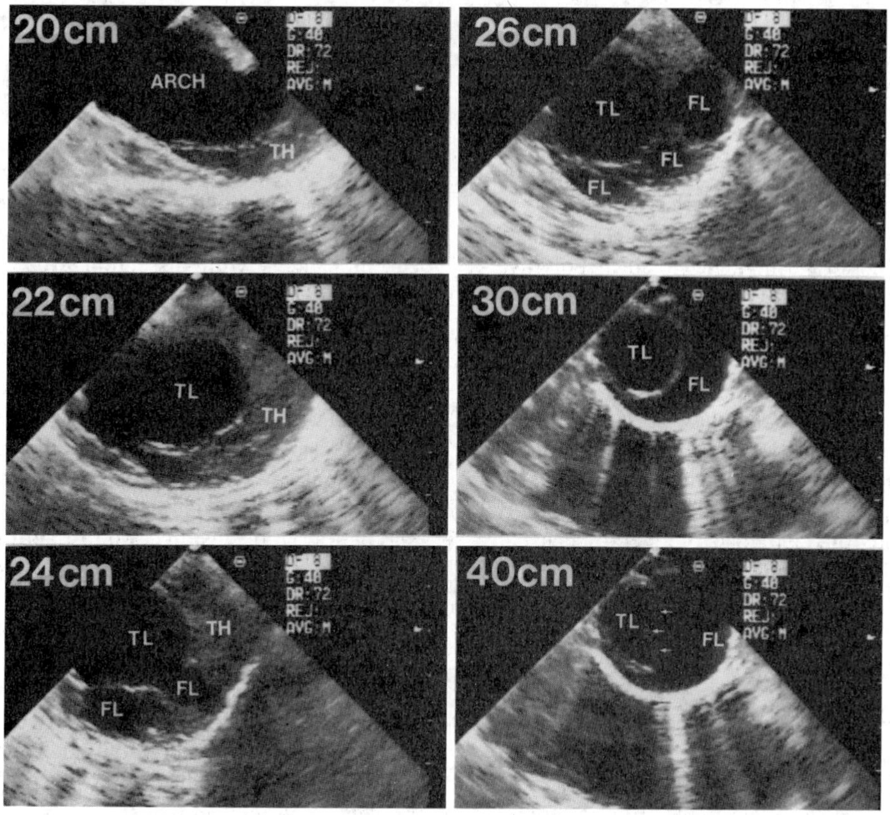

Fig. 21-4. Transesophageal echocardiography in a patient with type III acute aortic dissection. The proximal end of the dissection can be clearly identified at 20 cm, where the true lumen at the level of the aortic arch can be separated from the false lumen, which is obliterated by thrombus *(TH)* formation. At 22 cm, the centrally located true lumen is being surrounded by the thrombus-obliterated false lumen; at 24 and 26 cm, the false lumen is partially obliterated by the thrombus; at 30 cm, the false lumen is thrombus-free, suggesting free-flow circulation between the true lumen and the false lumen; at 40 cm, the dimensions of the false lumen are now larger than the true lumen and external compression of the intimal flap can be clearly appreciated *(arrows),* which is indicative of a hypertensive false lumen. At this latter level, the transesophageal transducer is beyond the diaphragm, that is, at the uppermost portion of the abdominal aorta. More distal imaging of the abdominal aorta is not possible because the aorta and the esophagus are no longer in contact.

iatic arthritis (Chapter 312), Reiter's syndrome (Chapter 312), relapsing polychondritis (Chapter 313), and enteropathic arthropathies (Chapter 313). The aortitis in each of these conditions may result in aortic dilatation and consequently in aortic regurgitation.

Cardiovascular symptoms occur in 3% to 10% of patients with ankylosing spondylitis and may be present before manifestations of arthritis are evident. Aortic regurgitation is the predominant cardiac manifestation of ankylosing spondylitis. Mitral regurgitation may be present but is rarely isolated or severe. Conduction abnormalities are usually not clinically important, but complete heart block has been reported.

Takayasu's arteritis (Chapter 307)

This type of vasculitis characteristically results in inflammation and obstruction of the aorta and its major branches. Panarteritis occurs during the active phase of the disease and is replaced by intimal proliferation. Wall scarring and intravascular thrombosis are late manifestations of the disease. The term *pulseless disease* is applied because of frequent severe obstruction of the innominate, left common carotid, and left subclavian arteries. Involvement of the abdominal branches of the aorta may produce gastrointestinal symptoms or renovascular hypertension. Obstruction of the iliofemoral arteries is rare.

The syndrome should be suspected in Asian females whose symptoms suggest proximal obstruction of upper extremity and head arteries. Examination reveals diminished or absent upper extremity and carotid pulses, with good preservation of lower extremity pulses. Bruits are frequently present. Contrast aortography may help to determine the extent and severity of obstruction and exclude the possibility of dissection of the aortic arch. Medical therapy includes anti-inflammatory and immunosuppressive agents during the acute phase, and anticoagulants during the late stage of the disease. Surgical bypass of critically narrowed arteries has been successfully performed.

Giant-cell arteritis (Chapter 307)

This vasculitis is characterized by focal granuloma involving all three layers of medium- and large-sized arteries throughout the body. Symptoms may range from the fatigue, morning stiffness, and myalgia noted in polymyalgia rheumatica syndrome to those resulting from obstruction of medium-sized arteries, especially the temporal and ophthalmic arteries. Aortitis with aneurysm formation, aortic branch obstruction, and aortic regurgitation is an uncommon finding. On laboratory examination, the erythrocyte sedimentation rate is markedly elevated and mild anemia may be present, but serum creatine kinase is normal. Although the disease is self-limited, it can result in arterial obstruction and infarction. Corticosteroid therapy is usually effective in controlling symptoms and progression of the inflammatory process.

ARTERIAL OBSTRUCTION

Occlusion of the terminal aorta may occur gradually, as a result of progressive atherosclerosis, or suddenly, secondary to arterial embolism. Symptoms and prognosis are related to the underlying disease and to the amount of collateral circulation.

Chronic aortic obstruction

Slowly progressive stenosis of the terminal aorta may occur over several years. Exercise-induced pain characteristically involves the low back, buttocks, and thighs and may progress to rest pain as the severity of stenosis increases. Inability to maintain penile erection is common. Absence of pulses in both femoral arteries and more distal locations is characteristic. Bruits are usually audible over the abdomen near the umbilicus and over both femoral arteries. Loss of lower extremity hair, atrophy of the skin and subcutaneous tissue, and loss of leg muscle mass are common in such patients; gangrene is a late manifestation of the disease.

Acute aortic obstruction

Systemic emboli are the primary cause. A cardiac source should be strongly considered. The presence of atrial fibrillation, mitral valve disease, cardiomyopathy, valve prostheses, or recent myocardial infarction makes emboli of cardiac origin more likely.

The severity of reduced arterial circulation to the lower extremities depends on the level of the occlusion, the competence of collateral circulation, the severity of acute arterial spasm, and the extent of thrombus propagation. Clinically, the patient notes the sudden onset of ischemic pain at the level of the occlusion. If collateral circulation is inadequate, cutaneous sensation and muscle strength are lost within the first hour. Severe muscle contractures may occur at 6 hours. Muscle swelling and skin discoloration signify prolonged ischemia. Initial improvement in symptoms may be followed by increased evidence of ischemia caused by proximal propagation of the arterial thrombus. On examination, the legs are cool, and the lower extremity pulses, including those of the femoral arteries, are absent. Muscle strength and cutaneous sensation are diminished. Muscle fasciculations and/or contractures may be present. Edema is a late finding. Similar clinical findings may occur in patients with dissection of the descending aorta. These patients are usually identified by the presence of severe back pain and asymmetrical extremity pulses.

Acute aortic obstruction is an emergency condition. The patient's life and the viability of both lower extremities depend on rapidly establishing the correct diagnosis and promptly instituting appropriate therapy. Doppler ultrasonographic measurement of lower extremity arterial pressures is useful in establishing the presence, severity, and site of arterial occlusion. Contrast aortography is necessary in acute distal aortic obstruction to exclude the presence of aortic dissection, to establish the site of obstruction, and to assess the adequacy of collateral circulation.

Prompt institution of intravenous heparin is essential as soon as aortic dissection is excluded. Surgical embolectomy or thrombectomy should be performed as soon as possible. Heparin therapy should be continued after surgery. Lifetime anticoagulation is indicated in the majority of patients to prevent recurrent embolism or propagation of arterial thrombus.

AORTIC TRAUMA

Injury to the aorta may result from penetrating wounds or from blunt trauma. Nonpenetrating injuries may lead to aortic rupture and produce meager or imperceptible evidence of chest wall trauma. Because of the forces produced by such acceleration-deceleration injuries, the most common site of tear or rupture is the aortic isthmus located just distal to the origin of the left subclavian artery where the mobile (ascending and arch) and fixed (descending) segments of the aorta join. Acutely, such patients present in shock from exsanguination. Occasionally, they complain of severe chest and back pain and have an increased upper extremity arterial pulse pressure and hypotension in the lower extremities. In survivors of aortic rupture, a periaortic thrombus may form, the aortic lumen may recanalize, and a pseudoaneurysm may develop just distal to the left subclavian artery. Because of the high incidence of spontaneous rupture of such aneurysms, surgical resection and repair should be performed immediately.

REFERENCES

Bergstein EF and Chan EL: Abdominal aortic aneurysm in high risk patients. Outcome of selective management based on size and expansion rate. Ann Surg 200:255, 1984.

Bulkley BH and Roberts WC: Ankylosing spondylitis and aortic regurgitation. Circulation 48:1014, 1973.

DeBakey ME, Cooley DA, and Creech O Jr: Surgical considerations of dissecting aneurysm of the aorta. Ann Surg 142:586, 1955.

Eagle KM and DeSanctis RW: Aortic dissection. Curr Probl Cardiol 14:227, 1989.
Erbel R et al: Echocardiography in diagnosis of aortic dissection. Lancet 1:457, 1989.
Gott VL et al: Surgical treatment of aneurysms of the ascending aorta in the Marfan syndrome. N Engl J Med 314:1070, 1986.
Hall S et al: Takayasu arteritis. A review of 32 North American patients. Medicine (Baltimore) 64:89, 1985.
Heggtveit HA: Syphilitic aortitis: a clinicopathologic autopsy of 100 cases: 1950-1960. Circulation 29:346, 1964.
Ishikawa K: Patterns of symptoms and prognosis in occlusive thromboaortopathy (Takayasu's disease). J Am Coll Cardiol 8:1041, 1986.
Lemon DK and White CW: Annuloaortic ectasia: angiographic, hemodynamic, and clinical comparison with aortic valve insufficiency. Am J Cardiol 41:482, 1978.
McDonald GR et al: Surgical management of patients with the Marfan's syndrome and dilated ascending aorta. J Thorac Cardiovasc Surg 81:180, 1981.
Miller DC: Acute dissection of the aorta: continuing need for earlier diagnosis and treatment. Mod Concepts Cardiovasc Dis 54:51, 1985.
Perruquet JL, Davis DE, and Harrington TM: Aortic arch arteritis in the elderly. An important manifestation of giant cell arteritis. Arch Intern Med 146:289, 1986.
Sterpnetti AV et al: Abdominal aortic aneurysms in elderly patients. Selective management based on clinical status and aneurysmal expansion rate. Am J Surg 150:772, 1979.
Szilagyi DE et al: Contribution of abdominal aortic aneurysmectomy to prolongation of life. Ann Surg 164:678, 1966.
Trinkle K: Management of thoracic trauma victims. Philadelphia, 1980, Lippincott.

CHAPTER

22 Diseases of the Peripheral Arteries and Veins

Peter C. Spittell
John A. Spittell, Jr.

The competent clinician should be familiar with peripheral vascular disorders, confident in making an accurate diagnosis, and knowledgeable regarding the available therapeutic options. Peripheral vascular disorders occur commonly, present important therapeutic opportunities, and often serve as valuable diagnostic clues to other significant conditions. Accordingly, a systematic and careful evaluation of the arterial and venous circulation should be included in the history and physical examination of every patient.

In this chapter the clinical aspects and management of acute and chronic occlusive peripheral arterial disease, arterial aneurysms, vasospastic disorders, arteritides, varicose veins, venous thrombosis, and chronic venous insufficiency are presented.

DISEASES OF THE PERIPHERAL ARTERIES

Peripheral arterial disease can be caused by one or more etiologic factors—aging, atherosclerosis, hypertension, infection, inflammatory disorders, degenerative disease, and trauma. Atherosclerosis is by far the most common cause of peripheral arterial disease, including both occlusive and aneurysmal disease; however, the less common types of occlusive arterial disease must also be considered since they often present important diagnostic and/or therapeutic opportunities. In addition to atherosclerotic occlusive disease and aneurysms, the peripheral arteries may be affected by vasospastic disorders, inflammation, and trauma.

Peripheral arterial disease, whether occlusive, aneurysmal, or vasospastic, is not difficult to diagnose since the peripheral arteries are easy to examine, and symptoms of peripheral arterial disease, when present, are fairly distinctive.

Examination of the upper extremity arteries (subclavian, brachial, radial, and ulnar), the abdominal aorta, and the lower extremity arteries (femoral, popliteal, posterior tibial, and dorsalis pedis) should be a part of every general medical evaluation. Auscultation over the major arteries for bruits is an additional important method for detecting proximal occlusive disease. The degree of any ischemia can be estimated at the bedside or in the office by the observation of elevation pallor (Table 22-1) and the time required for return of color and filling of the veins with dependency after elevation (Table 22-2).

The Allen test (Fig. 22-1, *A, B*) for assessing the adequacy of circulation in the hand is useful when there are symptoms or signs of peripheral arterial disease in the upper extremities, and routinely applying it before and after radial artery puncture is good practice. Another useful maneuver is palpation of the two radial arteries simultaneously; a delay in the pulsation of one may be noted when narrowing of the origin of the ipsilateral subclavian artery (not uncommon) occurs with consequent reversal of flow in the ipsilateral vertebral artery. In addition, compression of the subclavian artery in the thoracic outlet should be evaluated by the thoracic outlet maneuvers (Fig. 22-2, *A, B*).

Objectivity in the diagnosis of peripheral arterial disease has been aided by the development of noninvasive methods, which are useful for detecting occlusive arterial disease, aneurysmal disease, and vasospastic disorders.

Occlusive arterial disease in the lower extremities may be further evaluated by obtaining supine systolic brachial and ankle blood pressures, using a hand-held Doppler ve-

Table 22-1. Grading of elevation pallor*

Grade of pallor	Duration of elevation
0	No pallor in 60 sec
1	Definite pallor in 60 sec
2	Definite pallor in less than 60 sec
3	Definite pallor in less than 30 sec
4	Pallor on the level

From Spittell JA Jr: Recognition and management of chronic atherosclerotic occlusive peripheral arterial disease. Mod Concepts Cardiovasc Dis 50:19, 1981. With permission of American Heart Association, Inc.
*Elevation of extremity at angle of 60 degrees above the level.

Table 22-2. Color return and venous filling times

	Color return (sec)	Venous filling time (sec)
Normal	10	15
Moderate ischemia	15-20	20-30
Severe ischemia	40+	40+

From Spittell JA Jr: Recognition and management of chronic atherosclerotic occlusive peripheral arterial disease. Mod Concepts Cardiovasc Dis 50:19, 1981. With permission of American Heart Association, Inc.

locity transducer and a standard arm blood pressure cuff. Normally, the systolic pressure at the ankle equals or exceeds that at the brachial level; in the case of occlusive arterial disease in the lower extremity, the systolic pressure at the ankle is reduced. Determination of systolic brachial and ankle blood pressures before and after standard exercise is a more sensitive means of detecting occlusive arterial disease, providing an estimate of the degree of disability imposed by any intermittent claudication. Occlusive arterial disease in the upper extremity may be similarly evaluated by measuring systolic pressures in the arm and wrist. Using special cuffs and Doppler instruments, reproducible digital pressures can be determined as well.

More recently, duplex Doppler ultrasound imaging, which combines conventional B-mode ultrasound imaging with range-gated pulsed-wave Doppler, has been used to noninvasively estimate the degree of stenosis of the extracranial carotid and vertebral arteries, and potentially all superficially located peripheral arteries.

Noninvasive testing using 2D ultrasound is the diagnostic method of choice for aneurysmal disease involving the abdominal aorta, iliac artery, and femoral-popliteal arteries.

Although arteriography remains the best procedure for demonstrating the location and extent of occlusive arterial disease and the character of the arterial circulation proximally and distally, it is usually reserved for patients for whom restoration of pulsatile flow is being considered or when the etiology of the occlusive arterial disease is uncertain.

Raynaud's phenomenon can be confirmed by measuring the skin temperature of the digits before and after their immersion in ice water for 30 seconds. Normally, digital skin temperatures return to preimmersion levels in 3 to 10 minutes whereas in patients with a vasospastic disorder, the time required to reach preimmersion temperatures exceeds 10 minutes.

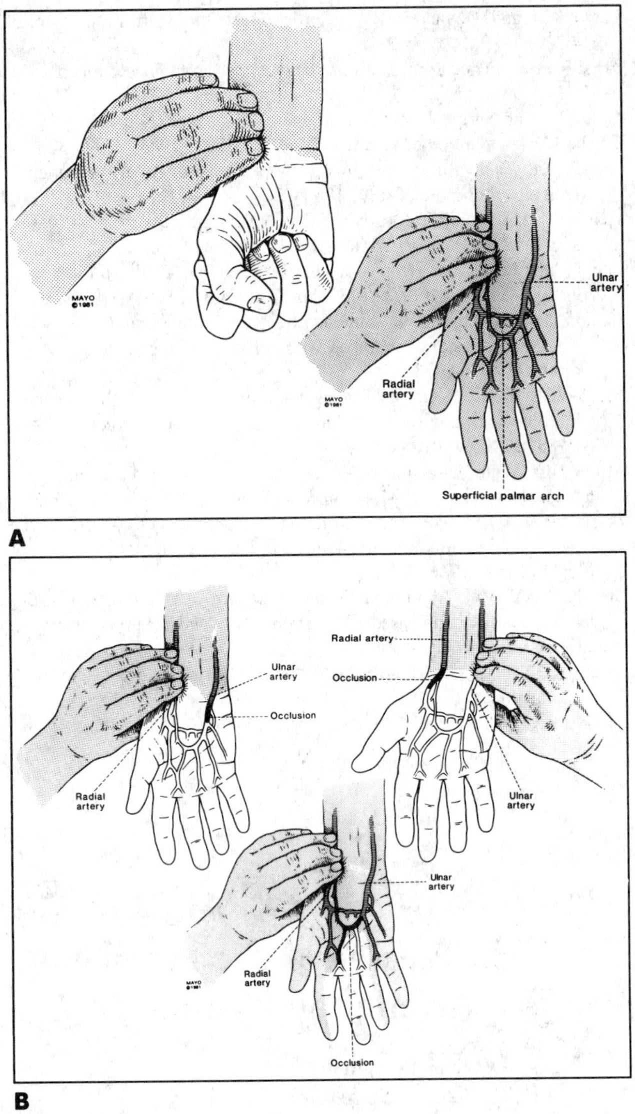

Fig. 22-1. The Allen test. **(A)** Normal (negative) result indicating patency of ulnar artery and superficial palmar arch. **(B)** Abnormal (positive) results caused by occlusion of ulnar artery *(left)*, radial artery *(right)*, and superficial palmar arch *(center)*. (From Spittell JA Jr: Occlusive peripheral arterial disease: guidelines for office management. Postgrad Med 71:137, 1982. With permission of McGraw-Hill Book Company, Inc.)

OCCLUSIVE PERIPHERAL ARTERIAL DISEASE

Occlusive peripheral arterial disease (OPAD), whether acute or chronic, results in ischemia to the affected limb(s) or digit(s) supplied by the affected artery. The symptoms and signs depend on the location and extent of the occlusion and the adequacy of the collateral circulation.

Acute occlusive arterial disease

The etiologies of acute arterial occlusion are enumerated in the box on p. 296. Acute peripheral arterial occlusion can be the initial or dominant manifestation of cardiac or systemic disease, as well as acute aortic dissection. The degree of ischemia depends on the size of the occluded artery and the adequacy of the collateral circulation. Associated arterial spasm, hypotension, and fragmentation of an occluding embolus also influence the impact of an acute arterial occlusion.

The clinical presentation of an acute arterial occlusion is variable and may include any or all of the "five P's"—pain, pallor, paresthesia, pulselessness, and paralysis. Oc-

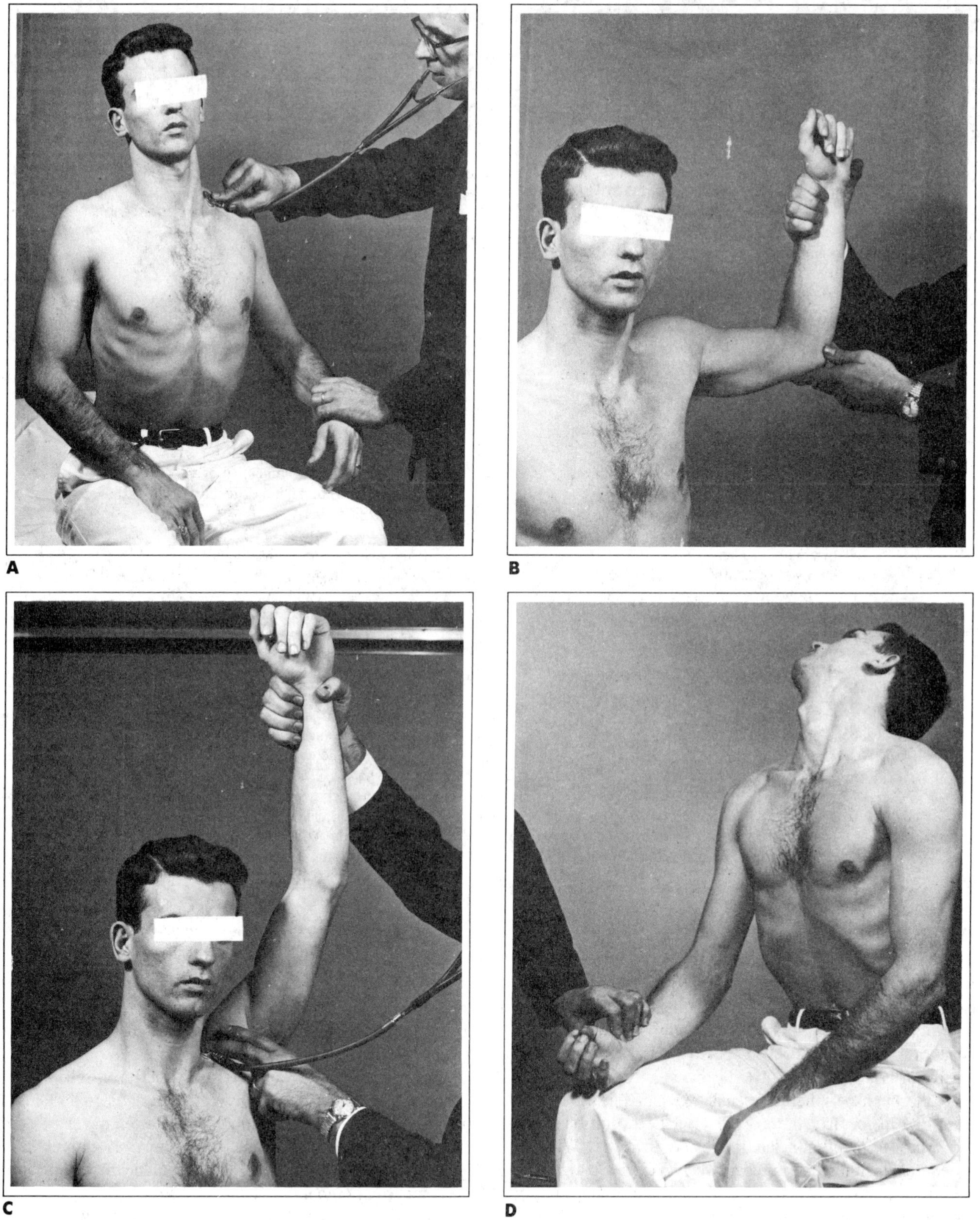

Fig. 22-2. **(A)** Costoclavicular maneuver, active. Auscultation over subclavian artery, above or below midportion of clavicle, may reveal systolic bruit as artery is being compressed. Radial pulse and bruit over subclavian artery disappear when complete compression of subclavian artery occurs. **(B)** Costoclavicular maneuver, passive. **(C)** Hyperabduction maneuver. Axillary artery may be completely or incompletely compressed by maneuver. In latter case, bruit may be heard above or below clavicle or, on occasion, deep in axilla. **(D)** Scalene or Adson's maneuver. This test is used in both cervical rib or anomalous first thoracic rib syndrome and scalenus anticus syndrome. Auscultation over subclavian artery being tested may reveal bruit when artery is partially compressed. (From Fairbairn JF, Campbell JK, and Payne WS: Neurovascular compression syndromes of the thoracic outlet. In Juergens JL, Spittell JA, and Fairbairn JF, editors. Peripheral vascular diseases, ed 5. Philadelphia, 1980, Saunders. With permission of Mayo Foundation.)

Classification of occlusive arterial disease

I. Acute arterial occlusion
  A. Thrombotic arterial occlusion secondary to
    1. Atherosclerosis
      a. Arteriosclerosis obliterans
      b. Atherosclerotic aneurysm
    2. Thromboangiitis obliterans (Buerger's disease)
    3. Arteritis resulting from
      a. Connective tissue diseases
      b. Giant-cell (temporal or cranial) arteritis
      c. Takayasu's arteritis
    4. Myeloproliferative disease
      a. Polycythemia vera
      b. Thrombocytosis
    5. Hypercoagulable states
      a. Complicating neoplastic disease
      b. Complicating ulcerative bowel disease
      c. Idiopathic ("simple") arterial thrombosis
    6. Trauma
      a. Arterial puncture and arteriotomy
      b. Secondary to fractures and bone dislocations
      c. Arterial entrapment
        (1) Lower extremity
          (a) Adductor tendon compression of superficial femoral artery
          (b) Popliteal artery entrapment
        (2) Upper extremity
          (a) Thoracic outlet compression
          (b) "Crutch" thrombosis
      d. Frostbite
  B. Embolic arterial occlusion (arising from thrombi of)
    1. Cardiac origin
      a. Valvular heart disease, including valvular prostheses
      b. Acute myocardial infarction
      c. Myocardial aneurysm
      d. Atrial fibrillation
      e. Cardiomyopathy
      f. Infective endocarditis
      g. Left-sided myxoma
    2. Proximal atherosclerotic plaques or arterial narrowing
    3. Proximal arterial aneurysms
      a. Atherosclerotic
      b. Poststenotic dilatation
      c. Fibromuscular dysplasia
  C. Miscellaneous causes
    1. Arterial spasm, secondary to
      a. Ergotism
      b. Trauma of blunt or penetrating type
      c. Intra-arterial injections
    2. Aortic dissection
      a. Luminal compression (by extension of the dissection into branch[es] of the aorta)
      b. Occlusion at site of reentry of dissection
    3. Foreign bodies
      a. Bullet embolism
      b. Guidewires and catheters

II. Chronic arterial occlusive disease
  A. Arteriosclerosis obliterans
  B. Thromboangiitis obliterans (Buerger's disease)
  C. Arteritis
    1. Connective tissue disorders
    2. Giant-cell (temporal or cranial) arteritis
    3. Takayasu's disease
  D. Trauma
    1. Blunt trauma
      a. Chronic occupational arterial occlusion in the hand
    2. Arterial entrapment
      a. Superficial femoral artery
      b. Popliteal artery
  E. Congenital arterial narrowing

From Spittell JA Jr: Office and bedside diagnosis of occlusive arterial disease. Curr Probl Cardiol 8:1, 1983. With permission of Year Book Medical Publishers, Inc.

casionally, abrupt shortening of the distance necessary to elicit claudication may be the presenting complaint of an acute arterial occlusion in the person with preexisting occlusive arterial disease.

A thorough peripheral vascular examination usually allows one to localize the site of an acute occlusion when the larger- or medium-sized arteries are involved. With arteriolar occlusions, livedo reticularis and cyanotic digits are the manifestations; when there is associated renal insufficiency and hypertension, atheroembolism from proximal atherosclerotic plaques or an aortic aneurysm should be suspected.

The diagnosis of acute arterial occlusion is usually readily apparent after a careful history taking and physical examination. Initial management includes protection of the extremity from trauma, plus pain relief, heparin anticoagulation, and immediate hospitalization. Arteriography and appropriate surgical therapy (thrombectomy or embolectomy) on an emergent basis are indicated to restore adequate circulation to the affected limb.

Embolic arterial occlusions can usually be relieved by embolectomy using a Fogarty catheter. It is important to identify the source of the emboli (most often the heart, less often a proximal arterial aneurysm), then to correct it, if possible, or to institute oral anticoagulant therapy to prevent recurrent embolic arterial occlusion.

Thrombotic arterial occlusion may be managed in several ways, depending on the size of the involved artery, the duration of the arterial occlusion, and the associated underlying disease. Thrombectomy, thrombolysis (often followed by balloon angioplasty [PTA]), and arterial bypass surgery are the available therapeutic options.

In the patient with atheroembolism (cholesterol embolization), surgical resection of the source of the atheromatous debris (aneurysm or atherosclerotic artery) is the only effective therapy; antiplatelet and anticoagulant therapy have not been effective in atheroembolism and at times may even precipitate atheroembolism.

Chronic occlusive arterial disease

Chronic occlusive peripheral arterial disease, most commonly caused by atherosclerosis, results in luminal narrowing of large and medium-sized arteries, especially of the lower extremities. Clinical recognition of chronic occlusive arterial disease, even in its early stages, is important since much of the limb loss that occurs results from preventable trauma to the ischemic limb.

Less common causes of chronic occlusive arterial disease such as thromboangiitis obliterans (TAO, Buerger's disease), trauma, arteritis, and extrinsic compression of arteries (e.g., popliteal artery entrapment) can be suspected at the time of initial evaluation of the patient (see box below). Thromboangiitis obliterans has distinct clinical features (see box at upper right) and deserves special mention because of its consistent relationship to tobacco use. If the patient with TAO abstains from using tobacco, the activity of the disease stops, but it recurs just as surely if tobacco use is resumed.

Differentiation of TAO and occlusive arterial disease of the hand caused by repetitive blunt trauma is also important and can present a diagnostic challenge in a person who smokes. Features suggestive of occlusive arterial disease of the hand caused by repetitive blunt trauma include unilateral symptoms and signs of digital ischemia and/or infarction, most commonly involving the dominant hand in a person whose occupation or leisure activity involves repetitive blunt palmar trauma. Arteriography is usually necessary to establish the diagnosis, and connective tissue disease and diabetes mellitus should be excluded. Treatment of occlusive arterial disease of the hand resulting from repetitive blunt trauma depends upon both the severity of the clinical manifestations and arteriographic findings. Conservative treatment includes protection of the hands from mechanical and thermal trauma, the use of padded gloves, and tobacco cessation. Calcium channel blockers and alpha-1 adrenergic receptor blockers (prazosin, doxazosin) can alleviate episodic digital vasospasm but are of no benefit in treating fixed obstructive arterial disease. For severe cases and those that are refractory to medical therapy, surgical sympathectomy and/or direct revascularization using microvascular techniques are indicated.

The clinical manifestations of chronic occlusive arterial disease are a direct result of ischemia of the tissues of the extremity supplied by the affected arteries. In milder cases there may be no symptoms, and the peripheral arterial examination may be nearly normal. The hallmark of symptomatic occlusive peripheral disease, intermittent claudication, is as typical in its occurrence with walking and its relief with standing still as angina pectoris is with exertion or stress. A careful history and physical examination usually allows differentiation of intermittent claudication from neurologic or musculoskeletal conditions. Pseudoclaudication, resulting from lumbar spinal stenosis, differs from true intermittent claudication in several respects. The patient with pseudoclaudication usually develops symptoms with long standing as well as with walking and only gets relief by sitting down or leaning over some object. Importantly, standing still will not relieve pseudoclaudication, although it does relieve true intermittent claudication.

When ischemia becomes more severe, the patient may develop pain at rest; this usually involves the toes and/or foot, is aggravated by cool temperatures, is often worse at night, and is relieved temporarily by dependency. Ischemic ulceration, commonly resulting from trauma, occurs most often on the toes, heel, or foot. An ischemic ulcer (Fig. 22-3) is painful and on examination has a discrete edge, a pale base, or is covered by an eschar.

All persons with occlusive peripheral arterial disease should be instructed in conservative measures. Avoidance of vasoconstrictive influences such as cold and certain pharmacologic agents (beta-blocking agents, ergot preparations, clonidine) and the complete cessation of tobacco use should be stressed. The need for tobacco cessation is of paramount importance for the patient with intermittent claudication. Epidemiologic studies have demonstrated that 5-year mortality, major amputation rate, and the need for revascularization are all significantly increased in persons who continue to smoke compared to those who stop smoking (27% versus 12%, 11% versus 0%, and 31% versus 8%, respectively).

Clinical features of thromboangiitis obliterans

More common in young (less than 30 years of age) males
Activity of disease correlates with tobacco use
Small arteries and veins of upper and lower extremities involved, producing
  Migratory superficial thrombophlebitis
  Claudication of arch and/or calf

Clinical features suggesting uncommon types of occlusive arterial disease

Person younger than age 40
Acute ischemia in the absence of prior evidence of occlusive arterial disease
Occlusive arterial disease confined to the upper extremity
Digital occlusive arterial disease, particularly if accompanied by systemic symptoms

From Spittell JA Jr and Spittell PC: Diseases of the aorta and peripheral arteries. In Parmley W and Chatterjee K, editors: Cardiology. Philadelphia, 1987, Lippincott. With permission.

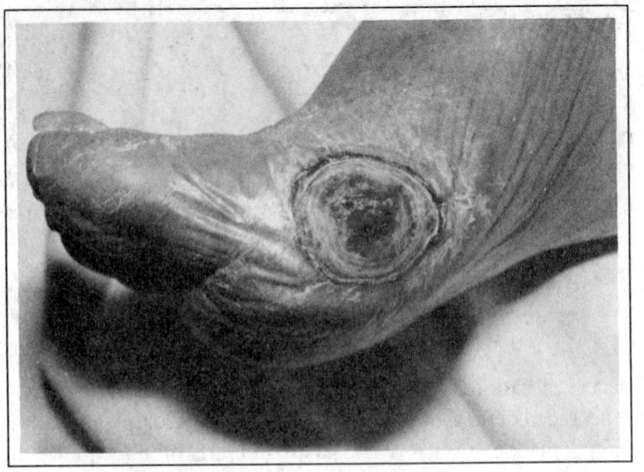

Fig. 22-3. Ischemic ulceration of the foot.

The risk factors for atherosclerosis such as obesity, diabetes mellitus, hyperlipidemia, and hypertension should also be modified. When intermittent claudication is the major complaint, a program of walking to the point of claudication, several times a day, may improve walking distance. Vasodilators are of no benefit in the symptomatic treatment of intermittent claudication. Pentoxifylline (a methylxanthine), which is reported to lower blood viscosity and decrease erythrocyte rigidity, may improve the walking distance of some patients with intermittent claudication. Recent data indicate that the likelihood of successful treatment with pentoxifylline is increased in a "target" population consisting of persons with a history of intermittent claudication for more than 1 year and an ankle/brachial index of 0.8 or less.

Reconstructive arterial surgery for chronic occlusive arterial disease has specific indications. These include the relief of disabling claudication (see box below), improved prognosis for limb survival in the diabetic patient (see box at upper right), as well as the need to relieve rest pain and to heal ischemic ulcerations. Percutaneous balloon angioplasty (PTA) provides a means of restoring pulsatile arterial blood flow with reduced morbidity, mortality, and cost when compared to arterial surgery. The indications for PTA are the same as for reconstructive arterial surgery except that PTA is most successful for focal lesions (less than 10 cm in length) in the iliac, femoral, and popliteal arteries. Surgical sympathectomy is reserved for the patient in whom restoration of pulsatile blood flow is not possible, as an aid to the healing of ischemic ulceration.

Restoration of pulsatile flow in chronic atherosclerotic occlusive arterial disease with rest pain or ischemic ulceration

1. The incidence of limb loss is relatively high without treatment.
2. It may permit a lower level of amputation.
3. The risks of the procedure are less than the risk of amputation

From Spittell JA Jr: Peripheral vascular disease: advances in diagnosis and management. Baylor Cardiology Series 7:1, 1984. With permission of Associates in Medical Marketing.

Elective restoration of pulsatile flow to limb in chronic atherosclerotic occlusive arterial disease with intermittent claudication

1. It does not affect longevity or ameliorate coronary or cerebrovascular disease.
2. The incidence of severe ischemia is relatively low.
3. Runoff should be adequate.
4. Complications of the procedure, though infrequent, do occur.
5. Reocclusion may occur.

From Spittell JA Jr: Peripheral vascular disease: advances in diagnosis and management. Baylor Cardiology Series 7:1, 1984. With permission of Associates in Medical Marketing.

PERIPHERAL ARTERIAL ANEURYSMS

Peripheral arterial aneurysms are most commonly caused by atherosclerosis; thus they are more common in males over 50 years of age. Less common causes of aneurysmal disease include inherited elastic tissue defects (Marfan, Ehlers-Danlos, and fragile X syndromes), infections, arteritides, congenital defects, and trauma. Regardless of etiology, aneurysmal disease is related to weakening of the media of the artery. Hypertension often coexists and directly or indirectly contributes to weakening of the arterial wall and expansion of the aneurysm.

Once initiated, aneurysmal dilatation tends to be progressive. Progressive enlargement of the aneurysm and slowing of flow contribute to the formation of laminated mural thrombus, which may progress to complete thrombosis of the lumen or be the source of emboli in the distal arterial circulation; as an aneurysm enlarges, it may exert pressure on surrounding structures and/or rupture.

When uncomplicated, aneurysms produce no symptoms or findings other than a pulsatile mass. Compression of surrounding structures, such as veins, may produce symptoms and signs of chronic venous obstruction. Rupture of an aneurysm presents acutely, usually with evidence of pain and bleeding. Less commonly, when rupture is into a companion vein, the acute development of signs of an arteriovenous fistula is the mode of presentation.

Ultrasound is currently the preferred method to detect and determine the size and extent of an abdominal aortic aneurysm. Computed tomography scanning with intravenous contrast is also an excellent, but more expensive, method of diagnosis. Aortography is usually reserved for patients in whom there is associated peripheral, renal, or mesenteric occlusive arterial disease.

The risk of rupture of an abdominal aortic aneurysm smaller than 4 cm is small but increases progressively as an aneurysm reaches 5 cm in diameter. Elective surgical resection is indicated in most patients with aneurysm diameter exceeding 4.5 cm, in the absence of other significant medical problems. Other indications for surgical intervention include a symptomatic (painful) aneurysm or an aneurysm enlarging under observation.

In the extremities, atherosclerotic aneurysms are most commonly found in the femoral and popliteal arteries. The aneurysm is bilateral in over half of the patients; more than 40% of patients with popliteal artery aneurysm have aneurysmal disease involving the abdominal aorta, femoral, or popliteal arteries. The most common complication of femoropopliteal aneurysms is thromboembolic. Surgical resection produces the best results when carried out before complications occur.

Atheroembolism occasionally complicates abdominal aortic aneurysms, producing a distinctive clinical picture of livedo reticularis, blue toes, hypertension, and renal insufficiency. Prompt recognition of this symptom complex is important because resection of the aneurysm is the only effective treatment. Unilateral atheroembolism—livedo reticularis and blue toes—may occur with femoropopliteal aneurysm; again, resection of the aneurysm is the only effective therapy.

Aneurysms involving the upper-extremity arteries are usually the result of blunt or penetrating trauma; in the subclavian artery they result from compression of the artery between the uppermost rib and clavicle. Thromboembolism from mural thrombus to the distal arterial circulation may be the first manifestation of aneurysms in the upper extremity.

VASOSPASTIC DISORDERS

The vasospastic disorders (see box below)—Raynaud's phenomenon, livedo reticularis, acrocyanosis, chronic pernio, and reflex sympathetic dystrophy—involve the small arteries and arterioles in the digits and skin, producing changes in skin color and temperature. The vasospastic disorders are transient, reversible, and precipitated by exposure to cold, emotional stress, or other vasoconstrictive influences (Table 22-3).

Raynaud's phenomenon, the most common vasospastic disorder, is defined as brief and intermittent color changes (usually triphasic—pallor, cyanosis, rubor) involving the digits and precipitated by exposure to cold or stress. Raynaud's disease (primary Raynaud's phenomenon) is a benign disorder; secondary Raynaud's phenomenon occurs with a broad spectrum of underlying disorders, and at times the Raynaud's phenomenon is the initial clue to the underlying disorder (see box, p. 300). An evaluation of the patient with Raynaud's phenomenon should consider the causes listed in the box on p. 300. If the initial evaluation is negative, the patient should be observed for a period of 2 years before a diagnosis of Raynaud's disease can be made. Management of all patients includes protection from cold and avoidance of causes of vasoconstriction (tobacco, trauma, and drugs). In addition, a trial of an alpha$_2$ blocker such as prazosin (1 to 2 mg b.i.d.) or of a calcium blocker such as nifedipine (10 mg t.i.d.) may be useful in reducing vasospastic episodes. Biofeedback is useful in younger patients and in those whose occupation precludes pharmacologic therapy. Sympathectomy is generally reserved for patients with Raynaud's disease who are refractory to the above therapies. In secondary Raynaud's phenomenon, results of sympathectomy are unfortunately less beneficial.

Livedo reticularis is a bluish-purple mottling of the skin of the extremities caused by spasm of dermal arterioles. Like Raynaud's phenomenon it is classified into primary and secondary forms. The differentiation of primary and secondary livedo reticularis is based on clinical and laboratory features (see box, p. 300). The management of idiopathic livedo reticularis includes protection from cold and reassurance; for more symptomatic patients, a trial of prazosin or nifedipine may be beneficial. Lumbar sympathectomy is reserved for ischemic ulceration not controlled by medication.

Chronic pernio is a vasospastic disorder of the toes seen most commonly in women with a prior history of cold injury. With the onset of cold weather each year, erythematous, cyanotic, and hemorrhagic vesiculation and/or ulcerative lesions of the toes occur. These resolve spontaneously

Vasospastic disorders

- Raynaud's phenomenon
  - Primary (Raynaud's disease)
  - Secondary
- Livedo reticularis
  - Primary
  - Secondary
- Acrocyanosis
- Reflex sympathetic dystrophy
- Chronic pernio

From Spittell JA Jr and Spittell PC: Diseases of the aorta and peripheral arteries. In Parmley W and Chatterjee K, editors: Cardiology. Philadelphia, 1987, Lippincott. With permission.

Table 22-3. Differential diagnosis of vasospastic and occlusive arterial disease

	Vasospastic disorders	Occlusive arterial disease
Arteries involved	Small	All
Color changes	+	±
Claudication	−	+
Absent pulses	−	+
Ischemic ulceration	±	±
Major gangrene	−	±

From Spittell JA Jr: The vasospastic disorders. Curr Probl Cardiol 8:1, 1984. With permission of Year Book Medical Publishers.

Conditions that may cause secondary Raynaud's phenomenon

A. After trauma
  1. Related to occupation
    a. Pneumatic hammer disease
    b. Occupational occlusive arterial disease of the hand
    c. Occupational acro-osteolysis
    d. Vasospasm of typists and pianists
  2. Following injury or operation
B. Neurologic conditions
  1. Thoracic outlet syndrome
  2. Carpal tunnel syndrome
  3. Other neurologic diseases
C. Occlusive arterial disease
  1. Arteriosclerosis obliterans
  2. Thromboangiitis obliterans
  3. Postembolic or postthrombotic arterial occlusion
D. Miscellaneous conditions
  1. Scleroderma
  2. Lupus erythematosus
  3. Rheumatoid arthritis
  4. Dermatomyositis
  5. Fabry's disease
  6. Paroxysmal hemoglobinuria
  7. Cold agglutinins or cryoglobulinemia
  8. Primary pulmonary hypertension
  9. Myxedema
  10. Associated with certain neoplasms
  11. Associated with hepatitis B antigenemia
  12. Pheochromocytoma
  13. Ergotism
  14. After combination chemotherapy for testicular cancer

Adapted from Spittell JA Jr: Vasospastic disorders: recognition and management. Cardiovasc Clin 10:279, 1980. With permission of F.A. Davis Co.

in the spring with warmer weather. Small doses of prazosin (1 mg once or twice daily) are extremely effective in preventing and treating symptomatic chronic pernio.

Acrocyanosis is a benign disorder resulting in almost constant coldness and bluish discoloration of the hands and fingers and occasionally the feet and toes. It is important not to confuse this disorder with the cyanotic phase of Raynaud's phenomenon. A right-to-left shunt and methemoglobinemia should be excluded. Reassurance that it is a benign condition is all that most patients need.

Although reflex sympathetic dystrophy is basically a neurologic disorder, vasospastic phenomena—coldness and cyanosis—are present and can be relieved by prazosin (1 mg once or twice daily), which aids in the rehabilitation process.

ARTERITIS

The arteritides known to involve the extremity arteries include scleroderma, systemic lupus erythematosus, periarteritis nodosa, giant-cell arteritis, and Takayasu's arteritis.

Procedures to evaluate recent Raynaud's phenomenon

History (include drugs)
Exam
  Thoracic outlet maneuvers
  Allen's test
Lab
  Blood count
  Sedimentation rate
  Protein electrophoresis
  Antinuclear antibody
  Cold agglutinins
  Cryoglobulin
  Urinalysis
  Other "indicated" by history or physical findings

From Spittell JA Jr and Spittell PC: Diseases of the aorta and peripheral arteries. In Parmley W and Chatterjee K, editors: Cardiology. Philadelphia, 1987, Lippincott. With permission.

Except for in the last two, arteriography is of little value in this group of disorders.

Takayasu's arteritis, or pulseless disease, is a chronic focal arteritis of the aorta and large elastic arteries seen predominantly in women less than 40 years of age. Aortic valve regurgitation is often present (Chapter 16). It involves the outer media and adventitia of the aorta and larger elastic arteries. Early in the disease nonspecific systemic manifestations such as malaise, low-grade fever, arthralgia, and weight loss are seen. Later, the symptoms of arterial insufficiency develop depending on the degree of arterial occlusion. Laboratory findings at the onset of the disease include an elevated erythrocyte sedimentation rate, mild anemia, and leukocytosis; later characteristic findings of occlusive arterial disease develop. Arteriography shows focal, segmental stenosis with smooth, tapered walls.

Management in the acute phase of Takayasu's arteritis includes adequate doses of corticosteroids; immunosuppressive agents have been used with success in some cases. In

Classification of livedo reticularis

Primary (idiopathic) livedo reticularis
Secondary livedo reticularis
  Connective tissue diseases
  Vasculitis
  Myeloproliferative disorders
  Dysproteinemias
  Atheroembolism (cholesterol embolization)
  After cold injury
  Use of amantadine hydrochloride (Symmetrel)
  Reflex sympathetic dystrophy

From Spittell JA Jr: Vasospastic disorders. Cardiovasc Clin 13:75, 1983. With permission of F.A. Davis Co.

the late inactive phase general measures for occlusive arterial disease are used, and arterial bypass grafting or balloon angioplasty can be used to relieve significant residual ischemia when the activity of the disease is suppressed. The overall prognosis is variable and depends on the arteries involved and the promptness and adequacy of treatment.

Giant-cell arteritis (cranial arteritis, temporal arteritis) is a granulomatous arteritis that affects segments of major arteries and the aorta, particularly branches of the carotid system, in persons more than 60 years of age. Although the most common symptoms of giant-cell arteritis are throbbing headaches and scalp tenderness and the major complication is loss of vision, involvement of other large arteries is being recognized with increasing frequency. Patients may develop intermittent claudication of the upper and/or lower extremities, and this may be a dominant feature. Arteriography is useful when there is peripheral arterial involvement; it shows smooth, tapering segmental stenosis in otherwise normal-appearing arteries. Definitive diagnosis is made by biopsy of a temporal or occipital artery and is recommended since corticosteroid therapy must sometimes be prolonged to control the arteritis. With steroid therapy the activity of giant-cell arteritis subsides; peripheral arterial involvement and resultant symptoms may require a prolonged course of corticosteroid therapy for control. Untreated, giant-cell arteritis is usually self-limited, lasting 1 to 5 years. A rare complication of giant-cell arteritis is aortic dissection.

DISEASES OF THE VEINS

Varicose veins are the most common peripheral vascular disorder affecting the lower extremity. Primary varicose veins are caused by a hereditary weakness of the vein wall and valves, whereas secondary varicose veins result from deep venous obstruction. Obesity, orthostatism, pregnancy, ascites, and right heart failure favor the formation of varicose veins. Symptoms vary from none to complaints of aching, heaviness, and swelling of the lower extremities. On examination dilated tortuous veins are seen with the patient standing, and there may be stasis changes of the skin of the medial aspect of the distal leg. The patient with primary varicose veins will usually describe disease that progresses distally from the upper thigh, whereas secondary varicose veins usually spread proximally from the lower leg. Nonspecific treatment of varicose veins includes adequate elastic support stockings. Sclerotherapy and surgical stripping of varicose veins are indicated for those who fail more conservative therapy or those with recurrent superficial thrombophlebitis or cosmetic problems caused by large varicosities.

Venous thrombosis complicates many types of surgical and medical illnesses and is a common cause of morbidity and mortality despite increased attention to early and accurate diagnosis. An increased incidence of venous thrombosis occurs in patients in the postoperative state and with trauma, congestive heart failure, malignant disease, myeloproliferative disease, obesity, oral contraceptives, tamoxifen, and inherited coagulapathies such as antithrombin III deficiency, protein C deficiency, and protein S deficiency.

Recurrent venous (and arterial) thrombosis is also associated with the presence of antiphospholipid antibodies, a heterogeneous group of autoantibodies to anionic phospholipids. Primary (idiopathic) and secondary (connective tissue and autoimmune diseases) antiphospholipid syndromes have both been associated with recurrent large- and small-vessel arterial and venous thrombosis, recurrent fetal loss, transient ischemic attack, cerebrovascular accident, cerebral venous thrombosis, thrombocytopenia, and livedo reticularis. Of note is the association of mitral and aortic valvular lesions, especially in persons with recurrent arterial thrombosis. The presence of antiphospholipid antibodies should be suspected in persons with unexplained recurrent venous and arterial thrombosis and in persons with an underlying connective tissue or autoimmune disease. Anticardiolipin antibodies can be readily identified using an enzyme-linked immunosorbent assay (ELISA). Therapy consists of treatment of the underlying disorder, if present, and long-term anticoagulation with warfarin in all patients with venous or arterial thrombosis associated with the presence of antiphospholipid antibodies. Subcutaneous heparin therapy may be an alternative in women of child-bearing age and during pregnancy.

Superficial thrombophlebitis presents as a firm, red, tender cord or nodule and is readily recognized on examination. It must be differentiated from acute lymphangiitis, cellulitis, and inflammatory nodular conditions such as erythema nodosum or vasculitis. The management of superficial thrombophlebitis includes warm, moist packs for pain relief and aspirin to decrease associated inflammation. For recurrent disease oral anticoagulant therapy may be used prophylactically.

The clinical presentation of deep venous thrombosis is highly variable and often necessitates the use of noninvasive and invasive diagnostic techniques for confirmation. Noninvasive diagnosis can be accomplished using Doppler flow-velocity studies and impedance plethysmography; these will confirm most deep venous thrombosis proximal to the calf veins. Duplex Doppler imaging can now reliably examine the deep venous system of the leg from the level of the common femoral vein to the distal popliteal vein and has become the noninvasive screening examination of choice for patients suspected of having deep venous thrombosis. The reported sensitivity of duplex Doppler imaging for detecting deep venous thrombosis in the femoral and popliteal veins is 89% to 100%, and the specificity is 97% to 100%. Limitations of duplex Doppler imaging for suspected deep venous thrombosis include poor visualization of the inferior vena cava and iliac veins as well as incomplete visualization of the numerous branches of the deep venous system of the calf. When results are equivocal, contrast venography remains the accepted standard in diagnosis. Pulmonary embolism remains the most serious complication and is seen most commonly with popliteal and thigh vein thrombosis, the latter posing a significantly higher risk.

Management of deep venous thrombosis begins with identification of patients with predisposing factors. Once identified, prophylaxis is accomplished by early ambulation, anticoagulant therapy, or intermittent calf compression in the patient at risk. Small-dose subcutaneous heparin (5000 units q8-12h) has proved effective in preventing deep venous thrombosis in general medical and surgical patients.

Once thrombosis has occurred, anticoagulant therapy is the treatment of choice, if no contraindications exist. Initial anticoagulation with intravenous heparin is followed by oral anticoagulant therapy, which is continued for 3 to 6 months. Thrombolytic therapy, with streptokinase or urokinase, followed by heparin and then oral anticoagulant therapy to prevent recurrent thrombosis, is the preferred treatment in extensive deep venous thrombosis (which is more likely to progress to chronic venous insufficiency if heparin therapy is used alone). As with anticoagulant therapy, the main contraindications to thrombolytic therapy relate to bleeding. Additional measures include bed rest with elevation of the involved extremity, along with the application of local warm packs. Surgical treatment of deep venous thrombosis is largely limited to inferior vena cava interruption in patients with a contraindication to anticoagulant or thrombolytic therapy, or in those who have recurrent pulmonary emboli despite adequate anticoagulant therapy.

Chronic venous insufficiency usually results from postphlebitic valvular incompetence or varicose veins with underlying dysfunction of venous valves. Recent investigation has implicated leukocyte trapping and "activation" in the microvasculature as a possible factor in the pathogenesis of venous ulceration. The clinical presentation of patients with chronic venous insufficiency is similar to that described for varicose veins, although the manifestations of venous stasis are usually more pronounced. Characteristic findings include dependent edema, cutaneous venous breakdown, and stasis changes (pigmentation, dermatitis, and ulceration). Therapy of chronic venous insufficiency includes adequate elastic support to prevent complications. Stasis dermatitis and stasis ulceration are both treated with bed rest, elevation of the foot of the bed, and intermittent moist dressings of normal saline; skin grafting is desirable for larger ulcers that require more than 2 or 3 weeks to heal. Additional measures include weight reduction in obese patients, low-sodium diets to help prevent leg edema, and adequate elastic support after healing. The overall outlook with chronic venous insufficiency is good with the regular use of adequate elastic support. Recently, the topical application of growth factors derived from homologous platelets has been shown to improve the healing rate of venous ulceration. Outpatient treatment with platelet-derived growth factors, applied topically to a wound twice a day for 8 weeks, can be accomplished using approximately 6 ounces of the patient's peripheral blood.

REFERENCES

Atri SC et al: Use of homologous platelet factors in achieving total healing of recalcitrant skin ulcers. Surgery 108:508, 1990.

Bickerstaff CK et al: Abdominal aortic aneurysms, the changing natural history. J Vasc Surg 1:6, 1984.

Carter SA: Arterial auscultation in peripheral vascular disease. JAMA 246:1682, 1981.

Cooke JB and Spittell JA Jr: Venous thromboembolism. Acute Care 12:118, 1986.

Doubilet P and Abrams HL: The cost of underutilization. Percutaneous transluminal angioplasty for peripheral vascular disease. N Engl J Med 310:96, 1984.

Hirsh J: Prophylaxis of venous thromboembolism. Mod Concepts Cardiovasc Dis 53:25, 1984.

Langsfeld M et al: The use of deep duplex scanning to predict hemodynamically significant aortoiliac stenoses. J Vasc Surg 7:395, 1988.

Lensing AWA et al: Detection of deep-vein thrombosis by real-time B-mode ultrasonography. N Eng J Med 320:342, 1989.

Lindgarde F et al: Conservative drug treatment in patients with moderately severe chronic occlusive peripheral arterial disease. Circulation 80:1549, 1989.

Love PE et al: Antiphospholipid antibodies: anticardiolipin and the lupus anticoagulant in systemic lupus erythematosus (SLE) and in non-SLE disorders. Ann Intern Med 112:682, 1990.

Pairolero PC et al: Subclavian-axillary artery aneurysms. Surgery 90:757, 1981.

Pederson OM et al: Compression ultrasonography in hospitalized patients with suspected deep venous thrombosis. Arch Intern Med 151:2217, 1991.

Rooke TW et al: Percutaneous transluminal angioplasty in the lower extremities: a 5 year experience. Mayo Clin Proc 62:85, 1987.

Smith C et al: Causes of venous ulceration: a new hypothesis. Br Med J 296:1726, 1988.

Spittell JA Jr: Abdominal aortic aneurysms. Hosp Pract 21:105, 1986.

Spittell JA Jr: Hypertension and arterial aneurysm. J Am Coll Cardiol 1:523, 1983.

Spittell JA Jr: Pentoxifylline and intermittent claudication. Ann Intern Med 102:126, 1985.

Spittell JA Jr: Some uncommon types of occlusive arterial disease. Curr Probl Cardiol 8:3, 1983.

Spittell JA Jr: Vasospastic disorders. Curr Probl Cardiol 8:1, 1984.

Spittell PC and Spittell JA: Occlusive arterial disease of the hand due to repetitive blunt trauma. A review with illustrative cases. Int J Cardiol (in press).

McDaniel MD and Cronenwett JL: Basic data related to the natural history of intermittent claudication. Ann Vasc Surg 3:273, 1989.

Wheeler HB: A modern approach to diagnosing deep venous thrombosis. Cardiovasc Med 5:217, 1980.

CHAPTER

23 Arterial Hypertension

Norman M. Kaplan

In the 1980s, the treatment of hypertension became the leading indication both for visits to physicians' offices and for the use of prescription drugs in the United States. In the 1990s, this growth will be further accelerated by the inclusion of elderly patients with isolated systolic hypertension now that treatment has been shown to be beneficial for them as well.

The major growth has had both positive and negative effects. The positive is the contribution that the reduction of blood pressure has made to the marked decrease in cardiovascular mortality in the United States since 1968. The more widespread treatment of hypertension has been responsible for much of the dramatic decrease in stroke and, to a lesser but uncertain extent, ischemic heart disease mortality.

On the other hand, the identification and drug treatment of millions more persons as hypertensives have had some undesirable consequences. First, many persons are being falsely labeled as hypertensive on the basis of initially elevated readings that do not remain high. As a result, they may carry psychological burdens that increase neurotic behavior and, more measurably, increase absenteeism from work. Second, many persons are being given drugs that may increase the risks of cardiovascular disease from various metabolic alterations at the same time that they reduce the risks for lowering the blood pressure, resulting in a stand-off or even a negative overall effect. Third, and probably considered least of all, the therapies of hypertension, both drug and nondrug, may interfere with the quality of life; thus, they may prolong life a bit but make it less worth living.

There is a need, then, to consider the evidence about the true frequency of hypertension, the risks of the untreated disease, and the rationale and practices of therapy in hopes of maximizing the benefits while minimizing the risks of treatment.

FREQUENCY OF HYPERTENSION

The frequency of hypertension rises progressively with the age of the population. The data in Fig. 23-1 were obtained in the 1976 to 1980 Health and Nutrition Examination Survey II (HANES II) of over 16,000 persons carefully chosen to be a representative sample of the American population. The criterion for the presence of hypertension was a systolic blood pressure of at least 140 mm Hg or a diastolic blood pressure of at least 90 mm Hg.

The rise in systolic blood pressure that is common in older persons is responsible for the progressive increase in the prevalence of hypertension as defined in the HANES II study after age 55. Among the general population, diastolic pressures tend to rise little after age 45, reflecting the usual appearance of primary (essential) hypertension by that time. Pure or predominant systolic hypertension should be considered separately from the combined systolic and diastolic elevations seen with primary hypertension. Although they share many risks, they are different in pathogenesis and management.

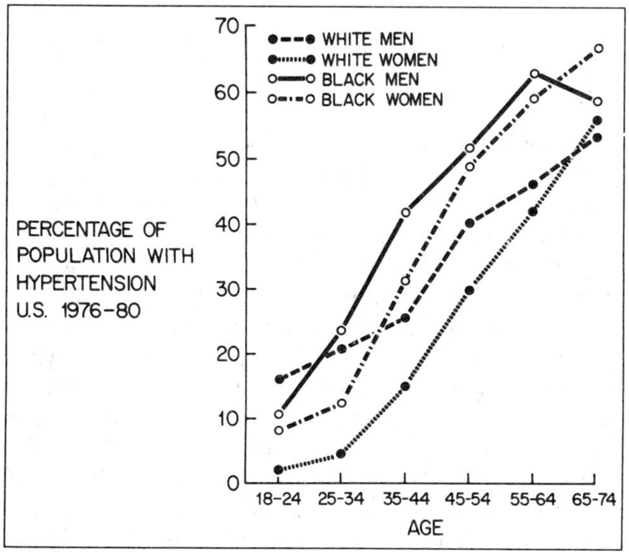

Fig. 23-1. The prevalence of hypertension among white and black men and women in the United States defined as systolic of 140 mm Hg and/or diastolic of 90 mm Hg or higher. (From Rowland M and Roberts J: Health and Nutrition Examination Survey II. Advance data, vital and health statistics of the National Center for Health Statistics, No. 84, October 8, 1982.)

Another problem with survey data such as those summarized in Fig. 23-1 is their reliance on single measurements in the face of a tendency for initial blood pressure readings to be higher than subsequent readings. For example, in the screening program for the Hypertension Detection and Follow-up Program (HDFP), among the white men whose second reading at the initial home visit was over 95 mm Hg diastolic, 44% were below 90 mm Hg at the second examination. Part of this tendency for repeated blood pressures to be lower reflects the regression toward the mean observed with repeated measurements of all biologic variables: outlying values, either high or low, tend to come toward the mean when repeated measurements are taken. A larger part of the tendency probably reflects the relief from some of the anxiety associated with initial examinations. Even after repeated visits, readings taken by a physician are usually higher than those obtained by a nurse and higher to an even greater degree than those obtained by the patient at home. The prevalence of "office" or "white-coat" hypertension is around 20% so that, if at all possible, out-of-the-office readings should be obtained both in diagnosing and monitoring hypertension.

Beyond the tendency for office readings to be higher, the blood pressure is markedly variable under ordinary conditions. This variability has been increasingly apparent with the wider use of ambulatory measurements over periods of 24 hours or longer. As seen in Fig. 23-2, readings vary a good deal during the day, mainly in relation to physical activity, and fall during sleep, only to rise abruptly upon arising. The early morning increase in sudden death, heart attacks, and strokes reflects, at least in part, this abrupt rise in blood pressure.

Precautions in measuring blood pressure

To minimize errors caused by variability, three readings should be taken each time and the average recorded. Additional precautions are given in the box on p. 305. Particular emphasis should be given to ensuring that the patient is as near basal level as possible, avoiding cigarettes, coffee, physical exertion, and anxiety-inducing activities. Attention should be paid to the use of properly functioning gauges and appropriately sized cuffs.

In the absence of automatic ambulatory recordings, multiple readings taken by the patient outside the physician's office may be used to establish the usual range of the blood pressure. The average of the readings taken under various circumstances may be taken since there is increasing evidence that the risks of hypertention are most closely pre-

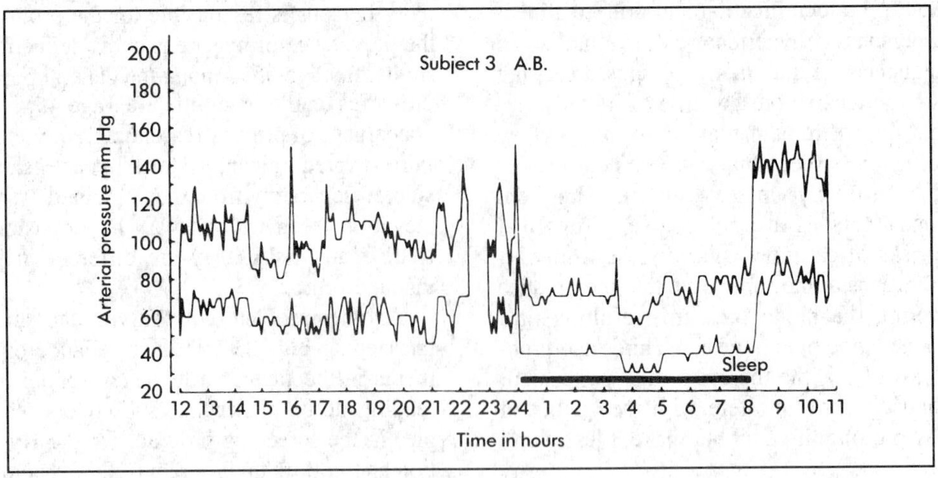

Fig. 23-2. Arterial pressure, plotted at 5 min intervals, of subject A.B. The period of sleep is shown by the horizontal bar. The high pressures shown at 16.00 and 24.00 hours result from a painful stimulus and coitus, respectively. (From Bevan AT et al: Clin Sci 36:329, 1969.)

dicted by the average of multiple out-of-the-office readings. In the study by Perloff, Sokolow, and Cowan of over 1000 patients, by far the majority had average ambulatory readings that were lower than those taken in their physician's office and they had significantly lower cardiovascular morbidity and mortality than did those whose ambulatory readings were as high as the office readings. Similarly, the degree of target organ damage, in particular the presence of left ventricular hypertrophy by echocardiography, has been shown to correlate better with the average ambulatory reading than with the office readings.

Definition of hypertension

Regardless of the problems in defining the usual or average blood pressure, there is a need for standard criteria to diagnose and categorize patients by. Despite the arbitrariness of the division, the upper limit of normal blood pressure is usually taken as 140/90 mm Hg in the office setting and as 160/95 mm Hg in community screening.

In view of the expected variability, a practical approach is to consider initial readings greater than 140/90 mm Hg as "suspicious" and to diagnose "hypertension" only if the average of readings at a third office visit is higher than 140/90 mm Hg. The term *labile* should be discarded. Patients with only occasional high readings may be called *borderline* and advised to keep close check on their blood pressure while also modifying their lifestyles to prevent a further rise. Since the systolic blood pressure tends to rise with the progressive large-vessel atherosclerosis that usually accompanies aging, a leve' greater than 160 mm Hg after age 60 seems to be an appropriate upper limit of normal.

For children, the recommendations of the 1987 Task Force on Blood Pressure Control in Children are based on readings persistently above the ninety-fifth percentile for age and sex (Table 23-1).

Table 23-1. Recommendations of the 1987 Task Force on Blood Pressure Control in Children based on readings above the ninety-fifth percentile for age and sex

Age (yr)	Significant hypertension (mm Hg)
3-5	116/76
6-9	122/78
10-12	126/82
13-15	136/86
16-18	142/92

Risks of hypertension

The level of the blood pressure remains the most direct risk factor for premature cardiovascular disease, every increment of pressure being associated with a greater overall risk for both stroke and coronary heart disease (Fig. 23-3). In the Framingham study, the systolic blood pressure was more closely correlated with risk than was the diastolic.

A number of other factors are also responsible for the development of the cardiovascular complications of hypertension. The patient's demographic features play a role. At any given level of blood pressure, women are at less risk than men, and blacks are at higher risk than whites. The elderly, who have more underlying atherosclerosis as a result of aging, develop complications more quickly than the younger in similar settings. However, all things being equal, the earlier the onset of hypertension, the greater the eventual likelihood of cardiovascular disease.

The degree of target organ damage that occurs in response to any given level of blood pressure varies considerably and obviously needs to be carefully assessed.

Guidelines in measuring blood pressure

I. Conditions for the patient
  A. Posture
    1. Some prefer readings after patient has been supine for 5 minutes. Sitting pressures usually are adequate.
    2. Patient should sit quietly with back supported for 5 minutes and the arm supported at the level of the heart.
    3. For patients who are over age 65, diabetic, or receiving antihypertensive therapy, check for postural changes by taking readings immediately and 2 minutes after patient stands.
  B. Circumstances
    1. No caffeine for preceding hour.
    2. No smoking for preceding 15 minutes.
    3. No exogenous adrenergic stimulants, for example, phenylephrine in nasal decongestants or eye drops for pupillary dilation.
    4. A quiet, warm setting.
    5. Home readings taken under varying circumstances; 24-hour ambulatory recordings may be preferable and more accurate in predicting subsequent cardiovascular disease.

II. Equipment
  A. Cuff size: The bladder should encircle and cover two thirds of the length of the arm; if not, place the bladder over the brachial artery; if bladder is too small, spuriously high readings may result.
  B. Manometer: Aneroid gauges should be calibrated every 6 months against a mercury manometer.
  C. For infants, use equipment employing ultrasound, for example, the Doppler method.

III. Technique
  A. Number of readings
    1. On each occasion, take at least two readings, separated by as much time as is practical. If readings vary by more than 5 mm Hg, take additional readings until two are close.
    2. For diagnosis, obtain three sets of readings at least a week apart.
    3. Initially, take pressure in both arms; if pressure differs, use arm with higher pressure.
    4. If arm pressure is elevated, take pressure in one leg, particularly in patients below age 30.
  B. Performance
    1. Inflate the bladder quickly to a pressure of 20 mm Hg above the systolic, as recognized by disappearance of the radial pulse.
    2. Deflate the bladder 3 mg Hg every second.
    3. Record the Korotkoff phase V (disappearance) except in children, in whom use of phase IV (muffling) is advocated.
    4. If Korotkoff sounds are weak, have the patient raise the arm, open and close the hand five to ten times, after which the bladder should be inflated quickly.

From Kaplan NM: Clinical hypertension, ed 5. Baltimore, 1990, Williams and Wilkins.

The presence of other risk factors along with hypertension may be the strongest and most important determinant of cardiovascular complications, particularly since it may be possible to modify them along with the blood pressure. The Framingham study clearly portrays the interaction between the blood pressure and the other major risk factors, namely hypercholesterolemia, cigarette smoking, abnormal glucose tolerance, and left ventricular hypertrophy on electrocardiography. For example, the likelihood of a major cardiovascular complication in the next 8 years for a 40-year-old man with a systolic blood pressure of 195 mm Hg rises from 4.6% in the absence of the other risk factors to 70.8% in the presence of all four of them.

TYPES OF HYPERTENSION

Hypertension may accompany numerous renal, hormonal, neurologic, and iatrogenic dysfunctions (see box on p. 307). In truly unselected populations, about 95% of hypertension is essential or primary, that is, without known cause. Of the secondary forms, excluding those related to alcohol, oral contraceptives, and other drugs, renal parenchymal disease is most common, responsible for 2% to 3%. Renovascular disease is the only other mechanism responsible for as much as 1% of hypertension. Among younger women, oral contraceptive use is the most common mechanism for secondary hypertension, but over all ages this mechanism accounts for less than 1% of all hypertension. The various adrenal hyperfunctions, medullary (i.e., pheochromocytoma) and cortical (i.e., Cushing's syndrome or primary aldosteronism), are involved in less than 0.5% of all hypertension.

PATHOGENESIS OF PRIMARY HYPERTENSION

The cause of primary (essential) hypertension is unknown. All the various factors known to affect the blood pressure have been implicated, and it is likely that many of these are involved, since if only one were responsible, the counterregulatory actions of the others should work to return the pressure to normal. In the search for causes, multiple hypotheses have been proposed, linking various factors directly or indirectly to the hemodynamic fault of established hypertension, namely an increased peripheral vascular resistance (Fig. 23-4).

The most widely held views implicate a renal defect in sodium excretion, possibly activated by stress, along with a certain threshold level of sodium intake. Some believe that stress by itself is sufficient. More recently, an inherited or acquired defect in sodium transport across cell membranes has been postulated. We will review the evidence for these mechanisms, with the awareness that, whatever else is responsible, heredity must be in the background. As much as half of the variability of blood pressure in the population can be ascribed to heredity, and the blood pressure tends to be similar in first-degree relatives. Inheritance appears to be polygenic.

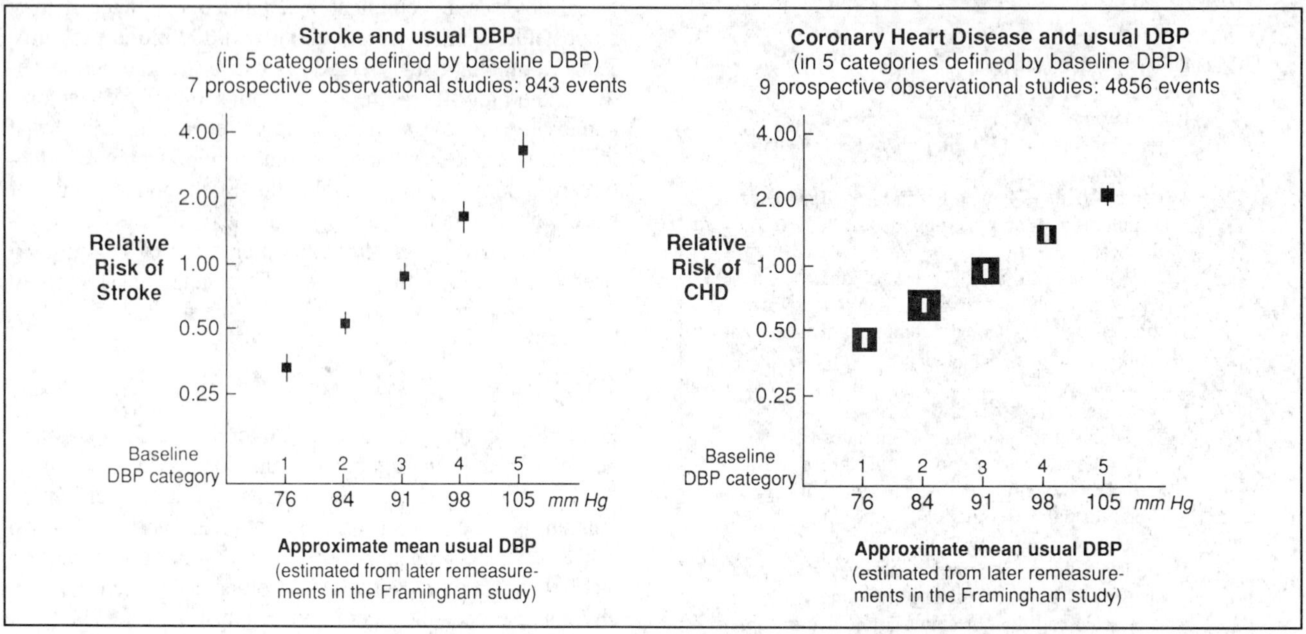

Fig. 23-3. The relative risks of stroke and of coronary heart disease, estimated from the combined results of the prospective observational studies, for each of five categories of diastolic blood pressure. (Estimates of the usual DBP in each baseline DBP category are taken from mean DBP values 4 years postbaseline in the Framingham study.) The solid squares represent disease risks in each category relative to risk in the whole study population; the sizes of the squares are proportional to the number of events in each DBP category, and 95% confidence intervals for the estimates of relative risk are denoted by vertical lines. (From MacMahon S et al: Lancet 335:765, 1990.)

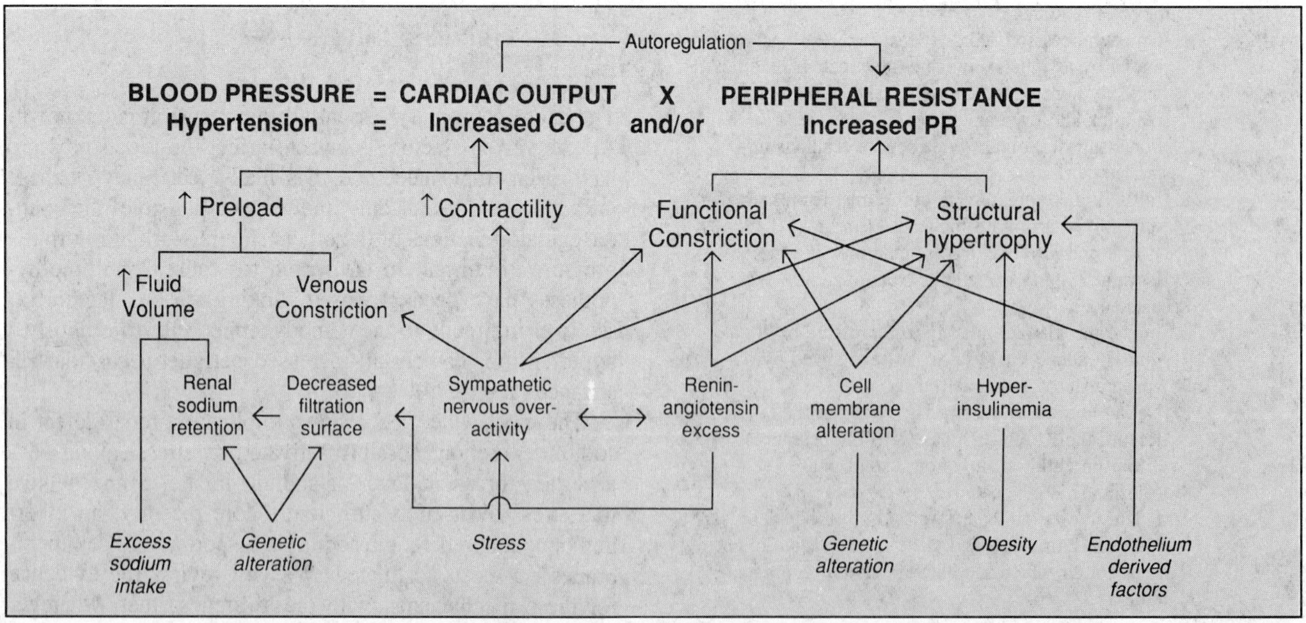

Fig. 23-4. Some of the factors involved in the control of blood pressure that affect the basic equation: Blood pressure = cardiac output × peripheral resistance. (From Kaplan NM: Clinical hypertension, ed 5. Baltimore, 1990, Williams & Wilkins.)

Types of hypertension

I. Systolic and diastolic hypertension
  A. Primary, essential, or idiopathic
  B. Secondary
    1. Renal
      a. Renal parenchymal disease
        (1) Acute glomerulonephritis
        (2) Chronic nephritis
        (3) Polycystic disease
        (4) Connective tissue diseases
        (5) Diabetic nephropathy
        (6) Hydronephrosis
      b. Renovascular
      c. Renin-producing tumors
      d. Renoprival
      e. Primary sodium retention (Liddle's syndrome, Gordon's syndrome)
    2. Endocrine
      a. Acromegaly
      b. Hypothyroidism
      c. Hyperthyroidism
      d. Hypercalcemia (hyperparathyroidism)
      e. Adrenal
        (1) Cortical
          (a) Cushing's syndrome
          (b) Primary aldosteronism
          (c) Congenital adrenal hyperplasia
        (2) Medullary: pheochromocytoma
      f. Extraadrenal chromaffin tumors
      g. Carcinoid
      h. Exogenous hormones
        (1) Estrogen
        (2) Glucocorticoids
        (3) Mineralocorticoids: licorice
        (4) Sympathomimetics
        (5) Tyramine-containing foods and monoamine oxidase inhibitors
    3. Coarctation of the aorta
    4. Pregnancy-induced hypertension
    5. Neurological disorders
      a. Increased intracranial pressure
        (1) Brain tumor
        (2) Encephalitis
        (3) Respiratory acidosis
      b. Sleep apnea
      c. Quadriplegia
      d. Acute porphyria
      e. Familial dysautonomia
      f. Lead poisoning
      g. Guillain-Barré syndrome
    6. Acute stress, including surgery
      a. Psychogenic hyperventilation
      b. Hypoglycemia
      c. Burns
      d. Pancreatitis
      e. Alcohol withdrawal
      f. Sickle cell crisis
      g. Postresuscitation
      h. Postoperative
    7. Increased intravascular volume
    8. Alcohol, drugs, etc.
II. Systolic hypertension
  A. Increased cardiac output
    1. Aortic valvular regurgitation
    2. Arteriovenous fistula, patent ductus
    3. Thyrotoxicosis
    4. Paget's disease of bone
    5. Beriberi
    6. Hyperkinetic circulation
  B. Rigidity of aorta

From Kaplan NM: Clinical hypertension, ed 5. Baltimore, 1990, Williams & Wilkins.

Increased peripheral resistance

Once initiated, the elevated pressure is maintained by an increased peripheral vascular resistance. Most of this resistance arises in small arteries and arterioles, whose proportionately large amount of smooth muscle provides a high wall/lumen ratio. When these smooth muscle cells contract or hypertrophy, relatively small decreases in luminal diameter induce marked increases in resistance. Folkow has postulated that those who are genetically predisposed have an exaggerated or reinforced pressor response to stress, which, by inducing an increase in perfusion pressure, leads to an immediate protective functional vasoconstriction to normalize tissue blood flow via the myogenic reflex mechanism, autoregulation. Soon thereafter, smooth muscle hypertrophy and the deposition of collagen and interstitial material lead to persistent structural thickening of resistance vessels.

Folkow's original hypothesis has been expanded to include the possible role of one or more trophic mechanisms that may cause hypertrophy directly (Fig. 23-5). Insulin is a likely candidate to be one of the trophic mechanisms in primary hypertension, particularly since high plasma insulin levels and resistance to insulin have been described in nonobese hypertensive patients as well as those who are obese.

In addition to various mechanisms that lead to increased contraction and hypertrophy, other forces are involved in relaxation of blood vessels (Fig. 23-6). One, an endothelium-derived relaxing factor (EDRF) that is now known to be nitric oxide (NO), may be deficient whereas endothelin, a potent vasoconstrictor, may be increased. The role of these and a number of other endothelium-derived relaxing and contracting factors may turn out to be important, but their place in the pathogenesis of hypertension remains uncertain.

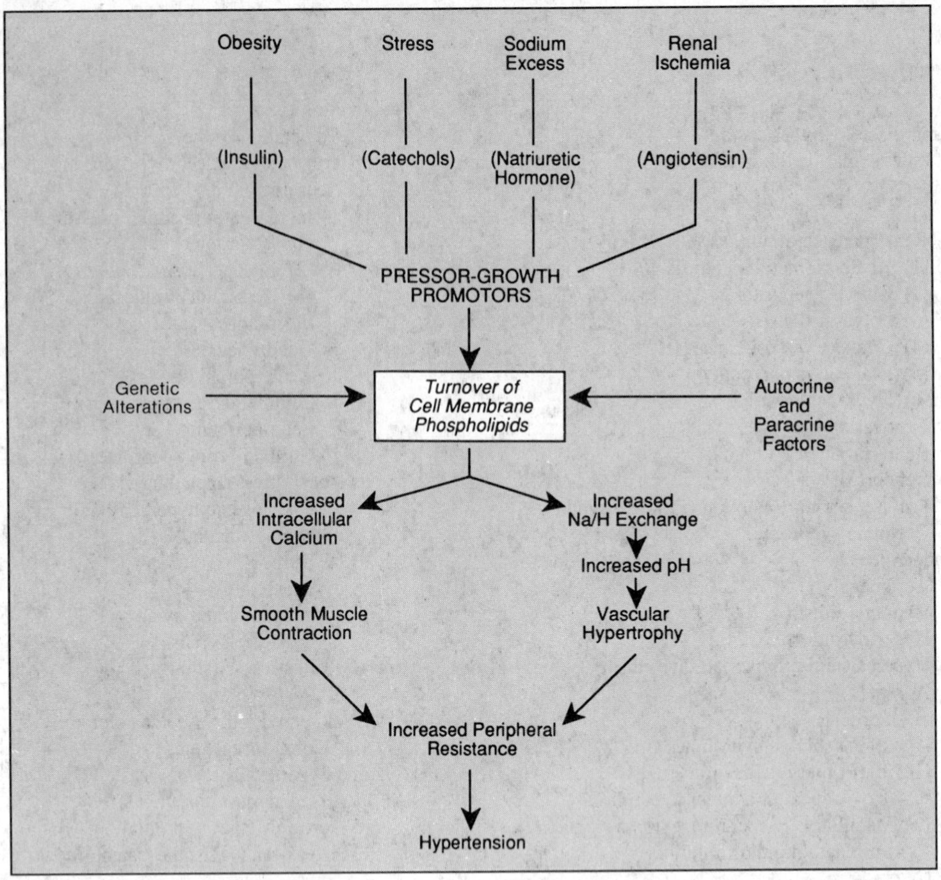

Fig. 23-5. Scheme for the induction of hypertension by numerous pressor hormones that act as vascular growth promotors. (From Kaplan NM: Clinical hypertension, ed 5. Baltimore, 1990, Williams & Wilkins.)

Stress and the sympathetic nervous system

As shown in Figs. 23-3 and 23-4, stress-induced activation of the sympathetic nervous system may lead to hypertension. Additional evidence for a direct mechanism is presented first. Then the evidence for an indirect path involving renal sodium retention is reviewed.

Persons under high levels of stress may develop more hypertension. Perhaps the best demonstration was by Cobb and Rose, who showed that highly stressed air traffic controllers had 5.6 times the annual incidence of hypertension of less-stressed weekend pilots who started with similar blood pressures and other characteristics. Less direct evidence indicates a higher prevalence of hypertension among American blacks and less-educated whites.

Stress may increase the release of epinephrine from the adrenal medulla and norepinephrine from adrenergic neurons activated by central nervous system (CNS) stimulation. High levels of circulating epinephrine mediate alpha-adrenergic effects including increases in heart rate and cardiac output. Epinephrine may also be taken up by $beta_2$ receptors on the presynaptic neuronal membrane and may enhance release of norepinephrine from storage granules. Thereby the transient epinephrine surge may produce considerably more prolonged vasoconstriction.

Higher levels of circulating epinephrine and norepinephrine have been found in hypertensives in the majority of carefully performed comparisons of matched normotensive and hypertensive persons. Moreover, the normotensive offspring of hypertensive parents have been shown to display an exaggerated pressor response to the stress of complex arithmetic problems compared with the similarly normotensive children of normotensive parents. Therefore all the ingredients suggested by Folkow are in place: increased stress, increased levels of circulating catechols, and increased pressor reactivity to stress. Whether these can directly lead to sustained hypertension by inducing structural hypertrophy of resistance vessels remains to be seen.

Renal sodium retention

The stress-induced activation of the sympathetic nervous system could also lead to hypertension via an indirect route, involving stimulation of renal sodium retention. One way or another, the renal retention of part of the daily sodium intake—at an absolute rate too small to measure—may be an essential part of the initiation of hypertension. Guyton has long argued that the kidneys have to reset their normal pressure-natriuresis relationship for hypertension to develop. Otherwise, whenever pressure might rise for what-

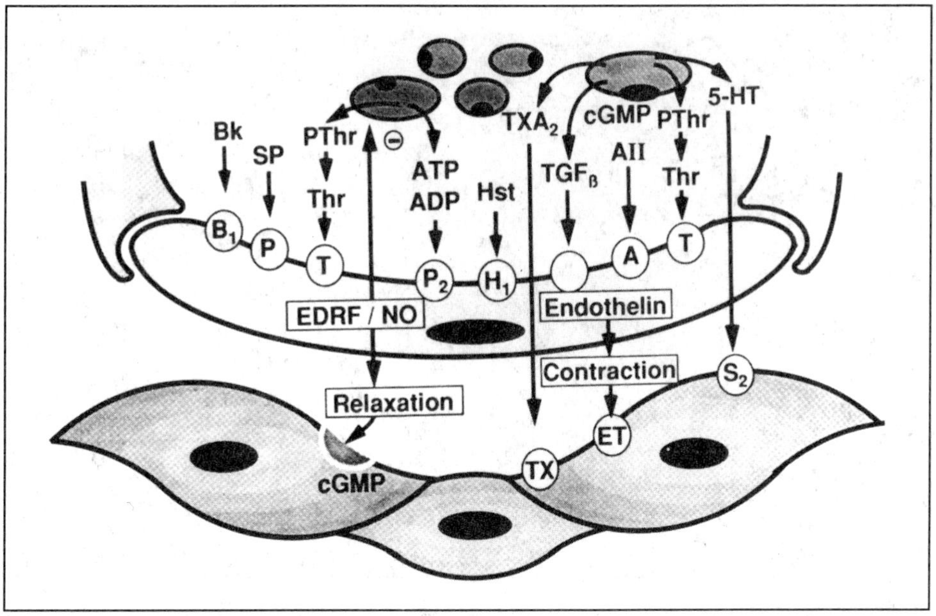

Fig. 23-6. Interactions among platelets, endothelial cells, and smooth muscle cells are complex. The interactions take place in the presence of activating/contracting/growth-promoting and deactivating/relaxing/growth-inhibitory endocrine and paracrine factors. *AII*, angiotensin II; *Bk*, bradykinin; *c*, cyclic; *EDRF*, endothelium-derived relaxing factor; *ET*, endothelin; *5-HT*, 5-hydroxytryptamine; *NO*, nitric oxide; *SP*, substance P; *TGF*, transforming growth factor; *Thr*, thrombin; *TX*, thromboxane. (From Bühler FR et al: J Hypertens 9(suppl 6):S28, 1991.)

ever reason, the prompt natriuresis that normally occurs in the face of higher pressure would promptly return the pressure exactly to normal.

This resetting could be explained by a greater constriction of the renal efferent arterioles, decreasing renal blood flow more than glomerular filtration and thereby increasing filtration fraction and eventually increasing sodium retention (Fig. 23-7). Body fluid volume would thereby be relatively expanded, not in an absolute amount but in excess for the level of blood pressure and the volume of the circulatory bed.

This higher-than-expected blood volume for the level of pressure could increase cardiac output, which according to the concept of autoregulation, would lead to an increased peripheral resistance. Such a pattern of high output changing over to high resistance has been documented by Lund-Johansen in a small number of hypertensives left untreated for 20 years. Whether this is the usual hemodynamic pattern for most patients is uncertain.

Some believe it is unnecessary to invoke an initially high cardiac output but rather hold to the view that peripheral resistance is primarily increased. Such an increase could come about very simply by an increase in the sodium and water content of vascular tissue, which could be a passive consequence of an expanded plasma volume. But in recent years, more active ways to explain an increase in intracellular sodium within vascular tissue have been proposed along with other explanations for the hypertension-inducing effect of the increased intracellular sodium.

Increased intracellular sodium and calcium

At least two distinct mechanisms have been proposed to explain the origin of increased intracellular sodium in hypertension. Both postulate a defect in the normal movement of sodium across the cell membrane, a process that preserves the usual sodium concentration within cells at around 10 mmol per liter with plasma at a concentration of 140 mmol per liter. One hypothesis proposes an acquired inhibitor of the ($Na^+ + K^+$)-ATPase pump, the major physiologic regulator of sodium transport (Fig. 23-7); the other proposes an inherited defect in one or more of the multiple sodium transport systems.

Acquired pump inhibitor. This hypothesis begins with the renal retention of sodium and water, which expands the total extracellular fluid volume or some portion of it, so that the secretion of a natriuretic hormone is activated in an attempt to shrink the expanded volume back to normal. In animal models, the source of this natriuretic hormone appears to be the AV3V region of the hypothalamus. After more than 30 years of active search in numerous laboratories, this putative hormone has only recently been identified as a ouabainlike substance. In the meantime, another natriuretic factor arising from cardiac atrial tissue has been identified and synthesized. This atrial natriuretic factor dilates the renal vascular bed while increasing sodium excretion but does not inhibit the ($Na^+ + K^+$)-ATPase pump nor affect sodium efflux from cells.

The inhibitory action of the ouabainlike natriuretic hormone on ($Na^+ + K^+$)-ATPase pump activity in the kidney

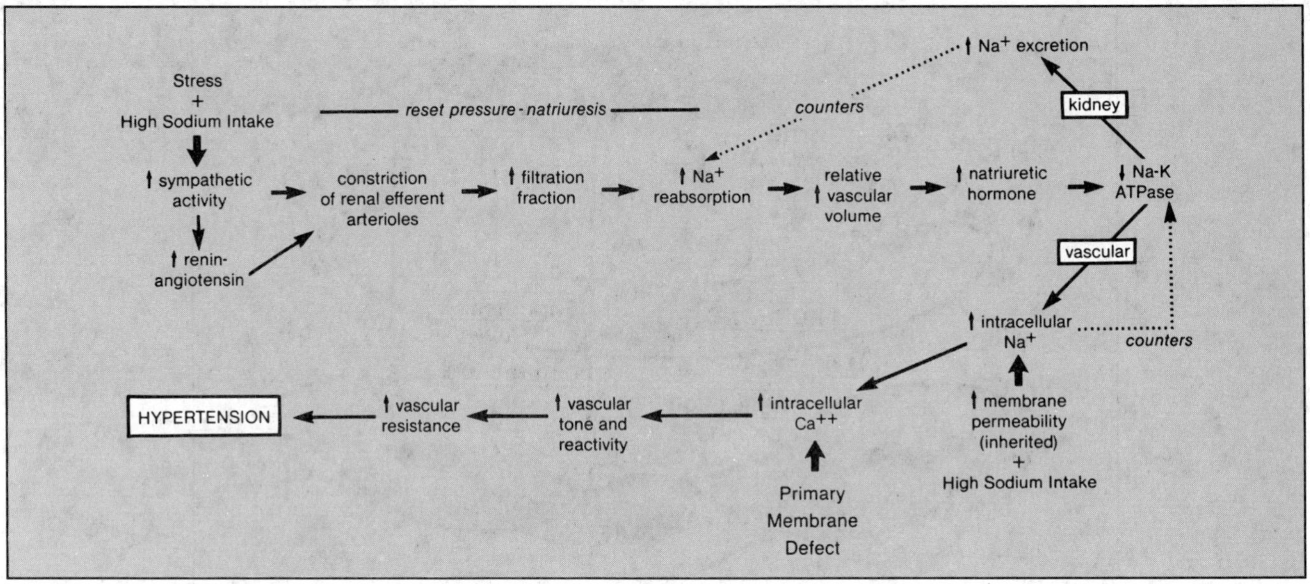

Fig. 23-7. Hypothesis for the pathogenesis of primary (essential) hypertension, starting from one of three points shown as heavy arrows. The first, starting on the top left, is the combination of stress and high sodium intake, which induced an increase in natriuretic hormone and thereby inhibits sodium transport. The second, at the bottom middle, suggests a primary membrane defect that directly leads to increased free intracellular calcium. The third, bottom right, is an increase in membrane permeability leading to increased intracellular sodium. (From Kaplan NM: In Braunwald E, editor: Heart disease. Philadelphia, 1988, Saunders.)

would induce a natriuresis, thereby countering the retention of sodium and returning the extracellular fluid to normal. At the same time, however, the inhibition of the pump in vascular smooth muscle would reduce sodium efflux, increasing intracellular sodium concentration. As postulated by Blaustein and Hamlyn, this would immediately increase the concentration of free calcium within these cells, causing an increase in tone and reactivity in response to any pressor stimulus. Thereby peripheral resistance is increased and hypertension induced.

Inherited defect in transport. Alterations in other membrane transport mechanisms for sodium have been measured in red and white blood cells both of patients with primary hypertension and of the normotensive children of hypertensive parents. Most investigators find an increased rate of Na^+, Li^+-countertransport, which may be a marker for Na^+-H^+ exchange. The field is confused with multiple assays, mostly involving highly artificial conditions, usually showing some alteration in most hypertensives. Beyond the confusion as to the type and frequency of alterations in sodium flux mechanisms, there remains the much more fundamental issue of their pathogenetic role in hypertension. None of these alterations have been measured in human vascular smooth muscle cells, so the role of this mechanism remains uncertain.

Increased concentrations of free intracellular calcium could also arise more directly from defective binding of calcium to the cell membrane, as shown by the Russian workers Postnov and Orlov (Fig. 23-7).

Increased sodium intake

Any theory about the pathogenesis of hypertension should account for the observation that the intake of increased amounts of dietary sodium is necessary but not sufficient in itself. The evidence for the involvement of sodium, although it remains circumstantial, is impressive. It includes (1) animal models in which hypertension develops in those genetically susceptible when they are given large sodium loads. (2) Multiple epidemiologic surveys correlating sodium intake and hypertension: those ingesting less than 50 to 75 mmol of sodium per day have little or no hypertension; those ingesting more than the threshold level of 100 to 150 mmol per day have a certain incidence of hypertension that is increased little if at all by higher levels of sodium intake. (3) Evidence that when groups of persons introduce more sodium into their diets, their mean blood pressures tend to rise. (4) Conversely, there is usually a 5 to 10 mm Hg fall in blood pressure when dietary sodium intake is reduced in patients with hypertension. (5) The induction of hypertension by the retention of sodium by exogenous mineralocorticoids or by the loss of renal function. (6) The demonstration that normotensive children of hypertensive parents tend to increase their blood pressure when given sodium loads and retain sodium during periods of emotional stress. To these may be added the previously noted increased concentration of sodium within blood cells and the vascular smooth muscle tissue of patients with hypertension.

All this evidence strongly supports a role for sodium.

Modern humans have been ingesting a high-sodium diet only in very recent times. Our ancestors consumed a naturally low-sodium, high-potassium diet. Much of what is attributed to the "unnatural" sodium load may be equally attributable to the "unnatural" reduction in potassium intake that has followed the substitution of processed foods for natural ones.

Other environmental mechanisms

Beyond too much sodium or too little potassium, a lower level of calcium intake, an excess of calories, and the ingestion of ethanol have also been found to be associated with hypertension. The data concerning calcium intake remain fragmentary and conflicting. Furthermore, no logical explanation as to how a reduced calcium intake could evoke a rise in blood pressure has been provided. Since increased concentrations of calcium in the blood or within cells raise the blood pressure, and since drugs that antagonize the entry or actions of calcium lower the blood pressure, skepticism remains appropriate.

The evidence for a connection between obesity and hypertension is much more solid. Although the specific mechanism is unknown, increased levels of plasma insulin may provide a common bond, particularly in those with predominately upper body obesity, the typical pattern in middle-aged males (Fig. 23-8). In addition to hypertension, dyslipidemias and type II diabetes often accompany the hyperinsulinemia of upper body obesity.

Of even greater interest, hyperinsulinemia secondary to resistance to insulin-mediated glucose utilization in peripheral muscles has been documented in about half of *nonobese* hypertensives. The role of insulin resistance and resultant hyperinsulinemia remains under intensive study. As will be noted later in this chapter, both nondrug and drug therapies may alter insulin sensitivity and these effects may prove to be important in the overall impact of therapy upon cardiovascular risk.

Ethanol, even in small amounts, exerts a pressor action. Those who consume an average of 2 or more ounces a day, as found in four to five bottles of beer, glasses of wine, or potions of 80-proof distilled spirits, may thereby develop considerable hypertension. In view of the large number of persons who consume that much or more, ethanol abuse is probably the most common form of rapidly reversible hypertension. On the other hand, ingestion of one to two drinks per day has been associated with less coronary disease.

Other postulated mechanisms

Hypertension may arise from either excessive pressor or deficient depressor mechanisms. As shown in Fig. 23-4, the renin-angiotensin system may be activated by stress along with the sympathetic nervous system. Laragh has long argued for a primary role of renin in the pathogenesis of primary hypertension. At the least, it is probably involved in those with high renin levels, since an elevated blood pressure would be expected to inhibit the release of renin through the juxtaglomerular baroreceptors so that low renin levels would be expected.

As noted previously, a host of endothelium-derived va-

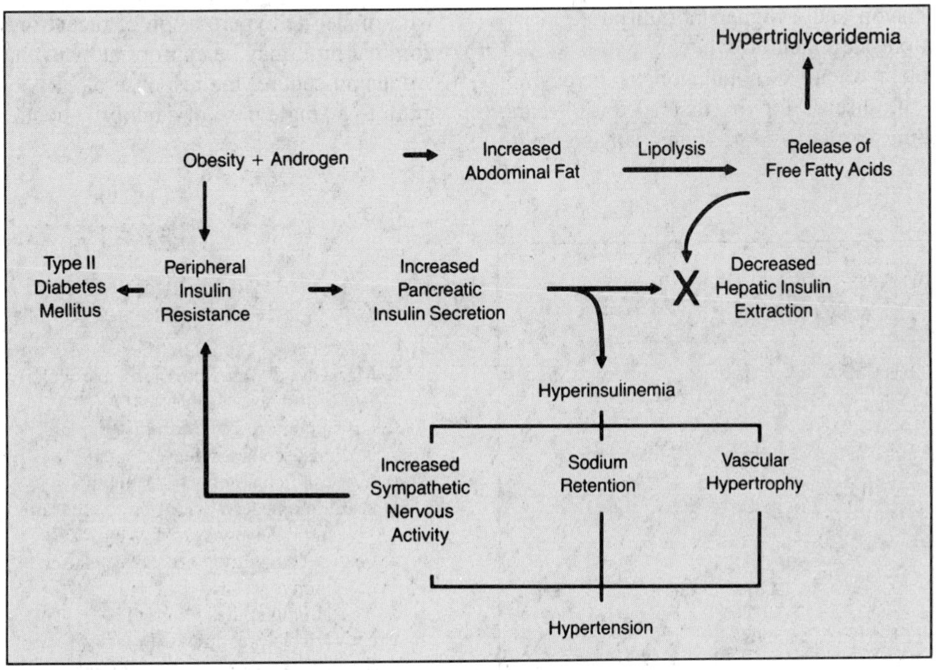

Fig. 23-8. Overall scheme for the mechanism by which upper body obesity could promote glucose intolerance, hypertriglyceridemia, and hypertension via hyperinsulinemia. (From Kaplan NM: Clinical hypertension, ed 5. Baltimore, 1990, Williams & Wilkins.)

soactive substances have been identified, and they may play an important role in the pathogenesis of hypertension (see Fig. 23-6). Too much vasoconstricting by endothelin or other constricting factors or too little vasodilation by nitric oxide, the major endothelium-derived relaxing factor, may be critical.

We are left with a mass of disparate data that may never fit together logically. However, while the search for the mechanisms continues, hints suggest preventive actions, including avoidance of obesity, moderate restriction of dietary sodium and increase in dietary potassium, and moderation of alcohol intake. As we shall see when the issue of treatment of asymptomatic mild hypertension is addressed, there may be risks associated with the active therapy of the disease once it appears.

NATURAL HISTORY OF ESSENTIAL HYPERTENSION

If left untreated, patients may proceed along the course shown in Fig. 23-9. Fewer are now proceeding into an accelerated malignant course, and the mortality, and probably the morbidity, from both coronary and cerebral vascular disease has been declining steadily in the United States since the late 1960s. We are uncertain, however, about the contribution of the greater recognition and treatment of hypertension to these improvements. Most analyses of the evidence suggest that there has been a fall in the incidence of coronary and cerebral vascular disease in addition to improved survival of patients after the complication develops.

Nonetheless, hypertension remains both common and poorly managed in much of the population. The problem is particularly prevalent among blacks, who have a higher incidence of hypertension and a higher mortality rate at every level of blood pressure than do whites.

Part of the problem among all populations is the asymptomatic nature of the disease for the first 10 to 20 years, while it is provoking cardiac and vascular damage. With use of more sensitive diagnostic procedures such as echocardiography, such damage is being recognized to be even more common than previously realized. Although some left ventricular hypertrophy may be either primary to the development of hypertension or essential for the maintenance of cardiac output in the face of an increased afterload, left ventricular hypertrophy has been observed by echocardiography in as many as half of young patients with asymptomatic, uncomplicated, mild hypertension.

Evaluation of the hypertensive patient

For most patients, only a hematocrit, urinalysis, automated blood chemistry study (electrolytes, glucose, creatinine, and cholesterol), and an electrocardiogram (ECG) are needed. More testing should be done on those with features that suggest secondary hypertension (see box below). Selectivity in the performance of screening tests is needed, since more false positives than true positives would be uncovered if procedures such as an intravenous pyelogram (IVP) or assay of plasma renin activity (PRA) were performed on all hypertensives.

Those found to have one or more features suggestive of a secondary form of hypertension during the initial screening by the history, physical examination, and routine laboratory work should have the additional confirmatory studies shown in Table 23-2 for the most common secondary causes. The choice and sequence of confirmatory tests will vary with the type of patient and circumstances. As an example, a young woman with significant hypertension and an abdominal bruit should probably immediately have a selective renal arteriogram, in view of the high likelihood of renovascular hypertension. On the other hand, an older man with moderate hypertension of recent onset who has an abdominal bruit may be appropriately evaluated by a less hazardous procedure, the response of PRA or an isotopic renogram to a single dose of captopril. In such a patient, a neg-

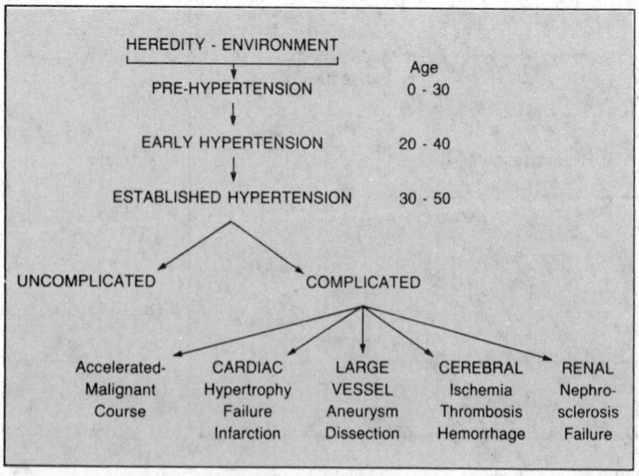

Fig. 23-9. A representation of the natural history of untreated essential hypertension. (From Kaplan NM: Clinical hypertension, ed 5. Baltimore, 1990, Williams & Wilkins.)

Features of "inappropriate" hypertension

1. Onset before age 20 or after age 50 yr
2. Markedly elevated pressures, particularly with grade III or IV funduscopic changes
3. Organ damage
   a. Funduscopic findings of grade II or higher
   b. Serum creatinine >1.5 mg/dl
   c. Cardiomegaly (on x-ray or echocardiogram) or left ventricular hypertrophy (on ECG)
4. Features suggesting secondary causes
   a. Unprovoked hypokalemia
   b. Abdominal diastolic bruit
   c. Variable pressures with tachycardia, sweating, tremor
   d. Family history of renal or endocrine disease
   e. Hematuria, palpable kidneys
   f. Decreased femoral pulses
5. Poor response to therapy that is usually effective

Table 23-2. Overall guide to workup of hypertension

Diagnosis	Diagnostic procedure	
	Initial	**Additional**
Chronic renal disease	Urinalysis, BUN or creatinine, sonography	Renin assay, renal biopsy, IVP
Renovascular disease	Bruit, isotopic renography and plasma renin before and 1 hr after 50 mg captopril	Aortogram, renal vein renins
Coarctation	Blood pressure in legs	Aortogram
Primary aldosteronism	Plasma potassium Plasma renin : aldosterone ratio	Urinary potassium; plasma aldosterone after saline
Cushing's syndrome	AM plasma cortisol after 1 mg dexamethasone at bedtime	Urinary cortisol after variable doses of dexamethasone
Pheochromocytoma	Spot urine for metanephrine	Urinary VMA and catechols; plasma catechols, basal, and after 0.3 mg clonidine

From Kaplan NM: Clinical hypertension, ed 5. Baltimore, 1990, Williams & Wilkins.
BUN = blood urea nitrogen; VMA = vanillylmandelic acid

ative captopril challenge excludes the less likely diagnosis of renovascular hypertension with virtual certainty.

Although the various secondary forms are present in no more than 5% of the hypertensive population, that segment may comprise some 2 million persons in the United States alone.

Secondary causes of hypertension

Oral contraceptive-induced hypertension. Most young women who take oral contraceptives have a rise in blood pressure of 2 to 4 mm Hg. In a survey of 23,000 pill users by the British Royal College of General Practitioners, the overall incidence of hypertension in 5 years was 5%, a figure 2.6 times that noted among 23,000 non–pill users. Though usually mild, the hypertension may on rare occasions be severe with resultant irreversible renal damage. The mechanism is uncertain. All women taking estrogens have an increase in renin substrate with increased levels of angiotensin II and aldosterone. Why hypertension develops only in some instances and whether this is hypertension produced de novo or simply uncovered at an earlier time remains unknown.

It should be possible to prevent serious problems from oral contraceptive–induced hypertension by these maneuvers:

1. Recheck the blood pressure every 3 to 6 months, with no refill of prescriptions permitted so that patients must return for observation.
2. Restrict estrogen use in women who are over 35, obese, smokers, or already hypertensive.
3. If hypertension develops, recommend other forms of contraception.

It should be noted that low-dose postmenopausal estrogen use is not a cause of hypertension.

Renal parenchymal disease. The diagnosis is simple, based on the presence of renal insufficiency and hypertension. Most patients start with primary hypertension that causes progressive renal damage. Among whites, hypertension is responsible for perhaps 20% of end-stage renal disease; in blacks, it is responsible for about 50%. Bilateral renovascular disease may be the underlying problem in a significant number of patients with refractory hypertension and azotemia; 39 of 106 such patients were reported in one series by Ying and colleagues.

Diabetics are particularly vulnerable to renal damage when hypertensive. Effective control of hypertension has been shown to slow the progression of their renal damage. Therefore, the diabetic hypertensive patient should be carefully monitored with measurements of urine protein excretion and serum creatinine and have even minimal hypertension treated vigorously, probably to a diastolic blood pressure level of less than 80 mm Hg (Chapter 355).

Recent advances in medical therapy of chronic renal disease may engender more hypertension: cyclosporine, erythropoietin, and perhaps extracorporeal shock wave lithotripsy.

Renovascular hypertension (also see Chapter 363). Many patients have renal artery lesions that are not functionally significant, the degree of stenosis being less than that required to activate renin release. It is therefore necessary to ensure the functional significance of a lesion before surgery and, to a lesser degree, before angioplasty. Among the usual clinical and laboratory features, only the presence of an abdominal bruit was of differential diagnostic value in the Cooperative Study on Renovascular Hypertension, being heard in 46% of those with renovascular hypertension and 9% of those with essential hypertension. The diagnosis can be made by the sequence of steps shown in the box on p. 314.

Particular attention should be given to any patient with severe hypertension as reflected in funduscopic changes of accelerated-malignant hypertension or refractoriness to potent therapy. A high frequency of renovascular hypertension among such patients, well beyond the 1% or less seen in the overall hypertensive population, has been documented. Most of them should have a renal arteriogram. Of the other procedures in the box on p. 314, the "captopril challenge test" measuring the rise of PRA and renal blood flow or GFR by isotopic renography 1 hour after a single 50 mg dose of captopril has been found to be a useful screening test to exclude the disease in those less likely to have renovascular hypertension.

Diagnosis of renovascular hypertension

Suggestive clinical features
1. Abdominal diastolic bruit
2. Hypertension of recent onset and rapid progression, particularly in young women and older men
3. Rapidly deteriorating renal function
4. Hypertension difficult to control medically

Screening studies
1. Evidence of renal ischemia
   a. IVP (rapid sequence)
   b. Isotopic renogram: 1 hr after 50 mg captopril
2. Demonstration of renin excess
   a. PRA in peripheral blood
   b. Response to captopril: 1 hr after 50 mg

Confirmatory studies
1. Visualization of renal arteries by angiography
2. Renal vein PRA from stenotic side increased more than 1.5 to 2.0 times; no increase from contralateral side above vena cava blood

The increasing availability of transluminal balloon angioplasty has made the search for functional renovascular disease even more attractive, since elderly and other persons who are poor risks for surgery probably can be successfully managed by that procedure. However, the place of angioplasty remains uncertain. Despite its low risk, it may not provide prolonged relief, particularly among those with atherosclerotic renovascular disease, who are by far the majority of patients. For now, reparative surgery is probably the best choice for those with proved renovascular hypertension, but angioplasty at the same time as renal arteriography may be used. Despite better antihypertensive efficacy with angiotensin converting enzyme (ACE) inhibitors, chronic use of these agents is generally not favored because of the distinct possibility of progressive loss of function in the ischemic kidney by removal of the support to perfusion provided by high levels of angiotensin II.

Renin-secreting tumors. Only a few dozen of these hemangiopericytomas of the juxtaglomerular cells have been reported. Most have been in young patients who have severe hypertension and markedly high renin levels with secondary aldosteronism manifested by hypokalemia and metabolic alkalosis. A similar but milder process may occur more commonly among patients with Wilms' tumor and other malignancies of the kidney.

Primary aldosteronism (also see Chapter 163). Aldosterone hypersecretion induces hypertension and renal potassium wastage, but hypokalemia may not always be present, making its recognition more difficult. In a series of 80 patients with primary aldosteronism seen at the Cleveland Clinic, although 75 had a history of hypokalemia, 22 were normokalemic when admitted to the clinic, and 10 remained normokalemic even when given sodium loads to increase potassium wastage. However, four of these patients had bilateral adrenal hyperplasia, and in such patients, the clinical manifestations tend to be milder. Little would be lost if they were not recognized, because they were not hypokalemic, and the therapy is medical, not surgical.

Conversely, adrenal masses are being found incidentally when abdominal computed tomography (CT) is performed for various reasons. Since as many as 8% of normotensive persons and 15% of hypertensives may have a nonfunctioning tumor, usually a lipoma, of the adrenal at autopsy, there is an obvious need to exclude the few functioning tumors that may require surgery from the larger number of nonfunctioning ones that should be left alone. The initial screening studies for the adrenal disorders shown in Table 23-2 should be performed on patients found by CT scan to have an adrenal mass. Surgery should only be done if hormone hypersecretion is proved.

In patients with aldosterone-producing adenomas, the hypertension may be of any degree of severity. In the Medical Research Council (MRC) series of 136 patients, the mean blood pressure was 205/123 mm Hg, and 31 had experienced either stroke or myocardial infarction. The diagnosis of primary aldosteronism can be best begun by measuring aldosterone and PRA in a single blood sample obtained whenever unexplained hypokalemia is observed. An aldosterone-to-PRA ratio of greater than 20:1 strongly suggests primary aldosterone. Most patients who have secondary aldosteronism (induced by diuretics, for example) have higher PRA and a ratio below 20:1. In addition to this simple screening test, the diagnosis should then be confirmed by finding more than 30 mmol of potassium per 24-hour urine collection *in the presence of hypokalemia*. The finding of less than 30 mmol suggests gastrointestinal losses or earlier use of diuretics, the more likely explanation in most hypokalemic hypertensive patients.

Once an elevated blood aldosterone and suppressed PRA are found along with renal wastage of potassium, the nature of the adrenal pathology must be determined by CT scan of the adrenals. Aldosterone-producing adenomas are usually small, but most can be differentiated from bilateral adrenal hyperplasia. The hyperplasia, which may arise in response to a still unidentified aldosterone-stimulating factor, usually causes milder degrees of the usual features: hypokalemia, renin suppression, and aldosterone hypersecretion. It must be recognized to avoid unnecessary surgery. Patients with hyperplasia should be treated with spironolactone; those with a tumor should have surgery.

The glycyrrhizic acid in licorice inhibits the 11β-OH-dehydrogenase enzyme responsible for conversion of cortisol, which exerts potent mineralocorticoid action in the kidney, to cortisone, which is much less potent, thereby inducing "apparent" mineralocorticoid excess.

Mineralocorticoid hypertension may rarely occur from 11-deoxycorticosterone-secreting adrenal tumors and more commonly in the 11- and 17-hydroxylase deficiency forms of congenital adrenal hyperplasia.

Cushing's syndrome (see Chapter 163). Hypertension may also be induced by the mineralocorticoid activity of high levels of cortisol. Hypokalemia is usually less prominent than with primary aldosteronism except in those with very high cortisol levels, as with ectopic adrenocorticotropic hormone (ACTH)-producing tumors. In the more common pituitary ACTH-induced bilateral adrenal hyperplasia, hypertension may be prominent and, if left untreated, may lead to serious cardiac damage.

Pheochromocytoma (see Chapter 164). The hypertension may be wildly episodic or fairly constant but is almost always accompanied by peculiar spells of profuse sweating, tremor, palpitations, headache, and various other symptoms. Although most recurrent spells are caused by anxiety-induced hyperventilation, menopause, or a number of other catecholamine-induced syndromes, the possibility of a pheochromocytoma can be easily excluded by the measurement of metanephrine in a single voided urine specimen. If the spot urine contains more than 1.2 μg of metanephrine per milligram of creatinine, 24-hour urine catecholamine levels should be determined. Plasma catechols may also be measured before and after an attempt to suppress them with the sympathetic inhibitor clonidine. Those with a pheochromocytoma have high plasma levels that cannot be suppressed by more than 50% or to a level of less than 400 pg per milliliter in the 3 hours after oral intake of 0.3 mg of clonidine.

Once the clinical signs have been confirmed by the biochemical assays, the pathology should be elucidated by abdominal CT scanning. Most pheochromocytomas—about 90%—are solitary and in an adrenal gland. About 10% are extra-adrenal, most along the abdominal sympathetic chain. About 10% are malignant, as ascertained by the finding of metastases. A few are associated with the type 2 multiple endocrine neoplasia syndrome or multiple neurofibromatosis.

After adequate alpha-adrenergic blockade, surgery is almost always indicated, with caution to avoid severe hypertension during induction of anesthesia and manipulation of the tumor.

Miscellaneous causes. As shown by the long list of secondary types of hypertension in the box on p. 307, numerous other mechanisms can induce hypertension. A variety of drugs and chemical agents may be responsible. Many of these, such as nasal decongestants and diet pills containing the sympathetic agonist phenylpropanolamine, are readily available and widely used. Nonsteroidal anti-inflammatory drugs (NSAIDs) have been found to interfere with the efficacy of numerous antihypertensive drugs. The potential of various drugs and chemical agents to induce or aggravate hypertension should be recognized in the evaluation of all patients.

TREATMENT OF HYPERTENSION

Many practitioners treat all persons with a diastolic pressure above 90 mm Hg and most with a systolic above 140 mm Hg. The reasons for this approach include the recognition that hypertension is common and, if left untreated, is a major risk factor for premature cardiovascular disease. After the benefits of antihypertensive drug therapy for the more severe degrees of hypertension were demonstrated in the late 1960s, the logical assumption was made that the millions with relatively milder degrees of hypertension should also be treated, particularly since medications became available that could be taken once or twice a day and seemed to be largely free of bothersome side effects. Therefore, more and more of the 80% of the hypertensive population who have mild hypertension (defined as a diastolic blood pressure between 90 and 104 mm Hg) have been begun on drug therapy; these include a large share of the 40% with diastolic blood pressure between 90 and 94 mm Hg. However, the extension of treatment to these less hypertensive patients began without proof that it was beneficial.

Results of clinical trials

Clinical trials of the therapy of mild hypertension were begun in the early 1970s. The results have provided both confirmatory evidence for the benefits of therapy in regard to the prevention of stroke and congestive heart failure and, at the same time, doubts about the benefits in regard to the most common and serious consequence of hypertension, coronary heart disease (Fig. 23-10). These figures are taken from an analysis by Cutler and colleagues of the nine randomized controlled trials that have examined the effects of drug therapy for mild to moderate hypertension (diastolic blood pressure 90 to 110 mm Hg) encompassing some 43,000 nonelderly patients with an average follow-up of 5.6 years. The figures show the relative differences with 95% confidence intervals in fatal events between the intervention and control groups in each study and the combined overall difference in all nine studies at the bottom.

Strokes were reduced by 38% overall and to a greater degree in the intervention groups of all but one study, the MRFIT, wherein 11 fatal strokes occurred in the intervention group and 9 in the control group. On the other hand, fatal coronary heart disease was *increased* in the intervention group in four of the nine trials, and the overall reduction of 8% was not statistically significant (CI of −21% to +6%). When the overall reductions in coronary heart disease and stroke observed in all of these trials taken together were compared with the reductions that were expected by the greater average fall in diastolic blood pressure of 5.8 mm Hg in the intervention groups, more than 90% of the expected reduction in stroke but less than 25% of the expected reduction in coronary heart disease was found. A similar pattern of protection against mortality from strokes but not from coronary disease was seen in a Swedish study of elderly hypertensives reported in late 1991.

Since the blood pressure was successfully lowered by therapy (or more therapy) in all of these trials, the inability to show clear protection against coronary disease may reflect the mode of therapy: high doses of diuretics were the first drug, and often the only drug, in all trials shown in Fig. 23-10 except in half of the MRC-treated group. Most of the excess coronary mortality seen in four of the nine trials was caused by sudden death, which may have been related to diuretic-induced hypokalemia. The MRC trial

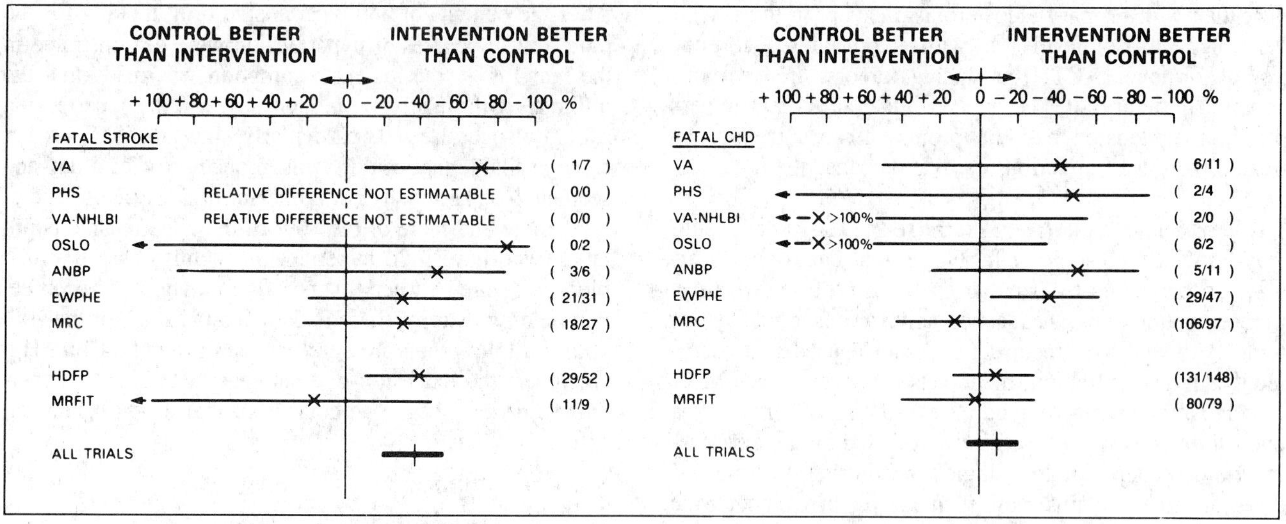

Fig. 23-10. The results of nine clinical trials of the treatment of mild hypertension, portraying the effects of antihypertensive therapy (intervention) versus placebo (control) in the top seven trials and more therapy versus less therapy in the bottom two. The effects are shown for fatalities from strokes *(left)* and coronary heart disease *(right)*. The X on each line represents the mean difference; the length of the line represents the 95% confidence interval. The actual number of events (intervention/control) is given on the right of each line. (From Cutler JA et al: Hypertension 13(suppl I):I, 1989.)

compared a thiazide diuretic to a beta blocker, propranolol. Both drugs protected against stroke, but coronary mortality was not reduced overall by either drug; only nonsmoking men who received propranolol had a reduced rate of coronary events.

These results have caused many to question the apparent wisdom of routinely treating mild hypertension and, even more, the manner by which it has been treated in the past. Many authorities, such as the British Hypertension Society, now advocate a somewhat more conservative approach of starting drug therapy in the majority of mild, low-risk hypertensives with diastolic blood pressure below 100 mm Hg only after 3 to 6 months of repeated blood pressure readings and nondrug therapy. The wisdom of this approach is shown by the results of the Australian trial: 48% of those who entered the trial with diastolic blood pressure between 95 and 109 mm Hg on the second set of readings had a fall to less than 95 mm Hg that persisted during the subsequent 4 years while they received no active drug (or nondrug) therapy. Most of this fall occurred in the first 4 months of observation.

Increasingly, the persistence of diastolic blood pressure above 95 mm Hg after this cooling-off period is being used as the decision point for institution of drug therapy. As shall be discussed later, the other major change in therapy, once decided on, is to minimize the use of diuretics and to use a number of other choices.

Part of the hesitation in starting drug therapy reflects the increasing awareness of the potential for any drug therapy to produce various side effects that may diminish the quality of life. In addition, the high cost of medications, particularly the newer angiotensin-converting enzyme inhibitors and calcium blockers, has prompted many to either withhold therapy or substitute less-expensive generic forms for others that may be preferable.

Nondrug therapies

One way to minimize or delay the need for drug therapy is by the use of various nondrug modalities, better called "lifestyle modifications." Although these, too, may interfere somewhat with the quality of life, they should have no bothersome side effects. These therapies should be continued and offered to all hypertensives whether they also need drugs or not. The hope is that these lifestyle modifications will lower blood pressure to levels wherein drugs are not required or, failing that, to reduce the amounts of medication needed. There is hope, but certainly no proof, that their widespread use could prevent the development of hypertension.

There is also no proof that these lifestyle modifications protect against cardiovascular complications or that they will be accepted by or effective in lowering the blood pressure for most hypertensives. But they do no harm, and they may do some good not only by lowering blood pressure but also by reducing other risk factors for cardiovascular disease. If the modifications are offered in a reasonable manner, as a gentle recommendation for gradual change rather than as a massive attack against current habits, most patients should be willing to at least try them.

Weight reduction. Weight gain clearly tends to raise blood pressure, and weight loss usually lowers blood pressure. The effect of reduced caloric intake is probably independent of concomitant sodium restriction. A 1- to 2-mm Hg fall in blood pressure usually accompanies each kg of weight loss.

Moderate sodium restriction. As documented in an analysis of data from over 70 controlled trials by Law and coworkers, a decrease of 50 mmol per day of sodium lowers blood pressure in many patients. Such a reduction to 2.4 g of sodium (6 g of NaCl or 100 mmol of sodium) per day can be accomplished simply by leaving out salt in cooking and avoiding heavily salted foods. In addition to lowering the blood pressure, diuretic-induced potassium wastage should be reduced. There is evidence that after a few months on a lower sodium intake, the taste preference for sodium decreases.

Other dietary changes. Supplements of three minerals, potassium, calcium, and magnesium, have been shown in limited trials to lower the blood pressure. It should not be necessary to give potassium supplements if a lower sodium intake is consumed. When natural, fresh foods are substituted for processed and canned foods, the intake of potassium rises markedly. As an example, canned peas have 236 mg of sodium and 96 mg of potassium per 100 grams; fresh peas have 2 mg of sodium and 316 mg of potassium.

Though the antihypertensive efficacy of calcium supplements has been found to be exceedingly small, the patient is advised not to reduce calcium intake by restricting milk and cheese consumption to reduce sodium intake.

Magnesium deficiency can be induced by diuretic therapy, but magnesium supplements have not been shown to lower blood pressure.

A few clinical studies have shown a lowering of the blood pressure by ingestion of a lacto-ovovegetarian diet, a low-saturated, high-polyunsaturated fat diet, or 2 to 3 g per day of omega-3-fatty acids. Such diets may reduce the blood pressure by increasing levels of vasodilatory prostaglandins.

Moderate alcohol consumption. Too little or too much alcohol may be harmful; too little by increasing the risks for coronary heart disease presumably through a lowering of high-density lipoprotein (HDL) cholesterol; too much by raising the blood pressure and, when carried further, by the ravages of alcohol abuse. Beyond 2 ounces per day, ethanol may raise the blood pressure and, in larger amounts, it is probably by far the most common cause of reversible, curable hypertension.

Exercise. Regular isotonic exercise may lower the blood pressure, perhaps through reduction of sympathetic nerve activity. Isometric exercise probably does no good for cardiovascular fitness and causes a reflex rise in blood pressure, so it should be avoided.

Relaxation. Various techniques to relieve tension and induce relaxation have been shown to lower the blood pressure, but in the majority of controlled studies, the effect is no greater than seen with placebo.

Drug therapy

Even if all of these lifestyle modifications are used, most hypertensives need antihypertensive drugs. As noted, the treatment of hypertension constitutes the largest single indication for drug use in the United States.

The choice of initial therapy. A diuretic has been the first drug chosen by most practitioners to treat most hypertensives. In the last few years, doubts about the routine use of diuretics have arisen for two reasons: first, the recognition that they may induce a number of biochemical aberrations, including hypokalemia, glucose intolerance, and hypercholesterolemia, which may add to cardiovascular risk; second, the realization that the use of diuretics—the first and often only drug used in the various clinical trials shown in Fig. 23-10—has not resulted in the degree of protection against coronary disease that was expected to follow the reduction in blood pressure. This observation is not to imply that, when used correctly in small doses and with proper attention to and correction of biochemical aberrations, diuretics may not be as safe and effective as any other drug. In trials comparing a diuretic to a beta blocker, elderly hypertensives, particularly those who are black, seemed to respond better to a diuretic, and that may remain the best initial choice for them. In the Systolic Hypertension in the Elderly Program (SHEP), diuretic-based therapy in small doses, starting with 12.5 mg of chlorthalidone, has been shown to reduce morbidity and mortality.

However, almost any of the drugs shown in Table 23-3 may be chosen for initial therapy with the expectation that about half of patients will have a 10% or greater fall in blood pressure, which will bring the diastolic blood pressure of most of those who start with fairly mild hypertension below 90 mm Hg, the usual goal of therapy. Drugs that tend to reduce renin-aldosterone activity such as beta blockers, ACE inhibitors, and calcium entry blockers may work particularly well in the absence of a diuretic.

Rather than a diuretic-first, step-ladder approach, adding drugs consecutively, most now recommend an individualized approach, largely based on the patient's other cardiovascular risks, for example hypercholesterolemia or glucose intolerance and concomitant conditions such as coronary artery disease or congestive heart failure (Table 23-4). If the initial choice is ineffectual or causes bothersome side effects, that drug should be discontinued and one from another class substituted.

Subsequent drug therapy. If the first choice is well tolerated but only partially effective, either increase the dose or add a second drug from another class. In about 10% of hypertensives, a third drug, usually a vasodilator, is needed. In the past, hydralazine was the usual choice, with minoxidil reserved for resistant cases. Calcium entry blockers will probably be used increasingly, since they are effective vasodilators of the systemic arteries as well as of the coronary arteries.

Table 23-3. Effective oral antihypertensive drugs

Drug	Trade name	Dose range mg/day (frequency)	Side effects
Diuretics (partial list)			
Hydrochlorothiazide	Hydrodiuril Esidrix	12.5-50(1)	Biochemical abnormalities: ↓ potassium, ↑ cholesterol, ↑ glucose Rare: blood dyscrasias, photosensitivity, pancreatitis
Chlorthalidone	Hygroton	12.5-50	
Metolazone	Mykrox, Diulo	0.5-10	
Indapamide	Lozol	2.5	Less if any hypercholesterolemia
Furosemide	Lasix	40-240	Short duration of action
Potassium-sparing agents (plus thiazide)			
Spironolactone	Aldactazide	25-100	Hyperkalemia, gynecomastia
Triamterene	Dyazide, Maxzide	25-100	Hyperkalemia
Amiloride	Moduretic	5-10	Hyperkalemia
Adrenergic inhibitors			
Peripherals:			
Reserpine	Serpasil	0.05-0.25(1)	Sedation, depression
Guanethidine	Ismelin	10-150	Orthostatic hypotension, diarrhea
Guanadrel	Hylorel	10-75	
Central alpha agonists:			
Methyldopa	Aldomet	500-3000(2)	Hepatic and "autoimmune" disorders
Clonidine	Catapres	0.2-1.2(2)	Sedation, dry mouth, "withdrawal"
Guanabenz	Wytensin	8-32(2)	Sedation, dry mouth, "withdrawal"
Guanfacine	Tenex	1-3(1)	Sedation, dry mouth, "withdrawal"
Alpha blockers:			
Doxazosin	Cardura	1-20(1)	Postural hypotension (mainly with first dose), lassitude
Prazosin	Minipress	2-20(2)	
Terazosin	Hytrin	1-20(1)	
Beta blockers:			
Acebutolol	Sectral	200-800(1)	Serious: bronchospasm, congestive heart failure, masking of insulin-induced hypoglycemia, depression
Atenolol	Tenormin	25-100(1-2)	
Betaxolol	Kerlone	5-20(1)	
Carteolol	Cartrol	2.5-10(1)	
Metoprolol	Lopressor	50-300(1-2)	Less serious: poor peripheral circulation, insomnia, fatigue, decreased exercise tolerance, hypertriglyceridemia, decreased HDL (except with ISA agents)
Nadolol	Corgard	40-320(1)	
Penbutolol	Levatol	10-20(1)	
Pindolol	Visken	10-60(2)	
Propranolol	Inderal	40-480(2)	
Timolol	Blocadren	20-60(2)	
Combined alpha and beta blocker:			
Labetalol	Normodyne Trandate	200-1200(2)	Postural hypotension, beta-blocking side effects
Direct vasodilators:			
Hydralazine	Apresoline	50-400(2)	Headaches, tachycardia, lupus syndrome
Minoxidil	Loniten	5-100(1)	Headaches, fluid retention, hirsutism
Calcium entry blockers			
Verapamil (SR)	Isoptin, Calan Verelan	90-480(1-2)	Constipation, conduction defects
Diltiazem (SR and CD)	Cardizem	120-240(1-2)	Nausea, headache, conduction defects
Dihydropyridines:			
Amlodipine	Norvase	2.5-10(1)	Flush, headache, local ankle edema
Felodipine	Plendil	5-20(1)	Flush, headache, local ankle edema
Isradipine	DynaCirc	5-20(2)	Flush, headache, local ankle edema
Nicardipine	Cardene	60-90(2-3)	Flush, headache, local ankle edema
Nifedipine (XL)	Procardia	20-120(1)	Flush, headache, local ankle edema
Converting-enzyme inhibitors			
Benazepril	Lotensin	5-40(1)	Cough, rash, loss of taste
Captopril	Capoten	25-150(2)	Rare: leucopenia, proteinuria
Enalapril	Vasotec	5-40(1-2)	Rare: leucopenia, proteinuria
Fosinopril	Monopril	10-40(1)	Rare: leucopenia, proteinuria
Lisinopril	Prinivil, Zestril	5-40(1)	Rare: leucopenia, proteinuria
Quinapril	Accupril	2.5-10(1)	Rare: leucopenia, proteinuria
Ramipril	Altace	1.25-20(1)	Rare: leucopenia, proteinuria

Table 23-4. Concomitant diseases and the choice of antihypertensive drug therapy

	Indications	Contraindications
Diuretics	Congestive heart failure Volume retention	Diabetes Gout Hypercholesterolemia
Central alpha agonists	Withdrawal from addictive behaviors (clonidine)	Liver disease (methyldopa) Autoimmune disease (methyldopa) Depression
Alpha blockers	Hypercholesterolemia High level of physical activity	Postural hypotension
Beta blockers	Coronary artery disease Tachyarrhythmias Migraine Anxiety	Asthma Diabetes requiring insulin Bradyarrhythmias Congestive heart failure Peripheral vascular disease Hypertriglyceridemia
ACE inhibitors	Congestive heart failure Renal insufficiency Peripheral vascular disease	Renal failure Renovascular hypertension Volume depletion Pregnancy
Calcium antagonists	Coronary artery disease Tachyarrhythmias (verapamil) Peripheral vascular disease	Bradyarrhythmias (verapamil)

Other guidelines

The goal of therapy should be to reduce the diastolic pressure to below 90 mm Hg, but caution is needed in reducing it below 85 mm Hg since that may induce myocardial ischemia; particularly in patients with preexisting coronary disease. The progressive fall in coronary mortality seen with progressive lowering of pressure is aborted at diastolic levels below 85 mm Hg and coronary mortality then begins to rise, producing a J-curve relationship as described by Cruickshank and analyzed by Fletcher and Bulpitt. In the elderly with predominantly systolic hypertension, the systolic pressure should be gently lowered toward 145 mm Hg. The failure of cerebral autoregulation may cause postural symptoms to appear in the elderly even with small falls in blood pressure.

In view of the significantly greater occurrence of cardiovascular catastrophes in the morning hours after arising from sleep, a time when blood pressure abruptly increases, it is vital to ensure that the antihypertensive effects of therapy be maintained at this time, preferably by having patients check their pressures soon after arising with home devices. Some agents approved for once-a-day dosing may not provide 24-hour control, so twice-a-day dosing may be needed or other longer-acting agents may be used once daily.

If the goal blood pressure has been reached on two or more drugs, the substitution of comparable combination tablets should be attempted. If the goal has been maintained for at least 1 year, the doses of drugs should be slowly reduced and, rarely, discontinued under careful surveillance.

Specific drugs

Diuretics. The most commonly used diuretics are listed in Table 23-3. The most appropriate choice for most patients is hydrochlorothiazide, with its 12- to 16-hour duration of action and mild, smooth effect, although the longer-lasting chlorthalidone may provide better efficacy. Patients on direct vasodilators or with renal insufficiency (i.e., serum creatinine above 2.5 mg/dl) may need more potent diuretics, either two or three doses per day of a loop diuretic, such as furosemide or bumetanide, or one dose a day of metolazone. Indapamide may have additional vasodilatory effects.

The side effects of diuretics largely reflect their pharmacologic actions (Fig. 23-11). Three of these metabolic changes may increase cardiovascular risk: the rise in serum cholesterol, up to 20 mg per deciliter; the fall in serum potassium, which averages 0.7 mmol per liter; and the worsening of glucose tolerance, which reflects greater insulin resistance. Efforts should be made to prevent hypokalemia by use of the smallest effective dose of diuretic, concomitant reduction in sodium intake, and generous use of potassium-sparing agents or supplemental potassium. Although microencapsulated potassium chloride tablets may be safely used, a level teaspoonful of a potassium chloride–containing salt substitute provides 40 mmol of potassium at less cost. Prudence suggests that a fall of serum potassium of more than 0.5 mmol per liter be reversed by the same measures.

The rise in serum uric acid and calcium levels shown in Fig. 23-11 need not be corrected unless the patient has concomitant gout or hyperparathyroidism. Although impotence has been considered unusual with diuretics, it was reported in 22% of men in the British MRC trial taking 10 mg per day of bendrofluazide, compared with 10% of those on a placebo and 13% on propranolol.

Adrenergic inhibitors. All of the agents shown in Table 23-3 lower the blood pressure about 10% and, if used with a diuretic, bring at least 80% of hypertensives to the goal of a diastolic blood pressure below 90 mm Hg. The choice between these drugs should be based on their propensity to induce metabolic mischief or bothersome side effects, although prescribing habits, in fact, largely determine the choice.

Peripheral inhibitors. Reserpine remains an effective, inexpensive, and generally well-tolerated drug. It can be effective in even smaller doses, 0.05 mg per day, than usually prescribed. Guanethidine is now reserved for resistant patients as a step 4 drug. Guanadrel is a shorter-lasting

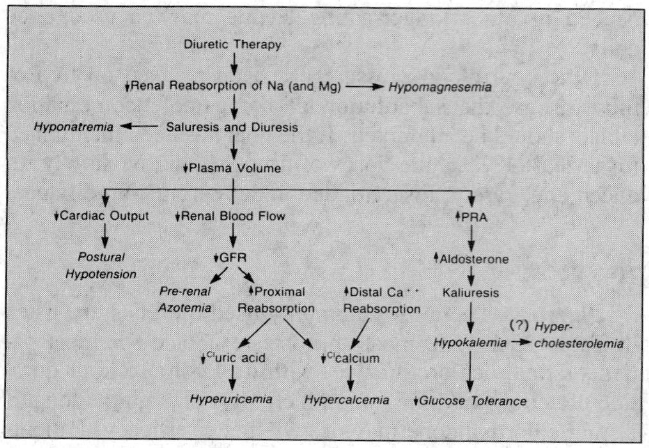

Fig. 23-11. The mechanisms by which chronic diuretic therapy may lead to various complications. The mechanisms for hypercholesterolemia remains in question, although it is shown as arising via hypokalemia. (From Kaplan NM: Clinical hypertension, ed 5. Baltimore, 1990, Williams & Wilkins.)

guanethidine-like agent, which seems to cause fewer side effects when used twice a day.

Central inhibitors. Clonidine, guanabenz, guanfacine, and methyldopa act in a similar manner to decrease sympathetic drive from the central nervous system. Other than for a variety of autoimmune syndromes with methyldopa, their side effects are similar, mainly sedation and dry mouth. All should be given twice daily. Guanabenz has been approved for monotherapy since it appears to induce less fluid retention.

Alpha blockers. Three are now available—prazosin, terazosin, and doxazosin—which act selectively on the postsynaptic $alpha_1$ receptor on the vascular smooth muscle. The most widely perceived side effect, first-dose hypotension, is seen infrequently, is seldom severe, and can be minimized by discontinuation of diuretic therapy for the day before and the day after start of the drug. Among this class of drug's advantages are the beneficial effects on plasma lipid levels and insulin resistance and the lack of interference with the ability to perform physical activity.

Beta blockers. These agents have been second in popularity to diuretics in the treatment of hypertension. Of those now available for use in the United States, equivalent doses probably exert similar antihypertensive effects. If one does not work, it is unlikely that another will but if one causes side effects, it may be worth trying another with different pharmacologic properties.

Beta blockers differ in three major ways: (1) *Relative $beta_1$ selectivity*. In the fairly large doses used to treat hypertension, the relatively greater $beta_1$ selectivity of acebutolol, atenolol, and metoprolol may not be enough to prevent $beta_2$-mediated side effects such as bronchospasm. (2) *Intrinsic sympathomimetic activity* (ISA). The greater ISA of pindolol and acebutolol may translate into less bradycardia, vasoconstriction, and alterations in lipid levels than are seen with the other beta blockers. (3) *Lipid solubility*. The lesser lipid solubility of atenolol and nadolol enables them to remain in the blood longer and they are slowly excreted, largely unchanged, through the kidneys. Because of the greater lipid solubility of metoprolol and propranolol, they are taken up and partially metabolized in the liver; hence it may take a while to reach sustained blood levels of free drug, and more than one dose per day may be needed to maintain steady effects.

The major side effects of beta blockers are largely a magnification of their pharmacologic $beta_1$- and $beta_2$-receptor blockade: decrease in cardiac output limiting exercise ability and, very rarely, inciting heart failure; bronchospasm; and the masking of the symptoms (except for sweating) while prolonging the duration of insulin-induced hypoglycemia. In addition, they may induce considerable fatigue, depression, and insomnia; these side effects may be less common with the lipid-insoluble beta blockers atenolol and nadolol, which do not enter the brain as much. All but pindolol and acebutolol may so constrict the peripheral circulation as to cause cold extremities and diminish the conversion of triglycerides into HDL cholesterol, raising the level of triglycerides and lowering the level of HDL cholesterol.

Combined alpha and beta blockers. Labetalol has both alpha- and beta-blocking effects, in an approximate 1:3 ratio, which results in even greater antihypertensive potency than an alpha or beta blocker alone with little reduction in cardiac output. Available for both oral and intravenous use, it has been used especially for severe hypertension. The most bothersome side effect is postural hypotension.

Vasodilators. A direct-acting vasodilator has usually been the third drug added for the 10% of patients who do not respond adequately to two. When added to a diuretic and an adrenergic inhibitor, the antihypertensive effect of all three is fully developed while their side effects are minimized. Hydralazine is the usual choice and need be given only twice daily. Beyond the expected side effects of direct-acting vasodilators of tachycardia, flushing, and headache, hydralazine may cause a febrile lupuslike reaction that is almost always totally reversible. Patients who inactivate the drug more slowly via acetylation may develop the reaction with total doses of less than 200 mg per day; fast acetylators rarely develop it with less than 400 mg per day.

Minoxidil, more potent than hydralazine, is usually reserved for those with renal insufficiency, near the end of their course. But, if given in small doses, it may provide excellent antihypertensive action on a once-daily schedule and not cause much hirsutism, the most common side effect. Significant fluid retention usually accompanies its antihypertensive action, often requiring the addition of potent diuretics.

Calcium entry blockers. These vasodilators may be used as first, second, or third drug. Of those now available, the dihydropyridines are the most potent peripheral vasodilators, but all lower blood pressure. The availability of verapamil, diltiazem, and some of the dihydropyridines in slow-release forms that provide once-a-day dosage adds to their attractiveness. Some find that calcium entry blockers are especially effective in the elderly hypertensive population.

Nifedipine as a liquid in a capsule has been found to be particularly useful for semiemergency situations in which very high blood pressure must be lowered within 20 to 30 minutes.

Angiotensin converting enzyme inhibitors. Angiotensin converting enzyme (ACE) inhibitors also act as vasodilators. By their inhibition of the enzyme that converts the inactive angiotensin I to the potent vasoconstrictor angiotensin II, the drugs are particularly effective in high renin-angiotensin forms of hypertension. They probably also work in other ways, so most patients with primary hypertension have some benefit from them. They work particularly well when renin levels are raised by concomitant diuretic therapy or sodium restriction.

In practice, the effects of ACE inhibitors are not much better than those observed with other antihypertensive agents, except in a few patients whose hypertension is very renin-dependent. Some of these, in turn, may depend on high levels of renin-angiotensin II to maintain renal perfusion. This dependence has been noted primarily in patients with stenoses in both renal arteries or in the one artery to a solitary kidney. When their renin support is removed by an ACE inhibitor, renal blood flow may fall precipitously, far below the level expected from the fall in systemic blood pressure.

These drugs are generally free of the CNS and cardiac-mediated side effects such as sedation, fatigue, and exercise limitation often seen with adrenergic inhibitors. By removing angiotensin II–mediated vasoconstriction, ACE inhibitors have proved to be particularly valuable in reducing afterload demands on a heart that has failed from prolonged hypertension. However, these drugs may cause side effects, such as cough, loss of taste, and rash, that are irritating, as well as some rare but serious problems such as angioneurotic edema.

Some special problems

Systolic hypertension in the elderly. Elderly persons often have isolated systolic hypertension caused by loss of elasticity in large arteries from atherosclerosis. They are at high risk for stroke and other cardiovascular catastrophes and, with publication of the results of the Systolic Hypertension in the Elderly Program (SHEP), antihypertensive drug treatment has been found to reduce these risks. Therefore, such patients should be treated in the same general way as described for systolic and diastolic hypertension in preceding portions of this chapter, but in a slower, more gentle manner toward a goal of a systolic blood pressure of 145 mm Hg.

All of the drugs listed in Table 23-3 may be used in the elderly; a low dose of the diuretic chlorthalidone, 12.5 mg, was the initial drug in the SHEP trial, and a low dose of the beta blocker atenolol, 25 mg, was the second. Special precautions are needed:

1. Diuretics may cause more volume depletion and hypokalemia.
2. Adrenergic inhibitors may cause more postural hypotension since the baroreceptor reflexes are less active. This sluggish baroreceptor response may allow for the use of hydralazine without an adrenergic inhibitor.
3. Any drug that effectively lowers the blood pressure may cause a fall in perfusion to the brain. Those that also cause sedation may lead to dementia in the elderly.
4. The widespread use of antidepressants and NSAIDs may block some of the expected effects of antihypertensive agents.

Hypertension in children. The 1987 report of the Second Task Force on Blood Pressure Control in Children says

> Nonpharmacological intervention strategies can be introduced as initial treatment and tailored to meet the needs of the individual patient. Traditional forms of antihypertensive drug therapy should be reserved for use in patients with severe hypertension or when BP remains markedly elevated after several weeks to months of nonpharmacological therapy. . . . Major questions still remain with regard to the long-term effects of drug treatment on children and adolescents. In particular, drugs altering peripheral or central adrenergic activity may adversely affect physical performance or cognitive function. Also, the recognized adverse effects of diuretics on glucose metabolism and of diuretics and beta-adrenergic blocking agents on lipid metabolism are of equal concern. Thus a definite need for treatment must be established before therapy with any of these agents is introduced during the first or second decade of life with the possibility of 50 to 60 years (or more) of continuous antihypertensive therapy.

Patients who need special care. Patients at higher risk from their hypertension need even more protection from effective antihypertensive therapy. This includes diabetics, blacks, and hypertensive patients with target organ damage affecting their brain, heart, or kidneys.

Of these patients, hypertensive diabetics are particularly vulnerable to rapidly progressive renal damage. They should be followed with frequent measurements of urine protein and creatinine clearance. If either is abnormal, intensive therapy to prevent hyperperfusion of remaining glomeruli by either hypertension or hyperglycemia may protect them from progressive sclerosis and thereby delay, if not stop, the hitherto inexorable progression to renal failure. Preliminary evidence shows that ACE inhibitors may be especially useful in reversing intraglomerular hypertension (Chapter 355).

Hypertensive crises. Several clinical circumstances require rapid reduction of the blood pressure. These circumstances include hypertensive encephalopathy, severe hypertension in the presence of rapidly developing target organ damage, and accelerated malignant-hypertension.

In most hypertensive crises the diastolic blood pressure is greater than 140 mm Hg. Funduscopic findings may include hemorrhages, exudates, and papilledema. The manifestations of encephalopathy include headache, confusion, somnolence, stupor, visual loss, focal defects, seizures, or coma. Cardiac findings include a hyperdynamic sustained left ventricular impulse, cardiac enlargement, and pulmonary venous hypertension. Oliguria and azotemia are usually present, as are symptoms of nausea and vomiting.

The drugs listed in Table 23-5 should provide as rapid and complete a reduction in markedly elevated pressures as needed. Oral nifedipine works very well for those not needing parenteral therapy who have only a hypertensive urgency, that is, severe hypertension but no immediate danger to vital organs. Intravenous nitroprusside is surely the most effective and certain way to lower dangerously high blood pressure, but it requires constant surveillance and blood pressure monitoring.

Maintaining adherence to therapy

Most patients for whom drug therapy is prescribed take the drug assiduously at first. But with the onset of either bothersome side effects or the natural tendency to lose motivation and forget, as many as half are not adhering to therapy a year later. The following practices should be helpful in improving patients' adherence to therapy:

1. Inform patients of their blood pressure and overall cardiovascular risk status by use of Framingham predictive data available from the American Heart Association's *Coronary Risk Handbook* or pharmaceutical companies' hand calculators.
2. Be gentle in trying to change unhealthy lifestyles, but insist on the need to do so.
3. Repeatedly emphasize the need to stop smoking, and to reduce calories, sodium, and saturated fat and to increase isotonic exercise, perhaps not all at one time but eventually.
4. Prescribe medications in the fewest number and lowest doses possible, slowly building up to required levels.
5. Go slow with medications to avoid symptoms of cerebral hypoperfusion, allowing the system to readjust by autoregulation to a lower blood pressure level. With the initial fall in blood pressure, even if not to "hypotensive" levels, cerebral blood flow may decrease. The range of blood pressure over which autoregulation maintains a normal cerebral blood flow is shifted to the right in chronic hypertensives; when blood pressure is lowered below the lower end of this range, but still at a level above 140/90 mm Hg, cerebral blood flow may fall, leading to postural dizziness, weakness, and fatigue.
6. Involve the patient (and, if acceptable, the spouse) in the process as a willing partner, not as a passive recipient. Use home blood pressure measurements, medication diaries, and self-determined behavioral goals. The currently available home blood pressure units with microphone detectors and digital readouts can be easily used by virtually every patient, and their

Table 23-5. Parenteral drugs for treatment of hypertensive emergency (in order of rapidity of action)

Drug	Dosage	Onset of action	Adverse effects
Vasodilators			
Nitroprusside (Nipride, Nitropress)	0.25-10 μg/kg/min as IV infusion	Instantaneous	Nausea, vomiting, muscle twitching, sweating, thiocyanate intoxication
Nitroglycerin	5-100 μg/min as IV infusion	2-5 min	Tachycardia, flushing, headache, vomiting, methemoglobinemia
Diazoxide (Hyperstat)	50-100 mg/IV bolus repeated, or 15-30 mg/min by IV infusion	2-4 min	Nausea, hypotension, flushing, tachycardia, chest pain
Hydralazine (Apresoline)	10-20 mg IV 10-50 mg IM	10-20 min 20-30 min	Tachycardia, flushing, headache, vomiting, aggravation of angina
Enalapril (Vasotec IV)	1.25-5 mg q 6 hr	15 min	Precipitous fall in BP in high renin states; response variable
Nicardipine	5-10 mg/hr IV	10 min	Tachycardia, headache, flushing, local phlebitis
Adrenergic inhibitors			
Phentolamine (Regitine)	5-15 mg IV	1-2 min	Tachycardia, flushing
Trimethaphan (Arfonad)	0.5-5 mg/min as IV infusion	1-5 min	Paresis of bowel and bladder, orthostatic hypotension, blurred vision, dry mouth
Esmolol (Brevibloc)	500 μg/kg/min for 4 min, then 150-300 μg/kg/min IV	1-2 min	Hypotension
Propranolol (Inderal)	1-10 mg load; 3 ng/hr	1-2 min	Beta blocker side effects, e.g., bronchospasm, decreased cardiac output
Labetalol (Normodyne, Trandate)	20-80 mg IV bolus every 10 min 2 mg/min IV infusion	5-10 min	Vomiting, scalp tingling, burning in throat, postural hypotension, dizziness, nausea

relatively low cost makes them accessible to most. Their use will provide a better idea of the usual range of the blood pressure, helping to establish the diagnosis and to make the decision to start treatment. Once patients are on therapy, it is particularly important to ensure dampening of the abrupt rise in pressure upon awakening that is responsible for the increased incidence of heart attacks and strokes in the early morning. If these postawakening pressures are not lowered, longer-acting medications or twice-a-day dosing may be needed.

7. Use nonphysician personnel for follow-up and psychological support. As physician extenders, they can be particularly effective in monitoring and encouraging the use of nondrug regimens.

The application of these maneuvers to improve adherence to treatment and the judicious use of both nondrug and drug therapies should make it possible to bring the blood pressure down to safe levels in virtually all patients with hypertension.

REFERENCES

British Hypertension Society Working Party. Treating mild hypertension. Agreement from the large trials. Br Med J 298:694, 1989.

Carlsen JE et al: Relation between dose of bendrofluazide, antihypertensive effect, and adverse biochemical effects. Br Med J 300:975, 1990.

Cruickshank JM: Coronary flow reserve and the J curve relation between diastolic blood pressure and myocardial infarction. Br Med J 297:1227, 1988.

Cutler JA, MacMahon SW, Furberg CD: Controlled clinical trials of drug treatment for hypertension. A review. Hypertension 13(suppl I):I, 1989.

Dahlöf B et al: Morbidity and mortality in the Swedish Trial in Old Patients with Hypertension (STOP-Hypertension). Lancet 338:1281, 1991.

Ferrannini E: Insulin and blood pressure: possible role of hemodynamics. Clin Exp Hypertens [A] 14:271, 1992.

Fletcher AE and Bulpitt CJ: How far should blood pressure be lowered? N Engl J Med 326:251, 1992.

Folkow B: Psychosocial and central nervous influences in primary hypertension. Circulation 76(Suppl. 1):I, 1987.

Guyton AC: Kidneys and fluids in pressure regulation. Small volume but large pressure changes. Hypertension 19(suppl I):I, 1992.

Horan MJ and Sinaiko AR: Synopsis of the report of the Second Task Force on Blood Pressure Control in Children. Hypertension 10:115, 1987.

Joint National Committee on Detection, Evaluation, and Treatment of High Blood Pressure. The 1993 report. Arch Intern Med in press.

Kaplan NM: Clinical hypertension, ed 5. Baltimore, 1990, Williams & Wilkins.

Kaplan NM: The deadly quartet: upper body obesity, glucose intolerance, hypertriglyceridemia and hypertension. Arch Intern Med 149:1514, 1989.

Law MR, Frost CD, and Wald NJ: III—Analysis of data from trials of salt reduction. Br Med J 302:819, 1991.

Lever AF: Slow pressor mechanisms in hypertension: a role for hypertrophy of resistance vessels? J Hypertens 4:515, 1986.

Lithell HOL: Effect of antihypertensive drugs on insulin, glucose, and lipid metabolism. Diabetes Care 14:203, 1991.

Lund-Johansen P: Central haemodynamics in essential hypertension at rest and during exercise: a 20-year follow-up study. J Hypertens 7(suppl 6):S52, 1989.

MacMahon S: Alcohol consumption and hypertension. Hypertension 9:111, 1987.

MacMahon S et al: Blood pressure, stroke, and coronary heart disease. Part 1, prolonged differences in blood pressure: prospective observational studies corrected for the regression dilution bias. Lancet 335:765, 1990.

Neaton JD and Wentworth D: Serum cholesterol, blood pressure, cigarette smoking, and death from coronary heart disease. Overall findings and differences by age for 316,099 white men. Arch Intern Med 152:56, 1992.

Perloff D, Sokolow M, and Cowan R: The prognostic value of ambulatory blood pressures. JAMA 249:2792, 1983.

Pickering TG et al: How common is white coat hypertension? JAMA 259:225, 1988.

SHEP Cooperative Research Group: Prevention of stroke by antihypertensive drug treatment in older persons with isolated systolic hypertension. Final results of the Systolic Hypertension in the Elderly Program (SHEP). JAMA 265:3255, 1991.

Shepherd JT: Increased systemic vascular resistance and primary hypertension: the expanding complexity. J Hypertension 8(Suppl 7):S15, 1990.

Treatment of Mild Hypertension Research Group. The treatment of mild hypertension study. A randomized, placebo-controlled trial of a nutritional-hygienic regimen along with various drug monotherapies. Arch Intern Med 151:1413, 1991.

Yanagisawa M et al: A novel potent vasoconstrictor peptide produced by vascular endothelial cells. Nature 332:411, 1988.

Ying CY et al: Renal revascularization in the azotemic hypertensive patient resistant to therapy. N Engl J Med 311:1070, 1984.

CHAPTER

24 Cardiac Tumors; Cardiac Manifestations of Endocrine, Collagen Vascular, and HIV Disease; and Traumatic Injury of the Heart

John S. MacGregor
Melvin D. Cheitlin

CARDIAC TUMORS

Primary tumors of the heart are relatively rare, but correct and timely diagnosis is important because surgical cure is often possible. Seventy-five percent of primary cardiac tumors are benign histologically; however, because of their location, they frequently produce life-threatening complications. Protean clinical manifestations, which are in part determined by the size and location of the tumor, have been described. They include chest pain, dyspnea, syncope, arrhythmias, murmurs, systemic and central nervous system emboli, and coronary artery and pulmonary artery emboli as well as pericardial effusion, cardiac tamponade, fever, weight loss, and edema. The diagnosis most often is made by two-dimensional echocardiography, and/or angiography. More recently it has been established with increasing fre-

Table 24-1. Incidence of primary cardiac tumors

	Percentage of primary cardiac tumors
Benign	
Myxoma	30.5
Lipoma	10.5
Papillary fibroelastoma	9.9
Rhabdomyoma	8.5
Fibroma	4.0
Hemangioma	3.5
Teratoma	3.3
AV node mesothelioma	2.8
Other benign tumors	2.1
TOTAL BENIGN TUMORS	75.1
Malignant	
Angiosarcoma	9.2
Rhabdomyosarcoma	6.1
Fibrosarcoma	3.2
Lymphoma	1.6
Other malignant tumors	4.8
TOTAL MALIGNANT TUMORS	24.9

Modified from McAllister HA and Fenoglio JJ: Atlas of tumor pathology. Washington, DC, 1978, Armed Forces Institute of Pathology.

quency by computer tomography or magnetic resonance imaging. The relative incidence of primary cardiac tumors is shown on Table 24-1.

MYXOMA

Myxomas account for about one third of primary cardiac tumors. They are much more common in adults, with the greatest incidence between the third and sixth decades. Most cases are sporadic, but familial autosomal dominant transmission has been reported. Rare cases have been associated with a syndrome that includes multiple pigmented skin lesions, myxomatous mammary fibroadenomas, and adrenocortical disease. The left atrium is the most common location for myxomas, accounting for about 80% of cases. Fifteen percent are located in the right atrium, with most of the remainder arising in the right ventricle. Left ventricular myxomas are exceedingly rare. Atrial myxomas are usually attached to the interatrial septum in the region of the limbus of the fossa ovalis. Less often they are attached to the posterior or anterior atrial walls or to the atrial appendage. Cardiac myxomas arise from multipotential mesenchymal cells present in subendocardial tissue. At the time of excision, they are usually 5 to 6 centimeters in diameter and project into a cardiac chamber on a short, broad-based fibrovascular stalk, which is in communication with the subendocardium. Characteristically, they have a polypoid and pedunculated appearance.

Although cardiac myxomas are generally considered to be benign, histologically, several reports have suggested that they may rarely possess a malignant potential. These include reports of distant metastasis with independent growth, local invasion, and local recurrence after excision.

Clinical manifestations fall into three major categories: hemodynamic compromise, embolization, and constitutional symptoms. The nature of the hemodynamic manifestations depends upon the size and location of the tumor. Left atrial myxomas commonly mimic mitral valve disease, especially mitral stenosis, in their clinical presentation. Symptoms are those of left-sided heart failure, including dyspnea and occasionally chest pain. Intermittent obstruction of the mitral outflow tract by a large mobile myxoma can lead to syncope or sudden death. Physical findings with left atrial myxoma may include a low-pitched, early to mid-diastolic sound known as a "tumor plop," and a diastolic murmur resembling that of mitral stenosis. Mitral valve disease can sometimes be distinguished from atrial myxoma on physical examination by identifying marked positional variation of the physical findings. The systolic murmur of mitral regurgitation may result from injury to the mitral valve caused by the tumor.

Right atrial myxomas produce hemodynamic symptoms, either by intermittently obstructing the tricuspid valve and mimicking tricuspid stenosis, or by damaging the valve and producing tricuspid regurgitation. Hemodynamic manifestations of right atrial myxoma include dyspnea, edema, hepatosplenomegaly, and elevated jugular venous pressure. These findings may be confused with cor pulmonale, constrictive pericarditis, and Ebstein's anomaly.

About 50% of patients with myxoma have embolic manifestations, including emboli to the central nervous system, coronary arteries, peripheral organs and viscera, and in the case of right atrial myxoma, to the lungs. Constitutional symptoms are common in patients with myxoma, and in some cases may dominate the presentation. Constitutional manifestations of myxoma include fever, fatigue, malaise, weight loss, arthralgias, myalgias, rash, Raynaud's phenomenon, leukocytosis, elevated erythrocyte sedimentation rate, abnormal serum proteins, and hypergammaglobulinemia. These symptoms result from an immunologic reaction to a "foreign" antigen. Typically, these systemic signs resolve after excision of the myxoma.

The diagnosis of myxoma is confirmed by either transthoracic or transesophageal two-dimensional echocardiography, which usually demonstrates the size and site of attachment of a myxoma (Chapter 5). Magnetic resonance imaging has been used to verify or exclude the presence of intracardiac tumors in cases where the echocardiographic diagnosis is equivocal. In most cases cardiac catheterization and cineangiography are not necessary to make this diagnosis. It may, however, be necessary to diagnose coexistent cardiac or coronary artery disease prior to surgery. When catheterization is required, direct catheterization of the chamber from which the tumor arises should be avoided, since it can lead to tumor dislodgement and embolization. Surgical excision including the portion of the atrium from which the tumor arises is usually curative, although local recurrence occasionally occurs. Operative mortality and morbidity are low, and the prognosis after excision is generally excellent, usually with total resolution of preoperative symptoms.

OTHER BENIGN CARDIAC TUMORS

Lipomas and papillary fibroelastomas each account for about 15% of benign cardiac tumors. Lipomas most often occur in the interatrial septum, where they grow as a non-encapsulated mass of adipose tissue, which bulges in the subendocardium into the right atrium. Lipomas develop by hypertrophy of adipose tissue, which is in continuity with epicardial fat, and are not true neoplasms. They are most commonly asymptomatic and are usually incidental findings at autopsy. Supraventricular arrhythmias, conduction disturbances, and hemodynamic compromise may be seen.

Papillary fibroelastomas arise from cardiac valves or adjacent endothelium. They are usually asymptomatic and, like lipomas, are usually incidental findings on postmortem examination. They occasionally cause symptoms either by embolization or by interference with valve function. Rarely they lodge in the ostium of one of the coronary arteries, resulting in sudden death. Rhabdomyomas are the most common benign cardiac tumor in children, 90% of cases occurring prior to age 15. Rhabdomyomas are thought to be hamartomatous growths derived from fetal cardiac myoblasts. They are multicentric in up to 90% of cases. They are found most commonly in the ventricles, but up to 30% involve the atria. This tumor usually grows deep within the myocardium but can also have intracavitary extension. There is a strong association between rhabdomyomas and tuberous sclerosis, a condition characterized by mental retardation and convulsions (Chapter 175). Clinical manifestations include tachyarrhythmias and heart failure. Surgical resection can be difficult because of multicentric growth, lack of encapsulation, and intramyocardial location, but it should be considered to relieve symptoms in suitable individuals.

Fibromas occur in both pediatric and adult patients but are more common in children. They are solitary and usually involve the ventricular septum. Symptoms relate to conduction system involvement and often include arrhythmias and sudden death. Surgical therapies have included tumor resection, and in the case of unresectable tumors, cardiac transplantation. Mesotheliomas are intramyocardial tumors, which most commonly occur near the atrioventricular node. They can cause conduction disturbances including complete heart block and sudden death. Antiarrhythmic agents and pacemaker implantation in selected patients with fibromas and mesotheliomas may be useful.

MALIGNANT PRIMARY CARDIAC TUMORS

Malignant tumors comprise about 25% of all cardiac tumors. Sarcomas account for almost all of the malignant tumors, with angiosarcomas and rhabdomyosarcomas being the most common histologic types. These tumors may arise in any cardiac chamber, but right-sided involvement is more common. Symptoms at presentation include rapidly progressive heart failure, arrhythmias, and hemopericardium with tamponade. At the time of diagnosis, advanced regional extension and distant metastasis are often present, precluding curative surgical excision. Surgery may be needed, however, to establish a tissue diagnosis to guide chemotherapy and radiation therapy, which may slow progression in some cases. The prognosis is poor with most patients dying within 1 year of the diagnosis.

METASTATIC TUMORS INVOLVING THE HEART

Metastasis of noncardiac tumors to the heart is a much more common cause of neoplastic heart disease than primary cardiac tumors. In a large autopsy series, up to 20% of patients dying of a malignancy had cardiac or pericardial metastases. Like metastasis elsewhere in the body, mechanisms of metastasis to the heart include direct tumor extension and lymphatic and hematogenous spread. The pericardium, myocardium, and endocardium may all be involved. The gross appearance of the metastatic tumor may be either diffuse and infiltrative or nodular.

The prevalence of cardiac involvement with several specific noncardiac primary tumors is shown in Table 24-2. Melanoma and leukemia commonly involve the heart, with a 45% and 33% incidence of cardiac metastasis diagnosed at autopsy, respectively. Lung and breast cancer account for the largest absolute number of cardiac metastases, accounting for 28% and 12% of all cardiac metastases, respectively. If cardiac involvement is present, widespread metastatic disease is usually present. With the advent of the adult immunodeficiency syndrome resulting from HIV infection, Kaposi's sarcoma and non-Hodgkin's lymphoma have become important tumors involving the heart. Cardiac symptoms attributable to metastases are present in only about 10% of the patients with metastatic tumors to the heart. Symptoms, when present, typically relate to heart failure, pericarditis, pericardial tamponade, and vena caval

Table 24-2. Prevalence of cardiac metastasis at postmortem examination in patients with various tumors

Tumor	Percentage with cardiac metastases*
Melanoma	45 (433)
Leukemia	33 (1345)
Lung	23 (3523)
Breast	21 (1639)
Non-Hodgkin's lymphoma	20 (953)
Hodgkin's lymphoma	8 (562)
Renal	10 (501)

Pooled data from 19 studies, modified from Weinberg BA, Conces DJ, and Waller BF: Clin Cardiol 12:289, 1989.

*Numbers in parenthesis indicate total number of autopsy examinations performed in each tumor category.

obstruction. The latter is seen frequently in tumors that can grow up from the kidney into the inferior vena cava and the right side of the heart.

A chest roentenogram showing an enlarged cardiac silhouette or evidence of mediastinal tumor may suggest the diagnosis of tumor metastasis to the heart. Echocardiography is useful for identifying pericardial effusion and confirming the presence of tamponade. Metastatic tumor masses may be seen with echocardiography, magnetic resonance imaging, or computed tomography. Large symptomatic malignant pericardial effusions can be effectively treated with drainage by a subxyphoid pericardial window under local anesthesia with minimal morbidity. Radiation therapy or treatment with a local sclerosing agent can be beneficial in controlling recurrence of malignant pericardial effusions (Chapter 18). Survival of patients with metastatic involvement of the heart depends on the extent and rate of progression of the primary disease. In one series, up to 50% of patients treated with a subxyphoid pericardiectomy were dead within 3 months.

CARDIOVASCULAR TRAUMA

Trauma to the myocardium, septum, valves, coronary arteries, aorta, and veins can occur with both penetrating and nonpenetrating injuries. In most instances of nonpenetrating cardiovascular trauma the patient has multiple injuries, and the cardiovascular trauma may be incidental and overlooked. This is especially true with nonpenetrating injuries, such as compression injuries in automobile accidents causing myocardial contusion. When a cardiac chamber is lacerated in nonpenetrating injury, the laceration is usually extensive and the injury fatal.

In penetrating trauma the amount of damage is related to the mass of the penetrating object and to its velocity. High-velocity missiles, as in gunshot wounds, cause extensive damage and are most frequently fatal. Low-velocity missiles, as in knife wounds, cause limited lacerations; if the bleeding is from a low-pressure chamber, such as the right ventricle or the right atrium, then pericardial tamponade occurs slowly enough for the patient to survive to receive medical care.

Pericardial tamponade must be suspected in every patient with a penetrating injury who has hypotension. If the intravascular volume is normal and tamponade occurs gradually, the patient may have the usual clinical picture of pericardial tamponade including tachycardia, increased central venous pressure, and hypotension. However, in trauma patients with hypovolemia caused by hemorrhage, pericardial tamponade must be suspected when the penetrating injury could have involved the heart and when there is hypotension despite fluid and blood replacement, even if the central venous pressure is not elevated. If the patient is hemodynamically stable, pericardiocentesis can be attempted. If the bleeding is rapid, however, blood often clots in the pericardium and is impossible to extract through a needle. In this case thoracotomy is necessary with extraction of the pericardial blood and clot. If the patient is hemodynamically unstable, immediate thoracotomy with relief of the tamponade and repair of the laceration is life-saving.

With nonpenetrating injury the commonest problem is myocardial contusion. This results from chest compression, as occurs with steering-wheel injuries, and also from sudden deceleration where the chest wall suddenly stops moving and the mediastinum crashes into the chest wall at the velocity that the vehicle had been travelling. The incidence of myocardial contusion at postmortem examination in fatal accidents involving thoracoabdominal trauma is about 15%. The incidence of myocardial contusion in survivors of nonpenetrating thoracoabdominal trauma is difficult to assess and depends on the criteria used to diagnose myocardial contusion.

Myocardial contusion results in intramyocardial hemorrhage and myocardial necrosis. Because of its location, the right ventricle is most frequently involved, followed in frequency by the left ventricle. The retrosternal right atrium and posterior left atrium are less commonly involved. Arrhythmias, both ventricular and atrial, are frequent; electrocardiographic changes, including ST-T wave changes and QRS changes, including those of acute myocardial infarction, are seen, as are varying degrees of AV block and bundle-branch block.

Myocardial contusion is difficult to diagnose. Pericardial friction rubs with pericardial effusion and congestive heart failure are good evidence for the presence of myocardial contusion. However, arrhythmias are less specific and can be seen with sympathetic stimulation and anxiety after injury. Electrocardiographic changes can be either preexisting or caused by hypoxia. Arrhythmias and ECG changes can be related to drugs that have been taken, such as alcohol or other therapeutic or illicit drugs involved in the precipitation of the accident. Hypotension can result from hemorrhage. Pulmonary edema on chest x-ray can actually be related to pulmonary contusion. None of these findings are specific for myocardial contusion. A rise in serum creatine kinase (CK) is usually caused by skeletal-muscle injury. A rise in CK-MB fraction is more specific for myocardial necrosis but also occurs with smooth-muscle injury and even with massive skeletal muscle necrosis. Imaging techniques such as radionuclide angiography or 2D echocardiography can show areas of hypokinesia or even akinesia in myocardial contusions and thus indicate that the ECG changes seen are probably related to myocardial contusion.

All the complications seen after acute myocardial infarction can occur after myocardial contusion, including rupture of the left ventricular free wall, rupture of the septum with the development of a ventricular septal defect, mitral regurgitation, fatal arrhythmias, congestive heart failure, and false and true ventricular aneurysms. However, if the patient has a suspected, uncomplicated myocardial contusion without tamponade and without heart failure, serious complications from the contusion rarely occur either in the hospital or on follow-up. In the absence of symptomatic arrhythmias the patient can safely be observed on a nonmonitored ward before discharge. Symptomatic arrhythmias should be observed in a monitored ward and treated with lidocaine. Late complications of uncomplicated myocardial contusion are very unusual.

On rare occasions penetrating and nonpenetrating injuries can injure the interventricular septum and cause an interventricular septal defect, or can rupture an aortic, mitral, or tricuspid valve cusp, or even rupture a papillary muscle, all resulting in valvular regurgitation, varying in degree from severe acute valvular regurgitation requiring afterload reduction and immediate surgery to mild degrees of valvular regurgitation that do not require surgery.

Coronary arteries can be injured, especially with penetrating injuries, and tamponade can occur from a laceration of the coronary artery. Injury to a coronary artery and coronary vein can result in a coronary arteriovenous fistula. Occasionally, coronary-cameral fistulas result from injury. All these can best be evaluated by coronary arteriography.

Of the great vessel injuries, traumatic rupture of the aorta is the most serious. It occurs most frequently in deceleration injuries in automobile accidents. The most common site of rupture is in the proximal descending aorta, just after the take-off of the subclavian artery, and about 15% of patients with ruptured aorta survive long enough to reach medical care and be diagnosed clinically. The second most common site of rupture is in the ascending aorta, just above the aortic valve; because of the intrapericardial position of the ascending aorta this almost always results in death from tamponade. Aortic rupture should be suspected on the basis of chest roentgenograms showing a widened mediastinum. Other signs such as fluid capping the left lung, left pleural effusion, and obscuration of the descending aorta by bleeding in the mediastinum should all alert the physician to possible rupture of the aorta. When suspected, immediate aortography followed by immediate repair is indicated. In false aneurysms caused by remote injury, repair is still indicated because false aneurysms can rupture at any time. In some centers, computed tomography (CT) scans are recommended as a screening test for ruptured aorta in patients with widened mediastinum. Transesophageal echocardiography (TEE) has also been used to make the diagnosis. In most hospitals aortography is the most immediately available diagnostic technique.

Slow-velocity missiles can enter the heart muscle or cardiac chambers or vessels and lodge there. These missiles can cause infection and damage to the chambers. Moreover, if they lie in the lumen of veins, arteries, or cardiac chambers they can migrate forward, the venous missiles lodging finally in the right heart or pulmonary artery and left heart or arterial missiles migrating distally causing obstruction. Another complication is the development of thrombus and fibrin, which can then embolize. Foreign bodies, especially in the left chamber of the heart or arteries, should be removed. If the missile is small and intramyocardial and causes no mechanical dysfunction, the patient can be observed without surgical removal.

Finally, the fastest growing cause of traumatic cardiovascular injury is iatrogenic trauma resulting from the increase in invasive medical procedures being performed. This includes laceration of arteries and veins, perforation of the right ventricle with a catheter resulting in tamponade, and cutting off of intravascular lines. These lost catheters usually can be removed with snare catheters without surgery.

ACQUIRED IMMUNODEFICIENCY SYNDROME (AIDS)

Infection with the human immunodeficiency virus (HIV), a retrovirus that invades the nucleus of the host cell and incorporates a copy of its DNA in the host genetic material, was first recognized in 1981 (Chapter 242). After a latent period, the virus releases into the cytoplasm double-stranded DNA copies of the virus, eventually killing the cell and invading other immune cells, usually T-helper lymphocytes, eventually compromising the immune defense mechanism of the host. This makes the host susceptible to opportunistic infections and unusual cancers such as Kaposi's sarcoma and non-Hodgkin's lymphoma from which the patient eventually dies.

In the United States, the populations at high risk are homosexual men, IV-drug-abusing patients, prostitutes, and patients receiving blood products, such as hemophiliacs. Heterosexual transmission occurs in women who are IV drug abusers and/or have sexual intercourse with infected men (Chapter 242).

Cardiovascular involvement in AIDS is usually clinically of little consequence, possibly because the myocardial cell lacks the CD-4 receptor necessary for the virus to enter the cell. Cardiovascular involvement is seen with opportunistic infections such as toxoplasmosis, *Candida, Cryptococcus,* and cytomegalovirus. Rarely, the patient can have a severe, clinically important myocarditis with toxoplasmosis. Pericarditis with pericardial effusion and tamponade is the commonest clinical cardiovascular problem in our experience; about a third of the patients with pericardial fluid develop tamponade requiring pericardiocentesis. Most often an etiologic agent is not found on culture of the pericardial fluid or biopsy of the pericardium. However, involvement with lymphoma and with *Mycobacterium tuberculosis* and *avium* is not uncommon.

Patients with severe pulmonary hypertension, right ventricular dilatation, and even right ventricular failure have been reported. This usually occurs in patients with multiple episodes of *Pneumocystis carinii* infections. Other cardiovascular abnormalities in patients with HIV infection have included thrombotic noninfectious endocarditis (marantic endocarditis) and mitral valve prolapse. When infective endocarditis is seen, it is usually in IV drug abusers.

The most interesting cardiovascular involvement seen is the patient with decreased left ventricular function, with or without left ventricular dilatation. This is not an uncommon echocardiographic finding, and wall motion abnormalities including hypokinesis are reported in 15% to 40% of patients with AIDS. At postmortem examination, focal collections of round cells in the myocardium—so-called focal myocarditis—can be seen in 20% to 40% of patients. Diffuse myocarditis, on the other hand, is rare. At autopsy, dilated cardiomyopathy is also rare, as is dilated cardiomyopathy with clinical congestive heart failure, which occur in approximately 1% of patients.

The etiology of cardiomyopathy is unknown, but there are probably multiple explanations. Myocarditis resulting from HIV infection is the most obvious explanation. Attempts have been made to demonstrate the HIV organism in the myocardium, with limited success. Calebrese reported culturing the HIV virus from a right ventricular myocardial biopsy from a patient with a normal left ventricular myocardium and no evidence of left ventricular disease. Lewis and colleagues have reported positive identification of portions of the HIV virion in the myocardium from people dying of AIDS by in-situ hybridization techniques. These positive findings were infrequent and from this technique it is not clear that the identified nucleic acid sequences were derived from myocytes. They could have been from endothelial cells, circulating lymphocytes, or tissue macrophages. Furthermore, the hearts of these patients were all normal without clinical or microscopic evidence of cardiac abnormality.

Other explanations of poor systolic contractile function have been suggested. These patients often are taking a wide variety of drugs, some of which are known cardiac depressants capable of causing cardiomyopathy. Such drugs as adriamycin, interleukin II, and interferon-alpha have all been reported to cause cardiomyopathy, which is at times irreversible. The patients with hypokinesis and poor contractile function on echocardiography have been described as improving when azidothymidine (AZT) is withdrawn, and a "drug holiday" has been advised in such patients. Another possible explanation for hypokinesis is cytokine production, either systemically or locally in the myocardium, which could produce myocardial depression.

If the patient has a known pathogen as the cause of the myocarditis or pericarditis, obviously treatment specific for the organism is indicated. The value of myocardial biopsy is limited in such patients, since the finding of round cell infiltration is not likely to alter treatment.

DIABETES

Patients with diabetes have increased cardiovascular mortality and morbidity (Chapter 168). Diabetes is an independent risk factor for the development of coronary artery disease, which is frequently more diffuse and severe than in patients without diabetes. Silent ischemia, or angina with atypical features, is more common in diabetics, probably resulting from autonomic and sensory neuropathies. Patients with insulin-dependent diabetes mellitus have an increased risk of developing congestive heart failure even in the absence of coronary artery disease, leading to the postulation of a diabetes-induced cardiomyopathy. Systolic and diastolic dysfunction have both been demonstrated in diabetics.

HYPERTHYROIDISM

Excess thyroid hormone stimulates the heart both through direct effects on cardiac muscle and by stimulating the sympathetic nervous system (Chapter 162). Cardiovascular manifestations of hyperthyroidism include palpitations, dyspnea, angina, heart failure, tachycardia, atrial fibrillation, hypertension, and increased cardiac output. Angina and congestive heart failure more commonly occur in patients with underlying heart disease, but they can occur in patients without coronary artery disease. In elderly patients, cardiovascular dysfunction, including atrial fibrillation and congestive heart failure, may be the only manifestations of hyperthyroidism. Therefore all elderly patients with these conditions should have laboratory determination of thyroid function. Findings on cardiac examination in hyperthyroid patients may include a wide pulse pressure, hyperdynamic precordium, accentuation of S_1 and S_2, and a pleuropericardial rub (Means-Lerman scratch) usually best heard in the second left intercostal space. Definitive therapy of hyperthyroidism is either surgical or pharmacologic ablation of the gland. Cardiac glycosides have been used to treat atrial arrhythmias; however, in hyperthyroidism there is frequently decreased sensitivity to conventional doses of these drugs. Beta-adrenoceptor antagonists are useful in controlling rapid atrial arrhythmias and may also decrease other symptoms related to thyrotoxicosis. In the presence of severe heart failure they must be used cautiously.

HYPOTHYROIDISM

Hypothyroid patients may present with bradycardia, dyspnea, and easy fatiguability (Chapter 162). Physical findings may include bradycardia, hypotension, distant heart sounds, edema, and rales. Cardiomegaly with global hypokinesis and four-chamber enlargement may be present in advanced cases. Pericardial and pleural effusion may be present, but pericardial tamponade is rare. Hypothyroidism is associated with hypercholesterolemia and hypertriglyceridemia and patients are at increased risk for atherosclerotic vascular disease. Cardiac dysfunction related to hypothyroidism can be totally reversible with thyroid replacement therapy. Repletion of thyroid hormone should be done slowly, especially in the presence of coronary artery disease, to avoid precipitating episodes of unstable angina or myocardial infarction.

OBESITY

Increased cardiovascular mortality and morbidity in obese patients is in part related to increased rates of hypertension, atherosclerosis, and glucose intolerance (Chapter 153). Hemodynamic effects of obesity include increased left ventricular filling pressures, increased left ventricular end-diastolic volume, and increased cardiac output. Some obese patients develop an eccentric left ventricular hypertrophy with chamber dilatation, which is associated with an increased incidence of ventricular ectopy and episodes of pulmonary edema. Weight reduction may have a salubrious effect on cardiac dysfunction related to obesity.

Some patients with extreme obesity hyperventilate causing hypoxia, hypercarbia, and respiratory acidosis, allpowerful stimulators of pulmonary vasoconstriction. This causes severe pulmonary hypertension and cor pulmonale. This has been called the Pickwickian syndrome (Chapter 190). The pulmonary hypertension is rapidly reversible with hyperventilation and the weight loss is the definitive treatment.

RHEUMATOID DISEASES

Cardiac manifestations of chronic rheumatoid diseases include pericardial effusion, pericarditis, myocarditis, arteritis, valvular abnormalities, conduction disturbances, heart failure, angina, and myocardial infarction. Systemic lupus erythematosus involves the heart in over 75% of patients; postmortem series demonstrate evidence of pericarditis in over two thirds of patients (Chapter 304). Pericardial tamponade and constrictive pericarditis are rare. Valvular pathology occurs in 30% to 50% of patients. Lesions include thickened valve leaflets with impaired function, which may lead to regurgitation or stenosis, and sterile Libman-Sacks vegetations. Myocarditis and coronary arteritis are sometimes seen. Accelerated or premature atherosclerosis may result in myocardial ischemia or infarction.

Necropsy series demonstrate cardiac involvement with rheumatoid arthritis in up to 50% of patients, pericarditis being the most common manifestation (Chapter 340). The clinical incidence of pericarditis is much lower than this, in the range of 5%, and is usually easily treated with steroids and anti-inflammatory agents. Tamponade and constriction are rare. Coronary arteritis is present at autopsy in about 20% of patients with rheumatoid arthritis and may rarely lead to severe luminal narrowing with development of angina or myocardial infarction. Rheumatoid arthritis patients also have a higher incidence of atherosclerosis. Granulomatous inflammation of the cardiac valves can result in deformity and valvular insufficiency.

Progressive systemic sclerosis carries a poor prognosis when there is cardiac involvement (Chapter 309). Diffuse myocardial fibrosis with congestive heart failure occurs late in the course of this disease. Pericarditis and coronary arteritis are often also present in patients with progressive systemic sclerosis.

Polyarteritis nodosa results in a necrotizing vasculitis of the coronary arteries in up to 50% of cases, often with the formation of multiple areas of aneurysmal dilatation (Chapter 307). Myocarditis and focal myocardial necrosis may follow the arteritis with subsequent development of congestive heart failure, a common cause of death in these patients. Valvular pathology is uncommon in patients with polyarteritis nodosa. Pericarditis is present in about 20% of these patients.

REFERENCES

Baroldi G et al: Echocardiography detects myocardial damage in AIDS: prospective study in 102 patients. Eur Heart J 9:887, 1988.

Cheitlin MD: The internist's role in the management of the patient with traumatic heart disease. Cardiol Clin 9:675, 1991.

Cristina S and Negri C: Focal lymphocytic myocarditis in acquired immunodeficiency syndrome (AIDS): a correlative morphologic and clinical study in 26 consecutive fatal cases. J Am Coll Cardiol 12:463, 1988.

Doherty NE and Siegel RJ: The cardiovascular manifestations of systemic lupus erythematosus. Am Heart J 110:1257, 1985.

Dubrow TJ et al: Myocardial contusion in the stable patient: what level of care is appropriate? Surgery 106:267, 1989.

Follansbee WP et al: Physiologic abnormalities of cardiac function in progressive systemic sclerosis with diffuse scleroderma. N Engl J Med 310:142, 1984.

Forfar JC et al: Abnormal left ventricular function in hyperthyroidism. N Engl J Med 307:1165, 1982.

Francis CK: Cardiac involvement in AIDS. Curr Probl Cardiol 15:571, 1990.

Hiatt JR, Yeatman LA Jr, and Child JS: The value of echocardiography in blunt chest trauma. J Trauma 28:914, 1988.

Hossack KF et al: Frequency of cardiac contusion in nonpenetrating chest injury. Am J Cardiol 61:391, 1988.

Kaul S, Fishbein MC, and Siegel RJ: Cardiac manifestations of acquired immune deficiency syndrome: a 1991 update. Am Heart J 122:535, 1991.

Khan AH and Spodick DH: Rheumatoid heart disease. Semin Arthritis Rheum 1:327, 1972.

Klein I and Levey GS: New perspectives on thyroid hormone catecholamines and the heart. Am J Med 76:167, 1984.

Lewis W: AIDS: cardiac findings from 115 autopsies. Prog Cardiovasc Dis 32:207, 1989.

Nihoyannopoulos P et al: Cardiac abnormalities in systemic lupus erythematosus. Circulation 82:369, 1990.

Potkin RT et al: Evaluation of noninvasive tests of cardiac damage in suspected cardiac contusion. Circulation 66:627, 1982.

Schrader ML, Hochman JS, and Bulkley BH: The heart in polyarteritis nodosa: a clinicopathologic study. Curric Cardiol 109:1353, 1985.

Trunkey DD and Cheitlin MD: Chest trauma. In Mills J, Ho MT, and Trunkey DD, editors: Current emergency diagnosis & treatment. Los Altos, 1983, Lange.

Van Hoeven KH and Factor SM: Diabetic heart disease: the clinical and pathological spectrum—part I. Clin Cardiol 12:600, 1989.

White RD and Davison MB: Cardiac tumors: diagnosis and management. Curr Probl Cardiol 17:78, 1992.

CHAPTER

25 Cardiac Transplantation

Lynne Warner Stevenson

CURRENT STATUS OF TRANSPLANTATION

Since the first cardiac transplant was performed in 1967, 20,000 have been performed in the world. Survival has improved from 25% at 1 year in 1970 to 80% at 1 year in 1991, and is now 60%-70% at 5 years (Fig. 25-1) for orthotopic transplantation (the new heart replaces the old, as opposed to heterotopic, where the new heart is attached

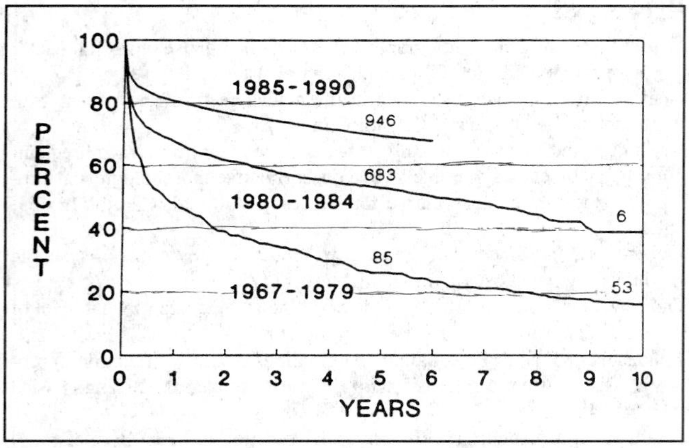

Fig. 25-1. Increasing survival after cardiac transplantation. The major differences are attributable to decline in early mortality with relatively parallel mortality after the first year, resulting in large part to accelerated coronary artery disease. (From Kriett JM et al: J Heart Lung Trans 10:491-498, 1991).

"piggy-back" to the old heart, a procedure rarely done now). The improving results of transplantation have expanded the pool of potential candidates, both to patients with less critical compromise and to older patients with other systemic medical problems.

The increasing number of patients referred for transplantation contrasts with the relatively fixed supply of donor hearts; fewer than 3000 hearts are available each year in the United States, compared to almost 3 million people with a diagnosis of heart failure. There are currently twice as many patients listed as transplanted each month. Paradoxically, the alternative medical therapy originally designed to stabilize patients before transplant now frequently rivals transplantation for improving the quality of life and survival for many patients with heart failure. The major current challenges are (1) to identify the patients who truly have no option except transplantation, (2) to select the patients with the greatest likelihood of doing well after transplantation, and (3) to prevent the accelerated arteriosclerosis that limits survival of the transplanted heart.

EVALUATION OF HEART FAILURE IN THE CANDIDATE

Etiology

Heart failure is the indication for transplantation in 95% of recipients. It is important to establish the underlying cause of heart failure, if possible (Chapter 10). Coronary artery disease accounts for approximately half of the heart failure in transplant candidates. In a few of these patients, revascularization of "hibernating" myocardium may result in gradual improvement of ventricular function in the native heart, thus avoiding transplantation.

Dilated nonischemic cardiomyopathy (Chapter 17) is the other major cause of transplant referral, while restrictive cardiomyopathy, valvular heart disease, and congenital heart disease together account for only 10% of primary transplant recipients. The causative factors of most concern during an evaluation for transplantation are those that are potentially reversible and those that influence posttransplant outcome. Patients with symptoms of less than 6 months duration, including those with peripartum presentation, have up to 50% chance of significant recovery of left ventricular function during the next 6-12 months, if transplant can be avoided during that time. Patients with a history of heavy alcohol consumption have a good chance of improvement with total abstention.

Medical therapy before transplantation

Multiple factors can contribute to decompensation even if they did not cause the heart failure (see box below). A central focus of assessment of potential heart transplant candidates is the adequacy of their previous care. Many physicians continue to perceive symptomatic heart failure as an untreatable disease terminated by early death or transplantation, and this perception is transferred to patients, who are often told that they have only a few months to live. However, many patients with heart failure can be stabilized on aggressive medical therapy and enjoy good functional capacity, quality of life, and survival similar to that achieved by transplantation.

Most patients referred for transplantation have severe symptoms of congestion, particularly orthopnea, anorexia, and abdominal discomforts, and dyspnea on minimal exertion. In most of these patients, the congestive symptoms have persisted despite previous therapy with diuretics, vasodilators, and digoxin, but they are not necessarily "refractory" to medical therapy.

Many patients with heart failure have not undergone adequate diuresis because of the old assumptions that (1) some

Evaluation of heart failure patients for potentially reversible factors of decompensation

Patient factors

- Extensive myocardial ischemia
- Recent viral infection
- Excessive alcohol consumption
- Frequent or incessant tachyarrhythmias
- Endocrine disorders
- Electrolyte disturbances
- Nutritional deficiencies
- Deconditioning

Health care factors

- Perception of "failure"
- Inadequate diuresis
- Reliance upon empiric vasodilator regimen
- Therapy with negative inotropic agents
- Therapy with prostaglandin inhibitors
- Excessive restriction of activity
- Incomplete patient education

elevation in filling pressures and thus symptomatic congestion is necessary to preserve cardiac output when the ejection fraction is low, and (2) filling pressures are not severely elevated if the lungs are clear. Many chronic heart failure patients can actually achieve their best cardiac ouputs with near-normal filling pressures. The major impact of unloading therapy once heart failure is advanced is reduction of the mitral and tricuspid regurgitation, which detract from forward output and lead to the congestive symptoms. A primary principle of therapy in these patients is to lower filling pressures to near-normal levels. Physical examination of the lungs is inadequate to rule out higher filling pressures resulting from compensation of the pulmonary lymphatic system in chronic heart failure. Orthopnea and elevated jugular venous pressure are the most reliable clinical indicators of excessive volume status, and diuresis should be pursued until both resolve.

Patients who cannot achieve adequate diuresis on combination diuretic therapy, because of poor diuretic response, declining renal function, or symptomatic hypotension, are not necessarily refractory, but need systematic and simultaneous adjustment of both filling pressures and systemic vascular resistance. This can be most efficiently achieved through hemodynamic monitoring during the standard transplant evaluation. Tailored therapy is initiated first with intravenous diuretics and nitroprusside, which is then weaned while the optimal hemodynamic profile is maintained with a tailored regimen of oral vasodilators and diuretics (see box below). The regimen generally includes angiotensin-converting enzyme inhibition and oral nitrates, a combination shown to prolong survival specifically for this population. High doses of captopril may be required for initial stabilization, usually 200-400 mg daily. After discharge, a loop diuretic once or twice daily is combined with intermittent metolazone, which is used for occasional increased fluid retention.

In addition to tailoring therapy, care must be taken to avoid potentially deleterious drugs (Chapter 10). Negative inotropic agents such as calcium channel blockers should be withdrawn unless nitrates cannot prevent angina. Beta-blocking drugs may be beneficial for some as yet unidentified subgroups but at this time should not be given to decompensated patients evaluated for transplant unless in controlled trials. Nonsteroidal anti-inflammatory agents can cause severe fluid retention and renal dysfunction in heart failure patients, who rely upon prostaglandins to vasodilate the afferent renal arterioles.

Prior to referral, many patients have been unable to comply with complicated medical regimens because of lack of education about their disease and drugs. The patients must participate actively to retain normal volume status by watching their fluid and salt intake and adjusting diuretic dosage in response to weight change. In addition, they must increase their exercise through a progressive walking program.

Tailored therapy has allowed stabilization according to current criteria (see box below) for 60% of heart failure patients referred with severe symptoms of heart failure despite previous therapy. Another 30% can be discharged but are unable to maintain stable status and may require frequent admissions for intravenous drug therapy. About 10% of potential candidates remain hospitalized in critical condition, frequently after an additional insult such as new myocardial infarction, cardiac arrest, open-heart surgery, or infection.

SELECTION FOR TRANSPLANTATION

Indications for transplantation

The definition of "unacceptable" quality of life and prognosis without transplantation (see box, p. 333) varies for each individual based on the relative risks and benefits of transplantation and alternative therapy, as perceived by the patient and the physician.

Patients who remain critically ill despite optimal medi-

Tailored therapy for advanced heart failure

1. Measurement of baseline hemodynamics
2. Intravenous nitroprusside and diuretics tailored to hemodynamic goals:
   - PCW $\leq$ 15 mm Hg — RA $\leq$ 8 mm Hg
   - SVR $\leq$ 1200 dynes-sec-cm^{-5} — SBP $\leq$ 80 mm Hg
3. Definition of optimal hemodynamics by 24-48 hours
4. Titration of high-dose oral vasodilators as nitroprusside weaned
   - captopril and isosorbide dinitrate
   - occasional addition of hydralazine
5. Monitored ambulation and diuretic adjustment for 24-48 hours
6. Maintenance digoxin levels 1.0-2.0 ng/dl if no contraindication
7. Detailed patient education including sodium restriction
8. Flexible outpatient diuretic regimen including intermittent metolazone
9. Progressive walking program
10. Vigilant follow-up

RA = right atrial pressure, PCW = pulmonary capillary wedge pressure, SBP = systolic blood pressure, SVR = systemic vascular resistance

Criteria for stability on medical therapy

Stable blood pressure (SBP $\geq$ 80 mm Hg)
Stable weight on flexible oral diuretic regimen
Stable creatinine and blood urea nitrogen (BUN $\leq$ 60 mg/dl)
Stable serum sodium (usually $\geq$ 132 mEq/L)
No angina
No recurrent sustained ventricular arrhythmias or syncope
No recurrent arterial emboli on anticoagulation
No serious drug side effects
Clinical status $\geq$ discharge
No congestive symptoms at rest
Ambulatory $\geq$ one city block

cal therapy clearly have unacceptable quality of life and survival. They need to be further evaluated only for contraindications (see below). While their early postoperative mortality is approximately twice that in patients without urgent need, their 1-year survival is still approximately 80%, compared to virtually no chance of 1-year survival without transplant (Fig. 25-2). Because the expected benefit (difference between transplant and no transplant) is so large, such patients should receive priority for the limited donor hearts.

Patients who are unstable have disabling symptoms and a poor prognosis, whether they are hospitalized or at home at any particular time. Evaluation for contraindications is the focus of further evaluation for these patients. Although the immediate risk is not as great as for the critically ill patients, there is still a major benefit of transplantation (Fig. 25-2). However, as the waiting list grows longer some patients will die before transplantation can be performed, while others will eventually achieve greater stability and should be re-evaluated after 6 months with the "stable" patients.

For patients who fulfill the criteria for stability, whether previously decompensated or not, it is unclear when transplantation is indicated. Even after they have presented for transplantation with symptoms of heart failure at rest (class IV), patients on tailored medical therapy can often improve to a quality of life, exercise capacity, and 1-year survival equivalent to that achieved after transplantation. Although these patients may have excellent survival after transplantation, the immediate expected benefit of transplantation is small or negative (Fig. 25-2).

The risk of major hemodynamic decompensation for patients followed closely after initial stabilization is approximately 10% per year and is highest in patients in whom pulmonary capillary wedge pressure initially cannot be reduced below 16-18 mm Hg, right atrial pressure cannot be lowered below 7–10 mm Hg, and serum sodium remains below 133. However, the major risk for patients who appear to be stable is sudden death, which may strike 10% to 30% per year. Risk factors specifically demonstrated for the transplant candidate population are listed in the box at far right.

A low left ventricular ejection fraction is neither a necessary nor a sufficient indication for transplantation. Severe angina in a patient without favorable coronary artery anatomy might confer a dismal prognosis and quality of life despite an ejection fraction above 25%. Patients with idiopathic restrictive myocardial disease (Chapter 17) may have refractory congestive symptoms without a severely reduced ejection fraction. While transplantation has been recommended for all patients with an ejection fraction less than 20%, there are too few donor hearts for all such patients, many of whom can do well without transplantation.

CONTRAINDICATIONS TO CARDIAC TRANSPLANTATION

Contraindications, listed in the box at right, were all considered "absolute" during the era when transplantation was an experiment, but many are now "relative" as the procedure is more widely available. Patients with heart failure resulting from chronic systemic illnesses such as scleroderma would be excluded. The benefit of transplantation for amyloidosis is questionable since the disease progresses after transplantation. Current experience with sarcoidosis is limited. Investigation continues regarding Chagas' disease,

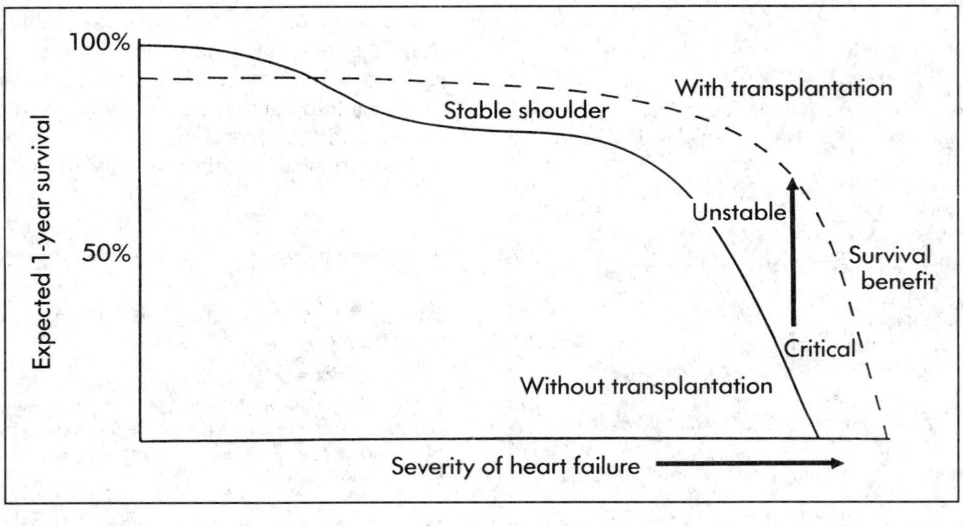

Fig. 25-2. Theoretical survival curves with and without transplantation according to severity of heart failure. Patients on the far left would do well with or without transplant, while patients on the far right have such severe compromise that death is inevitable with or without transplant. While absolute survival expected after transplant is slightly lower for more severely compromised patients, the expected improvement in survival is greatest in this group as long as absolute contraindications are avoided. (From Stevenson LW and Miller L: Curr Probl Cardiol 4:219, 1991.)

Selection for cardiac transplantation

Indications

Severe heart disease despite tailored medical therapy, causing (1) unacceptable quality of life from disabling symptoms of congestive heart failure, or (2) unacceptable risk of cardiac death within the next year, despite limited symptoms of congestive heart failure.

No other reasonable surgical option.

General eligibility

The patient must not have a noncardiac condition that would shorten life expectancy or increase the risk of death from rejection or from complications of immunosuppression, particularly infection.

Specific contraindications

Upper age limit 55-65 years (various programs).

Active infection.

Active ulcer disease.

Severe diabetes mellitus with end-organ damage.

Severe peripheral vascular disease.

Pulmonary function (FEV1, FVC) <60%* or history of chronic bronchitis.

Serum creatinine >2 mg/dl; creatinine clearance <50 ml/min.*

Bilirubin >2.5 mg/dl, transminases > 2× normal.*

Pulmonary artery systolic pressure >60 mm Hg.*

Mean transpulmonary gradient >15 mm Hg.*

High risk of life-threatening noncompliance:

- Inability to make strong, consistent commitment to transplant.
- Cognitive impairment severe enough to limit compliance.
- Psychiatric instability severe enough to jeopardize incentive for compliance.
- Recent history of alcohol or drug abuse.
- Failure to establish stable address.
- Previous demonstration of repeated noncompliance with medication or follow-up.

*May need to provide optimal hemodynamics with nitroprusside and/or dobutamine for 72 hours to determine reversibility of organ dysfunction caused by heart failure.

Potential risk factors for sudden death after referral for transplantation

Cardiac physiology

Left ventricular dimension index ≥ 40 mm/m^2

Persistently high filling pressures despite aggressive therapy

Ejection fraction <20%

Severe coronary artery disease

Arrhythmia substrate

History of syncope

Atrial fibrillation

High-grade ventricular ectopy

Therapy with type I antiarrhythmic drugs

Integrated profile

Class IV New York Heart Association functional class

Maximal oxygen consumption less than 11-14 ml/kg/min

Serum sodium less than 133 meq/l

which frequently recurs after transplantation. Age itself can be considered to limit life expectancy. Older patients have less rejection but more complications, and in the largest studies, have worse 5-year survival if over 50 years old. Diabetes mellitus was once an absolute contraindication but does not preclude transplantation if blood sugars are easily controlled and there is no evidence of neuropathy or retinopathy. Patients with a recent malignancy are excluded because immunosuppression may accelerate recurrence and progression.

The pulmonary pressures and resistance of all patients are measured. These factors may be elevated as a result of chronic left heart failure or unrecognized pulmonary conditions. Pulmonary hypertension that cannot be reversed pharmacologically can cause immediate failure of the right ventricle of the transplanted heart. The majority of elevated pulmonary pressures respond well to optimization of hemodynamics, which may take several days. Patients with refractory pulmonary hypertension are occasionally considered for heterotopic ("piggy-back") transplants, but the higher mortality of this procedure has discouraged its acceptance.

Evaluation of other organ systems is complicated by the effects of the compromised circulation, and often patients are accepted with some degree of renal or hepatic impairment that is expected to reverse after normal hemodynamics are restored by transplantation. Active infection remains an absolute contraindication to either transplantation or the insertion of a mechanical support device to "bridge" the patient to transplant.

A major cause of late deaths after transplant is patient noncompliance. The psychological and physical stresses after transplant, combined with the emotional lability resulting from steroid therapy, can precipitate fatal episodes of noncompliance. Evaluation by the psychiatrist and social worker includes consideration of previous noncompliance, substance abuse, and family support.

Most transplant centers find that approximately half of the patients who undergo complete evaluation are acceptable in terms of contraindications, although the indications for transplantation vary widely. Patients who await transplantation in a hospital with mechanical assist devices merit particular surveillance, because almost half develop contraindications such as infection or coagulopathy that preclude transplantation.

Selecting donors for transplantation

The heart, like the kidney and liver, must be harvested while still perfused after documentation of brain death. Criteria for brain death vary among states, but generally include cessation of all brain function. Most states have adopted the policy of "required request," which requires hospitals to offer the option of organ donation to the family.

Hemodynamic consequences of brain death include severe volume depletion from diabetes insipidus, sympathetic storm causing hypertension and tachycardia, and rapid depletion of tri-iodothyronine. Echocardiography is now widely used to assess ventricular function in donors. Coronary angiography is often performed in donors over 40 years old, whose hearts are being used more often than previously. Previous limits are also being extended for the ischemic time between harvest and implantation, but current data demonstrates decreased long-term graft survival when 5 hours is exceeded.

Donors are screened for evidence of HIV or hepatitis infections, which if present would exclude donation. Because of the potential "window" between infection and seroconversion, donors are also excluded if they have major risk factors for HIV infection.

Patients are matched to donors primarily on the basis of ABO blood group and body size. After potential recipients are screened for the presence of circulating antibodies to a random panel of antigens, those with elevated levels are frequently not transplanted unless a specific crossmatch to the donor blood is negative.

IMMUNOLOGY OF CARDIAC TRANSPLANTATION

Immune response

As soon as recipient blood perfuses the transplanted heart, the immune response begins. Antibodies, lymphocytes, monocytes, and cytokines all contribute to recognition and injury of the foreign organ. The major antigens recognized on the surface of an ABO-matched transplant appear to be the human leukocyte antigens (HLAs).

If preformed antibodies are already present in the recipient, hyperacute rejection can occur when these bind to the donor vessels. Such previous sensitization may result from blood transfusions or pregnancy. This rare response can cause immediate thrombosis and graft failure, leading to perioperative death, although in a few cases patients have been rescued with plasmapheresis.

The most common response is detected within the first 3-12 weeks. It is characterized by lymphocytes, which appear first in the perivascular areas, then infiltrate the myocardium. It is assumed that these lymphocytes recognize primarily HLA antigens of the donor. Cardiac myocytes can express these antigens but cannot present them to lymphocytes for recognition. The donor endothelium may play a crucial role in the initial immune response, because the endothelial cells can present as well as express their surface antigens. Class I HLA antigens are present on the graft endothelium initially and can be further up-regulated, while class II (DR) HLA antigens appear to require prior stimulation or injury for expression. Induction of class II antigen expression may be a critical event, determining the intensity and nature of the immune response, because the class II antigens are recognized primarily by CD4+ ("helper") T lymphocytes, which stimulate lymphocyte proliferation, antibody production, vigorous production of cytokines, and migration of cells, which can lead to a delayed-type hypersensitivity response.

There is increasing recognition of "vascular" or "humoral" rejection, which is characterized by immunoglobulin and fibrin deposition in the small vessel walls. This can occur with or without "cellular" rejection. Its presence is associated with a worse 1-year prognosis than with uncomplicated cellular rejection, and also with an increased incidence of accelerated graft arteriosclerosis.

Maintenance immunosuppression

Current immunosuppression is based on "triple therapy" with cyclosporin A, azathioprine, and varying corticosteroid doses. After introduction into clinical trials in 1982, cyclosporin A was heralded as a major advance, and indeed has decreased the severity of infection and rejection. It is a fungal endecapeptide that inhibits the message transcription for cytokines involved in T-cell activation and the inflammatory response. Original studies performed with cyclosporin A doses over twice current levels were associated with major nephrotoxicity. At current doses targeted to cyclosporin A levels, kidney function is detectably impaired but rarely severely enough to require drug discontinuation. Hypertension occurs in most patients on cyclosporin A partly as a result of direct sympathetic stimulation and perhaps from endothelin release. Cyclosporin A metabolism is affected by many drugs, such as erythromycin, calcium channel blockers, cimetidine, and ketoconazole, which increase levels, and Dilantin, isoniazid, nafcillin, sulfamethoxazole, and cholestyramine, which decrease levels. Hirsutism, tremor, hyperkalemia, and occasional gingival hyperplasia and seizures are well-recognized side effects.

Cytokine transcription is inhibited by corticosteroids, which also stabilize membranes and reduce local edema. Steroid therapy is initiated with methylprednisolone and subsequently maintained with prednisone, which is tapered rapidly to 5 mg/day by 3-6 months in patients without recurrent rejection. Steroid-free maintenance is attempted at varying times between programs, but eventual steroid-free maintenance is possible in 50% to 80% of transplant recipients, which reduces the incidence of infection, osteoporosis, obesity, and hyperlipidemia. Azathioprine is a purine antimetabolite converted hepatically to 6-mercaptopurine, which inhibits proliferation of lymphocytes. Addition of azathioprine adjusted to maintain white blood counts over $4000/cm^3$ allows lower doses of both steroids and cyclosporin A.

In some programs, antilymphocyte antibodies are used for 5-14 days to initiate immunosuppression, either with polyclonal antilymphocyte globulin or murine monoclonal antibody against the CD3 receptor on activated lymphocytes. These antibodies are also used for therapy of refractory rejection.

Attempts continue to increase the specificity of immunosuppression. Current agents under investigation include RS-61443, FK506, desoxyspergualine, anti-CD4 antibodies, cytokine antibodies, cytotoxic molecules binding to cytokine receptors, antibodies against adhesion molecules, and donor-specific HLA antigens or antibodies.

Diagnosis and therapy of rejection

The average incidence of rejection is 1.35 episodes per patient by the first year after transplant. Half of all patients have one episode of rejection, occurring within the first 6 months, while 25% of patients have no rejection and 25% have multiple episodes. The accepted standard for diagnosis is endomyocardial biopsy performed through a sheath in the right internal jugular vein. Using a bioptome, several pinhead-sized pieces are removed from the right ventricular septum. There is no discomfort from the biopsy sampling itself, although some patients describe a "tugging" sensation. Perforation with tamponade occurs in less than 0.1% of biopsies, more rarely than with native heart biopsies because of the encasing postoperative pericardial fibrosis.

The average patient undergoes 15-20 biopsies during the first year after transplant, with 2-4 each year thereafter. Rejection is characterized histologically by a lymphocytic and monocytic infiltrate of varying intensity and associated myocyte necrosis (Fig. 25-3). Occasionally light microscopy is nondiagnostic for cellular rejection, while immunofluorescence shows "vascular" rejection as described above.

Clinical evaluation is not as sensitive as biopsy for diagnosis of rejection episodes, 90% of which are asymptomatic. The other 10% of episodes are accompanied by atrial arrhythmias, decreased blood pressure, congestive symptoms, or vague malaise and low-grade fever. Frank cardiogenic shock occurs in about 5% of rejection episodes, frequently those precipitated by noncompliance. Hemodynamic compromise in these patients usually reflects not the degree of myocyte loss, but the reversible depression related to cytokines, intercellular edema, and local ischemia. Any transplant patient presenting with hemodynamic compromise should be rapidly evaluated with echocardiography and right-heart catheterization, to distinguish between rejection and sepsis. Corticosteroid therapy for severe rejection is frequently initiated prior to histologic confirmation.

Noninvasive assessment of rejection has involved multiple techniques. All of those adequately studied show no more than 70%-80% sensitivity for rejection. In the early days of transplantation, decreased electrocardiographic voltage was a reliable indicator of myocardial edema resulting from rejection, but this edema is decreased using cyclosporin A. Echocardiographic assessment suggests that rejection correlates with serial changes in ejection fraction and diastolic function. Nuclear imaging of antibodies to myocyte proteins may be helpful. Serial assessment of systemic immune activation such as by measuring circulating activated lymphocytes may allow biopsy frequency to be reduced.

Rejection resolves with bolus corticosteroid therapy in 90% of episodes. The remainder are treated with a second corticosteroid course or antilymphocyte antibodies. Patients presenting in cardiogenic shock usually receive corticosteroids and antilymphocyte sera simultaneously. After rejection, repeat biopsy is performed in 10-14 days to determine the response to therapy. Patients with recurrent or refrac-

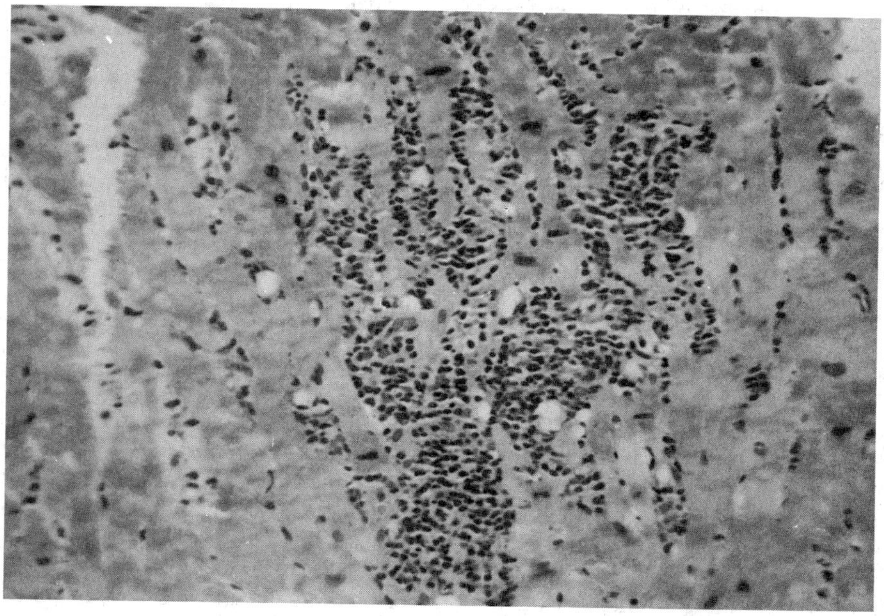

Fig. 25-3. Severe cardiac rejection with heavy infiltrate of mononuclear cells with occasional neutrophils, and myocyte necrosis with vascuolization and myofibrillar degeneration. (From Stevenson LW and Miller L: Curr Probl Cardiol 4:219, 1991.)

tory rejection may be considered for newer drugs or experimental therapies such as total lymphoid irradiation or photopheresis.

Accelerated transplant arteriosclerosis

While acute rejection and infection constitute the major events for the first year, subsequent graft function and survival are most threatened by accelerated coronary artery disease, also called "chronic rejection." The first long-term heart transplant survivor died after 19 months from coronary artery disease in the new heart, although both recipient and donor were under 25 years old and had previously been free of coronary artery disease. Most transplant recipients develop diffuse intimal thickening of the coronary arteries, which is evident on angiography in 50% of patients by 5 years, and more commonly observed by intracoronary ultrasound. Compared to native atherosclerosis, transplant arteriosclerosis is more diffuse and characterized by greater cellular infiltration (both of mononuclear and smooth muscle cells) but less lipid accumulation than native atherosclerosis.

Prolonged ischemic time, CMV infection (which increases surface antigen expression), and frequent rejection, particularly "vascular" rejection, are risk factors. Recipient age, hyperlipidemia, smoking, and obesity are implicated, but appear to be permissive factors rather than dominant as they are in native atherosclerosis. Therapy with HMG-CoA reductase inhibitors, if carefully monitored, can be safe and effective for lowering cholesterol levels in this population but it remains to be determined whether this intervention decreases transplant arteriosclerosis.

Activation of the endothelium after specific immune recognition by antibodies, lymphocytes, or monocytes, after nonspecific stimulation from cytokines during cellular rejection, or after viral infection with CMV, may be a central event in transplant arteriosclerosis. Such stimuli induce surface HLA II (DR) antigen expression for further recognition (see above) and stimulate production of antibodies, cytokines, and growth factors that attract mononuclear cells and stimulate smooth muscle proliferation. Cellular infiltration with lymphocytes and macrophages, lipid accumulation, smooth muscle proliferation, and possibly abnormal collagen production may all contribute to the diffuse sclerotic process that eventually compromises the coronary artery lumen. Alteration of the normal anticoagulant and vasodilatory properties of endothelium may also contribute to local thrombosis and ischemia.

Because the transplanted heart remains essentially denervated, the majority of patients with transplant coronary artery disease have no symptoms until ventricular function is markedly impaired, although rare patients have reported chest pain during a positive exercise stress test. The distal and diffuse nature of the disease limits the reliability of noninvasive testing. Baseline and yearly coronary angiography are the current standard for diagnosis, but will now be complemented by intracoronary ultrasound.

Once diagnosed, angioplasty or surgical bypass grafting are technically successful for "discrete" proximal lesions, but the disease usually progresses rapidly elsewhere. After diagnosis, survival is 67% at 1 year. Triple vessel disease is associated with a dismal 13% survival at 1 year. Symptoms of heart failure may recur, but most deaths are sudden. The major therapy for transplant arteriosclerosis has been retransplantation, with a 1-year survival of 61% compared to 80%-90% for first transplants.

INFECTION

The immunosuppression currently necessary to allow graft acceptance predisposes the transplant recipient to infection, which led to the death of the first human heart transplant recipient from pneumonia within the first month. The incidence of major infection is 0.83 episodes per patient by the end of the first year. Bacterial infections account for 45%, viral for 44%, and fungal and protozoal together 11% of episodes.

The approach to fever in the transplant recipient includes careful history and physical examination, complete blood count, chest x-ray, and cultures of blood, sputum, and urine. The lung is the most common site, involved in 22% of treated infections. Hypoxia or pulmonary infiltrates should be aggressively evaluated with bronchoscopy. Fever with gastrointestinal symptoms should usually be investigated with endoscopy to look for cytomegalovirus (CMV), candidal infection, or atypical presentation of lymphomas. Fever with any neurologic symptoms merits computerized axial tomography and lumbar puncture. The sinuses should not be overlooked.

In the early posttransplant period, bacterial infections are dominant, although cutaneous herpes can be troublesome. Systemic viral infections such as CMV often become apparent within the first 3 months. CMV accounts for 25% of all infections requiring therapy after transplant and ranges from an asymptomatic rise in antibody titer, usually not treated, to invasion of the lungs or gastrointestinal tract. Treatment with ganciclovir, which inhibits viral-induced DNA polymerase, can be life-saving. Later after transplant, Epstein-Barr virus can produce febrile syndromes or an insidious polyclonal lymphadenopathy, which in some cases may progress to lymphoma.

Infections occurring later after transplant include fungal infection such as *Aspergillus* and *Pneumocystis*. Additional organisms to consider are *Listeria, Legionella, Nocardia,* and *Toxoplasma*.

These patients do not have lymphopenia and are thus less vulnerable to opportunistic infections than patients with bone marrow transplants or acquired immunodeficiency syndrome. Face masks are recommended only for the first few weeks after transplant and during hospital visits. Patients are urged to avoid gardening or open construction areas. Prophylaxis with trimethoprim-sulfa is frequently given to prevent pneumocystis. Prophylaxis against CMV may help decrease the severity of infections in high-risk patients.

CARDIAC FUNCTION AFTER TRANSPLANTATION

Function of the transplanted heart is affected by denervation, acute rejection, arteriosclerosis, hypertension, and other side effects of immunosuppression. Vagal reinnervation does not appear to occur in humans, so drugs that normally alter vagal tone, such as digoxin, do not have the expected effect. Evidence for late sympathetic reinnervation has been demonstrated in some patients but most hearts function "independently" of the central nervous system, except for the effects of circulating catecholamines.

The cardiac output is usually within normal limits at rest, with a higher heart rate and lower stroke volume that is the product of a normal left ventricular ejection fraction and slightly reduced left ventricular volume. Right ventricular volume is generally slightly increased and right ejection fraction reduced compared to normal.

Maintenance of normal volume status frequently requires diuretic therapy, although at much lower doses than prior to transplant. The transplanted hearts do not provide the normal right ventricular-renal interaction and cardiac baroreceptor feedback that regulate volume. Fluid retention is also promoted by high steroid doses and some drugs used to treat the hypertension. The tendency to retain fluid occurs despite elevation of atrial natriuretic factor, which probably results from the abnormal geometry and stretch of the anastomosed atria. On appropriate therapy, resting ventricular filling pressures are frequently within normal limits in the absence of rejection. However, 10% to 20% of patients have persistently reduced compliance and elevated filling pressures despite adequate diuretic doses and normal systolic function. In most cases, these are patients who have had severe or repeated rejection episodes, which may cause either permanent myocyte loss or abnormal collagen synthesis. Many transplant recipients reveal mildly decreased ventricular compliance only during volume loading.

When the donor heart is anastomosed to the recipient, the back halves of the recipient atria are left in place so that the systemic and pulmonary veins do not have to be reattached. The joining of the old and new atria creates a "snowman" configuration (Fig. 25-4). The recipient sinus node remains, causing an extra "p" wave on the electrocardiogram, but absence of electrical continuity between the atria prevents this "p" wave from being conducted.

The response to exercise is delayed and blunted in the denervated heart. Heart rate does not increase until circulating catecholamines rise after 3-5 minutes of exercise and does not reach maximum levels predicted for the donor age. Although ejection fraction eventually increases as in normal hearts, compliance is reduced and the peak stroke volume is lower. Impaired right ventricular function may also be limiting.

Transplant recipients generally perform at 50% to 75% of maximal levels predicted for age, with oxygen consumption equivalent to that of patients with stable heart failure. However, transplant patients describe less limitation of routine activity, perhaps partly as a result of diminished exertional congestion.

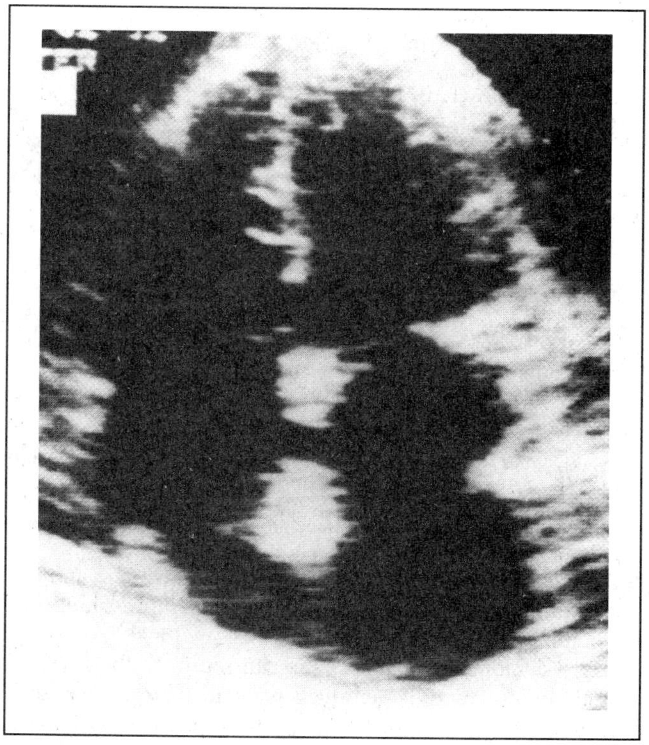

Fig. 25-4. Four-chamber view of the transplanted heart using two-dimensional echocardiography, showing the "snowman" atria created by the anastomosis of donor and recipient atria during orthotopic cardiac transplantation. Atria are at the bottom of the picture. (Stevenson LW: Am J Cardiol 60:119, 1987.)

LIFE AFTER TRANSPLANTATION

There are currently 12,000 patients alive after cardiac transplantation, 1800 alive more than 5 years and 60 more than 10 years. The longest documented survival is 21 years after transplant. The first 3 months are dominated by the highest frequency of complications, .83 rejection episodes/patient, and .53 infections. By the end of the first year, the average patient has had 1.35 rejections, .83 infections, and a creatinine of 1.3 mg/dl. Hypertension requires therapy in 70% of patients. Obesity, defined as weight 25% above ideal, occurs in 20% of recipients.

The occurrence of malignancy after transplantation is increased almost 100-fold over that of age-matched controls, presumably as a result of impaired immune surveillance. Approximately 5% of transplant survivors develop malignancy, which accounts for 12% of deaths occurring after 2 years. Cutaneous malignancy is most common, lung and intestinal tract being the next most common. Lymphoma is particularly common and may present in extranodal locations such as the gastrointestinal tract and central nervous system. The Epstein-Barr virus has frequently been implicated in these lymphomas, which may present within the

Table 25-1. Six months after transplant sample medical regimen*

Drug	Dosage
Cyclosporine	180 mg b.i.d.
Azathioprine	150 mg daily
Prednisone	5 mg daily*
Enalapril	10 mg b.i.d.
Diltiazem slow release	60 mg b.i.d.
Furosemide	40 mg daily
Lovastatin	20 mg daily
Trimethoprim-sulfasoxazole	4 times weekly
Aspirin	325 mg daily

*In absence of recent rejection. Patients with recent rejection would receive b.i.d. prednisone and antacids.

first year after transplant. Therapy with acyclovir and reduced immunosuppression can cause dramatic resolution of these tumors if diagnosed while still polyclonal.

By 3-6 months, most patients can return to the level of employment or activity enjoyed prior to their cardiac disability. Formal exercise training can improve peak capacity by 15% to 20%. Although they still do not achieve normal peak capacity, they are rarely physically limited except from heavy physical labor or competitive recreation. Their lives continue to be influenced by the complicated medical regimen. Biopsies are performed 15 to 20 times during the first year, but only 2 to 4 times yearly thereafter. Daily drug schedules continue to include 10 to 16 daily doses of medicines (Table 25-1).

Despite their good functional status, many patients do not return to employment. In some cases, they have chosen early retirement after previous disability. However, employers are often unwilling to hire these patients because of concerns about health insurance and liability. For many patients, the incentive to undergo transplantation reflects their desire to rejoin the work force as contributing members of society. Creative solutions are needed to allow them to do so.

THE FUTURE OF TRANSPLANTATION

The results of transplantation will continue to improve as the immune response can be better regulated, particularly with respect to accelerated arteriosclerosis. Transplantation of fewer than 3000 hearts yearly can have little impact, however, on the total heart failure population of 3 million in the United States, many of whom do well without transplantation. The excitement and glamor of transplantation and other experimental surgery such as cardiomyoplasty and artificial heart implantation should not divert attention from the more fundamental challenges of left ventricular dysfunction. Refinement of neurohumoral and hemodynamic modulation along with improved techniques for predicting and preventing sudden death will allow quality and length of life to be improved despite impairment of native heart function. Ultimately, elucidation of the myocardial responses to injury allow us to interrupt the progression to heart failure and limit the population for whom transplantation need ever be considered.

REFERENCES

Bourge RC et al: Risk factors for death after cardiac transplantation. J Heart Lung Trans 11:191, 1992.

Corcos T et al: Early and late hemodynamic evaluation after cardiac transplantation: a study of 28 cases. J Am Coll Cardiol 11:264, 1988.

Erickson KW et al: Influence of pre-operative transpulmonary gradient on late mortality after orthotopic heart transplantation. J Heart Transplant 9:526, 1990.

Fonarow GC et al: Effect of direct vasodilation vs angiotensin-converting-enzyme inhibition on mortality in advanced heart failure: the Hy-C trial. J Am Coll Cardiol 19:842, 1992.

Grattan MT et al: Eight-year results of cyclosporine-treated patients with cardiac transplants. J Thorac Cardiovasc Surg 99:500, 1990.

Hamilton MA et al: Sustained reduction in valvular regurgitation and atrial volumes with tailored vasodilator therapy in advanced congestive heart failure secondary to dilated cardiomyopathy. Am J Cardiol 67:259, 1991.

Kahan BD: Cyclosporine. N Engl J Med 321:1725, 1989.

Kavanagh T et al: Cardiorespiratory responses to exercise training after orthotopic cardiac transplantation. Circulation 77:162, 1988.

Keogh AM, Baron DW, and Hickie JB: Prognostic guides in patients with idiopathic or ischemic dilated cardiomyopathy assessed for cardiac transplantation. Am J Cardiol 65:903, 1990.

Kriett JM and Kaye MP: The registry of the international society for heart and lung transplantation. Eighth official report 1991. J Heart Lung Trans 10:491, 1991.

Mancini DM et al: Value of peak exercise oxygen consumption for optimal timing of cardiac transplantation in ambulatory patients with heart failure. Circulation 83:778, 1991.

Middlekauff HR, Stevenson WG, and Stevenson LW: Prognostic significance of atrial fibrillation in advanced heart failure: a study of 390 patients. Circulation 84:40, 1991.

Oaks TE et al: Combined registry for the clinical use of mechanical ventricular assist pumps and the total artificial heart in conjunction with heart transplantation: Fifth official report—1990. J Heart Lung Trans 10:621, 1991.

Penn I: Cancers following cyclosporine therapy. Transplantation 43:32, 1987.

Rose AG, Novitsky D, and Cooper DKC: Pathophysiology of brain death in the experimental animal: extracranial aspects/myocardial and pulmonary histopathologic changes. Transplant Proc 20:29, 1988.

Salomon RN et al: Human coronary transplantation-associated arteriosclerosis. Am J Pathol 138:791, 1991.

Stevenson LW et al: Exercise capacity for survivors of cardiac transplantation or sustained medical therapy for stable heart failure. Circulation 81:78, 1990.

Stevenson LW et al: Decreasing survival benefit from cardiac transplantation for outpatients as the waiting list lengthens. J Am Coll Cardiol 18:919, 1991.

Stevenson LW and Miller L: Cardiac transplantation as therapy for heart failure. Curr Probl Card 4:219, 1991.

Uretsky BF et al: Development of coronary artery disease in cardiac transplant patients receiving immunosuppressive therapy with cyclosporine and prednisone. Circulation 76:827, 1987.

PART TWO

Alimentary Tract, Liver, Biliary Tree, and Pancreas

ALIMENTARY TRACT

I PHYSIOLOGIC, BIOCHEMICAL, AND IMMUNOLOGIC PRINCIPLES

CHAPTER

26 Alimentary Tract Motor Function

Raj K. Goyal

The motor activity of the alimentary tract helps to prepare the food for digestion and facilitate absorption as the residues are carried caudally for final expulsion. The alimentary tract consists of functionally distinct segments such as the esophagus, the stomach, and the small and large intestines, each of which possesses distinctive motor activity. Despite major differences in function and motor control, the different segments have a similar overall structural organization. The wall of the alimentary tube consists of an outer layer of longitudinal muscle and an inner layer of circular muscle. Internal to these muscle layers is the submucosa, which is delimited by the muscularis mucosa. The mucosa lines the lumen and is separated from the muscularis mucosa by the lamina propria.

The motor activity of each part of the gut is designed to provide propulsion appropriate for the particular physical character and viscosity of food at its level of the alimentary canal. The distinctive motor activities of the different segments of the gut also permit performance of certain specialized functions. For example, the esophagus transports small chunks of swallowed food, whereas the stomach temporarily stores, digests, and grinds solid food into small particles and delivers them to the small bowel. The small bowel functions to allow digestion and absorption. The large bowel acts to retain food residues for several hours or days. Its motor activity allows absorption of water, so that watery food residues are converted to a semisolid or solid consistency. The large bowel also "turns over" residues, of which a small portion is expelled daily during defecation.

Various sphincters separate different segments of the alimentary tract. The sphincters act as one-way valves, normally allowing only forward flow. In addition to directing flow, some sphincters regulate the flow of volume and physical character of contents from one segment to another. Gastrointestinal motility is controlled by *myogenic, neural,* and *hormonal factors*. The distinctive motor activities of different segments of the gut and the sphincters are due to the heterogeneity and specializations of these controlling factors.

CONTROL SYSTEMS OF MOTOR ACTIVITY

Myogenic factors

Muscles are the ultimate mediators of motor function. While striated muscles have no myogenic tone, the smooth muscle of the gut possesses an intrinsic ability to generate tone or cause phasic contractions. Smooth muscle cells are normally in an electrically polarized state (i.e., the inside of the cell is negative in relation to the outside). The potential difference across the smooth muscle plasma membrane is called the *resting membrane potential* and is due to asymmetric distribution of charged cations and anions across the cell membrane. Muscle contraction is usually associated with depolarization, and inhibition of contraction is associated with hyperpolarization of the smooth muscle membrane. There is, however, marked heterogeneity in the specific electrical and mechanical behavior of smooth muscle in different regions of the gut.

The excitability of smooth muscle is determined by the resting membrane potential. Smooth muscles that have a less negative membrane potential *(depolarized)* are more excitable than those with a more negative membrane potential *(hyperpolarized)*. Smooth muscles in several regions of the gut exhibit oscillatory changes in the resting membrane potential. These oscillatory changes are called slow waves. Slow waves are not found in the esophagus but occur with remarkable consistency and regularity in the stomach and the small bowel. Slow waves occur irregularly and inconsistently in the colon.

The electrical activity associated with a contraction is called an *action potential*. The most obvious electrical activities associated with muscle contraction are rapid transient depolarizations called *spike potentials*. The spike potentials occur in bursts to cause phasic contractions, and they may occur continuously to cause sustained tonic contractions. Spike potentials are initiated when the cell membrane depolarizes to a value that is above the threshold for spike generation. Depolarization with superimposed spike potentials in many gastrointestinal smooth muscles occurs as a myogenic rebound following the hyperpolarizing action of inhibitory neurotransmitter substances released from the nerves. In smooth muscle cells that exhibit slow waves, spike bursts are more likely to occur during the depolarization phases of the slow wave (Fig. 26-1). Because each smooth muscle segment has its own characteristic slow wave frequency, the maximal rate of spike bursts is distinctive for each part of the gut. The slow waves are also called *pacesetter potentials* because they set the pace at which spike bursts will occur. They are also called *electrical control activities* because they determine the occurrence of a spike burst. The spike potentials in turn are called *electrical response activity*. An intense excitatory stimulus is associated with a large depolarization that may overwhelm the effect of a slow wave. With such stimuli, spike burst activity can occur regardless of the phase of the slow wave and can be prolonged to cover several slow wave cy-

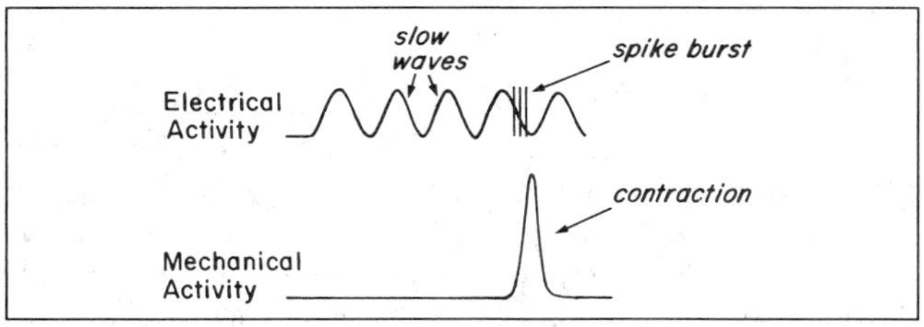

Fig. 26-1. Relation between electrical and mechanical activities in the small bowel. The electrical activity consists of slow waves (also called pacesetter potentials) and spike bursts. Spike bursts occur only on the depolarizing phase of the slow waves. Spike bursts, but not slow waves, are associated with muscle contraction.

cles. The frequency and amplitude of the spikes and the duration of spike bursts determine the amplitude and duration of contractions. A weak spike burst may not be associated with contraction.

Smooth muscle contraction can also occur in association with electrical activities other than spikes. Slow waves themselves may cause a small degree of contraction during their depolarization phases. In the stomach, excitatory agents may cause an increase in the amplitude of slow wave depolarizations, which in turn are associated with contractions. These depolarizations in the stomach are therefore also called action potentials. In the esophagus, spike bursts occur without an underlying slow wave. In colonic smooth muscle a prolonged spike burst covering several slow waves induces long-duration contractions.

Depolarization of gastrointestinal smooth muscle membrane results from influx of positively charged (Na^+ and Ca^{2+}) ions or efflux of negatively charged (Cl^-) ions. Depolarization also results from the inhibition of K^+ efflux. On the other hand, hyperpolarization results from either an increase in K^+ or a decrease in Cl^- efflux. Depolarization of the membrane leads to opening of the voltage sensitive Ca^{2+} channels and Ca^{2+} influx. Hyperpolarization serves to inhibit the voltage-dependent Ca^{2+} channels and, thus, inhibit Ca^{2+} entry into the cells. The coupling between electrical depolarization and muscle contraction is called *electromechanical coupling* and is caused by depolarization-induced increase in intracellular Ca^{2+}.

Sometimes smooth muscle contraction or relaxation can occur without any associated electrical events. Such mechanical phenomena are due to the direct action of endogenous neurotransmitters and hormones or exogenous pharmacologic agents on intracellular Ca^{2+} or other mediators of contraction. This phenomenon is called *pharmacomechanical coupling*. Because Ca^{2+} plays a critical role in the contraction of smooth muscles, calcium channel blockers serve as effective agents in inhibiting contractions of gastrointestinal smooth muscle. Intracellular messengers such as cyclic adenosine monophosphate (cAMP), cyclic guanosine monophosphate (cGMP), and phosphoinositols (PIs) are involved in the actions of hormones and neurotransmitters in the smooth muscle. These messengers act by modulating various ion channels and intracellular Ca^{2+} concentrations in the smooth muscles. In general, intracellular increases in both cAMP and cGMP lend to relaxation, and activation of the PI pathway leads to contraction of the muscles. However, there is marked heterogeneity in the cellular mechanisms of contraction in the different gastrointestinal smooth muscles.

Of the several muscle layers in the alimentary canal, contraction of the circular muscle is largely responsible for luminal occlusion and movement of food through the gut. These contractions occur either as a single monophasic contraction or as a train of contractions and may be either propagated or nonpropagated. The propagated waves may move forward, that is, caudally *(peristaltic contractions)*, or backward, that is, orally *(antiperistaltic contractions)*. The nonpropagated waves may occur as simultaneous contractions along a portion of the alimentary canal *(spastic contractions)* or as isolated contractions that occur randomly in time and space *(segmental contractions)*. Nonpropagated contractions help in digestion by facilitating mixing and absorption. Measurements that merely document the presence of intestinal contractions without indicating their propagational properties give no information about the movements of the intestinal contents. When contractions are spastic or segmental or when there are no contractions, there is little movement of intestinal contents. Only peristaltic contractions are associated with significant caudal movement of intestinal contents. In turn, antiperistaltic contractions cause retrograde movement.

The longitudinal muscle contractions also play an important role in the movement of luminal contents by sliding the intestine over the food in the lumen, just as one slides a pillowcase over a pillow. Contractions of the muscularis mucosa may be important both in the mixing of food and enzymes and in the expulsion of glandular secretions into the bowel lumen.

Neural control

The skeletal muscles at either end of the gastrointestinal tract connect directly with the central nervous system (CNS) through the lower motor neurons. The nervous system exerts total mastery over these muscles. When the nerves are destroyed, these muscles become paralyzed. The lower motor neurons cause muscle contractions by releasing acetylcholine at the motor end plate. Acetylcholine acts on the striated muscles via nicotinic acetylcholine receptors.

The neural control system for smooth muscle consists of extrinsic nerves composed of motor sympathetic and parasympathetic nerves, and intrinsic or "intramural" enteric nerves, which include the myenteric and submucous plexuses. The intrinsic nerves of the gut constitute the *enteric nervous system*, which can integrate and execute gastrointestinal function independent of the central nervous system. The neurons in the enteric nervous system exhibit morphologic, chemical, and functional characteristics that are similar to those of the central nervous system. The enteric nervous system represents the "local brain" of the gut, whereas the sympathetic and parasympathetic pathways provide connections between the central and enteric nervous systems. There are major differences in the anatomic details, chemical nature of transmitters, and organization of neural functions in the different regions of the gut.

Sympathetic nerves exert their effect by releasing norepinephrine and other catecholamines. The sympathetic nerves in general exert an inhibitory effect on the motor activity of the gut except in sphincters, which contract in response to sympathetic stimulation. Sympathetic overactivity may produce *adynamic ileus,* which is sometimes erroneously called *paralytic ileus,* a misnomer because there is no true muscular paralysis involved. On the other end of the spectrum, pharmacologic or surgical sympathectomy may cause diarrhea resulting from the increased propulsive activity in the gut.

Parasympathetic nerves exert a more discrete effect on the motor activity of the gut than do sympathetic nerves. Parasympathetic nerves have both excitatory and inhibitory effects on gastrointestinal smooth muscle. The vagus nerves mediate esophageal peristalsis and control gastric emptying. Vagal denervation impairs esophageal peristalsis and delays gastric emptying. Because the influence of parasympathetic nerves on the small bowel and colon is relatively small, nearly normal function continues in their absence. Sacral parasympathetic nerves exert an important influence on anorectal activity, and their lesions cause disorders of defecation.

The enteric motor nerves can exert both excitatory and inhibitory effects on the muscles. Stimulation of these nerves usually produces a biphasic response in the muscle consisting of hyperpolarization followed by depolarization produced by the release of inhibitory and excitatory neurotransmitters, respectively. The main inhibitory neurotransmitters are adenosine triphosphate (ATP), vasoactive intestinal peptide (VIP), and nitric oxide (NO) or a related product of the L-arginine nitric oxide pathway. The main excitatory transmitters are acetylcholine and substance P. A very large number of peptides and chemicals have been localized in the enteric nerves. These chemicals may serve other functions, such as modulation of neuromuscular transmission and afferent neural activity. The muscle inhibition and excitation work in concert to produce a wide spectrum of motor activity that is seen in different parts of the gut. The peristaltic contractions in the gut are based on the biphasic response of inhibition followed by contraction. The intramural neurons coordinate and organize activities such as peristalsis, sphincter relaxation, and more complex motor activities. Contractions can occur in smooth muscles in the absence of neural control; however, they are purposeless. Because extrinsic nerves exert their effects via the enteric neurons, lesions of enteric neurons may mimic some of the effects of extrinsic denervation in addition to producing some effects that are characteristic of lesions of the enteric nerves alone. Chagas' disease, which is due to the involvement of myenteric neurons by *Trypanosoma cruzi,* causes widespread derangement in gastrointestinal motility. This disease results in the loss of peristalsis in the esophagus as well as impaired relaxation of the lower esophageal sphincter, together producing the clinical picture of achalasia (Chapter 35), gastric stasis (Chapter 39), small intestinal pseudo-obstruction syndrome (Chapter 44), and megacolon resembling that of Hirschsprung's disease (Chapter 41).

Hormonal control

Almost two dozen circulating hormones have been shown to modify gastrointestinal motility, although their physiologic importance is not fully known. For example, gastrin increases lower esophageal sphincter pressure and delays gastric emptying. Secretin, VIP, somatostatin, and opioids delay gastric emptying and may decrease small bowel transit time. Calcitonin gene-related peptide may be involved in both the sensory and motor neural pathways. Although opioids cause constipation, motilin increases gastric emptying and enhances transit through the small intestine. Some of the same peptides that serve as circulating hormones may also act locally as neurotransmitters and response modulators. Some circulating hormones may affect certain muscle contractions directly, whereas others may activate or depress neurally organized activities. For example, in normal individuals, cholecystokinin delays gastric emptying and relaxes the lower esophageal sphincter by acting on inhibitory neurons. In patients with achalasia, however, who have degenerated inhibitory neurons in the sphincter, cholecystokinin causes sphincter contractions. The most important physiologic effects of cholecystokinin, however, are contractions of the gallbladder, relaxation of the sphincter of Oddi, and stimulation of pancreatic enzyme secretion.

MOVEMENT OF FOOD THROUGH VARIOUS GUT SEGMENTS

Oral cavity and pharynx

After food enters the mouth, it is prepared and formed into a bolus and is transported to the esophagus through the pharynx. The oral phase of swallowing is completely under voluntary control. As the bolus enters the oropharynx, an involuntary swallowing reflex is initiated by activation of sensory receptors on the posterior part of the oral cavity. The bolus enters the oropharynx, the nasal and laryngeal passages are occluded, and a wave of peristalsis sweeps the bolus ahead of it. The upper esophageal sphincter opens in anticipation of the arriving bolus. The pharynx and the upper esophageal sphincter are composed of striated muscles. They are innervated by lower motor neurons that accompany vagal and other cranial nerves. Neuromuscular disorders that involve these nerves or muscles cause pharyngeal paralysis. Pharyngeal paralysis produces the characteristic symptoms of dysphagia, nasal regurgitation, and tracheobronchial aspiration.

Esophagus

The peristaltic wave that starts in the pharynx continues through the esophagus at a speed of 3 to 4 cm per second, carrying the food bolus ahead of it. The normal transit time of a bolus of food through the esophagus is 5 to 6 seconds. The lower esophageal sphincter opens well before the arrival of the peristaltic wave so that food can pass into the stomach. When the bolus enters the stomach, the lower esophageal sphincter resumes the resting, contracted state.

Peristaltic contractions that occur in response to a swallow are called *primary peristalsis* and are always initiated in the pharynx. *Secondary peristalsis* occurs in response to esophageal distention and is not initiated by pharyngeal activity. The role of secondary peristalsis is to help clear the esophagus of food residue and materials that may reflux into it from the stomach.

The cervical esophagus is composed of striated muscle that is directly innervated by lower motor neurons. Primary as well as secondary peristalsis in the cervical esophagus are due to sequential activation in the brainstem of lower motor neurons that supply the progressively caudally placed musculature of the cervical esophagus.

The thoracic esophagus is composed of smooth muscle that is innervated by myenteric neurons, which are in turn innervated by vagal parasympathetic preganglionic fibers. In the thoracic esophagus primary peristalsis involves a vagally mediated central mechanism as well as a peripheral mechanism that involves myenteric neurons. Secondary peristalsis, however, is due entirely to local myenteric reflexes. The inhibitory neurotransmitters VIP and NO are involved in lower esophageal sphincter relaxation and the latency gradient of peristalsis.

Peristaltic contractions in the smooth muscle consist of a wave of hyperpolarization followed by depolarization. The peristaltic behavior is due to a progressive increase in the duration of hyperpolarizations aborally along the esophagus. In disease states the esophageal contractions may lose their peristaltic behavior coincident with the loss of aborally increasing hyperpolarizations. Such contractions are called *nonperistaltic* or *tertiary* contractions. The specific neurotransmitters that participate in peristalsis are not fully known, but it appears that multiple inhibitory and excitatory transmitters, including acetylcholine, substance P, and NO, are involved. Weak or absent esophageal contractions (as occur in esophageal scleroderma) cause dysphagia, whereas strong but nonperistaltic contractions (as occur in diffuse esophageal spasm) cause dysphagia and chest pain. Defective relaxation of the lower esophageal sphincter (as in achalasia) also causes dysphagia, whereas inappropriate relaxation or basal hypotension of the sphincter causes gastroesophageal reflux and esophagitis (Chapter 35).

Stomach

As swallowed food fills the stomach, the proximal stomach relaxes to accommodate the contents without causing an increase in luminal pressure. The distal stomach also becomes quiet, and any ongoing motor activity is inhibited. These responses are mediated by the vagus nerve along with intramural inhibitory neurons. Impaired gastric accommodation leads to symptoms of early satiety and enhanced gastric emptying of liquids.

A short time after a meal, peristaltic waves in the body and antrum of the stomach resume and then become stronger, carrying small bits of gastric contents into the terminal antrum. The terminal antrum contracts as a whole against a closed pylorus. This activity helps to grind coarse food into finer particles and mix it with gastric secretions. In the early phase of this activity the pylorus is partially open, allowing passage into the duodenum of small quantities of liquids and solid particles of less than 2 mm in size. However, such passage of food into the small bowel occurs only if small intestinal contractions at that precise time are inhibited. This requires coordination of antral and duodenal contractions. As the antrum continues to contract, larger particles of food are retropulsed into the main cavity of the stomach. The antrum then relaxes until the next peristaltic wave brings in another portion of food. Thus, the antrum and the pylorus act in a coordinated fashion to limit as well as to achieve the emptying of gastric contents. This mechanism is of primary importance in the grinding of digestible solid food and its eventual emptying from the stomach. Vagal inhibitory and excitatory pathways are involved in mediating these responses.

The rate of gastric emptying of liquids and small particulate solids (less than 2 mm) is dependent on the volume of gastric contents. The larger the volume, the faster the initial emptying rate. Gastric emptying is also regulated by the physicochemical properties of the chyme that enters the duodenum. The duodenal mucosa possesses sensory receptors that activate neurohumoral reflexes that influence gastric emptying. If the chyme coming out of the pylorus is drained so that it does not come in contact with the duodenum, gastric emptying increases markedly. Emptying is inhibited by increasing osmolarity, pH below 3.5, and products of fat digestion. Products of carbohydrate and protein digestion have only a small inhibitory effect. During the digestive period only liquids and small particles of ground digestible solids leave the stomach while large pieces of indigestible food are retained. One or two hours after a meal, all liquids and digestible solids leave the stomach. At this time, trains of contractions appear that occur at a rate of three to five per minute (which is the rate of gastric slow waves) and move across the stomach. Vagal nerves play an important role in these migratory contractions. Normally the stomach is emptied of all food materials in 2 to 4 hours.

Delayed gastric emptying occurs in a variety of disorders involving myogenic, neural, or hormonal control systems. Myopathic diseases of the gastric smooth muscle (e.g., scleroderma or visceral myopathy), and abnormalities of gastric slow waves such as tachygastria (fast rate of gastric slow waves) or gastric arrhythmia (disorganized gastric slow waves) lead to gastric stasis and symptoms of postprandial fullness, nausea, and vomiting. Similarly, bilateral vagotomy or a vagal neuropathy such as diabetic neuropathy also leads to gastric stasis. Stasis of indigestible solids in the stomach can lead to formation of gastric bezoars (Chapter 39). In diabetic gastroparesis, the intradigestive migrating activity front is particularly abnormal, leading to delayed emptying of indigestible solids as an early manifestation of the disease. Gastric prokinetic agents such as metoclopramide, domperidone, or cisapride improve delayed gastric emptying by increasing the amplitude of antral contractions, improving antroduodenal coordination, and initiating "migrating activity fronts." Macrolide antibiotics such as erythromycin act on motilin receptors to initiate migrating motor complexes and to improve gastroduodenal coordination to enhance gastric emptying.

Other factors can also lead to delayed gastric emptying such as sympathetic overactivity or increased levels of most of the gastrointestinal hormones, particularly cholecystokinin, secretin, glucagon, VIP, and somatostatin. On the other hand, motilin causes enhanced gastric emptying. Rapid gastric emptying can also occur after gastrectomy and may lead to symptoms of dumping syndrome (Chapter 38). The pyloric sphincter also acts to prevent duodenogastric reflux. An increased duodenogastric reflux may contribute to gastritis (Chapter 39) and gastric ulcer.

Small intestine

Liquids and finely ground food particles enter the small bowel with antral contractions. The pattern of small bowel motor activity observed when food is present in the small intestine is called the *fed pattern* and is characterized by segmental contractions. The segmental contractions are monophasic contraction waves that occur at different sites along the small bowel in a random fashion. Segmental contractions do not propagate in either an aboral or oral direction. These contractions are responsible for the mixing of food with digestive enzymes in intestinal, pancreatic, and biliary secretions. Additional stirring and mixing of the intestinal secretions and food are provided by the muscular activity movement of the villi. Mixing and stirring of intestinal contents are necessary not only for digestion but also for absorption of food. If segmental contractions are inhibited, as in certain disease states such as scleroderma or hollow visceral myopathy, intestinal digestion as well as absorption are impaired. In the absence of stirring, water layers develop between the intestinal mucosa and the food that is present in the lumen. The unstirred water layers impose a barrier between molecules of digested food and the intestinal mucosa.

Interspersed among the abundant segmental contractions during the fed pattern are also some contractions that propagate aborally for distances of several centimeters. These contractions help gradually to move the food as it is being digested and absorbed. Impaired transit of food throughout the small intestine has been shown to cause reflex inhibition of gastric emptying and may therefore contribute to early satiety, bloating, and anorexia.

After the digestion and absorption of food are completed, the pattern of small bowel motor activity is replaced by patterns of cyclic motor activity called *interdigestive migrating motor complexes*. Each migrating motor complex consists of periods of inactivity alternating with segmental or propulsive contractions (Fig. 26-2). The period of inactivity, which lasts around 20 to 60 minutes, is called *phase I*. Phase I inactivity is followed by irregular segmental contractions that last for a variable period and are called *phase II* activity. Phase II is followed by regular contractions of the activity front, which is designated *phase III*.

The activity front that is the hallmark of the migrating motor complex consists of an 8 to 10 minute cluster of regularly occurring contractions (Fig. 26-2). The rate of contraction varies in different parts of the small bowel and is determined by the intrinsic frequency of the slow wave in

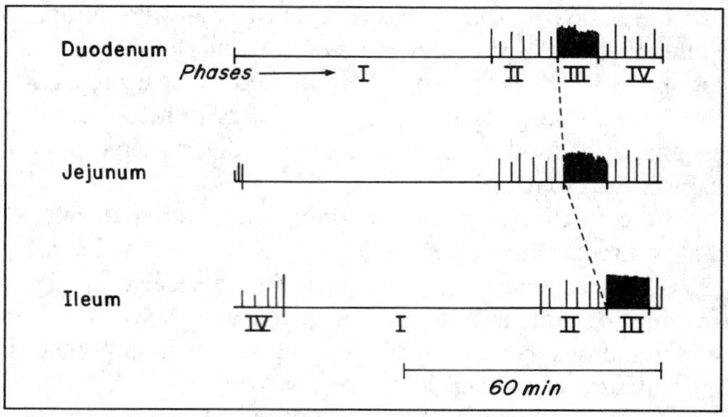

Fig. 26-2. Periodic activity in the small bowel in the resting state. Note aboral migration of phase III, also called the activity front. The migrating motor complex is present at rest and is interrupted promptly by feeding.

that segment of the intestine. The contraction rate in the activity front is around 12 per minute in the human duodenum. This rate decreases distally along the intestine, so that in the ileum the rate of contraction is 3 to 5 per minute. The activity front migrates toward the terminal ileum at a rate of 4 to 6 cm per minute and gradually decreases to 1 to 2 cm per minute as it approaches the terminal ileum. The activity front reaches the terminal ileum in 1½ hours, triggering a new activity front to begin in the duodenum. Activity fronts are inhibited by ingesting a meal and are thought to be initiated by the hormone motilin. The migrating motor complexes are responsible for the slow propagation of food residues through the small bowel and have been called the *interdigestive housekeepers* of the small intestine. Somatostatin can initiate migrating motor complexes; however, its overall effects on small bowel motility are not well understood. Somatostatin delays intestinal transit in normal subjects, but in patients with intestinal pseudo-obstruction a stable analogue of somatostatin has been shown to enhance small bowel transit.

Another type of propulsive contraction in the small bowel is the *giant peristaltic contraction,* which normally occurs periodically and only in the distal small intestine and the colon. These contractions are called *giant* because their amplitude is 1.5 to 2.0 times larger and their duration 4 to 6 times longer than the usual intestinal contraction. The electrical correlate of giant contractions is not known. Giant peristaltic contractions involve simultaneous contractions of a large (20 to 30 cm) segment of small intestine, and they propagate uninterrupted, aborally at a speed of 1 cm per second. Thus a giant peristaltic contraction can sweep food residues through the whole length of the intestine in a few minutes.

In certain disease states, giant peristaltic contractions can originate in the proximal small bowel and proceed aborally uninterrupted. These peristaltic contractions in the small intestine can be induced by intraluminal administration of agents such as vinegar or short-chain fatty acids. They can also be induced by administration of antibiotics such as erythromycin. Irradiation therapy and parasitic infections have been reported to cause an increase in the frequency as well as a more proximal origin of these contractions in the small bowel. Most of the manipulations that induce giant peristaltic contractions also cause diarrhea, and therefore it is reasonable to assume that these contractions may be involved in the pathogenesis of diarrhea. One of the interesting features of giant peristaltic contractions is their potential for producing painful abdominal cramps. These cramps are presumably related to vigorous, long-duration contraction involving large segments of the intestine. The occurrence of giant peristaltic contractions in the ileum is often associated with the perception of abdominal pain and cramps in patients with irritable bowel syndrome. The neurohormonal mechanisms responsible for giant peristaltic contractions are not known.

Gallbladder and sphincter of Oddi

Bile flows continuously from the liver into the biliary tract. Between meals the sphincter of Oddi largely remains closed, and bile is directed to the gallbladder. The gallbladder concentrates and stores bile. A small amount of bile is emptied into the duodenum as the gallbladder contracts and as the sphincter of Oddi relaxes during the interdigestive motor activity in the small bowel. After a meal, particularly a fatty meal, the gallbladder contracts vigorously, the sphincter of Oddi relaxes, and the bile is emptied into the duodenum (Chapter 51). This action is mediated by cholecystokinin, which is released by fat in the duodenum. Weakness of gallbladder contraction leads to enlargement of the gallbladder and stasis, which may predispose toward formation of gallstones. Impaired relaxation of the sphincter of Oddi may be responsible for biliary dyskinesia associated with pain and liver function abnormalities (Chapter 64).

Colon

The purpose of the motor activity of the colon is to mix, store temporarily, and propel food residues of semisolid to solid consistency very slowly. The main role of the ascending colon is to receive and store mostly liquid contents discharged through the ileocecal valve. The role of the left side of the colon is to store food residues for periodic expulsion into the rectum. Colonic motor activity is quite complex and promotes stasis and retropulsion in addition to infrequent but vigorous aboral propulsion of fecal material. Colonic motor activity consists of segmental contractions of either short (less than 10 seconds) or long (around 1 minute) duration. The short-duration contractions occur as a result of spike bursts in association with colonic slow waves. Because colonic slow waves occur irregularly at a frequency of 3 to 12 minutes, these contractions have a similar rate of repetition. The long-duration contractions occur without respect to slow waves and are associated with either long-duration spike bursts or oscillating potentials. The short- and long-duration contractions may occur singly, but more often they occur in trains. These trains of mostly nonpropulsive but sometimes retropulsive activity constitute a large portion of the motor activity of the colon. Segmental contractions in the left side of the colon are also associated with haustral contractions. The haustra are formed by thin, annular contractions that produce transitory septa, breaking up the lumen into saccules. Segmental contractions in the left colon provide resistance to distal movements of the contents; these contractions are increased in patients with constipation and are decreased in patients with diarrhea.

Slow and rapid caudal shifts of colon contents occur during its propulsive motor activity. Slow shifts of colonic contents occur with migrating trains of short- or long-duration contractions, which migrate at rates of 4 to 6 cm per minute and 0.5 to 2 cm per minute, respectively. The mean duration of these trains of contractions is 10 minutes, and they recur every 30 minutes. These migratory contractions move caudally over half the length of the colon. The migratory trains of contractions are separated by a period of quiescence, which may be interrupted by nonmigratory trains of short- or long-duration contractions. Rapid shifts of large volumes of colonic contents from the proximal colon to the middle or distal colon occur secondary to motor activity called *mass movement* or *giant peristaltic contractions* of the colon. Mass movements can occur without defecation or during defecation depending on their propagation through either a part or the entire length of the colon. The giant migrating contraction is two to three times larger in amplitude than are other colonic contractions, and its duration is around 1 minute. It propagates at a fast velocity of 0.2 to 3 cm per second. These contractions can occur singly or in trains of two or more contractions.

Mass movements are induced in the left colon as a reflex response to certain stimuli, such as eating (gastrocolic reflex) or rising in the morning (orthocolic reflex). During these movements, distal segments of the colon are relaxed to accommodate food residues that are pushed forward by the contractions. These reflexes are mediated by neurohumoral mechanisms and are affected by conditioning, but the precise role of neurohumoral control factors in the production of colonic motor activity is not fully understood. The gastrocolic reflex is heightened in some patients with the irritable bowel syndrome (Chapter 41). Weak colonic contractions lead to colonic stasis, megacolon, and constipation. Diminished mass movements also lead to constipation, whereas frequent mass movements may lead to frequent defecation. Increased segmental contractions may lead to abdominal pain and constipation. Prolonged haustral contractions may mold feces into fecal pellets like rabbit stools, which sometimes occur in patients with the irritable bowel syndrome. Defective relaxation of distal colonic segments also leads to functional obstruction of the passage of fecal contents and megacolon.

Defecation

The rectum is normally empty. Mass movement of the left side of the colon displaces feces into the rectum. When the rectum is distended with fecal matter, the defecation urge is experienced. It is associated with reflex relaxation of the internal anal sphincter and reflex contraction of the external anal sphincter. This urge may be suppressed, in which case both of the anal sphincters become contracted. Contraction of the rectum then propels the feces back into the colon, or the rectum simply accommodates the feces. However, if the subject decides to answer the call, the defecation reflex is activated. Intra-abdominal pressure is increased by contractions of the abdominal muscle and diaphragm. The external and internal anal sphincters remain relaxed, and feces are expulsed.

In Hirschsprung's disease, the internal anal sphincter and the aganglionic segment of the colon fail to relax causing constipation and megacolon (Chapter 41). Fecal incontinence occurs when liquid feces appear in the rectum, and the anal sphincters, particularly the external anal sphincter, are paralyzed. This may also occur when the threshold of rectal sensations becomes greater than the threshold of rectosphincteric inhibitory reflex, as may happen in patients with diabetic neuropathy.

REFERENCES

Furness JB and Bornstein JC: The enteric nervous system and its extrinsic connections. In Yamada T, editor: Textbook of gastroenterology. Philadelphia, 1991, JB Lippincott.

Goyal RK and Paterson WG: Esophageal motility. In Wood JD, editor: Handbook of physiology: the gastrointestinal system: motility and circulation, vol. 1. Bethesda, Md., 1989, American Physiologic Society.

Janssens J et al: Improvement of gastric emptying in diabetic gastroparesis by erythromycin. N Engl J Med 322:1028, 1990.

Kellow JE and Phillips SF: Altered small bowel motility in irritable bowel syndrome is correlated with symptoms. Gastroenterology 92:1885, 1987.

Reynolds JC: Prokinetic agents: a key in the future of gastroenterology. Gastroenterol Clin North Am 18:437, 1989.

Ryan JP: Motility of the gallbladder and biliary tree. In Johnson LR, editor: Physiology of the gastrointestinal tract, ed 2. New York, 1987, Raven Press.

Sanders KM: Electrophysiology of dissociated gastrointestinal muscle cells. In Wood JD, editor: Handbook of physiology: the gastrointestinal system: motility and circulation, vol 1. Bethesda, Md, 1989, American Physiologic Society.

Sanders KM and Ward SM: Nitric oxide as a mediator of nonadrenergic noncholinergic neurotransmission. Am J Physiol 25:G379, 1992.

Sarna SK: Motor correlates of functional gastrointestinal symptoms, Viewpoints Dig Dis 20:1, 1988.

Sarna SK: Physiology and pathophysiology of colonic motor activity. Dig Dis Sci 36:827, 998, 1991.

Soudah A, Hasler W, and Owyang C: Effect of octreotide on intestinal motility and bacterial overgrowth in scleroderma. N Engl J Med 325:1461, 1991.

Szurszewski JH: Electrophysiological basis of gastrointestinal motility. In Johnson LR, editor: Physiology of the gastrointestinal tract, ed 2, New York, 1987, Raven Press. pp. 383-422.

Wald A and Tunngunkla AK: Anorectal sensorimotor dysfunction in fecal incontinence in diabetes mellitus: modification with biofeedback therapy. N Engl J Med 310:1282, 1984.

Yamato S, Spechler S, and Goyal RK: Role of nitric oxide in esophageal peristalsis in the opossum, Gastroenterology 103:197, 1992.

CHAPTER

27 Gastric Secretion

Markus Goldschmiedt
Mark Feldman

The gastric mucosa secretes water, ions (mainly hydrogen, chloride, sodium, and potassium), intrinsic factor, pepsinogens, and mucus. Secretions originate from epithelial cells (surface cells and glands). Hydrochloric acid and intrinsic factor are secreted by parietal cells located in the fundus and body of the stomach (Fig. 27-1). Pepsinogens are secreted as inactive precursors by chief cells located in the fundus and body and also by mucus cells in the cardia, body, fundus, antrum, and pylorus (Fig. 27-1). In the presence of acid, pepsinogens are converted autocatalytically to pepsin, the active form of the enzyme. Gastric mucus is produced by surface epithelial cells and by mucous neck cells throughout the mucosa.

The stomach also secretes sodium bicarbonate. It appears that surface epithelial cells throughout the gastric mucosa are responsible for bicarbonate secretion. Bicarbonate secretion is thought to act in concert with the mucous gel layer to protect surface cells from injury by luminal acid-pepsin. The pH near the surface of the healthy gastric epithelium is approximately 7.0 even when luminal pH is around 2.0, presumably because of active bicarbonate secretion into the mucous gel.

Certain substances are secreted primarily into the circulation or tissue, but may also appear in the gastric lumen. Examples include the hormone gastrin (from gastrin cells in the antrum and pylorus) and histamine (from mast cells and enterochromaffin [ECL] cells in the lamina propria throughout the stomach). Other substances secreted into the lumen include immunoglobulin A (secreted by plasma cells in the lamina propria) and various blood group substances.

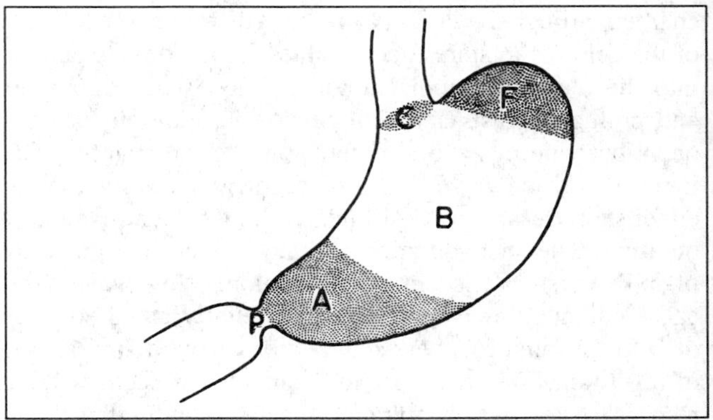

Fig. 27-1. Sites of secretion in the stomach. C, cardia; F, fundus; B, body; A, antrum; P, pylorus. Acid-secreting parietal cells are located in F and B; gastrin-secreting G cells are located in A and P.

The latter are mucoproteins secreted by approximately 80% of people. People who do not secrete blood group substances into gastric juice have a higher incidence of duodenal ulcer disease, whereas those who secrete blood group substance A are predisposed to gastric cancer. Plasma proteins also appear in gastric juice in small amounts, although in certain diseases (e.g., hypertrophic gastropathy [Ménétrier's disease]) large amounts of plasma protein can appear in the gastric lumen (Chapter 39).

In general, an agent or disease that increases or decreases gastric acid secretion has the same effect on secretion of intrinsic factor and pepsinogens. There are two notable exceptions. The hormone secretin decreases acid secretion but increases pepsinogen secretion. Also, patients with congenital intrinsic factor deficiency have deficient intrinsic factor secretion but secrete normal amounts of hydrochloric acid.

Most information on gastric secretion has come from studies of hydrochloric acid secretion. In the remainder of this chapter, normal physiology and pathophysiology of gastric acid secretion are discussed.

ACID SECRETION

Hydrogen ions are secreted by parietal cells into the gastric lumen against a 3 million/1 concentration gradient. Therefore this process requires energy (i.e., hydrogen ion secretion is active). Likewise, gastric chloride secretion is active, occurring against both a concentration gradient from plasma to lumen and an electrical gradient (potential difference of approximately −60 mV). During hydrochloric acid secretion there is a net exchange of one molecule of chloride from extracellular fluid or plasma for each molecule of bicarbonate generated in parietal cells from the hydration of carbon dioxide (CO_2).

Hydrochloric acid secretion by parietal cells is a result of activation of a unique proton pump. This proton pump, hydrogen-potassium ion adenosine triphosphatase, (H^+,K^+-ATPase), a magnesium-dependent enzyme, is found only on secretory membranes of parietal cells (apical plasma membrane, tubulovesicular membrane). It is composed of two polypeptide subunits: a larger alpha catalytic subunit that reacts with ATP and a smaller beta subunit that is closely associated with the catalytic subunit but of undefined function. This pump exchanges one potassium ion from the canalicular fluid for one hydrogen ion from the cytoplasm. The H^+,K^+-ATPase pump is distinct from the Na^+-K^+ATPase, the so-called sodium pump, which exchanges cytoplasmatic sodium ions for extracellular potassium ions and is present in all cells throughout the body. In contrast to the sodium pump, the proton pump in parietal cells is not inhibited by digitalis. Instead, the proton pump can be inhibited by compounds called substituted benzimidazoles (e.g., omeprazole, lansoprazole) and by potassium competitive antagonists such as SCH 28080. Omeprazole is a prodrug that is taken up by the parietal cell and, being a weak base, is concentrated in the acidic secretory canaliculi, where it is converted by acid to its active form, omeprazole sulfenamide, which reacts covalently with sulfhydryl groups of two cysteine residues on the extracellular domain of the alpha subunit of the H^+,K^+-ATPase. As a result of the formation of cysteinyl sulfenamides, the ability of the H^+,K^+-ATPase to push H^+ out of the cell and to pull K^+ back into the cell is lost and H^+ transport is blocked until new alpha subunits can be synthesized and inserted into the apical membrane of the parietal cell, a renewal process that requires more than 24 hours.

The rate at which parietal cells secrete acid is regulated by several substances, including histamine, gastrin, and acetylcholine (Fig. 27-2). *Histamine* in one of the most important endogenous stimulants of acid secretion. There is evidence that the ECL cell, rather than the mast cell, may be responsible for the phasic release of histamine after meals and other physiologic stimulants of acid secretion. Once histamine reaches the histamine-2 (H_2) receptor on the plasma membrane of the parietal cell, it activates the enzyme adenylate cyclase within the parietal cell, converting cytosolic adenosine triphosphate (ATP) to cyclic AMP. Gs, a guanine nucleotide-binding protein, and guanosine triphosphate (GTP) play a key role in this catalytic process. Cyclic AMP generated in parietal cells stimulates protein kinases that phosphorylate unidentified cellular proteins, and this ultimately results in activation of the proton pump. *Acetylcholine* is released from postganglionic, parasympathetic neurons near parietal cells (Fig. 27-2) in response to vagal stimulation. Acetylcholine stimulates the parietal cell by acting on a muscarinic M_3 cholinergic receptor. *Gastrin* is released from G cells in the antral and duodenal mucosa and reaches the parietal cells through the bloodstream (Fig. 27-2). Gastrin can act on the parietal cell directly but may also increase acid secretion by releasing histamine from ECL cells in the oxyntic mucosa.

Both acetylcholine and gastrin act by increasing the concentration of intracellular calcium ions in parietal cells (Fig. 27-2). Acute administration of exogenous calcium, introduced either orally or parenterally, increases acid secretion. This increase may be due to gastrin release by calcium or to calcium's direct effect on parietal cells. Patients with severe hypocalcemia are often achlorhydric. When hypocalcemia is corrected, acid secretion returns to normal levels.

Evidence that histamine and acetylcholine play physiologic stimulatory roles in acid secretion is derived primarily from studies in which specific antagonists of these compounds (e.g., cimetidine or atropine) are used. Evidence that gastrin plays a physiologic role in acid secretion is more direct because it is possible to measure serum gastrin concentrations by radioimmunoassay (see later discussion). There is evidence that other endogenous substances play a physiologic, inhibitory role in the regulation of acid secretion. These substances include prostaglandins, somatostatin, and secretin. Prostaglandins appear to act via a receptor on the parietal cell membrane that activates another guanine nucleotide-binding protein, Gi, which inhibits adenylate cyclase, thus reducing cyclic AMP. Whether somatostatin and secretin inhibit the parietal cell directly (via a receptor) or indirectly is not clear.

Gastric acid secretion can be measured under basal conditions, under conditions of maximum stimulation, or in response to a standard stimulus, such as a meal. Basal and

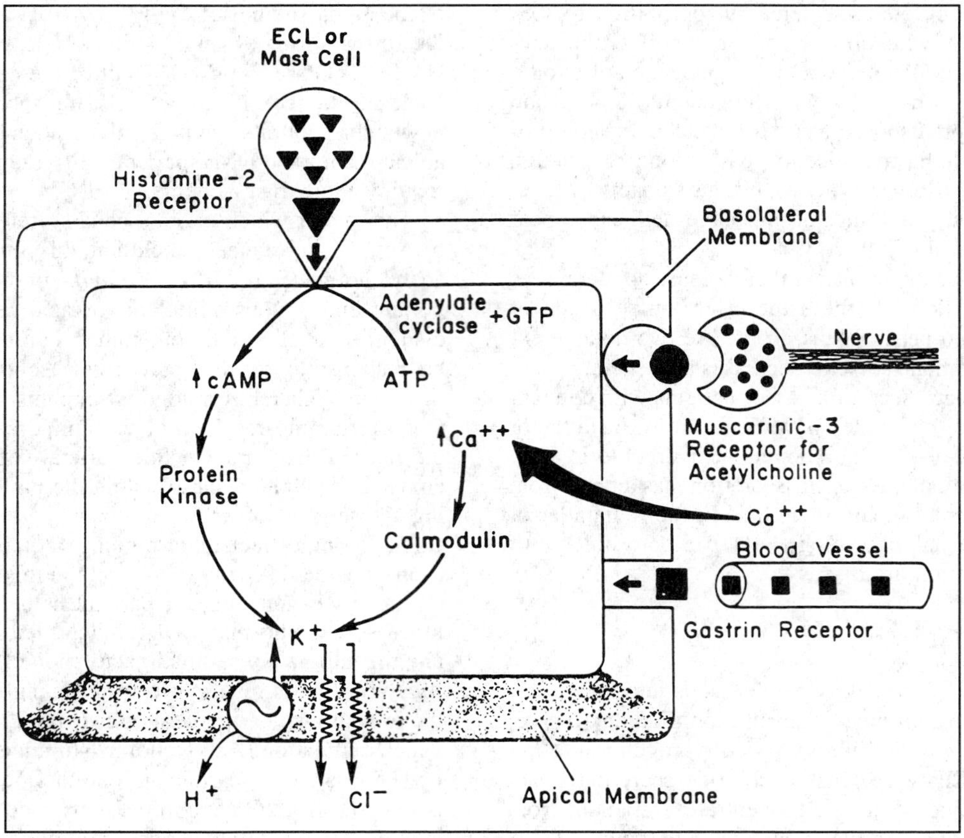

Fig. 27-2. Model for receptors on the basolateral membrane of the parietal cell and their intracellular mediators. Histamine from ECL or mast cells activates the proton pump *(shown on the apical membrane of the cell)* by increasing intracellular cAMP while acetylcholine from postganglionic nerves and gastrin from the blood act by increasing intracellular calcium. Although the increase in intracellular calcium is shown to arise from extracellular calcium, there is evidence that gastrin and perhaps acetylcholine release calcium from intracellular stores. Histamine may also increase intracellular calcium in addition to cAMP. cAMP, cyclic adenosine monophosphate.

maximum acid secretion are usually measured by aspirating gastric contents through a nasogastric tube (see Chapter 32). Aspiration techniques cannot be used to measure acid secretion while food is in the stomach. Instead, in vivo intragastric titration or indicator-dilution methods can be used. Using a combination of aspiration and in vivo intragastric titration methods, it has been shown that normal people secrete approximately 200 mmol gastric acid per day.

Maximum acid secretion

Maximum acid secretion is the maximum amount of acid that the stomach can secrete in response to large parenteral doses of histamine or gastrin (e.g., 6 μg per kilogram pentagastrin [Chapter 32]). MAO (or peak acid output [PAO]) correlates fairly well with the parietal cell mass of the stomach.

MAO or PAO is fairly constant when measured repeatedly in the same subject. Among subjects, however, there is wide variation in maximum acid secretion. PAO tends to be higher in men than in women and is correlated with lean body mass (Table 27-1). There is only a modest correlation between PAO and serum pepsinogen concentration, suggesting that parietal cell mass and chief cell mass are not tightly correlated.

Gastrin is trophic for parietal cells. Thus some patients with gastrinoma (Zollinger-Ellison syndrome) have a markedly increased parietal cell mass and PAO. Conversely, antrectomy removes gastrin-producing tissue (but few parietal cells) and leads to parietal cell atrophy and a fall in PAO. There is also evidence that the vagus nerve is trophic for parietal cells because excessive vagal stimulation in experimental animals increases PAO.

After vagotomy (truncal, selective, or highly selective), PAO decreases by approximately 50% (a range of 20% to 90%). This decrease occurs very quickly (within 24 hours) and is not caused by a decrease in the number of parietal cells present. It is unclear why PAO falls after vagotomy.

Basal acid secretion

Acid secreted in the absence of all intentional stimulation is called *basal acid secretion*. Unlike maximum acid

Table 27-1. Acid outputs in 365 healthy adult men and women*

	Mean BAO (range)	Mean MAO (range)	Mean PAO (range)	Mean BAO/PAO (range)
Women (n = 113)	2.1 ± 1.20 (0.0-13.5)	19.8 ± 0.86 (0.0-50.8)	24.9 ± 0.96 (0.0-52.6)	0.08 ± 0.01 (0.0-0.38)
Men (n = 252)	4.0 ± 0.24 (0.0-18.7)	29.7 ± 0.74 (0.0-72.4)	37.4 ± 0.84 (0.0-81.2)	0.10 ± 0.01 (0.0-0.42)

*Mean ± SE and range.

secretion, which is fairly constant in a given subject, basal acid output (BAO) varies considerably from day to day, for unclear reasons. Basal acid secretion tends to follow a circadian pattern, with lowest secretory rates occurring between 5 and 11 AM and highest rates between 2 and 11 PM.

BAO varies considerably among subjects (Table 27-1). This variation is due, in part, to differences in parietal cell mass (PAO). Factors other than PAO, however, are also responsible for differences in BAO because the BAO/PAO ratio (an estimate of the fraction of the parietal cell mass that is active basally) is highly variable (ranging from 0 to 0.42). Many factors, including vagal tone, histamine, and gastrin, probably contribute to the rate of basal acid secretion.

Although the average BAO is 3.4 mmol/hr, a few normal individuals have a BAO of 10 mmol or more/hr. Thus only a very high rate of basal acid secretion (greater than 10 mmol/hr) would be suggestive of a basal hypersecretory state (see later discussion). Moreover, because BAO/PAO can be as high as 0.42 in normal subjects, only a BAO/PAO considerably greater than 0.4 should be considered abnormal. As many normal subjects secrete no acid basally, absence of basal acid secretion has no pathologic significance, although a very high basal pH (> 5 in men and > 7 in women) is predictive of hypochlorhydria.

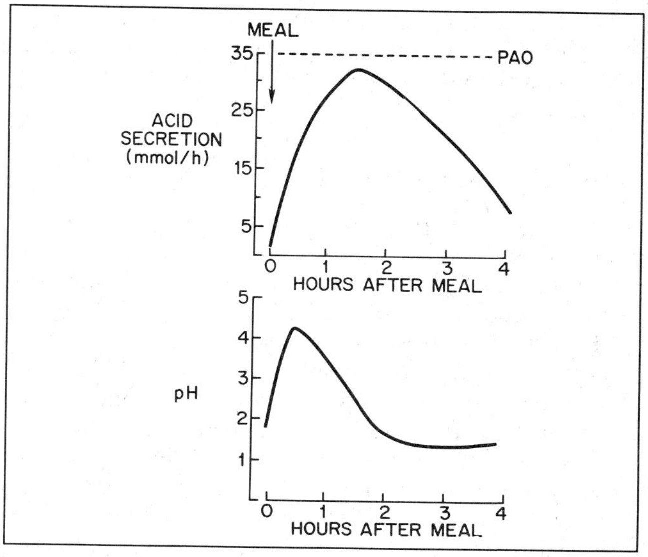

Fig. 27-3. The pattern of gastric acid secretion *(top)* and gastric pH *(bottom)* in response to a meal. Soon after a meal, pH within the stomach increases even though acid secretion is also increasing. Gastric pH increases because food in the stomach buffers the secreted acid. Within an hour or two, acid secretion rates are close to the maximum rate that can be attained with exogenous histamine *(PAO, dotted line)*. (From Luce JM, Tyler ML, and Pierson DJ: Intensive respiratory care. Philadelphia, 1984, Saunders.)

Meal-stimulated acid secretion

Food is the usual physiologic stimulus for acid secretion. When an appetizing meal is eaten, acid secretion increases from basal rates to nearly maximum rates within an hour or two (Fig. 27-3, *top*). Although acid secretion increases during the first hour after a meal, pH of gastric contents remains relatively high (more than 3.0) (Fig. 27-3, *bottom*), because protein in food buffers acid during this early postprandial period. This phenomenon probably explains why ulcer patients may experience symptomatic relief shortly after eating. During the second and third hours pH of gastric contents decreases as acid continues to be secreted at high rates and as food-buffer is utilized or emptied into the small intestine. At this time, ulcer patients may experience a recrudescence of symptoms.

Mechanisms that lead to an increase in acid secretion after eating include (1) cephalic-vagal stimulation, (2) gastric distention, and (3) chemical reactions of food with gastrointestinal mucosa. Although these mechanisms usually operate simultaneously, they are discussed separately.

Cephalic-vagal stimulation

The thought, sight, smell, and taste of appetizing food lead to stimulation of acid secretion that amounts to one third to one half of PAO. Thought and taste appear to be more potent stimulants than sight or smell. Because a successful vagotomy completely abolishes the acid-secretory response to sham feeding, it is generally believed that the cephalic phase of acid secretion is mediated solely via the vagus nerves. Cephalic-vagal stimulation elicits acid secretion by two mechanisms: (1) cholinergic stimulation of parietal cells by postganglionic neurons and (2) release of relatively small quantities of gastrin into the circulation. Whether vagal stimulation also releases histamine from mast cells or

ECL cells in the fundus and body of the stomach is uncertain.

Gastric distention

Distention of the stomach with a balloon or with an inert solution (saline, water) increases gastric acid secretion to one fourth to one half of PAO. The acid-secretory response to distention is mediated by reflexes that directly stimulate parietal cells (oxynto-oxyntic reflex) and that release gastrin (pyloropyloric reflex). The former reflex is probably cholinergic, whereas the latter may be beta-adrenergic because the gastrin response to distention can be blocked by propranolol. The acid-secretory response to distention is reduced but not abolished by vagotomy, implying that the distention-activated reflexes are both long (involving the vagi) and local.

Chemical reactions to food

The acid-secretory response to intragastric homogenized food (containing protein, carbohydrate, and fat) is much greater than the response to an equal volume of saline solution and amounts to 60% to 70% of PAO.

The major food constituent that stimulates acid secretion is protein. Undigested proteins are weak stimulants, whereas peptic digests (peptides, peptones, amino acids) are potent stimulants. Individual amino acids differ in their ability to stimulate acid secretion. The major mechanism by which amino acids and peptides elicit acid secretion is release of gastrin (both little gastrin, G17, and big gastrin, G34). Other mechanisms by which amino acids and peptides may increase acid secretion are (1) direct stimulation of parietal cells (either via the gastric lumen or via the circulation after intestinal absorption) and (2) release of a nongastrin secretagogue from the small intestine.

Dietary fats and carbohydrates reduce acid secretion. Although many peptide hormones are released from the small intestine by fats and carbohydrates, it has not been shown that any individual peptide is released in a sufficient amount to inhibit acid secretion. Thus the exact mechanism by which fats and carbohydrates reduce acid secretion is uncertain. Because intravenous fats and carbohydrates also reduce acid secretion under certain conditions, it is possible that the nutrients themselves act directly on parietal cells rather than through the release of a hormone from the small intestine.

Coffee and many other beverages (milk, beer, soft drinks) increase gastric acid secretion and release gastrin. Decaffeinated coffee stimulates about as much acid secretion as does regular coffee, indicating that coffee contains stimulants of acid secretion other than caffeine. The nature of coffee's noncaffeine stimulation of acid secretion is uncertain.

Regulation of gastrin release by luminal acid

As acid is secreted, gastric luminal pH decreases (Fig. 27-3, *bottom*). When pH decreases below 2.5 or 3.0, gastrin release from the antrum is inhibited, and, as a result, acid secretion decreases. The mechanism by which a low luminal pH reduces gastrin release is unclear. At low pH certain amino acids become ionized, reducing their uptake by gastrin cells. Reducing luminal acidity by administering antacids or antisecretory drugs or by performing a vagotomy can increase serum gastrin concentrations. Patients who have gastric atrophy and achlorhydria, with or without pernicious anemia, may have markedly elevated serum gastrin concentrations.

ABNORMALITIES OF GASTRIC SECRETION

Increased gastric acid secretion

Duodenal ulcer disease. Chronic duodenal ulcer disease is the most common disorder associated with increased gastric acid secretion. Duodenal ulcer patients as a group have a significantly higher PAO, BAO, and BAO/PAO than normal subjects, although there is considerable overlap among groups. In contrast, mean food-stimulated gastric acid secretion is no higher in duodenal ulcer patients than in normal subjects.

Zollinger-Ellison syndrome (gastrinoma). Patients with Zollinger-Ellison syndrome have elevated serum gastrin concentrations as a result of a gastrin-producing endocrine tumor, most often located in the pancreas. Increased serum gastrin concentration leads to increased basal acid secretion. Basal acid secretion is usually greater than 15 mmol/hr, and in some patients it may be as high as 150 mmol/hr. The BAO/PAO ratio is usually 0.6 or greater. This syndrome is associated with other endocrine tumors as part of multiple endocrine neoplasia, type I syndrome (MEN-I), in approximately 25% of patients (see Chapter 38).

Retained antrum syndrome. The rare retained antrum syndrome can develop after antrectomy and Billroth II gastrojejunostomy if the most distal antral and pyloric tissue is inadvertently not resected. Because of its new location at the end of the afferent loop, the retained antral and pyloric epithelium is continually bathed in alkaline secretions. Under these conditions, gastrin is continually released into the circulation from the antral and pyloric G cells, potentially leading to increased gastric acid secretion from remaining parietal cells and to recurrent peptic ulceration in some patients.

Other causes. In some patients with hyperparathyroidism, increased acid secretion and peptic ulcer disease may be due to a coexisting gastrinoma (MEN-I syndrome). There is no definite evidence for increased acid secretion in patients with hyperparathyroidism without gastrinoma. Less common causes of acid hypersecretion include extensive small bowel resection, central nervous system trauma or disease, and foregut carcinoid tumors. The latter disease may lead to acid hypersecretion by producing gastrin or histamine. Histamine overproduction is also the mechanism for acid hypersecretion in some patients with systemic mastocytosis and basophilic leukemia.

Decreased gastric acid secretion

Decreased acid and pepsin secretion are commonly observed in patients with gastric ulcer, gastric polyps, and gastric carcinoma. Patients with gastric atrophy and histamine-fast or pentagastrin-fast achlorhydria often have reduced or absent intrinsic factor secretion; in such individuals vitamin B_{12} deficiency may develop (Chapter 39). These latter patients may be at increased risk for gastric polyps and carcinoma. Other causes of reduced acid secretion include previous partial gastric resection and/or vagotomy and, on rare occasions, endocrine tumors that produce hormones that inhibit acid secretion (e.g., somatostatin or vasoactive intestinal peptide). Patients with acquired immunodeficiency syndrome (AIDS) often have reduced acid secretion.

Recent studies have not shown a significant reduction in gastric acid secretion with aging, and some found an increase in gastric acid secretion with age.

Helicobacter pylori and acid secretion

The effect of *Helicobacter pylori* (HP) on gastric acid secretion is controversial. Acute hypochlorhydria after ingestion of HP has been demonstrated in two uncontrolled case reports in previously healthy individuals. Some studies reported that chronic infestation with HP is associated with an increase in acid output; others have been unable to find a convincing relationship between gastric acid secretion and presence of HP.

The effect of HP on gastrin release is also controversial. Some studies did not find a relationship between the presence of HP and basal or postprandial serum gastrin concentrations. However, most studies have reported increased serum gastrin concentrations in healthy subjects and duodenal ulcer patients infected with HP. In addition, one study demonstrated a significant decrease in meal-stimulated gastrin release after treatment that eradicated HP.

REFERENCES

Brady CE et al: Acid secretion and serum gastrin levels in individuals with *Campylobacter pylori*. Gastroenterology 94:923, 1988.

Chen MCY et al: Prostanoid inhibition of canine parietal cells: mediation by the inhibitory guanosine triphosphate-binding protein of adenylate cyclase. Gastroenterology 94:1121, 1988.

Feldman M and Barnett C: Fasting gastrin pH and its relationship to true hypochlorhydria in humans. Dig Dis Sci 36:866, 1991.

Goldschmiedt M et al: Effect of age on gastric acid secretion and serum gastrin concentrations in healthy men and women. Gastroenterology 101:977, 1991.

Hakanson R and Sundler F: Histamine-producing cells in the stomach and their role in the regulation of acid secretion. Scand J Gastroenterol 26(suppl 180):88, 1991.

Sachs G and Wallmark B: The gastric H^+, K^+-ATPase: the site of action of Omeprazole. Scand J Gastroenterol 24(suppl 166):3, 1989.

Siurala M, Sipponen P, and Kekki M: *Campylobacter pylori* in a sample of Finnish population: relations to morphology and functions of the gastric mucosa. Gut 29:909, 1988.

Smith JTL et al: Inappropriate hypergastrinemia in asymptomatic healthy subjects infected with *Helicobacter pylori*. Gut 31:522, 1990.

Wagner S et al: *Campylobacter pylori* and gastric acidity. Am J Gastroenterol 84:201, 1989.

CHAPTER

28 Intestinal Absorption

Jerry S. Trier

The complex processes of digestion and absorption that take place in the stomach, small intestine, and colon of normal human beings are remarkably efficient. An adult who eats an average Western diet ingests approximately 100 g of fat, 400 g of carbohydrate, 100 g of protein, and 1.5 to 2.0 L of fluid per day. This diet also contains substantial amounts of sodium, chloride, potassium, and calcium as well as small amounts of other essential elements and vitamins. An additional load of roughly 7 L of endogenous fluids, including biliary, gastric, and pancreatic secretions, enters the intestine. These endogenous secretions contain substantial quantities of ions, protein, cholesterol, phospholipids, and bile salts. Normally, this massive load is reduced by absorption in the small intestine to a volume of 1.0 to 1.5 L, which enters the colon. Further water and ion absorption in the colon results in a stool mass of less than 200 g per day that contains 2 to 6 g of fat, 1 to 2 g of nitrogen, and less than 20 mEq each of sodium, potassium, chloride, and bicarbonate. In this chapter intestinal digestion and absorption are reviewed briefly, because an understanding of these processes is helpful in assessing alimentary tract diseases in which normal digestion and/or absorption is perturbed.

Because the intestine is a relatively narrow but long tube (12 to 20 ft) with many redundant loops, it uses its allocated space within the abdomen efficiently. Moreover, the surface specializations of the small intestine, which include circular or spiral folds (plicae circulares), microscopic mucosal villi, and ultrastructurally apparent apical microvilli on absorptive cells, amplify the surface presented to the luminal contents to approximately 1000 times that of a cylindrical tube with a flat surface (Fig. 28-1).

Digestion and absorption of most dietary lipids, proteins, and carbohydrates occur with remarkable efficiency in the duodenum and jejunum; therefore these nutrients are usually absorbed before the residual intestinal chyme reaches the ileum. However, substantial absorption of fats, carbohydrates, peptides, and amino acids may occur in the distal small intestine when digestion and absorption in the proximal intestine are compromised by disease. Absorption of calcium, food iron, and folic acid is most efficient in the proximal intestine, whereas absorption of most bile salts and vitamin B_{12} occurs in the ileum. The colon absorbs water, sodium, chloride, and bicarbonate efficiently. In patients with carbohydrate malabsorption, and, to a lesser degree in normal individuals, the colon also conserves carbohydrate by absorbing more than 50% of the breakdown products of bacterial carbohydrate metabolism.

During absorption, the end-products of digestion must first traverse the intestinal epithelial barrier to gain access to the terminal capillaries and lymphatics in the core of the villus for distribution to distant sites. This is accomplished

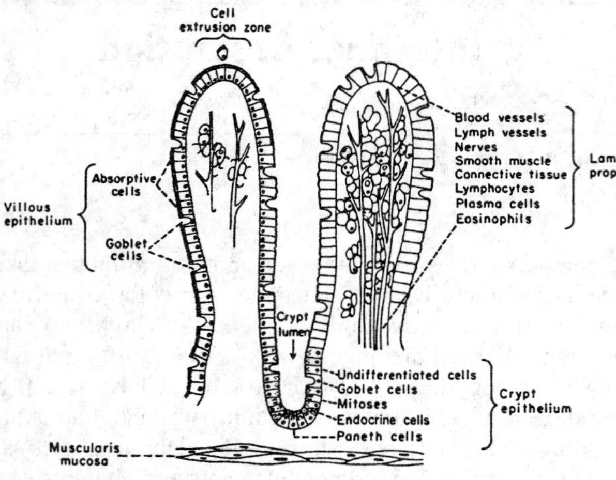

Fig. 28-1. Schematic diagram of histologic organization of the small intestinal mucosa.

by two major transport mechanisms: passive diffusion and active transport (Table 28-1). Substances absorbed by *passive diffusion* follow either a chemical gradient from a high to low concentration or, if the molecule is charged, an electrical gradient. Neither energy nor a membrane carrier is required for passive diffusion. Examples of substances absorbed by this mechanism include the products of triglyceride hydrolysis and, in the small intestine, potassium. Substances absorbed by *active transport* move against osmotic or chemical gradients from low to high concentrations and, if charged, against electrical gradients. During active transport, energy is expended, and selective carriers or pumps, presumably membrane proteins that facilitate transport across membranes against gradients, are required.

Two other transport mechanisms are facilitated diffusion and endocytosis. *Facilitated diffusion,* like passive diffusion, requires no energy and follows osmotic and chemical gradients but occurs more rapidly than passive diffusion, presumably because a carrier is present. Fructose appears to be absorbed by facilitated diffusion. *Endocytosis* permits bulk or receptor-mediated transport of large molecules such as intact proteins. During endocytosis, small regions of the apical plasma membrane first indent the absorptive cell cytoplasm. These regions then pinch off, forming small, membrane-bounded vesicles containing luminal contents that are then processed in the cell or that may traverse and then leave the cell cytoplasm by subsequent fusion of the vesicle membrane with the basolateral membrane. Endocytosis is important in transcellular calcium transport and in intestinal transport of colostral immunoglobulin in some neonatal mammals. Receptor-mediated endocytosis of regulatory peptides such as vasoactive intestinal peptide by the basolateral membrane of intestinal epithelial cells may be important in the regulation of certain intestinal transport processes such as electrolyte transport.

Table 28-1. Primary mechanism of absorption of some specific nutrients*

Active transport	Diffusion
Glucose	Short and medium chain fatty acids
Galactose	2-Monoglycerides
Amino acids	Lysophospholipids
Di- and tripeptides	Cholesterol
Na^+	Vitamins D, A, K, and E
Cl^-	K^+
HCO_3^-	H_2O
Iron	Fructose (facilitated diffusion)
Vitamin B_{12}	
Ca^{2+}	

*There is also substantial passive diffusion of Na^+ and Cl^-, especially in the upper small intestine.

ABSORPTION OF LIPIDS

Normally, most dietary fats consist of long-chain triglycerides, which, if not hydrolyzed and dispersed, are absorbed poorly by the small intestine. The steps involved in triglyceride digestion and absorption are summarized in Fig. 28-2. Triglyceride digestion begins in the stomach, where gastric peristalsis reduces the size of triglyceride droplets and facilitates contact with a lipase secreted by gastric chief cells. This gastric lipase is acid stable, with a pH optimum that ranges from 2.2 to 6. It releases fatty acids from triglycerides in the stomach. Initial intragastric lipid digestion is probably of substantial physiologic importance. Although its quantitative contribution to triglyceride hydrolysis in adults remains to be established, the fatty acids released by the process emulsify triglycerides and stimulate the release of cholecystokinin from the duodenal mucosa, which in turn stimulates secretion of pancreatic lipase and bile into the duodenal lumen. Gastric lipase is normally ineffective in the lumen of the intestine, because its pH optimum is exceeded and the enzyme is inhibited by bile salts. In patients with pancreatic exocrine insufficiency, it may account for the majority of intraluminal lipid hydrolysis.

As gastric contents enter the duodenum, hydrogen ions release from the duodenal mucosa secretin, which stimulates pancreatic and bile duct bicarbonate secretion. Secretion of bicarbonate normally maintains the intraluminal pH at approximately 6.5, an optimum level for intraluminal fat digestion and dispersion. Bile salts emulsify dietary fats to small droplets, increasing their surface area. Emulsification is important, because pancreatic lipase works only at the surface of the fat droplet. Pancreatic lipase hydrolyzes long-chain triglycerides at the alpha-ester linkages, releasing a mixture of free fatty acids and 2-monoglycerides. Colipase, a small protein also secreted by the pancreas, is necessary for this hydrolysis; it facilitates attachment of pancreatic lipase to the surfaces of the triglyceride droplets and blocks bile salt inhibition of pancreatic lipase. Dietary and biliary phospholipids such as lecithin are hydrolyzed intraluminally by phospholipase A_2 at their 2-ester linkage, whereas cholesterol esters and sev-

ity for absorption of ions and water may vary. For example, there is some evidence that villus absorptive cells normally absorb, whereas undifferentiated crypt cells may secrete water and ions in the small intestine. Net fluid and ion transport in the gut depends on the balance between net absorption and net secretion. Absorption predominates under normal conditions; however, in certain toxigenic enteric bacterial infections, with certain hormone-secreting tumors, and in some primary intestinal mucosal diseases, secretion may greatly exceed absorption, with devastating consequences.

There are two pathways by which small molecules, such as water and ions, may cross the mucosa: the paracellular and transcellular pathways. *Paracellular transport* requires penetration only of the tight junctions that connect adjacent epithelial cells at the apex of the lateral membrane, with subsequent diffusion along the lateral intercellular space. There is evidence that the tight junctions connecting adjacent small intestinal epithelial cells are quite permeable, especially to cations, and that the paracellular pathway is a major site of transepithelial water and ion transport. Transport via the paracellular pathway is passive and, therefore, follows electrochemical, osmotic, and hydrostatic gradients. Intestinal permeability is greater in the proximal than in the distal intestine. Recent studies suggest that tight junction permeability increases when the mucosa is exposed to an osmolar load as occurs during normal alimentation. *Transcellular transport* of ions requires their passage through two membrane barriers, the apical plasma membrane and the basolateral plasma membrane, as well as through the cytosol. Because plasma membranes are predominantly lipoidal, diffusion of hydrophilic molecules is limited, and membrane transporters facilitate transcellular ion movement.

Na^+ transport is both active and passive along the length of the small intestine and the colon. Several mechanisms are involved: (1) coupled neutral NaCl entry, which may involve Na^+-H^+ and Cl^--HCO_3^- exchange at the apical surface in the small intestine and colon; (2) Na^+ cotransport with sugars and amino acids in the small intestine; and (3) electrogenic Na^+ absorption at all levels of the small and large intestine that use Na-K-ATPase, which is located in the epithelial cell basolateral membrane. Unlike Na^+ transport, K^+ transport appears passive in the small intestine, but there are active absorption and secretion in the colon with secretion predominating. HCO_3^- appears to be secreted actively by the duodenum, ileum, and colon, whereas Cl^- is normally absorbed actively in the ileum and colon. Water movement is by passive diffusion throughout the intestine and follows osmotic and hydrostatic gradients. Water transport can contribute to ion transport by the mechanism of solvent drag. During this process, the solutes not filtered out by the cell membrane or tight junctions are carried along by the moving stream of solvent.

ABSORPTION OF IRON

To maintain iron balance the healthy adult male must absorb 0.5 to 1.0 mg per day, while the healthy adult female requires 1.5 to 2.0 mg per day during her reproductive years. Because normal iron intake in the Western diet averages 10 to 20 mg, the absorption of iron is a highly regulated process in which the gastrointestinal tract plays a major role in maintaining homeostasis, because intake exceeds needs. In iron deficiency, iron absorption increases; in iron excess, except in idiopathic hemochromatosis, iron absorption decreases. Heme iron from animal tissues is absorbed by the intestine more effectively than iron from cereals and vegetables. Inorganic iron is less avidly absorbed than food iron, but divalent ferrous ion is absorbed more efficiently than trivalent ferric ion.

Whereas the uptake of iron into epithelial cells occurs along the length of the small intestine, absorption, especially of inorganic iron, is most efficient in the duodenum. During the absorption of hemoglobin iron, the heme moiety is split from globin by intraluminal proteolytic hydrolysis and is absorbed intact after binding to a membrane receptor. Heme is then degraded within the absorptive cell, releasing inorganic iron into the portal circulation.

Within the gut lumen, inorganic iron forms chelates with ascorbic acid, amino acids, and sugar. In the case of ferric iron, this process is enhanced by hydrochloric acid in the stomach. Such chelation enhances the solubility of iron in the more alkaline environment of the duodenum. Inorganic iron then enters absorptive cells via a saturable process. The regulation of mucosal iron absorption remains incompletely understood but may involve mucosal iron content, ferritin, transferrin saturation, and erythropoietin.

Acute or prolonged excessive iron intake can overwhelm the mucosal regulatory process and result in acute iron toxicity or iron overload. Moreover, in patients with idiopathic hemochromatosis, the mucosal regulatory process may be defective, and amounts of iron greater than the body needs are absorbed. The importance of the duodenum in iron absorption is underscored by the high prevalence of iron deficiency in patients with mucosal lesions involving the proximal intestine (such as in celiac sprue) or in patients in whom the duodenum has been surgically bypassed (e.g., after partial gastrectomy with gastrojejunostomy).

ABSORPTION OF CALCIUM

Of the 1 g of calcium ingested daily in the average Western diet and the 300 mg added by endogenous secretions, 900 mg is excreted in the stool, resulting in a net normal gain of approximately 100 mg per day via the gut. In individuals who are not increasing or decreasing total body calcium, this 100 mg is excreted in the urine. Calcium is absorbed most avidly by the duodenum and jejunum, but it is also absorbed by the ileum by an active transport mechanism that is adaptable to the needs of the body. Thus the intestine is important in maintaining calcium homeostasis.

Vitamin D plays a key role in regulating calcium absorption. After its absorption from the gut or its production in the skin, vitamin D is hydroxylated in the 25 position in the liver and in the 1 position in the kidney to 1,25-dihydroxycholecalciferol. This active form of vitamin D then binds to a specific receptor in the small intestinal epithelium. There, it stimulates calcium transport by mechanisms that are not fully understood. During absorption, calcium appears to bind to one or more binding proteins (?calbindin D, ?calmodulin) at the microvillus membrane, is endocytosed, and is then transported to the basolateral membrane, most likely by vesicles via lysosomes. There is also evidence that there may be some transport of calcium via the paracellular pathway by a process that is not saturable or vitamin D dependent.

Mucosal lesions of the small intestine may result in direct impairment of calcium transport. Impaired intraluminal digestion and mucosal lesions also result in impaired vitamin D absorption. Steatorrhea facilitates formation of insoluble calcium soaps of fatty acids, decreasing the availability of soluble calcium for intestinal absorption.

ABSORPTION OF VITAMIN B_{12}

Although the requirement for vitamin B_{12} (cobalamin) is less than 2 μg per day, its absorption by the intestine is complex. After its release from foodstuffs of animal origin, vitamin B_{12} binds to several glycoproteins, or R-binders, found in saliva, gastric juice, and bile. In the upper small intestine, pancreatic proteases hydrolyze the R-binders, releasing vitamin B_{12}, which then binds to intrinsic factor (IF), a 44,000 dalton protein secreted in humans by gastric parietal cells. IF-B_{12} complex is resistant to intraluminal proteolysis and arrives intact in the distal ileum, where it binds to a specific receptor present only on the microvillus membrane of ileal absorptive cells. The mechanism involved in the subsequent transfer of vitamin B_{12} into and across the ileal epithelium and the mechanism of its release from IF are poorly understood. However, several hours after IF-B_{12} binds to the apical surface of ileal absorptive cells, B_{12} appears in the circulation complexed to transcobalamin II. Transcobalamin II delivers vitamin B_{12} to tissues and is the most important circulating B_{12} transport protein. A substantial amount of vitamin B_{12} is stored in the liver, normally enough to meet the body's needs for 4 to 5 years. Therefore factors inducing impaired B_{12} assimilation may be present for several years before B_{12} deficiency becomes evident.

Because of the complexity of vitamin B_{12} assimilation, abnormalities in several alimentary tract organs can impair its absorption. These include (1) gastric mucosal atrophy, which results in IF deficiency; (2) pancreatic exocrine insufficiency, which may, because of impaired intraluminal proteolysis, decrease B_{12} release from R-binders; (3) ileal mucosal disease, which results in decreased absorptive cell receptors for IF-B_{12}; and (4) conditions that result in long-term, intraluminal bacterial overgrowth in the small intestine, because bacteria in the small intestine may competitively bind and absorb B_{12}, reducing its availability for ileal absorption.

ABSORPTION OF FOLATES

Fruits, vegetables, liver, and yeast are important dietary sources of folates, of which roughly 90% are polyglutamate conjugates. Because pteroylmonoglutamate is absorbed much more effectively than pteroylpolyglutamates, deconjugation is an essential step in folate absorption. Folate conjugase is present in the microvillus membrane of duodenal and jejunal absorptive cells. The monoglutamate is then transported by the absorptive cell largely by a saturable process that appears to involve monoglutamate: OH^- exchange. The rate of hydrolysis greatly exceeds that of transport, which is rate limiting. The capacity for folate absorption is greatest in the duodenum and jejunum; consequently, the diseases in which mucosal lesions are most severe in the proximal intestine (e.g., celiac sprue) are frequently associated with folate deficiency. Unlike vitamin B_{12}, liver stores are usually sufficient to sustain body folate needs for only 2 to 3 months.

REFERENCES

Abrams CK et al: Gastric lipase: localization in the human stomach. Gastroenterology 95:1460, 1988.

Alpers DH: Digestion and absorption of carbohydrates and protein. In Johnson LR, editor: Physiology of the gastrointestinal tract, ed 2, New York, 1987, Raven Press, p 1469.

Davidson NO, Magun AM, and Glickman RM: Enterocyte lipid absorption and secretion. In Schultz SG, editor: Handbook of physiology, vol IV. Bethesda, Md, 1991, American Physiological Society, p 505.

Fondacaro JD: Intestinal ion transport and diarrheal disease. Am J Physiol 250:G1, 1986.

Gray GM: Dietary protein processing: intraluminal and enterocyte surface events. In Schultz SG, editor: Handbook of physiology, vol IV. Bethesda, Md, 1991, American Physiological Society, p 411.

Nemere I and Norman AW: Transport of calcium. In Schultz SG, editor: Handbook of physiology, vol, IV. Bethesda, Md, 1991, American Physiological Society, p 337.

Powell DW: Intestinal water and electrolyte transport. In Johnson LR, editor: Physiology of the gastrointestinal tract, ed 2. New York, 1987, Raven Press, p 1267.

Rose RC: Intestinal transport of water-soluble vitamins. In Schultz SG, editor: Handbook of physiology, vol IV. Bethesda, Md, 1991, American Physiological Society, p 421.

Wright EM et al: Molecular genetics of intestinal glucose transport. J Clin Invest 88:1435, 1991.

CHAPTER

29 Intestinal Immunity

Martin F. Kagnoff

The gastrointestinal tract contains approximately 25% of the lymphoid tissue in the body. Gut-associated lymphoid tissue (GALT) is exposed continually to materials from the external environment such as food antigens, bacteria, bacterial products, viruses, and parasites. In addition, the GALT is a key component of the more generalized mucosal immune system, which includes lymphoid tissue in the respiratory tract, genitourinary tract, and mammary glands. Intestinal immune reactions normally play an important role in host protection. However, abnormalities in intestinal mucosal immune function may contribute to allergic and autoimmune disorders and to specific intestinal diseases such as ulcerative colitis, Crohn's disease, and celiac disease (see Chapters 42 and 43). The importance of the intestinal immune system in host protection is perhaps best highlighted in the clinical syndromes that involve deficiencies in either immunoglobulin production (e.g., selective IgA deficiency, common variable immunodeficiency syndromes) or T cell function (e.g., acquired immunodeficiency syndrome).

GUT-ASSOCIATED LYMPHOID TISSUE

The immune system in the intestine has three major lymphoid components. These components are the Peyer's patches, the lamina propria lymphoid cells, and the intraepithelial lymphocytes. These three components are anatomically distinct and differ in their content of B and T lymphocyte subsets. Nonetheless, it is important to note that these three components are interrelated in terms of function.

Peyer's patches and lymphocyte migration

Peyer's patches are instrumental in the generation of the intestinal mucosal immune response. These lymphoid structures contain collections of lymphoid follicles and are present predominantly in the distal small intestine. Lymphocytes in Peyer's patches are separated from the intestinal lumen by epithelial cells that include specialized cells, termed *M cells*, that are scattered throughout the gut epithelium overlying the follicles of the Peyer's patch (Fig. 29-1). The M cells facilitate the transport of macromolecules from the intestinal lumen into the Peyer's patch.

B and T lymphocytes in Peyer's patches are activated by antigenic materials that enter from the intestinal lumen. Some of these cells then exit from this lymphoid structure, enter the lymphatic system, and undergo a migratory path that includes entry into the mesenteric lymph nodes, subsequent passage into the thoracic duct lymph and systemic circulation, and ultimate lodging in the intestinal mucosa. Many B lymphocytes that originate from Peyer's patches ultimately lodge in the lamina propria region of the intestinal mucosa. T lymphocytes lodge either in the lamina propria or between epithelial cells lining intestinal villi. Other B and T lymphocytes lodge in extraintestinal sites such as the salivary glands, mammary gland, female genital tract, and respiratory tract (Fig. 29-2).

Intraepithelial lymphocytes

Intraepithelial lymphocytes (IELs) are located between the intestinal epithelial cells close to the basement membrane (Fig. 29-3). These lymphocytes are abundant within the intestine. Thus, normally there is approximately one IEL for every six intestinal epithelial cells. The majority of IEL are T lymphocytes, most of which have the CD8 marker on their surface. Of IELs, 90% to 95% belong to the alpha/beta lineage of T lymphocytes, whereas approximately 5% to 10% belong to the gamma/delta lineage. Many IELs contain large cytoplasmic granules. IELs

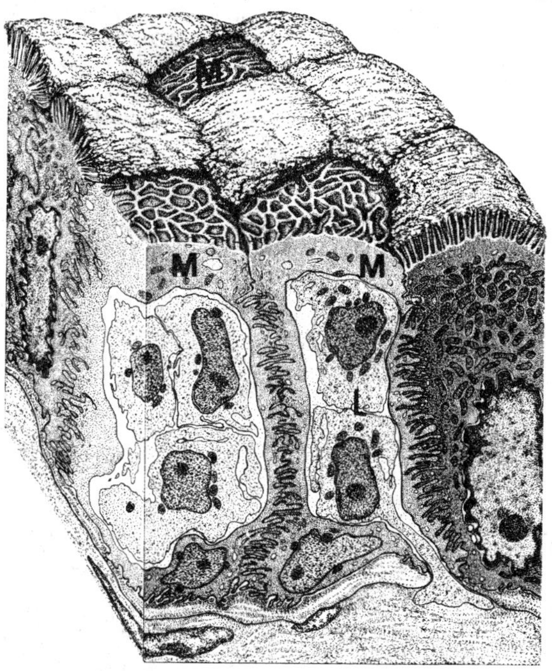

Fig. 29-1. M cells in the epithelium overlying a human Peyer's patch. Three M cells with luminal surface microfolds are shown schematically interdigitating with adjacent columnar cells over a Peyer's patch. The mononuclear lymphoid cells directly beneath the M cells may approach to within 0.3 μm of the intestinal lumen. M, M cells; L, lymphoid cells. (From Owen RL and Nemanic P: Scan. Electron. Microsc. 2:367, 1978.)

produce cytokines, but generally their other functions are not well characterized. However, IELs appear to be increased in diseases such as celiac disease and during infection with parasites such as *Giardia lamblia*, and, in the former, there is a marked increase in the proportion of IELs belonging to the gamma/delta T cell lineage. Nonetheless, knowledge of the ontogeny of IELs, the types of antigens they recognize, and the role of IELs in normal immune defense and in tissue-damaging mechanisms in disease is incomplete.

Lamina propria lymphoid cells

The lamina propria within intestinal villi contains B cells, plasma cells, and lymphocytes as well as other important mononuclear cells (macrophages, eosinophils, and mast cells) interspersed in a vascular and lymphatic-rich connective tissue (Fig. 29-3). Seventy to ninety percent of plasma cells in the intestinal lamina propria produce antibody of the IgA immunoglobulin class. Of note, the distribution of T cell subsets in the lamina propria differs markedly from that in the intraepithelial region. Thus, the ratio of T cells in the lamina propria that have the CD4 marker usually associated with helper/inducer T cells to those having the CD8 marker is similar to that seen in the peripheral circulation (i.e., a CD4/CD8 ratio of greater than 1.0).

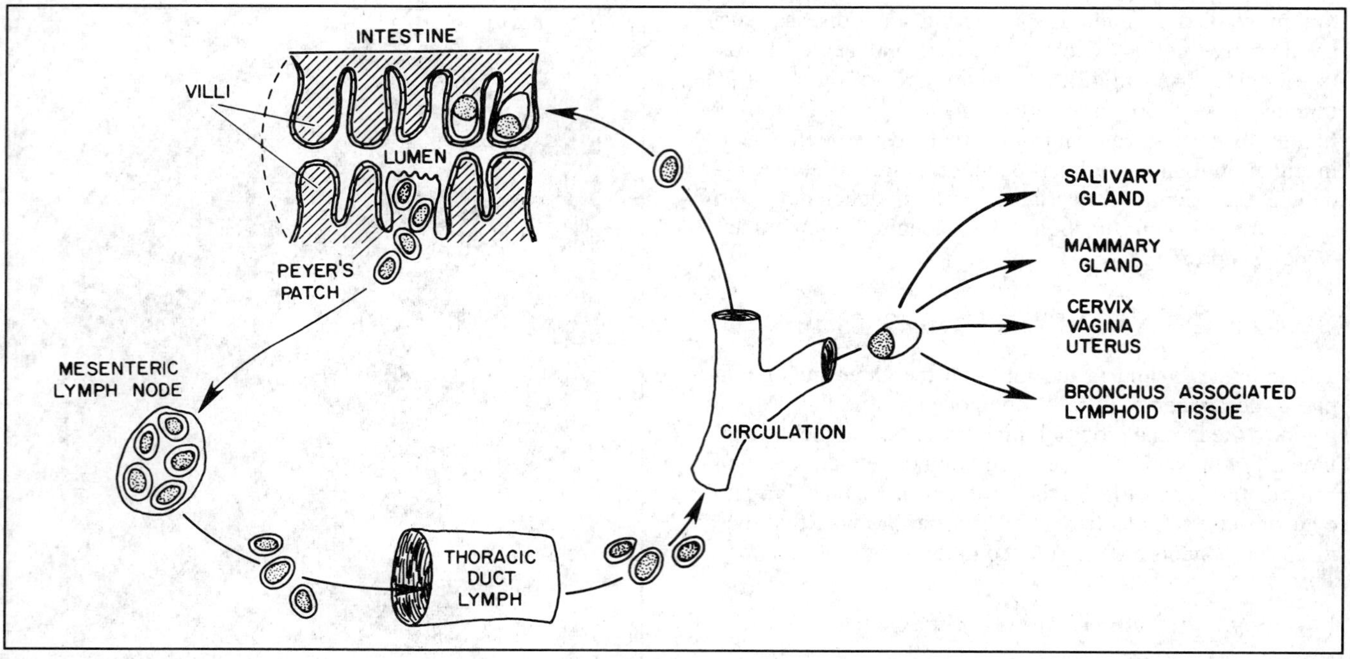

Fig. 29-2. Lymphocytes activated by antigen in Peyer's patches migrate to the mesenteric lymph node and thoracic duct lymph before entering the circulation. B cells disseminate to the lamina propria and T cells to the lamina propria and intraepithelial region of the intestine. Other cells leave the circulation and lodge in extraintestinal lymphoid tissues including the salivary glands, mammary glands, female genital tract, and respiratory tract. (From Kagnoff MF: Gastrointestinal disease, ed 5. Philadelphia, 1992, WB Saunders.)

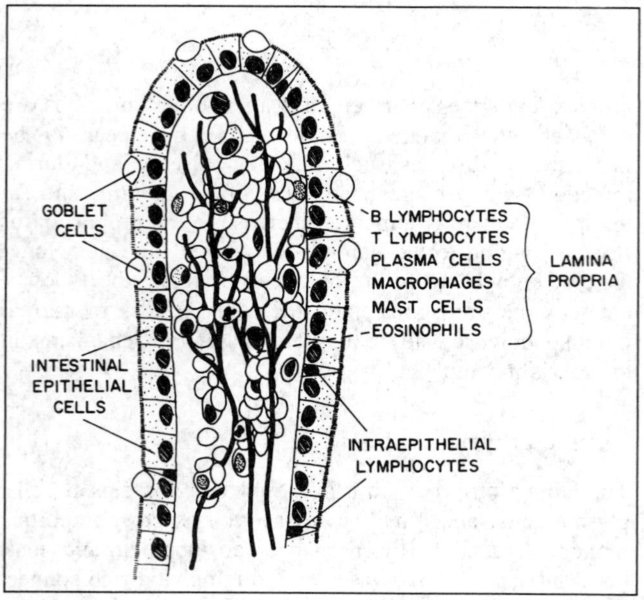

Fig. 29-3. Schematic representation of an intestinal villus demonstrating intraepithelial lymphocytes situated near the basement membrane between intestinal epithelial cells. The lamina propria within villi is rich in vasculature and lymphatics, and contains B lymphocytes, T lymphocytes, and plasma cells as well as macrophages, mast cells, and eosinophils. Intraepithelial T lymphocytes have predominantly the CD8 phenotype, whereas in the lamina propria CD4 T lymphocytes are more abundant than CD8 T lymphocytes. (From Kagnoff MF: Physiology of the gastrointestinal tract. New York, 1987, Raven Press.)

One additional point regarding the relationship between the intestinal lymphoid compartments warrants mention. A large proportion of Peyer's patch B cells is committed to the ultimate expression of the IgA immunoglobulin class. Thus, B cells that migrate out of Peyer's patches and lodge in the intestinal lamina propria and in other secretory sites (e.g., lungs, mammary gland) produce IgA in those sites after activation. This explains the predominance of IgA-producing cells in the intestinal lamina propria and at other secretory sites. Lymphocyte migration from the gut to the female breast explains why IgA antibodies in colostrum and milk can be directed against antigens encountered in the intestinal tract. As an example, breast feeding is known to protect the newborn against infection with enteric pathogens.

SECRETORY IGA

Structure

IgA secreted by the plasma cells in the intestinal lamina propria comprises the major immunoglobulin class in intestinal secretions. The adult human small intestine has as many as 10^{10} IgA-producing cells per meter and secretes more than 3 g of IgA per day into intestinal secretions. IgA in intestinal secretions differs from serum IgA in several important respects and is termed *secretory IgA (sIgA)*. Unlike monomer IgA, which has two heavy and two light chains and is produced largely in the bone marrow and other nonmucosal sites, IgA secreted into the intestinal juice is dimeric (four heavy and four light chains). In addition, sIgA has two extra polypeptide chains termed *secretory component* and *J chain* (Fig. 29-4).

Secretory component, also known as the *polyimmunoglobulin receptor*, is a transmembrane glycoprotein that is found on the basal and lateral surfaces of intestinal epithelial cells. This molecule functions as a receptor for the uptake and transport of dimeric IgA and other polymeric immunoglobulins (i.e., IgM) across the intestinal epithelial cell and into the intestinal secretions. During the transport process, secretory component binds covalently to IgA. Once in the intestinal lumen, the association between secretory component and IgA appears to stabilize the IgA molecule, making it less susceptible to proteolytic digestion (Fig. 29-5).

The J chain protein is produced by plasma cells in the lamina propria and is a component of all polymeric immunoglobulin (both IgA and IgM). This protein appears to be important in the process of immunoglobulin polymerization. Thus, IgA in intestinal secretions is a product of two different cell types, the plasma cell (IgA and J chain) and the intestinal epithelial cell (secretory component).

Function

The biologic functions of sIgA reflect its ability to bind antigen in the intestine. By binding to gut bacteria, sIgA can prevent bacterial attachment and penetration of intestinal epithelial cells. IgA also can bind to viruses and prevent viral colonization, and IgA can bind to macromolecules from food substances and prevent their passage across the intestinal mucosa.

Different immunoglobulin classes differ structurally and mediate different effector functions. IgA is not efficient at activating cell-damaging lytic mechanisms (e.g., complement activation) and in general does not participate in inflammatory reactions. However, the intestinal mucosa is exposed to a wide variety of antigenic materials that may enter the lamina propria of the normal or damaged intestine. Therefore, it is important not to produce in the gut significant amounts of immunoglobulin isotypes like IgG, which can participate in tissue-damaging immune reactions. Consistent with this, normally the intestinal tract contains few IgG-producing cells. However, in inflammatory bowel disease and celiac disease, IgG-producing cells are significantly increased in the intestinal mucosa and appear to play an important role in intestinal inflammation. Of note, there are increased numbers of IgE-producing cells in the normal intestinal tract relative to other sites. Although the function of those cells is not clear, IgE in the gut is known to be involved in host interactions with parasites and in intestinal allergic reactions. Further, IgE, acting through the release of mast cell mediators, may play a role in some diarrheal disorders by increasing intestinal fluid and electrolyte secretion.

IgA deficiency

(See also Chapter 42.) Humans have two subclasses of IgA: IgA1 and IgA2. Selective IgA deficiency is the most commonly recognized immunodeficiency (occurring in 1 in 500 to 1 in 700 of the population) and is usually associated with decreased levels of both IgA1 and IgA2. In addition, IgA deficiency may be accompanied by low levels of IgG2 and IgG4, is a frequent component of common variable immunodeficiency syndromes, and can be found together with abnormal cell-mediated immunity and/or IgE deficiency in diseases such as ataxia telangiectasia (Chapter 297). IgA1 and IgA2 are coded for by separate genes on chromosome 14. Rare individuals having selective IgA2 deficiency caused by a deletion of the IgA2 gene have been described.

In patients with celiac disease there is approximately a 10-fold increase in selective IgA deficiency over the numbers expected among the general population. Further, individuals with selective IgA deficiency have an increased prevalence of (1) autoimmune and connective tissue disease, (2) autoantibodies in the absence of overt autoimmune disease, (3) allergic disorders, and (4) malignancy. Such individuals frequently have circulating antibodies to food proteins and circulating immune complexes. This circumstance supports the notion that intestinal IgA plays a phys-

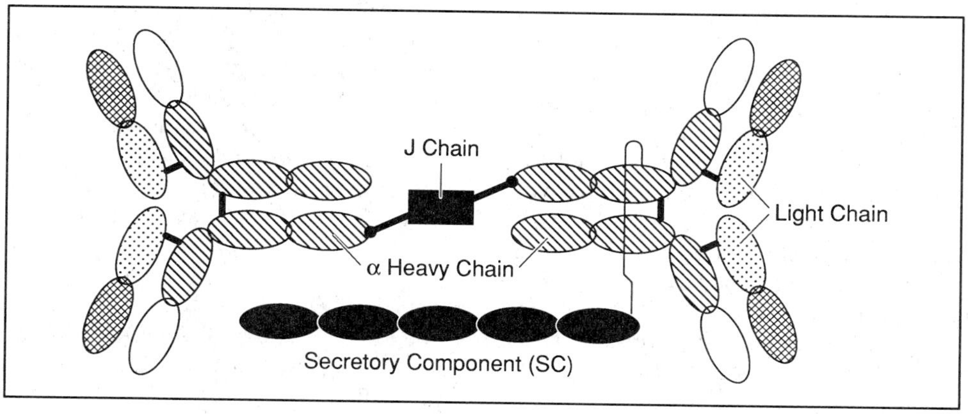

Fig. 29-4. Schematic representation of a secretory IgA molecule. Secretory IgA is a dimer that contains two monomer IgA subunits (each monomer subunit has two alpha heavy chains and two light chains) as well as two extra polypeptide chains, secretory component, and J chain. (From Kagnoff MF: Gastrointestinal disease, ed 5. Philadelphia, 1992, WB Saunders.)

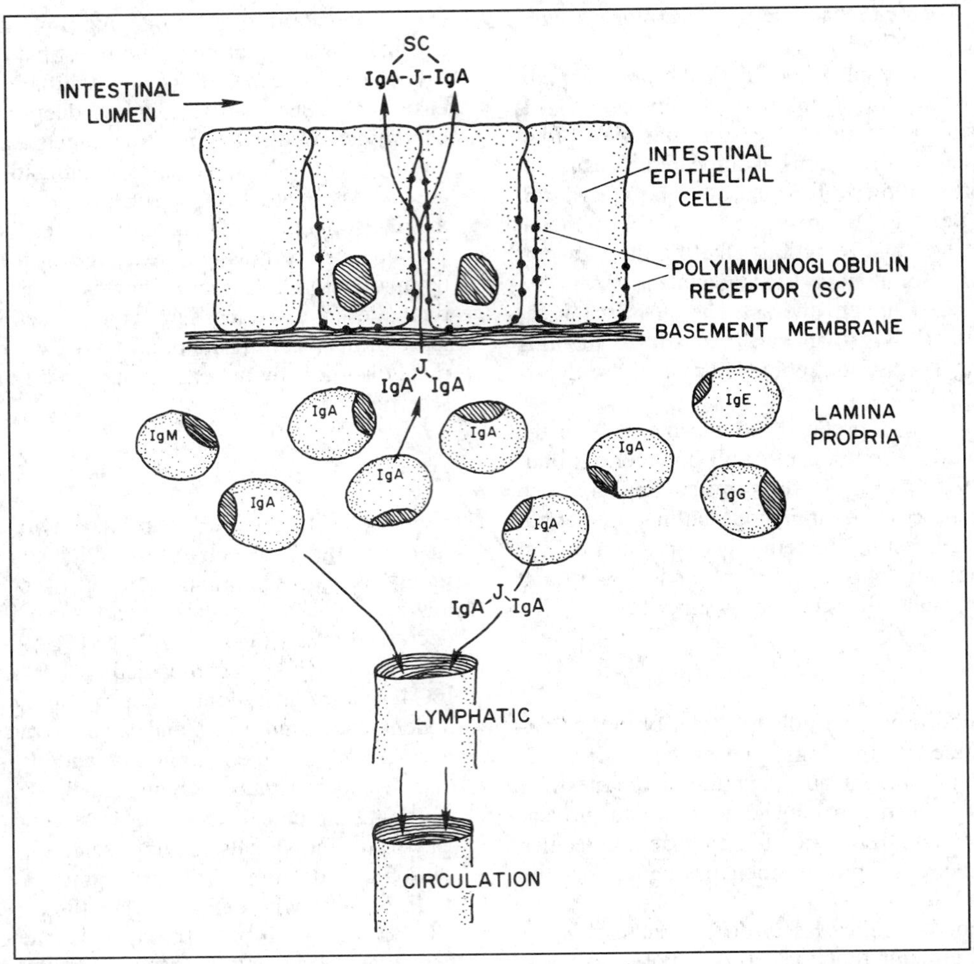

Fig. 29-5. Transport of IgA into intestinal secretions. Dimer IgA containing J chain is secreted by plasma cells in the lamina propria. This molecule couples with the polyimmunoglobulin receptor (also known as SC) on the basal and lateral surfaces of the intestinal epithelial cell. The IgA-SC complex is encytosed and transported through the intestinal epithelial cell and secreted into the intestinal lumen as sigA (dimer IgA plus J chain and SC). IgA produced in the lamina propria also can enter the draining lymphatics and circulation, and IgA producing cells can disseminate to extraintestinal secretory sites. IgA, immunoglobulin A. (From Kagnoff MF: Gastrointestinal disease, ed 5. Philadelphia, 1992, WB Saunders.)

iologic role in limiting the absorption of antigenic material from the gut.

Gastrointestinal manifestations vary among the different immunodeficiency syndromes. Gastrointestinal infections are not characteristic of selective IgA deficiency, a disorder in which increased numbers of IgM-producing cells often compensate for the IgA deficiency. When these individuals develop infections, they tend to be sinopulmonary. In contrast, gastrointestinal manifestations are frequent in the common variable immunodeficiency syndromes. This group of disorders is characterized by a low level of IgG together with diminished IgM and/or IgA levels. Diarrhea occurs in as many as 60% of these individuals, and 20% to 30% have mild to moderate malabsorption, often associated with infection with the protozoan parasite *Giardia lamblia* (Chapter 40). Common variable immunodeficiency syndromes may be accompanied by nodular lymphoid hyperplasia of the small intestine and occasionally of the stomach, colon, and rectum as well as by abnormalities in intestinal villous architecture. T cells also are important in host mucosal immunity. For example, persistent gastrointestinal infections with protozoal parasites such as *Cryptosporidium* or *Isospora belli* are seen with systemic and mucosal T cell deficiencies like those that occur in the acquired immunodeficiency syndrome (see Chapter 48).

Food allergy

Food allergy is a pathologic reaction that results from an immunologic response to ingested food antigens. As such, food allergy must be clearly differentiated from a broad spectrum of food intolerances. The latter represent adverse reactions to foods that are nonimmunologically mediated (e.g., reactions to toxins or pharmacologic mediators in foods, lactose intolerance). The diagnosis of food allergy frequently rests on the demonstration that clinical symptoms disappear when an offending food protein is eliminated from the diet and appear after ingestion of the food, ideally tested in a double-blind fashion. Unfortunately, tests commonly used to diagnose food allergy such as skin tests and radioallergosorbent (RAST) tests do not always correlate with clinical disease.

Immune reactions to foods such as milk and soy are relatively common in infancy and early childhood. However, food allergies also occur in adults and may result in a combination of gastrointestinal, respiratory, and cutaneous complaints. Colitis-like symptoms, protein-losing enteropathies, malabsorption syndromes, skin reactions such as urticaria and eczema, respiratory symptoms such as asthma and rhinitis, and acute anaphylactic reactions have all been attributed to food allergies. Allergy to cow's milk is the best studied example of food protein allergy. Other food substances frequently associated with allergy include eggs, chicken, fish, shellfish, nuts, and wheat products. Allergic reactions are caused by an IgE-mediated mechanism wherein mast cells coated with IgE degranulate and release biologically active mediators that act on local tissues to produce vasodilation, contraction of smooth muscle, and, at mucosal surfaces, secretion of mucus. Little is known about immune reactions to food proteins that are mediated by immunoglobulin classes other than IgE or by cell-mediated immune mechanisms.

ENTERIC IMMUNIZATION

The nature of the immune response evoked after immunization by the intestinal route depends on several factors. These include the type and dose of the immunizing antigen, the age of the immunized host, and whether or not the host has previously been exposed to the antigen used for intestinal immunization.

Immunization with replicating viruses (e.g., polio virus) or with bacteria that can invade the intestinal mucosa (e.g., *Shigella*) stimulates an IgA antibody response that mediates local protective immunity in the gut. The antibody response tends to be restricted to the region of the intestine that was exposed to the immunizing antigen rather than being generalized throughout the entire intestinal tract. Intestinal exposure to invasive bacteria and viruses also can stimulate a systemic antibody response.

Intestinal exposure to soluble proteins, nonviable particulate antigens, and nonreplicating viruses that are transported into Peyer's patches also may activate a local intestinal IgA response. However, in addition, those antigens may activate immune suppressor mechanisms that can markedly diminish the magnitude of the host's systemic immune response to the same antigen. This latter phenomenon is termed *oral tolerance*. This dual process that includes induction of intestinal immunity and concurrent systemic hyporesponsiveness to the same antigen may have an important physiologic role. Thus, secretory IgA in the intestine would decrease the absorption of the antigenic material from the gut. The concurrent suppression of the systemic immune response to the same antigen would prevent the development of an undesirable systemic immune reaction to an otherwise harmless antigenic material that may cross the intestinal mucosa.

REFERENCES

Branski D, Rozen P, and Kagnoff MF, editors: Gluten-sensitive enteropathy. In Frontiers of gastrointestinal research, vol 19. Basel, 1992, S. Karger.

Hanson LA and Svanborg Eden C, editors: Mucosal immunobiology: cellular-molecular interactions in the mucosal immune system. In Monographs in allergy. Basel, 1988, S. Karger.

Kagnoff MF, editor: Gut and intestinal immunology. Immunol Allerg Clin North Am 8 (3):1988.

Kagnoff MF: Celiac disease. In Yamada T, editor: Textbook of gastroenterology. Philadelphia, 1991, JB Lippincott.

Kagnoff MF: Immunology and inflammation of the gastrointestinal tract. In Fordtran et al, editors: Gastrointestinal disease, ed 5. Philadelphia, 1993, WB Saunders.

MacDermott RP and Elson CO, editors: Mucosal immunology. I. Basic principles. In Gastroenterology clinics of North America. Philadelphia, 1991, WB Saunders.

Strober W et al, editors: Mucosal immunity and infections at mucosal surfaces. New York, 1988, Oxford University Press.

Targan SR and Shanahan F, editors: Immunology and immunopathology of the liver and gastrointestinal tract. New York, 1990, Igaku-Shoin Medical.

DIAGNOSTIC PROCEDURES AND TESTS II

CHAPTER

30 Gastrointestinal Endoscopy

John F. Morrissey
Mark Reichelderfer

Gastrointestinal endoscopy is an area of medicine that has seen many important technologic developments in recent years beginning with the introduction of fiberscopes in the early 1960s. Fiberscopes that use bundles of very small (± 10 μ) glass fibers to transmit light to and carry images back from the gastrointestinal tract remain in widespread use at this time. They are being replaced in most institutions by videoendoscopes, which differ from fiberscopes in that the image is transmitted electronically from a tiny computer chip at the end of the instrument through a processing unit to a television screen. The resolution obtained is superior to that achieved with a fiberscope because a computer chip may have up to 100,000 light-sensitive points called pixels on which the image is focused. Both types of instruments have controls that move the tip and open channels for insufflation of air and water, suction, and insertion of a variety of accessory instruments such as polypectomy snares and biopsy forceps.

UPPER GASTROINTESTINAL ENDOSCOPY

Most endoscopists sedate patients for procedures and apply a local anesthetic to the pharynx. Survey examinations can be completed in 5 to 10 minutes. The risk of upper endoscopy to a patient in good general health is negligible. Most complications occur in patients with serious underlying cardiac or respiratory disease. Complications may be estimated at a morbidity of 0.13% and mortality of 0.004%.

Indications

Endoscopy in recent years has replaced the barium meal radiograph as the initial procedure for the evaluation of most patients with symptoms referable to the upper gastrointestinal tract when visualization of the small intestine is not considered essential (refer to the box below).

Dyspepsia and heartburn. Most physicians reserve endoscopy for dyspeptic patients who fail to respond to a 2 to 6 week trial of medical therapy. Mild symptoms of reflux esophagitis may never require endoscopic evaluation. The indications for endoscopy are stronger in older patients in whom malignancy is a greater risk.

Dysphagia and odynophagia. The symptoms of dysphagia and odynophagia mandate endoscopy in most patients. The procedure may lead to specific medical therapies through the diagnosis of reflux (Plate II-1) or candidal or herpetic esophagitis. It may result in specific invasive therapy of lesions such as lower esophageal rings (Plate II-2), peptic strictures, or achalasia (Chapter 35). If a stricture is found, malignancy must be excluded (see later discussion).

Bleeding. Endoscopy should be performed soon after admission in patients suffering major bleeding from the upper gastrointestinal tract (see also Chapter 34). The site of bleeding can be accurately localized in more than 90% of patients. Most endoscopists utilize one or more therapeutic techniques to attempt to stop bleeding and to prevent recurrent bleeding. Current techniques include bipolar electrocoagulation, Nd-YAG laser, heater probe, and injection of vasoconstricting or sclerosing drugs. Injection sclerotherapy or endoscopic application of rubber bands is used to control bleeding from esophageal varices (Chapter 34; Plate II-3).

Mass lesions. Patients with tumor masses, even those shown to be obviously malignant on radiographic examination, merit upper endoscopy (Plate II-4). Approximately 8% of malignant tumors of the stomach prove to be lymphomas. Patients with lymphomas require additional preoperative studies such as bone marrow aspiration and computed tomography. If disseminated disease is found, a combination of radiographic therapy and chemotherapy may be preferable to surgery. It is possible with biopsy and brush cytology to obtain a correct histologic diagnosis in more than 80% of patients with gastric tumors. As a general principle, surgery should not be performed for disease of the upper gastrointestinal tract without prior endoscopic examination.

Abnormal fold pattern. One of the indications for upper gastrointestinal examination is the radiographic finding of a very prominent rugal pattern in the stomach. Endoscopists frequently find that they can distend such a stomach with air, obliterating the abnormal fold pattern and revealing a normal stomach. In some cases large folds are nondistensible as a result of disease such as infiltrating carcinoma, lymphoma, or giant hypertrophy of the gastric mucosa. Differential diagnosis from the visual appearance alone can be difficult and it is often necessary to perform a deep biopsy of the mucosa using a small electrosurgical snare to sample the submucosa to identify the nature of the infiltrating process. On occasion, full-thickness surgical biopsy is needed to exclude malignant disease.

Ulcer craters and ulcer scars. Ulcerating lesions of the esophagus or stomach carry a significant risk of malig-

Indications for upper endoscopy

I. Primary endoscopy (no prior radiography)
  A. Dyspepsia
    1. Pain } unresponsive to a trial of therapy
    2. Heartburn }
  B. Persistent nausea or vomiting
  C. Dysphagia or odynophagia
  D. Hematemesis or melena
  E. Early satiety
  F. Noncardiac chest pain
  G. Iron-deficiency anemia—negative colon findings
  H. Caustic ingestion
  I. Chronic malabsorption and diarrhea—small bowel biopsy
II. Abnormal or equivocal radiographic findings
  A. Mass lesion
  B. Abnormal fold pattern
  C. Crater
  D. Stricture
  E. Deformity or scar
III. Surveys for malignancy
  A. Barrett's esophagus
  B. Familial polyposis or Gardner's syndrome
  C. History of adenomatous gastric polyp
IV. Therapeutic endoscopy
  A. Control of bleeding
  B. Sclerosis of esophageal varices
  C. Dilation of strictures and stomas
  D. Percutaneous gastrostomy
  E. Stenting esophageal tumors
  F. Laser obliteration of tumors
  G. Removal of foreign bodies
  H. Insertion of feeding tubes into duodenum
  I. Polypectomy

nancy. Endoscopy is indicated for most of these ulcers with the exception of small ulcers in young patients that appear benign on radiographic examination. Duodenal ulcers are almost never malignant, so endoscopic evaluation is not needed. A combination of visual and cytologic diagnosis with biopsy correctly identifies 80% to 90% of malignant ulcers. Symptomatic patients with a radiographic diagnosis of a persistent ulcer scar often merit endoscopic evaluation (Plates II-5 and II-6).

Esophageal strictures. Endoscopy is essential for diagnosing and treating esophageal strictures. Endoscopic biopsy and brush cytology are quite accurate in distinguishing between benign and malignant disease, provided the full length of the stricture is evaluated. Endoscopy assists the passage of dilators and guide wires through tightly strictured areas. Malignant strictures can be treated by endoscopic placement of a plastic stent to keep the esophageal lumen open. Nd-YAG lasers and BICAP tumor probes can be used to coagulate tumors that cannot be treated by other means, providing temporary palliation of esophageal obstruction.

Foreign bodies. Endoscopy is employed to remove foreign bodies that lodge in the esophagus and large or sharp foreign bodies that enter the stomach. A variety of grasping devices can be passed through the biopsy channel of the fiberscope to remove the foreign body. At times, the endoscope may be passed through an overtube to protect the airway and to remove sharp or multiple foreign bodies from the stomach more safely.

Percutaneous gastrostomy. It is possible to insert a plastic tube through the abdominal wall into the stomach under endoscopic guidance for feeding purposes. Such procedures are performed in patients with chronic conditions that prevent them from swallowing a normal diet. This simple endoscopic procedure has greatly reduced the need for the surgical performance of gastrostomy.

Surveys for cancer. Patients with long-standing reflux esophagitis in whom a significant portion of the lining of the esophagus has been replaced with metaplastic columnar epithelium (Barrett's epithelium) are at risk for the development of malignancy, and survey examinations at regular intervals are recommended by many. Multiple biopsy specimens are taken to look for intramucosal cancer and/or dysplasia. Gastric, esophageal, and duodenal cancer are so rare in the United States that surveys of other patient populations, with very few exceptions (such as selected familial polyposis syndromes), are not justified.

Chronic diarrhea and malabsorption. A small intestinal biopsy can be obtained endoscopically in patients with chronic diarrhea and malabsorption in whom mucosal disease of the proximal intestine is suspected. Such biopsies can also be obtained using suction biopsy tubes, which do not require endoscopy (Chapter 33).

ENDOSCOPIC ULTRASONOGRAPHY

Ultrasound has been used to examine the abdomen for many years with transducers applied to the skin. It is now possible to improve the accuracy of ultrasonic diagnosis by using an endoscope to move a transducer closer to the area of interest. Two systems are in use. The endoscope mounted system uses a dedicated fiberscope fitted with a rotating mechanical sector scanner at its tip. Contact with the mucosa is ensured by filling the stomach with water or using a water filled balloon attached to the endoscope. The second system uses a thin ultrasonic probe that is passed through the biopsy channel of a standard endoscope. The procedure is most useful for evaluating submucosal lesions, for determining the extent of invasion by tumors, and for imaging adjacent organs such as the pancreas or bile ducts.

ENDOSCOPIC RETROGRADE PANCREATOGRAPHY

Endoscopic retrograde cholangiopancreatography (ERCP) was developed in Japan in the late 1960s. The procedure is performed with a long, small-diameter, side-viewing fiberscope. The instrument is positioned in the second portion of the duodenum opposite the papilla of Vater, and a small 1.5 mm catheter is passed through the fiberscope and selectively into the common bile or main pancreatic duct. Contrast material is injected so that the duct systems of each organ can be seen. The procedure is technically quite difficult to perform. Only skilled endoscopists can achieve a cannulation success rate of 90% or better, and many do not fill the desired duct more than 80% of the time. Complications such as cholangitis and pancreatitis occur in 3% of examinations, and death in 0.2%.

Indications

Indications for ERCP are summarized in the box on p. 364.

Jaundice. It is essential to visualize the extrahepatic biliary system in all patients with jaundice except those with unequivocal hepatocellular disease (see Chapter 53). Visualization can be done either by ERCP or by percutaneous transhepatic cholangiography (PTC). ERCP is the most successful technique when there is a reasonable likelihood that a therapeutic endoscopic procedure may be needed. It is possible to open the end of the bile duct with electrosurgical current (papillotomy) to permit removal of bile duct stones, to bypass tumors of the papilla, and to relieve stenosis of the papilla. It is also possible to insert stents or balloon catheters to bypass obstructing lesions or to dilate strictured areas (Plate II-7). Procedures can be accomplished with a mortality that is less than that of comparable surgical procedures, while preventing the additional morbidity and cost of the surgical procedure.

Pancreatic disease. Endoscopic retrograde pancreatography can be used in conjunction with abdominal ultrasound and computed tomographic (CT) scanning to determine

Indications of endoscopic retrograde cholangiopancreatography

I. Jaundice; extrahepatic obstruction suspected
   A. Papillotomy available
      1. Past history of cholecystectomy
      2. Elderly, poor-risk patient
   B. Papillotomy not available or contraindicated (e.g., patient with hemorrhagic diathesis)
      1. CT or ultrasonic scan shows dilated ducts; PTC unsuccessful, incomplete, or contraindicated
      2. CT or ultrasonic scan shows normal-sized ducts
II. Pain, chronic or recurrent, suggestive of biliary or pancreatic origin
   A. Abnormal liver function studies
   B. Status after cholecystectomy
   C. History of documented pancreatitis
   D. History of lipase or amylase elevation
   E. Abnormal CT or ultrasonic scan
   F. Abnormal upper gastrointestinal x-rays
III. Ascites; elevation of amylase in the ascitic fluid

CT, computed tomography; PTC, percutaneous transhepatic cholangiography.

whether or not pancreatic disease is present (Chapter 54). This combined procedure shows abnormalities in 90% of patients with pancreatic cancer and in approximately 65% to 80% of patients with chronic pancreatitis. It is also possible to differentiate changes caused by pancreatitis from those caused by cancer in approximately 90% of patients. In patients with known chronic pancreatitis, the procedure is used to plan surgical therapy. Although it may be possible to fill a pseudocyst of the pancreas during endoscopic retrograde pancreatography, ultrasound is a much better and safer way of diagnosing and following such lesions.

The diagnostic yield of ERCP is very low in patients with abdominal pain and without other clinical evidence to suggest disease of the bile ducts or pancreas. The procedure is contraindicated in patients with recent acute pancreatitis unless a papillotomy with removal of an impacted common duct stone is planned. The major risk in endoscopic retrograde pancreatography is a flare of pancreatitis. If a pseudocyst is filled, bacteria may be introduced with the production of a pancreatic abscess. Endoscopic retrograde cholangiography, especially if duct obstruction is present, can be complicated by cholangitis. Sepsis is a much less frequent occurrence now that antibiotic prophylaxis is routinely used.

COLONOSCOPY

It is possible to examine the entire colon and the terminal ileum with long (130 to 180 cm) endoscopes very similar in appearance to those used for examining the upper gastrointestinal tract, but with enough flexibility and torque stability to facilitate passage of the instrument through the colon (Plates II-8 to II-10). Colonoscopy is a difficult technique that requires extensive experience for proficiency. A competent colonoscopist should be able to pass the instrument to the cecum in more than 90% of examinations in 15 to 45 minutes.

Although colonoscopy is more accurate than barium enema radiographic studies, detecting 90% to 95% of lesions 10 mm or larger (compared with the 80% to 85% detected by double-contrast-barium-enema examination), there are blind spots, especially at the flexures, that prevent complete visualization of the colon by the colonoscopist. Hence, if a colonic lesion is suspected but not found at colonoscopy, a barium enema should also be done.

Patients are prepared for colonoscopy either by 1 or 2 days of liquid diet, laxatives, and enemas or by lavage with an isotonic electrolyte solution (Golytely). Premedication is usually intramuscular meperidine and intravenous midazolam. The availability of fluoroscopy is occasionally an aid in passing a colonoscope, but it is not essential to the performance of the procedure. Colonoscopy is more hazardous than upper gastrointestinal endoscopy. The major hazards are perforation, hemorrhage, and cardiorespiratory complications. The overall complication rate is 0.43%, with a mortality of 0.02%.

Indications

Indications for colonoscopy are summarized in the box at upper right.

Polyps. A major use of colonoscopy is to diagnose and treat colonic polyps. Patients are usually referred for colonoscopy because a polyp is found on barium-enema radiography or proctoscopic examination. Most endoscopists believe that if a polyp is found in the distal colon by proctoscopy or flexible sigmoidoscopy, the patient should have an examination of the entire colon because of the frequency with which additional polyps are found in the proximal bowel of such patients. Polyps are removed either by a wire-loop electrosurgical snare or by "hot" biopsy forceps. After removal of colonic polyps, patients should be examined at regular intervals so that new polyps can be detected and removed as they appear (see Chapter 45 and Plate II-8).

Carcinoma. Patients who have radiographic evidence of carcinoma of the right colon or nonobstructing carcinomas of the left colon are usually referred for colonoscopy preoperatively because of the frequency with which synchronous carcinomas and synchronous polyps are detected by the colonoscopic procedure. Lesions that cannot be removed endoscopically can be removed at the time of the surgical procedure, saving the patient from the necessity of undergoing a second laparotomy. Many endoscopists follow up on patients after resection of colonic carcinomas by colonoscopy 1 year later and then at 2 to 3 year intervals to remove polyps, look for suture line recurrences, and detect metachronous carcinomas. Patients who have had one colonic carcinoma removed have a severalfold increase in risk of developing a second malignancy in the organ (Plate II-9).

Indications for colonoscopy

I. Abnormal radiographic and/or sigmoidoscopic findings
  A. Mass lesion
    1. ? Polyp
    2. ? Cancer
    3. ? Ischemia
  B. Stricture
    1. ? Cancer
    2. ? Inflammatory bowel disease
  C. Ulcerations
    1. ? Inflammatory bowel disease
  D. Diverticular disease
    1. ? Cancer or polyp
    2. ? Severity and activity
II. Radiographic result normal or not determined; sigmoidoscopic result normal
  A. Chronic diarrhea
    1. ? Inflammatory bowel disease
  B. Bleeding or iron deficiency anemia
    1. ? Cancer or polyp
    2. ? Angiodysplasia
III. Inflammatory bowel disease
  A. ? Diagnosis correct
  B. ? Activity, severity, and extent
IV. Acute massive bleeding, sigmoidoscopy result negative
V. Surveys for cancer
  A. Status postcolonic polypectomy
  B. Status postresection colon cancer
  C. Ulcerative colitis greater than 8 years' duration

Inflammatory bowel disease. Colonoscopy is very helpful in the evaluation of patients with inflammatory bowel disease (see Chapter 43). Determination of the severity and extent of inflammatory bowel disease is more accurate by colonoscopy than by radiographic examination. Patients suspected of having either ulcerative colitis or Crohn's disease and who have had negative radiographic and proctosigmoidoscopic examination results sometimes may have the diagnosis established by colonoscopy. Crohn's disease may present with multiple superficial ulcerations of the proximal colon, and rare patients with ulcerative colitis may not have rectal involvement. Colonoscopy is often helpful in planning surgical therapy in patients with Crohn's disease. Patients with ulcerative colitis of 8 to 10 years' or longer duration often are screened by colonoscopy at 1 to 3 year intervals to look for dysplastic or malignant changes. Colonoscopy is contraindicated in acute or very active ulcerative colitis (Plate II-10).

Other indications. Diverticulosis is a very common finding in older patients. When the disease process is severe, diagnosis by radiography of polyp or cancer within the involved segment of bowel is very difficult. Such lesions are much more easily recognized during colonoscopic examination. Acute diverticulitis is a contraindication for colonoscopy, but the procedure can be helpful in chronic cases.

Colonoscopy is difficult in the presence of massive bleeding. A 2 to 4 hour lavage with Golytely solution facilitates the examination. If is often preferable to localize the bleeding site first with an isotope scan. Both diagnostic and therapeutic colonoscopy are more likely to be successful if the site of bleeding is known (see Chapter 34).

A common clinical problem is diagnosis in the patient with symptoms and an indeterminate or somewhat unsatisfactory barium-enema examination. This situation frequently occurs in elderly patients, who can be quite difficult to prepare for barium-enema examination. Under these circumstances, it is often preferable to have a colonoscopy rather than to make repeated attempts to perform a radiographic study.

The isolated finding of abdominal pain is not a good reason to perform colonoscopy. A lesion large enough to produce pain usually does so by partially obstructing the colon. Such lesions are almost always detected by radiographic examination. Most patients with colonic pain and a negative radiographic examination result suffer from spasm secondary to an irritable colon. Colonoscopy is not needed to confirm this diagnosis.

PROCTOSIGMOIDOSCOPY

Proctosigmoidoscopy is by far the most commonly performed endoscopic examination of the gastrointestinal tract. Examination is performed with a rigid hollow tube measuring slightly less than 2 cm in diameter and made from metal or plastic. A smooth-tipped obturator is placed in the instrument to facilitate its passage into the rectum. The open lumen permits easy passage of forceps and snares. Patients with acute diarrhea or bright red rectal bleeding are examined without preparation. Other patients are prepared with a phosphosoda enema. The procedure is performed with the patient in the knee-chest or left lateral Sims's position. Examinations are facilitated if a special proctoscopic table that elevates the hips and places the patient in a head-down position is used.

Proctosigmoidoscopy is a valuable screening procedure because approximately 30% of carcinomas are located in the distal 25 cm of the bowel. Patients with multiple colonic polyps frequently have one within this area. The source of bright red rectal bleeding is within the anal canal in 90% of patients. The procedure is very helpful in the diagnosis of diarrheal diseases such as ulcerative colitis, acute amebiasis, and antibiotic colitis.

Proctosigmoidoscopy is an easy technique to learn. Most specialists in general surgery and general internal medicine and many family physicians perform the procedure routinely.

FLEXIBLE SIGMOIDOSCOPY

Most gastroenterologists and some primary care physicians prefer to examine the distal bowel with a shortened 30 or 60 cm fiberoptic or video colonoscope. The phosphosoda enema preparation given for rigid sigmoidoscopy has been found to clean the entire left side of the colon quite well, permitting its examination by the short fiberscope. Patient tolerance for the flexible instrument is similar to that for the rigid instrument, and examinations can be performed without premedication in nearly all patients. The new procedure adds 5 minutes to the examination time, but the yield in endoscopic abnormality findings is two to three times that of examination with the rigid instrument. With the longer flexible instrument, which most physicians prefer, the entire sigmoid can regularly be seen and usually the descending colon as well. The sigmoid is a difficult area to examine by barium enema because of the overlapping loops of bowel. Flexible sigmoidoscopy provides a good view of that portion of the sigmoid commonly involved by diverticulosis, and the endoscopist can easily differentiate inflammatory from neoplastic masses within the involved segment. In skilled hands, the risk of the procedure probably is no greater than that for rigid sigmoidoscopy. Many primary care physicians are being trained to use the flexible instrument, which then replaces the rigid instrument for most indications.

LAPAROSCOPY (PLATES II-11 TO II-12)

Laparoscopy (periteonoscopy) visualizes the peritoneal cavity by means of a short rigid telescope that is passed through a previously passed trochar. Safe passage of the trochar is facilitated by prior distention of the abdominal cavity with either carbon dioxide or nitrous oxide passed through a special blunt tipped spring-loaded Verres needle. Both lobes of the liver, the spleen, the gallbladder, and the peritoneal surfaces can be seen. The procedure has been in widespread use in Europe and South America for many years. It came into use in the United States in the 1970s, primarily for biopsy under direct vision of focal lesions in the liver by gastroenterologists. It has been largely replaced for this indication by biopsy with either ultrasound or computed tomography guidance by radiologists.

Gynecologists have used laparoscopy for many years to visualize and treat pelvic disease. In the late 1980s laparoscopic cholecystectomy by general surgeons began to have widespread use. In this procedure, in addition to inserting the laparoscope, the physician makes several small incisions in the abdominal wall for insertion of instruments, viewing a television screen during the procedure. The major advantage of the laparoscopic procedure is greatly shortened recovery time.

Table 30-1. Contraindications for endoscopy

Condition	Upper Endoscopy	ERCP	Colonoscopy
Recent myocardial infarction	+	+	+
Unstable cardiac rhythm	+	+	+
Severe chronic obstructive pulmonary disease	+	+	+
Suspected bowel perforation	+	+	+
Uncooperative patient	+	+	+
Comatose patient (unless intubated)	+	+	+
Bleeding diathesis	+	+	+
Acute pancreatitis	0	+	0
Acute diverticulitis	0	0	+
Acute ulcerative colitis	0	0	+
Immunosuppression	+	+	+
Previous abdominal surgery	0	0	0

ERCP, endoscopic retrograde cholangiopancreatography; +, contraindication; 0, no contraindication.

CONTRAINDICATIONS FOR ENDOSCOPIC PROCEDURES

Contraindications (most of which are relative, not absolute) for the major endoscopic procedures are summarized in Table 30-1.

REFERENCES

Blackstone MO: Endoscopic interpretation. New York, 1984, Raven Press.
Cotton PB and Williams CB: Practical gastrointestinal endoscopy, ed 3. Oxford, 1990, Blackwell.
Hunt RH and Waye JD: Colonoscopy. Chicago, 1981, Year Book.
Katon RM et al: Flexible sigmoidoscopy. Orlando, 1985, Grune & Stratton.
Morrissey JF and Reichelderfer M: Gastrointestinal endoscopy. N Engl J Med 325:1142, 1214, 1991.
Salem JH: Laparoscopy. Philadelphia, 1988, WB Saunders.
Schapiro M and Lehman GA: Flexible sigmoidoscopy. Baltimore, 1990, Williams & Wilkins.
Schiller KRF et al: A color atlas of gastrointestinal endoscopy. Philadelphia, 1987, WB Saunders.
Siegel JH: Endoscopic retrograde cholangio-pancreatography. New York, 1992, Raven Press.
Silverstein FE and Tytgat NJ: Atlas of gastrointestinal endoscopy. Philadelphia, 1987, WB Saunders.
Silvis S: Therapeutic endoscopy, ed 2. New York, 1990, Igaku-Shoin.
Sivak MV: Gastroenterologic endoscopy. Philadelphia, 1987, WB Saunders.
Waye JE et al: Techniques in therapeutic endoscopy. Philadelphia, 1987, WB Saunders.
Zucker KA, Bailey RW, and Reddick EJ: Surgical laparoscopy. St. Louis, 1991, Quality Medical.

CHAPTER

31 Evaluation of Esophageal Disease

Robert W. Summers
Konrad S. Schulze-Delrieu

ESOPHAGEAL SYMPTOMS

A careful consideration of symptoms can provide specific information about many functional and structural abnormalities of the esophagus. After a detailed history the physician can formulate the principal diagnostic possibilities and assess the need for specific diagnostic tests and treatments.

Dysphagia, odynophagia, and the globus sensation

Dysphagia is the sensation experienced when the passage of a bolus from the mouth to the stomach is slowed or arrested. Oropharyngeal dysphagia implies difficulty or inability in propelling a bolus from the mouth into the gullet; coughing, choking, or nasal regurgitation may result. Neuromuscular disorders of the pharynx frequently cause these problems and are often accompanied by nasal speech, dysphonia, or dysarthria. Esophageal dysphagia is the sensation provoked when a bolus sticks in the esophageal body. Symptoms may occur in the neck or the retrosternal region. Motility disorders of the esophagus usually interfere with the swallowing of both liquids and solids. Partial mechanical obstructions caused by mucosal webs, peptic strictures, and tumors primarily produce difficulty with the swallowing of solid boluses; patients adapt by changing to a soft diet and learn to wash foods down with liquids. Dysphagia that progresses over weeks or months from difficulties with solids to difficulties with liquids is typical of esophageal cancer. This sequence usually develops slowly over years with peptic stricturing.

The feeling of a lump in the throat that is not aggravated by swallowing is called the *globus sensation* or *pseudodysphagia*. There is no sense of difficulty in swallowing itself. A globus sensation in the absence of dysphagia or odynophagia is likely to relate to a process outside the oropharynx and esophagus (including choledocholithiasis, cardiovascular disease, emotional distress, and hysteria), although it may accompany gastroesophageal reflux disease.

When the mucosal lining of the esophagus is disrupted, swallowing may become painful. This symptom is known as *odynophagia*. If odynophagia occurs in an immunosuppressed patient, an opportunistic infection should be suspected. Infectious agents such as herpes simplex virus or candidiasis often produce soreness and pain in the mouth and hypopharynx. Odynophagia is atypical of gastroesophageal reflux unless a peptic ulcer of the esophagus has developed. Dysphagia and odynophagia are signs of serious esophageal disease, and their presence calls for detailed radiographic and endoscopic examination of the pharynx and esophagus (Fig. 31-1).

Regurgitation, aspiration, and waterbrash

Regurgitation is characterized by the unexpected, effortless appearance of gastrointestinal contents in the mouth, as both the upper and the lower esophageal sphincters fail. Regurgitation is often confused with vomiting; it differs from the latter in that it is not preceded by nausea. It does not involve forceful retching and is often postural. Regurgitation of undigested food indicates the accumulation of material in an area proximal to the stomach; this occurs with Zenker's diverticula and in achalasia of the esophagus. A sour taste implies mixing of the food with gastric acid; bitterness suggests mixing with bile from duodenal contents.

When patients have severe reflux, regurgitation of sour or bitter fluids occurs most frequently when they lie down or increase their abdominal pressure. Patients with easily

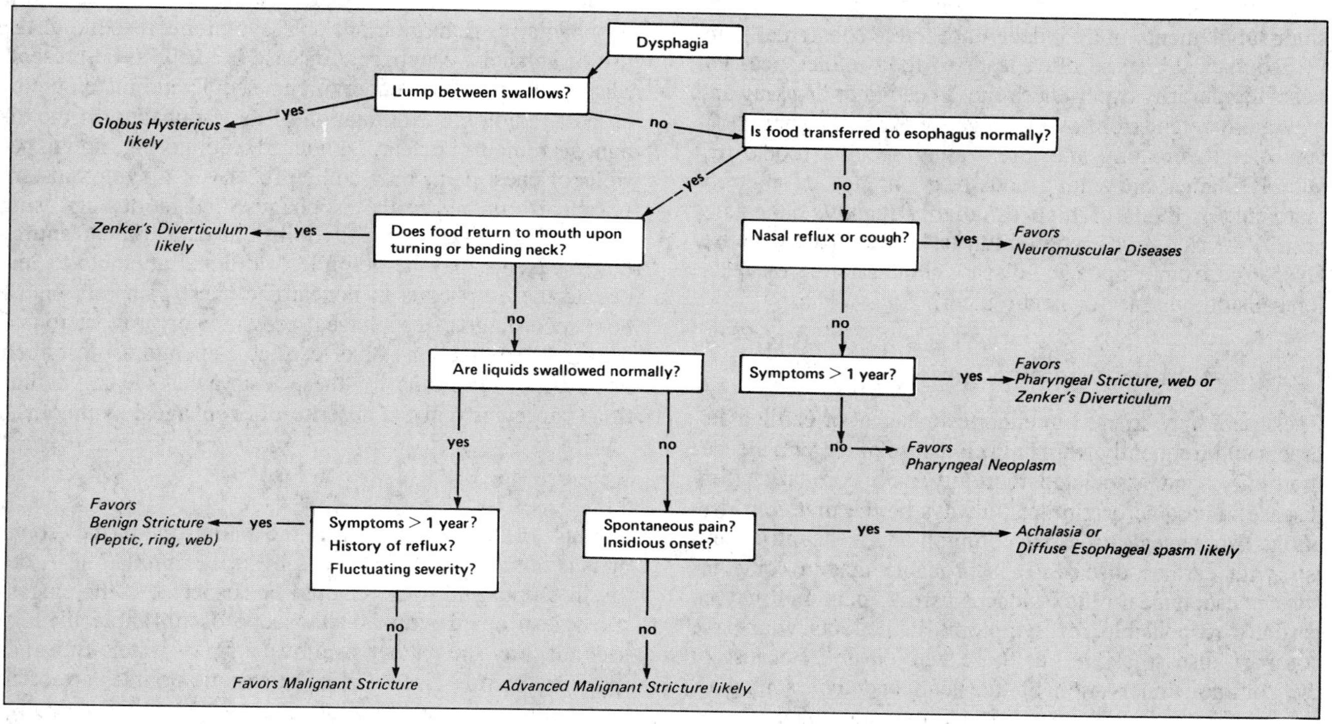

Fig. 31-1. An algorithm for the historical evaluation of dysphagia. (Modified from Edwards DAW: Scott Med J 15:378, 1970.)

provoked reflux and regurgitation are prone to severe esophagitis and should undergo diagnostic evaluation. These patients are at risk of nocturnal aspiration and should be specifically questioned about recurrent pneumonias, dyspnea, and cough during recumbency. Reflux may induce bronchospasm and asthma attacks through aspiration or reflex mechanisms. Hoarseness, otitis media, and dental injury are lesser known sequelae of reflux. Regurgitation that occurs only in the context of eructation after large meals is less serious and by itself is not an indication for full diagnostic testing. Coughing and choking with drinking of liquids but without dysphagia suggest the possibility of an esophageal-bronchial fistula.

Water brash is the outpouring of salivary secretions in response to gastroesophageal reflux as acidification of the esophagus stimulates oropharyngeal secretions through a vagally mediated reflex mechanism.

Heartburn and food intolerance

Heartburn (pyrosis) is the most common sensation experienced with gastroesophageal reflux. Depending on whether its burning or its pressure qualities predominate, patients describe it as "sour stomach" or "gas." Its character, intensity, and location vary: it may occur 1 or 2 hours after meals as a barely perceptible retrosternal warmth or burning sensation, gnawing, or pressure, or it may cause intense pain indistinguishable from myocardial ischemia (see later discussion). It characteristically increases with bending at the waist, lifting, or the supine position. Whereas mild heartburn is promptly relieved by antacids or other liquids, more intense episodes often respond poorly. Caustic substances, frequently pills such as tetracycline, quinidine, or potassium supplements, may induce unbearable substernal pain.

Esophageal disease often leads to food intolerance. Patients temporarily experience relief in eating or drinking and may gain weight from overindulgence. Later heartburn occurs after overeating and after eating specific foods; frequently blamed are acidic foods (e.g., orange or spicy tomato juice), foods of high osmolarity (candy, chocolate, pastry), or rich foods with a high fat content (fried foods). Dyspepsia from esophageal disease should not be mistaken for gallstone disease or peptic ulcer.

Chest pain of esophageal origin

Chest pain may arise from either esophageal or cardiac disorders and frequently from both. Because of the prevalence, morbidity, and associated mortality with coronary artery disease, a cardiac origin must always be the first consideration. Esophageal disease is common and frequently coexists with cardiac disease; it is probable that in some instances esophageal reflux induces cardiac pain and may be partially responsible for symptoms in patients who have coronary disease as well as those who do not. Because of the common innervation of the heart and the esophagus, over half of patients with substernal pain are unable to distinguish which is the origin of their symptoms. The description of esophageal pain is variable; squeezing, aching, and pressurelike discomfort often associated with anxiety are cited. Like cardiac pain (see Chapter 7), esophageal pain may radiate to the epigastrium, the neck, or the left arm; it may be exercise-induced; and it may respond to nitrates. A history of pyrosis, regurgitation, dysphagia, or relief with antacids may be a clue to an esophageal source. It is also important to remember that therapy with vasodilators (e.g., nitrates and calcium channel blockers) lowers sphincter pressure and aggravates reflux.

The mechanisms by which esophageal diseases cause chest pain are poorly understood but are often associated with mucosal injury and altered motility. Esophageal colic is a common manifestation of diffuse esophageal spasm and other motility disorders characterized by the excessive force of esophageal contractions (i.e., the hypertensive or "nutcracker" esophagus). Of hiatus hernias, only the rare paraesophageal type is currently accepted as a direct cause of esophageal pain. Esophageal stretch can also lead to spasm and chest pain: in bolus impaction the esophagus proximal to the obstruction dilates and contracts vigorously. The ingestion of ice cold liquids can also cause esophageal colic-like distress, but the esophagus is actually wide and flaccid in this situation. Esophageal pain may abate after the use of smooth muscle relaxants such as nitroglycerine. Not all noncardiac chest pain originates from the esophagus, and caution must be exercised in accepting minor changes in esophageal structure or function as causes of chest pain. Diseases of the mediastinum and chest wall and anxiety may all play a role.

If cardiac disease has been ruled out, a careful esophageal history is important to evaluate the cause of a patient's chest pain. If the symptoms are triggered by swallowing or by meals; if the patient experiences frequent heartburn, dysphagia, or regurgitation, or if symptoms respond to the use of antacids, esophageal disease is likely to be present. Such patients should undergo endoscopic and histologic or at least radiologic examination of the esophagus. If the diagnosis remains unclear, 24 hour pH monitoring, noting periods of chest pain, may be helpful. Even if symptoms are not clearly related to the esophagus, bedside testing using acid perfusion according to Bernstein or a trial of antireflux measures may be helpful. Additional attempts to implicate the esophagus in noncardiac chest pain rely on 24 hour recordings of esophageal pressures or provocation of abnormal contractions or of cardiac ischemia as described later. The indications for these tests await clearer definition, particularly in the absence of esophageal symptoms.

PHYSICAL EXAMINATION

Because of its position deep in the mediastinum, the esophagus is not accessible to direct physical examination. A delay in esophageal transit should be suspected if the epigastric splash heard with a stethoscope occurs more than 10 seconds after the patient swallows a sip of water. But findings of systemic disease or of metastatic nodules are often relevant to the assessment of esophageal problems. Malignancies involving the upper two thirds of the esophagus spread to cervical and supraclavicular nodes and may be palpable as firm fixed nodes. Metastases from tumors involving the lower esophagus may become palpable in the upper abdomen or the liver. Rarely, esophageal perforation produces subcutaneous emphysema and crepitus on palpation of the neck or thoracic wall. Findings of a pneumothorax or pleural effusion may also be present. Additional physical findings are due to underlying diseases that can cause esophageal dysfunction. They include pharyngeal thrush or vesicles in fungal or viral infections, oropharyngeal burns or ulcers in caustic ingestion, skin and joint findings in collagen vascular diseases, neurologic abnormalities in central nervous system diseases, and motor dysfunction in the muscular dystrophies. Esophageal dysfunction may also be associated with pregnancy, diabetes mellitus, amyloidosis, and iron deficiency.

DIAGNOSTIC TESTS

Radiographic and endoscopic examinations provide diagnostic information in most esophageal diseases. Often both tests should be performed because they provide complementary information. Radiographic examination of deglutition is the method of choice for the study of pharyngeal motility. If an esophageal motility disorder is suspected after the radiographic examination, this can be further defined by the aid of esophageal manometry. Endoscopy is indicated in all instances in which a tumor or mucosal disease is suspected after the radiographic examination (Chapter 30). Endoscopy provides the most accurate assessment of mucosal lesions. It provides tissue for histologic, cytologic, and microbial examination and often facilitates immediate treatment (e.g., dilation of the esophagus, extraction of foreign bodies, or control of variceal bleeding).

Radiographic and endoscopic examinations are useful to assess esophageal changes that result from reflux but are poor measures of the severity of gastroesophageal reflux itself. When reflux is suspected to be the cause of pulmonary or laryngeal complications in the absence of reflux esophagitis, esophageal pH monitoring and scintigraphic examination of reflux provide direct measures of the degree of reflux.

Barium contrast studies and fluoroscopic examination of deglutition

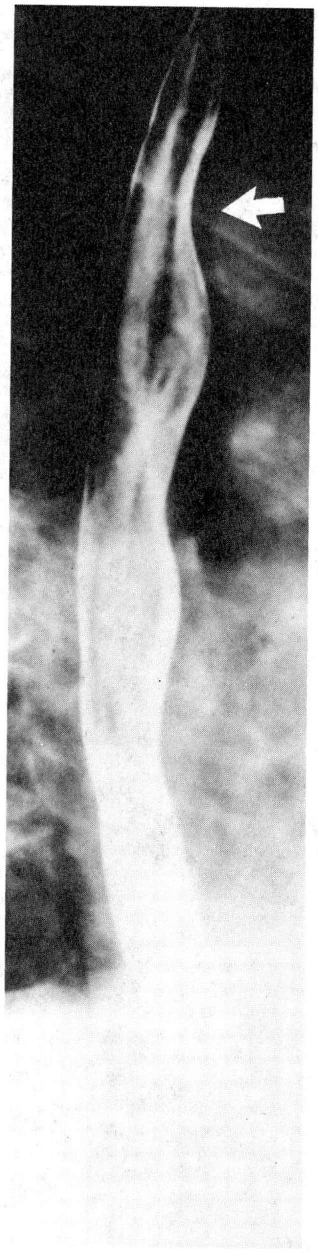

Fig. 31-2. Radiographic appearance of the normal esophagus. The proximal two thirds is demonstrated on this single contrast examination. The density of the barium *(lower one third)* can obscure mucosal abnormalities. The arrow points to the aortic impression; below it is the impression of the left main stem bronchus. (Radiograph courtesy of Charles C. Lu, MD.)

In the normal esophagus (Figs. 31-2 and 31-3) the mucosal outline is smooth and the walls are distensible. Video esophagrams aid in the evaluation of motility disorders. A small volume barium "cookie swallow" should be used in patients with pharyngeal paresis because of the risk of aspiration and the information about pharyngeal function it provides. Normally, the peristaltic contraction wave sweeps the barium bolus from the pharynx through the esophagus into the stomach within 10 seconds; esophageal contractions produce a sharp coning of the tail of the barium column. With ineffective peristalsis, the tail of the barium column is fuzzy and residual barium remains in the esophageal body. In diffuse spasm, disordered contractions squeeze the barium column into discrete segments or propel it in an orad direction. A barium soaked marshmallow, a piece of bread, or a 12 mm barium tablet aids in the demonstration of subtle strictures or motor abnormalities.

The radiographic examination serves to determine whether the esophagus has shortened or become strictured as a result of injury or malignancy. Shortening is recognized by the formation of transverse mucosal folds in the

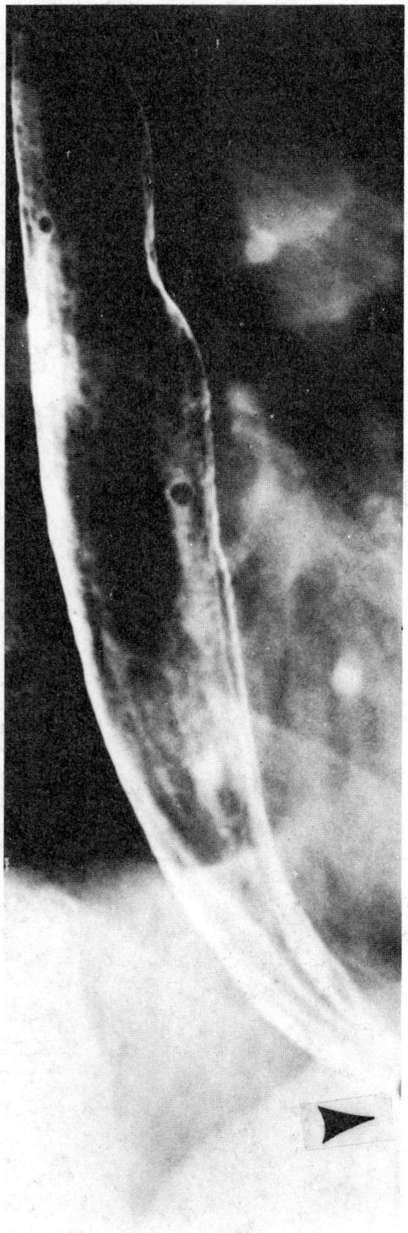

Fig. 31-3. The distal two thirds of the normal esophagus is demonstrated on this air *(double)* contrast esophagram. The esophagus distends well and its mucosal outline is smooth throughout. The two small round dark areas in the upper one half of the photo are air bubbles. The arrow points to the gastroesophageal junction just below the diaphragm; above it are the delicate longitudinal mucosal folds. (Radiograph courtesy of Charles C. Lu, MD.)

distal esophagus or by a persistent hiatal hernia. Webs and rings produce indentations of the barium column. Webs are more delicate and only a few millimeters thick. Strictures are short segments of the esophagus that lack normal distensibility. They are best demonstrated by maximal filling of the gullet and by viewing of the esophagus in several projections. Radiographic examinations provide only limited information about the severity of gastroesophageal reflux but are useful to determine the presence of complications such as a stricture or coexisting disease such as gastric outlet obstruction or peptic ulcer disease. Inflammation of the esophagus leads to mucosal irregularity and makes the esophageal walls less distensible. Small mucosal lesions are difficult to detect on radiographic examination of the esophagus and erosions are difficult to distinguish from varices.

Esophageal carcinomas produce irregular filling defects, disruption of the mucosal pattern, and ulcerations within the tumor mass; tumors existing outside the esophagus produce smooth mounds indenting the contour of the lumen. Computed tomography and endoscopic ultrasonography yield more information about extent of tumor spread and may help determine resectability.

If a perforation is suspected, barium should not be used because it may penetrate into paraesophageal tissue and produce severe mediastinitis. Only if no leak is detected with water-soluble contrast should thin barium be used because it is more sensitive in detecting small defects.

Other imaging studies may contribute to the understanding of esophageal problems. The scintigraphic evaluation of deglutition with the use of radioisotope labeled boluses provides some quantitative information about esophageal transit and gastroesophageal reflux. The technique, however, provides insufficient detail to detect anatomic abnormalities, it represents only one point in time and is not a reliable screening procedure. Computed tomography and magnetic resonance imaging are most useful to detect infection or to evaluate whether neoplastic diseases have spread beyond the wall of the esophagus.

Esophageal endoscopy, brushings, biopsies, and ultrasonography

Endoscopic examination is the best method to assess the mucosal diseases of the esophagus. It is also used to obtain brushings and biopsies for histologic and cytologic study of suspected abnormal tissue and samples for fungal, bacterial (including acid fast bacilli), and viral cultures in suspected infections. The pathologist must be provided information about the origin and description of the lesion being sampled. In all debilitated and immunosuppressed patients with esophageal symptoms, viral, bacterial, and fungal cultures should be obtained from abnormal mucosa and planted immediately on appropriate culture or transport media. Because over half of acquired immunodeficiency syndrome (AIDS) patients with esophageal symptoms have candida esophagitis, some recommend an empiric trial of antifungal therapy before resort to endoscopy. Alternatively, blind brushing to obtain specimens often yields good results. Details of endoscopic technique are described in Chapter 30.

Heartburn alone is not an indication for esophagoscopy. Only if pyrosis is severe, progressive, or refractory to antireflux therapy or if other symptoms such as bleeding, dysphagia, or odynophagia are present should endoscopy be done. Any stricture, ulcer, or mass involving the esophagus that is demonstrated radiologically should be visualized and a biopsy specimen taken to determine its cause. Benign-appearing strictures may be malignant; the radiographic appearance of achalasia may also be mimicked by infiltrating carcinomas at the gastroesophageal junction.

Esophageal lesions from reflux occur first at the gastroesophageal squamocolumnar junction, an irregular but sharply demarcated border where the salmon-colored gastric mucosa meets the more pearly pink esophageal mucosa. In the acute phase, the transparent mucosa becomes congested, obscuring the fine vascular network and making it friable. In more advanced stages, erosions and exudate occur on the crests of the folds and eventually the process spreads proximally and becomes confluent. In the chronic phase, longitudinal vessels become prominent. Mucosal metaplasia (Barrett's epithelium) appears as salmon-pink islands or tongues of columnar mucosa that extend into the squamous epithelium and may become confluent. Many patients with symptomatic reflux have no visible endoscopic changes. In the absence of gross lesions, biopsy specimens used to evaluate the effects of reflux should be taken 5 cm proximal to the lower sphincter, as histologic evidence of esophagitis may be present in the absence of visible abnormalities.

Follow-up endoscopy for reflux esophagitis is unnecessary unless symptoms do not respond to medical therapy, complications arise, or surgical therapy is contemplated. On the other hand, surveillance endoscopy is probably indicated for all patients with Barrett's esophagus, as the risk of esophageal adenocarcinoma appears to be increased at least 40-fold in this condition. Multiple biopsies at multiple levels are necessary to detect dysplasia or early cancer.

Endoscopic ultrasonography is increasingly used to evaluate submucosal lesions such as leiomyomas, but also to determine the extent of undermining or spread beyond the wall of esophageal cancers. The depth of neoplastic infiltration can be assessed with 90% accuracy and spread to lymph nodes with 80% accuracy. Its use preoperatively may eliminate the need for exploratory surgery in high-risk patients. The potential exists to determine blood flow in varices and other large vessels through the use of Doppler probes.

Acid perfusion of the esophagus (Bernstein test)

When the history alone does not allow the conclusion that symptoms are of esophageal origin, asymptomatic response to perfusion of the esophagus with acid often occurs when the esophageal mucosa is altered by injury. Esophageal mucosal injury can be due to reflux, infection, tumor, or chemical, thermal, or mechanical injury.

To perform the test a small-bore tube is introduced into the stomach and then withdrawn so that its tip lies at the junction of the middle and distal thirds of the esophagus. In most individuals, this corresponds to a distance of about 30 cm from the incisors. The esophageal tube is connected to two reservoirs, one containing 0.9 N sodium chloride, the other one 0.1 N hydrochloric acid. Perfusion is started at 1 ml/min with sodium chloride and is switched to hydrochloric acid without the patient's knowledge. All symptoms are recorded. Acid perfusion is stopped after 30 minutes or once symptoms have occurred. Symptoms should be promptly relieved by perfusion of saline solution or antacid, and symptoms should then be reproduced by repeated acid perfusion. Most patients with erosive esophagitis experience symptoms within 5 to 10 minutes after the start of the perfusion. The delay between the start of the perfusion and the onset of symptoms shortens with repeated perfusions.

Classically, the acid perfusion test is performed with the intent to convince patients and their physicians that the gullet rather than the heart is the source of pain. Patients are asked to compare symptoms during esophageal perfusion to those they experience spontaneously. The test finding is considered positive if spontaneous and provoked symptoms are identical. Patients with asthma and reflux disease may experience pyrosis and exacerbation of asthma during the test.

The conventional interpretation of the Bernstein test result assumes that esophageal symptoms are always alike and that past and present symptoms are easily compared. The prompt and reproducible production of symptoms by acid perfusion implies the presence of esophageal hypersensitivity. The test is about 90% specific for reflux disease, but not very sensitive (~35%). The test (and thus, possibly reflux) has been reported to reduce the threshold for electrocardiographic (ECG) changes of ischemia or of angina in some patients with coronary artery disease. The correlation between a positive acid perfusion test result and abnormal reflux determined by 24 hour monitoring is rather poor. Endoscopic and histologic evidence of esophagitis and long-term pH monitoring are more reliable indicators of reflux than a positive Bernstein test result. The Bernstein test, however, is less costly and can readily be performed by primary care physicians.

It has been claimed that some patients with noncardiac chest pain may have altered or abnormal sensitivity to normal stimuli and thus experience increased pain in response to acid, cold, or inflation of balloons in the esophagus. This approach may prove to be very important, but currently it is not standardized and cannot be used routinely. Acid perfusion (Bernstein test) should be thought of as a screening test and not a definitive test to establish the cause of chest pain. Others have reported that some of these patients have abnormal psychological profiles and should be tested with standardized tests. This information also may be quite important in the overall management of the patient's complaints.

Esophageal manometry

In esophageal manometry, the mechanical activity of the esophagus and of its sphincter is revealed by luminal pressure sensors. The normal human esophagus generates luminal pressures of 60 to 100 mm Hg in response to swallowing, the highest pressures being generated in the middle esophagus (Fig. 31-4). Pressure waves have a sequential progression from proximal to distal, and at any individual sensor, a single contraction wave does not nor-

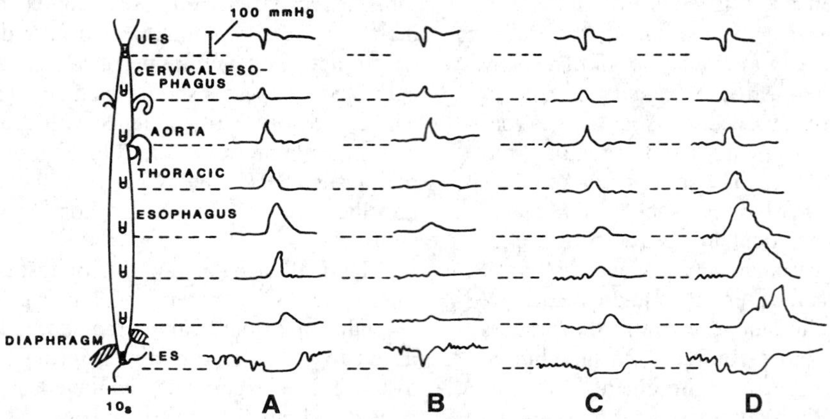

Fig. 31-4. Patterns of esophageal motility. In this semischematic drawing, the pressure sensors span the entire esophagus from the upper esophageal sphincter to the lower esophageal sphincter. **A,** In the normal state *(first panel),* both sphincters maintain a high pressure zone in which respiratory movements lead to pressure undulations. Swallowing leads to a brief relaxation of the upper esophageal sphincter and a longer relaxation of the lower esophageal sphincter. A contraction wave travels through the esophageal body; its amplitude is around 100 mm Hg and its duration about 4 seconds. Pressure patterns are abnormal in the distal two thirds of the esophagus in achalasia, systemic sclerosis, and esophageal spasm. **B,** In achalasia *(second panel),* the lower esophageal sphincter pressure is high and fails to disappear for an appropriate length of time on swallowing. Contractions in the esophageal body are weak and nonsequential. **C,** In systemic sclerosis *(third panel),* lower esophageal sphincter pressure is low; esophageal contractions are weak, but generally sequential. Similar abnormalities are often seen in erosive esophagitis and Barrett's esophagus. **D,** In esophageal spasm *(fourth panel),* esophageal contractions last more than 7 seconds and generate pressures above 150 to 200 mm Hg. Contractions may also be repetitive and nonsequential. UES, upper esophageal sphincter; LES, lower esophageal sphincter.

mally last more than 7 seconds. Most swallows lead to a complete peristaltic sequence, and repetitive esophageal contractions do not occur.

The resting pressure generated by the normal lower esophageal sphincter (LES) is 20 to 40 mm Hg and relaxes to near zero with the onset of a swallow. The sphincter is located at the point of respiratory reversal. Sphincter pressure tends to be higher and the sphincter fails to relax in achalasia and in some cases of esophageal spasm. In patients with severe esophagitis and scleroderma esophagus the high-pressure zone may be virtually abolished. A "common cavity phenomenon" (identical simultaneous waves at several sites) is observed with incompetence of the LES: increases of intragastric pressure are transmitted to the esophagus. Otherwise, manometry does not distinguish reliably between a competent and an incompetent LES. Similar waves may occur with straining, retching, or coughing.

Esophageal manometry is useful in the evaluation of achalasia, diffuse spasm, scleroderma, and other motility disorders. It is sometimes the only test that demonstrates those esophageal disorders that are characterized by excessive or reduced force of esophageal contractions. Abnormal contractions may not occur during short recording periods. Pharmacologic provocation of abnormal contractions with such agents as edrophonium and bethanechol may increase the sensitivity of manometric tests in evaluation of patients with suspected disorders of esophageal motility.

pH measurements

Gastroesophageal reflux can be monitored by introducing a pH probe into the distal esophagus and continuously recording luminal pH. Acid reflux is defined as being present when the intraluminal pH is 4 or less. The frequency, timing, and duration of reflux episodes are recorded and compared with the timing of heartburn and chest pain.

Long-term esophageal pH monitoring is useful to assess the reflux profile: 24 hour monitoring of the esophageal pH during regular activities and sleep has become a standard test to elucidate the role of reflux in chest pain, bronchospasm, laryngospasm, and laryngitis as well as in esophageal disease.

pH measurements suffer from the drawback that they assess reflux solely in terms of H^+ ion concentration at an arbitrary esophageal level. Measurements of the luminal pH provide little information on the volume of the refluxed bolus or on the presence of pancreaticobiliary secretions that can also damage the esophageal mucosa.

Monitoring the 24 hour intraluminal pressure profile simultaneously with the 24 hour profile and pain profile may document the existence of high-amplitude waves associated with chest pain episodes. Long-term concomitant Holter monitoring may identify periods of cardiac ischemia triggered by esophageal events and thus increases the reliability of monitoring.

REFERENCES

Benjamin SB: The relationship between esophageal motor disorders and microvascular angina. Med Clin North Am 74:1135, 1991.

Bonacini M, Young T, and Laine L: The causes of esophageal symptoms in human immunodeficiency infection: a prospective study of 110 patients. Arch Intern Med 151:1567, 1991.

Breumelhof R et al: Analysis of 24-hour esophageal pressure and pH data in unselected patients with non-cardiac chest pain. Gastroenterology 99:1257, 1990.

Browning TH: Diagnosis of chest pain of esophageal origin. Dig Dis Sci 35:289, 1990.

Cannon RO et al: Coronary flow reserve, esophageal motility, and chest pain in patients with angiographically normal coronary arteries. Am J Med 88:217, 1990.

Gelfand MD and Botoman VA: Esophageal motility disorders: a clinical overview. Am J Gastoenterol 82:181, 1987.

Ghillebert G et al: Ambulatory 24-hour intraoesophageal pH and pressure recordings vs. provocation tests in the diagnosis of chest pain of oesophageal origin. Gut 31:738, 1990.

Hewson EG et al: The acid perfusion test: does it have a role in the assessment of non-cardiac chest pain? Gut 30:305, 1989.

Jacob B, Kahrilas PJ, and Herzon G: Proximal esophageal pH-metry in patients with reflux esophagitis. Gastroenterology 100:3, 310, 1991.

Knuff TE et al: Histologic evaluation of chronic gastroesophageal reflux: an evaluation of biopsy methods and diagnostic criteria. Dig Dis Sci 29:194, 1984.

Reid BJ et al: Endoscopic biopsy can detect high-grade dysplasia or early adenocarcinoma in Barrett's esophagus without grossly recognized neoplastic lesions. Gastroenterology 94:81, 1988.

Richter JE, Barish CF, and Castell DO: Abnormal sensory perception in patients with esophageal chest pain. Gastroenterology 91:845, 1986.

Schindlbeck NE et al: Optimal thresholds, sensitivity and specificity of long-term pH-metry for the detection of gastroesophageal reflux. Gastroenterology 93:85, 1987.

Tio TL et al: Esophagogastric carcinoma: preoperative TNM classification with endosonography. Radiology 173:411, 1989.

CHAPTER

32 Evaluation of Gastroduodenal Diseases

Walter L. Peterson

A discussion of diagnostic procedures can no longer be simply a listing of tests with their sensitivities and specificities. Also included must be justification for employing such procedures. All too often, diagnostic procedures are performed routinely without consideration of cost or potential benefit to the patient. This chapter is a broad overview of time-honored and newly developed procedures for the evaluation of gastroduodenal diseases, with special emphasis on their value in patient management. For their use in specific diseases, the reader is referred to the chapters devoted to those topics.

UPPER GASTROINTESTINAL RADIOGRAPHY AND ENDOSCOPY

Barium contrast radiographic examination of the stomach and duodenum (upper gastrointestinal [UGI] series) and endoscopy of the UGI tract are the most frequently utilized procedures for evaluation of gastroduodenal diseases. The two major indications for one or both of these techniques are UGI hemorrhage and upper abdominal pain.

An air-contrast UGI series performed by a skilled radiologist is an inexpensive and, in many patients, accurate tool for the diagnosis of UGI hemorrhage. The only lesions not well seen in radiographic examination are superficial lesions such as Mallory-Weiss tears, superficial erosions, and vascular anomalies. On the other hand, there are several clinical situations in which endoscopy, a more expensive technique, is the preferred procedure. For patients whose bleeding continues despite gastric lavage, the physician would select endoscopy. He or she wants the most accurate technique to guide further therapy but does not want to preclude potential angiography by filling the stomach with barium. In patients whose bleeding has ceased, endoscopy is the procedure of choice when (1) high-quality air-contrast radiographs are not available; (2) portal hypertension is present, since patients with esophagogastric varices may bleed from other lesions; (3) endoscopic therapy (e.g., variceal sclerosis, endoscopic therapy of a peptic ulcer) is being considered; (4) the patient has had a gastric resection; and (5) an abdominal aortic graft is in place.

Compared with the UGI series, endoscopy is also more accurate in detecting organic causes of upper abdominal pain. For example, a UGI series may miss some gastric and duodenal ulcers, the latter particularly when the duodenal bulb is deformed from long-standing disease. It is not known, however, how often endoscopy actually facilitates diagnosis in patients with abdominal pain, or whether diagnosis benefits the patient. Is it worth the expense for all patients with abdominal pain to undergo endoscopy to find some unknown percentage of organic lesions, especially because it is not known that making a diagnosis is helpful? This question can be answered only by a controlled clinical trial. Until data are available, the following approach is logical for most patients. Many patients with mild symptoms of short duration may be treated empirically with antacids and/or H_2 blockers or sucralfate. If there are worrisome aspects to the history and physical examination (e.g., weight loss, occult stool blood) or if the patient does not respond to empiric therapy, an UGI series should be performed. If no diagnosis is made or if the UGI series discloses a lesion requiring documentation or biopsy, endoscopy can then be performed. Although such an approach may ultimately be discarded in favor of performing endoscopy in everyone, it is time honored and relatively inexpensive.

Most patients with documented duodenal ulcer disease need not undergo radiographic or endoscopic examination with each bout of pain, especially because active ulcer craters are often missed in deformed duodenal bulbs. Duodenal ulcer is a chronic disease with frequent recurrences (see Chapter 38) that may be treated empirically at the onset of symptoms. If there is a change in symptoms or if surgery is planned, endoscopic confirmation of the diagnosis is warranted. In contrast, most patients with gastric ulcer disease should undergo endoscopy for visual and histologic exclusion of malignancy. Exceptions to this policy occur when endoscopy is not readily available and the ulcer appears, on radiographic examination, to be benign. Endoscopy is clearly indicated in patients with suspected gastroduodenal malignancy (i.e., mass lesions, large folds, anatomic deformity seen on UGI series). Not only may visual inspection and biopsy results confirm or rule out malignancy, but histologic examination may also identify the type of malignancy.

GASTRIC BIOPSY AND CYTOLOGY

An important aspect of UGI endoscopy is its use in obtaining tissue for histologic and cytologic examination. Tissue is routinely obtained from patients with gastric ulcers or mass lesions to exclude or confirm malignancy. The procedure's usefulness in diagnosing malignancy primarily depends on three factors: (1) the number of specimens obtained, (2) the care with which they are collected and processed, and (3) the expertise of the pathologist examining the specimens. In most instances, if six to eight endoscopic biopsy specimens are obtained, malignant lesions of the stomach can be detected with 80% to 90% accuracy. In cases in which the biopsy result is benign, cytologic examination ("touch-preps" or brushings) increase accuracy to 95%. However, accurate cytologic findings depend on the expertise of the cytologist, and many institutions do not have such experts. In these situations, false-positive and false-negative results become a problem. In centers without expert cytologists, it appears prudent to rely on visual inspection of the lesion and perhaps more biopsy procedures than would otherwise be performed. Lavage cytologic examinations, done infrequently in the past, offer no advantage over endoscopically directed brush cytologic examinations.

Submucosal or nonulcerated lesions present a special problem, because often only normal mucosa is obtained by endoscopic pinch biopsies. In these instances, it may be helpful to perform suction biopsies, such as are obtained in the small bowel, or to use the "lift-and-cut" snare technique to obtain a large piece of gastric tissue (see Chapter 30). This technique may be especially helpful in evaluating patients with large gastric folds if the differential diagnosis includes lymphoma or Ménétrier's disease (Chapters 39 and 40). If this technique is not diagnostic and if the index of suspicion for infiltrative neoplasm is high, full-thickness biopsies of the stomach should be obtained by laparotomy.

GASTRIC ANALYSIS

Gastric analysis is not needed for most patients with peptic ulcers. However, it may be of potential benefit in four clinical situations. First, patients with gastric ulcers that are suspected to be malignant or that fail to show a reasonable progression of healing should undergo gastric analysis to detect achlorhydria. If histamine- or pentagastrin-fast achlorhydria is present, the likelihood is great that the ulcer is malignant. If acid is present in gastric juice retrieved at endoscopy, more extensive studies with stimulants are not needed. Second, gastric analysis may be of value in duodenal ulcer patients who are not responding to therapy with drugs designed to lower gastric acid secretion or in whom surgery is planned. Comparison of preoperative and postoperative gastric analyses provides evidence for the effectiveness of surgery in reducing gastric acid secretion. Third, patients with hypergastrinemia should have gastric analysis to differentiate between states of low acid secretion (i.e., gastric atrophy) and autonomous production of gastrin (i.e., Zollinger-Ellison syndrome). Fourth, some experts believe patients with Zollinger-Ellison syndrome should be treated with increasing doses of drugs until basal acid secretion falls below a certain level (e.g., 10 mmol/h). If this approach is taken, basal acid output should be measured during the hour just preceding the next scheduled dose of medication.

Measurement of gastric acidity and secretion

Gastric juice is collected in 15 minute samples through a sump-type nasogastric tube. Systemic medications designed to reduce acid secretion should be stopped 36 hours before gastric analysis, and no food or antacid is ingested for the 10 hours prior. (See Chapter 38 for special instructions in patients with suspected Zollinger-Ellison syndrome.) Gastric acidity of the samples may be determined either by a pH electrode or by titration to pH 7.0 with a base such as sodium hydroxide. Acid secretion in millimoles (or milliequivalents) per 15 minute is calculated by multiplying the acidity (mmol/L) times the volume (liters/15 min).

Basal acid output

Basal acid output (BAO) is the sum of acid secretion rates during four 15 minute collections, expressed as millimoles (or milliequivalents) per hour. BAO fluctuates from day to day but in normal subjects ranges from 0 to 12 mmol/hr, with a mean of 2 to 4 mmol/hr (Chapter 27).

Stimulated acid output

The stimulants most often used to determine the maximum ability of parietal cells to secrete acid are histamine, betazole hydrochloride (Histalog), and pentagastrin. Because pentagastrin has fewer side effects than histamine and because it elicits its effects more quickly than betazole hydrochloride, it is now the stimulant of choice. After determination of BAO, pentagastrin (6 μ/kg) is injected subcutaneously and gastric contents are collected during four 15 minute periods. Results may be expressed as maximum acid output (MAO) or peak acid output (PAO). MAO is the sum of the four 15 minute values. PAO is the sum of the two highest consecutive 15 minute values multiplied by 2. The PAO can be reproduced with repeated testing and in normal subjects ranges from about 10 to 80 mmol/hr, with a mean of 33 mmol/hr (Chapter 27).

Interpretation of basal acid output and peak acid output in disease

Acid secretory values in duodenal ulcer patients are, on average, higher than those in normal subjects. However, only approximately one third of duodenal ulcer patients have basal or peak acid outputs above the upper limit of normal. Patients with Zollinger-Ellison syndrome virtually always have a BAO greater than 12 to 15 mmol/hr and a BAO/PAO ratio of more than 60%.

Patients with gastric ulcers secrete, on average, less acid than normal subjects, but again there is overlap. Achlorhydria is defined by many as a PAO of 0, with pH of gastric contents never falling below 6.0 after stimulation. Benign peptic ulcer disease rarely occurs in achlorhydric patients. Thus a diagnosis of gastric carcinoma is suspected until disproved by endoscopy, biopsy, and/or cytologic examination.

Gastric analysis after ulcer surgery

An especially difficult clinical problem in which gastric analysis may provide useful information is the evaluation of patients with recurrent ulcers after gastric surgery. Most surgical procedures involve some form of vagotomy, and regardless of a patient's acid-secretory status, the crucial question usually revolves around the completeness of the vagotomy. If there is evidence that a vagotomy has been incompletely performed, a repeat vagotomy might be considered. If the vagotomy is judged adequate, some form of gastric resection may be in order. For many years, the only way of testing the adequacy of vagotomy was by insulin-induced or 2-deoxyglucose—induced hypoglycemia. These procedures are hazardous and may induce acid secretion by means other than vagal stimulation alone. Modified sham feeding, in which patients see, smell, taste, and chew (but do not swallow) food, is safe and is believed to stimulate acid secretion solely via the vagus nerve. Studies indicate that in the presence of a complete vagotomy, the 60 minute acid output by aspiration during 30 minutes of modified sham feeding plus 30 minutes after sham feeding is less than 10% of a patient's PAO. Values higher than this suggest that the vagus nerve is intact. This test may be useful in planning additional surgery for patients who have postoperative ulcer recurrence.

SERUM GASTRIN LEVELS

Normal fasting serum gastrin levels vary among different laboratories, but in most laboratories fasting values greater than 100 to 200 pg/ml are considered to be abnormal. The two most common causes of hypergastrinemia are the Zollinger-Ellison syndrome and atrophic gastritis (Chapters 38 and 88), two conditions that may readily be distinguished by gastric analysis. Other disorders reported to produce elevated fasting gastrin values include renal insufficiency and the short bowel syndrome.

Although a serum gastrin value above 1000 pg/ml in a patient who is not achlorhydric is virtually diagnostic of Zollinger-Ellison syndrome, values between 200 and 1000 pg/ml may be found in duodenal ulcer patients with and without Zollinger-Ellison syndrome. In the postoperative patient, the differential diagnosis also includes postvagotomy hypergastrinemia and the retained-antrum syndrome. In patients with only modest elevations in serum gastrin levels, the secretin infusion test may help differentiate among these conditions.

Two clinical units of GIH secretin per kilogram of body weight is injected intravenously over a 30 to 60 second period. Serum gastrin determinations are obtained twice just prior to secretin injection and at 2, 5, 10, 15, and 20 minutes after secretin injection. In all but patients with Zollinger-Ellison syndrome, secretin has little effect on serum gastrin levels. Rises of 200 pg/ml or more above basal levels are reported to be diagnostic of Zollinger-Ellison syndrome, although a few patients with proved Zollinger-Ellison syndrome may not exhibit a positive response to secretin.

A rare subgroup of duodenal ulcer patients has modestly elevated serum gastrin levels and negative secretin test results but exhibits substantial rises in postprandial gastrin concentration after a mixed test meal. These patients usually have antral G cell hyperplasia, which responds dramatically to antrectomy.

TESTS TO DETECT THE PRESENCE OF *HELICOBACTER PYLORI*

The most specific test for the presence of *Helicobacter pylori* is culture of the organism from gastric mucosal biopsy sections. A more sensitive test is histologic examination of mucosal biopsies, in which even small numbers of organisms can be seen with routine hematoxylin and eosin or Giemsa stains. *H. pylori* can be diagnosed indirectly by tests that detect the presence of urease, an enzyme produced by the organism. Mucosal biopsy specimens can be inoculated onto a urea-containing medium. If urease is present, the urea will be split into carbon dioxide and ammonia, the latter of which raises the pH of the medium and produces a color change of a pH sensitive indicator. Another means of detecting the presence of urease is a breath urea test. Urea labeled with ^{13}C or ^{14}C is ingested with a liquid meal. If urease is present, labeled carbon dioxide is split off, absorbed into the circulation, and expired into the breath, which is collected and analyzed. Tests for gastric urease are neither as sensitive nor as specific for the detection of *H. pylori* as culture and histologic examination. The easiest and least expensive test for *H. pylori* is determination of serum antibodies to the organism. This is a very specific test for the presence of *H. pylori* infection at some time in a person's life but may be less sensitive for current infection.

GASTRIC EMPTYING

Delayed gastric emptying can usually be diagnosed by means of a careful history and physical examination. If the patient reports vomiting recognizable food long after a meal and if a succussion splash is heard on examination, delayed gastric emptying may be the diagnosis. Response to therapy is best determined by resumption of the patient's ability to eat without discomfort or vomiting. Three tests—the saline load test, gastric isotopic scanning, and emptying of radiopaque markers—are available to provide objective confirmation of the diagnosis of delayed emptying and the response to therapy. Each test has its limitations, however, and none enables the clinician to differentiate between an obstructing lesion of the antral pyloric region, such as peptic ulcer or cancer, and primary motor disorders of the stomach, such as postvagotomy paresis. This differentiation must be accomplished by a UGI series or, preferably, endoscopy.

The saline load test is simple to perform and does not require expensive equipment. It has been validated only in patients with organic outlet obstruction and measures only the emptying of liquids, and therefore has limited clinical importance. Gastric isotopic scanning measures the emptying of both solids and liquids and is especially helpful in cases of suspected primary motor disorders. The radiopaque marker study measures the emptying of indigestible solids and may be more sensitive in some situations than isotopic scanning.

Gastric isotopic scanning

Gastric isotopic scanning accurately quantitates the ability of the stomach to empty its contents and is especially useful when endoscopy discloses no organic obstruction to explain delayed emptying. For example, patients with suspected diabetic gastroparesis or postvagotomy paresis may have a motility disorder that can be confirmed and quantitated by means of this test. Response to nasogastric suction or motility-enhancing drugs such as bethanechol chloride (Urecholine Chloride) or metaclopramide may also be assessed.

Isotopic scanning involves administration of a liquid or solid meal to which a radioisotope has been added. Isotopes employed include ^{51}Cr, ^{113m}In, and ^{99m}Tc. The isotope present at any time after administration of the meal is measured by a scintillation counter or a gamma camera. Although liquids are rather easily labeled with isotope, ingenuity has been required to label solids. One technique involves injecting chickens with ^{99m}Tc, which is rapidly incorporated into the liver. The harvested chicken liver is cooked, diced, and eaten by the patient. Because liquids and solids empty at different rates, investigators are now using meals with both liquid and solid components, with separate isotopes for each component. The major drawbacks to the procedure are that it requires expensive equipment and special expertise.

Emptying of solid radiopaque markers

A recent study suggests that the emptying of 1 cm segments of radiopaque plastic tubing (0.2 cm diameter), acting as indigestible solids, may be a simple and inexpensive means of detecting abnormal gastric motility. When 10 such markers are given with a meal to normal subjects, all the markers will be emptied (as determined by a plain abdominal radiograph) within 6 hours. In patients with diabetes mellitus, markers often are present in the stomach after 6 hours. Early studies suggest that this technique may be more sensitive than the more expensive gastric isotopic scan. Further work is needed to determine the clinical utility of this test.

OTHER TECHNIQUES

Patients with gastrointestinal bleeding are sometimes evaluated with ^{99m}Tc sulfur colloid or ^{99m}Tc-labeled red blood cells to detect the site of blood loss. Although at times of use in patients with obscure bleeding below the ligament of Treitz, these techniques have almost no value in patients with gastroduodenal bleeding.

Experimental modalities that may, in the future, be of benefit in the evaluation of gastroduodenal diseases include endoscopic Doppler studies to evaluate the patency (i.e., potential for further bleeding) of arteries eroded by peptic ulcers and endoscopic ultrasound techniques.

REFERENCES

Brady CE: Secretin provocation test in the diagnosis of Zollinger-Ellison syndrome. Am J Gastroenterol 86:129, 1991.

Feldman M: Gastric secretion. In Sleisenger MH and Fordtran JS, editors: Gastrointestinal disease, ed 4. Philadelphia, 1989, WB Saunders.

Feldman M, Richardson CT, and Fordtran JS: Experience with sham feeding as a test for vagotomy. Gastroenterology 79:792, 1980.

Feldman M, Smith HJ, and Simon TR: Gastric emptying of solid radiopaque markers: studies in healthy subjects and diabetic patients. Gastroenterology 87:895, 1984.

Graham DY et al: Prospective evaluation of biopsy number in the diagnosis of esophageal and gastric carcinoma. Gastroenterology 82:228, 1982.

Horowitz M and Dent J: Clinical relevance of disordered gastric emptying. Bailliere Clin Gastroenterol 5:371, 1991.

Morrisey JF and Reichelderfer M: Gastrointestinal endoscopy. N Engl J Med 325:1142, 1214, 1991.

Peterson WL: *Helicobacter pylori* and peptic ulcer disease. N Engl J Med 324:1043, 1991.

CHAPTER

33 Evaluation of Intestinal Diseases

Jerry S. Trier

The small and large intestines are subject to a large number of diseases with varied clinical manifestations. Judicious use of diagnostic studies can often clarify the nature of an underlying pathologic process, be it infectious, inflammatory, metabolic, immunologic, vascular, neoplastic, or neuromuscular. This chapter provides an overview of the usefulness of relevant available diagnostic studies in the differential diagnosis of diseases of the intestines.

A carefully elicited history and a thorough physical examination often provide important clues to guide the physician in selecting those studies most likely to provide information of diagnostic value. For example, the presence of nocturnal "stooling" that awakens the patient at night suggests an organic rather than a functional cause of diarrhea and should stimulate the clinician to pursue a diagnosis vigorously. Weight loss associated with normal or increased caloric intake suggests malabsorption. The diagnostic value of distinctive and characteristic historic features and physical findings in specific intestinal diseases is discussed in detail in the subsequent chapters that deal with individual diseases.

STUDIES OF FORMED BLOOD ELEMENTS

Changes in the formed elements of the peripheral blood accompany many diseases of the small and large intestines. Some of the more common abnormalities are summarized in Table 33-1.

Anemia accompanies many intestinal diseases. If microcytic, it may reflect impaired iron absorption associated with diffuse mucosal lesions of the proximal intestine such as celiac sprue and Whipple's disease or with chronic blood loss secondary to neoplasms, chronic specific or idiopathic inflammatory bowel disease, or vascular malformations. If macrocytic, anemia may reflect impaired folate absorption, which accompanies diseases that involve diffusely the proximal intestinal mucosa (celiac sprue, Whipple's disease, tropical sprue), or impaired vitamin B_{12} absorption caused by either primary ileal disease (Crohn's disease) or bacterial overgrowth in the lumen of the small intestine (scleroderma, jejunal diverticulosis). Dimorphic anemias are not uncommon in patients with diffuse mucosal lesions in whom iron, folate, and even vitamin B_{12} malabsorption may coexist. If normocytic, anemia may reflect acute blood loss from vascular malformations, diverticulitis, neoplasms, or acute enteritis or colitis.

Leukocytosis with increased neutrophils is common in invasive bacterial intestinal infections (shigellosis, salmonellosis, *Yersinia* or *Campylobacter* enterocolitis), severe idiopathic inflammatory bowel disease, appendicitis, *Clostridium difficile*–induced pseudomembranous enterocolitis, amebic colitis, and paraintestinal abscess formation in Crohn's disease or diverticulitis. Neutropenia is usually a complication of drug therapy (Table 33-1). Peripheral eosinophilia accompanies eosinophilic gastroenteritis and certain parasitic diseases such as roundworm and tapeworm infestations. Lymphopenia may accompany any of the many diseases that may cause excessive leakage of plasma protein into the gut, including idiopathic inflammatory bowel disease, Whipple's disease, and celiac sprue, but is most severe in primary or secondary intestinal lymphangiectasia. Thrombocytosis has been noted in celiac sprue, as a result of associated hyposplenism, and also in Whipple's disease and ulcerative colitis, in which the cause is unclear.

OTHER BLOOD TESTS

Abnormal serum electrolyte concentrations commonly accompany diarrheal diseases. If stool fluid losses are isotonic, serum Na^+ does not change unless losses are replaced with hypotonic solutions, causing hyponatremia. Hypernatremia develops if there is proportionally more water than Na^+ lost in the stool, as may occur in osmotic diarrhea caused by laxative abuse. Hypokalemia is a common manifestation of diarrheal diseases regardless of cause and may predispose the patient to systemic alkalosis. Hypokalemia may be out of proportion to the severity of diarrhea in patients with a history of chronic laxative abuse or with villous adenomas of the distal colon. If fecal loss of base (usually bicarbonate) is excessive, acidosis develops; if cation loss is out of proportion to bicarbonate loss, alkalosis develops. Low serum calcium, magnesium, and zinc concentrations may reflect increased fecal losses of these cations and are seen in severe, protracted malabsorption associated with massive resection, extensive Crohn's disease of the small intestine, and severe celiac sprue. Low serum calcium concentration may also reflect the hypoalbuminemia of exudative enteric protein loss or severely compromised nutrition.

Table 33-1. Some hematologic abnormalities in intestinal diseases

Test	Cause of increased level	Cause of decreased level
Hematocrit	Dehydration due to diarrhea	Bleeding from ulceration in idiopathic or infectious enterocolitis, neoplasm, vascular abnormalities, impaired coagulation of blood Malabsorption of iron, folate, and/or vitamin B_{12} Drug-induced hemolysis (sulfasalazine)
Neutrophils	Infectious enterocolitis Diverticulitis Appendicitis Idiopathic inflammatory bowel disease Other infections	Drug-induced marrow suppression (sulfasalazine, azathioprine, antineoplastic drugs)
Eosinophils	Eosinophilic gastroenteritis Selected parasitic infestations	
Lymphocytes		Intestinal lymphangiectasia and other causes of protein-losing enteropathy
Platelets	Celiac sprue Idiopathic inflammatory bowel disease Whipple's disease	Drug-induced marrow suppression (sulfasalazine, azathioprine, antineoplastic drugs, etc.)
Prothrombin activity		Malabsorption of vitamin K associated with impaired fat absorption

In severe protein-losing enteropathy, levels of several serum proteins are usually decreased (albumin and globulins, including transferrin). If only the albumin is decreased, poor nutrition, malabsorption without excess protein loss, or associated liver disease is more likely. Hypogammaglobulinemia is associated with or may predispose to several gastrointestinal ailments, including giardiasis, nodular lymphoid hyperplasia, intraluminal bacterial overgrowth, and, rarely, celiac sprue and idiopathic inflammatory bowel disease. Hence quantitative determination of serum immunoglobulin levels is useful in the evaluation of malabsorption and/or protracted diarrhea. Serum globulin levels may be elevated in intestinal inflammatory diseases or in malignant disease of the intestine or colon if protein-losing enteropathy is not associated. Serum immunoglobulin A (IgA) antigliadin and IgA antiendomysial antibody levels are useful screening tests for celiac sprue but are not sufficiently sensitive or specific to replace intestinal mucosal biopsy in establishing the diagnosis.

In intestinal malabsorption, serum cholesterol concentration is usually decreased; serum carotene concentration is also depressed, but the latter is of diagnostic value only if there has been recent ingestion of carotene-containing nutrients. Because vitamin K is fat soluble, the prothrombin time may be prolonged but should become normal after parenteral administration of vitamin K preparations. Serum alkaline phosphatase concentration may be increased in protracted malabsorption, reflecting osteopenic bone disease.

Low serum iron and ferritin levels commonly accompany diffuse mucosal lesions of the proximal intestine (celiac sprue, Whipple's disease) or chronic blood loss (idiopathic inflammatory bowel disease, neoplasm). Low serum folate levels may also reflect mucosal malabsorption or the use of drugs, such as sulfasalazine, that interfere with folate absorption. Low serum vitamin B_{12} levels may accompany ileal disease or resection or luminal bacterial overgrowth in the small intestine.

Determination of serum levels of certain hormones, including gastrin, vasoactive intestinal polypeptide (VIP), somatostatin, calcitonin, and thyroxine, may be useful in the evaluation of protracted diarrhea and/or malabsorption. Some gastrinomas are manifested by severe diarrhea and malabsorption in the absence of ulcer disease (Chapter 38). Excessive delivery of H^+ to the duodenum impairs intraluminal fat digestion and may cause diffuse damage to the mucosa of the proximal small intestine. VIP-secreting tumors also cause severe diarrhea but no steatorrhea. However, the sensitivity and specificity of serum VIP levels in diagnosis are suspect; serum levels do not correlate well with tumor mass, and elevated VIP levels have been noted in other diarrheal conditions such as laxative abuse. Somatostatin-secreting tumors produce diarrhea and steatorrhea by inhibiting pancreatic exocrine secretion. Calcitonin levels may be elevated in medullary carcinoma of the thyroid, which may cause severe diarrhea. Hyperthyroidism and hypoparathyroidism may induce diarrhea and mild to moderate malabsorption; therefore thyroid and parathyroid function should be evaluated in patients with unexplained diarrhea and malabsorption.

STUDIES OF THE STOOL AND URINE

There is no substitute for careful inspection of the patient's stool by the physician. Patients' descriptions of their feces are subjective and can be notoriously inaccurate. In our bowel-conscious society, one person's diarrhea may be another's constipation. In addition to assessing stool consistency, the physician should note the presence or absence of blood, mucus, or melena. Stool caliber should also be assessed, although the irritable colon syndrome causes narrow, pencil-like stools far more frequently than does colorectal carcinoma. The steatorrheic stool may be loose or formed but is bulky, pale, and greasy and has a characteristic rancid odor. Examination of a stool sample for occult blood should be an integral part of all complete physical examinations. Currently, the guaiac-impregnated paper slide test (Hemoccult) provides the most satisfactory compromise among convenience, sensitivity, and specificity. Ideally, patients should remain on a high-bulk diet free of rare red meat, peroxidase-rich vegetables such as turnips, and large amounts of vitamin C for 2 days, and three to six stools should be examined. HemoQuant, a test that detects heme-derived porphyrins in stools, appears to be highly sensitive and specific but is more expensive and less convenient than guaiac-impregnated paper slide tests.

Microscopic examination of methylene blue or Wright's stain of stool suspensions or anal or rectal swabs for polymorphonuclear leukocytes is of substantial value in the differential diagnosis of acute and chronic diarrhea (Table 33-2). Careful examination of stool and rectal mucus or exudate for ova and parasites may provide a rapid and unequivocal diagnosis but requires a knowledgeable examiner. For example, fecal leukocytes are often mistaken for amebic trophozoites by the inexperienced observer, although methylene blue staining minimizes such errors. Administration of antacids, enemas, or recent barium contrast studies of the intestine may preclude identification of offending ova and parasites for up to 10 days.

The Sudan stain of stool is a simple, rapid, inexpensive, and relatively sensitive screening test for steatorrhea that

Table 33-2. Association of pus cells in stool in some diarrheal diseases

Pus cells abundant	Pus cells absent or scarce
Salmonella enterocolitis	Viral gastroenteritis
Shigellosis	Enterotoxic *E. coli* infection
Campylobacter enterocolitis	*Vibrio cholerae* infection
Amebic colitis	Staphylococcal gastroenteritis
Invasive and cytotoxic *Escherichia coli* enterocolitis	*B. cereus* gastroenteritis
C. difficile–induced enterocolitis	Hormone-induced diarrhea
Idiopathic ulcerative colitis	Long-term laxative abuse
Crohn's enterocolitis	Celiac sprue

can easily be done by the physician in 3 to 4 minutes. A small amount of stool is homogenized on a glass slide, mixed with a few drops each of glacial acetic acid and Sudan III in ethanol, covered, heated to boiling, and examined while still warm. Some fat is present in normal feces, but the size and number of fat droplets are excessive in patients with steatorrhea. Because colonic bacteria rapidly hydrolyze triglycerides to free fatty acids, staining for neutral fat without prior acid hydrolysis is of limited value in differentiating impaired intraluminal digestion from impaired intestinal absorption. The presence of meat muscle fibers, identified by their cross striations, in fecal suspensions suggests maldigestion.

The definitive test for steatorrhea is the cumbersome quantitative determination of fat in 3 day pooled stool collections. Ideally, the patient should be placed on a known fat intake (usually 80 to 100 g) for a 2 day equilibration period, and the diet should be continued during the 3 day collection period. Excretion of more than 6% to 9% of ingested fat connotes steatorrhea. The collection must be complete and should be refrigerated to retard bacterial breakdown of long-chain fatty acids; nonabsorbable fats such as castor oil and mineral oil must not be ingested.

Protein-losing enteropathy is documented by determination of the clearance of alpha-1-antitrypsin from serum into stool. Obviously, gastrointestinal bleeding elevates alpha-1-antitrypsin clearance and the results must be interpreted with caution even in patients whose stools are hemoccult positive.

Determination of stool volume, electrolytes, and osmolarity is helpful in distinguishing secretory from osmotic diarrhea. In secretory diarrheas (VIP- or calcitonin-secreting tumors), stool volume usually exceeds 1 liter per 24 hour period, and stool osmolarity should be approximately twice the concentration of stool $Na^+ + K^+$. In osmotic diarrheas (maldigestion and malabsorption of ingested food, osmotic laxation, or severe lactase deficiency), stool osmolarity is substantially greater than twice the sum of stool $Na^+ + K^+$. When the patient with secretory diarrhea has fasted for 24 to 48 hours, diarrhea persists; osmotic diarrhea will cease when the offending, poorly absorbed solute is not ingested. Appearance of a pink color on alkalinization of diarrheal stool is indicative of ingestion of phenolphthalein-containing laxatives.

Stool cultures are, of course, crucial in the diagnosis of specific bacterial enterocolitides. Special efforts must be made to isolate recently recognized organisms such as *Escherichia coli* 0157:H7, *Aeromonas,* and *Plesiomonas* if the clinical picture is compatible with infections caused by these agents. Examination of the stool for *C. difficile* toxin is valuable in the assessment of diarrhea associated with antibiotic ingestion.

Urinary excretion of 5-hydroxyindole acetic acid and of histamine is increased in carcinoid syndrome and mastocytosis, respectively. Alkalinization of urine, like that of stool, may detect phenolphthalein abuse. Tests are also available for the detection in the urine of senna and bisacodyl and are useful in suspected laxative abuse.

ORAL ABSORPTION TESTS

Oral absorption tests are useful in the evaluation of chronic diarrhea and/or suspected malabsorption. The D-xylose absorption test helps distinguish malabsorption caused by impaired intraluminal digestion from malabsorption caused by small intestinal mucosal disease. After ingestion of a 25 g dose of D-xylose by a well-hydrated, fasting adult, 5 g or more is normally excreted in the urine in 5 hours, whereas blood levels reach 25 mg per deciliter 2 hours after the test dose. Because D-xylose requires no intraluminal digestion, low urinary excretion or blood levels suggest mucosal disease such as celiac sprue. An exception may occur in patients with bacterial overgrowth in the proximal intestine, because some strains of enteric bacteria metabolize D-xylose, although a mucosal lesion may also accompany bacterial overgrowth. The test is not foolproof; delayed gastric emptying, impaired renal function, urinary retention, and sequestration of D-xylose in ascites and edema may decrease urinary excretion. Instillation of D-xylose directly into the proximal intestine through a tube overcomes the vagaries of gastric emptying and increases the specificity of the test. The glucose tolerance test is not as useful as the D-xylose absorption test. Although blood glucose levels may fail to increase normally after an oral glucose load in patients with mucosal disease, the glucose tolerance test is insensitive and nonspecific in assessing malabsorption, because glucose metabolism may influence blood glucose levels. The lactose absorption test, like the lactose breath test (see later discussion), is of value in screening for intestinal lactase deficiency, although biochemical determination of mucosal lactase activity in biopsy tissue is more definitive. When a normal, fasting subject ingests 50 g of lactose, blood glucose should increase 20 to 30 mg/dl in the ensuing 2 hours. Pitfalls include delayed gastric emptying and abnormal glucose metabolism. The lactose absorption test does not distinguish between primary and secondary lactase deficiency.

Because the mechanism of vitamin B_{12} (cobalamin) absorption is unique (Chapter 28), B_{12} absorption tests are useful in evaluating intestinal function. Urinary excretion of radiolabeled vitamin B_{12} should be measured after its oral administration alone and with administration of intrinsic factor (IF). In patients with pernicious anemia or severe exocrine pancreatic insufficiency, free vitamin B_{12} is malabsorbed, but there is nearly normal absorption of IF-B_{12} complex in the absence of intestinal disease. In patients with (1) resection of the ileum, (2) severe infiltrative ileal disease, and (3) intraluminal bacterial overgrowth, absorption of both free B_{12} and IF-B_{12} is abnormal. Because there is substantial storage of vitamin B_{12} in the liver, abnormal B_{12} absorption study results often precede the appearance of low vitamin B_{12} blood levels by several years.

BREATH TESTS

Several breath tests are used to screen for steatorrhea, bacterial overgrowth, ileal disease, and lactase deficiency. The ^{14}C-cholylglycine breath test screens for bacterial overgrowth and impaired ileal absorption of conjugated bile salts. Normally, ^{14}C-cholylglycine is absorbed by the ileum and recycled via the enterohepatic circulation. In patients with bacterial overgrowth, the labeled glycine is removed by deconjugation in the lumen of the small intestine, absorbed, and metabolized, resulting in increased $^{14}CO_2$ excretion in the breath. In ileal disease, ^{14}C-cholylglycine enters the colon and is metabolized by colonic bacteria, again resulting in increased $^{14}CO_2$ excretion in the breath. To assess lactose malabsorption, 12.5 to 25.0 g of lactose is given to a fasting adult and breath hydrogen is quantitated. If lactose absorption in the small intestine is impaired, colonic bacteria ferment the lactose, releasing H_2 that is absorbed and excreted in the breath in excessive amounts. Lactulose, which is not absorbed, and glucose have been used as test substances, and breath H_2 is then measured to assess for bacterial overgrowth in the small intestine. Both lack sensitivity or specificity when compared to the gold standard, culture of jejunal contents. Measurement of breath $^{14}CO_2$ after ingestion of ^{14}C-D-xylose has been reported to be useful for detecting small intestinal bacterial overgrowth, but the test substance is not generally available.

Test substances labeled with the stable isotope ^{13}C in which breath $^{13}CO_2$ is quantitated with mass spectroscopy have been developed. These tests require sophisticated instruments. They do not expose patients to radioactivity and can be used without risk in children and pregnant women.

RADIOLOGIC STUDIES

Relevant radiologic findings for specific diseases are described in chapters dealing with those diseases, but a few principles will be emphasized here. Much can be learned from careful study of plain supine and erect or cross-table lateral films of the abdomen in patients with abdominal pain, vomiting, or diarrhea. Distention of only the small bowel with gas-fluid levels suggests mechanical obstruction of the small bowel. Distention of both small intestine and colon most often reflects ileus but may represent colonic obstruction with an incompetent ileocecal sphincter. Colonic distention in the absence of small bowel distention suggests a distal colonic obstruction with a competent ileocecal sphincter (Chapter 44). Nodularity or irregularity of the mucosal surface in distended colon suggests ischemic disease or inflammatory disease of the bowel wall. Linear streaks of air in the bowel wall suggest the possibility of necrosis produced by ischemia or inflammation (Chapter 46).

Barium contrast studies of the small intestine are a useful part of the evaluation of diarrhea, malabsorption, chronic abdominal pain, and alimentary tract bleeding of unknown cause. In malabsorption and diarrhea, diffusely thickened, coarse mucosal folds suggest infiltrative disease such as celiac sprue, eosinophilic enteritis, Whipple's disease, or amyloidosis. If the barium becomes less radiopaque as it progresses distally, net intestinal secretion of fluid is likely and may occur in a number of conditions, including celiac sprue, secretory diarrheas, or small intestinal obstruction. More localized mucosal defects may reflect inflammatory bowel disease (Crohn's disease, tuberculosis), neoplasm (lymphoma, carcinoid), or intramural bleeding caused by trauma or defective hemostasis. Enteroclysis, a technique in which barium and a radiolucent substance such as carboxymethylcellulose are instilled by tube into the small intestine, provides elegant contrast views of the mucosal surface and may show neoplasms and other mucosal abnormalities not apparent in routine barium contrast studies.

The barium enema is a valuable technique in the diagnosis of diseases of the colon and distal ileum. Indeed, retrograde reflux of barium into the ileum is often more sensitive for detecting distal ileal abnormality than barium administered orally. Utilization of air-contrast techniques greatly improves the sensitivity and specificity of the barium enema, increasing the detection rate for small neoplasms.

Viewing of the blood supply to the small and large intestines by angiography is of great value in defining sites of intestinal blood loss if the patient is bleeding 1 ml or more per minute (Chapter 34). If a bleeding site cannot be seen, candidate lesions such as vascular malformations, vascular neoplasms such as carcinoid or smooth muscle tumors, or vasculitis may be found, although such lesions may not prove to be the site of bleeding. It is particularly important to identify the site of blood loss in patients with suspected colonic diverticular bleeding. Such bleeding may occur from any portion of the colon; the origin is often not apparent at operation, and intra-arterial perfusion of vasopressin or embolization may control the bleeding. Angiography may be of diagnostic value in patients with suspected mesenteric ischemia, mainly to exclude occlusive lesions if the need for surgery is not obvious (Chapter 46). Occasionally, vascular endocrine cell tumors of the pancreas or small intestine are first detected angiographically in patients with unexplained severe diarrhea.

The specialized imaging techniques, abdominal ultrasound and computed tomography (CT), are of limited value in detecting intrinsic diseases limited to the small and large intestines. They are, however, of great value in detecting mass lesions and thickening of the bowel wall that may accompany primary intestinal disease. Examples include paraenteric and paracolonic abscesses that may be associated with Crohn's disease, diverticulitis, appendicitis, and neoplasms. Abdominal ultrasound and CT scanning are of substantial value in detecting pancreatic disease, which often enters into the differential diagnosis of patients with abdominal pain and/or diarrhea and malabsorption. Mesenteric, retroperitoneal, or intrahepatic metastases arising from primary intestinal malignancies can also be detected by these imaging techniques and by magnetic resonance imaging (MRI).

Scanning with technetium pertechnetate is of value in detecting Meckel's diverticula, which may present clinically as painless intestinal bleeding or mimic closely acute appendicitis. Scintiscanning with technetium sulfur colloid or technetium-labeled autologous erythrocytes can detect and localize intestinal bleeding that is not sufficiently brisk to be visualized angiographically. Unlike angiography, it does not permit definition of vascular abnormalities or concomitant therapeutic intervention (Chapter 34). Localized intra-abdominal abscesses contiguous with diseased intestine can be detected by gallium scanning or indium-labeled leukocyte scanning. Either procedure may complement abdominal ultrasound and CT scanning, especially in the absence of localizing physical findings.

ENDOSCOPY AND BIOPSY

The value of endoscopy in the evaluation of patients with alimentary tract symptoms is discussed in detail in Chapter 30. Upper gastrointestinal endoscopy is useful in defining the nature of localized disease of the duodenum, for it permits viewing of the lesions and directed biopsy of discrete lesions such as neoplasms and duodenal Crohn's disease. Enteroendoscopes for evaluating visually the length of the small intestine are still in the developmental stage.

Proctosigmoidoscopy is of enormous value in evaluating diseases that may involve the rectosigmoid, be they inflammatory, infectious, or neoplastic. It should be one of the first studies performed to evaluate diarrhea of unknown cause or lower intestinal bleeding. Seeing the mucosa often provides clues to the cause of diarrhea, and lesions can be readily subjected to biopsy. Mucosal exudate obtained at sigmoidoscopy is ideal for culture and microscopic examination for ova, parasites, and leukocytes. *Proctosigmoidoscopy is not performed often enough; it is necessary for virtually all patients in whom a barium enema radiographic examination is indicated.* The rectum, which is the site of much disease, is often poorly visualized by barium enema. Moreover, perforation, the most common serious complication of barium enema, may result from enema tip

Information provided by mucosal biopsy of small intestine

I. Disorders in which biopsy result is diagnostic: diffuse lesions
  A. Whipple's disease
    1. Lamina propria infiltrated with PAS-positive macrophages
    2. Characteristic bacilli in mucosa
  B. *Mycobacterium avium-intracellulare* enteritis: similar to Whipple's disease but bacilli are acid fast
  C. Severe immunoglobulin deficiency
    1. Mucosal architecture from normal to flat
    2. Plasma cells absent or markedly diminished in lamina propria
    3. Giardia trophozoites often present
  D. Abetalipoproteinemia
    1. Mucosal architecture normal
    2. Lipid-laden absorptive cells appear vacuolated

II. Disorders in which biopsy result may be diagnostic: patchy lesions
  A. Intestinal lymphoma
    1. Villi widened, shortened, or absent
    2. Malignant lymphoma cells in lamina propria and submucosa
  B. Intestinal lymphangiectasia
    1. Mucosal architecture normal
    2. Dilated lymphatics in lamina propria and submucosa
  C. Eosinophilic enteritis
    1. Mucosal architecture from normal to flat
    2. Patchy infiltration of lamina propria with eosinophils and neutrophils
  D. Mastocytosis
    1. Mucosal architecture from normal to flat
    2. Patchy infiltration of lamina propria with mast cells, eosinophils, and neutrophils
  E. Amyloidosis
    1. Mucosal architecture normal
    2. Amyloid in lamina propria and submucosa shown with Congo red stain
  F. Crohn's disease
    1. Mucosal architecture variable
    2. Noncaseating granulomata and inflammation in lamina propria and submucosa
  G. Giardiasis
    1. Mucosal architecture from normal to flat
    2. Trophozoites in lumen and on surface of absorptive cells
    3. Minimal to severe inflammation in lamina propria
  H. Coccidiosis
    1. Villi shortened
    2. Crypts hyperplastic
    3. Coccidial forms on surface of (cryptosporidosis) or within *(Isospora)* absorptive cells
    4. Inflammation of lamina propria

III. Disorders in which biopsy result is abnormal but not diagnostic
  A. Celiac sprue
    1. Villi shortened or absent
    2. Crypts hyperplastic
    3. Severe absorptive cell damage
    4. Inflammation of lamina propria
  B. Unclassified sprue: indistinguishable from celiac sprue
  C. Tropical sprue
    1. Mucosal architecture from nearly normal to flat mucosa (as in celiac sprue)
    2. Absorptive cell damage mild
    3. Inflammation of lamina propria
  D. Viral gastroenteritis: indistinguishable from mild to moderate tropical sprue lesion
  E. Intraluminal bacterial overgrowth: may be normal or indistinguishable from mild to moderate tropical sprue lesion
  F. Folate and/or B_{12} deficiency, acute radiation enteritis
    1. Shortened villi
    2. Hypoplastic crypts
    3. Megalocytic epithelium
    4. Diminished mitoses
    5. Inflammation of lamina propria

trauma or inflation of a balloon catheter in the presence of rectal disease (neoplasm, severe colitis). If the radiologist is aware of rectal disease that has been demonstrated at proctosigmoidoscopy, such perforations can often be prevented. If a biopsy of diseased rectosigmoid is obtained at the time of sigmoidoscopy, the barium enema should be done with extreme caution or, if possible, delayed for 4 to 7 days to allow healing of the biopsy site.

The substantial value of colonoscopy and mucosal biopsy of the large intestine in the diagnosis and treatment of colorectal disease is described elsewhere. (See Chapter 30 and chapters in which specific diseases are discussed.)

Mucosal biopsy of the small intestine is particularly valuable (see box) in the evaluation of patients with malabsorption and/or chronic diarrhea. Biopsy specimens can be obtained with forceps at the time of endoscopy or with dedicated suction biopsy tubes that are localized fluoroscopically. Each technique has advantages and disadvantages. Tube biopsy retrieves larger, less traumatized samples than those obtained with forceps. The biopsy tubes can readily be passed into the distal duodenum or proximal jejunum, avoiding Brunner's glands, which can confound interpretation by distorting mucosal architecture. Biopsy specimens obtained at endoscopy permit visualization of the esophagus, stomach, and proximal duodenum and facilitate sampling of focal lesions. Both techniques are safe, provided blood coagulation defects, if present, are corrected. Samples obtained with either technique should be oriented before fixation and then sectioned parallel to the plane of the villi to facilitate interpretation.

A few diseases are characterized by diffuse involvement of the proximal intestinal mucosa with a specific lesion. Examples include Whipple's disease and abetalipoproteinemia. Normal biopsy results in patients with intestinal symptoms virtually exclude these diseases from diagnostic consideration. Other diseases may have specific histologic abnormalities but may involve the proximal intestine in a patchy fashion. Examples include intestinal lymphoma, eosinophilic enteritis, and intestinal lymphangiectasia. Positive biopsy findings are immensely valuable, but negative findings do not exclude these illnesses, because normal mucosa adjacent to diseased mucosa may have been sampled. Other diseases are characterized by mucosal histologic abnormalities that are not specific. Examples are celiac sprue, tropical sprue, and viral gastroenteritis. Biopsy in such conditions, although not diagnostic, is still of great value, because it establishes the presence of mucosal disease unequivocally. The definitive diagnosis is then established by additional studies or by evaluation of response to specific therapy. The key abnormalities found in specific mucosal diseases are summarized in the box on p. 381.

MANOMETRIC STUDIES

Study of small intestinal and colonic motility is technically difficult and generally is available for diagnostic assessment in centers where it is also used investigatively. On the other hand, manometry of the anorectal sphincter and rectum is more commonly available and is of significant value in the assessment of chronic constipation and anal incontinence (Chapters 26 and 41).

REFERENCES

Ahlquist DA et al: Fecal blood levels in health and disease: a study using HemoQuant. N Engl J Med 312:1422, 1985.

Corazza GR et al: The diagnosis of small bowel bacterial overgrowth: reliability of jejunal culture and inadequacy of breath hydrogen testing. Gastroenterology 98:302, 1990.

Craig RM and Atkinson AJ, Jr: D-Xylose testing: a review. Gastroenterology 95:223, 1988.

Eherer AJ and Fordtran JS: Fecal osmotic gap and pH in experimental diarrhea of various causes. Gastroenterology 103:545, 1992.

Khouri MR et al: Sudan stain of fecal fats: new insight into an old test. Gastroenterology 96:421, 1989.

Lappas JC and Maglinte DDT: Enteroclysis: a technique for examining the small bowel. Crit Rev Diagn Imaging 30:183, 1990.

Perera DR, Weinstein WM, and Rubin CE: Small intestinal biopsy. Hum Pathol 6:157, 1975.

Schneider A et al: Value of the ^{14}C-D-xylose breath test in patients with bacterial overgrowth. Digestion 32:86, 1985.

Strygler B et al: α_1-antitrypsin excretion in stool in normal subjects and in patients with gastrointestinal disorders. Gastroenterology 99:1380, 1990.

Trier JS: Intestinal malabsorption: differentiation of cause. Hosp Pract 23(5):195, 1988.

Wright TL and Heyworth MF: Maldigestion and malabsorption. In Sleisenger MS and Fordtran JS, editor: Gastrointestinal, disease, ed 4. Philadelphia; 1989, WB Saunders, 263.

CLINICAL SYNDROMES AND SPECIFIC DISEASE ENTITIES II

CHAPTER

34 Gastrointestinal Bleeding

Gregory L. Eastwood

Throughout most of the gastrointestinal tract, the lumen of the gut is separated from the capillary blood supply by only a single layer of epithelial cells. Thus even minor injury to the epithelial lining may result in gastrointestinal bleeding.

Gastrointestinal bleeding ranges in severity from acute massive hemorrhage to chronic, intermittent, or nearly inconsequential blood loss. For the purposes of the following discussion, however, gastrointestinal bleeding is categorized as acute or chronic.

ACUTE GASTROINTESTINAL BLEEDING

Gastrointestinal bleeding is generally classified as either upper or lower in origin (Tables 34-1 and 34-2) because its source is only rarely in the "middle," that is, in the jeju-

Table 34-1. Diagnostic considerations in acute upper gastrointestinal bleeding and their relative frequencies

Diagnostic consideration	Relative frequency
Nasal or pharyngeal bleeding	Rare
Hemoptysis	Rare
Esophagitis	Occasional
Esophageal varices	Common
Esophageal carcinoma	Occasional
Esophagogastric mucosal tear (Mallory-Weiss syndrome)	Common
Esophageal rupture (Boerhaave syndrome)	Rare
Gastric erosions	Common
Gastric ulcer	Common
Gastric varices	Common
Gastric or duodenal neoplasms (carcinoma, lymphoma, polyps)	Occasional
Gastric mucosal vascular ectasia associated with cirrhosis	Occasional
Duodenitis	Occasional
Duodenal ulcer	Common
Anastomotic ulcer	Occasional
Submucosal neoplasms (leiomyoma, most common)	Occasional
Vascular-enteric fistula (usually from an aortic aneurysm or graft)	Occasional
Hemobilia	Rare

Table 34-2. Diagnostic considerations in acute lower gastrointestinal bleeding and their relative frequencies

Diagnostic consideration	Relative frequency
Hemorrhoids	Common
Anal fissure	Occasional
Proctitis	Common
Inflammatory bowel disease	Common
Infectious enterocolitis	Occasional
Carcinoma of the colon	Occasional
Rectal or colonic polyps	Occasional
Diverticulosis	Common
Ischemic colitis	Common
Radiation colitis	Occasional
Angiodysplasia	Common
Amyloidosis	Rare
Meckel's diverticulum	Occasional
Brisk bleeding from an upper gastrointestinal source	Occasional
Vascular-enteric fistula	Rare
Antibiotic-associated colitis	Rare

num or ileum, and also because the presenting symptoms and signs frequently are characteristic of either an upper or lower gastrointestinal source. Although diagnostic methods and specific therapies may differ for upper and lower gastrointestinal bleeding, the principles of initial management of all patients with acute gastrointestinal bleeding are the same (Fig. 34-1). The orderly sequence of history taking, physical examination, diagnostic evaluation, and treatment frequently is readjusted to meet immediate demands, and the important aspects of each step often commingle in the first critical moments of managing the acutely bleeding patient.

Initial management

History. Vomiting of red blood (hematemesis) or of dark material that looks like coffee grounds usually signifies a source of bleeding above the ligament of Treitz. Conversely, passage from the rectum of red blood (hematochezia) or of a dark, mahogany-colored stool is usually a sign of lower gastrointestinal bleeding. An important exception is the upper gastrointestinal lesion that bleeds profusely, such as ruptured esophageal varices or a bleeding peptic ulcer, in which a large volume of blood passes rapidly through the intestines and appears dark red or bright red at the anus. Stools may remain positive for occult blood for up to 12 days after an acute loss (1 liter or more) of blood from an upper gastrointestinal source. Passage of black stool (melena) usually indicates a loss of over 1 dl of blood from an upper gastrointestinal source, although bleeding from a source as low as the right colon occasionally can result in melena.

It may be important to determine whether the patient has a condition that could bleed, such as peptic ulcer disease, ulcerative colitis, diverticulosis, or polyposis. Cirrhotics may have vascular ectasias of the gastric mucosa and, of course, varices. However, this type of information sometimes is misleading. For example, more than half of acutely bleeding patients with known esophageal varices have another lesion in the upper gastrointestinal tract.

Recent ingestion of aspirin or other nonsteroidal antiinflammatory drugs or alcohol raises the possibility that gastric erosions may be the cause of upper gastrointestinal bleeding. With respect to lower gastrointestinal bleeding, knowledge of the patient's age makes certain diagnoses much more likely than others. The four most common causes of lower gastrointestinal bleeding in patients aged 60 and over are diverticulosis, ischemic bowel disease, angiodysplastic lesions of the colon, and carcinoma. None of these diagnoses is common in the young patient, in whom colonic polyps, ulcerative colitis, Crohn's disease, and enteric bacterial and parasitic bowel disease are more likely.

The physician should always inquire about concomitant illness. If the patient has known heart, liver, renal, or other serious disease, that information may be valuable in guiding medical and, if necessary, surgical decisions during the management of gastrointestinal bleeding.

Physical examination. The cardiovascular response to acute blood loss is manifested by changes in blood pressure and pulse rate. As the patient loses intravascular volume, cardiac output and blood pressure fall as a result of decreased venous return, and pulse rate increases. If, when the patient sits from a supine position, the pulse rate increases more than 20 beats per minute and the systolic blood

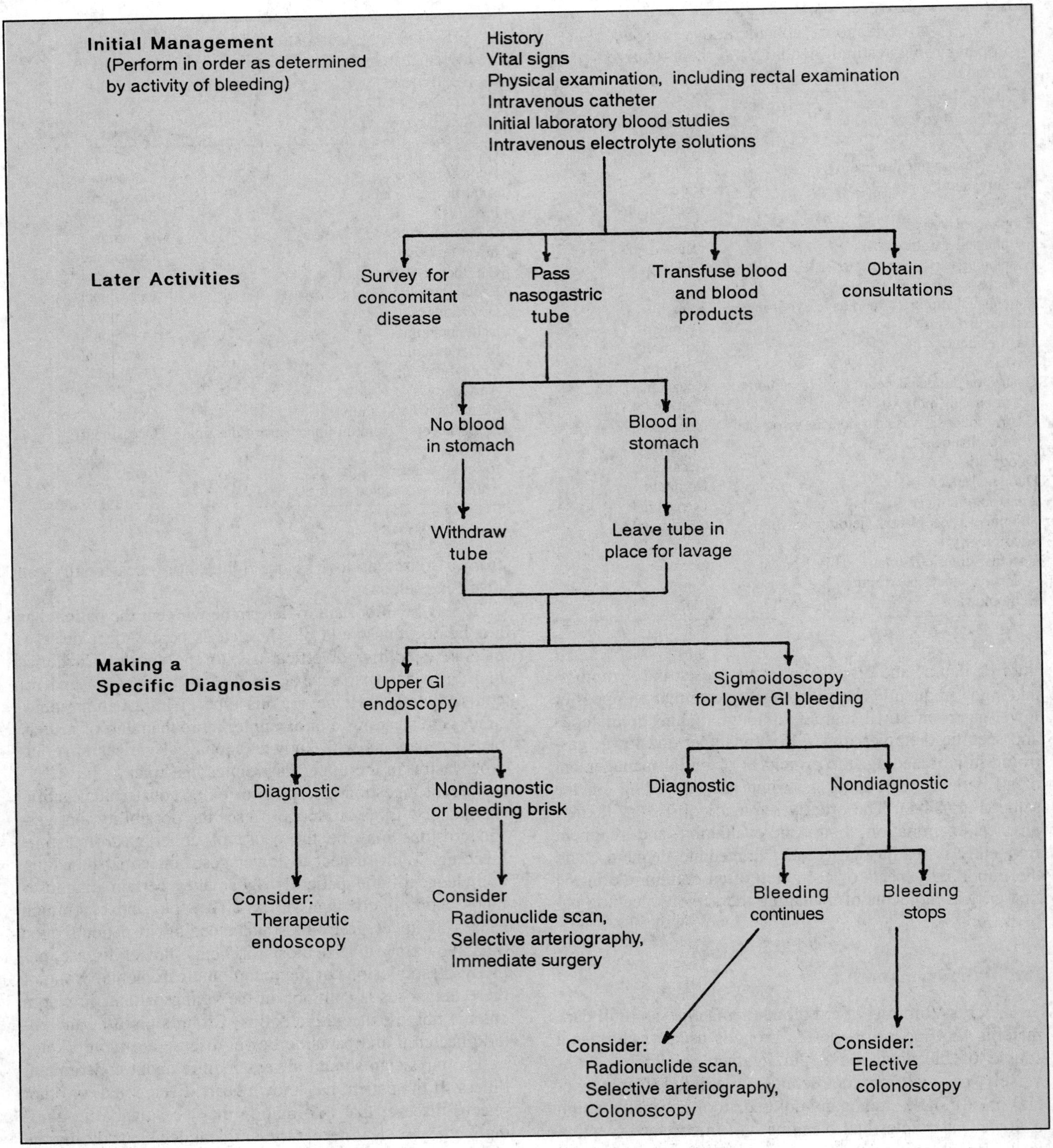

Fig. 34-1. Management of acute gastrointestinal bleeding.

pressure drops more than 10 mm Hg, it is likely that blood loss has exceeded 1 liter. Peripheral vasoconstriction may produce the typical "cold and clammy" extremities of the patient with major abrupt blood loss, and pallor of the conjunctivae, mucous membranes, nailbeds, and palmar creases may be seen.

The precise cause of bleeding is unlikely to be evident during the physical examination. Nevertheless, a mass in the abdomen, an abdominal bruit, or the physical signs of chronic liver disease may provide relevant information. The rectal examination provides direct access to the gastrointestinal tract and should not be omitted even in instances of seemingly obvious upper gastrointestinal bleeding. Aside from the information that can be gained about the anus, perianal area, and possible rectal masses, the character of the stool can be confirmed. If the patient has vomited blood or "coffee-grounds" material, yet the stool is brown or even if it contains no occult blood, bleeding may have been of brief duration.

Volume and blood replacement. A large-bore (14 to 16 gauge) intravenous catheter should be inserted promptly into a peripheral vein. Blood can be drawn at this time for laboratory studies (see later discussion). The catheter is then connected to normal saline solution, which is allowed to infuse rapidly until blood for transfusion, usually in the form of packed red cells, is available. Electrolyte solutions and clotting factors also may be necessary.

A single peripheral intravenous catheter may not be sufficient to provide adequate blood replacement in a profusely bleeding patient. In such instances, two or more venous catheters are needed, one of which should be placed in a central vein such as the jugular or subclavian. A central venous pressure catheter may also be necessary to evaluate the effects of volume replacement and the need for continued infusion of blood, particularly in elderly patients or in patients with cardiovascular disease. Finally, monitoring urine output provides a reasonable indication of vital organ perfusion.

Nasogastric intubation and gastric lavage. Blood from an esophageal or gastric source pools in the stomach, and in more than 90% of bleeding duodenal ulcers, it refluxed across the pyloric channel into the stomach. A nasogastric tube should be passed in all patients with acute gastrointestinal bleeding, unless the source is obviously the lower gastrointestinal tract. If the aspirate is clear or clears readily with lavage, the physician may elect to remove the nasogastric tube. If there is fresh blood or a large amount of old blood or retained material, the stomach should be lavaged by means of a large-bore sump tube or an Ewald tube in which additional side holes have been cut. Emptying the stomach facilitates subsequent endoscopy and may contribute to hemostasis by allowing the gastric musculature to contract.

The duration of nasogastric intubation must be individualized. Nasogastric intubation is usually uncomfortable and may predispose the patient to gastroesophageal reflux and aspiration. Moreover, the tube may irritate the esophagogastric junction and the gastric mucosa, creating mucosal artifacts and aggravating existing lesions. This may make accurate interpretation difficult at the time of endoscopy. Nasogastric tubes are used to identify the presence of and monitor the rate of upper gastrointestinal bleeding, to lavage and decompress the stomach, and to remove gastric acid. When these objectives are not important, the nasogastric tube should be removed.

Laboratory studies. Hemoglobin and hematocrit are usually low, and their level may have some relation to the degree of blood loss. However, some patients bleed so rapidly that there is not sufficient time for the blood volume to equilibrate, and the hemoglobin and hematocrit are normal or only slightly reduced. In the acutely bleeding patient, changes in blood pressure and pulse and direct evidence of massive bleeding are better indicators than hemoglobin and hematocrit for replacement of blood and administration of electrolyte solutions.

A low mean cell volume may mean that the patient is iron deficient and that the duration of blood loss has been prolonged. Elevated mean cell volume may indicate folate or vitamin B_{12} deficiency and raises the possibility of ethanol abuse, chronic liver disease, gastric cancer in association with pernicious anemia, or regional enteritis involving the terminal ileum.

Clotting status should be assessed with platelet count, prothrombin time, and partial thromboplastin time. If a defect in clotting exists, prompt correction of the deficiency is crucial. Extensive transfusion dilutes platelets and clotting factors, particularly factors V and VII. This problem can be treated by infusion of fresh-frozen plasma and platelets as necessary. Also, a high proportion of patients who bleed while taking therapeutic anticoagulants do so from a clinically significant lesion. Thus it is important to evaluate these patients for gastrointestinal abnormality in addition to correcting their clotting status.

Acute gastrointestinal bleeding may be associated with leukocytosis but usually not in excess of 15,000 per cubic millimeter. However, the physician should not attribute leukocytosis to acute blood loss without first seeking sources of infection.

Elevated blood urea nitrogen (BUN) level in a patient whose concentration has recently been normal or whose serum creatinine concentration is normal may indicate upper gastrointestinal bleeding if the site of bleeding is not apparent initially. The rise in BUN concentration results from digestion of blood in the small intestine and absorption of nitrogenous products. In contrast, impaired renal blood flow produced by hypovolemia usually causes an increase in both BUN and serum creatinine concentration. In patients with marginal liver function, the increased protein load from the hemoglobin in blood may be sufficient to induce hepatic encephalopathy. Thus gastric lavage and control of the bleeding are also important in these patients.

Because of rapid fluid shifts during gastrointestinal bleeding and subsequent infusion of blood, blood products, and other fluids, frequent assessment of serum electrolyte, calcium, and magnesium levels is necessary. In severely ill patients, arterial blood gases should be monitored.

The team approach. The appropriate management of acute gastrointestinal bleeding typically involves a team of physicians. Specific diagnostic studies, discussed later, usually require the expertise of a gastroenterologist or a radiologist. Furthermore, a surgeon who has been involved with the patient from the outset is in a much better position to make a decision regarding operative intervention.

Diagnostic and therapeutic studies

After the patient with acute gastrointestinal bleeding has been stabilized, specific diagnostic studies can be undertaken to identify the source of bleeding (Figs. 34-1, 34-2, and 34-3). Some diagnostic procedures, such as endoscopy and arteriography, also have therapeutic capabilities.

Endoscopy. (See also Chapter 30.) Endoscopy usually is recommended as the initial diagnostic procedure in patients with acute upper gastrointestinal bleeding because knowledge of a specific diagnosis may dictate a specific treatment regimen. For example, treatment of bleeding esophageal varices (see later discussion) is different from treatment of peptic ulcer, gastric erosions, or a Mallory-Weiss mucosal tear of the esophagogastric junction. Furthermore, the endoscopic identification of the so-called stigmata of recent hemorrhage (SRH) within an ulcer crater may have some prognostic and therapeutic significance. SRHs include a protruding visible vessel, an adherent clot, a black slough, and actual oozing or spurting of blood. Patients with SRH are more likely to have uncontrolled bleeding or recurrent bleeding and to require intervention by therapeutic endoscopic methods or by surgery.

The hope of endoscopists for decades has been not only to diagnose bleeding lesions of the gastrointestinal tract but also to treat them effectively, when appropriate, via the endoscope. Recently, that hope has been realized in several areas. Injection sclerotherapy of esophageal varices is as effective as or better than surgical procedures, such as portosystemic shunts and esophageal transection, in controlling acute variceal bleeding. The question remains whether sclerotherapy improves survival. With regard to endoscopic treatment of bleeding ulcers (Table 34-3), (1) multipolar electrocoagulation, laser photocoagulation, and injection of sclerosants or epinephrine all appear to be capable of controlling acute bleeding; (2) laser photocoagulation and electrocoagulation may reduce the need for emergency surgery and improve survival; (3) laser therapy is the most difficult to learn, whereas injection therapy is the least difficult; and (4) injection therapy appears to be the safest and the least expensive.

Because bleeding from upper gastrointestinal lesions stops spontaneously in 75% to 90% of patients, endoscopic treatment should not be used indiscriminately. In general, patients with actively oozing or spurting ulcers are candidates for endoscopic treatment. Most endoscopists would also treat a visible vessel, and, although this is controversial, some would even advocate dislodging an adherent clot to apply their method of endoscopic hemostasis. In all instances, the application of endoscopic therapy is dependent on accessibility. Thus some bleeding ulcers, particularly those within the duodenum, are in positions that are not readily amenable to endoscopic treatment.

The initial diagnostic procedure for acute lower gastrointestinal bleeding is proctosigmoidoscopy, using either a rigid or a flexible instrument. This procedure should be performed while the patient is bleeding actively to maximize the chance of making a diagnosis (Fig. 34-3). If the site of bleeding is not identified in the rectum, at least the appearance of the blood can be assessed.

The role of fiberoptic colonoscopy in massive lower gastrointestinal bleeding is not well defined. Some endoscopists advocate that an emergency colonoscopy be performed after cleaning the colon with osmotically balanced electrolyte solutions (e.g., Golytely) or saline solution, administered orally or by nasogastric tube. Others prefer initial selective arteriography, saving colonoscopy as an elective procedure.

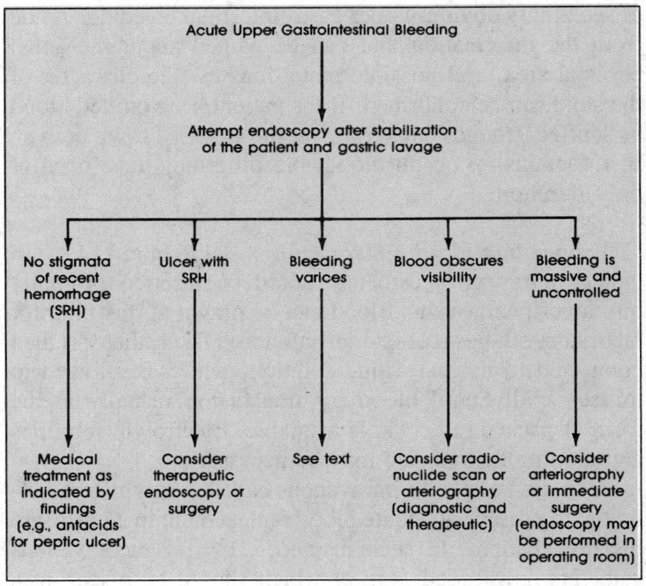

Fig. 34-2. Scheme for the diagnostic evaluation of acute upper gastrointestinal bleeding. Stigmata of recent hemorrhage are a visible vessel, fresh blood clot, black slough, and active bleeding. GI, gastrointestinal.

Selective arteriography. Selective arteriography of the celiac axis, superior mesenteric artery, inferior mesenteric artery, or their branches can be both diagnostic and therapeutic. A focal collection of extravasated dye indicates a bleeding arterial lesion. For this to occur, it has been estimated from animal studies that the rate of blood loss must be at least 0.5 ml per minute (750 ml/day). In hemorrhagic gastritis, a diffuse blush in the region of the stomach may appear. During the venous phase, esophageal, gastric, or small intestinal varices may be seen, although actual variceal bleeding usually cannot be documented by arteriography.

Infusion of vasopressin, 0.1 to 0.5 unit per minute into the artery supplying the bleeding site, has been effective in controlling arterial bleeding (Fig. 34-4). Diffuse hemorrhagic gastritis has been treated successfully by vasopressin infusion into the left gastric artery. Even variceal bleeding may be controlled by vasopressin infusion into the superior mesenteric artery, thereby diminishing splanchnic blood flow and reducing portal venous pressure. Infusion of vasopressin into a peripheral vein at a rate of 0.3 to 1.2 units per minute has been shown to be as effective as intra-arterial vasopressin infusion in the control of bleeding from esophageal varices, and the frequencies of cardiovascular side effects after peripheral and arterial vasopressin infusion are similar. The ease of administering

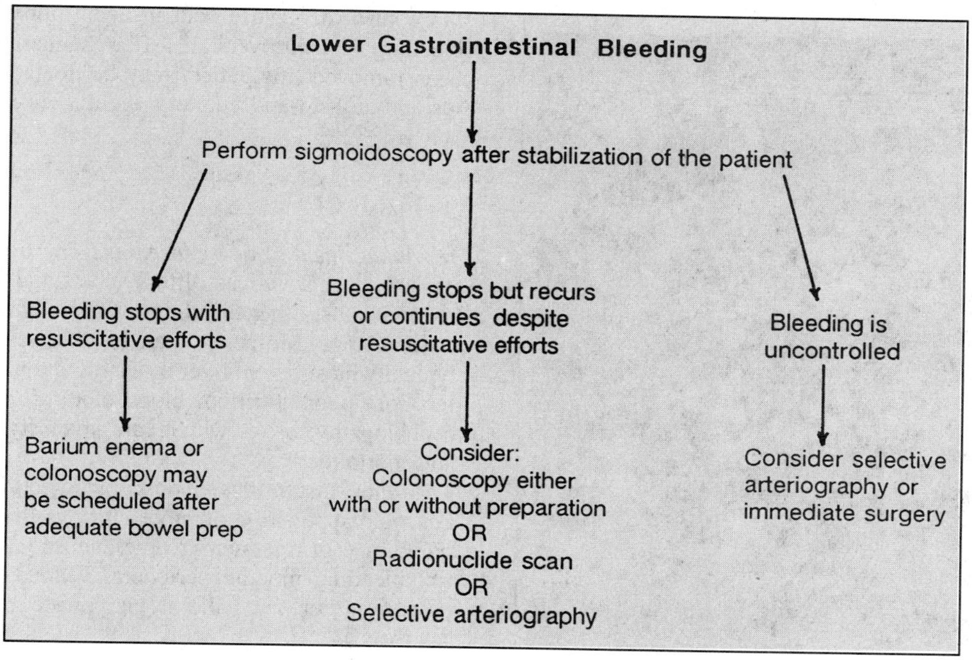

Fig. 34-3. Scheme for the diagnostic evaluation of acute lower gastrointestinal bleeding.

Table 34-3. Endoscopic treatment of bleeding ulcers

	Electrocoagulation	Laser photocoagulation	Injection therapy
Control of bleeding	Yes	Yes	Yes
Reduction in need for surgery	Yes	Yes	?
Reduction in mortality	Yes	Yes	?
Difficulty to learn	Intermediate	Most	Least
Safety	Intermediate	Least	Most
Expense	Intermediate	Most	Least

vasopressin peripherally makes it an early therapeutic choice in bleeding varices. Venous infusion of nitroglycerine may reduce the hazard of vasopressin in patients at risk for ischemic cardiovascular disease. Injection of autologous clot or small pieces of gel foam to embolize arteries supplying localized bleeding sites also has controlled bleeding in diverticulosis, angiodysplasia, and occasionally peptic ulcer disease.

Radionuclide scanning. Scanning the abdomen after intravenous injection of sulfur colloid or red blood cells labeled with ^{99m}Tc may indicate the site of bleeding and lead to more definitive diagnostic or therapeutic procedures. The radionuclide scan appears to be more sensitive than selective arteriography in detecting active bleeding because a positive scan result requires a lower rate of bleeding (0.1 ml/min versus 0.5 ml/min). However, the radionuclide scan is considerably less specific than arteriography in locating the site of bleeding.

Barium contrast radiography. Barium contrast studies of the upper or lower gastrointestinal tract usually are not recommended in the initial diagnostic evaluation of patients with acute gastrointestinal bleeding. Such studies have a lower diagnostic yield than endoscopic methods, and barium in the stomach or intestine can hinder endoscopic visualization and render an arteriogram uninterpretable.

Antacids and antisecretory agents

The reduction of intragastric acid in patients with upper gastrointestinal bleeding is helpful in two ways. First, the direct harmful effects of acid and pepsin on the bleeding site are diminished. Second, a less acid environment promotes platelet aggregation and clotting.

After the acute bleeding has abated and gastric lavage is no longer necessary, an appropriate initial regimen is administration of 30 ml of antacid by nasogastric sump tube every 2 hours. The tube is clamped for the first hour and

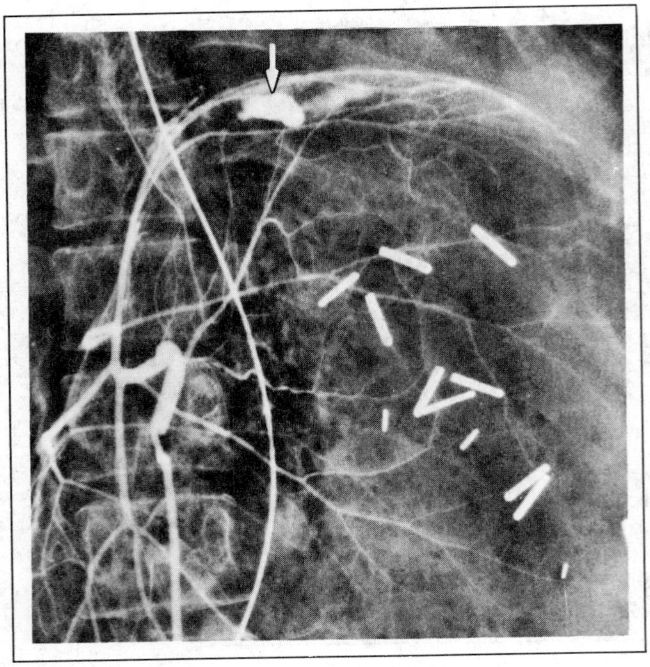

A

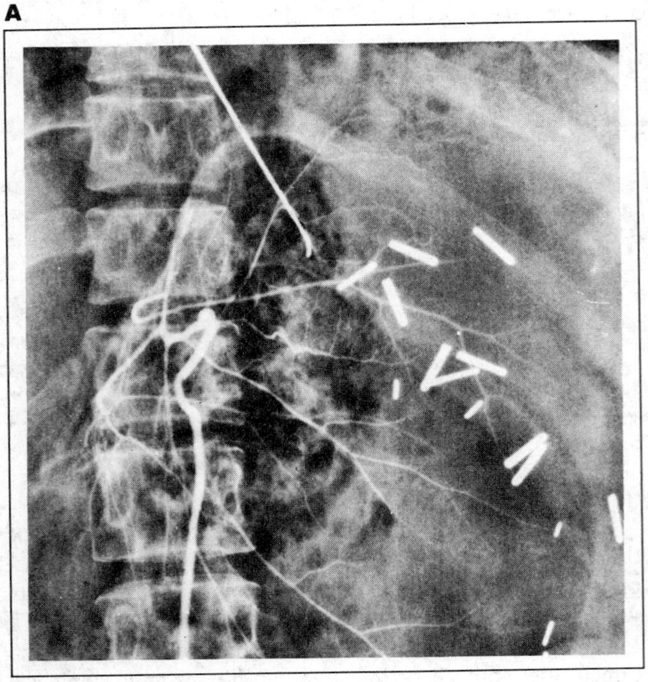

B

Fig. 34-4. Selective arteriogram from a woman with acute upper gastrointestinal hemorrhage. Endoscopy revealed a gastric ulcer of the fundus. **A,** Extravasation of dye in the fundus of the stomach (arrow). **B,** Infusion of vasopressin into the left gastric artery at 0.2 U per minute has resulted in a cessation of bleeding, manifested by disappearance of the extravasated dye. (Arteriograms courtesy of Frederick Keller, MD.)

suctioned for the second hour. Measurement of intragastric pH just before the next antacid dose indicates whether the frequency and dose of antacid should be increased. The intent is to maintain the intragastric pH above 4. Whether intravenous H_2 antagonists are as efficacious as antacids for the control of gastric acid in acute upper gastrointestinal bleeding is controversial. After the nasogastric tube has been removed, the patient may be treated with oral antacids and an acid-antisecretory agent.

Treatment of bleeding esophageal varices (See also Chapter 56)

Management of acute bleeding. The treatment of bleeding esophageal varices differs substantially from the treatment of most other bleeding lesions of the upper gastrointestinal tract. Moreover, patients with esophageal varices typically have severe liver disease and thus are likely to suffer from poor nutrition, blood clotting disorders, and encephalopathy, all of which can adversely affect morbidity and mortality.

In most institutions, endoscopic injection sclerosis or endoscopic application of rubber **0** rings (banding) is the initial choice of treatment. Some endoscopists prefer to control bleeding first by peripheral venous vasopressin (discussed earlier) or balloon tamponade before attempting sclerosis.

The triple-lumen Sengstaken-Blakemore tube is the prototype of several tubes that can compress gastroesophageal varices by balloon tamponade. One lumen is used to evacuate the stomach. The second and third lumens lead to the gastric and esophageal balloons, respectively. Some newer tubes have a fourth lumen that allows suction of blood and secretions from the esophagus. If the fourth lumen is not present, an accessory sump tube should be passed alongside the Sengstaken-Blakemore tube into the midesophagus.

If not used properly, the Sengstaken-Blakemore tube may terminate more lives than it saves! Prolonged or excessive compression of the mucosa by the balloons can cause ischemic necrosis. Also, because inflation of the gastric balloon obstructs the esophagogastric junction, secretions and blood from above can accumulate in the esophagus and may be aspirated into the lungs. Finally, the tube assembly itself may ride up in the esophagus to occlude the airway. Appropriate use of the Sengstaken-Blakemore tube, as described by Pitcher, minimizes these risks.

Because the surgical mortality is so high in patients with bleeding esophageal varices, emergency surgery (postacaval anastomosis or esophageal transection and reanastomosis) is an unwelcome last resort in the treatment of acute variceal bleeding.

Long-term management. After acute variceal bleeding has been controlled by endoscopic injection sclerosis, balloon tamponade, or vasopressin infusion, a decision regarding long-term management of the varices must be made because the risk of rebleeding is high. Beta-blockade therapy to reduce portal hypertension in patients with mild liver disease and little or no ascites may be effective. However, because enthusiasm for beta blockade has waned and long-term survival of some patients may be increased after either chronic endoscopic sclerosis or portasystemic shunt surgery, most patients should be considered for one of those treatments. The risk of encephalopathy is lower and the risk of rebleeding is higher in sclerosed patients than in shunted patients, but the short- and long-term survival and total health care costs are about the same with both methods of treatment. Chronic endoscopic sclerosis, consisting of repeated injections separated by 1 to 4 weeks, is a reasonable first choice. Complications include perforation of the esophagus, mucosal ulceration and necrosis, and stricture formation. Preliminary studies suggest that repeated banding of varices until they are obliterated may be associated with fewer complications. Patients who have recurrent variceal bleeding despite sclerotherapy or banding and are acceptable operative risks may benefit from portasystemic shunt surgery.

CHRONIC GASTROINTESTINAL BLEEDING

Most lesions that cause acute bleeding also can cause chronic bleeding from the gastrointestinal tract. Chronic bleeding usually is slow and may be intermittent, sometimes making diagnosis difficult.

If the history and physical examination do not strongly suggest an upper gastrointestinal site of bleeding, the usual first diagnostic study is a colonoscopy. When colitis is suspected, a balanced electrolyte bowel preparation or no preparation at all is preferred to a cathartic.

If no lesion of the large bowel is identified, upper gastrointestinal endoscopy should be performed to examine the esophagus, stomach, and proximal duodenum. Further evaluation is accomplished by radiologic examination of the small bowel by means of either a small bowel series or a small bowel enema (enteroclysis). The latter sometimes yields more diagnostic information than a conventional small bowel series and is performed by passing a tube by mouth into the proximal small intestine and then injecting barium and methylcellulose.

A small number of patients continue to bleed, usually intermittently, from a source that defies location, even after repeated hospital admissions. Unusual causes of bleeding must be considered in these patients, and sometimes extraordinary measures are required to make the diagnosis.

A ^{99m}Tc sulfur colloid scan may show a Meckel's diverticulum that contains gastric mucosa. Although only about 20% of Meckel's diverticula contain gastric mucosa, these are the diverticula that ulcerate and bleed. Thus a scan that reveals a Meckel's diverticulum in a bleeding patient who has no other identifiable site of bleeding is strong evidence that the diverticulum is the source.

Selective arteriography does not reveal the bleeding site by showing extravasation of dye in a chronically bleeding patient because the rate of bleeding is too slow. However, arteriography may suggest a tumor or an angiodysplastic lesion by showing an abnormal vascular pattern. Vascular lesions of the bowel, particularly in the ascending colon, are an important cause of gastrointestinal bleeding. These vascular lesions occur in all age groups but more frequently in the elderly and perhaps in patients with aortic stenosis. Arteriovenous shunts appear to develop as a normal consequence of aging, and their frequency in the asymptomatic elderly population is probably much greater than has been thought. Telangiectatic lesions anywhere within the gastrointestinal tract also may occur spontaneously, or they may be associated with hereditary telangiectasia (Osler-Rendu-Weber disease).

In some instances, obscure small intestinal lesions may be identified by passing an endoscope from above or below into the small intestine at the time of laparotomy. The surgeon advances the endoscope with ease throughout the small intestine by direct manipulation. Lesions can be visualized directly through the instrument by the endoscopist or may be transilluminated through the bowel wall and discovered by the surgeon.

Factitious gastrointestinal bleeding must be considered in some chronically bleeding patients. Self-injury, surreptitious phlebotomy, ingestion of blood, and rectal instillation of blood have all been used to simulate disease. Of such patients 90% are women, and they almost invariably have had work experience in a medically related field. Close supervision of the patient, alertness to unexplained needle marks, and a careful watch for hidden needles and syringes may suggest the diagnosis.

REFERENCES

Athanasoulis CA: Therapeutic applications of angiography. N Engl J Med 302:1117, 1174, 1980.

Burroughs AK et al: Controlled trial of propranolol for the prevention of recurrent variceal hemorrhage in patients with cirrhosis. N Engl J Med 309:1539, 1983.

Burroughs AK et al: A comparison of sclerotherapy with staple transection of the esophagus for the emergency control of bleeding from esophageal varices. N Engl J Med 321:857, 1989.

Caos A et al: Colonoscopy after golytely preparation in acute rectal bleeding. J Clin Gastroenterol 8:46, 1986.

Cello JP et al: Endoscopic sclerotherapy versus portacaval shunt in patients with severe cirrhosis and acute variceal hemorrhage: long-term follow-up. N Engl J Med 316:11, 1987.

Chojkier M et al: A controlled comparison of continuous intraarterial and intravenous infusions of vasopressin in hemorrhage from esophageal varices. Gastroenterology 77:540, 1979.

Chung SCS et al: Injection or heat probe for bleeding ulcer. Gastroenterology 100:33, 1991.

Fleischer D: Endoscopic control of upper gastrointestinal bleeding. J Clin Gastroenterol 12(suppl 2):S41, 1990.

Henderson JM et al: Endoscopic variceal sclerosis compared with distal splenorenal shunt to prevent recurrent variceal bleeding in cirrhosis: a prospective, randomized trial. Ann Intern Med 112:262, 1990.

Hui WM et al: A randomized comparative study of laser photocoagulation, heater probe, and bipolar electrocoagulation in the treatment of actively bleeding ulcers. Gastrointest Endosc 37:299, 1991.

Huizinga WK, Angorn IB, and Baker LW: Esophageal transection versus injection sclerotherapy in the management of bleeding esophageal varices in patients at high risk. Surg Gynecol Obstet 160:539, 1985.

Krejs GJ et al: Laser photocoagulation for the treatment of acute peptic-ulcer bleeding: A randomized controlled clinical trial. N Engl J Med 316:1618, 1987.

Laine L: Multipolar electrocoagulation in the treatment of active upper gastrointestinal tract hemorrhage. N Engl J Med 316:1613, 1987.

Lin HJ et al: Heat probe thermocoagulation and pure alcohol injection in massive peptic ulcer haemorrhage: a prospective, randomised controlled trial. Gut 31:753, 1990.

Markisz JA et al: An evaluation of 99mTc-labeled red blood cell scintigraphy for the detection and localization of gastrointestinal bleeding sites. Gastroenterology 83:394, 1982.

Matthewson K et al: Randomized comparison of Nd YAG laser, heater probe, and no endoscopic therapy for bleeding peptic ulcers. Gastroenterology 98:1239, 1990.

Pitcher JL: Safety and effectiveness of the modified Sengstaken-Blakemore tube: a prospective study. Gastroenterology 61:291, 1971.

Storey DW et al: Endoscopic prediction of recurrent bleeding in peptic ulcers. N Engl J Med 305:915, 1981.
Sugawa C: Injection therapy for the control of bleeding ulcers. Gastrointest Endosc 36:S50, 1990.
Wara P: Endoscopic prediction of major rebleeding: a prospective study of stigmata of hemorrhage in bleeding ulcer. Gastroenterology 88:1209, 1985.
Waring JP et al: A randomized comparison of multipolar electrocoagulation and injection sclerosis for the treatment of bleeding peptic ulcer. Gastrointest Endosc 37:295, 1991.

CHAPTER

35 Esophageal Diseases

Konrad S. Schulze-Delrieu
Robert W. Summers

Clinical problems arise commonly because of inflammation of the esophageal mucosa, tumors, or neuromuscular abnormalities that interfere with esophageal transit. Esophageal inflammation is often due to the reflux of corrosive gastrointestinal secretions and is sometimes caused by the ingestion of caustic agents or drugs. Viral or fungal infections may involve the esophagus, particularly in association with oropharyngeal or systemic infections. Esophageal dysmotility may be caused by systemic diseases that interfere with esophageal neuromuscular function (i.e., scleroderma, diabetes, Parkinson's disease) or by primary abnormalities in the intrinsic esophageal nerves and muscle (i.e., achalasia, spasm).

SYNDROMES OF CHRONIC GASTROESOPHAGEAL REFLUX AND REFLUX ESOPHAGITIS

The terms *hiatal hernia, reflux,* and *esophagitis* are often used interchangeably. The term *reflux* refers to the regurgitation of gastrointestinal contents into the esophagus without associated retching and vomiting. The contents may be gas, food, or gastrointestinal secretions. Brief episodes of reflux are common, particularly in the postprandial period, but rarely cause symptoms in healthy individuals. Abnormal reflux may manifest itself by ease of provocation (for instance, the regurgitation of gastric contents on stooping or lying down) or by frequency (for instance, the occurrence of heartburn after each meal). Long-term monitoring of esophageal pH (Chapter 31) is the best current means to document an abnormal reflux profile. *Gastroesophageal reflux disease* refers to manifestations of esophageal, laryngeal, or pulmonary injury related to the reflux of gastrointestinal contents. The most common manifestation is *reflux esophagitis;* the term should be reserved for instances in which reflux related changes in esophageal structure have been documented. Other problems in which gastroesophageal reflux disease has been implicated include dental deterioration, laryngitis, aspiration pneumonia, asthma, and interstitial pulmonary fibrosis.

Etiology and pathogenesis

The severity of gastroesophageal reflux disease depends on (1) the severity of the mechanical dysfunction, (2) the composition of the refluxate, and (3) the resistance of the target organ. Variations in these individual factors probably contribute to the development of laryngeal or respiratory tract complications from reflux in some patients in the absence of esophageal lesions.

Mechanical abnormalities. Abnormalities of lower esophageal sphincter (LES) function, of esophageal peristalsis and clearance, and of gastric motility are common in gastroesophageal reflux disease. Because the esophageal abnormalities may themselves be worsened by esophagitis and may improve as the esophagitis improves, it is at times difficult to distinguish cause from effect. In a few instances, abnormal reflux can be tracked to a specific cause such as gastric intubation, pregnancy, removal or destruction of the gastric cardia by operation, tumor, or systemic sclerosis. In some families, reflux complications occur at an early age in several individuals; it is possible that this reflux is due to an inherited defect in the antireflux barrier. An *incompetent LES* as defined by the virtual absence of a high-pressure zone and the presence of the "common cavity phenomenon" (Chapter 31) occurs in patients with scleroderma and severe esophagitis but otherwise is an inconstant finding in gastroesophageal reflux disease. Most episodes of gastroesophageal reflux occur across a competent sphincter that relaxes intermittently; the relaxation of the LES in these instances is thought to relate to inhibitory reflexes that can be triggered by gastric distention.

Esophageal clearance is impaired in many patients with gastroesophageal reflux disease. When there is significant inflammation of the esophageal mucosa, many swallows do not lead to the normal sequential contraction of the esophagus known as primary peristalsis. Swallowing ceases during sleep; combined with the horizontal position, this characteristic increases the time during which any refluxate is in contact with the esophageal mucosa.

Abnormalities of gastric emptying often compound the motility problems occurring with gastroesophageal reflux. Gastric retention from any cause aggravates reflux by increasing the volume of secretions available for reflux. Conditions that reduce the gastric storage capacity and increase postprandial intragastric pressure such as partial gastric resections also seem to increase the risk of reflux.

Corrosiveness of the refluxate. The composition of the refluxate is another determinant of injury. If the refluxate consists entirely of air and gas, the resulting belching would be considered harmless. It is also likely that neutral solutions refluxing back from the stomach would be of little importance to the esophagus but could have undesirable effects if aspirated into the respiratory tract. The hydrochloric acid and pepsin produced by the stomach are held primarily responsible for the corrosiveness of the gastric refluxate. Gastric secretions attack intercellular junctions and produce patchy, superficial lesions. Bile salts damage plasma membranes, thereby potentiating the corrosiveness of gastric secretions. Particularly severe esophageal injury can be produced by deconjugated bile salts in combination with trypsin. High gastric concentrations of bile salts have indeed been found in some patients with severe reflux esophagitis, and pancreaticobiliary secretions are held responsible for the esophageal reflux lesions that may occur in patients with achlorhydria or after total gastrectomy.

Resistance of the esophageal mucosa. The resistance of the esophagus to damage relates largely to the barrier functions of its mucosa. Important components of the barrier are (1) the glycoconjugate matrix in the extracellular space of the superficial layers of the squamous mucosa and (2) an antiport in the squamous cells that prevents cellular acidification and swelling. Alkaline mucosal and salivary secretions contribute to esophageal resistance by flushing the esophagus of residue and by neutralizing acid adherent to the esophageal mucosa. This function is impaired in the "sicca syndrome."

Indirect consequences of gastroesophageal reflux. Not all clinical manifestations of reflux are mediated by the direct exposure of tissues to the refluxate; gastroesophageal reflux stimulates esophageal nerves, which mediate reflex responses. Oropharyngeal secretions are triggered by esophageal acidification (leading to water brash). Esophageal distention and acidification lead to forceful contraction of the upper esophageal sphincter (cricopharyngeal spasm). Reflex responses as well as aspiration of refluxate are thought to be responsible for the bronchospasm, laryngospasm, and cricopharyngeal spasm that occur in some patients with gastroesophageal reflux.

Pathology of reflux esophagitis

Reflux can cause a variety of morphologic changes; acute injury is characterized by edema and necrosis, particularly of cells in the more basal layers of the squamous epithelium. The initial lesions occur in the distal esophagus; as the disease progresses, lesions spread to more proximal esophageal segments, and the distal esophagus may develop chronic changes. The major changes are (1) epithelial erosions, (2) squamous cell hyperplasia, (3) mucosal metaplasia (Barrett's esophagus), and (4) esophageal scarring (short esophagus, peptic esophageal stricture).

Esophageal erosions. Esophageal erosions are circumscribed areas of epithelial desquamation (compare Figs. 35-1 and 35-2). The mucosal blood vessels become congested, and the lamina propria and surrounding epithelium are infiltrated by leukocytes, many of which are eosinophils. Acute erosions are covered by a fibrinous exudate and have an erythematous margin. Erosions progress by involving ever-larger areas of the mucosal surface, but do not penetrate into the submucosa.

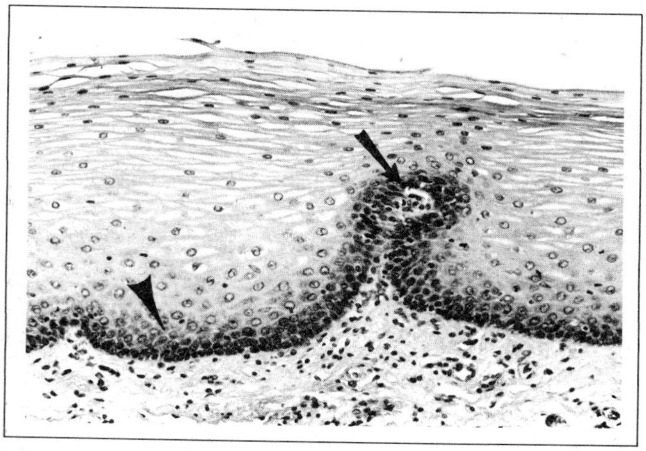

Fig. 35-1. Normal histologic appearance of the esophageal mucosa *(original magnification, ×50)*. The squamous epithelium is many layers thick and is supported by the lamina propria. Extensions of the lamina propria form papillae in the epithelium; the tips of the papillae reach about half the total epithelial height *(arrow)*. The germinative cells are recognized by their dark-staining nuclei. They are found in the basal cell layer, which contributes less than 15% of the total epithelial height *(arrowhead)*. (Photomicrograph courtesy of Frank Mitros, MD, Department of Pathology, University of Iowa.)

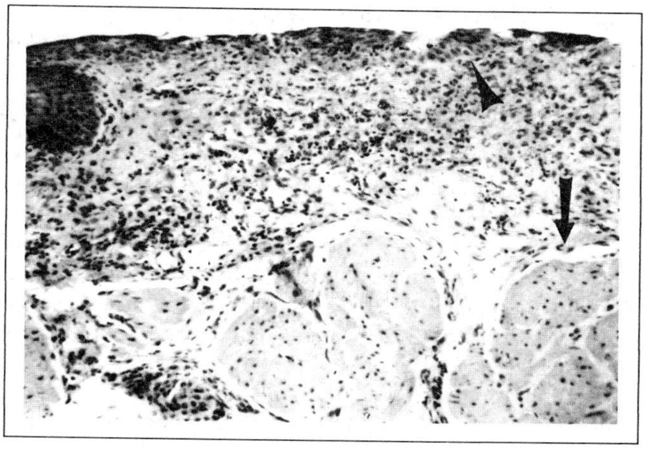

Fig. 35-2. Histologic abnormalities in reflux esophagitis *(original magnification, ×30)*. Esophageal erosion caused by esophageal reflux. Most layers of the epithelium have sloughed off, and only the basal cells remain *(arrowhead)*. The lamina propria is infiltrated by many inflammatory cells. The arrow points to the muscularis mucosae *(×100)*. (Photomicrograph courtesy of Frank Mitros, MD, Department of Pathology, University of Iowa.)

Squamous cell hyperplasia. The loss of superficial cells provokes regeneration in the basal cell layer or acanthosis (Figs. 35-3). Basal cells proliferate into the lamina propria, and the papillae remain covered only by relatively few layers of mature squamous cells. With long-standing recurrent injury, the bases of the papillae become narrow, and some papillae branch. *Epithelial hyperplasia* of the esophagus is present if the basal cells comprise more than 30% of total epithelial height and the papillae more than 75%. Precise

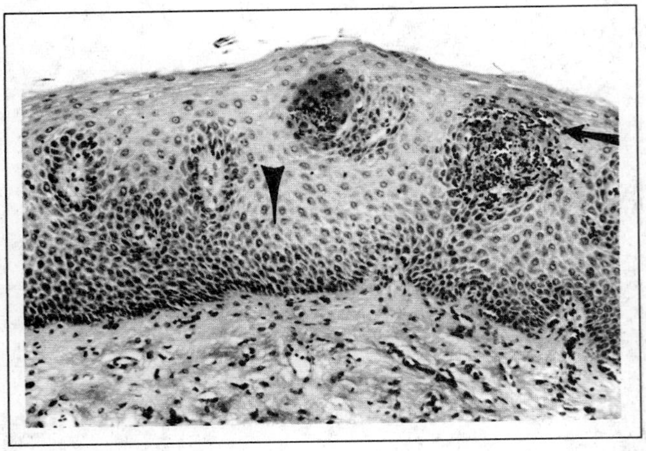

Fig. 35-3. Epithelial hyperplasia *(original magnification, ×40).* There is proliferation of basal cells *(arrowhead),* and the papillae reach through more than 75% of the total epithelial height *(arrow).* The blood vessels in the papillae are congested. (Photomicrograph courtesy of Frank Mitros, MD, Department of Pathology, University of Iowa.)

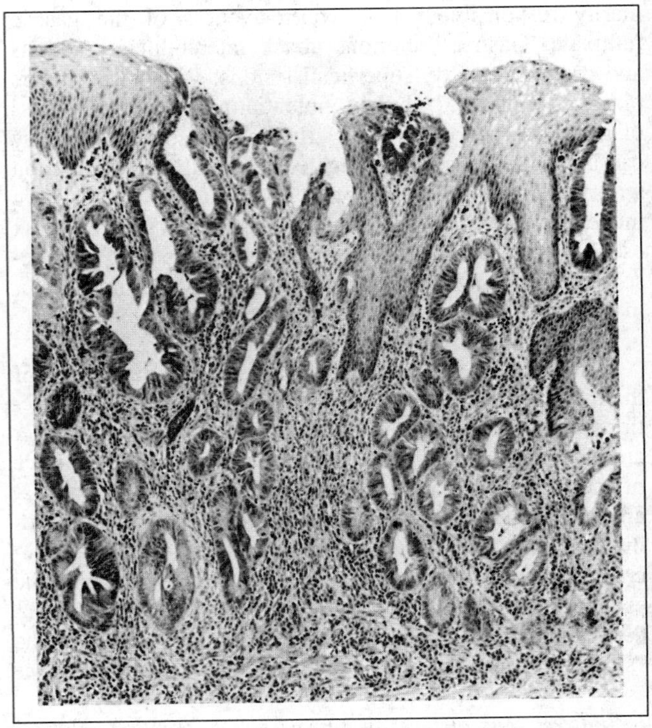

Fig. 35-4. Epithelial metaplasia *(original magnification, ×16).* The esophageal mucosa consists of columnar epithelium (Barrett's esophagus) intermixed with squamous epithelium. (Photomicrograph courtesy of Frank Mitros, MD, Department of Pathology, University of Iowa.)

diagnosis depends on the histologic examination of biopsy specimens; the diagnosis should be suspected in patients with severe heartburn whose esophageal mucosa appears grossly intact on endoscopy but shows a linear hyperemia from ectactic blood vessels.

Mucosal metaplasia (Barrett's esophagus). Replacement of the normal squamous epithelium by columnar epithelium is known as *Barrett's esophagus,* or mucosal metaplasia of the esophagus (Fig. 35-4). True peptic esophageal ulcers may develop in the metaplastic columnar epithelium. Ulcers form round-to-oval craters that reach the submucosa. Chronic injury leads to peptic esophageal strictures and may cause shortening of the esophagus. Peptic strictures are concentric and less than 1 cm long.

The most common type of epithelium in Barrett's esophagus is the so-called specialized columnar epithelium. This epithelium resembles intestinal mucosa because it forms villi and contains intestinal-type goblet cells. Less common types of metaplastic epithelium resemble the epithelium from the gastric cardia and from other parts of the stomach.

Most adenocarcinomas of the esophagus arise in metaplastic specialized columnar epithelium. Dysplasia, similar to that seen in long-standing ulcerative colitis, is thought to be the intermediate stage between metaplasia and neoplasia. It has been claimed that malignant transformation occurs in as many as 10% of all cases of Barrett's esophagus, but this reported high incidence has recently been challenged.

Clinical presentation and diagnosis

Three syndromes are associated with chronic gastroesophageal reflux: (1) chronic postprandial dyspepsia with minimal esophageal involvement, (2) erosive esophagitis, and (3) Barrett's esophagus (esophageal metaplasia). Individual syndromes may evolve one from the other during the course of the disease and overlap.

Gastroesophageal reflux with minimal esophageal changes (esophageal hypersensitivity, chronic esophagitis). Postprandial dyspepsia is a common complaint in middle-aged men and women; most have experienced heartburn and food intolerance since adolescence or early adulthood. Some patients become symptomatic especially after voluminous, greasy, or spicy meals. Epigastric pressure is often relieved by belching; thus the term *daytime bloaters*. In others, reflux symptoms may be triggered by mechanical factors, including exercise and recumbency *(night burners)*.

Acid perfusion of the esophagus (the Bernstein test) reproduces symptoms in most affected individuals (Chapter 31). LES pressure and esophageal contractions are typically normal. Increased frequency of reflux events is common during nighttime or postprandial recording periods. Endoscopic and histologic examination of esophageal mucosa shows erythema and basal cell hyperplasia only. This is the most common and least serious form of esophageal reflux disease.

Gastroesophageal reflux complicated by erosive esophagitis. Erosive esophagitis is apparently about as common as peptic ulcer disease. Many of these patients experience not simply heartburn but also high epigastric and substernal pain and regurgitation even when fasting. Dysphagia may result from muscle spasm or eventually from scarring with stricture formation. Occult blood loss is common, and severe bleeding occurs occasionally. Shortening of the esophagus with a persistent axial hiatal hernia may be present. LES pressure is low or normal, and esophageal contractions are often weak and abortive. The pH profile is severely abnormal, particularly for the increased duration of reflux periods during recumbency. The severity of esophagitis is best assessed by endoscopic examination of the longitudinal and circumferential extent of erosive changes (Plate II-1). Endoscopy is indicated in patients with dysphagia to exclude malignancy.

Gastroesophageal reflux complicated by esophageal metaplasia (Barrett's esophagus). Although most common in the middle-aged and elderly, the condition can be present in all age groups including infants. This condition manifests itself most often as dysphagia from an esophageal stricture or, less commonly, as a bleeding esophageal ulcer. The absence of heartburn despite a highly abnormal reflux profile in many of these patients may be linked to the special properties of the metaplastic epithelium.

Diagnostic studies reveal severe reflux and poor esophageal clearance. On radiographic examination, the esophagus may appear shortened, poorly distensible, and often strictured or ulcerated. Strictures are located at the junction of squamous and columnar epithelium, which is displaced proximally (thus the term *midesophageal stricture*) (Fig. 35-5, *C*). Typical erosive esophagitis with superficial ulcers is seen in the squamous mucosa proximal to this junction, whereas deep peptic "Barrett's ulcers" that resemble peptic gastric ulcers occur in the metaplastic epithelium distal to the junction. A "short esophagus" (brachyesophagus) is recognized by the formation of a permanent axial (or "sliding") hiatal hernia or by transverse mucosal folds in the distal esophagus.

Endoscopy, biopsy, and cytologic examination are essential for examination of the epithelial changes. Columnar cell metaplasia should be suspected when the esophageal mucosa is salmon-red and velvety in appearance instead of glistening smooth and pearly-pink with proximal displacement of the squamocolumnar interface. In columnar metaplasia, there is a risk of recurrent ulceration, stricture formation, and neoplastic transformation. Effective medical or operative treatment that controls reflux is thought to halt the progression of metaplasia. Yearly endoscopy with biopsy and cytologic evaluation for the early detection of dysplasia or cancer is currently recommended, although it remains to be determined whether this is cost-effective.

Treatment

Avoidance of esophageal injury is paramount. Many drugs, including calcium channel blockers, theophylline, and nitrates, may adversely affect the esophagus. Anticholinergic drugs are contraindicated in patients with gastroesophageal reflux, because they decrease LES pressure and delay gastric emptying. Abstinence from smoking and from drinking of alcohol and coffee is helpful.

Dietary and other symptomatic measures. Reduction of meal size and a diet that is low in fat, acidic foods, spices, and sweets provides relief in many patients with postprandial reflux symptoms. Taking fluids between rather than with meals is often advised. Avoidance of food or liquids for 2 hours before retiring for the night is desirable. Weight reduction is recommended in obese patients. Antacids are often helpful to alleviate heartburn or postprandial fullness. Alginic acid preparations are also popular, but their effectiveness is not established.

Postural measures. Esophageal clearance through gravity can be facilitated during sleep by elevating the head of the bed, which is best done by placing 4 to 6 inch blocks under the legs at the head of the bed; foam wedges that are long enough to elevate the entire chest can also be used. Postural measures are particularly helpful in patients with manifestations of recumbent reflux (i.e., nocturnal aspiration and cricopharyngeal spasm). Because of their inconvenience, postural measures are unlikely to be executed unless sleeping partners as well as patients understand their purpose.

Drugs

Antisecretory drugs. Antisecretory drugs (histamine H_2-receptor antagonists or proton pump inhibitors) improve the symptoms of gastroesophageal reflux and decrease the severity of esophagitis. If erosive esophagitis is documented, cimetidine (800 mg bid), famotidine (20 mg bid), or ranitidine/nizatidine (150 mg bid) should be administered for at least 3 months. Higher doses may be more effective. Omeprazole, 20 mg daily, is indicated for the treatment of severe erosive esophagitis or esophagitis refractory to other medical treatment. Favorable results can also be expected with use of the coating agent sucralfate, 1 g qid. Relapse is the rule after the drugs are discontinued. Long-term medical treatment is moderately effective and should be considered in patients with severe relapsing esophagitis or prominent nocturnal symptoms who are not candidates for operative treatment.

Gastrokinetic drugs. Gastrokinetic drugs (bethanechol, metoclopramide, cisapride) stimulate salivation, increase LES pressure, and improve esophageal clearance in the supine but not in the upright position. Nighttime dosing in conjunction with use of antisecretory or coating agents is especially indicated in conditions of nocturnal or alkaline reflux. Bethanechol may be gradually increased from 10 to 40 mg at bedtime if tolerated. Metoclopramide, 10 mg at bedtime if tolerated, is also helpful to alleviate nausea or vomiting. Cisapride, not yet available in the United States, is effective as well and does not produce the visceral cramps common with bethanechol or the dystonic reactions common with metoclopramide.

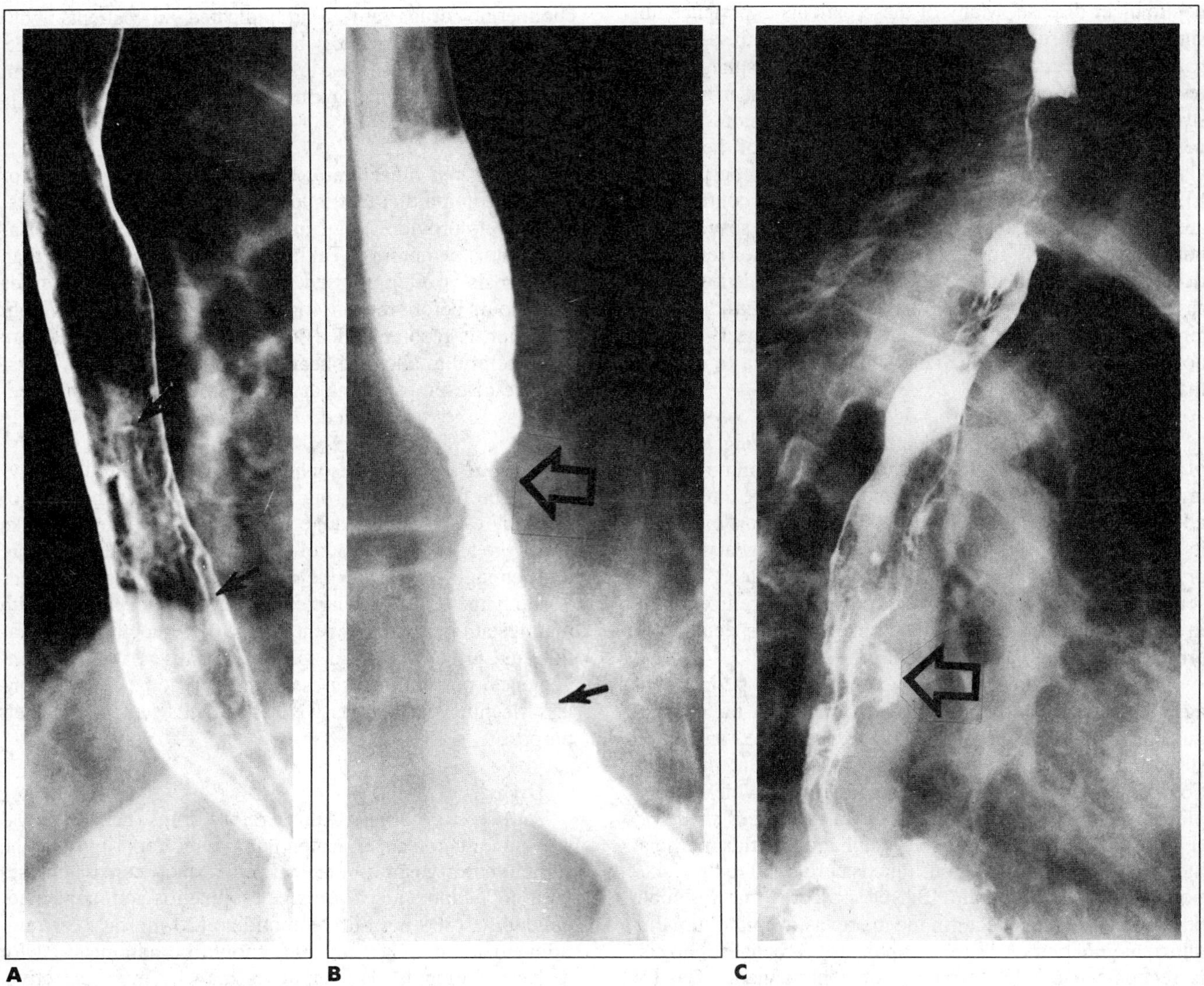

Fig. 35-5. A, Radiographic appearance of reflux esophagitis. This barium contrast study shows a linear erosion *(lower arrow)* and a circumscribed erosion *(upper arrow)*. **B,** Shortened esophagus with peptic stricture. Peptic strictures are fairly concentric, smooth, and narrow *(large arrow)*. Esophageal shortening has led to herniation of the stomach. The small arrow indicates the gastroesophageal junction. **C,** Peptic esophageal ulcer. The occurrence of an ulcer crater *(arrow)* in the esophagus is indicative of Barrett's esophageal mucosal metaplasia. (Radiographs courtesy of Charles C. Lu, MD, Department of Radiology, University of Iowa.)

Management of esophageal strictures

Any narrowing of the esophageal lumen may compromise nutrition and pose the risk of bolus impaction. Esophageal dilatation should be performed to the point where dysphagia resolves, generally at a luminal diameter in excess of 12 mm. Every attempt should be made to prevent recurrent stricture formation and to dilate strictures at an early stage.

Operative treatment

Fundoplication and similar operations can virtually eliminate gastroesophageal reflux and its symptoms. Healing of esophageal erosions and ulcerations is the rule, and strictures no longer recur. Although initial failure of the operation is rare in the hands of experienced surgeons, the likelihood of recurrent reflux increases after 5 to 10 years. Operative treatment is indicated in patients with serious complications of gastroesophageal reflux (i.e., recurrent aspiration pneumonia, peptic strictures, bleeding esophageal erosions or ulcers, and intractable symptoms) that fail to respond to rigorous medical management. Pyrosis alone may occasionally become an indication for fundoplication in patients who do not wish to depend on long-term use of acid-suppressing drugs. The use of fundoplication is controversial in patients with scleroderma and other diseases that permanently impair esophageal motility and clearance.

CHEMICAL AND PHYSICAL ESOPHAGEAL INJURY

As the first segment of the digestive tract, the esophagus is particularly prone to thermal, mechanical, and caustic injury. Drinking steaming hot beverages can produce serious esophageal injury and has caused the sloughing of entire mucosal casts. Sharp objects such as plastic or glass fragments, fish bones, or even corn chips can lacerate the esophageal mucosa or become embedded in its wall. Accidental ingestion of acids and alkalis by children and ingestion of such substances with suicidal intent by depressed persons cause severe esophageal injury. Iatrogenic esophageal injury ("pill esophagitis") results if certain drugs reside in the esophagus for an undue amount of time.

Esophageal injury from lye and related agents

Many household and industrial products such as lye contain sodium hydroxide, potassium hydroxide, ammonia, or various acids. Esophageal damage occurs in stages; in the immediate stage, liquefaction necrosis destroys the tissue and may produce perforation and mediastinitis. At the end of the first week, scarring begins as fibroblasts lay down collagen. Subsequently, mucosal re-epithelialization and scar retraction occur. Lye strictures usually develop within the first 3 months after the injury.

Ingestion typically leads to immediate burning of the mouth and attempts to spit out the material. Chest pain and odynophagia follow if the esophagus is injured. Not all patients who have ingested caustics and suffered oropharyngeal burns have esophageal or gastric lesions. The presence and the extent of esophageal and gastric lesions should be assessed by early endoscopy. The procedure is safe provided the endoscope is not advanced beyond the first caustic lesion.

If esophageal injury is present, food should be withheld and intravenous fluids administered. Antibiotics are primarily indicated for the treatment of septic complications, such as mediastinitis. Corticosteroids are often administered to prevent or reduce stricture formation, but proof of their efficacy is lacking. The best way to deal with strictures is by early detection and dilatation. Esophagograms should be made regularly between the second week and the third month after esophageal injury, and bouginage should be started as soon as a stricture is demonstrated. Caustic strictures may involve long esophageal segments and consist of dense collagen, making dilatation difficult. Long-term follow-up observation is recommended because of the risk of recurrent stricture formation and eventually esophageal cancer.

Esophageal injury caused by drugs (pill esophagitis)

Particularly when esophageal transit is delayed, bulky tablets or capsules may remain in the esophagus long enough to disintegrate and cause lesions. Patients who take pills while recumbent and without adequate liquids are at particular risk. Pills are most likely to lodge at the level of the aortic arch or the left main bronchus or proximal to the lower sphincter or an enlarged left atrium. Drug-induced esophageal lesions are manifested by sudden onset of odynophagia and retrosternal discomfort shortly after drug ingestion.

Doxycycline, other tetracyclines, and clindamycin are commonly implicated. Other responsible preparations include wax-matrix potassium chloride tablets, dental cleansing tablets, ascorbic acid, ferrous sulfate, quinidine, slow-release theophylline, and nonsteroidal anti-inflammatory agents. The acidity or alkalinity of a medication is a major factor in its caustic action. Doxycycline, tetracycline, and ferrous sulfate dissolved in water form solutions with pH values of 3.0 or less. At endoscopy, a circumscribed ulcer surrounded by normal mucosa is seen, typically in the midesophagus. Perforation and severe hemorrhage are rare. Treatment is symptomatic.

Caustic esophageal injury by drugs is preventable. Patients should always remain upright while taking tablets or capsules, and they should swallow them with adequate amounts of fluids (75 to 100 ml). Some patients prefer apple sauce or similar semisolid foods as carriers. Patients who have difficulty swallowing should be assisted into a sitting position and instructed to take sips of water even before swallowing the drug. The use of liquid preparations or crushed tablets is advisable in high-risk patients.

Radiation esophagitis

The esophagus may receive damaging doses of irradiation as part of radiotherapy for mediastinal tumors. Radiation injury is dose related but is enhanced by such chemotherapeutic agents as doxorubicin, bleomycin, and actinomycin D. Epithelial necrosis and mucosal ulceration and inflammation occur. They may be followed by superinfection with opportunistic organisms (especially candidiasis) and transmural inflammation. The mucosa becomes re-epithelialized 3 to 4 weeks after radiation is stopped. Motor abnormalities or strictures may occur months to years after the insult.

In the early stages of radiation esophagitis, patients experience odynophagia and substernal pain. Barium esophagram and esophagoscopy reveal fine serrated ulcers and edema of the mucosa. Local anesthetics, liquid diets, or parenteral fluid administration may be temporarily needed. Dysphagia occurs in the later stages because strictures form; these strictures should be dilated.

Bolus impaction and foreign bodies

Foreign bodies or poorly masticated food may become impacted in the esophagus. Infants and intoxicated or mentally ill individuals may swallow coins, pins, or batteries. At special risk for food impaction are edentoulous individuals or patients with a Schatzki's ring or other type of esophageal stricture. Patients experience substernal pain, excess salivation, and regurgitation. A chest radiograph is often sufficient to locate radiopaque objects. If the object is radiolucent, a contrast esophagram is required.

If the impaction is recent and caused by digestible food, spontaneous passage may occasionally be facilitated through the use of anticholinergic agents, glucagon, or carbonated beverages. Fiberendoscopy can be used for gentle attempts to push a digestible bolus into the stomach. If that fails, the bolus and all indigestible material should be removed with airway protection to prevent esophageal necrosis or obstruction elsewhere. To prevent recurrent impactions, patients should be evaluated and treated for any predisposing esophageal disease.

Mallory-Weiss laceration and Boerhaave syndrome

A mucosal laceration at the gastroesophageal junction leading to acute gastrointestinal hemorrhage is known as the *Mallory-Weiss syndrome*. This syndrome accounts for 5% to 15% of all upper gastrointestinal hemorrhages (Chapter 34). Severe retching and vomiting after an alcoholic binge are the most common causes of the laceration. Orogastric intubation, lifting and straining, abdominal trauma, and cardiopulmonary resuscitation have also been implicated. Most tears occur at the gastroesophageal junction. Lesions are rarely detected radiographically, and esophagoscopy is the preferred means of diagnosis.

Bleeding from Mallory-Weiss tears stops spontaneously in most cases. Endoscopic interventions (epinephrine injection or electrocautery), vasopressin infusion, or arterial embolization may obviate the need for surgical intervention in patients who cease to bleed spontaneously.

Boerhaave syndrome is an esophageal rupture caused by severe vomiting after excessive meals. Esophageal rupture can also be produced by physical trauma, including forceful epigastric compression to dislodge boluses impacted in the upper airway (Heimlich maneuver). Acute epigastric and substernal pain, dyspnea, tachycardia, cyanosis, and subcutaneous and mediastinal emphysema follow esophageal rupture. Mortality is high, even if the problem is promptly recognized and treated with surgical repair and antibiotics.

INFECTIOUS ESOPHAGITIS

Etiology and predisposing factors

Immunosuppression predisposes to esophageal infections. Those at most risk are patients with malignancies and the acquired immunodeficiency syndrome (Chapter 48) and those undergoing chemotherapy, organ transplantation, or treatment with corticosteroids. Infections also occur in patients with diabetes mellitus, after broad-spectrum antibiotic therapy, and with severe debilitating disease or advanced age. As a rule, infectious esophagitis differs by its diffuse involvement of the entire esophagus from reflux esophagitis, which leads primarily to circumscribed linear lesions of the distal esophagus.

Herpes viruses and the *Candida* fungal organisms account for most cases of infectious esophagitis. Mixed infections are common, and lesions are often secondarily infected with bacteria. In the herpes family, herpes simplex, varicella zoster, and cytomegalovirus may all cause esophagitis. Herpes simplex is commonly carried by human hosts. *Candida* species are found in the mouths of as many as 50% of normal individuals. *Candida albicans* is the most important fungal species causing esophagitis, although *C. krusei, C. tropicalis, Torulopsis glabrata,* and *Aspergillus* species have also been reported. Tuberculosis is the most common chronic bacterial infection of the esophagus; acute streptococcal infections may also involve the proximal esophagus.

Clinical and laboratory findings

The most prominent symptom is odynophagia (painful swallowing), which is often severe enough to interfere with eating and drinking. Dysphagia and substernal pain are common. Bleeding is usually absent or occult, but a few patients develop hematemesis and melena. Serious complications include esophageal obstruction, aspiration pneumonitis, esophageal perforation, and systemic dissemination.

The oropharynx should be examined for vesicles, ulcers, or thrush indicative of herpes or candidiasis. The barium esophagram typically reveals ragged mucosal ulcerations and plaques. Endoscopic examination plus mucosal biopsies, brushing, and cultures of biopsy tissue are necessary to determine the cause. Widely scattered vesicles or shallow discrete ulcers with a clean granular base and slightly raised margins are suggestive of herpes. Yellowish white pseudomembranes over shaggy hemorrhagic ulcers are suggestive of candidiasis. The endoscopic changes are not always typical, and nonspecific mucosal erythema, viability, erosions, or confluent ulcerations with exudate may be seen. Debris from either the ulcer base or the plaques often contains *Candida pseudohyphae* and other yeast forms that can be demonstrated microscopically by potassium hydroxide preparations or Gram stains from mucosal scrapings. In tissue sections, silver methenamine stains clearly demonstrate the yeast forms among desquamated epithelial cells (Fig. 35-6). The characteristic Cowdry type A inclusion, seen in cells from the margin of herpetic ulcers, is an eosinophilic intranuclear inclusion surrounded by a clear halo and a rim of chromatin. Both intranuclear and cytoplasmic inclusions occur with cytomegalovirus, and infected cells are characteristically related to blood vessels in the granulation tissue of the ulcer base. Cultures for *Candida* fail to distinguish commensals from pathogens; results of serologic tests are nonspecific. A rise in titer to complement-fixing antibody in patients with suspected herpetic esophagitis is helpful.

Treatment

Local anesthetics such as viscous lidocaine are useful to diminish odynophagia. If patients are unable to swallow, nutrition must be provided via enteral or parenteral feedings. Mild candidal esophagitis in immunocompetent patients usually responds to treatment with an oral nystatin suspen-

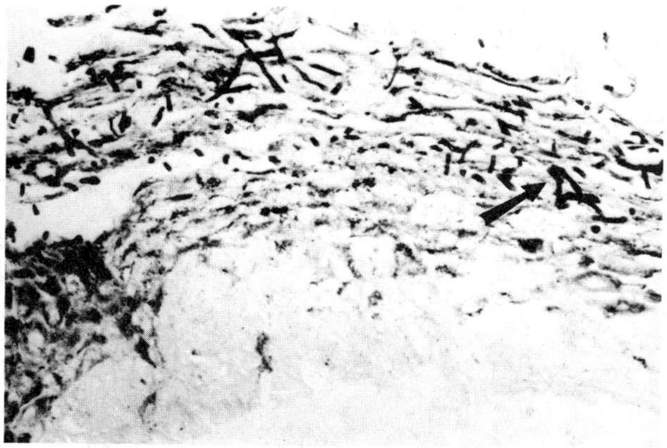

Fig. 35-6. This debris from a candidal ulcer shows mycelia stained with a silver stain *(arrow) (original magnification, ×100)*. (Photomicrograph courtesy of Frank Mitros, MD, Department of Pathology, University of Iowa.)

sion or clotrimazole lozenges. If local treatment fails, ketoconazole or fluconazole, 200 to 400 mg daily, is an alternative. In more severe infections and in systemic disease, amphotericin B in an intravenous dose of 0.3 to 0.5 mg/kg/day is effective.

Acyclovir is beneficial in systemic herpes infections and should be tried in patients with severe herpes esophagitis. In patients with mild herpes esophagitis, improvement often occurs when the immunosuppressive drug dose is reduced. Gauciclovir and foscarnet suppress cytomegalovirus esophagitis.

ESOPHAGEAL WEBS, RINGS, AND DIVERTICULA

Cervical webs and Schatzki rings

Esophageal rings and webs are thin membranous structures that cause focal narrowing of the esophageal lumen. They are a common cause of intermittent dysphagia for solids. In the cervical esophagus, single webs occur most commonly just below the cricoid muscle. They originate from the anterior wall of the esophagus opposite C6 or C7 (Fig. 35-7, *A*).

The formation of membranous webs is part of an inflammatory response. Irradiation of the esophagus can produce multiple esophageal webs. The triad of iron deficiency anemia, glossitis, and postcricoid web is known as either the *Plummer-Vinson* or the *Patterson-Kelly* syndrome. It occurs mostly in menstruating women of northern European extraction. Patients with this syndrome are at risk for developing carcinoma of the pharynx and cervical esophagus.

Mucosal diaphragms in the distal esophagus are referred to as *Schatzki* rings. They are located at the squamocolumnar junction and thus typically lie within the high-pressure zone generated by the LES and above the diaphragmatic hiatus. Rings 1.2 cm or less in diameter usually produce dysphagia, whereas those 2.0 cm or more in diameter rarely cause symptoms. Radiographic demonstration of even large diameter Schatzki rings is common if the esophagus is well distended (Fig. 35-7, *B*). Schatzki rings are easily demonstrable endoscopically if the distal esophagus is observed carefully during air insufflation (Plate II-2).

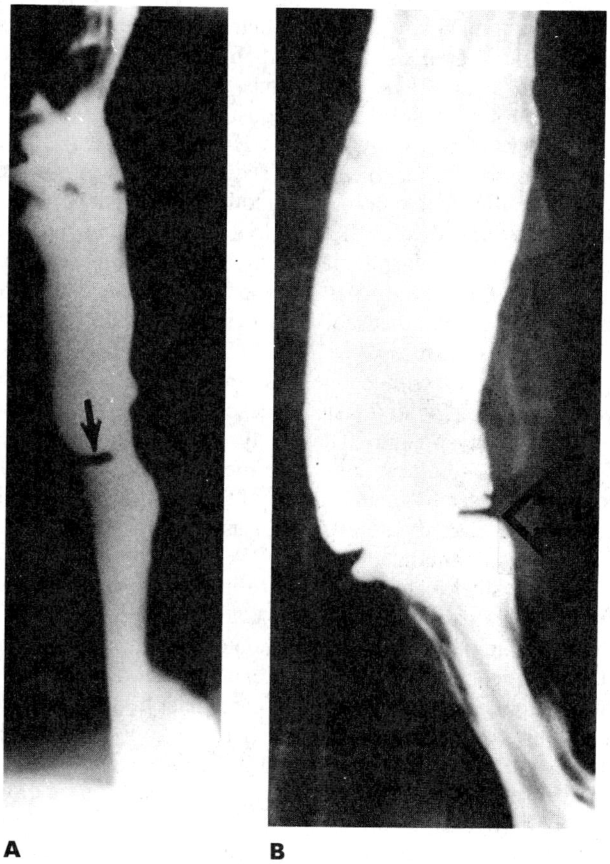

Fig. 35-7. **A,** Cervical web *(arrow)*. Cervical webs indent the lumen from the anterior esophageal wall at the level of the lower cervical spine. **B,** Schatzki ring *(arrow)* is a thin diaphragm at the gastroesophageal junction above a hiatal hernia. (Radiographs courtesy of Charles C. Lu, MD, Department of Radiology, University of Iowa.)

Symptomatic cervical webs and Schatzki rings should be dilated or ruptured with an endoscope with bougies. Iron deficiency, if present, should be treated.

Esophageal diverticula

Most esophageal diverticula are acquired and hence are more common in the elderly. Most diverticula do not contain any muscularis propria and probably form because of increased luminal pressure (i.e., they are pulsion diverticula). Esophageal diverticula are classified according to their location into (1) those occurring at the pharyngoesophageal junction (Zenker's diverticula), (2) those occurring in the vicinity of the tracheal bifurcation (midesophageal diverticula), and (3) those occurring close to the diaphragmatic hiatus (epiphrenic diverticula).

Zenker's diverticula. The muscle fibers of the pharynx and of the upper esophageal sphincter (UES) leave between them a weak area through which hypopharyngeal herniations can occur. These herniations occur most commonly on the left side, less commonly posteriorly and in the midline, and rarely on the right side. Hypertrophy of the UES is often associated with Zenker's diverticulum and is recognized radiographically as a smooth persistent indentation at the esophageal inlet. The "cricoid achalasia" syndrome is the pharyngeal dysphagia and globus sensation often observed in this setting. Hypertrophy interferes with the sphincter's compliance and hence its full opening during pharyngeal deglutition.

Most patients with Zenker's diverticula are male and 50 years or older. Patients usually describe an insidious onset of cervical dysphagia. They may regurgitate undigested food several hours or days after meals. Many patients try to empty the sac by manipulation of the neck or some bodily contortion. Patients are at risk for aspiration, and impaired nutrition is common.

On physical examination, gurgling and a lump may be found on palpation of the neck. Careful videoradiographic examination of deglutition is mandatory (Fig. 35-8). An endoscopic search for coexistent treatable lesions such as reflux esophagitis is valuable, but care must be taken to prevent perforating the diverticulum. Resection of the diverticular sac is recommended when it is more than 5 cm large and causes compression and regurgitation. Sectioning of the cricopharyngeal muscle is often added to diverticulectomy and is sometimes the only treatment needed when the diverticulum is small.

Midesophageal diverticula. Midesophageal diverticula occur over the bifurcation of the trachea. In the past they were associated with traction from inflamed mediastinal lymph nodes caused by tuberculosis or histoplasmosis. Presently, most midesophageal diverticula are associated with esophageal spasm and related motility disorders of the esophagus. Midesophageal diverticula rarely cause symptoms and should not be resected unless hemorrhage, impaction of food, or fistulization has occurred.

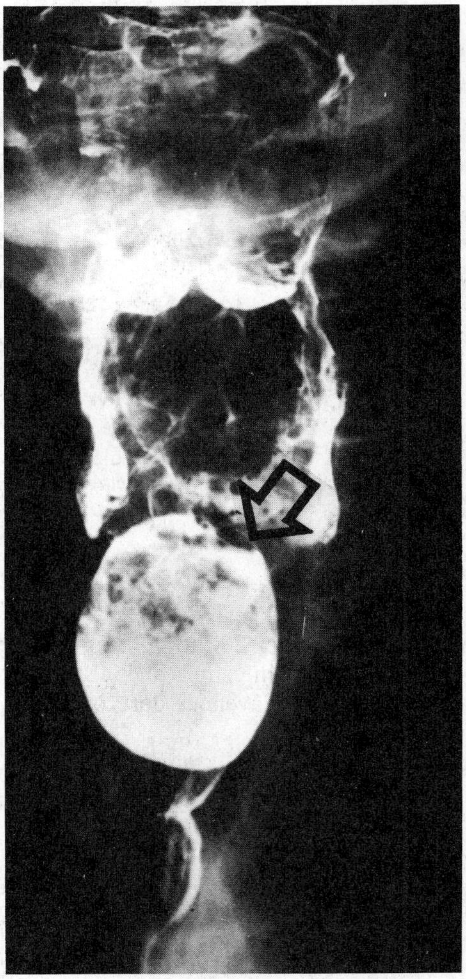

Fig. 35-8. This Zenker's diverticulum *(arrow)* is partially filled with food and impinges in the lumen of the cervical esophagus. It is in a posterior location. The most common location is left lateral. (Radiograph courtesy of Charles C. Lu, MD, Department of Radiology, University of Iowa.)

MOTILITY DISORDERS OF THE ESOPHAGUS

Achalasia

In achalasia, the LES fails to relax in response to swallowing, and the smooth muscle of the esophageal body fails to generate peristaltic contractions. Food and secretions accumulate in the esophagus. With time, the esophagus dilates and becomes tortuous. Stasis esophagitis may result, and there is an increased risk for the development of squamous cell carcinoma.

Esophageal achalasia is associated with destruction of nerve ganglia in the myenteric plexus of the esophagus. In South America, megaesophagus occurs as a consequence of infection by *Trypanosoma cruzi* (Chagas' disease), but in other parts of the world the cause is usually unknown. Occasionally, infiltrating carcinomas or lymphomas produce an achalasialike syndrome.

Achalasia presents at any age. Occurrence in members of the same family has been described, but most cases are isolated and idiopathic. Patients note dysphagia with both solids and liquids; they often swallow air and go through the Valsalva maneuver to empty their gullet. A substernal pressure sensation and weight loss are common. Chest pain is rarely severe. Regurgitation and aspiration dominate the clinical presentation in some patients.

Radiographic examination characteristically shows absence of the gastric air bubble and a long concentric narrowing at the gastroesophageal junction, with a variable degree of dilatation and elongation of the esophagus (Fig. 35-9). Poor clearance of barium paste, when the patient swallows in the supine position, is also characteristic. Esophageal manometry is helpful; the resting pressure of the LES is normal or high; swallows fail to produce com-

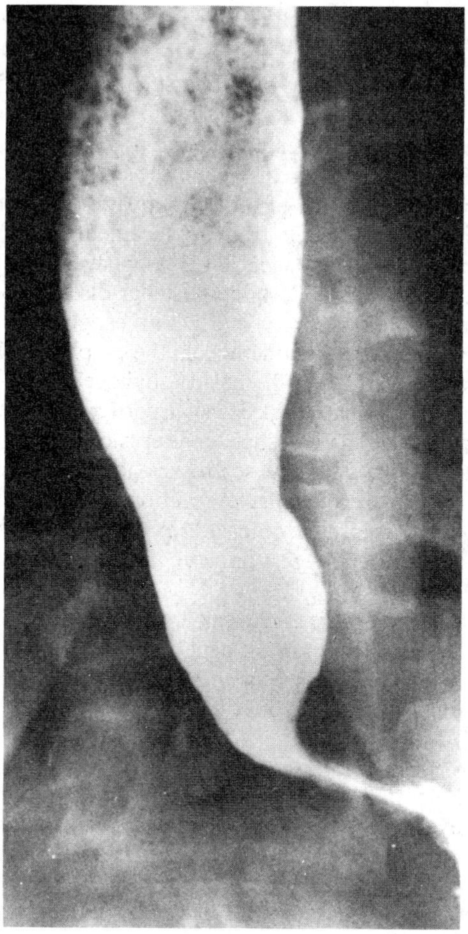

Fig. 35-9. Achalasia of the esophagus. Cardiospasm leads to a long, horizontal stricture *(beak)* at the gastroesophageal junction. The body of the esophagus is dilated and filled with food. (Radiograph courtesy of Charles C. Lu, MD, Department of Radiology, University of Iowa.)

plete and lasting reductions of LES pressure. Contractions of the distal two thirds of the esophageal body are of low amplitude and are nonsequential. Administration of a cholinergic agent leads to high-amplitude esophageal contractions (denervation hypersensitivity).

Because the motor abnormality in achalasia is occasionally the first manifestation of a tumor at the gastroesophageal junction, a careful endoscopic examination is mandatory in all cases of esophageal achalasia. In uncomplicated achalasia, the endoscope passes into the stomach easily, without resistance.

Treatment is aimed at lowering the resistance to passage of esophageal contents through the LES. In most cases, this can be achieved by forceful dilation of the LES; a balloon is placed in the gastric cardia under endoscopic or fluoroscopic control and inflated to a pressure sufficient to disrupt the sphincter. Operative section of the LES (Heller's myotomy) is indicated in instances when pneumatic dilatation has failed or is technically not feasible. Such successful abolition of LES closure is associated with the risk of esophagitis or stricture formation from gastroesophageal reflux. Patients should be advised to sleep with the head of the bed elevated and to follow other precautions against reflux (see earlier discussion).

Pharmacologic measures to decrease LES pressure have been advocated for those achalasia patients who are poor candidates for pneumatic dilatation or operative myotomy. The drugs used have included calcium channel-blocking agents, nitrates, and alpha-adrenergic receptor agonists. Administration of drugs before meals and by routes that bypass the esophagus is recommended. Unfortunately, to date no widely successful drug schedule has emerged.

Esophageal spasm and related motility disorder

In esophageal spasm and related motility disorder, esophageal contractions are of excessive force and duration. Esophageal clearance is typically poor even though no mechanical obstruction or organic lesion can be identified. Patients have intermittent dysphagia or chest pain, which may be intense. Some patients avoid eating in public for fear of being interrupted by bouts of pain or by forceful regurgitation of food. In most patients, the pain is brought on by meals or emotional stress although it may occur at any time, even during sleep. A detailed discussion of chest pain and its relation to esophageal pathophysiology is provided in Chapter 31.

On the basis of manometric findings, these disorders can be subdivided into classic (segmental or diffuse) esophageal spasm, vigorous achalasia with a hypertensive LES, and "nutcracker esophagus." It is not known whether these manometric subdivisions correspond to different disease entities or whether they represent different expressions of the same disease.

Classic esophageal spasm is characterized by the nonprogressive nature of esophageal contractions. Contractions involve long segments of the esophageal smooth muscle at the same time (thus the term *diffuse* or *segmental esophageal spasm*). There is hyperplasia of esophageal smooth muscle, which may be recognized radiographically as thickening of the esophageal wall. Other radiographic features of esophageal spasm are irregular "tertiary contractions" that are unrelated to swallowing (Fig. 35-10) and may give the esophagus a "corkscrew" appearance. On radiographic studies or radionuclide scanning, ineffective esophageal clearance resulting from to-and-fro movements of the bolus may be appreciated.

Manometric criteria for esophageal spasm include the presence of simultaneous contractions, repetitive contractions, and contractions of excessive force and duration (Chapter 31 and Fig. 31-4). LES function is normal in most patients with esophageal spasm, but occasionally distinguishing it from achalasia is rendered difficult by the presence of a hypertensive sphincter that fails to relax (this condition is referred to as *vigorous achalasia*).

Segmental esophageal spasm and vigorous achalasia are rare disorders. More common than segmental esophageal spasm is a variant of esophageal spasm, the so-called nut-

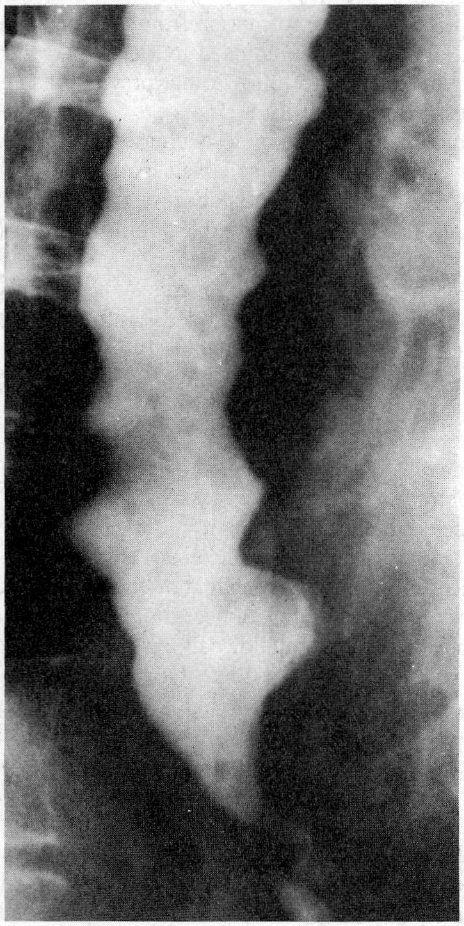

Fig. 35-10. Corkscrew esophagus characteristic of diffuse esophageal spasm. Tertiary contractions of the esophagus lead to the formation of many pseudodiverticula. (Radiograph courtesy of Charles C. Lu, MD, Department of Radiology, University of Iowa.)

cracker esophagus. In this disorder, esophageal contractions are progressive but are of excessive force or duration (Chapter 31). One problem with the diagnosis of esophageal spasm and its variants is that esophageal motility may be normal at the time of manometry, although provocative testing (Chapter 31) may demonstrate manometric abnormalities.

A search must be made to determine whether the motility disorder is precipitated by esophageal reflux, inflammation, or obstruction. Even if no discrete stricture is identified, esophageal bouginage may improve dysphagia. Similarly, measures to prevent reflux, even if this does not seem to be a severe problem, might prove more rewarding than pharmacologic manipulation of esophageal contractile activity. Tranquilizers, smooth muscle relaxants, nitroglycerin, and calcium antagonists provide some relief. Pneumatic dilation of the LES should be reserved for conditions associated with a hypertensive LES. Long surgical myotomy is occasionally advocated when nutrition is impaired but carries the risk of severe reflux esophagitis.

Esophageal motility disorders produced by systemic disease

Patients with progressive systemic sclerosis are particularly prone to severe reflux esophagitis and often develop recurrent esophageal strictures at a young age. Incompetence of the LES, poor esophageal clearance, and delayed gastric emptying all contribute to reflux esophagitis. The mechanical abnormalities result from replacement of esophageal smooth muscle by collagen. This esophageal fibrosis is a consequence of the underlying vascular disease.

Barium swallows show ineffective esophageal peristalsis. On manometry, contractions in the esophageal body are shown to be weak, and the gastroesophageal high-pressure zone may be absent (Fig. 31-4). Endoscopic examination often reveals extensive esophageal erosions.

Patients with systemic sclerosis and reflux esophagitis should observe strict reflux precautions and be maintained on antisecretory drugs, at least at night. It is doubtful that they can be helped by gastrokinetic drugs or operative treatment.

Poor LES pressure and weak, nonsequential esophageal contractions are common in patients with *diabetes mellitus* and diabetic neuropathy. Symptoms may be inconspicuous, yet treatment of an associated reflux esophagitis may be needed.

Dysphagia, both pharyngeal and esophageal, is a common problem in *Parkinson's disease*. Up to half of the patients have findings consistent with esophageal spasm; gastroesophageal reflux and poor esophageal clearance are common in the rest. Treatment of the Parkinson's disease with anticholinergics and levodopa often aggravates the dysphagia.

BENIGN TUMORS

Leiomyomas are the most common of the benign esophageal tumors. They are usually small and asymptomatic and are often discovered incidentally on a barium esophagram as smooth, round filling defects. Large tumors may cause dysphagia and rarely ulcerate and bleed. Endoscopically, they appear as firm, rounded mounds that usually have an intact overlying mucosa. Surgical resection of esophageal leiomyomas is indicated for severe pain, dysphagia, bleeding, compression of a vital structure, or progressive enlargement. Similar presentations may occur with other, less common benign tumors (lipomas, fibromas, and neurofibromas).

MALIGNANT NEOPLASMS

Incidence and risk factors

The incidence of esophageal carcinoma varies greatly among geographic regions. The risk is particularly high in northern Iran, central Asia, and southeastern Africa. The incidence in the United States is about 3 to 6 per 100,000 population per year, with a male predominance of approximately 3:1. The incidence is several times higher in blacks than in whites. This great variation in the incidence of esophageal carcinoma suggests that environmental factors are of great importance in its origin.

Alcohol and tobacco are risk factors for the development of squamous cell esophageal cancer in the Western world. In other regions, ingestions of hot beverages, mycotoxins from moldy or pickled food, combustion products of opium, or N-nitrosyl compounds appear to be associated with high rates of esophageal cancer. In addition, deficiencies of vitamins A, C, and riboflavin; trace minerals; and other nutrients may increase susceptibility. Peptic and lye strictures, webs, achalasia, and diverticula all cause esophageal stasis and have been implicated as risk factors for esophageal cancer. The familial condition of tylosis (hyperkeratosis of the hands and feet), celiac sprue, and the Plummer-Vinson syndrome are all associated with a high incidence of esophageal squamous cell carcinoma. The progression of reflux lesions to esophageal metaplasia and neoplasia is well recognized.

Pathology

Of primary esophageal cancers 90% to 95% are squamous cell or epidermoid cancers. However, the proportion of adenocarcinomas among primary esophageal cancers may be greater than that usually reported. Adenocarcinomas that involve the gastroesophageal junction are often considered extensions of primary gastric cancers; many of these cancers actually arise in dysplastic Barrett's epithelium.

The development of an epidermoid carcinoma is thought to be preceded by dysplasia of the squamous epithelium, whereas the development of adenocarcinoma is probably preceded by dysplasia of the metaplastic columnar epithelium. In squamous cell dysplasia, the basal zone shows increased mitotic activity, increased nuclear size, and hyperchromatism. In invasive carcinoma, cells break through the muscularis mucosae and form nests in the submucosa. Invasive squamous cell carcinoma produces a fungating (polypoid), ulcerating, or infiltrating pattern.

Because the esophagus has rich submucosal lymphatics, spread to the regional nodes occurs early in the course of the disease. Tumor cells spread to paraesophageal and upper abdominal lymph nodes in the distal esophagus, and to the posterior mediastinal, tracheobronchial, and deep cervical nodes in the proximal esophagus. Metastasis to the liver is common, but spread also occurs to the lung and pleura, aorta, adrenals, kidneys, bone, pancreas, and thyroid.

Clinical and laboratory findings

Dysphagia is the most common symptom for which patients seek medical attention. The dysphagia is progressive: over a few weeks to a few months, patients adopt a soft and then a liquid diet. Weight loss is prominent. Dull retrosternal and (sometimes) back pain occurs as the tumor enlarges. Bleeding occurs when the tumor ulcerates, but massive hemorrhage is rare. Aspiration caused by esophageal obstruction or tracheoesophageal fistula may cause coughing, other respiratory symptoms, and pneumonia. Cervical lymph nodes and the liver are enlarged when the disease is advanced.

Barium swallow typically reveals a ragged and asymmetric stenosis of the esophageal lumen (Fig. 35-11). Endoscopic examination is essential to inspect for surface irregularities, abnormal color, or associated Barrett's epithelium. Multiple biopsies and brushings for cytologic examination should be obtained. Endoscopic ultrasonography can provide information about the extent to which the tumor has invaded the wall and local lymph nodes. Other examinations for staging include endoscopic sonography, computed tomography, and magnetic resonance imaging of the thorax and upper abdomen. Bronchoscopy, mediastinoscopy, laparoscopy, or radioisotope scanning of the chest, abdomen, and bones may also be helpful.

Treatment

At the time of presentation, most esophageal cancers are widely metastasized and beyond cure. Local extension to the aorta, trachea, or other vital mediastinal structures often makes surgical resection impossible, and the operative

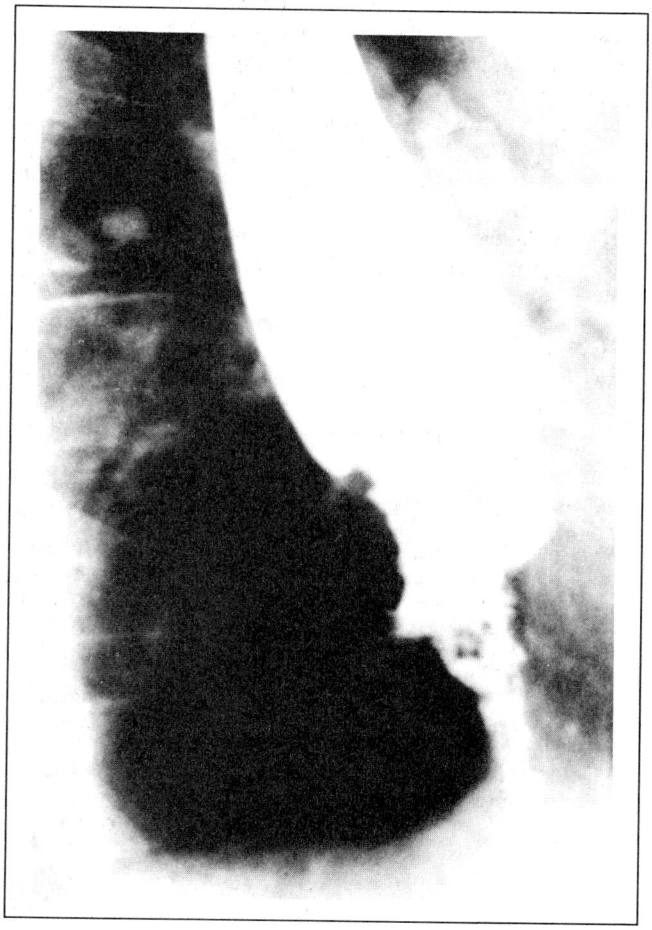

Fig. 35-11. Esophageal carcinoma. The tumor has led to an asymmetric, long stricture in the distal esophagus. The mucosal outline is shaggy. (Radiograph courtesy of Charles C. Lu, MD, Department of Radiology, University of Iowa.)

mortality is 10% to 20%. Curative therapy is rare, with an expected mean 5 year survival of no more than 5%. Survival rates for surgical and radiation therapy are about equal, but 5 year survival rates of up to 20% have been achieved with more radical operations in patients with early or suspected localized disease. Hence exact preoperative staging of the disease is important. In the lower esophagus, resection is preferred. Esophagectomy requires a reconstruction using a gastric tube, or, less desirably, a segment of jejunum or colon. Anastomotic leaks and early recurrences are frequent complications. Radiotherapy is the treatment of choice for squamous cell carcinoma in the upper esophagus. Curative doses are often complicated by radiation esophagitis, and care must be exerted to prevent radiation injury to the heart, lungs, and spinal cord. Some reports indicate that combined radiation therapy and chemotherapy (using 5-fluorouracil and *cis*-platinum or mitomycin C) is advantageous before operation.

Palliation is directed at relief of pain, dysphagia, and aspiration. Esophageal obstruction should be relieved by dilatation, laser therapy, or electrocautery as necessary to aid the managing of secretions and of nutrition. Jejunostomy may be required for access to enteral feeding. Endoscopic placement of a prosthetic stent is the treatment of choice for fistulas between the esophagus and trachea or bronchi. Bulky intraluminal tumors may be vaporized with an endoscopically delivered laser or reduced in size with a special electrocautery device or with radiotherapy. Combined radiotherapy and chemotherapy palliates dysphagia in up to 50% of patients with advanced disease. Bleomycin, methotrexate, cisplatin, and other agents have some activity against esophageal cancers, but given singly, they produce only temporary effects and do not prolong survival.

REFERENCES

Boyce GA: Palliation of malignant esophageal obstruction. Dysphagia 5:220, 1990.

Brindley JV, Jr et al: Carcinoma of the esophagus. Surg Clin North Am 66(4):673, 1986.

Castell DO: The esophagus. Boston, 1992, Little, Brown.

Cohen WJ: Esophageal motility disorders and their response to calcium channel antagonists. Gastroenterology 93:201, 1987.

Deschnere WK and Benjamin SB: Extraesophageal manifestations of gastroesophageal reflux disease. Am J Gastroenterol 84:1, 1989.

Dodds WJ: The pathogenesis of gastroesophageal reflux disease. Am J Roentgenol 151:49, 1988.

Goldstein JL et al: Esophageal mucosal resitance: a factor in esophagitis. Gastoenterol Clin North Am 19:565, 1990.

Janssen J, VanTrappen G, and Ghillebert G: 24 hr recording of esophageal pressure and pH in patients with noncardiac chest pain. Gastroenterology 90(6):1978, 1986.

Kikendall JW et al: Pill-induced esophageal injury: case reports and review of the medical literature. Dig Dis Sci 28(2):174, 1983.

Kitchin LI and Castell DO: Rationale and efficacy of conservative therapy for gastroesophageal reflux disease. Arch Intern Med 151:448, 1991.

Spechler SJ and the Department of VA Gastroesophageal reflux disease study group: Comparison of medical and surgical therapy for complicated gastroesophageal reflux disease in veterans. N Engl J Med 326:786, 1992.

Spechler SJ and Goyal RK: Barrett's esophagus. N Engl J Med 315:362, 1986.

Trier JS and Bjorkman DJ: Esophageal, gastric and intestinal candidiasis: proceedings of a symposium. Am J Med 77(40):39, 1984.

CHAPTER

36 Abdominal Pain

T. Edward Bynum

Abdominal pain is a common presenting complaint. It may be the symptom of a variety of intra-abdominal diseases or the major expression of diseases that reside primarily outside the abdominal cavity. The variety of diseases that cause abdominal pain and the tendency for both the location and the character of abdominal pain to be nonspecific make abdominal pain difficult to evaluate in some patients. This difficulty is compounded by unusual or bizarre types of abdominal pain that do not seem to have an organic basis (and may be psychosomatic), by "chronic pain syndrome," and by a less than discrete separation of functional and organic mechanisms in the generation of abdominal pain. This chapter presents current concepts relating to abdominal pain, an approach to evaluation of the patient who has abdominal pain, and an attempt to identify those types of abdominal pain most difficult to understand and diagnose.

CLASSIFICATION, CAUSES, AND PATHOPHYSIOLOGY

Abdominal pain is categorized as *visceral, somatic* (or *parietal*), and *referred*. The distinctions are somewhat artificial neurophysiologically, but they are useful clinically and conceptually. Visceral pain arises from an abdominal viscus; it is most commonly dull, cramping, or gnawing in quality, and not well localized to a specific region within the abdomen (usually midline). Pain is felt at the midline because bilateral dermatome innervation takes place at a stage in embryologic development in which the abdominal organs are a simple midline tube. This stage precedes the budding out that produces liver, biliary tree, and pancreas and precedes the elongation and rotation of the gastrointestinal tract. Somatic pain arises in the parietal peritoneum or structures of the body wall in the region of the abdomen. It is localized, aggravated by movement, and often characterized as sharp and discrete. Referred pain is perceived in areas remote from where it originates, usually because the diseased organ shares a neural segment with the area where pain is felt. Its character is usually similar to that of somatic pain.

Rapidly developing distention, stretching, or traction of an abdominal viscus and/or mesentery is the principal cause of visceral pain. Inflammation increases the sensitivity (lowers the threshold) of pain receptors, probably by releasing mediators such as histamine, prostaglandins, kinin polypeptides, serotonin, and potassium. Abdominal pain commonly occurs when normal or increased motor contractions affect an inflamed lesion. Thus distention, stretching, and traction generate pain in intra-abdominal organs in which obstruction, ulceration, ischemia, infection, or mass lesions exist.

The mechanisms involved in some causes of abdominal

pain are not well understood. Metabolic or toxic disorders such as porphyria and lead poisoning may be accompanied by severe and persistent abdominal pain but no demonstrated distention, altered contractions, or inflammation. Familial Mediterranean fever is characterized by severe abdominal pain, often with evidence for nonspecific peritonitis as part of a more general polyserositis, but the cause is not known beyond its geographic and genetic associations.

It is not clear whether patients who experience psychogenic or psychosomatic abdominal pain have markedly enhanced perceptions of normally occurring motor functions, which they perceive as "pains," or whether such patients have centrally mediated abnormalities in motor contractions, with or without transient local distention. Perhaps other, as yet unidentified phenomena may be involved. Diseases of the nerves, such as diabetic neuropathy, herpes zoster, and advanced syphilis, may cause the patient to perceive pain in the abdomen when there is no actual disease of intra-abdominal organs, peritoneum, or abdominal wall.

PATIENT EVALUATION

The first step in evaluating a patient with abdominal pain is to assess the severity and urgency of his or her situation and determine whether there may be associated conditions that represent a major threat to the patient. If the situation is urgent and potentially ominous, additional evaluation must be tailored to the patient's needs and to the clinical circumstances. Some therapy or management may be necessary before or during further evaluation. Fig. 36-1 summarizes the approach to the evaluation of patients with abdominal pain.

The initial assessment should establish whether the abdominal pain is acute or chronic. If pain is acute, the clinician must determine whether the situation is urgent. If pain is chronic, the clinician must determine whether there has been an acute (and perhaps urgent) exacerbation of the chronic condition. The perceptive clinician may pick up clues early in the evaluation that suggest a psychogenic basis for the abdominal pain. Early determination of psychogenic pain can eliminate costly, unnecessary, and perhaps risky procedures and enable the clinician to switch to an approach in which sympathetic listening and support are emphasized.

The signals of urgency are similar to those in other severe acute illness. At the extreme, they include coma, shock, and cardiac or respiratory arrest. Short of that, mental confusion, restlessness, sweating, pallor, and clamminess should cause concern. Careful attention should be given to the vital signs: greater clinical urgency is suggested by tachycardia, orthostatic hypotension, or high fever, which suggest massive hemorrhage or sepsis and require immediate therapeutic intervention. If the patient is free of these signs, a more systematic and standard approach to the evaluation is appropriate.

The history (as obtained from all available sources, including the patient or relatives, old medical records, and referring physicians) is extremely important. The history

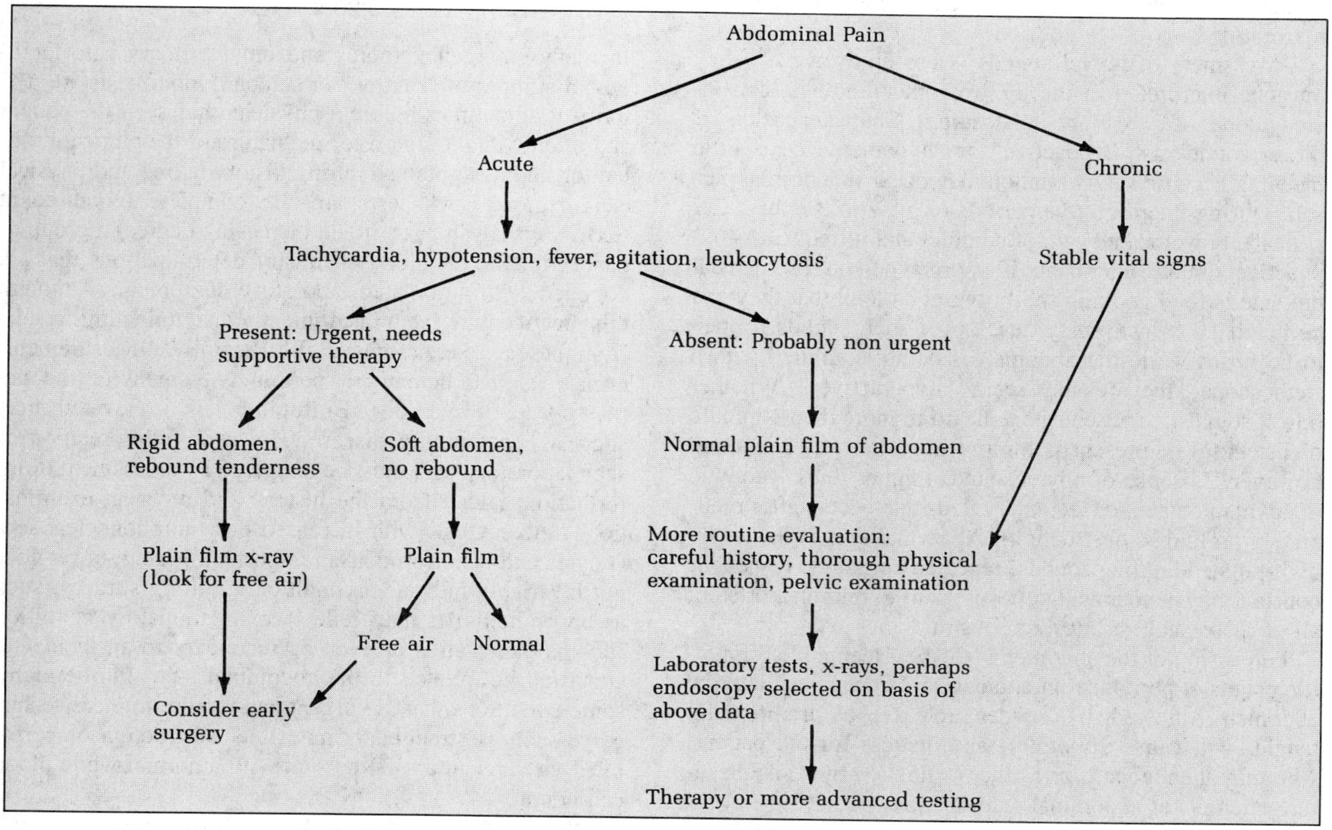

Fig. 36-1. Evaluation of patients with abdominal pain.

alone may allow functionally accurate diagnosis in a majority of patients, as high as 80% by some estimates. It often provides more essential information than do laboratory tests, radiographs, and other special tests. If the patient does not volunteer information about specific aspects of the pain, they must be elicited. Important aspects include intensity; character (dull, sharp, intermittent, constant, throbbing, burning, etc.); location; radiation; timing and setting; association with gastrointestinal functions (eating, defecation) or body positions; factors or events that contribute to exacerbation or relief; associated symptoms; use of narcotics or other medications; and relation to menstrual periods. The sequence of events is important and should be reconstructed as carefully as possible. Often, especially in evaluating patients with subacute or chronic abdominal pain, it is useful to ask what precisely caused them to seek medical attention at that particular time rather than earlier (or later). The usual pain patterns for specific conditions are described in the chapters that deal with these conditions.

If there is no indication of clinical urgency or if the patient has subacute or chronic abdominal pain (as is usually the case), a thorough and complete physical examination should be done, paying special attention to the abdomen. Even if the patient does not appear to be desperately ill and the vital signs are not dramatically abnormal, some findings indicate greater urgency: an extremely rigid abdominal wall related to marked involuntary contraction of the abdominal muscles (the "boardlike" abdomen) suggests peritonitis; marked abdominal distention with diffuse tympany (especially if located over the area of normal hepatic dullness) suggests intestinal obstruction, adynamic ileus, or perforation.

Assessment of bowel sounds is useful. However, they must be interpreted in the light of other findings; considered alone, they can be misleading. Characterization of bowel sounds as "hypoactive" or "hyperactive" has little meaning because such variation may occur in a normal person. During interdigestive periods (e.g., 2 to 3 hours after a meal), bowel sounds are often quiet and infrequent—hypoactive. On the other hand, if a normal person skips a meal but smells food cooking, borborygmi so loud that they can be heard 10 ft away may develop; if such sounds happen to be heard while the abdomen is being examined with a stethoscope, they would seem "hyperactive." Whether bowel sounds are absent (none heard in more than 1 minute of listening) or present is a more important determination however. Absence of bowel sounds implies ileus (paralytic or adynamic ileus, or secondary ileus that occurs after moderately prolonged obstruction). Abnormality is indicated by high-pitched tinkling sounds, repeated peristaltic rushes, or constant bowel sounds that never seem to diminish or stop; all of these suggest intestinal obstruction.

Percussion of the abdomen is the best technique for eliciting signs of peritoneal inflammation. A deep push into the abdomen followed by sudden release, as traditionally taught, will cause discomfort and distress for the patient, who may then jeopardize further evaluation by resisting future attempts at abdominal examination.

Rectal examination may help localize the site of pain, as, for example, in acute appendicitis or diverticulitis. Careful examination of the regions where hernias can occur (inguinal, femoral, umbilical, at the site of previous surgery, etc.) is essential for all patients who experience abdominal pain. Pelvic examination should not be neglected or deferred in female patients, particularly if the cause of abdominal pain is not apparent from the history and examination of the abdomen, because pelvic inflammatory disease and diseases of the ovaries often produce abdominal pain.

Potent analgesics (particularly narcotics and sedatives) should not be administered before initial history taking and physical examination, because they may considerably alter physical findings and the patient's ability to give verbal information. If feasible, such medication should be withheld if confirmation or elaboration of the physical examination by a senior colleague or surgical consultant is indicated. When appropriate, pain relief should be provided parenterally with, for example, meperidine (Demerol), 100 mg, or morphine, 10 mg. These medications must be used cautiously if there is any indication of decreased respiratory reserve.

If surgery is a possibility but not immediately necessary or certain, it is wise to obtain a surgeon's consultative participation at an early stage in the evaluation. Should the patient's condition suddenly deteriorate, the surgeon who has seen the patient earlier will better know how to proceed. If the patient is ill but the advisability of surgery is unclear, reevaluation at the bedside at frequent intervals is essential.

LABORATORY TESTS

In many emergency rooms and other primary care facilities, a number of "routine" or standard blood tests are performed, sometimes before a physician has seen the patient and often without regard for the nature of the clinical problem or findings obtained during history taking and physical examination. Such tests are the complete blood count (CBC), urinalysis, and (to an increasing degree) a group or panel of 12 to 24 blood chemistry determinations that are obtained with automated laboratory equipment. Although this practice may seem insufficiently discriminating, results from these tests are often helpful. Electrolyte measurement, urinalysis, and hematocrit permit assessment of the patient's state of hydration. Bilirubin levels, if elevated, may suggest hepatobiliary disease. However, interpretation of such laboratory data must be tempered by assessment of information gained from the history and physical examination. Leukocytosis with increased polymorphonuclear leukocytes and band forms is an important finding, but it does not invariably indicate a condition requiring surgery, such as appendicitis. It may reflect an inflammatory condition such as pancreatitis or even be secondary to an incidental condition not related to the abdominal pain. Furthermore, some conditions that are urgent and require immediate surgery, such as strangulated intestinal obstruction or perforated viscus, can at first present with a normal white blood cell count.

Other laboratory tests also need to be interpreted with

caution and in the clinical context. Serum amylase level can be moderately elevated in conditions other than pancreatitis and may be normal or only modestly elevated in acute pancreatitis (Chapter 54). Elevation of serum lipase level is more specific for pancreatitis than elevation of serum amylase level. If pancreatitis is suspected and blood urea nitrogen (BUN) (or serum creatinine) level is normal, a concomitant urine specimen tested for urine amylase concentration will show great elevation.

Diagnostic paracentesis with an 18 or 20 gauge needle, rather than with the large trocar that is part of many paracentesis sets, is valuable in patients with abdominal pain who have chronic ascites, sudden onset of ascites (which may be intraperitoneal hemorrhage or pancreatic ascites), suspected perforation of a peptic ulcer, or blunt trauma to the abdomen. If fluid is obtained, it should be analyzed for cell count, protein content, amylase, Gram's stain, routine cultures, anaerobic cultures, tuberculosis cultures, and, if enough fluid is available, cytologic evaluation.

RADIOGRAPHY

Plain flat (KUB) and upright radiographs are the most valuable tests, beyond the history and physical examination, in evaluation of patients with acute abdominal pain. The major radiographic findings pertinent to acute abdominal pain are free intraperitoneal air (Fig. 36-2) and dilated loops of intestine. In addition, an astute radiologist may be able to identify other pertinent findings such as air-fluid levels, abscess, ascites, enlarged intra-abdominal organs, masses, gallstones, air in the biliary tree, probable level of intestinal obstruction, intraluminal or extraluminal foreign bodies, calcifications, aneurysms, renal calculi, and possibly related bone fractures.

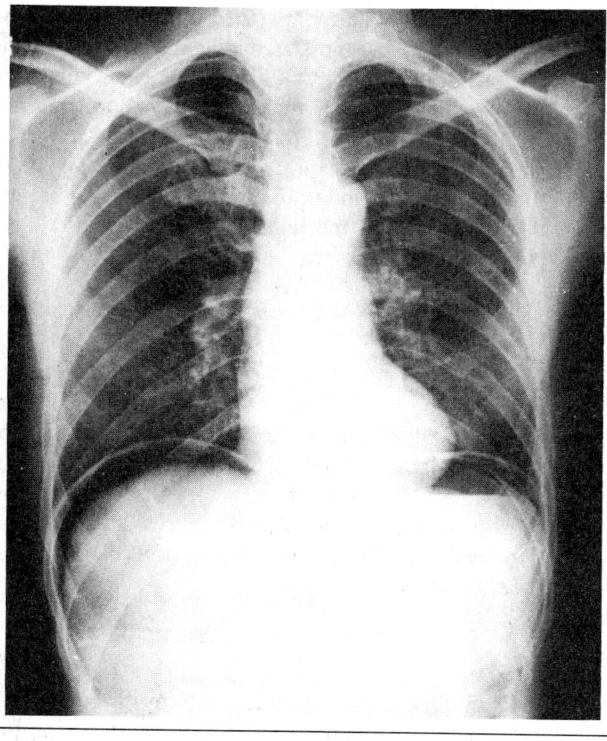

Fig. 36-2. Upright radiograph of the chest showing free intraperitoneal air beneath both sides of the diaphragm. The patient had a perforated peptic ulcer.

Free intraperitoneal air indicates perforation of a hollow viscus, provided the patient has not had abdominal surgery within the preceding 6 days or an even more recent laparoscopy (peritoneoscopy), or tubal insufflation test. If dilated loops of intestine are present, usually with air-fluid levels, the distinction between paralytic ileus and intestinal obstruction can be very difficult. In ileus, the entire bowel, both large and small intestines, is usually dilated. If this is so and if there is air in the rectum, the diagnosis is quite likely to be ileus. Both small and large bowel are dilated in distal sigmoid obstruction as, for example, in sigmoid volvulus or in distal sigmoid stricture from cancer or diverticulitis, but air is usually absent from the rectum. If the patient has ileus to a degree that shows obviously dilated loops of bowel on plain film, bowel sounds are almost always absent. If the patient has obstruction that has not been present for a prolonged period, abnormal bowel sounds usually are present or, less commonly, normal bowel sounds are present.

Contrast radiographic studies less often have a role in the evaluation of acute abdominal pain. If intestinal obstruction is a possibility, a gentle barium enema examination should be the initial contrast study. It may localize the site of obstruction in the colon or may clear the colon so that the small bowel can be examined safely. In some rare instances, the situation may be sufficiently confusing and the need for information sufficiently great that water soluble contrast material, meglumine diatrizoate (Gastrografin), is given orally (or by nasogastric tube) to elucidate possible perforation. Barium can be given orally to localize the level of small bowel obstruction if colonic obstruction and visceral perforation have been excluded. If indicated by previously accumulated information, an intravenous pyelogram may reveal the cause of the patient's pain.

Standard barium swallow radiography (the upper gastrointestinal series) has its greatest utility in evaluating patients with nonurgent acute or chronic abdominal pain. With regard to the patient with chronic or chronically recurrent abdominal pain, it is unlikely that repeated barium contrast studies will reveal any additional information if findings of earlier studies done for the same indication were negative. Certainly, such studies should generally not be repeated if the same study has been performed competently within the preceding 6 months.

OTHER STUDIES

Sonography

Abdominal sonography (ultrasonography, echography) is particularly appealing in that, in addition to being noninvasive, it does not expose the patient to radiation. Sonography is valuable and reliable in detecting stones in the gallbladder (Fig. 36-3) and abdominal aortic aneurysms. A skilled examiner often is able to detect dilated intrahepatic

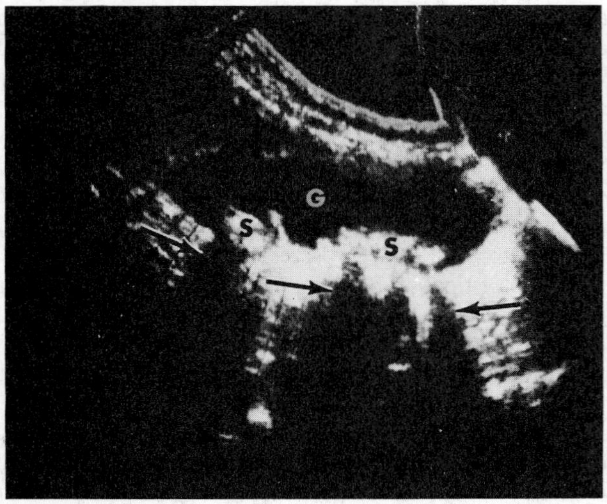

Fig. 36-3. Ultrasound view *(sonogram)* of right upper quadrant of the abdomen showing the gallbladder, which contains filling defects. The presence of acoustic shadows *(arrows)* confirms that these filling defects are gallstones. G, gallbladder; S, filling defects.

bile ducts; a thickened gallbladder wall; a dilated proximal common bile duct; intrahepatic, intra-abdominal, and pelvic abscesses; periappendiceal fluid; splenic hematomas; hydronephrotic kidneys; and masses greater than 2 to 3 cm in diameter. The value, reliability, and reproducibility of sonography are functions of the skill and experience of the sonographer.

Computed tomographic scan

Abdominal computed tomographic (CT) scans expose the patient to radiation but give excellent views of remarkably high resolution that are readily understood by anyone familiar with sagittal section anatomy. The CT scan is usually superior to sonography for evaluation of the pancreas (Fig. 36-4) and kidneys and for assessment for intra-abdominal or pelvic abscesses; sonography is more sensitive for detecting gallstones in the gallbladder.

The advent of sonography and CT scanning (as well as endoscopic retrograde cholangiography and percutaneous transhepatic cholangiography) has sharply reduced the role of radioisotope scans in the evaluation of abdominal disorders. In the patient with abdominal pain in whom acute cholecystitis is suspected but not established, failure to visualize the gallbladder during a ^{99m}Tc HIDA scan helps establish the diagnosis of acute cholecystitis (Chapter 65).

Arteriography

Abdominal arteriography is most useful in evaluating patients with abdominal pain secondary to blunt trauma. If an abdominal aortic aneurysm is suspected as the cause of the patient's pain (especially if there is clinical evidence of dissection), arteriography is often done to obtain additional, more detailed information prior to surgical therapy. Arteriography should be considered early in the evaluation of patients with suspected ischemic bowel disease because it may provide essential diagnostic information and has therapeutic potential (Chapter 46).

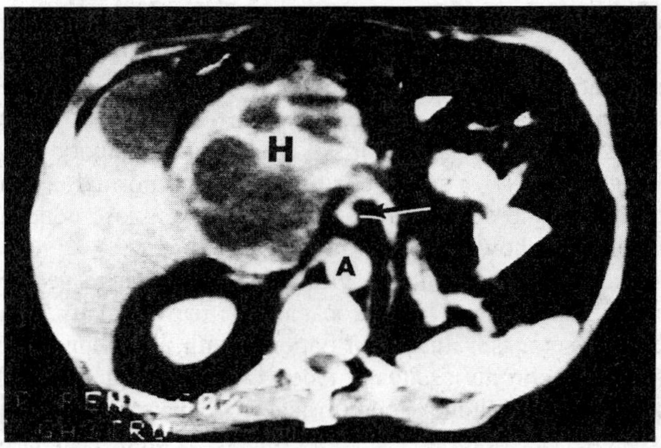

Fig. 36-4. CT scan of the abdomen in a patient with acute and chronic pancreatitis complicated by pancreatic pseudocysts. Cystic defects are evident in a massively enlarged pancreatic head. The aorta and superior mesenteric artery (arrow) are evident. H, head; A, aorta.

Endoscopy

Upper gastrointestinal endoscopy and colonoscopy seldom have a role in evaluation of patients with acute abdominal pain. In patients with nonurgent acute, subacute, or chronic abdominal pain that has not been diagnosed by the tests mentioned so far, endoscopy of the upper gastrointestinal tract may reveal an ulcer of the stomach or duodenum in 10% to 15% of patients in whom barium contrast radiograph results were negative. Only rarely can the endoscopist identify a colonic source of abdominal pain not seen on barium enema. An exception is the unusual patient with Crohn's disease whose diagnosis was not established by radiographs.

Laparoscopy

Laparoscopy is rarely used in evaluating abdominal pain. However, in selected cases of acute abdominal pain, such as blunt trauma, stab wounds, suspected ruptured ectopic pregnancy, or acute pelvic inflammatory disease, laparoscopy can give information not otherwise available that may reduce the need for exploratory surgery, thus reducing the cost of health care.

Surgery

Abdominal surgery (exploratory laparotomy) is required in some patients to establish the cause of acute abdominal pain, especially when the condition is urgent and disease that requires surgical therapy may be present. There is little if any role for exploratory surgery in the diagnosis of chronic abdominal pain. Unfortunately, many such patients have had previous abdominal surgery, which only complicates the evaluation and its interpretation. Adhesions by themselves do not cause pain. Adhesions may, however, cause obstruction, which is usually evident on plain film of the abdomen.

DIFFERENTIAL DIAGNOSIS

The clinical features, laboratory test results, and data from other tests and procedures that enable the specific distinction of one disease from another in the patient presenting with abdominal pain are not discussed here. The reader is referred to chapters dealing with specific disease entities and to the boxes below and on p. 408. The most common causes of abdominal pain and the most common extra-abdominal diseases that may present as abdominal pain are appendicitis, perforated viscus, diverticulitis, small bowel ischemia or infarction (including intestinal obstruction with strangulation of a loop of bowel), cholecystitis and cholangitis, fulminant pancreatitis, fulminant ulcerative colitis (often with toxic dilatation of the colon), atypical myocardial infarction, pulmonary embolus, ruptured ectopic pregnancy, and dissecting aortic aneurysm.

PSYCHOGENIC ABDOMINAL PAIN

In some patients with acute abdominal pain and in more with chronic abdominal pain, extensive evaluation fails to identify an organic lesion or definite malfunction that accounts for the pain. Such a negative evaluation represents "diagnosis by exclusion," which (although controversial) might be more appropriately labeled *failure of diagnosis,* in which all common and most rare or exotic diseases that can cause abdominal pain have been excluded. In this circumstance, the pain is interpreted as malingering, hysterical, imaginary, or psychogenic. Such a sequence or process may not be entirely invalid, but the interpretation and its connotations rarely, if ever, help the patient. Furthermore, it behooves physicians to keep in mind the fallibility of any diagnostic test as well as their own fallibility and at

Classification of acute abdominal pain

A. Urgent condition
  1. Appendicitis
  2. Abdominal aortic aneurysm
     a. Ruptured aneurysm
     b. Dissecting aneurysm
  3. Perforation
     a. Peptic ulcer (stomach, duodenum)
     b. Diverticulum of colon
     c. Meckel's diverticulum
     d. Diverticulum of duodenum, small intestine
     e. Duodenal stump (after gastric resection)
     f. Surgical anastomosis
     g. Boerhaave syndrome
     h. Crohn's disease
     i. Ingested foreign body (chicken bone, straight pin, etc.)
     j. Cecal volvulus
     k. Nonspecific ulcers of jejunum or ileum
     l. Lymphoma (especially *after* therapy)
     m. Gallbladder
     n. Ulcerative colitis (with toxic dilatation)
  4. Obstruction with strangulated loop of bowel
     a. Adhesions
     b. Hernias
     c. Cecal or sigmoid volvulus
     d. Gastric volvulus
  5. Ischemia of small intestine
     a. Occlusive ischemia
     b. Nonocclusive ischemia
  6. Acute cholecystitis, cholangitis
  7. Ruptured ectopic pregnancy
  8. Bacterial abscess of liver
  9. Pancreatic abscess
  10. Ruptured hepatic adenoma, hepatoma, or hemangioma
  11. Ruptured spleen

B. Less urgent condition
  1. Viral gastroenteritis
  2. Staphylococcal toxin gastroenteritis
  3. Peptic ulcer
  4. Hepatitis
     a. Viral
     b. Toxic
     c. Ischemic
  5. Spontaneous bacterial peritonitis
  6. Acute pancreatitis
  7. Diabetic neuropathy
  8. Crohn's disease
  9. Ulcerative colitis
  10. Pelvic inflammatory disease
  11. Infectious enterocolitis
  12. Mesenteric lymphadenitis
  13. Nephroureterolithiasis
  14. Budd-Chiari syndrome
  15. Veno-occlusive disease of liver
  16. Splenic infarction
  17. Twisted ovarian cyst
  18. Hemorrhage into uterine fibroid
  19. Fitz-Hugh–Curtis syndrome
  20. Endometritis
  21. Psychogenic
  22. Diverticulitis
  23. Intestinal obstruction
  24. Skeletal muscle spasm, hematoma, tear

C. Deceptive causes of abdominal pain
  1. Myocardial infarction
  2. Pulmonary embolus
  3. Adrenal insufficiency
  4. Herpes zoster
  5. Acute pyelonephritis
  6. Pneumonia
  7. Trauma to testicle
  8. Familial Mediterranean fever
  9. Porphyria

Causes of chronic abdominal pain

I. Inflammatory causes
  A. Chronic pancreatitis
  B. Pelvic inflammatory disease
  C. Crohn's disease
  D. Chronic ulcerative colitis
  E. Tuberculous peritonitis
  F. Chronic cholecystitis
II. Neoplastic causes
  A. Adenocarcinoma of pancreas
  B. Carcinoma of stomach
  C. Carcinomatosis peritonei
  D. Primary hepatocellular carcinoma
  E. Mesothelioma of peritoneum
  F. Carcinoma of kidney
  G. Intra-abdominal or retroperitoneal lymphoma
  H. Carcinoma of ovary
III. Metabolic causes
  A. Porphyria
  B. Lead poisoning
  C. Adrenal insufficiency
IV. Vascular causes
  A. Aortic aneurysm
  B. Mesenteric vascular insufficiency ("abdominal angina")
V. Other causes
  A. Irritable bowel syndrome
  B. Distended urinary bladder
  C. Fecal impaction
  D. Hydronephrosis
  E. Mesenteric cyst
  F. Endometriosis
  G. Ovarian cyst
  H. Psychogenic

least to consider the possibility that some pain-generating disease has been overlooked because of a laboratory error or because the disease is in too early a stage to be identified by current methods. If that possibility seems remote, in lieu of extending the evaluation to expensive and/or risky procedures or senselessly repeating tests, the physician might seek or become aware of positive evidence of psychological disturbance or emotional maladjustment. Such evidence is usually subjective and is often vague, but its presence allows the clinician to incorporate more "diagnosis by inclusion" into the evaluation. Depression is commonly a precursor of chronic abdominal pain. In actual clinical encounters, however, the dilemma may be whether the patient has abdominal pain because of depression or whether the patient has become depressed because of chronic abdominal pain for which no physician can find the cause and for which there has been no effective therapy.

If the abdominal pain is crampy, intermittent, exacerbated by stress, and associated with alternating constipation and diarrhea, it is reasonable to assume that the cause is irritable bowel syndrome. Irritable bowel syndrome is the most common gastrointestinal affliction in the United States and probably in all the industrialized nations (Chapter 41).

Organic disease subjects patients to social, occupational, and psychological complications and manifestations. This is particularly true for patients with pain. If, after evaluation, a patient's abdominal pain is not diagnosed, the physician must consider the pain to be real (even if psychogenic) and give that patient the same psychological support that is given the patient who has a diagnosed organic disease. The negative evaluation should be discussed gently but frankly, and the patient should be given the opportunity to react to this information. Then, while acknowledging the reality of the pain, the physician should suggest to the patient the possibility that it could be the manifestation of emotional disturbance, maladjustment, or stress rather than cancer or some other organic disease. If the patient has no insight or is at risk for narcotic dependency, the physician should consider referral to a unit or center that specializes in pain.

REFERENCES

Avorn J et al: The neglected medical history and therapeutic choices for abdominal pain. Arch Intern Med 151:694, 1991.
Bugliosi TF et al: Acute abdominal pain in the elderly. Ann Emerg Med 19:1383, 1990.
Drossman DA: Patients with psychogenic abdominal pain. Am J Psychiatry 139:1549, 1982.
Graham A et al: Laparoscopic evaluation of acute abdominal pain. J Laparoendosc Surg 1:165, 1991.
Gray DW and Collin J: Non-specific abdominal pain as a cause of acute admission to hospital. Br J Surg 74:239, 1987.
Irwin TT: Abdominal pain: a surgical audit of 1190 emergency admissions. Br J Surg 76:1121, 1989.
Lee PWR: The plain x-ray in the acute abdomen. Br J Surg 63:763, 1976.
Nauta RJ and Magnant C: Observation versus operation for abdominal pain in the right lower quadrant: roles of the clinical examination and the leukocyte count. Am J Surg 151:746, 1986.
Nemcek AA, Jr: CT of acute gastrointestinal disorders. Radiol Clin North Am 27:773, 1989.
Saclarides T et al: Abdominal emergencies. Med Clin North Am 70:1093, 1986.
Shafer N: Psychophysiologic diagnosis. Med Counterpt 5:42, 1973.
Silen W: Cope's early diagnosis of the acute abdomen, rev ed. New York, 1983, Oxford University Press.
Way LW: Abdominal pain. In Sleisenger MH and Fordtran JS, editors: Gastrointestinal disease, ed 4. Philadelphia, 1989, WB Saunders.
Wolf S, editor: Abdominal diagnosis. Philadelphia, 1979, Lea & Febiger.

CHAPTER

37 Nausea, Vomiting, and Anorexia

Makau Lee
Mark Feldman

Many diseases are associated with nausea, vomiting, and anorexia. These conditions include not only disorders of the gastrointestinal tract but also disorders of the thorax and central nervous system, endocrine and metabolic disturbances, and psychiatric illnesses. Although nausea, vomiting, and anorexia frequently coexist, they are discussed separately in this chapter.

NAUSEA AND VOMITING

Nausea can be defined as an unpleasant sensation, usually felt in the abdomen, associated with the desire to vomit. Unlike vomiting, which is a mechanical act that can be reproduced in experimental animals and therefore studied in the laboratory, nausea is a subjective symptom. Thus very little is known about the neural pathways that mediate nausea. Recent studies in human volunteers indicate that nausea is associated with release of vasopressin and pancreatic polypeptide. In general, a stimulus that produces nausea, if sufficiently intense or prolonged, results in vomiting.

Vomiting is defined as the forceful expulsion of gastric contents out of the mouth. The act of vomiting is usually preceded by retching. Vomiting is an important symptom for two major reasons. First, it can be the initial or predominant symptom in a number of conditions (e.g., gastric or intestinal obstruction, myocardial infarction, pregnancy, appendicitis, uremia, diabetic ketoacidosis, Addison's disease); and second, regardless of its cause, it can lead to life-threatening complications.

Emetic stimuli can cause vomiting by at least two mechanisms (Fig. 37-1). First, an emetic stimulus can activate afferent neural pathways that act directly on the vomiting center in the dorsal portion of the medulla oblongata. For example, orally ingested copper sulfate causes vomiting by this mechanism. In experimental animals, ablation of the vagus nerves and sympathetic pathways within the abdomen prevents vomiting induced by orally administered copper sulfate. It is likely that afferent impulses from parts of the body other than the gastrointestinal tract (e.g., the pharynx and heart) can also cause vomiting by directly activating the vomiting center.

A second mechanism by which an emetic stimulus can lead to vomiting is by activation of the chemoreceptor trigger zone (CTZ), which is located in the area postrema of the medulla in the floor of the fourth ventricle. Certain drugs that lead to vomiting, such as opiates and digitalis, are thought to activate the CTZ, which then stimulates the vomiting center. In experimental animals, the emetic response to intravenously administered apomorphine can be blocked by ablation of the CTZ (leaving the vomiting center intact). It is thought that stimulation of the CTZ is important in vomiting caused by labyrinthine stimulation, uremia, diabetic ketoacidosis, and drugs (including general anesthetics and certain antineoplastic agents).

Although the exact neurotransmitters that are released in the CTZ and vomiting center are not known, dopamine is likely involved. Thus levodopa and bromocriptine (a dopamine agonist) commonly cause nausea and vomiting, whereas dopamine antagonists, such as haloperidol, metoclopramide, and domperidone, are effective antiemetics. The latter two drugs appear to accelerate gastric emptying as well; this may be an additional advantage in certain patients with nausea and vomiting (e.g., diabetic patients with

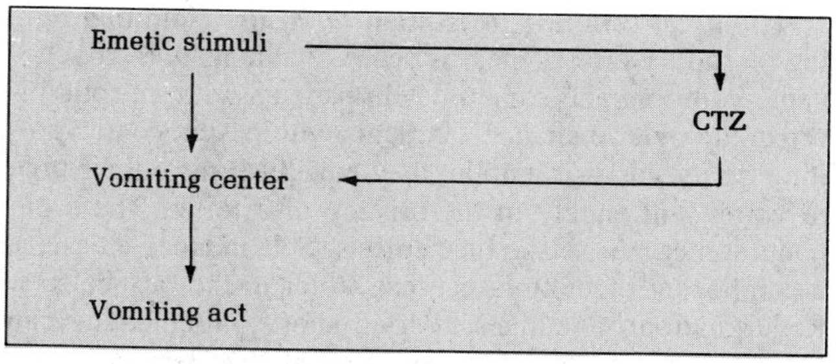

Fig. 37-1. Mechanisms by which stimuli can elicit the vomiting act. Stimuli can act directly on the vomiting center or indirectly through the chemoreceptor trigger zone (see text). CTZ, chemoreceptor trigger zone.

gastroparesis). In addition to dopamine, recent studies have suggested that the mammalian CTZ contains other neurotransmitters, including serotonin, norepinephrine, gamma amino butyric acid, and the neuropeptides substance P and enkephalin.

Regardless of the emetic stimulus or whether the CTZ is involved, the vomiting center is the anatomic location from which the act of vomiting is initiated and coordinated. The vomiting sequence can be summarized as follows: During nausea, gastric tone is reduced, while the tonus in the duodenum may increase, leading to reflux of duodenal contents into the stomach. During retching, there is to-and-fro movement of gastric contents into a dilated esophagus. The antrum and pylorus are contracted, the lower esophageal sphincter is relaxed, and, temporarily, the abdominal esophagus and gastric cardia herniate into the thorax. Vomiting occurs as a result of a forceful sustained contraction of the abdominal muscles and diaphragm while the cardia remains open and the pylorus remains contracted.

Clinical features

Because nausea and vomiting can be manifestations of many different illnesses, it is important to discern certain characteristics of the symptoms.

Duration of symptoms. If symptoms have been present for a brief period (hours or days), it is likely that the illness is due to an acute infection (especially of the gastrointestinal tract); to ingestion of a toxin, poison, or medication; to an acute inflammatory condition (e.g., appendicitis); or to pregnancy. Some patients with peptic ulcer disease, pancreatitis, cholecystitis, and myocardial infarction experience vomiting.

Nausea and vomiting that have been present for weeks or months suggest partial mechanical obstruction of the stomach or small intestine, carcinoma (especially of the stomach or pancreas), intracranial abnormality (e.g., brain tumor), or a psychogenic process. Less commonly, a motility disturbance such as gastroparesis diabeticorum or idiopathic intestinal pseudo-obstruction may be present. Some patients with long-standing nausea and vomiting have substantial weight loss.

Timing of vomiting in relation to meals. Vomiting during or shortly after a meal is seen in patients with psychogenic vomiting and sometimes in patients with a peptic ulcer in the pyloric channel. Patients with psychogenic vomiting rarely vomit in public; they usually control their urge to vomit until safely in the privacy of a toilet. These patients sometimes self-induce emesis. Self-induced emesis is a component of bulimia nervosa (refer to the box below). Regurgitation of undigested food shortly after eating can also be seen in patients with esophageal disorders (stricture, cancer, Zenker's diverticulum, achalasia). In these latter patients, regurgitation is not usually preceded by nausea; instead, the patient often experiences dysphagia.

Vomiting that occurs an hour or more after eating is characteristic of gastric-outlet obstruction or a gastric motor disorder. Physical findings can include a succussion splash and visible peristalsis.

Vomiting upon arising in the morning is characteristic of vomiting in pregnancy but may also be seen in uremia, alcoholism, alkaline reflux gastritis following peptic ulcer surgery, and in patients with increased intracranial pressure.

Content and odor of the vomitus. The presence of old food suggests gastric retention, assuming esophageal disorders and Zenker's diverticulum are excluded. Bile within the vomitus implies that there is an open communication between the duodenum and the stomach. The presence of blood in the vomitus is of obvious importance, although it must be remembered that vomiting of any cause may lead to a Mallory-Weiss laceration of the gastric or esophageal mucosa and thus to hematemesis or a bloody nasogastric aspirate (see later discussion). The odor of the vomitus may be feculent as a result of bacterial overgrowth secondary to gastric or small bowel stasis, obstruction, or ischemia.

Associated symptoms. Fever, weight loss, abdominal mass, menstrual irregularity, history of prior abdominal surgery, jaundice, headache, chest pain, and many other factors influence the clinical impression in a patient with vomiting.

Criteria for bulimia nervosa and anorexia nervosa

Bulimia nervosa

A. Recurrent episodes of binge eating (rapid consumption of a large amount of food in a discrete period).
B. A feeling of lack of control over eating behavior during the eating binges.
C. Regular engagement in either self-induced vomiting, use of laxatives or diuretics, strict dieting or fasting, or vigorous exercise in order to prevent weight gain.
D. A minimum average of two binge-eating episodes a week for at least 3 months.
E. Persistent overconcern with body shape and weight.

Anorexia nervosa

A. Refusal to maintain body weight over a minimal normal weight for age and height, e.g., weight loss leading to maintenance of body weight 15% below that expected; or failure to make expected weight gain during period of growth, leading to body weight 15% below that expected.
B. Intense fear of gaining weight or becoming fat, even though underweight.
C. Disturbance in the way in which one's body weight, size, or shape is experienced, e.g., the person claims to "feel fat" even when emaciated, believes that one area of the body is "too fat" even when obviously underweight.
D. In females, absence of at least three consecutive menstrual cycles that are otherwise expected to occur (primary or secondary amenorrhea).

American Psychiatric Association: Diagnostic and statistical manual of mental disorders-DSM-IIIR, Washington, DC, 1987, American Psychiatric Association.

Consequences of vomiting

The most common consequence of vomiting is the loss of water and electrolytes (especially chloride, hydrogen, potassium, and sodium ions) from the body. The result is a hypochloremic, hypokalemic, metabolic alkalosis. As the extracellular fluid volume shrinks, the concentration of bicarbonate in plasma increases, and as a result the renal threshold for bicarbonate reabsorption can be exceeded. This may lead to a transient sodium bicarbonaturia, which exacerbates sodium depletion. Thus a low urine chloride concentration ($<$ 10 mEq/L) is a more sensitive index for assessing the degree of salt depletion than the urine sodium concentration. In addition, the kidney may contribute to potassium losses and hypokalemia as a result of secondary hyperaldosteronism. In some patients, vomiting may be surreptitious or concealed. Thus the presence of a hypochloremic, hypokalemic, metabolic alkalosis should arouse suspicion that a patient has been vomiting. In addition to the loss of water and electrolytes, loss of ingested nutrients by vomiting contributes to weight loss and malnutrition.

Another serious sequela of vomiting is pulmonary aspiration, which usually occurs in patients with neurologic problems, such as head trauma, drug overdose, or cerebrovascular accident. Aspiration also can occur as a complication of vomiting during general anesthesia. The presence of hydrochloric acid in the terminal airways leads to an intense chemical pneumonitis. In addition, acid in the proximal airway can lead to laryngospasm and bronchospasm.

Mallory-Weiss syndrome is a complication of retching and vomiting. The lesion is a mucosal tear or tears, usually on the gastric side of the gastroesophageal junction, although the tear may extend to the esophagus. Many patients with the Mallory-Weiss syndrome have hiatal hernias. Although intraluminal bleeding stops in most cases, some patients require transfusions, endoscopic hemostatic therapy, or surgery. On rare occasions bleeding may dissect into the wall of the esophagus, leading to a hematoma that may cause difficulty in swallowing or chest pain. Postemetic esophageal hematomas resolve spontaneously in 5 to 7 days.

Vomiting may lead to life-threatening rupture of the

esophagus (Boerhaave's syndrome) or proximal stomach. The usual presentation of esophageal rupture is severe epigastric pain, cyanosis, dyspnea, left pleural effusion, and mediastinal and/or subcutaneous emphysema. Treatment usually consists of thoracotomy to repair the damaged esophagus plus administration of antibiotics.

Treatment of vomiting

If vomiting has been severe enough to lead to volume depletion and electrolyte disturbances, intravenous fluid and electrolyte replacement is warranted. When the cause of vomiting can be ascertained, this should be remedied if possible. For example, gastric-outlet or small bowel obstruction may require tube decompression or surgical intervention; adrenal (Addisonian) crisis requires hydrocortisone; and drug-induced vomiting requires a reduction in dosage or cessation of the medication. Antiemetic drugs may be helpful for temporary control of symptoms, but they should not be used in place of early definitive therapy. When the cause of nausea or vomiting is not known or when specific treatment is not available (e.g., viral gastroenteritis), it is often necessary to employ an antiemetic drug.

Antihistamines are useful in vomiting that is secondary to motion sickness and other vestibular disturbances. Phenothiazines and butyrophenones are useful with vomiting caused by radiation, gastroenteritis, or drugs. Because phenothiazines can cause blood dyscrasias, jaundice, or extrapyramidal-type reactions, they should be used cautiously. Prokinetic agents, such as metoclopramide, cisapride, and erythromycin, may be useful in patients with nausea and vomiting produced by gastroparesis syndromes. Tetrahydrocannabinol (dronabinol), a component of marijuana, is effective in prevention of vomiting induced by anticancer chemotherapy agents. Metoclopramide, domperidone, and dexamethasone are also effective in this setting. Selective 5-hydroxytryptamine$_3$ receptor antagonists, such as ondansetron, have recently been shown to be highly effective in controlling chemotherapy-induced emesis refractory to conventional therapy. Benzodiazepines (e.g., lorazepam) or behavior modification can be employed to reduce anticipatory nausea and vomiting, which may precede anticancer chemotherapy.

ANOREXIA

Anorexia can be defined as the lack of or loss of appetite. It is not to be confused with early satiety, in which patients experience hunger but, because of a problem with gastric filling or gastric emptying, stop eating prematurely. Anorexia is also not to be confused with sitophobia, in which a patient fears eating because pain or other unpleasant sensations are likely to occur (e.g., abdominal angina).

Very little is known about what regulates hunger and appetite. It is likely that the brain, liver, gastrointestinal tract, and ingested nutrients all are important. Psychological factors are also important in food intake. Thus, persons with profound depression may lose their appetite despite appropriate signals from the gut, liver, and/or bloodstream. There is also evidence to suggest that patients with cancer may develop learned aversions to specific foods eaten during the phase of tumor growth and/or nausea-producing chemotherapy.

Virtually any disorder of the gastrointestinal tract, liver, pancreas, or biliary tree can be associated with anorexia. In addition, many drugs, especially antineoplastic agents, lead to anorexia. There are many extraintestinal illnesses in which anorexia is a major feature. These include cancer; infections; endocrine disturbances (Addison's disease, panhypopituitarism, hyperparathyroidism); collagen vascular diseases; renal disease; pulmonary disorders (especially chronic obstructive lung disease); congestive heart failure; and psychiatric illness (especially depression). How these diseases cause anorexia is incompletely understood. Anorexia, if prolonged, leads to weight loss, protein-calorie malnutrition, and eventually death.

Anorexia nervosa

The disorder of anorexia nervosa is characterized by a distorted, implacable attitude toward eating that overrides hunger, warnings, and threats. As a result of decreased caloric intake, weight loss is profound and death may result. In most cases, the patient is a female below the age of 25 years. Because of a distorted body image, the patient strives to become thin and thus avoids food. There is evidence that these patients experience hunger but that they suppress the sensation because not eating is more pleasurable. Thus the term *anorexia nervosa* is a misnomer. Early in the disease amenorrhea develops, sometimes before weight loss occurs. Criteria for diagnosis are summarized in the box on p. 410.

Patients with anorexia nervosa may maintain an interest in food by becoming gourmet cooks or dietitians. Yet they will hoard food or throw it out rather than eat it. Intake of carbohydrate and fat is especially reduced. Some patients also have features of bulimia nervosa (see box). Thus patients may present with weight loss and a hypokalemic, hypochloremic alkalosis caused by vomiting. Other patients, who vomit more frequently and conspicuously, may be referred for evaluation of vomiting and weight loss. Patients with anorexia nervosa have slower than normal gastric emptying, although the connection between slow gastric emptying and anorexia and vomiting is unclear. Some patients abuse drugs such as diuretics, laxatives, and amphetamines (the latter to suppress hunger).

The cause of anorexia nervosa is not known, although most consider it a primary psychiatric disorder. The disease can be diagnosed after other diseases that lead to decreased food intake and weight loss have been excluded. It is important to exclude cancer and endocrine disturbances (especially panhypopituitarism and hypoadrenalism). Patients with anorexia nervosa are usually alert, active, and unaware that there is a problem. They may be exercise fanatics and deny that they are ill. Patients with panhypopituitarism are weak and lethargic and freely admit that they are not well.

Therapy for anorexia nervosa is both nutritional and psychiatric. In some cases, malnutrition may be so advanced that parenteral hyperalimentation may be necessary temporarily. Parenteral feedings should be started slowly, with a very gradual increase in calorie and volume load. As soon as possible, attempts should be made to supply calories, protein, and vitamins orally. Early in the course, psychiatric consultation should be sought. In some cases it may be helpful to institute a behavior modification program, with rewards for weight gain. Family group therapy sessions may be useful. The prognosis is generally good, although relapses are common and approximately 1 in 20 patients dies of the disease.

REFERENCES

Feldman M, Samson WK, and O'Dorisio TM: Apomorphine-induced nausea in humans: release of vasopressin and pancreatic polypeptide. *Gastroenterology* 95:721, 1988.

Halmi KA: Anorexia nervosa and bulimia. *Ann Rev Med* 38:373, 1987.

Janssens J et al: Improvement of gastric emptying in diabetic gastroparesis by erythromycin. N Engl J Med 322:1028, 1990.

Kurtzman FD et al: Eating disorders among selected student populations at UCLA. J Am Diet Assoc 89:45, 1989.

Lee M and Feldman M: Nausea and vomiting. In Sleisenger MH and Fordtran JS editor: Gastrointestinal disease, ed 5. Philadelphia, 1993, WB Saunders.

Marty M et al: Comparison of the 5-hydroxytryptamine$_3$ (serotonin) antagonist ondansetron (GR38032F) with high-dose metoclopramide in the control of cisplatin-induced emesis. N Engl J Med 322:816, 1990.

McCallum RW: Cisapride: a new class of prokinetic agent. Am J Gastroenterol 86:135, 1991.

Muraoka M et al: Psychogenic vomiting: the relation between patterns of vomiting and psychiatric diagnoses. *Gut* 31:526, 1990.

Tortorice PV and O'Connell MB: Management of chemotherapy-induced nausea and vomiting. Pharmacotherapy 10:129, 1990.

Worsley A et al: The weight control practices of 15 year old New Zealanders. J Paediatr Child Health 26:41, 1990.

CHAPTER

38 Peptic Ulcer Disease

Walter L. Peterson
Charles T. Richardson

Peptic ulcers occur in areas of the gastrointestinal tract exposed to acid and pepsin. The most common locations are the duodenal bulb and stomach, although lesions may also be found in the lower end of the esophagus. Rarely, peptic ulcers occur in other areas of the gastrointestinal tract. They can develop in the jejunum in patients with acid-hypersecretory states such as Zollinger-Ellison syndrome or in the ileum in patients with Meckel's diverticulum.

Peptic ulcers usually occur at or near mucosal junctions. For example, gastric ulcers are found near the junction of parietal cell (acid-secreting) and antral mucosa, whereas duodenal ulcers occur near the junction of antral (pyloric) and duodenal mucosa. Gastric ulcers are usually found on the antral side of the mucosal junction and rarely occur in acid-secreting mucosa. Presumably, ulcers occur in junction or border zones because the mucosa in these areas is less resistant to acid, pepsin, or other damaging factors. Ulcers are usually deep and penetrate the muscularis mucosae, in contrast to superficial erosions, which do not extend through the muscularis mucosae.

PREVALENCE

The lifetime prevalence of peptic ulcer is about 10%. Although at one time peptic ulcers occurred substantially more often in men than women, the ratio is almost equal now. Duodenal ulcers tend to be more frequent in men and gastric ulcers in women, but these ratios are also approaching equality.

Duodenal ulcer disease is rare before age 15, and the onset of symptoms most commonly occurs between the ages of 25 and 55 years (peak age, 40 years). On the other hand, gastric ulcers most commonly begin between the ages of 40 and 65 years (peak age, 50 years).

PATHOGENESIS

An ulcer is defined as a breach (with depth, as opposed to superficial erosions) of the gastric or duodenal mucosa (Fig. 38-1). Ulcers occur when mucosal integrity is disrupted in the presence of gastric acid and pepsin. Factors considered important in mucosal integrity and/or its disruption include *Helicobacter pylori (H. pylori)* gastritis, endogenous prostaglandin levels, mucosal bicarbonate secretion, genetic characteristics, and environmental factors such as psychological stress.

Gastric acid and pepsin secretion

Benign gastric or duodenal ulcers rarely develop in the absence of acid. However, the amount of acid produced by patients with peptic ulcer disease varies widely. As groups, patients with an ulcer of the gastric body secrete less acid

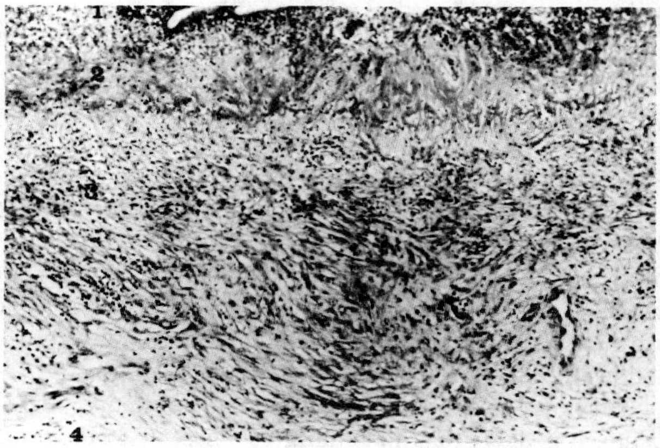

Fig. 38-1. Peptic ulcer with four microscopic layers. **1,** Acute inflammatory exudate; **2,** fibrinoid necrosis; **3,** granulation tissue; **4,** scar tissue. (Micrograph courtesy of Edwin Eigenbrodt, M.D.)

than normal and patients with more distal gastric or duodenal ulcers secrete more. When rates of acid secretion in individual patients are considered, however, the majority of patients fall within the normal range. Exceptions are patients with Zollinger-Ellison syndrome (ZES) or systemic mastocytosis whose stomachs produce above-normal amounts of acid. Variations in acid secretion can primarily be explained by the number of parietal cells (increased number = increased acid secretion) and the degree of gastritis involving the gastric body and fundus (increasing severity = decreasing acid secretion). Excess levels of the stimulants of parietal cells (e.g., increased gastrin in patients with ZES, increased acetylcholine in some patients with increased "vagal tone," and increased histamine levels from ECL cells or, in patients with systemic mastocystosis, mast cells), variation in the sensitivity of parietal cells to their stimulants, and variations in endogenous inhibitors of parietal cell function are also possibilities. Nevertheless, even very high levels of acid secretion can rarely produce ulceration without an initiating breakdown in mucosal integrity. Said another way, gastric acid is necessary, but not sufficient to produce ulceration.

Much less is known about the secretion of pepsin (as pepsinogen) in patients with peptic ulcers. The activity of this proteolytic enzyme is pH dependent (pH >4 leads to inactivation).

Decreased mucosal integrity

Several mechanisms are believed important in maintaining normal mucosal integrity in the stomach and duodenum. These mechanisms include production of mucus from surface and foveolar mucous cells, bicarbonate secretion from the same or similar cells, normal blood flow to the mucosa, and cell renewal and repair after injury. Mucus protects underlying mucosal cells, lubricates the mucosa, retains water and provides an aqueous environment for mucosal cells, and helps form an unstirred layer, impeding diffusion of hydrogen ions from the lumen of the stomach to the mucosal cell surface. Bicarbonate is believed to form an alkaline environment near the luminal surface of mucosal cells and assists in neutralizing hydrogen ions that come in proximity to the cell surface.

Prostaglandins are believed to play an important role in mucosal integrity. When exogenous prostaglandins are placed in the stomachs of animals, gastric mucosa is partially protected from damage from agents such as ethanol, boiling water, or nonsteroidal anti-inflammatory drugs. This ability of prostaglandins to protect the mucosa has been termed *mucosal protection*. Although it is assumed that endogenous prostaglandins function in a manner similar to that of exogenous prostaglandins in maintaining mucosal integrity, this has not been established with certainty. Recently, experiments performed in rabbits suggest a role for endogenous prostaglandins in ulcer pathogenesis. When rabbits were immunized actively with prostaglandin E_2 (PGE_2), ulcers developed in a relatively large percentage of animals and probably occurred as a result of production of antibodies that bound to and inactivated endogenous PGE_2. Additionally, passive transfer of plasma containing antibodies to PGE_2 to unimmunized rabbits also led to gastric lesions, further implying a role for endogenous prostaglandins in protecting against mucosal damage. Drugs that inhibit prostaglandin synthesis (aspirin and other nonsteroidal anti-inflammatory drugs [NSAIDS]) cause mucosal damage and may lead to ulceration in humans, providing indirect evidence that endogenous prostaglandins play a role in maintaining mucosal defense in humans.

Assuming that endogenous prostaglandins protect the gastric and duodenal mucosa, the mechanisms whereby this occurs are uncertain. Exogenous prostaglandins enhance mucus and bicarbonate secretion, increase mucosal blood flow, and play a role in cell repair after injury. Presumably, endogenous prostaglandins function by one or a combination of these same mechanisms to help maintain normal mucosal integrity.

Endogenous prostoglandin deficiency. Although results in animal models suggest that depletion of endogenous prostaglandins can lead to ulceration and there is an increased incidence of both gastric and duodenal ulcers in patients given NSAIDs, it has not been clearly shown that patients with non-NSAID-related ulcers actually have abnormally low levels of tissue prostaglandins. On the other hand, in several studies of normal volunteers older subjects, who have a greater incidence of peptic ulceration, have been shown to have decreased levels of tissue prostaglandins.

Decreased mucosal bicarbonate secretion. Normal gastric and duodenal mucosal cells secrete bicarbonate, which plays a role in protecting cells from gastric acid. Presumably, bicarbonate's beneficial effect is mediated by its ability to neutralize hydrogen ions near the mucosal cell surface. The mucosa of patients with duodenal ulcer disease responds to an acid load with significantly less bicarbonate secretion than the mucosa of normal control subjects. This may lead to localized areas of high acidity and predispose to ulceration. The mechanism of reduced bicarbonate secretion is not known but appears to be unrelated to prostaglandin levels.

Abnormal gastroduodenal mucus. Although much work has been carried out investigating both quantitative and qualitative abnormalities of gastroduodenal mucus in patients with peptic ulcer, no firm evidence exists that such abnormalities play a major role in the pathogenesis of peptic ulcer.

Mucosal blood flow. Maintenance of mucosal blood flow has been shown in experimental animals to be very important in preventing deep mucosal injury in response to injurious agents. Although abnormalities in mucosal blood flow are an attractive pathogenetic factor in the development of a peptic ulcer in humans, no good evidence exists either to prove or disprove the theory.

Mucosal growth factors. Evidence is available in experimental animals that mucosal growth factors (or their absence) may play an important pathogenetic role in the development of peptic ulcers. Their function in human peptic ulcer diseases remains unknown.

Gastroduodenal reflux. Reflux of duodenal contents into the stomach has been postulated as one cause of decreased mucosal integrity, and, in particular, bile salts and lysolecithin have been implicated as damaging agents. Solid data to support such a hypothesis in humans are not available.

***Helicobacter pylori* gastritis.** Evidence that *H. pylori* gastritis predisposes to the development of ulceration is indirect, but persuasive. First, *H. pylori* is present in virtually all patients with active duodenal ulcer and about 80% of those with gastric ulcer. Second, although not employing rigorous blinding, studies to date have consistently demonstrated that the recurrence rate of both duodenal and gastric ulcer is substantially reduced if the organism is eradicated. Questions remain as to the mechanism(s) by which gastritis leads to ulceration. Furthermore, even though *H. pylori* gastritis may be, like gastric acid, necessary for the development of ulceration, it also is not sufficient. In the majority of individuals infected with *H. pylori,* even those who produce substantial amounts of acid, ulcers never develop. Other factors, such as those discussed later, must also play important roles.

Other factors

Genetics. Hereditary factors probably play a role in the development of peptic ulcers in some patients. One study revealed that approximately 40% of patients with duodenal ulcers had at least one family member with ulcer disease. In addition, the prevalence of ulcers was greater in first-order than in second- or third-order relatives. Another study showed that 62% of children with peptic ulcers had a family history of ulcer disease. Studies in twins have shown a greater likelihood of concordance for peptic ulcers in identical than in fraternal twins.

How genetic influences determine ulcer susceptibility is not known. The effects may be mediated by increased secretion of acid and pepsin in some patients or by decreased mucosal defense in others. It is believed that ulcer disease represents a heterogeneous group of disorders and that different pathogenetic factors are operative in different families whose members have ulcers. In some members of families with multiple endocrine neoplasia type 1 (MEN-I) syndrome ulcers develop because of the presence of gastrinomas, which cause high serum gastrin concentrations. This high concentration, in turn, causes increased acid secretion (see Zollinger-Ellison syndrome). Other abnormalities of gastric function such as increased gastric emptying and enhanced serum gastrin response to food have been described in some families with ulcers.

Stress. Psychological stress has been postulated as a cause of peptic ulcers in some patients. A theory of how stress might lead to ulcer disease consists of three parts. First, a period of psychic conflict precedes ulcer disease by several months or years. Second, psychic conflict ultimately leads to ulcer disease by stimulating acid and pepsin secretion and/or by decreasing mucosal defense. Third, a stressful event occurs that accentuates the psychic conflict and further increases acid secretion or decreases mucosal defense. Results of a recent study suggest that patients with ulcer disease, as a group, are not exposed to more stressful life events than nonulcer patients but perceive these life events more negatively. Results of this study demonstrated strong associations among life events, stress, psychosocial factors, and peptic ulcer disease. Exactly how these variables interact to cause ulcers is unclear.

It is unlikely that there is one "ulcer personality." Just as several pathophysiologic abnormalities have been described in groups of ulcer patients, it is likely that a number of different personality or psychological traits exist in various ulcer patients. This likelihood does not mean, however, that these patients are abnormal or that specific personality or psychological traits are related to the development of ulcers.

Cigarette smoking. Cigarette smoking has not been shown to cause peptic ulcers, although there is evidence suggesting an association between the two. The incidence of both gastric and duodenal ulcers is higher in smokers than in nonsmokers; the death rate from ulcers is higher in smokers than in nonsmokers; ulcers are less likely to heal in smokers than in nonsmokers; and the recurrence of ulcers is higher in smokers than in nonsmokers. The mechanism(s) by which cigarette smoking contributes to the pathogenesis of peptic ulcer is unclear. It has been associated with decreased levels of tissue prostaglandins and nicotine may have effects on pancreatic and mucosal bicarbonate secretion.

CLINICAL MANIFESTATIONS

Pain, the most common symptom of peptic ulcers, is usually localized in the epigastric region, although it may be felt in the left or right upper quadrant. It may radiate to the back, the substernal region, or the lower abdomen. Words such as *nagging, aching, cramping, burning,* or *dull* have been used to describe ulcer pain. Not all ulcer patients experience pain, even if they have an active ulcer crater, and bleeding from an ulcer occasionally occurs as the presenting symptom.

Food relieves pain in most patients. However, some patients (about 25% of those with gastric ulcers) report that eating causes or aggravates ulcer pain. Nocturnal pain can occur in patients with gastric or duodenal ulcers and usually occurs within 1 to 2 hours after retiring.

Nausea and vomiting seldom occur in patients with ulcers unless gastric-outlet obstruction is present. Although weight loss is unusual in patients with duodenal ulcers, it may occur in patients with gastric ulcers. One study found that some weight loss occurred in as many as 50% of patients with benign gastric ulcers.

The findings of the physical examination in patients with uncomplicated peptic ulcers are usually unremarkable. Mild to moderate epigastric tenderness is occasionally present but is not specific for diagnosis of peptic ulcer disease.

DIFFERENTIAL DIAGNOSIS

Benign versus malignant gastric ulcer

It is difficult and, in most instances, impossible to differentiate a benign gastric ulcer from gastric cancer on the basis of signs or symptoms. Weight loss occurs more frequently and to a greater degree in patients with malignant ulcers but also occurs in patients with benign ulcers. Differentiation is usually made by radiographic examination, endoscopy with biopsy and cytologic evaluation, and response to medical therapy (Chapter 32).

Gastric versus duodenal ulcer

Differentiation between gastric and duodenal ulcers cannot be accomplished by history or physical examination but requires upper gastrointestinal radiographic or endoscopic examination.

Functional dyspepsia

Patients with functional (nonulcer) dyspepsia have symptoms compatible with ulcer disease but have no radiographic or endoscopic evidence of ulcers. It has been postulated that this condition is part of the spectrum of ulcer disease, but there is little evidence to support this. Symptoms usually are treated with antacids; however, response to antacids is inconsistent, as is response to H_2-receptor antagonists.

NATURAL HISTORY

Patients rarely experience a single occurrence of ulceration. Two recent developments have increased knowledge of the natural history of peptic ulcers. The first, the use of endoscopy, has allowed better documentation of ulcer recurrence. The second, controlled clinical trials performed to evaluate the effect of new drugs on ulcer recurrence, has included control groups of patients treated with a placebo. At least 50% of patients treated with placebo after initial ulcer healing experience a recurrent ulcer during the subsequent year. These results apply to the natural history of ulcer disease in patients who have undergone a course of medical therapy before entering a long-term study. The natural history of ulcer disease in patients who have never been treated is not known.

Spontaneous and permanent remissions occasionally occur in patients with gastric and duodenal ulcer disease. Thus, the saying "once an ulcer, always an ulcer" is not true for all patients.

DIAGNOSTIC APPROACH TO THE PATIENT WITH DYSPEPSIA

Dyspepsia is defined as abdominal pain, primarily epigastric, often relieved by food. This definition specifically excludes heartburn, pancreatitis, biliary colic, and irritable bowel syndrome. The majority of patients with dyspepsia do not have peptic ulcer disease but rather functional dyspepsia. The primary reasons to perform diagnostic tests in patients with dyspepsia are to exclude malignancy and to confirm the presence of peptic ulcer if there is consideration of long-term therapy. Thus diagnostic tests usually are not required for the younger (<40 years) patient with only occasional episodes of pain and no worrisome historical (e.g., weight loss, early satiety) or physical findings (e.g., abdominal mass, fecal occult blood). Such patients may be treated empirically with short courses of antiulcer medications (discussed later). For older patients, where the chance of malignancy is higher, or younger patients who display worrisome associated findings or who respond poorly to empiric therapy diagnostic studies are indicated.

Diagnostic studies (see Chapters 30 and 32)

Ulcers are diagnosed by either upper gastrointestinal radiographs or endoscopy. Several studies have shown that endoscopy is more sensitive than radiography in finding gastric or duodenal ulcers and more accurate in differentiating benign from malignant gastric ulcers.

On radiographic examination a benign gastric ulcer usually appears to have smooth margins and to extend beyond the wall of the stomach (Fig. 38-2). Malignant ulcers, on the other hand, usually have nodular or irregular margins, do not extend beyond the wall of the stomach, and may appear as an ulcer within a mass (Fig. 38-3). Sometimes it

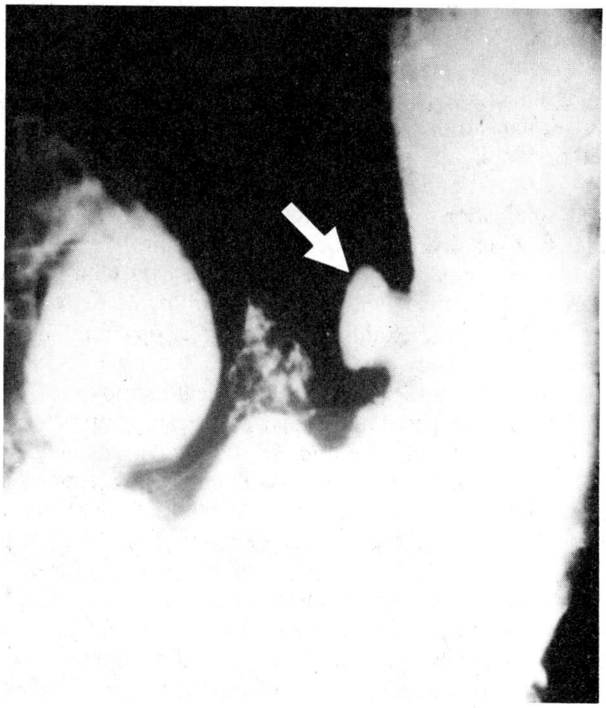

Fig. 38-2. Benign gastric ulcer *(arrow)*. The ulcer extends beyond the lesser curvature of the stomach.

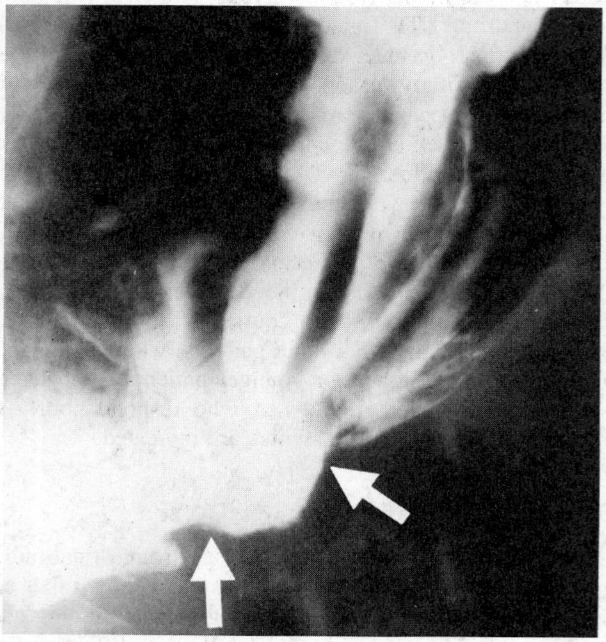

Fig. 38-3. Malignant gastric ulcer *(arrows)* that appears to be within a mass.

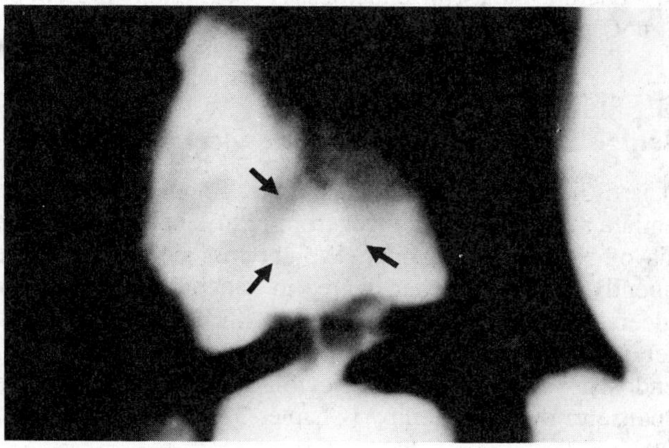

Fig. 38-4. Duodenal ulcer *(arrows)* with collection of barium in the ulcer crater.

is not possible to distinguish a benign from a malignant gastric ulcer by radiographic examination alone. Endoscopy with biopsy is a valuable additional study in differentiating benign from malignant ulcers (see Plate II-5). When radiographic examination and endoscopy with biopsy and cytologic evaluation are combined, malignant ulcers can be distinguished from benign ulcers in over 95% of patients.

Should all patients with gastric ulcers found by radiography undergo endoscopy with biopsy? Unfortunately there are no data to answer this question with certainty. In the authors' opinion, endoscopy with biopsy should be performed in all patients with gastric ulcers unless there is a contraindication to performing endoscopy in a particular patient such as a recent myocardial infarction.

If an ulcer is benign, it usually will heal with medical therapy. All patients with gastric ulcers should be followed with radiographic examination or endoscopy until the ulcers are completely healed. The repeat examination is usually performed after 8 weeks of medical therapy.

An acute duodenal ulcer appears, on radiographic examination, as an ulcer niche (Fig. 38-4). Because the incidence of cancer in the duodenal bulb is extremely low, endoscopic examination is not necessary in patients with duodenal ulcers, as it is in patients with gastric ulcers. Also, in patients with duodenal ulcers it is not necessary to repeat radiographic examinations during each episode of pain. If symptoms change, making the diagnosis uncertain, or if symptoms persist in spite of medical therapy, endoscopy may be indicated.

Gastric analysis. (See Chapters 27 and 32.) Because there is substantial overlap in acid-secretory rates among normal subjects and most patients with peptic ulcer, the indications for gastric analysis are limited: (1) If achlorhydria is documented in a patient with nonhealing gastric ulcer, gastric cancer should be strongly suspected, even if biopsy results have not revealed malignant tissue. (2) The adequacy of current therapy to reduce acid secretion in patients with nonhealing duodenal ulcer can be assessed by measuring basal acid output the hour before a scheduled dose of medication. (3) The success of ulcer surgery in reducing acid secretion can be assessed by gastric analysis. (4) In patients with elevated serum gastrin concentrations, a gastric analysis is helpful in differentiating gastric atrophy from Zollinger-Ellison syndrome. Patients with the former have achlorhydria or hypochlorhydria, whereas those with Zollinger-Ellison syndrome have markedly elevated basal acid output.

TREATMENT

Overview

The major goals of ulcer therapy are to relieve symptoms, heal ulcer craters, prevent recurrences, and prevent complications. Initially, all patients with uncomplicated active duodenal ulcers or benign gastric ulcers should be treated medically. Surgery should be reserved for patients who have complications of ulcer disease, intractable ulcer disease, or gastric cancer (discussed later).

Currently accepted medical treatment includes one of the following: (1) treatment with drugs that reduce gastric acidity, which can be accomplished either by neutralizing acid or by reducing acid secretion; (2) treatment with drugs that bind to and coat ulcer craters; (3) elimination of environmental factors such as nonsteroidal anti-inflammatory drugs and cigarette smoking; and (4) reduction of environmental stress.

Reduction of acidity

Gastric acidity can be reduced by drugs that either neutralize gastric acid (antacids) or inhibit acid secretion (histamine H_2-receptor antagonists, proton pump inhibitors, prostaglandins). Antimuscarinic drugs were used at one time to reduce acid secretion. However, proof of efficacy was never established and their side-effect profile was such that they are no longer considered useful in managing peptic diseases. Reduction of gastric acidity also reduces peptic activity, because acid is necessary for the conversion of pepsinogen to pepsin (the active form of the enzyme). If gastric pH is increased above 3.5, peptic activity is markedly reduced.

Antacids

Pharmacology. Antacids differ in chemical composition, relative potency, and rate of reaction with gastric acid. Most antacids contain various combinations of magnesium hydroxide, aluminum hydroxide, and/or calcium salts. Gastric acidity is reduced when a chemical reaction occurs between antacid constituents and hydrochloric acid. For example, magnesium hydroxide reacts with hydrochloric acid to form magnesium chloride and water.

Duration of antacid effect is determined primarily by the rate of emptying of antacid from the stomach. When antacids are taken on an empty stomach, their effect is brief (only 20 to 30 minutes) because, in the absence of food, antacid is emptied rapidly from the stomach. Thus if the stomach is empty, antacids must be taken frequently. In treating fasting patients, for example, patients in intensive care units, it may be necessary to prescribe antacids every 30 to 60 minutes to achieve adequate reduction of acidity. When antacids are taken after a meal, their effect is prolonged because food delays gastric emptying. Thus in treating ambulatory patients, antacids are prescribed to be taken after meals.

Treatment of active ulcers. The initial studies showing that antacids accelerated the healing of peptic ulcers utilized very large doses of liquid antacid taken seven times daily. Although very effective, such doses led to diarrhea in a substantial number of patients. The introduction of H_2-receptor antagonists, which were more convenient and produced fewer side effects, relegated antacids to adjunct therapy only. Ironically, recent studies suggest that much lower doses of antacids, which can be achieved with tablets four times daily, have no side effects, and are quite inexpensive, are as effective in healing ulcers as the original high doses of liquids. Nevertheless, it is unlikely that antacids will ever return to a position as primary therapy.

Histamine H_2-receptor antagonists

Pharmacology. Histamine stimulates gastric acid secretion by acting on a receptor located on the gastric parietal cell (Fig. 27-2). This receptor has been designated the histamine-2 or H_2-receptor. Drugs have been developed that block the action of histamine on H_2-receptors, just as the classic antihistamine drugs, such as diphenhydramine hydrochloride (Benadryl), block the action of histamine on H_1-receptors.

Cimetidine (Tagamet) was the first H_2-receptor antagonist to be developed. Currently, three additional H_2-receptor antagonists have been synthesized and are available for use in treating ulcer patients (Table 38-1). Each of these compounds reduces acid secretion effectively, although the drugs differ in structure, potency, and, to some extent, reported side effects. As far as structure is concerned, cimetidine contains an imidazole ring, ranitidine contains a furan ring, and famotidine and nizatidine contain a thiazole ring. On a molar basis famotidine is the most potent H_2-receptor antagonist. Ranitidine and nizatidine are similarly potent, and these two drugs are approximately five to six times more potent than cimetidine.

Treatment of active ulcers. The effects of cimetidine, ranitidine, famotidine, and nizatidine on healing of duodenal ulcers have been evaluated in a number of controlled clinical trials. Results of most studies have shown that treatment for 4 to 6 weeks with any of the four drugs is more effective than use of placebo in healing duodenal ulcers. The dosages and frequency of administration of the drugs are listed in Table 38-1. The incidence of healing of duodenal ulcers with any of the four drugs or any of the dosage regimens is approximately the same. In treating most patients with duodenal ulcers, bedtime dosages are preferable because patient compliance with single daily dose therapy is probably better. However, cost of therapy is one of the most important variables, and this frequently differs among hospitals and pharmacies. Physicians are encouraged to check the cost of medications and dosage regimens in their area and prescribe the most cost-effective regimen.

Gastric ulcers generally are larger than duodenal ulcers and for this reason may take longer to heal. Patients with gastric ulcers are treated usually for 8 to 12 weeks rather than the 4 to 6 week period needed to treat duodenal ulcers. It is important to document healing of gastric ulcers by either upper gastrointestinal radiography or endoscopy, although endoscopy is preferable. It is possible for a gastric ulcer to be malignant even though the appearance of the ulcer is benign on radiography or endoscopy and biopsy specimens from the ulcer crater also indicate benignity. Thus healing of a gastric ulcer provides additional evidence that the ulcer is benign.

Prevention of ulcer recurrence. Evidence suggests that continued medical therapy with cimetidine, ranitidine, famotidine, or nizatidine prevents duodenal ulcer recurrence in a large number of patients. For example, in patients who were treated for 6 months or a year with 400 mg of cimetidine or a placebo either at bedtime or twice daily, recurrences occurred in 15% to 25% of patients taking cimetidine and in 55% to 80% of patients taking placebo. Studies in which ranitidine, famotidine, or nizatidine have been evaluated have shown similar results. The recommended dosages of drugs for maintenance therapy of duodenal ulcer disease are as follows: cimetidine, 400 mg at bedtime, ranitidine, 150 mg at bedtime, famotidine, 20 mg at bedtime, and nizatidine, 150 mg at bedtime. None of the drugs has been approved by the FDA for maintenance therapy of benign gastric ulcer disease, although it is likely that these drugs are effective in preventing the recurrence of benign gastric ulcers in a relatively large number of patients.

Most patients with ulcer disease do not require long-term therapy with H_2-receptor antagonists. Chronic therapy

Table 38-1. Drugs used to treat patients with active peptic ulcers

	Generic name	Trade name	Duodenal ulcer* Dosages for adults (ml or mg/day)	Duodenal ulcer* Frequency of administration (times/day)	Gastric ulcer† Dosages for adults (ml or mg/day)	Gastric ulcer† Frequency of administration (times/day)
Drugs that inhibit acid secretion						
H_2-receptor antagonists	Cimetidine	Tagamet	300 mg	With each meal and at bedtime (four times daily)	300 mg	With each meal and at bedtime (four times daily)
			400 mg	Twice daily, in the morning and at bedtime		
			800 mg	Once daily at bedtime	800 mg	Once daily at bedtime
	Ranitidine	Zantac	150 mg	Twice daily, in the morning and at bedtime	150 mg	Twice daily, in the morning and at bedtime
			300 mg	Once daily at bedtime		
	Famotidine	Pepcid	40 mg	Once daily at bedtime	40 mg	Once daily at bedtime
	Nizatidine	Axid	300 mg	Once daily at bedtime	‡	‡
Proton pump inhibitors	Omeprazole	Prilosec	20 mg	Once daily	‡	‡
Drugs that coat the ulcer crater	Sucralfate	Carafate	1 g	Four times daily	‡	‡

*Most patients with duodenal ulcers are treated for 4-6 weeks (see text for more details).
†Most patients with gastric ulcers are treated for 8-12 weeks (see text for more details).
‡Not approved by U.S. Food and Drug Administration.

should be reserved for patients who have multiple recurrences of ulcer disease (three to four each year) or a complication of ulcer disease. Maintenance therapy with cimetidine, ranitidine, famotidine, or nizatidine also is beneficial in treating patients with acid-hypersecretory states such as Zollinger-Ellison syndrome (discussed later).

Although H_2-receptor antagonists are effective in preventing ulcer recurrence, chronic therapy has not changed the natural history of ulcer disease. Ulcer recurrence is prevented only as long as the medication is continued. Once the drug is stopped, ulcers recur at the same rate as if patients had been treated with a placebo. It is unclear how long patients should be treated with maintenance medical therapy. In most patients with recurrent duodenal ulcer disease, it seems reasonable to continue maintenance treatment indefinitely, especially if a complication has occurred.

Side effects. Considering the number of patients treated with H_2-receptor antagonists, adverse effects have occurred infrequently. The incidence of side effects has been greater in patients treated with cimetidine, although side effects have occurred in some patients treated with each of the drugs. The reader is referred to the prescribing information in the package inserts or *The Physicians' Desk Reference* for a complete listing of side effects of H_2-receptor antagonists.

Proton pump inhibitors. Proton pump inhibitors are compounds representing a new class of drugs that inactivate the hydrogen-potassium-adenosine triphosphatase (ATPase) enzyme (proton pump) on the luminal surface of parietal cells (Fig. 27-2). Inactivation of this enzyme leads to profound and prolonged inhibition of acid secretion: a single 20 mg dose of omeprazole (the first such compound approved for use in the United States) is roughly equivalent to 600 mg/day of ranitidine. Ulcer healing is somewhat more rapid than with standard doses of H_2-receptor antagonists, primarily as a result of the prolonged duration of time that gastric pH is maintained above 3.0. However, the clinical importance of such accelerated healing is modest. Because the cost of omeprazole may be higher than that of other forms of therapy, it should usually be reserved for situations where large doses of H_2-receptor antagonists would be needed (i.e., hypersecretory states or gastroesophageal reflux refractory to standard regimens). The profound reduction of gastric acidity leads, in some patients over time, to hypergastrinemia. This condition in rats has led to enterochromaffinlike cell hyperplasia and gastric carcinoid tumors, but has yet to be observed in humans. Nevertheless, long-term use in most patients with peptic ulcer disease is not recommended.

Prostaglandins. Synthetic prostaglandins were formulated with the goal of enhancing ulcer healing by means other than reduction of acid secretion (i.e., by "mucosal protection"). However, it became clear that this could not be accomplished and prostaglandins are considered antisecretory agents. As such, they are no more effective, and at times less effective, than H_2-receptor antagonists. Because use of prostaglandins frequently leads to diarrhea and abdominal cramps, they are not considered first-line therapy for active ulcers. Misoprostol, the first synthetic prostaglandin available, is approved by the FDA in a dose of 100 or 200 μg four times daily for the prevention of nonsteroidal anti-inflammatory drug (NSAID)-associated gastric ulcers. However, this therapy should be reserved only for patients at high risk of developing such ulcers (i.e., elderly patients with a history of prior peptic ulcer disease). It also should be noted that misoprostol, although reducing the rate of NSAID-associated gastric ulcers, in general, has not been found to prevent the complications of ulcer, such as bleeding.

Drugs that coat ulcer craters

Sucralfate (Carafate). Although sucralfate does form a protective coat over an ulcer crater, the means by which it accelerates ulcer healing is probably far more complicated than simply shielding the crater from acid and pepsin. Other mechanisms suggested include acting as a means of transporting growth factors to the ulcer, stimulating endogenous prostaglandins, stimulating mucus, and perhaps, mitigating the lipid peroxidation effects of oxygen radicals.

Results of several controlled clinical trials have shown that sucralfate (1 g four times daily, Table 38-1) is significantly better than placebo and as effective as cimetidine in healing duodenal or gastric ulcers. Sucralfate is also effective in preventing ulcer recurrence. Sucralfate is not recommended in treating patients with basal hypersecretory states, such as Zollinger-Ellison syndrome, because the drug does not reduce acid secretion.

Sucralfate is absorbed poorly from the gastrointestinal tract. Thus systemic side effects are rare. Constipation has occurred in a few patients treated with sucralfate.

Bismuth compounds. Bismuth compounds also coat ulcer craters. De-Nol (tripotassium dicitratobismuthate) is a bismuth compound used in other countries but is not currently available in the United States. Results of controlled clinical trials indicate that De-Nol is effective in treating patients with peptic ulcers and may be useful in preventing ulcer recurrence. Some investigators have suggested that bismuth compounds may lead to healing of ulcers because of their bacteriostatic effect on *Helicobacter pylori*.

Eradication of *Helicobacter pylori*

Evidence is accumulating that eradication of *H. pylori* will result in a reduction in the recurrence rate of duodenal ulcer and probably also of gastric ulcer. Eradication, however, is not easily accomplished. Bismuth alone results in eradication (defined as absence of the organism four or more weeks after cessation of therapy) in only about 10% of patients. When antibiotics are used alone, *H. pylori* becomes rapidly resistant and eradication cannot be accomplished. Rather, the current best therapy requires bismuth (i.e., in the United States bismuth subsalicylate [Pepto-Bismol] two tablets four times daily) plus at least metronidazole (250 mg three times daily) and perhaps a third antimicrobial agent such as tetracycline (500 mg four times daily). This triple therapy given for 14 days results in an eradication rate of 80% to 90%. Such therapy has side effects, however, and most patients with ulcer disease do well on periodic H_2-receptor antagonists or sucralfate. Therefore efforts directed at eradicating *H. pylori* should be reserved at this time for patients with frequent, severe recurrences despite maintenance therapy, patients who previously would have been candidates for surgery because of intractability.

Elimination of environmental factors

Patients should be advised not to take salicylate-containing drugs and should be provided with a list of medications that are known to contain salicylates. They also should be advised not to take other nonsteroidal anti-inflammatory drugs, especially while their ulcer is active. Patients should be advised to stop smoking cigarettes, because ulcers heal less well in smokers than in nonsmokers, and ulcer recurrences are more common in smokers. There is no convincing evidence that ulcer patients should avoid caffeine-containing beverages, because coffee without caffeine stimulates acid secretion to approximately the same extent as caffeine-containing coffee. There also is no evidence that alcohol intake should be eliminated, although moderation in alcohol ingestion seems advisable while an ulcer is active.

Reduction of psychologic stress

Evidence suggests that the level of anxiety in some ulcer patients may affect their response to medical therapy. In one study, 17 of 28 patients who had moderate to severe anxiety, as assessed by an interview during acute ulcer disease, had continued ulcer pain 6 months after therapy. This was in contrast to only 4 in a group of 36 patients who did not have anxiety at the beginning of therapy. Also, more of the patients with anxiety were still unable to work 6 months after treatment. It seems reasonable, therefore, to try to reduce psychological stress in ulcer patients.

The patient's physician should be the one to deal with stress. This usually can be accomplished by establishing a secure physician-patient relationship. The physician should be interested not only in the patient's ulcer but also in his or her emotional concerns. In other words, the physician must treat the patient as well as the disease. Patients should be encouraged but not forced to talk about their anxieties. Although there are no studies evaluating the effect of this approach in the treatment of ulcer disease, in practice it seems helpful. There is no evidence that formal psychotherapy is useful in treating patients with peptic ulcers.

Diet

Special diets have been advocated for many years in the treatment of ulcer disease; however, there is no evidence that they reduce gastric acidity to a greater extent than does a regular diet. Furthermore, four controlled clinical trials have shown that bland food and regular food have similar effects on the clinical course of peptic ulcers and that the incidence of ulcer healing is similar whether patients are on a bland or a regular diet. Patients should be advised to eat three meals a day, consisting of food of their own choosing. If certain foods cause symptoms, they should be avoided.

Medical therapy summarized

1. Patients with active duodenal ulcers should be treated initially for 4 to 6 weeks with an H_2-receptor antagonist or sucralfate (see Table 38-1 for dosage and frequency of administration). If symptoms resolve, no follow-up observation is necessary and medication can be stopped. If symptoms persist and endoscopy confirms a nonhealing duodenal ulcer, the patient should be switched to omeprazole.
2. Patients with active benign gastric ulcers should be treated for 8 to 12 weeks with an H_2-receptor antagonist (see Table 38-1 for dosage and frequency of administration). Healing of gastric ulcers should be documented by either barium radiography or endoscopy. If the ulcer has not healed and biopsy results indicate that the ulcer clearly is benign, it may be helpful to switch therapy to omeprazole although this approach is not yet approved by the U.S. Food and Drug Administration.
3. Patients should be advised not to take salicylate-containing drugs or other nonsteroidal anti-inflammatory drugs.
4. Patients should be told to stop smoking cigarettes.
5. Patients should eat three meals a day from a diet of their own choosing.
6. Long-term maintenance therapy at half doses of medication should be reserved for patients who have suffered a complication of ulcer such as bleeding or perforation or who have frequent recurrences necessitating several months a year of full-dose therapy.
7. Attempts at eradication of *H. pylori* should be reserved for patients who cannot take, choose not to take, or fail maintenance therapy.

COMPLICATIONS

Bleeding is the most frequent complication of ulcer disease, occurring in 15% to 20% of patients. Patients usually experience hematemesis, melena, or both. The management of patients with bleeding ulcer has been heavily influenced by the increasing body of data showing the efficacy of endoscopic therapy. Use of thermal therapy (i.e., heater probe, bicap electrocoagulation) or injection therapy with epinephrine or a sclerosing agent has been shown to stop active bleeding and, in patients with a visible vessel (see Plate II-6), prevent recurrent bleeding.

Perforation into the abdominal cavity is the second most common complication. Perforation causes the sudden onset of excruciating pain, and a patient usually can identify the exact moment that a perforation occurs. Immediate surgery is often required to repair the perforation.

Rather than perforating into the abdominal cavity, ulcers can penetrate into other organs such as the pancreas, omentum, biliary tract, liver, or colon. When ulcers penetrate into the pancreas, pancreatitis can develop (Chapter 67). Penetration can explain intractable ulcer pain.

Edema and scarring as a result of ulcer disease in or near the pylorus can cause gastric-outlet obstruction. When this occurs, patients usually have nausea and vomiting and may lose weight. Vomiting of food eaten 12 to 24 hours previously is characteristic of obstruction. A succussion splash is a common finding on physical examination. Initially, both penetration and obstruction are treated by nasogastric suction and an H_2-receptor antagonist. However, surgery is sometimes required.

Malignant gastric ulcers can also cause gastric-outlet obstruction, and endoscopy is often useful in determining whether obstruction is due to a benign or a malignant gastric ulcer. If obstruction is secondary to a malignant ulcer, surgery is required to relieve the obstruction.

INDICATIONS FOR SURGERY

Indications for surgery include (1) a single episode of brisk bleeding that does not cease with medical therapy within a reasonable period (*brisk bleeding* is usually defined as bleeding requiring 6 to 8 units of blood during a 24 to 36 hour period); (2) several episodes of upper gastrointestinal hemorrhage (surgery is usually recommended after two to three bleeding episodes); (3) perforated ulcers; (4) gastric-outlet obstruction that does not respond to medical therapy within a few days; and (5) malignant gastric ulcers. An occasional patient with frequent recurrence of ulcer who chooses not to take long-term maintenance therapy or who fails maintenance therapy may be a candidate for elective surgery. Many of these patients may choose a course of antimicrobial therapy aimed at eradicating *H. pylori* before undergoing an elective operation. Additionally, patients with nonhealing gastric ulcer may benefit from surgery to remove the ulcer and rule out malignancy.

Surgical procedures for ulcer disease include subtotal gastrectomy, vagotomy and antrectomy, vagotomy and pyloroplasty, vagotomy and gastrojejunostomy, and proximal gastric vagotomy (parietal cell vagotomy). A subtotal gastrectomy or vagotomy and antrectomy is usually performed to treat patients with gastric ulcers. If possible, the ulcer is also included in the resected portion of stomach. To treat patients with duodenal ulcers, a vagotomy and pyloroplasty or vagotomy and antrectomy is performed in most hospitals. In the authors' opinion, a proximal gastric vagotomy is the preferred procedure, however. In this operation the nerves to the antrum remain intact, and motor function of the distal stomach is preserved (Fig. 38-5). Thus postsurgical side effects are reduced with this operation (see later discussion).

POSTSURGICAL SYNDROMES

Surgical procedures for ulcer disease can lead to chronic postoperative problems. These complications are usually

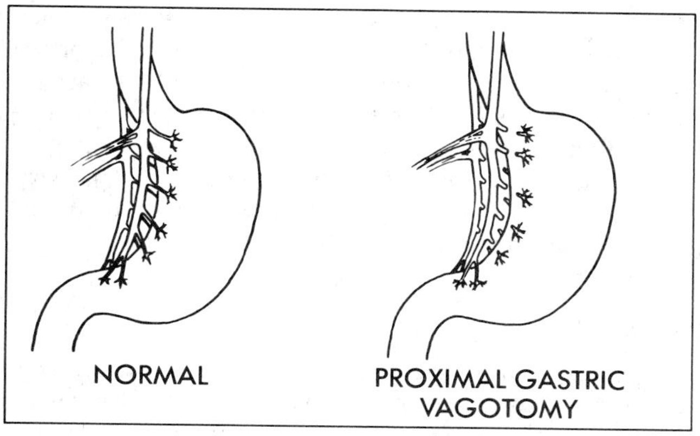

Fig. 38-5. Normal vagal innervation of the stomach *(left)* and vagal innervation following proximal gastric vagotomy *(right)*. Vagal innervation to the antrum remains intact with proximal gastric vagotomy.

called *postgastrectomy syndromes*. However, this term is a misnomer, because many of these problems can occur after either vagotomy and pyloroplasty or vagotomy and gastrojejunostomy without gastric resection. The most commonly encountered problems include diarrhea, malabsorption, dumping syndrome, weight loss or failure to gain weight after surgery, anemia, gastritis, and metabolic bone disease. Other, less commonly seen problems include bezoars, afferent loop obstruction, and stomal stenosis. As mentioned, the incidence of chronic postsurgical problems can be decreased if a selective proximal vagotomy rather than a truncal vagotomy is performed.

Diarrhea

Although diarrhea can occur after any of the surgical procedures mentioned, the incidence seems to be higher with truncal vagotomy (with or without gastric resection). The incidence ranges from 7% to 25%.

The cause of postsurgical diarrhea is not known, although several mechanisms have been postulated. These include disordered gastric emptying, increased output of bile acids, changes in bacterial population of the small bowel, and motility disorders of the small bowel secondary to truncal vagotomy. Sometimes diarrhea results from lactose intolerance that has been unmasked by surgical alteration of gastrointestinal anatomy.

Treatment of diarrhea should be limited initially to dietary manipulations similar to those employed in the treatment of dumping syndrome (see later discussion). Avoidance of lactose- and caffeine-containing foods is occasionally helpful. A variety of antidiarrheal drugs have been tried; however, they often are not successful in controlling postsurgical diarrhea. Cholestyramine has been prescribed with some success, but it is unclear whether the reduction in diarrhea is the result of decreased bile salts or of a nonspecific drug effect.

Malabsorption

The incidence of malabsorption after ulcer surgery varies with the degree to which normal anatomy is altered. For example, the incidence is higher after subtotal gastrectomy or vagotomy and antrectomy than after vagotomy and pyloroplasty. The incidence of clinically significant malabsorption (> 8% fecal fat excretion daily) is extremely low when a selective proximal vagotomy is performed.

The most common causes of postoperative malabsorption are poor timing and poor mixing of food with gastrointestinal juices (bile acids, pancreatic enzymes, etc.) Poor timing and poor mixing are also the most difficult causes to treat. Medical therapy usually includes prescription of antidiarrheal agents and antimuscarinic drugs (theoretically, to slow gastric emptying and allow more contact time among food, bile acids, enzymes, and the small bowel mucosa). Sometimes supplemental pancreatic enzymes will help.

Other, less common causes of malabsorption include bacterial overgrowth, unmasking of latent celiac sprue, gastroenterocolic fistula, and inadvertent gastroileostomy (rather than gastroduodenostomy or gastrojejunostomy). Bacterial overgrowth occurs because of decreased acid secretion and/or stasis, either in the afferent loop in a patient who has had a Billroth II anastomosis (Fig. 38-6) or stasis in the small intestine caused by postoperative adhesions. Bacteria deconjugate bile salts, making them less effective in aiding fat absorption. Bacterial overgrowth is usually treated with broad-spectrum antibiotics. Celiac sprue is treated with a gluten-free diet (Chapter 42), whereas gastroenterocolic fistula and inadvertent gastroileostomy must be treated surgically.

Vitamin and mineral malabsorption may also occur and lead to clinically significant problems. For example, in some patients calcium and vitamin D malabsorption may cause severe metabolic bone disease. Iron, folic acid, and/or vitamin B_{12} malabsorption may lead to anemia. Specific therapy is available for each of these vitamin and mineral deficiencies. Unfortunately, in the case of calcium and vitamin D malabsorption, the condition is often not recog-

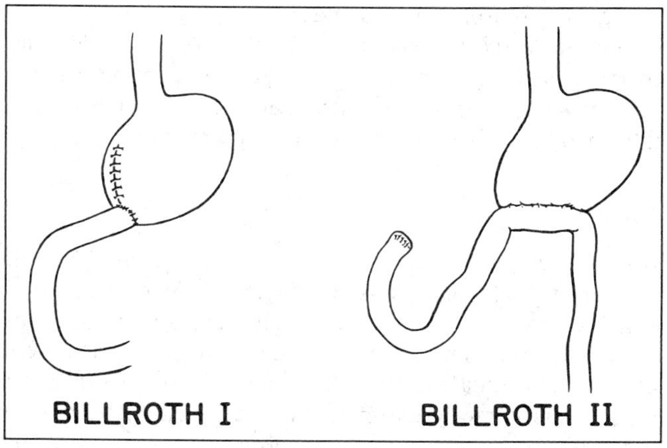

Fig. 38-6. Gastrointestinal anatomy following Billroth I and II anastomoses.

nized until severe bone disease is already present. For this reason, some physicians recommend prophylactic therapy with calcium and vitamin D in patients with subtotal or total gastrectomy or vagotomy and antrectomy.

Dumping syndrome

The term *dumping* was coined in 1922 by a physician who observed that barium emptied rapidly from the stomach of a patient after gastrojejunostomy. The patient's major symptoms were pain, vomiting, and weight loss. Today, the term *dumping syndrome* is used to describe a variety of postprandial symptoms, including epigastric fullness, a sensation of abdominal distention, nausea, borborygmi, drowsiness, fatigue, palpitations, and sweating. Patients usually have one or several but not all of these symptoms. In some patients, symptoms occur in the immediate postoperative period and then subside with time.

The cause of dumping is thought to be related to rapid emptying of hypertonic food products into the upper small bowel. This causes movement of plasma water into the gut lumen, which, in turn, leads to hypovolemia. Although a number of studies have shown that this sequence of events occurs after eating, it has not been established that it causes symptoms. Other postulated mechanisms include presence of hypoglycemia and release of vasoactive substances such as serotonin or bradykinin. Hyperglycemia commonly occurs during the immediate postprandial period in many patients who have undergone gastric resection, and in some patients hypoglycemia occurs 3 to 4 hours after a meal. Thus abnormal glucose tolerance test results are found in many postgastrectomy patients. Whether these blood sugar alterations are related to symptoms of dumping syndrome is controversial, because they can occur in patients with or without symptoms.

Only a few patients with dumping syndrome have symptoms severe enough to require treatment. Usually, symptoms can be controlled if patients eat frequent small meals (five to six times daily); follow a high-protein, high-fat, and low-carbohydrate diet; avoid extremely hot or cold foods; and drink liquids between rather than with meals. Some patients should avoid milk or milk products because lactose intolerance is sometimes unmasked by gastric surgery. In patients who fail to benefit from dietary therapy, antimuscarinic drugs are occasionally helpful. Surgical procedures such as narrowing of the gastric outlet and interposition of intestinal loops have been tried without much success.

Anemia

Anemia develops after gastric surgery as a result of iron, vitamin B_{12}, and/or folic acid deficiency. There are several reasons why these deficiencies might occur. First, food ingestion is often diminished after ulcer surgery. Thus there may be inadequate intake of vitamins and minerals, although this is rarely the main cause of anemia. Second, a few patients have chronic blood loss (e.g., from a recurrent ulcer) and lose excessive amounts of iron. Third, malabsorption of iron can occur after Billroth II anastomosis and can lead to iron deficiency. The small intestine may fail to absorb vitamin B_{12} as a result of intrinsic factor deficiency or if there is intraluminal overgrowth of bacteria in the proximal small intestine. Intrinsic factor deficiency may follow total gastrectomy or result from atrophic gastritis, which can develop after antrectomy or subtotal gastrectomy. All of these factors may contribute to the development of anemia in postoperative patients.

Bile reflux gastritis

Some patients may experience symptoms related to excess amounts of bilious fluid entering the stomach or gastric remnant after gastric resection. These symptoms include epigastric burning pain, heartburn, and bilious vomiting. Medical therapy, including use of cholestyramine, antacids, and H_2-receptor antagonists, has never been clearly shown to relieve such symptoms, although some enthusiasm has been generated recently for the use of ursodeoxycholic acid. Diversion of the bile stream via Roux-en-Y anastomosis aids some patients, especially those with bilious vomiting, but others do not benefit. It has been suggested that abnormally long retention in the stomach or gastric pouch of a radionuclide administered as a biliary scan might predict those patients who will benefit from biliary diversion.

Recurrent ulcers

Ulcers that occur after ulcer surgery usually develop in the duodenum in patients who have had a vagotomy and pyloroplasty, proximal gastric vagotomy, or partial gastrectomy with or without a vagotomy and Billroth I anastomosis. Recurrent ulcers usually occur in the jejunum in patients who have had a Billroth II anastomosis. Occasionally, recurrent ulcers develop in the stomach.

Causes of recurrent ulcers after ulcer surgery include incomplete vagotomy, basal acid hypersecretory states such as Zollinger-Ellison syndrome, ingestion of nonsteroidal anti-inflammatory drugs, and gastric cancer. Incomplete vagotomy is the most common cause of recurrent ulcer after ulcer surgery. Less common causes include retained antrum syndrome, which can occur in patients who have had a Billroth II anastomosis, and ulcers that occur in the area of retained surgical sutures.

Patients with postoperative recurrent ulcers should be questioned about the use of nonsteroidal anti-inflammatory drugs; serum gastrin concentration should be measured to rule out Zollinger-Ellison syndrome or retained antrum syndrome; and acid secretion should be measured to evaluate for Zollinger-Ellison syndrome or incomplete vagotomy. In evaluating for incomplete vagotomy, the acid secretory response to sham feeding should also be measured (Chapter 32).

Endoscopy should be performed in patients with recurrent ulcers, especially if the ulcer is in the stomach. Studies from Europe suggest that there is a higher incidence of gastric cancer occurrence 20 or more years after ulcer surgery in patients who have had partial gastrectomies or antrectomies compared with those who have not had gastric resection. These findings have not been confirmed by studies performed in patients in the United States, however. Endoscopy also is helpful in searching for retained surgical sutures as a cause of recurrent ulcers.

ZOLLINGER-ELLISON SYNDROME

Zollinger-Ellison syndrome, as originally described, consisted of a non-beta islet cell tumor of the pancreas, markedly increased gastric acid secretion, and severe peptic ulcer disease. Although it is believed that patients with Zollinger-Ellison syndrome have tumors, the tumors frequently cannot be found even after careful exploration of the abdominal cavity at the time of laparotomy. Thus in most patients, the diagnosis of Zollinger-Ellison syndrome is made on the basis of chemical criteria, which consist of an elevated fasting serum gastrin concentration, an exaggerated increase in fasting serum gastrin concentration following an intravenous injection of secretin, and basal acid hypersecretion. When a diagnosis of Zollinger-Ellison syndrome is made by chemical criteria, tumors are found in about 40% of patients at laparotomy. Although tumors are commonly located in the pancreas, they also may be found in the wall of the stomach or duodenum, the mesentery, the spleen, and lymph nodes. Because these tumors secrete gastrin, they are called *gastrinomas*. Tumors may be solitary or multiple and may vary in size from 2 mm to 20 cm or more in diameter. Over 50% of gastrinomas have malignant biologic activity, histologic appearance, or both. Approximately 30% of patients have tumors located in areas amenable to surgical resection. Not all of these patients are cured, however, by surgical removal of tumors.

Gastrinomas are often the only endocrine tumors in an individual patient. However, some patients have tumors in other endocrine organs. These patients have multiple endocrine neoplasia type I (MEN-I) syndrome and may have pituitary and adrenal tumors, other pancreatic islet cell tumors, and/or parathyroid hyperplasia or adenomas.

Clinical manifestations

As a result of the increased serum gastrin concentration, basal acid secretion is increased markedly in patients with Zollinger-Ellison syndrome. Gastrin also has a trophic effect on parietal cells. Thus parietal cell mass increases, as does stimulated or peak acid output (Chapter 27). Increased acid secretion often leads to severe peptic ulcer disease, and patients frequently have abdominal pain or a complication of ulcer disease such as bleeding or perforation. Ulcers usually occur in the duodenal bulb, although they often are found in unusual locations such as the postbulbar duodenum or jejunum. Some patients do not have ulcers even though serum gastrin concentration and acid secretion are increased. These patients presumably have enhanced mucosal defense, which prevents ulceration. Others have severe reflux esophagitis.

Diarrhea and steatorrhea also may be predominant signs and symptoms in some patients with Zollinger-Ellison syndrome. Diarrhea is caused primarily by the large volume of acidic fluid that flows from the stomach into the small intestine. Steatorrhea results from several abnormalities caused by acid hypersecretion, including inactivation of pancreatic lipase, precipitation of bile acids, and damage to the small intestinal mucosa. Kidney stones, bone disease, visual disturbances secondary to pituitary tumors, and lipomas are clinical features that may occur in patients who have a gastrinoma and MEN-I syndrome.

Diagnosis

Zollinger-Ellison syndrome should be suspected in (1) patients with unusually severe peptic ulcer disease, (2) patients with peptic ulcers located in the small intestine distal to the duodenal bulb, (3) patients with ulcer disease and severe diarrhea and/or steatorrhea, (4) patients with large mucosal folds in the stomach and thickened folds in the duodenum seen on upper gastrointestinal radiography, (5) patients who have a recurrent ulcer soon after ulcer surgery, (6) patients who have ulcer disease plus kidney stones or other manifestations of MEN-I syndrome, and (7) patients with unexplained diarrhea and steatorrhea.

Patients with suspected Zollinger-Ellison syndrome should have serum gastrin concentration measured as the initial diagnostic test (Chapter 32). A serum gastrin concentration of 600 pg/ml or greater in a patient with severe peptic ulcer disease is usually diagnostic of Zollinger-Ellison syndrome. However, increased serum gastrin concentration can also occur in patients with atrophic gastritis or gastric atrophy with or without pernicious anemia. Differentiation between Zollinger-Ellison syndrome and atrophic gastritis or gastric atrophy can be made by measuring gastric acid secretion (Chapter 32). Patients with Zollinger-Ellison syndrome have markedly increased acid secretory rates, whereas patients with the latter disease have hypochlorhydria or achlorhydria.

Basal acid output is usually greater than 15 mmol/hr, and the ratio of basal to peak acid output is frequently greater than 0.5:1.0 in patients with Zollinger-Ellison syndrome. If a patient has a basal to peak acid output ratio greater than 0.5:1.0 and an elevated serum gastrin concentration (>600 pg/ml), the diagnosis of Zollinger-Ellison syndrome is very likely. However, if the serum gastrin concentration is between 200 and 600 pg/ml, the diagnosis is less secure. Under such circumstances, a provocative test for gastrinoma, such as the secretin stimulation test, should be performed (Chapter 32). A combination of an abnormally elevated serum gastrin concentration, a positive secretin stimulation test result, an elevated basal acid secretion rate, and a high ratio of basal to peak acid output confirms the diagnosis of Zollinger-Ellison syndrome.

Treatment

There are two goals of therapy in patients with Zollinger-Ellison syndrome (ZES). The first is to control acid secretion to prevent end-organ damage and symptoms. For many years, the only means to achieve this goal was by total gastrectomy. Now, however, this can be accomplished with antisecretory medications. Using high doses of H_2-receptor antagonists or, preferably, omeprazole, basal acid secretion can be readily kept below 10 mmol/hr as measured during the hour before next administration of medication. Studies have shown that maintaining basal acid output below 10 mmol/hr in patients with ZES prevents recurrent ulceration. Numerous patients have been treated successfully and safely with omeprazole for several years.

The second goal of therapy is to control or cure the malignancy. Assuming preoperative evaluation with computed tomographic (CT) scan, with or without arteriography, does not disclose widespread metastatic disease, an exploratory laparotomy should be undertaken. A careful tumor search should be carried out, including transilluminating the duodenum, because some tumors are found in the duodenal wall. Initial studies using endoscopic ultrasonography for tumor localization are promising. All visible tumor that can be removed easily should be resected. Whether a patient should have a Whipple procedure to remove a tumor in the bed of the pancreas is controversial. After tumor resection, it also seems reasonable to perform a proximal gastric vagotomy to reduce acid secretion further. This may permit some patients to have the dose of antisecretory medication reduced, even if all of the tumor is not found or cannot be resected. Unfortunately, no more than 30% of patients achieve complete cure after surgery.

REFERENCES

Berg CL and Wolfe MM: Zollinger-Ellison syndrome. Med Clin North Am 75:903, 1991.

Blair JA, III et al: Detailed comparison of basal and food-stimulated gastric acid secretion rates and serum and gastrin concentrations in duodenal ulcer patients and normal subjects. J Clin Invest 79:582, 1987.

Feldman M and Burton ME: Histamine 2-receptor antagonists. N Engl J Med 323:1672, 1749, 1990.

Feldman M et al: Life events, stress and psychosocial factors in men with peptic ulcer disease. A multidimensional case-controlled study. Gastroenterology 91:370, 1986.

Graham DY: Prevention of gastroduodenal injury by chronic nonsteroidal antiinflammatory drug therapy. Gastroenterology 96:675, 1989.

Hunt RH: Peptic ulcer disease. Gastroenterol Clin North Am 19:1990.

Maton PN: Omeprazole. N Engl J Med 324:965, 1991.

McCarthy DM: Sucralfate. N Engl J Med 325:1017, 1991.

Peterson WL: *Helicobacter pylori* and peptic ulcer disease. N Engl J Med 324:1043, 1991.

Soll AH: Duodenal ulcer disease. In Sleisenger M and Fordtran JS, editors: Gastrointestinal disease: pathophysiology, diagnosis and management, ed 4. Philadelphia, 1989, WB Saunders.

Talley NJ and Phillips SF. Non-ulcer dyspepsia: potential causes and pathophysiology. Ann Intern Med 108:865, 1988.

Thirbly RC and Feldman M: Postoperative recurrent ulcer. In Sleisenger M and Fordtran JS, editors: Gastrointestinal disease: pathophysiology, diagnosis and management ed 4. Philadelphia, 1988, WB Saunders.

CHAPTER

39 Gastritis and Other Gastric Diseases

Gregory L. Eastwood

The term *gastritis* applies to a wide variety of hemorrhagic or inflammatory conditions of the gastric mucosa that differ in pathogenesis and clinical manifestations.

ACUTE GASTRITIS

Acute gastritis ranges from inflammation of the mucosa to multiple erosions and/or subepithelial hemorrhage throughout the stomach, with consequent loss of blood and tissue fluid. Erosions and subepithelial hemorrhages are defects that are confined to the mucosa. If erosions extend through the muscularis mucosae, frank ulcers are formed. Acute gastritis may involve the mucosa of the entire stomach, it may be limited to the fundic or antral mucosa only, or it may appear in a patchy distribution anywhere within the stomach. If erosions or subepithelial hemorrhages predominate, inflammation is often minimal. Predisposing conditions to acute gastritis are indicated in the box below.

Hydrochloric acid appears to be a requisite to the pathogenesis of acute erosive gastritis, regardless of what other agent or predisposing condition may be present. Aspirin, a weak organic acid, is nonionized and lipid soluble when it is in an acid milieu below its pK_a of 3.5. Consequently, aspirin, like other weak organic acids, diffuses rapidly into the gastric mucosa under these conditions and causes mucosal injury. Because prostaglandins are believed to be important in protecting the gastric mucosa, the inhibition of prostaglandin synthesis by aspirin also may contribute to the pathogenesis of aspirin-induced gastritis. Ethanol, which is lipid soluble at any pH, does not depend on acid to exert its harmful effects on the gastric mucosa, although an acid environment augments the injury caused by etha-

Conditions that cause acute gastritis

- Aspirin and other nonsteroidal anti-inflammatory drugs (NSAIDs)
- Bile, pancreatic secretions, and other duodenal contents
- Ethanol
- *Helicobacter pylori*
- Irradiation
- Ischemia
- Physiologic stress (e.g., shock, sepsis, burns, multiple organ system failure)
- Psychological stress?
- Trauma (e.g., nasogastric suction, therapeutic endoscopic techniques, large hiatal hernia)

nol. The ingestion of many of the nonsteroidal anti-inflammatory agents, such as indomethacin and ibuprofen, also is associated with acute gastritis.

Focal, but sometimes extensive, gastritis can develop as a result of trauma from nasogastric tubes; therapeutic endoscopic techniques, such as laser and electrocoagulation; and local mucosal irritation from pressure and movement in a hiatus hernia. *Helicobacter pylori* also now is recognized as a cause of acute gastritis.

In addition to the exogenous agents indicated, several endogenous conditions may predispose the gastric mucosa to acute gastritis. Reflux of bile and other duodenal contents may result from a poorly functioning pyloric sphincter and appears to be more common in patients with gastric ulcer disease. Free reflux of bile also occurs after phloroplasty or antrectomy with gastroenterostomy and is believed to predispose the gastric mucosa not only to acute erosive gastritis but also to the chronic gastritis that develops after gastric surgery (see late discussion). Furthermore, in patients who are under severe stress with sepsis, shock, burns, or renal, hepatic, or respiratory failure erosions or frank ulcers of the stomach may develop for reasons only partially understood. Alterations in mucosal blood flow, inhibition of gastric epithelial renewal, or impairment of the gastric mucosal defense mechanisms may play a major role in these conditions. Although acid continues to be an important pathogenic factor, many patients with acute gastritis secrete only small amounts of acid. The major complication of acute erosive gastritis is bleeding, which may be mild or severe and life threatening but is not often associated with pain.

Because the erosions and subepithelial hemorrhages of acute gastritis are superficial, barium contrast radiographic studies usually are not helpful. The definitive diagnosis of acute erosive gastritis is best made by early gastroscopy, which allows direct inspection and biopsy of the gastric mucosa.

The gastric mucosa is capable of rapid healing. Thus most patients who suffer the effects of acute gastritis recover promptly when the offending agent is removed. If the gastritis is related to a predisposing condition, that condition should be treated. Antacid therapy is indicated in addition to the other measures employed in the management of upper gastrointestinal bleeding (Chapter 34). H_2-receptor antagonists and sucralfate also have been used. Some patients, particularly those with severe predisposing disease, may respond poorly to treatment, continue to bleed from gastric erosions in spite of appropriate medical therapy, and require emergency surgery. The choice of operation is a difficult decision. Most patients improve after antrectomy and vagotomy; rarely is total gastrectomy necessary to control bleeding.

CHRONIC GASTRITIS

Chronic gastritis typically is not erosive and thus is not necessarily the consequence of long-standing acute gastritis. The histopathology of chronic gastritis involving fundic mucosa, which lines the body and fundus of the stomach, is a continuum that has been somewhat arbitrarily separated into three categories: chronic superficial gastritis, chronic atrophic gastritis, and gastric atrophy. A photomicrograph of normal fundic mucosa is shown in Fig. 39-1 for comparison with subsequent examples showing chronic gastritis.

In *chronic superficial gastritis,* the lamina propria is infiltrated with plasma cells, lymphocytes, and, in some instances, neutrophils and eosinophils (Fig. 39-2). This process may occur throughout the mucosa but typically is localized to the upper third of the mucosa in the region of the gastric pits. Below the pits, the lamina propria between

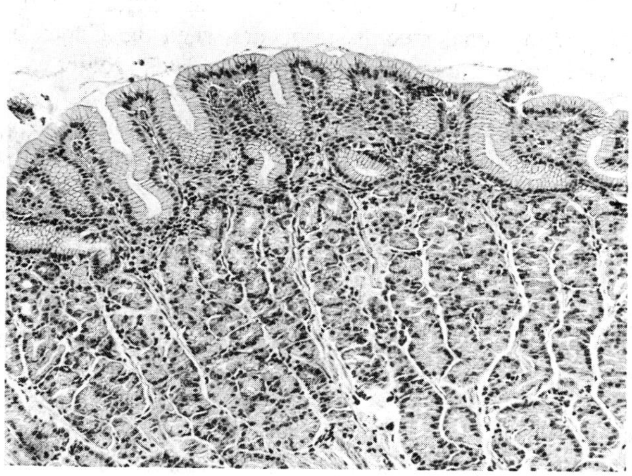

Fig. 39-1. Photomicrograph of normal human gastric fundic mucosa. Mucus-secreting epithelial cells cover the surface of the mucosa and extend down into the gastric pits. Beneath the pits and emptying into them are long, convoluted glands lined by acid- and intrinsic factor-secreting parietal cells and pepsinogen-secreting chief cells. The lamina propria between the pits and glands contains mononuclear cells and blood vessels.

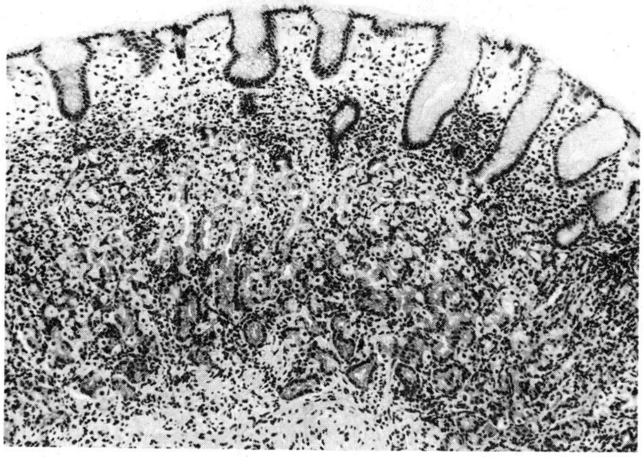

Fig. 39-2. Photomicrograph showing chronic superficial gastritis. The density of mononuclear cells within the lamina propria is increased throughout the mucosa, particularly in the upper third.

the gastric glands often appears normal except when the inflammation is extensive. The surface epithelial cells may be flattened, and some cells are necrotic.

Chronic atrophic gastritis is characterized by infiltration of plasma cells, lymphocytes, and, if severe, neutrophils, which is similar to that seen in chronic superficial gastritis but extends down to involve the fundic glands and the interglandular spaces. The glands become atrophic, so the spaces between them widen and the number of parietal and chief cells is reduced. The mucosal thickness decreases, although the muscularis mucosae becomes hypertrophied. In some instances, pseudopyloric or intestinal metaplasia develops. In pseudopyloric metaplasia, the glands lose their parietal and chief cells and become lined by mucus-secreting cells similar to those in normal pyloric (antral) mucosa. Intestinal metaplasia occurs when the glands become lined by intestinal-type absorptive cells, goblet cells, and Paneth cells (Fig. 39-3).

In *gastric atrophy,* the fundic glands have undergone pyloric or intestinal metaplasia so that few or no parietal or chief cells are visible. The mucosa is thin, and only minimal inflammatory cell infiltration is seen in the lamina propria, although some lymphoid aggregates may be present.

Chronic gastritis also develops in antral mucosa, but its appearance is somewhat different from that in fundic mucosa. Normal antral mucosa has deeper pits than fundic mucosa. The pits may occupy as much as half of the mucosal thickness, although total mucosal thickness in the antrum is less than in the fundus. In addition, there is more cellular infiltration in the lamina propria of the antrum than in the fundus of many normal subjects. Thus classification of the severity of gastritis based on the degree of inflammation is difficult. Antral gastritis may be graded as mild, moderate, or severe, on the basis of an evaluation of the degree of obliteration of the pyloric glands, the degree of infiltration of the lamina propria by inflammatory cells, and the presence and extent of intestinal metaplasia.

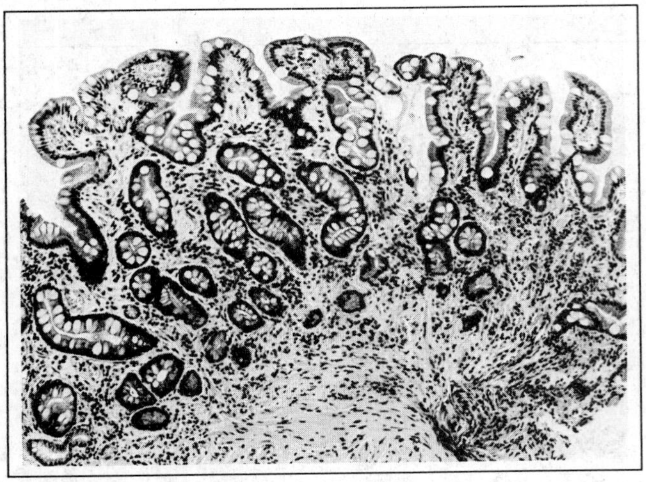

Fig. 39-3. Photomicrograph showing intestinal metaplasia of atrophic gastric mucosa. Villiform appearance and numerous goblet cells are characteristic. The number of gastric glands is diminished, parietal and chief cells are absent, and the thickness of the mucosa is reduced.

In some patients, superficial gastritis, atrophic gastritis, and gastric atrophy may represent different stages in the same disease. In other patients, atrophic gastritis or gastric atrophy seems to arise without prior progression through a stage of superficial gastritis. These differences in presentation may be explained by the diverse causes of chronic gastritis, which may include immunologic mechanisms as well as chronic exposure of the gastric mucosa to harmful agents.

Chronic gastritis that involves the body and fundus of the stomach and is associated with atrophic changes has been called type A. Patients with pernicious anemia have type A gastritis, although most patients with type A gastritis do not have pernicious anemia. Type A gastritis may be an autoimmune disorder. Humoral antibodies to the microsomal fraction of parietal cells are present in 20% to 50% of patients who have idiopathic atrophic gastritis and in up to 95% of patients with pernicious anemia, and antibodies to intrinsic factor are found frequently in patients with pernicious anemia. Defects in cell-mediated immunity also may be important in the development of chronic gastritis.

Type B gastritis, which is the more common type, primarily involves the antrum but may progress proximally to include fundic mucosa. *H. pylori* has been implicated as the cause of most cases of type B gastritis. *H. pylori* is in adherent mucus overlying antral mucosa in almost all individuals with type B gastritis yet is found only rarely in individuals with normal antral mucosa. The prevalence of *H. pylori,* like that of type B gastritis, increases with age in populations studied to date. Most patients with duodenal ulcers have *H. pylori*–associated gastritis (Chapter 38). On the other hand, the vast majority of individuals with *H. pylori*-associated gastritis, a very common entity, do not have peptic ulcer disease. How this noninvasive microorganism produces gastric mucosal inflammation is under intense investigation but is not yet understood. Chronic gastritis of varying degrees increases with normal aging as does the prevalence of *H. pylori.* Whether *H. pylori* is in any way related to the atrophic changes associated with type A gastritis is not known and will require further study.

Patients who have chronic gastritis typically have no symptoms that can be related directly to the gastric lesion. Hence treatment with antibiotics to eliminate *H. pylori* is not indicated in the absence of associated refractory duodenal ulcer disease. The diagnosis of gastritis is made by biopsy of the gastric mucosa. Most patients with atrophic gastritis who are achlorhydric do not have vitamin B_{12} malabsorption or pernicious anemia, although in some patients symptomatic associated conditions, such as pernicious anemia, iron deficiency anemia, gastric polyps, or gastric cancer, may develop. The diagnosis and treatment of these complications constitute the management of patients with chronic gastritis. Patients who have vitamin B_{12} deficiency with or without pernicious anemia should receive monthly 100 μ injections of vitamin B_{12}. Because patients with atrophic gastritis or gastric atrophy are at higher risk than normal of gastric cancer, they should be seen periodically by the physician to determine whether new signs or symptoms have developed. A special subgroup of atrophic gastritis patients are those who have undergone partial gastrectomy 20 or more years previously. Current evidence is conflicting as to whether these patients are at higher risk for gastric cancer.

OTHER TYPES OF GASTRITIS

Hypertrophic gastritis

Hypertrophic gastritis is characterized by large mucosal folds in all or part of the stomach. This condition is composed of two entities, Ménétrier's disease and hypersecretory gastropathy, but some patients show features of both. In Ménétrier's disease, hyperplasia of the gastric pits and superficial epithelium is the predominant histologic abnormality. Epigastric pain, vomiting, and upper gastrointestinal bleeding are common complaints. Massive loss of tissue protein from the gastric mucosa may lead to hypoproteinemia and edema. Acid secretion is normal or low. In the related condition, hypersecretory gastropathy, the hypertrophic mucosal folds are composed primarily of enlarged fundic glands that may contain increased numbers of parietal cells. High acid secretion is typical, whereas loss of protein is not. The hypoproteinemia of Ménétrier's disease is treated with a high-protein diet. Acid hypersecretion may respond to H_2-receptor antagonists or omeprazole. When these measures fail, surgical excision of the involved portion of the stomach may be indicated.

Other conditions that cause large gastric folds include carcinoma, lymphoma, and granulomatous disease. Parietal cell hyperplasia caused by the trophic effect of gastrin also produces large folds in the fundic mucosa of patients with Zollinger-Ellison syndrome.

Granulomatous gastritis

Virtually any disorder that is associated with granuloma formation can cause granulomatous involvement of the stomach. The most frequent causes of granulomatous gastritis include tuberculosis, sarcoidosis, Crohn's disease of the stomach, and syphilis. Also, eosinophilic granulomas may develop as a result of infestation with the nematode larva of *Anisakis marina,* or they may be idiopathic. Idiopathic eosinophilic granulomas of the stomach, which usually are nodular lesions of the antrum and are not associated with peripheral eosinophilia, should not be confused with eosinophilic gastroenteritis, in which the gastrointestinal tract may be infiltrated diffusely with eosinophils and in which peripheral eosinophil counts are high.

Patients with granulomatous gastritis may have epigastric pain, vomiting, and gastric-outlet obstruction as well as the signs and symptoms of the underlying disease. Treatment depends on the cause. When the cause of the underlying disease is itself unknown, such as in sarcoidosis, Crohn's disease, and idiopathic eosinophilic granuloma, corticosteroids may be beneficial. Occasionally, surgical removal of an obstructing or ulcerating lesion is necessary.

Eosinophilic gastritis

Eosinophilic gastritis is usually part of a more generalized eosinophilic infiltration of the gastrointestinal tract that is of unknown cause (Chapter 42). Peripheral eosinophilia is usually prominent. Patients have attacks of abdominal pain, vomiting, and diarrhea and may have protein-losing enteropathy. When the primary involvement is in the stomach, the radiologic appearance may resemble that of carcinoma, and symptoms may reflect gastric-outlet obstruction. Endoscopic biopsy of the stomach may establish the diagnosis, although occasionally surgical biopsy is necessary. Treatment with corticosteroids results in dramatic improvement in most patients, whereas elimination diets, from which foodstuffs suspected of causing an allergic response have been omitted, generally are unsuccessful (Chapter 42).

Corrosive gastritis

A wide variety of agents, if swallowed, can cause extensive injury to both the stomach and the esophagus (Chapter 35). Chief among these agents are lye, other strong alkalis, strong acid, and formaldehyde, as well as numerous household and commercial cleaners and solvents. The degree of injury depends on the amount and concentration of the substance swallowed and whether or not the stomach contains food. Patients generally experience severe abdominal pain and may have massive gastric bleeding. Perforation of the stomach or proximal bowel may occur. Fibrous stricture of the lumen of the stomach is a late complication. A cautious endoscopic examination is indicated to assess the extent of injury and to suction any remaining corrosive material (Chapter 35). Treatment consists of fluid, electrolyte, and blood replacement; antacid administration; and nasogastric suction. The efficacy of steroids in preventing late strictures is not established. Antibiotics may be indicated for complications such as aspiration. Indications for surgery include development of uncontrolled bleeding, gangrene, perforation, and obstruction caused by stricture during healing.

Infectious gastritis

Acute infection of the stomach may produce a diffuse phlegmonous, or suppurative, gastritis. This rare condition probably arises from preexisting disease of the stomach, such as damage by ethanol or noxious agents, chronic gastritis, trauma, or upper gastrointestinal surgery. The alpha-hemolytic streptococcus is the most common organism involved, although *Escherichia coli,* staphylococci, pneumococci, *Clostridium welchii, Proteus vulgaris,* and *Bacillus subtilis* also have been implicated. The disease, a medical emergency with a high mortality, requires surgical resection after appropriate treatment with fluids, electrolytes, and antibiotics.

H. pylori also causes acute gastritis of less severity and is recognized as the major cause of type B chronic gastritis that involves the antrum (see earlier discussion).

Fungal infection, notably candidiasis, can involve the

stomach in patients who take immunosuppressives, steroids, or antineoplastic agents or who are receiving radiotherapy. Gastric candidiasis also has been described as a superinfection in some patients who have been treated with cimetidine as well as in association with chronic gastric ulcers, although its significance in these conditions is unclear.

Irradiation gastritis

Irradiation causes both acute and chronic injury to the gastric mucosa. Within days or months after exposure to irradiation, varying degrees of mucosal inflammation, necrosis, and ulceration may occur in a dose-dependent fashion. Later, arterioles become narrowed as a result of swelling of the vessel walls and endarteritis. The mucosa usually regenerates, but submucosal fibrosis and edema and endarteritis often persist. A chronic gastric ulcer that is indistinguishable from a chronic peptic ulcer except for the presence of antral fibrosis and obliterative endarteritis may develop.

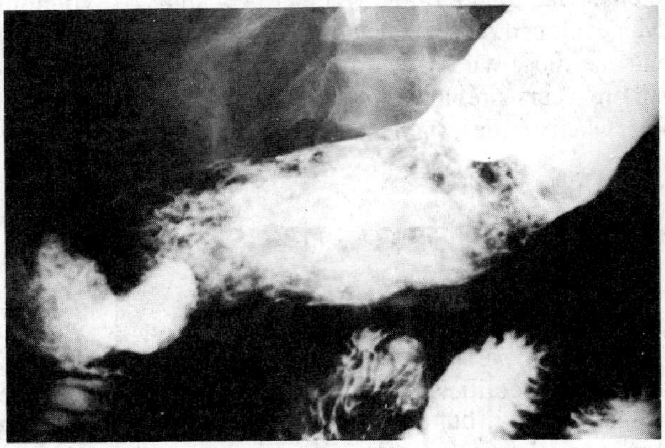

Fig. 39-4. Upper gastrointestinal radiograph series showing a large bezoar of the body of the stomach. The barium does not penetrate completely through the mass, resulting in an amorphous mottled appearance. (Radiograph courtesy of Murray Janower, MD)

MISCELLANEOUS DISORDERS OF THE STOMACH

Bezoars and foreign bodies

A *gastric bezoar* is a firm aggregation of nondigestible material that fails to pass into the small intestine. Bezoars are of two general types: trichobezoars, which are composed of hair, and phytobezoars, which are composed of plant products. Some bezoars contain elements of both. Bezoars can be associated with nausea, vomiting, abdominal pain, and a sensation of epigastric fullness, or they may be asymptomatic. Bezoars occur rarely in normal stomachs; they are most often associated with vagotomy and partial gastric resection or other conditions that induce gastric stasis, such as diabetic visceral neuropathy.

The diagnosis of gastric bezoar can be suspected if an upper gastrointestinal series shows an irregular mass in the stomach into which there is variable penetration of barium (Fig. 39-4). Upper gastrointestinal endoscopy with biopsy yielding hair or vegetable matter confirms the diagnosis. Bezoars may be disrupted by endoscopic manipulation. Phytobezoars may respond to cellulase, papain, or acetylcysteine enzyme treatment. A liquid diet and gastric lavage are also helpful. Phytobezoars that remain after medical therapy and nearly all trichobezoars may require surgical removal.

Hypertrophic pyloric stenosis

Hypertrophy and edema of the pyloric muscle is a condition most often seen in infants within the first month of life, but it also may occur in adults. In infants the cause is obscure, whereas in adults the disease may be idiopathic or associated with peptic ulcer disease, antral gastritis, or carcinoma.

In newborns with hypertrophic pyloric stenosis projectile vomiting develops, either immediately with the ingestion of food or after the stomach is filled. Because so little of what is ingested reaches the intestine, constipation is a frequent complication, and the infant fails to gain weight. Visible peristalsis and a firm mass in the right upper abdomen before the patient has eaten and a distended epigastrium in response to feeding are typical findings on physical examination. A plain film of the abdomen, taken as the infant is in the upright position, shows a large gastric air bubble and little or no air in the bowel. Upper gastrointestinal series shows a long, narrow pyloric channel, and the duodenal bulb and prepyloric antrum may be indented by the mass. The treatment of infantile hypertrophic pyloric stenosis is surgical division of the pyloric muscle from the serosa to the mucosa.

The signs and symptoms of adult hypertrophic pyloric stenosis are similar to those in the infant, except that a pyloric mass is rarely felt. Although surgical division of the pylorus is usually effective, the need to differentiate idiopathic disease from pyloric channel ulcer or gastric carcinoma makes local resection a more appropriate operation for most patients.

Diverticula

Seventy-five percent of gastric diverticula occur on the posterior wall within 2 cm of the esophagogastric junction. They are thought to be congenital. Diverticula that develop either as a result of peptic or neoplastic disease or as a result of surgery for those conditions are usually found in the prepyloric antrum. Rarely is a diverticulum, either idiopathic or acquired, located between these two extremes. Gastric diverticula are typically discovered as incidental findings on barium contrast studies. The vast majority are asymptomatic. Symptoms of pain, pressure, or dyspepsia, when they do occur, probably are related to other disease. However, bleeding and perforation of gastric diverticula have been reported and are treated surgically. Otherwise, no treatment is indicated.

Volvulus

Rarely, the stomach may twist on itself and cause either acute symptoms with severe pain, vomiting, and shock or the chronic, more subtle symptoms of mild pain and early satiety. Lengthy or lax ligaments are the major factors that predispose the stomach to develop gastric volvulus. Other predisposing factors include paraesophageal hernia, intrinsic lesions of the stomach, and adjacent masses or enlarged organs, which can distort the stomach and allow it to twist.

The diagnosis is suggested on the plain film of the abdomen, which shows two air-fluid levels in the left upper abdomen. Barium fails to pass into the stomach or, if it does, shows the twisted appearance of the organ. Decompression and relief of the volvulus can sometimes be accomplished by gentle passage of a nasogastric tube or endoscope and gastric suction. Acute strangulation of the stomach or recurrent or refractory volvulus must be treated surgically by gastropexy and repair of predisposing conditions.

Gastroparesis

Failure of the stomach to empty produced by a disturbance in gastric motility constitutes *gastroparesis*. The major causes are inflammatory conditions within the abdomen, scleroderma, diabetic neuropathy, vagotomy, and anticholinergic medications. Gastric emptying can also be delayed after gastric surgery and may be due to a combination of tissue swelling, vagotomy, and removal of the antrum, which is responsible for the major portion of gastric motility. Patients complain of epigastric fullness, and reflux or vomiting of gastric contents may occur. Obstructing lesions should be ruled out by barium contrast studies or gastroscopy. The treatment of gastroparesis begins with the treatment of the associated condition. Nasogastric suction may be necessary to decompress the stomach. Postoperative gastroparesis may not respond until nasogastric suction has been performed for several weeks. The smooth muscle agonist metoclopramide and the antibiotic erythromycin have been useful in promoting gastric emptying in some patients, provided mechanical obstruction is not present.

REFERENCES

Blaser MJ: Hypotheses on the pathogenesis and natural history of *Helicobacter pylori*-induced inflammation. Gastroenterology 102:720, 1992.

Dooley CP et al: Prevalence of *Helicobacter pylori* infection and histologic gastritis in asymptomatic persons. N Engl J Med 321:1562, 1989.

Glass GGJ and Pitchumoni CS: Atrophic gastritis. Hum Pathol 6:219, 1975.

Ivey KJ: Drugs, gastritis, and peptic ulcer. J Clin Gastroenterol 3(suppl 2):29, 1981.

Lundegardh G et al: Stomach cancer after partial gastrectomy for benign ulcer disease. N Engl J Med 319:195, 1988.

Parsonnet J et al: *Helicobacter pylori* infection and the risk of gastric carcinoma. N Engl J Med 325:1127, 1991.

Peterson WL: *Helicobacter pylori* and peptic ulcer disease. N Engl J Med 324:1043, 1991.

Schafer LW et al: The risk of gastric carcinoma after surgical treatment for benign ulcer disease: a population-based study in Olmsted County, Minnesota. N Engl J Med 309:1210, 1983.

Weinstein WM: The diagnosis and classification of gastritis and duodenitis. J Clin Gastroenterol 3(suppl 2):7, 1981.

CHAPTER

40 Tumors of the Stomach

Robert C. Kurtz

INCIDENCE AND EPIDEMIOLOGY OF GASTRIC ADENOCARCINOMA

Gastric carcinoma is the third most common gastrointestinal cancer in the United States, with approximately 23,000 new cases expected in the current year. Carcinoma of the stomach is rare in persons under 20 years of age, but the incidence rises gradually to over 110 cases per 100,000 per year in those above 50 years old. The disease occurs preponderantly in males; the male/female incidence is as high as 2:1 in certain age groups. The death rate from gastric cancer has been declining in the United States over the past several decades. Recent analysis of incidence data from the NCI Surveillance, Epidemiology and End Results (SEER) program have revealed sharply rising rates of adenocarcinoma of the gastric cardia and esophagus. Among white, middle-class males, adenocarcinoma of the cardia of the stomach accounts for about one half of the gastric cancers. In Japan, gastric cancer is a leading cause of cancer death. Other areas of the world in which there is a high prevalence of gastric cancer include Thailand, Finland, and the mountainous regions of Colombia, South America (but not the coastal regions). However, even in these countries the incidence has declined in recent years. Studies have shown that Japanese who emigrate reduce their chances of development of gastric cancer by 25%. Incidence in second-generation Japanese in the United States is reduced even further, by more than 50%. Variations in incidence of gastric cancer in different geographic locations and in migratory populations strongly suggest that environmental factors are important in the development of the disease. Such environmental factors may be carcinogens in food, but no one food that is common to all of the high-risk areas has been identified. Types of foods incriminated include cereal, dried foods, smoked fish, salted foods, and cured foods. Some foods thought to be protective are fresh fruits, lettuce, milk, and fatty foods.

Studies suggest a correlation between dietary nitrate intake and gastric cancer incidence. Nitrosamines are potent carcinogens in a number of animal species. These substances could play a role in the development of gastric cancer either by their presence in ingested food or by their in vivo production in the stomach of persons affected by nitrosation of secondary amines with nitrite. Human gastric juice contains a significant amount of amines that may be converted to nitrosamines in acid pH by nonenzymatic means or in neutral pH by certain bacteria. The previously widespread practice of salting foods and meats with a combination of sodium chloride and nitrate may have led to the substantially higher rate of gastric cancer seen in the United States before the widespread use of refrigeration. Additionally, the nitrate content of the soil is much higher in high-incidence geographic areas; for example, in Colombia the nitrate content is higher in the mountains than in the coastal areas.

Polycyclic hydrocarbons are another important group of compounds found in foods as well as in the environment. Studies of smoked foods in Iceland have shown that these foods contain large amounts of benzpyrene.

There have been familial aggregations of gastric cancer, but the influence of heredity in the development of the disease is not well understood. In one inbred Virginia family, 12 gastric cancer patients were identified in four generations. In relatives of gastric cancer patients the disease develops at a substantially high rate. Whether these family members have a genetic predisposition to gastric cancer or whether they have been exposed to common environmental factors is unknown.

In a large population-based study in Shandong, China, the risk of developing gastric cancer was influenced not only by dietary factors and cigarette usage, but by heredity. This risk rose by 80% among those with gastric cancer in a family member. Studies of the ABO blood groups show that blood type A is most commonly associated with gastric cancer. About 50% of patients with the diffuse type of gastric cancer have type A blood, whereas only 38% of the general population have this blood type. The reason for this difference is not known.

PREMALIGNANT CONDITIONS

Atrophic gastritis (see also Chapter 39)

Chronic atrophic gastritis is frequently seen in patients who have concurrent gastric cancer. Chronic gastritis is also associated with pernicious anemia, and it increases in frequency with increasing age. In severe chronic atrophic gastritis with hypochlorhydria or achlorhydria, "intestinalization" of the mucosa may occur.

Cell kinetic studies have shown that atrophic gastritis represents a hyperproliferative state in which the rapidly replicating proliferative compartment of the gastric gland has moved up to the luminal surface from its usual location in the gland neck. Although early such changes may be reversible, decrease in acid production, colonization by bacteria, and endogenous formation of nitroso compounds with potential mutagenicity may eventually lead to the development of cancer. However, although all patients with gastric cancer have underlying atrophic gastritis, the vast majority of people with atrophic gastritis never develop gastric cancer.

Pernicious anemia falls into the category of autoimmune chronic atrophic gastritis with associated "extragastric" features such as thyroiditis, diabetes mellitus, Addison's disease, and vitiligo. In 1955, a large study that followed over 1200 pernicious anemia patients at Boston City Hospital and found 28 patients with gastric cancer was published. This rate was considerably higher than the rate of gastric cancer in the general population in the state of Massachusetts at that time. More recent studies have suggested that the previously observed risk of gastric cancer in pernicious anemia is no longer seen. It is likely that the association of gastric cancer and pernicious anemia initially observed was a reflection of the high incidence of gastric cancer at that time.

A recent case-control study using a serologic test for *Helicobacter pylori* infection associated with chronic atrophic gastritis suggests that *H. pylori* infection is associated with an increased risk of gastric cancer and may represent a cofactor in its pathogenesis.

There have been a number of reports both supporting and rejecting the relationship between previous subtotal gastrectomy for peptic ulcer disease and later development of cancer in the gastric stump. These cancers have generally developed 20 years or more after the subtotal gastrectomy. The risk appears greater after a Billroth II than after a Billroth I anastomosis and may be etiologically related to the reflux of bile and pancreatic juice through the gastrojejunostomy. Because the risk of gastric cancer in the gastric remnant is low in areas where the incidence of gastric cancer is low, as in the United States, periodic endoscopic surveillance of these patients is not recommended.

Gastric polyps

There are a number of different types of gastric polyps, some of which are associated with gastric cancer. About 75% to 90% of all gastric polyps are hyperplastic. Hyperplastic polyps seem to be related to a regeneration of the gastric mucosa after injury and are not premalignant lesions. About 10% to 25% of gastric polyps are adenomatous. Adenomatous polyps are most commonly found in the antrum of the stomach and have malignant potential. Reported incidence of gastric cancer occurring in gastric adenomatous polyps greater than 2 cm in size varies widely (average incidence about 40%). Several syndromes of generalized polyposis of the gastrointestinal tract include gastric polyps. In the Peutz-Jeghers syndrome, hamartomatous gastric polyps occur with some frequency. Though their premalignant potential is low, Peutz-Jeghers syndrome polyps in the stomach and duodenum have occasionally developed into carcinomas. In adenomatous polyposis coli and Gardner's syndrome, adenomatous polyps of the stomach have been described, and there have been recent reports of gastric cancer developing in this setting.

When a gastric polyp is found, upper gastrointestinal endoscopy should be performed. The appearance of the polyp is often helpful. Hyperplastic polyps are covered by normal-appearing mucosa; adenomatous polyps appear more reddened. If a biopsy specimen shows hyperplasia, no further therapy need be considered. If the polyp is adenomatous, biopsy findings may be misleading, and the polyp should be removed by endoscopic polypectomy or surgery.

Immunodeficiency disorders

Gastric cancer has been described most commonly in patients who have common variable immunodeficiency. Approximately 50% of patients who have common variable immunodeficiency have achlorhydria, atrophic gastritis, and a pernicious anemia–like syndrome without autoantibodies to intrinsic factor and parietal cells. Gastric cancer has also been noted in patients with selective immunoglobulin A (IgA) deficiency.

PATHOLOGY

Gastric adenocarcinoma has been classified as diffuse and intestinal types. The intestinal type resembles small bowel mucosa. Cell cohesion is described as the morphologic cement that causes the neoplastic cells to attach to each other and form glandlike structures. When this cohesive element is absent, the malignant cells infiltrate the stomach wall, the so-called diffuse type of gastric adenocarcinoma. In high-risk areas of the world, the intestinal type of gastric cancer predominates. The diffuse cancer has a poorer prognosis, is more common in women and younger patients, and generally is not associated with the premalignant conditions noted previously. Because of the stomach's rich lymphatic supply, gastric cancer rapidly spreads to the regional lymph nodes.

Early gastric cancer, confined to the mucosa, is identified in more than one third of cases of gastric cancer in Japan. This is probably attributable to aggressive screening programs in that country. In Europe and the United States, early gastric cancer is found in only 5% to 10% of cases of gastric cancer. In Japan, over 90% of patients with early gastric cancer can be expected to survive 5 years. Improved survival is also seen in Europe and the United States with early gastric cancer but not yet to the same levels as in Japan.

Carcinoma of the stomach may occur as a superficial spreading tumor and may be difficult to diagnose. Superficial spreading gastric cancer involves only the mucosal surface and imparts to it a granular appearance. Occasionally, in more advanced cases, superficial spreading carcinoma can infiltrate the muscularis mucosae. Regional lymph nodes may show metastasis despite the superficial distribution.

CLINICAL FEATURES OF GASTRIC CARCINOMA

Most gastric cancers in the United States present at an advanced stage. Weight loss seems to be the most predictable symptom and is seen in 70% to 80% of patients. The second most common symptom is pain. This may be epigastric, substernal, or back pain, and it occurs in 70% of patients. Abdominal pain may mimic that of benign peptic ulcer disease, with relief of pain obtained by ingesting antacids, H_2-blockers, and food. In other patients, pain is worse after eating and anorexia and vomiting are present, especially if distal tumors cause pyloric obstruction. Patients frequently report a distaste for foods containing beef. Because of reduced dietary intake, constipation is common. Both acute and chronic upper gastrointestinal bleeding may occur, with hematemesis and melena, though frank hemorrhage occurs infrequently, usually in less than 10% of patients. Weakness and fatigue related to decreased dietary intake, weight loss, and anemia are also common complaints. Worsening angina pectoris and dyspnea may be related to progressive anemia. Dysphagia is an important symptom of adenocarcinoma of the fundus of the stomach, which involves the cardioesophageal junction. Jaundice may be present secondary to liver metastasis or extension of the cancer into the porta hepatis. Large bowel involvement by metastasis spreading through the gastrocolic ligament may be mistaken for primary colonic cancer and may cause large intestinal obstruction. Bone pain or neurologic symptoms of cord compression signal metastatic disease.

Physical examination may not reveal abnormality except in advanced disease. The physician may find signs of anemia, recent weight loss with temporal wasting and loss of muscle mass, and lymph node enlargement, particularly in the left supraclavicular area (or Virchow's signal node) or the left side of the neck. Physical findings may also include a palpable abdominal mass if the cancer is large, hepatic enlargement related to metastatic disease, gastric dilatation, and a succussion splash. Jaundice may be present if liver metastases are extensive or positioned at the porta hepatis. Malignant ascites can occur with metastatic gastric cancer. Rectal examination may reveal a rectal "shelf" (Blumer's shelf). Metastases are thought to spread by gravity to the true pelvis and form the shelf noted on rectal examination. Umbilical nodules indicate the presence of metastatic disease. Rarely, acanthosis nigricans may be found on examination of the patient's skin, particularly in the axillae or other body folds.

LABORATORY STUDIES IN GASTRIC CANCER

Between 40% and 50% of patients with gastric cancer are anemic at the time of presentation, usually as a result of chronic blood loss. The anemia is usually microcytic (iron deficiency), but it may be megaloblastic (pernicious) or mixed in type. Microangiopathic anemia has also been reported. The result of the stool test for occult blood is frequently positive, and melena occurs occasionally. Patients with atrophic gastritis, with or without gastric cancer, may have hypochlorhydria or achlorhydria. Decreased production of gastric acid occurs in some individuals during the aging process. Thus gastric secretory function should not be used as a diagnostic tool in gastric cancer detection. In patients who have chronic gastritis involving the proximal portion of the stomach but not the antrum, serum gastrin levels may be high. When gastritis involves the entire stomach, including the antrum, gastrin levels may be low or normal. Because they are so variable, serum gastrin levels are not useful as a screening test for gastric cancer.

DIAGNOSIS

A high index of suspicion is important in diagnosing gastric cancer. Early evaluation of patients for the possibility of gastric cancer is recommended if the family history reveals gastric cancer, gastric polyps, immunodeficiency, atrophic gastritis, pernicious anemia, or gastric ulcer disease. Barium radiographic examination of the upper gastrointestinal tract enables the physician to suspect the appropriate diagnosis in 75% to 80% of patients (Fig. 40-1). Abnormalities seen on radiographic examination include lack of distensibility of the stomach, an ulcerated mass or mass effect surrounding an ulcer, a mass in any portion of the stomach, enlarged gastric folds, and obstructing lesions at the cardioesophageal junction or at the pylorus.

Generally, the location of an ulcer is not important in assessing the possibility of malignancy, though ulcers within 1 cm of the pylorus are usually benign, and fundic ulcers are more likely to be malignant. Malignant ulcers may occur on both the greater and lesser curvatures.

Endoscopy, biopsy, and cytology

Upper gastrointestinal endoscopy provides the best overall method of diagnosing gastric cancer (see Plate II-4 and Chapter 30). Both biopsy and brush cytologic evaluation should be done, because they are complementary. In general, the more biopsies obtained, the higher the diagnostic yield. At least four to six biopsy specimens should be obtained from each separate lesion for maximum yield. For suspected submucosal lesions, multiple biopsy specimens can be obtained from the same site, with each successive sample being slightly deeper. In diagnosing exophytic gastric cancers, the combination of brush cytologic evaluation and biopsy is accurate in more than 90% of patients. When cancers are infiltrative, the accuracy of endoscopic brush cytologic evaluation and biopsy falls to about 50%. A technique utilizing endoscopic needle aspiration cytologic study may further increase the diagnostic yield. Overall, the diagnostic accuracy resulting from use of radiographic examination, endoscopy, biopsy, and cytologic evaluation is greater than 90%.

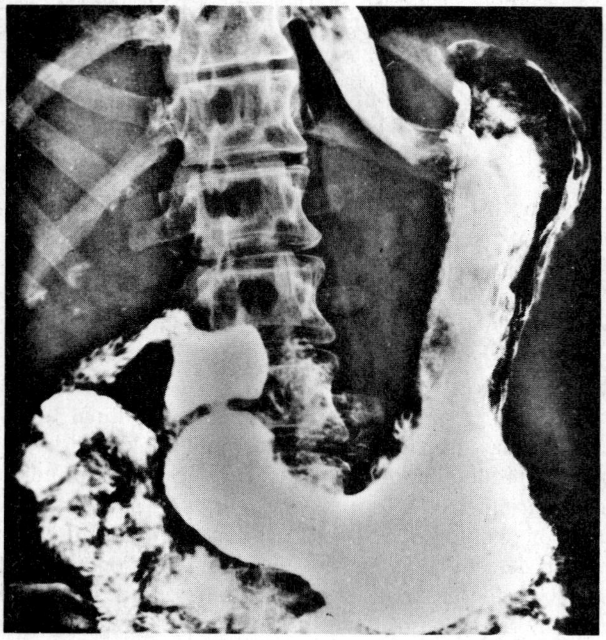

Fig. 40-1. Adenocarcinoma of the proximal stomach. Note the apparent rigidity and narrowing of the stomach with multiple filling defects.

Endoscopy is superior to diagnostic radiographic examination in differentiating benign from malignant gastric ulcers on the basis of appearance alone, and this advantage is substantially improved with the addition of biopsy and cytologic study techniques (Chapter 30). Should all patients with gastric ulcers undergo endoscopy? In one series, 3.3% of radiologically identified benign gastric ulcers were seen by endoscopy to be carcinomas. Other studies have demonstrated that up to 7% of radiologically benign gastric ulcers are actually malignant. Radiologic evidence of gastric ulcer healing on medical management is not sufficient to exclude the possibility that the ulcer is malignant. Early performance of endoscopy and biopsy is the best way to evaluate gastric ulcers. Even if the initial endoscopic examination reveals a benign gastric ulcer it should be followed endosopically at 6 to 8 week intervals until complete healing occurs. If the ulcer persists (Chapter 38) a repeat biopsy should be performed.

Computed tomography

Barium upper gastrointestinal radiography, endoscopy, and biopsy are almost always done before gastric cancer surgery. These diagnostic procedures give little information about the preoperative stage of this disease. Computed tomography (CT) has been successfully used to evaluate gastric wall thickness, direct extension of tumor into adjacent organs, regional and retroperitoneal lymph node enlargement, ascites, and liver metastases. CT has been shown to predict with reasonable accuracy which patients can undergo curative surgery and which tumors are unresectable. A substantial savings in time and resources should be realized as this modality is used more frequently for gastric cancer staging.

Endoscopic ultrasonography

Endoscopic ultrasonography (EUS) is a new technique that combines endoscopy and ultrasonography. High-frequency EUS can produce detailed images of the stomach wall allowing an accurate assessment of depth of tumor invasion (Fig. 40-2). CT produces only a measurement of total wall thickness and contour to estimate depth of tumor invasion. The accumulating data indicate that EUS represents a significant advance in the clinical staging of gastric cancer. Because of its limited depth of field, EUS cannot replace CT for detection of distant metastases. However, it is more accurate in assessing depth of cancer invasion and also ap-

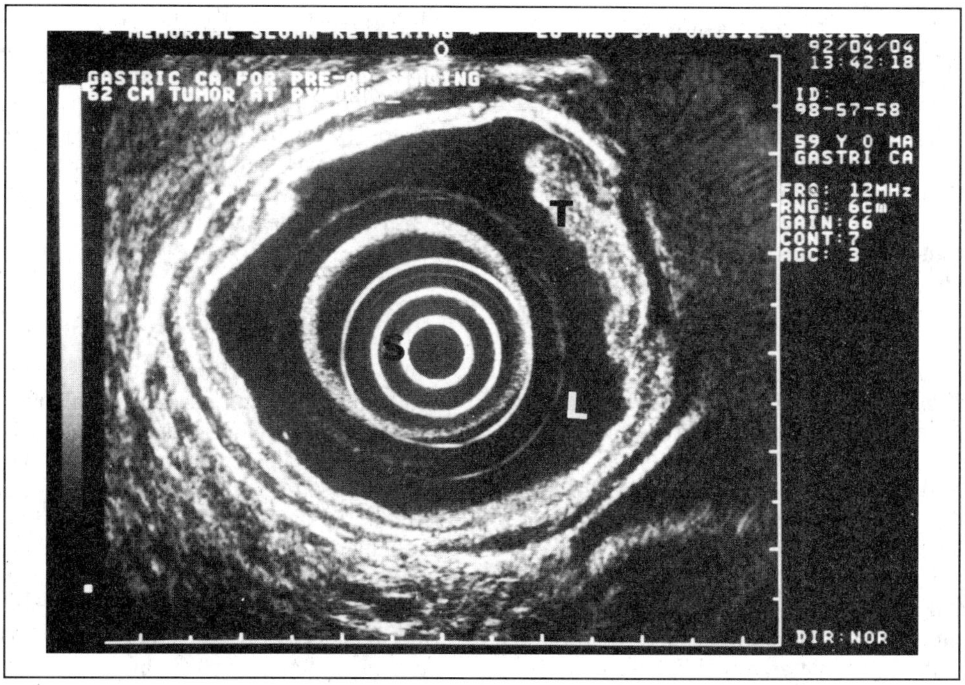

Fig. 40-2. An endosonogram of an early stage gastric cancer that does not penetrate the stomach wall. The lumen contains the endoscope with its associated sonographic artifact. T, early stage gastric cancer; L, lumen; S, endoscope. (Courtesy of Charles J. Lightdale, M.D.)

pears to be more accurate in determining cancer spread to regional lymph nodes. CT and EUS can judge nodal metastases by the size of imaged structures consistent with lymph nodes. EUS can image much smaller nodes (2 to 3 mm) and in addition can provide diagnostically helpful echo patterns. Malignancy is suggested if imaged lymph nodes are round, sharply demarcated, and hypoechoic.

In a study from Memorial Sloan-Kettering Cancer Center, EUS and CT were compared to surgical pathologic evaluation for staging gastric cancer preoperatively in 50 patients. Results showed that EUS agreed with surgical pathology in 88% versus 35% for CT in staging depth of tumor wall penetration ($p < 0.00005$), and in 72% versus 45% in staging nodal disease ($p < 0.02$). Endoscopic ultrasonography is also useful in identifying extraluminal recurrence of gastric cancer.

Other diagnostic tests

Evaluation of the bilirubin, alkaline phosphatase, and 5′-nucleotidase may indicate metastatic liver disease. If imaging studies suggest metastases, liver biopsy can confirm their presence. Carcinoembryonic antigen (CEA) concentration may be elevated in patients with gastric cancer, usually with advanced disease. If CEA level is elevated preoperatively and becomes normal after surgery, it can be used in follow-up evaluations. As in colonic cancer, CEA level frequently rises in recurrent gastric cancer months before the development of clinical recurrence. Beta subunit human chorionic gonadotropin (HCG) level is elevated in 20% of patients with gastrointestinal cancers, including gastric cancer. A few patients with gastric carcinoma have elevations of serum alpha fetoprotein level. Fetal sulfoglycoprotein antigen has been detected in the gastric juice of patients with gastric cancer. The sulfoglycoproteins of carcinomatous gastric juice have often been associated with blood group A activity.

TREATMENT

Surgery is the primary therapy for gastric cancer. If cancer is confined to the stomach, with extension only to the regional lymph nodes, curative procedures should be considered. If there is extension of the cancer beyond the stomach, for example, to the spleen, the spleen should be removed. If the cancer involves the upper third of the stomach, total gastrectomy and splenectomy is considered by many to be the procedure of choice. In Japan, with the use of radical surgery, including extensive lymph node dissection, even patients with advanced gastric cancer have a 5 year survival rate of over 40%. Total gastrectomy is rarely indicated for palliation. Instead, the bulk of the cancer is removed to control bleeding, obstruction, or pain. When a curative resection cannot be done, distal gastric exclusion or gastroenterostomy may relieve obstruction. Prosthetic tubes can be inserted to bypass obstructing lesions in the esophagus, at the cardioesophageal junction, and even farther distally in the stomach and small bowel. Laser therapy is useful to open obstructing cardioesophageal cancers. Feeding jejunostomy or gastrostomy is rarely indicated. Operative mortality varies, depending on the type of surgery performed, from approximately 7% with distal subtotal gastric resection to 23% for extended total gastrectomy.

Generally, conventional external radiation therapy has not been effective because of the radioresistance of gastric cancer. Implantation of radioactive materials into remaining tumor areas during surgery has met with varying results. Intraoperative radiation therapy (IORT) to the tumor bed is also being studied after curative and palliative surgical resection. In one report, the 5 year survival of patients who received IORT with advanced stage gastric cancer was better than that of those patients who did not.

Chemotherapy with 5-fluorouracil (5-FU), doxorubicin hydrochloride (adriamycin), and mitomycin-C or methyl-CCNU (chloroethyl cyclohexyl nitrosourea) may be useful in the management of patients with either residual, post-surgical disease or recurrent gastric cancer. Chemotherapeutic agents can be given as adjuvants to patients who are at high risk for development of recurrent disease. In North America, the Gastrointestinal Tumor Study Group (GITSG), in a randomized prospective trial, investigated the benefit of adjuvant chemotherapy using 5-FU plus methyl-lomustine given postoperatively for 2 years, compared with no postoperative therapy. An improvement of survival was noted but three similar trials failed to confirm the positive results. Because of lack of proven efficacy, and the potential toxicity of these drug regimens, adjuvant chemotherapy for gastric carcinoma remains investigational. Drugs capable of producing higher response rates and more durable, complete tumor responses as shown in patients with unresectable or recurrent gastric cancers will be needed for future adjuvant trials.

Numerous clinical trials of chemotherapy of advanced gastric carcinoma have appeared in the literature. The FAM regimen (5-FU, doxorubicin, and mitocycin C) has received most of the attention during the last decade, since its first report in 1979. Initial experiences suggested an objective response rate of 37% to 63%. In recent years, most centers have found that the response rate is about 20%, with complete response rates below 5%. More recently other protocols have yielded significantly higher response rates. One such proctocol consists of 5-FU, doxorubicin, and methotrexate, with leucovorin rescue (FAMTX protocol), and another of Etoposide, doxorubicin, and cisplatin (EAP protocol). Drug toxicities are moderately severe. Studies of these protocols are under way at a number of centers to corroborate these results.

The patient undergoing surgery coupled with chemotherapy or radiation therapy is at a tremendous disadvantage if nutrition is not maintained. Enteral nutrition is preferable, but if it is not possible, other measures, including intravenous hyperalimentation, must be made part of the treatment plan (Chapter 49).

PROGNOSIS OF GASTRIC CANCER

Early diagnosis affects the prognosis because, if a long period elapses from the onset of symptoms to diagnosis, lymphatic spread is more likely. If the cancer is limited to the mucosa, a 90% to 95% cure rate is possible. Resection of gastric cancer limited to the mucosa and submucosa has almost a 70% cure rate. If perigastric lymph nodes are involved with tumor, the 5 year survival rate is less than 15% despite resection. Linitis plastica and infiltrating lesions have a very poor prognosis compared with that of polypoid or exophytic lesions. Gastric cancer presenting as a peptic ulcer is associated with a 5 year survival rate of 25% to 35%.

LYMPHOMA OF THE STOMACH

Lymphomas of the stomach are less common than gastric adenocarcinomas and account for about 5% of gastric malignant lesions. Non-Hodgkin's lymphoma involves the stomach much more commonly than does Hodgkin's disease. The stomach can be involved by primary lymphoma or it may be involved secondarily, in conjunction with disseminated intra-abdominal or systemic lymphoma. The average age of patients with lymphoma is about a decade less than that of those with gastric adenocarcinoma. Males are affected more frequently than females. The most common symptom is pain, but bleeding, obstruction, and perforation may also occur, mimicking the manifestations of peptic ulcer disease. A palpable epigastric mass is a common presenting feature.

Gastric lymphoma often presents radiographically with bulky or prominent mucosal folds (Fig. 40-3). A mass may be seen, with ulceration and nodularity. It may be difficult to differentiate gastric lymphoma from adenocarcinoma, as gastric lymphoma may resemble linitis plastica or superficial spreading carcinoma. Many but not all gastric lymphomas can be diagnosed by gastroscopy with biopsy and brush cytology. Lymphomatous involvement of the stomach may

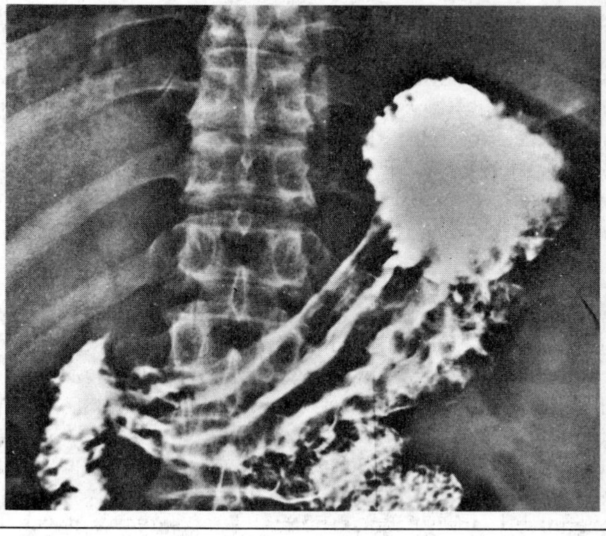

Fig. 40-3. Gastric lymphoma. Large rugal folds run through the body of the stomach. This is suggestive but not diagnostic of gastric lymphoma. Hypertrophic gastropathy (Ménétrier's disease) may also present this radiographic picture.

be confused with Ménétrier's disease (Chapter 39). Full-thickness surgical biopsy specimens obtained at the time of laparotomy may be needed to distinguish Ménétrier's disease from lymphoma. Endoscopic mucosal biopsy specimens are often inadequate, as the physician can never be sure that there is no underlying lymphoma or cancer.

Another gastric lesion that may confuse the diagnosis of gastric lymphoma is pseudolymphoma. This lesion accompanies some benign gastric ulcers and may represent an atypical inflammatory response in the region of the ulcer. Differentiating this lesion from true lymphoma, even in excised tissue, may be difficult for the pathologist.

Patients with lymphomas of the stomach have a significant incidence of non-neoplastic gastric lesions such as stress ulcers, erosive gastritis, and candidal gastritis (Chapter 39).

With a diagnosis of gastric lymphoma, the patient should undergo a thorough evaluation to determine the extent of the disease. In addition to the standard evaluation, chest and abdominal CT scan, bone marrow biopsy, and immunoglobulin analysis are performed. The results of these studies allow a tentative clinical staging of the disease into stomach involvement alone or stomach plus extragastric disease categories. This staging has implications for management as patients with extragastric disease would be candidates for chemotherapy in addition to surgery and radiotherapy. The 5 year survival rate for patients with primary lymphoma of the stomach following surgery is about 50% for non-Hodgkin's lymphoma and less for Hodgkin's disease, because Hodgkin's disease involving the stomach is almost never localized. The best prognosis is for small, well-differentiated lesions confined to the stomach, without lymph node involvement and with only superficial infiltration of the gastric wall.

OTHER MALIGNANT STOMACH TUMORS

Metastatic disease to the stomach from other primary tumor sites is uncommon. It occurs most often in lung cancer, breast cancer, and malignant melanoma. Adrenocortical steroids used in the treatment of breast cancer have been implicated in the spread of this disease to the stomach. Half the patients with ulcerated metastatic gastric lesions have severe gastric bleeding.

Leiomyosarcoma of the stomach comprises about 1% of gastric tumors and may present with a large intramural mass with central ulceration (Fig. 40-4). Massive bleeding or a palpable mass of which the patient is aware may be the presenting complaints. The tumor may be slow growing. After resection, the 5 year survival rate for patients with leiomyosarcoma of the stomach is about 50%. Metastases to the liver and nodes are common, but these patients have a better prognosis than those with most other metastatic tumors. Hepatoma, fibrosarcoma, myxosarcoma, and neurogenic sarcoma are extremely rare and present with features similar to those of leiomyosarcoma. Neurogenic sarcoma can be associated with von Recklinghausen's disease.

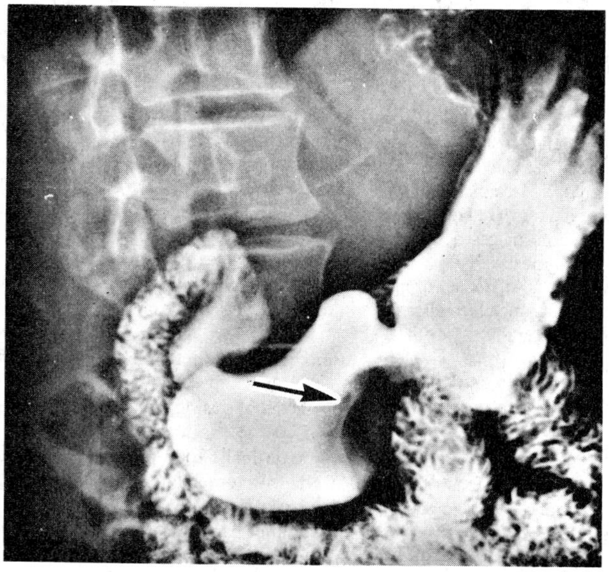

Fig. 40-4. Leiomyosarcoma of the body of the stomach. This tumor originates in the wall of the stomach *(arrow)* and has a characteristic radiologic appearance. It frequently has a central ulceration. It is often not possible to differentiate the benign from the malignant form of this tumor.

LEIOMYOMAS AND BENIGN GASTRIC TUMORS

Leiomyomas of the stomach are commonly found at postmortem examination and are rarely of clinical significance. They usually occur in the distal half of the stomach and may encroach on the lumen, efface the mucosa, and develop secondary ulceration. They may grow in the direction of the serosa, producing a mass that is predominantly extrinsic. Simultaneous inward and outward growth results in a dumbbell shape. This shape is also characteristic of leiomyosarcomas, and differentiation by radiographic examination (Fig. 40-4) or gastroscopy is difficult. Bleeding can occur, and epigastric pain may simulate peptic ulcer disease. Gastroscopic examination reveals effaced but normal mucosa overlying the mass. Biopsy is often unrewarding. Small, asymptomatic leiomyomas need not be removed, but symptomatic lesions, or those that are more than 3 cm in diameter, should be removed by surgery.

Neurofibromas, which are occasionally associated with von Recklinghausen's disease, neuromas, lymphangiomas, ganglioneuromas, lipomas, and carcinoids all can involve the stomach. Multiple gastric carcinoid tumors have been seen in a few patients with pernicious anemia or atrophic gastritis. One possible mechanism for the development of these tumors is achlorhydria and subsequent hypergastrinemia, with stimulation of the enterochromaffinlike cells in the gastric mucosa.

REFERENCES

Blot WJ et al: Rising incidence of adenocarcinoma of the esophagus and gastric cardia. JAMA 265:1287, 1991.

Botet JF et al: Preoperative staging of gastric cancer: comparison of endoscopic ultrasound and dynamic CT. Radiology 181:426, 1991.

Brooks JJ and Enterline HT: Primary gastric lymphomas: a clinicopathologic study of 58 cases with long-term follow-up and literature review. Cancer 5:701, 1983.

Bucholtz TW, Welch CE, and Malt RA: Clinical correlates of resectability and survival in gastric carcinoma. Ann Surg 188:711, 1978.

Carter DC: Cancer after peptic ulcer surgery. Gut 28:921, 1987.

Correa P: The epidemiology of gastric cancer. World J Surg 15:228, 1991.

Cunningham D, Hole D, and Taggart GJ: Evaluation of the prognostic factors in gastric: the effect of chemotherapy on survival. Br J Surg 74:715, 1987.

Erickson RA: Impact of endoscopy on mortality from occult cancer in radiographically benign gastric ulcers: a probability analysis. Gastroenterology 93:835, 1987.

Kurtz RC et al: Upper gastrointestinal neoplasia in familial polyposis. Dig Dis Sci 32:459, 1987.

Kurtz RC and Sherlock P: The diagnosis of gastric cancer. Semin Oncol 12:11, 1985.

LaCave A et al: An EORTC Gastrointestinal Group phase III evaluation of combinations of methyl-CCNU, 5-fluorouracil, and Adriamycin in advanced gastric cancer. J Clin Oncol 5:1387, 1987.

Lundegåardh G et al: Stomach cancer after partial gastrectomy for benign ulcer disease. N Engl J Med 319:195, 1988.

Parsonnet J et al: *Helicobacter pylori* infection and the risk of gastric cancer. N Engl J Med 325:1127, 1991.

Penston J and Wormsley KG: Achlorhydria: hypergastrinemia: carcinoids—a flawed hypothesis? Gut 28:488, 1987.

Remine WH: Gastric sarcomas. Am J Surg 120:320, 1970.

Shiu MH et al: Management of primary gastric lymphoma. Ann Surg 195:196, 1982.

Shiu MH et al: Influence of the extent of resection on survival after curative treatment of gastric carcinoma: a retrospective multivariate analysis. Arch Surg 122:1347, 1987.

Weissberg JB: Role of radiation therapy in gastrointestinal cancer (review). Arch Surg 118:96, 1983.

You WC et al: Diet and high risk of stomach cancer in Shandong. Chin Cancer Res 48:3518, 1988.

CHAPTER

41 Diarrhea, Constipation, and the Irritable Bowel Syndrome

Robin D. Rothstein
Ann Ouyong

DIARRHEA AND CONSTIPATION

Diarrhea and constipation are two of the most common complaints encountered in clinical medicine. An organized approach to these problems requires an understanding of normal and abnormal bowel habits in the general population and in the individual patient. The definitions of diarrhea and constipation used by the physician may not be those used by the patient. Because diarrhea and constipation are symptoms of many disorders, it is necessary to determine their underlying causes.

Diarrhea means a greater-than-normal fecal mass, often largely water, which is usually accompanied by increased stool frequency. The total volume of fluid that passes the ligament of Treitz daily is approximately 9 Ls, including oral intake and salivary, gastric, biliary, pancreatic, and small bowel secretions. Most of the fluid is absorbed in the jejunum and ileum. About 600 ml enters the colon, where all but about 150 ml is absorbed. A stool weight greater than 200 g per day is abnormal. Diarrhea is usually perceived by the patient as any change in bowel habits in which stool frequency or volume (or both) has increased or in which stool consistency has become more fluid.

Constipation is defined as stool frequency of less than three per week. This figure was derived from studies of the bowel habits of normal subjects in whom a frequency of bowel movements ranging from three per day to three per week was recorded. To patients, constipation is usually perceived as a change in bowel habits such that the stool frequency is decreased, or the stool is harder in consistency or more difficult to expel.

Diarrhea

Pathogenesis. Increased fecal water content can result from either a decrease in the amount of fluid absorbed or an increase in the secretion of fluid sufficient to overwhelm the absorptive capacity of the bowel distal to the secretory site. Decreased absorption of fluid can occur as a result of (1) inability to absorb osmotically active solutes, which subsequently retain water in the lumen of the gut (Chapter 42); (2) lack of contact between intraluminal contents and absorptive surfaces; (3) change in active ion transport; and (4) increase in tissue hydrostatic pressure. A change in net active intestinal ion transport causing diarrhea results from a combination of decreased sodium absorption and increased chloride secretion. These changes are mediated by increases in intracellular cyclic adenosine monophosphate (AMP), cyclic guanosine monophosphate, or calcium, by either a direct action on the intestinal epithelial cell or via intermediate steps.

The contribution of alterations in motility to the pathogenesis of diarrhea is less well understood. Many agents that cause diarrhea have been shown, experimentally, to be associated with changes in the motor activity of the bowel. Examples include the effects, in animals, of cholera toxin, enterotoxigenic *Escherichia coli,* ricinoleic acid, and prostaglandins. The importance of motor disturbances relative to the secretory effects of agents that cause diarrheal disease in human beings is not known. In irritable bowel syndrome and diabetic enteropathy, motor disturbances may result in frequent stools that may not have an increased water content but that are perceived as diarrhea by the patient.

The box at right outlines the major pathogenetic mechanisms and diseases in each category. In any disease, several mechanisms may be involved in causing diarrhea. For example, in Zollinger-Ellison syndrome, hypersecretion of gastrin results in increased gastric acid output and excessive acid leads to inflammatory mucosal injury of the small bowel. Gastrin is postulated to affect intestinal motility and transit directly.

Pathogenetic mechanisms of diarrhea

I. Decreased fluid absorption
  A. Inability to absorb osmotically active solutes
    1. Oral intake of poorly absorbable solutes (laxatives, some oral alimentation fluids)
    2. Maldigestion and malabsorption
      a. Diffuse mucosal disease (sprue, Whipple's disease, lymphoma, amyloidosis, ischemia)
      b. Patchy mucosal disease (viral, protozoal)
      c. Pancreatic insufficiency (chronic pancreatitis, pancreatic carcinoma, pancreatic resection, cystic fibrosis)
      d. Enzyme deficiencies (lactase, sucrase-isomaltase)
      e. Bile salt deficiency (biliary obstruction, bacterial overgrowth, ileal resection, Crohn's disease)
  B. Lack of contact of intraluminal fluid with absorptive surface
    1. Intestinal resection or bypass
    2. Enteroenteric fistulas (Crohn's disease)
  C. Deletion or inhibition of active ion absorption (congenital chloridorrhea)

II. Increased fluid secretion
  A. Passive secretion: increased hydrostatic pressure (obstruction of lymphatic drainage)
  B. Active secretion
    1. Secretory agent associated with activation of adenylate cyclase-cyclic AMP system
      a. Vasoactive intestinal peptide (watery diarrhea, hypokalemia, hypochlorhydria syndrome)
      b. Dihydroxy bile acids (acting on colon)
      c. Bacterial enterotoxins (*Vibrio cholerae* enterotoxin and *E. coli* heat-labile enterotoxin)
    2. Secretory agents associated with other intracellular second messengers
      a. Laxatives (bisacodyl, phenolphthalein, ricinoleic acid)
      b. Glucagon, substance P
      c. Toxins (staphylotoxin, *Clostridium perfringens* toxin, *E. coli* heat-stable enterotoxin, Aeromonas, Plesiomonas)
    3. Villous adenoma (? secretagogue)

III. Motor disturbances
  A. Irritable bowel syndrome
  B. Diabetic enteropathy
  C. Visceral scleroderma (results in bacterial overgrowth)
  D. Carcinoid syndrome

IV. Mucosal injury (multiple mechanisms involved)
  A. Bacterial (*Shigella,* invasive *E. coli*)
  B. Inflammatory bowel disease (Crohn's disease, ulcerative colitis, collagenous and lymphocyte colitis)
  C. Ischemic bowel disease

Drugs associated with diarrhea

Laxatives: e.g., cascara sagrada, bisacodyl, phenolphthalein, ricinoleic acid, lactulose
Magnesium-containing antacids
Antibiotics: clindamycin, lincomycin, ampicillin, cephalosporin; may be associated with *Clostridium difficile* toxin and pseudomembranes
Antiarrhythmic drugs: quinidine, propranolol
Digitalis
Antihypertensive drugs: guanethidine, propranolol
Potassium supplements
Artificial sweetners: sorbitol, mannitol
Chenodeoxycholic acid
Cholestyramine*
Sulfasalazine
Anticoagulants

*In patients with extensive ileal resection, bile salt depletion can result in malabsorption and diarrhea.

Acute diarrhea

Diarrhea is considered acute if less than 2 or 3 weeks duration in a patient without a prior history of similar complaints. Most episodes of acute diarrhea are self-limited, but it may be fatal if not treated promptly. Infectious diarrhea, drug-related disease, and inflammatory bowel disease are the three major causes of acute diarrhea. Acute diarrhea in patients with acquired immunodeficiency syndrome (AIDS) is discussed in Chapter 48.

Patients with infectious diarrhea are often systemically ill, with malaise, anorexia, and sometimes fever. A history of recent travel, contacts with patients with diarrhea, and ingestion of suspect foods should be sought. The type of food eaten may indicate the cause of the illness. Bacteria, including aeromonas and plesiomonas, have been implicated as foodborne and waterborne enteropathogens. *Bacillus cereus* has been associated with refried rice. Vomiting may suggest a toxin-related poisoning, possibly caused by staphylococcal toxin ingestion, but is unusual in *Salmonella*- or *Shigella*-induced diarrhea. Bloody diarrhea, suggesting mucosal invasion, may be due to *Shigella flexneri, Campylobacter jejuni,* or enteropathogenic *Escherichia coli*. In a homosexual male, venereal proctitis should be considered with the complaint of frequent stools.

Drugs besides laxatives may cause diarrhea by several different mechanisms. Systemic illness or bloody diarrhea is unusual in drug-induced diarrhea. Microscopic or gross blood may occur after antibiotic use if there is development of pseudomembranous colitis, an infectious diarrhea caused by overgrowth of *Clostridia difficile*. Some drugs that are implicated in the pathophysiology of diarrhea are listed in the box above.

Idiopathic inflammatory bowel disease may present as acute diarrhea, and the patient may be extremely ill. A patient experiencing bloody diarrhea related to ulcerative colitis or Crohn's disease of the colon is more likely to have acute diarrhea than is a patient with ileal Crohn's disease, who often has chronic or recurrent diarrhea and pain (Chapter 43).

Physical examination. The physical examination is important as a basis for both diagnostic and therapeutic decisions. The state of hydration should be determined by assessing tissue turgor and by checking for orthostasis. A rectal examination and stool examination for blood and inflammatory cells should be part of the physical examination. There may be nonspecific extraintestinal manifestations of inflammatory bowel disease, for example, the presence of perianal disease in Crohn's disease.

Diagnostic tests. The history and physical examination not only may suggest the diagnosis, but enables the physician to approach diagnostic testing in an organized fashion.

Fig. 41-1 outlines a diagnostic approach to patients with acute diarrhea. Most acute diarrheal attacks are self-limited, are probably viral in nature, and are usually not diagnosed

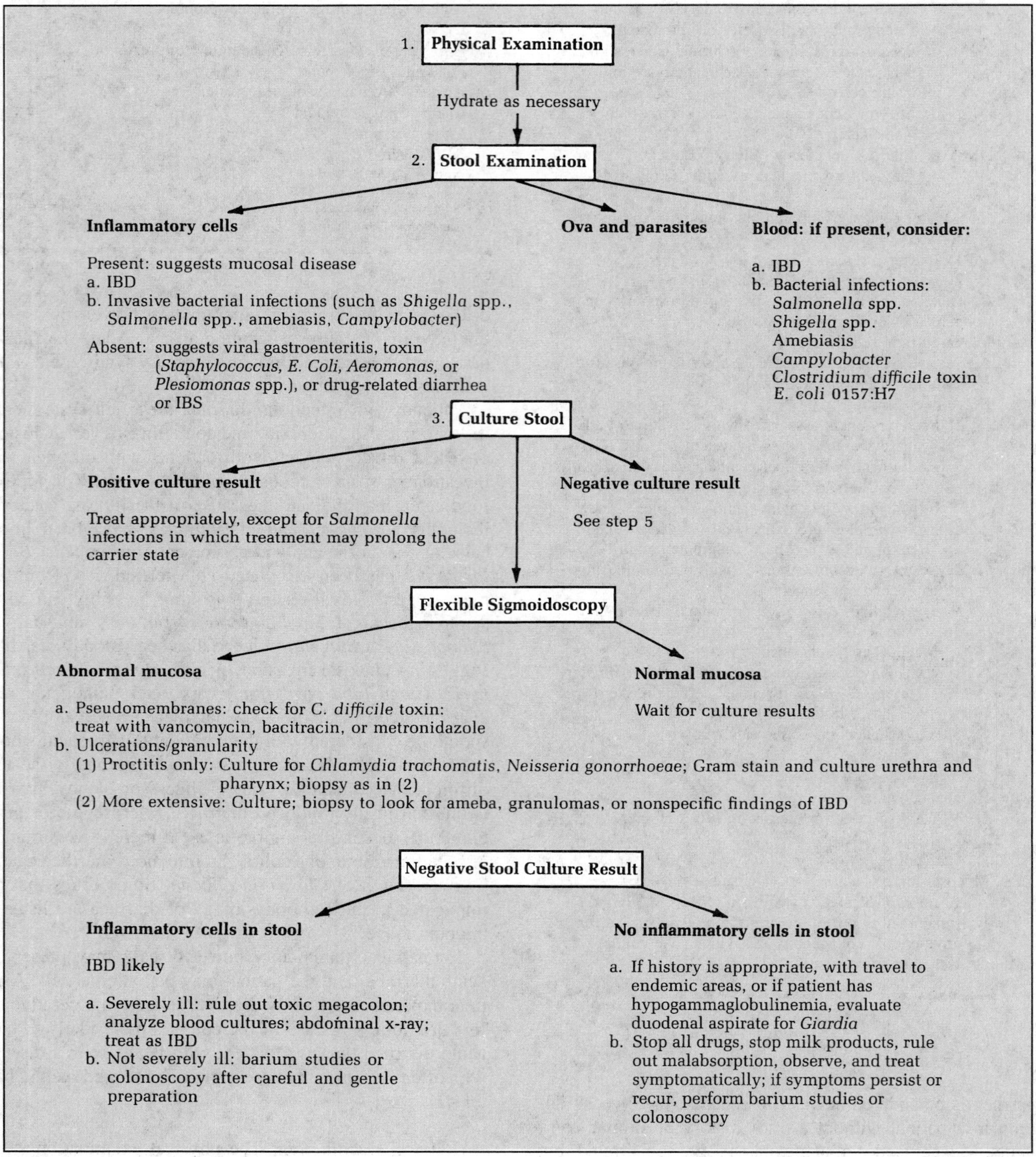

Fig. 41-1. Diagnostic steps in the assessment of acute diarrhea. IBD, inflammatory bowel disease; IBS, irritable bowel syndrome.

because of their self-limited nature. Viral gastroenteritis is not accompanied by bloody diarrhea or inflammatory cells in the stool. If the diarrheal illness is severe or is accompanied by the presence of fecal blood or inflammatory cells, further diagnostic studies are indicated. Flexible sigmoidoscopy allows for direct examination of the rectosigmoid mucosa. Findings of friability and ulcerations, although abnormal, are nonspecific features that can be noted in inflammatory or infectious causes of diarrhea. The presence of pseudomembranes suggests the diagnosis of *Clostridium difficile*-induced pseudomembranous colitis. The details of diagnostic tests for specific disease entities are covered in the appropriate chapters.

Chronic diarrhea

Chronic diarrhea is defined as recurrent diarrhea or diarrhea of greater than 3 weeks' duration. Apart from some infections, which are self-limited, most of the causes of diarrhea outlined in the box on p. 437 can cause chronic diarrhea. If the underlying pathogenesis is known, the physician can better choose which tests to use in the evaluation of chronic diarrhea. Information suggesting the likely diagnosis can often be obtained from the history and physical examination.

History. Drug ingestion is a common cause of chronic diarrhea. A history of laxative abuse by surreptitious ingestion is usually difficult to elicit. Other drug-related causes of diarrhea, however, may be evident from the patient's history of medication ingestion. Diarrhea may result from either a complication or a side effect of drug therapy, for example, excessive ingestion of antacids. (Please refer to the box on p. 437).

Systemic illnesses associated with diarrhea are often evident from the history. Chronic diarrhea is common in patients with AIDS and is discussed in detail in Chapter 48. Disorders such as diabetes are usually known by the patient. Others, such as scleroderma, may become evident when the patient is examined. Patients with carcinoid syndrome may have a history of flushing, or explosive diarrhea. In the absence of metastatic liver disease, diarrhea in patients with carcinoid tumors may be related to partial small bowel obstruction resulting from the dense desmoplastic reaction that these tumors may induce locally. Hyperthyroidism may present as diarrhea, and the patient may give a history of heat intolerance, irritability, or weight loss despite a good appetite.

An infectious cause of chronic diarrhea should be suspected in a patient with an appropriate travel history or with a history of eating foods that harbor parasites and that may not be adequately cooked. Giardiasis should be suspected in patients who have traveled to endemic areas, who are taking immunosuppressants, or who are male homosexuals. Bacterial proliferation in the small intestine, which causes malabsorption and diarrhea, should be suspected in patients who have a predisposition to gastrointestinal stasis, such as occurs (1) after vagotomy, with or without partial gastrectomy; (2) after intestinal surgery, with the formation of blind loops; (3) in scleroderma; and (4) in diabetes. The exact nature of any previous surgery is an important part of the patient's history.

Malabsorption syndromes (Chapter 42) should be suspected in patients who lose weight despite a good appetite. In some patients, diarrhea improves if they alter their diet in particular ways. Lactase deficiency is the most common cause of osmotic diarrhea. A history of chronic ethanol ingestion, recurrent attacks of pancreatitis, or surgical removal of the pancreas suggests pancreatic enzyme deficiency. A history of Crohn's disease or of surgical resection of the distal small bowel suggests bile salt depletion. Malabsorption syndromes usually present as large-volume, nonbloody diarrhea. The stool may be described by the patient as greasy, foul smelling, or floating, suggesting steatorrhea. Many diseases that produce malabsorption have extraintestinal manifestations, such as arthritis in Whipple's disease. Secretory diarrheas are more difficult to diagnose by history alone; the diagnosis is best established by demonstrating the excretion of large volumes of stool in the absence of oral intake.

Ulcerative colitis usually presents as bloody diarrhea. Tenesmus and small volume of diarrhea suggest involvement limited to the distal colon. Crohn's disease may present with a history suggestive of intermittent small bowel obstruction, with abdominal pain as a prominent feature. A history of previous perianal disease also suggests Crohn's disease. Extraintestinal manifestations, such as arthritis or skin lesions, may be present in both ulcerative colitis and Crohn's disease (Chapter 43).

Tumors of the colon may present with diarrhea and should be considered in the older patient, especially if there is blood in the stool. Irritable bowel syndrome (discussed later) usually occurs in the younger patient, is chronic, is often exacerbated by stress, and is not associated with blood in the stool or weight loss. Lymphocytic ("microscopic") and collagenous colitis are recently described entities that are associated with chronic watery diarrhea, and occur primarily in middle-aged women. The colon usually appears grossly normal, but histologic abnormalities such as subepithelial collagen deposition and inflammation are present.

Physical examination. The physical examination in patients with chronic diarrhea is important in assessing the degree of hydration and in suggesting associated systemic illness. For example, there may be resting tachycardia in hyperthyroidism, a pulmonary stenosis murmur or tricuspid regurgitation murmur in carcinoid syndrome, and evidence of autonomic neuropathy or peripheral neuropathy in diabetes. Scleroderma may be diagnosed if the characteristic facies and skin change of the hands are present. There may be evidence of nutritional deficiencies in patients with chronic diarrhea associated with malabsorption (Chapter 42). Abdominal examination may reveal tenderness or fullness, suggesting the matted loops of bowel characteristic of Crohn's disease. Perianal disease may also be evident. As in acute diarrhea, stool examination and sigmoidoscopic evaluation should be part of the physical examination.

Diagnostic tests. Diagnostic evaluation of the patient with chronic diarrhea is guided by the history and physical examination. It is important to determine whether there is an inflammatory component to the diarrhea by stool examination and/or flexible sigmoidoscopy.

Fig. 41-2 outlines a detailed, stepwise diagnostic approach to a patient with chronic diarrhea. Many steps may be omitted if the diagnosis is evident by history and physical examination. In the approach outlined in Fig. 41-2, the physician first determines whether the diarrhea is associated with inflammation of the mucosa and whether the cause is infectious or noninfectious. If no inflammation is demonstrable, an attempt is made to determine whether the diarrhea originates in the small or the large intestine. The volume of diarrhea is helpful in this determination. This framework suggests a rational approach to the ordering of appropriate tests to determine the underlying cause. A therapeutic trial of dietary manipulation (e.g., a lactose-free diet) may be considered in a stable patient before more invasive diagnostic studies are pursued. Specific treatment of causative diseases is discussed in the appropriate chapters.

Constipation

Pathogenesis. Constipation is caused by a decrease in the volume of fecal contents reaching the rectal ampulla or by a disorder of the normal defecation reflex that makes elimination of fecal contents difficult. The volume of fecal contents reaching the rectal ampulla can be decreased by mechanical obstruction, abnormal motility, or reduced volume of intraluminal contents. The box to the right outlines the causes of constipation. The diseases most likely to cause constipation are systemic and may be metabolic, endocrine, drug-related, or gastrointestinal.

Pathogenesis of constipation

1. Decreased fecal water content
   a. Dehydration
   b. Decreased oral intake
   c. Decreased bulk intake
2. Obstruction to flow
   a. Ileal
      (1) Constipation by prevention of normal passage of intraluminal contents
      (2) Presents with signs and symptoms of small bowel obstruction
   b. Colonic
      (1) Extraluminal (diverticular abscess, adhesions, distended urinary bladder, mesenteric tumor, etc.)
      (2) Intramural (intramural hematoma, etc.)
      (3) Intraluminal (carcinoma, polyp, intussusception, etc.)
   c. Anal
      (1) Extraluminal (fibrosis, etc.)
      (2) Intraluminal (tumors, etc.)
3. Decreased or altered motility
   a. Generalized (may present as acute ileus)
      (1) Drugs (opiates)
      (2) Hypothyroidism and other metabolic disorders
      (3) Intestinal pseudo-obstruction
      (4) Scleroderma, progressive systemic sclerosis
      (5) Diabetic enteropathy
      (6) Spinal cord injury (lumbosacral cord, paraplegia)
      (7) Bed rest
   b. Colonic: Irritable bowel syndrome
4. Altered defecation reflex
   a. Hirschsprung's disease (short segment in adults)
   b. Secondary to painful rectal or anal lesions
   c. Other causes of idiopathic constipation associated with abnormal anal manometric findings
   d. Psychiatric illness

History. Important points in the history are the duration of constipation and the presence of abdominal pain or weight loss. Acute onset of constipation is suggestive of either a drug-related problem or organic obstruction. A thorough history of any medications used is important in determining the cause of constipation. Pain often accompanies anatomic obstruction. Complete obstruction results in absolute constipation, with no passage of feces or flatus after the colon distal to the lesion has been emptied and with abdominal distention and cramping abdominal pain. Later in the course of the illness, vomiting may occur. An ileus may also present with absolute constipation and abdominal distention, but vomiting usually occurs early because of gastric and small intestinal paresis, and pain is a less common feature.

Events such as prolonged bed rest or spinal cord injury may cause constipation. Constipation resulting from systemic illnesses such as diabetes, scleroderma, and myxedema is more chronic, and an appropriate history of associated symptoms may be present. Electrolyte disturbances, such as hypokalemia or hypercalcemia, may present as constipation. A long history of obstructive symptoms and laparotomies should cause the physician to suspect intestinal pseudo-obstruction. Local anal lesions, particularly painful lesions such as an anal fissure, will be evident from the history and physical examination. A long-term history of constipation, frequent use of enemas, and abdominal pain is suggestive of either irritable bowel syndrome or short-segment Hirschsprung's disease. The onset of constipation in a middle-aged or older patient should always lead the physician to suspect the presence of colonic carcinoma.

Physical examination. The physical examination may enable the physician to determine whether the patient has acute ileus or acute anatomic obstruction. Ileus is usually accompanied by a quiet, often distended abdomen, with stool present in the rectum. Organic obstruction is usually associated with abdominal distention, initially with high-pitched bowel sounds or rushes on auscultation and often an empty ampulla on rectal examination. With time, the abnormal bowel sounds of acute obstruction may disappear.

In cases of chronic constipation, there may be evidence on physical examination, of an underlying systemic disease such as scleroderma or myxedema. The abdominal examination may reveal a mass suggesting a neoplasm. The rectal examination may demonstrate the presence of perianal or anal disease. There may be an empty ampulla, which,

1. Diagnostic Steps 1 to 4 as in Fig. 41-1

a. Results diagnostic for infectious diarrhea (uncommon in chronic diarrhea except for *Clostridium difficile* after antibiotics), inflammatory bowel disease, or overt drug-induced diarrhea

b. Results nondiagnostic; usually without inflammatory cells in stool

2. Stool Volume

a. Small volume: usually seen in infectious diarrhea or inflammatory bowel disease (consider colonoscopy), but can also be seen in malabsorption syndromes and irritable bowel syndrome

b. Large volume: suggests malabsorption syndromes, secretory diarrhea, or laxative abuse

3. Stool Sudan Stain

Positive

Suggests malabsorption syndrome: pancreatic insufficiency, bile salt insufficiency; or mucosal disease

Further studies, see Chaps. 31 and 40

Negative

See step 4

4. Oral Intake Stopped

Diarrhea continues

a. Secretory diarrhea: stool osmolality = stool $(Na^+ + K^+) \times 2$

b. Nasogastric suction
   (1) Diarrhea stops
      (a) Zollinger-Ellison syndrome: gastric analysis, gastrin, secretin stimulation
      (b) Laxative abuse: see step 5
   (2) Diarrhea continues
      (a) Secretory diarrhea: plasma VIP, calcitonin, urinary 5-HIAA abdominal ultrasound, computed tomography and/or selective mesenteric angiogram to identify tumor
      (b) Laxative abuse: see step 5

Diarrhea stops

a. Malabsorption syndromes: stool osmolality > plasma osmolality

b. Laxative ingestion: see step 5

c. Congenital chloridorrhea
   (1) Stool electrolytes: chloride concentration greater than the sum of sodium and potassium concentration in stool water
   (2) No fecal osmotic gap

5. Laxative Abuse Detection

a. Screening tests
   (1) Locker search
   (2) Add alkali to stool or urine (turns red or pink if phenolphthalein present)
   (3) Sigmoidoscopy and biopsy for melanosis coli
   (4) Barium enema: dilated, hypomotile "cathartic colon"

b. Specific tests
   (1) Urine screening test for senna
   (2) Chromatographic test for bisacodyl
   (3) Stool test for fecal sulfate and phosphate
   (4) Magnesium concentration in fecal water (atomic absorption spectrophotometry)

6. Radiologic Studies

Perform barium studies only after stool examination, culture, and studies requiring quantitative measurements of the stool have been completed.

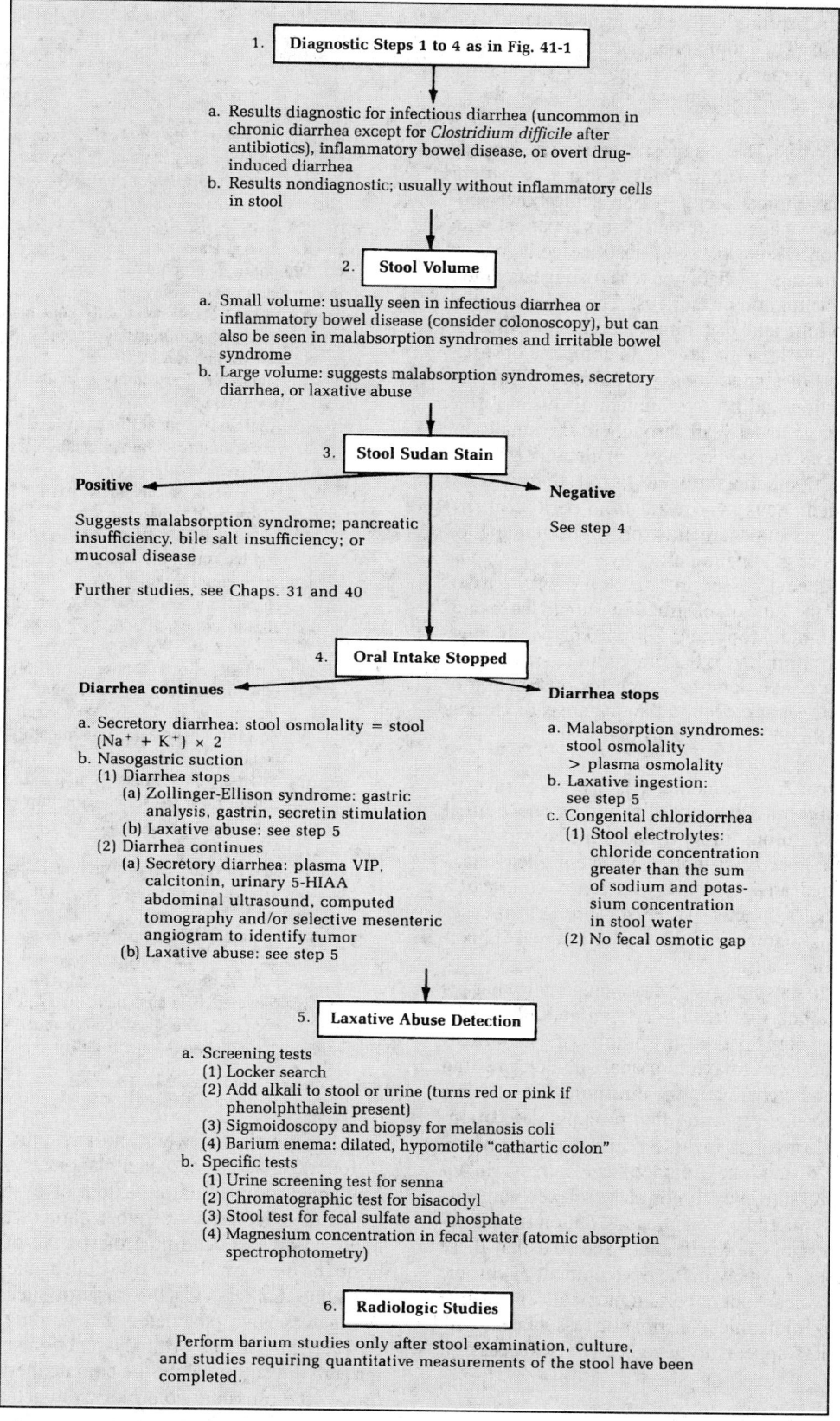

Fig. 41-2. Diagnostic approach to the patient with chronic diarrhea. VIP, vasoactive intestinal polypeptide; 5-HIAA, 5-hydroxyindoleacetic acid.

in the absence of enema administration, is suggestive of short-segment Hirschsprung's disease in a patient with chronic constipation. The stool should be tested for occult or frank blood. The presence of blood suggests a lesion involving the mucosa.

Diagnostic approach. The diagnostic approach depends on the historical and physical findings. Clearly, a patient presenting with the clinical picture of an acute bowel obstruction would be managed differently from a patient with chronic constipation. Acute onset of absolute constipation (i.e., absence of passage of flatus or feces) suggests either complete bowel obstruction or an ileus. The patient should undergo plain upright and decubitus abdominal radiography, which may show air-fluid levels. In complete obstruction, there may be distended loops of bowel proximal to the site of obstruction and no intraluminal air distal to the site. In ileus, there is usually air throughout the small and large intestines. The metabolic causes of ileus (i.e., electrolytes, calcium, blood urea nitrogen [BUN], thyroid tests) should be evaluated. Ileus may result from peritoneal irritation, such as occurs in pancreatitis, or from inflammation of adjacent organs (e.g., pneumonitis, pyelonephritis). The bowel should be decompressed in either case with a nasogastric tube, and the site of obstruction should be evaluated by proctosigmoidoscopy and barium enema. If these procedures reveal normalcy, a barium contrast small intestinal series can safely be done to search for obstruction of the small intestine. An approach to the diagnosis of chronic constipation is outlined in the box to the right.

Anal manometry. Anal manometry is useful for investigating lack of neuromuscular coordination of the normal defecation reflex, resulting in so-called outlet obstruction. In *normal* subjects, rectal distention induces reflex relaxation of the internal anal sphincter and reflex contraction of the external anal sphincter. In Hirschsprung's disease, or aganglionosis of segments of the colon, internal sphincter reflex relaxation is absent.

In addition to Hirschsprung's disease, manometry has reportedly revealed abnormalities in children and adults suffering from chronic constipation. In children, the abnormalities include an increased maximum anal sphincter resting closing pressure and a change in the threshold of rectal distention required for the sensation that prompts defecation. In adults, the abnormalities include a less-than-normal relaxation to rectal distention; a paradoxical increase in internal sphincter pressure, which normally relaxes with distention of the rectum; and spontaneous variation of sphincter pressures at rest in the anal canal. The role that these abnormal responses may play in the development of chronic constipation is not clear, but at certain medical centers anal myomectomy for idiopathic constipation associated with these varied findings appears to have been very successful.

Approach to the patient with chronic constipation

1. Systemic disease?
   a. Often suggested by physical examination or by history
   b. Helpful laboratory tests include: electrolytes, BUN, tests of thyroid function, calcium, blood sugar
2. History of
   a. Bed rest
   b. Spinal cord lesion
   c. Autonomic neuropathy
   d. Peripheral neuropathy
3. Drug history: stop all potentially constipating drugs
4. Assessment of gastrointestinal tract
   a. Rectal examination
      (1) Tight sphincter, empty ampulla (Hirschsprung's disease)
      (2) Anal and perianal disease (thrombosed hemorrhoid, fissure, fistulas, or abscess)
         (a) Treat and observe
         (b) Rule out associated Crohn's disease if perianal disease is present
      (3) Blood in stool: proceed to flexible sigmoidoscopy and barium studies or colonoscopy
   b. Flexible sigmoidoscopy
      (1) Normal mucosa: proceed to barium enema
      (2) Abnormal: carcinoma, polyp, etc: proceed with colonoscopy
   c. Barium studies or colonoscopy to rule out
      (1) Obstructing lesion (carcinoma, polyp, diverticular mass)
      (2) Stricture (neoplasm, inflammatory bowel disease, ischemia, radiation)
      (3) Short-segment Hirschsprung's disease
      (4) Small intestinal series if barium enema or colonoscopy normal to evaluate for small intestinal obstruction
   d. If cause of either an obstructing mass or stricture is not clear, perform colonoscopy for visual identification and biopsy
   e. If evidence for Hirschsprung's disease or if continued severe idiopathic constipation poorly responsive to medical therapy, perform anal manometry
   f. If no evidence of anal manometry abnormalities and no response to medical management, consider physiologic studies of colonic motility

Other physiologic studies

Recently, investigators have examined the physiologic abnormalities that may be seen in patients with chronic severe constipation in whom no anatomic abnormalities can be found. In addition to anal manometry, studies have been conducted to examine the extent of dysfunction of the colon or of involvement of other parts of the gastrointestinal tract. Studies to determine the transit of ingested material through the bowel have included the ingestion of radiopaque markers. On the basis of such studies, some investigators have postulated that chronic constipation may be seen in patients with dysfunction and delayed transit through the entire colon, the colonic inertia group; dysfunction of the proximal colon; or dysfunction of the rectoanal area, the outlet obstruction group. This classification has some usefulness in the management of patients, as those with functional outlet obstruction may respond to an anal sphincter myomectomy even though they do not have classical Hirschsprung's disease.

A small group of patients with chronic constipation appear to have motility abnormalities in several areas of the intestinal tract when studied carefully.

IRRITABLE BOWEL SYNDROME

The *irritable bowel syndrome* (IBS) is an intestinal motility disorder of unknown cause. It is characterized by its symptom complex and by the lack of either an anatomic abnormality or an identifiable infectious or metabolic cause. The symptom complex includes abdominal pain, a bloating sensation, and alterations in bowel habits, with diarrhea and/or constipation. The symptoms are generally intermittent and recurrent.

Incidence

IBS is one of the most frequently diagnosed disorders of the gastrointestinal tract and one of the most frequent conditions encountered by practicing physicians (40% to 70% of referrals to gastroenterologists). Surveys indicate that 14% to 22% of the general population who do not seek the advice of physicians complain of symptoms suggestive of IBS.

Pathophysiology

A variety of motility disorders that may have different pathophysiologic bases have been described in patients with IBS. Patients with IBS more often have abnormal personality patterns, including hypochondriasis, depression, and hysteria. Patients with IBS more often report themselves to be angry and hostile and more often negatively perceive life events than normal subjects. These studies are complicated by potential bias in patient reporting.

Exacerbation of symptoms in patients with IBS has been postulated to be temporally related to psychologic stress. Increased amplitude of esophageal contractions in patients with noncardiac chest pain occurs in response to experimental psychologic stress. Abnormal irregular contractions in the small intestine correlate with symptoms occurring during episodes of stress in IBS patients. At rest, colonic spike activity is increased in patients with IBS, and it increases more significantly when IBS patients are angered compared to controls. These data must be interpreted with caution as it is difficult to record and analyze myoelectrical activity and to select a homogeneous patient group. In addition, only a subset of IBS patients undergo evaluation. However, the relationship between motility and psychologic abnormalities needs further exploration.

The normal propulsive action of the bowel depends on the organized contraction of intestinal smooth muscle. Intestinal smooth muscle cells have an inherent property of cyclic membrane depolarization and repolarization. When depolarization reaches a threshold, rapid depolarization or action potentials are triggered, which in turn initiate contraction. Thus the rate of cyclic depolarization, or the *slow wave rate,* determines the maximum frequency of contractions. In human beings, recordings of colonic slow waves are present at two major frequencies, three and six cycles per minute. Comparison of slow wave rates in normal individuals and patients with IBS have resulted in disparate findings. In normal individuals a six cycle per minute frequency in the sigmoid and rectum accounts for 90% of recorded activity. In contrast, patients with IBS have three cycles per minute activity comprising 40% of slow wave activity, regardless of whether or not the patient has symptoms at the time of study. Patients with IBS during the resting, fasting state have no increase in contractile activity. After meal ingestion or exogenous administration of cholecystokinin, three cycle per minute contractile activity is significantly increased in IBS patients. Normal subjects respond to such stimulation with isolated contractions or low-amplitude contractions at a frequency of six cycles per minute.

Small bowel dysmotility has also been noted in patients with IBS. Interdigestive migrating myoelectric complexes have shorter cycling time in IBS patients with diarrhea. Ileal propulsive waves and clusters of jejunal activity are more often noted in patients with IBS and may coincide with abdominal complaints.

Many patients with IBS experience abdominal pain related to eating. In normal subjects, colonic spike activity increases with an increase in intraluminal pressure lasting for 40 minutes after a meal. Patients with IBS have a gradual increase in colonic spike activity response, which peaks 70 to 90 minutes after a meal. This delayed response may be largely related to the fat content of the meal. As the slow wave rate is a myogenic property, these differences in response suggest an intrinsic activity. Neural or hormonal mediators modulate spike activity and may be the cause of the abnormal contractile pattern in IBS patients.

Pain is a common symptom in patients with IBS. Patients with IBS have a lower tolerance for rectal balloon distention than normal individuals. Patients with IBS are more aware of intestinal events than normal subjects and may sense high-amplitude duodenal phase 3 activity. However, there is no difference in tolerance for holding one hand in ice water in normal and IBS patients, and patients with IBS are less likely to report a painful event from electrocutaneous stimulation than normal subjects. Thus perception of pain to nonvisceral sensations may be reduced in patients with IBS. There are no specific histopathologic findings in the bowels of patients with IBS.

Clinical presentation

Presentation of IBS is protean, and three broad subgroups have been identified on the basis of their major symptoms.

1. Abdominal pain predominant. In this group, pain is often related to meals. Altered bowel movements, although common, are not a major complaint.
2. Changes in bowel habit predominant. In this group, these changes usually take the form of alternating constipation and diarrhea. Abdominal pain is common but is not the major complaint.

3. Painless, watery diarrhea predominant. This is the least common type of symptom.

Attempts to identify these subgroups by colonic myoelectric studies or psychological testing have been unsuccessful. The ratio of female to male patients is about 2:1, although in children the ratio is more equal, with even a preponderance of males.

The most common presenting symptom is abdominal pain, often related to food ingestion and usually located in the left lower quadrant or suprapubically. Pain may worsen before defecation and improve afterward. Splenic flexure syndrome, a variant of IBS, may be associated with left upper quadrant pain precipitated by food ingestion. Abdominal films may demonstrate air in the splenic flexure.

Emotional stress, fear of cancer, anxiety, and depression may cause an exacerbation of symptoms. Treatment of depression may provide relief, although it remains unclear whether the response from antidepressants results from the drug's mood-altering effects or from the peripheral anticholinergic effects.

IBS in children presents as (1) painless diarrhea, usually at preschool age, or (2) abdominal pain in school age children. Diarrhea in the first group is usually watery or loose and occurs less than five times daily. In the second group, constipation is common and the stool may be hard and pelletlike. Pain is periumbilical or left lower quadrant, crampy, worse later in the day, and relieved with the passage of stool or flatus. Although there is a high familial incidence of functional bowel disease, the pathophysiology remains unclear.

Diagnostic studies

Diagnosis of IBS remains a process of exclusion, and major diseases to be ruled out include colonic neoplasms, diverticulosis, infectious causes of diarrhea, and inflammatory bowel disease. A typical history remains constant for years and might be that of a young women with a history of left lower quadrant pain with alternating constipation and diarrhea. Symptoms may become more severe with stress and are not associated with weight loss. A change of symptoms should alert the physician of some other possible process.

Questionnaires have been developed by the Local IBS Study Group to help the clinician differentiate IBS from organic disease. At present, these questionnaires have limited utility. Further refinement and validation of a scoring system for diagnosing IBS are needed.

Patients with suspected IBS should have a blood count, sedimentation rate, and occult blood testing of the stool. A barium enema should be performed in the adult if one has not been done for several years or since the onset of symptoms. An upper gastrointestinal barium study and an abdominal ultrasound should be considered in the patients who have upper abdominal complaints.

Management

The key to the management of a patient with IBS is a good patient-physician relationship. Emotional support is vital and the patient must be reassured that the physician does not think the symptoms are imaginary and that there is no life-threatening underlying illness.

Patients with IBS who seek medical attention may have a higher frequency of behavioral and personality problems and more often relate a history of traumatic events, including sexual abuse. If a psychiatric disorder is present, treatment and referral to a psychiatrist may be helpful. Stress management programs are useful for some patients.

The patient's diet should be designed to reduce intraluminal gas production and should limit legumes, cabbage, and artificial sweeteners. Legumes are gas producers as a result of the deficiency in human beings of alpha-galactosidase, which is necessary for the digestion of the sugars stachyose and raffinose. A trial of exclusion of dairy products should be undertaken as lactase deficiency is common in the adult population. Tight clothing should be avoided. Anticholinergics, despite the lack of proven clinical efficacy, may be tried in patients in whom pain and/or constipation is problematic. The anticholinergic clidinium bromide alters abnormal colonic spike activity in response to a meal in IBS patients.

If diarrhea is a major complaint, foods that may be poorly digested and may result in osmotic diarrhea should be avoided. Bulk agents, such as psyllium (plantago) seed, may add substance to the stool and decrease the number of bowel movements. Loperamide (Imodium) may be an effective agent, if an antidiarrheal agent is necessary, and is less addictive than other opiate derivatives.

The management of constipation is essentially the addition of bulk to the diet in the form of fiber, such as bran or bulk additives such as psyllium seed. Evidence that bran is effective varies.

Prognosis

IBS is a chronic problem, with remissions and exacerbations. Patients should be advised of this and assured that the disease will not alter their life expectancy.

REFERENCES

Diarrhea

Chopra S and Trier J: Diarrhea and malabsorption. In Chopra S and May RJ editors: Pathophysiology of gastrointestinal diseases. Boston; 1989, Little, Brown.

Fine KD, Krejs GT, and Fordtran JS: Diarrhea. In Sleisenger MH and Fordtran JS, editors: Gastrointestinal disease: pathophysiology, diagnosis and management, ed 4. Philadelphia, 1989, Saunders.

Greenberger NJ: Small intestine and colon. In Greenberger NJ, editor: Gastrointestinal disorders: a pathophysiologic approach, ed 3. Chicago; 1986, Year Book.

Keutch GT and Donowitz M: Pathophysiologic mechanisms of diarrhoeal diseases: diverse aetiologies and common mechanisms. Scand J Gastroenterol Suppl 84:33, 1983.

Constipation

Devroede G: Constipation. In Sleisenger MH and Fordtran JS, editors: Gastrointestinal disease: pathophysiology, diagnosis and management, ed 4. Philadelphia, 1989, Saunders.

Martelli H et al: Some parameters of large bowel motility in normal man. Gastroenterology 75:612, 1978.

Martelli H et al: Mechanisms of idiopathic constipation: outlet obstruction. Gastroenterology 75:623, 1978.

Meunier P, Marechal JM, and DeBeaujeu MJ: Rectoanal pressures and rectal sensitivity studies in chronic childhood constipation. Gastroenterology 77:330, 1979.

Read NW and Timms JM: Defecation and the pathophysiology of constipation. Clin Gastroenterol 15:937, 1986.

Irritable Bowel Syndrome

Bellentani S et al: Simple score for the identification of patients at high risk of organic diseases of the colon in the family doctor consulting room. The Local IBS Study Group. Fam Pract 7:307, 1990.

Creed F and Guthrie E: Psychological factors in the irritable bowel syndrome. Gut 28:1307, 1987.

Drossman DA et al: Psychosocial factors in the irritable bowel syndrome. Gastroenterology 95:701, 1988.

Kellow JE and Phillips SF: Altered small bowel motility in irritable bowel syndrome is correlated with symptoms. Gastroenterology 92:1885, 1987.

Schuster MM and Whitehead WE: Physiologic insights into the irritable bowel syndrome. Clin Gastroenterol 15:839, 1986.

Snape WJ, Jr et al: Evidence that abnormal myoelectric activity produces colonic motor dysfunction in the irritable bowel syndrome. Gastroenterology 72:383, 1977.

Welgan P, Meshkinpour H, and Beeler M: Effect of anger on colon motor and myoelectric activity in irritable bowel syndrome. Gastroenterology 94:1150, 1988.

Welgan P, Meshkinpour H, and Beeler M: Effect of anger on colon motor and myoelectric activity in irritable bowel syndrome. Gastroenterology 94:1150, 1988.

CHAPTER

42 Diseases of Intestinal Absorption

Jerry S. Trier

Intestinal malabsorption can occur in any of the many diseases in which there is impairment of one or more of the steps involved in normal digestion and absorption of nutrients. Thus diseases in which there is defective (1) intraluminal digestion and nutrient processing, (2) uptake and transport of nutrients across the epithelium of the small intestine, and (3) transport of nutrients from the mucosa to the systemic circulation can result in malabsorption. In some diseases, a clear-cut single abnormality impairs absorption. For example, in primary lactase deficiency, absence of lactase from the brush border of absorptive cells prevents lactose hydrolysis and thereby subsequent absorption of its constituent monosaccharides, whereas in abetalipoproteinemia, perturbation of apoprotein B production blocks chylomicron formation and the normal exit of absorbed fat from villus absorptive cells. In many diseases, several defects collectively produce malabsorption. For example, in conditions that produce bacterial overgrowth in the lumen of the proximal intestine, bile salt deconjugation and bacterial binding of vitamin B_{12} interfere with intraluminal events, and bacteria- and bile acid-induced damage to the mucosa may impair mucosal uptake and transport of available intraluminal nutrients.

CLINICAL FEATURES OF MALABSORPTION

Gastrointestinal manifestations

Certain clinical features are common to the many diseases of diverse origin that cause intestinal malabsorption of fat, carbohydrate, protein, water, electrolytes, and other nutrients (Table 42-1). Gastrointestinal symptoms may include diarrhea, weight loss, glossitis, stomatitis, flatulence, abdominal distention, cramps, and abdominal pain. Diarrhea is a common complaint, but the frequency and character of the stool may vary considerably from 10 or more watery stools per day to 1 stool daily or even every other day that may be voluminous and puttylike. Patients with the latter bowel habit may actually complain of constipation rather than diarrhea. However, stool mass is invariably increased. Unabsorbed nutrients contribute to stool mass and osmolarity. With steatorrhea, unabsorbed dietary fatty acids are delivered to the colon, where they are converted by bacteria to hydroxy fatty acids that impair absorption and induce colonic secretion of water and electrolytes. Similarly, colonic secretion is induced by unabsorbed bile acids in ileal disease or after ileal resection.

Weight loss is common in generalized malabsorption but varies with dietary intake and the severity of the absorptive defects. Patients with some diseases of malabsorption, such as celiac sprue, may compensate for excessive fecal wastage by consuming in excess of 5000 cal/day. In such situations, weight loss may be mild or absent. A thorough dietary history is therefore mandatory for meaningful interpretation of weight loss or its absence in patients with suspected malabsorption. Fatigue and lassitude may accompany weight loss.

Excessive flatulence is common in patients with malabsorption. Fermentation of dietary carbohydrate may result in excessive gas production, especially in patients with primary or secondary disaccharidase deficiency. Abdominal distention and bloating may reflect impaired absorption of intestinal contents, excessive gas formation, or actual net secretion of fluid into the intestinal lumen, which occurs in diffuse mucosal diseases such as celiac sprue and tropical sprue.

The prevalence and severity of abdominal pain vary among the various diseases and syndromes that produce malabsorption. Abdominal pain is common in patients with Crohn's disease, diffuse intestinal lymphoma, chronic pancreatitis, or pancreatic cancer with exocrine insufficiency but is relatively uncommon in patients with celiac sprue.

Extraintestinal manifestations

Patients with malabsorption may present initially with symptoms referable to organ systems other than the gastrointestinal tract (Table 42-1). Anemia may be present and represent impaired iron, folate, and/or vitamin B_{12} absorption. Purpura or frank hemorrhage may reflect hypoprothrombinemia. Osteopenic bone disease with bone pain and

Table 42-1. Clinical features of intestinal malabsorption

Organ system	Clinical feature	Cause
Gastrointestinal tract	Diarrhea	Nutrient malabsorption; small intestinal secretion of fluid and electrolytes; action of unabsorbed bile acids and hydroxy fatty acids on the colonic mucosa
	Weight loss	Nutrient malabsorption
	Flatus	Bacterial fermentation of unabsorbed dietary carbohydrates
	Abdominal pain	Distention of bowel, muscle spasm, serosal and peritoneal involvement by disease process
	Glossitis, stomatitis, cheilosis	Iron, riboflavin, niacin deficiency
Hematopoietic system	Anemia, microcytic	Iron, pyridoxine deficiency
	Anemia, macrocytic	Folate, vitamin B_{12} deficiency
	Bleeding	Vitamin K deficiency
Musculoskeletal system	Osteopenic bone disease	Calcium, vitamin D, and malabsorption
	Osteoarthropathy	Not known
	Tetany	Calcium, magnesium and vitamin D deficiency
Endocrine system	Amenorrhea, impotence, infertility	Generalized malabsorption and malnutrition
	Secondary hyperparathyroidism	Protracted calcium and vitamin D deficiency
Epidermal system	Purpura	Vitamin K deficiency
	Follicular hyperkeratosis and dermatitis	Vitamin A, zinc, essential fatty acids, niacin deficiency
	Edema	Protein-losing enteropathy, malabsorption of dietary protein
	Hyperpigmentation	Secondary hypopituitarism and adrenal insufficiency
Nervous system	Xerophthalmia, night blindness	Vitamin A deficiency
	Peripheral neuropathy	Vitamin B_{12}, thiamine deficiency

pathologic fractures may be due to impaired absorption of calcium and vitamin D. In severe malabsorption, acute calcium and magnesium loss may induce muscle cramps and even tetany. Protracted calcium deficiency may induce secondary hypoparathyroidism. Amenorrhea, impotence, or infertility may reflect malabsorption-induced malnutrition. Peripheral neuropathy may reflect thiamine and/or vitamin B_{12} deficiency. Follicular hyperkeratosis and night blindness may be due to vitamin A deficiency. Dependent edema and, less commonly, ascites may be caused by protein-losing enteropathy. Significant enteric protein loss caused by leakage of lymph or serum into the gut may be a prominent feature of a number of diseases that produce malabsorption, including primary and secondary intestinal lymphangiectasia, Crohn's disease, celiac sprue, tropical sprue, intestinal lymphoma, Whipple's disease, and eosinophilic gastroenteritis.

Physical findings

Physical findings vary tremendously depending on the severity and duration of malabsorption, because these characteristics influence extraintestinal manifestations. Fever may occur in some diseases (Whipple's disease, lymphoma, Crohn's disease). Tachycardia and skin pallor may reflect anemia. Hypotension and poor skin turgor may be caused by fluid and electrolyte depletion, whereas loose skin folds reflect weight loss. The skin may show dermatitis and ecchymoses (Table 42-1). Hypoproteinemia, especially when it is associated with lymphatic obstruction, may result in peripheral edema, ascites, and pleural effusion. Abdominal distention caused by increased gas and fluid in the intestinal lumen is common, but palpable mass lesions suggest malignancy or Crohn's disease. Bone tenderness may be prominent in association with osteopenia, especially if pathologic fractures are present. If hypocalcemia or hypomagnesemia is severe, Chvostek's or Trousseau's sign may be elicited. Loss of sensation in the extremities may reflect peripheral neuropathy.

Laboratory findings

Laboratory tests useful in evaluating intestinal disease are discussed in detail in Chapter 33. Those most often useful in evaluating patients with intestinal malabsorption are summarized in Table 42-2. Documentation of excessive stool fat excretion by qualitative or quantitative measurement establishes the presence of fat malabsorption but does not enable the physician to distinguish among impaired intraluminal digestion, primary mucosal disease, and impaired lymphatic drainage. However, a stool fat concentration of over 9.5% suggests maldigestion, whereas stool fat concentration of under 9.5% is common in mucosal diseases in which there is concomitant malabsorption of other nutrients. Abnormal xylose absorption, low serum iron concentration in the absence of blood loss, and/or a low serum folate concentration all suggest mucosal disease, which can often be confirmed and in some diseases diagnosed with specificity by peroral small intestinal biopsy (Chapter 33, box on p. 381). By contrast, in most patients with intraluminal maldigestion, serum iron and folate concentrations are normal, as are xylose absorption and intestinal mucosal structure. Pancreatic imaging and function tests, such as the secretin stimulation test, may document chronic pancreatic disease as the cause of intraluminal maldigestion (Chapter 54). Lymphatic obstruction can be suspected if small bowel biopsy reveals lymphatic dilatation in the presence of hypoproteinemia and lymphopenia, although thoracic and ab-

Table 42-2. Useful laboratory tests in evaluation of intestinal malabsorption

Test	Impaired intraluminal digestion	Mucosal disease	Lymphatic obstruction	Limitations
Stool fat (qualitative, quantitative)	Increased (concentration usually >9.5%)	Increased (concentration usually <9.5%)	Increased	False-negative result if inadequate ingestion of dietary fat or recent barium ingestion; false-positive result with castor oil or mineral oil ingestion
Serum carotene	Decreased	Decreased	Decreased	Low values may occur in normal subjects who ingest little dietary carotene
Serum cholesterol	Decreased	Decreased	Decreased	May be normal or increased in patients with untreated lipoprotein abnormality
Serum albumin	Usually normal, except with bacterial overgrowth	Often decreased	Often decreased	
Prothrombin activity	Decreased if severe	Decreased if severe	Decreased if severe	May also be decreased in liver disease, but parenterally administered vitamin K should induce normalization if caused by malabsorption
Serum iron	Normal	Often decreased	Normal	
Serum folate	Normal	Often decreased	Normal	
Xylose absorption	Normal, except with bacterial overgrowth	Abnormal, unless disease confined to distal small intestine	Normal	Requires normal gastric emptying and renal function
Lactose absorption (lactose tolerance test or breath hydrogen after lactose load)	Normal, except in some instances of bacterial overgrowth	Increase in plasma glucose <20 mg/dl; increased breath H_2	Normal	May be abnormal in all categories if patient has primary intestinal lactase deficiency
Vitamin B_{12} (Schilling test)	Decreased in bacterial overgrowth and exocrine pancreatic insufficiency	Decreased in extensive ileal disease	Normal	Requires good renal function
^{14}C-cholylglycine breath tests	Increased $^{14}CO_2$ excretion in bacterial overgrowth	Increased $^{14}CO_2$ excretion in ileal disease	Normal	Requires normal gastric emptying
Lactulose breath test	Early appearance of H_2 in breath in bacterial overgrowth	Normal	Normal	Requires normal gastric emptying; false-positive results may occur in patient with rapid small intestinal transit
Secretin/cholecystokinin stimulation tests	Abnormal in chronic pancreatic disease	Normal	Normal	Relatively low sensitivity
Peroral intestinal biopsy	Normal except in severe bacterial overgrowth	Often abnormal	Often abnormal	May miss patchy mucosal disease (see the box in Chapter 33)

dominal imaging studies and/or surgical exploration may be required to clarify the nature of the underlying disease process.

DISORDERS THAT PRODUCE INTRALUMINAL MALDIGESTION

Pancreatic and hepatobiliary diseases

Inadequate delivery into the intestinal lumen of lipase, proteases, and bicarbonate produced by the pancreas or of bile salts produced by the liver may perturb normal intraluminal digestion (Chapter 28). As a result, pancreatic diseases, such as pancreatitis, pancreatic cancer, and cystic fibrosis, or acute and chronic hepatobiliary diseases that produce cholestasis, such as primary biliary cirrhosis, acute hepatitis, sclerosing cholangitis, and carcinoma of the bile ducts, may produce significant malabsorption (Chapters 51 and 54). The clinical manifestations of these diseases are described elsewhere (Chapters 57, 58, 59, 60, 66, and 67). Although steatorrhea and its associated manifestations may be present, results of tests of intestinal mucosal function, such as D-xylose absorption and mucosal structure assessed by peroral intestinal biopsy, are usually normal (Table 42-2).

Intraluminal intestinal bacterial proliferation

Etiology. The lumen of the proximal small intestine normally contains less than 10^5 bacteria per milliliter of intestinal contents, most of which are derived from swallowed oropharyngeal flora. Two normal processes that prevent excessive growth of bacteria in the proximal intestine are (1) intestinal motor function and (2) gastric acid secretion. Any condition that predisposes the patient to intestinal stasis, whether it be a motor abnormality, as in visceral scleroderma, amyloidosis, diabetic visceral neuropathy, and intestinal pseudo-obstruction, or an anatomic abnormality, such as small intestinal diverticulosis or stricture, may be associated with malabsorption secondary to intestinal bacterial overgrowth (see the box below). Bacterial overgrowth also occurs occasionally in patients with profound hypochlorhydria or achlorhydria produced by gastric mucosal atrophy in the absence of altered intestinal motor function. Massive contamination of the proximal intestine with bacteria via a gastrocolic, jejunocolic, or ileojejunal fistula invariably produces malabsorption. Impaired immunoglobulin secretion into the intestinal lumen occasionally results in intraluminal bacterial overgrowth.

Pathophysiology and pathology. In bacterial overgrowth syndromes, bacterial hydrolysis of conjugated bile salts in the proximal intestine markedly interferes with normal intraluminal fat digestion and results in steatorrhea. Whereas conjugated bile salts are selectively absorbed by a specific transport process in the distal ileum (Chapter 51), the more lipid-soluble deconjugated bile acids are readily absorbed by passive nonionic diffusion in the proximal intestine, resulting in intraluminal bile salt deficiency. Moreover, unconjugated bile acids, unlike conjugated bile acids, are poorly soluble at the normal intraduodenojejunal pH and are less effective at dispersing dietary lipid. In many patients with bacterial overgrowth, a patchy, nonspecific lesion of varying severity develops in the proximal intestine. Villi are shortened, crypts are hyperplastic, and there is inflammation of the lamina propria. The bacteria produce glycosidases, proteases, and possibly toxins, which may damage the epithelium, especially brush border hydrolases. In addition, the unconjugated bile acids produced by bile salt deconjugation may be cytotoxic and contribute to the mucosal lesion, further compromising absorptive function. There is uptake of both free and intrinsic factor–bound vitamin B_{12} by the bacteria in the proximal intestine, preventing its normal absorption by the ileum.

Causes of bacterial overgrowth in proximal intestine

I. Motor abnormalities
   A. Scleroderma
   B. Amyloidosis
   C. Pseudo-obstruction
   D. Vagotomy
   E. Diabetes with visceral neuropathy (rare)
II. Structural abnormalities
   A. Diverticula
   B. Strictures
      1. Crohn's disease
      2. Vascular disease
      3. Radiation enteritis
   C. Adhesions causing partial obstruction
   D. Afferent loop stasis after Billroth II gastrectomy
   E. Fistulas
      1. Gastrocolic
      2. Jejunocolic
      3. Jejunoileal
III. Hypo- or achlorhydria
   A. Gastric atrophy with or without pernicious anemia
   B. Vagotomy and/or gastric resection
IV. Hypogammaglobulinemia or agammaglobulinemia

Clinical features and diagnosis. Symptoms may vary greatly, depending on the severity of bacterial overgrowth and the underlying predisposing cause (refer to the box on p. 454). Malabsorption may be severe, with prominent weight loss, steatorrhea, and diarrhea. Extraintestinal and intestinal manifestations may be prominent (Table 42-1). If untreated, megaloblastic anemia and neurologic manifestations identical to those found in pernicious anemia may ultimately develop. Patients with anatomic abnormalities, such as strictures or adhesions, may have symptoms of intermittent partial intestinal obstruction. In patients with visceral scleroderma, amyloidosis, or Crohn's disease, it may be difficult to distinguish symptoms caused by bacterial overgrowth from symptoms caused by the primary disease process.

The possibility of intestinal bacterial overgrowth should be considered in patients with unexplained diarrhea, documented steatorrhea, weight loss, or unexplained macrocytic anemia in the presence of predisposing conditions. These include previous gastric surgery (Chapter 38), Raynaud's phenomenon, heartburn or dysphagia suggestive of scleroderma, and apparently quiescent Crohn's disease of the small intestine. Quantitative culture of jejunal fluid is the most accurate diagnostic procedure but is difficult because of the fastidious growth requirements of the gut flora and therefore is available only in a few specialized bacteriology laboratories. In patients without ileal disease, demonstration of impaired absorption of both free and intrinsic factor–bound vitamin B_{12} permits a presumptive diagnosis of bacterial overgrowth. Abnormal lactulose, glucose, ^{14}C-xylose, or ^{14}C-cholylglycine bile acid breath test results with early and increased hydrogen or $^{14}CO_2$ excretion in the breath are helpful (Chapter 33), but their diagnostic sensitivity is low and their specificity is not fully established. When bacterial overgrowth in the proximal intestine has been documented, every effort should be made to establish the underlying cause, because the long-term therapeutic approach is not always the same.

Treatment. If bacterial overgrowth is associated with chronic motor abnormalities, achlorhydria, or structural abnormalities not readily amenable to surgical repair (multiple jejunal diverticula, some cases of Crohn's disease, or radiation enteritis), treatment with an orally administered broad-spectrum antibiotic such as tetracycline or ampicillin usually markedly improves both fat and vitamin B_{12} absorption. In some patients metronidazole is required to decrease anaerobes. In selected patients, a single 2 to 3 week course of treatment is adequate; more often, intermittent courses or even continuous antibiotic treatment is needed. Hence, therapy must be individualized. Gastrojejunal colic fistulas cannot be managed with antibiotics alone and usually require surgical repair. Surgery is also indicated in many patients with stasis caused by discrete, readily resectable strictures or adhesions.

DISORDERS THAT IMPAIR MUCOSAL ABSORPTION

Celiac sprue (gluten-sensitive enteropathy)

The hallmark of celiac sprue is a characteristic, though not specific, lesion of the small intestinal mucosa that, if extensive, may produce malabsorption of virtually all nutrients and that improves dramatically when wheat-, barley-, rye-, and oat-containing substances are withdrawn from the diet. Although the exact prevalence is not known, because subclinical disease is common, it has been estimated at 3 cases per 10,000 persons. In parts of Ireland, a prevalence as high as 1 case per 300 persons has been reported. The disease may present at any age but is most often diagnosed in young children or young to middle-aged adults; clinical symptoms generally decrease during adolescence, for unknown reasons.

Pathophysiology and pathology. In celiac sprue, gluten, the water-soluble protein moiety of the offending cereal grains, interacts with the mucosa of the small intestine to produce the characteristic lesion and, hence, perturb normal absorption. The exact nature of this interaction is not known, but there is increasing evidence that genetic factors and immune mechanisms participate although a metabolic defect has not been definitely excluded.

The prevalence of celiac sprue among first-degree relatives of probands with documented disease averages about 10% in available studies, a far greater percentage than is found in the general population. Many relatives have subclinical or "latent" disease; this emphasizes that celiac sprue is an "iceberg" disease in that patients who have clinical panmalabsorption represent only the tip. The importance of genetic factors is supported further by the association of certain human leukocyte antigen (HLA) antigens with celiac sprue. The class I antigen HLA-B8 and the class II antigen HLA-DR3 are found in 60% to 90% of patients compared to 20% of normal individuals. More recently, HLA-DQw2 has been observed in more than 90% of patients. Most patients who lack HLA-D3 are HLA-DR5/DR7 heterozygotes. As the same HLA-DQα/β heterodimer is present in D3 and DR5-DR7 patients encoded on the same chromosome (cis position) in DR3 and on opposite chromosomes (trans position) in DR5/DR7 patients, this heterodimer likely confirms susceptibility for celiac sprue and may actually bind toxic gluten peptides. However, the presence of associated HLA antigens is not the whole story because the majority of individuals with these haplotypes remain healthy, discordance for celiac sprue has been documented in some identical twins, and occasional celiac sprue patients lack DR3, DR5/DR7, and DQw2. It has been suggested that an additional as yet undefined susceptibility gene and/or an environmental trigger that sensitizes the mucosa to gluten such as a viral infection (adenovirus has been suggested) is needed. Other genetic markers including B cell surface alloantigens and an immunoglobulin G (IgG) heavy chain Gm allotype marker have been identified, but their role in pathogenesis, if any, is not clear.

In celiac sprue, the number of plasma cells and lymphocytes that infiltrate the mucosa of small intestine is increased. Circulating serum antibodies (IgA and IgG) to wheat gluten fractions (gliadens) are found in many but not all patients and antibodies to other dietary proteins may also be present. It has been shown that antigliaden antibodies are synthesized by diseased mucosa in sprue patients and that there is mucosal deposition of activated complement that may lead to epithelial cell damage. However, circulating antigliaden antibodies can be detected occasionally in individuals without overt intestinal disease as well as in patients with other diseases that damage the intestinal mucosa. There is evidence that some mucosal T lymphocytes are activated in untreated celiac sprue with resultant increased production of cytokines, including gamma-interferon. Class II HLA antigen expression by intestinal epithelial cells is increased and may facilitate lymphocyte-mediated damage to epithelium. However, whether these immunologic features represent primary defects or secondary phenomena, perhaps related to increased mucosal permeability to gluten peptides, is not established.

Evidence that celiac sprue is caused by a specific metabolic defect is less convincing. It has been demonstrated that relatively small glutamine-rich polypeptides obtained by controlled proteolytic digestion of wheat gluten are toxic when fed to patients with celiac sprue. This finding led to the hypothesis that a specific mucosal peptidase may be missing in patients with this disease and that this results in incomplete gluten digestion and formation of a toxic polypeptide intermediate. Whereas levels of mucosal peptidases and other mucosal hydrolases are reduced in untreated patients, enzyme levels revert toward normal after successful treatment and healing of the mucosal lesion. Because treated patients remain unable to tolerate noxious glutens in their diets, a mucosal peptidase deficiency, if causative, should be present in treated as well as untreated patients. Recent definition of the amino acid sequence of toxic gluten fractions should permit more definitive testing of the deficient peptidase hypothesis.

The relationship between celiac sprue and dermatitis herpetiformis is also of interest. Although patients with dermatitis herpetiformis may have no frank malabsorption, 90% or more have a mucosal lesion of the proximal intestine that is indistinguishable from the lesion of celiac sprue. This lesion improves when gluten is withdrawn from the diet. However, in most celiac sprue patients dermatitis herpetiformis does not develop. Like celiac sprue, dermatitis herpetiformis is associated with a high prevalence of HLA-B8, DR3, and DQw2 antigens.

The primary lesion in celiac sprue is confined to the mucosa of the small intestine. Villi are markedly shortened or absent. As a result, the mucosal surface often appears flat and is lined by severely damaged absorptive cells that are decreased in height, are vacuolated, and have a markedly attenuated striated border. Crypts are hyperplastic, with increased mitoses, and may extend to the flat mucosal surface (Fig. 42-1). The lamina propria is infiltrated with increased numbers of mononuclear cells and, in some instances, polymorphonuclear leukocytes, and the absorptive epithelium is heavily infiltrated with lymphocytes. Thus not only is the absorptive surface decreased by the architectural lesion, but what surface remains is lined by abnormal, damaged cells. The length of intestine involved varies substantially, but the lesion is always most severe in the proximal small intestine; involvement of the distal small intestine, with sparing of the duodenum or jejunum, does not occur. The lesion is not specific: identical histologic features can be observed in proximal intestinal biopsies of some patients with tropical sprue, Zollinger-Ellison syndrome, eosinophilic gastroenteritis, and intestinal lymphoma in mucosa overlying or adjacent to malignant infiltration.

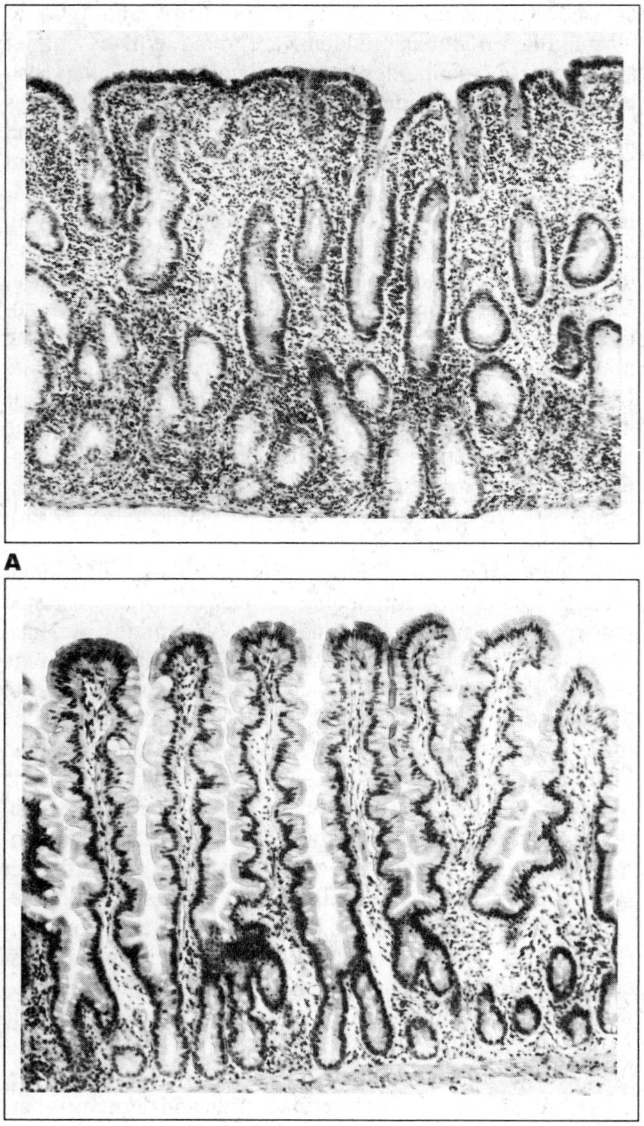

A

B

Fig. 42-1. **A,** Jejunal biopsy specimen from a patient with untreated celiac sprue. Villi are absent, crypts are hyperplastic, and cellularity of the lamina propria is markedly increased. **B,** Jejunal biopsy specimen from a normal adult, showing tall villi, shallow crypts, and normal cellularity of the lamina propria.

The severely damaged intestine in celiac sprue patients actually secretes rather than absorbs water and electrolytes, further increasing stool volume in patients with compromised absorption. There is evidence that release of cholecystokinin, secretin, and perhaps other enteric hormones from the damaged mucosa is impaired, reducing delivery into the gut lumen of bile salts and pancreatic enzymes, possibly compromising intraluminal digestive processes.

Clinical and laboratory features and diagnosis. The clinical and laboratory features of celiac sprue may vary enormously depending on the extent of intestinal involvement. A clinician need not be especially astute to suspect celiac sprue in patients with extensive intestinal involvement who exhibit devastating malabsorption, steatorrhea, diarrhea, weight loss, secondary extraintestinal symptoms (see Table 42-1), and many of the physical findings described at the beginning of this chapter. The challenge is to diagnose the disease correctly in those patients whose lesions are limited to the proximal small intestine and who may present with iron and/or folate deficiency anemia or symptoms of osteopenic bone disease in the absence of obvious intestinal symptoms and overt steatorrhea. Because of these subtleties, symptoms in many patients may wax and wane for several years before the correct diagnosis is finally made.

Like the clinical features, laboratory findings may vary considerably. At one extreme is the patient with involvement limited to the proximal intestine, with evidence of only an isolated deficiency such as microcytic anemia and low serum iron concentration. At the other extreme is the patient with involvement of the entire length of the intestine in whom there is laboratory evidence of steatorrhea, hypoalbuminemia, hypocalcemia, hypoprothrombinemia, impaired vitamin B_{12} absorption, and so on (see the box on p. 454).

The diagnosis rests on (1) demonstrating intestinal malabsorption by documenting steatorrhea (which may be absent in mild disease) and impaired absorption of xylose, (2) confirming the presence of the characteristic mucosal lesion by biopsy of the mucosa of the small intestine, and (3) documenting a clinical response and, ideally, histologic improvement of the intestinal lesion on withdrawal of noxious glutens from the diet. Barium contrast studies of the small intestine that show distortion or loss of mucosal folds, intestinal dilatation, and dilution of barium within the gut lumen (Fig. 42-2) are helpful but not specific, and these findings may be absent in patients with mild disease. De-

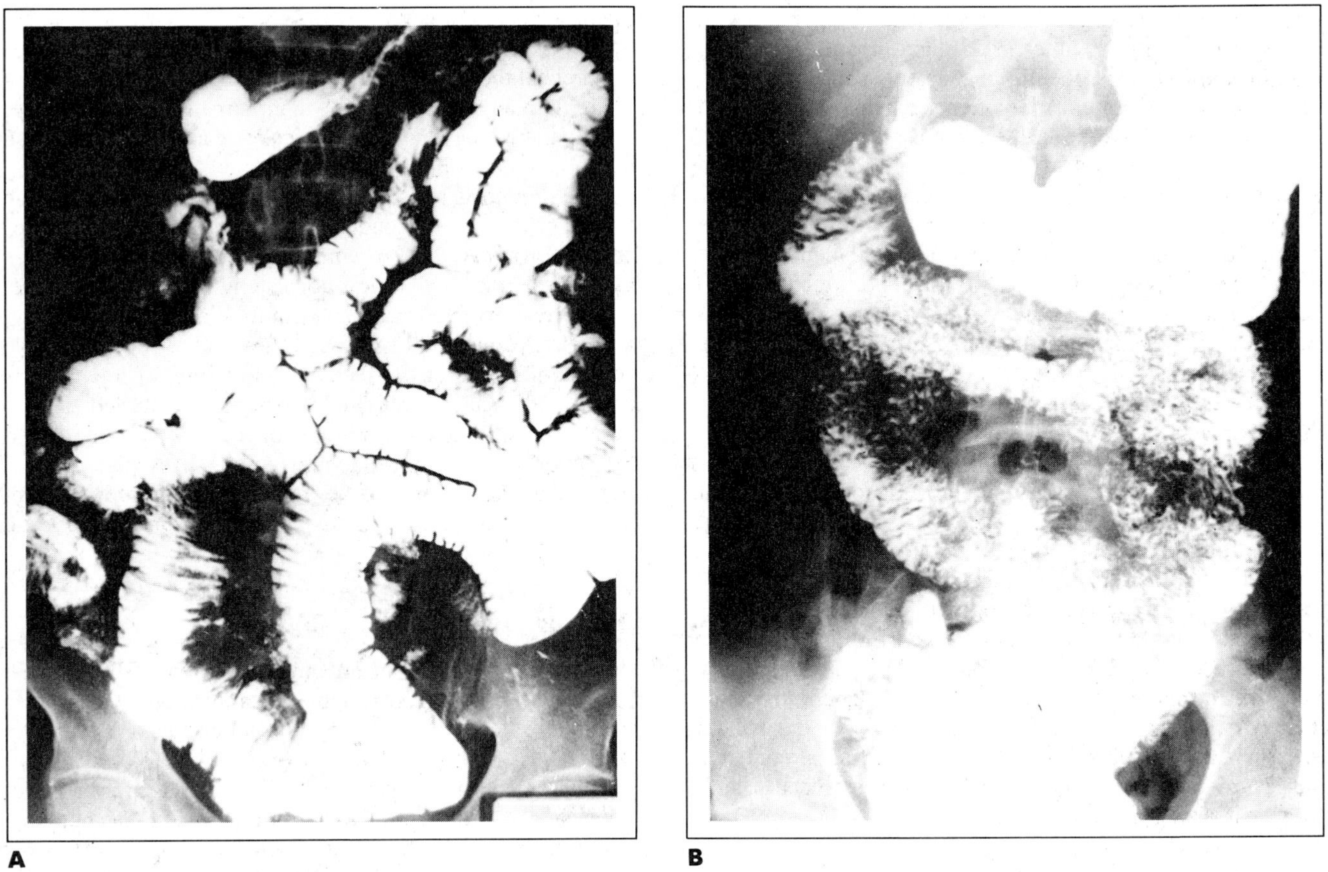

Fig. 42-2. **A,** Barium contrast small intestinal series from a patient with untreated celiac sprue. The small intestine is dilated, with loss of the normal mucosal fold pattern. **B,** Barium contrast small intestinal series from a normal adult. The caliber of the intestinal lumen is normal and the fine, feathery mucosal pattern is evident.

termination of serum antigliadin IgA and antiendomysial IgA are useful screening tests but no substitute for mucosal biopsy. These antibodies usually decrease in titer and disappear in patients compliant with a gluten-free diet.

Treatment. Elimination of all wheat, rye, barley, and oat gluten from the diet is the key to effective treatment. Corn and rice flour are not toxic and can be used as substitutes for conventional wheat flour. The clinical response to gluten withdrawal is usually dramatic and evident within 1 or 2 weeks. Absorptive cell structure also improves within that period, although reversion to normal of the architectural lesion may require months or years. The diet should be well balanced and contain normal amounts of fat, protein, and carbohydrate. Restriction of dairy products may be necessary initially because most patients have secondary lactase deficiency. Deficiencies of specific nutrients such as iron, folate, calcium, vitamin K, and vitamin B_{12} should be corrected with appropriate supplements. Because effective treatment requires lifelong elimination of noxious glutens, a "therapeutic trial" of gluten withdrawal, without histologic demonstration of the characteristic mucosal lesion, is not justified. Failure to respond to gluten withdrawal most often reflects inadvertent gluten ingestion. The prognosis is excellent, although the incidence of lymphoma, adenocarcinoma of the small intestine, and some extraintestinal carcinomas appears to be somewhat increased among patients with celiac sprue.

Unclassified sprue, collagenous sprue, and nongranulomatous ulcerative jejunoileitis

Occasionally, patients who have clinical features of celiac sprue, and an intestinal mucosal lesion histologically identical to that of celiac sprue and in whom other diseases that produce similar mucosal lesions are excluded, fail to respond to meticulous gluten exclusion from the diet. Because they do not respond to gluten withdrawal, these patients by definition do not have celiac sprue; their disease has been termed *unclassified* or *refractory sprue*. In a few instances, other offending dietary substances, such as soybeans, eggs, chicken, and tuna, whose withdrawal results in clinical and histologic improvement, have been identified. Rarely, previously responsive celiac sprue patients become refractory. About 50% of unclassified sprue patients respond to treatment with oral corticosteroids. If not, parenteral alimentation followed by addition of one foodstuff at a time, with careful monitoring of intestinal function and histology, may, in rare instances, identify a causative substance. With time, in a few unresponsive patients extensive deposition of collagen may develop in the lamina propria beneath the surface absorptive cells. This rare condition has been termed *collagenous sprue*. If there is no response to corticosteroids and no offending dietary constituent can be found, the prognosis in unclassified and collagenous sprue is very poor. Except for isolated case reports of improvement of unclassified sprue with other immunosuppressants such as azathioprine or cyclosporine, no other effective treatment has been identified.

Nongranulomatous ulcerative jejunoileitis is a rare condition characterized by abdominal pain, diarrhea, malabsorption, gastrointestinal bleeding, and protein-losing enteropathy. Pathologic features include a mucosal lesion that may be indistinguishable from the lesion of celiac sprue but that is often patchy, severe nonspecific mucosal and submucosal inflammation, and intestinal ulceration that may progress to perforation or scarring, with stricture formation. Whether this condition represents a specific disease entity is unclear; some patients in whom this diagnosis is initially made are in time shown to have intestinal lymphoma. Others may have a variant form of unclassified sprue or Crohn's disease. Immunosuppressive drugs, including prednisone and azathioprine, have been tried with little success, and the prognosis is generally grim.

Tropical sprue

Tropical sprue causes generalized intestinal malabsorption and is endemic in many but not all tropical countries located between the tropic of Cancer and the tropic of Capricorn. Devastating epidemics have been documented, especially in India. The disease affects not only the indigenous population but also travelers from temperate climates. In expatriates from the tropics symptoms may first develop months or even years after emigrating to temperate regions. The cause of tropical sprue is unknown. The epidemiology suggests that exposure to an infectious or other environmental agent is essential. There is some evidence that alterations in the intraluminal flora of the small intestine may be important. However, no specific causative organism has been identified.

The clinical features of tropical sprue include diarrhea, steatorrhea, abdominal pain, and weight loss. In contrast to celiac sprue, anorexia and low-grade fever are common. Anemia, usually megaloblastic, and other nutritional deficiencies develop within a few weeks to 6 months. Abnormal D-xylose and vitamin B_{12} absorption, vitamin B_{12} deficiency, and folate deficiency are characteristic laboratory features. Small intestinal biopsy reveals a wide range of mucosal abnormalities. Occasionally, severe lesions that resemble closely the histopathology of celiac sprue are found with absent villi and striking crypt hyperplasia. However, the majority of tropical sprue patients have milder, nonspecific lesions that may be patchy, with some shortening of villi, mucosal inflammation, and prominent infiltration of the absorptive epithelium with lymphocytes. Biopsy specimens obtained from asymptomatic residents of the tropics may reveal the same nonspecific milder mucosal lesions evident in many patients with symptomatic tropical sprue. Such patients may have subclinical disease, which has been termed *tropical enteropathy*.

The diagnosis is established by determining whether the patient (1) has been in endemic areas; (2) demonstrates malabsorption of fat, xylose, vitamin B_{12}, and/or folate; (3) has a mucosal intestinal lesion consistent with tropical sprue; and (4) responds to treatment with folic acid, 5 mg per day, and tetracycline, 250 mg four times daily. Nonabsorbable sulfonamides are also effective. One month of treatment is usually adequate in individuals who have returned to temperate zones, whereas 6 months of therapy may be needed by patients treated in endemic regions. Associated nutritional deficiencies should be treated with appropriate supplements such as fat-soluble vitamins, vitamin B_{12}, and iron.

Whipple's disease

Whipple's disease is an uncommon systemic disease that may affect many organ systems but almost always involves the small intestine, producing malabsorption. The cause is not fully understood. Involved organs are invaded by numerous small, gram-positive bacilli, suggesting an infectious cause. Although the associated organism has not been cultured, it recently has been identified as an *Actinobacter* using innovative molecular genetic techniques and has been designated *Tropheryma whipelli*. The extremely low incidence and lack of documented transmission among patients with Whipple's disease suggest that host factors must play an important pathogenetic role, but as yet no consistent or persistent immune defect has been identified, although there is a two- to threefold increase in the presence of the histocompatibility antigen, HLA-B27.

The pathologic features are quite specific. In the small intestine, large macrophages containing glycoprotein-rich lysosomes, which are magenta when stained with the periodic acid Schiff (PAS) technique, infiltrate the lamina propria and submucosa in concert with the *T. whipelli* bacilli, often distorting villous architecture (Fig. 42-3). Degenerating phagocytosed bacilli are found within the PAS-positive macrophage lysosomes (Fig. 42-4). Dilatation of mucosal and submucosal lymphatics is often prominent. The bacilli and PAS-positive macrophages are seen in other involved tissues, including mesenteric and peripheral lymph nodes, liver, spleen, heart, lung, eye, and central nervous system. Malabsorption is caused by the infiltrative mucosal lesion and by obstruction of lymphatics that is produced by involved mesenteric nodes. Bacilli and PAS-positive macrophages are also seen in the lamina propria of patients with acquired immunodeficiency syndrome (AIDS) complicated by intestinal *Mycobacterium avium* infection, but these bacilli are acid fast, whereas *T. whipelli* is not.

The clinical features of Whipple's disease are protean, depending on which organs are involved. Gastrointestinal symptoms are usually striking, resemble those seen in other

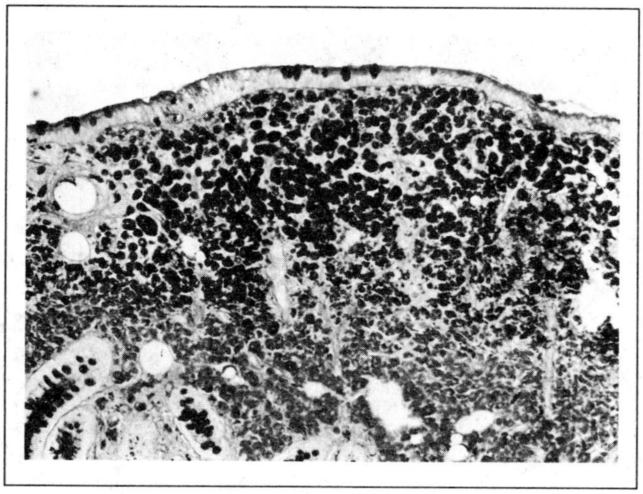

Fig. 42-3. Jejunal biopsy specimen from a patient with untreated Whipple's disease. The glycoprotein-containing, PAS-positive macrophages have virtually replaced the normal cellular elements of the lamina propria, markedly distorting normal mucosal architecture.

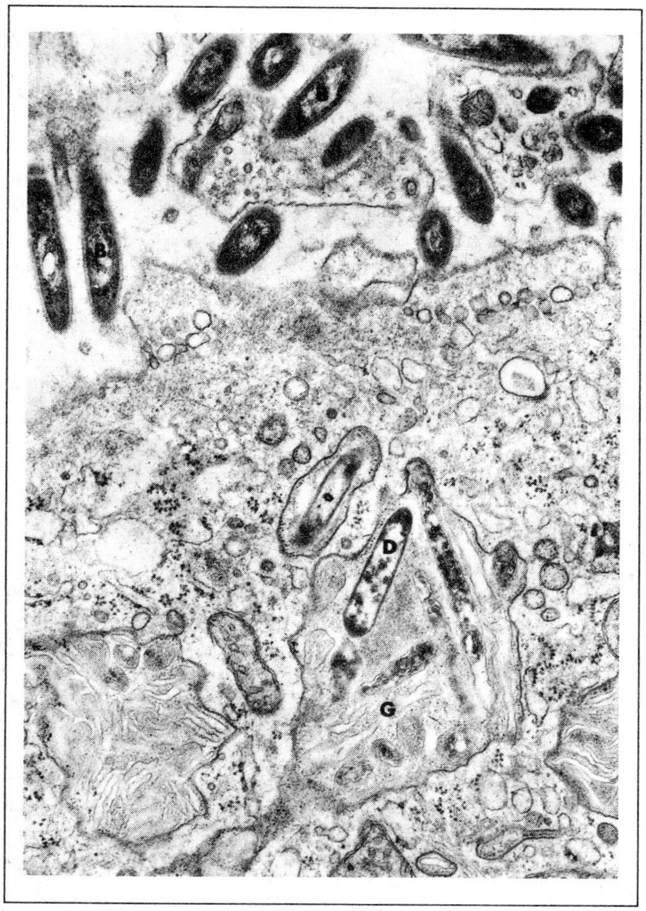

Fig. 42-4. Electron micrograph of jejunal lamina propria from a patient with untreated Whipple's disease. The typical bacilli (*B*) are seen in the intercellular spaces of the lamina propria. Additionally degenerating bacilli (*D*) are seen within the lysosomal PAS-positive granules (*G*) of a macrophage.

diseases that cause generalized malabsorption, and include diarrhea, weight loss, abdominal bloating, and abdominal pain (see earlier discussion). Peripheral edema is common, because protein leakage into the gut may be severe, especially when involved mesenteric nodes obstruct the lymphatic drainage from the gut. Fever, with or without chills, is present in over 50% of patients and may be the presenting symptom. Arthralgia and arthritis occur in over 60% of patients and may precede the onset of intestinal symptoms by several years. Central nervous system symptoms include confusion, loss of memory, bizarre behavior, and focal cranial nerve signs such as nystagmus and ophthalmoplegia. In addition to the physical findings characteristic of any generalized malabsorptive disease, lymphadenopathy, evidence of arthritis of peripheral joints, cardiac murmurs, or focal neurologic abnormalities suggest extraintestinal involvement. Anemia with occult bleeding, iron or folate deficiency, steatorrhea, malabsorption of D-xylose, hypoalbuminemia, and hypocalcemia are common laboratory features. Barium contrast study of the small intestine suggests an infiltrative process, often with striking thickening of the mucosal folds (Fig. 42-5).

The diagnosis is established by histologic examination of involved tissue. Mucosal small intestinal biopsy is the diagnostic procedure of choice, because the proximal small

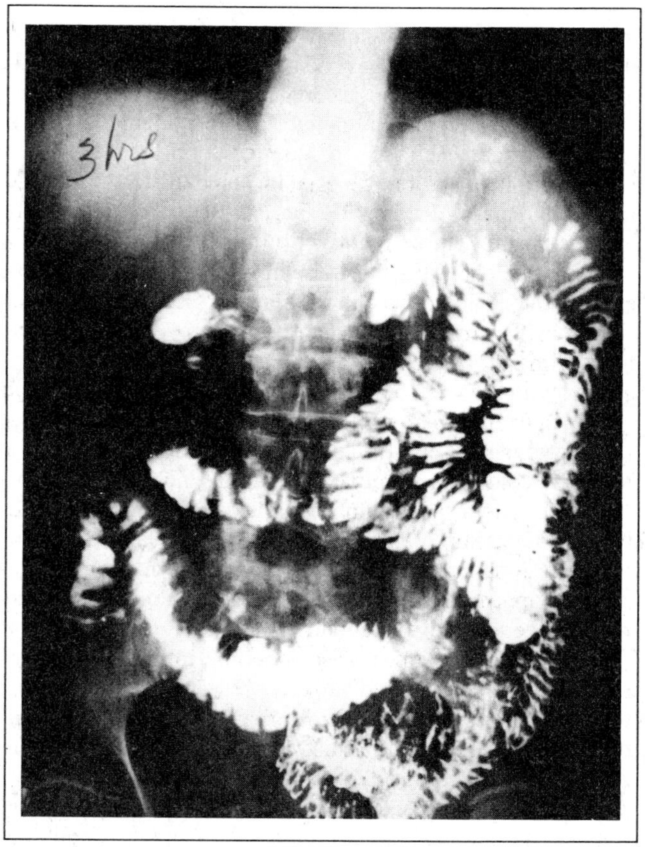

Fig. 42-5. Barium contrast small intestinal series from a patient with untreated Whipple's disease. The striking thickening of mucosal folds is shown, suggesting an infiltrative process.

intestine is involved in the vast majority of patients. Rarely, the intestine is spared or involvement is focal, and biopsy of other tissues such as peripheral or mesenteric lymph nodes is needed to establish the diagnosis.

Treatment with antibiotics effective against gram-positive organisms induces dramatic improvement. The optimal regimen is not known, but recently treatment with trimethoprim-sulfamethoxazole or chloramphenicol has been recommended, because these agents readily penetrate the blood-brain barrier and are likely to eliminate occult central nervous system (CNS) involvement. The ideal duration of treatment is not known, but 6 to 12 months of antibiotic treatment is generally given empirically. As in other diseases with malabsorption, replacement therapy designed to correct specific nutritional deficiencies is indicated. Relapses have occurred in patients treated with a variety of antibiotic regimens including tetracycline, penicillin with and without streptomycin, and erythromycin. Development of central nervous system symptoms may herald relapse and should be treated with antibiotics that cross the blood-brain barrier such as trimethoprim-sulfamethoxazole or chloramphenicol.

Spectrum of eosinophilic gastroenteritis

I. Focal muscle wall, submucosal, and subserosal involvement
   - A. Gastric antrum most commonly affected but small bowel and/or colon may be involved
   - B. Obstructive symptoms and pain are common
   - C. Radiologic features usually resemble those of malignancy, occasionally resemble those of Crohn's disease of stomach and proximal small intestine
   - D. Full-thickness biopsy may be required for definitive diagnosis

II. Mucosal and submucosal involvement
   - A. Diarrhea, mild to moderate steatorrhea, abdominal and back pain, nausea and vomiting, and edema are common
   - B. Stomach and/or small bowel usually involved in patchy fashion
   - C. Mucosal biopsy often diagnostic

III. Serosal and subserosal involvement
   - A. Eosinophilic ascites
   - B. Pleural effusions are sometimes present

IV. All types (I, II, and III) associated with
   - A. Peripheral eosinophilia
   - B. History of allergic disorders in many
   - C. Improvement or prolonged remission with corticosteroid therapy

Eosinophilic gastroenteritis

Eosinophilic gastroenteritis is a poorly understood, uncommon disease characterized by pronounced peripheral eosinophilia and infiltration of the wall of the stomach, small intestine, and/or colon with mature eosinophils. Many patients with eosinophilic gastroenteritis have or have had allergic disorders such as eczema, allergic rhinitis, or seasonal asthma. However, although IgE-dependent mast cell–mediated hypersensitivity to ingested foodstuffs has been implicated in the pathogenesis in some patients because many have an intolerance to a variety of foods, no specific allergic trigger can be identified in most patients.

The three patterns of eosinophilic infiltration in this disease produce distinctive clinical features (see the box, upper right). In the first pattern, there is extensive focal infiltration, primarily of the muscle wall and submucosa by eosinophils, with associated edema. The most common site is the gastric antrum, where muscle hypertrophy also occurs, but focal lesions may involve any level of the small intestine or even the colon. Obstructive symptoms, including abdominal pain, nausea, and vomiting are common presenting features, and barium contrast studies often reveal antral infiltrative lesions that resemble carcinoma or lymphoma in radiologic appearance. Laparotomy with full-thickness biopsy may be needed to exclude malignancy.

In the second pattern of eosinophilic infiltration, mucosal and submucosal involvement predominates. In adults, the small intestine is the major organ affected, but in children the gastric mucosa is also regularly involved. Mild to moderate malabsorption, diarrhea, abdominal and/or back pain, and edema caused by enteric protein loss are the more frequent symptoms. In addition to peripheral eosinophilia, laboratory findings may include iron deficiency anemia, hypoproteinemia, hypocalcemia, D-xylose malabsorption, and the presence of Charcot-Leyden crystals, as well as excess fat in the stools. In some patients whose symptoms increase when ingesting a particular food, serum IgE levels may increase after challenge with that substance. The architecture of the mucosa of the small intestine may vary from normal to flat, even in adjacent biopsy specimens. Infiltration of the mucosa or submucosa with sheetlike aggregates of eosinophils or the presence of eosinophilic microabscesses is of substantial diagnostic value (Fig. 42-6). However, mucosal eosinophilia, like the alterations in mucosal architecture, may be focal; therefore normal peroral jejunal biopsies do not exclude the diagnosis.

In the third and least common pattern of eosinophilic infiltration, eosinophilic inflammation is primarily subserosal and serosal and produces ascites and, in some instances, pleural effusions that contain many eosinophils.

Treatment with corticosteroids is remarkably effective in most patients with eosinophilic gastroenteritis. Sustained symptomatic remission may be induced with short (2 to 4 week) courses at moderate dosages (20 to 40 mg prednisone/day); other patients require repeated courses or continuous maintenance therapy, usually at substantially lower dosages. Elimination diets have been tried, primarily in patients with mucosal involvement who have histories that suggest a causative role for specific offending foodstuffs but are often disappointing in adults as sustained responses are uncommon.

Systemic mastocytosis

Although skin and cardiovascular manifestations are usually prominent in systemic mastocytosis, gastrointestinal symptoms may cause substantial morbidity and occasion-

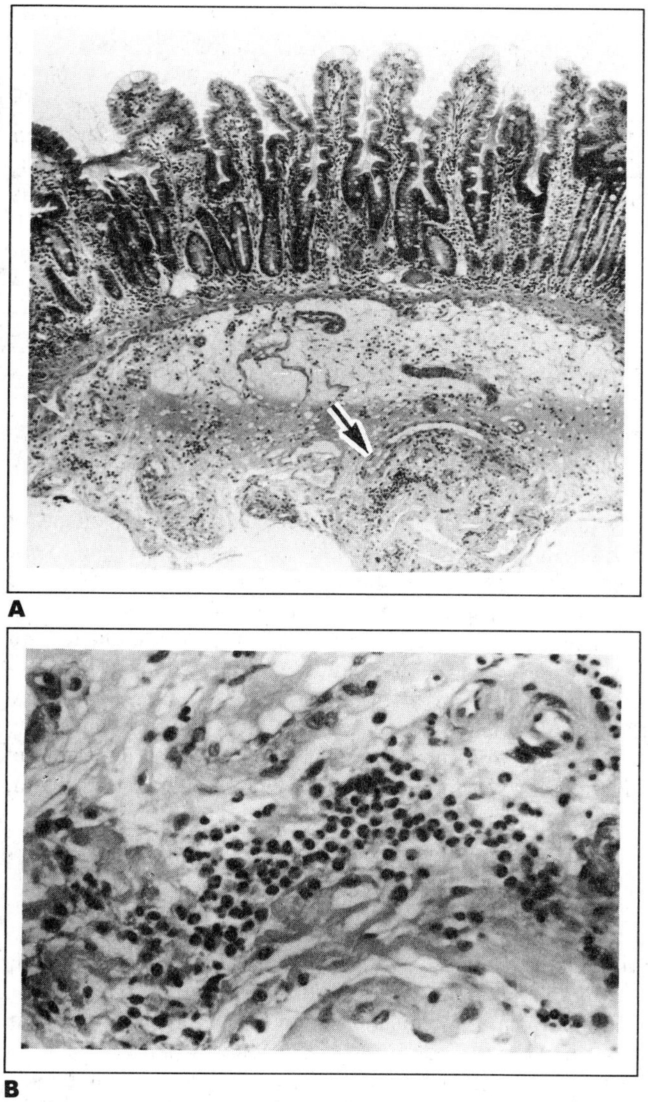

Fig. 42-6. A, Jejunal mucosal biopsy specimen from a patient with eosinophilic gastroenteritis. Villi, though present, are shorter than normal, and the crypts show moderate hyperplasia. **B,** The region designated by the arrow is shown at higher magnification and is heavily infiltrated with eosinophils.

ally occur in the absence of obvious skin lesions. The gastrointestinal symptoms, like those of other body systems, have been attributed to the release from mast cells of histamine and other humoral mediators such as prostaglandin D_2. There is increasing evidence that mucosal and connective tissue mast cells differ in regard to their structure, secretory regulation, and secretory products. Thus the relative importance of infiltrative mucosal lesions and the role of mediators released by connective tissue mast cells versus mucosal mast cells in the pathogenesis of gastrointestinal symptoms remains to be clarified.

Striking acid hypersecretion can occur, resulting in a high prevalence of peptic ulcer disease and contributing to diarrhea and steatorrhea, presumably by inactivating lipase and producing mucosal damage. Extensive infiltration of the intestinal mucosa with mast cells and eosinophils has been well documented and may be associated with architectural changes characterized by crypt hyperplasia and shortened to completely absent villi resembling closely the architectural features of the celiac sprue lesion. Improvement of gastrointestinal symptoms has been reported with administration of H_2-receptor antagonists and with oral cromolyn sodium therapy.

Radiation enteritis and colitis

Because of the rapid renewal rate of their epithelial linings, the small intestine and colon are particularly susceptible to acute radiation injury. In the small intestine, mucosal inflammation and shortening of villi caused by impaired crypt cell proliferation are regularly present during exposure to radiation. The acute mucosal lesion usually causes no symptoms and generally reverts to normal within 2 weeks after radiation therapy is terminated. In the colon and rectum mucosal inflammation and atrophy are seen, and symptomatic proctitis and colitis are not rare during acute radiation exposure. The clinical features resemble closely those of idiopathic ulcerative proctitis (Chapter 43), but the response to treatment with local corticosteroids in the form of enemas or suppositories and sulfasalazine is limited at best.

More serious cases of radiation enteritis and colitis occur weeks to many years after radiation therapy has been completed. This delayed lesion results in part from an obliterative endarteritis of submucosal arterioles and appears unrelated to the acute mucosal lesion. Fibrosis and edema of the intestinal or colonic wall develop, largely on an ischemic basis, and may produce strictures, obstruction of mucosal lymphatics, and secondary mucosal lesions, including ulceration. The threshold tissue dose for the delayed intestinal tissue lesion is in the range of 40 Gy, and the incidence of significant damage rises sharply at doses above 50 Gy. Malabsorption caused by involvement of the small intestine may reflect (1) bacterial overgrowth secondary to stricture-induced intraluminal stasis, (2) lymphatic obstruction, or (3) bile salt deficiency if ileal involvement is extensive. The clinical features of chronic radiation colitis or proctitis resemble those of idiopathic inflammatory or chronic ischemic disease of the large intestine, with diarrhea, abdominal pain, and hematochezia being prominent symptoms. Stricture formation may produce symptoms of partial or even complete intestinal obstruction (Chapter 44). Barium contrast studies of the colon and small intestine help characterize the extent of disease and localize the site of strictures but may resemble closely the radiologic features of other inflammatory or ischemic intestinal lesions.

Treatment is disappointing. Broad-spectrum antibiotic therapy may benefit patients with intraluminal stasis and bacterial overgrowth caused by strictures. Cholestyramine may reduce bile salt-induced diarrhea in patients with ileal disease but aggravate steatorrhea by further depleting the bile salt pool if the ileal disease is extensive. Dietary supplementation with medium-chain triglycerides and polymeric or elemental diet preparations may improve nutrition. In patients with mild colonic strictures, stool softeners and a low-residue diet may be helpful. If severe intestinal or colonic strictures or enterocolic, enterovesical, or rectovesical fistulas are present, surgery is needed. Surgery is associated with considerable morbidity, because the compromised vascular supply of the affected bowel may interfere with normal healing.

Regional enteritis

See Chapter 43.

Lymphoma

See Chapter 45.

Abetalipoproteinemia

In this rare disease, which is transmitted as an autosomal recessive trait, there is defective synthesis and/or secretion by intestinal absorptive cells of apoprotein B, an integral protein component of (1) chylomicrons, (2) very-low-density lipoproteins (VLDL), and (3) low-density lipoproteins (LDL). As a result, apoB-containing lipoproteins are absent from plasma. Although the products of dietary long-chain triglyceride digestion can enter absorptive cells, packaging of absorbed lipids into VLDL and chylomicrons does not occur; as a result, their normal exit along the basolateral membrane is prevented. The histopathology of the intestine is characteristic; mucosal architecture is normal, but villus absorptive cells are filled with fat and appear vacuolated in conventional paraffin-embedded sections.

Abetalipoproteinemia is usually evident in infancy or early childhood when steatorrhea is noted. Acanthocytic red cells appear early, whereas neurologic symptoms including ataxia, tremors, nystagmus, sensory abnormalities, and retinitis develop after several years in untreated patients. The diagnosis is established by documenting the absence in the blood of apoprotein B–containing lipoproteins and very low cholesterol and triglyceride levels. Treatment is supportive and should include (1) cautious substitution of medium-chain triglyceride supplements for normal dietary long-chain lipids (cirrhosis has been attributed to medium-chain triglycerides in a few patients); (2) supplements of fat-soluble vitamins, especially vitamin E, which prevent development and, if present, progression of retinitis and neurologic symptoms; and (3) psychologic support to help patients deal with their neuromuscular and visual disabilities.

In *chylomicron retention disease* (Anderson's disease) the intestinal epithelium appears to synthesize apolipoprotein B-48 yet is unable to transport absorbed lipid, which, as in abetalipoproteinemia, accumulates in absorptive cells. Although fasting serum triglyceride levels are normal and serum apoprotein B, though decreased, is present, the clinical features closely resemble those of abetalipoproteinemia, and the therapeutic approach is the same.

Intestinal lymphangiectasia

Intestinal lymphangiectasia may be *primary*, produced by congenital malformation of intestinal or more proximal lymphatic vessels, or *secondary*, produced by acquired lymphatic obstruction of mesenteric or more proximal lymphatic vessels caused by trauma, neoplasms, retroperitoneal fibrosis, or infectious diseases such as tuberculosis and Whipple's disease. The lymphatics distal to the obstruction become dilated and may rupture, with leakage of substantial quantities of lymph into the intestinal lumen. This lymph leakage results in protein-losing enteropathy, with exudation of serum proteins and concomitant loss of lymphocytes into the gut. If the lymphatics draining large segments of small intestine are obstructed, significant steatorrhea results. The characteristic histopathologic finding reveals dilatation of mucosal and submucosal lymphatics (Fig. 42-7), and, if enteric plasma protein loss is severe, edema of the bowel wall.

In patients with congenital lymphatic malformations, the onset of clinical features usually occurs shortly after birth. Asymmetric edema is common because of involvement of lymphatics draining one or more extremities. Acquired defects develop later in life, often with a history or clinical features that suggest the underlying cause, be it trauma, neoplasm, infection, and so on. Diarrhea, weight loss or growth failure, chylous ascites, pleural effusions, and peripheral edema are features common to both primary and acquired lymphangiectasia. Laboratory findings that help establish the diagnosis include lymphopenia and striking reductions of serum albumin, immunoglobulins, transferrin, and ceruloplasmin. Excessive intestinal clearance of alpha-1-antitrypsin pinpoints the alimentary tract as the site of protein loss (Chapter 33). Steatorrhea is usually present and may be severe, but D-xylose absorption is generally normal. Barium contrast studies of the small intestine usually reveal thickened edematous mucosal folds but are not specific. Lymphangiography may show obstruction or hypoplasia of major lymphatic channels, diminished or absent visualization of retroperitoneal nodes, and occasionally leakage of contrast material from mesenteric lymphatics into the intestinal lumen. Mucosal biopsy of the small intestine may be diagnostic, demonstrating tall villi but with dilated lymphatic vessels and widening of villi caused by edema (Fig. 42-7). Lymphangiectasia may involve the

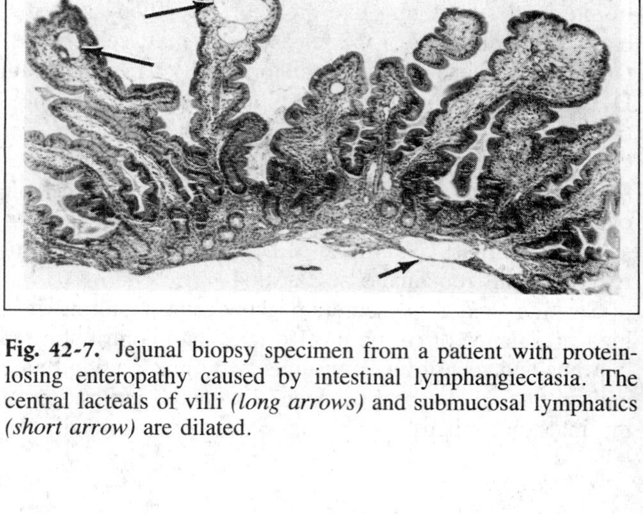

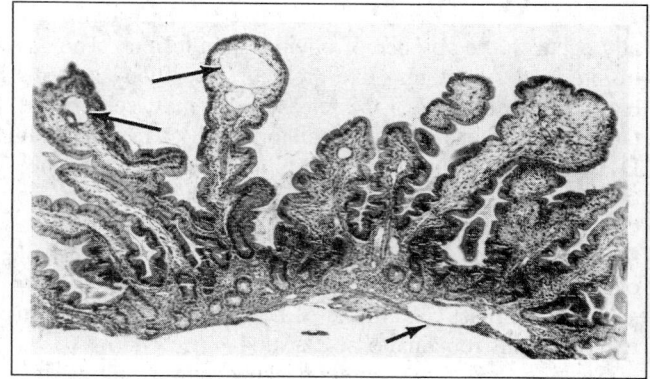

Fig. 42-7. Jejunal biopsy specimen from a patient with protein-losing enteropathy caused by intestinal lymphangiectasia. The central lacteals of villi *(long arrows)* and submucosal lymphatics *(short arrow)* are dilated.

small intestine in a patchy fashion or, rarely, may be confined to the colon. Therefore absence of dilated lymphatics in mucosal biopsy specimens does not exclude the diagnosis of lymphangiectasia.

Substitution of medium-chain triglyceride supplements for long-chain dietary fats reduces lymph flow. As a result, protein leakage into the gut is decreased and chylous effusions may disappear. Because medium-chain triglycerides, unlike long-chain triglycerides, are transported via the portal blood rather than the lymph, steatorrhea is reduced. If the lesion involves only a limited segment of the bowel, surgical resection of the segment can be beneficial but, in most instances, the process is too diffuse to permit this approach. Although the associated lymphopenia and hypogammaglobulinemia perturb immune function, severe or chronic infections are uncommon.

Immunoglobulin deficiency

Diarrhea and malabsorption are present frequently in patients with immunoglobulin deficiency. Several specific causes have been identified. Intestinal giardiasis is common in acquired hypogammaglobulinemia and has also been noted in X-linked hypogammaglobulinemia. Celiac sprue responsive to dietary gluten withdrawal and Crohn's disease with malabsorption have been associated with acquired hypogammaglobulinemia as well as with selective IgA deficiency. Intraluminal bacterial overgrowth may occur in acquired hypogammaglobulinemia, but whether this overgrowth is related directly to immunoglobulin deficiency or to the hypochlorhydria or achlorhydria that occurs in over 50% of these patients is not known.

Clinical evaluation of hypogammaglobulinemic patients with diarrhea and malabsorption should determine whether specifically treatable conditions are present. Stools should be examined for parasites; if test results are negative, duodenal contents and/or a mucosal small intestinal biopsy should be obtained to exclude giardiasis. If celiac sprue is suspected, mucosal biopsy should be performed to determine whether a characteristic lesion is present. Malabsorption of intrinsic factor–bound vitamin B_{12} suggests the coexistence of intraluminal bacterial overgrowth or the presence of a coexistent ileal lesion such as Crohn's disease (Chapter 43). Malabsorption of free vitamin B_{12} is observed often, because gastric hyposecretion and atrophy are common. A marked reduction or absence of plasma cells in the lamina propria is a characteristic feature of intestinal mucosal biopsy specimens obtained from patients with hypogammaglobulinemia. Many patients have hyperplasia of the lymphoid follicles of the intestinal mucosa, which may be evident in both mucosal biopsies and barium contrast studies of the small intestine and colon.

Treatment should be directed toward the underlying defect: quinacrine (Atabrine) or metronidazole for giardiasis, a gluten-free diet for celiac sprue, broad-spectrum antibiotics for bacterial overgrowth, and sulfasalazine and/or corticosteroids for associated inflammatory bowel disease. In the minority of patients, no specific coexistent disorder can be found even though the mucosal architecture of the small intestine may resemble that seen in celiac sprue. Some patients may improve with administration of gamma globulin or corticosteroids, but others are unresponsive to such therapy.

Intestinal resection

Resection of up to 50% of the mid small intestine is well tolerated, be it for ischemic disease, Crohn's disease, neoplasm, or trauma, provided that the remaining small intestine is free of disease. Resection or bypass of smaller lengths that include the duodenum or distal ileum and ileocecal valve frequently produces symptoms related to the selective absorptive function of the most proximal (iron, calcium, and folate) and most distal (conjugated bile salts and vitamin B_{12}) small intestine. Resection of 70% to 80% of the small intestine generally produces catastrophic malabsorption. Factors contributing to diarrhea and malabsorption are (1) a critical reduction in the absorptive surface; (2) acid hypersecretion, which occurs in some patients with massive resection, especially during the first several weeks or months following resection, and which results in lipase inactivation and acid-induced mucosal damage; (3) reduction of the bile salt pool and the presence of bile salt–stimulated colonic water and electrolyte secretion following ileal resection; and (4) induction of colonic secretion by hydroxy fatty acids produced by bacterial hydroxylation of unabsorbed fat.

In patients with massive resection, prompt and vigorous parenteral fluid and electrolyte replacement therapy is essential and lifesaving. It must be guided by careful monitoring of fluid losses and serial determination of serum electrolyte, calcium, and magnesium levels and body weight. Early implementation of parenteral alimentation with vitamin and mineral supplements is important (Chapter 49). Oral feedings should be initiated as early as possible, because oral alimentation may prevent atrophy and facilitate adaptive hyperplasia of the remaining intestinal mucosa by stimulating the secretion of trophic gastrointestinal hormones, pancreatic secretions, and bile. Commercially available elemental diets are helpful but should be diluted initially to reduce their high osmolarity. Fat intake should be supplemented with readily absorbable medium-chain triglycerides. If gastric hypersecretion is present, administration of an H_2-receptor antagonist is indicated. As intestinal adaptation occurs, the need for parenteral supplementation may diminish or disappear, and oral alimentation should be increased. Antidiarrheal agents, including opiates, diphenoxylate, and anticholinergics, are often useful. If 100 cm or less of ileum has been resected, administration of a bile salt–binding agent such as cholestyramine or aluminum hydroxide helps control bile salt–induced colonic secretion and diarrhea. If ileal resection has been more extensive, these agents may aggravate symptoms by further depleting the bile salt pool, which increases steatorrhea. The need for monthly vitamin B_{12} supplementation is determined by quantitating its absorption after ileal resection. Iron, folate, and calcium supplementation may be necessary, especially if the proximal intestine has been resected or bypassed. Vitamin supplements, especially those that are fat soluble, and trace metals such as zinc may be needed (Chapter 49).

Carbohydrate intolerance

Carbohydrate intolerance may be caused by (1) a deficiency of a specific disaccharidase, (2) impairment of the monosaccharide transport process in the small intestine, or (3) diffuse mucosal disease that results in low levels of several mucosal disaccharidases as well as impaired monosaccharide transport. In addition, sorbitol, a poorly absorbed polyalcohol sugar commonly used to sweeten "sugar-free" products such as gum, candy, and fruits, may cause symptoms in some individuals. Symptoms, which include bloating, excess flatus, crampy abdominal pain, and diarrhea, are produced by the osmotic effect in the gut lumen of the unabsorbed carbohydrates and by the production of gas and organic acids by intraluminal bacteria that ferment the unabsorbed carbohydrate.

Isolated acquired lactase deficiency is the most common cause of carbohydrate intolerance in adults. Low intestinal lactase levels are found in 5% to 20% of adult North American Caucasians, 50% to 99% of North American and African blacks, and up to 95% of Asians. Indeed, isolated acquired lactase deficiency is so common in many adult populations that the "defect" can hardly be considered abnormal. Adequate lactase levels are present in infancy but decrease in childhood or adolescence in those affected. In contrast, *congenital lactase deficiency,* like *congenital sucrase-isomaltase deficiency* and *congenital glucose-galactose malabsorption,* is rare and is evident at birth. Many but certainly not all lactase-deficient patients recognize their inability to tolerate dairy products, avoid them, and have few symptoms. Tolerance varies, and quite a few lactase-deficient individuals can ingest modest amounts of milk (150 to 240 ml) without symptoms.

The most direct and definitive means of establishing lactase deficiency is to determine biochemically the lactase content of intestinal mucosa obtained by mucosal biopsy. Histologic structure can be assessed concomitantly and, if normal, helps exclude secondary lactase deficiency caused by other mucosal diseases such as celiac sprue, tropical sprue, or acute gastroenteritis. However, biopsy is invasive and is often not necessary if (1) there is a history of milk intolerance, (2) if the lactose tolerance test produces symptoms and indicates abnormality (blood glucose normally should increase at least 20 mg/dl after a 50 to 100 g lactose challenge) or (3) if breath hydrogen excretion is excessive after a 50 g lactose challenge. However, the lactose tolerance and breath hydrogen tests may be influenced by abnormal gastric emptying and altered intestinal motor function as well as by glucose metabolism; therefore false-positive and, less often, false-negative test results occur.

Treatment consists of removal of lactose from the diet by eliminating dairy products and baked and processed foods that contain lactose. Sustained clinical improvement helps establish the diagnosis. In secondary disaccharidase deficiency, symptoms are often improved by restriction of dietary lactose until the primary disease responds to treatment; elimination of other disaccharides or monosaccharides from the diet is usually of little clinical benefit.

REFERENCES

Bayless TM et al: Lactose and milk intolerance: clinical implications. N Engl J Med 292:1156, 1975.

Beer WH, Fan A, and Halsted CH: Clinical and nutritional implications of radiation enteritis. Am J Clin Nutr 41:85, 1985.

Cherner JA et al: Gastrointestinal dysfunction in systematic mastocytosis: a prospective study. Gastroenterology 95:657, 1988.

Dobbins WO: Whipple's disease. Springfield, Ill, 1987, Charles C. Thomas.

Earnest DL and Trier JS: Radiation enteritis and colitis. In Sleisenger MH and Fordtran JS, editors: Gastrointestinal disease, ed 4. Philadelphia, 1989, WB Saunders, p 1369.

Hermans PE, Diaz-Buxo JA, and Stobo JD: Idiopathic late-onset immunoglobulin deficiency: clinical observations in 50 patients. Am J Med 61:221, 1976.

Heyman MB: Food sensitivity and eosinophilic gastroenteropathies. In Sleisenger M and Fordtran JS, editors: Gastrointestinal disease, ed 4. Philadelphia, 1989, WB Saunders, p 1113.

Hyams JS: Sorbitol intolerance: an unappreciated cause of functional gastrointestinal complaints. Gastroenterology 84:30, 1983.

Levy E et al: Steatorrhea and disorders of chylomicron synthesis and secretion. Pediatr Clin North Am 35:53, 1988.

Min KU and Metcalfe DD: Eosinophilic gastroenteritis. Food Allergy 11:799, 1991.

Relman DA et al: Identification of the uncultured bacillus of Whipple's disease. N Engl J Med 327:293, 1992.

Ryser RJ et al: Reversal of dementia associated with Whipple's disease by trimethoprim-sulfamethoxazole, drugs that penetrate the blood-brain barrier. Gastroenterology 86:745, 1984.

Simon GL and Gorbach SL: Intestinal flora in health and disease. Gastroenterology 86:174, 1984.

Trier JS: Medical progress: celiac sprue. N Engl J Med 325:1709, 1991.

Trier JS and Donnelly SM: A 78-year-old woman from the Dominican Republic with chronic diarrhea: case records of the Massachusetts General Hospital. N Engl J Med 322:1067, 1990.

Trier JS and Lipsky M: The short bowel syndrome. In Sleisenger MH and Fordtran JS, editors: Gastrointestinal disease, ed 4. Philadelphia, 1989, WB Saunders, p 1106.

Weser E, Fletcher JT, and Urban E: Short bowel syndrome. Gastroenterology 77:572, 1979.

CHAPTER

43 Idiopathic Inflammatory Bowel Disease

Fred H. Goldner
Sumner C. Kraft*

Idiopathic inflammatory bowel disease (IBD) refers primarily to two diseases, ulcerative colitis and Crohn's disease. Subcategories relate to the sites and extent of tissue involvement. *Ulcerative colitis* is essentially a mucosal disease limited to the large intestine and usually presents with bloody diarrhea. In contrast, *Crohn's disease* is a transmural process that may affect any point along the alimentary

*The opinions and assertions contained herein are those of the authors and are not to be construed as reflecting the views of the Department of the Army or Department of Defense.

canal, especially the distal ileum and proximal colon. Although diarrhea is common, additional features include obstruction, fistulas, and abscesses. Synonyms for Crohn's disease include descriptive terms such as *granulomatous, segmental, transmural,* or *regional enteritis* or *colitis*. The term *ileocolitis* is reserved for Crohn's colitis with concomitant involvement of the small bowel. Although Crohn's disease and ulcerative colitis represent an overlapping clinical spectrum, they will be discussed separately to a great extent.

ETIOLOGY

The etiology of IBD remains unknown. Infectious agents have been implicated, particularly in Crohn's disease, in which atypical mycobacteria have been identified in a small minority of patients. Clearly, Koch's postulates remain unfulfilled. Although various immunologic phenomena have been described (e.g., increase in cytokines or prostaglandins), many may be nonspecific phenomena or epiphenomena secondary to the inflammatory process. Indirect evidence of disturbed immunity includes the association of arthritis, erythema nodosum, episcleritis, uveitis, and vasculitis with these disorders as well as the beneficial response of many patients to immunosuppressive drugs. Genetic factors may contribute to the development of IBD as indicated by the 10-fold increased risk of disease in first-degree relatives of patients. The mode of inheritance is unclear, however, and no human leukocyte antigen (HLA) haplotype predominates. Interaction of genetic susceptibility with as yet undiscovered environmental factors is a distinct possibility. Smoking has been associated directly with an increased incidence of Crohn's disease, whereas an inverse relationship exists with ulcerative colitis.

INCIDENCE AND EPIDEMIOLOGY

The incidence and prevalence of IBD vary widely throughout the world: they are considerably higher in the United States and Europe than in Asia or Africa. In the United States and Europe most studies indicate a range of 4 to 8 new cases per 100,000 population per year. Although ulcerative colitis has generally been found to be more common in the past, the incidence of Crohn's disease appears to have increased. This seems to be a true increase rather than merely an increased awareness of the condition. Criteria for the diagnosis of IBD vary greatly among studies, however, and significantly affect incidence and prevalence data. For example, ischemic colitis has not always been excluded in older patients with alleged idiopathic IBD. Today, the total population with IBD in the United States is estimated to be 200,000 to 400,000, with 15,000 to 30,000 new cases occurring each year. IBD affects both sexes equally. The peak age of onset is in the second to fourth decades, but new cases in infants and octogenarians also occur. Other interesting observations of unclear significance include an increased occurrence of IBD among Jews, at least in North America, and a greater incidence in whites than in blacks.

CROHN'S DISEASE

Pathology

An important gross pathologic finding in Crohn's disease is its distribution along the intestine. Although it most commonly involves the ileocolic region, any level of the gut from mouth to anus may be involved. More than one area may be affected while the intervening bowel appears grossly normal, giving rise to so-called skip areas. Other typical gross findings are a thickened intestinal wall, mucosal fissuring, fistulas, inflammatory masses, and benign strictures. A "cobblestone" appearance results from edematous mucosa that is infiltrated with lymphoid cells and transected by communicating, deep fissures and linear ulcerations (Fig. 43-1).

A major histologic feature of Crohn's disease is the typical transmural involvement of the bowel wall. The submucosa is edematous and contains nodular aggregates and dense infiltrates of lymphocytes and plasma cells (Fig. 43-2). There may be lymphatic inflammation and secondary intestinal lymphangiectasia. Fibrosis may be extensive and may cause luminal narrowing, leading to bowel obstruction (Fig. 43-1). Ulcerations of various sizes and shapes may form, ranging from aphthous ulcers over the lymphoid nodules to deep, longitudinal fissures. The inflammation may extend completely through to the serosa, forming sinus tracts and fistulas. Even the mesentery may be edematous and thickened, with mesenteric fat wrapping around the bowel. Mesenteric lymph nodes become hyperplastic and are densely packed with chronic inflammatory cells.

Another characteristic feature of Crohn's disease is the formation of noncaseating, sarcoidlike granulomas (Fig. 43-2). These are present in about 30% to 40% of conventionally examined, resected intestinal specimens and may also be found in areas that appear normal grossly as well as in the mesenteric lymph nodes. Although the presence of granulomas is extremely helpful in making the diagno-

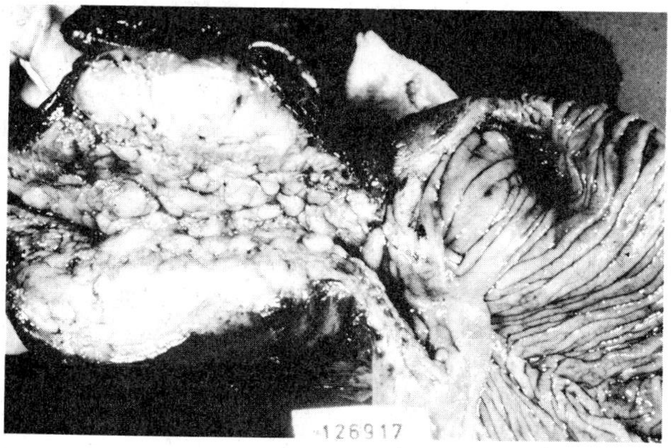

Fig. 43-1. Crohn's disease. Resected specimen of ileum showing transmural nature of inflammatory process, cobblestone mucosa on left, stricture in center, and normal but dilated proximal bowel on right.

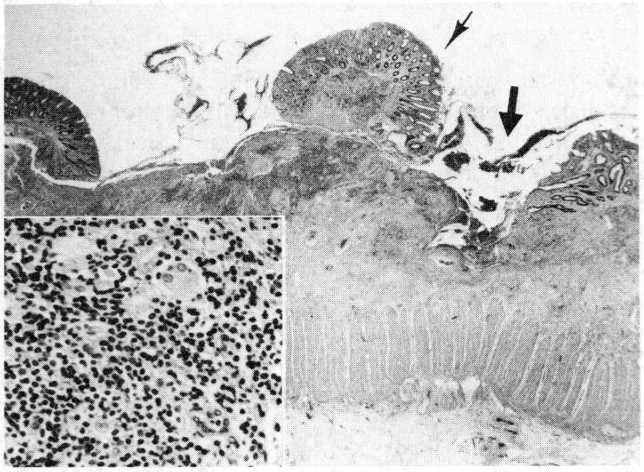

Fig. 43-2. Crohn's disease. Photomicrograph of resected specimen of colon showing residual mucosal nodule *(smaller arrow)* surrounded by ulceration. The deeper, fissured ulcer *(larger arrow)* may penetrate transmurally and result in fistulization. Insert shows multinucleated giant cells in a portion of a submucosal lymphoid follicle that contained sarcoidlike granulomas.

sis of Crohn's disease, their absence does not rule out this diagnosis.

Clinical and laboratory findings

The more common clinical features of Crohn's disease include diarrhea, abdominal pain, fever, and weight loss. Because the presentation may be extremely variable and the diagnosis far from obvious, there is an average 3 year delay from the onset of symptoms to diagnosis. The location of lesions in the gut influences the pattern of the clinical manifestations. Both the distal ileum and the proximal colon are diseased in 40% to 50% of patients, the small intestine alone in 20% to 30%, and the colon alone in 15% to 30%, whereas isolated anorectal disease occurs in only 3% of patients with Crohn's disease.

Diarrhea occurs in most patients with Crohn's disease and may have several possible causes. Disease of the terminal ileum may cause malabsorption of bile salts, leading to ion and water secretion by the colon (so-called cholorrheic enteropathy). After resection of more than 100 cm of distal ileum, greater degrees of bile salt loss may occur, resulting in a greatly diminished total bile salt pool and producing steatorrhea caused by impaired intraluminal micelle formation. Strictures of the small bowel may cause stasis, producing malabsorption that is the result of bacterial overgrowth (Chapter 42). Rectal involvement may lead to tenesmus, but hemochezia generally is not as prominent as in ulcerative colitis. Occasionally, however, a submucosal vessel is eroded, leading to massive bleeding in Crohn's disease; this may even be a presenting feature.

Abdominal pain is usually prominent. It is most often in the right lower quadrant, reflecting transmural involvement of the ileocecal area. If there is partial small bowel obstruction, the pain is often colicky and is aggravated by eating. A constant pain associated with spiking fever and leukocytosis should arouse suspicion of abscess formation and prompt a thorough evaluation for sepsis. Low-grade fever and malaise are common and may occur solely on the basis of bowel inflammation.

Perirectal disease, including abscess, fistulas, and anal fissures, may be a prominent feature of Crohn's disease. Such conditions may precede or occur concomitantly with intestinal disease and should alert the clinician to search for evidence of Crohn's disease elsewhere in the bowel. Perirectal abscess may result from rectal Crohn's disease, whereas fistulization may result from disease in the ileocecal and sigmoid regions.

Weight loss and malnutrition may be dramatic, producing extreme cachexia. Females often become amenorrheic. In children, growth retardation and delayed sexual maturation, sometimes to a striking degree, may occur even in the absence of or with only minimal abdominal symptoms. Multiple nutritional deficiencies may be caused by poor dietary intake, malabsorption, and increased catabolism caused by inflammation.

Physical examination of the abdomen may reveal either a tender, right lower quadrant mass caused by edematous, adherent loops of bowel or a chronic, walled-off abscess. Nutritional status can be assessed in part by measuring the triceps skinfold and upper arm muscle size and making comparisons with published norms (Chapter 49). Evidence of perirectal disease and extraintestinal manifestations of Crohn's disease must be carefully sought (see p. 468).

Laboratory findings are nonspecific. A complete blood count may show anemia, which is often multifactorial. For example, iron deficiency may be due to chronic blood loss or to iron malabsorption if the duodenum is diseased. Persistent intestinal inflammation may contribute to the anemia of chronic disease. Macrocytic anemia may develop if terminal ileal disease or bacterial overgrowth leads to vitamin B_{12} malabsorption. Rarely, medications may produce anemia. For example, sulfasalazine may induce folate deficiency or cause hemolysis. The total leukocyte count and erythrocyte sedimentation rate are often elevated but do not always correlate with disease activity. Absolute lymphopenia may be especially associated with small bowel disease, as well as malnutrition. Thrombocytosis may be marked and associated with thrombotic episodes. Fluid and electrolyte imbalance is common in patients with diarrhea and/or malabsorption. Malabsorption of fat-soluble vitamins may lead to low serum carotene levels (vitamin A), hypocalcemia (vitamin D), and prolonged prothrombin times (vitamin K). Decreased protein intake and absorption, combined with increased catabolism and protein exudation into the gut, result in low plasma protein and albumin values. Trace metal deficiencies (e.g., zinc) are known to occur.

Diagnosis

Because there is no single clinical feature or laboratory test that is diagnostic of Crohn's disease, it is important to be alert to the possibility of other conditions with similar manifestations, such as appendiceal abscess, cecal diverticulitis, tuberculosis, fungal diseases, amebiasis, and bacterial pathogens including *Salmonella, Shigella, Campylobacter,* and *Yersinia*. Culture and toxin assay for *Clostridium difficile* should be performed if there is a history of recent antibiotic treatment. Also to be considered are intestinal lymphoma, carcinoma, and ischemic bowel disease. However, in a young person with persistent or recurrent right lower quadrant abdominal pain, diarrhea, fever, and weight loss, together with an abdominal mass and perirectal abnormalities, the diagnosis of Crohn's disease is very likely.

Occasionally, the disease is diagnosed early when a patient with clinical features suggesting acute appendicitis undergoes laparotomy. The appendix looks normal but the terminal ileum and its mesentery are inflamed. Classic Crohn's disease develops in only 10% to 15% of such patients. When serologic testing is done in the remainder, this form of acute terminal ileitis often appears to be a self-limited *Yersinia enterocolitica* infection. If the cecum is grossly normal, the appendix may be safely removed to lessen confusion in the event of recurrent abdominal pain, but the terminal ileum should not be resected if it is only inflamed and there are no other complications (abscess).

In the more common elective evaluation, several fresh stools should be examined for ova and parasites and cultured for bacterial pathogens. A proctosigmoidoscopy should be performed to search for patchy mucosal nodularity and typical aphthous ulcers. A random rectal biopsy may be helpful. Although such rectal biopsies reveal granulomas in about 30% of cases in which there is gross colorectal disease, granulomas are detectable, if carefully sought, in a smaller but significant number of cases with more gross involvement limited to the small bowel.

The approach to suspected colonic disease generally begins with colonoscopy, which allows accurate assessment of inflammation as well as the option of tissue sampling (Plate II-10). If contrast radiography is performed, the double contrast technique is most sensitive unless the intent is to detect fistula tracts, in which case the single column method is preferred. The most common radiographic findings are mucosal nodules that cause a cobblestone appearance (Fig. 43-3), multiple ulcers, fissures, and strictures (Fig. 43-4). Fistula tracts, either within the intestinal wall or between loops of bowel (Fig. 43-5), may be apparent, but their exact site of origin is often difficult to determine. Patients who are acutely ill should have examination deferred or undergo a careful limited examination of the distal colon (flexible sigmoidoscopy) without prior catharsis to lessen the risk of toxic megacolon or perforation. Gastroduodenal examination with endoscopy or barium may be performed if indicated by upper intestinal symptoms. Crohn's disease may involve the duodenum in 5% to 10% of cases. Suspected small bowel disease remains the domain of the barium contrast small bowel examination. Edema and thickening of the bowel wall may lead to separation of the loops and a "string sign," classically seen as a manifestation of severe luminal narrowing in the terminal ileum (Fig. 43-6). Abscesses may cause displacement of bowel loops and extrinsic compression of the bowel wall.

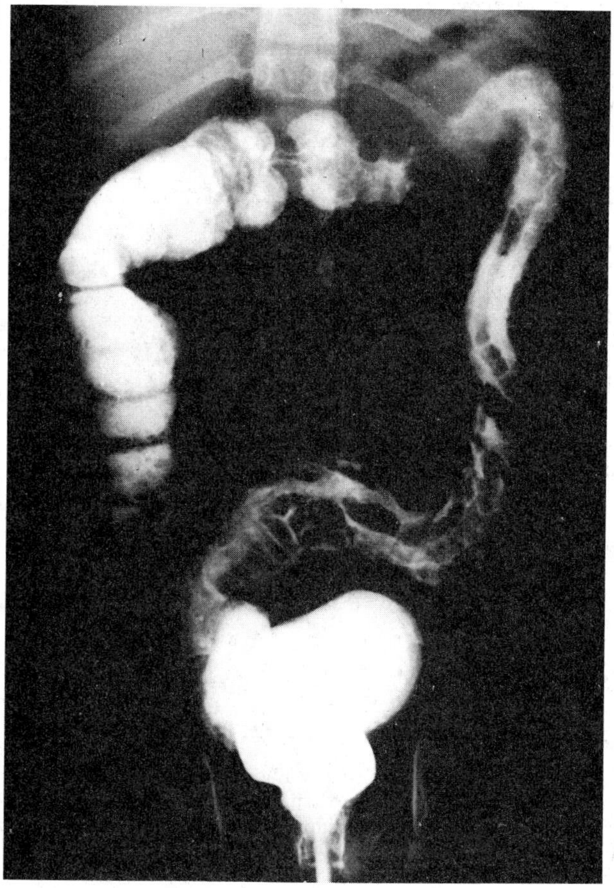

Fig. 43-3. Crohn's disease. Radiograph of colon showing multiple smooth-surfaced, ovoid, and elongated mucosal cobblestones, with relatively mild involvement of the rectum and right colon.

Suspected abscesses may be further defined by computed tomography (CT) scans or radionuclide scanning techniques using neutrophils labeled with indium-111.

Management

Great variation in the clinical course of Crohn's disease in individual patients makes evaluation of treatment programs difficult. Controlled trials, such as the National Cooperative Crohn's Disease Study, are therefore extremely useful. Such studies confirm that although Crohn's disease is often a relentless process, there may be long periods of spontaneous remission. Indeed, in this study one third of the patients with active regional enteritis who received a placebo entered clinical remission within 4 months, and half of this group was still in remission after 2 years.

The following suggestions are not intended as a standardized approach; rather, therapy should be individualized for a given patient. Although understanding and use of temporarily beneficial treatment programs have improved, therapy has not altered greatly the natural course of Crohn's disease.

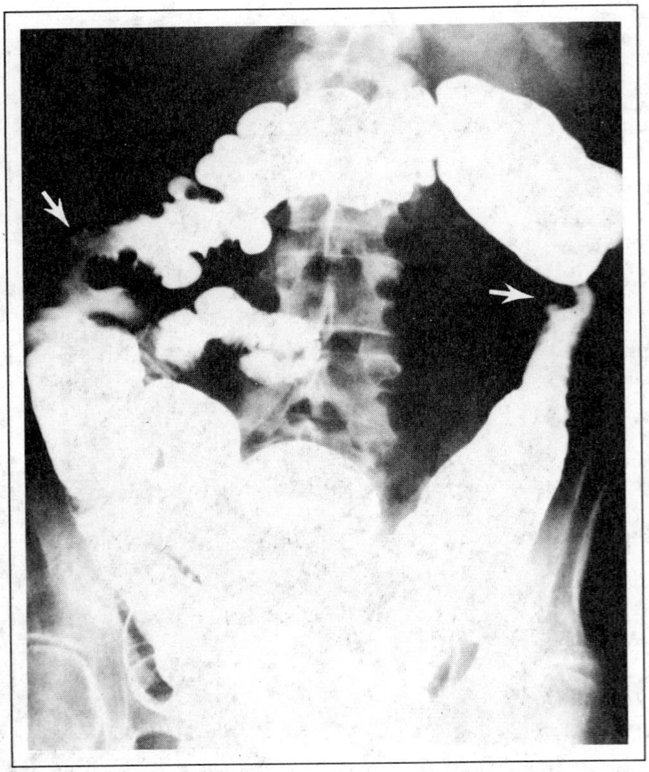

Fig. 43-4. Crohn's disease. Radiograph of colon showing two irregular inflammatory strictures *(arrows)* and less involved skip area. A pseudodiverticulum is seen in the descending colon.

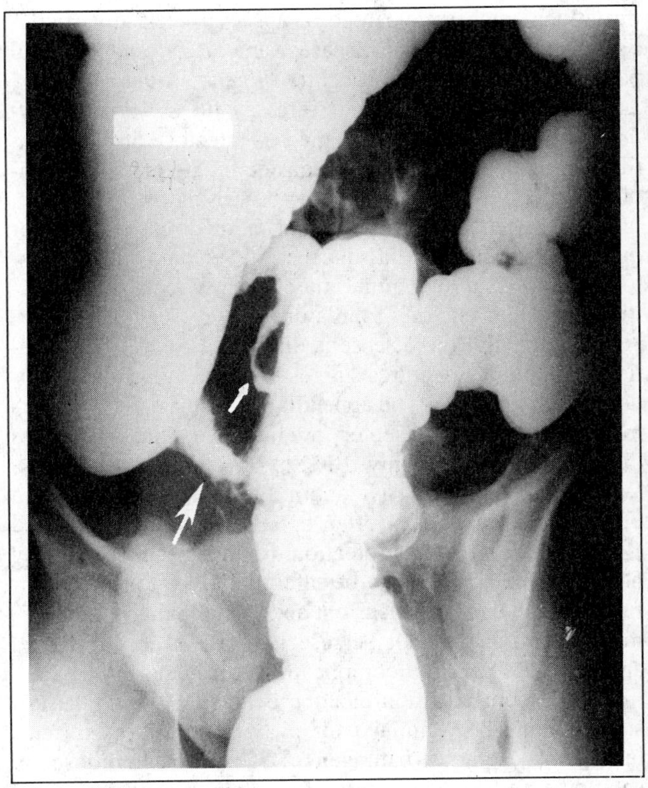

Fig. 43-5. Crohn's disease. Radiograph of colon showing wide fistula *(larger arrow)* between cecum and sigmoid colon and irregularly narrowed distal ileum *(smaller arrow)*.

Medical therapy

General therapy. Although medications are generally emphasized, it is important to consider the whole patient when devising a therapeutic plan. Adequate physical rest must be permitted and emotional support provided as anxiety and depression may be severe.

Nutrition. The importance of nutritional support cannot be overemphasized (Chapter 49). In addition to causing significant weight loss, malnutrition may hinder responses to other medications and increase both the risk of infection and the morbidity of surgery. In the adolescent patient, growth may cease. The patient should be allowed to choose foods that are palatable, with protein and calorie supplements taken as necessary. The occasional beneficial response to milk restriction may relate to the known occurrence of lactose intolerance in such patients. Specific replacement of fat-soluble vitamins, folic acid, calcium, iron, magnesium, and zinc may be needed. Vitamin B_{12} should be administered parenterally to patients with subnormal Schilling test results or after resection of the terminal ileum. Elemental or chemically defined diets may be useful as primary therapy in Crohn's disease, but their use remains controversial. In the presence of severe disease or multiple fistulas, parenterally administered nutrients may be needed. Although significant nutritional improvement usually ensues, this approach has no beneficial effect on the underlying disease. Long-term home parenteral nutrition is required in some patients.

Antidiarrheal measures. Treatment of diarrhea should primarily be directed at the underlying inflammatory process. Diphenoxylate, loperamide, and anticholinergics may provide symptomatic relief but should be used sparingly lest toxic dilatation of the colon ensue. If no intestinal obstruction exists, psyllium hydrophilic colloid may be tried to firm the stool. Because extensive (>100 cm) ileal disease or resection may lead to bile salt deficiency with steatorrhea, a low-fat diet supplemented with medium-chain triglycerides may be helpful, because the latter do not require bile salts for absorption. The anion-exchange resin cholestyramine may bind the unabsorbed bile salts and prevent them from inducing diarrhea, although steatorrhea may be aggravated if more than 100 cm of ileum is involved or resected (Chapter 42).

Anti-inflammatory agents. The cornerstone of medical therapy involves the rational use of sulfasalazine and corticosteroids. The literature abounds with anecdotal reports of the efficacy of these drugs, but despite the important information gained from the National Cooperative Crohn's Disease Study and other controlled trials, many important questions remain unanswered. The following represents a synthesis of recommendations from several studies.

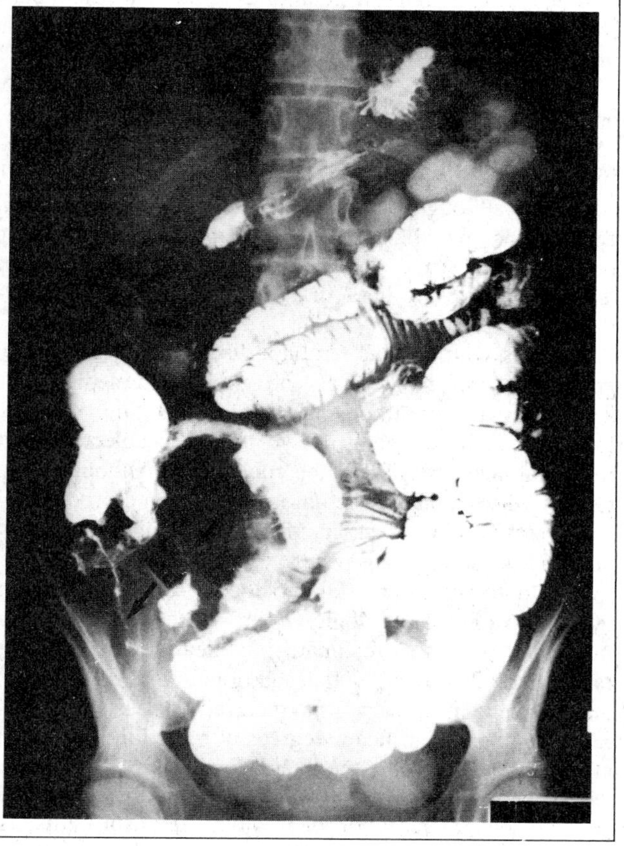

Fig. 43-6. Crohn's disease. Radiograph of gastrointestinal examination showing severe luminal narrowing *("string sign"; see arrows)* of an edematous, thickened, and irregular terminal ileum; there is also evidence of dilatation of more proximal small bowel.

Sulfasalazine (4 to 6 g/day) is an effective drug, particularly in ileocolonic or colonic Crohn's disease, but is less effective in patients with purely small bowel involvement. The activity of sulfasalazine in the distal bowel is explained by its metabolism by colonic flora to sulfapyridine and 5-aminosalicylic acid, the latter being the therapeutic moiety (for a more detailed discussion see p. 466).

Prednisone is an effective drug primarily for small intestinal Crohn's disease and should be considered initially for use in moderately to severely ill patients. The daily dosage may be adjusted according to disease severity, with a maximum of 1 mg per kilogram of body weight. High-dose intravenous methylprednisolone therapy may be indicated in extremely ill patients on a bowel rest program. If rectal Crohn's disease is present, steroid enemas twice daily may be helpful. Although systemically administered steroids are certainly useful, serious side effects such as diabetes, hypertension, cataracts, and osteoporosis often limit long-term administration. Alternate-day steroid therapy has been useful in children. The combination of sulfasalazine and prednisone does not appear to be more effective than either agent alone, and sulfasalazine does not provide a steroid-sparing effect.

A dilemma is presented by the Crohn's disease patient with fever, leukocytosis, and a palpable abdominal mass. It is usually best to treat such patients initially with intravenous antibiotics (e.g., ampicillin, aminoglycoside, or a second- or third-generation cephalosporin) rather than with high-dose corticosteroids for fear of producing septic complications.

Metronidazole appears to be an effective alternate drug in Crohn's disease; it is particularly useful for patients with ileocolonic or colonic involvement. For such patients, its efficacy is generally equivalent to that of sulfasalazine. Metronidazole also may be valuable in the management of perineal Crohn's disease. The dosage is 10 to 20 mg/kg/day, but beneficial effects may not be apparent before 4 to 6 weeks. Paresthesias, which may persist after metronidazole is discontinued, are a common side effect.

Immunosuppressive agents. Azathioprine and its metabolite 6-mercaptopurine (6-MP) have emerged in recent years as being clearly beneficial in Crohn's disease. Although not first-line agents, they are valuable in the treatment of refractory disease, problematic perianal disease, and fistulas. They also provide a steroid-sparing effect. When initiated at a dose of 50 mg, increasing to not more than 1.5 mg/kg body weight, azathioprine and 6-MP are safe and well tolerated. Of course, one must monitor for bone marrow suppression (2%) and pancreatitis (3%). Development of lymphoma is rare. A disadvantage of the use of azathioprine and 6-MP is the average wait of 3.1 months before an effect is seen. Cyclosporine, a suppressor of cell-mediated immunity, has shown promise in controlled trials of refractory Crohn's disease and has a relatively quick onset of action. Methotrexate is currently being evaluated in controlled trials, but its routine use cannot currently be recommended.

Maintenance of remission. When Crohn's disease goes into remission, corticosteroids should be tapered and stopped, because they probably do not prevent relapse when given on a long-term basis. There are, however, steroid-responsive patients who repeatedly relapse after the usual drug withdrawal sequence. In this subgroup, drug administration may have to be tapered very slowly (no more than 2.5 to 5.0 mg each 14 days) and maintained (5 to 15 mg of prednisone daily) for months to years. In contrast to corticosteroids and sulfasalazine, azathioprine or 6-MP may be used judiciously to extend the period of remission.

Surgical therapy for complications of Crohn's disease

Operative treatment is indicated in Crohn's disease only after failure of all reasonable attempts at medical control or for complications. Surgery should not constitute primary therapy because there is up to a 3% operative mortality. The incidence of disease recurrence is high, approaching 100% in patients with small intestinal involvement with long-term follow-up observation. However, if recurrence is defined only as disease significant enough to warrant reoperation, then rates of about 40% at 15 years pertain, being somewhat higher for ileocolonic disease. Despite these caveats, approximately 70% of patients with Crohn's disease ultimately require some form of surgery for this condition. Moreover, these operations can produce dramatic improvement when indicated as a required complement to medical management. Surgery itself does not appear to predispose the patient to earlier recurrence or to the need for further surgery. To procrastinate unduly while the patient is exposed to uncontrollable disease sequelae and drug side effects is a disservice to the patient.

The complications of Crohn's disease and therefore the indications for surgery vary with the location of the involvement. Obstruction is one of the most common problems and occurs mainly with ileal or ileocolonic disease. A short trial of intestinal decompression, parenterally administered steroids, and the balance of the bowel rest program may be helpful. If this fails, surgical therapy should involve resection of the minimum amount of bowel necessary. Strictureplasty, a method of treating short strictures without resection, is currently being evaluated with encouraging initial results.

Abscess formation often is a sequela of luminal narrowing and/or transmural involvement and thus is associated mostly with ileal and ileocolonic involvement. Although antibiotics should be instituted, they rarely are sufficient, and surgery often is required when a true abscess, rather than just matted loops of inflamed bowel, is present. A computed tomographic (CT) scan or ultrasonogram can help locate and define the abscess. Although guided percutaneous catheter drainage of abdominal abscesses has been successful in some patients, abscesses associated with Crohn's disease are often not amenable to this approach. The operative approach is difficult because many loops, including noninflamed bowel, may be matted together. The surgeon is obligated to save as much normal bowel as possible in order to prevent the short bowel syndrome. Temporary bypass with exclusion of the most severely diseased area may sometimes be prudent; the abscess may be drained through a separate incision. After inflammation subsides, the surgeon may resect bowel that cannot be salvaged and reestablish intestinal continuity. Permanent bypass procedures are to be avoided because they result in higher recurrence rates and higher risk of carcinoma in the bypassed segment many years later.

Fistula formation is also often associated with distal luminal obstruction or may occur without frank obstruction. Fistulas require surgery only if they are symptomatic or if enough bowel is bypassed to cause severe malnutrition or other deleterious effects. Unfortunately, enterocutaneous fistulas may follow fistulectomy. Fistulas may also involve the urinary bladder, vagina, psoas muscle, pelvic skeleton, and even the inferior vena cava; generally, these fistulas require surgical treatment.

Less common complications include free perforation, massive hemorrhage, multiple small bowel strictures with bacterial overgrowth, carcinoma, and obstructive uropathy. The latter may occur in the absence of an abnormality identified by urinalysis if an inflamed intestinal mass compresses the right ureter, a situation common enough to make abdominal ultrasound an indicated part of the evaluation in most patients with ileocolonic disease.

Perianal abscesses, often with associated fistulas, are quite common, occurring eventually in 50% of all patients, especially but not exclusively in those with colonic disease. External incision and drainage of the abscess are usually adequate, although occasionally a temporary diverting ileostomy also may be necessary. An aggressive surgical approach in which the surgeon attempts to remove all local disease may result in a draining, slow-healing perineal wound.

Patients with colonic Crohn's disease may require surgery because of the disease's intractability to medical management or the development of toxic dilatation of the colon. If the rectum remains grossly normal, a colectomy with ileorectal anastomosis may be considered. Although recurrence of disease in the rectum is common and proctectomy may eventually be necessary, the patient might not have to undergo ileostomy for several years.

The outcome after total proctocolectomy and conventional ileostomy for colonic Crohn's disease remains controversial. Although estimates of ileal recurrence rates range from 3% to 40% and additional surgery ultimately may become necessary, the recurrent disease is usually rather mild and significant degrees of resection are not usually necessary, making the overall prognosis for "cure" after colectomy for *colonic* Crohn's disease substantially better than that for resection of involved small intestine. Although ileostomy dysfunction occurs somewhat more frequently in Crohn's disease patients than in ulcerative colitis patients who require proctocolectomy, the difference between dysfunction in the two groups is not great. In any event, the risk of subsequent small bowel problems should not be a deterrent when the physician is faced with the necessity of performing total colectomy. However, continent ileostomies or ileoanal anastomoses should never be constructed in patients with documented or even suspected Crohn's disease.

ULCERATIVE COLITIS

Pathology

In acute ulcerative colitis, the colonic mucosa and on occasion the submucosa show striking histologic abnormalities. Findings include diffuse vascular congestion, edema, hemorrhage, distorted crypt architecture, and cellular infiltration with plasma cells, lymphocytes, neutrophils, and eosinophils. Goblet cells are usually depleted. A common problem is the need to distinguish acute ulcerative colitis from acute colitis of infectious cause (*Salmonella, Shigella, Campylobacter, E. coli 0157:H7,* and ameba). Although there are no pathognomonic features, the finding of distorted crypt architecture and the presence not only of neutrophils but also of increased numbers of plasma cells and lymphocytes in the lamina propria is highly suggestive of acute ulcerative colitis. Crypt abscesses, which may also be seen in Crohn's disease and in the infectious colitides, are common and consist of accumulations of neutrophils, eosinophils, and cellular debris (Fig. 43-7). The muscularis mucosae may be hypertrophic.

In *chronic ulcerative colitis,* inflammation, edema, muscular hypertrophy, and deposition of fibrous tissue and fat may cause thickening, contraction, narrowing, and shortening—a "lead pipe" appearance. Inflammatory polyps ("pseudopolyps") are common and represent mucosal remnants or accumulations of granulation tissue with or without overlying colonic epithelial cells (Fig. 43-8). Mucosal bridges may result from mucosal undermining or from the attachment of the free ends of inflammatory polyps to adjacent mucosa. Injury and healing proceed concurrently, so that different areas in the bowel may simultaneously manifest all stages of reaction from acute inflammation to epithelial regeneration. The mucosa rarely becomes histologically normal, despite the remission of symptoms and the disappearance of endoscopically and radiologically apparent abnormalities. Thus biopsies of the rectal mucosa during prolonged remissions may reveal persistent foci of chronic inflammatory cells and evidence of mucosal atrophy (e.g., a loss of parallelism, branching, and decreased numbers of rectal glands). Toxic dilatation and cancer of the colon in ulcerative colitis are discussed later.

Variant forms of chronic colitis include such conditions as microscopic or collagenous colitis. The hallmark of these processes is mucosal microscopic inflammation without endoscopic or radiographic abnormalities. Although hemochezia is not a feature, the diarrhea may respond to sulfasalazine, suggesting that these conditions may be part of the spectrum of chronic ulcerative colitis.

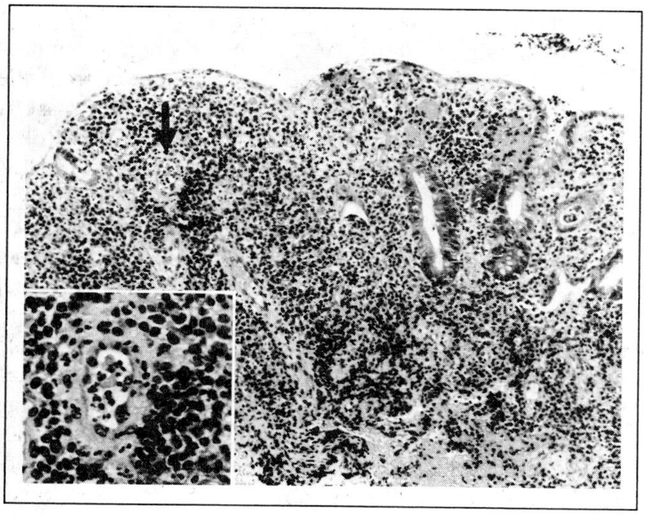

Fig. 43-7. Ulcerative colitis. Colonic mucosa with acute and chronic inflammatory cells, diminished crypts, and a thin layer of regenerating surface epithelium. The more highly magnified inset shows the crypt abscess indicated by the arrow in the main photograph and shows neutrophils infiltrating the crypt wall and many surrounding mononuclear cells.

Clinical and laboratory findings

The dominant symptoms of ulcerative colitis are diarrhea and hemochezia. In acute severe disease, the patient often is febrile and has 5 to 30 watery, bloody stools per day; dehydration; and anemia. Massive hemorrhage, requiring several daily blood transfusions to sustain an adequate blood volume, occurs in only 2% or 3% of patients. On the other hand, the onset may be mild and insidious, with one to four stools per day, minimal gross bleeding, and perhaps only vague abdominal discomfort. Associated symptoms include flatulence, rectal tenesmus, malaise, fatigue, anorexia, and loss of weight. Occasionally flares of colitis may be associated with constipation, perhaps as a result of inflammation-induced colonic dysmotility. Extracolonic complications (discussed later) involving the liver, skin, eyes, or joints may precede or accompany the colonic manifestations. In most patients ulcerative colitis is chronic, with exacerbations and remissions.

The physical examination may not reveal an abnormality, but fever, tachycardia, pallor, and wasting are common. The abdomen may be diffusely or locally tender and distended, perhaps with signs of peritoneal irritation, although the absence of abdominal findings is not unusual even in the presence of total colonic involvement. The presence of fever and colonic tenderness in a patient with chronic diarrhea is highly suggestive of IBD. Rectal examination may disclose perianal erythema, hemorrhoids, and fissures, but extensive anorectal complications such as the abscesses and fistulas common in Crohn's disease are rare in ulcerative colitis.

Laboratory findings include anemia caused by nutritional deficiency of iron or folic acid, blood loss, hemolysis, chronic inflammation, or combinations of these. The leukocyte count and erythrocyte sedimentation rate may be elevated, especially in the presence of complications, and thrombocytosis may indicate disease activity, especially in the absence of iron deficiency. Prolonged diarrhea may lead to depressed serum levels of potassium, chloride, sodium, and magnesium; diarrhea may also result in a metabolic acidosis. Low serum albumin levels may result from extensive protein loss into the gastrointestinal tract, and increased amounts of serum alpha-2 globulin and gamma globulin may be detected. Although the serum immunoglobulin levels are often within normal ranges, individual patients show wide variations. The feces usually contain no identifiable pathogenic bacteria or parasites, and occult blood may persist for long periods after subsidence of clinical symptoms.

Diagnosis

Chapter 41 describes the differential approach to acute and chronic diarrheal syndromes and outlines the specific conditions that may affect the colon and need to be ruled out in establishing a diagnosis of ulcerative colitis (e.g., amebiasis, bacterial colitis, ischemia, antibiotic-induced colitis, uremia, radiation colitis, Behçet's syndrome, and collagen-vascular diseases).

Proctosigmoidoscopy, although not specific, is a most valuable diagnostic procedure in ulcerative colitis. The mucosal appearance may range from that of mild hyperemia, fine granularity, petechiae, and minimal pinpoint bleeding after wiping with a cotton swab to moderate or severe abnormalities such as increased friability, edema, mucopurulent exudate, and frank ulceration with spontaneous bleeding. Inflammatory polyps, narrowing of the rectal ampulla, and stricture formation reflect both severity and chronicity. Biopsies may aid in the differentiation between benign and malignant strictures, between inflammatory and neoplastic polyps, and between ulcerative and Crohn's colitis. In mild to moderately severe cases, prompt healing with return to a grossly normal appearance may follow treatment. Colonoscopy may be useful in demonstrating the extent of mucosal involvement in selected cases; in documenting Crohn's colitis, which may not involve the rectosigmoid; and in excluding colonic carcinoma in selected patients. However, colonoscopy is hazardous in patients with active acute disease because it may produce perforation or precipitate toxic megacolon.

Colonic radiographs reveal abnormalities in approximately 90% of patients with ulcerative colitis and are valuable both for diagnosis and for delineating the extent of colonic involvement. However, barium enema examination should not be performed in a patient with very active or fulminant colitis. Mucosal detail is especially well seen with air-contrast barium enemas (Fig. 43-8). Mucosal ulceration may produce fine marginal serrations, a feathery outline, or well-circumscribed craters. Other common findings include diminished or absent haustrations, straightening, narrowing, shortening, an irregular mosaic pattern produced by mucosal edema, diminished distensibility, spasm, and an increase in the retrorectal soft tissue space. The latter finding by itself is not necessarily indicative of disease. The terminal ileum must be seen and, although often normal, may in the presence of contiguous colonic involvement show mucosal ulceration or irregularity ("backwash ileitis") with a lumen of increased or normal caliber, in contrast to the narrowing seen in Crohn's disease (Table 43-1). Partial or complete reversibility of the radiographic findings can occur in patients with ulcerative colitis in remission.

Strictures and inflammatory pseudopolyps may be difficult to differentiate from benign or malignant neoplasms without the aid of colonoscopy and biopsy. Benign strictures of the colon are found in 5% to 10% of patients with ulcerative colitis and are often related to hypertrophy of the muscularis mucosae; fibrosis is the usual cause of the more frequent benign strictures seen in Crohn's colitis. The benign strictures of ulcerative colitis are seldom multiple; generally form in the rectosigmoid; appear as smooth 2 to 3 cm long narrowed areas; and may obstruct the fecal stream. Features that may indicate the presence of malignant strictures include poor demarcation; flattened, rigid, tapered ("napkin-ring") margins (Fig. 43-9); irregular contours; an associated mass; a right-sided location; and multicentricity.

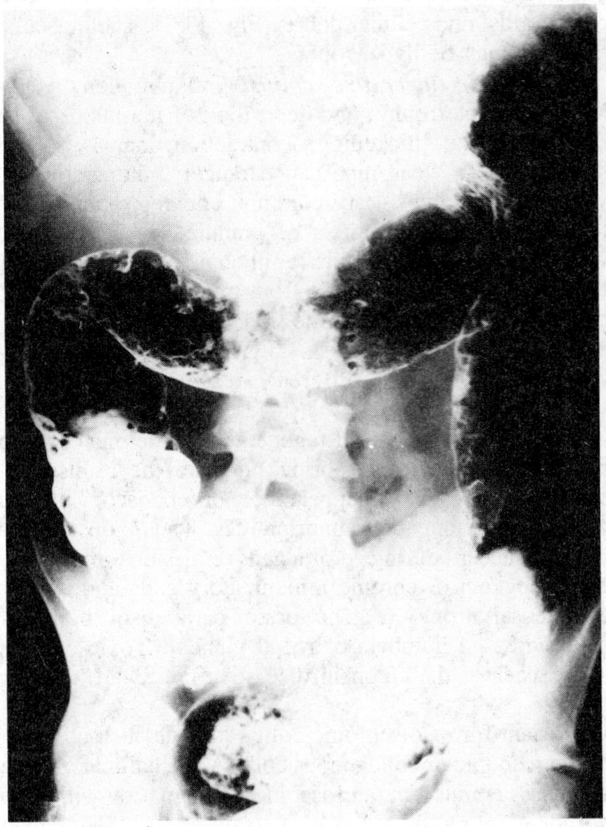

Fig. 43-8. Ulcerative colitis. Air-contrast radiograph of the colon showing absent haustrations and numerous inflammatory polyps.

Management

Current medical therapy uses an array of drugs to decrease mucosal inflammation as part of a broad program emphasizing adequate nutrition and emotional support from the family and physician. Diet in mild or quiescent disease is often unrestricted. If there is a question of lactose intolerance, dairy products should be avoided. In severe colitis parenteral nutrition may be necessary for short periods but does not improve the natural history of the disease.

The cornerstone of drug therapy in mild to moderate cases of ulcerative colitis has been sulfasalazine. The usual dose is 4 g/day for active disease and 2 g/day for maintaining remission. This drug is cleaved by colonic bacteria into its two components: sulfapyridine and 5-aminosalicylic acid (5-ASA). The therapeutic properties of sulfasalazine are due to 5-ASA; the problems with hypersensitivity (rash, arthritis, pancreatitis) and general intolerance (nausea, headache) are ascribed to the sulfapyridine moiety. To obviate the disadvantages of sulfapyridine, new forms and delivery systems of 5-ASA have been developed under the generic name mesalamine. A dimer of 5-ASA (olsalazine) that is likewise cleaved by colonic bacteria, freeing the active 5-ASA, is also available. In addition, mesalamine suppositories are available for treatment of ulcerative proctitis and

Table 43-1. Clinical and radiologic differentiation of ulcerative colitis and Crohn's colitis

Findings	Ulcerative colitis	Crohn's colitis
Clinical findings		
Hemochezia	Present in most patients	Present in 50% of patients
Abdominal pain	Mild, rarely severe	Severe in 50% of patients
Abdominal mass	None	Present in 10% of patients
Perianal lesions	Present in 20% of patients, rarely severe	Present in 80% of patients, often severe
Proctosigmoidoscopic findings	Distal involvement in virtually all patients	Distal involvement in 50% of patients
	Uniformly granular mucosa	Patchy granularity, cobblestones
		Discrete ulcers with or without normal intervening mucosa
Radiologic findings		
Distribution	Rectum involved in most patients	Rectum involved in 50% of patients
	Continuous disease	Often discontinuous disease
Contour	Bowel uniformly contracted and shortened	Bowel of varying diameter and rarely shortened
	Involvement usually concentric	Segmental, eccentric involvement
		Pseudodiverticula
	Absence of haustral pattern (late in disease)	Incomplete haustral loss
Mucosal detail	Generalized granular outline	Irregular, nodular, cobblestone pattern
	Loss of folds	Aphthous ulcers
	Diffuse shallow (<2 mm) ulceration, may be deeper	Deep, transverse, linear fissures (spiking)
		Longitudinal ulceration
	Pseudopolyps prominent	Pseudopolyps less extensive
Small bowel	Gaping ileocecal valve	Thickened ileocecal valve
	Terminal ileum may be dilated	Terminal ileum narrowed, irregular
	Backwash ileitis in 10% of patients	Involvement may be discontinuous
Internal fistulas	Vary rare, occasionally into vagina	Common
		Occasional intramural or pericolic abscesses

mesalamine enemas for disease distal to the splenic flexure. All forms of 5-ASA have proved beneficial in treating mild to moderately active disease and in maintaining remission. Although the newer preparations are better tolerated, they are no more effective but considerably more costly than sulfasalazine.

Corticosteroids continue to be valuable in moderate to severe disease either as initial therapy or as an alternative when sulfasalazine is not effective. In patients with mild disease who cannot tolerate sulfasalazine, the newer 5-ASA preparations should be tried rather than switching to corticosteroids with their attendant side effects. Oral prednisone (1 mg/kg/day) or parenteral methylprednisolone may be used depending on the clinical severity. Corticotropin appears to be an effective alternative but is expensive and more cumbersome to administer. For proctitis or left-sided colitis, corticosteroid enemas may be given but up to 20% of the dose may be absorbed, leading to systemic side effects. Newer, rapidly metabolized steroid enema preparations that do not have this effect are under development. Corticosteroids in any form are of no value in prolonging remission. The immunosuppressive agents azathioprine and 6-MP may have steroid-sparing effects, but their role in the treatment of ulcerative colitis is less certain than in Crohn's disease.

Surgery may be indicated in ulcerative colitis patients because of uncontrolled massive hemorrhage, obstruction from strictures, free perforation, toxic megacolon, carcinoma, severe mucosal dysplasia, or, more frequently, intractability (i.e., the disease's failure to respond to a truly comprehensive medical program while the patient is hospitalized). The most commonly performed operation is total proctocolectomy with ileostomy. Experience with ileoanal anastomosis in association with construction of a reservoir pouch has been increasing, and this is the preferred procedure in younger patients. When the rectal mucosa remains in situ, problems, including the risk of malignancy, persist. The presence of extracolonic complications per se is seldom an indication for colectomy, but some children with marked growth retardation and a few patients with severe progressive liver disease or severe pyoderma gangrenosum have benefited from this approach. Prophylactic colectomy has been recommended for ulcerative pancolitis of long duration because of the increased risk of colonic cancer, but this procedure has yet to gain more than limited acceptance for patients with only mild symptoms in the absence of severe dysplastic changes seen on multiple biopsies (see p. 470).

Prognosis

Prognosis for the initial attack of ulcerative colitis is affected by the severity and extent of the disease and by the age and physical condition of the patient. For example, the onset of ulcerative colitis in elderly or postpartum patients often is associated with a more stormy course. Factors as-

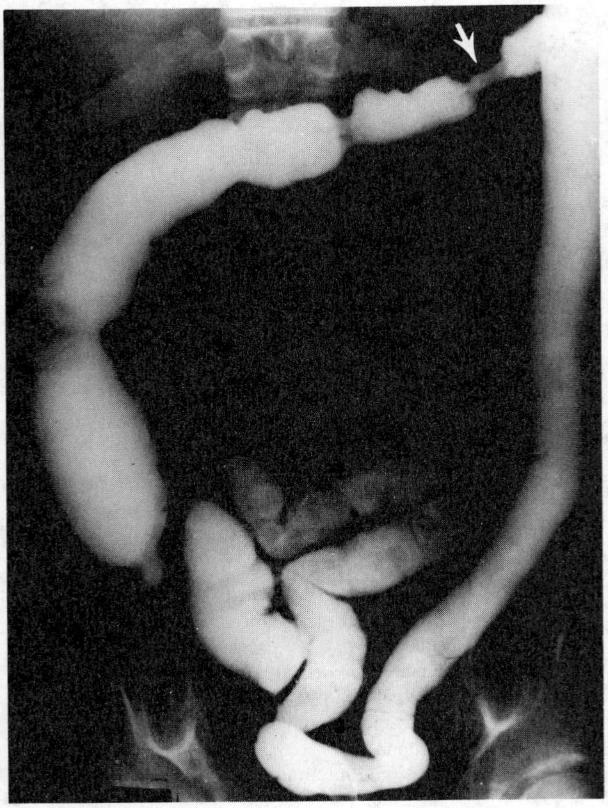

Fig. 43-9. Carcinoma in ulcerative colitis. Radiograph of colon showing diminished haustrations, generalized narrowing, and a malignant stricture *(arrow)* in the distal transverse colon.

sociated with poorer long-term prognoses are extensive involvement of the colon, severe initial attack, and onset either in childhood or after the age of 60 years. However, initial observations may not always accurately reflect the subsequent course, and the most severely ill patient may experience remarkable improvement. Exacerbations may be precipitated by upper respiratory infections, infectious gastroenteritis, other intercurrent illness, emotional stress, oral antibiotics, oral contraceptives, physical fatigue, and local anorectal surgery.

Unless the patient is currently ill, the disease is not a contraindication to becoming pregnant, and most pregnant patients with preexisting ulcerative colitis go on to a full-term normal delivery. Drug therapy (corticosteroids, sulfasalazine) does not appear to affect fetal development adversely. Although the pregnancy per se may not affect the course of the bowel disease, relapses occur in 25% to 50% of patients, especially during the first trimester and puerperium.

ULCERATIVE PROCTITIS

Ulcerative proctitis has the same pathologic process as ulcerative colitis but is limited to the rectum and distal sigmoid. This condition may constitute as much as 20% of all instances of ulcerative colitis in the general population. Proctitis usually runs a mild, intermittent course over many years and in most instances is not associated with serious local and systemic complications. Patients with ulcerative proctitis often have formed stools surrounded by blood, and rectal discharges consisting of blood and mucus (instead of true diarrhea). Indeed, constipation with or without bleeding may actually be the presenting complaint of patients with active ulcerative proctitis. Proctosigmoidoscopy and rectal biopsy show the typical findings of ulcerative colitis, but findings are limited to the distal 10 to 20 cm of the large intestine. Colonic radiographs may reveal normalcy or subtle findings of superficial inflammation limited to the rectum and distal sigmoid, narrowing of the rectal ampulla, or atrophy of rectal valves, and a lateral film of the rectum may show widening of the presacral space.

The differential diagnosis of ulcerative proctitis includes Crohn's colitis; ischemic, antibiotic-induced, or radiation proctitis; amebiasis; lymphogranuloma venereum; gonorrheal, syphilitic, or herpetic proctitis; and the effects of long-term trauma. Hyperemia, changes in vascular pattern secondary to diarrhea, or prior use of irritating enemas or cathartics may be confused with ulcerative proctitis.

The treatment of ulcerative proctitis is very similar to that of ulcerative and Crohn's colitis and includes nonspecific antidiarrheal agents such as diphenoxylate hydrochloride with atropine sulfate (Lomotil) or loperamide; sulfasalazine; and rectal corticosteroids or 5-aminosalicylic acid in the form of retention enemas or suppositories. The enemas or suppositories should be administered at bedtime to maximize retention. Systemic steroids are required much less frequently and should not be instituted as initial therapy.

Death directly attributable to ulcerative proctitis is rare and, although the disorder may persist for many years, it is not associated with an increased incidence of colorectal cancer. The process spreads beyond the rectum in only 10% to 30% of patients who are followed for 5 years or longer.

DIFFERENTIATION OF ULCERATIVE COLITIS AND CROHN'S COLITIS

Differentiating between ulcerative colitis and Crohn's colitis is important, because recurrence is more frequent after resection for Crohn's colitis. On the other hand, colonic cancer occurs much more frequently in ulcerative colitis patients, especially if the entire colon is involved. Making the distinction between these two conditions occasionally may be difficult even when a deep surgical biopsy of the rectal wall or a colectomy specimen is available. There is also substantial overlap with respect to epidemiologic factors, clinical manifestations, physical and laboratory findings, complications, and medical treatment. Indeed, on clinical grounds Crohn's colitis may on occasion be difficult to distinguish from diverticulitis coli or ischemic colitis. Table 43-1 summarizes the clinical and radiologic features by which ulcerative colitis and Crohn's colitis may be distinguished.

There is controversy about the prognosis of Crohn's colitis. Because in a number of patients with Crohn's colitis disease of the small bowel ultimately develops, the course and prognosis of regional enteritis are also pertinent here. Among the local complications of Crohn's colitis, free perforation and toxic dilatation of the colon are seen less frequently, and benign strictures more frequently, than in ulcerative colitis. Not only do sinus tracts predispose the colon to intramural or pericolic abscesses, but profound effects can follow internal fistulization to sites such as the urinary bladder and musculoskeletal tissues. Extraintestinal complications are similar to those of ulcerative colitis and are discussed later.

ADDITIONAL CONSIDERATIONS

Extraintestinal manifestations

Extraintestinal features are common and may even be the dominant or presenting manifestations of IBD. A useful classification relates these systemic problems to the major site of bowel involvement: (1) a "colitis-related" group, in which the severity of the extraintestinal disorder is more likely to vary directly with the activity of the bowel disease; (2) a group of disorders related to small bowel dysfunction; and (3) miscellaneous, nonspecific complications.

Of the colitis-related problems, seronegative arthritis or arthralgia is the most common (15% to 40%). The peripheral large joints (knees, ankles, wrists) are usually affected. The distribution may be monoarticular and asymmetric; in general, healing occurs without deformity. In contrast to this peripheral arthritis, ankylosing spondylitis more frequently presents years before the onset of bowel symptoms, may be severely incapacitating, and shows a striking association with the histocompatibility antigen HLA-B27. Skin manifestations affect about 15% of patients with IBD and are principally seen as pyoderma gangrenosum and erythema nodosum. Mouth lesions often present as aphthous ulcers. Crohn's disease itself may involve the oral cavity. Significant eye complications, occurring in about 5% of IBD patients, include conjunctivitis, episcleritis, iritis, and uveitis. Although these colitis-related features may disappear after colectomy, they persist in a sufficient number of patients that colectomy is rarely recommended for extraintestinal symptoms alone.

The second group of disorders is more closely related to small bowel dysfunction and impaired nutrition. For example, there is an increased incidence of gallstones, especially in regional enteritis, possibly as a result of bile salt malabsorption from terminal ileal disease or resection. Osteomalacia secondary to vitamin D deficiency may occur. Genitourinary complications include (1) uric acid stones related in part to excess fluid and bicarbonate loss through diarrhea and (2) oxalate stones caused by increased oxalate absorption from the colon in the presence of steatorrhea. Hydronephrosis may result from either ureteral obstruction by a mass of inflamed tissue or diffuse fibrosis in the pelvis, usually in Crohn's disease.

Nonspecific complications include liver disease. The most common histopathologic findings are mononuclear pericholangitis and an increase in parenchymal fat deposition. These lesions are not usually accompanied by symptoms and may be evident merely as a mild elevation of serum alkaline phosphatase concentration. Recently it has been appreciated that the incidence of sclerosing cholangitis is higher among patients with ulcerative colitis than previously believed (5% of patients with pancolitis), suggesting earlier consideration of biliary imaging studies. Cholangiocarcinoma is also more common in ulcerative colitis patients and is very difficult to distinguish from sclerosing cholangitis. Chronic active hepatitis is another condition associated with IBD.

In view of the spectrum of hepatic abnormalities associated with IBD, liver biopsy and procedures designed for viewing the bile ducts may be indicated. Although the incidence of peptic ulcer disease appears to be increased in patients with IBD, gastroduodenal Crohn's disease may exhibit similar signs and symptoms. Secondary amyloidosis occasionally is a late manifestation of Crohn's disease. As a result of the systemic nature of IBD, additional extraintestinal problems may include vascular disease (e.g., thrombophlebitis, arterial vasculitis, thrombosis) and bone disease (e.g., osteoporosis, hypertrophic osteoarthropathy).

Toxic dilatation of the colon

Toxic dilatation of the colon (toxic megacolon) is one of the most dreaded complications of IBD, with a mortality of about 25%. Although it is much more common in ulcerative colitis, it can also complicate Crohn's colitis. Although usually seen during exacerbations of chronic IBD, it may be part of the initial episode in patients having an acute fulminating course. In such cases it is crucial to exclude the infectious and other causes of colonic inflammation cited earlier. Clinically, the patient appears severely ill, with fever, leukocytosis, abdominal distention, direct and even rebound abdominal tenderness, and diminished bowel sounds. Concomitant severe hemorrhage is also present in about one third of such patients. Plain radiographs of the abdomen show a dilated, ahaustral colon and a diameter in the transverse colon exceeding 6 cm. Pathologically, the colon is characterized by mucosal denudation, necrotizing transmural inflammation, vasculitis, and thinning of the wall such that its consistency may approach that of wet tissue paper. The risk of imminent perforation is obvious. Precipitating factors may include use of opiates or anticholinergics, hypokalemia, and barium enema or colonoscopic examinations performed in the presence of very active disease. Although definitive therapy is usually total proctocolectomy, some patients do recover on medical therapy alone. Therefore if perforation or peritonitis is not evident, a short period (48 to 72 hours) of intensive parenteral therapy, including high-dose intravenous administration of corticosteroids and broad-spectrum antibiotics and nasogastric suction, is usually indicated. Close observation by both the internist and the surgeon is imperative, because the timing of surgery, if required, is very important. Once colonic perforation occurs, mortality may be as great as 80% to 90%. Although some patients with colonic dilatation who experience remission with medical management have relatively mild, easily controllable disease over the long term, the majority of ulcerative colitis patients who develop this complication ultimately require total proctocolectomy. If the toxic megacolon improves with medical therapy, surgery should be postponed because elective proctocolectomy done later will result in much lower surgical morbidity and mortality.

Bowel cancer

Although the risk of colonic adenocarcinoma is clearly increased in patients with ulcerative pancolitis, earlier studies may have exaggerated this threat. The incidence of cancer begins to increase (compared to that of the general population) after 10 years of disease, increasing by about 1% per year and reaching an absolute risk of 30% after 35 years of disease. The risk is somewhat higher when the onset of disease occurs before 15 years of age. These data apply only to patients with pancolitis, for those with disease confined to the rectum have little, if any, increase in risk of cancer. An intermediate risk exists for those with an intermediate extent of disease, but the limits of involvement cannot be adequately assessed in patients who have not undergone complete colonoscopy. Because most colonic cancers appear in patients with quiescent ulcerative colitis, severity of disease is not considered to be a contributing factor.

Carcinomas that complicate ulcerative colitis are different from adenocarcinomas that develop in otherwise normal colons in that the former are often flat, plaquelike lesions that may be difficult to recognize on barium enema or even colonoscopic examinations (Chapter 45). However, typical napkin-ring lesions also occur (Fig. 43-9). Colitis cancers are often multicentric, occur more commonly beyond the reach of the sigmoidoscope, and may not produce clear-cut symptoms before the neoplasm is advanced.

The preceding factors make cancer surveillance a difficult and important task. This involves careful examination of the mucosa endoscopically for gross evidence of neoplasia and histologic detection of dysplasia in random colorectal biopsies; these changes frequently are present when carcinoma exists nearby or elsewhere in the colon. Up to 50% of patients in whom severe dysplasia is seen in several biopsies may harbor colorectal cancers. Differences of opinion currently exist regarding the advisability of recommending proctocolectomy on the basis of severe dysplasia alone, but it is advisable that diagnoses be reviewed and confirmed in all cases of suspected high-grade dysplasia (an unequivocal neoplastic proliferation that includes carcinoma in situ). High-grade dysplasia in a lesion or mass is especially worrisome. Standardization of the histologic criteria for the different degrees of dysplasia and recent worldwide studies defining the specificity and sensitivity of dysplasia have improved the usefulness of this diagnostic and prognostic modality. In general, patients with pancolitis of greater than 8 to 10 years' duration should undergo colonoscopy every 2 years with multiple biopsies of both random sites and suspicious-appearing lesions. The benefits of this degree of surveillance have not yet been fully defined. Serial carcinoembryonic antigen determinations are of no predictive value.

Carcinoma also occurs more commonly in patients with ileal or colonic Crohn's disease than in the general population, although not nearly to the degree noted in patients with ulcerative pancolitis. Of particular concern is the higher rate of adenocarcinoma in diseased small bowel, especially bowel that has been surgically bypassed. The vigilant surveillance procedures for colonic carcinoma described have yet to be applied systematically to patients with Crohn's colitis.

REFERENCES

Block GE: Surgical management of Crohn's colitis. N Engl J Med 302:1068, 1980.

Collins RH, Feldman M, and Fordtran JS: Colon cancer, dysplasia, and surveillance in patients with ulcerative colitis. N Engl J Med 316:1654, 1987.

Dhar GJ and Kraft SC: Predicting outcome. In Gitnick G, editor: Inflammatory bowel disease: diagnosis and treatment. New York, 1991, Igaku-Shoin.

Farmer RG, Hawk WA, and Turnbull RB: Clinical patterns of Crohn's disease: a statistical study of 615 cases. Gastroenterology 68:627, 1975.

Jacoby RF and Kraft SC: Extraintestinal manifestations. In Gitnick G, editor: Inflammatory bowel disease: diagnosis and treatment. New York, 1991, Igaku-Shoin.

Kirsner JB: Inflammatory bowel disease. II. Clinical and therapeutic aspects. Disease-a-Month 37:673, 1991.

Kirsner JB and Shorter RG: Inflammatory bowel disease, ed 3. Philadelphia, 1988, Lea & Febiger.

Lock MR et al: Recurrence and reoperation for Crohn's disease. N Engl J Med 304:1586, 1981.

Malchow H et al: European Cooperative Crohn's Disease Study: results of drug treatment. Gastroenterology 86:249, 1984.

Pemberton JH et al: Ileal pouch-anal anastomosis for chronic ulcerative colitis: long term results. Ann Surg 206:504, 1987.

Peppercorn MA: Advances in drug therapy for inflammatory bowel disease. Ann Intern Med 112:50, 1990.

Present DH et al: 6-Mercaptopurine in the management of inflammatory bowel disease: short and long-term toxicity. Ann Intern Med 111:641, 1989.

Riddell RH et al: Dysplasia in inflammatory bowel disease: standardized classification with provisional clinical applications. Hum Pathol 14:931, 1983.

Singleton J et al: The National Cooperative Crohn's Disease Study. Gastroenterology 77:827, 1979.

Sitrin MD: Nutritional support in inflammatory bowel disease. Nutr Clin Pract 7:53, 1992.

Swift GL et al: A pharmacokinetic study of sulphasalazine and two new formulations of mesalazine. Aliment Pharmacol Ther 6:259, 1992.

CHAPTER

44 Intestinal Obstruction and Peritonitis

T. Edward Bynum

INTESTINAL OBSTRUCTION

Mechanical obstruction can occur at any site along the alimentary tract. In this chapter, the discussion is confined to obstruction of the small and large intestines, a complication that is often associated with intraperitoneal adhesions from previous abdominal surgery, colonic carcinoma, Crohn's disease, or diverticulitis. The intestine can be partially or completely obstructed by an extrinsic, intramural, or mucosal lesion that causes concentric or eccentric narrowing, ultimately leading to a severely reduced or obliterated lumen. Other ways the bowel can be obstructed are by volvulus or kinking of a loop, an intussusception, or a foreign body. See the box below for classification and differential diagnosis of intestinal obstruction.

Pathophysiology

Whatever the cause or mechanism of obstruction, the pathophysiology is similar. Initially, intestinal motor activity increases both above and below the site of obstruction. There is increased intestinal secretion by the intestine proximal to the obstruction to a degree that secretion often exceeds absorption. This leads to distention that, when combined with the increased motor activity, is clinically expressed as severe cramping abdominal pain, often recurring in waves. At this time, bowel sounds are very active and peristaltic rushes are often heard. The increased motor activity distal to the site of obstruction may lead to defecation, which does not relieve the pain. Later, bowel motor activity diminishes. During this phase, pain becomes more persistent, less severe, and less episodic, and bowel sounds may be normal or, more characteristically, continuous, and high pitched. Still later, bowel motor activity ceases entirely; the bowel proximal to the site of obstruction becomes dilated, with characteristic air-fluid levels that are seen on upright plain radiographs of the abdomen. Bowel sounds are often absent. This last phase has been called *obstructive ileus* (as opposed to *paralytic ileus*). If the site of obstruction is at or distal to the ascending colon, the cecum can become greatly dilated; when its transverse diameter exceeds 12 to 14 cm, there is danger of cecal perforation.

If obstruction is caused by a volvulus or kinked loop of bowel, it can become strangulated, with impaired blood supply, potential ischemic necrosis, and possible perforation. In some instances, strangulation is heralded by fever and leukocytosis.

Classification and differential diagnosis of intestinal obstruction

I. Paralytic ileus
II. Concentric narrowing
  A. Crohn's disease
  B. Neoplasm (lymphoma, adenocarcinoma, other)
  C. Diverticulitis
  D. Resolved ischemic enteritis
III. Kinking of a loop
  A. Postoperative adhesions
  B. Incarcerated hernia
IV. Twisting of a loop
  A. Cecal volvulus
  B. Sigmoid volvulus
  C. Midgut volvulus
V. Intussusception
  A. Spontaneous
  B. Secondary to polyp or mass
VI. Foreign body
  A. Ingested
  B. Gallstone
VII. Pseudo-obstruction

History

A patient who has obstruction usually gives a history of rather sudden onset of abdominal pain, the characteristics of which were described earlier, that may be accompanied by nausea and vomiting. After the patient has had obstruction of the jejunum or beyond for some time, usually several hours or longer, the emesis may become brownish and feculent, especially if the obstruction is located distal to the mid small intestine. Initially, the patient may have one or two urgent bowel movements, occasionally diarrhea, but then ceases to pass stool. One should inquire about previous abdominal surgery, recent (but less acute) changes in customary bowel habit, blood in the stool, family history of cancer or polyps, or previous symptoms or diagnosis of Crohn's disease.

Physical examination

If physical examination is performed early in the course, there may be few, if any, abnormal findings. Late in the course, the abdomen appears distended, with generally increased tympany to percussion, generalized tenderness, and often abnormal bowel sounds as previously described. If perforation complicates obstruction, there may be initial relief of pain. Pain subsequently returns, accompanied by rebound tenderness and fever as peritonitis develops fully.

Laboratory tests

Laboratory tests pertinent to intestinal obstruction itself are few. A rising white blood cell count may herald the development of strangulation, but strangulation may be present in the absence of leukocytosis, and leukocytosis may be due to other events not directly related to intestinal obstruction. Most other laboratory tests relate to specific diseases that can cause obstruction or to more general assessment of the patient's health, particularly with regard to the ability to tolerate surgical intervention. Electrolyte derangements and fluid depletion occur in prolonged obstruction consequent to sequestration of fluid and electrolytes in the bowel lumen or to severe emesis.

Radiographic studies

Radiographic studies are essential in the evaluation of a patient who may have intestinal obstruction. Plain films of the abdomen (KUB) show dilated loops of bowel (Fig. 44-1), often with air-fluid levels in upright views. The radiographic films can reveal these changes, for example, in a patient who has abdominal pain, before abdominal distention and hypertympany are present on physical examination. Sometimes, a sharp termination of dilated small bowel or colon can suggest a mechanical obstruction, whereas dilatation from duodenum to anus is more likely caused by nonspecific or paralytic ileus. Upright films of the abdomen or of the chest should be obtained also, to look for the free air under the diaphragm if a perforation has occurred (see Fig. 36-2).

Barium should never be given orally when intestinal obstruction might be present unless obstruction in the large intestine has been unequivocally excluded. If the obstruction is not very low in the rectum (if the proctosigmoidoscopic examination shows no obstruction), the next study is a gentle barium enema. This might safely reveal the obstructing lesion if it is in the colon or effectively exclude the colon as the site of obstruction and direct subsequent medical (or surgical) attention to the small bowel, which can then be studied radiographically with contrast media. Computed tomography or sonography (ultrasound) of the abdomen is not particularly helpful in this clinical situation.

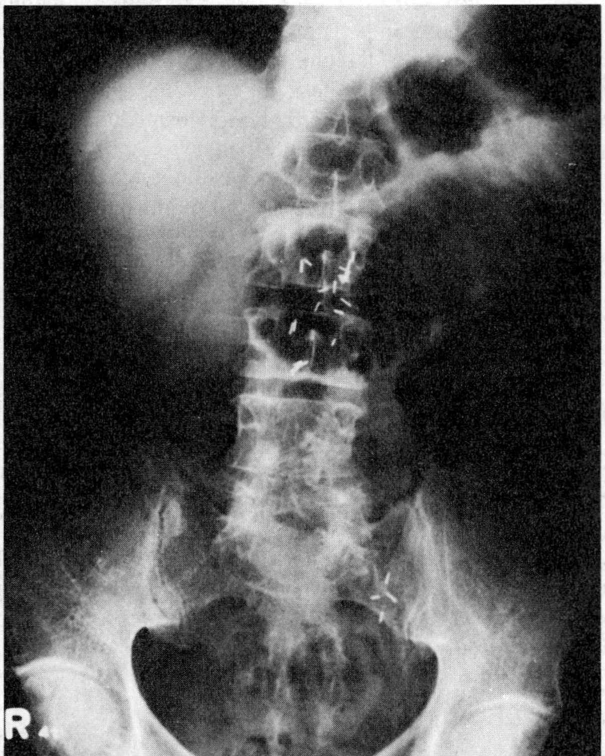

Fig. 44-1. Plain radiograph of abdomen showing dilated loops of small bowel. The patient had obstruction in the proximal ileum. *(The clips indicate previous abdominal surgery.)*

Endoscopy

Upper endoscopy and colonoscopy should not be performed if mechanical intestinal obstruction is suspected; these procedures require the introduction of air into the bowel to allow a field of view, which would further distend the bowel and possibly precipitate perforation. The exception is sigmoid volvulus, in which an experienced colonoscopist can often reduce the volvulus and relieve the obstruction.

Therapy

General therapy for intestinal obstruction is nasogastric intubation and intravenous administration of fluids, electrolytes, and glucose. Some advocate use of a long intestinal tube (such as the Miller-Abbott tube), but studies have demonstrated that nasogastric tube drainage results in decompression comparable to that achieved with longer tubes.

Patients with upper small bowel obstruction sometimes vomit large quantities of fluid. If this emesis is largely gastric juice, alkalosis and significant hypokalemia can result. If it is mostly upper intestinal and pancreatic secretions, the patient may become acidotic from loss of bicarbonate. Obviously, intravenous fluid and electrolyte replacement must be tailored to the individual patient's deficiencies and requirements. If the site of obstruction is the lower small bowel or colon, vomiting is usually minor and the volume of emesis low. Nevertheless, the patient can have major contraction of intravascular volume caused by sequestration ("third spacing") of remarkably large volumes of fluid in the dilated and secreting bowel.

Because of the danger of strangulation, with consequent ischemic necrosis, it is generally wise to consider surgery early in intestinal obstruction, particularly if there is evidence suggesting obstruction produced by adhesions, volvulus, or an incarcerated hernia and if the patient is a reasonable surgical candidate. In many instances in which obstruction is due to concentric narrowing such as in Crohn's disease, intestinal lymphoma, or acute diverticulitis, medical therapy that is more specific for the underlying disease may be sufficiently successful that obstruction is relieved without need for surgery.

Differential diagnosis

Patients with nonobstructive paralytic ileus frequently have clinical and radiographic findings that are indistinguishable from those of mechanical obstruction of the intestine in its mid or late phase. In ileus, bowel sounds are characteristically absent (but the same may be true very late in the course of mechanical obstruction). Paralytic ileus occurs in peritonitis (of any cause), pneumonia, hypokalemia, sepsis, head trauma, severe general trauma, anticholinergic or opiate drug overdose, pulmonary embolus, myocardial infarction, shock, toxic megacolon, pancreatitis, and myxedema and after many types of surgery, especially if general anesthesia is used. Mechanical obstruction caused by concentric narrowing occurs in Crohn's disease, neoplasms (lymphoma, adenocarcinoma, sarcoma, etc.), and acute or chronic diverticulitis. Kinking of a loop of bowel results from intra-abdominal adhesions (most commonly caused by previous abdominal surgery, even if performed decades prior to the onset of obstruction) and to incarceration of bowel in a hernia. Twisting of the bowel causes obstruction in midgut, cecal, or sigmoid volvulus. Intussusception (the invagination of proximal bowel into the lumen of immediately distal bowel) is often a spontaneous event in young children but is almost always associated with a leading intraluminal mass (such as a polyp or other local nonconcentric neoplasm) in adults. Foreign bodies only rarely cause intestinal obstruction; if something gets past the pylorus, it usually makes it all the way through. The distal ileum is the one region where an ingested foreign body or large gallstone may become stuck. Obstruction caused by a gallstone impacted in the lumen of the distal small bowel is (somewhat confusingly) referred to as *gallstone ileus* (Chapter 65). The classic, if rather rare, constellation of findings that, seen on an abdominal radiograph, indicate gallstone ileus is dilated loops of small bowel with air-fluid levels and air in the biliary tree.

INTESTINAL PSEUDO-OBSTRUCTION

Intestinal pseudo-obstruction is a blanket term used to describe an array of intestinal motor disorders that are characterized by hypomotility, often with dilatation of various portions of bowel. In the strictest sense, the term refers to a clinical syndrome in which the patient experiences abdominal pain, dilated loops of intestine (often with air-fluid levels), and diarrhea or constipation, all of which suggest obstruction—but no true mechanical obstruction exists. In the loosest sense, the term is a general classification under which the more specific diseases that may be responsible for the clinical presentation mentioned previously are included. This latter classification includes situations in which the clinical symptoms do not suggest obstruction but in which the findings on plain film resemble mechanical obstruction or ileus and situations in which there are other clinical manifestations (such as diarrhea or malabsorption caused by bacterial overgrowth) related to bowel hypomotility.

Intestinal pseudo-obstruction can be secondary to various disorders, such as scleroderma, amyloidosis, myxedema, muscular dystrophy, chronic renal failure, and hypokalemia, or can result from excessive drug therapy with anticholinergic agents or opiate narcotics (refer to the box at upper right). This condition overlaps with paralytic ileus. Idiopathic intestinal pseudo-obstruction includes sporadic and familial hollow visceral myopathy and a nonmyopathic disease in which the problem seems to reside in the autonomic innervation of the intestine.

Acute pseudo-obstruction of the colon characterized by massive colonic dilatation in the absence of mechanical obstruction in severely ill debilitated patients is commonly termed *Ogilvie's syndrome*. Predisposing conditions include recent surgery, neurologic disorders, serious infections, cardiorespiratory insufficiency, and metabolic disturbances, often coupled with the use of drugs that perturb colonic motility (anticholinergics or narcotics).

Classification of intestinal pseudo-obstruction

I. "Primary" (idiopathic intestinal pseudo-obstruction)
  A. Hollow visceral myopathy
    1. Familial
    2. Sporadic
  B. Neuropathic
    1. Abnormal myenteric plexus
    2. Normal myenteric plexus
II. Secondary
  A. Scleroderma
  B. Myxedema
  C. Amyloidosis
  D. Muscular dystrophy
  E. Hypokalemia
  F. Chronic renal failure
  G. Diabetes mellitus
  H. Drug toxicity caused by
    1. Anticholinergics
    2. Opiate narcotics
  I. Ogilvie's syndrome

Pathophysiology

Hypomotility and dilatation of bowel loops occur because the smooth muscle of the muscularis propria is incapable of contracting in normal fashion and is even incapable of maintaining tone. Hypomotility and dilatation are caused by intrinsic disease in the muscle fibers themselves (hollow visceral myopathy, muscular dystrophy), by impaired muscle metabolism (myxedema, hypokalemia), by infiltration of the muscle by some abnormal material (scleroderma, amyloidosis, myxedema), or by impaired autonomic neural regulation of smooth muscle function (neuropathic idiopathic intestinal pseudo-obstruction, anticholinergic toxicity).

Diagnosis

Surgery should be avoided in intestinal pseudo-obstruction. Patients who have symptoms or signs of intestinal obstruction or ileus may have pseudo-obstruction and should be evaluated for possible underlying disorders, especially those that can be readily corrected, such as drug toxicity, hypokalemia, and myxedema. If esophageal motility is also abnormal, consider scleroderma, amyloidosis, or idiopathic intestinal pseudo-obstruction. The diagnosis of idiopathic intestinal pseudo-obstruction becomes one of exclusion of those diseases that cause secondary pseudo-obstruction. Because of the more common occurrence of pain, hollow visceral myopathy more often requires exploratory surgery to exclude mechanical obstruction and, in some cases, to resect or bypass segments of bowel in an attempt to improve nutrition or control symptoms. The definitive diagnosis of hollow visceral myopathy (and of the abnormal myenteric plexus forms of idiopathic intestinal pseudo-obstruction) is a tissue diagnosis and requires careful evaluation of the histologic abnormalities of resected intestine.

Treatment

The therapy of some forms of secondary intestinal pseudo-obstruction such as renal failure and drug toxicity involves treatment of the underlying disorder. For other disorders, such as scleroderma, amyloidosis, and muscular dystrophy, there is no successful therapy for the primary disease that can be expected to reverse or ameliorate the pseudo-obstruction. There is no effective therapy that is specific for idiopathic intestinal pseudo-obstruction. Consequently, for those forms of pseudo-obstruction that are not readily amenable to cure, management consists of treating the complications. If the patient has bacterial overgrowth caused by intestinal stasis, manifested as diarrhea or malabsorption, recurrent cycles of broad-spectrum antibiotics can be successful, as in the treatment of other intestinal stasis syndromes (Chapter 42). Metoclopramide (Reglan) and erythromycin have the pharmacologic potential to increase propulsive intestinal motility in pseudo-obstruction and are worth a therapeutic trial in these patients. Overall effectiveness has not been great. Metaclopramide is limited by dystonic reactions and other central nervous system side effects. Obviously, anticholinergics and narcotics are contraindicated. Careful colonoscopic decompression has been useful in Ogilvie's syndrome.

If nutrition is impaired, oral administration of liquid, low-residue, complete nutrition preparations may achieve, and assist in maintaining, adequate nutrition. A rare patient may require long-term total parenteral nutrition.

As mentioned previously, surgical therapy is occasionally attempted to bypass severely dilated loops in an effort to improve oral nutrition and perhaps to relieve pain, but its effectiveness varies greatly from patient to patient.

PERITONITIS

Inflammation of the peritoneum can be classified as acute or chronic, or as infectious, chemical, or idiopathic, depending on the type of etiologic event that has resulted in peritonitis. Innervation of the peritoneum is rich in sensory receptors for pain. Therefore a patient may be able to indicate the specific site of local peritonitis such as that caused by contact with an adjacent inflamed intra-abdominal organ. This section concentrates on the more generalized forms of peritoneal inflammation.

The approach to the patient with acute peritonitis is described in Chapter 36. In patients with chronic peritonitis or forms of peritonitis that are rare or of obscure cause, important points from the history might be previous systemic disease or infection, type and timing of the onset of the symptoms, ethnic origin, and family history. On physical examination, tenderness, often with rebound tenderness, is characteristic for acute peritonitis. Patients with chronic peritonitis have little or no rebound tenderness. Paralytic ileus occurs frequently in acute peritonitis, so the absence of bowel sounds on auscultation of the abdomen is a common finding.

Plain film of the abdomen may appear unremarkable, may suggest ascites, or may show free air if peritonitis is secondary to perforation of a hollow organ. An upright film of the chest should be obtained in an effort to demonstrate free air under the diaphragm (Fig. 36-2).

Acute peritonitis commonly shows peripheral blood leukocytosis, but other blood tests are not likely to reveal an abnormality, except in patients with spontaneous bacterial peritonitis associated with cirrhosis and therefore abnormal liver chemical findings.

If ascites is present, diagnostic paracentesis is essential. The fluid in acute or chronic peritonitis is an exudate. The gross appearance of fluid obtained may help in the diagnosis. It may be purulent, feculent, hemorrhagic, or heavily bile stained. Fluid should be analyzed for cell count and differential, Gram stain, cultures (including those for tuberculous and anaerobic organisms), protein content, and amylase level.

After initial assessment and sometimes before all laboratory results are available, the physician must determine whether the patient has acute peritonitis related to a condition that requires early surgical intervention. If surgery is not indicated, further studies may be appropriate. One procedure that should be considered is laparoscopy, which can be done with local anesthesia with minimal risk and may make laparotomy unnecessary. Furthermore, it is the best method for obtaining biopsy specimens of the peritoneum. If expert laparoscopy is not available and diffuse and chronic peritonitis seems to be present, percutaneous needle biopsy of the peritoneum (with needle and technique similar to that used for pleural biopsy) is an adequate method for obtaining a tissue specimen. Sixty to seventy-five percent of patients with tuberculous peritonitis have caseating granulomas that can be seen in specimens obtained by percutaneous needle biopsy (Chapter 68).

Differential diagnosis

Infectious peritonitis can be caused by a wide array of organisms. If peritonitis results from rupture of a colonic diverticulum, cecal perforation secondary to colonic obstruction, toxic megacolon, ruptured appendix, or other type of colonic perforation, colonic organisms such as *Escherichia coli* or *Bacteroides* may predominate. If a patient has pre-existing ascites from whatever cause but especially from cirrhosis, spontaneous bacterial peritonitis may occur (Chapter 56). The infecting organism may be *E. coli* or other coliforms, but because this infection is blood-borne, pneumococcal peritonitis is common, especially during winter months, when pneumonia is common. Tuberculous peritonitis is frequently an indolent infection, and correct diagnosis requires that it be suspected in patients who are at high risk for tuberculosis. Tuberculosis and malignancy of the peritoneum are the most common causes of exudative ascites in patients without underlying liver disease. Gonococcal peritonitis occurs occasionally after massive gonococcemia. Chemical peritonitis occurs when the inflammation of the peritoneum is due primarily to the caustic effect of some substance rather than to infection by an organism. Offending substances are gastric acid, pancreatic fluid, bile, and starch. Miscellaneous or idiopathic peritonitis occurs in familial Mediterranean fever and in disease associated with vasculitis such as systemic lupus erythematosus and polyarteritis nodosa. Specific therapy for the various causes of peritonitis is discussed in the various chapters that deal with those diseases.

REFERENCES

Abbasi AA et al: Myxedema ileus. JAMA 234:181, 1975.
Achem SR et al: Neuronal dysplasia and chronic intestinal pseudo-obstruction. Gastroenterology 92:805, 1987.
Anuras S: Intestinal pseudo-obstruction syndrome. Annu Rev Med 39:1, 1988.
Borhanmanesh F et al: Tuberculous peritonitis. Ann Intern Med 76:567, 1972.
Bynum TE: Disorders of bowel motility. In Eastwood GL, editors: Core textbook of gastroenterology. Philadelphia, 1989, JB Lippincott.
Fabri PJ and Rosemurgy A: Reoperation for small intestinal obstruction. Surg Clin North Am 71:131, 1991.
Maddaus MA et al: The biology of peritonitis and implications for treatment. Surg Clin North Am 68:431, 1988.
Richards WO and Williams LF Jr: Obstruction of the large and small intestine. Surg Clin North Am 68:355, 1988.
Stranghellini V et al: Chronic idiopathic intestinal pseudo-obstruction. Gut 28:5, 1987.
Strodel WE and Brothers T: Colonoscopic decompression of pseudo-obstruction and volvulus. Surg Clin North Am 69:1327, 1989.
Wilcox CM and Dismukes WE: Spontaneous bacterial peritonitis. Medicine 66:447, 1987.

CHAPTER

45 Tumors of the Small and Large Intestines

Charles J. Lightdale

MALIGNANT TUMORS OF THE SMALL INTESTINE

That malignant tumors of the small intestine are quite uncommon is surprising considering the much higher frequency of malignancies originating in the large intestine and stomach. Liquidity of its contents, low bacterial population, rapid transit, rapid cell turnover, local immune responses, and active detoxifying enzyme systems, alone or in combination, have been suggested as contributing to the infrequency of small intestinal malignant tumors.

Epidemiology and incidence

There are about 2000 new cases of small bowel cancer per year in the United States. The majority are adenocarcinomas. The disease is rare before age 30, when incidence gradually begins to rise steadily, peaking in the sixth decade. There is a slight preponderance of incidence in males, but no marked social differential. The incidence of small bowel cancer in different geographic regions seems to parallel the incidence of colonic carcinoma. In the Middle East, the incidence of primary small intestinal lymphoma appears to exceed the incidence of other small intestinal malignancies.

Pathology

Adenocarcinomas arise from the crypts of the mucosa of the small intestine. They develop most commonly in the proximal small bowel and least commonly toward the ileum. Histologically, adenocarcinomas of the small intestine most often resemble colonic rather than gastric adenocarcinomas. Metastases to local lymphatics are common; hematogenous spread and peritoneal seeding also occur.

Lymphomas originate in lymphoid cells within and beneath the mucosa of the small intestine and are more common in the distal small intestine. Hodgkin's disease is the least common primary lymphoid malignancy of the small bowel. Small bowel lymphomas are often multifocal and may infiltrate beneath the mucosa over a wide area.

The "Mediterranean lymphoma" prevalent in the Middle East appears to be a distinctive pathologic entity. The small intestinal lesion is usually diffuse, and the cells that characterize this neoplasm often have features of plasma cells, histiocytes, and atypical lymphocytes. Mediterranean lymphoma *(immunoproliferative small intestine disease)* affects the duodenum and proximal jejunum more commonly than the ileum. It may be associated with the production of an abnormal circulating immunoglobulin A (IgA) immunoglobulin that contains only alpha chains (alpha chain disease), although not all diffuse mucosal lymphomas of the small intestine produce this immunoglobulin.

The smooth muscle layer of the muscularis externa of the small intestine may give rise to *leiomyosarcomas*. These are slightly more common in the proximal than in the distal small intestine. They metastasize by hematogenous spread to liver and lung and only rarely to regional lymph nodes.

Premalignant states and risk factors

Several conditions and diseases are associated with an increased incidence of small bowel adenocarcinoma or lymphoma.

Regional enteritis (Crohn's disease). Adenocarcinoma of the small bowel occurs more often in patients with regional enteritis than in age-matched controls and affects the ileum more often than the proximal bowel. Patients who have had segments of intestine bypassed surgically may be at higher risk.

Inherited polyposis syndromes. Several inherited intestinal polyposis syndromes are associated with an increased incidence of small intestinal adenocarcinoma. In familial adenomatous polyposis and Gardner's syndrome, adenomas and adenocarcinomas of the duodenum occur with increased frequency, particularly in the periampullary region (Chapter 66). Small intestinal (especially duodenal) adenocarcinoma has been reported in patients with Peutz-Jeghers syndrome, although the incidence is not high.

Celiac sprue. (Chapter 42). An increased incidence of malignancy, especially lymphoma of the small intestine, has been reported in patients with celiac sprue. These lymphomas, derived from intestinal T cells, occur most frequently in the proximal small intestine. The association of celiac sprue with lymphoma has been questioned, because a diffuse intestinal lymphoma can also cause malabsorption, but evidence for this association is increasing. There is one study indicating that strict adherence by celiac sprue patients to a gluten-free diet decreases the incidence of lymphoma.

Immune deficiency states. An increased incidence of lymphoma of the small intestine has been suggested in hereditary syndromes of decreased humoral and/or cellular immunity and also in acquired immunodeficiency. The latter group includes patients with acquired immunodeficiency syndrome (Chapter 48) and those treated with intensive radiation, chemotherapy, and immunosuppressives.

Clinical features

Any of the small intestinal malignancies may ulcerate and bleed into the bowel lumen. Blood loss is generally not massive and may be occult. Leiomyosarcomas may be particularly vascular and may be a cause of gross bleeding with melena or grossly bloody stools. Tumors proximal to the ligament of Treitz may occasionally cause hematemesis if they bleed rapidly.

Small bowel malignancies may narrow the intestinal lumen, creating partial obstruction that may cause cramping abdominal pain accompanied by loud peristaltic rushes and abdominal distention. Small bowel adenocarcinomas tend to create a ringlike constriction similar to that created by colonic adenocarcinomas. Small bowel tumors may also act as a lead point for an intussusception, producing intermittent obstruction. Higher grades of obstruction cause backing up of bowel contents, with nausea and vomiting; the vomiting may be feculent if the obstruction is in the distal small intestine and associated with stasis (Chapter 44).

Weight loss may be a prominent feature of small bowel malignancies. Malignant tumors in the abdomen frequently cause anorexia and decreased caloric intake. Abdominal pain due to partial bowel obstruction may be exacerbated by food intake, contributing to anorexia. Bacterial overgrowth in the obstructed small intestine may be a cause of malabsorption, producing steatorrhea and weight loss (Chapter 42). Malabsorption is common with diffusely infiltrating small intestinal lymphomas.

Small bowel malignancies can, on occasion, cause acute abdominal catastrophes such as perforation, massive hemorrhage, or acute intestinal obstruction.

Laboratory findings and diagnosis

Patients with small intestinal tumors may be anemic and have occult blood in their stools. They may be hypoalbuminemic as a result of protein loss from the tumor and obstruction of lymphatics, especially in lymphomas that may infiltrate the mesentery. Malabsorption may produce excess fat in the stool, abnormal Schilling and D-xylose test results, prolonged prothrombin time, and low serum calcium and magnesium concentrations (Chapter 33).

Most malignant tumors of the small intestine can be detected in carefully performed barium contrast studies. A common error in evaluating patients with abdominal symptoms is to perform only a barium enema and upper gastrointestinal series. These examinations usually demonstrate only the most proximal and distal small bowel loops; therefore a small intestinal series should be performed. The detection of small lesions in the small intestine by barium radiographic study requires a skilled, interested, and attentive radiologist. The use of enteroclysis, or small bowel enema, can provide increased accuracy. In this more invasive technique, barium is instilled directly into the intestine by passage of a tube through the nose or mouth.

Duodenal tumors may be detected and biopsy specimens obtained by upper gastrointestinal endoscopy. Modern fiberscopes may reach the third portion of the duodenum, and longer enteroscopes have been developed. Tumors of the terminal ileum may be revealed in some patients if the ileocecal valve is passed with a colonoscope. Peroral biopsy via tubes passed under fluoroscopic control may obtain a biopsy specimen of small bowel malignancy, particularly in diffuse or multifocal lymphoma. Frequently, the diagnosis of small bowel malignancy is made by the surgeon at the time of laparotomy, by palpation, and by biopsy.

Treatment

Surgery is usually the first-line therapeutic modality for small bowel malignancy. A localized neoplasm is resected widely to ensure that resection margins are free of tumor. In the case of adenocarcinoma, surgery is the only possibility for cure; recurrences are more likely if the cancer has penetrated the serosa and invaded regional lymph nodes. Chemotherapy and radiation therapy can provide temporary palliation in a few patients with unresectable disease.

Radiation therapy and chemotherapy are important modalities for small bowel lymphomas as primary treatment and as adjuvant therapy after surgical resection. Perforation of the gastrointestinal tract caused by rapid lysis of lymphomatous areas has been described after radiation therapy or chemotherapy. Thus surgical resection with curative intent is widely held as preferable. Involvement of local lymph nodes is generally an indication for postoperative irradiation or chemotherapy. In widespread, unresectable disease, chemotherapy is indicated.

Leiomyosarcomas are best treated with surgery. They are radioresistant, and chemotherapy has been largely ineffective.

CARCINOID TUMORS

Carcinoid tumors are an interesting group of neoplasms that has its origin in the endocrine argentaffin cells in the small intestinal mucosa (argentaffinomas). They are found incidentally in 0.50% to 0.75% of autopsies. Carcinoid tumors occur frequently in the ileum, where argentaffin cells are more abundant, and 20% of these tumors are multifocal. Histologic criteria do not help the physician to distinguish benign from malignant carcinoid tumors. The tumors are invariably small. About 80% of tumors more than 2 cm in size metastasize; those less than 1 cm in size are almost always benign. Metastases are to local lymph nodes, liver, lung, and bone. Carcinoid tumors may induce a reactive fibrosis in the bowel mesentery, sometimes creating an angulated intestinal segment. Even malignant and metastatic carcinoid tumors are indolent. More than 50% of patients with unresectable local metastases survive 5 years, as do about 30% of those with liver metastases. About 10% of individuals with liver metastases survive more than 10 years.

Carcinoid tumors of the small bowel do not often ulcerate and bleed and are usually too small to cause obstruction. They may, however, produce transient intussusceptions and cause cramping abdominal pain and diarrhea. These symptoms may be long-standing and intermittent, suggesting irritable bowel syndrome or Crohn's disease.

In about one third of patients with liver metastases, carcinoid syndrome, which occurs rarely with only nodal metastases, develops. *Carcinoid syndrome* is characterized primarily by episodes of flushing and diarrhea. The flush may produce a cyanotic appearance and, if attacks are prolonged, facial edema and telangiectasis may develop. The mediator of the carcinoid flush is unknown. Kallikrein, bradykinin, other kinin peptides, substance P, prostaglandins, serotonin, and histamine have been implicated. The flush has been precipitated by ingestion of a meal and by administration of ethanol, calcium, epinephrine, isoproterenol, and pentagastrin. The diarrhea and cramps in this syndrome appear to be related to the production of serotonin (5-hydroxytryptamine).

Bronchial spasm is often part of carcinoid syndrome, and wheezing may become a prominent feature. Right-sided heart lesions, particularly pulmonary and tricuspid valvular fibrosis, may develop with associated murmurs of pulmonary stenosis and tricuspid insufficiency. Right-sided congestive heart failure may produce further hepatomegaly, ascites, pulmonary congestion, and edema.

Diarrhea in carcinoid syndrome is usually watery, episodic, and associated with abdominal cramping and loud borborygmi. Gastric carcinoids that tend to produce more 5-hydroxytryptophan than serotonin and that also may produce histamine usually are not associated with diarrhea.

Most patients with carcinoid syndrome have liver metastases, which are usually evident on physical examination and liver scans. Carcinoid tumors with nodal metastases that produce the syndrome may cause a palpable abdominal mass. Ovarian carcinoid tumors are usually detected by abdominal or pelvic examination, and bronchial carcinoid tumors by chest radiography.

The biochemical marker for the carcinoid syndrome is increased urinary excretion of 5-hydroxyindoleacetic acid (5-HIAA). More than 30 mg of 5-HIAA is usually excreted in 24 hours by patients with carcinoid syndrome. Less striking increases in urinary 5-HIAA may be found in some patients with malabsorption such as occurs in celiac disease and bacterial overgrowth syndromes. Blood serotonin and 5-hydroxytryptophan levels can now be determined; the latter is helpful if gastric carcinoid is suspected. When urinary 5-HIAA excretion is being tested, patients should avoid drugs that may produce false-positive test results, most notably glyceryl guaiacolate, phenothiazines, and methenamine mandelate. Foods rich in serotonin should also be avoided. These include pineapples, bananas, avocados, and walnuts.

Carcinoid tumors may secrete a variety of other hormones, including insulin, adrenocorticotropic hormone, melanocyte-stimulating hormone, gastrin, and glucagon. The endocrine cells from which carcinoid tumors originate are part of the amine content, precursor uptake, and decarboxylation (APUD) family. Foregut carcinoid tumors have also been associated with pluriglandular adenomatoses (e.g., pituitary, adrenal, and parathyroid tumors) and with pancreatic gastrinomas.

Carcinoid tumors of the small bowel should be surgically resected. If metastatic disease is present, the approach remains the same as in other bowel malignancies. In patients with the carcinoid syndrome, all treatment must be carefully monitored and controlled to prevent precipitating a carcinoid crisis. Chemotherapy has had some benefit in unresectable disease, but treatment efforts, in general, should be tempered by the usually indolent growth of these tumors. A variety of antiserotonin agents, antihistamines, antiadrenergics, antiprostaglandins, and steroids have been helpful in the carcinoid syndrome, but benefits must be weighed against side effects. Intravenous somatostatin has been used to ameliorate acute symptoms, and subcutaneous somatostatin analog has been used successfully for long-term control.

BENIGN TUMORS OF THE SMALL INTESTINE

Most benign small intestinal tumors cause no symptoms and are incidentally found during radiographic or endoscopic examination, surgery, or autopsy.

Adenomas may be polypoid or sessile, similar to their colonic counterparts. The potential for malignant change, however, appears to be less for small intestinal than for colonic adenomas. Isolated adenomas may bleed intermittently, but because they are usually small and soft they rarely cause obstruction. Most occur in the upper small bowel and in some cases may be removed via cautery snare by an experienced endoscopist.

Leiomyomas, benign smooth muscle tumors, sometimes occur throughout the small intestine. They may have a rich blood supply and ulcerate and bleed profusely. They may also obstruct the lumen. Usually they produce a smooth filling defect, which can be seen on barium radiograph, as they grow beneath the bowel mucosa. Sometimes leiomyomas ulcerate, producing an umbilicated so-called target lesion, seen on barium radiographic examination as a mass with a central ulceration. Leiomyomas should generally be removed surgically if they cause symptoms.

Neurofibromas may arise as isolated lesions or as part of von Recklinghausen's disease, in which multiple tumors are often present. Neurofibromas tend to grow outward into the serosa and may become large, causing the intestine to twist around them and become obstructed.

Hamartomas are benign growths that may contain all of the cellular elements of the small bowel mucosa. Peutz-Jeghers syndrome is characterized by multiple hamartomatous polyps in the gastrointestinal tract. The polyps seem to increase in number as the patient gets older and may bleed, cause obstruction, or cause intussusception. If surgery is required for these complications, it is generally recommended that the length of resected bowel be kept to a minimum.

Duodenal glands (Brunner's glands) are submucosal and mucosal mucus-secreting glands that are most prominent in the duodenal bulb but may extend into the jejunum. Adenomas that develop in this tissue may form polypoid and even pedunculated tumors. A single adenoma may be associated with chronic gastric hyperacidity, but diffuse hyperplasia of Brunner's glands is more common. Duodenal gland adenomas may sometimes contain adipose tissue, in which case they are considered hamartomatous. Duodenal gland adenomas only rarely cause symptoms. Endoscopic observation and biopsy confirmation are usually all that is required for diagnosis; a pedunculated lesion can be removed endoscopically by cautery snare.

MALIGNANT TUMORS OF THE LARGE INTESTINE

Epidemiology and incidence

A striking feature of colonic cancer is its geographic variation in incidence. The disease seems to occur primarily in Western, industrialized countries. In the United States, the incidence has increased to more than 150,000 cases per year. Studies of migrant populations have shown fascinating changes in the incidence of colonic carcinoma. For example, in Japan, the incidence of colonic cancer is increasing but remains relatively low. In Japanese families who have emigrated to the United States, however, within one generation colonic cancer occurs at a rate similar to that in the general American population.

Carcinogenesis and its inhibition

Diets high in fat and refined carbohydrate and low in plant fiber, more typical in the industrialized West, have been implicated in higher colonic cancer rates. At least 20 different classes of chemicals, some of which occur naturally in food (e.g., calcium), seem to have a protective effect against colonic cancer in laboratory models.

Although the effects of environment continue to be studied and debated, genetic susceptibility to colonic cancer has become better defined. In certain groups, hereditary colonic cancer risk has been clearly established. In the hereditary polyposis syndromes, particularly in familial adenomatous polyposis and in Gardner's syndrome, the risk is very high. These diseases are inherited as autosomal dominants with high penetrance. Familial polyposis coli is characterized by the growth of numerous adenomatous polyps in the colon, most markedly in the distal colon. The polyps frequently begin in childhood and increase in number with the patient's age. The colon may become literally carpeted with adenomas. Gardner's syndrome is characterized by multiple soft tissue tumors, fibromas, and osteomas, as well as colonic adenomas. In every patient with familial polyposis coli or Gardner's syndrome a colonic carcinoma will develop, with risk increasing as the patient becomes older. Other syndromes involving colonic polyposis and increased cancer risk include Turcot syndrome, in which patients may have gliomas, and medulloblastomas, and Oldfield's syndrome, in which there are multiple sebaceous cysts. In the Peutz-Jeghers syndrome, characterized by abnormal pigmentation of the skin and mucous membranes and gastrointestinal hamartomas, there is a small increased risk of colonic adenocarcinoma.

Families have been identified with a marked hereditary increased risk of colonic carcinoma without florid polyposis, which has been called *hereditary nonpolyposis colorectal cancer* (HNPCC). Two groups have been recognized. In Lynch syndrome I, cancers occur at an earlier age on average than sporadic colon cancers, and are site specific to the colon. In Lynch syndrome II, there is an additional susceptibility to other forms of cancer, particularly of the endometrium and ovaries. These syndromes are dominantly inherited, may be related to an abnormality on chromosome 18, and are characterized by the occurrence of small "flat adenomas" in the ascending colon.

The actual gene responsible for familial adenomatous polyposis has been identified on the long arm of chromosome 5 and sequenced (APC gene), although its function remains unclear. Genetic research indicates a strong role as well for inherited susceptibility factors in sporadic colon adenomas and carcinomas. A variety of deletions of potential tumor suppressor genes have been identified in colon neoplasms on chromosomes 5, 17, and 18. Oncogenes, particularly K-ras mutations, also have been detected in human colonic adenomas and carcinomas.

Premalignant states

Patients with adenomatous polyps, especially villous adenomas, are considered to be at higher risk for colonic cancer. Evidence is mounting that there is a common sequence from adenoma to carcinoma. Invasive cancer has been frequently found in adenomatous tissue. Adenomas in patients with familial polyposis are similar to those in patients with single polyps. Several cases have been reported in which patients refused surgery for polyps that were subsequently observed over a period of years to become malignant. About one third of operative specimens from patients with colonic cancer also contain one or more adenomas.

With increasing size, polyps tend to show increasing villous change and increasing dysplasia. Precancerous dysplastic changes have been described in the colonic mucosa of patients with long-standing ulcerative colitis and Crohn's disease, in whom there is an increased risk of colonic cancer (Chapter 43).

In patients with colonic adenomas and carcinomas, the zone of cell proliferation at the base of the colonic crypts has been shown to expand upward. Cells continue to show evidence of deoxyribonucleic acid (DNA) synthesis and other evidence of immature cellular structure and function at the mucosal surface. Such changes have also been found in patients with inflammatory bowel disease.

Pathology

The location of cancers in the colon appears to be changing. Two decades ago, about two thirds of colonic cancers were reported to occur in the distal 25 cm of the rectosigmoid. More recently, this proportion has decreased to one half or less of colonic cancers.

Most colonic adenocarcinomas form hard, nodular areas that grow irregularly. They may be polypoid and fungate and ulcerate, producing exophytic, bulky masses, or they may infiltrate around the bowel lumen, causing the classic "napkin-ring" lesion. Histologically, colonic cancers may vary from well-differentiated cells that appear normal (grade I) to highly anaplastic cells (grade IV) and may contain a variable amount of mucin. Colonic cancers, which produce intracellular mucin (signet-ring type), tend to be particularly aggressive. The pathologic staging of colonic cancer is based on depth of invasion and absence or presence of lymph node or distant metastases. The Dukes' staging system is most widely used, but there is increasing acceptance of the TNM (tumor, node, metastasis) system proposed by the American Joint Committee on Cancer (AJCC) and the International Union Against Cancer (UICC) (Table 45-1).

Lymphomas, primarily the diffuse histiocytic type, may develop in the colon. These usually occur either in the cecal or rectal areas and, if polypoid, may be impossible to distinguish grossly from adenocarcinomas. They may also infiltrate diffusely, producing a nodular, thickened bowel wall with ulcerations. Although less common, sarcomas may occur in the wall of the colon and resemble in behavior those found in the stomach and small intestine (Chapter 40).

Clinical features

The incidence of colonic carcinoma is nearly the same in men and women, although incidence of rectal cancer is slightly higher in men, and overall incidence is slightly higher in women. Colonic cancer before age 40 is still quite uncommon, but there has been some tendency for the disease to occur more frequently in younger patients. The mean age at diagnosis is about 65 years.

Symptoms. The presenting symptoms vary according to the location of the neoplasm in the colon. Cancers that occur in the more voluminous and distensible cecum and right colon, where bowel contents are liquid, usually do not

Table 45-1. Relationship of the Dukes' staging classification and TNM staging proposed by the American Joint Committee on Cancer and the International Union Against Cancer

	AJCC/UICC			
	T*	N†	M‡	Dukes
Stage 0	Tis	N0	M0	
Stage I	T1	N0	M0	A
	T2	N0	M0	
Stage II	T3	N0	M0	B
	T4	N0	M0	
Stage III	Any T	N1	M0	C
	Any T	N2, N3	M0	
Stage IV	Any T	Any N	M1	

*T = depth of cancer invasion: Tis, carcinoma in situ; T1, invasion of submucosa; T2, invasion of muscularis propria; T3, invasion to the subserosa; T4, invasion of visceral peritoneum, other organs, or structures.

†N = lymph node metastases: N0, no lymph node metastases; N1, metastases to one to three pericolic lymph nodes; N2, metastases to four or more pericolic nodes; N3, metastases to nodes along a named vascular trunk.

‡M = metastatic disease: M0, no distant metastasis; M1, any distant metastasis.

cause obstruction. These cancers tend to grow to large size and ulcerate, producing a gradual chronic blood loss. In some cases, there is enough hemoglobin lost to produce melena. Passage of reddish-maroon stool sometimes occurs, indicating the diagnosis.

Large cecal masses may involve the ileocecal valve and produce apparent small bowel obstruction. Sometimes tumors of the ascending colon partially block the lumen. If the ileocecal valve is competent, the cecum becomes painfully dilated with gas and air, creating a tender right lower quadrant mass. Patients may massage this area and find relief as they force the trapped gas past the obstruction.

Cancers in the left colon, where the lumen is narrower and less distensible and the fecal stream is solid, commonly obstruct. This causes constipation and cramping abdominal pain. Sometimes, patients develop a paradoxical diarrhea as some colonic contents are forced past a partially obstructing cancer. Bleeding from left-sided lesions may be bright red but is generally not massive. Patients with rectal cancers in particular tend to have bright red bleeding as well as tenesmus and small-caliber stools. Colonic cancers that advance to the stage at which they invade through the bowel wall may perforate it and manifest peritonitis.

Anorexia and weight loss are common in advanced colonic cancer. Anorexia is intensified by partially obstructing lesions that may cause cramping abdominal pain associated with meals.

Colonic cancers may metastasize via lymphatic or hematogenous routes or both. Metastases to regional lymph glands, with intra-abdominal spread, are most common. Metastases to the liver are frequently found. Lung and bone are other sites of metastatic spread.

Physical findings. Digital examination of the rectum may reveal an unsuspected mass lesion. Thus the digital rectal examination becomes a crucial part of the physical examination and should not be omitted without reason. Abdominal mass lesions may be palpable at times. If there is metastatic spread to the liver, hepatomegaly may be noted, and the liver may feel hard and nodular and be slightly tender. Peritoneal metastases may cause ascites.

Sigmoidoscopy. Sigmoidoscopy with a rigid 25 cm sigmoidoscope should enable the physician to detect the 50% or so of colonic cancers that occur in the distal 25 cm of large bowel. In practice, however, sigmoidoscopy is not adequate for examining more than the distal 16 cm of bowel. Patient and physician resistance to routine rigid sigmoidoscopy has developed, and the examination is generally considered a failure for general screening. Sigmoidoscopy with flexible fiberoptic instruments has been developed and widely tested. The flexible sigmoidoscope is basically a shorter version of a colonoscope, and various lengths have been developed. With patients in the left lateral position, it is possible to examine the distal 30 to 60 cm of bowel comfortably in most patients (Chapter 30). Flexible sigmoidoscopy is a potential general screening procedure that promises increased compliance and improved diagnostic yield, albeit at a somewhat higher cost than rigid sigmoidoscopy.

Laboratory findings. Laboratory findings that suggest the presence of colonic neoplasm include hypoalbuminemia, iron deficiency anemia, and occult blood in the stool. The use of guaiac-impregnated slides to test for occult blood in the stool has been investigated as a means of detecting early, asymptomatic colonic cancers and adenomas. This may prove to be a sensitive screening test for colonic cancer in some population groups. A proposal for colonic cancer screening that begins with a fecal occult blood slide test is shown in Fig. 45-1.

Elevated alkaline phosphatase concentration suggests colonic cancer metastatic to liver or bone. In liver metastases, bilirubin concentration remains normal until late in the course, and transaminase levels are usually normal or only slightly elevated.

Diagnosis. Radiography and endoscopy are the primary means of establishing the diagnosis of large bowel cancer (Fig. 45-2, Plate II-9). Radiologists can detect fine mucosal details and small lesions with the air-contrast barium enema technique. It is a useful procedure for the identification of small polypoid lesions (Fig. 45-3) although colonoscopy may be more sensitive.

Colonoscopy is used instead of barium enema, or to confirm the presence of possibly cancerous lesions seen on barium enema and to document their nature by biopsy. With this information, appropriate therapy can be carried out with more assurance. In addition, synchronous colonic carcinomas that are not evident on barium enema examination can be detected; they occur in 1% to 5% of patients with colonic carcinoma. In addition, up to 40% to 50% of patients have synchronous adenomatous polyps. Colonoscopy is ad-

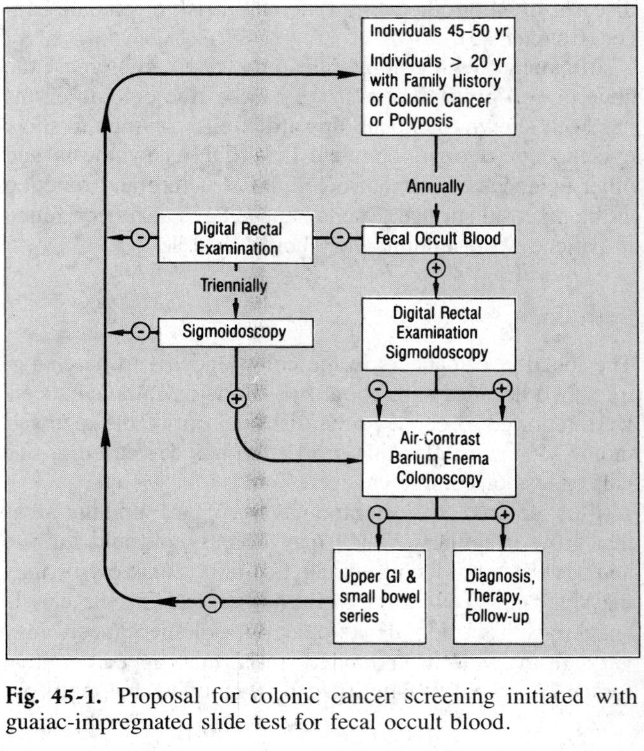

Fig. 45-1. Proposal for colonic cancer screening initiated with guaiac-impregnated slide test for fecal occult blood.

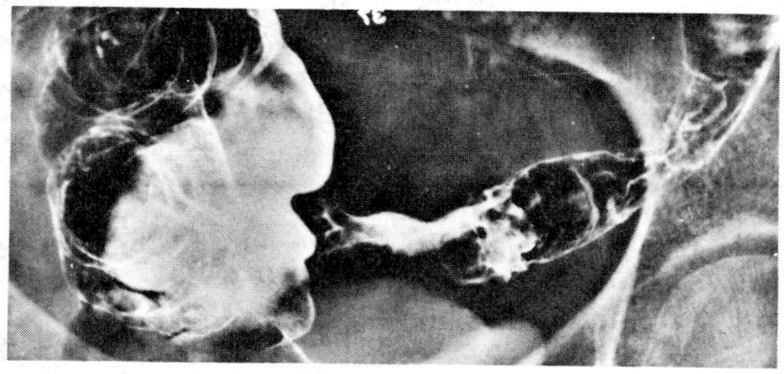

Fig. 45-2. Barium enema radiograph in a patient with carcinoma of sigmoid demonstrating apple core defect. (Radiograph courtesy of Memorial Hospital Diagnostic Radiology Department.)

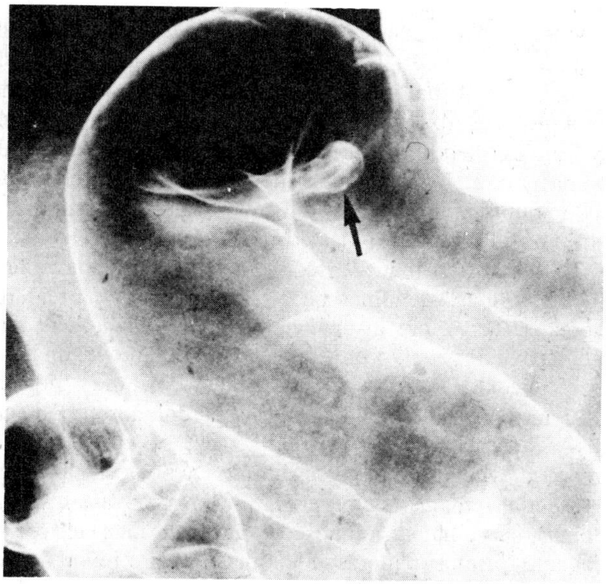

Fig. 45-3. Double contrast barium enema radiograph showing a small pedunculated polyp *(arrow)*. (Radiograph courtesy of American Society for Gastrointestinal Endoscopy Post-Graduate Course, 1976.)

vocated in postoperative surveillance of patients after partial colectomy for colon cancer for evaluation of anastomotic recurrence (rare) and for detection of additional polyps (20% to 40% risk). Annual examination is usually performed for the first 1 or 2 postoperative years and, if there are no further abnormalities, every 2 or 3 years thereafter. Periodic colonoscopic surveillance of individuals who have first-degree relatives with colon cancer has been advocated in view of the apparent increased risk.

There has been recent interest in searching for mutated oncogenes in fecal DNA as a screening test for colonic neoplasia. The serum immunoassay for carcinoembryonic antigen (CEA) was developed to provide a means of early detection of colonic cancer. However, it is too insensitive and nonspecific to be a useful screening test. CEA concentration may also be elevated with other cancers and with benign conditions such as inflammatory bowel disease, alcoholic liver disease, and pancreatitis. The test is most useful in assessing the results of surgery. If CEA concentration is elevated preoperatively and falls to normal after curative resection, a second rise is a good indication of recurrence and may develop long before the cancer can be detected clinically. Surgical "second look" procedures have been advocated in this circumstance, but it remains to be proved that they are of value. Also, when initially high, CEA concentration has been used to gauge patient response to chemotherapy for metastatic disease.

Differential diagnosis. Several conditions must be differentiated from colonic cancer. Diverticulitis may cause an inflammatory mass and obstruction that may resemble cancer, particularly in the sigmoid colon. Barium enema may sometimes not be sufficient for distinguishing between a perforated diverticulum and a perforated carcinoma. Colonoscopy with biopsy is valuable for distinguishing these disorders from one another once the infectious process has been controlled but can be difficult if muscle hypertrophy, spasm, and mucosal edema are present.

In patients with ulcerative colitis, inflammatory strictures may be difficult to distinguish from malignant strictures. Again, the colonoscope may not always be able to pass through the narrowed area. Frequently, however, a stricture has a component of muscle spasm, and such areas may be evaluated although they appear, on barium enema examination, to be too narrow for the colonoscope to pass. A cytology brush may be passed through the narrowed area, enabling the physician to detect malignant cells. Biopsy specimens from the proximal end of the stricture may not reveal a carcinoma present in the midportion or distal end. If there is any doubt, the stricture should be considered malignant until proved otherwise.

Benign-appearing polypoid lesions of the colon must be differentiated from carcinoma if they are larger than 0.7 mm in diameter. Simple biopsy of polyps may be misleading because a cancerous area may be missed as a result of sampling error. Cytologic specimens from polyps are not useful in practice because they do not permit differentiation of invasive carcinoma from the presence of atypical surface cells. Thus the best way to evaluate a polyp is to remove all of it by cautery snare. If a polypoid cancer with an involved margin is removed, resection of the involved segment of bowel and mesentery is usually indicated. Polyps 7 mm or smaller are not usually malignant and may be removed by fulguration ("hot") biopsy. In this technique, the polyp is destroyed by electrocoagulation while a biopsy specimen is obtained.

Treatment. The only known curative treatment for colonic adenocarcinoma is surgical resection. The prognosis for recurrence after resection depends on the degree of bowel wall invasion by the cancer and the presence of lymph node or distant metastases. If resection is adequate, in the Dukes' A group only 5% to 10% of patients will have recurrent cancer, as opposed to 20% to 30% in the Dukes' B group and to 50% in the Dukes' C group with cancer in the colon and 70% with cancer in the rectum.

Although the incidence of colonic cancer has steadily increased in the United States during the past decade, mortality has declined slightly. The observed decrease in mortality may be due in part to the widespread application of modern surgical principles but has also been attributed to increased awareness of the disease and diagnosis at an earlier stage.

Cancers in the right colon and left colon require right and left hemicolectomy, respectively. A wide margin should be taken with adequate resection of the mesentery and lymph nodes. Lesions in the rectosigmoid more than 6 to 8 cm from the anal verge may be treated by anterior resection, whereas sizable cancers below this level require combined abdominal-perineal resection with colostomy. Small low rectal cancers may sometimes be curatively removed by wide local excision. Full-thickness excision, with perirectal lymph nodes if possible, is preferable to electrofulguration for local treatment because it allows pathologic analysis. In unresectable rectal cancer, electrocautery or laser treatment may provide palliation, sometimes precluding the need for colostomy. Resection of colon cancer using laparoscopic "minimally invasive" technique has proved feasible on a trial basis, but long-term results that have been compared to those of standard laparotomy are not available and will require adequate follow-up studies.

Irradiation before surgery has been used in treating certain rectal cancers that, on digital examination, appear to be "fixed." An unresectable lesion occasionally becomes resectable after treatment with 2000 to 3000 rad. Some physicians have advocated the routine use of preoperative radiotherapy for rectal lesions, but the results of studies have been conflicting. Postoperative irradiation for patients with rectal cancer at risk for residual disease has been advocated, and radiation therapists are also evaluating a "sandwich" technique combining preoperative and postoperative treatment. In patients with advanced colorectal cancer, after resection of all gross disease, adjuvant therapy with a combination of 5-fluorouracil and levamisole has shown significantly improved survival rate compared to that of control subjects.

In patients with unresectable colonic cancer, both radiation therapy and chemotherapy have been widely used. Irradiation is usually employed for palliation and shrinkage of tumor masses in the pelvis. Chemotherapy remains unsatisfactory and experimental. 5-Fluorouracil has been the most widely used single agent: only about 15% to 20% of patients respond, most temporarily. Combination chemotherapy has not yet provided a noteworthy advance in colonic carcinoma treatment, although multiple-drug trials are currently in progress. A combination of radiation therapy and chemotherapy may have some increased benefit over either modality alone.

Infusions of 5-fluorouracil into the hepatic artery and/or portal vein have occasionally decreased hepatic metastases when systemic chemotherapy has failed. Patients with liver metastases have been treated with hepatic artery infusion via an implanted pump. A clear advantage over systemic treatment has not been demonstrated. A 5 year survival rate of about 20% has been reported in groups of patients who underwent surgical resection of localized liver metastases.

The judicious use of analgesics, sedatives, antidepressants, blood products, and nutritional supplements by a sympathetic physician can do much to enhance the quality of life for patients with metastatic colonic cancer.

BENIGN TUMORS OF THE LARGE INTESTINE

Adenomas of the colon comprise the great majority of polypoid lesions. The World Health Organization (WHO) has classified adenomas as (1) tubular, (2) villous, and (3) tubulovillous. Adenomas may be sessile, with a broad base, or have a large, thin pedicle containing fibrous tissue, blood vessels, and lymphatics. Polyps occur with greatest frequency in areas of the world where colonic cancer is common.

Most adenomas cause no symptoms. Bleeding from an adenoma may occur, more commonly with left-sided polyps. Bleeding usually is noted with bowel movements and is not profuse. Abdominal cramps may occur with large polyps. Intussusception of the large bowel from a benign adenoma is rare. Large villous adenomas may secrete copious amounts of potassium-rich mucus and cause diarrhea and hypokalemia when located in the distal large bowel.

It is estimated that 2% to 5% of single adenomas and 30% of villous adenomas become malignant, particularly if greater than 2 cm in diameter. Removing these benign tumors has been advocated as a means of preventing colonic cancer. Data from the National Polyp Study indicate that removal of all colonic adenomas at colonoscopy markedly decreases the expected incidence of colon cancer. However, whether removal of diminutive polyps ($<$0.3 cm) is essential remains controversial. After removal of all adenomas, surveillance colonoscopy at 3 year intervals seems adequate for most patients; adenomas that are found subsequently are usually small and tubular.

In familial polyposis coli and Gardner's syndrome, total proctocolectomy is recommended. In younger patients, a subtotal colectomy with ileorectal anastomosis is sometimes performed, with endoscopic surveillance of the remaining rectum and fulguration of polyps at least twice yearly. However, because cancers have developed in the rectal segment, a great responsibility is placed on the physician when a proctocolectomy is not done. Ileoanal anastomosis is an option to avoid ileostomy if the rectum is removed.

Hyperplastic polyps should be differentiated from adenomas. They are characteristically small (often only 2 to 3 mm) mucosal excrescences that are usually smooth and sessile, although occasionally they have a short stalk. They appear most often in the rectosigmoid and seem unrelated to colonic neoplasia.

Juvenile polyps, usually pedunculated hamartomas, may be seen in adults as well as children. They may ulcerate and bleed or cause obstruction. With time, they self-amputate spontaneously, but juvenile polyps that cause symptoms should be removed. Although there is no evidence that juvenile polyps undergo malignant change, there appears to be a higher incidence of cancer of the colon in patients and family members of patients who have had juvenile polyps.

Carcinoid tumors may occur in the colon and especially the rectum. As with carcinoid tumors in the small intestine, only tumors greater than 2 cm in size tend to metastasize. Carcinoid syndrome does not occur in patients with metastatic rectal carcinoid tumors.

Leiomyomas may occur in the colon but are much less common there than in the small bowel and stomach. *Lipomas* are the second most common benign colonic tumors. They are usually submucosal, and more than half are near the ileocecal valve. Lipomas may cause intussusception but are usually asymptomatic. They have a characteristic low-density appearance on CT scan. At colonoscopy they are seen to have a yellowish color and a soft, springy consistency and can be easily indented with a biopsy forceps, producing a "cushion" or "pillow" sign. Lipomas are usually sessile and, if asymptomatic, should be left alone.

REFERENCES

Burt RW et al: Dominant inheritance of adenomatous colonic polyps and colorectal cancer. N Engl J Med 312:1540, 1985.

Fearon ER and Vogelstein B: A genetic model for colorectal tumorogenesis. Cell 61:759, 1990.

Feldman JM: Carcinoid tumors and syndrome. Semin Oncol 14:235, 1987.

Holmes GKT et al: Malignancy in coeliac disease—effect of a gluten free diet. Gut 30:333, 1989.

Kemeny N: The role of chemotherapy in the treatment of colorectal cancer. Semin Surg Oncol 3:190, 1987.

Khojasteh A, Haghshenass M, and Hagnighi P: Current concepts in immunoproliferative small intestinal disease: a "third-world lesion." N Engl J Med 308:1401, 1983.

Lanspa SJ, Smyrk TC, and Lynch HT: The colonoscopist and the Lynch syndromes. Gastrointest Endosc 36:157, 1990.

Lightdale CJ, Koepsell TD, and Sherlock P: Small intestine. In Schottenfeld D and Fraumeni JF, editors: Cancer epidemiology and prevention. Philadelphia, 1982, WB Saunders.

Moertel BC et al: Levamisole and fluorouracil for adjuvant therapy of resected colon carcinoma. N Engl J Med 322:352, 1990.

Sugarbaker PH and Corlew S: Influence of surgical techniques on survival in patients with colorectal cancer. Dis Colon Rectum 25:545, 1982.

Winawer SJ, Schottenfeld D, and Flehinger BJ: Colorectal cancer screening. J Natl Cancer Inst 83:243, 1991.

CHAPTER

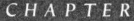

46 Vascular Diseases of the Intestine

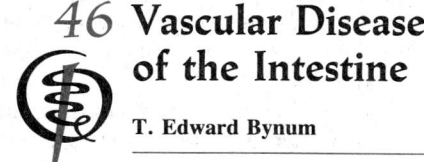

T. Edward Bynum

Mesenteric vascular disease is caused by the physical occlusion of a blood vessel (occlusive mesenteric vascular disease) or by low flow states in which either the vessels are normal or the luminal compromise is insufficient to impair significantly the flow of blood to the tissues (nonocclusive, or "hemodynamic," mesenteric vascular disease). Major-vessel occlusion can result from an embolus (e.g., from the left atrium, mitral valve, arterial thrombus elsewhere, paradoxical embolism) or from thrombus formation. An arterial thrombus usually forms on an atheromatous plaque or spontaneously, as may occur in young women who are taking birth control pills. Rarely, other events cause major artery occlusion (e.g., surgical accidents, abdominal trauma, or encroachment by a malignant neoplasm). Small-vessel occlusion at the level of the arterioles is associated with systemic diseases such as thrombotic thrombocytopenic purpura, disseminated intravascular coagulation, polyarteritis nodosa, and systemic lupus erythematosus.

Nonocclusive mesenteric vascular disease is more common than occlusive mesenteric vascular disease and occurs in such low flow and mesenteric vasoconstrictive states as severe congestive heart failure, aortic stenosis, shock (hemorrhagic, septic, cardiac), and cardiac arrhythmias and in concert with the use of vasoconstrictive drugs.

The incidence of mesenteric vascular disease is not known. Because of preterminal hypotension and rapid, postmortem autolysis of intestinal mucosa, the incidence figures obtained from autopsy series are overestimates. In the last 10 years, the incidence, especially that of nonocclusive disease, appears to be declining. Perhaps this decline is due to better recognition of the pathophysiologic characteristics of shock and of mesenteric vascular disease, less use of vasoconstrictive drugs, better drugs for support of cardiovascular function, and better methods that assist respiration and maintain oxygenation.

Pathophysiology

Ischemia or infarction of the intestine results when the bloodstream fails to carry oxygen and other nutrients in quantities sufficient for intestinal metabolic needs. This situation is obvious when a major artery supplying the intestine becomes completely occluded by an embolus or thrombus. The situation is less obvious, although more common, when there is no physical occlusion in the supplying vessels, as occurs in nonocclusive mesenteric ischemia and infarction. Nonocclusive mesenteric vascular disease is associated with a general threat to blood circulation such as hypovolemia (absolute or relative), hypotension, or shock. When effective circulating blood volume decreases, there is progressive vasoconstriction of mesenteric arterial vasculature, which shunts blood away from the splanchnic circulation into the general circulation. Teleologically, the less vital gastrointestinal tract is "sacrificed" in order to "protect" or "save" the more vital brain, heart, lungs, and kidneys. If vasoconstriction is combined with impaired cardiac output, severely depleted intravascular volume, or moderately compromised vascular channels, then a critical point may be reached at which the supply of oxygen falls below the minimum needed, and ischemia supervenes. If ischemia is severe or prolonged, infarction eventuates.

Intestinal villi are anatomically constructed so that the vessels within the villi can allow "countercurrent" exchange of oxygen. As a result, the villus tips are relatively hypoxemic even at full blood flow, so if there is a decline in intestinal blood flow, oxygen supply to the tips may rapidly become inadequate.

Fortunately, the gastrointestinal tract has a blood supply that is rich in collateral vessels, which provides considerable protection against occlusive vascular disease, especially when the occlusion develops slowly or involves the largest branches of the aorta. Chronic intestinal ischemia does not occur unless at least two of the three major mesenteric vessels (celiac axis, superior mesenteric artery, inferior mesenteric artery) are *completely* occluded. Unfortunately, this rich system of collaterals does not protect the gastrointestinal tract against nonocclusive vascular disease.

Infarction of the small intestine is associated with a high mortality, and the efficacy of therapy is low. Infarction of the colon is much more benign: the mortality is low and the colon frequently heals without residual complications.

Pathology

The earliest tissue changes in mesenteric ischemia are necrosis of villus tips in the small bowel and necrosis of the superficial epithelium in the colon. If the ischemic insult is more severe, deeper portions of the mucosa show hemorrhagic necrosis. Severe intestinal infarction is manifested by hemorrhagic necrosis of all layers of the bowel wall.

If blood flow is reinstituted, tissue injury becomes worse initially. Reperfusion actually increases cell necrosis because the reavailability of oxygen leads to the creation of toxic free radicals. However, the earliest lesion is fully reversible. Lesions of intermediate severity ulcerate or slough large areas of mucosa, after which repair takes place with ultimate re-epithelialization but often with fibrous scarring and possible stricture formation. Very severe acute lesions may be associated with massive bleeding or perforation or lead to irreversible shock and death (especially as a consequence of small bowel infarction).

Clinical presentation

Patients with mesenteric ischemia have abdominal pain that is cramping, generalized or periumbilical, and often severe. In early stages, the pain is not associated with any abnormalities evident on examination of the abdomen. Early in the course of intestinal ischemia, a patient's pain is "out of proportion" to any other physical findings, particularly in small bowel ischemia. Colonic ischemia may be heralded by rectal bleeding as well as by abdominal pain. Therefore timely diagnosis of mesenteric vascular disease requires a high index of suspicion. Objective physical findings in the abdomen, particularly peritoneal signs, are a relatively late manifestation of bowel infarction, and at such a stage often little can be done to reverse the process or rescue the bowel.

Occlusive mesenteric vascular disease should be suspected in patients with known cardiac disease, particularly if they have mitral valve disease, marked left atrial enlargement, or atrial fibrillation. In patients with severe generalized atherosclerotic and arteriosclerotic vascular disease, the major mesenteric arteries may gradually and progressively become occluded until there is chronic ischemia of the intestine. When this situation is manifested by abdominal pain following the ingestion of food, it is termed *abdominal angina*. In rare instances, patients may have mild to moderate malabsorption secondary to severe chronic mesenteric ischemia. However, most patients lose weight because of "cardiac cachexia" or because they stop eating to prevent pain.

The possibility of small-vessel occlusive disease is suggested by the presence of known multisystem disease (collagen-vascular or "autoimmune" disease) or in situations in which disseminated intravascular coagulation might occur.

Nonocclusive mesenteric vascular disease occurs with congestive heart failure, cardiac arrhythmias, hypotension, or shock. Sympathomimetic drugs and digitalis glycosides are potent vasoconstrictors of the mesenteric vasculature. Fortunately, adrenergic drugs are no longer widely used, and digitalis only has significant splanchnic vasoconstrictive action if it is administered parenterally. However, nonocclusive intestinal infarction may occur with digitalis toxicity. When ischemia and infarction occur in the distal small bowel or in the colon, the patient may have bloody diarrhea or bright red blood from the rectum.

The laboratory offers little to aid in the specific diagnosis of mesenteric vascular disease. With intestinal infarction, moderate to severe leukocytosis is common. Serum amylase and alkaline phosphatase concentrations can be mildly to moderately elevated, because these enzymes are present in the intestinal epithelium.

Diagnosis

It is very difficult to make the diagnosis of mesenteric ischemia or infarction with absolute certainty short of surgery or autopsy. Early diagnosis is mandatory and depends on the physician's high index of suspicion combined with an awareness of the clinical contexts in which the disease occurs. Mesenteric arteriography is helpful in documenting and locating a vascular occlusion. On the other hand, arteriograms may show radiographic evidence of vasoconstriction, or the arteries may appear entirely normal; either appearance is compatible with nonocclusive intestinal ischemia with or without infarction. If the arteriographic findings are compatible with nonocclusive disease, the catheter can be left in place for possible administration of a vasodilator drug intra-arterially.

In less urgent clinical situations, barium contrast radiographs of the alimentary tract are often made to evaluate abdominal pain. "Thumbprinting" (indentation of the barium column caused by submucosal hemorrhage and edema) is characteristic of mesenteric vascular disease (Fig. 46-1) but also occurs in uremia, thrombocytopenia, Crohn's disease, and *E. coli* O157:H7 colitis and after blunt trauma to the abdomen. Fibrous strictures may form in the colon after recovery from acute ischemia (Fig. 46-2).

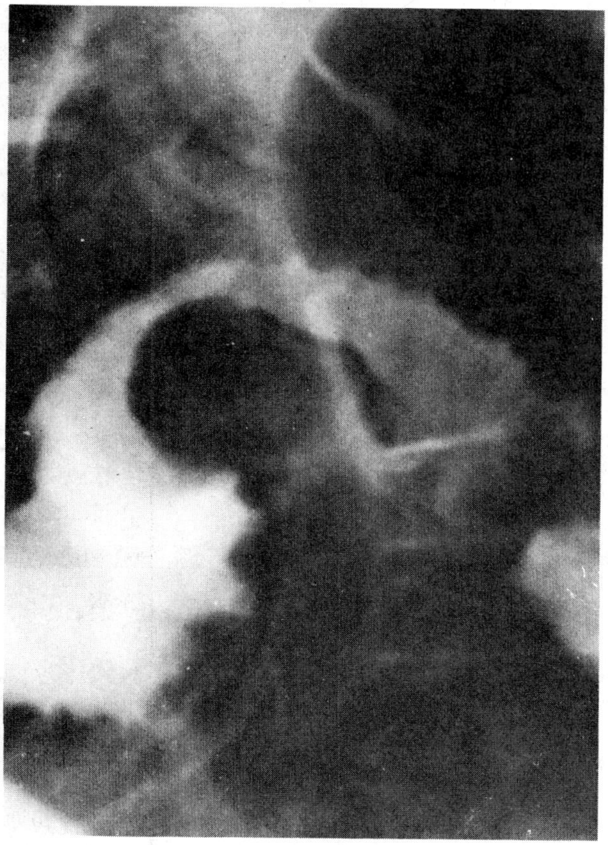

Fig. 46-1. Spot film of barium enema in a patient with ischemic colitis, showing a large thumbprint and mucosal irregularity with spicules of barium at the margins of the barium column *(indicating ulcerations).*

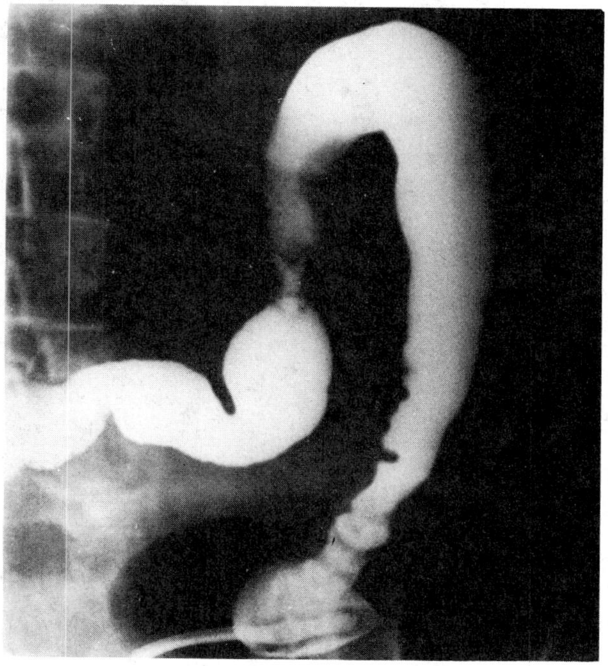

Fig. 46-2. Spot film of barium enema, showing a smooth, tapered stricture of the sigmoid colon in a patient who had an episode of ischemic colitis 15 months previously.

Treatment

If the small bowel becomes acutely ischemic but does not progress to infarction, and if good blood flow can be reestablished, the lesion is usually reversible and there are no clinical sequelae. Infarction of the small bowel is not reversible, and the outcome is usually death or surgical resection. Therefore chronic strictures of the small bowel produced by ischemia are extremely rare. If occlusive disease is documented by angiography or if there is clinical evidence of infarction, surgery is indicated. Prompt embolectomy or bypass of the obstructed vessel may prevent infarction. If infarction has already occurred, all of the infarcted bowel must be resected. If the patient subsequently recovers but has had so much bowel resected that nutrition cannot be maintained by oral alimentation, parenteral alimentation must be established and often maintained indefinitely. When nonocclusive disease is suspected or known to be present, general support and measures designed to correct or alleviate such possible underlying problems as hypovolemia, heart failure, or digitalis toxicity are crucial to restore circulating volume and enhance cardiac output. The goal is to restore perfusion of the intestine, reverse ischemia and tissue hypoxia, and prevent infarction. The diagnostic approach outlined in Fig. 46-3 is aggressive. However, mortality in patients with small bowel infarction is very high, and arteriography is quite safe when performed by experienced radiologists. Vasodilator drugs such as papaverine, glucagon, and the vasodilator prostaglandins can effectively increase mesenteric blood flow when administered intra-arterially via a catheter placed during mesenteric arteriography. Vasodilator therapy is generally safe if general circulating volume has been restored and is maintained.

In the colon acute ischemia is frequently reversible, and extensive bowel wall infarction (with resultant toxic dilatation or perforation) is rare. For the less than 15% of patients who have moderate ischemia of the colon that is not reversible, the outcome is a fibrous stricture (Fig. 46-2). If the patient with a postischemic stricture of the colon has significant obstructive symptoms, the stricture must be dilated endoscopically or surgically resected. However, if symptoms are minimal, or if the stricture is discovered on a barium enema made for other indications, it may be left alone; many cases have shown gradual improvement or disappearance of the stricture over 6 to 12 months.

Mesenteric venous thrombosis

There is no doubt that abdominal pain, intestinal ischemia, and perhaps intestinal infarction can result from thrombotic

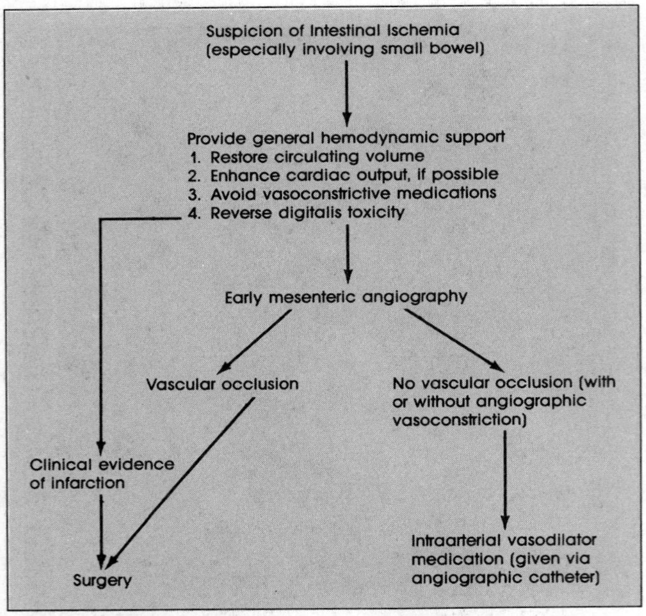

Fig. 46-3. Suggested evaluation and therapy of mesenteric ischemia.

occlusion of mesenteric veins. Individual cases have been well documented in young women taking birth control pills and in other patients with hypercoaguable states. However, the overall incidence of this problem or its proportion of all cases of mesenteric vascular disease is difficult to determine. The reason for the difficulty is as follows: mesenteric venous thrombosis, particularly of the small branches draining the intestine, sometimes occurs as a result of ischemia (or infarction) caused by failure of perfusion because of either occlusion of the arterial supply or nonocclusive reduction in arterial blood flow. Therefore if a patient actually has ischemia or infarction produced by nonocclusive disease, and thrombosis of mesenteric veins occurs secondarily, there has been a tendency to attribute the ischemia or infarction to the tangibly identified occlusion/thrombosis (i.e., that occurring in the mesenteric veins). Mesenteric vein thrombosis can be either the result of intestinal ischemia or infarction or the cause of it.

The largest vein draining the intestines is the portal vein. Complete occlusion of the portal vein is well known: portal vein thrombosis. The consequences of portal vein thrombosis are portal hypertension, esophageal varices, bleeding from varices, splenomegaly, and hypersplenism. Intestinal ischemia, intestinal infarction, malabsorption, or any measurable intestinal dysfunction does not result from portal vein thrombosis.

If mesenteric vein thrombosis is associated with infarction of the intestine, treatment is as outlined for infarction with prompt surgery after initial stabilization. Birth control pills should be discontinued if a woman is using that medication. If a hypercoaguable state is present, the treatment is that of the underlying disease and administration of anticoagulants.

REFERENCES

Bynum TE et al: The pathophysiology of nonocclusive intestinal ischemia. In Shepherd AP and Granger DN, editors: Physiology of the intestinal circulation. New York, 1984, Raven Press.

Bynum TE and Jacobson ED: Nonocclusive intestinal ischemia. Arch Intern Med 139:281, 1979.

Cooke M and Sande MA: Diagnosis and outcome of bowel infarction on an acute medical service. Am J Med 75:984, 1983.

Geelkerken RH et al: Chronic mesenteric vascular syndrome. Arch Surg 126:1101, 1991.

Grendell JH and Ockner RK: Mesenteric venous thrombosis. Gastroenterology 82:358, 1982.

Kaleya RN et al: Aggressive approach to acute mesenteric ischemia. Surg Clin North Am 72:157, 1992.

Reeders JWAJ et al: Ischaemic colitis. The Hague, Netherlands, 1984, Martinus Nijhoff Publishers.

Williams LF, Jr: Mesenteric ischemia. Surg Clin North Am 68:331, 1988.

CHAPTER

47 Diverticular and Other Intestinal Diseases

Michael D. Apstein

Diverticula, either congenital or acquired, can arise in any portion of the gastrointestinal tract; they frequently cause no symptoms. For example, in 15% of the general population, one to three diverticula are present in the second portion of the duodenum. Although periampullary diverticula are associated with an increased risk of pigment gallstones, the diverticula themselves rarely cause symptoms. In the rare instances when congenital diverticula involve the colon, they are found in the cecum.

MECKEL'S DIVERTICULUM

Meckel's diverticulum is the most frequent congenital anomaly of the gastrointestinal tract. The diverticulum is usually located in the distal ileum, within 100 cm of the ileocecal valve. It is found in 1% to 3% of the population but is symptomatic in less than half of those affected. Of those who become symptomatic, only half have ectopic, functional gastric mucosa lining the diverticulum. In these patients, acid-peptic secretion from the Meckel's diverticulum may cause bleeding or ulceration of the adjacent small bowel mucosa. Pain may occur and can mimic that of acute appendicitis. Occasionally, perforation of the bowel wall results. Regardless of the nature of its mucosal lining, a Meckel's diverticulum can induce symptoms of intermittent small bowel obstruction by causing either intussusception or internal herniation secondary to an accompanying mesodiverticular vascular band. Although 60% of patients who become symptomatic do so by 2 years of age, a Meckel's diverticulum should be considered in any young adult with melena, hematochezia, or small bowel obstruction. If the diverticulum contains ectopic gastric mucosa, the diagnosis can often be made by abdominal scanning after administration of radioactive technetium, which is concentrated and then secreted by gastric mucosa. Small bowel enteroclysis to visualize the diverticulum directly may be helpful in those patients who have intermittent, partial small bowel obstruction. The diagnosis may also be made at laparotomy. Treatment of a patient with a symptomatic Meckel's diverticulum is surgical excision.

MULTIPLE JEJUNAL DIVERTICULOSIS

Multiple jejunal diverticulosis is an acquired disease that usually manifests itself in adulthood. Some patients probably have a variant of progressive systemic sclerosis limited to the gastrointestinal tract or an idiopathic visceral myopathy or neuropathy. The smooth muscle or myenteric plexus abnormality, in turn, produces localized wall weakness and/or uncoordinated motor activity resulting in formation of diverticula.

Only 10% to 40% of patients with multiple jejunal diverticulosis are symptomatic. Their symptoms are usually those of chronic intestinal pseudo-obstruction (Chapter 44). The associated abnormal small intestinal motility and stasis within the diverticular lumens can result in bacterial overgrowth and malabsorption (Chapter 42). Additionally, there are isolated reports of inflammation, bleeding, or perforation of the diverticula.

Treatment is directed toward the underlying pathophysiologic process caused by the diverticula. Antibiotics are useful if bacterial overgrowth is present. Surgical resection of the involved diverticulum is the treatment of choice for perforation or uncontrollable bleeding but is of no use for chronic symptoms of intestinal pseudo-obstruction.

COLONIC DIVERTICULAR DISEASE

Prevalence and epidemiology

Prevalence rates of colonic diverticulosis vary tremendously depending on geographic area. For example, diverticulosis is so common in Western society that it almost could be considered a normal part of aging; 50% of individuals have colonic diverticula by age 70. However, diverticulosis is rare in Africa and other less industrialized parts of the world. This geographic variation in prevalence, the dramatic increase in prevalence in Western countries since 1900, and the appearance of the disease in Japanese immigrants to the West supports an environmental cause.

Many investigators believe dietary habits of a given population influence the prevalence of diverticulosis in that population. Diets low in fiber and other bulk and high in meat and refined carbohydrates have been implicated in the formation of colonic diverticula. The following statements offer support for this hypothesis: (1) Vegetarians have a lower prevalence of diverticulosis than age-matched nonvegetarian control subjects. (2) The increase in prevalence in Western society has paralleled the increased dietary consumption of refined carbohydrate. (3) Case-controlled studies have shown that patients with diverticula consume less dietary fiber than patients without diverticula. However, additional scientific evidence is needed before a true cause and effect relationship can be established.

Pathology

A colonic diverticulum is a herniation of mucosa and submucosa through or between fibers of the major muscle layer (muscularis propria). Colonic diverticula may involve all portions of the colon (Fig. 47-1). They form at the site where the vasa recta (intramural branches of the marginal artery) penetrate the circular muscle (Fig. 47-2). As a result, the lumen of the diverticulum is separated from the vasa recta and peritoneum by only a few millimeters of mucosa and submucosa.

Diverticulitis results from a microperforation of the diverticular mucosa, submucosa, and adjacent serosa into the surrounding pericolic fat. Thus diverticulitis is primarily a pericolitis, not a true colitis; there is only localized involvement of the mucosa without extensive or diffuse mucositis. The pericolic infection ranges from a well-contained microabscess to one large enough to form an intra-abdominal mass. Recurrent bouts of acute diverticulitis may lead to scarring, fibrosis, and stricture of the involved region.

Bleeding from colonic diverticula is caused by rupture of the underlying vas rectum. Data suggest that injurious factors in the diverticular lumen produce eccentric damage to the underlying artery. Progressive weakness of the arte-

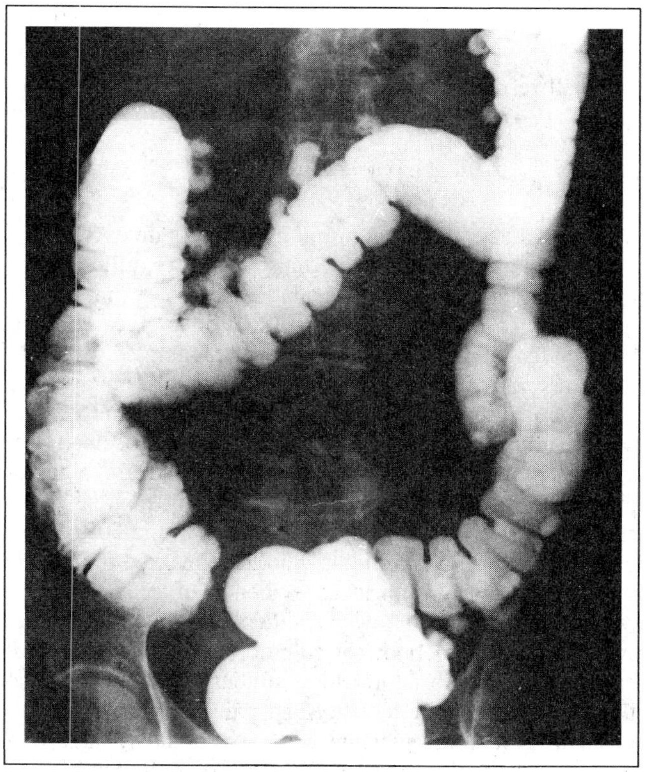

Fig. 47-1. Single-column barium enema radiograph showing numerous diverticula of the colon.

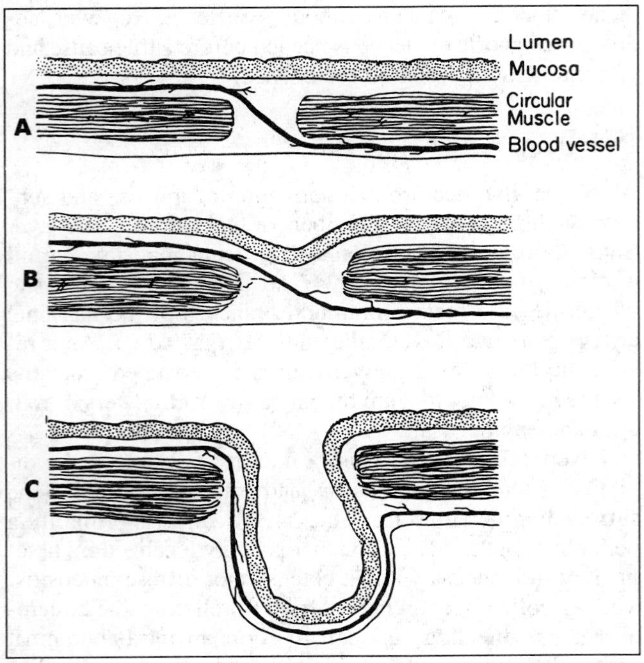

Fig. 47-2. Structural dynamics of diverticular formation and vascular relationships. **A,** The long branch of the vas rectum artery penetrates the colonic wall through a connective tissue gap in the circular muscle. **B,** Early mucosal protrusion widens the connective tissue gap. **C,** With transmural extension of the diverticulum, the vas rectum is displaced over it. As a result, the lumen of the diverticulum is separated from the vas rectum by only a thin layer of mucosa and submucosa. (Modified from Meyers MA et al: Gastroenterology 71:577, 1976.)

rial wall results in rupture into the lumen of the diverticulum (Fig. 47-3).

Pathogenesis

Diverticula develop when intraluminal pressure exceeds the focal resistance of the colonic muscular layer, allowing the mucosa and submucosa to herniate. Studies examining the role of increased intraluminal pressure have given conflicting results. Some have implicated exaggerated, nonsynchronous contractions (spasms) in the sigmoid in response to food or drugs that stimulate contraction of the colonic smooth muscle. Segmentation and localized occlusion of short segments of the sigmoid occur, producing high intraluminal pressures in these localized occluded areas of the sigmoid colon. These investigators point to the 50% of patients with colonic diverticula who have marked thickening of the muscularis propria as evidence of spasm-induced muscle hypertrophy. However, others have not found an association between abnormal colonic motility and the presence of diverticulosis. In these studies there is a correlation between colonic motility and pain, but not diverticulosis. In fact, most patients with diverticulosis have normal colonic motility patterns. Whether diverticulosis is part of the spectrum of irritable bowel disease is also controversial.

Clinical presentation and diagnosis

The overwhelming majority of patients with diverticulosis never have symptoms. Symptoms result from the complications of diverticulosis: microperforation and diverticulitis or arterial rupture. The clinical presentation of diverticulitis can vary and depends on the extent of the perforation. Most commonly, the patient has a walled-off microabscess and experiences abdominal pain, fever, and mild left lower quadrant tenderness and/or mass. Frequently, there is tenderness on rectal examination toward the area of inflammation. Laboratory tests usually reveal polymorphonuclear leukocytosis and an elevated sedimentation rate. Plain radiographs of the abdomen generally reveal normal results. This combination of findings is reminiscent of acute appendicitis; an older person who has "left-sided appendicitis" usually has diverticulitis.

Many patients with diverticulosis who experience cramping abdominal pain and irregular bowel movements have the irritable bowel syndrome and not diverticulitis. Diverticulitis should not be diagnosed in the absence of fever, tenderness, and in most instances, leukocytosis. Occasionally, patients present with an "acute abdomen" caused by peritonitis if the abscess has not been contained. An abdominal computed tomographic (CT) scan or a barium enema with gentle infusion of contrast at low pressure is indicated when the clinical setting or course is atypical. Abdominal CT scanning is particularly useful because it can detect other conditions, overlooked by barium enema, that may mimic diverticulitis. Frequently, during an acute attack the barium enema demonstrates diverticula only. Radiologic evidence of a fistula (Fig. 47-4), localized abscess, or colonic narrowing by a pericolic mass is consistent with diverticulitis. "Sawtooth" irregularity and narrowing correlate with thickening of the muscularis propria and do not indicate diverticulitis.

The differential diagnosis of acute diverticulitis includes localized Crohn's disease, colonic ischemia, or a perforated colonic cancer.

Colonoscopy is contraindicated early in the course of acute diverticulitis because of the risk of extending the microperforation. However, once the patient is stable, a barium enema, flexible sigmoidoscopy, or colonoscopy to exclude a perforated colon cancer is imperative.

Bleeding from a diverticulum characteristically involves sudden passing of bright red or dark red blood from the rectum. It is almost always painless or, at most, associated with mild cramping. Occasionally, blood loss may be massive, leading to hemorrhagic shock or even death. Fortunately, most instances are self-limited, and bleeding ceases before the patient's life is endangered (and often before a precise diagnosis is made). Because the bleeding from a diverticulum results from the acute rupture of an artery, patients almost never experience occult gastrointestinal blood loss. Occult blood in the stool should be attributed to diverticula only when all other possible causes (especially carcinoma of the cecum) have been confidently excluded. Diverticular bleeding occurs only very rarely in association with acute diverticulitis.

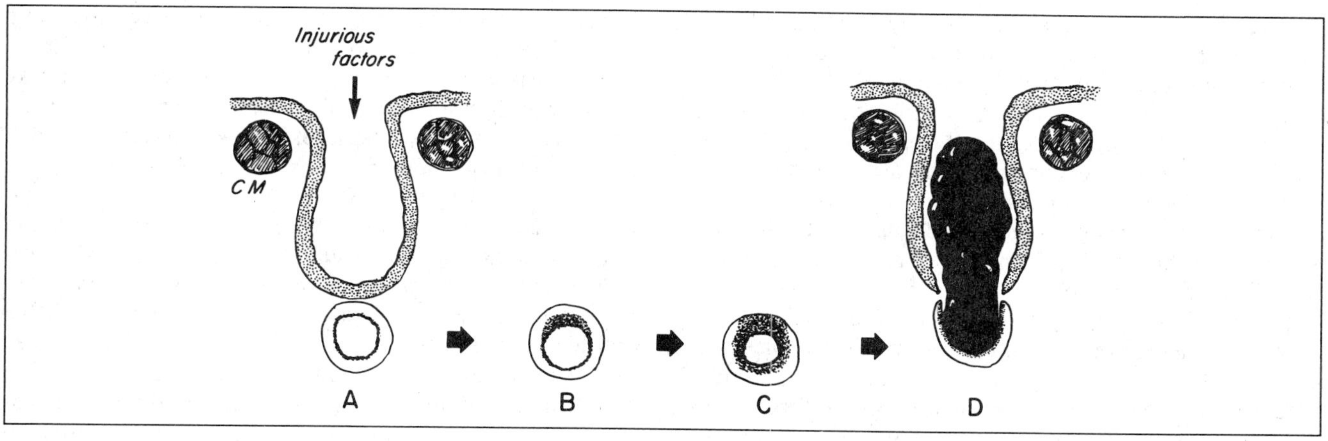

Fig. 47-3. Proposed pathogenesis of diverticular bleeding. **A,** A cross section through a diverticulum that has protruded between bands of circular muscle. Note the close apposition of the vas rectum artery to the dome of the diverticulum. Injurious factors in the lumen of the diverticulum cause initial damage to the vas rectum. CM, circular muscle. **B,** Eccentric intimal thickening of the vas rectum vessel follows. **C,** Concentric intimal thickening with luminal accentuation occurs. **D,** Eccentric, acute rupture of the vas rectum into the lumen of the diverticulum. (Modified from Meyers MA et al: Gastroenterology 71:577, 1976.)

Sigmoidoscopy should be done promptly in the evaluation of patients who are thought to be bleeding from a colonic diverticulum, to exclude another source of bleeding in the rectum or rectosigmoid. If sigmoidoscopy reveals that blood is coming from a location higher in the colon and if the patient continues to bleed briskly, the next diagnostic procedure should be a technetium-labeled red blood cell bleeding scan or a mesenteric arteriogram (Chapters 34 and 30). Colonoscopy is difficult during active lower gastrointestinal bleeding from any source; patients usually have not had a bowel-cleansing preparation, and blood mixed with even a small amount of feces cannot be removed adequately during colonoscopy to obtain a thorough examination. Furthermore, the risk of perforation is higher in the presence of diverticula. On the other hand, a 2 to 4 hour lavage with an osmotically balanced solution, such as GoLytely, administered orally facilitates localization of the bleeding site during colonoscopy in patients with acute colonic bleeding. Other diagnoses that need to be considered in the patient with brisk hematochezia are angiodysplasia (arteriovenous malformations) and, more rarely, colonic cancer or a massively bleeding lesion in the upper gastrointestinal tract. Angiodysplasia, small ectatic vascular lesions of the intestinal (frequently colonic) mucosa and submucosa, can be diagnosed with mesenteric angiography or with colonoscopy. Colonoscopy is more sensitive once the patient has stopped bleeding and the colon can be adequately prepared.

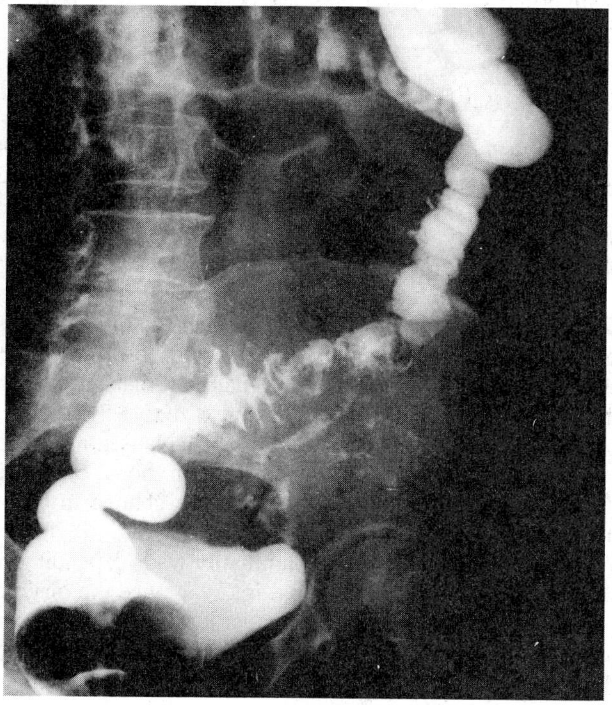

Fig. 47-4. Barium enema radiograph in a patient with diverticulitis, showing a fistula from the sigmoid colon to the bladder. *(The bladder is filled with barium, seen to the right of the rectum and rectosigmoid junction.)*

Treatment

Diets high in fiber have been recommended for patients with diverticulosis. Whereas these diets are probably beneficial in the irritable bowel syndrome, there is no conclusive evidence that any dietary changes will reduce the incidence of complications of diverticulosis or prevent additional diverticula from forming.

Some patients with mild diverticulitis can be treated as outpatients with a clear liquid diet and oral antibiotics such as ampicillin or tetracycline, 500 mg q6h. Addition of metronidazole to the regimen provides broader coverage for anaerobic bacteria. More symptomatic patients require hospitalization and bowel rest (nothing by mouth; intravenously administered fluid, electrolytes, and glucose; and nasogastric intubation if the patient has vomiting or ileus) in addition to antibiotics. The choice of antibiotics for the hospitalized patient depends on the severity of the illness. Choices include intravenous ampicillin alone or, for more severely ill patients, combined with an aminoglycoside and clindamycin or metronidazole. Immediate surgery is necessary if generalized peritonitis is present. If medical therapy fails as evidenced by a nonresolving or enlarging inflammatory mass, surgery is necessary. Preoperative percutaneous drainage of the mass (abscess) may reduce the need for colostomy and a "three-stage" operation. Elective surgery is indicated for recurrent attacks, fistula formation, or, rarely, inability to exclude carcinoma. Partial colonic obstruction can occur during acute diverticulitis, although it frequently resolves during medical treatment. Months or years after an episode of acute diverticulitis, however, chronic obstruction may develop from scarring and fibrosis and may require surgery or endoscopic dilation to relieve the obstruction.

Bleeding from a colonic diverticulum ceases spontaneously in most patients. Therefore the early management of diverticular bleeding is supportive, with replacement of red blood cells and intravascular volume as indicated. If the bleeding continues, selective intra-arterial infusion of vasopressin (0.2 to 0.4 unit/min) into the artery supplying the bleeding site (as determined by angiography) stops the bleeding in more than 80% of patients. Intravenous vasopressin has no role in the treatment of diverticular bleeding. There are anecdotal reports of a barium enema's stopping diverticular hemorrhage. However, the success of this "therapy" is probably no greater than the rate at which diverticula stop bleeding spontaneously. Furthermore, the presence of barium in the colon interferes with angiographic localization of the site of bleeding. If diverticular bleeding persists despite intra-arterial infusion of vasopressin, resection of the involved segment of colon is necessary. Twenty percent of patients who have had diverticular bleeding bleed again, whereas 50% rebleed if they have already bled twice. Therefore elective surgery is indicated for recurrent diverticular bleeding if the site can be localized with certainty. "Blind" hemicolectomy (right or left) in patients with recurrent lower gastrointestinal bleeding in whom no specific site of blood loss has been identified is not wise.

AGANGLIONIC MEGACOLON

Megacolon is characterized by massive colonic dilatation and constipation. It can be either congenital or acquired. In congenital megacolon (Hirschsprung's disease), the distal rectum lacks submucosal (Meissner's) and myenteric (Auerbach's) plexuses. The embryonic migration of ganglion cells to form these plexuses may be interrupted by intestinal ischemia secondary to structurally abnormal arteries or by an abnormal extracellular matrix microenvironment. The aganglionic segment may extend proximally for a variable distance from the distal rectum. Normal motor activity in this segment is lacking; the aganglionic segment is permanently contracted. As a consequence, the more proximal colon dilates secondary to the distal functional obstruction. In contrast, in acquired megacolon, which may be associated with Parkinson's disease, scleroderma, intestinal pseudo-obstruction, Chagas' disease, amyloidosis, and drug-induced or idiopathic constipation, the entire rectum and colon are usually dilated.

Hirschsprung's disease, more common in males than in females, occurs approximately once in 5000 births. Although the clinical presentation occurs most often in infants, the diagnosis of Hirschsprung's disease should be considered in any adolescent or young adult with a history of severe, often lifelong, constipation. Patients frequently complain of abdominal distention and inability to pass flatus. They may have symptoms of large bowel obstruction with crampy abdominal pain, nausea, and vomiting. Digital examination reveals no stool in the rectum, but occasionally, on withdrawal of the examining finger or at sigmoidoscopy, a mass of stool is evacuated. A barium enema demonstrating distal narrowing and proximal dilatation, most often at the level of the rectosigmoid, is characteristic. A lateral view frequently shows the transition zone best. Usually, definitive diagnosis can be made by rectal manometry (Chapter 41) and by suction biopsy that retrieves mucosa and submucosa, but a full-thickness rectal biopsy under general anesthesia may be necessary.

Surgery is the only treatment for Hirschsprung's disease. A temporary colostomy to relieve the functional obstruction may be indicated in some patients. However, several definitive procedures overcome the obstructing effect of the aganglionic segment yet preserve continence with minimal morbidity.

APPENDICITIS

Acute appendicitis most often occurs in adolescence and early adulthood, but no age is exempt. The cause is not known, although obstruction of the appendiceal lumen by a fecalith or hyperplasia of submucosal lymphoid tissue probably is a factor in promoting infection.

Clinically, the hallmark of acute appendicitis is the patient's history and progression of signs and symptoms. Classically, acute appendicitis starts with poorly localized epigastric or periumbilical abdominal pain that migrates to the right lower quadrant over the next 4 to 6 hours. The pain is always associated with anorexia. Nausea and vomiting occur in only 50% of patients and in those, only after the pain has begun. There is no specific change in bowel habits.

The findings on physical examination vary depending on the location of the appendix and interval since the onset of pain the patient is examined. Tenderness is always present at some time in the course of an attack and corresponds to the location of the appendix; the right lower quadrant most frequently but also the right upper quadrant or flank in the case of a retrocecal appendix. The patient's temperature may be normal or mildly elevated. Fever above 101° F suggests a perforated appendix or alternative diagnosis.

Laboratory data are not diagnostic. The white blood

count is usually but not invariably elevated. Values above 20,000 cells per cubic centimeter are rare and are consistent with a perforated appendix or other disease process.

Several other diseases may mimic symptoms and/or physical findings of acute appendicitis. The most common among these are pelvic inflammatory disease, Crohn's disease, ruptured or twisted ovarian cyst, and acute mesenteric adenitis. Occasionally, tubal pregnancy, right-sided diverticulitis, enteritis secondary to *Yersinia enterocolitica* infection, perforated duodenal ulcer, or acute pyelonephritis may mimic acute appendicitis. In addition, a perforated cecal carcinoma can mimic acute appendicitis in older individuals.

The classic course of acute appendicitis—epigastric pain that localizes to the right lower quadrant followed by nausea and vomiting—occurs in only 50% to 60% of individuals. Elderly patients and patients receiving immunosuppressive therapy may have blunted symptoms and physical findings, often delaying the diagnosis. This delay leads to an increased rate of rupture with attendant increased mortality.

If the clinical picture is not clear, abdominal ultrasonography may be helpful. Visualization of the appendix is consistent with the diagnosis of acute appendicitis. However, failure to visualize it does not exclude the diagnosis.

The accepted treatment for acute appendicitis is appendectomy, performed as soon as the diagnosis is apparent. Systemic antibiotic therapy has been effective in a number of patients with acute appendicitis but should be reserved for those who are unusually poor surgical risks.

Overlooked or delayed diagnosis of acute appendicitis can result in perforation of the appendix with subsequent increased immediate morbidity and mortality. Furthermore, the risk of subsequent tubal infertility increases sharply in women with a history of a perforated appendix. Very rarely does acute appendicitis resolve spontaneously without surgery or antibiotic therapy. Chronic appendicitis or recurrent acute appendicitis probably exists but must be extremely rare. Such a diagnosis should not be marshaled to account for chronic abdominal pain.

HEMORRHOIDS

Hemorrhoids are varicose veins of the anus and rectum. Most patients with hemorrhoids have no obvious predisposing factor. There is a familial tendency and an increased incidence in patients with irritable bowel syndrome who are constipated. Hemorrhoids develop frequently during pregnancy because the enlarging uterus obstructs veins that drain blood from the rectal area. In patients with portal hypertension, hemorrhoids (or dilated rectal veins that are clinically indistinguishable from hemorrhoids) are common, because this venous system participates in decompressing portal pressure.

In many patients, hemorrhoids are observed incidentally at the time of rectal, sigmoidoscopic, or colonoscopic examination and cause no symptoms. The major symptoms of hemorrhoids are bleeding, pain, itching, or rectal prolapse. Bleeding is usually painless. A patient may notice red blood on the toilet tissue or on the surface of formed stool, there may be dripping of blood into the water of the toilet bowl, or the patient's underclothing may become soiled with blood. Persistent, brisk bleeding is rare. Likewise, anemia resulting from hemorrhoidal bleeding is unusual and should prompt a more thorough investigation. Before any rectal bleeding can be attributed to hemorrhoids, sigmoidoscopy and a barium enema or colonoscopy should be performed to exclude other, more serious abnormalities. Pain is caused by thrombosis of a hemorrhoid. Itching represents low-order stimulation of pain fibers that occurs when a hemorrhoid becomes thrombosed. Itching may also be caused by fecal soiling, which irritates the perianal skin. This occurs if the presence of hemorrhoids causes mild sphincter incontinence in patients with loose stools.

Medical management of hemorrhoids requires treatment of any underlying condition. If a patient is constipated, a high-bulk diet and a hydrophilic substance such as psyllium seed mucilloid should be prescribed. Twice-daily sitz baths followed by insertion of an anesthetic hydrocortisone suppository are helpful. Patients should be advised to defecate when the urge is first experienced, avoid straining during defecation, and limit the amount of time spent sitting on a toilet. Although its effectiveness has not been evaluated objectively, witch hazel solution applied locally to the anus may reduce hemorrhoidal bleeding.

Indications for surgery are persistent bleeding and painful thrombosis not responding to medical therapy. A variety of surgical methods are used, including excision hemorrhoidectomy, rubber band ligation, cryosurgery, injection of sclerosing solutions, and extreme dilation of the anus. The rate of hemorrhoid recurrence is high after any method of surgical therapy.

SOLITARY ULCER SYNDROME

A single, usually large ulcer (often several centimeters in diameter) of unknown cause may occur in the cecum or in the midrectum. Solitary rectal ulcers have a high association with rectal prolapse and may be related to ischemia of a portion of the rectal mucosa produced by kinking or compression of the vasculature during prolapse.

Paradoxically, patients with solitary rectal ulcers rarely have rectal prolapse, possibly because they fail to notice the prolapse or because they are embarrassed to seek medical help. The usual presentation is rectal bleeding or, rarely, rectal pain. Because the ulcer is often large, with irregular edematous margins caused by granulation tissue, the lesion is often mistaken for carcinoma of the rectum after digital examination and/or sigmoidoscopy.

In patients with solitary rectal ulcers associated with rectal prolapse, the prolapse should be corrected surgically. Asymptomatic solitary rectal ulcers can be remarkably refractory, even to treatment with local adrenocorticosteroids. A stool softener and bulk agent (such as psyllium seed mucilloid) should be prescribed.

The patient with solitary cecal ulcer usually experiences lower gastrointestinal bleeding; very rarely, a cecal ulcer may be the source of colonic perforation. Entities to be excluded include Crohn's disease, carcinoma, or bleeding from some other site such as angiodysplasia or a diverticulum. Solitary cecal ulcers that cause symptoms require surgical resection.

ANAL FISSURE AND FISTULA

Stretching of the anal orifice during passage of a large, hard stool can tear the cutaneous-mucous membrane junction, resulting in a fissure. Anal inflammation secondary to any cause, such as herpes simplex type I or II, syphilis, or lymphogranuloma venereum, also facilitates formation of a fissure. On occasion, a fissure may bleed moderately. If it extends into a hemorrhoid, bleeding may become profuse. Most commonly, a patient with anal fissure complains of pain, particularly during defecation, with well-localized anal tenderness. The initial treatment is stool softeners (such as psyllium seed mucilloid) and sitz baths. If pain is severe, astringent-anesthetic solutions, ointments, or salves containing a local anesthetic may be added. Local corticosteroids can be used if infection can be excluded. If not associated with underlying inflammatory disease such as Crohn's disease or infection, fissures usually heal rapidly when the stools are softened.

Fistulas at or near the anus (rectal fistula, perineal fistula, or perianal fistula) are distressingly common complications of Crohn's disease and may be the first manifestation of that disease (Chapter 43). When perianal fistulas occur in Crohn's disease, there may not be obvious involvement of the rectal mucosa; the principal focus may be in distant bowel such as the terminal ileum. Short of local penetrating trauma, it is difficult to envision a cause for perianal fistula other than Crohn's disease. A perianal abscess can precede development of a perianal fistula. Patients with a perianal fistula have local pain, tenderness, swelling, and discharge of mucus, pus, or feces. The patient may have fecal incontinence if the fistula is severe and extends from rectal mucosa (and lumen) to perianal skin, bypassing the sphincter. If Crohn's disease is present, local surgery of the fistula may be followed by failure to heal and by further tissue breakdown. Therefore it is prudent to exclude conscientiously the possibility of otherwise occult or subclinical Crohn's disease before any local surgery is undertaken. Even then, better initial management might be prescription of antibiotics and stool softeners, local methylprednisolone injection, or, if the fistula is severe, bowel rest.

REFERENCES

Almy TP and Howell DA: Diverticular disease of the colon. N Engl J Med 302:324, 1980.

Barnes PRH et al: Hirschsprung's disease and idiopathic megacolon in adults and adolescents. Gut 27:534, 1986.

Brian JE, Jr and Stair JM: Noncolonic diverticular disease. Surg Gynecol Obstet 161:189, 1985.

Cho KC et al: Sigmoid diverticulitis: diagnostic role of CT comparison with barium enema studies. Radiology 176:111, 1990.

Ford MJ et al: Clinical spectrum of "solitary ulcer" of the rectum. Gastroenterology 84:1533, 1983.

Hughes LE et al: Local depot methylprednisolone injection for painful anal Crohn's disease. Gastroenterology 94:709, 1988.

Krishnamurthy S et al: Jejunal diverticulosis: a heterogeneous disorder caused by a variety of abnormalities of smooth muscle or myenteric plexus. Gastroenterology 85:538, 1983.

Meyers MA et al: Pathogenesis of bleeding colonic diverticulosis. Gastroenterology 71:577, 1976.

Mueller PR et al: Sigmoid diverticular abscesses: percutaneous drainage as an adjunct to surgical resection in 24 cases. Radiology 164:321, 1987.

Parikh DH et al: Abnormalities in the distribution of laminin and collagen type IV in Hirschsprung's disease. Gastroenterology 102:1236, 1992.

Puylaert JBCM et al: A prospective study of ultrasonography in the diagnosis of appendicitis. N Engl J Med 317:666, 1987.

Taguchi T, Tanaka K, and Ikeda K: Fibromuscular dysplasia of arteries in Hirschsprung's disease. Gastroenterology 88:1099, 1985.

Turgeon DK and Barnett JL: Meckel's diverticulum. Am J Gastroenterol 85:777, 1990.

Welch CE, Athanasoulis CA, and Galdabini JJ: Hemorrhage from the large bowel with special reference to angiodysplasia and diverticular disease. World J Surg 2:73, 1978.

CHAPTER

48 Gastrointestinal Manifestations of HIV Infection and AIDS

Donald P. Kotler

Gastrointestinal (GI) dysfunction is common in acquired immunodeficiency syndrome (AIDS). The GI tract and other mucous membranes have an inherent vulnerability to enteric pathogens, produced by the absence of a strong physical barrier. The GI tract also is in intimate contact with a multitude of potential pathogens in the external (luminal) environment. The defense of the GI tract includes an immune system that is homologous to but distinct from systemic immunity. Nonimmunologic factors also contribute to the defense of the GI tract. Deficiencies in either immunologic or nonimmunologic defenses leads to a series of disease complications. The aim of this chapter is to codify the effects of AIDS on the GI tract. Diagnosis and management are organized into a series of clinical syndromes.

The topic of mucosal immunity is reviewed in detail elsewhere. Mucosal immunity in individuals infected with the human immunodeficiency virus type 1, the etiologic agent of AIDS, has not been studied thoroughly, though there is ample clinical evidence and some confirmatory experimental evidence of mucosal immune deficiency. Immunohistochemical studies in AIDS patients demonstrated equivalent decreases in the helper T lymphocyte populations of blood and intestinal mucosa. Ultrastructural and flow cytometric evidence of lymphoid activation in the gut has been found. Evidence of immunoglobulin A (IgA) deficiency has been found in mucosal biopsy specimens and in saliva.

Several studies have demonstrated cellular reservoirs for

human immunodeficiency virus (HIV) in the GI tract. The evidence includes HIV deoxyribonucleic acid (DNA) by polymerase chain reaction and by in situ hybridization, HIV RNA by in situ hybridization, and HIV antigens by immunohistochemical staining and enzyme-linked immunosorbent assay (ELISA). In vitro infection of intestinal epithelial cell lines by HIV has been accomplished. Animal studies indicate that intestinal cells are reservoirs for retroviruses.

GENERAL PRINCIPLES OF EVALUATION AND TREATMENT

In HIV-infected individuals a wide variety of GI complications may develop (refer to the box below). Proper clinical management requires an appreciation of the different disease presentations in this group. The most striking difference between HIV-infected and other patients is the frequent coexistence of multiple enteric complications in AIDS patients. In most other circumstances, patients usually have a single disease entity, no matter how many or varied the symptoms: the so-called law of parsimony, or Occam's razor. Another aspect of the difference in disease presentations is that one organism may produce many different clinical syndromes while many organisms can produce identical syndromes. The implication is that investigations should be thorough and not necessarily stop once a single pathogen is found. The disease complications of AIDS are notable for their chronicity and, at present, susceptibility to suppression but resistance to cure. For this reason most treatments must be given chronically.

The specific pathogens producing disease in AIDS patients are different from those that usually affect immunocompetent individuals. However, HIV-infected individuals also are subject to common illnesses, such as appendicitis. In either case, the pathologic features usually match the clinical symptoms and physical findings, so that the inductive reasoning on which clinical diagnostics is based can be applied to gastrointestinal problems associated with HIV infection.

Gastrointestinal pathogens in AIDS patients

Parasites

Cryptosporidium parvum
*Enterocytozoon bieneusi**
Isospora belli
Giardia lamblia
Entameba histolytica
Blastocystis hominis†
Strongyloides stercoralis
Pneumocystis carinii

Bacteria

Salmonella sp.
Shigella sp.
Campylobacter sp.
Helicobacter pylori
Mycobacterium tuberculosis
Mycobacterium avium intracellulare
Clostridium difficile

Viruses

Human immunodeficiency virus†
Cytomegalovirus
Herpes simplex
Adenovirus
Epstein Barr virus†
Human papilloma virus
Hepatitis B
Hepatitis C
Hepatitis D

Fungi

Candida albicans
Torulopsis glabrata
Coccidioides imitis
Cryptococcus neoformans
Histoplasma capsulatum

*A second microsporidian species has been identified.
†Uncertain pathogenic potential.

CLINICAL SYNDROMES

Disorders of food intake

Oral candidiasis is the most commonly encountered complication in HIV-infected individuals and develops in more than three quarters of patients. The most common species is *Candida albicans,* which is part of the normal enteric flora. The presenting symptoms are sore throat and, if there is concomitant esophageal involvement, odynophagia, and substernal discomfort. Food intake may be decreased, and increased sensitivity of the oral mucosa to foods may be noted. Erosions and plaques on the gingiva, palate, hypopharynx, and/or esophagus are seen. Bronchial, gastric, and intestinal mucosae are not involved grossly or microscopically. In most cases, the diagnosis can be suggested by visual examination and confirmed by a response to treatment. Culture, biopsy, or brush cytology may be confirmatory.

Oral candidiasis can be successfully treated with topical or systemic agents; esophageal candidiasis requires systemically active agents. Topical therapies include nystatin and clotrimazole troches (Mycelex). Ketoconazole (Nizoral) and fluconazole (Diflucan) are effective systemic agents. A potential problem with treatment is decreased bioavailability of ketoconazole in the presence of hypochlorhydria, which has been documented in some AIDS patients. The infection is resistant to oral therapy in a small percentage of cases and must then be treated with intravenous amphotericin B.

Oral hairy leukoplakia is a whitish, verrucous excrescence that occurs along the sides of the tongue. Epstein-Barr virus has been found in the lesions by molecular hybridization studies as well as by electron microscopic examinations. There are few symptoms. Acyclovir or ganciclovir therapy causes resolution.

Painful ulcers or ulcerating neoplasms of the oral cavity, hypopharynx, or esophagus may cause significant impairment of food intake. Small aphthous ulcers in the oral cavity are common and may resolve spontaneously or after administration of topical steroids. Acute necrotizing ulcerative gingivitis (ANUG) is a focal, destructive process of uncertain cause that may extend to the bone. The most common viruses associated with ulceration are herpes simplex virus (HSV) and cytomegalovirus (CMV). If caused by HSV or CMV, the lesions respond to acyclovir and ganciclovir therapy, respectively.

Many esophageal ulcers in which no etiologic agent can be identified are seen. The presence of HIV in esophageal ulcers has been demonstrated, but its role in ulcer formation and progression is unknown. The ulcers are atypical in their large size and in the extensive undermining of the mucosa. The symptoms are refractory to antigastric secretory therapy and may respond poorly to opiates. Progressive malnutrition is the usual result in untreated cases. Corticosteroid therapy has been shown to produce symptomatic relief, weight gain, and ulcer healing in a substantial proportion of patients. Despite the potential hazards of steroid therapy, clinical experience has demonstrated that the treatment can be administered with relative safety.

Neoplasms, such as Kaposi's sarcoma or lymphoma, may affect food intake by interfering with mastication or swallowing. These lesions may respond to a variety of therapies.

In many cases, food intake is diminished in the absence of pathologic lesions. The causes are diverse but fall into several general categories: focal or diffuse organic neurologic lesions, altered release of cytokines caused by systemic illnesses, anorexia as an indirect effect of malabsorption, alterations in taste, nausea, and psychologic or psychosocial factors.

Dyspepsia

Nausea and dyspepsia are very common symptoms in AIDS but rarely dominate the clinical picture. These symptoms may be due to a variety of pathologic processes. The stomach may be involved by disseminated infections such as CMV, *Mycobacterium avium intracellulare* (MAI) and fungi, or tumors such as Kaposi's sarcoma, lymphoma, or adenocarcinoma. Symptomatic gastritis caused by *Helicobacter pylori* has been described but appears not to be common, possibly because of frequent antibiotic usage in AIDS patients. Some medications, such as nonsteroidal anti-inflammatory agents, promote gastric ulceration and produce dyspepsia. On the other hand, symptomatic peptic ulcer disease is uncommon in AIDS patients, possibly because of decreased gastric acid secretion. Dyspepsia is due to a low-grade pancreatitis in some patients and may precede the development of biliary tract disease (see later discussion).

The clinical symptoms are nonspecific. The presence of weight loss or fever implies a serious complication such as a systemic infection or ulcerating tumor. Treatment of dyspepsia depends on its cause. *Helicobacter pylori* in a symptomatic HIV-infected individual is treated in a similar manner to the infection in any other symptomatic patients. Diagnosis of CMV or MAI infection is an indication for anti-infective therapy. Widespread or ulcerating Kaposi's sarcoma is an indication for systemic chemotherapy, as is the presence of lymphoma.

Diarrhea and wasting

Diarrhea and weight loss are very common problems in AIDS patients, occurring in up to three quarters during the disease course. Symptoms are associated either with small intestinal injury and malabsorption or with enterocolitis. Although early studies reported large numbers of patients with unexplained diarrhea, an infectious agent can be found in the majority of AIDS patients, if a comprehensive evaluation is performed.

The clinical differentiation of malabsorptive from colitic disease is important in order to focus the diagnostic evaluation, though the possibility of multiple coexisting problems must be remembered. An algorithmic approach is shown in Fig. 48-1.

Parasites. *Cryptosporidium* is the most widely recognized enteric pathogen in patients with AIDS. The infection has a worldwide distribution and is responsible for 5% to 10% of cases of severe diarrhea in American AIDS patients. The parasite may infect immunocompetent individuals, who have a self-limited illness. Cryptosporidiosis has been implicated in traveler's diarrhea and in outbreaks of diarrheal disease in day care centers. Bidirectional infection of humans and animals has been reported. On the other hand, cryptosporidiosis usually is chronic and protracted in AIDS patients. Spontaneous remissions occasionally occur and may be related to a relatively high number of CD4+ lymphocytes or temporal rise in CD4+ lymphocyte counts.

A majority of affected AIDS patients have diffuse small intestinal disease without significant colonic involvement; others have an ileocolitis and no clinical or laboratory evidence of jejunal disease. Massive secretory diarrhea reminiscent of cholera occurs in a small percentage of patients with intestinal cryptosporidiosis and AIDS. The infection may spread to the biliary system, pancreas and gallbladder, and other areas.

Cryptosporidiosis can be diagnosed by special examination of stool specimens (Chapter 280) or intestinal biopsy specimens (Fig. 48-2). Therapeutic options for cryptosporidiosis are limited. Several antiparasitic agents are undergoing clinical trials. Immune bovine colostrum suppressed cryptosporidial infections in a child with a congenital agammaglobulinemia and in a few AIDS patients. Uncontrolled observations have demonstrated a positive clinical effect of paromomycin (Humatin, Parke Davis) in some patients.

Treatment of diarrhea caused by cryptosporidiosis may be difficult. Diet modification may help in patients with mild disase. Hydrophilic bulking agents generally are unhelpful. Opiates such as diphenoxylate, paregoric, or tincture of opium may be effective, though the amount required sometimes causes excessive sedation, and escalating doses may be required. Therapy with a somatostatin analogue

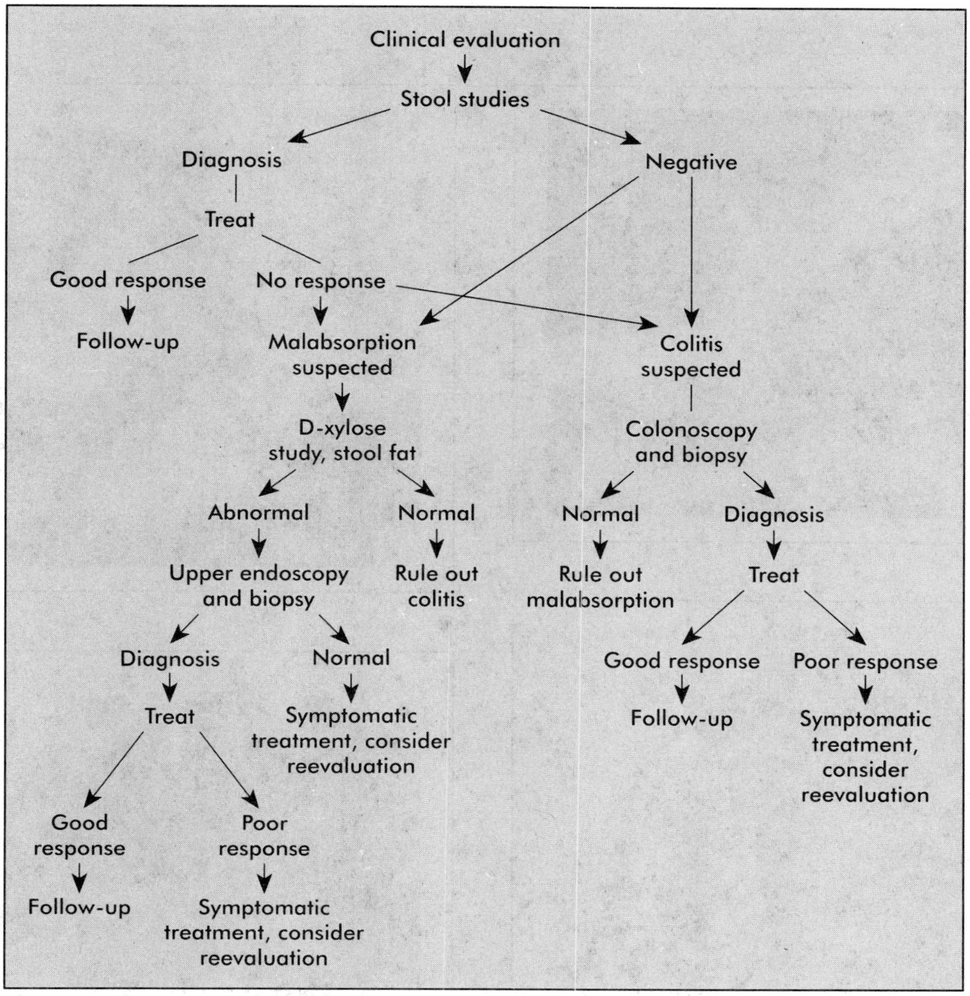

Fig. 48-1. An approach to the evaluation of diarrhea and wasting in AIDS patients.

may be successful. Despite these approaches, parenteral fluids often are required to maintain a normal state of hydration, and parenteral feedings may be required to maintain nutritional status.

Microsporidia have recently been recognized as a common cause of diarrhea in AIDS patients and may account for up to one quarter of cases of idiopathic diarrhea and progressive wasting. Two species producing intestinal disease have been identified. The majority of infections are caused by *Enterocytozoon bieneusi,* which is localized to the superficial epithelium. In most cases, the diagnosis requires electron microscopy of intestinal biopsy specimens for confirmation (Fig. 48-2), though microsporidial spores have been identified in stool specimens and intestinal aspirates. The second species, *Septata intestinalis,* can be distinguished ultrastructurally from *E. bieneusi.* In addition, the parasite may produce disseminated disease, as organisms have been found in the kidney, liver, and gallbladder.

Clinically, microsporidiosis resembles cryptosporidiosis and other diffuse small intestinal mucosal diseases; diarrhea is the major manifestation. There is no known effective therapy, though treatment trials are ongoing. Nutritional therapy is based on diet modification to decrease the fat and lactose content. Parenteral nutrition has been used in some patients.

Isospora belli has been reported frequently in AIDS patients from Haiti and West Africa, though fewer cases have been seen in northern climates. The symptoms are similar to those of cryptosporidiosis. Oocysts may be scarce in stool specimens (Plate V-1) and organisms rare in biopsy specimens (Fig. 48-2), so the diagnosis is more easily overlooked than is cryptosporidiosis. Successful disease suppression has been reported with trimethoprim sulfamethoxathole or pyrimethamine at various dosages but does not occur in every patient. Diarrhea often recurs on discontinuation of therapy so that chronic therapy with trimethoprim sulfamethoxathole, trimethoprim alone, or pyrimethamine and folinic acid is necessary.

Giardiasis (Fig. 48-2) is not a common cause of acute diarrhea in AIDS. Drug therapy with quinacrine or metronidazole is indicated if cysts or trophozoites are found, though suspicion of other causes should be high. Like gi-

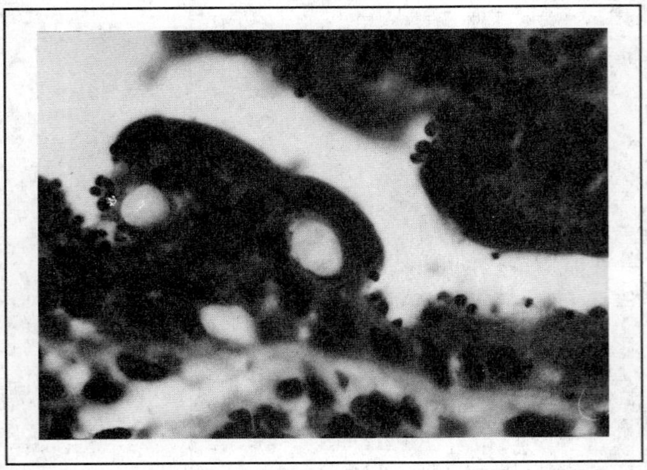

A

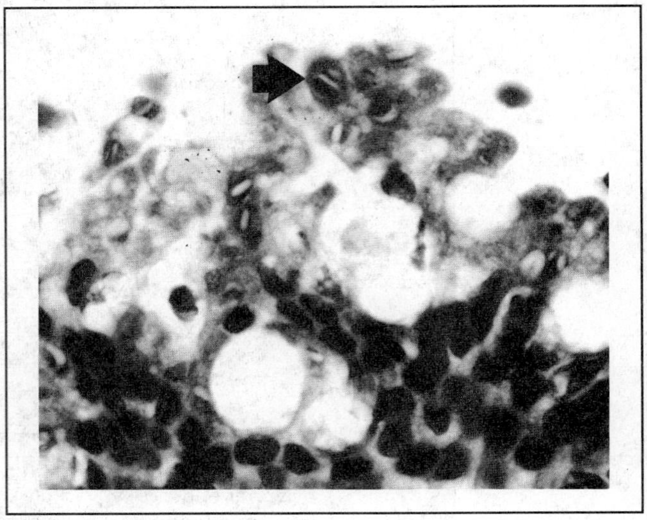

B

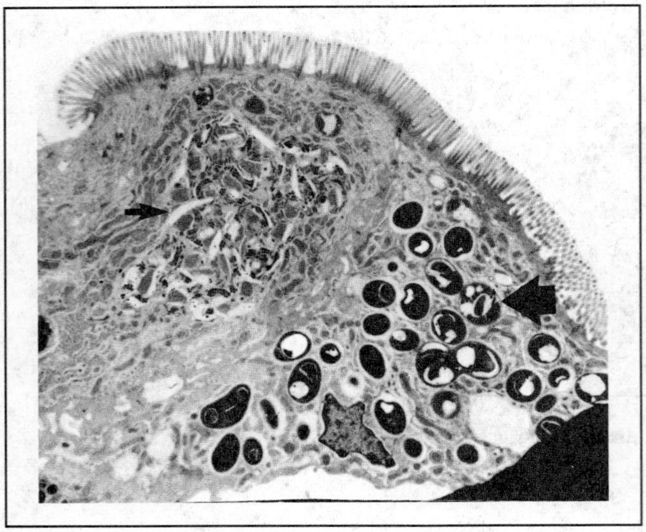

C

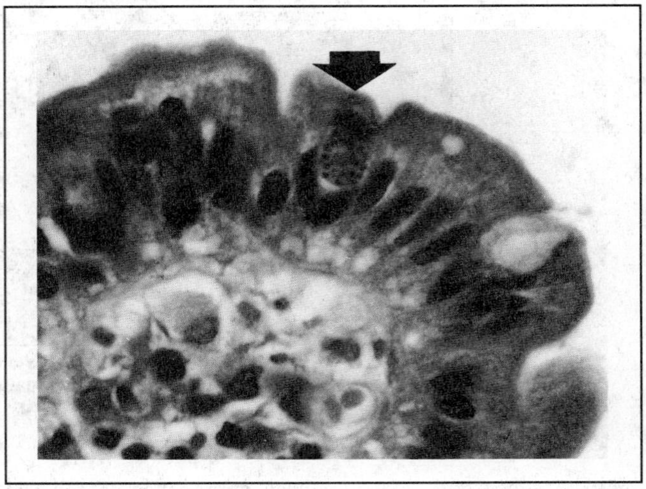

D

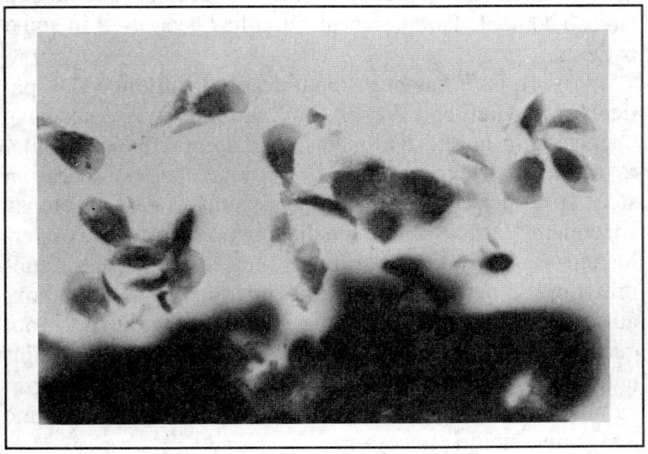

E

Fig. 48-2. A, Cryptosporidial organisms located at the epithelial brush border in the jejunum *(original magnification ×400);* **B,** Developing microsporidial organisms in sloughing cells at the jejunal villus tip *(arrow) (original magnification ×400);* **C,** Transmission electron microscopic photograph demonstrating developing organisms in one cell *(small arrow)* and mature spores in an adjacent cell *(large arrow) (×8000).* **D,** Microgametocyte of *Isospora belli (arrow)* in a jejunal epithelial cell *(original magnification ×400.* **E,** Trophozoites of *Giardia lamblia* adjacent to jejunal epithelium *(original magnification 400×).*

ardiasis, amebiasis is not a common cause of severe illness in HIV-infected patients. In the majority of cases, *Entameba histolytica* appears to act as a commensal organism. Although metronidazole therapy should be prescribed, the possibility of coexisting pathogens should be considered strongly. Other parasites have been reported, including *Strongyloides stercoralis,* which may produce a hyperinfection syndrome. *Blastocystis hominis,* which is considered by some but not by others to be an enteric pathogen, has been found in many HIV-seropositive people with diarrhea. Diarrhea may continue despite eradication of the organism.

Viruses. Cytomegalovirus (CMV) infection is common in HIV-infected individuals. Disseminated CMV infection is a progressive disease and contributes significantly to morbidity and mortality. Evidence of CMV infection is present in up to two thirds of autopsies, where the organs affected most commonly are the adrenals, lungs, and GI tract. CMV has been implicated in many GI syndromes and may infect any organ of the digestive system, but the most common presentation is CMV colitis. Patients complain of diarrhea, weight loss, and persistent fevers. In advanced cases, the diarrhea may become bloody. Development of severe abdominal pain may signal intestinal infarction or perforation.

The spectrum of endoscopic lesions in CMV colitis varies from essentially normal-appearing mucosa, to scattered groups of vesicles or erosions on an erythematous base, to broad shallow ulcerations that may coalesce. CMV often causes pancolitis but may be limited to a single area, especially in the right colon or ileocecal valve. Isolated deep ulcers caused by CMV also may occur in the absence of diffuse disease.

The diagnosis of CMV infection is made by histologic examination of tissue biopsy specimens. The key histopathologic feature is the characteristic intracellular inclusion. When inclusions are rare or atypical, immunohistologic or in situ hybridization techniques developed for clinical use may be helpful. Other available diagnostic techniques, such as viral culture and blood serologic analysis, generally are less useful.

Several agents are capable of inhibiting CMV replication. The most widely studied is ganciclovir. Clinical benefit from ganciclovir therapy in patients with serious CMV infection includes clinical stabilization, repletion of body mass, and prolonged survival. Ganciclovir is administered intravenously using an induction regimen followed by maintenance therapy, given through a chronic indwelling catheter. The drug has hematologic toxicity and may produce neutropenia. Foscarnet is an antiviral agent with activity against HIV as well as CMV. Evidence of clinical benefit has been reported. Like ganciclovir, foscarnet must be given by intravenous infusion. Other orally bioavailable antiviral agents with in vitro efficacy are being developed for clinical testing.

Adenoviruses are occasionally isolated from rectal swabs or biopsy specimens from AIDS patients with diarrhea and a stable or deteriorating course. Electron microscopic studies have demonstrated cytoplasmic inclusion bodies containing adenovirus in superficial epithelial cells.

The potential role of HIV as an enteric pathogen is undefined. A prospective study of HIV-infected subjects with abdominal complaints demonstrated significant correlations among altered bowel habits, altered histologic features, biochemical evidence of intestinal injury, and evidence of HIV production, which were independent of enteric pathogens. Mucosal content of an HIV-associated antigen, p24, was higher in HIV-infected individuals without AIDS than in AIDS patients. In a companion study, tissue content of inflammatory cells varied with HIV disease progression and was highest in a subgroup of non-AIDS patients. Mucosal lymphoid cellularity correlated with mucosal p24 content. These results suggest that inflammation and HIV expression in mucosa are related. An HIV-associated inflammatory bowel disease could be an important factor in the pathogenesis of the immune deficiency as well as a factor in disease transmission.

Bacteria. *Mycobacterium avium intracellulare* has been seen with increasing frequency in AIDS patients. The infection usually occurs late in the course of the disease in the setting of fever and progressive wasting. MAI rarely infects immunocompetent people. It is acquired orally or, possibly, by aerosol, and can disseminate widely in the liver, spleen, mesenteric and retroperitoneal lymph nodes, and intestinal mucosa. Nodes may undergo liquefaction necrosis and produce a syndrome that mimics an acute abdominal crisis. The intestinal lesion of MAI is the result of mucosal and submucosal infiltration with infected macrophages that block lymphatic flow and produce an exudative enteropathy.

Diagnosis is by culture or biopsy. Acid fast bacilli can be seen on stool examination, and their presence suggests possible intestinal involvement with MAI. Mucosal abnormalities on barium radiographs or thickening of the intestinal wall plus enlargement of mesenteric and retroperitoneal nodes on CT scan are characteristic though not diagnostic of MAI. Histologic demonstration of mycobacteria is straightforward, though molecular techniques are being developed to allow species identification on tissue sections. Recent studies have demonstrated clinical benefit of multidrug regimens.

Bacterial enteritides in HIV-infected persons include infections with salmonella, shigella, and campylobacter species. The incidence of serious disease is higher than in the general population. Bacterial enteritides in AIDS more frequently have a chronic, relapsing course, often with bacteremia. The diagnosis is straightforward with routine evaluation. Blood cultures as well as stool studies should be part of the evaluation of suspected infectious diarrhea with fever in an HIV-infected patient. Patients respond to antibiotic therapy with parenteral agents, though the incidence of disease recurrence after therapy is high. Chronic antibiotic administration may be needed.

C. difficile toxin–associated colitis is common in AIDS and resembles the clinical syndrome in non-AIDS patients. Suspicion should be raised by the clinical situation and diagnosis confirmed by stool toxin assay. Treatment with vancomycin or metronidazole is as effective in AIDS as in non-

AIDS patients. Residual symptoms can be managed with oral cholestyramine (Questran), which binds the bacterial toxin. Surveillance against recurrent colitis may be necessary in patients who require chronic antibiotic therapy.

Anorectal diseases

The anorectal region may be affected by ulcers, masses, warts, infections, and hemorrhoids. Anorectal ulcers may arise from stratified squamous epithelium in the anal canal, perianal and perineal skin, or rectal mucosa.

Herpes simplex virus (HSV) infections are common in HIV-infected individuals. The major clinical syndrome in AIDS is a slowly spreading, painful perineal or perianal ulcer. The primary lesion occurs at the pectinate line. Vesicles in the anal canal may be missed as they rupture during defecation or examination. Large, shallow, spreading perianal ulcers are recognized more commonly. Proctitis may occur but is more common in non-HIV-infected subjects. The diagnosis may be indicated by visual examination and confirmed by viral culture. Most patients respond to therapy with acyclovir. Parenteral acyclovir therapy is required for extensive lesions. Herpes simplex virus resistant to acyclovir has been demonstrated in patients with refractory ulcerations. The use of foscarnet or ganciclovir may bring resolution. Cytomegalovirus also can cause anorectal ulcerations. The diagnosis is established by biopsy and histopathologic findings. Ganciclovir or foscarnet therapy may be associated with clinical resolution.

A variety of classic venereal diseases can produce anorectal ulcerations. Diagnosis and therapy of *Neisseria gonorrhea* proctitis is similar in AIDS and non-AIDS patients. Syphilis may have an atypical presentation in HIV-infected subjects, and serologic diagnosis is affected by the presence of immunodeficiency. Darkfield examination or immunohistologic studies of clinical specimens may be needed to identify the spirochete (Plate V-2). Prolonged intravenous antibiotic therapy is required. *Chlamydia* are prevalent in sexually active groups, and the risk of infection rises with the level of sexual activity. Definitive diagnosis is made by cell culture. Usual therapy is oral tetracycline or doxycycline. The frequency of chancroid, caused by *Hemophilus ducrei,* in HIV-infected patients is unknown. The diagnosis usually is suggested on clinical grounds and confirmed after infection with *T. pallidum* is excluded. Therapy with either trimethoprim-sulfamethoxathole or sulfa drugs alone may be successful. Rectal spirochetosis has been recognized in homosexual men with or without HIV infections. The infection usually is asymptomatic and an incidental finding on evaluation.

Idiopathic ulcers of the anorectal region, similar to those occurring in the esophagus, are seen in AIDS patients. The pathogenesis of the painful ulceration is unknown. As with esophageal ulcers, they may contain evidence of HIV. The presence of CMV, HSV, human papilloma virus (HPV), acid fast bacilli, fungi, and other bacterial infections must be excluded by culture or histologic studies. Intralesional or systemic corticosteroids produce a prompt decrease in pain but have a variable effect on healing.

The incidence of anogenital neoplasms is increased in AIDS patients as it is in other immunosuppressed individuals. Kaposi's sarcoma and lymphoma in the form of mass lesions or ulcers are the most common neoplasms. Epidermoid cancers, including squamous cell and cloacagenic cancer, occur in anal skin and rectal glands, respectively. Although these cancers rarely metastasize in immunocompetent persons, they may do so in patients with AIDS. For these lesions, management after diagnostic biopsy includes excision, chemotherapy, or laser photocoagulation. Laser therapy of rectal Kaposi's sarcoma also is effective and may cause dramatic regression of bulky disease. The role of papilloma virus, the etiologic agent of condyloma acuminata (common venereal warts), in anorectal cancers is unclear. Specific serotypes of papillomaviruses are suspected as being cofactors for carcinogenesis in the anogenital region, and the incidence of squamous cell cancer of the anus was known to be increased in homosexual men before the recognition of AIDS. Leukoplakia of the anal canal, which is considered by some a premalignant lesion, is a common finding in HIV-infected homosexual men.

Hemorrhoids are common in HIV-infected persons. Factors predisposing to hemorrhoids may have predated the HIV infection. Severe diarrhea or proctitis may promote local thrombosis, ulceration, and secondary infection. Fleshy skin tags, resembling those seen in Crohn's disease, also are common.

Mass lesions

Kaposi's sarcoma in AIDS is indistinguishable, histopathologically, from classic Kaposi's sarcoma, endemic forms of Kaposi's sarcoma found in Africa, or the form that occurs during immunosuppressive therapy. Visceral involvement in AIDS patients with Kaposi's sarcoma is more common than in non-HIV-infected individuals with Kaposi's sarcoma. Visceral involvement may be asymptomatic. The diagnosis is made by visual inspection and confirmed by biopsy, though endoscopic biopsy may yield false-negative results if the tumor is in the submucosa. No treatment is needed in most cases. Kaposi's sarcoma is responsive to chemotherapy or radiation therapy, which can be used in symptomatic patients. Obstructive lesions can be treated effectively by laser ablation.

A high prevalence of extranodal high-grade non–Hodgkins B cell lymphomas has been noted in AIDS patients. The tumor occurs most commonly in the central nervous system and the gastrointestinal tract. Gastrointestinal lymphomas in AIDS, especially the Burkitt's lymphoma subtype, are biologically aggressive. The lesions may respond to chemotherapy, using combination therapies. There are few long-term survivors, however, because of the underlying immunodeficiency.

Sporadic reports of AIDS patients with carcinomas in the gastrointestinal tract have been published, but a higher incidence has not been documented convincingly.

Gastrointestinal hemorrhage

Gastrointestinal hemorrhage is not a common consequence of AIDS, but serious or life-threatening bleeding does occur. Bleeding may result from the same conditions that occur in the non-HIV-infected patient as well as from the tumors and ulcers seen in AIDS. Episodes of massive arterial hemorrhage have occurred in patients with acute or chronic intestinal ulcers or rapidly progressive Kaposi's sarcoma.

The basic concepts of diagnosis and treatment are the same in HIV-infected and noninfected individuals (Chapter 34). Bleeding lesions may be visualized by endoscopy and bleeding controlled locally. Angiographic localization of obscure lesions and pharmacologic control may be successful. If bleeding is related to a discrete ulcer, surgical excision may be indicated; surgery is less appropriate for patients with widespread disease. Proper management of bleeding neoplasms involves effective local control followed by systemic chemotherapy.

Complications requiring surgery

Disease complications requiring consideration of emergency surgical intervention occur in patients with AIDS. Perforated viscus occurs in AIDS, but the cause may more often be a solitary ulcer, CMV infection, or tumor rather than peptic ulcer disease or diverticulitis as in the case of patients without AIDS. Malignant obstruction usually is due to Kaposi's sarcoma or lymphoma rather than adenocarcinoma. Kaposi's sarcoma or lymphoma also may cause an intussusseption. Some patients with clinical peritonitis have had, at laparotomy, only mild fibrinous exudate without obvious perforation.

Though the physical findings of the acute abdomen are not significantly affected by the presence of AIDS, the laboratory evaluation differs markedly from expected. Elevated leucocyte counts with immature forms in the circulation may not be present, especially if there is pre-existing leukopenia or prior treatment with myelosuppressive drugs. Isotopic imaging studies such as an indium-labeled white blood cell study or gallium scan may yield false-negative results in the presence of severe leukopenia. Imaging studies such as CT scan with luminal contrast may be particularly valuable in detecting extraluminal collections of pus or fluid.

Although the indications for surgery are the same in AIDS patients and non-HIV-infected patients, the expected outcomes may differ. One can anticipate the possibility of unusual pathogens, prolonged recovery times, and impaired wound healing in AIDS patients. The incidence of postoperative complications and mortality was high in several series but was due to the seriousness of the underlying disease complications. Complete recovery after major abdominal surgery is possible in AIDS patients and may be followed by prolonged survival. Laparoscopic surgery has been used successfully in cases of chronic cholecystitis.

Hepatobiliary diseases

Three distinct clinical syndromes have been recognized: diffuse hepatocellular injury, granulomatous hepatitis, and sclerosing cholangitis. Many other patients with abnormal liver chemical findings have macrovesicular or microvesicular fatty infiltration or other nonspecific changes.

Diffuse hepatitis is most commonly a result of drug toxicity or hepatitis C or hepatitis D infection. Hepatitis B infection is clinically mild in most AIDS patients. Granulomatous hepatitis in AIDS patients is related to mycobacterial, fungal, or protozoal diseases or to drug toxicity. Fever and constitutional symptoms are prominent. Liver chemical test results demonstrate progressive elevations in the levels of alkaline phosphatase and gamma-glutamyl transpeptidase. Liver biopsy reveals poorly formed granulomas. Special stains can presumptively identify the causative organism. Peliosis hepatis has been described in AIDS patients and is associated with infection by a rickettsialike organism. A syndrome of sclerosing cholangitis has been frequently recognized in AIDS patients and resembles the non-AIDS variety. The pathogenesis is unknown, although cryptosporidia, microsporidia, and CMV inclusions have been observed in the biliary tract epithelium of some patients. Patients have nonspecific complaints and progressive cholestasis. Endoscopic retrograde examination demonstrates areas of narrowing and dilatation of the intrahepatic and/or extrahepatic ducts with mucosal ulceration. Endoscopic papillotomy, dilatation, or stent placement may give short-term relief. In long-term cases, progressive jaundice and liver failure may develop.

Pancreatic diseases

Pancreatic disease in AIDS has received little attention and may not be recognized before postmortem examination. The pancreas may be affected by systemic diseases, such as CMV, MAI, fungi, Kaposi's sarcoma, or lymphoma. Drug-induced pancreatitis is the most commonly recognized form. Hyperlipidemic pancreatitis has been observed. There are no reports of chronic pancreatitis as a specific complication of HIV infection. Pancreatic insufficiency is an uncommon cause of fat malabsorption in AIDS patients.

REFERENCES

Cappell MS: Hepatobiliary manifestations of the acquired immune deficiency syndrome. Am J Gastroenterol 86:1, 1991.

Cello JP: Acquired immunodeficiency syndrome cholangiopathy: spectrum of disease. Am J Med 86:539, 1989.

DeVito VT Jr, editor: AIDS: etiology, diagnosis, treatment, and prevention, ed 2. Philadelphia, 1988, JB Lippincott.

Glatt AE, Chirgwin K, and Landesman SH: Current concepts: treatment of infections associated with human immunodeficiency virus. N Engl J Med 318:1439, 1988.

Jacobson MA, and Mills J. Serious cytomegalovirus infection in the acquired immunodeficiency syndrome (AIDS): clinical findings, diagnosis and treatment. Ann Intern Med 108:585, 1988.

Knowles DM et al: Lymphoid neoplasia associated with the acquired immunodeficiency syndrome: the New York University Medical Center experience with 105 patients (1981-1986). Ann Intern Med 108:744, 1988.

Kotler DP: Gastrointestinal complications of the acquired immunodeficiency syndrome. In Yamada T, editor: Textbook of gastroenterology. Philadelphia, 1991, JB Lippincott.

Orenstein JM: Microsporidiosis in the acquired immunodeficiency syndrome. J Parasitol 77:843, 1991.

Ravalli S, Chabon AB, and Khan AA. Gastrointestinal neoplasia in young HIV antibody-positive patients. Am J Clin Pathol 91:458, 1989.

Rotterdam H and Sommers SC: Alimentary tract biopsy lesions in the acquired immune deficiency syndrome. Pathology 17:181, 1985.
Scannell KA: Surgery and human immunodeficiency virus disease. J Acq Immunodef Synd 2:43, 1989.
Smith PD et al: Gastrointestinal infections in AIDS: NIH Conference. Ann Intern Med 116:63, 1992.
Soave R and Johnson WD, Jr: Cryptosporidium and *Isospora belli* infections. J Infect Dis 157:225, 1988.
Young LS et al: Mycobacterial infections in AIDS patients, with an emphasis on the *Mycobacterium avium* complex. Rev Infect Dis 8:1024, 1986.

CHAPTER

49 Nutrition and Internal Medicine

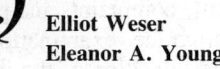

Elliot Weser
Eleanor A. Young

Nutrition plays an important role in the quality of life and in the prevention and treatment of disease. Many of the currently known nutrients are essential for life. Thus nutrition influences virtually every area of medicine.

Data from animal experiments indicate that the control of food intake by the central nervous system represents a basic integrative physiologic system. The existence of a "feeding center" in the lateral area of the hypothalamus and "satiety center" in the ventromedial nucleus of the hypothalamus is well established. Stimulation of the satiety center results in inhibiting food-eating behavior; ablation of the ventromedial nucleus (satiety center) results in hyperphagia. Numerous other reflexes associated with food intake are integrated and coordinated by these centers, resulting in a complex but basic system that regulates feedback control of nutrient intake. In addition, some enteric hormones are known to play a role in a gut-neural axis, which also affects eating behavior. Overriding this system in humans are cortical functions, such as psychologic influences, which add to the complexity of this regulation. Nevertheless, increased calorie consumption and obesity have been associated with hypothalamic injury or disease as well as frontal lobotomy and bilateral frontal cortical lesions, suggesting that this basic control system does operate in humans.

A complex array of metabolic, biochemical, and hormonal alterations occur within the host in response to systemic infection. These responses have nutritional consequences that vary in relation to the severity and duration of the illness. Both acute and chronic infections may deplete the body stores of nutrients and precipitate nutritional deficiency. This deficiency may result in greater susceptibility to secondary or superimposed infections as well as a general decrease in the ability to withstand the stress of disease. Additionally, severe protein-calorie malnutrition leads to impairment of nonspecific host defense mechanisms and specific forms of immune responsiveness, especially in hospitalized or ambulatory patients who have failed to maintain an adequate nutrient intake either as a result of disease or as a consequence of therapy (cytotoxic drugs, radiation, hemodialysis, etc.).

A close relationship also exists between nutrient intake and the gastrointestinal tract. Structural and/or functional changes within the small bowel may be produced by deficiencies in nutrient intake. Gastrointestinal disease may modify the digestion, absorption, and metabolism of nutrients and lead to secondary nutritional deficiencies (Chapter 28).

The liver is important in the utilization and storage of many nutrients. Abnormalities in the metabolism of protein, carbohydrates, fats, vitamins, and minerals often occur in liver disease and may have a significant impact on nutritional status. In time, this may affect the liver's ability to cope with further injury and contribute to the clinical complications of liver disease.

Epidemiologic studies suggest that 30% to 50% of all human cancers may be related at least in part to nutritional factors. The complexity of such relationships precludes an understanding of precise mechanisms at this time. On the other hand, a great deal of clinical experience is available for documenting the profound nutritional effects induced by cancer and the various modalities of therapy. Malnutrition may result from anorexia, impaired food intake (e.g., obstruction, nausea, reduced taste acuity), malabsorption, protein-losing enteropathy and disturbances of electrolyte and fluid balance. Radiation therapy, surgery, and/or chemotherapy used in neoplastic diseases frequently predispose the patient to nutritional problems precipitated by reduced taste acuity, dysphagia, bowel damage caused by radiation, direct toxic effect of drugs on the gastrointestinal tract, or resection of some portion of the gastrointestinal tract. Nutritional support therefore must be an essential component in the overall treatment plan for patients with cancer. This requires frequent assessment of the nutritional status of the patient, selection of appropriate nutritional therapy, and competent delivery of such support. Nutritional status, tumor growth, and antitumor treatment are interrelated, and the physician must have sufficient expertise to provide optimum medical management for cancer patients.

Nutritional status may be significantly compromised by chronic renal disease. Defective conversion of vitamin D_3 to 1,25-dihydroxycholecalciferol may cause decreased calcium and phosphorus absorption from the intestine, uremic osteodystrophy, and enhanced calcium reabsorption by the kidney. Renal disease may also affect the ability of the kidney to synthesize and catabolize certain hormones and amino acids; to degrade peptides and small proteins (e.g., insulin, glucagon, parathyroid hormone); and to produce or utilize certain amino acids (e.g., serine, alanine). Malnutrition can significantly affect renal function (e.g., glomerular filtration rate is decreased, as is the ability to concentrate and acidify urine). Thus nutritional therapy is an important consideration in the management of patients with renal disease. Hemodialysis or peritoneal dialysis may reduce the adverse effects of chronic renal insufficiency on nutritional status. However, inadequate protein and calorie intake may still contribute to malnutrition in patients undergoing dialysis. During dialysis, there are losses of free amino acids, peptides, bound amino acids, glucose, and water-soluble vitamins. Even in patients on maintenance dialysis therapy, body tissue wasting may continue as a result of catabolic effects related to complicating disease, endocrine disorders, blood loss, poor dietary intake, emotional depression, and anorexia.

Regulatory mechanisms of hormone action may alter metabolism and influence the distribution and utilization of nutrients within the body. Inappropriate hormonal secretion in some disease states may have profound nutritional consequences. Examples include diabetes mellitus; hypoglycemia; parathyroid-induced disorders of calcium, phosphorus, and magnesium metabolism; renal osteodystrophy; myxedema; and hyperthyroidism. Maturity-onset diabetes mellitus, the most common of the endocrine disorders, is frequently associated with obesity, elevated blood glucose and serum triglyceride levels, increased incorporation of triglycerides into prebetalipoproteins, elevated insulin levels, hypertension, and an accelerated rate of development of atherosclerosis. Restriction of calories to achieve and maintain desirable weight causes prompt reduction in serum insulin, blood glucose, and plasma triglyceride levels. Weight reduction and/or salt restriction may significantly improve hypertension in both diabetic and nondiabetic patients.

The nervous system tends to be more resistant to the effects of malnutrition than other body systems, and clinical manifestations occur only with an extreme degree and duration of nutrient depletion. Nutritional diseases of the nervous system are related to conditions of chronic stress, psychiatric disease, infection, hemodialysis, and alcoholism. Thiamine deficiency may lead to Wernicke's encephalopathy and Korsakoff's syndrome or to polyneuropathy. Deficiencies of niacin, pyridoxine (vitamin B_6), folate, and vitamin B_{12} may also lead to peripheral and/or central nervous system manifestations.

Anemia is probably the most common expression of nutritional deficiency in human beings. A deficiency of iron leading to hypochromic, microcytic anemia is widely recognized as the most important cause of anemia in the world. Depletion of body stores of folate or vitamin B_{12} leads to megaloblastic anemia. Anemia as a result of copper, vitamin E, and vitamin B_6 deficiencies has also been well described.

It is clear from these examples that nutritional deficiencies or excesses may be associated with a variety of diseases seen in the practice of clinical medicine. Malnutrition may precipitate or complicate existing disease states or be the end result of a disease process. The importance of nutrition requires that the physician be knowledgeable about its role in health and disease.

MALNUTRITION

Nutrition in health or disease is never an isolated phenomenon but is influenced by numerous, interrelated factors. Nutrition is the provision of adequate calories and essential nutrients to maintain health. In contrast, malnutrition refers to a state of bad or poor nutritional status. Although malnutrition is frequently considered strictly within the context of undernutrition, it is important that a broader view be taken in the practice of internal medicine.

One or a combination of several diseases may produce malnutrition. However, social, economic, psychologic, cultural, religious, and even political influences should be considered in the overall assessment of malnutrition. The five major factors contributing to malnutrition are undernutrition, overnutrition, imbalance of nutrients, increased nutrient requirements, and malabsorption.

Undernutrition

Undernutrition may result from inadequate intake of food or a deficiency of one or more specific nutrients.

Inadequate intake of food. Inadequate food intake may lead to a state of malnutrition depending on (1) the degree or severity of reduced food intake, (2) the duration of reduced food intake, (3) whether reduced food intake occurs during critical periods of rapid growth (infancy, adolescence, pregnancy), (4) the baseline body stores of nutrients, and (5) the presence of other factors such as fever, infection, immune status, and stress.

Primary chronic protein-calorie malnutrition is the predominant nutritional problem worldwide. In recent years significant progress has been made in preventing malnutrition in many areas, yet malnutrition remains a critical factor in disease prevention and health promotion in half of the countries of the world. The prevalence of protein-calorie malnutrition is directly related to inadequate food supply for the populations at greatest risk. It is estimated that 2 billion people, or about two thirds of the world's people, live in food deficit areas.[1]

Although protein-calorie malnutrition is much less prevalent in the United States, it does exist. The documentation of widespread malnutrition in the United States during the 1960s called forth development and expansion of federal food and nutrition programs to end hunger.[2] A great deal of progress toward this goal was achieved. However, currently the challenge of malnutrition is again a critical problem as a result of increased growth of the number of persons living below the poverty line, cutbacks of many federally subsidized nutrition programs, and growing numbers of persons seeking emergency food assistance. Substantive reports document evidence that there is a significant increase in hunger and malnutrition in the United States. The Physicians Task Force on Hunger reported (1985) that approximately 20 million Americans go hungry sometime during each month.

Documented protein-calorie malnutrition among hospi-

[1]WHO (Halfdan Mahler, Director-General). A Shift in the Wind. (No. 15), 1985.

[2]Panetta, L.E. Congressional Reports, Health and Medicine 2(3):18-19, 1984.

talized patients in the United States has been shown to range from 40% to 70%. These reports suggest that for hospitalized patients there are inadequate nutritional support, little or no attempt to reverse malnutrition, lack of concern and/or knowledge regarding nutritional status, and lack of clearly defined institutional goals regarding nutritional assessment.

Reduced total food intake is considered by many investigators as one of the major causes of weight loss leading to undernutrition in patients after total gastrectomy. After partial gastrectomy, approximately one half of patients lose weight and do not again achieve their ideal body weight. Reduced food intake may lead to malnutrition after small bowel resection and after jejunoileal or gastric bypass or volume reduction in markedly obese patients. Anorexia, loss of appetite, reduced food intake, and subsequent progressive tissue wasting are characteristically observed in patients with cancer.

Patients with anorexia nervosa experience significant weight loss and have an intractable negative attitude toward eating and weight gain that overrides hunger, admonitions, reassurance, and threats. Self-induced starvation results in cachexia, severe metabolic defects, and, if unchecked, in death (Chapter 37).

Other groups of patients at high risk for development of protein-calorie malnutrition are those with chronic alcoholism, renal disease, or draining abscesses, wounds, or fistulas and those receiving intravenous glucose support alone, with no oral intake.

Regardless of the cause of protein-calorie malnutrition, special attention should be given to nutrition in patients who are grossly underweight (weight/height ratio below 80% of standard) or who have recently lost 10% or more of their usual body weight.

Protein-calorie malnutrition should be further diagnosed as either marasmus (simple starvation) or kwashiorkor (acute visceral attrition). Table 49-1 indicates the comparative characteristics of kwashiorkor and marasmus. These two distinct forms of protein-calorie malnutrition differ in cause, pathophysiologic characteristics, symptom complex, and treatment requirements. For these reasons, differential diagnosis should be carefully made so that an appropriate nutritional support plan can be initiated.

Combined kwashiorkor and marasmus occurs when a chronically undernourished patient becomes acutely ill or stressed. This usually leads to a serious, life-threatening situation in which vigorous nutritional therapy is critical.

Overnutrition

Overnutrition is an excess intake of total calories or of a specific nutrient and represents another example of malnutrition.

Excessive intake of calories. Excessive intake of calories leads to obesity, a pathologic condition characterized by an accumulation of excess body fat. Obesity is the most prevalent form of malnutrition in the United States, afflicting approximately 40 to 80 million persons. Obesity alters a number of metabolic parameters and may complicate diseases encountered in clinical medicine.

Excessive intake of a single nutrient. Excessive intake of a single nutrient may produce an adverse effect, leading to malnutrition. Most vitamins and minerals are needed in only trace amounts. Usual therapeutic doses of water-soluble vitamins are normally excreted without ill effects. However, megavitamin therapy with pharmacologic doses of water-soluble vitamins may have toxic side effects. The fat-soluble vitamins are even more likely to be toxic.

Excess intake of minerals is much more likely to have a toxic effect than excess intake of vitamins. Hypermagnesemia has been reported in patients with renal insufficiency who are taking magnesium-containing drugs (e.g., antacids). High blood concentrations of magnesium (8 mEq/L) lead to central nervous system depression, pro-

Table 49-1. Comparative characteristics of kwashiorkor and marasmus

Kwashiorkor	Marasmus	Marasmic kwashiorkor
Edema; enlarged liver due to fat accumulation; hair: dry, brittle, easily pluckable; skin: scaly, hyperpigmented, erythematous	Obvious starved appearance; hair: sparse, thin, dry; skin: thin, dry, wrinkled	Combined clinical characteristics of kwashiorkor and marasmus Major features: (1) Edema of kwashiorkor with or without skin lesions (2) Muscle wasting and decreased subcutaneous fat of marasmus
Adequate fat reserves and muscle mass over short periods of adequate caloric but low protein intake	Severe fat and muscle wasting over prolonged periods of reduced caloric intake	
Depressed cellular immune functions Reduced wound-healing capacity Increased susceptibility to infection Lymphopenia: <1500 cells/mm^3 Serum albumin level: <2.8 g/dl Serum transferrin level: 150 mg/dl	Diminished skinfold thickness: <3 mm Height: weight ratio: $<80\%$ of standard Midarm circumference: <15 cm Serum albumin level: >2.8 g/dl Normal to low	Biochemical features of kwashiorkor and marasmus are seen. Alterations of severe protein deficiency usually predominate

found paralysis of the skeletal muscles, and respiratory distress.

Iron overload causing hemachromatosis and fluoride excess producing fluorosis are discussed in the sections on excess intake of minerals (Chapters 60 and 181).

Malnutrition produced by excess intake of trace metals is well documented. Excess iodide may lead to an inhibition of thyroid hormone synthesis, hypothyroidism, and iodide goiter. Acute copper intoxication in human beings causes nausea, vomiting, epigastric pain, diarrhea, headache, dizziness, and weakness. In severe cases, copper toxicity may lead to tachycardia, hypertension, coma, jaundice, hemolytic anemia, hemoglobinuria, uremia, and death. Toxic reactions generated by excess intake of manganese, cobalt, selenium, and cadmium have also been reported.

Imbalance of nutrients

Imbalance of nutrients may produce malnutrition. A protein's quality and biologic value are determined largely by the amino acids it contains. Low levels of essential amino acids or disproportionate ratios of amino acids alter the biologic value of a protein. Therefore in a diet limited largely to protein of vegetable origin, protein intake has to be greater than in a diet that includes protein of animal origin, because the amino acid ratio in animal proteins is more beneficial than that in vegetable proteins.

Heating a protein food in the presence of carbohydrate (Maillard reaction) produces an amino acid–carbohydrate complex that is not digested by human beings, with preferential binding of the essential amino acid lysine. This binding may result in an 80% loss of lysine, altering the amino acid ratio and decreasing the quality of protein present. This concept finds practical application in the processing of oral liquid formulas and solutions for total parenteral nutrition.

Folate therapy in a patient without adequate reserves of vitamin B_{12} can result in rapidly progressive subacute combined degeneration of the spinal cord, with neurologic deficits that may be irreversible.

Abnormalities of amino acid metabolism and urea formation are involved in the pathogenesis of hepatic encephalopathy (Chapter 56). The present therapy for hepatic encephalopathy produces a negative nitrogen balance, because it is based on decreasing the production of ammonia by reducing protein intake. In recent efforts to maintain nitrogen balance, a special mixture of amino acids has been used to normalize the amino acid pattern found in encephalopathy, and the keto analogs of amino acids have been used to offset hyperammonemia and negative nitrogen balance.

Many nutritional factors can increase urinary calcium, including increased vitamin D, magnesium, sodium, and vitamin A. Consumption of acids, ketogenic diets, and diets with a low calcium/phosphorus ratio causes hypercalciuria. Recent studies demonstrate that increased intake of dietary protein causes increased urinary excretion.

Nutrient imbalances other than deficiencies of iron, folate, or vitamin B_{12} have been shown to influence hematopoiesis. Anemia is often present in protein-calorie malnutrition and is thought to be due to an insufficient production of erythropoietin. Anemia characterized by neutropenia has been documented in copper deficiency. Vitamin B_6–responsive sideroblastic anemia is likely due to a defect in heme synthesis, although the exact location of the enzymatic block is not known. The hematologic effects of vitamin E deficiency in human beings have been debated. Hemolytic anemia has been clearly documented in premature babies maintained on tocopherol-deficient, high-polyunsaturated-fat formulas. It is suggested that in the absence of adequate vitamin E, polyunsaturated fats in the erythrocyte membrane structure are peroxidized.

Increased nutrient requirements

Increased nutrient requirements may lead to malnutrition unless intake of the specific nutrients required is similarly increased.

Fever and infection increase the need for nutrients. All infections result in aberrations of nutritional balance, with most notable effects on protein and nitrogen balance. Not only does the infectious agent block utilization of nutrients as an integral part of its attack on the host, but the host exhibits a series of metabolic reactions to infection that are detrimental to nutrition. Host defense responses include the synthesis of phagocytes and leukocytes, the production of immunoglobulins, and the synthesis of a variety of nonspecific proteins associated with the reaction to infection. Thus there are both increased losses of and increased requirements for nutrients, particularly protein, during infection.

Major injury, burns, undue stress, and fractures all increase the need for nutrients. For example, a severely burned patient may require about 6000 to 9000 kcal per day to maintain energy balance. In severe burns, weight loss during the recovery period may be 30% to 40% of the patient's preburn weight. Protein requirements may range from 3.2 to 3.9 g per kilogram of body weight (early catabolic phase) to 2.0 to 2.5 g per kilogram of body weight (early anabolic phase). Requirements for water and electrolytes are also elevated.

Nutrient requirements may also be increased by exposure to heat and to cold and by living at high altitudes. Athletes have increased demand for calories, but there is no evidence that protein, mineral, or vitamin needs are greater than in healthy nonathletes. Energy expenditure in the developmentally disabled patient or in the orthopedically handicapped patient may be increased or decreased, and caloric needs must be adjusted accordingly to prevent malnutrition.

Malabsorption of nutrients

Failure to absorb one or more dietary nutrients as a result of inadequate digestion or intestinal mucosal transport often produces severe malnutrition. Malabsorption may involve not only carbohydrates, fats, and proteins, but also water, electrolytes, calcium, magnesium, trace minerals, water-soluble and fat-soluble vitamins, and drugs (Chapter

42). By appropriate management of patients with malabsorption, malnutrition may be prevented.

OBESITY

It has been estimated that 25% to 40% of the adult population over the age of 30 years in the United States is more than 20% overweight. Although body weight that exceeds ideal standards as determined by age, sex, and height may be accounted for by greater bone or muscle mass, the majority of individuals who weigh more than 20% over their calculated ideal weight have excessive adipose mass. It is not yet certain whether the increase in regular exercise among various age groups in the population will significantly alter the incidence of obesity.

Although reduced longevity may not be associated with mild obesity, it is associated with extreme obesity. Increased susceptibility to cardiovascular disease (particularly hypertension), diabetes, pulmonary dysfunction, and gallstones is more often noted in the obese. Perhaps underemphasized are the psychologic, social, cultural, and occupational problems experienced by these patients (particularly in extreme obesity). The generally accepted increased risks of complications associated with anesthesia and major surgical procedures are additional considerations for the patient and physician. Obesity may affect the management of many disease states and requires attention in the total approach to the patient.

Causes

Various attempts have been made to classify obesity. An etiologic classification suggests four causes: (1) genetic transmission, (2) hypothalamic injury, (3) endocrine disorders, and (4) energy intake in excess of energy output.

Among experimental animals, several strains of mice with genetically inherited forms of obesity have been identified. Genetic causes of obesity in human beings are less clearly defined, and there has been consistent failure to demonstrate an inherited biochemical lesion that could explain obesity on a genetic basis. However, human population studies strongly suggest the existence of a genetic factor. Studies have shown that when both parents are of desirable weight, <10% of their children are obese. However, when one parent is obese, 50% of the children are obese, and when both parents are obese, over 80% of the children are obese. Correlations of parent-child weights comparing natural children with adopted children show significantly higher body weight correlations of natural parent–child weights. Studies of adopted children indicate that, relative to body weight, thin children tend to resemble their natural parents rather than their foster parents. Identical twins reared apart show higher weight correlations than do fraternal twins or fraternal siblings. None of these studies isolates genetic factors from environmental factors, an obvious limitation to gathering conclusive evidence of a genetic basis of human obesity.

Lesions of the hypothalamus induced by electrolytic, surgical, or chemical means can produce obesity in experimental animals, depending on the extent and location of the injury. There is an alteration of the set point at which body weight can be regulated, and excess weight gain is hypertrophic, caused mainly by enlargement of adipose cells with little change in the number of fat cells. There is clear evidence that injury to the hypothalamus can also produce obesity in human beings. Patients with obesity produced by hypothalamic injury are rare (about 100 such cases reported in the medical literature), and in such patients most hypothalamic injuries have been due to malignant tumors, inflammatory lesions, or trauma to the head.

The most striking form of obesity produced by endocrine abnormalities is seen in patients with Cushing's syndrome, insulinomas, or hyperinsulinemia associated with maturity-onset diabetes.

Obesity of specific genetic, hypothalamic, or endocrine origin is thought to account for <2% of all obesity. The overwhelming cause of obesity for most people is energy intake in excess of energy output, and a number of contributing factors are associated with this imbalance.

Restricted physical activity is a major cause of human obesity. Studies have demonstrated that obese persons are relatively inactive; however, there is no evidence that the obese are less active because of their obesity or that they are obese because they are less physically active. In either case, the effects of exercise on weight loss are clear. When energy expenditure is increased without a corresponding increase in food intake, body weight decreases. If food intake increases proportionately to exercise, body weight does not alter. With low levels of exercise, body weight and food intake tend to be higher than with moderate to high levels of exercise. Thus there is strong support for some form of physical activity as part of weight-reduction programs.

Subtle biochemical mechanisms may be operative in the development of obesity. An interlocking system of chemical reactions may lead to a futile cycle of thermogenesis. In this system, the thermal dissipation of food energy is much less marked in the obese than in the lean person. Thus in the obese person, more food energy is shunted into the body stores of fat than is dissipated as body heat. Occasionally, an obese person may consume approximately the same amount of calories as a lean person, yet remain obese. Recent studies have demonstrated that people differ with regard to energy requirements, ability to synthesize and dispose of fat, capacity to store fat, and appetite.

Socioeconomic factors may also contribute to obesity. Obesity has been shown to be 7 to 12 times more prevalent in lower socioeconomic population groups than in upper socioeconomic groups. Occupation, education, income, self-image, susceptibility to mass media influence, residential environment, and ethnic and cultural norms are all factors that may affect body weight.

Obese persons may be relatively insensitive to the internal hunger-satiety cues and excessively sensitive to the external cues of appearance, variety, aroma, and taste of foods. The obese person tends to overeat for nonphysiologic reasons, for when the external cues are removed, the obese person spontaneously decreases food intake and loses weight. The underlying mechanisms that trigger the "on" or "off" signals related to these cues require further study.

Frequency of food intake is another factor that may lead to energy intake in excess of energy expenditure. Controlled metabolic studies in human beings have demonstrated that when food intake is held both quantitatively and qualitatively constant, meal feeding (administration of total daily calories in a large meal rather than in small, frequent meals) is associated with increased lipogenesis, body fat, and cholesterol and insulin output and with decreased glucose tolerance.

Adipose cellularity may also be a significant factor leading to excess body fat. Studies of hyperplastic obesity (overweight condition related to an excessive number of fat cells) and hypertrophic obesity (overweight condition related to a normal number of fat cells of excessive size) have shown that (1) the number of fat cells can increase at any age; (2) once fat cells are made, they cannot be decreased in number by weight reduction; (3) the ability to attain normal body weight in relation to height is decreased in a person with an excess number of fat cells; and (4) when obese subjects lose and subsequently regain weight, the rate of weight gain is more rapid in subjects with hyperplastic obesity.

Dietary approaches

Caloric restriction and exercise are complementary approaches to weight reduction. A negative energy balance can be achieved by (1) decreasing caloric intake (approximately 3500 kcal equals 1 lb body fat) while keeping expenditure constant; (2) increasing caloric expenditure while keeping caloric intake constant; or (3) decreasing caloric intake and simultaneously increasing energy expenditure.

Although these thermodynamic facts are easy to understand, practical and realistic approaches to weight reduction are difficult for most obese patients and are strongly influenced by lifestyle, attitudes, knowledge, and understanding of the health-related risks of obesity, and a multitude of other biologic and social factors. Studies show that 15% to 20% of obese subjects are able to achieve a 20 lb weight loss by dietary means, while only 5% can achieve a weight loss greater than 40 lb. The percentage of patients who can maintain weight loss is substantially smaller.

Patients least likely to achieve weight reduction by dietary means (1) are morbidly obese, (2) have been obese since childhood or adolescence, (3) expect quick and dramatic results, (4) place the burden of success on the physician or on some special dietary manipulation, and (5) fail to realize that obesity is a serious disorder that is associated with significantly increased health problems.

There is no magic, miraculous, painless diet for weight reduction. The continual promulgation of new and faddish weight-reduction diets attests to this fact. The $39 billion diet industry (diet books, weight-reducing clinics, exercise equipment, diet pills, etc.) in the United States is considered by many to constitute a gigantic fraud on the American public. Most popular weight-reduction diets (Dr. Atkin's, Dr. Stillman's, Pritikin, Scarsdale, Last Chance, Air Force, Mayo, Drinking Man's) have not been tested in controlled long-term studies, thus making scientific appraisal difficult. No matter which diet is selected, certain general guidelines should be followed (refer to the box below).

Total fasting may be appropriate for patients with refractory obesity or for those who must reduce body weight quickly for medical reasons. Fasting should occur only with adequate medical supervision. The extent and rate of weight loss are directly proportional to initial weight, with greatest and most rapid losses occurring in the heaviest subjects. Men usually lose weight more rapidly, predictably, and linearly than women. Initial rapid weight loss is accounted for predominantly by decrease in body water level; a 2 to 11 lb weight loss may occur in the first 24 hours of fasting. Weight loss produced by decrease in body water level subsequently diminishes. Hunger is experienced by fasting patients for the first 2 to 4 days only, although many patients continue to be preoccupied with food. Prolonged fasting is accompanied by a number of physiologic and metabolic changes that should be continually monitored, including decreased body water level; electrolyte shifts produced by increased urinary loss of sodium, potassium, calcium, and magnesium; decreased volume of plasma and extracellular fluid; postural hypotension; continued negative nitrogen balance with loss of lean body mass; ketonemia; ketonuria; mild metabolic acidosis; hyperuricemia; hypoglycemia (40 to 50 mg/dl); decrease in serum cholesterol level; depletion of water-soluble vitamins (if not supplemented); and reduction in body fat stores.

With a semistarvation diet (400 to 600 kcal/day), some of the consequences of total fasting are ameliorated. Large losses of lean body mass can be prevented if 40 to 60 g protein is consumed, and this is one of the major advantages of partial over total fasting.

Short-term fasting interspersed with days of reduced caloric intake (fasting 1 or 2 days/week) may be an efficient approach to weight reduction. This approach has produced little adverse psychologic or physiologic stress; however, it should be based on a realistic weight-reduction plan.

A low-calorie (400 kcal) diet consisting of liquid pro-

Guideline for weight-reduction diets

1. Decide on rate of weight loss to be achieved. For most patients, a 1 to 2 lb weight loss per week is satisfactory.
2. Decrease caloric intake; 1 lb body fat = 3500 kcal.
3. Increase energy expenditure.
4. The percentage of calories should be 12% to 14% protein, <30% fat (with low-saturated fat), and 50% to 60% carbohydrate (with very low sucrose).
5. Provide for adequate intake of vitamins, minerals, and water. Supplementation may be needed when calories are restricted to less than 1000 kcal.
6. Provide for adequate and ongoing counseling and reinforcement aimed at behavior modification.
7. Salt restriction may decrease the tendency toward excessive fluid retention and may be effective in the prevention or reduction of hypertension.

tein hydrolysates, synthetic amino acids, or solid protein food has become popular over the past 10 years. This approach is based on the premise that complete elimination of carbohydrate from the diet enhances ketosis, eliminates hunger, improves compliance, and spares body protein. This approach is currently considered experimental, and the efficacy and potential risks have not been established. In some 50 patients who died while on protein-sparing diets, acute cardiac arrhythmia was suggested as the most common cause of death. Protein-sparing diets have not been shown to elicit greater patient compliance, and greater long-term acceptance remains unproved. Furthermore, weight loss on a hypocaloric pure-protein diet has not been found to be superior to that on a hypocaloric mixed diet.

Many popular diets are based on some alteration of the major energy components. Regardless of the claims made by proponents of such diets, well-controlled metabolic studies demonstrate that the most important single factor in weight loss is reduction of total caloric intake. On a long-term basis, the rate of weight loss is similar regardless of the ratio of carbohydrate, fat, and protein in the diet if total caloric intake is less than caloric expenditure. In patients on low-carbohydrate diets, initial weight loss is more rapid than in patients on carbohydrate-containing diets, but this initial weight loss is due mainly to loss of water.

Numerous one-food diets (egg diet, grapefruit diet, banana diet, etc.) have been in vogue for many years; however, compliance with such regimens is short-lived. In addition, no one food contains all of the essential nutrients, and the utilization of any one food for extended periods of time results in nutritional deficiencies.

A lecithin–kelp–vitamin B_6–cider vinegar diet continues to be widely published, although a well-controlled metabolic study indicated no advantage in weight reduction when use of capsules containing these ingredients was compared with use of a placebo.

Weight Watchers, TOPS (Take Off Pounds Sensibly), and other group approaches have been somewhat more successful than diet alone. These diet programs apply behavior-modification techniques and place emphasis on changes in lifestyle.

Exercise

A regular plan of exercise is an essential component of every weight-reduction program. Consideration should be given to the specifics of an exercise plan, including the type, duration, place, and time of exercise to be accomplished on a day-to-day basis. In order to enhance and encourage compliance, an evaluation of the exercise program should be included as a component of the medical assessment of the patient's progress. Elderly and/or physically disabled patients may benefit from assistance from a physical therapist regarding appropriate kinds of exercise. Aerobic expenditure of energy (e.g., walking briskly, running, swimming, bicycling) at a relatively constant but low level may have optimum effects on the cardiovascular system. Increased pulse rate and cardiac output should be reached and sustained for at least 15 minutes to achieve the greatest benefits from exercise.

Other approaches to weight reduction

Other approaches include behavior-modification, self-management training, external reinforcement, psychotherapy, psychiatric analysis, hypnosis, acupuncture, and ear lobe stapling. Most of these therapies have focused on helping patients achieve dietary self-control through understanding and modification of the conditions that affect their eating behavior. Recent reviews of studies using these methodologies indicate that they have greatly contributed to our understanding of the complexities of obesity. Most studies report changes that are clinically small, are variable, and usually cease at termination of formal therapy. Support for the effectiveness of these methods of therapy to produce long-term weight loss or behavioral change in the obese patient is yet to be demonstrated.

Numerous commercial gimmicks for weight loss such as sauna baths, body wraps, sweat suits, and vibrators have no known advantage in weight reduction and may precipitate adverse medical complications. These therapies are an economic fraud in addition to being ineffective in weight reduction.

Medical management

Although caloric restriction and increased energy expenditure are the basic treatment for obesity, the judicious use of amphetamines or other derivatives of phenylethylamine, particularly in the beginning phase of weight reduction, may be helpful. By stimulating the satiety center in the hypothalamus, amphetamines are thought to suppress appetite and inhibit intake. They are useful in patients with clear patterns of satiety and hunger. If the dose and timing of medication are correct, the patient may experience significant weight loss early in the diet and gain a sense of accomplishment as well as encouragement. In addition to suppressing appetite (and food intake), amphetamines stimulate the central nervous system, and patients may experience increased activity levels, which also contribute to weight reduction. Because these drugs have adrenergic effects on the heart and may cause serious arrhythmias, they should be used with caution in patients with heart disease, severe hypertension, hypothyroidism, glaucoma, agitated states, and history of previous drug abuse. An exception is fenfluramine, which has side effects of drowsiness, depression, and diarrhea, necessitating caution in its use in patients with depression or those taking central nervous system (CNS) depressants. Tolerance to amphetamines develops in approximately 4 to 6 weeks, and once tolerance develops they no longer adequately suppress the desire for food intake. Therefore amphetamine usefulness is short-lived, and they are best used in patients with recent onset of obesity. In a patient already receiving dietary and behavioral treatment, amphetamines may increase weight reduction by only an additional 10%.

Recently, numerous agents for weight reduction have become available as over-the-counter substances. These agents include phenylpropanolamine, benzocaine, bulk agents, spirulina, and a variety of food substances. Phenylpropanolamine is an active ingredient in many commercial products and is related chemically and pharmacologically to the phenylethylamines, although the side effects are generally milder. Nevertheless, the same precautions should be exercised in their use. The long-term effectiveness of these over-the-counter compounds is controversial and not medically proved.

Unless a patient has proven hypothyroidism, thyroid derivatives should not be used to produce weight loss. Dosages sufficient to cause weight reduction are likely to produce clinical hyperthyroidism. The use of human chorionic gonadotropin injections has also been advocated as a means of producing weight loss. Controlled studies have clearly shown that reduction in weight occurs only when this agent is used as an adjunct to caloric restriction. Resultant weight loss is completely accounted for by the ingestion of fewer calories.

Surgical therapy

It has been estimated that among men and women in the United States between 20 and 74 years of age, 4.9% and 7.2%, respectively, are severely obese as determined by skinfold thickness. In these persons, who are commonly referred to as the morbidly obese, the death rate may be up to 12 times that in a nonobese, matched population. Only 10% or less of extremely obese persons who do manage to lose significant amounts of weight (50% to 60% of initial body weight) by rigid dietary regimens are able to maintain weight loss for more than a few years. For these reasons, surgical approaches have been designed to decrease the ability to ingest food or to reduce its absorption significantly. Currently, there is still much debate about the overall medical usefulness, ethics, and research assessment of these procedures.

Lipectomy and wiring of the jaw have not proved adequate or effective on a long-term basis. Most experience has been acquired with the jejunoileal bypass, which essentially creates a short gut and results in impaired absorption. In most cases, significant weight loss results, usually about 40% of initial weight. Some regain the weight after 3 years. Two major factors influencing loss of weight are (1) degree of malabsorption, which is related to the length of unresected bowel and extent of adaptive changes, and (2) reduction in caloric intake. The latter may occur as a result of unpleasant intestinal symptoms precipitated by food intake and/or an altered taste acuity or desire to eat.

Numerous complications have been associated with the jejunoileal bypass (apart from the high surgical and anesthetic risks) for extremely obese individuals. These complications include oxalate stones and renal disease, liver necrosis and failure, malnutrition and intractable diarrhea, severe electrolyte imbalances, immune-complex arthritis, osteomalacia, proctitis and hemorrhoids, vitamin deficiencies, nausea and vomiting, intestinal pseudo-obstruction, and neuromyopathy. Because of the high incidence of these complications, jejunoileal bypass has largely been abandoned.

In recent years, gastric reduction surgery has replaced jejunoileal bypass as the preferred operation for morbid obesity. These procedures essentially create a gastric pouch that, because of its small size, limits the amount of food that can be eaten at any one time. Satisfactory weight loss appears to be well maintained in most patients. Although the metabolic complications associated with the jejunoileal bypass are not prevalent after these gastric procedures, they may result in complications, including bile reflux gastritis, staple dehiscence, anastomotic leaks, stenosis or ulceration, perforation of the gastric pouch, dumping syndrome, and failure to lose weight by patients who succeed in overcoming the limitations imposed by the gastric pouch. For some, malnutrition may also result from inadequate nutrient intake, too-rapid weight loss, and noncompliance in taking appropriate vitamin-mineral supplements. Nutrients most frequently reported to be deficient in patients with gastric reduction are thiamine, folate, vitamin B_{12}, vitamin A, and iron.

All surgical treatment for morbid obesity is palliative and not designed to treat the basic defect. The essential issue in obesity is behavioral, and completely satisfactory treatment must necessarily deal with this issue.

VITAMINS

Vitamins play an important role in health maintenance and in specific treatment of a variety of diseases. The initial awareness of vitamins resulted from identification of a group of vitamin-deficiency diseases (i.e., pellagra, beriberi, rickets, and scurvy), now essentially eliminated in the United States but still present in underdeveloped countries. Vitamins are biologically active organic compounds that are essential for normal growth, development, and health and that cannot be synthesized by the body. They must be obtained from exogenous sources, mainly dietary, and transported via the circulation in very low concentrations to a target organ. The vitamins may be separated into two groups, depending on their absorptive media. Vitamins A, D, E, and K are fat soluble and therefore intimately associated with lipid absorption. The nine water-soluble vitamins are thiamine (vitamin B_1), riboflavin (vitamin B_2), niacin, pyridoxine (vitamin B_6), folic acid, cyanocobalamin (vitamin B_{12}), ascorbic acid (vitamin C), pantothenic acid, and biotin. Four of the water-soluble vitamins are absorbed by active transport (thiamine, folic acid, ascorbic acid, and vitamin B_{12}) and the remaining five by passive diffusion through intestinal mucosa. The biochemical actions of the vitamins are listed in Table 49-2.

Vitamin-deficiency diseases

Vitamin A deficiency. Vitamin A deficiency from dietary causes is rare in North America and Western Europe, but represents an important cause of blindness in Southeast Asia, parts of Africa, and Central and South America. In these areas, the deficiency usually results from general malnutrition (often associated with kwashiorkor) in infants and young children. In the United States, vitamin A deficiency in adults is likely to be secondary to severe malabsorption (steatorrhea of diverse origin) or a restricted diet such as in anorexia nervosa. Low serum vitamin A levels are found in abetalipoproteinemia. Recent nutrition surveys in the

Table 49-2. Biochemical function of vitamins

Vitamin	Biochemical action
A	Stabilization of cell membranes Formation of visual pigments Synthesis of mucopolysaccharides
D	Increased intestinal calcium and phosphorus absorption Initiation of calcification of bone and activation of alkaline phosphatase Help in maintenance of serum calcium and phosphorus
K	Catalysis of synthesis of factors VII, VIII, IX, and X Cofactor in oxidative phosphorylation
E	Biologic antioxidant Protection of unsaturated fatty acid membranes
Thiamine (B_1)	Coenzyme in thiamine pyrophosphate Catalysis of decarboxylation of pyruvic acid and alpha-ketoglutaric acid
Riboflavin (B_2)	Coenzyme in flavoprotein enzyme system
Niacin	Coenzyme in nicotinamide dinucleotide Codehydrogenase for metabolism of alcohol, lactate, alpha-hydroxybutyrate
Pyridoxine (B_6)	Coenzyme in pyridoxal phosphate Activity in transamination, decarboxylation, deamination, desulfuration
Folic acid	Coenzyme in pyrimidine metabolism Transfer of single carbon units
Cyanocobalamin (B_{12})	Coenzyme in hydroxocobalamin Methyl biosynthesis, transmethylation, nucleic acid synthesis Activation of folic acid coenzymes
Ascorbic acid (C)	Antioxidant-reducing substance Hydroxylation of proline, tryptophan Iron reduction, absorption
Biotin	Coenzyme for carbon dioxide fixation (carboxylation)
Panthothenic acid	Conversion to coenzyme A

United States indicate significantly lower serum retinol levels in certain ethnic populations (e.g., Mexican-Americans in the Southwest).

The earliest symptoms of vitamin A deficiency are night blindness and xerosis (drying) of the conjunctivae. Xerophthalmia, or extreme dryness of the conjunctivae, may be associated with xerosis conjunctivae (Bitôt's spots), in the sclera, which are foamy, triangular white patches on the outer and inner sides of the cornea, consisting of shed corneal epithelium. The tarsal glands along the margin of the eyelid may enlarge and resemble a string of beads. Untreated, xerosis of the cornea, with photophobia, keratomalacia, corneal perforation, collapse of the iris, and lens extrusion, may occur. Abnormal keratinization of skin epithelium also occurs and may lead to folliculosis, follicular hyperkeratosis, and phrynoderma ("toad skin"). An early symptom is dry, rough, and pruritic skin.

In general, vitamin A deficiency responds rapidly to vitamin A–replacement therapy. If the eye lesions have progressed to the severe destructive stage, little can be done to restore vision. Mild cases of night blindness show rapid improvement (after the equivalent of 1000 units of vitamin A (as the vitamin itself or as fish liver oil). Keratomalacia, xerophthalmia, and advanced skin changes may require doses in excess of 100,000 units daily for several months.

Vitamin D deficiency. In the United States, vitamin D deficiency in infants and children has become a rare disease largely because of the enrichment of cows' milk with vitamin D and sufficient exposure to sunlight. As a result, deficient mineralization of growing bones leading to growth retardation and rickets is uncommon. Vitamin D deficiency in adults is usually related to intestinal malabsorption or altered vitamin D metabolism as seen in chronic hepatic and renal diseases.

Osteomalacia, with bone pain, widespread demineralization of bone, and microfractures or compression fractures, may be a presenting feature. Often, hypocalcemia is present and may cause tetany.

Treatment of vitamin D deficiency and osteomalacia in the presence of malabsorption may require doses of vitamin D in excess of 50,000 units daily. In addition, 15 g of calcium gluconate or lactate daily may also be necessary. Acute tetany requires immediate treatment with intravenously administered calcium gluconate, usually given as 10 to 20 ml of a 10% solution.

Vitamin K deficiency. It is unlikely that vitamin K deficiency occurs solely as a result of inadequate dietary intake. Amounts adequate to meet daily requirements are supplied not only from the diet but also from synthesis of vitamin K by intestinal bacteria. Inadequate absorption of vitamin K may occur in biliary obstruction and all other steatorrheic disorders, presumably because of its excretion with unabsorbed fat. Prolonged administration of antibiotics, particularly in children, may produce a deficiency that is probably related to altered or suppressed intestinal bacterial flora.

Hemorrhage is the clinical manifestation of vitamin K deficiency, which is usually indicated by decreased prothrombin activity in the blood not associated with concomitant liver disease. The hypoprothrombinemia is readily corrected by administration of vitamin K orally, 2 to 5 mg daily. Synthetic, water-soluble preparations are equally effective and particularly useful when bile duct obstruction or steatorrhea is present.

Vitamin E deficiency. Although vitamin E is essential in human nutrition, no clearly established deficiency syndrome has been consistently reported, although there is evidence that vitamin E replacement prevents the neurologic and visual complications that develop in patients with abetalipoproteinemia (Chapter 42). It has been suggested that vitamin E deficiency in premature and low-birth-weight infants causes hemolytic anemia and peripheral edema. There is no convincing evidence that vitamin E has any beneficial effects on the human reproductive system, habitual abortion, or in the treatment of myoneurogenic or cardiac diseases. Vitamin E does contribute an antioxidant role important in cancer prevention.

Thiamine (vitamin B_1) deficiency. Thiamine deficiency occurs in countries where polished rice is the staple dietary cereal or in instances of deprivation associated with dietary habits (food faddism, weight-reducing diets, anorexia nervosa, etc.). In the United States, thiamine deficiency is most commonly associated with chronic alcoholism. Partial deficiency coupled with increased requirements (rapid growth, pregnancy, lactation, hyperthyroidism, gastrointestinal disease, etc.) may also lead to clinical manifestations. In these instances, multiple deficiencies often occur together, particularly those of thiamine, riboflavin, and niacin.

Clinical manifestations of thiamine deficiency are related to the degree and duration of the deficit. Milder states of deprivation produce polyneuritis or dry beriberi. Greater degrees of thiamine deficiency cause beriberi, heart disease and, in severe cases, Wernicke's encephalopathy and Korsakoff's syndrome. In severely depleted alcoholic patients, glucose infusion without added thiamine may precipitate Wernicke's encephalopathy or cause an early form of the disease to progress rapidly. In general, B vitamins should be added with glucose solutions in all cases even though this complication is not due primarily to vitamin deficiency.

The early symptoms of thiamine deficiency may be nonspecific and undiagnosed. Intellectual impairment, emotional disturbances, reduced strength, weight loss, fatigue, difficulty walking long distances, insomnia, headache, and muscle tenderness may occur. The progression of impairment is variable, leading to dry, wet, or acute beriberi. Dry and wet beriberi are probably different manifestations of polyneuritis, although the pathogenesis of the edema is not clear. Early in the dry form, the patient may experience paresthesia, numbness, and muscle pain, leading to a slow and deliberate gait. Tendon reflexes may be exaggerated and later decrease or disappear. Muscle weakness may ensue, particularly in the lower extremities and torso. Ultimately, foot or wrist drop occurs, as does aphonia, which indicates paralysis of laryngeal muscles.

The wet form of beriberi is associated with peripheral edema and serous effusions. Although cardiac abnormalities are common at some stage of beriberi, edema may occur in the absence of heart disease. Certainly, heart failure with cardiac enlargement, tachycardia, cyanosis, and late pulmonary edema cause edematous fluid accumulation.

Acute, fulminant beriberi heart disease is typically accompanied by severe dyspnea, pronounced palpitations, and intense precordial chest pain. Heart failure of beriberi has been characterized as a high-output type during the earlier stages of the disease. If untreated, beriberi heart disease runs a progressive course, resulting in death usually within 1 year.

Wernicke's encephalopathy is characterized by altered mentation, eye muscle paralysis, weakness, and ataxic gait. Nystagmus is invariably present, as is paralysis of conjugate gaze. After treatment is begun with thiamine, Korsakoff's syndrome may become apparent. Memory of recent events is impaired and often associated with marked confabulation. There may be amnesia with regard to events during past months or years. Untreated Wernicke's encephalopathy results in high mortality; early treatment may effect complete recovery. Some features of Korsakoff's syndrome may not disappear, however.

The diagnosis of thiamine deficiency can be substantiated by measuring 24-hour urinary thiamine excretion. Values from 0 to 15 μ/24 hr have been found in beriberi. The usual dosage for adults with mild beriberi is 10 mg thiamine taken orally three times daily. In severe cases and in Wernicke's encephalopathy, 25 mg thiamine should be given intravenously, immediately and then two times per day. Patients with acute beriberi heart disease should receive higher doses (about 100 mg) along with other treatment for heart disease.

Riboflavin (vitamin B_2) deficiency. Riboflavin deficiency is found in all parts of the world, including the United States. Inadequate dietary intake is the principal cause, although intestinal malabsorption or poor utilization in patients with cirrhosis of the liver may also produce the deficiency.

The principal manifestations are cheilosis, angular stomatitis, seborrheic dermatitis, and glossitis. Photophobia, lacrimation, and itching of the eyes may also occur. Fissures may extend out from the angles of the lips onto the cheek or into the mouth in severe cases, and scars may remain after treatment and healing. Erythematous skin lesions of the scrotum and vulva may develop, with scaling and desquamation. The tongue may be deeply fissured and have a purple appearance. There also may be superficial vascularization of the cornea, ultimately producing punctate opacification and ulceration. Conjunctivitis and iritis may accompany the corneal lesions.

The diagnosis should be suspected from the history and clinical findings and can be confirmed if there is decreased 24-hour urinary excretion of riboflavin. Normal values are usually greater than 1000 μ/24 hr. Values less than 50 μ/24 hr are diagnostic of riboflavin deficiency.

In adults, administration of 2 to 5 mg riboflavin three times daily for several weeks usually results in rapid healing of the lesions. Some of the ocular symptoms may be relieved if vitamin A is given before riboflavin therapy, and even greater resolution results with riboflavin. Adequate dietary intake of milk, liver, meat, eggs, and some green leafy vegetables prevents recurrence.

Niacin deficiency. Niacin is a generic name for both nicotinic acid and nicotinamide, both biologically active and equivalent vitamins. The most prevalent cause of niacin deficiency (pellagra) in the United States is inadequate intake caused by chronic alcoholism. Often, increased requirements associated with physical labor or exposure to the sun may contribute to the clinical presentation. In areas of the world where corn is the staple, cereal pellagra is common among the poor. Corn is low in tryptophan, which is the amino acid precursor of niacin and also contains niacin in a bound and unusable form (niacytin). Niacin deficiency may also occur in patients with malignant carcinoid tumors, because a large amount of tryptophan is converted to 5-hydroxytryptamine (serotonin) instead of niacin. Isoniazid therapy has also been associated with niacin deficiency, presumably because of induced pyridoxine deficiency, which decreases the conversion of tryptophan to niacin.

Pellagra is characterized by dermatitis, diarrhea, inflammation of the mucous membranes, and mental symptoms. Early symptoms that may precede skin changes include anorexia, weight loss, mild digestive complaints, lassitude, irritability, depression, memory loss, anxiety, and confusion. Initially, dermatitis resembles ordinary sunburn, affecting particularly the parts of the body exposed to the sun. The affected skin may then become increasingly pigmented and clearly demarcated from uninvolved areas. Areas of irritation and trauma such as axillae, perineum, genitalia, elbows, and knees may also become involved. In chronic pellagra, the skin assumes a thickened, hyperkeratinized, deeply pigmented appearance.

Acute pellagra causes a sore, red, and swollen tongue, with painful swallowing. Inflammatory changes may occur throughout the entire gastrointestinal tract, producing heartburn, abdominal pain, severe diarrhea, and rectal pain. Achlorhydria is common. Other mucous membranes are affected, causing urethritis and vaginitis. Mental changes may progress to include severe confusion, disorientation, delusions, mania, delirium, hallucinations, dementia, and psychotic states. Death occurs within 4 or 5 years if pellagra is not treated.

The diagnosis is confirmed by demonstration of a decrease in the urinary excretion of niacin metabolites, usually 3 mg/24 hr. Niacin should be given orally, because intestinal absorption is slower, and blood concentrations remain elevated for longer periods. The usual dose is approximately 50 mg niacin or nicotinamide, 10 times daily. In severe cases, parenteral nicotinamide therapy may be advisable for several days, 100 mg per day.

Pyridoxine (vitamin B_6) deficiency. Pyridoxine deficiency from inadequate intake is rare in the United States and generally occurs only with other vitamin B deficiencies. In some patients receiving isoniazid, a potent pyridoxine antagonist, pyridoxine deficiency may develop, particularly if they are slow acetylators of the drug.

The principal manifestation of pyridoxine deficiency is peripheral neuritis, which may be particularly severe in alcoholic patients. Pyridoxine-responsive anemia is one of the pyridoxine-dependent syndromes (Chapter 91). Treatment of pyridoxine deficiency is administration of 10 to 150 mg pyridoxine daily. In patients receiving isoniazid, neuritis may be prevented (or treated) with doses of 50 to 100 mg pyridoxine daily.

Measurements of urinary vitamin B_6 and urinary 4-pyridoxic acid are useful in diagnosing deficiency. Excretion of less than 100 mg vitamin B_6 or 1.0 mg 5-pyridoxic acid should lead the physician to suspect pyridoxine deficiency. Tryptophan loading will also result in increased excretion of xanthurenic acid in the urine, because pyridoxine is a cofactor in normal tryptophan metabolism. In pyridoxine deficiency, the usual tryptophan metabolic pathway is blocked, and intermediates are converted into xanthurenic and kynurenic acids that are excreted in increased amounts into the urine.

Folic acid and vitamin B_{12} deficiency. Deficiencies of folic acid and vitamin B_{12} are relatively common and result from inadequate dietary intake, or are secondary to gastrointestinal disease or increased metabolic requirements. Clinical manifestations and treatment of these deficiency states are described in Chapter 88.

Ascorbic acid (vitamin C) deficiency. In adults, scurvy-producing ascorbic acid deficiency is seldom seen today. When it occurs, it does so primarily as a result of food faddism, chronic alcoholism, or psychiatric disorders. Scurvy usually develops after 4 to 7 months of vitamin C deprivation.

Nonspecific symptoms may be noted before any physical changes occur and include lassitude, irritability, weight loss, and aching pains in muscles and joints. Perifollicular hyperkeratotic papules may form on the buttocks, thighs, and legs, with fragmentation, coiling, and embedding of hairs in follicles. Petechiae occur around the hair follicles and may be most prominent on the legs. Hemorrhage appears in the skin, muscles, and gums, with progressive edema. These lesions may ulcerate, and scars from previous trauma may also break down. The gums become swollen, boggy, friable, hemorrhagic, and eventually infected, sometimes to the point of gangrene. Hemorrhage into tissues may produce hemarthroses, mucous membrane bleeding, gastrointestinal and genitourinary blood loss, nosebleed, and retinal and cerebral hemorrhages. Early in scurvy, radiographic examination may show interruption of the lamina dura, which, as gum tissue progressively deteriorates, leads to tooth loss. Anemia may develop because of chronic blood loss or impaired folic acid utilization.

By the time scurvy is clinically apparent, the plasma levels of vitamin C are usually zero. Although not readily available, the vitamin C content of white blood cells falls below 2 mg/100 g just before scurvy develops. Treatment with ascorbic acid produces rapid recovery. The usual dosage of 100 mg five to six times daily can be reduced to 100 mg three times daily after 4 or 5 days but should be continued until complete healing is apparent.

Biotin deficiency. It is doubtful that biotin deficiency can result solely from inadequate intake, because biotin is produced by intestinal bacteria. The rare deficiency described in adults has been associated with large consumption of raw eggs for a period of several months. Raw eggs contain avidin, which binds biotin and prevents its absorption.

The clinical picture is characterized by nonpruritic dermatitis, lassitude, somnolence, depression, muscle pains, and hyperesthesia. Later, anorexia, nausea, anemia, and hypercholesterolemia appear. All manifestations disappear within 2 to 5 days after parenteral treatment with biotin, approximately 200 μ daily.

Pantothenic acid deficiency. Pantothenic acid is so widely available from food sources that a deficiency state is extremely rare. Experimentally produced pantothenic acid deficiency causes fatigue, malaise, sleep disturbances, personality changes, numbness, paresthesia, and muscle cramps. In association with malnutrition, hyperhidrosis, burning feet, painful toes, and a flat-footed gait have been described.

The diagnosis should be suspected whenever malnutrition and coexistent vitamin deficiencies exist, particularly beriberi, pellagra, and ariboflavinosis. Treatment with 20 to 40 mg calcium pantothenate per day intramuscularly should produce complete recovery; paresthesia may be the last symptom to disappear.

Vitamin-dependent metabolic defects. A variety of rare diseases are characterized by a specific metabolic defect, usually an enzyme deficiency, in which the normal dietary vitamin content is not sufficient to prevent clinical manifestations. In patients with these metabolic defects, large doses of the specific vitamin may be effective in overcoming the metabolic block. Some vitamin-dependent metabolic diseases are listed in Table 49-3.

Therapeutic use of vitamins

A healthy adult consuming a wide variety of foods will ingest an adequate supply of vitamins to meet normal body requirements. Whenever dietary intake is curtailed for extended periods of time, supplemental vitamin therapy to prevent deficiency states seems justified. Curtailment of dietary vitamin intake is commonly associated with eating patterns in old age, debilitating illnesses, food faddism, food restriction for weight reduction, chronic alcoholism, anorexia nervosa, drug-nutrient antagonism, and insufficient supplementation during prolonged intravenous nutrition or long-term hemodialysis. A strict but carefully selected vegetarian diet can supply all the vitamins except vitamin B_{12}. This vitamin is found only in foods of animal origin and therefore needs to be ingested as a supplement.

Vitamin therapy may also be necessary in conditions associated with decreased absorption or increased need or utilization such as malabsorption, pregnancy, hyperthyroidism, carcinoid syndrome, or excessive urinary loss. Long-term use of certain drugs also increases the need for a specific vitamin (e.g., isoniazid and methyldopapyridoxine).

Megavitamin therapy. Apart from megadoses of specific vitamins required in the treatment of rare vitamin-dependent metabolic disorders, there is little reason for administration of large doses of vitamins. Such doses can cause vitamin toxicity, a serious clinical problem. Megadoses and toxicity of selected vitamins are listed in Table 49-4. Toxicity may be modulated by the biochemical form of the vitamin consumed, the dosage taken, and whether consumption was acute or chronic.

Hypervitaminosis A. In adults, chronic hypervitaminosis A may produce fatigue; weakness; anorexia; irritability; vomiting; lethargy; loss of body hair; brittle nails; constipation; dry, scaly, rough skin; peripheral edema; and mouth fissures. In addition, hepatosplenomegaly (with significant liver damage and cirrhosis), cortical bone thickening, and increased intracranial pressure have been reported. Serum concentration of vitamin A is usually above 100 μ per deciliter. With cessation of vitamin intake, clinical symptoms rapidly improve, with gradual resolution of the cortical bone changes. Recent reports confirm that the use during pregnancy of the vitamin A analog (13-cis-retinoic acid) for skin disorders may cause serious birth defects.

Vitamin D intoxication. Excessive doses of vitamin D, taken for several weeks, may produce polyuria, polydipsia, lethargy, nausea, vomiting, constipation, and hypertension. Increased intestinal absorption of calcium, hypercalcemia, and hypercalciuria lead to calcium deposition in the kidney and progressive renal insufficiency. Coma may result from hypercalcemia or hypertensive encephalopathy.

Table 49-3. Vitamin-dependent metabolic diseases

Disease	Biochemical defect	Vitamin
Hyperalaninemia and hyperpyruvic acidemia	Pyruvate decarboxylase	Thiamine
Maple syrup urine disease	Decarboxylation of ketoacid analogus of branched-chain amino acid	Thiamine
Thiamine-responsive lactic acidosis	Hepatic pyruvate decarboxylase	Thiamine
Hartnup disease	Tryptophan and neutral amino acid active transport system	Niacin
Cystathioninuria	Cystathionase	Pyridoxine
Xanthurenic aciduria	Binding of pyridoxal phosphate to kynureninase	Pyridoxine
Homocystinuira	Cystathionine synthase	Pyridoxine and vitamin B_{12}
Vitamin B_6–dependent infantile convulsions	?Defect in glutamic acid decarboxylase	Pyridoxine
Vitamin B_6–responsive anemia	?Defect in alpha-aminolevulinic acid synthetase	Pyridoxine
Folic acid malabsorption	Folic acid active transport system	Folic acid
Formiminotransferase deficiency	Formiminotransferase	?Folic acid
Methylmalonic aciduria	Formation of coenzyme B_{12}	Vitamin B_{12}
Beta-methylcrotonylglycinuria	Beta-methylcrotonyl-CoA carboxylase	Biotin

Table 49-4. Megadoses and toxicity of selected vitamins

Vitamin	Toxic levels
Vitamin A	>25,000 IU/day ingested chronically >660,000 IU ingested acutely (adults) >330,000 IU ingested acutely (children)
Vitamin E	>2200 IU/day
Vitamin D	>10,000 IU/day ingested chronically
Nicotinic acid	>3 g/day
Pyridoxine	>2-6 g/day
Ascorbic acid	>2-4 g/day

Ascorbic acid toxicity. Many claims have been made for the use of large daily doses of vitamin C, particularly for the prevention and treatment of the common cold and, more recently, for cancer. In numerous clinical trials, however, no significant benefits from vitamin C megadoses have been substantiated. There appear to be no significant toxic effects of megadoses of this vitamin in normal persons. However, abortion, fetal deformity, false-positive test results for glycosuria, augmentation of warfarin anticoagulation, high-altitude hypoxia, enhancement of uricosuria and oxalate renal stones, and increased hemolysis in glucose-6-phosphate dehydrogenase deficiency have all been reported as special side effects.

Niacin toxicity. The use of megadoses of niacin and some other vitamins in the treatment of schizophrenia has been publicized and referred to as orthomolecular psychiatry. There has been no clinical substantiation of the efficacy of such therapy, but it is known that toxic reactions may occur with large doses of niacin. These reactions include skin flushing, pruritus, hyperuricemia, hyperglycemia, postural hypotension, macular edema with loss of vision, and abnormal liver function test results.

Vitamin E toxicity. Finally, although many claims have been made for the use of megadoses of vitamin E, only recently have the results of clinical trials indicated that tocopherols may be of benefit in intermittent claudication. Vitamin E ingestion of more than 1200 IU per day has been reported to prolong prothrombin time, producing a "conditioned vitamin K deficiency."

Pyridoxine toxicity. Previously, megadoses of water-soluble B-complex vitamins were considered relatively harmless, because it was assumed that they were rapidly excreted from the body. Recent reports of the toxic effect of megadoses of pyridoxine (2 to 6 g/day, or 1000 to 2700 times the recommended daily allowance [RDA]) confirm that even water-soluble vitamins can be toxic and have direct adverse effects. The pathogenesis of the peripheral neuropathologic effect observed is not yet known with certainty.

MINERALS

About 4% of human body weight is composed of inorganic elements or minerals, and 17 of these are considered to be essential for life. As shown in Table 49-5, these minerals are conveniently subdivided into macrominerals (i.e., those needed in the diet at levels of 100 mg per day or more) and microminerals, or trace elements (needed in amounts less than 100 mg per day). The trace elements constitute less than 0.1% of the total body weight.

All inorganic minerals are derived from seawater, the earth's crust, and the biosphere. In fact, the mineral composition of the human body is very similar to that of the earth and the sea. Biologists and chemists have long been fascinated by the way evolution has selected certain elements as the building stones of living organisms, including humans, and virtually ignored others.

In recent years there has been a remarkable escalation of research into the role of the inorganic minerals in nutritional and biochemical processes that take place both in health and in disease. Seven macrominerals are known to be essential for human life: calcium, phosphorus, sodium, potassium, chlorine, magnesium, and sulfur. The essential microminerals are iron, copper, cobalt, zinc, manganese, iodine, molybdenum, selenium, fluoride, and chromium (Table 49-5). Above a defined level of intake, any one of these minerals is toxic. On the other hand, a deficiency of any one of these nutrients results in malnutrition. The minerals may share certain characteristics of biologic importance, frequently related to their proximity in the Periodic Table, substituting one element for another in specific reactions. Interactions among minerals may be antagonistic, with one element that inhibits the metabolic action of another. Interactions may also be additive or synergistic, causing an effect greater than either element alone. Many factors may influence the metabolism of minerals: stress, nutritional status, disease states, patterns of exposure, or excess, deficiency, or imbalance of minerals.

The functions of the minerals vary in biologic expression from the whole organism to the isolated subcellular organelle. The mechanisms of action are equally diverse: structural components of enzymes and vitamins; active components in the synthesis of amino acids, deoxyribonucleic acid (DNA), and ribonucleic acid (RNA); catalysts in enzyme reactions through substrate binding, activation of enzyme-substrate complexes, or formation of metalloenzymes; regulation of intracellular heme concentration, membrane transport, nerve conduction, muscle contraction, osmotic pressure, water, and acid-base balance.

Mineral deficiencies

There are numerous examples of deficiency states related to inadequate intake of minerals; however, only selected examples are given here to emphasize the importance of this concept.

Table 49-5. Minerals in medicine

Mineral	Absorption (%)	Mechanism of Action/Function
Macrominerals		
Calcium	20-30	Formation of bones, teeth Regulation of excitable tissues (striated, cardiac, and smooth muscles, nerves) Activation of some enzymes Blood clotting
Phosphorus	50-60	Mineralization of bones, teeth Component of DNA, RNA Regulation of acid-base balance Component of phosphorylated vitamins (thiamine, niacin, riboflavin, pyridoxine) and ATP Component of phospholipids
Sodium	≈ 100	Regulation of pH, osmotic pressure, water balance Conductivity or excitability of nerves, muscles Active transport of glucose, amino acids
Potassium	≈ 100	Regulation of osmotic pressure, acid-base balance Activation of number of intracellular enzymes Regulation of nerve and muscle excitability
Chlorine	≈ 100	Regulation of osmotic pressure, acid-base balance, water balance Component of gastric juice
Magnesium	35-40	Component of several enzyme systems involving ATP Maintenance of electrical potential in nerves and muscle membranes
Sulfur		Component of methionine, cysteine, cystine Component of vitamins: thiamine, pantothenic acid, biotin Component of insulin, glutathione, taurocholic acid Provides high-energy sulfur bonds (—SH)
Microminerals or trace elements		
Iron	5-15	Structural component of hemoglobin, myoglobin, cytochrome, and other enzymes
Copper	30-60	Cross-linking of elastin Required for mobilization of iron Component of ceruloplasmin Component of many enzymes (cytochrome C oxidase, tyrosinase, dopamine beta-hydroxylase)
Cobalt	80-95	Component of vitamin B_{12}
Zinc	10-40	Component of over 80 metalloenzymes (carbonic anhydrase, carboxypeptidases A and B, alkaline phosphatase, alcohol dehydrogenase) Wound healing Metabolism of nucleic acids (thymidine kinase)
Manganese	10-40	Formation of mucopolysaccharides Activation of many enzymes
Iodine	≈ 100	Constituent of thyroxine, triiodothyronine
Molybdenum	40-100	Structural component of xanthine oxidase, aldehyde oxidase
Selenium	35-85	Active component of glutathione peroxidase
Fluoride	75-90	Structural component of calcium hydroxyapatite of bones and teeth
Chromium	10-25	Component of glucose tolerance factor

Iron deficiency anemia (see Chapter 87). Iron deficiency anemia is probably the most prevalent nutritional deficiency that affects human beings. It is estimated that iron deficiency anemia may be present in approximately 50% of the population in some parts of the world. In the United States, prevalence figures indicate that approximately 20% of infants and children, 10% to 50% of women 15 to 45 years of age, and 15% to 58% of pregnant women are iron deficient. Inadequate iron intake is one of the major reasons for iron deficiency anemia. The average American diet contains about 6 mg iron per 1000 cal consumed. With a 2000 cal intake, one would ingest about 12 mg iron. This amount (12 mg) does not afford a sufficient margin of safety above the average physiologic requirement to cover variation among all individuals in the general population. A specific, concerted effort must be made to select iron-rich foods to meet requirements, or iron supplements may be needed by high-risk groups (e.g., infants, pregnant women). Increased menstrual bleeding and hemorrhage from the alimentary tract are the most common causes of iron deficiency.

Zinc deficiency. The trace metal zinc is closely associated with a variety of more than 80 zinc-containing proteins and enzymes. Zinc is essential for the catalytic functions and/or the structure of key enzymes that play a central role in metabolism, including alcohol dehydrogenase, alkaline phosphatase, carboxypeptidase, and carbonic anhydrase. Zinc deficiency has been reported in a variety of clinical circumstances, including acute inflammatory stress, some specific malignancies (e.g., leukemia), chronic infections (e.g., pneumonia, bronchitis), alcoholism, liver disease (e.g., cirrhosis), chronic renal disease, rheumatoid arthritis, inflammatory bowel disease, hemolytic anemias, and malabsorption syndromes. Zinc deficiency may also result from administration of zinc-chelating drugs (e.g., penicillamine), or total parenteral nutrition (TPN) without adequate zinc given in the solution. Acrodermatitis enteropathica was the first inherited zinc-deficiency disorder reported in human beings, and small amounts of zinc completely reverse all pathologic lesions and clinical manifestations. Other manifestations of zinc deficiency include poor wound healing, growth retardation, hypogonadism, impaired immune function, mental disturbances, diarrhea, altered taste and smell, and reduced night vision.

Mineral deficiencies associated with TPN. There has been increased awareness of deficiency states that may be precipitated by lack of a single mineral in the solutions used for TPN, including zinc, copper, selenium, and molybdenum. Mineral deficiencies occur with frequency in patients on TPN. The most common cause of trace mineral deficiency in such patients is the failure to provide a sufficient amount of each mineral to meet both losses from previous or ongoing illnesses or injury plus the normal maintenance requirements.

Mineral deficiencies associated with digestive disease. Abnormal conditions of the digestive tract may predispose to depletion of minerals, especially zinc. A deficiency of this mineral may occur as a result of geophagia; celiac diseases; short bowel syndrome; diarrheal fluid loss; ileostomy fluid loss; enterocolic, pancreaticocutaneous, or pancreaticocolic fistula; pancreatic insufficiency; and cystic fibrosis. Copper deficiency is less frequent than zinc deficiency and causes anemia, leukopenia, and neutropenia. Chromium deficiency is rare and occurs only in chronic TPN administration, usually manifested by an increase in glucose intolerance and peripheral neuropathy. Magnesium deficiency may be manifested by muscle cramps and sometimes tetany. Selenium deficiency after years of TPN usually is associated with myopathy or cardiomyopathy.

Excess intake of minerals

Excess intake of any one of the essential minerals may also lead to toxicity and malnutrition. In fact, excess mineral intake is more likely to have a toxic effect than excess vitamin intake because the upper and lower physiologic tolerances are within a narrower range.

Hypermagnesemia. Hypermagnesemia has been reported in patients with renal insufficiency who are taking magnesium-containing drugs (e.g., antacids). High blood concentrations of magnesium (8 mEq/liter) lead to central depression, profound paralysis of the skeletal muscles, and respiratory distress.

Iron toxicity. Iron overload can result from enhanced absorption, parenteral infusion, or a combination of these two factors and produce hemochromatosis. Prolonged intake of medicinal iron by patients who no longer need it may also lead to iron overload. Because iron preparations in the United States are widely advertised, available without prescription, and consumed in large quantities, one should consider the possibility of iron overload in appropriate clinical situations.

Trace mineral toxicity. Malnutrition caused by excess trace metals is well documented. Excess iodide may lead to an inhibition of thyroid hormone synthesis, hypothyroidism, and iodide goiter. Acute copper intoxication in human beings causes nausea, vomiting, epigastric pain, diarrhea, headache, dizziness, and weakness. In severe cases, copper toxicity may lead to tachycardia, hypertension, coma, jaundice, hemolytic anemia, hemoglobinuria, uremia, and death. Toxic reactions of excess intake of manganese, cobalt, selenium, and cadmium have also been reported. Fluoride excess has been studied extensively as a result of fortification of the public water supply of countries all over the world to decrease the prevalence of dental caries. It is well established that excess fluoride intake during the developmental period of the teeth leads to dental fluorosis but may also promote stabilization of newly synthesized bone matrix and inhibit bone resorption.

Mineral toxicity related to food contamination. The toxic potential of trace metals in foods and beverages should not be overlooked. Excess contamination of foods and beverages with lead, mercury, cobalt, and cadmium has been reported and in some instances has led to toxicity and death.

DRUG-NUTRIENT INTERACTION

Drugs may interfere with the effect or utilization of nutrients in many ways. In some instances, drug-nutrient interaction is an intentional effect. More often, drug-nutrient interaction impairs nutrient use and is undesirable. Drugs may decrease nutrient absorption, increase urinary excretion, directly compete with or antagonize nutrient action, displace the nutrient from a carrier protein, and interfere with the synthesis of an enzyme, coenzyme, or carrier essential for the metabolism of the nutrient. Some hormones may also alter nutrient metabolism, particularly those in oral contraceptives. Finally, substances present as components of a drug may produce alterations in nutrient status. Examples of drug-nutrient interactions are described in Table 49-6.

NUTRITIONAL ASSESSMENT

Advanced states of malnutrition may be recognized easily on visual inspection. Physical examination may reveal specific changes associated with malnutrition. However, a

Table 49-6. Some drug-nutrient interactions

Drug	Nutrients	Mechanism
Antacids	Iron, phosphates	Malabsorption, binding
Tetracyclines	Iron (antacids)	Chelation
	Calcium	Calcium binding in bones
Cholestyramine	Triglycerides, calcium, fat-soluble vitamins	Malabsorption, bile-acid sequestration
5-Fluorouracil	Protein	Malabsorption, reduced peptidases
Metformin	Vitamin B_{12}	Malabsorption, mucosal damage
Colchicine		
Para-aminosalicylic acid		
Ethanol	Folate	Uncertain
	Magnesium	?Malabsorption; increase in stool
	Zinc	Increased urinary loss
	Vitamin B_6	Reduced conversion to pyridoxal phosphate
Methyldopa	Vitamin B_6	Metabolic antagonism
Isoniazid	Vitamin B_6, tryptophan	Competition for active enzyme site
	Niacin	
Penicillamine	Vitamin B_6	Increased urinary loss
Diphenylhydantoin	Folate	Uncertain
Primidone		
Methotrexate	Folate	Direct antagonism: competition for active enzyme site
Pyrimethamine		
Triaminopteride		
Trimethoprim		
Coumadin	Vitamin K	Decreased synthesis
Barbiturates		Induction of warfarin inactivation
Oxyphenbutazone		Enhancement of warfarin action (displacement of albumin binding)
Oral contraceptives	Vitamin B_6	Altered metabolism
	Tryptophan	Increased protein binding
	Folate	Reduction in red cell levels

planned procedure of nutritional assessment enables the clinician to detect the presence of less obvious malnutrition. Nutritional assessment provides an objective characterization of nutritional status and should be a routine aspect of the clinical evaluation of every hospitalized patient.

No single assessment tool can adequately characterize nutritional status; thus a profile of tests and measurements should be used. Several assessment plans have been published. The four assessment parameters most useful in determining nutritional status are anthropometric, laboratory, clinical, and dietary. A list of the helpful anthropometric and laboratory parameters is shown in Table 49-7. Muscle or lean body mass may be estimated by determining the creatinine/height index. This index, which has proved to be particularly useful in assessing nutritional status, can be determined from comparison with the desirable weights and normal urinary creatinine excretion for given heights shown in Tables 49-8 and 49-9 respectively.

Calorie and nutrient requirements

The patient's diet is designed to provide adequate calories and essential nutrients. Caloric needs are best estimated as follows:

1. The basal metabolic rate is determined by first using a height-weight nomograph to obtain body surface area (Fig. 49-1). The metabolic rate for a given age

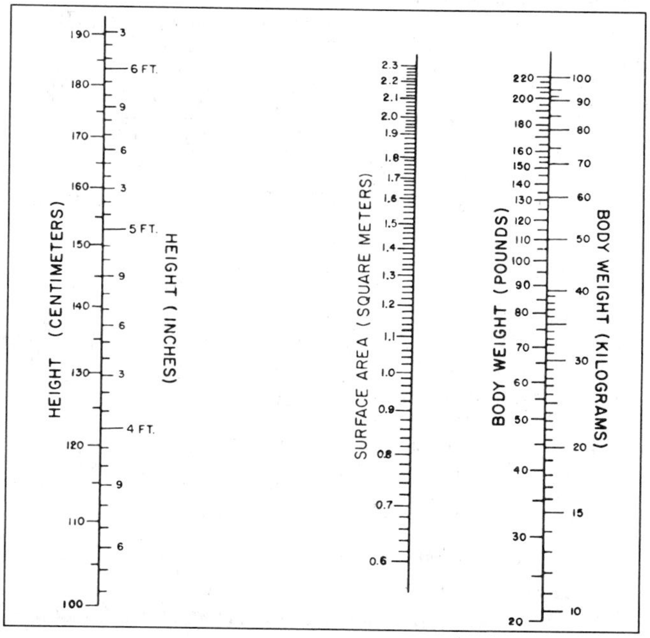

Fig. 49-1. Nomogram for determining body surface area from height and weight. To determine body surface area from height *(left-hand scale)* and weight *(right-hand scale)*, these points are connected with a straightedge and surface area is read from the middle scale. (From Wilmore DW: The metabolic management of the critically ill. New York, 1977, Plenum Medical.)

Table 49-7. Nutritional assessment

Measurement	Assessment
A. Anthropometric measurements	
1. Weight (kg)	Body weight status
2. Height (cm)	Desirable weight of adults (see Table 49-8)
3. Weight/height ratio	Body weight status
4. % Ideal body weight = $\frac{\text{actual weight}}{\text{ideal body weight}} \times 100$	
5. % Usual body weight = $\frac{\text{actual weight}}{\text{usual weight}} \times 100$	
6. % Weight change = $\frac{\text{usual weight} - \text{actual weight}}{\text{usual weight}} \times 100$	
7. Arm circumference (cm)	Body weight status
8. % Standard arm circumference = $\frac{\text{actual arm circumference}}{\text{standard arm circumference}} \times 100$	
9. Triceps skinfold (mm)	Body fatness Men: 8-23 mm Women: 10-30 mm
10. % Standard triceps skinfold = $\frac{\text{actual triceps skinfold}}{\text{standard triceps skinfold}} \times 100$	
11. Arm muscle circumference (mm) = arm circumference (mm) − 0.314 × triceps skinfold (mm)	Lean muscle mass Midarm muscle circumference (120-140 mm)
12. % Standard arm muscle circumference = $\frac{\text{actual arm muscle circumference}}{\text{standard arm muscle circumference}} \times 100$	Lean muscle mass
B. Laboratory measurements	
1. Total iron-binding capacity (TIBC)(μg/dl)	Labile or visceral protein status Protein-calorie malnutrition
2. Serum transferrin = (0.8 × TIBC) − 43, mg/dl	Visceral protein status Protein-calorie malnutrition
3. Serum albumin (g/dl)	Visceral protein status Protein-calorie malnutrition
4. White blood cell count (WBC/mm^3)	
5. Total lymphocyte count = $\frac{\text{percent lymphocytes} \times \text{WBC}}{100}$	Immune function
6. 24-hr urinary creatinine (mg)	Ideal urinary creatinine values (see Table 49-9)
7. Creatinine height index = $\frac{\text{actual urinary creatinine}}{\text{ideal urinary creatinine}} \times 100$	Muscle or lean body mass
8. 24-hr urinary nitrogen (g)	Body protein status
9. Nitrogen balance = $\frac{\text{protein intake}}{6.25}$ − (urinary urea nitrogen + 4)	Body protein status
10. Basal energy expenditure	Used to derive total caloric needs
11. Complete blood count (CBC)	Anemia: Normocytic Microcytic Macrocytic
12. Skin tests Purified protein derivative (PPD) Candida Dinitrochlorobenzene (DNCB)	Immune function

and sex shown in Table 49-10 is then multiplied by the body surface area to provide the basal metabolic rate. This calculation can be made easily by use of the nomograph in Fig. 49-2.

2. The energy required for the patient's activity level is estimated from Table 49-11. This is then added to the basal metabolic rate to obtain total daily caloric needs.

3. The patient's daily caloric requirements depend on whether weight reduction, maintenance, or weight gain is needed. Hypocaloric, nitrogen-containing diets usually provide 400 to 1800 kcal per day, which is about 1000 kcal below estimated metabolic rate. Maintenance diets provide calories sufficient to meet estimated energy needs. Hypercaloric diets generally provide 1000 kcal per day in excess of estimated

Table 49-8. 1983 Metropolitan Life Insurance Company height and weight table

Men*					Women†				
Height					Height				
Feet	Inches	Small frame	Medium frame	Large frame	Feet	Inches	Small frame	Medium frame	Large frame
5	2	128-134	131-141	138-150	4	10	102-111	109-121	118-131
5	3	130-136	133-143	140-153	4	11	103-113	111-123	120-134
5	4	132-138	135-145	142-156	5	0	104-115	113-126	122-137
5	5	134-140	137-148	144-160	5	1	106-118	115-129	125-140
5	6	136-142	139-151	146-164	5	2	108-121	118-132	128-143
5	7	138-145	142-154	149-168	5	3	111-124	121-135	131-147
5	8	140-148	145-157	152-172	5	4	114-127	124-138	134-151
5	9	142-151	148-160	155-176	5	5	117-130	127-141	137-155
5	10	144-154	151-163	158-180	5	6	120-133	130-144	140-159
5	11	146-157	154-166	161-184	5	7	123-136	133-147	143-163
6	0	149-160	157-170	164-188	5	8	126-139	136-150	146-167
6	1	152-164	160-174	168-192	5	9	129-142	139-153	149-170
6	2	155-168	164-178	172-197	5	10	132-145	142-156	152-173
6	3	158-172	167-182	176-202	5	11	135-148	145-159	155-176
6	4	162-176	171-187	181-207	6	0	138-151	148-162	158-179

*Weights at ages 25 to 59 based on lowest mortality. Weight in pounds according to frame (in indoor clothing weighing 5 lb, shoes with 1 in heels).
†Weights at ages 25 to 59 based on lowest mortality. Weight in pounds according to frame (in indoor clothing weighing 3 lb, shoes with 1 in heels).

needs. Patients with severe disease such as infection, sepsis, or cancer may require caloric intake significantly above daily metabolic rate to make up for existing defects or increased maintenance requirements.

4. The patient's nitrogen requirements can be determined from the nomograph shown in Fig. 49-3. Although healthy individuals maintain nitrogen balance with a nitrogen/total calorie ratio of 1:350, seriously ill patients benefit from a ratio of 1:150 because of their compromised protein status.
5. The appropriate route of feeding (oral, enteral, or parenteral) is determined from the patient's clinical condition. Route of intake usually influences selection of the diet's components.

Table 49-9. Ideal urinary creatinine values

Men*			Women†		
Height		Ideal creatinine	Height		Ideal creatinine
(in)	(cm)	(mg)	(in)	(cm)	(mg)
62	157.5	1288	58	147.3	830
63	160.0	1325	59	149.9	851
64	162.6	1359	60	152.4	875
65	165.1	1386	61	154.9	900
66	167.6	1426	62	157.5	925
67	170.2	1467	63	160.0	949
68	172.7	1513	64	162.6	977
69	175.3	1555	65	165.1	1006
70	177.8	1596	66	167.6	1044
71	180.3	1642	67	170.2	1076
72	182.9	1691	68	172.7	1109
73	185.4	1739	69	175.3	1141
74	188.0	1785	70	177.8	1174
75	190.5	1831	71	180.3	1206
76	193.0	1891	72	182.9	1240

From Margen S, Caan B, editors: The Medical Clinics of North America symposium on applied nutrition in clinical medicine, Philadelphia, 1979, Saunders.
*Creatinine coefficient (men) = 23 mg/kg of ideal body weight.
†Creatinine coefficient (women) = 18 mg/kg of ideal body weight.

Table 49-10. Metabolic rate

	kcal/m²/h	
Ages (years)	Men	Women
18	40.0	35.9
19	39.2	35.5
20	38.6	35.3
25	37.5	35.2
30	36.8	35.1
35	36.5	35.0
40	36.3	34.9
45	36.2	34.5
50	35.8	33.9
55	35.4	33.3
60	34.9	32.7
65	34.4	32.2
70	33.8	31.7
75 and over	33.2	31.3

Modified from Fleisch A: Helv Med Acta 18:23, 1951.

Table 49-11. Approximate energy output

Type of work	Calories added to basal rates (kcal/day)
Sedentary	400-800
Light work (professionals and business-persons)	800-1200
Moderate work (mechanical)	1200-1800
Heavy work (laborers and athletes)	1800-4500

Modified from Wilmore DW: The metabolic management of the critically ill. New York, 1977, Plenum.

6. Essential nutrients, including vitamins, minerals, and essential fatty acids, must be provided. The RDA (Tables 49-12 to 49-14) may serve as a guide, but special nutrient needs may require adjustment of daily doses above or below the RDA.

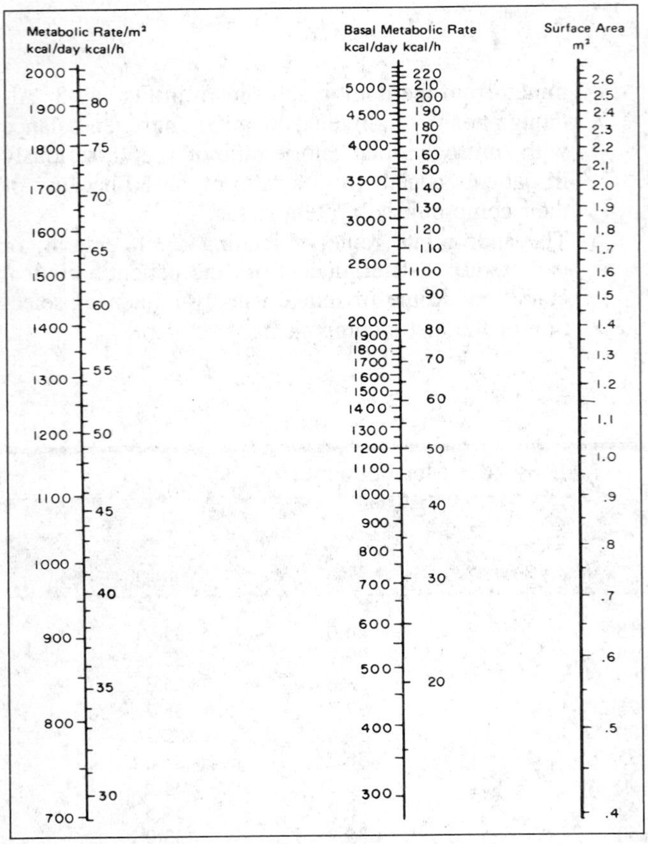

Fig. 49-2. Prediction of daily metabolic requirements per square meter of body surface *(right-hand scale)* for age and sex *(left-hand scale) (see Table 49-10)*. These points are connected with a straightedge, and the predicted daily or hourly requirements are read from the middle scale. (From Wilmore DW: The metabolic management of the critically ill. New York, 1977, Plenum Medical.)

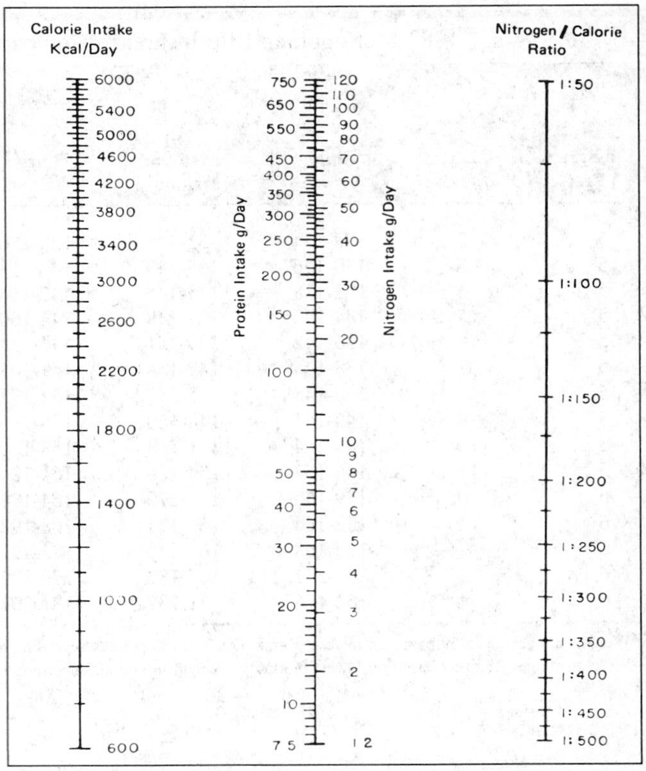

Fig. 49-3. Nomogram for determining daily nitrogen requirements. Daily calorie requirements are located on the left-hand scale, and a straightedge is used to connect this point with the point on the right-hand scale that indicates the desired nitrogen/calorie ratio *(1:150 for most patients)*. Nitrogen intake is read from the right-hand side of the center scale. (From Wilmore DW: The metabolic management of the critically ill. New York, 1977, Plenum Medical.)

7. Reassessment is necessary at frequent intervals to ensure the success of nutritional support and determine changing requirements.

NUTRITIONAL MANAGEMENT

Nutritional management is an essential part of therapy for specific disorders and is an important adjunct in the treatment of many diseases. The incidence of protein-calorie malnutrition may range from 25% to 50% in hospitalized medical and surgical patients. Awareness of this important problem has grown, but practitioners of internal medicine still do not give it sufficient attention. Physicians' failure to record and use data (height, weight, weight history, dietary history, etc.); failure to assign specific responsibility for nutritional assessment and treatment; tendency to overlook patients' nutritional needs while obtaining numerous diagnostic studies; and failure to provide nutritional support before malnutrition is overt have all contributed to nutritional problems. Nutrient and calorie requirements are dramatically influenced by disease or injury and can be strikingly increased in critically ill patients.

Total parenteral nutrition

Indications. It is now possible to provide partial or complete nutrition by intravenous infusion of nutrient solutions. If gastrointestinal absorption and delivery of nutrients are inadequate, impossible for prolonged periods of time, or contraindicated, nourishment should be provided parenterally. Specific conditions in which parenteral feeding is indicated include mechanical bowel obstruction, postoperative ileus, acute inflammatory bowel disease, acute pancreatitis, short gut syndrome, proximal intestinal fistulas, severe burns, cancer cachexia and adjunctive therapy, chronic debility, anorexia nervosa, and occasionally acute renal failure and hepatic or cardiac decompensation.

Nutrient solutions. The two most important sources of calories are carbohydrates and fats. Infusion of 100 to 250 g glucose daily prevents ketosis and decreases catabolism of protein. Hypertonic solutions of glucose in final concentrations of 20% to 30% have been the major source of calories in solutions used for TPN. These solutions require the use of a central venous catheter to prevent the complications of thrombophlebitis. The availability of fat emulsions has added to the capability of supplying adequate energy needs parenterally. One major advantage of fat emulsions is that they supply 9 kcal per gram, more than twice the kilocalories supplied by a gram of glucose. In addition, fat emulsions are isotonic and may be administered through a peripheral vein. In combination with glucose and amino acids, fat emulsions administered by peripheral vein infusion can meet the total nutritional requirements of some patients with limited metabolic needs. In patients receiving prolonged TPN, essential fatty acid deficiency may be prevented by fat emulsions. Fat emulsions contain either soybean or cottonseed oil and consist mainly of oleic or linoleic fatty acid. One preparation currently used widely in the United States is a 10% soybean oil emulsion with an egg yolk stabilizer.

Nitrogen for parenteral solutions consists of either protein hydrolysates or mixtures of crystalline amino acids. Both types have been used successfully, but crystalline amino acids are preferred because it is possible to alter the solution to meet more appropriately the metabolic requirements of patients with specific organic diseases (e.g., renal disease, hepatic insufficiency). These requirements depend on physiologic conditions and increase as protein catabolism increases. In general, it is necessary to infuse between 80 and 160 g protein equivalent per 24 hours to ensure positive nitrogen balance. For nitrogen to be usable for tissue synthesis (instead of energy), the calorie/nitrogen ratio should be about 150 to 250 cal to 1 g nitrogen. In most TPN protocols, calorie/nitrogen ratio is 150:1. It is important to provide appropriate amounts of essential and nonessential amino acids in these mixtures, usually in a ratio of about 1.0:1.5. The nonessential amino acids should include alanine, proline, arginine, glutamic acid, and histidine.

Sufficient electrolytes, vitamins, and minerals must be added to parenteral solutions to meet the needs of the patient. Additions may vary, depending on previous existing deficits, maintenance requirements (including daily losses), and deficiencies that may develop during prolonged therapy. For every 1000 cal infused, approximately 10 mEq sodium and chloride, 20 mEq potassium and phosphate, 8 mEq magnesium, and 5 mEq calcium is required just for metabolic utilization of nutrients in the solution. To these amounts should be added the daily basal losses of sodium, potassium, and chloride, so that the minimum daily requirement for common electrolytes is met. Cobalt, zinc, copper, manganese, and fluoride are required trace elements that must also be added to the solutions, although the precise daily requirements remain uncertain. Many hospital pharmacies compound a solution containing these trace minerals. The addition of water- and fat-soluble vitamins completes the basic solution. Usually, one ampul of a multiple vitamin preparation per day meets the daily recommended allowances, with the exception of those for folic acid, vitamin K, vitamin B_{12}, and iron. For maintenance, these compounds may be supplemented with parenteral injections at appropriate intervals. In some cases, insulin must be added to the solution to facilitate adequate utilization of the glucose present and to prevent hyperglycemia. A standard formula for basic parenteral nutrition administered through a central vein catheter is shown in Table 49-15. Variations in amounts of amino acids and sodium may be made to suit the needs of patients with renal, cardiac, and hepatic disease. Some incompatibilities or insolubilities are associated with these solutions. Addition of bicarbonate can form precipitates or cause inactivation of calcium, insulin, vitamin B complex, and vitamin C. If bicarbonate is required, it is usually given as the acetate salt of sodium or potassium. Exceeding the limits of calcium concentration may precipitate phosphate and sulfate salts. It is customary to begin total parenteral infusion at a rate of 10 dl per 24 hours and gradually increase the amount (by 10 dl) daily until estimated volume and calorie requirements are met.

Complications. Careful attention must be paid to preventing, detecting, and treating the many potential complications of TPN. Bacterial and fungal sepsis are major complications. Sepsis is usually associated with catheter placement, growth of organisms along the cutaneous-vascular route, and contamination of the closed system. Meticulous care must be taken of the insertion site, tubing, and filters, and a well-defined procedure must be established for documenting and treating infection. The central venous catheter should be used only for TPN: administration of "piggyback" medications, blood withdrawal, central venous pressure determination, and administration of other fluids or blood by this route should be prohibited. Mechanical malfunction of the central venous catheter also poses a risk for the patient. Embolism may occur with manipulation of the catheter or its connections, and thrombosis of the great veins may become a clinical problem if this produces emboli or sepsis. For these reasons, patients receiving TPN

Table 49-12. Recommended daily dietary allowances*

		Weight		Height			Fat-soluble vitamins		
	Age (years)	(kg)	(lb)	(cm)	(in)	Protein (g)	Vitamin A (μg R.E.)†	Vitamin D (μg)‡	Vitamin E (mg α-T.E.)§
Infants	0.0-0.5	6	13	60	24	kg × 2.2	420	10	3
	0.5-1.0	9	20	71	28	kg × 2.0	400	10	4
Children	1-3	13	29	90	35	23	400	10	5
	4-6	20	44	112	44	30	500	10	6
	7-10	28	62	132	52	34	700	10	7
Males	11-14	45	99	157	62	45	1000	10	8
	15-18	66	145	176	69	56	1000	10	10
	19-22	70	154	177	70	56	1000	7.5	10
	23-50	70	154	178	70	56	1000	5	10
	51+	70	154	178	70	56	1000	5	10
Females	11-14	46	101	157	62	46	800	10	8
	15-18	55	120	163	64	46	800	10	8
	19-22	55	120	163	64	44	800	7.5	8
	23-50	55	120	163	64	44	800	5	8
	51+	55	120	163	64	44	800	5	8
Pregnant						+30	+200	+5	+2
Lactating						+20	+400	+5	+3

From Food and Nutrition Board, National Academy of Sciences—National Research Council, Washington, 1980.

*The allowances are intended to provide for individual variations among most normal persons as they live in the United States under usual environmental stresses. Diets should be based on a variety of common foods in order to provide other nutrients for which human requirements have been less well defined. See Table 49-14 for heights, weights, and recommended intake.

†Retinol equivalents. One retinol equivalent = 1 μg retinol or 6 μg β-carotene.

‡As cholecalciferol. Ten μg cholecalciferol = 400 IU vitamin D.

§α-tocopherol equivalents. One mg d-α-tocopherol = 1 α-T.E.

‖N.E. (niacin equivalent) is equal to 1 mg of niacin or 60 mg of dietary tryptophan.

¶The folacin allowances refer to dietary sources as determined by *Lactobacillus casei* assay after treatment with enzymes ("conjugases") to make polyglutamyl forms of the vitamin available to the test organism.

#The RDA for vitamin B_{12} in infants is based on average concentration of the vitamin in human milk. The allowances after weaning are based on energy intake (as recommended by the American Academy of Pediatrics) and consideration of other factors such as intestinal absorption.

**The increased requirement during pregnancy cannot be met by the iron content of habitual American diets nor by the existing iron stores of many women; therefore, the use of 30-60 mg of supplemental iron is recommended. Iron needs during lactation are not substantially different from those of nonpregnant women, but continued supplementation of the mother for 2-3 months after parturition is advisable in order to replenish stores depleted by pregnancy.

are best cared for by a team that includes the physician, a specially trained nurse, and a nutritionist.

The patient's metabolism must be monitored daily and alterations corrected immediately. Metabolic alterations include hyperosmolar nonketotic hyperglycemia (with or without coma) and severe hypoglycemia, particularly if there is sudden cessation of administration of the concentrated glucose solution. Hyperchloremic metabolic acidosis may develop from excessive chloride and monohydrochloride present in crystalline amino acid solutions. When protein hydrolysates are used as the source of nitrogen, sensitivity reactions and hyperammonemia may result. Prerenal azotemia may result from an excessive total dose or rate of infusion of the protein hydrolysate or amino acid solution.

Essential fatty acid deficiency can be prevented with biweekly infusion of a fat emulsion via a peripheral vein. Hypocalcemia and hypophosphatemia may result from inadequate administration of calcium and phosphate. Hypercalcemia may occur from excessive calcium and vitamin D administration. Other metabolic hazards include hypo- and hyperkalemia, hypo- and hypermagnesemia, deficiencies of chromium and other trace metals, anemia, bleeding, hypervitaminosis A, cholestasis, and the frequent occurrence of abnormal liver enzyme levels. Ten types of nutrient deficiencies during TPN have been described: phosphate, essential fatty acid, copper, zinc, chromium, folic acid, selenium, vitamin A, biotin, and molybdenum. Under certain circumstances of TPN, especially when associated with chronic disease states, some nonessential nutrients may become limiting or deficient. Identification of five such substances that require vigilance are tyrosine, cysteine, taurine, choline, and carnitine.

Peripheral total parenteral nutrition

The objective of peripheral parenteral nutrition is to provide nutrition intravenously without inserting a central venous catheter. Peripheral infusion of amino acids, dextrose, and fat emulsion usually cannot provide adequate nonpro-

Table 49-12— con't.

Water-soluble vitamins							Minerals						
Vitamin C (mg)	Thiamine (mg)	Riboflavin (mg)	Niacin (mg N.E.)‖	Vitamin B_6 (mg)	Folacin¶ (μg)	Vitamin B_{12} (μg)	Calcium (mg)	Phosphorus (mg)	Magnesium (mg)	Iron (mg)	Zinc (mg)	Iodine (μg)
35	0.3	0.4	6	0.3	30	0.5#	360	240	50	10	3	40
35	0.5	0.6	8	0.6	45	1.5	540	360	70	15	5	50
45	0.7	0.8	9	0.9	100	2.0	800	800	150	15	10	70
45	0.9	1.0	11	1.3	200	2.5	800	800	200	10	10	90
45	1.2	1.4	16	1.6	300	3.0	800	800	250	10	10	120
50	1.4	1.6	18	1.8	400	3.0	1200	1200	350	18	15	150
60	1.4	1.7	18	2.0	400	3.0	1200	1200	400	18	15	150
60	1.5	1.7	19	2.2	400	3.0	800	800	350	10	15	150
60	1.4	1.6	18	2.2	400	3.0	800	800	350	10	15	150
60	1.2	1.4	16	2.2	400	3.0	800	800	350	10	15	150
50	1.1	1.3	15	1.8	400	3.0	1200	1200	300	18	15	150
60	1.1	1.3	14	2.0	400	3.0	1200	1200	300	18	15	150
60	1.1	1.3	14	2.0	400	3.0	800	800	300	18	15	150
60	1.0	1.2	13	2.0	400	3.0	800	800	300	18	15	150
60	1.0	1.2	13	2.0	400	3.0	800	800	300	10	15	150
+20	+0.4	+0.3	+2	+0.6	+400	+1.0	+400	+400	+150	**	+5	+25
+40	+0.5	+0.5	+5	+0.5	+100	+1.0	+400	+400	+150	**	+10	+50

tein calories to produce a positive nitrogen balance in adult patients under medical stress. Supplemental oral intake of these substances is necessary. Contraindications for peripheral parenteral nutrition include abnormalities in fat transport, uncontrolled diabetes mellitus (without insulin), liver disease, thrombocytopenia and/or coagulopathy, and severe chronic obstructive pulmonary disease. Basal requirements are usually met by infusing 1.5 liters of a 5% dextrose, 4.25% amino acid solution and 1.0 to 1.5 liters of a 10% fat emulsion daily. Appropriate electrolytes are also added to meet daily requirements. Additional calories can be provided only by increasing the volume of the dilute dextrose solution, thus limiting the amount of calories that can be added.

Defined-formula diets and other supplements

Special low-residue, liquid-formula diets composed of all nutrients known to be required by human beings have been developed over the past decade. These defined-formula diets ("elemental" or "chemically defined" diets) are being extensively used in clinical medicine for patients who are unable to eat solid foods but who have a partially or totally intact and functioning gastrointestinal tract. Specialized defined-formula diets are thought to be readily and almost completely absorbed in the upper small intestine. They facilitate minimum delivery of residue to the lower bowel and are free of lactose. If oral intake of food is contraindicated, maintenance of adequate nutrition by a defined-formula diet may be an alternative to parenteral feeding. If the gastrointestinal tract is functioning, defined-formula diets have decided advantages over parenteral nutrition, because entry of nutrients into the gut stimulates maintenance of structure and function of the mucosa. Patients who may benefit from defined-formula diets are those with cancer, severe and persistent anorexia, fistulas, severe malabsorption, coma, or impairment of swallowing mechanisms.

If the patient is unable to swallow, greatest tolerance is achieved if the liquid formula is delivered by continuous drip. Delivery may be by nasogastric or nasoduodenal tube or by gastrostomy or jejunostomy. Soft tubes made of silicone or polyurethane compounds are most acceptable. Care should be taken to follow recommended procedures for easy insertion and accurate placement of the feeding catheter.

Because all defined-formula diets are hyperosmolar, they are best tolerated if the concentration and rate of delivery are increased slowly. Accurate intake and output records must be kept, and the patient should be carefully monitored. Mechanical complications (e.g., aspiration, tracheoesophageal fistulas) and metabolic complications (e.g., hyperosmolar, hyperglycemic, nonketotic dehydration; fluid overload; nausea; vomiting; diarrhea) may occur and must be treated.

There are some contraindications for the use of defined-formula diets. Metabolic problems in patients with renal or hepatic disease may be exacerbated by the levels of protein, sodium, potassium phosphate, or magnesium present in the formula. Patients receiving corticosteroid treatment may not tolerate the amount of sodium in specific formulas. Patients with hypercalcemia may not tolerate the concentration of calcium.

Some currently available defined-formula diets are classified in Table 49-16. The nutrient composition of these di-

Table 49-13. Recommended dietary allowances: estimated safe and adequate daily dietary intakes of selected vitamins and minerals*

		Vitamins			Trace elements†						Electrolytes		
	Age (years)	Vitamin K (μg)	Biotin (μg)	Pantothenic acid (mg)	Copper (mg)	Manganese (mg)	Fluoride (mg)	Chromium (mg)	Selenium (mg)	Molybdenum (mg)	Sodium (mg)	Potassium (mg)	Chloride (mg)
Infants	0-0.5	12	35	2	0.5-0.7	0.5-0.7	0.1-0.5	0.01-0.04	0.01-0.04	0.03-0.06	115-350	350-925	275-700
	0.5-1.0	10-20	50	3	0.7-1.0	0.7-1.0	0.2-1.0	0.02-0.06	0.02-0.06	0.04-0.08	250-750	425-1275	400-1200
Children	1-3	15-30	65	3	1.0-1.5	1.0-1.5	0.5-1.5	0.02-0.08	0.05-0.10	325-975	550-1650	550-1500	
	4-6	20-40	85	3-4	1.5-2.0	1.5-2.0	1.0-2.5	0.03-0.12	0.03-0.12	0.06-0.15	450-1350	775-2325	700-2100
	7-10	30-60	120	4-5	2.0-2.5	2.0-3.0	1.5-2.5	0.05-0.20	0.05-0.20	0.1-0.3	600-1800	1000-3000	925-2775
Adolescents	11+	50-100	100-200	4-7	2.0-3.0	2.5-5.0	1.5-2.5	0.05-0.20	0.05-0.20	0.15-0.50	900-2700	1525-4575	1400-4200
Adults		70-140	100-200	4-7	2.0-3.0	2.5-5.0	1.5-4.0	0.05-0.20	0.05-0.20	0.15-0.50	1100-3300	1875-5625	1700-5100

From Food and Nutrition Board, National Academy of Sciences—National Research Council, Washington, 1980.

*Because there is less information on which to base allowances, these figures are not given in Table 49-12 and are provided here in the form of ranges of recommended intakes.

†Because the toxic levels for many trace elements may be only several times the usual intake, the upper levels for the trace elements given in this table should not be habitually exceeded.

Table 49-14. Mean heights and weights and recommended energy intake; recommended dietary allowances*

Category	Age (years)	Weight (kg)	Weight (lb)	Height (cm)	Height (in)	Energy needs (with range) (kcal)	Energy needs (MJ)
Males	11-14	45	99	157	62	2700 (2000-3700)	11.3
	15-18	66	145	176	69	2800 (2100-3900)	11.8
	19-22	70	154	177	70	2900 (2500-3300)	12.2
	23-50	70	154	178	70	2700 (2300-3100)	11.3
	51-75	70	154	178	70	2400 (2000-2800)	10.1
	76 +	70	154	178	70	2050 (1650-2450)	8.6
Females	11-14	46	101	157	62	2200 (1500-3000)	9.2
	15-18	55	120	163	64	2100 (1200-3000)	8.8
	19-22	55	120	163	64	2100 (1700-2500)	8.8
	23-50	55	120	163	64	2000 (1600-2400)	8.4
	51-75	55	120	163	64	1800 (1400-2200)	7.6
	76 +	55	120	163	64	1600 (1200-2000)	6.7
Pregnant						+300	
lactating						+500	

From Food and Nutrition Board, National Academy of Sciences—National Research Council, Washington, 1980.

*The data in this table have been assembled with desirable weights for adults given in Table 49-12 for the mean heights of men (70 inches) and women (64 inches) between the ages of 18 and 34 years as surveyed in the U.S. population (HEW/NCHS data).

The energy allowances for the young adults are for men and women doing light work. The allowances for the two older groups represent mean energy needs over these age spans, allowing for a 2% decrease in basal (resting) metabolic rate per decade and a reduction in activity of 200 kcal/day for men and women between 51 and 75 years, 500 kcal for men over 75 years, and 400 kcal for women over 75. The customary range of daily energy output is shown for adults in parentheses and is based on a variation in energy needs of ±400 kcal at any one age, emphasizing the wide range of energy intake appropriate for any group of people.

Energy allowances for children through age 18 are based on median energy intakes of children of these ages followed in longitudinal growth studies. The values in parentheses are 10th and 90th percentiles of energy intake, to indicate the range of energy consumption among children of these ages.

Table 49-15. Standard formulation for total parenteral nutrition*

Each 1000 ml contains:

Total calories:	**1000**
Amino acids: (4.25%, 180 cal)	**42.5 g**
Dextrose: (25%, 850 cal)	**250 g**
Nitrogen:	**6.25 g**
Vitamins:	**B complex (1 ml) and ascorbic acid equivalent (550 mg) every day; multivitamins (B group, A, D, E) (3.5 ml) and ascorbic acid equivalent (800 mg) once weekly**
Osmolarity:	**1900 mOsm**

Formula Type	K	Na	Mg as Sulfate	Ca	P (mM)	P (mg)	Cl	Acetate	Insulin (units)
Standard	12	21	8	4.5	13.4	415	8	25	0
With added sodium	12	51	8	4.5	13.4	415	24	43	0
With added insulin	12	21	8	4.5	13.4	415	8	25	15
With added sodium and insulin	12	51	8	4.5	13.4	415	24	43	15
With added potassium	40	21	8	4.5	17.3	536	16	43	0
With added potassium and sodium	40	51	8	4.5	17.3	536	32	53	0
With added potassium and insulin	40	21	8	4.5	17.3	536	16	43	15
With added potassium, sodium, and insulin	40	51	8	4.5	17.3	536	32	53	15

*Values expressed in milliequivalents unless otherwise noted.

ets varies widely; this should be taken into consideration in the selection of a diet for an individual patient.

Liquid formulas other than defined-formula diets may be effective for selected patients (Table 49-16). These formulas may be used to supplement regular food intake, to increase the intake of one or more nutrients, or to provide the combination and proportion of nutrients most beneficial for the patient. Supplements should be selected for specific reasons, and their use carefully monitored by the physician. Of particular interest are formulas designed for special medical indications, such as Amin-Aid for patients with renal disease; Lofenalac, a low-phenylalanine formula for

Table 49-16. Examples of commercial formulas for nutritional support

Formula	Grams per 1000 kcal			
	Protein	Fat	Carbohydrate	Lactose
Complete defined-formula diets				
Milk base: moderate residue, intact protein				
Carnation Instant Breakfast (Carnation)	55.2	27.6	124.1	84.0
Compleat (Sandoz)	40.2	40.2	119.6	24.4
Enfamil (Mead Johnson)	22.2	54.6	103.3	103.3
Meritene (Sandoz)	60.4	33.3	114.6	80.0
Sustacal (powder) (Mead Johnson)	57.0	25.9	133.3	93.0
Lactose-free, low-residue, intact protein, protein isolates				
Compleat-Modified (Sandoz)	40.1	32.0	130.8	0
Enrich (Ross)	36.1	34.8	147.3	0
Ensure (Ross)	35.1	35.1	136.8	0
Ensure HN (Ross)	41.9	33.4	133.2	0
Ensure Plus (Ross)	36.6	35.5	133.3	0
Ensure Plus HN (Ross)	41.7	33.3	133.3	0
Isocal (Mead Johnson)	32.1	41.1	126.2	0
Isocal HN (Mead Johnson)	41.5	42.4	116.0	0
Isomil (Ross)	26.4	54.4	101.5	0
Jevity (Ross)	41.9	34.7	143.1	0
Magnacal (Sherwood Medical)	35.0	40.0	125.0	0
Osmolite (Ross)	35.0	36.2	136.8	0
Osmolite HN (Ross)	41.9	34.7	133.2	0
Portagen (Mead Johnson)	34.6	47.5	114.8	0
Resource (Sandoz)	34.9	34.9	136.7	0
Prosobee (Mead Johnson)	30.0	53.0	100.0	0
Similac (Ross)	23.8	53.6	108.8	0
Sustacal (Mead Johnson)	60.3	22.8	138.6	0
Traumacal (Mead Johnson)	55.3	45.3	94.6	0
Ultracal (Mead Johnson)	41.5	42.4	116.0	0
Lactose-free, low-residue, hydrolyzed protein, amino acids				
Critical HN (Mead Johnson)	35.8	5.0	207.5	0
Nutramigen (Mead Johnson)	28.0	39.0	134.0	0
Pregestimil (Mead Johnson)	28.5	41.0	134.0	0
Reabilan (O'Brien/KMI)	31.0	39.0	131.0	0
Vital HN (Ross)	41.7	10.8	185.0	0
Vivonex T.E.N. (Sandoz)	38.2	2.8	206.0	0
Formula for special metabolic indications				
Amin-Aid (Kendall McGaw)	9.9	23.6	187.0	0
Hepatic-Aid II (Kendall McGaw)	37.5	30.8	143.3	0
Lofenalac (Mead Johnson)	32.5	39.8	129.2	0
Phenyl-Free (Mead Johnson)	50.0	16.8	162.5	0
Pulmocare (Ross)	42.0	61.3	70.7	0
Replena (Ross)	14.8	47.2	126.2	0
Travasorb Renal (Clintec)	17.1	13.3	202.7	0
Travasorb Hepatic (Clintec)	26.4	13.2	193.2	0
Supplementary feedings				
Casec (Mead Johnson)	237.6	5.4	0.0	0
Citrotein (Doyle)	60.5	2.6	184.2	0
Controlyte (Doyle)	0.0	48.0	143.0	0
MCT Oil (Mead Johnson)	0.0	120.5	0.0	0
Microlipid (Sherwood Medical)	0.0	111.0	0.0	0
Pedialyte (Ross)	0.0	0.0	250.0	0
Polycose (Ross)	0.0	0.0	250.0	0
Propac (Sherwood Medical)	189.9	20.5	0.0	0
Sumacal (Sherwood Medical)	0.0	0.0	250.0	0

infants and children with phenylketonuria; and Hepatic Aid, a special amino acid mixture containing relatively high amounts of branched-chain amino acids and relatively low amounts of aromatic amino acids used for patients with hepatic insufficiency.

REFERENCES

Brown ML, editor: Present knowledge in nutrition. Washington DC, 1990, International Life Sciences Institute—Nutrition Foundation.

Committee on Diet and Health, Food and Nutrition Board: Diet and health: implications for reducing chronic disease risk. Washington DC, 1989, National Academy Press.

Himes JH, editor: Anthropometric assessment of nutritional status. New York, 1991, Wiley-Liss.

Linder MD, editor: Nutritional biochemistry and metabolism with clinical applications, ed 2. New York, 1991, Elsevier.

McArdle WD, Katch FI, and Katch VL: Exercise physiology: energy, nutrition and human physiology, ed 3. Philadelphia, 1991, Lea & Febiger.

Rombeau JL and Caldwell MD, editors: Clinical nutrition: enteral and tube feeding, ed 2. Philadelphia, 1991, WB Saunders.

Rombeau JL and Caldwell MD, editors: Clinical nutrition: parenteral nutrition. Philadelphia, 1986, WB Saunders.

Rombeau JL et al, editors: Atlas of nutritional support. Boston, 1989, Little, Brown.

Shils ME and Young VR, editors: Modern nutrition in health and disease, ed 7. Philadelphia, 1988, Lea & Febiger.

Subcommittee on the Tenth Edition of the Recommended Dietary Allowances, Food and Nutrition Board: Recommended dietary allowances, ed 10. Washington DC, 1989, National Research Council, National Academy of Sciences.

LIVER, BILIARY TREE, AND PANCREAS

I PHYSIOLOGIC, BIOCHEMICAL, AND IMMUNOLOGIC PRINCIPLES

CHAPTER

50 Hepatic Metabolism

Seymour M. Sabesin

To consider the metabolic functions of the liver requires substantial discussion of the major biochemical processes in the body, particularly those that concern nutrient metabolism. The liver subserves central functions in the synthesis of proteins, carbohydrates, and lipids and is involved in many anabolic and catabolic reactions that regulate energy homeostasis in the fed and fasting states. The box provides an overview of the major metabolic functions of the liver and lists some specialized functions such as the storage of certain metals and vitamins. Only a few hepatic functions are discussed in detail in this chapter. Other functions of the liver are considered in other chapters and will be referred to in the text.

The liver is important in certain processes in addition to macromolecular synthesis; these include (1) energy production; i.e., the use of carbohydrates, proteins, and fats for aerobic respiration in hepatic mitochondria (tricarboxylic acid cycle); (2) the metabolism and detoxification of drugs, vitamins, and hormones; (3) ammonia metabolism, leading to ureagenesis; and (4) maintenance of blood glucose levels and ketogenesis.

It is appropriate to consider briefly the major anabolic and catabolic functions of the liver. Liver disease may be associated with derangements in these functions, although marked impairment does not occur unless there has been a substantial loss of hepatic parenchymal tissue. A detailed analysis of all the metabolic functions of the liver comprises a major aspect of biochemistry; the objective here is to highlight the most important functions emphasizing processes that are most important physiologically and that are deranged readily in liver disease.

AMINO ACID AND PROTEIN METABOLISM

The liver is the major site of plasma protein synthesis. The liver synthesizes and then secretes into the plasma a variety of proteins, several of which subserve very specific functions (coagulation factors, transport proteins, etc.) (see box). In addition to synthesizing export proteins, the liver synthesizes the structural proteins and enzymes required for the maintenance of hepatocellular function. About 50% of hepatic protein synthesis is synthesis of proteins for export. The 12 g of albumin synthesized daily represents 25% of total hepatic protein synthesis in human beings.

Total body protein in an average 70-kg adult is approximately 12 kg. In a steady state, protein turnover reflects the synthesis and degradation of equal amounts of protein. Total body protein turnover is 200 to 300 g/day. When dietary supply is normal, liver and muscle use amino acids released by local protein degradation for up to 50% of their synthetic requirements. With dietary protein restriction this figure may be increased to 90%. Thus the amino acid pool available for protein synthesis is derived from the degradation of about 250 g of body protein plus variable amounts of dietary protein. Total body protein turnover also includes endogenous secretion of enzyme proteins, exfoliated cellular protein, and protein exuded into the gastrointestinal lumen. In the intestinal lumen all of these proteins mix with amino acids of dietary origin and undergo a similar digestive-absorptive process. Amino

Hepatic functions

I. Protein synthesis
  A. Albumin
  B. Blood coagulation proteins
    1. Fibrinogen (factor I)
    2. Prothrombin (factor II)
    3. Factors V, VII, IX, X
  C. Synthesis of other proteins
    1. Haptoglobin
    2. Ceruloplasmin
    3. Transferrin
    4. Alpha and beta globulins
    5. Complement factors
    6. Hormone transport proteins (e.g., sex steroid-binding globulins)
  D. Glycoprotein synthesis
  E. Synthesis of structural proteins and intracellular enzymes
II. Lipid synthesis
  A. Triglyceride
  B. Cholesterol
  C. Phospholipids
  D. Lipoproteins (very-low and very-high-density)
  E. Bile acids
III. Metabolic functions
  A. Biochemical oxidations
  B. Carbohydrate metabolism
    1. Glycogenesis
    2. Glycogenolysis
    3. Gluconeogenesis
    4. Glucose clearance from blood
    5. Lactate clearance from blood
    6. Nonglucose hexose metabolism (e.g., fructose and galactose)
  C. Amino acid metabolism for protein, carbohydrate, and lipid synthesis
  D. Free fatty acid metabolism
  E. Ketogenesis
  F. Ureagenesis
  G. Bilirubin metabolism: conjugation and excretion of bilirubin
  H. Lipoprotein uptake and catabolism (e.g., chylomicron remnants, LDL)
  I. Hormone metabolism
    1. Insulin
    2. Glucagon
    3. Growth hormone
    4. Glucocorticoids
    5. Catecholamines
    6. Thyroxine
    7. Sex steroid hormones
  J. Conjugation, solubilization, and deamination of drugs
IV. Specialized functions
  A. Bilirubin and bile salt secretion
  B. Reticuloendothelial functions
    1. Phagocytosis
    2. Processing of antigens (bacterial, viral, dietary) absorbed from the intestine
  C. Receptor-mediated uptake and endocytosis of many ligands (e.g., LDL)
  D. Storage functions
    1. Fat-soluble vitamins (A, D, K)
    2. Vitamin B_{12}
    3. Metals (iron, copper)
  E. Maintenance of plasma volume and electrolyte concentrations

acids entering the portal vein originate from about 90 g of dietary protein, 50 g of exfoliated cellular protein, 16 g of secreted enzyme protein, and 2 g of exuded plasma protein.

The overall protein turnover rate is relatively stable, even with protein deprivation, reflecting compensatory changes in liver and muscle. With continued deprivation of exogenous amino acids, the mass of hepatic tissue protein decreases and the absolute rate of synthesis falls. In this way, the amino acid supply regulates the synthesis of proteins secreted by the liver into the plasma.

Most amino acids entering the liver via the portal vein are catabolized to urea in the Krebs-Henseleit cycle. The remainder are either utilized directly for protein synthesis (of either intracellular or plasma proteins), converted to special compounds (e.g., glutathione), or released into the blood as free amino acids. In the liver during a 12-hour absorptive period (12 noon to 12 midnight), 57% of incoming nitrogen is converted to urea, 6% is used for plasma protein synthesis, 14% is used for endogenous hepatic protein synthesis, and 23% is secreted into the circulation as free amino acids. During the nonabsorptive (fasting) period, the influx of amino acids in the portal blood is about one sixth of the absorptive level and is derived mostly from secreted and exfoliated protein. Plasma protein synthesis continues at the same rate as before, but amino acid release ceases and ureagenesis decreases by about two thirds. During fasting, hepatic tissue protein goes into a catabolic phase and, together with alanine (released from muscle), contributes to ureagenesis and gluconeogenesis. All of these metabolic changes are mediated by enzymes concerned with synthesis of nonessential amino acids, transamination, ureagenesis, and gluconeogenesis.

Turnover of plasma amino acids is rapid. The total plasma pool of amino acids is about one two-hundredths the size of the influx. The tissue amino acid pool is about half the size of the absorbed amino acid load. It is composed mostly of glutamic acid, glutamine, alanine, and glycine, indicating that the turnover of plasma amino acids is associated with rapid transamination as well as utilization for protein synthesis. The liver is selective in its uptake of amino acids. For example, the branched-chain amino acids valine, isoleucine, and leucine are metabolized predominantly by muscle.

Albumin synthesis

Albumin is synthesized exclusively in the liver at a rate in adults of 150 to 200 mg/kg/day. The half-life of albumin is 17 to 20 days but may be reduced with excessive losses from the body, as in protein-losing gastroenteropathy (Chapter 42) and massive proteinuria (Chapter 343). Albumin synthesis begins by association of messenger RNA with free ribosomal subunits in the hepatocyte cytosol. It is formed as a precursor molecule called *preproalbumin*. Portions of this molecule are subsequently removed within the hepatocyte, forming the final product, albumin, which is secreted from the cell. At the subcellular level, the time course for the assembly, intracellular transport, and secretion of albumin has been investigated by use of radioactively labeled amino acid precursors. The labeled amino acid is incorporated into the growing albumin chain within 1 minute. Sequentially, the radiolabeled albumin has its highest specific activity in the rough endoplasmic reticulum within 3 minutes, in the smooth endoplasmic reticulum within 6 minutes, and in the Golgi apparatus at 15 to 20 minutes. From the Golgi complex, the albumin molecules are packaged into secretory vesicles that migrate through the cytosol and fuse with the basolateral plasma membrane, thereby discharging the albumin into the perisinusoidal space of Disse.

About 0.3 to 0.4 mg of newly synthesized albumin per gram of liver tissue is present within hepatocytes. At a constant rate of synthesis and release, this quantity of albumin would turn over three times an hour; however, such a rate is two or three times greater than the normal synthetic rate of 150 to 200 mg/kg/day. Thus albumin synthesis and secretion operate at about one third of capacity.

Factors that regulate albumin synthesis are nutrition, hormonal balance, and osmotic pressure. Nutritional status is the prime factor, as albumin synthesis is very sensitive to the available supply of amino acids, particularly tryptophan. The livers of fasting animals produce less than half the amount of albumin that is synthesized by those of fed animals. The factors regulating albumin degradation are less well known. No organ has been implicated directly in albumin degradation. Fractional rates of albumin degradation are related directly to the albumin mass, serum albumin level, and dietary protein intake. When protein intake is limited, there is a low fractional rate of degradation.

Osmotic regulation of albumin synthesis is precise. The liver responds to reductions in extravascular osmotic pressure by increasing the rate of albumin synthesis. This effect is modulated by the osmotic pressure in the hepatic interstitial volume, only about one tenth of which is available for albumin distribution.

Hormones also influence hepatic protein metabolism, in part through their influences on nutrient metabolism. Examples of effects of hormones on hepatic protein synthesis include the anabolic effect of insulin on tissue and export protein synthesis and its anticatabolic effect on tissue protein degradation. Corticosteroids, growth hormone, and thyroid hormone stimulate albumin synthesis, whereas glucagon has an antianabolic effect on tissue and secretory proteins.

Ureagenesis

The formation of urea from ammonia is a unique hepatic function providing means by which the product of tissue and dietary nitrogen catabolism can be eliminated. Ureagenesis occurs in the Krebs-Henseleit cycle, which utilizes the four specific amino acids ornithine, citrulline, arginine, and aspartic acid to transform ammonia into urea. Urea is excreted primarily by the kidneys but also by the gastrointestinal tract (25%).

HEPATIC FORMATION OF SPECIALIZED PROTEINS

Coagulation factors (see Chapter 85)

The liver is the site of synthesis of many blood-clotting factors (see the box on p. 526). Factors II (prothrombin), VII, IX, and X are vitamin K responsive, and thus their synthesis is decreased if intestinal absorption of vitamin K is impaired. The half-life of several coagulation factors is quite short, varying from 4 hours for factor VII to 3 to 5 days for prothrombin. Prothrombin is synthesized as an inactive precursor whose conversion to an active coagulation protein requires vitamin K. The reduced form of vitamin K functions in the activation of an enzyme that removes gamma-carboxyglutamic acid from the precursor molecule. This reaction permits the conversion of prothrombin to thrombin, a process that requires factors V and X.

The liver synthesizes and degrades fibrinolytic factors and clears activated clotting factors from the circulation. Fibrinogen has a relatively constant fractional degradation rate, irrespective of plasma concentration. Alterations in fibrogen synthesis may occur in liver disease, possibly due to the formation of functionally abnormal fibrinogens with reduced clotting ability.

Transferrin

Transferrin, the iron-binding protein, is synthesized principally but not exclusively in the liver. Its synthesis may be increased in iron deficiency states. Transferrin synthesis is predominant in determining the plasma transferrin concentration.

Ceruloplasmin

Ceruloplasmin, important for copper transport and homeostasis, is synthesized in the liver. Plasma ceruloplasmin levels are decreased in Wilson's disease (Chapter 60).

Alpha$_1$ antitrypsin

Alpha$_1$ antitrypsin is synthesized by the liver, a process that is stimulated by acute stress. It is a serine protease inhibitor that may function to inactivate proteases released from intracellular sites. $Alpha_1$ antitrypsin is responsible for about 90% of the protease activity in plasma, but this is reduced to about 15% in patients with a hereditary defect in hepatic alpha-1 antitrypsin synthesis (Chapter 60).

Alpha-fetoprotein

Alpha-fetoprotein is a normal secretory product of human fetal liver. Normally not present in plasma, its appearance in association with hepatocellular carcinomas (Chapter 63) is thought to reflect the derepression of fetal genomes. Alpha-fetoprotein may be associated with hepatic regeneration, as it has been reported in plasma after viral or toxic hepatitis and massive hepatic necrosis.

Ferritin

Ferritin is the principal form of available stored iron. Serum ferritin originates in part as a hepatic secretory protein. Serum ferritin concentration correlates well with total body iron stores. Thus it provides a good screening test for iron overload or deficiency. Serum ferritin may also be elevated in association with acute liver injury or ongoing chronic active hepatocellular necrosis. The function of circulating ferritin is not known, but knowledge of its role in tissue as a storage protein for iron is well established.

LIVER AND LIPID METABOLISM

The liver is involved in many aspects of lipid synthesis and metabolism (Fig. 50-1). It is a major site of triglyceride, cholesterol, and phospholipid synthesis. Cholesterol and phospholipids are used in part as constituents of hepatocyte membranes. In association with triglycerides they are also assembled into certain classes of lipoproteins that are then secreted into the circulation. Cholesterol is also used for bile acid synthesis, a process confined to the liver (Chapter 51).

Cholesterol synthesis is derived from acetate via its conversion to beta-hydroxy-beta-methylglutaryl-CoA (HMG-CoA). Regulation of the activity of the enzyme HMG-CoA reductase that controls this step is quite complex, depending in part on the hepatic uptake of cholesterol from dietary sources in chylomicron remnants. The regulation of the body cholesterol pool, which is relatively constant, is determined by a balance between synthesis and loss in the gastrointestinal tract and from desquamating cutaneous cells. Factors that regulate hepatic cholesterol synthesis include dietary cholesterol absorption, bile acid homeostasis, and the uptake of cholesterol from lipoproteins during their catabolism.

Fatty acid uptake and utilization (see also Chapter 171)

Fatty acids liberated from adipose tissue are carried in the bloodstream bound to albumin. Approximately one third of the circulating fatty acids are removed by the liver, one third by skeletal muscle, and the rest by other tissues, especially myocardium. Hepatic triglyceride formation or accumulation is greatly affected by the rate at which fatty acids are presented to the liver. Fatty acids released from adipose tissue have a short half-life in the plasma, with a t½ of about 2 min. The liver can extract 30% of circulating free fatty acids in a single cycle.

After hepatic uptake, fatty acids may be oxidized or used for ketone body formation or for triglyceride and phospholipid synthesis (Fig. 50-1). Quantitatively, most of the fatty acids reaching the liver are resecreted into the bloodstream as triglycerides in the form of very-low-density lipoproteins (VLDL). After uptake of exogenously or endogenously derived fatty acids, hepatic triglyceride esterification occurs

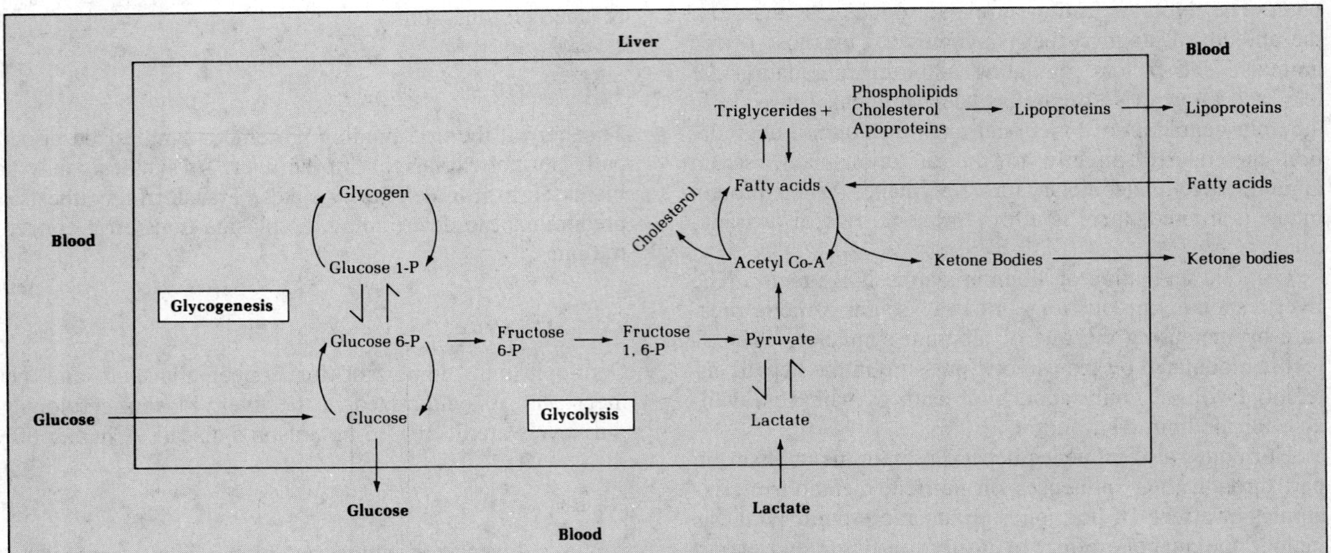

Fig. 50-1. Simplified scheme of carbohydrate and lipid metabolism in the liver.

rapidly. Thus within 2 minutes after injection of radiolabeled fatty acids, most fatty acids recovered from the liver are already esterified. Esterification is closely linked to hepatic oxidative phosphorylation and is dependent on a ready supply of alpha-glycerophosphate, the precursor of glycerol supplied almost exclusively from glucose, and the availability of fatty acyl CoA. Glucose and insulin are extremely important in the regulation of hepatic triglyceride formation. Insulin regulates the activity of glucokinase that is essential for glucose phosphorylation, increases fatty acid synthesis from glucose, and promotes hepatic triglyceride secretion.

During fasting or when metabolic demands are great, fatty acids are used for ketone body formation. Fatty acid oxidation is important in removing excess lipid from the liver so that accumulation does not ordinarily occur. Fatty acids incorporated into phospholipids are stored in the formed membrane lipids or in the exchangeable phospholipid pools.

The rate of hepatic triglyceride synthesis is usually regulated by approximately equal hepatic secretion of triglyceride, but acute stresses such as mobilization of fatty acids from adipose tissue or a rapid and prolonged increase in dietary chylomicron triglyceride can result in increased hepatic triglyceride synthesis. The liver may respond to an increased fatty acid influx by increasing the rate of lipoprotein and ketone body formation, but the extent to which the activity of these pathways can increase is limited. If the rate at which fatty acids are brought to the liver exceeds the ability of the liver to metabolize and/or resecrete the fatty acids into the circulation as lipoproteins, storage of fat within the hepatocytes will ensue.

Lipoprotein biosynthesis

The lipoproteins in fasting plasma are the metabolic products of newly synthesized (nascent) lipoproteins secreted by the liver or intestine. The liver contributes in many ways to the synthesis and metabolism of the plasma lipoproteins. Thus the liver synthesizes the major lipids and apoproteins of the plasma lipoproteins and secretes VLDL and high-density lipoproteins (HDL). VLDL and HDL are secreted as nascent particles whose lipid and apoprotein compositions are altered drastically in the plasma as a result of enzymatic transformations and exchange of lipids and apoproteins among various lipoprotein classes. These transformations, which are intrinsic to lipoprotein metabolism, are also dependent on other hepatic functions such as the synthesis of apoproteins C-II and A-I, which are the activators of lipoprotein lipase (LPL) and lecithin-cholesterol acyltransferase (LCAT), respectively. These enzymes are essential for the initiation of the lipoprotein metabolic pathways, as LPL is involved in the lipolysis of triglyceride-rich lipoproteins (chylomicrons and VLDL), and LCAT is responsible, in human beings, for all plasma cholesterol esterification. The liver is involved also in the uptake and degradation of chylomicron remnants, HDL, and LDL.

Significant advances have been made in lipoprotein metabolism in the past few years, with particular relevance to the role of the liver. This topic is discussed in Chapter 171.

Bile acid synthesis (see Chapter 51)

CARBOHYDRATE METABOLISM

The liver is essential for the regulation of carbohydrate metabolism, as it receives directly from the portal circulation most of the ingested carbohydrates and then, by hormonal regulation, controls the concentration of blood glucose in the fed and fasting states. The most important function of the liver in carbohydrate metabolism is its role in constantly regulating blood glucose levels, thereby providing a predictable supply of glucose for energy needs in tissues throughout the body (Fig. 50-1).

The metabolic actions of the liver with regard to carbohydrate metabolism and the maintenance of blood glucose levels are closely related to the liver's role in lipid (Fig. 50-1) and protein metabolism and to the fact that key hormones regulating carbohydrate homeostasis act mainly on the liver. These key hormones include insulin, glucagon, growth hormone, glucocorticoids, catecholamines, and thyroxine, all of which, except catecholamines, are catabolized by the liver. The liver's major role in carbohydrate metabolism can be subdivided into (1) functions that produce glucose, (2) functions that result in glucose storage as glycogen, and (3) the metabolism of hexoses and sugars other than glucose that are also derived from dietary sources. Processes involved in the maintenance of blood glucose concentration include (1) uptake and storage of glucose in the form of glycogen (glycogenesis), (2) conversion of stored glycogen into glucose (glycogenolysis), and (3) formation of glucose from noncarbohydrate sources (gluconeogenesis).

The main carbohydrates in the human diet are sucrose, fructose, lactose, and starch. Enzymatic hydrolysis of these substances yields glucose and fructose and smaller quantities of galactose. There is little fluctuation of blood glucose concentrations even after ingestion of large amounts of glucose. Glucose is disposed of rapidly and in large quantities, primarily by the liver. The importance of the liver in taking up a dietary glucose load is related not only to the anatomic location of the liver but also to the liver's sensitivity to insulin. Glucose disposal is autoregulated by glucose and insulin. Glucagon has short-term effects on glycogen breakdown but has a more sustained stimulatory effect on gluconeogenesis. Glucagon levels fall after glucose ingestion, and its effects are overcome by insulin. In contrast, glucocorticoids present in excess amounts can counteract the effects of insulin on glucose disposal in the liver. After its rapid diffusion into the liver, glucose is rapidly phosphorylated to glucose 6-phosphate by glucokinase. Most of the glucose is stored as glycogen. Glycolysis, from either glucose or glycogen, is relatively inactive in the liver, and less than 10% of glucose is disposed of by glycolysis. Glucose is also metabolized by the hexose monophosphate shunt.

The ingestion of glucose after fasting causes a rise in blood glucose levels and a concomitant release of insulin, which facilitates glucose uptake into cells. Approximately 60% of an oral glucose load is taken up by the liver and utilized for glycogen synthesis, triglyceride formation, and, in small amounts, for glycolysis (Fig. 50-1). About 25% of the glucose is used by the brain and by non-insulin-dependent tissues as an energy source. During fasting, the liver maintains glucose homeostasis by glycogenolysis and gluconeogenesis. These two processes occur in response to decreased blood insulin levels and corresponding increases in glucagon concentration. The liver's capacity for glycogen storage is limited, about 70 g. With fasting, hepatic glycogen stores are depleted after 1 day; however, glucose consumption continues at a constant rate, stimulating hepatic gluconeogenesis.

The liver is the major site of gluconeogenesis, which utilizes three types of nonsugar precursors: glycogenic amino acids, lactate, and glycerol phosphate. The pathways leading to gluconeogenesis include the transamination of glycogenic amino acids. The alpha-ketoacids formed by transamination enter the gluconeogenic pathway either directly (pyruvate, oxaloacetate derived from alanine, and aspartate) or after further metabolic conversions (alpha-ketoglutarate from glutamate). Glycogenic amino acids are used for gluconeogenesis when dietary protein is high and there is insufficient dietary carbohydrate. This process is stimulated by glucocorticoid hormones. When oxygen consumption is insufficient to keep up with glucose utilization, as with vigorous muscular exercise, lactate produced in muscle is used for gluconeogenesis. The pathway leading to glucose formation from lactate involves first the oxidation of lactate to pyruvate and then entrance of pyruvate into the pathway, leading to glucose formation from glucose 6-phosphate. Glucose production from lactate can exceed 60 μmol/g liver/hr; however this is very energy-demanding, consuming a considerable fraction of nucleotide triphosphates.

Lipid metabolism is important for glucose homeostasis, as the availability of glycerol phosphate for gluconeogenesis is derived from triglyceride and phospholipid metabolism. Triglyceride hydrolysis causes the release of free glycerol. The liver then converts glycerol to glycerol phosphate at the expense of adenosine triphosphate (ATP). In contrast, phospholipid hydrolysis leads directly to glycerol phosphate formation. Subsequently, glycerol phosphate is oxidized to dihydroxyacetone phosphate. When dietary carbohydrate is insufficient to maintain glucose homeostasis but fat intake is high, gluconeogenesis from the glycerol phosphate pathway takes place and the free fatty acids, released by triglyceride hydrolysis, are utilized for ketone body formation.

In short-term starvation the central nervous system (CNS) and peripheral nerves require glucose, whereas other tissues can use fatty acids and ketone bodies as energy substrates. The liver is essential to maintaining blood glucose levels, for it contains the enzyme glucose 6-phosphatase, which is necessary for the formation of glucose in the hepatocytes.

Lactate is the most important substance in gluconeogenesis, providing about 20% of total glucose after an overnight fast. More than 50% of the lactate is derived from glycogenolysis in extrahepatic tissues, principally muscle. Because muscle glycogen is derived from liver glucose, the utilization of lactate for gluconeogenesis does not represent a net increase in glucose synthesis. Gluconeogenesis from amino acids amounts to only about 6% to 12% of total glucose production after an overnight fast, but this percentage increases considerably if fasting continues. The principal amino acid for gluconeogenesis is alanine. Alanine is formed in peripheral tissues by transamination of pyruvate, but alanine is also synthesized from other amino acids. The regulation of gluconeogenesis is also sensitive to substrate availability; net glucose production increases with increasing precursor supply.

Most of the changes that occur in fasting can be attributed to alterations in the levels of circulating hormones that are superimposed on endogenous regulatory mechanisms. For example, as blood glucose concentrations fall, insulin secretion decreases and there are reciprocal elevations of glucagon secretion and increases in the concentrations of glucocorticoids, growth hormone, and catecholamines. The effects of glucocorticoids on peripheral tissues result in a release of alanine into the circulation, followed by an increased extraction of alanine by the liver, a process regulated by glucagon. The decrease in insulin lessens insulin's normal constraint on gluconeogenesis, which increases. At the same time glycogenolysis increases, due in part to lack of inhibition by glucose and insulin. With prolonged fasting there is an increase in adipose tissue lipolysis. This increase results in a marked increase in the uptake of free fatty acids by the liver, which results in increased ketone body formation, providing an alternative source of fuel for peripheral tissues and eventually for the CNS.

Metabolism of other hexoses

Fructose is an important caloric source. It is taken up and metabolized by the liver, where it is phosphorylated rapidly to fructose 1-phosphate. The latter enters the glycolytic/gluconeogenic pathway. Normally, about 70% of a fructose load appears as lactate, with the rest converted to glycogen. Galactose and other hexoses are also metabolized by the liver and are converted mostly to glucose or glycogen.

Ketogenesis

Ketone body formation, a process that occurs exclusively in the liver, is another essential hepatic function. Ketone bodies provide an energy source utilized by all tissues during starvation, and they are the only effective source of energy (other than glucose) for the CNS. The ketone bodies acetoacetate and beta-hydroxybutyrate are formed in the hepatocyte mitochondria from free fatty acids. This complex sequence of metabolic events depends in part on decreased insulin availability secondary to fasting or starvation. With insulin deficiency there is activation of lipolysis in peripheral adipose tissue, causing mobilization of free fatty acids. The rate of hepatic fatty acid oxidation is controlled by the activity of the carnitine acyltransferase system of enzymes that transports fatty acids into the mitochondria. During feeding, malonyl CoA, a potent inhibitor of carnitine acyltransferase I, prevents the transport of fatty acids into the mitochondria. This inhibition is removed during fasting by glucagon, which acts to lower the malonyl CoA concentration and increase the carnitine content of the liver. These changes enhance the capacity for fatty acid oxidation, and thus ketogenesis is activated. The rate of ketone body production is determined by the rate of delivery of free fatty acids from the periphery.

DETOXIFICATION

A major biochemical function of the liver is the detoxification and metabolism of drugs, vitamins, and hormones. The liver has a large capacity to modify exogenous and endogenous substances. Some compounds are metabolically converted to relatively inactive forms (e.g., steroid hormones), whereas others become more biologically active (e.g., vitamin D). Of prime importance in maintaining homeostasis and protecting the body against ingested toxins is the ability of the liver to metabolize and detoxify a wide variety of absorbed substances that reach it directly in the portal blood. Hepatic drug metabolism and drug-induced liver disease are considered in detail in Chapter 57.

HORMONE METABOLISM

The liver is involved in the metabolism of many hormones by virtue of its role in hormone biotransformation, inactivation, and excretion. In addition, many hormones exert direct effects on hepatic metabolic processes. Examples of the latter include the previously described effects of insulin, glucagon, and glucocorticoids on carbohydrate metabolism. The liver is particularly involved in steroid hormone metabolism. Steroid hormones are taken up from the circulation by the liver and then metabolized by hepatic enzymes, leading to their hydroxylation, oxidation, etc. The steroid hormones directly influence many of the liver's biochemical and physiologic functions. It is impossible to discuss all of the influences of hormones on the liver, because in some respects they encompass virtually all of its metabolic and physiologic functions. Therefore only examples of some key hormonal influences will be discussed.

The phagocytic function of the hepatic reticuloendothelial system is influenced directly by various steroid hormones. Estrogens stimulate phagocytosis, whereas glucocorticoids suppress reticuloendothelial function as assessed by the experimental inhibition of the clearance of infused particulate matter.

Insulin, glucocorticoids, estrogens, testosterone, thyroid hormone, and growth hormone are anabolic, increasing hepatic RNA synthesis and the rate of incorporation of amino acids into proteins. Hormones influence hepatic metabolism by regulating the synthesis of key enzymes involved in intermediary metabolism. There is considerable evidence that estrogens and progestins influence the plasma concentration of many proteins, presumably reflecting hormonal effects on hepatic synthesis, transport, and perhaps catabolism. Alteration in plasma concentration of certain proteins during pregnancy is an example of the physiologic regulation by hormones of hepatic protein production. Steroid hormones can induce key enzymes involved in porphyrin-heme synthesis, and by this means are important in the regulation of porphyrin and heme metabolism. The liver synthesizes special sex steroid-binding proteins and other globulins such as cortisol and thyroid-binding globulin (Chapter 147).

Hormones influence hepatic drug and chemical metabolism by their hormonal effects on hepatic enzymes involved in oxidative biotransformation and in drug conjugation. Sex hormones are particularly important in this regard, as evidenced by their effects on the oxidative capacity of the liver for certain drugs. Estrogens depress the rate of bile flow, and synthetic estrogens and progestins similarly depress the hepatic excretory capacity. The ability of the liver to excrete organic anions is compromised in pregnancy. Studies in pregnant women have demonstrated decreased capacity for the excretion of bilirubin and sulfobromophthalein sodium. The clinical counterpart of these hormonal effects is cholestasis, which sometimes occurs in pregnancy or after the use of oral contraceptives (Chapter 55). Steroid-induced cholestasis may also involve inhibitory effects on bilirubin conjugation, depressed bile salt synthesis, and other factors as yet poorly explained. The effects of liver injury on sex steroid biotransformation are discussed in Chapter 56.

REFERENCES

Cooper AD: Hepatic lipoprotein and cholesterol metabolism. In Zakim D and Boyer TD, editors: Hepatology. Philadelphia, 1990, WB Saunders.

Donohue TM Jr et al: Synthesis and secretion of plasma proteins by the liver. In Zakim D and Boyer TD, editors: Hepatology. Philadelphia, 1990, WB Saunders.

Glickman RM and Sabesin SM: Lipoprotein metabolism. In Arias I et al, editors: The liver: biology and pathobiology, New York, 1988, Raven Press.

Havel RJ: Structure and metabolism of lipoproteins. In Scriver CR et al, editors: The metabolic basis of inherited disease, New York, 1989, McGraw Hill.

Hellerstein MK and Munro HN: Interaction of liver and muscle in the regulation of metabolism in response to nutritional and other factors. In Arias I et al, editors: The liver: biology and pathobiology, New York, 1988, Raven Press.

Hoeg JM and Brewer HB Jr: Human lipoprotein metabolism and the liver. In Popper H and Schaffner F, editors: Progress in liver disease, vol 8, New York, 1986, Grune & Stratton.

Jones AL, Renston RH, and Burwen SJ: Uptake and intracellular disposition of plasma-derived proteins and apoproteins by hepatocytes. In Popper H and Schaffner F, editors: Progress in liver disease, vol 7, New York, 1982, Grune & Stratton.

Powers-Lee SG and Meister A: Urea synthesis and ammonia metabolism. In Arias I et al, editors: The liver: biology and pathobiology, New York, 1988, Raven Press.

Ratnoff OD: Disordered hemostasis in liver disease. In Schiff L and Schiff ER, editors: Diseases of the liver. Philadelphia, 1987, JB Lippincott.

Seifter S and Englard S: Energy metabolism. In Arias I et al, editors: The liver: biology and pathobiology, New York, 1988, Raven Press.

Shafritz DA and Panduro A: Protein synthesis and gene control in pathophysiologic states. In Arias I et al, editors: The liver: biology and pathobiology, New York, 1988, Raven Press.

Turley SD and Dietschy JM: Cholesterol metabolism and excretion. In

Arias I et al, editors: The liver: biology and pathobiology, New York, 1988, Raven Press.
Van Thiel DH: Endocrine function. In Arias I et al, editors: The liver: biology and pathobiology, New York, 1988, Raven Press.
Weisiger RA, Gollan JL, and Ockner RK: The role of albumin in hepatic uptake processes. In Popper H and Schaffner F, editors: Progress in liver disease, vol 7, New York, 1982, Grune & Stratton.
Zakim D: Metabolism of glucose and fatty acids by the liver. In Zakim D and Boyer TD, editors: Hepatology, Philadelphia, 1990, WB Saunders.

CHAPTER

51 Bile Production and Secretion

Martin C. Carey
Sander J. Robins

Bile is the "exocrine" secretion of the liver. Its solute composition is distinct, consisting principally of four kinds of lipids in an aqueous electrolyte solution. The lipids of bile possess differing degrees of water solubility but physically interact to be effectively solubilized and transported in bile and into the intestine. In the biliary tree, the function of bile is to aid the excretion of endogenous lipids, whereas in the intestine its principal function is to aid the absorption of dietary lipids. This chapter highlights the mechanisms of bile formation and secretion and focuses on its unique solute composition and properties.

COMPOSITION

The concentration by weight of solutes in bile varies, depending on the extent of water secretion and reabsorption at different anatomic sites in the biliary system. Average concentrations are 3% in the hepatic ducts and 10% in the gallbladder. The solute composition of bile is shown in Fig. 51-1. Two thirds of the total solute mass is composed of bile salts, a family of closely related detergent-like molecules. The phospholipids of bile are less than a quarter of the mass and consist mostly (95%) of lecithin (phosphatidylcholine); the sterols almost exclusively of unesterified cholesterol; and the bile pigments principally of bilirubin, which is conjugated predominantly with glucuronic acid. Present also are all the electrolytes of plasma and a variety of proteins of diverse origin, including plasma apolipoproteins, albumin, and secretory IgA; liver lysosomal and plasma membrane enzymes; and high-molecular-weight glycoproteins, most of which are secreted as gallbladder mucins. In addition, bile contains low concentrations of glutathione and trace amounts of heme, porphyrins, amino acids, vitamins, hormones, and many metals. Because of a high hepatic threshold for its secretion and avid resorption in the biliary ductules, bile contains no glucose. Hepatic bile contains a relatively high concentration of bicarbonate and maintains a pH of 7.0 to 8.0, whereas the secretion of protons and possibly resorption of bicarbonate in the gallbladder give gallbladder bile a pH of 6.2 to 7.4.

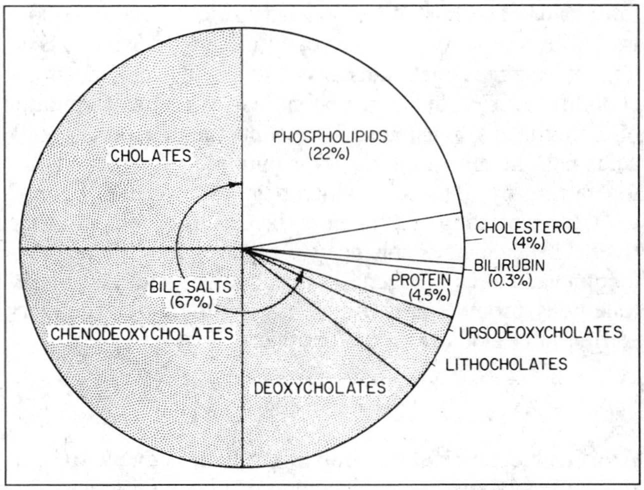

Fig. 51-1. Typical solute composition of human gallbladder bile by weight percentage.

BILE WATER PRODUCTION

In human beings, the volume of bile produced each day varies from 500 to 1200 ml. Bile water production is an entirely passive process that occurs in response to active secretion of a number of solutes and can be compartmentalized as shown in Fig. 51-2. Water transport occurs at hepatocellular, ductular, and gallbladder epithelial sites. Hepatocellular water production, generally referred to as *canalicular,* is mediated by the secretion of organic anions (predominantly bile salts) and by the electroneutral transport of inorganic cations (chiefly Na^+ and Ca^{2+}). In human beings, about 80% of secretion is canalicular in ori-

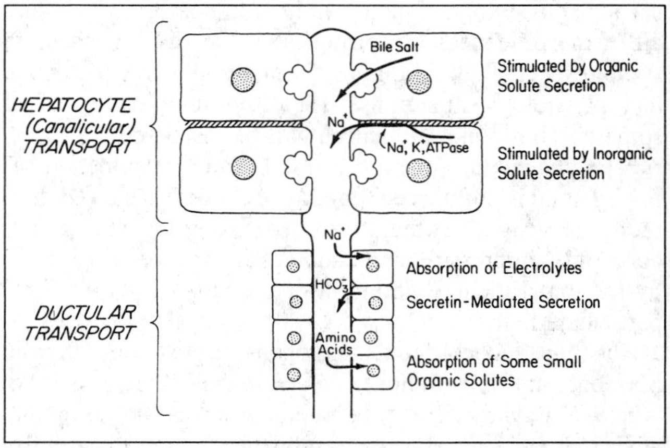

Fig. 51-2. Bile water production at different levels of the biliary system. Direction of water movement and principal stimuli for water transport shown by labeled arrows.

gin, 60% of which is bile salt dependent. Water secretion, which depends mainly on bile salt secretion, is directly proportional to the amount of osmotically active bile salts transported from the liver. Thus water secretion is less with native bile salts, which aggregate to form polymolecular aggregates called *micelles,* than with other organic anions, including highly hydrophilic synthetic bile salts, which may not aggregate extensively at biliary concentrations.

Bile salt-independent canalicular water flow that occurs chiefly in response to glutathione and Na^+ transport is mediated largely by the activity of $(Na^+ + K^+)$-ATPase located on the lateral plasma membranes of hepatocytes. By this process, Na^+-generated water is translocated into the paracellular spaces and then flows passively through low-resistance "tight" junctions into the canaliculi. Bile water is both secreted and reabsorbed by the epithelium of the bile ductules. Here, water production is stimulated chiefly by the gastrointestinal hormone secretin, which results in the formation of bicarbonate-rich bile. Resorption of water occurs along the entire length of the bile duct system, but chiefly in the gallbladder secondary to electrolyte absorption and, to some extent, to the absorption of small organic solutes (such as amino acids).

BILE LIPIDS

Bile salts and the enterohepatic circulation

Bile salts* have sharply defined hydrophobic (or nonpolar) and hydrophilic (or polar) regions and thus are soluble amphiphilic molecules that possess detergent-like properties. Structural transformations occur only on the polar plane of the bile salt surface (Fig. 51-3) and result in significant changes in the amphiphilic properties of the molecules. Thus by a shift in the ratio of ionized to acid form, of conjugated to nonconjugated form, or modifications by dehydroxylation and dehydrogenation, a bile salt molecule that is completely water soluble and readily forms micelles may be transformed to a water-insoluble molecule that is incapable of micelle formation. Thus bile salts must be considered a family of molecules whose physical-chemical properties are in a constant state of flux as a result of subtle biochemical alterations induced by bacterial enzymes and the variable H^+ ion concentrations in the gastrointestinal tract.

Cholic and chenodeoxycholic acids (Fig. 51-4) are termed *primary bile acids,* because they are synthesized de novo from unesterified cholesterol in the liver. Secondary bile acids are formed by removal or dehydrogenation of the 7-alpha-hydroxyl function on primary bile salts by anaerobic intestinal bacteria, whereas tertiary bile acids represent subsequent hepatic or bacterial modifications of the func-

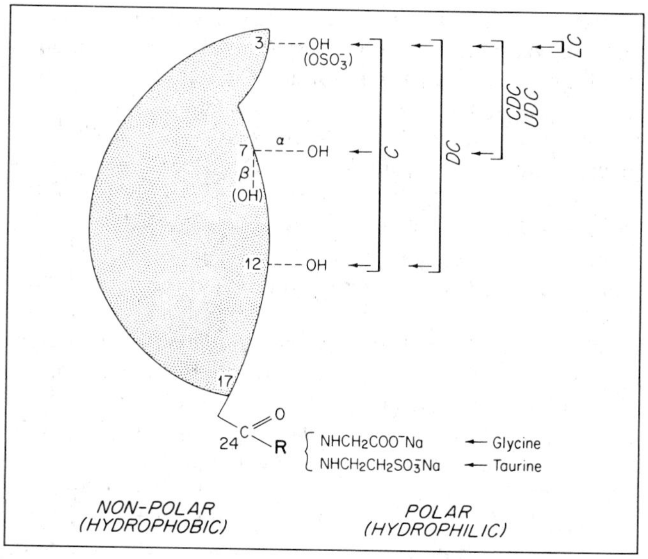

Fig. 51-3. Amphiphilic structure of common human bile salts. Arrows indicate position and number of polar substituents. *C,* cholates; *DC,* deoxycholates; *CDC,* chenodeoxycholates; *UDC,* ursodeoxycholates; *LC,* lithocholates; *R,* physiologic glycine or taurine conjugates found in bile and proximal small intestine. R is replaced by an OH group when bile salts are deconjugated in the colon. In UDC, the C-7 OH (β) group is equatorial, and in LC the C-3 OH group is predominantly sulfated.

tional groups on the steroid nucleus of secondary bile acids (Figs. 51-3 and 51-4). Cholesterol destined for bile acid synthesis is derived principally from newly synthesized cholesterol, but preformed cholesterol is drawn upon whenever synthetic demand increases.

Cholic and chenodeoxycholic acids are the end products

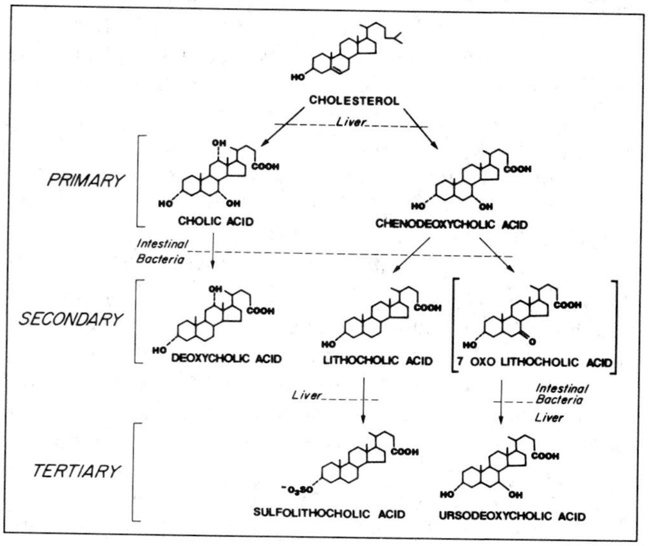

Fig. 51-4. Major bile acids in human beings. The primary bile acids are synthesized from cholesterol in the liver. Subsequent bacterial (and/or hepatic) modifications result in secondary and tertiary bile acids. Normally, 7-oxolithocholic acid is a trace constituent of bile.

*The terms *bile salt* and *bile acid* are used interchangeably in this chapter. It should be recognized, however, that the salt (ionized) form of these molecules, which is found in bile and small intestine, is more polar and more water soluble than the acid form, and thus is of greater physiologic importance. The sparingly soluble unionized bile acids are, in health, principally found only in the colon and in portal venous blood, but are converted completely to the salt form by conjugation during a single passage through the liver.

of a series of enzymatic reactions beginning with microsomal 7-alpha-hydroxylation of cholesterol. This reaction is rate-limiting in the overall synthetic process and is regulated by the magnitude of the return of bile salt to the liver in the portal venous blood. Downregulation of synthesis is much greater for hydrophobic bile salts (e.g., deoxycholates) than for hydrophilic bile salts (e.g., ursodeoxycholates) (Fig. 51-4). Subsequent synthetic steps involve additional hydroxylation to the steroid nucleus (principally by microsomal 12-alpha-hydroxylase), hydroxylation of the 27-carbon in the mitochondria (sterol 27-hydroxylase) and cleavage of the branched aliphatic side chain of the parent cholesterol molecule by β-oxidation to form a 24-carbon bile acid in the peroxisomes. Peripheral tissues are also believed to play an important but as yet unquantified role in bile acid synthesis in that plasma lipoproteins ferry 27-hydroxycholesterol from tissues to the liver where it can be converted to bile acids after 7α-hydroxylation.

Secretion of bile acids into bile requires that the acids be completely water soluble. To achieve water solubility, bile acids are conjugated (amidated) in the liver via a peptide bond with either taurine or glycine (Fig. 51-3). The conjugation reaction is a two-step process, involving a microsomal enzyme (bile acid: CoA ligase) followed by a cytosolic enzyme (bile acid-S-CoA: glycine/taurine N-acyltransferase). Conjugation lowers their pK_a values, thereby increasing the capacity of bile salts to remain ionized. As a result, their solubility at physiologic bile salt concentrations, calcium concentrations, and pH is also increased. In human beings, the normal pattern of bile salt conjugation results in a glycine/taurine ratio of approximately 3:1, but when excessive demands are placed on conjugation, such as increased de novo synthesis resulting from extensive bile salt malabsorption or with unconjugated bile acid therapy to effect gallstone dissolution, the ratio can increase to 10 to 20:1. An additional specialized form of conjugation occurs for the highly insoluble secondary bile salt lithocholate. In human beings, a small amount of this bile salt (about 20% of that synthesized by intestinal bacteria each day) is absorbed by the intestine and is returned to the liver, where it is rendered water soluble for biliary secretion by side-chain conjugation with glycine or taurine and, in 80% of the molecules, by sulfation at its single hydroxyl group (Figs. 51-3 and 51-4).

Three trace microsomal pathways involving glycosidic linkages of both amidated and nonamidated bile acids have been identified in healthy humans: nuclear hydroxyl or side-chain carboxylic glucuronidation, nuclear glucosidation, and nuclear N-acetylglucosaminidation. In cholestasis both sulfation and these specialized forms of glycosidation are induced, facilitating the elimination of all common bile acids in urine.

Deoxycholic and lithocholic acids, the physiologically important secondary bile acids (Fig. 51-4), are formed in the distal small intestine and colon by the action of strictly anaerobic bacteria. Subsequent bacterial or hepatic modifications of secondary bile salts result in tertiary bile salts (Fig. 51-4). Although bacterial enzymatic dehydroxylations and epimerizations result in the production of a large number of other molecular species, only those shown in Fig. 51-4 are resorbed into the portal circulation and have a continuing biologic life. The majority of bacterially transformed bile salts are water insoluble, poorly characterized derivatives that are excreted directly in the feces or, if absorbed, in the urine.

Bile salts undergo a highly efficient enterohepatic circulation (Fig. 51-5). After biliary secretion, 95% to 98% of the bile salts are absorbed by the small intestine (chiefly in the ileum), returned to the liver via the portal vein, effectively taken up by the liver, and resecreted into bile. Consequently, peripheral blood bile acid concentrations are extremely low (< 5 μM), and urinary excretion is trivial in healthy persons. Because the biliary secretion rate of bile salts calculated over the period of a day is appreciably larger than the size of the bile salt pool, it is clear that each bile salt molecule must recirculate a number of times each day.

In the normal steady state, hepatic bile salt synthesis just balances fecal bile salt loss, and the bile salt secretion rate remains constant. However, there may be considerable short-term variations in the bile salt secretion rate, which are contingent on several important physiologic events: (1) gallbladder sequestration of a large fraction of the bile salt pool during periods of fasting (such as during sleep); (2) intestinal transit time, which is responsible for the rate of delivery of bile salts to the sites of absorption; and (3) preferential absorption of bile salts of different polarities at different levels of the intestinal tract. Thus individual bile salts are absorbed and returned to the liver at different rates (Fig.

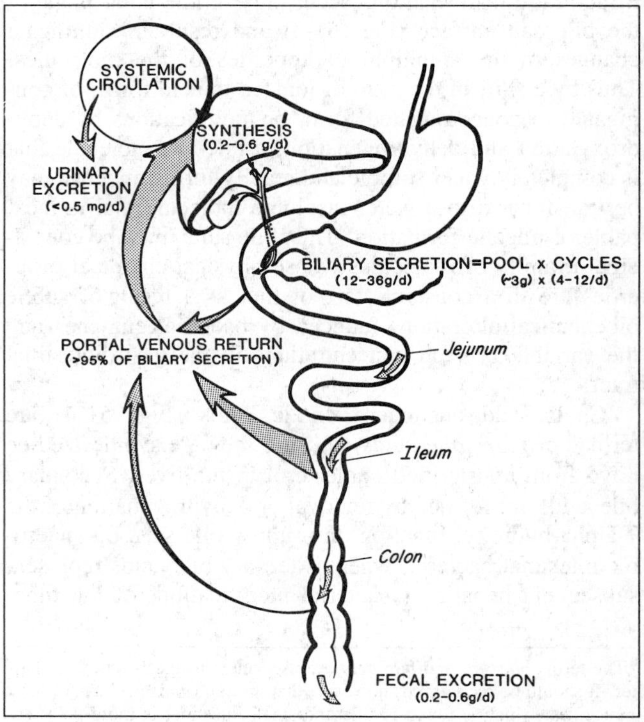

Fig. 51-5. Enterohepatic circulation of bile salts in normal human beings. Arrows indicate bile salt movement within the biliary tree, intestine, portal venous system, and liver with a small "spill-over" into the systemic circulation.

51-5). The glycine conjugates of dihydroxy bile salts are absorbed in appreciable amounts in the proximal small intestine by passive diffusion and recirculate most rapidly, whereas taurine conjugates are absorbed almost exclusively in the distal intestine by an active process and recirculate more slowly. The ileal bile salt transporter, which has been cloned from the hamster, is Na^+-dependent and saturable and has an apparent molecular mass of 99kDa. Certain anaerobic bacteria in the normal intestinal flora enzymatically hydrolyze the peptide bond of conjugated bile salts to liberate free bile salts, a process called *deconjugation*. When these "free" bile salts are protonated to form bile acids, as occurs at the ambient pH of the normal gut, they become extremely lipid soluble and are readily absorbed by passive diffusion at all levels of the intestine. In healthy persons, unconjugated bile acids predominate in the cecum and colon and therefore recirculate most slowly.

In portal venous blood, bile acids whether undissociated or ionized, conjugated (amidated, sulfated, glycosidated) or deconjugated, are transported to the liver bound to plasma albumin and high-density lipoproteins. First pass hepatic clearance is highly efficient. Hepatocellular uptake involves several sinusoidal plasma membrane transporters as well as nonionic diffusion of undissociated bile acids. Most proteins responsible for bile acid uptake and vectorial movement across hepatocytes accept a wide variety of other compounds, and all appear to be multifunctional enzymes. The principal sinusoidal bile acid transporter is a glycoprotein that binds Na^+ and ionized bile acids in equimolar stoichiometry. The transporter has a molecular mass of 49kDa and is identical apparently to epoxide hydrolase.

Expression cloning has revealed a second sinusoidal bile acid transport protein of molecular mass 35kDa, which is also Na^+-dependent. Only one Na^+-independent protein transporter has been identified. This protein has a molecular mass of 54kDa, transports undissociated bile acids, and is also responsible for hepatocytic uptake of unconjugated bilirubin (see later).

The soluble cytosolic proteins in hepatocytes that bind bile acids are dihydrodiol dehydrogenase, a 36kDa protein also known as 3-alpha-hydroxysteroid dehydrogenase, glutathione-S-transferase, and Z protein also known as fatty acid binding protein. Whether the principal hepatic bile acid binding protein is dihydrodiol dehydrogenase in human livers has not been determined.

The transcellular movement of bile salts is rapid and has been traced morphologically. Bile salts, after crossing the sinusoidal membrane, appear in part to reach the canalicular membrane by passing through the endoplasmic reticulum and Golgi apparatus and traversing a microtubular network. However, neither the precise physical form of the bile salts that traverse the hepatocyte nor the intracellular site at which bile salts entwine biliary cholesterol and lecithin molecules has been elucidated.

Bile acids are transported from hepatocellular cytosol into canalicular spaces against a chemical gradient. Three protein transporters are responsible and each requires energy because the intracellular concentrations of bile acids are believed to be in the 25 to 200 μM range, whereas canalicular concentrations are an order of magnitude higher. The first is a saturable Na^+-independent transporter with a molecular mass of 100kDa that drives bile salt movement uphill utilizing the negative intracellular electrical potential (−30 to −40 mV) of hepatocytes. The second, which may be related to the first, is a primary active ATP-dependent Na^+-coupled transporter with a molecular mass of 110kDa and which appears indentical to an ecto-ATPase on canalicular membranes. The third canalicular transport system, unlike the first two, is a multifunctional organic anion transporter (MOAT system), which mediates ATP-dependent Na^+-coupled primary active canalicular secretion of a wide variety of divalent organic anions, including sulfated and glucuronidated bile salts and bilirubin diglucuronide.

BILE LECITHIN SECRETION

Lecithin, the second most prevalent biliary solute, is also an amphiphilic molecule, with two long-chain fatty acids composing its nonpolar hydrophobic portion and phosphorylcholine composing its polar hydrophilic portion. Unlike bile salts, however, lecithin molecules possess no true water solubility. Instead, lecithin swells in water to form liquid crystals, which, in turn, can incorporate substantial amounts of unesterified cholesterol, which is also water insoluble.

Human and animal studies have demonstrated that (1) although bile lecithin is derived from the liver, the pattern of molecular species of bile lecithin (with predominantly palmitic acid in the C-1 position and linoleic or oleic acids in the C-2 position) is distinctly different (less hydrophobic in character) than the lecithin pattern found in the liver; and (2) bile lecithins do not originate from lecithins that have undergone an enterohepatic circulation or from lecithins on the surface coat of lipoproteins internalized by the liver, nor are they the direct result of de novo synthesis. Bile salts are necessary for eluting membrane lecithin and thus are required for biliary lecithin secretion into bile. Lecithin secretion increases in a curvilinear manner with increasing bile salt secretion over a wide range. However, lecithin secretion plateaus at high rates of bile salt output.

On the basis of in vitro studies, bile salt-mediated lecithin secretion can be conceptualized to take place as follows. It appears that lecithins from intracellular membranes are not recruited for biliary secretion solely by simple solubilization by bile salts. Rather, a specific lecithin-transfer protein present in cytosolic fraction of human liver becomes activated by cytosolic (submicellar) bile salt concentrations. This protein selects the more hydrophilic lecithin species from endoplasmic reticulum and transports them in a 1:1 complex to the inner leaflet of the canalicular membranes. From there lecithins may be translocated by a "flippase" to the outer (luminal) leaflet of the canalicular membrane. After canalicular secretion, ionized bile salt monomers apparently partition into the luminal monolayers of canalicular membranes and as these highly charged molecules cannot "flip-flop" to the inner leaflet, they build up a critical pressure in the outer leaflet, which results in selective vesiculation of the more hydrophilic lecithin species from the membrane. Vesicles of 600 to 800 Å in diameter have been identified in canalicular spaces of experimental animals.

BILE CHOLESTEROL SECRETION

As individual molecules, unesterified cholesterol is insoluble in water. In the hepatocyte, cholesterol is solubilized by phospholipids such as lecithin to form cellular membranes and is solubilized by bile salts (together with lecithin) in bile to form mixed micelles and small, closed membranelike fragments called *unilamellar vesicles*. Biliary cholesterol and lecithin secretion rates are not tightly coupled under physiologic conditions. Although cholesterol secretion is also stimulated by the transcellular flux of bile salts, it appears that cholesterol traffics independently of lecithins to the canalicular membrane. The mechanism is unknown but possibilities include binding to (1) phospholipid vesicles, (2) submicellar bile salt monomers, (3) the hepatocyte's nonspecific lipid transfer protein (sterol-carrier-protein-2) or the "sterol-rich organelle" that is identified in fibroblasts as the cholesterol transporter from endoplasmic reticulum to plasma membranes. Being without charge, cholesterol molecules can easily distribute across the canalicular bilayer by "flip-flop." It is believed that they are covesiculated with lecithin on the luminal side of the canalicular membrane by monomeric bile salts. The relation of cholesterol secretion to bile salt secretion is also curvilinear and plateaus at high bile salt secretion rates; for a constant bile salt secretion rate, however, this plateau is lower than that for lecithin. Because of these complex relationships, the relative concentrations of cholesterol in bile increase markedly in many individuals when bile salt secretion rates are low.

The immediate precursor source of biliary cholesterol is also from a preformed hepatic pool that is derived principally from the cholesterol of plasma lipoproteins. Cholesterol that is stored in the liver as esterified cholesterol and cholesterol that is newly synthesized by the liver make far smaller contributions to biliary cholesterol secretion.

The metabolic determinants of biliary cholesterol secretion (Fig. 51-6) are (1) the cholesterol mass taken up by the liver from lipoproteins, which is dependent on apolipoprotein B/E receptor activity as well as amounts, specific kind, and surface composition (specific apolipoproteins, phospholipids) of lipoproteins delivered to liver; (2) disposition of cholesterol within the liver, which is dependent on a) rate of esterification of free cholesterol to cholesteryl ester during formation of very-low-density lipoprotein (VLDL) and storage (catalyzed by acyl-CoA: cholesterol acyltransferase, ACAT), a process that is accelerated by increased triglyceride formation and inhibited by drugs such as progestogens, b) rate of the reverse reaction in which cholesteryl ester stores are hydrolyzed, a reaction catalyzed by neutral cholesteryl ester hydrolase (CEH), c) rate of conversion of free cholesterol to bile acids (catalyzed by cholesterol 7α-hydroxylase and stimulated principally by increased bile acid loss), d) availability of optimum solubilizing lipids (i.e., hydrophobic bile salts and hydrophilic lecithins); and (3) hepatic cholesterol synthesis catalyzed by the rate-limiting enzyme, hydroxymethylglutaryl-CoA reductase (HMG CoA Reductase).

In studies of prolonged duration, biliary cholesterol secretion in humans can be increased by increases in dietary cholesterol via hepatic chylomicron remnant uptake and during mobilization of peripheral cholesterol stores via low-density lipoprotein (LDL), as in obese patients during rapid weight loss as well as by drug therapy for hypocholesterolemia.

BILIRUBIN PRODUCTION AND SECRETION (See also Chapter 55)

Bilirubin is the major end product of the catabolism of heme (Fig. 51-7). Its production rate is about 350 mg/day, and it

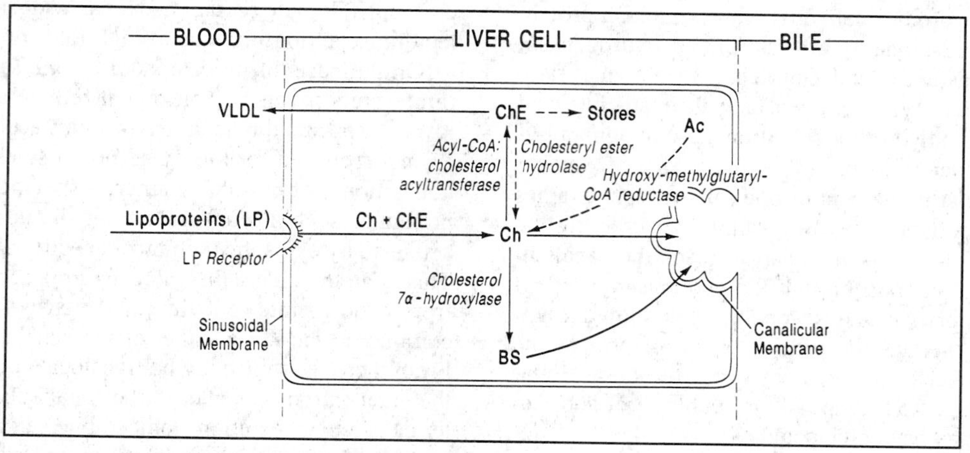

Fig. 51-6. Metabolic determinants of biliary cholesterol secretion. The rate-limiting enzymes are hydroxy-methylglutaryl-CoA reductase (cholesterol [*Ch*] synthesis), Acyl-CoA: cholesterol acyltransferase (cholesteryl ester [*ChE*] synthesis), cholesteryl ester hydrolase (ChE hydrolysis) and cholesterol 7-alpha-hydroxylase (bile salt synthesis). The major lipoproteins, LDL as well as VLDL remnants and chylomicron remnants are internalized by hepatocytes after binding to apolipoprotein B/E receptors.

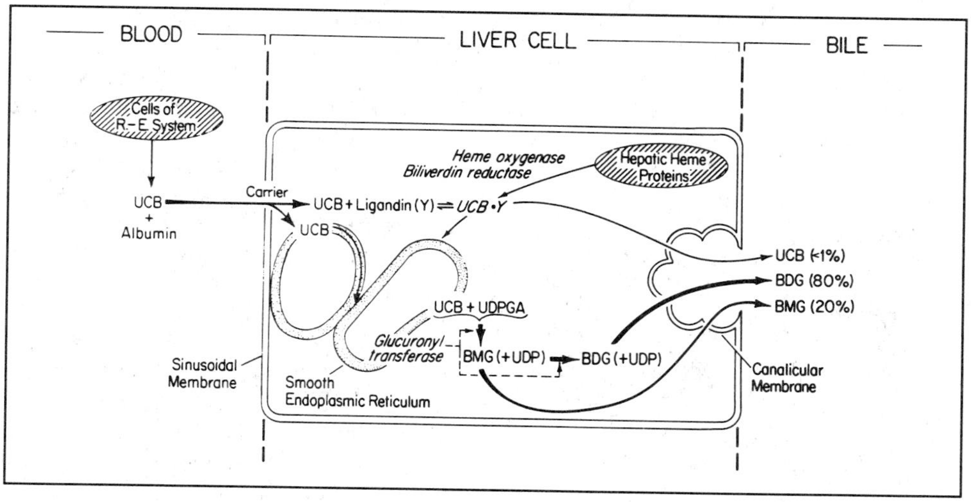

Fig. 51-7. Bilirubin formation, transport, uptake, conjugation, and secretion. *RE,* reticuloendothelial; *UCB,* unconjugated bilirubin; *BMG,* bilirubin monoglucuronide; *BDG,* bilirubin diglucuronide; *UDPGA,* uridine diphosphate glucuronic acid.

is derived principally (80%) from senescent red cell hemoglobin in the reticuloendothelial cells of the spleen and liver. The remainder is produced by destruction of newly synthesized heme in the bone marrow and from the turnover of myoglobin and heme-containing enzymes (e.g., catalase) and coenzymes (e.g., cytochrome P_{450}) in hepatic and extrahepatic tissues. Bilirubin formation is a two-step process: (1) oxidation of the α-carbon bridge of heme by microsomal heme oxygenase, releasing a molecule of carbon monoxide (the only metabolic source in human beings), iron, and a molecule of the green pigment, biliverdin; and (2) the quantitative reduction of the γ-methene bridge of biliverdin, catalyzed by the cytosolic enzyme biliverdin reductase to form the yellow-orange pigment, bilirubin. Because bilirubin is insoluble in water at pH 7.4, its transport to the liver, the secretory organ, takes place in plasma via tight noncovalent binding to serum albumin.

Hepatic uptake (see Fig. 51-7) of bilirubin is highly efficient. The process uses an Na^+-independent transporter of molecular mass 54kDa, which is shared with unconjugated hydrophobic bile acids but independent of ionized bile salt uptake and inhibited by other organic anions, such as fatty acids and iodipamide. Albumin itself is not taken up by the liver but appears to facilitate the process. Within the hepatocyte, bilirubin is bound first to an acceptor protein, termed *ligandin* (protein Y), or directly to membranes of the endoplasmic reticulum.

After intracellular binding, bilirubin is transported by cytosolic proteins or membrane diffusion to conjugating enzymes that are membrane-bound on the smooth endoplasmic reticulum. Here, uridine diphosphate-glucuronosyl transferase couples β-D-glucuronic acid (or, less commonly, β-D-glucose or β-D-xylose) in ester linkage to one or both propionic acid side chains of bilirubin. The resulting conjugates are all water soluble and are excreted rapidly in bile via the MOAT system (see earlier), which is shared with many other organic dianions including bile acid dianions (e.g., lithocholate glucuronide). Normally, the diconjugates (bilirubin diglucuronide with traces of bilirubin monoglucoside-monoglucuronide or monoxyloside-monoglucuronide diesters) predominate (80%), the monoconjugates (bilirubin monoglucuronide with traces of monoglucoside or monoxyloside) constitute about 20%, and unconjugated bilirubin constitutes less than 1% of total bile pigments.

Bilirubin conjugates are waste products with no certain physiologic function, although they may function as antioxidants in bile. In the adult, bilirubin conjugates are not reabsorbed from the intestine. However, the intraluminal bacterial flora of the colon deconjugate bilirubin and reduce the unconjugated form to a number of colorless urobilinogens. Urobilinogens are absorbed by passive diffusion from the colon, cycle enterohepatically in the portal vein, and, after uptake into the hepatocytes (95%), are excreted in bile or in the urine (5%).

ASSEMBLY AND STRUCTURE OF BILE

Compared with the large hydrocarbon portions of each of the major bile lipids (steroid nucleus or acyl hydrocarbon chains), the polar functions of these molecules are relatively weak. These amphiphilic molecules form true (monomeric) solutions only when very dilute (Fig. 51-8). Biliary lecithin and cholesterol molecules are extremely insoluble as monomers, whereas bile salts are soluble in the low millimolar range. In excess of their monomeric concentrations, each of these amphiphiles self-aggregates in a distinct manner: bile salt molecules self-associate via their hydrophobic portions to form small micelles. The solute concentration at which these micelles form is just above the maximum monomeric solubility (1 to 3 mM) and is operationally defined as the *critical micellar concentration*. Self-aggregates of cholesterol molecules are completely insoluble in water and precipitate as cholesterol monohydrate crystals, the major components of most gallstones. Self-aggregates of lecithin molecules are also insoluble in water, but are capable

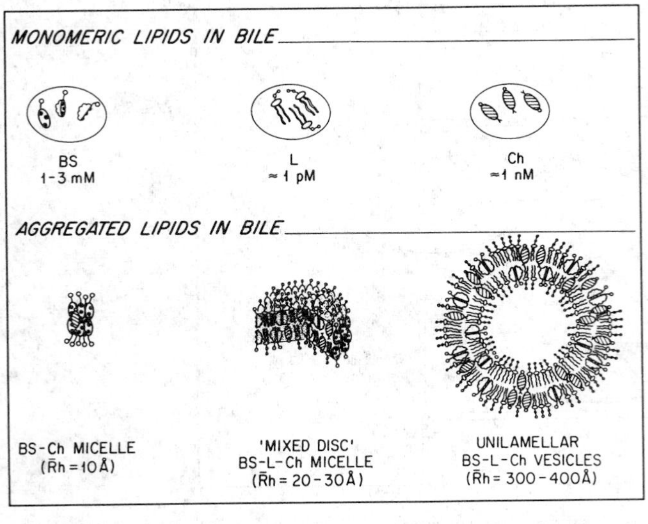

Fig. 51-8. Schematic models of the major biliary lipid molecules with depictions of the average sizes and structures of the mixed micelles and unilamellar vesicles found in human bile. *BS,* bile salt; *L,* lecithin; *Ch,* cholesterol; $\bar{Rh}$, mean hydrodynamic radius; *Å,* Ångstrom unit (10^{-10} m). Monomeric solubilities are given in SI units.

of becoming extremely hydrated, forming bilayers of lipid molecules interleaved with multilayers of water; these self-aggregates are called *liquid crystals.* When the solute concentration is low, lecithin liquid crystals can form closed structures of submicroscopic or macroscopic size; these structures are called *vesicles.*

In hepatic and gallbladder bile, the concentration of bile salt is usually well above its critical micellar concentration. The micelles formed have large capacities to bind and solubilize in mixed micelles both cholesterol and lecithin molecules secreted as vesicles. The solubilization process is not a simple transition but proceeds via another liquid crystalline structure, a rod-shaped particle that is a transient fragment of a hexagonal liquid crystalline phase. With typical biliary compositions (see Fig. 51-1), these globular micelles are not of uniform size, composition, or structure, but are composed of two distinct species: (1) bile salt—cholesterol micelles ("simple" mixed micelles), in which cholesterol is bound to the exterior surface; and (2) larger bile salt—lecithin-cholesterol micelles, in which a loosely organized fragment of a lecithin bilayer is both saturated with bile salt and enveloped on its perimeter by bile salt molecules (Fig. 51-8). In the latter, cholesterol is about five times more soluble than in simple micelles because it interdigitates between the liquid hydrocarbon chain of the lecithin molecules. All mammalian biles contain small unilamellar vesicles of lecithin-cholesterol and bile salt that are about ten times larger than the mixed micelles (Fig. 51-8). These small vesicles are found principally in hepatic bile and exhibit a greater capacity to solubilize cholesterol than either species of micelle. In animal bile, biliary vesicles that coexist with bile salt micelles are metastable and are continually undergoing transformation into unsaturated mixed micelles along the biliary tree. When bile salt micelles are saturated with cholesterol, a common occurrence in human hepatic and gallbladder bile, the biliary vesicles persist and become enriched in cholesterol by virtue of losing lecithin but not cholesterol molecules to bile salt micelles. In dilute human hepatic bile, these vesicles are relatively stable and may be responsible for carrying up to 80% to 90% of the total biliary cholesterol content. In concentrated gallbladder bile, vesicles although carrying much less total cholesterol, often become unstable, and crystallize their cholesterol, setting the stage for cholesterol gallstone formation.

Bilirubin conjugates self-associate at concentrations in the 1 to 2 μM range to form dimers and, at higher concentrations, larger aggregates *(multimers).* The proportion of bilirubin multimers depends on the pH of bile, increasing in number as alkaline hepatic bile is "acidified" in the gallbladder. In contrast to bile salt micelles, bilirubin aggregates have no capacity to solubilize lecithin or cholesterol molecules. However, most of the conjugated bilirubin molecules in bile become loosely attached to the hydrophilic parts of simple and mixed bile salt micelles as well as bile salt monomers to form mixed aggregates of bile salts and bilirubin conjugates. As a consequence, bilirubin conjugates have little or no osmotic activity in bile. The small quantities of unconjugated bilirubin in bile may be preferentially associated with the hydrophobic interiors of biliary micelles and unilamellar vesicles of bile.

PERTURBATIONS OF THE ENTEROHEPATIC CIRCULATION

Obstructed secretory apparatus

The secretion of biliary lipids may fail as a result of functional or mechanical obstruction of the bile secretory apparatus. Obstruction can occur at any anatomic site in the biliary tree from liver cell to duodenum. It has been shown that under these conditions the canalicular bile salt transporter becomes translocated to the sinusoidal membrane. The biliary lipids are shunted into the systemic circulation, leading to high levels of serum bile salt bound to albumin and all plasma lipoprotein classes, hyperbilirubinemia (jaundice), bilirubinuria, and the appearance of lipoprotein X, an abnormal, low-density lipoprotein containing biliary lecithin and unesterified cholesterol as unilamellar vesicles. In bile and blood, secondary bile salts disappear, and hepatic enzymes are induced to further hydroxylate, to sulfate, and glycosidate the primary bile salts, facilitating their renal clearance and urinary excretion. High levels of bile salts and perhaps other organic anions that are ordinarily secreted in bile and retained in blood and skin may also induce severe pruritus.

Defective bile salt synthesis

The bile salt pool may be reduced as a result of a congenital monoenzymatic defect or secondary to defective homeostatic mechanisms that are not fully understood. In these cases, hepatic bile salt synthesis is usually inappropriately low in the face of smaller than normal amounts of bile salt that are being recycled to the liver within the enterohepatic circulation. This is the situation in some nonobese cholesterol gallstone patients, in old age, and in the normal newborn. In adults, the shrunken bile salt pool may lead to a decrease in bile salt secretion rates, cholesterol- or calcium (hydrogen) bilirubinate-supersaturated bile, and a propensity for gallstone formation.

Contaminated small bowel

In the contaminated small bowel syndrome, bile salt-metabolizing anaerobic bacteria colonize the jejunum, deconjugate and dehydroxylate bile salts, and result in the formation of sparingly soluble unconjugated deoxycholic and lithocholic acids in the small intestine. Only rarely do these hydrophobic bile acids precipitate intraluminally to form bile acid-fatty acid stones (enteroliths). More commonly, the bile acids are absorbed by passive diffusion to enter portal venous blood and thereby short-circuit the enterohepatic circulation. Because intraluminal bile salt micelle formation is compromised, and unconjugated bile acids and anaerobic bacteria may injure the mucosa of the small intestine, malabsorption results (Chapter 42).

Increased fecal bile salt loss

Compensated loss. Small bowel disease that is not extensive and involves the ileum (or the administration of certain drugs that bind intraluminally to bile salt) can lead to increased bile salt loss in the feces. In these instances, fecal loss is sufficiently small so that the liver can compensate with increased de novo synthesis from cholesterol to maintain the content of bile salts in the proximal small intestine above their critical micellar concentrations. However, the high flux of bile salt through the colon leads to secretory diarrhea.

Decompensated loss. The causes of decompensated fecal bile salt loss are often the same as those of a compensated loss, but are more extensive and result in more severe clinical disease. In this situation, de novo synthesis of bile salt cannot keep pace with fecal loss, and a marked fall in the bile salt secretory rate results. This diminution in secretory rate leads to cholesterol- or calcium (hydrogen) bilirubinate-supersaturated bile with the risk of gallstone formation; fat malabsorption; both bile salt- and fatty acid-induced secretory diarrhea; and increased oxalate absorption, hyperoxaluria, and an increased incidence of calcium oxalate kidney stones.

REFERENCES

Cabral DJ and Small DM: Physical chemistry of bile. In Schultz SG et al, editors: Handbook of physiology—the gastrointestinal system III Section 6, Baltimore, 1989, Waverly Press.

Cahalane MJ, Neubrand MW, and Carey MC: Physical-chemical pathogenesis of pigment gallstones, Semin Liver Dis 8:317-328, 1988.

Carey MC and LaMont JT: Cholesterol gallstone formation. 1. Physical-chemistry of bile and biliary lipid secretion, Prog Liver Dis 10:139-163, 1992.

Carey MC and Duane WC: Enterohepatic circulation. In Arias IM et al, editors: The liver, biology and pathobiology, ed 3, New York, 1993, Raven Press.

Cohen DE, Angelico M, and Carey MC: Quasielastic light scattering evidence for vesicular secretion of biliary lipids, Am J Physiol 257:G1-G8, 1989.

Cohen DE and Carey MC: Physical chemistry of biliary lipids during bile formation, Hepatology 12:143S-148S, 1990.

Hay DW and Carey MC: Chemical species of lipids in bile, Hepatology 12:6S-16S, 1990.

Hofmann AF: Bile acid secretion, bile flow and biliary lipid secretion in humans, Hepatology 12:17S-25S, 1990.

LaMont JT and Carey MC: Cholesterol gallstone formation. 2. Pathobiology and pathomechanics, Prog Liver Dis 10:165-191, 1992.

Marzolo MP, Rigotti A, and Nervi F: Secretion of biliary lipids from the hepatocyte, Hepatology 12:134S-142S, 1990.

CHAPTER

52 Pancreatic Secretion

Vay Liang W. Go

The human pancreas is both an exocrine and an endocrine gland. This large, elongated retroperitoneal gland extends obliquely upward from the duodenum, behind the stomach, and across the posterior abdominal wall to the spleen at the level of the first and second lumbar vertebrae (Fig. 52-1). It is divided into three parts: the head, the body, and the tail. Exocrine tissue forms the greater mass of the gland, which secretes daily more than 1.5 to 3.0 liters of a colorless fluid containing digestive proenzymes and enzymes, electrolytes, and water. A major function of pancreatic juice is to adjust duodenal contents to an alkaline pH that will allow its digestive enzymes to act optimally on ingested food. Endocrine tissue accounts for less than 1% of the weight of the gland and consists of tiny islets embedded

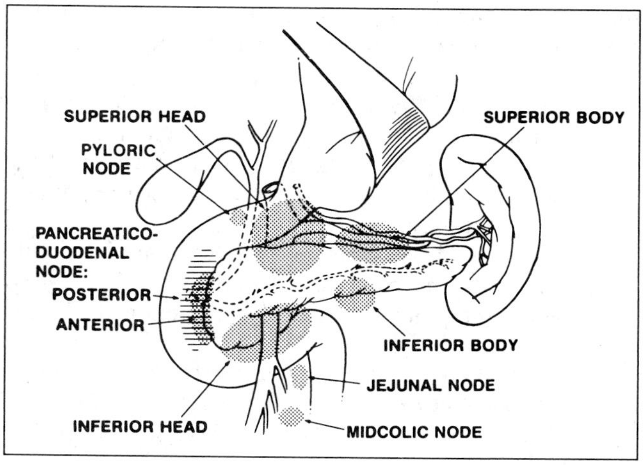

Fig. 52-1. Structural relationship between the pancreas and surrounding tissue and lymphatic drainage.

within the lobules of the acinar cells. These islets release their endocrine secretions, including insulin or glucagon, directly into the circulation. The hormones regulate the metabolism of absorbed nutrients.

Arterial blood supply to the pancreas is from the celiac and superior mesenteric arteries; the vein draining the pancreas generally accompanies the artery and empties into the splenic or portal veins. The pancreas has both parasympathetic and sympathetic nerves. The preganglionic parasympathetic nerve fibers reach the gland through the vagus nerve, pass through the celiac ganglia without making a synapse, and terminate at the intrinsic pancreatic ganglia. The postganglionic fibers are distributed between pancreatic lobules and around the acini and terminate in proximity to individual cells. The sympathetic nerve fibers reach the pancreas via the greater and lesser splanchnic trunks, which arise from the fifth to the ninth thoracic ganglia. The preganglionic fibers terminate at the celiac or superior mesenteric ganglia, and the postganglionic fibers accompany the blood vessels and are distributed primarily to blood vessels of the pancreas. In addition, peptidergic fibers containing vasoactive intestinal peptide, substance P, neuropeptide Y, enkephalin-related peptides, bombesin-like peptides, galanin, and calcitonin gene-related peptides have been identified in pancreatic tissue.

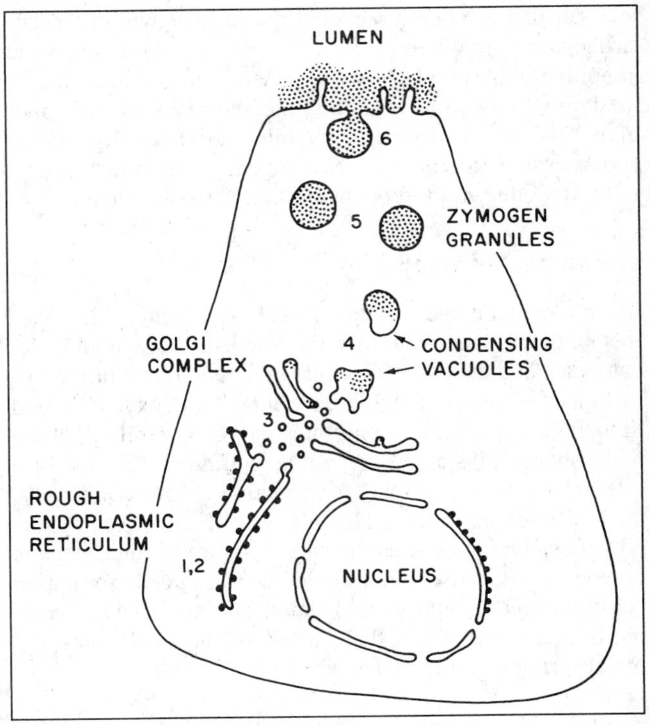

Fig. 52-2. Secretory pathway in a pancreatic acinar cell: 1 and 2, synthesis; 3 and 4, packaging; 5, transport; and 6, secretion. (From Scheele GA: Mayo Clin. Proc 54:420-7, 1979.)

STRUCTURAL CONSIDERATIONS OF EXOCRINE PANCREATIC FUNCTION

The exocrine pancreas consists of clusters of acini formed into lobules and separated by areolar tissue. The acinus is composed of a single layer of pyramidal cells, with the broad base of each cell resting on a thin basement membrane, while the narrow apex borders the ductal lumen with short, irregular microvilli (Fig. 52-2). The cytoplasm of an acinar cell has large zymogen granules, which vary in number and are located in the apex of the cell. The basal half of the cell contains a nucleus, extensive lamellar arrays of rough endoplasmic reticulum, and an elaborate supranuclear Golgi complex from which condensing vacuoles emanate. The pancreatic acinar cell is responsible for the synthesis and secretion of digestive enzymes. The secretory pathway of the pancreatic acinar cell can be divided into six general steps (Fig. 52-2).

1. Messenger RNA is formed on DNA in the nucleus and leaves the nucleus to attach to the membrane-bound ribosomes on the cytoplasmic surfaces of the rough endoplasmic reticular cisternae, where proteins are synthesized.
2. During synthesis, proteins are transported vectorially across the microsomal membrane and segregated within the cisternal space of the rough endoplasmic reticulum.
3. Segregated proteins are transported by an energy-dependent process from the rough endoplasmic reticulum to the Golgi apparatus, where they are modified.
4. Secretory proteins are sorted into secretory granules.
5. Proteins are stored within mature zymogen granules.
6. The proteins are discharged from the apical portion of the cell by exocytosis, which is energy-dependent and mediator responsive. (a) Secretory proteins are segregated within membrane-bound compartments and therefore are excluded from the cytosolic space; (b) transport of secretory proteins is vectorial and irreversible, proceeding from the basal portion of the cell to the apical portion of the cell through a series of membrane-enclosed compartments; and (c) transport is time-dependent, and under normal conditions approximately 30 minutes is required to position the secretory proteins for discharge into extracellular space.

All pancreatic digestive enzymes are believed to be synthesized, transported, and secreted in the acinar cells as described above. During a high rate of enzyme secretion, zymogen granules may be depleted, but enzyme secretion continues unabated. In short-term experiments in human beings, the relative concentrations of various pancreatic enzymes remain constant and, over a wide range of secretory rates, the various enzymes are secreted in parallel (parallel secretion). Some workers, however, claim to have observed significant deviation from parallel secretion in experimental animals such as the rabbit.

Each acinus is drained by a ductule. The ductular epithelium extends into the lumen of the acinus, forming the centroacinar cell. The ductule drains into the intercalated duct and joins the interlobular duct, which enters into the main duct of Wirsung. There is considerable evidence that the water and electrolytic components of pancreatic secretion are secreted by ductal and centroacinar cells.

COMPOSITION OF PANCREATIC SECRETION

Digestive enzymes

Enzymes and proenzymes comprise more than 90% of the protein in pancreatic juice; the remainder is made up of protease inhibitors, plasma proteins, and mucoproteins. It has been estimated that the human pancreas secretes as much as 6 g of protein every 24 hours. The acinar cells secrete digestive enzymes for every class of foodstuffs: a number of proteolytic enzymes (trypsin, chymotrypsin, carboxypeptidase A, carboxypeptidase B, elastase, and ribonucleases) for proteins, lipases for triglycerides, and α-amylases for carbohydrates. The proteolytic enzymes are secreted in inactive forms (proenzymes) and constitute more than 75% of the digestive enzymes secreted. Proenzymes are activated upon entering the duodenum. Enterokinase, a duodenal mucosal peptidase, converts trypsinogen to trypsin, which activates pancreatic phospholipase and other proteolytic enzymes. Lipase, amylase, and ribonuclease are secreted in their active forms by the acinar cells.

The exocrine pancreas has a tremendous reserve capacity, and the amount of digestive enzymes secreted into the duodenum far exceeds that needed for normal digestion. Regardless of the cause of pancreatic insufficiency, maldigestion of fat and protein usually does not occur until lipase and trypsin output is 10% of normal secretion.

Pancreatic juice also contains a colipase that combines stoichiometrically with lipase. Colipase, in the presence of bile salts, lowers the pH optimum for lipase to 6.5, the luminal pH of the proximal small intestine. Pancreatic juice also contains some lysosomal enzymes, trypsin inhibitors, endocrine peptides (e.g., insulin), and pancreatic polypeptides. Their physiologic significance is currently unknown, but their secretion can be altered during pathologic states.

Water and electrolyte secretion

Pancreatic juice is isotonic with extracellular fluid at all rates of secretion in both healthy and disease states. It has a pH of 8.0 to 8.5. Water enters the pancreatic juice passively according to osmotic gradients established by the active secretion of electrolytes and other solutes. The principal cations are sodium and potassium, which are secreted at fixed concentrations similar to those in extracellular fluid. Small amounts of calcium, magnesium, and zinc are also present in the pancreatic juice.

The principal anions are chloride and bicarbonate. The concentrations of these two anions vary reciprocally at different flow rates; together they total about 150 mE liter (Fig. 52-3). Bicarbonate concentration rises with an increase in flow rate, while chloride concentration decreases. This relationship is reversed with a decreased flow rate. Data from micropuncture study of the pancreatic ducts have provided evidence that the acinar fluid is rich in chloride, but becomes relatively richer in bicarbonate as the fluid passes down the duct. This effect is probably due to the activity of bicarbonate pumps in ductal cells, which concurrently exchange chloride for bicarbonate (Fig. 52-4). Pancreatic bicarbonate is formed from endogenous cellular carbon dioxide and through the action of carbonic anhydrase. Bicarbonate secretion across the apical pole of the duct cell is thought to occur via Cl^-/HCO exchange, with the Cl^- recycling across the apical membrane through a low-

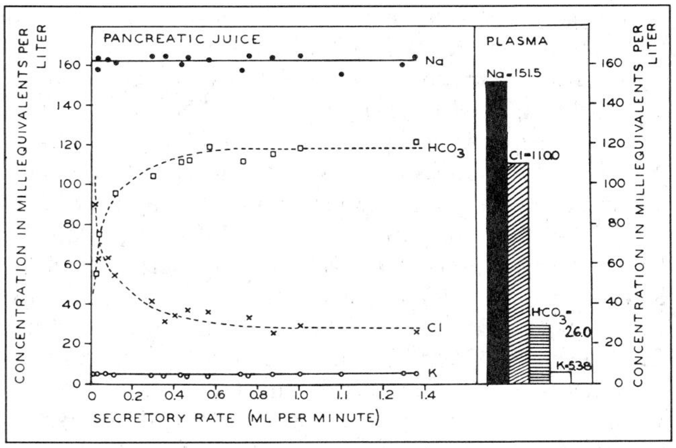

Fig. 52-3. Relation between the rate of secretion and the concentration of sodium, bicarbonate, chloride, and potassium in the pancreatic juice. (From Bro-Rasmussen F, Killmann S, and Thaysen JH: Acta Physiol Scand 37:97-113, 1956.)

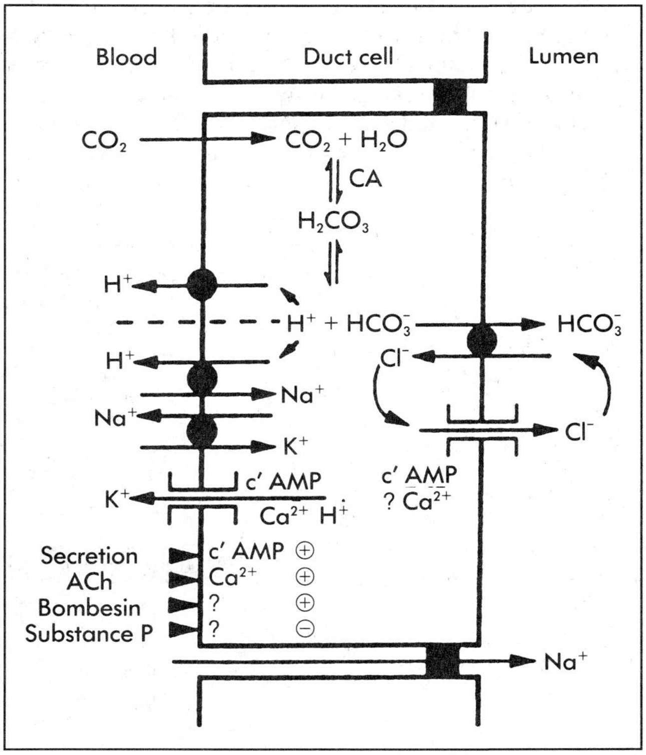

Fig. 52-4. Model of pancreatic duct cell bicarbonate and chloride secretion. *CA,* carbonic anhydrase; *ACh,* acetylcholine; *c'AMP,* cyclic AMP: +, stimulant of secretion; −, inhibition of secretion. (From Argent BE et al: Pancreas 7:408-413, 1992.)

conductance chloride channel. This channel is an amino acid polypeptide known as the *cystic fibrosis transmembrane conductance regulator (CFTR)* and is encoded by the cystic fibrosis gene. Activation of the CFTR channel by cyclic AMP-dependent phosphorylation is thought to be the primary event in secretory activation. The net effect is equal transport of HCO_3^- into the lumen and H^+ into the plasma (Fig. 52-4). The capacity of the normal pancreas to secrete HCO generally exceeds the acid secretory capacity of the human stomach. Stomach acid secretory capacity far exceeds pancreatic bicarbonate secretion in gastrinoma (Zollinger-Ellison syndrome), which results in an acidic environment ($pH < 4.0$) in the proximal duodenum. This environment can lead to peptic ulcer disease and inactivation of digestive enzymes, maldigestion, and malabsorption (Chapter 38).

REGULATION OF PANCREATIC SECRETION

Pancreatic exocrine secretion is regulated by neuronal and hormonal actions and by neurohormonal interactions (Fig. 52-5).

Neural control

Electrical stimulation of the vagus nerve produces a moderate flow of pancreatic juice high in enzyme but low in bicarbonate concentration. Parasympathomimetic drugs and insulin-induced hypoglycemia in human beings (presumably through vagal excitation) have similar effects. Additionally, a cholinergic enteropancreatic reflex can be activated by intraluminal chemical stimulation; its effect on pancreatic secretion is similar to that of vagal stimulation. Vagal transection reduces the pancreatic response to intestinal stimulants. Stimulation of the splanchnic nerves causes diminution of the blood supply to glandular tissue and thus inhibits pancreatic exocrine secretion.

Hormonal control

Hormones that regulate pancreatic exocrine secretion are secreted primarily by the endocrine cells in the upper gastrointestinal tract. Cholecystokinin (CCK) stimulates the pancreas to secrete a juice that is high in protein and enzymes but relatively low in bicarbonate and volume, an effect similar to that evoked by vagal stimulation. The hormone mainly responsible for fluid and electrolyte secretion in pancreatic juice is secretin, which is also a weak stimulus for protein secretion. These two major hormones are released in response to an intraluminal stimulant. Fatty acids, amino acids, and calcium are capable of stimulating CCK, and H^+ ion stimulates secretin release. Both secretin and CCK exert their full effects on the pancreas within minutes after entry into the bloodstream. Secretin and CCK augment each other's actions and show some degree of potentiation. A combination of secretin and CCK produces volume, bicarbonate, and enzyme outputs that exceed the rates of secretion observed when identical doses of each of the hormones are given alone.

The endocrine pancreas has long been known to affect pancreatic exocrine secretion. Insulin plays an important role in the action of secretin and CCK in both fasting and postprandial pancreatic secretion, whereas glucagon, which shares certain portions of its peptide structure with secretin, is an inhibitor of pancreatic volume and enzyme secretion. In contrast, vasoactive intestinal polypeptide (VIP), which is present in the peptidergic nerves of the pancreas, is structurally similar to secretin and glucagon and has secretin-like effects on pancreatic secretion. Somatostatin inhibits basal pancreatic exocrine secretion, whereas secre-

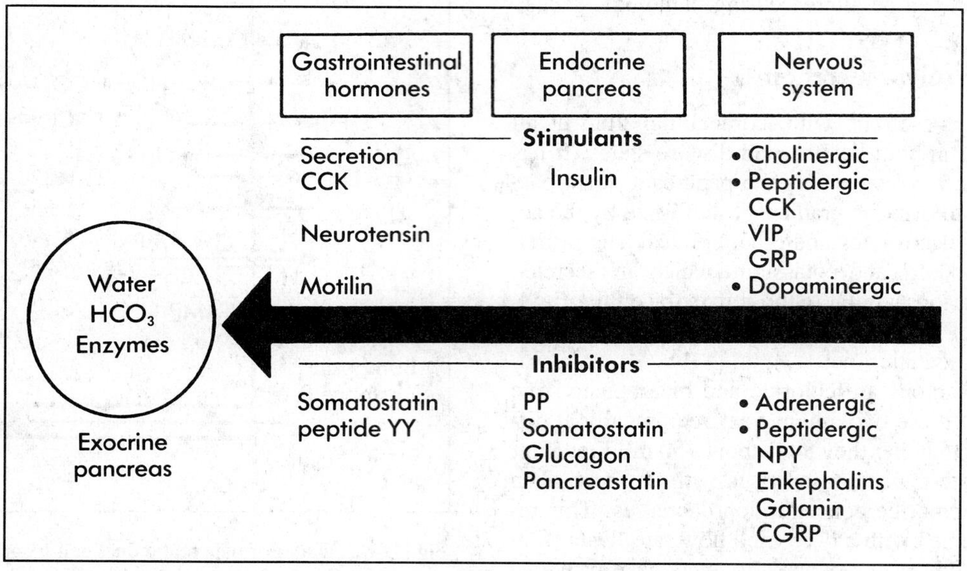

Fig. 52-5. Neurohormonal factors that regulate pancreatic exocrine secretion. (From Chey WY: Int J Pancreatol 9:7-20, 1991.).

tin and/or CCK stimulate such action. Stimulants such as neurotensin and motilin and inhibitors such as pancreatic polypeptide, neuropeptide y (NPY), and pancreastatin are among the other gut polypeptides released by intraluminal stimulants.

Integration of neurohormonal regulation in pancreatic acinar cells

Receptors on the surfaces of the acinar cells are classified according to their agonists as follows (Fig. 52-6): (1) cholinergic agents, (2) CCK and gastrin, and (3) secretin and VIP, and another class of membrane receptors of unknown physiologic significance, which includes (4) bombesin. The step following receptor occupancy that leads to secretion of either enzymes or ions is generally referred to as stimulus-secretion coupling. Operationally, it is divided into two components: (1) intracellular messengers ("second" messengers), which convey a message from the plasma membrane to the inside of the cell and include phospholipids, cyclic nucleotides, and calcium ions, and (2) effectors, which are system-activated by the intracellular messengers that bring about the secretory response and include enzymes such as protein kinases, phosphatases, and adenosinetriphosphatases and specific membrane ion channels. The result of interaction between intracellular messengers and effectors is the direct fusion of zymogen granules with the luminal plasma membrane and secretion of digestive enzymes (Fig. 52-6).

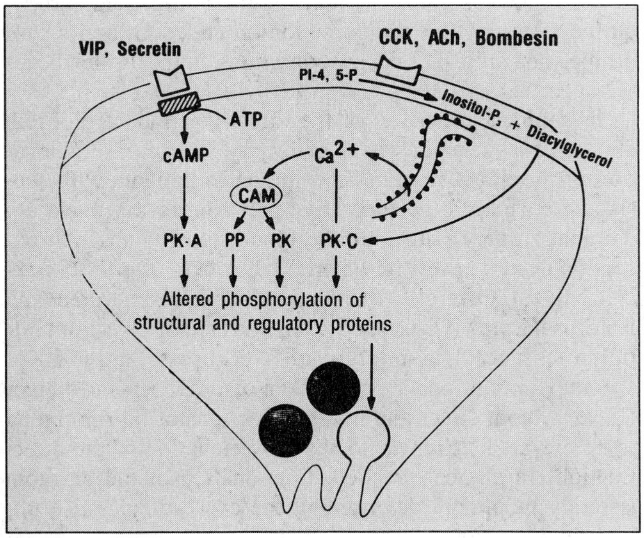

Fig. 52-6. Schematic diagram of stimulus-secretion coupling of pancreatic acinar cell protein secretion. *VIP,* vasoactive intestinal peptide; *CCK,* cholecystokinin; *ACh,* acetylcholine; *PK-A,* cyclic AMP-activated protein kinase; *CAM,* calmodulin; *PP,* protein phosphatase; *PK,* protein kinase; *PK-C,* phospholipid-dependent protein kinase; P1-4, 5-P, phosphatidylinositol-4,5-bisphosphate; inositol-P, inositol-1,4,5-trisphosphate. (From Williams JA and Hootman SR: Stimulus-secretion coupling in pancreatic acinar cells. In Go VLW et al, editors: The exocrine pancreas: biology, pathobiology, and diseases. New York, 1986, Raven Press.)

In the ductal cell, secretin activates ductal fluid transport via AMP pathways (see Fig. 52-4), whereas ACh increases intracellular Ca^{2+} by mobilization of intracellular stores and influx of Ca^{2+} across the plasma membrane. Substance P's inhibitory effect may be mediated through the increase in protein kinase C, whereas bombesin's intracellular messenger pathway has not yet been identified.

Interdigestive and digestive profile of pancreatic exocrine secretion

Human interdigestive pancreatic fluid and enzyme secretion usually begins after overnight fast when the upper gastrointestinal tract is empty of food. It is cyclical, recurring at 60- to 90-minute intervals and is integrated with the phases of upper gastrointestinal interdigestive motor activity (Chapter 26), gastric secretion, and gallbladder emptying. Maximum pancreatic secretion occurs just before the sweeping action of phase III of duodenal interdigestive motor activity (Fig. 52-7). The controlling mechanisms for this interdigestive exocrine pancreatic secretion are incompletely understood, although they are hypothesized to be under the influence of the cholinergic and adrenergic nervous systems. Ingestion of food interrupts interdigestive pancreatic secretion and converts it to a constant secretory pattern.

Enzyme output during the digestive phase is greater than during peak secretory output in phase III of the interdigestive period (Fig. 52-7). The rate of gastric emptying and meal composition play important roles in the regulation of digestive pancreatic secretion. The exocrine secretion continues as long as nutrients are emptied from the stomach into the duodenum. Mixed meals containing carbohydrate, fat, and protein stimulate maximal pancreatic enzyme secretion. Intraduodenal perfusion of long-chain fatty acids can stimulate maximal pancreatic enzyme secretion. In contrast, intraduodenal perfusion of essential amino acids yields only 50% maximal enzyme output, and carbohydrate causes minimal response.

The digestive profile of pancreatic secretion has custom-

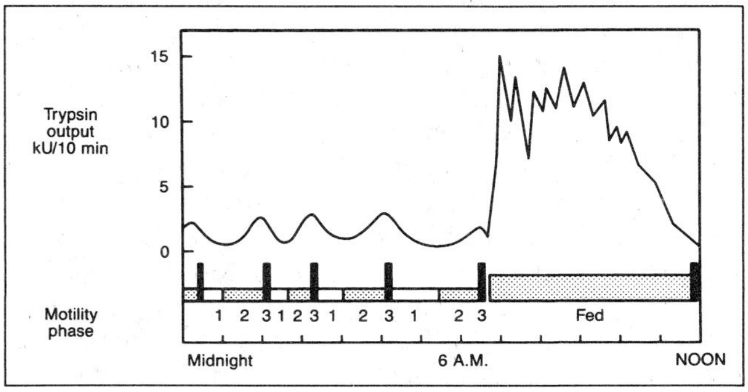

Fig. 52-7. Interdigestive and digestive profile of pancreatic enzyme secretion as represented by trypsin output in a healthy subject. The relation of the three phases of duodenal interdigestive motor activity (in numerical order) and the fed pattern (longest stippled bar) to the interdigestive and digestive pancreatic enzyme output is illustrated. kU = 1000 units.

arily been divided into cephalic, gastric, and intestinal phases. During the cephalic and gastric phases, vagal influences are important. As food enters the antrum and duodenum, however, hormonal secretions assume the principal role, although the release of CCK, secretin, and gastrin and their effects on the exocrine pancreas are modulated by neural mechanisms.

REFERENCES

Argent B et al: The pancreatic duct cell, Pancreas. 7:403-409, 1992.

Chey WY: Regulation of pancreatic endocrine secretion, Int J Pancreatol 9:7-20. 1991.

Creutzfeldt W, editor: The exocrine pancreas, Clin Gastroenterol 13(3):1, 1984.

Go VLW et al, editors: The pancreas: biology, pathobiology, and diseases, ed 2, New York, 1993, Raven Press.

Quinton, PM: Cystic fibrosis: disease in electrolyte transport. FASEB J 4:2709-2719, 1990.

Scheele, GA: Biosynthesis, segregation and secretion of exportable proteins by the exocrine pancreas, Am J Physiol 238:G467-G477, 1980.

Schulz I: Electrolyte and fluid secretion in the exocrine pancreas. In Johnson LR et al, editors: Physiology of the gastrointestinal tract, New York, 1987, Raven Press.

II DIAGNOSTIC PROCEDURES AND TESTS

CHAPTER

53 Evaluation of Hepatobiliary Diseases

Marshall M. Kaplan

LIVER FUNCTION TESTS

Liver function tests are blood tests used (1) to detect the presence of liver disease, (2) to distinguish among different types of liver disorders, (3) to gauge the extent of known liver damage, and (4) to follow the response of the diseased liver to treatment. Although liver function tests are very useful for these purposes, they have certain inherent shortcomings. Normal results may be obtained in patients with serious liver disease, and nonspecifically abnormal results may be obtained in patients with diseases that do not affect the liver. Finally, liver function tests rarely lead to a specific diagnosis of liver disease. Rather, they suggest a general category of liver disorder, such as cholestatic or hepatocellular disease, and direct the clinician toward the efficient use of other, more specific diagnostic tests.

No one liver function test enables the clinician to assess accurately the total functional capacity of the liver. The liver carries out thousands of biochemical reactions, most of which cannot be easily measured by blood tests. Liver function tests measure a very limited number of these reactions. In fact, many liver function tests do not measure liver function at all. Rather, they detect liver cell damage or bile duct patency.

Nevertheless, it is helpful conceptually to consider them as function tests and to group them into general categories. Although arbitrary, the currently used tests can be categorized as follows: (1) tests of the liver's excretory and detoxification capacity, (2) tests of the liver's biosynthetic capacity, (3) tests that detect injury to liver cells (most enzyme tests are in this category), and (4) tests that detect chronic inflammation in the liver or altered immunoregulation.

Tests based on detoxification and excretory functions

Serum bilirubin (See Chapter 55 for complete coverage). Serum bilirubin, a breakdown product of the porphyrin ring of heme-containing proteins, consists of two fractions, direct and indirect bilirubin. This fractionation is based on water solubility. Indirect bilirubin is insoluble in water and is unconjugated. Direct bilirubin (conjugated bilirubin) is water soluble and is conjugated to one or two glucuronic acids. A fraction of conjugated bilirubin may also be covalently bound to albumin but can only be detected by methods more sophisticated than simple water solubility. In most laboratories, the normal serum bilirubin concentration is considered to be less than 1.0 to 1.5 mg/dl. Less than 15% of the total is in the direct fraction.

Elevation of the indirect fraction of bilirubin alone is rarely due to liver disease. This elevation is seen primarily in hemolytic disorders, including serious inherited and acquired anemias, the benign condition called Gilbert's syndrome, and in a number of conditions found in newborns (Chapter 55).

In contrast, elevation of the direct fraction of bilirubin almost always implies liver or biliary tree disease. Elevation of the direct fraction is common in patients with sepsis and during the postoperative period after extensive abdominal surgery with multiple blood transfusions. An exception occurs in several inherited disorders of bilirubin excretion, for example, the Dubin-Johnson syndrome and Rotor syndrome (Chapter 55). An elevated direct serum bilirubin may occur in any type of liver disease and is never specific for just one type of liver disorder. In most liver diseases, both direct and indirect fractions of bilirubin tend to be elevated. It is rare to see only elevation of the direct fraction. In clinical practice, fractionation of the bilirubin is rarely helpful in determining the cause of jaundice unless the elevation is due solely to the indirect fraction. If the excretion of bilirubin were suddenly to fall to zero and bilirubin production were to remain constant, the serum bilirubin would increase by 2 to 3 mg/dl/day.

If the direct fraction of the serum bilirubin is elevated for any length of time, conjugated bilirubin may bind covalently to serum albumin. The albumin-bilirubin complex is included in the direct fraction if the serum is fractionated by conventional techniques. The serum half-life of the albumin-bilirubin complex (15 days) is much longer than that of direct bilirubin and closer to that of albumin. This fraction of the serum bilirubin accounts for the slower-than-expected decline in the serum bilirubin during convalescence from certain liver diseases such as successful surgical treatment of bile duct obstruction.

Urine bilirubin. Indirect bilirubin is tightly bound to albumin, is not filtered by the kidney and therefore is never present in the urine. Any bilirubin found in urine is direct bilirubin. Therefore bilirubinuria indicates an increased direct serum bilirubin concentration and consequently implies liver disease. This test is almost 100% accurate. Phenothiazines may give false-positive readings with the Ictotest tablet.

Blood ammonia. Ammonia is produced within the body by normal protein metabolism and by intestinal bacteria, primarily those in the colon. It is detoxified within the liver by conversion to urea and within skeletal muscle and brain by combining with glutamate to form glutamine (Chapter 56). Blood ammonia may be elevated in severe hepatocellular disease and in portal hypertension in which there is shunting of portal blood around the liver. Blood ammonia elevation has been used to detect hepatic encephalopathy. However, there is poor correlation between either the presence or the degree of acute encephalopathy and elevation of blood ammonia. If used, the test should be performed on arterial blood and processed immediately. An elevated blood ammonia level is characteristic of Reye's syndrome and is the major finding in patients with inborn errors of urea metabolism. It may be an important clue in a patient with dementia due to unsuspected occult liver disease and may occasionally be helpful in following the course of individual patients with difficult-to-manage chronic hepatic encephalopathy.

Serum bile acids. Conjugated bile acids are synthesized in the liver, secreted into bile, and then returned to the liver via the enterohepatic circulation (Chapter 51). Serum bile acids can be measured by sensitive radioimmunoassays and chromatographic techniques. Normal serum bile acid concentration, a mixture of primary and secondary bile acids, is approximately 1 to 2 μg/ml in the fasting state. Serum levels rise after a meal due to the increased enterohepatic recirculation of bile acids stored in the gallbladder. Measurement of the 2-hour postprandial serum bile acid concentration has been promulgated as a sensitive test of overall liver function. However, there has been little experience with this test, and there is no evidence that it is either more sensitive or more specific than other, more established liver function tests.

Other tests that estimate functional capacity of the liver. Isotopically labeled drugs, such as ^{14}C-aminopyrine and ^{14}C-phenacetin, have been used to measure hepatic function reserve. The principle is simple. These substances are metabolized almost exclusively in the liver. $^{14}CO_2$ is generated and can be trapped and measured in expired air. The rate and amount of $^{14}CO_2$ produced after administering these drugs are decreased in patients with hepatocellular diseases such as chronic active hepatitis, alcoholic hepatitis, and various types of cirrhosis. Results correlate well with other tests such as the serum albumin and serum prothrombin time and also with liver histology. Galactose and caffeine metabolism by the liver have also been used to measure functional hepatic mass. These tests eliminate the need to use radioisotopes. Galactose is administered intravenously and caffeine orally. Serial blood samples are then drawn at timed intervals and their rate of disappearance from blood measured. The results of these tests correlate well with the aminopyrine breath test. All of these tests have great theoretical value but are not generally available.

Tests that measure biosynthetic function of the liver

Serum albumin. Serum albumin, a protein of molecular mass of 69,000 daltons, is synthesized exclusively by hepatocytes. It is the most abundant plasma protein, accounting for 50% of all plasma proteins. Serum albumin has a long half-life—15 to 20 days. Approximately 4% is degraded per day. Its rate of synthesis is regulated by osmoreceptors whose nature and location are unknown. Albumin synthesis can be increased by as much as 100% by conditions that decrease the serum albumin or lower intravascular oncotic pressure. Corticosteroids and thyroxine appear to increase the rate of albumin synthesis, whereas malnutrition and chronic illness may lower it. The latter effect is mediated by interleukin-1 and tumor necrosis factor. Because of albumin's long half-life, only minimum changes are found in serum albumin values in acute liver conditions such as viral hepatitis. Low serum albumin values in patients with liver disease imply chronic hepatocellular disorders such as cirrhosis. Hypoalbuminemia, however, is not found exclusively in liver disorders. It also occurs in malnutrition, protein-losing enteropathy, inflammatory bowel disease, nephrotic syndrome and chronic infections that are associated with prolonged increases in serum interleukin-1 and/or tumor necrosis factor levels.

Serum globulins. The concentration of globulins in serum can be approximated by salt fractionation and determined precisely by serum protein electrophoresis. Gamma globulins are produced and secreted by B lymphocytes, whereas alpha and beta globulins are produced primarily in hepatocytes. Gamma globulins are increased in systemic disorders, such as chronic infections and inflammatory disorders, as well as in chronic liver diseases such as cirrhosis and chronic active hepatitis. In cirrhosis, increased serum gamma globulin concentration is due to the increased synthesis of antibodies, some of which are directed against intestinal bacteria. Increased antibody synthesis is due in part to the failure of the cirrhotic liver to sequester and degrade antigens that normally reach the liver through the portal circulation, either because of shunting of portal blood around the liver or because of the loss of Kupffer cell function. Those antigens that bypass the liver and reach the systemic circulation stimulate antibody production by lymphocytes in the spleen and lymph nodes.

Increases in the concentration of specific isotypes of immunoglobulins are often helpful in the recognition of certain chronic liver diseases. Diffuse polyclonal increases in IgG levels are common in autoimmune chronic hepatitis; increases greater than 100% should alert the physician to this possibility. Increases in IgM levels are common in primary biliary cirrhosis, and increases in IgA levels occur in alcoholic liver disease.

Specific antibodies are helpful in the diagnosis of liver disease. For example, antimitochondrial antibody is present in 85% to 95% of patients with primary biliary cirrhosis, in less than 20% of patients with chronic hepatitis, and rarely, if ever, in patients with obstructive jaundice or viral hepatitis. Smooth muscle antibody is less specific. It is present in up to 60% of patients with chronic hepatitis, but is also found in patients with acute viral hepatitis and different types of malignancies. Antibodies directed against determinants on the hepatitis A, B, C, and D viruses are helpful in the diagnosis of these disorders (Chapter 57).

Approximately 90% of the alpha-globulin fraction is made up of alpha$_1$ antitrypsin. Serum alpha$_1$ antitrypsin levels are increased in infectious and inflammatory disorders and absent in homozygous alpha$_1$ antitrypsin deficiency. An absence or marked diminution of the alpha$_1$ globulin band on serum protein electrophoresis should alert the physician to the presence of this inherited disorder. Many of the lipoproteins migrate in the beta-globulin fraction. Conditions that change the concentration of serum lipoproteins will be reflected in the beta-globulin fraction. The beta-globulin fraction may be increased in chronic cholestatic disorders.

Coagulation factors. With the exception of factor VIII, which is most likely synthesized in reticuloendothelial and vascular endothelial cells, the blood clotting factors are made exclusively in hepatocytes. They have a much shorter half-life in serum than does albumin, ranging from 6 hours for factor VII to 5 days for fibrinogen. Because of their rapid turnover, measurement of the clotting factors is valuable in the diagnosis and prognosis of acute parenchymal liver diseases such as hepatitis. Serum prothrombin time collectively measures factors II, V, VII, and X and is useful for this purpose. Biosynthesis of factors II, VII, IX, and X depends on vitamin K. The prothrombin time may be elevated in hepatitis and cirrhosis as well as in disorders that lead to vitamin K deficiency. These disorders include malabsorption, obstructive jaundice, and treatment with broad-spectrum antibiotics and vitamin K antagonists. Marked prolongation of the prothrombin time, greater than 5 seconds above control and not corrected by parenteral vitamin K administration, is a reflection of extensive liver necrosis and is a poor prognostic sign in acute viral hepatitis and other acute and chronic liver diseases. Any patient with a prolonged prothrombin time should be tested for vitamin K deficiency; 5 to 10 mg of vitamin K is administered parenterally and repeated 24 hours later. The return of prothrombin time to normal indicates vitamin K deficiency caused by a disorder other than hepatocellular disease.

Ceruloplasmin. Ceruloplasmin, a blue, copper-containing glycoprotein with oxidase activity, is an acute phase reactant. Ninety-five percent of patients with Wilson's disease will have serum ceruloplasmin concentrations of less than 20 mg/dl, as will 10% of heterozygous carriers. Elevated values are seen in patients with acute inflammatory diseases, chronic cholestatic disorders, and increased serum estrogen concentrations.

Ferritin. Ferritin, an iron-containing protein, can be measured accurately by radioimmunoassay. Serum values usually reflect the status of iron stores in the body. Serum ferritin values are low in iron deficiency and elevated in iron storage diseases such as hemochromatosis. Serum ferritin may also be transiently elevated in acute hepatocellular diseases because of leakage of ferritin from damaged hepatocytes.

Alpha$_1$ fetoprotein. Alpha$_1$ fetoprotein is a normal secretory product of human fetal liver. Its concentration is elevated in serum in more than 50% of patients with hepatocellular carcinoma. High concentrations have also been observed in some patients with massive hepatic necrosis.

Serum enzymes

The liver contains thousands of enzymes, some of which are also present in serum in very low concentrations. These enzymes have no known function in serum. Serum enzymes behave like other serum proteins. They are distributed in plasma and in interstitial fluid and have characteristic half-lives, usually measured in days. Very little is known about the catabolism of serum enzymes, although they are probably cleared by cells in the reticuloendothelial system, including hepatic sinusoidal cells. The elevation of a given enzyme activity in serum is thought to reflect primarily its increased rate of entrance into serum from damaged liver cells. Serum enzyme tests can be grouped into three categories: enzymes whose elevation in serum reflects generalized damage to hepatocytes, enzymes whose elevation in serum reflects cholestasis, and enzyme tests that do not fit precisely into either pattern.

Enzymes that reflect damage to hepatocytes. The aminotransferases (transaminases) are sensitive indicators of liver cell injury and are most helpful in recognizing acute hepatocellular diseases such as hepatitis. The aminotransferases are normally present in serum in low concentration, less than 40 International Units (IU) (< 0.67 μKat/L). Disorders that damage the liver cell membrane allow leakage of the aminotransferases into serum. Any type of liver cell injury may cause modest elevation in serum aminotransferase levels. Levels of up to 300 IU (5 μKat/L) are nonspecific and may be found in any type of liver disorder. Striking elevations, i.e., aminotransferase levels in the thousands, occur almost exclusively in disorders associated with extensive hepatocellular injury such as drug and viral hepatitis, acute heart failure, prolonged hypotension, and exposure to hepatotoxins such as carbon tetrachloride.

There is a poor correlation between the extent of liver cell necrosis and the elevation of serum aminotransferases. The absolute elevation of aminotransferases is of little prognostic significance in acute hepatocellular disorders. The aminotransferases are rarely elevated above 500 units (8.3 μKat/L) in obstructive jaundice and rarely above 300 units (5 μKat/L) in alcoholic hepatitis or cirrhosis. In most acute hepatocellular disorders, the alanine aminotransferase (ALT or serum glutamic pyruvic transaminase [SGPT]) is higher than or equal to the aspartate aminotransferase (AST or serum glutamic oxaloacetic transaminase [SGOT]). An AST/ALT ratio greater than 2:1 is suggestive of alcoholic liver disease. A ratio greater than 3:1 is rare in any condition other than alcoholic liver disease.

Measurement of serum lactic dehydrogenase provides little information about liver disorders not afforded by measurement of the aminotransferases. Lactic dehydrogenase comprises five isoenzymes, and only one of these, the slowest migrating band on electrophoresis, is increased in hepatocellular disorders.

Enzymes that reflect cholestasis. The activity of three serum enzymes, alkaline phosphatase, 5′-nucleotidase, and gamma glutamyl transpeptidase, is usually elevated in cholestasis. The elevated activity of these enzymes probably reflects their subcellular location within the liver. Alkaline phosphatase and 5′-nucleotidase are found in or near the bile canalicular membrane, while gamma glutamyl transpeptidase is located in the endoplasmic reticulum and in bile duct epithelial cells. Reflecting its more diffuse localization within the liver, gamma glutamyl transpeptidase elevation in serum is less specific for cholestasis than elevations of alkaline phosphatase and 5′-nucleotidase. Elevation of these three enzymes is not totally specific for cholestasis. Less than threefold elevations are nonspecific and may be seen in almost any type of liver disease. Alkaline phosphatase levels four times greater than normal occur primarily in patients with cholestatic liver disorders, infiltrative liver diseases such as cancer, and bone conditions characterized by rapid bone turnover. In bone diseases, the elevation is due to increased amounts of the bone isoenzyme. In liver diseases, the elevation is almost always due to increased amounts of the liver isoenzyme. If there is a question about the origin of the elevated serum alkaline phosphatase, its origin can be determined by measuring either the 5′-nucleotidase and gamma glutamyl transpeptidase or by fractionating the serum alkaline phosphatase by electrophoresis. Elevation of either 5′-nucleotidase or gamma glutamyl transpeptidase indicates that the elevated alkaline phosphatase is of liver origin. These two enzymes are rarely elevated by bone disorders.

In the absence of jaundice or elevated aminotransferases, an elevated alkaline phosphatase often, but not always, suggests early cholestasis or hepatic infiltrations by tumor or granulomata. Other conditions cause isolated elevations of alkaline phosphatase, such as stage I and stage II Hodgkin's disease, congestive heart failure, hyperthyroidism, diabetes, and inflammatory bowel disease.

The level of serum alkaline phosphatase is not helpful in distinguishing among the various types of cholestasis, either intrahepatic or extrahepatic. Measurement of 5′-nucleotidase and gamma glutamyl transpeptidase provides little additional information other than confirmation of the hepatic origin of elevated alkaline phosphatase.

Other enzyme tests. Gamma glutamyl transpeptidase may be disproportionately elevated in sera of patients who abuse alcohol, even in the absence of frank liver cell injury. The mechanism of the increase is not precisely known, and isolated increases in this enzyme may also be seen in patients taking medications such as phenobarbital and Dilantin. Hence, such elevations should be regarded as nonspecific. The presence of a disproportionately elevated serum gamma glutamyl transpeptidase and an AST/ALT ratio greater than 2:1 should alert the physician to the possibility of alcoholic liver disease.

A variety of other serum tests have been advocated as being either more specific or more sensitive in the diagnosis of liver disease than the enzyme tests above. These include leucine aminopeptidase, beta-glucuronidase, glutamate dehydrogenase, and alcohol dehydrogenase. There is little evidence to support these claims.

Use of liver function tests

Liver function tests provide little information if used individually. They are best used together, as shown in Table 53-1 and Fig. 53-1. Even then, the initial pattern may be nonspecific or confusing. Additional information is derived if these tests are repeated after days or weeks, depending on the severity of the clinical situation. A diagnostic pattern may then emerge. Table 53-1 provides characteristic patterns of liver function test results in different types of liver disorders. If, after the performance of these tests, the diagnosis is still uncertain, their results should facilitate efficient use of the additional diagnostic tests shown in Fig. 53-1. Liver function tests should always be used first because they are safe, inexpensive, and have no associated morbidity.

OTHER DIAGNOSTIC PROCEDURES

Ultrasonography

Ultrasonography uses narrowly focused, high-frequency sound waves of from 2 to 5 million cycles per second that are generated and detected by the same transducer. These high-frequency sound waves are partially deflected at interfaces between soft tissues of differing acoustic impedance. Images generated by the reflected waves are displayed on a cathode ray tube and may be photographed or recorded on videotape. The more homogeneous the tissue, the fewer the echoes generated. Fluid-filled tissues generate no echoes. Thus cysts or dilated bile ducts appear black. There is total reflection of high-frequency sound waves at gas-soft tissue interfaces and bone-soft tissue interfaces. Because the sound waves do not penetrate these interfaces, gas-filled loops of bowel, such as occur in ileus, or overlying bone structure limits the use of ultrasonography.

Table 53-1. Liver function test patterns in hepatobiliary disorders and jaundice

Type of disorder	Bilirubin	Aminotransferases	Alkaline phosphatase	Albumin	Globulin	Prothrombin time
Hemolysis Gilbert's syndrome	Normal to 5 mg/dl 85% due to indirect fractions No bilirubinuria	Normal	Normal	Normal	Normal	Normal
Acute hepatocellular necrosis (viral and drug hepatitis, hepatotoxins, acute heart failure)	Both fractions may be elevated Peak usually follows aminotransferases Bilirubinuria	Elevated, often >500 IU ALT ≥ AST	Normal to <3 times normal elevation	Normal	Normal	Usually normal. If >5s above control and not corrected by parenteral vitamin K, suggests poor prognosis
Chronic hepatocellular disorders	Both fractions may be elevated Bilirubinuria	Elevated, but usually <300 IU	Normal to <3 times normal elevation	Often decreased	Increased gamma globulin	Often prolonged Fails to correct with parenteral vitamin K
Alcoholic hepatitis Cirrhosis	Both fractions may be elevated Bilirubinuria	AST/ALT >2 suggests alcoholic hepatitis or cirrhosis	Normal to <3 times normal elevation	Often decreased	Increased IGA and increased gamma globulin	
Intrahepatic cholestasis Obstructive jaundice	Both fractions may be elevated Bilirubinuria	Normal to moderate elevation Rarely >500 IU	Elevated, often >4 times normal elevation	Normal, unless chronic	Gamma globulin normal Beta globulin may be increased	Normal If prolonged, will correct with parenteral vitamin K
Infiltrative diseases (tumor, granulomata); partial bile duct obstruction	Usually normal	Normal to slight elevation	Elevated, often >4 times normal elevation Fractionate, or confirm liver origin with 5′-nucleotidase, gamma glutamyl transpeptidase	Normal	Usually normal Gamma globulin may be increased in granulomatous disease	Normal

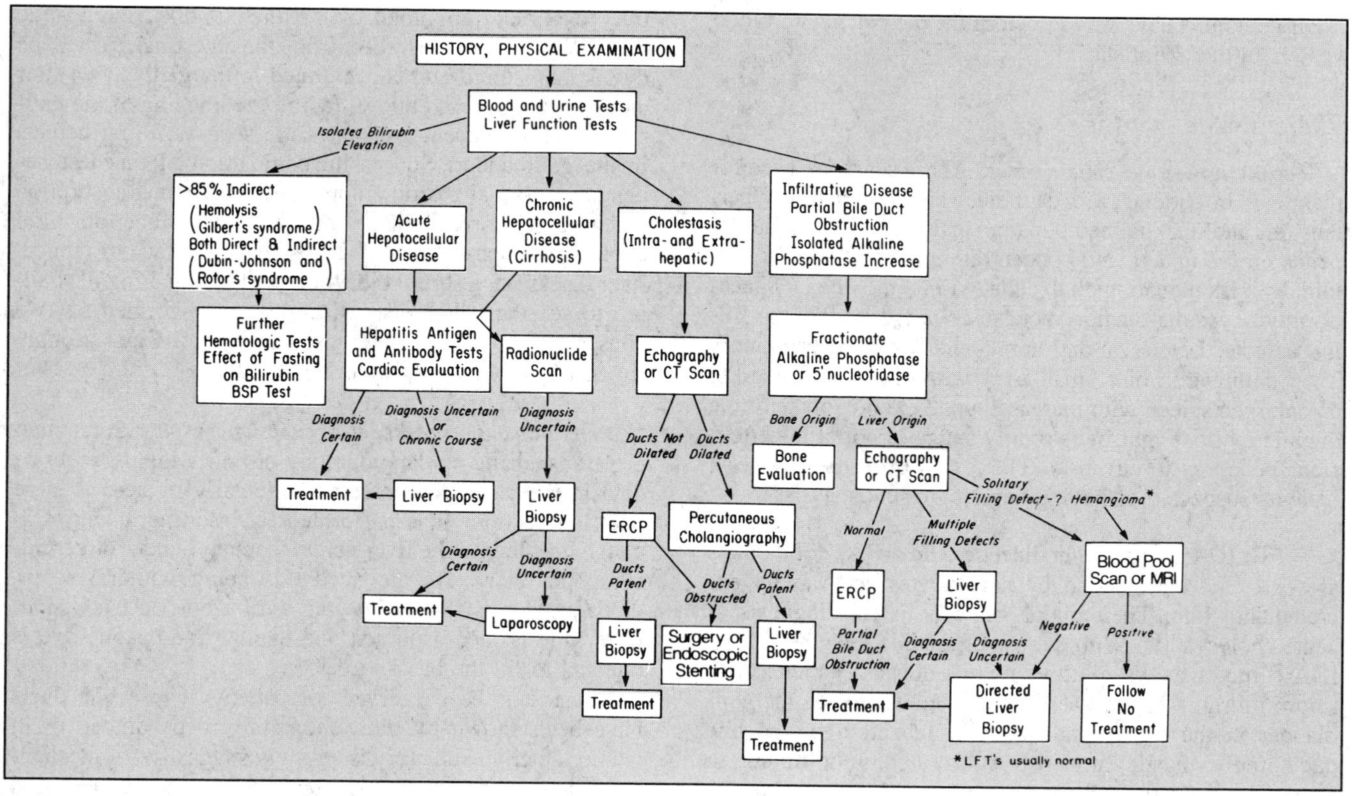

Fig. 53-1. Evaluation of jaundice and hepatobiliary disease. BSP, Bromsulphalein, CT, computed tomography; ERCP, endoscopic retrograde cholangiopancreatography; LFTs liver function tests.

Ultrasound has no known deleterious effects and is relatively inexpensive. Ultrasonography is the first diagnostic test to use in the patient whose liver function tests suggest cholestasis. By using current ultrasonic techniques, the clinician can accurately detect a dilated gallbladder or biliary tree. This information is then used to determine what other tests, such as percutaneous transhepatic cholangiography or endoscopic retrograde cholangiopancreatography, should be used. Ultrasonography will demonstrate gallstones as accurately as oral cholecystography and can do so if the gallbladder is nonfunctioning. In addition, it will show space-occupying lesions within the liver and enables the clinician to distinguish between cystic and solid masses in the liver previously detected by nuclide scanning. Aspiration of cystic lesions and percutaneous biopsies directed at previously detected masses within the liver are greatly facilitated by ultrasonographic scanning. Ultrasound with Doppler imaging can detect the patency of blood vessels in the abdomen and the direction of blood flow in them.

Computed tomography

Computed tomography (CT) uses x-irradiation to generate accurate transverse sectional views of the body. It provides information similar to that provided by ultrasonography. It is more expensive than ultrasonography and has the additional disadvantage of exposing the patient to ionizing radiation. Rapid-speed CT scanners provide sharper delineation of intra-abdominal lesions than does ultrasound, and neither gas nor bone interferes with its use. CT scanners can be programmed to measure accurately the density of individual lesions. Thus they can help to detect fatty livers and to distinguish between fluid-filled and solid lesions. CT will accurately measure liver size and demonstrate small amounts of ascites that cannot be detected by other means. It should be reserved for patients in whom ultrasonography fails to provide the necessary information.

The accuracy of CT scanning is increased if intravenous contrast dyes and dilute oral barium sulfate are administered during the scanning. This test can then be used to detect the size and patency of the portal vein and hepatic artery and to recognize space-occupying lesions within the liver such as neoplasms, cysts, and benign hemangiomas. Aspiration biopsy of such lesions can be greatly facilitated if done under CT guidance.

Recently developed CT scanners employ nuclear magnetic resonance imaging (MRI) rather than x-irradiation. There is no known risk associated with MRI exposure. Although expensive, this technique produces more information concerning infiltrative disorders of the liver and will recognize the accumulation within the liver of heavy metals such as iron and copper more clearly than other noninvasive tests. It is a sensitive way to detect benign hemangiomas and fatty infiltration of the liver, can usually recognize metastatic lesions in the liver with greater sensitivity and selectivity than other noninvasive tests, and is the most accurate noninvasive way to determine the patency of blood vessels in the abdomen.

Radionuclide scanning

Technetium sulfur colloid scans. These scans are used for diagnosis in patients with jaundice, signs of portal hypertension, and unexplained hepatomegaly. The technique depends on the uptake and concentration of ^{99m}Tc sulfur colloid by reticuloendothelial cells within the liver. Space-occupying lesions such as metastases or cysts appear as filling defects. Liver size and homogeneity can be estimated. The combination of a small liver with diminished uptake, an enlarged spleen with increased uptake, and uptake of the nuclide by bone marrow strongly suggests portal hypertension secondary to cirrhosis. The test is of limited value in patients suspected of having hepatitis or cholestasis.

^{99m}Tc IDA scans. Iminodiacetic acid (IDA) compounds are extracted from blood by hepatocytes and rapidly excreted into bile. Their major value is in the diagnosis of acute cholecystitis. With the use of nuclide imaging, ^{99m}Tc IDA compounds will outline the bile ducts in patients with serum bilirubin as high as 7 mg/dl. Failure to see the gallbladder in the face of adequate visualization of the bile ducts implies cystic duct obstruction, a common finding in acute cholecystitis. Ultrasonography and the cholangiographic techniques described later provide more accurate information.

^{99m}Tc blood pool scans. This test appears to be specific for benign hemangiomas of the liver. It should not be confused with ^{99m}Tc blood flow scans. Blood pool scans depend on the unusually slow blood flow through benign hemangiomas of the liver. The abdomen is scanned at intervals, 30 to 90 minutes after the intravenous administration of ^{99m}Tc technetium pertechnitate. Areas of residual nuclide uptake still visible within the liver after 30 minutes are indicative of benign hemangiomas. This test will detect hemangiomas as small as 2 cm in diameter.

Cholangiography

There are four widely available ways to see the biliary tree radiologically, two of which depend on the liver's ability to excrete a radiopaque dye into the biliary tree (oral cholecystography and intravenous cholangiography) and two of which depend on direct introduction of radiopaque material into the biliary tree (percutaneous transhepatic cholangiography and retrograde cholangiopancreatography). The diagnostic accuracy of the latter two procedures eliminates the need for exploratory laparotomy for diagnosis of biliary tract disease except in rare situations. Laparotomy therefore can be reserved for treatment of biliary tract disorders as well as for tissue diagnosis.

Oral cholecystography. Oral cholecystography is rarely used now and has been supplanted by ultrasonography for the detection of gallstones. It is based on the ability of the liver to extract from blood and secrete into bile a radiopaque dye that has been absorbed from the intestinal tract. The dye is then stored and concentrated in the gallbladder after an overnight fast and allows radiologic imaging of the gallbladder. Radiolucent gallstones are seen as filling defects in the gallbladder. Successful completion of this test depends on normal gastric emptying and intestinal absorption and nearly normal hepatic and gallbladder function. Oral cholecystography is rarely successful in the face of clinical liver disease or a serum bilirubin greater than 3 mg/dl. Failure to see the gallbladder if the test is performed on two consecutive days in an otherwise healthy individual strongly suggests gallbladder disease.

Percutaneous transhepatic cholangiography. Percutaneous transhepatic cholangiography provides highly accurate data in the jaundiced patient, particularly if there is large duct obstruction. It is performed by inserting a long, 23-gauge needle into the liver percutaneously, under direct fluoroscopic view. As the needle is being withdrawn, radiopaque dye is slowly injected until a bile duct is visualized. Bile is then aspirated and enough radiopaque dye is injected to fill the biliary tree.

The test is best reserved for patients whose bile ducts have been shown by ultrasonography to be dilated or in whom the clinical history is strongly suggestive of mechanical bile duct obstruction. If the bile ducts are dilated, the success rate is greater than 90%. The success rate is considerably lower in patients with intrahepatic cholestasis, as low as 50% in one prospective study.

If the biliary tree can be seen, diagnostic accuracy is very likely. In one large series, only 1% of the findings were false positive, and only 5% were false negative. Percutaneous transhepatic cholangiography can have uncommon though serious complications including bleeding, sepsis, and bile peritonitis. Sepsis and peritonitis occur in less than 1% of cases managed by experienced physicians, and bleeding occurs less often. Complications can be reduced if drainage catheters are left in place in patients with high-grade bile duct obstruction and systemic antibiotics are used or if these patients are operated on within hours after this procedure. This technique can be used to dilate and place stents through inoperable bile duct strictures and cancers and allows palliation of patients with inoperable bile duct obstruction.

Endoscopic retrograde cholangiopancreatography (see also Chapter 30). This test must be performed by an experienced endoscopist with special training. A side-viewing endoscope is guided into the duodenum perorally, and the ampulla of Vater located. A thin plastic catheter is then advanced into the ampulla and radiopaque dye injected. Both the pancreatic and the bile ducts can be visualized. The success rate ranges from 70% to 85%. Because the ability to see the biliary tree is independent of the caliber of the bile ducts, the success rate is similar in patients with extrahepatic or intrahepatic cholestasis. Endoscopic retrograde cholangiopancreatography has the added advantage of allowing viewing of the duodenum and biopsy of suspicious lesions in or near the ampulla. It is associated with a lower rate of serious complications than is percutaneous transhepatic cholangiography. It is the procedure of choice in jaundiced patients whose liver function tests suggest cholestasis and whose bile ducts are not shown by ultrasonography to be dilated. Another advantage of this procedure is that it allows peroral endoscopic papillotomy (sphincterotomy) and extraction of gallstones in those patients with demonstrable common bile duct stones as well as dilatation of bile duct strictures and placement of stents.

Percutaneous liver biopsy

Percutaneous needle biopsy of the liver is a safe procedure that can be performed at the bedside, with the use of local anesthesia. It provides an accurate tissue diagnosis and eliminates the risk of general anesthesia and laparotomy. Liver biopsy is of proven value in the following situations: (1) hepatocellular disease of uncertain cause; (2) prolonged hepatitis with a possibility of chronic active hepatitis; (3) unexplained hepatomegaly; (4) unexplained splenomegaly; (5) hepatic filling defects demonstrated by ultrasonography, CT, or radionuclide scanning; (6) fever of unknown origin; and (7) staging of malignant lymphoma.

Liver biopsy is most accurate in disorders causing diffuse changes throughout the liver and is subject to sampling error in focal infiltrative disorders such as hepatic metastases. Liver biopsy is associated with a high incidence of false-negative results in patients with macronodular cirrhosis, again because of sampling error. Liver biopsy should not be the initial procedure in the diagnosis of cholestasis. The patency of the biliary tree should first be established.

Contraindications for percutaneous liver biopsy include unexplained hemorrhagic diatheses, prothrombin time more than 5 seconds above control, and a platelet count of less than 80,000. It is wise to obtain a bleeding time in individuals with borderline clotting parameters. Some clinicians recommend that patients should always have their blood drawn and typed before liver biopsy, and blood should be held in the blood bank for possible cross-matching. The rate of serious bleeding following percutaneous liver biopsy is low, less than 0.3%, and the mortality is less than 0.1%. The most common complication is pain at the biopsy site, in the abdomen, or in the right shoulder. Pain usually lasts for several hours. Bile peritonitis is extremely rare in the patient with patent bile ducts. Liver biopsy is a safe procedure in the diagnosis of hepatic filling defects once the possibility of hemangioma has been ruled out by appropriate tests such as a ^{99m}Tc blood pool scan. Directed liver biopsy with ultrasound or CT guidance increases the diagnostic yield for focal lesions. The incidence of bleeding from vascular lesions, such as certain hepatomas and renal cell carcinoma, does not appear to be higher than in disorders such as cirrhosis. However, the presence of a loud bruit over a liver with filling defects is an indication for angiography before biopsy. Liver biopsy should not be performed if a hydatid cyst is suspected because of the risk of anaphylaxis.

Laparoscopy and minilaparotomy

These procedures are reserved for the patient whose x-ray films, scans, and liver biopsies fail to provide a diagnosis. Laparoscopy is 100% accurate in the diagnosis of cirrhosis, is more accurate than percutaneous liver biopsy in staging of lymphomas, and is useful in directing biopsies of the liver with malignant implants. Minilaparotomy provides similar information, with the added advantage of allowing direct cholangiographic viewing of the biliary tree. Minilaparotomy is rarely necessary in centers that use either percutaneous transhepatic cholangiography or endoscopic retrograde cholangiopancreatography.

Angiography

Angiography has limited value in the diagnosis of liver disease. Its earlier use in the diagnosis of metastatic disease of the liver has been replaced by radionuclide scanning, ultrasonography, CT, and MRI. These tests are safer and more accurate than angiography. Angiography need not be performed to evaluate hepatic filling defects unless there is a loud bruit over the liver. It is of value in judging the operability of patients with proven primary hepatocellular carcinoma, and it is useful to detect hemobilia, an uncommon complication of percutaneous cholangiography and liver biopsy.

Angiography is important in the evaluation of portal hypertension. Selected celiac angiography, through either a femoral or a brachial artery, may provide excellent delineation of the portal anatomy and demonstrate esophageal varices as well as occlusion of the portal or splenic veins. Another technique, percutaneous portography, provides even more accurate mapping of the portal system. As in percutaneous cholangiography, a 23-gauge needle is advanced percutaneously into the liver, and dye is injected until a branch of the portal vein can be seen. A plastic catheter may then be advanced over the needle into a larger portal vein radicle, and enough radiopaque contrast material injected to demonstrate the entire portal system. This technique is preferred by some vascular surgeons before portosystemic shunt surgery. Percutaneous portography must be used with great caution in the patient with impaired clotting function, ascites, or advanced cirrhosis because of the serious risk of intraperitoneal bleeding.

REFERENCES

Baron RL et al: The liver. In Moss AA, editor: Computed tomography of the body with magnetic resonance imaging, ed 2, vol 3, abdomen, Philadelphia, 1992, WB Saunders.

Clark RA and Matsui O: CT of liver tumors, Semin Roentgenol 18:149, 1983.

Engel MA et al: Differentiation of focal intrahepatic lesions with ^{99m}Tc-red blood cell imaging, Radiology 146:777, 1983.

Ferrucci JT: MR imaging of the liver, Am J Roentgenol 147:1103, 1986.

Freitas JW: Cholescintigraphy in acute and chronic cholecystitis, Semin Nucl Med 12:18, 1982.

Kaplan MM: Laboratory tests. In Schiff L and Schiff ER, editors: Diseases of the liver, ed 7, Philadelphia, 1993, JB Lippincott.

Lindsell DRM: Ultrasound imaging of pancreas and biliary tract, Lancet 335:142, 1990.

Mitchell DG and Stark DD: Liver. In Stark DD and Bradley WG Jr, editors: Magnetic resonance imaging, St Louis, 1992, Mosby–Year Book.
Morrissey JF and Reichelderfer M: Gastrointestinal endoscopy, N Engl J Med 325:1214, 1991.
Reichling JJ and Kaplan MM: Clinical use of serum enzymes in liver disease, Dig Dis Sci 33:1601, 1988.
Weiss JS et al: The clinical importance of a protein-bound fraction of serum bilirubin in patients with hyperbilirubinemia, N Engl J Med 309:147, 1983.

CHAPTER

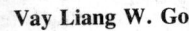

54 Evaluation of Pancreatic Diseases

Vay Liang W. Go

EVALUATION OF PANCREATIC DISEASES

In clinical practice, tests of pancreatic dysfunction include four main groups: those that (1) detect active pancreatic destruction, (2) estimate residual exocrine pancreatic function, (3) provide evidence of coincidental pancreatic endocrine dysfunction, and (4) permit imaging of the pancreas. Diagnosing pancreatic disease is difficult because of the inaccessibility of the pancreas for clinical examination, the time-consuming nature of the available diagnostic tests, and the lack of standardized procedures and criteria for detecting abnormal pancreatic function in human beings. In the past two decades, new methods for investigating the pancreas have focused on structural, as opposed to functional, changes in pancreatic disease. These methods include retrograde pancreatography, ultrasonic scanning, computed tomography (CT), arteriography, and magnetic resonance imaging (MRI). Imaging procedures and pancreatic function tests complement one another.

MEASUREMENT OF PANCREATIC ENZYMES IN BODY FLUIDS

Active pancreatic inflammation and/or destruction may be suspected when there is an increased concentration of pancreatic enzymes in body fluids such as blood, urine, and pleural, pericardial, and ascitic fluids. The underlying pathophysiologic factors involved include an active inflammatory process and/or an obstruction of the pancreatic duct, whereas acinar function remains relatively intact.

The enzymes commonly measured by their catalytic activity are amylase and lipase. Elevated concentrations of these enzymes suggest active pancreatic damage such as may be found in acute pancreatitis with or without necrosis, relapse of acute pancreatitis, or the early phase of relapsing chronic pancreatitis (Chapter 67). Measurement of amylase and lipase is generally not useful in the diagnosis of well-established chronic pancreatitis or of pancreatic cancer (Chapter 67).

Amylase

During uncomplicated acute pancreatitis, elevated serum amylase concentrations usually persist for 1 to 4 days (Fig. 54-1). Hyperamylasemia of longer duration often indicates more prolonged or severe pancreatitis or recrudescence of the initial acute process. Prolonged elevations of serum amylase for 1 to 3 months are most commonly due to the presence of a pancreatic pseudocyst. The height of serum amylase concentration does not correlate with the clinical severity of pancreatitis. Hyperamalasuria often persists for 7 to 10 days after serum amylase returns to normal. Thus urinary amylase may be elevated in the presence of normal serum levels, especially because the ratio of renal clearance of amylase to renal clearance of creatinine is increased early in acute pancreatitis. In spite of the advantages of urinary over serum amylase determination, urinary excretion of amylase depends on reasonably normal renal function.

Hyperamylasuria and hyperamylasemia are not always diagnostic of pancreatitis. Elevated serum and urine values may occur in biliary tract disease, perforated peptic ulcer disease, acute intestinal obstruction, tubal pregnancy, mumps, infective parotitis, and in some cases of pancreatic cancer. Elevated serum values but normal urine values may occur in macroamylasemia, in renal failure, and in

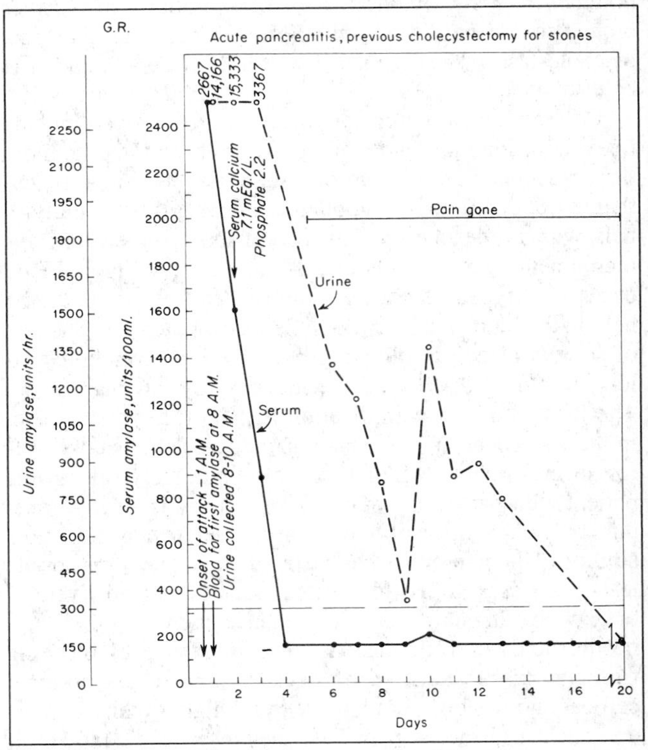

Fig. 54-1. Degree and duration of elevation of serum and urine amylase values in a patient with acute pancreatitis. (From Gambill EE and Mason HL: JAMA 186:24-28, 1963. Copyright 1963, American Medical Association.)

metabolic imbalances associated with burns and diabetic acidosis. Two modifications of the standard amylase procedure have been used in an attempt to improve the diagnostic accuracy of the amylase assay. These modifications include the measurement of renal clearance of amylase and the isoamylase analysis. The renal clearance of amylase (C_{am}) can be related to renal function by dividing C_{am} by the renal clearance of creatinine (C_{cr}), as determined by the following formula:

$$\frac{\text{urine amylase}}{\text{serum amylase}} \times \frac{\text{serum creatinine}}{\text{urine creatinine}} \times 100 = \frac{C_{am}}{C_{cr}}\%.$$

This amylase-creatinine clearance test is simple and requires only measurement of amylase and creatinine in simultaneously collected random samples of urine and serum. Thus errors related to incomplete recovery and inaccurate timing of urine collections are avoided. The ratio of C_{am}/C_{cr} averages 2.2% in normal subjects (Fig. 54-2), with a range of 1.0% to 4.0%. Similar values are obtained in patients with renal failure, indicating that C_{am} and C_{cr} are proportionally decreased in these patients. Early in the course of acute pancreatitis, C_{am}/C_{cr} is considerably above the normal range, with a mean value of 6.6%. In macroamylasemia, the ratio is reduced below normal, indicating that the hyperamylasemia is due to the presence of an unusual amylase in the serum that is cleared slowly by the kidney rather than due to an increased rate of release of amylase into the serum. The ratio usually remains normal in other conditions in which serum levels of amylase are elevated, but its specificity has been questioned because elevated ratios have been noted in some patients with diabetic acidosis, renal failure (especially in concert with hemodialysis), perforated peptic ulcers, severe burns, and pancreatic cancer. When present, increased amylase clearance appears to reflect defective renal tubular reabsorption of amylase and other proteins.

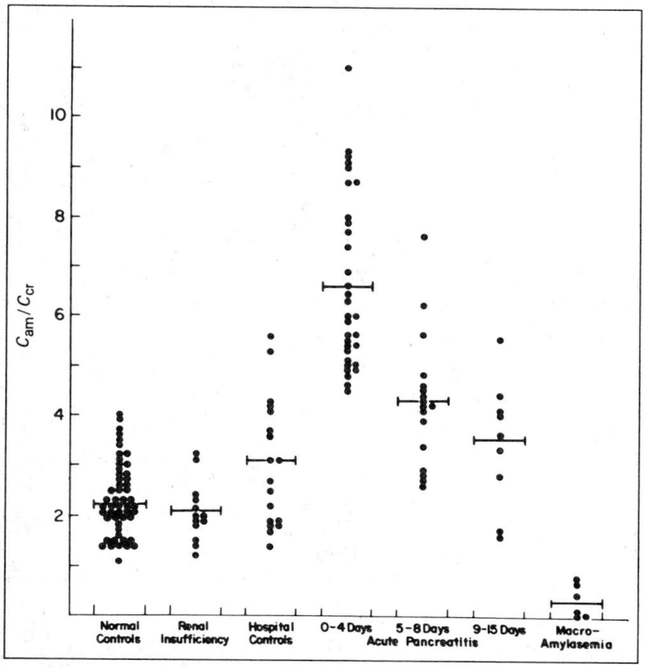

Fig. 54-2. Renal clearance of amylase (C_{am}) divided by the renal clearance of creatinine (C_{cr}). Acute pancreatitis patients are grouped according to number of days after onset of attack. (From Levitt MD: Mayo Clin Proc 54(7):428-431, 1979.)

The serum isoamylase analysis indicates whether hyperamylasemia is pancreatic (P-type), salivary (S-type), or macroamylasemic in origin. The discovery of an inhibitor to S-type amylase has rendered the enzymatic determination of serum amylase specific for pancreatic amylase. Similarly, the development of radioimmunoassay of S-type and P-type human amylase has improved the specificity of amylase determination. Currently, an elevated serum amylase has a 95% sensitivity and specificity in the diagnosis of acute pancreatitis.

Lipase

Because no nonpancreatic source of true serum lipase appears to exist and because serum lipase concentrations tend to follow the pattern of serum amylase, serum lipase concentrations may be a more specific indicator for pancreatitis. The advantage of determining serum lipase concentrations therefore is an increased overall specificity for pancreatic disease. Serum lipase concentrations are currently determined by a turbidimetric method using a synthetic substrate or through radioimmunoassay.

Trypsin and other proteases

Serum trypsin, as measured by radioimmunoassay, has been reported useful in the diagnosis of both acute and chronic pancreatitis. Because this test is expensive, however, it is not widely used. Serum trypsin is markedly elevated in acute pancreatitis, and the level is below the normal range in patients with pancreatic exocrine insufficiency. Nevertheless, although a low level of serum trypsin may indicate pancreatic exocrine insufficiency, the test has only limited sensitivity. Radioimmunoassay has been developed for measuring elastase, phospholipase A_2, and other proteases. The clinical utility of these measurements is presently being evaluated.

PANCREATIC FUNCTION TESTS

Pancreatic function tests can be classified as direct-stimulation tests, indirect-stimulation tests, fecal tests, and absorption tests, as outlined in the accompanying box. Direct-stimulation tests are those in which duodenal volume flow and bicarbonate and enzyme content are measured after appropriate hormones (secretin, cholecystokinin, or synthetic cholecystokinin octapeptide) have been administered parenterally. By contrast, indirect-stimulation tests require the feeding of test meals or the perfusion of nutrient substances, followed by measurement of duodenal enzyme and/or bicarbonate content. Unfortunately, all of these tests require intestinal intubation to recover pancreatic secretions and therefore are somewhat cumbersome.

Tests of pancreatic exocrine function

I. Direct-stimulation tests
  A. Secretin tests
    1. Submaximal secretin test (single IV injection, 1 CU/kg)
    2. Maximum secretin test
      a. Single injection (2-4 CU/kg)
      b. Continuous IV infusion (2-4 CU/kg/h)
    3. Augmented secretin test, bolus IV (1 CU/kg, then repeated with 4 CU/kg IV)
  B. Cholecystokinin (CCK)
    1. Single IV injection (3 CHR U/kg)
    2. Continuous IV injection (0.25 CHR U/kg/min)
  C. Combination of secretin and CCK tests
    1. Single injection
    2. Continuous IV infusion
II. Indirect-stimulation tests
  A. Lundh test meal
  B. ^{75}Se test meal, modification of Lundh test meal
  C. Duodenal perfusion of
    1. Essential amino acids
    2. Fatty acids
    3. Hydrochloric acid
  D. Synthetic peptide BZ-ty-PABA
III. Fecal tests
  A. Quantitative fecal fat and nitrogen
  B. Fecal excretion of ^{131}I-labeled triolein
  C. Fecal staining for fat
  D. Fecal examination for meat fibers
  E. Fecal enzyme determination
IV. Absorption tests
  A. ^{131}I-labeled triolein
  B. ^{131}I-labeled triolein and oleic acid
  C. Gelatin
  D. Starch
  E. Glucose

Direct-stimulation tests are the most specific for the detection of pancreatic insufficiency, and the results should indicate abnormality (reduced bicarbonate concentration and enzyme output) only in the presence of primary pancreatic disease, be it inflammatory or neoplastic. A noninvasive, indirect Bentiromide test using the synthetic peptide N-benzoyl-L-tyrosyl-p-aminobenzoic acid (BZ-ty-PABA) has been evaluated in the diagnosis of pancreatic disease. This synthetic peptide is administered orally and is specifically cleaved by pancreatic chymotrypsin in the intestinal lumen to BZ-ty and PABA. PABA is absorbed and excreted in the urine; thus the urine PABA concentration reflects intraluminal chymotrypsin activity. The BZ-ty-PABA test is a simple pancreatic function test but has limited sensitivity and specificity.

In primary chronic exocrine pancreatic insufficiency, direct and indirect stimulation should indicate abnormality because the target organ, the pancreas, is diseased and cannot respond with normal secretions despite the magnitude of the stimulus. Indirect tests are less specific for pancreatic disease, as their results may indicate abnormality in cases of malabsorptive disease in which the primary lesion is extrapancreatic. On the other hand, direct-test results usually indicate normality, whereas indirect tests may indicate may indicate abnormality. When the pancreas is normal in patients with extrapancreatic malabsorptive disease, the hormonal and neural influences that regulate pancreatic secretion are disturbed. Because indirect tests require an intact neurohormonal mechanism for normal pancreatic response, results may indicate abnormality. This "secondary" pancreatic insufficiency occurs in diseases of the small intestinal mucosa, such as celiac sprue in postgastrectomy or postvagotomy states and in patients with gastrimonias. In these cases, there may be decreased and/or delayed secretion of duodenal hormones as well as disease associated with excessive gastric acid secretion, resulting in impaired intraluminal digestion partly caused by inactivation of pancreatic enzymes.

Quantitative measurement of fecal fat is the standard and most accurate method for determining whether a patient has malabsorption. This measurement by itself, however, does not enable the clinician to differentiate among the many diseases that cause malabsorption (Chapters 33 and 42). Quantitation of fecal fat excretion is not a sensitive test for identifying impaired pancreatic function, as steatorrhea occurs only in advanced disease states in which enzyme output is decreased by 90% or more (Fig. 54-3). Therefore, values for fecal fat will be abnormal only in far advanced pancreatic insufficiency and will not measure mild or moderate pancreatic insufficiency. Qualitative determination of fat in stool (by microscopic examination after staining for fat) is useful, though perhaps less sensitive and less specific (Chapter 33). The presence of recognizable meat muscle fibers in the stool indicates intraluminal maldigestion but is not specific for pancreatic exocrine insufficiency.

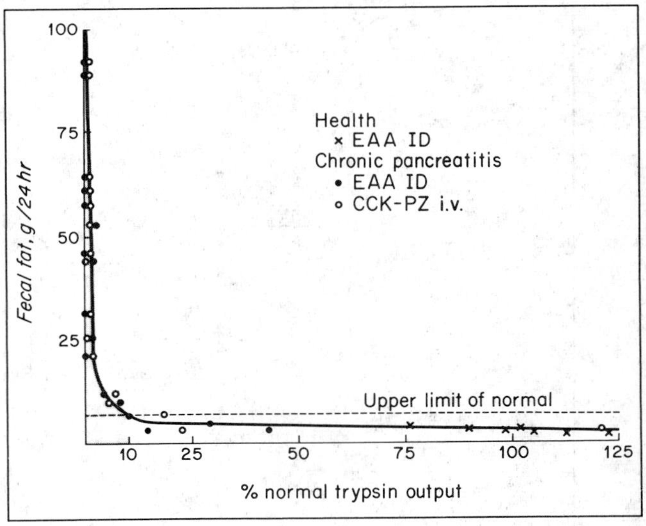

Fig. 54-3. Relation of trypsin output per hour to 24-hour fecal fat excretion in healthy subjects and in patients with chronic pancreatitis. Values above the horizontal dashed line denote steatorrhea (> 7 g fat excreted in 24 h). EAA ID, intraduodenal perfusion of essential amino acids solution; CCK-PZ i.v., intravenous cholecystokinin infusion. (From DiMagno EP, Go VLW, and Summerskill WHJ: N Engl J Med 288:813-815, 1973.)

Determination of the concentrations of chymotrypsin and trypsin in the stool has been used to identify pancreatic insufficiency, particularly because the specific synthetic substrates (n-acetyl-L-tyrosine-ethyl-ester [ATEE] for chymotrypsin and p-toluene-sulfonyl-L-arginine-methyl-ester [TAME] for trypsin) are now available. These substrates also allow easy enzyme determination with use of the pH-stat automatic titrator. However, fecal trypsin activity is an extremely unreliable indicator of pancreatic function because false-positive results are common. Although chymotrypsin activity is somewhat more specific, false-positive results occur in 10% of control subjects and false-negative results in more than 10% of patients with pancreatic exocrine insufficiency. This screening test for pancreatic exocrine insufficiency is used primarily in children.

Absorption tests utilizing starch, gelatin, and radiolabeled triglyceride have been advocated for distinguishing pancreatic from intestinal causes of steatorrhea. Unfortunately, these tests are not specific and have largely been discarded for differentiating pancreatic from intestinal diseases.

The glucose tolerance test, which assesses endocrine function of the pancreas, is abnormal in 60% to 70% of patients with chronic pancreatitis or pancreatic cancer. This test is limited, however, because glucose absorption may be impaired by intestinal disease.

Selection of pancreatic function tests

When considering the use of pancreatic function tests, the clinician usually is confronted by one of the following questions: (1) Does the patient have primary pancreatic disease? (2) Does the patient have malabsorption of pancreatic origin?

Does the patient have primary pancreatic disease? To answer this first question, the best tests to use are direct-stimulation tests of pancreatic function. The severity of the abnormality is assessed by direct-stimulation tests because their results are quantitatively expressed. Even when these tedious and time-consuming tests are administered, however, patients with pancreatic disease may exhibit "normal" pancreatic function. Patients with false-negative results may have subacute or resolving pancreatitis, chronic pancreatitis localized in the tail, carcinoma of the tail, or pseudocysts originating from the tail. Because function tests are not highly sensitive, even some patients with extensive pancreatic calcification may have normal direct-stimulation tests. Documentation of the presence of pancreatic disease may require a series of tests, including imaging techniques, and even then laparotomy may be required to resolve the issue.

Does the patient have malabsorption of pancreatic origin? First, the clinician must determine whether malabsorption is present. If malabsorption is documented by quantitative determination of fecal fat, the D-xylose absorption test in the presence of normal kidney function will help discriminate between intestinal mucosal disease and intraluminal maldigestion. Intestinal barium contrast radiography and peroral small intestinal biopsy may also be helpful in making this distinction (Chapter 33). In the absence of apparent small intestinal disease, a pancreatic function test should be useful unless pancreatic disease is obvious. Quantitative assessment of pancreatic secretion is preferable because quantitative tests are the most sensitive, and the severity of impaired pancreatic function can be correlated with the severity of steatorrhea.

RADIOLOGIC STUDIES

For many years, radiologic study of pancreatic disease was limited to indirect examinations, such as flat and lateral films of the abdomen, for identifying calcifications in the pancreatic bed and barium contrast studies of stomach, small intestine, and colon. In general, these procedures are insensitive, nonspecific, and imprecise in detecting small pancreatic lesions, whether inflammatory or neoplastic. However, barium contrast studies may reveal widening of the duodenal sweep and effacement of duodenal mucosal folds, suggesting the presence of an inflammatory or neoplastic mass in the proximal pancreas.

The use of ultrasonography, CT, endoscopy, and angiography has made major contributions important to our understanding of the structural changes in both pancreatic parenchyma and ducts. These imaging modalities, together with clinical and laboratory tests, can now be used to classify patients suffering from pancreatitis initially on admission with regard to etiology, morphology, and clinical severity. Imaging modalities are also used to monitor the hospitalized patient during the course of the disease for such potential complications of pancreatitis as necrosis, abscess, fistulae, pseudoaneurysm, or vascular thrombosis.

Ultrasonography of the abdomen is a noninvasive, safe, and relatively inexpensive procedure of considerable value in the investigation of suspected pancreatic disease. Cystic and mass lesions can be distinguished and detected with reasonable sensitivity, provided they are at least 2.5 cm in diameter. Pancreatic size can be assessed and echogenic calcifications are readily detected through ultrasound. In patients with suspected acute pancreatitis, the pancreas appears hypoechoic and edematous, with transudate also present, with or without infection. Abnormal ultrasonography has been reported to have a sensitivity and specificity ranging between 50% and 90% in the diagnosis of pancreatitis. It is also of value in the documentation of concurrent biliary tract stones.

CT complements ultrasonography in the assessment of the pancreatic bed and is particularly useful in patients with ileus or severe obesity, as these conditions often preclude adequate ultrasonic assessment of the pancreas but do not interfere with CT. Cystic lesions can be distinguished from mass lesions (see Fig. 67-8). Precise characterization of inflammatory lesions (pancreatic phlegmon versus pancreatic abscess) can be aided by guided needle aspiration. Similarly, if a mass lesion is found in the pancreas by ultrasonography or CT, its aspiration with a thin (22-gauge) needle with ultrasonic or CT guidance provides a cytologic specimen that may permit a definitive diagnosis of carcinoma. False-negative results are common; thus the test is of significance only if results are positive. Aspiration's major indication is in patients in whom exploratory surgery can be avoided if a definitive diagnosis of cancer is made by less invasive methods. CT scan, vascularly enhanced with intravenous bolus contrast, has added immeasurably to our understanding of the pathogenesis and history of pancreatitis and increased our ability to predict with success which acute pancreatitis patients will develop infections, necroses, or diabetes.

Selective angiography of the arterial vessels supplying the pancreas is useful in selected instances. Cystic lesions are avascular and distort the course of normal vessels. Pancreatic carcinoma may encase normal blood vessels, producing a narrowed and irregular lumen. Vascular neoplasms, such as islet cell tumors, may display a tumor blush. Because of its greater morbidity rate, selective angiography should be preceded by ultrasonography and/or CT in patients with suspected pancreatic disease. If a mass lesion is detected by the latter two techniques, the major role of angiography is to provide information before surgery regarding the potential resectability of the lesion.

Endoscopic retrograde cholangiopancreatography (ERCP) is an extremely useful means of visualizing the pancreatic and biliary ductal systems. ERCP is useful in the differential diagnosis of obstructive jaundice (Chapter 53). Moreover, visualization of the pancreatic ducts during ERCP often permits at least tentative differentiation between inflammatory and neoplastic disease. In chronic pancreatitis, the ducts may be irregular, with alternating areas of narrowing and dilatation, whereas, in carcinoma, isolated ductal stenosis or complete obstruction may be found. The procedure is discussed in detail in Chapter 30.

In selecting these specialized radiologic tests for the diagnosis of suspected pancreatic disease, the clinician must give preference to those methods with the least risks and greatest proven accuracy. Degrees of risk and accuracy often differ from institution to institution.

The application of MRI scanning is now established for various internal organs including the pancreas. The disadvantages of MRI as compared with CT are the relatively long scanning time and high expense. However, if this technology can develop beyond its current imaging capability, theoretically, this system permits the joint assessment of anatomy, metabolism, and biochemistry of the pancreas. In the future, further development of MRI may provide the single noninvasive approach for investigating the anatomy, physiology, biochemistry, and altered metabolic processes of the healthy and diseased pancreas.

REFERENCES

DiMagno EP and Go VLW: The exocrine pancreas. In Gitnick G, editor: Current gastroenterology, vol 4, New York, 1984, Wiley.

Frey CF: Classification of acute pancreatitis, Int J Pancreatol 9:39-49, 1991.

Go VLW et al, editors: The pancreas: biology, pathobiology, and diseases, ed 2, New York, 1993, Raven Press.

Gyr KE, Singer MV, and Sarles H, editors: Pancreatitis: concepts and classification, New York, 1984, Excerpta Medica.

Niederau C and Grendell JH: Diagnosis of chronic pancreatitis, Gastroenterology 88:1973, 1985.

Steinberg W, editor: Disorders of the pancreas, Gastroenterol Clin North Am 19:4, 1990.

CLINICAL SYNDROMES AND SPECIFIC DISEASE ENTITIES II

CHAPTER

55 Jaundice and Disorders of Bilirubin Metabolism

J. Donald Ostrow

Jaundice, or icterus, is the yellowish discoloration of the skin, sclerae, and mucous membranes caused by retention of bilirubin and/or its conjugates. Carotene and lycopene may also cause yellowing of the skin but not the sclerae.

Jaundice may be the first or sole manifestation of disease. It is most easily seen in the normally white sclerae but is more difficult to detect in artificial or dim light and in blacks. Because jaundice is not usually detectable clinically until total serum bilirubin levels are increased threefold to fourfold above normal, an elevation of this laboratory value on a blood chemistry screen is often the first indication of an abnormality in bilirubin metabolism.

NORMAL BILIRUBIN METABOLISM

Bilirubin is a yellow, tetrapyrrolic pigment that is the major product of heme catabolism. Due to internal hydrogen-bonding of all the polar groups in unconjugated bilirubin, the pK'a values of its two carboxyl groups are both above 8.0, and its interactions with water are limited, rendering it poorly water soluble. Like other poorly water-soluble organic compounds, bilirubin is transported in the plasma bound to albumin, which limits its renal excretion. Bilirubin is cleared mainly by hepatocytes, which convert the pigment to a variety of water-soluble conjugates *(conjugated bilirubin),* principally the monoglucuronides and diglucuronides. This biotransformation is necessary for the excretion of bilirubin, and only traces of *unconjugated bilirubin* appear in the bile. Under normal conditions, the conjugated bilirubin is efficiently excreted in bile, so that over 96% of the bilirubin in normal plasma is unconjugated. The excreted conjugated bilirubin then traverses the biliary tree to the intestine, where bacterial flora metabolize the pigments to a variety of products that are eliminated, predominantly in the stool, along with varied proportions of unchanged bilirubin.

Bilirubin metabolism can be divided into 10 successive steps (Table 55-1, Figs. 55-1 and 55-2).

Table 55-1. Specific steps in bilirubin metabolism and related abnormalities that affect them

Steps	Abnormalities
1. Formation of UCB* by catabolism of heme, mainly in reticuloendothelial cells	Overproduction of UCB: Hemolysis or ineffective erythropoiesis
2. Delivery of UCB in the circulation (mainly via the portal vein), bound to plasma albumin	Right-sided congestive heart failure Portosystemic shunts (cirrhosis, surgery)
Clearance	
3. Uptake of UCB across the basolateral membrane into the hepatocyte, after dissociation from albumin	Competitive inhibition of UCB uptake by drugs Gilbert's syndrome ?Fasting
4. Storage of UCB in the hepatocyte cytosol, bound to ligandin	Competitive inhibition of UCB storage by drugs Rotor's syndrome (storage disease) Fever
5. Conjugation of UCB in microsomes (endoplasmic reticulum) to form CB* (mostly glucuronides)†	Type I: Crigler-Najjar syndrome Type II: Arias' syndrome Gilbert's syndrome Inhibition of conjugation by drugs and progestogens
6. Secretion of CB into canalicular bile†	Hepatocellular jaundice (alcoholic, viral or toxic hepatitis ± cirrhosis) Dubin-Johnson syndrome Inhibition of CB secretion by 17α-alkyl steroids Rotor's syndrome (storage disease)
7. Flow of CB in bile down the biliary tree to the duodenum	Intrahepatic cholestasis due to estrogens, drugs, granulomas, tumors, sclerosing cholangitis, primary biliary cirrhosis, benign recurrent cholestasis, postoperative cholestasis, cholestasis of sepsis Extrahepatic cholestasis due to obstruction of ampulla or extrahepatic bile ducts
8. Intestinal transit of CB and catabolism by gut flora to UCB and urobilinogens	Ileus, bacterial overgrowth Absence of anaerobic gut flora neonates, antibiotic therapy
9. Enterohepatic recirculation via portal venous blood to the liver, to again undergo steps 3 through 8	Portosystemic shunting Acute cholecystitis Cholascos
10. Elimination in the feces	Obstipation

*UCB, unconjugated bilirubin; CB, conjugated bilirubin.
†Normally, step 5 or 6 may be rate-limiting.

The uptake, storage, conjugation, and secretion steps all apparently involve specific carriers or enzymes whose activity may be altered selectively by competitive or noncompetitive inhibition, induction, or genetic deletion. Disorders of the liver or biliary tree often preferentially involve one or more of these 10 steps, forming the basis for the classification and diagnosis of jaundice.

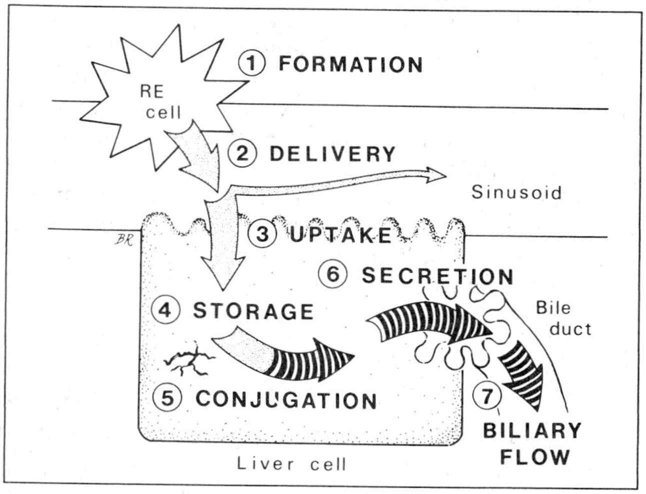

Fig. 55-1. Normal hepatic bilirubin transport showing sequence of the seven steps from formation in the reticuloendothelial (RE) cell to flow in the biliary tree. Stippled arrows, unconjugated bilirubin; striped arrows, conjugated bilirubin; squiggly figure, endoplasmic reticulum. (Modified from Ostrow JD et al: Unit I, Hepatic excretory function. Undergraduate teaching project, American Gastroenterological Association, Baltimore, 1975, Milner-Fenwick, Slide 26.)

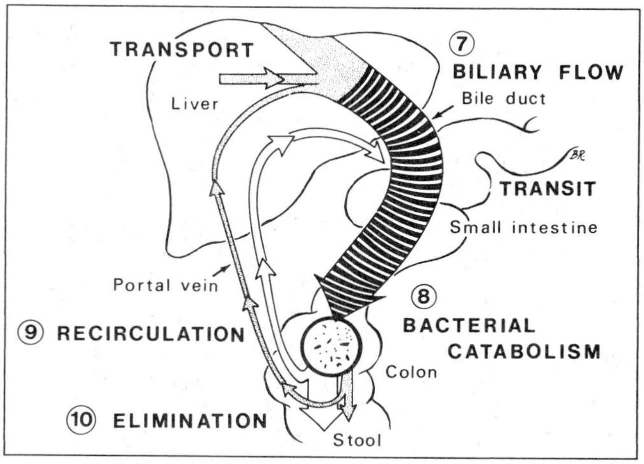

Fig. 55-2. The enterohepatic circulation of bile pigments. Symbols as in Fig. 55-1. Clear arrows, urobilinogens. (Modified from Ostrow JD et al: Unit I, Hepatic excretory function. Undergraduate teaching project, American Gastroenterological Association, Baltimore, 1975, Milner-Fenwick, Slide 22.)

INDIVIDUAL STEPS IN BILIRUBIN METABOLISM

Bilirubin formation

All bilirubin is derived from hemes and heme proteins (Fig. 55-3). Of the 3.8 ± 0.6 mg/kg of bilirubin produced per day, 75% to 80% derives from hemoglobin released during destruction of senescent red blood cells in the reticuloendothelial system. The remainder originates from nonhemoglobin heme proteins in the liver and from accelerated destruction in the marrow, spleen, and liver of immature or defectively formed red cells (ineffective erythropoiesis).

Regardless of the source, the normal pathways of heme catabolism involve its degradation by microsomal heme oxygenase to form carbon monoxide and biliverdin. Biliverdin is in turn converted to bilirubin by an enzyme in the cytosol, biliverdin reductase (Fig. 55-3). The heme oxygenase step is rate limiting. Both enzymes use NADPH as cofactor and are abundant in the hepatocytes, renal tubular epithelium, and reticuloendothelial cells.

Delivery of bilirubin

Unconjugated bilirubin passes into the plasma, where it is almost completely bound to two sites on plasma albumin, with dissociation constants of 2×10^{-8} and 2×10^{-7}M, respectively. Albumin, 4 g/dl, has the capacity to bind up to 85 mg of bilirubin per deciliter; consequently, a large fraction of unbound, unconjugated bilirubin rarely occurs clinically except in the neonate, in whom the capacity and affinity of albumin to bind bilirubin are less than in the adult. Conjugated bilirubin is also bound mainly to albumin, though with less affinity than unconjugated bilirubin. The 0.6% of circulating conjugated bilirubin that is not bound can filter at the glomerulus, leading to bilirubinuria in patients with diseases that cause retention of conjugated bilirubin. Normally, most of the bilirubin formed comes from the spleen to the liver via the portal venous blood.

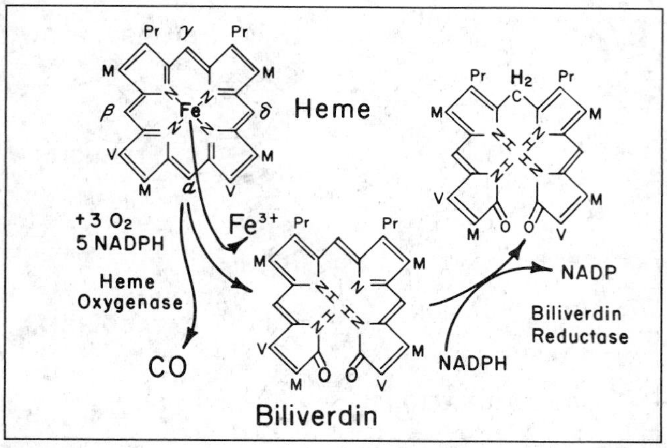

Fig. 55-3. The formation of bilirubin from heme by the sequential action of the enzymes heme oxygenase and biliverdin reductase. *M*, methyl; *V*, vinyl; *Pr*, propionic acid side chains. (Modified from Ostrow JD et al: Unit I, Hepatic excretory function. Undergraduate teaching project, American Gastroenterological Association, Baltimore, 1975, Milner-Fenwick, Slide 60.)

Hepatic clearance (uptake and storage)

In the liver, the bilirubin-albumin complex freely crosses the porous sinusoidal endothelium to reach the liver cell surface in the space of Disse, where bilirubin is detached from albumin and transported rapidly into the liver cell. Cellular uptake of bilirubin occurs by a Na^+-independent, facilitated diffusion process, mediated by at least three transporter proteins in the sinusoidal membrane of the hepatocyte. In the cytosol, unconjugated bilirubin is stored temporarily by binding to two groups of organic-anion binding proteins, which limits the passive reflux of bilirubin back into the plasma. Ligandin, the major bilirubin-binding protein, is the same as glutathione-S-transferase B.

In the steady state, the subsequent conjugation and active biliary secretion of bilirubin serve to maintain the gradient of unconjugated bilirubin from the blood to the liver cell. The net clearance of bilirubin from plasma, which is determined by the difference between the rates of uptake and reflux, is normally 0.68 ± 0.14 ml/kg per minute, or 5.4 ± 1.4% of the bilirubin load. A variety of other organic anions, but not conjugated bile salts, share affinities for both the uptake carriers and ligandin. These compounds include sodium sulfobromophthalein (BSP)*, indocyanine green (ICG), iopanoic acid, and the iminodiacetic acid derivatives used for hepatobiliary scintiscanning.

Conjugation of bilirubin

In the microsomes, unconjugated bilirubin is converted to water-soluble conjugates by covalent coupling with glucuronic acid, glucose, or xylose, and possibly sulfate (Fig. 55-4). Each sugar is first activated by enzymatic formation of a high energy bond with uridine diphosphate and then transferred to bilirubin by two specific bilirubin-UDP glucuronosyl transferases. Either one (monoconjugates) or both (diconjugates) of the carboxyethyl side chains of bilirubin may be thus coupled. The diglucuronide normally accounts for over 85% of the bilirubin conjugates in human bile, but the proportions of monoglucuronide and nonglucuronide conjugates increase in various hepatobiliary diseases.

Secretion of conjugated bilirubin into the bile

The transfer of bilirubin from blood to bile involves an active, energy-dependent, Na^+-independent process, mediated by a 100-kDa transporter in the canalicular membrane of the hepatocyte. This process is shared by many other organic anions but not by conjugated bile salts, which are excreted by an independent carrier system. The canalicular se-

*Although BSP is no longer available commercially, it is often mentioned throughout this chapter as many of the published physiologic studies were performed using this compound instead of bilirubin, which is more unstable and difficult to assay.

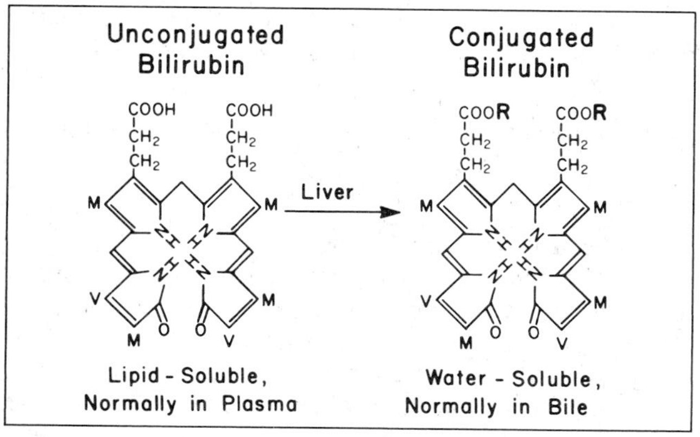

Fig. 55-4. Structures of unconjugated and conjugated bilirubins. *M*, methyl; *V*, vinyl; *R*, glycosides. Glucuronic acid, glucose, or xylose may be conjugated to acyl groups of one or both propionic acid side chains, yielding mono- and diconjugates, respectively. (Modified from Ostrow JD et al: Unit I, Hepatic excretory function. Undergraduate teaching project, American Gastroenterological Association, Baltimore, 1975, Milner-Fenwick, Slide 61.)

cretion of organic anions is driven in large part by the electrical gradient produced by the −35 mV negative intracellular potential generated by the Na^+/K^+-ATPase in the basolateral membrane of the hepatocyte. The energy-dependence of the secretory processes renders them susceptible to impairment during hypoxia, shock, and severe circulatory stasis. The less than 1% of the total bilirubin in normal bile that is unconjugated derives mainly from hydrolysis of excreted conjugates but may be the key to the formation of pigment (calcium-bilirubin) gallstones.

Flow of bilirubin down the biliary tree

Bilirubin conjugates, in large part bound to biliary mixed micelles, pass with the bile successively from the canaliculi through the bile ductules, the interacinar (portal) bile ducts, intrahepatic ducts of progressively increasing caliber, and the extrahepatic bile ducts. Between meals, the bile and bilirubin are stored mainly in the gallbladder, where conjugated bilirubin undergoes limited hydrolysis to unconjugated bilirubin, some of which may be absorbed. With feeding, the stored bile is emptied into the duodenum.

Intestinal catabolism, recirculation, and elimination of bile pigments

Conjugated bilirubin passes through the small intestine, with little reabsorption therefrom (see Fig. 55-2). Some hydrolysis to unconjugated bilirubin occurs owing to beta-glucuronidase in the intestinal epithelium; most of the intestinal catabolism of bile pigments, however, is mediated by ileocolonic flora except in the germ-free intestine of neonates or patients receiving broad-spectrum antibiotics. Three processes have been identified: (1) almost complete hydrolysis of conjugated to unconjugated bilirubin by bacterial beta-glucuronidase; (2) hydrogenation by intestinal anaerobes to form urobilinogens, a group of colorless tetrapyrroles that give positive results to Ehrlich's aldehyde test; and (3) oxidation to unidentified diazo-negative derivatives.

Probably over 90% of these products and some unchanged bilirubin are eliminated in the feces, there being limited passive intestinal reabsorption of unconjugated bilirubin and urobilinogens into the portal venous blood. After absorption, most of the pigments are cleared and reexcreted by the liver, the urobilinogens being transported without conjugation. Of the urobilinogen that escapes hepatic uptake, about one third filters across the glomerulus.

In the stool, some dehydrogenation of the central methylene bridge of the urobilinogens occurs, each yielding a corresponding urobilin. Urobilins are orange in color, yellow-green fluorescent, and diazo-negative. Together, the urobilinogens and urobilins in the feces account for about 30% to 80% of the bilirubin produced each day.

INITIAL CLASSIFICATION OF JAUNDICE

Conjugated versus unconjugated hyperbilirubinemia

Jaundice may be classified into two broad groups according to the predominant form of bilirubin, conjugated or unconjugated, that is retained in the plasma or tissues (Table 55-2). Unconjugated hyperbilirubinemia is caused by abnormalities in all steps up to and including the conjugation of bilirubin (steps 1 to 5). By contrast, impairment of secretion (step 6) or biliary flow (step 7) results in retention principally of conjugated bilirubin. In rare circumstances,

Table 55-2. Conjugated versus unconjugated hyperbilirubinemia

Finding	Unconjugated hyperbilirubinemia	Conjugated hyperbilirubinemia
Retained bilirubin	UCB	CB and UCB
Bilirubin in urine	No	Yes
Diazo reaction (direct/total)	<15%	>30% (usually >50%)
Abnormal steps	1-5 (Fig. 55-5)	6 or 7 (Fig. 55-6)
Usual causes	Hematologic, circulatory, or functional hepatic disorders	Hepatocellular or biliary tract disease
Compensatory mechanism	Catabolism of UCB to polar derivatives	Renal excretion of CB

CB, conjugated bilirubin; UCB, unconjugated bilirubin.

abnormalities of intestinal transit, catabolism, and recirculation of bilirubin may be implicated (steps 8 to 10).

Testing for bilirubinuria

The initial diagnostic test is a determination of whether the jaundice is of the conjugated or unconjugated type by checking the urine for bilirubin. Because there is normally no bilirubinuria, and only conjugated bilirubin is excreted into the urine, detection of bilirubinuria clearly indicates that conjugated hyperbilirubinemia is present. Due to some oxidation of bilirubin, the urine in such cases may vary from dark orange to reddish brown in color. Because the renal threshold for conjugated bilirubin is less than 1.0 mg/dl, bilirubinuria may occur without clinically visible jaundice. Moreover, discolored urine is often noticed by patients who do not notice that their skin and eyes are yellowed. Because other pigments may similarly discolor the urine, however, the presence of bilirubinuria must be confirmed chemically (Chapter 53).

Fractional diazo reaction of serum

The simple test for bilirubinuria usually is all that is needed to determine whether jaundice is of the conjugated or unconjugated type. This distinction, however, can be confirmed using the fractional diazo (van den Bergh's) reaction of serum bilirubin with a diazotized aromatic amine (Chapter 53).

Normally, the total bilirubin concentration should not exceed 1.0 mg/dl (17 μM), with less than 0.2 mg/dl (3.5 μM) reacting directly. In pure unconjugated hyperbilirubinemia, no more than 15% of the total serum bilirubin may give a direct diazo reaction. In both these circumstances, the direct reaction is not caused by conjugated bilirubin but by natural accelerators of the diazo coupling of unconjugated bilirubin or by other diazo-reactive substances.

In conjugated hyperbilirubinemia, more than 30%, and usually more than 50%, of the total serum bilirubin is direct reacting; there is also a significant indirect-reacting fraction, due mainly to unconjugated bilirubin formed by hydrolysis of the retained conjugates by tissue beta-glucuronidases. The direct-reacting fraction consists not only of diconjugates and monoconjugates but also of delta-bilirubin (BilAlb), a covalent conjugate of bilirubin to albumin. This amide conjugate, revealed by high-performance liquid chromatography (HPLC), forms whenever conjugated bilirubin is retained, through transesterification of the acylbilirubin from glucuronic acid to —NH groups on albumin.

A rapid, simple, sensitive multilayer film method has been developed for assay of unconjugated, conjugated, and delta bilirubins. At bilirubin concentrations below 3 mg/dl, the inaccuracies of the direct diazo reaction render it essential to use this film method or HPLC to measure bilirubin glucuronides and delta bilirubin, as their increase in serum is diagnostic of hepatobiliary dysfunction, even when total serum bilirubin level is normal. At total bilirubin concentrations above 3 mg/dl, measurement of the direct and indirect diazo fractions suffices for the clinical distinction of conjugated from unconjugated hyperbilirubinemia.

PATHOPHYSIOLOGY AND CLASSIFICATION OF UNCONJUGATED HYPERBILIRUBINEMIA

Unconjugated hyperbilirubinemia (Fig. 55-5) is characterized by retention exclusively of unconjugated bilirubin in the serum, without bilirubinuria, due to deficient hepatic clearance and/or conjugation of some of the bilirubin produced each day. In these conditions, retained bilirubin is in part oxidized by microsomal cytochromes P450-IA1 and -IA2, to polar derivatives that can be excreted in the bile without conjugation.

Unconjugated hyperbilirubinemia may be subclassified according to the step or steps in bilirubin metabolism that are deranged (Table 55-1). The most common etiologies are (1) overproduction of unconjugated bilirubin due to disorders of red blood cells; (2) impaired delivery of unconjugated bilirubin due to circulatory disturbances involving the liver; and (3) functional or hereditary defects in uptake, storage, or conjugation of bilirubin. Though the hematologic, circulatory, or functional disorders may be serious, the primary hepatic disorders that cause unconjugated hyperbilirubinemia are not life threatening except in patients with endogenous portosystemic shunting due to cirrhosis. Therefore liver biopsy and other invasive diagnostic studies are seldom indicated in these patients.

Overproduction jaundice

Excessive formation of bilirubin due to accelerated heme catabolism is a very common cause of unconjugated hyper-

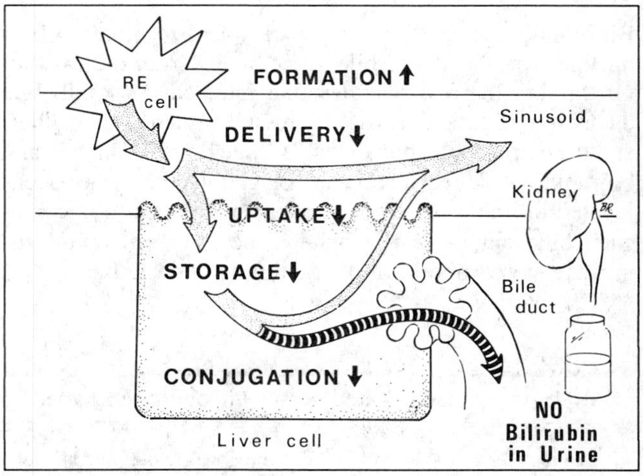

Fig. 55-5. Abnormal bilirubin transport in unconjugated hyperbilirubinemia: steps that may be deranged. Symbols as in Fig. 55-1. There is no bilirubinuria. Regurgitation of bilirubin conjugates may occur via tight junctions of bile canaliculi and/or ductules (not shown) as well as through the hepatocyte. (Modified from Ostrow JD et al: Unit I, Hepatic excretory function. Undergraduate teaching project, American Gastroenterological Association, Baltimore, 1975, Milner-Fenwick, Slide 27.)

bilirubinemia and often complicates and augments jaundice caused by other defects. Because the hepatic component of bilirubin formation constitutes a small fraction of normal heme turnover and can increase no more than fivefold, it is rarely itself a cause of clinical jaundice. Consequently, overproduction jaundice is usually due to an erythroid disorder, and the exact diagnosis rests mainly on hematologic studies.

Decreased delivery of bilirubin

Decreased delivery of bilirubin to the liver cells due to impairment of the hepatic circulation is the most common form of unconjugated jaundice. The delivery of other organic anion cholephiles is impaired also. This form of jaundice is most often due to right-sided congestive heart failure and clears as the heart failure is controlled. Another major cause is portosystemic shunting, due to either cirrhosis or surgical anastomosis, which diverts the bilirubin formed in the spleen directly into the systemic circulation.

Diminished hepatic clearance (uptake and storage)

Diminished hepatic uptake and/or storage of bilirubin may be acquired or hereditary. Acquired defects are often due to drugs, such as rifamycin, that competitively inhibit uptake and/or storage of bilirubin by binding to the same transporter and/or cytoplasmic storage proteins, respectively. The jaundice usually resolves within 3 days after the offending drug is discontinued. Hypothyroidism may impair hepatic uptake of bilirubin, although it also increases ligandin levels. Febrile illnesses may cause retention of unconjugated bilirubin, primarily because of decreased hepatic storage capacity and increased reflux of organic anions back into plasma.

Gilbert's syndrome is a group of hereditary disorders characterized by a chronic, often subclinical, fluctuating unconjugated hyperbilirubinemia that is due to dual impairment of the clearance and conjugation of bilirubin. Clearance is further (reversibly) impaired during fasting and stress, augmenting the severity of the jaundice. Up to half the subjects have associated hemolysis, with unconjugated bilirubin concentrations in the plasma in excess of the values predicted from the rates of bilirubin formation as estimated from the red blood cell life span.

Rotor's syndrome is characterized by severe impairment of the storage of bilirubin and other organic anions, associated with a moderate decrease in canalicular secretion of conjugated bilirubin, but the mild, chronic hyperbilirubinemia is predominantly of the conjugated type.

Impaired conjugation of bilirubin

Bilirubin-UDP glucuronosyl transferase activity in liver biopsy specimens is normal or increased in most hepatobiliary diseases. Exceptions are some patients with chronic persistent hepatitis, severe end-stage cirrhosis, acute hepatic failure, or Wilson's disease. Thus aside from impaired conjugation seen in neonates and patients with hyperthyroidism or caused by novobiocin or progestational steroids, most cases of impaired bilirubin conjugation are hereditary.

Gilbert's syndrome is the most common hereditary defect of bilirubin conjugation. The 50% to 90% decrease in the activity of bilirubin-UDP glucuronosyl transferase in liver biopsies is associated with impaired clearance of bilirubin and other organic anions (see later).

In addition, there are two rare forms of hereditary deficiency of bilirubin conjugation. In the homozygous recessive, Crigler-Najjar syndrome, type I, there is no detectable bilirubin-UDP glucuronosyl-transferase activity in the liver, and glucuronide conjugation of many phenolic substrates is also impaired. Jaundice is severe from the neonatal period, and kernicterus (bilirubin encephalopathy) is the rule. In the autosomal dominant, Crigler-Najjar type II (Arias' syndrome), some transferase activity is detectable but at less than 10% of normal levels. Jaundice begins usually in late childhood, is less severe, and seldom causes kernicterus (see later).

CHRONIC UNCONJUGATED HYPERBILIRUBINEMIAS

General considerations

Most cases of chronic unconjugated hyperbilirubinemia are related to partial deficiency of bilirubin-UDPGA transferase caused by Gilbert's syndrome (68%), erythroid disorders causing overproduction jaundice (12%), and portosystemic shunting due to cirrhosis (12%). The remaining 8% are related to surgical portacaval shunts, thyroid disorders, and Crigler-Najjar syndromes.

Overproduction jaundice

Etiology. Accelerated catabolism of heme to bilirubin, usually related to erythroid disorders, may be subclassified according to whether the increased heme turnover is related to the late or early peak of bilirubin formation. In hemolytic jaundice, there is an increased late bilirubin peak due to accelerated destruction of circulating erythrocytes, for example, in sickle cell disease, hereditary spherocytosis, polycythemia vera, and acquired hemolytic anemias (e.g., with sepsis, autoimmune mechanisms, hypersplenism, or intracardiac valve prostheses). The hemolysis is compensated by increased erythropoiesis, with an increase in early peak bilirubin formation also. Increased bilirubin production due to an enhanced early peak is almost always due to ineffective erythropoiesis, e.g., in megaloblastic anemias, thalassemia, lead poisoning, and congenital erythropoietic porphyria. Although a mild hemolytic component may also be present, the major source of added bilirubin is premature destruction of defective red cells in the marrow, liver, or spleen. In the rare familial "shunt hyperbilirubinemia," rapid turnover of hepatic hemes is the primary defect, but dyserythropoiesis contributes also, as serum bilirubin levels diminish after splenectomy. Porphyria cutanea tarda and erythropoietic protoporphyria are also associated with an increase in turnover of hepatic hemes and early-labeled bilirubin.

Pathophysiology and clinical features. A fixed fraction (5.4 ± 1.4%) of the bilirubin delivered is extracted by the normal liver regardless of the load. In the steady state, the rates of production and removal of unconjugated bilirubin are equal and proportional to its concentration in the plasma. Thus increased production and delivery of unconjugated bilirubin to the liver must result in an elevation of its concentration in the plasma. Because with a normal liver each threefold increase in bilirubin production results in a rise in serum bilirubin concentration of approximately 1.0 mg/dl, uncomplicated chronic hemolysis seldom elevates serum bilirubin concentrations above the level of 3.0 to 4.0 mg/dl that is usually necessary for clinically visible jaundice.

All forms of overproduction jaundice are accompanied by erythroid hyperplasia of the bone marrow and enhanced marrow uptake of ^{59}Fe from the circulation. The increased load of heme induces heme oxygenase in the liver and kidneys, resulting in augmented formation of bilirubin that is accommodated by enhanced uptake, conjugation, and excretion of bilirubin by the liver. The larger load of conjugated bilirubin presented to the intestinal bacteria results in greater output of urobilinogens in the feces. The increased bilirubin concentration in bile predisposes to pigment stone formation. Occasionally, significant retention of conjugated bilirubin may occur also if hemolysis is massive or if bilirubin secretion is diminished due to concomitant hepatobiliary disease.

In hemolytic jaundice, there is shortened survival of ^{51}Cr-labeled red cells and an increase in reticulocytes and incorporation of ^{59}Fe into circulating erythrocytes. In ineffective erythropoiesis, by contrast, red cell survival is at most mildly compromised, the reticulocyte count is low or normal, and incorporation of ^{59}Fe into circulating red cells is diminished.

Diagnosis and treatment. Usually, the presence of overproduction jaundice is revealed by findings of splenomegaly, anemia, or an abnormal peripheral blood smear. In some cases with compensated hemolysis, these tests are normal, and hemolysis is suggested by reticulocytosis or a disproportionate elevation of lactic dehydrogenase compared with transaminases in the serum. More specific diagnosis then rests on other hematologic studies, discussed fully in Chapter 73. A serum unconjugated bilirubin concentration in excess of that predicted for the rate of bilirubin production (assessed from ^{51}Cr-red cell survival) is evidence of an associated defect in unconjugated bilirubin transport or conjugation. Treatment is the therapy indicated for the underlying hematologic disorder.

Defects in bilirubin conjugation (Table 55-3)

Investigators have long been puzzled by the variable patterns and severity of defective conjugation of xenobiotics and bilirubin observed among subjects with bilirubin-UDP glucuronosyl transferase deficiency. These old observations have been explained by recent molecular biologic studies, which reveal that there are two bilirubin-UDP-glucuronosyl transferases, each encoded by a supergene that encodes also the transferases that form glucuronides of phenolic substrates. The downstream half of this gene contains four exons that are expressed in the mRNAs for all members of the family and includes the exon for the UDPGA-binding site. Mutations or deletions in this constant region of the gene will thus impair conjugation of phenols as well as bilirubin. The upstream half of the gene contains exons that code for the unique binding sites for each subgroup of substrates; mRNA encoded by one of these exons is alternatively spliced onto mRNA from the constant region during gene transcription, yielding an individual mRNA for the transferase for each class of subsubstrates. A mutation in one of these variable exons impairs the activity only of the transferase for the relevant substrates. A different supergene encodes the family of UDP-glucuronosyl transferases for steroids and bile acids, explaining why those substrates are conjugated normally by subjects with deficiency of bilirubin-UDP-glucuronosyl transferases.

Because conjugation of bilirubin is essential to its excretion in bile, deficient conjugation must be compensated by alternate routes for catabolism of unconjugated bilirubin. Studies in Crigler-Najjar I patients and the comparable animal model, the Gunn rat, reveal two major pathways: (1) oxidation of bilirubin by microsomal cytochromes P450 IA1 and IA2, to form polar (probably hydroxyl) derivatives that can be excreted in bile without conjugation and (2) dif-

Table 55-3. Disorders of bilirubin conjugation

Findings	Crigler-Najjar syndrome type I	Arias' syndrome type II	Gilbert's syndrome
Bilirubin-UDP glucuronosyl transferase	Undetectable	<10% of normal	10-50% of normal
Organic anion (ICG) kinetics	Normal	Normal	Usually abnormal
Serum bilirubin levels (mg/dl)			
Range (mean)	18-50 (27)	6-22 (13)	1-7 (3)
Bilirubins in bile	Trace UCB only	Mono-CB only	Mono-CB 30-76%
Inheritance (autosomal)	Recessive	May be dominant	May be dominant
Usual age of onset	1-3 days	1 day-10 years	10-30 years
Presence of kernicterus	Almost always	Occasionally	Never
Response to phenobarbital	None	Positive	Positive

Note: ICG, indocyanine green; UCB, unconjugated bilirubin; mono-CB, monoconjugates of bilirubin.

fusion of bilirubin directly across the intestinal wall with conversion to urobilinogens by intestinal bacteria. The relative importance of these two pathways and their function in patients with less severe defects in bilirubin conjugation are not known.

Gilbert's syndrome

Etiology. This syndrome of benign, mild, chronic unconjugated hyperbilirubinemia (1 to 7 mg/dl) is related to a 50% to 90% decrease in the activity of hepatic bilirubin-UDP glucuronosyl transferase combined with impaired clearance and/or overproduction of bilirubin (Table 55-3).

Prevalence. In asymptomatic populations, 3% to 7% of men and 0.6% to 2.0% of women have total serum bilirubin concentrations above 1.2 mg/dl without an increase in conjugated bilirubin. Most such subjects have Gilbert's syndrome. Among first-order relatives of probands, 27% to 55% of siblings and 16% to 28% of parents also exhibit mild unconjugated hyperbilirubinemia.

Pathophysiology. A 50% to 90% decrease in bilirubin conjugation is seldom sufficient by itself to produce hyperbilirubinemia and cannot in any case account for the decreased clearance of bilirubin seen in patients with Gilbert's syndrome. Thus an associated familial disorder of bilirubin production and/or clearance must be present for phenotypic expression of jaundice. As noted earlier, hemolysis with overproduction of bilirubin is present in the majority of cases. In addition, the relative contribution to total bilirubin uptake differs among the three basolateral membrane organic anion transporters, one or more of which may be defective in a given patient. These factors explain the variable penetrance of the apparently autosomal dominant gene for the conjugation defect.

Gilbert's syndrome has long been divided into four subtypes, according to which organic anions, bilirubin, BSP, ICG, and ursodeoxycholate, were defectively cleared by the individual patient. Recent work using lower doses of BSP, however, found that all of the patients with Gilbert's syndrome had delayed clearance of this dye. Recent knowledge concerning the bilirubin transporters suggest that, with appropriate kinetic studies over a full range of doses, all patients with defective bilirubin clearance will exhibit defective clearance of all the organic anions that share the same transporter(s). Immunologic/molecular biologic methods will likely be developed soon to permit rational subclassification of Gilbert's patients according to which of the three recently isolated transporters is defective, which will in turn account for the severity of the impairment in the individual patient.

Pathology. Except for decreased rough endoplasmic reticulum, hypertrophy of the smooth endoplasmic reticulum, and mild parenchymal iron deposition in patients with associated erythroid disorders, the liver in patients with Gilbert's syndrome is normal structurally.

Clinical features. Serum bilirubin concentrations are usually below the clinically detectable level of 3 to 4 mg/dl, and many subjects intermittently have normal values. Episodic increases in serum unconjugated bilirubin concentration occur with fasting, exertional or thermal stress, heavy alcohol intake, infections, or hemolysis, often unmasking previously subclinical jaundice. Hyperthyroidism, which impairs hepatic conjugation of bilirubin, also can aggravate jaundice from underlying Gilbert's syndrome.

The initial diagnosis is usually made in the second or third decade of life from test results obtained during investigation of unrelated conditions. Hepatic size is usually normal, but splenomegaly may be present in patients with associated erythroid disorders. Liver function test results are almost always normal except for hyperbilirubinemia. Characteristically, normal serum bile acid concentrations are helpful diagnostically. As evidence of associated erythroid disorders, ^{51}Cr-red cell survival is decreased in 50% to 60% of patients, and over 80% show impaired incorporation of ^{59}Fe into circulating erythrocytes. Diagnosis and treatment are discussed on p. 564 with other unconjugated hyperbilirubinemias.

Arias' syndrome (Crigler-Najjar syndrome II)

This rare syndrome (see Table 55-3) of moderate, chronic unconjugated hyperbilirubinemia, results from a decrease in the activity of bilirubin-UDP glucuronosyl transferase to less than 10 percent of normal. Conjugation of other aglycones, including menthol and o- and p-aminophenol, is deficient also. Hepatic transport of other organic anions is unaffected. In most families, it may be inherited as an autosomal dominant defect with variable penetrance, whereas in other families it may represent a double dose of the Gilbert's syndrome allele, as other relatives exhibit Gilbert's syndrome. Jaundice may appear initially in late childhood as often as in the neonatal period. Because serum bilirubin levels usually are 10 to 19 mg/dl (the range can be 6 to 22 mg/dl), kernicterus seldom develops. Bilirubin in the bile is virtually all monoglucuronide. Diagnosis and treatment are discussed on p. 564.

Crigler-Najjar syndrome I

This rare syndrome (Table 55-3), marked by severe unconjugated hyperbilirubinemia, is inherited as a homozygous recessive trait. No hepatic bilirubin-UDP glucuronosyl transferase activity is detectable, and the bile contains only traces of unconjugated bilirubin and nonglucuronide monoconjugates of bilirubin. There is usually associated severe but incomplete deficiency of the glucuronosyl transferases that conjugate salicylates, menthol, nitrophenols and aminophenols, but conjugation of steroid hormones and bile salts is usually normal. Heterozygous parents and siblings have normal serum bilirubin concentrations but exhibit a 50% decrease in their capacity to conjugate and excrete loads of unconjugated bilirubin and a variable impairment in glucuronide conjugation of other aglycones.

Hepatic histology and ultrastructure are normal. Jaundice in patients with Crigler-Najjar syndrome I is almost always manifested initially 1 to 3 days after birth, and serum unconjugated bilirubin concentrations plateau in excess of 20 mg/dl. Bilirubin encephalopathy (kernicterus) is almost inevitable, causing severe mental retardation, dysarthria, ataxia, spasticity, and usually death in infancy or early childhood. Diagnosis and treatment are discussed below.

Diagnosis of hereditary unconjugated hyperbilirubinemia

Routine examinations. Once the presence of unconjugated hyperbilirubinemia is established, causes of reversible, acquired unconjugated hyperbilirubinemia, such as fever and right-sided heart failure, should be sought by history, physical examination, and routine laboratory tests. If acquired conditions are not evident or if the jaundice does not resolve with appropriate therapy, one of the familial, functional disorders should be suspected. These syndromes can usually be distinguished by the patient's age at the onset of jaundice, the degree of elevation and variability of the serum bilirubin concentration, the presence or absence of kernicterus, and the presence of jaundice in parents or siblings (see Table 55-3). Patients may not be aware of jaundice in their relatives, so it is essential to assess serum bilirubin levels in other family members.

Serum bile acid levels. Serum bile acid levels are normal in all functional unconjugated hyperbilirubinemias, a fact that provides the best noninvasive method of excluding organic hepatobiliary diseases or portosystemic shunts.

Examination of the bile. Determination of the proportion of unconjugated bilirubin, monoglucuronide, and diglucuronide in duodenal bile, by either high-pressure liquid chromatography or analysis of azopigments, is of further assistance in making the differential diagnosis. Patients with Gilbert's syndrome usually have at least 30% monoglucuronide in the bile, compared with less than 15% in most normal subjects. Patients with Arias' syndrome have almost exclusively monoglucuronides in the bile. Patients with Crigler-Najjar type I syndrome show no glucuronide conjugates in the bile.

Effect on fasting on serum bilirubin. In all the syndromes associated with decreased hepatic bilirubin-UDP glucuronosyl transferase activity, more than 90% of males but only 40% to 50% of females whose caloric intake is limited to less than 400 kcal daily for 24 to 48 hours will have an increase in plasma unconjugated bilirubin concentration to at least twice baseline values (the mean increase is 135%). By contrast, normal subjects and patients with unrelated hemolysis or liver diseases usually have less than a 50% increase in serum bilirubin levels during fasting. The hyperbilirubinemia reverses within 6 hours of refeeding. The mechanisms are believed to involve (1) mobilization during lipolysis of unconjugated bilirubin stored in depot fats; (2) impaired hepatocellular uptake of bilirubin; (3) decreased ligandin concentrations; (4) inhibition of uridine diphosphoglucose dehydrogenase, thus decreasing the supply of UDPGA for bilirubin conjugation; and (5) absorption of unconjugated bilirubin from the stagnant intestine. The phenomenon is important in understanding the fluctuating jaundice in these patients but is too unreliable to be useful diagnostically.

Response to phenobarbital. Differentiation of complete from partial conjugation defects can be confirmed by administration of phenobarbital in doses of 2 to 5 mg/kg/day. Phenobarbital induces all the normal steps in hepatic bilirubin transport. Patients with Arias' or Gilbert's syndrome respond with a decline in serum bilirubin concentrations over 1 to 2 weeks to 30% to 50% of pretherapy values. By contrast, patients with Crigler-Najjar syndrome type I do not respond.

Percutaneous liver biopsy. Percutaneous liver biopsy is seldom necessary in the assessment of unconjugated hyperbilirubinemia except when fatty liver, malignancy, or cirrhosis is suspected or when unequivocal biochemical confirmation of decreased bilirubin-UDP glucoronosyl transferase activity is desired. Normal values average 1000 μg of bilirubin conjugated per gram of liver per hour, with a range of 500 to 1500 μg. Patients with Gilbert's syndrome have values ranging from 100 to 500 μg, and those with type II conjugation defects (Arias' syndrome) usually have values below 100 μg. In Crigler-Najjar Type I patients, there is no detectable bilirubin conjugation.

Treatment of unconjugated hyperbilirubinemia

Amelioration of jaundice depends mainly on treatment of the underlying hematologic, circulatory, metabolic, or hepatic disorder. Jaundice itself is not harmful except in the neonate and in Crigler-Najjar patients, in whom severe unconjugated hyperbilirubinemia may produce kernicterus. The cosmetic embarrassment of chronic jaundice may be alleviated with high-dosage, long-term phenobarbital therapy. Such treatment is ineffective if any of the steps in bilirubin metabolism and transport are completely defective, as occurs in Crigler-Najjar syndrome type I. In such patients, induction of alternate pathways with the nontoxic indole-3-carbinol found in cruciferous vegetables is a promising new therapy. Phototherapy with blue light is usually effective in young children and is the preferred treatment for neonatal jaundice. It acts by converting unconjugated bilirubin to geometric photoisomers that can be excreted in bile and urine without conjugation. Physical removal of bilirubin by exchange transfusion is still used to treat premature infants with severe jaundice who respond insufficiently to phototherapy. Extracorporeal removal of bilirubin by perfusion of plasma through albumin-agarose and reverse-phase columns or columns of immobilized bilirubin oxidase is under experimental evaluation. Another experimental approach is to administer tin protoporphyrin IX, a potent competitive inhibitor of heme oxygenase, which blocks bilirubin synthesis.

PATHOPHYSIOLOGY AND CLASSIFICATION OF CONJUGATED HYPERBILIRUBINEMIA

Conjugated hyperbilirubinemia (Fig. 55-6) is characterized by retention principally of conjugated bilirubin in the serum. There is also significant elevation of unconjugated bilirubin concentration, due in part to hydrolysis of retained conjugated bilirubin by tissue beta-glucuronidases and in part to associated hemolysis and/or impairment of delivery, uptake, and storage of unconjugated bilirubin with liver cell damage.

All forms of conjugated hyperbilirubinemia involve a partial or complete deficiency in the canalicular secretion or biliary flow of conjugated bilirubin. The retained conjugated bilirubin, and other components of bile, regurgitate into the plasma via the lymph in the space of Disse, traversing either the hepatocytes, where conjugated bilirubin is less tightly bound to ligandin than unconjugated bilirubin, or abnormally permeable canalicular and/or ductular tight junctions. The small fraction of retained conjugated bilirubin that is not bound to plasma albumin filters at the glomerulus, producing the bilirubinuria that is diagnostic of conjugated hyperbilirubinemia. This renal excretory route also constitutes the major alternate pathway for removal of conjugated bilirubin and other organic anions in the face of reduced hepatobiliary excretion.

With remission of hepatitis or relief of biliary obstruction, the urinary excretion of conjugated bilirubin terminates well before the serum level of "direct" bilirubin returns to normal. This occurs because delta-bilirubin is not excreted by the liver or kidneys and has the 14-day half-life of the albumin moiety, so it persists in the plasma after the glucuronide conjugates have been cleared.

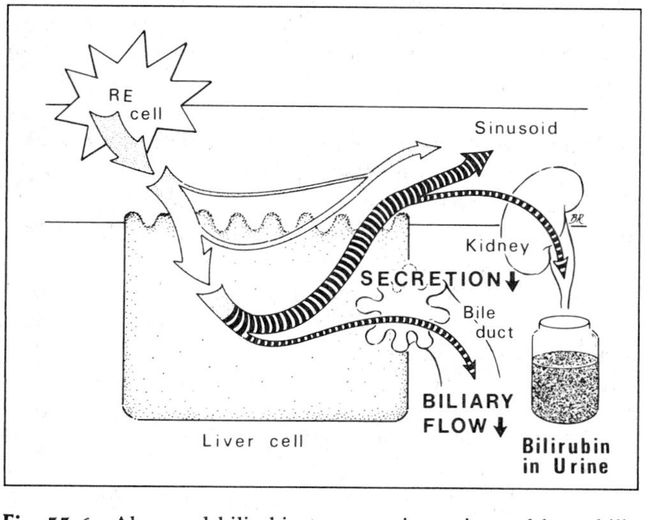

Fig. 55-6. Abnormal bilirubin transport in conjugated hyperbilirubinemia; steps that may be deranged. Symbols as in Fig. 55-1. Bilirubinuria is present. Regurgitation of bilirubin conjugates may occur via tight junctions of bile canaliculi and/or ductules (not shown) as well as through the hepatocyte. (Modified from Ostrow JD et al: Unit I, Hepatic excretory function. Undergraduate teaching project, American Gastroenterological Association, Baltimore, 1975, Milner-Fenwick, Slide 28.)

In contrast to unconjugated hyperbilirubinemia, jaundice with bilirubinuria almost always results from significant hepatobiliary disease, which may be classified further according to whether canalicular secretion or biliary flow is impaired. Defects in canalicular secretion are characteristic of hepatocellular diseases, whereas defects in biliary flow produce the syndrome of cholestasis. Combined defects are often present and lead to problems in differential diagnosis.

Step 6 defects: diminished canalicular secretion of bilirubin

Impairment of the system that transports conjugated bilirubin into the bile, with relatively less impairment of the secretion of bile acids, is characteristic of hepatocellular diseases. The most common of these are hepatitis and cirrhosis, caused by alcohol, drugs, toxins, or hepatitis viruses. ICG, gallbladder dyes, and iminodiacetic acid derivatives, which use the same transport system as conjugated bilirubin, are also excreted poorly. Because hepatocellular diseases also frequently affect the delivery, uptake, and storage of organic anions, plasma concentrations of unconjugated bilirubin and bile acids are usually increased as well.

The purest form of impaired conjugated bilirubin excretion is probably the Dubin-Johnson syndrome, which is believed to result from an autosomal recessive defect in the bilirubin carrier at the canalicular membrane. In another uncommon hereditary disorder, Rotor syndrome, impairment of canalicular transport of organic anions is less severe, but there is evidence of increased reflux of the conjugates from liver to plasma, so that the exact locus of the defect remains an enigma.

Step 7 defects: cholestatic jaundice

If any portion of the biliary tree from the canaliculi to the sphincter of Oddi becomes blocked or abnormally permeable, flow of bile is retarded, and excretion of all components of bile is decreased. This condition, known as *cholestasis,* may be distinguished from step 6 defects by the consequences of marked retention of bile acids: decreased hepatic synthesis of cholesterol, inhibition of hepatic catabolism of cholesterol to bile acids, and hypercholesterolemia. The retained bile acids also induce increased hepatic synthesis of alkaline phosphatase in the face of decreased hepatic excretion of this enzyme, leading to marked elevation of alkaline phosphatase concentration in the serum. Decreases of Na^+/K^+-ATPase at the sinusoidal membrane of the hepatocyte occur in many forms of cholestasis and may sometimes play a primary role. Damage to mitochondria, microfilaments, or microtubules in the hepatocyte, however, can cause cholestasis with intracellular as well as canalicular deposits of bilirubin.

Cholestatic disorders may be classified primarily according to the anatomic site of the damage to the biliary passages and secondarily according to the causative lesion or etiologic agent. Histologically and ultrastructurally, cholestasis is usually characterized by dilatation, sacculation, and bile plugging of canaliculi, with swelling and flattening of canalicular microvilli. The degree of disruption of canalicular membranes, associated hepatocyte necrosis and inflammatory reaction, and dilatation of larger ducts vary according to etiology and may be minimal despite laboratory evidence of severe cholestasis.

Canalicular cholestasis. Canalicular cholestasis is the most common form of intrahepatic cholestasis and involves injury primarily to the canaliculi (and ductules) but not to larger biliary channels. There is impairment of the canalicular secretory apparatus for bile salts, bilirubin, and other organic anion cholephiles, and the canalicular tight junctions may become abnormally permeable, allowing bile constituents to regurgitate into the intercellular extensions of the space of Disse.

Canalicular cholestasis is most often caused by drugs or steroid hormones, especially estrogens, but may occur in acute viral or alcoholic hepatitis. Drug-induced cholestasis usually occurs unpredictably in a few patients, may have many of the characteristics of an immunogenic reaction, and is usually associated with some degree of inflammation and hepatocellular necrosis, causing an associated increase in serum transaminase concentrations (hepatocanalicular cholestasis). Drugs most often implicated include phenothiazines, diazepoxides, sulfonylureas, and antithyroid preparations such as methimazole (Chapter 58).

Normal pregnancy or the administration of estrogens, 19-norprogestogens (19-nortestosterone derivatives), or $alpha_{17}$-alkyl anabolic steroids impairs maximum hepatic secretory capacity for organic anion cholephiles in almost all subjects but unpredictably engenders a full-blown cholestatic syndrome in a small proportion of patients. Mild to severe canalicular cholestasis may occur postoperatively after long, difficult procedures with multiple blood transfusions. A similar syndrome sometimes occurs during lobar pneumonia, severe infections with endotoxemia and/or septicemia, and sickle cell anemia crises. A rare hereditary syndrome, benign recurrent intrahepatic cholestasis, is characterized by intermittent prolonged episodes of pruritus, jaundice, and morphologic evidence of cholestasis, but hepatic morphology and liver function test results are normal during remissions. These syndromes are discussed individually later in this chapter.

Cholestasis due to damage to the interlobular bile ducts. Lesions in the ducts in the portal triads occur in the sclerosing pericholangitis that accompanies inflammatory bowel disease, in primary biliary cirrhosis, in about 20% of patients with postnecrotic cirrhosis, and in congenital intrahepatic biliary atresia. In biliary atresia and sclerosing pericholangitis, the larger intrahepatic and extrahepatic bile ducts are also usually affected. Some cases of intrahepatic atresia may be caused by hereditary defects in bile acid synthesis that result in the accumulation of unusual bile acids that may cause the ductal lesions.

Pericholangitis, with associated canalicular cholestasis, occurs in almost 40% of patients who are on total parenteral nutrition for more than 4 to 6 weeks. Most of these patients have thick, dark bile and biliary sludge, and about one fourth develop calcium bilirubinate gallstones. The lesions are believed to be due to a combination of infrequent gallbladder emptying plus accumulation of the toxic bile salt lithocholate in the biliary tree and liver. Frequent administration of cholecystokinin and therapy with metronidazole have been suggested as preventive measures.

Lesions of interlobular and larger intrahepatic bile ducts. These ducts probably are the major site of blockage with multifocal lesions of the liver, which include granulomas, metastatic tumors, lymphomas, and primary hepatocellular carcinomas. These lesions often cause striking elevation of the serum alkaline phosphatase concentration, with little or no hyperbilirubinemia until late in the disease. Less common lesions involving the larger intrahepatic radicles include sclerosing cholangitis, intraductal papillomatosis, intraductal lithiasis, and the varied permutations and combinations of congenital biliary ectasias (Caroli's disease) and cystic disease (congenital hepatic fibrosis). This group of diseases characteristically presents as recurrent episodes of acute cholangitis, sometimes unaccompanied by jaundice.

Extrahepatic cholestasis. Extrahepatic cholestasis, is most often caused by single focal lesions, especially carcinomas of the bile ducts, gallbladder, pancreas, or ampulla of Vater. Other common etiologies include choledocholithiasis, acute cholecystitis, and common duct strictures due to inadvertent injury to the duct during surgery. Less frequent causes are fibrosis and/or edema of the head of the pancreas due to chronic and/or acute pancreatitis, congenital choledochal cysts, pancreatic pseudocysts, and benign polypoid epithelial tumors of the bile ducts. Extrahepatic obstructive lesions are usually remediable surgically or by endoscopic manipulation but lead to progressive liver damage and secondary biliary cirrhosis if untreated. By contrast, intrahepatic forms of cholestasis usually should be treated medically.

Abnormalities of the enterohepatic circulation of bile pigments (steps 8 to 10). These abnormalities may simulate cholestasis owing to increased recirculation of bile pigments and other components of bile. Cholascos (leakage of bile into the peritoneal cavity) results in jaundice owing to the absorption of conjugated and unconjugated bilirubin as well as alkaline phosphatase and bile salts across the peritoneal membrane. In acute cholangitis or cholecystitis, bacterial deconjugation of conjugated bilirubin and increased permeability of the inflamed epithelium lead to increased absorption of conjugated bilirubin and unconjugated bilirubin from the gallbladder.

DIFFERENTIAL DIAGNOSIS OF CONJUGATED HYPERBILIRUBINEMIA

Distinction of hepatocellular from cholestatic jaundice (see Table 55-4)

Once the presence of conjugated hyperbilirubinemia has been established, the next steps in differential diagnosis are

Table 55-4. Cholestatic versus hepatocellular jaundice

Laboratory test	Cholestatic jaundice	Hepatocellular jaundice
Serum bile acids	Very high	Modestly elevated
Steatorrhea (insufficient micelles)	Common	Uncommon
Serum alkaline phosphatase	>Three times normal	<Three times normal
Serum cholesterol	Increased	Decreased
Serum transaminases (SGOTs*, SGPT†)	Mildly elevated, seldom >300 IU	Elevated, may be >1000 IU
Prothrombin-time response to parenteral vitamin K	Yes	No

*Serum glutamic oxaloacetic transaminase (aspartate aminotransferase).
†Serum glutamic pyruvic transaminase (alanine aminotransferase).

(1) to determine whether jaundice is hepatocellular or cholestatic and (2) to determine the level of the block to biliary flow if cholestasis is present (see also Chapter 53).

Itching, especially on the palms and soles, occurs in 75% of patients with intrahepatic or extrahepatic cholestasis and is virtually diagnostic. The responsible retained metabolite has not been identified. In those who do not itch, the presence of cholestasis may be surmised from an elevation of the serum alkaline phosphatase level more than threefold above normal, increased serum cholesterol level, absence of marked elevations of serum transaminases, and response to vitamin K in patients with an abnormal prothrombin time. Steatorrhea may result from insufficient biliary excretion of bile acids into the intestine.

It may not be easy to distinguish cholestatic from hepatocellular jaundice for several reasons:

1. Some agents that characteristically cause hepatocellular disease (e.g., alcohol and hepatitis viruses) sometimes also attack the canaliculi; drugs that characteristically cause intrahepatic cholestasis (e.g., chlorpromazine) may also damage the hepatocytes.
2. Prolonged cholestasis, especially extrahepatic obstruction, secondarily damages the liver cells, possibly due to the toxic effects of retained bile acids.
3. All forms of cholestasis and hepatocellular disease, if prolonged, may lead to cirrhosis and portal hypertension.

The criteria in Table 55-4 are not infallible. For example, serum alkaline phosphatase values less than three times normal occur in patients with cholestasis due to infections or estrogens, and in 15% of all patients with extrahepatic biliary obstruction, more commonly if the obstruction is incomplete or due to benign lesions. Serum transaminase and lactic dehydrogenase activities are occasionally markedly elevated in patients with hepatic cancer, biliary obstruction or cholangitis.

Determination of the site of blockage in cholestasis

Routine liver function tests are of absolutely no assistance in locating the site of a cholestatic lesion because all forms of cholestasis produce similar clinical, histologic, and biochemical abnormalities. Nonetheless, a careful epidemiologic history and physical examination can reveal the appropriate diagnosis in 85% to 90% of patients with jaundice.

Clues from the history or physical examination that suggest a diagnosis of intrahepatic cholestasis include (1) age less than 40 years (viral and drug hepatitis are most common in this age group); (2) liver span of more than 15 cm on percussion, especially if the liver is tender (this sign most often indicates alcoholic liver disease or malignancy but may be seen also in patients with primary biliary cirrhosis and sclerosing cholangitis); (3) drug addiction or homosexuality (high risk of transmission of hepatitis); and (4) history of alcoholism or recent treatment with drugs or hormones known to cause jaundice, especially estrogens. Moreover, a decreased serum cholesterol concentration in the presence of an otherwise typical cholestatic syndrome should strongly suggest viral or alcoholic hepatitis as the etiology.

Findings that favor a diagnosis of extrahepatic obstruction include (1) age greater than 60 years (in males in this age group, the obstruction is usually due to malignancy); (2) acholic stools persisting for more than 2 weeks; (3) colicky right upper quadrant pain and/or shaking chills compatible with choledocholithiasis and cholangitis; (4) severe jaundice without systemic symptoms (hepatocellular diseases with severe jaundice are almost always associated with severe systemic symptoms); and (5) a palpable (Courvoisier) gallbladder, an almost infallible sign of common bile duct obstruction, usually malignant.

With patients in whom diagnosis is difficult, watchful waiting is often valuable, accompanied by abdominal ultrasonography to see whether the extrahepatic and intrahepatic bile ducts are dilated. Ultimately, some patients require the more invasive special diagnostic techniques discussed in Chapter 53. If intrahepatic cholestasis is suspected clinically and ultrasonography reveals no dilated ducts, liver biopsy is the procedure of choice. If extrahepatic obstruction seems most likely, then transduodenal or percutaneous cholangiography is indicated.

BENIGN CHRONIC CONJUGATED HYPERBILIRUBINEMIAS

Dubin-Johnson syndrome

Etiology. Dubin-Johnson syndrome (Table 55-5) results from a hereditary autosomal recessive deficiency of the canalicular transporter that actively secretes organic anions other than bile salts into the canaliculus.

Incidence. Dubin-Johnson syndrome is found in about 1 of 1300 Iranian Jews. The incidence in Western populations is probably lower. Males are affected twice as often as females.

Table 55-5. Dubin-Johnson and Rotor syndromes

Finding		Dubin-Johnson syndrome	Rotor syndrome
Serum bilirubin	Total, mg/dl	1.8-9.9 in 90% of cases	2.9-7.9 in 90% of cases
	Direct: total (mean)	60%	60%
Organic anion kinetics	Secretory maximum (Tm)	<10% of normal	Mean 50% of normal
	Storage capacity	Normal	<20% of normal
	Late rise in conjugates	>90% of cases	Never present
Urinary coproporphyrin: total isomer		Normal	Very high
I/(I+III)		>80%	<65%
Hepatocellular pigment		Almost always present	Never present
Usual age of onset		10-40 years	<20 years
Gastrointestinal symptoms		>75% of cases	Seldom present
Hepatomegaly		>50% of cases	Rare
Gallbladder not seen on oral cholecystogram		>75% of cases	Usually seen

Pathophysiology. Analyses of plasma disappearance curves of bilirubin, BSP, ICG, ^{131}I rose bengal, and iodipamide indicate that the uptake and storage of these compounds are normal, but their secretory transfer maximum (Tm) is less than 10% of normal. After intravenous administration of BSP and bilirubin, the relatively normal initial plasma disappearance is followed in more than 90% of patients by a secondary rise in plasma concentration at 90 to 120 minutes due to reflux of unexcreted conjugates back into the plasma. This reflux occurs because the conjugated compounds are less well bound to cytoplasmic storage proteins than are the parent unconjugated substances. Kinetics, serum concentration, and biliary excretion of amidated bile acids are normal, but there is impaired secretion of ursodeoxycholic acid and bile acid 3-0-sulfates and glucuronides.

There is a high frequency of consanguinity, and about one third of tested siblings (but none of the parents) of children of Dubin-Johnson syndrome probands show increased serum conjugated bilirubin concentrations and delayed rise in plasma BSP conjugates. Patients with Dubin-Johnson syndrome also exhibit a markedly increased coproporphyrin I/coproporphyrin III ratio in their urine, though total urinary coproporphyrin excretion is normal. This phenomenon results apparently from differential impairment of the biliary excretion of the two isomers. Heterozygous relatives have normal serum bilirubin and BSP test results but show an increase in the urinary coproporphyrin I/coproporphyrin III ratio that falls between the ratios of normal and homozygous subjects.

Pathology. The liver is grossly black due to accumulation of a granular, melanin-like pigment in the lysosomes of the perivenular hepatocytes. Hepatic histology and ultrastructure are otherwise normal.

Clinical features. Jaundice is usually insidious in onset and begins in the second to fourth decades of life in 75% of patients. Serum bilirubin concentrations are less than 10 mg/dl in over 90% of patients, with an average of 60% direct-reacting bilirubin and a high proportion of δ-bilirubin. Bilirubin concentrations increase twofold to threefold during pregnancy, estrogen therapy, infections, trauma, or surgical procedures, often unmasking clinically latent jaundice.

For unexplained reasons, three fourths of patients with Dubin-Johnson syndrome have associated upper abdominal pain, nausea, or vomiting, and half have a palpably enlarged liver that is often tender. These symptoms, plus the fact that in 75% of oral cholecystogram examinations the gallbladder is not seen because of reduced secretion of iopanoic acid, have in the past suggested the mistaken diagnosis of choledocholithiasis. However, Dubin-Johnson syndrome is readily distinguished by the absence of itching, the infrequency of alcoholic stools, and minimal elevations of alkaline phosphatase (seen in less than 10% of Dubin-Johnson syndrome patients). Gallstones and dilated bile ducts are best excluded by ultrasonography or CT. Serum transaminases are almost always normal. Curiously, the prothrombin time is prolonged in two thirds and factor VII is deficient in 40% of patients.

Diagnosis. The family history should suggest whether the disorder is hereditary. Cholestasis is excluded if serum bile acid levels are normal, and biliary tract disease can be excluded by ultrasonography or ^{99m}Tc DISIDA (with delayed films). The diagnosis may be confirmed by the typical increase in the coproporphyrin I/coproporphyrin III isomer ratio in the urine, with normal total coproporphyrin levels. Liver biopsy is rarely needed and may be misleading, as some patients lack the pigment. There is no known treatment.

Rotor syndrome and hepatic storage disease

These two related syndromes (see Table 55-5), once thought to be variants of Dubin-Johnson syndrome because of their coexistence with it in some families, are chronic conjugated hyperbilirubinemias inherited in an autosomal recessive pattern. The dual defect involves severe impairment of storage of organic anions other than bile acids and a moderate defect in secretion.

Incidence. These syndromes are rare. Most reported cases have been in Hispanic families. The sexes are almost equally affected.

Pathophysiology. In contrast to the situation in Dubin-Johnson syndrome, the earlier portions of the plasma disappearance curves of unconjugated bilirubin, BSP, ICG, and iodipamide are markedly delayed, due to reduction of storage capacity to less than 20% of normal. Tm also is decreased but only to about one-half of normal values, and no late rise in plasma BSP conjugates is seen. It is thought that the impaired clearance of the multiple organic anions is due to a defect in storage, but ligandin levels have not been measured. The 50% reduction in Tm (biliary secretion) presumably accounts for the accompanying retention of bilirubin conjugates. Kinetic models that incorporate these dual defects in transport can reproduce the plasma disappearance curves obtained with BSP.

As in Dubin-Johnson syndrome, the ratio of coproporphyrin I/coproporphyrin III in the urine is elevated; by contrast, total urinary coproporphyrin is greatly increased owing to an average 20-fold increase in the output of isomer I and a mean fourfold increase in the output of isomer III. Heterozygotes handle bilirubin and BSP normally but show an intermediate increase in the coproporphyrin isomer ratio, with a twofold to threefold increase in excretion of isomer I.

Pathology. Hepatic histologic findings in Rotor syndrome and hepatic storage disease are normal, and there is no pigment.

Clinical features. Chronic, fluctuating jaundice usually develops in childhood or adolescence, with serum bilirubin concentrations usually in the range of 3 to 8 mg/dl; an average of 60% of serum bilirubin is direct reacting. In contrast to Dubin-Johnson syndrome, the oral cholecystographic findings are normal, there is no hepatic enlargement, abdominal pain is rarely present, and jaundice is not aggravated by pregnancy. Serum bile acids are normal. Hepatic storage disease may be distinguished from Rotor syndrome by the more severe impairment of BSP storage capacity and by the delayed oral cholecystographic visualization of the gallbladder.

Diagnosis. The same considerations apply as described for Dubin-Johnson syndrome, but the differences in BSP Tm and storage capacity and the high total urinary coproporphyrin levels are distinctive. No treatment is indicated.

INTERMITTENT CHOLESTATIC SYNDROMES

Estrogen-related cholestasis

Etiology. Although estrogens impair the Tm for BSP in all subjects, for unknown reasons a small proportion of women develop marked retention of bile acids and severe pruritus on prolonged exposure to high levels of estrogens. Such exposure may result from ingestion of oral contraceptive pills or from pregnancy. Twenty percent of affected patients also develop conjugated hyperbilirubinemia. Progestational steroids potentiate the effect of estrogens by inhibiting their conjugation and detoxification. Occurrence of the syndrome in about 15% of mothers and sisters of probands suggests a hereditary predisposition.

Incidence. In most countries, estrogen-related cholestasis occurs in less than 0.5% of women during pregnancy and/or oral contraceptive use. The incidence in Sweden, however, is about 2%, and in Chile it is about 10% among predominantly Caucasian probands and 28% among Araucanian Indians.

Pathophysiology. As in all forms of cholestasis, the etiology of the pruritus is not established. However, as in most steroid-related cholestases, alkaline phosphatase levels are rarely more than three times normal except in patients with jaundice. Estrogen metabolism in these patients is normal except for the decreased conversion of 16-hydroxy estrones to estriols that is seen with cholestasis of any cause. The reasons for the sensitivity to estrogens and the irregular occurrence of the syndrome during the different pregnancies of a given patient are not known. Estrogen administration reproduces the syndrome regularly in affected women, and the syndrome reverses spontaneously after parturition.

Pathology. Eighty percent of patients with estrogen-related cholestasis show the typical canalicular lesions of cholestasis, which include bile plugs, dilatation, and loss of microvilli. There is no evidence of liver cell degeneration or necrosis, inflammation, or fibrosis.

Clinical features. In women with estrogen-related cholestasis, pruritus begins without systemic prodromal symptoms, usually during the eighth or ninth month of gestation or within a few days of the start of estrogen therapy. If jaundice occurs, it usually develops 1 to 2 weeks later. Total serum bilirubin levels are rarely greater than 5 mg/dl; at least 50% of bilirubin is direct reacting. Serum transaminase levels are often elevated in the range of 100 to 200 units, and serum cholesterol is generally above 300 mg/dl. The liver and spleen are rarely enlarged. More than 50% of the patients, their mothers, and their sisters develop cholesterol gallstones.

Diagnosis. The family history and the relation of symptoms to pregnancy and oral contraceptive use should suggest estrogen-related cholestasis. The mild elevations of bilirubin, transaminases, and alkaline phosphatases and the absence of hepatomegaly, abdominal pain, fever, and systemic symptoms help to exclude viral hepatitis, choledocholithiasis, and the fearsome acute fatty liver of pregnancy. Abdominal ultrasonography can exclude biliary obstruction. X-ray examination and radioisotopic cholangiography are contraindicated in pregnancy.

Treatment. Discontinuing oral contraceptive use relieves the symptoms within 1 to 2 weeks. Cholestyramine may control itching; the effectiveness of phenobarbital and phototherapy has not been studied. S-Adenosylmethionine, 800 mg daily intravenously, reputedly reverses the syndrome in less than 1 week, but this finding is disputed.

Benign recurrent intrahepatic cholestasis (BRIC)

This syndrome of recurrent prolonged episodes of severe cholestatic jaundice is only sometimes familial and is usually unrelated to estrogen therapy or pregnancy. The etiology is unknown. Keto and ring-unsaturated bile acids appear during attacks, but their causal relationship is not established. Fewer than 75 cases of BRIC have been reported. Males are affected almost twice as often as females. Retention of bile acids and itching dominate the attacks, but the association of significant hepatocellular injury leads to severe jaundice and systemic symptoms and often prevents an increase in serum cholesterol levels. Anorexia, combined with steatorrhea from decreased excretion of bile acids into the intestine, results in weight loss during episodes. In addition to the typical lesions of canalicular cholestasis, there are also significant portal inflammatory infiltrates and hepatocellular lesions. Attacks usually begin in childhood or adolescence (before the age of 2 years in one third of patients) and often occur with regularity. Attacks typically begin with a prodrome of fatigue, malaise, and anorexia. Itching then begins, followed in 2 to 4 weeks by painless jaundice without fever. The liver is usually enlarged and is occasionally tender. Bilirubin concentrations usually plateau at 10 to 20 mg/dl. Transaminases may be elevated twofold to threefold. Attacks generally clear without sequelae in 1 to 4 months. Between episodes, liver function test results are normal. Diagnosis rests on the history of recurrent episodes of severe cholestasis from childhood and the limited abnormalities (other than marked bilirubinemia) revealed in liver function tests. Biliary obstruction can be excluded by abdominal ultrasonography and radiologic visualization of the biliary tree. Prednisolone therapy appears to shorten attacks in some patients, but its value is disputed. Cholestyramine may control itching, and oral and parenteral hyperalimentation may help to minimize weight loss. Fat-soluble vitamin supplements should be given to patients with steatorrhea.

POSTOPERATIVE CHOLESTASIS AND CHOLESTASIS RELATED TO SEVERE INFECTIONS

Mild to severe intrahepatic cholestasis may occur after long and difficult operations with multiple blood transfusions. The severe, less common form develops in 3 to 4 days and peaks 9 to 18 days postoperatively. It results from a combination of (1) a large bilirubin load from transfusion of many (usually more than 20) units of blood plus 1 to 2 liters from internal bleeding, (2) impaired hepatic transport of bilirubin due to hypotension and anoxia, and (3) acute renal failure, with impairment of the urinary route for excretion of conjugated bilirubin. These patients may have conjugated hyperbilirubinemia of 20 to 40 mg/dl and serum alkaline phosphatase levels three to five times normal. Centrilobular congestion and hemorrhagic necrosis with associated erythrophagocytosis are found at autopsy. The less severe form develops 1 to 2 days after prolonged surgery involving usually less than nine units of blood; shock, internal hemorrhage, and renal failure are absent. Serum bilirubin concentration is usually less than 10 mg/dl. Alkaline phosphatase levels are normal in 50% of patients and less than three times normal in the remainder. Histology reveals the canalicular dilatation and bile plugs typical of intrahepatic cholestasis. The syndrome resolves in 2 to 4 weeks unless additional complications supervene. Mild transaminase elevations exclude halothane or viral hepatitis, and the mild elevations of alkaline phosphatase in relation to bilirubin levels render extrahepatic obstruction unlikely. Treatment is directed at the underlying complications.

Similar syndromes occur with lobar pneumonia and severe infections, especially if accompanied by toxinemia and/or septicemia. Though endotoxin does produce cholestasis experimentally, its role in the human syndrome is not established. The more severe picture occurs only with septicemic shock. The usual, milder syndrome does not affect the prognosis of the patient, and its histologic features are similar to those of mild postoperative cholestasis with, in addition, necrosis of periportal hepatocytes and dilatation, plugging, and epithelial damage to the cholangioles.

REFERENCES

Primary source with extensive bibliographies

Ostrow JD, editor: Bile pigments and jaundice: molecular, metabolic and medical aspects, New York, 1986, Marcel Dekker.

Reviews

Berlin NI, and Berk PD: Quantitative aspects of bilirubin metabolism for hematologists, Blood 57:983, 1981.

Crawford JM, Hauser SC, and Gollan JR: Formation, hepatic metabolism, and transport of bile pigments: a status report, Semin Liver Dis 8:105, 1988.

Frank BB et al: Clinical evaluation of jaundice. A guideline of the Patient Care Committee of the American Gastroenterological Association, JAMA 262:3031, 1989.

Jansen PLM and Oude Elferink RPJ: Hereditary hyperbilirubinemias—a molecular and mechanistic approach, Semin Liver Dis 8:168, 1988.

Klaassen CD and Watkins JB: Mechanism of bile formation, hepatic uptake, and biliary secretion, Pharmacol Rev 36:1, 1984.

Maisels MJ: Neonatal jaundice, Semin Liver Dis 8:148, 1988.

McDonagh AF and Lightner DA: "Like a shriveled blood orange"—bilirubin, jaundice and phototherapy, Pediatrics 75:443, 1985.

Muraca M, Fevery J, and Blanckaert N: Analytical aspects and clinical interpretation of serum bilirubins, Semin Liver Dis 8:137, 1988.

Okolicsanyi L et al: Epidemiology of unconjugated hyperbilirubinemia—revisited, Semin Liver Dis 8:179, 1988.

Ostrow JD: Therapeutic amelioration of jaundice: old and new strategies (editorial), Hepatology 8:683, 1988.

Sieg A et al: Subfractionation of serum bilirubins by alkaline methanolysis and thin layer chromatography. An aid in the differential diagnosis of icteric diseases, J Hepatol 11:59, 1990.

Sorrentino D and Berk PD: Mechanistic aspects of hepatic bilirubin uptake, Semin Liver Dis 8:119, 1988.

Vore M: Estrogen cholestasis; membranes, metabolites or receptors? Gastroenterology 93:643, 1987.

CHAPTER

56 Principal Complications of Liver Failure

Steven Schenker
Anastacio M. Hoyumpa

The liver is a vital organ that has numerous anabolic (synthetic), catabolic (detoxifying), and storage functions and is the conduit by which portal blood enters the superior vena cava. Therefore liver failure may result in many derangements of normal body processes such as synthesis of protein; formation of glucose; detoxication of ammonia, various hormones, and drugs; storage of glycogen and certain vitamins; and maintenance of normal splanchnic blood flow. Many of these derangements are covered elsewhere in this book (Chapters 50 and 58); this discussion will concern only the following five cardinal manifestations of liver failure: hepatic encephalopathy, ascites, portal hypertension, the hepatorenal syndrome, and endocrine disturbances.

HEPATIC ENCEPHALOPATHY

Clinical features

Hepatic encephalopathy is a neuropsychiatric syndrome seen in some patients with liver failure. The disorder may be secondary to acute or chronic parenchymal liver disease, the latter frequently accompanied by spontaneous or surgically induced portosystemic shunting of blood. Rarely, encephalopathy may occur in children with congenital disorders of urea cycle enzymes and in patients with other types of hepatic dysfunction. The features common to all forms of hepatic encephalopathy are alterations of mental state, neurologic abnormalities, the presence of parenchymal liver disease, and, usually, certain characteristic but nonspecific laboratory findings. These clinical features are summarized in Table 56-1.

Hepatic encephalopathy can be considered as a spectrum of disorders. In acute liver failure, as seen in patients with fulminant viral or toxic hepatitis (i.e., due to acetaminophen or halothane) or with acute fatty liver of pregnancy, there are usually no obvious precipitants of encephalopathy. The course is explosive, with delirium, convulsions, and often cerebral edema and decerebrate rigidity. In about 80% of instances, the disorder is fatal.

By contrast, patients with chronic liver disease develop a more indolent type of neuropsychiatric disturbance, often called *portosystemic encephalopathy*. This disorder is often precipitated by specific events such as gastrointestinal hemorrhage, azotemia, or infection. The usual precipitating causes and their presumed mechanisms are shown in Table 56-2. Diagnosis of portosystemic encephalopathy depends on the identification of typical clinical features, the exclusion of other causes of encephalopathy, and, at times, a therapeutic trial.

As can be seen in Table 56-1, an abnormal mental state is the sine qua non of all types of hepatic encephalopathy. The mental abnormality may consist only of slight alterations in judgment and other intellectual processes, nonspecific personality changes, and inappropriate behavior. Motor skills (i.e., driving) may be especially impaired and can be assessed by psychomotor testing. A graphic or semiquantitative assessment of intellectual performance also can be obtained by following the patient's handwriting, by asking the patient to do simple manual construction such as reproducing a five-pointed star, or by administering a numbers-connection (Reitan Trailmaking) test in which the patient connects sequential numbers by lines during a timed interval. The score is the time in seconds necessary to complete the task. Rapid, inexpensive, simple, and accurate, the numbers-connection test is more sensitive than the star construction test and handier than the electroencephalogram or the use of event-related (visual, auditory, somatosensory) evoked potentials. With more severe portosystemic encephalopathy, progressive inversion of sleep pattern, staring, apathy, drowsiness, and eventually deep coma may occur. Hyperventilation and hypothermia may be seen before the onset of coma. In about 50% of patients with portosystemic encephalopathy, fetor hepaticus may be detected. This is a sweetish, musty odor of the breath believed to be caused by exhaled mercaptans, products of impaired hepatic metabolism of the sulfur-containing amino acid methionine.

Table 56-1. Stages of hepatic encephalopathy

Stage	Symptoms	Signs	EEG
Prodrome	Loss of affect, euphoria, depression, apathy, inappropriate behavior, altered sleep pattern	Asterixis ±, constructional apraxia, writing difficulty	±
Impending coma	Confusion, disorientation, drowsiness	Asterixis, fetor hepaticus	++
Light coma	Marked confusion, arousable from sleep, response to stimuli	Asterixis, fetor hepaticus, rigidity of limbs, hyperflexia, clonus, extensor response, grasping and sucking reflexes	+++
Deep coma	Unconsciousness, no response to stimuli	Fetor hepaticus, no muscle tone, flaccid limbs, depressed reflexes	++++

Note: ±, may or may not be present; +, abnormal finding showing decreased electrical activity. Separation into various stages is not necessarily sharp, and EEG changes may not always correlate with the severity of coma. Hypothermia may be seen in the early stages, and hyperventilation at any state, of encephalopathy.

Table 56-2. Precipitating causes of portosystemic encephalopathy

Cause	Presumed mechanism	Therapeutic implication
Azotemia (spontaneous or diuretic-induced)	Increased enterohepatic circulation of urea nitrogen, with increased ammonia production Direct sedative effect of uremia Diuretic-induced hypokalemic alkalosis, increased renal vein ammonia output, resulting in enhanced transfer of ammonia across blood-brain barrier Excessive diuresis, leading to hypovolemia, prerenal azotemia, decreased perfusion of vital organs Separate role of hypokalemia in cerebral function	Avoidance of excessive diuresis Avoidance of potentially nephrotoxic agents (i.e., aminoglycosides)
Sedatives, tranquilizers, analgesics	Direct depressant effect on brain Hypoxia from depression of respiratory center	Cautious use of these drugs if unavoidable, with careful monitoring of response and adjustment of dosage; ideally, select agent metabolized normally in presence of liver disease, with short half-life, inactive metabolites, and no enhanced effect on the site of action (cerebral sensitivity)
Gastrointestinal bleeding	Substrate for increased production of ammonia and other nitrogenous toxins; 1 dl blood = 15-20 g protein Hypovolemia, shock, and hypoxia that compromise hepatic, cerebral, renal function, the latter leading to increased activity of the enterohepatic urea nitrogen cycle and increased ammonia production Contribution of ammonia in stored blood	Prophylactic use of lactulose and evacuation of blood from the intestine in bleeding, noncomatose patients with liver disease; avoid gastrointestinal irritants (alcohol, NSAID*); measures needed to treat cough to minimize variceal bleeding from increased portal pressure during coughing or straining
Metabolic alkalosis	Diffusion of un-ionized ammonia across blood-brain barrier (see above)	K^+ replacement; in severe, unresponsive cases IV infusion of dilute HCl (1.5 dl 1 N HCl/1 L H_2O), 0.5-2.0 L/24 h
Excess dietary protein	Substrate for ammonia and other nitrogenous toxin production	Curtailment of dietary proteins, especially containing aromatic and sulfated amino acids and those with high ammonia-generating potential
Infection	Increased tissue catabolism, leading to more endogenous nitrogen load and increased ammonia production Dehydration and prerenal azotemia Hypoxia and/or hyperthermia that potentiates ammonia toxicity	Search for infection and early use of appropriate antibiotics
Constipation	Increased production and absorption of ammonia and other toxic nitrogen derivatives due to increased contact time between bacteria and nitrogenous substances Straining at stool that increases portal pressure, with subsequent variceal bleeding	Prophylactic use of stool softeners and laxatives

Modified with permission from Hoyumpa AM et al: Hepatic encephalopathy, Gastroenterology 76:184-195, 1979.
*Nonsteroid anti-inflammatory drugs.

The most characteristic neurologic sign of hepatic encephalopathy is a flapping tremor of the hands called *asterixis*. It is best seen with the arms outstretched, wrists hyperextended, and fingers separated. The flap is maximum with sustained posture, is usually bilateral but asynchronous, and is frequently preceded by a lateral tremor of the fingers. Asterixis, which can also be detected as unsustained clonus in the feet, in tightly closed eyelids, pursed lips, or protruded tongue, is thought to be due to improper integration of peripheral afferent information to the brainstem reticular formation. Asterixis is not specific for hepatic encephalopathy, however, because it occurs also in patients with uremia, pulmonary insufficiency, sedative overdose, and other metabolic neurologic derangements.

The other neurologic signs in classic hepatic encephalopathy are also believed to be caused by a metabolic rather than a structural brain disturbance. They are usually transient, changing (i.e., not localized), and potentially rapidly reversible. Thus early in portosystemic encephalopathy the patient may experience hyperreflexia, varying plantar extensor response, and spasticity. Later, with severe encephalopathy, depression of deep tendon reflexes is more common. In portosystemic encephalopathy, convulsions and decerebrate rigidity are rare. In some patients with portosystemic encephalopathy, two neurologic syndromes have been recognized. The first is called *hepatocerebral degeneration,* or pseudo-Wilsonian hepatic encephalopathy, as the neurologic signs resemble those of hepatolenticular degeneration. Prominent features include impairment of intellectual function, dysarthria, cerebellar ataxia, tremor, and athetoid movements. In contrast to Wilson's disease, however, there are no abnormalities of copper metabolism. The second syndrome, *spastic paraparesis,* consists of spasticity of the lower extremities, increased deep tendon reflexes, and extensor plantar responses. These motor disturbances are generally unaccompanied by sensory deficits or changes in cerebrospinal fluid pressure, protein concentration, or cell count. Unlike the more typical portosystemic encephalopathy, which responds to therapy in about 80% of instances, these less common neurologic syndromes are usually marked by slow, progressive deterioration, although improvement has been reported in a few patients with hepatocerebral degeneration treated with bromocriptine, a dopamine agonist, and once with hepatic transplantation, which resulted in normalization of the gait, disappearance of tremor, and marked improvement in mental function.

A number of abnormal laboratory findings are associated with hepatic encephalopathy. Changes in liver tests reflect an underlying hepatic disorder (Chapter 53). These tests do not, however, correlate with the presence or absence of hepatic encephalopathy, except for the prolonged prothrombin time in acute liver failure. Patients with hepatic encephalopathy, especially that secondary to chronic liver disease, also frequently show evidence of respiratory alkalosis due to hyperventilation and may have hypokalemic metabolic alkalosis due to diuretic overuse. Rarely, hypoglycemia is seen with fulminant liver failure. Abnormalities in nitrogen metabolism are characteristic. Arterial ammonia concentration is increased in about 90% of patients with hepatic encephalopathy. The arterial ammonia level, however, does not reflect well the degree of coma, probably because the assay is not fastidious enough, only single measurements are obtained, blood ammonia may not equate with brain ammonia, and ammonia is not the sole "toxin" causing hepatic encephalopathy. Serial measurements of ammonia may be more helpful in following the clinical course of hepatic encephalopathy in individual patients. Spinal fluid glutamine, which reflects brain ammonia metabolism, and is usually increased, has greater stability than ammonia but requires a spinal tap. Glutamine measurements may be very helpful in distinguishing portosystemic encephalopathy from nonhepatic coma. Except for these findings, the cerebrospinal fluid in most patients with hepatic encephalopathy is usually normal. Occasionally, the spinal fluid protein concentration is elevated, in which case other causes of coma must be sought. The spinal fluid pressure may be elevated in patients with cerebral edema. Finally, patients with hepatic encephalopathy usually have an abnormal serum amino acid profile. Patients with coma due to acute liver failure have markedly elevated levels of all amino acids, and the levels tend to correlate with the degree of hepatic necrosis. On the other hand, patients with portosystemic encephalopathy exhibit an increase in aromatic amino acids and methionine, whereas branched-chain amino acid levels are depressed. Short- and long-chain fatty acid levels are likewise elevated in the blood.

Electroencephalograms in patients with hepatic encephalopathy show characteristic but nonspecific changes. These changes consist of slowing of cerebral electrical activity and high-voltage waves, starting bifrontally and progressing posteriorly. Focal abnormalities are not seen in uncomplicated hepatic encephalopathy. Similar changes in the electroencephalogram are seen in patients with other metabolic encephalopathies, i.e., uremia, drug intoxication.

Diagnosis of hepatic encephalopathy is based on the presence of typical clinical features (see Table 56-1) and the exclusion of other causes of altered mental state. Imaging techniques (computed tomography [CT] or magnetic resonance imaging [MRI]) may be helpful in excluding disorders, such as subdural or intracerebral bleeding, that can cause coma in a patient with liver disease. In fulminant hepatic failure, these techniques may show cerebral edema, but this is not as sensitive as abnormal pupillary changes. Papilledema is usually a late finding. The diagnosis of hepatic encephalopathy is often supported by the characteristic laboratory findings mentioned earlier, but these are not specific (i.e., elevated ammonia concentration may be due to liver disease, while the coma may have a different cause) and are not essential for the diagnosis. At times, a trial of therapy is helpful in making a diagnosis of portosystemic encephalopathy and should be used, provided other causes of coma continue to be sought.

Pathogenesis

The pathogenesis of hepatic encephalopathy is incompletely understood, and the mechanism or mechanisms that cause coma accompanying acute and chronic liver failure (and even different types of portosystemic encephalopathy) may differ. Despite these reservations, certain unifying concepts about the pathogenesis of hepatic encephalopathy have emerged.

First, hepatic encephalopathy seems usually to be a metabolic and neurophysiologic disorder often not accompanied by structural lesions in the brain. Thus it is potentially fully reversible, except in some patients with hepatocerebral degeneration and spastic paraparesis whose dysfunction may be progressive and who may have evidence of necrosis in the basal ganglia and demyelination in the spinal cord, respectively. In other patients with hepatic encephalopathy, the brain is either free of lesions or demonstrates astroglial proliferation and hypertrophy and/or cerebral edema, which, because of their inconsistency, are felt to be consequences rather than causes of hepatic encephalopathy. It is not known what precise anatomic sites in the brain are affected by hepatic encephalopathy, although it has been suggested that maintenance of consciousness depends on normal function of the reticular activating system in the brainstem and the modifying influence of the cortex. Presumably, therefore, these sites are affected. There is some evidence for selective sensitivity of the brainstem to the toxic effects of ammonia.

Second, hepatic encephalopathy may be a multifactorial problem. It may be caused by a synergistic interaction at the cerebral level of various "toxins" such as excess ammonia, short- and long-chain fatty acids, and possibly by mercaptans, an abnormal amino acid and neurotransmitter balance or by lack of some undefined vital protective substance(s). Moreover, in portosystemic encephalopathy various insults and physiologic derangements such as azotemia, infection, and hypokalemic alkalosis may summate with putative toxins to precipitate hepatic encephalopathy (see Table 56-2). Patients with portosystemic encephalopathy may also have increased sensitivity to various insults (i.e., infection, sedatives) that may summate with other derangements to induce coma. In patients taking some sedatives, decreased drug metabolism with subsequent drug accumulation, increased penetration of the drug into the brain due to decreased drug binding to plasma proteins, and enhanced cerebral receptor sensitivity to the drug may combine to increase susceptibility to encephalopathy. The relative importance of toxins, physiologic derangements, and cerebral susceptibility may vary with the type of liver disease and among patients.

Third, although the precise molecular basis of hepatic encephalopathy is uncertain, the mechanisms to be considered include altered energy metabolism, a derangement of the neuronal membranes, altered synaptic transmission resulting from an imbalance in cerebral neurotransmitters, or some combination of these. The possible mechanisms by which the various accumulated toxins may induce hepatic encephalopathy are diverse and are listed in Table 56-3. None of these toxins, however, has been unequivocally proven to be the cause of hepatic encephalopathy. An imbalance of excitatory and inhibitory amino acid neurotransmitters may also contribute to encephalopathy and currently seems the best mechanistic explanation for hepatic coma. This imbalance may consist of decreased excitatory neurotransmitters (glutamate and aspartate) as a result of enhanced ammonia metabolism and increased gamma aminobutyrate (GABA) tone, an inhibitory effect. The latter does not appear to be due to greater influx of GABA into the brain (as originally proposed), but rather to the presence of a benzodiazepine-like substance that modulates the GABA receptor. This receptor (part of a supramolecular complex that also binds benzodiazepines and barbiturates) may also explain, at least partly, the cerebral sensitivity of patients with chronic liver disease to such sedatives. One major problem has been the inability to dissociate the causal from the casual neurochemical derangements; others are the difficulty in establishing valid experimental animal models of hepatic encephalopathy.

Table 56-3. Putative toxins and their mechanisms of action

Toxin	Possible mechanism(s) of action*
Ammonia†	Direct effects on neuronal membrane Alteration of cytoplasmic/mitochondrial NADH/NAD ratio and malate-aspartate shuttle Decreased excitatory neurotransmitters (glutamate, aspartate) Disturbance in energy metabolism
Mercaptans	Derangement of neuronal membrane activity via interference with $(Na^+ + K^+)$-ATPase activity Impairment of ammonia detoxication
Fatty acids	Impairment of ammonia detoxication Direct effects on neuronal/synaptic membranes Competition for intravascular binding of putative toxins
Various amino acids	Derangement of normal neurotransmitter status of brain Generation of ammonia Generation of mercaptans
Other substances	Benzodiazepine-like inhibitors

*Primary vs. secondary functional effects not defined.
†May especially affect glial function. Regional (i.e., brainstem) sensitivity may be present.
Modified from Hoyumpa AM et al: Hepatic encephalopathy, Gastroenterology 76:184, 1979.

Therapy

The management of patients with portosystemic encephalopathy involves (1) treatment of the underlying hepatic disease, if possible; (2) identification and removal of factors that may have precipitated the encephalopathy; and (3) reduction of the formation and influx of nitrogenous toxins into the brain by (a) alteration, reduction, or elimination of dietary protein; (b) use of lactulose, antibiotics, or both; and (c) intestinal cleansing. In addition, supportive care is provided to establish adequate caloric intake and to treat the complications of liver failure (i.e., hypoglycemia, gastrointestinal bleeding, and electrolyte abnormalities). Similar therapy is suitable for patients with coma due to acute liver failure, although its scientific basis and benefit for this group of patients are not as well documented.

Identification of precipitating causes of portosystemic encephalopathy (see Table 56-2) and their treatment frequently result in clinical recovery. Often, the same factor induces recurrent portosystemic encephalopathy in the same patient. Development of spontaneous portosystemic encephalopathy, without a precipitating event or evident worsening of liver function, is uncommon and warrants reevaluation of the initial diagnosis.

The major way to reduce the impact of nitrogenous toxins on patients with portosystemic encephalopathy is to reduce or eliminate dietary protein. The degree of protein restriction depends on the severity of the mental change. Patients with chronic liver disease require protein for hepatic regeneration; therefore complete withdrawal of dietary protein should be as brief as possible. Usually, with improvement of mental state, gradual increments of 10 to 20 g protein per day every 3 to 5 days are added and are adjusted to the clinical response. In addition to restriction of the quantity of ingested protein, changes in the quality of protein may be beneficial. Vegetable protein may be tolerated better than animal protein, probably because (1) the greater amount of fiber promotes increased incorporation of, and subsequent elimination of, nitrogen in fecal bacteria that ultimately results in lowering blood ammonia and (2) it has a laxative effect. Another approach has been the use of amino acid mixtures high in branched-chain amino acids and low in methionine and aromatic acids. This approach is based on the observation that patients with portosystemic encephalopathy usually have low serum branched-chain and high aromatic amino acids, which may promote greater entry of aromatic amino acids into the brain and formation therein of false (weak) neurotransmitters. Thus the rationale is to normalize the serum amino acid profile of these patients with portosystemic encephalopathy in the hope of improving the presumed altered cerebral neurotransmitter states (see Table 56-3) and possibly of enhancing the metabolism of ammonia by muscle. Other recent studies have suggested that nitrogen-free ketoanalogs of essential amino acids may provide the carbon skeleton for complete amino acids and be aminated with endogenous nitrogen in patients. These therapeutic alterations of nutritional nitrogen sources are theoretically promising, but further validating studies are needed before they become part of routine management.

Another standard therapeutic approach to portosystemic encephalopathy involves the use of lactulose, antibiotics, or both. Lactulose (a synthetic galactosidofructose), is given orally in doses of 60 to 120 ml of syrup per day in equally divided amounts so as to promote two to three soft stools daily with a pH of about 5.5. Low doses are given at first to determine patient tolerance and avoid diarrhea. Lactulose can also be given as an enema, 3 dl of lactulose syrup added to 7 dl of water. The drug, which is essentially not absorbed, (1) is broken down by gut bacteria to organic acids that lower colonic pH, thereby reducing the absorption of un-ionized ammonia and favoring the growth of low ammonia-producing bacteria, (2) serves as substrate for bacteria in utilizing ammonia, (3) promotes incorporation of fecal nitrogen by fecal bacteria, and (4) induces a more rapid evacuation of nitrogenous toxins from the bowel. Lactulose has few side effects, but gastric intolerance can occur, and large doses may produce osmotic diarrhea and occasional hypernatremia. Lactitol, a second-generation disaccharide in powder form, acts more promptly and has been shown to be as effective as lactulose but produces less diarrhea and flatulence. In populations with a high prevalence of lactase deficiency, lactose may be tried as an inexpensive substitute for lactulose. Recently, sodium benzoate, which combines with ammonia and is excreted as hippurate, has been used therapeutically.

Of the antibiotics, neomycin is the most commonly used. It is given in doses of 2 to 4 g per day orally or as a 1% enema. Oral treatment seems more reliable, except in the presence of ileus. The optimal dosage is not known, and the beneficial effect is presumed to be due to partial inactivation of bacteria that generate nitrogenous toxins from protein and urea. About 1% to 3% of neomycin may be absorbed from the upper and lower bowel. The drug may induce diarrhea by exerting a direct toxic effect on the gut mucosa or by altering the bacterial flora, although diarrhea usually occurs with higher dosages. Absorbed neomycin is excreted by the kidneys, and in patients with renal failure prolonged use of the drug may lead to its accumulation and to ototoxicity and nephrotoxicity. Metronidazole (250 mg QID) is another useful antibiotic, but it may produce peripheral neuropathy and central nervous system abnormalities, including convulsive seizures, especially with prolonged use.

Either neomycin or lactulose may be used to treat patients with portosystemic encephalopathy, although lactulose is preferred in the presence of renal or hearing impairment and for prolonged therapy. Theoretically, neomycin might decrease the effectiveness of concomitant lactulose use by depressing the bacterial flora of the gut, but there is evidence that in some patients treatment with both drugs may be more effective than treatment with either drug alone. Moreover, efficient lactulose fermenters like *Lactobacillus acidophilus* and *Clostridium perfringens* are resistant to neomycin. If both neomycin and lactulose are to be used, it would be prudent to check the stool pH and ascertain that addition of neomycin did not prevent the lactulose-induced decrease in stool pH, possibly obviating a beneficial effect of lactulose. A lactulose-metronidazole combination is probably undesirable because of metronidazole's activity against anaerobes. Bowel cleansing is an important adjunct for removing nitrogenous products from the bowel.

Degradation of endogenous protein should be prevented by provision of at least 1600 cal/day in the form of glucose. Adequate vitamins should also be supplied, as patients with chronic liver disease often have deficiencies of these nutrients. Electrolyte abnormalities, especially hypokalemic alkalosis, require appropriate treatment. Severe resistant metabolic alkalosis, which causes increased generation of un-ionized ammonia and its passage into the more acid milieu of the brain, may require administration of arginine hydrochloride or diluted hydrochloric acid. There is no good therapy for respiratory alkalosis.

The treatment of encephalopathy due to fulminant hepatic failure poses an even greater challenge. For the most part, management consists of intensive supportive care, with close monitoring of vital functions and laboratory parameters, to allow prompt management of sepsis and cardiac, respiratory, gastrointestinal, renal, and other life-threatening complications. The apparent better survival rates in recent years, in fact, may be due to improved intensive care methods rather than to any specific treatment. In patients with fulminant hepatic failure, hypoglycemia must be looked for early and treated with glucose. These patients often have a very prolonged prothrombin time and bleed easily. The incidence of gastrointestinal bleeding might be reduced by the prophylactic use of H_2-receptor antagonists, but these agents, especially in the elderly and those with concomitant renal failure and liver disease, may also cause mental obtundation. Infusion of fresh-frozen plasma may be beneficial, especially if bleeding is evident, but its effect is partial and transient and such therapy may lead to sodium and fluid overload and enhance consumptive coagulopathy. Heparin therapy for the consumptive coagulopathy that may accompany acute liver failure has not been helpful and may be risky. In acute liver failure, cerebral edema is a major cause of death. The precise pathogenesis of cerebral edema is still unclear. Altered permeability and inhibition of neuronal ($Na^+ + K^+$)-ATPase and osmolar changes due to ammonia metabolism have been cited as playing possible roles. Optimum therapy is uncertain. Initial encouraging results have been reported with mannitol.

There is no good evidence that corticosteroids, levodopa, or measures that provide temporary biologic support (e.g., exchange transfusions, absorbents) prolong the lives of patients with coma resistant to other measures, although improvement in the level of consciousness has been reported in some studies. Temporary liver assist measures are being studied. Hepatic transplantation has been shown to improve the survival rate of patients with fulminant or subacute hepatic failure and is discussed in detail in Chapter 64. The possibility that antagonists of benzodiazepine-like inhibitors will be effective therapy at the cerebral GABA receptor level is interesting and requires further study.

ASCITES

Clinical picture

The ease and accuracy with which ascites is detected depend on the amount of fluid accumulated and the examiner's experience. Small amounts (1 liter or less) may be missed by physical examination. Larger quantities may be perceived as abdominal distention, and initially as shifting dullness and then as a fluid wave on physical examination. As little as 200 ml may be detected as a puddle sign. Ascites may be seen radiologically as a diffuse haziness (ground-glass appearance) with separation of bowel loops. One hundred fifty milliliters or less can be appreciated ultrasonographically or by CT.

Pathogenesis

The accumulation of fluid in the peritoneal cavity of patients with cirrhosis results from an interaction of a number of factors. Those of principal importance are increased portal pressure and increased renal sodium reabsorption. Increased portal pressure, which is due principally to interference with portal flow in the cirrhotic liver and to increased total splanchnic plasma volume, disturbs the principle (Starling's hypothesis) that governs the normal interchange of fluid between the vascular compartment and tissue space and localizes the accumulation of fluid to the peritoneal cavity. The mechanism of increased reabsorption of sodium by the kidneys is uncertain but may be secondary to a decrease in "effective" plasma volume or more likely to hormonally mediated changes in sodium reabsorption in response to decreased perfusion of the renal cortex. Both portal hypertension and greater reabsorption of sodium are operative and interrelated in most patients with ascites, but there is debate as to which is the primary event. These interrelationships are shown schematically in Fig. 56-1 and are discussed in detail in Chapter 351. More recently, peripheral arterial vasodilatation with subsequent sodium and water retention has been proposed as the initiating basis of ascites.

Also important in the development of ascites is an im-

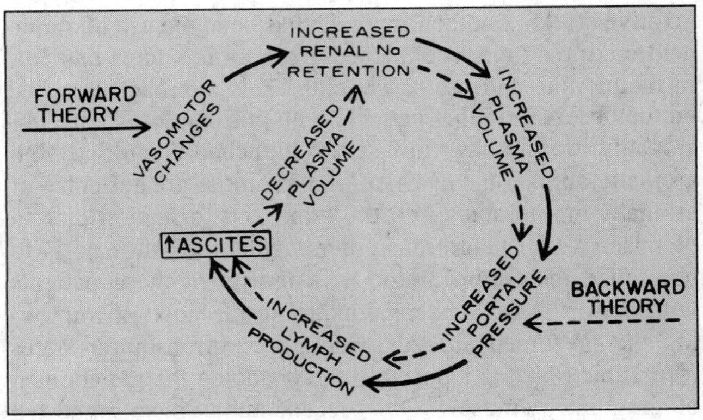

Fig. 56-1. Theories of ascites formation. According to the backward theory of ascites formation, the basic defect is portal hypertension; increased physical force drives fluid into the abdominal cavity, eventually lowering the effective plasma volume and causing increased (compensatory) renal sodium reabsorption. Because a decreased effective plasma volume is a prominent feature, this proposed mechanism is also known as the *underfill theory*. When lymphatic drainage is overwhelmed, ascites ensues. According to the forward (overflow) theory of ascites formation, excessive renal sodium retention precedes the development of ascites. Hemodynamic changes induced by vasomotor alterations induce renal salt conservation. These hemodynamic changes consist of increased arteriovenous shunts, decreased peripheral resistance, decreased renal cortical blood flow, and eventual enhanced renal sodium reabsorption. Increase in sodium reabsorption leads to increase in total body sodium, increase in body and plasma volume, rise in portal pressure, and eventual ascites when lymphatic drainage does not keep up with fluid retention. (From Galambos JT: Cirrhosis, Major Probl Intern Med 7:1, 1979.)

balance in the formation and removal of hepatic and gut lymph. When lymphatic drainage fails to compensate for increased lymph leakage, mainly due to elevated hepatic sinusoidal pressure, ascites develops. The fluid that leaves the hepatic sinusoids and seeps from the liver early in cirrhosis is generally rich in protein, while fluid escaping from the intestine later is low in protein because the intestinal capillaries are less permeable to protein than the hepatic sinusoids. Other nonrenal factors that contribute to ascites formation may include leakage of albumin into the abdominal cavity and impaired reabsorption of the fluid across a thickened peritoneal lining. Decreased oncotic pressure in plasma, contrary to earlier concepts, may not contribute significantly to ascites formation.

Differential diagnosis

The main causes of ascites are cirrhosis, peritoneal inflammation, malignancy, pancreatitis, heart failure, hepatic venous obstruction, nephrosis, peritoneal renal dialysis, and myxedema. Cirrhosis is the most common cause of ascites; and in cirrhotic patients it is worthwhile to rule out spontaneous bacterial peritonitis, pancreatitis, tuberculosis, and malignancy, as their presence affects management. Diagnostic paracentesis should be performed in patients with new-onset ascites or when there is unexplained fever, leukocytosis, altered mental state, abdominal pain, or deterioration of general condition. Coagulopathy is not a contraindication, and many believe that prophylactic fresh-frozen plasma need not be administered. At times ultrasonographically guided paracentesis is necessary to best localize the fluid. The fluid should be routinely examined with regard to protein and albumin concentration, cell count and type, amylase and cytology, and it should be cultured. An ascitic fluid/serum protein ratio of less than 0.5 suggests uncomplicated cirrhosis, whereas a larger ratio is more consistent with infection, cancer, or pancreatitis. There is substantial overlap, however, and high ascitic fluid protein may be seen in as many as 25% of cirrhotic patients with uncomplicated ascites. Such a condition may also be seen during effective diuresis. A low-protein ascites is reported in 30% of patients with malignant ascites. Thus use of total ascitic protein for diagnosis is hazardous.

The serum-ascites albumin concentration gradient, a measure of oncotic pressure gradient that indicates the presence or absence of portal hypertension, provides better discrimination between the ascites of cirrhosis and that of malignancy. A gradient of >1.1 favors cirrhosis and portal hypertension, whereas a lower value favors a noncirrhotic etiology such as a malignancy. The mean number of polymorphonuclear neutrophils in the uninfected ascites is $60/mm^3$. Neutrophil counts of $>250\ mm^3$ (total white blood cell count × % of neutrophils ÷ 100) indicate peritonitis. Predominantly, mononuclear fluid is suggestive of chronic infection, i.e., tuberculosis. An elevated serum lactic dehydrogenase level (>400 units) in ascites or an ascitic fluid/serum lactic dehydrogenase ratio of more than 6.0 suggests the presence of malignancy. The presence of blood in the ascitic fluid also suggests malignancy, which may be confirmed by a positive cytologic examination, although atypical mesothelial cells may yield false-positive interpretations. Pancreatitic ascites typically has a high specific gravity, a high protein concentration, increased numbers of polymorphonuclear leukocytes, and, almost invariably, an elevated amylase concentration. Increased triglycerides in ascitic fluid indicate chylous ascites and suggest the presence of lymphatic disruption due to tumor, infection, or trauma. Rarely, chylous ascites is seen in uncomplicated cirrhosis. Debris and high cell counts may produce a cloudy fluid (pseudochylous ascites).

Complications

Many complications of ascites result directly from increased intra-abdominal pressure and thus are proportional to the volume and rate of accumulation of the fluid. Complications include anorexia, vomiting, reflux esophagitis, dyspnea, ventral hernia, and leakage of ascitic fluid into the chest and along other tissue planes (e.g., into the scrotum). In addition, the increased pressure may contribute to esophageal variceal bleeding.

A common complication of ascites is the development of spontaneous bacterial peritonitis. It occurs in 10% to 27% of patients with alcoholic cirrhosis, but may be seen in other forms of liver disease as well. The full-blown clinical picture consists of an abrupt onset of fever, chills, abdominal pain with rebound tenderness, absent bowel sounds, and leukocytosis. However, the patient may be asymptomatic or may have only unexplained fever, hypothermia, hypotension, abdominal discomfort, encephalopathy, or unexplained deterioration. Diagnostic paracentesis as well as cultures of the ascitic fluid and blood should be obtained. In most instances, only a single organism is recovered, usually *Escherichia coli,* but a number of other bacteria have also been implicated. Three fourths are enteric organisms. In 70% of patients with acute bacterial infection, the blood culture is also positive. Anaerobic infection is rare. For optimal results, 10 ml of ascitic fluid should be inoculated into a blood culture bottle at the bedside. The sensitivity of this method is 93%. In contrast, if the usual method of inoculating 1 ml of fluid into agar plates or meat broth is used, the sensitivity is only 43%. Spontaneous bacterial peritonitis may be difficult to distinguish from peritonitis due to intestinal perforation in a patient with ascites. Favoring the latter are the following ascitic fluid features: protein > 1.0 g/dl, glucose < 50 mg/dl, lactic dehydrogenase > 225 IU, and recovery of multiple microorganisms on culture.

Many factors are involved in the pathogenesis of spontaneous bacterial peritonitis, including impaired ability of the hepatic reticuloendothelial system to filter enteric bacteria, decreased antimicrobial activity of the ascitic fluid because of low complement levels, and loss of opsonins and phagocytic activity of neutrophils. Spontaneous bacterial peritonitis is probably acquired by hematogenous spread of microorganisms from foci of infection elsewhere (urinary tract, skin), or bacteremia secondary to invasive procedures. Low ascitic fluid protein (i.e., low opsonins) predisposes cirrhotic patients to spontaneous bacterial peritonitis.

There are two variants of spontaneous bacterial peritonitis: culture-negative neutrocytic ascites, in which the ascitic fluid neutrophil count exceeds $250/mm^3$, and bacterascites, in which the ascitic fluid culture is positive but the neutrophil count is normal. These variants are otherwise similar clinically to the typical case and occur in the same clinical setting. They are managed as the main type.

Treatment of spontaneous bacterial peritonitis with a broad-spectrum antibiotic (cefotaxime) should be started promptly if the diagnosis is strongly suspected because of the high mortality, which may be as high as 78%. Narrower spectrum antibiotics can be substituted when the sensitivity results are obtained. Aminoglycosides in conjunction with ampicillin are no longer advocated because of the potential for nephrotoxicity. The optimal duration of antibiotic treatment is not known; most clinicians treat for 7 to 10 days, but as short a period as 4 days has been satisfactory. Follow-up paracentesis at 48 hours may be helpful in that a fall in the ascitic fluid white count implies response to therapy. Patients who have an increased ascitic fluid neutrophil count but a negative culture should be treated similarly. An associated positive blood culture requires a longer course of antibiotics. Antibiotic therapy for spontaneous bacterial peritonitis is generally successful, but the probability of recurrence is high, particularly in patients who have an ascitic fluid protein of ≤ 1 g/dl, serum bilirubin > 4 mg/dl, and prothrombin time ≤ 45% of normal. In patients likely to have a recurrence, prophylactic oral nonabsorbable antibiotics or norfloxacin (400 mg/day) may be of benefit.

Treatment

Because ascites is a complication of liver failure, management should start with attempts to improve hepatic function. Treatment for liver failure depends on the nature of the dysfunction and should include abstinence from alcohol, provision of nutrients for hepatic regeneration, and treatment with penicillamine for Wilson's disease or with corticosteroids for autoimmune chronic active hepatitis. In many instances, such therapy or spontaneous hepatic healing results in a decrease in ascites. It is also important to establish that ascites is not due to, or complicated by, another process; such verification is best accomplished by diagnostic paracentesis of 50 to 200 ml of fluid (see above). Measurements of baseline serum and urinary sodium concentrations are useful in deciding on further therapy of ascites. When urinary sodium is high (> 10 mEq/L), the patient is likely to respond well to therapy. Moderate periods of bed rest and initial restriction of dietary sodium intake to 500 mg/day may cause significant diuresis in such patients. Rest should not preclude physical activity that is adequate to prevent muscle atrophy, and the diet should not be so restrictive as to result in inadequate intake of nutrients.

If diuretics are required, it is wise to follow certain general principles. The maximum rate of peritoneal fluid reabsorption is only about 9 dl/day or less. Peripheral edema is mobilized more rapidly than ascites and tends to serve as a safety valve for fluid loss. Diuresis should not exceed 1 to 2 lb/day in the presence of edema and about 0.3 to 0.5 lb/day in the absence of edema. Otherwise, excessive diuresis may result in loss of plasma volume, with eventual azotemia, hyponatremia, hypokalemia, and encephalopathy. Thus the rate of diuresis, serum electrolyte concentration, and renal and mental function must be followed carefully, and the diuretic dosage adjusted according to response. Caution is particularly important when dry weight is approached and/or when larger doses of diuretics are needed to obtain a response.

When diuretics are used, it is reasonable to begin with spironolactone (Aldactone), 50 to 200 mg/day. This drug is an inhibitor of aldosterone-mediated distal tubular sodium reabsorption, and an effective dosage can be roughly titrated to urinary sodium excretion and overall diuretic response. Frequently, 200 mg/day is adequate, but if urinary sodium remains below 10 mEq/L and diuresis does not ensue, dosages of up to 300 to 600 mg/day may be used with success. The urinary sodium/potassium ratio may be helpful in adjusting the dose. Patients with a ratio of more than 1.0 are likely to respond to small doses (100 to 200 mg/day), whereas those with a lower ratio tend to need larger doses of spironolactone and to require loop diuretics. Spironolactone works slowly; diuresis begins in 3 to 4 days. This diuretic is not generally toxic, although gynecomastia in males, lactation in females, and hyperkalemia may be side effects.

More potent diuretics are available. Thiazides interfere with sodium reabsorption primarily in distal tubules. Both furosemide and ethacrynic acid impair sodium reabsorption in the loop of Henle. These drugs, which waste potassium, ideally should be used in conjunction with spironolactone, which conserves potassium. They should be administered intermittently and in the lowest effective dose so as to minimize the incidence of azotemia and electrolyte abnormalities. Some general and specific recommendations for diuretic therapy are shown in Table 56-4. In general, the higher the dose and the more potent the diuretic needed to obtain an effective response, the more severe the liver disease and the higher the complication rate from the drug. Diuretics should be stopped with the appearance of azotemia, encephalopathy, or electrolyte disturbances. Because the more potent loop diuretics may precipitate hypokalemic alkalosis, potassium supplements may be needed. Cirrhotic patients with ascites may also have significant hyponatremia, especially after treatment with diuretics. Although hyponatremia may rarely result from sodium loss via diarrhea or excessive diuresis, it is usually due to overhydration induced by impaired generation of free water in the distal nephron. Modest hyponatremia (125 to 132 mEq/L) that is dilutional and unaccompanied by neurologic symptoms can be treated with osmotic diuretics, such as mannitol, to induce diuresis of water in excess of electrolytes. More severe dilutional hyponatremia requires water restriction to the equivalent of insensible loss (500 to 700 ml) plus urine output. Rarely, sodium may have to be given cautiously if neurologic signs are evident.

There are instances when ascites is so tense as to cause great discomfort, respiratory distress, formation and rupture of umbilical hernia, negative effects on cardiovascular function, and perhaps variceal bleeding. Therapeutic paracentesis is indicated to relieve these symptoms or to treat ascites that is refractory to the usual medical management. Serial large-volume paracentesis (4 to 6 liters) with close

Table 56-4. Suggested stepwise treatment of ascites

Therapy	Dosage
Sodium restriction*	0.5-2.0 g/day
Bed rest	—
Spironolactone	50-600 mg/day
Furosemide† (or other loop diuretic) large volume paracentesis‡	40-400 mg/day
Peritoneovenous (LeVeen) shunt‡ or TIPS‡	—

Note: Usual procedure is to start with sodium restriction (often with low dosages of spironolactone) and gradually increase spironolactone dosage, eventually adding furosemide if ascites is refractory. Incidence of side effects increases with intensity of diuretic use.

*With substantially reduced serum sodium levels (see text), water restriction may become necessary.

†If used alone, supplemental potassium usually required.

‡See text.

monitoring of vital signs can be carried out safely. Large-volume paracentesis has been advocated also in patients who do not have tense ascites to relieve the ascites more quickly and to shorten the hospital stay, but the ascites often recurs unless subsequent control by diuretics and sodium restriction can be achieved. Alternatively, repeated large volume paracenteses are carried out. Most, but not all clinicians, advocate concomitant use of intravenous albumin with large volume paracentesis (40 g for each 5 liters removed) or equivalent and less expensive dextran to minimize any significant hemodynamic changes or deterioration of renal function. The role of paracenteses in lowering serum and ascitic complement and possible enhancement of spontaneous peritonitis requires further study.

Other measures have been tried to treat refractory ascites. In selected patients with good liver function, lowering of portal pressure with a side-to-side shunt has been used with some success. More recently, success has been reported with percutaneous placement of an intrahepatic shunt between portal and hepatic veins to lower portal pressure. This procedure is sometimes referred to as TIPS (transjugular intrahepatic portolsystemic shunt). Another procedure involves the reinfusion of ascitic fluid by a peritoneovenous (LeVeen) shunt. A one-way, pressure-activated valve interposed in a tube connecting the peritoneal cavity and the superior vena cava is implanted. This shunt allows ascitic fluid to flow into the systemic circulation when a positive pressure gradient is generated between the peritoneal and venous systems. Although resistant ascites may respond to peritoneovenous shunt placement, the response is usually transient, and this treatment carries a significant incidence of serious complications. These include consumptive coagulopathy, pulmonary edema, infection, shunt occlusion, and precipitation of variceal bleeding. The procedure is clearly contraindicated in patients with peritoneal sepsis, severe coagulation abnormalities, heart failure, a history of variceal bleeding, and acute, severe liver disease. There is no evidence that this procedure improves with the use of serial paracentesis or prolongs life.

PORTAL HYPERTENSION

Clinical features

Portal hypertension, which results from obstruction of portal blood flow due to extrahepatic or intrahepatic lesions, is manifested by splenomegaly, ascites, and formation of collateral veins, seen as prominent vessels in the anterior abdominal wall. Varices are collateral vessels that develop at the esophagogastric junction due to dilatation of the esophageal venous plexuses (esophageal varices) or short gastric veins (gastric varices). Portal hypertension may be asymptomatic or may lead to variceal bleeding, hypersplenism, or ascites. Portal hypertension is a common complication of chronic liver disease, but it may rarely be seen during acute hepatic decompensation in alcoholic or viral hepatitis. When it occurs in acute liver failure, portal hypertension may resolve as hepatic function improves. The clinical manifestations of portal hypertension may be the only overt evidence of chronic liver disease if hepatic fibrosis and cirrhosis are present without active hepatitis, or it may be accompanied by other signs of liver failure. In virtually all patients with clinically significant portal hypertension due to liver disease, careful clinical examination and laboratory tests reveal some hepatic abnormality.

Varices

Bleeding from gastroesophageal varices is the most important complication of portal hypertension. The presence of varices is best diagnosed by gastrointestinal endoscopy, which also reveals whether the varices are the site of bleeding (Chapter 30). Barium swallow and arteriography are less sensitive or desirable methods of diagnosis. Sometimes CT detects esophageal varices or other intraperitoneal venous collaterals. Occasionally, varices are also present in the peritoneal cavity and other parts of the bowel, i.e., small intestine, colonic, or rectal (hemorrhoidal) varices. Bleeding, however, usually is from the gastroesophageal area.

Variceal bleeding primarily reflects portal hypertension; acid reflux is not believed to contribute importantly to bleeding. There is no clear agreement as to whether bleeding correlates with increasing portal pressure, although some feel that hemorrhage is seen usually above a portal pressure of 12 mmHg. Portal pressure can be measured by percutaneous hepatic or splenic manometry, via catheterization of the umbilical or portal veins or by determining the net wedge hepatic vein pressure (wedge pressure minus free hepatic vein pressure).

Demonstration of bleeding gastroesophageal varices requires further elucidation of the cause of the varices. Most commonly, they are due to chronic parenchymal liver disease with postsinusoidal and sinusoidal obstruction of the portal blood flow into the liver secondary to portal fibrosis and regenerating cirrhotic nodules. Sometimes, bleeding gastroesophageal varices may be due to postsinusoidal obstruction from hepatic vein thrombosis, veno-occlusive disease, or to intrahepatic presinusoidal compression from sarcoidosis or schistosomiasis. These forms of portal hypertension can be confirmed by morphologic examination of liver tissue obtained by percutaneous or laparoscopic liver biopsy, by measurement of net wedge hepatic vein pressure, or by other techniques for determining postsinusoidal and sinusoidal pressure. It is essential to establish that the varices are not due solely to extrahepatic (presinusoidal) vascular obstruction caused by thrombosis, cavernomatous transformation of the portal vein, or by occlusion of the splenic vein due to pancreatitis, pseudocyst, or pancreatic carcinoma. The extrahepatic cause of the portal hypertension can be established by angiography, by finding a normal net wedge hepatic vein pressure, and by normal hepatic histology. The presence of gastric varices (which can mimic a gastric tumor) without associated esophageal varices suggests a segmental portal hypertension secondary to splenic vein obstruction. It is essential to recognize this condition because it is curable by splenectomy. Rarely, portal hypertension may be due to increased portal volume caused by splenic arteriovenous malformations, or it may have no apparent explanation. Portal hypertension may also contribute to development of congestive gastropathy, a common cause of gastric bleeding in these patients. Congestive colopathy also has been described.

Treatment

See the accompanying box for a treatment plan.

Medical therapy. The first step in the medical management of a patient with bleeding gastroesophageal varices is to ensure adequate circulation with transfusion of fresh-frozen plasma and packed cells. Because patients with liver disease often have a deficiency of clotting factors, at least some of the plasma should be fresh. After the vital signs are stabilized, it is mandatory to establish the cause of bleeding, as many patients with varices bleed from other causes (Chapter 34). The precise diagnosis is best established by endoscopic examination. Alternatively, if bleeding is too brisk to permit adequate endoscopic visualization of the upper gastrointestinal tract, angiography may be used to define not only the site of bleeding but also, in preparation for possible surgery, the vascular anatomy of the portal circulation.

After the diagnosis of bleeding varices is made, laxatives and enemas are given to evacuate blood from the intestinal tract. This strategy helps prevent the development of hepatic encephalopathy because blood in the gut is a source of nitrogenous toxins. Patients with severe liver disease who bleed into the gastrointestinal tract should receive short-term prophylactic treatment with lactulose. If the bleeding does not stop following gastric lavage, vasopressin (Pitressin) is given. There is no evidence that direct infusion of vasopressin into the superior mesenteric artery is more effective or less toxic than intravenous administration of the drug. Both routes of administration can lead to cardiac arrhythmia, sepsis, and other complications. Accordingly, the intravenous route is the preferred approach. There is no clear agreement about the optimal dosage and duration of treatment. One approach is to administer 0.4 IU/min for 12 hours with subsequent decrements of about 0.1 IU/min every 12 hours for a total of 24 to 36 hours. Another approach is to use this dose of vasopressin (or up to 0.9 IU/min if necessary) for only 2 to 4 hours and then change to other therapy, if needed, on an elective basis. Some have suggested lower doses, 0.2 IU/min for 48 hours to maximize effectiveness and decrease side effects. The addition of 0.4 mg sublingual nitroglycerin has been suggested as an adjunctive measure to reduce the toxic effects of vasopressin. Also shown to be effective is glypressin, which lacks the side effects of vasopressin. However, glypressin is not yet available for clinical use in the United States.

If administration of vasopressin does not stop the bleeding, there are several options. The patient can be evaluated for possible surgery, or an attempt can be made to tamponade the varices with a Sengstaken-Blakemore balloon or one of its modifications, and surgery can be considered if this therapeutic maneuver fails. Tamponade may be effective in stopping variceal bleeding, at least for a short time, and is useful in treating patients with vasopressin-resistant bleeding varices but is a difficult procedure with many serious complications (airway obstruction, arrhythmias, etc.) and therefore requires experienced medical and nursing personnel. There is a tendency to use endoscopic sclerosis of varices as the initial invasive therapy of choice. This procedure is generally easier to perform in patients in whom overt variceal bleeding has ceased. The approach varies with the clinical condition of the patient, the status of the liver, and with the experience and persuasion of the physician for these techniques. The techniques for sclerotherapy (vehicle, frequency, etc.) vary and are discussed in specialized texts. Endoscopic rubberband ligation is another promising approach and may cause few complications than sclerosis.

If bleeding stops, the condition of the patient and prior history of variceal bleeding usually define management. With a history of multiple prior bleeding and adequate hepatic reserve, some form of surgery to lower portal pressure may be indicated. With no prior bleeding and especially with concomitant severe liver disease an expectant approach may be adopted or beta blockers may be tried (see below).

If bleeding stops and then recurs, the options include repeat sclerotherapy or ligation, tamponade, and/or percutaneous placement of an intrahepatic shunt between the portal and hepatic veins to lower portal pressure rapidly; if

Stepwise management of bleeding esophageal varices

Blood replacement (fresh blood)
Gastric lavage (large-bore tube)
Evacuation of blood from gut
? Antacids or H_2-receptor antagonist*
Vasopressin (intravenous)

If bleeding stops	**If bleeding continues**
Endoscopic sclerosis†	Endoscopic sclerosis or tamponade‡
Surgery§	Percutaneous intrahepatic portal-hepatic vein shunt (TIPS;-see text)
	Coronary vein embolization‖
	Surgery§

*Benefit uncertain.
†May be used either as a temporary procedure to arrest bleeding in preparation for future elective surgery or as a definitive procedure, especially in patients with severe liver disease.
§Surgery may be especially considered in patients with less severe hepatic dysfunction. See text for types of surgery available, indications, and complications.
‡Exact place of tamponade in this schema is controversial. Some physicians avoid its use with mild hepatic dysfunction and go to surgery directly. Others use endoscopic sclerosis initially, even in acutely bleeding patients, at times before or together with vasopressin.
‖Procedure has significant side effects and is usually used only as second line of therapy.

these fail, other options include transhepatic coronary vein embolization or construction of a surgical shunt. The available data do not clearly favor any one of these approaches. Surgical shunting clearly prevents subsequent bleeding, but at the price of increased mortality during surgery and a greater risk of postoperative encephalopathy. Patients with less severe liver disease and those operated on electively do better. Continued sclerotherapy has a higher incidence of breakthrough bleeding and has its own risks (ulceration, perforation and mediastinitis, esophageal stenosis and bleeding, pleural effusions and fever). At times the initial approach may be sclerotherapy, followed by a surgical shunt when the sclerotherapy fails. Less rigorous surgical procedures (esophageal transection of varices by stapling) may be of temporary value but do not address the underlying portal hypertension, potential for delayed variceal bleeding, and eventual need for surgical shunt. The newest procedure, a percutaneous intrahepatic shunt between portal and hepatic veins is relatively easy to perform, even in patients with a severely decompensated liver, does lower portal pressure and allows hepatic transplantation at a later date. Its longer term outlook (potency, complications), however, is not known, and it has not been subjected to a controlled trial against other therapeutic modalities. Thus one must consider the chronic management of recurrent bleeding varices (especially in the setting of severe liver disease) as unresolved with several options available but without one in particular that has clearly been shown to prolong life in these very ill patients. In general, in patients with less severe liver disease who continue to bleed, some form of surgery, ideally elective, seems reasonable. In such patients with severe liver disease, an intrahepatic shunt might be tried, but no approach has been shown to be optimal. Hepatic transplantation is another alternative that addresses the whole problem at once (Chapter 64).

The difficult therapeutic challenge posed by bleeding varices has clearly not been fully met, and other invasive and noninvasive alternatives have been tried. One noninvasive approach is to lower portal pressure by pharmacologic means. Although the subject is still somewhat controversial, overall assessment of all the data suggests that beta blockers such as propranolol, given in doses of 20 to 180 mg twice a day, sufficient to lower resting cardiac rate by 25%, may decrease portal pressure and with it bleeding from varices and congestive gastropathy. This reaction seems to occur more in better compensated patients, but the subset that responds best is difficult to identify without actual measurement of portal pressure. It should be emphasized that propranolol metabolism is decreased in cirrhosis and the drug easily penetrates into the brain and may depress mentation so that careful monitoring and dose adjustment may be required. Other less lipophilic blockers may be better tolerated, but are less well studied.

Because the mortality from variceal bleeding is very high (25% to 65% in various patient populations) studies have been made of some form of prophylactic therapy, including prophylactic sclerotherapy, beta blockers, and even portacaval shunting. Although some favorable results have been reported, no consistent benefit (in terms of survival) from any of these procedures has been documented. Some investigators noted increased mortality with prophylactic sclerotherapy. Perhaps a critical subset of patients that may benefit has not yet been identified. Because only about one in four patients with varices bleeds from that site, prior detection of these individuals would be most helpful. This area is under active study. Endoscopy is useful to detect features predictive of future esophageal bleeding: (1) red color signs (cherry red spots, red wale markings, hematocystic spots), (2) gastric varices, and (3) large varices (> 5 mm). These endoscopic features, however, do not predict mortality.

Surgical therapy. Two main types of therapeutic shunts have been used. The first, consisting of portacaval or proximal splenorenal shunts, permits major diversion of portal flow into the inferior vena cava. This type of shunt has been shown to prevent subsequent variceal bleeding, but unfortunately has led to a high incidence of hepatic failure, and the long-term survival rate has not been prolonged in controlled studies. Portosystemic encephalopathy and hepatic iron overload (presumably due to enhanced iron absorption) have been postshunt complications.

The second type of shunt, distal splenorenal shunt, is more selective in that the varices are drained via a splenic-to-renal vein anastomosis, and superior mesenteric vein flow to the liver is maintained. The procedure, however, is technically difficult and is not advised in the presence of significant nonresponsive ascites, which it tends to worsen. Portal pressure is not lowered rapidly with this procedure; hence it may not be an option with acute bleeding. The distal splenorenal shunt may be initially associated with a lower incidence of hepatic encephalopathy, although in patients with alcoholic cirrhosis overall survival has not been enhanced. Ideally, the distal splenorenal shunt should be performed in patients whose hepatic portal flow a priori is good, as its diversion by a portacaval shunt might induce liver failure. Better techniques for measuring portal flow before surgery and correlation of portal flow with clinical outcome after surgery are needed to validate this concept. In patients with advanced liver disease, surgical transection of esophageal varices using the stapling gun has been performed with promising preliminary results but without alteration of the underlying problem of portal hypertension. Other, much less frequently used surgical procedures are usually reserved for patients with vascular anomalies or extensive prior surgery and complications that render the procedures discussed earlier technically impossible. These include transesophageal ligation of varices and gastric devascularization and splenectomy.

Hypersplenism

Obstruction to portal flow may cause hypersplenism, with increased destruction of all or some of the blood elements. These hematologic abnormalities are usually not severe and as a rule do not produce clinical problems or require therapy.

In the presence of a depressed platelet count, bleeding

time is a good index of adequacy of hemostasis. It is always important to rule out other causes of anemia, thrombocytopenia, and leukopenia (i.e., bone marrow suppression by drugs). The effect of surgical portal decompression on hypersplenism is unpredictable.

HEPATORENAL SYNDROME

Clinical picture

The development of unexplained progressive renal failure in a patient with liver disease should suggest the possibility of hepatorenal syndrome. This disorder is characterized by azotemia, usually oliguria, a concentrated urine with a urine/plasma osmolality ratio greater than 1.0, and a urinary sodium concentration of less than 10 mEq/L (often only 1 to 2 mEq/L). The urine is generally acid and may contain small amounts of protein, hyaline and granular casts, and a few erythrocytes. The syndrome usually appears in patients with decompensated cirrhosis and ascites, sometimes spontaneously but usually after forced diuresis, uncontrolled diarrhea, gastrointestinal hemorrhage, or other insults. Hepatorenal syndrome may also develop less commonly in acute liver failure due to alcoholism or viral or toxic hepatitis. This syndrome must be differentiated from other types of renal failure that may accompany liver diseases, including renal failure from exposure to toxins such as carbon tetrachloride or acetaminophen, leptospirosis or other infections, acute tubular necrosis due to hypotension from gastrointestinal bleeding or aminoglycoside ingestion, and obstructive uropathy. In patients with acute tubular necrosis, the urine has low, fixed specific gravity; urinary sodium excretion is usually high; and there may be a characteristic sediment (Chapter 347). The other entities require a careful history, examination, and culture of the urine and at times a radiographic evaluation for diagnosis. It should be appreciated that patients with cirrhosis may have subtle renal dysfunction not reflected by the serum creatinine. The latter may be falsely low due to large plasma volume and decreased muscle mass. The physician should be sure that the renal failure in cirrhosis is not due to simple volume depletion from diarrhea, excessive diuresis, or leakage of ascitic fluid. Renal failure in some patients who respond to fluid repletion is mistakenly diagnosed as hepatorenal syndrome. This illustrates the prevailing confusion concerning the pathogenesis of hepatorenal syndrome, which may be a spectrum of functional renal failures, the early manifestations of which are reversible with fluid replacement. Until the pathogenesis of this syndrome is elucidated, the term *hepatorenal syndrome* should apply only to renal failure occurring in patients with liver disease whose renal dysfunction is unresponsive to short-term intravenous fluid repletion and in whom other known causes of renal failure are excluded.

Pathogenesis

The exact pathogenesis of hepatorenal syndrome is unclear. It is generally agreed that it is a functional disorder of the kidneys caused primarily by liver disease. This agreement is based on the observations that (1) there are no important morphologic changes in the kidneys, (2) the kidneys regain normal function when implanted in a recipient without liver disease, and (3) renal function improves when liver disease abates or if a healthy liver is implanted in the patient. Most evidence suggests that the primary abnormality in the kidneys is altered renal blood flow. Causes postulated have included changes in "effective" blood volume and increased sympathetic tone, possibly due to accumulation of false neurotransmitters at nerve endings, and increased peripheral as well as renal arteriovenous shunting, possibly due to accumulation and alteration of the normal balance of humoral agents such as prostaglandins, vasoactive peptides, and kinins. At present, the relative roles of these possible mechanisms (which are not mutually exclusive) are uncertain, although the concept of an altered humoral milieu is popular. Recent studies in rats suggest the presence of a hepatorenal reflex. Glutamine infusion into the mesenteric vein, but not to the jugular or femoral vein, induces hepatocyte swelling and decreased renal function. Renal or hepatic denervation abolishes these adverse effects on renal function. Glucagon infusion into the mesenteric vein, but not into the jugular vein, prevents the renal effects of glutamine infusion; these findings suggest the existence of a substance, possibly released from the liver, that is capable of regulating renal function by way of the hepatorenal innervations. It may be that this syndrome reflects a continuum or spectrum of disorders, with a somewhat different mechanism for each type of dysfunction. A more likely possibility is that the hepatorenal syndrome starts with subclinical renal dysfunction due to decreased and/or unstable perfusion of the kidneys in many patients with severe liver disease, and that this is augmented in some patients by further liver failure and in most by various precipitants such as gastrointestinal hemorrhage. This possibility implies that a unitary underlying mechanism produces hepatorenal syndrome. The possible interaction in the genesis of this syndrome is shown in Fig. 56-2.

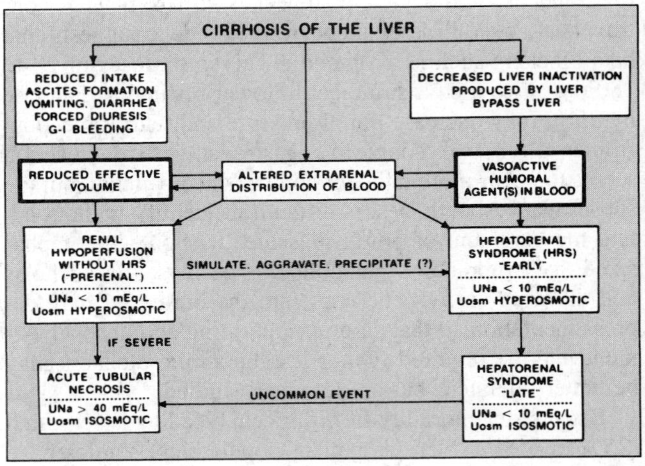

Fig. 56-2. A tentative formulation of the interrelationship of hypoperfusion and a humoral agent in the genesis of hepatorenal syndrome. UNa, urinary sodium concentration; Uosm, urinary osmolality. (From Papper S: The kidney in liver disease, New York, 1983, Elsevier.)

Prognosis and treatment

The prognosis of hepatorenal syndrome is very poor, indicating the lack of established, effective therapy. Defined rigorously (creatinine over 2.5 mg/dl), it is likely that mortality associated with this syndrome is 90% or more. The only favorable prognostic feature in one series of 30 patients was a urine volume of over 5 dl/24 hr.

Management of hepatorenal syndrome consists first of the exclusion of other, more treatable causes of renal failure such as infection, obstruction, or acute tubular damage. Another key approach is to identify, remove, or treat any factors known to precipitate renal failure in patients with severe liver disease; that is, diuretics should not be administered, blood volume lost via hemorrhage or dehydration should be replaced, correcting electrolyte problems should be corrected, and sepsis should be treated. Nonsteroidal anti-inflammatory agents should not be administered to patients with severe liver disease, as there is evidence that these inhibitors of prostaglandin synthesis may precipitate renal failure, because prostaglandins help to maintain effective renal blood flow. All patients with apparent hepatorenal syndrome should undergo a short trial of fluid replacement with albumin, plasma, or saline to increase plasma volume in those few patients in whom a decrease in plasma volume (total or effective) is present but inapparent. Administration of fluid must be monitored carefully (preferably by central venous pressure measurements) to document adequate volume replacement and to reduce the risk of precipitating heart failure or variceal hemorrhage with excessive fluid administration. Fluid should be discontinued if there is no clear diuretic response.

Numerous agents have been tried in the treatment of hepatorenal syndrome. Most have been used on the premise that this disorder is due to renal vasoconstriction. Unfortunately, no consistent benefit has been observed in these trials, in which phentolamine, acetylcholine, papaverine, aminophylline, metaraminol, phenoxybenzamine hydrochloride (Dibenzyline), prostaglandin E_1, and dopamine have been used. In most trials, only a few patients were studied.

In patients with potentially reversible liver disease, renal failure may be transiently controlled with dialysis to allow the liver to heal with the hope that renal function will benefit.

There are a few reports of recovery from hepatorenal syndrome after portacaval shunt and orthotopic liver transplantation, but these are drastic measures inapplicable to most patients with this disorder. Perhaps TIPS (see earlier) might be of benefit in patients who are not candidates for hepatic transplantation. The LeVeen shunt has been reported to benefit some of these patients. However, overall results from controlled studies have not been encouraging.

ENDOCRINE DISTURBANCES

(See also Chapters 157, 158, 165, and 166)

Clinical features

In patients with chronic hepatic failure, a number of endocrine disturbances may be observed, including raised fasting levels of plasma growth hormone, abnormal glucose tolerance test results despite normal or high insulin levels, decreased thyroxine values, increased aldosterone, cushingoid features, and changes in sex hormones. Of these, the most dramatic are the prominent manifestations of hypogonadism that affect both sexes and overt feminization in males. In females, gonadal failure is characterized by atrophy of the uterus and breasts. There may be loss of libido, and, in females of childbearing age, menstrual periods are erratic, excessive, diminished, or absent altogether. As a result, these women may be unable to conceive. In postmenopausal women, hypogonadism may have little clinical consequence. Gonadal failure in males is manifested by gross and histologic evidence of testicular atrophy (50% to 75%) associated with impotence (79%) and, in those capable of ejaculation, with a marked decrease in sperm counts. Moreover, males with cirrhosis have decreased body hair (47%), slower beard growth, a smaller prostate, and decreased incidence of benign prostatic hypertrophy. Histologically, the testes of men with alcoholic liver disease have reduced germinal epithelium and moderate peritubular fibrosis, but the Leydig cells may be normal. In addition, males with cirrhosis assume several feminine physical characteristics, most often gynecomastia (14% to 52%), which may be unilateral initially, but which eventually becomes bilateral. Occasionally, patients with fibrolamellar carcinoma of the liver, a distinct variant of hepatocellular carcinoma, may develop gynecomastia as the presenting symptom. Other, less dramatic signs of feminization include a female body habitus and escutcheon (64%), cutaneous vascular spider nevi (74%), and palmar erythema (51%).

Presumed mechanisms

There is a paucity of studies on the sex hormone changes in females. However, raised estrogen levels and impaired conversion of progesterone to pregnanediol have been noted in some females with cirrhosis. The precise mechanism of gonadal failure in females is still unclear. In contrast, more studies have been carried out to determine the mechanisms responsible for both hypogonadism and the overt feminization in male patients with cirrhosis. Therefore subsequent discussion will be confined mainly to hormonal changes observed in males.

The observation that in males with cirrhosis the urinary excretion of estrogens increases while that of testosterone decreases led to the theory that gynecomastia and the other endocrine features of cirrhosis were caused by an accumulation of estrogen due to impaired estrogen degradation by the liver. However, the clearance of estrogens in male cirrhotic patients may be normal; thus the matter is complex. Moreover, the available data are sometimes conflicting, perhaps because of differences in the methods of measuring the pertinent hormones and because of variations in the patient populations studied. Nevertheless, certain general remarks are warranted.

Androgen formation and regulation. Testosterone is converted by a series of biochemical steps from cholesterol, which may be synthesized de novo in the Leydig cells of the testes or extracted from the plasma pool. Only about 25 μg of testosterone is stored in normal testes, and to provide the average 6 mg secreted into the plasma in healthy young males, the total hormone content turns over approximately 200 times daily. Testosterone is transported in plasma, bound largely to a specific carrier protein (sex-hormone-binding globulin) and to albumin. Only 1% to 3% of testosterone remains free or unbound to plasma proteins, but it is this free fraction that is capable of combining with receptors to exert the biologic activity of the hormone. In the peripheral tissues, testosterone is converted to two active metabolites. Under the action of alpha$_5$-reductase, it is reduced to dihydrotestosterone, which possesses actions necessary for sexual differentiation and virilization. In addition, testosterone may be aromatized to estradiol. An estrogenic compound, estrone, which may be further converted to estriol, can also be derived form androstenedione, a testosterone precursor secreted principally from the adrenals. Primary liver cancer is capable of aromatizing androgens to estrogenic compounds, and this process may explain the feminization in patients with fibrolamellar carcinoma of the liver. Small amounts of dihydrotestosterone and estradiol may be derived directly from the testes and indirectly from the adrenal gland. Regulation of testosterone secretion is exerted largely by luteinizing hormone (LH) and to some extent by follicle-stimulating hormone (FSH), both from the pituitary. Testosterone in turn exerts a feedback influence on the pituitary to modulate the sensitivity of the gland to the LH-releasing hormone (LHRH) from the hypothalamus.

Hypogonadism. In male cirrhotic patients, the total testosterone concentrations in the plasma are significantly reduced. This hypotestosteronemia is associated with a marked increase in the sex-hormone-binding globulin. Consequently, the unbound testosterone fraction also falls. The low level of testosterone is due mainly to its diminished production by the testes. Despite an associated decrease in metabolic clearance, and notwithstanding peripheral conversion from androstenedione, which can provide up to 15% of the testosterone, normal plasma testosterone levels are not maintained. Plasma dihydrotestosterone is also low in cirrhosis.

That plasma androgen levels are low in cirrhosis appears to be accepted. The question then arises as to whether these low levels result from a local gonadal lesion or from a central hypothalamic-pituitary impairment. Some data suggest a double defect. The presence of low testosterone levels despite elevated LH and FSH concentrations in one third of patients suggests hyporesponsiveness of the testes to the stimulation of these gonadotropins. Furthermore, the rise of testosterone levels after the administration of human chorionic gonadotropin is less in cirrhotic patients than in healthy controls. This finding indicates a reduced Leydig cell reserve and suggests a gonadal defect. On the other hand, the presence of normal amounts of LH and FSH in two thirds of patients despite low testosterone levels implies a subnormal hypothalamic-pituitary response. Such a central defect, believed by some to play the more important role, is confirmed by the failure of cirrhotic patients to exhibit an adequate increase in LH and FSH secretion after the administration of clomiphene, a drug that interacts with estrogen-receptor sites to prevent the normal feedback inhibition of estrogens on the secretion of LH- and FSH-releasing hormones. The defect is further localized to the hypothalamus, as indicated by the either normal or supranormal pituitary response to the gonadotropin-releasing hormone in cirrhotic patients. The basis for the hypothalamic defect is not clear.

Feminization. The three principal estrogens found in the plasma of normal males are estrone, estradiol, and estriol. Of these, the most biologically potent is estradiol. Like testosterone, it is bound in the plasma to the sex-hormone-binding globulin and to albumin. Whereas the affinity of the sex-hormone-binding globulin is greater for testosterone than for estradiol, albumin has a greater affinity for estradiol than for testosterone. As a result, alterations in the sex-hormone-binding globulin may lead to greater changes in the level of unbound testosterone than in that of unbound estradiol. The effect of changes in plasma albumin concentrations on levels of unbound testosterone and estradiol is still to be determined.

Although the biochemical basis for hypogonadism in chronic hepatic failure is fairly well established, the mechanism for feminization remains controversial. While there may be a positive initial correlation between elevated estradiol level and the presence of spider nevi, palmar erythema, or gynecomastia in patients with cirrhosis, follow-up observations reveal that spider nevi and palmar erythema may appear and disappear without obvious correlation with clinical or hormonal status. Moreover, there are no simple correlations between the severity of the disease on one hand and plasma estradiol concentration or gynecomastia on the other, or between the degree of liver disease and testicular volume or plasma testosterone levels.

Results of plasma estradiol measurements in cirrhotic male patients are variable, ranging from normal to increased. Mean values, however, are significantly higher in cirrhotic patients than in controls. In addition, estrone levels may be elevated in cirrhotic male patients, with higher levels present in those with than in those without gynecomastia, perhaps as a result of increased estrone formation from androstenedione. The clinical significance of estrone elevation is unclear, as its biologic activity is weak. Nevertheless, these data provide some basis for the concept cited earlier that features of feminization are related to the accumulation of estrogen, at least in some patients with cirrhosis. The elevation of plasma estradiol is not easily explained, however, and estradiol levels in cirrhotic patients are not always high. The critical factor in feminization may be not the absolute level of estradiol but rather the level of free estradiol in relation to the unbound fraction of testosterone. The net result of a raised estrogen/testosterone ratio or free estradiol/free testosterone ratio is a tendency to feminization. When these ratios were compared in cirrhotic patients with and without gynecomastia, however, significant differences were found in some but not in other studies. This finding suggests that factors other than sex hormone levels or ratios may be important. These factors remain obscure. There is no correlation between estrogen receptor content or circulating hormone.

It has also been postulated that prolactin may be involved in the development of gynecomastia. Increased numbers of prolactin-secreting cells have been noted in patients dying of cirrhosis. Plasma prolactin levels are increased, with higher values in patients with gynecomastia than in those without it. Despite increased prolactin levels, galactorrhea is generally absent in cirrhotic males, with or without gynecomastia, raising questions regarding the clinical significance of such prolactin elevations. It has been proposed, however, that prolactin may potentiate the effect of estrogen by inducing or activating hepatic or other end-organ receptors for estrogens, thus contributing to the development of gynecomastia and enhancing the responsiveness of these receptors to estrogen action.

Malnutrition and alcohol. Many aspects of the relationship between the endocrine features and the hormonal abnormalities of cirrhosis remain obscure, and it is possible that other important factors are involved. At least two factors, malnutrition and alcoholism, are frequently associated with cirrhosis. Loss of libido, testicular atrophy, and suppression of gonadotropin and testosterone may be observed in malnutrition. Gynecomastia may be seen on refeeding, perhaps related to a rise in gonadotropin and estrogen secretion during recovery.

The role of alcohol consumption has been extensively investigated. Many of the endocrine abnormalities of chronic liver disease are noted in patients with alcoholic cirrhosis, but similar physical signs and hormonal changes may also be seen in patients with nonalcoholic cirrhosis. Unlike patients with alcoholic cirrhosis, however, males with viral liver disease of comparable histologic and biochemical derangements may have normal testosterone levels and show little evidence of gonadal failure. In addition, the responses to clomiphene or LHRH factor may be normal in nonalcoholic patients. There is also ample evidence that short-term alcohol consumption by nonalcoholic subjects fed an adequate diet leads to decreased testosterone levels without changes in LH levels. These findings suggest both an impairment of central hypothalamic-pituitary function and a local gonadal defect. Moreover, the metabolic clearance of testosterone in these subjects is increased, possibly related to enhanced A-ring reductase activity and decreased plasma binding capacity. More prolonged consumption of alcohol by these subjects is followed by a fall in LH. Thus alcohol itself may induce hormonal effects and perhaps even augment the influence of liver disease. Fig. 56-3 clearly illustrates this phenomenon. Finally, zinc deficiency, which may be seen in patients with alcoholic liver disease, may contribute to hypogonadism, probably by inducing Leydig cell failure.

Drugs. Gynecomastia related to drug use should be mentioned because one drug, spironolactone (Aldactone), is commonly used in the management of patients with cirrhosis. Spironolactone and cimetidine appear to be inhibitors of testosterone synthesis and both may suppress, in a competitive manner, the binding of dihydrotestosterone to its receptors. Other drugs that may induce gynecomastia include digitalis, marijuana, heroin, busulfan, ethionamide, methyldopa, tricyclic antidepressants, calcium-channel blockers, acetylcholine esterase inhibitors, penicillamine, and omeprazole. In patients with gynecomastia, occult Leydig cell tumor of the testes should be ruled out.

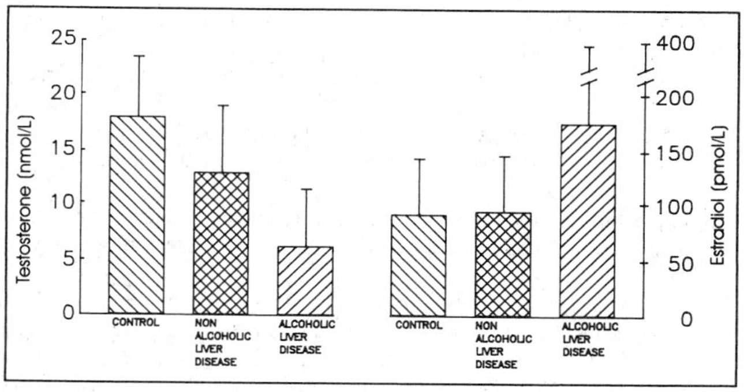

Fig. 56-3. Testosterone and estradiol levels in patients with comparable nonalcoholic and alcoholic liver disease. Statistical comparison reveals that the testosterone levels of both groups of patients are significantly lower than controls and that those with alcoholic liver disease have lower values than those with nonalcoholic liver disease; estradiol levels are higher in patients with alcoholic liver disease than in the two other groups in which values were similar. Thus liver disease causes changes in sex hormones, and these changes are made worse by alcohol. (Graphed from data reported by Bannister P et al: Q J Med 63:305, 1987.)

REFERENCES

Bannister P et al: Sex hormone changes in chronic liver disease: A matched study of alcoholic vs. non-alcoholic liver disease, Q J Med (new series) 63:305, 1987.

Cavanaugh J, Niewoehner CB, and Nuttall FQ: Gynecomastia and cirrhosis of the liver, Arch Intern Med 150:563-565, 1990.

Cello DP et al: Endoscopic sclerotherapy versus portacaval shunt in patients with severe cirrhosis and variceal hemorrhage, N Engl J Med 311:1589, 1984.

Conn HO et al: Propranolol in the prevention of the first hemorrhage from esophagogastric varices: a multicenter, randomized clinical trial, Hepatology 13:902-912, 1991.

De Franchis R et al: Prophylactic sclerotherapy in high-risk cirrhotics selected by endoscopic criteria, Gastroenterology 101:1087-1093, 1991.

Epstein M: Renal complications of liver disease, Clin Symp 37(5):31, 1985.

Galvaô-Tales A et al: Gonadal consequences of alcohol abuse: lessons from the liver, Hepatology 6:135, 1985.

Gines P et al: Paracentesis with intravenous infusion of albumin as compared with peritoneovenous shunting in cirrhosis with refractory ascites, N Engl J Med 325:829-835, 1991.

Gines P et al: Norfloxacine prevents spontaneous bacterial peritonitis recurrence in cirrhosis: results of a double-blind, placebo-controlled trial, Hepatology 12:716-724, 1990.

Herrera JL: Current medical management of cirrhotic ascites, Am J Med Sci 302:31-37, 1991.

Hoefs JC, and Jonas GM: Diagnostic paracentesis. In Stollerman GH et al, editors: Advances in internal medicine, vol 37, St Louis, 1992, Mosby–Year Book.

Hoyumpa AM, Jr and Schenker S: Perspective in hepatic encephalopathy, J Lab Clin Med 100:477, 1982.
Kleber G et al: Prediction of variceal hemorrhage in cirrhosis: a prospective follow-up study, Gastroenterology 100:1332-1337, 1991.
Maruyama Y et al: Mechanism of feminization in male patients with non-alcoholic liver cirrhosis: role of sex hormone-binding globulin, Gastroenterol Jpn 26:435-439, 1991.
Pinto PC et al: Large-volume paracentesis in non-edematous patients with tense ascites. Its effect on intravascular volume, Hepatology 8:207, 1988.
Prova Study Group: Prophylaxis of first hemorrhage from esophageal varices by sclerotherapy, propranolol or both in cirrhotic patients: A randomized multicenter trial, Hepatology 14:1016-1024, 1991.
Rocco VK et al: Cirrhotic ascites. Pathophysiology, diagnosis and management, Ann Intern Med 105:573, 1986.
Runyon BA: Spontaneous bacterial peritonitis: an explosion of information, Hepatology 8:171, 1988.
Runyon BA, Canawati HN, and Akriviadis EA: Optimization of ascitic fluid culture technique, Gastroenterology 95:1351-1355, 1988.
Schrier RW et al: Peripheral arterial vasodilation hypothesis: a proposal for the initiation of renal sodium and water retention in cirrhosis, Hepatology 8:1152, 1988.
Teres J et al: Sclerotherapy vs. distal splenorenal shunt in the elective treatment of variceal hemorrhage: a randomized controlled trial, Hepatology 7:430, 1987.
Terg R et al: Dextran administration avoids hemodynamic changes following paracentesis in cirrhotic patients. A safe and inexpensive option, Dig Dis Sci 37:79-83, 1992.

CHAPTER

57 Acute and Chronic Hepatitis

Douglas R. LaBrecque

Strictly speaking, the term *hepatitis* refers to an inflammation of the liver. A wide variety of agents and conditions can produce such inflammation, but in practice a physician who uses the term *hepatitis* is usually referring to one of the common forms of viral hepatitis: hepatitis A, hepatitis B, hepatitis C/non-A-non-B hepatitis, hepatitis D, and hepatitis E.

THE AGENTS OF VIRAL HEPATITIS

The agents of A, B, C, D, and E hepatitis account for about 95% of the cases of acute viral hepatitis. A number of other viruses, however, may also produce hepatitis, including the herpes viruses (Epstein-Barr, cytomegalovirus, herpes simplex, and varicella-zoster), yellow fever virus, rubella virus, coxsackievirus, and adenovirus. Other exotic viruses (e.g., Marburg, Ebola, and Lassa) may also choose the liver as their primary target.

Hepatitis A

The most common form of viral hepatitis worldwide is hepatitis A (also known as infectious or short-incubation hepatitis). The prevalence of hepatitis A varies inversely with the quality of hygiene and sanitation in a given population. Although in highly developed Western countries (e.g., the United States) antibodies to hepatitis A can be found in the serum of 50% to 60% of the population over 50 years of age, only 5% to 10% of those under 20 years of age have evidence of exposure to hepatitis A. In contrast, the prevalence of antibodies to hepatitis A often exceeds 95% in developing countries, where personal hygiene is difficult to maintain and public sanitation is poor. Most persons in these countries are infected before the age of 10 years and experience a mild, anicteric illness. Paradoxically, improved public hygiene measures have resulted in the proliferation of hepatitis A in many parts of Europe and Central and South America, where acquisition of hepatitis A infection has been delayed to adulthood, when the disease is frequently more serious. Although there are no sex or race differences in susceptibility to infection, certain groups are at greater risk, including those confined to custodial institutions or military barracks, children and staff of day care centers, overseas travelers, homosexual men, and intravenous drug users.

The hepatitis A virus is a small, icosahedral, single-stranded RNA virus belonging to the enterovirus genus of the picornavirus family, which includes such other human pathogens as the polio virus, coxsackievirus, and ECHO virus. As with other enteroviruses, infection occurs via the alimentary tract. Primary replication probably occurs there as well. The incubation period is 2 to 6 weeks, during which time virus infects the liver, is secreted into bile, and is excreted in the feces. Virus continues to be shed with the feces until clinical illness occurs. Once the patient is jaundiced, there is little risk of further transmission. Liver damage is probably not due to a direct cytopathic effect of the virus, but rather results from cell-mediated immune destruction of infected hepatocytes.

Diagnosis is made by the demonstration of IgM antibodies against hepatitis A (anti-HAV IgM). The anti-HAV IgM is detectable shortly after the patient starts shedding virus in the stool and is almost always positive by the time of clinical illness. Anti-HAV IgM is short lived and is superseded by the development of anti-HAV IgG (see box at upper right), which provides lifelong immunity to further infection with hepatitis A. The finding of anti-HAV IgG, but not anti-HAV IgM, in a patient with acute hepatitis indicates that the patient was previously exposed to hepatitis A, but *does not* indicate current infection with the hepatitis A virus (refer to the accompanying box). The serologic and clinical features of a typical patient with hepatitis A are portrayed in Fig. 57-1.

Hepatitis A causes less than half of all acute sporadic cases of viral hepatitis but is the usual cause of epidemic hepatitis in developed countries. In the latter case, infection usually can be traced to a contaminated water supply or an infected food handler, and transmission occurs by the fecal-oral route. Up to ten times as many anicteric cases as icteric cases will occur in a typical epidemic. Fortunately, fulminant hepatitis with a fatal outcome is very rare (less than 1/1000 cases), and *hepatitis A does not produce chronic hepatitis or a chronic carrier state*. Although the

Serologic markers in viral hepatitis

Hepatitis A

Anti-HAV-IgM: Marker of acute infection
Anti-HAV-IgG: Confers lifelong immunity

Hepatitis B

HBsAg: Hepatitis B surface antigen; positive during acute and chronic HB infection
Anti-HBs: Antibody to HBsAg; confers lifelong immunity
Anti-HBc-IgM: Antibody to HB core antigen; positive during acute infection and the "window period" when HBsAg and anti-HBs are both negative
HBeAg: Indicates viral replication and high risk of transmission
Anti-HBe: Indicates low or no viral replication and low risk of transmission
DNA polymerase: Specific HB polymerase; indicates viral replication
HBV-DNA: Best indicator of circulating viral particles

Hepatitis C

Anti-HCV: IgG antibody; becomes positive after 16 to 25 weeks; not useful in diagnosis of acute infection; does not confer immunity; high rate of false positivity
RIBA (Ortho)/HCV antibody neutralization test (Abbott): confirmatory test; RIBA simultaneously screens for antibody to several HCV antigens; low rate of false positivity; not yet FDA approved (9/92)
HCV-RNA: Most sensitive; positive early in illness; polymerase chain reaction (PCR) based test and available only in research labs

Hepatitis D

Anti-HD-IgM: Indicates acute infection
Anti-HD-IgG: Confers lifelong immunity

Hepatitis E

Anti-HE: Convalescent antibody; available through Centers for Disease Control, Atlanta, Ga

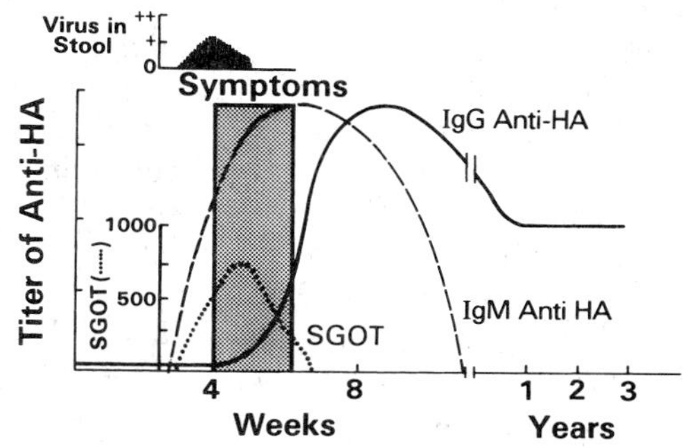

Fig. 57-1. Serologic events in a hypothetical patient inoculated with hepatitis A virus at time zero. Excretion of virus in stool occurs for approximately 1 week before onset of symptoms. Serum IgM hepatitis A antibody (anti-HAV IgM) develops soon after infection, disappears within several months, and serves as a marker of acute infection. Serum IgG hepatitis A antibody (anti-HAV IgG) persists indefinitely after infection and serves as a marker of previous exposure. SGOT = AST.

illness is usually brief with symptoms lasting only 1 to the 3 weeks, a prolonged illness of 3 to 6 months can occur with protracted cholestasis.

Hepatitis B

Hepatitis B, also known as serum or long-incubation hepatitis, is a major public health problem, with approximately 300 million chronic carriers of the virus worldwide. This chronic carrier state is responsible for much of the world's liver cirrhosis and is second only to tobacco as a worldwide human carcinogen, being implicated in 60% to 90% of hepatocellular carcinoma (HCC) cases in areas with a high prevalence of HCC. Although it ranks only twenty-fifth among cancers in the United States, hepatocellular carcinoma is the most common visceral malignancy worldwide, causing 250,000 to 1 million deaths per year.

The etiologic agent responsible is the prototype of a unique virus family, the HEPADNA viruses, which includes the human hepatitis B virus, the American woodchuck hepatitis virus, the Beechy ground squirrel hepatitis virus, the Pekin duck hepatitis virus, and the heron hepatitis virus.

The human hepatitis B virus is a 42 nm diameter DNA virus. The outer protein coat is made up of a complex lipoprotein, the hepatitis B surface antigen (HBsAg). Excess coat protein circulates in the plasma in 22 nm diameter spherical and tubular aggregates. It was the serendipitous discovery of this excess HBsAg, which Blumberg first identified as Australia Antigen in 1965, that formed the basis for the remarkable growth in our understanding of hepatitis over the past 25 years. The virus contains a central hexagonal core consisting of a core antigen (HBcAg), e antigen (HBeAg), a specific DNA polymerase, and a circular DNA (HBV-DNA), which is partially double stranded. The viral genome is among the smallest of all known viruses.

Hepatitis B serology. A variety of serologic tests are available for hepatitis B (see the box, upper left); however, only two are necessary to establish the diagnosis and chronicity of HBV infection: HBsAg and anti-HBc IgM. HBsAg is the first detectable evidence of infection with hepatitis B, appearing in serum within 3 to 4 weeks of exposure and 1 to 2 months before the onset of clinical disease. Its presence is pathognomonic of acute or chronic hepatitis B infection. Its level begins to fall with the development of jaundice, and it becomes undetectable during resolution of clinical illness, sometimes disappearing before other laboratory tests (bilirubin, transaminases) normalize and other times not until several weeks after other tests have normalized. A small percentage of patients will have already "cleared" HBsAg by the time they present to a physician with clinical hepatitis but will not yet have developed detectable anti-HBs. Because IgM antibodies to the core antigen (anti-HBc IgM) rise very shortly after onset of the illness and remain elevated for a number of months thereafter, the anti-HBc IgM test will be positive in this small subgroup of patients, allowing one to identify the illness as acute hepatitis B. The presence of anti-HBc IgM also indicates an acute hepatitis B infection and eliminates the possibility that the acute hepatitis is a superinfection by a second virus in a previously unsuspected chronic hepatitis B carrier. A typical clinical and serologic course in a patient with acute hepatitis B is shown in Fig. 57-2. Clearance of HBsAg generally indicates resolution of the infection. The development of antibodies to HBsAg (anti-HBs) provides immunity to future infections with hepatitis B.

The detection of hepatitis e antigen (HBeAg) suggests actively replicating virus and the presence of infectious virus in the blood. However, infection can occur even when antibodies to e antigen (anti-HBe) are present, and the best marker of a patient's relative infectiousness is the presence of circulating viral DNA (HBV DNA).

Outcome of hepatitis B infection. Of those patients infected with hepatitis B, 90% to 95% recover completely; 0.1% to 1.0% die within several weeks of disease onset from fulminant hepatitis; 5% to 10% become chronic carriers, unable to rid themselves of the virus. Asymptomatic carriers with normal transaminases usually do not progress to more serious forms of chronic liver disease. However, chronic carriers, with/or without symptoms, who have consistently elevated transaminases, may show mild nonspecific changes, chronic persistent hepatitis, chronic active hepatitis, and even cirrhosis when a liver biopsy is performed (see later). A small subgroup of patients from Mediterranean countries have been identified who carry a mutant form of hepatitis B that produces a more severe illness. These patients are HBsAg and HBV-DNA positive but HBeAg negative and anti-HBe positive. All chronic carriers are at a greater risk for the development of hepatocellular carcinoma, and those with circulating virus remain a potential source of transmission.

Epidemiology of hepatitis B. The prevalence of hepatitis B varies greatly worldwide, from areas of low endemicity, where less than 1% of adults are chronic carriers and less than 10% show evidence of prior hepatitis B exposure (United States, Canada, Western Europe), to areas of high endemicity, where 2% to 15% of adults are chronic carriers and 30% to 100% of adults have markers of prior hepatitis B infection (Africa, Asia, and Oceana). Over 75% of the world's population lives in areas of intermediate to high endemicity. Maynard and colleagues estimate that 1.3 million of the approximately 122 million babies born in these regions in 1985 will die of chronic sequelae of hepatitis B infection.

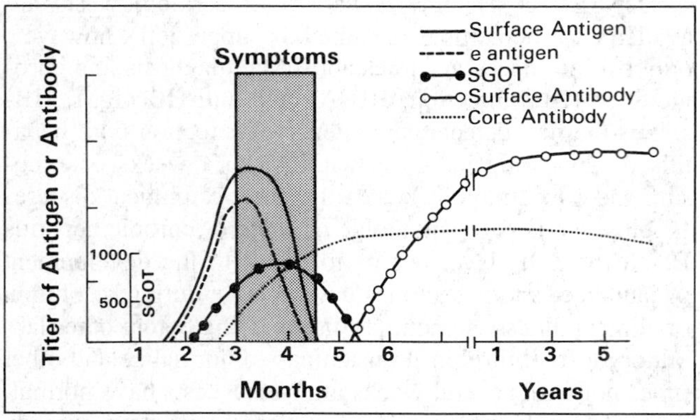

Fig. 57-2. Serologic events in acute hepatitis B. The first detectable evidence of infection is the appearance of surface and e antigens, followed by the rise in transaminases and onset of symptoms. Surface antibody persists indefinitely and protects against subsequent exposure. Core antibody is positive during the "window" period when both surface antigen and antibody are negative. SGOT = AST.

The risk of developing a chronic carrier state and the severity of illness is directly related to the age at which one acquires hepatitis B. This factor accounts for the high carrier rates in areas of high endemicity. In such countries, hepatitis B is usually acquired in early childhood by vertical transmission from a carrier mother or horizontal transmission by contact with a carrier through an open cut or skin lesion. In contrast in areas of low endemicity, transmission is primarily by sexual or parenteral exposure, and only 6% to 10% of those acquiring hepatitis B after the age of 6 years become chronic carriers. Individuals with an altered immune status, including chronic dialysis patients, those on immunosuppressive drugs, and IV drug users are also more likely to become chronic carriers.

In areas with low prevalence rates, selected populations have an increased risk of acquiring hepatitis B. Parenteral and sexual exposure are the primary modes of transmission in the United States. The highest risk groups include male homosexuals and IV drug users. Other high-risk groups are those likely to be exposed to blood (health care personnel, laboratory and blood bank technicians, dialysis patients, oncology and hemophilia patients receiving blood products); institutionalized individuals, including the mentally retarded and prisoners; and promiscuous heterosexuals. Several large hospitals that screened all entering patients for HBsAg found that 1% to 1.5% were positive; 80% to 90% were previously unsuspected carriers.

Hepatitis B is an extremely infectious agent. Approximately 10% of persons suffering an accidental needle stick from a carrier of hepatitis B develop hepatitis; 20% to 30% of health care personnel have evidence of prior hepatitis B infection compared to less than 10% of the general population. Despite meticulous screening of all blood products for the presence of HBsAg, approximately 5% of post-transfusion hepatitis continues to be caused by hepatitis B, presumably because quantities of this highly infectious virus sufficient to produce infection are below the level of detection of current assays.

Almost 50% of patients with acute hepatitis B do not give a history of exposure and are not in one of the high-risk groups. The mode of transmission is not clear but probably involves intimate contact with an unsuspected carrier. Oral transmission is probably extremely rare. No case has ever been traced to a food handler, and several studies have failed to show transmission by contaminated endoscopes. The virus, although present in tears, vaginal secretions, seminal fluid, breast milk, sweat, and urine, is not found in feces that are free of blood; and it is destroyed by gastric acid and pancreatic enzymes. It is possible, however, for it to enter the body via breaks in the oral mucosa, especially at the gum line. Inadvertent exposure via an accidental splash of blood or bodily secretions into the mucosa of the eye or through small cuts, abrasions, or hangnails is a frequent mode of transmission to health care personnel.

Non-A–non-B hepatitis

After serologic tests for hepatitis A and hepatitis B were developed, it rapidly became apparent that many cases of post-transfusion hepatitis, as well as many sporadic cases of hepatitis, were not caused by hepatitis A, hepatitis B, or any other known hepatitis-producing virus. As a diagnosis of exclusion, such cases were labeled non-A–non-B hepatitis, but careful epidemiologic studies soon made it clear that even non-A–non-B hepatitis was composed of several diseases with presumably different etiologic agents: post-transfusion non-A–non-B hepatitis; sporadic, community-acquired non-A–non-B hepatitis; and enterically transmitted or epidemic non-A–non-B hepatitis.

Hepatitis C

Non-A–non-B hepatitis accounts for 90% to 95% of all cases of post-transfusion hepatitis. In the United States 150,000 to 300,000 cases of post-transfusion hepatitis occur yearly. Prospective studies of the hepatitis risk after transfusion suggested that 1% to 6% of the volunteer blood donors in the United States might be chronic carriers of non-A–non-B hepatitis. Fifteen years of frustrating efforts to identify the agent of post-transfusion non-A–non-B hepatitis culminated with the cloning and sequencing of an RNA virus designated hepatitis C. This tour de force of molecular biology has provided an antibody test for hepatitis C virus (HCV) and a method to detect HCV-RNA using the polymerase chain reaction, but the virus itself has still not been visualized.

The hepatitis C virus is found throughout the world. This 50 to 60 nm RNA virus has a genome related to the flavivirus and pestivirus. Eighty to ninety percent of all post-transfusion non-A–non-B hepatitis cases are anti-HCV positive; 50% to 70% of sporadic community acquired cases of non-A–non-B hepatitis are also anti-HCV positive. In the United States, 1% of volunteer blood donors are anti-HCV positive and 90% of blood units found to have transmitted hepatitis are anti-HCV positive.

Up to 75% of post-transfusion cases are nonicteric and asymptomatic. The indolent nature of this infection initially led clinicians to assume that post-transfusion hepatitis C would have few sequelae. Unfortunately, this has not proved to be the case; 40% to 60% of post-transfusion hepatitis C cases become chronic, with 20% to 40% progressing to cirrhosis. Liver failure caused by chronic hepatitis C is a common reason for liver transplantation. Hepatocellular carcinoma (HCC) is also being reported as a consequence of this infection, which may be the major cause of HCC in Japan.

Transmission by parenteral exposure and needle-stick transmission is well documented. There is an annual attack rate of 2% to 6% in hemophiliacs and 3% to 6% in hemodialysis patients (1% in hemodialysis staff). The largest number of cases in the United States occurs in IV drug abusers, who make up 20% to 45% of all cases of hepatitis C. The risk of sexual transmission remains controversial but appears to be quite low. Several reports describe no evidence of the virus in semen samples by PCR analysis from anti-HCV-positive patients. It clearly occurs at a much lower frequency than with hepatitis B, probably because of lower circulating concentrations of the virus. Oral transmission of hepatitis C must be rare. A form of non-A–non-B hepatitis related to the enterically transmitted form of non-A–non-B hepatitis is transmitted orally. The agent has been identified as hepatitis E (see later).

Advances in our understanding of hepatitis C continue to be thwarted by the inability to isolate the virus and problems with false-positive serologic tests using the standard ELISA assay. Up to 60% of positive tests in volunteer blood donors are false positive (refer to the box on p. 587). Confirmatory tests, available on an experimental basis, will help to eliminate false-positive results, but the antibody tests do not become positive until 15 to 25 weeks after the onset of acute hepatitis C, making them of little use in the diagnosis of acute hepatitis C. Polymerase chain reaction (PCR) can identify hepatitis C RNA early in the acute illness, but is not available routinely.

Hepatitis D (δ hepatitis)

The delta agent was first described by Rizzetto in 1977. It is a unique 35 to 37 nm incomplete RNA virus that requires a "helper" virus to replicate. The delta agent is only found in patients with hepatitis B, and its outer coat is composed of HBsAg. Infection with the delta agent can occur concurrently with exposure to hepatitis B, producing acute hepatitis B and acute hepatitis D, or as a superinfection in a chronic carrier of hepatitis B. Infection with hepatitis D may be acute and short lived or become chronic.

Combined hepatitis B and D infections have a worse prognosis than hepatitis B alone, with an increased frequency of fulminant hepatitis. Superinfection of a chronic hepatitis B carrier is more likely to produce chronic hepatitis D as well. Diagnosis is made by the detection of IgM antibodies or rising titers of IgG antibodies to delta agent (refer to the box on p. 587). Hepatitis D should always be suspected in fulminant hepatitis B, where up to 30% to 50% of fulminant acute cases have been found to be coinfected with hepatitis D. A sudden exacerbation of hepatitis in a chronic carrier of hepatitis B also suggests a new, superimposed acute delta infection, although hepatitis A, hepatitis C, and other viral etiologies must also be considered.

Distribution of hepatitis D is worldwide, but prevalence varies greatly, even between different populations within the same and nearby geographic areas. As one would predict, prevalence of hepatitis D tends to follow that of hepatitis B, and transmission is usually by similar mechanisms, although there are exceptions. Thus in the Western world 33% to 66% of hepatitis B positive, IV drug users are also positive for antibodies to delta; however, male homosexuals, who also have a high prevalence of HB, do not have an increased prevalence of antibodies to the delta agent. In the Far East, where 5% to 20% of the population carries hepatitis B, superinfection with delta is uncommon (only 5% in Taiwan). When the delta agent is introduced into a susceptible community (e.g., a previously nonexposed IV drug user population), its spread can be epidemic. In areas where hepatitis D is endemic, transmission apparently occurs by intimate contact as well as parenteral exposure.

Hepatitis E (enterically transmitted or epidemic non-A–non-B hepatitis)

In some developing countries, more than 50% of acute viral hepatitis is unrelated to infection with the hepatitis A, B, or C viruses. Contaminated water has frequently been implicated as the source of infection, and epidemics have been reported in India, Nepal, Burma, Pakistan, Mexico, Somalia, Algeria, the Ivory Coast, and Russia. Outbreaks have been characterized by a high mortality rate in pregnant women, and the disease attacks primarily young to middle-aged adults. Hepatitis E is an RNA virus related to the Caliciviruses. Specific serologic tests are currently available through the Centers for Disease Control in Atlanta.

The mean incubation period is 6 weeks (2 to 9 weeks), and the clinical disease is very similar to hepatitis A except for severity. Mortality is 1% to 2% in the general population (0.1% in hepatitis A) and 10% to 20% in pregnant women (0.1% to 0.2% in hepatitis A). Sporadic cases of enterically transmitted hepatitis E also occur and may be the major cause of hepatitis in areas of the world where it is endemic. Enterically transmitted hepatitis E appears to be a self-limited disease with no chronic carrier state or long-term sequelae. Isolated cases have been reported in the United States in patients returning from underdeveloped countries.

Non-A–non-B–non-C hepatitis/hepatitis F?

As detailed previously, 5% to 10% of post-transfusion hepatitis cases, 30% to 50% of sporadic community acquired non-A–non-B hepatitis cases, and fulminant hepatitis caused by non-A–non-B hepatitis still cannot be accounted for by the viruses for which we currently have serologic tests. Improvements in HCV testing methods will no doubt pick up some of the cases, but it appears likely that one or more hepatitis viruses still await identification.

ACUTE VIRAL HEPATITIS

Clinical features of acute viral hepatitis

The development of jaundice is an infrequent complication of acute viral hepatitis. This is true with all forms of viral hepatitis, particularly hepatitis A and hepatitis C (Table 57-1). Most cases remain entirely asymptomatic and are diagnosed only serendipitously by the chance observation of an elevated transaminase level. Others demonstrate only slight malaise and gastrointestinal, influenza-like symptoms.

A typical icteric attack of viral hepatitis has a characteristic prodrome lasting from several days to several weeks. This period is marked by anorexia and nausea with, at times, severe vomiting; a characteristic loss of the desire to smoke or drink alcohol is frequently noted. Malaise and fatigue may be profound. Low-grade fever may be present. An ache or a dragging sensation in the right upper quadrant, along with a fullness in the right upper quadrant, is often noted by the patient. In hepatitis B, the patient may develop a serum sicknesslike syndrome with a symmetric, nonmigratory arthropathy of the small joints, or urticaria, due to circulating immune complexes containing HBsAg. Polyarteritis nodosum, glomerulonephritis, polymyalgia rheumatica, and essential mixed cryoglobulinemia may also be manifestations of acute hepatitis B. During the prodromal period the patient is quite ill and may not notice the initial darkening of the urine and lightening of the stool. With the onset of jaundice, symptoms often abate. On physical examination, the liver is palpable in 70% of patients, with a smooth, somewhat rounded, "full," and tender edge. The spleen is palpable in a minority of patients, and right posterior rib percussion produces a distinct sickening sensation. The presence of ascites, edema, evidence of hepatic encephalopathy, numerous spider nevi, or a large palpable spleen should suggest submassive or fulminant hepatitis or some form of chronic rather than acute liver disease.

Laboratory studies are characterized by transaminases elevated fivefold to 30-fold, with the serum alanine aminotransferase (ALT[SGPT]) somewhat more elevated than the aspartate aminotransferase (AST[SGOT]). Alkaline phosphatase, 5′ nucleotidase and gamma glutamyl transpeptidase are generally elevated only one to three times normal. Lactate dehydrogenase (LDH) is similarly elevated only two to three times normal, and a markedly elevated LDH should suggest a different diagnosis (e.g., malignancy, muscle necrosis, or hemolysis). Bilirubin levels are rarely above 10 mg/dl in uncomplicated hepatitis, with greater than 50% of the bilirubin conjugated or direct reacting. Serum albumin, prothrombin time, and ammonia levels should be normal, and abnormalities of these parameters suggest fulminant viral hepatitis or chronic liver disease. Prolongation of the prothrombin time, which is unresponsive to parenteral vitamin K administration, is a particularly ominous prognostic sign in acute viral hepatitis, as is the appearance of hepatic encephalopathy, ascites, or hypoglycemia. Prominent fever, rigors, leukocytosis, and a highly elevated sedimentation rate are unusual in hepatitis and should stimulate investigation for other causes, particularly ascending cholangitis and alcoholic hepatitis.

The more severe symptoms of acute viral hepatitis are usually short lived, and the course is generally one of gradual improvement. Although the patient's appetite and general feeling of well-being return rapidly, patients are frequently disappointed at the length of time their malaise and fatigue linger. Decreasing symptoms and liver test abnormalities usually occur in concert, leading to complete re-

Table 57-1. The ABCs of viral hepatitis

	Hepatitis A	Hepatitis B	Hepatitis C	Hepatitis D	Hepatitis E
Incubation period	2-6 wks	2-6 months	2-22 wks	4-8 wks	2-9 wks
Onset	Usually acute	Usually insidious	Usually insidious	Usually acute	Usually acute
Symptoms					
Nausea and vomiting	Common	Common	Common	Common	Common
Fever	Common	Uncommon	Uncommon	Uncommon	Uncommon
Jaundice	50%	33%	25%	?	10%-20%
Arthralgias	Rare	Common	Rare	Rare	Rare
Diagnosis	IgM Anti-HAV	HBsAg	Anti-HCV	IgM anti-HDV	Anti-HEV
Transmission					
Fecal-oral	Usual	Rare (not fecal)	Rare	?	Usual
Parenteral	Rare	Usual	Usual	Usual	No
Sexual	Yes	Yes	?Rare	?	?
Perinatal	No	Yes	?Rare	?	No
Sequelae					
Chronic carrier	No	5%-10%	Up to 60%	?Most	No
Chronic active hepatitis	No	Approximately 5%	?30%-50%	Up to 70%	No
Fulminant hepatitis	Approximately 0.1%	0.2%-1.0%	?	Up to 17%	2%-10%*
Recovery	Greater than 99%	85%-90%	?	?	90%-98%*
Epidemiology					
Sporadic cases	Mainly children in developing countries and adults in developed countries	Primarily males	40%-50% of sporadic hepatitis cases	—	Young to middle-aged adults
Epidemics	Foodborne or waterborne	Contaminated blood products (vaccines, dialysis machines, IV drug users)	Contaminated blood products	Contaminated blood products, IV drug users	Foodborne or waterborne
Post-transfusion	Extremely rare	Less than 5% of post-transfusion cases	85%-95% of post-transfusion cases	Possible	No
Prevention	ISG†	HBIG†, vaccine	? ISG†	Hepatitis B vaccine	?ISG† from endemic areas

*10%-20% fatalities in pregnant women.
†*ISG*, human immune serum globulin; *HBIG*, hepatitis B immune globulin.

covery in 3 to 6 weeks in acute hepatitis A and 4 to 10 weeks in acute hepatitis B. The malaise and fatigue may last considerably longer, however, and a small percentage of patients remain ill for 6 to 12 months. Abnormal liver tests or persistent HBsAg-positive serum beyond 6 months indicates chronic hepatitis and requires further investigation (see later). Hepatitis C is frequently characterized by multiple remissions and exacerbations with transaminases returning to normal, only to flare again several weeks or months later.

Management of uncomplicated acute viral hepatitis

Patients with uncomplicated acute viral hepatitis are best managed at home. Only those who require parenteral fluids because of severe nausea and vomiting, or who have physical or biochemical evidence suggesting fulminant hepatitis, require hospitalization (see later). The treatment of acute viral hepatitis is symptomatic and consists mainly of bed rest and diet. The effect of early ambulation on recovery from acute viral hepatitis remains controversial, but most experts agree that it is unlikely that such activity exacerbates the disease or produces more frequent relapses. Certainly, it does not increase the risk of developing fulminant hepatitis or chronic active hepatitis. Early in the disease, most patients have no desire to be active due to their severe weakness and fatigue. I encourage patients to increase activity gradually, as tolerated, remaining active up to the point of fatigue, but not beyond. It is important to limit the total bed rest to the shortest period necessary, with a gradual increase in activity thereafter to avoid the chronic weakness and fatigue experienced by any patient who has been bedridden for several weeks.

A low-fat, high-carbohydrate diet is generally the most

palatable for these anorexic patients, who appear to tolerate fatty foods less well than the normal patient. In general, the patient should be encouraged to maintain a high fluid intake and a high calorie intake, eating whatever foods are most attractive. Patients will generally adjust their diet according to their own tastes, which may be quite different from their normal preferences, until recovery is well underway.

No current therapy has been found to be beneficial, and there is no evidence that treatment with corticosteroids or interferon is of value in acute viral hepatitis. Patients should be followed on at least a weekly basis during the early symptomatic stage of the disease, with careful attention paid to the development of signs, symptoms, or laboratory changes suggestive of fulminant hepatitis or subacute hepatic necrosis (bridging hepatic necrosis). When the patient is well on the way to recovery, follow-up can be extended rapidly, but patients should continue to be checked until their enzymes have completely normalized and, in the case of hepatitis B, until HBsAg is lost and anti-HBs appears, confirming clearance of the infection.

About 90% to 95% of all cases of acute viral hepatitis caused by viruses other than the hepatitis C virus follow the course outlined here. Nevertheless, one must be aware of several occasional variations in presentation.

Potentially fatal variants of acute viral hepatitis

Fulminant hepatitis. Fulminant hepatitis is characterized by the rapid development of hepatic failure, resulting in severe coagulopathy and encephalopathy within 4 to 8 weeks of the onset of clinical disease. Viral hepatitis is the primary cause of fulminant hepatitis in the United States, with hepatitis B causing about 50% of all fulminant hepatitis cases; 30% to 50% of the fulminant hepatitis B cases demonstrate coinfection with hepatitis D. Non-A–non-B hepatitis causes most of the remaining fulminant viral hepatitis cases in the United States. These patients are negative for Anti-HCV and even PCR for HCV-RNA, so it is unclear what role hepatitis C plays in fulminant hepatitis. Rare contributions are made by hepatitis A, herpes simplex, Epstein-Barr virus, cytomegalovirus, and others. Drugs cause only 5% of acute hepatitis but 20% to 30% of fulminant hepatitis in the United States (Chapter 58). The pattern is reversed in Great Britain, where acetaminophen ingestion is a popular suicide method and drugs are the leading cause of fulminant hepatitis. Mushroom poisoning from *Amanita phalloides* remains a major problem in Europe.

The clinical course is characterized by worsening coagulopathy and deepening coma with the development of ascites, pulmonary complications, renal failure, cerebral edema, sepsis, and bleeding. Transaminases will initially remain in the 1000 to 2000 IU/L range. A falling transaminase can be quite misleading, sometimes inducing inappropriate optimism that the patient is starting to recover when, in reality, it indicates a declining number of viable hepatocytes. The presence of a rising bilirubin, increasing prothrombin time, and falling albumin and cholesterol levels presages a very poor prognosis. The development of hypoglycemia, producing abrupt deterioration of neurologic status and requiring massive amounts of IV dextrose to prevent further hypoglycemia, is usually a very late and ominous complication.

Treatment of fulminant hepatitis is frustrating and produces an average survival rate of only 30% to 40%. Corticosteroids, artificial liver support (charcoal and ion exchange columns), exchange transfusion, and other heroic measures have not been shown to increase survival. Therapy is supportive, requiring aggressive intensive care unit management with careful attention paid to fluids and electrolytes, blood gases, blood glucose, and prevention of nosocomial infection (Chapter 56). Routine use of fresh-frozen plasma to improve the prothrombin time is not recommended. H_2 antagonists have been shown to decrease the risk of gastrointestinal bleeding. All sedative/hypnotic drugs should be avoided. Lactulose should be used and protein restricted at the first hint of encephalopathy. Ultimately, many of these patients will require liver transplantation to survive (Chapter 64). However, this possibility must be considered early in the patient's illness so that transplantation can be discussed with the patient and the family while the patient is still alert, and arrangements can be made to transfer the patient to a transplant center while the patient is still in relatively good condition. Patients who are transfered after they are already in stage IV coma do considerably less well than those transfered earlier in the course of their illness.

Bridging hepatic necrosis (subacute hepatic necrosis). A small number of patients (1% to 4%) with acute viral hepatitis begin to resolve their illness normally but then appear to plateau. Thus as in most cases of acute viral hepatitis, symptoms and laboratory tests peak, remain markedly abnormal for several days, and then begin to improve rapidly. But whereas most acute hepatitis patients follow a fairly smooth curve to normal or near normal levels of laboratory tests and resolution of symptoms within 3 to 6 weeks of the peak of abnormalities, in this poorly defined subset, descriptively referred to as *subacute hepatic necrosis,* symptoms may or may not completely resolve and bilirubin frequently normalizes, but transaminases plateau in the 600 to 1000 IU/L range and fail to improve further. At the same time, serum albumin starts to fall, prothrombin time becomes prolonged, and physical signs of chronic liver disease may develop (spider angiomata, ascites, palpable spleen, encephalopathy). Clear-cut evidence of liver deterioration may not be obvious for 10 to 16 weeks, and these patients clearly fall somewhere between fulminant hepatitis and chronic active hepatitis. If a liver biopsy can be obtained, which is frequently difficult because of the developing coagulopathy, it invariably shows large zones of hepatocyte necrosis "bridging" adjacent terminal hepatic venules (central veins), central veins and portal triads, or adjacent portal triads. The development of the transjugular liver biopsy technique and a technique in which the biopsy tract is plugged with Gelfoam now make it possible to obtain a liver biopsy even in the face of markedly abnormal coagulation parameters.

Controversy continues concerning the prognostic significance of bridging hepatic necrosis. Although it is probably not predictive of outcome in drug hepatitis or during the first 4 to 16 weeks of acute hepatitis B, several studies have shown that the disease may be fatal in up to 20% of patients and produces chronic active hepatitis in another 30%, especially in those who are HBsAg negative and have autoimmune features.

There is rarely a reason to biopsy the liver earlier than 6 months after the onset of acute viral hepatitis. Development of the preceding clinical picture, however, should lead to an earlier biopsy at 3 to 4 months. At the present time, most authors would not advise steroid therapy of such patients. However, if the patient has non-A–non-B–non-C hepatitis, is severely symptomatic, and is steadily deteriorating, the author will usually initiate a trial of prednisone (40 to 60 mg/day) for 6 to 8 weeks with follow-up biopsy at that time. If there is not a clear-cut biochemical, clinical, and histologic response, steroids are rapidly tapered. At the very least, such patients merit close follow-up with repeat liver biopsy in 4 to 6 months and the recognition that, if they continue to deteriorate, liver transplantation may be required.

Benign variants of acute viral hepatitis

Cholestatic hepatitis. Cholestatic hepatitis is characterized by an unusually high bilirubin (often over 20 mg/dl) that persists for weeks to months and is often accompanied by severe pruritus, fever, twofold to fourfold elevations in alkaline phosphatase, and minimal twofold to fourfold elevations in transaminases. It is readily confused with obstructive biliary tract disease and can lead to unnecessary and hazardous surgery or interventional tests if the diagnosis is not considered. Most cases are associated with hepatitis A, and the presence in the serum of anti-HAV IgM will often suffice for a diagnosis.

If the question of biliary obstruction remains unresolved, dilated bile ducts should be readily detected by ultrasound examination or computed tomography (CT) in the presence of obstruction sufficient to produce a bilirubin of 20. The prognosis is complete recovery; however, because of the prolonged course of the disease and its sometimes severe accompanying pruritus, judicious use of corticosteroids in selected cases may be useful. An initial dose of 40 mg/day of prednisone for 4 days should produce a greater than 40% reduction in serum bilirubin. Steroids should then be tapered over 4 weeks to avoid an exacerbation caused by a too rapid withdrawal. If severe pruritus is the only problem, treatment with cholestyramine, 4 g, three times a day, may obviate the need to consider steroid therapy.

Prolonged viral hepatitis. This variant is also termed chronic lobular hepatitis and refers to slowly resolving cases that may last for 6 to 12 months or longer, with continued mild clinical symptomatology of anorexia, malaise and easy fatiguability, and persistent laboratory abnormalities. Definitive differentiation from chronic active hepatitis requires a liver biopsy, and treatment is reassurance.

Relapsing hepatitis. Usually, once a patient feels well and the laboratory tests have normalized, one can assure the patient that the disease is resolved and will not return. A small percentage of patients, however, will suffer a relapse 3 to 12 months later, often completely mimicking the original attack. The prognosis remains good and the illness usually resolves without sequelae. Hepatitis C is particularly bothersome in this respect, with multiple recurrences separated by weeks to months of normal laboratory tests and lack of symptoms. In a few patients, particularly those with hepatitis C, relapses may eventuate in chronic active hepatitis. Relapses have also been recently described with hepatitis A.

Differential diagnosis

The symptoms of hepatitis are nonspecific, and diagnosis is suggested by typical findings in the history and on physical examination. The diagnosis is confirmed by laboratory tests showing a parenchymal pattern of abnormalities (elevated transaminases and bilirubin with minimally increased cholestatic enzymes). A viral etiology is proved by a positive serologic test for hepatitis A, B, or C or one of the less common infectious causes described earlier. If these tests are negative, a number of other etiologies must also be considered before a diagnosis of non-A–non-B–non-C hepatitis is accepted.

Drug hepatitis. A number of drugs can produce typical acute hepatitis, cholestatic hepatitis, chronic active hepatitis, and fulminant hepatitis (Chapter 58). A careful drug history is essential in evaluating a patient with acute hepatitis, and all drugs should be discontinued if possible.

Alcoholic liver disease. Patients will often deny significant alcohol intake, thus misleading the examining physician. In contrast to viral hepatitis, in which the ALT is usually greater than the AST, the reverse is almost always true in alcoholic hepatitis (see also Chapter 59). If the AST/ALT ratio is greater than 1.5 to 2.0 and the gamma-glutamyltransferase (GGT), which is induced by alcohol, is significantly elevated, a diagnosis of alcoholic hepatitis must be seriously entertained; however, a note of caution is required in too quickly labeling a patient as having alcoholic hepatitis. The ALT rarely, if ever, rises above 250 to 300 IU/L in uncomplicated alcoholic hepatitis and, in a patient with an ALT >300 IU/L, a second, possibly additional diagnosis must be sought, even in the face of a history of massive alcohol intake.

Choledocholithiasis. Acute obstruction of the common duct with a stone may produce a transient rise in transaminases as high as 2000 IU/L. This level rapidly returns to normal over 3 to 4 days if the stone is passed or dislodged and floating. If the obstruction is relieved within 4 to 8 hours, elevated AST and ALT levels may be the only biochemical abnormalities. More prolonged obstruction will produce gradual rises in alkaline phosphatase and bilirubin levels as the transaminase levels fall. These patients usually can be differentiated from patients with acute viral hepatitis by the presence of accompanying fever, rigors, leukocytosis and right upper quadrant pain. Ultrasonography and even endoscopic retrograde cholangiopancreatography (ERCP) may occasionally be required to differentiate these patients. Dynamic hepatobiliary scanning is helpful if the bilirubin is less than 7.0 mg/dl.

Central passive congestion and hypoxia. Any condition that causes passive congestion of the liver with localized oxygen desaturation will produce pericentral hypoxia and cell necrosis. If this hypoxia is abrupt, as in myocardial infarction with congestive heart failure, shock, and the acute Budd-Chiari syndrome (hepatic vein obstruction), transaminases may rise to dramatic heights, exceeding 10,000 IU/L. Unlike viral hepatitis, the LDH will rise to similar very high levels, and this is quite useful in differential diagnosis. In most cases related to cardiac disease, symptoms and signs of the heart disease are obvious. With chronic diseases (e.g., constrictive pericarditis), however, changes may be more subtle and easily missed. The same is true with the chronic Budd-Chiari syndrome and hepatic veno-occlusive disease. A high degree of suspicion, plus appropriate tests to evaluate the above diseases (e.g., doppler ultrasonography) may be necessary. When the situation is unclear and there are no contraindications, a liver biopsy will readily demonstrate central passive congestion and point the way toward the correct diagnosis.

Prevention of viral hepatitis

Prevention of viral infections is classically managed in three ways: (1) elimination of the source of the infection, (2) passive immunization of exposed individuals with gamma globulin–containing antibodies to the virus, and (3) active immunization with vaccine. The availability of these different modalities varies for each of the forms of acute viral hepatitis and is summarized in Table 57-2.

Isolation procedures. Hepatitis A, in contrast to hepatitis B, is readily transmitted by intimate exposure. Fecal-oral transmission via contaminated food, shared glasses, shared bathroom facilities, etc. is the standard form of transmission, and immediate family members, or those who have eaten a meal prepared by the patient with acute hepatitis A during the 2 to 3 weeks before the onset of acute illness, should be considered at risk for acquisition of hepatitis A. Once the patient has developed clinical illness, he or she has generally stopped shedding the virus, and no significant isolation procedures are necessary, except for continued concern about exposure to the patient's stool. Such patients should not continue to work in a commercial food preparation area until they have cleared their jaundice, but appropriate handwashing should prevent transmission in the more localized home environment.

Hepatitis B is unlikely to be transmitted in normal everyday activities but is extremely infectious under certain circumstances. Transmission requires parenteral exposure to blood or bodily secretions (excluding feces), or exposure of a mucosal surface or a break in the skin to blood or bodily fluids. Thus sexual partners are at great risk, but other members of the household, including those eating food prepared by the individual with hepatitis B, are not at significant risk. An exception is young children, particularly those still in diapers. Health care personnel are not at risk from a patient with hepatitis B unless they have been directly exposed to the patient's blood or bodily secretions through a break in a skin or mucosal surface, and only needle and bodily secretion precautions are required.

Hepatitis C is probably transmitted almost exclusively via the parenteral route, and patients with hepatitis C require only needle and body secretion precautions. Sporadic cases may well be transmitted by intimate contact, and precautions, similar to those exercised with hepatitis B patients, should be taken. Similar precautions should be used for hepatitis B. Information is limited for hepatitis E, but recommendations parallel those made for hepatitis A.

Passive and active immunization. As discussed earlier, the development of good public sanitation and personal hygiene has reduced the prevalence of *hepatitis A* in children, from close to 100% in undeveloped countries to 5% to 10% in well-developed countries. However, this leaves most of the adult population at risk and minor epidemics of the disease continue to occur in adults. Because hepatitis A tends to be a more serious illness in adults, the reduction in attacks among children is a mixed blessing, particularly with the frequent travel of individuals from highly developed countries to developing nations. Standard human immune serum globulin, produced from a large pool of human donors, contains significant titers of antibodies against hepatitis A and provides protection against exposure for those traveling to high prevalence areas. For those who have had sexual, familial, or close intimate contact with a patient (such as a frequent playmate of a child or a client of the child's day care center), immune serum globulin is effective in preventing acquisition of acute hepatitis or ameliorating the severity of the acute attack, if given within 2 weeks of exposure. Two vaccines for hepatitis A have now been approved for use in Europe and Asia and are undergoing final, clinical trials in the United States. It is expected that a commercial vaccine will be available for use in the United States by 1993 or 1994. It will probably be recommended for use by the same individuals for whom hepatitis B vaccine is currently advised (see later), as well as those traveling to endemic areas. Whether it will ultimately be recommended as another of the routine childhood immunizations remains to be established.

Hepatitis B is best prevented by avoiding high-risk behaviors including sharing of needles with IV drug users, unprotected homosexual or heterosexual sex, sex with multiple partners, and indiscriminate use of blood products. Pooled human immune serum globulin contains variable quantities of antibodies against hepatitis B, but special gamma globulin prepared from multiply transfused individuals, which contains very high titers of hepatitis B surface antibody, called *hepatitis B immune globulin (HBIG)*, has

Table 57-2. Active and passive immunization against viral hepatitis

		Gamma globulin*		Vaccine*		
Virus	**Exposure**	**Dose**	**Timing**	**Recommendation**	**Timing**	**Comments**
A	Travel to endemic area	0.05 ml ISG/kg†	Repeat every 4-6 months	Yes	Vaccine should be available in United States in 1993 or 1994	0.02 ml ISG/kg sufficient for short visits
	Sexual or familial contact	0.02 ml ISG/kg	Within 7-14 days of exposure	Yes		
	Social or occupational contact	—	—	Yes	—	No prophylaxis recommended
B	Needle-stick or mucosal exposure	0.06 ml HBIG/kg†	Within 7 days of exposure	Yes	Immediately and at 1 and 6 months‡	Not necessary if recipient is HBsAg or anti-HBs positive
	Perinatal exposure to HBsAg (+) mother	0.50 ml HBIG	Single dose within 12 hours of birth	Yes	Within 12 hours of birth and at 1 and 6 months	HBIG and vaccine administered at separate sites
	Sexual or close personal contact with patient with acute HB	0.06 ml HBIG/kg	Single dose	No	—	Vaccine recommended if expect continued exposure to patient with chronic HB
	Familial or social contact with patient with acute HB	—	—	—	—	No prophylaxis recommended; vaccine recommended for young children of chronic carrier parent
C	Needle-stick or sexual exposure to hepatitis C	0.05 ml ISG/kg	Single dose	—	—	Generally recommended, although documentation of effectiveness is lacking

*Average dose is provided. Dosage of HBIG depends on titer of anti-HBs and should be in accordance with manufacturer's recommendations. Heptavax (plasma derived) and Recombivax and Engerix B (recombinant vaccines) are equally effective. Heptavax is no longer manufactured in the United States, and its use is restricted to hemodialysis patients and individuals who are immune compromised or have an allergy to yeast. Dosage should be in accordance with manufacturer's current recommendations.
†ISG, human immune serum globulin; HBIG, hepatitis B immune globulin.
‡A rapid immunization regimen has been approved for Engerix B in which vaccine is given immediately and at 1 and 2 months. A fourth, booster dose should be given at 12 months to achieve highest antibody titers.

been prepared for treatment of individuals exposed to hepatitis B.

Major indications for HBIG are in postexposure prophylaxis of individuals exposed via needle stick or intimate sexual contact. It is also used immediately postpartum in infants born in HBsAg-positive mothers. Because HBIG is expensive and available in limited quantities, it should be provided only to individuals who clearly require it. This goal may necessitate testing both the patient and the person exposed for the presence of HBsAg and anti-HBs. Gamma globulin is most effective if given within the first 7 days of exposure. If these tests will not be available within that time, standard human immune serum globulin should be given prophylactically. After the serologies are available, HBIG should then be given, if appropriate. With the newborn infant of a mother known to be HBsAg positive, HBIG is ideally given immediately in the delivery room. Because HBIG does not interfere with the patient's immune response, the single dose of HBIG is accompanied simultaneously, but at a different site, by the first dose of the hepatitis B vaccine. Surprisingly, the newborn infant is able to mount an excellent response to hepatitis B vaccine, and the combined regimen of HBIG and hepatitis B vaccine has reduced vertical transmission of hepatitis B from HBeAg-positive mothers to their children from 90% to 95% to less than 5%. This regimen is also recommended for the adult exposed by needle stick.

A major advance in the prevention of hepatitis B has been the development of the hepatitis B vaccine. The initial vaccine, an extremely pure preparation of HBsAg particles isolated from the plasma of chronic carriers, was shown to be extremely effective in preventing transmission of hepatitis B in all high-risk settings. Because of unfounded fears that this human-derived preparation might be contaminated with the virus for HIV, however, many individuals refused vaccination. Thus only some health care personnel at high risk for acquiring hepatitis B have been vaccinated. This most unfortunate fear of AIDS should now be obviated by the development and use of two second-generation vaccines prepared by recombinant DNA technology. These vaccines (Recombivax B and Engerix B), also pure preparations of HBsAg, are manufactured by inserting the gene for HBsAg into yeast. Clinical studies suggest that they are as effective as the human plasma-derived vaccine (Heptavax), and they are strongly recommended for use in the major high-risk populations: infants of HBsAg-positive mothers, accidental needle stick recipients, health care workers exposed to blood or blood products, hemodialysis patients, multiply transfused patients, promiscuous homosexual males, sexual partners of acute HB patients and household contacts of chronic HB patients, staff and residents of institutions for the mentally retarded, and certain groups of oncology and transplant patients.

The development of recombinant vaccines also holds out the promise of developing the massive quantities of vaccine necessary to initiate a worldwide program to eradicate hepatitis B. The potential to eliminate a viral infection for which human beings are the only reservoir carries with it the hope of eliminating a major worldwide disease. In addition, it provides the first opportunity to eliminate the largest cause of a major malignancy, hepatocellular carcinoma. Unfortunately, despite the availability of the plasma-derived vaccine in the United States since 1982 and recombinant vaccines since 1986 and 1988, the attack rate for hepatitis B has actually increased due to failure of high-risk groups to avail themselves of the vaccine. Accordingly, two additional steps have been recommended: (1) universal screening of all pregnant women and, more recently (2) universal vaccination of all newborn children.

Hepatitis C is best prevented at the present time by the use of an all-volunteer blood donor population and the careful screening of all blood products for the presence of anti-HCV. No vaccine is on the horizon, although this is an area of very active research.

Hepatitis D requires infection with hepatitis B and thus can be prevented by hepatitis B vaccination.

Hepatitis E prevention requires improved public sanitation. Passive protection by immune serum globulin collected from patients during the acute phase of the illness may be protective, but data are scanty; however, antibody titers appear to fall during convalescence. Neutralizing, protective antibodies may not be detected by the present assay- and more data are required before recommendations can be made. No vaccine is available.

CHRONIC HEPATITIS

Clinical and histologic criteria for the diagnosis, classification, and treatment of chronic hepatitis remain controversial. *Chronic hepatitis* is best defined as necroinflammatory liver disease which is continuously present for a period of 6 months or more. In clinical practice, the continuous elevation of serum transaminases for greater than 6 months provides a simple operational definition. Despite disagreement about a number of specific points, it has generally been accepted that chronic hepatitis presents in two major clinical forms: chronic persistent hepatitis and chronic active hepatitis (Table 57-3).

Chronic persistent hepatitis

Historically, chronic persistent hepatitis (CPH) has been considered to be benign. Patients are almost always asymptomatic, rarely have physical evidence of liver disease (jaundice, spider angiomata, palmar erythema, splenomegaly), and have only mildly elevated serum transaminases (1.5- to 5-fold). Alkaline phosphatase is normal to minimally elevated (onefold to twofold). Synthetic function (albumin, prothrombin time) and gamma globulin are usually normal.

Liver biopsy reveals little or no cell necrosis, although focal areas of cell dropout and necrosis may be seen. There is frequently a heavy portal infiltrate of mononuclear cells and little or no fibrosis is found.

Although the disease resolves spontaneously in only a few patients, CPH rarely if ever progresses to cirrhosis or liver failure. Because no specific treatment is required, liver biopsy is essential to histologically define the patient's form of chronic hepatitis. Treatment of CPH consists of reassuring the patient about its benign nature and yearly follow-up to look for changes. Repeat biopsy is indicated only if there are significant changes in the patient's disease state. At times it may be difficult to distinguish CPH from unresolved acute viral hepatitis on clinical, biochemical, or histologic grounds. Clinically, this is not a serious dilemma, however, because both are benign diseases and neither requires specific therapy. *Exceptions to this statement will be noted later (see specific etiologies).*

Chronic active hepatitis

Much debate continues concerning precise histologic definitions of chronic active hepatitis (CAH). In its initial description, emphasis was placed on the presence of "piecemeal necrosis," defined as ballooning degeneration and necrosis of hepatocytes along the edge (limiting plate) of portal tracts, fibrous septae, or zones of necrosis. Piecemeal necrosis came to be pathognomonic for CAH. Piecemeal necrosis, however, can also be found in a number of other forms of liver disease, including acute viral hepatitis, alcoholic hepatitis, primary biliary cirrhosis, sclerosing cholangitis, and Wilson's disease.

As prospective studies began to reveal the natural history of CAH, it became clear that the presence of piecemeal necrosis *alone* did not indicate a serious prognosis. Patients with this lesion rarely, if ever, progressed to cirrhosis and liver failure and probably do not require therapy. More useful prognostically was the finding of confluent areas of cell necrosis extending between portal areas or portal and central areas. This lesion of *bridging hepatic necrosis,* and the more extensive lesion in which whole lobules show parenchymal necrosis and collapse *(multilobular*

Table 57-3. Chronic hepatitis summary

Type	Etiology	Histologic subgroups	Prognosis	Treatment
Chronic persistent hepatitis	Autoimmune hepatitis (AIH) Hepatitis B virus Hepatitis C virus Hepatitis D virus Drugs	Chronic persistent hepatitis Unresolved acute hepatitis	Benign*	Reassurance and periodic followup for AIH Interferon alpha-2b for hepatitis B, ? for hepatitis C Withdraw potentially offending drugs
Chronic active hepatitis	Autoimmune hepatitis (AIH) Hepatitis B virus Hepatitis C virus Hepatitis D virus Drugs (isoniazid, methyldopa, nitrofurantoin)	1. Chronic active hepatitis without cirrhosis a. Piecemeal necrosis only b. Bridging hepatic necrosis or multilobular necrosis	1a. Probably not precir-rhotic† b. Definitely precir-rhotic	1a. Reassurance and periodic follow-up for AIH; interferon alpha-2b for hepatitis B and C b. Prednisone and Azathioprine for AIH; interferon alpha-2b for hepatitis B and C
		2. Chronic active hepatitis with cirrhosis	2. Already cirrhotic	2. Prednisone and azathioprine for AIH; interferon alpha-2b for hepatitis B and C
		3. Inactive cirrhosis	3. Already cirrhotic	3. Careful follow-up Withdraw potentially offending drugs

*An unknown percentage of patients with chronic persistent hepatitis C will progress to CAH and cirrhosis (see text).
†An unknown percentage of patients with chronic active hepatitis B and C will progress to CAH and cirrhosis (see text).

necrosis), are clearly precirrhotic and require therapy to prevent progression to cirrhosis and death from hepatic failure. Even if cirrhosis is already present, patients may still benefit from therapy if active necrosis is present. These closely held beliefs were developed based on four careful studies of patients with severe chronic liver disease. Subsequent evaluation of the data revealed that the studies contained very few patients with hepatitis B or post-transfusion hepatitis C, and the results cannot be extrapolated to these patient populations, as discussed later.

Etiology

Liver biopsy is essential in evaluating patients with chronic liver disease, not only to determine the histologic subtype, but also to rule out a number of other diseases that may cause chronic hepatitis. The liver has a limited repertoire of responses to damage, and many different forms of chronic hepatitis are indistinguishable on physical or biochemical grounds.

In this discussion viral and autoimmune etiologies are emphasized. In evaluating a patient with chronic hepatitis, however, the physician must always consider other potential causes, especially drugs, including isoniazid, nitrofurantoin, and methyldopa. In the young adult, Wilson's disease, a disorder of copper metabolism, must always be ruled out by obtaining a serum ceruloplasmin level and a slit lamp examination to look for Kayser-Fleischer rings. Wilson's disease is a potentially reversible disorder, which, while usually presenting with neurologic abnormalities, may present as chronic hepatitis in up to 25% of patients. Primary biliary cirrhosis, sclerosing cholangitis, and the "pericholangitis" associated with inflammatory bowel disease, alpha$_1$-antitrypsin deficiency, alcoholic liver disease, and hemochromatosis should also be considered. Because hemochromatosis is such a common disease (up to 1 in 400 in the population are hemizygotes), because it can be easily treated by phlebotomy to prevent complications if diagnosed before cirrhosis has developed, and because it is one of the most commonly missed diagnoses, special attention should be paid to the presence of iron in liver biopsies. Serum ferritin and transferrin saturation should be obtained if liver biopsy is not possible.

Chronic hepatitis B

Approximately 10% of patients with acute hepatitis B infection become chronic carriers. Most of them are asymptomatic and show minimal nonspecific changes or CPH on biopsy; 3% to 6% develop progressive liver disease. It is important to note that, as with all forms of chronic hepatitis, there are no clinical or biochemical tests which clearly differentiate CAH from CPH. The degree of clinical abnormalities do not necessarily correlate with the severity of histologic derangement, and liver biopsy is always required to determine etiology and prognosis as well as to determine therapeutic options.

Only about one third of patients with chronic hepatitis B recall a history of acute viral hepatitis. More typically, the patient presents with vague symptoms of malaise, fatigue, and anorexia, which may have been present for months before the patient sought medical help. Many patients, particularly older patients, will already have cirrhosis at the time of diagnosis. Symptoms and physical findings may range from anorexia and fatigue to abdominal pain, amenorrhea, ascites, jaundice, arthralgias, hepatosplenomegaly, bleeding varices, and hepatic encephalopathy. When the disease begins as acute hepatitis, the patient will initially appear to get better, often losing most or all symptoms and becoming anicteric. Transaminases remain elevated, however, although values may fluctuate from twofold to 20-fold above normal. HBsAg is virtually always positive along with anti-HBc. Rarely, HBsAg will be negative, but anti-HBc and HBV-DNA will be positive. Serologic markers suggesting an autoimmune response (antinuclear, antimitochondrial, and anti–smooth muscle antibodies) are rare, and their presence should raise serious questions about the diagnosis of chronic hepatitis B.

Prognosis is strongly correlated with underlying histology. Although 5-year survival rates for chronic hepatitis B patients were estimated at 97% for those with CPH and 86% for those with CAH and piecemeal necrosis only, patients with CAH and cirrhosis had only a 55% 5-year survival. Death was usually due to liver failure or its complications, with 10% to 13% dying of hepatocellular carcinoma. In a prospective study of the incidence of hepatocellular carcinoma in Taiwanese adult carriers of HBV who were infected at birth, the risk of developing hepatocellular carcinoma increased progressively with time and was approximately 96 times greater than in HBV-negative, matched controls.

Chronic active hepatitis C

Up to 60% of patients with post-transfusion hepatitis C develop chronic liver disease. Most often, the patient is only mildly symptomatic and nonicteric. Transaminases range from 200 to 800 and may show marked fluctuations, with rapid rises and falls and intervening periods of normality. Although post-transfusion hepatitis C affects men and women equally, 75% of those developing chronic hepatitis in one study were men. Similar to chronic hepatitis B, serum autoantibodies, hypergammaglobulinemia, and stigmata of chronic liver disease are rare, although a false-positive test for antinuclear antibodies may be present in some cases, leading to confusion with autoimmune hepatitis.

No good prospective histologic data are available in this group of patients, but CAH (usually without bridging or cirrhosis) is most common. Although it was initially thought that chronic active hepatitis C was a relatively benign disease, there is increasing evidence of slow progression to cirrhosis and liver failure. At least 20% of patients with CAH progress to cirrhosis within 5 to 10 years. Hepatitis C is the most common cause of cryptogenic cirrhosis and a common reason for liver transplantation in the United States. A strong association with the development of hepatocellular carcinoma is also recognized, with a particularly high correlation in Japan and Spain. *Hepatitis A and hepatitis E* do not produce CAH or CPH, and *hepatitis D* produces these lesions only in patients also infected with hepatitis B. In the latter instance, the frequency and severity of chronic hepatitis is greater than with hepatitis B alone.

CAH of unknown etiology ("auto-immune" or "lupoid" chronic hepatitis)

This classic form of CAH cannot be attributed to any known cause, and the original histologic classification referred to earlier was developed primarily in studies of this entity. First described by Waldenstrom in 1950 and Kunkel in 1951, the disease was thought to occur primarily in young women and demonstrated many autoimmune characteristics, including a positive lupus erythematosus (LE) cell phenomenon. It is now recognized that the disease occurs in persons of all ages and both sexes. Endocrine abnormalities (amenorrhea, hirsutism, acne, obesity, cushingoid facies, pigmented abdominal striae) and the LE cell phenomenon occur in only a small minority of patients and correlate with severity of disease rather than indentifying a unique subgroup. In contrast to chronic hepatitis B, which typically affects men, 70% to 80% of the patients are women. In one third of patients, the initial disease is identical to acute viral hepatitis. The remainder present insidiously with nonspecific symptoms of malaise, fatigue, and anorexia; are identified serendipitously on a random serum chemistry drawn for other reasons; or present with fully developed complications of advanced liver disease (ascites, variceal bleeding, hepatic encephalopathy). At least 85% of the patients have no history of exposure to jaundiced persons or other hepatitis risk factors.

Common clinical features on presentation include progressive jaundice, severe anorexia, malaise and fatigue, asymptomatic hepatosplenomegaly, and abdominal pain. Less common (20% or less) are epistaxis, acne, persistent fever, and tender hepatomegaly. Extrahepatic manifestations may occur in 20% to 25% of patients, with arthralgias and skin rashes the most common. Other abnormalities include thyroiditis, ulcerative colitis, pleurisy, pericarditis, myocarditis, and pulmonary complications, including fibrosing alveolitis. Isolated occurrences of lichen planus, mixed connective tissue disease, macroglobulinemia, and uveitis have been recorded. The multitude of disparate findings further support the likelihood of an immune origin for this disease, but it should be noted that some of these immune abnormalities (skin rashes, glomerulonephritis, arthritis) can be found in chronic hepatitis B due to immune complex desposition.

Laboratory studies are characterized by a fivefold to tenfold increase in transaminases, hypergammaglobulinemia, and the frequent presence of antinuclear (ANA), anti–smooth muscle and antiribosomal antibodies to titers of 1:160 or greater. ANAs to double-stranded DNA are negative, in contrast to their presence in patients with systemic lupus erythematosus (SLE). Abnormalities of other liver tests depend on the severity of disease at diagnosis.

Up to 20% of untreated patients will develop a spontaneous remission, but mortality rates are high in untreated patients with CAH and bridging hepatic necrosis. Nearly one third of untreated patients died over 3 years in the Mayo Clinic Study, 56% over 6 years at London's Royal Free Hospital, 28% over 2 years at King's College Hospital, and 65% over 5 years in Sydney, Australia.

In recent years, it has been recognized that many patients present with lesser increases in transaminases (onefold to threefold increased) and minor elevations in gamma globulin. Another subset of patients with negative ANA and anti–smooth muscle antibodies demonstrate antibodies to a liver-kidney microsomal antigen or a soluble liver antigen. The former is particularly a disease of children and may have a more aggressive course, occasionally even a fulminant one. Because these specialized antibody tests are not available in most hospital laboratories, the disease may be confused with fulminant non-A-non-B hepatitis.

Treatment

Immunosuppressive agents. The publication between 1969 and 1973 of four prospective, randomized, controlled therapeutic trials that demonstrated an improvement of symptoms and increased survival in patients treated with corticosteroids led to the belief that most forms of hepatitis and even cirrhosis could be treated effectively and a major disease brought under control. All patients with chronic hepatitis and a finding of "piecemeal necrosis" on liver biopsy were quickly placed on corticosteroids, but the high hopes that a serious disease process had been conquered were promptly dashed.

More careful analysis of these studies revealed that they had included almost exclusively symptomatic, HBsAg-negative, "autoimmune," chronic hepatitis patients with bridging or multilobular necrosis and/or active cirrhosis on liver biopsy. All of these qualifications have subsequently turned out to be important in determining the efficacy of immunosuppressive therapy. There is a broad consensus that therapy is appropriate in this select group with severe autoimmune chronic liver disease and that steroid treatment will improve 5-year survival from approximately 20% in untreated patients to 80% in those receiving steroids. This improved survival is produced by slowing progression to cirrhosis, if it is not already present, through an improvement in the histologic abnormality from CAH to CPH or even normal. Only approximately 15% achieve normal histology, however, and are able to remain in remission when therapy is discontinued.

Many factors must be considered in the decision to initiate steroid therapy in other forms of CAH. Chief among them are the presence of symptoms, histology, and the etiologic agent (see the accompanying box).

Most patients with CAH will have at least mild symptoms of malaise, lassitude, and fatigue. These symptoms may be difficult to ascribe purely to the patient's underlying liver disease and require a detailed and careful history. In most cases, therapy is not recommended in asymptomatic patients.

As discussed earlier, patients with autoimmune hepatitis who have CPH or CAH with "piecemeal necrosis" alone on their initial liver biopsy rarely, if ever, progress to cirrhosis or liver failure. Thus liver biopsy is required to be certain that therapy is necessary. Laboratory tests and imaging studies are not sufficient to make such a decision.

Use of corticosteroids in hepatitis

No benefit

Acute viral hepatitis
Fulminant viral hepatitis
Chronic persistent hepatitis
Chronic active hepatitis with piecemeal necrosis only
HBeAg positive chronic active HB

Possible benefit (requires 10 to 12 week trial and rebiopsy)

Subacute hepatic necrosis of undetermined etiology; symptomatic, anti-HBeAb(+), chronic active HB with bridging lesion or worse; symptomatic, chronic active hepatitis C with bridging lesion or worse that is unresponsive to interferon therapy

Definite benefit

Symptomatic, "autoimmune," or undetermined etiology chronic active hepatitis with bridging lesion or worse

In most cases, corticosteroids are not recommended for therapy of chronic hepatitis B or chronic hepatitis C. Corticosteroids increase replication of HBV and thus may increase the risk of transmission; however, HBV is not directly hepatotoxic, and the increased replication is not necessarily harmful to the patient. Some clinicians continue to use corticosteroids on a trial basis in patients with severe, rapidly deteriorating, symptomatic hepatitis B in whom interferon therapy is contraindicated (see later) and liver transplant offers no probability of long-term success. Beneficial results are occasionally seen in these highly selected patients. In addition two studies from Italy have reported clinical and histologic improvement in a subgroup of patients with chronic hepatitis B who were HBeAg negative and had antibodies to HBeAg. (Interferon treatment requires the presence of HBeAg to be successful.) I recommend corticosteroid use in chronic hepatitis B patients very rarely, on a case by case basis, and then on a *trial basis only* in those with severe, symptomatic, progressive disease who are anti-HBe positive and have a bridging or worse histologic lesion. Patients should be rebiopsied within 10 to 12 weeks and therapy discontinued if there is no clear-cut clinical, biochemical, and histologic improvement. Steroid therapy of post-transfusion hepatitis C has not been directly evaluated, but because it mimics hepatitis B in many ways, the same rigid approach to a therapeutic trial for this form of CAH seems rational. In most cases, except for those with severe decompensation, interferon is the drug of choice for chronic active hepatitis C (see later).

The immunosuppressive regimen is usually initiated with 30 to 40 mg of prednisone per day (occasionally as much as 60 mg/day). This dose is tapered over 4 to 8 weeks to a maintenance dose of 20 mg/day, with the goal of reducing transaminases to normal or, at worst, two times normal. After consolidating this response over 6 months, further decreases are titrated on a 4- to 6-week schedule to reach the lowest possible dose that will maintain the therapeutic response, ideally 10 mg or less, to reduce the risk of corticosteroid side effects. Therapy is usually continued for a minimum of 12 months. About 50% to 75% of patients will experience a flare of their hepatitis within several months of discontinuing therapy. These patients will usually respond to a second course of therapy and may require lifelong immunosuppression. Long-term follow-up of responsive patients has indicated that many whose histologic lesion improves to CPH but not normal will gradually develop cirrhosis, although this does not appear to increase mortality over a 10-year period.

Side effects of corticosteroids are frequent (up to two thirds of patients) and include moon facies, acne, abdominal striae, cataract formation, aseptic necrosis of the femoral head, and psychologic disturbances. These problems are minimized by achieving a low maintenance dose as quickly as possible. Further reduction can be achieved by combining prednisone with azathioprine, 50 mg/day. This combination allows one to reduce the prednisone dose by 50% and initiate therapy with 10 to 20 mg of prednisone. In one study, this regimen decreased steroid complications to 13% of patients. This combination regimen is particularly useful in patients in whom steroids are relatively contraindicated, including those with insulin-dependent diabetes mellitus, symptomatic osteoporosis, and postmenopausal women. Azathioprine is contraindicated in patients with fewer than 2500 leukocytes or 50,000 platelets or a past history of pancreatitis, which can be induced by azathioprine.

Table 57-4. Treatment of chronic hepatitis

Type	Steroids	Interferon alpha-2b
Chronic persistent hepatitis		
Autoimmune hepatitis	No	No
Hepatitis B	No	Yes
Hepatitis C	No	No
Chronic active hepatitis		
1. a. Piecemeal necrosis only		
Autoimmune hepatitis	No	No
Hepatitis B	No	Yes
Hepatitis C	No	Yes
b. Bridging hepatic necrosis		
Autoimmune hepatitis	Yes	No
Hepatitis B	No*	Yes
Hepatitis C	No	Yes
2. Chronic active hepatitis with cirrhosis		
Autoimmune hepatitis	Yes	No
Hepatitis B	No*	Yes
Hepatitis C	No	Yes
3. Inactive cirrhosis	No	No

See text for details of dose and duration of therapy.
*Trial worthwhile if anti-HBeAb(+) and symptomatic.

Antiviral therapy. Studies with a variety of antiviral agents, including vidarabine, acyclovir, deoxyacyclovir, and various types of human interferons, as well as additional immune-modulating agents, including transfer factor, levamisole, and thymosin, have generally been disappointing due to limited benefits and unacceptable side effects. Most studies have included very small numbers of patients and were frequently uncontrolled. Of the agents tested thus far, interferon alpha-2b has been by far the most successful and is the only antiviral or immune-modulating drug approved for the therapy of hepatitis B and hepatitis C. Its indications are summarized in Table 57-4. Thymosin has also shown some encouraging results in the treatment of chronic hepatitis B in limited preliminary trials. Interferon has both antiviral and immune-modulating effects, which may contribute to its observed benefits. Its effects on hepatitis B and hepatitis C are produced by different mechanisms. It appears to primarily modulate the body's own immune attack on the hepatitis B virus but has direct antiviral effects on the hepatitis C virus.

With both chronic hepatitis B and hepatitis C, one can expect 40% to 50% of patients to show a response. These responses are defined somewhat differently. For hepatitis C, a response is defined as normalization or near normalization of transaminases with an improvement in liver histology and, in most cases, disappearance of HCV-RNA by PCR testing. The response with hepatitis B is defined as the loss of circulating HBV-DNA and HBeAg with conversion to anti-HBeAg positivity. In most hepatitis B cases, surface antigen (HBsAg) is not lost. Approximately 50% of responding hepatitis C patients relapse within 6 months of discontinuing treatment. It is unclear whether the remaining patients (approximately 20% to 25% of the initially treated patients) represent cures or continued suppression of the disease. The response in hepatitis B patients appears to be durable with few relapses. Of particular interest is the recent report that many of the chronic hepatitis B patients who demonstrate a prolonged response eventually lose their HBsAg positivity and develop antibodies to B surface antigen. The standard, approved regimen for chronic hepatitis C infection is 3 million units of recombinant human interferon alpha-2b injected subcutaneously, three times a week for 24 weeks. Treatment of hepatitis B requires larger doses of interferon, 5 million units on a daily basis for 16 weeks.

Because it is unclear whether more than isolated patients with chronic persistent hepatitis C will progress to a more severe illness, most specialists do not currently treat this less aggressive lesion, preferring to follow these patients carefully, often repeating the liver biopsy within 1 to 2 years or earlier if their clinical situation changes. Treatment may be considered if the patient has significant associated symptomatology. If it becomes apparent through ongoing studies that a significant percentage of chronic persistent hepatitis C patients are progressing to cirrhosis and/or developing hepatomas, then this group will likely be recommended for therapy.

Chronic hepatitis B patients are generally treated regardless of histology because all are at risk of developing hepatoma, and a small number of those with more benign histology will progress to more severe disease over time. Some patients, however, predictably respond poorly to interferon therapy. Results from the controlled trials to date indicate that individuals with active, replicative disease are most responsive (detectable circulating HBV-DNA, but at levels less than 100 picograms/ml and transaminase values of greater than 100 IU/L). Individuals with very high circulating HBV-DNA levels, undetectable circulating HBV-DNA, or very low transaminase levels respond poorly. Similarly, individuals who acquired HBV at or around the time of birth are much less likely to respond than those who have had HBV for a short time and acquired it in adulthood. Limited studies suggest that a short rapid taper of steroid therapy, to increase the rate of replication of HBV, may increase responsiveness to interferon. This approach, however, is frought with danger, as it increases the activity of the disease and should, at present, be limited to ongoing controlled clinical trials.

Interferon has numerous side effects, and patients require considerable support during therapy. Most bothersome are the severe influenza-like symptoms of fever, malaise, fatigue, and chills experienced by the majority of patients. Pretreatment with acetaminophen, 30 to 60 minutes before the interferon injection, will decrease these symptoms, but usually not eliminate them entirely. Other significant side effects that require careful monitoring include bone marrow suppression with thrombocytopenia and neutropenia; psychologic disturbances, including irritability and depression; thyroid dysfunction, including hyperthyroidism and hypothyroidism; and moderate alopecia. Interferon therapy is not recommended for patients with decompensated liver disease, especially decompensated chronic hepatitis B, as it initially produces a flare in the hepatitis before the patient enters remission. In contrast, hepatitis C patients show a rapid improvement in transaminases without the initial flare. Careful screening for autoimmune disease must also be performed before initiating therapy, as interferon has been shown to exacerbate autoimmune disease, including autoimmune chronic active hepatitis. Any physician contemplating the use of interferon should read the product literature extremely carefully and follow meticulously the recommendations on pretreatment evaluation and follow-up during treatment.

Interferon therapy in its current form produces long-term benefits for only 20% or so of patients with chronic hepatitis B and C. Continued research to improve the response to interferon, as well as develop other modes of therapy, will be important to provide lasting help to those patients who do not respond to the currently available therapy.

REFERENCES

Balayan MS: HEV infection: historical perspectives, global epidemiology, and clinical features. In Hollinger FB, Lemon SM, and Margolis HS, editors: Viral hepatitis and liver disease, Baltimore, 1991, Williams & Wilkins.

Bernuau J, Rueff B, and Benhamou JP: Fulminant and subfulminant liver failure: definitions and causes, Semin Liver Dis 6:97, 1986.

Centers for Disease Control: Hepatitis B virus: a comprehensive strategy for eliminating transmission in the United States through universal childhood vaccination, MMWR 40(RR-13):1, 1991.

Cohen JI: Hepatitis A virus: insights from molecular biology, Hepatology 9:889, 1989.

Choo Q-L et al: Isolation of a cDNA clone derived from a blood-borne non-A, non-B viral hepatitis genome, Science 244:359, 1989.

Davis GL et al: Treatment of chronic hepatitis C with recombinant interferon α—a multicenter randomized controlled trial, N Engl J Med 321:1501, 1989.

Di Bisceglie AM et al: Recombinant interferon α therapy for chronic hepatitis C—a radomized, double-blind, placebo-controlled trial, N Engl J Med 321:1506, 1989.

Hoofnagle JH and Schafer DF: Serologic markers of Hepatitis B virus infection, Semin Liver Dis 6:1, 1986.

Hollinger FB and Ticehurst F: Hepatitis A virus. In Fields BN et al, editors: Virology, New York, 1990, Raven Press.

Kuo G et al: An assay for circulating antibodies to a major etiologic virus of human non-A, non-B hepatitis, Science 244:362, 1989.

LaBrecque DR: Medical ostriches, Infect Control Hosp Epidemiol 2:126, 1990.

Manns M: Autoantibodies in liver disease—updated, J Hepatol 2:272, 1989.

Maynard JE et al: Control of hepatitis B by immunization: global perspectives. In Zuckerman AJ, editor: Viral hepatitis and liver disease, New York, 1988, Alan R. Liss.

Perillo RP et al: A randomized, controlled trial of interferon alfa-2b alone and after prednisone withdrawal for the treatment of chronic hepatitis B, N Engl J Med 323(5):295, 1990.

Rizzetto M et al: Hepatitis delta virus infection: clinical and epidemiological aspects. In Zuckerman AJ, editor: Viral hepatitis and liver disease, New York, 1988, Alan R. Liss.

Sagnelli E et al: Effect of immunosuppressive therapy on HBsAg-positive chronic active hepatitis in relation to presence or absence of HBeAg and Anti-HBe, Hepatology 3:690, 1983.

Ticehurst J: Identification and characterization of hepatitis E virus. In Hollinger FB, Lemon SM, and Margolis HS, editors: Viral hepatitis and liver disease, Baltimore, 1991, Williams & Wilkins.

Werzberger A et al: A controlled trial of a formalin-inactivated hepatitis A vaccine in healthy children, N Engl J Med 327:453, 1992.

Wright EC et al: Treatment of chronic active hepatitis. An analysis of three controlled trials, Gastroenterology 73:1422, 1977.

CHAPTER

58 Drug- and Toxin-Induced Liver Disease

Hyman J. Zimmerman

A large number of chemical and biologic agents can induce hepatic injury (see the box on p. 602). Some hepatotoxins are plant or fungal products; some are minerals; and many are products, by-products, or wastes of the chemical and pharmaceutical industries.

Exposure to toxic agents can occur in domestic, occupational, or clinical settings. Some natural toxins, such as

Types of hepatotoxic agents

I. Inorganic agents
  A. Metals and metalloids (antimony, arsenic, beryllium, cadmium, copper, iron, lead, manganese, phosphorus, thallium)
  B. Hydrazine derivatives
  C. Iodides
II. Organic agents
  A. Natural agents
    1. Plant toxins (albitocin, cycasin, amanitin, icterogenin, indospicine, lantana, ngaione, nutmeg, phalloidin, pyrrolizidines, safrole, tannic acid)
    2. Mycotoxins, (aflatoxins, cyclochlorotine, ethanol, luteoskyrin, ochratoxins, rubratoxins, sterigmatocystins, griseofulvin, sporidesmin, tetracycline, and other antibiotics)
  B. Synthetic agents
    1. Nonmedicinal agents
      a. Haloalkanes and haloolefins
      b. Nitroalkanes
      c. Haloaromatic compounds
      d. Nitroaromatic compounds
      e. Organic amines
      f. Azo compounds
      g. Phenol and derivatives
      h. Various other organic compounds
    2. Medicinal agents (over 300 drugs used for treatment and diagnosis)

Note: Agents listed in this table vary considerably in their potential for causing hepatic injury.

the peptides of *Amanita phalloides* and related poisonous mushrooms, the pyrrolizidine alkaloids, and the toxin of the cycad nut, are taken as food or as folk medicine in ignorance of their toxicity. Other natural toxins, e.g., aflatoxin, are ingested because climatic conditions favor their presence as unsuspected contaminants of food. Synthetic hepatotoxins also may be ingested as accidental contaminants of food. Domestic exposure to hepatotoxins includes accidental or suicidal ingestion or inhalation of known toxins (e.g., CCl_4) or of large overdoses of medicinal agents (e.g., acetaminophen).

Occupational exposure to hepatotoxic agents has led to hepatic injury in the past; however, improved industrial hygiene seems to have reduced the incidence. Pollution of the environment by toxic industrial by-products and wastes is of great concern, but the magnitude of the hepatotoxic threat remains to be defined.

Drug-induced hepatic injury is the facet of hepatotoxicity of most relevance to clinicians. A large number of medicinal agents can produce liver damage. The importance of drug-induced hepatic injury rests on both its frequency and its character. Although reactions to drugs account for less than 10% of all cases of apparent hepatitis, they assume more importance with advancing age, accounting for up to 50% of cases of apparent hepatitis in patients over 50 years. Furthermore, drug-induced hepatic injury plays a prominent role in the causation of massive hepatic necrosis, accounting for about 25% of cases. The importance of drug toxicity as a cause of fatal hepatic necrosis stems from the gravity of the hepatocellular type of drug-induced injury.

Of increasing concern, but only vaguely substantiated, is the risk of acquiring chronic hepatic disease, particularly neoplasms, from prolonged occupational exposure to toxic chemicals or from ingestion of mycotoxins and other natural hepatotoxins. Drugs also can lead to chronic hepatic disease.

SUSCEPTIBILITY OF THE LIVER TO CHEMICAL INJURY

The great susceptibility of the liver to damage by chemical agents is presumably a consequence of its primary role in the disposition of foreign substances. The position of the liver as portal to the tissues for ingested agents and the concentration of xenobiotics in the liver may contribute to its special vulnerability. The role of the liver in the metabolic conversions of foreign compounds is even more relevant to its susceptibility.

Biotransformation of foreign compounds has been traditionally considered detoxifying. Such reactions, however, can also convert nontoxic agents to potentially toxic products. It has become clear that formation of reactive, toxic, metabolic intermediates within the hepatocyte accounts for the injury it sustains from many toxic chemicals and drugs.

Most of the biotransformations are catalyzed by the drug-metabolizing enzyme system called the *mixed function oxidase* (MFO) or *cytochrome P-450*. This enzyme consists of a number of isozymes, each of which has special catalyzing properties for different substrates.

Modification of the ability to metabolize foreign chemicals results from exposure to a number of compounds. Administration of phenobarbital and exposure to insecticides and many other agents enhance the ability of the liver to metabolize a large number of compounds. This phenomenon, which involves an increase in the amount and activity of cytochrome P-450, has been dubbed *induction*. Accordingly, induction enhances the hepatotoxicity of agents that are converted to toxic products by the isozyme of cytochrome P-450 that had been induced.

Among the agents that enhance the ability to metabolize foreign compounds and thereby increase the hepatotoxic effects of a number of toxic chemicals is ethanol. The increased susceptibility of alcoholics to hepatic injury from carbon tetrachloride or acetaminophen or isoniazid seems attributable, at least in part, to the enhancement of conversion of these agents to their toxic metabolites by the alcohol induction of the isozyme of cytochrome P-450 that is involved in the metabolism of these compounds. Conversely, inhibition of conversion of toxic agents to their active metabolic products by agents that inhibit the MFO may decrease the toxic effects of the drug. Cimetidine, for example, inhibits the MFO, thus decreasing the hepatotoxic effects of acetaminophen for experimental animals. (Effectiveness of cimetidine in poisoning in humans remains to be demonstrated.)

CLASSIFICATION OF HEPATOTOXIC AGENTS

Two main categories of agents produce hepatic injury: predictable (intrinsic) hepatotoxins and nonpredictable (idiosyncratic) "hepatotoxins." Idiosyncratic hepatotoxins produce hepatic injury only in unusually susceptible persons. The distinguishing characteristics of each type are listed in Table 58-1.

The division of hepatotoxic effects into intrinsic or idiosyncratic types is oversimplified. A spectrum of toxic potential exists, ranging from that of agents (e.g., phosphorus) that damage the liver of almost all members of a variety of species to drugs (e.g., penicillin) that hardly ever produce hepatic injury. The relative roles of host susceptibility and intrinsic toxicity of an agent might be portrayed as the two axes of a graph (Fig. 58-1).

Intrinsic hepatotoxins

There are two main types of intrinsic hepatotoxins, direct and indirect. Direct hepatotoxins destroy hepatocytes by direct physicochemical attack, i.e., peroxidation and denaturation of proteins or other destructive alteration of cell membranes. Indirect hepatotoxins divert or competitively inhibit essential metabolites, react selectively with and distort molecules essential for cell integrity, or in other ways interfere with specific metabolic or secretory functions of the hepatocyte. The effect of either type may be mediated by an active metabolite of the agent or by the native molecule.

Intrinsic hepatotoxins are either cytotoxic or cholestatic. Cytotoxic hepatotoxins produce steatosis, necrosis, or both. Steatosis results from interference with synthesis of apoprotein, with assembly of the lipoprotein complex required for transport of lipid from the liver, from impaired mitochondrial oxidation of fatty acids, and from other defects in lipid metabolism. Necrosis results from obscure mechanisms, presumably selective lesions of the membranes of the hepatocyte. Cholestatic hepatotoxins produce selective interference with mechanisms or structures involved in the excretion of bile or uptake of its constituents from the blood.

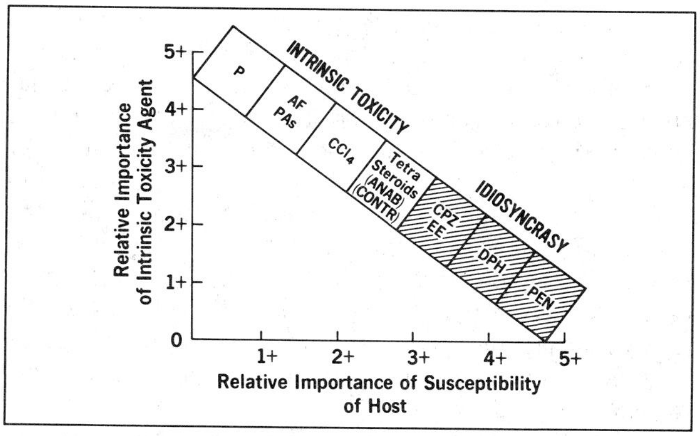

Fig. 58-1. Interplay between intrinsic toxicity of chemical agent and susceptibility of exposed persons in the production of hepatic injury. Interplay can be expressed as dichotomy or as spectrum. P, phosphorus; AF, aflatoxin; PAs, pyrrolizidine alkaloids; CPZ, chlorpromazine; EE, erythromycin estolate; DPH, diphenylhydantion (phenytoin). (From H J Zimmerman: Hepatotoxicity: adverse effects of drugs and other chemicals on the liver. New York, 1978, Appleton-Century-Crofts, p. 95.)

Idiosyncratic hepatic injury

Hepatic injury that occurs unpredictably in a small proportion of recipients of some drugs is an expression of a special susceptibility of the patient rather than of intrinsic toxicity of the agent. Idiosyncratic hepatic injury appears to be a manifestation of hypersensitivity or of aberrant metabolism of the drug.

The liver injury may be attributed to hypersensitivity if it is accompanied by clinical signs (fever, rash, eosinophilia) and histologic hallmarks (eosinophilic or granulomatous inflammation in the liver) of hypersensitivity. These characteristics, especially when supported by a prompt recurrence of the syndrome after a challenge dose, permit the inference that the hepatic injury is due to a drug allergy and that the drug or a metabolite has acted as a hapten. This form of injury usually develops after a "sensitization" period of 1 to 5 weeks.

Table 58-1. Features that distinguish intrinsic hepatotoxins from those that produce hepatic injury as idiosyncratic reactions

Basis for hepatic injury	Characteristics: Experimental reproducibility	Dose dependence	Incidence in human beings	Latent period
Intrinsic hepatotoxicity* (true, predictable hepatotoxic agents)	Yes†	Yes	High‡	Often short and relatively uniform
Idiosyncratic reaction* (nonpredictable hepatotoxic agents)	No§	No§	Low	Often long and quite variable

*Terms preferred by this author. Terms in parentheses are those used by other authors.
†May apply only to some species.
‡Depends on dosage.
§If due to metabolic idiosyncrasy, may be reproducible experimentally in specially manipulated animal models.

Lack of hypersensitivity and failure to evoke prompt recurrence of the hepatic injury with one or two challenge doses of the suspected drug suggest an alternative mechanism for the liver damage, presumably the production of hepatotoxic metabolites. This form of injury appears after widely variable latent periods ranging from weeks to months. For a number of drugs, evidence is strong that metabolic idiosyncrasy accounts for the injury they produce. Isoniazid, valproic acid, perhexiline maleate, and amiodarone produce hepatic injury that seems clearly ascribable to toxic metabolites that are produced to a greater degree by patients who develop hepatic injury than by those who remain uninjured.

Metabolic idiosyncrasy may also be the mechanism by which hypersensitivity develops. Phenytoin leads to injury that appears to be classically hypersensitivity provoked. The apparent hapten is a reactive metabolite (the arene oxide) of phenytoin that accumulates in patients who have an inborn defective ability to convert the arene oxide to a nonreactive metabolite.

Even among agents that produce hypersensitivity reactions there are several categories of association of hypersensitivity with hepatic injury (Fig. 58-2). Some drugs (e.g., phenytoin) produce hepatic injury only in association with systemic features of an allergic response. Others (e.g., chlorpromazine) produce hepatic injury that may or may not be accompanied by systemic features suggestive of drug allergy. Still other drugs that lead to generalized hypersensitivity (penicillin) do not necessarily cause hepatic injury. These observations, the high incidence of mild hepatic dysfunction among recipients of some drugs (e.g., chlorpromazine), and the toxic effects of these drugs in experimental animal models have led to the hypothesis that hypersensitivity leads to overt hepatic disease if the causative drug also has some intrinsic hepatotoxic potential.

Mechanisms of injury are classified in Table 58-2. Toxins encountered in the home or workplace are intrinsic, direct, or indirect. Medicinal agents have been included in each of the classifications, although known potent intrinsic hepatotoxins such as CCl_4 and chloroform are no longer in clinical use. Some intrinsic hepatotoxins, however, are still used in clinical medicine. Some, like acetaminophen, are usually hepatotoxic only in large overdoses or in patients whose susceptibility is enhanced by other factors (e.g., alcohol). Others lead to cytotoxic injury (e.g., tetracycline and oncotherapeutic agents) or cholestatic injury (anabolic and contraceptive steroids) even at doses in the therapeutic range.

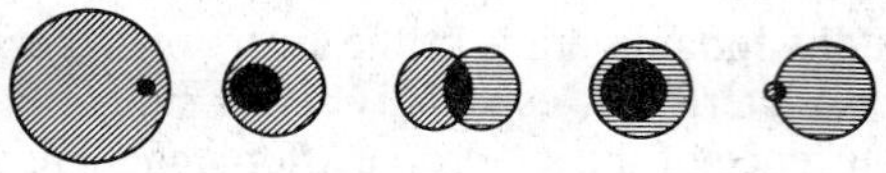

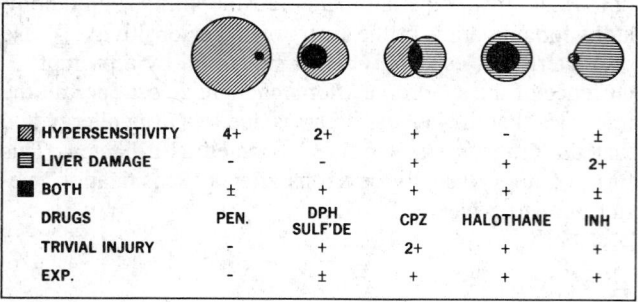

HYPERSENSITIVITY	4+	2+	+	-	±
LIVER DAMAGE	-	-	+	+	2+
BOTH	±	+	+	+	±
DRUGS	PEN.	DPH SULF'DE	CPZ	HALOTHANE	INH
TRIVIAL INJURY	-	+	2+	+	+
EXP.	-	±	+	+	+

Fig. 58-2. Relation between hypersensitivity and hepatic injury. Note that drugs like penicillin (PEN), despite a marked tendency to produce hypersensitivity reactions, very rarely lead to liver damage and then only in association with hypersensitivity. Other drugs, like phenytoin (DPH) and sulfonamides (SULF'DE), which are also prone to cause hypersensitivity, are much more likely to cause hepatic injury in association with hypersensitivity. A third group of drugs, represented by chlorpromazine (CPZ) and halothane, may produce liver damage with or without hypersensitivity, while a fourth group, represented by isoniazoid (INH), produces hepatic injury usually unaccompanied by hypersensitivity. All these drugs except penicillin produce a significant incidence of trivial injury in human beings and can produce injury in experimental animal models (EXP.). (From Zimmerman HJ: Drug hepatotoxicity: spectrum of clinical lesions. In Davis M, Tredger JM, and Williams R, editors: Drug reactions and the liver. London, 1981, Pittman, p. 43.)

CLINICAL ASPECTS OF CHEMICAL HEPATIC INJURY

Chemical hepatic injury has a broad range of clinical manifestations. It may occur as an unexpected idiosyncratic reaction to a therapeutic drug dosage or as the expected consequence of an agent's intrinsic toxicity. Hepatic injury may be acute or chronic. Liver disease may be the only clinical manifestation of the chemical's adverse effect, or it may be accompanied by evident injury to other organs or by systemic manifestations. Liver disease may develop within several days after ingestion of a toxic dose of a known hepatotoxin, after 1 to 5 weeks of taking a drug whose hepatic injury involves hypersensitivity, or after weeks to many months of taking a drug that causes injury as a result of metabolic idiosyncrasy.

Acute hepatic injury

Acute toxic hepatic injury may be (1) mainly cytotoxic, involving overt damage to hepatocytes; (2) cholestatic, involving mainly arrested bile flow; or (3) mixed, i.e., with prominent cytotoxic and cholestatic features (Table 58-3). Most intrinsic toxins produce mainly cytotoxic injury; only a few produce injury that is mainly cholestatic. Some drugs that produce idiosyncratic hepatic damage produce mainly cholestatic injury; others produce cytotoxic injury.

Cytotoxic injury includes necrosis, steatosis, or both. There are two types of cholestatic injury. One is accompanied by portal inflammation and evident, although slight, hepatocyte injury. This type is called sensitivity or hepatocanalicular cholestasis. The second type is accompanied by little inflammation and even less hepatocyte injury and is called steroid-induced, or canalicular, cholestasis. The hepatocanalicular type is exemplified by chlorpromazine jaundice and the canalicular type by anabolic or contraceptive steroid jaundice.

Clinical and biochemical features of toxic hepatic injury mirror the morphologic features. Hepatic necrosis leads to hepatocellular jaundice and a syndrome resembling that of viral hepatitis. Values for serum aspartate aminotransferase

Table 58-2. Classification of hepatotoxic agents and major characteristics of each group

Class of agent	Incidence	Experimental reproduction	Dose dependency	Mechanism	Histologic lesion	Example
Intrinsic toxicity	High	Yes	Yes			
Direct				Direct physicochemical distortion and destruction by peroxidation and related effects	Necrosis	
Cytotoxic					Hepatocytes	CCl_4
Cholestatic					Ducts	Paraquat
Indirect	High	Yes	Yes	Interference with specific metabolic pathways leading to structural injury by covalent binding or other metabolic distortion	Necrosis or steatosis	Acetaminophen
Cytotoxic						Tetracyclines
Cholestatic	High	Yes	Yes	Interference with excretory pathways leading to cholestasis	Bile casts	Anabolic steroids (C-17 alkylated)
Host idiosyncrasy						
Immunologic (hypersensitivity	Low	No	No	Drug allergy	Necrosis or cholestasis	Phenytoin Chlorpromazine Erythromycins
Metabolic	Low	No	No	Production of hepatotoxic metabolites	Necrosis or cholestasis	Isoniazid Valproic acid Benoxaproten

Table 58-3. Histologic types of acute toxic hepatic injury and associated biochemical and clinical aspects

Histologic lesion	Biochemical abnormalities of serum*			Clinical aspects	Examples†
	Aminotransferases (AST and ALT)	Alkaline phosphatase	Cholesterol		
Cytotoxic					
Necrosis					
Zonal	↑ (10-500X)	↑ (1-2X)	N, ↓	Hepatic and renal failure	CCl_4, MSH, ACM, HALO
Diffuse	↑ (10-200X)	↑ (1-2X)	N, ↓	Severe hepatitis-like disease	INH, methyldopa, HALO
Steatosis	↑ (5-20X)	↑ (1-2X)	↓	Resembles fatty liver of pregnancy and Reye's syndrome	Tetracycline, aspirin‡
Cholestatic					
With pericholangitis (hepatocanalicular)	↑ (1-10X)	↑ (3-10X)	↑	Resembles obstructive jaundice	CPZ, EE
Without pericholangitis (canalicular)	↑ (1-5X)	↑ (1-3X)	N, ↑	Resembles obstructive jaundice	Anabolic and contraceptive steroids
Mixed (mixture of cytotoxic and cholestatic)	↑ (10-100X)	↑ (1-10X)	N, ↑	May resemble hepatitis or obstructive jaundice	PBZ, PAS, sulfonamides, DPH

*Degree of abnormality indicated as times increase. N, normal; N, ↑ or ↓, normal or slightly abnormal.

†ACM, acetaminophen; CPZ, chlorpromazine; DPH, phenytoin; EE, erythromycin estolate; HALO, halothane; INH, isoniazid; MSH, poisonous mushrooms; PAS, para-aminosalicylate; PBZ, phenylbutazone.

‡Aspirin in therapeutic doses may contribute to development of Reye's syndrome in children exposed to influenza A, varicella, or other viral illness. A similar lesion is produced by poisonous overdose of aspirin.

(AST) and serum alanine aminotransferase (ALT) are often very high (see Table 58-3), 10 to 200 times the upper limit of normal (ULN), or even higher, and values for alkaline phosphatase are usually modestly increased (less than three times the ULN). The chief clinical manifestations are fatigue, anorexia, and nausea. Severe cases of toxic hepatic injury are manifested by deep jaundice, and hemorrhagic phenomena, coma, and death may develop. Indeed, the most important aspect of drug-induced hepatocellular jaundice is its tendency to result in fulminant hepatic failure. Fatality rates have ranged from 10% to 50%. Survival of the acute phase usually leads to complete recovery.

Acute steatosis, such as that caused by parenterally administered tetracycline or overdoses of aspirin leads to clinical and biochemical features resembling those of the acute fatty liver of pregnancy and of Reye's syndrome, which it also mimics histologically. (In these conditions, the steatosis is microvesicular, in contrast to the macrovesicular steatosis of alcoholic fatty liver.) Jaundice is usually relatively slight. Aminotransferase levels are usually somewhat lower than those in patients with hepatic necrosis (less than 20 times the ULN). The illness, however, is serious.

Cholestatic injury resembles extrahepatic obstructive jaundice. Jaundice and pruritus are the main clinical manifestations. Aminotransferase levels are only modestly elevated (usually less than eight times the ULN). There are biochemical counterparts to the two morphologic types of cholestasis. In the hepatocanalicular type, alkaline phosphatase levels are usually elevated to more than three times the ULN, and cholesterol levels are elevated; in the canalicular type, the values for alkaline phosphatase and cholesterol are normal or slightly elevated. Cholestatic injury, with a case fatality rate of less than 1%, has a far better prognosis than cytotoxic injury. In rare instances, however, cholestatic jaundice may fail to resolve and evolves into a syndrome resembling primary biliary cirrhosis.

The clinical syndrome of chemical hepatic injury may indicate liver disease alone or with systemic manifestations and evidence of injury to other organs (Table 58-4). Fever, rash, and eosinophilia are characteristic of reactions caused by some drugs, and in some instances these features are accompanied by lymph node enlargement, lymphocytosis, and "atypical" circulating lymphocytes, leading to a syndrome that resembles infectious mononucleosis and serum sickness ("pseudomononucleosis"). Bone marrow, lung, and skin may be involved in systemic reactions. Renal injury may be a component of generalized hypersensitivity caused by some drugs (e.g., phenytoin, sulfonamides) or the result of the nephrotoxic effect of a metabolite of a drug (e.g., methoxyflurane). Renal injury is particularly prominent in poisoning by CCl_4, phosphorus, and poisonous mushrooms.

Table 58-4. Systemic manifestations that may be associated with drug hepatotoxicity

Manifestations	Drugs
Allergic reactions	
Fever, rash, eosinophilia	Para-aminosalicylate, anticonvulsants
Pseudomononucleosis	
Lymph node hyperplasia	Oxyphenisatin
Lymphocytosis	
Autoantibodies	
LE factor	
Hemolytic anemia	Methyldopa
Bone marrow injury	Phenylbutazone, anticonvulsants
Renal injury	Sulindac, methoxyflurane
Gastrointestinal ulcer, pancreatitis	Phenylbutazone, tetracycline

Chronic liver damage

Chemical hepatic injury can also lead to chronic lesions. These lesions include chronic active hepatitis, steatosis, phospholipidosis, granulomatous disease, several vascular lesions, several forms of cirrhosis, noncirrhotic portal hypertension, and several types of hepatic tumors (Table 58-5). Chronic active hepatitis has occurred as a reaction to oxyphenisatin, methyldopa, nitrofurantoin, sulfonamides, propylthiouracil, clometacine, papaverine, and other drugs. The syndrome resembles the "autoimmune" type of chronic active hepatitis. Several drugs that lead to phospholipidosis also lead to hyaline degeneration of the alcoholic hyaline type. Amiodarone and perhexiline maleate have been incriminated in the production of a lesion that includes Mallory bodies and cirrhosis.

HEPATOTOXIC REACTIONS AND CIRCUMSTANCES OF EXPOSURE (See also Chapter 366)

A host of agents with hepatotoxic potential have been used in the munitions, rocketry, plastics, paint, cosmetic, pharmaceutical, and other chemical industries. Nevertheless, overt acute hepatic injury is a rare consequence of occupational exposure to toxic chemicals and is more likely to be acquired in the home (Table 58-6). The risk of chronic subtle injury continues to be a concern but there are scant data to support this. The toxicity of several of these agents warrants description in more detail.

Carbon tetrachloride poisoning

Instances of CCl_4 intoxication are now rare. Most victims are alcoholics because alcoholism enhances susceptibility by increasing transformation of CCl_4 to a toxic metabolite and leads to increased carelessness with its use. Inhalation or accidental ingestion has been the mode of exposure.

The clinical syndrome consists of hepatic failure accompanied by renal failure. Minutes to hours after exposure there are usually neurologic and gastrointestinal manifestations and a variable degree of vascular collapse. There may then be a period of abatement, followed by the appearance of hepatic injury within 2 to 4 days of exposure. The current mortality appears to be considerably lower than the 25% previously noted, presumably because of the improved

Table 58-5. Chronic hepatic disease caused by drugs

Lesion or syndrome	Causative agents
Cytotoxic	
Chronic necroinflammatory disease (chronic active hepatitis)	Oxphenisatin, iproniazid isoniazid, methyldopa, sulfonamides, nitrofurantoin, dantrolene, propylthiouracil
Subacute hepatic necrosis	Drugs listed above for chronic inflammatory disease, occupational toxins (e.g., TNT)
Steatosis	Ethanol, methotrexate antineoplastic agents, valproate, glucocorticoids
Phospholipidosis* and pseudoalcoholic disease†	Coralgil‡ perhexiline maleate amiodarone
Cholestatic	
Chronic intrahepatic cholestasis	Chlorpromazine, and several other phenothiazine, several tricyclic antidepressants, ajmaline; organ arsenical, tolben taniel throbedazole et al
Sclerosing cholangitis	Floxuridine
Cirrhosis	
Micronodular	Ethanol, methotrexate inorganic arsenical
Macronodular	Ethanol, methotrexate inorganic arsenical (also agents listed above for chronic inflammatory disease)
"Primary biliary"	See chronic intrahepatic cholestasisi
Congestive "cirrhosis"	Oral contraceptive steroids Thioguanine, pyrrolidizine alkaloids, urethan (x-ray)
Vascular lesions	
Peliosis hepatis and/or marked sinusoidal dilatation	Anabolic and contraceptive steroids, phalloidin, oxazepam, azathioprine
Hepatic vein thrombosis	Contraceptive steroids
Veno-occlusive disease	Pyrrolidizine alkaloids, urethan, thioguanine, and other antineoplastic drugs (x-ray)
Neoplasm	
Adenoma	Anabolic and contraceptive steroids
Carcinoma	
Hepatocellular	Anabolic and contraceptive steroids, Thorotrast
Cholangiocellular	
Angiosarcoma	Vinyl chloride, Thorotrast inorganic arsenicals
Other	
Hepatoportal sclerosis	Vinyl chloride, inorganic arsenicals
Centrilobular fibrosis	Vitamin A excess, methyldopa
Granulomas	Allopurinol, hydralazine, penicillin, phenylbutazone, quinidine, sulfonamides, sulfonylureas, and many other drugs

*Accumulation of phospholipids in lysosomes, with ultimate development of cirrhosis.
†Hyaline degeneration (Mallory bodies) resembling alcoholic liver disease. This lesion can lead to cirrhosis.
‡Trade name for 4,4′-diethylaminoethoxyhexesterol dihydrochloride (a drug formerly used in Japan to treat arteriosclerotic heart disease).

outlook provided by treatment of the renal failure with hemodialysis. Early treatment with acetylcysteine and hyperbaric oxygen have been proposed to have benefit.

Laboratory findings include neutrophilic leukocytosis, anemia, and azotemia. The urinary sediment reflects the acute tubular necrosis. Serum values of aminotransferases can reach astronomic levels.

Mushroom and phosphorus poisoning

A clinical syndrome somewhat similar to that seen with CCl_4 poisoning results from poisoning by the hepatotoxic mushroom *A. phalloides* and related species. The mortality, however, is about 25%. The patient presents with severe diarrhea, which is followed by a period of ameliorated symptoms and subsequently by severe hepatic and renal failure. In the liver, there is steatosis and centrilobular necrosis. The mortality rate is about 25%. A prothrombin concentration less than 10% of normal is strongly predictive of a fatal outcome, whereas a value above 40% of normal is predictive of survival.

Phosphorus poisoning is characterized by severe gastrointestinal symptoms and shock and by phosphorescence and garliclike odor of excreta and vomit. It leads to fulminant hepatic and renal failure, with a mortality also in excess of 50%. The liver shows mainly steatosis, at first at the periphery of the lobule and then throughout. Necrosis may be present and is also predominantly peripheral.

Acetaminophen poisoning

This mild analgesic has virtually no side effects when administered in the usual therapeutic doses. It produces severe centrilobular hepatic necrosis if large doses are ingested, usually in suicide attempts. Necrosis is produced by an active metabolite that binds covalently to tissue macromolecules. The small amounts of active metabolite normally formed from a therapeutic dose are readily detoxified by reacting with glutathione. Hepatic necrosis occurs only when the amount of active metabolite produced exceeds the binding capacity of glutathione. This occurs when the drug dose is large and especially in association with factors that increase the fraction of drug converted to an active metabolite (alcoholism, inducing drugs, stress) or that

Table 58-6. Known or potential* domestic hepatotoxic agents

Agent	Exposure	Lesion
Chlorinated hydrocarbons	Careless use; accidental; "solvent sniffing"	Centrilobular necrosis, steatosis
Phosphorus (yellow)	Suicidal or accidental	Steatosis, periportal necrosis
Toxic chemicals as inadvertent contaminants of food		
4′,4-Diaminodiphenylmethane	Contaminant of flour ("Epping jaundice")	Cholestatic jaundice
Hexachlorobenzene	Fungistatic added to wheat	Steatosis, necrosis, toxic porphyria
Chlorinated biphenyls	Contaminant of rice (Japan)	Steatosis, necrosis
Toxic foods of plant origin		
A. phalloides and related species	Ingested as food in ignorance of toxicity	Centrilobular necrosis, steatosis
Cycad nut	Ingested as food in ignorance of toxicity	Necrosis, steatosis, cirrhosis, hepatocellular carcinoma
Senecio, Heliotropium, Crotalaria and other plants that contain pyrrolizidine alkaloids	Ingested as additive to foods, as medicinal decoction, or as abortifacient	Centrilobular necrosis, venoocclusive disease, congestive cirrhosis, steatosis
Nutmeg	Ingested as abortifacient	Steatosis, midzonal necrosis
Ngaione	Potential food toxin	
Mycotoxins*		
Aflatoxins (*Aspergillus flavus* and related species)	Present mainly in legumes and other foods of vegetable origin when climatic conditions permit	Steatosis, necrosis, cirrhosis, hepatocellular carcinoma
Ochratoxin		
Luteoskyrin		
Other mycotoxins		

*Evidence for hepatotoxicity mainly epidemiologic and experimental.

decrease the availability of glutathione. Doses have exceeded 15 g in about 80% of such cases.

Acetaminophen also has been reported to produce hepatic injury as a therapeutic mishap. This effect has involved mainly alcoholics in whom severe hepatic injury developed because they had taken large therapeutic doses or in whom susceptibility to acetaminophen injury had been enhanced by the induction of cytochrome P-450 or by depletion of glutathione secondary to the alcoholism. Instances of nonalcoholic individuals in whom hepatic injury developed secondary to therapeutic doses of the drug or who have enhanced susceptibility also have been reported.

Clinical features. The clinical course of acetaminophen poisoning consists of three phases. The first, which comes within hours of intake, consists of acute gastrointestinal symptoms. The second phase, which continues for approximately 2 days, is characterized by abatement of symptoms. During this apparent subsidence, biochemical evidence of hepatic injury appears. Oliguria is usual. The third phase, that of overt hepatic damage, becomes clinically apparent 3 to 5 days after ingestion, with the appearance of jaundice. Renal failure may occur.

Biochemical changes. AST and ALT values are very high, reaching 20,000 units or more, but the bilirubin level is often only modestly elevated. Clotting abnormalities may be severe, and the one-stage prothrombin time is a useful prognostic indicator.

Histologic changes. The liver shows centrilobular (zone 3) necrosis and sinusoidal congestion. The kidney may show tubular necrosis.

Prognosis and treatment. Hepatic failure, as evidenced by hemorrhagic phenomena and hepatic encephalopathy, has occurred in up to one third of patients who develop jaundice. Many have died. The prognosis of an overdose of acetaminophen seems to correlate with blood levels of drug between 4 and 15 hours after ingestion. Early treatment with agents that replete glutathione has been effective in reducing the severity of hepatic injury. Indeed, acetylcysteine given within 16 hours of ingestion appears to prevent significant injury. Almost all patients so treated have survived. If it is administered after a longer interval, acetylcysteine seems to have little benefit.

Hepatic injury induced by other medicinal agents

Halothane. Halothane can cause serious hepatic disease. Despite a very low incidence of overt injury (estimated to be 1 in 2500 exposed), its severity (20% to 50% case-fatality rate in recognized toxicity) and widespread use make it an important cause of hepatic failure. The incidence is somewhat greater in females, is enhanced by obesity, and is low in children. Approximately 75% of patients in reported cases had prior exposure to the anesthetic. Many of the patients who developed jaundice had had fever after previous exposure. Onset of the syndrome is abrupt, usually with fever, and occurs a few days after exposure. Patients with fatal cases develop deepening jaundice, hemorrhagic phenomena, and coma. Aminotransferase levels are very high, leukocytosis is frequently present, and eosinophilia occurs in over 40% of patients. The mechanism appears to involve both hypersensitivity and a toxic metabolite. The centrilobular necrosis observed in many cases supports the likelihood that a hepatotoxic metabolite of halothane contributes to the injury.

Enflurane. This closely related anesthetic also has been reported to produce similar hepatic injury, although apparently the incidence is even lower. The lesser degree of biotransformation of enflurane appears to account for the lower incidence of injury. Isoflurane, also a related compound, has produced hardly any instances of hepatic injury. At this writing only two reported patients exposed to the drug have had injury that was convincingly attributed to isoflurane.

Methoxyflurane. This drug has led to similar instances of hepatic necrosis. It can also produce renal injury.

Chlorpromazine. Chlorpromazine, a phenothiazine widely used to treat psychosis and as a tranquilizer, can lead to hepatocanalicular jaundice in about 0.5% of recipients. A number of other phenothiazines produce similar injury. The mechanism for chlorpromazine-induced injury appears to involve both mild intrinsic toxicity and hypersensitivity (see description of idiosyncratic injury).

Phenytoin. Phenytoin and related anticonvulsants produce hepatocellular injury accompanied by sufficient evidence of cholestasis to warrant categorizing the lesion as a mixed hepatocellular injury. It is accompanied by prominent features of hypersensitivity and leads to a syndrome resembling serum sickness (see p. 604). Several other anticonvulsants have been incriminated in the production of hepatic injury. One of these drugs, valproate, has led to a number of instances of fatal hepatic disease characterized by microvesicular steatosis and necrosis. Encephalopathy and increased blood ammonia levels may precede other evidence of hepatic injury. The mechanism appears to be metabolic idiosyncrasy.

Drugs used to treat rheumatic and other musculoskeletal diseases. All of the many nonsteroidal anti-inflammatory drugs (NSAIDs) have been incriminated in the production of hepatic injury, although there are variations in potential for producing liver disease, in the mechanism for its production, and in the type of injury produced. Some agents produce hepatic injury accompanied by prominent hallmarks of hypersensitivity, and others appear to produce the injury as the result of a metabolic idiosyncrasy. Some NSAIDs produce hepatocellular injury, and others sometimes cause cholestatic jaundice. One recently abandoned agent (benoxaprofen) led to severe cholestasis and renal failure. Other drugs used in rheumatic disease (penicillamine, gold compounds) produce rare instances of idiosyncratic liver damage (usually cholestasis). The increasing use of methotrexate to treat rheumatoid arthritis has been expected to produce cases of steatosis and cirrhosis. The low dose used, however, has produced little evidence of hepatic injury. Salicylates have only recently been found to cause hepatic injury, despite almost a century of extensive clinical use. The injury, anicteric hepatocellular damage associated with high aminotransferase levels, occurs when blood levels are high (> 15 mg/dl). An important observation is the association of Reye's syndrome (Chapter 60) with aspirin use. Although this incrimination of aspirin has been debated, it seems convincing and also attributable to the conjoint adverse effects of the drug and viral infection.

Alkylated anabolic steroids and oral contraceptives. These agents are indirect cholestatic hepatotoxins. They lead to hepatic dysfunction and canalicular jaundice. The adverse effect is dose-related, and the incidence of jaundice is low at ordinary dosages. Contraceptive steroids have produced jaundice in a very small proportion of the millions of patients who have taken them. The higher incidence in patients with a personal or family history of jaundice of pregnancy and the clustering of cases in Chile and Scandinavia demonstrate that genetic susceptibility is relevant (Chapter 55).

Chronic lesions that can be induced by contraceptive and anabolic steroids include hepatic adenoma, peliosis hepatis, and carcinoma. The development of the Budd-Chiari syndrome in patients taking oral contraceptives seems to be attributable to the known thrombogenic effects of the estrogenic component (Chapter 61).

Isoniazid, rifampin, and amoxicillin. Isoniazid leads to hepatocellular jaundice in about 1% of recipients. The incidence is age-related. It approaches 3% in patients over 50 but is rare below the age of 20. Susceptibility appears to be enhanced by alcoholism. The inference that acetylator status affects susceptibility is controversial. The injury is apparently caused by toxic metabolites of isoniazid. Clinical features resemble those of severe acute viral hepatitis. Values for AST and ALT are often in the thousands. The case fatality rate for icteric patients exceeds 10%.

Minor elevations (below 200 units) of AST and ALT appear in 10% to 20% of patients during the first 2 months of isoniazid therapy and may subside despite continued administration of the drug. Perhaps this curious phenomenon represents metabolic adjustment with decreased production of toxic metabolites. Nevertheless, periodic measurement of aminotransferase levels, with withdrawal of the drug when values exceed three times the ULN, would probably serve to prevent serious hepatic injury. Administration of rifampin has been alleged to potentiate the ability of isoniazid to produce liver damage. Alone, rifampin leads to rare instances of hepatocellular jaundice. Presumably unrelated is the ability of rifampin to produce unconjugated hyperbilirubinemia. The drug apparently competes with other substances for excretion into bile or uptake from sinusoidal blood.

Amoxicillin in combination with the beta-lactamase inhibitor, clavulanic acid, has recently drawn attention as a cause of hepatic injury. The combination (trade name, Augmentin) has led to a number of instances of cholestatic jaundice.

Methyldopa. Methyldopa leads to hepatocellular jaundice in less than 1% of recipients. Aminotransferase levels are high, and serum alkaline phosphatase values are modestly elevated. The liver shows diffuse degeneration and necrosis. Death from hepatic failure has occurred in about 10% of reported cases. The mechanism of injury probably involves both hypersensitivity and toxic metabolites. A lesion resembling chronic active hepatitis has also been observed in recipients of methyldopa.

Methotrexate. Methotrexate has been in clinical use for 40 years. There have been many reports that it causes fatty liver and cirrhosis, especially in patients who have received it as long-term treatment for psoriasis. The development of chronic liver disease appears to depend on total dose, duration of therapy, and, particularly, the interval between doses. Significant liver disease seems far more likely to develop in patients who receive doses more frequently than once per week than in those who take the drug less frequently. Alcohol intake and diabetes appear to enhance susceptibility to methotrexate-associated hepatic injury. Unfortunately, the development of the histologic lesion is not reliably reflected in abnormal liver function test results or serum enzyme values. The mechanism for the production of the lesion is unclear, but it seems probable that methotrexate is an intrinsic hepatotoxin of the indirect type, with low potency and insidious effect.

DIAGNOSIS

Recognition that hepatic disease is due to drugs or other chemicals is most often based on circumstantial evidence. A history of exposure should be sought in every patient with hepatic disease. If such a history exists, its relevance should be judged according to the character of the hepatic disease and the known propensity of the agent for producing it.

A known toxin (e.g., CCl_4, acetaminophen) should be suspected as the cause of acute hepatocellular injury that progresses rapidly to hepatic failure, especially if hepatic failure is preceded by neurologic or gastrointestinal complaints, renal failure, and exposure to the toxin.

Drug-induced injury should be suspected as the cause of acute hepatic disease. If the hepatic injury is accompanied by fever and eosinophilia, the likelihood of drug-induced disease increases. Lack of these features, of course, does not exclude the diagnosis of drug-induced hepatic disease.

Distinction of drug-induced hepatocellular injury from viral hepatitis involves epidemiologic information, serologic studies to exclude hepatitis A, B, and C viruses, and a history that reveals exposure to a drug known to produce hepatocellular injury. Distinction of drug-induced cholestatic jaundice from extrahepatic obstructive jaundice may be difficult, and the special radiographic and sonographic techniques for distinction of intrahepatic cholestasis from extrahepatic obstruction may be needed (Chapter 50). The physician should strongly suspect that intrahepatic cholestasis is drug-induced. If liver biopsy reveals cholestasis with an eosinophil-rich portal inflammation, the diagnosis of the hepatocanalicular type of drug-induced jaundice is probable. Cholestasis without portal inflammation may be of the canalicular type (see Table 58-3).

Disappearance of hepatic abnormality after withdrawal of an incriminated drug and recurrence of hepatic dysfunction or hyperbilirubinemia after a test dose of it support the diagnosis of drug-induced injury. Failure of the liver to develop abnormalities on readministration, however, does not preclude the diagnosis of drug-induced injury; in some patients with drug-induced jaundice the liver may fail to show a recurrence of hepatic dysfunction after a test dose. Furthermore, some drugs reproduce the hepatic injury only after weeks of readministration.

Recognition that chronic disease is due to drug or other chemical injury is often more difficult. Awareness of the lesions that can be produced and of the agents that have been incriminated helps alert the physician to possible etiologic relationships. Reversal of lesions, for example those of chronic active hepatitis, after withdrawal of a suspected drug offers a helpful clue.

TREATMENT

Treatment consists in removal of the causative agent and provision of supportive care. Early detection of drug-induced injury and withdrawal of the offending agent may prevent the development of more severe hepatic disease. Supportive treatment for patients with hepatocellular injury is similar to that for patients with acute viral hepatitis. Large dosages of glucocorticoids have been used to treat the hepatic failure of drug-induced acute hepatocellular disease, but the effectiveness of this treatment remains to be proved.

Supportive treatment for patients with hepatocanalicular injury involves alleviation of pruritus and, if the syndrome is prolonged, treatment of malabsorption. Cholestyramine may alleviate the itching, as may phenobarbital. Glucocorticoid therapy appears to be of little benefit in the drug-induced cholestatic syndrome.

REFERENCES

American Academy of Pediatrics, Committee of Infectious Diseases: Aspirin and Reye's syndrome, Pediatrics 69:810, 1982.

Black M: Acetaminophen hepatotoxicity, Annu Rev Med 35:577, 1984.

Farber E and Fisher MM, editors: Toxic injury of the liver, New York, 1980, Dekker.

Gram L and Bentsen KD: Hepatic toxicity of antiepileptic drugs: a review, Acta Neurol Scand 68 (Suppl 97):81, 1983.

Kaplowitz N, editor: Recent advances in drug metabolism and toxicity. Semin in Liver Disease Vol 10.(4) Thieme Medical Publishers, New York, 1990.

Ludwig J and Axelson R: Drug effects on the liver. An updated tabular compilation of drugs and drug-related hepatic diseases, Dig Dis Sci 28:651, 1983.

Maddrey WC: Drug-related acute and chronic hepatitis, Clin Gastroenterol 9:213, 1980.

Mitchell JR et al: Metabolic activation: Biochemical basis for many drug-induced liver injuries, Prog Liver Dis 5:259, 1976.

Pessayre D and Larrey D: Drug-induced hepatitis, Baillieres Clin Gastroenterol 2:385, 1988.

Powell PR, Jackson JM, and Williams R: Hepatotoxicity to sodium valproate: a review, Gut 25:673, 1984.

Sharp JR, Ishak KG, and Zimmerman HJ: Chronic active hepatitis and severe hepatic necrosis associated with nitrofurantoin, Ann Intern Med 92:14, 1980.

Stricker BH, and Spoelstra P: Drug-induced hepatic injury, Amsterdam, 1985, Elsevier.

Wilson JHP: Drugs and the liver. In Arias IM, Frenkel M, and Wilson JMP editors: The liver annual, vol 4, Amsterdam, 1984, Elsevier.

Zimmerman HJ: Hepatotoxicity: adverse effects of drugs and other chemicals on the liver, New York, 1978, Appleton-Century-Crofts.

Zimmerman HJ: Effects of alcohol on other hepatotoxins, Alcohol Clin Exp Res 10:3, 1986.

Zimmerman HJ, and Maddrey WC: Toxic and drug-induced hepatitis. In Schiff L and Schiff ER, editors: Diseases of the liver, ed 6. Philadelphia, 1987, JB Lippincott.

CHAPTER

59 Alcoholic Liver Disease

Telfer B. Reynolds
Gary C. Kanel

Alcoholism is the most common cause of chronic liver disease in countries where alcoholic beverages are consumed extensively. Mortality from cirrhosis of the liver is increasing in Canada, England, and the United States, and most of the increase is due to alcoholic liver disease. Cirrhosis of the liver ranks as the third to fifth leading cause of death among urban men in the 25 to 64 age group in Canada and the United States. There is a close, direct correlation between per capita alcohol consumption and mortality for liver cirrhosis. For example, 1972 World Health Organization statistics show a range of annual mortality rates from 7.5 per 100,000 in Finland (annual per capita alcohol consumption, 5.1 liters) to 57.2 per 100,000 in France (alcohol consumption, 16.8 liters). Further proof of the relationship between quantity of alcohol consumed and liver disease comes from observed rapid falls in incidence of liver disease when wine was rationed in France in 1941 and when prohibition was instituted in the United States in 1920.

Though there is no doubt about the overall relationship between liver disease and quantity of alcohol consumed, there still is no clear concept of the pathogenesis of alcoholic liver disease. The type of beverage seems to play no important role, as liver disease is primarily related to wine ingestion in France and Italy, whiskey in the United States, and beer in Germany and Australia. There have been various estimates made of the "cirrhogenic dose" of alcohol. Available data indicate a progressively increasing risk of liver disease as daily consumption over a prolonged period rises above 120 g. Alcoholics usually provide unreliable histories and are difficult to observe scientifically, thus accounting for difficulty in deciding on the cirrhogenic dose. Not all alcohol abusers develop liver disease, so individual or racial susceptibility may be important. Women appear to be more susceptible than men, perhaps related to demonstrably lower levels of gastric alcohol dehydrogenase in women that result in a greater effective systemic dose of alcohol.

The actual pathogenesis of liver injury from alcohol remains a mystery, but several current lines of research appear promising. Acetaldehyde, the first product of alcohol metabolism, is potentially toxic because it forms adducts with body proteins that can damage hepatocytes directly or by acting as neoantigens that generate an immune response. In rats, the transfer of glutathione from cytoplasm to mitochondria is substantially slowed by alcohol feeding, leading to a lowered pool of mitochondrial glutathione and potential susceptibility to oxidant stress. Induction of the cytochrome P-450 microsomal ethanol oxidizing system (MEOS) by chronic alcohol consumption can increase susceptibility to the damaging effects of drugs such as acetaminophen, industrial solvents, and anesthetics, which are "toxified" by the same P-450 enzyme. Evidence from animal experiments demonstrates hypoxic hepatocyte damage in the perivenular area resulting from a sharp increase in hepatic oxygen consumption associated with alcohol metabolism.

Equally important to hepatocyte injury from alcohol is the remarkable predilection for collagen formation seen in alcoholic liver disease. Transformation of fat-storing parasinusoidal Ito cells into myofibroblasts with chronic alcohol exposure is an important line of current research as is the potential role of various cytokines such as tumor necrosis factor.

A serious handicap to research on alcoholic liver disease has been the lack of a suitable small animal model. In the past much work has focused on the production of fatty liver in small animals by alcohol feeding, but currently this theory has little relevance to alcoholic liver disease in human beings. In 1974, Rubin and Lieber reported the production of alcoholic liver disease in baboons fed a liquid diet containing all essential nutrients together with alcohol in an amount providing approximately 50% of total calories. After 9 months to 4 years of alcohol intake, 6 of 13 animals had histologic changes resembling either alcoholic hepatitis or cirrhosis. Alcohol intake at 4.5 to 8.3 g/kg/day was much higher than the average intake of human alcoholics, but so is the basal caloric intake of baboons. Limited additional work has been performed with this model because of its expense. In 1985, Tsukamoto et al. reported a rat model of intragastric ethanol infusion capable of producing hepatocyte necrosis, inflammation, and fibrosis in addition to steatosis. This model has great potential, and much has already been learned from it.

The results of the experiments with baboons and the Tsukamoto-French rat model suggest that alcohol metabolism can be directly hepatotoxic even in the presence of adequate nutrition. On the other hand, earlier alcohol-feeding experiments in humans with decompensated alcoholic liver disease failed to provide evidence that alcohol metabolism in a controlled environment with adequate nutrition slows recovery from alcoholic liver injury.

A potential clue to the pathogenesis of alcoholic liver disease is the "nonalcoholic steatohepatitis" that occasionally develops in obesity, early diabetes, and after intestinal bypass surgery. This liver disease has histologic similarity to alcoholic hepatitis with prominent fatty change, cell swelling and disruption, appearance of alcoholic hyalin, and deposition of intrasinusoidal collagen. Unfortunately for this line of research, intestinal bypass surgery for obesity has been appropriately replaced by various modifications of gastric stapling before pathogenesis of the liver injury could be identified.

ALCOHOL METABOLISM

The first step in alcohol metabolism is conversion to acetaldehyde in the cytosol of the hepatocytes by the enzyme alcohol dehydrogenase (ADH). Acetaldehyde is then converted to acetate by the mitochondrial enzyme acetaldehyde dehydrogenase. Lesser amounts of alcohol are metabolized by other hepatic enzyme systems, the microsomal ethanol oxidizing system, and catalase. The microsomal ethanol oxidizing system (MEOS) is usable at high blood ethanol levels and increases adaptively through induction of cytochrome P-450. It is generally agreed that the first step in alcohol metabolism, conversion to acetaldehyde, is rate limiting at concentrations of alcohol above 15 mg/dl, either because of the quantity of available ADH or because accumulation of excess reduced nicotinamide adenine dinucleotide (NADH) inhibits ADH activity. The usual figure given for the maximum rate of alcohol metabolism is approximately 100 mg/kg per hour, but there is wide variation in this rate among normal human beings, and there is evidence for adaptive increase in some alcoholic patients. In very severe liver disease, the maximum rate of alcohol metabolism often decreases.

The metabolism of alcohol causes an increase in the redox level (NADH/NAD ratio) in hepatic cytosol and mitochondria. This change in redox level has been blamed for (1) an increased lactate/pyruvate ratio, with hyperlactacidemia and resultant hyperuricemia; (2) decreased gluconeogenesis, with occasional hypoglycemia; (3) ketosis, with increased betahydroxybutyrate/acetoacetic acid ratio; and (4) decreased fatty acid oxidation from inhibition of the citric acid cycle, favoring fat accumulation in the liver.

Hypertriglyceridemia tends to occur with alcoholism, probably largely due to an increase in serum very-low-density lipoproteins (VLDL). At times, this can result in lactescent serum, with abdominal pain and mild hemolytic anemia (Zieve's syndrome).

STAGES OF ALCOHOLIC LIVER DISEASE

Alcoholic fatty liver

Pathogenesis. Moderate amounts of fat can be shown to accumulate in the human liver under experimental conditions in which protein and vitamin intake is normal and alcohol replaces carbohydrate at about 50% of total caloric intake. Whether production of severe fatty liver with clinical symptoms requires associated malnutrition or intermittent very high blood alcohol levels remains controversial. Factors thought to contribute to triglyceride accumulation in the livers of alcoholics include (1) decreased fatty acid oxidation from inhibition of the citric acid cycle, (2) increased fatty acid synthesis, and (3) decreased export of triglyceride from the liver.

Pathology. The alcoholic fatty liver is hypertrophic and may weigh as much as 5000 g. Grossly, it is yellow and has a smooth, stretched Glisson's capsule. The cut surface is uniformly yellow and greasy due to the marked accumulation of fat.

Microscopically, there is macrovesicular fatty change of the hepatocytes that typically affects cells centering around the terminal hepatic (central) veins. In more severe cases, however, cells in all zones of the lobule may be involved. Small amounts of intrasinusoidal collagen are present in the space of Disse, most prominently in the perivenular areas. Inflammatory infiltration and hyaline necrosis are typically absent.

Clinical features. Signs and symptoms of fatty liver vary markedly. Most patients have no symptoms directly attributable to liver disease, though they may have alcohol-related symptoms such as hypoglycemia, alcoholic ketoacidosis, or episodes of gout related to hyperuricemia. Other disorders that may bring the alcoholic patient to medical attention at this early stage of liver disease include delirium tremens, pneumonia, pancreatitis, and pyelonephritis. The liver is enlarged to percussion and is palpable and firmer than normal.

At the other extreme, patients with fatty liver may have jaundice, anorexia, and debility and may die with coma and hepatic failure. It is possible that such patients actually have alcoholic hepatitis with hepatocyte organelle damage that is obscured by the compressive effect of large fat vesicles in the cytoplasm.

Investigations. Many patients with alcoholic fatty liver have virtually normal hepatic tests except for mild transient increases in serum aspartate transaminase (AST) and gamma glutamyl transpeptidase (GGTP). The ratio of serum mitochondrial AST to total AST is often abnormally increased. Raised serum urate, lactate, or triglycerides may be present as clues to the alcoholic cause of liver enlargement. In patients with jaundice from fatty liver, both direct and indirect bilirubin are elevated, and AST is increased mildly or moderately. Serum alanine aminotransferase (ALT) is normal or nearly normal, alkaline phosphatase is moderately and occasionally markedly increased, GGTP is moderately increased, serum albumin is mildly to moderately decreased, and prothrombin is normal to moderately decreased.

Complications. Records from medical examiners' offices show that sudden death can occur at this stage of alcohol-induced liver injury. The mechanism of sudden death is unknown; suggestions have included withdrawal, hypoglycemia, and fat embolization to brain and lung. Postmortem blood alcohol levels are not consistent with alcohol overdose as the cause of death.

Prognosis. The prognosis is excellent for complete recovery from this stage of alcoholic liver injury if alcohol abstinence can be attained.

Treatment. There is no known treatment for alcoholic fatty liver beyond alcohol withdrawal and a nutritious diet. There is no proof of benefit from vitamin supplements or folic acid, though these are generally used because of the possibility of associated deficiencies. There is no evidence that more rapid fat mobilization from the liver occurs as a result of administration of lipotropic substances such as choline. Liver biopsy is important at this stage of alcoholic liver damage to establish the diagnosis firmly so that there can be no equivocation about the patient's need to cease drinking.

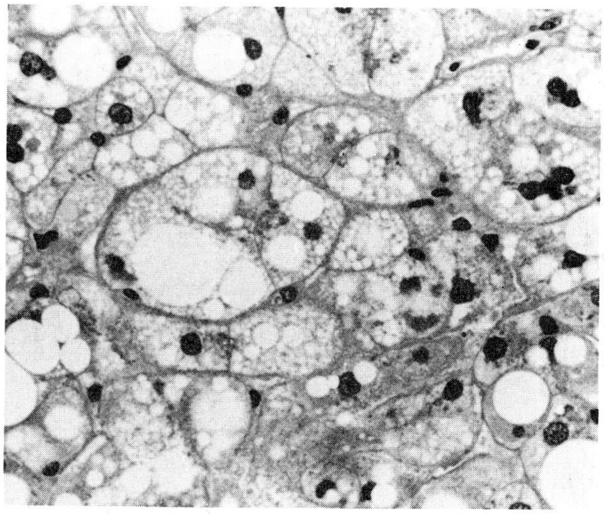

Fig. 59-1. Macrovesicular fat and microvesicular foamy fatty change (acute alcoholic liver disease).

Acute alcoholic hepatitis

Pathogenesis. Clearly, moderate hepatic fat accumulation can develop in human subjects on a nutritious diet in which alcohol replaces some of the carbohydrate. It has not been possible to prove that alcoholic hepatitis can occur under such circumstances; however, the demonstration by Rubin and Lieber in 1974 that baboons fed alcohol with adequate protein and vitamins can develop a lesion somewhat similar to that of human alcoholic hepatitis is strong evidence that this can happen.

Pathology. The hypertrophic alcoholic fatty liver may show no change other than large-droplet fat accumulation. However, in acute alcoholic liver injury a number of significant variations can be seen.

A classic change is sclerosing hyaline necrosis (acute alcoholic hepatitis). A marked arachnoid type of perivenular fibrosis occurs (Plate II-13) encroaching on and often closing off the terminal hepatic venules and establishing portal hypertension. Hepatocytes in this area exhibit hydropic degeneration. Many of these cells contain a ropy, eosinophilic cytoplasmic material known as Mallory bodies or alcoholic hyaline (Plate II-14). Neutrophils infiltrate the sinusoids and can often be seen surrounding individual hepatocytes. Cholestasis can be present. Occasionally, perivenular hepatocytes undergo a microvesicular foamy change (Fig. 59-1). Portal tracts usually demonstrate a neutrophilic and mononuclear inflammatory exudate.

Clinical features. Like alcoholic fatty liver, the term *alcoholic hepatitis* covers a wide pathologic and clinical spectrum. Asymptomatic patients with findings limited to palpable liver enlargement and, perhaps, a few vascular spiders may show pathologic changes of mild acute alcoholic hepatitis on biopsy. By contrast, the full-blown picture of acute alcoholic hepatitis (also called *acute sclerosing hyaline necrosis*) includes general debility, loss of muscle mass, jaundice, fever, abdominal pain, and often ascites (Table 59-1). Vascular spiders are common, as are parotid enlargement and palmar erythema. The liver is enlarged, firm, and often quite tender. Frequently, a systolic bruit can be heard over the liver if the bell of the stethoscope is pressed firmly against the liver surface. About 15% of patients have splenomegaly. Hepatic encephalopathy appears in the more seriously ill patients. Symptoms and findings often worsen for 2 to 3 weeks after hospitalization and cessation of alcohol intake. Temperatures as high as 103° F (39.4° C) can persist for several weeks in exceptional cases (Fig. 59-2). In patients with considerable abdominal pain, tenderness, and fever, the question of cholangitis or liver abscess may arise, particularly if there is substantial leukocytosis and alkaline phosphatase increase and, as sometimes happens, the patient denies alcoholism.

Acute alcoholic hepatitis may be superimposed on chronic alcoholic cirrhosis, in which case there may be

Table 59-1. Clinical findings in severe acute alcoholic hepatitis

Finding	Patients (percentage)
Hepatomegaly	84
Hepatic tenderness	67
Jaundice	100
Vascular spiders	62
Fever (over 100° F, 37.8° C)	63
Ascites	69
Encephalopathy	19
Gastrointestinal bleeding	33

Note: Findings in 112 patients at time of randomization to two controlled treatment trials in the University of Southern California Medical Center liver unit.

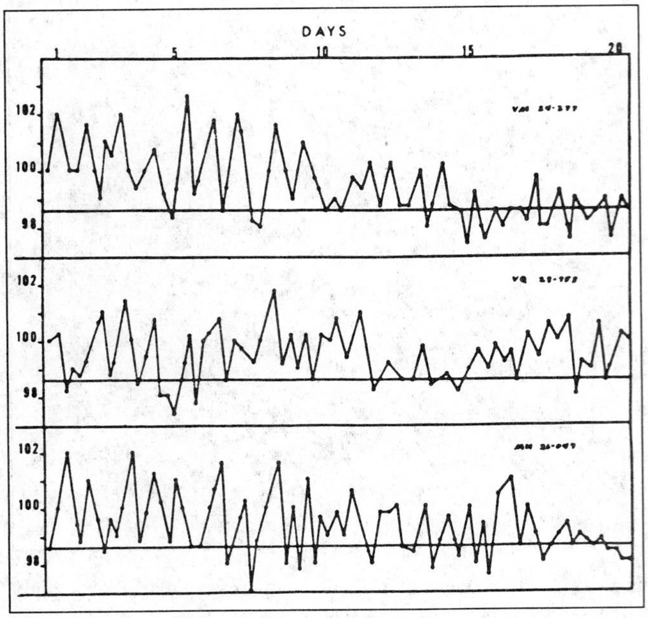

Fig. 59-2. Daily temperature charts of three patients with severe acute alcoholic hepatitis.

symptoms and signs of more long-standing liver disease, such as bleeding from esophageal varices or visible abdominal collateral veins. The liver usually is not enlarged if there is underlying cirrhosis.

Investigations. Laboratory test abnormalities correlate with the severity of the process and the presence of underlying cirrhosis. Table 59-2 shows the mean test results in 112 patients with severe alcoholic hepatitis who were chosen for two controlled trials in our liver unit. On biopsy or at autopsy, about 40% had evidence of underlying liver cirrhosis. Serum AST is increased, rarely to levels above 300 IU/L, and ALT is normal or mildly increased. Renal function is normal early in acute alcoholic hepatitis, but serum creatinine begins to rise during the second to fourth week of hospitalization in patients whose illness is progressive.

Table 59-2. Laboratory test results in severe acute alcoholic hepatitis

Test	Result
Bilirubin	17.8 mg/dl
Albumin	2.4 g/dl
Prothrombin	47%
White blood cells	15,700/mm^3
AST	145 IU/L*
ALT	26 IU/L*
Creatinine	1.3 mg/dl
Hemoglobin	10.8 g/dl

Note: Mean values in 112 patients at time of randomization to two controlled treatment trials in the University of Southern California Medical Center liver unit.
*Normal, less than 40 IU/L

Almost all who die have the hepatorenal syndrome (Chapter 56) before they expire. Anemia is present in most patients. It may be macrocytic or normocytic and normochromic with a low reticulocyte count; it rarely improves with folate administration. Low serum tri-iodothyronine level is common, though patients remain euthyroid. Serum cholesterol level is low and reflects the severity of the liver disease.

Electrolyte abnormalities are seen in acute alcoholic hepatitis even before treatment with diuretics. Hyponatremia related to reduction in free water clearance is common in severe cases with ascites. Hypokalemia is frequent at the time of admission to the hospital, presumably reflecting poor intake, vomiting, or diarrhea. Less frequently, hypomagnesemia occurs. Respiratory alkalosis is common in severely ill patients, may persist for weeks or months, and is the usual explanation for elevated serum chloride and depressed serum bicarbonate. Overt renal tubular acidosis is rare if it occurs at all; however, about 50% of patients have incomplete renal tubular acidosis, as indicated by poor urine acidification after administration of a calcium chloride load. Severe lactic acidosis is an occasional event in alcoholic hepatitis, and its pathogenesis is uncertain.

Urinary sodium content is low in patients who are forming ascites; a level over 20 mEq/L in the absence of diuretic administration suggests that spontaneous diuresis is occurring or will soon occur.

Endoscopy shows esophageal varices in many patients with severe alcoholic hepatitis, particularly if there is underlying cirrhosis. Wedge hepatic vein pressure is increased as is portal pressure when measured directly by transhepatic needling. Liver/spleen scan invariably shows redistribution of radionuclide to bone marrow and spleen—to a remarkable degree in severe cases (Fig. 59-3). Ultrasonography often shows enlarged hepatic arterial branches running parallel to portal vein branches in the hepatic parenchyma. We have called this the *pseudoparallel channel sign* to distinguish it from the *parallel channel sign* caused by enlarged intrahepatic bile ducts in mechanical bile duct obstruction. The *pseudoparallel channel sign* correlates well with the systolic hepatic bruit and presumably reflects increased hepatic arterial blood flow.

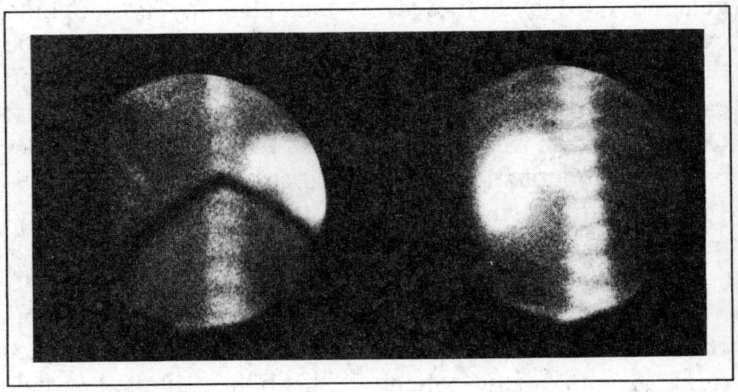

Fig. 59-3. Front *(left)* and back *(right)* views of ^{99m}Tc liver/spleen scan in a patient with severe alcoholic liver disease. Liver uptake of isotope is markedly reduced with increased visualization of spleen and bone marrow.

Complications (see also Chapter 56.)

Portal hypertension. Portal hypertension is probably present in all patients with symptomatic acute alcoholic hepatitis. Hepatocyte swelling and disruption, with intrasinusoidal collagen deposition, is maximum in the perivenular areas, and this is ideally situated for maximum interference with hepatic blood flow. The portal hypertension is reversible to some extent if there is histologic improvement with abstinence from alcohol. Well-developed esophageal varices are unusual in alcoholic hepatitis unless there is underlying chronic disease with cirrhosis; bleeding from gastric mucosal lesions is common, but variceal hemorrhage is unusual.

Ascites. Ascites develops in the majority of patients with severe alcoholic hepatitis. Often it is of brief duration if there is clinical improvement. In a few patients, ascites becomes refractory as progressive diffuse hepatic fibrosis develops.

Spontaneous bacterial peritonitis. This condition is relatively common in patients with ascites due to acute alcoholic hepatitis. Diagnostic paracentesis with white blood cell count and culture is indicated when patients with ascites are admitted to the hospital and whenever they take an unexplained turn for the worse.

Hepatic encephalopathy. Hepatic encephalopathy is a common complication of severe alcoholic hepatitis. When it develops spontaneously it is an ominous prognostic feature, and about half of such patients die with progressive hepatic failure. Common precipitants of hepatic encephalopathy in this setting are spontaneous bacterial peritonitis, gastrointestinal bleeding, use of diuretics, and use of sedatives such as diazepam.

Hepatorenal syndrome. Almost all patients who die of alcoholic hepatitis have hepatorenal syndrome. Rise in serum creatinine not related to diuretic use is an ominous prognostic feature, and only 15% to 20% of patients whose serum creatinine concentration exceeds 2 mg/dl survive. The most common reasons for creatinine increase not caused by the hepatorenal syndrome in this type of patient are vigorous diuresis and use of aminoglycoside antibiotics. Rarely, a patient has either severe pyelonephritis with renal papillary necrosis or creatinine increase due to use of a prostaglandin synthetase inhibitor.

Prognosis. Severe alcoholic hepatitis is associated with substantial mortality. In our patient population, mortality was 27% among 112 patients enrolled in two treatment trials and was nearly identical for controls and patients treated with corticosteroid or propylthiouracil. In a smaller group chosen for treatment because of the spontaneous development of hepatic encephalopathy during the first few days of hospitalization, mortality was 54%, again identical in treated patients (prednisolone) and controls. In other published controlled trials of treatment, mortality in controls has ranged from 19% to 100%. Prognostic indicators are the levels of prothrombin, serum bilirubin, and creatinine. In a controlled treatment trial involving 67 patients, we used the statistical technique of multivariate discriminant analysis in an attempt to detect prognostic features. Three findings that suggested a fatal outcome were (1) increase in white blood cell count of more than 7000 per cubic millimeter during the first 10 days of hospitalization, (2) increase in serum creatinine of more than 0.6 mg/dl, and (3) increase in serum bilirubin of more than 7 mg/dl during the same period. Findings that correlated well with recovery were (1) increase in serum total protein of more than 0.3 g/dl during the first 10 days, (2) increase in prothrombin of more than 15% during the same period, and (3) serum triiodothyronine above 80 ng/ml on admission to the hospital. These predictors need to be applied prospectively before they can be verified.

In patients with mild acute alcoholic hepatitis who stop drinking, there may be complete recovery, with normal or nearly normal hepatic histology within 6 months. In moderately severe disease, there may be marked histologic improvement, with substantial decrease in portal hypertension. More often there is progression to hepatic cirrhosis with nodular regeneration, even in patients who cease drinking and quite commonly in those who continue or resume drinking. Alternatively, the liver may show progressive increase in diffuse interstitial fibrosis without nodular regeneration. This type of lesion has a poor ultimate prognosis; refractory ascites with hepatorenal syndrome or bleeding esophageal varices often lead to a fatal outcome within a year or two.

Treatment. An effective treatment for alcoholic hepatitis that could reduce mortality and diminish hepatic collagen deposition would be an important development. Since an optimistic report in 1971, most attention has been given to corticosteroid treatment. Thirteen randomized controlled trials of prednisone or prednisolone treatment have been reported (Table 59-3). Four showed statistically significant reduction in mortality, and a fifth showed a faster rate of improvement in liver status test results with corticosteroid. In

Table 59-3. Results of controlled trials of treatment of acute alcoholic hepatitis with corticosteroids

Author	Mortality			
	Control group (%)		Corticosteroid-treated group (%)	
Helman et al (1971)	6/17	(35)	1/20	(5)
Porter et al (1971)	7/9	(77)	6/11	(55)
Campra et al (1973)	9/25	(36)	7/20	(35)
Blitzer et al (1977)	5/16	(31)	6/12	(50)
Lesesne et al (1978)	7/7	(100)	2/7	(29)
Shumaker et al (1978)	7/15	(47)	6/12	(50)
Maddrey et al (1978)	6/31	(19)	1/24	(4)
Depew et al (1978)	7/13	(54)	8/15	(53)
Theodossi et al (1982)	16/28	(57)	17/27	(63)
Mendenhall et al (1984)	18/88	(20)	19/90	(21)
Bories et al (1987)	2/21	(10)	1/24	(4)
Carithers et al (1989)	11/31	(35)	2/35	(6)
Ramond et al (1992)	16/29	(55)	4/32	(13)
Total	117/330	(35)	80/329	(24)

the liver unit at the University of Southern California, we have studied 143 patients in three separate randomized controlled trials; in each trial mortality was unaffected by corticosteroids. Though the negative trials outweigh the positive trials, there is a high possibility of a type II error in all of the negative studies except for the Veterans Administration Multicenter trial containing 178 patients reported in 1984. Meta-analysis of the first 12 trials shows a small (15%), statistically uncertain gain in survival with corticosteroid and a more definite benefit (28% increase in survival) in the subgroup of patients with spontaneous hepatic encephalopathy.

Centrilobular hypoxia related to a hypermetabolic state from alcohol metabolism has been proposed as a mechanism for hepatocyte injury. In rats chronically fed alcohol, reduction in hepatocyte damage from exposure to hypoxia was observed in propylthiouracil-pretreated animals compared to untreated controls. In a study of 310 patients with alcoholic liver disease, 157 were given propylthiouracil 300 mg daily for a mean period of 44 weeks in an outpatient setting. Cumulative mortality was significantly reduced from 25% to 13% with propylthiouracil. Analysis of mailed urine samples showed that the majority of patients continued to ingest alcohol during the trial. By contrast, we found no benefit from propylthiouracil treatment in a randomized controlled trial involving 67 hospitalized patients with severe acute alcoholic hepatitis. Mortality was 22.5% in propylthiouracil-treated patients compared to 19.4% in controls. Propylthiouracil may be of benefit in patients who are actively drinking either by the mechanism proposed above or by interfering with the toxic action of alcohol in some other way, perhaps analogous to its action in preventing acetaminophen toxicity in rats.

Other unproved but possible treatment modalities in alcoholic hepatitis include administration of penicillamine, colchicine, glucagon and insulin, androgenic steroids, parenteral nutrition, pentoxyfilline, polyunsaturated lecithin, and lathyrogenic substances to inhibit collagen formation or to enhance its dissolution.

CHRONIC LIVER DISEASE

Pathogenesis

As mentioned earlier, acute alcoholic hepatitis may progress to cirrhosis or to diffuse interstitial fibrosis. Many patients have an already well-established cirrhosis when symptoms and findings due to liver disease first develop. It is uncertain therefore whether acute alcoholic hepatitis is a necessary forerunner of cirrhosis. If so, the episodes in many patients must be asymptomatic or at least unrecognizable to the alcohol abuser. It would be very helpful to know more about the factors that stimulate collagen formation in alcoholic liver disease. Perhaps this would lead to more effective treatment.

Pathology

Whether the alcoholic has numerous clinical episodes of acute alcoholic hepatitis or whether there is subclinical, slowly progressive hepatocellular dropout and fibrosis, chronic alcoholic liver disease will ensue. If the regenerative activity of the liver is markedly decreased, a chronic sclerosing pattern, often with interstitial fibrosis, will occur. If there is significant regenerative activity, there will be nodule formation with resultant cirrhosis. In both cases, portal hypertension is a major sequela.

In progressive perivenular alcoholic fibrosis (in the past termed chronic sclerosing hyaline disease), the liver is eutrophic or atrophic. The surface is finely granular. On cut section, the parenchyma is extremely hard, and there is an absence of nodule formation. Microscopically, portal fibrosis and dense collagen surrounding and compressing the terminal hepatic veins can be seen (Fig. 59-4). Unless there is superimposed acute alcoholic hepatitis, no significant inflammatory change is seen. Liver cells show little regenerative activity. Often there is extensive intrasinusoidal collagen deposition throughout the lobule (diffuse interstitial fibrosis). Terminal hepatic venular areas and portal tracts are often connected by collagen.

However, when portal and perivenular fibrosis progress and there is regenerative hepatocellular activity, nodules arise, and cirrhosis eventually appears. At first the liver is hypertrophic, weighing 2000 to 4000 g, and has a fine, nodular external surface (Plate II-15). Cut section exhibits nodules a few millimeters in diameter that are distributed uniformly throughout the parenchyma (Plate II-16). As necrosis and inflammatory change continue, fibrosis increases and typical fibrous scars are produced. In more advanced stages of cirrhosis the liver becomes atrophic, and the nodules may become somewhat larger. Microscopically, they can be seen to have a uniform trabecular pattern. With time, paraplastic changes with a predisposition to hepatocellular carcinoma can occur.

Clinical features

Patients with chronic alcoholic liver disease present in a number of different ways. Most commonly, they appear in a decompensated state with a combination of jaundice, as-

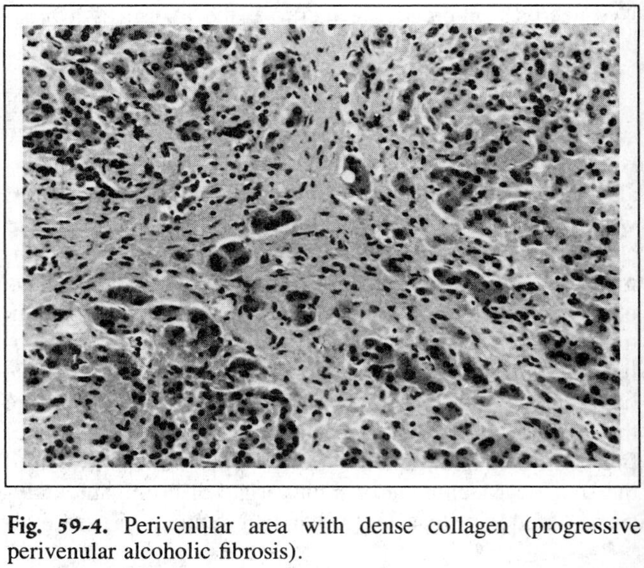

Fig. 59-4. Perivenular area with dense collagen (progressive perivenular alcoholic fibrosis).

cites, and debility. Inquiry will reveal some recent deterioration in health superimposed on a long history of alcohol abuse and its attendant social and medical problems. Often there is a loss of muscle mass and strength. Impotence or markedly reduced potency is the rule in men, whereas amenorrhea and loss of fertility are usually present in women (Chapter 56). Frequently, there is a history of hepatomegaly and/or mild liver abnormalities detected in the recent past, at which time the patient was warned to stop drinking. Patients with cirrhosis whose presenting features include substantial jaundice probably have some element of acute alcoholic hepatitis superimposed. A small proportion of patients present with ascites or with hemorrhage from esophageal varices as their first recognizable hepatic symptom.

Alcoholic liver disease may be suggested by physical findings or laboratory test abnormalities in patients undergoing routine physical examinations or seeking medical attention for alcohol-related problems like delirium tremens, pneumonia, pancreatitis, polyneuritis, or hemorrhage from gastric erosions. Additional symptoms common in patients with decompensated alcoholic liver disease that are not easily explained on a hepatic basis are diarrhea and irritating cough. These symptoms usually subside within a few days of hospital admission. Distressing gaseous abdominal distention with generalized bowel dilatation is an occasional unexplained finding in patients who also have ascites. Distention diminishes gradually in patients who survive.

Physical findings indicating chronic liver disease include firmness of the edge of the liver, splenomegaly (present in only 30% of patients with alcoholic cirrhosis), vascular spiders, palmar erythema, small soft testicles, ascites, and visible collateral veins on the abdominal wall (occasionally causing a continuous loud bruit and palpable thrill). Ankle edema may appear before ascites. Parotid enlargement is common, though this reflects chronic alcoholism rather than liver disease. Evidence of peripheral neuritis, particularly in the legs and feet, is common. Rarely, a patient has gynecomastia, which is more often unilateral than bilateral. Dupuytren's contracture and opaque fingernails have little diagnostic value, in our view. None of these except parotid enlargement and peripheral neuritis are of any value in determining that alcoholism is the cause of the liver disease.

Investigations

With the exception of leukocytosis, laboratory test abnormalities in chronic alcoholic liver disease are, in general, similar to those found in acute alcoholic hepatitis. Unless there is some element of superimposed acute alcoholic hepatitis, bilirubin concentration may be normal or only mildly increased. Elevation of AST is minimal in nonjaundiced patients, and ALT is usually normal. A frequent abnormality is substantial elevation of serum IgA. This is much more common in alcoholic liver disease than in other chronic liver diseases and is unexplained.

Though it would be unusual at presentation, it is possible for patients with established alcoholic cirrhosis who are not drinking to have entirely normal values for all of the standard laboratory tests. Postprandial serum bile salt level usually is elevated.

Differential diagnosis of alcoholic liver disease and other causes of cirrhosis depends mostly on liver biopsy, serum transaminase pattern, and the presence of serum markers for chronic infection with hepatitis B or C. Serum AST is rarely above 300 IU/L, and ALT rarely above 100 IU/L in alcoholic liver disease; values higher than this suggest that the cause of the cirrhosis is chronic hepatitis. Concomitant abuse of alcohol and intravenous drugs is increasingly common in the United States, so there is the potential for liver disease of dual causation. Even with liver biopsy, it may be difficult to decide which pathogenetic factor is most important. Hemochromatosis should always be considered in the differential diagnosis of alcoholic cirrhosis. Normal saturation of serum iron-binding capacity and normal serum ferritin levels exclude this diagnosis. High values point to it except in the jaundiced patient, in whom both tests may be unreliable. Quantitative determination of iron in a liver biopsy specimen is the definitive test (Chapter 60). Autoimmune liver disease is suggested by female sex, higher levels of transaminases and globulin, and positive tests for antismooth muscle and antinuclear antibodies. Serum ceruloplasmin should be measured to exclude Wilson's disease in the younger patient with presumed alcoholic cirrhosis. Alpha$_1$ antitrypsin deficiency is a rare cause of cirrhosis in adults and can be excluded if serum level is normal with MM phenotype (Chapter 60).

Complications

Jaundice and ascites are common complications of chronic alcoholic liver disease. Hepatic encephalopathy is frequent in the decompensated patient. If there is no obvious precipitating factor, the onset of encephalopathy may indicate hepatic failure and impending death. Patients who have undergone surgical portosystemic shunt frequently have recurring episodes of hepatic encephalopathy without obvious precipitating events. Recurring encephalopathy in the absence of a surgical shunt suggests the possibility of a large, spontaneous splenorenal shunt, which can be shown by celiac angiography, ultrasonography, or computed tomography. Hepatorenal syndrome is less common in cirrhosis than in acute alcoholic hepatitis but is still a relatively frequent terminal complication. Upper gastrointestinal bleeding is a common complication in cirrhosis; endoscopic observations indicate that from one third to one half of these episodes are due to ruptured esophageal varices, and the remainder are due to mucosal lesions (gastric erosions, portal hypertensive gastropathy, Mallory-Weiss tears, etc.). Spontaneous bacterial peritonitis is a frequent complication in cirrhotic patients who have substantial ascites, particularly those with an ascites total protein concentration below 1 g/dl.

Spur-cell anemia is an interesting red blood cell abnormality occasionally found in patients with advanced cirrhosis. It is characterized by a rise in serum bilirubin concentration that is predominantly indirect, moderate to marked anemia with reticulocytosis, a large spleen, and a low prothrombin level. Spur cells (acanthocytes) are found on blood smear. Prognosis is poor, even in patients who avoid alcohol, and most patients die within 1 year. Pathogenesis is uncertain, and there is no known treatment.

Hepatocellular carcinoma (Chapter 63) is a complication of advanced, longstanding alcoholic cirrhosis. It is most likely to be seen in a patient who has had a portacaval shunt, has stopped drinking, and has survived for 10 to 20 years after the initial diagnosis of alcoholic liver disease. It should be suspected when such a patient has an unexplained deterioration in health, with onset of jaundice and worsening of liver status test results.

Hypersplenism of varying degrees is usually evident when the spleen is large in alcoholic cirrhosis. Marked splenomegaly occurs in 15% to 25% of patients, less frequently than in those with nonalcoholic cirrhosis. Leukocyte count is often less than 5000 per mm^3, and platelet count less than 100,000 per mm^3. Anemia is moderate and usually not much more severe than in patients without hypersplenism. Bleeding phenomena and tendency to infection are not noticeably increased by the hypersplenism of cirrhosis, and splenectomy to relieve hypersplenism is not generally indicated.

Prognosis

The prognosis is largely dependent on two factors: (1) the degree of severity of the liver disease when detected and (2) whether the patient stops abusing alcohol. Soterakis, Resnick, and colleagues in 1973 interpreted their data as showing that alcohol abstinence had no favorable influence on survival once patients had reached the stage of bleeding from esophageal varices. Our data do not agree with theirs; we think that all but moribund patients have some chance for prolonged survival with sobriety. Unfortunately, permanent cure of alcoholism is the exception, and we estimate that only 15% to 20% of our patients with alcoholic liver disease achieve this goal.

Survival rates for patients with alcoholic liver disease were examined over 50 years ago by Ratnoff and Patek and about 25 years ago by Powell and Klatskin. One-year survival after the onset of ascites varied from 34% (Ratnoff and Patek) to 65% (Powell and Klatskin), and after the onset of upper gastrointestinal bleeding it averaged from 28% (Ratnoff and Patek) to 55% (Powell and Klatskin). Five-year survival of all patients with a diagnosis of alcoholic liver disease was 63% in those who stopped drinking and 40% in those who did not. More recent figures for survival after presumed variceal hemorrhage are available from controlled trials of portacaval shunt. Our own data show 50% survival at 2 years and approximately 25% survival at 5 years. Survival was improved in patients who had undergone portacaval shunt, but improvement was only marginal.

Treatment

Unfortunately, no treatment is available for alcoholic liver disease beyond helping the patient to achieve abstinence and treating the various complications when they arise. Prolonged hospital stay is undoubtedly beneficial for patients with decompensated disease, but this expensive care consists mainly of general support, antibiotics when needed, provision of a nutritious diet and appropriate electrolyte supplements, and enforced abstinence from alcohol. Corticosteroid therapy has been tried without benefit in a large study in Scandinavia. Penicillamine seemed mildly beneficial in one controlled trial, and colchicine caused significant improvement in another. Further trials of these two agents are indicated. Liver transplantation is an effective treatment in selected patients (Chapter 64). Treatment of the various complications of chronic liver disease are dealt with in detail in Chapter 56.

REFERENCES

Edmondson HA, Peters RL, and Reynolds TB: Sclerosing hyaline necrosis of the liver in the chronic alcoholic. A recognizable clinical syndrome, Ann Intern Med 59:646, 1963.

Fernandez-Checa JC et al: Impaired uptake of glutathione by hepatic mitochondria from chronic ethanol-fed rats, J Clin Invest 87:397, 1991.

Lieber CS: Biochemical and molecular basis of alcohol-induced injury to liver and other tissues, N Engl J Med 319:339, 1988.

Mendenhall CL et al: Short-term and long-term survival in patients with alcoholic hepatitis treated with oxandrolone and prednisolone, N Engl J Med 311:1464, 1984.

Orrego H et al: Long-term propylthiouracil treatment reduces mortality in alcoholic liver disease, N Engl J Med 317:1421, 1987.

Powell WJ and Klatskin G: Duration of survival in patients with Laennec's cirrhosis, Am J Med 44:406, 1968.

Ratnoff OD and Patek AJ Jr: The natural history of Laennec's cirrhosis of the liver: an analysis of 386 cases, Medicine (Baltimore) 21:207, 1942.

Ramond MJ et al: A randomized trial of prednisolone in patients with severe alcoholic hepatitis. N Engl J Med 326:507, 1992.

Reynolds TB, Benhamou J-P, Blake J et al: Treatment of acute alcoholic hepatitis, Gastroenterology 113:299, 1990.

Rubin E and Lieber CS: Fatty liver, alcoholic hepatitis and cirrhosis produced by alcohol in primates, N Engl J Med 290:128, 1974.

Tsukamoto H, Gaal K, and French SWJ: Insights into the pathogenesis of alcoholic liver necrosis and fibrosis: status report, Hepatology 12:599, 1990.

CHAPTER

60 Primary Biliary Cirrhosis, Wilson's Disease, Hemochromatosis, and Other Metabolic and Fibrotic Liver Diseases

Marshall M. Kaplan

PRIMARY BILIARY CIRRHOSIS

Primary biliary cirrhosis is an uncommon, progressive, and often fatal liver disease that occurs most frequently during the fourth to seventh decades of life. Clinically, primary biliary cirrhosis may mimic extrahepatic bile duct obstruction. Therefore the diagnosis of primary biliary cirrhosis should be considered in patients with unexplained chronic cholestasis or unexplained elevations of serum alkaline phosphatase so that appropriate diagnostic tests can be performed and an unnecessary operation avoided.

Incidence and etiology

Primary biliary cirrhosis was once considered a very rare disease. Improvements in diagnostic tests and increased awareness, however, have led to earlier and more frequent diagnoses of this condition. Its prevalence ranges from 3.7 to 14.4 cases per 100,000, and its incidence from 5.8 to 15 cases per 1 million per year. In some series, it accounts for almost 2% of deaths due to cirrhosis. The etiology is unknown but is thought to be related to altered immunoregulation. The evidence for this is indirect. Ninety percent of patients are women, a sex distribution similar to that of some other diseases of altered immunoregulation such as systemic lupus erythematosus. There is an increased prevalence of autoantibodies, including antimitochondrial, antinuclear, and antithyroid antibodies. Forty percent of primary biliary cirrhosis patients have granulomas in the liver or nearby lymph nodes. Many are anergic to tuberculin and dinitrochlorobenzene. Primary biliary cirrhosis patients have impaired lymphocyte transformation in response to phytohemagglutinin and impaired suppressor lymphocyte function. There is an increased association with other alleged autoimmune diseases such as thyroiditis, rheumatoid arthritis, scleroderma, and Sjögren's syndrome. Circulating immune complexes have been demonstrated in a small percentage of these patients, but they do not play a major role in the pathogenesis of primary biliary cirrhosis. Some of these patients have an unusually reactive IgM that gives false-positive results in many immune complex assays. This reactive IgM may account for the high prevalence of immune complexes reported from some centers.

Pathophysiology

Most of the signs and symptoms of primary biliary cirrhosis are due to long-standing cholestasis. The cholestasis is due to a gradual destruction of small intrahepatic bile ducts, which leads to a diminished number of bile ducts within the liver. This, in turn, results in retention of bile acids, bilirubin, copper, and other substances that are normally secreted or excreted into bile. The increased concentration of substances such as bile acids may cause further damage to liver cells. Other substances are regurgitated from the liver into blood and soft tissues, causing symptoms such as itching. The itching is almost certainly not due to the naturally occurring primary and secondary bile acids but to some other substance that is secreted in bile and binds to cholestyramine, a nonabsorbed quaternary ammonium resin. The striking hyperlipidemia and xanthoma formation in some primary biliary cirrhosis patients is also a consequence of long-standing cholestasis. Impaired secretion of bile causes a diminished concentration of bile acids within the intestinal lumen. The bile acid concentration is often below the critical micellar concentration and is inadequate for complete digestion and absorption of neutral triglycerides in the diet. This fact, plus the pancreatic insufficiency noted in patients with concomitant sicca syndrome, accounts for the striking fat malabsorption seen in some patients. In addition to fat malabsorption, there may be malabsorption of the fat-soluble vitamins A, D, E, and K and of calcium. The pathogenesis of the osteopenic bone disease that occurs in at least 25% of primary biliary cirrhosis patients is still unclear. Both osteoporosis and osteomalacia have been described. Although the osteomalacia is almost certainly due to vitamin D and calcium malabsorption, the clinically important disorder is osteoporosis. Its cause is not known.

Pathology

The liver is characteristically enlarged, smooth, and often bile stained early in the course of the disease. Primary biliary cirrhosis is divided into four pathologic stages. In stage I, there is a pathognomonic, florid, asymmetric destructive lesion of larger interlobular bile ducts (Plate II-17). These lesions are irregularly scattered throughout the portal triads and are often seen only on large surgical biopsies of the liver. The damaged bile ducts are usually surrounded by a dense infiltrate of mononuclear cells, most of which are lymphocytes. In stage II, the lesion is more widespread but less specific. There may be a reduced number of normal bile ducts within portal triads and increased numbers of atypical, poorly formed bile ducts with irregularly shaped lumens. There is diffuse portal fibrosis and mononuclear cell infiltrates within triads (Plate II-18). These may spill into the surrounding periportal areas. The cholestasis seen in stages I and II is characteristically periportal rather than pericentral. A diminished number of bile ducts in an otherwise unremarkable-appearing needle biopsy of the liver should alert the physician to the possibility of primary biliary cirrhosis. Stage III represents a more progressive lesion, with fibrous septa now extending beyond triads and forming portal-to-portal bridges. Nodule formation may be apparent. The portal triads are otherwise similar to those in stage II. Stage IV represents the end stage of the lesion, with frank cirrhosis and regenerative nodules. It is difficult to distinguish this late lesion from other types of cirrhosis.

Clinical and laboratory findings

The earliest complaint is usually unexplained pruritus, characteristically worse at bedtime, although disease in many patients is now detected because of fatigue or unexplained elevation of the serum alkaline phosphatase level. The pruritus may first occur during the third trimester of pregnancy and persist after delivery. Physical examination reveals hepatomegaly and increased skin pigmentation. The pigment is melanin, not bilirubin, at this early stage. Excoriations may be diffuse. Jaundice may occur weeks to months after the onset of pruritus but is usually present later in the course of the disease. Kayser-Fleischer rings have been observed in several primary biliary cirrhosis patients. Rarely, primary biliary cirrhosis may go undetected until late in the course of the disease, when patients present with either severe jaundice or bleeding from esophageal varices. During the course of the disease, malabsorption may develop in some patients, resulting in nocturnal diarrhea, frothy, bulky stools, or weight loss in the face of a voracious appetite and increased caloric intake. Xanthelasmas are common. Xanthomas develop in approximately 10% of patients and are found on the palms of the hands and soles of the feet, over extensor surfaces of the elbows and knees, in tendons of the ankles and wrists, and on the buttocks. Osteopenia occurs in at least 25% of patients with long-standing primary biliary cirrhosis. Bone pain is common, as are spontaneous collapse of vertebral bodies and hairline fractures of ribs. The underlying lesion is almost always severe osteoporosis.

Liver function tests in primary biliary cirrhosis patients reveal a cholestatic pattern. Serum alkaline phosphatase is disproportionately elevated. Serum aminotransferases (transaminases) are slightly elevated. Serum albumin, globulin, and prothrombin time are characteristically normal early in the course of the disease, although immunoelectrophoresis frequently reveals elevated IgM. Fractionation of the alkaline phosphatase reveals that it is of hepatic origin. 5′-Nucleotidase and gamma glutamyl transpeptidase parallel alkaline phosphatase and are markedly elevated. Serum bilirubin concentration may be normal early in the course of the disease but becomes elevated in 60% of patients as the disease progresses. Both direct and indirect fractions are increased. Despite strikingly high serum cholesterol values, occasionally 800 to 1600 mg/dl, the serum is always clear, never lactescent. Most of the cholesterol is in high-density lipoprotein. Atherosclerosis is uncommon. Antimitochondrial antibody is present in 85% to 95% of patients. The antigens against which antimitochondrial antibody is directed have recently been identified as pyruvate dehydrogenase and other enzymes in the 2-oxo-acid dehydrogenase complexes found in mitochondria. Serum ceruloplasmin is elevated, unlike in Wilson's disease, another disorder associated with increased retention of copper within the liver.

Diagnosis

Chronic cholestasis and the presence of antimitochondrial antibody make primary biliary cirrhosis the likely diagnosis. Percutaneous needle biopsy of the liver enables the physician to confirm the diagnosis and ascertain staging more accurately. Ultrasonography can be used to ascertain that bile ducts are patent in patients where the diagnosis is uncertain. Endoscopic cholangiography should be reserved for the patient with a negative antimitochondrial antibody test in whom other diagnoses such as sclerosing cholangitis are possible.

Treatment

The nonabsorbed resin cholestyramine relieves pruritus in almost all patients. It is given in 4-g doses with meals. Depending on the severity of cholestasis, from 4 to 24 g of cholestyramine per day may be required. Itching diminishes in 1 to 4 days. Commonly prescribed anti-itch medicines such as antihistamines are rarely helpful. Colestipol hydrochloride, an ammonium resin, is as effective as cholestyramine. Both medications may be unpalatable and are better tolerated if mixed with fruit juice or apple sauce. Large-volume plasmapheresis relieves pruritus in the rare patient whose itching does not respond to cholestyramine. Ultraviolet B (UVB) phototherapy, methyltestosterone, phenobarbital, rifampin, and cimetidine have relieved the itching in occasional patients who have not responded to cholestyramine.

Malabsorption of fat-soluble vitamins occurs most often in patients with jaundice and long-standing cholestasis. Consequently, such patients should be treated regularly with oral vitamin K_1, 5 to 10 mg/day; vitamin A, 10,000 to 25,000 1U/day; vitamin D, 50,000 IU twice per week; and supplemental calcium. Folic acid, 1 mg/day, is recommended in patients taking cholestyramine because of the occasional development of folic acid deficiency with this medication. Because cholestyramine may bind and inhibit the absorption of other drugs in the intestinal tract, these drugs should be given as far as possible from the time of cholestyramine administration.

Symptomatic steatorrhea may be treated by a low-fat diet supplemented with medium-chain triglycerides to maintain sufficient caloric intake. Primary biliary cirrhosis patients often develop iron deficiency anemia, which indicates either iron malabsorption or occult gastrointestinal blood loss. The anemia responds to iron taken orally. There is no effective treatment for the osteopenia.

Although there is no proved treatment for primary biliary cirrhosis, several drugs currently being evaluated, ursodeoxycholic acid, colchicine, and methotrexate, appear promising. Immunosuppressive agents such as corticosteroids and azathioprine are not effective. Corticosteroids have the serious disadvantage of hastening the onset of osteoporosis. Cyclosporine, another immunosuppressive drug, was minimally effective in slowing the rate of progression in a large, multicenter study; however, its renal toxicity and propensity to cause hypertension limit its value. D-penicillamine, a cupriuretic agent with some anti-inflammatory actions, was both ineffective and toxic in eight separate prospective controlled studies and should not be used in patients with primary biliary cirrhosis.

Ursodeoxycholic acid, 12-15 mg/kg body weight/day in divided doses, has been evaluated in a 2-year prospective double-blind trial. It lowered the aminotransferases and alkaline phosphatase significantly, stabilized serum bilirubin and albumin, decreased the severity of itching, and appeared to decrease the rate of clinical deterioration when compared to placebo. Colchicine, 0.6 mg twice daily, improved blood levels of the aminotransferases and alkaline phosphatase to a lesser (albeit significant) degree than ursodeoxycholic acid. It also stabilized the serum bilirubin and albumin but did not favorably affect itching or fatigue. Colchicine prolonged survival compared to placebo. Both drugs are safe. Although neither has been shown conclusively to affect the natural history of primary biliary cirrhosis, I believe that the potential benefits of using these drugs are greater than the risks of no treatment. Data suggest that methotrexate may be even more effective than ursodeoxycholic acid and colchicine. It appears to have induced clinical remissions in patients with precirrhotic disease and effectively relieve symptoms of itching and fatigue in most patients after 5 to 11 months. The dose is 0.25 mg/kg body weight per day taken orally. However, methotrexate is potentially more toxic than ursodeoxycholic acid and colchicine and is best used in controlled trials. Preliminary data suggest a 10% incidence of reversible but worrisome interstitial pneumonitis associated with methotrexate usage in primary biliary cirrhosis.

Prognosis

The outlook for patients with primary biliary cirrhosis is unpredictable but decidedly better than originally reported. Median survival in patients with symptoms ranges from 7 to 11 years in different studies and is longer in patients who are asymptomatic at the time of diagnosis. Most of these patients develop symptoms within 3 years. Granulomas are more common in the early stages of primary biliary cirrhosis and are associated with prolonged survival. A serum bilirubin greater than 10 mg/dl, a rapidly rising serum bilirubin, a decreased serum albumin, ascites, and symptomatic portal hypertension suggest a poor prognosis. In patients whose disease is progressive, the final year of life is marked by worsening liver failure, during which bilirubin concentration rises steadily. Pruritus and xanthomas often disappear, and the serum albumin level falls. Liver transplantation is accepted therapy in such patients (Chapter 64). One-year survival is approximately 85% in patients with end-stage primary biliary cirrhosis who undergo liver transplantation.

WILSON'S DISEASE

Wilson's disease is an inborn error of copper metabolism characterized by increased copper stores throughout the body. The disease occurs in individuals homozygous for an autosomal recessive gene, which is located on chromosome 13 and is tightly linked to the gene for the erythrocyte enzyme, sialic acid-specific D-acetylesterase (esterase D). The incidence is approximately 1 per 200,000 people. Once Wilson's disease has been diagnosed, it is mandatory to screen all the patient's siblings for the disease. Treatment with D-penicillamine will prevent expression of the disease in the asymptomatic patient whose condition is diagnosed early and will reverse neurologic and hepatic damage in those with more advanced disease.

Pathophysiology

Wilson's disease is caused by the chronic accumulation of excess copper within the body. The concentration of copper eventually reaches toxic levels and damages cells within which it has accumulated. Current evidence suggests that increased body stores are due to decreased excretion of copper into bile rather than to increased absorption of copper from the intestine. Copper initially accumulates in lysosomes within hepatocytes. With time, copper concentration increases, damages hepatocytes, and spills over and accumulates in other organs such as the kidney and brain. The increased copper concentration in renal tubules leads to renal tubular dysfunction and in the brain causes motor and psychiatric disorders. Deposits of copper in Descemet's membrane are recognized as Kayser-Fleischer rings. Copper toxicity may also cause hemolysis and inhibit normal bone formation, resulting in poor healing of bone fractures.

Ninety-five percent of patients with Wilson's disease have decreased serum concentrations of ceruloplasmin, a blue, copper-containing glycoprotein that is an acute phase reactant. This decreased concentration presumably reflects impaired synthesis and secretion of ceruloplasmin by the liver. However, the lowered serum ceruloplasmin concentration does not play any known role in the pathophysiology of the disease. Ten percent of heterozygotes also exhibit hypoceruloplasminemia, yet are healthy and will not develop Wilson's disease.

Pathology

The earliest lesion in Wilson's disease occurs in the liver. There is fatty infiltration within hepatocytes and glycogen inclusions within nuclei. As the disease progresses, frank hepatocellular necrosis occurs and the histologic lesion resembles that of chronic aggressive hepatitis. There is portal inflammation and fibrosis; piecemeal necrosis, with marked swelling and necrosis of periportal hepatocytes; and eventually frank cirrhosis. Intrahepatic inclusions similar to Mallory bodies may be seen in periportal areas. Histologic stains for copper demonstrate increased deposits of copper within the liver, renal tubule cells, and brain.

Clinical and laboratory findings

Approximately 40% of Wilson's disease patients present with signs and symptoms of chronic hepatocellular disease, either chronic hepatitis or cirrhosis. Many are asymptomatic and are recognized because of unexplained, moderate elevations of serum aminotransferase or bilirubin concentrations. Rarely, a patient presents initially with signs of advanced portal hypertension. Other uncommon presenting signs and symptoms include painless hematuria, glycosuria, hemolytic anemia, and, in the pediatric age group, a syndrome of acute hepatitis with liver failure, hemolysis, and renal insufficiency. Clinical manifestations of Wilson's disease are rare before age 6 years. Young patients whose disease is not detected at the stage of hepatic dysfunction may present in their teens or twenties with neuropsychiatric disorders. Approximately 10% of patients present with psychiatric problems and 35% with neurologic disorders. Neuropsychiatric problems range from subtle personality changes to overt depression and paranoia, deteriorating performance at school, tremor, rigidity, clumsiness of gait, slurring of speech, inappropriate and uncontrollable grinning (risus sardonicus), or drooling. While patients with hepatic involvement alone may not have a Kayser-Fleischer ring, every patient with a neuropsychiatric disorder exhibits this sign.

Diagnosis

Patients in whom Wilson's disease is suspected should have a slit-lamp examination performed by an experienced opthalmologist for detection of Kayser-Fleischer rings. Ninety-five percent of patients with Wilson's disease have serum ceruloplasmin levels below 20 mg/dl, and 80% have levels below 10 mg/dl. Ten percent of asymptomatic heterozygote carriers have serum ceruloplasmin levels less than 20 mg/dl. Thus this test alone is not diagnostic. Total serum copper is low, but free copper concentration is increased. Twenty-four-hour urinary copper excretion will be greater than 100 μg (normal ≤ 30 μg/24 hr). Twenty-four-hour urinary copper excretion in patients with Wilson's disease increases to greater than 1200 μg after 500 mg of D-penicillamine, whereas normal subjects excrete less than 500 μg. Quantitative hepatic copper determination in patients with Wilson's disease reveals more than 250 μg of copper per gram of dry weight (normal <50 μg). Special care must be taken to use copper-free needles and containers when quantitative tests of serum, urine, or liver biopsy copper concentration are performed. Patients often have evidence of renal tubular dysfunction manifested as glucosuria, aminoaciduria, and hypouricemia.

Treatment

D-Penicillamine is the drug of choice, 1000 to 2000 mg/day in four divided doses given 30 minutes before meals and at bedtime. Some physicians recommend a starting dose of 250 mg/day and increasing by 250 mg/day each week until the full dose is reached. This regimen may reduce the incidence of early adverse side effects such as fever and rash, but does not appear to reduce the incidence of late-onset toxicity such as nephrotic syndrome. Compliance is often a problem in children and can be ascertained by measuring 24-hour urinary copper levels or determining the presence of D-penicillamine in urine by amino acid analysis. The binding of copper to D-penicillamine is stoichiometric. Thus the amount of copper excreted in the urine will increase with increasing doses of D-penicillamine. Initially, cupruresis of 2000 μg of copper per day is desired. This level falls as copper stores are depleted. Because the tendency to accumulate excessive copper is lifelong, treatment also should be lifelong; however, the dosage of D-penicillamine can be lowered.

Liver function tests should be performed regularly. Serum ceruloplasmin commonly falls to lower levels during treatment, and values of zero may be seen. A complete blood count, platelet count, and urinalysis should be performed at monthly intervals initially because of possible bone marrow suppression and renal toxicity. Some patients with portal hypertension already have hypersplenism at the time of diagnosis, but this is not a contraindication for D-penicillamine therapy. The appearance of proteinuria may herald the onset of nephrotic syndrome, which may occur years after treatment begins. However, proteinuria up to 2 g/day usually can be tolerated and may not progress. The most common side effect is drug fever and rash. Patients with this type of D-penicillamine reaction may be desensitized if medication is stopped for 1 month. The drug is then restarted at a dosage of 25 mg/day. The dosage is then doubled at weekly intervals as long as it is tolerated. Nausea, vomiting, and anorexia are dose-related signs of gastric irritation and will disappear if dosage is reduced. Small doses of pyridoxine, 25 mg per day, should be given to patients taking D-penicillamine to prevent pyridoxal phosphate deficiency.

It is imperative that patients with Wilson's disease be on a low-copper diet and avoid liver, shellfish, nuts, dried fruits, chocolate, cocoa, and mushrooms. Agents such as potassium sulfide and carbacrylamine resins, which bind copper in the gastrointestinal tract, are not recommended. Triethylene tetramine dihydrochloride, another copper chelator, has been used successfully in patients unable to tolerate D-penicillamine and is now available in the United States. Dimercaprol (BAL), the first drug used successfully to treat Wilson's disease, is rarely used now. Oral zinc, 150 mg/day elemental zinc in six divided doses, has been used successfully to prevent the reaccumulation of copper in patients who have already responded to D-penicillamine and can no longer tolerate this agent. Zinc either inhibits copper absorption or promotes copper excretion in feces.

Prognosis

The prognosis is excellent in all but patients with very advanced Wilson's disease and those who present with the syndrome of rapidly progressive liver failure and hemolysis. Reduction of neurologic, psychiatric, and hepatic abnormalities occurs with treatment; and patients may become asymptomatic. Liver function test results usually return to normal. Treatment is most effective when it is applied early in the course of the disease. It is imperative therefore that the diagnosis be made as early as possible. Wilson's disease can be prevented in homozygotes who are identified before the disease has developed. Liver transplantation has been used successfully in patients with advanced disease in whom other forms of therapy have failed (Chapter 64).

HEMOCHROMATOSIS

Hemochromatosis is a liver disease associated with increased iron stores. There are at least two types: familial idiopathic hemochromatosis, which will be discussed here, and hemochromatosis due to secondary iron overload (see Chapter 87). Idiopathic hemochromatosis is an autosomal recessive inherited disease with an estimated gene frequency of 0.05 and a prevalence of approximately 2.5 per 1000. There is an increased incidence of the histocompatibility antigens HLA-A3, B7, and B14 in patients with idiopathic hemochromatosis, but HLA typing alone will not identify patients. Rather, HLA typing is used to identify siblings who are at risk for developing the disease.

Pathophysiology

Although the precise cause of idiopathic hemochromatosis is not certain, it is thought to be abnormal regulation of intestinal iron absorption and inappropriately high intestinal iron absorption. The human body has a limited ability to excrete iron. The average man can excrete up to 1 mg of iron per day and the menstruating woman up to 1.5 mg per day. In normal persons, intestinal iron absorption is carefully regulated to match iron excretion. In patients with idiopathic hemochromatosis, this regulation is lost. Instead, there is long-standing, inappropriately high intestinal iron absorption that leads to excess iron stores in the body. The intracellular iron concentration eventually reaches toxic levels and causes cellular dysfunction, necrosis, and fibrosis. Clinical symptoms rarely occur until total body iron stores reach 15 to 20 g (compared with <5 g in the normal human being). The heaviest accumulation of iron occurs in the liver and pancreas, where iron concentration is often 50 times greater than normal. Iron also accumulates in endocrine glands, the heart, and the skin.

Pathology

The most characteristic findings occur in the liver, which is enlarged and reddish brown in color. Microscopically, increased hemosiderin pigment can be seen, initially in periportal hepatocytes. As iron stores increase, hemosiderin becomes distributed widely within hepatocytes throughout the entire hepatic lobule and spills over into bile duct epithelial cells, Kupffer cells, and macrophages within fibrous tissue. Portal triads expand and form connecting bridges; eventually, true portal cirrhosis develops. Hemosiderin is also evident within acinar cells of the pancreas and, to a lesser extent, in the islets of the pancreas. It is also deposited in the conducting fibers of the atrioventricular node of the heart and in the adrenal, thyroid, parathyroid, and anterior lobe of the pituitary glands.

Clinical features

Symptoms of idiopathic hemochromatosis occur primarily in men, with a sex ratio of 5:1 (male/female). Symptoms most commonly begin in the fifth decade of life, although they may be present as early as the second or third decade. The most common initial complaints are lethargy, loss of libido, sexual impotence, and abdominal pain. Physical and laboratory examinations reveal the classic triad of pigmentation of the skin, hepatomegaly, and diabetes in less than one third of patients. Testicular atrophy is common. The skin may be bronze or bluish gray in color, due primarily to increased melanin pigment in the skin rather than to iron. Testicular atrophy is due to pituitary dysfunction rather than to increased iron deposition within the testes. Iron stores are normal or low in the testes.

Carbohydrate intolerance occurs in approximately 80% of patients, but overt diabetes mellitus is seen in only 60%. The severity of diabetes is variable, and there is an apparent coinheritance of diabetes in hemochromatosis. Complications of diabetes such as nephropathy, retinopathy, and peripheral neuropathy may occur, depending on the severity of the diabetes. Cardiac arrhythmias occur in up to 15% of patients. Severe heart failure is uncommon. As many as 50% of patients develop a characteristic arthropathy with deposits of both calcium pyrophosphate and iron in the synovium. Involvement of the metacarpophalangeal joints of the index and middle fingers is quite characteristic.

Cirrhosis is often present when hemochromatosis is diagnosed. Portal hypertension and liver failure usually develop if hemochromatosis is not treated effectively. The signs and symptoms of liver dysfunction in idiopathic hemochromatosis are similar to those in other types of chronic liver disease such as alcoholic or postnecrotic cirrhosis (Chapter 56). There is evidence that cirrhosis and hepatocellular carcinoma can be prevented if idiopathic hemochromatosis is detected and treated early.

Diagnosis

Diagnosis of idiopathic hemochromatosis is made on the basis of the preceding clinical features together with laboratory evidence of excess iron storage. The major diagnostic problem is in distinguishing patients with idiopathic hemochromatosis from those with iron overload secondary to other types of cirrhosis. Liver function tests are not specific, and results are similar to those in other types of cirrhosis (see Table 53-1). Serum iron concentration is usually greater than 175 μg/dl, and total iron-binding capacity is usually reduced to about 200 μg/dl. Thus transferrin is almost 100% saturated. Because serum iron tests do not enable the physician to distinguish idiopathic hemochromatosis from other types of cirrhosis with secondary iron overload, it is imperative that iron stores be quantitated more precisely and that familial incidence of iron overload be sought. Serum ferritin levels greater than 1000 ng/ml suggest significant iron overload as long as there is no evidence of active hepatocellular disease. Liver biopsy should be performed to estimate the extent of liver damage and to provide histologic evidence of iron overload. Quantitative chemical determination of iron content can also be performed on needle biopsy samples. If iron concentrations are expressed as an age-related index (hepatic iron concentration per year of age), values greater than 2 μmol/g per year are seen only in idiopathic hemochromatosis. All first-order relatives should be tested for features of iron overload. Liver function tests and measurement of serum iron, total iron-binding capacity, and serum ferritin levels are sufficient screening tests. Evidence of increased iron stores is usually seen in 25% to 50% of first-order relatives. Serum ferritin levels indicate increased iron stores in approximately 90% of families with idiopathic hemochromatosis.

In some instances, it is not possible to distinguish readily patients with idiopathic hemochromatosis from those with other types of cirrhosis and secondary iron overload. One way to accomplish this is to quantitate total body iron by weekly phlebotomy, 1 unit per week, until iron deficiency occurs. Total body iron can then be quantitated retrospectively. Each unit of blood contains approximately 250 mg of iron. Although there is no sharp separation between idiopathic and secondary hemochromatosis, patients with the former usually have more than 10 g of excess body iron, and phlebotomy improves their hepatic function. In patients with other types of cirrhosis, there is substantially less excess body iron, and phlebotomy has no effect on liver function.

Treatment

There is now adequate evidence that phlebotomy prolongs life and reverses much of the tissue damage in patients with idiopathic hemochromatosis. Five-hundred milliliter phlebotomies may be performed one to two times per week. Hematocrit should be checked before each phlebotomy, which should not be performed if hematocrit is less than 35. When hematocrit falls to this level and fails to increase after several weeks, excess iron stores have been removed. Most of the signs and symptoms of the disease will diminish. The exceptions are arthritis, diabetes, and testicular atrophy. These problems must be treated separately. After excess iron has been removed, 500 ml phlebotomies should be performed two to four times per year indefinitely to prevent the reaccumulation of iron and serum ferritin levels measured to monitor body iron stores.

Prognosis

Except for patients with end-stage liver disease, the prognosis is excellent with phlebotomy. There is considerable evidence that phlebotomy will prevent the disease manifestations in those treated in the precirrhotic stage. There is an increased risk of hepatocellular carcinoma in patients with cirrhosis who have responded to treatment, and there is evidence that hepatocellular carcinoma will not develop if the disease is treated in the precirrhotic stage.

GRANULOMATOUS HEPATITIS

Granulomatous hepatitis is an uncommon disease of unknown etiology that usually presents as fever of unknown cause and asthenia. The diagnosis is made when the many other conditions associated with hepatic granulomas have been ruled out.

Hepatic granulomas may be seen in tuberculosis, sarcoidosis, drug reactions, brucellosis, fungal infections, primary biliary cirrhosis, infectious mononucleosis, Hodgkin's disease, vasculitis, berylliosis, and parasitic infections. Patients with these conditions usually have systemic signs and symptoms of the underlying disease. Hepatic granulomas are part of the overall systemic disease and usually resolve when it is treated.

Pathogenesis

The cause of granulomatous hepatitis is unknown. It is thought to represent a host inflammatory response to some unknown stimulus.

Pathology

Liver biopsy generally reveals well-defined, noncaseating granulomas scattered throughout the parenchyma. There are usually increased numbers of mononuclear inflammatory cells within sinusoids, hepatocellular unrest with minor degrees of hepatocellular necrosis scattered throughout the hepatic lobule, and portal enlargement with mononuclear cell infiltration and fibrosis.

Clinical findings

Patients with granulomatous hepatitis usually present with fever of unknown cause. Temperature may exceed 105.8° F (41° C), and most patients experience chills and night sweats. Generalized asthenia is present in most individuals. Arthralgia, weight loss, abdominal pain, nausea, and vomiting are less frequent manifestations. More than 50% of patients have hepatomegaly, splenomegaly, or both. Signs of portal hypertension or liver failure are uncommon.

Laboratory findings and diagnosis

The sedimentation rate is greater than 100 mm/hr in 40% of patients with granulomatous hepatitis, and 25% may have anemia. Liver function test results are nonspecifically abnormal. Most patients have modest elevations of serum alkaline phosphatase, aminotransferases, and gamma globulins, while serum albumin may be minimally decreased. Jaundice is rare. The diagnosis is based on the presence of granulomas scattered throughout the hepatic lobule and on the exclusion of other diseases associated with hepatic granulomas.

Treatment

Granulomatous hepatitis invariably responds to corticosteroid treatment. An initial dosage of 30 mg/day of prednisone or its equivalent is usually adequate, but dosage must be adjusted on an individual basis. After clinical remission has occurred, the disease may be managed by corticosteroid treatment administered every other day. In some patients, the disease will remain in remission after prednisone is gradually tapered off and discontinued. In others, the disease will return, and further treatment will be necessary. Because of the difficulty in identifying *Mycobacterium tuberculosis* in liver biopsies and of culturing it from the liver, all patients with etiologically obscure granulomatous hepatitis should receive an initial trial of antituberculous therapy.

LIVER DYSFUNCTION SECONDARY TO HEART DISEASE

Liver dysfunction is commonly seen in patients with heart failure. The signs and symptoms of liver dysfunction depend on the nature of the heart disease (see also Chapter 10), whether it is acute or chronic, and whether it is primarily right- or left-sided.

Pathophysiology and pathology

The hepatic dysfunction is secondary to hepatic hypoxia, resulting from diminished hepatic blood flow. The pericentral area of the liver lobule is always more severely affected. The pericentral area receives blood after the rest of the liver lobule has been supplied. Oxygen tension is always lowest in the pericentral zone.

In predominantly right-sided heart failure, the liver is grossly enlarged and congested. The pericentral sinusoids and, at times, the central veins are dilated. The hepatocytes in the pericentral liver plates are attenuated. Central cholestasis may be present. Macrophages are common and are often filled with lipofuscin. In chronic heart failure, there may be degeneration of pericentral hepatocytes and replacement by bands of fibrous tissue. Very rarely, the bands of pericentral fibrous tissue coalesce to form nodules, as in cardiac cirrhosis.

In left-sided heart failure, evidence of congestion is lacking. Rather, there is a loss of hepatocytes from the pericentral hepatic plates and their replacement by red blood cells (Plate II-19). Red blood within the space of Disse is seen primarily in heart failure and Budd-Chiari syndrome.

Clinical and laboratory findings

In patients with chronic congestive heart failure, abundant evidence of liver dysfunction is generally found on physical examination. The liver is usually grossly enlarged and firm. There may be hepatojugular reflux. Serum aminotransferase levels and prothrombin time are moderately elevated. Bilirubin concentration is rarely greater than 3 mg/dl. Levels above 8 mg/dl are distinctly uncommon. Ten percent of such patients may have elevations of serum alkaline phosphatase, but values greater than two times normal are uncommon.

In acute right-sided heart failure or in chronic heart failure of unusual severity, abnormal liver function test results may be the most prominent findings. In this situation, the aminotransferases may be greater than 500 units, and the bilirubin concentration between 3 and 8 mg/dl. These patients occasionally present with severe right-sided abdominal pain due to the sudden stretching of Glisson's capsule. The signs of congestive heart failure are usually obvious. The heart is enlarged, neck veins distended, and the liver enlarged and occasionally pulsatile. Prominent hepatojugular reflux can usually be elicited. In patients with right-sided heart failure due to cor pulmonale, mitral stenosis with pulmonary hypertension, or restrictive cardiomyopathy, clinical signs of congestive heart failure may be more subtle. Rarely, patients with severe heart failure may develop changes in mental state indistinguishable from those in patients with hepatic encephalopathy. There may be confusion, somnolence, and, rarely, frank coma. A flapping tremor can often be elicited. Electroencephalography reveals the changes of metabolic encephalopathy.

Liver dysfunction frequently occurs in patients with isolated left ventricular failure. Patients without clinically obvious left-sided heart failure may present with a clinical picture indistinguishable from that seen in acute viral hepatitis. The serum aminotransferases may be disproportionately elevated, often greater than 1000 units, compared with the values of other liver function tests. Other liver function test results may be normal. Although the physical examination often fails to reveal signs of overt heart failure, there is almost always a history of underlying heart disease. Patients may complain of fatigue, anorexia, nausea, and vomiting. If the left-sided heart failure is chronic, there may be jaundice.

Diagnosis

The diagnosis of liver dysfunction in right-sided heart failure is almost always made on the basis of the history and physical findings. Liver function test results are confirmatory.

Liver dysfunction associated with isolated left-sided heart failure may be more difficult to recognize. Clinical signs of heart disease may be minimal or absent. In this case, liver function test results usually alert the physician to this possibility. The serum aminotransferases are disproportionately elevated, and other liver function test results are normal or minimally abnormal. Noninvasive cardiac function tests should be performed to document the severity of the underlying heart disease. If the diagnosis is uncertain, percutaneous needle biopsy of the liver will provide the correct diagnosis. The lesion is confined to the pericentral areas. In hepatitis, the histologic lesion is diffuse and demonstrates more inflammation and isolated liver cell necrosis.

Treatment and prognosis

Once the correct diagnosis is made, therapy should be directed at the underlying heart disease. Liver function improves if the underlying heart disease responds to treatment. The prognosis is that of the underlying heart disease.

ALPHA$_1$ ANTITRYPSIN DEFICIENCY

A deficiency of serum alpha$_1$ antitrypsin is associated with neonatal hepatitis and childhood cirrhosis. The identical deficiency is seen in adults with early-onset pulmonary emphysema (Chapter 204). Many of these patients also have cirrhosis, but it is typically asymptomatic and diagnosed only if sought.

Incidence and inheritance

Alpha$_1$ antitrypsin is an important serum protease inhibitor that migrates as an alpha$_1$ globulin on electrophoresis. Its concentration can be measured biochemically. Its inheritance is determined by a set of alleles at one gene locus. Although there are at least 30 different protease inhibitor (Pi) alleles detectable by electrophoretic techniques, the Pi^M allele is by far the most common, occurring with a gene frequency of 0.87. The allele responsible for childhood liver disease and adult lung disease is autosomal recessive and is termed Pi^{Z}. $Alpha_1$ antitrypsin deficiency diseases occur when Pi^{Z} exists in the homozygous state, Pi^{ZZ}. The prevalence of homozygous Pi^{ZZ} is as high as 1 per 1000 children in some parts of the United States.

Pathophysiology and pathology

Childhood hepatitis and cirrhosis occur in only 11% of children homozygous for Pi^{ZZ}. The remaining 89% reach adulthood without clinically apparent liver disease. Another genotype, Pi^{SZ}, is associated with low serum $alpha_1$ antitrypsin levels but rarely causes childhood liver disease. The presence of retained $alpha_1$ antitrypsin within liver cells, demonstrated as periodic acid Schiff (PAS)—positive, diastase-resistant globules in periportal hepatocytes, is a prerequisite for the development of liver disease (Plate II-20); however, not all persons with these globules develop liver disease. Asymptomatic Pi^{MZ} patients can also have PAS-positive, diastase-resistant globules in the liver. Current evidence indicates that the globules are $alpha_1$ antitrypsin that has been synthesized within the hepatocyte but that cannot be secreted into blood. Pi^{ZZ} $alpha_1$ antitrypsin differs from the Pi^{MM} inhibitor in that a glutamic acid residue is substituted for a lysine, and the normal complement of sialic acid is lacking. These molecular alterations may interfere with the secretion of the Pi^{ZZ} inhibitor by the hepatocyte. $Alpha_1$ antitrypsin deficiency appears to act as a "permissive" factor in the development of liver disease. Some additional, as yet unknown triggering factor is required.

The typical pathologic finding late in the course of the disease is advanced micronodular cirrhosis, with involvement of most hepatic lobules. Although bile duct proliferation within fibrous bands is most often seen at this stage, there are patients with a paucity of intralobular ducts. The only pathognomonic feature is the PAS-positive inclusion bodies.

Clinical findings

The hepatic manifestations of $alpha_1$ antitrypsin deficiency depend very much on the age of the patient at presentation. In the neonatal period, $alpha_1$ antitrypsin deficiency presents as acute hepatitis, with jaundice and moderately elevated serum aminotransferases. Alkaline phosphatase concentration may be greater than four times normal. Serum bilirubin usually returns to normal within 3 to 6 months, but aminotransferase and alkaline phosphatase levels remain elevated. Patients then remain asymptomatic until late childhood or early adolescence, when the clinical manifestations of advanced cirrhosis are recognized. The course is then progressive and downhill. Death usually results from liver failure. Liver function test results are often those of chronic cholestasis, with a markedly elevated alkaline phosphatase level.

Liver disease in adults with $alpha_1$ antitrypsin deficiency is most often asymptomatic macronodular cirrhosis. The disease is most often detected in homozygous Pi^{ZZ} adults with severe emphysema. There is also an increased incidence of hepatocellular carcinoma in these patients.

Diagnosis

$Alpha_1$ antitrypsin deficiency should be suspected in all young patients with neonatal hepatitis and juvenile cirrhosis and in adults with early-onset pulmonary emphysema. $Alpha_1$ antitrypsin normally makes up 90% of the serum $alpha_1$ globulin observed on routine serum electrophoresis. If this band is missing or is present in unusually low concentrations, the diagnosis of $alpha_1$ antitrypsin deficiency is suggested. A definite diagnosis can be made by chemically quantifying serum $alpha_1$ antitrypsin activity or by Pi typing using techniques such as acid starch gel electrophoresis followed by antigen-antibody crossed electrophoresis in agarose. The diagnosis is confirmed by liver biopsy, which will demonstrate PAS-positive, diastase-resistant inclusion bodies in periportal hepatocytes. Results of other liver function tests are nonspecific and typically present a cholestatic picture.

Treatment and prognosis

There is no known treatment for the liver disease associated with $alpha_1$ antitrypsin deficiency. The synthetic androgen danazol will increase serum antitrypsin levels up to 37% in Pi^{ZZ} patients. It is not yet known whether this agent will modulate the liver disease. Treatment currently is directed toward relieving symptoms and is similar to that used in other types of cirrhosis and liver failure (Chapter 56). There is no known contraindication to danazol usage in children with symptomatic $alpha_1$ antitrypsin deficiency, and it may be tried cautiously in this group. All family members should be screened for the presence of the Pi^{ZZ} genotype. Liver transplantation has been used successfully in patients with end-stage liver disease due to $alpha_1$ antitrypsin deficiency. Liver transplantation will correct the metabolic defect as well as the liver failure and portal hypertension. Portosystemic shunt surgery aimed at correcting symptomatic portal hypertension should be avoided because it makes subsequent liver transplantation more difficult and will not benefit the failing liver.

SCHISTOSOMIASIS

Schistosomiasis represents one of the major health problems of developing countries, affecting more than 200 million. (See also Chapter 282.) The liver disease is caused by infection with three species of the family of flatworms (Schistosomatoidea), *Schistosoma mansoni, S. mekongi,* and *S. japonicum*. The fourth species, *S. haematobium,* does not cause liver disease. *S. mansoni* is widely distributed throughout central Africa and is also found in Egypt and the Sudan. In the New World, it is found mainly in Brazil but also occurs in some of the Caribbean islands such as Puerto Rico and the Dominican Republic. *S. japonicum* is endemic to Japan, China, and the Philippines; and *S.*

mekongi to Indochina. The latter two cause an identical spectrum of disease.

Acute hepatic schistosomiasis

The schistosomes cause two types of liver disease, acute and chronic. The latter is much more of a health problem. Acute hepatic schistosomiasis occurs 20 to 60 days after exposure to and penetration of the skin by cercariae, a motile schistosome form that develops in certain types of aquatic snails. Patients experience fever, diffuse aches, chills, headache, and diarrhea. The disease is most likely caused by an allergic reaction to the large number of eggs found primarily in the large intestine during this stage of the disease. There is generalized lymph node enlargement, urticaria, and hepatosplenomegaly. Liver biopsy at this stage reveals granulomas in portal triads but no fibrosis. None of the drugs used to treat schistosomiasis is effective at this stage. The acute disease lasts several weeks and then gradually disappears.

Chronic hepatic schistosomiasis

Chronic hepatic schistosomiasis is seen most commonly in the United States, usually in Puerto Rican immigrants. Heavy worm burdens within the large intestine are a prerequisite for the development of clinically significant liver disease. Eggs are laid by adult worms living in the mesenteric and hemorrhoidal veins of the large intestine and are carried in portal blood to the liver. The eggs lodge in the smaller portal veins, where they evoke a granulomatous inflammatory reaction. There may be occlusion of these small portal veins by thrombi and eventually a characteristic pipestem type of fibrosis. Granulomas encompassing schistosome eggs may be seen on liver biopsy (Plate II-21). The parenchyma and bile ducts are not usually involved. As a consequence of portal vein fibrosis and narrowing, an intrahepatic block to portal blood flow occurs, with portal hypertension and portosystemic shunting. The hepatic lesion is presinusoidal. Thus wedge hepatic vein pressure is normal in the face of markedly elevated portal and splenic vein pressure.

Clinical findings. Initially, hepatomegaly is found. As fibrosis worsens, splenomegaly and frank portal hypertension develop. Patients are usually asymptomatic until sudden, unexpected hematemesis occurs due to rupture of esophageal varices. The bleeding may cease spontaneously and not return for years or may recur at frequent intervals. Patients with chronic hepatic schistosomiasis tolerate the bleeding much better than do patients with cirrhosis. Jaundice is almost never seen. Rarely, stigmata of chronic liver disease, such as spider nevi, palmar erythema, gynecomastia, and testicular atrophy occur. Hepatic encephalopathy is distinctly uncommon until end-stage liver disease develops. Hypersplenism, with a decrease in white blood cells and platelets, may occur but rarely causes complications.

Diagnosis. The diagnosis of chronic hepatic schistosomiasis is suggested by the presence of bleeding esophageal varices and signs of portal hypertension in a patient with relatively normal liver function test results who has lived in an endemic area. The diagnosis must always be confirmed by the presence of schistosome eggs in stool, rectal biopsy, or liver biopsy.

Treatment. Treatment is never undertaken until an unequivocal diagnosis has been made. Praziquantel, a new antiparasitic drug, has revolutionized the treatment of schistosomiasis. It is well tolerated and effective against all four species of human schistosomes. Cooperative studies throughout the world indicate that all patients with active chronic schistosomiasis can now be safely and effectively treated in 1 day. The drug may be given as one dose, 50 mg/kg body weight, or in three divided doses, 20 mg/kg body weight every 8 hours. Praziquantel results in death of the infecting schistosomes and is associated with parasitologic cure in close to 100% of infected patients. Therapy can be repeated in 2 to 3 months in the rare patient who does not respond initially. The drug is rapidly absorbed after an oral dose, undergoes first-pass biotransformation within the liver, and is rapidly excreted in urine. It is well tolerated in humans and has no known long-term toxicity.

In some patients, recurrent bleeding from esophageal varices becomes life threatening or so incapacitating that surgical portosystemic shunt becomes necessary. In general, patients tolerate recurrent bleeding so well that portosystemic shunt surgery is delayed as long as possible. Splenectomy produces only temporary lowering of the portal pressure. If surgery is necessary, the distal (Warren) splenorenal shunt is best tolerated and effective. The prognosis is better than that in patients with true cirrhosis who develop bleeding from esophageal varices.

CONGENITAL HEPATIC FIBROSIS

Congenital hepatic fibrosis is a rare disease inherited as a recessive autosomal disorder. It usually presents in children, rarely in adults, with abdominal distention, hepatomegaly, and signs of portal hypertension. Approximately one half of these patients have polycystic kidneys. On pathologic examination, the liver is markedly enlarged. Its normal architecture is distorted by dense bands of connective tissue that contain small, irregularly shaped cystic spaces lined by bile duct–like epithelial cells. The major clinical problem is recurrent gastrointestinal bleeding from esophageal varices. Liver function test results are normal, although alkaline phosphatase levels may be elevated. Jaundice, ascites, and hepatic encephalopathy are rare. The diagnosis is likely in a child or young adult who presents with gastrointestinal bleeding, obvious portal hypertension, and normal liver function test results and is confirmed by liver biopsy or laparoscopy. Frequently, the small specimen obtained by needle biopsy is inadequate to allow a definite diagnosis, and a larger, surgically obtained specimen is needed. Because hepatic function is normal, patients tolerate recurrent gastrointestinal bleeding very well. Portosystemic shunt surgery is reserved for those patients whose recurrent gastrointestinal bleeding becomes incapacitating or life threatening. Liver function test results are often worse after portosystemic shunt surgery, but the prognosis is much better than that in patients with true cirrhosis and bleeding esophageal varices. There appears to be an increased risk of bile duct cancer in adults.

METABOLIC STORAGE DISEASES OF THE LIVER

Lipid storage diseases

Niemann-Pick disease. Niemann-Pick disease, an inherited disorder of sphingomyelin metabolism, presents in early childhood as neonatal hepatitis. There is hepatosplenomegaly, with elevation of aminotransferase and alkaline phosphatase levels and, in more advanced cases, serum bilirubin concentration. Clinically, babies fail to thrive and have impaired motor and intellectual development. One half of afflicted children have a cherry-red spot of macular degeneration on funduscopic examination. All patients have pronounced hepatosplenomegaly. The disease is due to increased stores of sphingomyelin resulting from a deficiency of the enzyme sphingomyelinase. There are five distinct types of disease, each with a different type of enzyme abnormality. The liver is large, yellow, and fatty. Hepatocytes are vacuolated. There are many large, pale, foamy reticuloendothelial cells within sinusoids. Diagnosis is most readily made by bone marrow aspiration. Characteristic Niemann-Pick foam cells are usually abundant. There is no treatment, although temporary improvement occurred in one patient after the implantation of normal human amniotic epithelial cells. Death usually occurs before 4 years of age. One of the types is more benign than the others, does not involve the central nervous system, and allows affected individuals to reach adulthood.

Gaucher's disease. This lysosomal storage disease in which the cerebroside glucosylceramide accumulates in reticuloendothelial cells of the liver and spleen is due to a deficiency of the enzyme, glucosylceramide beta-glucosidase. There are three forms of the disease, each with a different degree of enzyme deficiency. Type II is most serious and occurs in infancy. There is progressive involvement of the central nervous system, and death usually occurs in the first year.

The most common form of Gaucher's disease, type I, is seen in adults. The nervous system is not involved; rather, the disease presents as unexplained hepatosplenomegaly, bone pain occasionally with pathologic fractures, and pingueculae. The onset is usually in childhood, but the patient may present with symptoms as late as age 60 years. Leukopenia and thrombocytopenia secondary to hypersplenism are common. Portal hypertension with bleeding from esophageal varices is rare.

The diagnosis is usually made by the finding of typical "wrinkled tissue paper" Gaucher's cells in bone marrow aspirates, liver biopsy specimens, or the resected spleen. The diagnosis can be confirmed by demonstrating a deficiency of the enzyme glucosylceramide beta-glucosidase in peripheral leukocytes. Serum acid phosphatase activity is elevated. Unlike the prostatic enzyme, it is not inhibited by L-tartrate.

Treatment and prognosis. The gene for the missing enzyme, glucocerebrosidase, has been cloned; and sufficient quantities of enzyme are now available for long-term replacement therapy. This treatment has revolutionized the therapy of Gaucher's disease. Most of the complications can be prevented with early diagnosis and aggressive enzyme replacement therapy. In the patient who already has painful splenomegaly at time of diagnosis, or symptomatic leukopenia or thrombocytopenia due to splenomegaly, splenectomy may be helpful. Even before enzyme replacement therapy was available, prognosis was good in patients with Gaucher's disease who had survived to adolescence. Portosystemic anastomosis has been curative in some patients with bleeding from esophageal varices and massive infiltration of the liver by Gaucher's cells. Splenectomy alone has been effective in others with normal livers whose portal hypertension was due primarily to massively increased splenic vein blood flow.

Glycogen storage diseases

There are 10 different genetically determined glycogen storage diseases, each due to the loss of or deficiency of a specific enzyme involved in glycogen metabolism. All types involve the liver and cause hepatomegaly, except for types V and VII, which involve muscle and/or red blood cells. Type I glycogen storage disease, von Gierke's disease, is the first inherited disease shown to be caused by loss of a specific enzyme activity, in this case glucose 6-phosphatase. In all of the eight glycogen storage diseases that involve the liver, glucose homeostasis is deranged because of the limited capacity of the liver to mobilize glucose from the hepatic glycogen stores. Under normal conditions, hepatic glycogen acts as the major carbohydrate reservoir in blood glucose homeostasis (see Chapter 50).

Von Gierke's disease and most of the other glycogen storage disorders present in infancy with hypoglycemia, often complicated by convulsions and mental retardation. Vomiting, acidosis, and diarrhea occur frequently. There is usually massive hepatomegaly. The histologic findings in the liver are not specific and consist of fatty infiltration of hepatocytes and prominent nuclear glycogenosis. Glycogen stores are also markedly increased in hepatocytes.

Laboratory findings. Fasting hypoglycemia is a constant feature. There is a diminished rise of blood sugar following intravenous administration of glucagon. Hyperlipidemia, hyperlactacidemia, and acidosis are also frequent features. The diagnosis is suspected on the basis of the clinical findings and these laboratory tests. Precise classification depends on demonstration of the specific enzyme defect.

Treatment. Hypoglycemia may be lessened by frequent feedings of carbohydrates. Glycogen storage disease is always worse in early childhood, and improvement is noted in those who survive beyond 5 years of age. Portacaval anastomosis has been effective in some patients with severe disease: hypoglycemia diminishes slightly, hyperlipidemia disappears totally, and growth rate increases. More recently, liver transplantation has been successfully performed in a patient with severe type I disease.

HEPATIC AMYLOIDOSIS

Although at least 70% of patients with amyloidosis have hepatic involvement demonstrable on biopsy or autopsy, symptoms of hepatic dysfunction are uncommon (Chapter 322). The liver is enlarged in 50% of patients and may be massively enlarged in some. In patients with massive enlargement, symptoms of abdominal fullness and early satiety may occur. Ascites is rare and more often reflects the severity of accompanying renal disease than hepatic dysfunction.

Pathology

The liver is large, pale gray, or pink in color and has a waxy, rubbery consistency. The microscopic appearance is striking. Amyloid appears as a pale, amorphous, eosinophilic material when stained with hematoxylin and eosin stains. It is characteristically located in the space of Disse, between endothelial cells and hepatocytes. Hepatocytes may be markedly compressed and shrunken because of the dense deposits of amyloid. Amyloid stains a salmon pink color with alkaline Congo red stain and has a blue green to yellow bi-refringence when viewed with polarized light.

There is no difference in the histologic appearances of primary and secondary amyloid. Primary amyloid is found in plasma cell dyscrasias such as multiple myeloma and light-chain disease. It has an amino acid sequence similar to that of the light chain of immunoglobulin. Primary amyloid most likely represents deposition of polymerized light chains. Secondary amyloid is found in patients with long-standing inflammatory diseases such as leprosy and rheumatoid arthritis. It is also seen in 25% of patients with familial Mediterranean fever. This type of amyloid is derived from serum protein A, a recently discovered acute phase reactant with a unique amino acid sequence. The pathogenesis of amyloid deposition is not known.

Clinical manifestations and diagnosis

Hepatic amyloidosis is usually an incidental finding in patients whose disease involves other organs such as the heart or kidney. However, striking hepatomegaly in a patient with vague symptoms, such as malaise and fatigue, is occasionally the first sign of amyloidosis. Jaundice occurs in less than 5% of patients. Alkaline phosphatase or serum aminotransferases are either at normal levels or minimally elevated. If hypoalbuminemia is present, it is usually secondary to proteinuria associated with the nephrotic syndrome rather than to liver dysfunction. Prothrombin time is usually normal.

The diagnosis is best made by fat pad or rectal biopsies. If these biopsies are normal and there is a suggestion of hepatic involvement, the diagnosis can be made by percutaneous needle biopsy of the liver. The risk of bleeding from percutaneous biopsy is no higher than in patients with other types of liver disease, unless the liver is massively enlarged, in which case liver biopsy is best avoided. Several case reports describe fatal hemorrhage after liver biopsy in such patients.

There is no specific treatment for amyloidosis. The disease occasionally regresses if the underlying disorder can be treated.

REYE'S SYNDROME

Reye's syndrome, first described in 1963, occurs almost exclusively in children younger than 16 years of age. It consists of acute encephalopathy accompanied by fatty infiltration of the liver, kidney, and, rarely, the heart and pancreas. Typically, Reye's syndrome occurs in a child recovering from a nonspecific viral illness, influenza B, or varicella. Its cause is unknown. Abnormalities of mitochondrial structure and function, defective oxidative phosphorylation, and inborn errors of ammonia metabolism have been noted in patients with Reye's syndrome. These abnormalities are most likely secondary to some other unknown primary disorder. Toxic, genetic, and infectious etiologies have been suggested. Epidemiologic data suggest that Reye's syndrome is related to aspirin use. The prevalence of Reye's syndrome has decreased dramatically since acetaminophen has replaced aspirin as the antipyretic of choice in children with viral infections.

Pathology

The brain and liver are the organs most seriously involved. The brain is usually edematous. There is neither inflammatory infiltration nor evidence of demyelination. The liver is enlarged, fatty, and pale, often appearing white on needle biopsy specimens. Microscopically, there is depletion of hepatic glycogen and marked fatty infiltration, usually microvesicular, so that the nucleus remains centrally located. Often, the presence and extent of the fatty infiltration are appreciated only if fat stains are performed on fresh-frozen specimens obtained by percutaneous needle biopsy.

Clinical manifestations and diagnosis

Reye's syndrome typically occurs in a child recovering uneventfully from a viral illness. Vomiting occurs initially and is followed by changes in the mental state. Lethargy and confusion may progress to delirium and frank coma. Convulsions occur in 30% of patients. Hypoglycemia and electrolyte abnormalities, usually acidemia, are common. Serum aminotransferases are typically elevated, with prolongation of the prothrombin time and elevated blood ammonia levels. Clinical jaundice is rare, and serum alkaline phosphatase is minimally elevated or normal.

The diagnosis can usually be made clinically. If there is uncertainty about the diagnosis, it can be confirmed by percutaneous needle biopsy with special fat stains of a frozen specimen.

There is no specific treatment for the underlying disease. Blood sugar should be monitored closely and hypoglycemia treated with intravenously administered glucose. Cerebral edema is treated with hypertonic mannitol or dexamethasone. Exchange transfusion is not efficacious. Continuous monitoring of intracranial pressure via an intraventricular catheter is useful.

ACUTE FATTY LIVER OF PREGNANCY
(See also Chapter 369)

Acute fatty liver of pregnancy (AFLP) is a potentially fatal, uncommon disorder that may complicate the third trimester of pregnancy. Until the late 1970s, both fetal and maternal mortality were as high as 85%. Prognosis has improved since then. Early recognition of the disorder and rapid treatment have brightened the outlook considerably. Fetal and maternal mortality are now as low as 23% and 18%, respectively.

Incidence

Once considered a rare disorder, AFLP now has an incidence of 1 per 13,000 deliveries. The most likely reason for the apparent increased prevalence is greater awareness and recognition of this disorder. Primiparas, particularly those carrying twins and/or males, are most often affected; however, the disorder can occur in any pregnant woman. AFLP usually occurs after the thirty-fifth week of pregnancy, although the disorder has been noted as early as the thirtieth week. Its time of onset is similar to that of preeclampsia and, like preeclampsia, AFLP is often associated with peripheral edema, hypertension, and proteinuria.

Pathophysiology and pathology

The cause of AFLP is unknown. It is clearly not an infectious disease, nor is it an inherited metabolic disorder. There are no familial cases, and subsequent pregnancies have been normal in those who survived the disorder.

Grossly, the liver is pale and small. Microscopically, hepatocytes, particularly those in the pericentral area, are swollen, pale, and infiltrated with microvesicular fat. The fat may not be recognized unless special fat stains such as Oil Red O are performed on fresh-frozen biopsy specimens. Inflammation and liver cell necrosis are uncommon.

Clinical and laboratory presentation

The symptoms of AFLP begin toward the end of the third trimester of pregnancy. The initial manifestations are nonspecific and may include headache, fatigue, malaise, nausea, vomiting, and abdominal pain. Back pain suggests pancreatitis, a recognized complication of AFLP. Jaundice, bleeding from puncture sites, hematemesis, seizures, and frank coma are later, more ominous manifestations.

The physical examination is rarely helpful. Patients are usually afebrile. Mild hypertension and peripheral edema suggest preeclampsia. Spider angiomas may be present but are not helpful because they also are common in normal pregnancy. Jaundice and hepatic encephalopathy occur later in the course of this disease and should immediately alert the physician to the possibility of AFLP. Abdominal tenderness is common but nonspecific. The liver is characteristically not palpable. Abdominal examination is difficult in any case because of abdominal tenderness and the enlarged uterus.

Because early recognition and prompt treatment of AFLP will improve both maternal and fetal survival, serum aminotransferases should be obtained immediately in any woman in the third trimester of pregnancy with the preceding symptoms. If the aminotransferases are elevated, a thorough laboratory evaluation should be rapidly performed. The white blood count is characteristically elevated, often above 15,000. The peripheral smear may show normoblasts, burr cells, fragmented red cells, and Howell-Jolly bodies. There is usually evidence of disseminated intravascular coagulopathy. The platelet count is low, the prothrombin time and partial thromboplastin time are elevated, and the fibrinogen is lower than the normally high levels of pregnancy. Fibrin split products are usually present. The blood urea nitrogen and creatinine levels may be modestly elevated, and the uric acid disproportionately increased compared with the creatinine. The aminotransferases are invariably elevated, usually around 300 IU but rarely greater than 500 IU. The bilirubin may be normal early in the course but will rise if the pregnancy is not terminated. The blood ammonia is usually increased. Alkaline phosphatase is elevated, but this finding is nonspecific because alkaline phosphatase is normally elevated in the third trimester. The blood sugar is often low, and profound hypoglycemia may occur.

Diagnosis

If the history, physical findings, and laboratory tests are consistent with AFLP, a liver biopsy should be performed as soon as possible and a fresh-frozen specimen taken for special fat stains. The finding of microvesicular fat is diagnostic of acute fatty liver of pregnancy. Treatment should begin immediately. If a liver biopsy cannot be performed safely, a presumptive diagnosis of AFLP may be made and treatment begun. Delay may endanger the life of the mother and child. Among the other causes of hepatic dysfunction in the third trimester of pregnancy, fulminant hepatitis most often poses a problem in the differential diagnosis. Liver disease may be present in preeclampsia (see below). However, jaundice is rare and the aminotransferases are minimally elevated unless the preeclampsia is severe, at which time they may reach 300 IU. Signs of liver failure are usually absent. Viral hepatitis is probably the most common cause of hepatic dysfunction in pregnancy, but is not usually associated with liver failure, disseminated intravascular coagulation, or signs of preeclampsia. Tetracycline hepatotoxicity can be diagnosed by the patient's history.

Fulminant hepatitis may be difficult to distinguish from AFLP, as both may present abruptly and rapidly progress to hepatic failure. Fulminant viral hepatitis, however, is usually associated with higher elevations of the serum aminotransferases, usually greater than 1000 IU, whereas these values are usually less than 500 in AFLP. Signs of preeclampsia, hypertension, and peripheral edema are common in AFLP and unusual in fulminant hepatitis. Elevated white blood counts and platelet counts below 100,000 are uncommon in fulminant hepatitis and occur in more than 80% of patients with AFLP. Percutaneous liver biopsy will clearly distinguish between these two entities but is often impossible because of the accompanying coagulopathy.

Treatment

Once the diagnosis of AFLP has been made or is strongly suggested, the pregnancy should be terminated as rapidly as possible. Patients with this condition may deteriorate suddenly, with danger to both fetus and mother. The disorder occurs so close to term that delivery does not endanger the baby. In addition, liver function usually improves in the mother after delivery. Blood sugar, hematocrit, platelet counts, prothrombin time, partial thromboplastin time, and mental status should be monitored closely before and after delivery. Any abnormalities should be corrected with intravenous administration of glucose, red blood cells, platelets, or fresh-frozen plasma. Hepatic encephalopathy should be treated as outlined in Chapter 56. Liver function is usually normal in babies born of mothers with AFLP; however, fetal hypoglycemia may occur and must be corrected with intravenous glucose. There have been no recurrences of AFLP in 12 women known to have had subsequent pregnancies.

Prognosis

Both fetal and maternal mortality have fallen dramatically since the late 1970s, from 85% to 23% and 18%, respectively. It is impossible to know whether this improvement represents a true response to early delivery and supportive therapy or merely reflects the recognition of milder forms of this disease.

LIVER DISEASE IN TOXEMIA OF PREGNANCY AND HELLP SYNDROME

Several other liver diseases are found only in pregnant women. In mild preeclampsia, 25% of women will have elevated serum levels of the aminotransferases. The pathologic process is thought to begin with vasospasm and result in localized areas of ischemia, fibrin deposition in small arterioles, and disseminated intravascular coagulation. The likelihood of aminotransferase elevations increases with the severity of the toxemia. The most dramatic hepatic complication of toxemia is frank rupture of the liver. The typical presentation of this rare complication is toxemia, right upper quadrant pain, and unexplained shock without overt blood loss. The treatment in patients who survive the initial rupture is hemodynamic support, blood replacement, and prompt delivery. Surgical repair of a ruptured Glisson's capsule is usually required.

The HELLP syndrome (hemolysis, elevated liver function tests, and low platelets) is thought to be a less severe complication of toxemia. Approximately 10% of women with severe toxemia have HELLP syndrome. There are usually signs of disseminated intravascular coagulation; aminotransferase levels may range from 300 to 4000 IU and bilirubin levels up to 5 mg/dl. Prognosis is related to the severity of the toxemia and accompanying liver disease. Treatment is directed at the toxemia. Early delivery will prevent serious complications.

REFERENCES

Bassett ML et al: Value of hepatic iron measurements in early hemochromatosis and determination of the critical iron level associated with fibrosis. Hepatology 6:24, 1986.

Brady RO: Glucosyl ceramide lipidosis: Gaucher's disease. In Stanbury JB et al: editors: The metabolic basis of inherited disease, ed 4, New York, 1978, McGraw-Hill.

Brewer GJ et al: Oral zinc therapy for Wilson's disease, Ann Intern Med 99:314, 1983.

Cohen A, Witzleben C, and Schwartz E: Treatment of iron overload, Semin Liver Dis 4:228, 1984.

Eriksson S et al: Risk of cirrhosis and primary liver cancer in alpha-1 antitrypsin deficiency. N Engl J Med 314:736, 1986.

Howell RR: The glycogen storage diseases. In Stanbury JB et al, editors: The metabolic basis of inherited disease, ed 4, New York, 1978, McGraw-Hill.

Kaplan MM: Liver dysfunction in the patient with congestive heart failure, Pract Cardiol 6:39, 1980.

Kaplan MM: Metabolic bone disease associated with gastrointestinal diseases, Viewpoints Dig Dis 1:9, 1983.

Kaplan MM: Primary biliary cirrhosis, N Engl J Med 316:521, 1987.

Kaplan MM et al: A prospective trial of colchicine for primary biliary cirrhosis, N Engl J Med 315:1448, 1986.

Kaplan MM and Knox TA: Treatment of primary biliary cirrhosis with low-dose weekly methotrexate, Gastroenterology 101:1332, 1991.

Kerr DNS, Okonkwo S, and Choa RG: Congenital hepatic fibrosis: the long-term prognosis, Gut 19:514, 1978.

Knox TA and Kaplan MM: Pregnancy and liver disease. In Taylor MB, editor: Gastrointestinal emergencies, Baltimore, 1992, Williams & Wilkins.

Kyle RA and Bayrd E: Amyloidosis. Review of 236 cases, Medicine (Baltimore) 54:271, 1975.

Mosse JO: Alpha-1 antitrypsin deficiency, N Engl J Med 299:1045, 1978.

Ong GB: Helminthic diseases of the liver and biliary tract. In Wright R et al editors: Liver and biliary disease, Philadelphia, 1979, WB Saunders.

Parker RI et al: Hematologic improvement in a patient with Gaucher disease on long-term enzyme replacement therapy: evidence for decreased splenic sequestration and improved red blood cell survival, Am J Hematol 38:130, 1991.

Pearson RD and Guerrant RL: Praziquantel: a major advance in anthelminthic therapy, Ann Intern Med 99:195, 1983.

Poupon RE et al: A multi-center, controlled trial of ursodiol for the treatment of primary biliary cirrhosis, N Engl J Med 324:1548, 1991.

Powell LW and Halliday JW: The liver and iron storage disorders. In Powell LW, editor: Metals and the liver, New York, Dekker.

Scheinberg IH et al: The use of trientine in preventing the effects of interrupting penicillamine therapy in Wilson's disease, N Engl J Med 317:209, 1987.

Simon HB and Wolff SM: Granulomatous hepatitis and prolonged fever of unknown origin: a study of 13 patients, Medicine (Baltimore) 52:1, 1973.

Walshe JM: Copper: its role in the pathogenesis of liver disease, Semin Liver Dis 4:252, 1984.

CHAPTER

61 Hepatic Veno-Occlusive Diseases

Stephen C. Hauser

Veno-occlusive diseases of the liver may involve either the portal venous system *(portal vein obstruction),* or the hepatic veins. Hepatic venous obstruction is subdivided on the basis of topographic and etiologic differences into the *Budd-Chiari syndrome,* which affects one or more of the major hepatic veins and/or the inferior vena cava and *veno-occlusive disease,* which involves microscopic centrilobular and small sublobular veins within the liver.

BUDD-CHIARI SYNDROME

Budd-Chiari syndrome is the result of an occlusive process, usually thrombotic, involving one or more of the three major hepatic veins (right, middle, and left), with or without extension of thrombus into the inferior vena cava. Moreover, any condition involving the inferior vena cava itself at or above the entrance of the hepatic veins, such as a web or tumor, also can produce the Budd-Chiari syndrome. Although severe right-sided congestive heart failure and constrictive pericarditis may present with a clinical picture similar to that of Budd-Chiari syndrome, a careful physical examination that includes evaluation of the jugular venous pulse should clarify the diagnosis.

Excluding webs, which most often occur in patients from the Orient and South Africa, an underlying disorder can be identified in approximately 70% of patients with the Budd-Chiari syndrome. Nearly 20% of patients are women who have been on oral contraceptives, are pregnant, or have recently delivered a child. It is likely that the hypercoagulable state present in each of these conditions is responsible for the hepatic vein thrombosis. Another 20% of patients with Budd-Chiari syndrome are found to have hematologic conditions characterized by hypercoagulable states, including myeloproliferative syndromes (polycythemia rubra vera, paroxysmal nocturnal hemoglobinuria), deficiencies of antithrombotic factors (antithrombin III, protein C, protein S), and the presence of circulating antiphospholipid antibodies. Other conditions associated with the Budd-Chiari syndrome include trauma to the liver, infections (bacterial, amebic or fungal abscess), malignant tumors (especially hepatoma), and other space-occupying lesions (adenomas, cysts). Many patients with so-called "idiopathic" Budd-Chiari syndrome eventually are found to have an occult myeloproliferative syndrome.

Budd-Chiari syndrome often presents as an insidious, chronic illness with nonspecific symptoms such as anorexia, nausea, vomiting, and generalized wasting. The three cardinal findings that suggest the diagnosis are *abdominal pain, hepatomegaly,* and *ascites*. The latter two findings eventually occur in nearly all cases. Some patients will develop splenomegaly, venous collaterals, and pedal edema. Large collaterals on the back suggest occlusion of the inferior vena cava. Symptoms and signs of cirrhosis are found in the late, preterminal stages of the disease. A few patients present with an acute illness mimicking fulminant hepatitis. In most cases, liver function test results are mildly elevated and are of little diagnostic value. The ascitic fluid may be either a transudate or an exudate. The usual natural history of untreated Budd-Chiari syndrome is one of gradual deterioration complicated by hepatic failure over a period of months to years. Given the nonspecific features of the illness, its insidious onset, and the lack of diagnostic value of standard laboratory tests, a high index of suspicion is prudent in patients with unexplained hepatomegaly, abdominal pain, and ascites.

Four noninvasive tests at present are useful in establishing the diagnosis of the Budd-Chiari syndrome: the liver-spleen scan, computed tomography (CT) with rapid intravenous contrast administration, real-time ultrasound with pulsed Doppler, and magnetic resonance imaging (MRI). Nearly half of the patients will have a peculiar central accumulation of colloid on the liver-spleen scan, due to caudate lobe hypertrophy (small veins that drain the caudate lobe directly into the inferior vena cava may be spared from thrombosis). Focal lesions such as hepatoma can be seen with the last three noninvasive tests mentioned. MRI and ultrasound are the more useful of the noninvasive tests because they do not require intravenous contrast and are readily able to demonstrate the presence or absence of flow in the hepatic veins and inferior vena cava. A liver biopsy of an affected area will demonstrate typical findings, including centrilobular congestion, sinusoidal dilatation, and atrophy of hepatocytes. Hepatic venography and visceral angiography are important to localize the precise areas involved by the thrombotic process and may help to elucidate the etiology. Whether the inferior vena cava, portal vein, or other adjacent structures are involved is critical in considering possible surgical treatment.

Treatment of the Budd-Chiari syndrome depends on the anatomic location and extent of the thrombotic process and the etiology. Predisposing conditions, such as polycythemia, should be treated, and oral contraceptives avoided. Antithrombotic treatment (heparin, warfarin, thrombolytic agents) has been of limited use. It is likely that by the time the diagnosis is made, the thrombotic process is well established. Medical treatment of ascites (Chapter 56) or the performance of a LeVeen shunt may diminish the ascites but will not ameliorate the detrimental effects of hepatic venous obstruction on the liver. In the rare case of a membranous web, balloon membranotomy (angioplasty) or surgical resection or bypass may eliminate the obstruction. In many cases, the surgical creation of a portosystemic shunt to decompress the liver will greatly benefit the patient. If the inferior vena cava is involved, grafts can be constructed from the portal-mesenteric system to the right atrium. In the future, transjugular intrahepatic portosystemic shunts (TIPS) may prove useful. Liver transplantation has been successfully performed in selected cases (Chapter 64).

VENO-OCCLUSIVE DISEASE

Veno-occlusive disease (VOD) is a nonthrombotic, fibrotic process that occludes and obliterates centrilobular and small sublobular veins in the liver. VOD occurs as a result of toxic injury secondary to pyrrolizidine plant alkaloids (i.e., herbal and "bush" teas derived from *Senecio, Crotolaria,* and *Heliotropium* genera), high-dose hepatic irradiation, and a number of chemotherapeutic and immunosuppressive agents (i.e., cyclophosphamide, cytosine arabinoside, azathioprine). VOD is most commonly a problem in patients given total body irradiation and/or high doses of cytotoxic agents in preparation for bone marrow transplantation. Hepatitis before transplantation, age greater than 15, and an underlying malignancy other than acute lymphocytic leukemia increase the risk for VOD, which overall is approximately 20%. Much like Budd-Chiari syndrome, VOD presents clinically with abdominal pain, hepatomegaly, and ascites. Posttransplant VOD usually occurs 1 to 3 weeks after the graft. Weight gain may be an early sign of impending VOD. Eventually, most patients develop jaundice. Serum transaminase and alkaline phosphatase levels may be normal or greatly elevated. VOD in post-transplant patients often pursues a rapid downhill course, with mortality rates of up to 50%, although many patients appear to have a mild illness and recover completely. A liver biopsy often will confirm the clinical diagnosis, demonstrating centrilobular congestion and hepatocellular necrosis as well as typical subendothelial fibrotic occlusion of central veins. Viral and fungal hepatitis, cholestatic hepatitis caused by drugs or parenteral nutrition, and unrecognized sepsis are the most important differential diagnoses to consider. Graft-versus-host disease usually occurs later. Unfortunately, no beneficial treatment has yet been found.

PORTAL VEIN OBSTRUCTION

Obstruction of the portal vein may occur at any point along its course, including small venous branches within the liver. Splenic and mesenteric veins also may be involved. In most cases of extrahepatic portal vein obstruction, collaterals bypass the occluded site, resulting in so-called cavernous transformation of the portal vein. Thrombosis of the extrahepatic portal vein may occur secondary to trauma (including surgical procedures in the upper abdomen), neoplasm, infection, inflammation, and thrombotic disorders. In neonates, umbilical sepsis may be a precipitating factor, although some cases may be congenital. Portal vein obstruction caused by cirrhosis, especially in the Orient, and occult myeloproliferative disorders, are being recognized more frequently. Overall, the etiology of extrahepatic portal vein obstruction remains unknown in up to half the cases. Noncirrhotic obstruction of small intrahepatic portal venous radicules may occur secondary to toxins such as arsenic, copper, vinyl chloride monomer, and cytotoxic drugs; or it may be idiopathic.

Acute obstruction of the portal vein may initially be accompanied by ascites, but this usually disappears or is minimal. Liver function test results in noncirrhotics usually remain normal. However, portal hypertension with varices, which may or may not bleed, is common. Children with varices may have bleeding episodes, especially around puberty, but the frequency of variceal hemorrhage often declines after puberty.

Angiography is crucial to identify the exact location and extent of the obstruction. Noninvasive tests such as real-time ultrasound with pulsed Doppler and magnetic resonance angiography also are useful. The presence of cirrhosis can be excluded by liver biopsy. Intrahepatic portal venous obstruction involving small venous radicules may be difficult to appreciate by angiography and in some cases even in percutaneous liver biopsy specimens. Treatment includes identification of the cause, endoscopic sclerotherapy for bleeding varices, and, in those few patients who continue to bleed from varices despite sclerotherapy, shunt surgery. Hypersplenism with thrombocytopenia, anemia, or pain rarely requires surgery.

REFERENCES

Bolondi L et al: Diagnosis of Budd-Chiari syndrome by pulsed Doppler ultrasound, Gastroenterology 100:1324, 1991.

Cohen J, Edelman RR, and Chopra S: Portal vein thrombosis: a review, Am J Med 92:173, 1992.

Gupta S et al: Comparison of ultrasonography, computed tomography and ^{99m}Tc liver scan in diagnosis of Budd-Chiari syndrome, Gut 28:242, 1987.

Lewis J, Tice HL, and Zimmerman HJ: Budd-Chiari syndrome associated with oral contraceptive steroids: review of treatment of 47 cases, Dig Dis Sci 28:673, 1983.

McDonald GB et al: The clinical course of 53 patients with veno-occlusive disease of the liver after marrow transplantation, Transplantation 39:603, 1985.

Mitchell MC et al: Budd-Chiari syndrome: etiology, diagnosis and management, Medicine 61:199, 1982.

Paglinca A et al: In vitro colony culture and chromosomal studies in hepatic and portal vein thrombosis—possible evidence of an occult myeloproliferative state, QJ Med 76:981, 1990.

Rollins BJ: Hepatic veno-occlusive disease, Am J Med 81:297, 1986.

Sparano J et al: Treatment of the Budd-Chiari syndrome with percutaneous transluminal angioplasty. Case report and review of the literature, Am J Med 82:821, 1987.

Triger DR: Extrahepatic portal venous obstruction (Editorial), Gut 28:1193, 1987.

CHAPTER

62 Liver Abscesses and Cysts

Sanjiv Chopra

LIVER ABSCESSES

Amebic liver abscess

Entamoeba histolytica is the only proved pathogen among the six species of amebas inhabiting the human colon. At increased risk for infection are persons living in custodial institutions, travelers, or immigrants from areas of the world with endemic amebiasis, and homosexuals. The hepatic manifestations (see also Chapter 280) include nonspecific hepatomegaly and amebic liver abscess. The nonspecific hepatomegaly is mild to moderate, is accompanied by tenderness, and occurs in the setting of apparent intestinal infection. This toxic response on the part of the liver is nonspecific; liver scans and biopsy findings indicate normalcy, and hepatic manifestations resolve after eradication of the intestinal infection.

Liver abscess, the most common extraintestinal complication of infection with *E. histolytica,* is observed in only 2% to 5% of patients with intestinal amebiasis. An abscess may occur months or years after the onset of intestinal infection, and in 50% of patients there is no history of diarrhea. Abscesses range in size from small to massive ($>$ 5 liters), are single or multiple, and occur more often in young and middle-aged men. Ninety percent are located in the right lobe. They can present as an acute inflammatory process or as a chronic indolent disorder with fever of unknown origin, suggesting malignancy as the probable etiology. Symptoms and signs include mild to severe right upper quadrant pain accompanied by fever. The pain is often pleuritic and referred to the right shoulder. Chills and night sweats are occasionally prominent and, with the pleuritic chest pain and nonproductive cough, may suggest primary pulmonary pathology. This constellation should suggest liver pathology but is not specific and may occur with pyogenic or amebic liver abscesses, necrotic hepatic tumors, or infected hepatic cysts.

Anemia, leukocytosis ($> 20{,}000/mm^3$ in 50% of patients) without eosinophilia, and hypoalbuminemia are common. The bilirubin level is elevated in 50% of patients, but values exceeding 10 mg/dl are unusual. Serum transaminases are elevated twofold to fourfold in 50% of patients, and similar range elevations in serum alkaline phosphatase are noted in 80% of patients. Clinical evidence of coexistent intestinal disease is uncommon, and amebas are recovered from the stool in only 15%. In contrast, serologic test results (indirect hemagglutination and/or gel diffusion precipitin) are positive in 95% of patients. Chest films show abnormalities in about 65% of patients and show elevation of the right hemidiaphragm, right lower lobe infiltrates, and a right pleural effusion. Hepatic scintiscanning with ^{99m}Tc sulfur colloid reveals focal cold lesions in more than 95% of patients, and gallium scanning may show increased uptake at the periphery of the defect. Ultrasonography is useful in detecting hepatic abscesses; however, a distinction between an amebic and pyogenic abscess cannot be made accurately on sonographic findings alone. There is evidence that ultrasonography, computed tomography (CT), and magnetic resonance imaging (MRI) are comparably effective in the detection of amebic liver abscess. Aspiration of abscess contents may reveal the characteristic chocolate-like or "anchovy-sauce" fluid. More important, the abscess content is not foul smelling, bacterial cultures are negative, and trophozoites are recovered in 20% to 50% of patients. Aspiration, ideally under ultrasound guidance, is indicated in the following situations: No clinical improvement within 72 to 96 hours, left lobe abscesses, abscesses greater than 10 cm in diameter, abscesses associated with severe pain or marked tenderness, and abscesses associated with negative serologic tests.

Complications include rupture into the pleural space, lung, pericardium, bowel, retroperitoneum, or skin. Bacterial superinfection, usually with enteric organisms, can occur spontaneously or after a drainage procedure and carries a poor prognosis. Very rarely, fulminant hepatic failure results as a consequence of massive hepatic parenchymal destruction accompanied by portal vein and hepatic vein occlusion. Treatment with metronidazole, 750 mg orally three times a day for 10 days followed by iodoquinol, 650 mg orally three times a day for 20 days, is usually effective. Alternatively, dehydroemetine followed by chloroquine phosphate and iodoquinol may be used (Table 62-1). Defervescence occurs rapidly, and 90% of patients are afebrile after a week of appropriate treatment. In the absence of serologic confirmation or diagnostic aspiration, caution should be exercised in interpreting the therapeutic response to metronidazole or chloroquine as being of diagnostic value. Metronidazole is effective against many anaerobes, and chloroquine is an antipyretic; and hence patients with pyogenic liver abscess or other intra-abdominal infections may respond favorably to these agents.

Pyogenic liver abscess

Pyogenic liver abscess, although more common in the United States than amebic abscess, is rare, with a reported autopsy incidence of less than 1%. In the past, it was highly prevalent in infants, children, and young adults, occurring as a sequel to umbilical sepsis and appendicitis. Early recognition and treatment of these disorders have resulted in a decline in the incidence of pyelophlebitis and subsequent liver abscess formation, so that pyogenic liver abscess is now seen predominantly in the middle-aged and elderly. A variety of clinical conditions are associated with the occurrence of pyogenic liver abscess (refer to box at right).

A principal source of infection is biliary tract obstruction due to gallstones or carcinoma of the pancreas or bile ducts. Biliary tract obstruction can result in either macroscopic or microscopic abscess formation. Other causes of macroscopic liver abscess formation include direct extension of infection from a contiguous site and nonpenetrating

Table 62-1. Chemotherapy of amebic liver abscess

Drug	Dosage	Comments
• Metronidazole or Tinidazole* followed by	750 mg po tid × 10 days	Tissue and luminal amebicide. Efficacy: > 90%. Side effects minor: metallic taste, nausea, disulfiram-like effect, rarely reversible neutropenia, ataxia, peripheral neuropathy
Iodoquinol	650 mg po tid × 20 days	Effective against luminal cysts. Side effects: rash, thyromegaly, optic atrophy
• Dehydroemetine followed by	1.0 to 1.5 mg/kg/day (maximum 90 mg/day) IM for 5 days	Tissue and luminal amebicide. Cardiotoxicity requires prudent use and close monitoring. Available from CDC Drug Service. Contraindicated in pregnancy
Chloroquine phosphate plus	1 g po daily × 2 days, then 500 mg po daily × 2-3 weeks	Tissue amebicide; not a luminal amebicide. Efficacy: 90%. Side effects significant: headache, incoordination, seizures, ECG changes, retinopathy
Iodoquinol	650 mg po tid × 20 days	See comment for Iodoquinol (above)

*A nitroimidazole similar to metronidazole but not marketed in the United States.

Pyogenic liver abscess: etiologic considerations and routes of infection

I. Biliary tract obstruction (40%)
  A. Benign (stone, stricture)
  B. Malignant
II. Hematogenous infection (30%)
  A. Infection via portal vein
    1. Diverticulitis
    2. Appendicitis
    3. Omphalitis
    4. Inflammatory disease of pancreas, spleen
  B. Infection via hepatic artery (bacteremia or septicemia from any cause)
III. Primary hepatic lesions (20%)
  A. Trauma (blunt abdominal trauma, penetrating liver injuries)
  B. Secondary bacterial infection of amebic abscess, cyst, or malignant lesion
IV. Cryptogenic infection (10%)

blunt abdominal trauma. Approximately 20% of pyogenic liver abscesses occur in patients with systemic bacteremia, who often develop microabscesses. Approximately 10% of all macroabscesses follow blunt trauma.

In older series, aerobic organisms were the major isolates from hepatic abscesses. With the advent of modern bacteriologic techniques, anaerobes have been isolated from up to 45% of pyogenic liver abscesses. Coliform bacteria and streptococci are seen in the majority and are most common in patients with biliary tract disease. Anaerobes are more common in cryptogenic infections and in those seeded via the portal system. *Staphylococcus aureus* and group A streptococci are seen in the setting of septicemia. In one study the organism most often recovered was *Streptococcus milleri*. *S. milleri* is a fastidious organism that grows well only in a carbon dioxide-enriched medium. Its presence in the blood of a febrile patient should alert the clinician to the possibility of an underlying liver abscess.

Patients present with a febrile illness of several days' to several months' duration. The duration of illness is generally shorter for patients with microabscesses than for patients with large abscesses. Fever is often associated with malaise, anorexia, and weight loss. Right upper quadrant pain is common, and patients with underlying biliary tract disease may have nausea and vomiting. Cough, pleuritic chest pain, dyspnea, and even hemoptysis may incorrectly suggest primary intrathoracic pathology. Tender hepatomegaly is present in only 50% of patients. Jaundice is seen in about 30% of patients, usually in those with multiple abscesses or biliary tract obstruction. Important complications include subphrenic abscess formation; rupture into the lung, pericardium, or peritoneal cavity; and hemobilia. Complications develop in 10% to 20% of patients.

Laboratory findings include anemia, leukocytosis, elevation of the sedimentation rate, and hypoalbuminemia. Serum alkaline phosphatase is elevated in over 90% of patients, whereas serum bilirubin is elevated above 2 mg/dl in 50%. Serologic tests are mandatory to exclude amebiasis in all patients with recognized liver abscess. Blood cultures are positive in 40% to 60% if obtained on several occasions and carefully cultured for aerobic and anaerobic organisms. Needle aspirates of the abscess should undergo Gram stain and culture. Microorganisms are recovered from the aspirated material in 80% of patients. X-ray abnormalities are evident in 50% of patients and include elevation or distortion of the right hemidiaphragm, basilar atelectasis, and right pleural effusion. Rarely, a gas-filled abscess with an air-fluid level is seen on a chest or abdominal film.

Scintiscanning reveals space-occupying lesions in about 90% of patients; simultaneous ^{111}In-labeled white blood cell scans and sulfur colloid scans may help differentiate abscess from tumor. Ultrasonography will enable the physician to identify most abscesses 2 cm or more in diameter as anechoic lesions (Fig. 62-1). CT can provide accurate anatomic localization and aid in percutaneous needle aspiration. MRI is also useful. Angiographic features include focal avascu-

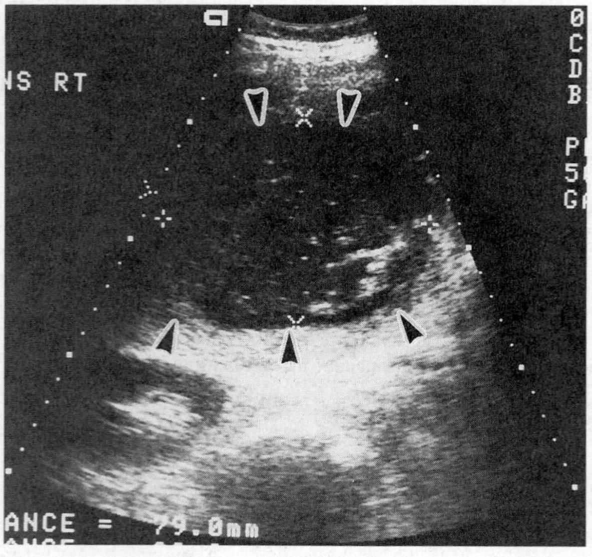

Fig. 62-1. Ultrasound reveals an 8 cm mass in the liver *(arrowheads),* with complex echogenic signals (debris) in a patient with pyogenic abscess. (Courtesy of Vassilios Raptopoulos, MD.)

lar masses with vessel displacement and a hypervascular periphery.

The principles of treatment include prompt drainage and effective broad-spectrum antibiotic therapy directed against both aerobic and anaerobic organisms. Antibiotics should be used for 4 to 8 weeks in patients with a solitary abscess and for 8 to 16 weeks in patients with multiple abscesses. Initial antibiotic therapy should include the use of a penicillin, an aminoglycoside, and either clindamycin or metronidazole. After blood and abscess culture results are available, antibiotic therapy can be adjusted accordingly. In the past, traditional therapy has consisted of surgical drainage of the abscess coupled with prolonged antimicrobial therapy. In recent years, the approach to treatment of pyogenic abscess has changed considerably. Although more than 60 patients have been successfully treated with antibiotics without drainage, it seems prudent to institute some form of drainage except under special circumstances, such as multiple small abscesses not amenable to drainage or a very favorable response to antibiotics given before the diagnosis of a pyogenic abscess has been established. A substantial number of patients have been successfully treated with percutaneous closed-catheter drainage of abscesses under ultrasonographic or CT guidance. Since percutaneous catheter drainage seems quite efficacious and is associated with a relatively low morbidity, this modality of treatment is currently favored over surgical drainage in patients who do not require laparotomy for other reasons. Complications of percutaneous catheter drainage include puncture of a viscus, septicemia, hemorrhage, and catheter displacement. Surgical drainage is clearly indicated in most patients in whom the hepatic abscess is secondary to biliary obstruction, a ruptured appendix, or any other intra-abdominal condition that merits surgical intervention.

In two studies published in 1984, with a total aggregate of 93 patients, the mortality rate was 25%. Poor prognostic factors include old age, severity of the underlying illness, hyperbilirubinemia, and hypoalbuminemia. In another study the overall mortality was 15% in patients with single abscesses and 41% in those with multiple abscesses.

HEPATIC CYSTS

The classification of hepatic cysts, which may be congenital or acquired, is shown in the box below.

Solitary cysts

Solitary cysts of the liver are most often unilocular and present in the right lobe. They may contain a few milliliters or more than a liter of fluid. Most cause no symptoms and are discovered incidentally at the time of diagnostic imaging or laparotomy performed for other reasons or autopsy. Among patients with symptoms, the most common complaints are vague abdominal discomfort, nausea, and vomiting. Hemorrhage, infection, strangulation, or rupture are rare complications. Treatment is indicated in patients with complications such as pain, infection, or hemorrhage into the cyst and consists of aspiration of the cyst and surgical excision or drainage into a jejunal loop.

Polycystic liver disease

Polycystic liver disease is characterized by the presence of a few to innumerable cysts ranging in size from a few millimeters to over 15 cm in diameter. Fifty percent of such patients have renal cysts (Chapter 358), and cystic lesions in the pancreas, lung, spleen, and other organs may be present, albeit rarely. Intracerebral aneurysms occur in 5% to 10% of patients with polycystic liver disease.

Hepatic parenchymal cysts appear to arise by gradual cystic dilatation of clusters of small intrahepatic ducts that

Classification of hepatic cysts

- I. Congenital hepatic cysts
  - A. Parenchymal cysts
    - 1. Solitary cyst
    - 2. Polycystic disease
  - B. Ductal cysts
    - 1. Localized dilatation
    - 2. Multiple cystic dilatations of intrahepatic ducts (Caroli's disease)
- II. Acquired hepatic cysts
  - A. Inflammatory cysts
    - 1. Retention cyst
    - 2. Echinococcal cyst
  - B. Neoplastic cyst
  - C. Peliosis hepatis

failed to involute during embryologic development of the liver.

Most patients with polycystic liver disease are asymptomatic, and their disease is diagnosed incidentally at laparotomy or because renal disease is recognized. Occasionally, abdominal discomfort is present because of stretching of the liver capsule. Fever may result from infection, hemorrhage into a cyst, or rupture of a cyst. Rare complications include jaundice due to compression of bile ducts by a large cyst and portal hypertension due to compression of the portal vein by enlarging cysts.

Liver function test results are generally normal. Liver scanning reveals multiple defects, the cystic nature of which can be documented by ultrasonography or CT (Fig. 62-2).

No treatment is required in most instances. Aspiration of large cysts may be required in the patient with troublesome complaints. Rarely, surgical decompression of portal hypertension may be necessary to control bleeding esophageal varices.

Echinococcal cyst

Echinococcal cyst is a common hepatic disorder in Kenya, Greece, France, Australia, and South America. In the United States, it is rare and occurs predominantly in immigrants from areas where the disorder is endemic. However, autochthonously acquired cases have been documented in California, Utah, and several other states. Two species of this cestode, *Echinococcus granulosus* and *Echinococcus multilocularis,* with human beings as the intermediate hosts, have been recognized (Chapter 358). Approximately 60% of patients have hepatic involvement and 20% have pulmonary involvement. The latent period can be many years, permitting the hydatid cysts to enlarge slowly before symptoms occur or a hepatic mass is detected.

In the liver, the hydatid cyst of *E. granulosus* is usually solitary, is located in the right lobe, and causes no symptoms. In contrast, the hydatid cyst of *E. multilocularis* is characterized by a germinal membrane that permits formation of new cysts on its outer surface. The developing scolices invade adjacent tissue as an infiltrative process and, on occasion, extend into blood vessels and metastasize to distant sites. A few patients present with abdominal pain or an abdominal mass. Complications include rupture (intrabiliary, intraperitoneal, and transdiaphragmatic), secondary bacterial infection, and allergic manifestations (urticaria and anaphylactic shock).

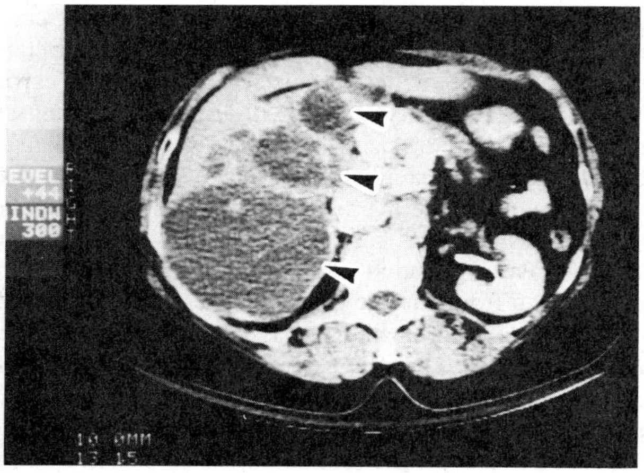

Fig. 62-2. Polycystic liver disease. Computed tomography with contrast enhancement showing several low-density lesions *(arrowheads).* (Courtesy of Joseph C. Sequeira, MD.)

The diagnosis is occasionally made incidentally at the time of laparotomy. Intrahepatic calcification is noted in over 50% of patients but is not specific. Eosinophilia is often present in patients with ruptured cysts but is otherwise inconstant. Casoni's skin test has limited utility because false-positive results are frequent, but the indirect hemagglutination and complement-fixation tests are positive in 90% of patients with hepatic involvement and are useful. Portable ultrasonography is being increasingly used in screening for hydatid cysts in nomadic populations with very high prevalence rates. Liver biopsy is contraindicated. Aspiration of the cyst has also been traditionally viewed as an absolute contraindication because leakage from the cyst may result in dissemination of daughter scolices and in fatal anaphylaxis. In recent years, however, this view has been challenged by some authors (see later).

In the past, surgery has been the only effective therapeutic approach. Small cysts should be enucleated, whereas large cysts should be extracted through a cryogenic cone device. Enucleation should be followed by instillation of silver nitrate or hypertonic saline solution into the residual exocyst space. Surgical mortality is less than 5%. Drugs being used for the treatment of echinococcal disease include mebendazole, albendazole, and praziquantel. Large control studies are needed to assess the optimal dosage, efficacy, and safety of these agents for echinococcal disease. Aspiration of hydatid cysts under ultrasound guidance and irrigation of the cyst cavity with 95% ethanol or hypertonic saline have been reported in a few recent series of small numbers of patients. There was a reduction in the size of cysts, and no major complications were noted. This modality of treatment may prove suitable for patients who refuse surgery or cannot undergo surgery.

Peliosis hepatis

Peliosis hepatis is characterized by the presence of blood-filled cystic lesions in the liver. A causal link to treatment with androgenic-anabolic steroids and oral contraceptives has been established. The duration of such treatment may be a few months or several years. Some patients are asymptomatic, and liver involvement is signaled by hepatomegaly or abnormal liver function. Progressive hepatic failure, with jaundice, impaired synthetic function, and encephalopathy can dominate the clinical picture, especially when the disorder is associated with androgenic-anabolic steroid administration. Fatalities have also occurred occasionally after spontaneous rupture of a subcapsular cyst with exsanguinating intra-abdominal hemorrhage. Liver scintiscanning reveals hepatomegaly or hepatosplenomegaly, with either discrete filling defects or patchy uptake of colloid in the liver. Percutaneous liver biopsy is often diagnostic but is potentially hazardous because of the vascular nature of the lesions. No specific treatment is available. Discontinuation of hormonal therapy is indicated and may result in complete regression of the peliotic lesions.

Both cutaneous bacillary angiomatosis and bacillary peliosis hepatitis have been reported in patients with HIV infection. The agent is likely a Rickettsia-like organism closely related to *R. quintana*. Patients may respond favorably to erythromycin.

REFERENCES

Acunas B et al: Purely cystic hydatid disease of the liver: treatment with percutaneous aspiration and injection of hypertonic saline, Radiology 182:541, 1992.

Anonymous: Man, dogs and hydatid disease, Lancet 1:21, 1987.

Barnes PF et al: A comparison of amebic and pyogenic abscess of the liver, Medicine 66:472, 1987.

Berger LA and Osborne DR: Treatment of pyogenic liver abscess by percutaneous needle aspiration, Lancet 1:132, 1982.

Chopra S et al: Peliosis hepatis in hematologic disease, JAMA 240:1153, 1978.

Davidson RA: Issues in clinical parasitology: the management of hydatid cyst, Am J Gastroenterol 79:397, 1984.

DelGuercio E et al: Esophageal varices in adult patients with polycystic kidney and liver disease, N Engl J Med 289:678, 1973.

Gibney EJ: Aemebic liver abscess, Br J Surg 77:843, 1990.

Greenstein AJ et al: Continuing changing patterns of disease in pyogenic liver abscess: a study of 38 patients, Am J Gastroenterol 79:217, 1984.

Halvorsen RA et al: The variable CT appearance of hepatic abscesses, Am J Roentgenol 141:941, 1984.

Kandel G and Marcon NE: Pyogenic liver abscesses: new concepts of an old disease, Am J Gastroenterol 79:65, 1984.

Macpherson CNL et al: Portable ultrasound scanner versus serology in screening for hydatid cysts in a nomadic population, Lancet 2:259, 1987.

McDonald MI et al: Single and multiple pyogenic liver abscesses. Natural history, diagnosis and treatment with emphasis on percutaneous drainage, Medicine (Baltimore) 63:291, 1984.

Milutinovic J et al: Liver cysts in patients with autosomal dominant polycystic kidney disease, Am J Med 68:741, 1980.

Perkocha LA et al: Clinical and pathological features of bacillary peliosis hepatitis in association with human immunodeficiency virus infection. N Eng J Med 323:1581, 1990.

Ralls PW et al: Amebic liver abscess: MR imaging, Radiology 165:801, 1987.

Reynolds TB: Medical treatment of pyogenic liver abscess, Ann Intern Med 96:373, 1982.

CHAPTER

63 Hepatic Tumors

Sanjiv Chopra

PRIMARY CARCINOMA OF THE LIVER

Incidence

The incidence of primary carcinoma of the liver (hepatocellular carcinoma, hepatoma) varies greatly in different parts of the world. It is relatively uncommon in the United States, accounting for less than 2.5% of all malignancies. In parts of Asia and Africa, it accounts for up to 50% of all malignancies. The tumor may arise from parenchymal cells (hepatocellular carcinoma), bile duct cells (cholangiocarcinomas), or from both cell types (mixed). The hepatocellular variety accounts for 80% to 90% of liver carcinomas.

Primary liver cancers occur 2 to 8 times more frequently in men than in women. Cirrhosis is present in 65% to 90% of autopsied patients with this tumor. Postnecrotic cirrhosis is most common, but patients with cirrhosis associated with alcoholic liver disease, hemochromatosis, or alpha$_1$ antitrypsin deficiency are also at increased risk of developing this tumor. Primary liver cancer is rare in patients with primary biliary cirrhosis, cardiac cirrhosis, and Wilson's disease, suggesting that factors other than cirrhosis are important in the pathogenesis of this tumor. Hepatocellular carcinoma occurs in 40% of children and teenagers with the chronic form of hereditary tyrosinemia. Incidence peaks in the fifth and sixth decades of life in the United States and Western Europe, but one to two decades earlier in parts of the world with a high prevalence of liver carcinoma.

Pathogenesis

An unequivocal association has been established between chronic hepatitis B virus infection and primary liver carcinoma. The incidence of primary liver carcinoma correlates with the presence of the chronic hepatitis B virus carrier state. Serologic markers of hepatitis B virus infection are more frequent in primary liver cancer patients than in matched controls. Familial clustering of hepatitis B virus infection and chronic liver disease in patients with hepatocellular carcinoma has been documented in Japan and Taiwan, and early infection with this virus, through vertical transmission from chronic carrier mothers, appears to play a critical role in the pathogenesis of hepatocellular carcinoma. The most compelling epidemiologic evidence linking hepatitis B virus infection and primary liver carcinoma is the observation of an apparent greater than 200-fold increased risk of this tumor in HBsAg-positive subjects compared with HBsAg-negative individuals in a prospective study of Chinese male civil servants in Taiwan. Studies have also described naturally occurring animal models of DNA virus infections (similar to chronic hepatitis B virus infections in humans), liver disease, and primary liver carcinoma. Examples include the eastern woodchuck, Peking duck, and ground squirrel. Virtually 100% of woodchucks raised in the laboratory develop primary hepatocellular carcinoma. Even in the United States, strikingly high prevalence rates of hepatitis B virus infection are present in patients with this tumor in the setting of nonalcoholic chronic liver disease. Direct oncogenicity of hepatitis B virus has not been established, but it has been shown that hepatitis B virus DNA is integrated into the genome of hepatocellular carcinoma cells of B virus carriers with hepatomas.

Recent studies have suggested that chronic hepatitis C virus infection is a risk factor for the development of primary liver carcinoma in many different parts of the world. Primary liver cancer has been documented to develop in follow-up studies of patients with chronic hepatitis C virus infection and in chimpanzees experimentally infected with hepatitis C virus. Hepatitis C virus antibody prevalence rates in patients with primary cancer of the liver have been reported to range from 28% among Italian patients to 53% in patients in Miami and approximately 75% in patients in Barcelona and Japan. So far, it appears that hepatocellular carcinoma in patients with chronic hepatitis C virus infection occurs only in those with underlying cirrhosis.

Mycotoxins, notably aflatoxins, are potent hepatocarcinogens in laboratory animals, including subhuman primates. Aflatoxins in high concentrations contaminate foods such as peanuts and corn in parts of Africa and Asia that have high prevalence rates of hepatocellular carcinoma. Recent studies suggest that aflatoxin may induce a specific G-T mutation at codon 249 of the p53 suppressor gene. Thorium dioxide (Thorotrast), used in the past as a radiologic contrast material, has been incriminated as a cause of hepatocellular carcinoma. This tumor has been reported in some patients on long-term androgen therapy. There have been a few reports of hepatocellular carcinoma in women taking oral contraceptives, but a cause-and-effect relationship has not been established. Other compounds implicated but not established as hepatocarcinogens include nitrosamines, azo compounds, *Senecio* alkaloids, and cycasin. Schistosomiasis and clonorchiasis may be important pathogenetic factors in parts of the world where these infestations are endemic.

Clinical features and diagnosis

Approximately one third of patients with primary liver carcinoma present with nonspecific symptoms of neoplasia such as malaise, weakness, anorexia, and weight loss. Another third have known cirrhosis and present with abdominal pain or deterioration of clinical status in the absence of known precipitating factors. Occasionally, patients present with signs of peritonitis caused by hemoperitoneum. Fever, abdominal pain, and jaundice may occur, simulating acute cholecystitis. Rare features include symptoms attributable to hepatic vein thrombosis (Chapter 61), fever of unknown origin, or one or more systemic manifestations associated with hepatocellular carcinoma such as hypoglycemia, polycythemia, hypercalcemia, porphyria, and dysglobulinemias. Hepatocellular carcinoma may present with symptomatic bone or pulmonary metastases. In about 10% of patients, the tumor is an incidental finding at the time of laparotomy or autopsy.

The liver is enlarged and often firm, nodular, and tender. A bruit or friction rub over the liver is suggestive of hepatocellular carcinoma. Ascites is present in approximately 50% of patients and often reflects preexisting portal hypertension. Exudative ascites or blood-tinged ascitic fluid suggests hepatic vein thrombosis or peritoneal metastases. Jaundice develops in less than 50% of patients and is an unusual presenting manifestation. Progressive jaundice is an ominous sign and suggests diminishing hepatic reserve or invasion of the bile ducts by tumor.

Anemia, leukocytosis, and elevations of serum transaminases, lactic dehydrogenase, and alkaline phosphatase are common laboratory findings. Alkaline phosphatase, 5′-nucleotidase, and gamma glutamyl transpeptidase are elevated in about 90% of patients, often disproportionately in relation to other liver function test results. Radiographs may reveal hepatomegaly, hepatic calcification, elevation or distortion of the right hemidiaphragm, right pleural effusion, or bone or lung metastases.

Ultrasonography is being increasingly used to screen high-risk populations and is probably the most useful and sensitive imaging modality for detecting very small tumors. Computed tomography (CT) reveals the extent of tumor and enables the physician to identify it in about 90% of patients (Fig. 63-1). Rapid sequential scanning after intravenous administration of contrast media may prove useful in determining patency of the portal vein or inferior vena cava. Ultrasonography and magnetic resonance imaging (MRI) can also provide valuable information about patency of these vessels (Fig. 63-2). The CT findings are not specific for hepatocellular carcinoma, and isodense lesions will be missed on examination. Celiac axis angiography reveals abnormalities such as enlargement of the hepatic arteries, neovascularity, arterio-

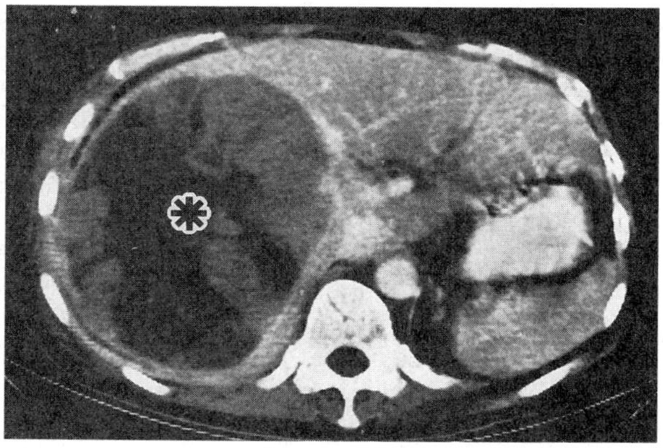

Fig. 63-1. CT scan showing a large well circumscribed mass *(*)* occupying the right lobe with irregular enhancement pattern in a patient with primary carcinoma of the liver. (Courtesy of Vassilios Raptopoulos, MD.)

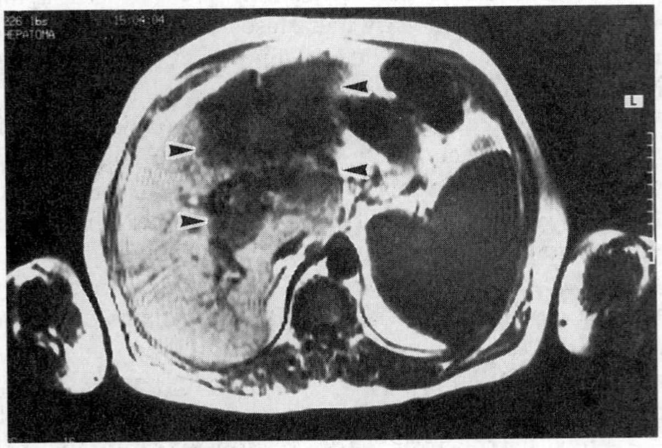

Fig. 63-2. MRI shows an irregular mass *(arrowheads)* with invasion of the portal vein on a T_1-weighted image in a patient with primary carcinoma of the liver. (Courtesy of Vassilios Raptopoulos, MD.)

venous shunting, and venous encasement in about 80% of patients. Differentiation of these abnormalities from vascular metastatic tumors, notably carcinoid, choriocarcinoma, and hypernephroma, as well as benign hepatic lesions such as focal nodular hyperplasia is not always possible. Angiography may be useful in defining the extent of tumor and delineating the anatomic blood supply in preparation for hepatic lobectomy. Liver scintiscanning with technetium-99m (^{99m}Tc) sulfur colloid may reveal discrete space-occupying lesions with decreased uptake of the isotope but does not enable the physician to distinguish between regenerating nodules in a chirrhotic liver and primary or metastatic malignancy. Gallium-67 (^{67}Ga) scans may show uptake of the isotope in primary hepatocellular carcinoma but not in regenerating nodules. However, hepatic abscesses and metastatic deposits in the liver may also show avidity for gallium.

Alpha fetoprotein, a unique alpha$_1$ globulin that is normally synthesized in large amounts by embryonic liver cells and in trace amounts by fetal yolk sac cells and the fetal gastrointestinal tract, is present in serum in high concentrations ($>$ 500 ng/ml by radioimmunoassay) in 70% of patients with hepatocellular carcinoma in the United States and in 85% of such patients in Africa and Japan. Highest concentrations are generally encountered in young patients and in those with poorly differentiated tumors. A proposed program for screening high-risk populations includes four to six monthly determinations of serum alpha fetoprotein together with ultrasonographic imaging of the liver. The utility of such a screening program has been challenged by some investigators, as it does not appear to appreciably increase the rate of detection of potentially curable tumors. Concentrations of alpha fetoprotein fall dramatically in patients in whom curative partial hepatectomy is carried out. Serial determinations aid in detecting early recurrence or in monitoring the response to chemotherapy. Patients with germ cell malignancies with yolk sac elements also may have high concentrations of serum alpha fetoprotein. Modest elevations are seen occasionally in association with gastrointestinal tumors, most often with metastatic spread to the liver, and transiently in up to 40% of patients with viral hepatitis. Levels up to 500 ng/ml are seen during pregnancy. Higher levels indicate fetal neural tube defects, fetal distress, fetal death, or multiple pregnancy.

Percutaneous needle biopsy of the liver is diagnostic in about 80% of patients. In patients with lesions in the left lobe of the liver, peritoneoscopy or laparotomy with open liver biopsy may be necessary. Peritoneoscopy may be useful for determining the extent of tumor and assessing resectability.

Prognosis and treatment

The usual clinical course of primary liver carcinoma is rapid deterioration and death. Average survival after diagnosis is 6 months. Common causes of death include cachexia, infection, hepatic failure, and gastrointestinal bleeding. Extrahepatic portal vein thrombosis is common and may aggravate portal hypertension, with resultant massive variceal bleeding. Massive hemoperitoneum secondary to rupture of the tumor occurs in about 10% of patients as a terminal event. Metastases to lungs, regional lymph nodes, and bones are common. Peritoneal implants develop in less than 5% of patients, explaining the low diagnostic yield of ascitic fluid cytology.

The only definitive therapy is complete excision of the tumors. Unfortunately, complete excision is feasible only in the rare patient who has no metastases and who has either a solitary tumor or tumor confined to one lobe. In addition, the other lobe should be noncirrhotic, and hepatic function should be well preserved. Surgical resection is indicated as the treatment of choice for small hepatocellular carcinoma especially in Child's Class A patients. The 5-year survival rate for surgically treated patients has been reported to be 10% to 30%. The modalities of selective intra-arterial infusion of chemotherapeutic agents, transcatheter embolization with autologous clot, and percutaneous injection of ethanol into the tumor appear promising and are being evaluated in clinical trials. Radiation therapy to the liver may afford palliation of pain in some patients. Liver transplantation has been attempted and carried out successfully in a few patients, but its usefulness is limited by the high rate of recurrence of tumor locally and at distant sites (Chapter 64).

Recently, several reports have emphasized the unique characteristics of a distinct histologic variety of primary hepatocellular carcinoma, termed fibrolamellar carcinoma. This unique tumor occurs with equal frequency in men and women and thus far has been reported only from the United States. Ninety percent of patients with this type of tumor are below the age of 40 years. Cirrhosis is distinctly rare, being present in less than 5% of patients. Seventy percent of the tumors are present in the left lobe of the liver.

Histologic features include deeply eosinophilic malignant cells interspersed with parallel laminated strands of collagen. Serum alpha fetoprotein levels are normal. Increased serum unsaturated vitamin B_{12}-binding capacity has been suggested as a marker of this tumor. Recognition of the fibrolamellar variant of primary hepatocellular carcinoma is important because the prognosis is relatively good, as reflected in a 50% operability rate and a 25% surgical cure rate. Additionally, liver transplantation is currently considered a reasonable option in selected patients with fibrolamellar hepatoma in whom partial hepatectomy is not on option.

Angiosarcoma

Angiosarcoma (malignant hemangioendothelioma, Kupffer cell sarcoma) is a rare, very vascular malignant tumor that accounts for less than 2% of all primary liver neoplasms. There is a high incidence of exposure to vinyl chloride, arsenic, or thorium dioxide. Tumors have typically occurred 15 to 25 years after exposure to thorium dioxide. In about 60% of patients, there is no history of exposure to these chemicals. Angiosarcoma occurs most often in men during their sixth or seventh decade. Patients present with nonspecific signs and symptoms of liver disease and hepatosplenomegaly. Most of the tumors are multicentric and involve both major lobes and branches of the portal and central veins. Hemoperitoneum occurs in 15% of patients. Metastatic spread to bones and lungs is common. Hematologic abnormalities include thrombocytopenia, disseminated intravascular coagulation, and thrombotic thrombocytopenic purpura. Alpha fetoprotein levels are normal. Diagnosis is best established by laparoscopic or open liver biopsy because percutaneous liver biopsy may be followed by fatal hemorrhage. There is no proved efficacious therapy, and most patients die within 3 to 6 months.

METASTATIC TUMORS

The incidence of metastatic malignant tumors in the liver is many times greater than that of primary carcinoma. Hepatic metastases are reported in up to 50% of patients dying from malignant disease. The liver is second only to lymph nodes as the most frequent site of metastases. Its large size, dual blood supply, and high rate of blood flow may explain its unique propensity to be the frequent site of metastases. Virtually all neoplasms except those originating in the brain metastasize to the liver. Those that metastasize to the liver most often originate in the gastrointestinal tract, pancreas, lungs, breasts, kidneys, ovaries, and skin. The lesions are most often multiple, involve both lobes, and have a characteristic umbilicated appearance on gross examination. Patients may have asymptomatic liver involvement; vague, nonspecific abdominal complaints; or features indicative of liver involvement such as abdominal pain, hepatomegaly, and ascites. Jaundice, even with massive replacement of liver tissue by tumor, is uncommon except as a preterminal event. Jaundice may be seen early if there is biliary tract compression by tumor at the porta hepatis; it is usually caused by colonic, breast, and bronchogenic carcinomas, some testicular neoplasms, malignant melanomas, and lymphomas.

Hepatomegaly, often tender, nodular, and very firm, is present in most patients. A friction rub may be audible. Portal hypertension and hepatic failure may occur as a consequence of widespread liver metastases. Elevated serum alkaline phosphatase and lactic dehydrogenase are common. Transaminase elevations are trivial in most patients. Rarely, transaminase elevations are striking and attain levels suggestive of acute viral or drug-induced hepatitis. Liver scintiscans disclose lesions greater than 2 cm in diameter. Ultrasonography, CT (Fig. 63-3), and MRI are valuable in detecting hepatic metastases. Blind liver biopsy is diagnostic in about 65% of patients with hepatomegaly or abnormal liver function test results. A 10% to 20% further increment may be attained by (1) using ultrasound or CT for guidance, (2) performing two or three passes, (3) performing cytologic examination of the aspirated fluid, and (4) examining multiple samples of sequential sections of the biopsy specimen.

For most patients, there is little effective treatment. Patients with solitary or localized multiple metastases may be candidates for partial hepatic resection if there is no evidence of metastatic spread elsewhere. Systemic chemotherapy may be palliative, depending on the nature of the primary neoplasm. The median survival after detection of hepatic metastases in untreated patients is less than 3 months.

BENIGN NEOPLASMS

Hemangiomas

Capillary and cavernous hemangiomas are the most common benign tumors of the liver and occur most often in females. They may be associated with hereditary telangiectasias in other organs. Their prevalence is as high as 7% in autopsy studies. Most hemangiomas are single, are located in the right lobe, and vary in diameter from a few millimeters to more than 30 cm. They may be calcified, and 10%

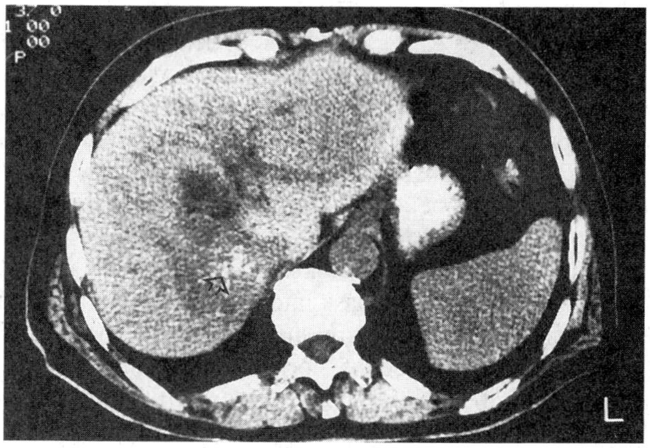

Fig. 63-3. CT scan reveals calcification *(arrow)* within a metastatic deposit to the liver in a patient with mucin producing colon cancer. (Courtesy of Vassilios Raptopoulos, MD.)

to 15% of the lesions are pedunculated. Most are asymptomatic and are usually discovered incidentally at the time of imaging, laparotomy or autopsy. In a few patients, abdominal pain ensues from thrombosis in the tumor or from rupture and intraperitoneal bleeding. Thrombocytopenia and hypofibrinogenemia may be seen in infants. In rare instances, arteriovenous communications are present and result in congestive heart failure.

Solitary, space-occupying lesions seen on scintiscan and appearing hyperechoic on ultrasonographic examination should raise the suspicion of hemangioma. Although angiography shows pooling of contrast material in a characteristic "cotton-wool" appearance, it is an invasive test. Technetium-tagged-RBC-SPECT (single photon emission computed tomography) scans and MRI are useful modalities for diagnosing hepatic hemangiomas. Percutaneous needle liver biopsy is contraindicated because of the danger of hemorrhage. Surgical excision is indicated for symptomatic lesions or if malignancy cannot be excluded. Corticosteroid therapy and/or hepatic artery ligation has been beneficial in children. Radiation therapy has been useful in treating multiple lesions.

Focal nodular hyperplasia

Focal nodular hyperplasia is probably not a true neoplasm but rather a reactive or a hamartomatous lesion. It is seen predominantly in women of childbearing age but occasionally occurs in children, older women, and males. Focal nodular hyperplasia is probably not causally related to oral contraceptive use. Most patients are asymptomatic. Liver function test results, including alpha fetoprotein levels, are usually normal. Calcification is virtually never present. Focal nodular hyperplasia may be associated with hepatic hemangiomas. In a recent study, 22% of patients with focal nodular hyperplasia were found to have associated hepatic hemangiomas. In the same study, hemangiomas were not found in any of the 27 patients with hepatic adenomas. Both CT and MRI show the lesion with its characteristic central stellate scar, but this finding is not specific and may be present in patients with fibrolamellar hepatocellular carcinoma. Technetium sulfur colloid scanning shows uptake in more than 50% of cases and hyperconcentration in approximately 10%. Angiography shows a hypervascular mass with the vascularity radiating peripherally in a "spoke-wheel" pattern; the diagnosis is definitively established by an open biopsy. Characteristically, the lesion is well circumscribed but nonencapsulated, varying from less than 1 cm to more than 15 cm. A stellate architectural configuration composed of central connective tissue with radiating septa that subdivide the mass into nodules is characteristic. Hemorrhage and necrosis are uncommon. Microscopically, the lesion is composed of normal-appearing hepatocytes without central veins or portal triads. Bile ductules and large blood vessels are prominent in the fibrous septa. There is no malignant potential and the prognosis is excellent. If the lesion is symptomatic and can be readily removed, resection is indicated.

Hepatic adenomas

Hepatic adenomas are encountered most often in women of childbearing age. Fifty percent to 75% of patients experience abdominal pain, and hemoperitoneum secondary to rupture has been reported in up to 25% of patients. Liver chemistries are usually normal, although slight elevations in alkaline phosphatase and aminotransferase levels occur in patients whose tumors have undergone hemorrhage or necrosis. Alpha fetoprotein levels are normal. An association with oral contraceptive ingestion appears established. Hepatic adenomas have also been described in patients with type 1a glycogen storage disease. Rupture of hepatic adenomas has coincided temporarily with menstruation, and inoperable adenomas have regressed after contraceptive medication was discontinued. Liver scintiscans with ^{99m}Tc most often show a cold defect. Angiography may reveal a fine reticular vascular pattern, with vessels entering from the periphery. In many instances, the lesions are hypovascular and show necrosis. Generally, the tumor is solitary, located in the right lobe, greater than 5 cm in diameter, and encapsulated. Microscopically, sheets of normal to slightly atypical hepatocytes without portal tracts or central veins are evident. Bile ductules are absent; and the characteristic septa, central scar, and thick-walled veins of focal nodular hyperplasia are absent. Currently, no evidence suggests that hepatic adenoma is a precursor of primary hepatocellular carcinoma, but some uncertainty regarding its malignant potential remains. For these reasons and because of the potential for hemorrhagic necrosis and rupture, hepatic adenomas should be surgically removed if cessation of oral contraceptives does not result in their regression. The prevention of hypoglycemia by dietary therapy in patients with glycogen storage disease may prevent the development of hepatic adenoma as well as cause regression in tumor size in those in whom the adenoma is already present.

REFERENCES

Beasley RP and Hwang L-Y: Hepatocellular carcinoma and hepatitis B virus, Semin Liver Dis 4(2):113, 1984.

Bennett WF and Bova JG: Review of hepatic imaging and a problem oriented approach to liver masses, Hepatology 12:761, 1990.

Blumberg BS and London WT: Hepatitis B virus and the prevention of primary hepatocellular carcinoma, N Engl J Med 304:782, 1981.

Bouwman DL and Walt AJ: Current status of resection for hepatic neoplasms, Semin Liver Dis 3(3):193, 1983.

Colombo M et al: Hepatocellular carcinoma in Italian patients with cirrhosis, N Engl J Med 325:675, 1991.

DiBisceglie AM, moderator: Hepatocellular carcinoma, Ann Intern Med 108:390, 1988.

Kerlin P et al: Hepatic adenoma and focal nodular hyperplasia: clinical, pathologic, and radiologic features, Gastroenterology 84:994, 1983.

Klatskin G: Hepatic tumors: possible relationship to use of oral contraceptives, Gastroenterology 73:386, 1977.

Nagasue N et al: The natural history of hepatocellular carcinoma: a study of 100 untreated cases, Cancer 54:1461, 1984.

Okuda K: Hepatocellular carcinoma: recent progress, Hepatology 15:948, 1992.

Ruffin MT: Fibrolamellar hepatoma, Am J Gastroenterol 85:577, 1990.

Simonetti RG et al: Hepatitis C virus infection as a risk factor for hepatocellular carcinoma in patients with cirrhosis, Ann Intern Med 116:97, 1992.

Tamburro FH: Relationship of vinyl monomers and liver cancers: angiosarcoma and hepatocellular carcinoma, Semin Liver Dis 4(2):158, 1984.

Weinman MD and Chopra S: Tumors of the liver other than primary hepatocellular carcinoma, Gastroenterol Clin North Am 16:627, 1987.

CHAPTER

64 Liver Transplantation

Michael F. Sorrell
Jeremiah P. Donovan

The rapid evolution of liver transplantation has revolutionized the field of liver disease. The responsible physician is now obligated to consider the possibility of liver transplantation when confronted with a patient suffering from end-stage liver disease for which an effective medical therapy is not available. After Starzl in Denver and Calne in Cambridge established the technical feasibility of liver transplantation, further progress was stymied by the lack of effective immunosuppression necessary for long-term survival. Survival after transplantation from the mid 1960s until 1980 never exceeded 25% to 30%. The advent of cyclosporine A in 1980, with the concomitant dramatic increase in survival rates to between 60% and 80%, signaled the beginning of a new era. Encouraged by these results, a National Institute of Health Consensus Conference in 1983 concluded that liver transplantation had become a proven therapeutic modality and was no longer an experimental procedure. This far-reaching recommendation resulted in a rapid proliferation of transplant centers, as insurance companies and Medicare could no longer deny payment based on the premise that transplantation was experimental. In 1992 approximately 100 centers performed liver transplantation in the United States. In busy centers, one can expect survival rates ranging from 60% to 90%, depending on the disease process and the recipient's clinical status before surgery. The debate has now shifted to donor availability, proper selection of recipients, timing of the transplant, and the place of transplantation in the overall scheme of financing health care. One should be reminded that the *raison d'être* for transplantation must include not only saving lives but also restoring quality of life. If properly selected, most patients should expect an improved and productive life after transplantation.

PATIENT SELECTION

As a general guideline, all patients with end-stage liver disease with an estimated life expectancy of 1 year or less should be considered as potential candidates for liver transplantation. The evaluation process is designed to answer specific questions surrounding the patient's candidacy (see the box below). Specific questions unique to a specific disease process must be answered, but overall the evaluation process is designed to uncover potential conditions that would preclude a successful transplant. As the field of transplantation has matured, one can responsibly recommend transplantation earlier in the disease process before complications ensue that lessen the chance for a favorable outcome.

INDICATIONS AND CONTRAINDICATIONS FOR TRANSPLANTATION

Indications

Specific diseases for which transplantation in the adult is indicated are listed in the box on p. 644. Liver transplantation has been performed for almost all chronic end-stage liver diseases, selected congenital metabolic diseases, and fulminant hepatic failure. However, transplantation is more debatable in neoplastic and non-neoplastic disease where the disease present in the native liver can predictably be expected to recur. Long-term survival after transplantation in patients with cancer of the liver and biliary tree, particularly for primary carcinoma of the bile ducts, has been disappointing. Improved survival awaits development of effective modalities of adjuvant chemotherapy. These patients should ideally be transplanted only as part of an experimental protocol. In most instances, transplantation of end-stage chronic hepatitis B in the United States has resulted in recurrence of hepatitis in the graft, with dismal graft and patient survival despite prophylaxis with immune hepatitis B globulin and/or interferon. More optimistic results have been reported from Europe using prophylactic intravenous hepatitis B immune globulin. Unfortunately, intravenous hepatitis B immune globulin is not available in the United States at the present time. Fulminant liver failure secondary to hepatitis B infection does not exhibit the same pro-

Evaluation process

- What is the patient's diagnosis and how well is it established?
- What complications does the patient have or is at risk of developing?
- How have the liver disease and its complications affected the patient's quality of life?
- Are there any contraindications to transplantation?
- Does the patient have any concomitant disease process that would complicate transplantation?
- Will the patient be compliant with therapy after the transplant, and does he or she have the necessary psychosocial support structures to undergo the stresses associated with transplantation?
- Is the patient an adequate operative risk?
- Is there adequate financial support for the transplant?
- How soon should a transplant be considered to best optimize the patient's survival and quality of life?

Indications for liver transplantation in adults

I. Irreversible advanced chronic liver disease
   A. Predominantly cholestatic liver disease
      1. Primary biliary cirrhosis
      2. Primary sclerosing cholangitis
      3. Secondary biliary cirrhosis
      4. Alagille syndrome
      5. Drug-induced biliary cirrhosis and cholestasis
      6. Caroli's disease
   B. Predominantly hepatocellular liver disease
      1. Chronic viral hepatitis
         a. Hepatitis B
         b. Hepatitis B with hepatitis D
         c. Hepatitis C
      2. Drug-induced liver disease
      3. Cryptogenic cirrhosis
      4. Autoimmune chronic active hepatitis with cirrhosis
      5. Alcoholic liver disease
      6. Wilson's disease
      7. Congenital hepatic fibrosis
   C. Vascular diseases that lead to hepatic dysfunction or portal hypertension, or both
      1. Budd-Chiari syndrome
      2. Veno-occlusive disease
II. Hepatic malignancies not resectable without hepatic replacement but confined to the liver
   A. Hepatocellular carcinoma
   B. Intrahepatic cholangiocarcinoma
   C. Hemangiosarcoma or other sarcomas
III. Fulminant hepatic failure
   A. Viral hepatitis (A, B, C, B+D)
   B. Wilson's disease
   C. Drug or toxin induced
IV. Inherited metabolic disorders
   A. Hemophilia A
   B. Homozygous familial hypercholesterolemia
   C. Primary hyperoxaluria type I
   D. Others

Contraindications for liver transplantation

Absolute contraindications

- Active sepsis outside the biliary tract
- HIV positive
- Extrahepatic malignancy
- Advanced cardiovascular disease
- Severe hypoxemia
- Active alcoholism
- Severe neurologic deficits

Relative contraindications

- Advanced age
- Biliary sepsis
- Extensive portal/mesenteric thrombosis
- Grade IV coma
- Hepatitis B positivity

clivity for reinfection and chronicity. Satisfactory results can be expected when such patients are transplanted. It is important to recognize other co-morbid, but not life-threatening, conditions related to the underlying liver disease, which may provide the impetus for early transplantation. Illustrative conditions would include severe osteopenic bone disease, intractable pruritus, and encephalopathy not responsive to medical therapy. Quality of life has become an increasingly important factor in timing the transplantation.

Contraindications

As transplantation science has developed and experience has accumulated, the number of contraindications have decreased. These contraindications are outlined in the box at upper right. Many of the original contraindications were related to technical problems such as portal and/or mesenteric vein thrombosis or extensive right upper quadrant surgery that made the performance of the transplant hazardous. Advances in surgical technique have largely obviated such problems in experienced centers. With accumulated experience, age has become less of a factor. Survival rates approaching 90% have been obtained in low-risk patients over the age of 60 years. It has become abundantly clear that increased survival rates are directly related to the condition of the patient at the time of transplantation. Shaw et al have demonstrated that when patients are stratified according to low, intermediate, and high-risk groups, 1 year actuarial survival rates of only 44.5% in 22 high-risk patients, compared with 85% and 90.5% for 27 intermediate and 52 low-risk patients, respectively, were obtained.

Specific indications in the adult

Alcoholic cirrhosis. Perhaps no single indication for liver transplantation has caused so much controversy as transplantation of the alcoholic. Much of the debate has centered around the question of potential recidivism in the recipient as well as the question of giving a scarce resource to a patient with a "self-inflicted" disease. What is clear, however, is that results from transplantation of the alcoholic parallels that of the nonalcoholic recipient. Several centers have reported less than 10% recidivism. Long-term follow-up will be necessary to confirm these early reports. According to UNOS (United Network Organ Sharing) data, the single most frequent indication for liver transplantation in 1991 was alcoholic liver disease.

Primary biliary cirrhosis. Historically, patients with primary biliary cirrhosis have been considered excellent candidates for transplantation. One- and 5-year survival rates of 90% and 70%, respectively, have been reported. Timing of the operation has been difficult because of the indolent and fluctuating course inherent in the disease. Predictive models based on selected laboratory and clinical features have been proposed to aid in decision making. Common indications for transplantation include variceal hemorrhage, recurrent encephalopathy, overwhelming fatigue, intractable pruritus, and hepatic osteodystrophy. The rare recurrence of primary biliary cirrhosis in the graft has been reported in one series but has not been confirmed by other centers.

Primary sclerosing cholangitis. In the majority of patients, primary sclerosing cholangitis occurs in association with ulcerative colitis. Rarely, the duct lesion will precede inflammatory bowel disease. Indications for transplantation are similar to those listed previously for primary biliary cirrhosis. Predictive models to aid in the timing of transplantation have been proposed but are not yet accepted clinically. One must be vigilant for the development of cholangiocarcinoma in these patients. In several series, cholangiocarcinoma was detected in 12% to 15% of patients in whom transplantation was considered.

Postnecrotic cirrhosis. The etiologic agents responsible for the development of postnecrotic or cryptogenic cirrhosis include hepatitis C and B plus Delta, as well as autoimmune hepatitis. A few cases are caused by drugs such as methotrexate. In most transplantation centers, hepatitis C–induced cirrhosis is one of the most frequent indications for transplantation. Hepatitis C frequently recurs after transplantation, but the subsequent course is often indolent. Management is often troublesome because of difficulty in distinguishing between recurrent hepatitis C and other causes of postoperative changes in liver function tests such as rejection or biliary tract problems. Further longitudinal experience with hepatitis C–transplanted patients will be necessary before accurate assessment of long-term outcomes can be estimated. Interferon is being used in various treatment protocols in the perioperative and postoperative period in an attempt to prevent or treat recurrent hepatitis C. Long-term efficacy of interferon therapy remains uncertain.

Fewer patients with autoimmune cirrhosis have been transplanted probably because of more effective treatment of the autoimmune process and the relative infrequency of the disease. There has been at least one reported case of recurrent autoimmune hepatitis after transplantation.

Budd-Chiari syndrome. The decision to perform liver transplantation in the patient with Budd-Chiari syndrome can be very difficult. Some patients can be treated with anticoagulation alone, whereas others with less advanced disease may benefit from portosystemic shunting. One must remember that what is possible is not obligatory. If the disease process is long-standing and cirrhosis is present, however, transplantation is the most feasible option. Outcome is usually excellent, although long-term anticoagulation is frequently necessary.

Fulminant hepatitis. Complex and difficult decisions surround the care of the patient with acute liver failure. In many instances, transplantation remains the best and often the only option in the desperately ill patient. The natural history of the well-characterized patient with fulminant failure and grade III to IV encephalopathy is such that one can predict, with a certain degree of confidence, mortality rates that exceed 80%. In these instances, transplantation can be life saving. Actuarial survival rates after transplantation in the most ill patients range from 50% to 65%. Recently, improved survival has been associated with the employment of intracranial pressure monitoring devices, as well as better selection and perioperative management of these patients.

PEDIATRIC TRANSPLANTATION

The most common cause for transplantation in children is biliary atresia. In the well-prepared child, 1-year survival rates exceed 85%. It is generally thought that if at all feasible, a Kasai (portoenterostomy) procedure should be performed before liver transplantation. If successful, this procedure will allow the child sufficient time to grow, thereby increasing the opportunity for obtaining a donor liver. Other indications for transplantation include alpha$_1$ antitrypsin deficiency, Wilson's disease not amenable to chelation therapy, and any number of congenital and metabolic diseases. The major challenge remains the scarcity of donor livers for the small child. The surgeons have responded to this problem in extremely inventive ways. The techniques of segmental and split liver grafts plus the recent development of living related donors have allowed for earlier and more optimum timing of transplantation.

THE DONOR LIVER

No discussion of liver transplantation would be complete without considering the donor liver. Donors are matched with recipients primarily by blood type and body size. The application of sophisticated tissue typing has not been clinically useful in the liver recipient as opposed to the kidney recipient. The improved survival in transplantation with the subsequent proliferation of centers has placed enormous demands on the donor pool. At the present time, over 2600 liver transplantations are performed each year. It is variously estimated that at any one time over 40,000 potential recipients could benefit from liver transplantation. With the realization that the liver ages very little and atherosclerotic vascular disease is unusual in the hepatic artery, the age limit for donation has been raised upward to 60 to 65 years. The problem is particularly acute in children as discussed earlier. Unfortunately, the use of reduced sized grafts in children has accentuated the shortage in adults. The encouragement of organ donation is everyone's responsibility.

POSTOPERATIVE COURSE

Any number of medical and surgical complications can occur in the postoperative period. The most catastrophic event is graft failure immediately after transplantation. Termed primary nonfunction, it happens in about 3% of cases and requires immediate retransplantation. As the result of technical problems, hepatic artery thrombosis occurs most frequently in children as compared to adults and may require retransplantation. Thrombosis of the hepatic artery may present under various guises including rapidly increasing transaminases, high bilirubin levels, bile duct strictures, or unexplained sepsis. Because the liver has a limited repertoire of response to injury, the transplantation team must always confirm their clinical impression by carefully selected diagnostic testing. When graft dysfunction develops after the transplant, to err in diagnosis or treatment can be disastrous.

Rejection

At least one episode of acute rejection can be expected in approximately 80% of patients undergoing transplantation. Acute rejection often occurs within the fifth to fourteenth postoperative day. When suspected, the diagnosis should be confirmed by percutaneous liver biopsy because many other causes of graft dysfunction can mimic rejection. Standard immunosuppressive therapy of rejection includes additional steroids, plus the use of intravenous anti-T cell monoclonal and polyclonal antibodies when indicated. In recalcitrant cases of acute rejection, newer immunosuppressive agents such as FK 506 are available on a compassionate use basis. An increasing number of drugs to treat rejection are in the investigational stage. The ideal immunosuppressive drug will prevent rejection without toxic side effects and without an increased susceptibility to infections.

Chronic rejection is clinically manifested by progressive, relentless cholestasis and histologically characterized by lymphocytic infiltration of the portal triads, arteriopathy, and disappearance of the interlobular bile ducts. It is estimated that chronic rejection develops in approximately 10% to 15% of transplants. It is not unusual for the patient to present with chronic rejection without previous evidence of acute rejection. Increased immunosuppression rarely will stay the course of documented chronic rejection. Retransplantation is often necessary.

Infection

In the postoperative period, the predominant cause of mortality and morbidity is infection. Early on, bacterial, viral, and opportunistic infections all play an important role. Cytomegalovirus infection, either primary or reactivation, is present in 20% to 30% of patients. The most serious complication is that of systemic fungal infection, in which mortality rates can exceed 90%. Bacterial infections account for over 90% of clinically important infections after the patient has returned home. The risk of infection is markedly increased in patients with difficult prolonged operations, an increased number of reoperations, and postoperative renal failure and in those who require increased immunosuppression for control of rejection.

Other considerations

Some impairment of renal function secondary to cyclosporine or FK 506 nephrotoxicity is a nearly constant feature in the post-transplantation patient. Occasionally the renal disease may become so severe that dialysis or renal transplantation will be required. The development of malignancies, primarily lymphoproliferative in nature, is thought to be caused by Epstein-Barr viral infection and related to immunosuppressive therapy. Some tumors will respond to reduction in immunosuppression and the concomitant use of acyclovir. Chemotherapy has not proved useful.

REFERENCES

Bismuth H and Sherlock DJ: Portasystemic shunting versus liver transplantation for Budd-Chiari syndrome, Ann Surg 214:581, 1991.

Lucey MR et al: Selection for and outcome of liver transplantation in alcoholic liver disease, Gastroenterology 102:1736-1741, 1992.

Martin P, Munoz SJ, and Friedman LS: Liver transplantation for viral hepatitis: current status, Am J Gastroenterol 87:409-418, 1992.

National Institutes of Health Consensus Development Conference Statement: Liver transplantation-June 20-23, 1983, Hepatology 4(suppl): 107s-110s, 1984.

Shaw BW Jr et al: Stratifying the causes of death in liver transplant recipients, Arch Surg 124:895-900, 1989.

Sorrell MF and Shaw BW Jr, editors: A primer of liver transplantation for the referring physician, Semin Liver Dis 9:159, 1989.

Starzl TE, Demetris AJ, and Van Thiel D: Liver transplantation, N Engl J Med 321:1014-1022, 1092-1099, 1989.

Stieber AC et al: The surgical implications of the post-transplant lymphoproliferative disorders, Transplant Proc 23:1477-1479, 1991.

Whittington PF and Balistreri WF: Liver transplantation in pediatrics: indications, contraindications, and pretransplant management, J Pediatr 118:169-177, 1991.

CHAPTER

65 Biliary Tract Stones and Associated Diseases

Michael D. Apstein
Martin C. Carey

Gallstones are extremely common throughout the Western world. In the United States, 15% of the population, 35 million individuals, are estimated to have gallstones. Every year in the United States, 1 million patients are newly diagnosed with gallstones; half undergo cholecystectomy at an estimated annual cost of $6 billion. Key issues for physicians include which patients should be treated and the roles of newer therapies, laparoscopic cholecystectomy and medical dissolution, and the experimental therapies, contact solvent dissolution and extracorporeal shock wave lithotripsy. A role for agents in preventing gallstones is emerging in patients who are at very high risk: those undergoing rapid weight loss or receiving total parenteral nutrition (TPN).

BILIARY TRACT STONES

Classification and composition

Cholesterol stones and pigment (calcium [hydrogen] bilirubinate) stones are the two major categories of gallstones.

Pigment stones are subdivided trivially as "brown" or "black." Black pigment stones are the more common pigment stones in Western populations and form principally under sterile conditions in the gallbladder. Brown pigment stones usually form de novo in infected, partially or intermittently obstructed bile ducts of patients following cholecystectomy. In Asians, brown pigment stones also form frequently in the intrahepatic bile ducts (hepatolithiasis) and also may involve the gallbladder.

The principal component of cholesterol stones is crystalline cholesterol monohydrate, usually greater than 70% by weight. Pigment stones are composed mostly of noncrystalline calcium (hydrogen) bilirubinate ("brown"), or polymer pigments ("black") derived from calcium (hydrogen) bilirubinate. Brown stones contain up to 30% cholesterol monohydrate, whereas black stones frequently contain none and only rarely as much as 10% cholesterol.

Both cholesterol and pigment stones always contain inorganic calcium salts. In the cholesterol and black pigment stones, these salts are predominantly one polymorph (distinct crystalline form) of calcium carbonate or calcium phosphate. If stones contain sufficient amounts of crystalline calcium carbonates and phosphates, they are radiopaque. Calcium fatty acid soaps are typically found in brown pigment stones and render them radiolucent (Table 65-1). These stones also contain dead bacteria and their secretions.

Another component invariably present in gallbladder and bile duct stones is a poorly characterized glycoprotein mixture, previously called *unmeasured residue,* which represents mucus and other biliary proteins. Mucin glycoproteins pigmented with bilirubinate salts are found at the nuclei of all gallstones. Bile acids, free fatty acids, phospholipids, heavy metals, gas, and water are present in only trace amounts of gallstones.

Because only cholesterol stones can be treated with nonsurgical therapies, identifying stone type by radiographic characteristics has practical importance even though it is imprecise and is now superseded by computed tomography (CT) scanning. Eighty percent of radiolucent gallstones and almost 100% with rim or central calcification are cholesterol stones; the remainder are brown pigment stones. Most diffusely calcified stones (70%) are black pigment stones. Overall, about 15% of gallstones are radiopaque on abdominal radiographs.

In addition to their chemical complexity, gallstones are physically heterogeneous. In appearance, cholesterol stones vary from yellow white to dark brown. If solitary (10%), they are usually round or mulberry shaped (Plate II-22). If multiple (90%), they are usually faceted and smooth (Plate II-23). Sizes range from less than 0.5 mm (gallsand) to 4 cm for solitary cholesterol gallstones. The cut surface demonstrates that the aggregated cholesterol monohydrate crystals have their long axes oriented radially to the nucleus. Mucin glycoproteins can be demonstrated in the nucleus and as a prosthesis dispersed throughout the stone. Solitary cholesterol stones always display pigmented centers composed of calcium (hydrogen) bilirubinate (Plate II-24). In the majority of cholesterol stones, discontinuous rings of calcium (hydrogen) bilirubinate, calcium salts, and amorphous material laminate the structure.

Black pigment stones almost always occur in multiples and are small (<5-10 mm), irregular in shape, often spiculated, and dark (usually black) in color (Plate II-25). Brown pigment stones are usually smooth, earthy to yellow in color, and often molded to the shape of the bile ducts. The content of mucin glycoproteins and other proteins in brown pigment stones is higher than that of cholesterol stones.

Pathophysiology

Gallstone formation, whether cholesterol or pigment, follows a logical pathophysiologic sequence: (1) Bile becomes supersaturated with the insoluble solute, e.g., cholesterol or calcium (hydrogen) bilirubinate, (the chemical stage); (2) if supersaturation is extreme, homogeneous (spontaneous)

Table 65-1. Classification of gallstones

	Cholesterol	Polymer calcium (hydrogen) bilirubinate ("black") pigment	Calcium (hydrogen) bilirubinate ("brown") pigment
Primary location	Gallbladder	Gallbladder	90% biliary tree 10% gallbladder*
Number	Solitary (~10%) Multiple (90%)	Multiple	Solitary or multiple
Size	Up to 4 cm	2 to 5 mm	2 to 20 mm
Appearance	White-Yellow-Brown	Shiny black	Earthy brown
Hardness	Hard	Hard	Soft
Clinical associations	Hypersecretion of biliary cholesterol	Increased bilirubin secretion and bile salt deficiency	Anaerobic biliary infection and biliary obstruction
Cholesterol content	> 70%	0-10%	< 30%
Calcium salts	Calcium carbonate or phosphate	Calcium phosphate carbonate and calcium (hydrogen) bilirubinate	Calcium (fatty acid) soaps, calcium (hydrogen) bilirubinate
Radiodensity	Lucent or rim calcification	70% opaque	Lucent

*Most likely secondary to prior episodes of healed, acute cholecystitis.

nucleation may occur; if supersaturation is modest, the biliary tree, especially the gallbladder, must produce an agent to induce nucleation (heterogeneous) and precipitation (the physical stage); and finally (3) stasis is required for the precipitates to agglomerate and grow to form macroscopic stones (the growth stage).

Cholesterol stones

Cholesterol supersaturation. Cholesterol and bile salt secretions into bile are the body's major excretory routes for cholesterol. Cholesterol is insoluble in water but is solubilized in bile by the other biliary lipids (i.e., the detergent-like bile salts and the phospholipid lecithin) to form macromolecular, water soluble complexes called mixed micelles and small unilamellar vesicles of lecithin and cholesterol (Chapter 51).

By plotting the relative molar compositions of bile salts, lecithin, and cholesterol in gallbladder and hepatic bile as a single point on triangular coordinates (Fig. 65-1), one can define the compositions in which the cholesterol is solubilized in mixed micelles or in the mixed micelles plus unilamellar vesicles. When plotted in this fashion, hepatic bile from both normal subjects and gallstone patients is "supersaturated" with cholesterol with respect to the solubilizing capacity of the micellar phase. However, a dilute bile system is extremely stable because the excess cholesterol is solubilized by metastable unilamellar vesicles, forming a two-phase (micellar and vesicular) system. Gallbladder bile from all cholesterol stone patients and approximately 50% of controls is also "supersaturated" with cholesterol with respect to the micellar phase. Bile from normal human beings contains relatively less cholesterol than that from gallstone patients. In gallstone subjects, the higher relative contents of cholesterol are solubilized in supersaturated micelles and unilamellar vesicles. In concentrated gallbladder biles, the vesicles become unstable and rapidly nucleate solid cholesterol crystals.

A relative excess of cholesterol molecules compared with molecules of the solubilizing lipids, bile salts, and lecithin must be present in bile before cholesterol gallstones can form. In this setting, cholesterol molecules can nucleate, crystallize, and precipitate from solution. In humans, this imbalance between cholesterol and bile salts plus lecithin (lithogenic bile) is caused by hypersecretion of biliary cholesterol, hyposecretion of biliary bile salts, or both. A deficiency of biliary lecithin has not been identified.

Nucleation. Cholesterol precipitates (nucleates) from bile as the unilamellar vesicles that carry excess cholesterol fuse and become unstable when concentrated in the gallbladder (Fig. 65-1). The control of nucleation by pronucleating and antinucleating factors is critical because most humans have supersaturated bile for hours during the day (fasting) yet do not form gallstones. A number of normal lipid and protein components of bile have been identified as pronucleating and antinucleating agents, but it is not known which ones are clinically relevant in normal and gallstone-forming biles. Gallbladder bile of persons with cholesterol stones precipitates cholesterol crystals about five times faster than do control gallbladder biles for the same degree of cholesterol supersaturation. Stimulation of the gallbladder mucosa by lithogenic bile induces hypersecretion of mucin glycoproteins. It is believed that mucin gel in the gallbladder lumen may be important in inducing nucleation. In fact, in lithogenic animal models, abnormal bile stimulates gallbladder mucin synthesis and secretion, whereas drugs that inhibit mucin production can prevent gallstones despite the persistence of supersaturated bile.

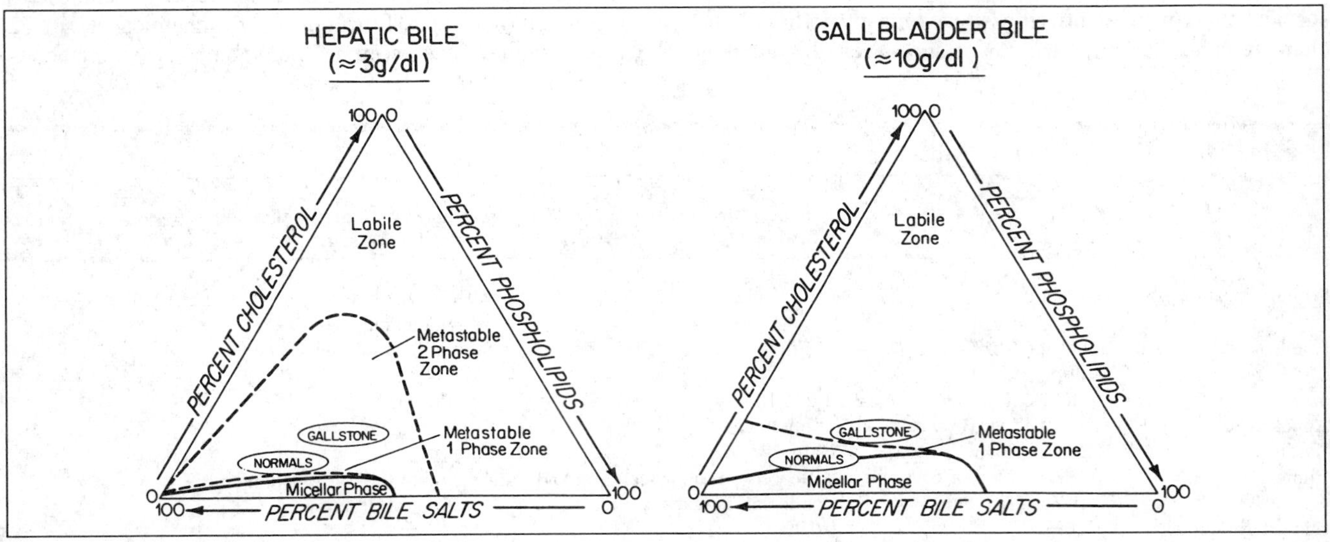

Fig. 65-1. Relative lipid compositions of hepatic and gallbladder bile in normal subjects and in patients with cholesterol gallstones. In the micellar phase, bile is unsaturated with cholesterol; in the one-phase metastable zones, micelles are supersaturated with cholesterol but do not nucleate readily. In the two-phase metastable zone, unilamellar vesicles cooperate with supersaturated micelles to solubilize cholesterol. Outside these zones, bile nucleates spontaneously.

Gallbladder dysmotility. Impaired gallbladder motility with increased gallbladder fasting and residual volumes (stasis) is an important primary defect predisposing to cholesterol gallstone formation. Animals fed a lithogenic diet demonstrate decreased gallbladder smooth muscle contractility and increased gallbladder fasting and residual volumes before gallstones develop. Furthermore, human gallbladder muscle contractility is reduced in patients with cholesterol gallstones compared to those with pigment stones. In cholesterol stone disease, gallbladder stasis allows cholesterol crystals to be entrapped by mucin glycoproteins, remain within the gallbladder, aggregate, and grow into macroscopic stones. Further, impaired gallbladder motor function is present in about 70% of gallstone patients consistent with the predominance of cholesterol stones.

Black pigment stones. Pathogenesis of black pigment gallstones is related to an increased biliary concentration of unconjugated bilirubin and ionized calcium, decreased biliary bile salt levels, and possibly gallbladder stasis. Both hepatic and gallbladder biles of black pigment stone patients without biliary infection or hemolytic states are supersaturated with calcium (hydrogen) bilirubinate and perhaps with calcium carbonate. The pigment supersaturation may result from (1) a defect in or overloading of hepatic conjugation with increased production of bilirubin monoglucuronides, (2) increased endogenous beta-glucuronidase activity within the biliary tree, or (3) a deficiency of bile salt-lecithin solubilizers. Biliary ionized calcium then forms a high affinity salt bond with two molecules of the acid species of unconjugated bilirubin, which precipitates and grows to form stones. Normally, bile salts both solubilize unconjugated bilirubin and bind ionized calcium. Consequently, decreased biliary bile salt levels strongly promote pigment stone formation by rendering more unconjugated bilirubin and free ionized calcium available for co-precipitation.

Very little is known about the nucleation or growth stage of black pigment stones, but it is likely that bilirubin and bile salt concentrations, biliary pH, calcium concentration, and gallbladder mucin glycoproteins play complementary roles. No work has been carried out on the polymerization of bile pigments. Because such stones occur predominantly in the gallbladder and always in noninfected bile, it is virtually certain that they form and grow by mechanisms chemically and physically distinct from those giving rise to brown pigment stones.

Brown pigment stones. Bacterial invasion is a prerequisite of brown pigment stone formation in both intrahepatic and extrahepatic bile ducts. Biliary tract infection results in high beta-glucuronidase, conjugated bile salt hydrolase, and phospholipase A_1 activities in bile. The microbial beta-glucuronidase, in contrast to the biliary tree enzyme, deconjugates bilirubin conjugates extremely rapidly at biliary pH and, as a result, the solubility of calcium (hydrogen) bilirubinate in bile is greatly exceeded. The conjugated bile salt hydrolase deconjugates bile salts and the phospholipase A_1 cleaves biliary lecithin, resulting in the formation of calcium bile salts and calcium soaps, respectively. Because of the limited capacity of human bile to solubilize any calcium salt and to maintain it in a metastable supersaturated solution, pigment stones can form in both intrahepatic and extrahepatic ducts. The appreciable cholesterol content in these stones results from depletion of the cholesterol solubilizers, bile salts and lecithin, by bacterial enzymatic hydrolysis.

Epidemiology. There is tremendous geographic variation in the prevalence as well as in the predominant type of gallstones (Table 65-2). Gallstones are much rarer in underdeveloped countries than in Western societies. In the West,

Table 65-2. Frequency of gallstone occurrence in selected groups and countries (autopsy series)

Very Common (10%-70%)	Common (10%-30%)	Intermediate (<10%)	Rare (0-1%)
United States (Indians)	United States (whites)	United States (blacks)	East Africa
South America (Indians)	Denmark	Japan (urban population)	West Africa
Ecuador	Norway	Thailand	New Guinea
Bolivia	United Kingdom	Northern India	Rural Japan
Chile	Italy	Canada (urban Eskimos)	Canada (rural Eskimos)
Mexico	New Zealand	China	Egypt
Canada (Indians)	Zimbabwe (whites)	Norway	Southern India
Sweden	Canada (whites)	Greece	
Czechoslovakia	Australia	Uzbekistan	
Germany	Finland	Indonesia	
	Japan	South Africa (Bantu)	
	South Africa (whites)		
	Russia		
	Ukraine		

Sources: Modified from Shaffer EA and Small DM: Gallstone disease; pathogenesis and management, Curr Probl Surg 13:1, 1976; after Lowenfels AB, Gut 21:1090, 1980, and Brett M and Barker DJP: Int J Epidemiol 5:335, 1976; Carey MC and O'Donovan MA: Gallstone disease: current concepts in the epidemiology, pathogenesis and management. In Harrison's Principles of Internal Medicine (Update V). New York, 1984, McGraw-Hill, 1984.

70% to 80% of gallstones are cholesterol, whereas pigment gallstones constitute the majority in rural areas of Japan, other Asian countries, and in certain parts of Latin America.

The prevalence of cholesterol and pigment gallstones has changed dramatically in parts of the Orient during this century. After World War II, gallstones were rare and usually of the pigment variety in Japan and China. Since 1950, the prevalence of cholesterol gallstones has increased markedly in these countries, and the prevalence of pigment gallstones has fallen.

With the advent of ultrasonography, numerous studies have determined the true prevalence rates of gallstones in ambulatory, healthy populations. The pivotal study was carried out, in the town of Sirimone, Italy in the early 1980s when males and females of all ages, 70% of the population, underwent abdominal ultrasonography. The prevalence of gallstones in women was shown to increase linearly with age from 2.9% in the 18- to 29-year-old group to 27% in the 50- to 65-year-old group. Prevalence in men was half that in women. Other ultrasonographic studies of Western populations—Great Britain, Denmark, Germany, and Russia—confirm that gallstones are very common, with considerable intercontinental variation, Germany having the highest prevalence rates in Europe. In the United States, rigorous studies of randomly selected samples of whites are lacking, but as is well known, certain US and Canadian Indian tribes (Pima, Navajo, Chippewa, and MicMac) have epidemic rates of gallstones. Hispanic populations have a higher prevalence of gallstones than do US whites.

Putative risk factors for gallstones

Cholesterol gallstones
- Female gender
- Parity
- Obesity
- Rapid weight loss
- Advancing age
- Family history
- American Indian heritage
- Gallbladder stasis syndromes
- Medication: fibrates, estrogens, anabolic steroids, octreotide
- Hypertriglyceridemia and low HDL cholesterol
- Inborn errors of bile salt synthesis
- Spinal cord injury

Pigment gallstones
- Hemolytic disorders
- Hepatic cirrhosis
- Advancing age
- Ileal disease/resection/bypass
- Stasis syndromes (TPN, postvagotomy)
- Chronic hypercalcemia
- Advanced AIDS
- Biliary infection

PUTATIVE RISK FACTORS FOR GALLSTONE FORMATION

Putative risk factors for gallstones are listed in the accompanying box and are summarized here.

Cholesterol gallstones

Gender. Women have twice the risk as men of developing cholesterol gallstones because estrogen increases biliary cholesterol secretion. Before puberty this risk is negligible and beyond the menopause the increased risk disappears.

Parity. Pregnancy is an independent risk factor for cholesterol gallstones. The risk increases with increasing parity, especially with more than two children. During pregnancy elevated estrogen and progesterone levels increase biliary cholesterol secretion. Elevated progesterone levels also inhibit gallbladder contractility. Forty percent of women develop "biliary sludge" in their gallbladder, a prestone condition, during pregnancy. Moreover, 12% of women form their first stones during pregnancy.

Obesity. Obesity is strongly associated with increased gallstone prevalence. The risk is proportional to the increase in total body fat. Obese people synthesize more cholesterol in both hepatic and nonhepatic tissues, transport it to the liver, and secrete more of it into bile, leading to bile that is often greatly supersaturated with cholesterol. Biliary cholesterol saturation reverts to normal after obese subjects achieve ideal body weight.

Rapid weight loss. Obese patients undergoing rapid weight loss (1% to 2% of body weight, or approximately 2 to 5 lb/week), either by very low caloric dieting or gastric stapling, have a 25% to 40% chance of developing gallstones within 4 months. During rapid weight loss biliary cholesterol saturation increases acutely as cholesterol is mobilized from adipose tissue and skin and secreted into bile.

Advancing age. Some but not all studies have demonstrated that biliary cholesterol saturation increases with advancing age as biliary cholesterol secretion increases and biliary bile salt synthesis decreases.

American Indians. Prevalence rates of gallstones among male and female Pima Indians are among the highest in the world: approximately 70% to 80% of men and women over 55 years of age have gallstones. In contrast to the low frequency of symptoms in whites or Pima men, 40% to 50% of Pima women over 35 years of age have symptoms or complications of gallstones.

Medications. Hypolipidemic drugs (clofibrate, gemfibrozil) that lower serum cholesterol by increasing biliary cholesterol secretion increase the risk of cholesterol gallstones by twofold to threefold. Sequestration of bile salts by drugs (cholestyramine, colestipol) does not result in an increased risk of gallstones because the liver compensates by increasing synthesis of bile salts to maintain normal bile salt secretion. Competitive inhibitors of 3-hydroxy-3-methylglutaryl coenzyme A (HMGCoA) reductase (lovastatin, simvastatin, pravastatin) *decrease* biliary cholesterol saturation. Estrogen therapy is associated with an increased risk of developing cholesterol gallstones in both men and women. Oral contraceptive steroids increase biliary cholesterol secretion and saturation but do not affect gallbladder motility.

Serum lipids. An *inverse* correlation exists between high-density lipoprotein (HDL) cholesterol and gallstone prevalence. In contrast, there is a very strong *positive* correlation between plasma triglyceride concentrations especially when combined with low HDL-cholesterol levels and gallstone prevalence.

Diet. Increased intake of calories, refined carbohydrate (sucrose, etc), cholesterol, and saturated fats have all been postulated to cause cholesterol gallstones. Patients with cholesterol gallstones secrete a greater fraction of dietary cholesterol into bile than normal subjects. A diet high in bran has been reported to decrease biliary cholesterol saturation and potentially prevent stones. However, there is no conclusive evidence, with the exceptions of obesity and weight loss, that dietary habits influence cholesterol gallstone formation.

Spinal cord injury. Patients with spinal cord injury have a 10% incidence of forming gallstones within the first year after injury. This high risk, which is 20 times normal, is believed to be secondary to abnormal gallbladder motility and probably biliary hypersecretion of cholesterol from the progressive reduction in body mass.

Primary biliary cirrhosis. Patients with primary biliary cirrhosis have an increased prevalence of gallstones. Stone analysis has not been performed, but the elevated cholesterol saturation of bile in these patients suggest that they form cholesterol stones. The underlying pathophysiologic defects are not known.

Diabetes mellitus. Despite obesity and increased total body cholesterol synthesis and decreased gallbladder motility seen in patients with diabetes, diabetes mellitus, per se, does not appear to be an independent risk factor for cholesterol gallstone disease. Studies describing such a correlation have failed to control for ethnic origin (e.g., American Indian), obesity, and hypertriglyceridemia.

Pigment gallstones

Chronic hemolysis. Inherited hemolytic anemias, sickle-cell disease, spherocytosis, thalassemia, chronic hemolysis associated with artificial heart valves, and malaria dramatically increase the risk of pigment stone formation because of increased biliary secretion of total bilirubin conjugates, especially bilirubin monoglucuronide at the expense of the bilirubin diglucuronides. The monoglucuronide is more easily hydrolyzed to unconjugated bilirubin in sterile bile than bilirubin diglucuronide, the predominant conjugate in healthy individuals.

Alcoholic cirrhosis. Patients with alcoholic cirrhosis have an increased prevalence of pigment gallstones, which is positively correlated with age and severity of liver disease. Thirty percent to 60% of alcoholic cirrhotics have gallstones, almost half of which are black pigment stones. The precise pathophysiologic defects have not been identified, but subclinical hemolysis, defective bilirubin conjugation, alcohol-induced biliary secretion of unconjugated bilirubin into bile, and/or defective bile salt synthesis associated with liver disease have all been suggested.

Age. Increasing age is a risk factor for both hemolytic and nonhemolytic pigment gallstone formation in high risk patients as well as the general population without any obvious risk factor for pigment stones. In fact, gallstones that recur after several cycles of successful gallstone dissolution appear to be age-related pigment stones.

Ileal disease, resection, and bypass. Patients with ileal dysfunction have a strikingly increased risk for developing gallstones. Provided the ileum is involved, gallstones develop in approximately 30% to 50% of patients with Crohn's disease; the risk correlates positively with the extent and duration of ileal dysfunction. Although ileal disease or resection leads to cholesterol supersaturation and cholesterol stone formation in some patients, careful studies now show that most patients with ileal dysfunction form black pigment, not cholesterol stones.

Biliary infection. In the Orient, brown pigment stones are frequently found in the intrahepatic bile ducts and are always associated with infection by colonic organisms (usually *Escherichia coli*) or parasitic infestation (*Clonorchis sinensis, Ascaris lumbricoides,* or other helminths). In Western patients, intraductal stones developing after cholecystectomy are invariably associated with bile stasis, biliary tree infection, and/or retained suture material. Diverticula near the ampulla of Vater are associated with pigment gallstones in the bile ducts, presumably because the colonized diverticulum alters ampullary muscular tone and allows the biliary tract to become repeatedly infected with anerobic bacteria.

Gallbladder stasis. Impaired gallbladder emptying is an essential early defect in both cholesterol and pigment gallstone formation. In cholesterol stone disease, gallbladder stasis occurs in women during pregnancy, in patients with somatastatinoma, or those receiving octreotide therapy, low fat-hypocaloric diets, and with spinal cord injury. Furthermore, increased fasting and residual gallbladder volumes have been demonstrated in the majority (70%) of white patients with gallstones.

For pigment stone disease, TPN is a powerful risk factor for gallstone formation. In one study, 100% of patients on TPN for longer than 6 weeks develop "biliary sludge" in their gallbladder. Routine ultrasonographic screening of adults on TPN for a mean of 23 months demonstrated that stones developed in 25% without and 39% with ileal disease. Gallstones form during TPN because of decreased gallbladder motility from lack of meal stimulated cholecystokinin (CCK) release, resulting in increased fasting and residual volumes. The daily intravenous administration of CCK-octapeptide (via the existing central venous catheter) in patients receiving TPN corrects the motility defect and prevents stone formation. A similar, though less severe, defect occurs after vagotomy and is associated with a threefold to fivefold increased risk of gallstone formation. Stone composition in patients after vagotomy has not been determined.

DIAGNOSTIC TESTS FOR BILIARY TRACT STONES

Calcified stones are visualized as radiopaque shadows in the right upper quadrant in supine, upright, and lateral abdominal films. Since 85% of stones are radiolucent, they are visualized only with an oral cholecystogram or by abdominal ultrasonography (see later). If radiopaque gallstones are seen elsewhere in the gut and/or air is present in the biliary tree, a spontaneous cholecystoenteric fistula should be suspected. If these patients have symptoms of intestinal obstruction, with air-fluid levels and dilated loops of small bowel, gallstone ileus is the most likely diagnosis. Air within the biliary system can also be seen in patients with an incompetent sphincter of Oddi, penetration of a chronic duodenal ulcer, or cholangitis with gas-forming organisms. In free perforation of the gallbladder, both gallstones and air may be seen free in the peritoneal cavity.

The time-honored radiologic examination of the gallbladder, oral cholecystography, has virtually been replaced by ultrasonography. Its major remaining use is to document gallbladder function in patients for whom medical dissolution therapy is contemplated. It is also used if ultrasound is technically not feasible. If the gallbladder is well visualized after ingestion of iopanoic acid the evening before, radiolucent stones may be detected (Fig. 65-2). Visualization of small stones may be enhanced by fatty food ingestion, which causes the gallbladder to contract. A number of factors such as gastric retention, vomiting, malabsorption, diarrhea, poor hepatic function, hyperbilirubinemia, and rarely, congenital absence of the gallbladder, may result in nonvisualization in the absence of gallbladder disease.

Abdominal real-time ultrasonography reveals gallbladder stones as small as 3 mm in 95% to 97% of patients. The precision of ultrasonic examination exceeds that of oral cholecystography. The diagnosis of gallstones with the use of ultrasonography is certain when (1) the stone is within the gallbladder, (2) the stone is mobile, and (3) it casts an acoustic shadow (Fig. 65-3). By this means, a solitary gallstone can be differentiated from the less common adenomyoma of the gallbladder. Because x-rays are not involved and because radiocontrast agents occasionally induces toxic or allergic reactions, we believe that ultrasonography should be the initial examination of choice for stones in the gallbladder and biliary tree in both acute and nonacute situations.

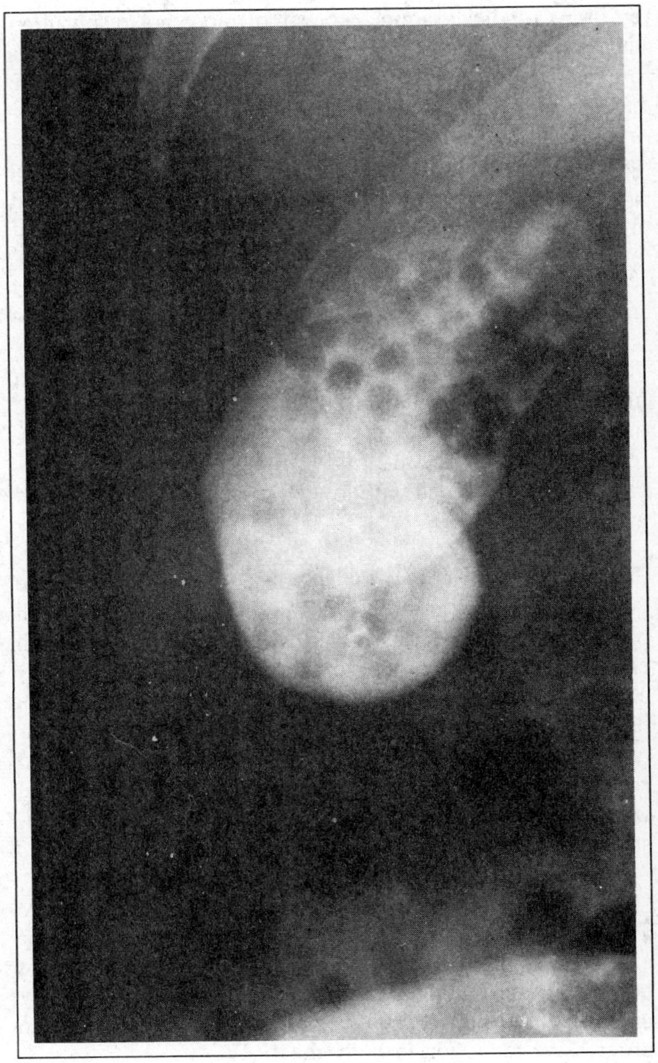

Fig. 65-2. Oral cholecystogram. Opacified gallbladder with multiple radiolucencies due to gallstones. The gallbladder has a phrygian cap (a common anomaly), giving rise to the double density.

Occasionally, ultrasonography gives false-negative results. If the clinical suspicion remains high, oral cholecystography should be administered.

The ultrasonographic examination, but not oral cholecystography, can detect "biliary sludge," multiple weak echoes without acoustic shadowing in the dependent part of the gallbladder. Biliary sludge is a mixture of mucin glycoproteins and microprecipitates of calcium (hydrogen) bilirubinate, liquid crystals of bile lipids, solid cholesterol monohydrate crystals, and microspheroliths of crystalline calcium carbonate or phosphate. Biliary sludge can form during prolonged fasting in debilitated hospitalized patients, during TPN, in the postoperative period, in patients with

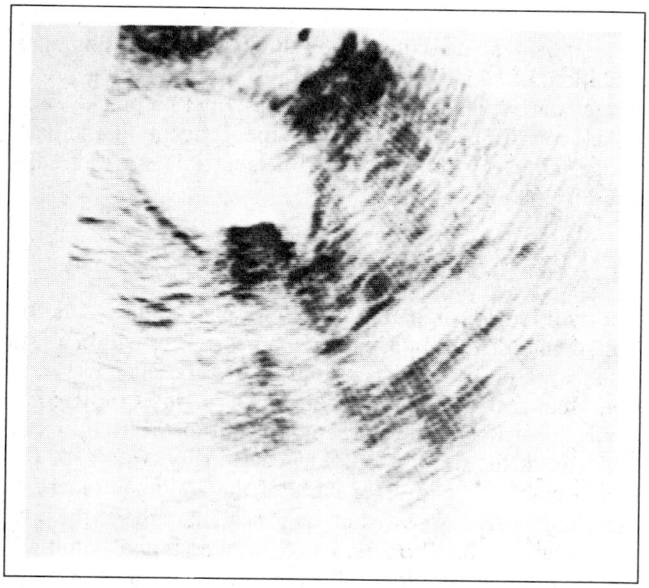

Fig. 65-3. Ultrasonogram demonstrating a large gallstone in a dilated gallbladder. Note acoustic shadowing.

extrahepatic biliary obstruction, and in 40% of women during the last trimester of pregnancy.

Ultrasonographic examination may also demonstrate intraductal stones and/or dilatation of the intrahepatic or extrahepatic ductal systems. Although false-positive results are considered rare, the impression that the duct is normal may be in error in about 15% of cases. Obstruction may not correlate with dilatation of intrahepatic ducts because cirrhosis or cholangitis may have caused scarring, thereby preventing ductal dilatation. Furthermore, small stones in a greatly dilated duct are easily missed.

For radionuclide scanning, a ^{99m}Tc-labeled iminodiacetic acid derivative (usually DISIDA) is injected intravenously. The isotope is efficiently extracted by the liver and secreted into the biliary tree even when serum bilirubin levels are 10 to 20 mg/dl. Surface counting of the gamma emission from the radionuclide source outlines the biliary tree, including the gallbladder, and demonstrates flow into the duodenum. Cholescintigraphy effectively excludes acute cholecystitis if the gallbladder is demonstrated. If the gallbladder is not visualized but the radionuclide scan demonstrates patency of the biliary tree and free flow into the duodenum, the diagnosis of cholecystitis is very likely in the appropriate clinical setting.

Endoscopic retrograde cholangiopancreatography (ERCP) permits visualization of the biliary tree by retrograde injection of radiographic contrast material directly into the common duct after cannulation at the ampulla via a flexible fiberoptic duodenoscope (Chapter 30). ERCP is the diagnostic procedure of choice for evaluating the bile ducts. It also allows visualization of the periampullary region of the duodenum and the pancreatic duct. Most important, therapeutic maneuvers, such as stone extraction, sphincterotomy, stent placement, can be performed via this approach (Chapter 30).

Transhepatic cholangiography is now reserved for patients whose bile ducts cannot be visualized by ERCP. Major complications are rare but include hemorrhage, cholangitis, and bile peritonitis.

Duodenal drainage can be useful in searching for occult gallstone disease when the patient's symptoms are typical but results of the other tests are negative or equivocal. A sample of gallbladder bile is obtained via a duodenal tube after the patient is given a substance (preferably cholecystokinin octapeptide) intravenously that contracts the gallbladder. The bile samples and the centrifuged sediments should be examined with a polarizing microscope. The presence of flat, rhombohedral birefringent plates with notched corners and angles of approximately 79 and 101 degrees is diagnostic of cholesterol monohydrate crystals (Plate II-26). These crystals are never observed in normal bile. Calcium bilirubinate forms amorphous, birefringent, golden-yellow precipitates (Plate II-26) and, when present, suggests pigment or pigmented cholesterol stones. Rounded "cart-wheel" birefringent crystals that are not compressible are pathognomonic for inorganic calcium, especially carbonate salts. They are often present with calcified cholesterol or black pigment gallstones. Birefringent liquid crystals of cholesterol esters and methyl sterol esters in bile are observed only with cholesterolosis of the gallbladder. The microscopic identification of these precipitates in bile requires considerable skill and experience. When found in association with a suggestive clinical history, crystals or precipitates indicate the presence of biliary tract stones or cholesterolosis. False-positive tests, however, have been reported in patients with hepatic and non-stone-related pancreatic diseases.

NATURAL HISTORY OF ASYMPTOMATIC VERSUS SYMPTOMATIC GALLSTONES

Asymptomatic (silent) gallstones are detected during routine screening or diagnostic evaluation of chest or abdominal pain with a more obvious etiology. Recent epidemiologic evidence from large well-designed ultrasonographic screening studies in various parts of the world suggests that up to 80% of whites with "silent" stones have never experienced biliary pain or complications. Ultrasonographic screening of a young population (2 to 18 years) with sickle cell anemia has demonstrated that although the prevalence of black pigment gallstones increases from approximately 10% in the 2- to 4-year-old age group to over 40% in the 15- to 18-year-old age group, only 22% of those with gallstones or sludge have biliary symptoms.

Recent data from typical Western populations suggest that the truly asymptomatic gallstone patient runs a relatively benign course, with only a 15% cumulative chance of developing symptoms over a 15-year period. In contrast, the mildly symptomatic patient (i.e., biliary pain not requiring hospitalization and no disruption of life-style) has a less benign course. These patients have a 20% chance of developing symptoms and complications over a 5-year period. Patients who are initially hospitalized for biliary pain have a greater than 50% chance of developing recurrent symptoms or complications over the next 20 years.

Gallstones may occasionally disappear. In about 7% of patients with multiple gallstones, but in less than 1% of patients with solitary cholesterol stones, the stones disappear spontaneously over a 10-year follow-up period, presumably via common bile duct migration into the duodenum. Spontaneous dissolution of stones is very rare.

Because of the benign course of patients with asymptomatic gallstones, the consensus of internists and surgeons is for expectant management only. A recent decision analysis demonstrated that prophylactic cholecystectomy for men with asymptomatic gallstones resulted in a *loss* of from 4 to 18 days of life expectancy depending on age. We advise these patients that they have a 10% to 30% chance of becoming symptomatic over the next 20 years, and they should be reevaluated only if symptoms occur.

Prophylactic cholecystectomy should be considered for several groups of patients with asymptomatic gallstones. One group is patients whose occupations require that they live for prolonged time periods in areas deficient in adequate medical facilities. In the past, because patients with diabetes who developed acute cholecystitis were thought to have a mortality rate as high as 15%, prophylactic cholecystectomies were recommended. Recent series suggest that other associated conditions, such as cardiovascular disease, are responsible for this increased mortality. Nonetheless, patients with diabetes are disproportionately represented in series of deaths from gallstone disease. Despite a decision analysis concluding that prophylactic cholecystectomy in patients with diabetes shortened life span from 2 to 8 months regardless of patient age, the issue remains unsettled. We believe that the presence of diabetes per se is not an indication for prophylactic cholecystectomy. Because patients with nonfunctioning gallbladders have a worse long-term course, however, we recommend prophylactic cholecystectomy for a diabetic with a nonfunctioning gallbladder by oral cholecystography. Gallbladder carcinoma is etiologically associated with gallstones and/or lithogenic bile, but its incidence in whites is very low (Chapter 66). Therefore, prophylactic cholecystectomy to prevent gallbladder carcinoma in asymptomatic stone patients is not recommended, except in two subgroups who have a fourfold to sevenfold increased risk: (1) American Indian women and (2) patients with solitary stones that exceed 3.0 cm in diameter. Dissolution therapy with ursodiol (see later) would be inappropriate in these settings, as the gallstones per se may not necessarily be the causative or even the promoting factor.

Four rare conditions require cholecystectomy even in the absence of gallstones because of the proven risk of gallbladder cancer: (1) gallbladder with a calcified wall ("porcelain" gallbladder), (2) gallbladder polyps >12 mm in absence of hyperplastic cholesterolosis in the remainder of the gallbladder, (3) anomalous pancreaticobiliary ductal junction, and (4) chronic *Salmonella typhosa* carriers.

The natural history of biliary sludge is variable. In many patients, biliary sludge in the gallbladder is innocuous and disappears soon after pregnancy or oral refeeding of the fasting patient. In others, however, biliary sludge may cause biliary pain, acute cholecystitis, or pancreatitis. The evolution of biliary sludge to gallstones has been documented during TPN, rapid weight loss, after pregnancy, and spinal cord injury and supports the concept that biliary sludge represents an early but still reversible stage of gallstone formation.

BILIARY "COLIC"

The traditional designation for biliary pain, biliary colic, is a misnomer. The pain usually becomes severe within a few minutes of onset and is constant (i.e., does not wax and wane like that of intestinal colic). The pain is most commonly located in either the epigastrium or the right upper quadrant at the time of onset. Occasionally, (<5% of patients) pain is felt in other parts of the abdomen or chest. Simultaneously referred pain in the scapular area or the posterior chest wall is common, as are nausea and vomiting, which often occur within 30 minutes of the onset of pain. Pain is usually intense for 1 to 4 hours and then resolves slowly, leaving the patient with a vague residual ache or soreness. As with renal "colic," the patient may have great difficulty lying still.

The timing of biliary colic is unpredictable, but the patient with known gallstones often associates its onset with the ingestion of a large or rich meal. Attacks may occur only once, every few years, or, in rare patients, daily. Patients with frequent episodes of pain should expect that pattern to continue in the future. It is believed that biliary pain is caused (1) by gallbladder contraction during transient cystic duct obstruction by a gallstone or (2) by common duct contraction during passage of a stone. Because pain is as common in patients with large solitary stones as in patients with multiple stones, however, it may also be related to stones in the infundibulum of the gallbladder or even to viscous mucus obstructing the neck of the gallbladder. Resolution occurs once the stone drops back into the fundus of the gallbladder or migrates out of the common duct into the duodenum. Fatty food intolerance, belching, postprandial bloating, "flatulent dyspepsia," heartburn, regurgitation, or painless nausea and vomiting do not correlate at all with the presence of gallstones, are more likely to have other causes, and are rarely relieved permanently by cholecystectomy.

Physical examination of a patient during an attack of biliary pain is usually normal or reveals only mild right upper quadrant tenderness. Fever or leukocytosis is absent; if they are present, acute cholecystitis should seriously be suspected.

Diagnosis

Ultrasonography is the test of choice for the diagnosis of gallstones in the acute setting. For technically inadequate ultrasonography, single- or double-dose oral cholecystography may be performed. As indicated earlier, up to 5% of adequately opacified gallbladders and technically valid ultrasonograms are falsely negative, either because the stones are too small, because they are the same density as the contract medium, or because they have migrated into the duodenum by the time of examination. In these patients, microscopy of an aliquot of bile obtained by duodenal drainage to look for crystals or precipitates may provide the only clue that gallstone disease is present (Plate II-26).

Other common causes of abdominal pain should be considered in the differential diagnosis of biliary pain, including peptic ulcer disease, lobar pneumonia, alcoholic hepatitis, pancreatitis, and radicular pain caused by spinal lesions that may mimic biliary colic. Just as biliary colic may occasionally (~ 5 percent of patients) be felt only in the precordium, angina pectoris may cause pain in the abdomen, usually a subxiphoid location, and may be associated with nausea, heartburn, and regurgitation. A common cause for recurrent nonspecific dyspeptic symptoms, including abdominal pain, is the irritable colon syndrome; but the pain is usually located in the left upper or lower quadrant, and bowel habits are usually abnormal. Other forms of abdominal pain, such as that of renal colic, intestinal colic, and pain that occurs in the early phase of acute appendicitis, are usually readily distinguishable from biliary pain by their location and character.

Treatment

Patients with more than one attack of biliary pain should be treated definitively to prevent (1) future attacks of biliary pain and (2) the complications of gallstones, including acute cholecystitis, cholangitis, and pancreatitis.

Although still the "gold" standard for gallstone disease, cholecystectomy via a subcostal incision is no longer the only therapy. Several surgical and medical treatment options are now available.

Cholecystectomy. Cholecystectomy is the treatment of choice for the majority of patients with biliary pain from gallstones. The operation relieves symptoms in greater than 85% of individuals. In the vast majority of the others, cholecystectomy fails because the operation was performed for inappropriate symptoms. Elective, traditional (open) cholecystectomy is very safe. Mortality is related to age, sex, preexisting medical conditions, and nature of the operation (emergency for complications or elective).

The National Halothane Study of 27,600 cholecystectomies performed in the early 1960s revealed operative mortality for elective procedures in women in moderately good health ranged from 0.05% below the age of 50 to 0.3% at age 70. Severe concomitant disease increased operative mortality to 1.3% and 1.7%, respectively. In all categories, men had roughly twice the operative mortality probably because of a higher prevalence of "silent" cardiovascular disease. Operative mortality doubled with emergency operations and quadrupled when the common bile duct was explored. The most serious morbidity was due to bile duct injury, occurring in 0.2% of patients. Recent surveys in the 1980s suggest that overall US mortality and morbidity is < 1% and < 5%, respectively.

Laparoscopic cholecystectomy has almost replaced open cholecystectomy, with up to 85% of elective operations being performed via this approach. However, no randomized studies have compared the safety of the two approaches. Clear advantages of laparoscopic cholecystectomy include: (1) far smaller scars, (2) reduced hospital stay (1 to 2 vs 5 to 6 days), and (3) earlier return to normal activities (7 vs 40 to 60 days). There is probably a higher rate of bile duct injury (0.8%) during laparoscopic than during traditional cholecystectomy but less overall morbidity. A relative contraindication is adhesions from previous abdominal surgery, which may prevent clear visibility of the gallbladder bed.

Cholecystectomy causes no digestive sequelae other than postprandial diarrhea or softer bowel movements in about 1% of patients. There is no malabsorption of fat and no special diet is ever indicated. Earlier epidemiologic evidence suggested that cholecystectomy doubles the risk of developing right-sided colonic cancer; however, recent studies deny this association. For the minority of patients who continue to experience abdominal discomfort after cholecystectomy, the term *postcholecystectomy syndrome* has been used. This is an unfortunate term, as it implies that symptoms occur only as a consequence of the operation. Many patients with this label, however, simply have persisting preoperative discomfort and/or pain. Thus the clinician must distinguish among postoperative complications such as bile duct injury, adhesions, or retained stones, and misdiagnosed preoperative diseases such as irritable bowel syndrome, neoplasms, peptic ulcers, and pancreatitis.

Medical dissolution therapy. The naturally occurring bile acid, ursodeoxycholic acid (ursodiol, Actigall) dissolves cholesterol gallstones by decreasing biliary cholesterol secretion and desaturating bile. Cholesterol molecules from the surfaces of gallstones are redissolved in newly desaturated micellar or vesicular solution.

Treatment with ursodiol is appropriate for mildly symptomatic patients with small, noncalcified cholesterol gallbladder stones. Additionally, selected patients who refuse or who are poor surgical candidates may be treated with ursodiol. Treatment with ursodiol is limited critically by the character and sizes of stones and severity of symptoms. The major disadvantages are that gallstones dissolve slowly (1 mm in diameter per month) and will recur in 50% of patients within 5 years of successful dissolution.

Before initiating ursodiol treatment, stone size, number, and calcium content must be determined by ultrasonography or OCG and abdominal flat plate. Small (<10 mm), noncalcified stones can be treated with 8 mg/kg of ursodiol administered in divided doses in the morning and at bedtime. Reassessment of stone size by either oral cholecystography (OCG) or ultrasonography after 6 months of therapy is the only specific follow-up required. Although a nonopacified gallbladder on initial OCG is *not* a poor prognostic sign, a nonvisualized OCG at follow-up predicts failure. Therapy should be discontinued if the patient develops a nonvisualized OCG or shows lack of dissolution at follow-up. Ursodiol should be continued for 3 months after complete stone dissolution has been confirmed by ultrasonography, not OCG. Frequent attacks of biliary pain occur rarely during dissolution therapy and surgery may be required.

After complete dissolution, patients should be reevaluated for recurrent gallstones only if biliary tract symptoms recur. Surveillance ultrasonography is not recommended. Maintenance therapy with either low-dose ursodiol, or a low-cholesterol, high-fiber diet, may prevent gallstone recurrence; but conclusive evidence is lacking. Ursodiol is remarkably free of side effects and, unlike its predecessor, chenodiol, does not cause hepatic injury, diarrhea, or elevation of serum cholesterol. Patients should be advised, however, that the drug is expensive and that a second course of therapy for symptomatic recurrence may be required.

Lithotripsy. Extracorporeal shock wave lithotripsy (ESWL) is still investigational. It should be used only in conjunction with ursodiol treatment to accelerate dissolution of cholesterol stones. The focusing of shock waves onto gallstones causes fragmentation, transforming a large stone into myriads of small stones and fragments, which then either migrate into the duodenum without obstruction or dissolve more rapidly in ursodiol-induced unsaturated bile. Mildly symptomatic patients with a single lucent 1 to 2 cm stone in a functioning gallbladder are the best candidates for combination ESWL and ursodiol therapy. They have an 80% to 90% chance of complete stone and fragment dissolution after ESWL and 1 year of ursodiol therapy. ESWL has limited overall applicability, as only 10% to 15% of gallstone patients will have a solitary noncalcified stone. Severe side effects of ESWL are uncommon and are related to transient obstruction of the cystic or common bile ducts resulting in acute cholecystitis or pancreatitis in 3% and 1%, respectively, usually within 48 hours of ESWL. Moreover, biliary pain occurs in 30% to 70% of patients during the first 3 months after lithotripsy.

Contact solvent dissolution. Methyl tert butyl ether (MTBE) is being evaluated for direct contact dissolution of gallbladder stones. It is a powerful cholesterol solvent that, when repeatedly instilled into the gallbladder via a percutaneous transhepatic catheter, dissolves cholesterol stones in 2 to 8 hours. In skilled hands, complications and side effects appear to be few and principally involve biliary leakage on withdrawal of the catheter. Because both inorganic and organic calcium salts and mucin glycoproteins of stones are insoluble in MTBE, many patients are left with biliary sludge containing calcium salts at the end of therapy. MTBE is still investigational, and its use is confined to a small number of skilled centers. This therapy should be reserved for patients who are very symptomatic but not amenable to ursodiol treatment or surgery.

Specific treatment recommendations. Patients with biliary pain should be treated in the following ways:

1. Young (<50 years of age) patients with *recurrent* attacks of biliary pain who are otherwise in good health should undergo elective cholecystectomy, as the operative risk is small (<0.1%). Fifty percent of these patients will continue to have attacks of pain or will develop complications of their gallstones during the next 20 years if not treated. They will have significantly higher operative risks at that time. Oral dissolution therapy with ursodiol has little role in healthy, young symptomatic patients.
2. Patients with diabetes should undergo elective cholecystectomy after only *one* episode of biliary pain before they develop complications of gallstones. These patients have an increased operative mortality for complications of gallstones, but not for elective cholecystectomy.
3. The management of nondiabetic patients after a single episode of biliary pain is controversial. In young, otherwise healthy patients, cholecystectomy is reasonable. An expectant watch-and-wait approach to observe the frequency of attacks and to confirm that they are due to gallstones is equally reasonable. Patients with small, radiolucent stones, especially if they developed during weight loss, recent pregnancy, or use of medications, would be ideal candidates for ursodiol therapy during the period of observation. In older patients, concomitant medical problems that increase operative mortality and reduce life expectancy make the treatment decision more difficult. The physician must balance the risks of deferring treatment and possibly performing emergent rather than elective surgery, versus the chance that the patient will remain asymptomatic and die from other causes.
4. Patients who refuse surgery can be treated only with expectant management or, possibly, medical therapy.

Prevention of gallstones

Patients receiving TPN for greater than 3 months not only invariably develop biliary sludge in their gallbladders, but also have more complications than would be expected in conventional populations with cholelithiasis. Therefore prophylactic medical therapy with daily administration of intravenous cholecystokinin-octapeptide (CCK-OP), which prevents gallbladder stasis, sludge, and gallstone formation, is indicated.

Standard ursodiol (8 to 10 mg/kg/day) administration during the period of rapid weight loss prevents stone formation. A lower ursodiol dose, or the oral intake of at least 10 g/day of long-chained triglyceride (i.e., corn, olive, or canola oil) may be effective and are being evaluated in clinical trials. Whether there is sufficient risk of gallstone formation in patients undergoing more moderate weight loss to justify ursodiol prophylaxis is unknown.

COMPLICATIONS OF GALLSTONES

Cholecystitis

Ninety-five percent of episodes of acute inflammation of the gallbladder are associated with obstruction of the cystic duct by a gallstone. Stone impaction, chemical inflammation, and superimposed bacterial infection occur in sequence. Early in the course of acute cholecystitis, the bile may be sterile (50%), but within a few days bacteria can be cultured from the bile of nearly all patients. Bacterial infection is responsible for all the serious sequelae of acute cholecystitis, particularly empyema and perforation. Acalculous cholecystitis, which accounts for approximately 5% of cases, most often occurs in the severely ill and is associated with trauma, operative procedures, extensive burns, immobility, and prolonged fasting. Although the etiology is unknown, it is probably caused by occlusion of the cystic duct with biliary sludge. Less commonly, acalculous cholecystitis is related to parasitic infestation of the gallbladder *(Clonorchis sinensis, Ascaris lumbricoides, Fasciola hepatica),* diabetes mellitus, torsion of the gallbladder, and vasculitis. The outcome for patients with acalculous cholecystitis is generally worse than for patients with gallstone cholecystitis, as perforation, empyema, and gangrene of the gallbladder often complicate the clinical picture in a patient already in a perilous medical state.

Pathology. The pathologic changes in the gallbladder during the evolution of acute cholecystitis reflect the duration of cystic duct obstruction and superimposed bacterial inflammation. The earliest pathologic findings are erythema and edema with a fibrinosuppurative exudate. Histologically, there is subserosal edema, hemorrhage, and inflammatory infiltration, which progress to mucosal ulcerations within a few days. In rapid sequence, mural gangrene and abscess formation may ensue. If the acute process resolves, collagen deposits appear in about 1 to 2 weeks. Eventually, the gallbladder becomes contracted and scarred around the enclosed gallstones, and a thick, pale wall forms. Because this lesion represents the healed stage of acute cholecystitis, it is not correct to label the condition chronic cholecystitis.

Empyema, by definition, indicates that the gallbladder is filled with pus, and results from suppurative cholecystitis. Its development often heralds gangrene of the gallbladder and/or perforation, which occurs most often at the fundus. When perforation occurs elsewhere, it is often the result of direct erosion by an impacted stone at the infundibulum. Because the greater omentum may become adherent to an acutely inflamed gallbladder, perforation may result in a pericholecystic abscess. If the inflamed gallbladder becomes adherent to an adjacent hollow viscus (usually the duodenum), a cholecystoenteric fistula may result. More commonly, perforation leads to free spillage of bile into the peritoneal cavity and bile peritonitis. Rarely, following chronic obstruction of the cystic duct, hydrops (mucocele) of the gallbladder develops.

Clinical findings. The patient with acute cholecystitis experiences initial symptoms typical of biliary colic. Because 80% of patients have previously experienced biliary colic, they may believe that this abdominal pain is caused by a repeat attack; however, the symptoms do not abate with time. As inflammation progresses, the pain becomes more severe and becomes localized in the right upper quadrant. Referred pain may radiate to the middle of the back, to the right infrascapular area, or to the right shoulder. As in biliary colic, the patient is often restless; but in contrast to biliary colic, the intensity of the pain in acute cholecystitis is affected by movement, including respiration. The severity of pain varies from patient to patient; in some, particularly those with diabetes, the aged, and patients receiving corticosteroids, pain may be minimal or absent.

Anorexia, nausea, and occasionally vomiting begin soon after the onset of acute cholecystitis. Fever is usually low grade (99.5 to 101.3° F, 37.5 to 38.5° C); in the elderly, fever may be the only clinical sign of acute cholecystitis. High fever and chills suggest a septic complication. In acute cholecystitis unassociated with choledocholithiasis, mild jaundice may develop due to edema of the nearby common bile duct and diffusion of bilirubin across the inflamed gallbladder mucosa. Nonetheless, hyperbilirubinemia of any magnitude in this setting should raise the possibility of choledocholithiasis.

In uncomplicated acute cholecystitis, bowel sounds may be diminished, and tenderness in the right upper quadrant of the abdomen or epigastrium is striking; palpation of the right upper quadrant may sharply aggravate pain and produce transient inspiratory arrest (Murphy's sign). A distended, tender gallbladder may be palpable in one third of patients, which suggests a first episode, as repeated attacks result in a scarred, nondistensible gallbladder. In the majority of patients, acute cholecystitis subsides spontaneously. Improvement is often noticeable within the first day or two, and the signs and symptoms gradually disappear in 1 to 4 days. If symptoms persist longer or increase in severity, the potential for perforation, gangrene, empyema, cholangitis, and septic shock requires prompt surgical therapy.

Laboratory findings and diagnostic tests. During acute cholecystitis, the leukocyte count is usually mildly elevated to 10,000 to 15,000/ml but may be higher. Serum transaminases and alkaline phosphatase may rise to two to four times normal, and bilirubin to 4 mg/dl. Dramatic hyperbilirubinemia and alkaline phosphatase elevations strongly suggest choledocholithiasis. Serum amylase may be elevated if stones pass through the common bile duct, with or without associated pancreatitis, or if vomiting is severe. Supine and upright abdominal films may demonstrate gallstones, an enlarged gallbladder, or air in the biliary system or peritoneal cavity. Ultrasonographic examination is the quickest, simplest, and most reliable method of determining the presence or absence of stones. Lack of visualization of the gallbladder with opacification of the common bile duct by ^{99m}Tc DISIDA cholescintigraphy strongly suggests the diagnosis in the proper clinical setting.

Differential diagnosis. In most patients, the presence of right upper quadrant abdominal pain and tenderness, nausea, vomiting, and mild fever permits an accurate clinical diagnosis. Myocardial infarction or angina pectoris may mimic acute cholecystitis. An electrocardiogram may enable the physician to differentiate between these conditions, but T-wave inversions in the inferior leads may be associated with acute cholecystitis. The symptoms of pancreatitis may resemble cholecystitis, but the patient with pancreatitis usually has more intense nausea and vomiting, with epigastric and periumbilical pain penetrating through to the back. Serum or urinary amylase concentrations may be increased in both conditions. Lipemic serum and hypocalcemia also suggest pancreatitis, but cholecystitis and pancreatitis occasionally occur simultaneously. Acute appendicitis may mimic cholecystitis, but pain in appendicitis is usually localized to the right lower quadrant. Acute alcoholic hepatitis may cause diagnostic confusion, especially if incidental calcified gallstones are present. A history of recent alcohol abuse, more diffuse nonspecific abdominal symptoms, marked hepatomegaly, and other physical and laboratory findings of chronic liver disease may help to distinguish between these two entities. Finally, both pyelonephritis and pneumonia can present with abdominal pain and simulate acute cholecystitis, so urinalysis and chest x-ray films should be obtained in all patients.

Treatment. In the majority of patients with cholecystitis, as with recurrent biliary colic, the treatment of choice is early surgery. With early surgery, the hazards of an emergency operation for worsening disease, the chances of missing a complication such as empyema or silent perforation; and the aggravation of preexisting cardiac, pulmonary, or renal disease can be reduced. Work absenteeism and the expenses associated with hospitalization for interval cholecystectomy (approximately 6 weeks) can also be greatly reduced. If patients are good surgical risks, a brief period of conservative therapy may be necessary for stabilization before cholecystectomy. In most cases, cholecystectomy can be scheduled as a routine procedure within 48 hours of hospitalization. The patient should receive intravenous fluid replacement to counter dehydration from vomiting and fasting, nasogastric suction to diminish hormonal stimuli to the biliary tree, sufficient analgesia to combat pain, and a third-generation cephalosporin. If sepsis or other complications supervene, a third-generation cephalosporin and an aminoglycoside should be administered intravenously, and the risks of surgery relative to the risks of continued delay must be assessed promptly. When emergency decompression becomes necessary, cholecystotomy, with evacuation of stones and pus followed by catheter drainage, may be the initial treatment of choice in such patients. Cholecystotomy is less risky than cholecystectomy and allows the acute infection to subside. Definitive surgery, however, is required 6 to 8 weeks later to remove the gallbladder to prevent a chronic mucous fistula and recurrent stone formation. Exploration of the common bile duct may also be necessary at the time of cholecystectomy if an intraoperative cholangiogram reveals ductal stones.

The natural history of patients with an episode of acute cholecystitis who do not undergo cholecystectomy is poor. Recurrences of biliary colic and complications are common, occurring in 50% of patients within 5 years. A nonfunctioning gallbladder by oral cholecystography doubles the risk of future complications in these patients.

Complications. The common complications of acute cholecystitis are empyema and perforation. Free perforation into the abdominal cavity may occur early in the course of cholecystitis and is associated with a high (approximately 30%) mortality rate, as it is often missed until bile peritonitis ensues. More often, perforation is localized by omental adhesions, producing a pericholecystic abscess, evident as a tender mass in the subhepatic region. Perforation into another hollow viscus (duodenum, colon, stomach, in that order) with fistula formation is less common. Many cholecystoenteric fistulas are discovered incidentally, as the acute perforation drains the gallbladder, relieving symptoms. However, cholecystocolonic fistulas may cause secretory diarrhea, fat malabsorption from diversion of bile, and profound bacterial contamination resulting in ascending cholangitis. A large gallstone ejected through a cholecystoduodenal fistula may obstruct the small intestine, causing gallstone ileus. Gallstone ileus should be suspected in the elderly and in patients with diabetes who present with acute, subacute, or intermittent small bowel obstruction. Abdominal x-ray films are typical of those seen in bowel obstruction and, in addition, reveal air in the biliary tree; in some cases a large, radiopaque gallstone may be evident in the right lower quadrant. The obstructing gallstones should be removed through an enterostomy. Cholecystectomy with repair of the fistula should be performed only if the patient subsequently has symptoms of biliary disease. Due to delay in making the diagnosis, the mortality of patients with gallstone ileus can be as high as 10% to 20%.

Choledocholithiasis

In Western countries, the vast majority of common duct stones have migrated from the gallbladder; consequently, most common duct stones are cholesterol stones. In patients younger than 60 years, the prevalence of common duct stones in association with gallbladder stones is about 8% to 15%. This prevalence increases to nearly 50% in patients aged 80 years and older. These data suggest that the longer stones are present in the gallbladder, the greater the likelihood they will migrate into the common bile duct. Nevertheless, most ductal stones are first discovered during exploration or intraoperative cholangiography at the time of cholecystectomy. Even after surgical exploration and removal of common duct stones, however, one or more stones, usually cholesterol, are left behind in 1% to 10% of patients. Stones that form in the duct (primary duct stones) are nearly always "brown" pigment stones. In the Western world, they are usually associated with cholangitis, which is often subclinical and caused by organisms producing beta-glucuronidase and other enzymes capable of hydrolyzing bile salts and lecithin (e.g., *E. coli*). Bile stasis caused by ductal obstruction contributes to their formation. Pigment stones in the ductal systems (often in the intrahepatic radicles) of Oriental patients with intact gallbladders is not uncommon, but this finding is rare in Western patients (see Table 65-1) except in those with sclerosing cholangitis. In the Orient, parasitic infestation, with accompanying bacterial infection, appears to be a major cause of choledocholithiasis.

Clinical findings. The natural history of choledocholithiasis is relatively benign in 50% of patients. Ten percent of patients with gallbladder stones pass them "silently" into the common duct and out into the intestines. In others, ductal stones are found incidentally during diagnostic evaluation or surgical exploration in patients with gallbladder stones. The natural history of stones that remain in the common bile duct is unpredictable and patients may present with (1) cholangitis, (2) intermittent or persistent obstructive jaundice with or without pain, (3) acute pancreatitis, and (4) biliary pain without other complications. Longstanding common bile duct obstruction with or without intermittent painless jaundice may lead to secondary biliary cirrhosis.

Patients with ascending nonsuppurative cholangitis may present with jaundice, biliary colic, and fever (Charcot's intermittent fever). The cholangitis is often transient or intermittent because most stones only partially obstruct the common bile duct. In a typical attack, a chill usually precedes fever and is followed by jaundice and dark urine from conjugated bilirubinuria. The pain is indistinguishable from that of classic biliary colic caused by gallbladder stones. Pain may be referred to the subxiphoid region, upper back, or shoulder and may be confused with that of pancreatitis, coronary disease, radicular neuritis, or lobar pneumonia. Usually, fever is moderate (100.4 to 102.2° F, 38 to 39° C), and pain and tenderness are localized to the right subcostal region. Symptoms usually subside within 24 to 48 hours with or without antibiotic administration, presumably because the stone is dislodged into a more capacious part of the common duct or is passed into the duodenum. The transient although often recurrent symptoms may not interfere with the patient's normal activities, so many patients first present after several weeks of mild recurrent fever. Most patients with jaundice due to choledocholithiasis do not have a palpable gallbladder because recurrent attacks of acute cholecystitis have left them with shrunken and fibrotic gallbladders. In contrast, patients who have a malignant process involving the distal biliary tree and who have not previously had cholecystitis usually have dilated and therefore palpable gallbladders (Courvoisier's law).

In acute suppurative cholangitis, ductal obstruction is usually complete, cholangitis is unremitting, and ductal contents are purulent. Mental confusion, lethargy, and bacteremic shock are common accompanying features and overshadow those of cholestasis. Fortunately, this form of acute cholangitis is rare. Because the overwhelming infection advances rapidly, emergency biliary drainage is essential. If delays occur, the patient may die from generalized sepsis and shock within a few hours, or inflammation may spread, giving rise to pericholangitis and multiple hepatic abscesses. The usual prognosis for neglected suppurative cholangitis, even with antibiotic treatment, is extremely poor.

Laboratory findings and diagnostic tests. In choledocholithiasis with or without cholangitis, the severity of jaundice varies, but serum bilirubin concentration is rarely greater than 15 mg/dl. Alkaline phosphatase, 5′-nucleotidase, and leucine aminopeptidase levels are substantially elevated, often paralleling serum bilirubin elevation. Hepatic transaminases are usually only mildly elevated to two or three times the upper limits of normal, but values as high as those reached in acute hepatitis are seen rarely, especially when there is associated ascending cholangitis. The leukocyte count is elevated to about 12,000 to 15,000 per milliliter, but may be much higher in suppurative cholangitis. Blood cultures are usually positive in patients with suppurative cholangitis. With suspected persistent cholangitis, diagnostic procedures should be few so that biliary tract drainage is not unduly delayed. In particular, if the patient is septic, with unequivocal signs and symptoms of suppurative cholangitis, prompt biliary tract decompression by endoscopic retrograde drainage and the administration of broad-spectrum antibiotics are desirable prior to definitive surgery. This approach has significantly reduced the mortality of acute suppurative cholangitis.

In contrast if the patient is clearly not septic and is stable, with or without evident obstructive jaundice, the investigation can proceed at a more measured pace. Ultrasonographic examination may show a dilated common bile duct with or without a stone. Its sensitivity is low (~25%), however, because cholangitis can occur without ductal dilatation. Furthermore, stones in the common duct are far more difficult to visualize by ultrasonography than are stones in the gallbladder. CT is useful only if ultrasonography is technically inadequate or a pancreatic neoplasm is suspected as causing the obstruction. ERCP is the definitive diagnostic test. If this test fails to demonstrate stones or duct dilatation, the stones have passed into the duodenum or the original diagnosis was in error.

Differential diagnosis. Differentiation among choledocholithiasis, benign biliary stricture, and periampullary and biliary neoplasms can, as a rule, be made with ERCP. In neoplastic biliary obstruction, jaundice is relatively painless, and ascending cholangitis is rare. The most important group of conditions that must be excluded are those that cause intrahepatic cholestasis, in which surgery is contraindicated. These conditions include drug-induced cholestasis, alcoholic hepatitis, viral hepatitis, and complications of pregnancy.

Therapy. Rehydration with intravenously administered fluids is often required, and broad-spectrum antibiotic treatment should be initiated promptly if there is evidence of cholangitis. Endoscopic sphincterotomy and drainage of the biliary tree is not only relatively safe and effective but also, in many, the only procedure that need be performed. For other patients, however, surgical exploration should be performed once the patient's condition is stable. The operative approach to definitive biliary decompression will depend on the nature of the ductal obstruction, and the presence or absence of the gallbladder. Before definitive surgery, the anatomy of the biliary tree and the nature of the ductal obstruction should be delineated by direct cholangiography, usually by ERCP. Patients with common bile duct stones and an intact gallbladder who are good operative candidates should undergo ERCP, sphincterotomy, and endoscopic removal of common duct stones followed promptly (1 to 2 days) by laparoscopic cholecystectomy.

Patients who are poor operative risks can be treated with sphincterotomy with removal of the common duct stone. With this treatment, they have only a 10% risk of developing subsequent cholecystitis of cholangitis. Patients with retained stones or newly formed stones after cholecystectomy should be treated by endoscopic sphincterotomy and stone extraction (Fig. 65-4). Even in those patients with a postoperative T tube, an endoscopic sphincterotomy rather than an attempt at Dormia basket retrieval via the T tube is preferable. The latter necessitates an 8- to 12-week wait for a fibrous tract to develop. Cholangitis or other complications could occur during this period. Endoscopic sphincterotomy is safe and effective, with a mortality rate of ~1% and a success rate of >85%. Relative contraindications include stones greater than 2 cm, bile duct stricture proximal to the ampulla, an ampulla situated in a duodenal diverticulum, and significant coagulopathy. ESWL (still investigational) to fragment large stones in the common bile duct coupled with endoscopic sphincterotomy will allow removal of almost all retained stones (Fig. 65-5). Surgical removal and exploration of the common bile duct should be considered as a last resort, but should be performed promptly if endoscopic sphincterotomy fails in a patient with an infected or obstructed biliary tree.

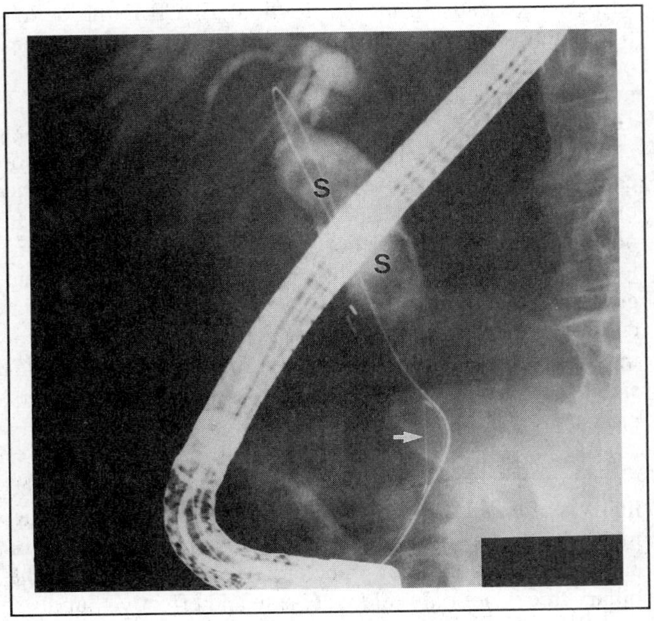

Fig. 65-4. ERCP. The endoscope is positioned in the duodenum. Contrast material has been introduced retrograde into the common bile duct. Radiolucent gallstones are demonstrated in the common bile duct. A sphincterotome is shown extending from the endoscope in preparation for a sphincterotomy at the site of the sphincter *(arrow)*. (Courtesy of Dr. David Carr-Locke, Boston.)

Attempted dissolution of retained common duct stones with T-tube infusion of cholesterol solvents, such as MTBE, monooctanoin (Capmul), or cholate is neither safe nor effective. Complete extraction of intrahepatic stones at ERCP may be technically impossible, especially in the brown pigment stone hepatolithiasis syndrome, in which proximal ductal strictures and cisternal dilatation are commonly present. Such patients may require choledochoduodenostomy or even hepatic lobectomy to ensure stone removal and adequate drainage of the intrahepatic biliary tree.

Gallstone pancreatitis

Evidence suggests that gallstones or biliary sludge migrating from the gallbladder through the common bile duct and into the duodenum can cause pancreatitis. The pathogenesis appears related to temporary impaction of a gallstone or biliary sludge in the common channel of the pancreatic and biliary ducts; the semipatent common channel allows activated pancreatic enzymes, bile, and lipid digestive products to reflux into the pancreas.

Although an acute attack of gallstone pancreatitis is indistinguishable from an episode of acute pancreatitis from any other cause, it carries a high (10%) mortality. However, gallstone pancreatitis, unlike alcoholic pancreatitis, rarely results in chronic pancreatitis or pancreatic insufficiency, even after recurrent attacks.

The diagnosis of gallstone pancreatitis is based on the finding of stones or sludge in the gallbladder or biliary tree in the presence of acute pancreatitis. The detection of gallstones by manual sieving or ultrasonographic examination of the feces is also diagnostic in the correct clinical setting. Furthermore, two thirds of patients with idiopathic pancreatitis have biliary precipitates found in samples of bile obtained by duodenal drainage and hence can be diagnosed as having gallstone pancreatitis. Therefore the search for these precipitates should be made before classifying the pancreatitis as idiopathic.

The immediate medical treatment of acute gallstone pancreatitis is the same as that for acute pancreatitis of any other etiology (Chapter 64). If the patient fails to improve within 24 to 48 hours, emergency ERCP and sphincterotomy are indicated to remove the impacted stone. An elective cholecystectomy and common bile duct exploration are recommended as soon as the patient recovers from an acute attack. If cholecystectomy is delayed, 25% of patients will experience another attack of potentially fatal acute pancreatitis within 30 days and 50% within 11 months. If biliary sludge alone is the cause, medical dissolution treatment with ursodiol is an acceptable alternative because it prevents recurrent attacks.

Cholesterolosis

This pathologic change in the gallbladder and cystic duct wall consists of submucosal macrophages filled with cholesterol esters and smaller amounts of free cholesterol,

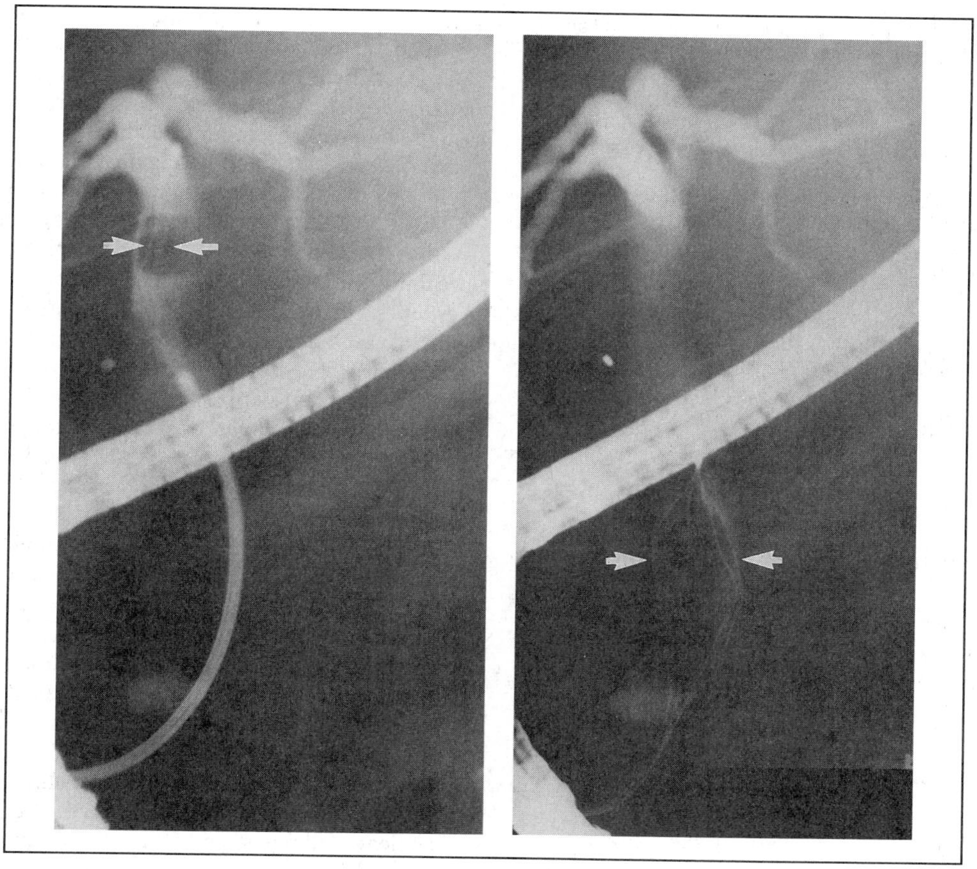

Fig. 65-5. An endoscopic sphincterotomy has been performed after visualization of the common bile duct via ERCP. Common bile duct stones are crushed and removed with the aid of a mechanical lithotriptor directed (*arrows*) into the common bile duct. (Courtesy of Dr. David Carr-Locke, Boston.)

triglycerides, fatty acids, and methyl sterols. The condition is extremely common, being found in up to 40% of gallbladders removed for uncomplicated gallstones, and is often the sole lesion at autopsy. The yellow pigmentation produced by cholesterol and methyl sterol esters on the red mucosal background produces an appearance similar to that of a ripe strawberry (strawberry gallbladder). The etiology is not clarified but appears to be secondary to enhanced transfer and esterification of lipids, particularly cholesterol, into the mucosa from bile. Grossly, the deposits are usually flat but may be raised and polypoid. If present as the sole gallbladder lesion, cholesterolosis usually causes no symptoms, although ill-defined episodic abdominal discomfort, which is probably unrelated, may occur. Oral cholecystography may be diagnostic if mucosal excrescences that do not move with change of position are present. More often, the oral cholecystogram is normal or exhibits decreased concentration of the contrast medium. The diagnosis may then be made if duodenal drainage is performed, followed by polarizing microscopy of the bile to look for birefringent liquid crystalline droplets composed of cholesterol esters. Relief of symptoms after cholecystectomy has been reported.

REFERENCES

Angelico M, DeSantis A, and Capocaccia L: Biliary sludge; a critical update, J Clin Gastroenterol 12:656-662, 1990.

Broomfield PH et al: Effects of ursodeoxycholic acid and aspirin on the formation of lithogenic bile and gallstones during loss of weight, N Engl J Med 319:1567-1572, 1988.

Cahalane MJ, Neubrand MW, and Carey MC: Physical-chemical pathogenesis of pigment gallstones, Semin Liver Dis 8:317-328, 1988.

Carey MC and LaMont JT: Cholesterol gallstone formation. 1. Physical chemistry of bile and biliary lipid secretion, Prog Liver Dis 10:139-163, 1992.

Friedman GD, Raviola CA, and Fireman B. Prognosis of gallstones with mild or no symptoms: 25 years of follow-up in a health maintenance organization, J Clin Epidemiol 42:127-136, 1989.

Friedman LS et al: Management of asymptomatic gallstones in the diabetic patient. A decision analysis, Ann Intern Med 109:913-919, 1988.

Gracie WA and Ransohoff DF: The natural history of silent gallstones. The innocent gallstone is not a myth, N Engl J Med 307:798-800, 1982.

Hay DW and Carey MC: Pathophysiology and pathogenesis of cholesterol gallstone formation, Semin Liver Dis 10:159-170, 1990.

LaMont JT and Carey MC: Cholesterol gallstone formation. 2. Pathobiology and pathomechanics, Prog Liver Dis 10:165-191, 1992.

Leuschner U et al: Gallstone dissolution with methyl tert-butyl ether in 120 patients, Dig Dis Sci 36:193-199, 1992.

Marks AJ et al: The sequence of biliary events preceding the formation of gallstones in humans, Gastroenterology 103:566-570, 1992.

May GR and Shaffer EH. Should elective endoscopic sphincterotomy replace cholecystectomy for the treatment of high-risk patients with gallstone pancreatitis? (editorial), J Clin Gastroenterol 13:125-128, 1991.
Ransohoff DF et al: Prophylactic cholecystectomy or expectant management for silent gallstones, Ann Intern Med 99:199-204, 1983.
Ransohoff DF et al: Outcome of acute cholecystitis in patients with diabetes mellitus, Ann Intern Med 106:829-832, 1987.
Ros E et al: Occult microlithiasis in "idiopathic" acute pancreatitis: prevention of relapses by cholecystectomy or ursodeoxycholic acid therapy, Gastroenterology 101:1701-1709, 1991.
Sackmann M et al: The Munich gallbladder lithotripsy study: results of the first 5 years with 711 patients, Ann Intern Med 114:290-296, 1991.
Schoenfield LJ et al: The effect of ursodiol on the efficacy and safety of extracorporeal shock-wave lithotripsy of gallstones: the Dornier National Biliary Lithotripsy Study, N Engl J Med 323:1239-1245, 1990.
The Southern Surgeons Club: A prospective analysis of 1518 laparoscopic cholecystectomies, N Engl J Med 324:1073-1078, 1991.

CHAPTER

66 Other Diseases of the Gallbladder and Biliary Tree

Stephen C. Hauser

A variety of diseases less common than cholelithiasis and choledocholithiasis (Chapter 65) that involve the gallbladder and biliary tree are discussed in this chapter. Patients with these disorders, like those with gallstone-related disease, may present with jaundice (sclerosing cholangitis, carcinoma of the bile ducts, benign stricture of the extrahepatic bile ducts, choledochal cyst, Caroli's disease), abdominal pain (carcinoma of the biliary tree, choledochal cyst, hemobilia, biliary dyskinesia), or fever (sclerosing cholangitis, Caroli's disease).

SCLEROSING CHOLANGITIS

Sclerosing cholangitis is a rare, chronic inflammatory, and fibrosing disorder of unknown etiology that usually involves both the extrahepatic and intrahepatic biliary ductal systems. It has been called primary sclerosing cholangitis when it is not associated with other disorders, and secondary sclerosing cholangitis when associated diseases such as ulcerative colitis, Crohn's disease, retroperitoneal fibrosis, or orbital pseudotumor also are present. This distinction, however, appears unimportant because the clinical course, response to therapy, and prognosis are identical in primary and secondary sclerosing cholangitis. Furthermore, in secondary cases, the natural history of the sclerosing cholangitis is independent of that of the associated disorder. For example, in patients with both sclerosing cholangitis and ulcerative colitis, medical or surgical treatment of the colitis does not affect the sclerosing cholangitis.

About half of all cases of sclerosing cholangitis are associated with ulcerative colitis. In contrast, only 1% to 4% of patients with ulcerative colitis have sclerosing cholangitis. Genetic factors, such as an increased frequency of HLA-B8, HLA-DR3, and HLA-DRw52a haplotypes; immunologic abnormalities including circulating immune complexes; autoantibodies against bile ductules; antineutrophil cytoplasmic antibodies and aberrant expression of HLA class II antigens on bile duct epithelial cells; and abnormal collagen metabolism all have been proposed as important factors in the pathogenesis of sclerosing cholangitis. Nevertheless, the etiology of this disorder remains unknown.

Sclerosing cholangitis can occur in young children or in the elderly, but it is most commonly diagnosed in the third to fifth decades, with a male/female ratio of about 2:1. Patients may be completely asymptomatic; or they may complain of fatigue, pruritus, jaundice, and epigastric or right upper quadrant pain. Symptoms of cholangitis may occur but are uncommon in the absence of bile duct manipulation (i.e., surgery or stents) or a complicating condition, such as choledocholithiasis or bile duct carcinoma. Hepatomegaly and splenomegaly on physical examination are common.

Laboratory tests demonstrate cholestasis, with elevated serum bile salt and alkaline phosphatase levels in nearly all patients, and conjugated hyperbilirubinemia and mild transaminase elevations in many patients. In the presence of cholangitis, leukocytosis with a left shift is seen, and blood cultures are often positive. Elevated serum IgM levels, antinuclear antibodies, and anti-smooth muscle antibodies occasionally are found; but the absence of antimitochondrial antibodies helps distinguish sclerosing cholangitis from primary biliary cirrhosis (Chapter 60). Thyroid dysfunction is not uncommon.

The diagnosis of sclerosing cholangitis is established by radiographic evaluation of the biliary tree, generally by endoscopic retrograde cholangiography. Cholangiography demonstrates multiple focal strictured areas with normal or dilated intervening ductal segments, producing a characteristic beaded appearance of involved ducts (Fig. 66-1). Diverticulum-like outpouchings also have been reported. In most patients both intrahepatic and extrahepatic ducts are involved, but in a few there is isolated intrahepatic duct involvement. Isolated extrahepatic duct involvement is rare. Percutaneous transhepatic cholangiography is often unsuccessful because the strictured intrahepatic bile ducts are difficult to puncture with a needle. Rarely, pancreatic duct and gallbladder involvement also have been described.

The radiologic findings of sclerosing cholangitis can be mimicked in several other disorders, including adenocarcinoma of the common bile duct, biliary tract infection with cytomegalovirus, cryptosporidia, Candida, Histoplasmosis, Fasciola, toxic/ischemic injury due to graft-versus-host disease, chronic rejection of a liver transplant, and hepatic artery infusion of fluorodeoxyuridine for treatment of cancer metastatic to the liver. Hence, these conditions should be considered in the differential diagnosis. It may be difficult to distinguish large-duct cholangiocarcinoma from sclerosing cholangitis, even at surgery and with multiple biopsies. In patients with immunodeficiencies, such as the acquired

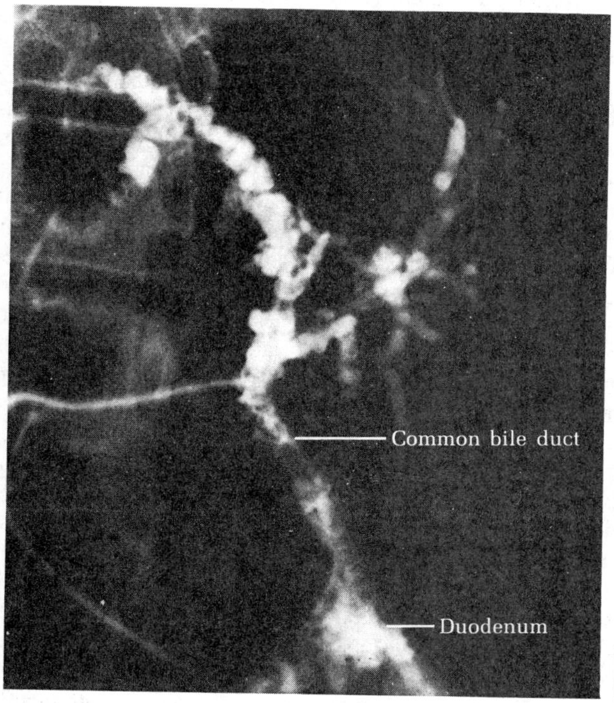

Fig. 66-1. Operative cholangiogram in a patient with sclerosing cholangitis.

immunodeficiency syndrome (AIDS), infections of the biliary tree may result in a clinical picture resembling sclerosing cholangitis. By definition, patients with a history of previous biliary tract surgery, choledocholithiasis, or congenital malformations are excluded.

A wide spectrum of nonspecific abnormalities can be demonstrated on liver biopsy, reflecting the variable degree and duration of small-and large-duct obstruction in these patients. Findings may include portal tract edema and infiltration with both mononuclear cells and neutrophils, periductal fibrosis and obliteration of small bile ducts, bile ductular proliferation, cholestasis, and in some patients, piecemeal necrosis and eventual secondary biliary cirrhosis. Thus there is no diagnostic lesion on liver biopsy in sclerosing cholangitis.

The term *pericholangitis,* which originally was described as a pathologic picture common to several disorders (e.g., some patients with primary biliary cirrhosis, extrahepatic biliary obstruction, and some infections), is now recognized as characteristic of the nonspecific chronic inflammatory changes found on liver biopsy in patients with idiopathic inflammatory bowel disease, especially ulcerative colitis. These morphologic findings can be indistinguishable from those described in liver biopsies from patients with sclerosing cholangitis. It is likely that pericholangitis, or small-duct sclerosing cholangitis, and large-duct sclerosing cholangitis are two extremes of a disease spectrum.

The natural history of sclerosing cholangitis is extremely variable. Some patients, identified by persistently elevated serum alkaline phosphatase levels and characteristic findings on cholangiography, remain asymptomatic for many years and often complete a normal life expectancy. In contrast, other patients die within a few years from complications of biliary cirrhosis, liver failure, portal hypertension, or cholangitis. Hepatomegaly and a serum bilirubin level of greater than 1.5 mg/dl at the onset of the disease have been identified as poor prognostic factors. Bile duct carcinoma may complicate the course of nearly 10% of patients but, as discussed previously, distinguishing cholangiocarcinoma from sclerosing cholangitis de novo can be difficult.

At present, there is no known effective medical therapy for sclerosing cholangitis. Given the variable and often prolonged clinical course of the illness and the apparent lack of correlation among patients between clinical, biochemical, histologic, and cholangiographic severity, investigation of specific therapeutic agents has been difficult. Corticosteroids, penicillamine, and a number of other immunosuppressive agents have been tried, all without apparent success. Preliminary data regarding the use of methotrexate and ursodeoxycholate appear promising. Symptomatic treatment of pruritus with cholestyramine, cholangitis with antibiotics, and malabsorption with fat-soluble vitamins and diets containing medium-chain triglycerides may be beneficial. Surgical, percutaneous transhepatic, or endoscopic dilatation of strictures and placement of stents may be of

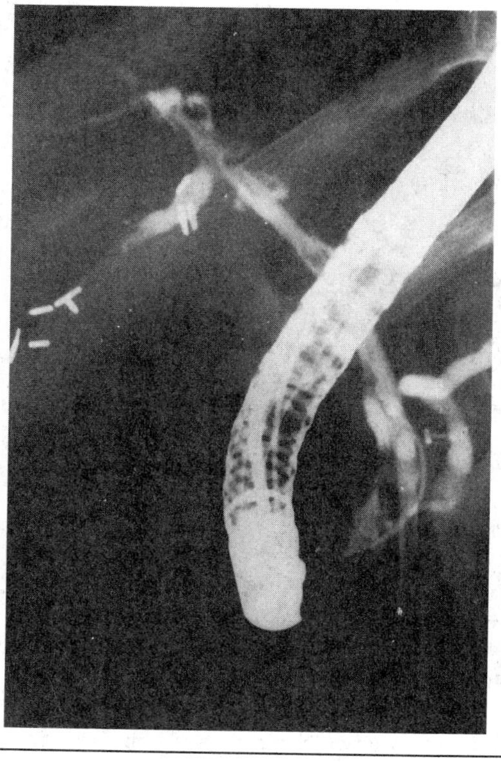

Fig. 66-2. Endoscopic retrograde cholangiogram in a patient with sclerosing cholangitis after placement of a stent.

use in selected patients, such as those with clinical deterioration and dominant strictures of the major biliary ducts (Fig. 66-2). Manipulation of the biliary tree may introduce bacteria and, in some cases, promote or worsen cholangitis. In addition, surgical procedures, but not endoscopic balloon dilatation or stenting of strictures, may increase the difficulty, morbidity, and mortality of a future liver transplantation, which in selected patients with progressive and advanced liver disease is a therapeutic option.

CARCINOMA OF THE BILE DUCTS

Primary adenocarcinoma of the bile ducts, or cholangiocarcinoma, accounts for the vast majority of tumors arising from the biliary ductal system. Anatomically, cholangiocarcinoma may originate in the intrahepatic bile ducts, in the hilar region where the hepatic ducts merge to form the common hepatic duct, or in the extrahepatic biliary tree, including the cystic duct and common bile duct. Intrahepatic bile duct carcinoma (peripheral cholangiocarcinoma) arises from very small bile ducts and is a rapidly growing tumor. Some carcinomas in this location consist of bile ductular as well as hepatocyte elements. Hilar cholangiocarcinoma, arising at or near the bifurcation of the common hepatic duct, is referred to as a Klatskin or bifurcation tumor (Fig. 66-3).

Cholangiocarcinoma is most common in the sixth decade and occurs with equal frequency in men and women. In persons from the Far East, chronic infestation with certain liver flukes, such as *Clonorchis sinensis* and *Opisthorchis viverrini,* has been associated with an increased incidence of cholangiocarcinoma, particularly the intrahepatic variety. The etiologic mechanism of this association is not known, but adenomatous proliferation of the ductular epithelium has been observed in the presence of these parasites. Interestingly, infestation with other flukes, including *Schistosoma mansoni, S. japonicum,* and *Fasciola hepatica,* has not been associated with cholangiocarcinoma. Other reported risk factors include chronic inflammatory bowel disease (usually ulcerative colitis, less often Crohn's colitis), sclerosing cholangitis, administration of anabolic steroids and thorium dioxide (Thorotrast), chronic biliary typhoid infections, familial polyposis coli, cancer family syndrome, and congenital cystic disorders of the biliary tree (choledochal cyst and Caroli's disease). Workers in the automotive, aeronautic, and rubber industries also have a higher incidence of cholangiocarcinoma, presumably due to exposure to environmental toxic substances.

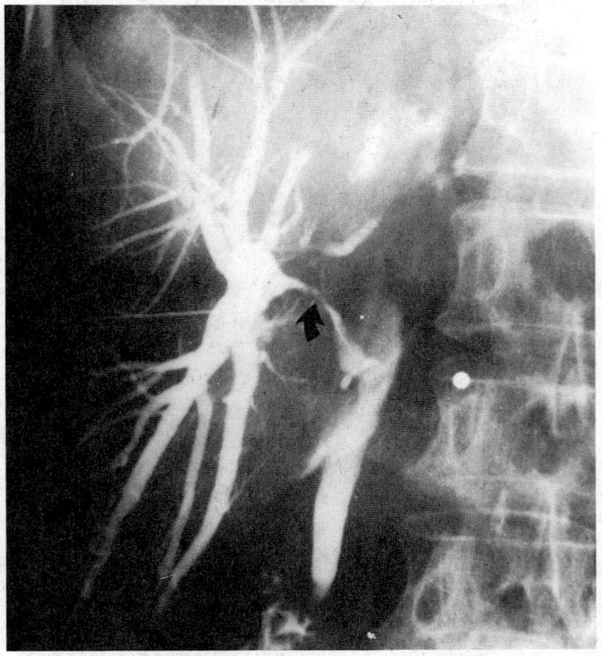

Fig. 66-3. Klatskin-type cholangiocarcinoma, involving the common hepatic duct (*arrow*), high in the porta hepatis close to the bifurcation, as demonstrated by percutaneous transhepatic cholangiogram. (The "skinny" needle is shown as a thin straight line of contrast material coming in from the left side of the x-ray.)

Patients with cholangiocarcinoma often present with symptoms of duct obstruction such as pruritus and jaundice, which may be intermittent early in the disease. Cholangitis is unusual, but anorexia, fatigue, abdominal pain, weight loss, and fever are common. Jaundice and hepatomegaly may be found on physical examination, and an enlarged gallbladder may occur with cholangiocarcinomas located below the common hepatic duct. Laboratory tests usually demonstrate cholestasis, with an elevated serum alkaline phosphatase level in most cases.

Noninvasive tests, including ultrasound, computed tomography (CT), and magnetic resonance imaging (MRI), may demonstrate dilated intrahepatic bile ducts proximal to the tumor, invasion of the adjacent liver parenchyma, and intra-abdominal lymph node involvement. However, noninvasive tests may not identify the tumor itself, and radiographic visualization of the biliary tree is crucial to define the exact location and extent of the tumor. This is particularly important with Klatskin tumors, which can be difficult to find at surgery in patients in whom the tumor is not localized preoperatively. Either percutaneous transhepatic cholangiography or endoscopic retrograde cholangiography can be used. It is important to visualize the entire biliary tree to avoid overlooking a small focal tumor. Cytology of material obtained by brushings, collecting bile, or fine-needle aspiration of the tumor site is diagnostic in about 50% of cases.

Most cholangiocarcinomas are unresectable, particularly when located at or above the hilus. Angiography and surgical exploration are required in selected patients to determine resectability. Palliative decompression of the obstructed biliary tree is useful. At present, this can be accomplished without surgical resection or bypass in many patients either by percutaneous transhepatic decompression, with placement of an endoprosthesis draining bile either externally or internally into the duodenum, or by endoscopic biliary decompression with nasobiliary or endoprosthetic stenting. Results with internal drainage are superior to those with external drainage. Radiotherapy can be useful for palliation in certain patients, whereas chemotherapy remains strictly investigational. Because many cholangiocarcinomas are slow growing, relief of biliary tract obstruction may prolong survival in some patients.

CARCINOMA OF THE AMPULLA OF VATER

Tumors in the vicinity of the ampulla of Vater may arise from the mucosa of the ampulla itself, the pancreatic duct, the distal common bile duct, or the duodenum. Nearly all of these tumors are adenocarcinomas. Noninvasive tests such as CT as well as invasive tests including endoscopic retrograde cholangiopancreatography and percutaneous transhepatic cholangiography are necessary to clarify the origin of adenocarcinomas in this region. This fact is important because patients with carcinoma of the ampulla of Vater, compared with other pancreatic, biliary tract, or small intestinal carcinomas, have a high 5-year survival rate (30% to 60%) after surgical resection of the pancreatic head and duodenum with pancreaticojejunostomy (Whipple's operation). Patients with familial polyposis coli, cancer family syndrome, and von Recklinghausen's disease are at increased risk for adenocarcinoma of the ampulla of Vater.

CARCINOMA OF THE GALLBLADDER

Nearly 5000 cases of gallbladder carcinoma are diagnosed in the United States annually. Over 80% of these are adenocarcinomas; the remainder are squamous cell and anaplastic carcinomas. The average age at presentation is 65, with a 2:1 female/male ratio. As many as 90% of gallbladder carcinoma patients also have gallstones, but the exact role of these stones, if any, in the etiology of gallbladder carcinoma is unclear. Because gallstones are so common and gallbladder carcinoma is so uncommon, the operative mortality of prophylactic cholecystectomy in the general population would be far higher than the number of deaths from gallbladder cancers that would be prevented. Specific groups of patients have been identified, however, in which prophylactic cholecystectomy is indicated. If left alone, about 50% of patients with porcelain gallbladders with patchy calcification of the gallbladder wall will develop gallbladder cancer. Chronic *Salmonella typhosa* carriers, women of American Indian heritage with gallstones, and patients with solitary gallstones larger than 3.0 cm in diameter are also at high risk of developing gallbladder cancer and should strongly be considered for prophylactic cholecystectomy.

The clinical presentation of gallbladder cancer is nonspecific and includes weight loss, pain, anorexia, nausea, and vomiting. A palpable mass, jaundice, fever, and chills also may occur. Laboratory findings also are nonspecific and include leukocytosis, anemia, and elevated serum alkaline phosphatase levels. Unfortunately, the tumor is usually silent until spread has occurred, and the diagnosis is rarely made when the tumor is still resectable. In fact, less than 20% of cases are diagnosed preoperatively. Ultrasound, CT, and MRI may demonstrate a mass as well as invasion of the liver. Survival beyond 1 year is uncommon. Occasionally, gallbladder carcinoma is found incidentally in gallbladders removed from patients with cholecystitis. If these have not yet penetrated the muscularis, they may be cured by surgery. Radiotherapy and chemotherapy are not effective in gallbladder cancer.

BENIGN STRICTURE OF EXTRAHEPATIC BILE DUCTS

Benign strictures of the extrahepatic bile ducts nearly always follow bile duct injury, most often as a result of surgery on either the ducts or the gallbladder. Inadvertent ligation of the extrahepatic bile duct may produce a symptomatic stricture in the immediate postoperative period, whereas more subtle injury may not produce symptoms until several years later. Depending on the degree of obstruction, the patient may be asymptomatic, jaundiced, or present with ascending cholangitis. Laboratory tests generally show evidence of cholestasis in symptomatic strictures with elevation of serum alkaline phosphatase and/or bilirubin levels. Ultrasound or CT may show dilated bile ducts proximal to the stricture. Chronic partial obstruction of the biliary tree may ultimately produce secondary biliary cirrhosis and portal hypertension. Percutaneous transhepatic cholangiography and endoscopic retrograde cholangiography are necessary to define the exact location of the stricture(s). In some instances, it may be impossible to exclude cholangiocarcinoma. To further complicate the picture, brown pigment gallstones can form secondary to stasis proximal to the stricture and precipitate obstruction (Chapter 65). Depending on the clinical circumstances, surgical bypass or repair of the strictured duct by a skilled and experienced surgeon or balloon dilatation and/or stenting of the stricture may be required. Long strictures of the distal common bile duct may develop in alcoholic patients with chronic pancreatitis owing to external compression of the duct by fibrosis and inflammation in the head of the pancreas. These patients require frequent cholangiographic evaluation as well as liver biopsies to determine when a biliary-enteric bypass procedure is indicated. If not corrected, partial biliary obstruction in this setting can result in secondary biliary cirrhosis within several months.

HEMOBILIA

Patients who bleed into the biliary tract often present with biliary colic and melena or hematemesis. The formation of clots within the biliary tree may cause jaundice. Hemobilia most often results from blunt or penetrating trauma to the abdomen. Transhepatic cholangiography, liver biopsy, biliary tract malignancy, and varices of the biliary tree may be complicated by hemobilia. In certain patients, the bleeding may not stop spontaneously, and either surgical intervention or therapeutic angiographic embolization may be required.

HYPERPLASTIC CHOLECYSTOSIS

Hyperplastic cholecystosis refers to a loosely defined group of disorders affecting the gallbladder that includes adenomyomatosis, gallbladder polyps, and phrygian cap. *Adenomyomatosis* is defined as a generalized or segmental hyperplasia of the gallbladder epithelium. When localized, it may assume the shape of a polyp, which can be visualized by ultrasonography or cholecystography. In the absence of gallstones, it is unlikely that adenomatosis produces symptoms. The same can be said for gallbladder polyps, most of which are cholesterol polyps, not true neoplasms. It is unknown if the phrygian cap deformity is congenital or acquired. For most patients with hyperplastic cholecystosis, therapy is not necessary, especially if the lesion is small (<10 mm) and does not change over time. However, if patients are symptomatic, have coexistent cholelithiasis or thickening of the gallbladder wall on ultrasound, or if the lesion increases in size, cholecystectomy is indicated.

BILIARY DYSKINESIA

A variety of dysmotility disorders of the biliary tract have been proposed to account for chronic abdominal pain that may resemble biliary colic in patients without gallstones. *Hyperkinesia* of the gallbladder is defined as excessive or abnormal contractility of the gallbladder after stimulation, such as after eating or after the administration of cholecystokinin. Gallbladder emptying can be studied by radionuclide scintigraphy with cholecystokinin octapeptide injection. Cholecystectomy may benefit selected patients. Dyskinesia refers to altered tonus of the sphincter of Oddi (usually increased pressure), disturbance in the coordination of contraction of the biliary ducts, and/or reduction in the speed of emptying of the biliary tree. Increased biliary ductal pressure secondary to diminished bile flow through the sphincter of Oddi may cause pain, transiently elevated results of liver function tests, dilatation of the ductal system, and delayed drainage of contrast after endoscopic retrograde cholangiography. Abnormal manometric pressure measurements of the sphincter of Oddi confirm the diagnosis, but it can be difficult to exclude organic papillary stenosis in some of these patients. Although endoscopic or surgical sphincterotomy may help selected patients with biliary dyskinesia, many patients with chronic abdominal pain syndromes suggestive of biliary dyskinesia probably suffer from the much more common irritable bowel syndrome. Hence objective findings such as manometric abnormalities or abnormal liver function test results are helpful in identifying patients who may benefit from surgery. Finally, it should be remembered that the presence of cholelithiasis and choledocholithiasis must be carefully excluded.

DEVELOPMENTAL ANOMALIES

Congenital abnormalities in the development of the biliary tract almost always present early in life. However, choledochal cysts and Caroli's disease, two conditions characterized by congenital dilatation of bile ducts, may become evident during adulthood. Choledochal cysts may present as a right upper quadrant mass, with pain and jaundice. Ultrasound, CT, radionuclide scintigraphy, and cholangiography all can be useful in making the diagnosis. Because of the age-related increase in the incidence of carcinoma complicating choledochal cysts, surgical removal of the cyst and biliary reconstruction are recommended if possible. Caroli's disease is characterized by multiple areas of cystic dilatation involving the intrahepatic and in some instances also the extrahepatic bile ducts. In some patients only the bile ducts of certain segments or a single lobe of the liver are affected. Congenital hepatic fibrosis may also be present (Chapter 60). Fever, pain, jaundice, cholangitis, and secondary intrahepatic choledocholithiasis and abscess formation may occur periodically in patients with Caroli's disease. Cholangiography as well as ultrasound and CT can establish the diagnosis. Surgical drainage of the affected biliary radicles, partial hepatectomy in patients with localized disease, and perhaps liver transplantation may benefit selected patients.

REFERENCES

Hogan WJ, Geenan JE, and Dodds WJ: Dysmotility disturbances of the biliary tract: classification, diagnosis and treatment, Semin Liver Dis 7:302, 1987.

Levin B: Diagnosis and medical management of malignant disorders of the biliary tract, Semin Liver Dis 7:328, 1987.

Lindor KD et al: Advances in primary sclerosing cholangitis, Am J Med 89:73, 1990.

May GR, Bender CE, and Williams HJ: Radiologic approaches to the treatment of benign and malignant biliary tract disease, Semin Liver Dis 7:334, 1987.

Nagorney DM, McIlrath DC, and Adson MA: Choledochal cysts in adults: clinical management, Surgery 96:656, 1984.

Nagorney DM and McPherson GAD: Carcinoma of the gallbladder and extrahepatic bile ducts, Semin Oncol 15:106, 1988.

Schneiderman DJ, Cello JP, and Liang FC: Papillary stenosis and sclerosing cholangitis in the acquired immunodeficiency syndrome, Ann Intern Med 106:546, 1987.

Slivka A and Carr-Locke D: Therapeutic biliary endoscopy, Endoscopy 24:100, 1992.

CHAPTER

67 Pancreatic Diseases

Patrick T. Regan
Vay Liang W. Go

ACUTE PANCREATITIS

Acute pancreatitis is a relatively common inflammatory process that can produce a spectrum of clinical manifestations ranging from the "acute abdomen," with shock, to mild and self-limited abdominal discomfort. Whether acute pancreatitis occurs as an isolated attack or is recurrent, there are no irreversible sequelae (i.e., diabetes, steatorrhea, calcification). Classification of acute pancreatitis can be based on etiology, clinical features, or pathologic changes (edematous, hemorrhagic).

Etiology

The most common causes of acute pancreatitis are chronic alcoholism and calculous biliary tract disease. Many other apparent clinical associations exist (Table 67-1), but a def-

Table 67-1. Acute pancreatitis

Common causes	Occasional causes	Rare causes
Biliary tract disease	Hyperlipemia	Pancreatic cancer
Alcoholism	Surgery	Cystic fibrosis
Idiopathic	Abdominal trauma	Ischemia
	ERCP*	Vasculitis
	Drugs (e.g., azathioprine)	Hereditary pancreatitis
	Infection	
	Peptic ulcer disease	
	Hypercalcemia	
	Renal transplantation	

*Endoscopic retrograde cholangiopancreatography.

inite etiologic relationship is often difficult to prove. Drugs are frequently implicated as causal factors, but there is strong supportive evidence for only azathioprine, thiazides, sulfonamides, valproic acid, metronidazole, tetracycline, and estrogens. Genetic hypertriglyceridemia can cause recurrent attacks of abdominal pain, but most often hyperlipemia seems to be the result of the pancreatitis itself. A particularly severe form of pancreatitis may occur in the postoperative state even if surgery has not been abdominal. Trauma and endoscopic retrograde pancreatography are relatively frequent precursors. The often mentioned relationship between acute pancreatitis and hypercalcemia, especially due to hyperparathyroidism, has been questioned. Infrequent etiologic factors include viral infections, complicated peptic ulcer disease, vasculitis or ischemia, primary or metastatic cancer of the pancreas, cystic fibrosis, hereditary pancreatitis, and structural anomalies of the pancreatic duct or the sphincter of Oddi. Biliary "sludge" is often discovered in idiopathic cases, and its presence appears to increase the likelihood of recurrent acute pancreatitis.

Pathology and pathophysiology

Substantial evidence supports the hypothesis that autodigestion occurs in acute pancreatitis. During the course of the illness, activated human pancreatic enzymes are present in the pancreas, pancreatic juice, and ascitic fluid. Some of these enzymes cause experimental pancreatitis in animals when injected into the pancreatic duct. The known physiologic effects of substances such as trypsin, phospholipase, elastase, lipase, unconjugated bile acids, and a variety of vasoactive agents such as kallikrein may then produce the observed pathologic changes of edema, hemorrhage, and fat and parenchymal necrosis.

Normally, trypsin is formed from its inactive precursor, trypsinogen, only after contact with the duodenal mucosal enzyme enterokinase (Chapter 52). Mechanisms proposed to explain the intrapancreatic activation of trypsin and other enzymes include reflux of duodenal secretions and/or bile into the main pancreatic duct, ductal obstruction by ampullary gallstones or protein precipitates induced by alcohol, direct toxic effects on the acinar or ductal cells, and ischemia induced by changes in the microcirculation of the gland. A current theory proposes that the mixing of zymogen and lysosomal hydrolases within the acinar cell itself leads to digestive enzyme activation. Although these hypotheses remain speculative, it is likely that the initiating insult is multifactorial. Presumably, the trypsin inhibitors normally present in both the pancreas and circulation are overwhelmed with a resultant vicious cycle of pancreatic inflammation and necrosis.

Clinical manifestations

The clinical manifestations of acute pancreatitis range from mild, nonspecific abdominal pain to profound shock with coma. Characteristically, a patient with biliary tract disease or chronic alcoholism complains of epigastric pain associated with nausea and vomiting, and abdominal tenderness is frequently the only physical finding.

Abdominal pain, the cardinal feature of acute pancreatitis, is usually sharp or boring, constant, and localized in the epigastrium, although it may be generalized or maximal in the subcostal or retrosternal regions. Radiation to the back is prominent in approximately 50% of patients. The onset of pain is often temporally related to eating or an alcoholic binge, and most patients experience discomfort for more than 24 hours. Typically, the pain is eased when the patient leans forward or assumes the knee-chest position. Rarely, patients may present in shock, with ileus and little or no abdominal pain. Nausea and vomiting occur in 75% of patients and may be severe and protracted.

On physical examination, the patient appears acutely ill and restless, and typically exhibits abdominal tenderness with muscular rigidity, distention, and hypoactive or absent bowel sounds. Frequently, low-grade fever, tachycardia, and hypotension are also present. Hectic or prolonged fevers suggest the presence of cholangitis, associated infection, or pancreatic abscess. Tachypnea and dyspnea are common, and auscultation may reveal evidence of atelectasis, pulmonary edema, pneumonitis, or pleural effusion. An abdominal mass may be palpable 5 to 10 days after the onset of the disease and represents an inflammatory phlegmon, pseudocyst, or abscess. Less common physical signs are jaundice, xanthomas, positive Chvostek's sign, subcutaneous nodules of fat necrosis, and flank or umbilical hemorrhagic skin discoloration, as described by Grey-Turner and Cullen.

Diagnosis

Diagnosis of acute pancreatitis is certain only when confirmed by surgical description or histology of the gland. In most cases, a detailed history and physical examination combined with ancillary laboratory and radiologic tests enable the physician to make a presumptive diagnosis.

Laboratory diagnosis relies heavily on analysis of serum amylase activity; serum amylase is derived primarily from the pancreas and salivary glands and is cleared by the kidneys. In acute pancreatitis, hyperamylasemia is detectable shortly after the onset of symptoms, and values usually re-

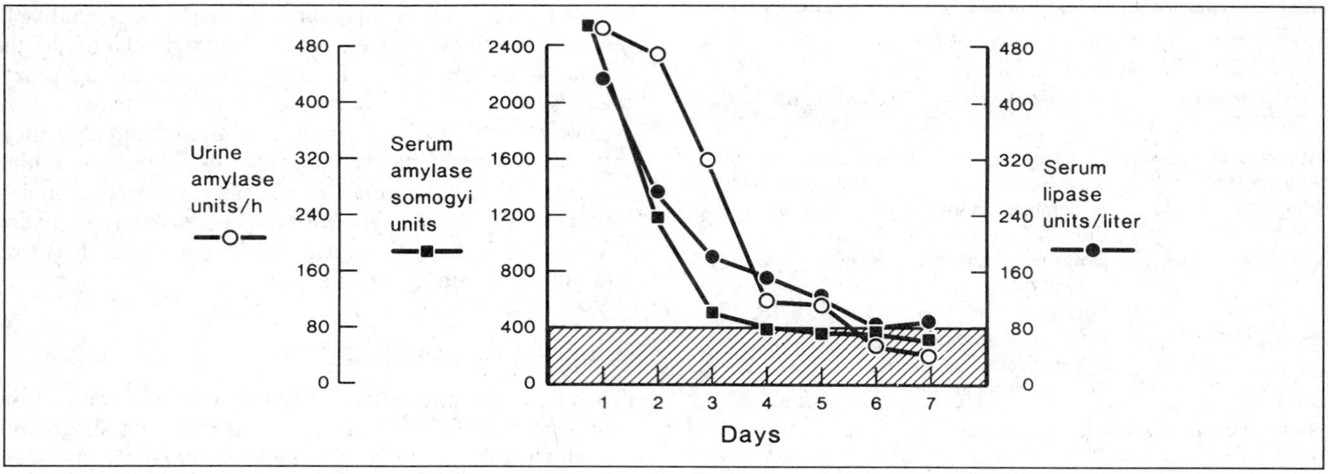

Fig. 67-1. Serum amylase, serum lipase, and urinary amylase values in typical acute alcoholic pancreatitis.

turn to normal within 1 to 4 days (Fig. 67-1). Prolonged hyperamylasemia suggests continuing pancreatitis, an associated pancreatic cancer, or a complication such as pseudocyst or abscess. The degree of serum amylase elevation does not correlate with the severity of pancreatitis.

Many nonpancreatic disorders may be associated with hyperamylasemia, including biliary tract disease, diabetic ketoacidosis, renal insufficiency, salivary disease, intestinal obstruction, perforation or ischemia, dissecting aneurysms, a variety of gynecologic disorders, and nonpancreatic tumors. Thus an increased serum amylase level supports but does not confirm a diagnosis of acute pancreatitis (Chapter 54). The serum amylase level may be falsely normal in the presence of hypertriglyceridemia.

Increased urinary amylase values may persist longer than hyperamylasemia (Fig. 67-1). Striking elevations of amylase content in pleural, pericardial, or peritoneal effusions may also be useful diagnostic factors.

Serum lipase assays are now available, reliable, and inexpensive. They confer the advantage of increased overall specificity for pancreatic disease. A recent study measured the serum lipase/amylase ratio (both expressed as a percent of normal values) in subjects with acute pancreatitis. A ratio greater than 2 was highly suggestive of an alcoholic etiology. Serum levels of pancreatic isoamylase, trypsin, and elastase are expensive and of unproven value.

Miscellaneous laboratory findings include leukocytosis, transient hyperglycemia, anemia, abnormal liver function test results, hypertriglyceridemia, and hypocalcemia. The latter generally suggests extensive and severe pancreatitis, especially in the absence of hypoalbuminemia.

The secondary effects of pancreatic inflammation may produce changes in adjacent organs that are visible on plain x-ray films of the abdomen. Ileus, generalized or localized in the jejunum ("sentinel loop") or colon ("colonic cutoff"), displacement of the stomach or duodenum, and gallstones are occasional findings in acute pancreatitis. A search for subdiaphragmatic air is mandatory to rule out visceral perforation.

Radiographs of the chest are often abnormal and may reveal elevation of the diaphragm, atelectasis, pneumonitis, pulmonary edema, or pleural effusion. Barium studies of the upper gastrointestinal tract may show duodenal loop mucosal changes or displacement, but these findings are not specific for acute pancreatitis.

Ultrasonography is primarily used for evaluation of the biliary tract. Contrast enhanced computed tomography (CT) is generally accepted as the best means for imaging the pancreas. Features of acute pancreatitis (Fig. 67-2) include enlargement and indistinct margins of the gland, alterations in enhancement patterns, phlegmon or fluid accumulations, and thickening of adjacent fascial planes. A normal CT ex-

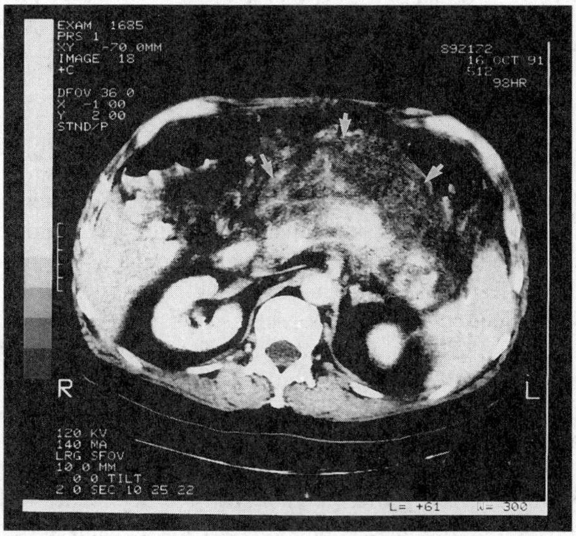

Fig. 67-2. CT of pancreas in acute pancreatitis. Edema and inflammatory infiltration of peripancreatic and mesenteric fat *(arrows)*.

cludes the presence of clinically severe acute pancreatitis. CT scans should be obtained early in the illness if the diagnosis is in doubt and if clinical improvement does not occur within 2 or 3 days. Recent studies support a role for urgent endoscopic retrograde cholangiopancreatography (ERCP) in the diagnosis (and subsequent treatment) of selected patients with acute gallstone pancreatitis.

Differential diagnosis

Nearly all of the common causes of acute abdominal pain can produce a clinical picture similar to that of acute pancreatitis (see the accompanying box), and the coexistence of hyperamylasemia may make accurate diagnosis in acute cases even more difficult. Acute cholecystitis with or without associated pancreatitis, peptic ulcer disease (especially with perforation or posterior penetration), intestinal obstruction or strangulation, and acute gynecologic disease (i.e., ectopic pregnancy, ruptured ovarian cyst) are the most common entities to be excluded. In the majority of cases, a detailed history and physical examination combined with the judicious use of diagnostic tests will clarify the diagnosis. Rarely, exploratory laparotomy may be required if the diagnosis remains uncertain.

Treatment

The mortality for an individual attack of acute pancreatitis is variable but low (~ 5%). Pancreatitis caused by biliary disease or occurring in the postoperative state more often results in excessive morbidity and mortality. The severity of acute pancreatitis is usually greatest in the first attack. Several authors have formulated multiple clinical scoring systems as a means of estimating disease severity and prognosis early in the course of the disease (Table 67-2). When three or more of these parameters are present in a patient within 48 hours of presentation, a severe clinical course with frequent complications and high mortality is likely.

Supportive management is the cornerstone of treatment. Relief of pain, maintenance of often severely depleted intravascular volume, and careful observation for complications result in complete and rapid recovery in nearly all patients. Energetic fluid replacement is the only treatment of proven value. Intravenous calcium or insulin and supplemental oxygen may be required. Parenteral hyperalimentation is essential in prolonged and severe cases.

No specific medical treatment has proved beneficial in acute pancreatitis. Although nasogastric suction clinically appears to reduce pain and relieve ileus, it does not alter the course of mild alcoholic pancreatitis and is not mandatory in all cases. Antibiotics do not prevent septic complications and should be administered only for coexistent obstructive biliary tract disease or when pancreatic abscess is proved or suspected. Glucagon, cimetidine, anticholinergics, somatostatin, and the enzyme inhibitor aprotinin have all been shown to be ineffective in controlled clinical trials.

Fulminant acute pancreatitis is an uncommon but troublesome problem that requires intensive therapy. Massive volume replacement, treatment of hypocalcemia, and support of the cardiorespiratory systems are necessary. Surgical intervention is clearly warranted when the diagnosis is uncertain and for definitive control of cholangitis or the complications of pseudocyst and abscess. Laparotomy with resection of necrotic tissue and sump drainage or peritoneal dialysis appear to be useful adjunctive measures in some critically ill patients, but overall survival is not clearly improved. For patients with severe or prolonged pancreatitis due to gallstones, endoscopic sphincterotomy is emerging as the therapeutic modality of choice (Fig. 67-3). In patients with mild disease and without choledocholithiasis, cholecystectomy (often via laparoscopy) can usually be performed during the same hospitalization. ERCP should be performed in most patients after recovery from the first attack of idiopathic acute pancreatitis in order to identify potentially treatable conditions such as gallstones, ampullary tumors or cysts, obstructed pancreatic duct, or pancreas divisum.

Diseases to be considered in the differential diagnosis of acute pancreatitis

- Acute cholecystitis
- Peptic ulcer disease
- Intestinal obstruction
- Acute gynecologic disorder
- Mesenteric vascular disease
- Appendicitis, diverticulitis
- Abdominal aneurysm
- Renal colic
- Splenic rupture
- Abdominal abscess
- Myocardial infarction
- Porphyria
- Familial Mediterranean fever

Table 67-2. Representative prognostic scoring systems in acute pancreatitis*

Ranson	Glasgow
Admission	
Age > 55 years	Age > 50 years
WBC > 20,000 cells/mm^3	WBC > 15,000
LDH > 350 IU/L	Glucose > 180 mg/dl
AST > 250 IU/L	BUN > 45 mg/dl
Initial 48 hrs	Po_2 < 60 mm Hg
Hematocrit decrease > 10%	Albumin < 3.2 g/dl
BUN increase > 5 mg/dl	Calcium < 8 mg/dl
Calcium < 8 mg/dl	LDH > 600 IU/L
Po_2 < 60 mm Hg	
Base deficit > 4	
Estimated fluid sequestration > 6 liters	

Modified from Ranson JAC et al: Surg Gynecol Obstet 143:209, 1976 and Neoptolemos VP et al: Lancet 2:979, 1988.

*Presence of 3 or more factors indicates poor prognosis.

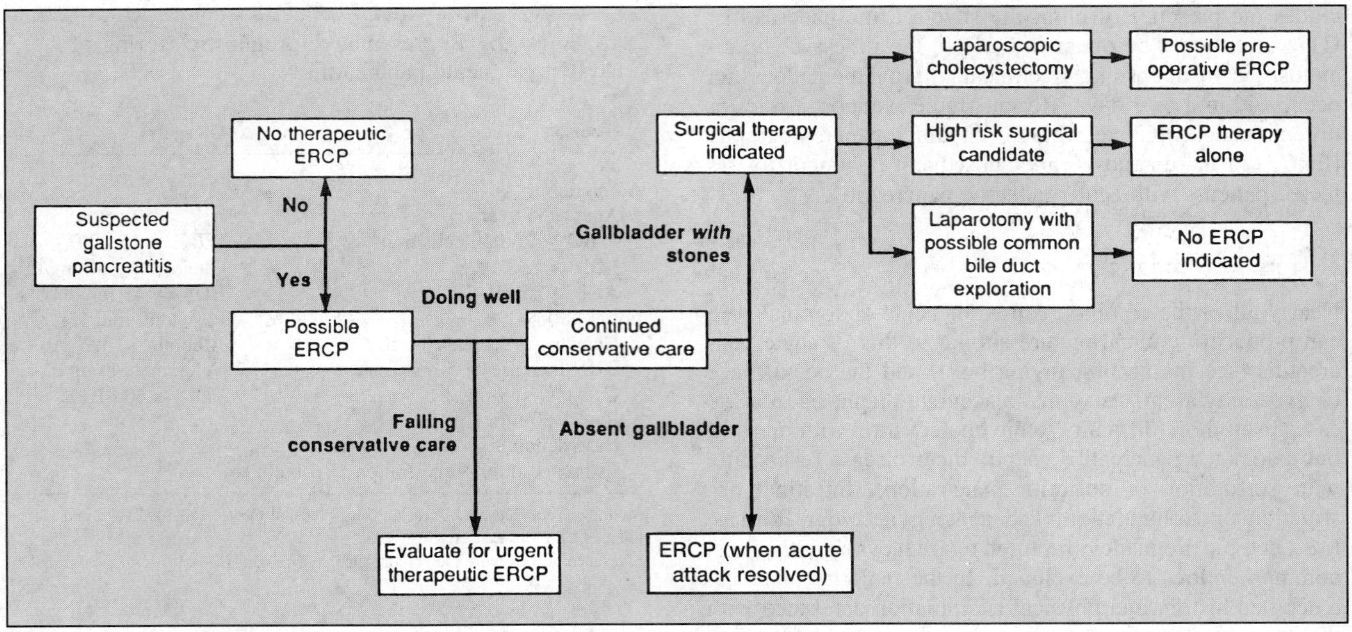

Fig. 67-3. Suggested approach to patients with suspected gallstone pancreatitis. (From Cello and Wilcox, Seminars in Gastroenterology 2:180, 1991.).

Complications

Systemic complications of acute pancreatitis include acute renal failure, cardiovascular collapse, respiratory insufficiency, gastrointestinal bleeding, infection, and metabolic sequelae such as electrolyte imbalance and hypocalcemia. Prevention and early treatment are the keys to successful management.

Pancreatic fistulas or ascites, splenic vein obstruction, or cholestasis due to inflammatory constriction of the common bile duct are infrequent local complications. An abdominal mass develops in 15% of patients, and 3 distinct entities must be differentiated: phlegmon, pseudocyst, and abscess. A *phlegmon* represents a swollen and inflamed pancreas, whereas a *pseudocyst* is a collection of fluid and necrotic debris without a true epithelial lining. Pseudocysts are typically located near the pancreas in the lesser sac, but occasionally may be present in atypical sites such as the pelvis or mediastinum. Clinical features include persistent or recurrent abdominal pain, a palpable (and often enlarging) mass in 50% of patients, fever, and persistent hyperamylasemia. Acute pseudocysts may be seen on ultrasonic examination in up to 50% of patients with acute pancreatitis and often resorb spontaneously. Chronic pseudocysts are larger, often associated with persistent abdominal pain and hyperamylasemia, and can be accurately diagnosed by use of CT or ultrasound (Fig. 67-4). Secondary infection, rupture, bleeding, and obstruction of an adjacent structure are potential serious complications. Internal surgical drainage (to the stomach or small bowel) is often required for persistent or enlarging lesions but is best delayed for at least 6 weeks if possible to allow maturation of the fibrotic walls. Percutaneous needle drainage may at times be appropriate.

A prolonged or hectic febrile course should suggest the presence of cholangitis due to gallstones or a pancreatic *abscess*. Abscesses are produced by enteric organisms and present with rapid clinical deterioration. Diagnosis is best made by use of ultrasound or CT. Guided needle aspiration is often helpful, and immediate surgical or effective catheter drainage is required. Prophylactic broad-spectrum antibiotic administration does not prevent septic complications of acute pancreatitis. Hemorrhagic complications

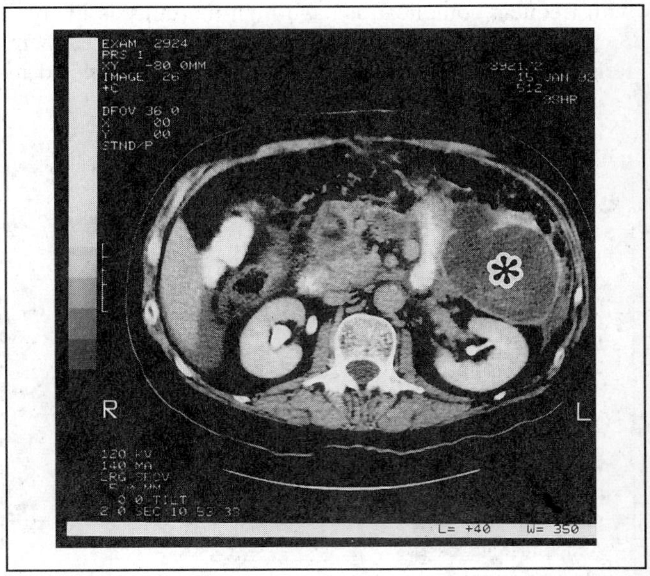

Fig. 67-4. CT demonstrates a large pseudocyst *(*)* in tail of pancreas. Head of gland is enlarged and edematous (pancreatitis).

(usually associated with infected pancreatic necrosis) are rare but frequently lethal.

Small amounts of exudative ascitic fluid are often present during the course of acute pancreatitis, and rarely there is massive ascites, usually associated with pancreatic ductal disruption or a leaking pseudocyst. Diagnosis is confirmed by the discovery of ascitic fluid with a very high amylase content at the time of paracentesis. Surgical or catheter drainage of the pseudocyst or rarely pancreatic resection may be necessary if conservative medical management that includes bowel rest with parenteral alimentation is unsuccessful.

CHRONIC PANCREATITIS

Chronic pancreatitis differs from acute pancreatitis in that irreversible histologic, clinical, or functional changes are always present. The resultant exocrine and/or endocrine pancreatic insufficiency may be subclinical or overt.

Etiology

In the United States, 75% of cases of chronic pancreatitis are due to chronic alcoholism of long duration. In fact, by the time initial symptoms of alcoholic pancreatitis occur, the characteristic pathologic changes are already widespread within the gland. Although cholelithiasis may coexist with pancreatitis, only rarely is biliary tract disease the primary cause of chronic pancreatitis. Hereditary pancreatitis is a rare, autosomal dominant disorder that causes repeated attacks of abdominal pain beginning in childhood and the eventual development of chronic calcific pancreatitis. Severe protein-calorie malnutrition, cystic fibrosis, hyperparathyroidism, and hyperlipemia are uncommon possible etiologic factors. In up to 25% of patients, no clear etiology can be identified. Some patients develop mild to moderate maldigestion after gastric surgery, presumably due to inadequate duodenal mixing of food and digestive enzymes (Chapter 38).

Pathology and pathophysiology

There appear to be two separate pathologic forms of chronic pancreatitis. Obstructive lesions (i.e., tumors, cysts, trauma) cause uniform changes of acinar atrophy and fibrosis distal to the duct obstruction. Calcification is usually absent and pancreatic structure and function often improve after relief of the obstruction. In chronic calcific alcoholic pancreatitis, the pancreas may be enlarged or atrophic, and dilated ducts are filled with a thick, protein-rich fluid. Microscopically, there is irregular ductal dilatation, and the epithelial lining is hyperplastic or metaplastic, with surrounding fibrosis (Fig. 67-5). Recent studies in both canine and human chronic alcoholism suggest that the initial physiologic defect is the secretion of pancreatic juice supersaturated with enzymatic proteins (Fig. 67-6). Protein plugs are formed in the smaller ductules, may calcify, and are thought to initiate a recurrent cycle of obstruction, inflammation, and fibrosis. Intraductal calcification, visible radiologically, is the end result. Deficient quantities of "pancreatic stone protein" (an inhibitor of calcium salt formation) may lead to stone growth. Reflux of duodenal contents into the pancreatic duct, hypersecretion of calcium, and nutritional deficiency may also be important pathogenetic fac-

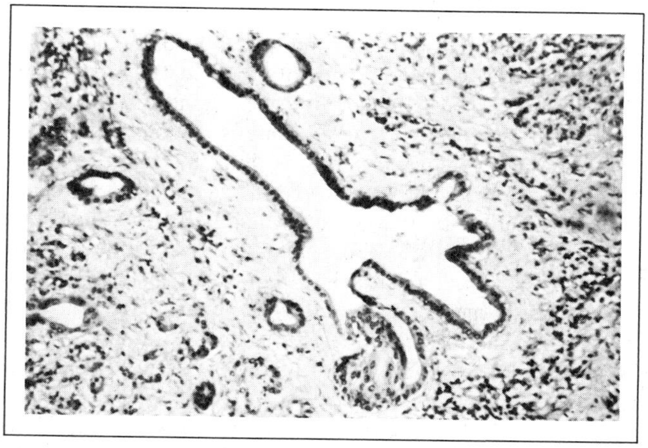

Fig. 67-5. Chronic calcific alcoholic pancreatitis revealing dilatation of large duct and surrounding fibrosis.

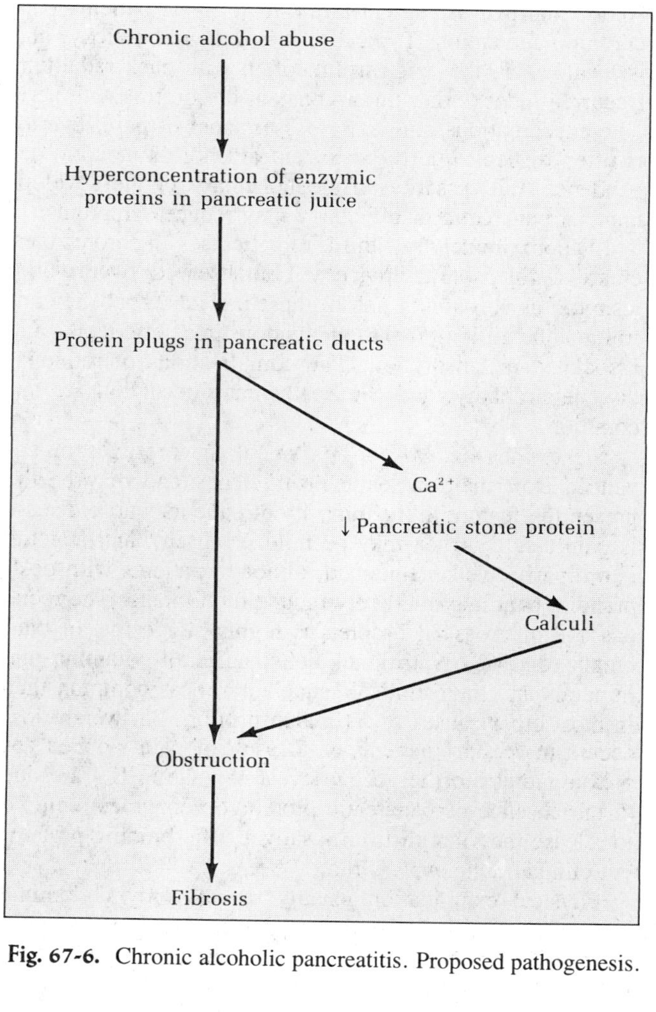

Fig. 67-6. Chronic alcoholic pancreatitis. Proposed pathogenesis.

tors. Pain is thought to result from increased intraductal pressure due to continued secretion with obstruction. The natural history of chronic alcoholic pancreatitis often consists of progressive clinical, functional, and histologic deterioration even when alcohol intake is discontinued.

The relation between pancreas divisum (failure of embryonic fusion of dorsal and ventral pancreatic segments) and pancreatitis remains controversial. This anomaly is present in 5% to 10% of the population, and relative stenosis of the minor papilla is the postulated defect. However, most subjects (even if they have pain) do not have ductal abnormalities characteristic of chronic pancreatitis on ERCP, and the response to surgical or endoscopic treatment is not predictable.

The reserve of the exocrine pancreas is very large, and malabsorption of dietary fat and protein occurs only when there is a reduction of 90% or more in the maximum secretion of lipase and trypsin. Patients with exocrine pancreatic insufficiency also exhibit decreased pancreatic bicarbonate secretion. As a result, in the postprandial state duodenal pH is reduced, leading to inactivation of orally administered exogenous enzymes and decreased micellar solubilization of bile salts.

Clinical features

Abdominal pain is present in the majority of patients with chronic pancreatitis. Typically, it is dull, not colicky, and is localized in the epigastrium, often with back radiation. Recurrent attacks of pain or constant discomfort with periodic exacerbations may exist. Assessment of pain severity is often difficult due to coexistent alcohol or narcotic dependence, but cessation of alcohol intake or the development of pancreatic insufficiency may reduce symptoms.

In approximately two thirds of patients with chronic pancreatitis, glucose intolerance will be observed; overt diabetes mellitus is found in half of these patients. Diabetic control may be difficult due to fluctuations in caloric intake and associated malabsorption. The complications of retinopathy, nephropathy, and neuropathy may occur but are uncommon.

Steatorrhea and azotorrhea signal the presence of advanced exocrine pancreatic insufficiency and may be the presenting feature in the minority of patients whose disease is painless. Diarrhea may be mild or absent, and appetite is ordinarily well maintained, although patients with postprandial pain may markedly reduce food intake. The rectal passage of gross oil droplets is highly suggestive of pancreatic disease. Nutritional deficiencies of vitamins and minerals and their clinical sequelae are less common than in most other causes of fat malabsorption, but weight loss occurs in 75% of patients as a result of pain-induced anorexia and steatorrhea. Low levels of vitamin B_{12} are due to the absence of pancreatic proteolytic enzymes required to release the vitamin from a salivary B_{12}-binding protein, but clinical deficiency is rare.

Physical examination usually reveals only abdominal tenderness, although the presence of a mass should suggest the possibility of a pseudocyst. Biochemical or overt jaundice may transiently occur during acute attacks of pain. Its persistence suggests concomitant biliary tract disease or fibrotic stricture of the intrapancreatic common bile duct.

Diagnosis

Hyperamylasemia may occur during an acute episode of inflammation, but in general routine laboratory tests are not useful in the diagnosis of chronic pancreatitis. Hyperglycemia reflects advanced pancreatic insufficiency, and abnormal liver function test results may be due to pancreatitis itself or to associated biliary tract disease or alcoholic liver disease.

In approximately 50% of patients, calcification of the pancreas can be seen radiologically (Fig. 67-7), and with rare exceptions this finding is specific for chronic pancreatitis. Displacement of the duodenal sweep or mucosal changes within it are nonspecific but may be seen with barium studies. Circumferential fibrous narrowing of the distal common bile duct is revealed by percutaneous transhepatic cholangiography or ERCP. Ultrasound and CT enable visualization of focal or diffuse enlargement or atrophy of the pancreas and calcifications. However, it may be difficult to distinguish carcinoma from chronic pancreatitis. Accurate diagnosis of pseudocyst and high-grade bile duct obstruction is usually possible with either modality. CT is the best diagnostic test for specific evaluation of the pancreas and surrounding retroperitoneal structures. Commonly observed changes include biliary or pancreatic ductal dilatation, calcifications, gland enlargement or atrophy, fluid collections, and peripancreatic fascial disruption. Angiography is performed infrequently but may aid in the distinction of inflammatory and neoplastic disease. ERCP is the most specific diagnostic test. The pancreatic duct is successfully visualized in over 90% of patients, and ductal tortuosity, dilatation, calcification, and pseudocysts can be seen (Fig. 67-8). There is no uniform relation between abnormal structure and function.

Fat and protein malabsorption is best documented by a quantitative, 72-hour fecal fat determination performed while the patient is ingesting a known amount of dietary

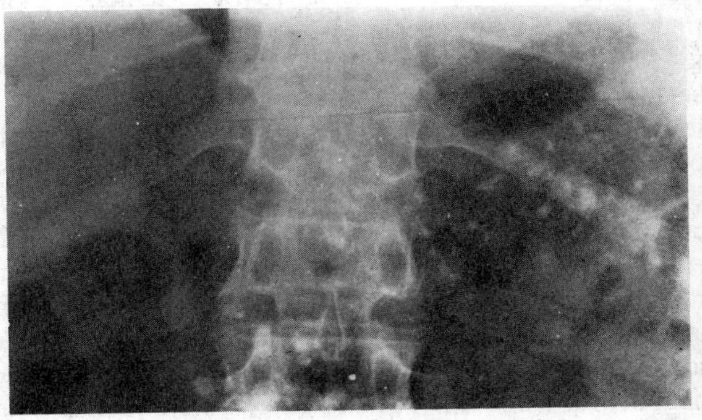

Fig. 67-7. Flat abdominal x-ray film. Diffuse pancreatic calcification visible.

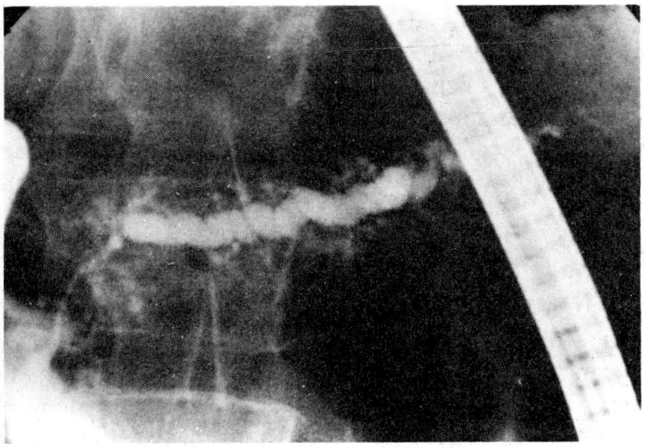

Fig. 67-8. Endoscopic retrograde cholangiopancreatogram in a patient with advanced alcoholic chronic pancreatitis, showing a diffusely dilated and tortuous main pancreatic duct.

fat (Chapter 33). D-Xylose absorption and small intestinal biopsies are characteristically normal in chronic pancreatitis. Measurement of the urinary excretion of para-aminobenzoic acid (specifically cleaved by pancreatic chymotrypsin from an orally ingested synthetic peptide) is now commercially available, but the test is insensitive in mild pancreatic insufficiency (Chapter 54). Pancreatic function tests measure pancreatic volume, bicarbonate, and enzyme secretion into the duodenum during stimulation by secretagogues such as secretin, cholecystokinin, or a test meal; but do not differentiate between insufficiency caused by pancreatic inflammation and cancer. ERCP enables the physician to differentiate carcinoma from pancreatitis and provides morphologic information useful in surgical management.

Differential diagnosis

A common diagnostic dilemma is the differentiation of chronic pancreatitis from carcinoma. In many instances, clinical features and noninvasive radiologic tests are sufficient; but ERCP, angiography, or exploratory laparotomy may be necessary to exclude carcinoma. It is occasionally difficult to provide histologic documentation of malignant disease even at the time of surgery.

Treatment

Management of abdominal pain in chronic pancreatitis often unsatisfactory, especially when coexistent narcotic addiction is present. The underlying cause, in most cases alcohol abuse, should be eliminated if possible. If attacks of inflammation and pain occur, treatment options are similar to those outlined for acute pancreatitis; but, once again, there is no definite proof of benefit. Splanchnic nerve blocks may be temporarily effective in relieving chronic continuous pain. There is some evidence that pain will spontaneously diminish as the disease progresses and as exocrine pancreatic insufficiency develops. A postulated feedback regulatory system (whereby duodenal trypsin inhibits exocrine pancreatic secretion) underlies the use of oral pancreatic enzymes to reduce pain. Preliminary studies suggest that chronic administration of large doses of these agents may be useful in selected patients with chronic pancreatitis.

Definitive surgery may be necessary for complications such as pseudocyst, pancreatic ascites, or biliary tract obstruction. Surgical intervention for chronic abdominal pain remains controversial, as it does not prevent or reverse pancreatic insufficiency and is not known to alter the natural history of the disease. The decision to perform surgery must be based on the severity and location of parenchymal disease and the anatomy of the ductal system as assessed by ERCP or operative pancreatography. When the main pancreatic duct is dilated, caudal or lateral drainage of the pancreatic duct into a loop of jejunum is most often performed. Resection of part or all of the gland (with or without islet cell autotransplantation) is favored for localized or diffuse pancreatitis without ductal dilatation, especially when exocrine insufficiency is already present. Biliary tract or sphincter surgery may also be indicated. Temporary or permanent relief of pain may occur in the postoperative state, but long-term prognosis is most closely related to the ability of the patient to discontinue alcohol intake. The long-term value of recently developed endoscopic techniques, such as biliary or pancreatic stent placement and endoscopic sphincterotomy with or without stone removal, are being evaluated.

Reduction in dietary intake of long-chain fats and supplemental intake of fat-soluble vitamins, especially vitamin D, are standard treatment measures; but administration of exogenous pancreatic extracts is the mainstay of treatment for steatorrhea with advanced exocrine pancreatic insufficiency. New enteric-coated formulations of oral pancreatic enzymes (i.e., Creon, Pancrease) are much more effective than older more crude preparations. Patients display considerable individual variation in enzyme requirements. Reduction of diarrhea and prevention of weight loss will occur in most patients, but steatorrhea is rarely totally corrected with this regimen. High cost and potential hyperuricosuria are negative aspects of enzyme-replacement therapy. Diabetes is managed with the standard measures and supplemental oral calcium intake is desirable in patients with persistent steatorrhea in an effort to minimize osteopenic bone disease.

Complications and prognosis

The metabolic complications of diabetes and malabsorption are frequent and treatable. Common bile duct obstruction and extrahepatic portal hypertension due to secondary thrombosis of the splenic or portal veins are rare but important sequelae that may require surgery. A pancreatic pseudocyst is clinically important in only 5% to 10% of cases, and abscess formation is unusual. Pancreatic ascites may present as a painless and often massive accumulation of exudative ascitic fluid rich in amylase. Pleural effusions may coexist, and leakage of pancreatic juice from a disrupted ductal system or pseudocyst can be documented by ERCP. Remission may occur with standard medical management or during treatment with somatostatin. Total parenteral nutrition therapy may be effective, but surgical resection or pseudocyst drainage is often necessary. The frequency of pancreatic cancer appears to be increased only in the hereditary form of chronic pancreatitis. Pseudoaneurysms of adjacent arteries may form and occasionally cause a highly lethal form of gastrointestinal bleeding.

More than 50% of deaths occur from direct complications of chronic alcoholism and are often unrelated to the pancreatitis itself. Prognosis is adversely affected by continued alcohol abuse.

EXOCRINE PANCREATIC TUMORS

Carcinoma of the exocrine pancreas is now the second most common cancer of the gastrointestinal tract and is the fourth leading cause of cancer deaths in the United States. A dramatic increase in age-adjusted mortality has occurred in recent decades, and the prognosis remains dismal, with survival after diagnosis averaging only 5 months.

Epidemiology and etiology

An increased incidence of pancreatic carcinoma is observed in males, in blacks, in developed countries, and with increasing age; but there is no clear relation of incidence to socioeconomic factors. The underlying cause is unknown, although chemical carcinogens are strongly suspected. These substances are postulated to reach the pancreas either hematogenously or by reflux of duodenal contents into the pancreatic duct. A variety of chemicals, including nitrosoureas and anthracene derivatives, induce cancer of the pancreas in experimental animals, but in these cases the tumors are of the acinar type. There is indirect evidence for the dose-dependent carcinogenic effect of cigarette smoke in human beings, and an increased frequency of carcinoma is reported in workers in some industries (i.e., chemists, metalworkers).

Pathology

Benign tumors of the pancreas are rare and usually cystic. Seventy percent of carcinomas originate in the head of the gland, with the remainder being diffuse or situated in the body or tail. It is important to differentiate periampullary cancers arising from the duodenum or common bile duct and the rare cystadenocarcinoma from pancreatic carcinomas, as these lesions have a better prognosis and should be treated with aggressive surgery.

Eighty percent of nonendocrine carcinomas develop from ductular epithelium and 1% from acinar cells; the remainder comprise a heterogenous group of unusual histologic types. Papillary, tubular, or acinar arrays of malignant cells with varying degrees of cellular differentiation are seen microscopically. Ductal epithelium at a distance from the cancer often exhibits papillary hyperplasia, and carcinoma in situ occurs in up to 20% of cases. Acute or chronic pancreatitis may exist distal to an obstructing cancer, but calcification is rare. Spread occurs by direct extension, with early neural and lymph node invasion. Visceral metastases are most common in liver, lungs, and bones. The pancreas can also be the site of secondary metastatic deposits, most commonly from breast, lung, or melanoma.

Clinical features

Men are affected by malignant exocrine pancreatic tumors twice as often as women, and the mean age at diagnosis is 55 years. Presenting symptoms and signs depend on the location and extent of the lesion (see the accompanying box), but nonspecific and vague complaints such as depression or anxiety are the earliest features in 50% of patients. The classic triad of abdominal pain, weight loss, and obstructive jaundice indicates a cancer situated in the head of the gland that is usually advanced and incurable. A palpably enlarged, nontender gallbladder in a jaundiced patient without biliary colic usually signifies malignant obstruction of the terminal bile duct (Courvoisier's law). Steatorrhea and severe weight loss may occur with proximal lesions. Cancer located in the body or tail may cause splenic vein obstruction, portal hypertension, and gastrointestinal bleeding. Otherwise, symptoms are similar no matter what the location of the tumor.

Abdominal pain is persistent, often postprandial and nocturnal, and is located in the upper abdomen. Weight loss is dramatic, progressive, and associated with aversion to food. Pruritus, ascites, hepatosplenomegaly, and constipation are other common features. Diabetes is observed in 25% of patients and may precede or follow other symptoms. Physical findings are variable but include jaundice, epigastric tenderness, and the presence of an abdominal mass or palpable gallbladder. Migratory thrombophlebitis and palpable subcutaneous fat nodules with polyarthralgias and prominent epigastric bruits due to compression of splanchnic vessels are unusual but striking manifestations. Pancreatic cancers may be associated with the ectopic production of hormones, resulting in hypoglycemia or hypercalcemia and Cushing's and carcinoid syndromes.

Diagnosis

Early diagnosis is not possible in the vast majority of patients with pancreatic cancer, as symptoms usually appear

Clinical syndromes in pancreatic cancer

Abdominal pain and weight loss
Obstructive jaundice
Malabsorption
Acute or chronic pancreatitis
Depression
Ectopic hormone syndromes

only when the neoplasm is widespread and there is no satisfactory screening test for asymptomatic persons. Blood tests such as those for serum amylase activity and carcinoembryonic antigen are not helpful in most cases. The value of serologic testing for diagnosis with the tumor antigen, CA 19-9, remains controversial. Levels are frequently normal in the early stages of pancreatic cancer, and elevations may occur in other conditions. Thus CA 19-9 is not a suitable screening test. Significant increases, however, may aid in the differentiation of benign and malignant pancreatic disease. The level of the antigen may also be useful in assessing prognosis and prediction of recurrence after surgery.

Abnormalities are observed in barium studies of the upper gastrointestinal tract in 50% of patients with symptoms, but the changes are of limited discriminative value and are usually seen only with large cancers. Diagnostic tests most commonly utilized currently are ultrasonography, CT, ERCP, and arteriography. A change in contour of the pancreas is accurately documented by the noninvasive methods of ultrasonography and CT, but it may be difficult to exclude inflammatory disease unless metastatic disease is documented (Fig. 67-9). Pancreatic function testing is also a nonspecific indicator of pancreatic disease. Initial studies with endoscopic ultrasonography are promising. The invasive procedures of ERCP and angiography are more specific in diagnosing pancreatic cancer. Extrinsic bile duct narrowing or abrupt and irregular obstruction of the pancreatic duct is seen in 90% of patients (Fig. 67-10). Because most pancreatic tumors are hypovascular, vessel deviation or encasement are the principal angiographic findings. Regardless of the diagnostic methods used to detect the tumor mass, cytologic, or histologic confirmation is important. Because of their relatively low sensitivity (≈50 percent false-negative results), duodenal or pancreatic fluid cytology studies are useful only when positive. CT or ultrasonography accurately demonstrates the presence of large hepatic metastases that can then be verified with percutaneous liver biopsy or laparoscopy. Percutaneous aspiration cytology of a pancreatic mass (guided by ultrasonography or CT) is an accurate diagnostic test (positive in 85% to 90% of cases), but should be reserved for those patients in whom surgery is not contemplated and in whom a diagnosis cannot be established by less invasive methods. Exploratory laparotomy may ultimately be necessary for diagnosis as well as treatment.

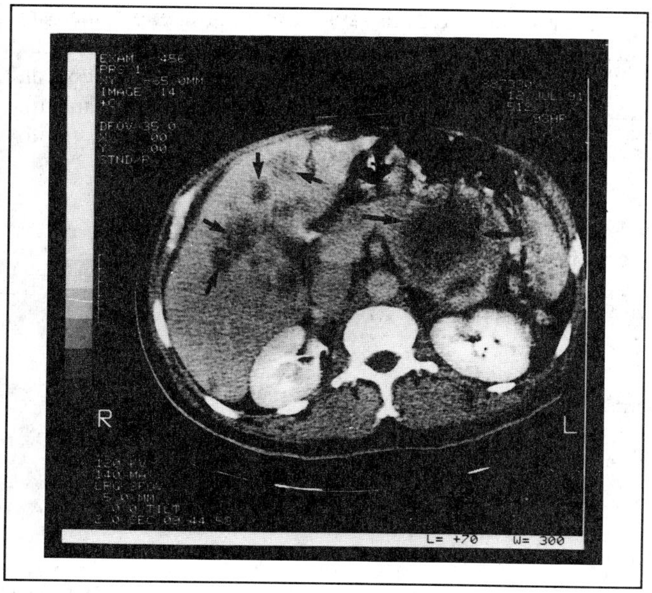

Fig. 67-9. CT scan in a patient with carcinoma of the tail of the pancreas. Necrotic pancreatic mass *(long arrows)* and hepatic metastases *(short arrows)* are evident.

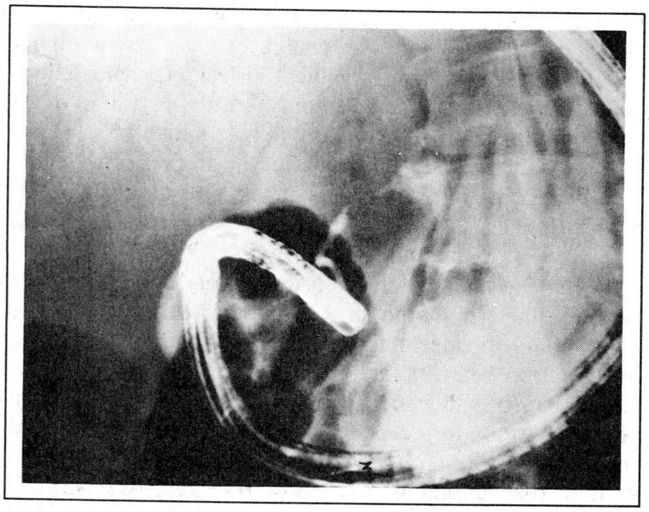

Fig. 67-10. Endoscopic retrograde cholangiopancreatogram showing abrupt, irregular obstruction of the main pancreatic duct by carcinoma.

Differential diagnosis

Chronic alcoholic pancreatitis is sometimes difficult to distinguish from carcinoma, and accurate diagnosis may require invasive tests or laparotomy. Patients with mesenteric vascular disease ("abdominal angina") may also present with abdominal pain and weight loss, and an identical clinical picture is occasionally observed with retroperitoneal lymphomas. In jaundiced patients, cancer must be differentiated from cholestatic liver disease, common bile duct stones, and ampullary or bile duct carcinoma.

Treatment and prognosis

Pancreatic carcinoma is a fatal disease, with 5-year survival less than 5%. Treatment therefore is palliative in the vast majority of patients. Surgical bypass procedures (cholecystojejunostomy and/or gastrojejunostomy) or endoscopic stenting or balloon dilatation transiently relieve biliary or gastric outlet obstruction, and splanchnic nerve blocks effectively reduce pain. Curative therapy is rarely possible for tumors of the body and tail, as local or distant metastases are almost invariably present at the time of diagnosis, and percutaneous fine needle aspiration is a recommended diagnostic procedure for such lesions. In cancers involving the head of the pancreas, radical surgery (pancreatoduodenectomy or total pancreatectomy) results in a high operative mortality, and 5-year survival is less than 15%. However, a Whipple operation can cure up to 30% of patients with carcinoma of the ampulla of Vater or the distal common bile duct (Chapter 65). Patients with metastatic disease are best treated nonsurgically.

Combined chemotherapy (5-fluorouracil) and high-dose radiation therapy may help relieve pain but does not alleviate biliary or intestinal obstruction. Whether intraoperative electron beam radiation therapy provides any advantage is being evaluated. Antiestrogen therapy, antagonism of cholecystokinin receptors, and radioimmunotherapy are speculative treatment modalities. The metabolic complications of diabetes mellitus and exocrine pancreatic insufficiency, whether caused by the tumor itself or by surgical treatment, can be effectively managed with insulin and pancreatic enzyme replacement (see p. 673).

ENDOCRINE PANCREATIC TUMORS

The rare tumors of the endocrine pancreas appear to arise from cells with a common embryologic origin and may be nonfunctioning (15%) or produce distinctive clinical syndromes characterized by excessive tissue and circulating concentrations of a variety of gastrointestinal hormones (Table 67-3). More than 30 different endocrine cell types have been identified. These cells produce peptides with neurocrine, paracrine, or endocrine effects. The tumors may occur in isolation or as part of the multiple endocrine adenomatosis complex and may secrete one or more peptide hormones. The tumors are variable in size, location, and degree of malignancy. Most are slow growing, vascular, and well differentiated.

Insulinoma

Insulin-secreting tumors of the endocrine pancreas are rare, often surgically curable, and characterized by recurrent fasting hypoglycemia and its neurologic sequelae. In 80% of cases, a single small benign tumor is demonstrated within the gland, but in 10% metastatic disease is evident at the time of diagnosis. Multicentric tumors occur in the remainder, and there is a high incidence of multiple endocrine adenomatosis syndrome in this subgroup.

Various combinations of headache, visual disturbances, confusion, weakness, and sweating and palpitations are characteristic, whereas convulsions or coma are unusual features of severe and prolonged hypoglycemia. Symptoms occur late in the postprandial state and are often confused with neurologic or psychiatric disease. Transient neurologic deficits may be observed during attacks.

Diagnosis requires repeated demonstration of hypoglycemia (< 40 mg/dl) concomitant with spontaneous or provoked symptoms, inappropriate hyperinsulinemia, and relief of symptoms after injection of carbohydrate. If attacks are infrequent, prolonged fasting or the intravenous tolbutamide test can be used to document hypoglycemia. Because up to one third of patients will have normal insulin levels, measurement of the insulin/glucose ratio (normal < 0.4) is important. Occasionally, levels of insulin secretory products (proinsulin and C-peptide) are required for confirmation. The absence of serum insulin antibodies rules out the surreptitious administration of insulin. CT and angiography are useful in localizing the site of the tumor. Percutaneous transhepatic portal venous sampling of hormone concentrations may help localize the site(s) of hormone production. Intraoperative and endoscopic ultrasonography is also useful in the diagnosis of this and other pancreatic endocrine tumors.

Surgical excision of the lesion is appropriate and usually curative. When unresectable metastatic disease is present, diazoxide may be effective in preventing hypoglycemic symptoms, and streptozotocin may cause partial tumor regression.

Subcutaneous administration of a long-acting somatostatin analog has been successful in the treatment of selected malignant endocrine tumors. By decreasing plasma concentrations of multiple peptide hormones (including insulin, gastrin, and glucagon), this agent may provide sympto-

Table 67-3. Clinical and diagnostic features of endocrine pancreatic tumors

Variables	Insulinoma	Gastrinoma	Pancreatic cholera	Glucagonoma	Somatostatinoma
Relative frequency	1	2	3	4	5
Clinical features	Fasting hypoglycemia	Ulcer disease, diarrhea	Diarrhea	Diabetes, rash	Steatorrhea, gallstones
Hormone secreted	Insulin	Gastrin	VIP	Glucagon	Somatostatin
Association with MEA	+	+	±	+	±
Rate of malignancy (%)	10	60	50	>50	>50
Provocative tests	+	+	−	±	±
Preferred treatment	Surgery, diazoxide, somatostatin	H_2-receptor antagonists, omeprazole, surgery	Surgery, somatostatin	Surgery, somatostatin	Surgery, chemotherapy

matic relief in patients in whom curative surgery is not possible. Current data do not support an antitumor effect of this drug.

Zollinger-Ellison syndrome

The pathophysiology, clinical features, and treatment of gastrinomas are discussed in detail in Chapter 38.

Pancreatic cholera

In recent years, a hormonally mediated syndrome of secretory diarrhea and hypokalemia has been described (Verner-Morrison syndrome). Constant clinical features of pancreatic cholera include profuse watery diarrhea and reduced or absent gastric secretion. Hypercalcemia, glucose intolerance, and urticarial skin lesions may occur in some patients. Fasting stool volumes are typically greater than 1 L/day, and there is no evidence of fat malabsorption or peptic ulcer disease. The syndrome appears to be caused by nonbeta islet cell tumors or hyperplasia of the pancreas. Increased amounts of the peptide hormone vasoactive intestinal polypeptide (VIP), which experimentally reduces gastric acid output and increases pancreatic and small intestinal secretion, are often found within the tumor and in the blood. Measurement of serum VIP levels should confirm the diagnosis, although secretion may be episodic. Diagnosis is often made by surgical exploration after other causes of chronic secretory diarrhea, especially laxative and diuretic abuse, have been excluded. Preoperative angiography or CT is diagnostic in only one third of cases. Surgical resection of any gross tumor (or blind subtotal or total pancreatic resection for hyperplasia or microadenomatosis) is curative in nearly 50% of reported cases. In unresectable disease, corticosteroid, phenothiazine, or somatostatin treatment may reduce diarrhea, and streptozotocin may cause residual tumor regression.

Glucagonoma and somatostatinoma

Hypersecretion of glucagon by the pancreatic alpha cells leads to diabetes mellitus, and a peculiar bullous and eczematoid dermatitis is a characteristic manifestation of glucagonoma. Anemia and weight loss are often present, and other endocrine abnormalities may coexist. A few cases of somatostatinoma have been reported, with clinical features of diarrhea and/or steatorrhea, glucose intolerance, exocrine pancreatic insufficiency, weight loss, and gallstones. These findings may be explained by the marked suppressive effects of somatostatin on the release of gastrointestinal peptides such as gastrin, cholecystokinin (CCK), and insulin. Documentation of a pancreatic tumor by angiography, CT, or at laparotomy and increased plasma levels of immunoreactive glucagon or somatostatin confirm the diagnosis. Surgical resection and, when necessary, chemotherapy with streptozotocin are appropriate modes of therapy. Somatostatin analogs are effective in reducing plasma glucagon levels.

MISCELLANEOUS PANCREATIC DISEASES

Cystic fibrosis

Cystic fibrosis is the most common lethal genetic defect observed in the white population of the Western world, and this autosomal recessive disease is estimated to occur in 1 of every 2000 live births. The early prognosis has improved dramatically in that up to 80% of patients now survive for more than 20 years. The recent genomic localization of the defect in cystic fibrosis to chromosome 7 has raised hopes for early diagnosis and prevention. The gene defect, however, is heterogeneous, and thus gene-based population screening is not yet feasible. Neonatal screening using serial immunoreactive trypsin levels may be a feasible alternative.

The affected gene appears to code for a membrane protein involved in transmembrane ion transport. In contrast to the normal state, the apical membrane chloride channels of airway epithelial cells in cystic fibrosis are not activated by cyclic AMP-dependent protein kinase. The resulting chloride impermeability could account for many of the clinical features of cystic fibrosis. Whether the same defect is present in pancreatic epithelial cells remains to be established; however, exocrine and mucous gland function are disturbed, and secretions of these organs are chemically altered. Thus the respiratory, gastrointestinal, and reproductive systems are affected, as well as the sweat and salivary glands. Recurrent pulmonary infections and the eventual development of chronic obstructive pulmonary disease account for much of the morbidity and almost all of the mortality of this disease.

Gastrointestinal symptoms occur in 85% to 90% of patients, and manifestations include pancreatic insufficiency, meconium ileus in infants, intestinal volvulus, rectal prolapse, recurrent fecal impactions, gallstones, and an unusual form of chronic liver disease characterized histologically as focal biliary cirrhosis. Strictures of the common bile duct may also be seen. In up to 20% of older subjects, recurrent small bowel obstruction occurs presumably due to inspissated secretions. Treatment with acetylcysteine or small-bowel lavage is usually successful. Increased doses of oral pancreatic enzymes may prevent this complication.

Cystic fibrosis is the most common cause of childhood exocrine pancreatic insufficiency in the United States. Nearly 90% of patients eventually require treatment for clinically significant maldigestion. Analysis of duodenal aspirates reveals a viscous solution of small volume with low concentrations of bicarbonate and enzymes. Little or no secretory response after secretin or CCK is characteristic. Even in the unusual subject without clinical evidence of pancreatic involvement, a marked reduction in bicarbonate secretion is noted.

Pancreatic damage appears to result from ductular obstruction with thick secretions and cellular debris and from resultant pressure necrosis of acinar structures. The end result is cystic dilatation of ducts filled with calcium-rich eosinophilic concretions and glandular fibrosis. Radiologically visible calcifications may be present. The islets of Langerhans are often spared until late in the course of the disease.

Clinical features consist of diarrhea with fat and protein malabsorption, although recurrent attacks of acute pancreatitis may occur. As expected, fecal fat loss is proportional to oral fat intake, and deficiencies of fat-soluble vitamins are common. Glucose intolerance is noted in nearly one third of cases, but overt diabetes mellitus is uncommon.

Diagnosis usually depends on the association of steatorrhea and respiratory disease developing in children or adolescents. Tests of exocrine pancreatic function are utilized as in adult-onset chronic pancreatitis (see previously), but a striking elevation of sodium content in sweat after pilocarpine iontophoresis remains the diagnostic hallmark of the disease. The occurrence of other gastrointestinal disorders should raise this diagnostic possibility even in older patients, for, in up to 2% of cases, the correct diagnosis is not made until the age of 18 years.

Treatment is supportive and consists primarily of maintaining adequate pulmonary function (Chapter 213) and nutrition. Reduction of dietary long-chain triglyceride intake with addition of medium-chain triglycerides and administration of oral pancreatic enzymes with meals are usually quite effective in reversing weight loss. Steatorrhea is rarely abolished by these measures, possibly due to a higher than expected frequency of gastric acid hypersecretion in these patients. Supplemental oral bicarbonate or H_2-receptor antagonists may be necessary in refractory cases. Fat-soluble vitamins and supplemental calcium are useful treatment adjuncts.

Congenital anomalies

Ectopic endocrine and/or exocrine pancreatic tissue is a common developmental anomaly that is rarely of clinical significance. The gastric antrum and proximal duodenum are the usual sites affected; but ectopia may also occur in the remainder of the small bowel, Meckel's diverticula, bile ducts, gallbladder, and the splenic hilum.

Annular pancreas results from an incomplete embryologic migration of the ventral pancreas, which instead encircles the second portion of the duodenum. Duodenal obstruction in the neonate is the usual presenting feature; but bile duct obstruction, pancreatitis, and duodenal ulcer may also occur. A smooth, symmetric constriction of the postbulbar duodenum with proximal dilatation is the characteristic radiologic feature, and surgical bypass is the treatment of choice. Preoperative confirmation is possible with endoscopic pancreatography.

Pancreas divisum results when the ventral and dorsal portions of the pancreatic ductal system fail to fuse. Drainage of pancreatic secretions into the duodenum then occurs primarily through the accessory papilla. This very common congenital defect (3% to 7% of the population) is discovered more often in patients undergoing endoscopic retrograde cholangiopancreatography for documented attacks of acute pancreatitis than in those subjects having the test performed for evaluation of biliary disease or chronic unexplained abdominal pain. Stenosis of the minor duct or accessory papilla is the proposed pathogenetic mechanism. Surgical transduodenal sphincteroplasty or endoscopic sphincterotomy of the accessory papilla is variably successful in preventing recurrent attacks of pancreatitis and should probably be considered only when other potential causes have been excluded and when radiologic evidence of minor duct dilatation is observed. In the occasional patient with irreversible chronic pancreatitis and pancreas divisum, sphincteroplasty has not been beneficial.

Pancreatic trauma

Traumatic injuries of the pancreas can occur after blunt or penetrating trauma or as a consequence of surgery. Penetrating abdominal wounds (i.e., gunshot and stab wounds) may lead to early lacerations, contusions, or hematomas of the gland or to the late complications of abscess, pseudocyst, or fistula. Associated major vascular and visceral injuries are common and result in the 20% mortality for pancreatic trauma. Elevated amylase levels in serum or paracentesis fluid are diagnostic, and early surgery with external drainage or pancreatic resection is usually required. Blunt abdominal trauma less commonly results in pancreatic damage but steering-wheel compression injuries are responsible for the uncommon entity of pancreatic transection. Postoperative acute pancreatitis usually occurs after biliary or gastric surgery, is difficult to diagnose, and results in a high mortality rate.

REFERENCES

Agarwal N et al: Evaluating tests for acute pancreatitis, Am J Gastroenterol 85:356, 1990.

Carter DC: Cancer of the pancreas, Gut 31:494, 1990.

Cello JP and Grendell JH, editors: Diagnosis and treatment of acute and chronic pancreatitis, Semin Gastrointest Dis. 2(3), July 1991.

Cello JP and Wilcox CM: Endoscopic therapy for pancreatitis and its complications, Semin Gastrointest Dis 2(3):177, 1991.

Cruickshank AH: Pathology of the pancreas, Great Britain, 1986, Springer-Verlag.

Glazer G and Ranson JHC, editors: Acute pancreatitis—experimental and clinical aspects of pathogenesis and management, London, 1988, Bailliere Tindall.

Go VLW et al, editors: The exocrine pancreas, New York, 1986, Raven Press.

Howard JM et al, editors: Surgical diseases of the pancreas, Philadelphia, 1987, Lea and Febiger.

Lee SP et al: Biliary sludge as a cause of acute pancreatitis, N Engl J Med 326:589, 1992.

Mannell A et al: Surgical management of chronic pancreatitis: long-term results in 141 patients, Br J Surg 75:467, 1988.

Mozell E et al: Functional endocrine tumors of the pancreas: clinical presentation, diagnosis and treatment, Curr Prob Surg V 27, No. 6, June 1990.

Neoptolemos VP et al: Controlled trial of urgent endoscopic sphincterotomy versus conservative treatment for acute pancreatitis due to gallstones. Lancet 2:979,1988.

Niederau C and Grendell JH: Diagnosis of chronic pancreatitis, Gastroenterology 88:1973, 1985.

Park RW and Grand RJ: Gastrointestinal manifestations of cystic fibrosis. A review, Gastroenterology 81:1143, 1981.

Ranson JHC et al: Prognostic signs and nonoperative peritoneal lavage in acute pancreatitis. Surg Gynecol Obstet 143:209, 1976.

Ranson JHC: The role of surgery in the management of acute pancreatitis, Ann Surg 211:382, 1990.

Singh M and Simsek H: Ethanol and the pancreas, Gastroenterology 98:1051, 1990.

Steinberg W, editor: Disorders of the pancreas, Gastroenterol Clin North Am V 19, No. 4, Dec. 1990.
Valenzuela JE et al, editors: Medical and surgical disease of the pancreas, New York, 1991, Igaku-Shoin.
Warshaw AL and Fernandez-del Castillo C: Pancreatic carcinoma, N Engl J Med 326:455, 1992.

CHAPTER

68 Diseases of the Peritoneum, Mesentery, and Omentum

Sanjiv Chopra

DISEASES OF THE PERITONEUM

Acute bacterial peritonitis

The clinical features, differential diagnosis, and approach to patients in acute bacterial peritonitis are described in Chapters 36 and 44.

Spontaneous or primary bacterial peritonitis

This process occurs in patients with ascites due to cirrhosis of the liver or nephrotic syndrome. It may also occur in patients with systemic lupus erythematosus receiving corticosteroids (see Chapter 56 for detailed discussion).

Bile peritonitis

Bile induces a chemical peritonitis, and facilitates secondary infection. Resorption of bilirubin and uptake of bacteria and toxins into the bloodstream results in hyperbilirubinemia, septicemia, and shock. Bile peritonitis following rupture of an inflamed gallbladder or following percutaneous needle biopsy of the liver in a patient with extrahepatic biliary obstruction is often followed by the rapid advent of severe abdominal pain and shock. The overall mortality is around 50%. Leakage of uninfected bile, as may occur consequent to abdominal trauma, often produces slowly progressive ascites with minimal abdominal pain. The treatment of bile peritonitis consists of appropriate fluid and electrolyte replacement, broad-spectrum antibiotic therapy, and, in most instances, early laparotomy.

Tuberculous peritonitis

See Chapters 44 and 276.

Fungal and parasitic peritonitis

Peritonitis secondary to infection with *Candida albicans* has been reported after peritoneal dialysis, perforation of peptic ulcers, and traumatic intestinal perforations. *Histoplasma capsulatum, Coccidioides immitis,* and *Cryptococcus neoformans* may rarely cause peritonitis. Parasitic infestation with *Schistosoma mansoni, Enterobius vermicularis,* and *Ascaris lumbricoides* can evoke granulomatous peritonitis and is clinically significant in that it may be mistaken for tuberculous or carcinomatous peritonitis at laparotomy. *Strongyloides stercoralis* and *Entamoeba histolytica* can cause more fulminant peritonitis. Treatment is geared toward eradication of the causative organism.

Granulomatous peritonitis

In addition to tuberculosis and the parasitic infestations mentioned previously, a variety of disorders can evoke a granulomatous inflammatory reaction of the peritoneum. These disorders include Crohn's disease, sarcoidosis, *immitis* infection, maternal meconium peritonitis, ruptured cystic teratomas, and adenocarcinomas. Starch peritonitis, another entity producing granulomatous peritonitis, is discussed later.

Gonococcal peritonitis

This entity is seen predominantly in young women. It produces severe abdominal pain, fever, and peritoneal signs often predominantly localized to the right upper quadrant. The gallbladder frequently is not visualized at the time of oral cholecystography, and minor abnormalities in liver function test results may occur, so that the clinical picture simulates that of acute cholecystitis (Fitz-Hugh–Curtis syndrome). Occasionally, a hepatic friction rub is audible. Although pelvic complaints may be overshadowed, the correct diagnosis is suggested by the presence of adnexal tenderness and demonstration of gonococci by a Gram stain and culture of cervical mucus. In advanced stages of gonococcal peritonitis, laparoscopy reveals perihepatitis with classic "violin string" adhesions between the parietal peritoneum and anterior surface of the liver; therapeutic benefit may result if these adhesions are transected during laparoscopic examination. Recently, *Chlamydia trachomatis* infection has been implicated in producing salpingitis and perihepatitis in a few patients. Additionally, infection with this organism can cause severe peritoneal infections with chronic ascites formation in women with Fitz-Hugh–Curtis syndrome. Appropriate antimicrobial therapy (Chapter 264) can lead to rapid resolution of symptoms.

Starch peritonitis

Granulomatous peritoneal reactions have been induced by foreign-body reactions to mineral oil used as a lubricant for surgical suture material, lint from surgical drapes, talc (magnesium silicate), and glove starch powder. Typically, symptoms appear 10 days to 4 weeks after laparotomy. Severe abdominal pain, fever, anorexia, nausea, and vomiting are common. Abdominal distention, tenderness, and a palpable abdominal mass may be present. The sedimentation rate is elevated, but leukocytosis or eosinophilia are inconstant features. At laparotomy, the peritoneal surface and omentum are seen to be covered with multiple nodules, mimicking peritoneal tuberculosis or carcinomatosis. Induration, thickening, and fat necrosis of the omentum are often mistaken for omental torsion and gangrene. Ascitic fluid is conspicuous, and examination under polarized light discloses starch granules with birefringent Maltese crosses. The diagnosis can be made by demonstration of these granules in fluid obtained by paracentesis or in tissue obtained by laparoscopic biopsy and will obviate a second operation. In some patients, treatment with corticosteroids or indomethacin produces a dramatic resolution of symptoms.

Retroperitoneal fibrosis

This entity is characterized by a well-delineated fibrous plaque centered around the sacral promontory, frequently enveloping the root of the aorta and extending laterally to the ureters and iliac vessels. Less commonly, the fibrotic process involves the kidneys, urinary bladder, duodenum, descending colon, spleen, pancreas, ovaries, and mesenteric blood vessels. Retroperitoneal fibrosis may occur in conjunction with other fibrotic processes such as mediastinal fibrosis, mesenteric fibrosis, sclerosing cholangitis, orbital pseudotumor, Dupuytren's contracture, Riedel's disease, and Peyronie's disease. Seventy percent of patients are in the fifth to seventh decades of life, and there is a 2:1 male predominance.

The etiology of retroperitoneal fibrosis is unknown in two thirds of patients. In a recent review, methysergide was responsible for approximately 12% of all cases. In 8% of cases, the process was associated with a malignant neoplasm, notably reticulum-cell sarcoma, lymphosarcoma, Hodgkin's disease, and carcinoid tumors. A picture simulating retroperitoneal fibrosis has been described in patients with abdominal aortic aneurysms (perianeurysmal fibrosis). Retroperitoneal injury resulting from any mechanism is capable of inciting retroperitoneal fibrosis.

Poorly localized abdominal or back pain is the most frequent presenting symptom. Other presenting symptoms are constitutional: anorexia, malaise, nausea, fever, and weight loss. Anuria is the sole manifestation in 10% of patients. Other symptoms include lower extremity edema, intermittent claudication, jaundice, gastrointestinal bleeding, and toxic megacolon.

A rectal or abdominal mass is palpable in 15% of patients. Anemia and elevation of the erythrocyte sedimentation rate and blood urea nitrogen are common findings. Although the inferior vena cava is often encased by the fibrous tissue, signs of obstruction are rare. Most deaths result from renal failure or an underlying malignant process. The diagnosis may be suggested by contrast urography: the classic triad consists of bilateral ureteral narrowing at the level of the fifth lumbar vertebra, medial deviation of the ureters, and dilatation of the ureter, calyces, and pelvis. Although computed tomography (CT) and magnetic resonance imaging (MRI) may disclose characteristic abnormalities, exploratory laparotomy is necessary to establish the correct diagnosis and permit ureterolysis.

Corticosteroid therapy has been used as an adjunct to surgical measures or as primary therapy in patients in whom all studies are consistent with the diagnosis of idiopathic retroperitoneal fibrosis and in whom the operative risks appear prohibitive. The long-term outlook is good, cumulative mortality being around 10%.

Periodic peritonitis

This disease, also called familial Mediterranean fever and familial recurring polyserositis, is inherited as an autosomal recessive trait and occurs predominantly in Sephardic Jews, Arabs, and Armenians. It is characterized by recurrent bouts of acute self-limited serositis, notably peritonitis, which develops eventually in more than 90% of patients. Eighty percent of patients are less than 20 years of age when they have their first attack. High fever, exquisite abdominal tenderness with marked rebound, and a rigid, boardlike abdomen lasting several hours and accompanied by leukocytosis mimic an "acute surgical abdomen" and often lead to surgical exploration. Arthritis, pleuritis, and pericarditis occur less frequently. Amyloid nephropathy, an almost uniformly fatal complication, occurs in about 25% of patients. Colchicine, 0.6 mg given two to three times daily by mouth, decreases the frequency and severity of attacks. Colchicine 1 to 2 mg daily appears to prevent amyloidosis. It also prevents additional deterioration of renal function in patients who have proteinuria but not the nephrotic syndrome. Intermittent colchicine treatment has been recommended for patients with infrequent attacks. In some of these patients, a short course of colchicine, instituted at the first premonition of an attack, will significantly ameliorate the characteristic acute pain and fever.

Peritoneal mesothelioma

This rare primary tumor of the peritoneum is associated with occupational exposure to asbestos in about 65% of patients. The development of peritoneal mesotheliomas has also been linked to exposure to thorium dioxide (Thorotrast). Exposure to asbestos need not be of long duration and often the latent period between exposure and development of the tumor is 30 to 40 years. Approximately 65% of mesotheliomas arise from the pleura, 25% from the peritoneum, and 10% from the pericardium. Men are affected more frequently than women, and the highest prevalence is in the sixth decade. The most frequent initial symptom is abdominal pain. Severe weight loss and ascites (occasionally very viscid) are almost universal features. Many patients have clubbing and respiratory signs associated with asbestosis. Symptomatic hypoglycemia has been reported on rare occasions. Diagnosis is established most often at the time of laparotomy or autopsy. Although the histologic features of peritoneal mesothelioma are quite variable and not necessarily specific, the tumor has distinctive ultrastructural features that are often extremely helpful in making a specific diagnosis. The course is virulent; there is no effective therapy, and most patients die 1 to 2 years after diagnosis.

Secondary carcinomatosis

Peritoneal involvement by malignant neoplasms is common. The vast majority are adenocarcinomas originating in the gastrointestinal tract, pancreas, or ovary. Patients with secondary carcinomatosis present with ascites, abdominal pain, and weight loss. Paracentesis yields fluid that is exudative and may be grossly bloody. The diagnosis is established by cytology, peritoneal biopsy, or peritoneoscopy. The prognosis is generally dismal. Some palliation may be achieved by repeated paracentesis, transperitoneal instillation of chemotherapeutic agents, or peritoneovenous shunting. Patients with malignant ascites due to ovarian carcinoma, breast cancer, and lymphoma can survive for years with appropriate treatment directed at the underlying malignancy.

Pseudomyxoma peritonei

This rare condition is characterized by the presence of gelatinous viscid material in the peritoneal cavity. The major causes are mucoceles of the appendix and mucinous cystadenocarcinomas of the ovary or appendix. Increasing abdominal girth in a patient with otherwise unimpaired general health is frequent. An abdomen distended with what appears to be fluid that does not shift may suggest the diagnosis. The correct diagnosis can be readily made at laparoscopy. Removal of the gelatinous material together with the primary tumor and omentum should be attempted at laparotomy; instillation of a chemotherapeutic agent may be beneficial.

Pneumatosis cystoides intestinalis

This rare condition is characterized by the presence of multiple air-filled cysts up to several centimeters in diameter in the intestinal wall and sometimes in the mesentery. The exact source of the gas is not clear; its composition is similar to that of atmospheric air. The intestinal flora has been implicated. In a large number of patients, pneumatosis cystoides intestinalis is an incidental finding. Associated diseases include obstructive pulmonary disorders, peptic ulcer diseases with outlet obstruction, scleroderma, inflammatory bowel disease, necrotizing enterocolitis, and ischemic colitis. The diagnosis is made by x-ray or sigmoidoscopic examination or at the time of laparotomy. The cysts may rupture and result in pneumoperitoneum. Treatment is directed toward the underlying primary disorder; occasionally antibiotic therapy with metronidazole or oxygen therapy is beneficial.

Eosinophilic ascites

Eosinophilic ascites is a rare entity characterized by the presence of large numbers of eosinophils (often greater than 50% of the total leukocyte count) in the ascitic fluid. It is seen in patients with eosinophilic gastroenteritis with predominantly subserosal and serosal disease (Chapter 42), vasculitis, lymphoma, ruptured hydatid cyst, and in patients undergoing chronic peritoneal dialysis. Patients with eosinophilic gastroenteritis usually respond dramatically to steroid administration with prompt and complete resolution of the ascites.

DISEASES OF THE MESENTERY

Mesenteric panniculitis

This condition (also called mesenteric Weber-Christian disease) presents in elderly patients, most often in men. About 60% of patients have abdominal pain, nausea, vomiting, weight loss, and low-grade fever. The remaining 40% are incidentally discovered to have an abdominal mass at the time of physical examination or laparotomy. Radiographic examination often reveals separation of small bowel loops, with kinking or angulation. The etiology is not known, but ischemia or infection may initiate the pathologic process that is characterized by thickening of the mesentery, infiltration of fat with foamy macrophages, and fat necrosis. Fibrosis and calcification occur in some patients and lead to a fibrotic and retracted mesentery (retractile mesenteritis). In the late stages, patients may have small bowel obstruction and intestinal lymphatic obstruction, producing protein-losing enteropathy, steatorrhea, and ascites. In general, the prognosis is good; many patients have spontaneous regression. Corticosteroids may afford symptomatic relief. Patients with retractile mesenteritis may have a fatal outcome.

Mesenteric fibromatosis

Mesenteric tumors develop in 10% to 18% of patients with Gardner's syndrome (Chapter 45). They are predominantly found in premenopausal women and frequently develop after colectomy. Although usually asymptomatic, the fibrous proliferation can be aggressive and lethal, causing severe ischemia due to involvement of the mesenteric blood vessels. Treatment with nonsteroidal anti-inflammatory drugs may be effective in reducing the size of the tumors and in affording pain relief.

Mesenteric hernia

A mesenteric hernia is an intraperitoneal herniation of a loop of bowel through a mesenteric defect. Most often the defect is single, 2 to 3 cm in diameter, and located in the mesentery of the small bowel. Mesenteric (internal) hernias account for 1% to 2% of intestinal obstruction in collected series of patients with intestinal obstruction. Patients may have a history of chronic intermittent abdominal distress. Complications include acute intestinal obstruction, volvulus, and gangrene of the bowel. A correct diagnosis is seldom made preoperatively, and mesenteric hernias can be missed at surgery. Treatment is surgical and consists in reduction of incarcerated bowel and repair of the defect together with resection of any nonviable bowel.

Mesenteric cysts

These rare lesions develop most often in the second decade of life. They present as smooth, painless masses that can be made to move freely at right angles to the line of attachment of the mesentery. Large cysts may mimic ascites. Rupture, hemorrhage, or infection occur rarely. Surgical excision is the preferred treatment.

Mesenteric tumors

Mesenteric tumors may be benign (fibromas, lipomas, myomas) or malignant (lymphomas). Physical signs are similar to those mentioned for mesenteric cysts, with the exception that the tumor mass is often solid. Most are locally invasive, and cure is effected by excision.

Mesenteric arteriovenous fistula

This entity occurs as a rare sequel to abdominal trauma. It also has been reported after percutaneous needle biopsy of the liver. The dreaded complication is portal hypertension.

DISEASES OF THE OMENTUM

The greater omentum has been called the"abdominal policeman," as it often limits the spread of intraperitoneal infections. Cysts and tumors of the omentum are similar in presentation to their mesenteric counterparts. By far the most dramatic disorder involving the omentum is torsion, which occurs predominantly in middle-aged, obese men. At laparotomy, gangrene of the omentum is found and bacterial peritonitis may be present. Treatment consists of omentectomy.

REFERENCES

Amis ES Jr: Retroperitoneal fibrosis, Am J Roentgenol 157:321, 1991.

Antman KH: Clinical presentation and natural history of benign and malignant mesothelioma, Semin Oncol 8(3):313, 1981.

Bayer AS et al: Candida peritonitis, Am J Med 61:832, 1976.

Bender MD: Diseases of the peritoneum, mesentery and diaphragm. In Sleisenger MH and Fordtran JS, editors: Gastrointestinal disease: pathophysiology, diagnosis and management, ed 4, Philadelphia, 1989, WB Saunders.

Durst AL et al: Mesenteric panniculitis, Surgery 81:203-211, 1977.

Janin Y, Stone AM, and Wise L: Mesenteric hernia, Surg Gynecol Obstet 150:747, 1980.

Kannerstein M and Churg J: Peritoneal mesothelioma, Hum Pathol 8:83, 1977.

Limber GK, King RE, and Silverberg SG: Pseudomyxoma peritonei, Ann Surg 178:587, 1973.

Marbet UA et al: Diffuse peritonitis and chronic ascites due to infection with *Chlamydia trachomatis* in patients without liver disease: new presentation of the Fitz-Hugh—Curtis syndrome, Br Med J 293:5, 1986.

McNabb BC et al: Transmural eosinophilic gastroenteritis with ascites, Mayo Clin Proc 54:119, 1979.

Meyerhoff J: Familial Mediterranean fever: report of a large family, review of the literature and discussion of the frequency of amyloidosis, Medicine (Baltimore) 59:66, 1980.

Reichert JA and Valle RF: Fitz-Hugh-Curtis syndrome: a laparoscopic approach, JAMA 236:266, 1976.

Tsukada K et al: Noncytotoxic drug therapy for intra-abdominal desmoid tumor in patients with familial adenomatous polyposis, Dis Colon Rectum 35:29, 1992.

Zemer D et al: Colchicine in the prevention and treatment of the amyloidosis of familial Mediterranean fever, N Engl J Med 314:1001, 1986.

Part Three

Hematology and Oncology

I BASIC PRINCIPLES

CHAPTER

69 Molecular and Cellular Biology of Hematopoiesis

Ronald Hoffman
David A. Williams

HEMATOPOIESIS

Human blood contains a variety of cells, each providing a vital function needed to sustain normal life. Red cells transport oxygen throughout the body, whereas platelets are required to promote clotting. White cells (granulocytes, monocytes, lymphocytes) combat attack by viruses, bacteria, fungi, and likely tumor cells. Quantitative or qualitative abnormalities of any of these blood cell types lead in a predictable manner to human disease. The life span of most blood cells is extremely short, ranging from hours to days, although some exceptions exist in the lymphoid compartment. The need for continued blood cell production requires the constant regeneration of the blood cell pool throughout life. In addition, various conditions such as bleeding or infection require that the bone marrow be able to respond quickly to produce additional cells. The term *hematopoiesis* refers to the system by which the body continuously produces blood cells. Blood cells ultimately arise from the bone marrow as the result of the proliferation and differentiation of primitive cells capable of maturation into all blood cell types. These primitive cells are termed *pluripotent hematopoietic stem cells*. Blood cell production is believed to be regulated in part by a series of glycoprotein hormones.

The vast majority of cells present in a healthy individual's bone marrow are bone marrow precursor cells (Color Plate III-1). From 60% to 70% of these cells are myeloid precursors, 20% to 30% are erythroid precursors, and the remaining 10% include lymphocytes, plasma cells, and macrophages. In addition, 4 to 5 megakaryocytes are normally found per 1000 nucleated bone marrow cells. The normal ratio of myeloid to erythroid precursors is 3 to 3.5:1. Alterations in these numbers are difficult to determine with bone marrow aspirates because of variations in dilution with peripheral blood. Bone marrow biopsy is the preferred method of quantitation of marrow cellularity and precursor frequency.

Hematopoietic stem cells

Hematopoiesis can be viewed as being composed of a continuum of functionally different cell populations with differing self-renewal, proliferative, and differentiation capacities (Fig. 69-1). The most primitive cell in this hierarchy is the pluripotent hematopoietic stem cell, which is characterized by its extensive self-renewal capacity and its capability of giving rise to all hematopoietic cell lineages. The stem cell is a quiescent cell that possesses self-renewal capacity during its life span, a characteristic that ensures the existence of an adequate pool of sustaining stem cells. Stem cells must undergo the *commitment process* to differentiate to different classes of progenitor cells, which are characterized by a progressive loss of self-renewal capacity and multipotentiality, leading to the production of multipotent, bipotent, and eventually unipotent progenitor cells. Unlike stem cells, a much greater proportion of progenitor cells are mitotically active. The decision to remain quiescent, undergo self-renewal, or proceed with commitment is a critical step in the determination of a stem cell's fate. Once the commitment decision is made, an irreversible movement toward production of blood cells occurs, which inevitably results in the loss of stem cell self-renewal capacity and ultimately stem cell "death." It remains unknown whether this decision is a random process *(stochastic hypothesis)* or whether it can be influenced by cytokines, matrix proteins, or marrow accessory cells present within the marrow microenvironment *(instructional hypothesis)*.

Several models have also been constructed that give insight into the clonal organization of hematopoietic cells. If stem cell self-renewal capacity is unlimited and stem cells are truly immortal, they could likely function for an individual's entire lifetime. Stem cell immortality would confer stability on the clonal composition of an animal's hematopoietic system. On the other hand, stem cell self-renewal capacity could also be much more limited. Under these circumstances, only a portion of the total stem cell population would be active at any given time, and new stem cells would be required to contribute to active blood cell production to replace dying cells. This constant turnover in the active stem cell populations would likely lead to changes in the clonal makeup of the different hematopoietic lineages over time. Hematopoiesis then would be maintained by a succession of short-lived clones *(clonal succession model)*. The concept of short-lived stem cells is supported by the finding that the hematopoietic systems of irradiated, reconstituted animals undergo clonal changes with time. Equally convincing evidence, however, indicates that at least a subpopulation of stem cells are long lived, able to function for prolonged periods, and able to expand clonally during the regeneration of a new hematopoietic system.

Resolution of these theories that deal with stem cell fate and life span is extremely important to further our understanding of the basic biologic properties of stem cells. Such accomplishments would allow further insight into the pathobiology of bone marrow failure and the origins of hematologic malignancies. Greater knowledge of the stem cell is likely necessary if the therapeutic potential of bone marrow transplantation and somatic gene transfer therapy is ever to be achieved. New insight into the biology of stem cells and progenitor cells will surely

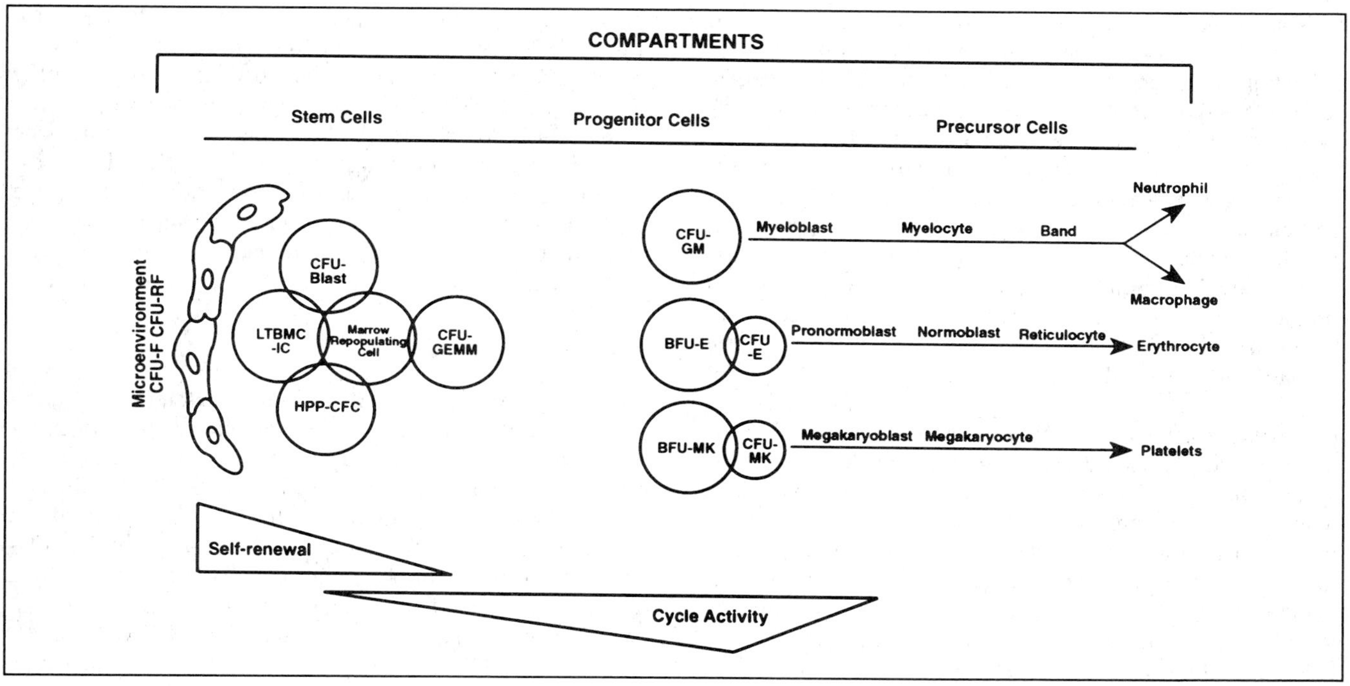

Fig. 69-1. Schematic presentation of cellular events that occur during normal human hematopoiesis. *CFU,* Colony-forming unit; *CFU-Bl, CFU-Blast* unit; *CFU-F,* CFU—fibroblast; *CFU-RF,* CFU—reticular fibroblast; *LTBMC-IC,* long-term bone marrow culture—initiating cell; *HPP-CFC,* high-proliferative-potential colony-forming cell; *CFU-GEMM,* CFU—granulocyte, erythrocyte, macrophage, megakaryocyte; *CFU-GM,* CFU—granulocyte, macrophage; *BFU-E* BFU—erythrocyte; *CFU-E,* CFU—erythrocyte, *BFU-MK;* BFU—megakaryocyte; *CFU-MK,* CFU—megakaryocyte.

occur with the recent ability of several research groups to obtain highly enriched populations of not only murine but also human stem cells.

Advances in our understanding of hematopoiesis have occurred following the development of several assays to measure stem cell and progenitor cell number and function. Stem cells and the numerous classes of marrow progenitor cells can be assayed using a variety of in vitro clonal assays performed in semisolid media (colony assays) or by using long-term marrow cultures. The time required for hematopoietic colonies to develop in vitro depends on the stage of differentiation of the cell from which they are derived. The most mature human progenitor cells produce small colonies after 7 days of incubation, whereas the more immature progenitor cells give rise to larger colonies after 14 to 28 days.

The overwhelming majority of morphologically identifiable cells within the marrow are precursor cells that have no self-renewal capacity, are unipotent, and are capable of limited mitosis. These cells exhibit well-described nuclear and cytoplasmic characteristics that allow the clinical hematologist to identify them as belonging to a particular cell lineage. Because of the quantity of precursor cells and their active engagement in mitosis, considerable amplification of cell numbers occurs at this stage of development, resulting in a steady supply of blood cells that egress from the marrow.

Hematopoietic microenvironment

Hematopoiesis occurs in a complex environment within the marrow cavity, termed the *hematopoietic microenvironment.* The marrow cavity is extremely vascular. Branches of a central longitudinal artery traverse the interior of the bone and cortex, either joining directly to venous sinuses or communicating indirectly through the haversian canals into bone cortex. These vascular connections define groups of developing hematopoietic cells termed *hematopoietic cords,* where stem cell self-renewal and commitment occur. Blood cells leaving the marrow cavity traverse the hematopoietic cords, pass through endothelial cells, eventually enter venous sinuses, and are rapidly transported into central longitudinal veins and arrive in the general circulation.

Various accessory cells contribute important functions to the hematopoietic microenvironment. Adventitial reticular cells cover most vascular surfaces and provide a reticular network that supports developing hematopoietic cells. Adventitial cells and preadipocytes probably also affect hematopoiesis by direct cell contact or local secretion of cytokines or other growth-regulatory proteins. Such marrow accessory cells normally contain fat and extend into the hematopoietic cord space. During periods of hematopoietic stress, these cells become flattened and devoid of fat globules, providing additional space for active hematopoiesis.

The hematopoietic microenvironment provides more than passive support for hematopoietic cells. Preferential localization of blood cell production to specific microenvironments is thought to affect stem cell differentiation, leading to the hypothesis that specific locations or "niches" within the marrow provide an inductive microenvironment for stem cell self-renewal and differentiation. The cellular and biochemical basis of such niches has yet to be defined, but the development of in vitro long-term marrow culture systems, which mimic the marrow microenvironment, has provided further insight into this process. Such cultures are composed of a complex adherent cell layer, termed the *stromal cell layer,* which contains endothelial cells, fibroblasts, macrophages, and preadipocytes. Hematopoiesis occurs within the adherent cell layer, and hematopoietic cells are continuously shed into the overlying media. Using this system, hematopoietic niches have been shown possibly to involve direct communication of stromal cells with stem cells through cell-to-cell contact, localization of growth factors and stem cells at the point of cell-to-cell contact, prevention of growth factor degradation by binding cytokines to extracellular matrix proteins, or secretion of growth factors that both stimulate and downregulate hematopoiesis. These interactions define a *local area network* (LAN) for hematopoiesis.

Stem cell assays

Attempts to assay stem cells began in the early 1960s, when Till and McCulloch injected lethally irradiated mice with marrow cells. These marrow cells contained CFU-S (colony-forming unit—spleen), which lodged in the spleens of these animals and formed macroscopic nodules within 7 to 12 days. The splenic nodules were derived from a single cell and consisted of differentiating cells belonging to several hematopoietic lineages. In addition, such splenic nodules contained cells capable of generating additional splenic colonies when transferred into secondarily irradiated hosts. Cells (CFU-S_{12}) that give rise to splenic nodules arising after 12 to 14 days contain larger numbers of CFU-S than splenic colonies that appear in 8 to 10 days (CFU-S_8). The biologic properties of the CFU-S led to speculations that this cell represented a hematopoietic stem cell. However, both CFU-S_8 and CFU-S_{12} have recently been shown to be a more differentiated class of stem cells. Stem cells are currently being defined by their marrow-repopulating ability.

Stem cell function is now thought to be best quantitated by such cells' ability to reconstitute hematopoiesis in lethally irradiated recipients. Marrow-reconstituting ability of stem cells is optimally measured by the use of long-term in vivo assays. The use of retroviral-mediated gene insertion has enhanced investigators' ability to track the progeny of individual stem cells in vivo. This approach has been useful in quantitating murine stem cells, but obviously the human system does not lend itself to this form of experimental freedom. In vivo xenograft systems, however, have been recently developed which may allow assay of the marrow-populating capacity of human stem cells. In vitro assays for various primitive hematopoietic progenitor cells that resemble stem cells have also been developed: the colony-forming unit—blast (CFU-Bl), the high-proliferative-potential colony-forming cell (HPP-CFC), and the long-term bone marrow culture—initiating cell (LTBMC-IC). These assays detect cells with self-renewal capacity and multilineage differentiation capacity. Using such in vitro and in vivo assays, human stem cells have now begun to be phenotypically characterized.

Erythropoiesis

The immediate progeny of differentiated stem cells committed to erythropoiesis is several classes of progenitor cells, including the colony-forming unit—granulocyte, erythrocyte, macrophage, megakaryocyte (CFU-GEMM) (Color Plate III-2); the burst-forming unit—erythroid (BFU-E); and the colony-forming unit—erythroid (CFU-E). This hierarchy of progenitor cells is characterized by a progressive loss of self-renewal capacity and further restriction in differentiation potential (CFU-GEMM→BFU-E→CFU-E). These progenitor cells each can be detected by their ability in semisolid media to form erythroid colonies in the presence of appropriate growth factors. Each of these assays requires the presence of erythropoietin. The most differentiated erythroid progenitor cells, CFU-E, then produces a variety of erythroid precursor cells.

The first identifiable and also largest erythroid precursor is the *pronormoblast* (Color Plate III-3, *A*), which has a diameter of 14 to 19 μ and a large, homogeneously staining (violet) oval nucleus with indistinct nucleoli. The cytoplasm is deeply basophilic, with lighter-staining areas usually near the nucleus, reflecting the position of the Golgi and lipid-containing mitochondria. Maturation to the basophilic normoblast is accompanied by reduction in cell size and pronounced changes in the nuclear chromatin structure. The *basophilic normoblast* (Color Plate III-3, *B*) is 12 to 17 μ in diameter, with basophilic cytoplasm and nuclear chromatin characterized by coarsening and prominent clumping, referred to as a "spoked wheel" or "cartwheel" appearance. Nucleoli are generally not visualized. The *polychromatic normoblast* (Color Plate III-3, *C*) is nearly the same size as the basophilic normoblast. The accumulation of hemoglobin is accompanied by progressively less basophilic and increasing muddy gray coloration of the cytoplasm on Wright-Giemsa staining. The nucleus is almost black because of further condensation. The most differentiated nucleated red cell precursor is the *orthochromatic normoblast* (Color Plate III-3, *C*). This cell's diameter approaches that of a reticulocyte (8 to 12 μ) and has an eosinophilic staining cytoplasm containing almost a complete complement of hemoglobin. The nucleus is fully condensed and pyknotic. Extrusion of the nucleus results in formation of a *reticulocyte,* a cell slightly larger than a fully mature erythrocyte. The reticulocyte is characterized by the presence of a fine granular or reticular network of ribosomal ribonucleic acid (RNA) (Color Plate III-4, *J*). Such cells are rarely present in peripheral blood but are increased in response to hemolysis or blood loss. The final stage of erythroid maturation is the *erythrocyte*. The cell is a biconcave, relatively flat, nonnucleated disc with a diameter of 7 to 8 μ.

Myelopoiesis

Neutrophils and monocytes are closely related cells that arise from a common committed progenitor cell, the colony-forming unit—granulocyte, macrophage (CFU-GM), which in turn gives rise to a CFU—granulocyte (CFU-G) or CFU—macrophage (CFU-M); these progenitors have a unipotential differentiation capacity. Progenitor cells of basophil-mast cells and eosinophils have also been identified.

The earliest identifiable precursor cell of the myeloid lineage is the *myeloblast*. The cell is approximately 12 to 14 μ in diameter, with a round or oval nucleus and a cytoplasm that lacks granules. Nuclear chromatin is fine, and nucleoli are easily visible and number one to five per cell. The nucleus often stains reddish. *Promyelocytes* are the most frequent and largest of the primitive myeloid precursors (Color Plate III-1). Promyelocytes are variable in nuclear shape, with less prominent nucleoli and coarse chromatin. The cytoplasm is deeply basophilic and contains variable numbers of peroxidase-positive granules. These granules distinguish the promyelocyte from the myeloblast. *Myelocytes* are characterized by round-to-oval nuclei with characteristic nuclear indentations, indistinct nucleoli, and unevenly stained, coarse chromatin structure. The cytoplasm stains pale gray-brown or pink-brown with numerous specific granules covering the nucleus and throughout the cytoplasm. The myelocyte is also characterized by the appearance of specific granules and is the final stage of myelopoiesis in which the cells are capable of cell division. The metamyelocyte, band neutrophil, and segmented neutrophil show progressive condensation and restriction of the nucleus. The *metamyelocyte* exhibits a characteristic bean-shaped nucleus, the *band neutrophil* a horseshoe-shaped or S-shaped nuclear structure without recognizable constrictions, and the *segmented neutrophil* the characteristic nuclear segmentations for which it is named that divide the nucleus into two to five lobes. These myeloid forms exhibit similar cytoplasmic characteristics to the myelocyte, with progressive reduction in overall cell size.

The marrow contains a large reserve of band and segmented neutrophils. In the peripheral blood, neutrophils are equally divided between circulating and marginal pools. A large reserve of neutrophils is therefore available in the marrow and the marginal pool to respond quickly to infection or inflammation. The mature neutrophil remains in the circulation for approximately 10 to 14 hours before entering tissues and performing its phagocytic function. This limited survival of granulocytes dictates that myelopoiesis be a highly dynamic biologic process.

HEMATOPOIETIC REGULATORY MOLECULES

Hematopoiesis is sustained by a family of glycoproteins, the hematopoietic growth factors. The term *cytokine* refers to a bioactive cell secretion, whereas the term *growth factor* refers to a growth-regulatory molecule and is a more specific term encompassing erythropoietin, the colony-stimulating factors, and the interleukins. Many cytokines serve as hematopoietic growth factors. The nomenclature of these growth factors was first defined operationally. The initial factors described were identified by their ability to stimulate progenitor cells to form in vitro colonies composed of particular types of cells and were therefore referred to as granulocyte colony-stimulating factor (G-CSF) or granulocyte-macrophage colony-stimulating factor (GM-CSF). The interleukins derived their names initially from their cellular sources as well as their actions on leukocytes. The biologic activity of erythropoietin was first detected using a variety of rodent animal models. Erythropoietin was subsequently shown to stimulate in vitro erythropoiesis. The genes for many of the hematopoietic growth factors have now been cloned and their respective recombinant proteins produced and purified. The availability of these purified recombinant biomolecules has permitted determination of their actions, cellular origins, and actual therapeutic use (Table 69-1).

Each of the hematopoietic growth factors exhibits multiple biologic activities, most affecting several hematopoietic lineages. GM-CSF, for example, promotes CFU-GM proliferation but also influences the development of CFU-GEMM, HPP-CFC, CFU-Bl, LTMBC-IC, and CFU megakaryocyte (CFU-MK). This cytokine stimulates the functional activation of such differentiated cells as eosinophils, macrophages, monocytes, and neutrophils. Many activities of the hematopoietic growth factors are either additive or synergistic. For example, both GM-CSF and interleukin-3 (IL-3) are capable of stimulating HPP-CFC–derived colonies, and their actions are additive. The c-kit ligand, on the other hand, has no colony-stimulating activity by itself but synergistically interacts with the combination of GM-CSF and IL-3 to optimize cloning efficiency of HPP-CFC in vitro, in addition to enhancing the cloning efficiency of many other classes of progenitor cells.

Some growth factors act directly on hematopoietic progenitors, whereas others induce the expression of a wide variety of other interleukins and growth factor genes by marrow accessory cells. Specific membrane receptors for various hematopoietic growth factors (IL-3, GM-CSF, G-CSF, erythropoietin, M-CSF, c-kit ligand) are restricted to undifferentiated and maturing cells of the appropriate target cell lineages. By contrast, other growth factors have no colony-stimulating activity but affect hematopoiesis indirectly. For instance, IL-1 has no known colony-stimulating activity itself but induces G-CSF and GM-CSF expression by a variety of cells, including fibroblasts, endothelial cells, thymic epithelial cells, and T lymphocytes. Such indirect-

Table 69-1. Potentially clinically useful hematopoietic growth factors

Growth factor	Potential clinical uses
Interleukin-1 (IL-1)	Radioprotective agent (decreases degree of granulocytopenia/thrombocytopenia); antitumor activity against renal cell carcinoma and melanoma with or without lymphokine-activated killer (LAK) cells
Interleukin-3 (IL-3)	Lessens degree of granulocytopenia/thrombocytopenia after bone marrow transplantation or chemotherapy
Interleukin-6 (IL-6)	Stimulates platelet production; lessens degree of granulocytopenia/thrombocytopenia after bone marrow transplantation or chemotherapy
Interleukin-11 (IL-11)	Stimulates platelet production; lessens degree of granulocytopenia/thrombocytopenia after bone marrow transplantation or chemotherapy
Granulocyte-macrophage colony stimulating factor (GM-CSF)	Lessens degree of granulocytopenia after bone marrow transplantation or chemotherapy; preparation of peripheral blood stem cell grafts
Granulocyte colony stimulating factor (G-CSF)	Lessens degree of granulocytopenia after bone marrow transplantation or chemotherapy; treatment of chronic neutropenic disorders
Macrophage colony stimulating factor (M-CSF)	Adjunctive therapy for fungal infections after bone marrow transplantation or chemotherapy; antitumor therapy when administered with monoclonal antibodies
Erythropoietin	Treatment of anemias of chronic renal disease, chronic inflammation cancer, and human immunodeficiency virus 1 (HIV-1) infection
c-kit ligand (stem cell factor [SCF])	Lessens degree of granulocytopenia/thrombocytopenia after bone marrow transplantation or chemotherapy; increases rate of in vitro gene transfer to hematopoietic stem cells; increases number of stem cells in marrow grafts; preparation of peripheral blood stem cell grafts

acting growth factors can have profound effects on in vivo and in vitro hematopoiesis.

Understanding growth factor physiology is an important step in optimizing their therapeutic use and furthering our knowledge of the biogenesis of many hematologic disorders. This information is available only for a few growth factors. Erythropoietin physiology is the best understood. Under steady-state conditions, erythropoietin is elaborated by either proximal tubules or peritubular cells of the kidney's inner cortex in response to a hypoxic stimulus or anemia. The oxygen sensor that monitors blood oxygen content is now thought to be a heme protein that controls the expression of erythropoietin messenger RNA (mRNA) in an unknown way and results in the elaboration of erythropoietin. With the correction of the hypoxia or anemia, erythropoietin production ceases, except in cells that constitutively produce this hormone. Inadequate elaboration of this growth factor results in anemia, whereas excessive erythropoietin production leads to polycythemia.

Cytokines act in an indirect way and play a role in the development of the hematologic consequences of several systemic diseases. IL-1 and tumor necrosis factor (TNF) have been shown to play important roles in producing the clinical features associated with acute and chronic inflammatory states and other serious illnesses, including septic shock and cachexia. For example, TNF and IL-1 produced by resident macrophages during an inflammatory response promote IL-6, G-CSF, and GM-CSF production by marrow accessory cells. These secondarily elaborated cytokines account for many hematologic consequences of bacterial infections. IL-6, G-CSF, and GM-CSF promote myelopoiesis, leading to granulocytosis and likely monocytosis. Increased IL-6 levels promote megakaryocyte maturation and contribute to the development of secondary thrombocytosis. Overexpression of IL-6 also plays a role in the biogenesis of Castleman's disease. TNF has been shown to be an important player in the biogenesis of the anemia of chronic inflammation. TNF directly suppresses erythroid development, leading to progressive anemia.

CONTROL OF CELL EXIT FROM MARROW

The movement of erythroid marrow cells from the marrow into the bloodstream has been studied using radiolabeled iron (Fe). After initial uptake of ^{59}Fe by the marrow, newly synthesized erythrocytes are released into the blood in 4 to 6 days. The generation time of proliferating erythroid precursors (pronormoblasts, basophilic and polychromatic normoblasts) averages about 24 hours at each stage of maturation. Nonmitotic erythroid precursor cells (orthochromatic normoblasts, reticulocytes) reside in the marrow cavity for approximately 48 hours each. The maturation process includes an average of four divisions and the generation of 8 to 16 cells from each pronormoblast. During periods of stress, red cells can exit the marrow prematurely after skipping several divisions. These cells maintain characteristics of more primitive red cells, such as macrocytosis, elevated fetal hemoglobin, and persistence of i (versus I) antigen on the cell surface. Red cell maturation time may also be shortened by decreasing the duration of each mitosis or by decreasing the maturation time of nondividing erythrocyte precursors. The red blood cell mass may be further elevated by increasing the number of erythrocytes actually entering the bloodstream. The last mechanism could result either from less destruction of red cell precursors (termed *ineffective erythropoiesis*) in the marrow cavity (normally about 10%) or from an expanded number of primitive cells entering the erythroid maturational sequence. The latter appears to be the usual mechanism of expansion of the erythroid compartment during times of increased requirement for red cells as a result of chronic hemolysis or blood loss.

Insight has recently been gained into the molecular basis of erythroid cells' movement out of marrow. Erythroleukemic cells have been shown to bind specifically to the extracellular matrix protein *fibronectin*. These cells' ability to adhere to fibronectin diminishes during their differentiation. Subsequent studies have demonstrated that binding to fibronectin involves a specific peptide in the fibronectin molecule, Arg-Gly-Asp-Ser (RGDS). This interaction is mediated by a receptor on the surface of erythrocytes, VLA-5, a member of the integrin supergene family of receptors. Loss of adhesion of differentiating erythrocytes is associated with the functional absence of this receptor at the reticulocyte stage. Similar interactions of maturing normal erythroid precursors are thought to play a role in red cell release.

The mechanisms responsible for the release of myeloid cells from the marrow have not yet been elucidated. However, it is clear that the marrow compartment consists of both a mitotic pool (consisting of myeloblasts, promyelocytes, and myelocytes) and a storage pool of granulocyte precursors (metamyelocytes and band forms) and granulocytes. Stress and steroid administration produce a mobilization of granulocytes into the blood. The storage pool in the marrow is significantly larger than the peripheral blood pool of granulocytes. The maturation time for cells of the neutrophil series is approximately 8 days. The peripheral blood pool of granulocytes is made up of both circulating and marginating compartments of cells, with a distribution of approximately 50% in each compartment. Administration of epinephrine and stress-related endogenous release of cortisol induce rapid demargination of neutrophils, with subsequent doubling of the peripheral leukocyte counts within 30 minutes.

In order for hematopoietic cells to egress from the marrow and gain entry into the venous system, hematopoietic cells must pass through or between the endothelial cells lining the marrow venous sinuses. The point at which hematopoietic cells move through the endothelial cell is frequently near endothelial cell junctions. Pores can be observed in the endothelial lining of the venous sinus, but it is unclear whether these are permanent features of the surface or are present in response to specific signals from departing cells. In addition, areas of marked attenuation of the endothelial cell thickness have also been observed in scanning electron micrographs. Cells departing the hematopoietic cord must deform to a considerable degree to gain entry into the venous sinus. These observations, along with physical measurements of cell deformability, have led to the theory that increasing deformability associated with differentiation in both the erythroid and the myeloid lineages is an important component of the normal physiology of hematopoietic cell egress from the marrow.

Effects of marrow disruption

Abnormalities in blood cell production can occur if significant qualitative or quantitative alterations take place in hematopoietic growth factor production, in the hematopoietic stem cell and progenitor cell pools, and in the marrow microenvironment. Aplastic anemia, a clinical disorder characterized by pancytopenia and an acellular or hypocellular bone marrow, results from the total failure of hematopoiesis caused by disruption in any of these processes. The etiology of this disorder is likely multifactorial and is discussed in more detail in Chapter 91. Single cell deficiencies, such as pure red cell aplasia, pure white cell aplasia, and selective amegakaryocytic thrombocytopenia, are associated with a normocellular marrow and a selective deficiency of single lineage of marrow precursors and the resultant cytopenia. These disorders can result from a variety of insults to the marrow progenitor cell and precursor pool, such as cytotoxic antibodies, viruses, suppressor T cells, or natural killer cells. By contrast, the anemia of chronic renal failure is caused by defective growth factor production. This inevitable consequence of chronic renal failure largely results from a deficiency in the production of the erythropoietin.

The hematopoietic microenvironment may also be important in pathologic conditions affecting hematopoiesis. Murine mutants exhibiting bone marrow failure, such as the *Steel* mouse, exhibit characteristics attributable to defective microenvironments, including the hematopoietic microenvironment. Phenotypically the *Steel* mouse is a black-eyed, white animal with reduced fertility and macrocytic anemia. Careful study has revealed defects in all hematopoietic lineages. The hematopoietic abnormalities of the *Steel* animal are not cured by transplantation of congenic normal marrow. However, the anemia can be partially corrected by transplantation of intact spleens into the peritoneal cavity, which indicates that the hematologic abnormality resides in the hematopoietic microenvironment. In support of this view, long-term marrow cultures from *Steel* mice do not support hematopoietic cells from normal congenic mice in vitro. The *Steel* mutation has recently been mapped to chromosome 10, the gene product of the *Steel* mutation cloned, and the molecular basis of the *Steel* mutation characterized.

The product of the *Steel* gene has now been shown to be a 28 to 35 kD growth factor. The protein product can thus be membrane bound or secreted, although the physiologic role of these different forms is unclear. The *Steel*-Dickie ($S1^d$) allele, which is known to be a nonlethal *Steel* mutation, is encoded by a *Steel* gene, with a deletion of the gene sequence encoding the protein's spanning portion. The resulting protein is secreted and plays an important role in hematopoiesis. The *Steel* gene product is now known to be the ligand for the c-kit proto-oncogene.

Although no congenital human bone marrow failure syndrome has been shown to result from a microenvironmental defect, the failure of engraftment of transplanted marrow in some patients with aplastic anemia suggests that such abnormalities may exist. The use of newer molecular methods, probes for growth-regulatory proteins, and more powerful genetic approaches to study affected kindreds may define abnormalities in the hematopoietic microenvironment associated with some congenital bone marrow failure syndromes.

CLINICAL IMPLICATIONS OF STEM CELL BIOLOGY

Knowledge of basic stem cell biology has influenced our understanding of the pathobiology of most hematologic malignancies, including the myeloproliferative disorders, the acute leukemias, and the lymphomas. The concept that a hematopoietic stem cell is capable of ultimately giving rise to each formed element of the blood has permitted further insight into the origins of each of these disorders. Using several techniques, such as analyses of blood cell isoenzymes, marker chromosomal abnormalities, and restriction fragment polymorphisms, normal hematopoietic cells have been shown to be replaced by a single neoplastic cell population that produces granulocytes, red blood cells, platelets, monocytes/macrophages, eosinphils, basophils, some B lymphocytes, and perhaps T lymphocytes, but not bone marrow fibroblasts, in each myeloproliferative disorder. The neoplastic cell population is clonally derived because it presumably arises following a series of oncogenic events affecting a single neoplastic hematopoietic stem cell. These events, leading to a neoplastic transformation, are thought to occur at the level of the stem cell, since only this primitive hematopoietic cell is capable of differentiating into multiple hematopoietic lineages.

Using similar investigative methods, acute myelogenous leukemia (AML) has been shown to also be a clonal disorder characterized by aberrant hematopoietic cellular proliferation and maturation. AML may involve each of the hematopoietic cell lineages, but it frequently has a more restricted pattern of involvement, presumably because of the distinct level of maturation along the hierarchy of hematopoietic development at which the initial oncogenic event occurs. In some elderly patients, peripheral blood granulocytes, red cells, and platelets possess the clonal features characteristic of the leukemia, indicating that the malignancy probably originated in a single hematopoietic stem cell. In other patients, predominantly children and young adults, red cells and platelets are frequently generated by normal residual stem cells. This situation likely comes about because the oncogenic event(s) has occurred in a more differentiated progenitor cell that does not have the multipotentiality of a stem cell. Alternatively, such limited lineage involvement in AML could result from the effect of the neoplastic process on the stem cell, resulting in its inability to commit to erythroid and megakaryocytic pathways. In support of the former hypothesis, data obtained by immunologically phenotyping AML progenitor cells have shown that some leukemic progenitors express a stem cell phenotype, whereas others resemble that of committed myeloid progenitor cells.

Both allogeneic and autologous marrow transplantation can be thought of as "stem cell rescue" of a patient who has received lethal doses of chemoradiotherapy (Chapter 78). The successful long-term engraftment of donor cells requires the transfer to the recipient of cells that possess marrow-repopulating ability. At present, at least two phases of engraftment are thought to occur after bone marrow transplantation. These phases are apparently caused by the graft being composed of both progenitor and stem cells. Early engraftment results from the transfer of donor committed progenitor cells in the graft. A second delayed but sustained engraftment then occurs, which is likely the result of stem cells within the graft. These two phases of engraftment usually overlap and are not clinically distinguishable. The phenomenon of late graft failure after either allogeneic or autologous marrow transplantation in the presence of large numbers of assayable progenitors within the graft probably is caused by an absence from the graft of stem cells responsible for establishing long-term hematopoiesis.

GROWTH FACTORS AS THERAPEUTIC AGENTS

The synergistic relationship during the last decade between protein chemistry, molecular biology, and hematopoiesis research has resulted in growing numbers of hematopoietic growth factors becoming available for clinical use (see Table 69-1). Erythropoietin, the physiologic regulator of erythropoiesis, is now used regularly to treat the anemia of chronic renal disease, anemia of chronic infection and inflammation, anemia of cancer, and anemia associated with HIV-1 infection. G-CSF, on the other hand, has had a major impact on accelerating granulocyte recovery after chemotherapy for neoplastic diseases and is used to treat several congenital neutropenic syndromes. This cytokine has resulted in the decrease in the number of life-threatening bacterial infections in patients with these diverse clinical conditions. GM-CSF is currently used for accelerating marrow recovery after autologous marrow transplantation. The use of GM-CSF in these patients has resulted in a decreased incidence of bacterial infections after marrow transplantation. Unfortunately, neither G-CSF nor GM-CSF accelerates platelet recovery after cytotoxic therapy. Currently a growing number of growth factors, such as IL-1, IL-3, IL-6, IL-11, and c-kit ligand, are undergoing evaluation in order to define their clinical uses. At present, combination therapy with several of these cytokines administered either simultaneously or in sequence is thought to be required pharmacologically to promote hematopoiesis optimally. The clinical use of these remarkably powerful agents will likely result in important advances in therapy.

REFERENCES

Bartelez SH, Andrews RG, and Bernstein ID: Uncovering the heterogeneity of hematopoietic repopulating cells. Exp Hematol 19:861, 1991.

Grush WW and Quesenberry PJ: Recombinant human hematopoietic growth factors in the treatment of cytopenias. Clin Immunol Immunopathol 62:525, 1992.

Long M: Blood cell adhesion molecules. Exp Hematol 20:286, 1992.

Spangrude GL et al: Murine hematopoietic stem cells. Blood 78:1395, 1991.

Witte ON: Steel locus defines new multipotent growth factor. Cell 63:5, 1990.

CHAPTER

70 Hemostasis and Fibrinolysis

James N. George
Michael A. Kolodziej

Normal hemostatic mechanisms can be divided into two basic reactions. Primary hemostasis involves the immediate response of platelet adhesion to exposed subendothelial fibers at the site of vessel injury. This is followed by aggregation of platelets and vessel contraction that can effectively seal a small lesion. Secondary hemostasis involves the formation of fibrin that reinforces the initial platelet aggregate, thereby preventing bleeding from larger lesions. Although this distinction is helpful as a framework for understanding the symptoms and signs of bleeding disorders, these reactions are intimately related. Platelets provide a critical surface on which the reactions occur to generate thrombin, which catalyzes the formation of fibrin from fibrinogen. Thrombin is also the most potent agonist for platelet secretion, and platelet secretion of fibrinogen and calcium provides the substrate and a cofactor for fibrin formation. Also, several platelet-secreted products cause blood vessel contraction, further promoting hemostasis.

Each of these reactions is regulated by effective control mechanisms. The integrity of the normal vascular endothelium prevents the interaction between circulating platelets and subendothelial fibers that initiate further aggregation and secretion. Plasma proteins, such as protein C and antithrombin III, can develop activity to inhibit fibrin formation. The formation of the enzyme plasmin by the fibrinolytic system exerts the final control mechanism, with the proteolysis of fibrin restricting the clot to its essential location and beginning the process of restructuring the vessel lumen.

PRIMARY HEMOSTASIS: PLATELETS AND BLOOD VESSELS

Blood platelets are continually involved in microscopic hemostasis, sealing the gaps that occur normally in capillary and venule endothelium. Because they are the least dense blood cells, platelets are displaced laterally by the flowing red cells and circulate adjacent to the endothelium. Their role in maintaining endothelial integrity is shown by the result of their absence: with sudden, severe thrombocytopenia, innumerable petechial hemorrhages quickly appear, concentrated in dependent regions where hydrostatic pressure within the superficial capillaries is greatest. Microscopic analysis of capillaries and venules in thrombocytopenic animals demonstrates diminished thickness of the endothelial cell layer and an increased frequency of gaps and fenestrations.

Disruption of vascular integrity results in a standard sequence of platelet reactions. First, platelets adhere to subendothelial fibers. This contact interaction causes platelets to change from their circulating shape as compact disks to a more spherical form with long, extended pseudopodia that facilitate further contact with the subendothelium and adjacent platelets (Fig. 70-1). As the platelets change shape, their secretory granules move to the cell's center, fuse with the deeply invaginated surface membrane of the open canalicular system, and discharge their contents.

Platelet development from megakaryocytes

Platelets are derived from marrow megakaryocytes, which in turn are derived from pluripotent hematopoietic stem cells. Therefore platelets share a common ancestry with red cells, granulocytes, and lymphocytes.

Megakaryocyte development appears to be regulated at multiple levels (Chapter 69). Pluripotent progenitor cells can mature through unclear mechanisms to cells committed to megakaryocyte development, or colony-forming unit—megakaryocyte (CFU-MK). At some point in megakaryocyte development, proliferation ceases and differentiation begins, manifested by nuclear endoreduplication, enlargement of cell size, and acquisition of complex membrane systems demarcating zones of nascent platelets. Multiple cytokines are important in promoting platelet production. Committed progenitor cells (CFU - MK) are stimulated to proliferate in response to stem cell factor (SCF), interleukin-3 (IL-3), and granulocyte-macrophage colony-stimulating factor (GM-CSF). IL-6, IL-11, and leukemia inhibitory factor (LIF) are among the cytokines capable of promoting subsequent megakaryocyte differentiation and increasing the platelet count in experimental animals. These latter cytokines are also capable of inducing the hepatic acute phase response, and IL-6 may be responsible for the thrombocytosis frequently observed in inflammatory states.

As megakaryocytes mature in the marrow, the vast amount of cytoplasm develops into several thousand distinct sections that correspond to individual platelets, each containing all the organelles present in mature platelets. Megakaryocyte maturation is also accompanied by expression of platelet-specific proteins important for normal platelet function. In the marrow, megakaryocytes occupy positions adjacent to vascular sinus walls, and some observations suggest that large portions of cytoplasm or even intact megakaryocytes move into the sinus and then to the pulmonary capillaries, where they are trapped and fragment into individual platelets. However, the mechanism and site of platelet release from megakaryocytes are unknown.

Once delivered to the circulation, platelets survive about 10 days. Within the normal circulatory system, about one third of platelets are transiently sequestered in the spleen. Some platelets may be randomly removed from the circulation at a young age, but most are only transiently and reversibly involved in aggregates. Repeated vessel wall encounters with loss of pseudopods and alteration of surface structures may contribute to platelet senescence.

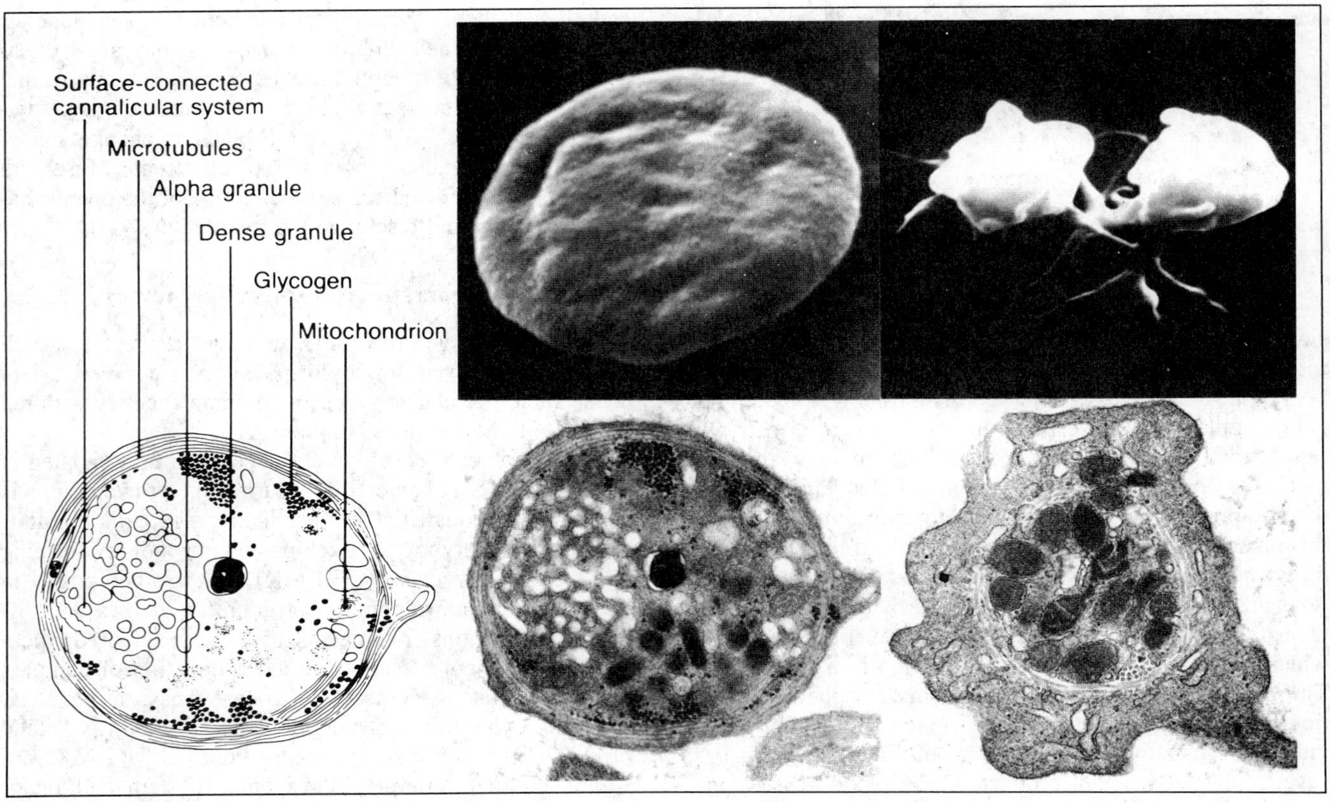

Fig. 70-1. Electron micrographs of resting and activated platelets. The top figures are scanning electron micrographs demonstrating the disk shape of normal circulating platelets (*left,* ×20,000) and the more spherical form of activated platelets with many long pseudopodia (*right,* ×10,000). The bottom left photograph is a transmission electron micrograph of the cross section of a resting platelet (×21,000) with a matched drawing *(far left)* labeling the normal subcellular structures. In the bottom right photograph (×30,000) of an activated platelet, the constriction of the microtubular ring around the centralized granules and the formation of pseudopodia can be seen. (Electron micrographs courtesy of James G. White, MD, and Marcy Krumwiede.)

Platelet structure and contents

Fig. 70-1 demonstrates platelet ultrastructure and the shape change that accompanies activation. Circulating platelets have a disk shape that is maintained by a coiled ring of microtubules. Microfilaments, composed primarily of polymerized fibrous actin, are seen in activated platelets, causing the shape change and pseudopod formation. Two distinct membrane systems are present within the cytoplasm of platelets. One, termed the *surface-connected canalicular system,* is merely an extension of the surface plasma membrane and results from deep, tortuous invaginations that communicate with the external milieu. The other, termed the *dense tubular system,* is located adjacent to the surface-connected canalicular membranes and contains specialized membranes that are the site of prostaglandin and thromboxane synthesis.

Three types of secretory granules are present in platelets: alpha granules, lysosomes, and dense granules. Alpha granules are the most numerous and account for the purple granular appearance of platelets on a stained blood smear. They contain a large variety of secreted proteins. Four of these proteins (fibrinogen, fibronectin, thrombospondin, von Willebrand factor) share physical and functional properties and are termed *adhesive proteins.* They are large and have rodlike or filamentous shapes; they are glycosylated, which facilitates their contact with other molecules; they are synthesized by a variety of cells, including megakaryocytes, endothelial cells, and vessel adventitial cells, and also are present in the plasma and vessel wall; and they are involved in platelet adhesion and aggregation reactions. Other secreted alpha-granule proteins include platelet factor 4 (a protein with strongly cationic regions that may bind to endothelial surface heparans and neutralize their repellent negative charge), platelet-derived growth factor, coagulation factor V, albumin, immunoglobulin G (IgG), immunoglobulin A (IgA), beta thromboglobulin, histidine-rich glycoprotein, high-molecular-weight kininogen, $alpha_2$ antiplasmin, and plasminogen activator inhibitor-1. Some alpha-granule proteins are the product of endogenous synthesis by megakaryocytes. Fibrinogen is not synthesized by megakaryocytes but is acquired by endocytosis after binding to its surface receptor, glycoprotein IIb-IIIa. Other plasma proteins within alpha granules, such as albumin,

IgG, and IgA, are acquired by pinocytosis, and their platelet concentration parallels their plasma concentration. Alpha-granule secretion occurs deep within the platelet into the long channels of the open canalicular system, providing for the secreted proteins a large area of surface-exposed membrane on which to rebind. The reassociation of some of these proteins on the platelet surface allows their concentration and organization to facilitate hemostatic reactions. Lysosomes, containing acid-hydrolase enzymes, are morphologically indistinguishable from alpha granules except when specific histochemical reactions are used to stain electron micrograph sections. The function of these enzymes is unknown, but they are probably involved in the clearance of cellular debris after hemostasis. Dense granules are the least frequent cellular organelle. They contain a high concentration of calcium and pyrophosphate ions (which cause the intrinsic electron density of these granules), as well as serotonin and adenine nucleotides. As with alpha granules, dense granules fuse with the plasma membrane after platelet activation. The exocytosed granule contents, particularly adenine nucleotides, in turn stimulate adjacent platelets, leading to amplification of the platelet response.

Platelet membrane glycoproteins represent a third important element necessary for normal platelet function. Although a number of such proteins have been identified, the best characterized are the surface receptors for the adhesive molecules von Willebrand factor and fibrinogen, glycoprotein Ib-IX and glycoprotein IIb-IIIa, respectively. These molecules are abundant components of the platelet membrane and serve the principal functions of platelets, adhesion and aggregation. Congenital absence of either glycoprotein Ib-IX (Bernard-Soulier syndrome) or glycoprotein IIb-IIIa (Glanzmann thrombasthenia) is associated with a significant bleeding diathesis. These molecules are also interesting because of their close structural resemblance with other adhesive protein receptors on other cells, making platelets the prototypical adhesive cell.

Platelet adhesion to subendothelium

The initial reaction of hemostasis is the adherence of circulating platelets to subendothelial fibers exposed by endothelial damage. Collagen is the principal fiber involved, and von Willebrand factor is required for platelet attachment. Von Willebrand factor is synthesized by both megakaryocytes, for storage within platelet alpha granules, and endothelial cells, from which it is secreted into the plasma and also back into the subendothelium. Through a poorly understood structural alteration, von Willebrand factor adsorbed onto a fibrillar surface becomes reactive and interacts with circulating platelets. The platelet receptor that binds von Willebrand factor to promote adhesion is the surface membrane glycoprotein Ib-IX. Therefore two different genetic disorders, von Willebrand's disease, caused by an abnormality or deficiency of von Willebrand factor, and Bernard-Soulier syndrome, caused by an abnormality or deficiency of platelet membrane glycoprotein Ib-IX, have similar clinical bleeding manifestations.

The localization of platelets to areas of endothelial injury promotes their exposure to various activating substances or agonists. Among these are collagen, adenosine diphosphate (ADP), epinephrine, and thrombin. These agonists probably act in concert, with ADP derived from dense-granule secretion and thrombin generated by coagulation factors Xa, Va, and prothrombin on the platelet surface. Early after exposure to these agonists, calcium is mobilized from platelet intracellular organelles into the cytoplasm. This allows actin polymerization into microfibrils and stimulates platelet shape change and the contractile events leading toward secretion. Arachidonic acid is liberated from membrane phospholipids and is then converted by cyclo-oxygenase and thromboxane synthetase to thromboxane A_2, an additional platelet agonist and vasoconstricting agent.

Platelet aggregation and secretion

Platelet aggregation involves the binding of firbrinogen to platelet membrane receptors, with resultant platelet-platelet bridging. These platelet-fibrinogen-platelet units comprise the backbone of the initial hemostatic plug. Platelet secretion is intimately associated with aggregation, both occurring within seconds of platelet stimulation. Without secretion, platelets are only transiently and reversibly aggregated by ADP and epinephrine. Secretion from dense granules provides additional Ca^{2+}, a necessary cofactor for aggregation, and ADP. Secretion from alpha granules provides additional fibrinogen, another required cofactor for platelet aggregation, which binds to its platelet surface receptor, glycoprotein IIb-IIIa. Therefore, as with platelet adhesion, platelet aggregation is defective in two different genetic disorders. Congenital afibrinogenemia, absence of the specific plasma protein, and Glanzmann thrombasthenia, an abnormality or deficiency of platelet membrane glycoprotein IIb-IIIa, both cause a lifelong bleeding disorder. With activation by ADP or thrombin, the surface membrane glycoprotein IIb-IIIa can also bind other platelet-secreted adhesive proteins—fibronectin and von Willebrand factor. These large proteins may also have a role in stabilizing the platelet aggregate.

Platelet involvement in thrombin generation

Platelets have long been recognized to play a role in coagulation by accelerating the generation of thrombin and the consequent formation of fibrin. This property, termed *platelet factor 3* 50 years ago, has been considered to reside in the phospholipid structure of the platelet membrane, providing a specific surface favoring the reactions leading to thrombin formation. Platelets, particularly platelet membrane microparticles shed during activation, can bind and organize the enzyme-cofactor-substrate complexes in two key coagulation reactions: (1) the activation of factor X by factor IXa (enzyme) plus factor VIIIa (cofactor) and (2) the activation of prothrombin by factor Xa (enzyme) plus factor Va (cofactor) (Fig. 70-2). The effectiveness of these platelet surface–dependent reactions is hundreds-fold

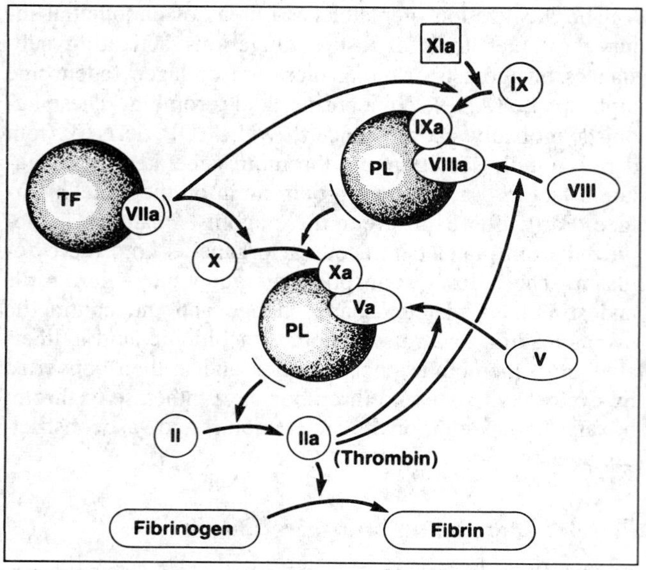

Fig. 70-2. Plasma coagulation reactions in normal hemostasis. In this diagram, factor XII, prekallikrein, and high-molecular-weight kininogen are omitted because they are not required for normal in vivo hemostasis. The role of factor XI is uncertain because some patients with absent plasma factor XI activity can have apparently normal hemostasis. The vitamin K–dependent factors are all similar in structure and are indicated by the small circles. Factors V and VIII, large molecules that are similar to each other in structure and function, are indicated by the ellipses. Three distinct reactions occur on lipoprotein surfaces that are shown as large spheres: the binding of factor VII to tissue factor *(TF)* on the surface of perivascular cells and the activation of factor X and prothrombin (factor II) on the surface of platelets *(PL)* or platelet membrane microparticles.

greater than a soluble reaction. The occurrence of thrombin formation on the platelet surface within the developing aggregate serves to protect the activated coagulation factors from their plasma inhibitors and to localize the fibrin formation to the immediate area of vessel damage. Platelets also have a specific surface receptor for thrombin, which is not only the key enzyme in coagulation reactions but also the most potent agonist for platelet activation and secretion.

SECONDARY HEMOSTASIS: COAGULATION

The reactions that lead to the formation of a fibrin clot, termed *coagulation,* are a cascade of sequential enzymatic reactions that are progressively amplified to generate the final key enzyme, thrombin. Within this sequence of reactions are many control loops; some accelerate thrombin formation, and others inhibit coagulation. The integration of these reactions and their controls effectively generates fibrin that is strictly localized to the site of hemostasis.

Traditionally, coagulation reactions have been divided into two pathways: one termed *intrinsic* because the major reactants are within the plasma, and the other termed *extrinsic* because the initiation requires tissue factor, a component not normally present within circulating blood. This distinction helps to define the laboratory assessment of hemostasis because the two basic clinical assays, the partial thromboplastin time and the prothrombin time, measure the components of the intrinsic and extrinsic systems, respectively (Chapter 76). A normal partial thromboplastin time also requires the presence of several proteins that are not necessary for in vivo coagulation: factor XII (Hageman factor), prekallikrein, and high-molecular-weight kininogen. For this reason, the coagulation scheme shown in Fig. 70-2, the sequence of in vivo coagulation, differs from that in Fig. 76-2, in vitro coagulation reactions measured by the standard laboratory assays. The proteins required for the development and control of normal plasma coagulation are described in Table 70-1.

Sequence of reactions leading to thrombin formation

Coagulation reactions are sequential activations of the plasma procoagulant proteins from their precursor (zymogen) form to active proteolytic enzymes, which are designated by a lowercase *a*. For example, factor X is the inactive zymogen found in normal plasma, and factor Xa is the active enzyme, a two-chain molecule resulting from the proteolytic cleavage by either factor VIIa–tissue factor or factors IXa-VIIIa (see Fig. 70-2). The triggering reaction that initiates blood coagulation in vivo is the exposure of tissue factor to plasma. Tissue factor, a cofactor for both factor VII activation and factor VIIa activity, is a specific cell surface protein that is constitutively expressed on perivascular fibroblasts, creating a hemostatic envelope poised to activate coagulation. At the site of vessel injury, exposed tissue factor selectively binds factor VII, causing it to become exquisitely sensitive for proteolytic activation by the normal trace plasma concentrations of factors VIIa or Xa. The tissue factor–factor VIIa complex then becomes the explosive force that activates factors IX to IXa and X to Xa. The coagulation system has many amplification steps: the appearance of factor Xa increases factor VII activation, and the first traces of thrombin convert cofactors V and VIII to more active forms (Fig. 70-2). The need for both pathways of factor X activation is demonstrated by the occurrence of bleeding disorders with deficiencies of factors VII, VIII, or IX. The sequence of coagulation is also consistent with the absence of clinical bleeding in patients deficient in factor XII, prekallikrein, or high-molecular-weight kininogen, even though they have very abnormal partial thromboplastin times. The role of factor XI is less clear because not all patients with severe plasma factor XI deficiency have significant bleeding problems. In vivo, factor XI may also be activated by thrombin, allowing an additional pathway of factor IX activation after tissue factor VIIa is inhibited by tissue factor pathway inhibitor.

Important similarities exist in the structural and complex-forming properties of the different coagulation factors. Four of these procoagulant proteins are vitamin K–dependent for normal functions: factors VII, X, IX, and prothrombin (also termed *factor II*). They are similar in size, and all become serine active-site proteases when activated from their zymogen form. Factor XIa is a larger molecule and is also a serine protease. Factors VIII and V are both very large molecules with extensive sequence homology. They do not have intrinsic enzymatic activity but function as cofactors for serine proteases (for factors IXa and Xa, respectively) in the form of a complex with phospholipid and Ca^{2+}.

Once formed, thrombin becomes the key coagulation enzyme in amplifying and promoting and also in inhibiting coagulation. Thrombin catalyzes the final steps in coagulation: the conversion of fibrinogen to fibrin and the activation of factor XIII to XIIIa, a transglutamase enzyme that converts the initial fibrin polymer to a covalently linked structure. It amplifies its own formation by directly activating cofactors VIII and V and also factor XI, and it stimulates platelet secretion and aggregation. In addition, thrombin, in combination with factor Va and an endothelial cell surface protein named *thrombomodulin,* activates plasma protein C, the zymogen of a coagulation inhibitor, to protein Ca (Fig. 70-3).

Fibrin formation

Fibrinogen is a large molecule present in high concentrations in plasma and platelet alpha granules. Its rod shape, made up of three pairs of polypeptide chains (designated alpha, beta, and gamma), allows it to polymerize spontaneously by both end-to-end and side-to-side hydrogen bonds after thrombin cleaves off four small peptides. These peptides are derived from the amino termini of the alpha and beta chains, at the center of the molecule, and are designated *fibrinopeptides A and B*. This initial fibrin polymer is neither properly oriented nor strong enough to provide permanent hemostasis or to allow clot retraction until the fibrin molecules are covalently linked by the transglutamase enzyme, factor XIIIa. Factor XIII zymogen is a molecule of a size similar to fibrinogen, consisting of a tetramer of two a chains and two b chains. In plasma, factor XIII circulates bound to fibrinogen, which allows it to be simultaneously activated by thrombin and directly incorporated into the fibrin clot. Platelets contain the factor XIII a chains, and it is the a-chain dimer that forms the enzyme, factor XIIIa. The active enzyme, factor XIIIa, but not the zymogen, binds specifically to thrombin-stimulated platelets, and this is an additional indication of the interactions between the fibrin clot and the platelet aggregate during hemostasis. Once the fibrin polymer is converted to a stable structure by the formation of covalent bonds between gamma chains and then alpha chains on adjacent molecules, the coagulation sequence is completed.

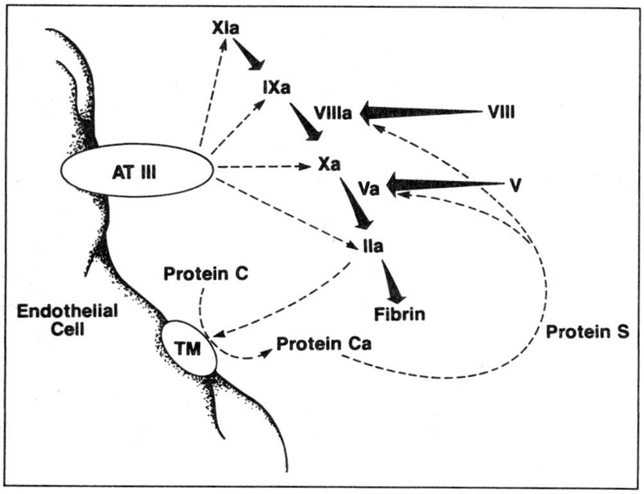

Fig. 70-3. Natural coagulation inhibitors: antithrombin III *(AT III)* and protein C. The solid arrows represent the procoagulant reactions; the broken arrows represent the inhibitory reactions. AT III inhibits the active serine protease enzymes, factors XIa, IXa, Xa, and IIa (thrombin). The inhibitory activity of AT III is greatly enhanced by heparin-like molecules on the endothelial cell surface. Factor VIIa is also inhibited by AT III, but it is more effectively neutralized by another plasma protein, tissue factor pathway inhibitor. Protein C is activated to a proteolytic enzyme, protein Ca, by thrombin with an endothelial cell protein, thrombomodulin *(TM),* serving as a cofactor. Protein Ca then specifically inactivates factors Va and VIIIa, with protein S as a required cofactor.

Controls of coagulation

Some activation of plasma coagulation factors occurs continuously, possibly by slight endothelial breaks or by circulation of plasma coagulation factors through extravascular tissues. This is normally controlled primarily by dilution in flowing blood and hepatic clearance of the activated enzymes. However, an enzymatic system that is as potentially explosive as these coagulation reactions must be regulated by a series of tight controls at each step. These control mechanisms are outlined in the box on p. 698 and Fig. 70-3. The increased risk for thrombosis associated with defects in these control mechanisms is shown in the box on p. 794 in Chapter 83.

An important control mechanism is the clearance and inactivation of the activated coagulation factors. Swiftly flowing blood is probably the most effective means of dispersing any activated factors not incorporated into the platelet aggregate and evolving clot. The protective effect of flowing blood is most clearly demonstrated by the increased risk for thrombosis associated with blood stasis. Circulation through the liver specifically removes activated coagulation factors from the plasma.

Antithrombin III and protein C are plasma proteins that are important for the inactivation of the activated coagulation factors generated during the coagulation reactions. Antithrombin III binds irreversibly to some serine protease enzymes (factors XIa, IXa, Xa, VIIa; and thrombin) and blocks their activity. Inhibition by antithrombin III alone is relatively slow, but its inhibitory activity is dramatically accelerated by heparin and heparinlike proteoglycan molecules. This acceleration is the basis for the therapeutic effect of heparin, and in normal hemostasis a similar role is performed by the proteoglycan heparan sulfate on the luminal surface of vascular endothelium.

Protein C is a vitamin K–dependent protein that is

Table 70-1. The major proteins of hemostasis and fibrinolysis*

Proteins	Primary tissue synthesis	Molecular weight (daltons)	Plasma concentration (mg/dl)	Plasma half-life (hours)	Structural properties	Function
Proenzymes of coagulation						
Factor XI	Liver	143,000	0.5	70	Unique	Activated by thrombin; activates IX
Factor IX	Liver	57,000	1.0	24	Vitamin K dependent	Activated by TF-VIIa and XIa; activates X
Factor VII	Liver	50,000	0.1	2-5	Vitamin K dependent	Activated by Xa and VIIa; activates IX and X
Factor X	Liver	59,000	1.0	36	Vitamin K dependent	Activated by TF-VIIa, and VIIIa-IXa; activates prothrombin
Prothrombin	Liver	72,000	2.0	72	Vitamin K dependent	Activated by Va-Xa; cleaves fibrinogen
Fibrinogen	Liver	340,000	300.0	96	Adhesive protein	Supports platelet aggregation; gels after thrombin cleavage
Factor XIII	Liver	320,000	3.0	240	Proenzyme of transglutamase	Covalently cross-links fibrin gel
Cofactors of coagulation						
Tissue factor (TF)	Perivascular cells	30,000	—	—	Transmembrane protein	Required for VII activation and VIIa activity
Factor VIII	Liver	330,000	0.1	12	Homologous to V; bound to VWF in plasma	Activated by thrombin; cofactor for IXa
Factor V	Liver	330,000	2.0	12	Homologous to VIII	Activated by thrombin; cofactor for Xa

Regulatory proteins of coagulation						
Thrombomodulin	Endothelium	75,000	—	—	Transmembrane protein	Required for protein C activation
Protein C	Liver	62,000	0.4	8	Vitamin K dependent	Activated by thrombin; digests VIII and V
Protein S	Liver	80,000	3.0	17	Vitamin K dependent; inhibited by C4b-bp†	Cofactor for protein C
Antithrombin III	Liver	54,000	20.0	24	Binds to endothelial heparan sulfate	Inhibits XIa, IXa, Xa, VIIa, thrombin in presence of proteoglycan
Tissue factor pathway inhibitor	Liver	36,000	0.009	1	Associated with plasma lipoproteins	Inhibits VIIa in presence of TF and Xa
Von Willebrand factor (VWF)	Endothelium, megakaryocytes	Subunit: 260,000 Molecule: 500,000-15,000,000	2.0	12	Giant filamentous adhesive protein; also component of perivascular matrix	Supports platelet adhesion; binds and stabilizes VIII in plasma: one VIII/30 to 60 VWF subunits
Enzyme/proenzyme of fibrinolysis						
Tissue plasminogen activator (tPA)	Endothelium	68,000	0.0006	0.1	Bound to PAI-1 in plasma	Activates plasminogen to plasmin
Plasminogen	Liver	86,000	20.0	50	Binds to fibrin and platelet surface	Activated by tPA; digests fibrinogen, fibrin, VIII, V, and other proteins
Regulatory proteins of fibrinolysis						
Plasminogen activator inhibitor-1 (PAI-1)	Endothelium	52,000	0.0005	0.1	Bound to vitronectin in plasma and platelet alpha granules	Binds to and inhibits tPA activity in plasma
$Alpha_2$ antiplasmin	Liver	60,000	5.0	60	Cross-linked to fibrin by XIIIa	Inactivates plasmin

*The principle structural and functional properties of selected proteins involved in hemostasis and fibrinolysis are presented. All are soluble plasma proteins except tissue factor and thrombomodulin, which are transmembrane proteins. Von Willebrand factor is both a soluble plasma protein and a component of the subendothelial matrix.

†C4b-bp, Plasma binding protein for the complement component 4b.

Control mechanisms for blood coagulation

I. Clearance of activated coagulation factors
   A. Dispersal by flowing blood
   B. Liver catabolism

II. Inactivation of activated coagulation factors
   A. Antithrombin III, a plasma protein, inactivates factors XIa, IXa, Xa, and VIIa and thrombin. This reaction is accelerated by complex formation with endothelial cell surface heparin-like molecules.
   B. Protein C, a plasma protein, is activated to a serine protease (protein Ca) by thrombin plus thrombomodulin. Thrombomodulin is a protein present on the luminal surface of endothelial cells. Protein Ca proteolytically inactivates both factors VIIIa and Va, with protein S as a cofactor.
   C. Heparin cofactor II, a plasma protein, inactivates thrombin in the presence of heparin or dermatan sulfate. In contrast to antithrombin III, it does not inactivate factors XIa, IXa, and Xa.
   D. Tissue factor pathway inhibitor (TFPI), a plasma protein synthesized by endothelium and liver, binds to and inhibits the function of the factor VIIa–tissue factor complex in the presence of factor Xa.
   E. Thrombin bound to thrombomodulin is inactive regarding its procoagulant and platelet activation effects.
   F. Fibrin binds thrombin and inhibits its proteolytic activity.

III. Fibrinolysis by plasmin degrades and clears the fibrin clot.

cleaved to form a serine protease, protein Ca, by thrombin when the thrombin is bound to an endothelial surface protein, thrombomodulin. Activated protein C inhibits factors VIIIa and Va by proteolytic degradation. The activity of protein Ca requires the presence of another vitamin K–dependent plasma protein, protein S, as a cofactor.

In addition to neutralization by antithrombin III, thrombin is also inactivated in its effect on factor V, fibrinogen, and platelets when it becomes bound to thrombomodulin on the endothelial surface or to the surface of polymerized fibrin.

Antithrombin III accounts for most of the plasma antithrombin activity, but another protein termed *heparin cofactor II* can also inactivate thrombin in the presence of heparin. In contrast to antithrombin III, heparin cofactor II requires higher concentrations of heparin; it can also be activated by another glycosaminoglycan, dermatan sulfate. Heparin cofactor II's inhibitory activity is restricted to thrombin; it has no effect on factors XIa, IXa, Xa, and VIIa. The association between a congenital deficiency of heparin cofactor II and an increased risk for thromboembolic disease has not been clearly established.

Tissue factor pathway inhibitor (TFPI) is synthesized and secreted constitutively by endothelial cells and binds firmly to the complex of factor VIIa and tissue factor in the presence of factor Xa and calcium. TFPI does not bind to factor VIIa or tissue factor individually, and binding requires the intact activated factor Xa molecule. This allows the newly formed factor Xa to feed back and control further activity of the factor VIIa–tissue factor complex. Sustained factor X activation may then require factor XIa and the intrinsic pathway. A deficiency of TFPI has not yet been recognized.

FIBRINOLYSIS

Digestion of the fibrin clot by the enzyme plasmin in the process of fibrinolysis is the ultimate coagulation control mechanism. This process helps to restrict the clot to the site of hemostasis and to clear away the fibrin as the process of wound healing begins. If the sequence of coagulation reactions is pictured as a cascade of enzyme activation resulting in the formation of thrombin, fibrinolysis can be pictured as a mirror-image cascade resulting in the formation of the proteolytic enzyme plasmin (Fig. 70-4). Plasmin has a broad spectrum of protein substrates. Plasmin is formed from a circulating zymogen, plasminogen, by an enzyme released from endothelial cells termed *tissue plasminogen activator* (tPA). Other enzymes are capable of activating plasminogen: urokinase (often designated uPA), which is present in most tissues; and streptokinase, a therapeutic ma-

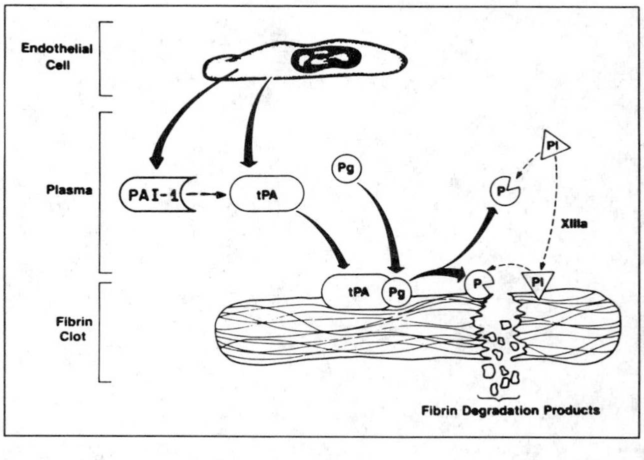

Fig. 70-4. Mechanism and control of endogenous fibrinolysis. Once the fibrin clot is formed, it becomes the active cofactor for its own dissolution by providing the specific surface on which fibrinolytic reactions occur. Tissue plasminogen activator *(tPA)* is secreted from endothelial cells. In plasma, tPA circulates in an active complex with another endothelial cell–secreted protein, plasminogen activator inhibitor-1 *(PAI-1)*. tPA binds avidly to fibrin, where it becomes a binding site for plasminogen *(Pg)* from the plasma. Thus plasminogen is converted to the active fibrinolytic enzyme plasmin *(P)* directly on the fibrin surface. Plasmin digests fibrin into multiple soluble fragments, termed *fibrin degradation products*. Any plasmin escaping into the plasma is immediately neutralized by $alpha_2$ plasmin inhibitor (*PI;* $alpha_2$ antiplasmin). $Alpha_2$ antiplasmin is also covalently linked to fibrin by factor XIIIa. Thus the complete sequence of plasmin production and control is organized within the developing fibrin clot. The solid arrows indicate the profibrinolytic reactions. The broken arrows indicate the reactions inhibiting fibrinolysis.

terial derived from streptococci. tPA appears to be the normal intravascular activator of plasminogen in the process of fibrinolysis. In contrast, the primary activity of urokinase appears to be the activation of plasminogen to plasmin in extravascular tissues, where proteolysis by plasmin is involved in such widely diverse functions as cell migration during inflammation and tumor cell metastasis, ovulation, and organogenesis and organ involution.

As in coagulation, surface binding of the reactants serves to localize the reaction to the specific site where the activated enzyme is required. In this case, fibrin itself serves as a potent cofactor for the action of tPA on plasminogen. tPA associates only weakly with soluble plasminogen and fibrinogen but binds strongly to fibrin. The complex of tPA with fibrin forms a site that in turn binds plasminogen with high affinity. Therefore plasmin is formed almost exclusively within the fibrin clot. As with coagulation, significant control mechanisms exist for the fibrinolytic reactions. These control mechanisms include the restriction of tPA activity to the fibrin surface and the presence of plasma inhibitors of tPA and plasmin. *Plasminogen activator inhibitor-1* (PAI-1) is synthesized and secreted by endothelial cells, and most tPA circulates in an inactive complex with PAI-1. Both tPA and PAI-1 appear to be released from endothelial cells constitutively as well as after a variety of stimuli. Among the several other plasminogen activator inhibitors that have been characterized, PAI-2, a selective inhibitor of uPA produced primarily by placental tissue, is notable because of its high concentrations in plasma during late pregnancy.

Any plasmin that escapes the fibrin clot is immediately neutralized by *alpha$_2$ antiplasmin,* a protein present in normal plasma. Plasmin bound to fibrin is 100-fold less sensitive to alpha$_2$ antiplasmin than when it is free in plasma. Other inhibitors of plasmin exist in plasma, but they may have no physiologic significance, since the congenital absence of alpha$_2$ antiplasmin causes a lifelong bleeding disorder characterized by excessive fibrinolysis. Some alpha$_2$ antiplasmin is bound to fibrin by factor XIIIa, where it acts as a more intimate check on plasmin activity. Both PAI-1 and alpha$_2$ antiplasmin are also secreted from platelet alpha granules, contributing to a higher concentration of these inhibitors in the milieu of hemostasis. These checks on the generation and activity of plasmin may protect the developing fibrin clot from premature dissolution.

REFERENCES

Bauer KA et al: Aging-associated changes in indices of thrombin generation and protein C activation in humans. J Clin Invest 80:1527, 1987.

Broze GJ Jr: Why do hemophiliacs bleed? Hosp Pract, March 1992, p 69.

Collen D and Lijnen HR: Basic and clinical aspects of fibrinolysis and thrombolysis. Blood 78:3114, 1991.

Coller BS: Platelets and thrombolytic therapy. N Engl J Med 322:33, 1990.

Davie EW, Fujikawa K, and Kisiel W: The coagulation cascade: initiation, maintenance and regulation. Biochemistry 30:10363, 1991.

Drake TA, Morrissey JH, and Edgington TS: Selective cellular expression of tissue factor in human tissues. Am J Pathol 134:1087, 1989.

Esmon CT: The protein C anticoagulant pathway. Arterioscler Thromb 12:135, 1992.

Furie B and Furie BC: Molecular and cellular biology of blood coagulation. N Engl J Med 326:800, 1992.

Gilbert GE et al: Platelet-derived microparticles express high affinity receptors for factor VIII. J Biol Chem 266:17261, 1991.

Krishnamurti C and Alving BM: Plasminogen activator inhibitor type 1: biochemistry and evidence for modulation of fibrinolysis in vivo. Semin Thromb Hemost 18:67, 1992.

Kroll MH and Schafer AI: Biochemical mechanisms of platelet activation. Blood 74:1181, 1989.

Mann KG et al: Surface-dependent reactions of the vitamin K–dependent enzyme complexes. Blood 76:1, 1990.

Rapaport SI: Inhibition of factor VIIa/tissue factor–induced blood coagulation: with particular emphasis upon a factor Xa–dependent inhibitory mechanism. Blood 73:359, 1989.

Sadler JE: von Willebrand factor. J Biol Chem 266:22777, 1991.

Vassalli JD, Sappino AP, and Belin D: The plasminogen activator/plasmin system. J Clin Invest 88:1067, 1991.

CHAPTER

71 Molecular and Cellular Biology of Cancer

Theodore G. Krontiris

Many physical and biologic agents of carcinogenesis have been identified in our environment. Until recently the cellular targets of such agents were poorly understood. The processes leading to malignant transformation, as well as the host genetic components of this transformation, remain obscure. In recent years, however, basic cancer research has identified a group of cellular genes that are the likely substrates of carcinogenesis. Although much remains to be learned, we now have insight into the genetic events that accompany malignant transformation. With this knowledge comes the potential for understanding how environmental agents might interact with host elements in the production of cancer. Ultimately, this work should benefit both the prevention and the treatment of neoplastic disease.

AGENTS OF CARCINOGENESIS

Physical agents

Ionizing radiation, in the form of x-rays or particle beams, causes cancer in direct proportion to the dose applied. Although the sensitivity of tissues varies, all forms of cancer can result from exposure to radiation. The mechanism by which neoplastic transformation is accomplished is the generation of lesions in deoxyribonucleic acid (DNA) molecules, leading to mutations when the lesions are repaired by cellular enzymes. Large-scale damage to chromosomes, with subsequent rearrangements and deletions of genetic material, may also be important. As discussed later, the mutation or rearrangement of cellular oncogenes can lead to unregulated cell proliferation.

Other physical agents are listed in the box below. Ultraviolet radiation induces skin cancer, including melanoma, again in direct proportion to the duration and intensity of the exposure. DNA damage with subsequent mutation is the probable mechanism. In disorders characterized by deficient DNA repair (e.g., xeroderma pigmentosum), ultraviolet-induced skin cancer is more prevalent.

Finally, foreign bodies are carcinogenic in some circumstances. Asbestos fibers are the most prominent example in this group. Squamous bladder carcinoma is strongly associated with the chronic inflammatory state induced by bladder infestation with *Schistosoma haematobium*. Implantation of prostheses has very rarely been associated with sarcoma. The mechanisms underlying foreign body carcinogenesis are not understood.

Chemical agents

Only a partial list of probable chemical carcinogens is provided in Table 71-1. Alcohol-related and tobacco-related cancers (head and neck, respiratory and upper gastrointestinal tracts, bladder) are among the most prevalent forms of malignant disease in the developed countries of the West. Such cancers are now increasing in the developing countries of Africa and Asia as well. Cancer risk from other chemicals was formerly associated only with industrial exposure (aniline dyes, benzols, vinyl chloride). However, environmental contamination from both sanctioned and illegal toxic waste sites may yield in the future a significant number of chemically induced cancers. It should be noted, however, that current epidemiologic data do not support the hypothesis that cancer incidence is now increasing because of these environmental sources of carcinogens.

In developing countries, aflatoxin-induced hepatocellular carcinoma, resulting from fungal contamination of grain stores, is a significant public health problem.

Biologic agents

With the exception of *S. haematobium,* the known biologic agents of cancer in human beings are viruses (Table 71-2). In the Western world, virus-induced cancer (with the possible exception of cervical carcinoma) is rare. In other parts of the world, however, viruses have been strongly implicated in the major forms of cancer. Hepatocellular carcinoma (hepatitis B virus) and nasopharyngeal carcinoma (Epstein-Barr virus) are the prominent examples.

Physical agents implicated in carcinogenesis

- Ionizing radiation
- Ultraviolet radiation
- Foreign bodies
  - Asbestos (glass fibers)
  - Implants
  - Schistosomiasis

Table 71-1. Chemical agents implicated in carcinogenesis

Agent	Site
Alcohol	Head and neck, esophagus, liver, breast
Tobacco (tars, metabolites)	Head and neck, lung, upper gastrointestinal tract, bladder
Metal compounds	
Cadmium	Kidney, prostate
Chromium	Lung
Nickel	Lung
Asbestos	Lung, pleura
Arsenic	Lung, skin
Aniline dyes	Bladder
Diethylstilbestrol	Uterus, vagina
Lye (strictures)	Esophagus
Phenytoin	Lymphoreticular system
Benzols	Hematopoietic system
Alkylating agents	Hematopoietic system
Aflatoxin	Liver
Vinyl chloride	Liver, blood vessels, lung

Recently, human retroviruses (human T cell leukemia viruses), have been described that induce T lymphocyte malignancies. Although many animal models of retrovirus-induced tumors are well characterized, the means by which human T cell leukemia viruses cause leukemia have not yet been determined. Papillomavirus, a DNA virus associated with cutaneous warts, is now strongly suspected as the etiologic agent of human cervical carcinoma.

MECHANISMS OF CARCINOGENESIS

Cell growth and differentiation are subject to both positive and negative regulatory influences. Genes that play positive, active, or dominant roles in the process of growth control are designated *proto-oncogenes,* or dominant oncogenes. Genes that function primarily in the inhibition or downregulation of growth are designated *tumor suppressor genes* (currently the preferred designation), antioncogenes, or recessive oncogenes. The interplay of these two regula-

Table 71-2. Biologic agents implicated in carcinogenesis

Agent	Associated cancer
Schistosoma haematobium	Squamous carcinoma of urinary bladder
T cell leukemia viruses (HTLV; HIV-III)	Leukemia/lymphoma
Epstein-Barr virus	Burkitt's lymphoma (Africa) Nasopharyngeal carcinoma (China)
Papillomavirus	Cervical carcinoma
Hepatitis B virus	Hepatocellular carcinoma

tory gene classes in the development of cancer is gradually being elucidated.

Cellular oncogenes

All the agents discussed in the first section must interact with some component(s) of the host cell to produce unregulated growth. Cellular genes with the potential for destabilizing growth regulation are the proto-oncogenes. When proto-oncogenes are activated by any one of various events discussed in this section, they become *oncogenes*.

The existence of specific cellular genes capable of directing malignant transformation was first established by the study of retrovirus-induced tumors. Retroviruses infect many vertebrate species and can rapidly produce a variety of leukemias, lymphomas, sarcomas, and carcinomas. At least 25 distinct viral genes have been identified in different retrovirus isolates; these *viral oncogenes* are directly responsible for the tumor-producing capability of retroviruses. It has been determined that each tumorigenic retrovirus acquired its oncogene by "capturing" a normal cellular gene of the host in which the virus grew. Therefore the cellular proto-oncogene, in its new association with the virus, was activated to become a viral oncogene. Other oncogenes have been identified by their association with specific chromosome abnormalities present in some human tumors (see later).

Oncogene/proto-oncogene function. Cellular proto-oncogenes have been highly conserved throughout evolution. For example, *ras* genes homologous to those present in the human genome are found not only in vertebrates but also in fruit flies and even yeast. Therefore proto-oncogenes must represent nature's solution to important problems of cell metabolism and have consequently been carefully maintained. Although we have only fragmentary evidence about the functions of proto-oncogenes in normal cells (see the box below), the data we do have suggest that these genes play a role in the regulation of cell proliferation by serving as elements of a multicomponent signal transduction apparatus.

Mitogenic signals from the microenvironment or from more distant influences are communicated to cells through many receptor structures associated with the plasma membrane. The most thoroughly studied of these are receptors with an external ligand binding domain, a transmembrane domain, and a cytoplasmic domain possessing tyrosine kinase activity (Fig. 71-1; see also following discussion). In addition to tyrosine kinase receptors, however, at least seven other distinct classes of molecules are thought to par-

Oncogene compendium*

Growth factors					
SIS	*egf*	*tgf-α*	*tgf-β* (many)	*fgf* (5)	*gro*
igf (2)	*wnt* (many)	Hematopoietic factors (many)			
Tyrosine kinases serving as transmembrane receptors					
ERBB1	*erbB2 (her/neu)*	*trk*	*KIT*	*ROS*	
FMS	*RET*	*sea*			
Tyrosine kinases associated with inner plasma membrane and cytoskeleton					
SRC	*YES*	*FGR*	*lck*	*ABL*	*FPS*
Serine-threonine kinases					
MOS	*RAF*	*pkc*	*pim-1*		
G proteins (guanosine triphosphate binding and hydrolysis)					
H-RAS	*K-RAS*	*N-ras*	*rho*	*gsp*	*gip*
Transcriptional regulatory factors					
MYC	*L-myc*	*N-myc*	*MYB*	*ERBA*	*rar-α*
FOS	*fosB*		*pbx*	*hox*	*scl*
JUN	*junC*	*junD*	*gli-1*	*vav*	*tal*
REL	*relB*		*max*	*SKI*	*lyl-1*
ETS-1	*ETS-2*	*spi*	*myl (pmi)*	*mdm*	
Others					
bcl-2	*bcl-3*	*bcr*	*dbl*	*mas*	*CRK*

*Oncogenes are classified according to their functional properties. Those listed in uppercase letters were discovered after their incorporation into retroviruses. Several oncogenes were discovered after their activation by the adjacent insertion of retroviruses (e.g., *pim*, several *wnt* genes, *mdm*). Members of oncogene families are boxed (e.g., *myc, L-myc, N-myc*).

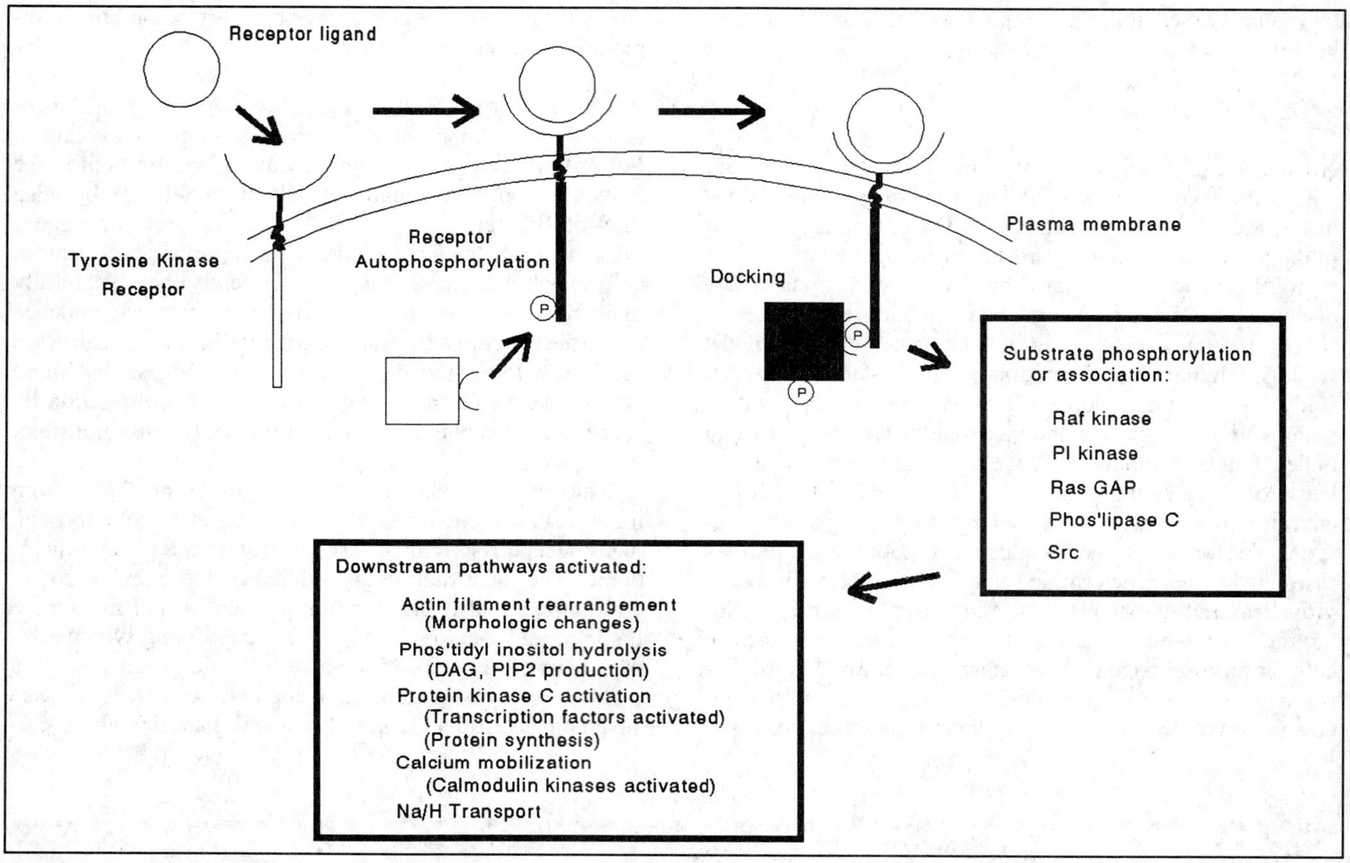

Fig. 71-1. Oncogenes in signal transduction. Binding of the growth factor representing the cognate ligand of a transmembrane receptor results in activation of the cytoplasmic domain of the receptor *(thin black rectangle)*. This activation is accompanied by autophosphorylation of several tyrosine residues. One of these activates the "docking" process, whereby cytoplasmic substrates of the receptor's kinase domain home in to the receptor and are themselves phosphorylated on tyrosine residues. Transmission of the signal continues by the resulting activation of the substrate *(solid black square)*. Recently identified substrates of tyrosine kinase receptors are listed in the right-hand box. Subsequent events in the signal cascade are listed in the center box. *Phos'lipase C,* Phospholipase C; *Phos'tidyl inositol,* phosphatidyl inositol.

ticipate in signaling. These include (1) receptors coupled to G proteins (distinct from the *ras* family), which modulate the activity of such entities as adenylate cyclase and ion channels; (2) ion channels themselves, which are activated by a variety of endocrine factors; (3) receptors with intrinsic guanylate cyclase activity; (4) receptors for many lymphokines, cytokines and growth factors (e.g., interleukin-1, interleukin-2, granulocyte-macrophage colony-stimulating factor [GM-CSF], erythropoietin), for which no mechanism has yet been determined; (5) receptors with phosphotyrosine phosphatase activity, which may represent a system antagonistic to the tyrosine kinase receptor class; and (6) the nuclear receptors of the steroid hormone receptor supergene family, which bind such ligands as estrogens, glucocorticoids, and thyroid hormone as the first step in the direct control of gene transcription. Finally, growing evidence suggests that adhesion molecules expressed on the surface of cells, such as the products of the integrin gene family, communicate with the microenvironment in ways that have very important consequences for cell growth and differentiation.

Signal transduction through a typical tyrosine kinase receptor is depicted in Fig. 71-1. Binding of a growth factor ligand results in activation of the cytoplasmic tyrosine kinase and autophosphorylation of that domain. For some receptors, such as that of platelet-derived growth factor (PDGF), ligand binding leads to receptor dimerization and intermolecular phosphorylation on key tyrosine residues. One of the consequences of tyrosine phosphorylation is the initiation of "docking" of kinase substrates, which are downstream elements of the signal apparatus (Fig. 71-1). These targets now recognize and bind to the cytoplasmic domain of the receptor through the newly phosphorylated tyrosine residue and are themselves subsequently phosphorylated. In this set of interactions the signal is thus transmitted from the extracellular to the cytoplasmic side of the plasma membrane.

Further stages of signal transduction require the participation of many proto-oncogenes with distinct functions. Although the identification and ordering of each step in signal transmission have not yet been elucidated, significant components can now be described. Many transmembrane receptors eventually communicate with G proteins. Chief among these for growth factor receptors are members of the *ras* proto-oncogene family. G proteins are activated to propagate signals by the binding of guanosine triphosphate (GTP); current evidence suggests the participation of still other proto-oncogenes, called *nucleotide exchange factors*, in the loading of G proteins with GTP. Signal transmission then occurs until G proteins hydrolyze the bound GTP to guanosine diphosphate (GDP). Inhibitory regulation of G proteins is presumably accomplished by interaction with a cognate GTPase activating protein (GAP). In upregulating the GTP hydrolytic activity of G proteins, GAPs remove them from the activated state. Therefore signal transmission depends on the balance between activation of a G protein by its binding of GTP (facilitated by nucleotide exchange factors) and inactivation of the protein by GAP-induced GTP hydrolysis. More distal events after Ras protein activation include the hydrolysis of phosphatidylinositol to yield diacylglycerol (DAG) and inositol diphosphates and triphosphates (PIP and PIP_2). These products continue signal propagation through DAG activation of protein kinase C (PK_C) and PIP_2 mobilization of intracellular calcium. As described next, PK_C may interact directly with transcription factors; changes in intracellular calcium lead to signal propagation through calmodulin kinases.

Propagation of a signal from this point requires activation of many transcriptional regulatory proteins. Several distinct mechanisms are recruited for this purpose. First, signals proceeding from growth factor receptors (e.g., that of PDGF) often result in the rapid onset of high-level messenger ribonucleic acid (mRNA) production for transcription factors such as *fos* and *jun*. The duration of this response is limited by the short half-lives of mRNA encoding these factors. In addition to augmenting the expression of transcriptional regulatory factors, mitogenic and differentiation signals often result in the posttranslational modification of pre-existing transcriptional regulatory proteins. Phosphorylation and dephosphorylation of various functional domains of both the Fos and the Jun proteins are required for full activation of these factors. In other cases, transcription factors sequestered in the cytoplasm by inhibitory binding proteins are released for translocation into the nucleus as the result of signaling. The *rel*-related product, NF-κB, is bound to an inhibitor, IκB, until signals mediated by PK_C result in phosphorylation and release of the inhibitor. NF-κB then migrates to the nucleus, where it binds specific DNA sequences near the promoters of genes that require this factor for transcription to occur. These few examples demonstrate the wide range of regulatory consequences that can be triggered by the signaling cascade.

The control of cell growth involves two other regulatory processes with relationships to signal transduction that are not completely understood. The first, *cell cycle regulation*, refers to control points at several critical boundaries between phases of the cell cycle. The most important of these are entrance into G_1 from the resting state, G_0; the passage from G_1 into DNA synthesis, S; and the transition from G_2 to mitosis. Several proto-oncogene products, such as Src and Mos, have recently been implicated in the function of these critical control points, particularly G_2/M. The products of several other genes (e.g., $p34^{cdc2}$, cyclins A and B) are also important in this regulatory process, as are several tumor suppressor gene products (see next section). Proto-oncogene products are also thought to play a role in another process of growth regulation, programmed cell death, or *apoptosis*. In many tissues, cells generated by the stem cell compartment proceed to terminal differentiation and ultimately to cell death. This process is particularly important in tissue with high cell turnover rates, such as hematopoietic and lymphopoietic organs and the gastrointestinal tract. Apoptosis results eventually in the cessation of cell division and the orderly degradation of the cell's genetic material. The 25 kD product of the *bcl-2* oncogene, located in the mitochondrial membrane, forestalls apoptosis, particularly in lymphoid cells. The continued expression of this oncogene (see later) is the key consequence of a pathogenetic chromosome translocation leading to human follicular lymphoma. The tyrosine kinase product of the *abl* proto-oncogene may also function in the control of apoptosis.

In the examples just described, each proto-oncogene product is considered to bear a single functional activity. Recently, proto-oncogene proteins with the apparent capability to perform multiple distinct functions have been defined. One of these, derived from the *bcr* proto-oncogene, possesses an N-terminal domain characteristic of a serine kinase, a C terminus with GAP homology, and an intervening domain with strong homology to the nucleotide exchange factor, Dbl. Although the precise roles of multifunctional proto-oncogenes have not yet been elucidated, it seems possible that they will function as bridges between distinct components of the mitogenic regulatory apparatus.

Tumor suppressor genes

Another important mechanism of tumorigenesis is the deletion of genes that repress cell proliferation. Such genes have been designated *suppressors* or *antioncogenes* because they can suppress, in a dominant fashion, the tumorigenic phenotype of activated oncogenes. The group of familial cancer syndromes characterized by autosomal dominant inheritance have yielded many distinct members of the suppressor gene category. The retinoblastoma gene *RB-1*, was the first of these to have been cloned and sequenced; it encodes a DNA-binding protein. Retinoblast differentiation, rather than proliferation, is the outcome of *RB-1* expression. When this gene is deleted, the absence of its tonic inhibitory function favors proliferation and, eventually, tumorigenic transformation. The tumor suppressor gene responsible for one variant of Wilms' tumor, *WT-1*, has also been isolated. The gene encodes a nuclear protein that possesses a so-called zinc finger domain governing DNA-binding specificity. The gene representing the *NF-1* locus, which is responsible for neurofibromatosis type I, has also been cloned and characterized. Unlike the products of the *WT-1* and *RB-1* loci, which encode DNA-binding proteins probably responsible for transcriptional regulation, the *NF-1* product bears homology to the GAPs described earlier. This is a very interesting and important result, since it demonstrates that tumor suppressor genes can also play a role in the inhibition of the cytoplasmic portion of the signal transduction apparatus. *NF-1* presumably functions by downregulating the activated state of its corresponding G protein. A candidate gene for polyposis coli, located on the long arm of chromosome 5, has also been recently isolated. Multiple endocrine neoplasia (all types), von Hippel-Lindau disease, and familial renal cancer all represent the inheritence of a deleted or otherwise inactive suppressor gene. The chromosome map positions of most of these loci are known, although the corresponding genes have not yet been isolated.

Another tumor suppressor gene with great importance for human carcinogenesis is *P53*. The product of this locus, a 53 kD nuclear protein, was originally described by virtue of its tight binding to the SV40 virus, large T antigen. It is now known that this binding results in the inactivation of p53 and direct tumorigenic consequences for the cell infected by this DNA tumor virus. Inherited mutations of the *P53* gene have been described in the Li-Fraumeni syndrome. Patients with this familial tumor syndrome are at risk for malignant tumors arising in a variety of organs. As with several other previously described tumor suppressor gene products, p53 is thought to regulate transcription of genes critical to the control of cell growth and differentiation.

Genetic alterations responsible for human cancers

In addition to oncogene activation, a variety of genetic lesions are responsible for the *inactivation* of tumor suppressor genes. The next three sections describe the principal mechanisms by which these pathogenetic changes are accomplished.

Oncogene activation. If proto-oncogenes function in normal cells, what changes take place to activate these genes in cancer cells? As discussed earlier, retroviruses can interact with proto-oncogenes to produce tumors in animals. However, retroviral activation of cellular proto-oncogenes is thought to occur very rarely, if at all, in humans. Activation by other types of viruses (hepatitis B virus, Epstein-Barr virus) has not been demonstrated but remains a possibility in the kinds of tumors discussed at the start of this chapter. Other, nonviral mechanisms have been defined in a broad spectrum of human cancers.

Three principal types of oncogene activation occur. In the first, a normal gene product is elaborated inappropriately by the cancer cell. The cell synthesizes too much of the protein or synthesizes it at the wrong stage of the cell cycle. Alternatively, the gene product may appear improperly at a given stage of differentiation. Finally, an otherwise normal oncogene product may appear in a cell type that does not usually express the gene. All these events lead to the same result: a stimulus for cell proliferation under inappropriate circumstances.

Cancer cells display several mechanisms for achieving the type of activation just described. Overexpression of an oncogene product may result from amplification of the gene. By increasing the number of copies of an oncogene, sometimes by more than 100-fold, protein production can be greatly augmented. This mechanism often leads to cytogenetic abnormalities, the double minutes (DMs) and homogeneously staining regions (HSRs) that are prominent features of tumor cell karyotypes. Amplification of the *myc* gene has been detected in leukemia and small cell lung carcinoma as well as in neuroblastoma and a neuroendocrine tumor of colonic origin. Neuroglial tumors demonstrate amplification of *erbB1,* which encodes the epidermal growth factor (EGF) receptor. An increased number of EGF receptors are detected on the cell surface in some of these tumors and also in some epidermoid carcinomas. The amplification of *erbB2* is associated with a poor prognosis in breast cancer.

Another important mechanism resulting in inappropriate expression is the rearrangement of oncogenes that occurs during the generation of chromosome translocations, inversions, and deletions. The *myc* gene is continuously transcribed in lymphoma cells bearing rearrangements of *myc* to chromosomes possessing immunoglobulin genes. Therefore these cells do not respond to whatever signals exist for the cessation of cell division. Continuous *myc* expression drives unceasing cell proliferation.

Other instances of overproduction or inappropriate production of oncogene proteins are known, although the means by which such aberrant expression occurs are not yet understood. For example, certain sarcomas elaborate PDGF, which in turn stimulates cell division within these tumors. Hematopoietic malignancies often produce many growth factors that are thought to provide mitogenic stimulation to tumor cells. The process whereby tumor cells synthesize and secrete growth factors to which they respond is called *autocrine* stimulation, a mechanism now recognized as assuming an increasingly more important role in tumor cell proliferation.

The second principal type of oncogene activation is DNA mutation. Physical and chemical carcinogens are known to be mutagens. Perhaps several of the viruses associated with human cancer also act as mutagens. In any event the result is the appearance of a qualitatively different oncogene product, not inappropriate expression of a normal product. The activation of *ras* genes in many different types of human tumors is the best known example of oncogene mutation. Specific point mutations in the DNA sequence encoding the *ras* G protein abolish its enzymatic activity. The precise consequence of this loss is not yet understood; perhaps the malfunctioning *ras* protein short-circuits any growth-inhibition signals from the cell surface or inappropriately prolongs growth-stimulatory signals. Several animal models of radiation and chemical carcinogenesis have demonstrated that *ras* mutation is the probable event by which these agents initiate malignant transformation.

The third mechanism for activation is a combination of the first two: namely, rearrangement of genetic material that, rather than augmenting the expression of a normal gene product, produces an entirely different one. Examples involving several oncogenes are discussed in the following section on chromosome translocations.

Tumor suppressor gene inactivation. Two common types of chromosome abnormalities in tumor karyotypes are interstitial deletions and translocations. Deletions are important in the inactivation of tumor suppressor genes. Such deletions may be inherited in a variety of familial tumor syndromes, such as Wilms' tumor [IIp(−)] or retinoblastoma [13q(−)]. However, characteristic, tumor-specific deletions also arise somatically in a wide range of human solid tumors. These include small cell carcinoma of the lung [3p(−)] and colon cancer [5q(−), 17p(−), 18q(−)]. With inherited deletions the lesions serve as markers for individuals at risk for developing the tumor. For example, individuals who inherit a 13q(−) chromosomal deletion have already had one lesion at the *RB-1* locus. According to Knudsen's "two-hit" hypothesis, they require only one more genetic lesion to inactivate the remaining "wild-type" allele. Such individuals are consequently at much higher risk for developing retinoblastoma than individuals with two wild-type alleles. The latter require two independent events to inactivate the suppressor effect of the *RB-1* locus before they can develop retinoblastoma (the so-called somatic version of the tumor).

An important consequence of cataloguing deletions in both inherited and somatic forms of the same tumor has been the realization that genes responsible for very rare forms of familial cancers are important in the pathogenesis of the sporadic forms of these same tumors. For example, the region affected in familial polyposis coli, 5q, is also frequently deleted in sporadic cases of colon cancer. Although inherited mutations of *P53* are associated with the Li-Fraumeni syndrome, many different types of sporadic tumors frequently bear inactivating deletions or mutations of *P53*. These include cancers of the bladder, colon, breast, esophagus, and lung.

In addition to interstitial deletions, inactivation of tumor suppressor genes can occur by point mutation. These mutations, particularly for *P53*, are often of the *dominant negative* form; that is, mutant protein may bind to and inactivate wild-type protein. Thus mutation of only one *P53* allele is sufficient to inactive both homologues of the gene. This is in contrast to deletion as an inactivating lesion; after deletion of one homologue, the remaining wild-type allele must still be damaged so that complete functional activity of the tumor suppressor locus is abrogated.

Chromosome translocations. One of the earliest observations about human tumors is that the number and appearance of chromosomes may become extremely abnormal. Changes in ploidy, loss and duplication of chromosomes, and the appearance of unusual chromatin bodies without centromeres (DMs) are all common karyotypic events. As techniques have improved for identifying particular chromosomes and delineating chromosomal substructure (e.g., banding pattern revealed by Giemsa staining or quinacrine fluorescence), much more reproducible data have emerged on specific chromosome defects occurring in association with particular human tumors (Table 71-3). The reliable appearance of certain abnormalities, such as the translocation involving chromosomes 9 and 22 in chronic myelogenous leukemia, has led to the hypothesis that movement, rearrangement, and deletion of genetic material in tumors can activate oncogenes.

During translocation a portion of one chromosome is transferred to another. The DNA present in the chromatin that has been transferred (the donor fragment) is covalently linked to the DNA in the recipient chromosome. This exchange is often reciprocal: fragments from two different chromosomes simply replace one another. Intuitively, we can see that the rearrangement resulting from translocation might drastically change the environment of an oncogene that happened to reside near the "breakpoint," that is, the junction between donor and recipient chromosome fragments. An oncogene lodged in a transcriptionally silent region of chromatin might be moved to a very active region of transcription, with obvious results. Conversely, active regulatory genes might be turned off.

In Burkitt's lymphoma the terminal portion of the long arm of chromosome 8 (8q) is involved in a reciprocal trans-

Table 71-3. Prominent chromosome abnormalities in human cancers*

Cancer	Chromosome abnormalities	Involved loci
Chronic myelogenous leukemia	t(9q;22q)	*ABL, BCR*
B cell lymphomas and leukemias	t(8q;14q)	*MYC*
	t(14q;18q)	*BCL2*
	t(1q;19p)	*PBX-1, E2A*
	t(14q;19q)	*BCL3*
	t(5q;14q)	*IL-3*
T cell lymphomas and leukemias	t(7q;19p)	*LYL-1*
	t(1p;14q)	*TAL, SCL, TCL*
	t(10p;14q)	*HOX*
	t(8q;14q)	*MYC*
Acute myelogenous leukemia	t(15q;17q)	*PML, RAR*
Retinoblastoma	13q(−)	*RB-1*
Wilms' tumor	11p(−)	*WT-1, WT-2*
Neurofibromatosis, type I	17q(−)	*NF1*
Polyposis coli	5q(−)	*FAP*
Li-Fraumeni syndrome and others	17p(−)	*P53*
Multiple endocrine neoplasia, type I	11q(−)	*MEN-1*
Colon carcinoma	18q(−)	*DCC*
Small cell lung carcinoma	3p(−)	?

*Autosomal chromosomes are assigned numbers from 1 through 22. The short and long arms of each chromosome are designated by the letters p and q, respectively; t stands for translocation and (−) for deletion. For example, in small cell carcinoma of the lung, tumors frequently demonstrate deletion of material from the short arm of chromosome 3. The tumor suppressor genes affected by the deletions in the lower portion of the table may also be inactivated by mutations.

fer to one of three sites: the long arm of chromosome 14, the long arm of chromosome 22, or the short arm of chromosome 2. Most tumors possess the t(8q;14q) translocation; 25% demonstrate t(2p;8q) or t(8q;22q). It is now known that the *myc* oncogene is located precisely at the 8q breakpoint of all Burkitt translocations. Furthermore, the regions on the recipient chromosomes represent the map positions of the kappa (κ) immunoglobulin light-chain gene (on 2p), the immunoglobulin heavy-chain locus (on 14q), and the lambda (λ) light-chain gene (on 22q). Therefore, in a B lymphocyte tumor, an oncogene is moved to a position of very active transcription, that is, one of the three immunoglobulin gene loci. The result of the translocation is not only the transcriptional activation of *myc* but also the uncoupling of its transcriptional regulation from events of the cell cycle. Signals go unheeded that might ordinarily result in the cessation of *myc* expression and cell division. Several other B lymphocyte lymphomas demonstrate translocations in which different oncogenes are brought into proximity of the heavy-chain locus (see Table 71-3). Once again, the result is transcriptional activation of previously silent genes. One prominent example, t(14q;18q) of follicular lymphoma, leads to the continued expression of *bcl-2*'s product, which, as described earlier, prevents the onset of programmed cell death (apoptosis). Translocations also occur that are T lymphocyte specific (see Table 71-3).

In addition to activating the expression of a pre-existing oncogene, chromosome translocations in tumors can result in the creation of entirely new genes. The Philadelphia chromosome of chronic myelogenous leukemia (CML) is one of the products of a reciprocal translocation of 9q and 22q. As a result, half the *bcr* oncogene on chromosome 22 is fused with half the *abl* oncogene from chromosome 9. When this chimeric gene is expressed, the gene product is a fusion protein consisting of the N-terminal half of the *bcr* protein and the C-terminal half of the *abl* protein. The new product has elevated tyrosine kinase activity. When translocation occurs further 5′ (upstream) in the *bcr* oncogene, acute lymphocytic leukemia results, rather than CML (Fig. 71-2). The fusion product of this latter translocation retains the tyrosine kinase of the *abl* parent at its C terminus and the serine kinase domain of the *bcr* parent at its N terminus. However, it now lacks the nucleotide exchange (*dbl*-like) domain present in the *bcr* parent and in the CML-specific translocation product. Evidently, this critical removal of internal amino acid residues represents the difference between an oncogene product with specificity for a myeloid cell that retains the ability to differentiate (giving rise to a chronic leukemia) and a shorter product with specificity for a lymphoid precursor that has lost its capacity to differentiate (giving rise to an acute leukemia). When the exact basis for this remarkable tropism is elucidated, we will have acquired a comprehensive understanding of the processes controlling growth and differentiation in lymphopoietic and hematopoietic tissues.

Several other spectacular examples show the power of

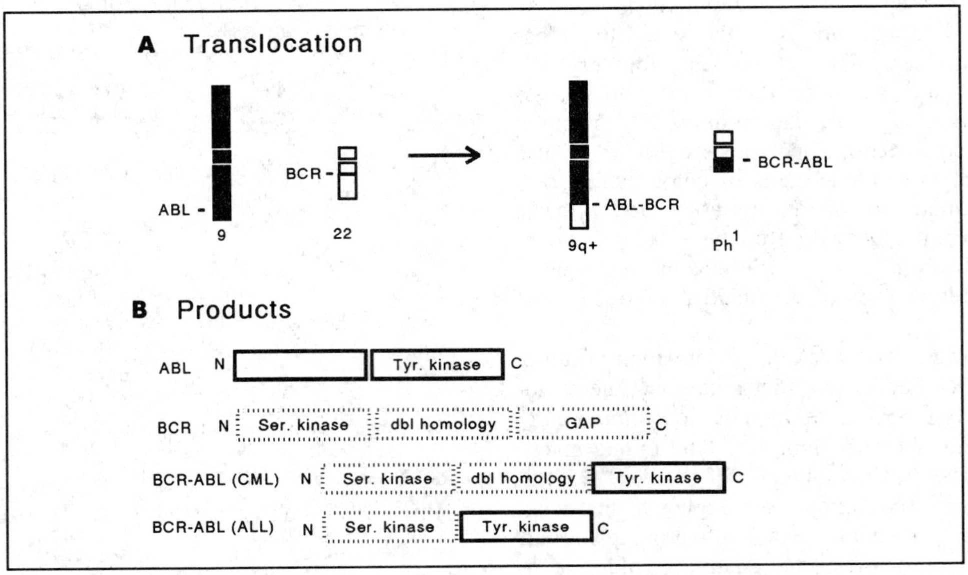

Fig. 71-2. Philadelphia chromosome translocation. **A,** Autosomomal chromosomes 9 and 22 undergo reciprocal exchange of genetic material through nonhomologous recombination. The Philadelphia chromosome [Ph[1];22q(−)] bears a head-to-tail fusion (*BCR-ABL*) of the *BCR* and *ABL* oncogenes. The reciprocal chromosome [9q(+)] also contains a gene fusion (*ABL-BCR*), but the pathogenetic significance of this hybrid product is unknown. **B,** The protein products of the proto-oncogenes, *BCR* and *ABL,* are depicted schematically, as well as the chronic myelogenous leukemia (CML) and acute lymphocytic leukemia (ALL) fusion proteins. *N* stands for N terminus; *C* for C terminus. Distinct functional domains are indicated by the rectangles. Because the ALL translocation occurs slightly more upstream in chromosome 22, the *dbl*-like domain of *BCR* is absent in the resulting fusion protein. The N-terminal domain of *ABL* may specify subcellular localization and/or substrate specificity.

translocation for creating new genes by fusing together fragments of pre-existing ones. In the t(15q;17q) translocation of acute promyelocytic leukemia, a retinoic acid receptor gene *(RARα)* is truncated and fused to the *PML* locus. The result is a chimeric product (PML-RARα) which is apparently capable of dominant negative interference with the function of *both* the parental (wild-type) products. In the t(1q;19p) translocation of acute pre–B cell leukemia, the gene encoding a B-cell-specific transcriptional regulatory factor, *E2A,* is fused to the homeobox gene, *PBX1*. Homeobox genes, bearing *homeodomains,* specify DNA-binding proteins important in development and differentiation. The PBX1-E2A fusion product therefore has the transcriptional activating potential of the B cell factor, E2A, fused to the DNA-binding domain of the homeobox gene. This redirects the transcriptional regulation of one gene *(E2A)* to the site of action, or gene targets, of the other *(PBX1)*. The general implications of these types of genetic rearrangements are twofold. First, regulatory domains of oncogenes may be mixed to produce new products with entirely distinct specificities, producing functional activity in entirely inappropriate cell lineages. The net result is often abnormal proliferation, accompanied by improperly timed or absent differentiation. The second implication is that fusion genes, being specific to the tumors in which they arise, potentially serve as targets for tumor-specific therapeutic strategies.

Stages of carcinogenesis and oncogene cooperation

The development of cancer has been considered a multistep process. Histopathologic observations, for example, have documented the sequence of changes from hyperplasia or dysplasia through carcinoma in situ to invasive metastatic cancer for a number of different tumors. In addition, genetic and epidemiologic analyses have suggested that multiple events are required for expression of the malignant phenotype. Recent oncogene research has supported the multistep hypothesis and provided a pathogenetic framework for further investigation.

Molecular clones of oncogenes have been obtained by employing recombinant DNA technology. As a result, detailed analysis of oncogene structure and function has been facilitated. In particular, the possession of molecular clones has made it possible to transfer activated oncogenes to cells with normal growth properties to determine what combination of oncogenes is required to generate a cancer cell. Several independent studies have shown that a cell that harbors a mutated *ras* gene may assume the abnormal morphologic features of a cancer cell but is not fully tumorigenic when inoculated into animals. The further addition of an activated *myc* gene is required for tumor formation to occur in vivo. More generally, for tumorigenic transformation of normal cells to occur, an activated oncogene with a product located in the cytoplasm requires the cooperation of an oncogene with a product located in the nucleus.

Interestingly, even two oncogenes are not sufficient for generating the full-blown cancer phenotype. The tumors resulting from transfer of activated *myc* and *ras* into normal cells do not invade and metastasize. Clearly, further steps and, presumably, other genetic alterations are required. The frequent appearance of deletions and mutations inactivating tumor suppressor genes strongly suggests that these changes must also accompany oncogene activation. The most compelling evidence for this hypothesis comes from the correlation of genetic lesions with distinct stages in the progression of colon cancer. As noted earlier, frank carcinomas of the colon frequently demonstrate deletion at 5q, 17p, and 18q. Mutations of *Kras* and, to a lesser extent, of *Nras* also often occur. However, in precursor lesions (adenomas less than 1 cm) very few *ras* mutations can be detected. Furthermore, early adenomas infrequently demonstrate deletions of 17p and 18q but do contain lesions involving 5q. Only advanced adenomas and carcinomas possess frequent changes in 18q. Finally, 17p deletions are almost always confined to frank carcinoma. It is now known that the 17p changes represent inactivating lesions of *P53*. From these correlations, we conclude that oncogene activation must be accompanied by the orderly progression of genetic changes that inactivate other (minimally, three) growth regulatory genes.

REFERENCES

Bishop JM: Molecular themes in oncogenesis. Cell 64:235, 1991.
Cantley LC et al: Oncogenes and signal transduction. Cell 64:281, 1991.
Hollstein M et al: p53 mutations in human cancers. Science 253:49, 1991.
Hunter T: Cooperation among oncogenes. Cell 64:249, 1991.
Rabbitts TH: Translocations, master genes, and differences between the origins of acute and chronic leukemias. Cell 67:641, 1991.
Vogelstein B et al: Genetic alterations during colorectal-tumor development. N Engl J Med 319:525, 1988.

CHAPTER

72 Principles of Treatment of Cancer

Robert L. Capizzi

Neoplastic diseases and their complications are the second most common cause of death among Americans. The approach to the therapy of neoplastic diseases, whether for cure or for palliation, is predicated on the biology of these diseases. Neoplasms produce clinical disease by local growth and disruption of normal organ function, by dissemination to distant sites with subsequent growth of metastases, or by the synthesis and secretion of biologically active products that can cause a variety of paraneoplastic syndromes. Thus the physician's approach to the treatment of patients with cancer varies depending on the following features: organ of origin, histology and stage, paraneoplastic syndromes, age of the patient and presence of other morbid diseases, and ultimate therapeutic intent, that is, cure or palliation.

Before discussing specific therapeutic approaches, it is worthwhile to review the general magnitude of the cancer problem. An estimated 1.1 million new cases of cancer will be diagnosed in the United States in 1992. The organ systems of origin of these cancers are shown in Fig. 72-1. A common misconception among the public is that "cancer" is one disease. Cancer represents hundreds of diseases with many causes. Although each disease may share certain general features with others, the approach to therapy for a given problem will vary. At presentation, approximately 64% of patients will have clinically localized cancers amenable to local therapy such as surgery and/or radiation therapy. Two thirds of these patients will in turn be cured, and one third will have recurrent disease, either locally advanced or metastatic. Today, many of these patients with localized disease are candidates for adjuvant chemotherapy, that is, the administration of drugs in the perioperative period when there is no overt metastatic disease but rather a high probability of recurrence despite local therapy. Clinical trials to date indicate that adjuvant chemotherapy is useful for some forms of cancer. At presentation, the remaining 36% of patients will have either locally advanced cancers that are not amenable to surgery or radiation therapy or will have overt metastatic disease. Provided that effective drugs or suitable clinical trials exist, these patients are candidates for systemic chemotherapy, possibly followed by surgery and/or radiation therapy.

The decision about what constitutes appropriate therapy for a given patient is a function of the organ of origin and the stage of the cancer. The latter is frequently influenced by certain biologic features of the tumor, such as histology and degree of differentiation of the neoplastic cells. For example, patients with clinical stage I non–small cell cancer of the lung may be cured with surgery or radiation therapy. However, the cure rate of patients with clinical stage I small cell carcinoma of the lung is considerably less than that for most stage I cancers, since small cell lung cancer has a propensity to metastasize early and widely. One concludes that the repeated failure of local or regional therapy to cure patients with clinical stage I small cell carcinoma of the lung reflects the presence of micrometastases that defy detection at the time of original diagnosis and staging.

It should be recognized that for most patients, optimum therapy is still in a state of evolution. Although the basic principles of cancer surgery were developed in the early 1900s, important new concepts, such as curative surgery for metastatic disease and limited surgery as part of a multimodality approach to the cure of breast cancer, were introduced in the 1970s and 1980s. Likewise, improved means for delivering radiation therapy became available only in the 1960s, and the use of radiation sensitizers and protectors is still under investigation. Chemotherapy was introduced in the 1950s and 1960s, primarily for palliation

CANCER INCIDENCE AND DEATHS BY SITE AND SEX—1992 ESTIMATES

CANCER INCIDENCE BY SITE AND SEX*

PROSTATE 132,000	BREAST 180,000
LUNG 102,000	COLON & RECTUM 77,000
COLON & RECTUM 79,000	LUNG 66,000
BLADDER 38,500	UTERUS 45,500
LYMPHOMA 27,200	LYMPHOMA 21,200
ORAL 20,600	OVARY 21,000
MELANOMA OF THE SKIN 17,000	MELANOMA OF THE SKIN 15,000
KIDNEY 16,200	PANCREAS 14,400
LEUKEMIA 16,000	BLADDER 13,100
STOMACH 15,000	LEUKEMIA 12,200
PANCREAS 13,900	KIDNEY 10,300
LARYNX 10,000	ORAL 9,700
ALL SITES 565,000	ALL SITES 565,000

*Excluding nonmelanoma skin cancer and carcinoma in situ.

CANCER DEATHS BY SITE AND SEX

LUNG 93,000	LUNG 53,000
PROSTATE 34,000	BREAST 46,000
COLON & RECTUM 28,900	COLON & RECTUM 29,400
PANCREAS 12,000	PANCREAS 13,000
LYMPHOMA 10,900	OVARY 13,000
LEUKEMIA 9,900	UTERUS 10,000
STOMACH 8,000	LYMPHOMA 10,000
ESOPHAGUS 7,500	LEUKEMIA 8,300
LIVER 6,600	LIVER 5,700
BRAIN 6,500	BRAIN 5,300
KIDNEY 6,400	STOMACH 5,300
BLADDER 6,300	MULTIPLE MYELOMA 4,500
ALL SITES 275,000	ALL SITES 245,000

Fig. 72-1. Cancer incidence and deaths by site and sex, 1992 estimates. (Reprinted with permission from American Cancer Society: Cancer facts and figures—1992.)

of acute leukemias, lymphomas, and certain childhood malignancies. Drugs were used at first as single agents. Combinations of drugs administered with curative intent were introduced in the mid-to-late 1960s and were used as part of a multimodal approach to solid tumors in the 1970s. The newest modality of cancer treatment is biotherapy, or the use of biologic response modifiers. Effective agents in this modality became commercially available in the 1980s.

Although certain forms of cancer, including some that are locally advanced and metastatic, are now within the realm of cure, the great majority of the more common malignancies are not curable. Thus the principles outlined in this chapter indicate current approaches, all of which are subject to modification and change to take into account the results of ongoing clinical investigations.

STAGING

At times the opportunity to cure cancer (e.g., breast cancer) resides in the first therapeutic attempt. Thus adequate staging and employment of the appropriate modality at the outset are of critical importance. For reliable staging, the therapist must be familiar with the sensitivity, specificity, accuracy, and roles of various maneuvers (history and physical examination, blood chemistries, radiographs, scans, imaging procedures, surgical staging). Briefly, the *sensitivity* of a test defines the number of positive tests discovered among patients with the abnormal condition (i.e., ideally, there are no false-negative results); the *specificity* of a test refers to the number of negative tests in a truly normal situation (i.e., ideally, there are no false-positive results); and lastly, *accuracy* reflects the number of correct tests in the total population tested. Implicit in the outcome of the staging exercise and therapeutic plan is prognosis. Given the general public view of cancer, most patients and their families will ask or want to ask about prognosis: "Can I be cured?" "How long will I live?" "What kind of symptoms from the disease or therapy do I need to look out for?" The physician must have as much information as possible to answer these questions, not only for proper treatment planning but also for proper psychosocial management of the patient and family.

As shown in Table 72-1, a substantial decline has occurred in the mortality of patients with certain types of neoplastic disease. This is the direct result of systematic clinical trials that have tested various laboratory advances and/or clinical hypotheses. These trials often assign the patient to one treatment or another by random allocation. Proper *stratification,* that is, the comparable assignment of patients to each treatment group according to known prognostic variables, is important to ensure the validity of the study's conclusions. Patient eligibility for the trial and proper stratification require adequate staging. For some cancers, international agreement exists about staging features and nomenclature, for example, stage IA lymphocytic predominant versus stage IVB lymphocytic depleted Hodgkin's disease. These stages and histologic classifications immediately indicate the type of therapy and the prognosis for the patient and, just as importantly, facilitate communication of the results of new clinical trials. Manuals prepared by the American Joint Committee for Cancer Staging and End Results Reporting outline the criteria for staging classifications; these criteria are updated and refined as new information becomes available.

Table 72-1. Trends in survival according to site of cancer and race: patients diagnosed in 1970-1973 and 1981-1986

	Relative 5-year survival (%)			
	White		Black	
Site	1970-73*	1981-86†	1970-73*	1981-86†
All sites	43	52	31	38
Stomach	13	16	13	18
Colon	49	57	37	48
Rectum	45	54	30	41
Larynx	62	69	—	52
Breast (female)	68	78	51	64
Prostate gland	63	75	55	62
Testis	72	92	—	92
Urinary bladder	61	79	36	59
Hodgkin's disease	67	76	—	74
Non-Hodgkin's lymphoma	41	51	—	45
Leukemia	22	36	—	29

From American Cancer Society: Cancer facts and figures—1991. Data from Cancer Statistics Branch, National Cancer Institute.

*Rates are based on End Results Group (American Joint Committee) data from a series of hospital registries and one population-based registry.

†Rates are from the SEER Program, based on data from population-based registries in Connecticut, New Mexico, Utah, Iowa, Hawaii, Atlanta, Detroit, Seattle-Puget Sound, and San Francisco-Oakland. Rates are based on follow-up of patients through 1986.

A broad categorization of neoplasms is based on the embryonic origin of the involved tissues. Thus *carcinomas* arise in tissue of epithelial origin, *adenocarcinomas* arise in glandular (adeno-) epithelium, and *sarcomas* arise in tissue of mesenchymal origin. Leukemias and lymphomas are also of mesenchymal origin. In general, these broad categorizations indicate certain patterns of growth and spread.

The prognosis of patients with neoplastic diseases is influenced by the general features outlined in the box on p. 710. The organ site and histologic classification obviously influence the treatment plan and prognosis (e.g., squamous cell versus small cell carcinoma of the lung). The specific features related to stage for most solid tumors are a function of their TNM characteristics: tumor size and local invasion (T), lymph nodal metastases (N), and metastases to other organs (M) (see the box on p. 710). Although far from perfect, the TNM stage is included as an important parameter for stratification in clinical trials. Other features that bear on prognosis or choice of therapy may include degree of cellular differentiation, nuclear grade and DNA ploidy, absence or presence of hormone receptors (in breast cancer), and so on. Finally, certain clinical parameters listed in the box on p. 710 also must be factored into the prognostic equation because these may influence the choice and aggressiveness of therapy.

Clinical features that may influence the prognosis of a given type and stage of cancer

Age
Performance status
Nutritional status
Immunologic status
Comorbid, nonneoplastic conditions that may influence the choice or aggressiveness of therapy (e.g., heart, lung, kidney, or liver disease)

On a statistical basis, cancers are diseases of elderly persons. This fact, coupled with the reduced mortality from heart disease and stroke and the increasing median age of the U.S. population, means that physicians will be caring for more patients with neoplastic diseases, whose numbers will be augmented by the rising incidences of lung cancer in men and women. The reasons for these rising incidences are probably multifactorial, but two prominent features are prolonged carcinogen exposure, especially tobacco use, and decreasing immune function with age.

At age 25 years, only 1 in 600 individuals develops cancer; in contrast, the frequency is 1 in 10 at age 70. Unfortunately, no effective screening method exists for the early detection of the most common cancer in the U.S. population, lung cancer. Thus, prevention (smoking cessation) is the most prominent public health issue. Early detection of colorectal cancer through periodic testing of the stool for occult blood, of breast cancer through breast self-examination and mammography, of cervical cancer with Pap smears, and of prostatic cancer with digital examination and testing of prostate-specific antigen should be part of every general medical evaluation. These tests are cost-effective and save lives.

Care of the elderly patient with cancer is complicated by the presence of comorbid diseases that often prohibit aggressive multimodality therapy shown to be effective in younger patients. Nevertheless, elderly patients should be staged adequately and therapy offered with appropriate consideration of the risk/benefit ratio.

General features for classification and staging of neoplastic diseases

Organ site of origin
Histologic classification
Size of primary tumor and extent of local invasion (T)
Location and extent of lymphatic (nodal) metastases (N)
Metastases to other organs (M)

TUMOR MARKERS

There has been an ongoing search for a single, inexpensive blood test that will assist in the early detection of cancer and thus will increase the cure rate. Although certain tumor markers in the blood are useful in cancer medicine, none precisely attains this goal for several reasons: (1) usually, tumor markers are elevated only when the disease has advanced beyond the possibility of cure by local therapy (i.e., low sensitivity); (2) most lack specificity for a given type of tumor; and (3) blood levels may be increased by nonmalignant diseases.

The type and utility of typically employed tumor markers are noted in Table 72-2. Five major types of tumor markers are used in clinical practice: (1) oncofetal proteins, (2) hormones, (3) serum enzymes, (4) immunoglobulins, and (5) tumor-associated antigens.

The *oncofetal proteins* exist as major normal proteins during embryonic or fetal life that regress to very low levels in the normal adult. However, the blood level of these proteins increase in certain malignant and nonmalignant disease states. Two such proteins are well established in clinical practice: carcinoembryonic antigen (CEA) and alpha fetoprotein (AFP).

In the fetus, CEA peaks during the second to sixth months and is primarily produced in the gastrointestinal track, pancreas, and liver. Its appearance in tumors is believed to be either a function of genetic derepression or a natural product of the primitive stem cells that give rise to the tumor. The initial expectation for CEA was that it might prove useful in the early detection of colorectal cancer. However, as was subsequently learned, serum CEA may be elevated by several nonmalignant diseases. Even when serum CEA is elevated in neoplastic diseases, it does not identify the cancer's site of origin. Currently, the main use of the CEA and other markers is in serial measurements during follow-up of a patient who has been treated for cancer. For example, patients with breast or colon cancer whose CEA was moderately elevated preoperatively and then falls to normal levels postoperatively have a statistically better disease-free survival than patients with persistently elevated values. Likewise, a rising value during serial follow-up may be the first clue to recurrent disease and thus may be reason for further evaluation. The same principle pertains to other markers.

Because of the amino acid homology between AFP and adult albumin, it is believed that in the fetus, AFP functions as the fetal counterpart of adult albumin in the circulation. After birth, AFP gradually disappears and is replaced by albumin. In the fetus, AFP is produced by the yolk sac, liver, and gastrointestinal tract. Since the plasma half-lives are 6 to 8 days and 5.5 days for CEA and AFP, respectively, the time necessary for abnormally elevated values to return to normal after complete removal of an oncofetal protein–producing tumor can be calculated. The failure of these values to return to normal indicates residual tumor and the need for further, perhaps alternative, therapy.

Human chorionic gonadotropin (HCG) and various other

Table 72-2. Tumor markers

General uses:

1. Monitor serial titers before and after therapy. For example, a high preoperative CEA titer that falls to the normal range postoperatively is associated with a better prognosis in breast or colon cancer than is one that remains elevated after local therapy.
2. Serial values are also of use in monitoring (a) the clinical course of disease after local therapy and (b) the response to systemic chemotherapy. A decline in elevated values is usually consistent with tumor regression. Tumor markers are most valuable in monitoring disease not readily assessable by physical examination or simple radiographs.

			Conditions in which elevated serum/plasma concentrations occur	
	Characteristics	**Presence in normal serum/plasma**	**Neoplastic**	**Nonneoplastic**
I. Oncofetal proteins				
1. Carcinoembryonic antigen (CEA)	Glycoprotein (MW 200,000)	<2.5 ng/ml	Gastrointestinal, breast, lung cancers	Inflammatory bowel disease, pancreatitis, gastritis, smoker's chronic bronchitis, alcoholic liver disease, hepatitis
2. Alpha fetoprotein (AFP)	Alpha globulin (MW 70,000)	<40 ng/ml	Hepatoma, nonseminomatous testicular cancers	Pregnancy, regenerating liver tissue after viral hepatitis, chemically induced liver necrosis, partial hepatectomy
II. Hormones				
1. Human chorionic gonadotropin, beta subunit (β-HCG)	Glycoprotein (MW 45,000); beta subunit provides specificity versus LH, FSH, TSH	0	Choriocarcinoma, nonseminomatous testicular cancer, giant cell carcinoma of lung	Pregnancy
2. Ectopic hormones	ACTH, ADH, PTH		Lung, breast, head and neck, cervical cancers	
III. Serum enzymes				
1. Prostatic acid phosphatase (PAP)	Radioimmunoassay detects prostatic isozyme and distinguishes it from acid phosphatases of other organs (e.g., liver, spleen, kidney, small intestine), red and white blood cells, and platelets	0	Prostatic carcinoma	
2. Placental alkaline phosphatase	Biochemically and immunologically similar to that produced by the placenta	0	Seminoma, ovarian cancer	Pregnancy
3. Lactic dehydrogenase (LDH)	Tetramer, two distinct polypeptide chains: H (heart) and M (muscle)		Lymphoma	Hepatitis, myocardial infarction, muscle injury
IV. Immunoglobulins	Monoclonal elevation (M spike) of complete protein, light or heavy chain, or portions		Multiple myeloma, B cell lymphoma	Monoclonal gammopathy of unknown significance (M-GUS)
V. Tumor-associated antigens				
1. CA-125			Ovarian, lung cancers	Benign gynecologic disease, cirrhosis
2. CA-15.3			Breast, ovarian, lung cancers	
3. Prostate specific antigen	Glycoprotein (MW 30,000-40,000)		Prostatic carcinoma	Benign prostatic hypertrophy

MW, Molecular weight; LH, luteinizing hormone; FSH, follicle-stimulating hormone; TSH, thyroid-stimulating hormone; ACTH, adrenocorticotropic hormone; ADH, antidiuretic hormone; PTH, parathormone (parathyroid hormone).

ectopic polypeptide *hormones* are produced by some tumors. Some ectopic hormones, such as adrenocorticotropic hormone (ACTH), antidiuretic hormone (ADH), and parathormone (PTH), may produce signs and symptoms of hormone excess. Elevated plasma levels of HCG are found in virtually all women with choriocarcinoma and in approximately 60% of young men with nonseminomatous testicular carcinoma. The plasma half-life of HCG is 1.5 to 2 days, which allows the rapid assessment of the efficacy of therapy. As with several other polypeptide hormones, HCG is composed of both an alpha and a beta subunit. Whereas the alpha subunit is shared by follicle-stimulating hormone (FSH) and luteinizing hormone (LH), the beta subunit imparts biologic and immunologic specificity to each of these hormones. Consequently, antibodies made to the beta subunit of HCG allow its measurement by radioimmunoassay. This is important because normal serum in nonpregnant individuals should have nondetectable HCG levels, whereas the pituitary hormones FSH and LH are measurable. If β-HCG is elevated in an adult male, the most likely cause is a testicular tumor (see Table 72-2).

The tumors most frequently associated with ectopic hormone secretion are small cell lung cancer (ACTH, ADH) and epidermoid carcinoma of the lung, head and neck, cervix, and breast (PTH-like substance). The polypeptides may not be exactly homologous with the natural hormone and may be larger prohormone proteins or fragments of these. The endocrine function of these polypeptides may vary.

Normal *serum enzymes* typically produced by the affected organ may be extremely elevated in neoplastic conditions. Prostatic acid phosphatase (PAP) is normally secreted by the normal prostate gland. Although abnormally elevated plasma levels of PAP reflect the extension of prostate cancer beyond the prostatic capsule, the value per se is not a good reflection of tumor burden and is not a useful screening method for prostate cancer (see next paragraph). Placental alkaline phosphatase can be distinguished from its isozymes derived from liver or bone by various laboratory methods. Elevation of either or both of the latter two isozymes usually indicates metastases to these organs. The serum value of lactic dehydrogenase (LDH) has prognostic significance in certain types of lymphoma and is a useful measure to monitor during therapy. Protein electrophoresis showing a monoclonal spike (M protein) coupled with typical signs and symptoms of disease is pathognomonic for the diagnosis of multiple myeloma or certain B cell lymphomas. The amount of the M spike can be quantifiably linked with tumor burden and provides an excellent marker for response to therapy and follow-up. Certain *immunoglobulins* may be associated with serum hyperviscosity, which may present as a medical emergency.

There is an ongoing search for *antigens* that display absolute specificity for a given cancer. The development of monoclonal antibodies to such antigens would have obvious diagnostic, prognostic, and therapeutic uses. No antigen discovered to date has this property. However, several tumor-associated antigens have substantial usefulness in patient care. These include CA-125, CA-15.3, and prostate-specific antigen. CA-125 is especially useful for monitoring response to therapy in women with ovarian cancer; it is elevated in approximately 80% of women with tumors measuring less than 2 cm after debulking surgery. Likewise, CA-15.3 may be used to follow the course of patients with breast, ovarian, lung cancers. Prostate-specific antigen appears to be more sensitive than PAP in the management of men with prostate cancer. This antigen's usefulness for screening for this common tumor is diminished because it may be elevated in men with benign prostatic hypertrophy.

GENERAL CONSIDERATIONS

The biology of a given tumor and its location, together with its associated signs and symptoms, determine its presentation. Early versus late presentation of disease affects stage of disease, and in turn, stage and location have substantial impact on the choice of optimum therapy. The goal of therapy, palliation versus cure, affects choice of modality(ies), timing, and intensity of therapy. In theory, most tumors derive from a single mutated cell that has been stripped away from normal growth regulatory processes. Detailed studies of the malignant transformation of normal human colonic mucosa describe a multistep process that can occur in the general population, a process that is accelerated in populations who may have a genetic predisposition for the development of neoplastic diseases. Detailed clinical and laboratory studies describe a spectrum of genetic events giving rise to cellular hyperplasia, to benign adenomas, to carcinoma in situ, to local and regional invasion, and to frank metastases. It is hoped that an early understanding of this process will lead to more effective means for prevention, early detection, and treatment.

Experimental studies have defined patterns of tumor growth that, when coupled with clinical observations of the natural history of diseases, have enhanced overall cure rates. A crude estimate of the overall cure rate for all types of cancer in the United States, as reflected in the overall 5-year survival figures, has increased from approximately 42% 20 years ago to 50% today. The specific tumors affected by this process are shown in Table 72-1. The general public is mostly unaware of this progress because the tumor with the highest frequency and mortality in the United States, lung cancer, has generally not been affected. Indeed, the frequency of lung cancer has increased greatly (Fig. 72-2), a statistic largely attributable to cigarette smoking.

Established tumors have three broad categories of cells. Stem cells propagate the tumor mass, invade local/regional tissues, and metastasize. The stem cell pool is composed of proliferating and nonproliferating (dormant) cells in G_0 or G_1 phases of the cell cycle. Various stimuli can engage dormant cells into active cellular multiplication. Any curative modality(ies) must eradicate the stem cell pool. The cellular composition of the largest components of the tumor mass consists of nonproliferating end-stage viable cells, dead cells, and stroma. These cell populations account for signs and symptoms of organ dysfunction, obstruction, bleeding, and so on.

The therapeutic index should determine the selection of

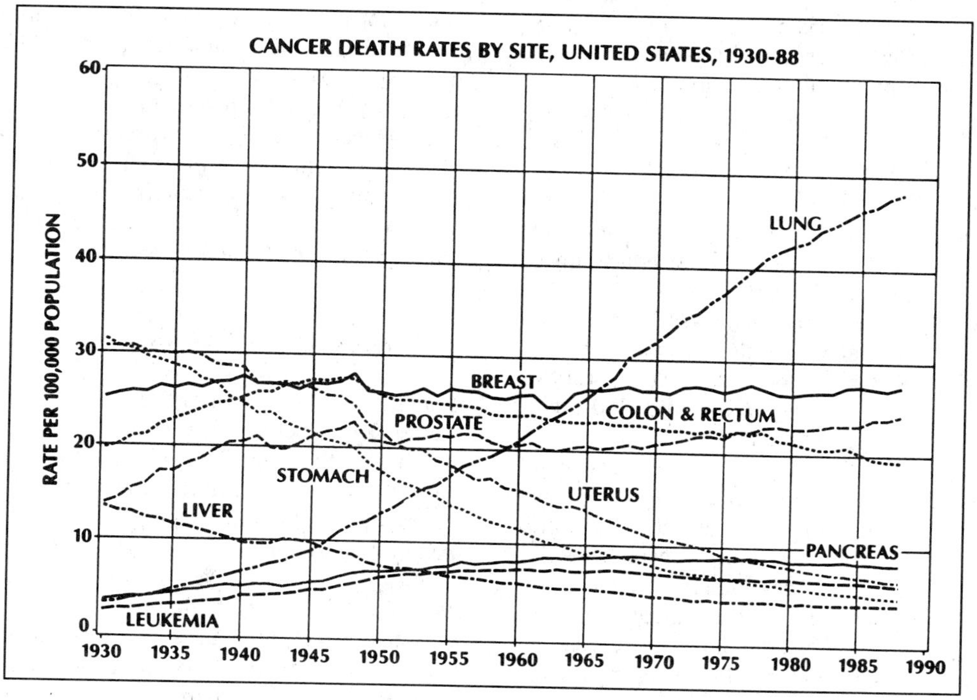

Fig. 72-2. Cancer death rates by site, United States, 1930 to 1988. (Reprinted with permission from American Cancer Society: Cancer facts and figures—1991.)

appropriate curative therapy. For example, equal cure rates for certain stages of laryngeal cancer can occur from radiation treatments or surgery. In this case, preservation of the voice leads one to select radiation therapy.

Effective surgery removes all tumor stem cells. Radiation therapy and chemotherapy destroy tumor stem cells, and host physiology then removes the debris of dead cells. Major clinical decisions associated with the selection of radiation therapy and/or chemotherapy involves the selection of dose, frequency, and duration of therapy. The cell-kill associated with these cytotoxic treatments follows first-order kinetics; that is, each treatment causes the same fractional cell-kill regardless of the tumor mass. Thus the same treatment intensity is required to reduce a small tumor burden from 10^3 cells to 0 (i.e., cure) as to reduce a large tumor mass of 10^{11} cells (100 g) to 10^8 cells (100 mg). The latter condition (10^8 cells) is undetectable by current clinical measures and is consistent with what is termed as a *complete remission*.

As tumor cells grow, they have a high propensity for mutations that affect both the biology and the therapeutic response of tumors. This mutational process gives rise to the observed "tumor heterogeneity" in response to radiation or chemotherapy.

One of the most important understandings of tumor biology during the past 20 years is the concept of *micrometastases* (i.e., the presence of clinically undetectable microscopic metastases at the time of diagnosis of an apparently localized tumor). This becomes evident by the appearance of distant metastases some time after the complete removal of a local tumor (e.g., the appearance of distant metastases months or years after radial mastectomy for stage II breast cancer). Detailed clinical observation has defined various prognostic determinants that indicate a high probability of distant micrometastases despite the only evident clinical disease being totally eradicated by surgery and/or radiation therapy. The validation of this hypothesis is provided from the results of randomized clinical trials that indicated the effectiveness of adjuvant chemotherapy or hormonal agents administered for a time after surgery and/or radiation therapy. Successes for adjuvant chemo/hormonal therapy include breast cancer, Duke's C colon cancer, rectal cancer, and various pediatric neoplasms.

The term *neoadjuvant* or *primary chemotherapy* refers to the use of chemotherapy before local surgery or radiation therapy. The intent of primary chemotherapy is not only to affect distant micrometastases but also to shrink the size of the primary tumor so as to facilitate local therapy.

The effects of therapy are defined by several terms. A *complete remission* refers to the complete eradication of all clinical evidence of disease, including evidence from physical examination, radiographs, and scans; normalization of well-defined tumor markers; and the patient's return to a premorbid performance status. A *pathologic*, or *histopathologic, complete remission* refers to the further verification of the complete remission by second-look surgery and rebiopsy of prior known locations of disease. A clinical *partial remission* or *response* is the reduction of measurable tumor masses by at least 50%; a tumor mass is measured as the product of its longest diameter (M_1) and the diameter perpendicular to this diameter (M_2). Thus the product of M_1 and M_2 after therapy must be at least 50%

less than the pretherapy measurement. A *pathologic partial response* refers to the presence of histologic or microscopic disease in a biopsied clinical complete remission site.

SURGICAL ONCOLOGY

Surgeons have a multifaceted role in the care of the cancer patient. Although prevention of disease and education of patients are part of all medical practice, the surgeon has several unique roles in cancer prophylaxis. These include the follow-up of individuals with multiple endocrine neoplasia, prophylactic colectomy in patients with a history of familial polyposis or juvenile ulcerative colitis, and orchiectomy in patients with cryptorchidism.

In every instance the diagnosis of cancer resides in proper histopathologic examination. Obtaining the proper amount of tissue and placing it properly in the correct preservative for electron or light microscopy, receptor analysis, immunologic phenotyping, and other procedures are crucial for adequate diagnosis, staging, and treatment planning. Various biopsy procedures, ranging from needle aspiration to excision, may be indicated, depending on the tumor's location and size. The proper surgical procedure, with or without the integration of radiation therapy and/or chemotherapy, depends on meticulous, thorough staging. A complete knowledge of both the natural history of disease and the patterns and modes of spread are critical to reliable staging. The surgeon may be assisted in this regard by the results of prior lymphangiography, computed tomography, or other scans.

The basic principles of surgical cure of patients with any cancer are tumor removal with adequate tumor-free margins surrounding the tumor and avoidance of seeding the operative field with tumor cells. Although the largest proportion of surgical cures occur in patients with local or local/regional cancers, certain patients with an isolated metastasis may be cured or may have a longer disease-free survival after surgical removal of the metastasis. These include patients with pulmonary metastases from bone or soft tissue sarcomas, isolated hepatic metastasis from colorectal cancer, residual masses after chemotherapy for testicular cancer, and isolated cerebral metastasis from melanoma or lung cancer.

The effects of radiation therapy and chemotherapy may be improved after the removal of large tumor masses such as those associated with ovarian cancer and sarcomas. Likewise, relief of symptoms of spinal cord or nerve root compression, correction of obstruction or perforation of a hollow viscus, control of bleeding, or drainage of an abscess will enhance the quality of life. At times, management of the compromised host will require open lung or liver biopsy to establish a diagnosis. Removal of the spleen may be important in the control of cytopenias associated with certain hematologic disorders. Palliation of breast or prostate cancer with relief of bone pain and other symptoms of metastatic disease may follow castration. Proper venous access is critical to the therapy and supportive care of many patients. The use of central venous catheters and implantable pumps has increased comfort by improving venous access for ease of drug administration and allowing greater mobility of patients.

Finally, since the most dramatic successes in overall cure rates for certain neoplastic diseases have resulted from an integrated therapeutic approach combining surgery, radiation therapy, and/or chemotherapy, further successes are sure to follow with continued research. The coordinated participation of all health care providers in this regard is critical.

RADIATION THERAPY

Radiation is used as a single modality or combined with surgery and/or chemotherapy with either curative or palliative intent. Since the curative potential of radiation, as with surgery, depends on effective therapy delivered to the diseased area, meticulous staging is of paramount importance. Again, this requires a thorough knowledge of the natural history of disease as well as the sensitivity and specificity of various diagnostic techniques.

Ionizing radiation used in cancer therapy either is derived from decay of radioactive isotopes (gamma radiation), such as cobalt-60, radium, radon, or iridium, or is electrically generated (roentgen rays). The ability of radiation to ionize air is measured in roentgens (R). The unit of measurement used in clinical medicine is the *rad* (*r*adiation *a*bsorbed *d*ose), which indicates the amount of energy absorbed per unit of mass measured in joules per kilogram. The term in current clinical use is the *gray* (GY); 1 gray = 100 rad. Ionizing radiation produces biologically active intermediates within the cell, such as free radicals that damage deoxyribonucleic acid (DNA) and interfere with its replication. Partial (sublethal) damage to DNA may be mutagenic, thus creating long-term complications such as carcinogenesis or leukemogenesis. Although the physical and chemical changes induced in tissues by irradiation take place almost instantaneously (10^{-12} to 10^{-14} second), the biologic effects may not be observed for weeks (e.g., tumor necrosis), years (carcinogenesis), or decades (genetic change).

The type of equipment used in therapy has a significant impact on the therapeutic and toxic effects. Orthovoltage machines deliver the maximum radiation dose superficially, and skin burns are the dose-limiting immediate toxic result. In contrast, the higher-energy supervoltage equipment delivers maximum radiation at greater depths, consequently sparing the skin. The most frequently used means for delivering radiation to tissues is by external beam (teletherapy), wherein the desired area to be treated is mapped out with appropriate shielding of vital organs such as heart, lungs, and kidneys. This composite of treated and lead-shielded areas is called the *port* or *treatment field*. The total dose of radiation to be given over a time is divided into a series of small doses that cumulatively equal the desired total dose. This is called *dosage fractionation*. At times the total dose delivered to the central tumor is increased by a *coned-down boost*. For example, the treatment field or port is reduced for additional external beam therapy, or radioactive implants such as radium or radon are inserted directly into the tissue. The intent of the boost is to cure.

Selection of the proper dose of radiation takes into account the tumor's radiosensitivity, that is, the dose required to sterilize the tumor mass so that the cancer cells can neither replicate nor metastasize. A tumor's radioresistance is relative because any tumor cell can be destroyed with a sufficiently large dose of radiation. Some features that affect a tumor's radiation sensitivity include oxygen tension, cellular content of endogenous thiols, and proliferative capacity. Because of the relatively poor vascularity of tumors, oxygen delivery is grossly impaired. This relative hypoxia diminishes the content of radiation-induced oxygen-free radicals that damage DNA. Certain tumors have a higher content of endogenous thiols, which act as free-radical scavengers, a process that also diminishes DNA damage. More rapidly proliferating tumors are usually more radiosensitive; however, these same tumors have a higher propensity for early widespread metastases. The limitation that prevents total kill of tumor is radiation damage to normal organs. In an attempt to improve the selective effect of radiation on tumors, clinical trials of drugs with radiation-sensitizing properties that concentrate in tumors or, conversely, drugs that protect normal tissues are currently under way.

Curative radiation therapy rather than surgery is usually considered when surgery would be either technically difficult or extremely mutilating (e.g., in laryngeal cancer and, more recently, early-stage breast cancer). Radiation with curative intent requires that the radiation dose sterilize the tumor while producing reversible and tolerable toxicity to the surrounding normal tissues. The radiosensitivity of tumors decreases from lymphoproliferative malignancies and leukemias to carcinomas to sarcomas. Consequently, local eradication of lymphomatous masses can be achieved with a significantly smaller total dose than is required to eradicate breast cancer. Local control of breast cancer requires both the removal of the gross tumor (lumpectomy or partial mastectomy) and a large total dose of radiation delivered by both external beam and interstitial implant. An understanding of the radiosensitivity of a particular neoplasm is important in selecting the best modality for its treatment. For example, spinal cord compression from lymphoma responds well to radiation, thus sparing the patient a surgical procedure. Conversely, the same problem caused by metastatic non–small cell carcinoma of the lung might best be treated by surgery because of the tumor's radioresistance.

Thus the approach to the patient must consider the type of tumor, its intrinsic radiosensitivity, its location, its stage, requirement for debulking, size of treatment field and total dose of radiation, and obviously, whether the ultimate goal is cure or palliation. Radiation may have substantial palliative potential, as indicated in the box at upper right. The use of palliative radiation therapy must be tempered with the need for systemic chemotherapy in patients with frank metastatic disease. Because of the possibility of additive side effects, some cytotoxic drugs cannot be given concurrently with radiation therapy. Also, irradiation of bone destroys normal bone marrow when successive areas of active marrow are included in the radiation ports. Extensive irradiation of marrow, perhaps coupled with myelophthisis from the tumor, may reduce marrow reserves, thus limiting the use of cytotoxic drugs necessary to control systemic disease. Clinical judgment must thus be used in the selection of sequential therapies.

Indications for radiation therapy in treatment of patients with cancer

Curative intent

Alone or in combination with surgery and/or chemotherapy; relevant diseases: Hodgkin's disease, head and neck cancer, Wilms' tumor, seminoma, rhabdomyosarcoma, early-stage breast cancer

Palliation

For example, for treatment of (1) pain—bone pain and pathologic fractures; (2) obstruction of airway, intestine, ureter, bile duct, lymphatic channel, blood vessels (e.g., superior vena caval obstruction) or spinal cord or nerve root compression; (3) bleeding (e.g., gastric, intestinal, bladder, carcinoma); and (4) intracranial or leptomeningeal metastases

Prophylaxis

For example, for treatment of pharmacologic sanctuaries, such as the brain and testes in childhood acute leukemia and brain in small cell lung cancer

Side effects of radiation therapy may be either immediate (days to weeks) or long term (months to years) (see the box on p. 722). When considering the implications of the side effects of radiation, one must consider the type of neoplastic disease, the radiation dose, and the geometry of the irradiated field. For example, symptoms of hypothyroidism may occur years after the cure of Hodgkin's disease by irradiation of fields that included the neck.

HORMONAL THERAPY

Hormone deprivation through castration was one of the earliest therapeutic approaches for the treatment of men and women with metastatic cancers of the prostate and breast, respectively. With a demonstrated effect from this surgical maneuver, successive surgical ablation of the adrenal and pituitary glands provided additional palliation. In selected patients, oophorectomy after mastectomy (adjunctive castration) in premenopausal women improved the cure rate.

Various drugs have largely replaced these surgical ablative procedures. An added advantage to the pharmaceutical approach is that the hormonal agents cause less morbidity than cytotoxic drugs and, for selected patients, provide excellent quality of life. Approximately 75% of women whose breast cancers possess receptors for both estrogen and progesterone significantly benefit from therapy with the antiestrogen, tamoxifen. Likewise, 80% of men with metastatic prostate cancer respond to therapy with luteinizing hormone releasing hormone (LHRH) agonists, which reduce the pro-

Table 72-3. Drugs used in treatment of cancer

Drug	Route of administration	Acute toxicity	Intermediate or delayed toxicity*	Precautions
I. *Alkylating agents*. The alkyl group of these molecules forms covalent bonds with DNA and thus interferes with its replication. This interference not only is cytotoxic, but also is potentially mutagenic and carcinogenic				
A. Mustard derivatives				
Mechlorethamine, nitrogen mustard (Mustargen)	IV, Intrapleural	Nausea and vomiting, local phlebitis; chemical cellulitis and tissue necrosis if drug extravasates	Bone marrow suppression; alopecia	Administer through a running IV infusion; must be given immediately on reconstitution because of short physical half-life.
Cyclophosphamide† (Cytoxan), ifosfamide (IFEX)	IV, oral	Nausea and vomiting with intermittent high dose	Bone marrow suppression; chemical cystitis; alopecia; syndrome of inappropriate antidiuretic hormone (SIADH)	Use forced hydration to induce polyuria to avoid *cystitis* (metabolites of drug irritate the bladder). Mesna (see under miscellaneous) is administered with IFEX to prevent hemorrhagic cystitis.
Chlorambucil (Leukeran)	Oral	Daily doses well tolerated; may be slight nausea and vomiting	Bone marrow suppression	None
Melphalan (Alkeran)	Oral, IV (experimental)	Daily doses well tolerated; may be slight nausea and vomiting	Bone marrow suppression	None
B. Alkyl sulfonate				
Busulfan (Myleran)	Oral	None	Bone marrow suppression; *pulmonary fibrosis*, hyperpigmentation of skin, gynecomastia	None
C. Ethylenimine				
triethylenethiophosphoramide (Thiotepa)	IV	None	Bone marrow suppression	None
D. Triazene				
Dacarbazine (DTIC)	IV	Nausea and vomiting that lessens with repetitive doses; occasional flulike syndrome; pain and tissue damage if extravasated	Bone marrow suppression, hepatic toxicity	Avoid extravasation.

E. Nitrosoureas				
Carmustine (BiCNU)	IV	Burning pain along vein, facial flushing, nausea and vomiting within 4 to 6 hours	Bone marrow suppression 3 to 6 weeks after administration, occasional renal and hepatic toxicity	Slow infusion rate to prevent local pain; cumulative bone marrow suppression may occur.
Lomustine (CeeNU)	Oral	Nausea and vomiting	As for carmustine	
Streptozocin (Zanosar)	IV	Nausea and vomiting, renal tubular acidosis, renal failure	Diabetes mellitus	Inject through running IV infusion; avoid extravasation.
F. Platinum analogs				
Cisplatin (Platinol)	IV	Nausea and vomiting; mild bone marrow suppression	High-frequency hearing loss, distal sensory neuropathy	Forced saline hydration can prevent renal damage; otherwise, irreversible renal failure may occur.
Carboplatin (Paraplatin)	IV	Nausea and vomiting, bone marrow suppression, especially thrombocytopenia	Thrombocytopenia, possibly cumulative	Dosage may be adjusted according to renal function.
G. Altretamine (Hexalen)	Oral	Mild nausea and vomiting, mild marrow suppression	Peripheral neuropathy	Avoid concurrent monoamine oxidase inhibitors.
II. *Antimetabolites*. Structural analogs of normal metabolites that compete with normal metabolites in the synthesis of RNA and/or DNA. This interferes with normal cellular replication.				
A. Folate analogs				
Methotrexate (MTX)	Oral, IV, SC, IM, IT	Nausea and vomiting with high doses	Bone marrow suppression, stomatitis, vasculitis, "MTX lung," cirrhosis with long-term use	Measure blood urea nitrogen, creatinine; creatinine clearance *must* be measured before instituting therapy and periodically thereafter. Dosage adjustment is obligatory if the creatinine clearance is not normal. Saline hydration and $NaHCO_3$ administration to alkalinize the urine is indicated for doses of 3 g/m^2 or greater to prevent MTX crystalluria with consequent renal failure.
B. Purine analogs				
6-Mercaptopurine† (6-MP) (Purinethol)	Oral	Nausea and vomiting, anorexia rare	Bone marrow suppression, rare hepatocellular toxicity	*Allopurinol* may prevent drug catabolism; therefore 6-MP dose should be reduced to two-thirds to one-third the usual dose if given with allopurinol.

Continued.

Table 72-3. Drugs used in treatment of cancer—cont'd

Drug	Route of administration	Acute toxicity	Intermediate or delayed toxicity*	Precautions
Thioguanine† (6-TG) (Tabloid)	Oral	Rare gastrointestinal intolerance	Bone marrow suppression	None
Fludarabine (Fludara)	IV	Bone marrow suppression	High doses associated with central nervous system toxicity, coma, cortical blindness	None
C. Pyrimidine analogs				
5-Fluorouracil† (5-FU)	IV	Occasional nausea and vomiting	Bone marrow suppression, stomatitis, cerebellar ataxia, diarrhea	Monthly loading regimens may be more toxic than weekly doses; accumulates in effusions; decrease dose with severe liver disease.
Cytarabine,† cytosine arabinoside, arabinosylcytosine, ara-C (Cytosar)	IV, SC, IM, IT	Nausea and vomiting with intermediate or high doses; repetitive high doses possibly associated with central nervous system, hepatic, pulmonary, and skin toxicity	Bone marrow suppression	None
III. *Plant alkaloids*. Interfere with mitotic spindle of the cell.‡				
Vincristine (Oncovin)	IV	Severe inflammatory reaction from extravasated drug	Loss of deep tendon reflexes; constipation; impotence; paresthesia; neurotoxicity, possibly leading to foot or wristdrop or cranial nerve palsies; alopecia; rare abdominal, chest, or jaw pain; bone marrow suppression minimal	Inject through running IV infusion; avoid extravasation.
Vinblastine (Velban)	IV	Inflammatory reaction from extravasated drug	Bone marrow suppression, alopecia, occasional mild peripheral neuropathy	Inject slowly into vein or through running IV infusion.
IV. *Epipodophyllotoxins*. Inhibit topoisomerase II, DNA-processing enzyme.				
VP-16-213, etoposide (VePesid)	IV, oral (50% bioavailability)	Occasional nausea and vomiting; hypotension with rapid IV injection; rare anaphylaxis	Bone marrow depression; leukopenia more prominent; alopecia; mild peripheral neuropathy (may be additive with vincristine); mild diarrhea; abnormal liver function tests	Infuse drug over 30 minutes or longer; cardiovascular precautions for hypotension.

V. *Antibiotics*				
Dactinomycin, actinomycin D (Cosmegen)	IV	Severe inflammatory reaction from extravasated drug; nausea and vomiting, occasional cramps and diarrhea	Bone marrow suppression, stomatitis, diarrhea, erythema, hyperpigmentation with occasional desquamation in areas of previous irradiation, alopecia	Administer through running IV infusion.
Doxorubicin (Adriamycin)	IV	Severe inflammatory reaction from extravasated drug; local phlebitis, nausea and vomiting, red urine (drug)	Bone marrow suppression, alopecia, *radiation recall, cardiac toxicity* related to cumulative doses (>500-550 mg/m^2), stomatitis	Inject through running IV infusion. Use with caution in patients with history of heart disease. Monitor left ventricular ejection fraction. Intractable ventricular failure may occur and is dose related. Reduce dosage with renal or hepatic impairment.
Daunorubicin, daunomycin, rubidomycin (Cerubidine)	IV	Same as for doxorubicin	Same as for doxorubicin except no radiation recall; *cardiotoxic* dose approximately 1000 mg/m^2	Same as for doxorubicin
Mitoxantrone (Novantrone)	IV	Occasional nausea and vomiting; serum and urine with possible green tint	Bone marrow depression; alopecia (less common than with anthracyclines); diarrhea; stomatitis; potential cardiotoxicity as function of cumulative dose; mild liver function test abnormality	Cardiac toxicity is function of *total cumulative* dose of *prior anthracyclines* plus dose of mitoxantrone. Drug precipitates with heparin.
Bleomycin (Blenoxane)	IV, IM, SC	Fever, chills, nausea and vomiting; immediate hypersensitivity in lymphoma patients	Striae and hyperpigmentation of skin, sore or ulcerated fingertips, rash, alopecia; diffuse pulmonary interstitial infiltrate leading to irreversible *pulmonary fibrosis,* especially with cumulative doses of 400 mg or greater; toxic dose possibly lower with previous radiation to lung or presence of other pulmonary toxins (e.g., methotrexate)	Immediate hypersensitivity with first 1 to 2 doses in lymphoma patients; follow serial pulmonary function tests, especially diffusion capacity.
Mitomycin (Mutamycin)	IV	Nausea and vomiting; inflammatory reaction from extravasated drug	Bone marrow suppression, stomatitis, alopecia, skin ulceration	Administer through running IV infusion.
Mithramycin (Mithracin)	IV		Bone marrow suppression, hepatotoxicity with reduced synthesis of clotting factors, nephrotoxicity, hypocalcemia	Low therapeutic index; a severe bleeding diathesis can occur and may be fatal.

Continued.

Table 72-3. Drugs used in treatment of cancer—cont'd

Drug	Route of administration	Acute toxicity	Intermediate or delayed toxicity*	Precautions
VI. *Miscellaneous*				
L-Asparaginase (Elspar)	IV, IM, SC	Immediate hypersensitivity reactions, fever, anorexia, nausea and vomiting	Hepatic dysfunction, decreased synthesis of liver proteins (albumin, clotting factors), decreased synthesis of insulin with nonketotic hyperglycemia and coma, pancreatitis	Potential for *immediate hypersensitivity* reaction must be considered; IV line must be in place and epinephrine at bedside.
Procarbazine (Matulane)	Oral	Nausea and vomiting, especially if dose is escalated too rapidly; improves after first few days	Bone marrow depression after 3 to 4 weeks, lethargy, drowsiness, fever, myalgia, arthralgia	Decrease dose in patients with hepatic, renal, or marrow dysfunction; synergism with central nervous system depressants (phenothiazine, barbiturates) may be seen, as well as *Antabuse-like reaction* with ethanol. Monoamine oxidase inhibitory activity sometimes occurs. Sympathomimetic drugs, cheese, and bananas should be avoided.
Hydroxyurea (Hydrea)	Oral	Anorexia, nausea	Bone marrow depression, megaloblastic anemia; stomatitis, diarrhea, and alopecia are less common	Decrease dose in patients with marrow and renal dysfunction.
Mesna (Mesnex)	IV	Nausea and vomiting, bad taste in mouth		Incompatible with cisplatin; false-positive urinary ketone test may occur.
VII. *Steroids*				
Glucocorticoids	Oral, IV, IT	Epigastric distress	Weight gain, truncal obesity, striae, skin fragility, moon facies, euphoria and psychosis, peptic ulcers, osteoporosis; enhanced risk of infection, diabetes, and hypertension	Consider prophylaxis for tuberculosis in patient with history of or exposure to tuberculosis or with lymphomas; use antacids for gastric distress.

Estrogens	Oral	Nausea and vomiting with large doses; slow *escalation* of dose	Gynecomastia in men, breast tenderness in women; *high doses* have been implicated in *increased cardiovascular deaths* in men with prostate cancer	*Steroid flare:* serum calcium levels can rise rapidly in breast cancer patients shortly after therapy is started, especially in those with bony disease; edema may occur with poor cardiac function.
Progestational agents	Oral, IM, SC	None	Occasional liver function abnormalities, alopecia, and hypersensitivity reactions	Use with care in presence of liver dysfunction; may be teratogenic to fetus; increases risk of thromboemboli.
Androgens	Oral	Occasional nausea and vomiting more frequent at higher doses	Fluid retention, virilization (increased facial hair, acne, deepening of voice, clitoral hypertrophy), hypercalcemia, liver function abnormalities with rare jaundice, increased red cell mass	Use with care in elderly patients with cardiac, liver, or renal disease with nephrotic syndrome. Acute hypercalcemia may occur in immobilized patients.
Antiandrogen Flutamide (Eulexin)	Oral	Nausea and vomiting, hot flashes	Gynecomastia, impotence	
Gonadotropin-releasing hormone agonist Leuprolide (Lupron)	SC, IM	Steroid flare, hot flashes	Gynecomastia, impotence	
Aromatase inhibitor Aminoglutethimide (Cytadren)	Oral	Nausea and vomiting	Hypoadrenalism	
VIII. *Biologic response modifiers*				
Interferon alpha-2a (Roferon-A)	IM, SC	Flulike symptoms	None	
Lymphokine (interleukin-2)	IV	Capillary leak syndrome, flulike syndrome	Anaphylaxis	

*The teratogenic and abortifacient properties of most anticancer drugs must be kept in mind when treating women of childbearing age. Many anticancer drugs have been shown to be carcinogenic in laboratory animals.

†Inactive in this commercial form; must be metabolized in vivo to the active drug.

‡Plant alkaloids, epipodophyllotoxins, and antibiotics are typically referred to as *natural products,* that is, derived from nature.

IV, Intravenous; SC, subcutaneous; IM, intramuscular; IT, intrathecal; RNA, ribonucleic acid; DNA, deoxyribonucleic acid.

Complications of radiation therapy

Within hours to days

Systemic
- Malaise
- Nausea and vomiting

Gastrointestinal
- Anorexia
- Nausea and vomiting
- Stomatitis
- Diarrhea

Within days to weeks

Cystitis
Cutaneous erythema
Alopecia
Bone marrow suppression

Within months to years

Bone necrosis
Pneumonitis and lung fibrosis
Nephritis
Hepatitis
Bowel stenosis
Transverse myelitis
Memory loss
Learning disabilities
Leukemogenesis
Carcinogenesis
Hypothyroidism
Cataracts
Xerostomia
Sterility

duction and release of gonadal hormones. Inhibitors of 5-alpha-reductase interfere with the production of dihydrotestosterone. Continued palliation with other hormonal therapies, such as progestins (medroxyprogesterone, megestrol acetate) and inhibitors of the aromatase enzyme (aminoglutethimide), is possible after the development of refractoriness to the preceding hormonal therapy for women with breast cancer. Details of these approaches are discussed in Chapters 97 and 99.

Awareness of the so-called steroid flare in patients with breast or prostate cancer is of importance. In the initial days of therapy with any of the hormonal agents in women or therapy with LHRH agonist in men, an exacerbation of the symptoms of metastatic bone disease may cause incapacitating pain. Also of concern is a possible acute rise in the serum calcium level, which could be life-threatening. This "flare" of symptoms usually portends a good response but requires appropriate supportive care measures and close observation of the serum calcium level until signs and symptoms abate.

CHEMOTHERAPY

Approximately 35 cytotoxic drugs have been approved in the United States for the treatment of patients with cancer (Table 72-3). The classification of these drugs has not conformed to a systematic method. The drugs have been variously grouped according to their chemical structure, pharmacology, or origin. For example, chemical structure defines the alkylating agents, pharmacology defines the antimetabolites, and origin defines the plant alkaloids, epipodophyllotoxins, and antibiotics. These are defined in each major heading in Table 72-3. General biologic effects of cytotoxic drugs are similar to those described previously for radiation therapy and are further defined in Table 72-4.

Because of the many biochemical similarities between neoplastic and normal cells, the actual chemotherapy of cancer, that is, the chemically induced cytodestruction of a tumor with preservation of normal cells, was thought to be an impossibility. However, two rather fortuitous occurrences and subsequent clinical trials based on intuitive reasoning sparked interest in the possible chemical or drug treatment of cancer. The first was the observation that mustard gases used as chemical weapons in World Wars I and II caused lymphopenia and splenic involution in exposed troops. This led the noted pharmacologists Goodman and Gilman to suggest these gases' use as therapeutic agents in lymphoproliferative malignancies; indeed, the first clinical therapeutic attempt with nitrogen mustard proved its usefulness in patients with lymphomas refractory to radiation. Similarly, the observation of megaloblastosis in children with acute lymphoblastic leukemia suggested to the pathologist Sidney Farber that perhaps leukemia was a vitamin deficiency disease. When the administration of folic acid to these patients actually worsened their disease, the idea of synthesizing an antifolate was conceived. Aminopterin, the predecessor of methotrexate (amethopterin), was tested and found to induce complete remissions in children with acute lymphoblastic leukemia.

Thus it was shown that drugs could alter the natural history of malignant disease and that selectivity of drug action was possible; the tumor could be destroyed to clinically imperceptible levels with reversible toxicity to normal organs. However, the therapeutic index was narrow, and drug resistance emerged rapidly. Subsequent to these early observations, laboratory studies of tumor biology and cancer drug pharmacology suggested certain hypotheses that have been tested in clinical trials. These are outlined in Table 72-4. It must be remembered that these concepts are still under active laboratory and clinical investigation and are subject to further development.

Drugs are the therapeutic tools of the internist. As in all areas of internal medicine, the physician must be fully cognizant of the therapeutic and toxic potential of drugs, their optimum doses and schedules, and drug interactions. Given the relatively narrow therapeutic index for most anticancer drugs, these features assume special significance because the dose-response effect is also rather steep; that is, apparently small modifications in dose, up or down, may have substantial impact on response or lack of response. Table 72-3 details the important clinical features of currently available anticancer drugs. Expanded details can be found in the referenced texts. Special attention should be given to the precautions. Of special note are the (1) potential for

Table 72-4. Biologic and pharmacologic principles underlying clinical cancer chemotherapy

Laboratory observations	Therapeutic observations
1. The major target of most therapeutically useful anticancer drugs is DNA.	1. Rapidly proliferating tumors (i.e., cells actually synthesizing DNA) are most sensitive to the drugs.
2. Cell-killing (cytocidal) effects of drugs follow first-order kinetics; that is, per unit of dose the same *fractional* number of cells are destroyed, rather than an absolute number.	2. It takes the same dose to reduce a tumor burden from 10^9 (1 billion) cells to 10^6 (1 million) as it does to reduce the tumor burden from 10^3 cells to 10^0 (1 cell).
3. (a) As a tumor population increases, the growth fraction decreases (i.e., that fraction of the total number of tumor cells that are replicating their DNA and actively dividing). The total number of cells is composed of a dividing population, a dormant (G_0-state) population (i.e., those cells capable of division but in a resting state), and an end-stage population (i.e., those cells not capable of division). As a corollary to this, resting cells, as created by nutritional deficiency, are temporarily resistant to most drugs, especially antimetabolites. (b) Restoration of growth restores drug sensitivity. (c) There is a high frequency of spontaneous mutation to drug resistance, and thus the tumor population is heterogeneous with regard to drug-sensitive and drug-resistant cells.	3. (a) Small tumors and micrometastases are more readily curable than clinically evident tumors. (b) Drug sensitivity of large tumors can be restored by reducing the tumor mass ("tumor debulking") with surgery and/or radiation. (c) Despite an initial response (tumor shrinkage, complete response), drug-resistant populations will emerge from large populations of tumor cells (large tumors).
4. Combined use of drugs with different mechanisms of action and different toxicities to normal organs is possible, even in (near) full dosage. In populations of cells with heterogeneity in drug sensitivity, these combinations of drugs are more cytocidal than single agents. Drug resistance takes longer to emerge.	4. Similar generic observations in cancer medicine.
5. Cytocidal effects display a dose-response relationship.	5. Similar generic observation in cancer medicine. This feature must be kept in mind despite the narrow therapeutic index for most drugs. Appropriate supportive care must be available to offset life-threatening side effects of high doses of drugs.
6. Duration of drug exposure and schedule of drug administration may have a profound effect on the therapeutic index.	6. Similar generic observations in cancer medicine.
7. Complete clinical remissions in animals are the hallmark of cure.	7. Similar generic observations in cancer medicine. Drugs that produce a high frequency of complete remissions as single agents result in cures when combined together.
8. Use of alternating non-cross-resistant combinations increases the cure rate.	8. Similar generic observations in cancer medicine.
9. Chemically induced cytodifferentiation may occur with minimum or no cytotoxicity. The differentiated cell loses the capacity to divide.	9. Clinical evidence suggests that this may occur in humans; under current clinical investigation.

Modified from Skipper HE: Cancer 21:600, 1968; Cancer Chemother 1:1, 1978; and Cancer Chemother 9:1, 1980.

chemical cellulitis and thus the requirement for a free-flowing intravenous route for the administration of nitrogen mustard, vincristine, actinomycin D, doxorubicin, and daunorubicin; (2) hydration to avoid cyclophosphamide-induced or ifosfamide-induced cystitis and cisplatin nephrotoxicity; (3) adequate glomerular filtration with methotrexate therapy; (4) monitoring of left ventricular function and total cumulative dose of the anthracycline antibiotics, doxorubicin and daunorubicin, to avoid anthracycline-induced cardiomyopathy; (5) monitoring of pulmonary diffusion capacity and total cumulative dose of bleomycin to avoid pulmonary fibrosis; and (6) monitoring of symptoms and serum calcium levels in patients with bony metastases from breast cancer treated with hormones and antihormones for early diagnosis of the "steroid flare."

Three major goals underlie the use of anticancer drugs in clinical medicine: cure, palliation, and research to develop more effective therapy. Since 20 years ago, when only one form of disseminated cancer (gestational choriocarcinoma) was curable with systemic chemotherapy, new drug development and multimodal approaches tested in controlled clinical trials have provided evidence for the potential curability of various disseminated malignancies (see the box on p. 724). The details of therapy for these diseases can be found in the appropriate chapters.

Unfortunately, most patients with metastatic disease currently cannot be offered the possibility of cure. However, substantial improvement in the quality of life for all patients and the duration of life for some patients can be achieved with the judicious use of chemotherapy and with attention to appropriate supportive care. The indications for chemotherapy in the presence of metastatic disease are twofold: (1) documented efficacy of a drug or drug combination and (2) enrollment in a clinical trial searching for new or im-

Fourteen cancers in which a fraction of patients can be cured with chemotherapy

Choriocarcinoma	Ovarian carcinoma
Acute lymphocytic leukemia in children	Acute myelogenous leukemia
Hodgkin's disease	Wilms' tumor
Diffuse histiocytic lymphoma	Burkitt's lymphoma
Nodular mixed lymphoma	Embryonal rhabdomyosarcoma
Testicular carcinoma	Ewing's sarcoma
Breast carcinoma	Colorectal carcinoma

proved therapy. The second aspect deserves substantial emphasis. Large-scale, multi-institutional, randomized clinical trials were first introduced in oncology. Our ability to cure some patients with disseminated malignancies is the legacy of the patients who willingly participated in earlier clinical trials. By participating in clinical trials available from regional cancer centers, community physicians can offer their patients the most up-to-date therapy, which in many instances can be offered at home in liaison with the cancer center. For many patients, the best therapy is an investigative protocol. Diseases for which drugs may produce substantial regression with relief of symptoms are listed in the box below. Specific details regarding their therapy can be found in the appropriate chapters.

Dose intensity

Most anticancer drugs have a narrow *therapeutic index,* that is, the dosage necessary to produce tumor reduction versus the dose associated with normal organ toxicity. Consequently, subjective and objective toxicities, patient compliance, and physician attitudes may have a strong bearing on the dosage and frequency of drug treatment. A recent analysis of the outcome of therapy for several malignancies has strongly suggested that a steep dose-response relationship exists. This analysis formulated the concept of dose intensity, defined as the amount of drug given per unit time, usually mg/m^2/week. Such retrospective analysis of grouped clinical trials indicates steep dose-response effects for 5-fluorouracil in the treatment of metastatic colon cancer; vincristine in breast cancer; VP-16 (etoposide) in small cell lung cancer; and cisplatin in ovarian, endometrial, and small cell lung cancer. These data strongly suggest that adherence to protocol, close patient monitoring, and the use of drugs to the point of patient tolerance are of importance for optimum results. Adherence to these concepts is especially important with chemotherapy use in adjuvant settings when the drugs' immediate effect on disease is not evident.

Advanced cancers in which a fraction of patients respond to chemotherapy and improved survival is demonstrable*

Breast carcinoma	Gastric carcinoma
Chronic myelogenous leukemia	Malignant insulinoma
Chronic lymphocytic leukemia	Endometrial carcinoma
Nodular poorly differentiated lymphocytic lymphoma	Adrenal cortical carcinoma
Multiple myeloma	Medulloblastoma
Small cell carcinoma of lung	Neuroblastoma
Soft tissue sarcomas	Polycythemia vera
	Prostatic carcinoma
	Glioblastoma

Data from DeVita VT, Hellman S, and Rosenberg SA: Cancer: principles and practice of oncology. Philadelphia, 1982, Lippincott.

*The cancers listed above account for about 40 percent of all new cancers per year and about 30 percent of all cancer deaths.

Combination chemotherapy and combined modality therapy

As noted, great strides have been made in the past 20 years with the demonstration that drugs can produce dramatic regressions, that is, clinical complete remissions in patients with overt disseminated cancer. These complete remissions are the herald of cure. Only one form of disseminated cancer, choriocarcinoma, is cured with single-agent chemotherapy (methotrexate); all others require combinations of drugs and, with increasing frequency, multimodality therapy.

The origin of combination chemotherapy for cancer was based on earlier experiences with combinations of drugs to treat serious bacterial disease such as tuberculosis. The basis for the use of these combinations is twofold: (1) the narrow therapeutic index of individual drugs, which prohibits dose escalation to achieve more effective systemic drug concentrations; and (2) the rapid emergence of drug resistance to single-agent chemotherapy.

The initial principles of combination chemotherapy for cancer included the dicta that each component had to have demonstrated activity against the candidate disease as a single agent; had to have a different mechanism of action mediating its cytotoxic effect; and had to have nonoverlapping toxicities to normal organs, so that the drugs could be given at or near full therapeutic doses. These basic principles met with early success with the combination of prednisone, vincristine, and daunorubicin in the treatment of acute lymphoblastic leukemia and with the MOPP regimen—mustargen (nitrogen mustard), Oncovin (vincristine), prednisone, and procarbazine—for the treatment of Hodgkin's disease. These initial successes, confirmed in many subsequent clinical trials, have stimulated additional trials in almost every human neoplasm, with varying degrees of success.

Further laboratory and clinical investigation has provided an expanding data base in cancer pharmacology, which has led to several exceptions to the basic tenets previously enumerated. For example, the basic requirement for each drug to have therapeutic activity alone is not necessarily a hard-and-fast rule, if other reasons exist for inserting a drug in a combination. This includes the use of the reduced form of the vitamin folic acid, folinic acid (citrovorum factor, leucovorin), as an antidote to toxicity; the delayed administration of folinic acid after methotrexate (MTX) has allowed the use of substantially higher doses of MTX to overcome various mechanisms of drug resistance (see following section). These higher doses of MTX in turn have proved useful in the treatment of osteosarcoma and, for pharmacokinetic reasons, as prophylaxis against central nervous system leukemia in patients with acute lymphoblastic leukemia (ALL). Many preclinical pharmacologic investigations attest to the biochemical basis for selectivity of drug action with the use of high-dose MTX with so-called leucovorin rescue, in that substantial therapeutic effects have occurred, with sparing of normal organs.

Substantial laboratory data also indicate that folinic acid potentiates the effect of 5-fluorouracil (5-FU) by enhancing its binding to the target enzyme, thymidylate synthetase. Clinical trials indicate that the combination of 5-FU and folinic acid has improved therapeutic efficacy compared with 5-FU alone in the treatment of patients with advanced colon cancer.

Ongoing laboratory investigations of multidrug resistance (see next section) suggest that this phenomenon may be reversed by the combination of calcium channel blockers, such as verapamil, with the chemotherapeutic agent. In this case the calcium channel blocker has no antineoplastic effects of its own.

The dictum that drugs of the same pharmacologic class should not be used in combination is also undergoing reinvestigation. Preliminary laboratory and clinical investigations suggest that combinations of alkylating agents may be useful.

The major limitation in using combinations of drugs that have overlapping toxicity profiles is the requirement for dose reduction to avoid toxic side effects. Such dosage reduction may also proportionately reduce therapeutic effects to the point where the effects of the combination are no better than those achieved from optimum doses of individual drugs.

Various strategies of combination chemotherapy have been used in an attempt to perturb the cell cycle of the cancer cell to enhance the overall efficacy of a second drug that is *cell cycle phase specific*. Although such a strategy can be very effective in the laboratory, its practical application in clinical trials has many logistical problems.

Several examples from laboratory and clinical research indicate significant schedule dependency in outcome when two or more drugs are administered in combination. Sufficient drug-drug interaction may occur such that the outcome may be pharmacologic synergy or antagonism, with either outcome a function of the dose and schedule of administration of the component drugs (i.e., concurrent or sequential). Schedule dependency is most evident with antimetabolites used alone, used in combination with another antimetabolite, or used with a member of another class of drugs. Examples include the combinations of MTX + 5-FU, MTX + asparaginase, ara-C + asparaginase.

In multimodality therapy, combinations of drugs are integrated with surgery and/or radiation therapy in a therapeutic strategy designed to improve on the cure rate achieved with either modality alone. The sequence of employing these modalities depends on the type and nature of the disease.

It is now well recognized that many patients with seemingly localized cancers at diagnosis have micrometastases in various organs throughout the body. Excellent local control of such cancers with surgery and/or radiation cannot cure these patients. This is now clearly evident with breast carcinoma and certain pediatric cancers, such as rhabdomyosarcoma, osteosarcoma, and Wilms' tumor. In these cancers, eradication of the primary disease is possible with surgery and/or radiation therapy. However, despite excellent local eradication of the cancer, patients die from metastatic disease, which usually becomes evident within 1 to 5 years. Current diagnostic methods cannot detect the location of these micrometastases, but a constellation of clinical and laboratory prognostic factors places such patients at high risk for subsequent recurrence. The use of these prognostic factors has guided the design of controlled clinical trials that have demonstrated the utility of systemic chemotherapy in enhancing the overall cure rate. Such chemotherapy consists of combinations of drugs administered in different strategies with surgery and/or radiation. For example, combinations of drugs administered after effective local treatment of breast cancer, Wilms' tumor, osteosarcoma, or rhabdomyosarcoma have had a major impact on disease-free survival. In other instances, preoperative chemotherapy in patients with bladder and ovarian cancer has resulted in sufficient reduction in tumor bulk so as to allow more effective surgical removal of local disease. Likewise, treatment of patients with metastatic testicular, ovarian, and bladder cancers has resulted in substantial tumor reduction, to the point where surgical removal of residual disease has converted chemotherapy-induced partial regressions to surgical complete regressions. This new strategy has engendered new jargon: "clinical complete remission," after chemotherapy; and "pathologic complete remission," after surgical pathologic verification of disease-free status. This practice has had a definite impact on disease-free survival. The test of time will validate its curative potential. Nevertheless, these early successes have stimulated clinical trials in other disease areas.

Drug resistance

Drug resistance is the most important obstacle to therapeutic success in the medical management of patients with cancer. The box on p. 726 lists major mechanisms of resistance to anticancer drugs, and Table 72-5 lists various ways to approach the causes of clinical refractoriness to drug therapy. Clinical drug resistance to therapy may be evident from the outset or may be manifest after a period of responsiveness. The former situation is generally referred to as *natural* drug resistance, the latter as *acquired* drug re-

Resistance to anticancer drugs

- Biochemical genetic
  - Natural
  - Acquired
- Pharmacologic
  - Pharmacokinetic
    - Dose, schedule
    - Blood/organ barrier
  - Drug-drug interactions
- Biologic
  - Low growth fraction

sistance. A considerable gray zone may exist between the two. It is now well recognized that tumors are quite heterogenous in biologic, biochemical, and pharmacologic properties. Thus the manifestation of acquired drug resistance after a period of responsiveness could imply an adaptation phenomenon; that is, sublethal drug damage may engender enzyme induction or somatic mutation that will alter the vulnerable target so as to make it less vulnerable to drug effect. For example, mutation to an isoenzyme form of an enzyme that is the target of drug action may result in a reduced binding affinity of the drug for that enzyme, and therefore a reduced pharmacologic effect. Many anticancer drugs are themselves mutagenic and can theoretically induce a mutation to drug resistance. Acquired drug resistance may also be a manifestation of tumor heterogeneity. The selective removal of the drug-sensitive component of a heterogenous tumor may provide sufficient selective pressure to allow the overgrowth of a subpopulation of resistant tumor cells. From the outset these cells were "naturally" resistant or acquired resistance by various adaptation phenomena. A partial listing of mechanisms shown to make tumors resistant to various cancer drugs is given in Table 72-5.

Antimetabolites and several alkylating agents enter the cell by a carrier-mediated process, sharing the carrier with various normal metabolites: MTX using the folate carrier, nucleoside analogs using the corresponding normal nucleoside carrier, and alkylating agents using the carrier of certain amino acids. Laboratory studies have shown that certain tumor cells develop resistance by deleting the drug carrier. This information has provided leads for new drug development. With transport resistance to MTX, the development of an antifol that enters the cell by a different process can restore drug effect; in this case, lipid-soluble antifols such as trimetrexate may enter the cell by a passive diffusion mechanism.

Higher doses of the drug in question may be useful in circumventing resistance caused by several mechanisms, including transport resistance; higher drug concentrations entering the cell by passive diffusion rather than using the carrier; gene amplification resulting in increased synthesis of the target enzyme; and somatic mutation resulting in the synthesis of an altered enzyme with decreased binding to the drug. These general mechanisms have been most extensively studied with MTX. Amplification of the gene that codes for the protein dihydrofolate reductase (DHFR) has resulted in a marked increase in DHFR synthesis, to the point where it may constitute 5% of the total cellular protein. Use of considerably higher doses of MTX is possible because of the availability of the reduced folate, folinic acid

Table 72-5. Some mechanisms of tumor cell resistance to anticancer drugs and possible means for their circumvention

Drugs	Possible means for circumvention of resistance
I. Alkylating agents	
A. Decreased membrane transport capacity	Increase dose; switch to alternate agent that does not share the same transport carrier.
B. Increased DNA repair mechanisms	Use inhibitors of DNA repair in combination with alkylating agent.
II. Antimetabolites	
A. Antifols	
1. Decreased membrane transport capacity	Increase dose; switch to alternate agent that does not share the same transport carrier.
2. Amplification of the gene for dihydrofolate reductase (DHFR)	Increase dose.
3. DHFR with altered drug-binding capacity	Increase dose; use alternate antifols with improved binding capacity.
4. Reduced polyglutamylation	Increase dose and/or duration of exposure.
B. Pyrimidine antagonists	
1. Decreased membrane transport capacity (nucleosides only)	Increase dose.
2. Impaired anabolism	Increase dose.
3. Increased catabolism	Increase duration of exposure.
III. Multidrug resistance (drugs derived from natural sources such as plants, fungi, bacteria; see text)	
A. Enhanced efflux of drug out of cell	Coadminister inhibitors of efflux pump.
B. Enhanced detoxification mechanisms	

(citrovorum factor), the delayed administration of which protects normal cells from MTX toxicity. Further details of this strategy can be found in the cited references.

Recent laboratory research on drug resistance has shed new light on broader aspects of clinical drug resistance. Prolonged treatment of various experimental cell lines in culture to drugs derived from natural products (see Table 72-3; those drugs derived from plants, fungi, and bacteria) will elicit the emergence of a drug-resistant subline. Subsequent exposure of this same resistant subline to another natural product of different origin, structure, and mechanism of action will result in cross-resistance. For example, the development of acquired resistance in the murine leukemia P388 to the anthracycline antibiotic doxorubicin (Adriamycin) will elicit cross-resistance to other natural products, such as the *Vinca* alkaloids vincristine, and vinblastine, the podophyllotoxin derivatives VP-16 and VM-26, and actinomycin D, despite that the parental cell line is sensitive to these drugs and that the resistant cell line only was exposed to doxorubicin. This phenomenon, called *pleiotropic* or *multidrug resistance* (MDR), has now been shown to occur in a variety of human and nonhuman cell lines, although the degree of resistance may vary from cell line to cell line. It appears that a common denominator in all these cell lines is decreased drug accumulation in the cell as a result of increased activity of an energy-dependent efflux pump. This in turn has been related to an increased concentration in the cell membrane of a phosphoglycoprotein (molecular weight, 170,000 daltons) called the *P-170 protein*. Further studies showed amplification of the gene that codes for the P-170 protein (MDR-1 gene). The drugs with MDR characteristics have been shown to bind to the P-170 protein, which then mediates the efflux of the drug out of the cell. Recent investigations have shown that more than one species of membrane glycoprotein have been overexpressed in addition to the P-170 protein.

Related research on multidrug resistance has provided additional information of potential clinical importance, including (1) the detection of increased P-170 protein and amplified MDR gene in human tumor specimens and their correlation with drug resistance; (2) the potential abrogation of enhanced drug efflux by using unrelated drugs that competitively bind to the P-170 protein; and (3) the identification of enhanced P-170 protein expression in normal organs after exposure to noxious, potentially carcinogenic agents. In the laboratory, three calcium channel blockers—verapamil, nifedipine, and diltiazem—enhance the cellular accumulation of MDR drugs and thereby lessen resistance or restore drug sensitivity. Unfortunately the concentrations of these drugs necessary to elicit this effect in the laboratory are too high for clinical use. The role of calcium channel blockade in this process is also in question.

Many cellular biochemical changes associated with the development of MDR occur in normal organs after exposure to a variety of carcinogens. Consequently, it has been hypothesized that the common human epithelial cancers of the lung and colon are resistant to chemotherapy because of prior exposure to carcinogens, with the elicitation of various cellular detoxification processes similar to those that occur in the development of MDR. These biochemical changes are especially prominent in the mucosa of the small and large intestines, liver, kidneys, and adrenal glands. Their development has been viewed as a normal function intended to rid the body of cytotoxic molecules. Ongoing research into this type of drug resistance may provide a means for its circumvention.

Other means by which tumors might manifest drug resistance are listed in the box at far left. Knowledge of the systemic and cellular pharmacokinetics of drugs may suggest changes in dose and schedule of drug administration that may elicit a therapeutic response when none previously existed. An example is the clinical efficacy of high-dose ara-C in patients with acute myelogenous leukemia (AML) who had failed to respond to conventional doses.

Tumors in certain locations may fail to respond to systemic chemotherapy because of poor penetration of the drug into the organ. Such organs have been termed *pharmacologic sanctuaries;* the central nervous system (CNS) and testes are the most common examples. Thus the therapeutic strategy in patients with ALL requires deliberate therapy to the CNS with intrathecal chemotherapy and/or CNS radiation and, in high-risk males, radiation of the testes.

Various drug-drug interactions provide laboratory examples of pharmacologic antagonism. These usually involve combinations of antimetabolites such as MTX and 5-FU, MTX and ara-C, MTX and asparaginase, ara-C and asparaginase. The biochemical details of these interactions are found in the cited references.

Finally, since most anticancer drugs directly or indirectly affect DNA synthesis, the tumor's growth state will influence outcome. Most tumors at diagnosis have a low *growth fraction,* that is, the proportion of cells in the tumor populations actively undergoing cellular replication. Consequently, the use of inhibitors of DNA synthesis or inhibitors of various enzymes involved in DNA synthesis or processing is likely to have little or no effect in patients with advanced disease. The reduction in tumor burden with surgery and/or radiation may enhance drug effect by "recruiting" cells into active proliferation. This phenomenon is well documented in the laboratory and may be a factor in the efficacy of surgical adjuvant chemotherapy for breast cancer, osteosarcoma, and other cancers.

BIOTHERAPY

The box on p. 728 lists various therapeutic approaches that are broadly defined as biotherapy or biologic therapy of cancer. Extensive laboratory research has shown that a variety of chemicals, including certain widely used anticancer drugs, can cause terminal differentiation of subhuman and human tumor cells propagated in vitro. This chemically induced differentiation results in loss of the malignant phenotype and stabilization of the process. Until recently, this chemically induced differentiation remained as a laboratory tool until the demonstration of actual cytodifferentiation of acute promyelocytic leukemia cells in patients after treatment with all-*trans* retinoic acid. Although unfortunately not permanent, this clinical demonstration provides impe-

Biological therapy of cancer

1. Drugs that cause cellular differentiation
2. Immunotherapy
   a. Active
   b. Passive
   c. Cell mediated
   d. Biologic response modifiers: interferons, interleukins
3. Monoclonal antibodies
   a. Laboratory diagnosis: radioimmunoassay, fluorescent microscopy
   b. Imaging
   c. Therapeutic
4. Cytokines
   a. G-CSF (granulocyte colony-stimulating factor)
   b. GM-CSF (granulocyte-macrophage colony-stimulating factor)
   c. Erythropoietin

tus to the continued laboratory research for better understanding and improvements of this therapeutic approach.

Similarly, research into the immunotherapy of cancer has been extensively pursued for a number of years. Whereas excellent preclinical data indicate that animals can be actively or passively immunized against various experimental neoplasms, to date this approach has not demonstrated reproducibly consistent, useful therapeutic effects in patients, with perhaps one exception, the intravesicular application of BCG (bacille Calmette-Guérin) as therapy for bladder carcinoma in situ. Despite this efficacy, definitive data indicating an immunologic mechanism do not exist. Another putative stimulant of the immune system, levamisole, has been shown in a randomized clinical trial to prolong the survival of patients with Duke's C colon cancer when given in conjunction with 5-FU after surgical removal of the tumor. Again, definitive data indicating an immunologic mechanism are lacking. Other approaches in active immunotherapy using various tumor vaccines remain experimental.

The most effective passive immunotherapeutic approach to date is adoptive immunotherapy, in which lymphocytes from peripheral blood or those enmeshed in the patient's tumor (so-called tumor-infiltrating lymphocytes, or TIL cells) are propagated ex vivo in the presence of interleukin 2 and/or other lymphokines. After a period of growth in vitro, these lymphokine-activated killer cells, or LAK cells, are then transfused back to the same patient. Using this approach, impressive regressions of metastatic melanoma and renal cell carcinomas have been noted. However, the procedure is associated with considerable toxicity to the patient. Also, debate surrounds whether this labor-intensive, costly process results in superior therapeutic benefit above that achieved by the systemic use of the lymphokines. Such research is being actively pursued. Large-scale commercial development of lymphokines, interferons, and cytokines for therapeutic uses has been greatly facilitated by recombinant DNA technology.

The most extensively developed agents for biologic therapies to date are the interferons, derived from three major sources: leukocytes (alpha interferons), fibroblasts (beta interferons), and mitogen-stimulated lymphocytes (gamma interferons). Interferons have a broad range of biologic activities, the mechanisms of which are poorly understood. These include antiviral, growth-regulatory, and direct cytotoxic properties. Remarkable therapeutic effects have been seen in patients with hairy cell leukemia, a relatively rare disease, as well as in patients with other B cell neoplasms, including non-Hodgkin's lymphoma and multiple myeloma. Of substantial interest, alpha interferon has caused the regression of the Philadelphia (Ph^1) chromosome in patients with chronic myelogenous leukemia. The Ph^1 chromosome is the hallmark of the malignant phenotype, and its deletion has been correlated with prolonged remissions. No other therapy to date has caused the loss of the Ph^1 chromosome. Thus this association with interferon therapy is of substantial clinical and biologic interest.

Extensive research is being conducted with monoclonal antibodies (MoABs) for diagnostic and therapeutic uses. Spleen cells from mice immunized with human tumor cells are fused with myeloma cells in culture. The growth of these fused hybrid cells in culture (hybridomas) are then screened for their antibody production. Testing for antibody specificity allows the selection of the appropriate clone for large-scale propagation of the MoAB. Experimentally, MoABs have multiple uses, including (1) diagnostic use in radioimmunoassays for the detection of antigens in serum or other body fluids, such as an assay for various tumor markers (e.g., CEA, CA-125); (2) conjugation with fluorescein for use in fluorescent microscopy to delineate tumor cell invasion of normal bone marrow or other tissues not otherwise visible by light microscopy; (3) isotopic (e.g., ^{131}I, ^{99}Tc, ^{111}In) labeling of the MoAB for imaging studies to detect tumor metastases not otherwise discernible with other scanning techniques, such as use of radiolabeled anti-CEA MoAB to detect occult colorectal carcinoma; (4) linkage of the MoAB with cytotoxic drugs, toxins (e.g., ricin), or radioisotopes (e.g., ^{90}Y, ^{131}I) for direct delivery of the toxic ligand to the tumor; and (5) systemic use of the MoAB to cause tumor cell lysis through interaction with complement or through antibody-dependent cellular cytotoxicity. All these approaches are in various stages of clinical development and use. Various pitfalls associated with their clinical use, such as development of human antimouse antibodies (HAMA response) as well as other technical and biologic problems, are active areas of research.

Recombinant DNA technology has greatly facilitated the clinical development of various cytokines. Hematopoietic growth factors (G-CSF, GM-CSF, erythropoietin) are now commercially available for various supportive care needs not only for patients with cancer, but also for those with other marrow-suppressed states (e.g., anemia of chronic renal failure). The availability of these cytokines has greatly reduced the need for blood product transfusion and the hazards associated with such transfusions.

REFERENCES

Capizzi RL, editor: Pharmacologic basis of cancer chemotherapy. Semin Oncol 4:131, 1977.

Moscow JA and Cowan KH: Multidrug resistance. J Natl Cancer Inst 80:14, 1988.

Neville AM, editor: Proceedings of a workshop on the biochemical and immunologic diagnosis of cancer. Tumor Biol 8:158, 1987.

Pater JL, editor: Implications of dose intensity for cancer clinical trials. Semin Oncol 14(suppl 4):1, 1987.

Pritchard KI and Sutherland DJA: The use of endocrine therapy. Hematol Oncol Clin North Am 3:765, 1989.

Sell S: Cancer markers of the 1990's—comparison of the new generation of markers defined by monoclonal antibodies and oncogene probes to prototypic markers. Clin Lab Med 10:1, 1990.

Skipper HE: Biochemical, biological, pharmacologic, toxicologic, kinetic, and clinical (subhuman and human) relationships. Cancer 21:600, 1968.

Skipper HE: Reasons for success and failure in treatment of murine leukemias with the drugs now employed in treating human leukemias. Cancer Chemother 1:1, 1978.

Skipper HE: Concurrent comparisons of some 2-, 3-, and 4-drug combinations delivered simultaneously and sequentially (L1210 and P388 leukemia systems). Cancer Chemother 9:1, 1980.

II LABORATORY TESTS

CHAPTER

73 Evaluation of Cells in Peripheral Blood and Bone Marrow

Robert V. Pierre

AUTOMATED TECHNOLOGY FOR COMPLETE BLOOD AND DIFFERENTIAL COUNTS

Automated complete blood count (CBC) and differential instruments (ACBCD) give inexpensive, fast, precise, and accurate red blood cell (RBC), white blood cell (WBC), and platelet (PLT) counts on small quantities of whole blood. The ACBCD also permits the use of closed-tube sampling, bar code sample identification, and bidirectional communication with laboratory computers. Four technologies are used for the leukocyte differential count (LDC) by different instrument manufacturers:

1. Simultaneous aperture impedance with direct current (DC) and radiofrequency (RF) current and laser light scatter (LLS) (Coulter STKS)
2. Combined aperture resistance with DC and RF with selective cell lysis (Sysmex NE-8000)
3. Electro-optical scatter and absorption combined with cytochemistry and LLS (Technicon H*2)
4. Aperture resistance with multiple-angle scatter and polarized orthogonal LLS (Abbott Cell-Dyne 3000)

These instruments generate histograms, scatterplots, and scattergrams that may have characteristic patterns helpful to the identification of selected abnormalities (Table 73-1).

The ACBCD results are used in three basic ways:

1. Detection of specific abnormalities that establish a specific diagnosis (e.g., detection of sickle cells, blasts, malarial parasites)
2. Detection of a nonspecific abnormality that aids in differential diagnosis or suggests the direction of additional diagnostic tests (e.g., anemia, erythrocytosis, hypochromia, neutropenia)
3. Use of parameters to "track" the course of a disease, response to therapy, or recovery of marrow function (e.g., serial neutrophil and PLT counts in patients receiving chemotherapy)

The ACBCD is almost universally used and appears justified as a routine test in the initial workup of an ill patient. The eye-count LDC is an expensive, inaccurate, and imprecise method. Clinical sensitivity studies of the 100-cell eye-count LDC compared with the National Committee for Clinical Laboratory Standards (NCCLS) reference method have demonstrated the inaccuracy of classification (Table 73-2).

The automated differential has a very low false-normal rate compared with the eye-count method, which makes it an excellent screening method. A routine differential count should not be requested in patients being screened by an ACBCD instrument. These instruments can also be used very effectively to "track" patients and provide only pertinent parameters such as the WBC, neutrophils, lymphocytes, or PLT counts without review of a blood film. The ACBCD instruments are unable to give accurate results in a variety of situations. Fortunately, these situations occur infrequently and should be recognized by good laboratory practices so that the erroneous instrument results are not reported. Examples would include hyperlipidemia, EDTA-induced or cold agglutinin–induced PLT or leukocyte agglutination, and partially clotted specimens.

The peripheral blood film examination remains an essential element in the evaluation of patients with hematologic disorders.

The ACBCD is blind to certain morphologic abnormalities of RBC, WBC, and PLT. The MCV (mean RBC [corpuscular] volume) is a valuable tool, especially when combined with the RDW (RBC distribution width), but neither can identify specific RBC shape abnormalities. ACBCD instruments are relatively blind to spherocytes, sickle cells, target cells, acanthocytes, elliptocytes, keratocytes, RBC inclusions, fragmented RBCs, and other shape abnormalities (Color Plate III-4). They are also blind to many specific WBC abnormalities, such as Pelger-Huët, hypersegmented, or toxic neutrophils. Blast populations are flagged accurately by the instruments, but identification of the type of blasts and stages of neutrophil or lymphocyte matura-

Table 73-1. Median/central 95% reference ranges for automated complete blood count (CBC) and differential instruments and eye-count differential

	Coulter STKS	Sysmex NE-8000	Technicon H*2	Eye count (400 cell)
Males				
WBC	5.8/3.9-7.9	5.71/3.85-7.84	5.16/3.39-7.04	
RBC	4.86/4.27-5.31	4.89/4.30-5.27	5.02/4.39-5.46	
HGB	14.9/13.0-15.9	15.1/13.3-16.2	14.7/13.1-15.7	
MCV	88.5/83.8-94.3	87.8/82.4-95.1	84.9/79.6-91.9	
RDW	12.5/11.0-16.3	12.5/12.0-16.0	12.7/11.7-15.4	
PLT	248/179-316	247/177-324	226/166-287	
NEUT%	56.0/44.97-68.26	61.05/48.7-73.1	55.3/45.0-67.9	58.75/42.75-74.25
LYMPH%	29.86/17.82-41.54	30.85/18.5-43.1	33.8/18.3-43.6	32.00/19.00-48.50
MONO%	9.83/4.86-14.78	4.65/2.70-10.10	7.4/4.8-10.6	7.00/3.00-11.00
EOS%	2.92/1.24-6.59	2.5/0.9-6.2	2.4/0.9-6.2	2.50/0.50-8.00
BASO%	0.405/0.00-0.980	0.7/0.2-1.5	0.8/0.4-1.4	0.50/0.0-1.50
NEUT#	3.28/1.88-4.74	3.44/1.89-4.77	2.94/1.67-4.34	
LYMPH#	1.74/0.94-2.73	1.80/0.99-2.80	1.70/0.91-2.70	
MONO#	0.58/0.33-0.91	0.27/0.15-0.54	0.37/0.25-0.60	
EOS#	0.165/0.07-0.39	0.14/0.06-0.37	0.12/0.05-0.31	
BASO#	0.02/0.00-0.07	0.04/0.01-0.07	0.04/0.02-0.08	
Females				
WBC	6.3/3.4-10.5	6.1/3.44-10.21	5.59/3.1-9.48	
RBC	4.37/3.61-4.97	4.35/3.60-4.85	4.48/3.72-5.10	
HGB	13.2/11.3-14.8	13.5/11.4-14.6	13.3/11.5-14.4	
MCV	89.0/81.4-96.3	89.7/83.4-95.6	86.6/80.0-92.9	
RDW	—	—	—	
PLT	265/153-410	274/165-432	242/141-377	
NEUT%	58.08/44.37-70.9	61.5/49.9-72.4	58.24/46.0-71.5	60.25/45.50-75.75
LYMPH%	28.91/19.15-41.33	29.9/19.5-40.4	32.85/20.30-44.5	31.00/19.5-49.0
MONO%	8.36/4.72-13.49	4.2/2.0-7.7	6.3/4.2-10.2	7.00/3.00-11.0
EOS%	2.46/0.82-7.17	2.2/0.8-6.1	2.0/0.7-7.2	2.50/0.50-8.00
BASO%	0.43/0.03-2.17	0.8/0.0-2.0	0.7/0.3-1.5	0.5/0.0-1.50
NEUT#	3.48/1.69-6.57	3.76/1.87-6.70	3.095/1.56-5.83	
LYMPH#	1.91/1.15-2.88	1.865/1.120-2.730	1.83/1.12-2.66	
MONO#	0.52/0.30-0.93	0.22/0.11-0.57	0.36/0.18-0.65	
EOS#	0.145/0.05-0.50	0.13/0.05-0.28	0.115/0.04-0.25	
BASO#	0.03/0.00-0.09	0.04/0.00-0.13	0.04/0.01-0.08	

WBC, White blood cells; RBC, red blood cells; HGB, hemoglobin; MCV, mean RBC (corpuscular) volume; RDW, RBC distribution width; PLT, platelets; neut, neutrophils; lymph, lymphocytes; mono, monocytes; eos, eosinophils; baso, basophils.

tion requires examination of a stained blood film (Color Plates III-5 and III-6). The use of absolute cell counts as opposed to the proportional count eliminates frequent misinterpretation of LDC results. The automated LDC is an effective screening method for determining which patient requires examination of a stained blood film examination by a technologist, hematologist, or pathologist. It is critical that the individual reviewing the blood film have access to the ACBCD results and the instrument displays of the RBC, WBC, and PLT populations.

The reticulocyte count (RETIC) is also a labor-intensive, inaccurate procedure if done by microscope eye-count methods. The College of American Pathology (CAP) proficiency survey results show that the coefficient of variation (CV) of RETIC in the normal range is almost 50%. A reticulocyte is defined by the CAP as a supravitally stained anucleate RBC containing more than one granule (Color Plate III-4).

The flow cytometry methods for determination of RETIC can produce a CV of 5% in the normal range. Heilmeyer recognized the importance of classification of reticulocyte maturation stages and devised a classification based on morphology of the reticulocytes. In flow cytometry instruments, maturation stages can be based on the ribonucleic acid (RNA) content of the reticulocytes by measurement of laser excitation fluorescence of various dyes. The time required for reticulocytes to lose their reticulin in the peripheral blood correlates well with the severity of anemia. Attempts to correct the RETIC for the hematocrit and maturation time in the peripheral blood have resulted in indices such as the reticulocyte maturation production index (RMI). The RMI can be calculated from median fluorescence in-

Table 73-2. Eye count compared with NCCLS reference method (800-cell differential)

	100-cell eye count (%)	Coulter S-Plus IV (%)
Agreement	52.7	71.0
Distributional false abnormal	8.8	3.3
Distributional false normal	29.9	2.3
Morphologic false abnormal	0.0	21.7
Morphologic false normal	18.6	1.7

tensity, as measured by flow cytometry. The RMI appears to have clinical usefulness in predicting marrow recovery from bone marrow aplasia resulting from chemotherapy and for prediction of recovery of marrow erythropoiesis in neonates. The automated absolute RETIC, with its greater precision and accuracy, is an important tool for distinguishing defects in RBC production from hemolysis or blood loss.

BONE MARROW EXAMINATION

Indications

1. If there are changes in the peripheral blood counts or film that can only be interpreted by bone marrow examination (BME)
2. In the absence of hematologic abnormalities, the presence of unexplained bone pain, a high sedimentation rate, or bony lesions on x-ray films
3. Diagnosis and accurate classification of the acute leukemias
4. Presence of unexplained lymphadenopathy or splenomegaly
5. When staging of lymphoma or other neoplastic diseases is required and the presence of marrow involvement alters the therapeutic approach
6. Assessment of the response to therapy in patients with acute and chronic leukemias and malignant lymphomas as well as marrow involvement by solid tumors
7. Evaluation of patients with fever of undetermined origin (possible indication)
8. Evaluation of patients with single cytopenias or pancytopenia to establish the etiology
9. Bone marrow biopsy (BM BX) is indicated in patients in whom an adequate aspirate cannot be obtained. It is becoming increasingly common practice to obtain a biopsy routinely with BM aspirate

Special stains may be of value in the interpretation of the BM aspirate or biopsy. An iron stain on the BM aspirate and biopsy should be routinely obtained (Color Plate III-7). Special stains of value on BM aspirates consist of cytochemical and immunocytochemical stains to differentiate the acute and chronic leukemias and lymphomas; these stains are discussed in Chapters 93 and 94. Stains for organisms, particularly acid-fast organisms, may be done on both aspirate and biopsy. Stains for amyloid may also be done on both BM aspirates and biopsies. BM BX should be stained for reticulin content, particularly if a hypocellular aspirate was obtained.

Role in disease evaluation

The BME is not a good screening test for diagnostic problems. Unless specific indications exist for a BME, fruitful results are infrequent.

Anemia. Hypochromic microcytic anemias caused by iron deficiency or thalassemic disorders and the anemia of chronic infection or inflammation do not require BME, nor do rare causes of hemoglobin loss through the kidney in disorders such as paroxysmal nocturnal hemoglobinuria (PNH) and chronic intravascular hemolysis from defective cardiac valves. Diagnostic evaluation of hypochromic anemias associated with siderocytes in the peripheral blood (Color Plate III-4) and/or with dyspoietic changes in any cell lines should include a BME to exclude the possibility of a hereditary or acquired sideroblastic anemia (Color Plate III-8).

In most patients with hypomicrocytic anemias suspected to result from iron deficiency, a BME is not indicated. Serum, iron, and ferritin studies are usually conclusive. The BME is of value in clinical situations when the clinical picture is complicated by disorders that can interfere with normal iron metabolism, such as chronic inflammatory disorders, particularly rheumatoid arthritis. These disorders are frequently further complicated by possible reasons for blood loss, such as anti-inflammatory drugs. The iron stain on the BM aspirate and BM BX is often helpful (Color Plates III-7 and III-8). If the BM aspirate shows normal or increased amounts of stainable iron, little reason exists to perform an iron stain on the biopsy. However, a negative iron stain on the aspirate should always be followed by an iron stain on the biopsy. If the assessment of iron stores is significant to the patient's clinical management, BME is indicated.

Macrocytic anemias can be divided into two types, round and oval. Round macrocytosis of the premature infant or neonate, liver disease, or regenerative macrocytes do not require a BME. Oval macrocytes are an indication for BME because they indicate dyserythropoiesis. The BM aspirate is more useful in the detection of dyserythropoiesis than the BM BX.

BME cannot distinguish between hereditary and acquired hemolytic spherocytic anemias. In acquired hemolytic spherocytic anemias the indication for a BME is suspicion of an underlying lymphomatous process. In nonspherocytic hemolytic anemias caused by hereditary enzymopathies, unstable hemoglobin disorders, and PNH, the BME has no value. Hemolytic anemias may be associated with specific RBC abnormalities, such as parasitic inclusion, schistocytes, keratocytes, stomatocytes, sickle cells, elliptocytes, pyropoikilocytes, and red cell agglutination. The only subtype in which a BME is indicated is fragmented RBCs to rule out thrombotic thrombocytopenic purpura or marrow metastatic disease.

In normocytic or macrocytic anemia with decreased

reticulocyte count and no abnormalities of the leukocytes or platelets, a BME is indicated. The diagnostic indications are idiopathic pure RBC aplasia or B19-parvovirus infection. Parvovirus infection is characterized by the presence of giant rubriblasts, which have a distinctive appearance. The BM BX offers no additional information.

Isolated leukopenia or neutropenia. Isolated neutropenias have limited causes. There are rare hereditary forms and rare cases of dysmyelopoietic syndromes (DMPS); however, most result from drugs or immune mechanisms. The BM aspirate is done to determine whether neutropenic precursors are absent (a rare situation) or a "maturation defect" of granulopoiesis is present. An adequate BM aspirate is sufficient to answer the question.

Isolated thrombocytopenia. Isolated thrombocytopenias may be hereditary in nature or may be caused by drugs or immune disorders. The purpose of the BME is to determine whether megakaryocytes are normal, decreased, or increased in number, with or without maturation abnormalities. An adequate BM aspirate is usually sufficient to answer the question, and the biopsy contributes little.

Peripheral blood bicytopenia or pancytopenia. Patients with peripheral blood bicytopenia or pancytopenia require BME.

Acute leukemias. The diagnosis of the acute leukemias invariably follows the discovery of peripheral blood abnormalities, usually the presence of blasts or pancytopenia (Color Plates III-5 and III-6). A BM aspirate is always done in patients with acute leukemia, even when the peripheral blood is unequivocally diagnostic. Accurate classification is best made on the BM aspirate. The criteria for acute leukemia subtypes established by the French-American-British Cooperative (FAB) Group (Chapter 93) are BM criteria. If an adequate BM aspirate is obtained, the BM BX contributes little information. In the event of an inadequate BM aspirate because of technical failure, the presence of myelofibrosis, marrow necrosis, or a "packed marrow, the BM BX is of value. Acute megakaryocytic leukemias often present with marked myelofibrosis with a "dry" tap. The BM BX is done routinely in most leukemia centers despite its relative lack of value. In patients with refractory anemias with excess blasts (RAEB, RAEBIT) or in those suspected of having early acute leukemia, the biopsy occasionally shows large infiltrates of blasts and influences the diagnosis that is made. The BM BX is indispensable in the diagnosis of hypoplastic acute leukemias and in distinguishing them from myelodysplastic syndrome (MDS), aplastic anemia, or other causes of leukoerythroblastic clinical pictures. Two forms of acute leukemia particularly are frequently accompanied by myelofibrosis: acute lymphoblastic leukemia (ALL) and acute megakaryoblastic leukemia. Thirty percent of adults with ALL and 60% of children with ALL have some degree of myelofibrosis at diagnosis. The most useful aspect of the BM BX in acute leukemia is in following therapy. Inadequate BM aspirates are often obtained after therapy, but the biopsy may clearly show pockets of persistent blasts or foci of recovering marrow. An immunostain for cytoplasmic hemoglobin is helpful to determine whether the foci of blasts are early recovery of erythroid cells or persistent leukemic blasts. In MDS the role of BM BX is similar to that in acute leukemia. If a cellular BM aspirate can be obtained with good morphology, a biopsy is of little value. The biopsy is valuable in distinguishing MDS from aplastic anemia or from an MDS with myelofibrosis.

Chronic lymphocytic leukemias. The diagnosis of chronic lymphocytic leukemia (CLL) is usually based on the presence of 10,000 lymphocytes or more in the peripheral blood (Color Plate III-5, *D*) and/or demonstration of a clonal population of B or T lymphocytes.

The BM aspirate shows an increase in lymphocytes of moderate to marked proportions, and such marrow involvement is essential for the diagnosis of at least the B cell variants.

The BM BX is playing an increased role in the diagnosis of CLL. The marrow patterns of CLL are interstitial, nodular, mixed, or diffuse. There is a progressive infiltration pattern in CLL from interstitial and nodular to mixed and diffuse, and these patterns can be reversed by treatment.

Plasmacytic myeloma and amyloidosis. The diagnosis of plasmacytic myeloma is based on BME (Color Plate III-9). The aspirate is usually conclusive in the diagnosis. A minimum of 10% of malignant plasma cells are required for the diagnosis. Because myeloma is a spotty disease, the occurrence of a BM aspirate with less than 10% plasma cells and the presence of foci, clumps, or sheets of plasma cells on the BM BX that clearly identify the patient as having myeloma are not unusual. Biopsy should be done routinely in patients with myeloma at the time of suspected diagnosis. The demonstration of a monoclonal population of plasma cells by immunostaining is possible on biopsy by use of kappa and lambda light-chain staining. Although amyloid can be demonstrated in BM aspirates, it is frequently difficult to detect and is often missed. Staining for amyloid on the BM BX is more useful.

Chronic myeloproliferative disorders. The classification of chronic myeloproliferative disorders (CMPDs) has expanded in recent years from the traditional "big four" of polycythemia vera, myelofibrosis, idiopathic thrombocythemia, and chronic myelogenous leukemia. Many authors now also include undifferentiated CMPDs, as defined by the Polycythemia Vera Study Group; chronic neutrophilic leukemia; chronic monocytic leukemia; chronic myelomonocytic leukemia; the hypereosinophilic syndrome; and chronic basophilic leukemia. The CMPDs are not strictly morphologic diagnoses. In the absence of clinical history, physical examination, and peripheral blood findings, it may be impossible to differentiate the early stages of polycythemia vera, idiopathic thrombocythemia, the cellular phase of myelofibrosis, and chronic myelogenous leukemia on either BM aspirate or biopsy.

Malignant lymphomas. The primary value of BME is in the staging of lymphoma, that is, the demonstration of marrow involvement. A typical problem in this situation is to distinguish normal lymphoid follicles from lymphomatous involvement. The resolution of this problem almost always depends on immunostains on the biopsies.

Mast cell disease. Mast cell disease can frequently be suspected on BM aspirate because of an increase in large mast cells with round nuclei in the aspirate. However, the BM BX is needed to confirm the diagnosis by demonstration of the typical perivascular and paratrabecular areas of involvement.

Metastatic tumors. Although it is commonly believed that BM BX is more often productive in diagnosis of metastatic carcinoma, several studies have shown the BM aspirate to be just as effective from a statistical standpoint. However, using both the aspirate and biopsy seems prudent. In patients in whom the metastatic disease is associated with myelofibrosis, the biopsy is clearly superior.

Infectious disorders. Although organisms may be detected on BM aspirates in the presence of massive infection, granulomata are more easily detected on BM BX.

Storage disorders. The storage disorders, such as Gaucher's disease, Niemann-Pick disease, and sea-blue histiocytosis, are more easily recognized on the BM aspirate. Because these disorders may form masses of cells, however, their presence may be more readily noticed on the BM BX.

REFERENCES

Davis BH and Bigelow NC: Flow cytometric reticulocyte quantification using thiazole orange provides clinically useful reticulocyte maturation index. Arch Pathol Lab Med 113:684, 1989.

Hillman RS: Characteristics of marrow production and reticulocyte maturation in normal man in response to anemia. J Clin Invest 48:443, 1969.

Koepke JA, Dotson NA, and Schifman MA: A critical evaluation of the manual/visual differential leukocyte counting method. Blood Cells 11:173, 1985.

Pierre RV et al: Comparison of four leukocyte differential methods with the National Committee for Clinical Laboratory Standards (NCCLS) reference method. Am J Clin Pathol 87:201, 1987.

CHAPTER

74 Molecular Diagnostics

Robert V. Pierre

The mainstay of the diagnosis of malignant neoplasms is light microscopy by a well-trained observer. Most malignant neoplasms have microscopic features that are distinctive and permit the accurate identification and classification of the tumor sufficient for clinical purposes. However, some neoplastic diseases may prove difficult or impossible to distinguish from nonmalignant disorders by conventional light microscopic techniques, even with the addition of cytochemical or immunostains. Examples are the myelodysplastic states, reactive or atypical lymphoid hyperplasia, and solid tumors that resemble benign tumors. Molecular diagnostic techniques have brought major advances to the solution of many of these problems in hematologic and oncologic practice. Their major uses have been:

1. To establish clonality in a tumor or cell line
2. To identify specific cell types, such as subtyping of acute lymphoblastic leukemias, lymphomas, and metastatic tumors for diagnostic, staging, and prognostic purposes
3. To detect the presence of specific genes or altered gene sequences by deoxyribonucleic acid (DNA) studies, DNA fingerprinting, or DNA probes

The demonstration of clonality in a tumor or cell line can often determine whether the process is malignant. A variety of molecular and other techniques can be used to demonstrate clonality:

1. Cytogenetic studies
2. Proto-oncogene mutations
3. Study of glucose-6-phosphate dehydrogenase (G6PD) phenotype in patients who are heterozygotes for G6PD isoenzymes A and B
4. Restriction fragment length polymorphism (RFLP) analysis

CYTOGENETICS AND NEOPLASIA

The story of cytogenetic abnormalities and human disease began in 1959 with the description of trisomy 21 in Down syndrome by Lejeune and colleagues. The findings of the Philadelphia chromosome in chronic myelogenous leukemia (CML) in 1960 by Nowell and Hungerford and the 14q+ in Burkitt's lymphoma by Manolov and Manolov in 1972 generated an explosion of interest and investigation of cytogenetic abnormalities in leukemia and lymphomas. Another landmark was the description of a deletion of chromosome 13 in retinoblastoma. With this discovery came the concept that deletion of a specific gene might lead to a specific neoplasm. Rapid advances have occurred in the field of cytogenetics of neoplasms. Many thousands of specific chromosomal abnormalities have been described, and correspondence to specific disease states has been established in a limited number.

Cytogenetic studies of the acute myelogenous leukemias (AMLs) and acute lymphoblastic leukemias (ALLs) have the following clinical uses:

1. Demonstration of a clonal chromosomal abnormality. Two metaphases with identical structural abnormalities (e.g.,t[9;21][q34;q11]) or three metaphases with loss or gain of a specific chromosome (e.g., 47,XX,+8) can identify the neoplastic nature of a myeloid or lymphoid disorder.
2. Specific chromosomal abnormalities are characteristic of some myeloid and lymphoid disorders, such as the t(9;21) with CML, t(15;17) with AML-M3, and

t(1;19) in pre–B cell ALL (see Table 71-3 for a more complete listing).

3. The extent of involvement gives prognostic information for response to therapy and survival. If all metaphases of a bone marrow specimen from patients with AML and ALL show the same clonal abnormality (AA), the prognosis for survival is poorer than if there is a mixture of normal and abnormal metaphases (AN) or all normal metaphases (NN). Complete remissions are less frequently attained in AN and AA patients.
4. The immunoglobulin (Ig) gene locations for heavy chains at 14q32, kappa light chain at 2p11, and lambda light chain at 22q11. The *c-myc* oncogene is located at 8q24. Translocations that result in location of the *c-myc* oncogene next to a portion of the heavy-chain or light-chain genes occur in B cell leukemias and lymphomas. Correspondence exists between the site of the *c-myc* translocation and the type of Ig made by the tumor cells; for example, B cell lymphoma cells with the t(2;8) produce kappa light chains.
5. In T cell ALL, several of the specific translocation chromosome breakpoints are located at or near the site of T cell receptor genes. The alpha-chain receptor is located at 14q11-12, the beta-chain receptor at 7q32-36, the delta-chain receptor at 14q11.2, and the gamma-chain receptor at 7p15. The T cell receptor genes rearrange during T cell differentiation, analogous to the changes in Ig genes during B cell differentiation. Translocation abnormalities have been described with breakpoints at the T cell receptor gene sites in patients with T cell ALL.

In malignant lymphoma the diagnostic and prognostic value of cytogenetic studies have been established. Correlations between cytogenetic abnormalities and specific histologic subtypes have been made, for example, the t(8;14) in Burkitt's lymphoma and the t(14;18) in small cleaved-cell type of B cell lymphoma. Some are similar to those just described in the acute leukemias. Breakpoints involving the Ig genes on chromosome 14 have been described in B cell lymphomas, and breakpoints involving the *TCR* genes have been described in T cell lymphoma. Several putative oncogenes have been described, *tcl-1,2,3,4,5,6* and *bcl-1,2,2a,4,* which occur at breakpoints seen in malignant lymphoma. Cytogenetic studies in Hodgkin's disease have not been as successful or informative to date. This may relate to the infrequency of the neoplastic cells in Hodgkin's disease or other technical factors.

Plasmacytic myeloma is a difficult tumor to study cytogenetically because of the low mitotic index of the tumor cells; however, clonal chromosomal abnormalities are described. Abnormalities of 14q occur often, but other abnormalities are observed as well. The presence of chromosomal abnormalities and the degree of involvement has prognostic significance. AA patients essentially die within 1 year, whereas AN or NN patients survive longer.

B cell chronic lymphocytic leukemia (CLL) is the most common hematologic malignancy. Only 10% of CLL cases are T cell in origin. Trisomy 12 is the most frequent abnormality observed in B cell CLL. The second most frequent abnormality is a 14q+ marker. A t(11;14)(q13;q32) is the most common cause of a 14q+ marker. The breakpoint on 14 is at the Ig gene, and the site on 11 has been postulated to contain a cellular oncogene, *bcl-1*. A variety of other abnormalities have been described in B cell CLL. The presence of chromosomal abnormalities in CLL also appears to have prognostic significance for survival. Various cytogenetic abnormalities have also been described in patients with T cell CLL, the most frequent being inv(14) and +8q.

The adult T cell leukemia associated with human immunodeficiency virus III (HIV-III) infection seen in Japan and limited other areas also shows a variety of cytogenetic changes. The most frequent abnormalities involve chromosome 14 and a +3 abnormality.

Cancer susceptibility genes appear to exist that are hereditary and therefore germ-line mutations. Retinoblastoma occurs in both sporadic and hereditary forms. Chromosome 13q14 is deleted in many patients with the hereditary form of the disease. It has been postulated that all retinoblastomas occur as a result of two mutational events. In the hereditary form, the first is germinal in origin. The second mutation occurs in the somatic cells, with loss of the normal allele resulting in homozygosity for the retinoblastoma gene (loss of heterozygosity). A similar mechanism has been proposed for Wilms' tumor occurring in patients with the AGR triad (aniridia, gonadal dysplasia, mental retardation) for a gene located at 11p13.

PROTO-ONCOGENE MUTATIONS

Cellular proto-oncogenes are primitive genes that arose early in metazoan evolution and have been retained virtually unaltered in humans; for example, *ras* proto-oncogenes occur in similar form in yeast genomes. It is presumed that these proto-oncogenes are involved in regulating normal cell growth and differentiation and cannot be substantially altered or lost, although this hypothesis remains unproved. Each cellular proto-oncogene is composed of a regulatory and a structural region. The *regulatory region* modulates the expression of the gene during development or in response to physiologic stimuli, whereas the *structural region* encodes for the amino acid sequence of a functional cellular protein. Alterations in the regulatory portion of the gene can lead to inappropriate levels of production of the cellular protein, such as a growth-inducing protein. Structural mutations, however, lead to synthesis of a protein that has an aberrant structure and function.

An example of activation of a cellular proto-oncogene by structural alteration is seen in the *ras* proto-oncogenes, in which point mutations occur at codons 12, 13, or 61. These simple mutations may be produced by chemical carcinogens or radiation. The point mutation results in change of a single amino acid residue in the *ras* protein. The normal *ras* protein is involved in the binding and hydrolysis of guanosine triphosphate (GTP). Alteration in this protein compromises the ability of the *ras*-coded protein to hydrolyze GTP, thereby trapping this molecule in a state in which

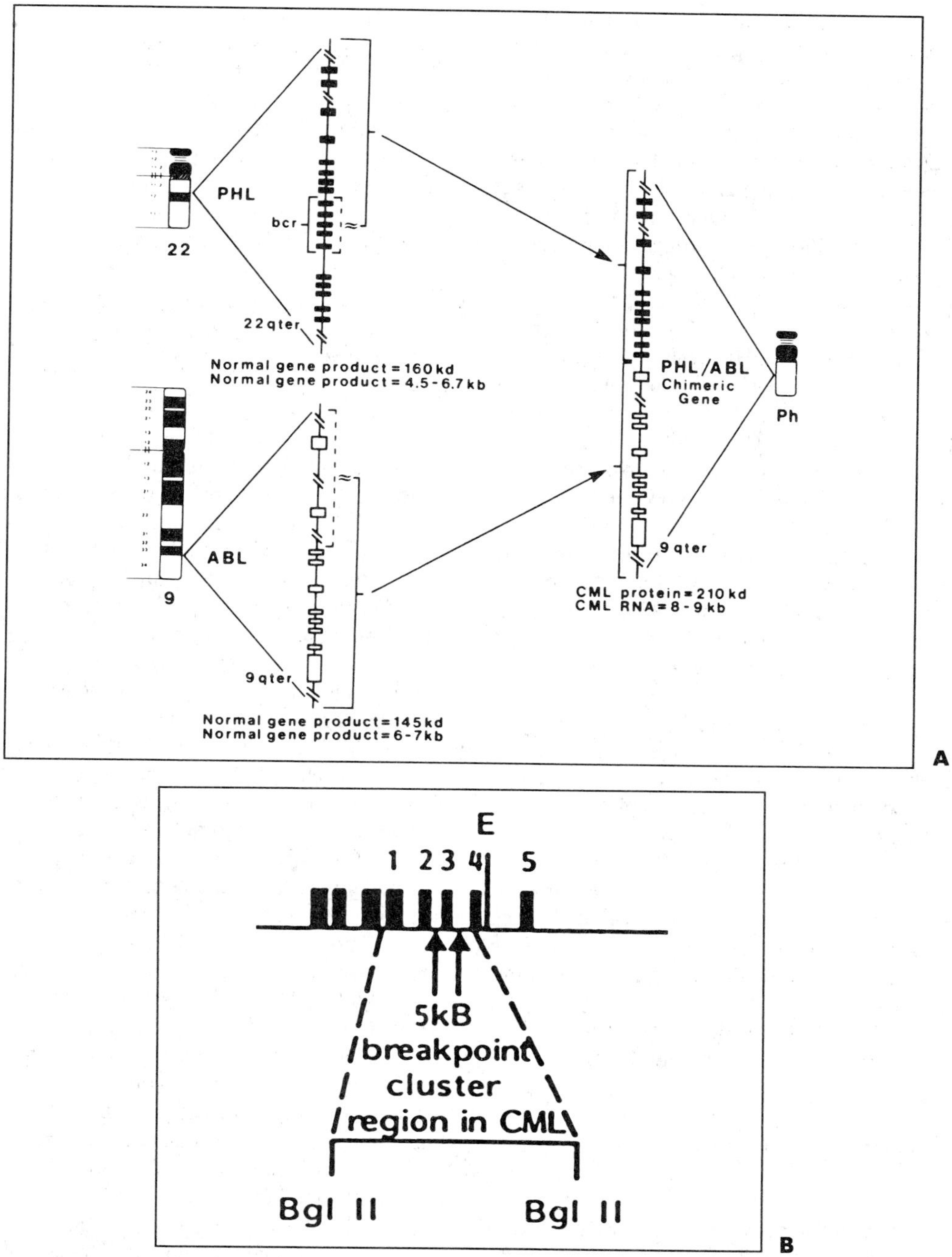

Fig. 74-1. A, Schematic presentation of the normal PHL gene on chromosome 22, the ABL gene on chromosome 9, and the fusion gene on the Philadelphia (Ph^1) chromosome. The sizes of the gene products are indicated in kilodaltons (kD) for the proteins and in kilobases (kb) for the encoding RNA. **B,** Detailed view of the breakpoints in the major breakpoint cluster region of the ABL gene typical of chronic myelogenous leukemia (CML). *E,* EcoRI restriction enzyme cleavage site; *Bgl II,* Bgl restriction enzyme cleavage site. (From Sandberg AA: The chromosomes in human cancer and leukemia, ed 2. New York, 1990, Elsevier. With permission from the author.)

it constitutively sends out growth-stimulating signals. The physiologic effect of the *ras* oncogene mutation can now be understood in terms of this change of protein structure. Mechanisms of the proto-oncogene effect are as follows:

1. Activation of the *ras* oncogene results from the point mutation. This can be demonstrated by transfection of DNA containing the mutant gene into benign target cells, which will then produce tumors when injected into nude mice.
2. A chromosome translocation may result in the *myc*

oncogene regulatory area replacing the regulatory sequence derived from the Ig gene, resulting in inappropriately regulated production of a normal protein.

3. Amplification of an oncogene may occur, with the amplified gene seen as a homogeneous staining region of a chromosome or as amplified copies that are not integrated into a chromosome (double minutes). Amplification of *n-myc* is frequently found in neuroblastoma. The amplified gene produces greatly increased quantities of the encoded protein.
4. The translocation of a portion of the abelson protooncogene *(abl)* on chromosome 9 to the breakpoint cluster region *(bcr)* of the PHL gene on chromosome 22 results in a fusion gene, with production of a unique 210 kD protein with tyrosine kinase activity. This defect is the hallmark of CML. The detection of the *abl-bcr* translocation is done by Southern blot analysis of DNA extracted from blood or bone marrow cells hydrolyzed by restriction endonucleases (Fig. 74-1). Various DNA probes directed against the major *bcr* (a small 5.8 kb region of the PHL gene in which most breaks on chromosome 22 occur) can be used that will hybridize with the germ-line *bcr* or with rearranged fragments of the *bcr* region.

GLUCOSE-6-PHOSPHATE DEHYDROGENASE

The gene for G6PD is located on the X chromosome. The enzyme has two isoenzyme forms, A and B. Black females who are heterozygotes for the isoenzymes A and B would be expected to have a mixture of blood cells containing either the A or B form of the enzyme because of the normal random inactivation of one of the X chromosomes. If such a double-heterozygote female should develop a clonal bone marrow disorder, all red cells would come from one common ancestor cell and would exhibit only one enzyme type. This tool for demonstration of clonality is obviously of limited use because it can only be used in double-heterozygote females.

RESTRICTION FRAGMENT LENGTH POLYMORPHISMS

RFLPs have been used to determine clonality based on common RFLPs on X-chromosome-linked genes (PGK, HPRT).

POLYMERASE CHAIN REACTION

Polymerase chain reaction (PCR) is an enzymatic method of amplifying the amount of a specific segment of DNA. This technique permits detection of specific DNA sequences from very small amounts of DNA or small numbers of cells. Coupled with RFLP analysis or the use of specific DNA probes to specific genes, it can be used to increase greatly the sensitivity of detection of specific DNA segments for diagnosis or detection of residual disease.

The use of DNA probes to sequences on specific chromosomes linked to compounds with different fluorescent colors has allowed "chromosome painting." Different chromosomes can be stained different colors in the same chromosome preparation. This can make chromosome translocations between specific chromosomes very apparent. This technique can also be used to detect monosomy or trisomy of specific chromosomes in interphase cell preparations. This also has the possibility of detecting minimum residual disease in patients with known chromosome abnormalities that can be detected by this technique.

MONOCLONAL REAGENTS AND SURFACE MARKERS OF LYMPHOID CELLS: APPLICATIONS TO LYMPHOID MALIGNANCIES

A discussion of lymphoid cell differentiation is found in Chapter 283. The differentiation of T cell and B cell lymphocytes is accompanied by the appearance of antigens on the cell surface. Monoclonal antibodies have been developed to these differentiation antigens and can be used to characterize both acute and chronic lymphoid disorders. These monoclonal antibodies can be used in several ways: labeling of cells for flow cytometry, staining of cells on blood films by immunocytochemical techniques, and immunohistochemical techniques for identification of cells in tissue sections.

In ALL the following markers of lymphoid cells are used; the use of flow cytometry or slide-based immunostains or cytochemistry is based on the particular clinician's preference and expertise. The immunophenotype and cytogenetic subtype of ALL is of greater prognostic significance and therapeutic significance than the morphologic classification. Although some laboratories use an all-inclusive battery approach to classification of ALL, a sequential use of tests is more cost-effective, if the test results can be made rapidly available. Morphologic diagnosis of ALL by Romanowsky-stained blood films is unreliable because many cases cannot be distinguished from AML, particularly M1. Also, most cases cannot be reliably differentiated into T cell or B cell subtype. The first step in characterization of a morphologically indeterminate acute leukemia is performance of peroxidase (or Sudan black B) and esterase stains (Color Plate III-6) to rule out acute nonlymphocytic leukemia of granulocytic or monocytic subtype. A determination terminal deoxynucleotidyl transferase (TdT) is the next logical step. If it is positive, then subtyping of ALL should be done. In the presence of a negative TdT with negative peroxidase and esterase stains, the possibility of a B cell ALL should be considered and ruled out by use of either surface immunoglobulin (SmIg) stain or anti-CD19 or anti-CD20 monoclonal stains. In the presence of a peroxidase-, esterase-, TdT-, and SmIg-negative acute leukemia, other subtypes to consider are acute erythroblastic leukemia, acute megakaryocytic leukemia, and acute basophilic leukemia.

In the presence of a positive TdT test, the leukemia must be divided into the B cell or T cell lineage. The major antibodies used to subdivide the types of acute lymphoblastic leukemia are shown in Table 74-1. A recent proposal for

Table 74-1. Major antibodies used as diagnostic reagents to subdivide types of acute lymphoblastic leukemia (ALL)

	Monoclonal antibody					
Subtype of B cell ALL	**TdT**	**HLA-DR**	**CD19**	**CD10**	**CyIg**	**SmIg**
Early B precursor	Pos	Pos	Pos	Neg	Neg	Neg
Common	Pos	Pos	Pos	Pos	Neg	Neg
Pre-B	Pos	Pos	Pos	Pos	Pos	Neg
B-ALL	Neg	Pos	Pos	Pos	Pos	Pos
				Neg	Neg	

Subtype of T cell ALL	**TdT**	**CD7**	**CD2/E receptor**
Early T precursor	Pos	Pos	Neg
T ALL	Pos	Pos	Pos

Table 74-2. Proposal for classification of chronic lymphoid leukemias

	Immunophenotype of chronic B cell leukemias									
Category of CLL	**SmIg**	**CyIg**	**MRFC**	**CD5**	**CD19 CD20**	**HLA-DR**	**CD22**	**CD10**	**CD25**	**CD38**
CLL	Wk	−	++	++	++	++	−/+	−	−	−
PLL	Strg	−/+	−	−/+	++	++	++	−/+	−	−
HCL	Strg	−/+	−/+	−	++	++	++	−	++	−/+
FCL	Strg	−	−/+	−	++	++	+	+	−	−/+
IL	Mod	−	−/+	++	++	++	+	−/+	−	−
Lymphoma										
SLVL	Strg	−/+	−	−	++	++	++	−	−/+	−/+
PCL	Neg	++	−	−	−	−	−	−/+	−	++

	Immunophenotype of chronic T cell leukemias						
Category of CLL	**CD2**	**CD3**	**CD5**	**CD7**	**CD4**	**CD8**	**CD25**
T-CLL	++	++	−	−	−	++	−
T-PLL	++	+	++	++	+	−/+	−
ATLL	++	++	++	−	++	−	++
Sézary syndrome	++	++	++	−	++	−	−

Modified from Bain BJ: Leukaemia diagnosis: a guide to the FAB classification. New York, 1990, Gower.

CLL, Chronic lymphocytic leukemia; PLL, prolymphocytic leukemia; HCL, hairy cell leukemia; FCL, follicular center cell leukemia; IL, intermediate lymphoma; SLVL, splenic lymphoma with villous lymphocytes; PCL, plasma cell leukemia; T-CLL, T cell chronic lymphocytic leukemia (large granular lymphocyte leukemia); T-PLL, T cell prolymphocytic leukemia; ATLL, adult T cell leukemia/lymphoma; Strg, strong; Wk, weak; Mod, moderate. The frequency with which a marker is positive in >30% of cells is indicated by ++, 80%-100%; +, 40%-80%; −/+, 10%-40%; −, 0%-9%.

the classification of the chronic lymphoid leukemias is shown in Table 74-2. The most common and important types of chronic lymphoid leukemia are chronic lymphocytic leukemia (CLL in Table 74-2) and hairy cell leukemia (HCL in Table 74-2). There is increasing recognition that the chronic B cell and T cell leukemias are composed of distinct entities that have different clinical manifestations.

REFERENCES

Bennet JM et al: The French-American-British (FAB) Cooperative Group. J Clin Pathol 42:567, 1989.

Fialkow PJ, Jacobson RJ, and Papayannopoulou T: Chronic myelocytic leukemia: clonal origin in a stem cell common to the granulocyte, erythrocyte, platelet and monocyte/macrophage. Am J Med 63:125, 1977.

Knudson AG Jr: Mutation and cancer: statistical study of retinoblastoma. Proc Natl Acad Sci USA 68:820, 1971.

Lee MS et al: Detection of minimal residual cells carrying the t(14;18) by DNA sequence amplification. Science 237:175, 1987.

Lejeune J, Gautier M, and Turpin R: Etude des chromosomes somatiques de neuf enfants mongolians. CR Acad Sci (D) (Paris) 248:1721, 1959.

Manolov G and Manolov Y: Marker band in one chromosome 14 from Burkitt lymphomas. Nature 237:33, 1972.

Nowell PC and Hungerford DA: A minute chromosome in human chronic granulocytic leukemia. Science 132:1497, 1960.

Sawyers CL et al: Molecular relapse in chronic myelogenous leukemia patients after bone marrow transplantation detected by polymerase chain reaction. Proc Natl Acad Sci USA 87:563, 1990.

Schiffer CA et al: Prognostic impact of cytogenetic abnormalities in patients with de novo acute nonlymphocytic leukemia. Blood 73:263, 1989.

Solomon E, Borrow J, and Goddard AD: Chromosome aberrations and cancer. Science 254:1153, 1991.

Vogelstein B et al: Clonal analysis using recombinant DNA probes from the X-chromosome. Cancer Res 47:4806, 1987.

CHAPTER

75 Evaluation of Monoclonal Proteins in Serum and Urine

Robert A. Kyle

Each monoclonal protein (M protein, paraprotein) consists of two heavy-chain polypeptides of the same class and subclass and two light-chain polypeptides of the same type (Chapter 285). The different monoclonal proteins are designated by capital letters that correspond to the class of their heavy chains, which are designated by Greek letters: γ in immunoglobulin G (IgG), α in IgA, μ in IgM, δ in IgD, and ϵ in IgE. Their subclasses are IgG1, IgG2, IgG3, and IgG4, or IgA1 and IgA2, and their light-chain types are kappa (κ) and lambda (λ).

A monoclonal protein is characterized by a narrow peak (resembling a church spire) (Fig. 75-1, *A*) or a localized band on electrophoresis; by a thickened, bowed arc on immunoelectrophoresis; and by a localized band on immunofixation. Many different entities are associated with monoclonal proteins (monoclonal gammopathies) (see the box at upper right).

In contrast to a monoclonal protein, a polyclonal protein consists of one or more heavy-chain classes and *both* light-chain types. A polyclonal protein is characterized by a broad peak or band, usually of γ mobility, on electrophoresis (Fig. 75-1, *B*); by thickening and elongation of all heavy- and light-chain arcs on immunoelectrophoresis; and by the absence of a localized band on immunofixation. A list of the conditions in the differential diagnosis of polyclonal gammopathies is given in the box at right.

Although monoclonal proteins have long been considered abnormal, studies during the past several years have strongly suggested that they are only excessive quantities of normal immunoglobulins. Each heavy-chain subclass and light-chain type in a monoclonal protein has its counterpart among normal immunoglobulins and among antibodies. Monoclonal proteins are individual antibodies and are products of a single clone of plasma cells. Although some monoclonal proteins represent known antibodies, most do not; however, it is almost certain that more mono-

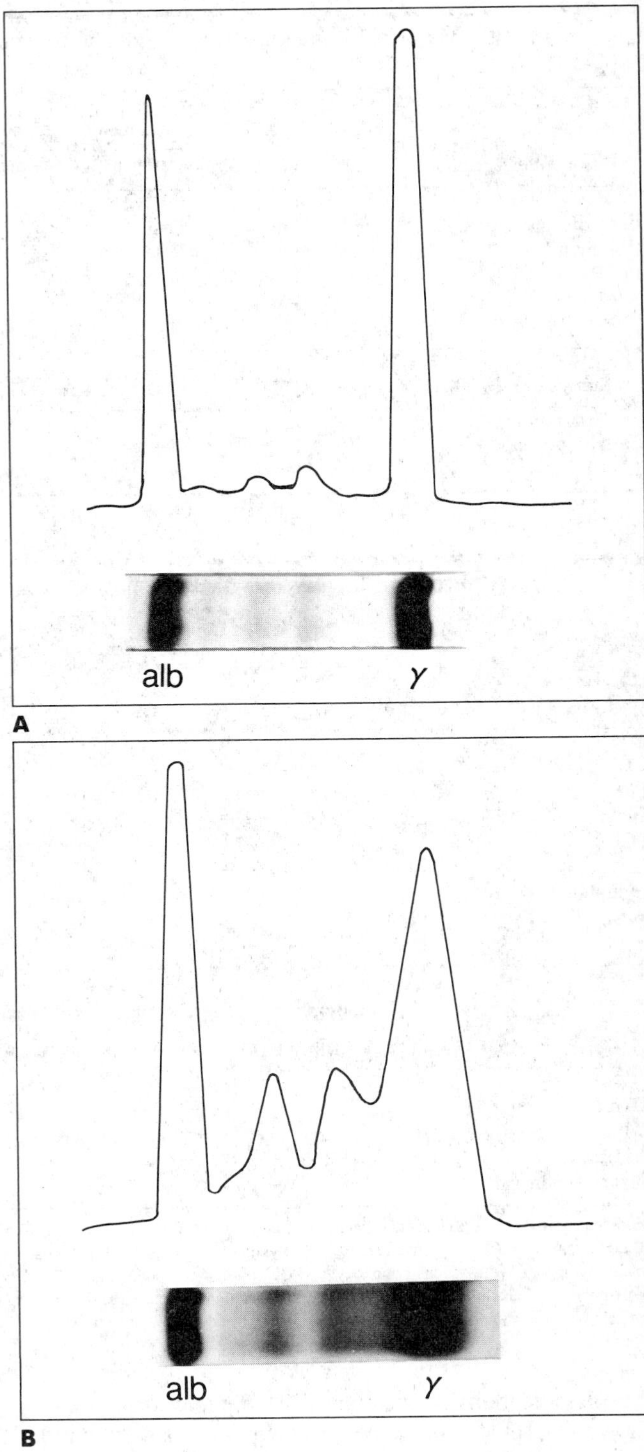

Fig. 75-1. A, *Top,* Monoclonal pattern of serum protein from densitometer tracing after electrophoresis on cellulose acetate (anode on *left*): tall, narrow-based peak of γ mobility; *bottom,* monoclonal pattern from electrophoresis of serum on cellulose acetate (anode on *left*): dense, localized band representing monoclonal protein in γ area. **B,** *Top,* Polyclonal pattern of serum protein from densitometer tracing after electrophoresis on cellulose acetate (anode on *left*): broad-based peak of γ mobility; *bottom,* polyclonal pattern from electrophoresis of serum on cellulose acetate (anode on *left*): γ band is broad. (From Kyle RA and Garton JP: Semin Oncol 13:310, 1986. Reproduced with permission of WB Sanders.)

Differential diagnosis of monoclonal gammopathies

I. Malignant monoclonal gammopathies
   A. Multiple myeloma (IgG, IgA, IgD, IgE, and free light chains)
      1. Overt multiple myeloma
      2. Smoldering multiple myeloma
      3. Plasma cell leukemia
      4. Nonsecretory myeloma
      5. Osteosclerotic (POEMS) myeloma
   B. Plasmacytoma
      1. Solitary plasmacytoma of bone
      2. Extramedullary plasmacytoma
   C. Malignant lymphoproliferative diseases
      1. Waldenström's (primary) macroglobulinemia
      2. Malignant lymphoma
   D. Heavy-chain diseases
      1. Gamma heavy-chain disease
      2. Alpha heavy-chain disease
      3. Mu heavy-chain disease
   E. Amyloidosis
      1. Primary
      2. With myeloma
      (Secondary, localized, and familial amyloidoses have no monoclonal protein.)
II. Monoclonal gammopathies of undetermined significance (MGUS)
   A. Benign (IgG, IgA, IgD, IgM, and, rarely, free light chains)
   B. Associated with neoplasms of cell types not known to produce monoclonal proteins
   C. Biclonal gammopathies of undetermined significance (BGUS)

From Kyle RA: In Rose NR, Friedman H, and Fahey JL, editors: Manual of clinical laboratory immunology, ed 3. Washington, 1986, American Society for Microbiology. By permission.

Differential diagnosis of polyclonal gammopathies

Connective tissue (autoimmune) diseases
Chronic liver disease, especially chronic active hepatitis
Chronic infections
Lymphoproliferative diseases
Normal

clonal proteins will be found to have antibody activity. The generation of antibody diversity is complex (Chapter 285). The one-cell one-immunoglobulin concept is supported by almost all individual plasma cells containing either κ or λ light chains, but not both.

Analysis of the serum and urine for monoclonal proteins requires a sensitive, rapid, dependable, inexpensive screening method to detect the monoclonal protein and a specific assay to identify its heavy-chain class and light-chain type. Electrophoresis on cellulose actetate membrane is satisfactory for screening, although agarose is more sensitive than cellulose acetate in detecting small monoclonal proteins. After screening, immunoelectrophoresis or immunofixation, or both, should be used to confirm the presence of a monoclonal protein and distinguish its immunoglobulin class and light-chain type (Fig. 75-2).

ANALYSIS OF SERUM FOR MONOCLONAL PROTEIN

Electrophoresis

In electrophoresis the basic principle is that particles in solution migrate according to their charge, albumin toward the anode (positive pole) and globulin toward the cathode (negative pole). Serum protein electrophoresis should be done on all patients in whom multiple myeloma, macroglobulinemia, or amyloidosis is known or suspected. The test is also indicated for any patient with unexplained weakness or fatigue, anemia, elevation of the erythrocyte sedimentation rate, back pain, osteoporosis or osteolytic lesions or fractures, immunoglobulin deficiency, hypercalcemia, Bence Jones proteinuria, renal insufficiency, or recurrent

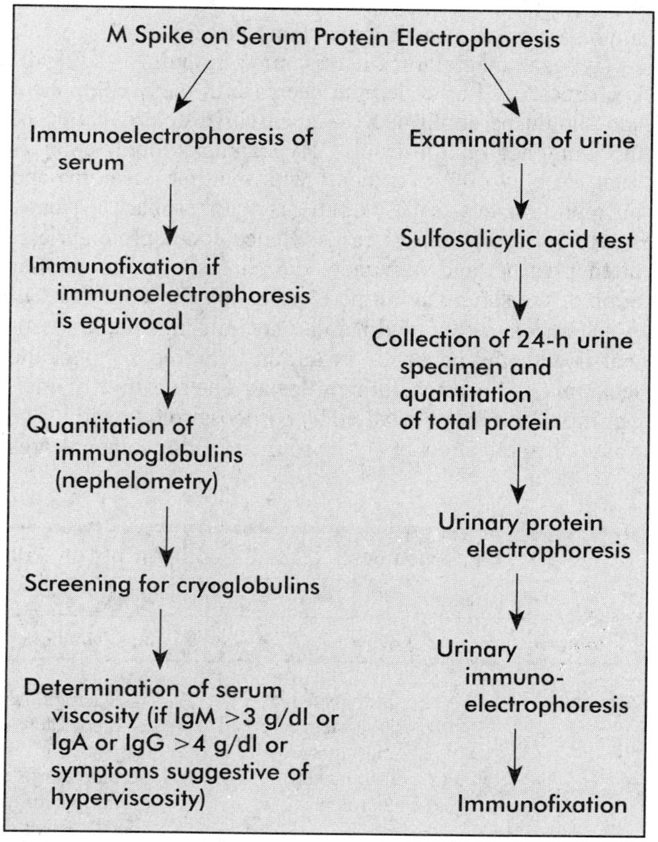

Fig. 75-2. Sequence of immunologic testing for monoclonal proteins.

infections. Because a localized band or spike is strongly suggestive of primary amyloidosis, serum protein electrophoresis also should be performed on adults with peripheral neuropathy, carpal tunnel syndrome, refractory congestive heart failure, nephrotic syndrome, orthostatic hypotension, or malabsorption.

Several proteins are found in each of the peaks on electrophoresis (Table 75-1). Although immunoglobulins (IgG, IgA, IgM, IgD, IgE) make up the γ component, they are also found in the β-γ and β regions, and IgG extends to the α_2-globulin area. Thus an IgG monoclonal protein may range from the slow γ region to the α_2-globulin region.

The α_1-globulin component is usually decreased because of a deficiency of α_1-antitrypsin. The decrease may be associated with recurrent pulmonary infections and chronic obstructive pulmonary disease. A large peak in the α_2-globulin area may represent free hemoglobin–haptoglobin complexes resulting from hemolysis. In this situation the serum is often pink. Large amounts of transferrin in patients with iron deficiency anemia may produce a peak in the β region.

Fibrinogen appears as a discrete band between the β and γ peaks. It may be present because the sample has not clotted completely or the patient has received heparin. Therefore the specimen should be examined for a clot; if there is no clot, either thrombin should be added to the sample or fibrinogen may be detected by immunodiffusion using fibrinogen antisera. If no evidence of fibrinogen is found, immunoelectrophoresis should be done because the β-γ band might represent a small monoclonal protein.

Hypogammaglobulinemia (gamma globulin <0.6 g/dl) is characterized by a definite decrease in the γ component and should be confirmed by quantitative determination of the immunoglobulin levels. Hypogammaglobulinemia is seen in about 10% of patients with multiple myeloma and in approximately 25% of patients with primary systemic amyloidosis. In both diseases, Bence Jones proteinuria is often present, and immunoelectrophoresis or immunofixation of the serum and urine is necessary for identification. Also, hypogammaglobulinemia may be congenital or associated with the nephrotic syndrome, chronic lymphocytic leukemia, lymphoma, protein-losing enteropathy, or malnutrition; or it may be caused by corticosteroid therapy. The point of application of the specimen in the cathodal area may be confused with a monoclonal protein. In 3% of sera, an additional monoclonal protein of a different immunoglobulin class is seen; this condition is designated *biclonal gammopathy* (Chapter 95).

A monoclonal protein may be present when the total serum protein concentration, β and γ globulin levels, and quantitative immunoglobulin levels are normal. The cellulose strip must be examined visually because the densitometer tracing may not detect a small monoclonal protein. A small monoclonal protein also may be concealed among the β or γ components and be missed. A monoclonal light chain (Bence Jones proteinemia) is rarely seen on the cellulose acetate tracing. In IgD myeloma the serum peak sometimes is small or not evident. Occasionally a sharp peak is seen in mu heavy-chain disease but is never seen in alpha heavy-chain disease. In gamma heavy-chain disease a broad band is often seen on electrophoresis. A monoclonal protein may appear as a rather broad band on the cellulose acetate membrane or as a broad peak in the densitometer tracing and can be mistaken for a polyclonal increase in immunoglobulins. Presumably the broad band is caused by aggregates or polymers. Therefore immunoelectrophoresis or immunofixation is necessary to identify a monoclonal protein.

For follow-up after the diagnosis of a monoclonal protein in the serum, one should use a densitometer tracing of the cellulose acetate electrophoresis or quantitation of the immunoglobulins. The quantitative immunoglobulin level may be 2000 mg/dl or more than that in the densitometer tracing. It is essential to follow the size of the monoclonal protein with serum protein electrophoresis or quantitation of the immunoglobulins, but one should not change from one method to another.

Immunoelectrophoresis

This test should be performed when a sharp peak is found on the cellulose acetate tracing or when myeloma, macroglobulinemia, amyloidosis, or a related disorder is suspected (Fig. 75-2). The serum sample is placed in wells on microscope slides covered with 1% agar or agarose. Electrophoresis separates the various proteins, and a trough is cut parallel to the line of migration and filled with monospecific antisera. Proteins from the electrophoresed sample (antigen) and from the antisera (antibody) are then allowed

Table 75-1. Constituents of major components of serum electrophoretic pattern*

(anode)← Albumin	α_1-Globulin	α_2-Globulin	β-Globulin	→(cathode) γ-Globulin
Albumin	α_1-Antitrypsin	α_2-Macroglobulin	β-Lipoprotein	IgG
	α_1-Lipoprotein	α_2-Lipoprotein	Transferrin	IgA
	α_1-Acid glycoprotein (orosomucoid)	Haptoglobin	Plasminogen	IgM
	α-Fetoprotein	Ceruloplasmin	Complement	IgD
		Erythropoietin	Hemopexin	IgE
		Lactate dehydrogenase		

*Immunoglobulins may migrate from the slow γ-globulin to the α_2-globulin region.
Modified from Kyle RA and Griepp PR: Mayo Clin Proc 53:719, 1978. By permission of Mayo Foundation.

to diffuse toward each other and form precipitin lines or arcs where they meet. In multiple myeloma, monospecific antisera to IgG, IgA, IgD, IgE, κ, or λ produce a localized thickening or bowing of both the heavy-chain arc and the light-chain arc (Fig. 75-3).

In Waldenström's macroglobulinemia, IgM antisera produce a bowed, thickened arc, and a similar arc is seen with monospecific κ or λ antisera. Occasionally, no diagnostic light-chain arcs are seen, and a mistaken diagnosis of mu heavy-chain disease may be considered. Immunofixation is usually diagnostic in this situation. Another approach is to use a reducing agent such as dithiothreitol (DTT), which often makes an IgM κ or an IgM λ monoclonal protein identifiable with immunoelectrophoresis. Occasionally a monoclonal IgM protein may precipitate (euglobulin) near the application well without producing diagnostic arcs. The problem may be solved by repeating immunoelectrophoresis with a buffer of lower ionic strength, by adding a reducing agent (e.g., DTT), or by immunofixation.

If a bowed κ or λ arc is seen without an accompanying abnormality of the IgG, IgA, or IgM arcs, one must consider the possibility of a free monoclonal light chain or an IgD or IgE monoclonal protein. Bence Jones proteinemia is more common than an IgD or an IgE monoclonal protein. Ouchterlony immunodiffusion with IgD and IgE antisera should be performed when only a monoclonal light chain is found. All sera that form a precipitin band should then be studied by immunoelectrophoresis with monospecific antisera to IgD and IgE as well as to κ and λ. The presence of an additional light-chain arc (double bowing) without a similar change in the heavy-chain arc indicates a free monoclonal light chain (Bence Jones proteinemia) or a component of a biclonal gammopathy in which the associated heavy-chain arc has not been detected. Immunofixation is often useful in this setting.

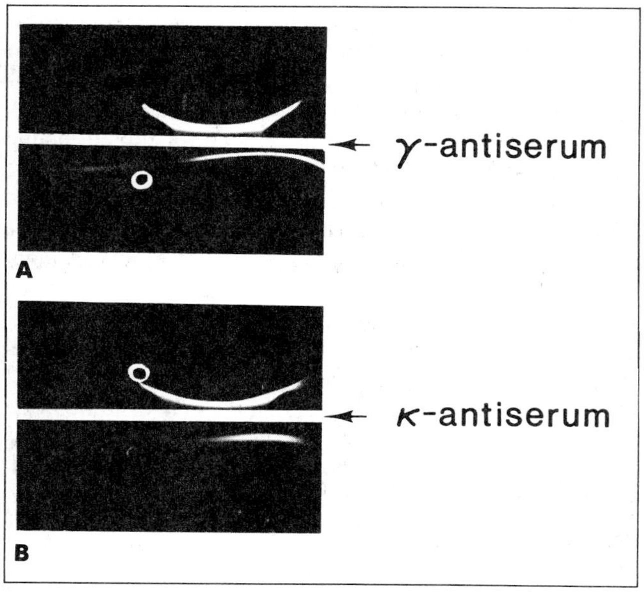

Fig. 75-3. Immunoelectrophoretic pattern obtained in myeloma. **A,** Antiserum to IgG (γ) shows thickened arc from a patient's serum *(top well);* for comparison, normal arc from normal serum is also shown *(bottom well).* **B,** Antiserum to κ chains shows thickened arc that is similar to IgG arc *(top well);* for comparison, note normal arc from normal serum *(bottom well).* Conclusion: patient's serum contains IgG (κ). (From Kyle RA and Greipp PR: Mayo Clin Proc 53:719, 1978. Reproduced with permission of Mayo Foundation.)

Immunofixation

Immunofixation is often useful when results of immunoelectrophoresis are equivocal. An appropriately diluted serum sample is placed in a small trough in 1% agarose. Electrophoresis is performed, and immediately afterward, monospecific antiserum is placed over the electrophoresed proteins. The excess protein is removed by washing, and bands corresponding to an antigen-antibody complex remain. The preparation is stained and read. A sharp, well-defined band with a single heavy-chain class and light-chain type is indicative of a monoclonal protein. A polyclonal increase in immunoglobulins appears as a broad, diffuse, heavily stained band with all heavy-chain antisera and both κ and λ antisera. Care is necessary because overdilution of the sample results in loss of a monoclonal band, whereas an inadequate dilution may obscure the presence of a small monoclonal heavy or light chain in serum with normal background immunoglobulins. A prominent polyclonal band may be misinterpreted as a monoclonal protein.

Immunofixation is helpful when one suspects a monoclonal protein and finds only bowing of a single heavy-chain class or a single light-chain type on immunoelectrophoresis. A bowed light-chain arc may be absent when a monoclonal IgG, IgA, or IgM arc is present. Immunofixation is most helpful in the recognition of a biclonal gammopathy (Fig. 75-4) and for the detection of a small monoclonal protein in the presence of normal or polyclonal immunoglobulins. It is particularly useful in successfully treated myeloma or macroglobulinemia when no spike occurs on electrophoresis, in suspected amyloidosis, or in an apparently solitary plasmacytoma after radiation.

Immunofixation is more sensitive than immunoelectrophoresis and therefore helpful in recognizing small monoclonal proteins. Despite the obvious advantages of immunofixation, immunoelectrophoresis is useful as the initial procedure because it is technically easier and less expensive.

Identification of monoclonal proteins with a rate nephelometer

Monoclonal proteins can be identified without immunoelectrophoresis or immunofixation. The rate nephelometer, with use of monospecific anti-κ and anti-λ and the appropriate heavy-chain antisera, has been used successfully to detect the light-chain type of large monoclonal gammopathies. However, small monoclonal proteins will have a normal κ:λ ratio and will not be recognized. Thus one must be aware that small monoclonal proteins, particularly IgG κ, may be overlooked in a determination of κ:λ ratios with a rate nephelometer. Furthermore, in patients with biclonal gammopathy, the diagnosis frequently will be incorrect.

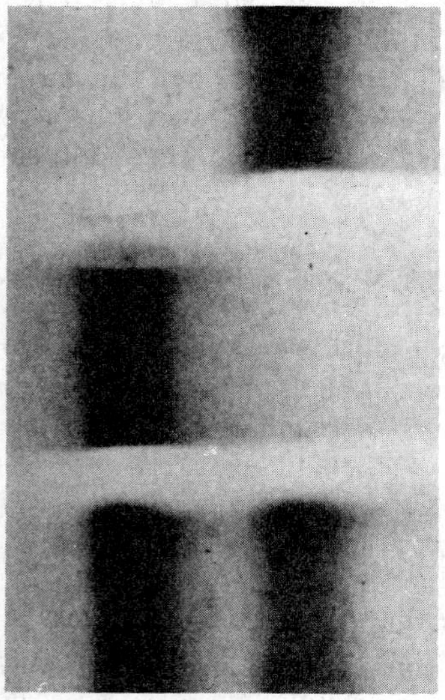

Fig. 75-4. Immunofixation of serum. *Top,* Dense band with IgG (γ) antiserum; *middle,* dense band with IgA (α) antiserum; *bottom,* two dense bands with κ antiserum. This patient has biclonal gammopathy (IgG κ and IgA κ). (From Kyle RA and Garton JP: Semin Oncol 13:310, 1986. Reproduced with permission of WB Sanders.)

Immunoblotting

In combination with high-resolution electrophoresis on agarose, immunoblotting may detect monoclonal proteins in concentrations as low as 0.5 mg/L. In one series, immunoblotting detected a monoclonal protein in three fourths of patients older than 95 years in whom electrophoresis and immunofixation failed to find a monoclonal protein.

Quantitation of immunoglobulins

For the diagnosis of hypogammaglobulinemia, the quantitation of immunoglobulins is more useful than either immunoelectrophoresis or immunofixation. The use of a rate nephelometer is practical for quantitation of immunoglobulins. In this system the degree of turbidity produced by antigen-antibody interaction is measured by nephelometry in the near-ultraviolet region. Because the method is not affected by molecular size of the antigen (as is radial immunodiffusion), the nephelometric technique accurately measures 7S IgM, polymers of IgA, and aggregates of IgG.

Radial immunodiffusion is tedious and subject to spurious abnormalities and is not recommended. For example, low-molecular-weight (7S) IgM will produce a spuriously elevated value because its rate of diffusion is greater than that of the 19S IgM used as a standard. Alternatively, spuriously low levels for IgA may occur because of polymeric IgA, which produces less diffusion than the 7S IgA used as a standard.

Serum viscometry

Serum viscometry should be measured in every patient with more than 3 g/dl of IgM monoclonal protein or more than 4 g/dl of IgA or IgG protein and in any patient with oronasal bleeding, blurred vision, or neurologic symptoms suggestive of a hyperviscosity syndrome. The Ostwald-100 viscometer is a satisfactory instrument for this purpose. Distilled water and serum are made to flow separately through a capillary tube; the quotient of the flow duration (serum divided by water) is the viscosity value (normal, <1.6). The Wells-Brookfield viscometer is preferred because it is more accurate and requires less serum (about 1.0 ml) and because the procedure can be done quickly and performed at different shear rates and different temperatures. Symptoms of hyperviscosity are rare unless the value is more than 4 centipoises (normal, <1.8). Some patients with a value of 10 centipoises or more do not have symptoms of hyperviscosity.

ANALYSIS OF URINE FOR MONOCLONAL PROTEINS

Screening tests

When patients with serum gammopathies are studied, the urine should also be analyzed (Chapter 339). The use of sulfosalicylic acid, or Exton's test, is best for the detection of protein. Sulfosalicylic acid detects albumin and globulin, Bence Jones protein, polypeptides, and proteases. False-positive reactions may be induced by penicillin or its derivatives, tolbutamide metabolites, sulfisoxazole metabolites, and organic roentgenographic contrast media.

Dipstick tests are used in many laboratories to screen for protein. The dipstick is impregnated with a buffered indicator dye that binds to protein in the urine and produces a color change proportional to the amount of protein bound to it. However, dipsticks are often insensitive to Bence Jones protein and should not be used when a possibility of Bence Jones proteinuria exists. Almost from the time of the discovery of the unique thermal properties of urinary light chains (Bence Jones protein), screening tests have been used for their detection. All such tests have serious shortcomings, and the heat test is not recommended. Both false-positive and false-negative results occur. The diagnosis of Bence Jones proteinuria depends on the demonstration of a monoclonal light chain by electrophoresis and either immunoelectrophoresis or immunofixation of an adequately concentrated aliquot from a 24-hour urine specimen (see Fig. 75-2).

Electrophoresis

Electrophoresis of urine should be performed on all patients with a large monoclonal serum protein or the diagnosis of suspected multiple myeloma, macroglobulinemia, amyloidosis, or related diseases.

Before electrophoresis, a 24-hour urine collection is needed to determine the total amount of protein excreted

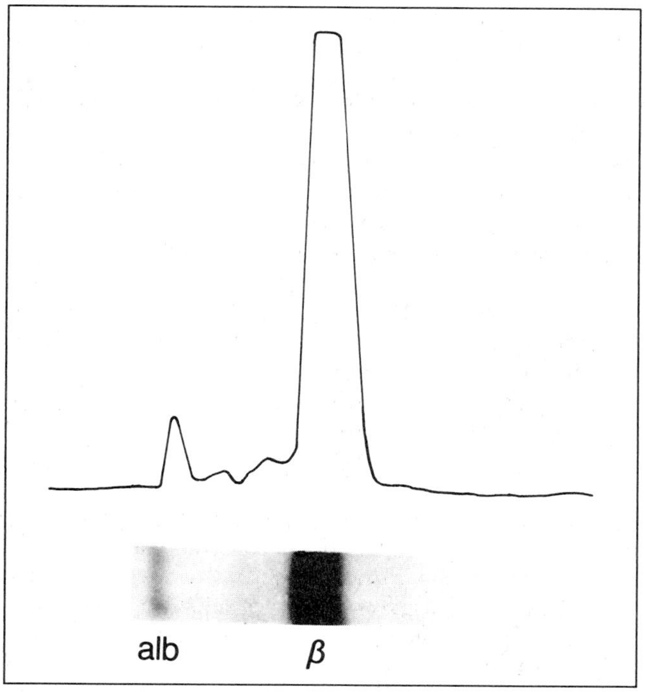

Fig. 75-5. Monoclonal urine protein. *Top,* Densitometer tracing showing a tall, narrow-based peak of β mobility; *bottom,* cellulose acetate electrophoretic pattern showing a dense band of β mobility. This is consistent with a monoclonal urine protein (Bence Jones protein). (From Kyle RA and Garton JP: Semin Oncol 13:310, 1986. Reproduced with permission of WB Sanders.)

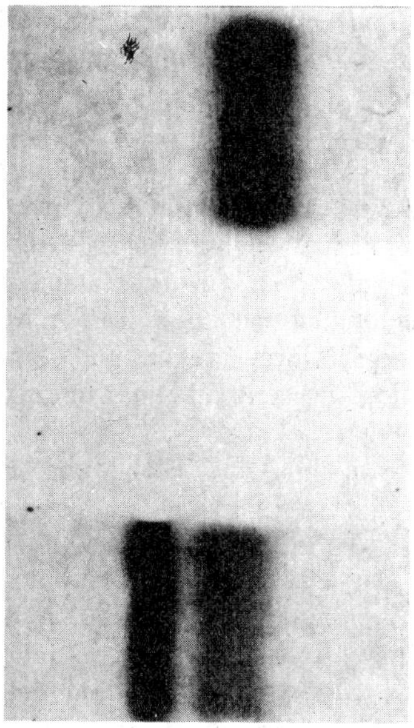

Fig. 75-6. Immunofixation of urine. *Top,* Narrow, localized band with IgA (α) antiserum; *middle,* no reaction with κ antiserum; *bottom,* two discrete bands with λ antiserum. This patient has a monoclonal λ protein plus an IgA λ fragment. (From Kyle RA and Garton JP: Semin Oncol 13:310, 1986. Reproduced with permission of WB Sanders.)

per day. This collection is important when following the course of a patient because the amount of urinary monoclonal protein (size of spike on densitometer tracing × g protein/24 hr) correlates directly with the size of the plasma cell burden.

A urinary monoclonal protein appears as a dense, localized band on the cellulose strip and as a tall, narrow peak on the densitometer tracing (Fig. 75-5). Occasionally, two discrete globulin bands are seen, and these may represent either monomers and dimers of the monoclonal light chain or a monoclonal light chain plus a monoclonal immunoglobulin fragment from the serum (Fig. 75-6). Rarely, two monoclonal light chains (κ and λ, biclonal) have been found in the urine.

Immunoelectrophoresis or immunofixation

Either of these techniques should be performed on the urine of any patient with a serum monoclonal protein and on the urine of all patients with suspected monoclonal gammopathy, even if the sulfosalicylic acid test is negative. The tests should also be performed on the urine of every adult in whom a nephrotic syndrome of unknown cause develops. Most patients with a nephrotic syndrome and a monoclonal light chain in the urine have primary systemic amyloidosis (usually λ) or light-chain deposition disease (usually κ). Immunofixation is more sensitive than immunoelectrophoresis and is most helpful when a monoclonal light chain is present with a polyclonal increase in light chains. Immunofixation is also useful in detecting monoclonal heavy-chain fragments in the urine.

REFERENCES

Howerton DA, Check IJ, and Hunter RL: Densitometric quantitation of high resolution agarose gel protein electrophoresis. Am J Clin Pathol 85:213, 1986.

Jones RG et al: Use of immunoglobulin heavy-chain and light-chain measurements in a multicenter trial to investigate monoclonal components. I. Detection. Clin Chem 37:1917, 1991.

Kyle RA: Classification and diagnosis of monoclonal gammopathies. In Rose NR, Friedman H, and Fahey JL, editors: Manual of clinical laboratory immunology, ed 3. Washington, 1986, American Society for Microbiology.

Kyle RA and Greipp PR: Amyloidosis (AL): clinical and laboratory features in 229 cases. Mayo Clin Proc 58:665, 1983.

Kyle RA, Robinson RA, and Katzmann JA: The clinical aspects of biclonal gammopathies: review of 57 cases. Am J Med 71:999, 1981.

Radl J, Wels J, and Hoogeveen CM: Immunoblotting with (sub)class-specific antibodies reveals a high frequency of monoclonal gammopathies in persons thought to be immunodeficient. Clin Chem 34:1839, 1988.

Roberts RT: Usefulness of immunofixation electrophoresis in the clinical laboratory. Clin Lab Med 6:601, 1986.

Whicher JT et al: The laboratory investigation of paraproteinaemia. Ann Clin Biochem 24:119, 1987.

Whicher JT, Wallage M, and Fifield R: Use of immunoglobulin heavy- and light-chain measurements compared with existing techniques as a means of typing monoclonal immunoglobulins. Clin Chem 33:1771, 1987.

Wolf PL: Interpretation of electrophoretic patterns of serum proteins. Clin Lab Med 6:441, 1986.

CHAPTER

76 Evaluation of Hemostasis and Thrombosis

James N. George
Michael A. Kolodziej

The laboratory methods used to confirm the clinical diagnosis of a bleeding disorder are well established, and a specific etiology should be detected in every patient with severe bleeding. Patients with mild bleeding disorders may be difficult to define by laboratory studies, but newer information is allowing more insight into these problems. In contrast, laboratory evaluation of patients with excessive thrombosis is less likely to yield an explanation for the abnormality, even when the history clearly indicates a recurrent, severe disease. Recent investigations have more clearly defined the natural control mechanisms of coagulation, and congenital abnormalities of this control system that cause an increased risk for thrombosis are now being diagnosed with increased frequency.

PLATELETS AND PLATELET FUNCTION

Platelet number

The normal platelet count is about 250 $\times$ 10^9/L, with a range of 150 to 350 $\times$ 10^9/L. With the use of automated particle counters for all blood cell counts, including platelets, many more patients are being detected with mild asymptomatic thrombocytopenia. However, the automated particle counters may report falsely abnormal platelet counts. Falsely low platelet counts can occur with in vitro clumping caused by innocent antibodies that agglutinate platelets in the presence of the standard EDTA anticoagulant or at temperatures less than 37° C. Also, the particle counter may not detect very large platelets in patients with hereditary giant platelet syndromes. Falsely high platelet counts may occur if other cellular fragments, such as leukocyte fragments in leukemia, are not distinguished from platelets by the particle counter. Therefore examination of a routine stained blood smear is essential to confirm an abnormal platelet count. On the proper area of the smear, where the red cells just begin to overlap and their morphology is best, there should be about 7 to 20 platelets per oil immersion ($\times$1000) field. This figure is derived from the fact that in this area, there should be about 200 red cells per oil immersion field and that the normal red cell/platelet ratio in whole blood is about 10 to 30:1.

Evaluation of thrombocytopenia

The first step must be to distinguish decreased marrow production from increased peripheral destruction or splenic sequestration as the cause of thrombocytopenia. To obtain this information, an examination of the bone marrow must be done. In some disorders of increased platelet destruction the appearance of large platelets on the peripheral blood smear has been reported, but this observation is not reproducible or clear enough to be an alternative to bone marrow aspiration. Megakaryocytes, the large precursor cells of platelets, are easily identified on marrow smears, but they cannot be quantified without special techniques. However, estimates of megakaryocyte frequency are sufficient. If megakaryocytes are difficult to locate in an adequately cellular marrow smear, thrombocytopenia is most likely caused by decreased production. If megakaryocytes are plentiful, it can be assumed that they are functioning normally and that thrombocytopenia is caused by peripheral platelet destruction or splenic sequestration. Megakaryocyte morphology has no clinical significance in this evaluation.

Bleeding time

The template bleeding time is performed with devices that can make a reproducible skin incision 1 mm deep and several millimeters long. With these small wounds, the primary hemostatic mechanisms involving platelets and blood vessels can stop the bleeding almost independently of coagulation reactions. For standardization, a blood pressure cuff is inflated to 40 mm Hg to cause capillary filling and to ensure bleeding. Normal values are about 3 to 8 minutes. A platelet count of more than 75 $\times$ 10^9/L is sufficient to allow a normal bleeding time. A bleeding time test is rarely indicated when the platelet count is less than this because bleeding time is often prolonged and rarely yields clinically useful information. A normal bleeding time provides confidence that platelet function is normal.

Prolonged bleeding times are difficult to interpret. Elderly or malnourished patients may have a long bleeding time because of poor cutaneous elasticity. Some normal people may have a prolonged bleeding time because of aspirin or certain antibiotics and yet have a normal hemostatic response to surgical trauma. Although the bleeding time is clearly an important *diagnostic* aid for disorders affecting platelet function, such as von Willebrand's disease, its value in *predicting* the risk of bleeding in normal subjects is unknown. In some typical situations, such as uremia and the use of high doses of penicillin and related beta-lactam antibiotics, a prolonged bleeding time does *not* predict an increased risk for hemorrhage.

Evaluation of von Willebrand factor concentration, structure, and function

Abnormal platelet function may result from an intrinsic platelet defect or a deficiency or abnormality of plasma von Willebrand factor, which is required for normal platelet adhesion to subendothelium. Therefore investigation of a disorder of primary hemostasis must include an evaluation of plasma von Willebrand factor. Von Willebrand factor is a very large multimeric protein, reaching the enormous molecular size of 12 million daltons and potential length, 1.5 μm! The concentration of von Willebrand factor in plasma can be measured by immunoassays. In some genetic variants of von Willebrand's disease, the highest-molecular-weight multimers—the most hemostatically effective molecules—are missing, even though the plasma concentration is in the normal range. This can be assessed by sodium dodecyl sulfate agarose gel electrophoresis of the plasma sample and identification of the von Willebrand factor multimers by autoradiography after incubating the gel with ^{125}I-labeled anti–von Willebrand factor. Fig. 76-1 demonstrates this technique and illustrates the abnormalities of von Willebrand factor in different variants of von Willebrand's disease.

The function of von Willebrand factor is assessed indirectly by the use of ristocetin-induced platelet agglutination. Ristocetin is an antibiotic that was withdrawn from clinical use more than 30 years ago because of its association with thrombocytopenia. Later it was recognized that ristocetin in vitro agglutinated all platelets except those from subjects with a severe deficiency of von Willebrand factor and subjects with Bernard-Soulier syndrome, who lack platelet membrane glycoprotein Ib-IX, a receptor for von Willebrand factor. Ristocetin-induced platelet agglutination using the patient's platelet-rich plasma can be used as a screening test. The standard ristocetin concentration of 1.5 mg/ml should cause rapid agglutination of normal platelets. Paradoxically, in some variant forms of von Willebrand's disease, such as type IIB, increased reactivity with ristocetin is clearly abnormal; platelet agglutination is strong at ristocetin concentrations of 0.3 to 0.5 mg/ml, well below the concentrations necessary to induce the agglutination of normal platelets.

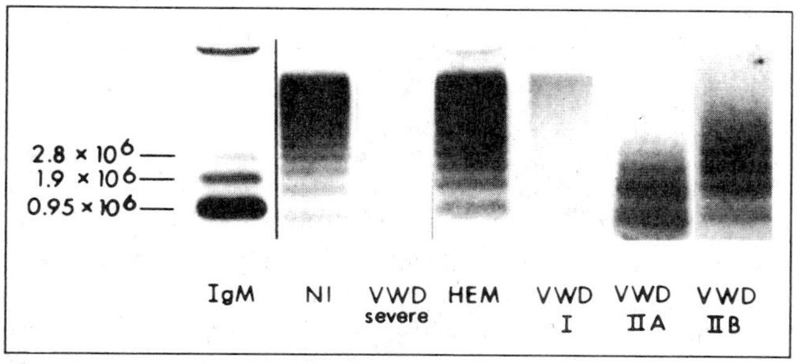

Fig. 76-1. The polymer pattern of human plasma von Willebrand factor analyzed by sodium dodecyl sulfate (SDS)–agarose electrophoresis. The migration of proteins proceeds from the top to the bottom of these gels, with smaller molecules moving farther toward the bottom. Immunoglobulin M (IgM) and IgM polymers are shown in the left gel, and their molecular weights are noted. After electrophoresis of plasma samples, the gels were incubated with ^{125}I-labeled rabbit anti–human von Willebrand factor, and the plasma von Willebrand factor was identified by autoradiography. From the left, these plasma samples are from (1) a normal individual *(NI),* with a predominance of high-molecular-weight polymers; (2) a patient with severe von Willebrand's disease *(VWD)* and no demonstrable plasma von Willebrand factor; (3) a patient with severe hemophilia A *(HEM),* factor VIII deficiency, and normal plasma von Willebrand factor; (4) a patient with type I VWD and a diminished concentration of plasma von Willebrand factor that has the normal polymer size distribution; (5) a patient with type IIA VWD with a selective deficiency of the large and intermediate-size polymers of plasma von Willebrand factor; and (6) a patient with type IIB VWD with a selective deficiency of the largest polymers of plasma von Willebrand factor. (From Hoyer LW: Blood 58:1, 1981. Reproduced with permission.)

Von Willebrand factor function is more accurately evaluated by measurements with the patient's plasma, referred to as *ristocetin-cofactor assays.* Normal platelets fixed with formalin provide a stable reagent. (The term *agglutination* is used because ristocetin causes clumping of formalin-fixed platelets, in contrast to *aggregation,* which requires active metabolic participation of the platelets.) In this assay the washed normal formalin-fixed platelets are mixed with a dilution of patient plasma and ristocetin, and platelet clumping is evaluated by aggregometer tracings or simply by determining the time required for the formation of visible clumps. The principle is the same as that used for assays of coagulation factors except that the end-point is platelet clumping rather than fibrin clot formation. By comparing different dilutions of patient plasma with normal plasma, a result can be expressed as a percentage of normal ristocetin cofactor (von Willebrand factor) activity. The rare patients with acquired inhibitors of (antibodies to) von Willebrand factor can be detected by mixing patient plasma and normal plasma, similar to coagulation assays. If an inhibitor is present, normal plasma will not correct the deficient ristocetin cofactor activity.

Platelet aggregation studies

Normal platelets can be aggregated by several physiologic agonists: adenosine diphosphate, epinephrine, collagen, and thrombin. The platelet response to each of these agents is similar: shape change from the normal compact disk to a spiny sphere, fibrinogen binding to the platelet surface, aggregation, and secretion. These studies are performed in platelet-rich plasma prepared from citrate-anticoagulated whole blood, which is placed in a cuvette and mechanically stirred at 37° C. The response is detected by an increase in light transmission through the cuvette as the platelet clumping causes clearing of the plasma. Platelet aggregation studies are performed in patients who have a prolonged bleeding time and a normal or near-normal platelet count. In some patients, two phases of platelet aggregation, termed *primary* and *secondary,* can be distinguished on the light transmission response. The primary wave occurs because of direct interaction between the platelets and agonists and is reversible. The secondary wave occurs with endogenous granule secretion and is irreversible. Collagen causes only a secondary wave of aggregation after a lag phase.

Aspirin and other inhibitors of platelet thromboxane synthesis prevent normal platelet secretion by low concentrations of agonists and cause defective secondary aggregation. Since aspirin has an irreversible effect on platelets, patients must be studied after they have refrained from taking aspirin or related drugs for 10 days, the survival time of normal platelets. This is a difficult requirement because aspirin is ingested so frequently. Platelet defects associated with impairment of secretion or with a deficiency of granule contents may be associated with aggregation abnormalities similar to those caused by aspirin. The most striking abnormality occurs in the rare hereditary platelet membrane glycoprotein defect, Glanzmann thrombasthenia, in which no macroscopic aggregation occurs in response to any of these four agonists.

Although they are popular in many laboratories, the usefulness of platelet aggregation studies is difficult to assess. The ubiquitous use of aspirin must be emphasized, and platelets from some normal people may not respond well to epinephrine or collagen. Moreover, various collagen preparations cause different responses, and the responses to each of the agonists depend on the agonist concentration. No standardized method of quantitation exists. Finally, it is not known if abnormal aggregation predicts an increased risk for clinically important bleeding.

Platelet coagulant activity

With certain in vitro conditions in which platelets are disrupted or activated by contact with a foreign surface, platelet-rich plasma clots more rapidly than platelet-free plasma. Part of this platelet property seems attributable to membrane phospholipid and is possibly related to the specific interaction between platelets and coagulation factors VIIIa and IXa in the activation of factor X and factors Va and Xa in the activation of prothrombin. Tests of platelet coagulant activity are widely used, but they can be interpreted only qualitatively.

The simplest test to perform in a clinical laboratory, and therefore the best screening assay, is the serum prothrombin time (PT), which seems to reflect primarily the platelet contribution to coagulation. The PT is measured in serum after whole blood is allowed to clot in a glass tube for 1 hour at 37° C. In normal subjects the serum PT is more than twice as long as the PT time in plasma (i.e., >25 seconds), whereas in disorders of platelet coagulant activity, the serum PT may be similar to the PT time with plasma. In another common test, referred to as *platelet factor 3 availability,* citrate-anticoagulated platelet-rich plasma is activated by kaolin, and the clotting time is measured after recalcification.

PLASMA COAGULATION

Laboratory evaluation of plasma coagulation is based on a series of tests that activate the coagulation sequence at different sites. The activating substances have been developed empirically and their use established by clinical experience. However, it should never be forgotten that these in vitro assessments of plasma coagulation are useful artifacts and that they may be very different from the in vivo events. The coagulation scheme as tested by typical coagulation assays is shown in Fig. 76-2. Note the differences from the coagulation scheme presented for normal in vivo hemostasis in Fig. 70-2. The activators used for the partial thromboplastin time (PTT) initiate the reaction at factor XII, and a normal PTT requires three factors that are unnecessary for hemostasis in vivo: factor XII, prekallikrein, and high-molecular-weight kininogen. Moreover, platelets are not required in these reactions because exogenous phospholipid is supplied. The PTT and the PT have different sensitivities to the same defect in their common pathway. For example, the PTT is more sensitive to the inhibitory effect of heparin (which inactivates thrombin and factor Xa, as well as factors IXa, XIa, and VIIa) and the inhibitor that occurs in systemic lupus erythematosus (which inhibits the reaction of factors X, V, and II), whereas the PT is often more sensitive to the abnormalities in liver disease (which reduce the concentration of most coagulation factors). In addition, the sensitivities of the PTT and PT to coagulation factor deficiencies also vary, depending on the commercial source of the reagents. Despite these problems, both tests are valuable contributors to the evaluation of hemostasis because they provide useful information: they usually become abnormal at levels of coagulation factor deficiencies that are associated with clinical bleeding.

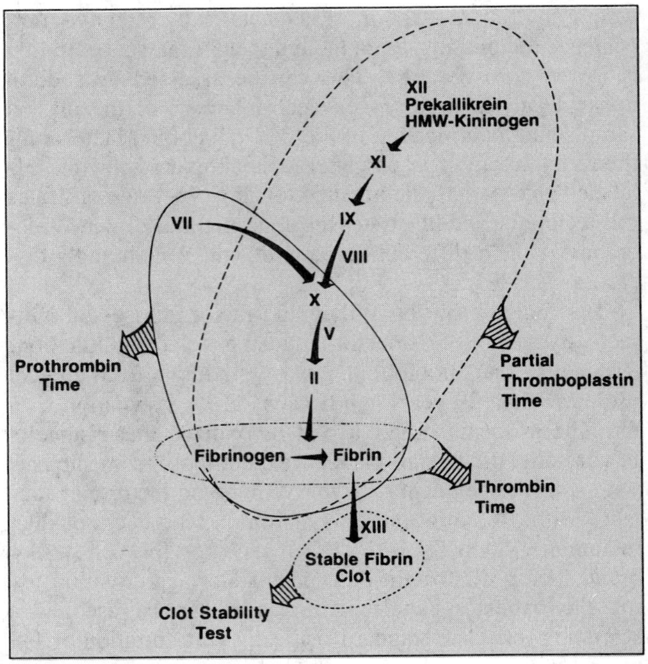

Fig. 76-2. Plasma coagulation reactions in in vitro laboratory assays. Note the differences between this diagram and Fig. 70-2. Factor XII, prekallikrein, and high-molecular-weight kininogen are required for a normal partial thromboplastin time but not for normal in vivo hemostasis. Also, plasma factor XI may not always be required for normal in vivo hemostasis. Platelets and tissue factor are required for normal in vivo hemostasis but are supplied by exogenous reagents in the laboratory assays. This diagram outlines the coagulation factors required for each of four basic tests.

For all coagulation assays, blood collection is critical. Citrate anticoagulant is used to provide mild calcium chelation. EDTA reduces the calcium concentration to a level that irreversibly inactivates factors V and VIII and thereby prevents subsequent assessment of plasma coagulation. Heparin, an inhibitor of coagulation, is unsatisfactory. Since some coagulation factors are labile, the assays must be performed promptly on fresh or fresh-frozen plasma. Normal control plasma is always simultaneously assayed because these tests are vulnerable to artifacts of technique and their results cannot be expressed in absolute units.

Partial thromboplastin time

The name of this test was derived from studies of various "thromboplastins" more than 40 years ago, when it was thought that these coagulation-stimulating tissue extracts represented materials actually involved in in vivo coagulation. Therefore, when certain extracts were shown to correct the coagulation defect of hemophilic plasma, it was thought that missing factors were replaced, and these materials were termed *complete thromboplastins*. Extracts that did not correct the hemophilic defect were termed *partial thromboplastins*. Subsequently, these tissue extracts were shown to activate the coagulation sequence at different points, factors VII and XII, respectively.

The current standard test is referred to as an *activated* PTT because of the inclusion of a reagent (e.g., silica) that activates factor XII. This is a distinction from the original PTT assays, which depended on the glass tube to induce activation and were subject to much greater variability. The PTT is a good screening test for coagulation abnormalities except for factors VII and XIII. Its level of sensitivity is best known for factor VIII because it is usually prolonged when factor VIII levels are below 20%. Since this is also the factor VIII concentration associated with a risk of bleeding after trauma, the PTT is a good screening test for detecting mild hemophilia and is presumably also an effective screening test for other coagulation disorders. However, patients with mild hemophilia, who may have significant bleeding after trauma, may sometimes have a normal PTT. The normal values for the PTT depend on the specific reagent used and the incubation conditions, and the normal range is relatively broad, usually about 20 to 40 seconds. The significance of an abnormally fast PTT is unclear, but in some cases it may result from activated coagulation factors in the plasma and may be associated with an increased risk for thrombosis.

Prothrombin time

The PT was originally described by Quick in 1935, when the other factors involved in this test (factors VII, X, and V) were unknown. This is a highly reproducible assay with a normal value of 9 to 13 seconds using the conventional American tissue factor reagent, an acetone extract of rabbit brain that is very rich in tissue factor. In most laboratories a difference of more than 3 seconds from the control value is significant. Based on Fig. 76-2, a combination of an abnormal PT with a normal PTT appears to be diagnostic of a factor VII abnormality. This is not necessarily true, however, and this observation is common in patients with liver disease or vitamin K deficiency in whom multiple coagulation factors are deficient. The only explanation is the difference in inherent sensitivities of these two assays.

The PT is used for the control of warfarin anticoagulation because the results are very reproducible. However, commercial PT thromboplastin reagents vary widely in their sensitivity to warfarin-induced deficiencies of factors II, VII, IX, and X activity. Therefore all reagents are now standardized, and an accurate description of the intensity of warfarin anticoagulation must express the PT as an International Normalized Ratio (INR) (Chapter 86).

Thrombin time

The thrombin time is simply the measurement of the fibrin clotting time after the addition of bovine thrombin. In theory this test may seem to be unnecessary, since both the PTT and the PT involve fibrin formation. In fact, the thrombin time is much more sensitive than either of the other two assays to abnormalities of the thrombin-fibrinogen interaction and subsequent fibrin polymerization. For example, the thrombin time is very sensitive to heparin anticoagulation (too sensitive to be clinically useful), deficiencies of fibrinogen, and abnormalities of fibrin polymerization such as those caused by fibrin degradation products, myeloma paraproteins, or congenital dysfibrinogenemias.

Fibrinogen concentration

The plasma concentration of fibrinogen is frequently and rapidly measured by comparing the thrombin time of various dilutions of patient plasma with a control plasma sample of known fibrinogen concentration. When heparin is present or abnormalities of fibrinogen are suspected, immunoassays can be done.

Clot stability test

All the standard coagulation tests measure the time needed to form a fibrin clot. The subsequent conversion of this fibrin polymer into a permanent, covalently bonded structure is essential to form a firm clot in vivo but is not required for normal clotting times. The clot stability test evaluates the function of factor XIII, the enzyme that catalyzes the formation of covalent bonds within the fibrin polymer. Citrate plasma is clotted by thrombin, and the clot is then incubated with urea or monochloroacetic acid, agents that can dissolve the hydrogen bonds of the initial fibrin polymer but cannot break covalent bonds. This test may also be abnormal in the presence of inhibitors of factor XIII or with abnormal fibrin polymerization.

Specific coagulation factor assays

These assays are based on the PTT (for prekallikrein, high-molecular-weight kininogen, factors XII, XI, IX, and VIII) or the PT (for factors VII, X, V, and II). In each case the assay requires a plasma sample that is deficient in the single coagulation factor to be measured. Then various dilutions of the patient plasma or a normal control plasma are added, and the clotting time is measured. Curves are constructed, and the activity of the patient plasma is compared with the normal control, which is assigned an arbitrary value of 100%, or 1.0 U/ml of the coagulation factor. For example, to assay factor VIII, a series of PTTs is performed. Each assay tube contains plasma from a patient with severe hemophilia (less than 1% of normal factor VIII activity) and dilutions of normal or patient plasma, usually between 1:10 and 1:500. If the patient has a 50% level of factor VIII (0.5 U/ml), the clotting time with a 1:10 dilution of plasma will be the same as the clotting time of a 1:20 dilution of normal plasma. If the patient has a 5% level of factor VIII (0.5 U/ml), the clotting time of his or her 1:10 diluted plasma will be the same as the clotting time of normal plasma diluted 1:200.

Screening test for coagulation inhibitors

An abnormality of any coagulation factor can be caused by a lack of activity of the factor or by an inhibitor of the activated factor. The inhibitors may be antibodies to a coagulation factor, heparin-like molecules, or proteins that interfere with fibrin polymerization, such as fibrin degradation products or myeloma paraproteins. In some patients, both a deficiency and an inhibitor are present, as in the 10% of patients with severe hemophilia who develop antibodies to normal factor VIII after repeated transfusions. The detection of an inhibitor is critical because replacement therapy is difficult or impossible when an inhibitor is present. For example, a patient with a very prolonged PTT may have a deficiency of factor VIII and/or an acquired inhibitor of factor VIII. When the PTT is repeated using a 1:1 mixture of patient and normal plasma, the abnormality is corrected if only a deficiency exists and the clotting time is similar to that of a 1:1 mixture of normal plasma and saline (see the box on p. 792 in Chapter 83). An inhibitor will inactivate some or all of the factor VIII activity in the normal plasma, just as it will the factor VIII in the patient's plasma, and therefore the clotting time of the mixture will be prolonged.

Screening test for fibrinolysis: measurement of fibrin degradation products

Plasmin activation is most easily assessed by measuring the products of plasmin digestion of fibrin. The simplest assays are based on most fibrin degradation products not being incorporated into a fibrin clot and remaining soluble in serum. Therefore the blood samples are collected in special tubes that have excess thrombin to ensure complete clotting, plus an inhibitor of in vitro fibrinolysis. Serum is collected, and fibrinogen-related antigens are measured by an immunoassay. This is not an entirely satisfactory assay, however, and the artifacts that may occur during serum preparation can be avoided by performing the immunoassays on whole plasma, using antibodies that recognize new antigens that are formed or exposed during plasmin digestion of fibrin and are specific for fibrin degradation products.

SCREENING TESTS FOR THROMBOTIC DISORDERS

Risk factors for thrombotic disease are primarily abnormalities of blood flow or blood vessels; abnormalities of blood coagulation are less apparent. In most persons with thrombosis, specific laboratory variations indicating blood coagulation abnormalities cannot be identified. However, in some patients, screening tests for abnormal regulation of coagulation may be indicated: patients with recurrent thrombotic disease without clinically apparent risk factors, with thrombosis in an unusual site, with thrombosis at an early age, or with a familial tendency for recurrent thromboembolism. Even in these carefully defined populations, however, abnormalities of the blood coagulation system that may contribute to an increased risk for thrombosis are identified in less than 10% of patients.

Among the coagulation factors recognized as important for the regulation of hemostasis, commercially available assays are available for antithrombin III, protein C, and protein S. These assays generally measure the plasma protein concentration of these factors rather than their functional activity, although the more important functional assays are becoming available. Assays for plasminogen and antiphospholipid antibodies, including the "lupus anticoagulant," are also frequently employed in the evaluation of persons with recurrent thrombotic disease. In many laboratories, this battery of tests is referred to as a *hypercoagulable profile*. Unfortunately, interpretation of these assays' results can be equivocal, and indiscriminate use must be discouraged. For example, levels of antithrombin III fall after administration of therapeutic heparin, and levels of protein C and protein S fall after therapeutic administration of warfarin. Analysis of these proteins' levels after therapeutic anticoagulation therefore is difficult, if not impossible. A second major problem is that abnormalities of these proteins have been well documented in normal asymptomatic subjects. Thus the identification of an isolated abnormality raises the difficult question of the need for anticoagulation therapy. In fact, the need for therapy must be determined on the basis of clinical, not laboratory, data.

Newer laboratory assays that measure the activity of the coagulation system are being developed for evaluation of patients prone to thrombosis. An example is the measurement of the plasma concentration of peptides released on enzymatic activation of coagulation factors, such as measurement of a peptide fragment designated $F_{1.2}$, which is released from prothrombin when it is converted to thrombin. The objective of these assays is to assess the procoagulant reactions, which may be increased in patients with thrombotic disease. The clinical roles of these screening tests are not yet known.

REFERENCES

Bauer KA and Rosenberg RD: The pathophysiology of the prethrombotic state in humans: insights gained from studies using markers of hemostatic system activation. Blood 70:343, 1987.

Garcia-Suarez J et al: EDTA-dependent pseudothrombocytopenia in ambulatory patients: clinical characteristics and role of new automated cell-counting in its detection. Am J Hematol 39:146, 1992.

George JN and Shattil SJ: The clinical importance of acquired abnormalities of platelet function. N Engl J Med 324:27, 1991.

Lind SE: The bleeding time does not predict surgical bleeding. Blood 77:2547, 1991.

Mielke CH: Aspirin prolongation of the template bleeding time: influence of venostasis and direction of incision. Blood 60:1139, 1982.

Onder O, Weinstein A, and Hoyer LW: Pseudothrombocytopenia caused by platelet agglutinins that are reactive in blood anticoagulated with chelating agents. Blood 56:177, 1980.
Rodgers RPC and Levin J: A critical reappraisal of the bleeding time. Semin Thromb Hemost 16:1, 1990.
Suchman AL and Griner PF: Diagnostic uses of the activated partial thromboplastin time and prothrombin time. Ann Intern Med 104:810, 1986.

III SPECIAL TOPICS

CHAPTER

77 Blood Transfusion

Jay E. Menitove

WHOLE BLOOD AND RED CELL TRANSFUSION

Whole blood

Whole blood units contain approximately 500 ml and have hematocrits of 35% to 40%. Red blood cells (RBCs), or packed cells, are prepared by removing plasma from whole blood and adding 100 ml of a solution containing saline and nutrient. The resultant volume is approximately 325 ml and the hematocrit 55% to 65%. The expected posttransfusion hematocrit or hemoglobin increase for adults is 3% or 1 g/dl, respectively, per unit.

Whole blood is indicated for symptomatic patients requiring concomitant correction of oxygen-carrying and intravascular volume deficits not corrected by previous administration of crystalloid or colloid solutions. RBC transfusions are indicated when a deficiency in oxygen-carrying capacity exists and compensatory mechanisms are insufficient to alleviate signs and symptoms of anemia, such as syncope, dyspnea, postural hypotension, tachycardia, angina, or cerebral hypoxia.

In the past, clinicians used a preset number, or "transfusion trigger," as the basis for transfusing RBCs, such as the "10/30" rule, a hemoglobin of 10 g/dl or a hematocrit of 30%. This obsolete approach was supplanted by an emphasis on transfusion avoidance in the absence of symptoms attributable to anemia. Treatment with iron, vitamin B_{12}, folate, or in selected patients, recombinant erythropoietin should precede transfusion unless anemia renders the patient unstable. Patients with cardiovascular disorders, advanced age, significant pulmonary disease, or cerebrovascular insufficiency may show symptoms at higher levels, but most patients tolerate hemoglobin concentrations of 7 to 10 g/dl.

Leukocyte-depleted red blood cells

Adhesion filters or "third-generation" leukocyte reduction filters remove at least 99% to 99.9% of the 2 to 5 $\times$ 10^9 leukocytes contained in each unit of RBCs. This is at least a tenfold greater reduction than is needed to prevent febrile, nonhemolytic transfusion reactions. The filters effectively deter transmission of cytomegalovirus by cellular blood components. However, it is unproved if they preclude or delay alloimmunization against HLA antigens (human leukocyte antigens) in patients with acute leukemia or aplastic anemia.

Washed red blood cells

Washing RBCs with normal saline by manual or semiautomated techniques removes all but small amounts of plasma and reduces the number of leukocytes to approximately 5 $\times$ 10^8/unit RBC. Saline-washed RBCs are used for patients with recurrent or severe anaphylactic or allergic reactions. They should not be used for leukocyte reduction because adhesion filters are significantly more effective.

Frozen deglycerolized red blood cells

RBCs are prepared for frozen storage at $-65°$ C for up to 10 years by adding a cryoprotective agent, glycerol. They are used predominantly to ensure availability of blood with "rare" phenotypes for patients with alloantibodies against frequently occurring RBC antigens. Occasionally, blood collected for autologous purposes is frozen, if the scheduled surgical procedure is postponed.

Autologous transfusion

Autologous transfusion involves collection and subsequent reinfusion of a patient's own blood by one or a combination of three techniques: (1) preoperative blood donation, (2) perioperative blood salvage, or (3) acute normovolemic hemodilution. Preoperative collections should begin at least 2 weeks before a scheduled surgical procedure and can be repeated every 3 days provided the patient's hemoglobin level is greater than 11 g/dl. Patients most likely to benefit from autologous predonation programs include orthopedic, cardiac, and vascular surgery patients and obstetric patients with placenta previa. Preoperative blood donation poses little risk to selected elderly and pediatric patients.

Perioperative *blood salvage* involves the collection and reinfusion of blood lost during and immediately after surgery. Several commercially available instruments are available for providing washed or unwashed blood for reinfusion. Intraoperative blood salvage is not used if the operative field is contaminated by bacteria or tumor.

Acute *normovolemic hemodilution* entails removal of blood immediately before surgery with simultaneous infusion of crystalloid or colloid solutions to maintain vascular volume. After surgery the removed blood is reinfused. This option is not offered to patients with anemia, renal dysfunction, or limited ability to increase cardiac output.

Directed donation

A directed or designated donation refers to blood provided by donors selected by the patient, usually family members or friends. Although many patients believe blood supplied by these donors is less likely to transmit bloodborne infections than that from the general blood supply, available data are not consistent with this hypothesis.

Compatibility testing

Compatibility testing includes determining donor and recipient blood grouping, testing the recipient for RBC alloantibodies, and performing all clerical and documentation procedures. This is accomplished by incubating the patient's serum with RBCs from a donor unit or, more frequently, by screening patient sera for "unexpected" antibodies with reagent RBCs. If unexpected antibodies are not present, blood is released for transfusion after demonstrating the absence of ABO incompatibility. If unexpected antibodies, such as anti-K, $-Jk^a$, $-Fy^a$, or those directed against Rh antigens, are detected, a crossmatch using donor sera and patient RBCs is performed.

PLATELET TRANSFUSION

Platelet concentrates are prepared by separating platelets from a single unit of whole blood or by apheresis techniques using semiautomated blood cell separators. Therapeutic doses for the recipient are prepared by pooling 1 U of platelet concentrates for each 10 kg of the recipient's body weight or by providing a similar number of platelets collected from a single donor by apheresis. The ABO blood group of platelet donor and recipient should be compatible, although this is not required. Compatibility testing is not performed routinely. The expected posttransfusion platelet count increment in the recipient is approximately 50×10^9/L per transfusion.

Platelet transfusion efficacy is related directly to the etiology of thrombocytopenia. Patients with bone marrow hypoplasia are most likely to benefit from a platelet transfusion, whereas those with immune or nonimmune platelet destruction are least likely to achieve significant posttransfusion platelet count increments.

Platelet transfusions are used to control active bleeding or to prevent hemorrhage associated with thrombocytopenia. In general, patients undergoing surgical or other invasive procedures are not considered at risk for significant microvascular bleeding if the platelet count is greater than 50×10^9/L and thrombocytopenia is the sole abnormality.

Prophylactic platelet transfusions are used to prevent bleeding in patients with severe thrombocytopenia secondary to aplastic anemia, acute leukemia, or other disorders. Several cancer chemotherapy protocols consider a platelet count less than 20×10^9/L as an indication for platelet transfusion. This may be appropriate in patients with severe mucositis, emesis, and other acute toxic effects of chemotherapy. However, a stable patient may tolerate platelet counts as low as 5 to 10×10^9/L without significant hemorrhage.

Posttransfusion platelet counts should be obtained 10 to 60 minutes after transfusion and the next day. The immediate posttransfusion platelet count provides information about platelet recovery and is diminished in alloimmunized patients and those with splenomegaly. The posttransfusion platelet count after 18 to 24 hours provides information about platelet survival and is decreased in patients with consumptive processes such as disseminated intravascular coagulation, sepsis, fever, and other inflammatory states.

Alloimmunization and refractoriness to platelet transfusion

Approximately one half of patients requiring long-term platelet support develop antibodies against HLA antigens and become refractory to platelet transfusions. Adequate posttransfusion platelet increments are restored by collecting platelets by apheresis from donors who are HLA-matched to the patient.

Intensive investigation is under way to determine feasible mechanisms for preventing alloimmunization by reducing leukocyte content, restricting donor exposures, using ultraviolet B irradiation, or employing a combination of these methods.

PLASMA TRANSFUSION

Plasma separated from whole blood and frozen within 8 hours of collection contains all coagulation factors.

Fresh-frozen plasma (FFP) is used to increase clotting factor levels in patients with demonstrated deficiencies: a prothrombin time or partial thromboplastin time greater than 1.5 times normal. FFP rapidly reverses the anticoagulant effect of warfarin but should be reserved for patients who are actively bleeding or require emergent surgery and cannot wait approximately 12 hours for the therapeutic effect of vitamin K. FFP is appropriate for patients receiving massive blood transfusion replacement provided laboratory evidence supports a coagulation factor deficiency. FFP is the preferred replacement fluid for patients undergoing therapeutic plasma exchange therapy for thrombotic thrombocytopenic purpura.

GRANULOCYTE TRANSFUSION

Granulocytes are collected by apheresis. Each transfusion contains more than 1.0×10^{10} granulocytes suspended in approximately 200 ml of plasma. Significant numbers of lymphocytes, platelets, and 20 to 50 ml of RBCs are also present.

Currently, granulocyte transfusions are used infrequently because antibiotic therapy is effective and the transfusion dose is relatively small compared with normal daily neutrophil production. Granulocyte transfusion therapy is provided to neutropenic patients (absolute granulocyte count $<0.5 \times 10^9$/L) with documented sepsis who do not respond initially to antibiotic therapy. Transfusions are infused daily for at least 4 days until the infection is controlled or there is evidence of granulocyte recovery.

THERAPEUTIC APHERESIS

Therapeutic apheresis involves the removal of plasma or blood cells for treatment of a disease process.

Plasma exchange

Plasmapheresis combined with infusion of normal saline, plasma protein fraction, albumin, FFP, or a combination of these solutions is referred to as a plasma exchange procedure. A one-volume plasma exchange procedure, which removes two thirds of the initial plasma volume, can be completed in 2 to 3 hours. Procedures are repeated at intervals of 1 to 2 days. Conditions for which therapeutic plasma exchange is considered acceptable therapy include cryoglobulinemia, coagulation factor–inhibitor reduction, Goodpasture's syndrome, Guillain-Barré syndrome, homozygous familial hypercholesterolemia, hyperviscosity syndrome caused by multiple myeloma or Waldenström's macroglobulinemia, myasthenia gravis, posttransfusion purpura, Refsum disease, and thrombotic thrombocytopenic purpura.

Patients in whom plasma exchange therapy is reported to be beneficial as a second-line therapy include those with chronic inflammatory demyelinating polyneuropathy, cold agglutinin disease, hemolytic uremic syndrome, pemphigus vulgaris, rapidly progressive glomerulonephritis, and systemic vasculitis related to rheumatoid arthritis or systemic lupus erythematosus. Drug overdose and poisoning with agents that are bound to proteins are also treated by plasma exchange. Efficacy is not conclusively demonstrated for treatment of patients with ABO-incompatible organ or marrow transplantation, maternal therapy for maternal-fetal incompatibility, thyroid storm, multiple sclerosis, progressive systemic sclerosis, pure RBC aplasia, warm autoimmune hemolytic anemia, or transfusion refractoriness caused by alloantibody.

Current experience indicates a lack of efficacy of plasma exchange for treatment of acquired immunodeficiency syndrome (AIDS), amyotrophic lateral sclerosis, aplastic anemia, fulminant hepatic failure, chronic idiopathic thrombocytopenic purpura, lupus nephritis, polymyositis and dermatomyositis, psoriasis, renal transplant rejection, rheumatoid arthritis, and schizophrenia.

Table 77-1. Acute transfusion reactions

Adverse effect	Signs/symptoms	Approximate frequency per component
Hemolytic reaction	Fever, fever and chills, nausea, vomiting, chest pain, facial flushing	1:6000-25,000
Febrile, nonhemolytic reaction	Fever and chills, headache, chilliness, rigor 15 to 60 minutes after transfusion	1:200
Transfusion-related lung injury	Dyspnea, cyanosis, cough, blood-tinged sputum, fever, chest pain within 4 hours of transfusion	1:5000
Allergic reactions	Hives, pruritus	1:100-300
Anaphylactic reactions	Apprehension, chest pain, facial flushing, urticaria, laryngeal edema, wheezing, dyspnea, hypotension	1:150,000
Bacterial sepsis	Severe chills, rigors, nausea, vomiting, lethargy, fever	Rare

Cytapheresis

Cytapheresis involves the reduction of cellular blood components for disorders such as leukemia with hyperleukocytosis syndromes, sickle cell syndromes (with the possible exception of prophylactic use in pregnancy), and systemic thrombocytosis. Cytapheresis is probably effective in the treatment of a cutaneous T cell lymphoma, hairy cell leukemia, fulminant malaria, peripheral stem cell collection for hematopoietic reconstitution, and rheumatoid arthritis. Anecdotal reports suggest that cytapheresis may play a role in the treatment of patients with life-threatening hemolytic transfusion reactions, multiple sclerosis, and organ transplant rejection and as prophylactic therapy for pregnant patients with sickle cell disease. Lack of efficacy has been demonstrated in patients with leukemia without hyperleukocytosis, hypereosinophilia, and polymyositis or dermatomyositis.

ADVERSE EFFECTS OF TRANSFUSION THERAPY

Acute reactions (Table 77-1)

These complications occur within minutes to hours after infusion of blood or components. Significant overlap in presenting signs and symptoms prevents an accurate assessment of the diagnosis in the absence of appropriate laboratory testing.

Hemolytic reactions. Fever (elevation of at least 2° F [1° C]) or fever and chills are seen in almost all patients with a hemolytic transfusion reaction. The antibodies responsible for causing most hemolytic reactions include anti-A, anti-B, anti-K, anti-Jk^a, anti-Fy^a, anti-D, anti-C, and anti-E.

If a hemolytic reaction is suspected, the infusion must be stopped immediately. The transfusion service must perform a clerical check to ascertain the patient was given the intended unit. A direct antiglobulin test should be performed. Since destruction of only 5 to 10 ml of RBCs renders a hemolytic hue to plasma, a postreaction serum or plasma sample should be examined for a pink or red tinge. In addition, a urine specimen should be examined for the presence of free hemoglobin.

Acute intervention is directed at correction of hypotension, control of bleeding, and prevention of acute tubular necrosis.

Febrile nonhemolytic reactions. These reactions are characterized by fever and chills without hemolysis and are caused by antibodies against transfused lymphocytes, granulocytes, or platelets. The "threshold" leukocyte content for evoking a chill/fever reaction in susceptible patients is approximately 2×10^8 to 2.5×10^9 cells per component. Since the initial manifestation of a hemolytic transfusion reaction is similar to a chill/fever reaction, the transfusion should be discontinued and a laboratory evaluation for hemolysis initiated. A diagnosis of a febrile nonhemolytic reaction is made on the basis of the clinical findings, the absence of hemoglobinemia, and a negative direct antiglobulin test in the postreaction specimen. Treatment consists of supportive measures, including orally administered antipyretics. Since only 15% of patients with a febrile reaction have a recurrence, components with reduced numbers of leukocytes are not provided until a second reaction occurs.

Lung injury. Passive infusion of antibody against recipient leukocytes occasionally causes a noncardiogenic pulmonary edema–like syndrome. The patients require respiratory support, but recovery usually occurs within 48 hours.

Allergic reactions. Hives and pruritus, usually without fever, occur occasionally after a plasma-containing blood component is infused. Treatment with an antihistamine is usually sufficient to alleviate symptoms. Removal of plasma from RBCs and/or platelet transfusions by washing with saline prevents recurrence in severely affected patients.

Anaphylactic reactions, mediated by anti-IgA antibody, require immediate treatment with sympathomimetic drugs. If subsequent transfusions are required, cellular components should be washed to remove plasma.

Bacterial sepsis. Between 1986 and 1991, the U.S. Food and Drug Administration (FDA) received 29 reports of transfusion-related fatalities caused by bacterial contamination; seven involved RBC components infected with *Yersinia enterocolitica*. Contaminated platelets resulted in the death of five patients in 1990 and six in 1991. An aliquot from the component should be examined for bacteria by appropriate staining and culture techniques. Broad-spectrum antibiotics and supportive measures should be administered promptly.

Table 77-2. Delayed transfusion reactions

Adverse effect	Signs/symptoms	Approximate frequency per component
Delayed hemolytic reaction	Anemia, fever, recent transfusion (within 3 to 21 days)	Serologic: 1:300-1600 Hemolytic: 1:1500-8000
Grafts-versus-host disease	Fever, erythema, diarrhea, liver function abnormalities, pancytopenia 4 to 30 days after transfusion	Uncommon
Iron overload	Endocrine, cardiac, and liver dysfunction	Chronically transfused patients (~ 120 units of blood)
Immunosuppression	? Decreased survival after tumor resection ? Increased postoperative infection rate	Unknown

Delayed transfusion reactions (Table 77-2)

Hemolytic reactions. Delayed hemolytic transfusion reactions are the result of alloantibody-mediated RBC destruction by an antibody that is not detected at the time pretransfusion testing is performed. Alloantibody, usually a secondary or amnestic response, is produced 6 to 8 days (range, 3 to 21 days) after transfusion. Fortunately the consequences of the reaction are non-life-threatening, and only supportive therapy is required.

Graft-vs-host disease. Graft-vs-host disease (GVHD) is a result of infused lymphocytes recognizing and reacting against host tissues. The syndrome usually occurs in immunosuppressed patients with conditions such as severe combined immunodeficiency and Wiscott-Aldrich syndrome or in bone marrow transplant patients. Premature newborns and neonates undergoing exchange transfusion who previously received intrauterine transfusions and patients undergoing chemotherapy for Hodgkin's disease, non-Hodgkin's lymphoma, acute leukemia, and neuroblastoma may be at increased risk for transfusion-associated GVHD. Immunocompetent patients who have received transfusions from donors with closely matched HLA types (e.g., blood relatives) may develop GVHD. The mortality rate is approximately 90%. Prevention is accomplished by irradiating blood and components with 2500 rad (25 Gy).

Iron overload. Adult patients infused with 60 to 210 (mean, 120) units of blood may develop endocrine, cardiac, and liver dysfunction as a result of iron overload. Iron chelation therapy has been used successfully to decrease iron stores in some patients.

Immunosuppressive effects. Evidence suggests, but not definitively, that blood transfusion causes impairment of immune function. An increased frequency of tumor recurrence after surgical resection of malignant tumors and an increased incidence of postoperative infection have been reported in transfused patients. Investigation is ongoing to determine whether these postulated effects are causally related to transfusion.

Transfusion-transmitted diseases (Table 77-3)

Hepatitis. The incidence of posttransfusion hepatitis declined from approximately 10% of transfused patients in the late 1970s to approximately 4% in the early 1980s, to 1.5% after introduction of alanine aminotransferase (ALT) and

Table 77-3. Transfusion-transmitted diseases

Disease	Approximate frequency per component
Hepatitis A	Rare
Hepatitis B	1:25,000-200,000
Hepatitis C	1:4000-5000
HIV-1	1:60,000-400,000
HIV-2	No transfusion-associated cases reported
HTLV-I	1:50,000
Cytomegalovirus	?
Syphilis	Rare
Lyme disease	No transfusion-associated cases reported
Babesiosis	Rare
Malaria	Rare
Chagas' disease	Rare

HIV, Human immunodeficiency virus; HTLV, human T cell leukemia/lymphoma virus.

anti–hepatitis B core antigen (anti-HB_c) tests in the mid-1980s, and to approximately 0.6% after introduction of the first-generation anti–hepatitis C virus (HCV) tests in May 1990. Second-generation or multiantigen tests for detecting antibody to HCV were introduced in March 1992. They detect more than 90% of donors potentially infectious for HCV. Despite use of anti-HCV testing, blood donors will continue to be screened for ALT because this liver function test becomes abnormal approximately 2 months before anti-HCV seroconversion.

Occasionally, patients with posttransfusion hepatitis A and hepatitis B are reported. Anti–HB_c testing should interdict donations from donors infected with hepatitis B whose HB_sAg (hepatitis B surface antigen) levels are below detectable levels.

Retroviruses. Blood collection agencies currently test all donated blood for the presence of antibodies to human immunodeficiency viruses 1 and 2 (HIV-1, HIV-2). A recently introduced test detects immunoglobulin M (IgM) in addition to IgG antibodies against HIV-1 and is reactive sooner than tests for IgG alone, since IgM antibody formation precedes IgG production. Blood donor history screening procedures are in place to deter persons at risk for HIV from donating in the "window" period between infection and seroconversion. Of note, fewer than 25 patients with HIV infection attributed to screened blood were reported to the Centers for Disease Control (CDC) between spring 1985 and mid-1992 among an estimated 22 million persons who received transfusions.

Anti-HIV-2 testing was introduced in spring 1992 despite no transfusion-associated infections among the 32 HIV-2 infected patients in the United States at that time.

Human T cell leukemia/lymphoma viruses 1 and 2 (HTLV-1, HTLV-2) are transforming retroviruses that cross-react serologically. Testing for these agents was introduced in December 1988. HTLV-1 infection poses a lifetime risk of approximately 4% for adult T cell leukemia or tropical spastic paraparesis. HTLV-2 infection is not linked conclusively to a symptomatic illness. Approximately 40% to 60% of HTLV seropositive blood donors are infected with HTLV-2. Transmission of HTLV-1 and HTLV-2 by transfusion is restricted to cellular components.

Cytomegalovirus. Immunocompetent patients rarely have significant illness as a result of cytomegalovirus (CMV) infection through transfusion. Patients at risk for a significant CMV infection include premature infants weighing less than 1200 g born to CMV-seronegative mothers, CMV-seronegative recipients of allogeneic bone marrow transplantation from CMV-negative donors, and possibly CMV-seronegative patients receiving renal, heart, liver, or lung transplants from CMV-seronegative donors. In addition, CMV poses a risk to CMV-seronegative pregnant women because a primary CMV infection places the fetus at risk.

Methods for reducing CMV transmission through transfusion include serologic testing to identify donors not previously infected with CMV (i.e., seronegative), leukocyte depletion by third-generation filters, or frozen, deglycerolized RBC components. Transmission has not been documented after infusion of plasma or cryoprecipitate.

Spirochete infections. Syphilis is an extremely infrequent complication of blood transfusion as a result of blood donor testing and the organism's lack of viability for more than 24 to 96 hours at 4° C. Transfusion-transmitted Lyme borreliosis has not been reported.

Parasitic infections. Transfusion-transmitted malaria occurs infrequently. To reduce the risk of obtaining blood from asymptomatic carriers, donations are not accepted from persons who traveled to malarious areas within the previous 12 months. Transfusion-associated babesiosis is a potentially fatal complication in immunocompromised, asplenic, or elderly patients. Potential donors with a history of babesiosis are deferred indefinitely from donating blood. Several cases of acute Chagas' disease *(Trypanosoma cruzi)* have been attributed to transfusion in North America; transfusion-associated Chagas' disease has been a long-standing problem in South America. Development of appropriate laboratory tests and procedures for screening U.S. blood donors, in light of significant immigration of Central and South Americans to the United States, is under investigation.

REFERENCES

Dodd RY: The risk of transfusion-transmitted infection. New Engl J Med 327:419, 1992.

Lane TA et al: Leukocyte reduction in blood component therapy. Ann Intern Med 117:151, 1992.

National Blood Resource Education Program Expert Panel: The use of autologous blood. JAMA 263:414, 1990.

Office of Medical Applications of Research: Fresh-frozen plasma: indications and risks. JAMA 253:551, 1985.

Office of Medical Applications of Research: Platelet transfusion therapy. JAMA 257:1777, 1987.

Office of Medical Applications of Research: Perioperative red blood cell transfusion. JAMA 260:2700, 1988.

Schiffer CA: Prevention of alloimmunization against platelets. Blood 77:1, 1991.

Welch HG, Meehan KR, and Goodnough LT: Prudent strategies for elective red blood cell transfusion. Ann Intern Med 116:393, 1992.

CHAPTER

78 Bone Marrow Transplantation

Frederick R. Appelbaum

The first suggestion that marrow transplantation might be possible was made in 1949, when Leon Jacobson demonstrated that if a mouse spleen was shielded during total body irradiation, the otherwise lethal myelosuppressive effects of the radiation could be averted. Shortly thereafter, a similar radioprotective effect was demonstrated when bone marrow from one mouse was given intravenously to a radiated recipient of the same strain. By the mid-1950s, several laboratories, using cytogenetic markers, had shown that the radioprotective effect of bone marrow was accompanied by replacement of the original hematopoietic system of the host with cells of donor origin. The extent of replacement was shown to include all myeloid, lymphoid, and macrophage elements. The potential clinical implications of marrow transplantation were immediately obvious, but the application of this technique had to await a better understanding of the major histocompatibility complex in humans and the development of improved methods of intensive supportive care. Advances in both these areas have been accompanied by a steady increase in the number of long-term healthy recipients of marrow transplants and the application of marrow transplantation to an increased number of diseases.

INDICATIONS

Marrow transplantation has been used to treat a variety of nonmalignant and malignant diseases.

Immunodeficiency states

Marrow grafting can successfully establish a normal immune system in infants with all forms of severe combined immunodeficiency. Similarly, the lymphoid and platelet abnormalities of the lethal sex-linked disorder, the Wiskott-Aldrich syndrome, can be corrected with transplantation.

Nonmalignant disorders of hematopoiesis

Patients with acquired severe aplastic anemia can achieve long-term survival in 70% of cases if previously transfused or 80% if not transfused. Similarly, marrow transplantation can cure more than 70% of children with β-thalassemia and has been successfully used as treatment for sickle cell anemia, other hereditary hemoglobinopathies, and various congenital aregenerative anemias.

Enzymatic disorders

Marrow transplantation has been used to provide patients with normal enzyme systems in such disorders as the mucopolysaccharidoses and Gaucher's disease.

Malignant diseases

Patients with acute myelogenous leukemia or acute lymphoblastic leukemia in relapse after failure of combination chemotherapy or in blastic crisis of chronic myelogenous leukemia can still be cured in 10% to 30% of cases with marrow transplantation. If transplantation is carried out earlier in the course of these diseases, the results are better. For patients with acute myelogenous leukemia or acute lymphoblastic leukemia in first remission or chronic myelogenous leukemia in the chronic phase, 5-year disease-free survival is seen in at least 50% of cases. Transplantation has been successfully applied to patients with myelodysplastic syndromes, non-Hodgkin's lymphoma, Hodgkin's disease, hairy cell leukemia, myelofibrosis, multiple myeloma, and neuroblastoma. Experimental studies are being conducted in patients with other chemosensitive tumors such as breast cancer.

DONOR SELECTION

Three forms of transplantation are possible. With *autologous* transplantation, a portion of the patient's own marrow is removed, the patient is treated with intensive chemotherapy and/or radiotherapy, and the patient's marrow is reinfused. Autologous transplantation has generally been used as a means of treating patients for malignancies with higher doses of chemoradiotherapy than would normally be tolerated. *Syngeneic* transplantation refers to transplantation of marrow from a normal genetically identical twin. *Allogeneic* transplantation is transplantation of marrow from a normal genetically different donor.

Most allogeneic transplants have been performed between siblings with identical human leukocyte antigen (HLA). HLA identity implies identity for HLA-A and HLA-B, as determined by serotyping, and identity for HLA-D, as demonstrated by nonreactivity in mixed leukocyte culture (MLC) (Chapter 284). The HLA genes are located on chromosome 6. Because their products are codominantly expressed, the chance that any two siblings will be HLA identical is one in four. Because patients have an average of slightly more than one sibling, the chances that a matched sibling can be identified for any one patient are 30% to 40%. Efforts to expand the donor pool include using donors who are genotypically identical for one HLA haplotype but only partially matched for the other. Also, donors who are totally unrelated to the patient but are matched for HLA-A, HLA-B, and HLA-D have been used with promising results.

The formation of a National Bone Marrow Donor Registry has led to an increase in the use of matched unrelated donors. Currently, more than 500,000 normal individuals have volunteered to serve as marrow donors in the United States alone. With the use of partially matched and unrelated donors, the proportion of patients for whom transplantation is a reasonable option has increased significantly. Major ABO incompatibility is not a barrier to successful transplantation. However, to avoid hemolysis, incompatible red blood cells must be removed from the marrow inoculum by centrifugation or sedimentation, or alternatively, isoagglutinins must be removed from the patient's blood by immunoadsorption or plasma exchange.

PREPARATIVE REGIMEN

The form of treatment administered to the patient directly before transplantation depends on the disease being treated. Patients with severe combined immunodeficiency often require no pretransplant therapy because there is no malignant cell population to eradicate and the patients are, by the nature of their disease, so immunoincompetent that they rarely reject the infused marrow. In other patients who are relatively immunocompetent, the preparative regimen must be immunosuppressive enough to prevent the patient from rejecting the marrow. In treating a patient with aplastic anemia when there is no malignancy to eradicate, high-dose cyclophosphamide is often used as the preparative regimen. When transplantation is applied to the treatment of leukemia or other malignancy, the regimen must be both immunosuppressive and capable of eradicating the malignancy. In these patients, other forms of therapy (e.g., high-dose total body irradiation) or chemotherapeutic agents (e.g., busulfan) are added to cyclophosphamide for their cytotoxic effects.

MARROW ASPIRATION AND INFUSION

Marrow is usually obtained from the donor's anterior and posterior iliac crests using standard aspiration needles with the donor under general or spinal anesthesia. To obtain as many marrow cells with as little peripheral blood contamination as possible, each aspirate site is limited to 3 to 5 ml. Approximately 10 to 15 ml of marrow per kilogram body weight is obtained, so for a normal adult male donor, this means 700 to 900 ml of marrow and 100 to 200 aspirations. The marrow is placed in heparinized tissue culture media and then filtered through screens of 0.30 and 0.20 mm diameter to remove bony spicules and fat globules. The marrow is then either cryopreserved for later autologous transplantation or, in the case of allogeneic transplantation, taken to the patient's room and infused intravenously. In certain experimental studies the marrow may be treated before infusion, for example, to test whether removal of T cells from the marrow can prevent graft-versus-host disease (GVHD) or whether tumor cells can be removed from marrow before autologous transplantation. The risk associated with marrow donation is small; among 1220 marrow donations in Seattle, no fatal complications were seen, but six serious complications occurred (three cardiopulmonary, two infectious, one cerebrovascular accident). Although small, this risk must be weighed carefully when considering the use of matched unrelated donors.

Hematopoietic stem cells circulate in the peripheral blood, although in very small numbers. During recovery from drug-induced cytopenias or after exposure to hematopoietic growth factors such as granulocyte-macrophage colony-stimulating factor (GM-CSF), the number of hematopoietic progenitor cells in the peripheral blood increases dramatically. With the use of these mobilizing techniques followed by leukapheresis, it is possible to collect sufficient stem cells from the peripheral blood to permit successful autologous transplantation. Peripheral stem cell transplantation is indicated for patients who are otherwise candidates for autologous marrow transplantation but have bone marrows that are unsuitable for the procedure, either because of prior radiotherapy to the marrow or histopathologic evidence of tumor involvement. Peripheral stem cell transplantation is not used for allogeneic marrow transplantation, partly because of the high proportion of T cells compared with progenitor cells in the peripheral blood.

ENGRAFTMENT

After the preparative regimen, a period of profound myelosuppression ensues. Within 1 to 2 weeks of transplant, however, the peripheral leukocyte count begins to increase, signifying engraftment (Fig. 78-1). The granulocyte count reaches $0.1 \times 10^9/L$ in about 16 days and $1.0 \times 10^9/L$ by about day 26. Administration of GM-CSF can accelerate the recovery of peripheral granulocyte counts by as much as 1 week. The platelet count recovers simultaneously with or shortly after the recovery of granulocytes. Engraftment of allogeneic marrow can be documented using cytogenetic techniques or red cell antigens and isoenzymes. Cytogenetics is most easily done when donor and recipient are of different sexes. When they are of the same sex, unique chromosomal polymorphisms can be identified by banding techniques, thus allowing for the identification of chromosomes as being of host or donor origin in approximately half of same-sex donor-recipient pairs. With the use of deoxyribo-

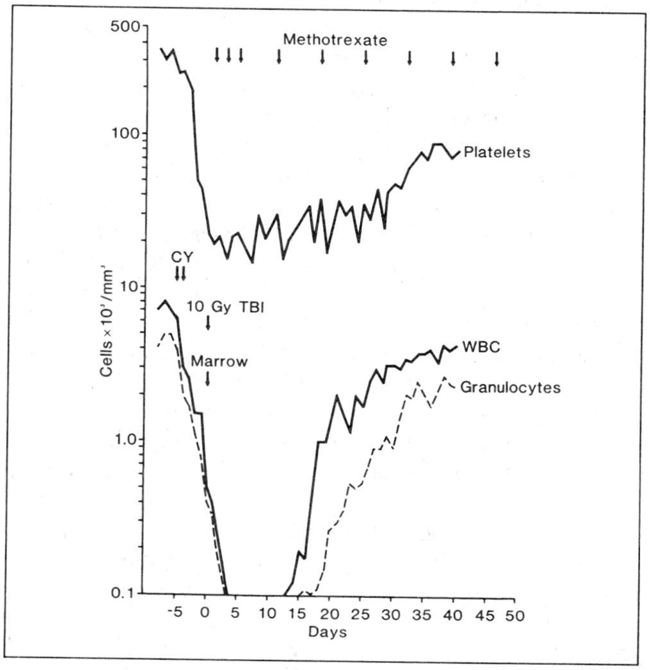

Fig. 78-1. Peripheral blood counts of a patient treated for acute leukemia with cyclophosphamide, total body irradiation, and marrow transplantation from an HLA-identical sibling. Platelet transfusions were administered from day 3 through day 24; methotrexate was given in an effort to reduce or prevent graft-versus-host disease.

nucleic acid (DNA) restriction fragment length polymorphisms, the origin of a population of cells can now be determined in virtually all cases. Polymorphic red cell enzymes can be used to monitor engraftment provided the patient has not received recent red cell transfusions.

COMPLICATIONS

Graft rejection

In some patients the transplanted marrow graft functions briefly, but after a period of days or weeks, marrow function is lost, and myeloid elements are absent on marrow biopsy. In most patients, marrow graft rejection is thought to be the result of residual host immunity to the donor. Graft rejection occurring in recipients of HLA-identical marrow is thought to be the result of the patient having been sensitized to unshared non-HLA antigens of the donor by prior transfusions. Among recipients of HLA-identical marrow, graft rejection is seen most often when the patient has received prior transfusions and when the preparative regimen is less immunosuppressive, such as with the use of cyclophosphamide alone before transplantation for aplastic anemia. If patients are not transfused or if total body irradiation is used, graft rejection occurs less frequently.

Graft-versus-host-disease

GVHD is thought to be the result of allogeneic T cells that were transfused with the graft or developed from it and reacted against targets of the genetically different host. Acute GVHD develops within the first 3 months of transplantation and presents with characteristic lesions of the skin, liver, and gastrointestinal tract. An erythematous maculopapular skin rash that favors the palms and soles is usually the first sign of GVHD (Color Plate III-3). This is followed by diarrhea, often with abdominal pain and ileus, and liver disease characterized by rises in bilirubin, transaminases, and alkaline phosphatase. Pathologic features include lymphocytic and monocytic infiltration into perivascular spaces in the dermis and the dermoepidermal junction of the skin, into the epithelium of the oropharynx, tongue, and esophagus, into the base of the intestinal crypts of the small and large bowel, and into the periportal areas of the liver with secondary necrosis of cells in infiltrated tissues. In animal models, immunosuppressive therapy given immediately after transplantation can diminish or prevent GVHD, and based on these studies, in the past most patients have been treated after transplantation with methotrexate. Despite methotrexate prophylaxis, 20% to 50% of patients receiving HLA-identical marrow from family member donors will develop acute GVHD, and 20% to 40% of those will die of GVHD and/or associated infections. GVHD is more frequent and more severe in older individuals and in recipients of partially matched marrow or marrow from matched unrelated donors.

Recently, other immunosuppressive agents such as steroids, antithymocyte globulin, or cyclosporine have also been used in attempts to prevent GVHD. Randomized trials have shown that cyclosporine is as effective as methotrexate and that the use of both agents in combination is more effective than the use of either agent alone. With the combination of methotrexate and cyclosporine, lethal acute GVHD is the exception in HLA-identical transplants, occurring in fewer than 10% of patients. Another approach to prevention of acute GVHD, based on animal studies, is removal of T cells from donor marrow.

Methods of treating established acute GVHD have included prednisone, antithymocyte globulin, cyclosporine, cyclophosphamide, and monoclonal antibodies against T cells. Responses have been seen with each, but no one approach has yet been shown to be superior.

Chronic GVHD affects 20% to 40% of patients surviving more than 6 months after transplantation and resembles a collagen vascular disease, with skin changes that include malar erythema, sclerodermatous changes, and cutaneous ulcers, alopecia, sicca syndrome, polyserositis, and liver dysfunction characterized by bile duct degeneration and cholestasis. Two factors that are closely associated with the development of chronic GVHD are increasing age and a preceding episode of acute GVHD. Prednisone alone or in combination with either azathioprine or cyclophosphamide is effective in controlling chronic GVHD in 50% to 70% of patients. Thalidomide results in a complete response in 30% of patients not responsive to conventional therapy. Patients with chronic GVHD are susceptible to bacterial infections and should receive antibiotic prophylaxis (see following section).

Infectious complications

The first 2 or 3 weeks after transplantation are complicated by severe granulocytopenia, fever, and in about 50% of patients, at least one episode of bacteremia. Therefore, at virtually all transplant centers, febrile granulocytopenic patients are treated empirically with broad-spectrum antibiotics, and in many centers, antibiotics are begun once patients become granulocytopenic, even if afebrile. Fungal infections also occur often among this group of patients. The use of fluconazole prophylaxis reduces the incidence of both superficial and invasive fungal infections. Patients who become or remain febrile despite broad-spectrum antibiotics and have no obvious source of infection are usually treated with amphotericin. Both prophylactic granulocyte transfusions and laminar airflow isolation have been demonstrated to be effective in preventing early infections, but neither has been shown to affect survival. With current methods of supportive care, the risk of death from infection during the early granulocytopenic posttransplant period is about 5%.

Herpes simplex (HSV) infection can contribute to the severity of early oral mucositis and in some patients can result in esophagitis, bronchopneumonia, and rarely, encephalitis. Systemic acyclovir, 250 mg/m^2 every 8 hours intravenously, is highly effective in the treatment of established HSV infection after marrow transplantation. If used as prophylaxis starting 1 week before transplant and continuing for 4 weeks after transplant, acyclovir can prevent HSV reactivation in more than 90% of seropositive patients.

If patients have detectable antibody to cytomegalovirus (CMV) before transplantation, in 50% to 75% of cases the virus can be recovered from the throat, urine, or stool during the first 100 days after transplant. In approximately 50% of these patients, CMV reactivation is asymptomatic, but in the other 50%, reactivation of CMV is followed by the development of CMV pneumonia or CMV gastrointestinal disease. In the past, CMV pneumonia occurred in about 15% of patients receiving an allogeneic marrow transplant and had a case fatality rate of 80%. Primary CMV infection in patients with no detectable antibody to CMV before transplant can be prevented by the sole use of CMV-seronegative blood products. In patients with antibody to CMV before transplant, the use of prophylactic ganciclovir, starting either at the time of initial engraftment or at the time of CMV reactivation, can substantially reduce the risk of CMV disease.

Pneumonia caused by *Pneumocystis carinii,* although previously a problem seen in 5% to 10% of transplant recipients, can be prevented by treating patients with oral trimethoprim-sulfamethoxazole for 1 week before transplant and resuming treatment 2 days per week once the granulocyte count exceeds 0.5×10^9/L.

Late infections (more than 3 months after the transplant) are usually caused by varicella-zoster virus (VZV) or, in patients with chronic GVHD, recurrent bacterial or fungal infections. The use of prophylactic trimethoprim-sulfamethoxazole and/or penicillin can reduce the incidence of late bacterial infections.

Chemoradiotherapy toxicities

After the standard cyclophosphamide–total body irradiation preparative regimen, the immediate toxicities include nausea, vomiting, fever, parotitis, and mild skin erythema. Unusual toxicities associated with high-dose cyclophosphamide include hemorrhagic cystitis and, rarely, acute hemorrhagic carditis. Five to seven days after total body irradiation most patients develop oral mucositis, and by 2 weeks most patients have developed complete but reversible alopecia. Also by this time, all patients are profoundly pancytopenic, with the resultant risks of bleeding and infection.

Veno-occlusive disease (VOD) of the liver can be seen within 1 to 4 weeks of transplantation and presents with ascites, tender hepatomegaly, and jaundice. VOD is seen in approximately 10% of transplant recipients and is fatal in one third of these. Patients with abnormal liver function before transplant have a higher incidence of VOD.

Idiopathic interstitial pneumonia, which is thought to be a direct chemoradiotoxicity, is seen in 5% to 10% of patients between 30 and 90 days after transplant. The disease has an approximately 50% case fatality rate; no clearly effective therapy exists. Increasing age, pre-existing lung disease, and prior exposure to chest radiotherapy increase the incidence of this complication, whereas the use of fractionated instead of single-dose irradiation decreases its incidence.

Late complications attributable to the cyclophosphamide–total body irradiation preparative regimen include decreased growth velocity in children and delayed development of secondary sex characteristics. Most postpubertal women develop ovarian failure, and few men regain spermatogenesis. Approximately 40% of patients develop cataracts within 2 years of transplantation, although this incidence may be less if fractionated irradiation is used. Thyroid dysfunction, usually well compensated, has been reported as well.

PATIENT REFERRAL

On encountering a patient who may be a candidate for a marrow transplant, the physician should contact a marrow transplant center as soon as possible. The center can provide the physician with valuable information about the relative risks and benefits of transplantation, the process by which a donor may be identified, and the mechanism of transferring the patient for transplantation. For patients with nonmalignant disorders, marrow grafting should be considered early in the course of disease before multiple transfusions have been given. Transfusions from family members should especially be avoided because of the increased risk of graft rejection. For patients with leukemia, the best results have also been obtained if transplantation is carried out early in the course of disease.

The ultimate choice of whether and when to undergo transplantation rests with the patient. Therefore the physician is obligated to provide the patient and family with up-to-date, reliable information to help in making the decision.

REFERENCES

Anasetti C et al: Effect of HLA compatibility on engraftment of bone marrow transplants in patients with leukemia or lymphoma. N Engl J Med 320:197, 1989.

Antman K and Gale RP: Advanced breast cancer: high-dose chemotherapy and bone marrow autotransplants. Ann Intern Med 108:570, 1988.

Appelbaum FR et al: Bone marrow transplantation for patients with myelodysplasia: pretreatment variables and outcome. Ann Intern Med 112:590, 1990.

Armitage JO: Bone marrow transplantation in the treatment of patients with lymphoma. Blood 73:1749, 1989.

Beatty PG et al: Marrow transplantation from HLA-matched unrelated donors for treatment of hematologic malignancies. Transplantation 51:443, 1991.

Cheson BD et al: Autologous bone marrow transplantation: current status and future directions. Ann Intern Med 110:51, 1989.

Nemunaitis J et al: Recombinant granulocyte-macrophage colony-stimulating factor after autologous bone marrow transplantation for lymphoid cancer. N Engl J Med 324:1773, 1991.

Ramsay NK and Kersey JH: Indications for marrow transplantation in acute lymphoblastic leukemia. Blood 75:815, 1990.

Santos GW: Marrow transplantation in acute nonlymphocytic leukemia. Blood 74:901, 1989.

Storb R et al: Methotrexate and cyclosporine compared with cyclosporine alone for prophylaxis of acute graft versus host disease after marrow transplantation for leukemia. N Engl J Med 314:729, 1986.

Storb R et al: Marrow transplantation for severe aplastic anemia and thalassemia major. Semin Hematol 28:235, 1991.

Thomas ED and Clift RA: Indications for marrow transplantation in chronic myelogenous leukemia. Blood 73:861, 1989.

CHAPTER

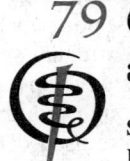

79 Complications of Cancer and Cancer Therapy

Stanley P. Balcerzak
Eric H. Kraut

Cancer describes a process rather than a single disease. Since any cell capable of replication has the potential to undergo neoplastic transformation, the manifestations of cancer are protean. Even within the same organ, the natural history of cancer differs greatly based on the cell of origin; contrast the biologic behavior of malignant melanoma with squamous cell carcinoma of the skin, non–oat cell with oat cell carcinoma of the lung, or polycythemia vera with acute myelogenous leukemia. For the physician, the challenge in management and treatment is twofold: (1) detailed knowledge of the pathophysiology of each malignancy, which is available in general oncology textbooks, and (2) awareness of the more general clinical problems encountered in patients. This chapter discusses these common complications and is organized into clinical problems as they are encountered in patients.

PAIN

Pain is almost synonymous with cancer in the minds of the public and physicians. Ironically, the lack of pain in the early stages of cancer often compromises current therapy by delaying diagnosis. Pain, whether acute or chronic, may be assigned to one of three etiologic categories: (1) malignancy related, (2) treatment related, or (3) unrelated to either of these.

Assignment of pain to one of these three categories may be difficult, but a correct diagnosis is necessary for proper management of the problem. For example, an elderly woman receiving adjuvant tamoxifen after mastectomy for localized carcinoma of the breast may develop severe back pain caused by collapse of a vertebral body. Determining whether this pain is secondary to metastatic carcinoma or is related to the patient's pre-existing osteoporosis has major therapeutic and prognostic implications. An even more serious situation may occur when the cause for pain at a particular location changes and this change is unrecognized by the physician or the patient. Thus a patient with rib pain or pleural pain from metastatic disease may assume that the new pleuritic pain from a pulmonary embolus is still directly related to the cancer and not alert the physician to this significant change. Confusion regarding the etiology of pain in patients with cancer contributes significantly to failure in the management of their pain.

Management of pain in the patient with cancer continues to test the physician's skill despite significant advances in the understanding of pain transmission and modulation. Pain in the patient with cancer may be considered as two major types. The first is pain that may be expected to improve with therapy or with natural healing. Management of pain in these patients requires a relatively short-term strategy. The second type of pain is chronic and is not expected to improve. Management of such pain requires a long-term strategy.

Resolution of bone pain by radiotherapy for metastatic disease, healing of mucositis caused by chemotherapy, or subsidence of nerve root pain associated with herpes zoster are examples of pain that, although possibly severe, may be expected to improve with time. When the physician identifies the patient's pain as likely to be of limited duration, the physician needs to be certain that the patient understands this fact. The expectation of complete pain relief provides more comfort than morphine. Patients without the probability that their pain will be temporary need to know that this pain can be ameliorated.

Analgesic drugs provide the principal mode of pain relief in the cancer patient. These agents may be grouped in three categories: nonnarcotic analgesics, narcotic analgesics, and adjuvant analgesics. The nonnarcotic analgesics include aspirin, acetaminophen, and the nonsteroidal anti-inflammatory drugs. These drugs are appropriate for mild to moderate pain and represent the initial agents used in the treatment of cancer pain. If inadequate for pain control when used alone, these agents will produce additive analgesia when used in combination with narcotic analgesics.

Narcotic analgesics produce their effects by binding to receptors in the central nervous system (CNS). Unlike the analgesic effect of nonnarcotic drugs such as aspirin, narcotic agents such as morphine produce increasing pain relief with increasing dose, without a limit on the analgesic effect until loss of consciousness. Other side effects, however, usually provide an upper limit of a narcotic's dose. These side effects include sedation, anorexia, nausea, vomiting, constipation, confusion, and CNS excitation.

Because of the subjective nature of pain, use of analgesic drugs requires good rapport between physician and patient. The patient needs to feel certain about the physician's clinical ability and compassion so that he or she will be confident that the physician is attempting to find an analgesic regimen that will provide maximum pain relief and minimum side effects. This confidence is especially necessary as the analgesia is being started and when abrupt changes occur in the level of pain. Because of significant individual variation in response to analgesic agents, the patient should play a major role in evaluating the effectiveness and toxicity of analgesia without being made to think the physician has abandoned responsibility. The physician must employ medical knowledge and judgment to the fullest in interpreting the patient's complaints; a thorough knowledge of the analgesic's pharmacology is particularly important.

Morphine is the prototype analgesic drug used for severe pain. When given intramuscularly (IM), 10 mg of morphine reaches a peak level in ½ to 1 hour; its plasma half-life is 2 to 3½ hours; and its duration of analgesia is 4 to 6 hours. IM doses of other drugs used in quantities sufficient to give the same analgesia as 10 mg of morphine exhibit similar peak and duration of analgesia values.

IM doses equivalent to 10 mg of morphine are as follows: meperidine (Demerol), 75 mg; methadone (Dolophine), 10 mg; levorphanol (Levo-Dromoran), 2 mg; hydromorphone (Dilaudid), 1.5 mg; and codeine, 130 mg. The same narcotics given orally in doses that achieve the same level of analgesia reach peak levels in 1 to 2 hours and produce analgesia for 4 to 7 hours. These drugs differ, however, in their plasma half-lives. Given IM, most have half-lives of 2 to 4 hours, but methadone has a much longer half-life of 15 to 30 hours and levorphanol, 12 to 16 hours. Thus, with repeated dosing at the 4- to 6-hour intervals necessary for adequate analgesia, methadone and levorphanol may accumulate, causing excessive sedation and respiratory depression. Similarly, narcotics with shorter half-lives also may accumulate in the presence of impaired renal or hepatic function.

The pharmacology of meperidine deserves special mention. Although its plasma half-life is 3 to 4 hours, meperidine is metabolized to normeperidine. Because of a 15-hour half-life, normeperidine accumulates with repetitive dosing and causes CNS irritability that may lead to multifocal myoclonus and seizures. This is especially a problem in patients with impaired renal function. Toxic doses of all narcotics may produce CNS irritability, but normeperidine is more often associated with this problem.

With continued use, patients are likely to develop tolerance to a narcotic. Intravenous (IV) administration of narcotics is especially likely to lead to rapid development of tolerance; therefore the use of oral narcotic analgesics should be encouraged for this reason as well as for convenience. Tolerance may be managed by increasing dose and frequency, keeping in mind the drug's pharmacology. The size of the dose should not be of primary concern to the physician as long as the therapeutic/toxic ratio remains high. Another approach to tolerance involves switching from one narcotic to another because cross-tolerance is incomplete. The new narcotic should be given initially at an analgesic equivalent dose that is significantly less than that of the original narcotic. Combinations of drugs (e.g., narcotic with aspirin or acetaminophen, narcotic with an amphetamine) may also increase analgesia without requiring additional narcotic.

A narcotic not only should be given in sufficient dose to control pain, but usually should be given regularly. Regular administration of narcotics helps maintain pain at a tolerable level and reduces patient anxiety. It frequently reduces the daily consumption of narcotics. Slow-release morphine is frequently successful in achieving this more prolonged analgesia through the oral route. Other, more complicated methods for maintaining persistent pain control include continuous subcutaneous, IV, and epidural or intrathecal narcotic infusions with the aid of portable or nonportable pumps.

Although nonnarcotic and narcotic drug therapy is the mainstay of pain management in patients with cancer, the armamentarium available to the physician is extensive and varied. Psychology plays an important role in pain management. As mentioned previously, the patient's attitude toward pain is crucial. If the patient can be made to feel in control of the pain, drug therapy is likely to be more effective in that the patient will use the narcotic specifically for pain reduction rather than an escape from a feeling of helplessness. Other psychologic approaches beyond the immediate physician-patient relationship include the assistance of family, friends, nursing personnel, patient groups, psychologists, psychiatrists, and other support groups to help the patient face the reality of the situation in the most positive way possible. Specific techniques, such as hypnosis or biofeedback, may be useful in certain patients.

In addition to drug therapy, psychology, and local and spinal anesthetics, neurosurgical methods may be very effective in patients with well-defined localized pain. Because cancer pain is often not localized or may become diffuse, procedures such as nerve blocks, epidural blocks, dorsal rhizotomy, and cordotomy have limited application.

Localized pain in the mouth from drug-induced mucositis, herpes simplex, or bacterial infection consequent to granulocytopenia may be significantly relieved by Zilactin, a hydroxypropylcellulose-based topical medication. Zilactin forms an adhesive film on oral mucosal ulcerations and may provide relief for several hours.

Each patient with cancer pain is unique not only in regard to the specifics of pathophysiology, but also in regard to psychologic and social setting. Successful management of an individual cancer patient's pain requires understanding of the entire patient by a well-informed, compassionate physician capable of mature judgment regarding the appropriate interventions to control pain.

WEIGHT LOSS

The mechanism of weight loss in cancer patients is complex and only partially understood. Factors that contribute to this problem include decreased caloric intake and systemic effects of cancer, which may increase basal metabolic rate or alter substrate utilization.

Many possible reasons exist for the decrease in daily food intake. Anorexia is present in 15% to 25% of patients at the time of diagnosis and affects almost all patients with advanced disease. One proposed mediator of anorexia and increased catabolism in cancer and inflammatory disease is the polypeptide hormone *cachectin,* or tumor necrosis factor. This hormone, which is produced by macrophages in response to endotoxin and probably other stimuli, may also be made autonomously by dedifferentiated tumor cells.

Other factors affecting food intake include nausea and vomiting, mechanical obstruction of the gastrointestinal (GI) tract, or malabsorption. Nausea and vomiting may be related to treatment with radiation or with drugs such as chemotherapeutic agents or narcotics but also may occur with increased intracranial pressure, hypercalcemia, stress ulcers of the stomach, or neoplastic involvement of the stomach, liver, or retroperitoneal nodes.

Mechanical obstruction of the GI tract from intrinsic tumors of the head and neck, esophagus, stomach, small bowel, and large intestine may cause vomiting. Extrinsic obstruction from ovarian carcinoma may involve multiple sites of the GI tract and contribute significantly to morbidity and mortality of these patients. Adhesions resulting from surgery for intra-abdominal malignancy also may cause mechanical obstruction.

Malabsorption may occur with lymphomatous involvement of the small intestine or secondary to a deficiency of pancreatic or biliary excretions because of pancreatic or biliary neoplasia. Amyloidosis with involvement of the small intestine in association with multiple myeloma is a rare cause of malabsorption.

Coupled with decreased food intake are cancer-induced metabolic abnormalities. Tumors are associated with increased protein turnover. The daily protein need for positive nitrogen balance in cancer patients is double that of malnourished patients without cancer. Energy requirements for a malignancy are met primarily by glucolysis. When the supply of glucose from the diet is inadequate, as it often is, as a result of cancer-related anorexia or other causes previously discussed, gluconeogenesis from amino acids and lactate is enhanced in the liver.

Hyperalimentation has been used in several randomized trials in an attempt to treat the weight loss of cancer. None has shown benefit in regard to survival or reduction in marrow toxicity from myelosuppressive chemotherapy, although weight gain occurred in four of seven trials. The length of hyperalimentation, however, was brief in these trials. Possibly a more sustained way of improving nutrition in cancer patients is with the agent hydrazine sulfate. This drug is an inhibitor of gluconeogenesis at the level of phosphoenolpyruvate carboxykinase and thus is thought to interrupt host energy wasting caused by the augmented gluconeogenesis associated with cancer. Randomized, placebo-controlled, double-blind studies have reported statistically significant improvement in weight gain and survival in cancer patients. This drug is still being evaluated in active clinical trials.

Megestrol acetate, a progestational agent, has been studied for the treatment of anorexia and weight loss in patients with cancer and acquired immunodeficiency syndrome (AIDS). These studies demonstrated improved appetite, food intake, and weight gain in patients taking megestrol acetate, and dose-response studies are now being done.

NAUSEA AND VOMITING

The pathophysiology of nausea and vomiting is discussed in Chapter 37. The vomiting center is located in the lateral reticular formation of the medulla and receives signals from (1) the GI tract, (2) midbrain receptors of intracranial pressure, (3) the labyrinthine structure, (4) higher CNS centers such as those that respond to psychologic factors, and (5) the chemoreceptor trigger zone in the floor of the fourth ventricle. The chemoreceptor trigger zone responds to stimuli in the cerebrospinal fluid as well as in the blood. Previously, it was thought that dopamine receptors in the brain and GI tract were mediators of the vomiting reflex. It has been demonstrated that the neurotransmitter serotonin (5-hydroxytryptamine, or 5-HT) is involved in nausea and vomiting, and the 5-HT receptor now appears to be the principal mediator of the emetic reflex. This observation resulted in the development of a new class of compounds, the serotonin antagonists, which are highly effective in combating chemotherapy-induced nausea and vomiting.

The basic principle in the treatment of nausea and vomiting is to identify the underlying cause if possible and to treat the patient before symptoms develop. Patients with malignancies have nausea and vomiting primarily because of therapy, but other important causes the physician needs to consider include GI inflammation or obstruction, brain metastases, and hypercalcemia. These disease-related problems may be the sole cause of nausea and vomiting or may exacerbate treatment-related nausea and vomiting.

Nausea and vomiting occur as part of the toxicities of certain, but not all, chemotherapeutic agents and radiotherapy. Table 79-1 lists frequently used chemotherapy drugs associated with nausea and vomiting and attempts to rank them in regard to severity. Cisplatin, dacarbazine, nitrogen mustard, and actinomycin D often cause severe nausea and vomiting. Cisplatin and actinomycin D usually produce vomiting after a few hours, whereas nitrogen mustard often causes immediate vomiting. Tolerance of each chemotherapeutic agent, however, varies from patient to patient and is affected by dose.

Several compounds are effective antiemetics for chemotherapy-induced nausea and vomiting. These include the phenothiazines, benzodiazepines, butyrophenones, cannabinoids, corticosteroids, substituted benzamides, and serotonin antagonists. For mild nausea and vomiting the phenothiazines are most often used, including prochlorperazine (Compazine), perphenazine (Trilafon), and thiethylperazine (Torecan). Extrapyramidal reactions and agitation are known side effects of the phenothiazines, and antihistamines may be added to prevent this. Droperidol (Inapsine) and haloperidol (Haldol) are butyrophenones that are also effective alone in alleviating mild nausea and vomiting and may have less extrapyramidal toxicity. Corticosteroids such as dexamethasone have some activity alone in combating nausea and vomiting, but they are typically used in combination with the neurotransmitter blocking drugs.

Table 79-1. Relative emetic potential of chemotherapeutic agents

Emetic potential	Chemotherapeutic agent
High likelihood of emesis ↓	Cisplatin
	Dacarbazine (DTIC)
	Actinomycin D
	Nitrogen mustard
	Mithramycin
	Doxorubicin
	Cyclophosphamide
	Cytosine arabinoside
	Procarbazine
	Etoposide
	Methotrexate
	5-Fluorouracil
	Vincristine
	Hydroxyurea
Low likelihood of emesis	Chlorambucil

The benzamide, metoclopramide (Reglan), acts centrally on the chemoreceptor trigger zone and peripherally on the GI tract. It may do so by blocking not only dopamine, but also 5-HT receptors. Metoclopramide is often used for severe nausea and vomiting in combination with corticosteroids.

The serotonin antagonists such as ondansetron have quickly become the most frequently used antiemetics for moderate to severe vomiting. These drugs have fewer side effects than the other antiemetics and appear to be more active.

Regardless of the antiemetic agents used, the regimen should begin before the administration of the chemotherapeutic agents because prevention of nausea and vomiting is easier than treatment of existing nausea and vomiting. Prevention also helps to reduce the occurrence of anticipatory vomiting. The antiemetic regimen should be given on a scheduled basis in an attempt to prevent vomiting. The exact schedule and duration require individualization.

MUCOSITIS

Mucositis has become one of the more frequent complications seen in cancer patients because of increased dose intensity of radiation and chemotherapy. It is especially important not only because of its effects on patient comfort and nutrition, but also because it may allow pathogenic organisms to enter the bloodstream. Mucositis may occur directly because of injury from chemotherapy or radiation involving the GI and genitourinary tracts or indirectly because of impaired immunity and subsequent mucosal infection. Chemotherapeutic agents typically associated with mucositis from direct injury of the mucosa include methotrexate, fluorouracil, doxorubicin, and bleomycin, but such injury may occur with other chemotherapeutic agents as well. These agents and radiotherapy involving the mucosa probably cause a reduction in the renewal rate of the basal epithelium and consequent mucosal atrophy.

Because the renewal rate of the mucosa is rapid, symptoms of stomatitis, esophagitis, gastroenteritis, and vaginitis usually occur 3 to 7 days after direct mucosal injury from chemotherapy or radiation. Indirect mucosal injury most often occurs 10 to 14 days after chemotherapy with myelosuppressive drugs because this is the interval when granulocytopenia and lymphocytopenia are most severe. Mucositis develops at this time because of infection, most often bacterial, caused by gram-negative organisms, but also fungal, from *Candida albicans,* or viral, from herpes simplex or varicella. Measures to ameliorate mucositis include the use of (1) chlorhexidine mouthwash, which may limit oral microflora; (2) locally acting antibacterial and antifungal agents; (3) systemic prophylactic antibacterial, antifungal, and antiviral agents; and (4) growth factors such as granulocyte colony-stimulating factor (G-CSF), which may not only decrease the duration and severity of neutropenia but also of mucositis after chemotherapy.

PARANEOPLASTIC SYNDROMES

The adverse effects of cancer in the patient usually result from local growth of the primary tumor or spread to distant tissues through the lymphatics or the blood. These local effects may produce signs and symptoms caused by obstruction, hemorrhage, or organ destruction. Tumors may also produce effects at distant sites without direct involvement by malignant cells. These more indirect effects are referred to as paraneoplastic syndromes. They may be endocrine or nonendocrine in type. Paraneoplastic syndromes are reported in most series to occur in less than 10% of patients. Despite this infrequent occurrence, their recognition is important for the following reasons:

1. They may be the first manifestation of a malignancy and thus alert the physician to search for a primary tumor.
2. The activity of the paraneoplastic syndrome may parallel the course of the tumor and thus may be used as a marker of response to therapy or evidence of early relapse. Paraneoplastic syndromes, however, may develop independent of the tumor's course.
3. They may be confused with the cancer's direct effects or even the side effects of therapy. It is important to distinguish between these pathophysiologic mechanisms because the paraneoplastic syndromes may be effectively treated, thus improving the patient's clinical status even though the malignant lesion is unchanged.

Pathogenesis

The manifestations of the paraneoplastic syndromes are many and may include endocrine, neurologic, hematologic, renal, GI, rheumatic, and cutaneous abnormalities. They may develop by several different mechanisms. The tumor may produce biologically active peptides or proteins, including hormones and their precursors, prostaglandins, or immunoglobulins. These may be normal products of the tumor's tissue of origin but may be produced in unusually large amounts, such as in adrenocortical carcinoma, which releases excessive amounts of corticosteroids. Ectopic production may arise after neoplastic transformation of tissue that usually does not produce that hormone. The hormone may be authentic to that produced normally or may be structurally different but functionally similar.

The number of hormones produced by tumors is extensive, but the number proved to cause paraneoplastic syndromes is limited. Usually these hormones are peptides or glycoproteins. Using radioimmunoassay techniques, investigators have identified the hormones and their precursor molecules responsible for various paraneoplastic syndromes. These include adrenocorticotropic hormone (ACTH), antidiuretic hormone (ADH), parathormone (PTH), erythropoietin, gastrin, and vasoactive intestinal peptide. At times the material demonstrated immunologically is not identical to the natural hormone. For example, in PTH-related protein (PTH-rP), which is produced by tumor cells, 8 of its first 13 amino acid residues are identical to the natural parathyroid hormone. This is sufficient to mimic PTH biologically and immunologically, but PTH-rP appears to be encoded by human chromosome 12, whereas the PTH gene has been located on chromosome 11.

Evaluation of many cancer patients with radioimmunoassays has demonstrated that ectopic hormone production occurs more frequently then previously realized. Frequently the substances released from the tumors are large-molecular-weight precursors, fragments, or substrates that are biologically inactive. Thus, although they may not cause clinical problems, they still may be good markers of tumor growth. In addition, they may have prognostic importance; for example, the presence of the hormone ACTH in small cell carcinoma of the lung may portend a poor response to therapy.

Table 79-2 illustrates some of the more common paraneoplastic syndromes associated with malignancy and ectopic hormone production. The reader is referred to the appropriate chapters in this book for further description of these disorders.

In addition to occurring secondary to excessive hormone production, paraneoplastic syndromes may result from release into the circulation of tissue enzymes normally excluded from the systemic circulation, such as placental alkaline phosphatase. These substances may induce antigenic reactions, inappropriately initiate normal physiologic functions, or cause other toxic reactions.

Tumor cells also may shed proteins or antigens from their surface, leading to the formation of antigen-antibody complexes. Immune complexes may damage organs such as the kidney. Besides, damage from immune complexes, tumors, or their products may stimulate autoimmune injury caused by cross-reactivity with normal cell surface proteins. The box, upper right, lists a few of the many nonendocrine syndromes associated with malignancy.

Nonendocrine paraneoplastic syndromes

- Cutaneous
  - Dermatomyositis
  - Acanthosis nigricans
  - Sweet's syndrome
  - Erythema gyratum repens
  - Systemic nodular panniculitis (Weber-Christian disease)
- Renal
  - Nephrotic syndrome
  - Nephrogenic diabetes insipidus
- Neurologic
  - Subacute cerebellar degeneration
  - Progressive multifocal leukoencephalopathy
  - Subacute motor neuropathy
  - Sensory neuropathy
  - Ascending acute polyneuropathy (Guillain-Barré)
  - Myasthenic syndrome (Eaton-Lambert)
- Hematologic
  - Microangiopathic hemolytic anemia
  - Migratory thrombophlebitis (Trousseau's syndrome)
  - Anemia of chronic disease
- Rheumatologic
  - Polymyalgia rheumatica
  - Hypertrophic pulmonary osteoarthropathy

OTHER COMPLICATIONS

The complications of cancer are legion and occur much more frequently than paraneoplastic syndromes. An incomplete list of other complications includes fever unrelated to infection (Chapter 227), infections from impaired defense

Table 79-2. Endocrine paraneoplastic syndromes

Syndrome	Mediator	Associated malignancy
Hypercalcemia	Parathyroid hormone (parathormone, PTH) or PTH-like substance Osteoclast-activating factors Prostaglandins Tumor growth factor (TGF), alpha Interleukin-1 (IL-1) Tumor necrosis factor Lymphotoxin	Breast cancer Squamous cell carcinoma of lung, head and neck, esophagus Multiple myeloma Renal cell carcinoma
Syndrome of inappropriate secretion of antidiuretic hormone (SIADH)	Antidiuretic hormone (ADH)	Small cell carcinoma of lung Head and neck carcinomas Hodgkin's disease Non-Hodgkin's lymphoma
Hypoglycemia	Insulin Insulin-like peptides	Insulinoma Mesenchymal tumors, including mesothelioma, fibrosarcoma, neurofibrosarcoma, rhabdomyosarcoma
Zollinger-Ellison syndrome	Gastrin	Gastrinoma
Ectopic secretion of human chorionic gonadotropin	Human chorionic gonadotropin (HCG)	Germ cell tumors containing trophoblastic elements
Cushing's syndrome	Adrenocorticotropic hormone (ACTH)	Lung carcinoma

mechanisms (Chapter 229), changes in platelet counts or white counts in nonhematologic malignancies (Chapter 81), effusions (Chapter 218), CNS metastases (Chapter 136), bony metastases (Chapter 188), and superior vena cava obstruction (Chapter 219).

SIDE EFFECTS OF THERAPY

Chemotherapy and radiation are often used as part of an intensive program to control or cure cancer. These modalities, however, affect all rapidly proliferating cells, whether normal or malignant. Normal cells that proliferate rapidly include cells of the bone marrow, GI tract, skin, and genitourinary tract. The extent of injury to these tissues depends not only on the amount of radiation or drugs to which they are exposed but also on their ability to regenerate. Alopecia, for example, is usually transient with exposure to chemotherapeutic agents, and hair returns when the offending agent is stopped, whereas alopecia from radiation is usually permanent.

In addition to these expected effects of therapy, individual chemotherapeutic drugs may have idiosyncratic effects resulting in such complications as renal insufficiency, pulmonary fibrosis, diabetes, myocardiopathy, or CNS dysfunction. The physician needs to be aware of these complications and appreciate the most common ones seen after therapy (Table 79-3).

As seen in Table 79-3, chemotherapeutic drugs may cause multiple adverse effects. This table gives only a partial list of potential side effects. Cisplatin and methotrexate can cause interstitial nephritis with severe renal insufficiency. Although protection may be provided by adequate hydration before treatment, cumulative toxicity may still occur. Bleomycin induces an interstitial pneumonitis and consequent pulmonary fibrosis, which frequently can be prevented because it is often related to total drug dose administered. Many other drugs may also be associated with pulmonary toxicity, including cyclophosphamide and mitomycin.

The anthracycline drugs such as doxorubicin can cause both acute and chronic effects on the heart. Cumulative doses of doxorubicin greater than 450 mg/m^2 are associated frequently enough with significant loss of cardiac function and subsequent heart failure that doses greater than this level are usually not given. Prolonged continuous infusion (48 to 96 hours) of doxorubicin reduces cardiotoxicity compared with bolus injection without compromising antitumor efficacy.

CNS damage is less often seen because most chemotherapeutic drugs do not cross the blood-brain barrier. Drugs such as cytosine arabinoside and methotrexate, however, cross into the brain when administered in high doses and can cause acute or chronic demyelinating processes associated with frontal lobe or cerebellar dysfunction.

Table 79-3. Organ-specific toxicities of chemotherapy

Organ	Injury	Drugs
Heart	Cardiomyopathy	Anthracyclines such as doxorubicin (Adriamycin)
Lungs	Pneumonitis and interstitial fibrosis	Bleomycin Mitomycin Cyclophosphamide Methotrexate
Kidneys	Interstitial nephritis	Cisplatin
	Acute renal failure	High-dose methotrexate
Liver	Hepatitis or hepatic dysfunction	Procarbazine Dacarbazine (DTIC) Cytosine arabinoside
Central nervous system	Cerebellar degeneration	High-dose cytosine arabinoside
	Dementia	High-dose methotrexate
	Neuropathy	Vincristine Cisplatin
Bone marrow	Myelosuppression	Most chemotherapeutic drugs except for bleomycin, vincristine, and usual doses of cisplatin
Gastrointestinal tract	Mucositis	5-Fluorouracil
	Nausea and vomiting	Methotrexate Doxorubicin Cisplatin
Skin	Alopecia	Nitrogen mustard Doxorubicin Cyclophosphamide Vincristine
	Ulceration at site of extravasation	Nitrogen mustard Doxorubicin Mitomycin C Vincristine

Chemotherapy, especially alkylating agents and combination therapy, has a major impact on gonadal function. Although cancer itself may alter normal reproductive function, as exemplified in almost one third of men with untreated Hodgkin's disease who have marked reduction in sperm count and viability, the major effects on reproductive function result from treatment. Thus patients intensively treated for Hodgkin's disease demonstrate gonadal dysfunction in up to 80% of men and 50% of women, with recovery occurring less often in the men. Since gonadal function in young women is less susceptible to injury by chemotherapy than in men, pregnancy is often achieved when therapy is stopped. New chemotherapeutic drug programs have been introduced that have decreased the incidence of gonadal dysfunction.

Radiation administered in doses greater than 100 cGy to the testicles causes decreased testicular function and azoospermia that may be irreversible. Ovarian function is less sensitive to radiation, although reduction in menses may occur, but pregnancy is often still possible.

Radiation causes tissue injury and long-term organ damage according to the total dose used and sensitivity of the organ treated (see the box below). The organs often affected include the lungs, with development of pneumonitis and fibrosis; heart, with development of pericarditis or accelerated atherosclerosis; thyroid gland, with development of hypothyroidism; CNS, with development of memory loss or progressive dementia; and spinal cord, with transverse myelitis.

Despite the adverse effects of radiation and drugs on normal tissues, fetal survival and development appear to be minimally affected after the first trimester of pregnancy. When chemotherapy or radiotherapy is given during the first trimester, a real but poorly quantifiable risk of congenital abnormalities exists.

Complications of radiation therapy

Acute (days to weeks)

Mucositis
Cystitis
Enteritis
Alopecia
Bone marrow suppression

Late effects (weeks to years)

Pneumonitis, fibrosis
Constrictive pericarditis, accelerated atherosclerosis
Development of secondary malignancies
Hypothyroidism
Cataracts
Sterility
Memory loss and dementia
Transverse myelitis
Bone necrosis

SECONDARY MALIGNANCIES

Both radiation and certain forms of chemotherapy are mutagenic. Recent follow-up of successfully treated cancer patients has demonstrated that the risk of treatment-induced malignancy is significant and can reach 20% at 15 years. During the first several years, acute myelogenous leukemia and non-Hodgkin's lymphoma may be seen, with an increasing number of solid tumors demonstrated after 5 years.

The type of therapy may influence the type of malignancy, with chemotherapy causing a higher incidence of acute leukemia and radiation alone usually associated with solid tumors. Especially important is the increased incidence of lung cancer after radiation, suggesting that such patients should avoid other potential carcinogens such as cigarette smoking.

REFERENCES

Barrett AP: A long-term prospective clinical study of oral complications during conventional chemotherapy for acute leukemia. Oral Surg Oral Med Oral Pathol 63:313, 1987.

Byrne J: Fertility and pregnancy after malignancy. Semin Perinatol 14:423, 1990.

Bunn PA Jr and Minna JD: Paraneoplastic syndromes. In Devita VT, Hellman S, and Rosenberg SA, editors: Cancer principles and practices in oncology, ed 3. Philadelphia, 1989, Lippincott.

Doll D, Ringenberg S, and Yarbro J: Antineoplastic agents and pregnancy. Semin Oncol 16:337, 1989.

Foley KM: The treatment of cancer pain. N Engl J Med 313:84, 1985.

Gralla RJ et al: The management of chemotherapy-induced nausea and vomiting. Med Clin North Am 17:289, 1987.

Hohl RJ and Schilsky RL: Non malignant complications of therapy for Hodgkin's disease. Hematol Oncol Clin North Am 3:331, 1989.

Kerr ID et al: Continuous narcotic infusion with patient-controlled analgesia for chronic cancer pain in outpatients. Ann Intern Med 108:554, 1988.

Marty M et al: Comparison of the 5-hydroxytryptamine (Serotonin) antagonist ondansetron (GR 380 32F) with high dose metoclopramide in the control of cisplatin induced emesis. N Engl J Med 322:816, 1990.

Nixon DW, editor: Nutrition and cancer. Hematol Oncol Clin North Am 5, 1991.

Palma G: Paraneoplastic syndromes of the nervous system. West J Med 142:787, 1985.

Perry MC, editor: Toxicity of chemotherapy. Semin Oncol 19:453, 1992.

Tucker MA et al: Risk of second cancer after treatment for Hodgkin's disease. N Engl J Med 318:76, 1988.

V CLINICAL SYNDROMES

CHAPTER

80 Abnormal Hematocrit

Emmanuel N. Dessypris

Under normal conditions the production of red blood cells (RBCs) is closely regulated so that the hematocrit remains in the range of 38% to 48% in women and 40% to 52% in men. The production of RBCs is controlled by *erythropoietin,* a glycoprotein hormone produced by the interstitial cells in the kidneys. The concentration of erythropoietin in the blood is inversely related to the degree of oxygen delivery to the tissues by the blood. Hypoxia resulting from a decreased RBC mass leads to increased synthesis and release of erythropoietin by the kidney, which in turn stimulates RBC production by the bone marrow, thus restoring the RBC mass and tissue oxygenation back to normal levels. Under normal conditions the serum level of erythropoietin is low, but it is adequate to maintain a stable hematocrit.

The red cell *mass* is defined as the volume of RBCs per kilogram of body weight and can be accurately measured by the dilution technique using intravenously injected, autologous radiolabeled RBCs. By this technique the RBC mass is found to be 26 ml in women and 30 ml in men of RBCs per kilogram body weight, with a 10% variation among normal individuals. *Anemia* is a pathologic condition in which an absolute decrease occurs in the RBC mass. *Polycythemia* is an absolute increase of the RBC mass.

In clinical practice the RBC mass is assessed by the concentration of the hemoglobin in the blood or by the hematocrit, which measures the ratio of the RBC volume to the plasma volume. In general a close agreement exists between the RBC mass and the hematocrit or the hemoglobin concentration, except when a significant change occurs in the plasma volume. Thus dehydration of a patient with a normal RBC mass may lead to an elevation of hematocrit that may falsely be interpreted as a sign of polycythemia, whereas dehydration of an anemic patient may result in a normal hematocrit that drops precipitously on rehydration. In contrast, expansion of the plasma volume, as typically occurs during pregnancy, may result in an inappropriately low hematocrit in the presence of a normal RBC mass. In this chapter the terms *low* or *high* hematocrit refer to those circumstances in which the patient's hydration status and plasma volume are normal, so they can be considered synonymous with anemia and polycythemia, respectively.

LOW HEMATOCRIT

Anemia is one of the most common manifestations of disease. It should always be considered as a sign of an underlying disease and not a diagnosis in itself. Anemia can result from a reduction in the rate of RBC production, from an increase in the rate of RBC destruction in the peripheral blood, or from acute blood loss (Fig. 80-1). Blood loss can be easily ruled out by the history and clinical examination. Differentiation between decreased production and increased destruction of RBCs relies on the reticulocyte count. *Reticulocytes* are young RBCs that have recently been released from the bone marrow (Color Plate III-4), and their number is expressed as a percentage of RBCs. Under normal conditions, only 1% to 2.5% of the RBCs are reticulocytes. In the presence of anemia, high levels of erythropoietin stimulate the marrow, and the release of reticulocytes increases many-fold. A reticulocyte count should be corrected for the degree of anemia. This correction is performed by multiplying the reticulocyte count by the patient's hematocrit and dividing by 45, which represents the average normal hematocrit. Using automated technology, the absolute number of reticulocytes in blood can be determined with great accuracy and is less labor intensive than manual methods (Chapter 73). Fig. 80-2 shows a diagnostic approach to the patient with a low hematocrit.

Decreased reticulocyte count

A corrected reticulocyte count of less than 1% or a low absolute number of reticulocytes is strong evidence that the anemia is caused by underproduction of RBCs by the bone marrow. This may result from erythropoietin deficiency secondary to renal failure, subnormal marrow response in the presence of an endocrinopathy, chronic inflammation or neoplasia, nutritional deficiencies (e.g., iron, folate, vitamin B_{12}), or a primary hematologic disease (e.g., marrow aplasia, dysplasia, myeloproliferation, leukemia). In the absence of abnormal white blood cell (WBC) or platelet counts, which usually indicate a primary hematologic disease and the need for bone marrow examination, further differentiation between nutritional deficiencies and other

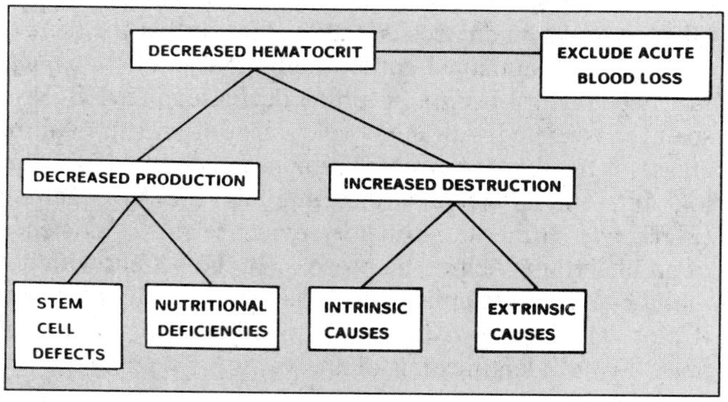

Fig. 80-1. Simplified classification of anemias.

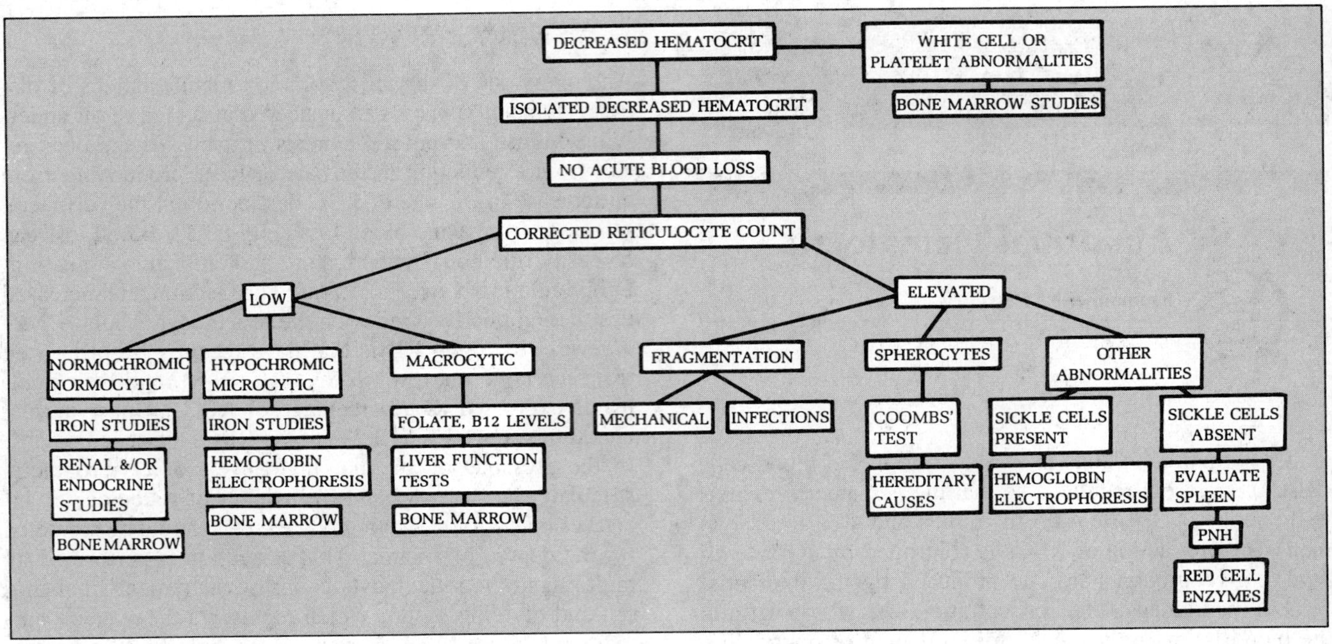

Fig. 80-2. Evaluation of a patient with a low hematocrit.

causes of underproduction anemia can be based on RBC size. Evaluation of RBC size requires both examination of the peripheral blood smear and direct measurement of mean corpuscular volume (MCV) by an electronic cell counter (Chapter 73). In iron deficiency the RBCs are microcytic and hypochromic, whereas in folate or B_{12} deficiency they are macrocytic and elongated (macro-ovalocytes). In general, other causes of reduced RBC production are associated with RBCs with a normal or near-normal MCV (*normocytic* RBCs) (see the box on the right).

Increased reticulocyte count

An elevated corrected reticulocyte count (> 3%) or elevated absolute reticulocyte count in excess of 100,000 per μl indicates that the marrow has responded appropriately to anemia with an increase in RBC production and that the basic mechanism of anemia is accelerated destruction of the RBCs in the peripheral blood. Under normal conditions the RBCs survive in the blood for about 120 days. If their life span decreases to as low as 20 days, the bone marrow can produce RBCs in an accelerated manner so that the hematocrit can be maintained within the normal limits *(compensated hemolytic anemia)*. A further decrease in the RBC life span is associated with the development of anemia. An increase of the serum bilirubin, disappearance of serum haptoglobin, and an elevation of serum lactate dehydrogenase (LDH) add further confirmatory evidence to the existence of an underlying hemolytic process. In the patient with hemolytic anemia, examination of the peripheral blood smear (Color Plate III-4) provides very important information that helps in the identification of the cause of hemolysis (see Table 90-1). Fragmented RBCs (schistocytes) are frequently seen in microangiopathic hemolytic anemia caused by the presence of a prosthetic heart valve or by disseminated intravascular coagulation. Spherocytes are seen in congenital spherocytosis and in acquired immune hemolytic anemia. The antiglobulin test (Coombs' test) is negative in congenital spherocytosis and positive in autoimmune hemolytic anemia. The presence of sickle cells or severe anisocytosis with microcytosis or target cells suggests the pres-

Disorders associated with decreased production or increased destruction of red blood cells (RBCs)

Decreased production

Renal failure
Chronic diseases (infectious, inflammatory, neoplastic)
Nutritional deficiencies (iron, folate, vitamin B_{12})
Myelodysplasia
Pure RBC aplasia
Endocrine hypofunction (thyroid, pituitary)
Hemoglobin with low oxygen affinity

Increased destruction

Hemolytic transfusion reaction
Infections
Immune hemolysis
RBC fragmentation
Hereditary spherocytosis
Hemoglobinopathies
Hypersplenism
RBC enzyme defects (G6PD, pyruvate kinase deficiency)
Paroxysmal nocturnal hemoglobinuria
Miscellaneous (severe burns, fresh water drowning)

ence of hemoglobinopathy, and a hemoglobin electrophoresis should be performed. In the absence of any prominent RBC morphologic abnormalities, one should consider the possibility of an RBC enzyme defect, hypersplenism, or of paroxysmal nocturnal hemoglobinuria. Glucose-6-phosphate dehydrogenase (G6PD) deficiency, an X-chromosome-linked enzymopathy, is the most common RBC enzyme defect and should be considered in patients with hemolysis appearing during the course of infections or after ingestion of a variety of oxidant drugs.

Borderline low hematocrit

A common clinical problem is a borderline low hematocrit without another abnormality in the peripheral blood or without signs of systemic disease. The extent to which such a laboratory abnormality should be investigated depends on the patient's age and sex. A careful history, a complete physical examination, and testing of stools for occult blood should be performed in all patients. Patients older than 70 years may have a slightly lower-than-normal hematocrit as a result of aging; however, malignancies, nutritional deficiencies, and myelodysplasia also occur quite frequently in this group of patients. Examination of the peripheral smear, a reticulocyte count, and assessment of the renal function should be performed in every patient. Depending on the size of RBCs, iron studies should be done in the presence of microcytes or hypochromia, and RBC folate and serum B_{12} should be measured in the presence of macro-ovalocytes or hypersegmented neutrophils. If these studies do not provide an explanation for the cause of anemia, the patient should be re-evaluated every 3 to 6 months with a complete blood count (CBC). If the drop of hematocrit is progressive, one should proceed with a complete workup of anemia regardless of its severity.

Men of younger age should always have a complete investigation of a borderline low hematocrit. During their reproductive period, women frequently develop iron deficiency, which may present initially as a borderline low hematocrit. In the absence of any other abnormality, a therapeutic trial with oral iron is justified. If the hematocrit does not normalize within a period of 4 to 8 weeks, a full investigation of anemia should be initiated.

Abnormal red cell indices in nonanemic patient

Occasionally in a patient with a normal hematocrit, the RBC size is found to be abnormal. Such a finding must be confirmed by examination of the peripheral blood smear. Microcytosis without iron deficiency is a common manifestation of heterozygous thalassemia. In β-thalassemia, this can be confirmed by quantification of hemoglobin F and A_2. In α-thalassemia trait, hematologic studies of the patient's family members may confirm the familial nature of this finding. Isolated macrocytosis may be an early manifestation of folate or vitamin B_{12} deficiency, alcoholic liver disease, hypothyroidism, or myelodysplasia. Pseudomacrocytosis may occasionally be seen in patients with severe reticulocytosis resulting from compensated immune hemolytic anemia due to cold agglutinins with clinically insignificant thermoamplitude, and with cryoglobulinemia. Examination of the peripheral blood smear and measurement of folate and B_{12} are usually necessary for the patient's initial evaluation. In the absence of any abnormal finding indicating further investigation, the patient should be re-evaluated with a CBC at 3- to 6-month intervals.

HIGH HEMATOCRIT

A high hematocrit can result from hemoconcentration or an increased rate of RBC production by the bone marrow, which may be either autonomous or secondary to high serum erythropoietin levels. With hemoconcentration the RBC mass is normal, and the increased hematocrit is caused by decreased plasma volume. *Polycythemia* is defined as an absolute increase in the RBC mass that is appreciated clinically by a high hematocrit. In the absence of dehydration, a hematocrit greater than 60% is always associated with an increase of RBC mass and is diagnostic of polycythemia. For hematocrit values of 50% to 60%, the diagnosis of polycythemia requires direct measurement of the RBC mass. An RBC mass greater than 32 ml/kg in women and 35 ml/kg body weight in men confirms the diagnosis of polycythemia. A classification of polycythemia is shown in the box below. Fig. 80-3 illustrates a diagnostic approach to the patient with a high hematocrit.

In *relative* or *stress polycythemia,* the patient has a high hematocrit because of decreased plasma volume, but the RBC mass is found to be normal. In this sense the "stress" or "relative" polycythemia is a misnomer. This condition most often appears in anxious males, older than 50 years, who frequently are hypertensive and smokers with a high incidence of thrombotic episodes. Smoking and high blood pressure have been considered to be the cause of plasma

Classification of polycythemia

I. Relative polycythemia (stress, spurious, Gaisböck's syndrome)
II. True polycythemia
    A. Polycythemia vera
    B. Secondary polycythemia
        1. Decreased tissue oxygenation
            a. Chronic pulmonary disease
            b. Smoking
            c. Congenital cyanotic heart disease
            d. Hemoglobin with high oxygen affinity
        2. Normal tissue oxygenation
            a. Benign renal lesions (renal artery stenosis, renal cysts, hydronephrosis, nephrocalcinosis, transplant rejection, etc.)
            b. Neoplasms (renal, hepatic, ovarian, adrenal, cerebellar)
            c. Endocrinopathies (Cushing's syndrome, pheochromocytoma)
            d. Idiopathic

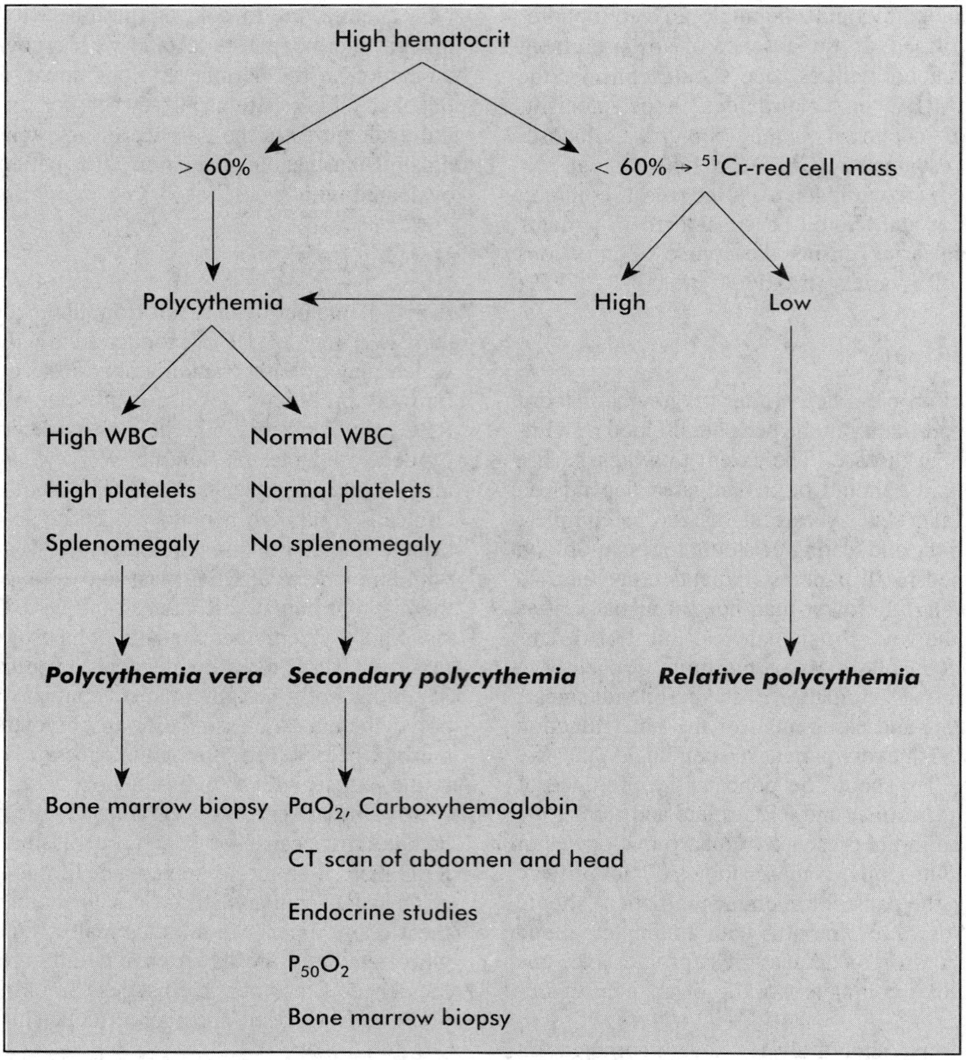

Fig. 80-3. Evaluation of a patient with a high hematocrit.

volume contraction. Cessation of smoking, correction of hypertension, or switching from a diuretic to another antihypertensive medication may lead to normalization of the hematocrit. If these measures are not successful, and in the presence of any symptoms or signs of vascular insufficiency, treatment with phlebotomies to reduce the hematocrit to less than 45% is warranted.

Once the diagnosis of true polycythemia is established, the major differential diagnosis centers between polycythemia vera and secondary polycythemia (Table 80-1). *Polycythemia vera* is a myeloproliferative disorder in which the production of RBCs is not controlled by and is independent of erythropoietin (Chapter 93). Besides an elevated hematocrit, patients with this disease also have leukocytosis, thrombocytosis, splenomegaly, and a hypercellular bone marrow with trilinear hyperplasia (Color Plate III-11). In early stages, however, a high hematocrit may be the only manifestation.

In *secondary polycythemia* the high hematocrit is always secondary to elevated levels of circulating erythropoietin, and the bone marrow remains normocellular. Neither leukocytosis nor thrombocytosis occurs, and the spleen size remains normal. Measurement of serum erythropoietin levels may help occasionally in the differential diagnosis. With a high hematocrit, a significantly elevated serum erythropoietin level favors the diagnosis of secondary polycythemia; however, a normal or mildly elevated value by itself cannot exclude the diagnosis of secondary polycythemia. Without an underlying disease or condition that can possibly cause hypoxia and elevated serum erythropoietin levels, and if the white cell and platelet counts are normal and the spleen size is not increased (as documented by spleen scan or abdominal computed tomography [CT]), examination of bone marrow is the only diagnostic procedure that can differentiate polycythemia vera from secondary polycythemia.

In secondary polycythemia the increase in the RBC mass is caused by an elevated serum erythropoietin level. This

Table 80-1. Differentiation among relative polycythemia, polycythemia vera, and secondary polycythemia

	Relative polycythemia	Polycythemia vera	Secondary polycythemia
Hematocrit	H	H	H
Red cell mass	N	H	H
White blood count	N	H	N
Platelet count	N	H	N
Spleen size	N	H	N
Marrow cellularity	N	H	N

H, High; N, normal.

may represent a normal response to tissue hypoxia or may result from autonomous production of erythropoietin. Therefore the investigation of secondary polycythemia should focus on the identification of the cause of increased erythropoietin production. Chronic pulmonary disease resulting in a decrease of arterial oxygen tension (Pao_2) to less than 67 mm Hg is a frequent cause of secondary polycythemia. In patients with chronic obstructive lung disease and polycythemia in whom the Pao_2 is higher than 67 mm Hg while awake, oximetry during sleep may be necessary to detect periods of severe hypoxia during sleep. Severe cardiovascular disease may also lead to the development of hypoxia and polycythemia, particularly after years of chronic pulmonary congestion. Congenital cyanotic cardiac disease is a frequent cause of secondary polycythemia in children but is rare in adults.

In the absence of chronic lung disease, smoking by itself can cause polycythemia. Smoking not only causes an elevated level of carboxyhemoglobin (greater than 1%) but also shifts the oxyhemoglobin dissociation curve to the left, which results in an increased affinity of hemoglobin for oxygen (O_2). The latter is probably much more important in the pathogenesis of smokers' polycythemia than the conversion of a small percentage of hemoglobin to carboxyhemoglobin. The magnitude of the effect of smoking on O_2 delivery from hemoglobin to tissues can be more accurately assessed by measuring the $P_{50}O_2$, which is usually less than 25 mm Hg. Rarely, secondary polycythemia is caused by an abnormal hemoglobin with high affinity for O_2. The presence of a positive family history for polycythemia appearing at an early age should lead to the measurement of $P_{50}O_2$. If abnormal, the type of abnormal hemoglobin can be identified by hemoglobin electrophoresis.

In some patients with secondary polycythemia, the elevation of serum erythropoietin levels is not the result of tissue hypoxia and thus is considered to be physiologically inappropriate. Such an elevation of erythropoietin leading to polycythemia has been described as a paraneoplastic manifestation of a variety of malignant or benign tumors, including tumors of the kidneys, liver, adrenal glands, ovaries, and cerebellum. More frequently, such an inappropriate elevation of serum erythropoietin is caused by benign focal lesions in the kidney that result in focal hypoxia stimulating erythropoietin production. Renal cysts, renal artery stenosis, hydronephrosis, nephrocalcinosis, transplant rejection, and a variety of other renal lesions may cause secondary polycythemia through this mechanism. Endocrinologic disorders characterized by high levels of androgenic steroids or catecholamines, such as Cushing's syndrome and pheochromocytoma, respectively, may directly or indirectly stimulate erythropoietin production by the kidney, resulting in polycythemia. In the absence of any clinically obvious cause of hypoxia, a CT scan of the abdomen is necessary for detection of pathology in the kidneys, liver, adrenal glands, or ovaries. If clinically indicated, a CT scan of the head and measurement of serum or urine 17-ketosteroids and catecholamines may be necessary. Even after the most thorough investigation, however, the exact cause of polycythemia may not be found.

The treatment of polycythemia vera is described in Chapter 93. The management of secondary polycythemia first should be directed toward the primary underlying disease. Cessation of smoking, long-term O_2 therapy, removal of a tumor, or correction of a surgically amenable renal lesion may be all that is needed to restore the hematocrit to normal. If these measures are not effective, the aim of therapy is to reduce the hematocrit to levels that will reduce blood viscosity, improve blood flow to the tissues, reduce symptoms from vascular insufficiency, and reduce a possibly increased risk of thrombotic episodes. This can be obtained by repeated phlebotomy of 250 to 400 ml of blood every other day until the hematocrit drops to 45%. Thereafter the frequency of phlebotomy should be individualized so that the hematocrit is kept within the normal range. Phlebotomy should be performed with caution in older patients with underlying cardiovascular disease. Usually the volume of removed blood should be replaced by an equal volume of colloids or oral fluids.

Borderline high hematocrit

At times the physician faces the dilemma of how extensively to investigate a borderline high hematocrit. Generally, if the hematocrit is 48% to 54%, only a repeat examination and follow-up are necessary. If the hematocrit remains stable or fluctuates between normal and slightly elevated levels, and if the clinical history, physical examination, and routine urine analysis are normal, the patient should be followed-up at regular intervals. If the hematocrit increases to levels of 55% or higher, a complete workup is warranted.

REFERENCES

Berlin NI: Diagnosis and classification of polycythemias. Semin Hematol 12:339, 1975.

Finch CA and Cook JD: Iron deficiency. Am J Clin Nutr 39:471, 1984.

Golde DW: Polycythemia: mechanisms and management. Ann Intern Med 95:71, 1981.

Herbert V: Megaloblastic anemias. Lab Invest 52:3, 1985.

Kellermeyer RW: General principles of the evaluation and therapy of anemias. Med Clin North Am 68:533, 1984.

CHAPTER

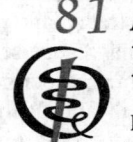

81 Abnormal Nucleated Blood Cell Counts

David H. Boldt

Patients frequently have alterations in numbers of leukocytes or abnormal nucleated blood cells in the peripheral circulation. Sometimes these changes may be discovered unexpectedly in an individual being seen for a routine examination. At other times the finding may be sought as part of the evaluation of a patient with debilitating systemic illness. In either case, blood is uniquely accessible and easily examined for the presence of underlying hematopathology. This chapter considers causes, clinical features, and approaches to diagnosis in patients who have abnormal peripheral nucleated blood cell counts. An overview is given in the box to the right. Specific disease entities are the subjects of other chapters.

QUANTITATIVE ALTERATIONS IN NORMAL NUCLEATED CELLS

Quantitative alterations—increases or decreases—in circulating leukocyte counts are encountered most often in clinical practice. Clinically important types of leukocytoses include neutrophilia, eosinophilia, basophilia, lymphocytosis, and monocytosis. The leukopenia of highest clinical importance is neutropenia because of both the frequency of its occurrence and its effects on host susceptibility to infection. By contrast, eosinopenia and basopenia have no known adverse effects, and so few blood basophils normally are present that a reduction in their numbers is difficult to detect. Monocytopenia may be observed with stress, acute infections, or hairy cell leukemia. Its clinical significance is unknown. Lymphocytopenia occurs in chronic debilitating conditions and is often associated with malnutrition. Lymphocytopenia is a prominent hematologic manifestation of both congenital and acquired immunodeficiency syndromes, including AIDS.

Increases in circulating leukocytes

Neutrophilia. The neutrophil count of each individual is tightly regulated so that under usual circumstances little day-to-day variation occurs. However, a small normal diurnal variation and age-related changes that are characteristic for each sex have been described. In females the neutrophil count normally fluctuates with the menstrual cycle.

Neutrophilia may be defined as an increase in circulating neutrophils to more than 8.0×10^9/L. Neutrophil counts in excess of this level do not always indicate underlying pathology because certain "physiologic" causes of neutrophilia are recognized. These include stress, physical exercise, and pregnancy. The neutrophilia observed with stress reflects elevated blood levels of catecholamines and

Abnormal white blood cell counts: diagnostic considerations

I. Quantitative abnormalities
  A. Increases in circulating leukocytes
    1. Neutrophilia
      a. Reactive: infections, inflammatory disorders, tissue destruction, malignancies, drug induced, hemorrhage, hemolysis, diabetic ketoacidosis
      b. Primary myeloproliferative disorders
      c. Physiologic
      d. Idiopathic
    2. Eosinophilia
      a. Reactive: allergies and hypersensitivity reactions, parasitic infections, immunologic disorders, malignancies
      b. Primary: hypereosinophilic syndromes
      c. Adrenal insufficiency
    3. Basophilia: myeloproliferative disorders
    4. Monocytosis
      a. Reactive: malignancies, immunologic disorders, infections
      b. Primary: monocytic leukemia
    5. Lymphocytosis
      a. Reactive: infection, especially viral, pertussis, acute infectious lymphocytosis, immunologic disorders
      b. Primary: lymphoproliferative diseases
  B. Decreases in circulating leukocytes
    1. Neutropenia
      a. Decreased production: bone marrow injury caused by ionizing radiation or drugs, marrow replacement, nutritional deficiencies, congenital stem cell defects
      b. Increased destruction/utilization/sequestration: hypersplenism, immune mechanisms, overwhelming infection
    2. Lymphocytopenia
      a. Decreased production: primary immunodeficiency diseases
      b. Increased destruction/utilization/loss: collagen vascular disease, acute infections or stress, ionizing radiation, cytotoxic drugs, antilymphocyte globulin, loss of lymph
      c. Unknown mechanism: malignancies, chronic infection
II. Qualitative abnormalities
  A. Immature granulocytes: leukemoid reactions, leukemia, myeloproliferative syndromes
  B. Morphologic alterations in granulocytes: toxic granulations, Döhle's bodies, vacuoles, Chédiak-Higashi syndrome, Pelger-Huët anomaly
  C. Abnormal lymphocytes
    1. Atypical lymphocytes: viral infections, immunologic reactions, toxoplasmosis
    2. Plasmacytoid lymphocytes: viral infections, immunologic reactions, Waldenström's macroglobulinemia
    3. Lymphoblasts: acute lymphoblastic leukemia
    4. Lymphosarcoma cells: lymphoma
    5. Sézary cells: cutaneous lymphomas
    6. Hairy cells: hairy cell leukemia
    7. Prolymphocytes: prolymphocytic leukemia

glucocorticosteroids. The leukocytosis associated with all these conditions may be striking. For example, white blood cell counts in excess of 50.0×10^9/L have been documented in long-distance runners immediately after exercise. After several hours of rest the white count returns to normal. A minority of uncomplicated pregnancies are associated with leukocytosis, which occurs chiefly during the last trimester. However, the physician must remain alert to the possibility that the development of neutrophilia during pregnancy signifies a serious complication such as eclampsia or bleeding. Neutrophilia in the absence of apparent pathology also may be seen in heavy cigarette smokers, although it is not clear whether subclinical bronchopulmonary infection contributes to this elevation. Finally, a group of individuals with mild chronic neutrophilic leukocytosis (neutrophil counts in the range of 12.0 to 20.0×10^9/L) has been described. This condition, termed *chronic idiopathic neutrophilia,* occurs both as a familial disorder and sporadically. It is considered benign in nature and may represent the extremes of the normal range, but chromosomal abnormalities and organomegaly have been reported in some of these individuals. Some have also developed diseases such as vasculitis, rheumatoid arthritis, and Hodgkin's disease after prolonged follow-up. In other patients, however, long-term follow-up has failed to reveal evidence of any systemic illness.

Although neutrophilia may be a common host response to a variety of physiologic stimuli, it is more frequently encountered as a reaction to an underlying disease process (see the box on p. 770). The three major classes of disorders associated with neutrophilia are (1) infections and inflammatory diseases; (2) tissue destruction, as in myocardial or pulmonary infarction, major surgery, or shock; and (3) malignant disease. Other miscellaneous causes include hemorrhage, hemolysis, diabetic ketoacidosis, thyroid storm, eclampsia, or the administration of drugs such as lithium or glucocorticosteroids. Usually the underlying condition is obvious and the neutrophilia properly recognized as reactive.

Occasionally, however, neutrophilia may be the presenting sign of an occult process, and the physician must search for its cause. A diagrammatic approach to assessment of a patient with neutrophilia is given in Fig. 81-1. Bacterial infection is the most common cause of a neutrophilic leukocytosis, but neutrophilia may also be seen in fungal, viral, and parasitic infections. Presence of toxic granulations, Döhle's bodies, and/or cytoplasmic vacuolization in circulating neutrophils favors an infectious process, although none of these changes is specific. Occult sources of infections should be considered when diagnosis is difficult. These include bacterial endocarditis, deep-seated abscesses especially in the abdomen, chronic fungal or mycobacte-

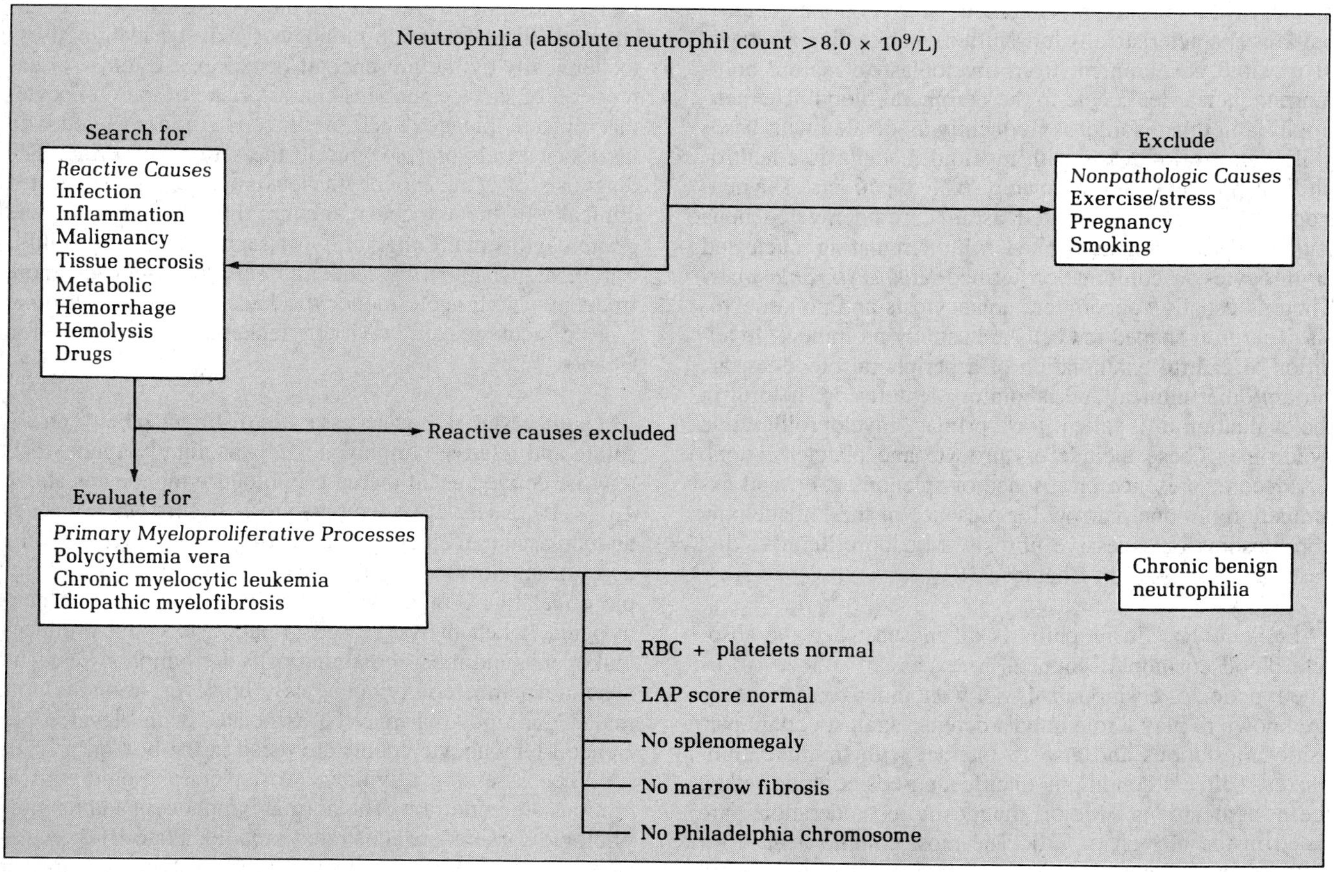

Fig. 81-1. General approach to neutrophilia.

rial infections, and ascending cholangitis. In hospitalized patients, indwelling tubes and catheters are potential sites of infection.

Usually infection is accompanied by a *left shift* on the peripheral blood smear. This term refers to the presence in the circulation of increased numbers of neutrophil precursors. Two patterns of left shift may be encountered. In one form there are increased numbers of band forms (more than 0.45×10^9/L); in the other form, neutrophilic metamyelocytes, myelocytes, or promyelocytes are present. Cells less mature than band forms are not normally present on the peripheral smear. A granulocytic "leukemoid" reaction may be considered an extreme form of a reactive, left-shifted neutrophilia in which a very high neutrophil count and/or abundant neutrophil precursors may simulate the appearance of true leukemia in the peripheral blood. Features that aid in differentiation of such a leukemoid reaction from chronic myelogenous leukemia are listed in Table 93-3. Cytogenetic testing, leukocyte alkaline phosphatase (LAP) score, and presence of basophilia are the most helpful discriminating points. Granulocytic leukemoid reactions are seen most often in association with infections and malignancies.

When reactive neutrophilia has been excluded, consideration should be given to a primary myeloproliferative process. A neutrophilic leukocytosis consisting predominantly of mature segmented and band forms is a common feature of polycythemia vera and reflects that this disorder is a panmyelosis. In chronic myelogenous leukemia the neutrophilia is characteristically left-shifted, manifesting all stages of myeloid development from myeloblast to mature polymorphonuclear leukocyte in the peripheral blood. The neutrophilia in this disorder is frequently associated with basophilia. In myelofibrosis with myeloid metaplasia a neutrophilia is present in approximately 80% of patients. The neutrophilia, usually left-shifted as in chronic myelogenous leukemia, is often associated with circulating nucleated erythrocytes, a combination termed *leukoerythroblastosis*. There is usually concomitant anisocytosis and poikilocytosis. Teardrop-shaped red cells are usually prominent. In addition to careful examination of a peripheral blood smear, certain other clinical and laboratory features are helpful in the evaluation of a patient for a primary myeloproliferative syndrome. These include erythrocyte and platelet counts, LAP score, presence or absence of splenomegaly, and examination of bone marrow for presence of the Philadelphia chromosome or excessive fibrosis. Myeloproliferative diseases are discussed in Chapter 93.

Eosinophilia. Eosinophilia is diagnosed when the absolute blood eosinophil count is in excess of 0.5×10^9/L. The function of eosinophils is not well understood, but they are known to play a role in host defense against certain parasitic infestations and also to interact with immune complexes. Clinical conditions manifesting eosinophilia reflect these associations. Major diagnostic considerations are listed in the box on p. 770. The most common cause for mild eosinophilia in hospitalized patients is drug allergy. Hypereosinophilic syndromes (Chapter 92) are associated with the most marked elevations of eosinophil counts.

Basophilia. Basophilia is rarely encountered. Its presence may be helpful in diagnosing a primary myeloproliferative disorder such as chronic myelogenous leukemia, polycythemia vera, or myelofibrosis.

Monocytosis. Peripheral blood monocytes are precursors of the tissue macrophages. The monocyte-macrophage system serves an important role in the body economy that may be summarized as (1) antigen uptake and presentation for generation of immune responses; (2) immune regulation; (3) phagocytosis and killing of microorganisms, macrophages being the first line of defense against various intracellular parasites such as *Mycobacterium tuberculosis, Listeria,* and *Brucella;* and (4) secretion of biologically active molecules, including complement, interferon and various cytokines, and hematopoietic growth factors. The presence of monocytosis (monocyte count in excess of 0.70×10^9/L) generally indicates an underlying neoplastic process, immunologic disease, or chronic inflammatory process (see the box on p. 770). Monocytosis also may be associated with several primary hematologic disorders. These include drug-induced and other forms of neutropenia, hemolytic anemias, and dysmyelopoietic syndromes (preleukemia). In addition, monocytosis may be a feature of the early phase of bone marrow recovery from myelosuppression. Certain primary and secondary myelodysplastic syndromes as well as certain types of acute nonlymphoid leukemias may be characterized by the presence of abundant, well-differentiated monocytic cells in the circulation. When less well differentiated, these leukemic monocytes may be identified cytochemically by the presence of nonspecific esterase or expression of surface antigens characteristic of the monocyte-macrophage lineage. Their presence is also associated with increased levels of lysozyme in the serum and urine. The diagnosis of acute monocytic leukemia may be suggested clinically by the associated anemia, thrombocytopenia, and granulocytopenia. Gingival hypertrophy secondary to infiltration of the gums by leukemic cells is associated more frequently with acute monocytic leukemia than with other types of acute leukemia. (Acute leukemias are discussed in Chapter 93.)

Lymphocytosis. It is necessary to distinguish between absolute and relative lymphocytosis. Absolute lymphocytosis may be defined as an increase in blood lymphocytes above 4.0×10^9/L. Relative lymphocytosis occurs when there is an increased percentage of circulating lymphocytes, but the absolute number does not exceed 4.0×10^9/L. An example of relative lymphocytosis occurs in patients with neutropenia, when the decreased granulocyte count produces leukopenia and most remaining cells are lymphocytes. The absolute number of lymphocytes, however, remains normal. Conditions that may be associated with elevated peripheral lymphocyte counts are listed in the box on p. 770.

When assessing a lymphocytosis, morphologic considerations are important. The normal lymphocyte and its morphologic variants are illustrated in Color Plate III-5. A variety of morphologically distinct types of lymphocytes can be seen in normal peripheral blood. Approximately 80% of normal lymphoid cells are small lymphocytes 6 to 9 μ in diameter. These cells are characterized by nuclei containing compact clumps of chromatin surrounded by thin rims of clear blue cytoplasm. Most of the remaining lymphoid cells are of intermediate size, 10 to 15 μ in diameter, with more abundant cytoplasm and less compact nuclear chromatin. Some of these cells, referred to as *large granular lymphocytes* (LGLs), contain prominent intracytoplasmic azurophilic granules. LGL is the predominant cell type that mediates natural killer (NK) activity (Chapter 286). From 0.5% to 1% of lymphocytes are large, blastlike cells, up to 25 μ in diameter, whose nuclei may contain several nucleoli and finely dispersed chromatin. Frequently the cytoplasm of these cells may appear deeply basophilic and may contain vacuoles. Intermediate- and large-sized lymphoid variants including classic atypical lymphocytes are often referred to as *reactive lymphocytes*. Moderate increases in reactive lymphocytes are seen as a characteristic response to viruses and other infections, especially in children. Increases also occur in a wide variety of other situations, including primary and secondary immune responses, hypersensitivity reactions, and autoimmune disorders.

The differential diagnosis of marked lymphocytosis composed solely of normal small lymphocytes is limited in scope. In the adult the major consideration is chronic lymphocytic leukemia. This diagnosis may best be confirmed by demonstrating the monoclonal B cell nature of the proliferation and coexpression of the CD5 antigen by appropriate lymphocyte surface marker studies. In childhood and adolescence the chief considerations are pertussis and acute infectious lymphocytosis. In pertussis the lymphocyte count regularly reaches levels of 10.0 to 50.0 $\times$ 10^9/L during the early phase of the disease. Acute infectious lymphocytosis is a mild, asymptomatic, self-limited disease of childhood and adolescence. When symptoms do occur, they are transitory in nature and may include fever, rash, coryza, cough, pharyngitis, or gastrointestinal complaints. Lymphocytosis may reach 100 to 150 $\times$ 10^9/L and generally persists for 3 to 5 weeks. Red blood cell and platelet counts are normal, and lymphadenopathy or hepatosplenomegaly does not occur. These features, as well as the mature morphology of the circulating lymphocytes, aid in differentiating acute infectious lymphocytosis from acute lymphoblastic leukemia. The absence of reactive or atypical lymphocytes and the extreme elevation of the lymphocyte count in acute infectious lymphocytosis allow its ready differentiation from infectious mononucleosis and other infectious conditions. The age distribution contrasts greatly with that of chronic lymphocytic leukemia, which is a disease of elderly persons. No treatment is indicated because the disease is uniformly self-limiting.

Lymphocytosis has been described in association with certain endocrine disorders, especially thyrotoxicosis and adrenal insufficiency. A small percentage of patients with thyrotoxicosis may display a relative lymphocytosis, sometimes associated with lymphoid hyperplasia, including splenomegaly. Lymphocytosis, usually relative, is seen in approximately half of patients with untreated Addison's disease. Lymphocytosis rarely may be impressive enough to simulate a lymphoid malignancy. Lymphoproliferative disorders associated with peripheral lymphocytosis are discussed later in this chapter.

Decreases in circulating leukocytes

Neutropenia. Neutropenia exists when numbers of circulating neutrophils are reduced below the normal range. Although neutrophil counts less than 2.0 $\times$ 10^9/L occur infrequently in normal individuals, some healthy, resting adults, particularly blacks and Yemenite Jews, may have counts as low as 1.0 $\times$ 10^9/L without evidence of disease.

Neutropenia may occur as an isolated condition or in association with decrease in other circulating elements, as in pancytopenia (Fig. 81-2). In either case the neutropenia is caused by one of two major pathologic mechanisms: (1) de-

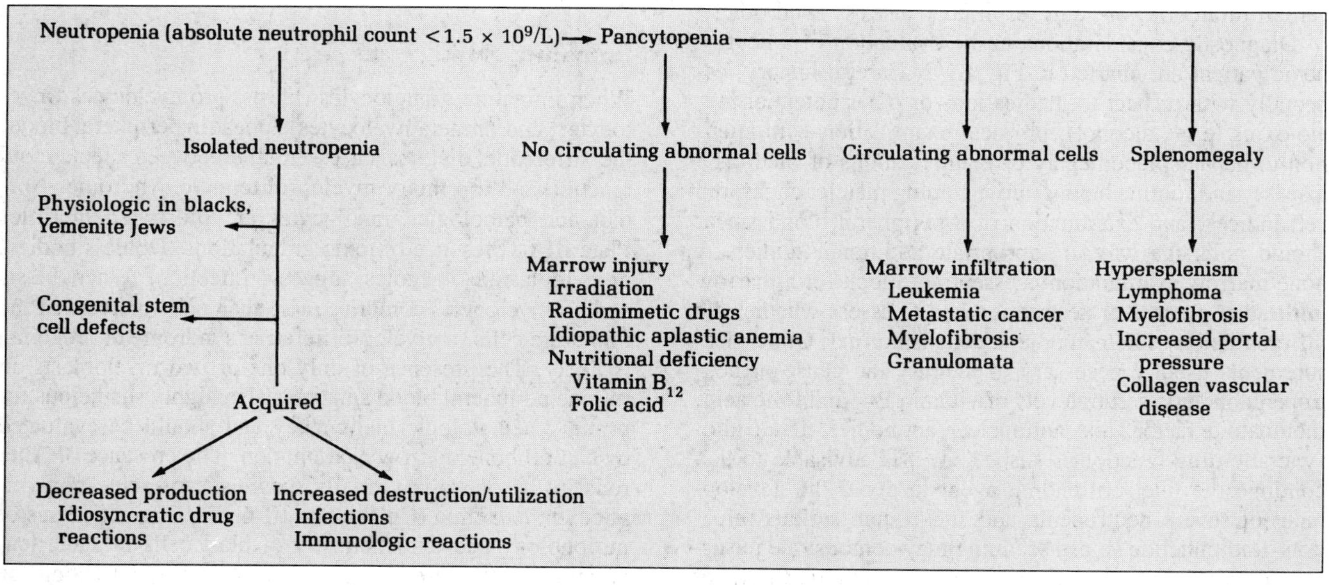

Fig. 81-2. General approach to neutropenia.

creased production (i.e., a bone marrow problem) or (2) increased destruction or removal from the circulation.

Decreased production may be secondary to ionizing irradiation, cytotoxic drugs such as nitrogen mustard or other alkylating agents, or idiopathic causes, as in aplastic anemia. Bone marrow replacement by leukemia, metastatic tumor, fibrosis, or granulomata is an additional consideration. Decreased production may result from nutritional deficiencies, particularly of vitamin B_{12} or folic acid. Hypersplenism is a cause of pancytopenia related to peripheral destruction or sequestration. This concept is discussed in Chapter 82.

The occurrence of isolated neutropenia secondary to failure of myelopoiesis implies a defect in the myeloid stem cell or in a committed progenitor such as the CFU-GEMM or CFU-GM. Such a defect may be acquired, as in patients with certain idiosyncratic drug reactions, or it may be congenital, as in those with cyclic neutropenia. There are a variety of other poorly understood congenital disorders of myelopoiesis. Some of these disorders are associated with other abnormalities and constitute well-recognized clinical syndromes. In these congenital diseases, neutropenia is generally recognized during infancy, and fatal infections may supervene. A thorough drug and medication history should be obtained from all patients with acquired neutropenia. Idiosyncratic drug-induced neutropenia is discussed in Chapter 92.

Isolated neutropenia may be a sign of overwhelming infection, in which case it is caused by both rapid egress of neutrophils from blood to tissue sites and suppression of myelopoiesis. In certain instances, isolated neutropenia may be caused by immunologically mediated granulocyte destruction. Recently, complement-induced granulocyte aggregation has been suggested as a cause of leukopenia in Felty's syndrome (neutropenia and splenomegaly in association with rheumatoid arthritis) and systemic lupus erythematosus. It might also be a mechanism for tissue damage caused by leukostasis in such diverse clinical settings as pulmonary dysfunction in hemodialyzed patients, myocardial infarction, or adult respiratory distress syndrome.

Diagnostic considerations in the evaluation of a neutropenic patient are charted in Fig. 81-2. Careful history, especially with respect to medications or other potential myelotoxins (e.g., alcohol), physical examination with attention to hepatosplenomegaly or manifestations of rheumatic disease, and routine hemogram including platelet count, red cell indices, and examination of a peripheral blood smear should point the way to appropriate additional studies. A bone marrow examination is essential to look for a marrow infiltrative process or destruction and to assess whether the differentiation of hematopoietic cells is normal. Other measurements usually necessary to identify the cause of neutropenia include serum levels of vitamin B_{12} and folic acid, rheumatoid factor, and antinuclear antibodies. If an idiosyncratic drug reaction is suspected, it is advisable to discontinue the likely offending agent to avoid the development of severe neutropenia and subsequent serious infection. Radionuclide spleen scanning may demonstrate unsuspected splenic enlargement or help to resolve questions of equivocal splenomegaly. These relatively straightforward tests will resolve 90% of clinically encountered cases of neutropenia. Further evaluation requires expertise and research procedures generally available only at specialized centers.

Lymphocytopenia. An absolute lymphocytopenia occurs when the peripheral lymphocyte count is less than 1.5×10^9/L in adults, or less than 3.0×10^9/L in children. Major causes include immunodeficiency disorders, malignancy, collagen vascular diseases, and chronic infections (see the box on p. 770). The most common cause of sustained lymphocytopenia is malignancy, followed by collagen vascular disease. Currently, AIDS and AIDS-related complex (ARC) have emerged as additional important causes. Transient decreases in blood lymphocyte counts also occur often and may be noted in association with acute infections or other stressful situations. Lymphocytopenia in these patients is thought to reflect redistribution of lymphocytes into the tissues in response to increased serum levels of glucocorticosteroids. Lymphocyte destruction may follow treatment with or exposure to ionizing radiation, chemotherapy with alkylating agents, or antilymphocyte globulin. Lymphocytes may be lost from the body during thoracic duct drainage or in conditions associated with excessive loss of intestinal lymph. These include Whipple's disease, intestinal lymphangiectasis, mechanical obstruction of intestinal lymphatics by tumor or fibrosis, and severe right-sided congestive heart failure.

ABNORMAL NUCLEATED CELLS IN PERIPHERAL BLOOD

Under normal circumstances in the adult, only mature anucleate erythrocytes, mature granulocytes (including stab or band forms), monocytes, and lymphocytes (80% small nonreactive, 20% reactive) are seen in the peripheral circulation. The appearance of immature or abnormal cells in the circulation is indicative of underlying hematopathology and demands explanation.

Immature granulocytes

When immature granulocytes (blasts, promyelocytes, myelocytes, and/or metamyelocytes) appear in peripheral blood, the differential diagnosis is essentially between a leukemoid reaction and a primary myeloproliferative syndrome. Normal and pathologic granulocytes are illustrated in Color Plate III-6. Presence of toxic granulations, Döhle's bodies, or cytoplasmic vacuoles suggests infection. When blasts and promyelocytes comprise more than a few percent of the immature cells, a myeloproliferative syndrome or leukemia is likely. The presence of only one or two myeloblasts on routine peripheral blood smears is also highly suspicious for primary hematologic malignancy and should be evaluated by careful bone marrow examination. The presence of Auer rods in the blasts is virtually diagnostic of acute nonlymphocytic leukemia (Color Plate III-6, *E*). Characteristics of morphology and cytochemistry of blast cells in acute leukemias are discussed in Chapters 74 and 93. It should be remembered that in acute leukemias the total leukocyte count may be elevated, normal, or low. It has been said that leukopenia is as suggestive of leukemia as leukocytosis. The peripheral blood smear in chronic myelogenous leukemia resembles a smear of bone marrow because all stages of myeloid maturation from blast through mature polymorphonuclear neutrophil leukocyte (PMN) can be found (Color Plate III-6, *D*). A basophilia may also be present. Leukocyte alkaline phosphatase and cytogenetic analysis can confirm the diagnosis of chronic myelogenous leukemia.

In idiopathic myelofibrosis, immature myeloid cells are usually present in the setting of a leukoerythroblastic blood smear. A leukoerythroblastic blood picture may also be seen in other marrow infiltrative processes, such as tumor, granulomata, or myelofibrosis secondary to certain drugs.

The Pelger-Huët anomaly (Color Plate III-6, *C*) is a hereditary condition in which mature granulocytes have two nuclear segments only. This condition has no pathologic significance because the granulocytes are normal in number and function. An acquired Pelger-Huët anomaly sometimes develops in myeloproliferative disorders, dysmyelopoietic syndromes, and severe infections.

Abnormal lymphoid cells

The variety of morphologic types of lymphoid cells that may be seen in normal blood has been discussed. The proportion and absolute number of reactive lymphocytes in the circulation may increase with certain conditions, such as infections and allergic reactions. It is important to distinguish such normal reactive variants from the variety of lymphoid cells that may enter the blood in malignant lymphoproliferative disorders (Table 81-1). Some of the malignant lymphocytes are illustrated in the photomicrographs in Color Plate III-5, which allows for their comparison with normal and reactive lymphocytes. Table 81-1 lists some laboratory

Table 81-1. Differential diagnosis of abnormal lymphocytes in peripheral blood

Lymphocyte type	Usual disease association	Cytologic features	Laboratory features	Clinical features
Small lymphocyte	Chronic lymphocytic leukemia	B cell surface markers with low concentration of surface immunoglobulin, CD5 antigen	Hypogammaglobulinemia in 50%; positive direct Coombs' test in 15%; on node biopsy, diffuse, well-differentiated lymphocytic infiltrate	Elderly adults; presentation runs gamut from asymptomatic with lymphocytosis only to bulky disease with adenopathy, splenomegaly, and "packed" bone marrow
Atypical lymphocyte	Infectious mononucleosis, other viral illnesses	Suppressor T cell markers	Heterophil agglutinin; positive serology for Epstein-Barr virus, cytomegalovirus, toxoplasma, HBsAg	Pharyngitis, fever, adenopathy, rash, splenomegaly, palatal petechiae, jaundice
Plasmacytoid lymphocyte	Waldenström's macroglobulinemia	Cytoplasmic IgM, periodic acid-Schiff (PAS) positivity	IgM paraprotein, rouleaux, cryoglobulins	Adenopathy, splenomegaly, absence of bone lesions, hyperviscosity syndrome, cryopathic phenomena
Lymphoblast	Acute lymphoblastic leukemia (ALL)	Terminal transferase positivity, common ALL antigen	Anemia, granulocytopenia, thrombocytopenia, hyperuricemia, diffuse bone marrow infiltration	Peak incidence in childhood, acute onset, bone pain frequent
Lymphosarcoma cell	Lymphocytic lymphoma	B cell surface markers with high concentration of surface immunoglobulin	Nodular, or diffuse, poorly differentiated lymphocytic lymphoma on node biopsy, patchy, peritrabecular bone marrow involvement	Middle-aged to older adults, generalized adenopathy, constitutional symptoms
Sézary cell	Cutaneous lymphomas	T lymphocyte surface markers	Skin biopsy is diagnostic	Exfoliative erythroderma, cutaneous plaques or tumors
Hairy cell	Hairy cell leukemia	B lymphocyte markers, cytoplasmic projections, tartrate-resistant acid phosphatase, interleukin-2 receptors, CD11 antigen	Pancytopenia	Middle-aged males, moderate to marked splenomegaly without adenopathy
Prolymphocyte	Prolymphocytic leukemia	B cell surface markers with high concentration of surface immunoglobulin	Marked lymphocytosis (frequently $>100 \times 10^9$/L)	Elderly adults, massive splenomegaly, minimum adenopathy, poor response to therapy

and clinical considerations helpful in assessing patients who are found to have abnormal lymphoid cells on peripheral blood films. Additional information is provided in Chapter 74. The lymphoproliferative disorders with which these cells are associated are discussed in Chapters 93 to 95.

The small lymphocyte has a deeply stained, round nucleus of densely aggregated chromatin (Color Plate III-5, *A*). The nuclear membrane is distinct, and occasionally one or two nucleolar remnants may be seen. The nucleus is eccentrically located in the blue cytoplasm, which is scanty compared with the nucleus; often only a thin rim is seen. Atypical lymphocytes are larger, approximately 1½ to 3 times the size of a small lymphocyte, with more abundant cytoplasm (Color Plate III-5, *B*). The chromatin is less condensed than that of a normal lymphocyte. Nucleoli may be present. Although the cytoplasm may be foamy, more often it has no distinctive features other than denser staining at the periphery and the characteristic scalloping where the membrane contacts other cells.

Lymphoblasts, the characteristic cells of acute lymphoblastic leukemia, are large (15 to 20 μ) but variable in size (Color Plate III-5, *F*). The chromatin is finely distributed and threadlike. One or two indistinct nucleoli are always present. The cytoplasm is scanty. It is important to distinguish an atypical lymphocytosis such as occurs frequently with infectious mononucleosis syndromes or other viral illnesses in infancy and childhood from acute lymphoblastic leukemia (ALL), which has its peak occurrence in these same age groups. Additional similarities are that both infectious mononucleosis and ALL may be acute in onset and may be associated with lymphadenopathy and splenomegaly. In addition to careful evaluation of a peripheral blood film for the morphologic features just discussed and shown in Color Plate III-5, useful discriminatory points are the frequent presence in leukemia of anemia, granulocytopenia, and thrombocytopenia, as well as hyperuricemia and bone pain caused by accelerated cell turnover. Serologic features of the infectious mononucleosis syndromes are diagnostic. Diagnostic features of infectious mononucleosis are summarized in the box to the right. Cytochemical and immunologic features of lymphoblasts include presence of the enzyme terminal deoxynucleotidyl transferase (TdT) and/or the detection of the common ALL antigen at the cell surface (Table 81-1).

Circulating lymphoma cells are sometimes seen in the peripheral blood of patients with non-Hodgkin's lymphoma. When these cells are so abundant as to cause a leukemic peripheral blood picture, the term *lymphosarcoma cell leukemia* has been applied. Various forms of lymphosarcoma cells have been described. These range from lymphoid forms, slightly larger and less mature looking than the usual forms, to blastlike cells that may be difficult to distinguish from the blasts of ALL. A characteristic morphologic feature of lymphosarcoma cells is a cleaved folded nucleus, which has led to the descriptive term *buttock cell* (Color Plate III-5, *E*). Often there is a single, large, prominent nucleolus demarcated by a dense periphery of condensed chromatin. Lymphosarcoma cell leukemia frequently develops in middle-aged or older individuals as a late manifestation of lymphoma. In such patients its recognition and proper diagnosis are not difficult. At other times, lymphosarcoma cell leukemia may be an initial manifestation of lymphoma. In this setting it must be differentiated from chronic lymphocytic leukemia (CLL) (Color Plate III-5, *D*) and prolymphocytic leukemia (Color Plate III-5, *H*) on the one hand and ALL (approximately 20% of adult acute leukemias) on the other (Color Plate III-5, *F*). The differentiation from CLL is best done by lymph node biopsy, whereas lymphocyte surface marker analysis, cytochemistry (TdT), and bone marrow examination in addition to lymph node biopsy will aid in the differentiation from ALL (Table 81-1). In ALL, bone marrow is diffusely infiltrated by the abnormal cells, whereas in lymphosarcoma cell leukemia, marrow involvement is patchy and has a characteristic distribution in association with bony trabeculae. In prolymphocytic leukemia the abnormal cells superficially may resemble lymphosarcoma cells but on close in-

Diagnostic features of infectious mononucleosis syndromes

I. Clinical
   A. Fever, exudative tonsilitis, lymphadenopathy (98%-100%)
   B. Splenomegaly (50%-75%)
   C. Palatal petechiae (30%-50%)
   D. Periorbital edema (30%)
   E. Hepatomegaly (10%-20%)
II. Hematologic
   A. Relative and absolute lymphocytosis
   B. Atypical lymphocytes 20% or greater
III. Etiologic agents
   A. Epstein-Barr virus (EBV) (90%) (Chapter 251)
   B. Cytomegalovirus (CMV) (5%) (Chapter 251)
   C. *Toxoplasma gondii* (Chapter 280)
   D. Other viruses (e.g., adenovirus, hepatitis viruses, rubella)
IV. Serologic diagnosis
   A. For EBV syndrome, presence of one or more of the following:
      1. Heterophil antibodies (Monospot test)
      2. IgM antibodies to viral capsid antigen (VCA) that decline during convalescence
      3. Fourfold or greater rise in IgG antibodies to VCA
      4. Transient antibody response to the diffuse component of the virus early antigen (anti-D)
   B. For CMV syndrome, negative heterophil plus one or more of the following:
      1. Seroconversion from anti-CMV negative to positive
      2. Fourfold or greater rise in anti-CMV antibodies
      3. Positive CMV buffy coat culture
   C. For other heterophil-negative syndromes, specific serologic tests for the following:
      1. *Toxoplasma gondii* (Chapter 280)
      2. Hepatitis viruses (Chapter 57)
      3. Adenovirus (Chapter 253)
      4. Rubella (Chapter 246)

spection appear intermediate in development between the cells of CLL and those of lymphosarcoma cell leukemia (Color Plate III-5, *H*). Prolymphocytes lack the characteristic cleaved nucleus of lymphosarcoma cells. Patients with prolymphocytic leukemia typically are elderly and manifest marked splenomegaly without adenopathy and very high lymphocyte counts ($>100 \times 10^9$/L). Prolymphocytic leukemia may present de novo or as "prolymphocytoid" transformation in a patient with CLL.

In mycosis fungoides and other cutaneous lymphomas, characteristic *Sézary cells* may appear in the circulation (Color Plate III-5, *I*). These cells may represent only a small percentage of circulating cells in these patients (1% to 20%) or, more rarely, may be the predominant peripheral cell present, leading to a leukemic peripheral blood picture. The Sézary cell is large and contains a prominent, characteristic nucleus that occupies three fourths or more of the cell. The nucleus is lobulated and convoluted with numerous folds and clefts. The cytoplasm is deep blue and may contain multiple small, round vacuoles sometimes rimming the nucleus. Electron microscopy is useful in demonstrating the convoluted pattern of the nucleus. Sézary cells are derived from T lymphocytes and express mature T cell markers. The recognition of circulating Sézary cells in patients with advanced mycosis fungoides is not difficult. Conversely, the appearance of classic Sézary cells in the peripheral blood of patients with nonspecific dermatologic lesions should suggest the possibility of cutaneous T cell lymphoma. Definitive diagnosis should be pursued by biopsy of the appropriate lesions for histopathologic study.

The characteristic cell of hairy cell leukemia may also be confused with other lymphoid variants. The hairy cell is a large cell with an eccentrically located nucleus containing lacy-appearing chromatin (Color Plate III-5, *G*). Nucleoli may be easily seen. The cytoplasm appears pale grayish blue and usually contains no granules. Characteristic fine filamentous projections are observed at the cytoplasmic border and may give the cell margins a serrated or fragmented appearance. These cells are prone to smearing artifacts with spreading and fusing of the cytoplasmic projections and loss of the hairy appearance. Furthermore, they may comprise only a small percentage of peripheral mononuclear cells in any given patient and thus may escape detection. Conversely, artifactual hairy cells may be created on normal blood smears when blood is drawn and allowed to stand before smears are made. This is especially true if the blood is kept refrigerated. The diagnosis of hairy cell leukemia thus requires a high index of suspicion and careful examination of a peripheral blood smear. The typical patient is a middle-aged man with pancytopenia and splenomegaly. Hairy cells are best demonstrated in wet mounts with supravital stains. Cytochemical staining for the tartrate-resistant isoenzyme of acid phosphatase can provide important confirmatory information. In about 50% of patients the cells contain peculiar cylindric cytoplasmic inclusions termed *ribosome lamella complexes*. As with the small lymphocyte of CLL, the lymphosarcoma cell, and the prolymphocyte, the hairy cell usually is of B lymphocyte origin. The characteristic hairy cell may be distinguished from other neoplastic B cells by the presence of receptors for the lymphokine interleukin-2 (T cell growth factor) and expression of the CD11 antigen on surfaces of hairy cells.

Plasmacytoid lymphocytes may appear during infections (Color Plate III-5, *C*) and are also the characteristic malignant cell seen in Waldenström's macroglobulinemia. The diagnosis of Waldenström's macroglobulinemia is confirmed by demonstration of an IgM paraprotein by serum protein electrophoresis and immunoelectrophoresis. Patients with this disease frequently complain of cryopathic phenomena or give evidence of hyperviscosity syndrome (Chapter 95). Erythrocyte rouleaux are present on blood films (Plate III-4, *F*), and a cryoglobulin may be detected in plasma and serum during routine blood processing. Mature plasma cells are not normally present in the circulation. A small number may be seen in association with multiple myeloma, and their presence in large number is diagnostic of plasma cell leukemia, a rare complication of multiple myeloma.

Nucleated red blood cells

Nucleated red blood cells are not normally present in peripheral blood but may appear when the bone marrow is subjected to intense stimulation, as in response to acute hemorrhage, hypoxemia, or hemolytic anemia (see the box below). They may also be seen in asplenic individuals who lack the normal "pitting" function of the spleen. When present in substantial numbers, nucleated erythrocytes may produce spurious elevation of the leukocyte count because automated cell counters do not distinguish between nucleated red and white cells. Examination of a peripheral blood smear will readily resolve such a discrepancy. Nucleated red blood cells also enter the blood in marrow infiltrative processes, which may result in a leukoerythroblastic blood picture. In the absence of a clear cause for nucleated red cells in the blood, bone marrow biopsy is indicated.

Circulating nucleated erythrocytes: diagnostic considerations

I. Reactive secondary to intense erythropoietic stimulus
   A. Acute hemorrhage
   B. Hypoxemia
   C. Hemolytic anemia
   D. Megaloblastic anemia
II. Infiltrative processes in the bone marrow
   A. Metastatic malignancies
   B. Primary hematologic malignancies
   C. Myelofibrosis, either primary, secondary, or drug related
   D. Granuloma
III. Asplenic individuals

REFERENCES

Bessis M: Blood smear reinterpreted. New York, 1977, Springer Verlag.

Gurwith MJ et al: Granulocytopenia in hospitalized patients. I. Prognostic factors and etiology of fever. Am J Med 64:121, 1978.

Maldonado JE and Hanlon DG: Monocytosis: a current appraisal. Mayo Clin Proc 40:248, 1965.

Mintzer DM and Hauptman SP: Lymphosarcoma cell leukemia and other non-Hodgkin's lymphomas in leukemic phase. Am J Med 75:110, 1983.

Schlossberg D, editor: Infectious mononucleosis. In Praeger monographs in infectious disease, vol I. New York, 1983, Praeger.

Ward PC: The lymphoid leukocytoses. Postgrad Med 67(2):217, 1980.

Ward PC: The myeloid leukocytoses. Postgrad Med 67(1):219, 1980.

CHAPTER

82 Lymphadenopathy and Splenomegaly

David H. Boldt

The immune system consists of various highly specialized cell types involved in carrying out the reactions of cell-mediated and humoral immunity (Chapter 283). These cells include the lymphocytes (T cells, B cells, and non-T, non-B cells), plasma cells, and mononuclear phagocytes. Most are produced in the bone marrow, but the lymphocytes may undergo programming in central lymphoid organs such as the thymus during fetal and neonatal life. After their differentiation has been completed, these cells populate peripheral lymphoid organs such as the lymph nodes and spleen. Anatomic localization in organs provides an organization to the immune system and serves to promote the generation of an immune response after antigenic challenge. Lymph nodes and spleen have blood and lymphatic supplies as well as internal architectures that facilitate antigen processing and cellular interactions, two prerequisites for normal immunologic function.

Because the immune system plays a central role in host defense against microbial and antigenic challenge, abnormalities of lymphoid organs are encountered frequently in clinical practice. Lymphadenopathy and splenomegaly are prominent features of a wide variety of diseases and in many instances serve as a focal point for subsequent clinical investigation. This chapter discusses the structure and function of lymph nodes and spleen as a basis for understanding clinical abnormalities, then focuses on etiologic considerations and guidelines for evaluation of patients with lymphadenopathy and/or splenomegaly.

LYMPHADENOPATHY

Lymph node structure and function

Lymph node are distributed in clusters along the courses of lymphatic vessels throughout the body. They are ovoid in shape and normally range in size from a few millimeters to more than a centimeter. Their architecture facilitates efficient filtration of lymph and promotes internal migration of cells, primarily lymphocytes and mononuclear phagocytes (Fig. 82-1). A lymph node consists of three anatomic zones. In the cortex of the node adjacent to the subcapsular sinus are aggregates of B lymphocytes termed *lymphoid follicles*. Some of the follicles contain germinal centers, areas of plasma cells, macrophages, and rapidly dividing lymphocytes actively engaged in protein synthesis. Among and adjacent to the follicles is the paracortical zone, consisting of sheets of T lymphocytes. Beneath the paracortex and occupying the central portion of the node is the medulla. Here the lymphocytes are arranged in cordlike arrays, termed *medullary cords,* that converge on the hilus.

Antigen is carried into the node by the afferent lymphatics and is engulfed and processed by cortical macrophages. A specialized type of cell, termed *dendritic cell,* is believed to play a major role in antigen presentation to lymphocytes. Within the node, antigen is concentrated at the interface between paracortex and lymphoid follicles, a location where T and B lymphocytes are normally in close apposition. The lymph node serves to bring together all the elements necessary for initiating an immune response. It is within the cortex of the node that sensitized T lymphocytes are produced and antibody is first formed. An intense immunologic reaction, as in a secondary immune response, will lead to proliferation of lymphoid follicles and formation of germinal centers. An increase in the number and size of lymphoid follicles secondary to such an immune response frequently results in clinically apparent lymphadenopathy.

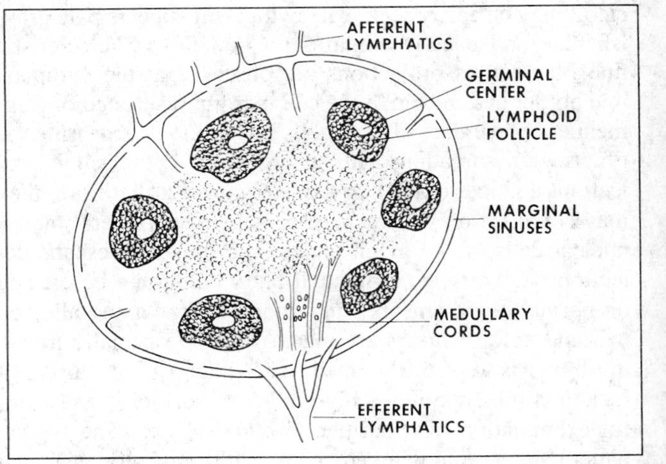

Fig. 82-1. A lymph node. At the surface of the node the reticular fibers form a dense fibrous capsule. Afferent lymphatic vessels enter the node by piercing the capsular surface and empty into a subcapsular sinus. From there lymph flows inward along the channels formed by the reticular network and exits the node at the hilus via a single efferent lymphatic vessel. The lymphoid follicle consists of aggregates of B lymphocytes. Germinal centers are areas of plasma cells, macrophages, and rapidly dividing lymphocytes. Among and adjacent to the follicles is the paracortical zone of T lymphocytes.

The patient with lymphadenopathy: general considerations

When one encounters a patient with lymphadenopathy, several considerations are important. One is the patient's age. The possibility that peripheral lymphadenopathy is caused by a benign process decreases with age. Reactive hyperplasia of lymphoid tissue in response to infectious or inflammatory processes is characteristic of infants and children. In a study of 925 adult patients undergoing diagnostic lymph node biopsies, approximately 80% of the lesions were benign in patients younger than 30, but only 40% were benign in patients older than 50. Conversely, 20% of lesions were malignant in patients under 30, and 60% were malignant in patients over 50.

Two questions are of primary importance in assessing lymphadenopathy. Is lymphadenopathy localized or generalized? What is the time course of its appearance? Lymphadenopathy in certain regions takes on special clinical significance. For example, palpable supraclavicular nodes are frequently associated with intrathoracic or intra-abdominal malignancies, and therefore demand careful evaluation. By contrast, isolated occipital lymphadenopathy seldom represents a malignant condition and usually reflects an infectious process of the scalp, such as ringworm or insect bites. Progressive enlargement of nodes over several weeks, especially if associated with complaints of fever, chills, night sweats, or weight loss, is suggestive of serious systemic illness such as chronic mycobacterial or fungal infection or a malignant lymphoproliferative disease.

Nodal tenderness is suggestive of an infectious process but does not adequately distinguish malignant from nonmalignant causes. For example, rapid lymph node enlargement in acute lymphoblastic leukemia may be associated with considerable discomfort. A peculiar symptom occasionally reported in association with Hodgkin's disease is the development of pain in enlarged lymph nodes after alcohol ingestion.

The consistency of enlarged nodes to palpation can provide clues to etiology. Tender, warm, erythematous nodes associated with fluctuance or lymphangitic streaking of adjacent skin are associated with local infectious processes. Stony, hard nodes fixed to the adjacent tissues are highly suggestive of malignancy, especially metastatic carcinoma or sarcoma, whereas rubbery, mobile nodes are suggestive of lymphomas. Conditions that may be associated with lymphadenopathy are listed in the box at upper right.

Causes of lymphadenopathy

I. Infections: bacterial, mycobacterial, fungal, viral, or parasitic
II. Immunologic disorders
  A. Rheumatic disorders
  B. Serum sickness
  C. Sarcoidosis
  D. Drug reactions: hydantoins
III. Malignancies
  A. Hematologic
  B. Nonhematologic
IV. Miscellaneous or unknown etiology
  A. Atypical lymphoproliferations of unknown cause: angioimmunoblastic lymphadenopathy, angiofollicular lymph node hyperplasia (Castleman's disease), sinus histiocytosis with massive lymphadenopathy
  B. Dermatopathic lymphadenopathy
  C. Endocrinopathies: thyrotoxicosis, adrenal insufficiency
  D. Lipidoses

The patient with regional lymphadenopathy

Fig. 82-2 presents a clinical approach to patients with regional lymphadenopathy. Evaluation of a patient with localized adenopathy depends on knowledge of both the lymphatic drainage patterns of various portions of the body and the pathologic processes most likely to affect these areas. Lymphadenopathy in certain regions takes on special clinical significance that may allow for efficient direction of diagnostic investigation.

Cervical lymph nodes. Enlarged nodes confined to the neck may result from occult infection or malignancy. Because the cervical lymph nodes receive lymphatic drainage from the head, neck, and oropharyngeal cavities, infections that must be considered include soft tissue infections of the face, dental abscesses, otitis externa, and bacterial pharyngitis. Careful ears, nose, throat examination and bacterial throat cultures, including use of special media and plating conditions for gonococci if recent orogenital contact is suspected, will aid in diagnosis. Infectious mononucleosis may also present with localized cervical lymphadenopathy and may be diagnosed by appropriate serologic tests and examination of a peripheral blood film for atypical lymphocytes (Chapter 81). The disorder is most common in young adults and is very rare after the age of 30. The occurrence of typical clinical and hematologic findings of infectious mononucleosis in the face of a negative heterophil reaction should suggest the possibility of infection by cytomegalovirus; another virus such as hepatitis, adenovirus, or rubella; or *Toxoplasma*. Diagnostic features of infectious mononucleosis syndromes are given in Chapter 81 (box on p. 776). Malignancies frequently presenting as localized cervical lymphadenopathy include Hodgkin's disease, non-Hodgkin's lymphomas, and squamous cell carcinomas arising from nasopharyngeal or laryngeal structures.

Axillary nodes. Localization of lymphadenopathy to the axilla suggests a different spectrum of diagnostic possibilities. Axillary nodes drain the lymphatics of the upper extremities and the breasts. Axillary adenopathy should suggest infectious processes such as cat scratch fever, sporotrichosis, tularemia, and staphylococcal or streptococcal infections. Examination of the upper extremities for scratches, bites, suppurative lesions, or lymphangitis may provide important diagnostic clues. Malignancies that may

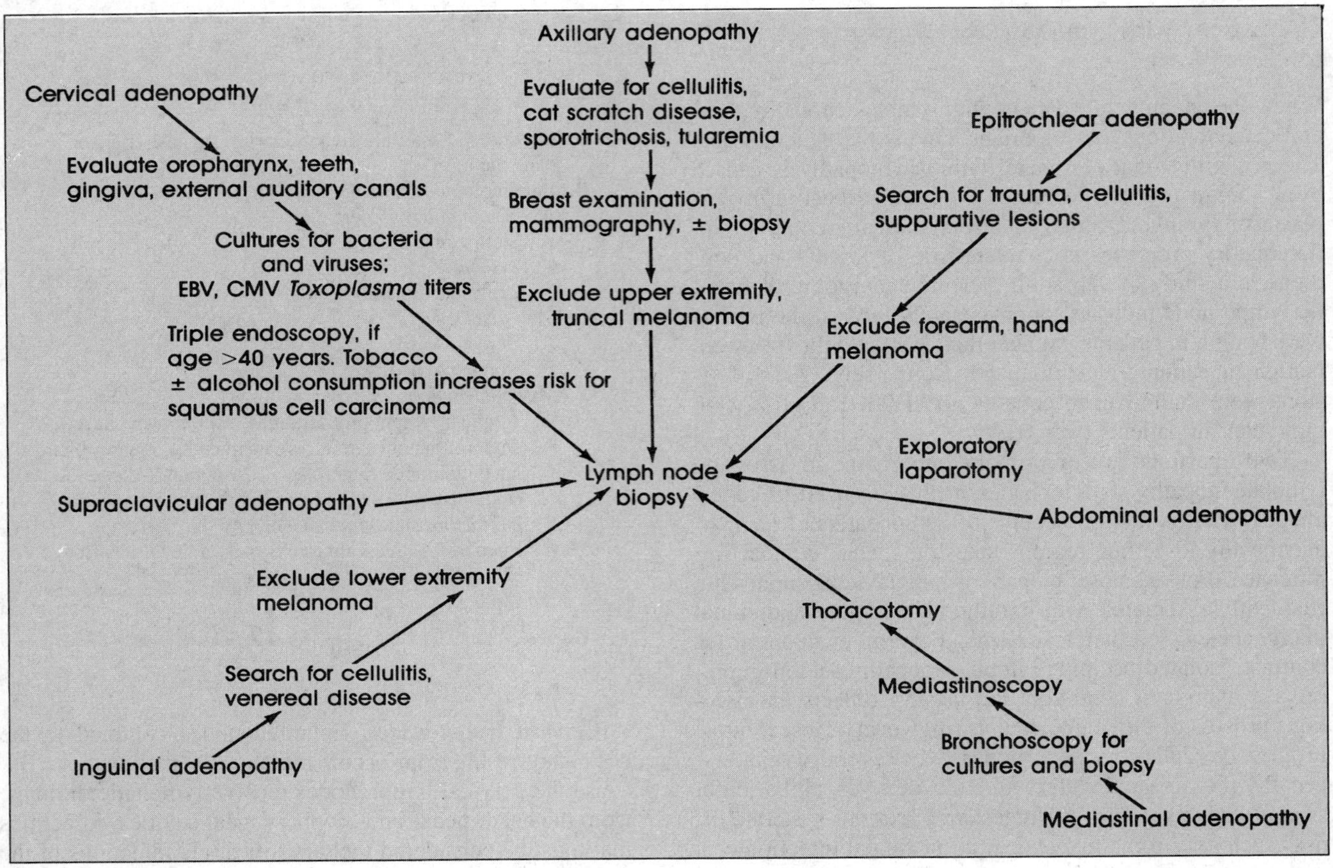

Fig. 82-2. Clinical approach to the patient with localized lymphadenopathy.

present with localized axillary adenopathy include lymphoma, melanoma, and carcinoma of the breast.

Epitrochlear nodes. Bilateral, painless, epitrochlear lymphadenopathy may occur as a result of repeated minor trauma and/or infections in manual laborers. Its occurrence in other settings is suggestive of lymphoma.

Supraclavicular nodes. Palpable supraclavicular lymph nodes are of ominous significance because of their frequent association with intrathoracic and intra-abdominal malignancies and with breast cancer in women. Lymphatic drainage of the chest and mediastinum is to the supraclavicular nodes bilaterally. The thoracic duct carrying abdominal lymphatic drainage empties into the left innominate vein in the left supraclavicular region. This anatomic feature accounts for the well-known phenomenon of a left supraclavicular sentinel node (Virchow's node) that heralds the presence of an occult abdominal neoplasm. Intrathoracic infections, usually chronic mycobacterial or fungal infections, may also present with localized supraclavicular lymphadenopathy, as may sarcoidosis. However, bacterial pneumonias or bronchial infections do not present in this manner. Early biopsy of localized enlarged supraclavicular nodes to establish a definitive diagnosis is usually indicated.

Inguinal nodes. Localized inguinal lymphadenopathy may be most difficult to evaluate because virtually all adults manifest some degree of inguinal node enlargement as a consequence of repeated trauma and minor infections involving the genitalia and lower extremities. The inguinal nodes provide lymphatic drainage for the lower extremities and the skin of the lower abdomen, genitals, and perineum. An important point is that the internal pelvic organs and testes drain via the iliac nodes into the para-aortic chain so that deep pelvic infections or malignancies do not usually present as inguinal lymphadenopathy. Infectious considerations in a patient with inguinal lymphadenopathy include cellulitis of the lower extremities and venereal infections such as syphilis, chancroid, genital herpes, or lymphogranuloma venereum. Malignant conditions include lymphomas, metastatic melanomas arising in the lower extremities, and squamous cell carcinomas from primary sites in the penis or vulva.

Internal nodes. Internal lymphadenopathy may come to the physician's attention on radiologic examination, for example, hilar or mediastinal adenopathy on chest radiographs. These nodes may be the principal manifestation of bronchogenic carcinoma or lymphoma. Hodgkin's disease is more often associated with hilar or mediastinal lymphadenopathy than are non-Hodgkin's lymphomas. Sarcoidosis, tuberculosis, or fungal infections are important nonmalignant conditions that must be considered in the differential diagnosis. Bacterial infections in the lung are not usually associated with lymphadenopathy. Because there are so many different causes of intrathoracic adenopathy, aggressive workup, including bronchoscopy and/or mediastinoscopy for biopsy and establishment of a histopathologic diagnosis, is indicated.

Intra-abdominal lymphadenopathy may be detected as a palpable mass on physical examination or it may come to attention indirectly, through obstruction or pressure effects on some adjacent organ such as a ureter. Various radiographic techniques must usually be employed to delineate fully the extent of intra-abdominal or retroperitoneal lymphadenopathy. These include the intravenous pyelogram, lymphangiogram, ultrasonography, and/or computed tomography. If lymphadenopathy is confined to the abdomen and peripheral tissue is not available, exploratory laparotomy may be indicated to establish a diagnosis. Intra-abdominal lymphadenopathy frequently signifies a malignant process such as Hodgkin's disease or a non-Hodgkin's lymphoma. Hodgkin's disease typically involves pelvic and retroperitoneal nodes, while sparing mesenteric nodes. By contrast, non-Hodgkin's lymphomas frequently involve mesenteric nodes as well. Tuberculous mesenteric lymphadenitis may produce large, suppurative, abdominal lymph nodes that may calcify or rupture.

Superficial nodes. Patients with a variety of dermatologic disorders, especially exfoliative dermatitis, may develop regional superficial lymphadenopathy. This condition, termed *dermatopathic lymphadenopathy,* is self-limited and regresses with improvement of the skin disease. On biopsy the involved nodes are characterized by the presence of large numbers of atypical reticulum cells and foamy cells containing lipoid material or melanin.

The patient with generalized lymphadenopathy

Fig. 82-3 presents a clinical approach to patients with generalized lymphadenopathy. In the adult, generalized lymphadenopathy usually signifies the presence of serious systemic illness, either infectious, immunologic, or malignant in nature. Prompt biopsy of an involved lymph node is usually indicated. Nonetheless, it is important to exclude the possibility that the lymphadenopathy is related to drug ingestion. This relationship is best recognized in association with the phenytoin group of anticonvulsant drugs, hydralazine, and allopurinol. Clinical findings may include fever, rash, lymphadenopathy, hepatosplenomegaly, arthritis, and jaundice, all of which generally disappear rapidly once the offending agent has been discontinued. The clinical picture strongly resembles an immunologically mediated hypersensitivity reaction. Lymph nodes obtained at biopsy have architectural features that may be difficult to differentiate from malignant lymphoma. These atypical histologic findings have led to the use of the term *pseudolymphoma* for these lesions. Although true malignant lymphomas have developed in some of these patients, an etiologic relationship

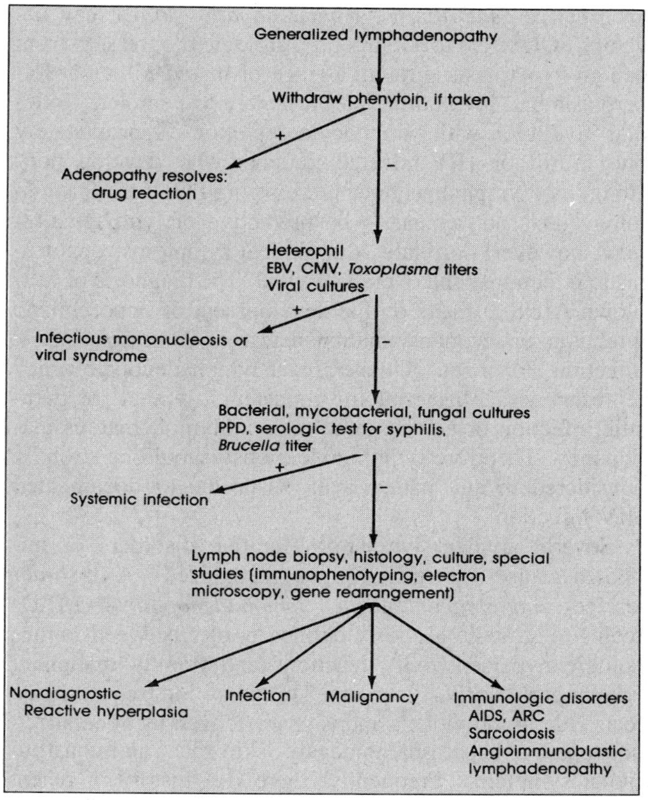

Fig. 82-3. Clinical approach to the patient with generalized lymphadenopathy.

between the malignant transformation and either anticonvulsant therapy or the hypersensitivity reaction is not established.

Generalized adenopathy may be caused by systemic infections. The most common of these are probably the infectious mononucleosis syndromes, including those caused by Epstein-Barr (EB) virus, cytomegalovirus, other viruses, and *Toxoplasma*. Otherwise, generalized lymphadenopathy occurs infrequently in adults with infections except those who have tuberculosis, fungal infections such as histoplasmosis or coccidioidomycosis, brucellosis, bacterial endocarditis, infectious hepatitis, or secondary syphilis. Immunologic disorders to be considered in patients with generalized lymphadenopathy include sarcoidosis, rheumatoid arthritis, systemic lupus erythematosus, the acquired immunodeficiency syndrome (AIDS), and AIDS-related complex (ARC).

Generalized or localized lymphadenopathy may occur during the course of infection with the human immunodeficiency virus (HIV), the causative agent of AIDS. HIV infections are discussed in Chapter 252. After infection, an initial asymptomatic period during which subjects exhibit serologic evidence of HIV may evolve into the symptomatic state ARC. ARC frequently is associated with a syndrome of generalized lymphadenopathy characterized by reactive lymph node hyperplasia on microscopic examination. In some of these patients a histopathologic syndrome of *progressive generalized lymphadenopathy* (PGL) may develop. PGL refers to a temporal histologic progression from benign hyperplasia through a stage of mixed follicular hyperplasia and involution and ultimately to complete follicular involution with lymphocyte depletion. Approximately one fourth of HIV-infected patients who develop non-Hodgkin's lymphomas have pre-existing PGL, but this histology does not appear to be predictive of lymphoma. It may, however, correlate with clinical symptoms, opportunistic infections, and overall survival. The diagnosis of full-blown AIDS is made on the development of opportunistic infections or secondary malignancies. At this stage of HIV infection, localized or generalized lymphadenopathy may represent viral, bacterial, mycobacterial, fungal, or parasitic infection or a lymphoma or a nonlymphomatous malignancy. Therefore lymph node biopsy should be strongly considered in any patient with suspected or documented HIV infection.

Several atypical lymphoproliferative disorders of unknown cause are increasingly recognized. A disorder termed *angioimmunoblastic lymphadenopathy* (AILD) seems to straddle a poorly defined border between immunologic hypersensitivity reactions and frankly malignant lymphoproliferative disorders. This condition frequently affects elderly individuals and is characterized by generalized adenopathy, hepatosplenomegaly, skin rash, and constitutional symptoms. Frequently, there is a history of recent drug exposure, insect bite, immunization, or other potential immunologic stimuli. Laboratory evaluation may reveal Coombs-positive hemolytic anemia and polyclonal hypergammaglobulinemia. Histologic examination of the lymph nodes demonstrates a mixed cellular infiltration with immunoblasts, lymphocytes, plasma cells, and eosinophils. A characteristic feature is proliferation and arborization of small capillary blood vessels. Recent studies have identified clonal populations of T cells in AILD specimens, raising the concern that many cases actually may represent T cell lymphomas. Patients with AILD usually follow a progressive downhill course, with a median survival of approximately 3 years. No effective treatment exists. In some patients the disease evolves into a true malignant lymphoma that is generally refractory to therapy.

Angiofollicular lymph node hyperplasia (Castleman's disease) usually presents with mediastinal lymphadenopathy. Two variants are recognized: hyaline vascular type (90%) and plasma cell type (10%). Often the disease is asymptomatic and discovered only by routine chest x-ray examination. Most cases are self-limited. Other cases may be associated with systemic symptoms of fever, sweats, fatigue, or weight loss and with anemia and hypergammaglobulinemia. The plasma cell variant tends to be more aggressive and may be associated with multicentric lymph node involvement and a progressive clinical course. Some cases may evolve into overt lymphoma. No effective therapy exists.

Malignant conditions associated with generalized lymphadenopathy include leukemias (especially acute lymphoblastic leukemia in children and chronic lymphocytic leukemia in elderly adults) and lymphomas.

Lymph node biopsy

Lymph node biopsy is an important diagnostic procedure, and in many instances it becomes the definitive technique by which to establish or confirm a diagnosis. Biopsy should be undertaken without delay in any patient in whom lymphadenopathy not obviously resulting from an infectious cause such as infectious mononucleosis or in whom some localized infective focus has persisted for a week or more. Persistent enlargement of peripheral nodes is frequently associated with serious, potentially lethal systemic disease; early diagnosis with rapid initiation of appropriate therapy may spell the difference between cure and a fatal outcome.

When the decision is made to perform a diagnostic lymph node biopsy, it is important to select a representative node in an area where extraneous processes are unlikely to confuse the histologic picture. For example, nodes from inguinal, femoral, or upper cervical regions are often useless because they demonstrate reactive hyperplasia caused by repeated localized infectious processes. It is important to obtain an intact node with preservation of the capsule, particularly if one is dealing with the possibility of lymphoma. The architectural features that enable specific diagnosis and typing of a lymphoma require an intact lymph node. Because the histologic subtype of lymphoma conveys important prognostic and therapeutic information, this is not a trivial consideration. It should be emphasized that adequate classification of lymphomas can only be done on nodal tissue. Extranodal involvement by lymphoma can be diagnosed by biopsy, but the specimen is generally inadequate for detailed classification of the lymphoma. Needle biopsies of lymph nodes are seldom useful and should be avoided.

At the time of node biopsy, a portion of the specimen is preserved in formalin for routine pathologic examination. Adequate material must be obtained for bacterial, fungal, and mycobacterial cultures, for special stains for these organisms, and under certain circumstances for special cytochemical stains and analysis of lymphocyte surface markers. In some instances, as in undifferentiated malignancies, electron microscopy may be helpful and a specimen may be preserved in special fixatives for this procedure. Several studies have demonstrated that lymph node biopsy will lead to a specific diagnosis in approximately two thirds of patients in whom it is undertaken.

Problem of nondiagnostic lymph node biopsy

In one-third of lymph node biopsies, no specific diagnosis is established. Lymph nodes with atypical features suggestive but not diagnostic of malignancy are a continuing problem for the surgical pathologist. Traditionally this type of difficult biopsy has been called *atypical hyperplasia*. It is instructive to consider the fate of patients who have this diagnosis. In a 1957 study by Moore and others, 158 of 379 lymph node biopsies were nondiagnostic at the first attempt. Among these undiagnosed patients, 63 individuals developed either a malignancy or a rheumatic disorder over the ensuing decade. At the end of a decade, 47 of the 158 were alive and well, 56 were alive with serious disease, and 55 were dead. In a more recent study published in 1979 by Schroer and Franssila, 21 of 70 patients whose initial lymph node biopsy demonstrated atypical hyperplasia developed a malignant lymphoproliferative disorder during a follow-up period of 2 to 13 years. Clearly, persistent lymph node enlargement is frequently associated with serious, often fatal, systemic illness and careful follow-up of patients with nondiagnostic lymph node biopsies is essential.

SPLENOMEGALY

Spleen structure and function

The spleen is the largest lymphoid organ in the body. It is well designed for accomplishing its major functions as a filter of the blood and generator of immune responses. When a fresh spleen is cut, it appears to consist of the relatively avascular white pulp and the vascular red pulp. The white pulp, where immunologic function resides, consists of lymphoid aggregates associated with a central arteriole. This lymphoid tissue is organized into periarteriolar sheaths that are collections of T lymphocytes analogous to the paracortical regions of lymph nodes and lymphoid follicles that are collections of B lymphocytes. The marginal zone, a loosely organized collection of lymphocytes and reticuloendothelial cells, surrounds periarteriolar sheaths and follicles and is thought to play a major role in antigen uptake and processing. Antigenic challenge results in changes in the white pulp of the spleen analogous to those that occur in lymph nodes. There is hyperplasia of lymphoid follicles and formation of germinal centers, reflecting generation of immunologically competent T and B lymphocytes. These phenomena cause splenic hyperplasia and may result in palpable splenomegaly.

The red pulp occupies the largest portion of the spleen. It is within the unique vasculature of this region that the spleen's filtration function is accomplished. Here terminal arterial vessels empty into a reticular meshwork containing large numbers of macrophages. Blood cells must traverse this region to reach the venous sinuses, which they enter by passing between sinusoidal endothelial cells. In order to negotiate its passage through the red pulp, a cell must be sufficiently deformable to squeeze through the cords and sinuses and return to the systemic circulation. Inability to accomplish this passage results in sequestration of the cell in an environment of low oxygen tension and its ultimate phagocytosis and destruction by splenic macrophages. This is the normal mechanism for removal *(culling)* of effete erythrocytes or other cells that have been damaged by physical or immunologic mechanisms, or those that contain nuclear remnants, siderotic granules, denatured hemoglobin (Heinz bodies, Color Plate III-4, *P*), or parasites such as malarial organisms. In certain instances, inclusions such as these may be removed from the red cell without its destruction, a process termed *pitting*. Absence of these normal pitting and culling functions of the spleen accounts for the characteristic peripheral blood picture of splenectomized patients. Nucleated red cells and Howell-Jolly bodies are frequently seen (Color Plate III-4, *K*). In fact, absence of nucleated red cells and Howell-Jolly bodies from the peripheral blood of a patient who has had a splenectomy is evidence of a functional accessory spleen. The spleen normally contains large amounts of storage iron because of its role in red cell destruction. The spleen also plays a role in phagocytosis and disposal of foreign particles and microorganisms. It is normally the site of blood formation in utero, but after birth the presence of extramedullary hematopoiesis in the spleen always signifies a pathologic condition.

Patient with splenomegaly

A list of conditions associated with splenomegaly is given in the box below. The normal spleen weighs 150 g and is located in the left upper abdominal quadrant against the diaphragm and close to the abdominal wall. As enlargement occurs, the spleen retains its superficial location just beneath the abdominal wall so that deep palpation is usually not necessary to detect splenomegaly. However, substantial splenomegaly can occur in the absence of a palpable spleen by physical examination. Radionuclide scanning may be useful in resolving presence or absence of splenomegaly when the question is in doubt.

In evaluating causes of splenomegaly, it is convenient to divide them into two categories, depending on whether lymphadenopathy is present. Fig. 82-4 presents a clinical approach to patients with splenomegaly. In general, any condition that can cause generalized lymphadenopathy can cause splenomegaly. These conditions include the chronic infections and the inflammatory and immunologic disorders discussed previously. In any of these conditions, splenomegaly may occur as an isolated finding without accompanying lymphadenopathy. Diagnostic considerations and approach to management of patients with both splenomegaly and lymphadenopathy are the same as approaches to lymphadenopathy discussed earlier in this chapter. Diagnosis is based on blood counts, morphology of cells in the peripheral blood, serologies, appropriate cultures, and in many instances, examination of a lymph node obtained at biopsy.

Differential diagnosis of splenomegaly

I. Associated with generalized lymphadenopathy
  A. Infections
  B. Inflammatory and immunologic diseases
  C. Hematologic malignancies
II. Not associated with lymphadenopathy
  A. Any condition listed above
  B. Hematologic disorders: chronic hemolytic anemias, megaloblastic anemias
  C. Congestive splenomegaly: portal hypertension or severe congestive heart failure
  D. Infiltrative processes: amyloidosis, storage diseases
  E. Other causes: splenic cysts, arteriovenous malformations, splenic artery aneurysms, splenic abscess
  F. Normal variation in young adults

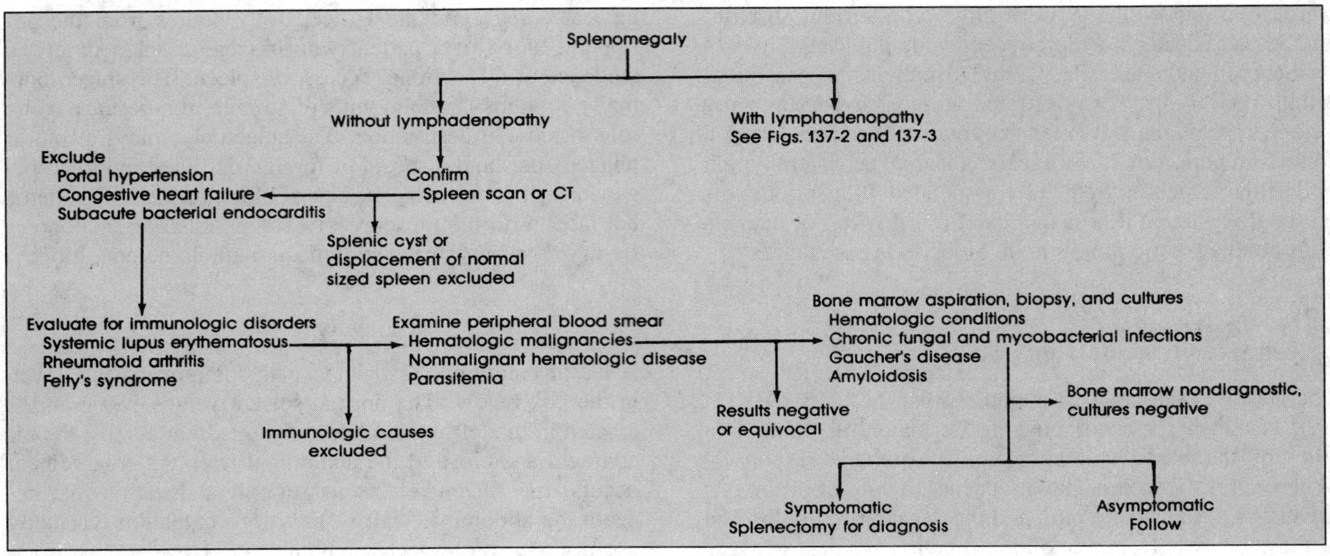

Fig. 82-4. Clinical approach to the patient with splenomegaly.

In certain parasitic infections such as malaria or schistosomiasis, splenomegaly is frequently seen in the absence of significant lymphadenopathy. In kala-azar (leishmaniasis), massive splenomegaly may accompany modest lymphadenopathy. The occurrence of splenomegaly and leukopenia in association with rheumatoid arthritis is known as Felty's syndrome.

Malignancies associated with splenomegaly are predominantly the myeloproliferative or lymphoproliferative disorders. Hairy cell leukemia and prolymphocytic leukemia are examples of disseminated lymphoproliferative diseases marked by prominent splenomegaly without lymphadenopathy. Careful examination of the peripheral blood should allow recognition of these disorders. Although metastases to the spleen have been found in up to 50% of patients who died of carcinoma, these usually occur as a late event in the course of the disease and seldom cause clinically detectable splenomegaly. Splenomegaly in a setting of metastatic carcinoma is usually caused by portal hypertension secondary to obstruction by tumor deposits in the liver or elsewhere.

Splenomegaly in the absence of lymphadenopathy may be caused by nonmalignant hematologic disorders. These conditions are primarily hemolytic anemias such as congenital erythrocyte enzyme defects, hereditary spherocytosis, immune hemolytic anemia, or hemoglobinopathies. This has led to the concept of *work hypertrophy* of the spleen, which has been supported by experimental evidence. According to this hypothesis, the increased workload in terms of phagocytosis and destruction of erythrocytes imposed on the spleen by a chronic hemolytic state leads to reticuloendothelial hyperplasia, a subsequent further increase in hemolysis, which may be followed by more hyperplasia and so on. For this reason, splenectomy may confer substantial benefit in many chronic hemolytic disorders. Other nonmalignant hematologic diseases that may be accompanied by splenomegaly are the megaloblastic anemias caused by nutritional deficiencies of folic acid or vitamin B_{12} (Chapter 88). Iron deficiency is associated with splenomegaly in the older literature, but this association is rarely, if ever, observed today. Besides these nonmalignant hematologic disorders, the other major cause of splenomegaly without lymphadenopathy is congestive splenomegaly. This type of splenomegaly is caused by portal hypertension, caused in turn by hepatic cirrhosis or, rarely, by severe congestive heart failure.

Evaluation of patients with isolated splenomegaly in the absence of lymphadenopathy is straightforward. Approximately 3% of adolescents and young adults have a palpable spleen as a normal finding on careful physical examination. Presence of chronic hemolysis, portal hypertension, or congestive heart failure usually is determined from the history and physical examination. Laboratory evaluation for hemolysis is discussed in Chapters 73 and 90. Rarely, isolated splenomegaly will be an incidental finding in an otherwise healthy adult. Such an individual may be screened for serious underlying pathology by careful examination of a peripheral blood film (to rule out asymptomatic chronic lymphocytic or chronic myelocytic leukemias), spleen scan to look for splenic cyst or extrasplenic mass causing displacement of the spleen, and a noninvasive procedure such as sonography or abdominal computed tomography to search for occult abdominal masses, as in lymphoma.

Concept of hypersplenism

The term *hypersplenism* refers to the occurrence of splenomegaly and peripheral cytopenias (anemia, leukopenia, or thrombocytopenia alone or in any combination) in the presence of normal or increased bone marrow activity, and the correction of the hematologic abnormalities by splenectomy. Any condition known to cause splenomegaly may be associated with hypersplenism, but conversely, splenomegaly is not always associated with the syndrome of hypersplenism.

The causes of the peripheral cytopenias in hypersplenism

are multifactorial. Anemia is caused both by the dilutional effect of an increased splanchnic blood volume and also by a shortened survival of erythrocytes damaged during splenic pooling. Thrombocytopenia results mainly from splenic pooling, whereas granulocytopenia appears to reflect increased margination of granulocytes in the blood vessels of the spleen.

Splenectomy for treatment or diagnosis

The physician managing a patient with splenomegaly must decide whether splenectomy is indicated and if so, when the procedure should be performed. It is important to recognize that most patients with splenomegaly will not require specific treatment directed toward an underlying disease. Four indications for splenectomy can be identified. First, splenectomy is an important treatment option for those patients with life-threatening cytopenias in whom the spleen may be responsible for persistence of the cytopenia. These conditions include hemolytic anemias, immune thrombocytopenia, myeloproliferative and lymphoproliferative diseases, and miscellaneous disorders such as Felty's syndrome. Indications for splenectomy in specific disease entities are discussed in the appropriate chapters. Splenectomy for hematologic diseases is not curative but may provide significant amelioration of symptoms by reducing or eliminating transfusion requirements and may improve prognosis by reducing the risk for complications such as sepsis or bleeding. In general, past experience provides the best guide to the utility of splenectomy in specific disease settings. Radionuclide studies to assess splenic sequestration or destruction of blood cells are not sufficiently reliable to provide useful information on which to base the decision for or against splenectomy. A second indication for splenectomy is the occurrence of a vascular or traumatic accident involving the spleen. Splenectomy may be life-saving in the setting of traumatic rupture of the spleen, and with splenic infarction it may provide symptomatic relief as well as prophylaxis against spontaneous splenic rupture. A third indication for splenectomy is mechanical encroachment by the enlarged spleen on other intra-abdominal organs. Most often affected is the stomach with resultant symptoms of early satiety and sometimes prominent weight loss. Less frequently, obstruction to the left renal collecting system may occur. A fourth indication for splenectomy is for diagnosis. Evaluation of the patient with isolated splenomegaly or with splenomegaly and lymphadenopathy is discussed earlier (see Fig. 82-4). In some patients with isolated splenomegaly, careful evaluation by noninvasive means may fail to provide a diagnosis. In these patients, exploratory laparatomy for splenectomy and diagnostic lymph node and liver biopsies may be indicated. Three fourths of such patients will prove to have significant pathologic conditions approximately equally divided among lymphoproliferative diseases, inflammatory diseases, and congestive splenomegaly.

Asplenic patient

Susceptibility to overwhelming infection is a well-recognized complication of splenectomy. Although this risk is magnified for splenectomy done in infancy or early childhood, it remains significant in the adult. The incidence of overwhelming postsplenectomy infection is approximately 1.5% when splenectomy is done for trauma and may be much higher in other conditions such as treated Hodgkin's disease. Overwhelming postsplenectomy infection may occur many years after splenectomy. The mortality rate is approximately 50%. Because pneumococci are the causative agents in more than half the patients, penicillin prophylaxis and pneumococcal vaccination have been recommended for patients who undergo splenectomy. Evidence suggests that in children these modalities are effective in reducing the incidence of overwhelming postsplenectomy infection, but comparable data for adults are not available.

Removal of the spleen results in characteristic blood cell changes that are readily identifiable on the peripheral smear. These changes include abnormalities in red blood cell shape, including appearance of target cells, acanthocytes, and fragmented cells. Red cells may contain nuclear remnants, termed *Howell-Jolly bodies* (Color Plate III-4, *K*), and nucleated erythrocytes may be seen. Transient leukocytosis and thrombocytosis occur after splenectomy in the absence of underlying hematologic disease. In patients with myeloproliferative disorders or hemolytic anemia, marked thrombocytosis may persist.

REFERENCES

Abrahms DI: AIDS-related lymphadenopathy: the role of biopsy. J Clin Oncol 4:126, 1986.

Bowdler AJ: Splenomegaly and hypersplenism. Clin Haematol 12:467, 1983.

Eichner ER and Whitfield CL: Splenomegaly: an algorithmic approach to diagnosis. JAMA 246:2858, 1981.

Fijten GH and Blijham GH: Unexplained lymphadenopathy in family practice. J Fam Pract 27:373, 1988.

Greenfield S and Jordan MC: The clinical investigation of lymphadenopathy in primary care practice. JAMA 240:1388, 1978.

Moore RD, Weissberger AS, and Bowerfind ES: An evaluation of lymphadenopathy in systemic disease. Arch Intern Med 99:751, 1957.

Schroer K and Franssila KO: Atypical hyperplasia of lymph nodes: a follow-up study. Cancer 44:1155, 1979.

CHAPTER

83 Excessive Bleeding and Clotting

James N. George

Michael A. Kolodziej

Although the evaluation of patients who have excessive bleeding or thrombosis (or both simultaneously) is usually considered from the perspective of laboratory assessment, this chapter emphasizes that (1) the history and physical examination are the most important diagnostic aids, (2) laboratory studies are confirmatory and must be used selectively, and (3) laboratory analyses are necessarily artificial and may be misleading.

The initial discussion of bleeding disorders is organized in relation to the physiologic sequence of hemostasis. First, disorders of primary hemostasis, involving platelets and small vessels, are discussed, followed by disorders of secondary hemostasis involving plasma coagulation factors. The nature of the bleeding in these two categories of abnormalities can be clearly distinguished by the history and physical examination. In contrast to patients with bleeding disorders, evaluation of patients whose primary problem is an increased tendency toward thrombosis is often less clear. However, better understanding of the natural control mechanisms of hemostasis and their abnormalities in thrombotic diseases is improving the ability to diagnose specific abnormalities. The assessment of patients anticipating surgery and the interpretation of laboratory assays of coagulation related to the risk of bleeding represent a special problem for hemostasis: not merely the diagnosis of an abnormality but the assurance of normality. Here the sophistication of the laboratory evaluation is guided by the suspicion of a bleeding abnormality from the history. Finally, this chapter discusses the problem of patients who have a laboratory abnormality of hemostasis but no clinical bleeding, observations that further emphasize the importance of the clinical examination and the artificial nature of laboratory assays.

The clinical approach to a patient with a bleeding disorder is outlined in the box on the right. The history and physical examination should allow a distinction to be made between disorders of platelets and small blood vessels (primary hemostasis), characterized by mucocutaneous bleeding, petechiae, and superficial purpura, from disorders of coagulation (secondary hemostasis), characterized by delayed, recurrent oozing and hematoma formation. From the history and physical examination, a preliminary diagnosis can be made based on the type of bleeding, the history (indicating a congenital or acquired disorder), and the expected frequency of certain diseases (see the box).

DISORDERS OF PRIMARY HEMOSTASIS: PLATELETS AND BLOOD VESSELS

Clinical evaluation

Purpura, or "easy bruising," resulting from increased fragility of small blood vessels or a decrease in blood platelets is the most common hemostatic abnormality; milder thrombocytopenias not associated with purpura occur even more frequently. Normal blood platelets may function continuously to seal the small gaps in vascular endothelium that normally occur. Evidence for this is the sudden, asymptomatic appearance of innumerable petechiae around the feet, ankles, and lower legs when severe thrombocytopenia develops (Color Plate III-12, *A*). This distribution of petechiae in dependent regions parallels intravascular hydrostatic pressure and the greater vulnerability of these small vessels to endothelial breaks. This occurrence also emphasizes that disorders of platelets and blood vessels must be considered together and may initially be indistinguishable. The evaluation of patients with a suspected disorder of primary

Clinical evaluation of a bleeding patient

I. History
   A. Type of bleeding
      1. Mucocutaneous, petechiae: suggests platelet disorder or vasculitis
      2. Delayed, recurrent oozing; hematoma: suggests plasma coagulation disorder
      3. Menorrhagia or gastrointestinal bleeding possible in either type of disorder
   B. Duration of bleeding
      1. Lifelong: indicates congenital defect of a single factor; confirm with family history of bleeding or presence of consanguinity for suspected recessive traits
      2. Recent onset: indicates an acquired disorder, usually defects of multiple factors; confirm by history of no bleeding with past trauma, surgery, teeth extractions, menses
   C. Systemic illnesses associated with bleeding: liver disease, malignant disease
II. Physical examination
   A. Petechiae and superficial mucocutaneous bleeding
      1. Dependent distribution, asymptomatic: indicates thrombocytopenia
      2. Clusters of palpable, pruritic petechiae: indicates vasculitis
   B. Deep hematomas or hemarthroses, which may be associated with extensive superficial purpura: indicates a coagulation disorder
III. Preliminary diagnostic categories
   A. Mucocutaneous bleeding, platelet-vessel defect
      1. Congenital
         a. von Willebrand's disease most likely
         b. Well-defined platelet function defects rare; mild, poorly defined platelet defects possibly more common
         c. Thrombocytopenia rare
         d. Afibrinogenemia rare
      2. Acquired
         a. Severe thrombocytopenia most likely caused by autoimmune thrombocytopenic purpura (ITP)
         b. Mild or moderate thrombocytopenia caused by splenic pooling in liver disease common
         c. Other thrombocytopenias caused by peripheral destruction (thrombotic thrombocytopenic purpura, disseminated intravascular coagulation [DIC], sepsis) or marrow failure less common
         d. Mild congenital von Willebrand's disease possible in an adult.
   B. Hematomas and delayed bleeding, coagulation defect
      1. Congenital
         a. Hemophilia A most likely, hemophilia B one-tenth as frequent
         b. Other coagulation defects rare
         c. Homozygous von Willebrand's disease with severe factor VIII deficiency rare
      2. Acquired
         a. Liver disease common
         b. DIC, vitamin K deficiency, coagulation factor inhibitors, anticoagulant therapy
         c. Mild congenital hemophilia possible in an adult
IV. Proceed to laboratory evaluation

hemostasis may initially present an important but difficult differential diagnosis between normal and abnormal bleeding. Control groups in clinical studies have consistently documented that about 20% of subjects with normal hemostasis report mild to moderate bleeding symptoms. Easy bruising, epistaxis, gingival bleeding, and bleeding after trauma that may seem excessive are both the hallmarks of abnormal primary hemostasis and part of the spectrum of normal bleeding.

The characteristic lesion of thrombocytopenia or vasculitis is the petechia. This dot hemorrhage does not blanch with pressure and will evolve over days from bright red to yellow to brown with the catabolism of extravasated heme. These characteristics, although obvious, are critical in distinguishing petechiae from the vascular telangiectasias that are common in normal people. Petechiae are tiny because the endothelial lesion is contained by supporting perivascular tissue (Color Plate III-12, *A*). However, if the same endothelial lesion occurs in an area of very loose tissue (buccal mucosa, conjunctiva), the small hemorrhage can readily dissect into a larger hemorrhagic bulla measuring a centimeter or more in diameter (Color Plate III-12, *B*). In contrast, regions with stronger connective tissue support of small vessels have fewer petechiae, such as the sole of the foot in Color Plate III-12, *A*. The distinction between thrombocytopenic and primary vasculitic petechiae is best made by the history and physical examination. With thrombocytopenia, the appearance of petechiae is totally asymptomatic, whereas in vasculitis there are often prodromal symptoms of burning or stinging in the skin before the appearance of petechial hemorrhages. In addition, the petechiae of vasculitis may be palpable and may occur in clusters that are not necessarily distributed in dependent regions. Acute thrombocytopenia is usually unassociated with other systemic symptoms or diseases, whereas acute vasculitis usually occurs with symptoms in other organ systems, a drug reaction, or other systemic disease. Whereas vasculitis usually causes only superficial petechiae, severe thrombocytopenia can cause severe and fatal internal hemorrhage. Thrombocytopenic bleeding may occur without trauma in the more vascular organs, resulting in nosebleed, gingival bleeding, menometrorrhagia, hematuria, and cerebral and gastrointestinal hemorrhage. Large, slowly developing hematomas in less vascular regions, such as the retroperitoneum, and hemarthroses, which are so characteristic of coagulation disorders, do not occur.

Purpura may refer to the appearance of many petechiae and is also frequently used to describe larger superficial hemorrhages. Purpura is distinct from the term *hematoma,* which implies a substantial mass of extravasated blood. The most common cause of purpura is the vascular fragility caused by atrophy of subcutaneous supporting tissue. *Senile purpura* is not a disease associated with other bleeding problems but an inevitable accompaniment of aging. The appearance of large, superficial, nonpalpable purple blotches on the back of the hands and forearms is predictable with thin, shiny, inelastic skin and the vulnerability of these areas to minor trauma. The same lesions accompany the cachexia of chronic illness and the peripheral subcutaneous atrophy of cortisol excess.

Laboratory evaluation

The laboratory evaluation of congenital and acquired disorders of primary hemostasis is outlined in Figs. 83-1 and 83-2. The initial step in both evaluations is an estimation of platelet number; the absolute number obtained by a platelet count with confirmation by examination of a peripheral blood smear. A platelet count less than 150×10^9/L is abnormal, but bleeding does not occur from thrombocytopenia alone until the platelet count is less than 50 to 100×10^9/L, and spontaneous bleeding with many petechiae does not occur until the platelet count is less than 10×10^9/L. If thrombocytopenia is documented, the next diagnostic study is a bone marrow aspiration to determine the presence or absence of megakaryocytes. Their presence is interpreted as evidence that the thrombocytopenia is caused by excessive peripheral platelet destruction or splenic pooling, and their absence or severe decrease indicates marrow failure as the cause of thrombocytopenia.

Congenital thrombocytopenias are rare; some are associated with specific disorders of platelet function (Bernard-Soulier syndrome) or abnormalities such as nephritis and deafness (Epstein's syndrome), granulocyte inclusions (May-Hegglin anomaly), or immunodeficiency (Wiskott-Aldrich syndrome), whereas others manifest only a low platelet count. Since the most common acquired thrombocytopenia, idiopathic (autoimmune) thrombocytopenic purpura (ITP), is essentially diagnosed by excluding other etiologies, and since mild to moderate thrombocytopenia may cause minimum bleeding symptoms, congenital thrombocytopenia must be considered in the differential diagnosis of ITP. This is particularly important in the unusual cases of children who are thought to have chronic ITP.

The most common abnormality among congenital disorders of primary hemostasis is von Willebrand's disease. The incidence of von Willebrand's disease is hard to define because in mildly affected patients, laboratory tests may be variably abnormal, and even all tests may be normal at some times in some patients. Also, the pattern of laboratory abnormalities is not always consistent among family members, an unusual occurrence in a hereditary disease. In typical type I (heterozygous) von Willebrand's disease (defined and discussed in Chapter 85), the platelet count is normal but the bleeding time is prolonged because of a deficiency of the von Willebrand factor required for platelet adhesion to the damaged vessel wall. The von Willebrand factor deficiency can be measured by both immunoassays and functional assays (Chapters 76 and 85 for a full description). In plasma, von Willebrand factor functions as a carrier molecule for factor VIII, and therefore the plasma factor VIII concentration may also be decreased. Patients with type III (homozygous or doubly heterozygous) von Willebrand's disease have severe abnormalities of all these parameters. Because of their very low factor VIII concentration, these patients may also have clinical bleeding problems characteristic of a coagulation defect. Other well-defined diseases among the group of congenital primary hemostasis disorders are rare (see Fig. 83-1).

With rare exceptions, acquired disorders of primary hemostasis are caused by thrombocytopenia. The suspected

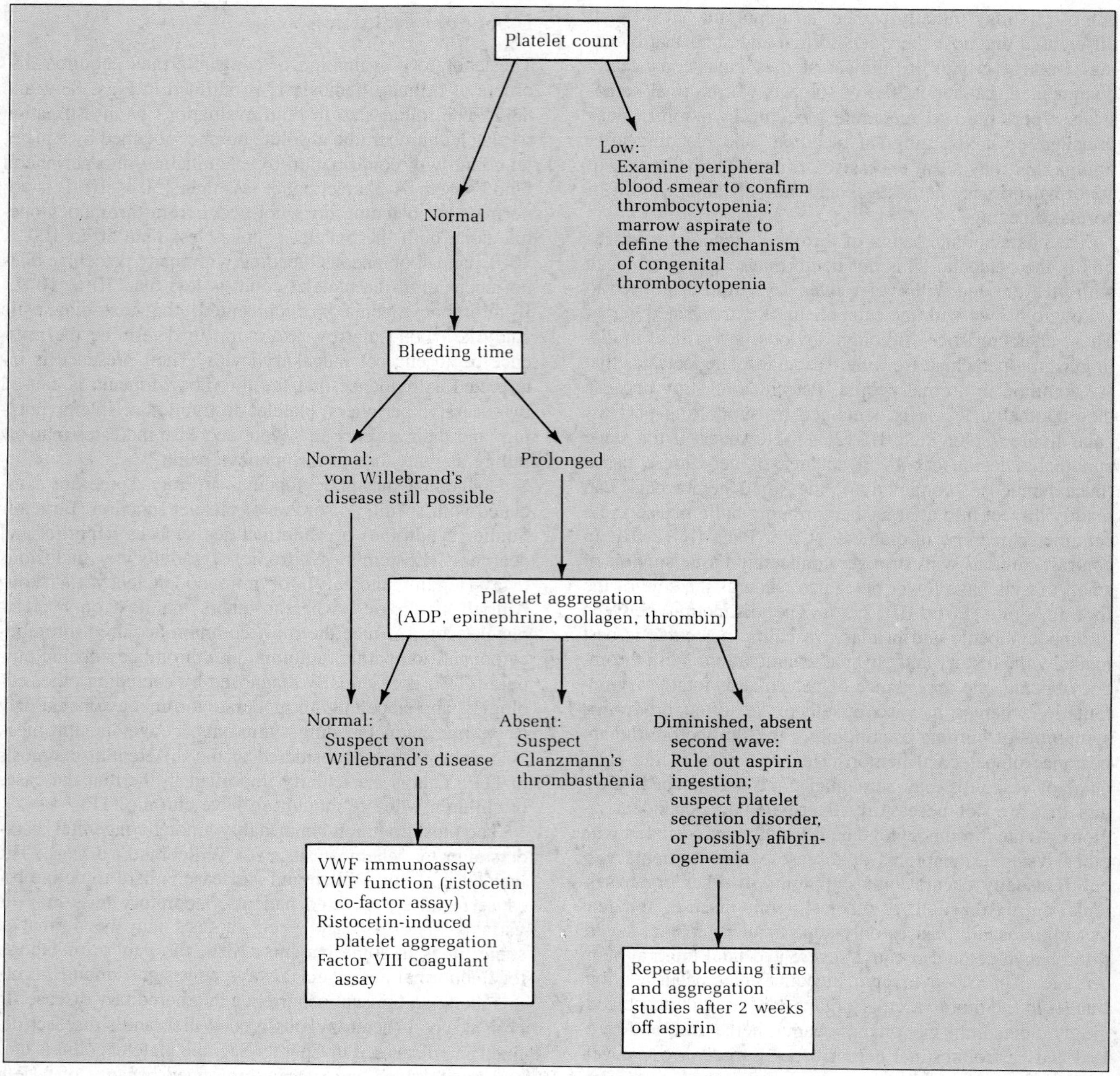

Fig. 83-1. A diagram for the laboratory evaluation of a patient with a bleeding disorder in whom the history and physical examination suggest a congenital disorder of platelets or small vessels.

etiology depends on the associated medical problems. In an otherwise healthy person, thrombocytopenia caused by increased peripheral platelet destruction is most common, and ITP is the most likely diagnosis. Thrombocytopenia resulting from marrow failure, with rare exceptions, is associated with other evidence of marrow disease. In patients with chronic liver disease the spleen becomes congested because of portal hypertension and thrombocytopenia occur because of splenic pooling. In these patients the platelet count is rarely less than 50×10^9/L. Finally, patients with marrow involvement by a malignant disease or folic acid or vitamin B_{12} deficiency or those who are receiving marrow-suppressive chemotherapy have expected thrombocytopenia, and these may be the most common causes of thrombocytopenia among hospitalized patients. The diagnostic approach to a patient with thrombocytopenia depends on the clinical setting: in otherwise healthy patients, bone marrow aspiration is essential to determine if platelet production is adequate; in patients with known chronic liver disease or marrow suppression, bone marrow aspiration is typically not indicated.

Mild thrombocytopenia with no bleeding manifestations must be very common. Viral infections and acute alcoholism both can cause thrombocytopenia because of marrow

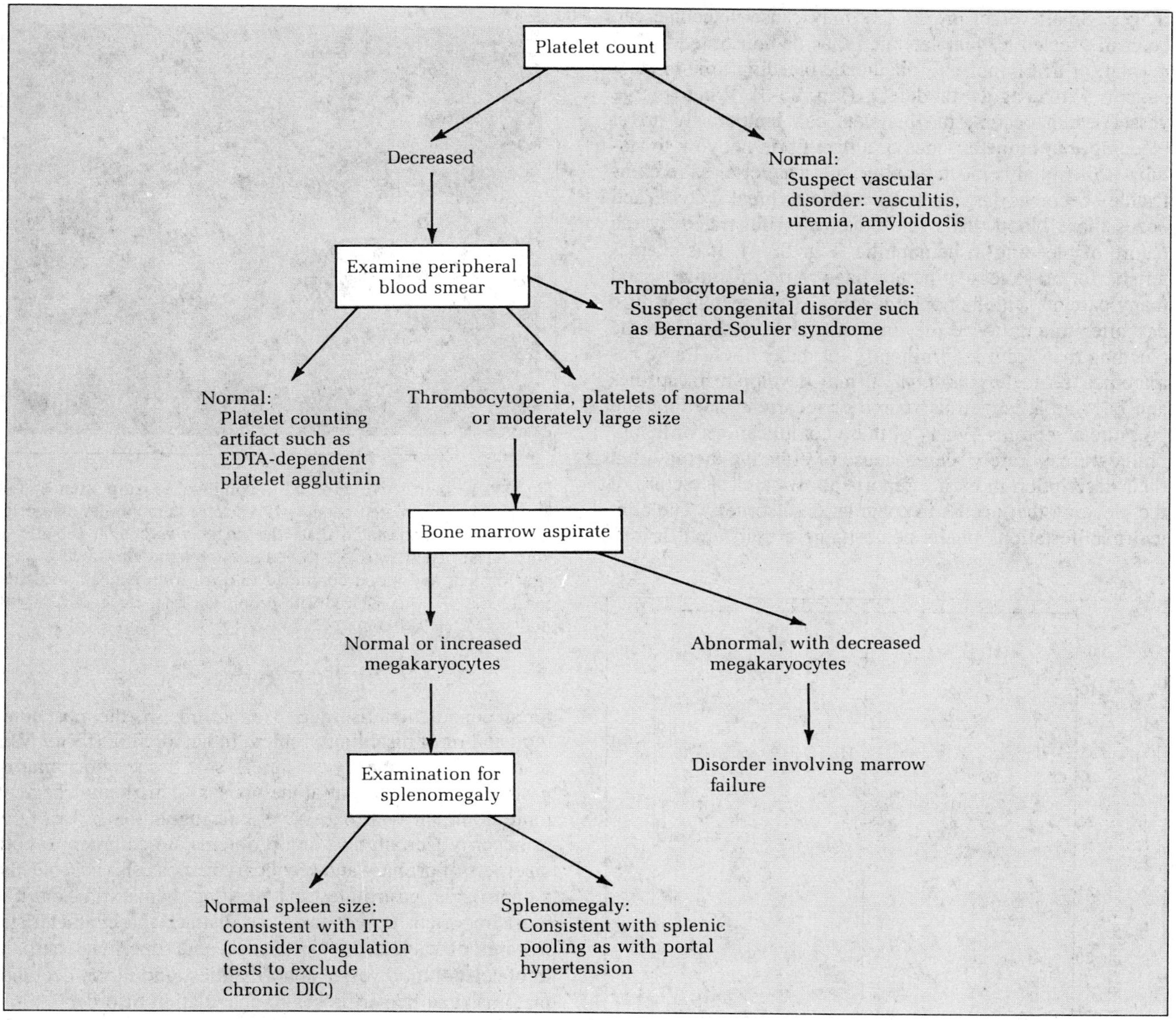

Fig. 83-2. A diagram for the laboratory evaluation of a patient with a bleeding disorder in whom the history and physical examination suggest an acquired disorder of platelets or small vessels.

suppression with decreased megakaryocytes. It has been documented that most children receiving live attenuated viral vaccines develop mild thrombocytopenia, although petechiae do not occur. These mild thrombocytopenias may be clinically significant when they occur concurrently with another hemostatic abnormality.

An enormous number of drugs, foods, and spices can cause abnormal platelet function, but of these, only aspirin has been documented to cause a significantly increased frequency of bleeding. Even with aspirin, abnormal clinical bleeding is difficult to document, and most studies of major surgery on patients taking aspirin demonstrate minimally increased bleeding compared with control groups. Chronic renal failure also causes abnormal platelet function, but whether this causes clinically significant bleeding is unknown. In a patient who has a history and clinical signs of a disorder of primary hemostasis but a normal platelet count and normal platelet function, vasculitis should be suspected, and a cause of associated illness should be apparent. Rarely a biopsy of the petechial lesion to demonstrate the vasculitis directly may be helpful. Primary amyloidosis may cause more brittle tissue support for fine vessels with resulting purpura.

DISORDERS OF SECONDARY HEMOSTASIS: COAGULATION

Clinical evaluation

The nature of excessive bleeding in patients with coagulation disorders is distinct from the bleeding that occurs with platelet–blood vessel abnormalities. A few large, deep tissue hematomas occur rather than innumerable tiny hemorrhages. Small vessel breaks that may cause petechiae can be easily sealed by platelets alone, as demonstrated by the normal, or nearly normal, diagnostic bleeding time in most patients with coagulation defects (Fig. 83-3). When a large vessel lesion occurs, the platelets can temporarily arrest bleeding, but in the absence of a firm fibrin network to stabilize this initial hemostatic plug, the platelet mass remains friable, becomes larger, and eventually breaks down and oozes more blood. This is dramatically illustrated by the nature of bleeding in hemophilia (Fig. 83-4). It is characteristic for no excessive hemorrhage to occur initially, and many patients with hemophilia consider the second or third day after trauma to be the time of greatest risk. Then the bleeding may recur intermittently for many days. Large hematomas, termed *pseudotumors,* may develop firm capsules and become a dangerous source of recurrent bleeding and pressure symptoms. Many of these complications of hemophilia are now rarely seen because of effective therapy, but their description in earlier reports allows a clear picture of the bleeding that occurs in coagulation disorders. The clinical manifestations of the hemorrhage are different in different coagulation disorders. Hemarthrosis is the most common and most disabling problem in hemophilia (factor VIII or factor IX deficiency), whereas soft tissue hematoma or gastrointestinal or central nervous system hemorrhage is more common with excessive anticoagulation by warfarin or heparin. Certain bleeding problems are common to both disorders of primary and secondary hemostasis (nosebleeds, menorrhagia, gastrointestinal bleeding, hematuria), but it is most important to recognize the distinct and characteristic features of each defect: petechiae and superficial purpura in platelet–blood vessel abnormalities, and large, deep hematomas and hemarthroses in coagulation disorders.

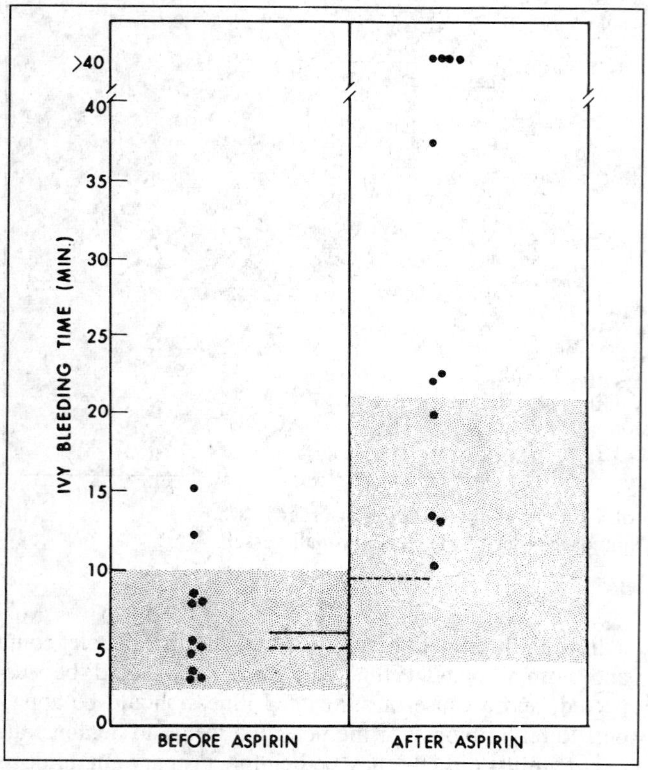

Fig. 83-3. Ivy bleeding time in 11 patients with severe classic hemophilia (factor VIII deficiency) before and 2 hours after ingestion of 1 g of aspirin. The shaded areas represent the range of normal subjects. The dotted straight line is the normal mean, and the solid straight line is the mean for the patients. After aspirin ingestion, bleeding continued in four of the patients when the test was stopped at 40 minutes. In five patients, control of continued bleeding or rebleeding from the incisions eventually required the administration of either plasma or factor VIII concentrate. (Reproduced with permission from Kaneshiro MM et al: N Engl J Med 281:1039, 1969.)

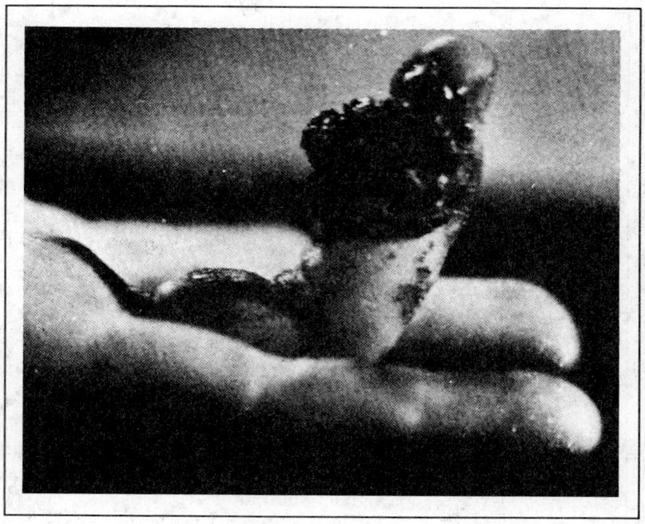

Fig. 83-4. Ineffective clot with continual oozing after minor trauma in an untreated patient with severe hemophilia. The original figure legend stated that "the finger was cut on a blade of grass. The patient was put to bed and the hand elevated. A large clot formed, and blood continued to ooze from beneath the crust for 12 days." (Reproduced with permission from Birch CL: Univ Ill Bull 34, March 9, 1937.)

It is most common for congenital defects to involve only a single coagulation factor, whereas acquired defects involve multiple factors. Congenital disorders should be apparent from a lifelong history of bleeding problems and the presence of similar problems in other family members. Congenital coagulation disorders such as hemophilia may be very mild, and therefore a history specifying the amount of bleeding associated with circumcision, teeth extractions, menstruation, lacerations that require sutures, trauma, or surgery is necessary to document adequately the presence or absence of a clinically significant defect. However, some patients with mild congenital defects may be totally asymptomatic despite active lives until some more severe trauma occurs in adult life.

Laboratory evaluation

The evaluation of a suspected congenital disorder of hemostasis is diagrammed in Fig. 83-5. Of all the possible disorders, hemophilia A is by far the most common, hemo-

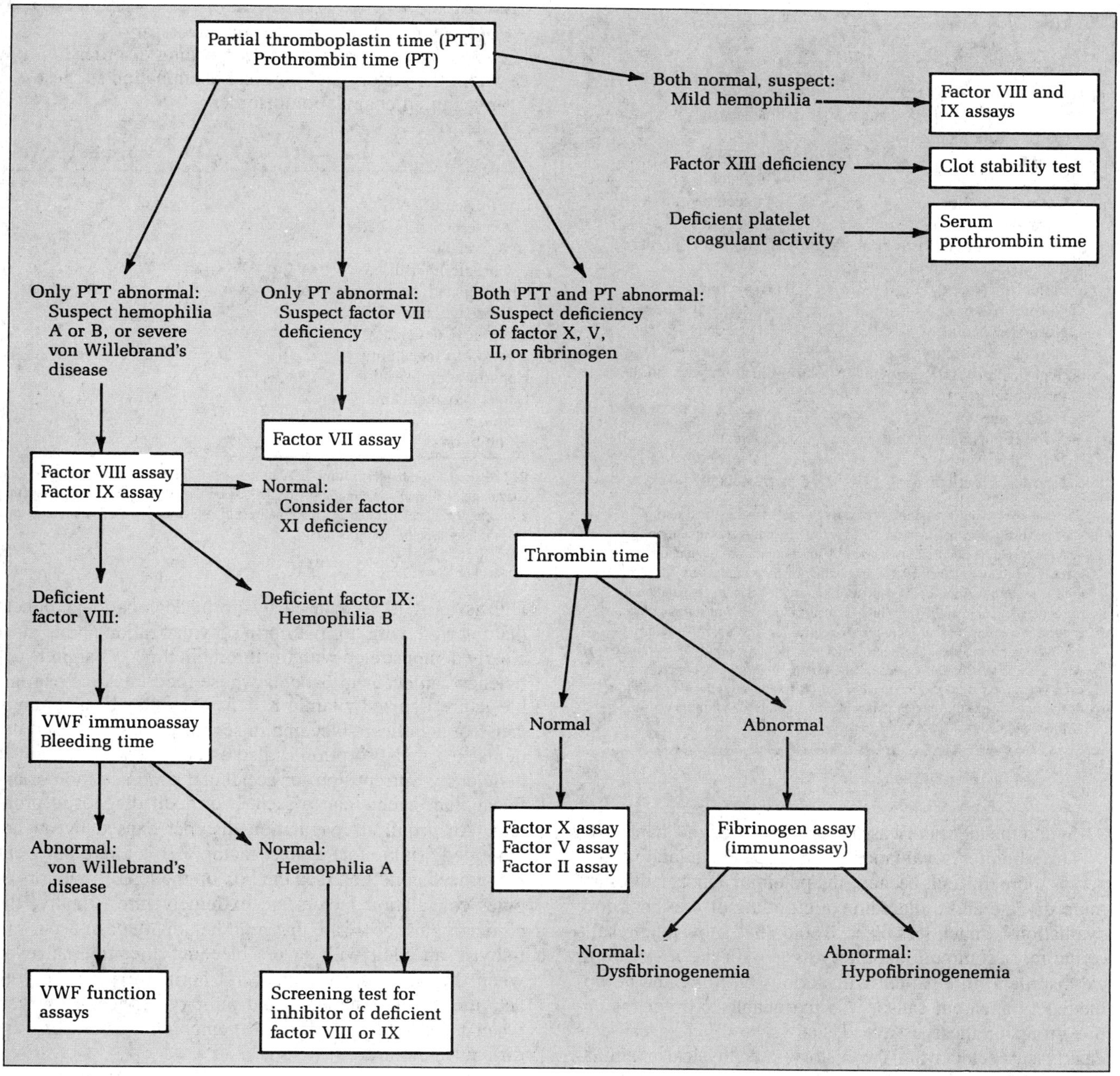

Fig. 83-5. A diagram for the laboratory evaluation of a patient with a bleeding disorder in whom the history and physical examination suggest a congenital coagulation disorder.

philia B being one-sixth to one-tenth as common. The other disorders are rare. The basic screening tests, partial thromboplastin time (PTT) and prothrombin time (PT), are sufficient to initiate the workup, although specific assays for factors VIII and IX are often ordered simultaneously when a history of an X-linked congenital coagulation disorder is clear. It is reasonable to perform assays for both factors VIII and IX to provide additional certainty of the diagnosis, since the coagulation factor replacement therapy is different for these two diseases. It is possible for the PTT to be normal or very close to normal in patients with mild hemophilia and plasma concentrations of factor VIII or IX of more than 10%. The finding of factor VIII deficiency necessitates additional studies to rule out von Willebrand's disease. Because coagulation inhibitors, antibodies to the transfused factor that are recognized by the recipient as foreign antigens, occur in 5% to 10% of patients with hemophilia, a screening test for an inhibitor (see the box on p. 792) should be performed. This test should be repeated before any elective procedure for which factor VIII or IX replacement therapy may be required. The identification of other congenital coagulation disorders is outlined in Fig.

Demonstration of coagulation inhibitors

Patient 1: hemophilia A (factor VIII deficiency), no inhibitor (partial thromboplastin time)	
Patient plasma	82 seconds
Normal plasma	36 seconds
Normal + saline	44 seconds
Normal + patient	41 seconds
Patient 2: acquired postpartum factor VIII inhibitor (partial thromboplastin time)	
Patient plasma	110 seconds
Normal plasma	40 seconds
Normal + saline	51 seconds
Normal + patient	85 seconds
Patient 3: lupus anticoagulant (prothrombin time with dilute thromboplastin)	
Patient plasma	63 seconds
Normal plasma	28 seconds
Normal + saline	33 seconds
Normal + patient	52 seconds

These assays, using a mixture of equal volumes of patient and normal plasma, distinguish between an abnormality caused by a coagulation factor deficiency and an abnormality caused by an inhibitor of coagulation. To identify inhibitors of factor VIII, incubation of the samples at 37° C for an hour is required. Addition of patient plasma with a severe coagulation factor deficiency may slightly prolong the coagulation time of normal plasma even in the absence of an inhibitor. A control for this is a mixture of normal plasma plus saline. The lupus anticoagulant may initially be confused with a factor VIII inhibitor because the prothrombin time is often normal even when the partial thromboplastin time is prolonged. However, dilution of the thromboplastin reagent makes the prothrombin time more sensitive to this abnormality.

Table 83-1. A diagram for the laboratory evaluation of a patient with a bleeding disorder in whom the history and physical examination suggest an acquired coagulation disorder

	PTT	PT	TT	Inh	FDP	Plt
Liver disease						
Acute hepatitis, early liver disease		A				
Chronic liver disease	A	A	A	A	A	A
Disseminated intravascular coagulation (DIC)	A	A	A	A	A	A
Vitamin K deficiency, warfarin ingestion	A	A				
Heparin administration	A	A	A	A		
Lupus anticoagulant	A	A*		A		
Acquired factor VIII inhibitor	A			A		

PTT, Partial thromboplastin time; PT, prothrombin time; TT, thrombin time; Inh, coagulation inhibitor screening test (see the box on the left); FDP, fibrin degradation products; Plt, platelet count; A, abnormal result; A*, often the PT is abnormal only when dilute thromboplastin is used.

83-5, and the laboratory assays are described in Chapter 76.

The laboratory evaluation of acquired coagulation disorders is more difficult because the potential abnormalities are more diverse and a diagrammatic outline of the laboratory evaluation is much less clear. Table 83-1 shows the results of the most common laboratory assays for the major clinical disorders. In a patient with serious bleeding and no immediately apparent cause, it is reasonable to order the entire group of these assays. Usually, however, a cause is clearly suspected from the history and physical examination. Liver disease occurs often, and since all coagulation factors are synthesized by the liver, this is the most common cause of acquired coagulation disorders. In acute liver disease, such as infectious hepatitis, a coagulation abnormality may be manifest only by a prolonged PT. No explanation exists for a simultaneously normal PTT other than the artifactual sensitivity of these tests and their reagents. As liver disease progresses to severe chronic cirrhosis, all studies become abnormal. The synthesis of all plasma coagulation factors is diminished. Thrombocytopenia is the result of excessive pooling in an enlarged, congested spleen. Chronic disseminated intravascular coagulation (DIC) and fibrinolysis may occur in chronic liver disease because of the liver's failure to clear activated coagulation factors and because of a deficiency of plasmin inhibitors. DIC from other causes is discussed later. The coagulation inhibition that may be present in chronic liver disease and DIC is most likely caused by fibrin degradation products that interfere with normal fibrin polymerization and is most clearly demonstrated with the thrombin time. Vitamin K deficiency can occur in patients whose food intake is negligible. Unrecognized vitamin K deficiency may be a common cause of significant bleeding in severely ill hospitalized patients. Fat malabsorption is also associated with vitamin K deficiency. Surreptitious or accidental administration of anticoagulant agents can present a difficult diagnostic problem. An acquired coagulation disorder caused by an autoantibody (inhibitor) against factor VIII is a rare but well-recognized condition (see the box on the left). Inhibitors of other coagulation factors are extremely rare. Finally, the clinician must be aware that mild hemophilia can occur initially in an adult with severe bleeding after trauma, even when the past history indicates a normal experience with activities such as athletics and military service. However, when bleeding begins in mild hemophilia, it can be very difficult to control.

BLEEDING DISORDERS WITH MULTIPLE HEMOSTATIC DEFECTS

Bleeding problems resulting from multiple causes are seen frequently in hospital practice. An example is postoperative bleeding, in which it is often difficult to distinguish normal from excessive amounts and whether excessive bleeding is caused by a hemostatic abnormality or a structural defect such as an unligated vessel or broken suture. If the patient has received many units of transfused blood, platelets and the labile coagulation factors (factors V and VIII) may be deficient. If, in addition, the patient has had significant episodes of hypotension, tissue necrosis will have occurred, releasing thromboplastic material that provokes DIC. DIC may also result from bacteremia, which often complicates major trauma requiring surgery. A simpler example of the problems associated with defects in both primary and secondary hemostasis is illustrated in Fig. 83-3. In this study, aspirin significantly prolonged the bleeding time in a group of normal subjects but not to a clinically relevant degree. Patients with severe hemophilia had, as expected, a normal or nearly normal bleeding time. However, when these patients took three aspirin tablets and the bleeding time was repeated 2 hours later, 4 of the 11 patients were still bleeding when the test was terminated at 40 minutes. This remarkable observation demonstrates that both platelet–blood vessel and coagulation components are required for normal hemostasis; if one of these components is normal, the other can compensate, but when both components are impaired, hemostasis is severely compromised.

DISORDERS ASSOCIATED WITH AN INCREASED TENDENCY FOR THROMBOSIS

Contributing factors to thromboembolic disease are outlined in the box below. The three major categories are often termed Virchow's triad, in reference to the proposal by Rudolph Virchow in 1845 that these abnormalities were the principal mechanisms of thrombotic disease. Vessel wall damage can expose subendothelial matrix cells that constitutively display tissue factor on their membrane surfaces, and this, plus a trace amount of factor VIIa, can effectively trigger coagulation. Vessel surface abnormalities such as atherosclerosis and prostheses may initiate thrombosis by activating coagulation and/or causing formation of platelet aggregates, which then dislodge to obstruct distal circulation. Venous stasis contributes to thrombosis by less effective dilution and clearing of activated coagulation factors. Cardiac abnormalities may cause sufficient stasis to allow formation of ventricular wall thrombi. Turbulent arterial circulation may increase the risk for thrombosis because the high shear forces can damage endothelium and activate platelets. The portal-systemic shunting of chronic liver disease causes less effective catabolism of activated coagulation factors. This can be a critical problem when procoagulant material enters the circulation, as during malignant disease or obstetric complications, or with infusion of concentrates of the coagulation factors II, VII, IX, and X, which may contain activated coagulation factors or other procoagulant material. Patients with malignancies may be predisposed to severe recurrent thromboembolic disease, a condition known as *Trousseau's syndrome*. In certain malignant diseases the cause is clear: secretion of thromboplastic mucin into the circulation by adenocarcinomas or release of procoagulant material from the cells of acute promyelocytic leukemia. Women with abnormal placental separation from the uterine wall at the time of delivery may have thromboses that are related to the presence of thromboplastic material from the placenta in the circulation.

Increased risk for thrombosis: pathophysiologic mechanisms

I. Abnormalities of the vessel wall
   A. Acute
      1. Vasculitis, caused by inflammation or infection
      2. Tissue necrosis, caused by trauma or hypotension
   B. Chronic
      1. Atherosclerosis
      2. Prosthetic heart valve or vascular graft

II. Abnormalities of blood flow
   A. Stasis
      1. Peripheral venous stasis
      2. Arterial or intracardiac stasis
   B. Liver disease with portal-systemic shunting

III. Abnormalities of blood coagulability
   A. Injection of procoagulant material
      1. Malignant disease
      2. Uterine-placental abnormalities
      3. Tissue necrosis
      4. Therapeutic infusions
   B. Hematologic abnormalities
      1. Deficiency of coagulation inhibitor
      2. Diminished fibrinolytic activity
      3. Excess or abnormality of procoagulant factor

The recognized clinical conditions that can predispose to thrombosis are outlined in the box on p. 794. Defects of three proteins involved in the control of coagulation reactions—antithrombin III, protein C, and protein S—appear to allow increased thrombosis because of failure to inhibit activated coagulation factors (see the box on p. 794). Some heterozygous deficient subjects develop recurrent venous thromboembolism. The rare patients with homozygous protein C or protein S deficiency develop fulminant and potentially fatal thromboses in infancy. Abnormalities of other coagulation inhibitors, heparin cofactor II and tissue factor pathway inhibitor, have been less well or not yet described. Congenital abnormalities of fibrinogen and the fibrinolytic system have also been associated with an increased frequency of thrombosis because of the absence of effective fibrinolysis to control a developing clot.

Sickle cell anemia can predispose to thrombosis by the vascular obstruction caused by irreversibly sickled cells. Homocystinuria is associated with vessel wall damage that can result in venous or arterial thrombosis and accelerated atherosclerosis.

The acquired disorders that can increase the risk for thrombosis are much more frequent. Several of these factors often may coincide to result in a thromboembolic complication. For example, an elderly patient with congestive heart failure who is confined to bed has a significantly increased risk for thrombosis. Thrombocytosis may be associated with thrombosis, but also many patients have extreme thrombocytosis (platelet counts of over $1000 \times 10^9/L$) for years with no evidence of thromboembolic complications. Paradoxically, heparin-induced thrombocytopenia has been associated with arterial thromboses. The lupus anticoagulant is an antibody to phospholipid-bound prothrombin that was originally described in patients with systemic lupus erythematosus, but also occurs in other subjects with or without accompanying illnesses (see the box on p. 792). These patients do not have excessive bleeding unless there is concomitant thrombocytopenia or a coagulation abnormality, but they do have an increased risk for thrombosis. The reason for this risk is unknown.

Increased risk for thrombosis: clinical conditions

I. Congenital disorders
   A. Deficient coagulation inhibitor activity
      1. Antithrombin III
      2. Protein C
      3. Protein S
   B. Deficient fibrinolytic activity
      1. Deficiency or abnormality of plasminogen
      2. Abnormality of plasminogen activator/plasminogen activator inhibitor balance
      3. Dysfibrinogenemia
   C. Blood or vessel wall disease
      1. Sickle cell anemia
      2. Homocysteinuria
II. Acquired disorders
   A. Primary hematologic disorders
      1. Proliferative diseases
         a. Myeloproliferative diseases with erythrocytosis and thrombocytosis
         b. Acute promyelocytic leukemia
         c. Paroxysmal nocturnal hemoglobinuria
         d. Macroglobulinemia, cold agglutinin disease
      2. Adverse reactions to therapy
         a. Factors II, VII, IX, X concentrates
         b. Fibrinolysis inhibitors (e.g., EACA)
         c. Heparin-induced thrombocytopenia/thrombosis
         d. Warfarin-induced protein C and S deficiency
      3. Diverse etiologies
         a. Lupus anticoagulant
         b. Thrombotic thrombocytopenic purpura
         c. Disseminated intravascular coagulation
   B. Nonhematologic conditions
      1. Malignant disease
      2. Cardiac abnormalities (e.g., prosthetic valve, dilated cardiomyopathy, ventricular aneurysm, congestive heart failure)
      3. Pregnancy, oral contraceptives
      4. Nephrotic syndrome
      5. Extremes of age
      6. Immobility

The number of specific abnormalities that may be associated with an increased risk for thrombosis is large and growing. As in the assessment of bleeding disorders, clinical evaluation must be the primary basis of diagnosis. For example, a discrete arterial embolism suggests a cardiac origin, and histology of the embolus may reveal a diagnosis of endocarditis or tumor. An isolated occurrence of deep venous thrombosis in the lower leg may have no apparent predisposing cause but not warrant a thorough investigation for a hemostatic defect. However, a recent onset of recurrent severe thromboembolic complications suggests the possibility of an underlying malignancy, and a thorough workup is indicated. Patients with congenital hemostatic disorders that predispose to thrombosis often do not have a history of lifelong symptoms; many patients have a thrombotic episode only after a triggering event such as trauma or enforced bed rest. Affected relatives may then be identified who have had no apparent problems. For example, a recent survey of a normal population suggested a prevalence of protein C deficiency of 1 in 250, although none of the identified subjects had a history of thrombotic disease. A thorough laboratory evaluation should be reserved for patients who have recurrent thromboembolic disease with no obvious cause. Even with these selected patients, less than 10% will have an identifiable laboratory abnormality.

Diffuse (also called disseminated) intravascular coagulation

One clinical syndrome associated simultaneously with both hemorrhage and thrombosis is DIC. The clinical spectrum of DIC extends from clinically insignificant laboratory abnormalities to uncontrollable hemorrhage and thrombosis. DIC has innumerable specific etiologies, but all are related to vascular damage with activation of plasma coagulation factors or entry of tissue thromboplastic material into the blood. Occasional patients have peripheral, symmetric infarction of fingertips and toes, or renal failure may occur with thrombosis of small renal cortical vessels. Bleeding is the most prominent clinical problem, and cerebral hemorrhage is the most common cause of death. Two mechanisms contribute to the bleeding. First, the most apparent abnormality is the consumption of platelets and certain coagulation factors by DIC. In severe DIC, thrombocytopenia and fibrinogen deficiency may be extreme. The coagulation abnormalities are comparable to the changes found in normal serum after in vitro clotting of whole blood: platelets, fibrinogen, prothrombin, and factors V and VIII are decreased; other coagulation factors may be decreased or may be present with even greater activity than in plasma. In the second mechanism, as a consequence of DIC, systemic fibrinolysis is activated, clot lysis is accelerated, and the soluble products of plasmin proteolysis of fibrin and fibrinogen are present in plasma. During severe DIC, $alpha_2$ antiplasmin can be consumed and allow fibrinolysis to be unchecked.

Laboratory evaluation of coagulation in DIC demonstrates abnormalities in the PTT, PT, and thrombin time (TT). Among these, the TT is the most sensitive test and is most prolonged because of interference with fibrin polymerization by the fibrin degradation products. A TT performed on a mixture of patient and normal plasma yields results consistent with a coagulation inhibitor (see the box on p. 792) produced by the fibrin fragments.

PREOPERATIVE ASSESSMENT TO ENSURE A PATIENT'S NORMAL HEMOSTASIS

A special problem in hemostasis is determining the clinical approach to the patient whose primary illness requires surgery and in whom evaluation must be effective to ensure normal hemostasis. Although this problem is often considered primarily from the laboratory perspective of screening assays, a careful history and physical examination are much more helpful and important. First it is necessary to be sure that the patient has no current disease typically associated with acquired hemostatic defects, such as chronic liver disease. Previous bleeding episodes must be carefully documented, and specific questions are essential: menses (number of days and number of pads); teeth extractions (number of hours or days of bleeding, requirement for sutures or repacking); previous surgery (wound hematoma, reexploration, any requirement for transfusion). The history of any extraordinary bleeding in the family is important. Finally, the physical examination should focus on physical signs of a hemostatic defect or a systemic disease that could be associated with a hemostatic defect. If the history and physical examination are normal, only three basic laboratory tests are necessary to provide adequate reassurance of normal surgical hemostasis: platelet count, PTT, and PT. Several studies have documented that preoperative laboratory screening is not helpful in predicting postoperative hemorrhage in asymptomatic adults with a normal history. The obvious flaw in extrapolating these studies to everyday practice is that careful histories frequently are not performed. If the history suggests the existence of a significant bleeding problem, surgery must be postponed even if the primary laboratory evaluation is normal. A more thorough laboratory evaluation must then be done. However, it must be noted again that rare patients with mild congenital bleeding abnormalities may be normal by this evaluation but have serious bleeding complications after surgery.

LABORATORY ABNORMALITIES OF HEMOSTASIS NOT ASSOCIATED WITH CLINICAL BLEEDING PROBLEMS

Since laboratory studies of hemostasis are often ordered as part of an evaluation for another problem, unexpected abnormalities are occasionally found in patients who have no indication of any problem with excessive bleeding (see the box, upper right). These observations further emphasize the artificial nature of these coagulation assays.

"Pseudothrombocytopenia" has been described as a result of an EDTA-activated or cold-activated, platelet-agglutinating antibody. Since EDTA is the conventional anticoagulant for laboratory platelet counts, the platelets agglutinate in the blood sample and the count is falsely low. Platelets are normal in number and morphology on the peripheral blood smear made from finger-stick blood, and platelet counts are normal in blood anticoagulated by heparin. This is one example of the importance of examining the peripheral blood smear to confirm the presence of thrombocytopenia. These agglutinins may occur in any patient and also in normal subjects. They have no clinical significance.

The initial coagulation reactions required for a normal PTT involve three proteins that are unnecessary for normal hemostasis in vivo: factor XII, prekallikrein, and high-molecular-weight kininogen. The association of each of these proteins with in vitro coagulation was originally recognized by the observation of a prolonged PTT in a subject with entirely normal hemostasis. A similar observation has been made in some patients with plasma factor XI deficiency, although other patients may have a severe bleeding abnormality. Also, some patients with severe factor VII deficiency have no abnormal bleeding. The lupus anticoagulant also causes a significant in vitro coagulation abnormality (see the box on p. 792) but no clinical bleeding, although it is associated with an increased risk for thrombosis (described earlier).

A simpler in vitro artifact is the abnormality of coagulation tests reported in patients with extreme erythrocytosis. A common example is the finding of an abnormal PTT and PT as screening tests before cardiac catheterization in a patient with cyanotic congenital heart disease and a hematocrit greater than 65%. In these samples the ratio of the liquid sodium citrate anticoagulant to plasma is too great, and the standard amount of calcium added for the coagulation assay is inadequate. This problem can be corrected by removing an appropriate amount of the anticoagulant from the commercially prepared tube.

Laboratory abnormalities of hemostasis not associated with clinical bleeding problems

I. Spurious thrombocytopenia caused by EDTA-activated platelet agglutinins
II. Coagulation abnormalities
   A. Prolonged PTT caused by deficiencies of factor XII, prekallikrein, or high-molecular-weight kininogen. Some patients with factor XI deficiency and rare patients with factor VII deficiency have normal hemostasis
   B. Prolonged PTT and PT (the latter abnormality is often present only when the thromboplastin reagent is diluted) caused by the "lupus anticoagulant," an antibody against phospholipid
   C. Prolonged PTT and PT caused by extreme erythrocytosis resulting in an increased ratio of citrate anticoagulant to plasma

PTT, Partial thromboplastin time; PT, prothrombin time.

REFERENCES

Abilgaard CF et al: Serial studies in von Willebrand's disease: variability versus "variants." Blood 56:712, 1980.
Alperin JB: Coagulopathy caused by vitamin K deficiency in critically ill, hospitalized patients. JAMA 258:1916, 1987.
Aster RH: Pooling of platelets in the spleen: role in the pathogenesis of "hypersplenic" thrombocytopenia. J Clin Invest 45:645, 1966.
Bell WR et al: Trousseau's syndrome: devastating coagulopathy in the absence of heparin. Am J Med 79:423, 1985.
Bolan DD and Alving BM: Pharmacologic agents in the management of bleeding disorders. Transfusion 30:541, 1990.
Gastineau DA et al: Lupus anticoagulant: an analysis of the clinical and laboratory features of 219 cases. Am J Hematol 19:265, 1985.
George JN, Caen JP, and Nurden AT: Glanzmann's thrombasthenia: the spectrum of clinical disease. Blood 75:1383, 1990.
George JN and Shattil SJ: The clinical importance of acquired abnormalities of platelet function. N Engl J Med 324:27, 1991.
Kaplan EB et al: The usefulness of preoperative laboratory screening. JAMA 253:3576, 1985.

Kitchens CS: Occult hemophilia. Johns Hopkins Med J 146:255, 1980.
Kitchens CS: Concept of hypercoagulability: a review of its development, clinical application, and recent progress. Semin Hemost Thromb 11:293, 1985.
Kleiner GS et al: Defibrination in normal and abnormal parturition. Br J Haematol 19:159, 1970.
Macpherson DS, Snow R, and Lofgren RP: Preoperative screening: value of previous tests. Ann Intern Med 113:969, 1990.
Miletich J, Sherman L, and Broze G Jr: Absence of thrombosis in subjects with heterozygous protein C deficiency. N Engl J Med 317:991, 1987.
Oski FA and Naiman JL: Effect of live measles vaccine on the platelet count. N Engl J Med 275:352, 1966.
Rapaport SI: Preoperative hemostatic evaluation: which tests, if any? Blood 61:229, 1983.
Rodeghiero F, Castaman G, and Dini E: Epidemiological investigation of the prevalence of von Willebrand's disease. Blood 69:454, 1987.
Schafer AI: The hypercoagulable states. Ann Intern Med 102:814, 1985.
Suchman AL and Mushlin AI: How well does the activated partial thromboplastin time predict postoperative hemorrhage? JAMA 256:750, 1986.
Zwaal RFA et al: Lupus anticoagulant IgG's are not directed to phospholipids only, but to a complex of lipid-bound human prothrombin. Thromb Haemost 66:629, 1991.

V Specific Diseases

CHAPTER

84 Thrombocytopenia and Disorders of Platelet Function

Andrew I. Schafer

DISORDERS OF PLATELET FUNCTION

Etiology

The formation of a hemostatic platelet plug at a site of vascular injury is initiated by disruption of the monolayer of endothelial cells that normally covers the intimal surfaces of blood vessels. This exposes circulating platelets to subendothelial structures such as collagen and leads to the process of platelet *adhesion* (platelet-vascular interaction), in which platelets seal the site of vascular damage. Platelet adhesion is mediated by von Willebrand factor, which binds to platelet surface receptors localized on membrane glycoprotein Ib (GpIb) to attach platelets to the subendothelium. After adhesion, platelets undergo the *release* reaction, during which they degranulate (secreting constituents of specific storage granules such as fibrinogen and adenosine diphosphate [ADP]) and also rapidly synthesize thromboxane A_2, a potent vasoconstrictor and platelet-activating derivative of arachidonic acid. Released granule constituents and thromboxane A_2 act in concert to mediate the process of platelet *aggregation* (platelet-platelet interaction), in which platelets stick to each other to form a platelet plug that occludes the damaged vessel lumen. Fibrinogen and von Willebrand factor mediate aggregation, binding to platelet surface receptors localized on the membrane glycoprotein complex IIb-IIIa (GpIIb-IIIa). Several disorders of platelet function are caused by specific defects in each of these steps in platelet plug formation, as shown in Fig. 84-1.

The most common disorder of platelet adhesion is *von Willebrand's disease,* an inherited (or rarely, acquired) quantitative deficiency or qualitative defect in plasma von Willebrand factor (Chapter 85). The platelet counterpart of von Willebrand's disease is the *Bernard-Soulier syndrome,* a rare autosomal recessive disorder of platelets in which adhesion is defective because of a structural or functional loss of receptors for von Willebrand factor on platelet membrane GpIb. This intrinsic platelet abnormality, the clinical manifestations of which mimic those of von Willebrand's disease, is associated with mild thrombocytopenia and circulating giant platelets. Using in vitro models of perfused vessels, platelet adhesion to subendothelium is greatly impaired in both von Willebrand's disease and Bernard-Soulier syndrome; however, the release reaction and the platelets' capability to aggregate remain preserved in these disorders.

Defects in the platelet release reaction can be caused either by the structural loss of platelet storage granules (i.e., *storage pool disease*) or by a *functional release defect* that is most often caused by impaired thromboxane A_2 formation. Both types of release defects can be either congenital

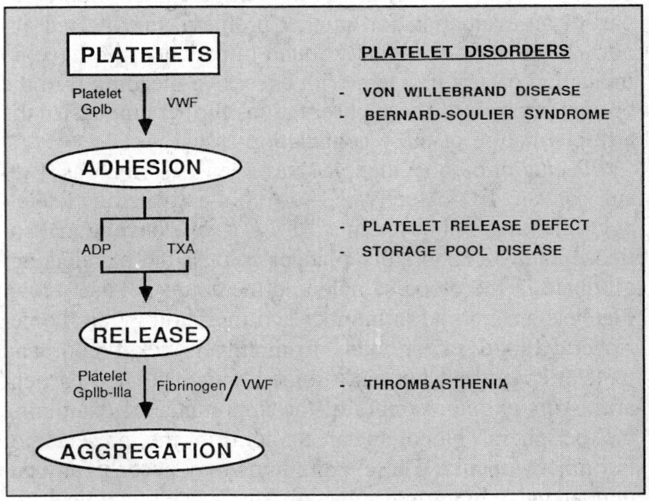

Fig. 84-1. Biochemical basis of disorders of platelet function. Platelet adhesion is mediated by von Willebrand factor *(vWf)* binding to platelet GpIb: defective adhesion is found in von Willebrand's disease (a plasma defect) and Bernard-Soulier syndrome (a platelet defect). The release reaction is mediated by adenosine diphosphate *(ADP)* and thromboxane A_2 *(TXA);* abnormal release is found in platelet-release defects (aspirin-like defects) and storage pool disease. Platelet aggregation is mediated by fibrinogen and vWf binding to platelet GpIIb-IIIa; defective aggregation is found in Glanzmann's thrombasthenia.

or acquired. Some patients with congenital storage pool disease have associated abnormalities, such as oculocutaneous albinism in the Hermansky-Pudlak syndrome and immunodeficiency in the Wiskott-Aldrich syndrome. Acquired storage pool disease may develop in the course of various disorders, including the myeloproliferative disorders and transiently in patients undergoing cardiopulmonary bypass. Functional platelet release defects caused by impaired production of thromboxane A_2 most frequently result from drugs that inhibit platelet cyclo-oxygenase. This enzyme oxygenates arachidonic acid to cyclic endoperoxides, which are then converted in platelets by thromboxane synthase to thromboxane A_2. *Aspirin* acetylates cyclo-oxygenase and irreversibly blocks its activity. Therefore, since platelets are incapable of resynthesizing new uninhibited enzyme, the aspirin-induced platelet release defect persists for the lifetime of the affected platelet (i.e., 7 to 10 days). A single, low dose of aspirin (one children's aspirin) thus produces a defect in platelet function for several days. *Nonsteroidal anti-inflammatory agents* inhibit platelet cyclo-oxygenase reversibly, and their effects on platelet function are therefore lost with the clearance of the drugs from the circulation (i.e., within hours). Diets rich in omega-3 fatty acids or dietary supplementation with fish oils can produce a similar platelet release defect. They exert this action in part by causing the release of eicosapentaenoic acid (EPA) to compete with arachidonic acid (AA) for cyclo-oxygenase, producing EPA-derived functionally inactive thromboxane A_3 rather than AA-derived active thromboxane A_2. Rare cases of congenital cyclo-oxygenase deficiency, thromboxane synthase deficiency, and deficiency of platelet receptors for thromboxane/endoperoxides have also been described. The platelets of patients with storage pool disease and functional release defects are able to adhere normally to damaged vessels and can also aggregate normally in response to certain potent stimuli that bypass the requirement for the release reaction.

Functional platelet abnormalities that are specifically caused by defective aggregation are rare. Quantitative or qualitative disorders of fibrinogen, including afibrinogenemia and dysfibrinogenemia, are sometimes associated with abnormal platelet aggregation. *Glanzmann's thrombasthenia* is an unusual autosomal recessive disease involving an intrinsic platelet abnormality that is characterized by a structural or functional loss of receptors for fibrinogen and von Willebrand factor on the platelet membrane GpIIb-IIIa complex. The platelet count and morphology are normal in this disorder.

Some acquired clinical conditions are associated with qualitative defects of primary hemostasis and platelet function, in which the pathophysiology of bleeding is more complex and poorly understood. The hemorrhagic disorder of *uremia* is characterized by a prolonged bleeding time, but no specific, reproducible functional platelet abnormalities can be demonstrated in vitro. Easy bruising is the most frequently encountered symptom, but more severe bleeding can occur. The hemostatic defect appears to be caused, at least in part, by dialyzable uremic toxins, since dialysis transiently improves or even completely corrects the prolonged bleeding time and the clinical bleeding tendency. For unclear reasons, amelioration of the anemia of renal failure, either by red cell transfusion or by administration of recombinant erythropoietin, also leads to improved hemostasis. Cryoprecipitate, deamino-8-D-arginine vasopressin (DDAVP), and conjugated estrogens have also been shown to have beneficial effects in uremic bleeding, although their mechanisms of action are largely unknown.

Bleeding and thrombosis are major causes of morbidity and mortality in the *myeloproliferative disorders* (Chapter 93). The thrombocytosis that occurs in many of these patients is generally not causally linked to the hemostatic complications. A variety of metabolic and biochemical platelet abnormalities have been identified in patients with myeloproliferative disorders, and these qualitative platelet defects that occur independently of platelet count are more likely to be responsible for the bleeding and thrombotic problems. Lowering of the platelet count in asymptomatic patients with even extreme thrombocytosis is generally not indicated. However, cytoreduction with hydroxyurea or interferon may benefit patients with thrombocytosis who have recurrent hemostatic complications, and aspirin can promptly improve microvascular thrombotic manifestations in the cerebrovascular or peripheral circulation. Qualitative platelet abnormalities also occur in patients with acute leukemia and myelodysplasia and may exacerbate a bleeding tendency when they coexist with thrombocytopenia.

Platelet dysfunction occurs in patients with *dysproteinemias* (Chapter 95), including multiple myeloma and Waldenström's macroglobulinemia, in whom the hemostatic problems tend to be related to the level of paraprotein and are improved by plasmapheresis. The bleeding problems in these patients may be complicated by other associated coagulopathies, including defective fibrin polymerization, thrombocytopenia, and hyperviscosity. The bleeding diathesis of chronic *liver failure* is highly complex and multifactorial, including components of thrombocytopenia secondary to hypersplenism, multiple coagulation factor deficiencies, dysfibrinogenemia, impaired clearance of activated coagulation factors causing intravascular coagulation, and increased fibrinolytic activity. Poorly defined defects in platelet function related to extracorpuscular plasma factors may contribute to these patients' hemorrhagic tendency. In addition to aspirin and nonsteroidal anti-inflammatory agents, a variety of other drugs interfere with platelet function in vitro; however, only a few of these drugs have demonstrable clinical effects on hemostasis. Ticlopidine exerts potent platelet inhibitory actions by producing a thrombasthenia-like defect. High doses of penicillins, cephalosporins, and related antibiotics, including penicillin G, carbenicillin, ticarcillin, ampicillin, and moxalactam, cause prolongation of the bleeding time and interfere with platelet function by binding to platelets and blocking recognition of platelet membrane agonist receptors. Platelet dysfunction caused by antibiotics can contribute to serious bleeding complications when administered in the clinical setting of coexisting illnesses (e.g., renal and hepatic failure, malignancy, concomitant use of anticoagulants), which themselves may independently cause a bleeding diathesis. Alcohol, which itself does not affect the bleeding time, enhances the effect of aspirin on prolongation of the bleeding time.

Clinical features

Patients with disorders of platelet function generally develop bleeding complications that are clinically distinguishable from those seen in patients with coagulation factor deficiencies. In contrast to the bleeding patterns associated with coagulopathies, which usually involve deep tissue and visceral hemorrhage and which often occur in a delayed manner after trauma, patients with platelet disorders characteristically exhibit superficial hemorrhage that develops either spontaneously or immediately after injury. Superficial bleeding may involve mucosal hemorrhage (e.g., epistaxis, gastrointestinal or genitourinary tract bleeding) or cutaneous hemorrhage in the form of ecchymoses (common bruises) and purpura. Petechiae are more typically seen in severe thrombocytopenic states. Patients with platelet adhesion or aggregation abnormalities generally have more severe bleeding tendencies than do those with platelet release defects.

Laboratory features

The most valuable laboratory screening test of primary hemostasis is the *bleeding time*. This is determined by measuring the time to cessation of bleeding from a standardized incision on the volar aspect of the forearm. The bleeding time is prolonged in patients with (1) thrombocytopenia (platelets < 100,000/μl), (2) disorders of platelet function, and (3) primary vascular defects. Generally, it is unnecessary to perform this test in patients with thrombocytopenia unless an associated qualitative platelet abnormality is suspected, in which case the bleeding time would be expected to be disproportionately prolonged for the degree of thrombocytopenia (Fig. 84-2). The bleeding time is usually unaffected by coagulation factor deficiencies or pharmacologic anticoagulation. Although it is a valuable diagnostic test, the bleeding time is prone to both falsely abnormal or falsely normal results when performed by improper technique. Furthermore, in patients without a known clinical history of bleeding problems, the bleeding time has been found to be unreliable as a routine screening test to predict the risk of excessive surgical hemorrhage.

In patients who exhibit a prolonged bleeding time associated with a normal platelet count, the presence of an intrinsic qualitative platelet defect can be evaluated by platelet aggregation studies. In vitro platelet aggregation induced by the addition of specific agonists to platelet-rich plasma is monitored by a turbidometric method in an aggregometer. The normal platelet response to epinephrine and certain concentrations of ADP demonstrates a biphasic pattern of aggregation, the second wave of which results from the release reaction; a single wave of aggregation is generally noted in response to collagen, arachidonate, and ristocetin (Fig. 84-3). In patients with adhesion defects (von Wille-

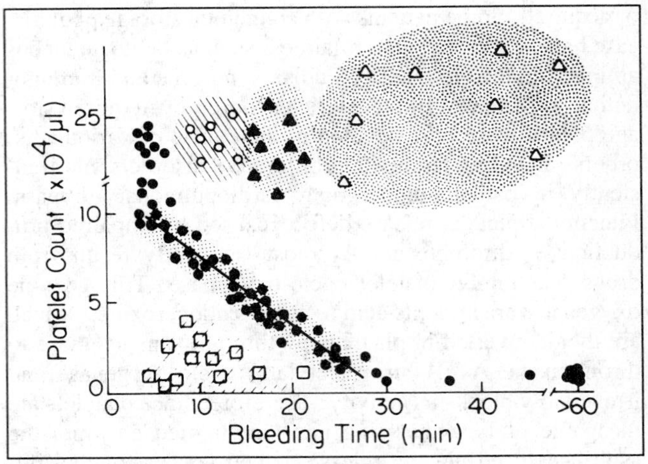

Fig. 84-2. Relationship of bleeding time to platelet count. The bleeding time is inversely related to circulating platelet count in patients with thrombocytopenia because of decreased production (*closed circles*, which also include eight normal subjects) when the count is between 100,000 and 10,000/μl. Platelet function defects (without thrombocytopenia) are represented by subjects taking aspirin *(open circles)* and patients with uremia *(closed triangles)* and inherited severe von Willebrand's disease *(open triangles)*. Patients with idiopathic thrombocytopenic purpura may have platelets with increased hemostatic competence *(open squares)*. (Reproduced with permission from Thompson AR and Harker LA: Manual of hemostasis and thrombosis. Philadelphia, 1983, FA Davis.)

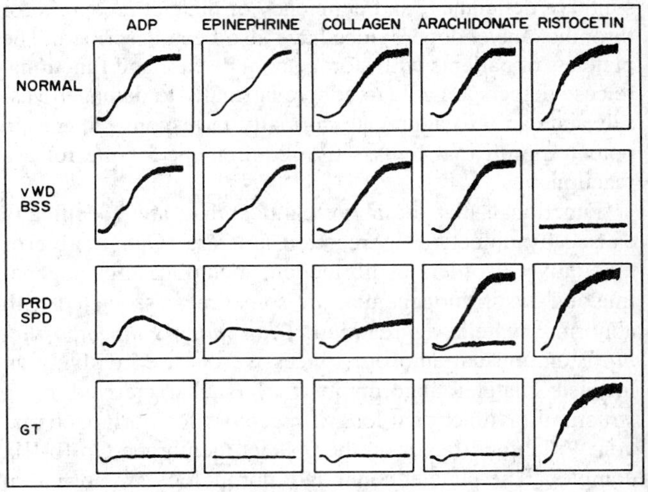

Fig. 84-3. Normal and abnormal patterns of platelet aggregation in response to ADP, epinephrine, collagen, arachidonate, and ristocetin. In classic (type I) von Willebrand's disease *(vWD)* and Bernard-Soulier syndrome *(BSS)*, platelet aggregation is normal with all agents except ristocetin. In platelet release defects *(PRD)* and storage pool disease *(SPD)*, only first-wave aggregation occurs in response to ADP and epinephrine, and collagen-induced aggregation is greatly blunted; arachidonate-induced aggregation may or may not be abnormal but is always lost after aspirin ingestion. In Glanzmann's thrombasthenia *(GT)*, the initial shape-change remains normal, but aggregation is completely inhibited in response to all agents except ristocetin.

brand's disease or the Bernard-Soulier syndrome), only ristocetin-stimulated platelet aggregation may be affected. In patients with release defects caused by storage pool deficiency or a functional release abnormality (e.g., after aspirin ingestion), second-wave aggregation in response to epinephrine or ADP is lost, and arachidonate-induced aggregation may be entirely absent, particularly in subjects taking aspirin. In patients with thrombasthenia, complete loss of aggregation to all agonists is characteristically found. Specific patterns of abnormal aggregation can be pursued with more specialized platelet function studies, such as serotonin uptake and release, measurements of platelet adenine nucleotide content, or electron microscopy, but these tests are rarely necessary for clinical management.

Nonthrombocytopenic patients with prolonged bleeding times but with normal platelet aggregation studies pose difficult diagnostic problems. Unless they are using potentially implicated medications, they should be evaluated for (1) von Willebrand's disease, even when ristocetin-induced aggregation is normal, (2) renal failure, (3) hepatic dysfunction, and (4) dysproteinemia. Unfortunately a substantial number of patients remain with unexplained prolongations of the bleeding time, possibly because of a primary vascular disorder. In these patients, clinical management must depend on empiric therapeutic trials of platelet transfusions, DDAVP, cryoprecipitate, or occasionally, brief courses of corticosteroids.

Treatment

Most patients with disorders of platelet function do not require chronic treatment, and avoidance of the use of aspirin or other platelet inhibitory drugs may be the only intervention recommended. The prophylaxis or management of surgical or traumatic bleeding depends on the clinical severity and the specific type of qualitative platelet abnormality. Patients undergoing elective surgery should be advised to avoid aspirin-containing medications for at least 1 week before surgery. The definitive treatment for severe bleeding from an intrinsic platelet disorder is the transfusion of normal platelets. Cryoprecipitate may ameliorate bleeding and shorten the prolonged bleeding time not only in von Willebrand's disease, but also in uremia. The arginine vasopressin analog, DDAVP, infused intravenously at a dose of 0.3 μg/kg body weight over 15 to 30 minutes immediately before surgery, has been shown to shorten the bleeding time and improve hemostasis in patients with type I and, to a lesser extent, type IIA von Willebrand's disease. This drug has also demonstrated efficacy in shortening the bleeding time of some patients with uremia, as well as those with a variety of functional platelet disorders. The mechanism of clinical action of DDAVP is not clear, but it stimulates the release of von Willebrand factor from vascular endothelial cells and may also exert nonspecific vasoactive effects to improve hemostasis. Rapid tachyphylaxis tends to occur, and second infusions of DDAVP 12 hours after the initial treatment generally result in suboptimum responses. Therefore, although DDAVP can obviate the need for blood products in many of these patients, its hemostatic actions tend to be short-lived. More sustained improvement in the prolonged bleeding time of uremic patients may be achieved with the use of conjugated estrogens. Partial correction of the anemia of renal failure (to a hematocrit of about 27% to 31%) with either red cell transfusions or erythropoietin is sufficient to normalize the bleeding time of most such uremic patients.

THROMBOCYTOPENIA

Thrombocytopenia is defined as a platelet count less than 150×10^9/L. The major causes of thrombocytopenia are outlined in the box below. These can be broadly divided into three categories on the basis of platelet kinetics. Thrombocytopenia may be caused by (1) impaired production of platelets by the bone marrow, (2) platelet sequestration from splenomegaly, or (3) increased destruction of platelets in the peripheral circulation that exceeds the approximately eightfold capacity of the bone marrow to compensate by accelerated production. In patients receiving large volumes of rapidly administered platelet-poor blood products, thrombocytopenia may also develop on a dilutional basis. The destructive thrombocytopenias can be further subdivided into nonimmune and immune-mediated disorders; immune thrombocytopenias, in turn, may be caused

Major causes of thrombocytopenia

I. Decreased platelet production
   A. Megakaryocyte hypoplasia
      1. Aplastic anemia
      2. Myelofibrosis
      3. Leukemia
      4. Marrow invasion by metastatic tumor, granulomas
      5. Viral infection
      6. Radiation myelosuppression
      7. Toxic agents, drugs, antineoplastic chemotherapy
   B. Ineffective thrombopoiesis
      1. Vitamin B_{12} deficiency
      2. Folate deficiency

II. Splenic sequestration, hypersplenism

III. Increased platelet destruction
   A. Non-immune-mediated platelet destruction
      1. Disseminated intravascular coagulation (DIC)
      2. Prosthetic intravascular devices
      3. Extracorporeal circulation
      4. Thrombotic thrombocytopenic purpura (TTP)
   B. Immune-mediated platelet destruction
      1. Drug-induced immune thrombocytopenia
      2. Alloimmune thrombocytopenia
         a. Neonatal
         b. Posttransfusion purpura
      3. Autoimmune thrombocytopenia (ITP)
         a. Idiopathic thrombocytopenic purpura
         b. Secondary to rheumatic diseases, infections, lymphoproliferative disorders

by drug-induced antibodies, alloantibodies, or autoantibodies.

The clinical bleeding manifestations of thrombocytopenia depend on the severity of thrombocytopenia, its cause, and possible associated coagulation defects. In general, abnormal bleeding is unusual even after surgery or trauma, when the platelet count is greater than 100×10^9/L, unless complicating coexisting conditions are present. Patients with platelet counts of 20 to 100×10^9/L are at risk of excessive posttraumatic bleeding, whereas those with platelet counts less than 20×10^9/L may bleed spontaneously. For any given degree of thrombocytopenia, bleeding tends to be more severe when the cause is decreased production rather than increased destruction of platelets; in the latter situation, accelerated platelet turnover results in the circulation of younger, larger, and hemostatically more effective platelets. The types of clinical bleeding manifestations of thrombocytopenia are similar to those described previously for functional platelet abnormalities. In addition, severe thrombocytopenia is typically associated with the appearance of mucous membrane and cutaneous petechiae (Color Plate III-12), particularly over dependent parts of the body (e.g., lower legs).

The laboratory evaluation of thrombocytopenia must begin with a careful examination of the peripheral blood smear. "Pseudothrombocytopenia" occurs when platelets clump in the test tube, leading to an artifactually low platelet count reading by automated machines that exclude large platelet aggregates. This phenomenon in some patients may be caused by the EDTA anticoagulant in tubes used for blood counts or a clinically insignificant platelet cold agglutinin that functions only at room temperature. Pseudothrombocytopenia should be suspected in patients who have unexpected reports of very low platelet counts in the absence of bleeding problems; it is confirmed by the finding of platelet clumps on the peripheral smear. In these patients, platelet counts obtained by finger-stick, from blood drawn into tubes containing alternative anticoagulants, or in promptly processed samples will reveal a normal concentration of platelets. Examination of the peripheral smear may also provide critical clues to the etiology of the thrombocytopenia (e.g., fragmented red cells in thrombotic thrombocytopenic purpura).

Certain laboratory tests may provide guidance to the broad kinetic category of thrombocytopenia. In general the occurrence of a severe, selective thrombocytopenia (in the absence of anemia or leukopenia) strongly suggests that the etiology involves increased peripheral platelet destruction by either a non-immune-mediated or immune-mediated mechanism. The finding of large platelets on the blood smear may likewise be an indication of increased platelet turnover. In patients with low platelet counts because of peripheral platelet destruction, an increased number of megakaryocytes is typically seen in the bone marrow, and bone marrow examination can often directly reveal the cause of thrombocytopenias caused by decreased platelet production (e.g., aplastic anemia, myelofibrosis, leukemia, tumor infiltration). Platelet survival studies, tracing the fate of autologous chromium-51-labeled platelets infused intravenously (Fig. 84-4), can be instructive but are rarely necessary clinically. A cruder but more practical clinical approach to this kinetic diagnosis of thrombocytopenia is the serial testing of platelet counts after a platelet transfusion. An expected level and duration of rise in the platelet count suggests that the thrombocytopenia results from decreased platelet production, whereas failure of an expected response suggests a mechanism involving increased platelet clearance.

Thrombocytopenia caused by decreased platelet production

Patients with congenital thrombocytopenia caused by decreased platelet production are rarely seen; they include those with constitutional aplastic anemia (Fanconi's syndrome) and congenital amegakaryocytic thrombocytopenia, which may be associated with skeletal malformations. Acquired disorders of platelet production are caused by either (1) hypoplasia of megakaryocytes or (2) ineffective thrombopoiesis. Megakaryocytic hypoplasia can result from a variety of conditions, including *marrow aplasia* (including idiopathic forms or myelosuppression by chemotherapeutic agents, toxins, or radiation therapy), *myelofibrosis, leukemia,* and invasion of the bone marrow by *metastatic tumor* or *granulomas*. In most of these patients, red cell and leukocyte production are also affected, and the diagnosis can be made on bone marrow biopsy. In some situations, *toxins, infectious agents,* or *drugs* may interfere with thrombopoiesis relatively selectively. Examples include transient thrombocytopenias caused by alcohol and certain viral in-

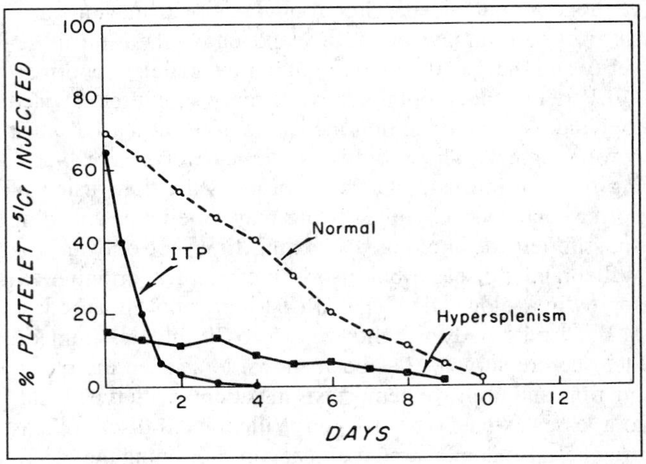

Fig. 84-4. Platelet survival measured by chromium-51-labeled autologous platelets. Normal platelet survival is 10 days. The recovery of labeled platelets in the general circulation 2 hours after infusion is approximately only 70%. The remainder are reversibly sequestered in the spleen. In patients with immune thrombocytopenia the initial recovery may not be changed, but platelet survival is greatly shortened. In patients with hypersplenism the initial platelet recovery is decreased because of platelet pooling within the spleen, but platelet survival is normal. (Reproduced with permission from Aster RH: In Williams WJ et al, editors: Hematology. New York, 1972, McGraw-Hill.)

fections and mild thrombocytopenia associated with the administration of thiazide diuretics. Finally, ineffective thrombopoiesis secondary to megaloblastic processes (*folate* or *vitamin B_{12} deficiency*) can cause thrombocytopenia, usually with coexisting anemia and leukopenia.

Effective treatment of thrombocytopenias caused by decreased platelet production depends on identification and reversal of the underlying cause of the bone marrow failure. Platelet transfusions are generally reserved for patients with serious bleeding complications or for coverage during surgical procedures, since isoimmunization may lead to refractoriness to further platelet transfusions. Mucosal bleeding resulting from severe thrombocytopenia may be ameliorated by the oral or intravenous administration of an antifibrinolytic agent such as epsilon aminocaproic acid. Thrombotic complications may develop, however, if antifibrinolytic agents are used in patients with disseminated intravascular coagulation (DIC).

Thrombocytopenia caused by splenic sequestration

Splenomegaly from any cause may be associated with mild to moderate thrombocytopenia. This phenomenon of *hypersplenism* results from expansion of the splenic platelet pool. This is a largely passive process of splenic platelet sequestration, in contrast to the active destruction of platelets by the spleen in patients with immune-mediated thrombocytopenia (discussed later). Although the most common cause of hypersplenism is congestive splenomegaly from portal hypertension caused by alcoholic cirrhosis, other forms of congestive, infiltrative, or lymphoproliferative splenomegaly are also associated with thrombocytopenia. Platelet counts generally do not fall below 50×10^9/L as a result of hypersplenism alone, and coexisting anemia and leukopenia frequently occur. The size of the spleen does not clearly correlate with the degree of thrombocytopenia. Splenectomy, which is rarely indicated solely because of the thrombocytopenia, leads to an unpredictable rise in the platelet count.

Thrombocytopenia caused by non-immune-mediated platelet destruction

Thrombocytopenia can result from the accelerated destruction of platelets by various nonimmunologic processes. Disorders of this type include DIC, prosthetic intravascular devices, extracorporeal circulation of blood, and thrombotic microangiopathies such as thrombotic thrombocytopenic purpura (discussed in the next section). In all these situations, circulating platelets that are exposed to either artificial surfaces or abnormal vascular intima are either consumed at these sites or are damaged so that they are then prematurely cleared by the reticuloendothelial system. DIC is discussed in Chapter 85. A localized consumptive coagulopathy occurs in patients with *giant cavernous hemangiomas,* termed the *Kasabach-Merritt syndrome,* in which thrombocytopenia is usually associated with laboratory evidence of intravascular coagulation. *Intravascular prosthetic devices,* including cardiac valves and intra-aortic balloons, can cause a mild to moderate destructive thrombocytopenia. Finally, transient thrombocytopenia in patients undergoing *cardiopulmonary bypass* or *hemodialysis* may result from consumption or damage of platelets in the extracorporeal circuit. Successful treatment of these types of thrombocytopenia depends on the correction or removal of the underlying cause.

Thrombotic thrombocytopenic purpura

Thrombotic thrombocytopenic purpura (TTP) is a rare form of thrombocytopenia caused by widespread platelet thrombi that form in the microcirculation. This is a syndrome of largely unknown and probably multiple diverse etiologies that occurs predominantly in adults without evidence of antecedent illness. Although infectious, genetic, or immunologic etiologies have been suspected in some patients, the cause of TTP usually is unknown. Some laboratory observations have indicated that TTP may be caused by a primary endothelial cell disorder in which the thromboresistant properties of normal vascular intima are defective; this has been suggested by the finding of decreased endothelium-derived prostacyclin (PGI_2), impaired protein C activation, and defective fibrinolysis. A plasma defect has been implicated by the finding of a circulating platelet agglutinating factor in the plasma of some patients with TTP and the appearance in plasma of unusually large multimers of von Willebrand factor during remission in patients with chronic relapsing TTP.

The major clinical manifestations of TTP are attributable to the disseminated occlusive microvascular platelet thrombi: (1) thrombocytopenia, which may be very severe and associated with bleeding; (2) microangiopathic hemolytic anemia, caused by red cell fragmentation during passage of blood through the disrupted microcirculation; (3) neurologic symptoms and signs, including nonspecific headache, mental changes, seizures, coma, and focal neurologic signs; (4) renal abnormalities, ranging in severity from proteinuria and microscopic hematuria to frank renal failure; and (5) fever. Not all these major manifestations of TTP may be present simultaneously. Other clinical features may include abdominal pain, nausea, vomiting, malaise, and weakness. The onset of symptoms is frequently abrupt, and the disease course may be fulminant and self-limited or fatal. Other patients may be characterized by an insidious onset or a chronic, relapsing course.

In patients with typical, acute disease the diagnosis of TTP should not pose difficulty. The constellation of laboratory findings include thrombocytopenia, red cell fragmentation on peripheral smear, evidence of intravascular hemolysis (including reticulocytosis, elevated indirect serum bilirubin and lactate dehydrogenase, decreased haptoglobin), proteinuria, abnormal urinary sediment, or uremia. No activation of the coagulation system occurs in TTP, and therefore laboratory manifestations of DIC should not be found. Diagnostic problems may arise in patients with more subtle disease, particularly when other conditions coexist to which some of the clinical and laboratory features could be attributed. Associated DIC, malignant hypertension, eclampsia or pre-eclampsia, or vasculitis may mimic some of the features of TTP. A tissue diagnosis, most conveniently obtained by gingival biopsy, is rarely necessary and should not delay therapy in fulminant cases. The characteristic pathologic features of TTP, consisting of microvascular hyaline thrombi, should be clearly distinguishable from the changes of vasculitis whenever the differential diagnosis is in doubt.

The design of rational therapy has been hindered by the lack of understanding of etiology, the unpredictable natural history, and the rarity of patients with TTP. Nevertheless, prompt treatment of TTP has dramatically reduced mortality from rates of more than 90% in historically untreated patients. In acute, fulminant TTP, two major therapeutic interventions are generally used simultaneously. First, prednisone at a dose of 1 to 2 mg/kg/day is started. Second, plasma exchange is begun without delay. Plasmapheresis is usually performed with a 2 to 3 L exchange daily for at least 7 days, using fresh-frozen plasma as replacement. In some patients who fail to respond to this treatment, the substitution of cryosupernatant for fresh-frozen plasma in the plasma exchange procedure has been found to be effective. Plasma exchange has been demonstrated to be more effective than simple plasma infusion in the treatment of TTP. Other, second-line treatments of largely unproven efficacy may include heparin, antiplatelet agents (aspirin, dipyridamole, prostacyclin), vincristine, and splenectomy. Platelet transfusions are contraindicated, even in the presence of severe thrombocytopenia, because transfused platelets may "fuel the fire" to exacerbate the thrombotic microangiopathy.

Several syndromes that are clinically and pathologically similar to TTP have been described. The *hemolytic-uremic syndrome* (HUS) is typically encountered in children and frequently follows viral infections. Gastroenteritis caused by a verotoxin-producing serotype of *Escherichia coli* or by *Shigella* may also cause a similar syndrome. Thrombocytopenia and microangiopathic hemolytic anemia are prominent manifestations of HUS, but neurologic symptoms are unusual and renal complications, including frank renal failure, are more predominant features of HUS than TTP. Treatment of patients with HUS also centers around the use of plasma exchange. During the late stages of pregnancy, a pre-eclamptic TTP-like syndrome of microangiopathic hemolysis, elevated liver enzymes, and low platelet counts has been give the acronym "HELLP." Finally, an either fulminant or slowly progressive thrombotic microangiopathy that resembles TTP/HUS has been observed in some patients receiving chemotherapy with certain agents, including mitomycin, cyclosporine, and cisplatin.

Drug-induced immune thrombocytopenia

More than 100 drugs have been implicated in immunologically mediated thrombocytopenia. However, only a small number of these, notably quinidine, quinine, gold, sulfonamides, cephalothin, and heparin, have been well characterized. The mechanism of drug-induced immune platelet destruction depends in part on the offending agent. It may be mediated either through the binding of the drug (hapten)-antibody complex to platelets with subsequent complement fixation and platelet damage or, alternatively, the drug's binding to platelets to induce new and unstable immunogenic platelet surface antigens that are expressed only in the drug's presence and are stabilized on reaction with antibody. The mechanism of heparin-associated thrombocytopenia is unusual in that the antibodies to heparin or the heparin-antibody complex cause platelet aggregation.

Drug-induced thrombocytopenia is frequently very severe and typically occurs precipitously within days while patients are taking the sensitizing medication. These idiosyncratic reactions are generally not drug-dose dependent. For example, severe quinine-induced thrombocytopenia may be precipitated by drinking tonic water. Although clinical manifestations of drug-induced thrombocytopenias are common to the bleeding complications encountered in other forms of thrombocytopenia, heparin-associated thrombocytopenia has unusual features. As many as 10% of patients receiving heparin may develop thrombocytopenia, but this is usually dose related, not immune mediated, and mild, stable, and asymptomatic. The idiosyncratic form of heparin-associated thrombocytopenia, in contrast, tends to be more severe and precipitous and may be triggered by even the small doses included in intravenous flushes. These latter patients may develop serious venous or arterial thrombosis, presumably on the basis of *in vivo* platelet aggregation mediated by heparin-induced antibody. The thrombotic complications of heparin may also be related to heparin-dependent antibodies targeted to vascular endothelial cells. In most patients with any drug-induced thrombocytopenia, rapid recovery of the platelet count occurs within 7 to 10 days of removal of the offending agent. With some drugs that are metabolized and eliminated slowly, particularly gold, recovery may take weeks or even months. In the latter patients, the possible coexistence of autoimmune thrombocytopenia caused by the underlying rheumatic disease may complicate and confuse the clinical picture.

Specific laboratory tests may confirm the diagnosis with certain types of drugs; in vitro platelet immunoinjury or, in the case of heparin, platelet aggregation may be found when target platelets, patient serum (or plasma), and the suspected drug are mixed. However, the definitive demonstration is prompt recovery after withdrawal of the immunizing agent.

Treatment of drug-induced thrombocytopenia depends on immediate discontinuation of any suspected medication. In patients with severe disease and bleeding complications, a short course of prednisone (1 to 2 mg/kg/day) may be of benefit. Platelet transfusions are indicated only for critical or life-threatening hemorrhage, since the transfused platelets are likely to be destroyed as rapidly as the recipient's own platelets. The management of patients with heparin-associated thrombocytopenia poses special problems if alternative antithrombotic treatment is required after discontinuation of the heparin or in choosing anticoagulation for the thrombotic complication caused by the heparin itself. Institution of an oral anticoagulant and interim antithrombotic therapy with a fibrinolytic agent has been suggested as one approach. Low-molecular-weight heparin, which causes fewer problems with thrombocytopenia than does unfractionated heparin in currently used commercial preparations, has been suggested as alternative anticoagulant treatment of patients with this complication. However, the appropriate management in these situations is not clearly established.

Alloimmune thrombocytopenic purpura

Neonatal alloimmune thrombocytopenia and posttransfusion purpura are disorders of alloimmune platelet destruction that usually involve patients whose platelets lack the platelet-specific antigen Pl^{A1}. About 2% of the normal population is platelet Pl^{A1} negative. In *neonatal alloimmune thrombocytopenia* the Pl^{A1}-negative mother carrying a Pl^{A1}-positive fetus develops antibodies against this antigen, and transplacental transmission of the antibodies causes temporary immune platelet destruction and thrombocytopenia in the neonate. This syndrome is a platelet counterpart of hemolytic disease of the newborn. Until the maternal anti-Pl^{A1} antibodies are cleared from the neonatal circulation, the newborn frequently requires support with transfusions of platelets from a Pl^{A1}-negative donor, who is most conveniently the unaffected mother herself.

Posttransfusion purpura is a rare disorder of Pl^{A1}-negative adult recipients of blood products containing Pl^{A1}-positive platelets. Affected patients are typically multiparous females who have been previously sensitized to the platelet antigen. The mechanism of thrombocytopenia is unclear in this disorder. It has been considered that Pl^{A1} antigen or Pl^{A1}-positive platelet fragments in the transfused blood bind to anti-Pl^{A1} antibody, and these immune complexes are then adsorbed onto the surfaces of the Pl^{A1}-negative platelets of the transfusion recipient, effectively converting them to Pl^{A1} positivity. The clinical consequences are the development of acute, profound thrombocytopenia in some of these patients 7 to 10 days after the transfusion. Platelet counts generally return to normal within 10 to 14 days. During the period of thrombocytopenia, transfusions of either Pl^{A1}-negative or Pl^{A1}-positive platelets are usually ineffective. Intravenous gamma globulin is the treatment of first choice in this life-threatening disease. Plasmapheresis, in patients who fail to respond to intravenous gamma globulin, and prednisone may also improve the thrombocytopenia and bleeding tendency.

Immune (autoimmune) thrombocytopenic purpura

Immune thrombocytopenic purpura (ITP) in adults is a chronic disease characterized by autoimmune platelet destruction. The autoantibody is usually immunoglobulin G (IgG) that may or may not fix complement, although other immunoglobulins have also been reported. Although the autoantibody of ITP has been found to be associated with platelet membrane GpIIb-IIIa, the platelet antigen specificity has not been identified in most patients. Extravascular destruction of sensitized platelets occurs in the reticuloendothelial system of the spleen and liver. Although more than half of all cases of ITP are idiopathic, many patients have underlying rheumatic or autoimmune diseases (e.g., systemic lupus erythematosus) or lymphoproliferative disorders (e.g., chronic lymphocytic leukemia). ITP is also increasingly recognized as a complication of human immunodeficiency virus (HIV) infection.

Childhood ITP appears to be a distinctly different clinical entity. This is an acute and self-limited disorder, usually resolving spontaneously within a few weeks. It frequently follows minor viral infections, and the deposition of resultant immune complexes on platelets is considered to be the major mechanism of immune platelet destruction in these patients. There is no absolute separation of the two clinical forms of ITP by age; occasionally, adults may develop acute "childhood" ITP, and children may have chronic ITP.

The onset of bleeding problems in patients with chronic ITP may be either insidious or abrupt and fulminant. The hemorrhagic complications of ITP are indistinguishable from those associated with other types of thrombocytopenia described earlier. Besides signs of bleeding, the physical examination is generally unremarkable. The finding of splenomegaly is distinctly unusual in idiopathic forms of ITP and strongly suggests the presence of an underlying rheumatic or lymphoproliferative disease.

Laboratory studies usually reveal a selective thrombocytopenia. In rare patients, autoimmune hemolytic anemia may coexist with ITP (an association known as *Evans's syndrome*). Bone marrow examination, which is not indicated in all patients, is typically normal except for the presence of an increased number of megakaryocytes that is characteristic of other types of destructive thrombocytopenias. Several laboratory tests for the detection of antiplatelet antibodies have been developed. However, interpretation of the results of many of these assays is complicated by both false-positive tests (e.g., from platelet adsorption of immunoglobulin in patients with hypergammaglobulinemia) and false-negative tests. In making the diagnosis of ITP, other types of destructive thrombocytopenias must be rigorously excluded. DIC can be ruled out in most patients by the presence of a normal prothrombin time, partial thromboplastin time, and fibrin degradation products. TTP can be ruled out by the absence of red cell fragmentation on the peripheral smear and the lack of renal or neurologic involvement. Drug-induced thrombocytopenia must be ruled out by the discontinuation of any suspected medications.

The therapeutic approach to patients with ITP is dictated by the severity and urgency of the clinical situation. Some adult patients with only mild to moderate chronic thrombocytopenia and no bleeding problems may require no treatment. However, such patients may experience transient precipitous decreases in platelet counts at times of even trivial viral infections. The standard approach in patients requiring treatment is to begin prednisone at a dose of 1 to 2 mg/kg/day as initial therapy. Even before a demonstrable platelet response to prednisone is noted, clinical bleeding manifestations are often promptly ameliorated, presumably by the beneficial effects of corticosteroids on microvascular fragility. Although some patients obtain a prolonged complete remission after a short course of prednisone, in most patients the response is either incomplete, or relapse occurs when the prednisone dose is decreased. Splenectomy should be performed in patients who fail to respond after 2 to 3 weeks of prednisone or do not achieve sustained responses after discontinuation of prednisone. Patients who have even a transient response to prednisone tend to have better results with splenectomy. Splenectomy removes the major site of platelet destruction and a major source of autoantibody production in most patients. This procedure results in prolonged, treatment-free remissions in about two thirds of patients. The use of intravenous gamma globulin (IV IgG) has now been established as highly effective treatment and is particularly useful when rapid correction of the thrombocytopenia is required (e.g., with the threat of serious bleeding or for surgical coverage). The usual dose of IV IgG is 0.4 g/kg/day infused on 3 to 5 consecutive days. Platelet counts frequently begin to rise after only 2 to 3 days of this treatment. The emergency regimen of IV IgG is 1 g/kg, which can be repeated with a second dose on the following day. IV IgG has been found to be effective in patients with ITP refractory to prednisone or splenectomy and may be used as maintenance therapy in such patients. In patients who fail to respond to these therapies, second-line treatment modalities include other immunosuppressive drugs (azathioprine, vincristine, cyclophosphamide) and the synthetic androgen danazol (600 to 800 mg/day).

The response to treatment of ITP in HIV-infected patients is not significantly different from that used in uninfected patients. However, long-term corticosteroid therapy may cause further immunologic suppression in such patients. Furthermore, thrombocytopenia in HIV-infected patients may be caused by factors other than immune destruction of platelets, including the suppressive effects of the viral infection on hematopoiesis, bone marrow infiltration with opportunistic microorganisms (e.g., tuberculosis, *Mycobacterium avium-intracellulare*), or tumor (e.g., lymphoma) and TTP. Many patients with HIV-associated thrombocytopenia have been found to respond to zidovudine (azidothymidine, AZT) with a significant increase in platelet count.

The management of pregnancy and delivery in patients with chronic ITP, which is not rare because ITP most frequently affects women of childbearing age, poses special problems. Maternal antiplatelet autoantibodies cross the placenta and can cause fetal platelet destruction. No reliable correlation exists between the maternal and neonatal platelet counts. Even mothers in apparent remission from ITP (e.g., after splenectomy) may give birth to severely thrombocytopenic infants. Unless a prenatal fetal platelet count can be obtained, delivery should be performed by cesarean section to prevent the possibility of intracranial hemorrhage caused by head trauma during vaginal delivery. If a safe fetal platelet count can be ensured before delivery by percutaneous umbilical or fetal scalp vein blood sampling, vaginal delivery can be performed.

REFERENCES

Berchtold P and McMillan R: Therapy of chronic idiopathic thrombocytopenic purpura in adults. Blood 74:2309, 1989.

Berkman N et al: EDTA-dependent pseudothrombocytopenia: a clinical study of 18 patients and a review of the literature. Am J Hematol 36:195, 1991.

Burrows RF and Kelton JG: Incidentally detected thrombocytopenia in healthy mothers and their infants. N Engl J Med 319:142, 1988.

Eisenstaedt R: Blood component therapy in the treatment of platelet disorders. Semin Hematol 23:1, 1986.

George JN and Shattil SJ: The clinical importance of acquired abnormalities of platelet function. N Engl J Med 324:27, 1991.

Karpatkin S: HIV-1-related thrombocytopenia. Hematol Oncol Clin North Am 4:193, 1990.

Kelton JG: Advances in the diagnosis and management of ITP. Hosp Pract 20:95, 1985.

Kwaan HC: Clinicopathologic features of thrombotic thrombocytopenic purpura. Semin Hematol 24:71, 1987.

Leung L and Nachman R: Molecular mechanisms of platelet aggregation. Annu Rev Med 37:179, 1986.

Lind SE: The bleeding time does not predict surgical bleeding. Blood 77:2547, 1991.

Mannucci PM: Desmopressin: a nontransfusional hemostatic agent. Annu Rev Med 41:55, 1990.

Moake JL: TTP—desperation, empiricism, progress. N Engl J Med 325:426, 1991.

Rao AK: Congenital disorders of platelet function. Hematol Oncol Clin North Am 4:65, 1990.

Rodgers RP and Levin J: A critical reappraisal of the bleeding time. Semin Thromb Hemost 16:1, 1990.

Samuels P et al: Estimation of the risk of thrombocytopenia in the offspring of pregnant women with presumed immune thrombocytopenic purpura. N Engl J Med 323:229, 1990.

Schafer AI: Bleeding disorders: finding the cause. Hosp Pract 19:88K, 1984.

Smith ME et al: Binding of quinine- and quinidine-dependent drug antibodies to platelets is mediated by the Fab domain of the immunoglobulin G and is not Fc dependent. J Clin Invest 79:912, 1987.

CHAPTER

85 Disorders of Blood Coagulation

Gilbert C. White II

CONGENITAL DISORDERS

The most common inherited disorders of blood coagulation are the two sex-linked disorders, hemophilia A (factor VIII deficiency, classic hemophilia) and hemophilia B (factor IX deficiency, Christmas disease), and the autosomal disorder von Willebrand's disease (vWD). These disorders account for more than 95% of congenital disorders of blood coagulation. Deficiencies of other clotting factors are inherited in an autosomal recessive manner and are quite rare. These disorders are summarized in Table 85-1. The clinical and laboratory approach to the bleeding patient is discussed in Chapters 76 and 83.

Hemophilia A

Hemophilia A (classic hemophilia) is caused by a deficiency or abnormality of factor VIII procoagulant activity

Table 85-1. Congenital disorders of blood coagulation

Coagulation factor	Inheritance	Incidence (per million)	Bleeding symptoms	Abnormal screening tests	Biological half-life of protein (hours)	Treatment
I (fibrinogen)	Autosomal recessive	1	Umbilical bleeding at birth, posttrauma hemorrhage	PT, PTT, TT	100	Cryoprecipitate
II (prothrombin)	Autosomal recessive	1	Similar to hemophilia	PT, PTT	72	FFP, rarely prothrombin complex concentrates
V	Autosomal recessive	1	Similar to hemophilia	PT, PTT	24	FFP, possibly platelet concentrates
VII	Autosomal recessive	1	Similar to hemophilia	PT	4-6	Recombinant VIIa
VIII (hemophilia)	Sex-linked recessive	100 (milder disease is much more common)	Hemarthrosis, hematoma, bruising, severe postoperative bleeding	PTT	12	VIII concentrates or cryoprecipitate
vWf (von Willebrand's factor)	Autosomal dominant or recessive	Probably as frequent as hemophilia A	Epistaxis, gingival bleeding, bruising, menorrhagia, severe postoperative bleeding	PTT	4-6, for correction of bleeding time	Cryoprecipitate, DDAVP
IX (hemophilia B)	Sex-linked recessive	20	Identical to hemophilia	PT, PTT	24	Prothrombin complex concentrates
X	Autosomal recessive	1	Similar to hemophilia	PT, PTT	50	FFP, rarely prothrombin complex concentrates
XI	Autosomal recessive	1	Mild; however, severe postoperative hemorrhage can occur	PTT	60	FFP, level of 25% adequate for hemostasis
XII	Autosomal recessive	1	None	PTT	60	None
XIII	Autosomal recessive	1	Umbilical bleeding at birth, posttrauma hemorrhage, poor wound healing	—	120	FFP monthly, since level of 2% is adequate for hemostasis
Alpha$_2$ antiplasmin	Autosomal recessive	Unknown	Similar to hemophilia	—	Unknown	FFP
Plasminogen activator inhibitor (PAI-1)	Unknown	Unknown	Severe postoperative and posttrauma bleeding	—	Unknown	EACA
Passovoy	Autosomal dominant	Unknown	Similar to factor XI	PTT	Unknown	FFP

FFP, Fresh-frozen plasma; PT, prothrombin time; PTT, partial thromboplastin time; TT, thrombin (clotting) time; DDAVP, 1-deamino-8-D-arginine vasopressin; EACA, epsilon aminocaproic acid.

(VIII; see Table 85-2 for a definition of factor VIII activities). Factor VIII, as measured by clotting activity, is diminished. In most patients, factor VIII procoagulant antigen (VIII:Ag) is diminished and is proportional to VIII activity, although some patients have levels of VIII:Ag in excess of VIII clotting activity and are said to have cross-reacting material (CRM$^+$). von Willebrand factor (vWf) and vWf:Ag activities are normal in hemophilia A. The bleeding time is usually normal or only minimally prolonged.

Diagnosis. The diagnosis of hemophilia A is suggested by a prolonged partial thromboplastin time (PTT) in association with a normal prothrombin time (PT) and thrombin

Table 85-2. Factor VIII and von Willebrand factor (vWf) activities

Factor/antigen	Activity
VIII	Factor VIII procoagulant activity. Clot-promoting activity of factor VIII as determined by a coagulation assay. Circulates in plasma complexed with vWf.
VIII:Ag	Factor VIII procoagulant antigen. Antigenic expression of factor VIII as detected by monoclonal or patient antibodies.
vWf	Von Willebrand factor activity. Supports platelet–vessel wall and platelet-platelet interactions. Most often measured by platelet agglutination in the presence of the antibiotic ristocetin, but also reflected in tests such as the bleeding time and platelet adhesion to glass bead columns. Previously called *factor VIII–von Willebrand factor activity* (VIIIR:WF) and *ristocetin cofactor activity* (VIIIR:RCoF). Circulates in plasma complexed with VIII.
vWf:Ag	Von Willebrand factor antigen. Antigenic expression of vWf as detected by heterologous antibodies. Previously called *factor VIII–related antigen* (VIIIR:Ag).

Table 85-3. Characteristics of hemophilia and von Willebrand's disease (vWD)

	Hemophilia	vWD
Clinical bleeding	Joint, soft tissue	Mucous membranes
VIII	↓	↓
vWf	nl	↓
vWf:Ag	nl	↓
Bleeding time	nl	↑
Inheritance	X-linked	Autosomal
De novo synthesis	No	Yes

↓, Reduced factor levels in plasma; ↑, prolongation of bleeding time; nl, normal. This table is a comparison of clinical and laboratory findings in patients with hemophilia A and vWD. Clinical bleeding refers to the characteristic location of hemorrhages in each disorder. De novo synthesis refers to the delayed rise in factor VIII activity after administration of cryoprecipitate that is characteristic of vWD but does not occur in hemophilia. Although this has been termed *synthesis,* little evidence indicates whether the delayed rise results from synthesis, activation, or some other mechanism.

(clotting) time (TT). Factor VIII activity assay is required for a specific diagnosis. One unit of VIII activity is defined as the activity present in 1 ml of a standard normal plasma pool. Levels in normal individuals range from 0.6 to 1.5 U/ml. In patients with hemophilia A, VIII levels are decreased (i.e., less than 0.5 U/ml). Because VIII can also be diminished in vWD (Table 85-3), vWf:Ag and vWf levels and a bleeding time should be determined in patients with no clear history of sex-linked hemophilia. In patients with mild VIII deficiency, a factor V level should also be measured to exclude combined factor V and VIII deficiency.

Molecular defects. Factor VIII is synthesized as a linear polypeptide of 330,000 molecular weight. It circulates as a two-chain, calcium-linked molecule that consists of a variable heavy chain of 90,000 to 200,000 molecular weight and a light chain of 80,000 molecular weight (Fig. 85-1). Three structural domains have been identified. The A domain consists of three triplicated segments, each 350 amino acids in length, that are homologous with similar domains in the copper-binding protein ceruloplasmin and that may play a role in calcium binding. The C domain consists of two duplicated segments, each 150 amino acids in length, that may be important in phospholipid binding. The B domain is proteolytically removed from VIII during activation by thrombin.

Among more than 500 individuals with hemophilia who have been studied, the molecular defect responsible for hemophilia has been identified at the level of the gene in over 50. The defects identified so far consist of either deletions of part or all of the molecule or of point mutations. Defects in all three domains of factor VIII have been reported.

Genetics and carrier state. Because hemophilia A is an X-linked disorder, almost all symptomatic individuals are males (X^hY). All daughters of affected males are obligate carriers (X^hX), whereas sons, who receive their father's Y chromosome, are unaffected. Daughters of carriers have a 50:50 chance of being carriers, and sons of carriers have a 50:50 chance of having hemophilia.

Traditional methods for carrier detection are based on two observations: (1) the abnormality in hemophilia is a deficiency of VIII, whereas vWf:Ag is normal; and (2) only one X chromosome in a given cell is expressed. Thus, in a carrier who possesses a hemophilia gene (X^h) from her father and a normal gene (X) from her mother, some of the VIII-producing cells (X) make normal amounts of VIII, whereas the rest of these cells (X^h) make no VIII. Thus, if there are equal numbers of X and X^h cells, the ratio of VIII to another unrelated protein such as vWf:Ag will be 0.5 in a carrier, whereas the ratio in a normal woman will be 1.0. However, according to the Lyon hypothesis, inactivation of the X chromosome in each cell is a random process, so that frequently an unequal number of X-active and X^h-active

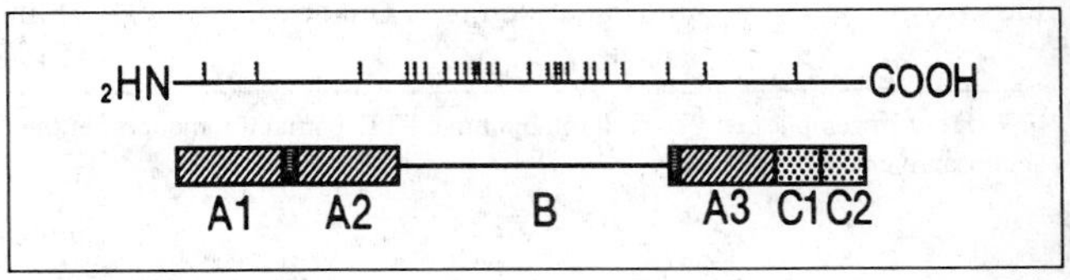

Fig. 85-1. Factor VIII molecule. Linear representation of the factor VIII molecule. Carbohydrate chains are indicated by the curved lines. The hatched boxes indicate the segments of the A domain *(A1, A2, A3)*. The stippled boxes indicate the segments of the C domain *(C1, C2)*. The B domain separates the A2 and A3 segments of the A domain.

cells results. Furthermore, the assays have an inherent variability. For these reasons, the ratio of VIII to vWf:Ag in carriers may vary from 0.1 to more than 1.0, whereas the ratio in normal persons may vary from 0.5 to 1.5 or more. Because of this overlap, the laboratory data are used to determine the likelihood that a subject is a carrier, and then that likelihood ratio is combined with pedigree information to arrive at a final statistical probability that she is a carrier. These carrier detection tests are 90% to 95% accurate, but they are more accurate against normal than against carrier women.

New molecular biology techniques using deoxyribonucleic acid (DNA) probes hold the promise of more precise carrier detection. One approach using DNA probes has been called *gene detection*. With this technique, a probe specific for the defective portion of the genomic sequence for VIII is used to study an individual's DNA. This technique depends on recognition by the probe of the specific genomic defect, whether a deletion or a nucleotide change, and has the advantage of not requiring samples from family members if the precise defect has been established in the family in question. A second approach, termed *gene tracking*, takes advantage of restriction polymorphisms linked to the hemophilia gene. The DNA probes in this case identify independently segregating restriction polymorphisms close to a hemophilia A gene. Since the probe is not directed at the VIII gene, it is not necessary to know the specific genomic defect. The disadvantages of this technique is that key family members have to be available and that the mother must be heterozygous for the restriction polymorphism. A weakness of the method is that only 50% of mothers are heterozygous for a specific polymorphism.

The object of carrier detection is to assist family planning and to allow the putative or obligate carrier the option of prenatal diagnosis during pregnancy. Two procedures are now available to help with prenatal diagnosis. First, *amniocentesis* and karyotyping can be performed to determine fetal sex. This can be done from weeks 13 to 16 of pregnancy. If the fetus is female, no further testing is required, although the female infant may prove to be a carrier, a fact that might possibly be specifically determined by one of the DNA methods just described. If the fetus is male, amnionic cells can be used for DNA analysis. DNA can be obtained earlier in pregnancy (between 9 and 12 gestational weeks) by *chorionic villus sampling*. If amniocentesis indicates the fetus is male but the DNA studies fail to establish a diagnosis of hemophilia, *fetal blood sampling* may be undertaken by either ultrasound-guided needle aspiration or fetoscopy. Fetal blood is tested by measuring VIII (usually VIII:Ag) and vWf:Ag ratios in fetal blood. The affected family members must first be tested to ensure that they have the type of hemophilia A in which VIII:Ag is reduced. Fetal morbidity with these procedures is 0.5% to 1.0%.

In cases of extreme inactivation of the normal (X) gene (termed *extreme lyonization*), VIII levels in carriers may be as low as 0.1 U/ml and may result in hemorrhage after major surgery, trauma, or tooth extractions. Factor VIII levels should therefore be obtained on all potential carriers so that treatment may be instituted as necessary.

Clinical features. Patients with hemophilia A are classified clinically as severe, moderate, or mild, depending on the frequency of hemorrhage, the severity of the hemorrhage, and the degree of trauma producing the hemorrhage. Clinical severity is usually related to the plasma level of VIII. Severely affected individuals may have two or three bleeding episodes per month, may frequently bleed spontaneously without noticeable trauma, may bleed profusely unless treated, and may have VIII levels of less than 0.01 U/ml (less than 1% of normal). Moderately affected individuals bleed perhaps five or six times per year but may have prolonged periods free of bleeding, usually bleed only with trauma, and have VIII levels of 0.01 to 0.05 U/ml (1% to 5% of normal). Mildly affected individuals bleed rarely, if at all, and then only with significant trauma or surgical stress. The disease in many of these individuals is so mild that it is undetected throughout their lives. Factor VIII levels are usually greater than 0.05 U/ml (5% of normal).

Although clinical symptoms closely parallel plasma levels of VIII, an occasional patient is clinically moderate or mild yet has VIII levels of less than 0.01 U/ml. Conversely, patients with VIII levels of 0.05 to 0.10 U/ml occasionally, if trauma occurs, develop a joint bleed that recurs and becomes a "target joint" mimicking joint bleeds seen in severe hemophiliacs.

Hemarthroses are the most characteristic and among the most disabling of the hemorrhages that occur in hemophilia A. Any joint can be involved, but those most frequently affected in adults are the knees, elbows, and ankles. According to most hemophiliac persons, the initial manifestation of a joint hemorrhage is a "tingling" or "bubbling" sensation in the joint. This then progresses over a matter of hours to swelling and pain. Joint range of motion becomes limited. Since the joint is a closed space, bleeding is confined to the joint. Vessel and nerve compression do not occur, and the acute consequences of the joint bleeding are primarily pain and limitation of motion. When proper treatment is started, the hemorrhage abates promptly, and resolution of the joint hematoma is related to the quantity of the blood that accumulates in the joint.

The chronic consequences of joint hematomas are caused by the biochemical responses to blood in the joint space and are very similar pathophysiologically to joint changes in rheumatoid arthritis. Clinically, recurrent hemorrhages in the joint lead to proliferation of synovial tissue, which results in a swollen, boggy joint. The vascular synovial tissue has an increased tendency to hemorrhage, and the joint bleeding becomes cyclic. Eventually, collagenolytic enzymes begin to attack the joint, resulting in progressive loss of joint space. The final result is a collapsed joint with marked limitation or complete loss of motion (Fig. 85-2).

Muscle hematomas occur less often than joint hemorrhages but have more acute effects. Muscles of the arms and legs tend to be common sites. The initial manifestation is pain and swelling of the involved muscle. If the bleeding continues, a compartment syndrome may occur with compression of nerves and/or vessels.

Bleeding into the iliopsoas and iliacus muscles, called *retroperitoneal hematomas*, deserves special comment be-

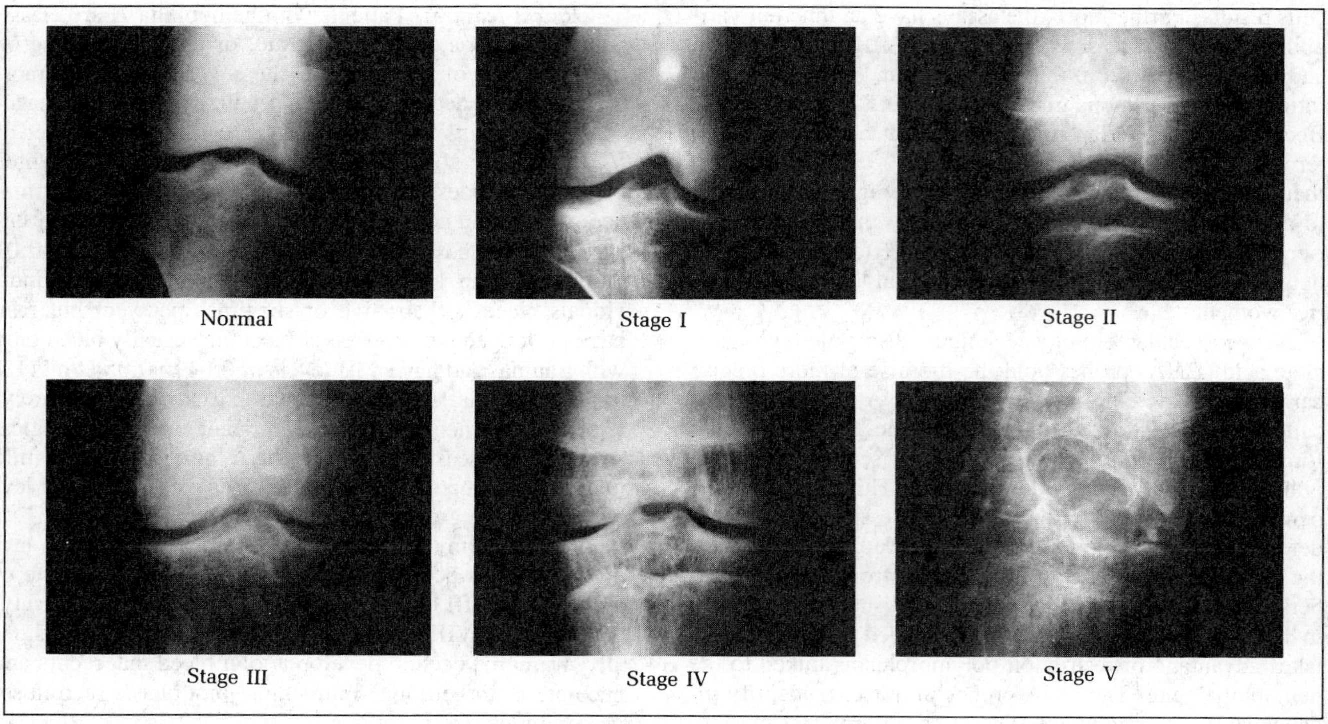

Fig. 85-2. Radiologic joint changes in hemophilia A. Knee joints illustrating the various stages of hemophilic arthropathy.
Stage I: no skeletal abnormalities; soft tissue swelling caused by bleeding in and around joint
Stage II: osteoporosis and epiphyseal overgrowth; joint space intact; no bone cysts
Stage III: subchondral cysts; minor irregularities of the joint surface; joint space is preserved
Stage IV: cysts and joint surface irregularities more prominent; joint space is narrowed as a result of cartilage damage.
Stage V: loss of joint space; marked epiphyseal overgrowth) (Radiographs courtesy of Bonner Guilford, MD.)

cause these particular hemorrhages tend to cause nerve compression. The anatomic relation of the iliopsoas and iliacus muscles to the ischium means that hemorrhages in this muscle are prone to compartmentalization, which results in femoral nerve or lateral cutaneous nerve palsy.

Intracranial bleeds are among the most common causes of death in hemophiliac patients, and prompt treatment of possible intracranial hemorrhage is one of the main goals of home therapy. Any unusual or persistent headache in a person with severe hemophilia should arouse the strong suspicion of an intracranial bleed.

Hematuria occurs frequently, and whereas abnormalities of the collecting system by intravenous pyelogram may be seen during the acute episode and may sometimes persist, abnormalities of renal function occur infrequently.

Inhibitors to VIII develop in approximately 15% of patients treated with VIII. These inhibitors are antibodies that are identified by their ability to specifically inactivate VIII in coagulation assays. In the United States the Bethesda unit is used for inhibitor quantitation. One Bethesda unit is that amount of inhibitor that will inactivate half the VIII in 1 ml of normal plasma in 2 hours at 37° C. Several clinically distinct types of inhibitors may be observed. In a small number of patients with inhibitors, the level of inhibitor is low (less than 10 Bethesda units) and remains low despite challenge with VIII. Other patients have *high-response inhibitors*. These are inhibitors that remain at low levels until stimulated by exposure to VIII. This exposure then leads to an anamnestic increase in antibody level, frequently to very high levels (up to 1000 to 2000 Bethesda units). The antibody level then starts to fall and continues to fall until the next exposure to VIII. In some individuals the inhibitor may become undetectable before the next treatment. A final group of patients have antibody levels that are high (greater than 20 Bethesda units) and remain high even in the absence of VIII administration.

Antibodies should be described according to their anamnestic response to VIII (high or low response) and by their level (high or low titer). Thus an inhibitor that is currently 5 Bethesda units but has previously been shown to increase to 200 Bethesda units after administration of VIII is a *high-response, low-titer inhibitor*. After treatment with VIII, the inhibitor in this patient might rise to 125 Bethesda units and, accordingly, be termed a *high-response, high-titer inhibitor*.

Although it was initially postulated that inhibitors would be found in patients with deletions of the VIII gene, who would therefore "see" VIII as a foreign protein, present data indicate that inhibitors can occur in patients who have partial deletions of the VIII gene as well as in patients with point mutations.

Patients with inhibitors are subject to the same type and frequency of hemorrhage as are patients without inhibitors, but they differ in that when the antibody level is greater than 10 Bethesda units, they respond poorly, if at all, to treatment with VIII. Patients should be tested for inhibitors when a surgical procedure is contemplated or response to therapy is diminished.

Treatment. Treatment consists of replacement VIII. In the United States, this is accomplished with fresh-frozen plasma, a blood bank–prepared cryoprecipitate fraction of fresh plasma, or commercial concentrates of VIII. Several different types of commercial concentrates have now been developed (Table 85-4), and recent advances in the purification of VIII and genetic engineering hold the promise of synthetic VIII in the future. In contrast to plasma and cryoprecipitate, which must be frozen, commercial concentrates are lyophilized and are stable at ambient temperatures. More than 90% of the VIII given in the United States is in the form of commercial concentrate because of its high potency and ease of administration.

Calculation of the dose of VIII is performed as follows:

$$VIII_i = (VIII_f - VIII_s) \times PV$$

where VIII_i is the amount of VIII to be infused in units; VIII_f is the desired peak VIII level in units per milliliter; VIII_s is the initial VIII level in units per milliliter; and PV is the plasma volume in milliliters, which is calculated as 5% of body weight. The half-life of VIII in plasma is approximately 12 hours. To maintain a specific level of VIII usually requires that half the loading dose be administered every 12 hours. Factor VIII may be administered by either intermittent boluses or continuous infusion.

The following are intended as general guidelines for replacement therapy for patients with severe disease. Relatively minor bleeding episodes such as hemarthroses are treated with sufficient concentrate to bring the VIII level to 0.30 U/ml (30% of normal). If bleeding continues, the dose is repeated in 12 to 24 hours. Minor muscle bleeds may be treated the same way, but muscle bleeds with incipient neurovascular compromise and retroperitoneal bleeds should be treated with higher doses to bring the VIII level to 0.5 to 1.0 U/ml (50% to 100% of normal) for up to 5 to 7 days. Intracranial hemorrhage and hemorrhage in the neck or throat with potential airway compromise are major medical emergencies and are treated with sufficient concentrate to raise the VIII level to 1.0 U/ml (100% of normal) for 10 to 14 days.

Patients with severe hemophilia can best treat minor bleeding episodes at home. The advantage of home therapy is that treatment can be instituted as soon as the patient suspects bleeding. It is not yet certain if the development of joint deformities can be avoided by this approach. However, it reduces time away from work or school and has clear advantages in potentially life-threatening bleeds such as intracranial and neck bleeds. Because of the great cost of the commercial concentrates, the cost of treatment for a patient with severe hemophilia can easily exceed $50,000 per year.

Patients with mild forms of hemophilia A may occasionally need treatment for surgery or traumatic injuries. Although concentrates or cryoprecipitate may be used, there is still a small risk of hepatitis and/or acquired immunodeficiency syndrome (AIDS). Intravenous infusion of a

Table 85-4. Comparison of various sources of factors VIII and IX

	Volume to 100%	Ease of use	Risk of hepatitis	Risk of AIDS	Risk of hemolysis	Risk of thrombosis
Factor VIII						
Plasma	3000	—	+	+	±	—
Cryoprecipitate	750	+	+	+	±	—
VIII Concentrate						
Solvent	50	4+	—	—	4+	—
Monoclonal	50	4+	—	—	—	—
Recombinant	50	4+	—	—	—	—
Factor IX						
Plasma	6000	—	+	+	±	—
PCC heated	50	4+	4+	?	—	4+
IX Concentrate						
Solvent	50	4+	—	—	—	—
Monoclonal	50	4+	—	—	—	—

± to 4+, Degree of increasing risk or ease of use; —, no risk.

This table is a general assessment of the relative risks of treatment sources available for treating hemophilia A and B. Plasma and cryoprecipitate are usually obtained from the American Red Cross or blood banks, whereas VIII and IX concentrates are usually obtained commercially. Solvent-detergent extracted factor VIII and IX concentrates are treated to remove coated viruses, including HIV-1 and hepatitis B and C viruses. Monoclonal factor VIII and IX concentrates are ultrapure products prepared using affinity chromatography and viral inactivation steps. Recombinant factor VIII is a synthetic product prepared in Chinese hamster ovary cells. PCC, prothrombin complex concentrates. Heated PCC refers to product prepared from donors screened for human immunodeficiency virus I (HIV-I) antibodies and heated at 56° to 68° C during the manufacturing process to inactivate heat-sensitive viruses such as HIV-I.

vasopressin analog, 1-deamino-8-D-arginine vasopressin (DDAVP), increases VIII levels twofold or threefold and provides an alternative to plasma products and their risks. DDAVP is the treatment of choice in patients with mild hemophilia who require treatment.

The type of treatment of bleeding episodes in patients with inhibitors is determined by the titer of the antibody at the time treatment is required, the antibody response to administration of VIII, and the severity of the bleed. Patients with low-response inhibitors can be treated with VIII for all bleeding episodes, although doses of up to 4000 U or more may be required to achieve VIII levels of 30%. In patients with high-response, high-titer inhibitors, it becomes impossible to infuse sufficient VIII to achieve hemostasis. For these individuals, several alternative treatment modalities are available, including porcine VIII, activated or nonactivated prothrombin complex concentrates, plasmapheresis, and immunosuppressive agents, although none works as well as VIII in patients without inhibitors. Patients with high-response, low-titer inhibitors can be treated with human VIII, but this treatment is likely to result in an anamnestic increase in inhibitor titer. For this reason, use of VIII in these patients is often reserved for life-threatening bleeding episodes. For other hemorrhages, such as joint bleeds or hematuria, treatment with prothrombin complex concentrates is sometimes effective but is less likely to produce an anamnestic increase in inhibitor titer. Patients with inhibitors should generally be referred to specialized centers for care.

Complications of treatment. Transfusion-associated *hepatitis* occurs in a large percentage of hemophiliac patients receiving replacement therapy. Almost 80% of hemophiliac patients demonstrate at least intermittent abnormalities of liver function tests, although only about 10% offer a history of symptoms. The chronic consequences of transfusion-associated hepatitis—cirrhosis, hepatosplenomegaly, portal hypertension, esophageal varices, hypersplenism, and hepatocellular carcinoma—occur in a small number of those at risk. Both hepatitis B and non-A, non-B hepatitis viruses have been implicated in the liver disease in hemophilia.

Treatment of hepatitis in hemophiliac patients should conform to the guidelines outlined in Chapter 57. Patients should continue to take VIII as needed. In chronic hepatitis, thrombocytopenia from hypersplenism may be especially troublesome because of the underlying bleeding defect. Hepatitis B virus vaccine should be given to patients who have never been treated before or who demonstrate negative hepatitis B serology. Current VIII concentrates, including solvent-detergent-extracted VIII, monoclonal VIII, and synthetic preparations, when available, appear to be free of hepatitis B and non-A, non-B hepatitis.

Before the development of heat treatment and donor screening, factor VIII concentrate use was associated with infection with human immunodeficiency virus (HIV). Thus many patients with hemophilia are HIV antibody positive, and many have developed AIDS. Current VIII concentrates are free of HIV.

With intermediate-purity VII concentrates, antibodies to red cell blood group substances are isolated with VIII and can cause red cell *hemolysis* in intensively treated patients. Blood typing should be performed before intensive treatment, and concentrates containing low isoagglutinin titers should be used in susceptible individuals.

Hemophilia B

Hemophilia B (Christmas disease), as with hemophilia A, is an X-linked recessive disease. However, hemophilia B is caused by an abnormality in factor IX, one of the vitamin K–dependent factors. Factor IX protein (as detected by immunologic tests) may be absent (CRM^-), present in reduced amounts (CRM^r), or present in normal amounts but with greatly decreased clot-promoting activity (CRM^+). The molecular defect responsible for hemophilia B has been determined in more than 500 patients.

Diagnosis. As in hemophilia A, the PTT is prolonged, and the PT and TT are normal. The diagnosis of hemophilia B is made by specific factor IX assay. As in hemophilia A, the factor IX levels are predictive of the severity of the bleeding tendency. The normal level of factor IX is 1.0 U/ml. Levels less than 0.01 U/ml indicate severe disease, levels of 0.01 to 0.05 indicate moderate disease, and levels greater than 0.05 indicate mild disease.

Carrier state. Hemophilia B is an X-linked disorder, and all affected males are X^hY and carriers are X^hX. All daughters of affected males are carriers, and daughters of carriers have a 50:50 chance of being carriers. Because of random inactivation of the X chromosome, carriers have a spectrum of factor IX activity levels that ranges from levels as low as those in patients with mild hemophilia (0.10 U/ml) to normal levels. Diagnosis of the carrier state can sometimes be made on the basis of factor IX activity levels alone. Detection of carriers may be improved by measuring factor IX antigen levels in families that have a CRM^+ defect, but measuring the antigen adds no useful information to measuring the activity alone in CRM^- kindred. Carriers of hemophilia B are more likely to be symptomatic from low IX levels than are carriers of hemophilia A from low VIII levels.

Carrier detection by gene detection or gene tracking is also applicable to hemophilia B and with appropriate probes should permit carrier assignment in CRM^-, CRM^r, and CRM^+ variants.

Clinical features. The types and complications of hemorrhages in hemophilia B are similar to those in hemophilia A.

Inhibitors to factor IX occur infrequently, in approximately 3% of severely affected individuals. Preliminary studies suggest that those most likely to develop inhibitors are CRM^- individuals who demonstrate partial or complete deletion of the factor IX gene.

Treatment. Factor IX concentrates, prothrombin complex concentrates, which are rich in factor IX, and fresh-frozen plasma are available for treatment of hemophilia B (see Table 85-4). Although more expensive, IX concentrates appear to be safer than PCC with less risk of thrombosis and hepatitis. Because factor IX distribution is approximately twice the plasma volume, it takes twice as much factor IX as VIII to achieve a given level. The half-life of factor IX is approximately 8 to 14 hours, so maintenance treatment is needed twice a day. Factor IX concentrate should be given as intermittent bolus treatment every 12 hours and not by continuous infusion.

Commercial prothrombin complex concentrates are associated with a risk of hepatitis, both hepatitis B and non-A, non-B hepatitis. In addition, prothrombin complex concentrates are potentially thrombogenic. Hemolytic reactions do not occur with prothrombin complex concentrates. Factor IX concentrates appear to have little risk of hepatitis or thrombosis. As a result, factor IX concentrates are the current treatment of choice in hemophilia B.

von Willebrand's disease

This is probably the most frequently diagnosed inherited bleeding disorder in adults. The exact prevalence of vWD is unknown because precise criteria for its diagnosis and classification are only now being evolved.

Inheritance. In contrast to hemophilia A and B, vWD is inherited in an autosomal manner (see Table 85-3). The vWf gene is located on chromosome 12. The more common varieties (types I and II) are autosomal dominant. However, the most severe form of this disorder is recessive and is expressed only in homozygous or doubly heterozygous subjects.

von Willebrand factor. vWf is currently thought to circulate in plasma as a complex with VIII. Its role in hemostasis is to act as a carrier for VIII and to promote adhesion of platelets to the subendothelium and to one another. Thus vWf plays an important role in primary hemostasis. Abnormalities of vWf are expressed as an abnormality of platelet function, as reflected in a prolonged bleeding time. vWf is present in endothelial cells, megakaryocytes, platelets, and plasma. The subunit protein has a molecular weight of 220,000, but it is found in cells and in plasma as multimers ranging in molecular weight from approximately 800,000 to between 10 and 14 million or more, in increments of 800,000 to 1 million (Chapter 76). Factor VIII appears to be able to complex with any size of multimer. However, the large-molecular-weight multimers are the most effective in supporting the interaction between platelets and the vessel wall and are necessary for a normal bleeding time.

Diagnosis. The diagnosis of vWD should be suspected in patients who demonstrate an abnormality of one or more of the following: bleeding time, VIII, vWf, and vWf:Ag (see Table 85-3). Because these tests may be somewhat variable in vWD and because an isolated bleeding time prolongation and isolated reduction in VIII may be confused with a platelet defect and hemophilia, respectively, testing patients should be performed on more than one occasion in cases that are unclear. Different forms of vWD can be distinguished using vWf multimer analysis and other special tests (Fig. 85-3).

Type I. Type I vWD results from decreased production of a structurally normal vWf molecule. The most common form of vWD, it is inherited in an autosomal dominant pattern. Plasma levels of vWf, vWf:Ag, and VIII are variably reduced, usually concordantly. All sizes of vWf multimers are present but are reduced in concentration. Type I variants with anomalous patterns of individual multimers or alterations in platelet vWf have been reported.

Type IIA. This variant form of vWD is inherited as an autosomal dominant trait and is characterized by an absence of the large and medium-sized multimers from plasma and platelets. vWf activity is greatly reduced and is lower than vWf:Ag and VIII, which may be decreased or normal. Ristocetin-induced platelet aggregation is reduced.

Type IIB. In this variant, only the high-molecular-weight multimers are absent from plasma. All multimers are present in platelets, and the plasma levels of vWf, vWf:Ag, and VIII may be normal or decreased. The distinguishing characteristic of type IIB vWD is the finding that ristocetin-induced aggregation is increased rather than decreased. This observation and the finding that type IIB vWf demonstrates increased ristocetin-induced binding to normal platelets has suggested that the defect in type IIB disease is a qualitative abnormality of vWf causing increased affinity of the large-molecular-weight multimers for cellular binding sites on platelets. Therefore deficiency of the large multimers results from increased utilization, not reduced production. Inheritance of type IIB disease is autosomal dominant.

Type IIC. This rare variant is inherited in an autosomal recessive pattern. The high-molecular-weight multimers are absent from plasma and platelets, and the pattern of the smaller multimers is abnormal electrophoretically. Plasma levels of vWf, vWf:Ag, and VIII are decreased or normal, and ristocetin-induced platelet aggregation is decreased or normal.

Other variants. Single-case reports of other variants of vWD (designated IID, IIE, IIF, IIG, IIH) have been described. As with the other forms of type II vWD, these are generally characterized by an absence of large-molecular-weight multimers. There are also unique structural abnormalities of the individual multimers.

Type III. This is severe homozygous or doubly heterozygous, autosomal recessive vWD. Plasma levels of vWf and vWf:Ag are undetectable, and VIII levels are less than 10%. The bleeding time is invariably prolonged. Ristocetin-induced platelet aggregation is absent. Bleeding in this form may be severe and may involve joints and soft tissues.

Pseudo–von Willebrand's disease. This condition is similar in many respects to type IIB vWD. There is a deficiency of the high-molecular-weight multimers in plasma but not in platelets. Plasma levels of vWf, vWf:Ag, and VIII are decreased or normal. Ristocetin-induced aggregation is increased. However, vWf from these patients does not demonstrate increased binding to normal platelets. Instead, platelets from these patients show increased ristocetin-

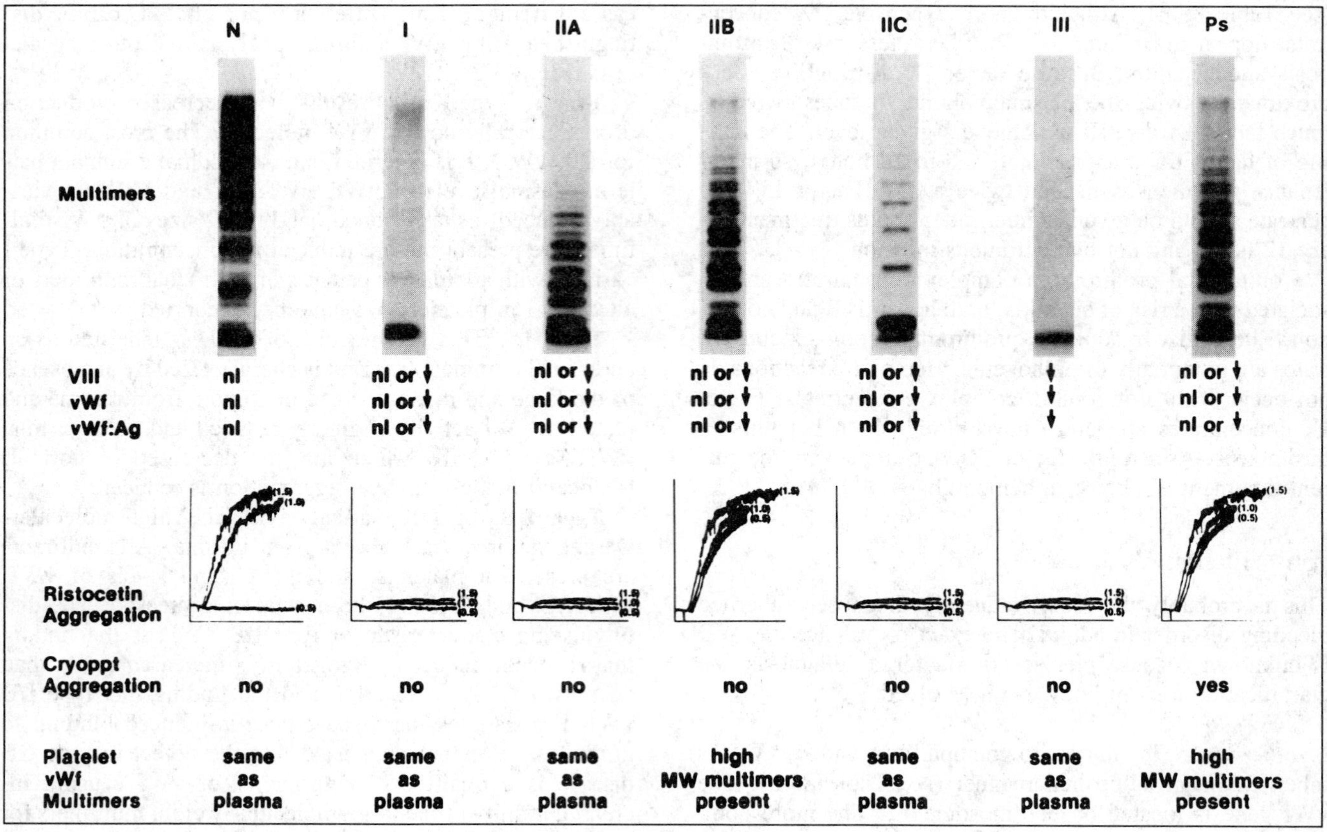

Fig. 85-3. Classification of von Willebrand's disease (vWD). Multimeric von Willebrand factor (vWf) patterns; levels of VIII, vWf, and vWf:Ag; patterns of ristocetin aggregation; response of patient platelets to normal cryoprecipitate in vitro; and the multimeric pattern of vWf in patient platelets are shown for normal, type I vWD, variant vWD (types IIA, IIB, IIC), type III or homozygous vWD, and pseudo-vWD or platelet-type vWD, individuals.

In type I individuals the characteristic laboratory findings are variably reduced vWf, vWf:Ag, and VIII. The multimeric pattern and ristocetin aggregation abnormalities are proportional to the reduction in vWf, vWf:Ag, and VIII.

In type IIA individuals the characteristic finding is the absence of high- and middle-molecular-weight multimers. Factor VIII, vWf, vWf:Ag, and ristocetin aggregation abnormalities may be indistinguishable from those in type I individuals.

In type IIB individuals the characteristic finding is absence of the high-molecular-weight multimers and increased ristocetin aggregation.

In type IIC individuals the high-molecular weight multimers are absent and the triplet pattern is aberrant.

Type III individuals show a profound reduction in VIII, vWf, and vWf:Ag, and this profound reduction is reflected in the pattern of vWf multimers and ristocetin aggregation.

In pseudo-vWD the distinguishing feature is aggregation of patient platelets by normal cryoprecipitate. Otherwise, this variant is similar to type IIB vWD.

(The vWf multimer patterns courtesy of ZM Ruggeri and TS Zimmerman, MDs.)

induced binding of normal vWf. The presumed defect is a platelet abnormality, and the absence of large vWf multimers results from increased utilization, as in type IIB vWD. Two additional features that help to distinguish this condition from type IIB vWD are (1) many pseudo-vWD patients have chronic or intermittent thrombocytopenia, and (2) cryoprecipitate causes aggregation of pseudo-vWD platelets in vitro but not of platelets from type IIB.

Clinical features. The bleeding in vWD is usually much less severe than that in hemophilia. Massive bleeding into joints and tissues occurs only in patients with type III forms of the disease, but bleeding from mucous membranes (nasal, intestinal, uterine mucosa) and easy bruising are common and are characteristic of patients with other forms of the disease. Bleeding typically follows minor injury or surgery. Major surgical procedures or trauma may result in serious bleeding. The tendency to bleed appears to decrease later in life.

Menorrhagia may be severe and may lead to iron deficiency and anemia. Oral contraceptives may reduce menorrhagia and increase plasma levels of vWf, vWf:Ag, and

VIII in some forms of vWD. *Angiodysplasia* of intestinal vessels may lead to recurrent intestinal bleeding. Demonstration of the site of bleeding is often difficult because of the lack of radiologically detectable structural lesions and the intermittent nature of the bleeding. Endoscopic procedures sometimes reveal telangiectasia of the bowel mucosa. *Mitral valve prolapse* has been reported in patients with vWD, but whether this is more common in vWD than in the general population is questionable.

Treatment. Several agents are used in the treatment of patients with vWD. The traditional treatment has been with cryoprecipitate that contains all the multimers of vWf and is effective therapy for all forms of vWD. However, since cryoprecipitate is derived from plasma but has no virus inactivation step, it has a small but finite risk of transmitting hepatitis or HIV infection. Concentrates of factor VIII contain large amounts of vWf: Ag, but most lack the larger vWf multimers and therefore have little effect on the bleeding time in vWD. Two products, Humate-P and Koate-HS, have some large vWf multimers and can be used to treat patients with vWD. Both are treated to inactivate hepatitis and HIV viruses. In addition, concentrates of vWf are being developed and should be useful. DDAVP, the synthetic vasopressin analog, releases vWf from storage sites in endothelial cells and thus provides an endogenous source of vWf.

The form of treatment is dictated by the type of vWD. In patients with type I disease, DDAVP increases plasma levels of VIII and vWf of all multimeric sizes. Levels of VIII and vWf can be increased twofold to threefold. In patients with type IIA or IIB disease, the defect is production of an abnormal vWf molecule. Thus, in variant forms of vWD, VIII or vWf concentrates (when available) are the treatment of choice. VIII or vWf concentrates are also the treatment of choice in type III disease because DDAVP is ineffective in increasing vWf release. In pseudo-vWD the platelet is defective, and treatment should be with platelets. Administration of VIII concentrate, vWf concentrates, or DDAVP to these patients may trigger sudden aggregation of platelets and cause severe thrombocytopenia.

Treatment of vWD, when required, is aimed at correction of both the bleeding time and the VIII level. If major surgery is undertaken, VIII level and bleeding time should be monitored. Treatment should be aimed at keeping both within normal limits in the perioperative period.

Complications of treatment. DDAVP may cause water retention and lead to symptomatic hyponatremia. Plasma sodium levels should be monitored. Inhibitors (antibodies) to vWf develop only in the most severely affected individuals.

Congenital deficiencies of factors II, V, VII, and X

Deficiencies of these clotting factors are inherited as autosomal recessive traits and are quite rare. Deficiencies may reflect either absence of the clotting factor or its presence in a dysfunctional form.

Diagnosis. A deficiency of any one of these clotting factors results in a prolonged PT. With factors II, X, and V, the PTT is also prolonged. However, in factor VII deficiency, the PTT is normal. Diagnosis is made by specific factor assays.

Clinical features. The severity of symptoms varies considerably among individuals, and severity does not uniformly correlate with factor levels.

Treatment. Milder episodes are best treated with fresh-frozen plasma, even though plasma levels can only be brought to 20% because of the limitation of the volume of plasma that can be infused. The prothrombin complex concentrates used to treat factor IX deficiency also contain variable quantities of factors VII, X, and II, and higher plasma levels can be obtained with them. However, the risk of hepatitis and thrombosis is significant. These concentrates do not contain significant quantities of factor V. Platelet transfusions have been used to treat factor V deficiency.

Deficiency of factor XI and Passovoy defect

Factor XI deficiency is the result of a decreased quantity of this protein in some individuals; the presence of an inactive clotting factor appears to be responsible in others. It is inherited in an autosomal recessive manner. The abnormality in patients with Passovoy defect is not known at this time, but it is presumed to be a deficiency of an as-yet unidentified plasma protein. Passovoy defect appears to be inherited in an autosomal dominant manner.

Diagnosis. The PT is normal and the PTT is prolonged in both disorders. Precise diagnosis of factor XI deficiency requires a specific factor assay.

Clinical features. The clinical picture in both disorders is similar. Many patients are asymptomatic throughout their lives, and others have relatively mild bleeding problems. However, postoperative bleeding may be severe even in patients without previous hemorrhagic symptoms. Inhibitors to factor XI in patients with factor XI deficiency have been described but are rare.

Treatment. Treatment for factor XI deficiency is usually required only for surgery. Fresh-frozen plasma is the only modality available. Fortunately, levels of 30% appear adequate for hemostasis. Repeat doses need be given only every third day because of the unusually long half-life of factor XI (64 hours).

Deficiencies of factor XII, prekallikrein, and high-molecular-weight kininogen

These three factors are all involved in the contact activation of blood coagulation, fibrinolysis, and kinin generation. Deficiencies are inherited in an autosomal recessive fashion.

Diagnosis. The PTT is prolonged in the absence of any of these factors. Specific factor assays are required for precise diagnosis.

Clinical features. No clinical abnormalities have been associated with deficiency of any of these proteins. However, correct diagnosis is necessary to exclude other causes of a prolonged PTT.

Factor XIII deficiency

The function of factor XIII is to cross-link fibrin monomers to one another by transamidation, thus stabilizing the fibrin clot. Factor XIII also cross-links fibronectin (cold-insoluble globulin, LETS protein) to fibrin and to collagen. The latter process is important for migration of macrophages into sites of injury, and absence of this function may be responsible for the poor wound healing sometimes seen in factor XIII deficiency.

Inheritance of factor XIII deficiency is clearly autosomal recessive in some families. In others the only affected individuals have been males, suggesting a sex-linked pattern.

Diagnosis. The PTT, PT, and TT are normal in factor XIII deficiency. The diagnosis is suggested by demonstrating solubility of the fibrin clot in either 5 M urea or 1% monochloroacetic acid.

Clinical features. Clinical features differ from those of hemophilia A and B in that hemarthroses are rare. Bleeding after separation of the umbilical cord is characteristic of this disorder. Intracranial hemorrhage, often fatal, has been reported in several patients. Spontaneous abortions have been a serious problem in adult females. Bleeding is common after trauma but is often delayed. Wound healing may be poor, with resultant gaping scars.

Treatment. Treatment is relatively simple because the half-life of factor XIII is relatively long (4.7 days), and levels of only 2% of normal provide satisfactory hemostasis. Monthly plasma transfusions are therefore sufficient to prevent spontaneous bleeding.

Fibrinogen abnormalities

Congenital disorders of circulating fibrinogen include both quantitative (afibrinogenemia or hypofibrinogenemia) and qualitative (dysfibrinogenemia) defects. Qualitative disorders may also be acquired and are discussed elsewhere in this chapter.

Diagnosis. Patients with severe fibrinogen abnormalities may have prolonged PTT, PT, and TT, since all three depend on formation of a fibrin clot as an end-point, but these screening tests are only sensitive to fibrinogen levels less than approximately 100 mg/dl (normal fibrinogen levels in most laboratories are 150 to 250 mg/dl). The diagnosis of a quantitative abnormality is confirmed by direct measurement of fibrinogen by clotting, chemical, or immunologic techniques. In patients with congenital dysfibrinogenemias, the clotting screening tests may be normal or abnormal, or the abnormality may be limited to the TT, which is the most sensitive screening test of fibrinogen defects. The diagnosis depends on either the demonstration of reduced functional levels of fibrinogen with normal levels by physiochemical or immunologic techniques, or, in patients with normal clotting times on screening tests, the demonstration of a functional or electrophorectic defect.

Genetics. Congenital afibrinogenemia is an autosomal recessive disorder. Affected individuals are homozygous or doubly heterozygous; heterozygous individuals are clinically asymptomatic, although some may have mild or moderately reduced plasma fibrinogen levels. Congenital dysfibrinogenemias, on the other hand, are inherited in an autosomal dominant manner in most patients, although in a few cases a recessive pattern of inheritance has been suggested.

Clinical features. Clinical symptoms in patients with abnormal fibrinogens are highly variable. Patients with congenital afibrinogenemia have a moderately severe bleeding diathesis. Spontaneous hemorrhage in soft tissues and from mucous membranes occurs, and bleeding caused by trauma or surgery may be severe. Clinical symptoms in dysfibrinogenemias range from those described in patients with afibrinogenemia to none at all. Defects in wound healing with wound dehiscence and subsequent keloid formation are prominent in some dysfibrinogenemias. A small number of patients with dysfibrinogenemias have been reported to have a thrombotic tendency. Fibrinogen inhibitors are rare. Platelet function tests may be abnormal in afibrinogenemia. In approximately 25% of reported cases, mild thrombocytopenia has been described.

Treatment. Bleeding problems in the afibrinogenemic patient are treated with transfusions of cryoprecipitate. In most patients the fibrinogen circulates with a normal half-life. Normal hemostasis in congenital afibrinogenemia is achieved with fibrinogen levels of 100 mg/dl or higher.

Hemorrhagic disorders associated with inherited deficiencies of protease inhibitors

Recently, deficiencies of $alpha_2$ plasmin inhibitor and plasminogen activator inhibitor (PAI) have been reported in association with a severe bleeding disorder. Presumably, bleeding is the result of dissolution of fibrin clots by plasmin. The diagnosis is suggested by rapid lysis of whole blood clotted in a glass tube. Specific diagnosis may be made by immunologic measurement of $alpha_2$ plasmin inhibitor or PAI concentration. At present, infusions of fresh-frozen plasma are the only therapy.

ACQUIRED DISORDERS

Vitamin K deficiency

Vitamin K is a fat-soluble vitamin that catalyzes the post-ribosomal modification of glutamic acid residues in certain proteins to γ-carboxyl glutamic acid (Gla). Proteins known to contain Gla residues include clotting factors II, VII, IX, and X (called vitamin K–dependent clotting factors); protein C and protein S (involved in the control of coagulation); protein Z; protein M; and the skeletal proteins, bone Gla protein (osteocalcin) and bone matrix Gla protein. Vitamin K–dependent clotting factors that contain Gla residues bind ionic calcium and, as a result, are able to efficiently assemble procoagulant complexes on the surface of platelets (Chapter 70). How the vitamin K–dependent proteins are targeted for postribosomal modification by vitamin K is not completely understood; protein sequences in both the pre-pro portion of the protein and in the Gla-rich domain of the mature protein may be involved. For example, hemophilia $B_{Cambridge}$ is a CRM^+ factor IX variant characterized by mutation of Arg to Ser at position −1 in the propeptide and by defective γ-carboxylation of glutamic acid. Similarly, hemophilia $B_{San\ Dimas}$ and hemophilia B_{Oxford} are CRM^+ variants characterized by mutation of Arg to Gln at position −4 in the propeptide and by defective γ-carboxylation of glutamic acid.

Several forms of vitamin K exist. Vitamin K_1, or phytonadione (2-methyl-3-phytyl-1,4-naphthoquinone), is a naturally occurring compound that has a 20-carbon side chain attached to the naphthoquinone nucleus. It is found primarily in green leafy plants and vegetables. Vitamin K_2, or menaquinone, has a 20-60-carbon side chain and is produced by bacteria as a metabolic product. Vitamin K_3, or menadione, has no side chains. Vitamin K is absorbed in the small intestine and transported to the liver, where the vitamin is obligatorily oxidized by a microsomal enzyme, vitamin K epoxidase, to vitamin K-2,3-epoxide (Fig. 85-4). The vitamin is stored in the liver as the epoxide. To become catalytically competent, vitamin K must be reduced

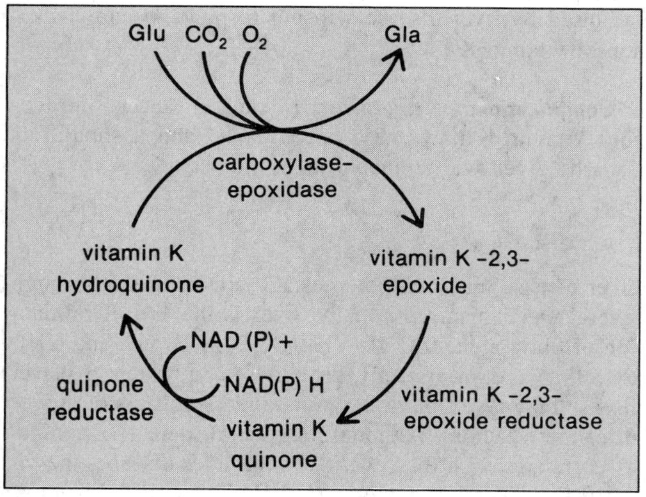

Fig. 85-4. The vitamin K cycle. γ-carboxylation of glutamic acid *(Glu)* residues to γ-carboxylglutamic acid *(Gla)* residues is catalyzed by a hepatic microsomal carboxylase in a reaction that is coupled to the conversion of vitamin K hydroquinone to vitamin K-2,3-epoxide by vitamin K epoxidase. Vitamin K-2,3-epoxide is reduced by a series of reactions involving vitamin K-2,3-epoxidase, vitamin K quinone reductase, and NAD(+). Both vitamin K-2,3-epoxide reductase and vitamin K quinone reductase appear to be inhibited by coumarin drugs.

by other microsomal enzymes, vitamin K-2,3-epoxide reductase and quinone reductase, to vitamin K_1, which is the active form of the enzyme. Vitamin K_1 catalyzes the γ-carboxylation of glutamic acid by a hepatic carboxylase.

Etiology. The causes of vitamin K deficiency are listed in the box below. Most cases are acquired and result from either reduced absorption of the vitamin or a block in the metabolism of vitamin K.

Hemorrhagic disease of newborn. In the newborn, levels of vitamin K–dependent clotting factors are lower than in adults, perhaps in part because of poor transplacental transfer of maternal vitamin K, the absence of vitamin K–synthesizing intestinal flora, and immature hepatic protein synthesis. In a small number of infants, especially premature infants and those who are breast-fed, severe reduction of one or more of the vitamin K–dependent clotting factors to levels of less than 10% may occur with the development of severe hemorrhagic symptoms. Onset of bleeding occurs typically within 2 or 3 days of birth and may be severe, with a significant risk of intracranial hemorrhage. Before institution of routine prophylactic administration of vitamin K to newborns, hemorrhagic disease occurred in up to 1% of births, with a mortality of up to 30%. Today, however, hemorrhagic disease of the newborn occurs rarely and almost exclusively in infants who have not received vitamin K prophylaxis.

Drug induced. The therapeutic administration of coumarin drugs in patients with venous or arterial thrombosis is the most common cause of vitamin K deficiency. Coumarin and its various congeners act as anticoagulants by interfering with the regeneration of vitamin K_1 from vitamin K-2,3-epoxide. As a result, II, VII, IX, and X cannot be γ-carboxylated, and inactive, decarboxy forms of the vitamin K–dependent clotting factors circulate in plasma. Surreptitious use of coumarin drugs, especially in health care workers and poisoning by administration of rat poison are other causes of coumarin-associated coagulopathy and should be considered in the differential diagnosis of vitamin K deficiency. Hydantoin anticonvulsants and salicylates are also vitamin K antagonists.

Causes of deficiency of vitamin K–dependent clotting factors

Abnormal or inadequate absorption

Hemorrhagic disease of newborn
Dietary deficiency
Parenteral nutrition
Malabsorption
Biliary tract obstruction
Liver disease
Drugs (broad-spectrum antibiotics)

Abnormal metabolism

Congenital
Drugs (coumarins, hydantoin)

Broad-spectrum antibiotics suppress vitamin K–synthesizing intestinal flora and may cause vitamin K deficiency. However, in most patients taking antibiotics, dietary sources of vitamin K are sufficient to maintain body levels and prevent vitamin K deficiency. Vitamin K deficiency is most likely to result when broad-spectrum antibiotics are given in conjunction with limited intake of food or a vitamin K–deficient diet. In vitro evidence indicates that cephalosporins may also affect vitamin K metabolism in the liver.

Defective absorption. Since vitamin K is fat soluble and requires bile salts for its absorption, biliary tract obstruction frequently causes vitamin K deficiency. Malabsorptive syndromes, such as celiac sprue, pancreatic insufficiency, ulcerative colitis, regional ileitis, and short bowel syndrome, produce vitamin K deficiency, but less frequently.

Inadequate dietary intake. Since vitamin K is derived from dual sources (i.e., dietary and intestinal flora), vitamin K deficiency caused by dietary deficiency alone is unusual. Vitamin K is found in all green leafy vegetables and is plentiful in a normal diet. Dietary deficiency of vitamin K combined with concomitant therapy with oral antibiotics or disease of the gastrointestinal tract will generally produce clinical evidence of vitamin K deficiency within 1 to 3 weeks.

Congenital defects. Congenital γ-carboxylation defects involving the vitamin K–dependent clotting factors are rare. Patients demonstrate variable deficiency of II, VII, IX, and X with levels from less than 1% to 50%. In general, all four factors are reduced proportionately. Levels respond poorly or not at all to large doses of vitamin K_1. The defect is presumed to be in the vitamin K cycle, either in the epoxidase/carboxylase or the reductase step. Inheritance appears to be autosomal recessive.

Diagnosis. The hallmark of vitamin K deficiency is a prolonged PT and PTT with a normal TT. Since factor VII has a half-life of approximately 4 hours and the other vitamin K–dependent clotting factors have longer half-lives, patients with early or mild vitamin K deficiency may demonstrate only minimum prolongation of PT (14 to 17 seconds with control of 12 seconds). With more advanced deficiency, both the PT and PTT are prolonged. In severe cases, prolongation of the PT and PTT may be marked. Measurement of clotting factor levels will reveal variably reduced levels of II, VII, IX, and X, depending on the degree of vitamin K deficiency.

The differential diagnosis of prolonged PT and PTT includes liver disease, the lupus inhibitor, and deficiency of clotting factors of the final common pathway such as V and X. Liver disease can be identified by tests of liver function (Chapter 53), but liver disease and vitamin K deficiency may coexist, especially in alcoholics and in patients with metastatic disease to the liver. In such patients the only way to demonstrate vitamin K deficiency may be to administer a trial of vitamin K.

Clinical features. With mild vitamin K deficiency, bleeding is minimal, and oozing after venipuncture or easy bruising may be the only manifestation. With more severe deficiency, spontaneous hemorrhage may be evident. Hematomas, hematuria, gingival bleeding, and gastrointestinal bleeding may occur.

Treatment. Deficiency of vitamin K is treated with vitamin K_1, either orally or parenterally. For patients with mild prolongation of the PT and no hemorrhagic tendency, 5 mg oral vitamin K_1 daily for 3 days is usually sufficient to restore vitamin K levels to normal. The dose can be repeated at weekly intervals if it is anticipated that deficiency will persist. For mild hemorrhage, administration of larger doses of vitamin K_1 (15 to 20 mg) usually results in cessation of hemorrhage within 24 to 36 hours. For intracranial and other serious hemorrhages, 25 mg of parenteral vitamin K_1 should be administered immediately by the subcutaneous or intramuscular route. Vitamin K may be administered intravenously but should not be given in doses greater than 1 mg and only when other routes are not feasible. In addition, since vitamin K_1 may take 6 to 24 hours to have an effect, 2 units of fresh-frozen plasma should be given to provide an immediate source of II, VII, IX, and X. Fresh-frozen plasma should be given every 4 to 6 hours until the PT and PTT demonstrate response to vitamin K. Prothrombin complex concentrates, which contain II, VII, IX, and X, should be avoided because of a high frequency of hepatitis and because they have been reported to cause thrombosis and diffuse intravascular coagulation. In patients with coumarin drug overdose, the same general rules just described apply, except that it may be advantageous to avoid administration of vitamin K_1 if coumarin anticoagulation is to be continued.

Hemorrhagic disease of the newborn is prevented by parenteral administration of 1 mg of vitamin K_1 to the child on the day of birth. Patients in whom prolongation of PT is caused by liver disease will not respond to administration of vitamin K_1.

Complications of treatment. In rare instances, intravenous vitamin K may cause anaphylaxis, and it should always be given with epinephrine at the bedside.

Liver disease

Liver disease may cause hemostatic abnormalities through several mechanisms. First, the liver is the site of production of fibrinogen, II, VII, VIII, IX, X, XI, XII, and XIII, as well as antithrombin III, protein C, and protein S. Liver disease may result in variably impaired synthesis of any or all of these factors. Although in general, defective synthesis correlates with the severity of the liver disease, the vitamin K–dependent factors, II, VII, IX, and X, are most sensitive to hepatocellular disease and may be the only abnormalities in mild forms of liver disease. In contrast, V and VIII are most resistant to hepatocellular disease and are only decreased in fulminant hepatitis and severe liver failure. Synthesis of both procoagulant and anticoagulant proteins may be affected, resulting in hemorrhagic or thrombotic tendencies. Second, deficiency of plasminogen or alpha$_2$ plasmin inhibitor may cause alterations in plasma fibrinolytic activity and increased levels of fibrin(ogen) degradation products (FDP). Third, vitamin K deficiency may occur in liver disease, especially in binge alcoholics with limited nutritional intake. In addition, in severe hepatic parenchymal disease with severe jaundice, intrahepatic biliary obstruction may be present and cause vitamin K deficiency. Fourth, synthesis of functionally abnormal molecules of fibrinogen characterized by increased sialic acid content occurs in some forms of liver disease, especially hepatocellular carcinoma, chronic active hepatitis, and some types of cirrhosis. Functionally, these abnormal molecules, called dysfibrinogens, demonstrate delayed fibrin monomer polymerization, resulting in marked prolongation of TT. Fifth, small amounts of activated clotting factors generated during normal homeostasis are cleared through the activity of the hepatic reticuloendothelial system. In liver disease, clearance of these activated factors may be impaired, and circulation of these factors may predispose to diffuse (disseminated) intravascular coagulation (DIC) or thrombosis. Sixth, in patients with cirrhosis and increased portal pressure, splenomegaly occurs and may cause sequestrational thrombocytopenia. In addition, alcohol itself may have a suppressive effect on thrombopoiesis and cause thrombocytopenia, as may nutritional defects, especially folate deficiency. Finally, qualitative platelet defects may occur in liver disease with bleeding times that are mildly or moderately prolonged in the absence of or out of proportion to the degree of thrombocytopenia.

Diagnosis. The diagnosis of hemostatic abnormalities in liver disease is based on routine screening tests of coagulation: the PT, PTT, TT, and tests of platelet function. In *acute liver failure,* which may occur in toxic or fulminant viral hepatitis, the PT, PTT, and TT are all extremely prolonged. The PTT mix is normal, but the TT mix may be prolonged by FDP. Assays for specific coagulation factors show severely reduced levels of those factors synthesized in the liver, including V and VIII. Levels of FDP are initially very high but may decrease as levels of fibrinogen decrease from synthetic failure and fibrinolysis. The platelet count is moderately decreased. In *chronic liver disease* a spectrum of coagulation abnormalities may occur. The PT, PTT, and TT may be variably prolonged or may be normal. Since the vitamin K–dependent factors are more sensitive to hepatocellular disease, PT is often more prolonged than PTT. Measurement of clotting factor levels in patients with chronic liver disease will often reveal reduced levels even when the screens are normal. In contrast, VIII may be increased in patients with less severe liver disease. Finally, in *acute hepatitis,* the coagulation screening tests are usually normal. Prolongation of the PT in patients with acute hepatitis is a bad prognostic sign.

Although hemostatic abnormalities can be simply diagnosed with routine screening tests, the nature of the abnormality can be difficult to determine. For example, since II, VII, IX, and X are sensitive to hepatocellular disease, it may be difficult to diagnose vitamin K deficiency in patients with liver disease. In many patients a trial of vitamin K may be needed to make the diagnosis. It is also difficult to diagnose DIC in patients with liver disease. Since V and VIII are resistant to hepatocellular disease and are rapidly consumed in DIC, reduced levels of these factors may suggest the presence of DIC. Another way to diagnose DIC in liver disease is to measure serial platelet counts and levels of fibrinogen, V, and VIII. Progressive decline in these parameters is consistent with DIC. Patients with the lupus inhibitor have a prolonged PT and PTT, but such patients can be distinguished from those with coagulopathy of liver disease because the TT is normal and the PTT mix is prolonged.

Clinical features. Bleeding in patients with acute liver failure may be catastrophic. Spontaneous hemorrhage from mucous membranes, skin, and other sites can be prominent, and bleeding from varices, gastritis, Mallory-Weiss tears, and other structural sites may be greatly aggravated by the hemostatic abnormalities in liver disease. Bleeding is typically from multiple sites. Petechiae may be present in patients who are thrombocytopenic or have a qualitative platelet defect. In patients with chronic liver disease, bleeding signs are less prominent.

Treatment. Treatment of hemostatic defects in liver disease is complicated by the defect's global nature and the short half-life of some clotting factors, especially VII. To maintain correction of the hemostatic defect may require administration of 2 to 4 units of fresh-frozen plasma every 3 to 4 hours. This and the administration of other products, such as platelet concentrates, cryoprecipitate, and red cells, can quickly lead to severe volume overload in patients who already have difficulty with fluid balance. For this reason, a major question in the treatment of hemostatic defects in liver disease is often not how to treat but whether to treat.

For patients who are not actively bleeding, vitamin K should be administered orally; treatment with fresh-frozen plasma and other products should be reserved for bleeding episodes. In such patients, minor procedures, such as liver biopsy, should be covered with 2 units of fresh-frozen plasma immediately before the procedure. Platelets may also be given for minor procedures if the platelet count is less than 50,000, and cryoprecipitate if the fibrinogen is less than 75 mg/dl. A single bag of cryoprecipitate contains approximately 150 mg of fibrinogen and will raise the plasma concentration of fibrinogen by about 5 mg/dl.

For patients with significantly abnormal coagulation screening tests who have generalized or severe localized bleeding, therapy should be considered. Vitamin K and folate should be administered initially. Two units of fresh-frozen plasma are given and the coagulation screens repeated after the second bag. This therapy is then repeated until the bleeding stops or the screens are normal. For patients with severe fluid retention, plasma exchange should be considered. Red cells and platelets are given as needed, and cryoprecipitate is given if the fibrinogen level is decreased. Prothrombin complex concentrates have been associated with a high incidence of DIC or thrombosis in liver disease, and their use is best reserved for life-threatening bleeding unresponsive to other agents.

Diffuse intravascular coagulation (DIC)

Diffuse intravascular coagulation (also called disseminated intravascular coagulation or DIC) is a catastrophic bleeding disorder caused by the generation of excessive thrombin in the circulation. DIC has innumerable specific etiologies (see the box on p. 819), but all are related either to (1) vascular damage with activation of plasma coagulation factors, leading to thrombin generation by the intrinsic coagulation pathway, or (2) entry of tissue thromboplastic material into the blood and generation of thrombin by the extrinsic coagulation pathway.

The consequences of thrombin generation in blood on the coagulation system are shown in Fig. 85-5. Thrombin causes platelets to aggregate, converts fibrinogen to fibrin, activates coagulation factors V and VIII, activates protein C, converts plasminogen to plasmin, activates factor XIII, and combines with and is inactivated by antithrombin III. Thus thrombin simultaneously promotes thrombosis by activating platelets, fibrinogen, V, VIII, and XIII; promotes the dissolution of any thrombi that form by generating plasmin; and inhibits hemostasis by producing thrombocytopenia and by consuming fibrinogen, V, and VIII. The net effect is a hemorrhagic tendency from deficiency of the consumed coagulation factors. For this reason, DIC is also called *consumptive coagulopathy*.

Diagnosis. Laboratory evaluation of coagulation in DIC demonstrates abnormalities in PTT, PT, and TT. Among these, TT is the most sensitive test and is most prolonged because of interference with fibrin polymerization by FDP.

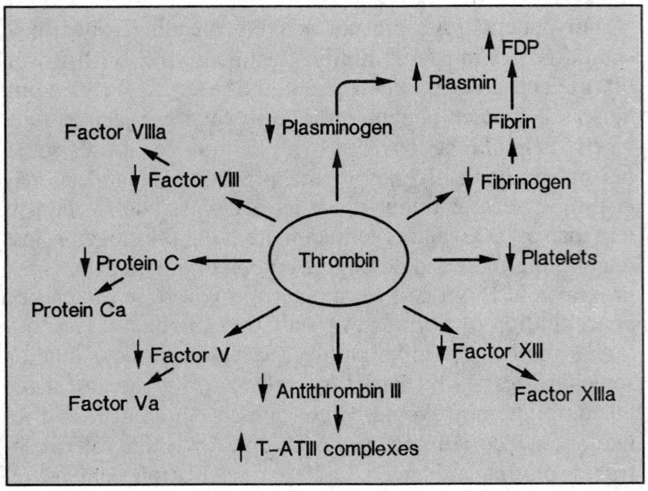

Fig. 85-5. Consequences of thrombin generation in diffuse (disseminated) intravascular coagulation (DIC). Thrombin has multiple effects on the coagulation system, activating cellular, humoral, and fibrinolytic components. Down arrows indicate reduced plasma concentrations of factors. Up arrows indicate increased plasma concentrations of factors.

A TT performed on a mixture of patient and normal plasma yields results consistent with a coagulation inhibitor produced by the fibrin fragments. Platelets are also decreased, sometimes to very low levels; this is often an early indicator of DIC. The blood smear may show fragmented red blood cells, called *schistocytes,* in about half of patients. The diagnosis is confirmed by factor assays showing a decreased fibrinogen, V, and VIII and elevated FDP, although the latter may be increased with surgery and trauma and in other patients and are therefore not specific for a diagnosis of DIC.

Clinical features. The clinical spectrum of DIC ranges from clinically insignificant laboratory abnormalities in mild cases to uncontrollable hemorrhage in patients with severe disease. The bleeding manifestations of DIC are very characteristic. In contrast to structural bleeding, hemorrhage in DIC is typically from multiple sites. Bleeding from small wounds, such as venipuncture sites, continues without stopping for hours or days. In contrast to patients with thrombocytopenia alone, the bleeding in patients with DIC is not arrested with local pressure that would normally allow fibrin formation. Even in patients with severe thrombocytopenia, bleeding from a deep wound such as that caused by marrow aspiration is easily controlled with local pressure. In contrast to patients with only a defect in coagulation, the bleeding in DIC is not initially delayed and is not arrested intermittently by platelet aggregates.

Rarely, patients with DIC have peripheral, symmetric infarction of fingertips and toes, or renal failure may occur with thrombosis of small renal cortical vessels. In these patients the fibrinolytic component appears to be either deficient or insufficient, and microthrombi develop. These unusual patients demonstrate the importance of the fibrinolytic component in DIC and provide a strong argument against the use of antifibrinolytic agents in the treatment of DIC.

Treatment. When DIC occurs, it is important to remove the provoking cause: correct the hypotension, control the sepsis, or deliver the placenta or dead fetus. The treatment of DIC itself consists of replacement of consumed coagulation factors and alpha$_2$ antiplasmin with fresh-frozen plasma, replacement of fibrinogen with cryoprecipitate, and platelet transfusions. Because of the short half-life of some of the clotting factors, fresh-frozen plasma must be given as often as every 30 minutes or so to patients with severe DIC. Antithrombin III concentrates are now available and may be used in the treatment of DIC. Intravenous heparin is also used to increase neutralization of thrombin, but it should be used in very low doses and may increase the bleeding in patients with DIC.

Acquired inhibitors of blood coagulation

Acquired inhibitors are endogenous substances, usually polyclonal antibodies, that interfere with normal blood coagulation. Most are IgG immunoglobulins, but some are IgM or mixtures of IgG and IgM. In most patients the an-

Causes of diffuse (disseminated) intravascular coagulation (DIC)

Obstetric complications
Amniotic fluid embolism
Abruptio placentae
Retained dead fetus
Eclampsia
Septic abortion
Induced abortion
Hydatidiform mole

Shock
Hemorrhagic
Traumatic
Septic
Anaphylactic

Carcinoma
Prostate
Lung
Pancreas
Stomach
Ovary
Colon
Sarcoma

Infections
Bacterial (gram positive and negative)
Viral (herpes)
Rickettsial (Rocky Mountain spotted fever)
Fungal (aspergillosis)
Parasitic (malaria)
Granulomatous (tuberculosis)

Vascular and pulmonary
Pulmonary embolism
Hyaline membrane disease
Crush syndrome
Malignant hypertension
Cardiopulmonary bypass pump
Thoracic surgery
Giant hemangioma
Fat embolism

Hematologic
Promyelocytic leukemia
Acute leukemia
Tranfusion reaction
Acquired hemolytic anemia
Sickle cell crisis

Renal
Transplant rejection
Glomerulonephritis
Acute renal failure

Miscellaneous
Hepatic cirrhosis
Acute pancreatitis
Allergic drug reaction
Snakebite
Decompression sickness
Amyloidosis
Heatstroke

tibody is directed against a site at or near the active site of a single coagulation factor and either inhibits the participation of that factor in coagulation or interferes with normal circulation of the protein. Most acquired inhibitors are directed against VIII, but antibodies to fibrinogen, II, V, IX, X, XI, XIII, and vWf have been reported.

Factor VIII inhibitors. Spontaneous inhibitors of factor VIII have been reported in a variety of clinical settings (see the box on p. 820). More than half of spontaneous inhibitors occur in individuals over the age of 40 without any associated underlying disorder. Autoimmune disorders, including rheumatoid arthritis, systemic lupus erythematosus, temporal arteritis, dermatomyositis, polymyositis, myasthenia gravis, and Sjögren's syndrome, may be found in 10% to 15% of patients with VIII inhibitors. Inhibitors occur infrequently in patients with neoplasms, particularly lymphoproliferative disorders and cancer of the prostate and lung, and may be the initial manifestation of a malignancy. It is therefore important to search for occult malignancies in otherwise asymptomatic patients with inhibitors. Postpartum factor VIII inhibitors typically appear after the birth of a normal child, usually the first. The inhibitor becomes manifest weeks to months after delivery, but intervals of up to 1 year have been reported. In about half of such patients the anticoagulant disappears within 12 to 18 months and does not recur during subsequent pregnancies. Other conditions associated with VIII inhibitors include ulcerative colitis; dermatologic disorders such as psoriasis, pemphigus, and exfoliative dermatitis; asthma, especially when treated with corticosteroids; and drugs, including penicillin, sulfa, diphenylhydantoin, and phenylbutazone.

The course of VIII inhibitors is variable. Low-titer inhibitors and those in postpartum women may disappear spontaneously or after a course of corticosteroid therapy. It has been estimated that approximately one-third may disappear spontaneously within 2 years. High-titer inhibitors and inhibitors in patients with autoimmune disorders are more persistent and are unlikely to spontaneously resolve. Some will improve or disappear after treatment with corticosteroids in combination with alkylating agents.

Lupus inhibitor. The "lupus anticoagulant" is an antibody with affinity for negatively charged phospholipids, perhaps in a complex with beta$_2$ glycoprotein I, that inhibits phospholipid-dependent coagulation reactions by pre-

Conditions associated with coagulation inhibitors*

Factor VIII inhibitors
Autoimmune disorders (SLE, RA, TA)
Neoplasms (lymphoma, prostate, lung)
Postpartum
Inflammatory bowel disease
Skin diseases (psoriasis, pemphigus, exfoliative dermatitis)
Drugs (penicillin, sulfa, phenylbutazone)
Asthma
Idiopathic

Acquired von Willebrand's disease
Lymphoma
Autoimmune disorders (SLE)
Idiopathic

Factor XI inhibitor
Autoimmune disorders (SLE)
Drugs (prednisone)
Idiopathic

Factor V
Drugs (streptomycin)
Surgery

Fibrinogen
Ulcerative colitis?
Sarcoidosis?

Factor XIII
Drugs (isoniazid, diphenylhydantoin)

Lupus inhibitor
Autoimmune disorders (SLE, RA, Raynaud's disease)
Acquired immunodeficiency syndrome
Drugs (phenothiazines)
Hypothyroidism
Neoplasms
Atherosclerotic cardiovascular disease
Idiopathic

SLE, Systemic lupus erythematosus; RA, rheumatoid arthritis; TA, temporal arteritis.
*Excluding inhibitors occurring in inherited coagulopathies.

venting the normal interaction of clotting factors with the phospholipid surface. Thus the phospholipid-dependent conversion of prothrombin to thrombin and factor X to Xa is inhibited. Recent studies indicate that although the lupus inhibitor inhibits the catalytic action of the negatively charged phospholipids used in the PTT and PT, it may have little effect on the catalytic action of the platelet surface in these reactions. This may explain why the lupus inhibitor is an in vitro inhibitor but does not have anticoagulant effects in vivo.

Clinically, patients with the lupus inhibitor have a thrombotic tendency. Up to 50% of patients with the lupus inhibitor have clinically detectable thrombosis. In addition, in women of childbearing age the lupus inhibitor is associated with a syndrome of recurrent spontaneous abortions. A strong correlation exists between the presence of the lupus inhibitor, the tendency to thrombosis, and the presence of antibodies to cardiolipin, the lipid used in most serologic tests for syphilis. Based on retrospective studies, cardiolipin antibodies have been shown to predict thrombosis correctly in nearly 90% of patients, but the specificity of the test is lower (approximately 70%). In women with the lupus inhibitor and the syndrome of recurrent spontaneous abortions, the risk of abortion is related to the level of anticardiolipin antibody.

A corollary of the presence of anticardiolipin antibodies is that many patients with the lupus inhibitor have a false-positive test for syphilis. Tests based on detection of treponemal antigens (i.e., fluorescent treponemal antigen, or FTA) should be used to distinguish a false-positive from a true-positive serology.

Although the lupus inhibitor may be seen in the absence of any underlying disorder, several associated diseases have been described (see the box on the left). Nearly half of patients with the lupus inhibitor have systemic lupus erythematosus (but only 10% of patients with systemic lupus erythematosus have the lupus inhibitor). The lupus inhibitor has also been reported in patients with drug-induced lupus, rheumatoid arthritis, rheumatic fever, Raynaud's phenomenon, hypothyroidism, AIDS, neoplasms, prostatic hypertrophy, and atherosclerotic cardiovascular or peripheral vascular disease.

Other inhibitors. The prevalence of inhibitors directed against coagulation factors other than factor VIII is much lower. With a single exception, all reported examples of inhibitors of factor V have appeared in patients who were previously normal. The persistence of the inhibitor is usually short. The occurrence of inhibitors to factor V seems to be associated with surgical procedures or the administration of streptomycin or penicillin. Inhibitors to either factor XIII activation or factor XIII transamidase activity have been described, especially in association with antituberculous drugs. Inhibitors against vWf also have been described. The blood of some patients with dysproteinemias also demonstrates inhibition of various tests of blood coagulation (and platelet function). This apparently results from an interaction between an abnormal protein and certain plasma proteins involved in blood coagulation. In contrast to the previously described examples of circulating anticoagulants, in this instance inhibition results from a presumed physicochemical rather than an immunologic interaction. Hemorrhagic symptoms are seen only rarely and are more likely caused by increased blood viscosity secondary to high levels of abnormal proteins or decreased platelet function.

Clinical features. Patients with spontaneous VIII inhibitors typically experience the sudden appearance of a severe hemorrhagic defect when they were previously free of a bleeding tendency. Bleeding is usually spontaneous and profuse. Bleeding is primarily from mucous membranes, the gastrointestinal tract, and genitourinary tract. Joint bleeds occur less frequently than in patients with hemophilia A.

The lupus inhibitor may become manifest in several ways. In many patients the presence of the inhibitor is an incidental finding in a patient admitted for other reasons. There may or may not be a history of remote thrombosis. Patients with the lupus inhibitor may also have thrombosis. Both deep venous thrombosis, primarily in the lower extremities, and superficial venous thrombosis may occur. Arterial thrombosis, especially cerebral thrombosis, is less often encountered but may also occur. Finally, women with the lupus inhibitor may have spontaneous abortion or a history of recurrent spontaneous abortion. Patients with the lupus inhibitor and systemic lupus erythematosus may bleed when thrombocytopenia or a coexisting specific inhibitor to VIII, XI, or other clotting factors is present.

Diagnosis. Diagnosis of an inhibitor to a specific coagulation factor is suggested by a history of a coagulopathy of recent onset and the presence of an abnormal screening test. In such patients, it is important to try to obtain the results of past clotting tests to ascertain that the abnormality is new. The pattern of abnormal screening tests depends on the clotting factor to which the antibody is directed and will be similar to the pattern seen in deficiency of that factor (see Table 85-1). For example, an inhibitor to VIII is characterized by a prolonged PTT and normal PT and TT, whereas an inhibitor to XIII is characterized by a normal PTT, PT, and TT. The presence of an inhibitor is confirmed by demonstration of an abnormal mixing test. When plasma from a patient with an inherited clotting factor deficiency is mixed with normal plasma, the normal plasma supplies sufficient amounts of that clotting factor to correct the clotting time in the deficient plasma. In contrast, when plasma from a patient with an inhibitor is mixed with normal plasma, the inhibitor neutralizes the target clotting factor in the normal plasma, and the clotting time of the mixture remains prolonged. With most inhibitors, this neutralization is rapid, and abnormal mixing studies are immediately apparent. With VIII inhibitors, however, the neutralization of VIII in the normal plasma is enhanced by incubation of the mixed plasmas at 37° C for 2 hours. The specificity of the inhibitor is determined by demonstrating reduced levels of the target clotting factor by specific assay.

Diagnosis of the lupus inhibitor is based on the presence of a prolonged PTT with an abnormal mix, a variably prolonged PT, and normal TT. The PTT is typically two or three times the control value but may be minimally prolonged. Individual clotting factor assays may be normal or slightly reduced and show an inhibitory pattern. Numerous clotting tests have been proposed for the specific diagnosis of the lupus inhibitor. The platelet neutralization procedure is based on the ability of platelet phospholipids to correct the PTT. Other tests include the kaolin clotting time, the dilute Russell's viper venom time, and the tissue thromboplastin inhibition index, but the number of tests that have been used attests to the uncertainty of each.

Treatment. Bleeding in patients with spontaneous inhibitors to VIII can be treated according to the guidelines outlined for treatment of hemophilic inhibitors in the previous section on hemophilia A. The same principles apply except that the patient usually has not been previously exposed to plasma products, and immunization with hepatitis B vaccine should be started before administration of plasma products. Treatment of the inhibitor itself should be considered. Although some inhibitors may disappear without therapy, a course of corticosteroids may hasten disappearance of the inhibitor. Intravenous gamma globulin has also been reported to be effective in some patients with acquired VIII inhibitors. For patients who do not respond to corticosteroids or intravenous gamma globulin, a trial of alkylating agents may be considered. When an underlying disease or drug is associated with a circulating anticoagulant, therapy should be directed at the basic disease or discontinuation of the potentially causative drug.

Patients with inhibitors to V or XIII have been successfully treated with either plasma or transfusion of platelet concentrates. Those with inhibitors to II, IX, and X may respond to prothrombin complex concentrates. Patients with inhibitors to vWf may respond at least transiently to intravenous gamma globulin. Treatment of the associated disease may result in permanent disappearance of the inhibitor.

Thrombosis associated with the lupus anticoagulant can be successfully controlled with anticoagulants. In women with recurrent spontaneous abortions, corticosteroids and antiplatelet agents have been reported to improve fetal mortality. Coumarins appear to be less effective and can produce fetal malformations, especially if administered during the first trimester.

REFERENCES

Aledort LM: Blood clotting abnormalities in liver disease. Prog Liver Dis 5:350, 1976.

Antonarakis SE et al: Hemophilia A: detection of molecular defects and of carriers by DNA analysis. N Engl J Med 313:642, 1985.

Aoki N and Harpel PC: Inhibitors of the fibrinolytic enzyme system. Semin Thromb Hemost 10:24, 1984.

Branch DW et al: Obstetric complications associated with the lupus anticoagulant. N Engl J Med 313:1322, 1985.

Brettler DB and Levine PH: Factor concentrates for treatment of hemophilia: which one to choose. Blood 73:2067, 1989.

Collen D: On the regulation and control of fibrinolysis. Thromb Haemost 43:77, 1980.

Fass DN and Toole JJ: Genetic engineering and coagulation factors. Clin Haematol 14:547, 1985.

Kasper CK: Management of inhibitors to factor VIII. Prog Hematol 12:143, 1981.

Mammen EF: Congenital coagulation disorders. Semin Thromb Hemost 9:1, 1983.

McGraw RA et al: Structure and function of factor IX: defects in hemophilia B. Clin Haematol 14:351, 1985.

Perkins HA, MacKenzie MR, and Fudenberg HH: Hemostatic defects in dysproteinemias. Blood 35:695, 1970.

Rao AK and Walsh PN: Acquired qualitative platelet disorders. Clin Haematol 12:201, 1983.

Roberts HR and Cederbaum AI: The liver and blood coagulation: physiology and pathology. Gastroenterology 63:297, 1972.

Shapiro SS and Hultin M: Acquired inhibitors to the blood coagulation factors. Semin Thromb Hemost 1:336, 1975.

Shapiro SS and Thiagarajan P: Lupus anticoagulants. Prog Hemost Thromb 6:263, 1982.
Smith JK and Bidwell E: Therapeutic materials used in the treatment of coagulation defects. Clin Haematol 8:183, 1979.
Suttie JW: Mechanism of action of vitamin K: synthesis of gamma carboxyglutamic acid. CRC Crit Rev Biochem 8:191, 1980.
White GC II and Shoemaker CB: The factor VIII gene and hemophilia A. Blood 73:1, 1989.
Zimmerman TS and Ruggeri ZM: Von Willebrand factor and von Willebrand disease. Blood 70:895, 1987.

CHAPTER

86 Thrombosis and Anticoagulation

Russell D. Hull
Graham F. Pineo
Gary E. Raskob

This chapter provides an overview of the management of patients with arterial and venous thromboembolic disease (Chapter 22) and reviews the role of heparin, oral anticoagulant therapy, thrombolytic therapy, and venous interruption procedures in the treatment of patients with established thromboembolism.

VENOUS THROMBOEMBOLISM

Etiology and pathogenesis

Venous thromboembolism (venous thrombosis and/or pulmonary embolism) usually complicates the course of sick, hospitalized patients but may also affect ambulatory and otherwise apparently healthy individuals. Pulmonary embolism remains the most common preventable cause of hospital death and is responsible for approximately 150,000 to 200,000 deaths per year in the United States. Most patients who die from pulmonary embolism succumb suddenly or within 2 hours after the acute event, before therapy can be initiated or can take effect. Effective prophylaxis against venous thromboembolism is now available for most high-risk patients. The use of prophylaxis is more effective for preventing death and morbidity from venous thromboembolism than is treatment of the established disease.

Venous thrombi are composed predominantly of fibrin and red cells with a variable platelet and leukocyte component. The formation, growth, and dissolution of venous thromboemboli represent a balance between various thrombogenic stimuli and several protective mechanisms. The factors that predispose to the development of venous thromboemboli are venous stasis, activation of blood coagulation, and vascular damage. The protective mechanisms that counteract these thrombogenic stimuli include (1) the inactivation of activated coagulation factors by circulating inhibitors (e.g., antithrombin III, $alpha_2$ macroglobulin, $alpha_1$ antitrypsin, protein C), (2) clearance of activated coagulation factors and soluble fibrin polymer complexes by the reticuloendothelial system and by the liver, and (3) dissolution of fibrin by fibrinolytic enzymes derived from plasma, endothelial cells, and circulating leukocytes.

Various risk factors predispose to the development of venous thromboembolism (see the box below). Other conditions that have been reported to be associated with a high risk of venous thromboembolism include homocystinuria, polycythemia vera, paroxysmal nocturnal hemoglobinuria, and the presence of the lupus inhibitor.

Pulmonary embolism originates from thrombi in the deep veins of the leg in 90% or more of patients. Other less common sources of pulmonary embolism include the deep pelvic veins, renal veins, inferior vena cava, right side of the heart heart, or axillary veins. Most clinically important pulmonary emboli arise from thrombi in the popliteal or more proximal deep veins of the leg (proximal-vein thrombosis). Pulmonary embolism occurs in 50% of patients with objectively documented proximal-vein thrombosis; many of these emboli are asymptomatic. Usually only part of the thrombus embolizes, and 50% to 70% of patients with angiographically documented pulmonary embolism have detectable deep vein thrombosis of the legs at presentation. The clinical significance of pulmonary embolism depends on the size of the embolus and the patient's cardiorespiratory reserve.

Clinical features

The clinical features of venous thrombosis include leg pain, tenderness and swelling, a palpable cord (i.e., a thrombosed vessel that is palpable as a cord), discoloration, venous distention and prominence of the superficial veins, and cyanosis. The clinical diagnosis of venous thrombosis is highly

Risk factors predisposing to development of venous thromboembolism

Clinical risk factors

Surgical and nonsurgical trauma
Age (>40)
Previous venous thromboembolism
Immobilization
Malignant disease
Heart failure
Myocardial infarction
Leg paralysis
Obesity
Varicose veins
Estrogens
Parturition

Inherited abnormalities

Antithrombin III deficiency
Protein C deficiency
Protein S deficiency
Dysfibrinogenemia

nonspecific, because none of the symptoms or signs is unique, and each may be caused by nonthrombotic disorders. The rare exception may be the patient with phlegmasia cerulea dolens, in whom the diagnosis of massive iliofemoral thrombosis usually is clinically obvious; this syndrome occurs in less than 1% of patients with symptomatic venous thrombosis. In most patients who have clinically suspected venous thrombosis, the symptoms and signs are nonspecific, and in more than 50% of these patients the clinical suspicion of venous thrombosis is not confirmed by objective testing. Further, patients with relatively minor symptoms and signs may have extensive deep venous thrombi, whereas in patients with florid leg pain and swelling, suggesting extensive deep vein thrombosis, objective testing may produce negative results. Thus objective testing is mandatory to confirm or exclude a diagnosis of venous thrombosis.

Pulmonary embolism may present clinically in a variety of ways, depending on the size, location, and number of emboli and on the patient's underlying cardiorespiratory reserve. The clinical manifestations of acute pulmonary embolism generally can be divided into several syndromes that overlap considerably: (1) transient dyspnea and tachypnea in the absence of other associated clinical manifestations; (2) the syndrome of pulmonary infarction or congestive atelectasis (also known as *ischemic pneumonitis* or *incomplete infarction*), including pleuritic chest pain, cough, hemoptysis, pleural effusion and pulmonary infiltrates on chest radiographs; (3) right-sided heart failure associated with severe dyspnea and tachypnea; (4) cardiovascular collapse with hypotension, syncope, and coma (usually associated with massive pulmonary embolism); and (5) a variety of less common and highly nonspecific clinical features, including confusion and coma, pyrexia, wheezing, resistant cardiac failure, and unexplained arrhythmia. For a detailed discussion of the clinical features and diagnosis of suspected acute pulmonary embolism, refer to Chapter 217.

It is now widely accepted that the clinical diagnosis of pulmonary embolism is highly nonspecific. Multiple studies indicate that in more than half of all patients with clinically suspected pulmonary embolism, this diagnosis is not confirmed by objective testing. Therefore objective testing is mandatory to confirm or exclude the presence of pulmonary embolism.

Laboratory features

Various laboratory abnormalities have been associated with venous thromboembolism, including a decrease in the activated partial thromboplastin time (APTT), increased levels of fibrinopeptide A and fibrin/fibrinogen degradation product (FDP) E, and a group of nonspecific laboratory changes that make up the acute phase response to injury. Tissue injury is associated with a systemic response, including elevated levels of fibrinogen, factor VIII, and $alpha_1$ antitrypsin and increases in both the leukocyte and the platelet counts. Tissue injury is also associated with systemic activation of blood coagulation and fibrin formation, a decrease in the APTT, and increases in the levels of fibrinopeptide A and FDP E. All the above changes are highly nonspecific and may occur as a result of surgical or nonsurgical trauma, infection, inflammation, or infarction. Patients with venous thromboembolism frequently have other comorbid conditions, and it is not surprising that the laboratory changes reported to be associated with venous thromboembolism are highly nonspecific. Currently no evidence exists to indicate that any of the reported laboratory changes associated with venous thromboembolism can be used to predict the development of venous thromboembolism.

Two blood tests, the fibrinopeptide A assay and the assay for fibrin/fibrinogen fragment E, are highly sensitive to venous thromboembolism in symptomatic patients but are nonspecific. Both the fibrinopeptide A assay and the assay for fragment E are performed by radioimmunoassay and require technical simplification for routine clinical use. If simplified, however, either of these assays possibly could be used to exclude a diagnosis of venous thromboembolism in symptomatic patients, but this would require formal evaluation in adequately designed and executed clinical trials. The assay for fragment D–dimer of fibrin may overcome the technical limitations of the previous assays of fibrinopeptide A and fragment E.

Differential diagnosis

The differential diagnosis in patients with clinically suspected venous thrombosis includes muscle strain (usually associated with unaccustomed exercise), muscle tear, direct twisting injury to the leg, vasomotor changes in a paralyzed leg, venous reflux, lymphangitis, lymphatic obstruction, Baker's cyst, cellulitis, internal derangement of the knee, hematoma, and venous insufficiency. An alternate diagnosis is frequently not evident at presentation, and without objective testing, it is impossible to exclude venous thrombosis. The cause of symptoms can often be determined by careful follow-up once a diagnosis of venous thrombosis has been excluded by objective testing (Table 86-1). In some patients, however, the cause of pain, tenderness, and swelling remains uncertain even after careful follow-up.

Table 86-1. The alternative diagnosis in 87 consecutive patients with clinically suspected venous thrombosis and negative venograms*

Diagnosis	Patients (%)
Muscle strain	24
Direct twisting injury to leg	10
Leg swelling in paralyzed limb	9
Lymphangitis, lymphatic obstruction	7
Venous reflux	7
Muscle tear	6
Baker's cyst	5
Cellulitis	3
Internal abnormality of knee	2
Unknown	26

*The diagnosis was made once venous thrombosis had been excluded by the finding of a negative venogram.

The differential diagnosis of the clinical features of acute pulmonary embolism is shown in the box below (see also Chapter 217).

Treatment

General considerations. The objectives of treatment in patients with venous thromboembolism are (1) to prevent death from pulmonary embolism, (2) to prevent recurrent venous thromboembolism, and (3) to prevent the postphlebitic syndrome.

Initial therapy with intravenous (IV) heparin is the treatment of choice for most patients with pulmonary embolism or proximal-vein thrombosis. IV heparin given in doses that maintain the APTT greater than 1.5 times the control value is highly effective and associated with a low frequency (2%) of recurrent venous thromboembolism. Failure to follow the initial course of heparin with adequate long-term anticoagulant therapy exposes patients with proximal-vein thrombosis to a 40% to 50% risk of recurrent venous thromboembolism. This risk is reduced to 2% with adequate long-term anticoagulant therapy with warfarin sodium. Adjusted subcutaneous heparin is an effective alternative to warfarin sodium for long-term treatment, with a low risk (2%) of bleeding, and is preferred in selected patients (see section on long-term subcutaneous heparin therapy).

Thrombolytic therapy is indicated in patients with life-threatening massive pulmonary embolism and in selected patients with acute massive proximal-vein thrombosis (e.g., phlegmasia cerulea dolens with impending venous gangrene). Besides these indications, the role of thrombolytic therapy remains uncertain.

The relative and absolute contraindications to anticoagulant therapy are listed in the box below. Inferior vena caval interruption, using a transvenously inserted filter (Greenfield filter), is the management of choice for preventing pulmonary embolism in patients with proximal-vein thrombosis in whom anticoagulant therapy is absolutely contraindicated, as well as in the very rare patient in whom anticoagulant therapy is ineffective. In patients with proximal-vein thrombosis who have relative contraindications to anticoagulant therapy, the preferred treatment is carefully controlled continuous IV heparin, maintaining the anticoagulant effect near the lower limit of the therapeutic range (see later discussion), or interruption of the inferior vena cava.

The optimum management of patients with calf vein thrombosis has not been completely resolved. Two approaches are currently available: (1) initial heparin therapy followed by long-term anticoagulant therapy or (2) surveillance with serial objective testing for proximal-vein thrombosis (e.g., using impedance plethysmography or duplex ul-

Differential diagnosis of clinical features of pulmonary embolism

Dyspnea
Atelectasis
Pneumonia
Pneumothorax
Acute pulmonary edema
Acute bronchitis
Acute bronchiolitis
Acute bronchial obstruction

Acute right-sided heart failure
Myocardial infarction
Myocarditis
Cardiac tamponade
Acute respiratory infection
Complicating chronic lung disease

Pleuritic chest pain
Pneumonia
Pneumothorax
Pericarditis
Pulmonary neoplasm
Bronchiectasis
Subdiaphragmatic inflammation
Myositis
Muscle strain
Rib fracture

Cardiovascular collapse
Myocardial infarction
Acute massive hemorrhage
Gram-negative septicemia
Cardiac tamponade
Spontaneous pneumothorax

Hemoptysis
Pneumonia
Bronchial neoplasm
Bronchiectasis
Acute bronchitis
Mitral stenosis
Tuberculosis

Contraindications to anticoagulant therapy

Absolute contraindications
Subarachnoid or cerebral hemorrhage
Serious active bleeding (postoperative, spontaneous, or associated with trauma)
Recent brain, eye, or spinal cord surgery
Malignant hypertension

Relative contraindications
Recent major surgery
Recent cerebrovascular accident (stroke)
Active gastrointestinal hemorrhage
Severe hypertension
Hemorrhagic diathesis
Bacterial endocarditis
Severe renal failure
Severe hepatic failure

trasound) to detect and treat those patients who develop proximal extension. If untreated, approximately 20% of calf vein thrombi extend into the proximal venous segment. Pulmonary embolism is unlikely in the absence of proximal-vein thrombosis. Recent prospective clinical trials in patients with suspected venous thrombosis indicate that anticoagulant therapy can be safely withheld if the results of the impedance plethysmography (which is insensitive for calf vein thrombosis, but highly sensitive for proximal-vein thrombosis), remain negative on repeated testing over 10 to 14 days. Negative findings by serial impedance plethysmography are associated with a low risk of clinically important pulmonary embolism (less than 1%) or recurrent venous thrombosis (2%). Thus surveillance with serial impedance plethysmography can be used to separate the 20% of patients with calf vein thrombosis who develop proximal extension (and require treatment) from the 80% who do not extend, in whom the risks and costs of anticoagulant therapy may outweigh the benefits. If impedance plethysmography is not available to monitor for extension, patients with calf vein thrombosis should be treated initially with heparin and then with adequate long-term anticoagulant therapy.

Anticoagulant therapy for venous thromboembolism

Heparin. Heparin continues to be the initial treatment of choice for most patients with venous thrombosis or pulmonary embolism because it is both effective and relatively safe. Heparin can be administered intravenously or subcutaneously. Continuous IV infusion is the preferred approach. Intermittent IV injection is associated with a greater risk of bleeding and should be reserved for patients in whom continuous infusion and anticoagulant monitoring is not possible. A practical intermittent IV regimen is 5000 units (U) every 4 hours (30,000/24 hr). Interest has reawakened in the use of subcutaneous (SC) injection for initial heparin therapy, but further clinical trials are required to establish the effectiveness of this approach and to define the optimum regimen.

Recent clinical trials have improved our knowledge of the relations among heparin dose, anticoagulant response, and effectiveness of heparin therapy for preventing recurrent venous thromboembolism. Low doses of SC heparin (5000 U every 12 hours) provide effective prophylaxis against venous thromboembolism in moderate-risk to high-risk general surgical patients but are not effective for preventing recurrent venous thromboembolism in patients with established proximal-vein thrombosis. This difference in the dose of heparin required for the prevention and treatment of proximal-vein thrombosis is probably caused by the biochemical amplification that occurs with each successive step in the blood coagulation pathway. Consequently, much lower doses of heparin are required to prevent thrombin generation and the formation of venous thrombi than are required to inhibit thrombin activity and to prevent extension or recurrence of established thrombosis.

The findings of a randomized trial comparing intermittent SC heparin with continuous IV heparin infusion for the initial treatment of proximal-vein thrombosis strongly suggest a relation between the intensity of anticoagulant response and the effectiveness of initial heparin therapy. Eleven of 57 patients (19%) given SC heparin developed symptomatic recurrent venous thromboembolism confirmed by objective testing, whereas only 3 of 58 patients (5%) given IV heparin ($p = 0.024$) did so. In the group given SC heparin (15,000 U every 12 hours), 36 of 57 patients (63%) had an APTT response of less than 1.5 times control during the initial 24 hours or more, compared with 17 of 58 patients (29%) receiving continuous IV heparin ($p < 0.001$). All but one of the recurrences occurred in patients with an inadequate initial anticoagulant response (APTT less than 1.5 times control) (Table 86-2). Recurrent venous thromboembolism occurred in 25% of patients with an inadequate initial anticoagulant response but was virtually eliminated in both treatment groups in patients whose anticoagulant response was greater than the lower limit of the therapeutic range (APTT greater than 1.5 times control) (Fig. 86-1). (The mean APTT responses during the first 5 days of initial heparin therapy in the SC and IV heparin groups for patients with and without recurrent venous thromboembolism, respectively, are shown in Fig. 86-1.) Thus the episodes of recurrent venous thromboembolism observed in this trial were associated with, and likely the result of, an inadequate anticoagulant response. These results strongly suggest that an adequate initial anticoagulant response (APTT of 1.5 or more times control) is required to prevent recurrent venous thromboembolism and support the clinical practice of monitoring heparin therapy with the APTT to ensure an adequate anticoagulant response is obtained.

Heparin is usually administered for 7 to 10 days, followed by a course of long-term anticoagulant therapy. Multiple randomized clinical trials have indicated that this approach is associated with a low frequency (less than 5%) of recurrent venous thromboembolism. An alternative approach is to commence heparin and oral anticoagulants together at the time of diagnosis and to discontinue heparin on the fourth or fifth day. If the latter approach is effective, it would avoid 4 to 5 days of unnecessary hospitaliza-

Table 86-2. Frequency of recurrent venous thromboembolism according to whether activated partial thromboplastin time (APTT) response was above or below 1.5 times control

Treatment group	Frequency of recurrent venous thromboembolism (no. of patients [%])		p value
	APTT response <1.5	APTT response ≥1.5	
Subcutaneous	10/36 (27.8)	1/21 (4.8)	0.041
Intravenous	3/17 (17.6)	0/41	0.022
All patients*	13/53 (24.5)	1/62 (1.6)	<0.001

From Hull R et al: N Engl J Med 315:1109, 1986. Reprinted with permission.
*The relative risk of recurrent venous thromboembolism was 15 times higher in patients with an APTT response below the lower limit (1.5 times control) of the prescribed range for 24 hours or more from the start of therapy than in patients with an APTT response at or above the lower limit.

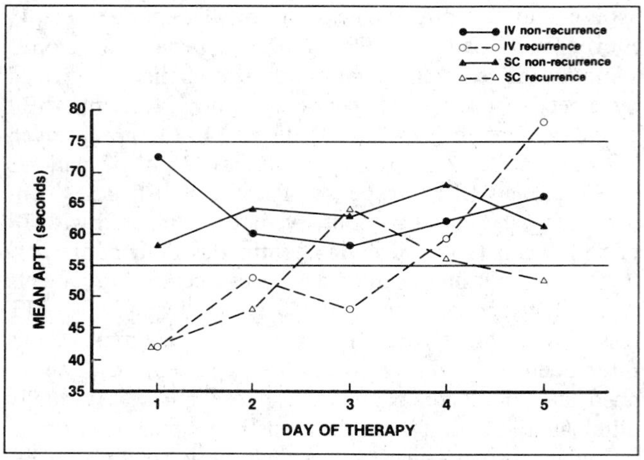

Fig. 86-1. Mean values for activated partial thromboplastin time *(APTT)* during initial therapy with intravenous *(IV)* or subcutaneous *(SC)* heparin in patients with and without recurrent venous thromboembolism. On day 1 the mean values in the subcutaneously and intravenously treated groups were 57.7 and 73.4 seconds, respectively, in patients without recurrent venous thromboembolism ($p = 0.002$), and 42.3 and 42.3 seconds, respectively, in patients with recurrent venous thromboembolism; the difference in mean APTTs between patients with and without recurrence was significant ($p = 0.006$). (From Hull R et al: N Engl J Med 315:1109, 1986. Reprinted with permission.)

tion in many patients and reduce the cost of initial heparin therapy. A recent randomized trial indicates that 4 to 5 days of initial heparin therapy is effective and safe in patients with submassive venous thromboembolism. This approach must be evaluated by further randomized clinical trials before it is routinely recommended for patients with extensive proximal-vein thrombosis.

Heparin currently in use clinically is polydispersed unmodified heparin, with a mean molecular weight ranging from 10,000 to 16,000 daltons. In recent years, low-molecular-weight derivatives of commercial heparin have been prepared that have a mean molecular weight of 4000 to 5000 daltons. Recent pharmacologic studies with low-molecular-weight SC heparin indicate that some of these heparin fractions have greater bioavailability and have a longer duration of anticoagulant effect (anti-Xa activity) than does SC unfractionated heparin. The anticoagulant response (anti-Xa activity) to SC low-molecular-weight heparin is highly correlated with body weight.

Several different low-molecular-weight heparins and one heparinoid are available for study, and five low-molecular-weight heparins have been approved for prophylactic use in Europe. A number of trials of deep vein thrombosis prophylaxis have been carried out in general and orthopedic surgery in both Europe and North America. A recent analysis indicates that the low-molecular-weight heparins are as effective as unfractionated heparin in the prevention of deep vein thrombosis, with the added convenience of once-daily administration. However, the incidence of postoperative bleeding may be somewhat higher than with low-dose unfractionated heparin. A recent multicenter trial comparing low-molecular-weight heparin with unfractionated heparin in the initial management of proximal-vein thrombosis revealed a significant decrease in recurrent thromboembolic events throughout the trial and decreased major bleeding in the trial's initial phase in the low-molecular-weight heparin group. The incidence of major bleeding was higher in the low-molecular-weight heparin group during the long-term warfarin treatment phase. This suggests that unfractionated heparin, with its greater tendency to cause bleeding in the initial phase of treatment, probably unmasked underlying bleeding lesions early, whereas these only became evident in the low-molecular-weight heparin group during long-term treatment. Low-molecular-weight heparin offers the convenience of daily SC administration and no dosage adjustment. When these agents become available, they will undoubtedly replace IV unfractionated heparin in the initial management of patients with proximal-vein thrombosis, as well as in the management of other patients in whom IV heparin is currently used.

Initial intravenous heparin protocol. Heparin is given as an initial IV of 5000 U, followed by a maintenance infusion of 30,000 to 40,000 U/24 hr. Laboratory monitoring with the APTT (or heparin level) is performed 4 to 6 hours after the initial bolus injection to ensure that an adequate anticoagulant response is obtained. A sufficient 24-hour heparin dose should be administered to maintain the APTT greater than 1.5 times the control value; in most patients, this anticoagulant response is equivalent to 0.3 to 0.5 U heparin/ml using protamine sulfate neutralization. If the APTT response is less than 1.5 times control, the 24-hour heparin dose should be augmented by 2000 to 4000 U and the APTT repeated 4 to 6 hours later. If the APTT shows very little or no prolongation, an IV heparin bolus of 2000 to 5000 U can also be given to obtain an immediate effect. If the APTT response is greater than 2 times control, the maintenance infusion is stopped for 1 hour and restarted with the total daily (24-hour) heparin dose reduced by 2000 to 4000 U. The APTT should be repeated 4 to 6 hours after restarting the infusion. Once the patient's APTT response and heparin dose requirements are stabilized, the APTT is measured daily for the duration of initial treatment.

A protocol has been reported for the IV administration of unfractionated heparin that guarantees that the optimum therapeutic range with respect to APTT is reached within the first 24 hours of treatment and maintained within that range throughout the course of treatment. The incidence of recurrence was low. The PTT was greater than the therapeutic range in a significant number of patients, but the incidence of bleeding did not correlate with the supratherapeutic values. Bleeding, however, was closely related to the pretreatment assessment of bleeding risk, corroborating previous observations that bleeding in patients receiving heparin is related to underlying risk rather than the PTT level. An interesting diurnal variation in the PTT values was observed, with the peak levels occurring early in the morning. This circadian rhythm was unrelated to any change in heparin dosage. This periodicity could result in inadvertent administration of an inadequate heparin dose if an incorrect adjustment of the heparin infusion is made in response to the early-morning PTT value.

Long-term subcutaneous heparin therapy. Adjusted-dose SC heparin is the long-term anticoagulant regimen of choice in pregnant patients, patients at high risk of bleeding, and patients who return to geographically remote areas in which long-term anticoagulant monitoring is unavailable or impractical (in whom the heparin dose is adjusted during the first few days of long-term therapy and then fixed). The starting dose of long-term SC heparin is determined from the patient's initial IV heparin dose requirement. A starting SC dose equivalent to one third of the patient's 24-hour IV heparin dose is administered every 12 hours. For example, if the patient required 30,000 U/24 hr of continuous IV heparin to maintain the APTT greater than 1.5 times the control value, the starting dose of long-term SC heparin would be 10,000 U every 12 hours. The SC dose is adjusted during the first few days of long-term therapy to maintain the midinterval APTT (determined 6 hours after injection) at 1.5 times the control value. This level of anticoagulant response is usually achieved with a dose of 8000 to 12,000 U every 12 hours (mean dose, 10,000 U every 12 hours). In pregnant patients, larger doses may be required, and continued monitoring is desired because of changes in heparin requirements throughout the course of pregnancy.

Adverse effects of heparin therapy. The side effects of heparin therapy include bleeding, thrombocytopenia, arterial thromboembolism, hypersensitivity, and osteoporosis.

Bleeding, the most common side effect of heparin, occurs in 5% to 10% of patients during initial continuous IV heparin therapy. At particular risk are those patients who have been exposed to recent surgery or trauma and those with an underlying hemostatic defect or predisposing clinical risk factor (e.g., unsuspected peptic ulcer or occult carcinoma). The risk of bleeding complications is greater in patients who receive IV heparin by intermittent injection than in those who receive continuous infusion.

The onset of thrombocytopenia, now a well-recognized complication of heparin therapy, usually occurs 7 to 10 days after heparin treatment is commenced but may be earlier in patients previously exposed to heparin. This complication has been seen with the low-molecular-weight heparins as well, although the exact incidence with these agents is as yet undetermined. Heparin-induced thrombocytopenia occurs more often in patients receiving beef-lung heparin than in those receiving porcine-gut heparin. The thrombocytopenia may be moderate or severe. The precise mechanism of heparin-induced thrombocytopenia is currently unknown but probably involves immune mechanisms, particularly in the severe forms. Although the severe form is less common than the moderate form, it is currently unknown how frequently patients with moderate thrombocytopenia may progress to the severe form with the added complication of arterial thrombosis. This may precede or coincide with the fall in platelet count. Heparin-induced thrombocytopenia with arterial thrombosis results in a high-incidence of limb amputation and mortality. It is therefore mandatory that heparin in all forms be discontinued when heparin-induced thrombocytopenia is diagnosed. Alternate approaches to treatment include insertion of an inferior vena caval filter or the use of Arvin (ancrod), a defibrinogenating extract of snake venom that produces effective anticoagulation while oral anticoagulants are being instituted. A heparinoid consisting mainly of dermatan sulfate along with heparan and condroitin sulfate (ORG 10172; Lomoparin) does not cross-react with heparin using in vitro immunoassays and has been used effectively in a few patients with heparin-induced thrombocytopenia.

Osteoporosis occurs rarely in patients receiving long-term SC heparin therapy (>15,000 U/day for longer than 6 months). The earliest clinical manifestation of heparin-associated osteoporosis is usually the onset of nonspecific low-back pain primarily involving the vertebrae or ribs; patients may also have spontaneous fracture in these areas.

Hypersensitivity to heparin occurs infrequently and may take the form of a skin rash or, less often, anaphylaxis. Alopecia has been reported as a rare complication of heparin. Serum transaminase levels may be moderately raised. Rarely, a bluish discoloration of the toes, associated with a burning sensation, has been reported.

Antidote to heparin. The anticoagulant effect of heparin can be immediately neutralized by the IV injection of protamine sulfate. The appropriate neutralizing dose depends on the dose of heparin, its route of administration, and the time it is given. If protamine sulfate is used within minutes of an IV heparin injection, a full neutralizing dose (1 mg protamine sulfate/100 U heparin) should be given. Because the plasma half-life of IV heparin is approximately 60 minutes, an injection of protamine sulfate in a bolus of more than 50 mg is seldom required. An occasional hypotensive response to protamine sulfate has been reported; therefore it should be injected slowly over 10 to 30 minutes. Treatment with protamine sulfate may need to be repeated because protamine is cleared from the blood more quickly than heparin. After an SC injection of heparin, repeated small doses of protamine may be required because of prolonged heparin absorption from the SC depot.

Oral anticoagulant therapy. There are two distinct chemical groups of oral anticoagulants; the 4-hydroxy coumarin derivatives (e.g., warfarin sodium) and the indane-1,3-dione derivatives (e.g., phenindione). The coumarin derivatives are the oral anticoagulants of choice because they are associated with fewer nonhemorrhagic side effects than are the indanedione derivatives (see later section on adverse effects).

Oral anticoagulants produce an anticoagulant effect by inhibiting the vitamin K–dependent γ-carboxylation of coagulation factors II, VII, IX, and X. This results in the synthesis of immunologically detectable but biologically inactive forms of these coagulation proteins. Oral anticoagulants also inhibit the vitamin K–dependent γ-carboxylation of proteins C and S. Protein C circulates as a proenzyme that is activated on endothelial cells by the thrombin/thrombomodulin complex to form activated protein C. Activated protein C inhibits activated factor VIII activity directly, and in the presence of protein S, it also inhibits activated factor V. Therefore vitamin K antagonists such as warfarin sodium create a biochemical paradox by producing an anticoagulant effect because of the inhibition of procoagulants (factors II, VII, IX, X) and a potentially thrombogenic effect by impairing the synthesis of naturally occurring inhibitors of coagulation (proteins C and S).

The anticoagulant effect of the vitamin K antagonists is delayed until the normal clotting factors are cleared from the circulation, and the peak effect does not occur until 36 to 72 hours after drug administration. With a 40 mg loading dose, factor VII levels usually fall rapidly to less than 20% of normal, and sometimes to less than 10% of normal for as long as 3 to 4 days. In some patients, suppression of factor VII to this level is seen within 24 hours. Sick patients with impaired liver function or reduced vitamin K stores are particularly susceptible to large loading doses. Equilibrium levels of factors II, IX, and X are not reached until about 1 week after the initiation of therapy. The equilibrium levels of these factors are not achieved more quickly by using a large loading dose (e.g., 40 mg). Therefore the use of small initial daily doses (e.g., 10 mg) is the preferred approach for initiating warfarin treatment.

A 4- to 5-day overlap with IV heparin during the initiation of warfarin sodium therapy is important. In a recent trial comparing IV heparin plus oral warfarin with oral warfarin alone, the incidence of recurrent thromboembolic events was shown to be excessively high in the warfarin group. Experimental evidence indicates that the maximum antithrombotic effect of warfarin is delayed for as long as 5 days, even though the anticoagulant effect, reflected by an increase in the prothrombin time (PT; mainly caused by a reduction in factor VII), may be evident within 2 to 3 days. Factor VII and protein C have similar short half-lives (approximately 4 to 5 hours). During the first 24 to 48 hours of warfarin sodium therapy, the levels of functional factor VII and protein C fall while the levels of functionally active factors II, IX, and X remain relatively normal. Thus, during the first 24 to 48 hours of therapy, oral anticoagulants have the potential to be thrombogenic, since the anticoagulant effect of low functional factor VII is counteracted by the potentially thrombogenic effect of low levels of functional protein C, with near-normal levels of functional factors II, IX, and X. After 72 to 96 hours the levels of functional factors II, IX, and X fall, and the optimum anticoagulant activity of warfarin therapy is expressed. For these reasons, it is important to overlap oral anticoagulant therapy with heparin therapy for 4 to 5 days, even though the PT may be prolonged into the therapeutic range after 2 to 3 days.

The laboratory test most often used to measure the effects of warfarin is the one-stage PT, which is sensitive to reduced activity of factors II, VII, and X but is insensitive to reduced activity of factor IX. The optimum therapeutic range for oral anticoagulant therapy monitored using the PT has been controversial because, until recently, it had not been adequately evaluated in clinical trials. Further confusion about the appropriate therapeutic range occurred because the different tissue thromboplastins used for measuring the PT vary considerably in sensitivity to the vitamin K–dependent clotting factors and in response to warfarin. Rabbit brain thromboplastin, which is widely used in North America, is less sensitive than is standardized human brain thromboplastin, which has been widely used in the United Kingdom and other parts of Europe. A PT ratio of 1.5 to 2.0 using rabbit brain thromboplastin (i.e., the traditional therapeutic range in North America) is equivalent to a ratio of 4.0 to 6.0 using human brain thromboplastin. Conversely, a twofold to threefold increase in the PT using standardized human brain thromboplastin is equivalent to a 1.25-fold to 1.5-fold increase in the PT using a rabbit brain thromboplastin such as Simplastin or Dade-C.

The optimum therapeutic range for oral anticoagulant therapy in patients with venous thrombosis has recently been established. The findings of randomized trials indicate that venous thrombosis can be treated effectively and more safely with a therapeutic range of 1.25 to 1.5 times the control value using a rabbit brain thromboplastin such as Simplastin or Dade-C, rather than the range of 1.5 to 2.0 times control conventionally recommended in North America.

To promote standardization of the PT for monitoring oral anticoagulant therapy, the World Health Organization (WHO) has developed an international reference thromboplastin from human brain tissue and has recommended that the PT ratio be expressed as the International Normalized Ratio (INR). The INR is the PT ratio obtained by testing a given sample using the WHO reference thromboplastin. For practical clinical purposes, the INR for a given plasma sample is equivalent to the PT ratio obtained using a standardized human brain thromboplastin known as the Manchester Comparative Reagent, which has been widely used in the United Kingdom. The currently recommended therapeutic range of 1.25 to 1.5 times control using a rabbit brain thromboplastin such as Simplastin or Dade-C corresponds to an INR of 2.0 to 3.0.

Oral anticoagulant (warfarin sodium) protocol. Warfarin sodium is administered in an initial dose of 10 mg/day for the first 2 days, and the daily dose is then adjusted according to the PT. Heparin therapy is discontinued on the fourth or fifth day after initiation of warfarin therapy, providing the PT is prolonged into the therapeutic range (PT 1.25 to 1.5 times control value, INR 2.0 to 3.0).

Once the anticoagulant effect and patient's warfarin dose requirements are stable, the PT is monitored weekly throughout the course of oral anticoagulant therapy. However, if factors exist that may produce an unpredictable response to warfarin (e.g., concomitant drug therapy), the PT should be monitored more frequently to minimize the risk of complications caused by poor anticoagulant control.

Attempts have been made to improve the control of oral anticoagulants while at the same time decreasing the risk of bleeding complications. These have included the use of warfarin protocols to predict dosing requirements, the development of anticoagulant clinics, or the use of a prothrombin home monitor device. An alternative to PT measurement is the use of an immunoassay to detect native prothrombin antigen. Early clinical trials indicate that ultra-low-dose warfarin therapy may be effective prophylaxis in certain patients. Such treatment does not significantly prolong the PT, and other methods must be used for control, such as the measurement of prothrombin fragments 1.2 or an assay of activated factor VII.

Adverse effects of oral anticoagulants. The major side effect of oral anticoagulant therapy is bleeding. This is discussed in detail in Chapter 85. Bleeding during well-controlled oral anticoagulant therapy is usually caused by surgery or other forms of trauma or by local lesions such as peptic ulcer or carcinoma. Spontaneous bleeding may occur if warfarin sodium is given in an excessive dose, resulting in marked prolongation of the PT; this bleeding may be severe and even life-threatening. The risk of bleeding can be substantially reduced by adjusting the warfarin dose to achieve a less intense anticoagulant effect than has traditionally been used in North America (PT 1.25 to 1.5 times control using a rabbit brain thromboplastin such as Simplastin or Dade-C, INR 2.0 to 3.0).

Nonhemorrhagic side effects of oral anticoagulants differ according to whether the coumarin derivatives (e.g., warfarin sodium) or indanediones are administered. Nonhemorrhagic side effects of coumarin anticoagulants occur infrequently, and the coumarins are the oral anticoagulants of choice. Nonhemorrhagic side effects occur more frequently with the indanedione derivatives and include skin necrosis, dermatitis, and a syndrome of painful blue toes. Hypersensitivity reactions have been reported to occur in 1% to 3% of patients receiving indanedione derivatives and include rash, fever, hepatitis, leukopenia, renal failure, and diarrhea; these side effects are sometimes fatal. The indanedione derivatives also produce red discoloration of the urine in many patients, which may be confused with hematuria.

Coumarin-induced skin necrosis is a rare but serious complication that requires immediate cessation of oral anticoagulant therapy. It usually occurs 3 to 10 days after therapy has commenced, is more common in women, and most often involves areas of abundant subcutaneous tissues such as the abdomen, buttocks, thighs, and breast. The mechanism of coumarin-induced skin necrosis, which is associated with microvascular thrombosis, is uncertain but appears to be related, at least in some patients, to the depression of protein C. Patients with congenital deficiencies of protein C may be particularly prone to the development of coumarin skin necrosis.

It has recently been shown that oral anticoagulants may affect bone mineral metabolism. Two major components of bone matrix require vitamin K for γ-carboxylation (osteocalcin and matrix Gla-protein [MGP]), and levels of these proteins and mean bone mass are decreased in patients receiving long-term oral anticoagulant therapy when compared with age-matched control subjects. Many patients with osteoporosis and fracture of the femur or vertebral bodies have decreased levels of circulating vitamin K, and the administration of vitamin K will correct low osteocalcin levels. Studies are currently under way to assess further the impact of oral anticoagulants on bone mineral metabolism, particularly in elderly females or patients being administered lifelong oral anticoagulants.

Oral anticoagulants cross the placenta and may cause fetal malformations when used during pregnancy. Two specific fetopathic syndromes are associated with oral anticoagulant administration during pregnancy. Treatment with oral anticoagulants during the sixth to twelfth weeks of gestation may induce the syndrome of *warfarin embryopathy* in the fetus. This syndrome consists of skeletal abnormalities ranging from stippled epiphyses to frank skeletal hypoplasia. Although most reported cases have occurred in infants of mothers receiving warfarin, it has also been reported as a result of phenindanedione or acenocoumarin administration. Oral anticoagulant administration during the second or third trimester of pregnancy may result in central nervous system abnormalities in the fetus, including abnormalities of the ventricular system (Dandy-Walker malformation), dorsal midline dysplasia, and optic atrophy. Therefore the use of oral anticoagulants is contraindicated at any time during pregnancy, and they should not be used in women planning a pregnancy.

Oral anticoagulants may be secreted in the milk of nursing mothers, and the use of these agents in lactating women remains controversial. Recent studies in small numbers of patients have indicated that the PT and levels of factors II, VII, and X in breast-fed infants were normal, even though the nursing mother received therapeutic doses of warfarin sodium. Further studies are required to make firm clinical recommendations about the use of warfarin in lactating women.

A recent report assessed quality of life parameters in patients receiving low-intensity warfarin compared with those not taking warfarin. Oral anticoagulants did not affect quality of life parameters except in those patients with bleeding complications. The patients in this study were older (mean age, 68 years), and the outcomes may not be applicable to younger patients receiving long-term anticoagulants, who may experience more inconvenience and lifestyle changes.

Factors that interact with effect of oral anticoagulant therapy. Many drugs interact with oral anticoagulants and may produce either a prolongation or a reduction in the anticoagulant effect (see the box on p. 830). Special care should be taken to adjust the dose of oral anticoagulant during the time that other drugs are being taken to minimize the risk of inadequate anticoagulant control.

Increased sensitivity to oral anticoagulants occurs in vitamin K deficiency, impaired liver function, and thyrotoxicosis because of the more rapid metabolism of the vitamin K–dependent clotting factors.

Antidote to oral anticoagulants. The antidote to the vitamin K antagonists is vitamin K_1. If the PT is excessively prolonged, treatment depends on the degree of prolongation and whether or not the patient is bleeding. If the prolongation is mild (i.e., less than three times the control value) and the patient is not bleeding, no specific treatment is necessary other than reduction in the warfarin dose. The PT can be expected to decrease during the next 24 hours with this approach. With more marked prolongation of PT in patients who are not bleeding, treatment with small doses of vitamin K_1, given either orally or by SC injection (2.5 to 5.0 mg), could be considered. With very marked prolon-

Drug interactions with oral anticoagulants

Increase anticoagulant effect

Allopurinol
Anabolic steroids
Chloramphenicol
Clofibrate
Co-trimoxazole (trimethoprim and sulfamethoxazole)
Dextrothyroxine
Disulfiram
Mefenamic acid
Neomycin
Nortriptyline
Oxyphenbutazone
Phenylbutazone
Phenyramidol
Quinidine
Salicylate
Sulfaphenazole
Sulfafurazole (sulfisoxazole)
Sulfinpyrazone

Decrease anticoagulant effect

Barbiturates
Cholestyramine
Dichloralphenazone
Diuretics
Estrogens
Glutethimide
Griseofulvin
Heptabarbitone
Phenytoin
Rifampicin

gation of the PT, particularly in a patient who is either actively bleeding or at risk of bleeding, vitamin K_1 should be given.

Second-generation rodenticides known as "super warfarins" have an extremely long half-life. Accidental or intentional consumption of these agents requires repeated injection of vitamin K and fresh-frozen plasma for up to 1 to 2 years to overcome their effects completely.

Reported side effects of vitamin K include flushing, dizziness, tachycardia, hypotension, dyspnea, and sweating. IV administration of vitamin K_1 should be done with caution to avoid inducing an anaphylactoid reaction. The risk of anaphylactoid reaction can be reduced by giving vitamin K_1 slowly, at a rate no faster than 1 mg/min IV. In most patients, IV administration of vitamin K_1 produces a demonstrable effect on the PT within 3 to 4 hours and corrects the prolonged PT within 6 to 8 hours. Because the half-life of vitamin K_1 is less than that of warfarin sodium, a repeat course of vitamin K_1 may be necessary. If bleeding is very severe and life-threatening, vitamin K therapy can be supplemented by using concentrates of factors II, VII, IX, and X.

Thrombolytic therapy for venous thromboembolism. The frequency of clinically evident recurrent venous thromboembolism is very low during anticoagulant therapy, and this remains the treatment of choice in most patients. Theoretically, anticoagulant therapy is not ideal, however, because it does not induce thrombolysis. Thus, although anticoagulant therapy is highly effective in reducing the important immediate complications of venous thromboembolism, it may be relatively ineffective at preventing the late sequelae (e.g., postphlebitic syndrome). For these reasons, thrombolytic therapy is recommended in selected patients with acute massive venous thrombosis or massive pulmonary embolism.

Advocates of thrombolytic therapy point out that it may achieve the following objectives of ideal management: (1) lysis of the thrombi and emboli with circulation restored to normal, (2) rapid reduction of hemodynamic disturbances, and (3) prevention or minimizing of damage to the pulmonary vascular bed, reducing the likelihood of persistent pulmonary hypertension. In patients with venous thrombosis the use of thrombolytic therapy is based on the premise that thrombolysis can minimize or prevent venous valvular damage and prevent the postphlebitic syndrome. Unfortunately, this may not be the case, since the critical factor in the development of the postphlebitic syndrome appears to be venous valve damage, which occurs early in the formation of the venous thrombus and may not necessarily be restored by thrombolysis.

Thrombolytic agents currently available for clinical use in patients with venous thromboembolism include streptokinase and urokinase. Streptokinase, a product of hemolytic streptococci, combines with plasminogen, producing a conformational change that exposes an active site, which in turn converts noncomplexed plasminogen to plasmin by proteolytic cleavage. Streptokinase is antigenic in humans and stimulates the production of neutralizing antibodies. Urokinase, which is isolated from human urine or from cultures of human embryonic kidney cells, is nonantigenic. Newer thrombolytic agents (e.g., tissue plasminogen activator, tPA) are currently undergoing clinical evaluation for treatment of venous thromboembolism.

Thrombolytic therapy with streptokinase, urokinase, or tPA is more effective than heparin for inducing rapid resolution of recent venous thrombi and pulmonary emboli. In patients with massive pulmonary embolism, the degree of lysis can be striking. The use of streptokinase or urokinase for 12 to 24 hours followed by conventional anticoagulant therapy is indicated in patients with massive pulmonary embolism. Thrombolytic therapy should also be considered in patients with pulmonary embolism and underlying severe cardiac or pulmonary disease in whom even a small or moderate embolus may be life-threatening.

Thrombolytic therapy may benefit selected patients with acute massive venous thrombosis, such as those with phlegmasia cerulea dolens. In most patients with acute deep vein thrombosis, however, the indication for thrombolytic therapy remains controversial. Currently, randomized clinical trials have yielded no definitive evidence that thrombolytic therapy is associated with improved benefit by prevention of the postphlebitic syndrome.

The following guidelines are recommended for patient selection for thrombolytic therapy:

1. The presence of an appropriate clinical indication, including an objectively documented diagnosis and evidence that the venous thromboembolic event is of recent origin (less than 7 days)
2. Careful evaluation of contraindications (see the box below).

Before thrombolytic therapy is begun, the diagnosis of venous thromboembolism should be established by objective means. If pulmonary angiography is performed to confirm a diagnosis of pulmonary embolism, the angiography catheter should be inserted into an arm vein, where hemostasis is easier to achieve than in the femoral vein.

Complications of thrombolytic therapy. The major complication of thrombolytic therapy is hemorrhage. Thrombolytic therapy produces lysis of fibrin in hemostatic plugs in wounds, and therefore bleeding occurs more frequently than with heparin. Review of the published data suggests that the risk of major hemorrhage or intracerebral hemorrhage with streptokinase is approximately twice that associated with heparin therapy. Bleeding complications occur in 30% or more of patients treated with streptokinase infusions for more than 12 hours. The risk of hemorrhage increases with the length of the infusion and occurs most often from sites of previous surgery or trauma or from sites of vascular invasion, such as needle puncture wounds and cutdown sites for catheterization. In about one third of patients, bleeding commences during thrombolytic therapy; in the remainder, it is first noted after completion of thrombolytic therapy and during anticoagulant therapy. Bleeding may also occur from the genitourinary or gastrointestinal tract; occasionally, cerebral bleeding occurs. Bleeding complications can be reduced by careful selection of patients and avoidance of treatment of those with contraindications.

Fever occurs in approximately 25% of patients receiving streptokinase. Allergic reactions occur in 10% of patients treated with streptokinase, usually in the form of pruritus or urticaria, but approximately 1% to 2% of patients may develop anaphylactic reactions. The allergic reactions to streptokinase can be promptly reversed by standard therapy, including epinephrine, IV corticosteroids, and antihistamines.

Antidote to thrombolytic therapy. If bleeding is life-threatening, the fibrinolytic process can be rapidly reversed by the infusion of 5 g of epsilon-aminocaproic acid (EACA, Amicar), given over a half-hour period and followed by 1 g/hr until hemostasis has been achieved. Antifibrinolytic therapy with EACA frequently must be supplemented with transfusions of fresh plasma or cryoprecipitate.

Contraindications to thrombolytic therapy

Absolute contraindications

Active internal bleeding
Recent (within 2 months) cerebrovascular accident or other active intracranial processes

Relative major contraindications

Recent (<10 days) major surgery
Recent obstetric delivery
Recent organ biopsy
Recent previous puncture of noncompressible vessels
Recent serious gastrointestinal bleeding
Recent serious trauma
Severe hypertension (systolic >200 mm Hg, diastolic > 110 mm Hg)

Relative minor contraindications

Recent minor trauma, including cardiopulmonary resuscitation
High likelihood of left-sided heart thrombus (e.g., mitral stenosis with atrial fibrillation)
Bacterial endocarditis
Diabetic hemorrhagic retinopathy
Pregnancy
Age >75 years

Management of massive pulmonary embolism. Most patients who die from pulmonary embolism do so within 2 hours. In patients who survive for more than 2 hours, the prognosis with standard anticoagulant therapy is usually excellent, and invasive procedures such as pulmonary embolectomy have little or no place. Thrombolytic therapy produces rapid lysis of pulmonary emboli and helps patients with cardiorespiratory decompensation by promoting more rapid resolution of the pulmonary emboli during the first few days than does standard anticoagulant therapy.

Inferior vena caval interruption. Inferior vena caval interruption by intraluminal or extraluminal approaches should be used in the following circumstances:

1. In the patient with acute venous thromboembolism and an absolute contraindication to anticoagulant therapy (see the box on p. 824)
2. In the rare patient with massive pulmonary embolism who survives but in whom recurrent embolism may be fatal
3. In the very rare patient who has objectively documented recurrent venous thromboembolism during adequate anticoagulant therapy

Inferior vena caval interruption has the potential for increasing the risk of long-term sequelae (e.g., more severe postphlebitic syndrome), and it may be ineffective in preventing late embolic recurrence because of the development of collaterals that bypass the inferior vena caval interruption. The frequency of these late complications can be reduced by using the Greenfield filter (a transvenously inserted filter), which is associated with a very low frequency of loss of patency.

MANAGEMENT OF SUPERFICIAL THROMBOPHLEBITIS

Superficial thrombophlebitis may occur with or without associated deep venous thrombosis. In the absence of associated deep vein thrombosis, the treatment of superficial thrombophlebitis is usually confined to symptomatic relief with analgesia and rest of the affected limb. The exception is the patient with superficial thrombophlebitis involving a large segment of the long saphenous vein, particularly when it occurs above the knee; these patients should be treated with either heparin therapy or superficial venous ligation.

Patients in whom superficial thrombophlebitis occurs in association with deep vein thrombosis should be treated with full-dose heparin therapy followed by long-term oral anticoagulant therapy (see previous sections on heparin protocol and oral anticoagulant protocol).

ARTERIAL THROMBOEMBOLISM

Etiology and pathogenesis

Arterial thrombi (white thrombi) are composed predominantly of platelets and fibrin, in contrast to venous thrombi (red thrombi), which consist primarily of red cells and fibrin. Arterial thromboemboli usually occur when platelets come into contact with exposed subendothelium at the site of vascular injury or with a prosthetic surface. The platelets adhere, undergo the release reaction, and aggregate; if these aggregates are sufficiently large or if the atherosclerotic stenosis is severe, an occlusive thrombus may form. Frequently, however, the platelet aggregates embolize to obstruct the arterial circulation distally. Thus the clinical manifestations of arterial thromboembolism may be the result of occlusive thrombus formation (e.g., acute coronary thrombosis), which usually occurs on a background of ruptured or ulcerated atherosclerotic plaque, or the result of peripheral embolization of platelet-fibrin aggregates (e.g., transient cerebral ischemic attacks).

Systemic embolism is an important clinical sequela of arterial thrombosis. Prosthetic cardiac valves, prosthetic vascular grafts, and implanted catheters are sites for arterial thrombus formation and are important sources of systemic emboli. The introduction of a prosthetic material into the circulation exposes blood to a foreign surface that may induce platelet adhesion, aggregation, and embolization of the aggregated platelets. Furthermore, foreign surfaces may induce the activation of blood coagulation. Systemic embolism also occurs from left ventricular thrombi that form secondary to transmural myocardial infarction. Atrial fibrillation and valvular heart disease (e.g., rheumatic mitral stenosis) may also lead to systemic embolism (Chapter 16). Thrombi originating in the right side of the heart or on the surface of central venous catheters may lead to pulmonary embolism.

The various risk factors for atherosclerosis and arterial thromboembolism that have been identified include age, sex, hypertension, diabetes mellitus, smoking, obesity, hypercholesterolemia, and the inherited hyperlipidemic disorders.

A tendency to arterial thrombosis, which may be massive, may be seen in patients with the anticardiolipin syndrome or in those who develop heparin-induced thrombocytopenia and thrombosis.

Clinical features

The clinical manifestations of arterial thromboembolism are organ specific and depend on the particular area of the circulation affected.

Atherosclerotic narrowing of the coronary arteries with ruptured or ulcerated plaque may lead to thrombus formation; if a sufficient area of the lumen is occluded, myocardial infarction may result (Chapter 14). Left ventricular mural thrombosis frequently complicates the course of patients with transmural anterior myocardial infarction and poses the risk of systemic embolism.

Severe atherosclerosis of the carotid artery may progress to thrombotic occlusion and subsequent cerebrovascular accident (CVA, stroke); the junction of the vertebral and basilar arteries and the main bifurcation of the middle cerebral artery are also common sites for thrombosis (Chapter 120). Atherosclerotic narrowing of the carotid arteries may serve as a nidus for repeated formation and embolization of platelet aggregates to the cerebral circulation or to the eye. Repeated "showers" of platelet-fibrin emboli result in transient and reversible episodes of cerebral ischemia or episodes of amaurosis fugax (Chapter 120). These emboli usually lyse and disperse spontaneously, with resolution of the neurologic deficit during a period of hours.

Atherosclerosis frequently affects the large to medium-sized arteries of the lower limbs (e.g., distal aorta; iliac, femoral, and popliteal arteries); these lesions may serve as foci for the development of occlusive thrombi or as a source of distal embolization. Acute thrombotic occlusion of the large or medium-sized arteries of the leg results in limb-threatening ischemia; untreated, it may progress to ischemic necrosis. Distal embolization of platelet-fibrin thrombi from the proximal arteries of the leg may result in multiple discrete areas of localized tissue necrosis.

For a detailed discussion of the clinical features associated with atherosclerosis and thromboembolism in the coronary arteries, cerebral vasculature, and peripheral vessels, see Chapters 13, 120, and 22, respectively.

Laboratory features

A variety of laboratory abnormalities have been reported in patients with arterial thromboembolism, including elevated plasma levels of beta thromboglobulin and platelet factor 4 (indicating that platelets have undergone the release reaction) and elevated plasma levels of thromboxane B_2 (indicating that the platelet prostaglandin pathway has been activated). The continuous process of platelet adhesion, aggregation, and embolization may result in an increased platelet turnover (decreased survival), which can be detected by measuring the survival of isotopically labeled platelets injected intravenously. Although these laboratory tests have been useful research techniques that have provided important information about the pathophysiology of arterial thromboembolic disease, they currently have no role in patient management. Furthermore, these laboratory changes are nonspecific because many nonthrombogenic stimuli (e.g., trauma, infection, inflammation, infarction) may interact with platelets, inducing platelet release and prostaglandin formation and producing decreased platelet survival.

Treatment

Role of anticoagulant therapy. The objective of treating patients with arterial thromboembolism with anticoagulants is to prevent the clinical sequelae that occur as a consequence of thrombosis and systemic embolism. In contrast to the treatment of venous thromboembolism, the role of anticoagulant therapy in the management of patients with arterial thromboembolism is less certain. The exception is the prevention of systemic embolism, for which anticoagulant therapy is effective. The role of anticoagulant therapy in the management of individual clinical disorders of arterial thromboembolism is discussed in the next sections.

Traditionally, patients with arterial thromboembolism have been treated using a more intense oral anticoagulant regimen (PT 2.0 to 2.5 using rabbit brain thromboplastin, INR 4.0 to 10.0) than that used with patients with venous thromboembolism. Randomized clinical trials support the use of a less intense therapeutic range (INR 2.0 to 3.0) for the prevention of systemic embolism in patients with myocardial infarction, atrial fibrillation, and prosthetic cardiac valves.

Myocardial infarction. Anticoagulant therapy was recommended as part of the routine management of patients with myocardial infarction in the 1950s but later fell into disrepute because of the fear of bleeding complications and doubt about its effectiveness. The objectives of anticoagulant treatment in patients with myocardial infarction are (1) to improve survival; (2) to prevent recurrent infarction, mural thrombosis, and systemic embolism; and (3) to prevent the complication of venous thromboembolism (Chapter 14). Although there is consensus that anticoagulant therapy should be used for preventing systemic embolism, the use of long-term anticoagulant therapy for improving survival and preventing recurrent infarction has been controversial. The findings of recurrent randomized clinical trials have reopened this longstanding debate and have rekindled interest in the role of long-term anticoagulant therapy after myocardial infarction. The Sixty-Plus Reinfarction Study Research Group reported a 50% reduction in fatal and nonfatal reinfarction in elderly patients (over 60 years) treated with long-term oral anticoagulant therapy after myocardial infarction. In a more recent trial, warfarin treatment was associated with a 24% reduction in total mortality over 3 years (from 20% to 15.5%). The beneficial effect of warfarin persisted in patients who were also taking beta blockers on a long-term basis. Both trials evaluating long-term warfarin therapy after myocardial infarction used relatively intense warfarin therapy (INR 2.7 to 4.8), and trials are currently underway using less-intense warfarin or very-low-intensity warfarin plus low-dose acetylsalicylic acid (ASA, aspirin) in this setting.

Anticoagulant therapy is effective for preventing systemic embolism in patients with myocardial infarction. Cerebral embolism occurs in 2% to 4% of nonanticoagulated patients after myocardial infarction. Patients with transmural anterior myocardial infarction are at particularly high risk of mural thrombosis (30%) and systemic embolism (2% to 6%) and should be treated with anticoagulant therapy for the period of risk. Full-dose continuous IV heparin followed by warfarin sodium for up to 1 year is a current practical regimen. Further studies are required to establish definitively the most appropriate duration of anticoagulant therapy. Heparin is administered in full therapeutic doses to maintain the APTT at 1.5 to 2.0 times the control value; the protocol for heparin administration and the adverse effects of heparin are the same as those outlined previously for the treatment of venous thromboembolism. Therapeutic doses of heparin are used because the effectiveness of low-dose SC heparin for preventing systemic embolism is currently uncertain. Warfarin sodium is overlapped with IV heparin for 4 or 5 days and then continued long-term. Warfarin is administered according to the protocol outlined previously for venous thromboembolism to maintain the INR between 2.0 and 3.0.

Antiplatelet agents, primarily ASA, have been used in patients with cardiovascular diseases as an adjunct to thrombolytic therapy, in the prevention of myocardial infarction in patients with unstable angina, as secondary prophylaxis after an initial myocardial infarction, and as primary prophylaxis. When compared with placebo or no treatment, ASA has been shown to be superior in all these situations. A meta-analysis performed by the Antiplatelet Trialists Collaboration Group reviewed 25 randomized trials of antiplatelet treatment in patients with a history of transient ischemic attacks, occlusive CVA, unstable angina, or myocardial infarction. Vascular mortality and occurrence of a nonfatal vascular event (CVA or myocardial infarction) were reduced. The addition of dipyridamole to aspirin had no benefit. A larger meta-analysis of antiplatelet drug therapy is currently under review by the same group.

Cerebrovascular disease. For practical purposes, patients with thromboembolic cerebrovascular disease can be divided into three categories: (1) those with attacks of transient cerebral ischemia, (2) those with CVA-in-evolution (progressing thrombotic CVA), and (3) those who have had a completed CVA (thrombotic infarction).

The aim of treating patients who have had transient ischemic attacks with anticoagulants is to prevent further episodes of transient cerebral ischemia, to prevent CVA, and to improve survival (Chapter 120). The use of anticoagulant therapy in patients with transient ischemic attacks is highly controversial because of doubt about its effectiveness and the fear of bleeding complications. Further clinical trials are required to establish definitively the role of anticoagulant treatment in patients with transient ischemic attacks. Antiplatelet therapy with aspirin is partially effective for preventing CVA and death in men with transient ischemic attacks. The effectiveness of antiplatelet therapy with aspirin in women is currently uncertain.

In patients with CVA-in-evolution, the objectives of treatment with anticoagulants are to arrest the thrombotic process, prevent its progression to completed infarction, and improve survival. The effectiveness of anticoagulant therapy for these purposes is currently uncertain. In patients with completed CVA, anticoagulant therapy is without benefit and is potentially dangerous.

Review of the published literature indicates that the risk

of bleeding complications associated with long-term anticoagulant therapy in patients with established cerebrovascular disease ranges from 12% to 40% (mean, 29%). Importantly, the risk of fatal bleeding ranges from 2% to 7% (mean, 5%); most fatal bleeding episodes are caused by intracranial hemorrhage. The risk of cerebral bleeding is increased approximately 2.5-fold in patients with documented hypertension.

Because of the lack of effectiveness and the documented high risk of both fatal bleeding and serious major hemorrhage, long-term anticoagulant therapy should be reserved for patients who have systemic embolism and should not be used routinely for preventing further episodes of arterial thrombosis and CVA in patients with established cerebrovascular disease.

Prosthetic cardiac valves. The goal of anticoagulant therapy in patients with artificial cardiac valves is to prevent thrombus formation on the valve surface and subsequent systemic embolism (Chapters 16 and 120). In the absence of anticoagulant treatment, patients with prosthetic cardiac valves have a yearly risk of systemic embolism of approximately 5% to 30% or more, depending on the type of valve and its position. Mechanical valves are associated with a higher frequency of systemic embolism than are tissue (bioprosthetic) valves. Mitral prosthetic valves are associated with a greater risk of systemic embolism than are aortic valves. The risk of systemic embolism appears to be increased by the presence of coexistent atrial fibrillation. The frequency of systemic embolism in anticoagulated patients with mechanical valves is approximately 4% per year for valves in the mitral position and 2% per year for aortic placement.

The clinical practice of treating patients with prosthetic heart valves with long-term oral anticoagulant therapy is now well established. The use of warfarin sodium to maintain an INR of 2.0 to 3.0 has been the standard approach for patients with bioprosthetic (tissue) valves. In the past an INR of 3.0 to 4.5 has been recommended for patients with mechanical valves, particularly if they have been complicated by systemic embolism. However, lower-intensity regimens of warfarin alone (INR 1.9 to 3.6) or warfarin (INR 2.0 to 3.0) plus ASA and dipyridamole have been shown to be as effective as higher-dose warfarin, with fewer bleeding complications. The addition of aspirin, 100 mg/day, to warfarin (INR 3.0 to 4.5) when compared with warfarin alone resulted in a marked improvement in efficacy without an increase in major bleeding or cerebral hemorrhage.

The role of antiplatelet therapy, either as a substitute for anticoagulant therapy or in addition to treatment with anticoagulants, is currently uncertain, and further clinical trials are necessary to determine its place in the management of patients with prosthetic cardiac valves. Dipyridamole in addition to warfarin may be of benefit in patients who have systemic embolism during adequate warfarin treatment.

Oral anticoagulant therapy reduces the risk of CVA and systemic embolism in patients with nonvalvular atrial fibrillation when compared with either aspirin or placebo. Furthermore, less intense warfarin therapy (INR 2.0 to 3.0) is as effective as higher-intensity warfarin therapy, without the added risk of bleeding. Ambulatory patients with atrial fibrillation are usually started on warfarin therapy without the addition of heparin, and this appears to be safe in such patients who have no ongoing thrombotic process.

The risk of bleeding complications associated with long-term anticoagulant therapy in patients with prosthetic heart valves has been reported to range from 1%-11% (mean, 6%). The risk of bleeding appears to be increased by the addition of aspirin to oral anticoagulant therapy.

In pregnant patients with prosthetic heart valves, SC heparin in therapeutic doses (e.g., 15,000 U every 12 hours) that maintain the APTT to 1.5 to 2.0 times the control value is a practical anticoagulant regimen that avoids the risk of fetopathic effects associated with warfarin therapy during pregnancy. To date, however, the effectiveness of this regimen for preventing systemic embolism in patients with prosthetic valves has not been formally evaluated by randomized clinical trials. A recent study indicates that lower doses of SC heparin (5000 U every 12 hours) are ineffective in preventing valve thrombosis and systemic embolism in pregnant women with prosthetic cardiac valves. The use of long-term SC heparin exposes the patient to the potential risk of osteoporosis (see previous section on adverse effects of heparin).

Peripheral vascular disease. The role of anticoagulant therapy in the management of patients with arterial occlusive disease of the legs is limited. Anticoagulant therapy is effective in preventing recurrent distal embolism in patients with acute arterial occlusion. Continuous IV heparin (see previous heparin protocol) should be commenced immediately in patients with acute arterial occlusion of the limb and continued postembolectomy until full therapeutic oral anticoagulation with warfarin is accomplished (see next section). The role of long-term anticoagulant therapy in the management of patients with intermittent claudication or ischemic rest pain is uncertain. Anticoagulant therapy may be effective in improving the long-term patency of peripheral arterial bypass procedures (e.g., femoropopliteal bypass), particularly procedures involving prosthetic graft materials, but further studies are required to adequately assess its role in this context. A recent randomized trial suggests that long-term oral anticoagulant therapy improves survival after femoropopliteal bypass surgery by reducing mortality from associated cardiovascular disease (e.g., coronary artery disease).

Systemic embolism. Anticoagulant therapy is effective in preventing recurrent embolism in patients who have had an episode of systemic embolism. Recurrent embolism occurs early in the clinical course of patients with systemic embolism. In the absence of anticoagulant therapy, approximately 10% to 15% of patients with cerebral embolism from a defined source have a second embolic event within 2 weeks. For this reason, anticoagulant therapy should be commenced immediately once a diagnosis of systemic embolism is established. In patients with cerebral embolism, computed tomographic scanning should be performed immediately and before commencing anticoagulant therapy to exclude the presence of hemorrhagic infarction.

Full-dose continuous IV heparin is the preferred approach to achieve an immediate and sustained anticoagulant effect; the heparin dose is adjusted to maintain the APTT at 1.5 to 2.0 times control. The protocol for administering heparin is the same as that outlined previously for the treatment of venous thromboembolism. Heparin therapy is continued for 5 to 6 days and is followed by long-term oral anticoagulant therapy, with warfarin sodium adjusted to maintain the INR between 2.0 and 3.0.

Role of thrombolytic therapy. The role of thrombolytic therapy in the management of patients with arterial thromboembolism has not been definitively established. The objective of treating these patients with thrombolytic therapy is to restore vessel patency by inducing rapid lysis of thrombi and emboli.

The application of thrombolytic therapy in the management of patients with acute myocardial infarction has been the subject of intensive investigation in recent years. Recent studies have shown that IV thrombolysis is effective in inducing coronary thrombolysis and reperfusion and reducing mortality in patients with acute myocardial infarction of recent onset ($<$ 6 hours). The relative effectiveness of streptokinase, anisoylated plasminogen-streptokinase activator complex (APSAC), and tPA in patients with myocardial infarction should be determined over the next few years. (For further details on thrombolytic therapy of acute myocardial infarction, see Chapter 14.)

REFERENCES

Altman P et al: Comparison of two levels of anticoagulant therapy in patients with substitute heart valves. J Thorac Cardiovasc Surg 101:427, 1991.

The Boston Area Anticoagulation Trial for Atrial Fibrillation Investigators: The effect of low-dose warfarin on the risk of stroke in patients with non-rheumatic atrial fibrillation. N Engl J Med 323:1505, 1990.

Clouse LH and Comp PC: The regulation of hemostasis: the protein C system. N Engl J Med 314:1298, 1986.

Connolly SJ et al: Canadian Atrial Fibrillation Anticoagulation (CAFA) study. J Am Coll Cardiol 18:349, 1991.

Duke RJ et al: Intravenous heparin for the prevention of stroke progression in acute partial stable stroke: a randomized controlled trial. Ann Intern Med 105:825, 1986.

Gallus AS et al: Safety and efficacy of warfarin started early after submassive venous thrombosis or pulmonary embolism. Lancet 2:1293, 1986.

Goldhaber SZ et al: Randomized controlled trial of tissue plasminogen activator in proximal deep venous thrombosis. Am J Med 88:235, 1990.

Hirsh J: Oral anticoagulant drugs. N Engl J Med 324:1965, 1991.

Huisman MV et al: Serial impedance plethysmography for suspected deep-vein thrombosis in outpatients. N Engl J Med 314:823, 1986.

Hull R et al: Warfarin sodium versus low-dose heparin in the long-term treatment of venous thrombosis. N Engl J Med 301:855, 1979.

Hull R et al: Adjusted subcutaneous heparin versus warfarin sodium in the long-term treatment of venous thrombosis. N Engl J Med 306:189, 1982.

Hull R et al: Different intensities of oral anticoagulant therapy in the treatment of proximal vein thrombosis. N Engl J Med 307:1676, 1982.

Hull R et al: Continuous intravenous heparin compared with intermittent subcutaneous heparin in the initial treatment of proximal-vein thrombosis. N Engl J Med 315:1109, 1986.

Hull R et al: Heparin for 5 days as compared with 10 days in the initial treatment of proximal venous thrombosis. N Engl J Med 322:1260, 1990.

Italian Group for the Study of Streptokinase in Myocardial Infarction: Effectiveness of intravenous thrombolytic treatment in acute myocardial infarction. Lancet 1:397, 1986.

Iturbe-Alessio I et al: Risks of anticoagulant therapy in pregnant women with artificial heart valves. N Engl J Med 315:1390, 1986.

Kretschmer G et al: Influence of post-operative anticoagulant treatment on patient survival after femoropopliteal vein bypass surgery. Lancet 2:797, 1988.

Lagerstedt EI et al: Need for long-term anticoagulant treatment in symptomatic calf-vein thrombosis. Lancet 2:515, 1985.

Marder VJ and Sherry S: Thrombolytic therapy: current status. N Engl J Med 318:1512, 1988.

Moser KM and LeMoine JR: Is embolic risk conditioned by location of deep venous thrombosis? Ann Intern Med 94:439, 1981.

Petersen P et al: Placebo controlled, randomized trial of warfarin and aspirin for prevention of thromboembolic complications in chronic atrial fibrillation. Lancet 1:175, 1989.

Pineo GF and Hull RD: Adverse effects of coumarin anticoagulants. Drug Safety, 1993 (in press).

Salzman EW et al: Management of heparin therapy: controlled prospective trial. N Engl J Med 292:1046, 1975.

Saour JN et al: Trial of different intensities of anticoagulation in patients with prosthetic heart valves. N Engl J Med 322:428, 1990.

Serneri GGN et al: Effectiveness of low-dose heparin in prevention of myocardial reinfarction. Lancet 2:937, 1987.

Sixty-Plus Reinfarction Study Research Group: A double-blind trial to assess long-term anticoagulant therapy in elderly patients after myocardial infarction. Lancet 2:989, 1980.

Smith P et al: The effect of warfarin on mortality and reinfarction after myocardial infarction. N Engl J Med 323:147, 1990.

Turpie AGG et al: Randomized comparison of two intensities of oral anticoagulant therapy after tissue heart valve replacement. Lancet 1:242, 1988.

Urokinase-Streptokinase Pulmonary Embolism Trial: Phase II results: a cooperative study. JAMA 229:1606, 1974.

Warkentin TE and Kelton JG: Heparin-induced thrombocytopenia. In Coller BS, editor: Progress in hemostasis and thrombosis, vol 10. Philadelphia, 1991, Saunders.

CHAPTER

87 Iron Deficiency Anemia, the Anemia of Chronic Disease, Sideroblastic Anemia, and Iron Overload

David A. Lipschitz

As a central component of the heme molecule, iron plays an essential role in oxygen transport in red cells and in virtually every aspect of intermediary metabolism. Interest in iron metabolism was stimulated because iron deficiency constitutes a major worldwide health problem. A great deal of information has accumulated on the biochemistry and physiology of iron metabolism as well as insights into the consequences and clinical manifestations of both iron deficiency and iron overload.

NORMAL IRON METABOLISM

Iron absorption

In normal subjects the total iron content of the body remains relatively constant. To maintain iron balance, body losses must be matched by the absorption of an equal amount of dietary iron. No physiologic mechanism exists for regulating iron excretion, so that maintenance of homeostasis is exclusively regulated by altering iron absorption. Iron losses from the body have been calculated to be approximately 0.6 mg/day for men and 1.2 mg/day for menstruating women; the difference is a consequence of iron loss through menstrual flow. Physiologic control over iron balance is normally maintained by the regulation of iron absorption. The average intake of iron in the American diet is about 6 mg/1000 cal or 10 to 18 mg/day. Approximately 10% of dietary iron is in the form of heme or myoglobin, which is more readily absorbed than the nonheme iron contained in other foods. Nonheme iron absorption is markedly affected by dietary composition. The presence of meat enhances food iron absorption, whereas phytates, phosphates, soy protein, tea, and bran limit absorption through the formation of insoluble complexes. The stimulating effect of ascorbic acid on iron absorption is partly related to the fact that it reduces iron to the more soluble ferrous form. The simultaneous administration of iron salts with tetracycline may result in a gross impairment of absorption of both substances caused by the formation of unavailable iron chelates in the gastrointestinal lumen. Reduced gastric acid secretion also exerts an effect on iron available for absorption.

Iron is virtually exclusively absorbed in the duodenum and proximal jejunum. A distinct pathway exists for heme iron absorption, whereas a separate pathway is involved for nonheme iron. Heme is removed from its apoprotein by gastric juices and is absorbed intact into the mucosal cell, where it is further metabolized. Three separate processes appear to be involved in nonheme iron absorption. These are (1) uptake of iron by the brush border membrane of intestinal epithelial cells, (2) binding of iron to intracellular carrier proteins or other complex agents, and (3) transfer across to the serosal surface where the iron binds to transferrin. If iron requirements increase, the entire process of transfer through the mucosal cell is enhanced. When iron demands are decreased, iron uptake is reduced, as is iron transfer through the mucosal cell. Iron that is not transported to transferrin remains in the mucosal cell and, when the cell is sloughed, is eventually lost.

Internal iron exchange

Within the circulation iron is bound entirely to transferrin, which has two binding sites each able to bind one atom of iron. Although chemical and physical differences between the binding sites have been clearly demonstrated, functional differences in the delivery of iron either to red cell precursors or to iron stores have not been confirmed. Transferrin is responsible for the delivery of iron either to erythroid precursors for new heme synthesis or to iron stores located in the hepatocyte (Fig. 87-1). Virtually all the iron bound to transferrin is transported to the bone marrow and is delivered to red cell precursors through transferrin receptor sites on the cell's surface. Iron-loaded transferrin attaches to these receptors and transfers its iron into the cell. Within the red cell, iron is transported through the cytoplasm to the mitochondria, where it combines with protoporphyrin-9 to form heme. The heme molecule then enters the cytoplasm, where it forms complexes with globin chains to form hemoglobin. A small amount of iron in red cell precursors does not bind to heme. It is diverted to the cytoplasm, where it is incorporated into the iron storage protein ferritin. In approximately 10% of normal red cell precursors iron granules are visible in the cytoplasm. These cells are referred to as *normal sideroblasts*.

The mature red cell leaves the bone marrow, entering the peripheral blood as a reticulocyte (Fig. 87-1). Approximately 10% of young circulating red cells have visible iron granules and are referred to as *siderocytes*. Early in its lifespan, iron not contained in hemoglobin is removed from red cells during their transit through the spleen.

At the end of their lifespan of approximately 120 days, senescent red cells are phagocytosed by reticuloendothelial cells in the liver, spleen, and bone marrow. The engulfed red cell is broken down to its constituent amino acids, bilirubin and iron (Fig. 87-1). The iron is transported back to the cell membrane, where it combines with transferrin and is recircuited to the marrow for reincorporation into heme

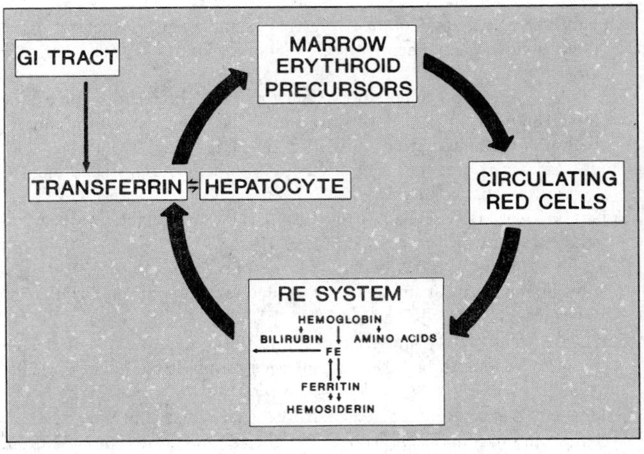

Fig. 87-1. Internal iron exchange. The iron cycle involves the release of iron from reticuloendothelial cells and hepatocytes to transferrin in the plasma, which transports it to marrow erythroid precursors for incorporation into heme. Reticulocytes leave the marrow, and after approximately 120 days they become senescent and are phagocytosed by the reticuloendothelial system, and the iron is recircuited back to transferrin. Approximately 30 mg of iron passes through the plasma pool each day. The 1 to 2 mg absorbed from the GI tract is balanced by equal daily iron losses. Increased body demands for iron result in mobilization of iron from stores in reticuloendothelial cells and hepatocytes, as well as increased iron absorption. When body demands decrease, iron is diverted to stores and iron absorption is reduced.

in erythroid precursors. Approximately 30 mg of iron moves through the plasma pool each day, virtually all being derived from recircuited senescent red cell iron. One to two milligrams of iron is mobilized from iron stores or from absorbed iron and is matched by equal daily iron deposition in stores and losses from the body. This process is referred to as the iron cycle. Iron flow through the plasma pool has the capacity to increase up to 10-fold if marrow demands for iron increase. The degree to which the cycle can increase is dependent virtually exclusively on iron supply, which is determined largely by the availability of iron derived from red cell breakdown. Iron stores or dietary iron only contributes minimally to internal iron exchange.

In recent years a great deal of information has been obtained on the mechanism whereby transferrin transfers iron into a cell. Iron containing transferrin attaches to a specific receptor on the cell membrane, then the transferrin/receptor complex enters the cell by endocytosis. As the pH of the endocytotic vesicle decreases, iron is released into the cell. The vesicle then returns to the cell membrane and the apotransferrin is released back to the circulation. When iron supply is inadequate or when the cell's requirements for iron increase, an upregulation of transferrin receptor number occurs, thus increasing its ability to obtain iron. The concentration of transferrin receptors is markedly increased in rapidly growing tissues and in erythroid precursors that are rapidly producing hemoglobin. Receptor numbers decrease when requirements for iron are reduced. Thus by altering transferrin receptor number, cells play an active role in regulating iron uptake and in regulating internal iron exchange.

Iron stores

Approximately 80% of the body's iron content is located in circulating red cells, averaging 4 g in men and 2.5 g in women. In addition to iron circulating in red cells, a small fraction is located in heme enzymes, and approximately 1000 mg in men and 300 mg in women is located in tissue iron stores. Tissue iron stores are divided equally between the parenchymal cells of the liver and reticuloendothelial cells in the spleen, liver, and bone marrow. Fifty percent of the iron is stored in ferritin, which is a protein made up of approximately 20 polypeptide subunits arranged as an envelope around a central storage cavity. Variable amounts of iron are present in the storage cavity as microcrystals of ferrous hydroxyphosphate. Iron moves freely into and out of ferritin through channels in the protein envelope, is easily available for metabolic use, and can be mobilized when body demands for iron increase. Conversely iron can be diverted into ferritin, if demands are decreased (Fig. 87-1). Individual ferritin molecules are too small to be seen by light microscopy.

The remaining 50% of storage iron is contained in hemosiderin, which is made up of precipitated aggregates of ferritin with largely degraded protein components. These granules are large enough to be visible by light microscopy and hence are used histologically to grade tissue iron content. Like the iron in ferritin, hemosiderin iron is also readily available. If demands for iron increase, iron is readily mobilized. Iron accumulates in hemosiderin, if demands for iron diminish.

IRON DEFICIENCY ANEMIA

Iron deficiency is the single most common cause of anemia in humans, as well as the most common global nutritional deficiency. Although the prevalence has been decreasing in the Western world, the disorder remains epidemic in developing countries. The causes of iron deficiency anemia are listed in the box below. They result from blood loss, inadequate dietary iron intake, malabsorption of iron, urinary losses of hemosiderin associated with intravascular hemolysis, and diversion of body iron stores to the fetus during pregnancy.

Blood loss is the single most common cause of iron deficiency. In women, excessive menstrual blood loss accounts for the majority of iron deficiency anemia. The

Etiology of iron deficiency anemia

I. Blood loss
  A. Menstrual
  B. Gastrointestinal
    1. Stomach
      a. Hiatal hernia
      b. Esophageal varices
      c. Peptic ulcer disease
      d. Acute gastritis
      e. Drugs
      f. Carcinoma of the stomach
    2. Large bowel
      a. Carcinoma of the colon/rectum
      b. Benign polyps
      c. Angiodysplasia
      d. Diverticular disease
      e. Ulcerative colitis
    3. Small bowel
      a. Hookworm
      b. Crohn's disease
      c. Milk allergy
  C. Other
    1. Epistaxis
    2. Hematuria
    3. Coagulopathy
    4. Blood donation
    5. Chronic hemodialysis
II. Malabsorption
  A. Achlorhydria
  B. Total gastrectomy
  C. Gastrojejunostomy
  D. Celiac disease and spruelike syndromes
  E. Pica
III. Inadequate intake or increased requirements
  A. Dietary (rare)
  B. Pregnancy and lactation
  C. Growth and development
IV. Miscellaneous
  A. Pulmonary sequestration of iron (Goodpasture's syndrome)
  B. Hemosiderinuria

amount of blood loss with menstruation varies markedly, averaging approximately 45 ml of blood per cycle. In approximately 10% of women, blood loss may exceed 80 ml/cycle (30 mg of iron). Frequently a woman who has iron deficiency anemia caused by menstrual blood loss does not complain of excessive menstrual bleeding. Limited availability of dietary iron in the face of even moderate menstrual blood losses places many women in precarious iron balance and explains the very high prevalence of iron deficiency anemia. In adult males and in postmenopausal women iron deficiency is most commonly caused by gastrointestinal blood loss (refer to the box on p. 387). The importance of iron deficiency as the initial manifestation of colorectal cancer cannot be overemphasized. The presence of iron deficiency in postmenopausal women and in men must be considered to be a consequence of a gastrointestinal cancer until proved otherwise. Additional gastrointestinal causes to be considered include peptic ulceration, hiatal hernia, gastritis, and drug ingestion. In children, milk allergy is a common cause of occult blood loss from the gut. In the elderly, angiodysplasia of the large bowel frequently results in iron deficiency anemia. In approximately 50% of individuals above the age of 70 with iron deficiency anemia, the cause of gastrointestinal blood loss is never identified. On a worldwide basis hookworm infestation is the most common cause of iron deficiency anemia.

Chronic hemodialysis is associated with significant blood loss. The routine use of prophylactic parenteral iron therapy has been recommended in these patients but may result in iron overload and tissue damage. Dialysis patients should be appropriately evaluated before treatment with iron. Additional causes of iron deficiency anemia produced by blood loss include multiple blood samples for investigative purposes, frequent blood donations, hematuria, epistaxis, and self-induced bloodletting.

Iron deficiency anemia is a particular problem in pregnancy. The iron requirements of the fetus, blood loss during delivery, and lactation average approximately 900 mg. If iron supplementation is not given during pregnancy, significant iron deficiency becomes a serious clinical problem, occurring in 85% to 100% of pregnant women. For this reason, prophylactic iron should be given orally to all pregnant women.

Malabsorption of iron is a rare cause of iron deficiency. This has been described in the presence of achlorhydria after gastrectomy or proximal small bowel resection. A variety of small bowel syndromes associated with malabsorption can cause iron deficiency anemia. Additional rare causes of iron deficiency include chronic loss of hemosiderin in the urine associated with intravascular hemolysis and iron sequestration in pulmonary macrophages (Goodpasture's syndrome).

Manifestations

The major clinical feature of iron deficiency is the presence of microcytic anemia. The red cells are small, pale, irregularly shaped, and hypochromic (Plate III-4, B). Patients with iron deficiency anemia occasionally show fatigue that is out of proportion to the degree of anemia. It has been suggested that this may be related to depletion of iron-containing muscle enzymes. Studies have shown that iron depletion is associated with diminished work performance. Manifestations occasionally seen in very severe iron deficiency anemia include glossitis, koilonychia (spooning of the nails), and rarely a syndrome associated with esophageal web and dysphagia. This is referred to as the *Plummer-Vinson syndrome*. It must be emphasized, however, that the majority of patients with iron deficiency anemia are asymptomatic.

Pathophysiology

There are three phases in the pathogenesis of iron deficiency. The first is iron depletion, during which storage iron is mobilized to meet the increased needs of the bone marrow for iron. Provided iron stores are present, erythropoiesis remains normal. Second, when iron stores are totally depleted, iron deficient erythropoiesis develops. This is characterized by significant reductions in the serum iron level and inadequate iron delivery to meet the needs of red cell precursors. Inadequate iron delivery to red cell precursors results in elevations of the red cell free erythrocyte protoporphyrin and the development of hypochromia and microcytosis, which are recognizable before the development of anemia. Finally, the hemoglobin and hematocrit begin to decrease and iron deficiency anemia develops.

LABORATORY PARAMETERS EMPLOYED TO EVALUATE IRON STATUS

Serum ferritin

The concentration of the ferritin in serum can be measured radioimmunologically. The serum ferritin level varies in direct proportion to body iron stores and is markedly reduced in iron deficiency anemia when iron stores are absent. The level is significantly increased in disorders associated with iron overload. A serum ferritin value of less than 12 ng/ml is characteristic of uncomplicated iron deficiency anemia (Fig. 87-2). Serum ferritin values of less than 50 ng/ml in anemic subjects should be regarded as suggestive, but not diagnostic, evidence of iron deficiency. Disproportionate elevations of the serum ferritin level occur in the presence of inflammation, liver disease, or hemolysis. The measurement is also used to diagnose disorders associated with iron overload, in which the concentration is usually above 1000 ng/ml.

Bone marrow iron

Iron status can be examined in bone marrow aspirates by determining the presence or absence of storage iron in Prussian blue stained bone marrow aspirate or biopsy specimens. Hemosiderin granules stain a bluish green color on exposure to prussian blue (Plate III-7). Hemosiderin granules accumulate in reticuloendothelial cells and are absent in iron deficiency anemia. Using standard grading procedures, bone marrow iron stores can be absent (0), depleted (+), normal (++), or increased (+++). The presence of

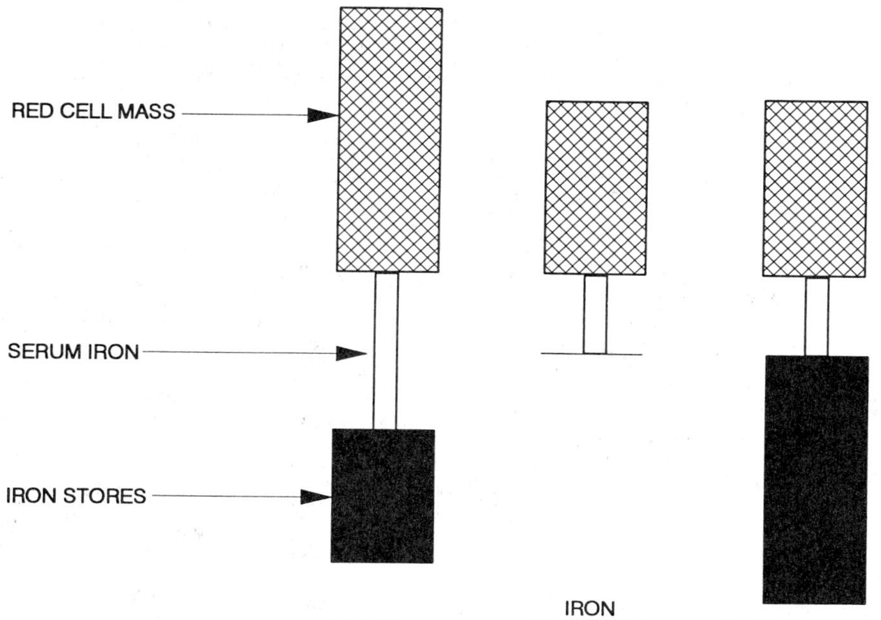

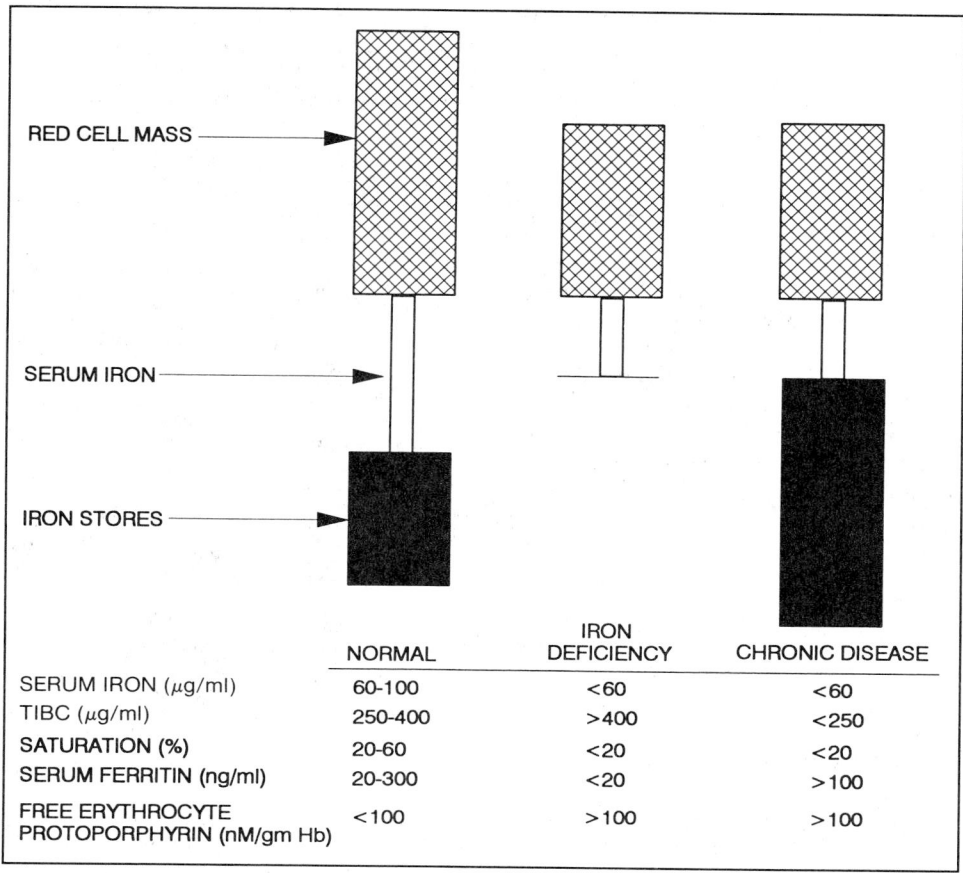

	NORMAL	IRON DEFICIENCY	CHRONIC DISEASE
SERUM IRON (μg/ml)	60-100	<60	<60
TIBC (μg/ml)	250-400	>400	<250
SATURATION (%)	20-60	<20	<20
SERUM FERRITIN (ng/ml)	20-300	<20	>100
FREE ERYTHROCYTE PROTOPORPHYRIN (nM/gm Hb)	<100	>100	>100

Fig. 87-2. Hematologic profile, red cell mass, tissue iron stores, and laboratory parameters in normal subjects and in patients with anemia caused by iron deficiency or chronic disease. Both disorders demonstrate laboratory evidence of iron deficient erythropoiesis. Iron stores are absent in iron deficiency but are increased in the anemia of chronic disease.

iron granules in red cell precursors can also be evaluated. As indicated previously, under normal circumstances approximately 10% to 15% of marrow normoblasts have up to 10 visible iron granules scattered in their cytoplasm and are referred to as sideroblasts. The absence of sideroblasts is a cardinal feature of iron deficient erythropoiesis. Abnormal sideroblasts can also be detected (Plate III-8). A ringed sideroblast is pathologic, reflects iron deposits in mitochondria, and is diagnostic of sideroblastic anemia (see later discussion). An abnormal nonringed sideroblast containing more than 10 granules randomly located in the cytoplasm is frequently seen in the thalassemia syndromes and in lead poisoning.

Serum iron, total iron binding capacity, and transferrin saturation

The serum iron concentration is usually low in untreated iron deficiency anemia although values in the normal range are occasionally observed. The total iron binding capacity (TIBC) measures the amount of transferrin present in circulating blood. Generally there is sufficient transferrin to bind between 250 and 450 μ/dl of iron. Thus with an average serum iron concentration of 100 μ/dl, the circulating transferrin is approximately 30% saturated. The transferrin saturation appears to be a far more accurate measure of iron deficient erythropoiesis than the serum iron determination and a value below 20% is highly suggestive of deficient iron supply for normal erythroid function. The level of circulating transferrin varies inversely with tissue iron stores, tending to be increased when iron stores are diminished and decreased when they are elevated. Thus in classic iron deficiency anemia the TIBC is above 400 μ/dl. Elevations of circulating transferrin are also noted during pregnancy and use of oral contraceptives. In general, reductions in the TIBC are invariable in the anemia of chronic disease (see later discussion). Transferrin functions as an acute phase reactant and is diminished in the presence of acute-stress. Inadequate supply of protein to the liver, as occurs in protein-energy malnutrition, also results in decreases in the TIBC.

Free erythrocyte protoporphyrin

The free erythrocyte protoporphyrin level is elevated in disorders of heme synthesis. It is elevated in iron deficient erythropoiesis but is also increased in lead poisoning, sideroblastic anemias, and various other conditions. It is a very useful and simple tool for mass screening for iron deficiency anemia.

Red cell morphology

A feature of iron deficient erythropoiesis is the presence of microcytosis and hypochromia (Plate III-4, B). These changes in erythrocyte volume and hemoglobin concentration are reflected in reductions in the mean corpuscular volume, which in iron deficiency is usually less than 80 fl (Chapter 73). The mean corpuscular hemoglobin concentration also decreases, but it only becomes significant in the severest form of iron deficiency and is thus of little value diagnostically. Characteristically, the reticulocyte count is normal or decreased in iron deficiency and the reticulocyte production index is invariably below 2.

Serum transferrin receptor

Recently, the specific receptor to which transferrin binds on cells has been purified and cloned. As a consequence, methods have been developed to measure the number of transferrin receptors on cells. In addition, employing sensitive immunoradiometric techniques, measurable concentrations of transferrin receptor can be identified in the serum. Preliminary studies have shown significant increases in circulating serum transferrin receptor concentrations in patients with iron deficiency anemia and in those in whom the rate of erythropoiesis was markedly increased. In contrast, serum transferrin receptor concentrations are markedly reduced in individuals who have aplastic anemia, in whom erythropoiesis is absent or markedly decreased. In the future this measurement may have utility as a measure of iron supply for erythropoiesis and in the quantitation of red cell mass.

ANEMIA OF CHRONIC DISEASE

An anemia frequently accompanies a variety of chronic disorders, including chronic inflammation, malignancy, and connective tissues diseases such as rheumatoid arthritis. The anemia is hypoproliferative in type, is associated with iron deficient erythropoiesis, and is commonly confused with iron deficiency anemia produced by blood loss. Anemia, with an identical hematologic profile, is also common in acute inflammatory disorders and in protein-energy malnutrition (refer to the box at upper right).

Diseases associated with the anemia of chronic disease

- Acute infections
  - Bacterial, fungal, or viral
- Chronic infections
  - Tuberculosis
  - Infective endocarditis
  - Chronic urinary tract infection
  - Coccidioidomycosis and other chronic fungal diseases
- Chronic noninfectious inflammatory disorders
  - Osteoarthritis
  - Rheumatoid disease
  - Collagen vascular disease
  - Polymyalgia rheumatica
  - Acute and chronic hepatitis
  - Decubitus ulcer
- Malignancy
  - Metastatic carcinoma
  - Hematologic malignancies
    - Lymphoma
    - Leukemia
    - Myeloma
- Protein-energy malnutrition

Mechanism

A cardinal feature of the anemia of chronic disorders appears to be an impaired ability of the reticuloendothelial cell to recirculate the iron derived from previously phagocytosed senescent red cells. As a result, the serum iron level is low, iron supply to the marrow is inadequate, and iron deficient erythropoiesis develops. In contrast to iron deficiency, tissue iron stores in the anemia of chronic disease are normal or increased rather than absent.

Although iron supply for erythropoiesis is compromised, recent studies have shown that this defect does not account for the anemia. A significant increase in macrophage proliferation occurs. The macrophages release a number of cytokines, including interleukin-1α, tumor necrosis factor and interferon. These cytokines have been shown to suppress erythroid growth directly. Other abnormalities that contribute to the anemia include a modest reduction in red cell survival and an inappropriately low serum erythropoietin level for the degree of anemia.

Clinical manifestations include a mild to moderate anemia; a hemoglobin concentration below 10 g/dl is extremely unusual. Red cell morphology is usually normocytic and normochromic, although a close analysis of red cell size and shape reveals a relative reduction in hemoglobin concentration within the cell. The anemia usually is manifested in an individual in whom the primary disease is obvious. Rarely, the anemia of chronic disease may be the initial manifestation of an occult disorder requiring investigation. It must be emphasized that this disorder produces clinical and laboratory manifestations that make an accurate diagnosis possible. The anemia of chronic disease must be distinguished from iron deficiency and other causes of anemia. Failure to make an accurate diagnosis frequently leads to inappropriate investigations and unnecessary treatment with oral iron.

DIFFERENTIAL DIAGNOSES OF ANEMIAS ASSOCIATED WITH IRON DEFICIENT ERYTHROPOIESIS

A number of approaches can be employed in defining the cause of an anemia in which iron deficient erythropoiesis is suspected. Because menstrual blood loss is almost always the cause of a mild iron deficiency anemia in otherwise healthy premenopausal women, a therapeutic trial of oral iron to confirm the diagnosis is rational provided the history and physical examination are completely normal and no coexisting hematologic problems can be identified on routine complete blood count (CBC). After a 2 to 3 week trial of oral iron a 1.5 g/dl or greater rise in the hemoglobin concentration should have occurred. Failure of the hemoglobin to increase warrants further investigation. A therapeutic trial is not appropriate for postmenopausal women or for men of any age.

The first step in the laboratory differential is to determine that the anemia is of the hypoproliferative type as evidenced by a corrected reticulocyte count of less than 1% (Chapter 80). The presence or absence of iron deficient erythropoiesis should then be determined (Fig. 87-3). The first clue is the presence of microcytosis. Microcytosis can be caused by inadequate iron supply for erythropoiesis, but it is also caused by disorders associated with defective globin synthesis, such as the thalassemias, or abnormalities in heme synthesis that characterize the sideroblastic anemias or lead poisoning. Mild iron deficiency anemia can easily be confused with other microcytic disorders, particularly the mild form of beta-thalassemia trait or the two deletion form of alpha thalassemia (Chapter 89). In general, microcytosis is more severe in the thalassemias and hypochromia is less obvious. Thus the presence of a normal MCHC and an elevated red cell count in the face of severe microcytosis favors a diagnosis of thalassemia. Irrespective of whether the anemia is microcytic or normocytic, the presence of iron deficient erythropoiesis must be confirmed by the detection of a low serum iron level or, more importantly, a transferrin saturation of less than 20% (Fig. 87-3). An elevated free erythrocyte protoporphyrin level provides further evidence for iron deficient erythropoiesis. Free erythrocyte protoporphyrin levels are also elevated in the sideroblastic anemias and in lead poisoning, but in these conditions the serum iron and the transferrin saturation are not reduced. Once iron deficient erythropoiesis has been diagnosed, iron deficiency anemia can be distinguished from the anemia of chronic disease by demonstrating the absence of iron stores in the former and normal or increased iron stores in the latter. A serum ferritin value less than 20 ng/ml is essentially diagnostic of iron deficiency anemia (Fig. 87-3). Similarly a serum ferritin value greater than 100 ng/ml associated with a TIBC of less than 250 μg/ml is generally diagnostic of the anemia of chronic disease. Frequently, the serum ferritin level and TIBC yield equivocal results. This is particularly likely to occur in patients in whom chronic disease and blood loss may coexist, for example, an individual with rheumatoid disease who also has drug-induced gastrointestinal blood loss. In these or other similar circumstances, a bone marrow aspirate with Prussian blue stain for iron shows absent sideroblast and marrow iron stores in iron deficiency anemia. In the anemia of chronic disease, sideroblasts are absent, but iron stores are normal or increased.

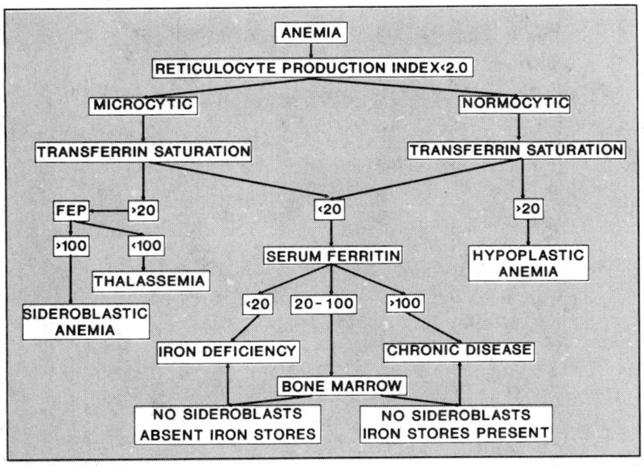

Fig. 87-3. A rational approach to the laboratory diagnosis of iron deficiency anemia and the other common disorders that must be considered in the differential diagnosis.

TREATMENT

Iron deficiency anemia

The treatment of iron deficiency anemia is replacement of iron, which may be administered orally as simple iron salts or parenterally as an iron-carbohydrate complex. For the vast majority of patients, oral ferrous sulfate, in either tablet or liquid form, is the drug of choice; the usual dose is 300 mg (60 mg elemental iron) three times per day. Approximately 5% of patients suffer significant gastrointestinal side effects. These include abdominal discomfort, nausea, vomiting, and, occasionally, diarrhea. The side effects may be minimized if the iron tablets are given with meals. The use of slow release iron tablets, which are far more expensive than ferrous sulfate, has not been proved to diminish the incidence of gastrointestinal discomfort.

In response to oral iron treatment, a gradual increase in the hemoglobin concentration occurs. Minimal reticulocytosis may be observed after approximately 10 days of treatment. Within 2 to 3 weeks the hemoglobin concentration should have increased approximately 1.5 g/dl. Oral iron therapy should continue for approximately 6 months after the hemoglobin level has returned to normal to allow repletion of body iron stores. It must be emphasized that an important part of management is to correct the cause of iron deficiency. Appropriate attention should be paid to minimizing menstrual blood loss or to identifying and initiating therapy for gastrointestinal or other causes of bleeding.

Failure to respond to oral iron is most frequently caused by lack of patient compliance. Other considerations include the possibility that the diagnosis is incorrect, that excessive blood loss is continuing, or that gastrointestinal malabsorption of iron exists.

Parenteral iron is rarely needed for the management of iron deficiency anemia. It should be considered in the unreliable, noncompliant patient with severe iron deficiency anemia, in individuals with obvious gastrointestinal malabsorption of iron, and in those rare subjects who are intolerant of oral iron therapy. Iron dextran is the parenteral iron of choice and can be given either intravenously or intramuscularly. It is very important to recognize that occasional severe anaphylactic reactions occur with parenteral iron therapy. To minimize this possibility, a small test dose has been recommended. It is unlikely that this approach will assist in the detection or prevention of adverse reactions. A high level of awareness and close observation are both essential and prudent.

Intravenous injection with administration of the total dose in a single infusion or infusion of divided doses at regular intervals is the method of choice. Formulas through which the total dose of iron required to correct the defect can be calculated are available. Because of pain and the risk of skin staining, intramuscular injections should be avoided.

Anemia of chronic disease

At the current time there is no specific therapy for anemia of chronic disease. The use of oral iron in this disorder is of no benefit in correcting the anemia. Attention should be paid to management of the underlying disease accounting for the anemia. In the future, recombinant erythropoietin may prove to be of value in increasing the hemoglobin concentration in selected patients who have this anemia.

THE SIDEROBLASTIC ANEMIAS

Sideroblastic anemias are characterized by the presence of ineffective erythropoiesis associated with large numbers of ringed sideroblasts in the bone marrow (Plate III-8). A cardinal feature of the peripheral blood is "dimorphism" in which a population of microcytic hypochromic red cells coexist with morphologically normal red cells. An additional unique feature of these disorders is their relationship to pyridoxine metabolism. Some sideroblastic anemias show a partial response to pharmacologic doses of pyridoxine, whereas frank pyridoxine deficiency results in a anemia that is fully reversible through appropriate treatment.

The abnormal sideroblast is characterized by the presence of microscopically visible iron granules in the mitochondria of red cell precursors. Their location in the perinuclear region gives rise to the appearance of an iron granule ring surrounding the nucleus. Iron loaded mitochondria are distorted and morphologically abnormal. The iron appears not in the form of ferritin, but as abnormal crystal iron complexes. Except when caused by iron deficiency, abnormalities in heme synthesis at the point of incorporation of iron into protoporphyrin 9 result in mitochondrial iron accumulation and frequently lead to sideroblastic anemia. The exact mechanism resulting in this abnormality is not clear, but it may be the result of inadequate synthesis of protoporphyrin, deficiency in the heme synthetic pathway, or abnormality of globin synthesis. There clearly is a relationship between pyridoxine metabolism and development of sideroblastic anemia. Pyridoxal-5-phosphate is a necessary coenzyme for the initial reaction of protoporphyrin synthesis, acting as a cofactor to the enzyme delta-aminolevulinic-acid synthetase. Deficient biosynthesis of pyridoxal-5-phosphate may be important in some sideroblastic anemias. Frequently, a universal defect in hematopoiesis exists with significantly abnormal myeloid and megakaryocytic elements.

The box below classifies the various sideroblastic anemias on the basis of their causes and their responsiveness to pyridoxine therapy. Congenital and acquired varieties occur, both of which may or may not demonstrate a response to pyridoxine treatment.

The acquired sideroblastic anemias

Idiopathic. Acquired sideroblastic anemia, the most common form of sideroblastic anemia, is invariably refractory and chronic in nature with a protracted clinical course. The anemia is characteristically produced by ineffective erythropoiesis as evidenced by a highly significant increase in marrow erythroid precursors with marked intramedullary destruction of functionally abnormal erythroid cells. A modest reduction in red cell survival is frequently noted.

The disease is particularly common in the elderly, although it may occur in individuals of any age. Presenting symptoms include weakness, dyspnea, angina, and pallor. Splenomegaly is frequently present and hepatomegaly is common. The anemia develops insidiously and may be profound at time of presentation.

Laboratory findings. A moderate to severe anemia is the cardinal feature. Generally, it is normocytic although microcytosis may be noted. As indicated, a dimorphic pattern is the most striking morphologic change. The white cell count may be normal, but leukopenia and neutropenia are common. The platelet count is usually normal, although thrombocytopenia or thrombocytosis is present on occasion.

Classification of the sideroblastic anemias

- Hereditary
  - X-Linked—recessive
    - Pyridoxine responsive
    - Pyridoxine refractory
  - Autosomal recessive
- Acquired
  - Idiopathic
    - Pyridoxine responsive
    - Pyridoxine refractory
  - Secondary
    - Carcinoma
    - Hematologic malignancy
    - Chronic infections
    - Chronic noninfectious inflammatory diseases
    - Lead poisoning
  - Drug-induced (pyridoxine reversible)
    - Alcohol
    - Chloramphenicol
    - Isoniazid
    - Cycloserine
    - Pyrazinamide

The bone marrow is characterized by an intense erythroid hyperplasia with megaloblastic erythroid and myeloid precursors. The cardinal diagnostic feature is the presence of ringed sideroblasts (Plate III-8).

The serum iron and transferrin saturation are generally elevated. The free erythrocyte protoporphyrin level is almost always moderately increased. Special investigations show variable abnormalities in the heme-synthetic protoporphyrin pathway.

Secondary sideroblastic anemias. Sideroblastic anemia has been reported in a wide array of hematologic and nonhematologic disorders (see the box at lower left). Why it occurs in some patients with these diseases and not in others remains unknown. Most commonly, the secondary sideroblastic anemias arise from exposure to drugs or toxins that interfere with ALA synthetase activity. Reversible sideroblastic anemia after acute alcohol ingestion is very common. Examination of these patients' bone marrows frequently shows megaloblasts, vacuolated normoblasts, and ringed sideroblasts that disappear within a few days of cessation of alcohol intake. Alcohol is thought to inhibit pyridoxal kinase and hence synthesis of pyridoxal 5′-phosphate from nonphosphorylated precursors. Sideroblastic anemia is common in patients who take isoniazid, which is known to inhibit pyridoxine metabolism. Ringed sideroblasts are also occasionally seen after chloramphenicol ingestion. Lead intoxication may also produce a sideroblastic anemia; the defect is more severe in children than in adults.

Hereditary sideroblastic anemia. The hereditary forms of sideroblastic anemia are heterogeneous. The majority are inherited as X-linked recessive traits and, hence, occur virtually exclusively in males. Close examination of female family members demonstrates minor abnormalities in erythrocyte morphology. Very rarely the disorder is inherited as an autosomal recessive trait. It usually becomes apparent in young adults, although occasionally it may be seen at birth or in early childhood. The major complication of this disorder is the development of iron overload, which can, on occasion, be particularly severe. Hepatomegaly and splenomegaly may be present and occasionally diabetes and myocardial failure develop as a consequence of iron overload (see later discussion).

The laboratory features of the hereditary sideroblastic anemias are very similar to those described for the acquired variety. Ineffective erythropoiesis is present, and the serum iron and free erythrocyte protoporphyrin levels are elevated. The diagnosis is made on histologic examination of the bone marrow.

Differential diagnosis of the sideroblastic anemias. The first step in differential diagnosis is to distinguish the sideroblastic anemias from other causes of anemia associated with microcytic red cells. Elevated serum iron level, transferrin saturation, and serum ferritin level distinguish sideroblastic anemias from iron deficient erythropoiesis associated with either iron deficiency or chronic disease (Fig. 87-3). The thalassemia syndromes are associated with a normal free erythrocyte protoporphyrin concentration and an abnormal hemoglobin by hemoglobin electrophoresis. The diagnosis of sideroblastic anemia is confirmed by examination of bone marrow aspiration and biopsy (Plate III-8). Because megaloblastic features may be seen on bone marrow examination, the determination of serum folate and vitamin B_{12} levels may be indicated to differentiate between nutritional megaloblastic and sideoblastic anemias. The primary, or idiopathic, variety of sideroblastic anemia can only be diagnosed when appropriate testing has excluded the secondary causes of the disorder. Most importantly, it is imperative that hematologic malignancy, solid tumor, or inflammatory disease be excluded. Primary acquired sideroblast anemia may be difficult to distinguish from preleukemia or the early stages of acute myelogenous or monocytic leukemia. When leukocyte immaturity is present, it is essential that the patient be followed closely for a number of months to ensure that a frank leukemia is not evolving. The disease can mimic other myelodysplastic syndromes in which ineffective erythropoiesis and refractory anemia occur without sideroblasts. Sideroblastic anemia may be mistakenly thought to be one of these disorders, if Prussian blue stains of the bone marrow are not examined. The hereditary sideroblastic anemias are usually suspected on the basis of presentation in late childhood or in young adulthood, family history, and most importantly, evidence of iron loading.

Therapy of the sideroblastic anemias. For both the idiopathic acquired and hereditary forms of sideroblastic anemia oral pyridoxine at doses of 50 to 200 mg/day should be administered. These doses are clearly pharmacologic and far greater than the daily physiologic pyridoxine requirement of 1.5 to 2.0 mg. In approximately 50% of individuals a partial response to pyridoxine treatment is noted. A mild reticulocytosis is followed by a significant increase in the hemoglobin concentration. A return of the hemoglobin to normal levels is unusual. These patients remain dependent on pyridoxine, and the anemia worsens when the drug is stopped. The remaining patients are refractory to pyridoxine and demonstrate no response to therapy. In these individuals continued use of the vitamin is not indicated. Irrespective of the response to pyridoxine, repeat bone marrow examination usually demonstrates disappearance of the ringed sideroblasts, while the patient is on pyridoxine.

If megaloblastic changes are present, folic acid therapy should be considered. This frequently leads to normoblastic maturation but rarely elevates the hemoglobin concentration. For those individuals with moderate to severe iron overload, approaches to reducing body iron stores should be considered (see later discussion).

Treatment of the secondary sideroblastic anemias is related to the nature of the associated disease. When the disease can be cured or relieved, the sideroblasts may disappear from the marrow and the anemia may lessen or disappear without any therapy. This has been noted when infectious diseases are treated and or when the hematologic malignancies go into remission. Pyridoxine should be given to patients with chronic disorders that are not amenable to curative therapy. Like those who have the idiopathic varieties, approximately 50% of these individuals respond to pyridoxine by a definite improvement in the anemia.

When sideroblastic anemia is caused by a drug, the problem can be corrected by cessation of therapy and administration of physiologic doses of pyridoxine. It has been suggested that pyridoxine therapy should always be given to patients receiving isoniazid for tuberculosis. There is concern that pyridoxine replacement may interfere with the antituberculous activity of the drug, although this has not been proved.

IRON OVERLOAD

Because no mechanism exists for the physiologic excretion of iron, any disorder associated with excessive iron entry into the body causes a progressive increase in iron stores. If the increased iron uptake persists for extended periods, significant iron overload develops and frequently leads to mortality and morbidity. *Hemochromatosis* describes a group of disorders associated with pathologic iron overload, specifically the accumulation of iron in parenchymal cells such as the liver, heart, and endocrine system, resulting in iron-induced organ damage. Iron overload may be caused by excessive iron absorption from the gastrointestinal tract as a consequence of excessive absorption of iron from a normal diet or of marked elevation in dietary iron content. Multiple blood transfusions or injection of parenteral iron dextran can also lead to severe iron overload.

Idiopathic hemochromatosis

Idiopathic hemochromatosis is discussed in detail in Chapter 60.

Secondary hemochromatosis

The iron loading anemias. Iron overload is common in individuals with aplastic and other hypoproliferative anemias requiring multiple blood transfusions. Alternatively, in patients with disorders associated with hyperplastic marrow and ineffective erythropoiesis iron overload can develop as a consequence both of transfusion and of increased dietary iron absorption occurring in association with the increased plasma iron turnover. This condition has been described in patients with ineffective erythropoieses such as thalassemia major and sideroblastic anemia. Increased absorption of iron also occurs in the hemolytic anemias. Iron overload tends to be particularly severe in patients with ineffective erythropoiesis as a large fraction of the excess iron is deposited in parenchymal tissues. The mechanism of the increased iron absorption in ineffective erythropoiesis is ill understood. Most current data suggest a direct positive correlation between iron absorption and plasma iron turnover. When the plasma iron turnover is high, a great deal of iron is absorbed and together with transfused iron is deposited in parenchymal tissues. Parenchymal iron accumulation in the liver, heart, and endocrine glands accounts for the major symptoms and signs of hemochromatosis, including cirrhosis, diabetes, and other endocrinopathies. Iron deposition in the heart results in a cardiomyopathy that is characterized by arrhythmia and congestive heart failure. In the aplastic anemias, the plasma iron turnover is reduced. Excessive iron derived from transfused red cells accumulates predominantly in the reticuloendothelial system. Although this frequently leads to modest hepatosplenomegaly, the development of cirrhosis, diabetes, or myocardial disease is quite rare.

Laboratory diagnosis. The most useful tests to detect increases in body iron stores are the transferrin saturation and serum ferritin concentration, both of which are markedly elevated in secondary hemochromatosis. The transferrin saturation is usually above 70% and frequently is greater than 90%. A serum ferritin concentration above 700 ng/ml is strongly suggestive of iron overload. In patients with symptomatic hemochromatosis, values in excess of 3000 ng/ml are usual. The diagnosis of significant parenchymal iron overload should be suspected if liver function is abnormal, if diabetes or other endocrinopathies are present, or if there is evidence of myocardial disease. Liver biopsy confirms the presence of significant increases in hepatocyte iron content. Hepatocellular damage or frank micronodular cirrhosis may also be detected. Determination of urinary iron excretion after the injection of the iron chelating agent deferoxamine, is occasionally performed. The 24 hour urinary iron excretion normally should not exceed 2 mg when a dose of 15 mg/kg of deferoxamine is injected intramuscularly; in contrast, values above 10 mg are usually found in patients with hemachromatosis.

Therapy. The treatment of choice for idiopathic hemochromatosis is phlebotomy therapy (Chapter 60). Unfortunately, in patients with the iron-loading anemias it is usually not possible to remove excess iron by phlebotomy. At the current time the most effective approach to treating iron overload uses deferoxamine. Recent studies have shown that when this drug is administered by slow intravenous or subcutaneous infusion, 10 mg or more of iron can be excreted from the body each day. Using subcutaneous infusion by means of a portable pump to administer the drug over 12 hr/day, studies in patients with thalassemia have shown that iron overload can be not only prevented but reversed. The amount of iron excreted after deferoxamine injection is affected by ascorbic acid metabolism. Because ascorbic acid deficiency is very common in individuals with iron overload, the simultaneous administration of high doses of ascorbic acid can significantly increase deferoxamine urinary iron secretion. Supportive care of the complications of iron overload includes management of diabetes, cirrhosis, and cardiac disease. In individuals who have hypogonadism, testosterone therapy may be of value.

Hypertransfusion treatment has been employed extensively in the management of patients with severe ineffective erythropoiesis, as occurs in thalassemia major and occasionally in X-linked hereditary sideroblastic anemia.

Maintaining an above normal hemoglobin concentration allows normal growth and development in affected children and reduces plasma iron turnover. This minimizes excessive gastrointestinal absorption of iron. A combination of hypertransfusion and deferoxamine therapy currently enables individuals with severe iron-loading anemias to survive well into adult life.

REFERENCES

Bottomley SS: Sideroblastic anemia. Clin Haematol 11:389, 1982.

Brown EB: Recognition and treatment of iron overload. Adv Intern Med 26:159, 1980.

Charlton RW, and Bothwell TH: Iron absorption. Annu Rev Med 34:55, 1983.

Cook JD: Clinical evaluation of iron deficiency. Semin Hematol 19:6, 1982.

Cook JD and Lynch SR: The liabilities of iron deficiency. Blood 68:803, 1986.

Finch CA: Clinical aspects of iron deficiency and excess. Semin Hematol 19:1, 1982.

Finch CA and Cook JD: Iron deficiency. Am J Clin Nutr 39:471, 1984.

Finch CA and Huebers H: Perspectives in iron metabolism. N Engl J Med 306:1520, 1982.

Gordeuk VR, Bacon BR, and Brittenham GM: Iron overload: causes and consequences. Annu Rev Nutr 7:485, 1987.

Huebers HA and Finch CA: Transferrin: physiologic behavior and clinical implications. Blood 64:763, 1984.

Kohgo Y et al: Serum transferrin receptor as a new index of erythropoiesis. Blood 70:1955, 1987.

Lee GR: The anemia of chronic disease. Semin Hematol 20:61, 1983.

Lipschitz DA, Cook JD, and Finch CA: A clinical evaluation of serum ferritin as an index of iron stores. N Engl J Med 290:1213, 1974.

Propper RD et al: Continuous subcutaneous administration of deferoxamine in patients with iron overload. N Engl J Med 297:418, 1977.

Roodman GD: Mechanism of erythroid suppression in the anemia of chronic disease. Blood Cells 13:171, 1987.

Schafer AI et al: Clinical consequences of acquired transfusional iron overload in adults. N Engl J Med 304:319, 1981.

Stevens RG et al: Body iron stores and risk of cancer. N Engl J Med 319:1047, 1988.

Weatherall DJ, Pippard MJ, and Callender ST: Iron loading in thalassemia-five years with the pump. N Engl J Med 308:456, 1983.

CHAPTER

88 Megaloblastic Anemias

Aśok C. Antony

The term *megaloblastosis* describes a process in which all proliferating cells are affected by a primary defect in deoxyribonucleic acid (DNA) synthesis without significant alterations in ribonucleic acid (RNA) and protein synthesis (nuclear-cytoplasmic dissociation/asynchrony). This results in unbalanced cell growth and impaired cell division (usually involving the blood elements first) leading to megaloblastic anemia. The most common causes of megaloblastosis are *true cellular deficiencies* of vitamin B_{12} (cobalamin [Cbl]) or folate, which are essential for DNA synthesis. There are three stages in the diagnostic approach to the patient: (1) recognizing megaloblastosis, (2) determining whether folate and/or Cbl deficiency led to megaloblastosis, and (3) defining the underlying disease and mechanism. Because folates cure the megaloblastosis of folate/Cbl deficiency but aggravate the neuropsychopathology of Cbl deficiency, specific replacement is mandatory. Thus folate/Cbl physiology is an appropriate starting point in any discussion of megaloblastosis.

Cobalamin (Cbl)

Cobalamin (vitamin B_{12}) is a family of compounds, two of which, methyl-Cbl (CH_3-Cbl) and deoxyadenosyl-Cbl (Ado-Cbl), are cofactors for methionine synthase (MS) and L-methylmalonyl-CoA (MMCoA) mutase, respectively. Cbl is only produced in nature by microorganisms that contaminate plants. Humans receive Cbl (directly or indirectly) solely from their diet, and animal protein is a major source. A Western diet contains 5 to 10 μg/day of Cbl, which adequately sustains normal Cbl equilibrium (1 μg/day is excreted) because Cbl is exceptionally well stored in body tissues (of 2 to 5 mg in adults, ~ 1 mg is in the liver). It takes approximately 3 to 4 years to deplete Cbl stores when dietary Cbl is abruptly malabsorbed by the terminal ileum, but it may take longer to develop nutritional Cbl deficiency because of an efficient enterohepatic circulation. Food-Cbl is usually in coenzyme form (Ado-Cbl and CH_3-Cbl), bound to physiologic enzymes. Thus proteolysis at low (gastric) pH is a *prerequisite* for food-Cbl release. On release, Cbl preferentially binds to a salivary protein (R protein) even in the presence of parietal cell-released intrinsic factor (IF). In the duodenum, pancreatic proteases degrade Cbl-bound R proteins, but not IF, which then binds both biliary and R protein-released-Cbl. Next, IF receptors for the IF-Cbl complex on microvilli of distal ileal mucosal cells bind and internalize the IF-Cbl. After 3 to 5 hours, Cbl appears in the portal blood largely (>90%) bound to transcobalamin II (TC II), which it encounters in ileal enterocytes. More than 90% of *recently* absorbed/injected Cbl is bound to TC II, which is a specific transport protein for rapid delivery of Cbl to tissues. Whereas TC II bound-Cbl accounts for 10% to 30% of the total Cbl in serum, the remaining Cbl is mostly bound to a storage form, TC I. A third protein, TC III, probably removes unphysiologic Cbl forms via the liver. Cell surface TC II receptors bind and internalize the TC II-Cbl complex, then Cbl is reduced before conversion to CH_3-Cbl and Ado-Cbl. Mitochondrial MMCoA mutase in the presence of Ado-Cbl converts MMCoA to succinyl CoA, thereby converting the products of propionate metabolism, MMCoA, into easily metabolized products. Cytoplasmic CH_3-Cbl is a coenzyme for MS, which catalyses transfer of **methyl (-CH_3)** groups from CH_3-Cbl to homocysteine (HC) to form methionine; CH_3-Cbl is thereby reduced to Cob(I)alamin. The -CH_3 of 5-methyltetrahydrofolate (5-CH_3H_4PteGlu) is donated to Cob(I)alamin, thus regenerating CH_3-Cbl and H_4PteGlu (Fig. 88-1).

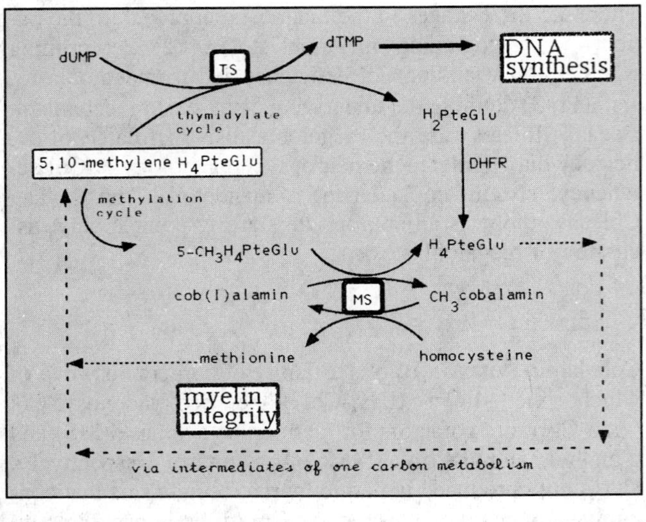

Fig. 88-1. Major biochemical reactions involving cobalamin and folate intracellularly. TS, thymidylate synthase; MS, methionine synthase; DHFR, dihydrofolate reductase. See text for additional discussion.

Folates

Folic acid (pteroylmonoglutamate [PteGlu]) is the parent compound for more than 100 derivatives collectively referred to as folates. PteGlu consists of three components, a pteridine ring, para-aminobenzoic acid (PABA), and a glutamic acid residue to which multiple glutamic acids can be added ($PteGlu_{(n)}$, polyglutamates). When PteGlu is reduced to **H_4PteGlu**, it can accept several different "one-carbon units" such as methyl-, formyl-, formimino-, hydroxymethyl-, methenyl-, and methylene- in its N^5 and/or N^{10} positions, which are then donated during numerous critical enzyme reactions in amino acid and nucleotide metabolism. Thus folates, like Cbl, are coenzymes. Folates are widely distributed in nature in green vegetables and are synthesized by microorganisms and plants. The daily requirement of folate is 50 μg for adults *and* children, but 300 to 400 μg for pregnant and lactating women. Food-$PteGlu_n$ is broken down to -$PteGlu_1$ before rapid absorption via a carrier-mediated uptake system in the jejunal brush border. It is then reduced to the **tetrahydro**folate (H_4PteGlu) form, methylated, and released within 2 hours into the circulation as **5-CH_3**-H_4PteGlu. The serum folate level is maintained constant by dietary folates and an intact enterohepatic circulation (90 μg/day). Serum folate is rapidly cleared by cell surface folate receptors that are expressed in amounts that ensure the presence of sufficient intracellular folates to support deoxyribonucleic acid (DNA) synthesis. In the cell, **5-CH_3**-H_4PteGlu is reduced via **Cbl-dependent MS** to **H_4**PteGlu (Fig. 88-1), which ensures its polyglutamation, cellular retention, and participation in one-carbon metabolism. In contrast, PteGlu must be reduced by dihydrofolate reductase (DHFR) to **H_2**PteGlu and then to **H_4**PteGlu before it is used. **H_4**PteGlu is converted via one-carbon metabolism to **5,10-methylene**-H_4PteGlu, which can be used in either (1) the ***thymidylate cycle*** via thymidylate synthase (TS) for thymidine and DNA synthesis or (2) the ***methylation cycle*** to form **5-CH_3**-H_4PteGlu, which, via MS, forms methionine and H_4PteGlu. Perturbation of either pathway thus affects DNA synthesis. TS catalyzes the transfer of the formyl group from 5,10-methylene-H_4PteGlu to deoxyuridylate; in this process 5,10-methylene-H_4PteGlu is reduced to H_2PteGlu (Fig. 88-1)

Cbl-folate interrelationships.. Cbl deficiency does not allow the MS reaction to proceed, leading to (1) an excess buildup (trapping) of 5-CH_3-H_4PteGlu, which is not polyglutamated and leaks out of the cell, leading to intracellular H_4PteGlu deficiency, and (2) a reduction in generation of methionine, an essential amino acid for protein synthesis and myelin integrity (Fig. 88-1). The overall consequences of a reduction of cellular H_4PteGlu from folate/Cbl deficiency are a shutdown of one-carbon metabolism and a net decrease in 5,10-methylene-H_4PteGlu. This interrupts TS, which converts deoxyuridine monophosphate (dUMP) to deoxythymidine monophosphate (dTMP), that is, causes thymidine deficiency and a marked increase in dUMP/dTMP ratio. Thus deoxyuridine monophosphate (dUMP) and thereby deoxyuridine triphosphate (dUTP) levels increase. Because DNA polymerase cannot distinguish between dUTP and deoxythymidine triphosphate (dTTP), the elevated dUTP level promotes misincorporation of uridine residues into DNA. A DNA editorial enzyme, however, recognizes the faulty misincorporation of dUTP (instead of dTTP) and excises dUTP out of the growing DNA chain. With continued deficiency of dTTP, this cycle is repeated many times over in several regions of the replicating DNA strand. Repeated DNA strand breaks lead to its fragmentation and leakage out of the cell. Thus affected cells cannot complete DNA synthesis and are arrested in cell cycle in prophase of the mitotic cycle and G_2. Many cells have DNA contents between 2N and 4N, which appear morphologically (Plate III-13) as "hypercellularity" with numerous "mitotic figures"; these cells are, however, not proliferating and die prematurely. There is an apparent direct correlation between the proliferative status of a cell and its propensity to megaloblastosis.

The neuropsychopathology of Cbl and folate deficiency. The clinical disorder of Cbl and folate-deficient megaloblastosis are indistinguishable. However, whereas folate deficiency commonly leads to cognitive defects and depression, only Cbl deficiency results in an unexplained demyelination process with cerebral abnormalities and subacute combined degeneration of the spinal cord. The patchy demyelinating process involves swelling of the myelin sheath and its breakdown, leading to axonal and secondary Wallerian degeneration. Progressive coalescence of microscopic foci of demyelination, usually beginning in the dorsal columns in the thoracic segments of the spinal cord, leads to early loss of vibration (256 cycle/sec tuning fork) and proprioceptive senses. Demyelination then contiguously involves corticospinal, spinothalamic, and spinocerebellar tract dorsal root/celiac ganglia and Meissner's/Auerbach's plexus. This indicates that Cbl-deficient neuropsychopathology rivals neurosyphilis as being one of "the great imitators" in clinical neurology.

PATHOGENESIS OF COBALAMIN (CBL) DEFICIENCY

Strict lacto-ovovegetarians and food faddists of almost any age may experience nutritional Cbl deficiency (see the box below), mild megaloblastosis, and neurologic manifestations. Food faddists often consume unconventional foods, which may have an anti-Cbl effect. Folate supplementation during ongoing nutritional Cbl deficiency leads to pure neurologic presentations. Prophylaxis with Cbl (50 μg/day) tablets suffices.

Because food Cbl is bioavailable only after proteolysis, patients with hypochlorhydria or achlorhydria (gastrec-

Megaloblastic anemias

I. Etiopathophysiologic classification of cobalamin (Cbl) deficiency
   A. Nutritional Cbl deficiency (insufficient Cbl intake) vegetarians, vegans, breast-fed infants of mothers with pernicious anemia
   B. Abnormal intragastric events (inadequate proteolysis of food Cbl) atrophic gastritis, partial gastrectomy with hypochlorhydria
   C. Loss/atrophy of gastric oxyntic mucosa (deficient IF molecules) total or partial gastrectomy, pernicious anemia (PA), caustic destruction (lye)
   D. Abnormal events in small bowel lumen
      1. Inadequate pancreatic protease (R-Cbl not degraded, Cbl not transferred to IF)
         (i) Insufficiency of pancreatic protease—pancreatic insufficiency
         (ii) Inactivation of pancreatic protease—Zollinger-Ellison syndrome
      2. Usurping of luminal Cbl (inadequate Cbl binding to IF)
         (i) By bacteria—stasis syndromes (blind loops, pouches of diverticulosis, strictures, fistulas, anastomoses); impaired bowel motility (scleroderma, pseudo-obstruction), hypogammaglobulinemia
         (ii) By *Diphyllobothrium latum*
   E. Disorders of ileal mucosa/IF receptors (IF-Cbl not bound to IF receptors)
      1. Diminished or absent IF receptors—ileal bypass/resection/fistula
      2. Abnormal mucosal architecture/function—tropical/nontropical sprue, Crohn's disease, TB ileitis, infiltration by lymphomas, amyloidosis
      3. IF-/post IF-receptor defects—Immerslund-Gräsbeck syndrome, TC II deficiency
      4. Drug-induced effects (slow K, biguanides, cholestyramine, colchicine, neomycin, PAS)
   F. Disorders of plasma Cbl transport (TC II-Cbl not delivered to TC II receptors)
      1. Congenital TC II deficiency, defective binding of TC II-Cbl to TC II receptors (rare)
   G. Metabolic disorders (Cbl not utilized by cell)
      1. Inborn enzyme errors (rare)
      2. Acquired disorders: (Cbl oxidized to cob[III]alamin)—N_2O inhalation

II. Etiopathophysiologic classification of folate deficiency
   A. Nutritional causes
      1. Decrease dietary intake—poverty and famine (associated with kwashiorkor, marasmus)/institutionalized individuals (psychiatric/nursing homes)/chronic debilitating disease/goat's milk (low in folate), special diets (slimming)/cultural/ethnic cooking techniques (food folate destroyed) or habits (folate-rich foods not consumed)
      2. Decreased diet and increased requirements
         (i) *Physiologic:* pregnancy and lactation, prematurity, infancy
         (ii) *Pathologic:* intrinsic hematologic disease (autoimmune hemolytic disease, drugs, malaria; hemoglobinopathies (SS, thalassemia), RBC membrane defects (hereditary spherocytosis, paroxysmal nocturnal hemoglobinopathy); abnormal hematopoiesis (leukemia/lymphoma, myelodysplastic syndrome, agnogenic myeloid metaplasia with myelofibrosis); infiltration with malignant disease; dermatologic—psoriasis
   B. Folate malabsorption
      1. With normal intestinal mucosa
         (i) Some drugs (controversial)
         (ii) Congenital folate malabsorption (rare)
      2. With mucosal abnormalities—tropical and nontropical sprue, regional enteritis
   C. Defective cellular folate uptake—familial aplastic anemia (rare)
   D. Inadequate cellular utilization
      1. Folate antagonists (methotrexate)
      2. Hereditary enzyme deficiencies involving folate
   E. Drugs (multiple effects on folate metabolism)—alcohol, sulfasalazine, triamterine, pyrimethamine, trimethoprim-sulfamethoxazole, diphenylhydantoin, barbiturates
   F. Acute folate deficiency

III. Miscellaneous megaloblastic anemias (not caused by Cbl or folate deficiency)
   A. Congenital disorders of DNA synthesis (rare)-orotic aciduria, Lesch-Nyhan syndrome, congenital dyserythropoietic anemia
   B. Acquired disorders of DNA synthesis
      1. Thiamine-responsive megaloblastosis (rare)
      2. Malignancy—erythroleukemia
         —refractory sideroblastic anemias
         —*all* antineoplastic drugs that inhibit DNA synthesis
      3. Toxic-alcohol

tomy) malabsorb food Cbl. Loss or atrophy of gastric oxyntic mucosa leads to loss of IF and to Cbl deficiency in approximately 5 years (2 to 10 years) often associated with iron deficiency. IF deficiency can also be caused by partial gastrectomy (10% to 20%, 8 years later), pernicious anemia, or caustic (lye) ingestion.

Pernicious anemia (PA), which is the most common of several causes of Cbl deficiency, is a disease involving atrophy of the gastric parietal cells leading to absent IF and HCl secretion. Despite an incidence of approximately 25 new cases/yr/100,000 persons older than 40 years, PA affects individuals of all ages, races, and ethnic origins and there is a positive family history in up to 30% of patients. The association of PA with several autoimmune diseases (Graves disease [30%], Hashimoto's thyroiditis [11%], vitiligo [8%], Addison's disease, hypoparathyroidism, and hypogammaglobulinemia) is striking. The steroid-responsive gastric abnormality also resembles autoimmune-type lesions. Among several autoantibodies, only anti-IF antibodies are specific for PA (60% in serum, 75% in gastric juice; 90% have antibodies in either serum or gastric juice). Intestinal anti-IF antibodies can interfere with IF-Cbl binding or IF-Cbl interaction with ileal IF receptors to accelerate Cbl deficiency. There is altered cellular immunity and a twofold to threefold increase in gastric carcinoma (despite correction of Cbl deficiency). Collectively, these observations suggest that the pathogenesis of PA is heterogeneous with a combined genetic, autoimmune, and acquired basis.

Because 30% of patients with severe pancreatic insufficiency fail to degrade R proteins, they can malabsorb Cbl, which responds to exogenous pancreatic extract. Pancreatic proteases are also inactivated by the massive gastric hypersecretion in Zollinger-Ellison syndrome, and if the pH of the ileal contents is less than 5.4, interference with IF-Cbl interaction with IF receptors results. Disorders conducive to relative stasis predispose to bacterial colonization. Thus Cbl may be usurped before it can bind to IF (correctable by 7 to 10 days of antibiotic therapy). Rarely, fish tapeworms, *Diphyllobothrium latum* (in poorly cooked infected fish), are found in the jejunum, where they can avidly usurp Cbl, causing Cbl deficiency in 3% of infected individuals (expulsion of the worms and therapy with Cbl are curative).

Loss of only 1 to 2 ft of terminal ileum results in a net decrease in IF receptor numbers and malabsorption of Cbl. Some drugs also impair transepithelial transport of Cbl. A heterogeneous group of congenital disorders in children causing selective Cbl malabsorption involving IF- or post-IF-receptor defects leading to megaloblastosis associated with mild, nonspecific proteinuria (in 90%) is known collectively as *Immerslund-Gräsbeck syndrome*. Other congenital defects of intracellular Cbl utilization (enzymopathies) also appear in childhood, but intermittent "shotgun" therapy can delay presentation into young adulthood (simulating multiple sclerosis). Nitrous oxide (N_2O) exposure functionally inactivates coenzyme forms of Cbl by oxidizing the fully reduced Cob(I)alamin to Cob(III)alamin. High-risk blue/white collar individuals who suffer acute or chronic (surreptitious, accidental, and/or occupational) N_2O exposure may experience acute megaloblastosis and/or Cbl-deficient neuropsychopathology, respectively.

PATHOGENESIS OF FOLATE DEFICIENCY

Folate deficiency (see the box on p. 847) arises from decreased intake/absorption/transport/utilization or increased requirement/destruction/excretion, alone or in combination in the patient. The body stores of folate are adequate to sustain normal function for approximately 4 months after removal of folate from the diet. Because 38,000 children die every day of hunger or starvation related illness, folate deficiency in the setting of general malnutrition is very common. Decreased availability of folate-rich foods (in winter), poverty, various cultural/ethnic diets/cooking techniques that destroy food folate, and chronic illness–related anorexia lead to folate deficiency. Anorexia/bulimia, food faddism, alcoholism, and slimming diets often lead to decreased folate intake in the young and middle-aged, whereas the edentulous, infirm, or neglected elderly and psychiatric patients are also particularly at risk for dietary folate deficiency.

Pregnancy and lactation with poor folate intake and increased requirements commonly cause megaloblastosis, but dimorphic (folate and iron) deficiency is the most common presentation worldwide in this group. It is now well established that *periconceptional* folate supplements protect the majority of infants from developing neural tube defects (NTDs) (spina bifida, encephalocele, meningocele) of normal mothers as well as 72% of infants of mothers at risk as a result of prior delivery of a child with NTD. Likewise, cleft lip is also folate-responsive periconceptionally. Twin/multiple frequent pregnancies and hypermesis gravidarum also predispose to folate-deficiency-induced low-birth-weight and premature infants. Folate requirements are increased in hemolytic diseases, abnormal hematopoiesis, and marrow infiltrative states. Folate deficiency during hemolytic states can lead to an acute aplastic crisis warranting routine folate prophylaxis.

Folate malabsorption accompanies the early generalized nonspecific malabsorption of sprue syndromes (Chapter 42), but after more than 2 years, Cbl deficiency supervenes. The response of tropical sprue to folate and antibiotics suggests a close interplay among a pathogen, endogenous flora, and the enterocytic folate status.

Many conventional cancer chemotherapeutic agents (antimetabolites, alkylating agents, etc.) kill malignant cells by interfering with DNA synthesis. However, limitation in dosage of such drugs because of toxicity is in part due to megaloblastosis-induced effects on normal proliferating tissues. Methotrexate binds to dihydrofolate reductase (DHFR) and thereby interferes with generation of H_4PteGlu; the ensuing megaloblastosis can be reversed by 5-formyl-H_4PteGlu (leucovorin). Although the sulfa drugs, trimethoprim and pyrimethamine, bind with higher affinity to bacterial than human DHFR, patients with underlying folate deficiency are more susceptible to megaloblastosis from these drugs. Sulfasalazine decreases conversion of $H_4PteGlu_{(n)}$ to $H_4PteGlu_1$ and can induce Heinz body hemolytic anemia (Plate III-4,P) and anticonvulsants also probably impair folate absorption. Ethanol affects several steps in folate metabolism, but the relative extent of its effects in a given patient has not been quantitated; it is also directly toxic to hematopoietic precursors.

The cause of 5-formyl-H_4PteGlu (leucovorin)-responsive acute folate deficiency with acute megaloblastosis and thrombocytopenia is unknown. Patients are usually acutely ill, in subclinical negative folate balance, and are placed in intensive care units. The combination of additional insults (decreased intake, dialysis, surgery, sepsis, drugs) somehow provokes frank megaloblastosis in the bone marrow, often unaccompanied by other morphologic/biochemical evidence for folate deficiency in the peripheral blood.

APPROACH TO DIFFERENTIAL DIAGNOSIS OF MEGALOBLASTOSIS

Clinical issues

In general, the cause of folate deficiency is found in the recent past history of the patient (<6 months), whereas Cbl deficiency has a more insidious onset of approximately 3 to 12 years. With widespread use of multivitamins containing folic acid, the megaloblastosis of Cbl deficiency may be substantially attenuated, leading to pure neurologic presentations. Common features of folate deficiency include a blunted affect with evidence of depression, irritability, forgetfulness, and sleep deprivation. All other neuropsychiatric manifestations are due to Cbl neuropathy. The physical examination may reveal different features in well-nourished patients (Cbl-deficient vegetarians or pernicious anemia patients) and poorly nourished (folate deficient) individuals with weight loss or other stigmata of multiple deficiency produced by "broad-spectrum" malabsorption. Megaloblastic manifestations of folate and Cbl deficiency are the same; they may necessitate hematologic (pancytopenia with megaloblastic marrow), cardiopulmonary (anemia), gastrointestinal (megaloblastosis with or without malabsorption), dermatologic (skin pigmentation), genital (megaloblastosis of cervical epithelium), reproductive (infertility/sterility), and psychiatric (depression) evaluation. Megaloblastosis per se in rapidly proliferating GI tract cells leads to visible changes in the oral cavity (beefy-red tongue) and functional defects, including malabsorption of folates (if the condition is uncorrected for more than 2 to 3 years, Cbl deficiency supervenes). Thus it is an axiom that megaloblastosis begets more megaloblastosis! Cbl uniquely has additional neuropsychiatric manifestations, and associated autoimmune diseases (with PA) can complicate the overall presentation. With few exceptions, Cbl deficiency is produced by Cbl malabsorption, but folate deficiency may be due to several causes, often in combination. Therefore first establish that the patient does have megaloblastosis by evaluation of the peripheral smear and a bone marrow aspirate.

Morphologic evaluation of megaloblastosis

The characteristic morphologic features of megaloblastosis are best appreciated by examination of the bone marrow aspirate (Plate III-13). It is important to perform the bone marrow aspiration as soon as possible, because megaloblastosis reverts to a normal state in approximately 24 hours of folate replenishment from average hospital meals. There are a few cases in which bone marrow aspiration may be delayed, which are primarily related to the urgency and degree of symptoms and signs (as in mild megaloblastosis). Whereas the classical megaloblastic changes are striking in orthochromatic megaloblasts (as opposed to normoblasts) in the bone marrow, leukopoiesis is also abnormal, characterized by giant metamyelocytes and "band" forms that are pathognomonic for megaloblastosis. Although hypersegmented polymorphonuclear neutrophils (PMNs) enter the circulation, the majority of megaloblastic hematopoietic precursors die in the bone marrow (intramedullary hemolysis). If these forms enter the circulation (via extramedullary hematopoiesis), their morphologic characteristics can simulate acute erythroid/myeloid leukemia and the bone marrow findings may be rather convincingly misleading. The lack of hemoglobinization of orthochromatic normoblasts (reduced iron/globin synthesis) usually leads to an overall smaller size of cells. Thus with reduced hemoglobinization and superimposed folate/Cbl deficiency, these cells are not larger than those expected in pure megaloblastosis resulting in masked megaloblastic morphologic features; iron therapy alone unmasks megaloblastosis. Megaloblastic leukopoiesis is, however, unaffected by superimposed problems with hemoglobinization.

The earliest manifestation of megaloblastosis in the peripheral blood smear is an increase in mean corpuscular volume (MCV) with macro-ovalocytes (up to 14 μm). Because these cells have adequate hemoglobin, the central pallor that normally occupies about one third of the cell is decreased, whereas in *thin macrocytes* the central pallor is increased (Plate III-4, C). Macrocytosis without megaloblastosis is seen with reticulocytosis, liver disease, aplastic or myelodysplastic syndrome ($5q^-$), hypothyroidism, myeloma, and hypoxemia and in smokers. It is spurious when a high MCV (by Coulter counter) (Chapter 73) is not substantiated on the peripheral smear (cold agglutinins, hyperglycemia, leukocytosis). Nuclear hypersegmentation of PMNs (one PMN with six lobes or 5% with five lobes) strongly suggests megaloblastosis when associated with macro-ovalocytosis (Fig. 88-2). The intramedullary hemolysis of megaloblastic erythroid cells is reflected by a low absolute reticulocyte count, increased bilirubin (<2 mg/dl) level, decreased haptoglobin level, increased LDH (often > 1000 units/ml level, and reduced red blood cell (RBC) lifespan.

Biochemical evaluation

Once megaloblastosis is confirmed, distinguishing whether it is due to Cbl/folate deficiency can be done by Cbl, folate, MMA, and HC levels (Table 88-1).

Serum homocysteine and methylmalonic acid. Among the earliest evaluable manifestations of cellular nutrient deficiency are increased serum methylmalonic acid (MMA) and homocysteine (HC) levels caused by substrate buildup when

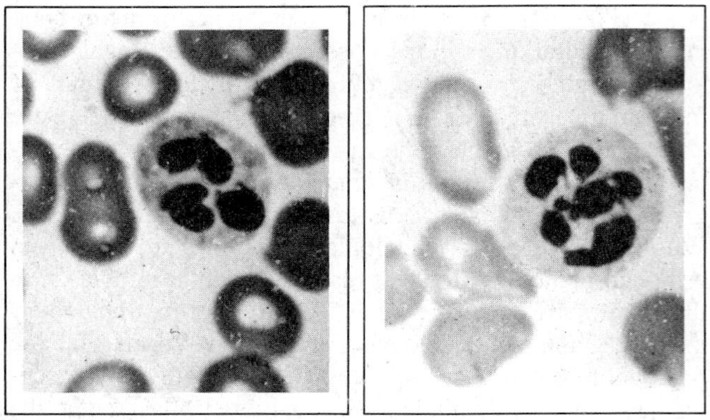

A B

Fig. 88-2. Normal and hypersegmented neutrophils on peripheral blood smears. **A,** Normal; **B,** abnormal. Hypersegmentation is seen in polymorphonuclear leukocytes from patients with folate or cobalamin (vitamin B_{12}) deficiency and in those treated with drugs such as 6-mercaptopurine that inhibit the synthesis of DNA or its percursors.

Table 88-1. Diagnostic patterns of vitamin assays

Deficiency	Serum cobalamin	Serum folate	Red blood cell folate
Cobalamin	Low	High or normal	Low or normal
Folate	Normal (low in 30%)	Low	Low
Both vitamins	Low	Low	Low

the coenzyme Cbl forms are unavailable to drive the enzyme reaction forward (Fig. 88-1). Deficiency of either Cbl or folate is reflected by elevated serum levels of HC, which can now be routinely obtained from reference laboratories. Recently, 77 of 78 patients with confirmed Cbl deficiency had elevated HC level and 74 of 78 also had increased serum MMA level, which correlated with clinical parameters of Cbl deficiency. Similarly, 18 of 19 with folate deficiency had elevated HC level but normal MMA level. Thus MMA and HC levels can distinguish Cbl from folate deficiency.

Serum cobalamin. Low serum Cbl level only suggests Cbl deficiency. However, reports of Cbl-deficient neuropsychopathology despite the absence of anemia and normal/minimally depressed Cbl suggest that these conventional tests are not infallible. The serum Cbl may be low in the absence of true Cbl deficiency in one third of patients with folate deficiency and also in multiple myeloma, TC I deficiency, and megadose vitamin C therapy. Furthermore, if the patient's serum contains ^{99m}Tc or ^{67}Ga, these radioisotopes can interfere with Cbl assays and can be interpreted as falsely low Cbl level. Thus low serum Cbl is not synonymous with Cbl deficiency. Falsely raised Cbl values are seen when Cbl binders are nonspecifically increased (myeloproliferative states, active liver disease/tumors, autoimmune diseases, lymphomas).

Serum and RBC folates. The serum folate is labile and highly influenced by folate intake. Tissue folate deficiency develops after hepatic folate stores are depleted (>4 months) and is marked by a decrease in RBC folate. Thus in folate deficiency both serum and RBC folate levels are low whereas Cbl levels are normal. Because RBC folate levels are 30-fold higher than those of serum folates, a hemolyzed specimen can falsely raise serum folate levels. In Cbl deficiency, the RBC folate level is often low because the trapped 5-CH_3-H_4PteGlu leaks out of the cell; therefore serum folate levels in Cbl deficiency may/will be normal. If a combined folate and Cbl deficiency coexists, results of all three tests will be low. Thus routinely performing all three tests at the outset in every patient (Table 88-1) distinguishes negative folate balance from a single deficiency of Cbl, folate, or combined Cbl and folate deficiency.

Clinical evaluation of Cbl absorption—the Schilling test

The Schilling test helps identify the mechanism of Cbl malabsorption: under normal conditions, oral crystalline CN-[^{57}Co]Cbl first binds R protein, which on degradation by pancreatic proteases releases the labeled Cbl for IF binding and absorption via ileal IF receptors. If the blood contains an excess of Cbl (from a "flushing" injection of exogenously administered Cbl), more than 8% of CN-[^{57}Co]Cbl is excreted in the urine in the next 24 hours (stage I test). If there is a decrease in endogenous IF level (as in PA), less than 8% of the radiolabel is excreted; however, if IF is given together with CN-[^{57}Co]Cbl, this abnormality can be corrected (stage II test). Bacterial usurping of CN-[^{57}Co]Cbl results in decreased absorption of CN-[^{57}Co]Cbl+IF, and prior therapy with antibiotics (7 to 10 days) corrects Cbl malabsorption (stage III test). If antibiotics have no corrective effect, then (with rare exceptions) the Cbl malabsorption can be localized to an ileal cause. If the stage I test result is normal in the presence of a low serum Cbl level and megaloblastosis, the problem may be inability to release Cbl from food. This commonly occurs in older patients with hypochlorhydria or achlorhydria and is an indication to order the ovalbumin-CN-[^{57}Co]Cbl absorption test, whose result will be abnormally low.

The most common cause of an abnormal Schilling test result is incomplete urine collection. Other causes include renal failure, use of some drugs (see the box on p. 847), and technical errors during the test. Because Cbl/folate deficiency causes megaloblastosis of intestinal cells, the stage I, II, and III test findings may be abnormal in florid Cbl/folate deficiency and suggest an ileal cause of Cbl malabsorption in 25% to 75% of patients. Therefore repeat stage II test after 2 months of Cbl replacement can identify those with true IF deficiency.

PRACTICAL ISSUES IN DIAGNOSIS AND THERAPY

If the patient's cardiovascular system is decompensated or if decompensation is imminent, careful slow transfusion of 1 unit (or even $<$ 1 unit) of packed RBC (with diuretic coverage) is appropriate. Both Cbl and folate should be administered in full doses and tests for Cbl absorption can be deferred until the patient is more stable.

If the patient is well compensated, check the peripheral smear for evidence of megaloblastosis and rule out macrocytic anemias (thin macrocytes with a normoblastic marrow). If there are macro-ovalocytes, bone marrow aspiration can confirm megaloblastosis within 1 hour. If the marrow does not reveal megaloblastosis but iron stores are absent, review the morphologic features again for subtle evidence of masked megaloblastosis. The serum and RBC folate, and serum Cbl and/or MMA and HC levels can sort out in a few days whether a folate/Cbl or combined deficiency led to megaloblastosis. If there is no urgency, these tests can obviate the need for bone marrow examination, provided the results are unequivocal. If the patient has been empirically treated or if there is neurologic disease with minimal anemia, serum MMA and HC levels can distinguish Cbl deficiency (increased MMA and HC level) from pure folate deficiency (increased HC but normal MMA level). However, pure Cbl deficiency cannot be distinguished from combined Cbl and folate deficiency (increased MMA and HC levels in both conditions). Normal MMA and HC levels nevertheless rule out megaloblastosis caused by Cbl or folate deficiency. A low reticulocyte count confirms the hypoproliferative state and documents the patient's response to replacement, and studies to document intramedullary hemolysis may be performed.

Once megaloblastosis is established, try to determine the underlying mechanism of Cbl/folate deficiency. If pure folate deficiency has been prolonged, expect associated Cbl deficiency to ensue. If Cbl deficiency is present, then proceed with the Schilling test and test for serum anti-IF antibodies to differentiate PA from other causes. (The Schilling test per se initiates reticulocytosis by day 2 to 3 in pure Cbl deficiency and produces a partial response in pure folate deficiency). A therapeutic trial is invaluable when diagnostic resources are limited. A positive response to physiologic doses of Cbl (1 to 2 μg/day) or folate (100 μg/day) is manifested by reticulocytosis. If subnormal responses are obtained by either vitamin, the other can be added. If in doubt, treat with full doses of Cbl and folate pending definitive diagnosis elsewhere.

Replacement therapy

An appropriate regimen for Cbl replenishment is 1 mg of intramuscular CN-Cbl/day (week 1), 1 mg twice a week (week 2), 1 mg/wk for 4 weeks, and then 1 mg/month *for life*. Oral folic acid (1 to 5 mg/day) produces adequate absorption (despite intestinal folate malabsorption), restores megaloblastosis to normal, and replenishes stores. Routine folate supplementation for all normal women periconceptually and throughout pregnancy and lactation, as well as in higher doses periconceptionally for those mothers whose infants are at risk for neural tube defects, and for premature infants, is well established. After replenishment of stores, long-term oral Cbl (1000 μg/day tablets), is an appropriate alternative provided normal serum Cbl levels are ensured.

Appropriate vitamin replacement returns megaloblastosis to normal within approximately 24 hours, and by 48 hours the only evidence of prior megaloblastosis may be the persistence of hypersegmented PMNs (delay of diagnostic bone marrow aspiration is to be avoided for this reason). Accelerated turnover of normal DNA in erythroid precursors is associated with an increase in serum urate level, which usually peaks by day 4; increased cellular phosphate uptake for nucleotide synthesis; and increased potassium flux intracellularly. This can precipitate gout or hypokalemic arrhythmias. The reticulocyte count increases by day 2 to 3 and peaks by day 5 to 8, and the hemoglobin level eventually normalizes in approximately 2 months, irrespective of the initial degree of anemia. If the RBC count is not greater than $3 \times 10^6/\mu l$ by the third week, underlying iron deficiency, hemoglobinopathy, chronic disease, or hypothyroidism should be suspected. In response to Cbl, progression of neurologic damage and dysfunction is inhibited. In general, the degree of neurologic recovery is inversely related to the extent of disease and duration of signs and symptoms. If these have been of less than 3 months' duration, they are usually completely reversible; with longer duration, there is invariable residual neurologic dysfunction. Follow-up visits every 6 months ensure adequate maintenance of hematopoeisis and diagnosis of other diseases commonly associated with the Cbl/folate deficiency state.

REFERENCES

Antony AC: The biological chemistry of folate receptors. Blood 79:2807, 1992.

Beck WS: Diagnosis of megaloblastic anemias. Annu Rev Med 42:311, 1992.

Czeizel AE and Dudás I: Prevention of the first occurrence of neural-tube defects by periconceptional vitamin supplementation. N Engl J Med 327: 1832, 1875(Editorial), 1992.

Healton EB et al: Neurologic aspects of cobalamin deficiency. Medicine 70:229, 1991.

Herbert V: Nutrition science as a continually unfolding story: the folate and vitamin B_{12} paradigm. Am J Clin Nutr 46:387, 1987.

Lindenbaum J et al: Frequency of neuropsychiatric disorders caused by cobalamin deficiency in the absence of anemia or macrocytosis. N Engl J Med 318:1720, 1988.

Stabler SP et al: Clinical spectrum and diagnosis of cobalamin deficiency. Blood 76:871, 1990.

CHAPTER

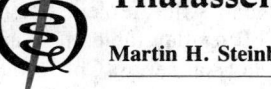

89 Hemoglobinopathies and Thalassemias

Martin H. Steinberg

The genetics and molecular abnormalities of hemoglobin (Hb) disorders are understood in detail. The chromosomal locations of the globin genes have been pinpointed and the genes cloned and sequenced. *Cis*-acting elements and *trans*-acting transcription factors that control globin gene expression are being identified.

Genes for the gamma chains of fetal hemoglobin (HbF), the delta chain of HbA_2, and the beta chain of adult hemoglobin (HbA) are located in a closely linked cluster on the short arm of chromosome 11 (Fig. 89-1, *A*). The duplicated alpha-globin genes (Fig. 89-1, *B*) are present as two identical coding sequences that are at the telomere of the short arm of chromosome 16. Interspersed among active globin genes are pseudogenes that represent inactive remnants of ancient gene duplications (Fig. 89-1). The chromosomal milieu in which these gene clusters are imbedded has been defined as the beta- or alpha-gene cluster haplotype. This is delineated by a collection of polymorphic restriction endonuclease cleavage sites within and about these genes. Globin genes share the characteristics of most eukaryotic genes; their translated, or protein-coding, regions are interrupted by non-coding, untranslated nucleotides called introns, or intervening sequences (Fig. 89-2). Globin genes are compact and contain two introns. Gene transcription is dependent on a series of phylogenetically conserved nucleotides 5′ to the coding portion called promoters. These ensure the fidelity and influence the rate of gene transcription (Fig. 89-2). Remote from the epsilon gene and zeta gene in the 5′ direction lies the locus control region (LCR), a group of DN'ase hypersensitive sites and recognition sites for ubiquitous and erythroid-specific transcription factors (Fig. 89-1). The LCR interacts with the proximal promoters of the globin genes, permitting access to transcription factors and allowing high levels of gene expression. Erythroid-specific transcription factors have been identified. The most active is called GATA-1, after the nucleotides that the core of its recognition sequence comprises. The gene for this factor is on the X-chromosome. GATA-1 plays an important role in the transcription of other erythroid-specific proteins as well as the globin genes.

The steps involved in synthesis of a globin polypeptide chain from the gene are shown in Fig. 89-2. Gene transcription results in a large intranuclear pre-messenger ribonucleic acid (pre-mRNA) (Fig. 89-2, *A*). This is processed to a smaller mRNA by excision of introns, splicing together the translated sequences, or exons, and adding special nucleotides 5′ and 3′ to the coding sequence (Fig. 89-2, *C*). The latter enhance the translatability and stability of the mRNA. Processed mRNA is exported to the cytoplasm, where, on polyribosomes, it is enzymatically translated into

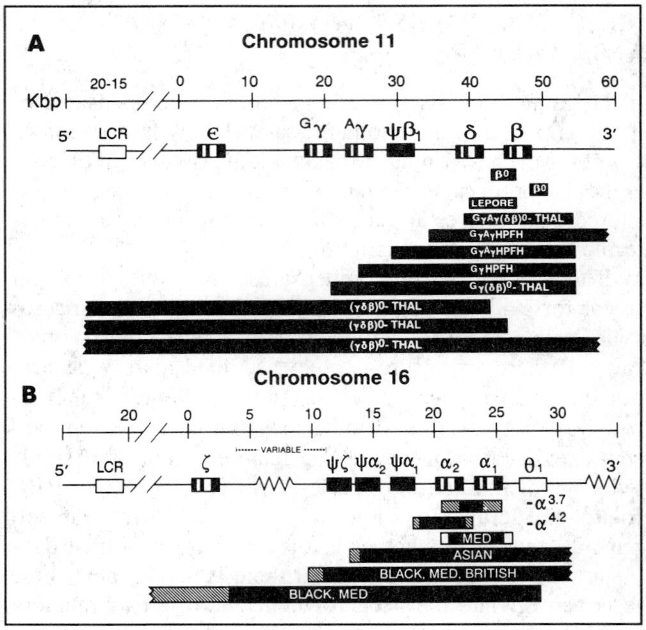

Fig. 89-1. Globin gene arrangement and deletion types of thalassemia. **A,** The betalike genes, epsilon, ^{G}gamma, ^{A}gamma, delta, and beta, are found in a 50 kb cluster on the short arm of chromosome 11. About 20 kbp 5′ to the epsilon-gene lies the LCR, which interacts with the betalike gene promoters to permit high-level gene expression. The pseudo beta gene is not expressed, the epsilon gene is expressed in the embryo, and the paired gamma genes are active mainly in fetal life. The gamma-globin gene products differ by a single amino acid at residue 136: glycine (^{G}gamma) or alanine (^{A}gamma). The deletions described in some forms of HPFH, Hb Lepore, and delta-beta thalassemia, as well as a type of beta^{0} thalassemia found in Asian Indians and small deletions in the 5′ portion of the beta gene that are associated with very high HbA_2 levels, are shown below. **B,** The alpha-gene cluster including the zeta gene, pseudogenes, the paired alpha-globin genes and the theta gene are on the short arm of chromosome 16. The alpha-LCR works in an analogous fashion to the beta-LCR. The extensive homology between alpha-globin genes makes crossing over and gene deletion common. The zeta gene is expressed only in embryonic and fetal life. A theta-gene product has not been detected. The extent of deletion in alpha-thalassemias is shown below. The two uppermost deletions remove only one gene (alpha-thalassemia-2, α^{+}); the remainder delete both genes: alpha-thalassemia-1, α^{0}). LCR, locus control region; HPFH, hereditary persistence of fetal Hb; Med, Mediterranean population; Asian, Southeast Asian population. (Modified from Weatherall and Clegg: Cell 29:7, 1982)

protein. Alpha and beta chains are produced on separate ribosomes in nearly equal quantities. Globin chains acquire heme groups and form heterodimers, which rapidly self-associate, forming a tetrameric hemoglobin molecule.

Both globin gene clusters undergo developmental switches in utero (Fig. 89-3). The embryonic globin chains, epsilon and zeta, are normally made only in the earliest stages of gestation. The epsilon-globin chain is soon replaced by gamma- and beta-globin, constituents of the predominant hemoglobin of the fetus (HbF) and adult (HbA), respectively. The alpha-globin chain, common to all adult

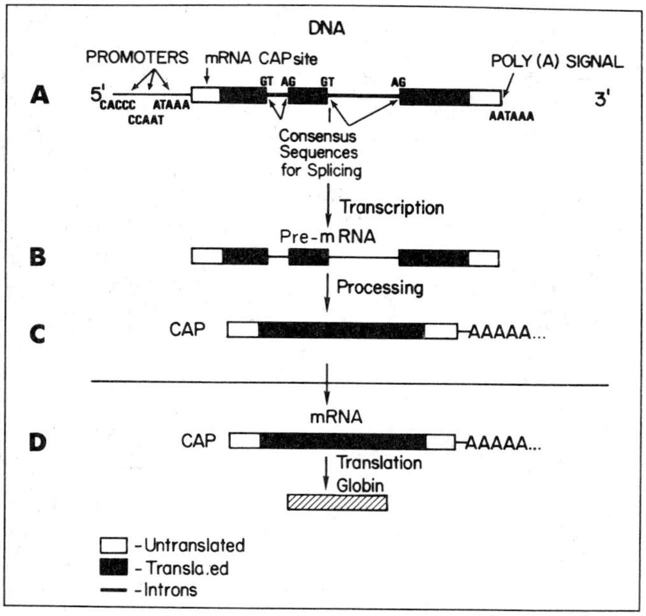

Fig. 89-2. Molecular aspects of globin biosynthesis. **A,** Globin coding sequences, or exons, are arranged in three blocks, interrupted by two noncoding intervening sequences, or introns. A series of nucleotides located 5′ to the mRNA capping site are the cis-acting promoters of gene expression that may bind transacting regulators. At the 3′ end are signals for chain termination and mRNA polyadenylation. The removal of introns is dependent in part on conserved GT and AG dinucleotides at their 5′ (donor) and 3′ (acceptor) extremities. **B,** The entire gene is enzymatically transcribed into a pre-mRNA containing untranslated sequences and introns. **C,** mRNA is processed by excision of introns and ligation of exons, capping of the 5′ end by a special nucleotide, and polyadenylation. The latter two processes enhance the translatability and stability of mRNA; mRNA is then exported to the cytoplasm for translation. **D,** mRNA is translated to a globin polypeptide on ribosomes via the interplay of groups of initiation and elongation factors and transfer RNAs that convey amino acids to the growing polypeptide. Completed alpha and beta chains acquire heme groups and associate to make a completed hemoglobin tetramer. RNA, ribonucleic acid; mRNA, messenger RNA. (Modified from Steinberg MH and Adams JG: Am J Pathol 113:396, 1983.)

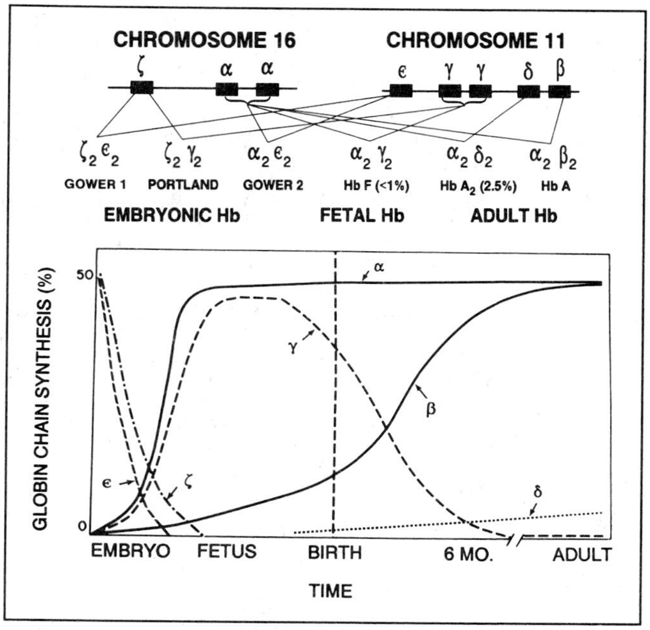

Fig. 89-3. Developmental switching of globin synthesis and the globin chain composition of human hemoglobins. Switching of gene expression within the beta-like and alpha-like gene clusters leads to the synthesis of different hemoglobins in the embryo, fetus, infant, and adult. **Top,** The globin gene-containing chromosomes and their contributions to the hemoglobin molecules of the embryo, fetus, and adult. **Bottom,** Embryonic epsilon and zeta chains rapidly disappear and are replaced by fetal gamma and adult alpha-chains. Gamma-chain synthesis peaks in midgestation and reaches its adult level at 6 months of age. There is a progressive rise in beta-chain synthesis from the first trimester to its peak at 6 to 12 months. The small amounts of delta chain synthesized peak at about 12 months.

and fetal hemoglobins, begins accumulating during the first trimester and persists at high levels throughout life (Fig. 89-3). In normal adults, hemoglobin A, composed of two alpha and two beta globin chains, comprises about 97% of the total hemoglobin. Therefore, in adults, only abnormalities affecting the alpha- or beta-globin chain have clinical significance. Although the general features of all globin genes are similar, differences in their coding sequences exist. The similarities among the beta-like genes are greater than those between the beta-like and alpha-genes. Hemoglobin switching during development may be governed by competitive interactions of the LCR with different globin gene promoters as well as the interplay of positive regulatory factors and gene "silencers."

Hemoglobin is a tetrameric globular protein with a molecular weight of about 64,000 (Fig. 89-4). Oxygen transport is mediated by the heme groups, which are cradled within a protected niche of each globin chain. All heme groups do not acquire or release their oxygen simultaneously. Rather, this is accomplished sequentially, so that the loading or unloading of each oxygen molecule is dependent on the number of oxygen molecules already bound. This property of hemoglobin is termed *cooperativity,* or *heme-heme interaction*. It is a result of specific interactions among the four globin chains of the tetramer. Cooperativity is responsible for the familiar sigmoid shape of the hemoglobin-oxygen dissociation curve. It permits blood to be oxygenated in the lungs and then to release oxygen to the tissues. The point on this curve where hemoglobin is half saturated with oxygen is called the P50. A dimeric globin molecule, such as myoglobin, does not have the property of cooperativity. Neither does a tetramer of a single type of globin chain, such as HbH (beta-4) or Bart's Hb (gamma-4). Some hemoglobin mutants have an abnormal P50, and this alters oxygen transport and erythropoiesis. Temperature, pH, erythrocyte metabolism, 2,3-biphosphoglycerate (2,3-BPG) levels, and blood phosphate concentration may all influence the P50 of normal hemoglobin.

The expression of globin disorders is usually not clinically significant unless the affected person is a homozygote

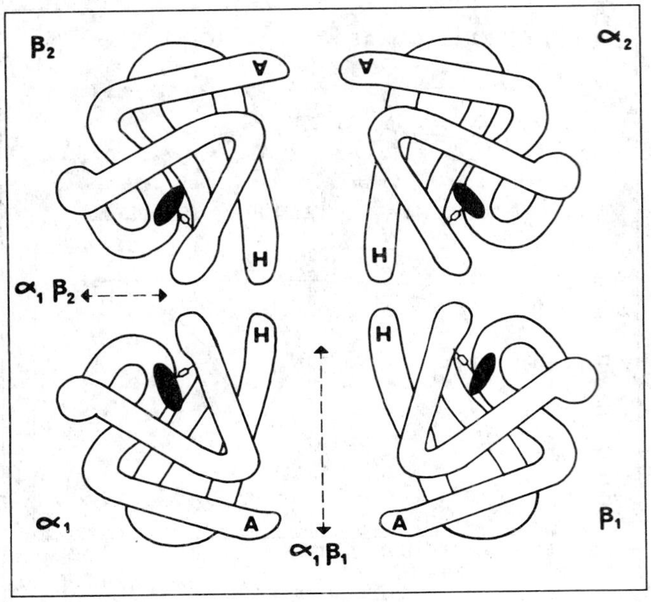

Fig. 89-4. A schematic diagram illustrating the relationships of the four globin chains and heme groups to form the hemoglobin tetramer. Each chain consists of eight helical segments (A-H) joined by short nonhelical regions. The important areas of contact, alpha$_1$, beta$_1$, and alpha$_1$, beta$_2$, are noted by the arrows. Blackened ovals within each chain represent heme groups. (From White JM and Dacie JV: Prog Hematol 7:69, 1971.)

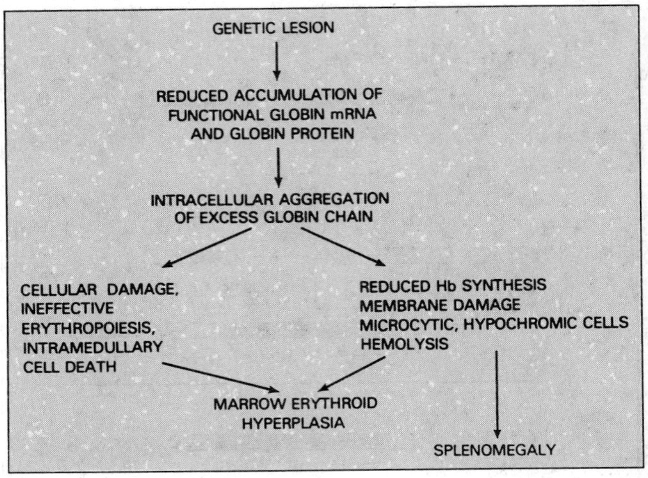

Fig. 89-5. The pathophysiology of thalassemia. The genetic lesion of thalassemia results in absent or insufficient accumulation of globin mRNA and absent or reduced globin synthesis. The redundant globin chain, a product of the nonthalassemic genes, causes injury to the developing and mature cells by virtue of their aggregation into insoluble Heinz bodies and promotion of oxidant-induced damage to the cell membrane and contents. The damaged cells either undergo intramedullary cell death or are removed from the circulation by the spleen. mRNA, messenger RNA.

or mixed heterozygote. However, in cases of unstable hemoglobins, or variants with altered oxygen affinity, heterozygotes are affected clinically. Clinical expression thus depends on the globin-gene product, which, in turn, is usually readily detectable by widely available tests. These disorders are transmitted autosomally and their inheritance obeys mendelian laws.

BETA THALASSEMIA

The beta thalassemias are widely distributed throughout the world population and result from a reduction or absence of normal beta-globin synthesis. Some regions of Italy, Greece, and Southeast Asia have carrier frequencies of nearly 20%, but beta thalassemia may appear sporadically in any ethnic group. In the United States, beta thalassemia is found mainly in descendants of immigrants from these areas of high disease prevalence. About 0.5% to 1% of blacks are beta thalassemia heterozygotes.

The thalassemic phenotype encompasses microcytosis, hypochromia reticulocytosis, anemia, ineffective erythropoiesis, and splenomegaly. Depending on the thalassemia-causing mutations that are present, these features may be insignificant or flagrant.

Etiology

In all beta thalassemias, the reduction in beta-globin synthesis leads to redundant alpha-globin chains. These are insoluble, precipitate intracellularly as Heinz bodies, and damage the developing cell, leading to intramedullary hemolysis and ineffective erythropoiesis. Unbalanced hemoglobin synthesis and membrane injury, caused in part by oxygen radical generation and Heinz bodies, curtail the erythrocytes' life span. These cells are destroyed in the spleen, which in turn hypertrophies to meet the demand for removing abnormal cells from the circulation (Fig. 89-5). Within each broad category of beta thalassemia (refer to the box at upper right) there is considerable clinical and hematologic heterogeneity. This heterogeneity can be accounted for by the numerous thalassemia-causing mutations so far discovered. Patients may be heterozygotes, homozygotes, or mixed heterozygotes for these mutations.

Beta thalassemia either totally prevents (beta^0) or partially inhibits (beta$^+$) the production of normal beta globin. Over 100 molecular lesions have so far been associated with beta thalassemia. Particular mutations are often the predominant causes of beta thalassemia in certain populations. The beta^{39} nonsense mutation (CAG→TAG) is the predominant cause of beta^0 thalassemia in Sardinians, and a promoter mutation at position -29 5′ to the beta gene(ATA→ATG) often produces mild beta$^+$ thalassemia in blacks. Restriction enzyme site polymorphisms in and about the beta globinlike gene cluster identify haplotypes associated with particular thalassemia mutations. But even within an ethnic group, there is an imperfect correlation between haplotype and mutation. Haplotype analysis has shown that certain mutations have arisen on more than one occasion in different ethnic groups. A small number of beta-thalassemia mutations are usually the predominant cause of disease in a given racial or ethnic group. The phenotype of severe beta

The thalassemias

I. Beta thalassemia
   A. Beta$^+$ thalassemia (suboptimal beta-globin synthesis)
   B. Beta^0 thalassemia (total absence of beta-globin synthesis)
   C. Delta-beta thalassemia (total absence of both delta- and beta-globin synthesis)
   D. Lepore hemoglobin (total absence of normal delta- and beta-globin synthesis with synthesis of small amounts of a fused delta-beta-globin chain)
   E. HPFH (reduction or absence of delta- and beta-globin synthesis and increased Hb F synthesis)
II. Alpha thalassemia
   A. Silent carrier, heterozygous alpha thalassemia-2 (three alpha-globin genes present; $-\alpha/\alpha\alpha$)
   B. Alpha thalassemia trait, heterozygous-alpha thalassemia-1, homozygous alpha thalassemia-2 (two alpha-globin genes present; $-\alpha/-\alpha$ or $--/\alpha\alpha$)
   C. Hb H disease (one alpha-globin gene present; $-\alpha/--$)
   D. Hydrops fetalis (no alpha-globin genes present; $--/--$)
   E. Hb Constant Spring (elongated alpha-globin chain; α^{cs})
III. Thalassemic hemoglobinopathies
   A. Hb Terre Haute, Hb Quong Sze (reduced synthesis produced by extreme instability)
   B. Hb E, Hb Knossos (reduced hemoglobin synthesis produced by abnormal mRNA splicing)

Table 89-1. Molecular causes of beta-thalassemia

Mutation class	Location	Phenotype
Nonsense mutations	Codon 39 C→T	beta^0
	Codon 121 G→T	beta^0
Frameshift mutations	Codon 6, A deleted	beta^0
mRNA Processing mutants	IVS-1, G→A	beta^0
	IVS-2, A→G	beta^0
	IVS-1 pos 5, G→C	beta$^+$
	IVS-1 pos 110, G→A	beta$^+$
Transcriptional mutants	−88 C→T	beta$^+$
mRNA Cleavage site mutants	AATAAA→AACAAA	beta$^+$
Hyperunstable globins	Codon 106 T→G (leu→arg)	beta^0

thalassemia can be caused by mixed heterozygosity as well as homozygosity for beta-thalassemia-causing mutations.

The various molecular mechanisms of beta thalassemia can modify nearly every point of the globin biosynthetic pathway and, by doing so, interfere with the accumulation of beta globin chains (Fig. 89-2). A partial list of the point mutations causing beta-thalassemia is presented in Table 89-1. Conceptually, the simplest form of beta thalassemia to understand is that produced by total or partial deletion of the beta-globin gene (Fig. 89-1). However, gene deletion is a relatively uncommon cause of beta^0 thalassemia. Gene transcription may be impaired by point mutations in the promoter elements of the gene. These mutations generally cause mild beta$^+$ thalassemia. This class of mutations is a common cause of beta thalassemia in blacks and accounts for the mildly affected homozygotes who have the phenotype of thalassemia intermedia. To assemble a functional mRNA, the introns must be excised from the initial transcript and the exons ligated to produce a contiguous coding sequence. Mutations that involve the splicing sites at the intron-exon borders can thwart this process, either totally or partially, and cause beta^0 or beta$^+$ thalassemia. Mutations that introduce a premature termination codon (nonsense mutation) into the coding region may occur, leading to a truncated and useless globin. The discovery of mutations that simultaneously produce a structurally abnormal hemoglobin and a thalassemia phenotype has blurred the distinction between thalassemias and hemoglobinopathies. These disorders have been called thalassemic hemoglobinopathies. They are often caused by mutations that occur in the third exon of the globin gene and create a globin with such marked instability that no detectable protein accumulates. The severe abnormality caused by heterozygosity for these mutations, in distinction to thalassemia trait caused by heterozygosity for the more common mutations, is due to the deleterious effects of both the abnormal, unstable globin and the globin chain in excess. Lepore hemoglobins, resulting from nonhomologous crossing over between the delta-and beta-globin genes, are characterized by a delta-beta fusion chain and deletion of the normal beta-globin gene from the affected chromosome. The fusion gene is under the regulation of the weak delta-gene promoter and is poorly expressed.

At times the fetal hemoglobin level is found to be increased, with or without a thalassemic phenotype. Most delta-beta thalassemias and pancellular hereditary persistence of fetal hemoglobin (HPFH) syndromes result from large deletions that remove both the beta- and delta-globin-genes. Homozygotes have 100%, and heterozygotes, 10% to 30% HbF. A class of HPFH is produced by a variety of mutations in the promoters of the gamma genes. These mutations lead to increased transcription of either the ^{G}gamma or the ^{A}gamma gene, in contrast to the deletion forms of HPFH, where, usually, both gamma-chains are increased. The HbF levels range from 3% to 20% and as the beta-gene in *cis* is expressed, "nondeletion" HPFHs are not accompanied by a thalassemia phenotype.

Clinical features

Heterozygous beta thalassemia is usually innocuous. The sole consistent finding is microcytosis and hypochromia (Plate III-4, M), and with "mild" mutations even this may be marginal. These individuals are called silent carriers. They may have severely affected offspring when their "mild" allele interacts with a more "severe" mutation. In beta-thalassemia trait, anemia is not often found and when present, is minimal. Few indicators of hemolysis are seen, but slight reticulocytosis and splenomegaly may occur. Clinical features depend on the type of thalassemia mutation, so that, for example, blacks with a mild beta$^+$-thalassemia gene may have slight microcytosis only, whereas Italians with a beta-0-thalassemia gene may have mild anemia, reticulocytosis, and splenomegaly.

Homozygous beta thalassemias (Thalassemia major, Cooley's anemia, or Mediterranean anemia) are characterized by intense chronic hemolytic anemia, evident within months of birth, and dependency on transfusion to sustain life. Undertreated homozygous beta thalassemias present the most flagrant display of the consequences of hemolysis. Marked intramedullary and extramedullary expansion of bone marrow causes deformity of the skull and typical "mongoloid" facial characteristics, bowing and rarefaction of long bones, and extension of marrow into paraspinal or intra-abdominal tumors. Massive enlargement of the liver and spleen can occur. Iron overload, produced by excessive intestinal absorption and transfusion, leads to cardiac failure and endocrinopathies that include diabetes mellitus and hypogonadism. Growth is retarded, infections common, and gallstones prevalent. When untreated, patients with homozygous beta thalassemia die within the first two decades of life. With modern management, this tragic spiral to dissolution need not transpire.

Thalassemia intermedia is caused by combinations of beta and alpha thalassemia, mixed heterozygosity for beta-thalassemia and Hb Lepore, and homozygosity for mild beta$^+$ thalassemia alleles. Many patients do not require transfusion, and some need it only occasionally. The evidence of iron overload, growth retardation, marrow expansion, and hypersplenism is generally less obvious than in severely affected patients, but bone disease can be prominent.

Mixed heterozygotes with beta thalassemia and a gene for beta-globin structural variants, such as HbS or HbC, are commonly found (see Table 89-2).

Laboratory features

Erythrocytes of the beta-thalassemia heterozygote have an MCV of 55 to 80 fl and a corresponding reduction in MCH. The RDW (Chapter 73) is normal in contrast to iron deficiency anemia, in which it is high. People who are silent carriers can have a normal MCV value. The red cell count is often elevated and the blood film commonly shows target cells and basophilic stippling (Plate III-4, M). Reticulocyte counts may be elevated (2% to 3%), but this is an inconsistent finding. Detection of most heterozygotes is simplified by the presence of an elevated HbA_2 level (4% to 6%), which is most accurately measured by column chromatography. HbF level may be slightly increased (1% to 3%). In delta-beta-thalassemia carriers, the HbA_2 level is normal or reduced, and the HbF concentration is increased (5% to 20%).

Homozygotes are severely anemic with hemoglobin levels of less than 5 g/dl in the absence of transfusion. MCV and MCH are reduced, and the reticulocyte count strikingly elevated. The blood film findings are characterized by nucleated red cells, Pappenheimer and Howell-Jolly bodies, marked anisocytosis, poikilocytosis, and polychromatophilia (Plate III-4, L). The bone marrow is hypercellular with marked erythroid hyperplasia and increased iron stores. Heinz bodies can be demonstrated by special staining methods (Plate III-4, P). Fetal hemoglobin is the major hemoglobin component, with absent or very reduced levels of HbA. The HbA_2 level shows considerable variation. Other indicators of chronic hemolysis are present, such as unconjugated hyperbilirubinemia, elevated LDH level, and decreased haptoglobin. Radiography of the skull may show the "hair on end" appearance of an enlarged diploic space, and other bones may appear osteoporotic.

Differential diagnosis

The heterozygous beta thalassemias may be confused with iron deficiency and other microcytic anemias (Fig. 89-6 and Chapter 87). There are few disorders that may be confused with the severe homozygous beta thalassemias. Improperly managed patients with serious growth retardation, impaired nutrition, and marked hepatosplenomegaly superficially resemble individuals with advanced cirrhosis of the liver or malignancy.

Treatment

Heterozygous beta thalassemias require only recognition, so that iron is not injudiciously administered, and carriers can be offered counseling. Screening programs, based on the detection of microcytosis and presence of elevated HbA_2 levels, are practical in groups with a high disease prevalence. When a family is at risk for having homozygous offspring, prenatal diagnosis is possible. In parts of Greece, Italy, and Cyprus, screening, counseling, and prenatal diagnosis have led to a nearly 100% reduction in the numbers of homozygotes born.

Intensive transfusion therapy and chelation of excessive iron have improved the management of severe disease. When transfusion is started very early in life and the hemoglobin levels are kept at 9 to 10 g/dl, erythropoiesis is suppressed, marrow expansion does not occur, severe hemolysis is not present, and growth and development are near normal. Besides the usual complications of transfusion, such as alloimmunization and transmission of retroviral infection, the iron burden, deposited in tissues as a result of the destruction of transfused blood, must be removed by chelation to prevent the development of transfusion-induced hemochromatosis. Desferrioxamine (Desferal), a chelating agent, is given by prolonged subcutaneous or intravenous infusion, 8 to 12 hours nightly, 5 to 6 days weekly, at doses of 2 to 6 g/day, using a portable infusion pump. The regimen must be tailored to each individual as the amount of iron excreted varies. Although optimum chelation therapy can induce negative iron balance, the ultimate effects of this treatment are not yet known. When treatment is started after significant iron accumulates, the cardiomyopathy may not always be reversible and is a leading cause of death, although intense chelation may reduce the prevalence of arrhythmias and congestive failure. Ideally, chelation should be started in young children before the acquisition of excessive iron stores. Low doses of vitamin C may increase the excretion of iron by desferrioxamine and can be used in vitamin C depleted individuals while they are receiving chelation treatment. An effective oral chelating agent that provides relief from the arduous regimen of subcutaneous infusion may soon be available.

Splenectomy may be performed when the red cell survival shortens. This reduces the excessive red cell destruction and cytopenias of hypersplenism and lengthens the interval between transfusions. Severe postsplenectomy infection is a risk that must be weighed and argues for delaying surgery as long as possible. Polyvalent pneumococcal, *Haemophilus influenzae* and *Neisseria meningitidis* vaccine should be given before surgery and prophylactic penicillin afterward.

Bone marrow transplantation has been employed in severe beta thalassemia and considerable experience has been gained in Italian centers. It is the sole way to eradicate the disease. However, the best candidates are the youngest children, as older, more heavily transfused patients are less likely to become engrafted and have higher morbidity and mortality. Because transfusion and chelation can allow normal development and a decent quality of life for many years, and because bone marrow transplantation still has appreciable short-term mortality, the decision to recommend this therapy has been very difficult. However, in children who have little or no liver disease as a result of efficient chelation, transplantation using haploidentical donors results in a disease-free survival rate of 95%. If these results are replicable, then early transplantation may be the most efficacious and cost-effective method of treatment and free the patient from the lifelong burden of parenteral chelation therapy. If the promise of an effective oral chelating drug is realized, the arguments regarding early transplantation may have to be reconsidered.

Preliminary studies have suggested that hydroxyurea may increase the level of HbF and raise the hemoglobin level in some individuals with severe beta thalassemia. This therapy may be enhanced by the administration of erythropoietin. These are exciting experimental observations but await further study before their use can be recommended. Further over the horizon are other HbF-inducing agents, such as butyrate analogs, and means of altering the genetic defects of thalassemia by gene therapy.

ALPHA THALASSEMIA

Etiology

Alpha thalassemia results from a reduction in the synthesis of alpha chain so that insufficient amounts are available for combination with non-alpha globins and for assembly of hemoglobin. The usual cause of alpha thalassemia is deletion of alpha-globin genes. Combinations of chromosomes with one- or two-gene deletions give rise to the different alpha thalassemias (refer to the box on p. 855). Point mutations cause alpha thalassemia less commonly. A common cause of alpha thalassemia in Asians is a mutation in the normal termination codon of the 5′-alpha gene. This allows continued translation of mRNA until the next termination codon is encountered. The variant alpha-globin produced, Hb Constant Spring, is elongated by 31 amino acids and is made in greatly diminished quantities. In the heterozygote, Hb Constant Spring mimics alpha thalassemia-1 caused by gene deletion. Triplicated alpha loci have been found. Although the additional gene appears to be expressed, the clinical effects are minimal. Alpha thalassemia may be the most common genetic disease of humankind. Fortunately, most instances are trivial clinically.

There are two forms of "nongenetic" alpha thalassemia that resemble HbH disease (see later discussion): one that is seen with myeloproliferative disorders and another with mental retardation. Some of the alpha thalassemia–mental retardation syndromes are X-chromosome-linked.

Clinical features

The prevalence of a single deleted alpha-globin gene ($-\alpha/\alpha\alpha$) may be near 90% in some Southwest Pacific Island populations and is 30% in blacks. Clinically significant disease is seldom seen in blacks because of the rarity of the chromosome lacking two alpha genes (α^0 or $--/$). Some Southeast Asians have a high prevalence of both the $-\alpha/$ and $--/$ chromosomes. Therefore the clinically important alpha thalassemias, HbH disease and hydrops fetalis, are most often seen in patients from this region. However, HbH disease is found in Mediterranean populations and occurs rarely in blacks.

The lack of a standard nomenclature for alpha thalassemia is reflected in the clinical and genetic terminology of the box on p. 855.

Loss of one or two alpha-globin genes is inconsequential clinically. Single gene deletions are virtually undetectable, and loss of two genes results in microcytosis only. HbH disease, in which only a single alpha-gene is active, is a mild to moderately severe hemolytic anemia with microcytic erythrocytes and splenomegaly. Total loss of four functional alpha-genes is incompatible with life and causes stillbirth of hydropic fetuses. Pregnancies carrying hydropic fetuses are complicated by a high incidence of toxemia.

Laboratory features

Diagnosis of mild forms of alpha thalassemia is hindered by lack of a simple test. In populations where the prevalence of this disorder is high, suspicion of its presence can be raised by finding microcytosis and a normal RDW (Chapter 73) with minimal or no anemia, in the absence of iron deficiency or beta thalassemia (Fig. 89-6). Hb Barts and HbH are produced by tetramerization of excessive gamma and beta chain, respectively. They have very high oxygen affinity and are of no value in oxygen transport. The levels of Hb Barts in cord blood of individuals with alpha thalassemia are proportionate to the reduction of functional alpha-genes, but considerable overlap in levels precludes this from being a facile method of diagnosing alpha thalassemia in neonates. In HbH disease, HbH can be de-

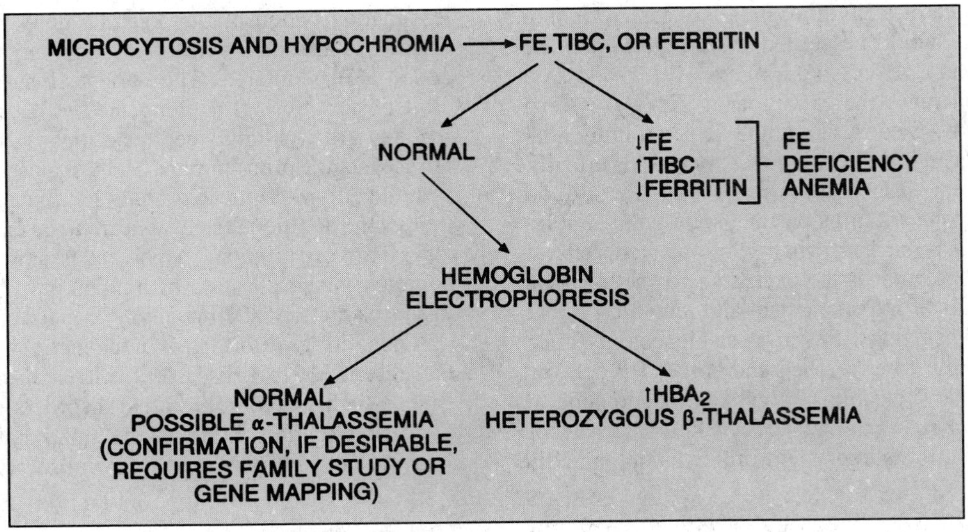

Fig. 89-6. The evaluation of microcytosis and mild thalassemias. Microcytosis, best detected by electronic cell counters, may result from a number of causes. Iron deficiency is excluded by measuring serum iron level and iron binding capacity or ferritin level. If these values are normal, hemoglobin electrophoresis should be done, with measurement of the level of HbA_2 and HbF. An elevated HbA_2 level is consistent with heterozygous beta thalassemia. If HbA_2 and HbF levels are normal, microcytosis, with minimal or no anemia, suggests alpha thalassemia. This diagnosis is more likely in populations where the prevalence of this disorder is high.

tected by electrophoresis and by special staining of erythrocytes. Hb Barts and HbH predominate in hydropic fetuses.

Restriction endonuclease mapping of the alpha-globin genes provides definitive detection of alpha-gene deletion. The technique is time consuming and expensive, and best reserved for instances involving prenatal diagnosis or special circumstances that call for a definitive diagnosis. Alpha thalassemia has been reported to prevent the development of macrocytosis in individuals with megaloblastic anemias, impairing the diagnosis of these disorders.

Treatment

Mild alpha thalassemias need no treatment or follow-up care. The injudicious use of iron to reverse a nonresponsive microcytosis should be resisted. HbH disease is best managed by periodic observation so that any increase in the degree of anemia, for example, from a supervening aplastic crisis or enlarging spleen, can be properly treated. HbH disease can be clinically heterogeneous depending on its molecular causes, and some patients may need blood transfusion. In individuals from populations where the α^0 or −−/ chromosome is common, screening can identify couples at jeopardy for hydropic fetuses. Pregnancies at risk should have prenatal diagnosis and, if a hydropic fetus is found, be terminated.

SICKLE CELL DISEASE

Sickle hemoglobin [HbS]; beta-6 glu→val) results from a GAG to GUG mutation in the codon for the sixth amino acid of beta globin. Molecular genetic evidence suggests that this mutation occurred several times during human history. The high prevalence of heterozygotes for HbS in blacks and selected other ethnic groups results from the survival advantage of the heterozygote under the selective pressure of *Falciparum malaria* infestation. Natural selection has also led to the high prevalence of alpha and beta thalassemia, HbC and HbE, ovalocytosis, and glucose-6-phosphate dehydrogenase deficiency in areas where malaria is endemic.

Etiology

HbS polymerizes on deoxygenation. Accumulation of HbS polymer within the erythrocyte distorts the cell and injures the membrane. Potassium and water leak from the cell, and it becomes dense and inflexible. Travel through the microcirculation, where capillary diameter is often only 2 to 3 μ, is slowed because considerable cellular deformability is a requisite for successful passage. Lodging of cells retards flow, reducing oxygen tension and causing further hemoglobin polymerization and tissue ischemia or infarction. These events may be initiated by subpopulations of dense cells within the community of sickle erythrocytes. In contrast to normal erythrocytes, the erythrocytes in sickle cell anemia are very heterogeneous, with a spectrum of density, deformability, membrane injury, hemoglobin content, and lifespan.

Adherence of some cells to endothelium may permit vaso-occlusion to take place before their escape into large vessels. Polymerization of HbS after its deoxygenation is reversible. But, after an unspecified number of sickleunsickle cycles, permanent membrane damage occurs, leaving the cell distorted regardless of the quantity of intracellular polymer. These irreversibly sickled cells (ISCs) are seen on the blood film (Plate III-4,H), and their numbers are related to the intensity of hemolysis. The number of ISCs varies quite widely among patients. For each individual, the number of ISCs remains relatively constant, but they may diminish early in the course of a painful episode.

Clinical features

Sickle cell trait (HbAS; heterozygotes for the beta^S gene) is present in about 8% of black Americans but is asymptomatic. Carriers have none of the hemolytic or vaso-occlusive events typical of patients with sickle cell anemia (HbSS) or other severe sickling disorders (Table 89-2). Their sole clinical complication is hematuria, which is usually mild and self-limiting and needs no treatment. Hyposthenuria is also present but is clinically unimportant. Both renal abnormalities result from sickling that may occur in the hypertonic, hypoxic, acidotic environment that typifies the normal renal medulla. There is no valid reason to restrict the activities or occupation of individuals with HbAS.

HbSS is present in about 1 in 600 American black newborns, and HbSC disease is found in 1 in 800. The appreciable early mortality rate of sickle cell disease reduces its prevalence in adults. The beta^S gene is often present in mixed heterozygotes with genes for beta thalassemia or other beta-globin mutants, such as HbC, HbD, HbE, and HbO. In addition, alpha thalassemia may be found in individuals with HbAS and HbSS (Table 89-2). Examples of the inheritance of HbSS and HbS-beta^0-thalassemia are shown in Fig. 89-7 and illustrate the mendelian transmission of all globin gene abnormalities. The pathophysiologic and clinical features of sickling disorders can be separated into those that result from hemolysis of sickle cells and those that result from vaso-occlusive episodes. The former are common to all chronic hemolytic anemias, are amenable to management, and are generally benign. The latter typify the sickling disorders, are difficult to manage, and are the major cause of morbidity and mortality.

HbSS

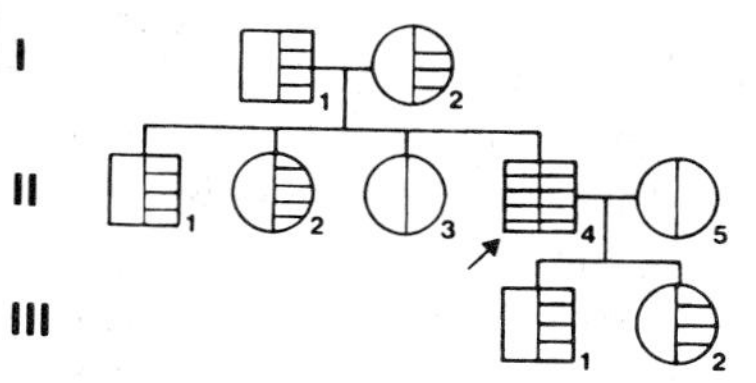

	HbA	HbS	HbA$_2$	MCV
I-1	60	40	2.5	90
I-2	60	40	2.5	90
II-1	60	40	2.5	90
II-2	60	40	2.5	90
II-3	100	0	2.5	90
II-4	0	90	2.5	90
II-5	100	0	2.5	90
III-1	60	40	2.5	90
III-2	60	40	2.5	90

HbS-β^0-THALASSEMIA

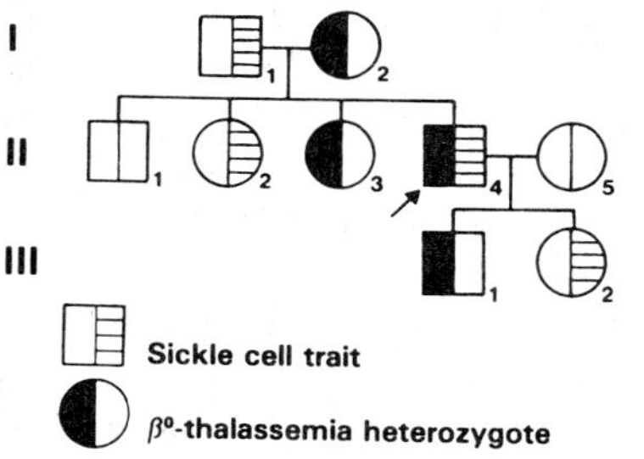

	HbA	HbS	HbA$_2$	MCV
I-1	60	40	2.5	90
I-2	100	0	5.0	65
II-1	100	0	2.5	90
II-2	60	40	2.5	90
II-3	100	0	5.0	65
II-4	0	90	5.0	70
II-5	100	0	2.0	90
III-1	100	0	5.0	65
III-2	60	40	2.5	90

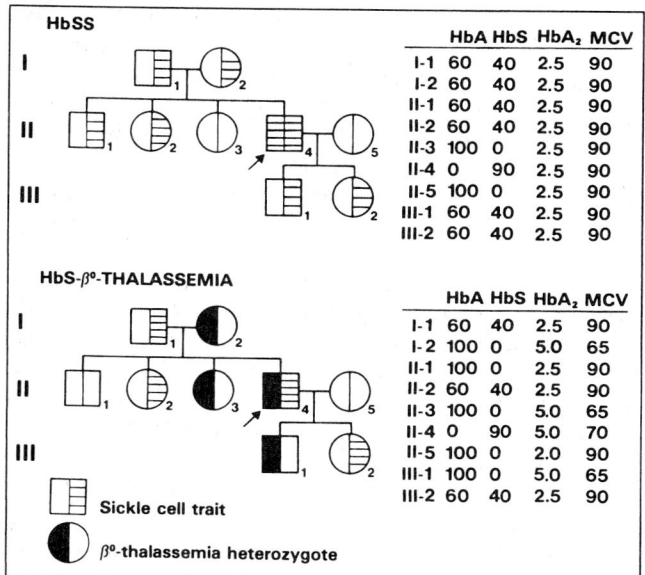

Fig. 89-7. Genetics of sickle cell disease. Pedigrees and hematologic data in two typical families with a proband who has the "Hb S only" pattern on hemoglobin electrophoresis. In the first family, the proband (↗) is homozygous for the beta^S gene and has sickle cell anemia. Both his parents have the sickle cell trait. In the idealized family of four offspring, two have the sickle trait, one is normal, and one has Hb SS. All offspring of the proband have the sickle trait, given a normal spouse. In the second family, the proband (↗) is a mixed heterozygote for the beta^S gene and a beta^0 thalassemia gene (Hb S-beta^0 thalassemia). One parent has sickle trait and the other has heterozygous beta^0 thalassemia. The idealized family of four offspring contains one normal, one sickle trait, one beta^0 thalassemia trait, and one Hb S-beta^0 thalassemia individual. The offspring of the proband, given a normal spouse, have either sickle trait or beta^0 thalassemia trait.

Hemolysis in sickle cell disease occurs largely extravascularly and even in HbSS is usually only of moderate severity. The symptoms of anemia per se are not the hall-

Table 89-2. Sickle hemoglobinopathies

	Hematocrit	MCV (fL)	HB A(%)	Hb S(%)	Hb A_2(%)	Hb F(%)	Vaso-occlusive severity
Sickle trait	Normal	Normal	60	40	2.5	<1	0
Sickle trait alpha thalassemia	Normal	70-80	65-75	25-35	2.5	<1	0
Sickle-beta$^+$ thalassemia	25-40	60-75	10-30	70	>3.5	<3	++
Sickle cell anemia	15-30	80-100	0	>85	2.5	5-15	++++
Sickle-beta^0 thalassemia	20-35	60-80	0	>85	>3.5	5-15	++++
Sickle cell anemia alpha thalassemia	20-35	70-90	0	>85	>3.5	5-15	++++
Sickle-delta-beta thalassemia	25-35	60-80	0	>80	2.5	10-20	++
Sickle-hereditary persistence of HbF	Normal	80-90	0	>70	2.5	20-30	0
Hb SC disease	25-45	70-90	0	50	2.5	1-5	+++
Normal	38-55	80-95	97	0	2.5	<1	0

mark of this disease. Severely anemic patients commonly have an element of renal failure, or the anemia develops acutely because of acquired marrow failure. Plasma volume in HbSS may be expanded 20% to 40%, making it difficult to predict the red cell mass from the hemoglobin level. Persistent hyperbilirubinemia, a consequence of hemolysis, is associated with a high prevalence of gallstones. These may appear at a remarkably young age and are found in nearly half of all adults.

Vaso-occlusive events of the sickling disorders can occur acutely, producing dramatic clinical findings, or be more chronic but nevertheless disabling (Table 89-3). The recurrence and duration of painful episodes vary markedly among patients. Some have monthly episodes that last for 3 to 10 days and require hospitalization for their management. Other patients never describe a serious pain crisis. The frequency of painful episodes is directly related to the total hemoglobin concentration and inversely related to the HbF level. Numerous painful crises are a poor prognostic sign.

The heart is usually enlarged and systolic murmurs are common. Overt congestive heart failure is not common, but there is reduced compliance of the ventricular myocardium. In children with sickle cell disease "hand-foot" syndrome, a sickling-induced periostitis of metacarpal and metatarsal bones that mimics acute rheumatoid arthritis, may develop.

The hemoglobin level remains quite constant over time unless erythropoiesis is depressed, indicating little fluctuation in the intensity of hemolysis. Bacterial infection may transiently reduce erythropoiesis. Dramatic but transient falls in hemoglobin level can occur in association with infection by the human B19 parvovirus, which preferentially attacks erythroid precursors, and is the major cause of aplastic crisis. In aplastic crisis the bone marrow has few primitive red cells and reticulocytes may be absent. Recovery occurs in 1 to 2 weeks. Children with HbSS and splenomegaly, and less often adults with HbSC disease or HbS-beta thalassemia, may have splenic sequestration crisis—the sudden pooling of red cells in the spleen. The spleen rapidly enlarges as the hemoglobin level plummets, and transfusion may be lifesaving. Rarely, megaloblastic arrest of erythropoiesis is found when severe anemia develops. This is usually due to marginal nutrition that causes folic acid deficiency.

Infection is the major cause of death in children in the first years of life, and the most common offending agent is *Streptococcus pneumoniae*. Sepsis produced by this bacterium claims a quarter of its victims. Osteomyelitis, caused by *Salmonella,* is typical of sickle cell disease. During the course of HbSS, and to a lesser extent in HbSC and HbS-beta thalassemia, splenic function decreases and is ultimately lost, as a result of repetitive infarction. Early in life the spleen may be large but hypofunctional. It then atrophies and disappears. The rate of splenic regression is related to the natural reduction in HbF levels that occurs during postnatal development and can be readily detected by the appearance of intraerythrocytic inclusions such as Howell-Jolly bodies (Plate III-4, K). Hyposplenic patients are susceptible to infection with encapsulated bacteria such as *S. pneumoniae* and *H. influenzae*. Sepsis, pneumonia, meningitis, and otitis are most frequent, and infection can progress with devastating rapidity. Sepsis in adults is often due to *Escherichia coli* and associated with urinary tract infection. Defects of the alternative complement pathway, other opsonins, and the antibody response to capsular polysaccharides may also increase the susceptibility to infection. Causes of death in adults are more varied. Death may be related to organ failure but is often sudden and unexplained. In developed countries, many patients with HbSS survive beyond the third and fourth decades, but survival past childhood is still unusual in underdeveloped lands.

A general feature of sickle cell disease is its clinical heterogeneity. Some patients have very mild disease and some

Table 89-3. Vaso-occlusive consequences of sickle cell disease

Event	Incidence	Features
Acute		
Painful episodes	Over 50% of patients with Hb SS and Hb S-beta thalassemia	Mild to severe pain, one or several areas
Chest syndrome	10%-20% of adults	Difficult to distinguish from pneumonia; may involve entire lung
Priapism	10%-40% of males	Can have a more chronic form; causes impotence
Cerebrovascular accidents	1%-10% of children	Usually subarachnoid bleeds in adults
Hepatopathy	<2% of adults	Bilirubin may reach level >80 mg/dl
Chronic		
Aseptic bone necrosis	10%-25% of adults	Hips and shoulders: also seen in Hb SC
Proliferative retinopathy	50% of adults with Hb SC, <5% Hb SS	Can lead to retinal detachment
Leg ulcers	10%	Can be severe and disabling
Functional asplenia and autosplenectomy	Starts in infancy >90% of adults with Hb SS	Predisposes to sepsis
Nephropathy	Renal failure in older patients	Nephrotic syndrome, renal failure

suffer from most or all of its complications. We still do not fully understand the reasons for this, but most likely they are due to associated genetic and environmental modulators.

Laboratory features

Typical hematologic findings in sickle cell diseases are listed in Table 89-2. The cornerstone of diagnosis is hemoglobin electrophoresis. The hemoglobin solubility test can confirm the presence of HbS but should not be relied on for primary diagnosis. The blood film (Plate III-4, H) shows ISCs, Howell-Jolly bodies, and Pappenheimer bodies in most patients with HbSS. In HbSC disease, only target cells may be seen (Plate III-4, *D* and *N*), and in HbS-beta thalassemia, hypochromia, microcytosis, and target cells are present (Plate III-4, *M*). For the evaluation of mixed heterozygous conditions (Table 89-2; Figure 89-7), family studies are vital.

Differential diagnosis

Diagnosis of sickle hemoglobinopathies is not difficult, but in some cases, differentiating these disorders can be confusing. Some useful points of distinction are shown in Table 89-2. The broad range of clinical events that occur in these patients makes sickling-induced complications a great mimic of many other diseases.

Treatment

Sickle cell disease is a chronic disorder, and attention should be given to good nutrition, immunizations, and avoidance of extremes of temperature and activity. Nonexertional work should be encouraged. Increased rates of red cell production and inadequate nutrition have led to the routine use of supplemental folic acid, 1 mg daily. Although polyvalent pneumococcal vaccine provides only limited protection in children, it should be used. Its value in adults is not proved. *H. influenza* vaccine should also be employed in infancy. Prophylactic penicillin, starting at 3 to 4 months of age and continuing for an indefinite period, decreases the incidence of pneumococcal sepsis and death. Children less than age 3 should receive 125 mg of an oral penicillin twice a day, and older children, 250 mg orally twice a day.

Painful episodes may be mild and managed at home with oral hydration and analgesics. More severe episodes may require intravenous hydration and liberal use of parenteral narcotics. In some settings, patient controlled analgesia has been effective in reducing pain. Newer oral nonnarcotic analgesics such as ketorolac (Toradol) are currently enjoying widespread use. Infection often precipitates crisis. It is best to be liberal with the decision to use antibiotics if the possibility of infection is present. Differentiating lung infection from infarction is often not possible. The choice of an antimicrobial agent need not deviate from the general practice in nonimmune suppressed individuals. However, it should be recalled that pneumococcal infection is the scourge of childhood, salmonella osteomyelitis has a high incidence in HbSS, and gram-negative infections may occur in adults.

The treatment of all vaso-occlusive episodes is directed at alleviation of symptoms because there is currently no therapy available that directly attacks the fundamental problems of HbS polymerization or occlusion of vascular flow.

Replacement of sickle with normal blood is the most specific form of treatment available. Unfortunately, the problems of transfusional hemosiderosis, alloimmunization, venous access, viral infection, and expense limit this approach. However, transfusion of red cells at times can be lifesaving and at other times may be useful. Anemia alone is rarely an indication for transfusion. Hemoglobin levels fall with aging, and with the onset of incipient renal failure, severe anemia may become symptomatic. Transfusion may then become necessary. Preliminary studies have shown that the judicious use of very high doses of erythropoietin, aimed at restoring the hemoglobin level to values customarily seen in HbSS, may substitute for transfusion in this expanding group of patients with renal insufficiency.

Packed red cells are often needed during the acute and very severe anemia of aplastic and splenic sequestration crisis. In splenic sequestration, normal erythrocytes appear to reverse the hypoxic injury to the splenic vasculature. Sequestration crises do recur, and splenectomy is indicated after the first recurrence. Repeated thrombotic cerebrovascular accidents can be prevented by prophylactic transfusion. Here the aim is to reduce the proportion of HbS to 20% to 30% of total hemoglobin. It is not clear how long prophylactic transfusion should be continued or what is the lowest effective HbA concentration. After keeping the HbS percentage at 20% to 30% for several years, some authorities believe that the frequency of transfusion may be readjusted to maintain about 50% HbS. Transcranial Doppler measurement of cerebral blood flow may be capable of identifying patients at greatest risk for stroke. If this finding proves to be true, then patients at risk could be candidates for primary stroke prevention by transfusion. Hemorrhagic stroke is the most prevalent form of cerebrovascular accident in adults. The value of prophylactic transfusion in this condition is unknown. Intensive transfusion to reduce HbS levels should be done before angiographic studies of the cerebral vasculature.

Transfusions are often used without the benefit of critical studies that confirm their value. Refractory severe leg ulcers may respond to intensive transfusion but often recur when the HbS level rises. Severe sickle hepatopathy and episodes of acute chest syndrome with hypoxia have also been managed by transfusion. Reduction of the HbS level is most easily achieved by red cell exchange using a cell separator to prevent hypervolemia. The goal of 20% to 30% HbS concentration can then often be achieved by transfusion of 1 or 2 units of packed red cells every 2 to 4 weeks. Alloimmunization occurs in about a quarter of frequently transfused patients. In the presence of multiple alloantibodies it may be difficult to find compatible blood. This high incidence of alloimmunization is a result of underrepresentation of blacks in the blood donor pool and antigenic differences that exist between erythrocytes of white donors and black recipients. To minimize the risk of sensitization if a prolonged regimen of transfusion seems likely, the recipient's red cell antigen phenotype should be determined and the most compatible blood provided. An alternative is to transfuse racially identified blood, as this will reduce the chance of exposure to units containing new antigens. The use of transfusion before surgery under general anesthesia is currently the subject of a large national study. Until it is completed, it seems wisest to individualize treatment. Patients who are undergoing prolonged surgeries, or who have antecedent pulmonary or cardiovascular problems might best receive transfusions. Rather than transfusing of 1 or 2 units just before surgery, merely to raise the hemoglobin, it is best to plan ahead and reduce the HbS level to 20% to 30%. Increasing the hemoglobin level without reducing the number of HbS containing cells may have a deleterious effect on blood viscosity. Use of random transfusions for painful episodes and other acute or chronic events is not helpful and exposes the patient to the previously discussed risks.

Pregnancy in HbSS and HbSC disease has a 10% to 20% incidence of spontaneous abortion even with the best management. This is presumably a result of placental insufficiency. It is not clear whether programs of intensive intrapartum transfusion decrease the incidence of miscarriage when compared to meticulous obstetric care alone. There is no general indication for sterilization or interruption of pregnancy in women with HbSS. Folic acid should be given, iron supplements employed if there is evidence of reduced iron stores, and transfusions given only when the clinical and hematologic status indicates their necessity. The usual methods of birth control can be used, although contraceptive pills might be avoided by older women.

The management of gallstones is problematic. As many events can provoke right upper quadrant pain in HbSS, making a firm diagnosis of cholecystitis is often difficult. When stones are asymptomatic or symptoms and laboratory findings are equivocal, it is probably best not to perform cholecystectomy. Laparoscopic cholecystectomy has been performed successfully in HbSS and could, because of its minimal morbidity, change the approach to stones.

There is considerable interest in the use of cell cycle–specific drugs such as hydroxyurea to increase the level of HbF in HbSS. A placebo-controlled, double-masked trial of the efficacy of hydroxyurea is under way. This drug can increase HbF levels in most patients with HbSS. The abnormal erythrocyte characteristics of HbSS are improved, the hemoglobin level may rise, and when hydroxyurea is carefully monitored, the toxicity is minor. Combining hydroxyurea with erythropoietin and iron may be more efficacious than using hydroxyurea alone. Efforts to minimalize the effective dose of hydroxyurea seem justified because the long-term employment of a drug that may have carcinogenic potential may be hazardous. At this time there is no proof of the efficacy of hydroxyurea, and until this is at hand, the drug should be used only in controlled clinical investigations.

Bone marrow transplantation is being studied as a means of definitively treating HbSS. The early results are encouraging, but studies indicate that parental acceptance of this procedure may be low. Current trials focus on young patients with the poorest prognosis, such as individuals who have had a stroke.

PRENATAL DIAGNOSIS AND SCREENING

Prenatal diagnosis of thalassemia and hemoglobinopathies is a feasible option in the United States and many parts of the world where these disorders are common. Prenatal diagnosis should be carried out in the context of a program of screening and education of high-risk groups. The major goal of screening for heterozygotes is family counseling regarding the risks and potential outcomes of pregnancy. This screening should be accompanied by easily understandable information about the medical problems that might occur in the heterozygote, although these are minor in HbAS and thalassemia trait. Cord blood screening programs, in contrast, are directed at the detection of offspring at risk for one of the clinically severe sickle hemoglobinopathies. These programs are cost-effective in high-risk populations. Early detection permits the institution of care that might prevent the early mortality and severe morbidity rates associated with these disorders and targets those infants who should receive prophylactic penicillin. Nearly 40 states currently screen neonates for sickle hemoglobinopathies.

Recombinant DNA technology has revolutionized prenatal diagnosis of thalassemias and is likely to be the method of the future for sickle cell screening programs. Earlier techniques relied on the placental aspiration of fetal blood, radiolabeling of globin, and chromatographic separation of globin chains. This approach is only applicable at 18 weeks of pregnancy and occasionally produces results that are difficult to interpret. It is associated with a 5% risk of miscarriage. Prenatal diagnosis can now be done on fetal DNA from amniotic fluid cells at 16 weeks of gestation or from chorionic villi that can be obtained at 10 weeks. The risk of fetal loss of the former is about 1% whereas that of the latter is near 5%. Homozygosity for HbS can be detected by use of restriction endonucleases that cut at the site of the HbS mutation or by direct examination of the HbS mutation using allele-specific oligonucleotide probes. Alpha thalassemia hydrops fetalis can be detected by the complete absence of alpha genes when DNA is probed with alpha-globin gene-specific probes. Because beta-thalassemia-causing mutations cluster in different racial and ethnic groups, direct detection of the mutations in fetal DNA, using gene amplification and groups of oligonucleotide probes specific for the mutations common in the patients' ethnic group, has become the standard means of detection. Unusual or new mutations can be ascertained by direct nucleotide sequencing of DNA that lacks a mutation represented in the group of probes employed. Quantum leaps in technology have characterized the past decades' work in molecular biology. There is ample reason to be-

Table 89-4. Clinical syndromes produced by hemoglobinopathies

Syndrome	Examples	Clinical and hematologic findings	Diagnosis
Unstable hemoglobin	Hb Zurich	Hemolytic anemia	Hb electrophoresis
	Hb Koln	May be drug-induced	Heat instability
		Heinz bodies	Isoproponol test
			Often a new mutation
High O_2 affinity	Hb Chesapeake	Polycythemia	Hb electrophoresis
	Hb Yakima	Normal MCV	Hb-O_2 dissociation curve (P_{50})
		Normal WBC	
Methemoglobinemia	Hb M-Boston	Cyanosis	Hb electrophoresis
	Hb M-Iwate	Mild hemolysis	Hb absorption spectra

lieve that the future will see even greater advances as the power of computer-based data acquisition, processing, and automation is applied to molecular techniques and analysis. It is well within our current expectations that most common genetic diseases will be rapidly and inexpensively ascertainable before or at birth.

OTHER HEMOGLOBINOPATHIES

Several other categories of hemoglobinopathies can produce clinical disorders. These are summarized in Table 89-4. Of the several hundred hemoglobinopathies that have been characterized, those causing clinically recognizable disorders are a minority. Amino acid substitutions involving residues that bind heme may lead to methemoglobinemia and cyanosis as a result of irreversible iron oxidation. Substitutions at points of contact between globin subunits may alter the affinity of hemoglobin for oxygen. When hemoglobin-oxygen affinity is increased and less oxygen is available in tissues, erythropoietin production is enhanced and erythrocytosis results. Anemia or cyanosis can be the consequence of variants with reduced hemoglobin oxygen affinity. Hemolytic anemia caused by hemoglobin instability may result from several molecular mechanisms, including introduction of proline residues into the alpha helix, substitutions near the heme ring, and deletion or addition of amino acids.

HbC ($beta^6$glu→lys) and HbE ($beta^{26}$glu→lys) are common beta-globin variants. The former is present in about 2% of blacks, and the latter is seen in Asians; its prevalence in Southeast Asians may reach 60%. Heterozygotes with either mutation are asymptomatic. Even homozygotes for these variants have virtually no clinical disease, only mild hematologic abnormalities such as microcytosis, target cells, and in the case of HbC, mild anemia. When HbE and beta thalassemia interact, a syndrome similar to homozygous beta thalassemia is produced as a consequence of the intrinsically "thalassemic" nature of the HbE gene. HbE heterozygotes have the phenotype of mild beta-thalassemia trait. In certain Southeast Asian groups in which HbE, alpha, and beta thalassemia are prevalent, screening for heterozygotes can identify couples likely to have severely affected offspring.

REFERENCES

Eaton WA and Hofrichter J: Hemoglobin S gelation and sickle cell disease. Blood 70:1245, 1987.

Hebbel RP: Beyond hemoglobin polymerization: the red blood cell membrane and sickle disease pathophysiology. Blood 77:214, 1991.

Kazazian HH, Jr: The thalassemia syndromes: molecular basis and prenatal diagnosis in 1990. Semin Hematol 27:209, 1990.

Nagel RL: Severity, pathobiology, epistatic effects, and genetic markers in sickle cell anemia. Semin Hematol 28:180, 1990.

Piomelli S and Loew T. Management of thalassemia major (Cooley's anemia). In Nagel RL, editor: Hematology-oncology clinics of North America, vol 5, number 3. Philadelphia, 1991, Saunders.

Platt OS et al: Pain in sickle cell disease-rates and risk factors. N Engl J Med 325:11, 1991.

Steinberg MH: Prospects of gene therapy for hemoglobinopathies. Am J Med Sci 302:298, 1991.

Steinberg MH: The interactions of α-thalassemia with hemoglobinopathies. In Nagel RL, editor: Hematology-oncology clinics of North America, vol 5, number 3. Philadelphia, 1991, Saunders.

Vichinsky EP et al: Alloimmunization in sickle cell anemia and transfusion of racially unmatched blood. N Engl J Med 322:1617, 1990.

CHAPTER

90 Hemolytic Anemia

G. David Roodman

The lifespan of the red blood cells in the circulation is 100 to 120 days. At the end of this period the oldest red cells are selectively removed by the reticuloendothelial system. The process by which the oldest red cells are removed is not well understood but may reflect changes in red cell membrane elasticity and acquisition of an autoantibody directed against the senescent cell antigen on older red cells. These antibody coated red cells are then removed by splenic macrophages. However, the lifespan of the red blood cell in the circulation can be prematurely shortened and the red cells destroyed by a variety of pathologic processes. Destruction of red cells, hemolysis, can result from (1) intrinsic defects in the red cell capacity to handle oxidative stress or to carry out anaerobic glycolysis and produce adenosine triphosphate (ATP), (2) defects in the red cell membrane, (3) abnormalities in hemoglobin synthesis or the hemoglobin produced, or (4) extrinsic causes that result in destruction of red cells within the circulation or the reticuloendothelial system. These extrinsic causes include (1) immune destruction of red cells by coating of the red cells with antibody or complement and subsequent removal of these cells from the circulation by the reticuloendothelial system, (2) infectious agents that directly invade the red cell, or (3) disease processes that activate the coagulation cascade or cause changes in the microvasculature. The defects responsible for hemolytic anemias can be hereditary or acquired and may or may not affect red cell structure (Table 90-1). Thus a family history and examination of the blood smear for abnormal red cell structure are critical in the diagnostic evaluation of these patients and provide important clues for planning further studies to determine the cause of their hemolytic anemia (Fig. 90-1).

HEREDITARY HEMOLYTIC ANEMIAS

Enzyme defects

Hereditary hemolytic anemias result from abnormalities in red cell enzymes that make the red cells more vulnerable to oxidative or osmotic stress or to abnormalities in the red cell membrane, which lead to red cell destruction. Patients with hereditary red cell enzymopathies who have chronic hemolysis, but whose red cells are normal in shape, are classified as having a congenital nonspherocytic hemolytic anemia (Table 90-2). A variety of mechanisms have been implicated to explain the decreased red cell survival in patients with these enzyme defects. Superoxide anions, hydroxyl radicals, and electron-avid compounds are constantly generated in the red blood cell around the iron-oxygen bond. These agents cause damage by oxidizing thiol groups on the proteins and by generating lipid peroxides in the membrane. Superoxide dismutase, vitamin E, and oxidation-reduction reactions coupled to the hexose monophosphate shunt in the red cell serve to protect red cells from oxidative damage. The hexose monophosphate shunt carries electrons from glucose-6-phosphate and 6-phosphogluconate to NADP and converts it to NADPH. NADPH in turn reduces glutathione, which then donates electrons to hydrogen peroxide, a product of the superoxide dismutase reaction. The box at lower right lists several disorders in which the red cell is damaged by oxidation either by exposure to oxidizing agents or by a defect in the endogenous enzyme pathways that protect the red cell from

Table 90-1. Peripheral blood morphology (Wright's stained smears)* as a guide to evaluation of patients with suspected hemolytic disease

	Differential diagnosis		
Blood smear findings	**Congenital**	**Acquired**	**Further tests (in order of priority)**
Spherocytes	HS, Hb CC	Immune, burns	Direct Coombs, osm. fragil., Hb electrophoresis
Elliptocytes, poikilocytes	HE, HPP	Myelodysplasia	Osm. fragil., specialized membrane studies
Hypochromic microcytes, "leptocytes"	Thalassemia, Hb Lepore, sideroblast	Iron defic., lead poisoning sideroblast	Fe/TIBC, Hb A_2 and F, Hb electrophoresis, marrow, DNA probes
Sickle cells	SS, SA, SC	—	Hb electrophoresis
Target cells (normocytic)	AC, SC, CC	Obstructive jaundice, post splenectomy	Hb electrophoresis
Acanthocytes	PK defic., abetalipoproteinemia	Liver disease	PK screen, LFTs, lipid panel
Stomatocytes	Hydro-cytosis or xerocytosis, Rh null	Liver disease, alcohol	Red cell Na/K and water content
Erythrophagocytosis, clumped RBC	—	Immune	Direct Coombs, D-L test, cold agglutinins
Schistocytes	Kasabach-Merritt syndrome	TTP, DIC, heart valve defects, myelodysplasia	Cardiac auscultation, coagulation tests
Blister cells, eccentrocytes	G6PD defic., unstable Hb	Oxidant poisoning	G6PD screen, test for unstable Hb
Heavy basophilic stippling	pyr-5′-nucleot. defic.	Lead poisoning	Lead screen, specialized enzyme assay
Nondescript or no changes	G6PD, most glycolytic defects	PNH, internal bleeding†, recovering marrow†	Sucrose lysis test, acid lysis test, G6PD screen, PK screen, specialized enzyme assays

*Many of these abnormalities are illustrated in Plate III-4.

†These conditions may simulate hemolytic disease because both feature the combination of anemia and a high reticulocyte count.

HS, hereditary spherocytosis; HE, hereditary elliptocytosis; HPP, hereditary pyropoikilocytosis; osm. fragil., osmotic fragility; sideroblast., sideroblastic anemia; Hb, hemoglobin; SS, SA, SC, CC, A_2, F, hemoglobin variants; Fe/TIBC, iron and iron-binding capacity; PK, pyruvate kinase; defic., deficiency; LFTs, liver function tests, D-L test, Donath-Landsteiner test; TTP, thrombotic thrombocytopenic purpura; DIC, disseminated intravascular coagulation; G6PD, glucose-6-phosphate dehydrogenase; pyr'5′-nucleot, pyrimidine-5′-nucleotidase; PNH, paroxysmal nocturnal hemoglobinuria; Rh null, congenital absence of Rh antigens.

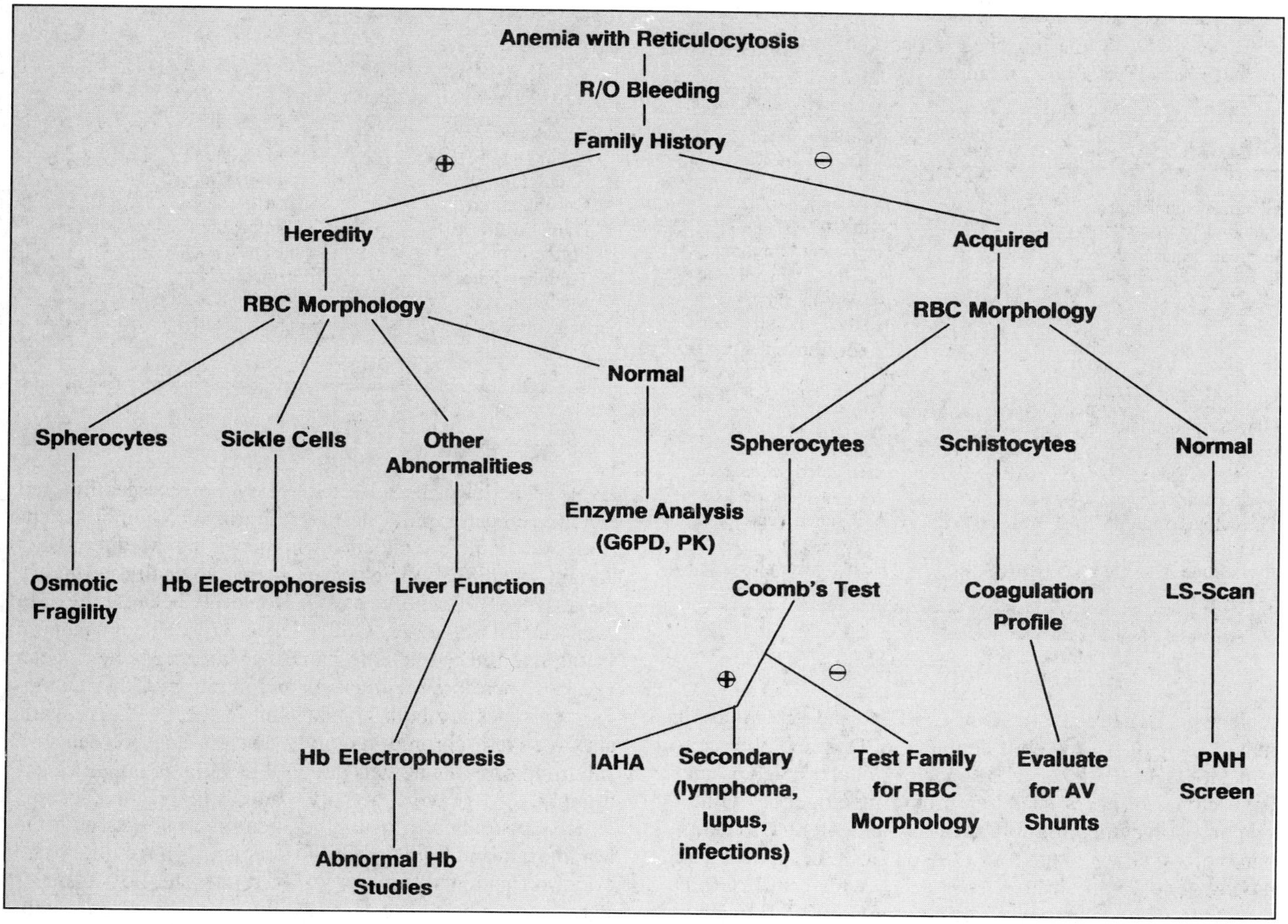

Fig. 90-1. Evaluations of patients with hemolytic anemia. LS, liver spleen; AV, arteriovenous; PNH, paroxysmal nocturnal hemoglobinuria; IAHA, idiopathic autoimmune hemolytic anemia; Hb, hemoglobin.

oxidative stress. Patients with enzyme defects in the hexose monophosphate shunt or in other reactions normally responsible for maintaining reduced glutathione level usually have episodic hemolysis when exposed to oxidative stress. In contrast, patients with defects in the Embden-Meyerhof pathway, whose red cells do not generate sufficient amounts of adenosine triphosphate (ATP), usually have chronic hemolysis and decreased red cell survival.

Glucose-6-phosphate dehydrogenase deficiency. The most common enzyme deficiency that results in oxidative damage to the red cell is glucose-6-phosphate dehydrogenase (G6PD) deficiency. It is the most common known human enzymopathy and affects approximately one tenth of the world's population. Approximately 300 electrophoretically separable variants of G6PD have been reported. The normal "wild type" enzyme is termed G6PD-B. Two common variants of G6PD occur in blacks, G6PD-A and G6PD-A^-. G6PD-A is characterized by nearly normal levels of catalytic activity, but G6PD-A^- becomes increasingly unstable with increased red cell age and is associated with hemolytic episodes. The gene frequencies for G6PD-A and A^- among American blacks are 20% to 25% and 10% to 13%, respectively. Because the G6PD gene is located on the X chromosome, males with G6PD deficiency are hemizygotes and may be more severely affected than females, who can be either homozygotes or heterozygotes. In a fe-

Oxidative disorders resulting in hemolytic anemia

- Ingestion of exogenous agents that catalyze the generation of oxidant species in normal red cells, e.g., alpha naphthol (mothballs)
- Unstable hemoglobins, including the unmatched globin chains of thalassemia
- Vitamin E deficiency
- Pentose shunt defects, including glucose-6-phosphate deficiency and other rare conditions

Table 90-2. Some inherited red cell enzymopathies that lead to hemolytic anemia

Enzyme affected	Mode of inheritance	Comments
Glucose-6-phosphate dehydrogenase	SL	Most common; see text discussion
Pyruvate kinase	AR	Next most common; echinocytes may be seen on blood smear; possible benefit from splenectomy
Hexokinase	AR	
Glucose phosphate isomerase	AR	
Triose phosphate isomerase	AR	Associated severe neuromuscular disease
Phosphoglycerate kinase	SL	Associated neurologic disease
Pyrimidine-5′ nucleotidase	AR	Heavy basophilic stippling of red cells.

SL, sex-linked; AR, autosomal recessive.

Drugs known to cause hemolysis in patients with G6PD deficiency

Acetanilid	Sulfacetamide
Nalidixic acid	Sulfapyridine
Nitrofurantoin	Trinitrotoluene
Phenylhydrazine	Primaquine
Sulfanilamide	Niridazole
Toluidine blue	Pentaquine
Methylene blue	Sulfamethoxazole
Naphthalene	Thiazolesulfone
Pamaquine	

male who is heterozygous for G6PD-A and -B, approximately 50% of her red cells contain G6PD-A and 50% contain G6PD-B. Patients who are G6PD heterozygotes and have clonal diseases such as chronic myelogenous leukemia and polycythemia rubra vera (Chapter 71) have malignant cells that are either G6PD-A or G6PD-B, rather than having equal proportions of cells with both G6PD isozymes. The geographic distribution for G6PD deficiency coincides with that of tropical malaria, suggesting that red cells deficient in G6PD may be more resistant to *Plasmodium falciparum* infection than normal red cells.

The normal African isozyme (G6PD-A) results from a single amino acid substitution and has normal catalytic activity and other biochemical properties of G6PD-B. The G6PD-A$^-$ variant differs by an additional amino acid substitution that markedly decreases the catalytic activity and alters its biochemical properties. The Mediterranean isozyme is the most common G6PD variant in white populations, and this variant is associated with favism. The Mediterranean variant has markedly decreased catalytic activity, but hemolysis is only seen in patients exposed to certain drugs, infections, surgery, or fava beans. The box at upper right lists drugs known to cause hemolysis in patients with G6PD deficiency.

Clinical features. Black patients with G6PD-A$^-$ usually have normal red cell survival. Hemolysis only occurs when these patients are exposed to a drug that induces oxidative stress in the red cell, are infected, have diabetic ketoacidosis, or develop hepatitis. In patients with G6PD-A$^-$ the enzyme activity rapidly declines in mature red cells, whereas in reticulocytes the enzyme activity is normal. Thus when patients with G6PD-A$^-$ have a hemolytic episode and large numbers of reticulocytes subsequently appear in their circulation, measurement of G6PD may reveal near normal levels of activity, because the older, more susceptible red cells have been rapidly destroyed during the hemolytic episode. In contrast, patients who have the Mediterranean variant of G6PD deficiency are hematologically normal in the absence of oxidative stress. However, because they are catalytically defective, G6PD levels are deficient in both young and old red cells in patients with the Mediterranean variant. Therefore the intensity and duration of their hemolytic episodes are both greater than in the G6PD-A$^-$ variant. A severe chronic hemolytic anemia can be seen in a subgroup of patients with rare G6PD variants that have extremely low enzyme activity. Interestingly, fava beans, which cause intense hemolytic anemia in patients with the Mediterranean variant of G6PD deficiency, have little or no effect on patients with the A$^-$ variant. The box at upper right lists drugs that can be safely given to patients with G6PD A$^-$ deficiency.

Patients with G6PD deficiency have variable signs and symptoms. These range from an intermittent mild anemia to a life-threatening episode of hemoglobinuria, shock, and renal shutdown. Hemizygotes for G6PD deficiency are believed to be particularly vulnerable to the lethal consequences of infections with Rickettsia rickettsiae, the cause of Rocky Mountain spotted fever.

Laboratory features. Most clinical laboratories can rapidly screen for G6PD deficiency by measuring enzyme activity in hemolysates. As noted, patients with G6PD-A$^-$ deficiency may have nearly normal levels of G6PD activity after a recent hemolytic episode because the susceptible older red cells, which have low levels of G6PD and were sensitive to oxidative stress, were lysed during that episode. Reticulocytes, which have near-normal levels of G6PD activity, are proportionately increased. The blood smear of patients who are undergoing hemolysis may have "blister cells" with a lopsided distribution of hemoglobin (Plate III-4, O), spherocytes, poikilocytes, and reticulocytes. If hemolysis has been severe, nucleated red cells may be seen. Heinz bodies, which represent precipitated hemoglobin adhering to the red cell membrane, are usually not seen in Wright stained blood smears but can be seen with supravitally stained peripheral blood using methylene blue or brilliant cresyl violet (Plate III-4, P). In patients with in-

Drugs that can be safely given to patients with G6PD deficiency of the A^- type

Acetaminophen	Probenecid
Acetophenetidin	Procainamide
Ascorbic acid	Pyrimethamine
Aspirin	Quinidine
Chloramphenicol	Quinine
Chloroguanidine	Streptomycin
Chloroquine	Sulfacytine
Colchicine	Sulfadiazine
Diphenhydramine	Sulfaguanidine
Isoniazid	Sulfamerazine
Levodopa	Sulfamethoxypyridazine
Menadione	Sulfisoxazole
Menaphthone	Trimethoprim
p-Aminobenzoate	Tripelennamine
Phenylbutazone	Vitamin K
Phenytoin	

tact spleens, Heinz bodies may not be seen, but bite cells may be present.

Management. The primary treatment of patients with G6PD deficiency is prevention of exposure to agents that trigger hemolysis. Once hemolysis has begun, patients should be kept well hydrated and the inciting agent removed. Splenectomy is of little value in most patients with common types of G6PD deficiency because they have periodic acute hemolytic episodes that are usually self-limited. Splenectomy has been helpful in some patients, usually caucasian, with chronic hemolytic anemia caused by severe G6PD deficiency.

Pyruvate kinase deficiency. Pyruvate kinase catalyzes the conversion of phosphoenolpyruvate to pyruvate with the generation of two molecules of ATP. Inhibition of pyruvate kinase activity results in loss of ATP, elevated concentrations of 2,3 diphosphoglycerate, and decreased NAD^+/NADH concentrations. Severe pyruvate kinase deficiency usually is manifested as a chronic hemolytic anemia early in childhood and may cause hydrops fetalis. The severity of the anemia may vary from a mild anemia to a severe transfusion dependent anemia. Clinical manifestations include splenomegaly, icterus, indirect hyperbilirubinemia, decreased haptoglobin level, and reticulocytosis with marrow erythroid hyperplasia. Infections, pregnancy, and surgery can exacerbate the chronic hemolysis. Parvovirus infections may result in an aplastic crisis in these patients. Splenectomy has been used to treat these patients and has frequently resulted in decreased transfusion requirements.

Other enzyme defects. In addition to pyruvate kinase deficiency there are other very rare enzyme deficiencies, such as hexokinase deficiency, glucose phosphate isomerase deficiency, triose phosphate isomerase deficiency, phosphoglycerate deficiency, and pyrimidine 5′ nucleotidase deficiency, that cause hemolytic anemia. These patients usually have chronic hemolysis that can vary in severity from mild to severe. Except for phosphoglycerate kinase deficiency, they have an autosomal recessive pattern of inheritance. Severely affected patients may require transfusional support.

Red cell membrane defects

An important characteristic of the red cell is its capacity to deform reversibly in the microcirculation. A reticular network of proteins directly beneath the inner surface of the lipid bilayer of the plasma membrane is believed to be responsible for the red cell's capacity to deform reversibly. The major building blocks for this protein network are spectrin and actin. The proteins are held together by a protein named band 4.1, and the membrane cytoskeleton that is formed is anchored to proteins in the lipid bilayer by ankyrin. Defects in any of these membrane components can cause hemolytic anemia. The two most common hereditary hemolytic anemias caused by membrane defects are hereditary spherocytosis and hereditary elliptocytosis.

Hereditary spherocytosis and hereditary elliptocytosis. Several different biochemical defects can cause hereditary spherocytosis (HS). The most common variety results from a molecular defect in ankyrin and displays autosomal dominant inheritance. In the recessive form of hereditary spherocytosis, defects in alpha spectrin and band 4.2 have been reported. Red cells in patients with HS have a decreased amount of all cell membrane components with a resultant decrease in their surface area. A closely related membrane defect results in deficiency in band 4.1. This interferes with the normal association of spectrin molecules with band 4.1. The consequent disorder is hereditary elliptocytosis, where elliptical red cells, rather than spherocytes, are formed. The elliptocytic configuration is thought to arise from the inability of cells to recover from molding in small capillaries. Because of the limited deformability of red cells in patients with hereditary spherocytosis or elliptocytosis, red cells are more likely to be trapped in the microcirculation of the spleen and removed from the circulation.

Clinical features. In patients with HS, the intensity of hemolysis is directly proportional to the amount of surface area lost by the red cell. Some patients may have a mild well-compensated hemolytic anemia that may never be diagnosed, and others may have severe life-threatening hemolysis. In all these patients, the spleen is often enlarged as a result of the chronic hemolysis. Increased splenic trapping, infections that suppress red cell production, or folate deficiency occurring in pregnancy may further exacerbate the hemolysis in patients with HS and can lead to an aplastic crisis. Bilirubin gallstones may develop at an early age, and, rarely, patients may have chronic leg ulcers. The mode of inheritance of HS can be either autosomal dominant or autosomal recessive; the autosomal dominant variant is by far the most common form of the disease.

Laboratory features. Evidence of accelerated red cell destruction with reticulocytosis is present in these patients.

Serum levels of lactate dehydrogenase and unconjugated bilirubin are elevated, and serum haptoglobin level is decreased. The degree of abnormality of these parameters parallels the severity of the hemolytic process. Spherocytes are easily identified on the peripheral blood smear and are characterized by a lack of central pallor, decreased mean corpuscular diameter, and increased density (Plate III-4, G). Red cell indices show an increase in MCHC and a decrease in MCV. Tests for red cell osmotic fragility, by placing red cells in hypotonic solutions, demonstrate that the cells in these patients have an increased propensity to lyse compared to normal red blood cells. The increased osmotic fragility results from the decreased amounts of membrane per red cell and increased membrane rigidity. Thus these red cells cannot compensate for the increase in intracellular volume that occurs in hypotonic solutions. Increased osmotic fragility is a characteristic of all spherocytic anemias and is not unique to HS. The increased osmotic fragility persists in patients who have undergone splenectomy, because splenectomy does not change the basic membrane defect. In patients who have very mild spherocytosis, overnight incubation of the cells at 37° C may be required to demonstrate the increased osmotic fragility. Bone marrow examination is not required to make this diagnosis so long as the reticulocyte count is elevated.

Management. Bilirubin gallstones are found in approximately 50% of patients with HS and frequently are present in patients with very mild disease. Therefore periodic ultrasonic evaluation of the gallbladder should be performed for these patients. Megaloblastic crisis can develop during pregnancy or if red cell turnover is high, so that folate acid supplementation may be required. Parvovirus infection can induce an aplastic crisis in patients with chronic hemolytic anemia and can be seen in patients with HS who have not undergone splenectomy. Splenectomy is the treatment of choice for patients with HS and is curative in most patients with the disease, although the indications for splenectomy are not always clear. After splenectomy, red cell survival remains slightly shorter than normal, and spherocytosis and increased osmotic fragility persist. However, the increase in red cell survival allows the patients to maintain a normal hematocrit. The morbidity of splenectomy is generally low in patients with HS. Candidates for splenectomy include younger patients who suffer growth retardation and individuals who have gallstones or a history of gallstones. Splenectomy should not be performed until after the age of 3 or 4 years because of the increased incidence of postsplenectomy infections with encapsulated organisms such as *Streptococcus pneumoniae* and *Haemophilus influenzae* in young children. Gallbladder evaluation should be part of the preoperative evaluation in patients undergoing splenectomy to determine whether cholecystectomy also should be done. Patients should be immunized against *Streptococcus pneumoniae, Haemophilus influenzae,* and *Neisseria meningitidis* at least 1 month before splenectomy. Patients at increased risk for these types of infections should be considered as candidates for lifelong treatment with prophylactic penicillin. Patients with hereditary elliptocytosis probably require no treatment.

ACQUIRED HEMOLYTIC ANEMIAS

Erythrocyte fragmentation syndromes

Microangiopathic hemolytic anemia. Fragmentation of red cells occurs when they pass through abnormal microvasculature, abnormal cardiac valves, or arteriovenous malformations. The normal red blood cells are broken on fibrin strands or by severe shear generated in damaged valves or malformed arteries. The fragmented cells are irregular in shape and rigid. They are called *schistocytes* (Plate III-4, E) and are easily recognized on the peripheral blood smear.

Clinical features. The most common cause of microangiopathic hemolytic anemia is disseminated intravascular coagulation ([DIC,] Chapter 85), associated with infections or tumors. In this syndrome the coagulation system is activated by endotoxin, tumor products, or bacterial enzymes, causing deposition of fibrin strands in the microvasculature. Red cells pass over these fibrin strands and are sliced into pieces as they traverse the circulation. The red cell membrane is relatively elastic and not very leaky so that little or no hemoglobin is released into the circulation. These damaged red cells are then removed in the spleen by the reticuloendothelial system. Thus there are little change in haptoglobin levels and little evidence of intravascular hemolysis, unless the red cell damage is severe. A variety of other diseases can cause disseminated intravascular coagulation (Chapter 85).

Fragmentation can also result from mechanical damage to the red cell by abnormal heart valves, usually through an aortic prosthesis where blood regurgitates around the artificial valve, or by a prosthetic patch in an endocardial cushion defect. Usually the hemolysis is minimal. Mechanical damage to red cells can also occur after stressful exercise. March hemoglobinuria was first described by Fleischer in 1891 in a soldier who passed dark urine after a long and vigorous field march. It also occurs in joggers after running on hard surfaces or after karate or conga drumming. Anemia is rare and reticulocytosis is uncommon, although iron deficiency may develop, if iron is persistently lost through hemoglobin in the urine. Treatment of March hemoglobinuria involves having the patient change to better shoes. Resolution of hemolytic anemia caused by mechanical trauma by a heart valve requires replacement of the abnormal valve. However, if the valve cannot be replaced and the anemia is severe, iron supplementation may cause marked improvement. An occasional blood transfusion may be required. If the patient's diet is poor, folate supplementation should be added. Other types of trauma to red cells include heat denaturation. This can be seen in patients who have sustained intense burns. In rare patients a febrile inflammatory response, pulmonary decompensation, and hemoglobinemia from lysis of red cells during cardiopulmonary bypass can develop. This is most probably caused by complement activation because the red cell ghosts found in these patients are coated with complement complex C5b-C9.

Freshwater drowning has also been associated with hemolysis. This is caused by severe decrease in the osmolality in the lung blood vessels resulting in osmotic shock and lysis of the red cells. Similarly, osmotic shock and lysis of red cells can occur during transurethral resection of the prostate, when the prostatic bed is washed with large amounts of distilled water.

Laboratory features. The severity of the clinical findings in patients with microangiopathic hemolytic anemia is proportional to the severity of their underlying disease. The peripheral blood smear consistently shows fragmented red cells and occasional microspherocytes (Plate III-4, E). The reticulocyte count is usually elevated and occasional nucleated red blood cells can be seen. In patients with sepsis, the leukocyte count may be elevated. The platelet count is reduced if consumption of platelets is an associated feature. If the hemolytic process is severe, there is evidence of intravascular hemolysis with elevated plasma hemoglobin levels, decreased or absent haptoglobin levels, and presence of hemoglobin and hemosiderin in the urine. A characteristic finding in patients with march hemoglobinuria is hemosiderin in the urine. They usually are not anemic and do not have an elevated reticulocyte count. On rare occasions these patients may have iron deficiency anemia caused by iron loss in their urine. In DIC there is evidence of a consumptive coagulopathy with elevation of the prothrombin and activated thromboplastin times and decreased fibrinogen levels.

Differential diagnosis. The differential diagnosis of erythrocyte fragmentation syndromes is usually evident from the clinical presentation. Patients with prosthetic heart valves or arteriovenous malformations can be identified through physical examination. The clinical picture of thrombotic thrombocytopenic purpura ([TTP] Chapter 84) or hemolytic uremic syndrome ([HUS], Chapter 84) is usually dramatic and acute and is diagnosed by presence of renal failure, microangiopathic hemolytic anemia, neurologic findings, and fever. Pregnant patients with pre-eclampsia, eclampsia, or HELLP syndrome can be readily diagnosed. These conditions may be life-threatening and are treated by delivery of the fetus. In addition, some drugs, such as cyclosporin and mitomycin C, can produce microangiopathic hemolytic anemia.

Management. Treatment of microangiopathic anemia is treatment of the underlying disease process. Removal of the abnormal valve, repair of the arteriovenous shunt, delivery of the pregnant patient, or plasmapheresis in patients with TTP/HUS stops the hemolytic process. In patients whose underlying disease cannot be treated, transfusions and iron and folate replacement may be required.

Hemolytic anemia caused by infectious agents and environmental factors

As noted, hemolysis can occur in the course of a variety of infectious diseases in which disseminated intravascular coagulation is present with deposition of fibrin strands in the microvasculature. Some of these infections are also associated with splenomegaly, which may be responsible for the increased destruction of red cells. Several infectious agents invade the red cell and destroy the red cell membrane. Malaria is the most common cause of hemolytic anemia in the world (Chapter 280). It is transmitted by the *Anopheles* mosquito. The merozoites enter the erythrocytes and grow intracellularly. The osmotic fragility of the red cell is increased in uninfected as well as infected cells. The infected red cells are removed by the spleen, and splenomegaly is a common finding in chronic malarial infections (tropical splenomegaly). Infection with falciparum malaria is sometimes associated with severe hemolysis and may result in the syndrome of black water fever, in which patients pass dark urine and have high fever. The diagnosis of malaria requires the demonstration of the parasites on blood film. Treatment of malaria includes quinine, chloroquine, sulfones, and pyrimethamine. Care should be take in administering these drugs to black patients who may have G6PD deficiency, because they may induce a hemolytic episode in G6PD deficient patients. Other infections that can cause hemolysis include Bartonellosis, which is transmitted by the sandfly. This organism infects the red blood cell by adhering to the cell membrane rather than growing within the cell. The infected red blood cells are rapidly removed from the circulation by the spleen and liver. Infection with *Bartonella* responds appropriately to antibiotics. *Clostridium perfringens* infection can induce massive hemolysis as a result of the production of an enzyme, lecithinase (Chapter 262).

Hemolysis associated with liver disease

The peripheral blood smear of patients with severe liver disease may display a variety of red cell shapes. Frequently, patients have round macrocytes and target cells (Plate III-4, D). Target cells are caused by an increased ratio of surface area to surface volume, as a consequence of increases in both the cholesterol and the phospholipid content of the membrane bilayer, compared to normal. These target cells probably do not have a shortened red cell survival. Spur cells are another red cell abnormality seen with liver disease that can result in marked hemolysis. Patients with spur cell anemia have large numbers of acanthocytes that are rapidly removed by the spleen. Splenectomy may be considered as therapy in persistent severe hemolysis. Zieve and coworkers have described a syndrome characterized by alcoholic fatty liver, hypertriglyceridemia, and hemolytic anemia. Hemolysis most probably results from acute congestive splenomegaly, which is observed frequently in patients with fatty livers, rather than from changes in the composition of the red cell membrane.

Acute alcoholism can cause low levels of serum phosphate with subsequent depletion of ATP in the red cell. Low ATP levels increase red cell rigidity, and this process may lead to fragmentation, loss of surface area, and splenic entrapment of the cells. The diagnosis of hemolytic anemia associated with liver disease can be made on the basis of the clinical setting, examination of the blood smear for spur cells, elevated liver enzyme levels, and, if the liver disease is severe, abnormalities in coagulation parameters. In patients with end-stage liver disease, treatment of the hemolytic anemia is frequently difficult and transfusion of red cells may be necessary.

Hemolytic anemia caused by drugs, chemicals, and toxins

A wide variety of chemicals and drugs can induce hemolytic anemia. Lead poisoning causes a modest shortening of the red cell lifespan and interferes with normal production of erythrocytes. Lead blocks several enzymes of the heme synthetic pathway, especially ALA dehydrase and heme synthetase. Lack of heme probably causes abnormal synthesis of alpha and beta globin chains. Blockade of heme synthetase probably is responsible for elevation of free erythrocyte protoporphyrin in these patients. Examination of the peripheral smear reveals coarse basophilic stippling, which represents abnormally aggregated ribosomes in the red cells. The diagnosis of lead poisoning can be made by finding basophilic stippling on the peripheral blood smear coupled with the presence of lead lines on the teeth at the gumline. Other chemicals that can cause hemolysis include copper, which can interfere with glucose metabolism by inhibition of hexokinase; arsine gas, generally associated with industrial accidents; chloramines, which may contaminate water used in hemodialysis; sodium and potassium chlorate; nitrobenzene; and aniline dyes.

Hemolysis can also occur after bee and wasp stings, and snake and spider bites when the venoms contain enzymes that can degrade the red cell membrane. The venom of the cobra contains phospholipases that lyse red cells; other snake venoms induce DIC (Chapter 85) with an associated microangiopathic/hemolytic anemia.

A variety of drugs can induce oxidative hemolysis by generating methemoglobin. Methemoglobin cannot reversibly bind oxygen and oxygen radicals. Continued oxidation leads to irreversibly oxidized hemoglobin intermediates which precipitate and form Heinz bodies (Plate III-4, P). Heinz bodies can destroy membrane function and cause oxidation of the membrane protein and lipids. The peripheral blood smear shows bite cells that appear as if a macrophage has taken a bite from the cell. Similar findings can be seen in patients with G6PD deficiency, as noted.

Paraquat ingestion can induce profound cyanosis with methemoglobinemia and Heinz body hemolytic anemia. Isobutyl nitrates that are abused as recreational drugs or used in suicide attempts can also induce methemoglobinernia. Transfusion of methylene blue (1 to 2 mg/kg), which reduces methemoglobin to hemoglobin, is the treatment for unacceptably elevated levels of methemoglobin.

Hypersplenism

In pathologically enlarged spleens, cell transit time is increased; the increase can cause the reduction of one or more of the circulating blood elements. Splenomegaly can result from a large number of disease processes and may decrease red cell mass. Hypersplenism is discussed in Chapter 82.

Paroxysmal nocturnal hemoglobinuria

Paroxysmal nocturnal hemoglobinuria (PNH) is an acquired stem cell defect in which the cell membrane of all three myeloid cell lines (red cells, granulocytes, and platelets) shows increased sensitivity to activated complement. This disorder may occur without a precipitating event but also may follow marrow injury. Patients have intravascular hemolysis with absent serum haptoglobin, varying degrees of hemoglobinemia and hemoglobinuria, and presence of hemosiderin in their urine. The degree of hemolysis depends on the relative sensitivity of the red cells to complement.

Autoimmune hemolytic anemias

Autoimmune hemolytic anemias result from the binding of autoantibodies against antigens on the red cell membrane, which causes premature removal of the red cells from the circulation. Three major types of antierythrocyte antibodies cause these diseases: (1) warm antibodies that bind to the red cell membrane at 37° C, (2) cold agglutinins that are usually immunoglobulin M (IgM) antibodies and clump red blood cells at temperatures below 37° C, and (3) Donath-Landsteiner antibodies that are IgG, fix to red cell membranes in the cold, and then activate the complement cascade when the cells are warmed to 37° C. Autoimmune hemolytic anemias can be primary and occur as isolated disease processes or can be secondary and associated with hematologic malignancies, autoimmune diseases, or adverse drug reactions. Approximately 25% of autoimmune hemolytic anemias are primary and have no associated predisposing condition. Of autoimmune hemolytic anemias 60% to 65% are secondary and are associated with either systemic autoimmune diseases such as lupus erythematosus or lymphoproliferative diseases or viral infections. Among cases of autoimmune hemolytic diseases 10% to 15% are drug-induced and are cured by stopping the drug. About 75% of anti–red cell antibodies are warm antibodies of the IgG subclass and about 25% are cold reacting antibodies.

Warm antibody hemolytic anemia

Clinical features. Warm antibody autoimmune hemolytic anemia is the most common type of autoimmune hemolytic anemia. Symptoms in these patients are directly related to the severity of the hemolytic process. Many patients have splenomegaly, and in patients who have secondary autoimmune hemolytic anemia, the signs and symptoms of the underlying disease (lymphoma, systemic autoimmune diseases, etc.) are present. The autoantibody is an IgG that does not fix complement and reacts with the portion of the Rh locus common to all Rh phenotypes. This disorder is diagnosed by the Coombs' test, which can detect the presence of IgG and/or complement on the red cell surface. This disorder is more common in women than in men, occurs most frequently in midlife, but can occur at all ages. The incidence of warm antibody induced autoimmune hemolytic anemia is approximately 10 cases per 1 million population. On presentation the patient may complain of increasing shortness of breath, decreased exercise tolerance, or other symptoms of anemia. Physical examination may rarely reveal signs of congestive heart failure, but this is usually in patients in whom autoimmune hemolytic anemia has developed rapidly. Splenomegaly is found in approximately one third of patients. Signs of the underlying disease such as fever, lymphadenopathy, rash, petechiae, and hematuria may be present.

Laboratory features. Microspherocytes are the hallmark of this process and can be seen on examination of the peripheral blood smear (Plate III-4, G). The reticulocyte count will be increased. In severe cases the peripheral blood smear may reveal polychromatophilia, microspherocytes, occasional red cell fragments, and nucleated red blood cells (Plate III-4, E). Examination of the bone marrow is not usually indicated but will show erythroid hyperplasia. The indirect serum bilirubin level is elevated as a sign of hemolysis. Hemolysis is usually extravascular. Signs of intravascular hemolysis may be present with increased levels of serum lactic dehydrogenase and decreased levels of plasma haptoglobin. In severe cases of intravascular hemolysis plasma free hemoglobin level may be elevated and hemoglobinuria may be present. The direct Coombs' test yields a positive result for the presence of Ig and/or complement on the surface of the red cell. The IgG autoantibodies present on the red cells in warm antibody hemolytic anemia are usually IgG_1 or IgG_3 subclasses. In addition, the proteolytic fragment of C3 of the complement cascade may also be bound to the red cells. If the direct Coombs' test result is positive, it should be repeated with more specific reagents against IgG or complement. In about 10% of the patients who have warm antibody autoimmune hemolytic anemia, the standard Coombs' test result is negative, because insufficient numbers of antibody molecules are bound to the red cell surface to be detected. In patients who have both IgG and C3 bound to the red cell membrane, the diagnosis of systemic lupus erythematosus should be considered. In about 80% of patients with autoimmune hemolytic anemia, autoantibodies are present in the serum as well as on the red cell membrane. The indirect antiglobulin test can detect the presence of these antibodies in the patient's serum. In this test, the patient's serum is mixed with normal type O red blood cells at 37° C, the cells are washed, the antiglobulin reagent is added, and the tube is examined for red cell agglutination.

In warm antibody hemolytic anemia, the interaction between macrophage surface receptors for the Fc portion of IgG and the IgG coated red cells results in ingestion and destruction of red cells. Such extravascular hemolysis is particularly prominent in the spleen, where blood cells are trapped in the hemoconcentrated microcirculation and bind to the Fc receptors on splenic macrophages. Most commonly, the macrophages only remove small bits of the erythrocyte membrane, producing a microspherocyte. These microspherocytes have a more rigid cell membrane and are more prone to osmotic lysis than normal red blood cells and can lyse more easily during repassage through the slow circulation of the spleen. The amount of antibody bound to the red cell surface, which depends on the avidity of antibody for the erythrocyte autoantigen, and the capacity of the antibody to fix complement contribute to the rapidity and efficiency of red cell clearance by the splenic macrophages.

In rare patients, autoantibodies may be directed against red cell precursors as well as mature red cells and produce pure red cell aplasia. Despite ongoing destruction of erythroid cells, the reticulocyte count is low. Pure red cell aplasia is difficult to treat and carries a serious prognosis.

Management. Glucocorticoids are the primary therapy for patients with autoimmune hemolytic anemia. Oral prednisone is usually given at doses of 1 to 2 mg/kg/day. Most physicians begin with a single dose of 60 mg/day and increase the prednisone to 100 mg/day, if no improvement is seen within several days. Prednisone is continued until a response becomes evident, usually within 10 days to 3 weeks. Responses are detected by an increase in the hematocrit and fall in the reticulocyte count. Prednisone decreases both the expression and the function of macrophage Fc receptors, and this accounts for the early effects of prednisone. Prednisone also decreases autoantibody production, but because the half-life of IgG in the circulation is approximately 3 weeks, the early response to prednisone most likely reflects its interference with macrophage function. Once a response is noted, prednisone dosage is slowly tapered over the next 2 to 3 months, and the patient is monitored closely. Approximately 75% of patients who have the primary form of autoimmune hemolytic anemia respond to large doses of prednisone. Approximately 25% of these patients maintain a sustained remission after glucocorticoids have been tapered to zero dose, and 50% require continued maintenance therapy with 5 to 20 mg of prednisone per day. The remainder of patients require relatively high doses of prednisone to maintain a satisfactory hematocrit. These adult patients, as well as adults who initially fail glucocorticoid therapy, should undergo splenectomy. Splenectomy removes a major site of red cell destruction and also eliminates a source of autoantibody production. Of patients 50% to 60% have a good initial response to splenectomy and will require less than 15 mg of prednisone per day to maintain an adequate level of hemoglobin. However, complete remission is uncommon after splenectomy, and patients generally must be maintained on low doses of glucocorticoids.

Approximately 10% of patients are unresponsive to glucocorticoids or splenectomy and require immunosuppressive drugs such as azathioprine, cyclophosphamide, or vinca alkaloids to impair macrophage function and decrease antibody production. However, immunosuppressive agents that are cytotoxic can induce numerous side effects, including marrow suppression. Therefore danazol, a synthetic androgen that has been found to be beneficial in some patients by an unknown mechanism of action, is usually tried before cytotxic agents and is given in doses of 400 to 600 mg/day. Danazol has benefited a limited number of patients with refractory hemolytic anemia, with remissions lasting for up to 1 year. In case reports, intravenous gamma globulin has been used in a similar fashion as it is used in immune thrombocytopenia. Intravenous IgG therapy appears to be effective in some patients with autoimmune hemolytic anemia associated with lymphoproliferative diseases.

In patients with life-threatening hemolytic anemia, transfusion of red cells may be necessary. Transfusion therapy is not without risk in these patients. Clinicians must supervise the transfusions carefully, because the blood bank is usually unsuccessful in finding compatible blood. The patient's autoantibody generally reacts with the basic component of the Rh locus, common to all Rh phenotypes. In patients with life-threatening hemolysis, the most compatible unit of red cells should be infused and the transfusion stopped if adverse reactions occur. Relatively small quantities of red cells may alleviate the signs and symptoms of anemia (½ to 1 unit of packed red cells), so that large amounts of blood need not be transfused in these patients. The major goal of transfusion therapy is to support the patient until other forms of treatment can control the hemolytic process.

Cold agglutinin disease

Cold agglutinins are complement fixing IgM antibodies that react with the Ii antigen system on red cells. Normal individuals have low titers of cold agglutinins (less than 1:16 at 4° C) that have low thermal amplitude and do not bind to red cells at 20° to 37° C. In cold agglutinin disease, the antibody titers measured at 4° C are greatly increased (up to $1:1 \times 10^6$) and the thermal amplitude of the antibody is increased so that the antibody binds to the surface of red cells at temperatures as high as 28° to 32° C. Cold agglutinins associated with lymphoproliferative diseases are usually monoclonal; cold agglutinins associated with *Mycoplasma* pneumonia or lupus erythematosus are polyclonal. Patients with cold agglutinins usually have a moderate anemia and attacks of acrocyanosis that are precipitated by exposure to the cold. This acrocyanosis usually results from intra-arterial agglutination of red cells in the tips of the fingers, toes, ear lobes, and nose. Most patients with chronic cold agglutinin disease are elderly (70 to 80 years of age) and many have lymphomas, Waldenstrom's macroglobulinemia, or chronic lymphocytic leukemia. Uncommonly, patients with cold agglutinin disease may exhibit Raynaud's-like reactions or hemoglobinuria. Splenomegaly is less common than in warm antibody autoimmune hemolytic anemia, and hemolysis is usually extravascular, with varying degrees of intravascular hemolysis. The peripheral blood smear shows reticulocytosis, polychromatophilia, and spherocytosis. The serum indirect bilirubin and lactate dehydrogenase levels are elevated. Anemia in patients with cold agglutinin disease is usually stable because the C3b inactivator in serum limits the extent of cold agglutinin induced complement activation on the red cell membrane. The severity of the anemia in these patients is directly correlated with the thermal amplitude of the autoantibody. The higher the temperature at which the cold agglutinin can react with the red cell, the more rapid the destruction of the cell. The direct Coombs' test result is positive because the red cells are coated with C3b. Results of tests with the anti-IgG reagents are usually negative, as is the result of the indirect Coombs' test. Extravascular hemolysis occurs because membrane receptors for C3b on hepatic macrophages allow binding and ingestion of C3b coated red cells. Hepatic clearance of these cells predominates because there is no plasma C3b to inhibit macrophage binding competitively.

A subset of patients have cold agglutinin disease of acute onset associated with *Mycoplasma pneumoniae* or infectious mononucleosis. These patients tend to be younger than those who have the chronic form of the disease and usually have an abrupt onset of hemolysis as the infection wanes. The cold agglutinin produced in patients with *Mycoplasma pneumoniae* has anti-I specificity, whereas the antibody in infectious mononucleosis has anti-i specificity. These cases of cold agglutinin disease improve as the patient recovers from the infection.

Prednisone is usually not useful in treatment of cold agglutinin disease because corticosteroids do not impair macrophage binding of C3b coated red cells. Splenectomy usually is not beneficial because hepatic clearance of red cells predominates. No treatment is usually required for the self-limited episodes associated with this disease except avoidance of cold. If the patient requires transfusion of red cells, the cross-match must be done at 37° C to find compatible units of blood. The blood must be warmed to body temperature before transfusion. Rapid infusion of blood at room temperature results in dramatic hemolysis because the autoantibody reacts well at low temperatures. Immunosuppressive agents are sometimes used to reduce cold agglutinin titers in patients with B cell malignancies.

Paroxysmal cold hemoglobinuria

Paroxysmal cold hemoglobinuria (PCH) has been reported in patients with tertiary congenital syphilis and in children who have viral infections. It is an extremely rare disease and accounts for less than 2% of cases of acquired hemolytic anemia. It is now most often associated with chicken pox and mumps. The Donath-Landsteiner antibody responsible for paroxysmal cold hemoglobinuria is of the IgG subclass. It binds to red cells at 4° C and fixes complement at 37° C. It has an anti-P specificity and does not agglutinate red cells in the cold. Patients with PCH have a positive Coombs' test result. The antibody is hemolytic in vivo and in vitro and can bind to red cells at temperatures as high as 32° C. Symptoms of patients with paroxysmal cold hemoglobinuria include fever, malaise, anorexia, and flank pain. The urine contains hemoglobin, and paroxysms of hemolysis are followed by jaundice. Treatment consists of bed rest and treatment of the primary disease process. Prednisone therapy is not useful.

Drug-induced immune hemolytic anemia

Drug-induced immune hemolytic anemia is produced by three different mechanisms. In the first, the drug acts as a hapten and binds the red cell membrane. Circulating antibodies that are directed against the drug then develop, and the drug-antibody interaction occurs on the red cell surface (e.g., penicillin) and causes red cell destruction. The red cell is thus an innocent bystander. The patient's antidrug antibodies may fix complement and cause severe anemia and hemoglobinuria. These episodes of hemolysis usually occur during the first 3 weeks of therapy with the drug but may occur after longer intervals. In the case of penicillin, hemolytic anemia occurs only with administration of large doses of the drug. With lower doses of penicillin, a positive direct Coombs' test result without hemolytic anemia is not unusual. Discontinuation of the drug stops the hemolytic process. In this innocent bystander type of hemolytic anemia, antibodies eluted from the patient's red blood cells do not react with a panel of red blood cells from normal donors, showing that the antibodies are not directed against normal red cell antigens. Diagnosis is often proved by showing that the antibody eluted from the patient's red cells and the patient's serum itself reacts with penicillin-coated red cells.

The second mechanism responsible for drug-induced hemolytic anemia is immune complex deposition on the red cell surface. The offending drug often binds to plasma Ig, forming an immune complex. This complex then binds to the red cell membrane, and the antidrug antibody that is present may bind complement. The clinical picture may include intravascular hemolysis with hemoglobinemia, hemoglobinuria, and rarely renal failure. This is the most common type of drug-induced immune hemolytic anemia. In this type of drug-induced hemolytic anemia, the direct Coombs' test result reveals complement bound to the red cell surface. The patient's serum reacts with red cells in the presence of the offending drug. The patient's red cell eluate usually does not react with normal red cells. Therapy is discontinuation of the offending drug.

The third mechanism involved in drug-induced hemolysis is induction of authentic autoantibodies against red cell antigens by a drug. Methyldopa is the classic example, in which patients develop a red cell autoantibody with specificity against the Rh system. The serologic findings in these patients are indistinguishable from those of primary autoimmune hemolytic anemia. Patients have positive direct Coombs' test and indirect Coombs' test results, and their serum reacts with normal erythrocytes. In 15% to 20% of patients who take alpha methyldopa a positive direct Coombs' test result develops, but hemolytic anemia develops in few. The Coombs' test result demonstrates IgG alone on the red cell surface. Patients who have this disorder usually have been taking alpha-methyldopa for several months. The antibody that binds to the red cells does not fix complement. Once the drug is stopped, the hemolysis often improves over 1 to 2 weeks. However, the titer of the autoantibody declines slowly and it requires 3 to 6 months before the Coombs' test result becomes negative. Other drugs in addition to alpha-methyldopa can also cause induction of red cell antibodies. Therapy for these drug induced autoantibodies to red cells is to discontinue the drug. Patients may require transfusions, if the anemia is severe. It may take several months for the Coombs' test result to return to normal.

REFERENCES

Arese P and De Flora A: Pathophysiology of hemolysis in glucose-6-phosphate dehydrogenase deficiency. Semin Hematol 27:1, 1990.

Fries LF, Brickman CM, and Frank MM: Monocyte receptors for the Fc portion of IgG increase in number in autoimmune hemolytic anemia and other hemolytic states and are decreased by glucocorticoid therapy. J Immunol 131:1240, 1983.

Garratty G: Effect of cell-bound proteins on the in vivo survival of circulating blood cells. Gerontology 37:68, 1991.

Morse EE: Toxic effects of drugs on erythrocytes. Ann Clin Lab Sci 18:13, 1988.

Sokol RJ and Hewitt S: Autoimmune hemolysis: a critical review. Crit Rev Oncol Hematol 4:125, 1985.

Thurn J: Human parvovirus B19: historical and clinical review. Rev Infect Dis 10:1005, 1988.

Valentine WN, Tanaka KR, and Paglia DE: Hemolytic anemias and erythrocyte enzymopathies. Ann Intern Med 103:245, 1985.

CHAPTER

91 Bone Marrow Failure

Frederick R. Appelbaum

The term *bone marrow failure* describes the clinical situation in which peripheral blood cytopenias develop because of the failure of bone marrow stem cells to produce mature progeny. A wide range of diseases can result in bone marrow failure (refer to the box below). This chapter discusses three relatively specific categories of bone marrow failure: bone marrow failure associated with aplastic anemia, with the myelodysplastic syndromes, and with myelofibrosis.

APLASTIC ANEMIA

Definition

Aplastic anemia is defined by presence of pancytopenia in the peripheral blood and bone marrow that is markedly hy-

Causes of pancytopenia

1. Pancytopenia with hypocellular bone marrow
   a. Acquired aplastic anemia (see the box on p. 874)
   b. Constitutional aplastic anemia (see the box on p. 874)
   c. Exposure to chemical or physical agents including ionizing irradiation and chemotherapeutic agents
   d. Some hematologic malignancies including myelodysplasia and aleukemic leukemia.
2. Pancytopenia with normal or increased cellularity of hematopoietic origin
   a. Some hematologic malignancies, including myelodysplasia, and some leukemias, lymphomas, and myelomas
   b. Paroxysmal nocturnal hemoglobinuria
   c. Hypersplenism
   d. Vitamin B_{12}, folate deficiencies
   e. Overwhelming infection
3. Pancytopenia with bone marrow replacement
   a. Tumor metastatic to marrow
   b. Metabolic storage diseases
   c. Osteopetrosis
   d. Myelofibrosis

pocellular and largely replaced by fat. Although a similar condition regularly occurs in patients receiving chemotherapy or radiotherapy for malignant disease, such patients quickly recover and are not considered to have aplastic anemia. Aplastic anemia may be categorized as mild or severe. *Severe aplastic anemia* has been defined by the International Aplastic Anemia Study Group as: (1) a marrow of less than 25% marrow cellularity and (2) at least two of the following three peripheral blood values: granulocytes less than 0.5×10^9/L, platelets less than 20×10^9/L, anemia with reticulocytes less than 1% (corrected for the hematocrit). *Mild aplastic anemia* is defined as marrow hypoplasia with cytopenias in two or more cell lines, but not severe enough to meet the preceding criteria.

Etiology

In the majority of cases the cause of aplastic anemia is unknown. In others a possible cause can be identified on the basis of a statistical or temporal relationship. However, the existence of such a relationship is not equivalent to proving cause and does not explain the mechanisms involved. An etiologic classification of aplastic anemia is presented in the box below.

Drugs. Two types of marrow suppression produced by drugs can be distinguished. Many drugs have the potential to suppress proliferation of one or more cell lines in all individuals in a dose-related fashion, a form of suppression that is not considered as aplastic anemia. Rather, drug-induced aplastic anemia is an idiosyncratic reaction that occurs relatively independently of dose and affects only a very small population of patients receiving the drug. The true incidence of drug-induced aplastic anemia is unknown. But in about 20% of cases of severe aplastic anemia a suspected agent can be identified. Historically, the broad-spectrum antibiotic chloramphenicol has been the most commonly identified drug. Severe aplastic anemia is estimated to occur in 1 in every 20,000 to 30,000 exposed individuals, which is 10 to 20 times the risk in unexposed individuals. Marrow aplasia cannot be anticipated or prevented by hematologic monitoring during chloramphenicol therapy and often occurs after cessation of the drug. The other drugs with the strongest association to aplastic anemia are phenylbutazone, quinacrine, sulfonamides, phenytoin (Dilantin), and gold salts. Gold salts deserve special mention because when they are given a falling neutrophil count may presage the development of aplasia and careful monitoring of blood counts may prevent the disease.

Chemicals. Benzene and benzene-containing compounds such as kerosene and carbon tetrachloride cause marrow damage that may take the form of aplastic anemia, myelodysplasia, or acute leukemia. The frequency of marrow damage is related to the extent of benzene exposure. Benzene is widely used in industry, particularly in organic synthesis and as a solvent, and makes up 1% of unleaded gasoline. Exposure to a number of other chemicals has been temporally associated with the development of severe aplastic anemia, particularly the insecticides DDT and lindane, and derivatives of toluene.

Viral. Approximately 5% of cases of aplastic anemia occur in the wake of a preceding viral infection. The strongest association is with non-A, non-B hepatitis, but on occasion aplasia has been associated with hepatitis A and, rarely, hepatitis B. Other viral infections, including Epstein-Barr virus and human immunodeficiency virus (HIV), have been implicated in aplastic anemia. Parvovirus B19 can cause temporary cessation of red cell production but is not generally considered to be a cause of aplastic anemia.

Immunologic. In immunodeficient children and other immunosuppressed individuals who receive unirradiated blood products and have graft-versus-host disease caused by the inadvertent engraftment of donor T cells, aplasia may develop. Aplastic anemia also rarely develops in association with other immunologically based diseases, such as systemic lupus erythematosus, myasthenia gravis, and eosinophilic fasciitis.

Congenital. Fanconi anemia is the most common inherited form of aplastic anemia and is caused by one of several autosomal recessive genes. The disorder is associated with a broad spectrum of congenital abnormalities, the most consistent of which are small stature; skeletal defects, especially hypoplastic thumbs or radii; and renal abnormali-

Classification of aplastic anemia by cause

- Idiopathic
- Drugs
  - Chloramphenicol
  - Phenylbutazone and related anti-inflammatory drugs
  - Quinacrine and related antiprotozoals
  - Sulfonamides
  - Cimetidine
  - Gold salts
  - Hydantoins
- Chemicals
  - Benzene and benzene-containing solvents
  - Insecticides including DDT
- Viral
  - Hepatitis
  - Epstein-Barr virus
  - Human immunodeficiency virus
- Immunologic
  - Graft-versus-host disease
  - Systemic lupus erythematosus
  - Eosinophilic fasciitis
  - Thymoma
- Pregnancy
- Congenital
  - Fanconi anemia
  - Dyskeratosis congenita
  - Shwachman-Diamond syndrome
  - Reticular dysgenesis

ties. Patients frequently have pancytopenia during the first or second decade of life and also have a high incidence of myelodysplasia and leukemia. Patients with Fanconi anemia have a defect in deoxyribonucleic acid (DNA) repair and are particularly sensitive to the toxic effects of chemotherapy. Some investigators believe the incidence of Fanconi anemia may be higher than generally appreciated and recommend that all young patients with aplastic anemia be screened for Fanconi anemia before undergoing marrow transplantation. If evidence of Fanconi anemia is found, the doses of chemotherapy in the transplant preparation regimen should be reduced. Rare cases of aplastic anemia are associated with dyskeratosis congenita, Shwachman-Diamond syndrome, or reticular dysgenesis.

Pathogenesis

The mechanisms by which the previously mentioned agents or conditions cause aplastic anemia are poorly understood. In perhaps 50% of cases it seems likely that an ongoing immunologic mechanism is responsible. Evidence for this view includes the observation that about 50% of patients respond to therapy with immunosuppressants such as antithymocyte globulin (ATG) or cyclosporine, and that only about 50% of patients with aplastic anemia who receive infusions of bone marrow cells from their normal genotypically identical twin without intensive preconditioning recover. In the other 50% of cases the mechanisms leading to aplastic anemia are less well understood, but a direct toxic insult to marrow stem cells is generally assumed. In occasional cases of otherwise typical aplastic anemia, clonal hematopoiesis has been demonstrated, suggesting that in those cases the disease might be due to the replacement of normal stem cells by a clone of cells incapable of normal proliferation and differentiation.

Clinical features

The clinical features of aplastic anemia are the consequences of the anemia, neutropenia, and thrombocytopenia that result from bone marrow failure. Anemia leads to weakness, easy fatiguability, and pallor. Neutropenia may result in recurrent infections, most frequently of the gingiva, throat, and perirectal area. Petechiae, easy bruising, bleeding from the nose and gums, and heavy menses in females are results of thrombocytopenia. Findings other than those attributable to marrow failure are rare. Thus bone pain, lymphadenopathy, or hepatic or splenic enlargement suggests a disease other than aplastic anemia. The clinical history should carefully document all exposures to drugs, solvents, or other causative agents and any symptoms related to previous viral illnesses. A family history of anemia or congenital abnormalities may disclose unsuspected cases of Fanconi anemia.

Laboratory findings

Patients with severe aplastic anemia have less than 0.5×10^9 neutrophils/L, less than 20×10^9 platelets/L, a corrected reticulocyte count less than 1%, and a hypoplastic or aplastic bone marrow biopsy result (Fig. 91-1). The anemia is usually normocytic and normochromic with normal-appearing red cells. Likewise, the neutrophils and platelets, though severely diminished in number, are normal in their individual structure. The bone marrow biopsy result shows less than 25% of normal cellularity. There is, on occasion, an increase in plasma cells, but marrow fibrosis or replacement by malignant cells is not seen. Occasionally, foci of active hematopoiesis persist and by chance may undergo biopsy. In such cases repeat biopsy procedures may be required to establish the diagnosis. Although not usually required, magnetic resonance imaging can provide an accurate method of determining the extent of fatty replacement of the marrow. Cytogenetic studies of bone marrow are useful to distinguish aplastic anemia, which has normal cytogenetic findings, from hypoplastic myelodysplasia, in which clonal abnormalities such as trisomy 8 or monosomy 7 may be seen.

Differential diagnosis

As listed in the box on p. 873, mild to moderate pancytopenia occurs in many situations, but severe pancytopenia is markedly less common. The diagnosis of aplastic anemia generally rests on the marrow biopsy specimen's demonstration of the characteristic findings mentioned. The most difficult distinction is between severe aplastic anemia and hypoplastic myelodysplasia. Cytogenetic study may be helpful in making the distinction.

Therapy

An important first step in therapy is determining whether patients have mild or severe aplastic anemia, because the prognosis differs so greatly. If aplasia is judged to be mild, the appropriate course is to remove any possible offending agents and provide supportive care as necessary. Most patients spontaneously recover; in others mild aplasia remains for years. However, in some patients mild aplasia may progress to severe aplastic anemia. Those patients who are judged to have severe aplasia, on the other hand, have a poor prognosis if no specific therapy is given. Fifty percent of patients die within 3 months of diagnosis and the overall mortality rate is estimated to be approximately 80%. As for mild aplastic anemia, a first step in therapy is removal of offending agents. The next steps are providing supportive care and then administering specific therapy designed to restore normal hematopoiesis.

Supportive care. Anemia is easily reversed with packed red cell transfusions. Thrombocytopenia can likewise be reversed, at least temporarily, with platelet transfusions. However, with repeated transfusions of random donor platelets most patients become sensitized to human leukocyte antigen (HLA) and other antigens on the platelet surface, leading to rapid destruction of the transfused platelets. In most cases, with the use of carefully selected HLA-matched platelet donors, good platelet increments can be produced even in sensitized patients. Platelet transfusions are obviously warranted for any patient with thrombocyto-

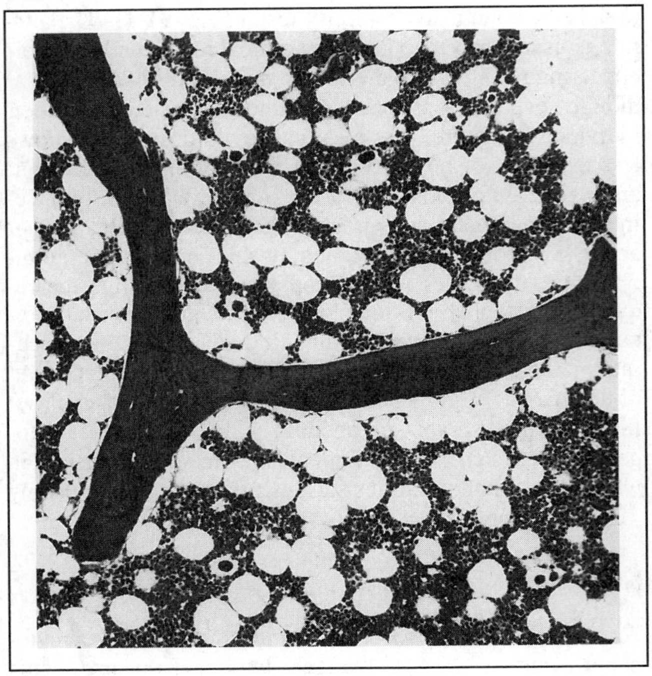

A

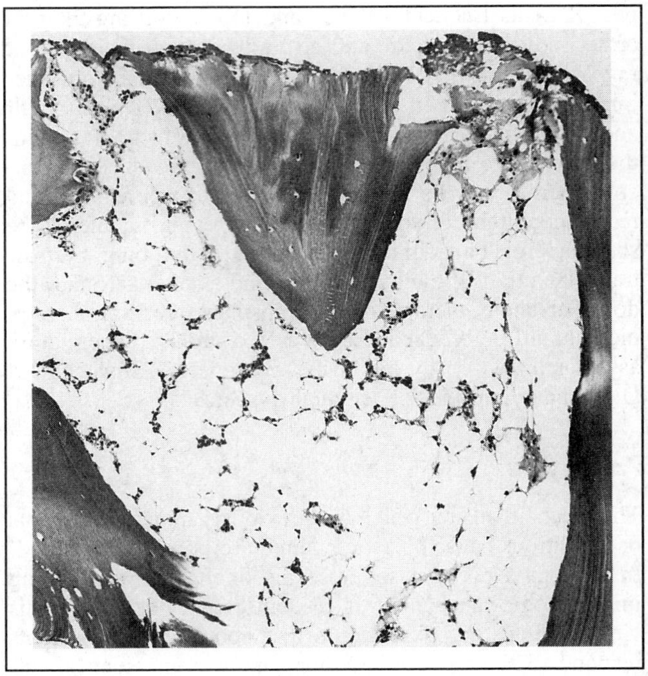

C

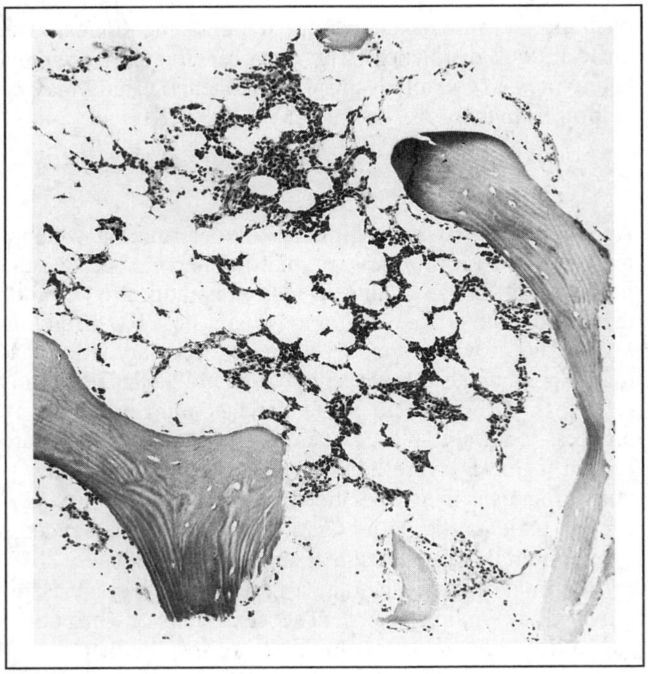

B

Fig. 91-1. Bone marrow biopsy specimens. **A,** a normal person. **B,** From a person with mild aplastic anemia. **C,** From a person with severe aplastic anemia. In the normal individual the marrow cavity between bony trabeculae contains approximately 50% nucleated cells and 50% fat. Megakaryocytes are large and easily seen. Hematopoietic cells are absent in the aplastic marrow.

penia and signs of bleeding. Whether platelets should be given prophylactically is less settled, but such transfusions can generally be recommended for patients with a demonstrated bleeding tendency and in those with less than 20×10^9 platelets/L and a count that is rapidly falling. Granulocyte transfusions may be useful temporarily in the granulocytopenic patient with severe infection. However, there is no role for prophylactic or long-term granulocyte transfusion support. If bone marrow transplantation is a possibility, the approach to transfusion support is affected. The best results with marrow transplantation are seen in the untransfused patient. Thus it may be appropriate to defer transfusions, if possible, until it is determined whether marrow transplantation is possible. If transfusions are required, family member donors should be avoided and as many white blood cells as possible should be removed from transfused red cells and platelets to prevent sensitization and subsequent graft rejection. Leukocytes can be removed by a variety of methods, including using frozen washed red cells and in-line blood filters.

Prevention of infection. Unfortunately, there are no methods to prevent infection that are both effective and practical. Simple procedures, such as the use of prophylactic trimethoprim-sulfamethoxazole, modified diets, or nonabsorbable oral antibiotics, have not been shown to be effective. Total decontamination and laminar airflow isolation, although effective, are impractical in the long run. Patients who have fever require an intensive diagnostic and therapeutic approach. Once bacteremia develops in patients with severe aplastic anemia, even if it is successfully treated, the outlook is particularly grave.

Drug therapy. A number of drugs, including glucocorticoids, androgens, etiocholanolone, and lithium, have been proposed as marrow stimulants. None of these agents is of proven benefit in severe aplastic anemia, but modest responses have been reported in some patients with milder forms of aplasia. Among this group of agents, oral androgens and, in particular, oxymetholone at 3 mg/kg/day or norethandrolone, 1 mg/kg/day, have been most commonly used. Prolonged androgen use can cause hepatic toxicity. None of the agents listed should substitute for more definitive therapy.

Hematopoietic growth factors. There is as yet no clearly established role for the use of hematopoietic growth factors in patients with aplastic anemia. Treatment with G-CSF and GM-CSF may produce a modest increase in granulocyte levels in some patients, but these responses are temporary and are not accompanied by changes in platelets or red cells. Further, these responses have mostly been seen in patients with some residual hematopoiesis and are rarely observed in patients with complete aplasia. Experiments with hematopoietic growth factors with broader activities, such as interleukin-3 (IL-3) and the c-kit ligand, are under way.

Bone marrow transplantation. Bone marrow transplantation is the treatment of choice for patients with severe aplastic anemia who are age 50 or less and who have a histocompatible sibling donor. If such patients undergo transplantation before receiving transfusions, the likelihood of long-term disease-free survival is at least 80%. If patients have had previous transfusion, long-term survival rate is slightly poorer, around 70%, largely as a result of an increased incidence of graft rejection (Fig. 91-2). Patients less than age 50 who lack an HLA-identical sibling can still be cured with transplantation using either a partially matched family member or a matched, unrelated donor. However, the likelihood of a successful outcome is considerably less with these alternative donors, and such transplantations should be restricted to patients for whom immunosuppressive therapy with ATG and/or cyclosporine has failed. The principles of marrow transplantation are presented in Chapter 78.

Immunosuppressive therapy. For patients who are not candidates for immediate transplantation, because they either are above age 50 or lack an HLA-identical sibling donor, immunosuppression has emerged as the treatment of choice. Approximately 50% of patients treated with either antithymocyte globulin (ATG) or cyclosporine (CSP) respond with an increase in granulocytes to a safe level and an increase in platelets and red cells to levels no longer requiring transfusion (Fig. 91-2). Recent studies suggest that combining ATG with cyclosporine produces more responses and better survival rate than either agent alone. With the combination, 60% to 80% of patients can be expected to survive at least 3 years. ATG is usually administered intravenously at a dose of 15 mg/kg/day for 8 days. ATG binds to peripheral blood cells, and therefore platelet and granulocyte numbers usually fall during treatment. Serum sickness often develops about 10 days after initiation of ATG therapy, but it is self-limited. Cyclosporine is administered orally at a dose of 12 mg/kg/day with subsequent adjustments according to blood levels. Nephrotoxicity and hypertension are the most common side effects of cyclosporine. Response to either drug, if it occurs, is usually seen between 30 and 90 days after treatment. Although most responses are sustained, in approximately 10% of patients aplasia recurs. These patients sometimes respond to retreatment with immunosuppression. In addition, in another 10% of patients (higher in some studies), clonal evolution is seen with the subsequent development of paroxysmal nocturnal hemoglobinuria, myelodysplasia, or acute myelogenous leukemia. Clonal evolution is rarely seen after marrow transplantation for aplasia. The mechanisms by which immunosuppressants work are unclear. An overall schematic approach to the management of patients with aplastic anemia is presented in Fig. 91-3.

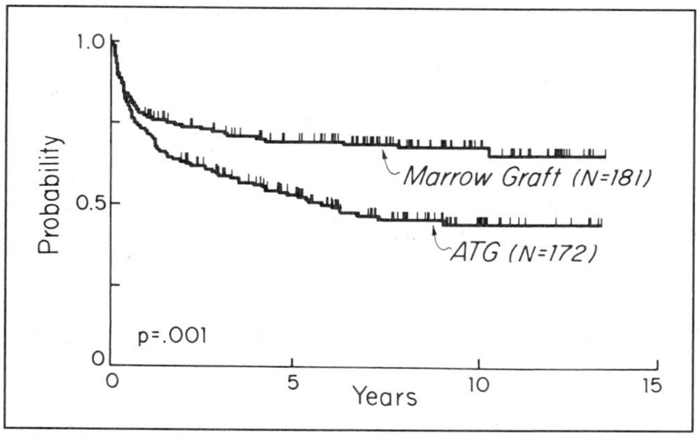

Fig. 91-2. Survival of patients with severe aplastic anemia less than 51 years of age given either immunosuppressive therapy with ATG or marrow transplantation. ATG, antithymocyte globulin.

APLASIAS OF SINGLE CELL LINEAGES

In contrast to aplastic anemia, in which all three cell lines are affected, patients sometimes have aplasia restricted to a single cell lineage. Such patients lack both the marrow precursors and the mature circulating cells of the affected lineage, a situation different from those syndromes such as

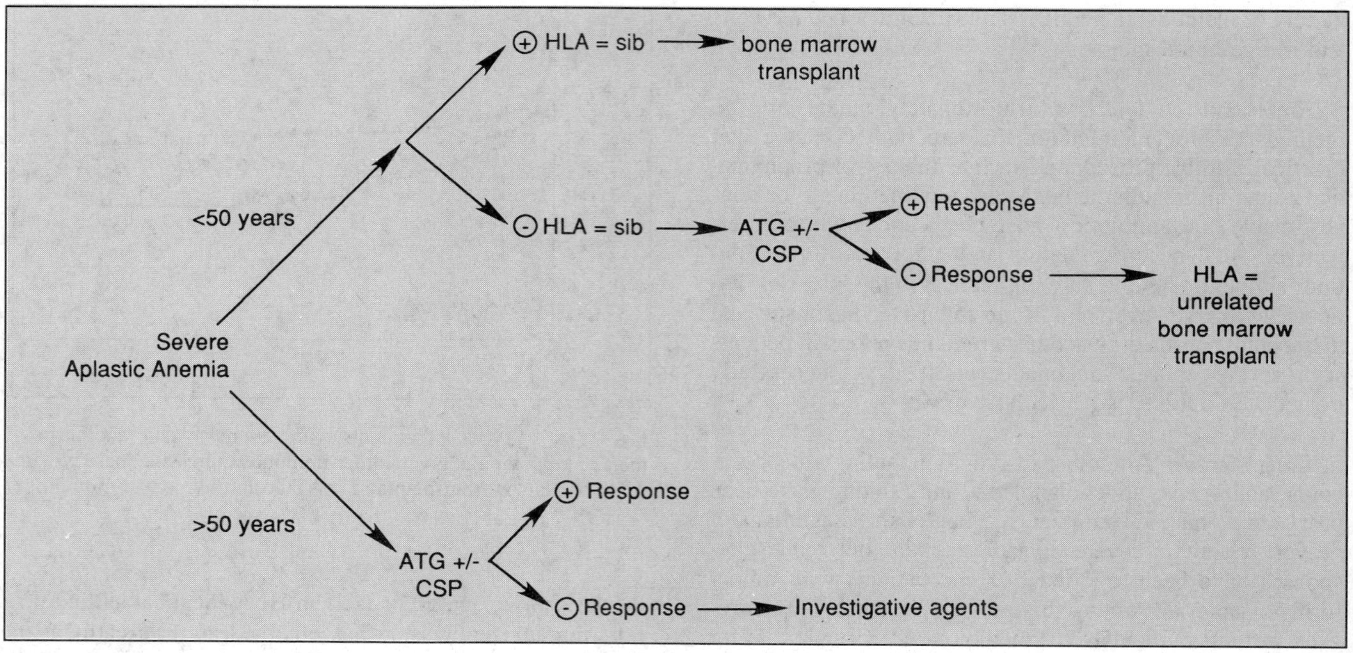

Fig. 91-3. Management of patients with severe aplastic anemia. Appropriate therapy depends on patient age, availability of an HLA-identical sibling (HLA = sib), and response to ATG therapy. ATG is combined with cyclosporin (CSP) is some treatment regimens. HLA, human leukocyte antigen; ATG, antithymocyte globulin; CSP, cyclosporine.

hemolytic anemia or immune-mediate thrombocytopenia in which the problem is one of destruction of the mature blood element rather than its production.

Pure red blood cell aplasia

Pure red blood cell aplasia (PRCA) occurs as a congenital or acquired syndrome. The congenital form, Diamond-Blackfan syndrome, usually is manifested as an isolated anemia during the first 2 years of life. The disease is thought to be transmitted as an autosomal recessive trait and in 25% of cases is associated with other minor congenital anomalies. The disorder responds to glucocorticoids in 50% to 75% of cases and occasional patients who fail glucocorticoid therapy respond to other immunosuppressants. Marrow transplantation has been used in steroid-resistant patients and can cure the disease.

Primary acquired pure red cell aplasia has both acute and chronic forms. The acute form of PRCA is most often seen in young patients with underlying hemoglobinopathy or hemolytic anemia. The disease often follows a relatively mild viral infection, most often with parvovirus. The disease is usually self-limited, and therefore the appropriate management involves maintaining an adequate hemoglobin level with red cell transfusions during the period of severe anemia and administration of folic acid 1 mg/day during the regenerative phase to prevent folate deficiency. The chronic form of PRCA is usually seen in patients aged 20 to 50 and as a slowly progressive anemia. Thymomas are found in 20% to 40% of cases of PRCA. Most often these tumors are of the spindle cell type and behave as benign tumors. PRCA is sometimes associated with other diseases, such as chronic lymphocytic leukemia or systemic lupus erythematosus, and rarely co-occurs with the same groups of drugs associated with aplastic anemia. In many patients complement-fixing immunoglobulin G (IgG) selectively cytotoxic to marrow erythroblasts can be detected and is thought to be causative. Management of patients with PRCA begins with discontinuation of any suspected offending agent followed by a search for a thymoma. Thymectomy induces remission in 50% of patients with an enlarged thymus but is not effective in those with normal-sized thymuses. For patients without thymoma or for whom thymectomy fails, a trial of immunosuppressive therapy is warranted. Glucocorticoid or cyclosporine is usually the first agent of choice; ATG and cytotoxic immunosuppressants such as cyclophosphamide and azathioprine are reserved for treatment failures.

Pure white cell aplasia

Pure white cell aplasia is a very rare condition with parallels to PRCA in that it appears to have an immune basis and is sometimes associated with thymoma, whereas in other cases it appears to be drug-related. Management, like that of PRCA, involves removal of any identified offending agent, thymectomy if an enlarged thymus is found, and immunosuppressive therapy with glucocorticoids or cyclosporine for patients in whom the first two maneuvers are inappropriate or unsuccessful.

Pure amegakaryocytic thrombocytopenic purpura

Pure amegakaryocytic thrombocytopenic purpura (PATP) is a rare syndrome characterized by severe thrombocytopenia associated with a total absence or a marked reduction of bone marrow megakaryocytes. Changes in other cell lines are minimal or absent. PATP has been attributed to viral infections, toxin or drug exposure, or immune mediated suppression of megakaryocytopoiesis. Patients generally have symptoms caused by cutaneous or mucus membrane hemorrhage. Physical examination findings are otherwise normal. Laboratory evaluation findings reveal severe thrombocytopenia with normal or small platelets, as opposed to the large platelets of ITP, and bone marrow that is normal except for the virtual absence of identifiable megakaryocytes. Therapy is directed at removal of all possible offending agents and administration of platelet transfusion support. Responses to other therapies, such as those using corticosteroids, gamma-globulin infusions, cyclosporine, and cyclophosphamide, are largely anecdotal.

MYELODYSPLASIA

The myelodysplastic syndrome (MDS) includes a group of clonal hematopoietic diseases characterized by impaired maturation of hematopoietic precursors with the development of progressive peripheral cytopenias. MDS is now understood to be the result of the neoplastic transformation of a cell at a level of differentiation close to that of the hematopoietic stem cell. Unlike in acute leukemia, the abnormal clone expands only gradually and retains the ability to differentiate, albeit not entirely normally. With time, the abnormal clone completely suppresses normal hematopoiesis and becomes increasingly abnormal, a process referred to as clonal evolution that reflects the inherent genetic instability of the abnormal clone. The final result is development of either progressively severe and ultimately fatal pancytopenia or progression to an acute leukemialike state.

Etiology

The cause of the defect leading to MDS is, in the majority of cases, unknown. A number of cases of MDS arise 3 to 7 years after exposure to chemotherapy, particularly with alkylating agents. Other cases have been seen after exposure to irradiation and exposure to benzene and other marrow toxins.

Clinical features

MDS has previously been considered to be a relatively rare disease with a reported incidence of around 1 per 100,000 per year, but recent studies suggest a much higher incidence. The disorder is much more common in the elderly, with a median age of onset of about 60, but MDS is seen even in young children. Symptoms are usually related directly to the consequences of bone marrow failure, so that fatigue, pallor, infection, and bruising or bleeding are the most common chief complaints. Physical findings are likewise restricted to the consequences of bone marrow failure, although occasional patients, perhaps 15% to 20%, may have splenomegaly.

Laboratory features

The laboratory hallmarks of MDS are peripheral pancytopenias and dysplastic features of the marrow including dyserythropoiesis often with ringed sideroblasts, dysgranulopoiesis with hypogranulation, and dysmegakaryocytopoiesis with micromegakaryocytes. The French/American/British Cooperative Group (FAB) recognizes five distinct forms of MDS, which are based predominantly on pathologic findings (see Table 91-1). In refractory anemia (RA), anemia is invariably seen and the reticulocyte count is usually low. Peripheral blood granulocytes and platelets may be normal or diminished. Leukemic blasts are rarely seen in the periphery and make up less than 5% of marrow cells. Refractory anemia with ringed sideroblasts (RARS) has features essentially like those of RA except that ringed sideroblasts make up 15% or more of the marrow cellularity. In refractory anemia with excess blasts (RAEB), blasts make up from 5% to 20% of the marrow cells and can comprise up to 5% of the peripheral white cells. Thrombocytopenia is common. RAEB in transformation (RAEB-t) is similar to RAEB, but the blast count is greater than 5% in the peripheral blood or greater than 20% but less than 30% in the marrow. If more than 30% marrow blasts are seen, the diagnosis of acute leukemia is made. Chronic myelomonocytic leukemia (CMMoL) shows features similar to those of RAEB, but circulating monocytes are greater than 1.0 $\times 10^9$/L.

Table 91-1. Classification of MDS by the FAB Cooperative Group

Classification	% Marrow blasts	% Peripheral blood blasts	Ringed sideroblasts >15% of BM	Monocytes >1000/μl
Refractory anemia	< 5	≤1	–	–
Refractory anemia with ringed sideroblasts	<5	≤1	+	–
Refractory anemia with excess blasts	5-20	<5	–/+	–
Refractory anemia with excess blasts in transition	20-30	>5	–/+	–/+
Chronic myelomonocytic anemia	≤20	<5	–/+	+

Clonal chromosomal abnormalities are found in 50% to 75% of patients. The most common abnormalities are loss of part or all of chromosome 7, trisomy 8, isochrome 17, 5q−, and 20q−. These abnormalities are also seen in some cases of AML and in that setting are associated with a poor prognosis.

Course and treatment

The prognosis of patients with MDS is extremely variable: some patients survive beyond a decade, whereas others die within the first year of diagnosis. Patients with RA and RARS have a much better prognosis than those with RAEB, RAEB-t, or CMMoL. Those who have a particularly unfavorable prognosis include those with greater than 10% blasts in their marrow at diagnosis, with platelets less than 40×10^9/L or with granulocytes less than 1.0×10^9/L. These patients have a median survival rate of less than 1 year. The cause of death in MDS is usually related either to the consequences of pancytopenia or to the evolution to an acute leukemia. Once leukemia occurs, response to treatment is poor and survival is short. Patients with RAEB and RAEB-t have a much higher likelihood of progression to leukemia, with an incidence of 50% within 2 years of diagnosis.

The category and stage of MDS dictate the appropriate therapy. Patients with RA or RARS with adequate granulocytes and platelets with anemia as their only problem are best treated with transfusion support alone. Once increased numbers of blasts (> 5%) are seen in the marrow or either granulocytopenia or thrombocytopenia develops, more aggressive intervention should be considered. The only curative therapy for MDS is bone marrow transplantation (BMT), which results in long-term disease-free survival in 40% to 50% of transplanted patients. Most of the experience with BMT for MDS has been in patients less than age 50 with HLA-matched sibling donors. Recent studies are exploring the use of partially matched and matched unrelated donors as well as the use of BMT in older patients.

A number of therapeutic approaches have been explored for patients who are not candidates for BMT. Glucocorticoids and androgens have been studied but are probably of no benefit. Although occasional responses have been reported after treatment with differentiating agents such as 13-cis retinoic acid, controlled randomized studies have failed to show any advantage with their use. Low-dose subcutaneous cytosine arabinoside (20 mg/m^2/day) has been studied extensively. A survey of numerous reports and the results of one randomized study indicate a complete response rate to low-dose cytosine arabinoside of about 15%, but these studies have failed to find any effect on overall survival. Patients with RAEB or RAEB-t have a slightly higher response rate to this therapy. Intensive combination chemotherapy, similar to that used in acute myelogenous leukemia, results in complete responses in 30% to 60%. The highest CR rates occur in younger patients with primary MDS. The average duration of complete response is less than 12 months and few patients are cured. These results are inferior to what is seen with the use of similar chemotherapeutic approaches in patients with de novo acute myelogenous leukemia.

More recently, the use of hematopoietic growth factors has been studied in patients with the hope that these factors might increase normal counts in pancytopenic patients both by stimulating normal cell production and by inducing abnormal progenitors to differentiate more normally. Both granulocyte and granulocyte macrophage colony-stimulating factor appear to have some of these effects in that their use significantly increases the granulocyte counts in the majority of neutropenic MDS patients. Improvements in red cell or platelet counts, however, are unusual, and occasional patients treated with hematopoietic growth factors experience a sudden increase in the number of circulating blasts, a change that is usually, but not always, reversed when administration of the growth factor is discontinued.

MYELOFIBROSIS

Myelofibrosis is characterized by fibrosis of the bone marrow space with development of extramedullary hematopoiesis. These changes can occur as a response to other disorders or as a primary hematologic disease. Cancer metastatic to the bone marrow; infectious agents such as fungi, mycobacterium, or leishmaniasis; granulomatous disorders such as sarcoidosis; and metabolic disorders such as Gaucher's disease have all been reported to cause myelofibrosis. The following section deals predominantly with primary myelofibrosis, also termed idiopathic myelofibrosis (IMF) or agnogenic myeloid metaplasia with myelofibrosis (AMM). This disorder is now understood to be the result of a clonal proliferation of an abnormal hematopoietic progenitor and as such is usually categorized as one of the myeloproliferative disorders.

Etiology

The cause of IMF is unknown, but as in the other myeloproliferative syndromes an increased incidence is seen after exposure to irradiation, benzene, and other marrow toxins. Although marrow fibrosis is the hallmark of the disease, recent studies have demonstrated that the disorder is a result of a clonal proliferation of cells of hematopoietic origin and that the fibroblasts seen, although increased in numbers, are not clonal. This suggests that the abnormal hematopoietic clone produces a substance or substances that result in the reactive proliferation of otherwise normal fibroblasts.

Clinical features

The majority of patients with IMF are in their mid-fifties, but occasionally children are affected. The disease evolves slowly; as many as 25% of patients are asymptomatic and diagnosis is made because an abnormality is found during a routine physical examination or blood count. In most patients the chief symptoms are produced by anemia with weakness and/or pallor; others have abdominal fullness caused by an enlarged spleen. Fever, night sweats, anorexia, and weight loss are other common complaints. The most common physical findings are pallor and splenomegaly: splenomegaly is present in 90% of cases, and in 50% the spleen extends at least 6 cm below the rib cage. In an occasional patient, the spleen may be remarkably large, filling most of the abdomen. Hepatomegaly is present in 50% to 70% of cases. Purpura caused by thrombocytopenia occurs in 10% to 20% of cases. Often patients have mild jaundice produced by low-grade hemolysis.

Laboratory features

Most patients have mild to moderate anemia that becomes more severe as the disease progresses. The anemia is due to a combination of ineffective erythropoiesis and low-grade hemolysis. The peripheral leukocyte count is increased in approximately half of patients, is normal in about one quarter, and is low in the remainder. Immature myeloid precursors including blasts are usually present in the blood smear, platelets are increased in one third of patients, and the same fraction are normal or thrombocytopenic. As the disease progresses, thrombocytopenia becomes more severe. The peripheral smear invariably demonstrates a leukoerythroblastic pattern with teardrop poikilocytosis, nucleated red cells, and immature myeloid elements all present. Bone marrows are usually not aspirable, and on bone marrow biopsy, bone marrow fibrosis and osteosclerosis are the rule. Large numbers of blast cells are usually not seen in the marrow and if present suggest that the diagnosis might instead be M7 acute myelogenous leukemia, a disease that in the past has sometimes been called acute myelofibrosis or acute myelosclerosis. Although no single cytogenetic abnormality is associated with IMF, approximately 40% of patients have a clonal chromosomal abnormality, frequently of chromosomes 1, 5, 7, 9, 11, or 13. A new, second abnormality often heralds the conversion to an acute leukemia-like condition.

Differential diagnosis

The clinical findings of pallor and splenomegaly, along with a complete blood count and smear showing a leukoerythroblastic pattern, usually suggest a diagnosis of IMF, and a biopsy specimen of the marrow disclosing diffuse fibrosis helps confirm that impression. Fibrosis secondary to other diseases must be excluded. Hairy cell leukemia (Chapter 93) may be characterized by splenomegaly, neutropenia or pancytopenia, and a dry tap when the marrow is aspirated. Hairy cell leukemia can be excluded by examination of the blood and staining of the blood and marrow lymphocytes for tartrate resistance acid phosphatase. Chronic myelogenous leukemia (CML) with fibrosis can look very much like IMF, but a decreased leukocyte alkaline phosphatase score and the presence of the Ph chromosome distinguish CML from IMF. Large numbers of myeloblasts in the marrow help distinguish M7 AML from IMF. More rapid disease onset and lack of splenomegaly also favor a diagnosis of M7 AML.

Course and treatment

Survival after the diagnosis of IMF is quite varied, ranging from 1 to 30 years and averaging approximately 5 years. Not surprisingly, a poor prognosis is associated with the presence of increasingly severe anemia, thrombocytopenia, hepatomegaly, and B symptoms at diagnosis. Many investigators view the disease as comprising two groups: one with a fulminant course and a median survival of less than 2 years, and a separate group accounting for about half the patients, with a median survival of approximately 10 years. The asymptomatic patient with IMF requires no treatment. Therapy of the disease is aimed at treating the anemia, the thrombocytopenia, and the problems associated with an enlarged spleen, including pain, portal hypertension, and hypersplenism. Anemia is usually treated with transfusion therapy, and in one third of patients androgens appear to decrease transfusion requirements. Corticosteroids are used in patients with a hemolytic component of the disease. Patients with IMF may have difficulty with either thrombocytosis or, later in their disease, thrombocytopenia. If thrombocytosis is severe and thrombosis occurs, platelet count can be lowered by platelet pheresis, by the administration of oral hydroxyurea at 500 to 1500 mg/day, or by the use of anagrelide (Chapter 93). Patients with thrombocytopenia are treated with platelet transfusions, but long-term effective replacement is usually not possible because of poor transfusion increments, in part as a result of hypersplenism, as well as development of alloimmunization. Treatment of splenic enlargement in IMF is controversial, and splenectomy, splenic irradiation, and administration of busulfan and alpha interferon have all been used. Splenectomy is effective in alleviating splenic pain and portal hypertension in most patients, but only about 50% of patients experience improvement in either red cell requirements or platelet counts. Irradiating the spleen may result in a transient decrease in spleen size and alleviation of splenic pain but only rarely has a beneficial effect on anemia and thrombocytopenia. Busulfan, likewise, can control splenic pain, but leads to a decrease in peripheral counts. Marrow transplantation has been used in a handful of patients, and long-term survival has been reported in several of them. In most patients with IMF, refractory thrombocytopenia and neutropenia eventually develop, leading to death from bleeding or infection. Approximately 15% to 20% of patients die after evolution to an acute leukemia-like state.

REFERENCES

Anasetti C et al: Marrow transplantation for severe aplastic anemia: long term outcome in fifty "untransfused" patients. Ann Intern Med 104:461, 1986.

Appelbaum FR et al: Bone marrow transplantation for patients with myelodysplasia: pretreatment variables and outcome. Ann Intern Med 112:590, 1990.

Frickhofen N et al: Treatment of aplastic anemia with antilymphocyte globulin and methylprednisolone with or without cyclosporine. N Engl J Med 324:1297, 1991.

Hows JM: Severe aplastic anaemia the patient without a HLA-identical sibling. Br J Haematol 77:1, 1991.

Young NS: The problem of clonality in aplastic anemia: Dr. Dameshek's riddle, restated. Blood 79:1385, 1992.

CHAPTER

92 Abnormalities of Phagocytes, Eosinophils, and Basophils

David H. Boldt

Granulocytes-neutrophils, eosinophils, basophils, and monocytes together account for the majority of leukocytes circulating in the blood of normal individuals. These cells pass through the blood during their migration from the bone marrow to the tissues, where they carry out their specific roles in host defense. Neutrophils and monocyte-macrophages constitute the two major phagocytic systems in the body. Although the functions of eosinophils and basophils are not so well understood, many important clinical disorders are associated with abnormalities of these cell types.

ABNORMALITIES OF NEUTROPHILS

Abnormalities of neutrophils are listed in the box at right. They are divided conveniently into three groups: (1) quantitative abnormalities—neutropenia or neutrophilia, the most frequently encountered group of neutrophil disorders; (2) qualitative abnormalities—inherited or acquired functional defects in spite of normal neutrophil numbers; (3) neoplastic abnormalities—as in the myelocytic leukemias. Diagnostic considerations and approaches to patients with neutropenia or neutrophilia are addressed in Chapter 81.

Neutropenia

Neutropenia refers to a reduction below the normal range of absolute numbers of circulating neutrophils. In the adult, this is generally below 2.0×10^9 per liter.

Clinical features. The clinical manifestations of neutropenia result from an increased susceptibility to infection. Generally, no increase in infection occurs until the neutrophil count falls below 1.0×10^9 per liter; the risk of infection is moderately increased when the count is 0.5 to 1.0 $\times 10^9$ per liter and greatly increased when the count is below 0.5×10^9 per liter. Infections in neutropenic patients are most often caused by encapsulated gram-negative or gram-positive bacteria, which normally are controlled by opsonization and phagocytosis. When the course of neutropenia is prolonged beyond a few weeks, opportunistic infections caused by fungi such as *Candida* or *Aspergillus* become increasingly prevalent.

Because neutrophils are responsible for most clinical findings during acute infection, the classic signs of infections may be diminished or absent in a severely neutropenic patient. Evaluation for infections should include extensive cultures for both bacteria and fungi. During examination of the neutropenic patient, particular attention should be given to the sinuses, skin, and perirectal region in addition to the usual sites of lung, nasopharynx and oropharynx, urinary tract, and central nervous system. Because of the potential for rapid and fatal progression of any infection, broad-spectrum antibiotic coverage should be provided the febrile, neutropenic patient pending the outcome of cultures, at which point a more specific therapeutic regimen may be devised. In addition, treatment with the hematopoietic growth factors, granulocyte colony-stimulating factor (G-CSF), or granulocyte-macrophage colony-stimulating factor (GM-CSF) may shorten the period of severe neutropenia in some patients with transient marrow suppression (as in drug-induced cases) or ameliorate the clinical severity in patients with chronic neutropenia. The CSFs also have the potential benefit of enhancing the phagocytic and cytotoxic activities of neutrophils. At this time blanket recommendations about the use of CSFs in neutropenic patients cannot be made, but their application should be individualized on a case-by-case basis. The management of the neutropenic patient is discussed in detail in Chapter 229.

Etiology. Causes of neutropenia are listed in the box at right. Pathophysiologically, these can be broadly divided into two groups: (1) decreased production and (2) excessive destruction, utilization, or sequestration.

Drug-induced neutropenia. There are two types of drug-induced neutropenia. First, predictable neutropenias, usually occurring in association with anemia and thrombocytopenia, are regularly caused by many agents used for cancer chemotherapy or immunosuppression. These drugs inhibit cellular proliferation and include alkylating agents, antimetabolites, nitrosoureas, antibiotics, and certain vinca alkaloids (Chapter 72). Irradiation of the bone marrow and exposure to benzene also have predictable myelotoxicity. Examination of the bone marrow of affected individuals reveals hypoplasia with decreased or absent neutrophil precursors.

The second type of drug-induced neutropenia is an idiosyncratic reaction to drug administration. A hallmark of this disorder is its unpredictable occurrence. As a general rule, any drug should be considered capable of causing neutropenia in a susceptible individual, but certain agents have been especially prominent. These are the phenothiazines, phenylbutazone, antithyroid drugs, sulfonamides, and chloramphenicol.

Two basic mechanisms are believed to account for drug-induced neutropenia. These are (1) direct marrow suppression and (2) immune-mediated granulocyte destruction. In drug-induced marrow suppression the onset is insidious and occurs in subjects who have been receiving the drug over an extended period, usually many weeks. The classic example is the neutropenia associated with phenothiazine administration. Typically, the neutropenia occurs 2 to 10 weeks after initiation of the drug and after a total dose of 10 to 20 g. By contrast, immune-mediated granulocyte destruction often begins abruptly after 1 to 2 weeks. Symp-

Abnormalities of neutrophils

- I. Quantitative abnormalities
  - A. Neutropenia (Chapter 81)
    - 1. Decreased production
      - a. Predictable drug-induced marrow suppression
      - b. Irradiation injury
      - c. Idiosyncratic drug-induced marrow suppression
      - d. Bone marrow replacement by tumor, hematologic neoplasm, granulomatous reaction, or myelofibrosis
      - e. Nutritional deficiencies: malnutrition, starvation, vitamin B_{12} or folic acid deficiencies
      - f. Immunologically mediated marrow suppression caused by antibodies or T lymphocytes
      - g. Stem cell defects (hereditary): cyclic neutropenia, Kostman's hereditary neutropenia, reticular dysgenesis, Schwachman-Diamond syndrome, dyskeratosis congenita, lazy leukocyte syndrome, cartilage-hair hypoplasia, Chediak-Higashi syndrome
    - 2. Excessive destruction, utilization, or sequestration
      - a. Idiosyncratic drug-induced granulocyte destruction (usually immunologically mediated)
      - b. Immunologically mediated granulocyte destruction: isoimmune neonatal neutropenia, autoimmune neutropenia (primary or secondary)
      - c. Overwhelming infection (utilization)
      - d. Hypersplenism
      - e. Sequestration in lungs or spleen caused by complement activation during hemodialysis, sepsis, adult respiratory distress syndrome
    - 3. Unknown or multiple causes: chronic idiopathic neutropenia, Felty's syndrome
  - B. Neutrophilia (Chapter 81)
    - 1. Infections
    - 2. Malignancies
    - 3. Inflammatory disorders: rheumatoid arthritis, vasculitis, inflammatory bowel disease, gout
    - 4. Hematologic disorders: acute hemolysis, transfusion reactions, rebound from myelosuppression, postsplenectomy state
    - 5. Drugs: corticosteroids, epinephrine, etiocholanolone, lithium
    - 6. Metabolic conditions: diabetic ketoacidosis, thyroid storm
    - 7. Tissue destruction: myocardial infarction, pulmonary infarction, bowel infarction
    - 8. Pregnancy
    - 9. Physiologic: exercise, stress
    - 10. Chronic idiopathic neutrophilia
- II. Qualitative abnormalities (Chapter 223)
  - A. Intrinsic
    - 1. Chronic granulomatous disease
    - 2. Job's syndrome
    - 3. Myeloperoxidase deficiency
    - 4. Chediak-Higashi syndrome
    - 5. Lazy leukocyte syndrome
  - B. Extrinsic
    - 1. Complement and immunoglobulin abnormalities
    - 2. Hypophosphatemia
    - 3. Sickle cell anemia
    - 4. Diabetes mellitus
    - 5. Alcoholism
    - 6. Corticosteroid administration
- III. Neoplastic abnormalities (Chapter 93)
  - A. Acute nonlymphocytic leukemia
  - B. Chronic myeloproliferative disorders: chronic myelogenous leukemia, polycythemia vera, idiopathic myelofibrosis

toms including fever, chills, arthralgias, and prostration may be due to neutrophil lysis.

Bone marrow examination in the patient with idiosyncratic drug-induced neutropenia may reveal either hypoplasia or a hypercellular marrow. Myeloid precursors may be absent, normal, or increased. Because of their rapid release from the marrow, mature neutrophils are often markedly reduced, giving a false picture of maturation arrest. A hypercellular marrow containing an abundance of myeloid precursors suggests that neutropenia is due to peripheral destruction, utilization, or sequestration.

Management of patients with suspected drug-induced neutropenia consists in withdrawal of all drugs that are not absolutely essential, particularly those known to be associated with neutropenia. The condition then usually resolves within 2 to 3 weeks. Some patients may benefit from treatment with hematopoietic growth factors to shorten the period of severe neutropenia.

Felty's syndrome. In Felty's syndrome (Chapter 304) neutropenia is associated with rheumatoid arthritis and splenomegaly. Hypersplenism, circulating antineutrophil antibodies, complement-mediated granulocyte aggregation, inhibitory T lymphocytes, and bone marrow failure may all be involved in causing the neutropenia. The degree of neutropenia in Felty's syndrome is variable but may be profound, and infectious complications may be frequent and severe. Splenectomy leads to improvement of the neutrophil count in about half the patients. Such improvement is most likely to occur in patients with normal or hypercellular bone marrows and is less likely to occur in patients with hypocellular marrows or marrows infiltrated with lymphocytes. Responses to corticosteroids or lithium therapy have also been reported.

Human cyclic neutropenia. Human cyclic neutropenia is a unique disorder characterized by regular oscillations of the blood neutrophil count with periodic disappearance of neutrophils from the circulation. The oscillations are based on cyclic changes in bone marrow production and release of neutrophils. The diagnosis of cyclic neutropenia rests on the demonstration of regular, recurrent episodes of profound neutropenia. The periodicity is usually about 21 days but may be as short as 14 days or as long as 30 days. It is not unusual for neutrophil counts to fall to zero and to remain below 0.2×10^9 per liter for 3 to 5 days. The disease is often familial, and clinical manifestations usually occur before the age of 10 but can occur later in life. An association has been noted between adult-onset cyclic neutropenia and increased numbers of large granular lymphocytes. Symptoms attributable to infection typically occur during the period of neutropenia and last from 3 to 10 days. Treatment of infections with antibiotics decreases their severity and reduces the likelihood of dissemination and death. Recent data from a multicenter, randomized, controlled trial indicate that long-term treatment with G-CSF can be effective in cyclic neutropenia. Previous reports indicated that androgens, lithium, or splenectomy may be successful in selected cases. In addition, corticosteroid therapy may correct neutrophil cycling in some patients with the adult-onset form of the disease.

Chronic idiopathic neutropenia. The term *chronic idiopathic neutropenia* has been used to refer to patients in whom blood neutrophil counts of less than 2.0×10^9 per liter persist for months or years and in whom other known causes of neutropenia are excluded. Some subjects follow a benign clinical course and no specific therapy is required. In this condition, referred to as chronic benign neutropenia, patients can mobilize neutrophils from the bone marrow reserve pool in response to corticosteroid administration, an occurrence that may account for their ability to deal appropriately with infections. Other subjects have a more aggressive clinical course marked by frequent and severe infections. These patients do not respond to corticosteroid administration with an increased neutrophil count, and they may benefit from treatment with hematopoietic growth factors.

Neutrophilia

Causes of neutrophilia are listed in the box on p. 883. Evaluation of patients with neutrophilia is discussed in Chapter 81.

Qualitative neutrophil abnormalities

Functional defects of neutrophils may be hereditary or acquired, extrinsic or intrinsic to the cell. Some of these abnormalities are discussed in Chapter 223.

Neoplastic abnormalities of neutrophils

Myeloid leukemias and myeloproliferative diseases are discussed in Chapter 93.

Immunologically mediated neutropenia. In certain instances, neutropenia may be due to immunologic mechanisms that cause granulocyte destruction or that interfere with neutrophil production by interacting with precursor cells in the bone marrow. Antibody-mediated neutrophil destruction analogous to immune thrombocytopenia or immune hemolytic anemia has been described. It may occur as a primary condition or as a complication of an underlying lymphoproliferative disorder or collagen-vascular disease. Secondary immune neutropenia may respond to appropriate therapy of the underlying condition. Primary immune neutropenia has been managed by administration of short intensive courses of corticosteroids and/or splenectomy. However, such therapy is risky, and the indications are not well established.

Inhibitory T lymphocytes have been shown to be responsible for granulopoietic failure in 20% of a large group of patients with neutropenia and hypocellular bone marrows. Affected patients had a variety of underlying conditions, including rheumatic diseases, preleukemic syndromes, acquired or congenital immunodeficiency diseases, and idiopathic acquired neutropenia. A high percentage of subjects with T cell–mediated neutropenia responded to corticosteroids.

The association of lymphocytosis of large granular lymphocytes (LGLs) with neutropenia has been described. Anemia is also common in affected patients with red cell precursors decreased or absent from the bone marrow. In vitro tests often demonstrate suppression of erythroid progenitor growth by the LGL in this condition, but similar suppression of myeloid progenitors has been difficult to demonstrate. Affected patients generally follow a chronic course marked by hyperlymphocytosis, neutropenia, and frequent, mild infections. The syndrome often occurs in association with rheumatoid arthritis, and patients may have positive rheumatoid factor and antinuclear antibody test findings as well as polyclonal hypergammaglobulinemia. Lymphocytes in this disorder express the CD8 surface antigen characteristic of the cytotoxic suppressor T lymphocyte subset, and the cells may display antibody-dependent cellular cytotoxicity and variable natural killer activity. In some cases the lymphocyte proliferation is monoclonal and the disease may manifest some features of a malignancy, such as organ infiltration; but in other cases the disease is polyclonal and organ infiltration does not occur. Treatment of this syndrome with corticosteroids or cytotoxic agents has been largely ineffective.

ABNORMALITIES OF MONOCYTES AND MACROPHAGES

Abnormalities of monocytes and macrophages are listed in the box at right. Similar to neutrophil disorders, quantitative, qualitative, and proliferative abnormalities are recognized. In addition, storage disorders resulting from inability of the monocyte-macrophage properly to dispose of organic materials may lead to accumulation of tissue macrophages containing an overabundance of various ingested substances. These storage disorders, caused by hereditary deficiencies of certain lysosomal enzymes, are discussed in Chapter 174. Monocytosis and reactive hyperplasia of macrophages are the abnormalities most commonly encountered. In general, diseases that cause a peripheral blood monocytosis are also associated with macrophage proliferation in tissues. Causes of monocytosis and reactive macrophage hyperplasia are given in the box below.

Proliferative abnormalities of monocytes and macrophages may be benign or malignant. The latter category includes monocytic and myelomonocytic variants of acute myelogenous leukemia (Chapter 93), true histiocytic lymphoma (Chapter 94), and malignant histiocytosis. The clinical behavior of malignant histiocytosis resembles that of the malignant lymphomas. Common features are fever, weight loss, lymphadenopathy, hepatosplenomegaly, and progressive pancytopenia. Diagnosis is based on demonstration of malignant macrophages in involved tissues. In many patients abnormal histiocytes may be seen by examination of the peripheral blood. Untreated, the disorder is rapidly fatal but recent studies report successful treatment with combination chemotherapy. In such patients the 5 year actuarial survival rate is approximately 40%.

Langerhans cell histiocytosis is the currently preferred terminology for the group of histiocytic syndromes formerly known as eosinophilic granuloma, Hand-Schuller-Christian disease, Letterer-Siwe disease, and histiocytosis X. These disorders most commonly affect infants and young children but may be seen in adults. The signs and symptoms vary, depending on which organs are infiltrated by histiocytes. In addition to the usual visceral sites, involvement of bones and skin may be especially troublesome. For example, involvement of the skull may lead to dental impairment, chronic otitis media, loss of vision, or diabetes insipidus. Extent of involvement ranges from solitary bone lesions to massive systemic involvement with multiorgan failure. Prognosis is related to age, extent of disease, and presence of organ dysfunction. Treatment must be tailored to the needs of individual patients and may require no or only supportive care, irradiation therapy of solitary lesions, systemic corticosteroids, or single- or multiagent chemotherapy. Young age (less than 2 years), involvement of four or more organ systems, and dysfunction of three organ systems—lungs, liver, and bone marrow—are poor prognostic features. Approximately 25% of all patients die of disease progression or complications of treatment such as infections. Most of the remaining patients respond to therapy and eventually stabilize without need for further treatment. Long-term follow-up observation is required for these patients to manage disabilities resulting from the histiocytic syndrome itself and to observe for secondary malignancies that may be associated with chemotherapy and/or radiotherapy.

Abnormalities of monocytes and macrophages

I. Monocytosis and reactive macrophage hyperplasia
   A. Infectious diseases: especially tuberculosis, syphilis, brucellosis, malaria, leprosy, listeriosis, schistosomiasis, leishmaniasis, histoplasmosis, cryptococcosis, toxoplasmosis, bacterial endocarditis
   B. Neoplastic diseases: myelomonocytic leukemia, lymphoproliferative and myeloproliferative disorders, preleukemia, other malignancies
   C. Hematologic diseases or conditions: hemolytic anemia, recovery from neutropenia, postsplenectomy state
   D. Rheumatic disorders: rheumatoid arthritis, systemic lupus erythematosus, others
   E. Gastrointestinal disorders: inflammatory bowel disease, cirrhosis
   F. Miscellaneous disorders: sarcoidosis, drug reactions, reactive macrophage hyperplasia to chemicals such as beryllium, silica, or organic substances

II. Proliferative disorders
   A. Neoplastic: monocytic and myelomonocytic leukemia, histiocytic lymphoma, malignant histiocytosis
   B. Reactive or of uncertain cause: Langerhans cell histiocytosis, sinus histiocytosis with massive lymphodenopathy, virus-associated hemophagocytic syndrome

III. Storage diseases (Chapter 174), Gaucher's disease, Niemann-Pick disease, Tay-Sachs disease, Fabry's disease, sea-blue histiocyte disorders

IV. Monocyte-macrophage dysfunction syndromes
   A. Congenital: chronic granulomatous disease, myeloperoxidase deficiency, Chediak-Higashi syndrome
   B. Acquired: alveolar macrophages in smokers, macrophages in lepromatous leprosy, miliary tuberculosis, disseminated fungal infections

Sinus histiocytosis with massive lymphadenopathy is a benign condition characterized by painless and massive lymphadenopathy usually involving cervical lymph nodes. Other node groups and extranodal sites also may be involved. The cause is unknown. Lymph node biopsies show sinusoidal dilatation and follicular hyperplasia with abundant foamy histiocytes and multinucleated giant cells within the sinuses. A characteristic finding is "emperipolesis," the presence of intracellular lymphocytes apparently engulfed by histiocytic cells. As disease manifestations commonly resolve spontaneously, no treatment is usually necessary. However, massive adenopathy in strategic locations may cause serious or fatal complications, such as trachael or epidural compression, and treatment may become necessary under special circumstances. In these instances, local excision, irradiation, corticosteroids, or chemotherapy may be used but results have been inconsistent.

A virus-associated hemophagocytic syndrome has recently been described in immunosuppressed subjects with herpes virus infections. It may also occur in some previously healthy subjects. Clinically the disorder may mimic histiocytic medullary reticulosis with hepatosplenomegaly, lymphadenopathy, skin rash, and pancytopenia. Involved tissue shows macrophage infiltration with prominent erythrophagocytosis. Differentiation from histiocytic medullary reticulosis is based on the morphology of the macrophages. They are malignant and poorly differentiated in histiocytic medullary reticulosis but well differentiated and reactive in the hemophagocytic syndrome. The hemophagocytic syndrome is a self-limited disorder and usually resolves within several weeks or months when patients are given appropriate supportive care.

ABNORMALITIES OF EOSINOPHILS AND BASOPHILS

Eosinophils and basophils are the least numerous of the circulating leukocytes. Clinically important disorders of these cell types are eosinophilia and basophilia (refer to the box below). In most of these conditions the eosinophilia or basophilia is a reactive phenomenon and may result from secretion by activated lymphocytes or other cells of hematopoietic growth factors that stimulate production of eosinophils (IL-3, IL-5, GM-CSF) or basophils (IL-3).

A small subset (approximately 5%) of patients with acute myelogenous leukemia (AML) have a variant termed acute myelomonocytic leukemia with abnormal eosinophils (M4Eo). In addition to myeloblasts with characteristic features of FAB class M4 (Chapter 93), bone marrows of these patients are infiltrated by up to 30% atypical eosinophils. The abnormal morphologic and cytochemical features of these eosinophils suggest that they may be derived from the leukemic clone, but this has not yet been rigorously proved. M4Eo typically is associated with cytogenetic abnormalities of the long arm of chromosome 16. Patients with the M4Eo variant of AML have a favorable prognosis for response and survival with current therapies.

The idiopathic hypereosinophilic syndrome appears to represent a primary disorder of eosinophils. It may be defined according to the following three criteria: (1) persistent eosinophilia of at least 1.5×10^9 per liter for longer than 6 months or fatal termination within 6 months; (2) lack of evidence of parasitic, allergic, or other known causes of eosinophilia (see the box at lower left); (3) signs and symptoms of organ involvement or dysfunction either directly related to eosinophilia or unexplained in the given clinical setting.

The onset of disease typically occurs between the ages of 20 and 50 years, and there is a strong male predominance. Involvement of the heart and nervous system is responsible for the most important clinical findings. Cardiac involvement produces congestive heart failure, valvular dysfunction, conduction defects, and myocarditis. Congestive heart failure secondary to endocardial fibrosis is a frequent cause of death. Central neurologic findings may include altered behavior and cognitive function, spasticity, and ataxia.

Prognosis in the idiopathic hypereosinophilic syndrome historically has been poor, with median survival of approximately 1 year. However, chemotherapy has recently been reported to produce 70% survival at 10 years.

A recently described disorder, eosinophilia-myalgia syndrome, is a chronic multisystem disease with a spectrum of clinical manifestations ranging from self-limited myalgias and fatigue to a progressive, occasionally fatal illness characterized by scleroderma-like skin changes, peripheral and central nervous system abnormalities, and pulmonary hypertension. Peripheral eosinophilia is a universal feature. The illness has been related to ingestion of L-tryptophan. Corticosteroids may ameliorate acute symptoms, but they have not been consistently effective, and their role in the long-term management of patients with progressive disease is undefined.

Basophilia refers to an increase in the absolute peripheral basophil count above 0.15×10^9 per liter. Basophilia can accompany myxedema, ulcerative colitis, Hodgkin's disease, and hemolytic anemias. Significant basophilia is also seen with the myeloproliferative disorders—chronic myelogenous leukemia, polycythemia vera, and myeloid metaplasia. Basophilic leukemia is a very rare disorder.

Causes of eosinophilia and basophilia

I. Eosinophilia
   A. Metazoan infestation, especially amebiasis, ascariasis, schistosomiasis, strongyloidiasis, trichinosis, visceral larva migrans
   B. Allergic conditions: bronchial asthma, allergic rhinitis, eczema, acute allergic reactions to drugs or food, insect bites
   C. Skin diseases: especially atopic dermatitis, acute urticaria, pemphigus, pemphigoid, eczema
   D. Pulmonary eosinophilias: tropical eosinophilia, visceral larva migrans, ascariasis, fungal infections, inhalation of allergens, Churg-Strauss allergic granulomatosis
   E. Neoplastic diseases: acute myelogenous leukemia, Hodgkin's and non-Hodgkin's lymphomas, solid tumors, especially carcinoma of the lung
   F. Immunologic disorders: polyarteritis nodosa, rheumatoid arthritis, angioimmunoblastic lymphadenopathy
   G. Idiopathic hypereosinophilic syndrome
II. Basophilia
   A. Allergic conditions: drugs, foods, inhalants
   B. Myeloproliferative disorders
   C. Miscellaneous conditions: myxedema, ulcerative colitis, systemic mast cell disease
   D. Basophilic leukemia

Mastocytosis

The mast cell is a connective tissue cell widely distributed throughout the body. Mast cells are involved in allergic reactions and immunoglobulin E (IgE)-mediated immune phenomena. Although the basophil and mast cell share many histologic, biochemical, and physiologic properties, they probably represent two distinct cell lines. Abnormalities of mast cells include urticaria pigmentosa and systemic mastocytosis. Urticaria pigmentosa is a benign, self-limiting disorder characterized by focal cutaneous infiltrates of mast cells. Bone lesions may also occur. In systemic mastocytosis infiltration of mast cells occurs in many organ systems. Signs and symptoms reflect this multisystem involvement and may include weight loss, fever, flushing, bronchospasm, hypotension, diarrhea, gastrointestinal bleeding, rhinorrhea, palpitations, and dyspnea. When large numbers of mast cells appear in bone marrow and peripheral blood the condition is designated mast cell leukemia. Treatment of systemic mast cell disorders is usually symptomatic with the aim of alleviating symptoms. Antihistamines, H_2 receptor blockers, and cromolyn sodium may be effective for this purpose. Prognosis is quite variable. Some patients follow a prolonged stable course. However, mast cell leukemia and clinically aggressive mast cell disorders do not respond to conventional chemotherapeutic regimens. The prognosis in this setting is poor with rapid progression of disease and death.

REFERENCES

Bagby GC, Jr, Lawrence HJ, and Neerhout RC: T-lymphocyte-mediated granulopoietic failure. N Engl J Med 309:1073, 1983.

Fauci AS et al: The idiopathic hypereosinophilic syndrome: clinical, pathophysiologic, and therapeutic considerations. Ann Intern Med 97:78, 1982.

Glaspy J and Golde D: Clinical trials of myeloid growth factors. Exp Hematol 18:1137, 1990.

Osband ME and Pochedly C: Histiocytosis-X. Hematol Oncol Clin North Am 1:1, 1987.

Reynolds CW and Foon KA: T-gamma lymphoproliferative disease and related disorders in humans and experimental animals: a review of the clinical, cellular, and functional characteristics. Blood 64:1146, 1984.

CHAPTER

93 The Leukemias and Polycythemia Vera

John J. Hutton

LYMPHOID LEUKEMIAS

Lymphoproliferative disorders may originate either in the bone marrow or in extramedullary sites such as lymph nodes and thymus. Those primarily involving bone marrow are classified as lymphoid leukemias and are discussed in this chapter. The remainder are classified as lymphomas and are discussed in Chapter 94. Three of the most common lymphoid leukemias are presented here. Of these, acute lymphoblastic leukemia, if untreated, is rapidly fatal, whereas chronic lymphocytic leukemia and hairy cell leukemia run a more indolent clinical course.

Acute lymphoblastic leukemia

Etiology. The clonal origin of acute lymphoblastic leukemia has been demonstrated by studies of cytogenetic abnormalities, immunoglobulin and T-cell receptor gene rearrangements, and glucose-6-phosphate dehydrogenase isoenzymes in leukemic cells. The concept of clonality is discussed in Chapters 69 and 74.

The cause of malignant transformation of a normal lymphoid cell to a leukemic cell is not known. Retroviruses have long been implicated in the induction of leukemia and lymphoma in animals. There is no evidence that typical human acute lymphoblastic leukemia is caused by a retrovirus, although a member of the family of human T cell lymphotropic viruses, human immunodeficiency-related retrovirus (HIV-III), is consistently associated with an aggressive T cell lymphoma (Chapter 94) that can have a leukemic phase. The malignant T cell in this disease is more differentiated than is typical of blasts in acute lymphoblastic leukemia. The clinical presentation of the acute adult T cell leukemia/lymphoma syndrome resembles that of mycosis fungoides-Sézary syndrome (Chapter 96). Patients with subclinical infection are almost entirely asymptomatic. Human T cell leukemia-lymphoma is not considered further in this chapter.

Chromosomal translocations are commonly seen in leukemic cells (Table 93-1). Genes located near the breakpoint of a translocation are in a new environment. This may affect the regulation of gene expression so that its products are made inappropriately, thereby affecting cellular proliferation and differentiation. There is a concordance between the breakpoint of translocations or deletions and the chromosomal locations of cellular oncogenes that control the synthesis of growth factors or receptors for growth factors. The exact relationship between the rearrangements of genes and leukemogenesis is unclear, but it is likely that the rearrangements are the cause of the leukemia rather than a

Table 93-1. Classification of acute lymphoblastic leukemia (ALL)

Type of leukemia	Approximate percentage of patients	Markers present*	Common cytogenetic abnormalities†	Ig genes rearranged
Common ALL	50	CALLA, terminal transferase, may have cytoplasmic IgM	t(1;19), t(9;22)	+
T cell ALL	20	T cell antigens, terminal transferase	t(11;14)	–
B cell ALL	5	Surface Ig	t(2;8), t(8;14), t(8;22)	+
Null	25	Terminal transferase may be present	t(4;11)	±

*Markers included terminal transferase, surface and cytoplasmic immunoglobulin, T cell antigens, and the common ALL antigen (CALLA). Markers not listed as present are absent.

†The letter *t* indicates a chromosomal translocation. For example, a translocation involving the long arm of chromosome 1 and the short arm of chromosome 19 is called t(1;19). The locus of the immunoglobulin heavy-chain gene is on chromosome 14 at a region commonly involved in the translocations seen in lymphoid malignancies. The c-myc oncogene is located on chromosome 8 and immunoglobulin genes are on chromosomes 2, 14, and 22. Translocations involving c-myc and an immunoglobulin are commonly found in β-cell ALL.

result of the abnormal cellular proliferation seen in the disease. For example, blasts from certain patients with acute lymphoblastic leukemia have been found to have a reciprocal translocation between chromosomes 9 and 22. The breakpoint on chromosome 22 occurs within the breakpoint cluster region (bcr) of the PHL gene, and the breakpoint on chromosome 9 occurs within the c-abl proto-oncogene. This creates a hybrid gene with juxtaposition of bcr and c-abl deoxyribonucleic acid (DNA) sequences. The abnormal c-abl proto-oncogene messenger ribonucleic acid (RNA) that is produced encodes a protein that might affect cell proliferation and differentiation, that is, be leukemogenic. Causes of cancer are further discussed in Chapter 71.

Clinical features. Signs and symptoms of acute leukemia are caused by infiltration of normal tissues by leukemic cells. Marrow infiltration is most prominent and results in the failure of normal hematopoiesis. Fatigue, weakness, pallor, and weight loss are common. Easy bruising and bleeding develop in patients with thrombocytopenia. Pneumonia, urinary tract infection, and perirectal abscess occur in those with granulocytopenia. Enlargement of the spleen, thymus, liver, and lymph nodes is common. Meningeal leukemia with headache and cranial nerve dysfunction is seen in 5% to 10% of patients.

The differential diagnosis of acute lymphoblastic leukemia includes infections and other malignancies. Infections that produce lymphocytosis and lymphadenopathy include toxoplasmosis and viral infections such as cytomegalovirus and infectious mononucleosis (Chapter 251). These infections do not seriously distort bone marrow structure. Analysis of viral antibody titers and the results of the heterophil and monospot tests should establish the correct diagnosis. Malignant diseases that may mimic acute lymphoblastic leukemia include acute myelogenous leukemia, neuroblastoma, small cell or oat cell carcinoma of the lung, Ewing's sarcoma, chronic lymphocytic leukemia, non-Hodgkin's lymphoma in leukemic phase, and lymphoid transformation of chronic myelogenous leukemia.

Laboratory features. Leukemia is diagnosed on the basis of laboratory tests rather than clinical findings. The hallmark of acute leukemia is the presence of an increased percentage (generally a minimum of 30%) of blasts in the bone marrow. In most patients with acute lymphoblastic leukemia, the peripheral white blood cell count exceeds 10.0×10^9 per liter, but it ranges from 1.0 to 1000.0. An occasional patient is leukopenic. Unlike the situation in acute myelogenous leukemia, the blasts in lymphoblastic leukemia do not tend to aggregate, so that high leukocyte counts are rarely associated with signs of leukostasis in the patient. Anemia, granulocytopenia, and thrombocytopenia are common.

Lymphoblastic and myelogenous leukemias are distinguished on the basis of the cytochemical and immunologic features of the leukemic blasts (Chapter 74). The distinction is critically important because of differences in therapy. Lymphoblasts do not contain myeloperoxidase or Auer rods. This means that they do not stain for peroxidase and do not contain granules that stain with the lipophilic dye, Sudan black. Lymphoblasts, but not myeloblasts, typically contain clumps of material that stain with the periodic acid–Schiff reagent (PAS reaction). Examples of the cytochemical properties of blasts are shown in Plates III-5 and III-6.

Acute lymphoblastic leukemia can be further classified according to immunologic reactivity, presence or absence of terminal transferase, and arrangement of immunoglobulin genes. The subgroups appear to represent clonal expansions of lymphocytes that are partially blocked in their capacity to differentiate. They differ in prognosis and may require different types of treatment (Table 93-1). The prognostic relevance of the immunologic subtypes varies with type of therapy and is continuously changing as therapy evolves. Markers are most commonly defined by commercially available monoclonal antibodies directed against antigens such as those characteristic of T and B cells (Chapter 74). They are usually detected by flow cytometry. Classifications by immunologic subtype have changed over time. For example, cases previously classified as "null" are now known to be pre-B in phenotype. The enzyme terminal deoxynucleotidyl transferase helps to distinguish myelogenous from lymphoblastic leukemias. It is present in most lymphoblasts, but not in myeloblasts. Finally, immunoglobulin genes are rearranged from germ line configuration in blasts corresponding to stages of B cell differentiation, but not T cell differentiation. Conversely, T cell receptor genes rearrange during T cell differentiation in a way that is analogous to the changes in immunoglobulin genes during B cell differentiation. It is through studies of gene rearrangements that most non-T, non-B marked acute lymphoblastic leukemias (common and null ALL of Table 93-1) have been proved to represent clonal proliferation of committed precursors of B lymphocytes. The leukemic blasts always possess rearranged immunoglobulin heavy (H) chain genes, and approximately half also have light (L) chain rearrangements. The recombination of individual segments from multiple alternative variable (V), diversity (D), and joining (J) gene segments generates a specific rearrangement pattern unique to each patient's disease.

Treatment. Prolonged survival in patients with acute leukemia is correlated with the ability to eradicate detectable leukemic cells. This is termed a complete remission. Initial attempts to achieve a remission, termed the induction phase, involve the administration of multiple drugs over weeks to months. Most induction regimens include vincristine, prednisone, and an anthracycline. If a remission is achieved, the next step is to attempt to prolong its duration by the cyclic administration of additional drugs. This is referred to as the consolidation phase. Subsequently, lower doses of drugs may be given over months to years during the maintenance phase. Other phases of treatment may include late intensification and central nervous system prophylaxis. The entire treatment regimen is extraordinarily toxic and must be carried out in specialized centers.

As the intensity of therapy has increased, the proportion of patients achieving a complete remission and the median duration of complete remission have increased. The continuation of therapy in remission of acute lymphoblastic leukemia appears to be essential, although the optimal intensity and duration of such therapy are not known. Current regimens require intensive therapy for 2 to 3 years after achievement of complete remission and include central nervous system prophylaxis.

Approximately 90% of adults with acute lymphoblastic leukemia achieve complete remission when intensively treated. Approximately 40% remain free of disease at 5 years, when optimally managed. Relapse of disease is a grim prognostic indicator, and essentially all adults who experience relapse die of their disease, unless transplanted. Survival is worse in patients over the age of 35 years and is particularly poor in those over 60 years. Other indicators of a poor prognosis include mature B cell phenotype and presence of chromosomal translocations t(9;22) or t(4;11). Extramedullary masses, a high initial blast count, and T marked blasts were associated with a poor prognosis in regimens developed several years ago but are not always detrimental with more recent intensive treatment regimens.

Chemotherapy reduces spermatogenic activity in males and secondary follicles in females. Patients who have been treated for leukemia usually recover gonadal function and may have a normal child, particularly if they do not have chemotherapy for several years.

Allogeneic bone marrow transplantation has not proved superior to chemotherapy alone in primary treatment of adults with acute lymphoblastic leukemia. Broader use of allogeneic bone marrow transplantation has been hindered by the morbidity and mortality of graft-versus-host disease, the poor ability of patients over the age of 50 years to tolerate the procedure, and the high frequency of relapse in patients prepared for grafting by total body irradiation (Chapter 78). However, because patients who relapse while receiving primary chemotherapy have such a poor prognosis with secondary chemotherapy, they should be considered candidates for allogeneic transplantation.

Hairy cell leukemia

Etiology. Hairy cell leukemia is a rare neoplasm but is important because it responds well to appropriate treatment. It was formerly called *leukemic reticuloendotheliosis*. The cause of the leukemia is not known. There is no association with exposure to chemicals or radiation, and it is not hereditary. In most patients the disease appears to represent the clonal expansion of a cell committed to the B lymphocyte lineage. The best evidence for this is the rearrangement of immunoglobulin genes in hairy cells in a way thought to be pathognomonic of B cell differentiation. These cells circulate in the blood, where they have prominent cytoplasmic projections. They also infiltrate the bone marrow and spleen in a characteristic fashion.

Clinical features. The typical patient with hairy cell leukemia is a middle-aged man with a palpable spleen. The median age of occurrence is the midfifties, although the disease occurs in patients from 20 to 80 years of age. There is a 4:1 male predominance. In half of patients the presenting complaints are vague weakness, lethargy, and fatigue. In one fourth of patients the presenting complaints are severe infection or bruising. These symptoms are related to the neutropenia and thrombocytopenia that are so characteristic of the disease. In the remainder of patients the diagnosis of hairy cell leukemia is made incidentally, usually as a result of a routine blood count.

The characteristic physical finding is palpable splenomegaly, which is found in 90% of patients. Mild hepatomegaly may be present. Peripheral lymphadenopathy and infiltration of skin are not characteristic.

Laboratory features. At least 80% of patients have a cytopenia of one or more elements of blood. The differential diagnosis of peripheral cytopenias is discussed in Chapter 81. A pancytopenia involving erythrocytes, neutrophils, and platelets is most common, although isolated cytopenias of one element may occasionally occur. The cytopenias are secondary to both increased destruction by hypersplenism and decreased production because of marrow infiltration by hairy cells. Hairy cells account for 2% to 80% of cells in the peripheral blood, but they are easily missed. Hairy cells are large cells with irregular, fine, filamentous cytoplasmic projections that can be seen by both light and electron microscopy (Plate III-5, G). The projections are redundant plasma membranes. Hairy cells are best demonstrated in wet mounts with supravital stains. Cytochemical staining for the tartrate-resistant isoenzyme of acid phosphatase can provide confirmatory information, although it is not diagnostic. The enzyme is present in hairy cells from 95% of patients. It can sometimes be seen in other lymphoproliferative disorders such as Sézary syndrome and chronic lymphocytic leukemia. In about 50% of cases the hairy cells contain peculiar cylindrical cytoplasmic inclusions termed ribosome-lamella complexes that are best seen by electron microscopy. Hairy cells can also be distinguished from other neoplastic B cells by the presence of receptors for interleukin 2 and by the expression of the CD-11 antigen. The differential diagnosis of abnormal lymphocytes in peripheral blood is listed in Table 81-2.

Bone marrow biopsy is recommended as a diagnostic procedure in all patients. Bone marrow aspiration usually results in a nondiagnostic "dry tap." The biopsy shows the presence of hairy cells as well as other specific morphologic changes. The histopathology of spleen is also diagnostic. Because of splenomegaly, the spleen is frequently removed before the underlying diagnosis of hairy cell leukemia has been made. The correct diagnosis is usually made by an experienced pathologist, even if the diagnosis has not been suspected clinically.

Treatment. Hairy cell leukemia is a chronic disorder. The clinical course of the disease is extremely variable, and treatment must be individualized. Approximately 10% of patients have minimal splenomegaly and mild cytopenias. They may remain asymptomatic for many years with minimal progression and no need for therapy. The remaining 90% require therapy at some time during the course of their disease. In the past, the accepted indications for therapy have included an absolute neutrophil count below 0.5 × 10^9 per liter, a platelet count below 50.0 × 10^9 per liter, symptomatic anemia requiring red cell transfusions, life-threatening infection, symptomatic splenomegaly, or splenic infarction. Splenectomy has been the treatment of choice under these circumstances and produces a return of all blood counts to the normal range in 40% of patients. Most of the remaining patients show objective improvement. The size of the spleen does not indicate whether the response to splenectomy will be favorable. Heavy infiltration of the bone marrow with hairy cells seems correlated with a poor response to splenectomy and a generally poor prognosis. Approximately one third of patients show progressive disease at intervals from months to years after splenectomy. Long-term survival is common: 40% live longer than 8 years after diagnosis. The most common cause of death is infection. Although most infections are bacterial, fungal and mycobacterial infections are common and should always be suspected in patients who do not respond promptly to specific antibacterial therapy.

Three agents (alpha interferons, deoxycoformycin, and 2-chlorodeoxyadenosine) have substantial activity in treatment of hairy cell leukemia and have been in clinical trial over the past decade. They have changed the approach to therapy in two ways. First, therapy is initiated earlier in the course of the disease to eliminate the need for repeated transfusions of blood products and, second, splenectomy is playing a rapidly decreasing role as primary therapy. The adenosine deaminase resistant deoxyadenosine analog, 2-chlorodeoxyadenosine (2-CdA), shows the most promise in therapy. The recommended dose for patients with significant cytopenias who need treatment is 0.1 mg 2-CdA/kg/day as a continuous intravenous infusion for 7 consecutive days. Using this protocol approximately 50% of patients show a complete hematologic response with normal peripheral blood counts and no hairy cells in their bone marrows. Approximately 90% of patients who are treated have a complete or partial response. The most common adverse effects are fever and infection. The average duration of complete responses is 8 months, although some patients achieve very long remissions of their disease. Patients who relapse generally respond to retreatment with 2-CdA.

Significant hematologic improvement also occurs in the majority of patients treated with interferon alpha. Two recombinant proteins, α2a-IFN (Roferon; Roche) and α2b-IFN (Intron A; Schering), have been studied extensively. In a typical treatment protocol, symptomatic patients receive a dose of 2 × 10^6 units/m^2 of body surface area subcutaneously three times a week. Patients are generally treated for 1 year, with weekly to monthly complete blood counts and monthly chemistry profiles. After 1 year, they are taken off treatment. They can be retreated at relapse of disease. Under this protocol, approximately 10% of patients achieve complete and 70% partial hematologic remission. Duration of remissions is not yet well defined. Transient myelosuppression may occur during the first month or two of therapy. Administration of interferon produces constitutional symptoms in all patients. These include a flu-like syndrome, fatigue, and anorexia, which become less severe with continuation of therapy.

2′-Deoxycoformycin, an inhibitor of adenosine deaminase, is approved for the treatment of hairy cell leukemia. At doses of 4 mg/m^2 of body surface area given intravenously as a bolus every other week for 3 to 6 months it has induced, with minimal toxicity, complete hematologic remissions in 60% of patients. It appears to be equally effective in previously untreated patients and in those who have progressive disease after splenectomy and administration of interferon. Clinical trials that will establish with certainty the relative merits of 2-chlorodeoxyadenosine, alpha interferon, and deoxycoformycin in therapy of hairy cell leukemia have not yet been completed. Of particular importance are the duration of responses that will be achieved with each agent and a test of their effectiveness when administered in combination with one another.

Chronic lymphocytic leukemia

Etiology. Chronic lymphocytic leukemia is a disease of the elderly and is the most common type of leukemia in the population aged 50 and over. In more than 95% of patients the disorder represents the accumulation of slowly proliferating, long-lived B lymphocytes derived from a single clone. The remainder of patients have an aggressive T cell leukemia that is refractory to therapy and rapidly fatal. The T cell disorder is not discussed here further.

The cause of B cell chronic lymphocytic leukemia is unknown. It is not associated with prior exposure to radiation or chemicals. A trisomy of chromosome 12 is present in malignant cells from 40% of patients and may play some role in causing the disordered cellular kinetics that characterize the disease.

Humoral immunodeficiency occurs in all patients with chronic lymphocytic leukemia and becomes worse as the disease progresses. There is an expansion of the peripheral T cell pool. Because most of the additional cells are suppressor cells, the helper/suppressor T cell ratio is much lower than normal. The relative increase in suppressor cell activity may account for the immunodeficiency. Autoimmune disorders are frequently observed in chronic lymphocytic leukemia. For example, 10% to 25% of patients have autoimmune hemolytic anemia at some time during the course of their disease.

Malignant lymphocytes can invade the blood of patients with poorly differentiated lymphocytic lymphoma and other types of non-Hodgkin's lymphomas (Table 81-2). The resulting leukemia is usually called lymphosarcoma cell leukemia and may be confused with, but is not, chronic lymphocytic leukemia (Plates III-5, D and E).

Clinical features. Ninety percent of patients with chronic lymphocytic leukemia are above the age of 50 years. Twice as many males as females are affected. The presenting symptoms and signs of chronic lymphocytic leukemia are extremely variable. In one fourth of patients the diagnosis is made incidentally at the time of a routine physical examination or blood count. Common presenting complaints are fatigue, weight loss, repeated infections, and enlarged lymph nodes. On physical examination the most common abnormality is lymphadenopathy, usually generalized with small, discrete, movable, nontender nodes. Localized masses of matted nodes may also be seen. Bone marrow failure is common in the advanced stages of the disease, so that signs of anemia and thrombocytopenia occur. Signs of infection, mostly pyogenic, are also common because of humoral immunodeficiency that becomes worse as the disease progresses. Relationships between clinical and laboratory features of the disease and survival are outlined in Table 93-2.

Laboratory features. Chronic lymphocytic leukemia is a laboratory diagnosis. The minimal requirement is a sustained absolute increase of well-differentiated lymphocytes in the peripheral blood and bone marrow not attributable to other causes (Table 81-2 and Plate III-5, D). Disorders most commonly confused with chronic lymphocytic leukemia include non-Hodgkin's lymphoma, hairy cell leukemia, Waldenström's macroglobulinemia, and viral infections. There is controversy about the degree of sustained lymphocytosis necessary to make the diagnosis. A minimum of 5.0×10^9 per liter lymphocytes in peripheral blood is accepted in some schemes; 15.0×10^9 per liter is required in others. If a sustained peripheral lymphocyte count of 10×10^9 per liter is present, then documentation of either bone marrow involvement or a B cell phenotype typical of chronic lymphocytic leukemia serves to make the diagnosis. If the peripheral count is less than 10×10^9 per liter, then both bone marrow involvement and a typical B cell phenotype should be documented. For bone marrow, 30% or more of the nucleated cells must be well-differentiated lymphocytes. The abnormal lymphocytes in the marrow and peripheral blood are fragile and easily traumatized, resulting in the presence of ruptured "smudge" cells on the peripheral blood smear. Surface immunoglobulin is present on the surface of the leukemic lymphocyte and is decreased in amount compared with normal B lymphocytes. The SIg is usually IgM, frequently with coexpression of IgD, and is rarely IgG. Because the population is clonal, the light chain is either lambda or kappa, not both. There is clonal rearrangement of heavy- and light-chain immunoglobulin genes. The concentration of immunoglobulins in the serum is markedly decreased. The Coombs' antiglobulin test result is positive in 15% of patients. The majority of these patients do not have signs of hemolysis, although autoimmune hemolytic anemia is a well-known complication of chronic lymphocytic leukemia.

Table 93-2. Clinical staging of chronic lymphocytic leukemia

Rai Stage	Features	Median survival from diagnosis (mos)
0	Lymphocytosis of peripheral blood (lymphocytes $>5.0 \times 10^9$/L) and bone marrow only	>150
I	Lymphocytosis plus enlarged nodes	101
II	Lymphocytosis plus enlarged spleen and/or liver; nodes may or may not be enlarged	71
III	Lymphocytosis plus anemia (hemoglobin <11 g/dl); nodes, spleen, and liver may or may not be enlarged	30
IV	Lymphocytosis plus thrombocytopenia (platelets $<100.0 \times 10^9$/L); nodes, spleen, and liver may or may not be enlarged; anemia may or may not be present	30

These criteria for clinical staging of chronic lymphocytic leukemia are a modification of those first proposed by Rai KR et al: Blood 46:219, 1975.

Treatment. Chronic lymphocytic leukemia cannot be cured by current therapy, so palliation is the goal. The course of the disease varies from patient to patient. Because the patients cannot be cured, it is critically important to observe each patient over a period to ascertain the pace of the disease. This information is necessary if therapeutic interventions are to be made at appropriate times without increasing the patient's morbidity.

Criteria for assessing the stage of disease at diagnosis are listed in Table 93-2. The stage is related to prognosis. Stages 0, I, and II do not require treatment if the patient is asymptomatic. Randomized clinical trials have shown that treatment of such good prognosis patients with daily chlorambucil slows the progression of the disease to more advanced stages, but ultimate survival is shorter. Early treatment is harmful because treated patients have short survival after disease progression and an increased incidence of fatal epithelial cancers, when compared to untreated patients. Indications for treatment include progressive marrow failure, debilitating symptoms such as weakness, symptomatic bulky disease, autoimmune phenomena such as hemolytic anemia, and progressive lymphocytosis with a peripheral lymphocyte count above 100.0×10^9 per liter. Stages III and IV generally do require treatment. Some patients may initially exhibit stage III or IV disease, whereas others may progress to these stages from earlier stages. Initial therapy is usually an alkylating agent such as chlorambucil, 6 to 10 mg/day orally for 1 to 2 weeks, followed by maintenance at lower doses, such as 2 to 6 mg/day. Approximately 75% of patients respond to therapy, but in only 10% to 20% is there complete remission. Response is usually slow and is monitored both in the peripheral blood and by the size of the lymph nodes. The peripheral lymphocytosis should decrease; the platelet count and hematocrit should increase. Because bone marrow function is compromised, the possibility of dangerous marrow suppression by chemotherapy must be borne in mind. The most serious toxicity is usually progressive thrombocytopenia, which is a relative contraindication to further therapy with alkylating agents. Some clinical trials have produced evidence that chlorambucil given as a pulse of 0.4 to 0.6 mg/kg of body weight once every 2 to 4 weeks induces remissions with less toxicity than daily dosage produces. If chlorambucil therapy is inadequate or if autoimmune phenomena occur, a glucocorticoid (typically prednisone 60 mg/day initially, tapering to 10 to 20 mg every other day) is added to the alkylating agent. Local radiotherapy may be used to treat isolated symptomatic masses of nodes. Progressive advanced disease may respond to combination chemotherapy, but the long-term prognosis is grim, with a median life expectancy of 1 to 2 years. Relatively small clinical trials have suggested that CHOP combination chemotherapy (Table 94-7) in which the dose of intravenous doxorubicin is reduced to 25 mg/m^2 produce remissions in 30% to 50% of patients with advanced disease: median survival was greater than 4 years. Fludarabine monophosphate is a newly approved drug that may be useful in the treatment of chronic lymphocytic leukemia. Precise doses and indications are not yet well defined, but it has produced complete remissions in some patients. Most patients die of infection, usually bacterial, but sometimes mycobacterial or fungal. In patients with IgG levels below 50% of the lower limit of normal or with a history of serious bacterial infection, intravenous immunoglobulin G (400 mg/kg of body weight) every 3 or 4 weeks reduces the frequency of infection. Treatment, however, is extremely expensive and inconvenient and results in very little increase in life expectancy. Transformation of chronic lymphocytic leukemia to an immunoblastic sarcoma (Richter's syndrome) or to an acute leukemia is rare but can occur. Each is resistant to therapy.

MYELOPROLIFERATIVE DISORDERS

The myeloproliferative disorders are clonal neoplasms arising in a pluripotent hematopoietic stem cell and characterized either by excessive production of phenotypically normal mature cells (chronic myeloproliferative disorders) or by impaired or aberrant maturation of hematopoietic precursor cells (acute myeloproliferative and myelodysplastic disorders) (refer to the box at upper right).

The evidence for the clonal nature of these disorders is derived from studies on the expression of isoenzymes of glucose-6-phosphate dehydrogenase (G6PD) and from chromosomal analyses. Women who are heterozygous for isoenzymes of G6PD have two populations of cells, one containing type A isoenzyme and the other type B. When a neoplastic disease develops, cells containing only one enzyme (A or B) are present, indicating that the neoplasm is derived from a single cell. In the myeloproliferative disorders, single isoenzymes are present in granulocytes, erythrocytes, monocytes, and megakaryocytes, indicating that the neoplasms arise in a stem cell common to the different cell lineages. In some, the single enzyme is also present in lymphocytes, indicating that the disease arises in a more primitive pluripotent stem cell common to both the myeloid and lymphoid cell lines. Similarly, identical marker chromosomes are present in erythroid, myeloid, and megakaryocytic precursor cells, but not in marrow stromal fibroblasts.

The exact nature of the defects is unknown but differs in the two groups of disorders. In the chronic disorders, there appears to be a loss of regulatory signals that control the production of mature cells, whereas in the acute disorders the major defect is in cell maturation. The differential diagnosis of an elevated blood neutrophil count is discussed in Chapter 81.

Classification of the myeloproliferative disorders

I. Chronic myeloproliferative disorders (excessive production of mature cells)
   A. Chronic myelogenous leukemia (chronic granulocytic leukemia)
   B. Idiopathic myelofibrosis (agnogenic myeloid metaplasia)
   C. Essential thrombocythemia (essential thrombocytosis)
   D. Polycythemia vera
II. Acute myeloproliferative and myelodysplastic disorders (impaired maturation or dysplasia of hematopoietic cells)
   A. Acute myelogenous leukemia (acute nonlymphocytic leukemia)
   B. Myelodysplastic syndromes
      1. Refractory anemia
      2. Refractory sideroblastic anemia
      3. Chronic myelomonocytic leukemia
      4. Refractory anemia with excess blasts (RAEB)
      5. Refractory anemia with excess blasts in transformation

Chronic myeloproliferative disorders

The chronic myeloproliferative disorders include chronic myelogenous leukemia (CML), essential thrombocythemia (ET), polycythemia vera (PV), and idiopathic myelofibrosis. Distinguishing features are listed in Table 93-3. This chapter focuses on CML, ET, and PV; myelofibrosis is discussed in Chapter 91. These are clonal neoplasms of a pluripotent stem cell with an overproduction of one or more formed elements of the blood. The variation in patterns of cellular proliferation and differentiation can be explained by a clonal mutation of pluripotent stem cells with different

Table 93-3. Distinguishing features of chronic myeloproliferative disorders

	CML	IMF	PV	ET
Leukocytes	↑↑↑	↑/N/↓	↑	N/↑
Hematocrit	↓	↓	↑↑↑	N
Platelets	↑↑	↑/N/↓	↑↑	↑↑↑
LAP score	↓	↑/N/↓	↑↑↑	N/↑
Teardrop RBC	−	↑↑↑	−	−
Marrow fibrosis	±	↑↑↑	−	−
Ph[1] chromosome	+	−	−	−

CML, chronic myelogenous leukemia; IMF, idiopathic myelofibrosis; PV, polycythemia vera; ET, essential thrombocythemia; LAP, leukocyte alkaline phosphatase. ↑↑↑, marked increase, ↑↑, moderate increase; ↑, slight increase; ±, variable; +, present; −, absent; N, normal; ↓, decrease.

lineage potentials. PV arises from a stem cell with a high erythroid potential, and CML may arise in a stem cell with a high neutrophil potential. Stem cells with equal potential for neutrophils and megakaryocytes may be involved in CML and ET. The diseases are interrelated, and one may evolve into another during its course. PV and ET may evolve into myelofibrosis, and all may evolve into acute leukemia.

Chronic myelogenous leukemia

CML is a clonal neoplasm, arising in a pluripotent stem cell, that is characterized by extreme leukocytosis with an increase in immature and mature granulocytes and by splenomegaly. It occurs most frequently in young and middle-aged adults, with a slightly higher incidence in males. A distinctive chromosome abnormality, the Philadelphia (Ph^1 or Ph) chromosome, a shortened G-22 chromosome resulting from the reciprocal translocation of genetic material between chromosomes 9 and 22, appears in 95% of patients with CML. This abnormality is present in granulocytes, erythrocytes, and megakaryocytes, indicating that CML arises from a pluripotent stem cell. The disease follows two distinct courses: a mild chronic phase lasting approximately 3½ years and an acute phase (blast crisis) that results in death in 90% of patients within several months.

Etiology. The cause of CML is unknown, but its incidence is increased in atom bomb survivors and in patients who have received irradiation for ankylosing spondylitis. Of significance is that the breakpoint of the translocation between chromosomes 9 and 22 occurs in the region of the cellular oncogene, c-abl on chromosome 9. The oncogene, c-sis, is on chromosome 22 at some distance from the breakpoint. C-abl is the cellular homolog of the transforming gene of the Abelson murine leukemia virus, which causes pre-B cell leukemia in mice. C-abl is translocated to a specific region of chromosome 22, the breakpoint cluster region (bcr). This translocation results in a hybrid bcr/abl gene that is unique to CML. Its product is a 210 kD protein with greater tyrosine phosphokinase activity than normal. The abnormal kinase may be responsible for the development of the disease. The cause of cancer is discussed further in Chapter 71.

In 5% of patients with features resembling CML, the Ph^1 chromosome is not detected. In some of these patients there is a translocation between chromosomes 9 and 22, even though there is no detectable chromosomal abnormality, and in most, there is rearrangement of the bcr gene. A number of patients considered to have Ph^1-negative CML were found on re-evaluation to have features more consistent with a myelodysplastic disorder (chronic myelomonocytic leukemia) than with CML.

The Ph^1 chromosome is found in a number of adults and children with acute lymphoblastic leukemia (ALL). Some of these may represent CML presenting in the acute phase.

Clinical features. The chronic phase of CML is characterized by a stable overproduction of leukocytes. The acute phase (blast crisis) is an aggressive form of the disease similar to acute myelogenous leukemia, and 90% of patients with CML die as a consequence of transformation to the acute phase. Transformation occurs at a rate of 25% per year after the first year after diagnosis but can occur at any time during the disease. Survival from diagnosis of the chronic phase is approximately 3½ years.

Chronic phase. The onset of CML is insidious, and 20% of patients are asymptomatic at the time of diagnosis. Most symptoms are related to anemia (fatigue, weakness) or to splenomegaly (discomfort or a mass in the left upper quadrant of the abdomen). Less common are bleeding or thrombotic episodes, arthralgias, and bone pain. Some patients have fever, sweating, and weight loss produced by hypermetabolism. Splenomegaly and pallor are the major findings on examination. The spleen is palpable in more than 90% of patients and ranges in size from those that are barely palpable to those that fill the entire left side of the abdomen. Spleen size is directly correlated with the height of the peripheral leukocyte count. In 50% of patients the liver is enlarged at diagnosis; 20% have purpura; and a few have lymphadenopathy or infiltration in the skin.

Acute phase. Onset of the acute phase (blast crisis) occurs randomly, but most often at about 3½ years after diagnosis. Transformation to the acute phase may be insidious, occurring over several months, or abrupt. Any change in symptoms or signs, or in blood findings during the chronic phase that are unrelated to chemotherapy, usually indicates that transformation to the acute phase has occurred (Table 93-4). Symptoms usually include fever, weight loss, increasing size of the spleen, worsening anemia and thrombocytopenia, bone pain, and purpura. Additional cytogenetic abnormalities are commonly seen such as a second

Table 93-4. Findings associated with onset of the acute phase of CML

Clinical observations
Rapidly increasing spleen size
Resistance to previously effective doses of chemotherapy
New and unexplained fever
Lymph node enlargement
Skin infiltration
Lytic bone lesions
Laboratory data
Progressive basophilia
Progressive thrombocytosis
Thrombocytopenia
Progressive anemia
Normalization of the leukocyte alkaline phosphatase (LAP) score
Progressive myelofibrosis
Increasing percentage of blast forms in peripheral blood and bone marrow
Cytogenetic clonal evolution
Hypercalcemia

Ph[1] chromosome, monosomy 7, trisomy 8, and trisomy 19. Transformation in most patients is to acute myelogenous leukemia or to one of its variants. In 20% transformation is to an acute lymphoblastic leukemia.

Laboratory features of CML. Leukocytosis is the most prominent feature; the peripheral leukocyte count ranges between 50×10^9 per liter and 200×10^9 per liter at the time of diagnosis but can exceed 1000×10^9 per liter. The entire spectrum of neutrophils from myeloblasts ($<5\%$) to mature polymorphonuclear leukocytes is present (Plate III-6, D). Numbers of eosinophils and basophils are increased. Most patients have a normochromic normocytic anemia resulting from decreased erythropoiesis. Platelet numbers are increased in 50% of patients; they function normally, and thrombotic events are uncommon. The marrow is hypercellular, with a marked increase in the ratio of myeloid to erythroid cells caused by the marked increase in granulocytes and their precursors. The marrow contains more immature granulocytes than the blood, but the concentration of blasts is less than 5% in the chronic phase. In some patients, mild fibrosis of the marrow is present and may increase during the course of the disease.

Leukocyte alkaline phosphatase (LAP) is decreased in neutrophils in more than 90% of patients. It may return to normal after treatment or increase with acute transformation. The serum B_{12} level and B_{12} binding proteins are increased and correlate with the degree of leukocytosis. Hyperuricemia may result from increased cell turnover.

The acute phase is accompanied by a variety of changes in the blood and marrow (Table 93-4), including an increase in blasts and promyelocytes in the blood and marrow, worsening of the anemia and increasing leukocytosis, thrombocytosis or thrombocytopenia, increase in basophils, and increase in fibrosis of the marrow. The Ph chromosome persists, and additional chromosomal abnormalities may be detected.

Treatment. The chronic phase of the disease is well controlled by chemotherapy, which induces a remission of symptoms and a decrease in the leukocytosis and size of the spleen. Busulfan and hydroxyurea are the most widely used drugs to treat CML. Busulfan is an alkylating agent and can be given intermittently or continuously. It is given in a dose of 4 to 6 mg/day orally until the peripheral leukocyte count decreases to 10 to 15×10^9 per liter, at which time it is discontinued. The disease may be controlled for months after a single course of therapy, and patients may receive repeated courses of treatment. Side effects of busulfan include myelosuppression, increased skin pigmentation, pulmonary fibrosis, and, rarely, adrenal insufficiency. Hydroxyurea is an active agent affecting cells in DNA synthesis; continuous oral administration of 1 to 3 g/day is required to control the disease. Higher doses can be administered when a very high leukocyte count must be quickly reduced. Leukocyte counts increase and decrease rapidly as doses of hydroxyurea are modified so that frequent peripheral blood counts are necessary during therapy. With either drug, a remission in symptoms and blood counts occurs, but the Ph chromosome persists in cells in the marrow. Treatment with aggressive combination chemotherapy in an attempt to eradicate the leukemic clone has not resulted in an increase in survival. Treatment with recombinant alpha interferon can induce hematologic remissions in the chronic phase, although most patients become refractory to therapy after 4 to 12 months.

Bone marrow transplantation is increasingly performed in good-risk patients with CML who have an identical twin, a human leukocyte antigen–(HLA)–compatible sibling, or a compatible unrelated donor (Chapter 78). Of patients who receive allogeneic bone marrow, approximately 60% who had transplantation in chronic phase and 40% who had transplantation in accelerated phase survive 5 years or more. Most of these long-term survivors are probably cured.

Patients who do not receive bone marrow transplantation eventually progress to myelofibrosis with bone marrow failure (Chapter 91) or to "blast crisis," a form of acute leukemia; 80% have myeloid blasts and 20% have lymphoid blasts. Treatment of the acute phase ("blast crisis") of CML is unsatisfactory, and the disease is less responsive to therapy than the de novo acute myelogenous or acute lymphoblastic leukemias. The overall median survival from onset of blast crisis is approximately 18 weeks unless bone marrow transplantation can be performed.

Essential thrombocythemia

Essential thrombocythemia (essential thrombocytosis [ET]) is the least common of the myeloproliferative disorders and is characterized by a marked increase in circulating platelets, usually in excess of 1000×10^9 per liter. It occurs most frequently in the fifth and sixth decades and affects men and women equally. With the advent of automated platelet counts, the disorder is seen with increasing frequency as an incidental diagnosis in young adults. The major criteria for a diagnosis of ET are (1) persistent elevation of platelet count, usually more than 1000×10^9 per liter; (2) marked increase in megakaryocytes in the marrow; (3) absence of other chronic myeloproliferative disorders; and (4) absence of an underlying condition responsible for reactive thrombocytosis, such as infection, chronic inflammatory disease, iron deficiency, malignancy, or prior splenectomy.

Clinical features. Symptoms are related to thromboembolic phenomena in one third of patients and to bleeding in two thirds. Bleeding results from abnormal platelet function and may take the form of easy bruising, nosebleed, or gastrointestinal bleeding. Thrombotic events often include vascular ischemia of the central nervous system, manifested by transient ischemia attacks, dizziness, visual problems, and headaches; or peripheral vascular ischemia, including deep vein thrombosis, pulmonary emboli, and emboli of digital vessels leading to painful ischemia of the toes. In approximately 40% of patients the spleen is palpably enlarged, although not to the extent seen in other myeloproliferative disorders.

Laboratory features. Platelet counts are increased to more than 600 × 10^9 per liter, usually exceed 1000 × 10^9 per liter, and can be as high as 5000 × 10^9 per liter. Platelet function is abnormal. The leukocyte count is elevated in 50% of patients but seldom exceeds 40 × 10^9 per liter. Leukocyte alkaline phosphatase level is normal or increased, but not to the extent seen in polycythemia vera (PV). Megakaryocytes are markedly increased in the marrow. Serum B_{12} and uric acid levels are usually increased. Pseudohyperkalemia may result from the increase in circulating platelets that release potassium during the preparation of serum.

Treatment. Treatment is directed at controlling the platelet level and relieving symptoms. In asymptomatic patients with mild thrombocythemia (less than 600 × 10^9 per liter), treatment is not indicated. However, treatment should be given if platelets exceed 1000 × 10^9 per liter or if patients are symptomatic at lower levels. The disorder is not benign even in young people; nearly 40% of patients have bleeding or thrombosis or both. Previously, treatment included administration of alkylating agents and radioactive phosphorus (^{32}P). Although these are effective forms of therapy, they are associated with an increased risk of leukemia or other neoplasm. Therefore, it seems more appropriate to treat patients with hydroxyurea or anagrelide. Hydroxyurea at an oral dose of 1 to 3 g/day generally maintains the platelet count at near-normal levels. The dose of hydroxyurea must be adjusted to prevent inducing severe neutropenia and anemia. The peripheral blood count should generally be checked every week or two for patients receiving hydroxyurea because the drug can rapidly change the blood count. If hydroxyurea is ineffective, anagrelide can be used. This is a relatively new drug that appears to have few side effects. Induction doses of 1 mg every 6 hours orally usually reduce the platelet count to near-normal levels within 1 to 2 weeks. Maintenance doses generally range from 1 to 4 mg/day. Anagrelide is not cytotoxic to bone marrow. Side effects are generally mild but can include headache, nausea, palpitations, fluid retention, and diarrhea.

The course of the disease in most patients is rather benign and resembles that of PV. ET may evolve into other myeloproliferative disorders and in some cases into acute leukemia.

POLYCYTHEMIA VERA

Polycythemia vera in most cases can be easily distinguished from secondary polycythemia by the presence of leukocytosis, thrombocytosis, basophilia, splenomegaly, and trilinear hyperplasia of the marrow with clustering of megakaryocytes. The polycythemias are discussed in Chapter 80. Polycythemia vera is a clonal disease in which the primary production of increased red cells by the bone marrow depresses erythropoietin levels to normal or below normal values (<30 mU/ml). The clonal cells overgrow the normal population of red cell precursors that may still be present as a minority of cells. The incidence of polycythemia vera is highest in patients who are 60 to 70 years old, but it may occur in individuals ranging in age from adolescence to 90 years. The male to female ratio is 1.2:1.0, and all races are affected. Some reports indicate a higher than expected incidence in Jews. In addition to the signs and symptoms common to all cases of polycythemia, there is a severe pruritus that may be related to elevated blood levels of histamine and/or increased numbers of skin mast cells. Thrombotic and hemorrhagic complications are frequent as a result of the high blood viscosity, and some patients with virulent disease have marked symptoms of hypermetabolism. Clinical gout can result from hyperuricemia accompanying increased hematopoietic cell turnover.

Treatment. With optimum therapy, mortality resulting from the hyperviscosity can be greatly reduced, allowing patients with polycythemia vera to have prolonged median survival times of 10 to 15 years. In 15% of patients acute leukemia eventually evolves. This is most often myelogenous but may occasionally be monocytic or lymphocytic. The incidence of leukemia is much higher in patients who have been treated with alkylating agents than in those who receive phlebotomy alone. Fifteen to thirty percent of cases evolve into myelofibrosis with myeloid metaplasia (Chapter 91). The evolution may take the form either of a primary marrow fibrosis with consequent pancytopenia or of a rampant myeloid metaplasia with extramedullary hematopoiesis throughout the body that produces marked splenomegaly and hepatomegaly with portal hypertension. In this case, a marked leukocytosis may produce a blood state like that of chronic myelogenous leukemia. A variety of cytogenetic abnormalities have been reported, but none is characteristic.

Because patients with polycythemia vera who have not been treated have an extremely poor prognosis (median survival, 1.5 years), caused by massive thrombotic and hemorrhagic complications, it is extremely important to reduce the hematocrit. Because thromboembolic events increase precipitously in patients with polycythemia vera when the hematocrit is greater than 44%, this level is the therapeutic end-point for therapy. Patients undergoing surgery without such control have extremely high morbidity and mortality rates, whereas those whose hematocrits have been under good control for more than 3 months have a normal course.

Patients 40 years old or less without evidence of severe vascular disease whose primary manifestation is erythrocytosis and whose hematocrit can be controlled by phlebotomy should continue to have this form of therapy. The administration of aspirin or dipyridamole has been recommended to reduce thrombosis, but clinical trials show that these anti–platelet aggregating agents do not reduce the incidence of thrombotic events associated with phlebotomy. They do increase morbidity from bleeding. Older individuals with poor blood vessels have a very high incidence of thrombotic complications and should be treated with chemotherapy in addition to phlebotomy to suppress the bone marrow activity. This therapy produces better long-term control of the disease than phlebotomy alone. Hydroxyurea is recommended because it has not been reported to increase the frequency of acute leukemia, unlike phosphorus 32 and the alkylating agents. During the first week 30 mg/kg/day of hydroxyurea is given orally in divided doses, followed by 15 mg/kg/day orally the second week, and the dose is then individualized to maintain normal blood counts. Periodic phlebotomy is continued as necessary to keep the hematocrit in the normal range. Hydroxyurea can produce marrow aplasia in a short time, and patients taking it must be followed very carefully. Marrow suppression is reversible. Other indications for starting chemotherapy are severe pruritus not controlled by H_1-, H_2-receptor blocking agents (either alone or in combination), symptomatic splenomegaly, severe hypermetabolism, or history of thrombotic or hemorrhagic events.

ACUTE MYELOPROLIFERATIVE AND MYELODYSPLASTIC DISORDERS

In contrast to the chronic myeloproliferative disorders, which are characterized by excessive production of mature functional cells, the acute myeloproliferative disorders are marked by a defect in maturation of hematopoietic precursors (refer to the box on p. 892). Generally, by the time the diagnosis of the disorder is made, the clone of abnormally maturing cells has suppressed the normal marrow cells. This results in symptoms of bone marrow failure and cytopenias. If failure of maturation occurs rapidly, immature precursor cells (blasts) may be dominant in the marrow with features of acute myelogenous leukemia (AML). Alternatively, defects in maturation may be minimal initially and progress slowly over many years, with the marrow showing only variable degrees of dysplasia. In some of these patients, clonal evolution occurs with increasingly more malignant characteristics in the marrow until, eventually, a large number of blasts are present, as in classical AML.

Acute myelogenous leukemia

Acute myelogenous leukemia, also referred to as acute nonlymphocytic leukemia (ANLL) or acute myeloblastic leukemia, is a malignant disorder arising in a stem cell capable of differentiating along the granulocytic, erythrocytic, and megakaryocytic cell lines. In some patients the malignant clone is expressed in all three cell lines, whereas in others expression may be restricted to erythrocytes and granulocytes or to granulocytes and macrophages. Malignant transformation occurs at different stages of differentiation, leading to morphologically different subtypes. These are listed in Table 93-5, as classified by a French-American-British group (FAB).

In all subtypes the malignant clones of immature myeloid cells (primarily blasts) proliferate but do not differentiate to mature functional end cells. Blasts eventually replace the marrow, circulate in the blood, and invade most tissues in the body. Suppression of normal hematopoiesis by leukemic cells or their products results in anemia, neutropenia, and thrombocytopenia. These cytopenias are responsible for the symptoms of the disease. All subtypes except acute promyelocytic leukemia are similar in regard to course and response to treatment. In untreated cases, survival is less than 3 months. With therapy, prolonged survival and cure can be achieved. Although AML may occur at any age, the incidence increases with advancing years. The disease is more common in males.

Etiology. The exact cause of AML is unknown, but certain factors are associated with an increased incidence of the disease. These factors include exposure to ionizing radiation (atom bomb survivors), chemicals (benzene), or chemotherapy with alkylating agents and nitrosoureas. Genetic factors also predispose to AML. Identical twins have an increased incidence of disease that occurs before the age of 6. Diseases with chromosome instability, including Down's syndrome, Bloom's syndrome, Fanconi's anemia, neurofibromatosis, and Wiskott-Aldrich syndrome, convey greater risk for developing leukemia. Chronic myeloproliferative diseases may evolve to AML, as may the myelodysplastic syndromes. Acute promyelocytic leukemia (APL) is associated with a specific chromosomal abnormality, the translocation of a portion of the long arm of chromosome 17 onto the long arm of chromosome 15. The chromosomal breakpoints from several patients have been clustered within the gene on chromosome 17 that encodes the nuclear retinoic acid receptor (RAR-alpha) and within the myl gene on chromosome 15. The translocation results in the production of a hybrid fusion messenger RNA that contains portions of both the RAR-alpha and the myl transcripts. This fusion transcript appears to represent an abnormal transcription factor that affects the expression of genes in myeloid cells. The results are abnormal growth and differentiation of myeloid precursors with consequent clin-

Table 93-5. Subtypes of acute myelogenous leukemia

Subtype	Predominant cell in marrow	FAB classification	Prevalance (%)
Myeloblastic (AML)	Myeloblast	M1, M2	45
Promyelocytic (APL)	Promyelocyte	M3	10
Myelomonocytic (AMML)	Myeloblasts, monoblasts	M4	30
Monocytic (AMMOL)	Monoblasts, promonocytes	M5	10
Erythroleukemia (AEL)	Pronormoblasts, myeloblasts	M6	5
Megakaryocytic (AMgL)	Megakaryoblasts	M7	3

ical APL. Remission of APL can be induced by treatment of patients with all-trans-retinoic acid, a ligand that binds to the receptor encoded by RAR-alpha. Presumably the retinoic acid binds to the abnormal transcription factor in APL cells and inhibits its ability to induce abnormal growth and differentiation of myeloid precursors.

Clinical features. Signs and symptoms are similar in all subgroups of AML and result from suppression of normal hematopoiesis. Symptoms are usually present for less than 3 months and are related to anemia (fatigue, pallor, tachycardia, dyspnea), neutropenia (infection), or thrombocytopenia (bruising, bleeding, petechiae). Several of the subgroups are associated with distinctive features. Acute promyelocytic leukemia (M3) is associated with disseminated intravascular coagulation (DIC) and bleeding caused by procoagulants released from the cytoplasmic granules of promyelocytes. Myelomonocytic (M4) and monocytic (M5) subtypes are associated more frequently with skin infiltration and gum hypertrophy. The spleen is enlarged in approximately one third of patients, and rarely there is enlargement of the liver or nodes. Approximately 25% of patients with AML have a history of myelodysplasia or "preleukemia."

Laboratory features. Anemia, neutropenia, and thrombocytopenia are present in most patients and may be severe. The peripheral nucleated blood cell count is increased in 50% of patients, and this increase is nearly always due to circulating blasts. The blasts may contain Auer rods (rod or string-shaped abnormal aggregation of lysosomal granules in the cytoplasm) (Plate III-6, E and Figs. 93-1 and 93-2), which are pathognomonic for AML. The marrow is usually hypercellular, with blasts being the predominant cell type. Differentiation of AML subtypes and acute lymphocytic leukemia is based on morphology and uses specific cytochemical stains or monoclonal antibodies. Serum uric acid level may be increased, and serum and urine muramidase levels are increased in the monocytic and myelomonocytic subtypes.

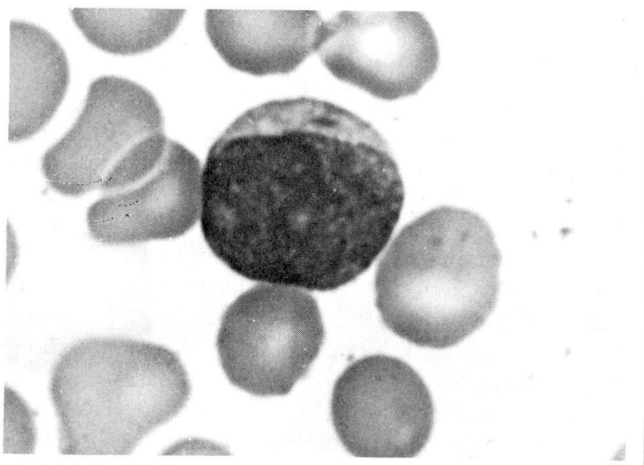

Fig. 93-1. Stained smear of blood from a patient with acute myelogenous leukemia. The nucleated cell is a myeloblast that contains a dark-staining cytoplasmic body known as the Auer rod.

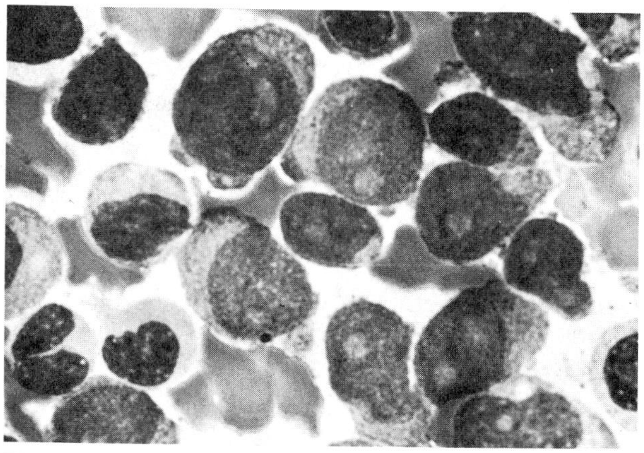

Fig. 93-2. Stained bone marrow aspirate from a patient with acute myelogenous leukemia. The predominant cell type, the myeloblast, has a high nuclear/cytoplasmic ratio and has large nucleoli (compare with normal marrow, Plate III-1).

Nonrandom chromosome abnormalities are found in more than 80% of patients with AML. Specific abnormalities are associated with certain morphologic subtypes and are correlated with prognosis. For example, chromosomal translocation t(15;17) is associated with M3 and inverted 16 with M4. These have a better response to treatment and a longer duration of survival than do those with translocation t(9;11) or deletions of portions of chromosomes 5 or 12.

Treatment. The goal of treatment is to induce a complete remission by eradication of the leukemic clone and restoration of normal hematopoiesis. A *complete remission* is defined as disappearance of signs and symptoms related to AML and a return to normal of blood counts and marrow, with less than 5% blasts in the marrow. The two most effective agents for inducing a remission are daunorubicin, an anthracycline antibiotic, and cytosine arabinoside, a pyrimidine antimetabolite (Chapter 72). In a typical treatment protocol, induction therapy, given in a 7-day schedule as illustrated in Table 93-6, results in complete remission after one or two cycles of therapy in 60% to 80% of patients. Duration of survival depends on the length of the first remission, which usually lasts between 12 and 18 months. Cure is a possibility, but only 20% of patients survive 5 years or more. Attempts to prolong the duration of remission and survival are carried out through various programs of "maintenance" therapy or "consolidation" therapy for periods ranging from several months to 1 to 2 years. Repeated courses of multidrug consolidation over a period of 4 to 8 months have resulted in 30% to 40% disease-free survival rates at 3 to 5 years. These results are encouraging and suggest that all patients should receive postinduction consolidation therapy. There is little evidence to indi-

Table 93-6. Drugs commonly used to induce a remission in AML

Drug	Dose (mg/m^2)	Route	Schedule*
Cytosine arabinoside	100-200	iv	Continuous infusion days 1-7 of 7 day cycle
Daunorubicin	30-60	iv	Single dose, days 1, 2, 3, of 7 day cycle

*May require two cycles to induce a complete remission.

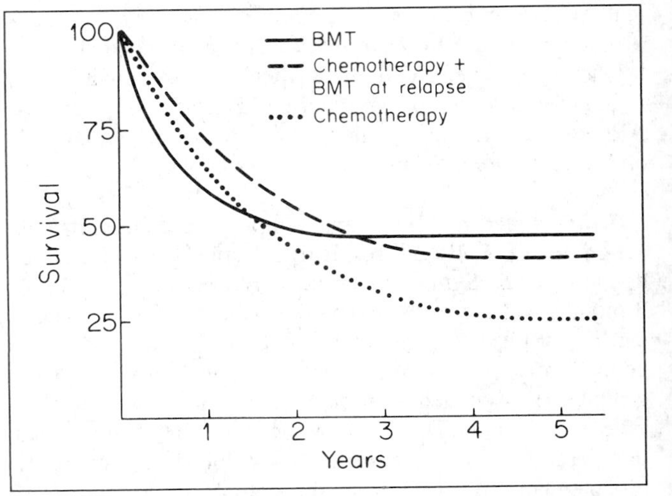

Fig. 93-3. Survival of adults with acute myelogenous leukemia receiving either allogenic bone marrow transplants in first remission, postremission chemotherapy, or postremission chemotherapy with bone marrow transplants at relapse. (From Champlin RE and Gale RP: Semin Hematol 24:55, 1987.)

cate that maintenance therapy has improved the duration of remission or survival.

In nearly all instances the marrow must be made aplastic to achieve a remission with induction therapy, because the chemotherapeutic agents do not distinguish between leukemic and normal cells. The exception is acute promyelocytic leukemia, in which complete remission can be induced without marrow aplasia. During periods of marrow aplasia (2 to 3 weeks) aggressive support must be given to prevent fatal infections or bleeding. Infections with gram-negative bacilli or gram-positive cocci and fungi are common in patients with severe neutropenia. Neutropenic and febrile patients should receive broad-spectrum antibiotic coverage with an aminoglycoside and a semisynthetic penicillin (Chapter 229). If fever persists or recurs after 1 week of antibiotics, amphotericin B should be given, because Aspergillus and Candida infections are common in this setting. Platelet transfusions must be given to prevent bleeding, and platelets should be maintained above 20×10^9 per liter (Chapter 77). If patients become sensitized to random donor platelets, single-donor or HLA-matched platelets must be given.

A different approach to therapy has proved effective in acute promyelocytic leukemia. Tretinoin (all-trans-retinoic acid) administered orally at a dose of 45 mg/m^2 of body surface area per day induces a complete remission in more than 80% of patients. Aplasia of the bone marrow does not occur and abnormalities of coagulation (DIC) resolve promptly. Patients eventually experience relapse. Ongoing clinical trials must define the roles of conventional chemotherapy, treatment with all-trans-retinoic acid, and allogeneic bone marrow transplantation. The aim is to cure a higher percentage of patients with APL who generally have a more favorable prognosis than patients with other types of acute myelogenous leukemia.

Bone marrow transplantation (BMT) is an effective therapy for AML, with a 50% long-term survival rate and probable cure. This option is limited primarily to those patients less than age 55 with an identical twin or an HLA-identical sibling, although use of HLA-matched unrelated donors is increasing (Chapter 78). The morbidity and mortality rates associated with BMT are significant because of graft-versus-host disease, interstitial pneumonitis, and other infections. This raises the question of when a BMT should be performed. The best results are obtained in patients less than 30 years of age during first remission. Compared to chemotherapy, BMT in first remission appears to improve survival rate. Results are also encouraging for BMT in very early relapse. Therefore because of the increasing survival and possible cure in some patients with chemotherapy, it may be appropriate to defer BMT until the first sign of relapse. A comparison of survival rate after chemotherapy or BMT in adults is illustrated in Fig. 93-3. As BMT procedures and techniques are further improved and complications are better controlled, BMT should become available to more patients. Results with autologous transplants after removal of the marrow and cleansing with monoclonal antibodies or cytotoxic agents in vitro have been associated with prolonged survival in several reports. However, the latter procedure requires further study and a longer follow-up period of observation.

Myelodysplastic syndromes

The myelodysplastic syndromes (MDSs) are stem cell disorders characterized by a defect in maturation of hematopoietic precursors to functionally mature cells. The defect in maturation leads to ineffective hematopoiesis, which results in variable degrees of cytopenia or even pancytopenia, leading to infection and hemorrhage. There may be gradual expansion of the abnormal clone of cells over many years, with concomitant suppression of normal hematopoiesis. In some cases, the clonal evolution increases with progressive malignant characteristics in the marrow. Eventually, there is a large number of blasts and consequently, a classic picture of acute myelogenous leukemia. The classification of MDS is complex and confusing. MDS encompasses disorders ranging from those with a low likelihood of evolution to leukemia (refractory anemia, refractory sideroblastic anemia) to those with a high propensity for developing into leukemia (refractory anemia with excess blasts in transformation). Myelodysplastic syndromes are seen in older adults, occur at a median age of 60 years, and are more frequent in males. Because chronic failure of hematopoiesis with anemia, leukopenia, and thrombocytopenia is prominent, these syndromes are discussed in Chapter 91.

REFERENCES

Champlin R and Gale RP: Acute lymphoblastic leukemia: recent advances in biology and therapy. Blood 73:2051, 1989.

Champlin RE and Golde DW: Chronic myelogenous leukemia: recent advances. Blood 65:1039, 1985.

Dighiero G et al: B-cell chronic lymphocytic leukemia: present status and future directions. Blood 78:1901, 1991.

Goldman JM et al: Bone marrow transplantation for patients with chronic myeloid leukemia. N Engl J Med 314:202, 1986.

Horowitz MM et al: Chemotherapy compared to bone marrow transplantation for adults with acute lymphoblastic leukemia in first remission. Ann Int Med 115:13, 1991.

Kantarjian HM et al: Chronic myelogenous leukemia in blast crisis. Am J Med 83:445, 1987.

Landaw SA: Polycythemia vera and other polycythemic states. Clin Lab Med 10:857, 1990.

Mastrianni DM, Tung NM, and Tenen DG: Acute myelogenous leukemia: current treatment and future directions. Am J Med 92:286, 1992.

McGlave PB et al: Therapy for chronic myelogenous leukemia with unrelated donor marrow transplantation. Blood 75:1728, 1990.

Mitus AJ et al: Hemostatic complications in young patients with essential thrombocythemia. Am J Med 88:371, 1990.

Ramsay NKC and Kersey JH: Indications for marrow transplantation in acute lymphoblastic leukemia. Blood 75:815, 1990.

Saven A and Piro LD: Treatment of hairy cell leukemia. Blood 79:1111, 1992.

Silverstein MN et al: Anagrelide: a new drug for treating thrombocytosis. N Engl J Med 318:1292, 1988.

Tallman MS et al: A single cycle of 2-chlorodeoxyadenosine results in complete remission in the majority of patients with hairy cell leukemia. Blood 80:2203, 1992.

Thomas ED and Clift RA: Indications for marrow transplantation in chronic myelogenous leukemia. Blood 73:861, 1989.

Warrell RP et al: Differentiation therapy of acute promyelocytic leukemia with tretinoin (all-trans-retinoic acid). N Engl J Med 324:1385, 1991.

CHAPTER

94 Hodgkin's Disease and Non-Hodgkin's Lymphoma

Thomas P. Miller
Thomas M. Grogan

Lymphomas are malignant tumors that arise from cells of the lymphoreticular system. They are divided into two broad categories—Hodgkin's disease and the malignant lymphomas. The malignant lymphomas are about three times more common than Hodgkin's disease and can potentially involve any site in the body. All lymphomas have many features in common, such as lymphadenopathy, mediastinal masses, abdominal masses, enlarged spleen or liver or both, and, not uncommonly, constitutional symptoms (fevers, night sweats, weight loss). Although patients with different lymphomas may have some common features, the clinical characteristics of each of these diseases are so distinct that it is often possible to predict the type of lymphoma from the clinical presentation.

The proper treatment of patients with lymphoma is predicated on an accurate diagnosis and complete staging to determine the extent of disease. Many of the lymphomas are curable when properly treated (refer to the box below), and it is extremely important to recognize the curable lymphomas so that these patients have the best opportunity to survive their illness. Other forms of lymphomas, although common, may not be curable and require different (palliative) therapeutic approaches. Mistakes in histologic diagnoses are common. In general, these are uncommon tumors, and the improper handling of lymph node material or inexperience of the pathologist may lead to erroneous diagnoses. If there is any question about the diagnosis, it is always preferable to send the histologic material to an experienced hematopathologist for review.

Because many patients with lymphomas have lymphadenopathy or enlarged mediastinal or abdominal masses, a few general principles about selecting a site for biopsy should be kept in mind. With respect to selecting the lymph node most likely to yield a diagnosis, the largest node should be chosen. Moreover, deep lymph nodes are preferable to superficial lymph nodes (which may be reactive), and axillary, cervical, or supraclavicular lymph nodes are preferable to inguinal lymph nodes. If a mediastinal mass or abdominal mass is chosen for biopsy, the clinician should make sure that adequate tissue has been given to the pathologist so that a diagnosis can be made. It is often impossible to make an accurate diagnosis of lymphoma on the basis of a needle biopsy or a small piece of tissue. If at all possible, the pathologist should be alerted to the suspicion of a lymphoma. Touch imprints of the fresh lymph node on microscopic slides are a useful adjunct to routine histologic studies. Portions of the fresh unfixed lymph node should be set aside for snap freezing so that tissue section

Lymphomas that may be curable

Hodgkin's disease (all subtypes and stages)
Malignant lymphoma
- Childhood lymphomas
- Diffuse small noncleaved cell
- Lymphoblastic
- Diffuse large cell (including immunoblastic)
- Diffuse mixed
- Follicular large cell (?)*
- Follicular mixed (?)*

*(?) Controversial data exist.

immunohistochemical evaluation or molecular analyses (Chapter 74) can be performed later if needed. In addition, a piece of the lymph node should be set aside for cell suspension immunologic techniques or electron microscopy. At the present time, routine histologic evaluation remains the mainstay of proper diagnosis, and this requires prompt and thorough fixation (often 24 hours is needed to fix all of the tissue completely), cutting the blocks with a sharp knife to prevent artifacts, and thin sectioning (4 μ).

HODGKIN'S DISEASE

Etiology

The cause of Hodgkin's disease is unknown. Historically, it was thought to be an infectious illness. Hodgkin's disease occasionally is seen in clusters, either geographic or familial, leading to speculation that there might be a causative virus. Recently, the Epstein-Barr virus (EBV) has been implicated as an etiologic agent by finding both elevated serologic features and EBV genomic material in the neoplastic Reed-Sternberg cells using in situ hybridization techniques. Whether EBV is playing a primary pathologic or secondary "passenger-stand-by" role is not certain. There is evidence of a genetic susceptibility because an occasional relationship between Hodgkin's disease and certain human leukocyte antigens (HLA) has been found. However, the overall risk of Hodgkin's disease in members of affected families is only slightly higher than that in the general population.

Histology

The diagnosis of Hodgkin's disease is based on pathologic review of a tissue biopsy specimen, usually of a lymph node. Hodgkin's disease is unique among neoplasms in that only a small proportion of cells are malignant. The great majority of cells are normal reactive cells (lymphocytes, plasma cells, fibroblasts, and eosinophils, Fig. 94-1). The diagnostic malignant cells are large, polylobated, and lymphoreticular with large nucleoli known as Reed-Sternberg cells (Fig. 94-1) and generally constitute less than 1% of the total cell population. The diagnosis cannot be made without finding a Reed-Sternberg cell in the proper reactive lymphoid background (Figs. 94-1 and 94-2). The exact nature of the Reed-Sternberg cell remains uncertain, although recent evidence suggests that it may be derived from a primary lymph node lymphoreticular cell with an unusual hybrid of lymphocytic, granulocytic, and reticulum cell antigens (see later discussion). This unusual phenotype may represent a lymph node stem cell defect or a lymphoreticular cell with aberrant gene expression. That Reed-Sternberg–like cells are seen in other conditions, such as large cell lymphomas, infectious mononucleosis, and cytomegalovirus infections, emphasizes the importance of finding the cells in the correct histologic context. Reed-Sternberg cells and variant cells are clearly malignant on the basis of karyotypic abnormalities, clonal growth, and growth and tumorgenicity in the "nude" mouse.

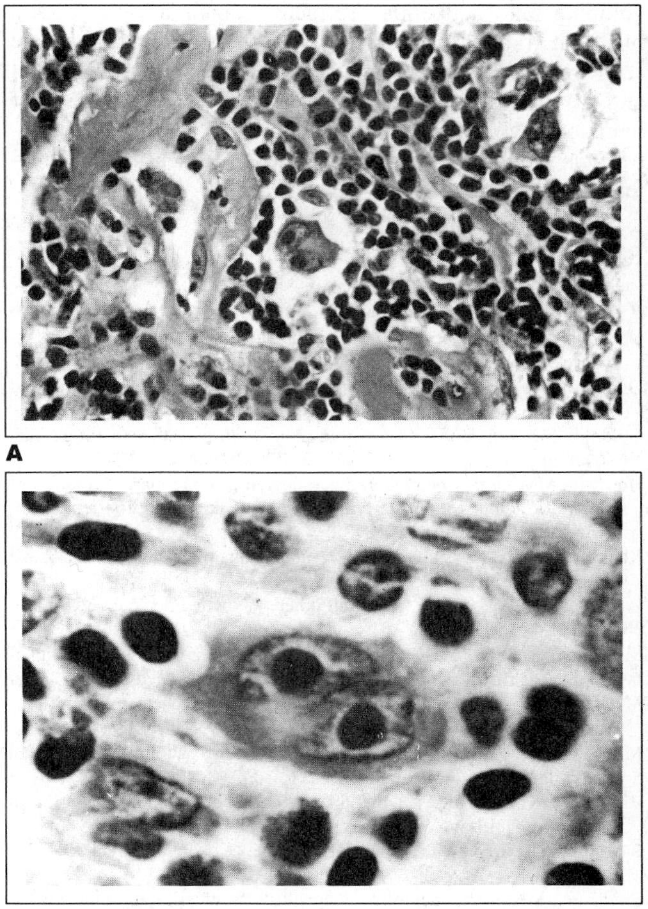

A

B

Fig. 94-1. A, Reed-Sternberg cell in "proper" cellular background consisting of small round lymphoid cells and plasma cells. ×400. **B,** High-power details of Reed-Sternberg cell. Note prominent nucleoli, distinct nuclear envelopes, and polylobated nucleus. ×1000.

Because diagnostic Reed-Sternberg cells constitute a small minority population of the tumor, it is often difficult to establish the diagnosis on limited tissue (needle biopsy specimens) or tissue obtained from extranodal sources (e.g., liver biopsies, bone marrow biopsies). If there is no prior diagnosis of Hodgkin's disease, it is essential to obtain an entire lymph node for examination. If the diagnosis remains in doubt, repeat lymph node biopsy should be done. In some cases, Reed-Sternberg cells may be very sparse and hard to find. The pathologist may need to make 30 or 40 cuts through the lymph node in order to identify a diagnostic cell. Such a rigorous search for the diagnostic cell is not possible with small tumor samples. Some of the more common sources of error in histologic or clinical diagnosis are summarized in the box at upper right.

There are four major histologic types of Hodgkin's disease (Table 94-1). Nodular sclerosis and mixed cellularity are by far the most common types, constituting 90% of all

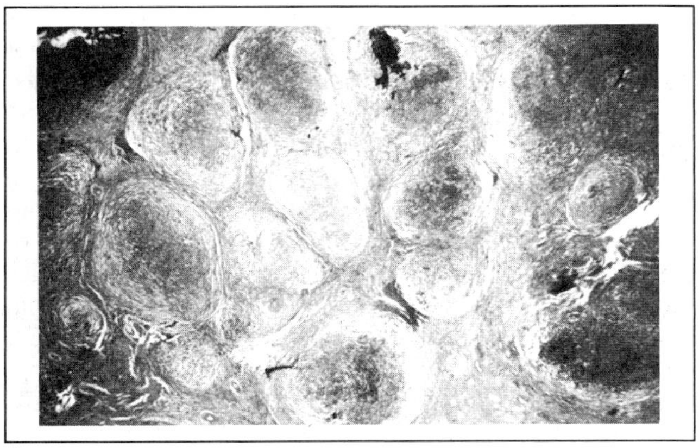

A

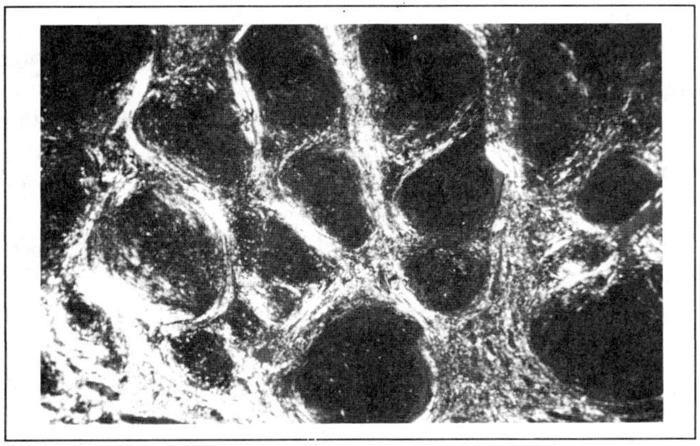

B

Fig. 94-2. **A,** Low-power view of nodules in nodular sclerosing Hodgkin's disease. × 100 **B,** Polarized light demonstrates birefringent collagen surrounding nodules. × 100.

Hodgkin's disease: sources of pathologic or clinical errors of diagnosis

Suspicious pathologic diagnosis if one of the following exists:
- Only extranodal tissue is available for review
- Reed-Sternberg–like cells or mononuclear variants are present but other features are lacking (may be confused with pleomorphic large cell lymphoma or anaplastic carcinoma)
- Reed-Sternberg cells and fibrosis are present without other features (may be confused with large cell lymphoma with compartmentalizing fibrosis)
- Slides are inadequate for interpretation (e.g., poor fixation, excessive thickness, cut with dull knife)

Suspicious clinical diagnosis if one of the following exists:
- Unusual sites of presentation (e.g., extranodal tissue: thyroid, bone, gastrointestinal tract, tonsil, skin)
- Noncontiguous pattern of spread (occurs in only 10% to 15% of patients with Hodgkin's disease)
- Subdiaphragmatic presentation (occurs in only 15% of patients with Hodgkin's disease)
- Elderly patient population (non-Hodgkin's lymphomas are more common)

cases. Historically, there was a difference in prognosis related to the histologic subtype of Hodgkin's disease, but with modern treatment this difference has been largely obliterated.

Immunohistochemical analysis is a major aid to diagnosis and provides a useful adjunct to light microscopy, thereby reducing errors in diagnosis. Using immunohistochemical techniques, the neoplastic Reed-Sternberg cells and variants have been shown to have a complex array of phenotypic properties including sometimes coexpression of lymphoid activation (CD30, Ki1), granulocyte (CD15, Leu M1), and reticulum cell antigens. The neoplastic cells in Hodgkin's disease are characteristically positive for Ki1 and Leu M1 and negative for leucocyte common antigen (CD45). This CD 30+15+45-phenotype occurs in 80% of Hodgkin's disease cases. A majority of Hodgkin's disease of the lymphocyte predominant subtype cases show Pan-B cell antigen (CD20) expression, indicating that some

Table 94-1. Clinical and pathologic features of Hodgkin's disease subtypes (Lukes-Butler classification)*

Histologic subtype	Frequency (%)	Usual clinical features	Relative prognosis
Lymphocytic predominance—lymphocytic infiltrate; rare Reed-Sternberg cells	5-10	Often quite localized in cervical regions; teenage males predominate	Excellent
Nodular sclerosis—broad bands of fibrosis (collagen); "lacunar" cells; rare Reed-Sternberg cells	40-70	Usually localized; 70% have mediastinal masses; young women predominate	Usually excellent
Mixed cellularity—abundant Reed-Sternberg cells, histiocytes; can be confused with diffuse large cell lymphoma	20-40	Tends to be widespread; occurs in older population; males predominate	Usually good
Lymphocytic depletion—fibrosis; abundant Reed-Sternberg cells; may be easily mistaken for diffuse large cell lymphoma; very rare	5	Frequent in older patients; often widespread at discovery	Good to poor

*The comments regarding prognosis associated with particular types of Hodgkin's disease illustrate only a general relationship and may not apply to individual patients. Effective treatment may be curative in patients with any stage or type of Hodgkin's disease.

Hodgkin's disease subtypes may be specifically of B cell origin.

Clinical features

Hodgkin's disease primarily affects younger patients than does malignant lymphoma. The majority of patients are between the ages of 15 and 40, and a second, smaller peak occurs about age 50. Hodgkin's disease can occur in childhood. The presenting symptom is usually an enlarged lymph node, often in the cervical or supraclavicular regions. Only about 15% of patients have subdiaphragmatic disease. Lymph nodes characteristically are firm, mobile, and "rubbery." Lymph nodes 2 cm or larger suggest the diagnosis of lymphoma, particularly when they are located in the supraclavicular or axillary region. Hodgkin's disease rarely involves epitrochlear or popliteal lymph nodes. Tender lymph nodes more often have infectious or inflammatory causes than lymphomas, but occasionally rapidly enlarging lymph nodes can be tender. Rock-hard or fixed lymph nodes are more common with carcinoma than with lymphoma. The evaluation of patients with lymphadenopathy is fully discussed in Chapter 82.

Hodgkin's disease frequently involves mediastinal and/or hilar lymph nodes. Patients may have cough or shortness of breath. Hemoptysis and the superior vena cava syndrome are very rare. Pleural effusions are sometimes found in association with mediastinal involvement but rarely contain malignant cells.

Because Hodgkin's disease generally spreads to contiguous lymph node regions, abdominal lymph nodes may also be involved. Within the abdomen, the disease often first involves the spleen, although the spleen rarely is massively enlarged. With splenic involvement the splenic hilar lymph nodes commonly are involved; so too, eventually, are the paraaortic lymph nodes. The disease may spread farther down the lymph node chains to involve the iliac or inguinal lymph nodes or farther up the lymph node chains to involve celiac or porta hepatis nodes. Mesenteric lymph node involvement, even with widespread Hodgkin's disease, is rare. Eventually, Hodgkin's disease may involve the liver and bone marrow. The frequency of visceral sites of involvement found during pretreatment staging is shown in Table 94-2.

Table 94-2. Approximate frequency of involvement by Hodgkin's disease of various sites

Mediastinal lymph nodes	40%-70%
Hilar lymph nodes	25%-50%
Abdominal lymph nodes	
Paraaortic	40%
Mesenteric	5%
Portal	5%
Splenic hilar	30%-40%
Liver	10%
Spleen	35%-40%
Bone marrow	5%

Symptoms associated with Hodgkin's disease are nonspecific. Three symptoms are considered "constitutional" or "B" symptoms: unexplained fever, drenching night sweats, and weight loss of more than 10% of body weight. Occasionally, fever is periodic (Pel-Ebstein fever). These constitutional symptoms may mimic an infectious disease. In addition, generalized pruritus may be a presenting symptom of Hodgkin's disease, but it does not constitute one of the B symptoms and does not influence prognosis. Pruritus abates with satisfactory treatment of disease. Rarely, patients may experience a peculiar syndrome of alcohol-induced pain at sites involved by disease. This rare symptom is virtually pathognomonic for Hodgkin's disease.

A severe defect in cell-mediated (T cell) immunity exists in patients with even the most limited forms of Hodgkin's disease. This T cell defect leads to anergy and a propensity for infection with opportunistic organisms, particularly tuberculosis, fungi, and viruses. Herpes zoster is commonly seen during the course of Hodgkin's disease and can be a life-threatening illness. In addition, patients who have undergone splenectomy as part of staging are at increased risk of overwhelming bacterial septicemia (Chapter 82). Despite successful treatment of Hodgkin's disease, the immune defect persists for life. Patients should be cautioned against receiving live virus vaccinations, such as smallpox or yellow fever, that might prove fatal. Some of the clinical features that are uncommon in Hodgkin's disease and may lead to an erroneous clinical diagnosis are summarized in the box on p. 901.

Laboratory features

No specific laboratory abnormalities are associated with Hodgkin's disease. Routine peripheral blood evaluation often indicates a mild neutrophilic leukocytosis, a slightly increased platelet count, and a mild normochromic normocytic anemia. Very rarely, a Coombs' test positive hemolytic anemia is found. A number of nonspecific serum protein abnormalities are present and account for an increased erythrocyte sedimentation rate and increased ceruloplasmin and copper levels. None of these abnormalities is diagnostic or particularly useful in following patients. Mild abnormalities of liver function are sometimes noted. With bulky disease, hyperuricemia may be present, but it is less common than with non-Hodgkin's lymphomas. Hypercalcemia is not a feature of Hodgkin's disease except occasionally as a terminal event. Rare patients may experience nephrotic syndrome. Because bone marrow involvement is uncommon, pancytopenia caused by marrow replacement is rare.

Differential diagnosis

Hodgkin's disease may mimic many infectious diseases. In addition, other malignancies including leukemia and carcinoma can sometimes be characterized by lymphadenopathy, and the diagnosis can be established only through biopsy and histologic review. The most important differential diagnosis is between Hodgkin's disease and other malignant lymphomas. In particular, pleomorphic large cell lymphomas with scattered Reed-Sternberg–like cells may be histologically problematic. In such a circumstance, snap-frozen tissue section phenotyping can be useful.

Staging

The proper treatment for patients with Hodgkin's disease is predicated on knowledge of the exact extent of disease before treatment and the potentially adverse prognostic features that might influence the type of treatment. The usual pretherapy evaluation includes a careful history and physical examination, paying particular attention to all of the lymph node areas and the abdomen. Routine chest radiographs are quite accurate for showing the presence of mediastinal or hilar adenopathy. If such involvement is found, whole lung and mediastinal tomography or a computed tomographic (CT) scan of the chest is indicated to define better the extent of disease and to rule out pulmonary nodules not apparent on plain chest radiographs. For patients with B symptoms or evidence of at least stage III disease (Table 94-3), a bone marrow core biopsy is useful for ruling out involvement of the bone marrow. An abdominal imaging procedure should be performed to rule out abdominal lymph node involvement. CT scanning of the abdomen has increasingly been used to screen for enlarged paraaortic or iliac lymph nodes. Ultrasonography is somewhat less reliable for screening for enlarged abdominal lymph nodes. Neither ultrasonography nor CT scanning can reliably detect involvement of the liver or spleen. Bipedal lymphangiography remains an extremely useful procedure in defining paraaortic and iliac lymph node involvement in Hodgkin's disease. The results of this initial evaluation usually provide enough information to make a decision about the most appropriate form of initial therapy, although staging laparotomy and splenectomy are required in many patients, as indicated in Table 94-4. In general, radiotherapy with curative intent is utilized for patients with limited disease without potentially adverse prognostic features (refer to the box on p. 904). Alternatively, chemotherapy with curative intent is employed for patients with more advanced stages of disease. Certain special situations require the use of radiotherapy and chemotherapy together (combined modality treatment).

The staging evaluation should be designed to discover those prognostic factors that have a potentially adverse impact on the results of radiotherapy (see the box on p. 904). Patients with these features generally have a much worse prognosis if treated with radiotherapy alone and probably should be managed with chemotherapy or chemotherapy plus radiotherapy. Thus a patient without B symptoms and with a normal lymphangiogram who has enlarged bilateral supraclavicular lymph nodes and a mediastinal mass that measures less than one third of the chest diameter should probably be evaluated surgically with a staging laparotomy and splenectomy (Table 94-4). If no evidence of extensive disease was found within the abdomen at the time of surgery, this patient would then receive appropriate radiotherapy with curative intent. Conversely, if extensive splenic disease or liver involvement was discovered, the patient would receive chemotherapy. If the patient has obvious advanced stage III or IV disease, then initial staging laparotomy is probably not indicated, and the guidelines for staging would be those indicated in Table 94-4.

For most patients with apparently localized Hodgkin's disease who might receive radiotherapy with curative intent, a careful staging laparotomy is now standard. This includes splenectomy (so that the pathologist can carefully "breadloaf" the spleen, looking for tiny nodules), wedge as well as needle biopsies of both lobes of the liver, and biopsies of the splenic hilar, paraaortic, and any other suspicious lymph nodes. In addition, oophoropexy can be performed if pelvic radiotherapy is being considered.

Table 94-3. Ann Arbor staging* classification of Hodgkin's disease

Stage I	Involvement of a single lymph node region (I) or single extralymphatic site (I_E)
Stage II	Involvement of two or more lymph node regions on the same side of the diaphragm (II), which may also include the spleen (II_S), localized extralymphatic involvement (II_E), or both (II_{SE}), if confined to the same side of the diaphragm
Stage III	Involvement of lymph node regions on both sides of the diaphragm (III), which may also include the spleen (III_S), localized extralymphatic involvement (III_E), or both (III_{SE})
Stage IV	Diffuse or disseminated involvement of extralymphatic sites (e.g., bone marrow, liver, or multiple pulmonary metastases), with or without lymph node involvement

*The presence of fever, night sweats, or unexplained weight loss of 10% or more of body weight over 6 months is designated by the letter *B*. The letter *A* indicates absence of these symptoms.
Clinical staging (CS) refers to the use of noninvasive tests; pathologic staging (PS) refers to staging based on invasive or surgical procedures (e.g., laparoscopy or laparotomy with splenectomy). Thus, a patient with CSIIA Hodgkin's disease may prove to have $PSIV_{S+He+}$ on the basis of positive liver and splenic biopsies.

Table 94-4. Initial surgical or clinical staging of Hodgkin's disease based on most likely primary therapy

Radiotherapy as most likely initial treatment	Chemotherapy as most likely initial treatment
Staging including lymphangiogram and full exploratory laparotomy with splenectomy	Staging excluding lymphagiogram; employ other noninvasive procedures instead: CT scan of the abdomen or abdominal ultrasound examination After completion of initial treatment, thorough restaging should include a lymphangiogram and strong consideration for exploratory laparotomy and splenectomy

Potentially adverse prognostic features of Hodgkin's disease to be defined through careful staging

- Constitutional or B symptoms (fever, night sweats, weight loss)
- "Bulky" disease (usually defined as a mediastinal mass greater than one third of the chest diameter on a chest radiograph or an abdominal mass greater than 10 cm in diameter)
- Hilar adenopathy
- Extranodal (E) spread
- Extensive splenic involvement (more than four nodules of Hodgkin's disease)
- Substage III_2 (pelvic node involvement)

After careful staging, about half of patients are found to have localized disease (stage I, II, or II_E; see Table 94-3), and the remainder have advanced disease (stages III or IV).

Therapy

With the development of modern radiotherapy (Fig. 94-3), localized Hodgkin's disease has been treated successfully, with cure rates of 60% to 90% depending on the experience of the radiotherapist and the presence or absence of several prognostic indicators (see the box above). Radiotherapy should be performed only in centers in which the radiation oncologists have extensive experience with Hodgkin's disease to minimize acute and long-term side effects as well as to optimize the chances for cure.

The prognostic factors listed in the box above are usually believed to have an adverse impact on the outcome when radiotherapy is employed as the only treatment modality. Thus the ideal patients for treatment with radiotherapy alone are those without the adverse factors listed in this table, and cure is achieved in 70% to 80% of patients. If any of the adverse factors listed in the table is present, the chance of cure with radiotherapy alone drops significantly, and consideration should be given to chemotherapy or chemotherapy plus radiotherapy (combined modality treatment). For patients with stage III_2, IIIB, or IV disease, chemotherapy is the mainstay of treatment. Some groups advocate the use of radiotherapy along with chemotherapy. Chemotherapy is curative in 50% to 70% of patients with advanced Hodgkin's disease.

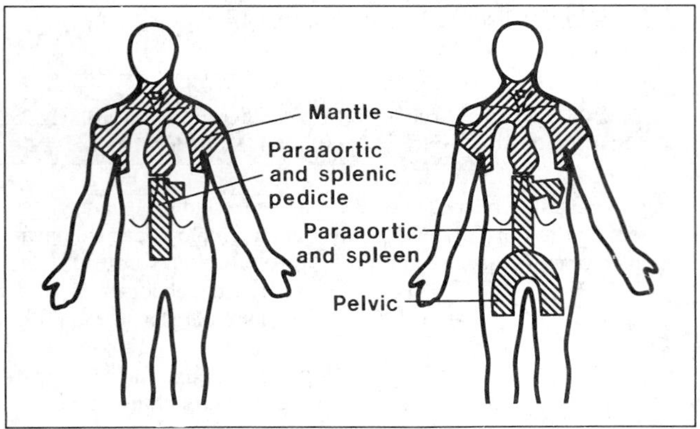

Fig. 94-3. Standard radiotherapy ports used for treating Hodgkin's disease with curative intent (with [left] or without [right] splenectomy).

In the 1960s, the major form of treatment for recurrent or advanced Hodgkin's disease was single-agent chemotherapy, but complete responses were rarely observed. A major breakthrough in the drug treatment of Hodgkin's disease occurred in the mid-1960s, when investigators at the National Cancer Institute combined four agents (nitrogen mustard, vincristine, procarbazine, and prednisone) in what is now known as the MOPP program. In patients without prior chemotherapy, complete remissions are regularly achieved in 70% to 80% of patients with 6 to 10 courses (months) of therapy. Among patients who achieve complete remission, approximately 70% remain in long-term remission and are cured. Since the first reports of treatment with the MOPP regimen appeared, considerable clinical research has been invested in attempts to define new or improved regimens to supersede MOPP. The first of these alternative regimens combined doxorubicin, bleomycin, vinblastine, and dacarbazine (ABVD). The ABVD regimen has been shown to be effective in patients relapsing after MOPP treatment and appears to be more active than MOPP in the previously untreated patients. Further, the ABVD regimen causes less long-term toxicity, including a decreased frequency of treatment-related leukemia, ovarian failure, and sterility. Over the past decade investigators have combined MOPP and ABVD in attempts to exploit the advantages of each regimen, reduce the toxicities of each, and overcome multidrug resistance. The MOPP regimen has been alternated with the ABVD regimen and the combination (MOPP/ABVD) has been shown to be better than MOPP alone. Two hybrids formed by combining elements of MOPP and ABVD (MOP-BAP and MOPP-ABV) have also been tested. The MOP-BAP regimen was shown to be better than MOPP in a randomized trial and the MOPP-ABV regimen was recently compared to MOPP followed by ABVD. Further follow-up evaluation of patients is required in this latter study. However, it appears that regimens containing doxorubicin and vinblastine are superior to and less toxic than classical MOPP. Drug doses and schedules for several of these regimens are shown in Table 94-5. This type of intensive multiagent chemotherapy is associated with considerable acute toxicity, such as nausea, vomiting, myelosuppression, hair loss, and predisposition to infection. The use of these multidrug regimens is complicated and should be overseen by only experienced physicians. In addition to acute toxicity, two important types of long-term toxicity are associated with combination chemotherapy—sterility and carcinogenesis. Sterility occurs in about 50% of women and in 80% to 90% of men. Secondary malignancies occur in about 1% of long-term survivors, although in certain high-risk groups, the projected actuarial risk of

Table 94-5. Chemotherapeutic regimens useful in the treatment of Hodgkin's disease

Regimen*	Dose	Schedule (days)														
MOPP		1	2	3	4	5	6	7	8	9	10	11	12	13	14	
M = nitrogen mustard	6 mg/m² iv	x							x							
O = vincristine (Oncovin)	1.4 mg/m² iv	x							x							
P = procarbazine	100 mg/m² po	x	x	x	x	x	x	x	x	x	x	x	x	x	x	
P = prednisone	40 mg/m² po	x	x	x	x	x	x	x	x	x	x	x	x	x	x	
ABVD		1	2	3	4	5	6	7	8	9	10	11	12	13	14	15
A = doxorubicin (Adriamycin)	25 mg/m² iv	x														x
B = bleomycin	10 mg/m² iv	x														x
V = vinblastine	6 mg/m² iv	x														x
D = dacarbazine (DTIC)	375 mg/m² iv	x														x
MOPP/ABVD	Monthly courses alternating two regimens															
MOP-BAP		1	2	3	4	5	6	7	8	9	10	11	12			
M = nitrogen mustard	6 mg/m² iv	x														
O = vincristine (Oncovin)	1.4 mg/m² iv (max. 2 mg)	x							x							
P = procarbazine	100 mg/m² po		x	x	x	x	x	x		x	x	x	x			
B = bleomycin	2 mg/m² iv	x							x							
A = doxorubicin (Adriamycin)	30 mg/m² iv								x							
P = prednisone	40 mg/m² po		x	x	x	x	x	x		x	x	x	x			
MOPP-ABV (repeat every 4 weeks)		1	2	3	4	5	6	7	8	9	10	11	12	13	14	
M = nitrogen mustard	6 mg/m² iv	x														
O = vincristine (Oncovin)	1.4 mg/m² iv (max. 2 mg)	x														
P = procarbazine	100 mg/m² po	x	x	x	x	x	x	x								
P = prednisone	40 mg/m² po	x	x	x	x	x	x	x	x	x	x	x	x	x	x	
A = doxorubicin (Adriamycin)	35 mg/m² iv								x							
B = bleomycin	10 mg/m² iv								x							
V = vinblastine	6 mg/m² iv								x							

*MOPP is the standard regimen most often used, and ABVD is the regimen most often used for MOPP failures. MOPP/ABVD is a program that has produced superior results to MOPP alone in one trial. MOP-BAP was shown to be superior to MOPP-bleomycin in one trial. MOPP-ABV is commonly used, but a comparative trial with MOPP has not been completed. In general, each regimen is repeated on a 4 week basis. Most physicians administer a maximum of 2 mg of vincristine per dose in these regimens.

leukemia or undifferentiated lymphomas may be as high as 8%.

Hodgkin's disease has become a model of a curable neoplasm. Its cure depends on close cooperation among a team of experienced cancer specialists, including hematopathologists, diagnostic radiologists, surgeons, medical oncologists, and radiation therapists. Should Hodgkin's disease recur after initial therapy, often a second and perhaps even a third major treatment effort may result in cure.

MALIGNANT LYMPHOMAS

Etiology

A specific cause of most malignant lymphomas cannot be identified. However, several distinct types of non-Hodgkin's lymphomas have been associated with a viral cause (Chapter 71). For example, the Burkitt's lymphoma of Africa is a unique clinical entity that is strongly associated with the Epstein-Barr virus. More recently, a family of T lymphotropic retroviruses has been isolated from humans, and one member of this family, the human immunodeficiency-related retrovirus (HIV-III), is strongly associated with a distinct type of lymphoma called adult T cell leukemia-lymphoma. HIV-III is endemic in southern Japan, the Caribbean islands, Africa, and the southeastern United States, and there is strong seroepidemiologic evidence linking HIV-III and the adult T cell leukemia-lymphoma. A second member of this retrovirus family, HIV-I, has been linked to the pathogenesis of acquired immunodeficiency syndrome (AIDS), an immunodeficiency disease that frequently predisposes to life-threatening infections, Kaposi's sarcoma, and lymphoma (Chapters 96 and 252). Malignant lymphomas can develop in association with a wide range of other immunologic disorders. In as many as 10% of patients with Sjögren's syndrome lymphoma eventually develops. Immunosuppressive therapy for heart, liver, or kidney transplant patients using azathioprine plus prednisone or cyclosporine is associated with development of malignant lymphoma in approximately 4% to 10% of patients.

The addition of anti–T cell serum to these immunosuppressive drugs greatly increases the risk of development of lymphoma and the risk is related to the dosage of the immunosuppressive agent(s) used. The Epstein-Barr virus genome is associated with lymphomas that develop in both the posttransplant immunosuppressed patient and the human immunodeficiency viral syndrome patient. Whether the virus is causative or simply an associated finding in immunocompromised hosts is unclear. Malignant lymphomas are also rarely observed as a second malignancy after chemotherapy for Hodgkin's disease. Finally, there is indirect evidence that chronic "immunostimulation" such as occurs with inflammatory bowel disease, with drugs such as phenytoin, or with lymphoproliferative disorders such as angioimmunoblastic lymphadenopathy may predispose to the development of malignant lymphomas.

Table 94-6. Nomenclature of non-Hodgkin's lymphomas

New Working Formulation	Old Rappaport Classification
Low grade: favorable types	
1. Small lymphocytic	1. Diffuse, lymphocytic, well-differentiated
2. Follicular, small cleaved cell	2. Nodular, poorly differentiated lymphocytic
3. Follicular, mixed small cleaved and large cell	3. Nodular, mixed, lymphocytic and histiocytic
Intermediate grade: unfavorable types	
4. Follicular, large cell	4. Nodular, histiocytic
5. Diffuse, small cleaved cell	5. Diffuse, poorly differentiated lymphocytic
6. Diffuse, mixed small and large cell	6. Diffuse mixed, lymphocytic and histiocytic
7. Diffuse, large cell	7. Diffuse, histiocytic
High grade: unfavorable types	
8. Large cell immunoblastic	8. Diffuse, histiocytic
9. Lymphoblastic	9. Lymphoblastic
10. Small noncleaved cell	10. Burkitt's undifferentiated

Histology

The diagnosis of malignant lymphoma is based on the morphologic appearance of an excised lymph node. The normal architecture of the lymphomatous lymph node is frequently replaced by a monomorphic infiltrate of neoplastic lymphoid cells. However, the pathologic diagnosis is often complicated by the finding of incomplete effacement of the lymph node and residual follicles with normal-appearing architecture. In addition, the infiltrate may be polymorphic, and the degree of cellular atypia may be subtle. In such cases it is often difficult to determine whether the lymph node represents neoplastic growth or benign reactivity. At other times a lymph node may be replaced with such an extreme degree of cellular atypia that the lymphoid nature of the neoplasm cannot be determined on the basis of morphologic characteristics alone. In such difficult cases, the diagnosis often requires expert review by an experienced pathologist, or application of newer diagnostic processes such as immunohistochemical or molecular biologic techniques to demonstrate gene rearrangements.

In the majority of instances, the diagnosis of a non-Hodgkin's lymphoma is made on morphologic criteria, and the histologic subtype is classified according to the Working Formulation. Until recently, many systems were used to classify non-Hodgkin's lymphomas. All of these systems are based on the morphologic appearance of the lymphoma, and all have some clinical utility for determining response to treatment and prognosis. The Working Formulation is an attempt to accommodate the terminology of these different systems. Before adoption of the Working Formulation, the Rappaport classification was most often used in the United States. Many textbooks and journal articles still use the terminology of the Rappaport classification. Table 94-6 summarizes these two systems and divides the histologic subtypes of each system into two clinically useful subgroups based on prognosis. The terms favorable and unfavorable have gained wide clinical acceptance and are useful for discussing general aspects of these complex diseases.

Morphologically, malignant lymphomas may appear as follicular (nodular) or diffuse (Fig. 94-4). This difference in architecture is both the most reproducible histologic feature and the most important variable affecting survival. Approximately 50% of patients have lymphomas with a follicular pattern, and these patients in general have a more favorable prognosis. In addition to the architectural pattern, malignant lymphocytes can be categorized on the basis of size as small (lymphocytic) or large (histiocytic) (Fig. 94-5). This distinction is helpful but does not suffice to subdivide patients into groups with different prognoses. Finally, malignant lymphocytes can be characterized as to their degree of cellular atypia (poorly differentiated or well differentiated). These three morphologic determinations (architectural pattern, cell size, and cellular atypia) determine the histologic subtype of the lymphoma.

Immunophenotypic and genetic analysis has further subdivided lymphomas into biologically relevant subgroups. Immunohistochemical evaluation of snap-frozen biopsy tissues, in particular, has delineated specific clinicopathologic entities. As an example, high-grade lymphoblastic lymphomas were initially separated from the lower-grade small cleaved cell category on the basis of an immature T cell phenotype that mimics the chemical characteristics of immature cortical thymocytes found in the thymus. Clinically, lymphoblastic lymphomas commonly occur in the mediastinum (thymic area) in teenage males consistent with their thymic lineage. As another example, the follicular lymphomas have immunoglobulin and pan–B cell antigen expression consistent with their origin from germinal centers. Typically, there is a monoclonal immunoglobulin-bearing

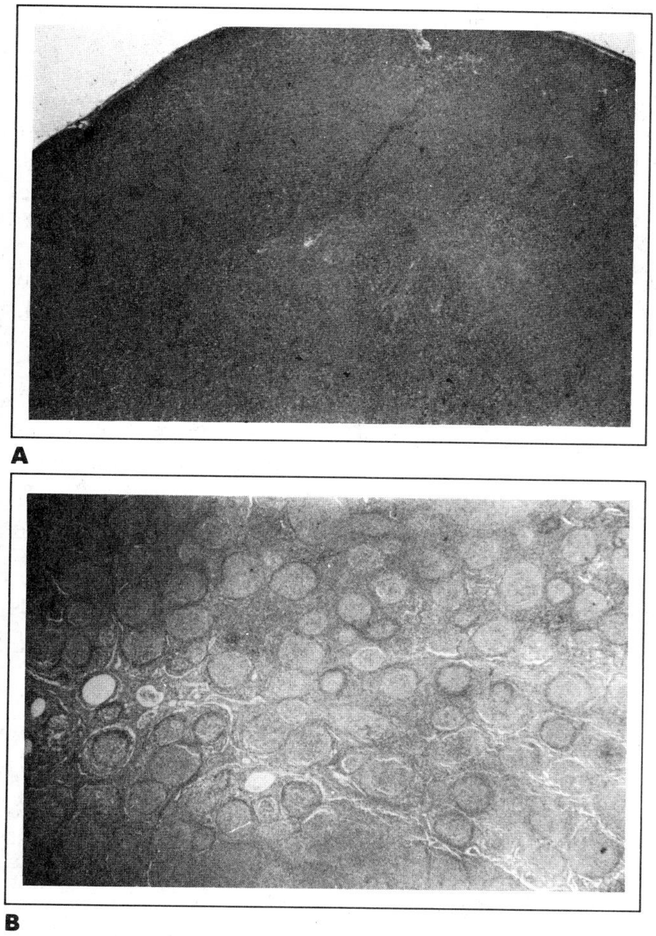

Fig. 94-4. **A,** Diffuse effacement of node by lymphoma. ×100. **B,** Follicular effacement of node by follicular (nodular) lymphoma. ×100.

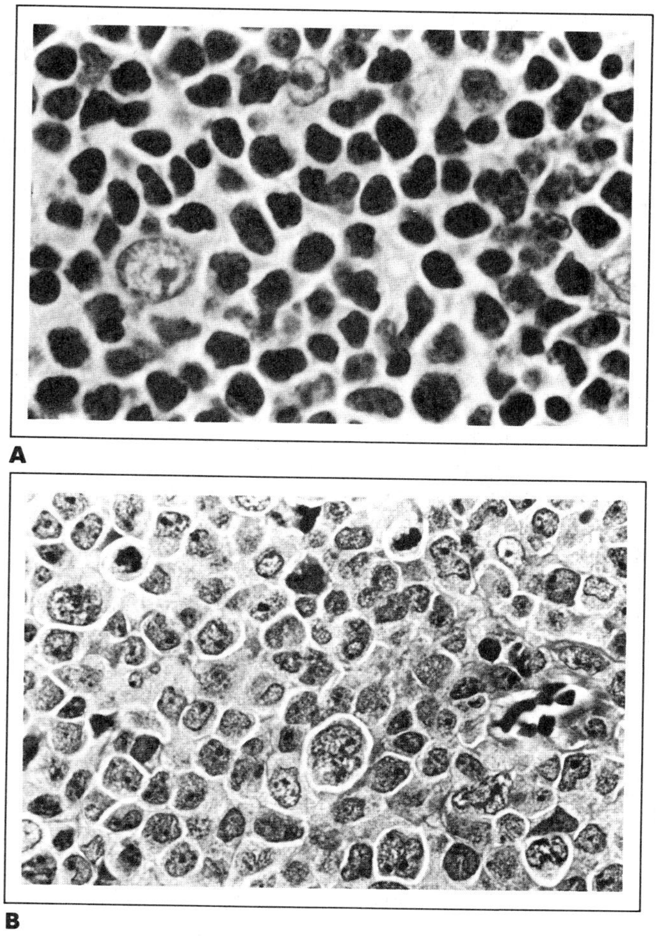

Fig. 94-5. Small cleaved cell lymphoma. ×600. **B,** Large cell lymphoma. Note mitoses. × 600.

pattern with light and heavy chain restriction. Genotypic assay using Southern blotting reveals a comparable monoclonal rearrangement of the immunoglobulin genes. Beside B and T cell lineage, other markers are useful in lymphoma categorization, including markers of (1) proliferative status, (2) histocompatibility (HLA) status, (3) cell adhesion molecule and "homing" receptor status, and (4) immunosurveillance status as measured by the quantity of infiltrating T cytotoxic/suppressor cells. For example, the proliferative status varies from 1% to 3% in low-grade categories to greater than 80% in high-grade categories. A proliferative rate of 20% to 25% identifies patients with low-grade lymphomas having a poor prognosis. Genotypic markers have also proved relevant to biologic subcategorization. In particular, the BCL-2 oncogene product, which in physiologic circumstances confers long-lived status on "memory B cells" by preventing normal B cell death, may be overexpressed in some of the low-grade lymphomas. BCL-2 overexpression in these lymphomas immortalizes the neoplastic lymphoid cells in the resting state. The overexpression of BCL-2 in low-grade lymphomas has been specifically related to a distinct chromosomal translocation t(14, 18), which results in a fusion gene readily detected by immunoblotting and the polymerase chain reaction. At the other end of the proliferative spectrum are the high-grade lymphomas. In this instance, the greater than 80% proliferative rate may be associated with a translocation t(8, 14), and upregulated expression of the MYC oncogene. The upregulated MYC oncogene is a nuclear mitogenic factor accounting for the loss of proliferative control. Immunoblotting may also be used to detect MYC rearrangement or amplification.

Clinical features

Malignant lymphomas are a group of diseases having as a common feature the malignant transformation of a lymphocyte. The diseases are, however, relatively distinct with regard to clinical presentation and natural history.

The favorable histologic subtypes of malignant lymphomas are most often seen in older patients and are present in equal frequency in both sexes. The median age of onset is during the sixth decade, and the diseases are rare in patients less than 30 years. Patients usually seek medical attention because of unexplained or persistent adenopathy. These patients often feel well, but systemic symptoms may be present in 15% at the time of diagnosis. Frequently, patients recall having enlarged lymph nodes for months or even years before diagnosis. The adenopathy is frequently generalized and may involve any peripheral lymph node site including the epitrochlear, inguinal, and femoral lymph node. Less commonly, patients present with symptoms related to anemia that is usually caused by bone marrow involvement with lymphoma, which is present in 50% to 70% of patients at diagnosis. Involvement of other extranodal sites of disease at the time of diagnosis may occur in 15% to 30% of patients, frequently including the liver, spleen, or, less often, the gastrointestinal tract. Follicular small cleaved-cell lymphoma is the most common type of lymphoma with favorable histologic features. After diagnosis, the course of disease may be variable but is often indolent (i.e., does not require treatment for periods of time). In 20% to 30% of patients, these diseases are slowly progressive or occasionally undergo spontaneous regression (decrease in size of the involved lymph nodes). When treatment is required, these diseases are often quite responsive, sometimes for years. Eventually they become more aggressive and refractory to treatment. A repeat lymph node biopsy at such a time frequently reveals a change in morphology to a more aggressive histologic subtype. Documentation of this transition from a favorable to an unfavorable lymphoma portends a poor prognosis and requires a change in treatment strategy. The median survival of patients with favorable histologic subtypes of malignant lymphoma is approximately 6 years, and as many as 25% of patients are alive after 12 years.

The unfavorable histologic subtypes of malignant lymphomas can occur at any age, including childhood. However, the majority of patients are older, and the median age of onset is in the sixth decade. These diseases affect males more often than females. Patients frequently seek medical attention because of symptoms related to a rapidly enlarging tumor mass. The disease usually begins in a recognized lymph node area but may form an extranodal mass in 20% of patients. After a thorough evaluation, extranodal disease can be documented in 75% of patients. The most common sites of extranodal involvement, in decreasing order of frequency, include the gastrointestinal tract, bone marrow, liver, spleen, nasopharynx, lung, and skin. Any extranodal site can be involved with malignant lymphoma, and case reports abound describing patients who have lymphoma involving such organs as the thyroid gland, testicle, kidney, and ovary.

Patients may have diffuse adenopathy at presentation, but clinically localized disease is much more common in patients with unfavorable histologic types than in those with the more indolent histologic features. Approximately 30% to 40% of patients are found to have localized disease (stages I or II; see Table 94-3) after careful clinical staging. The malignant lymphomas of unfavorable histologic types are characterized by a rapid doubling time and a propensity for early hematogenous spread. Consequently, even patients with clinically localized disease at the time of diagnosis frequently have microscopic metastatic disease. The clinical course of these patients is rapidly progressive, and very few patients survive 2 years without treatment. However, combination chemotherapy has substantially affected the prognosis of these patients, and a discussion of the natural history is no longer relevant unless one includes an assessment of the impact of treatment. The major determinant of prognosis for patients treated with systemic chemotherapy is the extent of disease at the time of diagnosis. The most common unfavorable histologic subtype is diffuse large cell lymphoma (Fig. 94-5, *B*). The cure rates are 90% to 95% of patients with stage I diffuse large cell lymphoma, 75% to 85% of patients with stage II disease, and 30% to 50% of patients with stage III or IV disease. In general, patients who respond to treatment do so quickly, and detectable disease completely disappears within 2 or 3 months. Relapses after 5 years of follow-up observation can occur but are unusual. Patients who do not respond to initial therapy or who relapse after completion of therapy most often die of their disease. Second-line therapy using standard drug regimens is rarely successful. Consequently, these patients are often considered for experimental approaches, including high-dose chemotherapy with autologous marrow rescue, new cytotoxic drugs, or immunomodulators. Relapses after therapy may occur at any site but most frequently involve sites of initially bulky disease.

The unfavorable histologic subtypes of malignant lymphoma may involve the central nervous system. Rarely, diffuse large cell lymphomas may appear as a localized brain mass. More frequently, these lymphomas involve the central nervous system during the course of therapy with diffuse meningeal involvement, resulting in symptoms of headache and multiple cranial nerve palsies. The histologic subtypes most likely to have meningeal involvement are lymphoblastic lymphoma and diffuse large cell lymphoma.

LABORATORY FEATURES

No laboratory findings are specific or diagnostic of non-Hodgkin's lymphoma. However, several laboratory features are variably present and may be important in determining prognosis or helpful in managing complications of therapy. The peripheral blood counts are usually normal at the time of diagnosis, but anemia, leukopenia, or thrombocytopenia may occur. Abnormalities of the peripheral blood counts are usually the result of bone marrow infiltration with lymphoma. Occasionally lymphoma cells are found in the peripheral blood (leukemic phase) at diagnosis but more commonly as a terminal event. However, excessive destruction of any blood cell line may occur, most commonly through immune mediated destruction or hypersplenism. Increases in serum enzyme levels usually reflect involvement of bone or liver with lymphoma but are not sensitive indicators of involvement of these organs. Elevation of the serum lactic dehydrogenase (LDH) level is nonspecific, but higher levels have been associated with a worse prognosis, particularly in large cell lymphoma. Hyperuricemia is common in patients with high tumor burdens or rapidly proliferating tumors. Rarely, bulky disease may cause jaundice or azotemia. Hypercalcemia is unusual at the time of diagnosis except in patients who have lymphoma associated with the HIV III virus. Hypogammaglobulinemia or serum monoclonal protein spikes are occasionally observed.

Staging

The extent of disease before treatment is determined in patients with malignant lymphoma to assess prognosis, to establish a baseline for gauging response to treatment, and to make certain that tumor masses have not compromised organ function. Because malignant lymphomas have a propensity for early hematogenous spread and are usually systemic at the time of diagnosis, staging has less importance for determining proper treatment than in Hodgkin's disease. The stage of disease is usually assigned as in Hodgkin's disease (see Table 94-3). All patients should have a careful history and physical examination, a chest radiograph, a complete blood count, and measurements of serum enzyme levels. Bone marrow aspiration should be done and a biopsy obtained, because they frequently reveal lymphoma. A computed tomographic (CT) scan of the abdomen should be performed; it is preferred to a lymphangiogram because the mesenteric lymph nodes and visceral organs within the abdomen are involved relatively frequently. A lumbar puncture with a cytocentrifuge preparation for morphologic examination is recommended for patients with unfavorable histologic subtypes if central nervous system symptoms are present. More invasive procedures such as a liver biopsy or staging laparotomy are generally not required, and patients are usually assigned a stage on the basis of clinical findings.

Treatment

Before initiating treatment it is imperative to establish an accurate histologic diagnosis and to determine carefully the extent of disease. Because the non-Hodgkin's lymphomas have a propensity for early hematogenous spread, locally or regionally directed treatment such as surgery or radiotherapy is infrequently used. The majority of patients receive chemotherapy as the initial therapy. The intensity of the initial chemotherapy is determined primarily by the presenting histologic diagnosis. For this reason it is emphasized that the diagnosis must be established with certainty, usually by a pathologist who has considerable experience with lymphomas. Patients with low-grade or favorable histologic subtypes almost always have systemic disease (stages III or IV) at the time of diagnosis. The favorable histologic subtypes are not thought to be curable with currently available chemotherapy or radiotherapy (see Table 94-6), and consequently the goal of therapy is palliation of symptoms. Some patients with these histologic types have a very indolent disease course. Palpable lymph nodes may remain stable, wax and wane in size, or even regress spontaneously. These patients may not require any treatment for months or even years. Once it is established that therapy is indicated, single-agent chlorambucil or cyclophosphamide is usually well tolerated and effective in the majority of patients. Combination chemotherapy with CVP (cyclophosphamide, vincristine, and prednisone; Table 94-7) is also usually well tolerated and probably offers a higher response rate but no survival advantage over single-agent chemo-

Table 94-7. Chemotherapeutic regimens useful in the treatment of malignant lymphomas

Regimen*	Dose	Schedule (days)														
CVP (repeat every 21 days)		1	2	3	4	5	6	7	8	9	10	11	12	13	14	15
C = cyclophosphamide	400 mg/m² po	x	x	x	x	x										
V = vincristine	1.4 mg/m² iv (max. 2.0 mg)	x														
P = prednisone	100 mg po	x	x	x	x	x										
C-MOPP (repeat every 28 days)		1	2	3	4	5	6	7	8	9	10	11	12	13	14	15
C = cyclophosphamide	650 mg/m² iv	x								x						
O = vincristine (Oncovin)	1.4 mg/m² iv	x								x						
P = procarbazine	100 mg/m² po	x	x	x	x	x	x	x	x	x	x	x	x	x	x	
P = prednisone	40 mg/m² po	x	x	x	x	x	x	x	x	x	x	x	x	x	x	
CHOP (repeat every 21 days)		1	2	3	4	5										
C = cyclophosphamide	750 mg/m² iv	x														
H = doxorubicin (Adriamycin)	50 mg/m² iv	x														
O = vincristine (Oncovin)	1.4 mg/m² iv	x														
P = prednisone	100 mg iv	x	x	x	x	x										

*CVP and single-agent chlorambucil are the standard regimens most often used for favorable histologic subtypes of malignant lymphoma. CHOP is the standard regimen most often used for intermediate grades of unfavorable histologic subtypes. C-MOPP is useful for patients with unfavorable histologic types who have pre-existing heart disease, for whom doxorubicin may be contraindicated. Regimens for the high grades of unfavorable histologic subtypes have not been standardized.

therapy. Other drug combinations do not have any proven advantage over CVP. A systemic form of radiation (total body irradiation [TBI]) has been advocated by some, but its use is not widespread. At some point in time, usually after several years of observation and palliative therapy, in most patients with favorable histologic subtypes a more aggressive clinical course develops. Previously responsive areas of disease may develop clinical resistance to drugs, existing sites of tumor may begin growing rapidly, or new sites of disease may develop in spite of ongoing chemotherapy. These are all indications for a repeat biopsy to determine whether histologic transformation to a more aggressive form of lymphoma has occurred. Histologic progression usually portends a rapidly fatal course. However, some patients benefit from a change in chemotherapy to one of the more aggressive drug regimens that are used for treating the unfavorable histologic types of lymphoma.

Malignant lymphomas of favorable histologic type occur in localized forms (stages I or II) in only 10% of cases. Accordingly, the approach to localized disease is less well defined than the approach to disseminated disease. Observation without treatment, involved field radiotherapy, total nodal radiotherapy, and chemotherapy have all been advocated, but none is clearly the treatment of choice for localized disease. Involved field radiotherapy is probably the least harmful of these approaches.

Treatment of advanced stages of malignant lymphoma of unfavorable histologic subtype (stages III and IV; some experts would include patients with stage II disease in the "advanced" stage category) requires chemotherapy with drug regimens of proven curative potential. These drug regimens usually include doxorubicin and cyclophosphamide (see Tables 94-7 and 94-8). The most commonly used regimen is the CHOP (cyclophosphamide, Adriamycin, Oncovin, prednisone) combination, which produces a complete response rate of 50% to 68%. For patients who achieve a complete response, treatment is normally discontinued after 6 months. After treatment with CHOP, approximately 30% to 50% of patients experience a relapse and eventually die of their disease. Most relapses occur within the first 2 years, and relapses after 5 years are uncommon. Maintenance chemotherapy has not been shown to be helpful for prolonging the complete response. In recent years there have been a number of attempts to improve on the complete response rate and the duration of response achieved using the CHOP combination (Table 94-8). The results of initial pilot studies of such regimens as m-BACOD, ProMACE-CytaBOM, and MACOP-B are encouraging; approximately 80% of patients achieve a complete response, and 70% to 80% of the complete responses are durable. These more aggressive regimens are associated with increased morbidity and a treatment-related mortality as high as 6%. However, a recently completed national cooperative group study directly comparing CHOP to m-BACOD, ProMACE-CytaBOM, and MACOP-B demon-

Table 94-8. Developmental chemotherapeutic regimens frequently used to treat malignant lymphomas of unfavorable histology

Regimen*	Dose	Schedule (days)
m-BACOD (repeat every 21 days)		
m = methotrexate (followed by leukovorin rescue)	200 mg/m^2, iv	8,15
B = bleomycin	4 mg/m^2, iv	1
A = doxorubicin (Adriamycin)	45 mg/m^2, iv	1
C = cyclophosphamide	600 mg/m^2, iv	1
O = vincristine (Oncovin)	1.4 mg/m^2, iv	1
D = dexamethasone	6 mg/m^2, po	1-5
ProMACE-CytaBOM (repeat every 21 days)		
Pro = prednisone	60 mg/m^2, po	1-14
A = Adriamycin (doxorubicin)	25 mg/m^2, iv	1
C = cyclophosphamide	650 mg/m^2, iv	1
E = etoposide	120 mg/m^2, iv	1
Cyta = cytarabine	300 mg/m^2, iv	8
B = bleomycin	5 mg/m^2, iv	8
O = Oncovin (vincristine)	1.4 mg/m^2, iv	8
M = methotrexate (followed by leukovorin rescue)	120 mg/m^2, iv	8
MACOP-B (one 12-week course)		
M = methotrexate (followed by leukovorin rescue)	400 mg/m^2, iv	8,36,64
A = Adriamycin (doxorubicin)	50 mg/m^2, iv	1,15,29,43,57,71
C = cyclophosphamide	350 mg/m^2, iv	1,15,29,43,57,71
O = Oncovin (vincristine)	1.4 mg/m^2, iv (max. 2.0 mg)	8,22,36,50,64,78
P = prednisone	75 mg/m^2, po	1-84
B = bleomycin	10 mg/m^2, iv	22,50,78

*These regimens are frequently used to treat unfavorable histologic features of non-Hodgkin's lymphomas. However, a study directly comparing these regimens to CHOP has recently been completed demonstrating similar response rates and overall survival, but with increased toxicity and costs. The schedules are complex, and morbidity rate can be significant. Thus, expert consultation is required to adjust doses, prescribe prophylactic antibiotics, and administer the leukovorin rescue.

strated remarkable similarity among regimens. In this randomized study of 1138 patients, response rates, failure-free survival rate, and overall survival rate were similar. However, CHOP was associated with the fewest fatal toxicities (1%) and is the least expensive regimen to administer.

Malignant lymphomas of unfavorable histologic subtypes appear as apparently localized disease (stages I or II) in approximately 30% to 40% of patients. Traditionally, these patients have been treated with radiotherapy alone, with a cure rate of approximately 40% to 50%. More recently, the strategy of using chemotherapy of proven curative potential in advanced disease, such as CHOP, as initial therapy for localized disease has increased the proportion of patients who are apparently cured of disease to approximately 80%. Patients with very localized disease (stage I) can be treated with initial chemotherapy after clinical staging or with involved field radiotherapy after pathologic staging with equal success. Approximately 90% to 95% of these patients are cured of disease.

There are many exceptions to the general guidelines for treatment as outlined. For example, patients with T cell lymphoblastic lymphoma are seldom cured using conventional drug regimens such as CHOP. These patients frequently have bone marrow involvement. Standard regimens often fail because central nervous system disease develops. More successful approaches to these patients include intensive induction therapy and central nervous system prophylaxis similar to the treatment strategies used in acute lymphoblastic leukemia (Chapter 93). The intensive multiagent chemotherapy programs used to treat childhood malignant lymphomas have resulted in a marked improvement in prognosis for these adult patients.

REFERENCES

Croce CM and Nowell PC. Molecular basis of human B cell neoplasia. Blood 65:1, 1985.

Diel V et al: The cell of origin in Hodgkin's disease. Semin Oncol 17:660, 1990.

Grogan TM and Miller TP: New biologic markers in non-Hodgkin's lymphomas. Hematol Oncol Clin North Am 5:925, 1991.

Horning SJ and Rosenberg SA: The natural history of initially untreated low-grade non-Hodgkin's lymphomas. N Engl J Med 311:1471, 1984.

Miller TP, Byrne GE, and Jones SE: Mistaken clinical and pathologic diagnoses in Hodgkin's disease. Cancer Treat Rep 66:645, 1982.

Miller TP et al: P-glycoprotein expression in malignant lymphoma and reversal of clinical drug resistance with chemotherapy plus high dose verapamil. J Clin Oncol 9:17, 1991.

Urba WJ and Longo DL. Hodgkin's disease. N Engl J Med 326:678, 1992.

CHAPTER

95 Multiple Myeloma and the Dysproteinemias

Robert A. Kyle

Multiple myeloma (plasma cell myeloma, myelomatosis, Kahler's disease) and related disorders are characterized by a neoplastic or potentially neoplastic proliferation of a single clone of plasma cells engaged in the production of a specific immunoglobulin. This immunoglobulin is monoclonal—one class of heavy chains (gamma, alpha, mu, delta, or epsilon) and one type of light chains (kappa or lambda)—and often is referred to as monoclonal protein (*M* protein or paraprotein). This group of disorders is classified in the box below.

MULTIPLE MYELOMA

Etiology and epidemiology

The cause of multiple myeloma is unknown. Radiation may be a factor in some cases. Exposure to asbestos, benzene or industrial and agricultural toxins, a genetic element, and viruses have all been considered possible causes, but proof is meager.

Multiple myeloma accounts for about 1% of all types of malignant disease and slightly more than 10% of hematologic malignancies. The incidence of multiple myeloma is 4 to 5 per 100,000 per year. The apparent increase of rates in recent years is probably related to increased availability and utilization of medical facilities and improved diagnostic techniques.

Multiple myeloma and related disorders

I. Multiple myeloma
II. Variant forms of myeloma
  A. Smoldering myeloma
  B. Plasma cell leukemia
  C. Nonsecretory myeloma
  D. Osteosclerotic myeloma
  E. Solitary plasmacytoma of bone
  F. Extramedullary plasmacytoma
III. Waldenström's macroglobulinemia
IV. Heavy-chain diseases
  A. Alpha heavy-chain disease
  B. Gamma heavy-chain disease
  C. Mu heavy-chain disease
V. Monoclonal gammopathy of undetermined significance (MGUS, benign monoclonal gammopathy)
VI. Biclonal gammopathies
VII. Cryoglobulinemia
VIII. Primary amyloidosis (Chapter 322)

Clinical findings

The onset of multiple myeloma usually occurs in older persons with a median age of approximately 65 years. Only 3% of patients are younger than 40 years. It is slightly more common in men than in women. The incidence of multiple myeloma in blacks is almost twice that in whites. At diagnosis, bone pain, particularly in the back or chest, is present in more than two thirds of patients. Pain is usually induced by movement and does not occur at night, except with change of position. Weakness and fatigue are common and often are associated with anemia.

Some renal insufficiency occurs in about half the patients. This is often due to "myeloma kidney," in which the distal and collecting tubules become obstructed by large laminated casts consisting mainly of Bence Jones protein (Chapter 356). Hypercalcemia is also a common preventable cause of renal insufficiency. Hyperuricemia, amyloid deposition, acute or chronic pyelonephritis, infiltration of the kidney by plasma cells, and increased blood viscosity may all contribute to renal insufficiency. Acute renal failure has occurred after dehydration, infection, hypercalcemia, and intravenous urography.

Neurologic involvement is most often manifested by root pain from nerve compression. Compression of the spinal cord or cauda equina, usually produced by myeloma arising in the marrow cavity of a vertebra and extending to the extradural space, occurs in about 5% of patients with myeloma. This compression produces back pain with radicular features, weakness or paralysis of the lower extremities, and bowel or bladder incontinence. Peripheral neuropathy may occur but is usually associated with amyloidosis.

Patients with multiple myeloma have an increased susceptibility to bacterial infections, particularly pneumococcal pneumonia, although the incidence of gram-negative infections has recently increased. The greatest risk of infection occurs during the first 2 months after the initiation of chemotherapy. The incidence of herpes zoster is increased in myeloma. Bleeding may be a prominent feature. Qualitative platelet abnormalities, inhibition of coagulation factors from the monoclonal protein, and thrombocytopenia are major causes. Intravascular coagulation, amyloid deposition, and hepatic or renal insufficiency also may contribute to bleeding.

Pallor is the most common physical finding. The liver is palpable in about 20% of patients and the spleen in 5%. Extramedullary plasmacytomas are uncommon except in the late stages of the disease. Amyloidosis, which occurs in 10% of patients, may produce such diverse findings as defects of cardiac conduction, congestive heart failure, macroglossia, swelling of the joints, and peripheral neuropathy.

Laboratory findings

At diagnosis, two thirds of patients have a hemoglobin value less than 12 g/dl. A normocytic normochromic anemia eventually occurs in nearly every patient with multiple myeloma. The anemia is due mainly to inadequate production of red cells. Increased plasma volume from the osmotic effect of a large amount of monoclonal protein may produce a spurious decrease of hemoglobin and hematocrit values.

Serum electrophoresis reveals a peak or discrete band in 80% of cases, hypogammaglobulinemia in 10%, and no apparent abnormality in the remainder. A monoclonal protein is detected in the serum in about 90% of cases. The laboratory evaluation of monoclonal proteins is discussed in Chapter 75. Approximately 50% are immunoglobulin G (IgG), 20% IgA, 17% light chain only (Bence Jones proteinemia), 2% IgD, and 1% biclonal. Electrophoresis of urine shows a globulin peak in 80% of cases, mainly albumin in 5%, and a normal pattern in 15%. Immunoelectrophoresis or immunofixation shows a monoclonal protein in 75% of cases. The kappa/lambda ratio is 2:1. Nearly all (99%) patients with multiple myeloma have a monoclonal protein in the serum or urine.

The serum creatinine level is elevated initially in about one half of patients and is greater than or equal to 2 mg/dl in one fourth. The serum calcium level is elevated in 30% of patients at diagnosis, and 15% have a calcium value of more than 11 mg/dl. Conventional radiographs show abnormalities consisting of punched-out lytic areas, osteoporosis, or fractures in 75% of patients at diagnosis. The vertebrae, skull, thoracic cage, pelvis, and proximal humeri and femurs are the most frequent sites of involvement. There is a positive correlation between the production of osteoclast-activating factor by bone marrow cells and the extent of skeletal destruction. Technetium-99m bone scans are inferior to conventional radiographs for detecting lesions in myeloma. Computed tomography or magnetic resonance imaging is helpful in patients with myeloma who have skeletal pain but normal radiographic findings.

The peripheral blood of patients with myeloma shows a reduction of $OKT4^+$ cells (helper T lymphocytes) and an increased percentage of $OKT8^+$ cells (suppressor T lymphocytes). An aneuploid myeloma cell population is found in approximately three fourths of cases. Chromosome abnormalities are detected in about half of patients, but no specific abnormality has been demonstrated.

The demonstration of the monoclonal protein idiotype and the production of the patient's monoclonal protein by peripheral blood lymphocytes or plasma cells indicate that they are part of the malignant clone. This is supported by the demonstration of heavy- and light-chain immunoglobulin gene rearrangements in circulating blood cells.

Interleukin-6 (IL-6) is an important growth factor for myeloma cells. It induces a polyclonal proliferation of plasma cells. Elevated levels of IL-6 have been reported in patients with active multiple myeloma, in contrast to those with benign monoclonal gammopathy.

Differential diagnosis

The differential diagnosis of monoclonal gammopathies is listed in Chapter 75. Bone pain, anemia, and renal insufficiency constitute a triad that is strongly suggestive of multiple myeloma. The diagnosis depends on the demonstration of increased numbers of plasma cells in the bone marrow (Plate III-9). Identification of a monoclonal immunoglobulin in the plasma cells by immunofluorescence or immunoperoxidase is useful in differentiating multiple myeloma from reactive plasmacytosis and also in recognizing myeloma cells that have unusual morphologic features. Minimal criteria for the diagnosis of multiple myeloma are listed in the box at right. Because of differences in prognosis and therapy, variant forms of myeloma, such as smoldering multiple myeloma (SMM), and monoclonal gammopathy of undetermined significance (MGUS), must be distinguished from typical progressive multiple myeloma.

Minimal criteria for the diagnosis of multiple myeloma

Bone marrow with ≥10% plasma cells OR
Plasmacytoma plus one of the following:
- Monoclonal protein in serum (>3 g/dl)
- Monoclonal protein in urine
- Lytic bone lesions

Usual clinical features of myeloma
Exclude connective tissue diseases, chronic infections, carcinoma, lymphoma, and leukemia

Prognosis

The plasma cell labeling index (LI) using a monoclonal antibody to 5-bromo-2-deoxyuridine is helpful in distinguishing patients with overt multiple myeloma from those with stable monoclonal gammopathies. LI is low in MGUS, in SMM, and in successfully treated multiple myeloma (plateau phase) but is usually elevated in overt multiple myeloma at the time of diagnosis and in patients with myeloma in relapse.

In 1975, Durie and Salmon devised a clinical staging system based on a combination of factors that correlated with the myeloma cell mass (Table 95-1). The median survival is approximately 5 years in patients with stage IA disease and approximately 3 years in those with stage IIIA disease. Renal insufficiency is associated with shorter survival. Patients with stage IIIB disease have a median survival of slightly more than 1 year.

Elevation of the plasma cell labeling index and the uncorrected beta-2-microglobulin level are two very important independent prognostic factors in multiple myeloma. In addition, elevations of thymidine kinase, lactic dehydrogenase, and C-reactive protein levels; advanced age; plasmablastic morphology; hypodiploidy; low RNA content of plasma cells; elevation of serum creatinine level; hypercalcemia; and stage IIIB disease are all associated with shortened survival.

Table 95-1. Clinical staging system for multiple myeloma

Stage I	Low cell mass ($<0.6 \times 10^{12}/m^2$)
	All of the following:
	Hb >10 g/dl; IgG <5 g/dl; IgA <3 g/dl; calcium normal
	Urinary Monoclonal protein <4 g/24 hr
	No generalized lytic lesions
Stage II	Intermediate (neither stage I nor stage III)
Stage III	High cell mass ($>1.2 \times 10^{12}/m^2$)
	Any one of the following:
	Hb <8.5 g/dl; IgG >7 g/dl; IgA >5 g/dl; calcium >12 mg/dl
	Urinary Monoclonal protein >12 g/24 hr
	Advanced lytic bone lesions
Subclasses	A if creatinine level is <2 mg/dl and B if level is ≥2 mg/dl

From Durie BGM and Salmon SE: Cancer 36:842, 1975.

Treatment

Chemotherapy is the preferred initial treatment for overt symptomatic multiple myeloma. Patients with SMM or MGUS (benign monoclonal gammopathy) should not be treated. The patient's symptoms, physical findings, and all laboratory data must be considered when determining whether to begin chemotherapy. If there is doubt in the physician's mind, it is usually better to withhold therapy and to re-evaluate the patient in 2 or 3 months.

In most instances, analgesics, together with chemotherapy, can control the pain. This combination is preferred to local irradiation because the bone marrow reserve of many patients is limited and focal irradiation does not benefit systemic disease. The major controversy is whether a single alkylating agent or a combination of alkylating agents should be used.

The oral administration of melphalan (Alkeran) (0.15 mg/kg daily for 7 days) and prednisone (20 mg three times a day) for the same 7 days every 6 weeks is a satisfactory regimen that produces objective responses in 50% to 60% of patients. Leukocyte and platelet counts must be determined at 3 week intervals and the dose of melphalan altered to achieve modest cytopenias at midcycle, because the absorption of melphalan is variable.

Because of the obvious shortcomings of melphalan and prednisone therapy, various combinations of therapeutic agents have been tried. A useful combination, VBMCP (M-2), consists of vincristine (1.2 mg/m^2 intravenously on day 1), BCNU (20 mg/m^2 intravenously on day 1), melphalan (8 mg/m^2 orally on days 1-4), cyclophosphamide (400 mg/m^2 intravenously on day 1), and prednisone (40 mg/m^2 orally on days 1-7). In a recent meta-analysis of 18 published trials, no difference in efficacy was shown between melphalan/prednisone and combination chemotherapy. However, there was an implication that melphalan and prednisone therapy was superior for patients with a good prognosis and inferior to combination chemotherapy for those with a poor prognosis.

Chemotherapy should be continued until the patient

reaches a plateau phase, which is defined as a stable monoclonal protein in the serum and urine and no evidence of progression of myeloma. The plateau state is prolonged and relapses are fewer with administration of alpha-2 interferon, but overall survival rate is probably not altered. Chemotherapy must be reinstituted when relapse occurs.

The highest response rates reported for patients with multiple myeloma that are resistant to alkylating agents have been with VAD: vincristine (0.4 mg/day) plus Adriamycin (doxorubicin) (9 mg/m^2/day) by continuous infusion for 4 days, plus dexamethasone (40 mg each morning for 4 days beginning on days 1, 9, and 17 of each 28 day cycle). Most of the activity of VAD is from dexamethasone. If the patient has pancytopenia or does not want to take VAD, methylprednisolone in a dosage of 2 g intravenously three times weekly for a minimum of 4 weeks produces a response in about one third of refractory patients. We find fewer side effects from methylprednisolone than from dexamethasone. If there is a response, administration of methylprednisolone is reduced to once or twice weekly. VBAP (vincristine, BCNU [carmustine], Adriamycin [doxorubicin], and prednisone) has produced some benefit in approximately 40% of patients.

Newer therapeutic approaches

In a pilot study, a combination of alternating cycles of alpha$_2$ interferon with VBMCP produced an objective response in 80% of previously untreated patients with myeloma. Thirty percent had a complete response. The overall median survival was 42 months.

A reversal of resistance to chemotherapeutic agents is an important area of research. The use of verapamil or quinine to reverse the resistance to doxorubicin has been disappointing, and other agents must be sought. The use of monoclonal antibodies to IL-6, a potent growth factor for plasma cells, has produced some response in patients with advanced multiple myeloma and plasma cell leukemia.

The capacity of granulocyte-macrophage colony-stimulating factor (GM-CSF) and granulocyte-colony-stimulating factor (G-CSF) to shorten the duration of neutropenia after high-dose chemotherapy is being studied. Administration of these growth factors is beneficial in the collection of hemopoietic peripheral blood stem cells for autologous peripheral stem cell rescue of patients with myeloma after lethal chemotherapy or total body irradiation.

Bone marrow transplantation from an identical twin donor (syngeneic) has been associated with occasional prolonged survival, but most patients die of their myeloma. Allogeneic bone marrow transplantation from an HLA-compatible donor is possible in approximately 5% to 7% of patients with multiple myeloma. A significant early mortality rate, risk of graft-versus-host disease, and eventual relapse make allogeneic bone marrow transplantation of limited use. Autologous bone marrow transplantation is applicable to more patients because the age limit is higher and a matched donor is unnecessary. Two major problems exist: (1) eradication of multiple myeloma from the patient may not occur even with large doses of chemotherapy and irradiation and (2) reinfusing autologous marrow contaminated by myeloma cells or their precursors is a major concern. Purging of the marrow in vitro with a combination of monoclonal antibodies and cytotoxic agents is not yet effective for routine clinical use. Peripheral blood stem cells have successfully reconstituted the marrow of patients with multiple myeloma treated with high-dose chemotherapy, and this approach is being vigorously pursued in several institutions. The eventual role of this procedure is yet to be determined.

Management of complications

Hypercalcemia must be suspected if the patient has anorexia, nausea, vomiting, polyuria, increased constipation, weakness, confusion, stupor, or coma. Treatment is urgent because renal insufficiency commonly develops. Hydration, preferably with isotonic saline, is essential. In addition, oral prednisone in an initial dose of 25 mg four times daily should be given, but the dose must be reduced and discontinued as soon as possible. If these fail to control the hypercalcemia, pamidronate disodium (Aredia), etidronate disodium (Didronel), gallium nitrate, mithramycin, or calcitonin is useful. Maintenance of a high fluid intake (3 L/24 hr) is important in preventing renal failure. Allopurinol is necessary if hyperuricemia is present. Patients with acute renal failure should be treated promptly with fluid and electrolyte correction and then with hemodialysis if indicated. Peritoneal dialysis is preferable in some patients. Plasma exchange may be helpful for regaining renal function, but patients with severe myeloma cast formation or other irreversible renal changes are less likely to benefit from plasmapheresis. Renal transplantation for myeloma kidney has been followed by prolonged survival.

Prompt and appropriate treatment of bacterial infections is necessary. Pneumococcal and influenza vaccines should be given to all patients despite their suboptimal antibody response. Intravenously administered gamma globulin may be helpful for patients with recurrent infections, but it is very expensive for long-term therapy. Prophylactic daily oral penicillin often benefits patients with recurrent streptococcal pneumonia infections. Patients should be encouraged to be as active as possible because confinement to bed increases demineralization of the skeleton. Trauma must be avoided because even mild stress may result in multiple fractures. Fixation of long bone fractures or impending fractures with an intramedullary rod and methyl methacrylate has given excellent results. Diphosphonates, sodium fluoride, calcium supplementation, and vitamin D may be of some benefit for demineralization of the skeleton. Erythropoietin is helpful for most patients with symptomatic anemia when the plateau state has been reached.

Symptoms of hyperviscosity include oronasal bleeding, blurred vision, neurologic symptoms, and congestive heart failure. Hyperviscosity is more common in IgA myeloma than in IgG myeloma. Vigorous plasmapheresis will promptly relieve the symptoms of hyperviscosity. If spinal cord compression is suspected, magnetic resonance imaging (MRI), computed tomography (CT), or myelography must be done immediately to determine whether an extradural mass is causing the symptoms. Radiation therapy to the mass is usually beneficial.

VARIANT FORMS OF MYELOMA

Smoldering multiple myeloma (SMM)

The diagnosis of SMM depends on the presence of a monoclonal protein concentration of greater than 3 g/dl in the serum and more than 10% atypical plasma cells in the bone marrow and on the absence of anemia, renal insufficiency, and skeletal lesions. Often, a small amount of monoclonal protein is found in the urine, and the concentration of uninvolved immunoglobulins in the serum is decreased. Clusters or aggregates of plasma cells are often seen in the biopsy specimen of the bone marrow. The plasma cell labeling index is low. These patients should be observed without treatment because, in some, overt symptomatic multiple myeloma has not developed for years. Biologically, patients with SMM have a "benign" monoclonal gammopathy (MGUS), but it is difficult to accept that diagnosis initially when the monoclonal protein is greater than 3 g/dl and the bone marrow contains more than 10% plasma cells.

Plasma cell leukemia

Plasma cell leukemia is characterized by more than 20% plasma cells in the peripheral blood and an absolute plasma cell count of at least 2000/μl. It is classified as primary when it is diagnosed in the leukemic phase (60%) and as secondary when there is leukemic transformation of a previously recognized multiple myeloma (40%). Patients with primary plasma cell leukemia are younger and have a greater incidence of hepatosplenomegaly and lymphadenopathy, a higher platelet count, fewer lytic bone lesions, a smaller serum monoclonal protein component, and a slightly longer survival than those who have secondary plasma cell leukemia. Treatment is generally unsatisfactory, but administration of melphalan and prednisone or combinations of alkylating agents frequently produces a response; however, the median survival is only 7 to 9 months. Secondary plasma cell leukemia rarely responds to chemotherapy because the patients have already been treated for myeloma and are resistant.

Nonsecretory myeloma

In approximately 1% of patients with multiple myeloma, a monoclonal protein cannot be detected in either the serum or the urine; this disorder has been designated nonsecretory myeloma. To confirm the diagnosis, a monoclonal protein should be identified in the plasma cells by the use of immunoperoxidase or immunofluorescence. More than a dozen patients with nonsecretory myeloma have been reported in whom a monoclonal protein cannot be found within the cells—a finding that suggests a lack of synthesis. Patients with nonsecretory myeloma have longer survival times than do those with typical multiple myeloma.

Osteosclerotic myeloma

Osteosclerotic myeloma (POEMS syndrome) is characterized by *p*olyneuropathy, *o*rganomegaly, *e*ndocrinopathy, *m*onoclonal protein, and *s*kin changes (POEMS). The major clinical features are a chronic inflammatory-demyelinating polyneuropathy with predominantly motor disability and sclerotic skeletal lesions. The diagnosis is confirmed by the finding of a plasmacytoma on a biopsy specimen of a bony lesion. Hyperpigmentation and hypertrichosis may be striking. Gynecomastia, atrophic testes, and clubbing of the fingers and toes may occur. Papilledema is common. Hepatomegaly, splenomegaly, and lymphadenopathy may develop. In contrast to that in multiple myeloma, the hemoglobin level is usually normal or polycythemia is present. Thrombocytosis occurs in more than half of patients. A monoclonal protein is found in the serum in most patients, but it is usually small and is almost always of the lambda class. IgA is common. The presence of a monoclonal light chain in the urine is infrequent; when it is present, it is of modest amount. The bone marrow usually contains less than 5% plasma cells. Renal insufficiency and hypercalcemia are rare. Irradiation for single or multiple lesions in a limited area benefits more than half of patients. If the patient has widespread osteosclerotic lesions, chemotherapy with melphalan and prednisone may be helpful.

Solitary plasmacytoma (solitary myeloma) of bone

The diagnosis of solitary plasmacytoma of bone depends on histologic confirmation, absence of other lesions in the skeletal radiographs, no evidence of multiple myeloma in the bone marrow, and absence of or small amounts of monoclonal protein in the serum or urine. More than one half of patients have involvement of the vertebral column. Treatment consists of radiation to the local lesion in the range of 45 Gy (4500 rad). The patients must be closely followed because in approximately half overt multiple myeloma develops and in approximately 10% new bone lesions or local recurrence develops. Progression usually occurs within 3 to 4 years. Approximately half of patients survive 10 years. There is no evidence that adjuvant chemotherapy affects the incidence of conversion to multiple myeloma.

Extramedullary plasmacytoma

Extramedullary plasmacytoma is a plasma cell tumor that arises outside the bone marrow. The upper respiratory tract, including the nasal cavity and sinuses, nasopharynx, and larynx, is the most frequent site, but it may also occur in the gastrointestinal tract, central nervous system, urinary bladder, breast, testes, thyroid, parotid gland, and lymph nodes. Epistaxis, rhinorrhea, and nasal obstruction may occur. There is a predominance of IgA monoclonal protein in extramedullary plasmacytomas. The diagnosis is based on the finding of a plasma cell tumor in an extramedullary site and on the absence of multiple myeloma (determined from bone marrow examination, skeletal films, and examination of the blood and urine). Treatment consists of tumoricidal irradiation (40 to 50 Gy). The prognosis is favorable; regional recurrences develop in 25% of patients. Development of typical multiple myeloma is uncommon.

WALDENSTRÖM'S MACROGLOBULINEMIA

This malignant lymphoplasma cell proliferative disorder produces a high concentration of IgM monoclonal protein. The condition bears similarities to multiple myeloma, lymphoma, and chronic lymphocytic leukemia.

Etiology

Although the cause of Waldenström's macroglobulinemia is unknown, the disease may be more frequent in certain families. Studies of relatives of patients with macroglobulinemia reveal an increased frequency of IgM monoclonal proteins as well as quantitative abnormalities.

Clinical findings

Macroglobulinemia has a predilection for older men, and the onset is usually insidious. Weakness, fatigue, and bleeding (especially oozing from the oronasal region) are common presenting symptoms. Blurring or other impairment of vision affects one third of patients. In contrast to multiple myeloma, bone pain is rare. Dyspnea, weight loss, recurrent infections, or congestive heart failure may occur. Pallor, mild splenomegaly, hepatomegaly, and peripheral lymphadenopathy are the most frequent physical findings. Retinal abnormalities, including hemorrhages, exudates, and venous congestion with vascular segmentation ("sausage" formation), may be striking.

Pulmonary involvement is manifested by diffuse pulmonary infiltrates, isolated masses, or pleural effusion. These lesions consist of plasmacytoid lymphocytes. Peripheral neuropathy may be the initial symptom and usually involves both sensory and motor modalities. Sudden deafness, progressive spinal muscular atrophy, and multifocal leukoencephalopathy have all been noted. Renal failure rarely occurs. Systemic amyloidosis may be associated with Waldenström's macroglobulinemia.

Laboratory findings

Almost all patients have a normocytic, normochromic anemia. Spuriously low hemoglobin and hematocrit levels may result from the increased plasma volume produced by a large amount of monoclonal protein. Occasionally, there is a Coombs'-test-positive hemolytic anemia. Rouleau formation is striking on the peripheral blood smear (Plate III-4, *F*), and erythrocyte sedimentation is greatly increased. Mild lymphocytosis or monocytosis is not uncommon. The serum cholesterol value is frequently very low. The bone marrow aspirate is usually hypocellular, but fixed sections are hypercellular and extensively infiltrated with lymphoid and plasma cells. The number of mast cells is usually increased.

An IgM monoclonal protein, often more than 3 g/dl, is found in all cases. Approximately 75% of light chains are kappa. Both 7S and 19S IgM are present. About 10% of macroglobulins are cryoprecipitable. Most often, the bones are normal, but diffuse osteoporosis may be seen, and in rare instances lytic lesions develop. Almost 80% of the patients have a monoclonal light chain in the urine but the amount is usually small. Elevation of serum viscosity is common, but most patients have no symptoms of hyperviscosity.

Differential diagnosis

The combination of typical symptoms and physical findings, IgM monoclonal protein, and lymphoplasma cell infiltration of the bone marrow provides the diagnosis of Waldenström's macroglobulinemia. The major problem in the differential diagnosis centers around the distinction from multiple myeloma, chronic lymphocytic leukemia, lymphoma, undifferentiated lymphoproliferative disease, and monoclonal gammopathy of undetermined significance (MGUS) of the IgM type. To differentiate MGUS of the IgM class from early Waldenström's macroglobulinemia, the patient must be carefully observed for an indefinite period.

Treatment

Specific treatment should be directed against the abnormal proliferation of lymphocytes and plasma cells. Therapy should be withheld until the patient is symptomatic. Chlorambucil, in an initial daily oral dose of 6 to 8 mg, is an effective agent. The dosage of chlorambucil must be altered, depending on the results of leukocyte and platelet counts, which should be determined every 2 weeks. Chlorambucil also may be given in a dosage of 0.3 mg/kg daily for 7 days plus prednisone in a dosage of 60 mg daily for the same 7 day period and repeated every 4 to 6 weeks. The dosage must be altered depending on the leukocyte and platelet levels. Alpha-2 interferon and fludarabine have both been reported to be beneficial in about half of patients who are resistant to an alkylating agent. Cyclophosphamide or combinations of alkylating agents such as the M2 protocol (vincristine, BCNU, melphalan, cyclophosphamide, and prednisone) also have been beneficial. Chemotherapy should be discontinued when the patient's monoclonal protein level decreases and reaches a stable state and there is no other evidence of active disease. Transfusions of packed red cells should be given for symptomatic anemia. Erythropoietin may be of benefit for patients in the plateau state with symptomatic anemia. Patients must be followed up and treatment reinstituted in the event of relapse. The symptoms of hyperviscosity must be treated with vigorous plasmapheresis. The median survival is approximately 5 years after diagnosis.

HEAVY-CHAIN DISEASES

Gamma heavy-chain disease

This lymphoplasma cell proliferative syndrome produces a monoclonal gamma heavy chain with extensive deletions of amino acids. The median age at diagnosis is approximately 60 years, although the condition has appeared before the age of 20 years. Patients with gamma heavy-chain disease usually have a lymphoma-like illness, although the clinical findings are diverse, ranging from an aggressive lymphoproliferative disease to an asymptomatic state. Hepatosplenomegaly and lymphadenopathy occur in about 60% of patients; anemia occurs in about 80%. Serum electrophoresis frequently shows no localized band or spike. Proteinuria consisting of gamma heavy chains is usually modest in amount. Increased numbers of plasma cells, lymphocytes, or plasmacytoid lymphocytes are seen in biopsy specimens of bone marrow and lymph node. Treatment is not indicated for the asymptomatic patient. The combination of cyclophosphamide, vincristine, and prednisone (CVP) useful in the treatment of lymphoma (Chapter 94) has been beneficial. If there is no response to this regimen, doxorubicin should be added (CHOP).

Alpha heavy-chain disease

The majority of patients with alpha heavy-chain disease are from the Mediterranean area and have involvement of the digestive tract with severe malabsorption, loss of weight, diarrhea, and steatorrhea. The duodenum and jejunum are almost always involved. The diagnosis is most often made in persons who are in the second and third decades of life, and approximately 60% of patients are men. The serum protein electrophoretic pattern is normal in half the cases; in the remainder, an unimpressive broad band may appear in the alpha-2 or beta region. Bence Jones proteinuria does not occur. The diagnosis depends on the recognition of a monoclonal α heavy chain. Alpha heavy-chain disease must be differentiated from immunoproliferative small intestinal disease (IPSID) or "Mediterranean" lymphoma. Most often, alpha heavy-chain disease is progressive and fatal, but responses occur with antibiotics or with chemotherapy, such as melphalan, cyclophosphamide, and prednisone.

Mu heavy-chain disease

In mu heavy-chain disease, chronic lymphocytic leukemia or a lymphoma-like pattern is most common. The presence of vacuolated plasma cells in the bone marrow may be a helpful finding. A stable, asymptomatic state also has been noted. The clinical spectrum of mu heavy-chain disease should broaden, as it has in gamma heavy-chain disease. Serum electrophoresis usually reveals hypogammaglobulinemia; a localized spike occurs in less than half of patients. Bence Jones proteinuria has been found in two thirds of patients. Treatment with alkylating agents and corticosteroids has produced some benefit. The course of mu heavy-chain disease is variable; median survival is approximately 2 years.

MONOCLONAL GAMMOPATHY OF UNDETERMINED SIGNIFICANCE (MGUS) (BENIGN MONOCLONAL GAMMOPATHY)

Serum monoclonal proteins have been found without evidence of myeloma, macroglobulinemia, amyloidosis, or related diseases in approximately 3% of persons more than 70 years of age in Sweden and the United States. Currently at the Mayo Clinic, of the patients with newly recognized monoclonal proteins, only 13% have multiple myeloma, whereas nearly two thirds have MGUS.

Of 241 patients with monoclonal protein but no evidence of multiple myeloma, macroglobulinemia, amyloidosis, or lymphoma (benign monoclonal gammopathy) who were followed for more than 20 years, in 24.5% myeloma, macroglobulinemia, amyloidosis, or related diseases developed; 9.5% had an increased monoclonal protein to more than 3 g/dl, but myeloma and macroglobulinemia did not develop; 47% died of unrelated causes; and only 19% had no increase in the monoclonal protein and fulfilled the criteria for the diagnosis of benign monoclonal gammopathy.

The actuarial rate for the development of multiple myeloma, macroglobulinemia, amyloidosis, or a malignant lymphoplasma proliferative process at 10 years was 17% and was 33% at 20 years. There was no difference in the actuarial rate for development of serious disease with IgG, IgA, or IgM proteins.

The interval from the recognition of monoclonal gammopathy to the diagnosis of multiple myeloma ranged from 2 to 29 years (median, 10 years). After multiple myeloma was diagnosed, the median survival was 34 months. The median interval from the recognition of monoclonal gammopathy to the diagnosis of macroglobulinemia was 8 years, whereas the median interval from the recognition of monoclonal gammopathy to the diagnosis of systemic amyloidosis was 9 years.

Differential diagnosis

Patients with MGUS have less than 3 g/dl of monoclonal protein in the serum and no or small amounts of Bence Jones proteinuria, less than 5% plasma cells in the bone marrow aspirate, and no anemia, hypercalcemia, renal insufficiency, or osteolytic lesions (unless caused by other diseases). The only basis for deciding that the patient has MGUS is the absence of an increase in the monoclonal protein or the development of a lymphoplasma cell proliferative disease during long-term follow-up observation. The differentiation of benign monoclonal gammopathy from myeloma or macroglobulinemia is very difficult at the time when the monoclonal protein is found. The following may be helpful: the amount of the serum monoclonal protein, levels of normal polyclonal or background immunoglobulins, the presence and amount of Bence Jones proteinuria, the number of plasma cells in the bone marrow, the presence of osteolytic lesions, plasma cell labeling index, the serum beta-2 microglobulin level, the presence of J chains in plasma cells, and the presence of circulating plasma cells.

At the time of recognition of a monoclonal protein, patients in whom multiple myeloma and related disorders will develop cannot be differentiated from those with MGUS on the basis of age, sex, presence of organomegaly, the initial hemoglobin level, size of the serum monoclonal protein peak, IgG subclass type, levels of uninvolved immunoglobulins, serum albumin level, presence of small amounts of monoclonal light chain in the urine, and number of plasma cells in the bone marrow. The most reliable means of distinguishing a benign course from a malignant one is serial measurement of the monoclonal protein. Periodic examinations must be performed to determine whether the disorder is benign or the initial manifestation of multiple myeloma, systemic amyloidosis, macroglobulinemia, or other malignant lymphoproliferative disorders.

Although MGUS frequently exists without any other abnormalities, certain diseases are associated with it, as would be expected in an older population. Therefore, studies of such an association must include a control group to determine whether the association is merely a coincidence. Monoclonal proteins have been noted in lymphoma, leukemia, and a wide variety of hematologic conditions. Rheumatic diseases and neurologic disorders such as peripheral neuropathy have been seen. Lichen myxedematosus has frequently been noted with an IgG lambda monoclonal protein, whereas pyoderma gangrenosum is often associated with an IgA monoclonal protein.

The monoclonal protein may exhibit high specificities to dextran, antistreptolysin O, antinuclear activity, von Willebrand factor, thyroglobulin, insulin, double-stranded DNA, apolipoprotein, thyroxin, various antibiotics, actin, calcium, and copper.

Biclonal gammopathies

Two monoclonal proteins (biclonal) occur in approximately 4% of patients with a gammopathy. Electrophoresis often shows only a single localized band, and the second monoclonal protein is recognized only when immunoelectrophoresis or immunofixation is done. IgG and IgA are the most frequent combinations, followed in frequency by monoclonal IgG and IgM. The clinical findings are similar to those seen in monoclonal gammopathy, and most patients have a biclonal gammopathy of undetermined significance. Approximately one third of patients have multiple myeloma, macroglobulinemia, or other malignant lymphoproliferative disease. Triclonal gammopathies have been found.

Cryoglobulins

Cryoglobulins are proteins that precipitate when cooled and dissolve when heated. To test for cryoglobulins, 5 ml of fresh centrifuged serum, kept at 37° C, is placed in a graduated centrifuge tube and incubated at 1° C (in an ice bath in a refrigerator or cold room) for 7 days. The precipitate is washed, and immunoelectrophoresis is performed.

Cryoglobulins may be classified as type I (monoclonal, consisting of IgG, IgM, IgA, or rarely, free light chains), type II (mixed, two or more immunoglobulins, of which one is monoclonal), or type III (polyclonal, no monoclonal protein found).

In most cases, monoclonal cryoglobulins are IgM or IgG, but IgA and Bence Jones cryoglobulins have been reported. Unexpectedly, many patients with large amounts of cryoglobulin are completely asymptomatic, whereas others with monoclonal cryoglobulin levels of 1 to 2 g/dl may, because of high thermal insolubility, have pain, purpura, Raynaud's phenomenon, cyanosis, and even ulceration and sloughing of skin and subcutaneous tissues on exposure to the cold. Cryoglobulinemia may produce a spurious elevation of the leukocyte count on the model S Coulter counter. Monoclonal cryoglobulins are associated with multiple myeloma, macroglobulinemia, lymphoproliferative disease, and benign monoclonal gammopathy.

Most commonly, mixed cryoglobulins (type II) consist of IgM-IgG, but IgG-IgG and IgA-IgG combinations have been reported. Usually, the quantity of mixed cryoglobulin is less than 0.2 g/dl and may not reach maximal amounts for 7 days. The serum protein electrophoretic pattern either is normal or shows diffuse hypergammaglobulinemia. Patients with mixed cryoglobulinemia frequently have vasculitis, glomerulonephritis, or lymphoproliferative or chronic infectious processes. Hepatic dysfunction and serologic evidence of previous infection with hepatitis B virus are common.

Type III (polyclonal) cryoglobulinemia is not associated with a monoclonal component. It is found in many patients with infections or inflammatory diseases and is of no clinical significance.

REFERENCES

Dimopoulos MA et al: Curability of solitary bone plasmacytoma. J Clin Oncol 10:587, 1992.

Durie BGM and Salmon SE: A clinical staging system for multiple myeloma: correlation of measured myeloma cell mass with presenting clinical features, response to treatment, and survival. Cancer 36:842, 1975.

Fermand J-P et al: Gamma heavy chain "disease": heterogeneity of the clinicopathologic features: report of 16 cases and review of the literature. Medicine 68:321, 1989.

Gahrton G et al: Allogeneic bone marrow transplantation in multiple myeloma. N Engl J Med 325:1267, 1991.

Gregory WM, Richards MA, and Malpas JS: Combination chemotherapy versus melphalan and prednisolone in the treatment of multiple myeloma: an overview of published trials. J Clin Oncol 10:334, 1992.

Greipp PR et al: Immunofluorescence labelling indices in myeloma and related monoclonal gammopathies. Mayo Clin Proc 62:969, 1987.

Jagannath S et al: Autologous bone marrow transplantation in multiple myeloma: identification of prognostic factors. Blood 76:1860, 1990.

Kelly JJ, Jr et al: Osteosclerotic myeloma and peripheral neuropathy. Neurology (NY) 33:202, 1983.

Kyle RA: Multiple myeloma: review of 869 cases. Mayo Clin Proc 50:29, 1975.

Kyle RA: 'Benign' monoclonal gammopathy—after 20 to 35 years of follow-up. Mayo Clin Proc 68:26, 1993.

Kyle RA and Garton JP: The spectrum of IgM monoclonal gammopathy in 430 cases. Mayo Clin Proc 62:719, 1987.

Kyle RA and Gertz MA: Second malignancies after chemotherapy. In

Perry MC, editor: The chemotherapy source book. Baltimore, 1992, Williams & Williams, pp 689-702.
Kyle RA and Greipp PR: Smoldering multiple myeloma. N Engl J Med 302:1347, 1980.
Kyle RA and Greipp PR: Plasma cell dyscrasias: current status. CRC Crit Rev Oncol Hematol 8:93, 1988.
MacLennan ICM et al: Combined chemotherapy with ABCM versus melphalan for treatment of myelomatosis. Lancet 339:200, 1992.
Mandelli F et al: Maintenance treatment with recombinant interferon alpha-2b in patients with multiple myeloma responding to conventional induction chemotherapy. N Engl J Med 322:1430, 1990.
Noel P and Kyle RA: Plasma cell leukemia: an evaluation of response to therapy. Am J Med 83:1062, 1987.
Rambaud JC et al: Immunoproliferative small intestinal disease (IPSID): relationships with α-chain disease and "Mediterranean" lymphomas. Springer Semin Immunopathol 12:239, 1990.
Wahner-Roedler DL and Kyle RA: μ-Heavy chain disease: presentation as a benign monoclonial gammopathy. Am J Hematol 40:56, 1992.

CHAPTER

96 Melanoma, Kaposi's Sarcoma, and Mycosis Fungoides

James J. Nordlund
Debra L. Breneman
Nancy J. Pelc
A. Daniel King

MELANOMA

Etiology and epidemiology

The incidence of melanoma has increased yearly since the 1940s. The lifetime risk for melanoma is projected to reach 1 per 100 individuals by the year 2000 compared to 1 per 1000 in the 1950s. The desirability for tanned skin and the popularity of outdoor activities have been implicated in the rising incidence of melanoma. Exposure to sunlight is one risk factor. Outdoor workers such as farmers and sailors have a low incidence of melanoma. People working indoors who enjoy occasional exposure to intense sunlight that causes severe burns are at risk for development of melanoma. Sunlight and sunburn increase the risk of melanoma for an individual only by a factor of 2 to 4. Excessive sun exposure is the most well known risk factor over which individuals and the medical profession have some control. Genetic factors seem to carry the higher risk. Individuals who exhibit Celtic features such as red hair, blue eyes, and freckles (types I and II skin) are at much greater risk than deeply colored individuals. Age is a major risk factor. Prepubertal children and adolescents under the age of 20 years very rarely have melanomas. All individuals acquire nevocellular nevi (moles). At the age of 45 years, the typical white person has approximately 40 to 50 nevi. Some individuals exhibit two to four times more nevi. Those individuals with over 100 nevi have an 8- to 20-fold higher risk for melanoma than those with few nevi. Currently, such nevi (moles) are subcategorized as either normal or atypical (dysplastic). Atypical moles are characterized by large size (> 5 mm diameter), haphazard colors, irregular borders, and histologically atypical nevus cells. Whether atypical moles alone are a risk factor for melanoma is not clear. Individuals with atypical nevi are usually Northern European in ancestry and have numerous nevi, often 100 or more. The number of nevi and clinically atypical features seem to be inherited as autosomal dominant traits. The most predictive factor for melanoma is family history. Individuals who have three or more members of their primary kinship with a history of melanoma have an extremely high probability of development of a melanoma. If they have a large number of atypical nevi, the relative risk for development of melanoma might approach 10%. In summary, environmental factors such as sunlight may constitute less risk than genetic factors.

Clinical features

Most melanomas are pigmented. A few are amelanotic. Typically a melanoma exhibits irregularity: of color (blues, browns, blacks, reds, gray, and white); of outline (notches or protuberances); and of topography. The surface has areas that are macular, verrucous, papular, and/or nodular.

Clinically, cutaneous melanomas have been categorized into four types: superficial spreading, nodular, lentigo maligna, or acral lentiginous. The importance of classifying cutaneous melanomas is to alert the clinician to the different appearances of melanomas. Early detection and removal assure a cure. The most common type of melanoma is the superficial spreading type (80% to 85%) (Plate III-14, *A*). Nodular melanomas (5% to 10%) present as blue-black nodules (Plate III-14, *B*). The lentigo maligna begins as a fawn-colored macule that slowly enlarges and acquires extreme variation in color and outline. These latter tumors are usually found on the face. Lentigo maligna is defined as a melanoma in situ and the malignant cells are confined above the basement membrane of the epidermis. After the cells have invaded into the dermis, the lesion is called a lentigo maligna melanoma. The acral lentiginous melanoma is located on the palms, on the soles, or around or under the nails.

The prognosis for a melanoma can be predicted with moderate statistical accuracy. It is determined by the depth of penetration into the dermis (the Clark level) and/or the Breslow thickness (the distance from the stratum granulosum to the deepest tumor cell) (Table 96-1). The clinical type (i.e., nodular, superficial, or lentigo maligna melanoma) is not an indicator of prognosis. Melanomas with the same thickness carry the same prognosis.

Melanomas with a Breslow thickness of 0.75 mm or less are curable in 98% or more of individuals. As the thickness increases from 0.75 to 2 mm, the rate of metastasis increases to about 20% to 30%. Melanomas greater than 4 mm carry a probability of metastasis as high as 70% to 80%. Even the thickest melanomas have a 5% to 10% cure rate.

Table 96-1. Prognostic parameters for melanoma

Staging	Approximate Breslow measurement	Estimated 5-year survival after excision
Level (Clark system)		
I. Epidermis	< 0.75 mm	Premalignant
II. Papillary dermis	0.4-1.25 mm	70%-98%
III. Papillary-reticular dermis interface	1.25-2.5 mm	45%-65%
IV. Reticular dermis	2.5-4.0 mm	30%-50%
V. Subcutaneous tissue or deeper	> 4.0 mm	5%-30%
Stage (UCCC system)		
I. Primary with or without satellite lesion at the primary site		70%
II. Regional lymph node involvement		15%-20%
III. Disseminated melanoma		<5% (median <6 if extracutaneous disease)

The tumor must also be staged. A stage I melanoma is confined by all clinical parameters and imaging techniques to the primary site. A stage II melanoma has spread to the regional draining lymph nodes. Stage III indicates distant metastasis. Common sites for metastasis are the skin, lungs, brain, liver, heart, and intestine.

Diagnosis and staging

The most important diagnostic technique is histologic examination of the primary lesion by a dermatopathologist knowledgeable in the nuances of distinguishing a true melanoma from melanoma simulative. Preferably the primary lesion is excised in its totality for histologic examination. However, often a lesion is too large or located where a large excision would cause cosmetic disfigurement. In these or similar situations, a deep incisional biopsy is proper. If the diagnosis is confirmed, the patient should have a thorough physical examination with careful attention to the local lymph nodes, the skin, and other sites commonly involved by metastasis. A chest radiograph is helpful. Any sign or symptom suggestive of metastasis should be evaluated by appropriate imaging techniques.

Laboratory features

The histopathologic characteristics of cutaneous melanomas can be straightforward or very subtle. Usually the specimen exhibits large, epithelioid cells, singly or in nests, scattered throughout all layers of the epidermis. Spindle cells may also be present. If the cells are confined to the epidermis, the lesion is considered a melanoma in situ and is premalignant. Dermal invasion is a sign of advanced malignancy. Cells in the deep dermis might contain the pigment melanin. A dense lymphocytic infiltrate is common. The malignant cells exhibit the pleomorphic, hyperchromatic, and bizarre nuclei of malignancy. Amelanotic melanomas may require electron microscopy or special stains such as for the S100 protein to distinguish them from other undifferentiated malignancies. The pathologist must provide the clinician with an accurate assessment of both the Clark and Breslow levels.

Laboratory studies

No laboratory studies are required or specific for the evaluation of a patient with primary melanoma. Before the removal of the primary tumor, a chest radiograph is usually obtained, as well as a complete blood count, urinalysis, and a stool test for occult blood. A more intensive evaluation by imaging techniques depends on the detection of signs on the physical examination that suggest the presence of metastasis.

Treatment and natural history

The treatment of choice is complete excision of the primary tumor. The excision generally is down to the deep fascia unless the tumor is confined to the epidermis. The excision must always extend beyond the depth of the deepest hair follicles. The margin of excision should extend about 5 to 10 mm beyond the entire primary lesion if the lesion is thin (i.e., less than 1 mm in thickness). A larger margin of 2 to 3 cm, especially on the proximal side of the lesion toward the draining lymph nodes, is recommended for thicker (> 1 mm or Clark level III) lesions. The size of the excision probably does not alter ultimate survival but minimizes the probability of local recurrence.

The resection of local lymph nodes is not recommended for thin lesions (i.e., those less than 1 mm in thickness). For individuals with thicker lesions, lymph node resection is indicated if the nodes are involved either by clinical examination or by imaging procedures. About 20% of patients with stage II disease survive for a long period after excision of the local lymph nodes. Prophylactic or blind resection of nodes is controversial. The prevailing recommendation is not to resect local lymph nodes if the patient has a very thick lesion (> 4 mm Breslow thickness). Some, but not all, investigators believe prophylactic resection of intermediate levels (1.0 to 4 mm) is useful. Cutaneous metastases should be excised, if possible. The procedure is not curative but prevents significant morbidity.

Patients with melanoma should be examined at 3 month intervals for the first year after excision and at 6 month intervals for the subsequent 2 years. Over 90% of metastasis occurs within 3 years of the diagnosis. Thereafter, annual examination is essential with particular care given to inspection of the entire integument. In about 4% of individuals a second primary melanoma develops.

Chemotherapy has not been successful in prolonging the life of individuals with metastatic disease. Dacarbazine (DTIC) is the standard agent used for treatment of metastasis. About 20% of patients show regression of the tumors, but the duration of survival probably is not altered and the morbidity from chemotherapy is significant. Numerous new combinations of chemotherapy and various types of innovative immunotherapy are on trial throughout the United States and other countries. Irradiation therapy can relieve pain caused by metastasis or ameliorate the symptoms from intracranial tumors. It is not curative and should not be used as a therapy of the primary lesion.

KAPOSI'S SARCOMA

Epidemiology

Kaposi's sarcoma (KS) is a neoplasm that apparently begins in the skin but involves other organs. The malignancy most likely is of endothelial origin. There are epidemic and endemic patterns of KS. There are two forms of endemic KS: The classical form is rare; it affects elderly men of Mediterranean or Eastern European ancestry. The second endemic type is found in tropical Africa and affects children and adults, especially males.

Epidemic KS was one of the first diseases associated with the acquired immunodeficiency syndrome (AIDS). Epidemic KS predominantly affects homosexual and bisexual men with AIDS (95% of cases). The incidence of KS in AIDS patients has declined from 40% to 15% over the past decade. KS has been observed sporadically in homosexual and bisexual men in the absence of laboratory evidence of human immunodeficiency virus (HIV) infection and rarely in patients who are immunosuppressed or who have a lymphoproliferative malignancy.

Etiology

The cause of all types of KS and the cause(s) of its association with AIDS are not known. HIV by itself or a coinfection with a second retrovirus that is transmitted with HIV has been implicated. HIV itself seems unlikely to be the direct cause of KS, but it may have an indirect role by causing production of growth factors for KS by HIV-infected lymphocytes. The preponderance of KS in homosexual and bisexual men with HIV, but not in drug users or hemophiliacs with HIV infection, suggests a role for a second infection, possibly another retrovirus.

Immunosuppression facilitates spread of KS in the AIDS and organ transplant populations. Partial or complete regression of KS has been noted after restoration of immune function.

Clinical features and course

Manifestations of KS vary from isolated red-brown macules to fungating cutaneous tumors. Patients may exhibit patches, papules, plaques, or nodules (Plates V-40 and VI-24). Their color can be pink, red, or purple in early lesions, or dark brown in older lesions. The size of lesions ranges from millimeters to centimeters. Lesions may enlarge, coalesce, or regress. Although usually asymptomatic, the lesions can be pruritic or painful and ulcerated lesions can become secondarily infected.

The epidemic form associated with HIV infection is characterized by aggressive skin lesions and visceral involvement. Widely distributed erythematous patches, infiltrated plaques, and nodules on skin or on the oral mucosa, typically the hard palate, are characteristic. Involvement of viscera occurs occasionally in the absence of cutaneous involvement. Opportunistic infections are more frequently the cause of death for patients with AIDS than for those with KS.

The endemic KS found in Africa consists of four forms: nodular, aggressive, florid, and lymphadenopathic. The nodular form is similar to classic epidemic KS. The most common endemic type usually presents a solitary round plaque, nodule, or patch on the lower extremities. Visceral involvement occurs uncommonly. The course is indolent. In the aggressive type, large exophytic nodules and fungating tumors occur on the lower extremities and invade adjacent tissues, including bone. The florid form is characterized by widely disseminated cutaneous nodules with lymph node and visceral involvement. The fourth type, lymphadenopathic, affects lymph nodes and viscera, but not skin. Both the florid and lymphadenopathic forms are rapidly fatal.

Diagnosis and staging

A patient who has a clinically suspicious lesion should have a biopsy taken to confirm the diagnosis. The differential diagnosis is extensive. Macular KS may resemble ecchymosis, hemangioma, nevus, or melanoma. Plaque KS may look like an arthropod reaction, sarcoidosis, metastatic cancer, or secondary syphilis. Nodular KS resembles hemangioma, angiosarcoma, melanoma, metastatic cancer, pyogenic granuloma, or bacillary angiomatosis. No staging system is consistently used in the assessment of KS.

Laboratory features

Histopathology. The histologic characteristics vary, depending on the structure of the lesion. The patch form consists of a proliferation of irregularly shaped and thin-walled blood vessels that follow a haphazard course. Extravasated red blood cells and hemosiderin deposition may be observed. In the plaque type, aggregates of spindle cells are present with extravasated red blood cells and hemosiderin deposition may be observed. In the plaque type, aggregates of spindle cells are present with extravasated red blood cells. The vascular component is less pronounced. Nodules are characterized by a predominance of spindle cells in parallel array with interspersed extravasated red blood cells. Cellular atypia is not pronounced in any form.

Laboratory studies

There are no characteristic laboratory abnormalities. Patients infected with HIV have laboratory abnormalities associated with AIDS.

Treatment and natural history

In most cases of sporadic and in some cases of endemic Kaposi's sarcoma, the disease appears limited, nodular, and indolent. Such disease tends to be radiosensitive and can be treated with low-dose radiation therapy (often electron beam), which gives high response rates and long-term control. In florid or infiltrating Kaposi's sarcoma unrelated to AIDS syndrome, local radiation is of palliative benefit, but relapse is common. Chemotherapy may be useful for short-term palliation, but eventual failure is common.

In the epidemic form the disease is disseminated. Radiation therapy, although useful palliatively for troublesome lesions, does not provide overall disease control. Chemotherapy may evoke temporary remissions in roughly one-half of patients, and useful agents include vinblastine, vincristine, and etoposide (VP-16-213). Response rates of 40% have been achieved using recombinant alpha-2 interferon. Most responses have been observed in patients without a history of opportunistic infection. Localized, nonvisceral Kaposi's sarcoma in AIDS not accompanied by opportunistic infection can frequently be managed with observation alone, with survival exceeding 2 years not uncommon.

Many of these patients have disease that is resistant to therapy and ultimately fatal, whereas other patients with active and progressive Kaposi's sarcoma die of other causes. Patients with sporadic or endemic nodular Kaposi's sarcoma may survive with indolent but persistent disease until they die of competing causes, whereas patients with epidemic AIDS-related Kaposi's sarcoma may die of opportunistic infection. Additionally, second malignancies are common, occurring in perhaps 30% or more patients with sporadic Kaposi's sarcoma. In AIDS-related Kaposi's sarcoma, the period of risk for a second malignancy may be less because of poorer overall survival. Nevertheless, second malignancies, particularly malignant lymphomas, have been commonly observed.

MYCOSIS FUNGOIDES

Etiology and epidemiology

Mycosis fungoides belongs to a spectrum of diseases referred to as cutaneous T cell lymphomas, in which malignant clones of T cells have a marked predilection for the skin. Also included in this disease spectrum are Sézary syndrome, Ki-1+ lymphoma, adult T cell leukemia/lymphoma, and a variety of others that form a heterogeneous group. Mycosis fungoides is more common among men, blacks, and older individuals and is increasing in incidence. The cause is unknown, but environmental, infectious, and genetic factors have all been postulated to play a role in the development of this disease.

Clinical features

The natural history of mycosis fungoides is widely variable: some patients have protracted preclinical phases followed by prolonged survival with relatively little morbidity; others have a fulminant course with rapid development of systemic dissemination and death. Mycosis fungoides generally evolves through three distinct cutaneous phases, from patch to plaque to tumor, sequentially over time. In the patch stage, the lesions are flat, nonpalpable, and erythematous or hyperpigmented and may be scaly. There is a predilection for covered areas of the skin. Lesions often assume unusual shapes and may have angulated borders. In a variant of this stage called poikiloderma vasculare atrophicans, the lesions are atrophic in appearance with mottled pigmentation, erythema, and telangiectasia. In the plaque stage the lesions are elevated above the surrounding skin surface and are erythematous, light brown, or violaceous in color. Unusual shapes such as arcuate or serpiginous are common. Tumor stage lesions are farther elevated above the skin surface. These may arise de novo or develop within existing plaques. Ulceration of cutaneous tumors is common and may lead to development of secondary infection (Plate III-15). The disease may progress to the development of an exfoliative erythroderma in which the skin becomes diffusely red and scaly. In this stage there are often severe pruritus and chilling caused by poor body temperature homeostasis.

Recent studies have indicated that extracutaneous dissemination probably occurs early in the course of the disease, often before diagnosis. The sites of dissemination are varied; disease is identified in virtually every organ system. Lymphadenopathy is present in about one half of all patients and in 80% to 90% of erythrodermic patients. Gross involvement of the peripheral blood occurs late. There is a strong association between gross lymph node and/or peripheral blood involvement and visceral disease. Dissemination to the bone marrow, liver, spleen, lungs, bones, central nervous system, and other organs generally occurs late in the disease and may be detectible only at autopsy.

Laboratory features and staging

The diagnosis of mycosis fungoides is generally established by skin biopsy. The cellular infiltrate of mycosis fungoides consists of malignant T helper cells admixed with variable numbers of inflammatory cells. In early lesions cellular atypism is often not pronounced. The atypical cells vary from small cells with hyperchromatic convoluted nuclei, referred to as cerebriform cells, to large cells with pale staining vesicular nuclei. In early lesions the cellular infiltrate is located predominantly in the superficial part of the dermis, is often arranged in a bandlike distribution, and characteristically extends into the epidermis with the formation of small groups of cerebriform cells called Pautrier microabscesses. With tumor formation the infiltrate extends deeper into the dermis and subcutaneous fat, and a higher proportion of atypical cells is found. In cases with extracutaneous involvement, the lesions have a cellular composition that closely resembles that found in the skin. Immunologic phenotyping and tests for monoclonality of lymphocytes by assay of antigen receptor gene rearrangements may be helpful in establishing a diagnosis in uncertain cases (Chapter 74).

On the average, 5 years elapse between the onset of

symptoms and the time a definitive diagnosis is made. Several skin biopsy procedures are often necessary to make a histologic diagnosis. If diagnostic biopsies cannot be obtained, the patient should be followed at regular intervals with repeat biopsies. Skin lesion mapping is helpful in determining the percentage of skin surface area involved. A complete blood count with particular note of the percentage of atypical convoluted cells should be performed (Plate III-5, I). A chest radiogram reveals gross pulmonary involvement, if present. An abdominal CT scan may be helpful in evaluating patients with advanced disease. Lymph node histologic characteristics often, but not always, correlate with the extent of skin involvement and the presence or absence of palpable lymph nodes. A bone marrow biopsy may be helpful in staging patients with advanced disease and occasionally may show evidence of involvement in patients with otherwise limited disease. Further evaluation of specific organ systems is performed as indicated by the results of the initial evaluation. A staging system using both clinical and histopathologic findings is shown in Table 96-2.

Differential diagnosis

The differential diagnosis of early cutaneous mycosis fungoides includes chronic dermatitis and parapsoriasis en plaque. Plaque and tumor stage of mycosis fungoides should be differentiated from pseudolymphoma, cutaneous B cell lymphoma, and leukemic infiltrates. Erythrodermic mycosis fungoides should be distinguished from other causes of erythroderma. Other types of cutaneous T cell lymphoma should also be considered in the differential diagnosis.

Table 96-2. Staging system for mycosis fungoides

Definitions

T Stage	***Adenopathy***
T1: Limited patch/plaque (<10%)	Ad^{+}: Palpable adenopathy
T2: Generalized patch/plaque (≥10%)	Ad^{-}: No palpable adenopathy
T3: Cutaneous tumor	
T4: Erythroderma	
Lymph node class (biopsy)	***Visceral***
LN1: Reactive node	V^{+}: Positive visceral biopsy finding
LN2: Dermatopathic node, small clusters of convoluted cells	V^{-}: Negative visceral biopsy finding
LN3: Dermatopathic node, large clusters of convoluted cells	***Blood***
LN4: Lymph node effacement	B^{+}: Positive blood smear result
	B^{-}: Negative blood smear result

Stages

IA: T1; Ad^{-}; LN1,LN2; V^{-}	III: T4; $Ad^{\pm}$: LN1,LN2; V^{-}
IB: T2, Ad^{-}: LN1,LN2; V^{-}	IVA: T1-T4; $Ad^{\pm}$, LN3 or LN4; V^{-}
IIA: T1, T2; Ad^{+}; LN1,LN2; V^{-}	IVB: T1-T4; $Ad^{\pm}$; LN1-LN4; V^{+}
IIB: T3; $Ad^{\pm}$; LN1,LN2; V^{-}	

From Sausville EA et al: Ann Intern Med 109:372, 1988.

Treatment and prognosis

The best approach for treatment of these patients is not agreed upon. Many treatments are initially effective, but subsequent relapse and dissemination of tumor are common. Treatment can be divided into two basic approaches, those aimed primarily at the cutaneous disease and those with systemic effect. Cutaneous patches and plaques are more responsive to topical treatment modalities than are tumors. Early cutaneous disease may respond to treatment with topical or intralesional corticosteroids or ultraviolet B irradiation. Total skin electron beam radiation is the single most effective treatment for cutaneous disease, and continuous complete remissions have been reported in approximately 40% of stage IA patients. Frequent remissions and occasional sustained long-term disease-free intervals have been reported in patients treated with photochemotherapy using oral 8-methoxypsoralen and ultraviolet A radiation (PUVA), and with topical mechlorethamine. The nitrosourea BCNU (carmustine) may be used topically in patients who are allergic or unresponsive to mechlorethamine. Local irradiation is useful in treating plaques or tumors unresponsive to other forms of treatment. Treating patients with advanced cutaneous disease or with visceral involvement often requires a systemic approach. Although many of these patients exhibit a response to cytotoxic chemotherapy, responses are generally of short duration and chemotherapy alone is not curative. Cytotoxic chemotherapy for lymphoma is discussed in more detail in Chapter 94. Other systemic agents that have been used in the treatment of mycosis fungoides include interferon alpha, fludarabine, cyclosporine, 2′-deoxycoformycin, and the retinoids. Photopheresis, in which the patient's lymphocyte-enriched blood obtained by leukapheresis is irradiated with ultraviolet A after ingestion of 8-methoxypsoralen and subsequently returned to the patient, is useful in some erythrodermic patients.

The survival of patients with mycosis fungoides is directly related to the type of skin involvement and the presence or absence of extracutaneous disease. Although the natural history is often long with slow disease progression, 70% of patients die of causes directly related to their disease. Death may result from infection, with sepsis usually originating in the skin, or from overwhelming infiltration of vital organs.

REFERENCES

Dover JS and Johnson RA: Cutaneous manifestations of human immunodeficiency virus infection. Arch Dermatol 127:1383, 1991.

Elder DE: Dysplastic nevus syndrome—biological significance. Semin Oncol 15:529, 1988.

Friedman-Kien AD and Saltzman BR: Clinical manifestations of classical, endemic African, and epidemic AIDS-associated Kaposi's sarcoma. J Am Acad Dermatol 22:1237, 1990.

Greene MH et al: High risk of malignant melanoma in melanoma-prone families with dysplastic nevi. Ann Intern Med 102:458, 1985.

Kemme DJ and Bunn PA: State of the art therapy of mycosis fungoides and Sezary syndrome. Oncology 6:31, 1992.
Koh HK: Cutaneous melanoma. N Engl J Med 325:171, 1991.
Zackheim HS: Cutaneous T-cell lymphomas: a review of the recent literature. Arch Dermatol 117:295, 1981.

CHAPTER

97 Breast Cancer

C. Kent Osborne

ETIOLOGY AND EPIDEMIOLOGY

Breast cancer is the leading cause of cancer death in women in the United States and Western Europe. In one of every nine women born in the United States breast cancer will develop during her lifetime. An estimated 170,000 new cases were detected in the United States in 1992, and an estimated 40,000 women die of the disease. Surprisingly, breast cancer is the most common cause of death of disease in young women between the ages of 25 and 35, and the most common cause of death of all causes in women between the ages of 35 and 50. In older women breast cancer mortality rate is second only to death caused by cardiovascular disease. Death from lung cancer now exceeds that from breast cancer in women in certain areas of the United States.

The cause of breast cancer is unknown, although a variety of risk factors have been identified that provide clues to its genesis (Table 97-1). Hormonal regulation of the breast is clearly related to the development of breast cancer, but the mechanisms are poorly defined. Early menarche or late menopause prolongs exposure to estrogen and is associated with increased risk. Prolonged estrogen administration for menopausal symptoms, particularly when combined with progesterone, is also associated with a slightly increased risk of breast cancer, although an increased risk has not yet been observed consistently with use of oral contraceptives. In contrast, early castration reduces the risk of breast cancer. Parity and age at the time of the first full-term pregnancy are also related to breast cancer risk. Early pregnancy reduces the incidence, whereas nulliparity and, especially, late pregnancy increase the risk. These data, together with studies in experimental model systems, suggest that sex steroid hormones may act as tumor promoters or cocarcinogens in concert with initiating agents to induce malignant change. For unclear reasons obese and/or tall women are at increased risk for breast cancer. This risk may relate to dietary or hormonal factors.

Table 97-1. Risk factors influencing the occurrence of breast cancer

Risk of breast cancer	Factor
Increased	Increasing age
	Early menarche
	Late menopause
	Nulliparity
	Late pregnancy (above age 30)
	Interrupted first pregnancy
	Western culture (? diet)
	Family history of breast cancer
	Benign breast disease with atypical epithelial hyperplasia
	Obesity
	Ionizing radiation
	Prolonged postmenopausal use of estrogens
	Prior diagnosis of breast cancer, colon cancer, endometrial cancer, major salivary gland cancer
	Alcohol intake
Decreased	Full-term pregnancy (before age 24)
	Early oophorectomy
No effect	Breast feeding (lactation)
	Oral contraceptive use
	Benign breast disease without atypical epithelial hyperplasia

Living in Western societies also increases the risk of breast cancer. Specific factors have not been identified, although high dietary intake of fat and dairy products and/or high-caloric intake has been implicated. Immigrants to the United States from areas of low breast cancer incidence have little change in incidence rates, but with succeeding generations the incidence rate approaches that of the U.S. female population.

Family history of breast cancer increases the risk to a variable extent. In first-degree relatives (mother, sister, or daughter) the risk is a function of whether the cancer was bilateral (5.4-fold increase) and whether it occurred during the premenopausal (3-fold increase) or postmenopausal (1.5-fold increase) period. The highest risk (8.8-fold increase) is observed in relatives of patients with bilateral breast cancer that develops in the premenopausal years. Obviously these women require careful monitoring because of the high risk of breast cancer development at a relatively young age.

Exposure to ionizing radiation also increases breast cancer risk. Survivors of atomic bomb exposure in Japan have an elevated incidence of breast cancer, especially if exposure occurred during adolescence. Children and older women appeared to be unaffected. Early exposure to radiation to the head (acne), neck, or chest (thymus) may also increase the risk of breast cancer. Moderate alcohol intake has been shown in several studies to be a risk factor for breast cancer.

BIOLOGY

The majority of breast carcinomas arise from large-, medium-, or small-sized duct epithelium. Tumors originating from duct epithelium but still confined to the duct lumen without invasion into adjacent stroma are called intraductal, or ductual carcinoma *in situ* (DCIS) tumors. These tumors rarely metastasize, and they have a high cure rate with local therapy. Carcinomas invading adjacent stromal tissues are called infiltrating duct carcinomas. These tumors have a propensity for early metastasis and a worse prognosis.

The concept of how a primary breast carcinoma spreads to distant sites has changed during the past 20 years. In the late nineteenth century, when William Halsted developed the radical mastectomy, it was assumed that breast cancer spread through the lymphatics, under the skin, and along fascial planes to involve the regional lymph nodes first. The lymph nodes were thought to provide a temporary barrier to further dissemination. With these principles in mind, Halsted reasoned that "en bloc" dissection of the primary tumor, adjacent normal tissue, and the regional lymph nodes (radical mastectomy) would result in a high cure rate. It is now clear that the major contribution of this procedure was a reduction in the local-regional recurrence rate with little impact on overall survival rate. In about half of all women with primary operable breast cancer and nearly 90% of those with significant numbers of axillary lymph nodes involved with cancer at the time of radical mastectomy recurrent disease in distant metastatic sites eventually develops, indicating early hematogenous dissemination of the tumor. Thus breast cancer is already a systemic disease in the majority of women at the time of presentation. Ultimate survival of patients depends on the net interaction between tumor and host defense factors. This concept led to the development of two new alternative treatment strategies—conservative breast cancer surgery to improve the cosmetic result and adjuvant chemotherapy after local therapy to attempt to eradicate distant micrometastases.

The natural history of breast cancer varies considerably from patient to patient. The disease can be indolent and slowly progressive with about 5% of patients surviving 10 years even without treatment. In other patients the disease takes a fulminating, relentless course resistant to all therapy and resulting in death within a few months of diagnosis. Several variables have been recognized as important prognostic factors for individual patients. The most important prognostic marker is axillary lymph node status. The actual number of positive lymph node findings represents a continuum of rising risk for later recurrence of disease after mastectomy. Histopathologic evidence of the degree of tumor differentiation is another important prognostic factor. Tumors displaying morphologic features reminiscent of those of normal breast tissue carry a lower risk of recurrence. Tumor size also correlates with risk of recurrence.

The presence of hormone receptors for estrogen and progesterone is biochemical evidence of tumor differentiation and indicates a relatively good prognosis. Abnormal deoxyribonucleic acid (DNA) content (aneuploidy) determined by flow cytometry reflects poor tumor differentiation and a higher risk for recurrence. Finally, an index of the proliferative potential of the tumor can be obtained by cell kinetic analysis to determine the fraction of cells in S phase of the cell cycle. Patients with high S fraction tumors have a higher risk for recurrence and a shorter survival. Certain cellular oncogenes have also been identified in human breast cancer tissue. Amplification or overexpression of the c-erb B-1 oncogene, which codes for the membrane receptor for epidermal growth factor, or the related c-erb B-2 (HER-2/neu) oncogene are associated with a higher risk of recurrence after mastectomy. Tumor content of the lysosomal protease cathepsin D, which has been implicated in tumor invasiveness, may also have prognostic significance. Knowledge of these prognostic factors is playing an increasing role in the design of appropriate therapy for the patient with breast cancer.

METHODS OF EARLY DETECTION AND SCREENING

Evidence suggests that the earlier a breast cancer is detected, the better the survival prospect of the patient. Preinvasive intraductal carcinomas are highly curable, and patients with small invasive cancers have a better survival rate than those with large tumors. Numerous methods have been developed to detect breast cancer at an early, potentially curable stage. However, the only screening method for asymptomatic women with documented survival benefit is mammography combined with regular physical examination of the breast by physician and patient. It is clear that this technique can detect cancers in the preinvasive and nonpalpable stage. Thermography, ultrasound, computed tomography, magnetic resonance imaging, and diaphanography have not yet proved useful as screening tools and remain experimental. The widespread use of screening mammography has been controversial because of cost considerations and because of the potential for carcinogenesis with repeated exposure to radiation. However, with modern equipment and proper expertise the radiation dose to the breast is low, and the estimated carcinogenic risk is infinitesimally small relative to the natural risk of the disease. A prudent approach is to obtain a baseline mammogram at age 35 and then to begin annual mammography in women after age 50. Women between the ages of 40 and 50 should be considered for periodic mammography every 1 or 2 years, depending on the presence of risk factors outlined in Table 97-1. Extremely high-risk women (multiple risk factors, previous breast cancer) may be considered for periodic mammography and close physician follow-up observation at an earlier age. In general, however, mammography is less useful in younger women because of increased breast density, and because the younger breast may be more susceptible to the carcinogenic effects of radiation.

HISTOLOGIC FEATURES

Most breast cancers are infiltrating adenocarcinomas that arise from the ductal or lobular epithelium (Table 97-2). These carcinomas have similar prognoses, whereas medullary carcinoma, colloid carcinoma, tubular carcinoma, and papillary carcinoma have a slightly better prognosis. Paget's disease of the breast is characterized by eczematoid changes in the nipple caused by neoplastic involvement of the epidermis. Inflammatory carcinoma is an uncommon clinical entity characterized by extensive erythema, edema, and induration of the breast caused by invasion of the dermal lymphatics by tumor cells. Prognosis is so poor that it must be treated as a systemic disease even when it is ap-

Table 97-2. Comparison of histologic types of infiltrating breast carcinoma in women

Histologic type	Percent of total cases of breast cancer	Average age at diagnosis (years)	Average size at diagnosis (cm)	Regional nodes involved at diagnosis (% of patients)	Median survival of treatment failures (years)	Crude survival (%)	
						5-year	10-year
Ductal carcinomas with fibrosis	78.1	50.7	3.1	60	3.75	54	38
Lobular carcinoma	8.7	53.8	3.5	60	3.25	50	32
Medullary	4.3	49.0	3.4	44	2.25	63	50
Colloid	2.6	49.7	3.8	32	4.3	73	59
Tubular carcinoma	4.6	48.6	3.9	32	2.7	73	58
Papillary	1.2	51.9	3.4	17	5.0	83	56

From a long-term follow-up study of 1458 patients with infiltrating breast carcinomas, all of whom were treated with a radical mastectomy at the Memorial and James Ewing Hospitals, 1940-1943. The histologic and statistical analyses were done by Drs. J. Berg and GF Robbins as reported in 1968 in McDivitt, et al: Atlas of Tumor Pathology, 2nd series, fascicle 2. Washington, DC, 1968, Armed Forces Institute of Pathology.

parently localized. Pure tubular carcinomas are also uncommon, but these very well differentiated tumors have an excellent prognosis.

CLINICAL FEATURES

Breast cancer is usually discovered by the patient as a painless mass in the breast. Although it may appear as a vague thickening in what is otherwise an area of physiologic nodularity, most carcinomas are hard and have an irregular border that can be relatively well defined. The term dominant mass is sometimes used to identify highly suspect lesions that have distinct character and margins. Breast pain, skin dimpling, nipple discharge, retraction, or erosions occasionally lead to diagnosis. Fixation of the cancer to the skin or pectoral fascia, skin edema or ulceration, satellite nodules, and presence of large axillary metastases are all signs of more advanced breast cancer and are uncommon at presentation. Rarely, patients show signs of metastatic disease without a palpable mass in either breast.

LABORATORY FEATURES

The diagnosis of breast cancer may be suggested by the presence of a hard, irregular dominant mass or by suspect mammographic findings. Confirmation of the diagnosis depends on histologic examination of tissue obtained by needle aspiration cytologic evaluation, needle biopsy, or incisional or excisional biopsy. With the advent of breast conservation surgery, the biopsy should be performed with the ultimate definitive therapeutic options in mind, so that appropriate tissue can be obtained without compromising the optimal cosmetic results and eliminating the need for repeated general anesthesia. Needle aspiration cytologic testing has become popular for patients desiring breast conservation. In experienced hands this technique is accurate and rapid and can be done under local anesthesia on outpatients.

Except when lesions are very small, tumor tissue should always be sent for estrogen receptor (ER) and progesterone receptor (PgR) analyses. Knowledge of receptor status provides important prognostic information and serves as a guide to treatment strategy if the patient should relapse. Growing evidence also suggests that cell kinetic analysis by flow cytometry and tritiated thymidine labeling index and oncogene expression are helpful prognostic indicators. In the near future these techniques will be widely applied, although currently they should still be considered experimental.

Tumor markers measured in serum are not helpful in establishing the diagnosis of breast cancer. No markers specific for breast cancer have been discovered, and those currently available lack the sensitivity and specificity for early detection of disease. Carcinoembryonic antigen (CEA), the breast cancer–associated antigen CA 15-3, human chorionic gonadotropin (HCG), and ferritin levels are elevated in some patients with primary breast cancer and in the majority with metastatic disease and are sometimes helpful in monitoring response to therapy.

DIFFERENTIAL DIAGNOSES

Many benign lesions of the breast may mimic clinically the symptoms and signs of breast carcinoma (see the box at upper right). Acute bacterial mastitis may easily be confused with inflammatory cancer. Fat necrosis may appear as a firm irregular dominant mass. Mammary dysplasia usually presents diffuse changes (lumps) in the breast but may present a single suspicious mass. Benign tumors can also be confused with carcinoma clinically. The majority of breast lumps prove to be benign, especially those in premenopausal women. Nevertheless, if there is any clinical question of the diagnosis, evaluation, including biopsy, should continue. Mammography and ultrasound are sometimes helpful in differentiating benign from malignant breast disease. It is important to emphasize, however, that suspicious masses should receive biopsy evaluation even if the mammogram finding is unremarkable. Ten to twenty percent of cancers cannot be seen mammographically. Needle aspiration of suspected cysts is also helpful. If fluid is obtained and the lump regresses with aspiration, the physician can be confident that the process is benign. The rare cystic carcinoma can sometimes be detected by cytologic

Differential diagnosis of breast mass

- Inflammatory disease
  - Acute bacterial mastitis
  - Chronic mastitis
  - Fat necrosis
- Mammary dysplasia (benign breast disease)
  - Adenosis
  - Cystic disease
  - Duct ectasia
- Benign tumors
  - Fibroadenoma
  - Papilloma
- Malignant tumors

evaluation of the cyst fluid. Solid dominant masses usually require definitive tissue diagnosis by aspiration cytologic examination, needle biopsy, or open excisional biopsy. These can be done as outpatient procedures. If the biopsy result is positive for carcinoma, a second definitive procedure can be planned after discussion with the patient. This two-step procedure is preferred to the older one-step operation in which women with suspicious lumps went to the operating room for general anesthesia with biopsy, frozen section diagnosis, and definitive surgery. Many patients found this process psychologically debilitating. Patients with "lumpy" breasts who have associated breast cancer risk factors pose a difficult management problem. Regular breast self-examination coupled with frequent breast examination, including detailed mapping of all lesions by an experienced physician, is required. Mammography may not be helpful in such patients because of the density of the breast tissue. Some patients require repeated biopsy procedures over a period of years to exclude malignant change.

STAGING AND PROGNOSIS

Once a histopathologic diagnosis of breast cancer has been established, the physician must determine the stage of the disease before planning therapy. Tables 97-3 and 97-4 summarize the relationship between the stage of disease and prognosis. The extent of staging before treatment of the primary tumor depends on the initial clinical stage of the patient. In a patient with clinical stage I disease without symptoms of metastases, chest radiography, mammography, complete blood count, and screening panel of blood chemical features (such as an SMA-12) are sufficient. Bone and liver radionuclide scans are not required unless symptoms or laboratory tests suggest metastases. In patients with clinical stage II disease a bone scan is sometimes recommended, but a liver scan is not necessary unless symptoms or liver function tests suggest metastases. For patients with clinical stage III or IV disease, bone scans are recommended, as well as any other tests required to assess symptoms or abnormal laboratory values. Bone marrow biopsy is generally unnecessary unless the patient has unexplained bone marrow dysfunction, such as the presence of anemia or nucleated red cells on the peripheral blood film.

Table 97-3. Survival of women with breast cancer relative to clinical stage

Clinical staging (American Joint Committee)	Crude 5-year survival (%)	Range of survival at 5 years (%)
Stage I	85	82-94
Tumor less than 2 cm in diameter		
Nodes, if present, not believed to contain metastases		
Without distant metastases		
Stage II	66	47-74
Tumors less than 5 cm in diameter		
Nodes, if palpable, not fixed		
Without distant metastases		
Stage III	41	7-80
Tumor more than 5 cm		
Tumor any size with invasion of skin or attached to chest wall		
Nodes in supraclavicular area		
Without distant metastases		
Stage IV	10	—
With distant metastases		

From Henderson I and Canellos GP: N Engl J Med 302:17, 1980.

Table 97-4. Survival of women with breast cancer relative to histologic stage

Histologic staging (National Surgical Adjuvant Breast Project)	Crude survival (%) 5-year	Crude survival (%) 10-year	5-year survival (%)
All patients	63.5	45.9	60.3
Negative axillary lymph nodes	78.1	64.9	82.3
Positive axillary lymph nodes	46.5	24.9	34.9
1-3 positive axillary lymph nodes	62.2	37.5	50.0
More than 4 positive axillary lymph nodes	32.0	13.4	21.1

From Henderson I and Canellos GP: N Engl J Med 302:17, 78, 1980.

TREATMENT OF LOCALIZED BREAST CANCER

Twenty years ago radical mastectomy was performed immediately after biopsy and frozen section diagnosis in the majority of women with primary localized breast cancer. With the change in our understanding of the mechanisms of breast cancer metastases and the recognition that survival is predetermined in most patients by distant micrometastases, clinical trials of more conservative, cosmetically appealing local therapies were initiated. Modified radical mastectomy has now become the most frequent operation performed in the United States in women with clinical stage I or II breast cancer. This procedure still involves en bloc removal of the breast and axillary contents, but the preservation of the pectoral muscles and the horizontal scar result in a more normal appearance of the upper chest wall. There is also convincing evidence now from retrospective studies as well as prospective randomized clinical trials that even less radical breast conservation procedures provide excellent local control without jeopardizing survival. Segmental mastectomy or lumpectomy involves excision of the breast mass, usually with a small rim of adjacent normal tissue. Axillary dissection must be done on all patients treated by breast conservation operations both for local control in the axilla and for pathologic staging purposes. Radiation therapy to the breast frequently with a "boost" dose to the area of excision is then given. With proper planning, patient selection, and technical expertise, these procedures can produce excellent cosmetic results. Patients with very large tumors, small breasts, or multicentric lesions identified by mammography are poor candidates for segmental mastectomy and are best treated by modified radical mastectomy followed by reconstructive surgery for optimum cosmetic results. Patients with active collagen vascular diseases are also poor candidates for breast irradiation because of increased risk of local complications. Most authorities now agree that postoperative chest wall and regional lymph node irradiation is not necessary for most patients undergoing modified radical mastectomy. Exceptions might be patients at very high risk for local recurrence such as those with tumor involvement at the margin of surgical resection, those with extension into the axillary fat from grossly involved axillary lymph nodes, or those with large central or medial primary tumors with more than four positive axillary lymph nodes. Combined surgery plus irradiation is useful for local control in patients with more advanced stage III or IV primary tumors.

ADJUVANT CHEMOTHERAPY FOR PRIMARY BREAST CANCER

On the basis of the concept that breast cancer is frequently already a systemic disease at the time of diagnosis, which assumes that many patients with stage I and especially stage II disease have micrometastatic disease in occult sites, the practice of early administration of systemic therapy after surgery to eradicate micrometastases has evolved. This treatment, commonly called adjuvant chemotherapy, involves the administration of chemotherapy and/or endocrine manipulation in patients at high risk for early recurrence and poor survival. More than 100 clinical trials in both axillary node positive and negative patients have been completed in the past 20 years.

The first-generation studies now have a minimum of 15 years of patient follow-up observation, and several conclusions can be drawn. First, combination chemotherapy using three to five drugs together is superior to the use of single agents. Evidence suggests that aggressive therapy with high drug doses is required for optimal results. Second, the optimal duration of therapy has not yet been established for all regimens, although 6 months appears adequate for the popular CMF regimen (cyclophosphamide, methotrexate, and 5-fluorouracil), and 3 to 4 months of doxorubicin regimens may suffice. Third, disease-free and overall survival rates are significantly improved by treatment, although many patients continue to relapse despite therapy. In the initial clinical trials, benefit of adjuvant chemotherapy was confined to premenopausal women. More recent trials, however, suggest that postmenopausal patients also benefit from adjuvant chemotherapy. In contrast, postmenopausal patients receive the most benefit from adjuvant endocrine therapy with the antiestrogen tamoxifen. Fourth, the ER and PgR status of the primary tumor may be useful in identifying high-risk patients requiring intensive therapy (receptor-negative) as well as patients who may benefit from the addition of endocrine therapy (receptor-positive). Clinical trials involving chemotherapy combined with endocrine therapy are promising, but it is premature to draw firm conclusions. Early results from adjuvant therapy trials in node-negative patients who have a lower natural risk for recurrence are also encouraging. A statistically significant improvement in recurrence rate with adjuvant therapy has been observed in several studies. Definitive conclusions about the risk/benefit ratio await longer follow-up study. A recent overview analysis of all randomized trials suggests that about one in four to one in three deaths at 10 years can be prevented by appropriate adjuvant therapy. The toxicity of adjuvant chemotherapy is acceptable: nausea, vomiting, alopecia, and myelosuppression are common but reversible, and death caused by drug toxicity is rare. Permanent ovarian dysfunction is an important long-term side-effect that occurs in some premenopausal patients. An increased incidence of second malignancy has not yet been observed after adjuvant chemotherapy. Commonly used adjuvant chemotherapy regimens are similar to those used for advanced disease and are shown in Table 97-5.

SYSTEMIC TREATMENT OF METASTATIC BREAST CANCER

The two major kinds of systemic therapy for the treatment of metastatic breast cancer are endocrine manipulation and cytotoxic chemotherapy. Other systemic therapies, such as immunotherapy or whole body hyperthermia, remain experimental. Similarly, the use of cytotoxic drugs combined with endocrine therapy has not yet proved superior to the sequential administration of each modality and thus should still be considered an experimental approach. Tables 97-5, 97-6, and 97-7 list the endocrine therapies and cytotoxic regimens most commonly used in the treatment of advanced breast cancer. Choosing between endocrine therapy and cytotoxic chemotherapy requires an understanding of the natural history of the disease and careful evaluation of the individual patient. The hormone receptor status of the patient's tumor is of paramount importance in making this choice. Only about 30% of all breast cancers are hormone dependent and respond to endocrine therapy. Hormone manipulation is unlikely (less than 10% response rate) to benefit a patient whose tumor lacks ER or PgR. If the tumor is

Table 97-5. Commonly used chemotherapy regimens

Regimen	Dose	Schedule
CMF* (repeat every 28 days)		
C = cyclophosphamide	100 mg/m^2 po	Days 1-14
M = methotrexate	40 mg/m^2 iv	Days 1 and 8
F = 5-fluorouracil	600 mg/m^{2}iv	Days 1 and 8
CMFVP (continuous for 1 year)		
C = cyclophosphamide	60 mg/m^2 po	Daily
M = methotrexate	15 mg/m^2 iv	Weekly
F = 5-fluorouracil	400 mg/m^{2}iv	Weekly
V = vincristine	0.625 mg/m^{2}iv	Weekly × 10 weeks only
P = prednisone	30 mg/m^2 po	Days 1-14
	20 mg/m^2 po	Days 15-28
	10 mg/m^2 po	Days 29-42, then discontinue
AC (repeat every 21 days)		
A = Adriamycin	60 mg/m^2 iv	Day 1
C = cyclophosphamide	600 mg/m^2 iv	Day 1
FAC (repeat every 21 days)		
F = 5-fluorouracil	500 mg/m^2 iv	Days 1 and 8
A = Adriamycin	50 mg/m^2 iv	Day 1
C = cyclophosphamide	500 mg/m^2 iv	Day 1

*Prednisone is sometimes used at a dose of 40 mg/m^2 po days 1-14. The CAF regimen is identical except Adriamycin 30 mg/m^2 iv days 1 and 8 is substituted for methotrexate.

ER-positive, the patient has a 50% chance of responding. If the tumor has a high concentration of ER and/or also contains PgR, the chance of response is increased to 70% to 80%. Patients with receptor-positive tumors also tend to have a more indolent course with prolonged survival, and

Table 97-6. Cytotoxic regimens useful in the treatment of advanced breast cancer

	Objective response rate (%)
Single agents	
Cyclophosphamide	34
Methotrexate	34
5-Fluorouracil	26
Phenylalanine mustard	22
Chlorambucil	20
Vincristine	21
Vinblastine	40
Doxorubicin	35
Mitomycin-C	21
Taxol	50
Combinations*	
CMF	34-62
CMFP	63
CMFVP	48-73
FAC	43-82

*C, cyclophosphamide; M, methotrexate; F, 5-fluorouracil; P, prednisone; A, Adriamycin (doxorubicin).

Table 97-7. Endocrine therapies useful in the treatment of advanced breast cancer

Therapies	Dose
Additive therapy	
Estrogens	
Diethylstilbestrol	5 mg po, tid
Ethinyl estradiol	1 mg po, tid
Antiestrogens	
Tamoxifen	10 mg po, bid
Progestins	
Megestrol acetate	40 mg po, qid
Androgens	
Fluoxymesterone	10 mg po, tid
Medical adrenalectomy	
Aminoglutethimide plus	250 mg po, qid
hydrocortisone	20 mg pohs, 10 mg po AM and PM
Ablative therapy	
Oophorectomy	
Surgical adrenalectomy*	
Hypophysectomy*	

*Major ablative procedures that have now been supplanted by less toxic medical treatments.

they have a predominance of bone and soft tissue metastases compared to those with ER-negative tumors, who have frequent visceral metastases and shorter survival. Care must be taken in interpreting the receptor assay results. False-negative values may arise from assay of very small tissue biopsy specimens, or from hormone receptor occupancy in patients taking exogenous estrogens, or in premenopausal patients with high endogenous progesterone levels during the luteal phase of the menstrual cycle.

A variety of other factors in addition to the hormone receptor status of a tumor may affect the choice of therapy. These factors include the length of time between removal of the original primary tumor and its recurrence (disease-free interval), site of metastatic disease, age of patient, and response to previous therapy. For example, it is widely recognized that a short disease-free interval (less than 2 years) between primary treatment and subsequent metastatic disease is associated with a rapidly growing tumor. Such patients tend to respond poorly to hormonal manipulation and may be more appropriately treated with cytotoxic chemotherapy. Conversely, a very long disease-free interval is often associated with a better response to hormonal manipulation than to cytotoxic chemotherapy. The site of metastatic disease may influence the choice of systemic treatment. Metastatic disease in the soft tissues, skin, regional lymph nodes, pleural space, or bone may respond well to endocrine manipulation, whereas metastatic tumor involving abdominal visceral organs or the brain rarely responds to such treatment. Endocrine manipulation may be especially effective in elderly women, whereas cytotoxic chemotherapy tends to be poorly tolerated by this group of patients. A good response to oophorectomy or other hormonal manipulation is also useful in predicting a good response to other kinds of endocrine treatment. Indeed, patients may pass successively from one form of endocrine manipulation to another when the disease is relatively indolent and restricted to either soft tissues or bone.

Before specific programs of treatment are discussed, several general principles underlying the management of patients with disseminated breast cancer must be stressed. First, cure is not possible with current treatment modalities, so that optimal palliation with the least toxicity is the primary therapeutic goal. Second, only one form of therapy at a time is employed. An exception to this rule is irradiation of a destructive lesion in a weight-bearing bone in combination with other modalities of treatment. Third, therapy is changed only if the disease is advancing, not if it is static or regressing. This approach is especially important in patients with bone metastases only, because such lesions are notoriously difficult to evaluate. Fourth, endocrine therapy might even be considered in ER- or PgR-negative patients despite the small chance of benefit especially in the elderly patient or the patient with indolent disease who cannot tolerate or who is no longer responsive to chemotherapy. Endocrine therapy should be considered for initial therapy in most receptor-positive or receptor-unknown patients, unless life-threatening visceral metastases are present. Fifth, after initiating endocrine therapy, patients should be observed for a minimum of 6 to 12 weeks. Tumor regression may be quite delayed in certain patients. Sixth, patients failing an initial course of endocrine therapy usually should be considered to have endocrine-unresponsive tumors that require chemotherapy. An exception to this rule is the patient with an indolent receptor-positive tumor that is not life-threatening. About 20% of such patients may respond to a second attempt at hormone manipulation. In contrast, patients responding to an initial course of hormone therapy should be considered for sequential second- or third-line therapies when the disease progresses. Such patients have an excellent chance for additional responses, although the duration of remissions tends to become shorter with each treatment. Initial responses generally last from 10 months to 2 years; occasional patients have remissions lasting many years. Seventh, newer forms of endocrine therapy such as antiestrogens or medical adrenalectomy have largely replaced the need for the more radical major ablative procedures of surgical adrenalectomy and hypophysectomy. Finally, some patients demonstrate a transient "flare" in their disease with hypercalcemia or increased bone pain during the first 2 weeks of additive hormonal therapy. Therapy should not be stopped in such patients (unless the flare is life-threatening); patients should be observed and symptoms controlled, and many enjoy tumor regression with continued therapy.

ENDOCRINE MANIPULATION

Menopausal status determines the precise type of endocrine therapy for patients whose tumors are known to be ER-positive and those whose receptor status is unknown. The initial choice of endocrine manipulation is commonly called primary hormonal manipulation. Subsequent manipulation is called secondary or even tertiary therapy. Doses of drugs for these regimens are summarized in Table 97-7.

Premenopausal patients

Patients who are menstruating or who are within 1 year of their last menstrual period are considered premenopausal.

Primary endocrine manipulation. Bilateral oophorectomy is still an acceptable initial therapy in premenopausal patients with metastatic disease who are candidates for endocrine therapy. This treatment is presumed to work by the ablation of ovarian estrogen and estrogen precursors that may stimulate the growth of breast cancer. Oophorectomy causes objective regression in approximately one third of all premenopausal women. The response rate is approximately 50% in those who have ER-positive disease and less than 10% in those who have ER-negative disease. Castration can also be achieved medically with the use of superagonists or antagonists of luteinizing hormone-releasing hormone. These agents may supplant surgical castration in the future when comparative studies are completed.

Some clinicians consider the antiestrogen tamoxifen to be preferable to oophorectomy as initial treatment. The frequency of response to tamoxifen is similar to that of oophorectomy. Patients who fail to respond to tamoxifen are less likely to benefit from oophorectomy. Thus tamoxifen may represent an effective initial therapy that may be supplemented subsequently by oophorectomy in responding patients whose disease progresses later.

Secondary endocrine manipulation. Patients who do not respond to oophorectomy usually proceed to treatment with cytotoxic drugs. Those who respond to oophorectomy and then relapse may respond to antiestrogens. These compounds block the effects of residual estrogens that may be stimulating the tumor after oophorectomy by competitively binding to and functionally inactivating ER. An alternative to use of antiestrogens in this setting is medical adrenalectomy with aminoglutethimide plus hydrocortisone. This therapy further reduces serum estrogen levels in postmenopausal patients (surgical or natural) by blocking production of adrenal androgens and by inhibiting the enzyme aromatase, which converts androgens to estrogens in peripheral tissues. This regimen may also be used as tertiary therapy in patients responding to tamoxifen. Other effective secondary or tertiary therapies use megestrol acetate or fluoxymesterone. Patients who no longer respond to endocrine manipulations or in whom rapidly progressing visceral disease develops are candidates for chemotherapy.

Postmenopausal patients

Patients whose last menstrual period occurred more than 1 year before the development of metastatic disease are considered postmenopausal. A subgroup of patients who are 1 to 5 years postmenopausal may also be identified as perimenopausal.

Primary endocrine manipulation. The initial treatment of choice for most postmenopausal women with metastatic breast cancer who are candidates for endocrine manipulation is tamoxifen. A response rate of 16% to 52% has been reported, with an average of 32% for unselected women. In patients with ER-positive tumors the response rate is approximately 50%. Conversely, fewer than 10% of ER-negative tumors respond. In the past, diethylstilbestrol (DES) was used to treat these patients. However, tamoxifen is less toxic than DES and has largely supplanted the older agent.

Secondary endocrine manipulation. Patients who respond to tamoxifen and then experience a relapse are candidates for secondary endocrine manipulation. Medical adrenalectomy, DES, megestrol acetate, or androgens are effective secondary and/or tertiary therapies. The choice of treatment is partially dependent on the individual patient and the relative toxicities of the agents. Younger women may reject androgen therapy because of the virilizing effects. Elderly patients, especially those with cardiovascular disease, are not good candidates for DES because of fluid retention and other cardiovascular side effects.

CHEMOTHERAPY

Cytotoxic chemotherapy is the initial treatment of choice for most patients with ER-negative tumors or individuals who have aggressive, life-threatening disease, regardless of receptor status. In patients with receptor-positive or receptor-unknown tumors, chemotherapy is withheld until the patient is shown to be refractory to endocrine treatment. Although partial responses can be obtained frequently with cytotoxic chemotherapy in advanced breast cancer, complete responses are uncommon, and chemotherapy rarely induces a long-term disease-free state.

Single agents

A variety of single agents with different mechanisms of action and different toxicities are effective in this disease (see Table 97-6). Among the most active and frequently used agents are doxorubicin (Adriamycin), cyclophosphamide, methotrexate, and 5-fluorouracil. Single agents usually induce remission durations of only a few months, and complete remissions are rare. Taxol is a new agent with response rates approaching 50%.

Combination chemotherapy. Combination chemotherapy was developed on the rationale that combining agents with different mechanisms of action and different toxicities might increase the response rate without increasing morbidity. It has had considerable success, particularly in the hematologic malignancies. Combination chemotherapy for advanced breast cancer has been studied extensively since 1969, when Cooper reported a high response rate to the five-drug combination of cyclophosphamide, methotrexate, 5-fluorouracil, vincristine, and prednisone (CMFVP). This report generated numerous clinical trials testing CMFVP or a modification of it against single agents. In general, the response rate, particularly the complete response rate, is higher for the combination regimens (Table 97-7). However, clear survival advantage has not been consistently demonstrated for the combination regimens compared to that for sequential use of the same agents except in patients with extensive visceral involvement. Nevertheless, combination chemotherapy has become standard for the initial treatment of advanced breast cancer in this country. Although there are numerous modifications of the original CMFVP regimen, no major differences in response rate or duration exist. Objective response rates range between 34% and 73%, and median response durations are consistently less than 1 year. Complete response rates average about 15%. Side-effects of these regimens include transient bone marrow suppression, occasional mucositis, alopecia, and nausea and vomiting. Doses of drug are modified according to individual patient characteristics and toxicity encountered. Cytotoxic drugs should be given only by physicians experienced in their administration. Commonly used regimens are described in detail in Table 97-5.

The introduction of doxorubicin (Adriamycin) is considered to be a major advance by some oncologists. However, the incorporation of this agent into combination regimens (such as FAC) has failed to achieve a significant improvement in response rate, response duration, or duration of survival despite its high activity as a single drug (Table 97-7). Nausea, vomiting, and alopecia are more severe with the Adriamycin regimens, and cardiac toxicity is a potential dose-limiting problem. There are no convincing data demonstrating that one combination regimen is superior to another in advanced breast cancer.

Patients who fail initial combination chemotherapy or who are not candidates for this more aggressive approach may be treated with single agents used alone in sequence. The use of drug combinations as second-line treatment offers no proven advantage. In general, secondary chemotherapy for advanced breast cancer is of modest benefit: responses usually last no more than a few months. The use of high-dose chemotherapy with autologous bone marrow transplantation has shown promise in the treatment of metastatic and high-risk primary breast cancer, but its role needs to be defined by additional study.

INTEGRATION OF TREATMENT MODALITIES

The management of breast cancer is in a state of flux; recommendations must be made within the context of the results of current therapeutic research. The evolving nature of the situation makes for some disagreement among experienced physicians about the specific management of some patient groups. In addition, it should be remembered that each patient has a distinct socioeconomic and psychologic background, spectrum of associated organ dysfunctions, and stage of disease activity. The tumor may also be distinctive in terms of the rate of growth, areas of dominant disease, and presence or absence of estrogen and progesterone receptors. The experienced physician individualizes therapy when appropriate. Nevertheless, it is useful to have a generalized approach to treatment as a guide. Figure 97-1 presents one such scheme.

PSYCHOLOGIC FACTORS AND REHABILITATION

Through the Reach to Recovery Program, the American Cancer Society has pioneered efforts to help the woman who has undergone mastectomy adjust to an altered body image. Breast reconstruction should also be considered in some patients who are not candidates for breast conservation procedures to augment psychologic adaptation. Whatever approach to rehabilitation is chosen, it is critical to employ a sensible and attentive manner in dealing with a patient's emotional concerns. Most patients do adjust, but the speed of adjustment can be markedly influenced by an attentive and sensitive physician.

MALE BREAST CANCER

Although rare, breast cancer in men nevertheless comprises approximately 1% of all breast carcinomas. The fact that men have approximately 1% as much breast tissue as women suggests that the difference in incidence of breast cancer in men and women may relate to the volume of tissue susceptible to neoplastic change. There are multiple reports of familial male breast cancer, and altered estrogen metabolism has been proposed as a possible etiologic factor. However, with the exception of idiopathic gynecomastia and Klinefelter's syndrome, predisposing conditions for the development of male breast cancer are poorly defined.

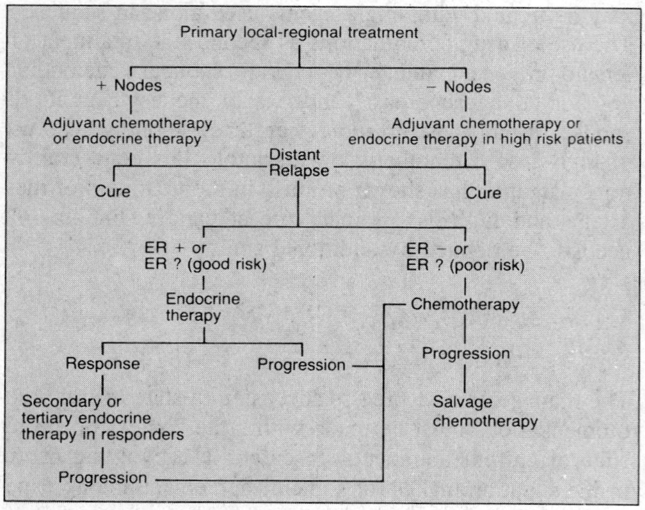

Fig 97-1. A sequential program of treatment for women with breast cancer. Key: + nodes, regional lymph nodes contain metastatic carcinoma; − nodes, regional nodes free of tumor; ER +, the tumor contains estrogen receptor in its cytoplasm; ER −, the tumor has either very low or no detectable estrogen receptor; Er ?, estrogen receptor status is unknown. (Modified from Haskell CM, Sparks FC, and Thompson RW, Breast Cancer. In Haskell CM, editor: Cancer Treatment. Philadelphia, 1980, Saunders.)

Numerous reports have confirmed a high frequency of estrogen receptors and progesterone receptors in male breast cancer tissue. Furthermore, the disease mimics female breast cancer in histologic features, clinical presentation, and tendency to metastasize to bone. Therapeutic considerations are also similar, although complete concordance does not exist. Specifically, it would appear that men with breast cancer should be treated with endocrine manipulation as the initial approach, even in fairly advanced disease. Primary endocrine manipulation in the male generally consists of orchiectomy. As an alternative, one may consider tamoxifen and, less frequently, androgens or DES. Hypophysectomy and adrenalectomy may also be considered in selected patients, although pharmacologic manipulations are replacing these operative procedures in men as they are in women. Although few data exist, combination chemotherapy seems to provide the same benefit to men as to women.

REFERENCES

Bonadonna G and Valagussa P: Chemotherapy of breast cancer: current views and results. Int J Radiat Oncol Biol Phys 9:279, 1983.

Bonadonna G et al: Ten-year experience with CMF-based adjuvant chemotherapy in resectable breast cancer. Breast Cancer Res Treat 5:95, 1985.

Clark GM et al: Progesterone receptors as a prognostic factor in stage II breast cancer. N Engl J Med 309:1343, 1983.

Early Breast Cancer Trialists' Collaborative Group: Systemic treatment of early breast cancer by hormonal, cytotoxic, or immune therapy. Lancet 339:1, 71, 1992.

Fisher B et al: Ten-year results of a randomized trial comparing radical mastectomy and total mastectomy with or without radiation. N Engl J Med 312:674, 1985.

Fisher B et al: Five year results of a randomized clinical trial comparing total mastectomy and segmental mastectomy with or without radiation in the treatment of breast cancer. N Engl J Med 312:665, 1985.

Fisher B et al: The pathology of invasive breast cancer: a syllabus derived from findings of the National Surgical Adjuvant Breast Project (protocol No. 4). Cancer 36:1, 1975.

Fisher B et al: Ten year results from the National Surgical Adjuvant Breast and Bowel Project (NSABP) clinical trial evaluating the use of L-phenylalanine mustard (L-Pam) in the management of primary breast cancer. J Clin Oncol 4:929, 1986.

Henderson IC and Canellos GP: Cancer of the breast: the past decade. N Engl J Med 302:17, 78, 1980.

Ingle JN et al: Randomized clinical trial of diethylstilbestrol versus tamoxifen in postmenopausal women with advanced breast cancer. N Engl J Med 304:16, 1981.

Miller AB: Screening for breast cancer. Breast Cancer Res Treat 3:143, 1983.

Miller AB and Bulbrook RD: Special report: the epidemiology and etiology of breast cancer. N Engl J Med 303:1246, 1980.

Osborne CK et al: Modern approaches to the treatment of breast cancer. Blood 56:745, 1980.

Osborne CK et al: The value of estrogen and progesterone receptors in the treatment of breast cancer. Cancer 46:2884, 1980.

Santen RJ et al: Aminoglutethimide as treatment of post-menopausal women with advanced breast carcinoma. Ann Intern Med 96:94, 1982.

Veronesi U et al: Comparing radical mastectomy with quadrantectomy, axillary dissection, and radiotherapy in patients with small cancers of the breast. N Engl J Med 305:6, 1981.

CHAPTER

98 Gynecologic Cancers

Vicki V. Baker

Cancers of the endometrium, cervix, and ovary are diagnosed in approximately 68,000 women each year and result in 22,000 cancer-related deaths. Cancer screening, prompt recognition of symptoms, and advances in therapy have reduced the mortality rate attributable to these diseases. Coordination of care by a gynecologic oncologist, an individual specifically trained to operate on, administer chemotherapy to, and manage the surgical and medical complications experienced by women with cancer of the female reproductive tract, is also an important component of the comprehensive care of these women.

ENDOMETRIAL CANCER

Epidemiology and etiology

Among cancers of the female genital tract, adenocarcinoma of the endometrium is the most common and is also associated with the best overall survival rate. It is primarily a disease of postmenopausal women although one fourth of cases are diagnosed in premenopausal women.

This neoplasm has been associated with a number of different risk factors (see the box below), many of which are associated with excessive stimulation of the endometrium by estrogen. However, this cancer also occurs in women who do not exhibit any of these risk factors, suggesting that other variables are also operative in the pathogenesis of this disease.

Clinical features

Painless postmenopausal vaginal bleeding, regardless of the amount or duration, is the sentinel warning sign of endometrial cancer. Premenopausal and perimenopausal women may experience menstrual irregularities and intermenstrual spotting. Advanced stage disease is often associated with anemia secondary to vaginal bleeding, inguinal adenopathy, lymphedema and deep venous thromboses of the lower extremities, urinary retention resulting from suburethral metastases, and weight loss.

The symptom of abnormal vaginal bleeding should always prompt further evaluation. A pelvic examination is performed in an effort to localize the site of bleeding. A Papanicolaou smear should be obtained although this test is not specific for endometrial cancer. Endometrial cancer cells are detected in only approximately 50% of cervical cytologic specimens obtained from women with endometrial cancer. Endometrial biopsy, which is routinely performed as an office procedure, should always be part of the diagnostic evaluation. This procedure compares favorably with formal uterine dilation and curettage performed in the operating room in terms of diagnostic accuracy, sensitivity, and specificity.

After the histologic diagnosis of endometrial cancer, chest radiography is performed to provide a baseline study and to exclude metastatic disease. Because the patient who has uterine cancer is at increased risk of breast cancer, mammograms should be obtained. In addition, patients with any change in bowel habits or those with stools positive for occult blood should undergo evaluation of the colon because the risk of colon cancer is also increased in patients with endometrial cancer.

Risk factors for endometrial cancer

- Obesity
- Unopposed estrogen hormone replacement therapy
- Diagnosis of colon cancer
- Diagnosis of breast cancer
- Chronic anovulation
- Low parity
- Late menopause
- Adult onset diabetes mellitus
- Hypertension
- Complex atypical hyperplasia of the endometrium

Treatment

The staging and primary treatment of endometrial cancer are surgical, consisting of abdominal hysterectomy, bilateral salpingo-oophorectomy, and selected biopsies of pelvic and para-aortic lymph nodes. Peritoneal washings should be obtained for cytologic study. Radiation therapy as primary treatment is reserved for those patients who are not surgical candidates.

Prognosis is directly related to stage of disease (Table 98-1). Other prognostic indicators include steroid hormone receptor status, ploidy, S-phase fraction, and overexpression of the HER-2/neu proto-oncogene by the malignant cells. After surgery, recommendations for additional ther-

Table 98-1. Staging and 5 year survival rate in endometrial cancer

Stage	Description	5-year survival (%)
I	Tumor confinement to uterine corpus	75
II	Tumor extension to endocervix or cervical stroma	55
III	Tumor extension to uterine serosa, retroperitoneal node biopsies positive for metastatic disease, vaginal metastases, positive peritoneal cytologic findings	30
IV	Tumor invasion of the bladder or bowel or presence of distant metastases	10

apy are based on the presence of high-risk factors such as poorly differentiated or deeply invasive neoplasms, positive surgical margin findings, metastatic disease, and positive peritoneal cytologic results.

In an effort to control extrauterine pelvic disease, whole pelvic radiation therapy, consisting of 45 to 50 Gy, is administered over a 4 to 5 week period in an outpatient setting. Chemotherapy is reserved for patients with distant metastatic disease and for those who experience recurrence after radiation therapy. Single-agent chemotherapy is associated with modest response rates of variable duration. Clinical responses in as many as 42% of patients treated with cisplatin (50 mg/m^2 IV once every 3 weeks) have been reported. Adriamycin (50 mg/m^2 IV once every 3 weeks) is associated with an objective response rate of 37%. 5-Fluorouracil (1000 mg/m^2 IV once every 3 to 4 weeks) is associated with a response rate of 23%, and cytoxan (1000 mg/m^2 IV once every 3 to 4 weeks) induces a response rate on the order of 21%. There is no evidence that combination chemotherapy is superior to single-agent therapy. Although complete response rates may be achieved with aggressive chemotherapy in a small number of patients who have advanced or recurrent disease, this rarely translates into curative therapy.

Hormonal therapy with high-dose progestational therapy, such as Megace (80 mg po bid) or antiestrogen therapy with Tamoxifen (20 mg po bid) may benefit patients with metastatic disease. Response rates of 13% to 42% are reported, although this therapy is not considered curative.

CERVICAL CANCER

Epidemiology and etiology

Invasive cervical cancer is preceded by a premalignant phase, cervical dysplasia. The transit time between the premalignant and malignant conditions is estimated to be 5 to 10 years in most cases. This interval, which gives ample opportunity for therapeutic intervention, in addition to accessibility of the cervix for inspection and testing, has contributed to the decline in the number of deaths secondary to invasive cervical cancer.

Risk factors for cervical cancer include young age at first sexual encounter, multiple male partners, or a male partner with multiple consorts. These observations provide circumstantial evidence that cervical cancer is a sexually transmitted disease. The identification of specific subtypes of human papillomavirus (HPV), which is a sexually transmitted disease, in a significant proportion of both dysplastic and neoplastic lesions of the cervix has strengthened this hypothesis. Although it has been postulated that HPV is the causative agent of cervical dysplasia and neoplasia, there is no conclusive evidence to support this contention. In addition, the dramatic increase in HPV infections of the cervix noted during the past decade has not been accompanied by a parallel increase in the number of premalignant and malignant lesions, suggesting that other causative factors contribute to the development of neoplastic cervical disease. Possible cofactors include the mutagens found in cigarette smoke that are selectively concentrated in cervical mucus, nutritional deficiencies, and the use of oral contraceptives. Alterations of the host immune system also appear to play an important role in predisposing patients to the development of cervix dysplasia and neoplasia. As an example, renal transplant patients exhibit a 40-fold increased risk of cervical cancer, emphasizing the need for periodic gynecologic examinations and Papanicolaou smears in these patients. There are also recent reports suggesting that the incidence of cervical dysplasia and neoplasia may be increased in patients infected with human immunodeficiency virus (HIV).

Diagnosis

Largely as a result of effective cervical cancer screening programs using the Papanicolaou smear, the goal of which is premalignant disease detection, the incidence of invasive cervical cancer and the number of deaths attributable to this disease have demonstrated a steady decline over the past two decades. Current recommendations by the American College of Obstetricians and Gynecologists concerning the frequency of Papanicolaou smear screening are provided in the box below.

To obtain a Papanicolaou smear, an unlubricated speculum is inserted into the vagina to expose the cervix. An Ayre spatula is rotated 360 degrees around the cervix to sample ectocervical cells, which are then promptly smeared onto a clean glass slide. A cytobrush is inserted into the endocervical canal and rotated to collect endocervical cells, which are also transferred to a glass slide. Once the cells are placed on the slide, they must be promptly fixed to prevent drying artifact.

A Papanicolaou smear is considered adequate when sufficient numbers of endocervical cells and squamous cells are present. The diagnosis of cytologic abnormalities is based on alterations in cell morphologic character, size, and nuclear appearance. The nomenclature for cervical cytologic reports is detailed in Table 98-2. Although the Papanicolaou smear currently provides the best cancer screening test available, a variable percentage of cases of dysplasia and carcinoma is not detected. Improper preparation of the smear, inaccurate interpretation, and presence of inflammatory cells or red cells that obscure visualization of the cervical cells contribute to false negatives. It is important that any suspicious appearing lesion on the cervix re-

Current recommendations concerning cervical cancer screening

- Annual Papanicolaou smears after age 18 or the onset of sexual activity, whichever occurs first
- After three consecutive normal smear results, subsequent screening is based on the presence of risk factors for cervical dysplasia/neoplasia
- "At risk" patients should be screened annually
- Low-risk patients should be screened every 3 years

Table 98-2. Nomenclature for cervical cytologic reports

Bethesda system	WHO system
Normal	Normal
Reactive or reparative changes	Atypia
Squamous epithelial abnormality of undetermined significance	Dysplasia
	Mild
Low-grade intraepithelial lesion (includes mild dysplasia and HPV)	Moderate
	Severe
High-grade intraepithelial lesion (includes moderate and severe dysplasia and carcinoma in situ)	Carcinoma in situ
	Invasive squamous cell carcinoma
Squamous carcinoma	Adenocarcinoma
Glandular cell abnormalities	

ceive biopsy evaluation regardless of the cervical cytologic finding report.

Treatment of dysplasia is never based solely on the results of a Papanicolaou smear. Colposcopy with directed biopsies of the cervix must first be performed to obtain a histologic diagnosis. Colposcopy involves inspection of the cervix at fourfold to sixfold magnification after the application of 3% acetic acid solution to the cervix. Biopsy specimens should be obtained from areas demonstrating abnormal vascular patterns such as punctation and mosaicism as well as areas of white epithelium, all of which are often associated with dysplastic epithelial changes. In addition, an endocervical curettage is performed to evaluate the endocervical canal for the presence of dysplasia.

Both cervical dysplasia and early invasive carcinoma of the cervix are asymptomatic conditions. Patients with more advanced disease may have vaginal discharge, postcoital spotting, and intermenstrual spotting. Patients with disease beyond the cervix may experience profuse vaginal bleeding, malodorous vaginal discharge, unilateral lower extremity edema or pain, and weight loss. Uremia secondary to bilateral ureteral obstruction caused by advanced disease extension into the paracervical tissue is not uncommon.

Treatment

After histologic confirmation of the diagnosis of dysplasia, the treatment options include cryotherapy, laser vaporization, excision of the transformation zone, and hysterectomy. The location and extent of the lesion seen at the time of colposcopy and the patient's wishes concerning future fertility determine which option(s) is appropriate.

In order to formulate a treatment plan after the diagnosis of invasive cervical carcinoma, the extent of disease must first be determined. In addition to a careful pelvic examination to assess the palpable extent of disease, select radiographic tests are helpful. A radiograph of the chest is obtained to detect pulmonary metastases. An intravenous pyelogram is performed to detect hydronephrosis or a nonfunctioning kidney, either one of which indicates advanced stage disease. Patients with large lesions that extend anteriorly beneath the bladder or posteriorly toward the rectosigmoid should be further evaluated by cystoscopy and sigmoidoscopy, respectively. Although computed tomography (CT) and magnetic resonance imaging (MRI) studies provide additional information about the extent of disease, this information is not incorporated into the clinical staging system currently used for cervical cancer (Table 98-3).

In general, cervical cancer is treated with radiation therapy. Whole pelvic radiation, consisting of 50 to 60 Gy, is given in 1.8 to 2 Gy fractions per day, 5 days a week for a total of 4 to 5 weeks. Intracavitary irradiation, in which radioactive sources are placed in close proximity to the cervix and parametriae, is also incorporated into the treatment plan.

Patients with small lesions confined to the cervix, who are surgical candidates, may be treated by radical hysterectomy and pelvic lymphadenectomy. These patients exhibit

Table 98-3. FIGO staging and 5 year survival in cervical cancer

Stage		Description	5 year survival
0		Carcinoma in situ	100%
I		Carcinoma confined to uterus	90%
	Ia	Preclinical invasive carcinoma, diagnosed by microscopy	
	Ia1	Minimal stromal invasion	
	Ia2	Invasion < 5 mm in depth and < 7 mm horizontally	
	Ib	Any lesion > Ia2	
II		Carcinoma beyond uterus, but not to sidewall or to lower third of vagina	70%
	IIa	No parametrial invasion	
	IIb	Parametrial invasion	
III		Carcinoma to sidewall or to lower third of vagina	44%
	IIIa	Tumor extension to lower third of vagina, but not to pelvic sidewall	
	IIIb	Tumor extension to pelvic sidewall or hydronephrosis or nonfunctioning kidney	
IV		Distant disease or invasion into adjacent organs	<14%
	IVa	Tumor invasion of bladder or rectum	
	IVb	Distant metastases	

comparable 5 year survival rates to those who are treated with radiation therapy.

After completion of therapy, patients should be seen at 3 to 4 month intervals for the first 2 years, followed by visits at 6 month intervals for the next 3 years. At each visit, a careful physical examination, including pelvic examination and Papanicolaou smear, should be performed. The value of periodic chest radiographs, intravenous pyelograms, and computed tomography has not been established.

Recurrent disease is most commonly diagnosed in the first 2 years after completion of therapy. Treatment options are determined by the location and extent of the recurrence and the patient's general medical condition. Recurrent disease in the nonirradiated pelvis is treated with radiation therapy with salvage rates of 30% to 40%.

When radiation therapy is not an option, recurrent disease in the pelvis that is surgically resectable may be treated by pelvic exenteration, in which the uterus, cervix, vagina, bladder, and rectosigmoid are removed. Although the morbidity and mortality rates of this operation are appreciable, it represents the patient's only realistic chance for cure.

Treatment of metastatic and recurrent, surgically unresectable disease with cisplatin chemotherapy (50 to 100 mg/m^2 IV every 3 weeks) is associated with response rates that range from 10% to 30%, but cures are anecdotal.

In summary, the 5 year survival of cervical cancer is directly related to stage of disease at the time of diagnosis (Table 98-3). Implementation of Papanicolaou smear testing has been the single greatest advance in the management of this disease, permitting disease diagnosis in premalignant stages when the cure rates approach 100%.

OVARIAN CANCER

Clinical features

Ovarian cancer holds the distinction of being the most lethal gynecologic cancer. Approximately 17,000 new cases of ovarian cancer were diagnosed in 1993 and 12,000 women died of this disease. A woman's cumulative lifetime risk of development of ovarian cancer is 1 in 76. Epithelial ovarian cancer, which is the most common histologic type, is generally a disease of postmenopausal women, although this cancer is also diagnosed in women during the third and fourth decades of life. The use of oral contraceptives is associated with a decreased risk of ovarian cancer. Factors associated with increased risk of epithelial ovarian cancer include low parity, delayed childbearing, and diagnosis of breast cancer. Hereditary factors increase the risk of ovarian cancer in a small subset of women. Approximately 5% of women with ovarian cancer can be classified by a currently recognized inherited ovarian cancer syndrome.

Less common ovarian neoplasms include germ cell and stromal cell tumors of the ovary. Germ cell tumors usually occur in prepubescent and adolescent patients with the exception of dysgerminoma, which is more common in the third decade. Stromal cell tumors are diagnosed in reproductive age and postmenopausal women.

Survival in ovarian cancer is clearly a function of stage of disease (Table 98-4). The disparity between 5 year survival rate of women with stage I and II disease and that of those with stage III and IV disease provides the rationale for the development of effective methods of early disease detection. As a cancer screening method, pelvic examination is insensitive and nonspecific. Although transabdominal and transvaginal ultrasound are useful radiographic tests that aid in the differentiation of benign and malignant pelvic masses, the applicability of these tests to cancer screening in the general population has not been demonstrated. Similarly, ovarian cancer screening tests based on measurement of serum tumor antigens such as the CA125 antigen, which is produced by over 85% of nonmucinous epithelial neoplasms of the ovary, exhibit sensitivities and specificities that are unacceptably low, given the limited prevalence of ovarian cancer in the general population. At this time, no screening strategies for ovarian cancer have been endorsed as public health policy.

Unfortunately, no pathognomonic signs are associated with neoplasms of the ovary. The detection of asymptomatic, early stage ovarian cancer is usually serendipitous. Patients with advanced stage ovarian cancer typically have a variety of nonspecific signs and symptoms, including abdominal distention, early satiety, nausea and vomiting, and weight loss.

The differential diagnosis of an ovarian mass is in part determined by the patient's age although considerable overlap occurs (Table 98-5). In general, young girls are at risk for malignant germ cell tumors and postmenopausal women are at risk for epithelial neoplasms. However, ovarian cancer of virtually every cell type has been diagnosed in females of all ages. The radiographic characteristics of the mass also assist in the preoperative differentiation of benign versus malignant masses. In general, malignant epithelial ovarian neoplasms are bilateral, exhibit cystic and solid components, and may be associated with ascites. When ovarian cancer is considered the likely diagnosis, it is advisable to consult a gynecologic oncologist to assist with the preoperative evaluation, surgery, and postoperative chemotherapy.

Table 98-4. Staging and 5-year survival rate for epithelial ovarian cancer

Stage	Description	5-year survival rate (%)
I	Carcinoma limited to ovaries	55
II	Carcinoma with extension to pelvis	40
III	Carcinoma with implants outside the pelvis or positive retroperitoneal nodes	5
IV	Distant metastases (positive pleural effusion, lung metastases, hepatic parenchymal metastases)	<5

Table 98-5. Differential diagnoses of ovarian masses with respect to age

Neonate	Prepubescent/adolescent	Reproductive age	Postmenopausal	Masses are
Simple cyst	Mature teratoma (dermoid) Cystadenoma	Functional cyst Endometrioma Mature teratoma	Fibroma Thecoma Cystadenoma	Benign
Primary ovarian cancer very rare	Germ cell tumors	Epithelial ovarian neoplasm Germ cell tumors Sex cord/stromal tumors	Epithelial ovarian neoplasm	Malignant

Treatment

The cornerstone of therapy for women with ovarian cancer is surgery, consisting of abdominal hysterectomy, bilateral salpingo-oophorectomy, omentectomy, surgical staging, and resection of all obvious disease. Because of the low incidence of bilaterality, unilateral adnexectomy and surgical staging without hysterectomy may be appropriate for patients with germ cell tumors when future fertility is of concern.

With the exception of stage I, well-differentiated ovarian neoplasms in patients who have undergone a thorough and complete staging operation, all ovarian neoplasms require additional therapy after surgery. Traditionally, cisplatin-based combination chemotherapy has been the first-line treatment for patients with epithelial ovarian cancer. A standard regimen includes 50 to 100 mg/m^2 of cisplatin and 1000 mg/m^2 of cyclophosphamide administered intravenously every 3 weeks for six to eight cycles of therapy. More recently, carboplatin, which is a cisplatin analog, has been used with cyclophosphamide as first-line therapy for epithelial ovarian cancer. The clinical results achieved with cisplatin and carboplatin regimens are comparable, but the reduced toxicity profile favors the use of carboplatin. Regimens for germ cell tumors include vincristine-actinomycin D-cyclophosphamide, vinblastine-bleomycin-cisplatin, and bleomycin-VP16-cisplatin.

Response to chemotherapy is assessed by monitoring of serum tumor marker levels when applicable in addition to pelvic examination before each cycle of therapy. The use of radiographic studies such as computed tomography and magnetic resonance imaging must be individualized. Second-look laparotomy to assess response to chemotherapy is generally reserved for patients participating in clinical research protocols.

Germ cell tumors were once considered uniformly lethal, but the administration of aggressive combination chemotherapy has resulted in striking improvements in prognosis. Although there is some reason for cautious optimism for the patient diagnosed with a germ cell tumor, that is not the case for the patient with epithelial ovarian cancer. In spite of aggressive, multiagent chemotherapy, most such women suffer persistent or recurrent disease. Although a variety of agents are used to treat these women, response rates are modest, ranging from 20% to 35%, and cures are rare. Death is usually the result of starvation secondary to a carcinomatous ileus.

REFERENCES

Lindahl B: Endometrial carcinoma: current concepts and future perspectives. Crit Rev Oncol Hematol 10:315, 1990.
Ozols RF, editor: Ovarian cancer. Semin Oncol 18:177, 1991.
Trope CG and Makar AP: Epidemiology, etiology, screening, prevention, and diagnosis in female genital cancers. Curr Opin Oncol 3:908, 1991.

CHAPTER

99 Cancer of the Testis and Prostate

C. Kent Osborne

TESTICULAR CANCER

Previously, the management of patients with malignant tumors of the testis fell primarily into the domain of the urologic surgeon and radiation therapist. However, over the past 20 years dramatic advances in chemotherapy have propelled the internist into a major role in the treatment of these diseases. Testicular cancer is now one of the malignancies most likely to be cured.

Epidemiology and etiology

Testicular cancer is uncommon, with only about 6000 cases annually in the United States. This contrasts with the annual incidence of breast or lung cancer of more than 150,000 cases. Although uncommon, testicular cancer is the most frequent solid tumor in males aged 15 to 35 years. These tumors are quite rare in both American and African blacks and in Asian peoples, suggesting a genetic causative factor.

The cause of testicular cancer is unknown, but several

factors may be important. Testicular maldescent results in a marked increase in incidence that may be reduced by orchiopexy in early childhood. A history of trauma to the testis is frequently obtained, but its role in carcinogenesis is not clear. Trauma to an established tumor may facilitate its spread. Animal studies suggest that endocrine factors may also be involved. A higher incidence has been reported in twins, suggesting the presence of genetic factors.

Classification

Tumors of the testis can be divided into several groups: gonadal stroma tumors, tumors of the spermatic cord and epididymis, germ cell tumors, lymphoma, and metastatic lesions. Lymphomas are the most common primary testicular neoplasm in men above the age of 55 years. Germ cell tumors, which are the most common in younger men, are the focus of the discussion in this chapter.

Germ cell tumors may develop along unipotential lines to form a seminoma or along totipotential lines to form a teratoma, embryonal carcinoma, choriocarcinoma, or yolk sac tumor. Tumors frequently contain more than one of these elements.

Clinical features

The presenting symptoms and signs, the appropriate diagnostic evaluation, and the staging classification can all be easily remembered if one understands the typical pattern of metastases for germ cell tumors of the testis. Most patients have a painless testicular mass. Occasionally the mass is quite tender, simulating epididymo-orchitis. A few patients experience symptoms from metastatic disease without a palpable testicular mass. Ultrasound of the testis may help to reveal an occult primary. Testicular cancer spreads in a predictable fashion. In most patients the first site of metastasis is the retroperitoneal lymph nodes. Enlargement of these nodes can be massive, resulting in back pain, sciatica, ureteral obstruction, renal failure, or obstruction of the inferior vena cava with edema formation in the lower extremities. Metastases can also progress up the lymphatic channels to involve mediastinal lymph nodes with symptoms and signs related to compression of mediastinal structures. Supraclavicular lymph nodes are also occasionally involved, and their enlargement may be the presenting manifestation of the disease. Hematogenous dissemination also occurs with germ cell tumors of the testis. The lung is by far the most frequent organ involved, providing the rationale for a complete diagnostic evaluation before radical surgery and during the course of the disease. The brain is also a frequent site of hematogenous dissemination, especially with choriocarcinoma. Necrosis with hemorrhage is common with choriocarcinoma and may result in a stroke-like syndrome. Occult testicular tumors may also have the manifestations of the ectopic production of human chorionic gonadotropin. A young adult male with gynecomastia should be thoroughly evaluated for the presence of a germ cell tumor.

Differential diagnosis and staging

The differential diagnosis of a testicular mass includes a hydrocele, spermatocele, varicocele, hematocele, periorchitis, and epididymo-orchitis. Most of these disorders can be excluded by a careful history and physical examination by an experienced urologist. If there is any doubt about the diagnosis, immediate surgical exploration with a high inguinal orchiectomy should be performed. Palpation should be kept to a minimum and a biopsy avoided because these may facilitate hematogenous spread. Testicular cancers proliferate very rapidly, and the chance for cure declines as the body tumor burden increases. Delay in diagnosis and treatment is a major problem and is usually attributed to lack of education of both physicians and patients.

After the diagnosis is made, a staging evaluation based on the typical pattern of spread of the tumor is performed to determine the extent of disease for treatment planning. This evaluation should include serial determination of tumor markers, chest radiograph, and computed tomography of the chest, abdomen, and pelvis. Bipedal lymphangiography is also advocated by some experts, especially when follow-up observation only is being considered in lieu of retroperitoneal lymph node dissection in clinical stage A patients. However, a false-negative finding rate of about 20% in detecting intra-abdominal involvement has prompted most urologists to perform routine radical retroperitoneal lymph node dissection in patients with nonseminomatous germ cell tumors, as both a diagnostic and a therapeutic modality. A "nerve sparing" node dissection prevents the complication of infertility caused by retrograde ejaculation.

The staging classification used by most physicians in the United States is shown in Table 99-1. Proper staging is important for its prognostic significance and for the design of appropriate treatment. The recurrence rate after orchiectomy and lymph node dissection varies according to the preoperative tumor burden (stage).

Tumor markers

A major advance in the management of testicular cancer came with the development of sensitive radioimmunoassays for alpha fetoprotein (AFP) and human chorionic gonadotropin (hCG) levels. AFP is a glycoprotein normally produced by fetal yolk sac, liver, and gastrointestinal tract. In addition to germ cell tumors with yolk sac or embryonal

Table 99-1. Staging classification for testicular cancer

Stage	Involvement	Recurrence rate (%)
A (I)	Confined to the testis	10
B (II)	Retroperitoneal nodes	50
C (III)	Supradiaphragmatic or visceral	—

elements, other tumors such as hepatoma and gastrointestinal malignancies may secrete AFP. Fortunately, AFP level is increased in only a limited number of benign conditions including parenchymal liver disease and ataxia telangiectasia. hCG is a glycoprotein hormone composed of alpha and beta subunits. A radioimmunoassay for the beta subunit (beta-hCG) does not cross-react with the pituitary glycoprotein hormones. hCG is normally produced by the placenta. It is also frequently elevated in patients with gestational tumors, germ cell tumors containing trophoblastic elements, and occasionally tumors of the liver, breast, stomach, pancreas, and lung.

The frequency and degree of elevation of AFP and hCG levels are proportional to the stage of disease. More than 90% of patients with extensive stage C disease have elevation of levels of one or both markers. Because of the high specificity, an elevated marker in a patient with a testicular mass is diagnostic of the presence of a germ cell neoplasm. In addition to their diagnostic implications, serial marker measurements are invaluable in the management of patients with germ cell tumors. They are critical for determining the presence of residual subclinical disease and monitoring for recurrence after surgical resection. Furthermore, these markers are helpful in evaluating response to chemotherapy in patients with advanced disease, and in localizing tumors in patients with occult residual disease. Lactate dehydrogenase (LDH) is also a valuable marker in this disease.

Therapy

Treatment of testicular cancer can be divided into local regional modalities, including surgery and radiation therapy, and systemic chemotherapy. Treatment depends on the extent of disease and whether the tumor is a pure seminoma or a nonseminomatous subtype.

Seminomas. Seminomas frequently are manifested as local-regional disease only, and 90% of patients have either stage A or B disease. The orderly lymphatic spread of these tumors and their exquisite sensitivity to radiation therapy have led to the routine use of radical orchiectomy followed by radiation therapy to involved and adjacent, clinically uninvolved lymph nodes. With these techniques, 95% of patients with stage A seminoma and 90% of patients with stage B are cured of their disease. Chemotherapy for advanced or recurrent seminoma is similar to that for the nonseminomatous subtypes.

Metastatic nonseminomatous germ cell tumors. Metastatic nonseminomatous germ cell tumors generally proliferate rapidly, and before effective chemotherapy, most patients died within a few months. Developments in chemotherapy, however, have made a dramatic impact on survival from this aggressive neoplasm.

Testicular cancer has long been known to be sensitive to cytotoxic drugs. During the past 20 years continued progress has been made as new drugs have been developed. The most active single agents include alkylating agents, actinomycin-D, vinblastine, bleomycin, and cisplatinum. Combination chemotherapy is clearly superior to single-agent therapy, and the historic development of several regimens is shown in Table 99-2. Today, more than 60% of patients with advanced testicular germ cell tumors can be cured of their disease. Not surprisingly, the success of therapy depends heavily on the tumor burden at the time of chemotherapy; nearly all patients with minimal disease (elevated marker levels only or small tumor masses) have prolonged survival, whereas less than half with bulky disease remain disease-free. This emphasizes the need for early diagnosis and therapy. Prolonged therapy is not required in this disease. Only three or four monthly courses of platinum-based combination chemotherapy are necessary for most patients. Regimens combining platinum and etoposide are as effective as and less toxic than those using vinblastine, at least in low-tumor-burden patients. More-intensive therapy is being investigated in the poor-prognosis patients with large tumor burdens. Maintenance therapy has not yet proved valuable. Common chemotherapy regimens used for testicular cancer are listed in the box on p. 940.

Table 99-2. Chemotherapy of testicular germ cell tumors

Year	Drugs	Complete response (%)	Cured (%)
1960	Chlorambucil, actinomycin-D, methotrexate	15	10
1970	Vinblastine, bleomycin	33	25
1972	Vinblastine, actinomycin-D, bleomycin	14	—
1974	Vinblastine, actinomycin-D, bleomycin, cis-platinum	50	24
1976	Vinblastine, actinomycin-D, bleomycin, cis-platinum, cyclophosphamide	63	44
1976	Cisplatinum, vinblastine, bleomycin	70	60
1986	Cisplatinum, etoposide, +, − bleomycin	70	60

An intriguing observation has been made since the development of effective chemotherapy for testicular cancer. A few patients have a significant reduction in the size of the tumor, but a residual mass persists. When these patients are taken to surgery for removal of residual disease, about one third have persistent tumor, one third have fibrosis only, and another third have benign teratoma. The mechanism for the conversion to a benign neoplasm is not clear but may be related to selective resistance of benign elements present in the original malignant tumor to chemotherapy, or differentiation of malignant to benign cells over time. In any event, surgical resection of localized residual masses should be considered in all patients with nonseminomatous germ cell tumors achieving only a partial remission with chemotherapy. Growing evidence suggests that second-look

Chemotherapy regimens for testis cancer

PEB
- Etoposide 100 mg/m^2, days 1-5, IV
- Bleomycin 30 units, days 1, 8, 15, IV
- Cisplatin 20 mg/m^2, days 1-5, IV
  - Repeat every 3 weeks for three cycles (good risk)
  - Repeat every 3 weeks for four cycles (poor risk)
  - Repeat every 3 weeks for four cycles without Bleomycin (good risk)

VIP (VelP) (generally used as salvage therapy)
- Cisplatin 20 mg/m^2, days 1-5, IV
- Ifosphamide 1.25 g/m^2, days 1-5, IV
- Mesna 400 mg 1, 4, and 8 hours after ifosphamide, days 1-5, and either:
- Etoposide 75 mg/m^2, days 1-5, IV, or
- Vinblastine 6 mg/m^2, days 1 and 2, IV

surgery is not required in patients with pure seminoma, although large residual masses may harbor viable tumor.

To obtain these excellent results, intensive chemotherapy is required. Thus these patients should be treated only in centers with the necessary expertise and supportive care facilities. Although treatment-related mortality is uncommon, toxicity can be life-threatening. The major toxicities observed with the active agents include nausea and vomiting, weight loss, alopecia, myalgias, constipation or ileus, and granulocytopenia. Bleomycin can cause fatal lung toxicity and pulmonary function should be assessed during treatment. However, the survival benefit in these young men far outweighs the risks of therapy.

Local-regional nonseminomatous germ cell tumors. The treatment of stage A or B disease remains controversial. Radical orchiectomy is the undisputed therapy for the primary tumor. Most physicians in the United States also favor surgical treatment of the retroperitoneal nodes, because of the relative radioresistance of nonseminomatous tumors and because of the additional prognostic information that a radical lymph node dissection provides. However, a "dry" ejaculate and sterility accompany radical lymph node dissection. Although this can be avoided by using the nerve-sparing procedure, some physicians prefer initial chemotherapy for patients with stage B disease and reserve lymph node dissections for those with residual masses. Some experts now withhold all treatment of the retroperitoneal nodes in patients with clinical stage A disease because of the relatively low risk for recurrence and the excellent salvage rate in those patients who do experience relapse. Those with embryonal elements or vascular invasion in the primary tumor are at high risk for nodal involvement.

The role of chemotherapy after appropriate local-regional treatment is also controversial. The recurrence rates for patients with stage B disease vary from 30% to 75%, depending on the extent of lymph node involvement. A randomized trial has demonstrated that for appropriate compliant patients, careful follow-up observation with delayed chemotherapy given to those who relapse is equivalent to immediate adjuvant chemotherapy. The high cure rate in patients with minimally advanced disease suggests that this strategy may be the optimum approach. In any event, it appears that with either therapy more than 90% of patients with stage B disease are cured.

PROSTATE CANCER

Adenocarcinoma of the prostate requires more than a casual understanding by internists, because of its high incidence in the older male population, because of medical complications associated with the disease process, and because medical treatment plays a major role in patients with metastatic disease.

Epidemiology and etiology

Whereas testicular cancer is the most common tumor in young men, cancer of the prostate is the most common tumor in elderly males in the United States. It ranks second to lung cancer in the male population. Prostate cancer is rare in men younger than 50, but the incidence steadily rises with age thereafter. The autopsy incidence of the disease is as high as 50% in older age groups, indicating that this tumor may remain clinically silent in a large segment of the population. Another striking feature of this neoplasm is the racial difference in occurrence. In this country the incidence in blacks has been rising for more than 40 years and is now more than 50% higher than in the white population. Internationally, the incidence of prostate cancer is highest in developed Western countries and lowest in the Far East. These geographic variations suggest that an environmental factor may be related to the development of the disease, but a clear cause has not been defined. Obesity, dietary fat, and meat consumption have been associated with increased risk for this disease.

Pathology

More than 95% of cancers of the prostate are adenocarcinomas. Sarcomas are rare. Histologic grading to quantify the degree of tumor differentiation is of important prognostic significance.

Clinical features

Unfortunately, prostatic cancer rarely causes symptoms until it is locally advanced or widely disseminated. Occasionally the diagnosis is suggested by the presence of a nodule confined to the prostate or diagnosed from a surgical specimen from a patient with benign prostatic hypertrophy. Early symptoms may be due to bladder outlet obstruction. Many patients with metastatic disease complain primarily of bone pain. Screening tests of proven value to detect the tumor at an earlier stage have not yet been developed.

Serum-prostate-specific antigen (PSA) level is elevated in benign prostatic disease, making its use as a screening test for malignancy difficult.

Nevertheless, periodic screening with rectal examination and PSA level determination, sometimes combined with rectal ultrasound, is gaining popularity. PSA values above 10 ng/ml or a rising PSA level (even in the normal range) over time may signify the presence of occult cancer that theoretically should be at a more curable stage. Mortality data using this approach, however, are lacking at present.

Diagnosis and staging

Appropriate diagnostic procedures are listed in the box below. The typical pattern of metastases from carcinoma of the prostate involves local invasion, regional lymph node involvement in the pelvic and para-aortic chains, and spread to bone. Visceral organs such as lung or liver may be involved but much less frequently. Parenchymal brain metastases are rare, although brain compression from skull lesions is not uncommon. Thus the pelvis, retroperitoneum, and bone are emphasized in the staging evaluation. Before radical surgery or radiation for clinically localized disease, many urologists now perform a pelvic lymphadenectomy to document the stage of disease accurately. Although androgen receptors have been identified in cancers of the prostate, their role in the clinical management of these tumors remains to be defined. The staging classification used by most physicians in the United States is shown in Table 99-3.

Table 99-3. Prostate cancer: staging classification

Stage	Sites of involvement
A	Confined to prostate, no nodule palpable
B	Palpable nodule confined to gland
C	Local extension
D	Regional lymph nodes or distant metastasis

Therapy

Localized prostatic cancer. Surgery and radiation therapy are the modalities used in the treatment of localized prostatic cancer, and a detailed discussion of these is not warranted in a textbook of medicine. Briefly, patients with stage A disease require no therapy, unless there is extensive microscopic involvement of the prostate, or unless the tumor is poorly differentiated. Younger patients should also be considered for treatment. The treatment of these patients, as well as those with stages B and C disease, remains controversial. Traditionally, the treatment has been surgical, with a staging pelvic lymphadenectomy followed by a total retropubic or perineal prostatectomy if the lymph nodes do not contain tumor. Complications include stricture, incontinence, and, most importantly, impotence. The new technique of "nerve-sparing" prostatectomy preserves potency in many patients. Radiation therapy is also an option for patients with localized cancer of the prostate, especially stage C. External beam radiation therapy and interstitial implants have been used, and results may be equivalent to those with surgical treatment, although follow-up time on these studies has been shorter. Complications include cystitis and proctitis; impotence occurs in only one third of patients initially, but with time the incidence rises. Extensive pelvic irradiation may compromise bone marrow reserve, making chemotherapy more difficult to administer if the tumor recurs. The exact role for these modalities remains to be defined. A large randomized prospective study is needed to assess these alternatives definitively.

Prostate cancer: diagnostic procedures

History and physical examination
Transrectal needle biopsy or TURP
Prostatic acid phosphatase, PSA, CEA, alkaline phosphatase level determination
Prostatic ultrasound (transrectal)
Computed tomography or magnetic resonance imaging
Radionuclide bone scan
Bone marrow biopsy
Pelvic lymphadenectomy
Tumor androgen receptor?

Advanced prostatic cancer. Therapy of patients with metastatic prostatic cancer often involves several treatment modalities. Surgical transurethral resection of prostatic tissue is often necessary for relief of obstructive urinary symptoms. Radiation therapy may be used for local palliation of bone pain.

The major treatment used in patients with stage D cancer of the prostate is endocrine therapy (see the box on p. 942). Traditionally bilateral orchiectomy or estrogen therapy with diethylstilbestrol (DES) has been used, but treatment with progestational agents, and more recently antiandrogens, is probably as effective. Luteinizing hormone-releasing hormone (LHRH) agonists and antagonists, which induce medical castration, without or with antiandrogens are effective treatments. These drugs are expensive and require daily subcutaneous injections. A randomized clinical trial suggests that "total androgen blockade" with an LHRH agonist combined with an antiandrogen (Flutamide) offers some advantage in disease control compared with medical castration alone.

About 70% of patients with advanced disease benefit from endocrine therapy. Although research evaluating the usefulness of measuring androgen receptors in cancer tissue is in progress, currently there is no method of predicting the androgen dependence of the tumor in a manner analogous to that for estrogen receptors in breast cancer. Most patients treated with endocrine therapy survive for 2 or 3

Systemic therapy for prostate cancer

Endocrine therapy

Orchiectomy
LHRH agonists
  Lupron depot 7.5 mg, IM, monthly
  Zoladex 3.6 mg, SC, monthly
Flutamide* 250 mg, PO, three times daily
DES 1-3 mg, PO, daily
Ketaconazole 400 mg, PO, every 8 hours
Stilphostrol 0.5-1.0 g, IV, daily (acute management only)

Chemotherapy

Cyclophosphamide 1 g/m^2, IV, every 3 weeks
Doxorubicin 20 mg/m^2, IV, weekly, or 40-60 mg/m^2, IV, every 3 weeks
5-Fluorouracil 600 mg/m^2, IV, weekly
Cis-platinum 60-100 mg/m^2, IV, every 3 weeks

*Flutamide administration may be combined with orchiectomy or one of the LHRH agonists.

Complications of prostatic cancer

Obstructive uropathy with renal failure
Spinal cord compression
Disseminated intravascular coagulation (DIC)
Pathologic fracture
Bone pain

years, although survival may be considerably shorter or longer in a few patients.

Most oncologists reserve endocrine treatment for patients with symptomatic stage D or refractory locally invasive disease. The term *symptomatic* includes bone pain, bone marrow compromise, ureteral or bladder outlet obstruction, or evidence of other organ failure or dysfunction related to tumor involvement. Reserving treatment for symptomatic patients is based on the observation of a Veterans Administration study that survival was not improved by initiating treatment earlier in the asymptomatic patient. Castration is considered to be the endocrine treatment of choice by many physicians, with additive hormonal therapies or LHRH analogs reserved for patients who refuse the surgical approach. This prejudice is probably related to the occasional morbidity and mortality observed with estrogen therapy. These complications include painful gynecomastia, fluid retention precipitating congestive heart failure in these elderly patients, thromboembolic disease, and an increase in deaths caused by cardiovascular disease. The increased death rate was observed in the VA study in patients treated with 5 mg per day of DES. This complication was not observed with a dose of 1 mg per day, a reduction that did not diminish antitumor activity. Interestingly, many physicians now use 3 mg per day of DES because of the observation that this dose (but not 1 mg per day) consistently lowers serum testosterone levels to orchiectomy levels. Patients on 3 mg per day of DES have not been evaluated systematically for an increased risk of early cardiovascular death. The recent development of synthetic antiandrogens such as Flutamide and LHRH analogs that have a low incidence of toxicity offers an alternate approach to the endocrine therapy of these patients.

Although endocrine therapy is palliative for many patients, the tumor eventually recurs, requiring additional treatment. Secondary endocrine therapy, in contrast to use in breast cancer, is not commonly beneficial in patients with prostatic cancer. Aminoglutethimide combined with hydrocortisone to inhibit adrenal androgens is sometimes beneficial in patients who have previously had an orchiectomy. Occasional subjective responses are obtained. For this reason, studies using cytotoxic chemotherapy were initiated. Success has been limited to date, although a few patients obtain temporary palliation, including 10% to 20% with objective tumor regression. There is no evidence that chemotherapy prolongs survival, and it should still be considered experimental. Cyclophosphamide, 5-fluorouracil, doxorubicin (Adriamycin), and cisplatinum all have modest antitumor activity (refer to the box at upper left). Combination chemotherapy has not yet proved superior to the use of single agents. The results of chemotherapy should be interpreted in the context of the clinical setting in which they have been given, to patients with far-advanced disease and large tumor burdens. Studies using chemotherapy earlier in the course of the disease are now underway.

Complications. Prompt recognition and treatment of potential complications of this disease may improve the quality of life for many patients. Several important complications are shown in the box above). Because of the relative radioresistance of prostatic cancer cells, rapidly progressing spinal cord compression should be approached surgically with decompression laminectomy.

REFERENCES

Blackard CE: The Veterans Administration Cooperative Urological Research Group's studies of carcinoma of the prostate: a review. Cancer Chemother Rep 59:225, 1975.

Catalona WJ et al: Measurement of prostate-specific antigen in serum as a screening test for prostate cancer. N Engl J Med 324:1156, 1991.

Crawford ED et al: A controlled trial of leuprolide with and without flutamide in prostatic carcinoma. N Engl J Med 311:1281, 1984.

Einhorn LH and Donohue JP: Cis-diamminedichloroplatinum, vinblastine, and bleomycin combination chemotherapy in disseminated testicular cancer. Ann Intern Med 87:293, 1977.

Einhorn LH et al: The role of maintenance therapy in disseminated testicular cancer. N Engl J Med 305:727, 1981.

Klein LA: Prostatic carcinoma. N Engl J Med 300:824, 1979.

Labrie F et al: New approach in the treatment of prostate cancer: complete instead of partial withdrawal of androgens. The Prostate 4:579, 1983.

Lange PH et al: Serum alpha fetoprotein and human chorionic gonadotropin in the diagnosis and management of non-seminomatous germ cell testicular cancer. N Engl J Med 295:1237, 1976.

The Leuprolide Study Group: Leuprolide versus diethylstilbestrol for metastatic prostate cancer. N Engl J Med 311:1281, 1984.
Logothetis CJ et al: Primary chemotherapy for clinical stage II nonseminomatous germ cell tumors of the testis: A follow-up of 50 patients. J Clin Oncol 5:906, 1987.
Mendenhall WL et al: Disseminated seminoma: re-evaluation of treatment protocols. J Urol 126:493, 1981.
Paulson DF: Carcinoma of the prostate: the therapeutic dilemma. Annu Rev Med 35:341, 1984.
Peckham MJ et al: Orchidectomy alone in testicular stage I nonseminomatous germ-cell tumors. Lancet 2:678, 1982.
Richardson RL et al: The unrecognized extragonadal germ cell cancer syndrome. Ann Intern Med 94:181, 1981.
Scott WW et al: Hormonal therapy of prostatic cancer. Cancer 45:1929, 1980.
Torti FM et al: Weekly doxorubicin in endocrine-refractory carcinoma of the prostate. J Clin Oncol 1:477, 1983.
Torti FM and Carter SK: The chemotherapy of prostatic adenocarcinoma. Ann Intern Med 92:681, 1980.
Williams SD et al: Treatment of disseminated germ-cell tumors with cisplatin, bleomycin, and either vinblastine or etoposide. N Engl J Med 316:1435, 1987.
Williams SD et al: Immediate adjuvant chemotherapy versus observation with treatment at relapse in pathological stage II testicular cancer. N Engl J Med 317:1433, 1987.

CHAPTER

100 Head and Neck Cancer

Daniel D. Von Hoff

Cancer of the head and neck comprises a heterogeneous group of tumors that includes a large number of different sites as well as different histologic types of malignancies (Table 100-1). Because of this heterogeneity, the natural history of tumors at each site varies considerably. As can be seen from Table 100-1, the majority of the tumors are squamous cell. In 1991 in an estimated 43,000 people head and neck cancer developed, and 12,000 died of the disease.

The male-to-female ratio of cases is 3:1. In addition to their high frequency, the impact of tumors in this anatomic region on the quality of life of patients is quite substantial, with defects in facial features, speech, and swallowing. Therefore early diagnosis to preserve both life and cosmetic appearance is of the utmost importance. Note that thyroid, parathyroid, and esophageal cancer are discussed in other portions of this textbook and are not covered here.

Table 100-1. Site and histologic characteristics of head and neck cancer

Site	Histologic varieties	Percent of head and neck cancers
Skin	Squamous cell, basal cell, adenocarcinoma	Variable
Oral cavity (lip, tongue, floor of mouth, buccal mucosa, gums, hard palate)	Squamous cell	40
Pharynx (nasopharynx, oropharynx, hypopharynx [excluding larynx])	Squamous cell, lymphoepithelioma	15
Larynx	Squamous cell	25
Paranasal sinuses (maxillary, ethmoid, sphenoid, frontal)	Adenocarcinoma	Variable
Salivary glands	Adenocarcinoma, adenoid cystic carcinoma, mucoepidermoid, malignant mixed	7

SQUAMOUS CELL TUMORS

Etiology and epidemiology

The exact cause or causes of squamous cell cancer of the head and neck are unknown. However, tobacco use is clearly associated with an increased risk. For people smoking two packs per day, the risk of developing head and neck cancer is two to five times that of a nonsmoking population. The use of chewing tobacco and the practice of dipping snuff have also been associated with premalignant lesions such as leukoplakia.

Alcohol consumption is a risk factor for head and neck cancer. The risk of developing head and neck cancer is 3 to 11 times higher for alcohol drinkers (3 oz of whiskey or 12 oz of beer per day) than for nondrinkers. When a person both consumes alcohol and smokes there appears to be a synergism between the risk factors. The risk of developing head and neck cancer for a smoker and drinker appears to be 15 to 16 times higher than it is for a nonsmoker and nondrinker.

Carcinoma of the nasopharynx has been associated with infection by the Epstein-Barr (EB) virus. A high correlation between the presence of the tumor and the presence of antibodies to EB virus in the host has been established. In addition, nasopharyngeal carcinoma cells frequently contain EB viral deoxyribonucleic acid (DNA). The EB virus also causes infectious mononucleosis (Chapter 251), a benign disease. It is not understood how presumably the same virus can cause two quite different diseases.

Other factors that seem to predispose to development of head and neck cancer include sunlight (lip), asbestos exposure (larynx), shoe, wood, or textile work (nasal cavity), furniture and nickel work (nasal cavity, maxillary sinus), betel nut chewing (tongue, oral cavity), syphilis (tongue), poor oral hygiene, ill-fitting dentures (oral cavity), and Plummer-Vinson syndrome (hypopharynx).

Precancerous lesions

The head and neck are relatively easy areas to examine. Despite this, most head and neck cancers are quite advanced at the time of diagnosis. Therefore during the routine examination of the head and neck, the internist must search carefully for both premalignant and malignant lesions, particularly in high-risk populations. For example, among patients at a Veterans Administration Hospital, one asymptomatic carcinoma is found in every 200 to 250 routine oral examinations. The anatomic areas at highest risk for premalignant or malignant change include the floor of the mouth, the ventrolateral aspect of the oral tongue, the anterior pillars, and the lingual aspects of the retromolar trigone. At least 90% of early carcinomas are found in these particular areas.

Leukoplakia and erythroplasia are two distinctive findings that are important in the oral examination. Leukoplakia is a thick, whitish plaque that can be either benign hyperkeratosis or an area where malignant change has already occurred. Malignant transformation of leukoplakia is seen in only 2% to 10% of instances. Erythroplasia is an asymptomatic area of granular red or smooth nongranular, velveteen appearance that is really an asymptomatic carcinoma. Usually such lesions have minimal depth of invasion. Biopsies should be done of areas of leukoplakia and erythroplasia to ascertain whether or not they contain carcinoma. Of great interest is a recent report of the use of 13-*cis*-retinoic acid to treat premalignant lesions of the oral cavity.

Some patients have multiple areas of precancerous and cancerous lesions. They are referred to as having field cancerization and pose difficult management problems.

Clinical and laboratory features

Unfortunately, a large number of patients are asymptomatic until the carcinoma has become quite large. Common symptoms include a sore that will not heal, dysphagia, hoarseness, loosening of teeth, dentures that will not fit, earache, and disturbances in hearing. Clinical signs include hoarseness (laryngeal carcinoma), cranial nerve abnormalities (nasopharyngeal, paranasal sinus carcinomas), trismus (tonsillar tissue tumors—a very bad prognostic sign), or chronic sinusitis (sinus carcinoma). Physical examination must include both inspection and palpation. A normal surface examination is incomplete without palpation. A small area of induration or nodularity may be readily felt, although it cannot be seen. If a tumor of the nasopharynx is being examined, palpation of any polypoid mass must be done very cautiously because severe hemorrhage can occur if a juvenile angiofibroma is torn.

The laboratory findings are not particularly helpful. Approximately 3% of patients have hypercalcemia as a very late manifestation of disease.

Evaluation and staging

When an area suspected of having malignancy is discovered, it is important to subject this area to biopsy examination. It is important to remember that a surgical excisional biopsy is better than a surgical incisional biopsy because for an excisional biopsy there is a lower incidence of recurrence than for an incisional biopsy. If the mass (or lymph node) is so large that excision is difficult, a needle biopsy of the lymph node is preferred. If on biopsy the diagnosis is malignancy, then formal staging must be performed to determine the extent of disease. Careful staging is very important both for decisions about treatment and for estimation of prognosis. Of particular note is the fact that multiple primary cancers (mostly of the lung but occasionally of the esophagus) are found in 10% of patients with head and neck cancer. In addition, multiple head and neck cancers are found in 10% to 20% of patients with a primary head and neck cancer. Of interest is the recent report that treatment of patients who have had one malignancy of the aerodigestive tract with 13-*cis*-retinoic acid can significantly decrease the risk of developing a second malignancy elsewhere.

On physical examination the tumor and involved lymph nodes must be measured. The extent of tumor involvement occasionally has to be determined by multiple biopsies around the tumor. For optimal staging of oropharyngeal cancer it is preferable for the patient to have a triple endoscopic examination (bronchoscopy. esophagoscopy, and laryngoscopy) with both examination and biopsy performed under one period of anesthesia. Radiologic evaluation may include films of the adjacent bony structures (e.g., mandible or base of the brain) and a computed tomography (CT) scan to define soft tissue masses. The search for metastases should include chest radiography. Bone scans and liver scans are indicated only if the patient has nodal disease and abnormal liver function test results or elevation of bone alkaline phosphatase levels.

The staging system currently used by most centers is the system of the American Joint Committee on Cancer. Table 100-2 details the T (tumor), N (nodes), and M (metastases) classifications. This is the general staging classification; it is slightly different for each tumor site. Once the T, N, and M classification of the patient is known, the stage can be determined as noted in Table 100-3. Identifying the correct stage of disease is the key to the future management of the patient.

Management

To determine the best method of management, consultation among specialists involved in the treatment of patients with head and neck cancer, including surgery, radiation therapy, and medical oncology, is necessary. Specialists should examine the patient, preferably in the setting of a staging conference, and arrive at a joint plan for optimum management. Coordinated treatment by all three modalities is termed combined modality management. A general scheme for management is shown in Fig. 100-1. Patients with stage I or II disease (Fig. 100-1, box 1) are usually treated with surgery alone, radiation therapy alone, or occasionally both. Depending on the important prognostic factors outlined later, the outlook is usually quite good, with 5 year survival rate for stage I disease approaching 75% to 100%

Table 100-2. American Joint Committee TNM classifications for squamous cell head and neck cancer (oral cavity)

Tumor		Nodes*		Metastases	
T_x	No information available on primary tumor	N_0	No clinically positive nodes	M_x	Not assessed
		N_1	Single clinically positive homolateral node ≤3 cm in diameter	M_0	No distant metastasis
T_0	No evidence of primary tumor			M_1	Distant metastasis present
T_{is}	Carcinomas in situ				
T_1	Tumor 2 cm or less in greatest diameter	N_2	Single, clinically positive homolateral node >3 cm but ≤6 cm in diameter, or multiple, clinically positive homolateral nodes ≤ 6 cm in diameter		
T_2	Tumor greater than 2 cm but ≤4 cm				
T_3	Tumor greater than 4 cm in diameter				
T_4	Tumor greater than 4 cm with deep invasion involving antrum, pterygoid muscle, root of tongue, or skin of neck	N_3	Massive homolateral node(s) bilateral nodes or contralateral node(s)		

*Note: Cervical nodal classifications are more extensive than the abbreviated form shown here. For more complete detail, please refer to the American Joint Committee citation listed in the References.

Table 100-3. American Joint Committee stages for head and neck cancer (squamous cell)

Stage	TNM Inclusion
I	T_1 N_0 M_0
II	T_2 N_0 M_0
III	T_3, N_0 M_0
	T_1, T_2 or T_3 N_1 M_0
IV	T_4, N_0 or N_1, M_0
	Any T, N_2 or N_3, M_0
	Any T, and N, M_1

and for stage II disease, 60% to 75%. For patients with stage III or IV disease who are judged operable (Fig. 100-1, box 2), the standard treatment is surgery followed by radiation therapy. Because the results of surgery followed by radiation therapy have been disappointing (5 year survival rates of 10% to 30%), there has been a great deal of investigation into using chemotherapy before surgery, to shrink the tumor. Surgery is then followed by radiation therapy to destroy any remaining viable tumor cells. There is no question that combination chemotherapy (e.g., *cis*-platinum combined with 5-fluorouracil) can dramatically shrink large tumors. In some instances, there has been no histologic evidence of tumor in the surgical specimen. However, randomized trials of chemotherapy used before surgery and radiation versus no chemotherapy used before surgery and radiation have not yet shown that preoperative chemotherapy has any effect on the disease-free interval or on patient survival. Because the prognosis is so poor and this is an area of active investigation, patients should be offered participation in relevant ongoing clinical trials.

Recently in one important type of head and neck cancer the initial use of chemotherapy to shrink patients' tumors has been reported to have a major impact on quality of life. The Veterans Administration Research Group reported a study in which patients with operable stage III and IV squamous carcinoma of the larynx were randomized either to receive standard treatment (laryngectomy followed by radiation therapy) or to receive chemotherapy first, followed by radiation therapy (with no laryngectomy). A laryngectomy was only performed as a salvage procedure for patients with recurrent disease in the larynx or for those who did not achieve control with the chemotherapy and radia-

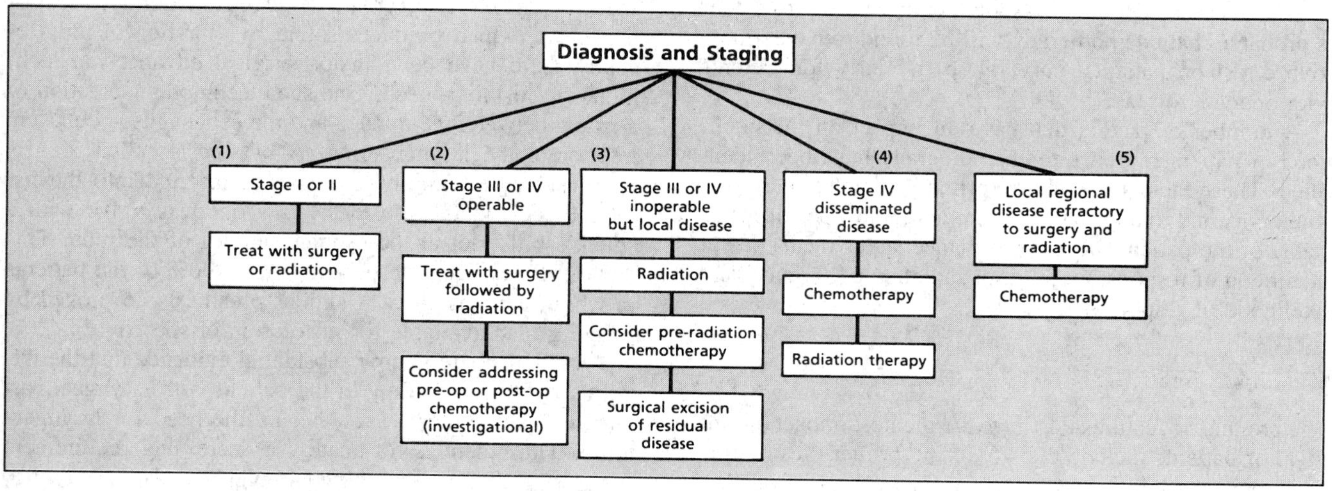

Fig. 100-1. Scheme for management of a patient with head and neck cancer.

tion therapy. Of note is that there was no difference in survival rate in the groups. This is a very important finding because it is the first study that clearly demonstrates that use of chemotherapy as initial treatment can lead to preservation of an important organ for quality of life, the larynx.

For patients with inoperable stage III or IV disease (Fig. 100-1, box 3), the usual treatment is radiation therapy by either external beam or brachytherapy, or both. However, with this approach there are very few 5 year survivors (approximately 10%). In an attempt to improve these results, chemotherapy has been given before radiation. Chemotherapy can cause dramatic shrinkage of tumors, making them more amenable to treatment with radiation. Again, however, it has not been conclusively demonstrated that shrinkage by chemotherapy has a positive impact on survival of patients. This approach is an area of active investigation, and patients with inoperable stage III or IV head and neck cancer should be offered participation in ongoing clinical trials. Use of chemotherapy given concurrently with radiation is another area of active investigation, as is the use of intra-arterial chemotherapy to shrink the tumor and make it more amenable to radiation or radiation followed by surgery.

Patients who have disseminated malignancy or advanced local regional recurrences that are refractory to surgery and radiation are usually treated with chemotherapy (Fig. 100-1, boxes 4 and 5). Basically, four standard agents are available for treatment of patients with advanced head and neck cancer: methotrexate, *cis*-platinum, 5-fluorouracil, and bleomycin. When used alone, each of these agents has a 10% to 30% response rate (i.e., it shrinks the tumor by ≥ 50%). Complete disappearance of disease is unusual. Until recently there has been no evidence that combinations of these chemotherapeutic agents improved the response rate or the percentage of cases of complete disappearance of disease. However, recently developed combination regimens of *cis*-platinum plus 5-fluorouracil or *cis*-platinum plus 5-flourouracil plus leucovorin seem to have substantially improved the response rate (60% to 90%). In addition, the percentage of patients achieving complete disappearance of disease has also improved (40% to 60%). If the incidence of complete responders can be improved, it is probable that chemotherapy will be found to have a positive effect on patients' survival, particularly for patients with operable disease.

A number of factors that have an impact on the likelihood of patient response to chemotherapy have been identified. These factors include the primary site of disease (nasopharynx and hypopharynx are unfavorable), performance status of the patient (poor performance status means lower likelihood of response), and prior radiation or surgery (less likelihood of response).

Prognostic features

The prognostic features that have the greatest impact on survival of patients include the site of the primary lesion (nasopharyngeal cancer is worse than cancer of the oral cavity), stage (higher stage is worse), degree of differentiation (poorly differentiated is worse), performance status (nonambulatory patients do worse), nutritional status (malnourished do worse), and prior therapy (patients who have failed prior therapy do worse).

Natural history

As noted, prognosis is most closely related to stage of disease. For stages I and II disease, the 5 year survival rate ranges from 75% to 100%, depending on prognostic factors. For patients with stages III and IV disease, the prognosis is poor, with a 10% to 40% 5 year survival. If the patient's local disease cannot be controlled, a significant number of clinical problems develop. A tumor in the larynx can grow, necessitating an emergency laryngectomy to prevent suffocation. Tumor infiltration of the tongue or pharyngeal wall can cause swallowing difficulties and aspiration of food into the lungs, resulting in an aspiration pneumonia. Tumor invasion of major arteries can cause massive hemorrhage and death.

For patients in whom good local and regional control of disease is obtained, there is the threat of development of distant metastases. Most distant metastases occur within the first 18 months after definitive surgery or radiation therapy. Patients at greatest risk of developing distant metastases are those with nasopharyngeal or hypopharyngeal lesions. Distant visceral metastases are most common in the lung (20%) and the liver (8%). Bone is the second most common site of distant metastasis (14%). It seems that with greater success in control of primary local or regional disease, there is actually an increase in the incidence of distant metastases. This is related to the fact that patients are now living long enough for metastases to grow to visible size.

Rehabilitation

The patient with a laryngectomy has a most devastating defect that needs to be addressed. Preoperatively and postoperatively the patient can be instructed in the technique of esophageal speech. However, only about 60% of laryngectomy patients are able to develop ability to produce intelligible esophageal speech. An alternative to esophageal speech is the electrolarynx, a device held externally against the throat, which produces sound by vibration of air. Recently there have been major surgical advances in techniques to restore speech. One such technique is creation of a fistula between the trachea and the esophagus about 1 cm inferior to the laryngostoma. A prosthesis called Singer-Blom voice restoration prosthesis is inserted into the fistula. Basically, the prosthesis is a one-way valve with a "duck's bill" slot at the esophageal end of the tube. This device allows fluent speech in 70% to 90% of the patients in whom it is inserted. A similar prosthesis developed by Pange is also available for restoration of speech.

As noted, there is now substantial evidence that the initial use of chemotherapy in the patient with laryngeal carcinoma can, in most cases, negate the need for laryngectomy. Thus there is fortunately a decreasing requirement for prostheses in patients with laryngeal cancer because they can now keep the larynx.

NONSQUAMOUS CELL TUMORS

Salivary gland tumors

Tumors of the salivary glands may be either malignant or benign and constitute about 7% of all head and neck tumors. Tumors of the major salivary glands (parotid, submaxillary, and sublingual) are usually benign, whereas the majority of tumors of the minor salivary glands (present in the palate, tongue, pharynx, tonsils, and nasal cavity) are malignant. This section deals only with malignant salivary gland tumors. Their cause is unclear, although survivors of the atomic bomb blasts did have a higher than usual incidence of salivary gland tumors. Neither tobacco nor alcohol seems to play a role in their development.

Histologic types of salivary gland tumors include mucoepidermoid, adenoid cystic carcinomas (cylindromas), and adenocarcinomas. Mucoepidermoid tumors have a good prognosis, particularly if they are low grade and have a preponderance of mucinous elements. However, higher-grade tumors do recur locally and metastasize. Adenoid cystic carcinomas are slow-growing tumors with a great propensity for perineural invasion beyond the field of obvious tumor involvement. The tumor frequently metastasizes to lung, bone, and brain, but many patients survive 10 to 15 years even with evidence of widely disseminated disease.

Treatment of malignant salivary gland tumors is usually surgical. Patients with disease that is too locally advanced for surgery should receive radiation therapy, although these tumors are not highly radiosensitive. Experience with chemotherapy is very limited, but complete responses have been documented.

Basal cell carcinoma

Basal cell carcinomas are the most common form of human cancer. They are discussed in detail in Chapter 326. Eighty-five percent of basal cell carcinomas appear on the head and neck. The tumor is generally locally invasive and nonmetastasizing. The interval between diagnosis of the primary and metastatic disease is 7 to 43 years. The most common pattern of metastasis is to the regional lymph nodes. A solitary metastasis is frequently the only manifestation of metastatic disease. Basal cell carcinoma is usually treated by surgical excision. Recurrent disease is usually treated by repeat excision and/or radiation therapy. The tumor is also responsive to chemotherapy with *cis*-platinum.

Verrucous carcinoma

Verrucous carcinoma is a variant of squamous cell carcinoma. It is a low-grade malignancy that is often associated with leukoplakia and is common in tobacco chewers. Macroscopically, the tumor is an exophytic fungating mass with large fronds. Microscopically, the well-differentiated squamous carcinoma cells are covered by a thick keratinizing layer. The treatment of choice is surgical excision. There is controversy about the use of radiation therapy.

REFERENCES

American Joint Committee on Cancer: Staging of cancer of head and neck sites and of melanoma. Chicago, 1980, American Joint Committee on Cancer.

Biller HF and Lucente FE: Conservation surgery of the head and neck. Semin Oncol 4:365, 1977.

Fedder M and Gonzalez MF: Nasopharyngeal carcinoma. Am J Med 79:365, 1985.

Fletcher GH: Place of irradiation in the management of head and neck cancers. Semin Oncol 4:375, 1977.

Forastiere AA: Review: management of advanced stage squamous cell carcinoma of the head and neck. Am J Med Sci 291:405, 1986.

Hong WK et al: The effectiveness of 13-*cis*-retinoic acid (13-CRA) in the treatment of premalignant lesions in the oral cavity. N Engl J Med 315:1501, 1986.

Hong WK et al: Prevention of second primary tumors with isotretinoin in squamous-cell carcinoma of the head and neck. N Engl J Med 323:795, 1990.

Kish JA et al: A randomized trial of cisplatin (CACP) + 5-fluorouracil (5-FU) infusion and CACP + 5FU bolus for recurrent and advanced squamous cell carcinoma of the head and neck. Cancer 56:2740, 1985.

Malefatto JP et al: The clinical significance of radiographically detected pulmonary neoplastic lesions in patients with head and neck cancer. J Clin Oncol 2:625, 1984.

Mashberg A and Barsa P: Screening for oral and oropharyngeal squamous carcinomas. Cancer 34:262, 1984.

McKenna RJ: Tumors of the major and minor salivary glands. Cancer 34:24, 1984.

Mead GM and Jacobs C: Changing role of chemotherapy in treatment of head and neck cancer. Am J Med 73:582, 1982.

Panje WR: Prosthetic vocal rehabilitation following laryngectomy—the voice button. Ann Otol Rhinol Laryngol 90:116, 1981.

Pratt LL: Workup and staging of patients with head and neck cancer. Semin Oncol 4:357, 1977.

Rothman K and Keller A: The effect of joint exposure to alcohol and tobacco on risk of cancer of the mouth and pharynx. J Chronic Dis 25:711, 1972.

Singer MI and Blom ED: An endoscopic technique for restoration of voice after laryngectomy. Ann Otol Rhinol Laryngol 89:529, 1980.

Wolf et al: Induction chemotherapy plus radiation compared with surgery plus radiation in patients with advanced laryngeal cancer. N Engl J Med 324:1685, 1991.

Wynder EL and Hoffman D: Tobacco and health: a societal challenge. N Engl J Med 300:894, 1979.

CHAPTER

101 Lung Cancer

Duane Sigmund

The epidemiologic features and causes, general clinical picture, and diagnostic considerations in primary lung cancer are discussed in Chapter 214. The focus of this chapter is on staging, treatment, and prognosis.

STAGING

The fundamental purpose of staging in any disease is to determine the most appropriate therapy for a given patient and to assist in the determination of the patient's prognosis. Staging represents a quantitative assessment of disease burden. A secondary benefit is that accurate staging allows comparisons of outcome of therapy across many groups of patients and improves the interpretation of clinical trials. Accurate staging is of critical importance in patients with lung cancer.

Non–small cell lung cancer

Squamous cell carcinoma, adenocarcinoma, and large cell carcinoma of the lung generally are classed together under the heading of non–small cell lung cancer (NSCLC) for the purposes of staging and treatment because of similarities in clinical behavior. Collectively, these histologic types account for 75% to 80% of all primary lung neoplasms seen in the United States. Surgical resection remains the mainstay of treatment for NSCLC. The International Staging System, developed by the American Joint Commission on Cancer in conjunction with the International Union against Cancer, is a reflection of that fact. Staging is based on assessment of the size, location, and extent of invasion of the primary tumor (T), the degree of lymph-node invasion (N), and the presence or absence of distant metastatic disease (M). Each increase in T, N, or M correlates with a worsening prognosis, as does each increment in stage (Table 101-1).

Once a diagnosis of NSCLC has been made, the cost-effective staging process begins with an accurate history and physical examination. Nearly one half of patients have surgically unapproachable disease at the time of presentation and only about one third have cancers that ultimately prove to be resectable. Squamous cell tumors tend to arise more centrally and often are quite advanced at the time of presentation compared with other NSCLCs. Adenocarcinomas and large cell tumors tend to arise more peripherally and invade the pleura and chest wall. Adenocarcinomas may metastasize earlier in their development than squamous cell tumors. Constitutional symptoms such as weight loss

Table 101-1. Staging of carcinoma of the lung

TNM definitions

Primary tumor (T)

T_X Tumor proved by the presence of malignant cells in bronchopulmonary secretions but not visualized roentgenographically or bronchoscopically, or any tumor that cannot be assessed as in a retreatment staging

T_0 No evidence of primary tumor

T_{IS} Carcinoma in situ

T_1 A tumor that is 3 cm or less in greatest dimension, surrounded by lung or visceral pleura, and without evidence of invasion proximal to a lobar bronchus at bronchoscopy

T_2 A tumor more than 3 cm in greatest dimension, or a tumor of any size that either invades the visceral pleura or has associated atelectasis or obstructive pneumonitis extending to the hilar region; at bronchoscopy, the proximal extent of demonstrable tumor must be within a lobar bronchus or at least 2 cm distal to the carina; any associated atelectasis or obstructive pneumonitis must involve less than an entire lung

T_3 A tumor of any size with direct extension into the chest wall (including superior sulcus tumors), diaphragm, or mediastinal pleura or pericardium without involving the heart, great vessels, trachea, esophagus, or vertebral body, or a tumor in the main bronchus within 2 cm of the carina without involving the carina

T_4 A tumor of any size with invasion of the mediastinum or involving heart, great vessels, trachea, esophagus, vertebral body or carina or presence of malignant pleural effusion

Nodal involvement (N)

N_0 No demonstrable metastasis to regional lymph nodes

N_1 Metastasis to lymph nodes in the peribronchial or the ipsilateral hilar region, or both, including direct extension

N_2 Metastasis to ipsilateral mediastinal lymph nodes and subcarinal lymph nodes

N_3 Metastasis to contralateral, mediastinal lymph nodes, contralateral hilar lymph nodes, ipsilateral or contralateral scalene or supraclavicular lymph nodes

Distant metastasis (M)

M_0 No (known) distant metastasis

M_1 Distant metastasis present—specify site(s)

Stage grouping of TNM subsets

Occult carcinoma	T_X	N_0	M_0
Stage 0	T_{IS}	Carcinoma in situ	
Stage I	T_1	N_0	M_0
	T_2	N_0	M_0
Stage II	T_1	N_1	M_0
	T_2	N_1	M_0
Stage IIIa	T_3	N_0	M_0
	T_3	N_1	M_0
	$T_{1\text{-}3}$	N_2	M_0
Stage IIIb	Any T	N_3	M_0
	T_4	Any N	M_0
Stage IV	Any T	Any N	M_1

(>10% of baseline) and bone pain raise the likelihood of disseminated disease and in themselves worsen the prognosis. Palpable adenopathy and organomegaly may direct attention to sites of metastatic disease and spare the patient unnecessary invasive diagnostic procedures. Fine-needle aspiration of suspected metastatic disease is widely available and should be used to confirm the presence of metastases.

Baseline laboratory investigations are desirable and may further guide the diagnostic evaluation. A posteroanterior (PA) and lateral chest roentgenogram, complete blood count, coagulation studies, serum calcium level, liver function studies, and alkaline phosphatase level are appropriate and complement the history and physical examination.

If disseminated disease is not suspected after initial evaluation of the patient, then additional testing is indicated. The goal is to identify patients who may benefit from surgical resection, primarily those with stages I, II, and IIIa disease. Routine radionuclide scans are not of general value in the absence of specific physical findings, symptoms, or abnormal laboratory findings. The role of computed axial tomography (CT scan) of the chest for evaluation of the mediastinal lymph nodes remains controversial.

CT scanning is of limited benefit in the staging of patients with NSCLC because of its low specificity (88%) and sensitivity (71%). CT scanning also is not capable of distinguishing the presence or absence of malignant chest wall involvement. Despite the deficiencies of CT scans, their use remains popular. An emerging consensus is to omit mediastinoscopy and proceed with definitive surgery in those patients whose mediastinum is "uninvolved" in terms of chest CT scan criteria, but to proceed with mediastinal node sampling in patients whose mediastinal nodes are "abnormal" as indicated by CT scan. Enlargement of mediastinal nodes is caused by benign processes approximately as often as neoplastic processes. Patients should not be denied definitive surgical therapy without histologic confirmation of metastatic disease as the cause of enlarged mediastinal nodes. In many institutions, the adrenal glands can be included in the chest CT scanning, which may be of benefit. Asymptomatic adrenal metastases may be present in 10% to 15% of patients with NSCLC, more commonly in patients with adenocarcinoma and poorly differentiated tumors than with squamous cell carcinomas. Solitary adrenal masses may be benign adenomas or metastases. Fine-needle aspiration may be required to establish the diagnosis. CT scanning of the abdomen generally is not helpful but may be indicated in patients with abnormal screening blood evaluation findings or disease that appears to be locally advanced in the chest.

All patients without known stage IV disease should be offered bronchoscopy, if not already performed for diagnosis. Rigid bronchoscopy remains a valuable tool, although flexible fiber optic bronchoscopes have become increasingly popular. Bronchoscopy permits an accurate assessment of the proximal extent of endobronchial involvement and thus assists in determination of the appropriate T designation. Tumors more than 2 cm from the carina are designated T_2; those less than 2 cm from the carina, but not involving it, are T_3. Tumors that involve the carina are classified T_4, which establishes the patient's disease as at least stage IIIb and therefore not appropriate for surgical cure, except in highly selected cases.

For patients with tumors T_3 or less, nodal biopsy procedures are generally indicated. The purpose of such biopsies is to identify those patients who have N_3 disease (stage IIIb) and who therefore are not surgically curable. Mediastinoscopy and anterior mediastinotomy for lesions on the left side remain the most popular methods; many centers use cervical mediastinoscopy for direct evaluation of the paratracheal, tracheobronchial, and anterior subcarinal nodes. In skilled hands, these procedures have low morbidity rates. Those patients with N_2 or less advanced disease are candidates for surgical exploration via thoracotomy. Multiple node sampling at the time of operation completes the staging process. Meticulous lymph node dissections for the purpose of cure remain of questionable value.

Small cell lung cancer

Approximately 20% of primary lung cancers are so-called small cell tumors. These tumors differ from the other histologic subtypes of primary lung cancers in that early and widespread hematogenous dissemination is the rule, not the exception. In addition, small cell lung cancer is not considered to be a surgically treatable disease, except in the infrequent case when it is manifested as a solitary pulmonary nodule (Chapter 215). This fact was established more than 20 years ago by a Medical Research Council Study that randomized patients to surgical excision or chest irradiation without surgery. Surgery did not improve the survival rate. Thus except in very unusual circumstances, surgical treatment is not indicated. TNM staging has not been prognostically or therapeutically valuable in cases of small cell lung cancer and generally is not applied. Rather, small cell cancer is "staged" on the basis of its extent vis-à-vis the thoracic cavity. "Limited stage" small cell cancer consists of disease confined to the ipsilateral hemithorax and/or the regional lymph node drainage. All of the disease should fit within a single radiation port. The presence of a malignant pleural effusion does not increase the patient's stage. "Extensive stage" cancer encompasses all other patients who have small cell lung cancer that is not classified as "limited."

A careful history and physical examination are as important in cases of small cell lung cancer as in those of NSCLC. Particular attention should be paid to the central nervous system because of the high frequency of metastases to the brain. About 8% of patients have asymptomatic central nervous system metastases at the time of diagnosis. Routine CT scanning of the head is less popular than in the past because of data that overall survival rate and quality of life are not affected by early whole brain irradiation. Fine-needle aspiration cytologic study of suspicious findings can establish the presence of disease outside the chest. Bone marrow examination may be indicated if no other sites of spread are identified by physical examination or screening laboratory tests. Unilateral aspiration and core biopsy of bone marrow are adequate; bilateral sampling increases the yield by only about 5%. The presence or absence of anemia does not correlate with marrow involvement, but nucleated red blood cells may be present on the peripheral blood smear when tumor is in the marrow. Radionuclide bone scanning can be helpful in detecting metastatic lesions and should be obtained in most patients.

THERAPY

Non–small cell lung cancer

Patients with stage I and II NSCLC are candidates for surgical resection (Fig. 101-1 and Table 101-2). Intraoperative histologic assessments are required to determine the appropriate scope of the surgery. The optimal extent of resection remains controversial. Some believe that wedge resection is adequate for early stage disease, whereas other clinicians consider lobectomy the minimum procedure required. More extensive procedures may preclude reresection for recurrences because of compromised pulmonary reserve. Several randomized clinical trials in progress are evaluating this issue. Postoperative chemotherapy or radiotherapy has no proven benefit for patients with stage I or II NSCLC and cannot be considered standard therapy at this time.

Cases of stage III disease are more problematic. Increasingly, these patients are being offered neoadjuvant treatment with chemotherapy and/or radiation. At the present time, research data do not support routine use of such therapy. Patients interested in such therapy should be referred for entry into one of the clinical trials that aim to establish the role of adjuvant therapy.

Not all individuals with IIIa disease are likely to benefit from surgical resection. Patients may be grouped according to whether the N_2 extent is clinically apparent on chest radiography or at bronchoscopy. Those patients without clinically apparent N_2 disease whose diagnosis is made at the time of resection have a high rate of complete resection and a 5 year survival rate of around 30%. Those patients with clinically apparent N_2 disease, on the other hand, have only a 14% chance of complete resection and a dismal 6% survival rate at 5 years.

Early chest irradiation for stage IIIa patients and in lieu of surgery for stage IIIb patients remains controversial.

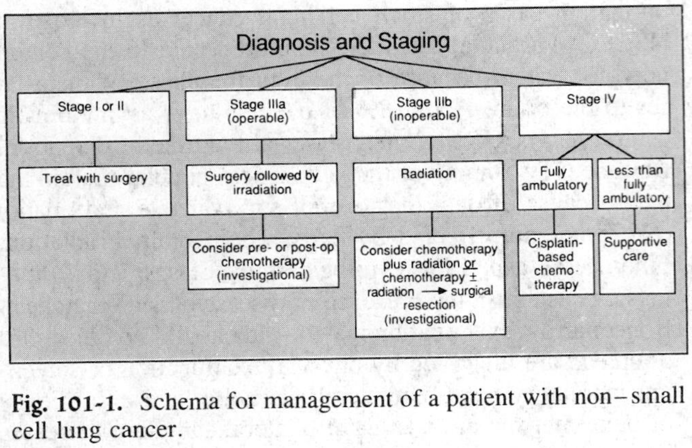

Fig. 101-1. Schema for management of a patient with non–small cell lung cancer.

Table 101-2. Surgical staging by TNM and survival in non–small cell lung cancer at 5 years with surgery ± radiation therapy

		Survival at 5 years (%)
Stage I	$T_1N_0M_0$	60
	$T_2N_0M_0$	50
Stage II	$T_1N_1M_0$	40
	$T_2N_1M_0$	30
Stage IIIa	$T_3N_0M_0$	20
	$T_3N_1M_0$	15-20
	$T_{1-3}N_2M_0$	15-20

Doses in the range of 45 to 65 Gy give local control to most patients; distant failure is the most common cause of death. Survival rate does not appear to be improved by radiotherapy. Many have argued that prior trials of radiotherapy did not use adequate doses or modern techniques and that the true benefit of this treatment is not known. However, Johnson et al. recently reported a randomized crossover trial of single agent vindesine versus vindesine plus megavoltage radiotherapy of 60 Gy to the primary tumor for patients with locally advanced NSCLC. The 5 year survival rates for 272 evaluable patients were 3% with radiation alone, 3% with radiation plus vindesine, and 1% with vindesine alone. In light of such evidence, withholding radiotherapy in asymptomatic patients with locally advanced NSCLC can be justified.

Much interest currently is focused on the addition of chemotherapy to chest radiotherapy in patients with locally advanced NSCLC, but such an approach remains investigational and is best used in the setting of an appropriate clinical trial.

Resectable tumors but inoperable patients

Resectability refers to the anatomic extent of disease and the fact that a surgical cure can be accomplished; *operability,* on the other hand, is the patient's ability to withstand the procedure required to remove all of the cancer. A patient's tumor might be anatomically removable with a lobectomy, but because of poor pulmonary or cardiac reserve the patient may not be able to tolerate more than a wedge resection. Such a patient would be resectable, but inoperable. Preoperative evaluation of pulmonary function and cardiac reserve is as important as accurate staging in the care of patients with lung cancer. Patients with lung cancer often suffer from intercurrent cardiac or pulmonary disease that significantly reduce their operability.

Some patients with stage I and II NSCLC may have tumors that can be resected but are not able to withstand the required surgery for medical (usually cardiac) reasons or refuse surgery. For such patients "curative" radiotherapy is a reasonable option. Doses of at least 60 Gy are preferred and involved field treatment probably is adequate. Talton et al. reported the following survival rates for 77 patients treated with 60 Gy target dose in 30 fractions over 6 weeks: 1 year, 57%; 2 years, 36%; 4 years, 17%; and 5 years, 17%.

Stage IV

Metastatic NSCLC carries a poor prognosis. Median survival ranges from 6 to 9 months. The search for chemotherapy regimens that can improve these dismal figures has been frustrated by a lack of drugs with substantial antitumor activity. Carefully performed studies that demonstrate improved survival in treated patients have been published, but the improvements are measured in weeks or, at best, a few months. Improved survival is not the only goal of treatment, however, and slow progress has been made in the palliation of patients with metastatic lung cancer.

Cisplatin based combinations have emerged as the most active therapies for metastatic lung cancer, frequently in combination with VP-16 and/or other agents (refer to the box below). Objective response rates to platin based combinations cluster around 35% with significant toxicity in some patients from delayed nausea, diminished appetite, and malaise.

The National Cancer Institute of Canada completed a series of studies in patients with stage IV NSCLC. The purpose of these studies was to determine which of two commonly used regimens was more active and whether combination chemotherapy afforded any survival advantage. Patients were randomized to receive either cyclophosphamide, doxorubicin, and cisplatin (CAP), cisplatin and VP-16 (VP), or best supportive care (BSC). Patients randomized to BSC could receive palliative radiation therapy. Entrants were stratified according to histologic features, performance status, and weight loss in the 3 months before entry onto the study. The median survival rates for the three groups were as follows: BSC, 17 weeks; CAP, 24 weeks; and VP, 32.6 weeks. A second study suggested that chemotherapy was cost-effective when compared with BSC when the cost for the entire illness was considered. Nonetheless, other studies have not found significant survival advantages for chemotherapy treated patients.

Several principles that can guide the use of chemotherapy in patients with metastatic NSCLC have emerged. Patients should understand that the goal is relief of symptoms and that most who receive treatment will not respond. Treatment is of most benefit when started before the patient is debilitated. Several studies have established that those who have a poor performance status (Karnofsky, <70%) at the beginning of chemotherapy have low response rates and increased toxicity when compared with patients with good performance status at the time of treatment. Patients with poor performance status are not likely to benefit from chemotherapy. Cisplatin is the most valuable agent available at the present time and is the cornerstone of treatment, most commonly in combination with VP-16. Platin is poorly tolerated by many patients. Finally, responses can be assessed after a relatively short period of treatment, usually one or two cycles of therapy. Patients who do not respond promptly probably will not have a meaningful response. Continuation of treatment for prolonged periods in the absence of response is of questionable value.

The role of radiation therapy in the palliation of patients with metastatic NSCLC cannot be overlooked. Improvement may be achieved in chest symptoms, such as dyspnea, cough, and hemoptysis, with relatively low morbidity. Pain from bony and hepatic metastases often is alleviated in a relatively short period. Paralysis from epidural spinal cord compression and devastating neurologic deficits from cerebral metastases also may be prevented if treatment is promptly instituted. Because of the wide availability of radiotherapy equipment and the low morbidity rate associated with limited treatment ports, few patients are unable to be treated.

Common regimens for chemotherapy of non–small cell lung cancer

VP regimen

Cisplatin
 100 mg/m^2 IV day one
VP-16 (Etoposide)
 100-120 mg/m^2 IV days 1-3
Repeat every 3-4 weeks for 4-6 cycles

or

Cisplatin
 50 mg/m^2 IV day 1 and day 8
VP-16 (Etoposide)
 50 mg/m^2 IV day 1 to day 5
Repeat every 3-4 weeks for 4-6 cycles

CAP regimen

Cyclophosphamide
 400 mg/m^2 IV day 1
Doxorubicin
 20 mg/m^2 IV day 1
Cisplatin
 40 mg/m^2 IV day 1
Repeat every 4 weeks for 4-6 cycles

Small cell lung cancer

Chemotherapy is the mainstay of treatment for small cell lung cancer, regardless of stage (refer to the box on p. 952). Rapid responses associated with large "cell kills" put patients at risk for the tumor lysis syndrome. Hydration to establish a high urinary output, administration of allopurinol to block formation of uric acid, and frequent monitoring of serum potassium and phosphate levels with appropriate interventions are common practices during the first cycle of therapy.

Limited disease

Cyclophosphamide, doxorubicin (Adriamycin), and vincristine (CAV) was one of the first effective combinations used for the treatment of small cell lung cancer and remains in wide use today (see the box on p. 952). Complete response rates around 40% and partial response rates around 30% yielded overall response rates in the 60% to 70% range. The median duration of response is approximately 40 weeks with median survival of about 1 year. The sub-

Common regimens for chemotherapy of small cell lung cancer

CAV regimen	CEV regimen
Cyclophosphamide 750-1000 mg/m² day one IV Doxorubicin 40-50 mg/m² day one IV Vincristine 1.4 mg/m² day one IV Single intravenous dose every 3 weeks for 4-6 cycles	Cyclophosphamide 1000 mg/m² day one IV VP-16 (Etoposide) 50 mg/m² day one IV VP-16 (Etoposide) 100 mg/m² day 2 to day 5 PO Vincristine 1.4 mg/m² day one IV Repeat every 3-4 weeks for 4-6 cycles

stitution of VP-16 (etoposide) for doxorubicin (CEV) (see the box above) led to a slight increase in response rate and improvement in survival. The use of VP-16 permits simultaneous application of chemotherapy with chest irradiation that is precluded with doxorubicin because of potentiation of toxicity. Cisplatin in combination with VP-16 (see the box above) has become popular, particularly for patients with "limited" stage disease because of improved response rates to radiation that can be given simultaneously with chemotherapy without a significant increase in toxicity.

The role of irradiation to the primary tumor and mediastinum in patients with limited stage small cell cancer appears established. Prevention of local recurrence and improved long-term survival rate have been established in several trials. The optimum technique to use is less clear. Some prefer the so-called sandwich technique, in which several cycles of chemotherapy are given initially, followed by a break for irradiation, and chemotherapy resumed at the end of irradiation. Others are inclined toward the simultaneous use of chemotherapy and radiation therapy.

Prophylactic whole brain irradiation in a dose of 30 Gy has been standard treatment for patients with limited disease who have a complete response to therapy. The long-term morbidity rate associated with neurologic problems, most commonly dementia, can be considerable, and some have questioned the wisdom of routine use of this treatment.

For patients who complete the planned chemotherapy and radiation therapy for limited stage small cell lung cancer, perhaps 10% to 15% remain alive and disease-free more than 2 years after the end of treatment. Unfortunately, late relapses continue to occur.

Innovative approaches to therapy of small cell lung cancer continue to be reported. For example, the NCI reported a trial of twice a day chest irradiation concurrent with VP-16 and *cis*-platin chemotherapy followed by chemotherapy selected by in vitro drug sensitivity testing. Platin was given on days 1 and 27 and VP-16 on days 1 to 3 and 27 to 29. Chest irradiation was given at 15 Gy twice daily Monday through Friday on days 5 to 24. Patients then were given two more cycles of cisplatin/VP-16 followed by four cycles of individualized chemotherapy, or empiric vincristine, doxorubicin, and cyclophosphamide, if in vitro testing could not be performed. The complete response rate was 81% and the remaining 19% of patients had a partial response. The median survival of 27 months is more than twice the period generally seen.

Extensive disease

Chemotherapy is the initial treatment for patients with extensive small cell lung cancer. Generally the same regimens are used as for limited disease. Responses are less common in extensive than in limited disease; however, 6% to 14% attain complete and 35% to 41% partial response, for overall response rates in the range of 45% to 49%. Median duration of response is shorter than for patients with limited disease (24 to 32 weeks), as is overall survival (31 to 38 weeks). Two year survival is uncommon for patients who have extensive disease.

Irradiation to the primary tumor and mediastinum does not improve overall response or survival rate and is not indicated. Similarly, whole brain irradiation is reserved for those patients in whom symptomatic brain metastases develop.

REFERENCES

Armstrong JG and Mindky BD: Radiation therapy for medically inoperable Stage I and II non-small cell lung cancer. Cancer Treat Rev 16:247, 1989.

Ihde DC and Minna JD: Non-small cell lung cancer. II. Treatment. Curr Prob Cancer 15:105, 1991.

Johnson DH et al: Thoracic radiotherapy does not prolong survival in patients with locally advanced, unresectable non-small cell lung cancer. Ann Intern Med 113:33, 1990.

Mantravadi RYP et al: Unresectable non-oat cell carcinoma of the lung: definitive radiation therapy. Radiology 172:851, 1989.

Miller JD, Gorenstein LA, and Patterson GA: Staging: the key to rational management of lung cancer. Ann Thorac Surg 53:170, 1992.

Rose LJ: Neoadjuvant and adjuvant therapy of non-small cell lung cancer. Semin Oncol 18:536, 1991.

Talton BM, Constable WC, and Kersh CR: Curative radiotherapy in non-small cell carcinoma of the lung. Int J Radiat Oncol Biol Phys 19:15, 1990.

CHAPTER

102 Carcinoma of Unknown Primary Site

John D. Hainsworth
F. Anthony Greco

Patients with metastatic cancer and no obvious primary site account for 1% to 5% of all cancer patients. These patients have a variety of tumor types, and specific guidelines for diagnostic evaluation, staging, and treatment are difficult to formulate. Because effective therapy is currently available for many types of advanced cancer, patients with metastatic neoplasms of unknown primary site can no longer be routinely consigned to receive supportive care only. The clinician must therefore be aware of the neoplasms for which effective treatment exists (refer to the box at right) and must approach the patient with carcinoma of unknown primary site with two objectives: (1) to identify treatable malignancies by performing the necessary diagnostic studies and (2) to prevent superfluous, uncomfortable, and costly evaluation.

Most metastatic neoplasms of unknown primary site are carcinomas, and routine light-microscopic examination is usually sufficient to make the diagnosis. However, other types of neoplasms (e.g., lymphomas, sarcomas) are occasionally difficult to exclude by histologic criteria, particularly when they are poorly differentiated. Because some of these neoplasms are very responsive to treatment, further pathologic tests (electron microscopy, cell immunotyping, immunochemistry) should be performed when uncertainty exists.

Patients with the diagnosis of carcinoma on the initial biopsy can be further subdivided into three groups: adenocarcinoma, squamous carcinoma, and poorly differentiated carcinoma. These histologic diagnoses can be used to guide diagnostic evaluation and treatment, because these three groups are often distinct with respect to clinical presentation, management, and prognosis (Table 102-1).

ADENOCARCINOMA OF UNKNOWN PRIMARY SITE

Histologic features

The diagnosis of well-differentiated or moderately well-differentiated adenocarcinoma is based on the formation of glandular structures by neoplastic cells. This diagnosis is usually made without difficulty by light microscopy. Unfortunately, specific histologic features that enable precise identification of the site of tumor origin are rarely present. Immunoperoxidase staining for prostate specific antigen is quite specific for prostate carcinoma and should be considered for men who have suggestive clinical features. However, in most cases specialized pathologic evaluation (i.e., use of special stains, electron microscopy) does not provide useful additional information.

Unlike the diagnosis of well-differentiated adenocarcinoma, the diagnosis of poorly differentiated adenocarcinoma is sometimes difficult to make by light-microscopic features alone. Often, this diagnosis is made in tumors that have little or no glandular differentiation but that show positive staining results for mucin. Poorly differentiated adenocarcinomas more closely resemble poorly differentiated carcinomas than well-differentiated adenocarcinoma in their tumor biologic characteristics and responsiveness to treatment. Patients with poorly differentiated adenocarcinoma of unknown primary site should therefore be evaluated and treated in a manner similar to that described for patients with poorly differentiated carcinoma.

Advanced cancers effectively treated with chemotherapy

Potentially curative therapy available

Hodgkin's disease
Non-Hodgkin's lymphomas
Testicular cancer and other germinal malignancies
Acute leukemia
Childhood malignancies (Wilms' tumor, Ewing's sarcoma, other sarcomas)
Small cell lung cancer
Ovarian cancer

Effective palliative therapy available

Breast cancer
Prostate cancer
Gastric cancer
Bladder cancer
Sarcoma
Multiple myeloma/plasmacytoma
Chronic leukemia
Carcinoid tumors
Islet cell tumors

Clinical features and natural history

Although metastatic adenocarcinomas can involve any organ, the most common sites of involvement are the liver, lungs, and bones. More than 50% of patients have more than one site of metastasis at the time of diagnosis. Symptoms are related to sites involved by tumor.

In most patients with adenocarcinoma of unknown primary site, the clinical course is dominated by symptoms at metastatic sites. In only 15% to 20% of patients does the primary site become obvious during the clinical course. At autopsy, the primary site can be detected in 75% to 80% of patients; in the remainder, the primary site is never established. Approximately 75% of primary sites are located below the diaphragm. The pancreas is found to be the primary site in 20% of patients and is the most commonly identified primary site. Other gastrointestinal sites (colorectal, gastric, hepatic) are also relatively frequent. The lung is the most frequent site above the diaphragm and accounts for 15% to 20% of patients. Adenocarcinomas of the breast, ovary, and prostate, which occur frequently in the general population, are infrequently identified in this group of patients.

Diagnostic and staging evaluation

After histologic documentation of metastatic adenocarcinoma, the clinician is frequently tempted to perform an exhaustive search for a primary site. This type of extensive evaluation is not recommended, because in most patients a primary site is not identified even with multiple radiologic procedures. In addition, identification of a primary site does not have specific therapeutic implications in most patients.

Table 102-1. Profile of typical clinical characteristics, recommended evaluation, and prognosis

Histologic type	Age	Etiologic factors	Common sites of involvement	Recommended evaluation (in addition to routine history and physical examination, blood counts, serum chemical evaluations)	Response to treatment; prognosis
Adenocarcinoma	Elderly	None known	Liver, bone, lung	Chest radiography, CT scan of abdomen. Men: prostate specific antigen level; Women: mammograms. Additional radiologic studies to evaluate abnormal symptoms, signs, laboratory values	Poor response to chemotherapy, short median survival (3-6 months), unless in specific subgroup (see text)
Squamous carcinoma	Middle-aged, elderly	Cigarette, alcohol use	Cervical, supraclavicular lymph nodes	Chest radiography, panendoscopy, fiberoptic bronchoscopy	30%-50% long-term survival rate with radical surgery and/or radiotherapy
Poorly differentiated carcinoma	Variable—young patients frequent	None known	Variable—mediastinum, retroperitoneum, lymph nodes frequently involved	Chest radiography, CT scan of abdomen. Tumor markers: hCG, alpha-fetoprotein. Additional radiologic studies to evaluate abnormal symptoms, signs, laboratory values	High response rate to cisplatin-based chemotherapy. Approximately 15% long-term survival rate

The recommended evaluation for this group of patients is outlined in Table 102-1. All patients should have a thorough history and physical examination (including careful pelvic examination in females). In addition, standard laboratory screening tests, including a complete blood count, SMA-12 determination, and urinalysis, should be performed. Chest radiography should be performed in all patients. Serum prostate specific antigen determinations should be made for all males, and women with axillary adenopathy or other clinical features suggestive of breast cancer should have mammography. Additional radiologic evaluation should be designed to evaluate abnormal findings identified by history, physical examination, or routine laboratory studies. Radiologic examination of the gastrointestinal tract should be performed when patients have new bowel symptoms or are found to have occult blood in the stool. Patients with hematuria should have genitourinary tract evaluation by intravenous pyelography and in some cases renal angiography and cystoscopy.

Although data are limited, computed tomography (CT) of the abdomen appears to be of significant diagnostic value in these patients. In one series, abdominal primary sites were identified in 15 of 46 patients (33%) on the basis of CT findings, and other unsuspected metastatic sites were identified in an additional 65%.

Treatment and prognosis

Although treatment is ineffective in many cases of adenocarcinoma of unknown primary site, optimum management of this group of patients requires identification of several clinical subgroups with specific therapeutic implications. Breast cancer should be suspected in all women who have adenocarcinoma involving axillary lymph nodes. Documentation of estrogen receptors in the tumor tissue is strong supportive evidence for this diagnosis. Women who have no evidence of other metastatic sites (on the basis of the evaluation recommended) may have stage II breast cancer and are therefore potentially curable with appropriate therapy. Mastectomy reveals a breast primary site in 50% to 65% of patients, even when physical examination and mammogram findings are normal. Primary treatment should include either modified radical mastectomy or high-dose radiation therapy to the breast and axilla. Adjuvant systemic therapy (chemotherapy or hormonal therapy) using guidelines established for stage II breast cancer should be considered. Females with positive axillary lymph node findings and evidence of other metastatic sites should also be suspected of having metastatic breast cancer; those with positive estrogen receptor results often have prolonged responses to hormonal therapy. An empiric therapeutic trial of combination chemotherapy that is effective in metastatic breast cancer should be considered in women who are estrogen receptor negative (Chapter 97).

The diagnosis of metastatic ovarian cancer should be considered in women with diffuse peritoneal involvement with adenocarcinoma, particularly in those with no evidence of visceral metastases. All women with this distribution of tumor should be treated as if they had ovarian cancer; initial aggressive cytoreductive surgery should be followed by combination chemotherapy with a platinum-based regimen. Complete responses and long-term survival after combination chemotherapy have been reported not only in women with no primary tumor demonstrated in the ovary but also in those with a history of previous oophorectomy (Chapter 98).

Male patients with adenocarcinoma and blastic bone metastases or elevated serum prostate specific antigen level should be suspected of having prostatic adenocarcinoma. Although the prostatic primary site in these patients is usually demonstrable, a trial of palliative hormonal therapy should be considered even when evaluation of the prostate is unrevealing (Chapter 99).

Unfortunately, most patients with metastatic adenocarcinoma of unknown primary site do not fit into any of these subsets. Treatment of these patients is usually ineffective. Most empiric chemotherapy trials have used 5-fluorouracil either as a single agent or in combinations (e.g., 5-fluorouracil, doxorubicin, mitomycin-C [FAM]) developed for the treatment of gastrointestinal malignancies. These regimens have produced responses in less than 30% and have had little or no impact on median survival. Cisplatin-based regimens have not substantially improved these results. The poor response to systemic therapy is not surprising, because most patients have primary tumors that are unresponsive to chemotherapy. The prognosis of these patients is poor: median survival is 3 to 4 months.

SQUAMOUS CARCINOMA OF UNKNOWN PRIMARY SITE

The identification of squamous carcinoma in the biopsy of a metastatic site is unusual; in such patients, evaluation and treatment depend on the site of involvement.

Cervical lymph nodes

Patients found to have squamous carcinoma in an upper or midcervical lymph node should be suspected of having a primary tumor in the head and neck region (Chapter 100). Evaluation should include a careful examination of the oropharynx, hypopharynx, and larynx by indirect laryngoscopy. Suspicious sites should receive biopsy examination. If no primary site is demonstrated, the patient should undergo direct laryngoscopy with random biopsy examination. In addition, the nasopharynx should be visualized and a biopsy should be done if no other primary site has been identified. Patients with squamous carcinoma involving the lower cervical or supraclavicular lymph nodes are more likely to have an unsuspected lung primary site and should be evaluated with fiberoptic bronchoscopy if the head and neck examination and chest radiograph results are unrevealing.

A thorough diagnostic evaluation will reveal a primary site in most patients, and appropriate therapy can be administered. Patients in whom no primary site is identified can also benefit greatly from treatment of the involved neck, with high-dose radiotherapy, radical surgery, or a combination of these modalities. In patients with high or midcervical adenopathy, 3 year survival rate after appropriate therapy ranges from 35% to 59%. These patients presumably have clinically undetectable primary sites in the head and neck, which are effectively treated along with the metastatic disease. Patients with involvement of the lower cervical and supraclavicular lymph nodes have a poorer prognosis, because many of them have lung primary sites that later become manifest; only 10% to 15% of these patients are long-term survivors after local treatment to the cervical area.

Inguinal lymph nodes

Squamous carcinoma found in the inguinal lymph nodes is almost always metastatic from the genital or anorectal area. Females should undergo careful examination of the vulva, vagina, and cervix, with biopsy of any suspect areas. Uncircumcised males should have careful inspection of the penis. In addition, the anorectal area should be examined carefully with digital examination and anoscopy in both sexes, with biopsy of suspicious areas. These procedures almost always identify a primary site, and appropriate therapy can then be initiated. When no primary site is identified, patients with tumor localized to the inguinal region should undergo lymph node dissection or local radiation therapy; some of these patients are long-term survivors.

Other metastatic sites

Patients who are found to have metastatic squamous carcinoma in other visceral sites almost always have metastatic lung cancer. These patients should have careful examination of the chest radiograph; bronchoscopy should be considered even in those with normal chest radiography findings. Systemic therapy is usually unrewarding in these patients (Chapter 101).

POORLY DIFFERENTIATED CARCINOMA OF UNKNOWN PRIMARY SITE

The patient with poorly differentiated carcinoma of unknown primary site poses a very difficult management problem; in addition to the uncertainty regarding the site of tumor origin, the pathologic findings are nonspecific and often fail to narrow the diagnostic spectrum. Although less common than adenocarcinomas of unknown primary site, poorly differentiated carcinomas have consistently accounted for 10% to 15% of all carcinomas of unknown primary site and are therefore not rare. Careful diagnostic evaluation and appropriate treatment in this patient group are imperative, because many of the patients are young, and several types of potentially curable malignancies can sometimes masquerade as poorly differentiated carcinomas. These include undifferentiated lymphomas, germinal malignancies (both gonadal and extragonadal), small cell lung cancer (intermediate cell subtype), and a variety of "childhood" malignancies.

Clinical characteristics

Detailed analyses of the clinical characteristics in this diverse group of patients have not been reported. The median age of these patients is lower than that of patients with adenocarcinoma of unknown primary, although there is a wide age range. Metastatic tumor may involve any site; however, predominant involvement of the mediastinum, retroperitoneum, or peripheral lymph nodes is more common than in patients with adenocarcinoma. Often patients have evidence of multiple sites of metastatic involvement. There is frequently a history of rapid progression of symptoms and/or objective evidence of rapid tumor growth.

Pathology

Because routine light-microscopic examination provides inadequate information in these patients, more specialized pathologic studies are imperative. Histochemical staining for mucin or mucicarmine usually yields negative findings, but strong positive results suggest adenocarcinoma. Immunoperoxidase staining has greatly aided in diagnosis and is now widely available. Lymphomas can be reliably identified by means of the stain for leukocyte common antigen (LCA). The diagnosis of carcinoma can be confirmed with a positive staining result for cytokeratin. Other tumors, such as melanoma or sarcoma, can also be suggested with the use of appropriate stains. However, few of these stains are entirely specific, and staining results must be interpreted in conjunction with histologic and clinical features. At present, identification of a specific primary site is rarely possible.

Electron microscopy can also provide important information and should be used when the diagnosis remains unclear after immunoperoxidase staining. The identification of certain ultrastructural features provides important clues concerning the nature of the malignancy. The important distinction between lymphoma and carcinoma can be reliably made in almost all cases on the basis of electron microscopic findings. Other important ultrastructural findings include neurosecretory granules (small cell lung cancer, carcinoid tumors, neuroblastoma), premelanosomes (melanoma), and intracellular lumina and microvilli (adenocarcinoma).

Patient evaluation

The diagnostic evaluation of the patient with poorly differentiated carcinoma of unknown primary site should be similar to that described for patients with adenocarcinoma of unknown primary site. A careful history, physical examination, routine laboratory evaluation (hemogram, SMA-12, urinalysis), chest radiograph, and CT scans of the abdomen should be performed. In addition, determination of the serum tumor markers human chorionic gonadotropin (hCG) and alpha fetoprotein is essential in all patients, because elevated levels of these substances suggest the diagnosis of a germ cell neoplasm. Other radiologic procedures should be performed to evaluate abnormalities detected with routine evaluation; further exhaustive radiologic search for a primary tumor site is not indicated.

Because pathologic evaluation in these patients is difficult, the clinician should make certain that the pathologist is provided with adequate biopsy specimens. Needle biopsies generally provide inadequate amounts of tissue for complete pathologic evaluation. Often rebiopsy, or biopsy of additional metastatic sites, is appropriate to provide the pathologist with additional material for specialized studies.

Treatment

Patients in whom a specific diagnosis is made on the basis of specialized pathologic studies should be treated appropriately. In particular, those patients who have high-grade lymphomas should receive intensive chemotherapy, which is potentially curative (Chapter 94). Patients with clinical features suggestive of extragonadal germ cell tumor (young men, mediastinal or retroperitoneal tumor, elevated serum hCG, and/or alpha fetoprotein level) should receive intensive combination chemotherapy with a regimen used for testicular cancer (e.g., cisplatin, etoposide, bleomycin), even if the histologic diagnosis of germ cell tumor cannot be made (Chapter 99).

In many patients, no specific diagnosis is made even after all appropriate studies have been performed. In some, no distinguishing ultrastructural features can be identified by means of electron microscopy, and a diagnosis more specific than "poorly differentiated carcinoma" cannot be made. In others, a diagnosis such as "neuroendocrine tumor" or "poorly differentiated adenocarcinoma" is made on the basis of electron microscopic findings, but the exact nature of the tumor remains unclear. Patients with neuroendocrine features demonstrated by electron microscopy or immunoperoxidase staining usually have highly responsive tumors; they should be treated with combination chemotherapy (e.g., cis-platinum, etoposide) similar to that which is effective in the treatment of small cell lung cancer. Some other patients with poorly differentiated carcinomas of unknown primary site also have highly responsive neoplasms. In this group, empiric therapy with cisplatin-based regimens (cisplatin/vinblastine/bleomycin or cisplatin/etoposide ± bleomycin) have produced complete responses in 26% of patients, with 16% long-term disease-free survival rate. Several clinical and pathologic features have been found to be predictive of highly responsive tumors: (1) predominant tumor in the retroperitoneum or peripheral lymph nodes, (2) tumor limited to one or two metastatic sites, (3) lower age, (4) no smoking history, and (5) neuroendocrine features. However, these features do not identify all responsive patients. A brief trial of cisplatin-based chemotherapy is therefore appropriate in all patients with poorly differentiated carcinoma or poorly differentiated adenocarcinoma of unknown primary site. Patients with responsive tumors can be identified after one or two courses of therapy and treatment should continue for four courses.

REFERENCES

Ashikari R et al: Breast cancer presenting as an axillary mass. Ann Surg 183:415, 1976.

Coker DD et al: Metastases to lymph nodes of the head and neck from an unknown primary site. Am J Surg 134:517, 1977.

Didolkar MS, et al: Metastatic carcinomas from occult primary tumors. Ann Surg 186:625, 1977.

Fromm GL, Gershenson DM and Silva EG: Papillary serous carcinoma of the peritoneum. Obstet Gynecol 75:89, 1990.

Goldberg RM et al: 5-Fluorouracil, Adriamycin, and mitomycin in the treatment of adenocarcinoma of unknown primary. J Clin Oncol 4:395, 1986.

Greco FA, Vaughn WK, and Hainsworth JD: Advanced poorly differentiated carcinoma of unknown primary site: recognition of a treatable syndrome. Ann Intern Med 104:547, 1986.

Hainsworth JD, Dial TW, and Greco FA: Curative combination chemotherapy for patients with advanced poorly differentiated carcinoma of unknown primary site. Am J Clin Oncol 11:138, 1988.

Hainsworth JD, Johnson DH, and Greco FA: Poorly differentiated neuroendocrine carcinoma of unknown primary site: A newly recognized clinicopathologic entity. Ann Intern Med 109:364, 1988.

Hainsworth JD, Johnson DH, Greco FA: Cisplatin-based combination chemotherapy in the treatment of poorly differentiated carcinoma and poorly differentiated adenocarcinoma of unknown primary site: results of a twelve year experience at a single institution. J Clin Oncol, in press.

Hainsworth JD et al: Poorly differentiated carcinoma of unknown primary site: clinical usefulness of immunoperoxidase staining. J Clin Oncol 9:1931, 1991.

Hainsworth JD et al: Poorly differentiated carcinoma of unknown primary site: Correlation of light microscopic findings with response to cisplatin-based combination chemotherapy. J Clin Oncol 5:1275, 1987.

Jesse RH, Perez CA, and Fletcher GH: Cervical lymph node metastasis: unknown primary cancer. Cancer 31:854, 1973.

Nystrom JS et al: Metastatic and histologic presentations in unknown primary cancer. Semin Oncol 4:53, 1977.

Patel J et al: Axillary lymph node metastasis from an occult breast cancer. Cancer 47:2923, 1981.

Strnad CM et al: Peritoneal carcinomatosis of unknown primary site in women: a distinctive subset of adenocarcinoma of unknown primary site with specific therapeutic implications. Ann Intern Med 111:213, 1989.

Woods RL et al: Metastatic adenocarcinomas of unknown primary site. N Engl J Med 303:87, 1980.

Part Four

Neurologic Disorders

I CLINICAL AND LABORATORY EVALUATION OF THE NERVOUS SYSTEM

CHAPTER

103 Neurologic History and Examination

Jock Murray

Every patient who has a medical examination should receive a neurologic examination to identify any evidence of abnormality in the nervous system. This should be a practical, efficient survey with high-yield examination techniques that best identify most neurologic abnormalities. A more complex and detailed neurologic examination, if abnormalities are identified, can be found in textbooks of neurology (see References).

The neurologic examination is aimed at helping the clinician determine whether a neurologic problem is present; if so, at what level (muscle, myoneural junction, nerve, spinal cord, brainstem, cerebral or cerebellar hemisphere); the likely process involved (pathologic condition); the likely cause; and whether urgent management is required (therapy). Infrequent application of the neurologic examination results in a disuse atrophy of skills, competence, efficiency, and confidence in assessing neurologic problems. Clinicians must develop a brief, efficient, and reliable examination that can be made on every patient, so that accuracy and confidence are maintained.

Although the term *neurologic examination* reflects the clinical testing of the patient, the most important diagnostic device is a careful history. Experienced clinicians are seldom surprised by the results of a neurologic examination and they use it to confirm and qualify the conclusions derived from a careful history. Such a detailed interview is not merely the hobbyhorse of an obsessive-compulsive neurologist. It is an important means of developing a relationship with the patient that will be important in subsequent management, and it provides an understanding of the person in the circle of family, fellow workers, and community. Osler taught us that it was more important to know what kind of person has the disease than what kind of disease the person has.

ELEMENTS OF THE NEUROLOGIC EXAMINATION

The elements of the neurologic examination can be divided into the general observation and specific tests. The general observation is often the most informative and sometimes suggests the diagnosis of many disorders before the patient has taken a seat.

The specific tests can be subdivided into the categories of examination of the mental status, cranial nerves, motor and sensory function, reflexes, and the assessment of stance and gait.

Observation

We see what we look for. From the time the patient enters the office, diagnostic observations can be made. The portraits of depression, Parkinson's disease, movement disorders, muscle weakness, myotonic dystrophy, and many other conditions can often be observed. In those initial moments and in the subsequent interview, the perceptive and sensitive clinician can receive a great deal of information about the patient and the patient's condition.

General observation is best to recognize the patient's emotions and responses, but many specific neurologic signs can be observed during the interview, sometimes better than on the formal examination. These signs include subtle facial weakness, speech difficulties, memory disturbances, and aspects of denial and insight.

Mental status

Most of the elements of the mental status examination can be observed in the interview, but again, these characteristics may be seen only if the clinician looks for them. If there is a suspicion of intellectual change or memory abnormality, a few simple tests will confirm these abnormalities in most instances: (1) testing orientation, (2) the 100-7 test, (3) asking the patient to remember four simple objects in 2 minutes, and (4) asking him or her to spell *world* or *pencil* backward.

Cranial nerves

Although there are 12 cranial nerves, a few are particularly important to examine because they are indicators of serious disease or are commonly involved if disease is present. This examination should include assessment (1) of the optic discs, (2) of ocular movements and tests for nystagmus, (3) of sensory function over the face, and (4) of motor asymmetry of the face.

Motor system

Is there any weakness, and if so, is it due to a lesion of the upper or lower motor neuron? Also, is there any alteration of muscle tone or coordination, or any abnormal movement? By the time the patient has entered the office and taken a chair, the physician already knows a great deal about the patient's motor system.

On formal testing, look for any signs of facial weakness. Test motor power in the shoulder muscles, elbow flexors and extensors, wrists, and grip. In the legs, examine hip, knee, and ankle flexors and extensors and ask the patient to walk on the heels and toes. The two most subtle and high-yield tests for upper motor neuron weakness are to ask the patient, with eyes closed, to hold the hands extended, palms upward, for 1 minute and later to elevate both legs off the bed at the same time. When there is mild weakness, the hand begins to drop and pronate. The weak leg elevates more slowly and to a lower level.

Tone is tested in the arms by shaking the wrists or by gripping the hand and rapidly rotating the forearm. Tone of the legs can be best judged by suddenly lifting the leg from under the knee. In the normal relaxed limb, the heel drags along the examining table, whereas the heel rises off the bed if there is increased quadriceps tone.

Muscle power can be graded on a scale that rates total paralysis as (0), a flicker of contraction (1), movement only if gravity is eliminated (2), movement against gravity only (3), movement that can be overcome by resistance (4), and full power (5).

Coordination can be observed in the patient's walking and spontaneous movements, and also by the finger-nose, rapid alternating movements of the hand, and heel-shin tests and tandem walking.

Sensory examination

A scanning survey sensory examination should be made quickly but accurately to identify whether there is any sensory difference on one side of the body from the other, and distal compared with proximal. Pin-prick, touch, and temperature can be tested on the arms and legs and compared with those on the opposite side, and then the same is done for proximal and distal areas of the limbs. It is much more accurate to compare areas with an area that the physicians is satisfied is normal than to use the coarse test of whether the patient feels the pin as sharp or dull. A sensory level (i.e., decreased sensation caudally below a certain body level) should be sought in a patient with a suspected spinal cord lesion. Vibratory sense should be examined over the feet, and the Romberg test is a good measure of proprioception.

If there is any evidence of sensory change on one side, cortical sensation should be tested by two-point discrimination, palm writing, stereognosis, and bilateral simultaneous stimulation.

Reflexes

An examiner becomes reliable and efficient at testing reflexes only by doing them so often and by thinking about them as they are being done. The major reflexes to be tested are the biceps (C5, C6), quadriceps (L3, L4), and ankle (S1) jerks. The most important superficial reflex is the plantar response, seeking a Babinski sign. If the patient is very sensitive over the feet, use the Chaddock sign or gently and repeatedly do both together, using two halves of a broken tongue depressor.

Gait

The patient should be observed walking into the office, but there is often not enough time or distance to allow one to judge the normal stride. Unfortunately, offices are not designed to test gait, although it is one of the most important aspects of the neurologic examination. If necessary, the physician should ask the patient to walk in a hallway after he or she is dressed. Watch for the smoothness, the arm swing, and the pace of gait. Most important, observe the smoothness on quick turning.

CONCLUSION

The skills of neurologic examination can easily be learned, but reliability and confidence come only from continued application to each patient examined. A well-performed high-yield neurologic examination not only enables the physician to identify and solve neurologic problems but also gives one confidence that the patients do not have neurologic disease.

REFERENCES

Matthews PM and Arnold DL, editors: Diagnostic tests in neurology New York, 1991, Churchill Livingstone.

Pryse-Phillips W and Murray TJ: Essential neurology, ed 4. New York, 1992, Elsevier.

CHAPTER

104 Psychologic Testing

William E. M. Pryse-Phillips

Psychologic (or "psychometric") tests provide valid and reliable data about a patient's mental status. A variety of psychometric tests can be used to determine whether important personality or cognitive variables are similar to those in a target population. There are four main categories of test:

1. Personality tests. Personality tests provide information about an individual's motives and emotional stability and usually involve completion of a self-administered questionnaire. One such test, the Eysenck Personality Inventory, measures personality along two scales (stability/neuroticism and introversion/extroversion), which allows various patient groups to be characterized. For example, anxiety-neurotics are high on the neuroticism scale and low on the extraversion scale. Many other personality inventories and projective tests are available (e.g., the Minnesota Multiphasic Personal Inventory [MMPI] and the Rorschach test). They are used when information on the presence or degree of depressive ill-

ness is sought; in patients with behavioral disturbances, such as suspected conversion reactions; and in patients with chronic pain problems.

2. Aptitude, interest, and achievement tests. These tests measure global skills or interests in an effort to clarify an individual's vocational potential. Again, they compare a person's performance with the mean scores of large defined groups. Normative data collected from individuals well established in different careers provide such comparisons. The use of this type of test in diagnosis of medical or neurologic states is less common than in counseling.
3. Mood assessment. Tests for depressive illness are most often employed. The best-known short scales are those devised by Hamilton, Zung, or Beck, in each of which the individual is assessed for both psychologic and physical symptoms either by the examiner at interview or by the subject filling in a self-rating scale. Hamilton's Depression Rating Scale provides both a checklist to help to structure the interview and a semiquantitative score to assist in diagnosis.
4. Neuropsychologic tests. These standardized scales are designed to test relatively pure cognitive skills and thus allow assessment of the presence and site of organic neurologic disease. To achieve this, neuropsychologists typically employ a variety of instruments, selected to examine such cognitive abilities as memory, language, visuospatial or constructional skills, and basic sensory and motor skills. One can assess both global psychometric functions (e.g., intelligence and memory quotients) and specific functions (e.g., finger agnosia and receptive language skills). A neuropsychologic report can provide much psychometric information in addition to a detailed interpretation of any particular pattern of results. Such tests refine and deepen the formal bedside examination of highest cerebral function.

Thus whereas tests in group 2 describe abilities or skills that are then compared with those of a population of normal individuals, group 4 tests try to determine how specific abilities are being affected by brain disorders in order to localize such disease. The Wechsler Adult Intelligence Scale (WAIS) is composed of 11 subtests performing most of these functions and offering a scale of global intellectual ability as well as providing figures for verbal, performance, and full-scale intelligence. In subjects with acquired diseases, impaired performance test results with relatively retained verbal skills are often noted, whereas some varieties of brain dysfunction may result in unique patterns; thus a left hemisphere stroke lowers verbal rather than performance scores. The Token Test is widely used to examine receptive language skills. Here the patient is required to follow a simple set of instructions that become progressively more complex ("Touch a square. . . . In addition to touching the yellow square, touch the blue circle"). The patient's score can suggest to what degree his or her receptive language abilities are impaired.

The tests most likely to be used by internists or neurologists are those that assess the presence, degree, or nature of the dementias. Among these the Mini-Mental state examination (MMSE) or its variant, the modified MMS (3MS), are useful screening instruments. They examine orientation, learning capacity, remote memory, attention, calculation, praxis, and aspects of language function and are both valid and reasonably reliable, though affected by previous educational standards. The 3MS, although currently less well validated, nevertheless does include a greater range of cognitive functions than the MMSE and is almost as easy to administer.

The severity of dementing diseases may be determined by using semiquantitative scales such as the Clinical Dementia Rating Scale. This instrument allows the rater to assign scores for memory orientation, judgment and problem solving, community interaction, function in the home, and personal care abilities on the basis of impressions received during interviews of the patient and a caregiver. It thus acts as a template for the interview, the responses to which may be scored in a defined way, rather than providing a standardized series of questions. Other means of rating disturbance in function include scales for rating a person's ability to perform the usual activities of daily living, both personal (ability to feed, bathe, go to the toilet, dress, transfer, and move about) and instrumental (abilities to use the telephone, shop, handle money, cook, or do housework). Dysfunction in such areas correlates well with cognitive impairment, and as the data are obtained from a caregiver and can be given by telephone, they provide a simple and reasonably objective assessment of the degree of impairment experienced. Other accepted instruments include the Mattis Dementia Rating Scale, the Brief Cognitive Rating Scale, and the Alzheimer Disease Assessment Scale, all of which are rather more complex and sometimes require the use of standard test materials but are valid and easily administered after mnimal practice by any physician.

These assessment procedures can be extremely useful. However, the physician should be aware that whatever technique is used, the outcome is a probability statement about a given patient's scores resembling those of an identified group of normal subjects or of those with the same disease. But they are not specific; a patient who has chronic organic pain problems could well score in the same range as a population of hysteria patients on the MMPI. All that can reasonably be concluded in such a case is that the patient has a tendency to focus on somatic complaints to a much greater extent than the normal population. This does not indicate that the patient is malingering. A psychologist would use additional assessment techniques to discriminate between organic and nonorganic components of the patient's reported pain.

Common and appropriate reasons for requesting a neuropsychologic evaluation are (1) assessment of mental status after brain insults such as head injury or stroke; (2) early diagnosis, assessment of severity, follow-up observation, and counseling in patients with suspected dementia; (3) differentiation of the relative part played by functional and by organic components in disease states; (4) detection and evaluation of cognitive deficits in cases of learning disability, mental retardation, and so forth; and (5) counseling of patients and their families regarding the management of acquired cognitive deficits.

REFERENCES

Beck AT et al: An inventory for measuring depression. Arch Gen Psychiatry 4:561, 1961.

Berg L: Clinical dementia rating (CDR). Psychopharmacol Bull 24:637, 1988.

Boll TJ: The Halstead-Reitan neuropsychological battery. In SB Filskov and TJ Boll, editors: Handbook of clinical neuropsychology. New York, 1981, Wiley-Interscience.

Folstein MF, Folstein SE, and McHugh PR: "Mini-mental state": a practical method for grading the cognitive state of patients for the clinician. J Psychiatr Res 12:189, 1975.

Hamilton M: Development of a rating scale for primary depressive illness. Br J Soc Clin Psychol 6:278, 1967.

Hamilton M: A rating scale for depression. J Neurol Neurosurg Psychiatry 23:56, 1960.

Lezek MD: Neuropsychological assessment, ed 2. New York, 1983, Oxford University Press.

Mattis S: Mental status examination for organic mential syndrome in the elderly patient. In Bellck R and Karasu B, editors: Geriatric psychiatry. New York, 1976, Grune & Stratton.

Mohs RC, Cohen L: Alzheimer's disease assessment scale (ADAS). Psychopharmacol Bull 24:627, 1988.

Reisbert B and Ferris SH: The brief cognitive rating scale (BCRS). Psychopharmacol Bull 24:629, 1988.

Wechsler D: Wechsler intelligence scale for children manual, revised ed. New York, 1974, The Psychological Corporation.

Wechsler D: WAIS-R Manual. New York, 1981, The Psychological Corporation.

Zung WWK: A self-rating depression scale. Arch Gen Psychiatry 12:63, 1965.

CHAPTER

105 Spinal Fluid Examination

J. Donald Easton

The introduction of a needle into the lumbar subarachnoid space (lumbar puncture [LP]) allows one to measure the cerebrospinal fluid (CSF) pressure and obtain CSF for examination. There are normally free flow of fluid and transmission of pressure between the intracranial and intraspinal subarachnoid space. Although some differences exist between the CSF constituents in these two spaces, they are usually minor.

The lumbar puncture is primarily a diagnostic procedure. It is most useful in identifying abnormal intracranial pressure, subarachnoid hemorrhage, and meningeal inflammation and neoplasia. In addition, various abnormal antigens, antibodies, and other abnormal proteins may be present, suggesting specific disease processes (e.g., syphilis, cryptococcosis, and multiple sclerosis).

The patient generally is placed horizontal, in the lateral decubitus position, and a 20 gauge needle is introduced into the L4-L5 intervertebral space. A manometer is used to measure the opening pressure after the patient is relaxed. In the first tube, 2 ml of fluid is collected for sugar and protein concentration determinations; 5 ml of fluid is collected in a second tube. This tube should be labeled properly and set aside in the refrigerator; it can be used should any of the determinations require repeating, or unexpected findings in the first sample suggest the need for additional studies. If the circumstances warrant it, additional fluid should then be obtained for Gram, India ink, Wright, and Ziehl-Neelsen stains; for bacterial, fungal, or viral cultures; for serologic or special protein studies; and for detection of malignant cells. One milliliter should be collected in the last tube for a cell count. If blood is discovered in the CSF, a cell count on the first tube also should be obtained. The color and clarify of the fluid should be recorded. If low CSF sugar (hypoglycorrhachia) concentration is suspected, and the circumstances warrant it, CSF should be collected after the patient has fasted for at least 4 hours. The blood sugar concentration is then stable and "equilibrated" with the CSF sugar concentration; therefore if the concentration is less then 60% of the serum value, hypoglycorrhachia is present.

If the CSF pressure unexpectedly is found to be high (greater than 200 mm CSF) and the possibility of an intracranial mass lesion exists, only enough fluid to perform the necessary assays should be removed (slowly). The stylet should be replaced, and neurologic assistance should be sought. There will be a substantial pressure gradient between the CSF and the extra-arachnoid space, and if the needle is removed, fluid will continue to leak from the needle hole in the meninges. In benign intracranial hypertension with papilledema, a lumbar puncture may be therapeutic, and a persistent leak leading to a gradual decompression may be desirable. The risk of brain herniation exists, however, if there are differential pressure gradients within the CSF spaces, caused by either a mass lesion or obstruction of CSF pathways.

Whenever pink or frankly bloody spinal fluid is observed, it is important to distinguish true subarachnoid hemorrhage from a "traumatic tap." Even when the procedure goes smoothly, it is possible for a punctured vessel to bleed and produce a traumatic tap. Usually with a traumatic puncture, the CSF clears gradually as it is removed, and the red blood cell count diminishes in each successive tube. One tube should be centrifuged immediately, and the supernatant separated and observed for discoloration. A pink or yellow fluid (provided the CSF protein is less than 150 mg/dl) represents hemoglobin degradation products and indicates that blood has been present for 2 hours or more. If the protein concentration in the CSF is higher than 100 to 150 mg/dl, for any reason, the fluid appears yellow.

The LP procedure should be recorded in the medical record. The recording includes the position of the patient, the type and dose of local anesthetic used, the spine interspace entered, and the size of the needle used. The opening pressure, appearance of the fluid and amount collected in each tube, and tests ordered on each tube should be recorded.

The therapeutic lumbar puncture provides a route of administration for antibiotics, antineoplastic agents, and anesthetics, as well as a means of relieving the increased pressure in benign intracranial hypertension or subarachnoid hemorrhage.

The main risk in lumbar puncture is brain herniation. This may occur whenever there is an intracranial mass, or obstruction to CSF flow, causing a pressure gradient between two brain compartments. High degrees of obstruction or displacement of the ventricular system are associated with increased risk of brain herniation. All patients with papilledema, focal neurologic signs, or obtundation should be considered for conditions that may cause brain herniation after LP, even though most will not have such conditions. A computed tomographic (CT) or magnetic resonance imaging (MRI) brain scan is useful in making this assessment. Other serious risks of LP are less common. Bleeding disorders (including therapeutic anticoagulation) and blood platelet counts below 20,000 to 30,000 may lead to intraspinal hemorrhage and cauda equina or spinal cord compression. Infection of skin at the puncture site may result in bacterial meningitis.

The most common complication of lumbar puncture is the post-LP headache. It may appear several hours to a day after the puncture. When a sharp small-bore needle is used (20 gauge or smaller) and a single puncture is successful, the incidence of this complication is approximately 10% to 15%. When a large-bore needle is used or several puncture attempts are necessary, the incidence is probably higher. The headache is typically bifrontal or generalized, is worse when the patient is upright, and is diminished when he or she lies flat. The headache appears to be due to a loss of CSF that results in intracranial hypotension. Displacement and stretching of pain-sensitive structures then occur when the patient is upright. Maintaining the patient prone (or supine) in the flat, or even in the Trendelenberg position, for 30 to 60 minutes after the procedure diminishes the CSF pressure at the needle puncture site and presumably decreases the persistent leakage of fluid from the subarachnoid space that occurs when the needle is withdrawn.

REFERENCES

Fishman RA: Cerebrospinal fluid in diseases of the nervous system, ed 2. Philadelphia, 1992, Saunders.

Marton KI and Gean AD: The spinal tap: a new look at an old test. Ann Intern Med 104:840, 1986.

Samuels MA: Manual of neurologic therapeutics, ed 4. Boston, 1990, Little, Brown.

CHAPTER

106 Electroencephalography and Evoked Responses

Rodney D. Bell
Sabrina G. Beacham

ELECTROENCEPHALOGRAPHY

The electroencephalogram (EEG) is a record of the electrical activity of the brain obtained by the standardized placement (International 10-20 system) of recording electrodes on the scalp (Fig. 106-1, *A*). Traditionally the EEG is recorded to paper with a chart recorder; however, newer computer technology has enabled the electrical signals to be digitized and stored on various devices such as optical disks and digital audiotape. With the digitization of the EEG, the potential for developing new ways of viewing the electrical signals of the brain is possible, along with the advantage of decreasing the storage space required for paper hard copy.

The EEG is obtained by recording from these scalp electrodes in a standard pattern of electrode connections called montages. The montages used may vary among individual laboratories (Fig. 106-1, *A* and *B*). The EEG is useful in providing information about the electrical physiologic processes of the brain. Electroencephalography constitutes the single most valuable laboratory test in the evaluation of patients with epilepsy. It is a safe, noninvasive, and readily repeated procedure by which patients can be followed and evaluated during the interictal or ictal periods. It is important to realize that a normal interictal EEG result does not exclude the presence of epilepsy. An initial EEG reveals an epileptiform (suggestive of epilepsy: i.e., containing spikes or sharp waves) abnormality in about 55% of cases. This percentage can be increased to approximately 80% by obtaining serial EEGs over a prolonged length of time (i.e., a minimum of three EEGs at intervals of several months). The EEG is also more likely to reveal epileptiform activity in younger patients (below 10 years of age, 80%) than in older patients (above age 40, 30%). Sleep recording and cerebral activation procedures such as hyperventilation and photic stimulation also increase the percentage of "positive" EEG results. Sleep deprivation for 24 hours results in activation (production of an epileptiform abnormality) of the EEG in about 40% of patients. In general, withdrawal of anticonvulsant medication for the purposes of obtaining an abnormal EEG result in a patient with the clinical diagnosis of epilepsy is not warranted, because it may precipitate seizures or status epilepticus. Repeating the EEG in a patient with clinical epilepsy is more likely to yield a "positive" EEG finding and is far less dangerous to the patient. If, however, the diagnosis of epilepsy is in question, and the EEG result has been repeatedly normal, it is reasonable to taper and stop anticonvulsant medication and repeat the EEG.

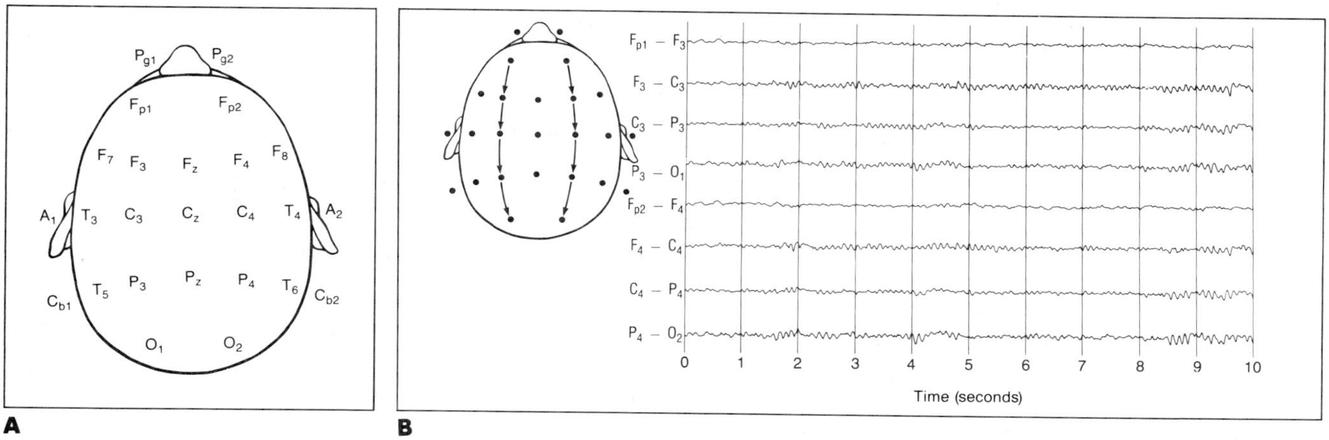

A **B**

Fig. 106-1. A, The International 10-20 system of electrode placement. Right-sided placements are indicated by even numbers, left-sided placements by odd numbers, and midline placements by z. The C_b notation refers to an electrode placed midway between the posterior temporal and occipital electrodes. C_b was originally part of the International 10-20 system but is seldom used, as it does not accurately reflect cerebellar activity. A, arricular; C, central; F, frontal; F_p, frontal polar; P, parietal; P_g, nasopharyngeal; T, temporal; O, occipital. The electrodes can be connected in various arrays, called montages. The most common montage is straight lines from front to back or transverse across the head. **B,** 8-Channels of normal electroencephalogram. Note the well-organized occipital rhythms (0_1 and 0_2) at 8 to 10 Hz; this represents the normal alpha rhythm. The letters and numbers are the standard designations, odd numbers on the left, even on the right. The montages *(electrode connections)* used here are from the front of the head to the back of the head *(occipital)*. The first four channels are from the left side of the head, the second four from the right. Current clinical practice of electroencephalography commonly uses 16 to 21 channels of EEG. The distance between each of the vertical lines represents 1 second *(10 seconds for the recording shown).*

The predominant abnormalities seen in epilepsy are the spike (an evanescent electrical event lasting less than 70 milliseconds) and the sharp wave (a transient electrical event lasting between 70 and 200 milliseconds). Examples of these events are shown in Fig. 106-2. Spikes and slow waves can occur in adults and children. "Classic" 3 Hz spike-and-slow-wave complexes are seen in children with absence seizures. Bursts of multiple spikes, followed by a slow wave repeating at rates of every 2 to 3 seconds, occur in patients with myoclonic seizures. Paroxysmal rhythmic slow-wave activity (1 to 3 Hz) can also be associated with epilepsy.

Computed tomography (CT) scanning and magnetic resonance imaging (MRI) have gained widespread acceptance, making the EEG far less important in screening patients for structural disease of the nervous system and in localizing structural brain abnormalities. The EEG is generally not as sensitive as the CT/MRI scan in identifying structural abnormalities. Nevertheless, in certain instances (e.g., herpes simplex encephalitis and strokes), the EEG usually reveals an abnormality long before the CT/MRI scan. This example is particularly relevant because early detection and treatment of this disease are vital. Thus the EEG is complementary to the CT/MRI scan in the identification of structural disease.

Clinical electroencephalography is based on the recognition of electrical patterns. Certain patterns are relatively specific (e.g., spikes for epilepsy), whereas others, such as diffuse slowing (implying diffuse neuronal dysfunction from any cause), are nonspecific. Certain disorders produce patterns that, although nonspecific, help to suggest, support, or establish a diagnosis. Specific patterns with clinical relevance are discussed later.

Hypoxia

Cardiopulmonary arrest is a common clinical problem. The EEG (and serial EEGs) can provide useful physiologic and prognostic information about patients who have suffered cardiopulmonary arrest. The main effects of progressive hypoxia on the EEG are reduction and slowing of the normal background alpha activity (8 to 13 Hz), increased theta activity (4 to 7 Hz), generalized delta slowing (1 to 3 Hz), and, finally, suppression of all activity. After a hypoxic insult to the brain, several patterns that have prognostic significance can emerge. These patterns have been most thoroughly studied after a minimum of 6 hours has elapsed after the insult. To use the EEG as a prognostic indicator, at least this amount of time should have passed.

An EEG showing a normal background, reactivity to external stimuli, and sleep patterns usually indicates the potential for clinical improvement. Patterns indicating a poor prognosis after a hypoxic insult are (1) alpha coma, which is an EEG pattern that looks very much like a normal awake tracing but is nonreactive to stimulus (alpha coma is also seen with brainstem lesions); (2) burst suppression, which is a pattern in which the EEG background varies between periods of relative flattening and bursts of higher-voltage

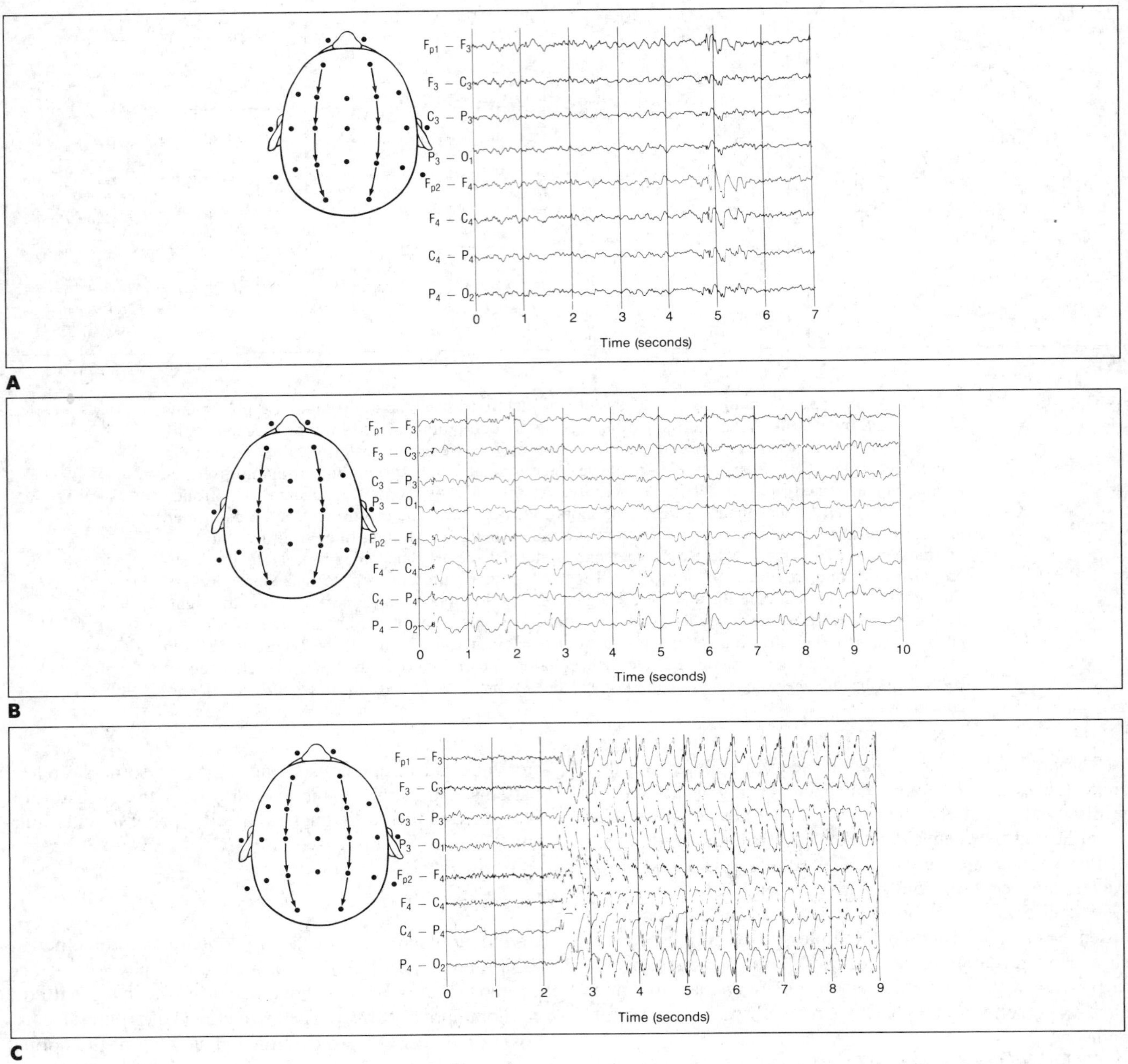

Fig. 106-2. **A,** Spike-and-slow wave in a 25-year-old man. **B,** Sharp wave in a 9-year-old boy. **C,** Three-hertz spike and wave in a 1-year-old child with "classic" absence seizures.

slow or sharp activity; (3) periodic spike-wave activity with isoelectric intervals, which is a pattern generally associated with myoclonic jerks; and (4) electrocerebral inactivity, which is present in patients with brain death (Fig. 106-3).

Hepatic disease

In hepatic stupor or coma, as with any metabolic encephalopathy, the EEG result is generally abnormal by the time there is any alteration of consciousness. In the early stages of hepatic encephalopathy, the EEG shows progressive slowing until a triphasic pattern appears. Triphasic waves do not occur in every patient with hepatic coma, nor are they specific for this disease. However, when they do occur, they suggest a hepatic cause of the coma. Triphasic waves consist of medium-to-high-voltage broad waves, occurring rhythmically or in trains of 1 to 2 Hz in a symmetric fashion over both hemispheres (Fig. 106-4, *A*).

Herpes simplex encephalitis

The EEG is frequently the first abnormal laboratory test finding in herpes simplex encephalitis. The earliest changes are focal, temporal slow waves generally in the delta range

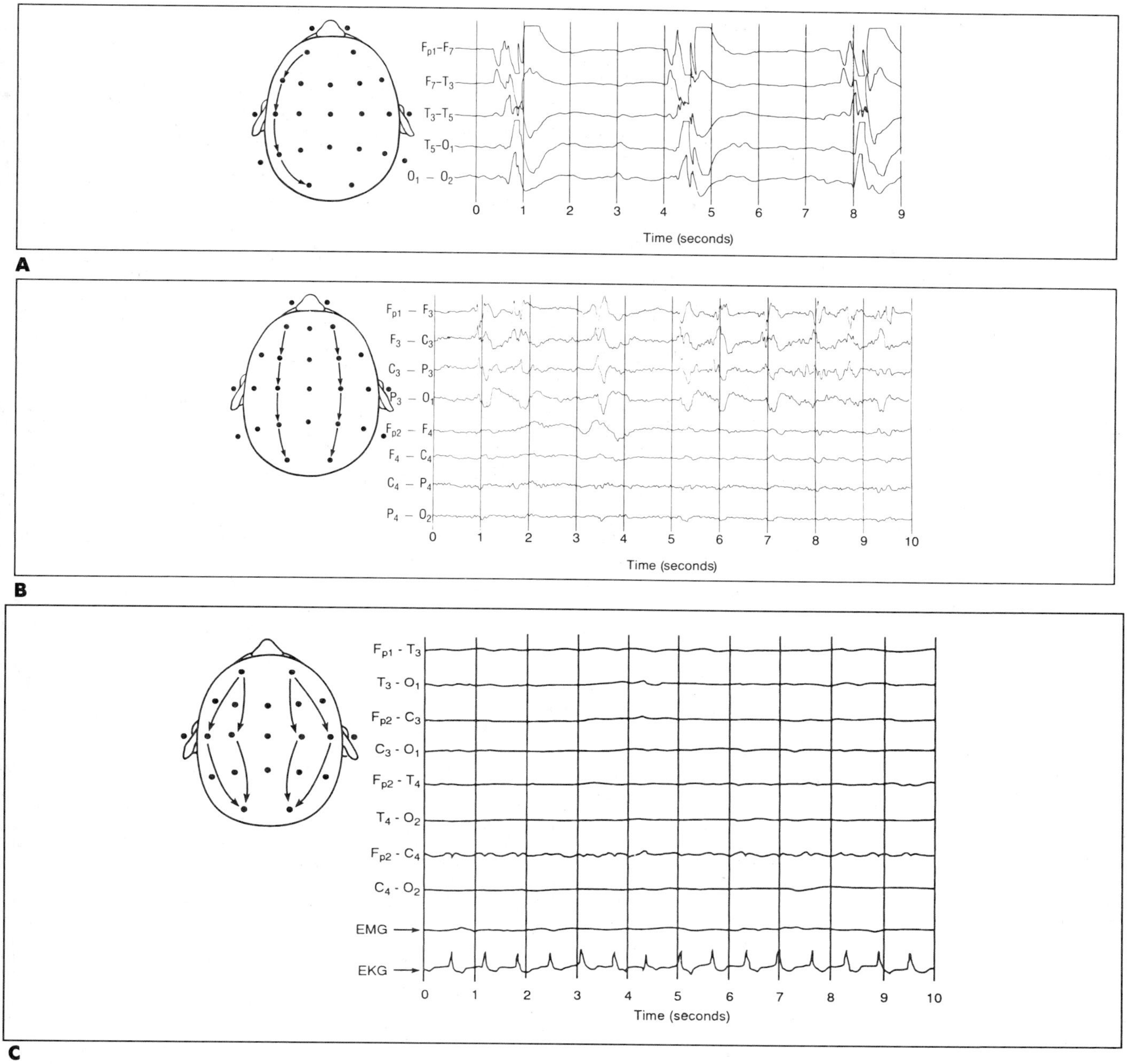

Fig. 106-3. **A,** Burst suppression pattern in a 49-year-old man after cardiac arrest. **B,** Periodic spike wave associated with myoclonic jerks of the arm. **C,** Electrocerebral silence in a patient with brain death. Double electrode distance is used as well as a EMG electrode and ECG monitoring.

(1 to 3 Hz). These waves are frequently followed by large sharp waves, which appear over the affected region and occur with a periodicity of 2 to 4 seconds. These sharp waves can occur bilaterally (Fig. 106-4, *B*).

Creutzfeldt-Jakob disease

Creutzfeldt-Jakob disease is a rare dementing disease caused by an atypical infectious agent. The classic EEG findings consist of periodic complexes that may be unilateral, are often triphasic, and repeat every 0.5 to 4.0 seconds. In sleep these discharges tend to disappear. The periodic patterns may or may not be associated with myoclonus.

Subacute sclerosing panencephalitis

Subacute sclerosing panencephalitis is a rare progressive inflammatory disease in young children and adolescents believed to be caused by a variant of the measles virus. The

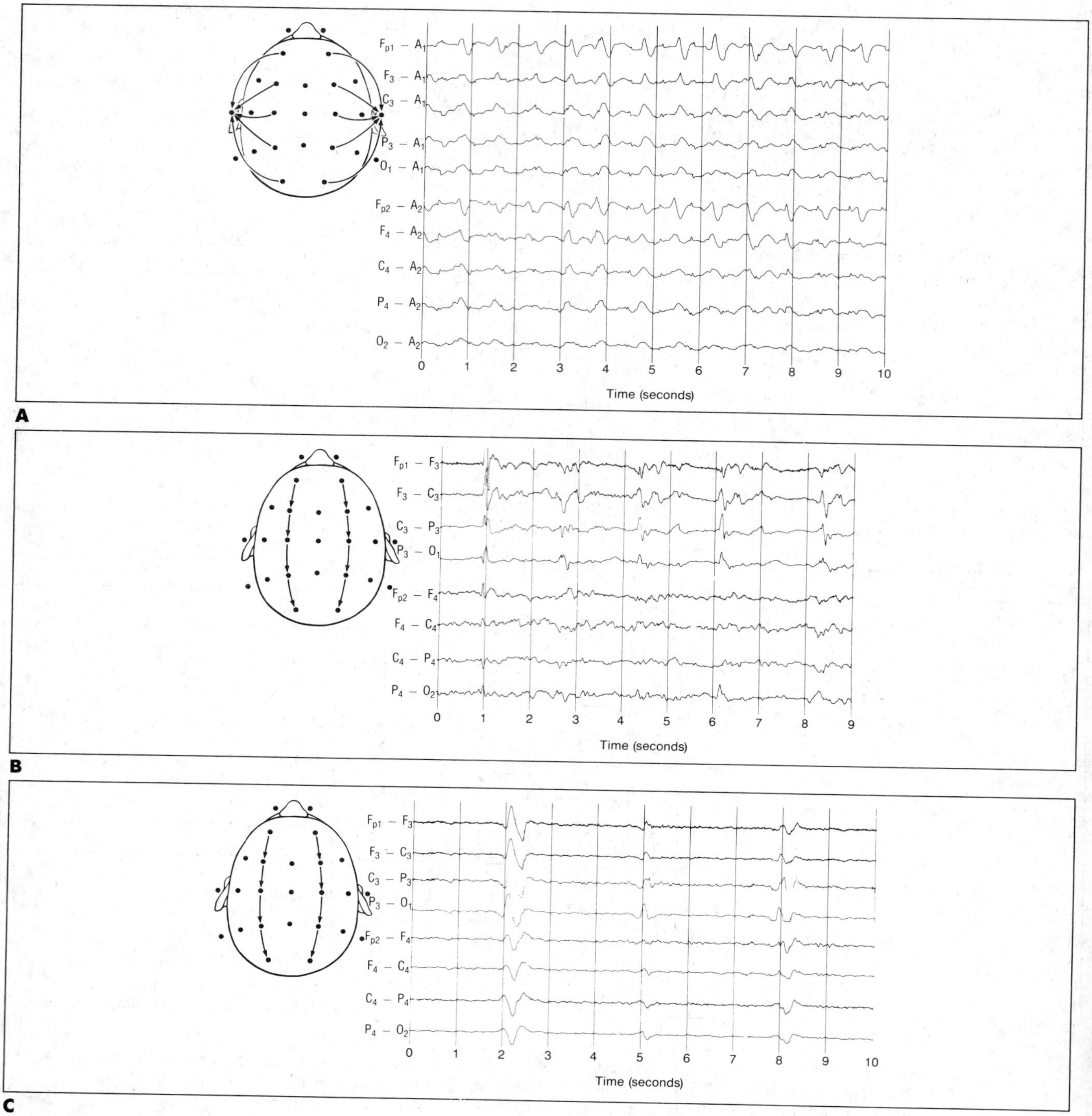

Fig. 106-4. A, Triphasic waves in a 48-year-old patient with hepatic coma. In this instance, all electrodes are referenced to the ear. **B,** Burst of sharp waves in a 29-year-old woman with biopsy-proven herpes simplex encephalitis. **C,** High-voltage periodic complexes in a 6-year-old patient with subacute sclerosing panencephalitis.

disease is characterized by progressive intellectual deterioration, a variety of abnormal movements, and a characteristic EEG pattern. The EEG pattern consists of periodic, high-voltage, repetitive polyphasic and sharp-and-slow-wave complexes, ranging from 0.5 to 2.0 seconds in duration and occurring every 4 to 15 seconds (Fig. 106-4, *C*).

Dementia

Senile dementia and Alzheimer's disease in the early stages cause very little alteration in the EEG. Therefore an abnormal EEG result is more suggestive of a specific structural problem or of a treatable form of dementia, suggesting the need for more extensive clinical investigation. In the late stages of Alzheimer's disease, the EEG pattern generally is diffusely slow (Fig. 106-5, *A*).

Metabolic encephalopathy

Any metabolic derangement, including hypoglycemia or hyperglycemia, hyponatremia or hypernatremia, hypocalcemia or hypercalcemia, uremia, or drug intoxication, that alters sensorium can affect the EEG result. The changes in each of these metabolic derangements are not specific and generally consist in a slowing of the background rhythms from the normal alpha frequency (8 to 13 Hz) to the theta range (4 to 7 Hz). As the derangement becomes more profound, the EEG slows further into the delta range (1 to 3 Hz) (Fig. 106-5, *B*).

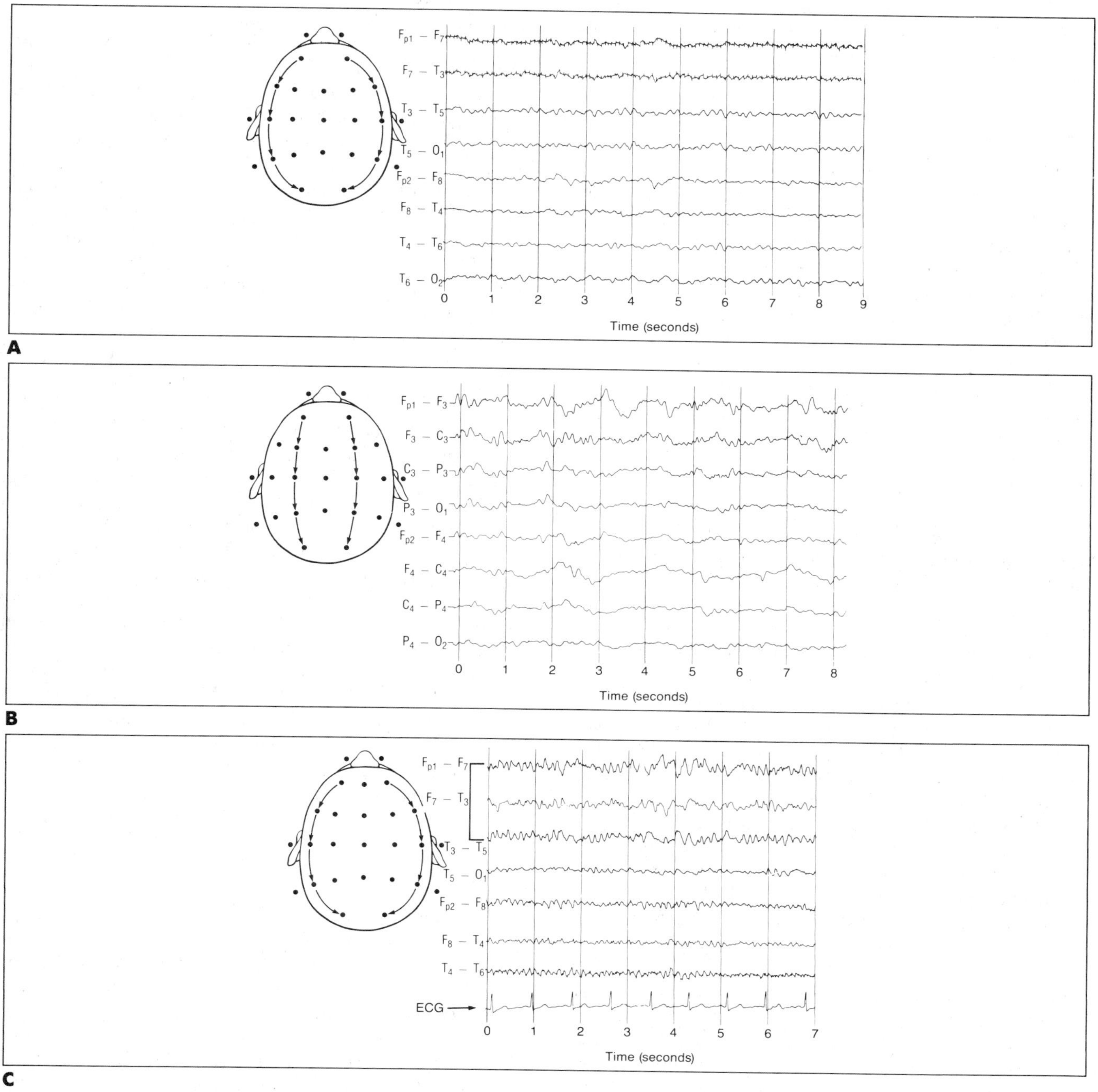

Fig. 106-5. A, An EEG from a 67-year-old patient with senile dementia, Alzheimer's type. The EEG shows mild slowing. **B,** An EEG from a patient with hyponatremia. This type of EEG can be seen in any form of metabolic derangement. **C,** An EEG from a patient with a brain tumor. Note the focal slowing indicated by the bracket.

In patients with renal failure, the slowing of the EEG generally parallels the degree of alteration of consciousness. In patients who have the dialysis disequilibrium syndrome, however, the EEG may reflect the shifts in osmolality with high-voltage paroxysmal activity.

Dialysis dementia is a progressively fatal disorder characterized by slowly progressive dementia, speech disturbances, myoclonus, abnormal movements, and convulsions. The EEG can aid in this diagnosis, because there is a characteristic pattern of slowing of the background activity with superimposed bursts of high-amplitude slow waves, triphasic contoured waves, sharp waves, or spike-and-slow-wave complexes.

Focal structural disease

The EEG is neither as specific nor as sensitive as the CT scan in the diagnosis of focal structural disease of the brain. Nevertheless, in either early strokes or small, focal structural disease of the brain, the EEG can reveal positive information not available from the CT scan. EEG features characteristic of focal structural disease include (1) continuous focal delta waves (1 to 3 Hz), which are irregular in waveform; (2) intermittent delta waves, which are regular in waveform; (3) depression or absence of usual background activity in the vicinity of the local slowing; and (4) epileptiform discharges, which remain or begin focally (Fig. 106-5, *C*).

EVOKED RESPONSES

Advances in microprocessing in the early 1970s and commercialization of signal-averaging computers made possible the measurement of small changes in the electrical activity of the brain caused by an external stimulus. These signs, small in voltage as compared to EEG, are not obtainable without the aid of a computer that detects and averages the electrical signal and retains it in memory. To average, a sensory stimulus is given that triggers the computer to record a sample of brain electrical activity over a fixed length of time, generally from 10 to 500 milliseconds. The stimulus is repeated several hundred or thousand times, and each evoked potential (or evoked response) is averaged by the computer. The background activity (essentially the EEG) tends to average to a straight line, leaving the recorded evoked potential from the sensory stimulus.

There are presently three types of evoked responses used in clinical medicine: brainstem auditory evoked potentials, visual evoked potentials, and somatosensory evoked potentials. They are used (1) to demonstrate abnormal sensory system function when the history and neurologic examination findings are equivocal; (2) to reveal the presence of a clinically unsuspected malfunction in the sensory system when demyelinating disease is suggested by symptoms and signs in another area of the nervous system; (3) to help define the anatomic distribution of a disease process; and (4) to monitor changes in a patient's status objectively over time.

Visual evoked potentials

The pattern-reversal visual evoked potential (VEP) is a widely used and reproducible response. It is generally performed by using small checks, usually subtending the eye 28 minutes to 1 degree of an arc. These checks appear on a monitor or television screen that has a specific known luminance. The size check fills a 3 degree span of foveal vision and produces a response that is nearly as large as a signal that covers 10 to 20 degrees. The checks are reversed (i.e., black to white) at a specific rate and the monocular response is recorded over the visual cortex from occipital electrodes 0_1, 0_z, and 0_2. The major potential in this technique is a large positive wave seen at about 100 milliseconds, usually maximally from the midoccipital electrode 0_z (Fig. 106-6). This potential is referred to as the P100 response. Measurements usually taken are the (1) absolute latency, (2) interocular absolute latency difference, (3) amplitude, and (4) interocular amplitude difference ratio. Both the shape and the latency of PVEPs are significantly affected by stimulus parameters including luminance, check and pattern size, rate of reversal, and nature of the stimulator as well as such factors as visual acuity, body temperature, age, and gender.

A prolongation of the latency of the P100 response, an interocular difference of greater than 6 milliseconds (each laboratory must establish its own normal values), and a difference greater than 50% in amplitude of the P100 response are suggestive of an abnormality anterior to the optic chiasm (Fig. 106-6). However, this test is not specific, and the difference between a demyelinating lesion as seen in multiple sclerosis and a compressive lesion involving the optic nerve cannot be ascertained on the basis of this test.

The major clinical use for PVEPs at the present time is in the diagnosis of subclinical optic neuritis or multiple sclerosis. About 90% of patients who have a clear history of optic neuritis have abnormal PVEPs, regardless of the interval since the clinical episode of neuritis. Abnormalities occur in 75% to 97% of patients with definite multiple sclerosis, including those without visual symptoms.

Abnormalities of the PVEP are not specific for optic neuritis or multiple sclerosis (see the box on p. 972). Prolonged latencies can occur in diseases that resemble multiple sclerosis clinically, such as the spinocerebellar degenerations.

Brainstem auditory evoked potential (BAEP)

The preferred stimulus for evaluation of the brainstem auditory system is a high-frequency click produced by a high-quality earphone given at a fixed stimulus rate and intensity. Signals generated from this stimulus can be recorded from scalp and ear electrodes. In normal subjects, a total of seven short-latency waves can be defined within 10 milliseconds of the click each measured for absolute latency and compared to that of normal controls (Fig. 106-7, *A*). Wave I arises in the distal portion of the acoustic nerve; wave V is thought to arise near the inferior colliculus. The generators for the other waves are less clearly defined but

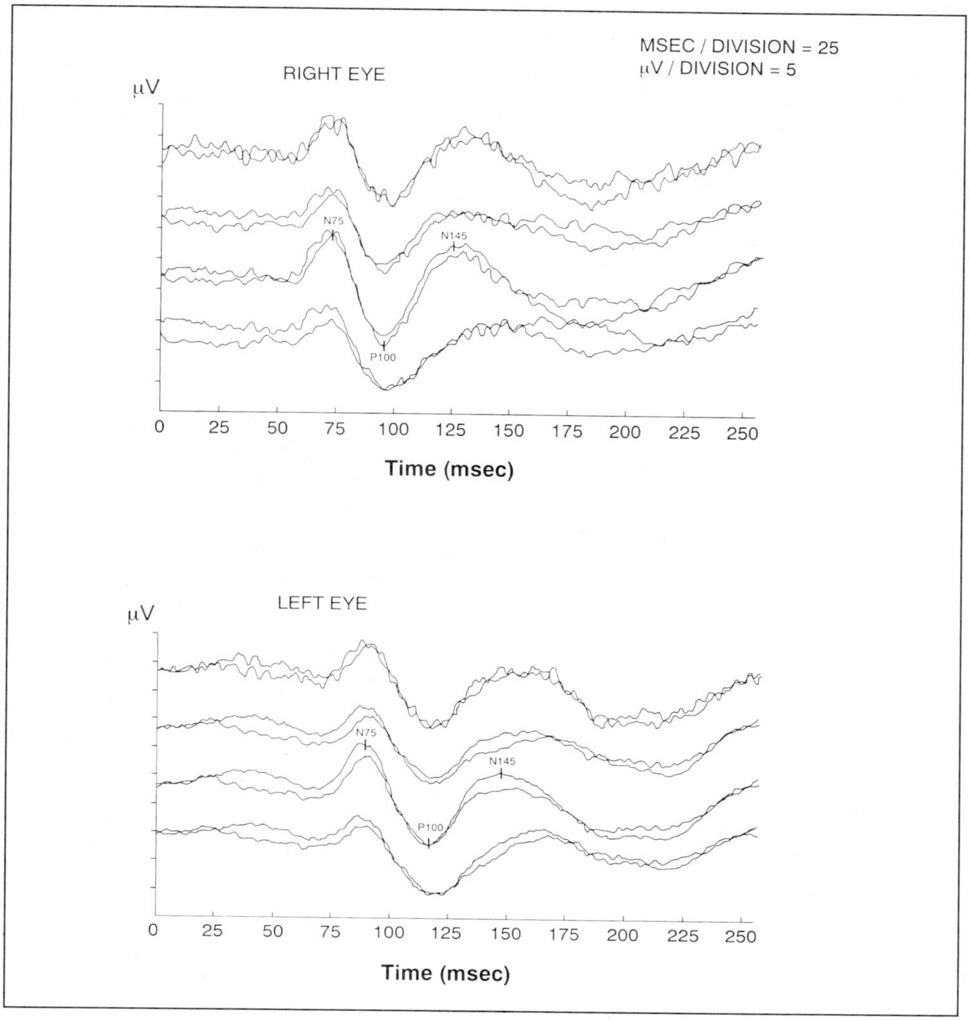

Fig. 106-6. Normal pattern-reversal visual evoked response (PVEP) with the P100 response at 100 milliseconds in the right eye. The left P100 response is prolonged more than 6 milliseconds as compared with the right. This patient has multiple sclerosis. Microvolts *(μV)* are in multiples of 5.0. N75 and N145 indicate the major negative deflections before and after the P100 response with their corresponding approximate latency.

can be thought of as follows: wave II, cochlear nucleus and proximal acoustic nerve; wave III, superior olivary complex; wave IV, tract or nuclei of the lateral lemniscus. Many clinicians believe that with the exception of wave I, all waves of the short-latency BAEP originate from a complex interaction of numerous generators in the brainstem and cannot be separated anatomically.

Stimulation rate, click polarity, and intensity are critical parameters in recording the BAEP. Therefore these parameters must be specified in any recording and normal values defined for each rate, type of click polarity, and intensity above threshold that is used.

BAEPs are the best noninvasive laboratory tests for the detection of acoustic neuromas. There are a true-positive rate of 98% and a false-positive rate of about 1%. The BAEP patterns found with acoustic tumors are not specific. Most commonly, wave I is present and all other waves are delayed or absent (Fig. 106-7, *B*). Small lesions produce a prolongation of the I-III interpeak latency, and large lesions compressing the brainstem may produce a prolongation of the III-V interpeak latency in the contralateral ear.

BAEPs are also useful in the diagnosis of multiple sclerosis. Abnormalities in BAEPs occur in 21% to 55% of patients without brainstem symptoms or signs. The most common abnormalities are low-amplitude wave V and prolongation of the III-V interpeak latency. BAEPs are also useful in the early diagnosis of hearing loss in young children who cannot cooperate for formal audiometric testing. They are particularly valuable in evaluating the possibility of hearing loss in children with meningitis (Fig. 106-7, *C*). A partial list of other diseases in which BAEP result has been abnormal is seen in the box on p. 973.

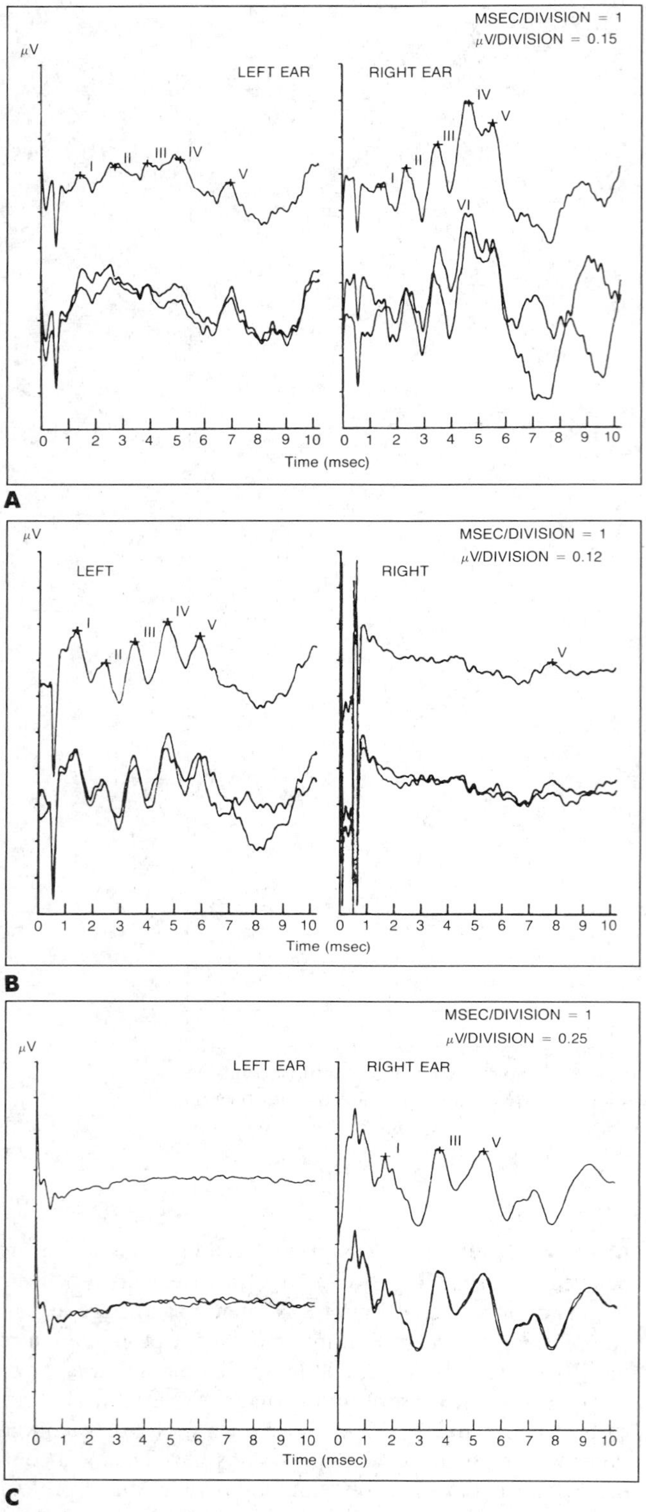

Fig. 106-7. **A,** A normal brainstem auditory evoked response (BAEP) is shown in the right ear. The left BAEP response is abnormal as a result of the prolongation of left I-V and I-III interpeak latencies. This patient has a cerebellopontine angle tumor. Microvolts *(μV)* are in multiples of 0.15. **B,** A BAEP from a patient with an acoustic neuroma on the right. There is essentially no response on the right. Microvolts *(μV)* are in multiples of 0.12. **C,** A BAEP from a child with meningitis. Note the normal response on the right ear and the lack of response in the left ear even at high-stimulus intensities, indicating that hearing is impaired on the left. Microvolts *(μV)* are in multiples of 0.25.

Some diseases that produce abnormalities in the pattern-reversal visual evoked response

Compressive lesions of the anterior visual pathways
Extrinsic and intrinsic tumors
Pseudotumor cerebri

Generalized CNS diseases
Parkinson's disease
Pernicious anemia
Sarcoid
Neurosyphilis
Renal failure
Spinocerebellar degenerations
Charcot-Marie-Tooth disease
Phenylketonuria
Adrenoleukodystrophy

Spinal cord diseases
Chronic progressive myelopathy

Large refractive errors
Glaucoma
Toxic amblyopia
Amblyopia ex anopsia
Hydrocephalus
Central serous retinopathy
Factitious prolongation of latency

Somatosensory evoked potential

Somatosensory evoked potentials (SEPs) are produced by repetitively stimulating with brief electrical pulses peripheral nerves and recording at various locations along the nervous system to the sensory cortex. Although this technique has been studied for many years, there is some lack of uniformity in the recording techniques and the neuroanatomic substrates of the responses obtained with various amounts of stimulation. Therefore, in 1985 the American Electroencephalographic Society published guidelines for clinical evoked potentials to help address this issue. The most widely used are the median nerve SEP and posterior tibial nerve SEP. By convention, positive waves are designated with a capital P followed by a number. The number refers to the number of milliseconds following the stimulus where the waveform occurs, for example, P_{38}. Similarly, a negative wave is designated by a capital N followed by a number representing the number of milliseconds following the stimulus, for example, N_{11}.

Some diseases that produce abnormal brainstem evoked responses

Lateral pontomedullary junction infarcts
Brainstem gliomas
Multiple sclerosis
Neonatal hearing loss
Vitamin B_{12} deficiency
Acoustic neuromas
Brain death
Friedreich's ataxia
Charcot-Marie-Tooth disease
Hereditary cerebellar ataxia
Metachromatic leukodystrophy
Adrenoleukodystrophy
Pelizaeus-Merzbacher disease

Some diseases that produce abnormalities of somatosensory-evoked potentials

Peripheral nerve lesions
Brachial plexus and cervical root trauma
Thoracic outlet syndrome
Cervical radiculopathies
Spinal cord trauma
Multiple sclerosis
Lumbar radiculopathies
Thalamic tumors
Cerebral and brainstem hemorrhages and infarctions
Coma secondary to head trauma
Pelizaeus-Merzbacher disease
Adrenoleukodystrophy
Friedreich's ataxia
Spinocerebellar degenerations
Myelodysplasias

Median nerve SEP. Median nerve SEPs are generally recorded by placing electrodes over Erb's point, the cervical spine over the C_5 or C_2 process, and over the somatosensory cortex on the scalp. Using a repetitive stimulation rate of 4 to 7/sec waveforms are generated and represent volleys traversing the posterior columns, medial lemnisci, and spinocerebellar tracts. The waveform recorded over Erb's point is generated from the brachial plexus; the waveform that appears at approximately 11 milliseconds (N_{11}) is generated in the cervical cord root entry zone or posterior columns; the waveform recorded from the C_5 or C_2 ($N_{13\text{-}14}$) process is generated in the dorsal column and dorsal column nucleus; the scalp-recorded wave at about 20 milliseconds (N_{20}) is generated in the thalamus or thalamocortical radiations; and the waveform occurring at 22 milliseconds (P_{22}) is considered to be of cortical origin (Fig. 106-8, *A*).

SEPs are sensitive to lesions of the dorsal column–medial lemniscus systems and are generally not affected by isolated involvement of the spinothalamic tract. Abnormalities are generally defined by a prolongation of the interpeak wave latency compared with empirically established normal values or by a side-to-side difference of greater than 1 millisecond. A prolonged interpeak latency between Erb's point and the dorsal column (N_{11}) suggests a lesion located between the proximal portions of the brachial plexus and the dorsal column nuclei. An abnormal latency between the dorsal column and the thalamus and cortex (N_{20}-P_{22} suggests a lesion located between the medulla and the thalamocortical systems. Cerebral lesions usually abolish N_{20} and P_{22} rather than prolonging their latencies. Median nerve short-latency SEPs have been reported to be abnormal in 63% to 87% of patients with definite multiple sclerosis, many of whom appear to lack signs of sensory dysfunction on the appropriate side.

Lower-limb SEP. For testing the lower limb (tibial and peroneal nerves), the reference point for latency measurements is the time when the volley of stimuli passes through the cauda equina and lower spinal cord. Activity in these structures is generally referred to as the lumbar potential. Although additional recording sites can be added anywhere along the neuroaxis, recordings are usually limited to the lumbar potentials (LPs) and scalp recordings over the somatosensory cortex. The posterior tibial nerve is used most frequently because of the greater ease of stimulation. The waveform recorded from the cervical spine at about 30 milliseconds (N_{30}) after stimulation of the posterior tibial nerve is presumably generated in the nucleus gracilis. The waveform recorded from the scalp at about 37 milliseconds (P_{37} is thought to be generated in the cortex (Fig. 106-8, *B*).

One of the major uses for lower limb SEPs is the monitoring of the spinal cord and brainstem structures during surgery. The SEP can provide information about neurologic function during both anesthesia and an operation that would otherwise be available only through clinical assessment of the unanesthetized patient. Operative manipulation of neural or vascular structures can alter the SEP, as can pressure on neural structures from surgical retractors. SEPs may be affected by manipulation of a spinal cord tumor or by obliteration of vessels feeding an arteriovenous malformation of the spinal cord. Instrumentation can likewise alter the SEP. During operations on the spine, the surgeon can respond to a deterioration of the SEP by altering the spinal curvature, replacing retractors, or repositioning a bone graft or Harrington rod. Likewise, the anesthesiologist can reverse hemodilution or raise the arterial blood pressure. Therefore the SEP in the anesthetized patient can provide useful physiologic information about the functional integrity of the nervous system that would otherwise be unavailable.

As with other evoked potentials, an abnormal SEP finding indicates only an anatomic lesion that disrupts the normal physiologic mechanisms of that system, and not a specific disease process (see the box at lower left).

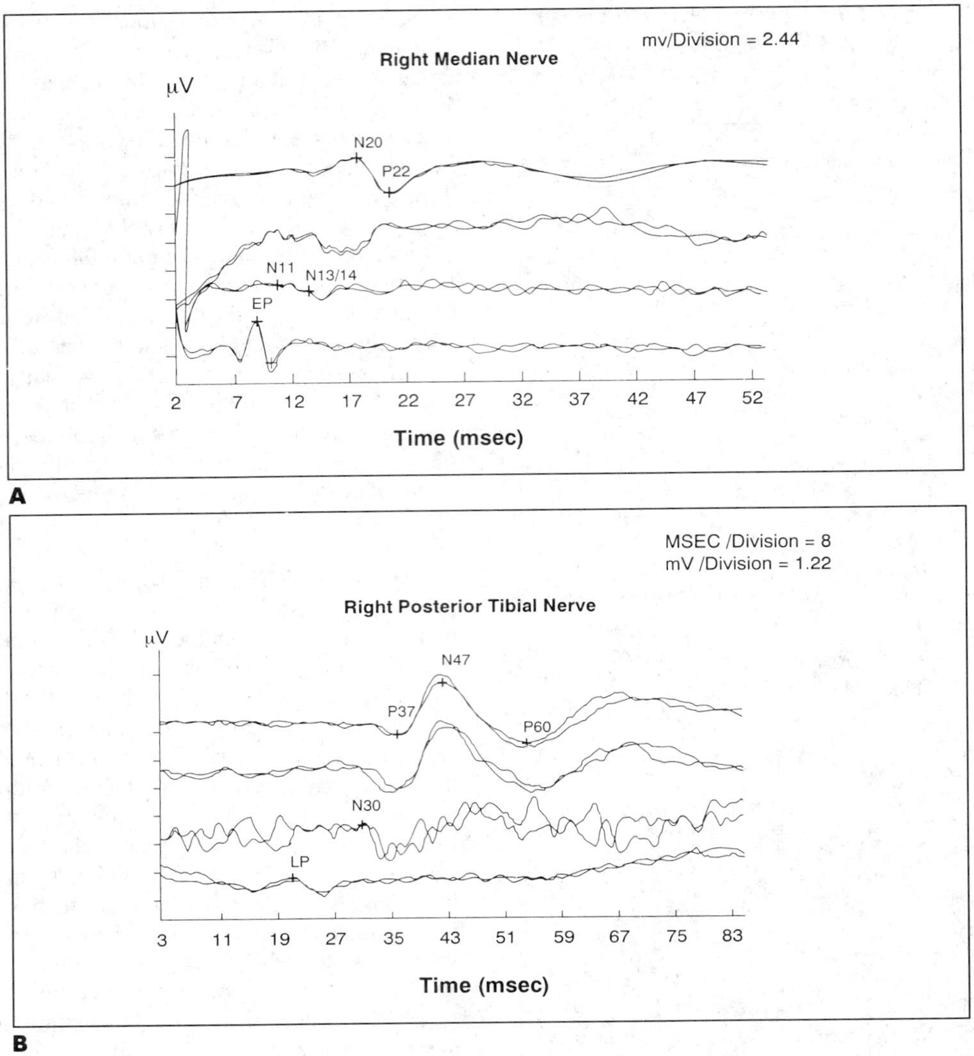

Fig. 106-8. A, A normal median nerve somatosensory evoked potential. The waveforms are thought to represent the following: **1,** Erb's, the brachial plexus; **2,** N_{11}, cervical cord root entry zone; **3,** $N_{13\text{-}14}$, dorsal columns and cuneate nucleus; **4,** N_{20}, the thalamus or thalamocortical radiations; **5,** P_{23}, the cortex. **B,** A normal posterior tibial somatosensory evoked potential. The waveforms shown are thought to represent the following: **1,** LP, the entry zone for lumbar potentials; **2,** N_{30}, the thalamus; **3,** P_{37}, cortex.

REFERENCES

American Electroencephalographic Society: Guidelines for clinical evoked potential studies. J Clin Neurophysiol 1:3, 1984.

Chiappa KH: Evoked potentials in clinical medicine, ed 2. New York, 1990, Raven Press.

Daly DD and Pedley TA: Current practice of clinical encephalopathy, ed 2. New York, 1990, Raven Press.

Hecox KE et al: Brainstem auditory evoked response in the diagnosis of pediatric neurologic disease. Neurology 31:832, 1981.

Niedermeyer E and Lopes da Silva F, editors: Electroencephalography: basic principles, clinical applications, and related fields, ed 2. Baltimore, 1987, Urban & Schwazenberg.

Tyner FS, Knot JR and Myer WB: Fundamentals of EEG technology. vol 2. Clinical correlates. New York, 1989, Raven Press.

CHAPTER

107 Electromyography

Allen B. Gruber
Richard J. Barohn

Electromyography (EMG) is the electrophysiologic assessment of the neuromuscular system. This assessment consists of a nerve conduction study (NCS), a needle electromyography study, and other miscellaneous tests. Thus *EMG* may be used as an inclusive term to describe all of these tests, or at times it may refer to the more restricted needle electromyographic study.

The basic principle of EMG is that a moving wave of an electric potential from either nerve or muscle is measured with a recording device. This is the same physiologic basis for recording electrical potentials from the heart (ECG) and brain (EEG). For nerve conduction studies, a nerve is depolarized with an electrical stimulator. The electric potential is measured either over the muscle (motor NCS) or nerve (sensory NCS). For needle EMG, the patient voluntarily contracts a muscle, and a needle electrode inserted directly into the muscle records the electrical wave of muscle depolarization.

Often the physician who is familiar with the patient's history and physical findings is not the one performing the EMG. Therefore specific information concerning the history and physical findings should be conveyed to the EMG laboratory. The electromyographer can then tailor the examination to answer the questions of the referring physician. Electromyographers usually corroborate the history and physical findings to help guide their study, but electromyography should not be considered to constitute a neuromuscular consultation.

Different techniques and equipment are used by each EMG laboratory. An EMG laboratory should state its normal values for each test, taking into account variables such as age, skin temperature, and height. In individuals less than 5 years or more than 60 years of age, nerve conduction velocities are slower, and nomograms must be consulted. Some laboratories use normative data for each decade of age. Prominent slowing of nerve conduction can occur with a cold extremity. For a NCS, an extremity should be warmed to a surface temperature of 34° C or more. An EMG report should include the raw data and offer an electrodiagnostic interpretation considering technical limitations, such as cooperation of the patient.

For a motor NCS, a nerve is supramaximally stimulated with a surface stimulator placed over it at various locations. Electric activity is recorded with a surface electrode over the belly of a standard muscle innervated by the nerve being studied. For example, in a median motor NCS (Fig. 107-1, *A*), stimulation is typically just above the wrist and at the elbow. The recording electrode is placed over the belly of the abductor pollicus brevis muscle. The evoked muscle potential (also known as the compound motor action potential [CMAP] is displayed on an oscilloscope screen and is usually permanently recorded. The amplitude of the CMAP is recorded in millivolts. Amplitudes can be measured either from the peak to the baseline or from the peak to the trough of the potentials, depending on the laboratory convention. For each point of stimulation, a latency is measured (in milliseconds), which represents the time elapsed from the delivery of the stimulus to the appearance of the muscle potential. The latency recorded from the most distal point of stimulation is referred to as the distal latency. In addition to measuring the time of conduction in the distal nerve, the distal latency includes the time of transmission across the neuromuscular junction and the conduction time of the muscle action potential through the muscle. If a standardized distance from the recording electrode is used for the distal stimulation, a normal range for the distal latency is available. A conduction velocity (CV) can be calculated by dividing the distance (in millimeters) between two points of stimulation by the time it takes to travel between these two points. Thus

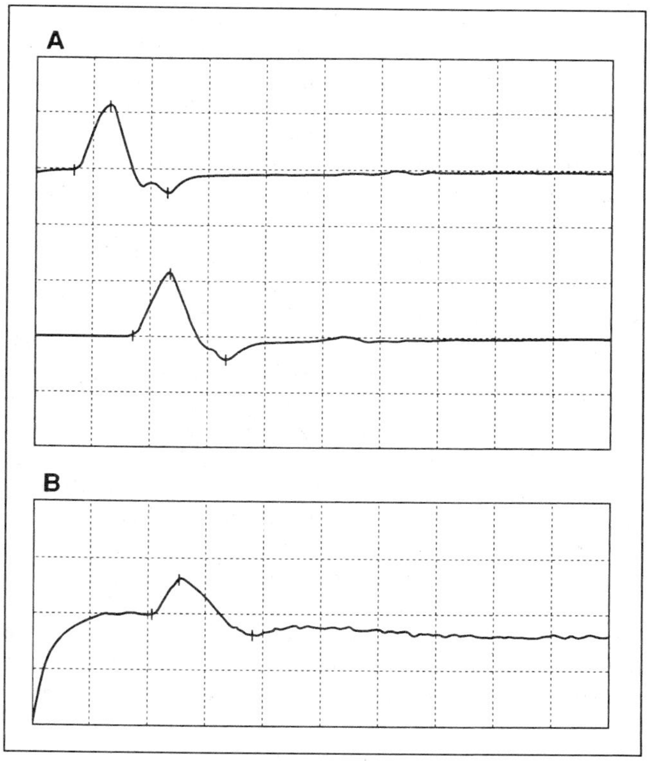

Fig. 107-1. **A,** Motor nerve conduction study. Median nerve stimulated at the wrist *(top)* and elbow *(bottom)*. Recording made over the thenar eminence. Sweep speed: 5 ms/division. Gain: 5 mV/division. **B,** Sensory nerve conduction study. Median nerve stimulated at the wrist and recorded with ring electrode over the index finger. Sweep speed: 1 ms/division. Gain: 50 μV/division.

$$CV\ (m/sec) = distance\ (mm) \div (proximal\ latency - distal\ latency\ [msec])$$

In the example of a normal median motor NCS given in Fig. 107-1, *A*, distal latency = 3.0 milliseconds, proximal latency = 6.3 milliseconds, distance from elbow to wrist = 293 mm. Therefore

$$CV = 293 \div (6.3 - 3.0) = 88.79\ m/sec$$

The amplitude of the CMAP is 6.0 mV proximally and distally. Commonly measured motor nerves are the median, ulnar, peroneal, and tibial.

For sensory nerve conduction studies, either antidromic (opposite to the physiologic direction of current flow; proximal stimulation at different sites and distal recording) or orthodromic (in the physiologic direction of current flow; distal stimulation and proximal recording at different sites) techniques are used. Again, supramaximum surface stimulation is usually employed. The recording is made directly over nerve fibers, with rings around a finger, or with disk electrodes taped over the wrist (for median and ulnar nerves) or the lateral ankle (for the sural nerve). For the sensory fibers of the median nerve, stimulation can be given in the palm, at the wrist, and at the elbow, and a recording is typically made over the index finger. For sensory nerves, a relatively lower amount of voltage output is needed to reach supramaximum stimulation, the potentials are much smaller than motor potentials (microvolts rather than millivolts), and they usually appear sooner than any volume-conducted motor potential. As with motor nerves, the parameters measured consist of the amplitude, latency, and conduction velocity. Because recordings are made directly over nerves, a conduction velocity can be calculated for the most distal part of the sensory nerve by dividing the distance from stimulation to recording site by the latency. Some laboratories, however, simply report distal latencies without calculating velocity. Latencies can be measured to the onset or to the peak of the potential, depending on the laboratory, and the amplitude is measured either from the peak of the potential to the baseline or peak-to-trough. Commonly measured sensory nerves are the median, ulnar, radial, sural, and plantar nerves. In the example given (Fig. 107-1, *B*), this normal median sensory nerve action potential was obtained by wrist stimulation and recording over the index finger. The amplitude (peak to trough) is 49 μV and the distal latency is 2.6 milliseconds. Because potentials can be quite small, especially in the feet, an average of multiple stimulations may be needed.

In addition to motor and sensory nerve conduction studies, F waves and H reflexes can be helpful. Measurement of these potentials provides some indication of conduction in the proximal portion of the nerve. F waves are small-amplitude, long-latency responses produced by supramaximal stimulation of a motor nerve with the cathode directed antidromically (directed away from the muscle that is being recorded). An F wave represents the muscle potential produced by an alpha motor neuron depolarized by the antidromic stimulus. The latency and shape of the F wave can vary from stimulus to stimulus with a fixed arrangement of stimulating and recording electrodes. Typically, at least 10 F waves are recorded at one stimulus site, and the shortest latency, measured to the onset of the F wave, is recorded. F wave amplitude is not a clinically useful measurement. Some institutions report only the latency of the F waves, using nomograms relating this value to the height of the individual. Others measure the distance over which the F wave travels and calculate a velocity.

An H reflex is a large-amplitude potential produced by submaximum stimulation. Typically, sensory fibers (IA afferents) of the posterior tibial nerve are stimulated in the popliteal fossa, and the muscle potential of the gastrocnemius-soleus muscle, caused by the reflex excitation of anterior horn cells, is recorded. The H reflex is an electrophysiologic correlate of an ankle jerk. The latency is measured to the onset of the H reflex. The absolute latency for the H reflexes is reported, and in most laboratories this value is then compared to the normal range based on the patient's height or leg length.

The interpretation of nerve conduction studies can provide information regarding the location and the pathologic characteristics of a particular neuropathy. Diffuse symmetric NCS abnormalities reflect a generalized polyneuropathy, whereas isolated focal changes indicate a mononeuropathy. The NCS may determine whether the neuropathy is purely motor, only sensory, or mixed. For axonal polyneuropathies, the electrophysiologic hallmark is an amplitude reduction of the motor and sensory action potentials, whereas distal latencies and conduction velocities may be only mildly abnormal. This amplitude reduction generally reflects a loss of motor or sensory axons that are available for stimulation. In demyelinating neuropathic conditions, prolonged latencies and very slow conduction velocities are encountered, and the amplitude of potentials is reduced only if there is conduction block (see later discussion). Conduction velocity slowing to greater than 70% of the lower limit of normal is usually attributed to segmental demyelination. For most laboratories, a motor conduction velocity below 35 m/sec in the arms and 30 m/sec in the legs fulfills this criterion for demyelination. However, often generalized neuropathies do not fit neatly into electrophysiologic demyelinating and axonal paradigms and other clues from the neurologic examination, spinal fluid analysis, and other laboratory tests (including possibly nerve biopsy) may be needed. Also, results of nerve conduction studies can be normal in small-fiber sensory neuropathy characterized by pure sensory or autonomic symptoms. In a radiculopathy, in which root compression occurs proximal to the dorsal root ganglion cell bodies, the sensory nerve action potentials are always normal. A focal entrapment palsy or mononeuropathy can be manifested by slowing over a particular nerve segment (prolonged latency or slowed velocity) or by a conduction block (failure to conduct above a locus with normal conduction below). Partial motor conduction block may be present if the amplitude of distal stimulation at the wrist or ankle is 50% higher than the amplitude with stimulation above the elbow or knee, respectively. Often, the potentials with proximal stimulation are also prolonged and polyphasic, so-called temporal dispersion, implying a delay in conduction across a focally demyelinated nerve segment. Common examples of entrapment palsies are the carpal tunnel syndrome and the cubital tunnel syndrome (ulnar entrapment at the elbow). In carpal tunnel syndrome, the most common NCS finding is a prolonged distal latency of the median nerve motor and sensory potentials with stimulation across the wrist.

F wave and H reflex latencies (long latencies) may complement the routine NCS study. In early polyneuropathies, F waves may be slowed long before there are demonstrable changes in the routine nerve conduction velocities. F waves are also abnormal when there is a proximal abnormality with relative sparing of the more distal parts of the peripheral nervous system, as in the Guillain-Barré syndrome. In addition, F waves may occasionally be abnormal in focal proximal neuropathic disorders such as a plexopathy. H reflexes can be used to assess conduction over the large sensory fibers of the leg as well as over proximal nerve fibers, as in an S1 radiculopathy. An H reflex may be prolonged or absent in an S1 radiculopathy even before the ankle reflex is depressed or lost on the physical examination.

After appropriate nerve conduction studies, a needle EMG examination is done. Electrodes are inserted into various muscles, and electric discharges are displayed on an oscilloscope screen and simultaneously heard on the speaker. Concentric needle electrodes or monopolar needle electrodes (with separate referential electrodes) are used, depending on the laboratory. Recently, disposable needle electrodes have become available. For detailed motor unit analysis, motor unit potentials are stored, and the oscilloscope screen is repeatedly triggered off a recurrent motor unit potential. In a typical examination, the initial insertional activity is recorded. The muscle is then observed at rest for spontaneous discharges and then during minimal, moderate, and full contraction. The patient then voluntarily contracts the muscle and motor units are analyzed for their amplitude, duration, and number of phases (two normal motor units, Fig. 107-2, *A*). The rate and characteristics of motor unit recruitment and the final interference pattern are noted. All observations must be analyzed in light of the normal range of variation for the muscle being studied.

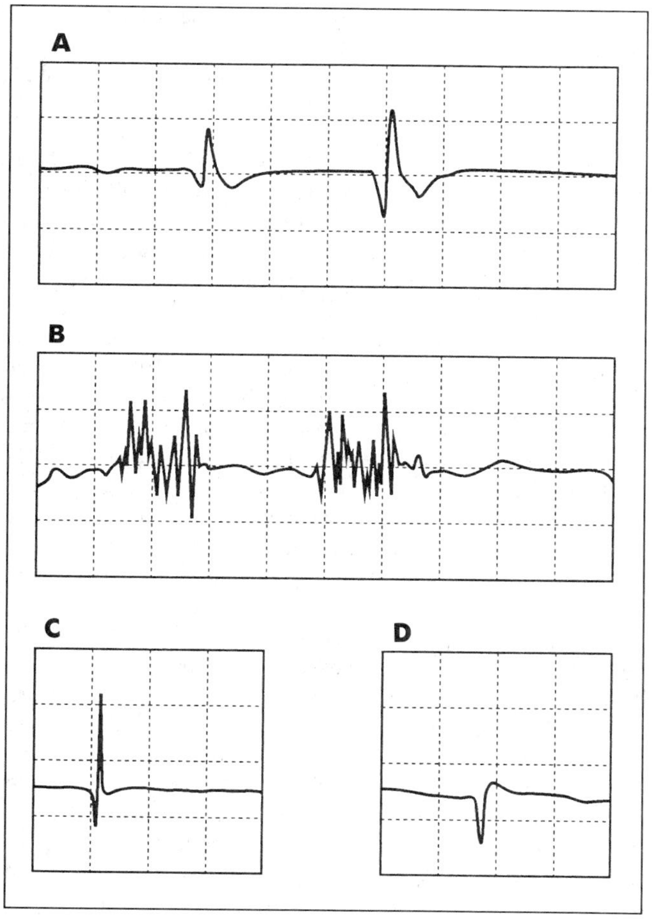

Fig. 107-2. A, Normal motor unit potentials. Gain 0.5 mV/division. **B,** Polyphasic, long-duration rapidly firing motor unit potential. Gain 1 mV/division. **C,** Fibrillation potential. Gain 50 μV/division. **D,** Positive sharp wave. Gain 50 μV/division. All sweep speeds 10 ms/division.

Prolonged insertional activity is often a nonspecific finding suggesting irritability of the muscle. In isolation, the finding of prolonged insertional activity should not be overinterpreted. Normally, there is no electric activity at rest. Fibrillations (Fig. 107-2, *C*) and positive sharp waves (Fig. 107-2, *D*) occur at rest when the patient is not voluntarily contracting the muscle and represent spontaneous discharges of individual muscle fibers disconnected from their nerve axons. Fibrillations are stereotyped diphasic or triphasic potentials with a small initial down slope followed by a larger upward deflection. Positive sharp waves are biphasic potentials with a prominent sharp initial down slope, followed by a prolonged phase back to the baseline. The positive sharp wave is believed to represent a fibrillation-type potential that is not propagated over the site of the needle recording. Fibrillations and positive sharp waves are typical of a denervating (neuropathic) process but can occur in myopathic disease. In inflammatory myopathy, there is often a profusion of fibrillations and positive sharp waves. On the other hand, if these potentials are present in the setting of a neuropathic process, this implies some degree of axonal damage and therefore the neuropathy is not purely demyelinating. These spontaneous potentials have to be distinguished from those normally encountered in the end-plate zone.

Fasciculations are usually large-amplitude potentials that are simple, are diphasic or triphasic, and resemble normal motor units, or they are large-amplitude polyphasic potentials. They represent the spontaneous discharge of a motor unit, which is a group of muscle fibers of the same histochemical type under control of a single anterior horn cell. Although they are not clearly abnormal discharges and occur in many normal patients, a profusion of fasciculations in association with other abnormalities is suggestive of an anterior horn cell or a nerve root disorder. Certain peculiar spontaneous discharges can be observed. One typical pattern occurs with myotonia; it has the sound of a dive bomber, caused by gradually increasing and then decreasing amplitude and frequency of the individual potentials in the discharge. Another pattern is a complex repetitive discharge (or pseudomyotonia) that abruptly starts and stops, and the component potential has a complex waveform. The former pattern usually occurs in the myotonic syndromes (Chapter 125), and the latter is less specific and can occur in both chronic neuropathies and myopathies.

In evaluating motor units, the electromyographer evaluates their morphologic features and recruitment. Two morphologic patterns are commonly observed. "Neuropathic" potentials are often increased in amplitude ($>$ 5 mV), increased in their phases (polyphasic), and often increased in duration ($>$ 10 mseconds) (Fig. 107-2, *B*). "Myopathic" potentials are small, brief polyphasic potentials ($<$ 4 mseconds). These are generalizations, and there are many examples of denervating illnesses that produce myopathic potentials and vice versa. A mixed pattern is not unusual. In regard to motor unit recruitment, a few patterns emerge. In a neuropathy, rapidly firing motor units are often recruited early, and often a full interference pattern is not accomplished (so-called decreased recruitment). Normally, early recruited motor units fire at less than 10 Hz (Fig. 107-2, *A*) and therefore initial units firing faster than 20 Hz are clearly abnormal (Fig. 107-2, *B*). This indicates a loss of motor units with a compensatory increased rate in the remaining units. In a myopathy, multiple motor units are recruited early, and a full interference pattern is obtained at a level of activity lower than normal. A decreased number of motor units without a compensatory increase in the firing rate of remaining units usually indicates lack of effort, or possibly a upper motor neuron lesion, but not a neuropathy. The abnormalities can be interpreted as either a generalized myopathy (which predominantly involves proximal muscles); a generalized neuropathy (which predominantly involves distal muscles); a radiculopathy, plexopathy, mononeuropathy, or mononeuritis multiplex; or an anterior horn cell disease. The distribution of the findings and the needle EMG findings helps in making the final assessment. For example, anterior horn cell disease (amyotrophic lateral sclerosis) usually produces diffuse needle EMG abnormalities in three or four extremities, but motor and sensory NCSs are normal.

There are many pitfalls to the interpretation of needle EMG. In acute lesions such as radiculopathy or traumatic palsy, denervation potentials appear only after 1 to 2 weeks, so timing of a study is important. In certain illnesses, an EMG is not the most sensitive test, as extreme abnormality may be necessary to produce electric changes clearly outside the normal range. For example, in amyotrophic lateral sclerosis, the EMG result of a clinically uninvolved extremity may be normal, whereas the biopsy finding of a muscle in that extremity may show the characteristic changes of the illness, albeit at an early stage. In various forms of muscular dystrophy that are long-standing, the electric changes may be hard to interpret and a muscle biopsy will give more diagnostic information. In general, for most myopathic disorders, both dystrophic and inflammatory, a muscle biopsy is more specific and sensitive than an EMG. One exception to this are the myotonic disorders, in which the EMG result does nearly always exhibit the typical myotonic discharges, but a muscle biopsy result may be only minimally and nonspecifically abnormal. Many electromyographers are hesitant to read changes in foot muscles such as the extensor digitorum brevis because of the large percentage of fibrillations and motor unit changes in this muscle in normal individuals. Some muscles, such as the extensor digitorum communis in the forearm, normally have motor units firing at 20 to 25 Hz. Needle EMG of paraspinal muscles is often rewarding, but most electromyographers restrict their interest to the presence of denervation potentials as motor units are notoriously difficult to interpret in this muscle. After a laminectomy, fibrillations can persist for years in paraspinous muscles and therefore may not indicate persistent root compression. In trying to distinguish an L5 radiculopathy from a peroneal palsy, it is important to sample the gluteus maximus and the tensor fasciae latae, which are only involved in the former process. Also, the short head of the biceps femoris (peroneal nerve above the fibular head) should be sampled to localize the site of a potential peroneal palsy. In spite of these pitfalls, an EMG allows several muscles to be sampled, and it can be very helpful in characterizing a neuromuscular illness.

In evaluation of the neuromuscular junction, repetitive stimulation and single-fiber EMG studies are most useful. For repetitive stimulation, a series of supramaximal stimuli are given to a nerve (typically at the rate of 3 per second for 2 seconds), and the amount of decrement of the amplitude of the evoked compound muscle action potential is recorded. A decrease of greater than 10% of the fourth potential's amplitude as compared with that of the first is considered significant. This test is easiest to perform on distal muscles of the upper extremity, but it can also be performed on facial and proximal arm muscles. If an abnormality is seen, the ability of edrophonium hydrochloride to reverse it is sometimes investigated. A standard protocol involves a measurement of baseline responses, a period of 60 seconds of sustained exercise of the relevant muscles, and then a repeat series of stimuli given at 1 minute intervals for up to 5 minutes.

In single-fiber EMG, a small needle is inserted into a muscle, and, using special techniques, the relationship of two muscle fibers within one motor unit is examined. The fluctuation in the time lag between the excitation of the two fibers can be recorded and is known as the jitter (often reported a mean value of consecutive differences [MCD]). The muscles most extensively studied are the extensor digitorum communis in the forearm and the orbicularis oculi in the face.

Repetitive stimulation studies and single-fiber EMG are often used to substantiate a diagnosis of myasthenia gravis. In a classic case, there is a decrement of the amplitude of the compound muscle action potential after repetitive stimulation; the CMAP amplitude increases transiently after exercise (postexercise facilitation) and then progressively decreases (postexercise exhaustion). Some or all of these phenomena may be seen in individual patients, but the most sensitive measurement is that of postexercise exhaustion. However, repetitive stimulation may show a decrement in only 50% to 75% of myasthenia gravis patients. In single-fiber EMG, there is an increased jitter suggestive of variable transmission in the neuromuscular junction in an otherwise normal muscle. Blocking, which represents intermittent failure of excitation of the second fiber of the pair, can also occur. This technique is highly sensitive and may yield an abnormal result in 95% of patients with myasthenia gravis. In the Eaton-Lambert syndrome, there may be a mild decrement to repetitive stimuli at slow rates (2 to 3 Hz). However, the initial potentials are small and are greatly increased by exercise. Repetitive stimulation at fast rates (20 to 50 Hz) produces an incremental response. The pattern in botulism may be similar, but exercise produces facilitation only at a certain stage of the disease. In organophosphate poisoning and intoxication with antibiotics such as neomycin, there may be a myasthenic pattern. Single-fiber EMG, although a sensitive test for myasthenia gravis and related diseases, is less specific than repetitive stimulation, as it can produce abnormal results in various neuropathies and myopathies.

The blink reflex is obtained by stimulation over the supraorbital nerve, with surface recording over both ipsilateral and contralateral orbicularis oculi. This study is used to assess trigeminal and facial nerve function, including their central connections, and can document lesions in diseases such as Bell's palsy, trigeminal neuropathy, and multiple sclerosis.

REFERENCES

Barry DT: Basic concepts of electricity and electronics in clinical electromyography. Muscle Nerve 14:937, 1991.

Brown F and Bolton C: Clinical electromyography. Boston, 1987, Butterworths.

Daube JR: Needle examination in clinical electromyography. Muscle Nerve 14:685, 1991.

Dawson DM, Hallet M, and Millender LH: Entrapment neuropathies, Boston, 1990, Little, Brown.

Donofrio PD and Albers JW: Polyneuropathy: classification by nerve conduction studies and electromyography. Muscle Nerve 13:889, 1990.

Johnson EW: Practical electromyography. Baltimore, 1988, Williams & Wilkins.

Kimura J: Electrodiagnosis in diseases of nerve and muscle: principles and practice. Philadelphia, 1989, Davis.

Sethi R and Thompson LL: The electromyographer's handbook. Boston, 1989, Little, Brown.

CHAPTER

108 Neuroradiologic Studies

Ashwani Kapila

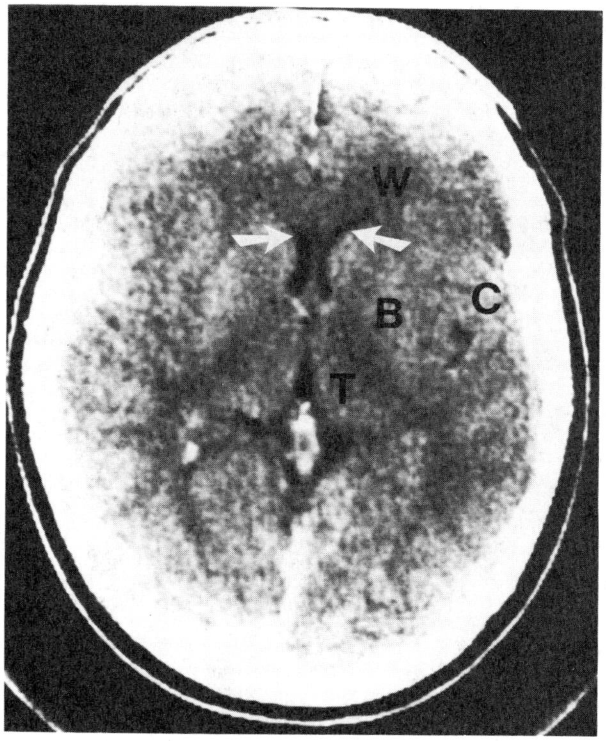

Fig. 108-1. CT scan of the head of a normal individual. The white matter is a slightly darker shade of gray than the gray matter of the cortex, basal ganglia, and thalamus on this contrast-enhanced scan done at the level of the frontal horns *(arrows)* of the lateral ventricles. W, white matter; C, cortex; B, basal ganglia; T, thalamus.

COMPUTED TOMOGRAPHY

Computed tomography (CT) is a cross-sectional imaging technique that since its introduction in 1972 has greatly advanced the ability of clinicians to diagnose and manage neurologic diseases. The CT scanner consists of an x-ray tube and an array of movable or fixed x-ray detectors. The body part of interest is exposed to a narrowly collimated x-ray beam of predetermined slice thickness. The transmitted radiation is detected by the radiation detectors. These data are collected in various projections and channeled into a computer, which by mathematical computation reconstructs the cross-sectional CT image. The various tissues of the head and body are displayed in various shades of gray depending on the x-ray attenuating properties of that particular tissue, which in turn are dependent on their electron density (physical density) and atomic number. Air is black, and fat, cerebrospinal fluid (CSF), white matter, gray matter, blood, and bone are progressively whiter (Fig. 108-1). Brain CT slices are typically 3 to 10 mm thick; spine CT slices are usually 2 to 5 mm thick. Several consecutive slices are obtained to display the entire region of interest. An entire scan of the brain can be obtained in 1 to 10 minutes, depending on the type of scanner, slice thickness, and desired resolution. Acquisition time for a CT scan of the spine is somewhat longer and depends on the extent of the spine to be scanned.

CT scanning of the head is usually done without contrast in patients with acute head trauma, in the diagnosis of hydrocephalus and monitoring of ventricular size in shunted patients (Fig. 108-2), in the diagnosis of intracranial hemorrhage (Fig. 108-3), in distinguishing hemorrhagic from bland infarcts, in evaluating diseases of the skull base, and in detecting and displaying complex craniofacial anomalies. Contrast enhanced CT with intravenously administered iodinated contrast medium is, however, required for adequate evaluation of a number of intracranial diseases. Contrast enhancement has an intravascular component that enhances normal vessels and abnormal vascular structures such as aneurysms and vascular malformations; and an extravascular component where contrast leaks out of vessels into areas of blood brain barrier disruption such as brain tumors (Fig. 108-4), cerebral infarction, and various inflammatory processes. The need for intravenous contrast enhancement in CT has diminished with the acceptance of magnetic resonance imaging (MRI) as the superior imaging modality for most neurologic disease. Contrast enhancement of cerebrospinal fluid (CSF) in the subarachnoid space or in the ventricles by injection of contrast material by lumbar, cervical, or ventricular puncture was used for a variety of in-

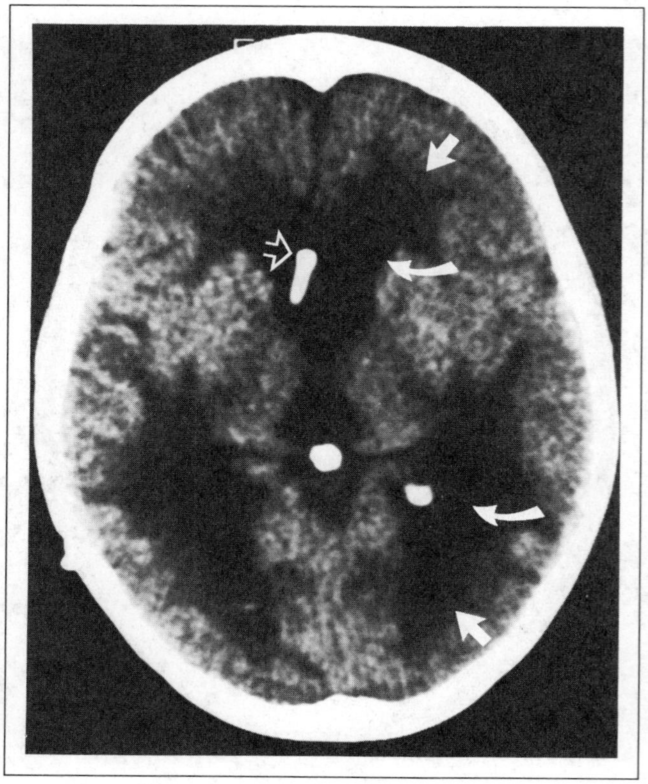

Fig. 108-2. CT scan showing marked enlargement of the lateral ventricles *(curved arrows)* and periventricular lucency representing CSF edema *(straight arrows)* in a patient with shunted hydrocephalus who developed shunt failure. The ventricular end of the ventriculoperitoneal shunt is identified in the right lateral ventricle *(open arrowhead)*. CSF, cerebrospinal fluid.

tracranial abnormalities before the advent of MRI but is rarely used now other than for the evaluation of CSF rhinorrhea.

CT of the spine is used for a large number of spinal disorders including spinal stenosis, degenerative disk disease (Fig. 108-5), vertebral and paraspinal tumors and inflammatory lesions, vertebral fractures, and congenital abnormalities. For detailed evaluation of spinal anatomy and disease CT is often performed with intrathecal contrast enhancement (Fig. 108-6), usually in association with plain film myelography.

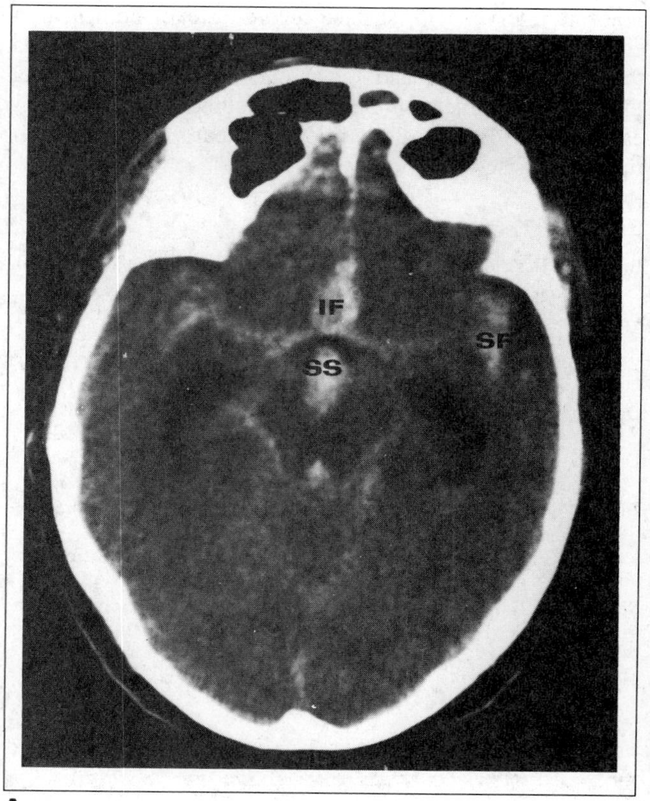

A

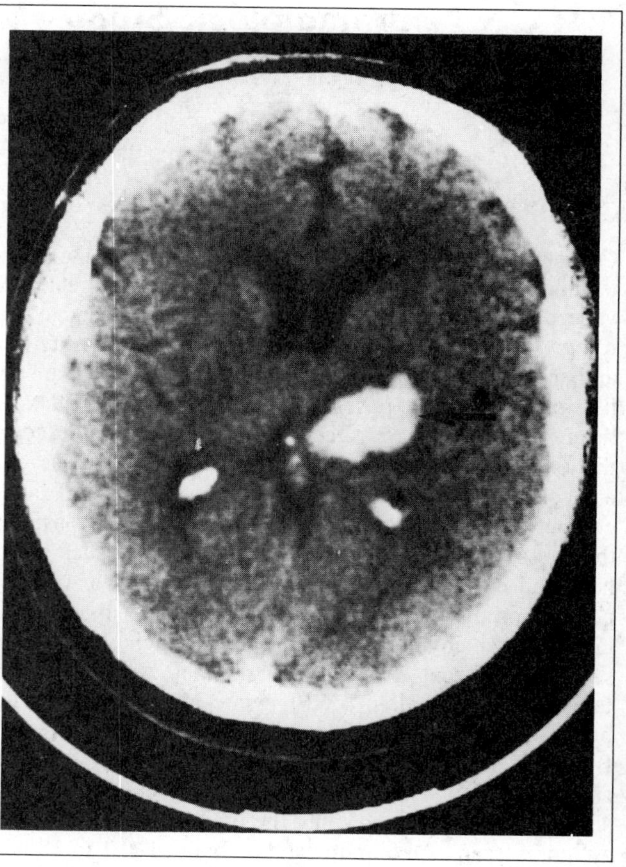

B

Fig. 108-3. Intracranial hemorrhage. **A,** CT scan showing a subarachnoid hemorrhage. Rupture of an anterior communicating-artery aneurysm has produced a massive subarachnoid hemorrhage, seen as a high-attenuation *(white)* area in the suprasellar cistern, the anterior interhemispheric fissure, and the Sylvian fissures. The aneurysm cannot be seen separately for the hematoma in the interhemispheric fissure. SS, suprasellar cistern; IF, interhemispheric fissure; SF, sylvian fissures. **B,** CT scan showing a hypertensive hemorrhage. A hematoma *(arrow)* is seen in the left thalamus and in the posterior part of the basal ganglia—a classic location for hypertensive hemorrhages.

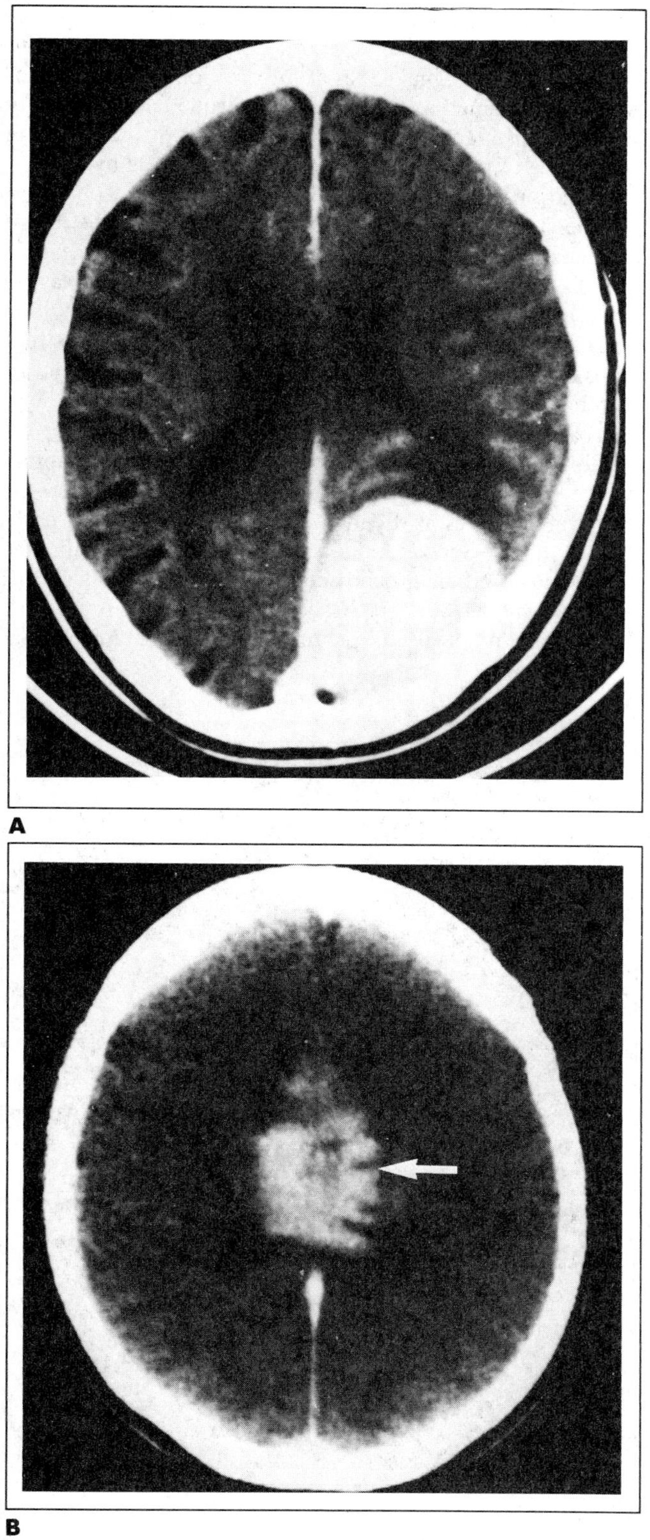

Fig. 108-4. Brain tumors. **A,** Meningioma. Contrast-enhanced CT scan showing a uniform density contrast-enhancing meningioma abutting the falx and the calvarium in the left occipital region. **B,** Lymphoma. Contrast-enhanced CT scan showing an enhancing lesion of the corpus callosum *(arrow)*. The location and the absence of surrounding edema or mass effect are characteristic of primary CNS lymphoma. CNS, central nervous system.

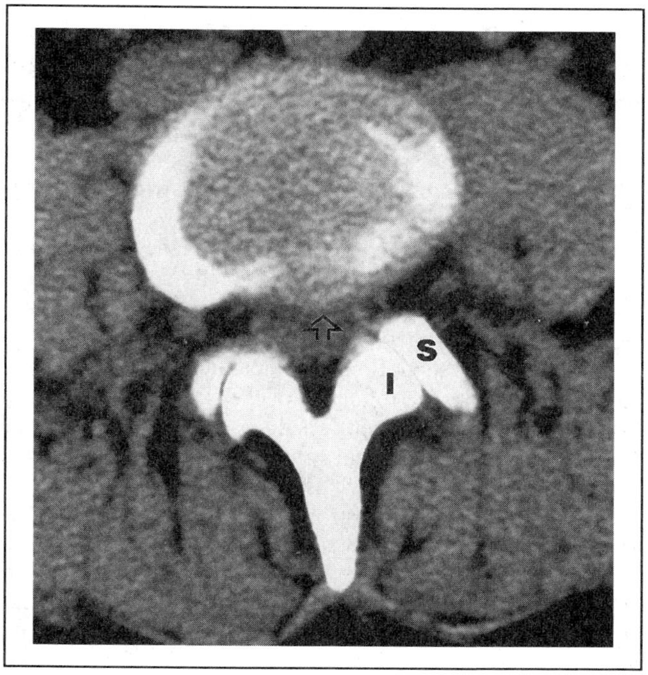

Fig. 108-5. Lumbar intervertebral disk herniation. CT scan of the lumbar spine at the L3-L4 level showing posterior disk herniation centered just to the left of midline *(arrow)*. S, superior facet of L4; I, inferior facet of L3.

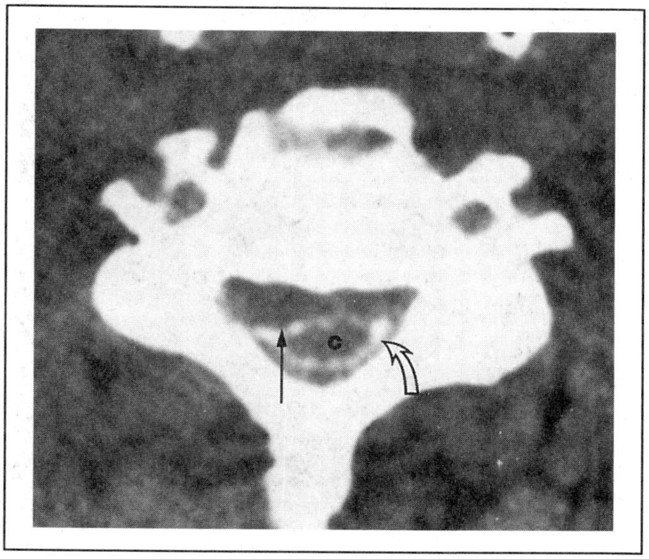

Fig. 108-6. Cervical epidural abscess. CT scan of the cervical spine at the C5 level after myelography with water soluble contrast medium showing subarachnoid space opacified with contrast *(curved arrow)*, and ventral extradural abscess appearing as a soft tissue mass larger on the right side *(arrow)*. Cord compression is demonstrated as mild degree of flattening of the cervical cord at this level. c, cervical cord.

MAGNETIC RESONANCE IMAGING

MRI is a cross-sectional imaging modality that has greater sensitivity than CT for detecting pathologic processes and is superior for displaying normal and altered anatomic relations in the brain and spine. MRI has displaced CT as the primary neurodiagnostic imaging modality in most diseases of the brain and spine.

Various elements exhibit nuclear magnetic resonance (NMR) properties; however, current clinical MRI is limited to hydrogen nuclear (proton) imaging. In essence, proton MRI is a hydrogen map of the tissue in the volume of interest that reflects not only the quantitative hydrogen distribution but also the influence of the surrounding physical and chemical environment on these various hydrogen atoms. The process of image generation in MRI is complex, and the scheme that follows is an extreme simplification of basic MR imaging. In a strong magnetic field, the hydrogen protons, which act like small magnets, are aligned parallel to the main magnetic field and then are energized by applying a radiofrequency pulse of the appropriate energy (resonant frequency). The excited protons return to the ground state or equilibrium (relaxation) by emitting radiofrequency energy, which is recorded by a receiver and constitutes the MR signal. Spatial information for image generation is obtained by producing a controlled nonuniformity of the main magnetic field and subsequently determining the source of the various radiofrequency signals by a mathematical process called Fourier transformation.

The strength of the MR signal in each part of the image depends on the proton density and the relaxation times (T1 and T2) of the tissue in the area of interest as well as on the effects of motion, including flow and pulsation of blood and CSF. The MR signal generated by various normal structures or pathologic processes can be manipulated by choosing the appropriate scanning technique and adjusting imaging parameters to enhance their proton density, T1 or T2, or flow characteristics selectively (Fig. 108-7). The ability of the operator to modulate the effect of these factors on the scan helps tailor MR imaging to solve the clinical problem at hand. Special flow-sensitive sequences using the technique of gradient echo scanning form the basis of MR angiography (MRA). The tissue relaxation times in turn can be modified by the use of paramagnetic contrast media. Ga-

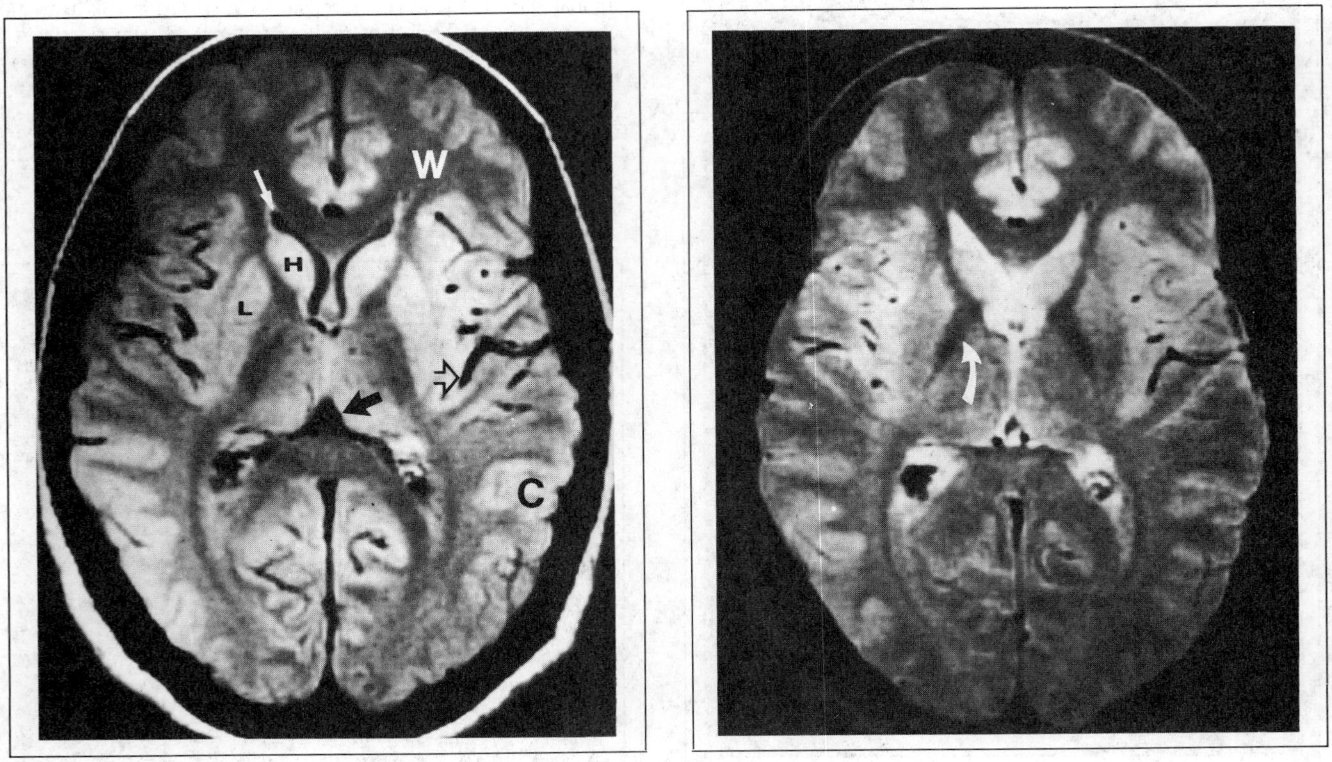

A B

Fig. 108-7. Normal MRI of the head. These two transverse scans are at the same location, done in the same imaging sequence. **A,** The proton density scan *(TR 2000 milliseconds; TE 25 milliseconds)* shows relatively high-intensity cortex, caudate, and lentiform nuclei; lower intensity in the white matter; and low intensity of the CSF in the frontal horns *(white arrow)*. There is flow void in the Sylvian vessels *(open arrowhead)* and internal cerebral veins *(black arrow)*. C, cortex; H, caudate nucleus; L, lentiform nucleus; W, white matter; CSF, cerebrospinal fluid. **B,** The T2-weighted scan shows high intensity of the CSF. The low intensity seen in the medial part of the globus pallidi *(curved arrow)* is a normal phenomenon caused by increased iron in this region.

dopentetate dimeglumine (Magnevist) is used widely in clinical practice because of the T1 shortening it produces in clinical doses. Other paramagnetic contrast agents with similar properties are on the threshold of FDA approval. These agents have a pharmacologic distribution similar to those of conventional iodinated contrast media used for CT, though the mechanism of enhancement is different. However, contrast enhancement of tissues with blood brain barrier disruption and of extracerebral tumors yields an appearance similar to that of CT contrast enhancement. Signal changes in vascular structures are primarily governed by intrinsic flow parameters and scanning sequence and are only secondarily affected by paramagnetic contrast media. Agents that primarily modify T2 show promise in evaluating brain perfusion but are not currently in routine clinical use.

MRI has a number of advantages over CT scanning other than its considerably greater capability of displaying anatomic details and superior sensitivity in detecting abnormality: it (1) does not use ionizing radiation and has no apparent adverse biologic effects, (2) is not subject to bone artefact, (3) allows coronal and sagittal imaging with ease and with excellent resolution, (4) requires contrast enhancement less often than CT, and (5) uses contrast agents, which are generally considered safer than agents used for CT scanning. There are also limitations to the use of MRI in its present state of evolution that prohibit it from completely replacing CT. MRI (1) is more expensive than CT; (2) is limited in acutely ill patients on life support because of interactions between the magnetic field and life support equipment; (3) is often unacceptable to claustrophobic patients; (4) cannot be used in patients with ferromagnetic intracranial aneurysm clips, metallic structures in or around the eyes, pacemakers, cochlear implants, or neurostimulator devices; (5) has limited utility when the area of clinical interest is located close to ferromagnetic surgical hardware; and (6) is inferior to CT in detecting acute subarachnoid hemorrhage and in evaluating calcified lesions.

MRI is currently the imaging procedure of choice in the majority of diseases of the brain and spine. It is especially useful in evaluating white matter diseases (Fig. 108-8), cryptic vascular malformations and hemangiomas, neuronal migration anomalies, abnormalities of larger arterial and venous structures, syringomyelia, and intervertebral disk disease. MRI is also the imaging test of choice in most developmental, ischemic, inflammatory, degenerative, neoplastic, and subacute or chronic posttraumatic processes of the brain (Figs. 108-9, 108-10, 108-11) or spinal cord (Figs. 108-12, 108-13). When performed with intravenous contrast enhancement, MRI has very high sensitivity in de-

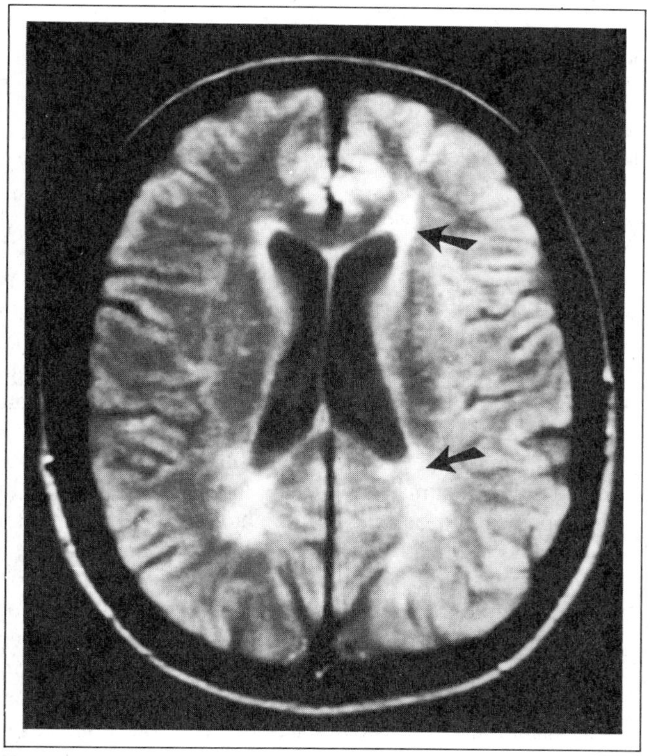

A

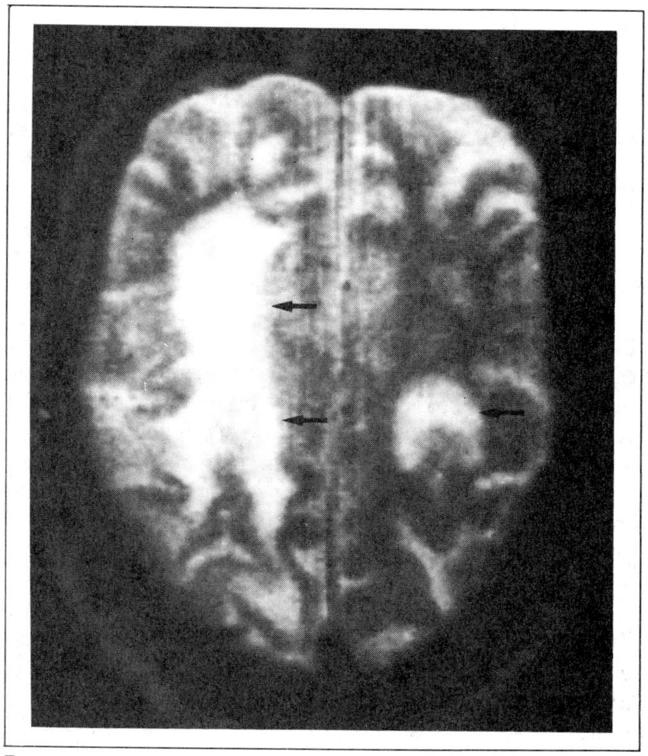

B

Fig. 108-8. MRI of the head in demyelinating disease. **A,** Multiple sclerosis. This transverse proton density scan shows abnormal high intensity *(arrows)* in the periventricular white matter bilaterally in a pattern characteristic of multiple sclerosis. **B,** Progressive multifocal leukoencephalopathy. This transverse T2-weighted scan *(TR 2500 milliseconds; TE 100 milliseconds)* shows bilateral high-intensity foci *(arrows)*. The white matter distribution of the lesion and the patient's history of an immunosuppressed state were instrumental in making this diagnosis.

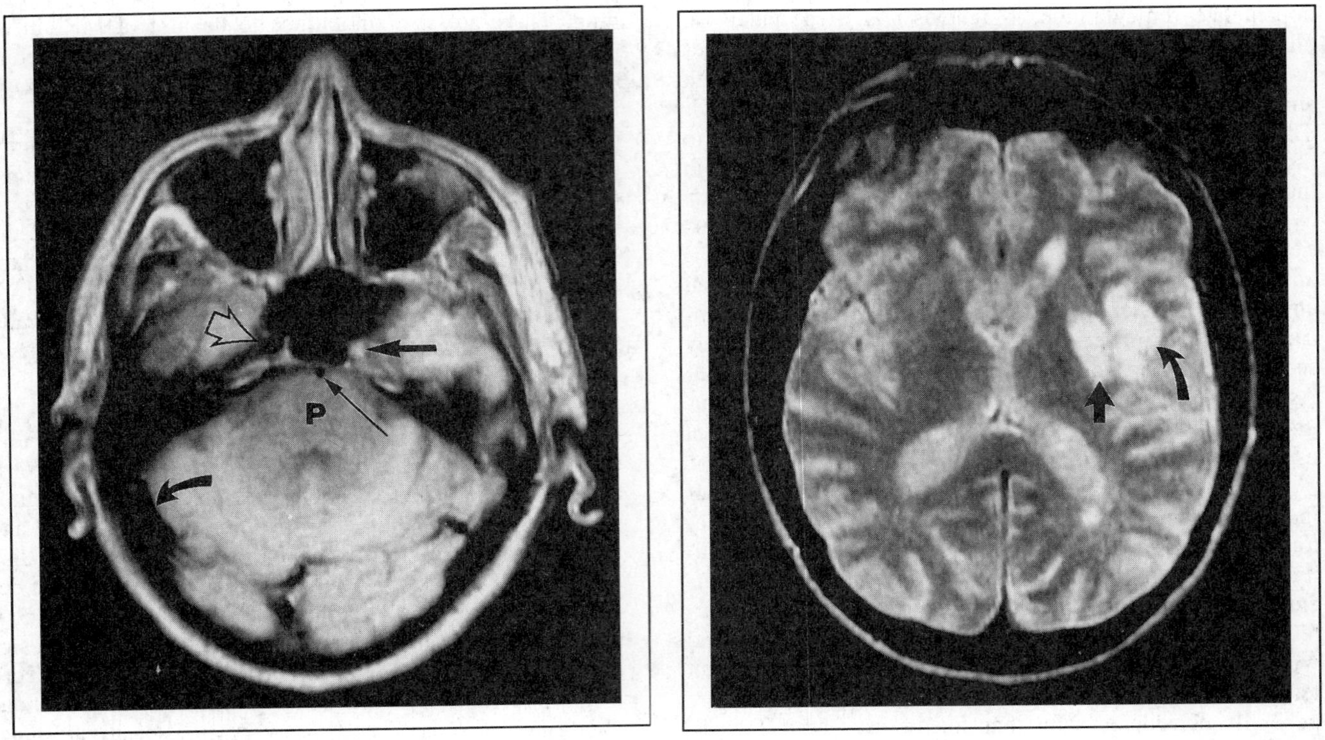

A B

Fig. 108-9. Cerebral infarction. **A,** MRI scan weighted for proton density *(TR 2300 milliseconds; TE 25 milliseconds)* showing slightly increased signal in the left precavernous internal carotid artery *(thick arrow)*, a finding representing thrombus in the occluded vascular lumen. Rapidly flowing blood in the right internal carotid artery *(empty arrow)*, basilar artery *(thin arrow)*, and right transverse sinus *(curved arrow)* appears black, the so-called signal void sign. **B,** MRI scan on the same patient at a higher level using T2 weighting *(TR 2300 milliseconds; TE 90 milliseconds)* showing increased signal intensity representing infarction in the left insula *(curved arrow)* and lentiform nucleus *(straight arrow)*.

tecting leptomeningeal involvement by neoplastic or inflammatory processes. Contrast enhancement also increases the sensitivity of MRI in detecting small intraparenchymal or extraparenchymal lesions and early cerebral infarction, helps in choosing the appropriate biopsy or resection site for spinal cord and brain tumors, and provides greater diagnostic specificity for lesions that are also seen without contrast such as in distinguishing recurrent disk herniation from epidural fibrosis.

CONVENTIONAL RADIOGRAPHY

The use of skull radiographs as a routine screening procedure in patients with headaches, seizures, and transient or fixed neurologic deficits is not indicated, because of extremely low diagnostic yield. Careful selection of patients for skull radiographs, however, may yield useful diagnostic information. Most skull radiographs are currently performed (1) on emergency room patients with relatively mild head trauma and without neurologic findings, to detect fractures and to screen patients for CT examination; and (2) on patients with facial injury, lacerations to the head, or penetrating missile injury. In patients suspected of having severe intracranial injury, skull radiographs are superfluous, and immediate CT is indicated. Skull radiographs can also provide useful information in the assessment of congenital craniofacial abnormalities, palpable lesions in the scalp, and inflammatory conditions of the paranasal sinuses and mastoids.

Plain films of the spine are useful in patients with suspected spinal trauma, and supine lateral cervical spine radiographs should be made in comatose patients with signs of injury to the head and neck before transporting them, to prevent further injury to the spinal cord. Other indications for spine radiographs include scoliosis, congenital anomalies of the spine, back pain, point tenderness, and most conditions for which spine CT or MRI is performed. Flexion and extension views of the spine are often used to diagnose instability and to evaluate adequacy of spinal fusion procedures. Spine radiography is also used to evaluate and follow placement and results of surgical instrumentation.

MYELOGRAPHY

Myelography is radiographic examination of the spinal canal and spinal cord by means of iodinated water soluble

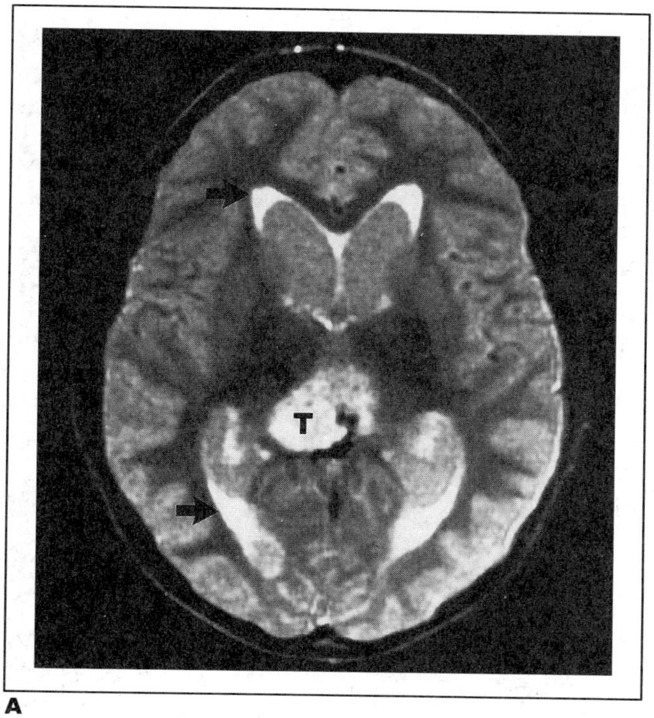

A

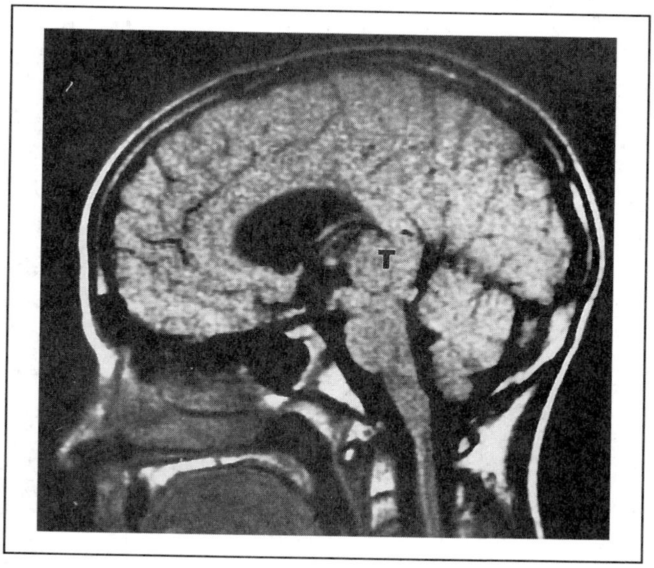

B

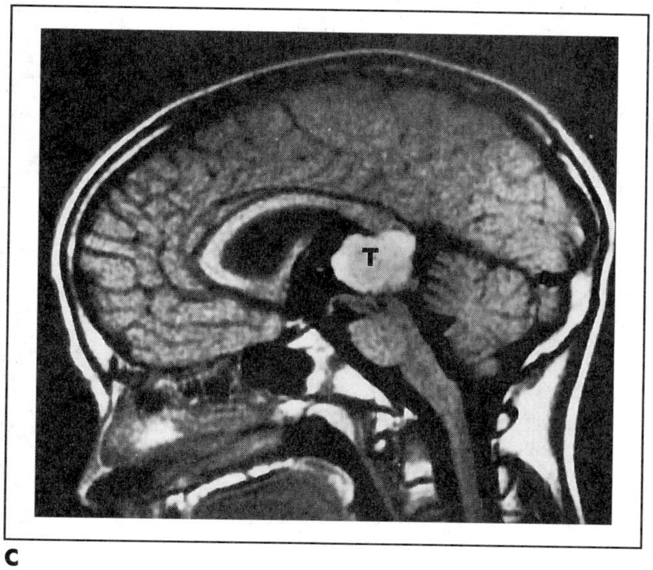

C

Fig. 108-10. Brain tumor. MRI scan showing pineal tumor in 11-year-old with upgaze paresis and headache. **A,** T2 weighted *(TR 2300 milliseconds; TE 90 milliseconds)* axial scan showing tumor mass (T) in region of pineal gland, lateral ventricular enlargement, and an abnormal periventricular rim of high signal *(arrows)* representing CSF edema secondary to hydrocephalus. T, tumor mass; CSF, cerebrospinal fluid. **B,** Midsagittal T1 weighted scan *(TR 500 milliseconds; TE 30 milliseconds)* showing isointense tumor mass in the region of the pineal gland. **C,** Midsagittal T1 weighted scan after contrast enhancement with Magnevist showing fairly intense but slightly inhomogenous enhancement of the tumor, clearly delineating its margins.

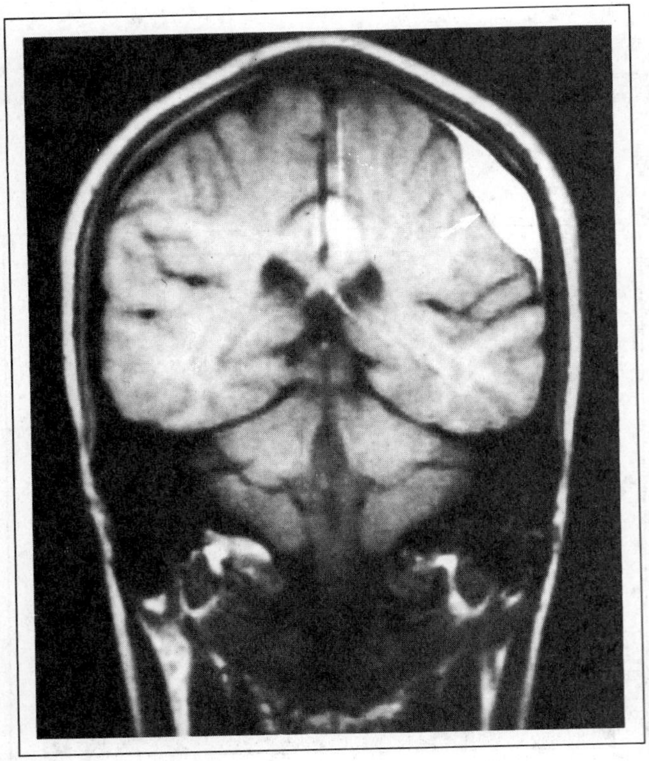

A

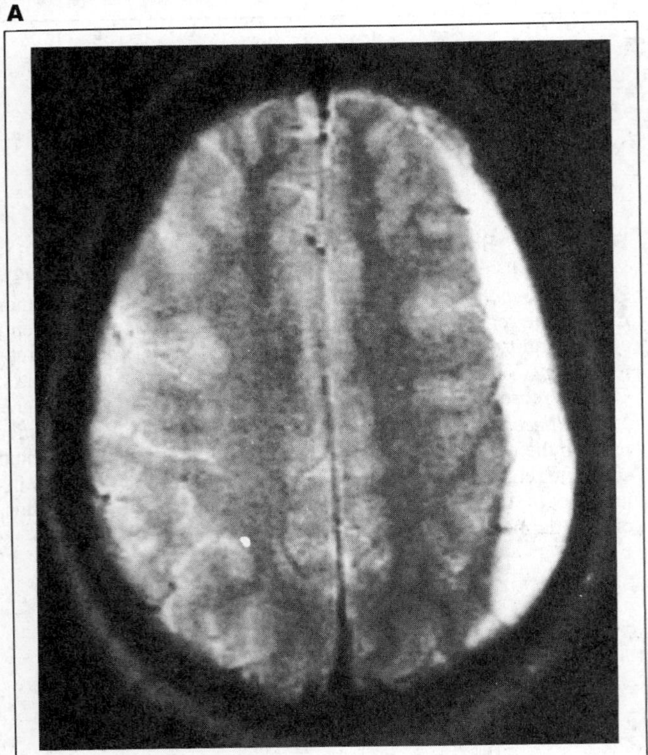

B

Fig. 108-11. MRI of a chronic subdural hematoma. **A,** The coronal T1-weighted scan *(TR 550 milliseconds; TE 20 milliseconds)* shows a high-intensity extracerebral biconvex collection over the midconvexity *(arrow)*. **B,** The transverse T2-weighted scan *(TR 2500 milliseconds; TE 90 milliseconds)* of the same patient shows a large, crescent-shaped, high-intensity abnormality on the same side. These findings are characteristic of a subdural hematoma, estimated to be between 1 week and several months old.

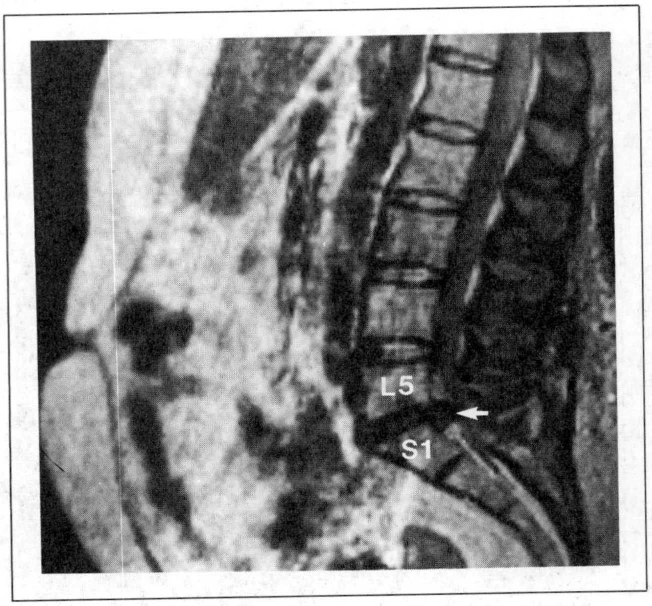

A

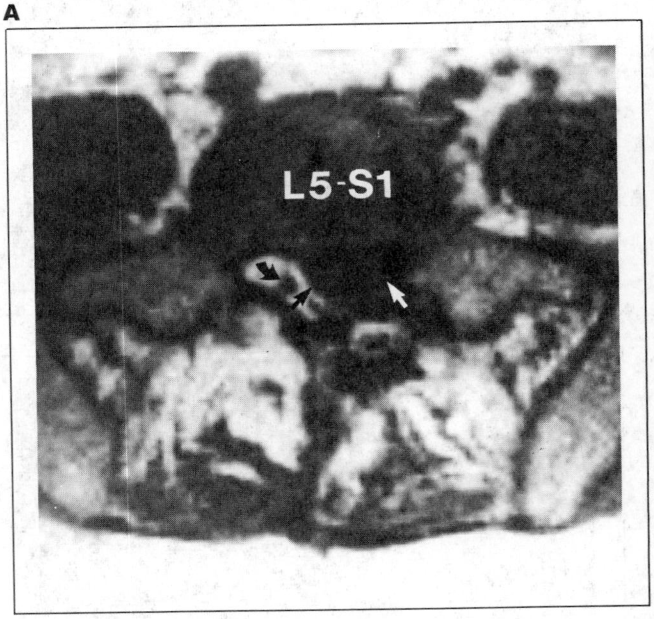

B

Fig. 108-12. MRI of lumbar intervertebral disk herniation. **A,** This sagittal paramidline proton density scan *(TR 2500 milliseconds; TE 30 milliseconds)* shows low intensity in the L5-S1 disk space with marked posterior protrusion of the disk *(arrow)* into the spinal canal. **B,** The transverse T1-weighted scan *(TR 366 milliseconds; TE 20 milliseconds)* shows the herniated disk *(arrows)* at the corresponding level. The opposite first sacral root *(curved arrow)* is seen surrounded by normal high-intensity epidural fat. The nerve root on the side of the disk herniation cannot be separated from the herniated disk material.

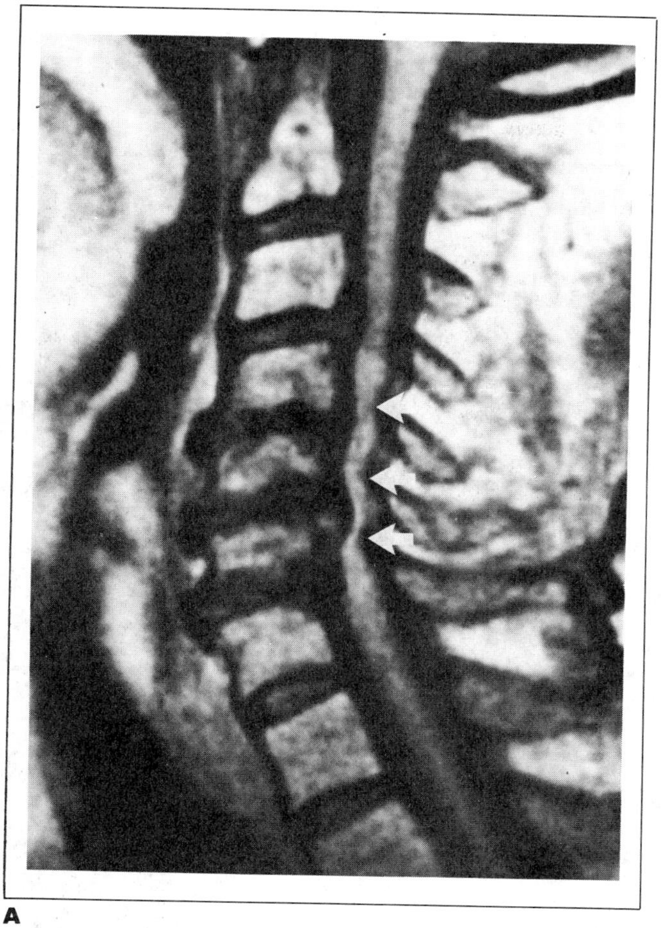

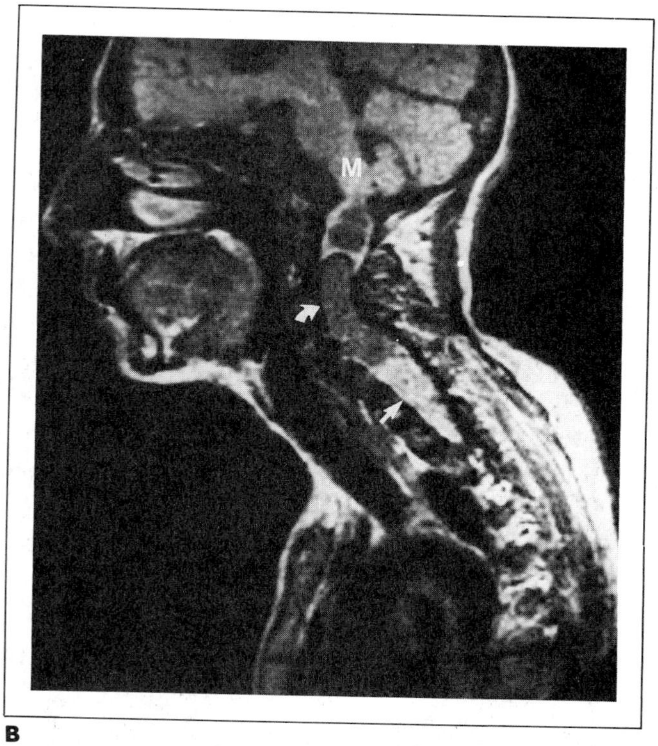

Fig. 108-13. MRI of cervical spine. **A,** Cervical spondylosis. This sagittal T1-weighted scan shows multiple levels of narrowing of the anteroposterior dimensions of the spinal canal, with compression of the cord at the same levels *(white arrows)*. **B,** Cervical cord astrocytoma. This sagittal proton density image *(TR 1500 milliseconds; TE 40 milliseconds)* shows a cord mass with solid *(straight arrow)* and cystic *(curved arrow)* components extending above the foramen magnum into the medulla. M, medulla.

nonionic contrast media. The contrast medium is introduced into the subarachnoid space via lumbar puncture in most instances. Occasionally lateral cervical puncture at the C1-C2 level is required. Introduction of the contrast medium is monitored fluoroscopically and spot radiographs are exposed to verify extradural or intradural abnormalities, nerve root asymmetries (Fig. 108-14), obstruction to CSF flow, and cord compression. Although relatively safe, myelography remains an invasive procedure with a number of side-effects including headache, nausea, vomiting, and vasovagal episodes. Seizures, hypersensitivity reactions, bleeding, aseptic meningitis, infection, and cardiovascular complications can also occur. The incidence of adverse reactions can be reduced by screening out potentially allergic patients, performing hydration before and after the procedure, administering seizure prophylaxis with barbiturates, limiting intracranial entry of contrast medium, and adhering to the manufacturer's dosage specifications.

Despite the generally superior information provided by MRI, myelography remains a useful procedure in selected cases especially when followed by postmyelographic CT. Nerve root compromise by bony or soft tissue structures, facet joint disease, neural foramina and central spinal canal stenosis, extent of cauda equina compression, communication of the thecal sac with adjacent cystic structures, and presence and extent of certain types of spinal vascular malformations can usually be assessed with a greater degree of confidence with the combination of myelography and postmyelography CT scanning than with MRI.

ANGIOGRAPHY

Conventional or catheter cerebral angiography uses x-rays to image intra-arterially injected iodinated contrast material. The image may be made on radiographic film by using a film screen combination, or alternatively the radiographic data may be digitized and electronically subtracted from another exposure obtained during contrast injection. This latter technique, known as digital subtraction angiography, was initially developed to study vascular structures by peripheral or central venous injection but has since become an adjunct of catheter angiography. The angiographic catheter is introduced through the femoral artery and occasionally through the axillary artery over a guide wire. Multihole catheters are used for aortic arch injections to evaluate the origins of the great vessels. End-hole catheters are

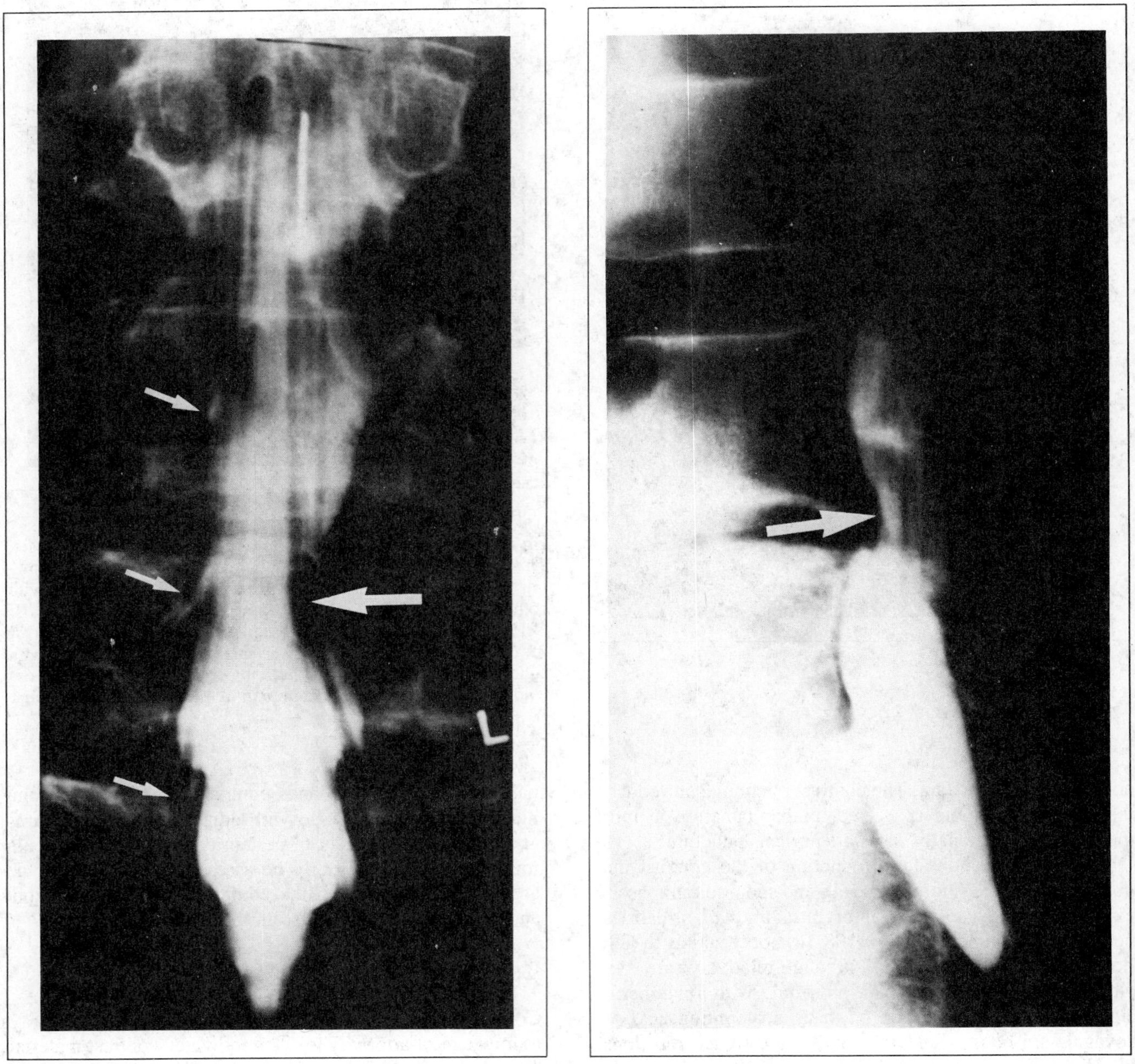

A **B**

Fig. 108-14. Lumbar intervertebral disk herniation. Anteroposterior and lateral views of this lumbar myelogram show an extradural defect anteriorly at the L4-L5 level on the lateral view *(large arrow)* and on the left side on the anteroposterior view *(large arrow)*. The contrast outlines the normal lumbar and sacral nerve roots *(short arrows)*. The left fifth root does not fill with contrast, because of impingement on the root by the herniated disk. **A,** Anteroposterior view. **B,** Lateral view.

used for injections into the carotid and vertebral arteries for detailed angiographic evaluation of their respective territories without overlap of other vascular structures. Conventional cerebral angiography is used in the diagnosis, presurgical evaluation, and occasionally intraoperative and postsurgical assessment of aneurysms (Fig. 108-15), vascular malformations and fistulas (Fig. 108-16); in evaluation of arterial stenoses, occlusions, and collateral circulation in vascular occlusive diseases including atherosclerosis (Fig. 108-17), trauma, and vasculitis; and in evaluation of vascular intracranial (Fig. 108-18) and skull base tumors. Spinal angiography is used for diagnosis of and for preembolization or presurgical mapping of spinal arteriovenous malformations and occasionally for vascular tumors such as hemangioblastomas. Complications of catheter cerebral angiography may be local (hematoma, infection, pseudoaneurysm, fistula, arterial occlusion), systemic (allergic reaction, renal failure), or neurologic (transient neurologic deficit, stroke, cortical blindness). Observation of the patient in the hospital overnight or for several hours after the procedure is essential to monitor neurologic status and prevent serious local hemorrhagic complications.

Magnetic resonance angiography (MRA) is the use of flow effects inherent to MRI to image vascular anatomy using the MR scanner. Vascular images are generated either by simultaneously suppressing signal from static tissue while maximizing signal in inflowing blood (time-of-flight angiography) or by modifying magnetic field gradients to use information present in radiofrequency phase changes in flowing blood (phase contrast angiography). Data collected by these mechanisms can be displayed in a format resembling that of conventional angiography. Currently MRA is used as a screening examination for extracranial cerebrovascular disease (Fig. 108-19) and is being scrutinized for a number of intracranial applications. Although desirable to the patient because of its noninvasive nature and safety, MRA is currently limited in its application by its high cost, sensitivity to patient motion, various artefacts and techni-

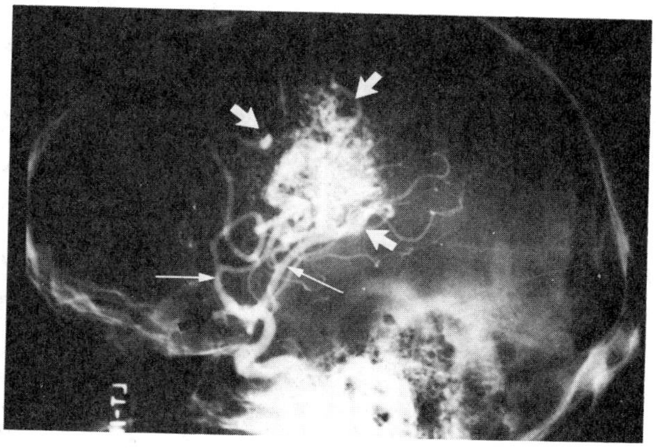

Fig. 108-16. Vascular malformation. This lateral view of an internal carotid angiogram shows a large arteriovenous malformation *(thick white arrows)* fed by enlarged branches of the middle cerebral artery *(thin white arrows)*. A middle cerebral artery aneurysm is also present *(black arrow)*.

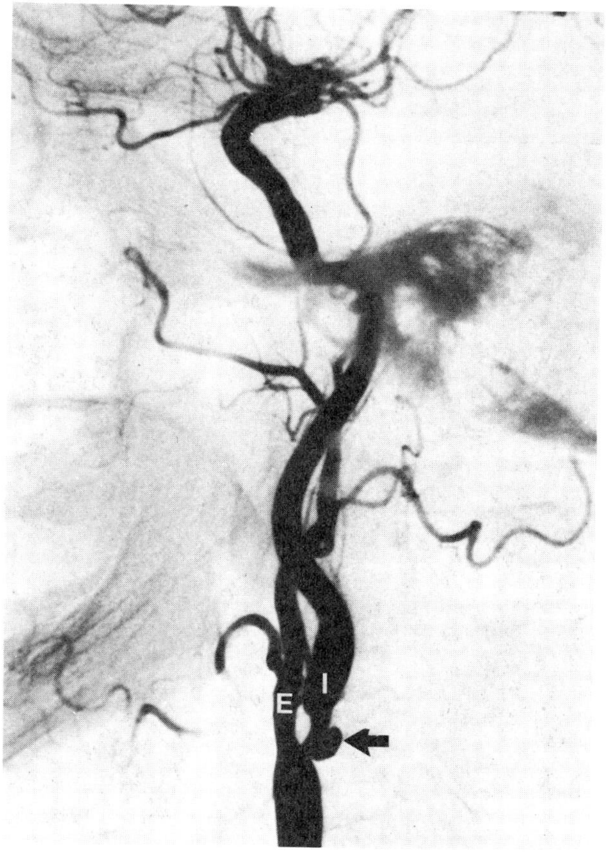

Fig. 108-17. Cerebral angiogram demonstrating an ulcerated atherosclerotic plaque. This lateral subtraction neck view of the carotid bifurcation shows an atherosclerotic plaque at the origin of the internal carotid artery with a central ulcer *(arrow)*. The internal and external carotid arteries are labeled. I, internal carotid artery; E, external carotid artery.

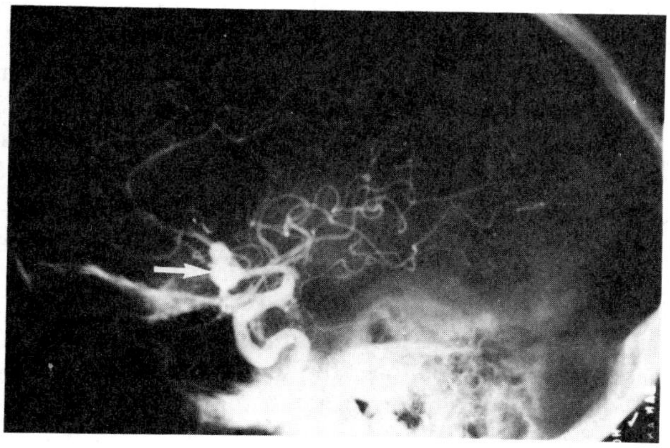

Fig. 108-15. Aneurysm. This lateral view of a selective internal carotid angiogram shows a large bilobed aneurysm at the anterior communicating artery *(arrow)*.

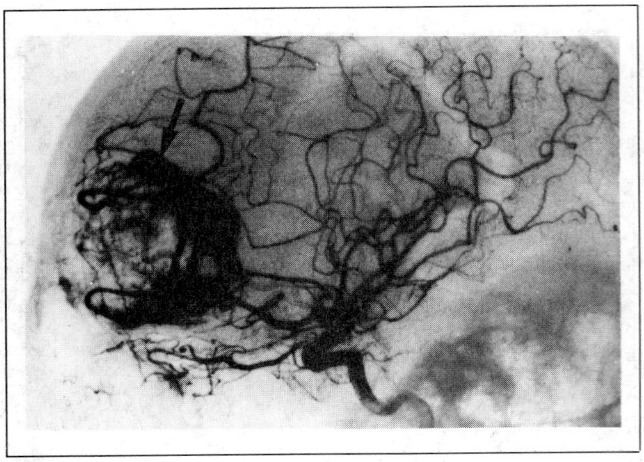

A

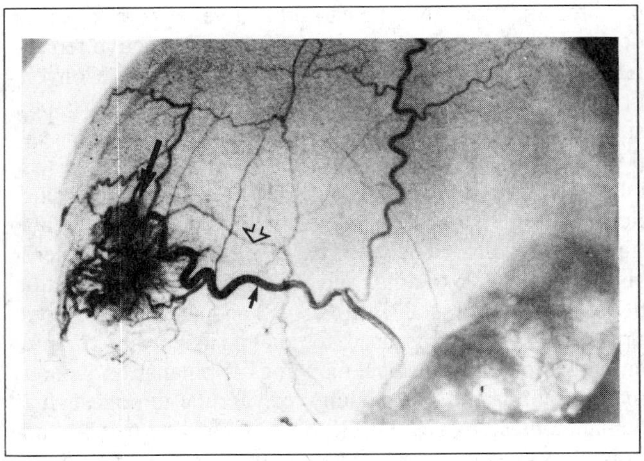

B

Fig. 108-18. Cerebral arteriogram demonstrating a meningioma. Lateral subtraction views of the internal and external carotid arteries show a vascular tumor stain in the frontal region *(large arrows)*. **A,** Internal carotid artery. **B,** External carotid artery. The peripheral part of the tumor is supplied by internal carotid branches, whereas the central part is supplied by the superficial temporal *(small arrow)* and middle meningeal *(open arrowhead)* branches of the external carotid artery.

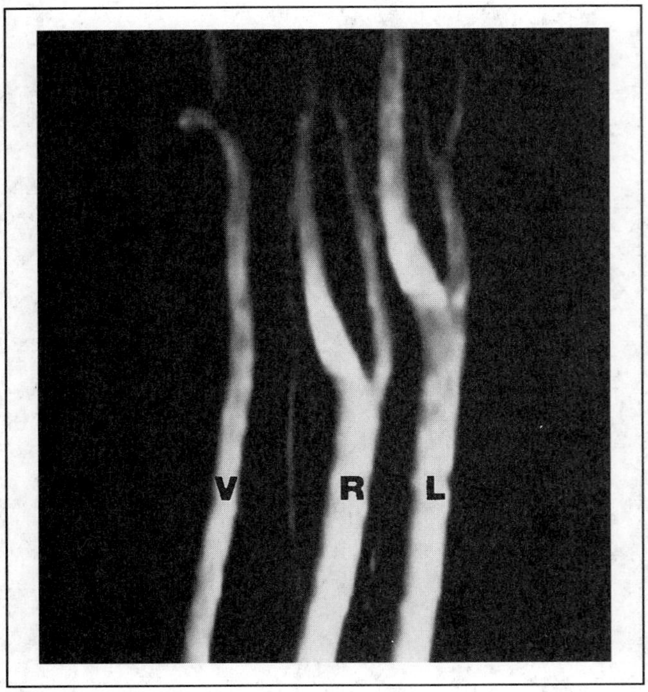

Fig. 108-19. Carotid bifurcation MRA. Two-dimensional time-of-flight MRA of the neck showing normal right and left carotid arteries and respective bifurcations and normal right vertebral artery. The left vertebral artery was not definitively demonstrated and may be congenitally absent or occluded. MRA, magnetic resonance angiogram; R, right carotid artery; L, left carotid artery; V, vertebral artery.

cal limitations that have not been completely resolved, and lesser spatial resolution than conventional angiography.

RADIONUCLIDE STUDIES

Conventional radionuclide (RN) brain scans were obtained by intravenously administering a radiopharmaceutical that did not cross the blood-brain barrier and recording the gamma emissions from the head with a scintillation camera (gamma camera) to demonstrate areas of blood-brain barrier disruption. This has been replaced by CT and MRI and is only rarely used now other than occasionally to confirm the presence of brain death.

Radionuclide cisternography is performed by injecting a radiopharmaceutical, usually indium-111 diethylene triamine pentaacetic acid (DTPA), into the subarachnoid space via lumbar puncture, then scanning the head to detect its presence and to demonstrate its distribution. Communicating hydrocephalus, commonly called normal pressure hydrocephalus, can be diagnosed by demonstrating intraventricular entry and retention of the radiopharmaceutical (Fig. 108-20). RN cisternography can be used to complement iodinated contrast CT cisternography in the detection and localization of CSF rhinorrhea. Ventriculoperitoneal shunt function can also be assessed by injecting the radiopharmaceutical into the ventricular system or into the shunt reservoir.

The current emphasis in RN imaging of the central nervous system (CNS) is on radioisotope labeled agents that cross the blood-brain barrier and accumulate in various regions of the brain depending on regional cerebral blood flow and energy metabolism, and on the techniques used to compute and image their distribution. Positron emission tomography (PET) and single-photon emission computed tomog-

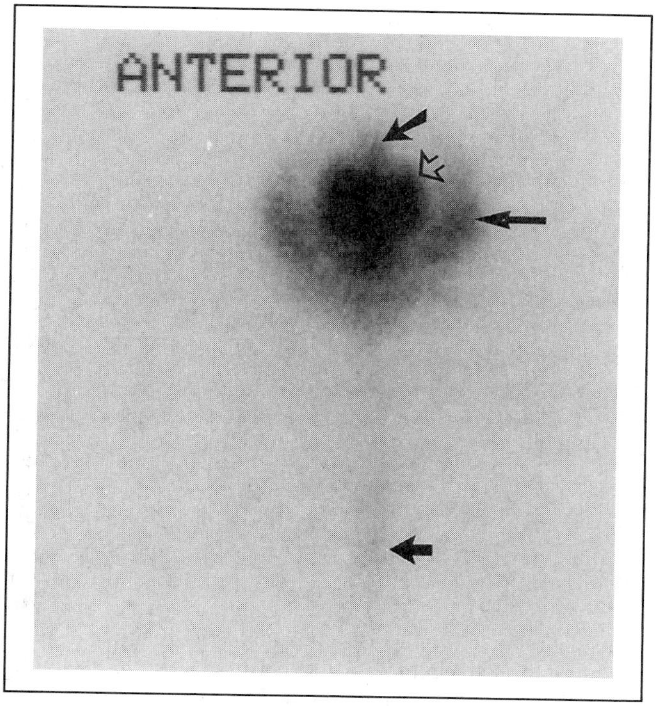

Fig. 108-20. Communicating hydrocephalus demonstrated by RN cisternogram. Anterior view of the head made 24 hours after radionuclide injection by lumbar puncture showing marked intraventricular reflux of the radionuclide *(open arrow)*. Note presence of smaller amounts of radionuclide activity in the Sylvian fissure *(long straight arrow)*, interhemispheric fissure *(slanted arrow)*, and spinal canal *(short arrow)*. RN, radionuclide.

raphy (SPECT) use positron (positively charged electron) emitting and photon (gamma ray) emitting substances, respectively, as radioactive tracers, whose distribution is displayed in tomographic fashion by a backprojection reconstruction process similar to that used in radiographic CT. PET uses synthetic, short-lived, proton-abundant isotopes of biologically active atoms to radiolabel compounds that enter physiologic processes in the brain. PET researchers have shown oxygen-15 to be of major importance in the regional measurement of blood flow, blood volume, and oxygen metabolism, and fluorodeoxyglucose (F-18) to be a useful indicator of the local cerebral metabolic rate for glucose. With the use of these and other radioactive tracers, a large amount of research data has been compiled in normal patients and in those with epilepsy, brain tumors, stroke, dementias (including Alzheimer's disease and Huntington's disease), Parkinson's disease, and psychiatric disorders. Because of its high cost, as well as the necessity for an onsite cyclotron and a skilled support staff for a successful operation, PET use is still limited to a few university centers. SPECT imaging is relatively inefficient by PET standards, and quantitative blood flow data and metabolic information available from PET are more difficult to obtain with SPECT, and less accurate. Iodine-123 labeled amines and technitium-99m labeled hexamethylpropylene-amineoxime (HMPAO) are used for evaluating cerebral blood flow by means of SPECT. Low cost of operation relative to PET, new therapeutic developments for cerebrovascular disease, and interest in neuroreceptor localization could help make it an exciting and clinically useful took in the future.

CAROTID ULTRASONOGRAPHY

Duplex scanning, a technique that combines the information provided by high-resolution real-time ultrasonography with the physiologic data obtained by pulse gated Doppler, is used as a screening procedure for extracranial vascular disease primarily at the carotid bifurcation. Real-time sonography is used to detect atherosclerotic plaques and to evaluate plaque morphologic features. Changes in the frequency of the sound wave produced by flowing blood are recorded during the cardiac cycle and constitute the Doppler waveform. The quantitative frequency shift during the various phases of the cardiac cycle provides a velocity profile of blood flow in the vessel being examined. Stenotic lesions alter the normal velocity profile, and the extent of stenosis can be determined from the Doppler waveform by comparing the systolic and diastolic velocity measurements with known standard values (Fig. 108-21). With color Doppler the velocity induced frequency shifts in vascular structures are color coded for direction of flow and velocity. This allows easy identification of the flow abnormality and fa-

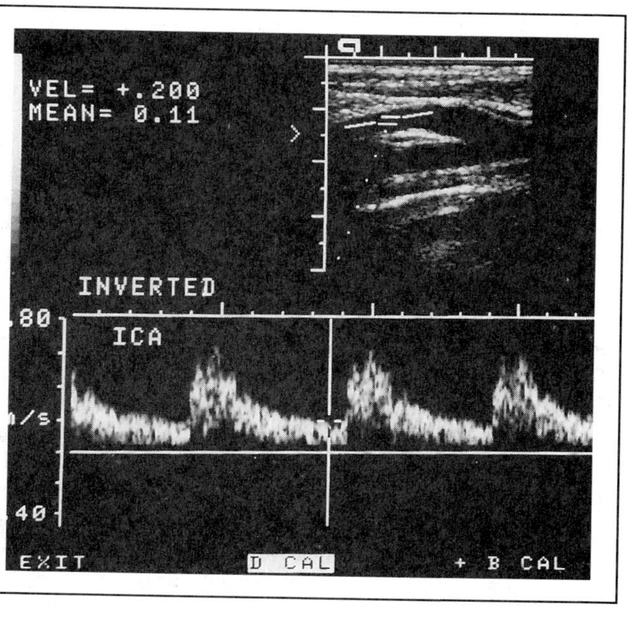

Fig. 108-21. Carotid sonogram. Duplex sonogram of the carotid bifurcation showing essentially normal carotid bifurcation in the upper right corner of illustration. Pulsed Doppler examination of the proximal internal carotid artery *(short parallel lines over proximal internal carotid artery indicate sample window)* produces normal Doppler tracing shown at bottom of illustration. Maximal measured diastolic velocity of 0.2 m/sec from this tracing indicated in the upper left corner of illustration is normal.

cilitates the examination by letting the sonographer quickly choose the best site for Doppler sampling to determine maximal stenosis. Although totally noninvasive and safe, carotid sonography is an operator dependent technique requiring a fair amount of skill and experience, is of limited utility for disease above the region of the carotid bifurcations, and is subject to errors of interpretation in cases of high-grade stenoses or complete occlusion.

REFERENCES

Hillman BJ and Newell JD II: Digital radiography. Radiol Clin North Am 23(2):1, 1985.

Newton TH and Potts DG: Advanced imaging techniques. San Anselmo, CA, 1983, Clavadel Press.

Newton TH and Potts DG: Computed tomography of the spine and spinal cord. San Anselmo, CA, 1983, Clavadel Press.

Osborn AG: Introduction to cerebral angiography. Hagerstown, MD, 1980 Harper & Row.

Shapiro R: Myelography, ed 4. Chicago, 1984, Year Book.

Stark DD and Bradley WG: Magnetic resonance imaging. St Louis, 1988, Mosby.

Taveras JM and Ferruci JT: Radiology: diagnosis-imaging-intervention. Philadelphia, 1986, Lippincott.

CHAPTER

109 Autonomic Nervous System

Roy Freeman

The autonomic nervous system is the principal innervator of visceral and vascular smooth muscle, endocrine and exocrine glands, the immune system, viscera, and certain soft tissues. This division of the neuraxis is almost entirely self-governing and mediates moment-to-moment homeostatic adjustments to the external and internal milieu. The efferent division of the autonomic nervous system has sympathetic and parasympathetic components that are mutually antagonistic in many tissues. The sympathetic nervous system is anatomically widespread and its reactions, best characterized by the "flight or fight response," tend to involve many organ systems simultaneously. In contrast, the parasympathetic nervous system is anatomically more discrete, and its reactions are more localized. The autonomic nervous system also transmits afferent impulses mediating visceral sensation.

The autonomic nervous system is integrally connected to neocortical regions, the limbic system, and somatosensory pathways. It is also subject to neurohumoral influences. Thus such diverse situations as stress, postural change, hypovolemia, pain, fear, and anxiety can activate the appropriate physiologic responses. These reactions are rapid in onset and usually of short duration, in contrast to the longer-lasting effects of the endocrine system.

NEUROANATOMY

The hypothalamus plays a central role in the integration of autonomic function. Projections from the hypothalamus descend to the midbrain and other brainstem structures and then spread in a cascading fashion throughout the spinal cord. The peripheral autonomic nervous system consists of two neurons. The cell body of the first (or preganglionic) neuron, which is found within the central nervous system, sends out an axon that synapses with a ganglion in the periphery. From this ganglion a second (postganglionic) neuron supplies an effector organ. The exception to this scheme is the adrenal gland, where the adrenal medulla functions as a second neuron.

Preganglionic sympathetic neurons extend from the first thoracic to the second lumbar levels of the intermediolateral column in the spinal cord. Myelinated sympathetic axons leave the anterior roots as white rami communicantes, forming the paravertebral sympathetic chain and ganglia that extend from the base of the skull to the coccyx. These axons synapse with 10 to 20 postganglionic neurons at various segmental levels in the sympathetic chain, and postganglionic axons return to the peripheral nerve as lightly myelinated gray rami communicantes (Fig. 109-1). Alternatively, preganglionic axons may pass through the sympathetic chain forming the superior, middle, and inferior splanchnic nerves en route to abdominal and pelvic sympathetic ganglia or the adrenal gland. This anatomic arrangement provides the framework for the diffuse, widespread response mediated by the sympathetic nervous system (Fig. 109-2).

The parasympathetic nervous system has its origin in the brainstem and sacral spinal cord. The preganglionic parasympathetic neurons of the brainstem emanate from the cranial nerve nuclei of the oculomotor, facial, glossopharyngeal, and vagus nerves. The sacral division originates in the intermediolateral column of the second, third, and fourth sacral segments of the spinal cord and supplies abdominal and pelvic viscera via the pelvic nerves. These neu-

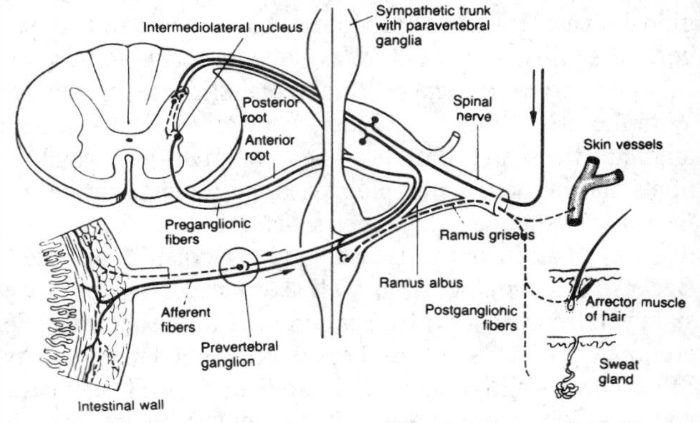

Fig. 109-1. The course of preganglionic and postganglionic sympathetic fibers and the organization of the sympathetic trunk. (From Duus P: Topical Diagnosis in Neurology. New York, 1983, Thieme-Stratton.)

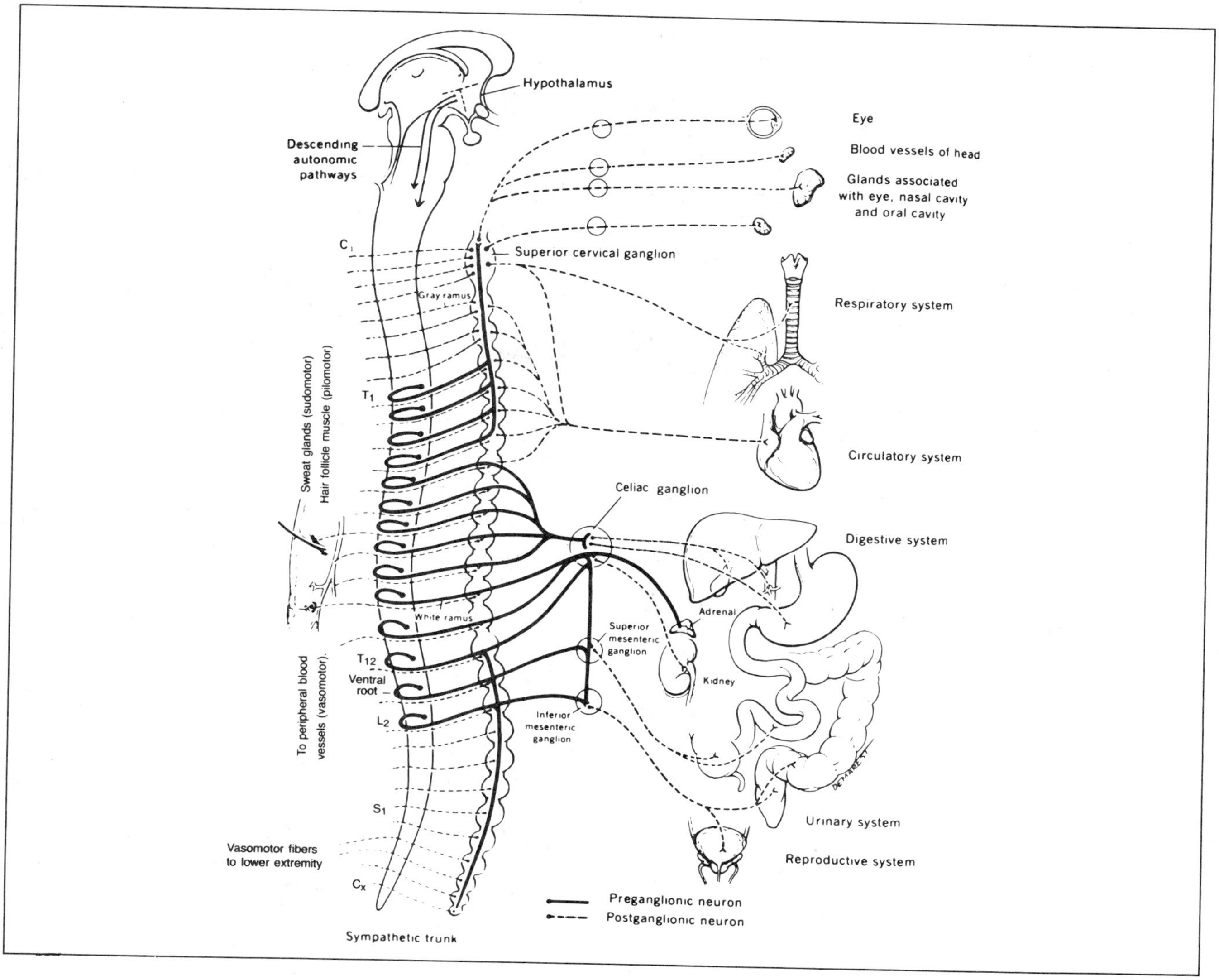

Fig. 109-2. The sympathetic division of the autonomic nervous system. (From Novak CR, Demarest RJ: The Human Nervous System, ed 2. New York, 1975, McGraw-Hill.)

rons form a postganglionic synapse close to the end-organ, often within the visceral wall (Fig. 109-3).

NEUROCHEMISTRY

Acetylcholine is the neurotransmitter released at the preganglionic synapse in both the sympathetic and parasympathetic divisions of the autonomic nervous system. It is also the neurotransmitter released by postganglionic parasympathetic nerve terminals, postganglionic sympathetic nerves to eccrine sweat glands, and possibly nerves to blood vessels supplying skeletal muscle.

Acetylcholine is derived by the enzymatic acetylation of choline with acetylcholine coenzyme A by choline acetyltransferase. Acetylcholine is then stored in vesicles within the axon terminal and, after an action potential, is extruded by exocytosis into the synaptic cleft.

The catecholamine norepinephrine is the neurotransmitter released at the remaining sympathetic postganglionic nerve terminals. The adrenal gland (which is the equivalent in function to a postsynaptic neuron) releases epinephrine and smaller quantities of norepinephrine into the circulation in response to preganglionic nerve impulses.

Norepinephrine is formed within postganglionic nerve terminals by the enzymatic conversion of catecholamine precursors. The aromatic amino acid tyrosine is actively taken up by the nerve terminal and is hydroxylated to dihydroxyphenylalanine (DOPA). This is decarboxylated to form dopamine (DA), which is then converted by dopamine beta hydroxylase (DBH) within the synaptic vesicle to form norepinephrine. Phenylethanolamine-N-methyltransferase, an enzyme present in the adrenal gland, allows conversion of norepinephrine to epinephrine (Fig. 109-4).

Norepinephrine is stored within vesicles in the nerve terminals and is released into the synaptic cleft with dopamine

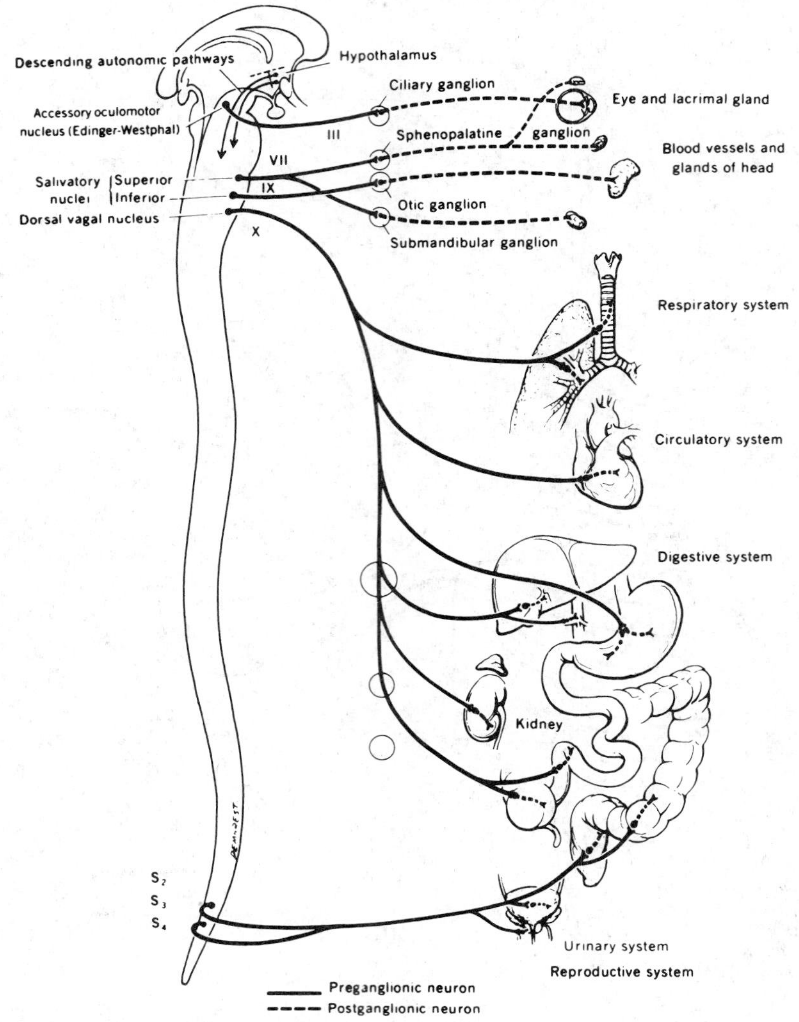

Fig. 109-3. The parasympathetic division of the autonomic nervous system. (From Novak CR and Demarest RJ: The Human Nervous System, ed 2. New York, 1975, Mcgraw-Hill.)

beta hydroxylase by exocytosis in response to a nerve impulse. Norepinephrine activates presynaptic or postsynaptic receptors, producing an effect that is dependent on the nature and site of the receptor.

Released norepinephrine can be actively taken up by the presynaptic neuron (uptake I), where it is either stored in vesicles ready for rerelease or oxidatively deaminated by intramitochondrial monoamine oxidase (MAO). Norepinephrine can also be actively taken up by the postsynaptic cell or (after diffusion into the circulation) by other tissues (uptake II). Norepinephrine is then degraded by catechol-O-methyltransferase (COMT). The major metabolic end-products of norepinephrine and epinephrine include vanillylmandelic acid (VMA), dihydroxyphenylglycol (DHPG), 3-methoxy-4-hydroxyphenylglycol (MHPG), normetanephrine (NMN), and metanephrine (MN).

Our understanding of autonomic neuroeffector transmission has undergone a major revision in recent years. It is now accepted that most autonomic neurons contain more than one neurotransmitter. These cotransmitters include purines (e.g., adenosine 5′-triphosphate and adenosine), peptides (e.g., neuropeptide Y, vasoactive intestinal peptide, somatostatin, and calcitonin gene-related peptide), aminoacids, and possibly nitric oxide. These agents may modify neurotransmission at the neuroeffector junction by prejunctional modulation of the amount of neurotransmitter released or by postjunctional modulation of the duration of action of the neurotransmitter. The process of chemical coding, whereby the specific combinations of different neurotransmitters in autonomic neurons are established, is thus responsible for the remarkable heterogeneity of the human autonomic nervous system.

AUTONOMIC PHYSIOLOGY

Cardiovascular regulation

The autonomic nervous system mediates immediate cardiovascular homeostatic adjustments, whereas long-term

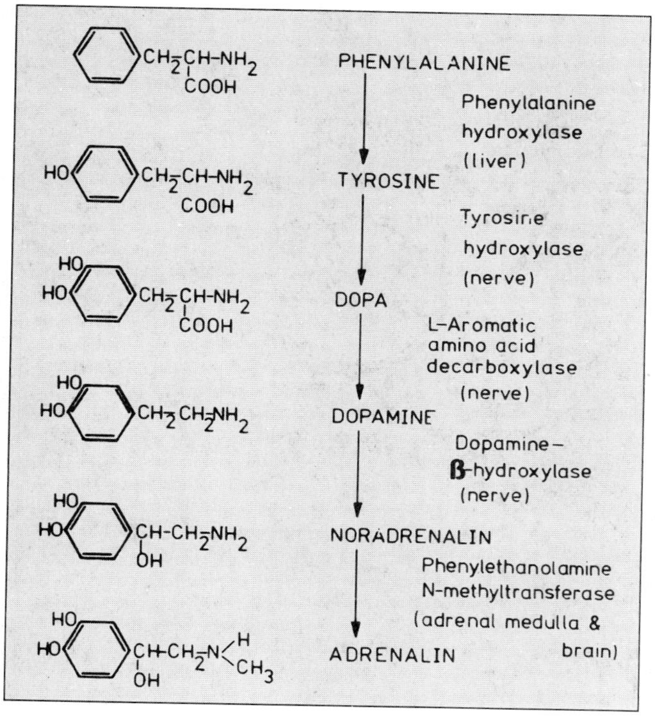

Fig. 109-4. Catecholamine metabolism. (From Bannister R, editor: Autonomic Failure. Oxford, 1982, Oxford University Press.)

changes are mediated by the endocrine system—in particular, the renin-angiotensin-aldosterone system of the kidney. The short-term changes in cardiac function and vasomotor tone are regulated by a group of brainstem nuclei that integrate information from a variety of neural and humoral sources. Important sites of afferent information for these brainstem centers include the arterial and cardiopulmonary baroreceptors, the cerebral cortex, the limbic cortex, and the hypothalamus.

The baroreceptor reflex arc extends from the cardiopulmonary volume receptors of the great vessels (via the vagus nerve) and the pressure receptors of the carotid sinus and aortic arch (via the glossopharyngeal nerve) to the nucleus of the solitary tract in the ventrolateral medulla. This is an inhibitory pathway and responds to changes in blood pressure. Thus a fall in blood pressure decreases baroreceptor impulses to the nucleus of the solitary tract and other brainstem autonomic nuclei. Parasympathetic pathways extend from the nucleus of the solitary tract to the nucleus ambiguus and dorsal motor nucleus of the vagus. Efferent fibers from these brainstem nuclei then synapse in the heart and the postganglionic neurons innervate the myocardium, sinoatrial (SA) node, atrioventricular (AV) node, and bundle of His. The nucleus of the solitary tract and associated brainstem autonomic nuclei also give rise to sympathetic fibers passing via the upper thoracic segments of the intermediolateral column to the heart. These mutually antagonistic pathways mediate the changes in heart rate and contractility.

The sympathetic nervous system provides the innervation of the vascular tree. It predominantly supplies the smaller vessels—particularly, small arteries and the arterioles. The most common adrenergic receptor is the $alpha_1$ receptor, which causes vasoconstriction when stimulated. Vasodilating $beta_2$-adrenergic receptors and vasoconstricting $alpha_2$-adrenergic receptors are also found. Cholinergic axons possibly cause dilatation of skeletal muscle blood vessels, and purine derivatives and peptides also play a role in mediating vascular tone.

An important aspect of autonomic circulatory function involves the regulation of the cardiovascular response to postural change. The act of standing, with the resulting gravitational-induced pooling of blood in the lower extremities and splanchnic circulation, produces a decrease in the venous return and ventricular filling, with a consequent reduction in stroke volume and cardiac output and thus a fall in blood pressure. The baroreceptors respond by decreasing their inhibitory afferent impulses to the vasomotor centers in the brainstem, provoking immediate adjustments in arterial tone (increasing peripheral vascular resistance) and venular tone (increasing venous return) that occur simultaneously with an increase in heart rate and myocardial contractility. These interrelated physiologic mechanisms maintain blood pressure in the erect position. When these homeostatic reflexes fail, a postural fall in blood pressure or orthostatic hypotension occurs. As a result of inadequate cerebral perfusion, lightheadedness, fatigue, visual blurring, and syncope may ensue.

The pupil

The pupil best exemplifies the mutual antagonism of the sympathetic and parasympathetic nervous systems—dilating in response to sympathetic impulses and constricting in response to parasympathetic impulses.

Sympathetic fibers en route to the pupil pass through the posterolateral hypothalamus, midbrain, pons, and lateral medulla, descending to the intermediolateral column and leaving the spinal cord after forming a synapse at spinal segments C8-T2. The preganglionic neuron ascends in the sympathetic chain (looping over the subclavian artery and crossing the lung apex) to the superior cervical ganglion located at the bifurcation of the common carotid. The postganglionic neuron extends from the superior cervical ganglion to the eye via a nerve plexus surrounding the internal carotid artery and to the eccrine sweat glands of the face via a plexus surrounding the external carotid artery (Fig. 109-5).

Oculosympathetic paralysis (Horner's syndrome of ptosis, miosis, and anhidrosis) can thus occur with a lesion affecting the primary neuron (e.g., a brainstem stroke, tumor, or syrinx); the preganglionic neuron (e.g., trauma to the brachial plexus, and tumors or infections of the lung apex); or the postganglionic neuron (e.g., a dissecting carotid aneurysm, carotid artery ischemia, migraine, or a middle cranial fossa neoplasm). The lesion site can be determined by pharmacologic testing of the pupil (Table 109-1).

The pupil receives parasympathetic innervation from the

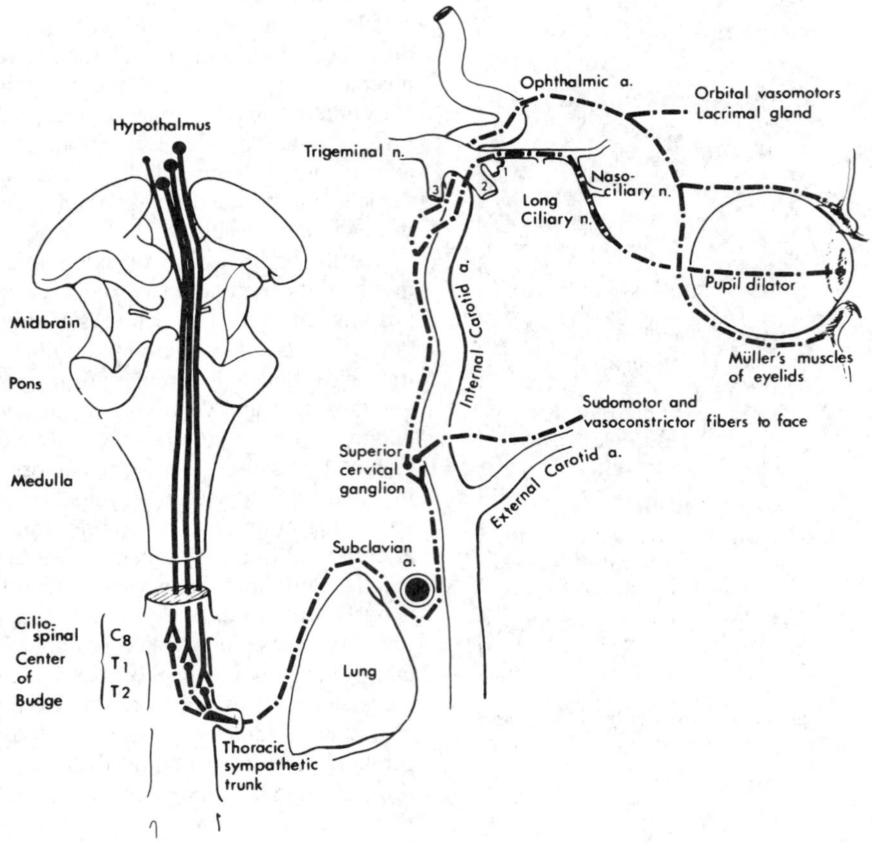

Fig. 109-5. Ocular sympathetic pathways. (From Glaser JS: Neuro-ophthalmology, ed 2. Philadelphia, 1990, Lippincott.)

Table 109-1. Pharmacologic testing of the pupil

Pharmacologic agent	Normal response	Abnormal response	Mechanism
Cocaine (2%-10%)	Dilatation	No response	Blocks presynaptic norepinephrine uptake
Hydroxyamphetamine (1%)	Dilatation	No response if lesion is in postganglionic neuron; normal response if postganglionic neuron is intact	Releases norepinephrine from postganglionic neuron
Phenylephrine (1%)	No response or minimal response	Dilates abnormal pupil, especially if postganglionic lesion is present	Pupil supersensitive because of denervation
Pilocarpine			
(0.125%	No response	Constricts Adie's pupil	Pupil sensitive because of denervation
1%	Constriction	No response if pupil is pharmacologically dilated	Pharmacologic blockade
Methacholine (2.5%)	No response	Constricts Adie's pupil	Pupil supersensitive because of denervation

third cranial nerve. These parasympathetic pupillomotor fibers originate in the Edinger-Westphal complex of the third cranial nerve nucleus, located in the midbrain, and travel to the ciliary ganglion with the third cranial nerve. The postganglionic short ciliary nerves directly innervate the pupil.

Thus mydriasis produced by parasympathetic dysfunction can result from a central process affecting the Edinger-Westphal nucleus or third cranial nerve fasciculus (e.g., strokes or tumors of the midbrain); a preganglionic lesion affecting the third cranial nerve (e.g., compression by an enlarging posterior communicating artery aneurysm, transtentorial herniation a mononeuropathy affecting the third cranial nerve or trauma); or a postganglionic process (e.g., Adie's pupil, a third cranial nerve mononeuropathy, pharmacologic blockade of the pupil or trauma).

Sweating

Sweating is the thermoregulatory response to an increase in central core temperature and is mediated by heat regulator centers in the anterior hypothalamus. Sweating also occurs in response to gustatory and emotional stimuli. Two types of sweat glands are found. The eccrine glands are innervated by sympathetic nerves with cholinergic synapses at both the preganglionic and postganglionic neuron. The apocrine glands, found in the axilla, the genital region, and the nipples, are not under neurologic control. They respond to circulating humoral factors and produce apocrine secretions, primarily in response to emotional stimuli.

Bladder

The bladder is composed of three layers of interdigitating smooth muscle (the detrusor muscle) and serves as a receptacle for the storage and appropriate evacuation of urine. The detrusor muscle forms the internal sphincter at the junction of the bladder neck and urethra. This sphincter is not anatomically discrete and functions as a physiologic sphincter. In contrast, the external sphincter is formed from the striated muscle of the urogenital diaphragm and is a true anatomic sphincter.

Higher centers involved in bladder control include the anterior and medial frontal lobes, limbic regions, basal ganglia, thalamus, hypothalamus, and brainstem. These regions receive afferent fibers from and send efferent fibers to "micturition centers" in the lower spinal cord.

The bladder has parasympathetic, sympathetic, and somatic innervation. The parasympathetic nerves originate in the intermediolateral column of the second, third, and fourth sacral segments of the spinal cord. Passing through the ventral nerve roots, these fibers form pelvic nerves that synapse with postganglionic neurons on the surface of the bladder. These muscarinic cholinergic postganglionic nerves produce detrusor muscle contraction. The sympathetic nerve supply to the bladder originates in the intermediolateral column of spinal segments T12-L2. These nerve fibers pass through the sympathetic ganglia and reach the hypogastric plexus via the splanchnic nerves. Postganglionic sympathetic neurons then innervate the dome of the bladder (beta-adrenergic receptors) and the internal sphincter (alpha-adrenergic receptors) via the hypogastric nerves. The striated muscle of the external urethral sphincter is innervated by the pudendal nerves, which originate from the anterior horn cells of the second, third, and fourth sacral segments. This sphincter is under voluntary control but undergoes reflex relaxation during micturition. Afferent fibers mediating bladder sensation and reflex bladder contraction are carried by both the sympathetic and the parasympathetic nerves to the spinal cord (Fig. 109-6).

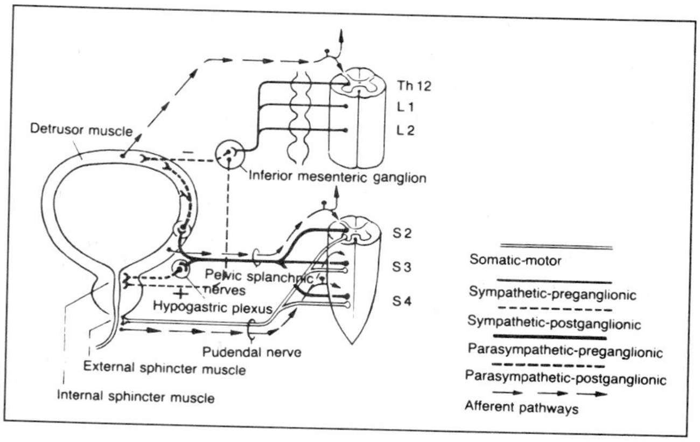

Fig. 109-6. The innervation of the urinary bladder. (From Duus P: Topical Diagnosis in Neurology. New York, 1983, Thieme-Stratton.)

Normal voluntary micturition is most likely coordinated by pontomesencephalic centers and modulated by higher cerebral regions. This act entails a complex sequence of neural activity, including voluntary relaxation of the striated external sphincter, increased intra-abdominal pressure produced by abdominal wall tension, and detrusor muscle contraction with subsequent relaxation and opening of the internal sphincter. Micturition ceases after voluntary contraction of the external sphincter.

Genital system

Normal sexual function involves the integration of several psychologic and physiologic processes. These include appropriate sexual drive (libido) and sexual arousal, penile erection, orgasm, and ejaculation in the male, and genital vascular engorgement in the female. The neurologic control of sexual function thus involves a complex coordination of higher centers with sympathetic, parasympathetic, and somatic nervous activity.

Penile erection is produced by vascular engorgement of the corpus spongiosum and corpora cavernosa caused by arterial vasodilatation, venous constriction, and closure of arteriovenous shunts. Local stimuli (bowel or bladder distention and tactile stimulation of the external genitalia) provoke this response via a spinal reflex (reflexogenic erections), whereas psychogenic erections are provoked by stimuli to higher centers. Erections are mediated by the parasympathetic pelvic nerves (nervi erigentes) from spinal segments S2-4. The sympathetic nervous system (segments T12-L2) via the hypogastric nerves plays an accessory role, particularly in the production of psychogenic erections. Recent evidence has suggested that nitric oxide,vasoactive intestinal peptide, and neuropeptide Y may also have a role in erectile function.

Ejaculation is a complex reflex mediated by the hypogastric sympathetic nerves (which cause contraction of the smooth muscle of the seminal vesicles, vas deferens, epididymis, and ejaculatory ducts) and somatic pudendal nerves (which produce contraction of the ischiocavernosus and bulbocavernosus muscles).

Less is known about the autonomic control of the female genital system. Parasympathetic pelvic nerves stimulate vaginal secretions and mediate vascular engorgement of the vulva, vagina, and clitoris during sexual arousal. The pudendal nerves mediate contraction of the vaginal and pelvic floor muscles during orgasm.

Because sexual function involves vast neural territories and intricate interactions among the sympathetic, parasympathetic, and somatic nervous systems, dysfunction may occur at several levels as a result of diverse psychologic, neurologic, medical, and endocrinologic causes.

GENERALIZED AUTONOMIC DISORDERS

Autonomic overactivity

A wide range of disorders produce generalized overactivity of the autonomic nervous system. This appears most frequently as tachycardia, raised blood pressure, perspiration, tremor, and hyperventilation associated with anxiety and panic attacks. A more ominous presentation of increased autonomic activity is the Cushing response, a triad of increased blood pressure, bradycardia, and respiratory irregularity produced by the compression of brainstem autonomic centers by raised intracranial pressure. Space-occupying masses confined to the brainstem may produce a similar response due to local effects, even in the absence of raised intracranial pressure. In addition, strokes, trauma, subarachnoid hemorrhage, and meningitis can all produce signs of autonomic hyperactivity. The electrocardiographic changes associated with these neurologic diseases are also mediated by autonomic overactivity and may represent microscopic myocardial abnormalities.

Symptoms of autonomic overactivity such as hypertension, sweating, flushing, anxiety, changes in heart and respiratory rates, salivation, abdominal cramps, and pupillomotor responses may occur as manifestations of a seizure. Temporal lobe seizure foci provide the most frequent source of such symptoms. Rarely, central lesions in the region of the third ventricle, thalamus, and hypothalamus also produce this symptom complex. This has been called diencephalic epilepsy. However, rather than a true epileptic phenomenon it is more likely due to pressure on brainstem autonomic centers or release of those centers from cortical and subcortical control. The propensity of seizure foci to affect the autonomic nervous system may well be reflected in the increased incidence of sudden death in patients with epilepsy.

A "mass reflex" of autonomic overactivity, with signs such as hypertension, cardiac arrhythmias, piloerection, and sweating, frequently follows spinal cord injury. Afferent impulses, such as pain or bladder distention, usually provide the provocative stimulus for this response, which most commonly occurs after cervical and high-thoracic-cord lesions.

Sedative or alcohol withdrawal is a common cause of sympathetic nervous system overactivity. In its most florid form, this state consists of agitation, confusion, hypervigilance, hallucinosis, and tremulousness, with autonomic accompaniments such as mydriasis, tachycardia, tachypnea, and sweating. Although these symptoms usually abate gradually after several days, in extreme cases the withdrawal syndrome can be fatal.

Pheochromocytoma and other tumors of chromaffin cell origin produce a picture of autonomic hyperactivity characterized by paroxysmal hypertension, sweating, flushing, tachycardia, and anxiety, generated by intermittent catecholamine release (Chapter 164).

Although peripheral neuropathies customarily produce symptoms of autonomic hypoactivity, acute inflammatory demyelinating neuropathy (the Guillain-Barré syndrome) may produce periodic autonomic overactivity, often alternating with symptoms and signs of reduced autonomic function. Acute intermittent porphyria can produce a similar clinical picture of increased autonomic activity associated with an acute progressive neuropathy (Chapters 121 and 123). For a complete list of those disorders that produce autonomic overactivity, see the box below.

Autonomic failure

Autonomic failure produces a wide array of symptoms and may be caused by a diverse group of disorders. Orthostatic hypotension, the most debilitating of these symptoms, ini-

Autonomic overactivity

1. Central nervous system
- Raised intracranial pressure
- Temporal lobe epilepsy
- Diencephalic epilepsy
- Cerebrovascular disease
- Head trauma
- Meningitis
- Encephalitis
- Spinal cord injury
- Tetanus
- Familial dysautonomia
- Poliomyelitis
- Neuroleptic malignant syndrome

2. Peripheral nerve
- Acute pandysautonomia
- Porphyria
- Acute inflammatory demyelinating polyneuropathy
- Toxic neuropathies

3. Tumors
- Pheochromocytoma
- Neuroblastoma
- Ganglioneuroblastoma
- Ganglioneuroma
- Carotid body tumor

4. Drugs
- Monoamine oxidase inhibitors
- Sympathomimetic agents
- Sedative or alcohol withdrawal

Modified from Johnson RH, Lamby DG, and Spalding JMK: The autonomic nervous system. In Baker AB and Joynt RJ, editors: Clinical neurology, vol 4. Philadelphia, 1986, Harper & Row.

tially is characterized by occasional lightheadedness or dizziness, usually provoked by sudden standing, a warm environment, or large meals. Patients may also have associated visual disturbances reflecting retinal or occipital lobe ischemia and neck pain caused by ischemia of trapezius and other neck muscles. Eventually, severely afflicted patients are unable to maintain erect posture and may be confined to bed. Frequently, supine hypertension produced by baroreceptor dysfunction accompanies orthostatic hypotension.

Bladder symptoms are a common complaint of patients with autonomic dysfunction. Central nervous system disease usually produces detrusor hyperreflexia, with such symptoms as frequency, urgency, nocturia, and incontinence. This often occurs in conjunction with sphincter dysynergy—a failure to coordinate bladder contraction with sphincter relaxation. Peripheral nervous system disease, on the other hand, customarily produces detrusor muscle areflexia, with such symptoms as difficulty in initiating urination, failure to maintain an adequate stream of urine, urinary retention, and overflow incontinence. Such patients are often subjected to unnecessary prostatic surgery, which usually exacerbates the clinical condition by producing further incontinence.

Impotence, diminished libido, ejaculatory dysfunction, and failure to attain orgasm may be early symptoms of autonomic dysfunction, although patients often do not seek immediate medical attention for these problems. Depression, secondary to the debilitating symptoms of autonomic failure, may at times be the primary cause of impotence.

Generalized anhidrosis with attendant thermoregulatory dysfunction occurs late in the clinical course of those conditions producing autonomic failure. At an early stage, patchy or partial anhidrosis is accompanied by hyperhidrosis in other areas in an attempt to maintain normal thermoregulation. Some patients complain of excess sweating associated with eating.

Gastrointestinal complaints of patients with autonomic failure include nausea, vomiting, early satiety caused by gastroparesis, constipation, diarrhea, and incontinence. Symptoms referable to other organ systems include difficulty adapting to changing light conditions, produced by decreased pupillomotor function; and respiratory difficulties, caused by paralysis of the abductors of the larynx. Obstructive and central apneic episodes and other disorders of central respiratory control may also occur.

Shy and Drager first described a syndrome of progressive autonomic failure in conjunction with dysfunction in the extrapyramidal, pyramidal, and cerebellar systems. Extraocular movement abnormalities and disturbances in respiratory, bulbar, and peripheral motor neuron function may also occur. This clinical condition, known as the Shy-Drager syndrome or multiple system atrophy, is progressive and culminates in death after several years. The pathologic hallmark of this disorder is extensive loss of the cellular elements in the intermediolateral columns of the spinal cord. Accompanying pathologic changes appear in the striatum, cerebellum, pyramidal system, anterior horn cells, and autonomic nuclei of the brainstem, including the locus ceruleus, nucleus of the tractus solitarius, nucleus ambiguus, and dorsal motor nucleus of the vagus. The norepinephrine content of the basal ganglia, septal nuclei, hypothalamus, locus ceruleus, and nucleus accumbens is reduced. Autonomic failure may also accompany Parkinson's disease, olivopontocerebellar atrophy, and striatonigral degeneration.

Various disorders affecting the peripheral nervous system result in autonomic dysfunction. Pure autonomic failure, or idiopathic orthostatic hypotension, is a disorder characterized by progressive autonomic dysfunction that usually occurs without clinical evidence of central nervous system disease or an obvious peripheral neuropathy. This disorder is most likely due to degeneration of the postganglionic peripheral autonomic neuron. Recent investigations have indicated that some pathologic and physiologic preganglionic autonomic nervous system involvement also occurs in this disease.

Acute and subacute presentations of pure autonomic neuropathy occur. Patients with these disorders, which are most likely a form of inflammatory polyneuropathy confined to the autonomic nerves, generally recover autonomic function.

In 20% to 40% of patients with diabetes evidence of autonomic dysfunction develops as a consequence of small fiber damage (Chapter 168). This usually occurs late in the illness, although subclinical autonomic involvement may be detected in newly diagnosed and teenage diabetics. Cardiovascular autonomic abnormalities associated with diabetes include orthostatic hypotension, resting tachycardia, fixed heart rate, and a tendency to painless myocardial infarction. Insulin may exacerbate the orthostatic hypotension. Other symptoms of autonomic dysfunction include gastroparesis (with nausea, vomiting, early satiety, and postprandial abdominal discomfort), nocturnal diarrhea, constipation, incontinence of feces, sweating abnormalities, bladder dysfunction, and unawareness of hypoglycemia. In one prospective study, autonomic dysfunction, as defined by abnormal cardiovascular reflexes, was associated with a mortality rate of 56% at 5 years.

The peripheral neuropathies associated with amyloid, alcoholism uremia, porphyria, and Fabry's disease are other prominent causes of autonomic dysfunction. Disorders of the peripheral nervous system with autonomic involvement are listed in the box on p. 1000.

LOCAL AUTONOMIC DISORDERS

Several diseases are due to or associated with local autonomic nervous system dysfunction. These diseases are listed in the box on p. 1000. Details of these disorders are covered elsewhere in the text.

TESTING THE AUTONOMIC NERVOUS SYSTEM

The anatomic location of the autonomic nervous system renders it relatively inaccessible for direct clinical testing. Furthermore, because most autonomic fibers are unmyelinated and therefore conduct nerve impulses slowly, conventional neurophysiologic techniques are inadequate means of

Autonomic failure

Disorders of the central nervous system
- Multiple system atrophy (Shy-Drager syndrome)
- Parkinson's disease
- Olivopontocerebellar degeneration
- Striatonigral degeneration
- Brain tumors (brainstem, cerebellum, diencephalon)
- Wernicke's disease
- Multiple infarcts
- Syringomyelia and syringobulbia
- Hydrocephalus
- Multiple sclerosis
- Myelopathies
  - Traumatic
  - Inflammatory
  - Pernicious anemia
  - Degenerative
  - Tabes dorsalis
- Familial dysautonomia
- Menke's syndrome
- Mitral valve prolapse

Disorders of the peripheral nervous system
- Pure autonomic failure (idiopathic orthostatic hypotension)
- Peripheral neuropathies
  - Diabetes
  - Amyloid
  - Guillain-Barré syndrome
  - Chronic inflammatory polyneuropathy
  - Acute pandysautonomia
  - Fabry's disease
  - Pernicious anemia
  - Chagas' disease
  - Porphyria
  - Uremia
  - Alcoholic neuropathy
  - Paraneoplastic neuropathy
  - Toxic neuropathies
    - Vincristine
    - Perhexilene maleate
    - Vacor
    - Acrylamide
    - Thallium
    - Arsenic
    - Mercury
  - HIV neuropathy
- Surgical sympathectomy
- Botulism
- Adie's syndrome
- Dopamine beta hydroxylase deficiency

Miscellaneous disorders
- Medications
  - Antihypertensive agents
  - Tricyclic agents
  - Monoamine oxidase inhibitors
  - Antipsychotic agents
- Aging (?)
- Hyperbradykinism
- Endocrine
  - Adrenocortical deficiencies
  - Pheochromocytoma
  - Hyperaldosteronism

Local autonomic disorders

Head and neck
- Baroreceptor denervation
- Carotid endarterectomy
- Migraine
- Cluster headache
- Melkersson's syndrome
- Spastic dysphonia
- Carotid sinus hypersensitivity
- Horner's syndrome

Limbs
- Raynaud's phenomenon
- Acrocyanosis
- Angioneurotic edema
- Causalgia
- Reflex sympathetic dystrophy
- Erythromelalgia
- Hyperhidrosis
- Anhidrosis

Trunk
- Cystic fibrosis
- Asthma
- Spastic colon
- Chronic intestinal pseudoobstruction

Modified from Johnson RH, Lamby DG, and Spalding JMK: The autonomic nervous system. In Baker AB and Joynt RJ, editors: Clinical neurology, vol 4. Philadelphia, 1986, Harper & Row.

studying autonomic function. A battery of tests assessing autonomic function and dysfunction has been established to circumvent these problems by measuring end-organ responses to various physiologic and pharmacologic perturbations; by determining the levels of autonomic neurotransmitters and neuromodulators in blood, cerebrospinal fluid, and urine; and by quantifying autonomic receptor density and affinity.

The most frequently used tests are described below.

CARDIOVASCULAR REFLEXES

R-R interval variation

A reflex increase in the heart rate occurs with inspiration and is followed by a reflex decrease in heart rate with expiration. This response is mediated by the vagus nerve and is abolished by atropine. When breathing at a rate of six breaths per minute normal subjects display a difference between the maximum and minimum heart rates of more than 10 beats per minute. Alternatively, a ratio can be calculated between the sum of the longest R-R intervals occurring on each of six expirations and the sum of the shortest R-R interval occurring on each of six inspirations. This is known as the expiration-inspiration (E-I) ratio. Because there is a progressive decline in the amplitude of heart rate variation (and most other tests of autonomic function) with increasing age, age-based norms should be established.

The Valsalva maneuver

The patient is requested to exhale against a resistance of 40 mm Hg for 20 seconds while heart rate and blood pressure are monitored. Four discrete phases occur. In phase 1 the increase in intrathoracic and intraabdominal pressure causes aortic compression and an increase in peripheral resistance that results in a transient increase of blood pressure and decrease in heart rate. In phase 2 the increase in intrathoracic pressure produces decreases in venous return, left ventricular filling pressure, and cardiac output. This causes a fall in pulse pressure, which is terminated after several seconds by reflex vasoconstriction mediated via the baroreceptor reflex pathways. During this phase there is compensatory increase in heart rate. Phase 3 begins with the cessation of forced expiration. In this phase there is a further drop in blood pressure as the aortic compression ceases. In phase 4, blood pressure increases ("the overshoot") as a result of the "postrelease" increase in cardiac output and persisting peripheral vasoconstriction. This blood pressure increase causes a reflex bradycardia.

The Valsalva maneuver tests both the sympathetic and parasympathetic divisions of the nervous system. With sympathetic dysfunction the tachycardia in phase 2 and blood pressure increase at the start of phase 4 are attenuated. The fall in blood pressure occurring in phase 2 may not be terminated by vasoconstriction. With parasympathetic dysfunction the baroreceptor-mediated reflex bradycardic response to the elevated blood pressure in phase 4 does not occur.

The Valsalva maneuver is best tested by measuring blood pressures with an arterial line; however, a Valsalva ratio—an indirect measure of the blood pressure response—can be calculated by comparing the longest R-R interval in phase 4 to the shortest R-R interval in phase 2. The recent availability of noninvasive beat-to-beat blood pressure recordings permits the direct measurement of this reflex.

Heart rate response to standing

On moving from a supine to a standing position a relative tachycardia occurs, usually maximizing around the 15th beat after standing is initiated. This is followed by a relative bradycardia that is maximum at approximately the 30th beat. This biphasic response is mediated by afferent impulses from muscle, the vagus nerve, and the baroreflex arc. It does not occur with passive tilting and is blocked by atropine. The ratio of the R-R interval at the 30th beat to the R-R interval at the 15th beat (the 30:15 ratio) may be used as a measure of this reflex.

Blood pressure response to standing

On moving from the horizontal to the vertical position, blood pressure is maintained by reflex vasocontriction and an increase in heart rate. A fall in systolic blood pressure of greater than 20 to 30 mm Hg or diastolic blood pressure of 10 to 15 mm Hg is abnormal.

The cold pressor test

The patient immerses his or her hand in cold water (4° C) for 60 seconds. A normal response, mediated by afferent sensory pathways and efferent sympathetic pathways that bypass the baroreceptors, is a systolic blood pressure increase of approximately 10 to 15 mm Hg.

Isometric hand grip

The patient squeezes a hand grip dynamometer at 30% of his or her maximum strength for 3 minutes. A normal response is a diastolic blood pressure increase of approximately 15 mm Hg or greater.

Other cardiovascular reflexes

Other cardiac reflexes include the vagally mediated bradycardiac response to apneic facial immersion in cold water, the tachycardia and blood pressure increase in response to mental stress, the blood pressure and heart rate response to passive tilting or lower-body negative pressure, and the bradycardic response to carotid sinus massage.

Power spectral analysis

Power spectral analysis of the resting heart rate produces several prominent peaks. A number of animal and human experiments with pharmacologic blockade of the autonomic nervous system have shown that the sympathetic and parasympathetic nervous systems mediate heart rate fluctuations in different frequency bands. Heart rate fluctuations at frequencies greater than 0.15 Hz are mediated by changes in vagal efferent activity alone, whereas heart rate fluctuations at less than 0.15 Hz are mediated by changing levels of both vagal and sympathetic activity. In normal subjects the move from supine to upright position produces a shift in the power spectrum from high to low frequencies. This shift in spectral power, induced by postural change, is reduced by betareceptor blockade and reflects a change in the balance of sympathetic and parasympathetic efferent activity. Indices derived from the power spectrum thus provide a potential measure of both sympathetic and parasympathetic nervous system function.

Pupillometry

The integrity of the autonomic innervation of the pupil can be simply determined by use of pharmacologic agents. The sympathetic supply to the pupil is tested by using cocaine (2% to 10%) and hydroxyamphetamine (1%). The normal pupil dilates after the instillation of cocaine eyedrops, which prevent norepinephrine reuptake by the presynaptic neuron. However, there is no response to cocaine eyedrops if there is a lesion anywhere in the sympathetic pathway to the eye. Both a normal pupil and a miotic pupil (as a result of preganglionic lesion) dilate in response to the instillation of hydroxyamphetamine, which releases intraneuronal norepinephrine from the postganglionic axon terminal. A lesion of the postganglionic neuron distal to the superior cervical ganglion prevents dilatation after hydroxyamphetamine instillation. The use of these two agents provides a simple means of diagnosing and localizing the site of neuronal injury responsible for sympathetic ocular paralysis.

Dilute pilocarpine is used to assess parasympathetic postganglionic pupil dysfunction. The normal pupil does not constrict to dilute pilocarpine (0.125%); however, the dilated denervated supersensitive pupil (e.g., produced by Adie's syndrome or other postganglionic neuronal dysfunction) rapidly becomes miotic. In contrast, pharmacologically induced mydriasis, producing a fixed dilated pupil, can be demonstrated by the use of 1% pilocarpine. This surprisingly frequent clinical phenomenon, which could be confused with imminent transtentorial herniation, is due to the accidental or deliberate contact of sympathomimetic agents with the conjunctival surface. Medication-induced mydriasis does not respond to 1% pilocarpine.

An infrared pupillometer with an attached television camera provides an accurate and sensitive, although expensive, means of assessing a number of aspects of pupil function.

Sweat testing

Testing the eccrine sweat glands provides a useful means of assessing the sympathetic nervous system. The simplest of the available clinical tests—the thermoregulatory sweat test—entails raising the body temperature with an external thermal source. The sweat response is assessed by measuring the color change in an indicator such as iodine with starch, quinizarin, or alizarin-red. Skin bioelectric recordings measuring the electrodermal potential (the sympathetic skin response), skin conductance (the galvanic skin reflex), or skin resistance provide an alternate measure of sweating. These tests examine both central and peripheral aspects of the afferent sympathetic nervous system.

The integrity of the postganglionic sympathetic neuron can be determined by measuring sweat output after iontophoresis or intradermal injection of cholinergic agonists such as pilocarpine or acetylcholine. The response can be quantified by using a sudorometer or by measuring the size of an imprint formed by the sweat droplets.

Catecholamine measurements

The advent of assays for catecholamines and catecholamine metabolites has provided a quantitative biochemical index of sympathetic nervous system activity. These compounds can now be measured with sensitivity and specificity in plasma, urine, and cerebrospinal fluid.

Plasma norepinephrine level doubles on movement from a supine to an erect position. A substantial further increase occurs after isometric or isotonic exercise. Patients with orthostatic hypotension caused by central nervous system disease have a normal resting norepinephrine level, because the postganglionic peripheral sympathetic neuron is intact. The normal norepinephrine increase in response to postural change or other stressful stimuli does not occur, because the central nervous system is unable to activate the postganglionic neuron. In contrast, patients with hypotension produced by peripheral nerve injury have a low resting norepinephrine level, which results from the postganglionic peripheral sympathetic nerve dysfunction. These patients also have no postural or stress-induced increase in plasma norepinephrine.

Catecholamines and their metabolites can also be measured in the cerebrospinal fluid (CSF) and urine. Although these determinations are not widely used clinically (with the exception of urinary catecholamine level measurements to diagnose pheochromocytoma), our understanding of many neurologic, psychiatric, and endocrine diseases has been enhanced by such measurements, which may well have future therapeutic applications.

Pharmacologic testing

Pharmacologic agents can be used systemically to determine the status of specific regions of the autonomic nervous system. The postsynaptic receptor agonists are generally used to demonstrate the state of enhanced sensitivity that a receptor develops when its presynaptic neuron degenerates (denervation supersensitivity). In this way, norepinephrine and phenylephrine can be used to determine alpha$_1$-receptor function, and isoproterenol and epinephrine can be used to determine beta$_1$- and beta$_2$-receptor function. The oral ingestion of yohimbine and clonidine, the respective antagonist and agonist of the alpha$_2$ receptor, can be used to assess alpha$_2$-adrenoreceptor function. Tyramine, which induces norepinephrine release from the intact postganglionic noradrenergic neuron, provides a useful means of assessing postganglionic neuronal integrity by measuring norepinephrine output. The cholinergic system can be assessed by an intravenous infusion of atropine.

Urodynamic testing

Current technologies available to most investigators allow for detailed physiologic evaluation of bladder, urethra, and sphincter function. The simplest yet most important of these investigations, the measurement of residual urinary volume, entails only transurethral catheterization immediately after micturition. This provides a measure of bladder evacuation and can also gauge the effectiveness of any therapeutic interventions.

The cystometrogram documents intravesical pressure and sensation as the bladder is progressively distended, usually by a transurethral water or carbon dioxide infusion. The perception of bladder filling occurs at 100 to 200 ml, and patients normally feel a strong desire to void at 400 to 500 ml. Patients with detrusor hyperreflexia caused by upper motor neuron disease display inhibited bladder contractions at volumes considerably lower than this. In contrast, the large-capacity atonic bladder produced by lower motor neuron disease shows no increase in intravesical pressure despite the introduction of large volumes of fluid. The coordination of bladder contraction and sphincter relaxation can be determined by carrying out simultaneous sphincter electromyography.

The voiding cystourethrogram is a radiologic study that provides structural and dynamic measures of bladder function. The patient is requested to void after the introduction of contrast material. Radiography carried out during micturition displays bladder size and shape, sphincter function, and urinary flow.

The selected use of these studies permits accurate diagnosis and appropriate therapy of bladder disturbances.

REFERENCES

Appenzeller O: The autonomic nervous system: an introduction to basic and clinical concepts, ed 4. New York, 1990, Elsevier Science.

Bannister R editor: Autonomic failure, ed 3. New York, 1992, Oxford University Press.

Bannister R and Oppenheimer DR: Degenerative disease of the nervous system associated with autonomic failure. Brain 95:457, 1972.

Burnstock G and Hoyle CHV, editors: Autonomic neuroeffector mechanisms, Chur, Switzerland, 1992, Harwood Academic.

Ewing DJ, Campbell IW, and Clarke BF: The natural history of diabetic autonomic neuropathy. QJ Med 49:95, 1980.

Johnson RH, Lamby GD, and Spalding JMK: The autonomic nervous system. In Baker AB and Joynt RJ editors: Clinical neurology, vol 4. Philadelphia, 1986, Harper & Row.

Loewy AD and Spyer KM, editors: Central regulation of autonomic functions. New York, 1990, Oxford University Press.

Low PA: Quantification of autonomic responses. In Dyck PJ et al, editors: Peripheral neuropathy. Philadelphia, 1984, Saunders.

McLeod JG and Tuck RR: Disorders of the autonomic nervous system. I. Pathophysiology and clinical features. Ann Neurol 21:419, 1987.

McLeod JG and Tuck RR: Disorders of the autonomic nervous system. II. Investigation and treatment. Ann Neurol 21:519, 1987.

McLeod JG: Autonomic dysfunction in peripheral nerve disease. Muscle Nerve 15:3, 1992.

Polinsky RJ et al: Pharmacologic distinction of different orthostatic hypotension syndromes. Neurology 31:1, 1981.

Thomas PK: Autonomic involvement in inherited neuropathies. Clin Autonom Res 2:51, 1992.

I CLINICAL SYNDROMES

CHAPTER

110 Sleep and Its Disorders

Jean K. Matheson

Sleep is an active, clinically important behavior, during which many physiologic processes of the organism changes. These processes are temporally organized under cerebral influence. Sleep abnormality may represent a primary disorder of mechanisms regulating sleep, or failure within a specific organ system that manifests in a unique way during sleep. Thus it is important that sleep complaints are not ignored or treated empirically with pharmacologic agents. More often than not, disordered sleep is a symptom of underlying disease.

PHYSIOLOGY

There are two sleep states, rapid eye movement (REM) and non-REM (NREM) sleep. REM sleep was discovered by Aserinsky and Kleitman in the early 1950s. By waking subjects during REM, they also established that vivid dreaming occurs during this sleep state. Soon thereafter Dement recognized that episodes of REM sleep alternate with NREM sleep in cycles lasting approximately 90 minutes throughout the night.

Recordings derived from electroencephalograms (EEG), eye movements (EOG), and chin tone (EMG) are necessary to distinguish sleep states. Polysomnography is the technique used to record multiple physiologic variables during sleep. In clinical practice several other physiologic measures are typically recorded, including respiratory effort from chest and abdomen, oral and nasal airflow, cardiac rhythm, and electromyographic activity in the anterior tibialis muscles of the legs.

NREM sleep is divided into four sleep stages, numbered I, II, III, and IV. The waking EEG with the eyes closed reveals the characteristic "alpha rhythm," which is a posteriorly predominant 8 to 12 Hz rhythm that attenuates with eye opening. Stage I sleep is characterized by the gradual disappearance of the alpha rhythm, which is replaced by slower, 2 to 7 Hz, activity, and some fast 12 to 14 Hz low-voltage activity. Stage II is distinguished by the presence of spindles (bursts of 12 to 14 Hz activity lasting at least 0.5 seconds, with a "spindle" appearance) and K complexes (high-voltage biphasic negative/positive waves best seen at the vertex, usually associated with spindles). Stages III and IV are defined by the presence of high-voltage slow-wave activity of 2 Hz or less. An epoch of 30 seconds is measured: if 20% to 50% of the record shows high-voltage slow activity, it is termed stage III; more than 50% high-voltage slow activity is termed stage IV. Stages III and IV are often described together as "slow wave sleep" or "delta sleep." Delta sleep can be characterized as "deep sleep," because during this stage subjects are difficult to arouse. Detailed dreaming does not occur, but subjects awakened during this sleep stage have reported "thinking."

The normal subject descends in an orderly progression through the four NREM sleep stages. Delta sleep appears 30 to 45 minutes after sleep onset. The first REM period follows this delta sleep, about 70 to 90 minutes after sleep onset.

The polysomnogram during REM shows dramatic changes. There is a sudden loss of EMG in the chin muscles, which reflects generalized skeletal muscle atonia. Except for the eye muscles and respiratory muscles, the subject is paralyzed. Rapid eye movements occur in phasic bursts. The EEG shows mixed frequencies similar to those of stage I and waking. Characteristic sawtooth waves sometimes occur during eye movements. Respiration and heart rate are irregular.

The first REM period is short—approximately 10 minutes. The end of the first REM period ends the first sleep cycle. Thereafter NREM continues to alternate with REM; there are 4 to 6 cycles in the healthy young adult (Fig. 110-1). Sleep architecture is the organization of sleep stages and cycles. The normal young adult spends approximately 5% of the night in stage I, 50% in stage II, 12% in stage III, 13% in stage IV, and 20% in REM. Delta sleep is concentrated in the first third of the night, whereas REM episodes become progressively longer later in the night. Delta sleep decreases as a function of age, but REM percentage is relatively stable after early childhood. Of the newborn's daily 17 to 18 hours of sleep 50% is REM. Children and early adolescents sleep 10 to 11 hours. Most adults prefer to sleep 7 to 8 hours per day, but sleep needs vary. Short sleepers are classified as those individuals who feel adequately rested with less than 6 hours of sleep; long sleepers require more than 9 hours.

Sleep efficiency is defined as the time spent asleep divided by the time spent in bed. Sleep efficiency decreases in old age, as both the number of arousals and time spent in bed increase. This does not necessarily represent "normal" aging. Arousals usually have a cause (see Sleep Disorders).

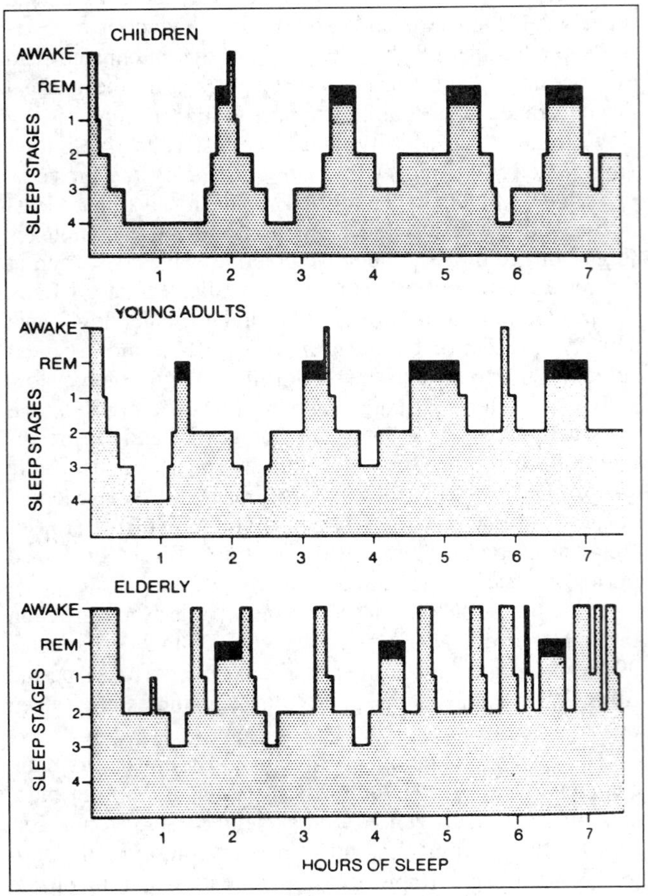

Fig. 110-1. Sleep architecture. REM sleep alternates with NREM in cycles approximating 90 minutes in all age groups. Delta sleep is prominent in childhood and decreases in old age as awakenings and wake time increase. (From Kales A and Kales JD: N Engl J Med 290:487, 1974.)

If there are frequent external or internal disrupters of sleep, the sleep patterns change. After arousal, the patient develops stage I sleep, followed by stage II sleep, repetitively, and the percentages of delta sleep and REM sleep decrease. Drugs can also inhibit REM and delta sleep. Monoamine oxidase inhibitors and tricyclic antidepressants, for example, decrease the percentage of REM sleep dramatically. Alcohol and caffeine increase arousal. If patients are deprived of either REM or delta sleep, "rebound" is usually seen on recovery nights. REM rebound can be intrusive and frightening, with an abundance of vivid dreams. Chronic partial sleep deprivation results in inattentiveness in monotonous tasks, deterioration of mood, irritability, and even mild paranoia.

REM sleep and NREM sleep differ physiologically. REM sleep is characterized by both phasic and tonic changes. The drop in baseline EMG correlates with a tonic change. Rapid eye movements correlate with phasic changes. Tonic physiologic changes also include impaired thermoregulation, hypotension, bradycardia, increased cerebral blood flow and intracranial pressure, increased respiratory rate, and penile erection. Intercostal and upper-airway muscles become atonic, but the diaphragm maintains activity. Phasic changes include vasoconstriction, increased blood pressure, tachycardia, and further increases in cerebral blood flow and respiratory rate. During NREM, physiologic state is more stable, but blood pressure, heart rate, cardiac output, and respiratory rate decrease. Growth hormone is secreted during stages III and IV, in the first third of the night. Many other rhythms occur during sleep, but these need not be directly tied to sleep, as discussed later.

REM sleep can be abolished by lesions restricted to the pons, but the generator of REM/NREM cycling has not been established. The neurotransmitters serotonin, norepinephrine, and acetylcholine all appear to play some role in the regulation of sleep. "Hypnogenic" peptides have been isolated, including delta sleep—inducting peptide (DSIP), substance S, a muramyl peptide, and interleukin-1.

Chronobiology is the science of the temporal organization of physiologic processes. Circadian rhythms are bodily rhythms that occur approximately every 24 hours. Sleep is the most obvious example of a circadian rhythm. There are multiple other circadian rhythms, including body temperature, growth hormone secretion, and cortisol secretion. In an environment free of external time cues, human beings have a "free-running" period of approximately 25 hours; the subject tends to go to bed 1 hour later each day. This means that if a regular schedule is maintained, circadian clocks are "reset" backward approximately 1 hour each day by environmental cues. It follows that it is easier to delay, rather than to advance bedtime, because circadian rhythms move in the direction of daily delay. In the free-running environment, rhythms that usually occur together may desynchronize. The sleep/activity cycle can become longer than the body temperature rhythm, which remains at about 25 hours. Two separate pacemakers emerge, termed X (body-temperature driven) and Y (rest/activity driven). REM sleep and cortisol secretion follow the X pacemaker, whereas slow-wave sleep and growth hormone follow the Y pacemaker. The Y pacemaker is thought to reside in the suprachiasmatic nucleus of the hypothalamus. The location of the X pacemaker is unknown.

SLEEP DISORDERS

In 1972 the Association of Sleep Disorders Centers established a diagnostic classification system of sleep and arousal disorders. The nosology served to unify clinical definitions across medical and research disciplines. The disorders were classified by presenting complaint rather than by cause into four major categories: disorders of initiating and maintaining sleep (DIMS), or insomnias; disorders of excessive somnolence (DOES); disorders of the sleep-wake schedule; dysfunctions associated with sleep, sleep stages, or partial arousal (parasomnias). This organization is helpful in approaching differential diagnosis. However, for statistical and research purposes the classification is inadequate because one disorder may be characterized by more than one symptom. Thus the classification was revised in 1990, as the International Classification of Sleep Disorders (ICSD) (see the box on p. 1006) and is now based on broadly defined pathophysiologic mechanisms rather than presenting symptoms.

The major divisions of the ICSD classification are the (1) dyssomnias, (2) parasomnias, (3) sleep disorders associated with medical and psychiatric disorders, and (4) proposed sleep disorders.

Dyssomnias

The dyssomnias are primary sleep disorders that produce either *difficulty initiating and maintaining sleep* or *excessive daytime sleepiness.*

Difficulty initiating and maintaining sleep (DIMS, insomnia). Inability to sleep may take the form of prolonged initial latency to sleep, recurrent nocturnal awakenings, or early morning awakening without the ability to return to sleep. Insomnia is an extremely common complaint that causes high levels of frustration and significant misery. For reasons that are inexplicable, insomnia is frequently trivialized by the clinician and treated pharmacologically without attention to the underlying cause of the complaint. Inability to initiate or maintain sleep is a symptom that must be explored with the same approach the clinician uses to assess other medical complaints. As in most disorders, a careful history is the most significant diagnostic tool. Exploring the patient's daily schedule in an orderly fashion is often markedly revealing. A sleep log helps document patterns that suggest specific disease. The schedule of daily activities gives insight into the patient's personality and discloses habits that contribute to poor sleep hygiene. All medical history is relevant, and illnesses that may cause nocturnal arousal are particularly important. A family history of sleep disorder and history of childhood sleep behavior are useful. A review of drug use, including prescription medications, home remedies, caffeine, alcohol, and illicit drugs, is critical.

Excessive daytime sleepiness (DOES). Excessive daytime sleepiness is defined as the tendency to fall asleep inappropriately when sedentary. Patients with excessive daytime sleepiness may or may not demonstrate hypersomnolence: that is: excessive sleep during a 24 hour period. Patients with chronic disorders of excessive daytime sleepiness often accept their sleepiness as normal. The clinician should look for a history of excessive daytime sleepiness in any situation presenting as chronically reduced performance, including dementia, or in situations suggesting episodic inattention, such as automobile accidents. Instead of complaining of sleepiness, many patients cite blackouts, forgetfulness, poor concentration, automatic behavior, and amnestic spells. Children may have poor school performance or behavioral problems, including apparent hyperactivity. These situations require the taking of a sleep history that includes questioning the patient as to whether or not sleeping occurs during sedentary activities, social activities, driving, and eating. Sleepiness needs to be distinguished from fatigue and disorders of consciousness secondary to encephalopathy.

Within the classification of the dyssomnias, the sleep abnormalities must be fundamental to the existence of the disorder. Psychiatric and medical disorders that influence sleep, as only one component of the clinical presentation, are not included in the ICSD definition of dyssomnia. The dyssomnias are further divided into three groups: the intrinsic sleep disorders, the extrinsic sleep disorders, and the circadian rhythm sleep disorders. Intrinsic sleep disorders are thought to originate within the body; examples are narcolepsy and obstructive sleep apnea. Extrinsic sleep disorders originate outside the body; these include poor sleep hygiene and environmental disruption. Circadian rhythm sleep disorders represent disorders of the timing of the sleep-wake cycle within the 24 hour day.

Intrinsic sleep disorders. "*Psychophysiologic insomnia* is a disorder of somatized tension and learned sleep-preventing associations that results in a complaint of insomnia and associated decreased functioning during wakefulness." These patients usually do not have evidence of underlying psychiatric disease but may be highly focused on their insomnia. Overconcern with the process of going to sleep is alerting, induces increased tension, and becomes a sleep-preventing association. The precipitant for this disorder may be a period of acute insomnia associated with an external stress (see the discussion of adjustment sleep disorder). A characteristic pattern emerges: inability to obtain satisfactory sleep for a few nights induces fear that another sleepless night will follow. Patients report that they feel

---

Classification and quoted definitions (throughout this chapter) reproduced with permission from Diagnostic Classification Steering Committee, Thorpy MJ, Chairman: International classification of sleep disorders: diagnostic and coding manual. Rochester MN, 1990, American Sleep Disorders Association.

International classification of sleep disorders

Classification outline

1. Dyssomnias
   - A. Intrinsic sleep disorders
   - B. Extrinsic sleep disorders
   - C. Circadian rhythm sleep disorders
2. Parasomnias
   - A. Arousal disorders
   - B. Sleep-wake transition disorders
   - C. Parasomnias usually associated with REM sleep
   - D. Other parasomnias
3. Medical/psychiatric sleep disorders
   - A. Associated with mental disorders
   - B. Associated with neurologic disorders
   - C. Associated with other medical disorders
4. Proposed sleep disorders

---

1. **Dyssomnias**
   - A. Intrinsic sleep disorders
     1. Psychophysiologic insomnia
     2. Sleep state misperception
     3. Idiopathic insomnia
     4. Narcolepsy
     5. Recurrent hypersomnia
     6. Idiopathic hypersomnia
     7. Posttraumatic hypersomnia
     8. Obstructive sleep apnea syndrome
     9. Central sleep apnea syndrome
     10. Central alveolar hypoventilation syndrome
     11. Periodic limb movement disorder
     12. Restless legs syndrome
     13. Intrinsic sleep disorder not otherwise specified (NOS)
   - B. Extrinsic sleep disorders
     1. Inadequate sleep hygiene
     2. Environmental sleep disorder
     3. Altitude insomnia
     4. Adjustment sleep disorder
     5. Insufficient sleep syndrome
     6. Limit-setting sleep disorder
     7. Sleep-onset association disorder
     8. Food allergy insomnia
     9. Nocturnal eating (drinking) syndrome
     10. Hypnotic-dependent sleep disorder
     11. Stimulant-dependent sleep disorder
     12. Alcohol-dependent sleep disorder
     13. Toxin-induced sleep disorder
     14. Extrinsic sleep disorder NOS
   - C. Circadian rhythm sleep disorders
     1. Time zone change (jet lag) syndrome
     2. Shift work sleep disorder
     3. Irregular sleep-wake pattern
     4. Delayed sleep phase syndrome
     5. Advanced sleep phase syndrome
     6. Non-24-hour sleep-wake disorder
     7. Circadian rhythm sleep disorder NOS
2. **Parasomnias**
   - A. Arousal disorders
     1. Confusional arousals
     2. Sleepwalking
     3. Sleep terrors
   - B. Sleep-wake transition disorders
     1. Rhythmic movement disorder
     2. Sleep starts
     3. Sleep talking
     4. Nocturnal leg cramps
   - C. Parasomnias usually associated with REM sleep
     1. Nightmares
     2. Sleep paralysis
     3. Impaired sleep-related penile erections
     4. Sleep-related painful erections
     5. REM sleep-related sinus arrest
     6. REM sleep behavior disorder
   - D. Other parasomnias
     1. Sleep bruxism
     2. Sleep enuresis
     3. Sleep-related abnormal swallowing syndrome
     4. Nocturnal paroxysmal dystonia
     5. Sudden unexplained nocturnal death syndrome
     6. Primary snoring
     7. Infant sleep apnea
     8. Congenital central hypoventilation syndrome
     9. Sudden infant death syndrome
     10. Benign neonatal sleep myoclonus
     11. Other parasomnia NOS
3. **Sleep disorders associated with medical/psychiatric disorders**
   - A. Associated with mental disorders
     1. Psychoses
     2. Mood disorders
     3. Anxiety disorders
     4. Panic disorder
     5. Alcoholism
   - B. Associated with neurologic disorders
     1. Cerebral degenerative disorders
     2. Dementia
     3. Parkinsonism
     4. Fatal familial insomnia
     5. Sleep-related epilepsy
     6. Electrical status epilepticus of sleep
     7. Sleep-related headaches
   - C. Associated with other medical disorders
     1. Sleeping sickness
     2. Nocturnal cardiac ischemia
     3. Chronic obstructive pulmonary disease
     4. Sleep-related asthma
     5. Sleep-related gastroesophageal reflux
     6. Peptic ulcer disease
     7. Fibrositis syndrome
4. **Proposed sleep disorders**
   1. Short sleeper
   2. Long sleeper
   3. Subwakefulness syndrome
   4. Fragmentary myoclonus
   5. Sleep hyperhidrosis
   6. Menstrual-associated sleep disorder
   7. Pregnancy-associated sleep disorder
   8. Terrifying hypnagogic hallucinations
   9. Sleep-related neurogenic tachypnea
   10. Sleep-related laryngospasm
   11. Sleep choking syndrome

From ICSD—International Classification of Sleep Disorders: Diagnostic and Coding Manual. Diagnostic Classification Steering Committee. Thorpy MJ, Chairman. Rochester, MN, American Sleep Disorders Association 1991.

alert as soon as they try to initiate sleep. They toss and turn, watch the clock, and become frustrated and angry that they are unable to sleep. Often sleep is better in a new environment that is free of the usual external sleep-onset associations.

Psychophysiologic insomnia can be treated with relaxation techniques in combination with methods that "decondition" the patient's negative associations with sleep onset. A technique known as "stimulus-control therapy," proposed by Bootzin, is highly effective. The patient is instructed to (1) go to bed only if sleepy; (2) use the bed only for sleeping and sexual relations, not as a place to read, write, or watch television; (3) get up and leave the bedroom if not asleep within 10 to 15 minutes and engage in a nonstimulating activity until sleepiness is perceived; (4) repeat this step as many times as necessary throughout the night; (5) maintain a fixed schedule of awakening each morning; (6) take no naps during the day.

"*Sleep state misperception* is a disorder in which a complaint of insomnia or excessive sleepiness occurs without objective evidence of sleep disturbance." There is a small but distinct group of patients who complain of insomnia because of inability to recognize that they have slept. These patients are most clearly identifiable when there is a report of absolute lack of sleep. Polysomnographic recording reveals normal sleep latency, a normal number of arousals and awakenings, and normal sleep duration, but the patient perceives poor or absent sleep. This disorder needs to be distinguished from the phenomenon of paradoxic improvement in sleep during overnight recording in the sleep laboratory, which occurs in patients with psychophysiologic insomnia. In the latter disorder, sleep may improve in a novel environment, such as the sleep laboratory, and this improvement is appreciated by the patient.

Sometimes patients report sleepiness that cannot be verified on objective testing with the multiple sleep latency test ([MSLT] discussed later), and this may be a sleep state misperception. Sleepiness, however, is more difficult to measure than presence or absence of sleep.

The underlying pathophysiologic mechanisms of sleep state misperception are not understood. Many patients who report near-absence of sleep are mistakenly treated with hypnotic medications for years without improvement. The existence of this disorder underscores the importance of polysomnographic evaluation of patients with chronic sleep complaints.

"*Idiopathic insomnia* is a lifelong inability to obtain adequate sleep that is presumably due to an abnormality of the neurological control of the sleep-wake system." This disorder may also be termed *childhood-onset insomnia*. Unlike "short sleepers" who feel rested despite short sleep duration, patients with this disorder complain of chronically poor performance caused by poor sleep. Polysomnographic evaluation reveals increased sleep latency, decreased efficiency, and increased arousals, but the cause of the disrupted sleep is not apparent. Because of the chronicity of the disorder, secondary sleep disorders such as psychophysiologic insomnia and hypnotic dependence often develop. There is no effective treatment except directing attention to conditions that may aggravate the underlying insomnia.

"*Narcolepsy* is a disorder of unknown etiology which is characterized by excessive sleepiness that typically is associated with cataplexy and other REM sleep phenomena such as sleep paralysis and hypnogogic hallucinations." Narcolepsy was first defined as a distinct disorder in 1880 by Gelineau, who described the syndrome as a "rare, little known neurosis characterized by imperative need to sleep." It is now known that the disorder is not rare. The prevalence is estimated at between 2 and 16 per 10,000 persons. The onset of symptoms occurs typically in the second or third decades, and both sexes are equally affected. A family history is noted in approximately one third of cases.

The discovery of REM sleep was followed by the finding that patients with narcolepsy have abnormal REM physiology. It is now accepted that the major manifestations of narcolepsy represent a disorder of control mechanisms that regulate REM sleep. Episodes of REM occur at the wrong time, intruding on wakefulness, and the physiologic components of this sleep state dissociate and appear independently. These major symptoms are referred to as the *narcolepsy tetrad:* (1) excessive daytime sleepiness, (2) cataplexy, (3) hypnogogic hallucinations, and (4) sleep paralysis. Few patients report all of these symptoms, especially in the early stages of the disorder, but almost all patients have evidence of excessive daytime sleepiness.

The cardinal symptom of narcolepsy is excessive daytime sleepiness, and approximately 10% of patients complain of this symptom alone. The tendency to sleep inappropriately may have a gradual or an abrupt onset. History taking typically reveals that patients remember brief lapses of attention in sedentary situations years before presentation to a physician. With time, sleepiness is evident in clearly inappropriate situations, such as during driving, attending business conversations, eating, or engaging in sexual intercourse. Patients are frequently able to recognize impending drowsiness and take measures to alert themselves. Irresistible sleep attacks are characteristic, however, and tend to occur when the urge to sleep has been delayed. Two features are unique to the naps of narcoleptics: (1) dreaming during naps is common and (2) brief naps of 5 to 10 minute duration are remarkably refreshing.

Cataplexy is a sudden, usually brief, loss of muscle tone induced by emotion. The presence of cataplexy is considered diagnostic of narcolepsy, but only 60% to 80% of patients experience this symptom, and it may occur years after the onset of sleepiness. Rarely, cataplexy is the presenting symptom of the disorder. Idiopathic cataplexy may exist but is poorly described. Laughter and anger are the most common precipitants, but the emotional trigger may be specific to the patient. The weakness that develops usually involves the muscles of the face or the supporting muscles of the legs; it may be so mild as to give only the sense that the face will not move properly or so profound as to cause a sudden fall. The appearance of facial tremulousness can be confused with seizure activity. Occasionally, patients have difficulty speaking. Consciousness is maintained during a cataplectic episode, but prolonged episodes may be immediately followed by REM sleep. Cataplexy is the result of sudden skeletal muscle atonia sparing extraocular eye movements and diaphragm. Deep tendon reflexes during the episode are absent. This atonia is similar to that which occurs during normal REM sleep. Cataplexy thus seems to represent a dissociation of normal REM phenomena, occurring inappropriately during waking.

In hallucinations occurring at the onset of sleep, referred to as *hypnogogic hallucinations*, the sensory events associated with normal dreaming occur during perceived wakefulness. These hallucinations are a manifestation of the sudden onset of inappropriate and dissociated REM sleep. Hallucinations may involve any sensory system and are frequently visual, auditory, or vestibular.

Sleep paralysis is an inability to move skeletal muscles voluntarily during sleep-wake transitions. Normal subjects may experience the sensation awakening from REM, but narcoleptics typically complain of sleep paralysis at sleep onset. The episodes can be associated with extreme fear, especially when they are accompanied by threatening hypnogogic hallucinations. Sleep paralysis is thought to be another manifestation of REM-related atonia.

Two other symptoms are typical of narcolepsy: automatic behavior and disrupted nighttime sleep. Patients with automatic behavior complain that they perform complex, often routine activities "automatically" with partial amnesia and evidence of inattention during the behavior. "Microsleeps" or poor attentiveness caused by sleepiness may be the cause of this behavior. Just as patients have difficulty maintaining alertness because of intrusion of sleepiness during the day, narcoleptics complain of inability to maintain sleep at night. The narcoleptic's sleep tends to be punctuated by frequent awakenings and vivid dreams. Periodic movements in sleep syndrome and sleep apnea are more common in narcoleptics and contribute to poor-quality sleep.

Cataplexy, hypnogogic hallucinations, and sleep paralysis are episodic symptoms that may resolve. Complaints of automatic behavior, poor memory, and disturbed sleep often worsen with age. The degree of sleepiness remains relatively constant over the years.

The underlying pathogenesis of narcolepsy is not understood. Polysomnographic studies demonstrate two major features: (1) excessive daytime sleepiness, as measured in multiple daytime naps; and (2) the tendency to develop REM sleep within minutes of sleep onset in daytime and nocturnal recordings. Normal patients do not show sleep-onset REM unless they are sleep deprived, on an irregular sleep-wake cycle, or withdrawing from REM-suppressing medication. Recordings during periods of cataplexy and sleep paralysis show the sudden onset of muscle atonia characteristic of REM sleep.

Narcolepsy is highly associated with the HLA antigens DR2 and DQw1. More than 90% of white narcoleptics are DR2 and DQw1 positive. The association is less good for DR2 in nonwhites but holds for DQw1. DQw1 negative patients are rare, and it appears that the DQ, rather than the DR gene, is a marker for susceptibility to narcolepsy.

Occasionally narcolepsy and/or cataplexy occurs in association with other neurologic disorders, in which case it is called symptomatic narcolepsy. Both narcolepsy and cataplexy have been described in patients with tumors in the region of the third ventricle and upper brainstem. Cataplexy has also been described in Niemann-Pick disease. Occasionally narcolepsy is said to follow head trauma and encephalitis. Patients with symptomatic narcolepsy also have been reported to have a high prevalence of the DR2 antigen.

The diagnosis of narcolepsy is secure if excessive daytime sleepiness is associated with unequivocal cataplexy. The diagnosis can be confirmed in these patients—and especially in those without a clear history of cataplexy—with polysomnographic studies. The current standard of diagnosis is the multiple sleep latency test (MSLT), which measures the tendency to sleep and the type of sleep the patient obtains in brief naps scheduled throughout the day. The mean latency to sleep is usually less than 5 minutes. The diagnosis of narcolepsy requires that two of five naps include REM sleep. A polysomnogram on the night preceding the multiple sleep latency test is preferred, to exclude sleep deprivation as a cause of short daytime latencies and to identify other sleep disorders.

Excessive daytime sleepiness is treated with CNS andrenergic stimulant medication. Nonamphetamine stimulant medications, such as pemoline and methylphenidate, have fewer side effects than do amphetamines and are effective in most patients. The goal of treatment is to use the lowest effective doses of stimulant medication that will maintain adequate alertness to perform day-to-day activities. Stimulants used late in the day may increase nocturnal sleep deprivation and, paradoxically, increase excessive daytime sleepiness. Codeine is reported to increase subjective alertness without significantly changing sleep parameters.

Cataplexy is treated with tricyclic antidepressant drugs, particularly those with prominent anticholinergic properties. Clomipramine is the most effective anticataplectic drug currently available. Protriptyline is also highly effective and widely used.

Nonpharmacologic techniques include the use of "strategic napping." Brief naps during the day, during periods of maximum fatigue or before periods of required alertness result in decreased sleepiness and decreased total daily dose of stimulant medication. Attention is directed to maintenance of nocturnal sleep by avoidance of stimulant drugs, caffeine, and alcohol in the evening. Because patients with narcolepsy have a higher incidence of sleep-disordered breathing than normal individuals, the clinician should remain vigilant to the possibility that sleep-disordered breathing is contributing to excessive daytime sleepiness and treat that disorder appropriately.

"*Recurrent hypersomnia* is a disorder characterized by recurrent episodes of hypersomnia that typically occur weeks or months apart." Kleine-Levin syndrome is the prototype of these disorders. This is usually thought of as a disorder of young men, but young women are also affected in a male/female sex ratio of 3:1. In a large series, median age of onset was 16.0 for males and 19.5 for females. Daily sleep durations of 18 to 20 hours are associated with behavioral abnormalities including hyperphagia and lack of sexual inhibition. During periods of wakefulness, the patient appears apathetic and irritable. Delusions and hallucinations occasionally occur. Electroencephalograms (EEGs) may show background slowing and bursts of high-voltage slow waves. Spontaneous remission is typical. A thorough neurologic evaluation is appropriate to exclude structural abnormalities of brain.

"*Idiopathic hypersomnia* is a disorder of presumed central nervous system cause that is associated with a normal or prolonged major sleep episode and excessive sleepiness consisting of prolonged (1-2 hours) sleep episodes of non-REM sleep." This disorder has also been termed non-REM narcolepsy and CNS hypersomnolence. Patients demonstrate excessive sleepiness on the MSLT, but there is no evidence of sleep-onset REM. The all-night polysomnogram should not show nocturnal disruption induced by sleep-disordered breathing, leg movements, or other causes. Psychiatric and medical conditions that might contribute to sleepiness are absent. Thus the diagnosis is one of exclusion. However, a group of these patients, when restudied, have been shown to demonstrate subtle evidence of sleep disordered breathing (discussed later), which has been termed "upper airway resistance syndrome." Brain tumors, especially those in the region of the third ventricle, may induce sleepiness as a primary symptom. Magnetic resonance imaging (MRI) or computed tomography (CT) of the brain is an appropriate screening technique in patients whose hypersomnia is unexplained.

"*Posttraumatic hypersomnia* is excessive sleepiness that occurs as a result of a traumatic event involving the central nervous system." Subtle derangements of neurologic function often follow head trauma, and there may be disruption of usual sleep patterns. It is critical, however, to exclude life-threatening conditions such as subdural hematoma and atlantoaxial dislocation. The latter condition has been associated with sleep attacks that may be secondary to brainstem ischemia or involvement of medullary respiratory centers.

"*Obstructive sleep apnea syndrome* is characterized by repetitive episodes of upper airway obstruction that occur during sleep, usually associated with a reduction in blood oxygen saturation."

"*Central sleep apnea syndrome* is characterized by a cessation or decrease of ventilatory effort during sleep usually with associated oxygen desaturation."

"*Central alveolar hypoventilation syndrome* is characterized by ventilatory impairment, resulting in arterial oxygen desaturation that is worsened by sleep, which occurs in patients with normal properties of the lung."

When decreased ventilation and irregular breathing patterns result in sleep disruption and/or hypoxemia, the patient may be said to have sleep-disordered breathing. These syndromes are discussed in detail in Chapter 190. Most of these patients, particularly those with obstructive sleep apnea, demonstrate excessive daytime sleepiness as the primary complaint. Others, especially those with central sleep apnea, including Cheyne-Stokes respirations, complain of insomnia—usually difficulty maintaining sleep.

In patients with sleep-disordered breathing, treatment of the insomnia symtomatically with hypnotic medications can be life-threatening, because of respiratory depression and increased atonia of the upper airway muscles. Sleep-disordered breathing is a ubiquitous problem. The important risk factors are listed in the box below. Patients who have any of these risk factors should never receive hypnotic drugs for symptomatic treatment of insomnia. In this group, a polysomnogram should be used for diagnosis of the underlying sleep disorder. Oximetry alone may be helpful. Even bedside observation, although not ideal, may be diagnostic.

"*Periodic limb movement disorder* is characterized by periodic episodes of repetitive and highly stereotyped limb movements that occur during sleep."

"*Restless legs syndrome* is a disorder characterized by disagreeable leg sensations, usually prior to sleep onset, that cause an almost irresistible urge to move the legs." It is an extremely annoying, aching, crawling sensation affecting predominantly the legs when sedentary, especially when trying to initiate sleep. The subject feels the overwhelming urge to move the legs continually to abort the sensation. All patients with restless legs syndrome have another disorder, periodic limb movement disorder (also termed periodic leg movements or nocturnal myoclonus). Periodic limb movement disorder may also occur without restless legs. Patients show recurrent, periodic leg jerks involving flexor muscles of the legs, analogous to the withdrawal reflex. Upper extremity movements may also occur. Leg twitches occur approximately every 20 to 40 seconds episodically throughout the night. Hundreds of leg jerks may occur, unknown to the patient but often witnessed by the bed partner. The repetitive movements result in arousal. Patients with these disorders may have difficulty initiating and maintaining sleep or excessive daytime sleepiness. Restless legs syndrome is sometimes familial. Periodic limb movements can be exacerbated and possibly induced by drugs, especially tricyclic antidepressants. Both disorders may be intermittent and related to an underlying metabolic abnormality, such as uremia, iron deficiency, or chronic alcohol use. Symptoms may be worse during pregnancy. Periodic limb movements may also accompany other primary sleep disorders, including sleep apnea and narcolepsy. Often no cause is discovered. Both carbidopa-levodopa and bromocriptine reduce leg movements and ameliorate the

Risk factors for sleep-disordered breathing

- Advanced age
- Loud snoring
- Obesity
- Upper-airway abnormality (e.g., tonsillar hypertrophy, micrognathia, macroglossia, nasal obstruction)
- Pulmonary disease
- Muscular weakness (e.g., muscular dystrophy, myasthenia, polymyositis, Guillain-Barré syndrome)
- Brainstem lesions (Shy-Drager syndrome, infarct)
- Cheyne-Stokes respiratory pattern (congestive heart failure, bihemispheric cerebral disease)

sensation. A small dose of the controlled-release formulation of carbidopa-levodopa before bedtime has proved the most effective treatment to date. Clonazepam and codeine may also be used with moderate success.

Extrinsic sleep disorders. "*Inadequate sleep hygiene* is a sleep disorder due to the performance of daily activities that are inconsistent with the maintenance of good quality sleep and full daytime alertness." Many types of daily behavior are inconsistent with obtaining good-quality sleep. Frequent daytime napping, inattention to maintenance of regular sleeping hours, and use of caffeine, nicotine, or alcohol are the most common offenders. Poor sleep secondary to this or another disorder may perpetuate the maladaptive habits. For example, insomniacs frequently insist on maintaining caffeine intake or daytime naps to counteract the effects of sleep deprivation.

The presence of at least one of the following is necessary for the diagnosis of inadequate sleep hygiene by ICSD standards: "(1) daytime napping at least two times each week; (2) variable wake-up times or bedtimes; (3) frequent periods (two to three times per week) of extended amounts of time spent in bed; (4) routine use of products containing alcohol, tobacco, or caffeine in the period preceding bedtime; (5) scheduling of exercise too close to bedtime; (6) engaging in exciting or emotionally upsetting activities too close to bedtime; (7) frequent use of the bed for nonrelated activities (e.g., television watching, studying); (8) sleeping on an uncomfortable bed (poor mattress, inadequate blankets, etc.); (9) bedroom that is too bright, too stuffy, too cluttered, too hot, too cold, or in some way nonconducive to sleep; (10) performance of activities demanding high levels of concentration shortly before bed; (11) occurrence in bed of such mental activities as thinking, planning, or reminiscing."

"*Environmental sleep disorder* is a sleep disturbance due to a disturbing environmental factor that causes a complaint of either insomnia or excessive sleepiness." External physical factors are temporally associated with the development and resolution of the sleep complaint. The elderly appear to be at more risk for this disorder. Attention to the quality of the sleep environment may prevent needless trials of hypnotic medication. Perhaps nowhere is this more apparent than in the hospitalized setting.

"*Altitude insomnia* is an acute insomnia, usually accompanied by headaches, loss of appetite and fatigue, that occurs following ascent to high altitudes." This insomnia is associated with a periodic (Cheyne-Stokes) respiratory pattern caused by low inspired oxygen pressure. Arousals are associated with the hyperventilatory phase of the periodic breathing (Chapter 190).

"*Adjustment sleep disorder* represents sleep disturbance temporally related to acute stress, conflict, or environmental change causing emotional arousal." Inability to initiate sleep in the presence of an acute stressor is a nearly universal experience. Occasionally the opposite is true: patients note excessive sleepiness in response to a stressful situation. Symptoms are generally short lived and resolve with removal of the stressor.

"*Insufficient sleep syndrome* is a disorder that occurs in an individual who persistently fails to obtain sufficient nocturnal sleep required to support normally alert wakefulness." A large percentage of the population suffers from self-imposed sleep deprivation. Sleep logs help document the disorder for the patient who is unwilling to recognize the problem. A history reveals that symptoms resolve during vacations and weekends when sleep duration increases. Symptoms resolve if the patient chooses to prolong nocturnal sleep.

"*Limit setting disorder* is a predominantly childhood disorder that is characterized by the inadequate enforcement of bedtimes by a caretaker, with resultant stalling or refusal to go to bed at an appropriate time." The disorder is characterized by persistent struggle between the caretaker and child, with sleep disruption for both. Irregular sleep-wake cycles may develop. The disorder resolves with the institution of firm limits. The underlying psychosocial factors that may foster the lack of limit setting are several, and deserve exploration.

"*Sleep onset association disorder* occurs when sleep onset is impaired by the absence of a certain object or set of circumstances."

"*Food allergy insomnia* is a disorder of initiating and maintaining sleep due to an allergic response to food allergens." Onset of this disorder is usually within the first 2 years of life, especially after the introduction of cow's milk into the diet. The disorder may also occur in adults. Sleep is characterized by frequent arousals and awakenings. Symptoms of allergy, such as wheezing, abdominal pain, or itching, need not be present.

"*Nocturnal eating (drinking) syndrome* is characterized by recurrent awakenings with the inability to return to sleep without eating or drinking." This disorder occurs predominantly in early childhood in association with breast or bottle feeding. Large amounts of fluid consumed during the night contribute to repeated awakenings and excessive urination. An adult variant of this disorder is unusual but striking in its presentation. Patients wake fully and engage in uncontrolled binge eating without evidence of similar behavior during daytime hours.

"*Hypnotic-dependent sleep disorder* is characterized by insomnia or excessive sleepiness that is associated with tolerance to or withdrawal from hypnotic medications." Hypnotic medications are to be avoided whenever possible. The benzodiazepines are the safest sleep-inducing medications but should be reserved for short-term use in patients with transient, usually situationally induced insomnia. Hypnotics are discouraged for several reasons. The underlying cause of the insomnia may be masked or exacerbated, as in sleep-disordered breathing. Tolerance to the benzodiazepines develops with regular use, and the medication becomes ineffective, resulting in escalation of dose. Half-lives of the benzodiazepines and their active metabolites vary widely. Drugs with long half-lives accumulate and impair performance during waking, especially in the elderly. Withdrawal effects are more evident with shorter-acting drugs. Rebound insomnia follows withdrawal, leading the patient to overestimate the underlying sleep disorder.

"*Stimulant-dependent sleep disorder* is characterized by a reduction of sleepiness or suppression of sleep by central stimulants and resultant alterations in wakefulness following drug abstinence." Use of stimulants is an obvious cause of difficulty initiating and maintaining sleep but can be easily overlooked in the history. Caffeine is the most common stimulant, in the form of coffee, tea, soft drinks, or chocolate. Decongestants and bronchodilators are often-forgotten offenders. Nonamphetamine stimulants prescribed for attention deficit disorder and narcolepsy such as pemoline and methylphenidate may produce insomnia as a major side-effect, usually because of dosage taken too late in the day. Prolonged periods of sleeplessness followed by excessive sleep are seen in amphetamine and cocaine abuse.

"*Alcohol-dependent sleep disorder* is characterized by the assisted initiation of sleep onset by the sustained ingestion of ethanol that is used for its hypnotic effect." Alcohol usually causes fragmentation of sleep and frequent arousal, contrary to the popular belief that it helps induce sleep. It also exacerbates sleep-disordered breathing. Many patients become alcohol-dependent in attempting to treat insomnia of other causes with nocturnal use of alcohol; in fact it exacerbates the problem.

"*Toxin-induced sleep disorder* is characterized by either insomnia or excessive sleepiness produced by poisoning with heavy metals or organic toxins."

Circadian rhythm sleep disorders. The activities of modern society allow for marked variations in the patterns of day-to-day activity. Air travel and shift work are common. Nighttime activities are no longer limited by darkness. Continuous activity with the potential for disrupting sleep-wake cycles is particularly evident in the hospitalized setting. When the timing of sleep is disrupted, the patient is said to have a circadian rhythm sleep disorder.

"*Time zone change (jet lag) syndrome* consists of varying degrees of difficulties in initiating or maintaining sleep, excessive sleepiness, decrements in subjective daytime alertness and performance, and somatic symptoms (largely related to gastrointestinal function) following rapid travel across multiple time zones."

"*Shift work sleep disorder* consists of symptoms of insomnia or excessive sleepiness that occur as transient phenomena in relation to work schedules."

An abrupt change in the sleep schedule induced by travel across time zones or a change in work shift results in transient disorders of the sleep-wake cycle. Circadian rhythms are out of phase with the imposed sleep schedule. Subjects note difficulty in both initiating and maintaining sleep, as well as sleepiness during waking hours. Schedules that result in an "advance" of the sleep cycle, as in eastward flight, are more poorly tolerated. A natural endogenous rhythm of 25 hours makes it easier to delay, rather than advance, bedtime. Symptoms resolve after circadian rhythms entrain to the new schedule, which may take more than a week.

If the sleep-wake cycle changes constantly, because of either travel or shift work, no entrainment occurs and the circadian rhythm disorder becomes persistent.

"*Irregular sleep-wake pattern* consists of temporally disorganized and variable episodes of sleep and waking behavior." The sleep pattern of the patient with irregular sleep-wake cycle is erratic. Unlike those of patients with non–24 hour sleep-wake syndrome (discussed later), sleep logs reveal no underlying periodicity. This disorder usually occurs in patients with developmental or degenerative abnormalities of the brain. Prolonged illness with enforced bed rest and absence of attention to daily routines may be precipitating factors. Patients complain of chronic fatigue. Neither sleep nor wakefulness is well maintained. This disorder is treated by external reinforcement of a normal sleep-wake cycle but usually recurs.

"*Delayed sleep phase syndrome* is a disorder in which the major sleep episode is delayed in relation to the desired clock time that results in symptoms of sleep-onset insomnia or difficulty in waking at the desired time." Patients habitually adopt a late bedtime and wake late in the day. The amount of sleep and its quality are normal. The patient is symptomatic when attempts to advance the bedtime to an earlier hour fail. These patients appear to be less able to advance their circadian rhythms to reset the body's natural tendency to delay endogenous rhythms or to compensate for occasional schedule changes. Bright-light therapy is the most effective treatment. Patients are exposed to bright light in the range of 2500 to 10,000 lux during morning hours, which serves to advance endogenous rhythms and allow earlier sleep onset.

"*Advanced sleep phase syndrome* is a disorder in which the major sleep episode is advanced in relation to the desired clocktime, that results in symptoms of compelling evening sleepiness, an early sleep onset, and an awakening that is earlier than desired." This disorder is commonly seen in the elderly. Advanced sleep phase may explain the physiologic changes seen in endogenous depression, including early REM latency and early morning awakenings. Patients with advanced sleep phase syndrome alone generally do not complain of the disorder. When symptoms are bothersome, patients can be treated with progressive delay of bedtime or bright-light therapy in the evening.

"*Non–24 hour sleep-wake syndrome* consists of a chronic steady pattern comprised of 1-2 hour daily delays in sleep onset and wake times in an individual living in society." Patients with this disorder have what appears to be an erratic sleep-wake cycle. However, sleep logs demonstrate a non–24 hour periodicity in the sleep-wake cycle. This disorder mimics the prolongation of the sleep cycle that can be seen in experimental environments in which subjects are isolated from time cues and are said to be "free-running." In patients who do not attend to environmental cues, including the blind, this syndrome may develop.

Parasomnias

The term *parasomnia* refers to undesirable physical events that occur during sleep or are exacerbated by sleep. These phenomena are often sleep-stage specific. Subdivisions of the parasomnias are (1) the arousal disorders, (2) the sleep-wake transition disorders, (3) the parasomnias usually associated with REM sleep, and (4) the other parasomnias.

Arousal disorders. Arousal disorders are characterized by confusion and automatic behavior after sudden arousal from delta sleep. The tendency to arouse from delta sleep spontaneously is a familial trait unrelated to epilepsy. Most patients have an affected first-degree relative; the co-occurrence of these disorders in the same patient is common. Onset in childhood and resolution by adolescence are typical, but episodes may recur or occur for the first time with greater severity in adolescence and adulthood. Stress, sleep deprivation, and any factors that may contribute to sleep disruption are clear exacerbants. Sleep-disordered breathing and nocturnal alcohol consumption are common precipitants of arousal in the predisposed adult population. Psychopathologic abnormality—especially anxiety, depression, obsessive compulsive behavior, and phobicness—is said to be more common in the symptomatic adult.

"*Confusional arousals* consist of confusion during and following arousals from sleep, most typically from deep sleep in the first part of the night." These episodes are most commonly seen in forced arousals from delta sleep, particularly in individuals with a family or personal history of sleepwalking or sleeptalking, and in children below the age of 5. Amnesia for the events during the arousal is typical. This is predominantly a problem for individuals, such as physicians, who are called at night and must react appropriately.

"*Sleepwalking* consists of a series of complex behaviors that are initiated during slow wave sleep and result in walking during sleep." Sleepwalkers characteristically arouse during the first third of the night from delta sleep, leave the bed in a confused state, and perform complex, automatic acts. Some episodes of sleepwalking are initiated by sleep terror (discussed later), in which case the behavior exhibited may be violent, as the subject tries to combat a perceived threat. More routine behavior, such as eating and urinating, may be performed in a remarkably stereotyped fashion idiosyncratic to the subject. The patient may awaken during the behavior embarrassed and bewildered. Most often the patient returns to bed and has no memory of the episode. Patients with this disorder are at risk of injuring themselves and their bed partners. Care must be taken to secure the sleep environment to prevent falling from heights. Occasionally dangerous objects, such as knives and guns, need to be made inaccessible. Although sleepwalking is frequently perceived as amusing, it may entail social stigma, especially when there is associated violence. Murders have been committed during apparent sleepwalking, and serious personal injury occurs frequently.

"*Sleep terrors* are characterized by a sudden arousal from slow wave sleep with a piercing scream or cry, accompanied by automatic and behavioral manifestations of intense fear." Typically, the individual arouses within the first 2 hours of sleep, sits bolt upright, and screams. Marked tachycardia, mydriasis, and sweating may be evident. The subject is agitated, confused, and difficult to console or arouse fully. There is no detailed dream recall, but a single terrifying image, such as a demon, insect, or intruder, may be reported. Generally sleep is resumed in a few minutes with amnesia for the entire episode the next morning.

In patients with arousals from delta sleep, polysomnography may show characteristic high-voltage synchronous deltal activity followed by arousal, even in the absence of a clinical episode. Most patients can recognize factors that tend to exacerbate their sleep terrors or sleepwalking. If episodes persist after attempts to control the underlying precipitants, a small nightly dose of clonazepam is usually effective.

Sleep-wake transition disorders. "*Rhythmic movement disorder* comprises a group of stereotyped, repetitive movements involving large muscles, usually of the head and neck, which typically occur immediately prior to sleep onset and are sustained into light sleep." This disorder is predominantly recognized as headbanging or rocking in children, with onset at about 6 months and resolution, in most cases, by the age of 4. Persistence into adulthood is sometimes seen.

"*Sleep starts* are sudden, brief contractions of the legs, sometimes also involving the arms and head, which occur at sleep onset." Also called hypnic jerks, these episodes are often associated with the sensation of falling and are considered normal unless they occur so frequently as to interfere with sleep onset. When episodes are disruptive, sleep-onset epilepsy should be considered. Periodic limb movement disorder may induce arousal at sleep onset, but the movements are less generalized, and polysomnographic study reveals persistent movements during sleep.

Parasomnias usually associated with REM sleep. "*Nightmares* are frightening dreams that usually awaken the sleeper from REM sleep." Because nightmares occur during REM sleep, the subject arouses easily and has detailed dream recall. Episodes typically occur later in the night, when REM is more predominant. Autonomic activation and confusion are not characteristic features of the nightmare. Commonly, the episodes are recurrent in the same night during each REM period. Nightmares occur normally in childhood. In adults, recurrent nightmares may represent underlying psychiatric disorders, especially anxiety and depression, or REM rebound secondary to drug withdrawal. Sometimes, recurrent nightmares seem to be induced by physiologic disruptions occurring during REM sleep, such as sleep-disordered breathing or arrhythmia.

"*Sleep paralysis* consists of a period of inability to perform voluntary movements either at sleep onset (hypnagogic or predormital form) or upon awakening either during the night or in the morning (hypnopompic or postdormital form)." Sleep paralysis represents a partial arousal or entry into REM sleep such that the atonia of REM sleep is present, but the cerebral cortex is awake. This is a common symptom of narcolepsy (discussed earlier), especially at sleep onset. Normal subjects may have occasional episodes of sleep paralysis on awakening. A familial disorder characterized by sleep-onset sleep paralysis without other features of narcolepsy has been described. Sleep paralysis is particularly common in patients taking REM modifying drugs, especially MAO inhibitors.

"*REM sleep-related sinus arrest* is a cardiac rhythm disorder that is characterized by sinus arrest during REM sleep in otherwise healthy individuals." Asystole may be prolonged, lasting as long as 9 seconds. This arrhythmia responds to atropinergic drugs. Most patients have been treated with artificial pacemakers, because the natural history of the disorder and the risk of sudden death are unknown.

"*REM sleep behavior disorder* is characterized by the intermittent loss of REM sleep electromyographic (EMG) atonia and by the appearance of elaborate motor activity associated with dream mentation." Lack of the usual atonia of REM sleep allows the patient to enact dreams. Patients typically run, punch, kick, or leap from bed. Vocalization consistent with the dream activity is usual. This disorder predominantly affects men in late middle age. Forty percent of cases have been associated with neurologic disease, most commonly dementing illnesses of unknown cause, as well as olivopontocerebellar degeneration, Parkinson's disease, and subarachnoid hemorrhage. A familial predisposition may exist. Diagnosis is made by polysomnography, which shows excessive EMG tone during REM associated with dream enactment. Treatment with a nightly dose of clonazepam is highly effective.

Other parasomnias. "*Sleep bruxism* is a stereotyped movement disorder characterized by grinding or clenching of teeth during sleep." This is a common disorder that is sometimes correlated with stress. It results in disrupted nocturnal sleep, temporomandibular joint dysfunction, damage to teeth, and morning headache. Bruxism is inhibited by the use of a nocturnal tooth guard.

"*Sleep enuresis* is characterized by recurrent involuntary micturation that occurs during sleep." Bedwetting after the age of 5 years is considered abnormal. There may be a delay in toilet training without the development of continence during sleep, termed primary enuresis. Secondary enuresis refers to the development of bedwetting after toilet training is complete. Symptomatic enuresis is secondary to underlying medical disease—for example, urogenital disorder or nocturnal seizure. Some cases of enuresis follow arousal from delta sleep, but enuresis may occur in any sleep stage. If no underlying medical cause is identified, the disorder is treated with bladder training, behavioral techniques, and, if these fail, imipramine.

"*Nocturnal paroxysmal dystonia* is characterized by repeated dystonia or dyskinetic (ballistic, choreo-athetoid) episodes that are stereotyped and occur during NREM sleep." Both short- and long-lasting episodes have been described and appear to have different mechanisms. Short episodes often respond to carbamazepine, and there is debate as to whether these episodes may represent seizure activity that is unrecordable with surface electrodes. Long-duration episodes have been observed in one patient in whom Huntington's disease later developed.

"*Sudden unexplained nocturnal death syndrome (SUND)* is characterized by sudden death during sleep in healthy young adults, particularly of Southeast Asian descent."

Medical/psychiatric sleep disorders

Associated with mental disorders. Disordered sleep is typical of most psychiatric disorders. Unipolar depression is characteristically associated with a disorder of initiating and maintaining sleep, most commonly early morning awakening. The patient may fall asleep easily but wake a few hours later, alert and unable to return to sleep. This can be the earliest symptom apparent to the patient. Sleep studies in some of these patients demonstrate an earlier-than-normal REM latency and increased phasic REM activity early in the night. In contrast, the sleep in bipolar depressive disease is characterized by prolonged periods of inability to sleep during the manic phase and excessive sleep during the depressive phase. Most actively psychotic patients have difficulty maintaining sleep, but some may be hypersomnolent at the onset of their psychosis. Patients with panic disorder may wake suddenly at night with panic; polysomnographic evaluation is sometimes useful to distinguish these episodes from sleep terror or seizure. The treatment of sleep disorders of psychiatric cause is directed to treatment of the underlying illness. Improvement in sleep is often a sensitive measure of the effectiveness of treatment.

Associated with neurologic disorders. *Cerebral degenerative disorders, dementia, parkinsonism.* Sleep disruption is a prominent, but not well studied, symptom in all of the degenerative diseases of the brain. Patients with degenerative disease of the brain are at particular risk for sleep-disordered breathing produced by Cheyne-Stokes respirations, abnormal chest wall and upper airway muscle tone, brainstem dysfunction, and use of sedating medications. The resulting hypoxemia can contribute to episodes of nocturnal confusion. In the disorders involving motor systems, sleep fragmentation also occurs secondary to rigidity, tremor, myoclonus, and periodic limb movements. Brainstem involvement induces REM sleep abnormalities, including REM sleep behavior disorder. Circadian rhythm disorders are frequent and probably represent derangement of neurologic control mechanisms, coupled with the secondary effects of disrupted sleep and medication.

Sleep-related epilepsy seizures are facilitated by sleep, particularly stage II sleep. Hypoxia secondary to sleep apnea also precipitates seizures. Some types of seizure disorders, especially complex partial seizures with temporolimbic symptoms, closely mimic sleep terrors and sleepwalking. Usually the clinician is alerted by features that would be atypical of delta sleep arousals, including recurrent episodes during the same night, history of seizures, or abnormal neurologic examination. Nocturnal wandering secondary to epilepsy tends to be less well organized and goal directed. Grand mal seizures are suggested by falls from bed, incontinence, bitten tongue, and morning confusion.

Sleep-related headaches are of various types. Cluster headache is a severe unilateral orbital headache associated with ipsilateral rhinorrhea and tearing. The headache is frequently nocturnal and appears to be exacerbated specifically by REM sleep. Chronic paroxysmal hemicrania, a similar headache disorder, more frequent in women and responsive to indomethicin, is also REM-related. Increased blood flow and hypoxemia during REM may be etiologic factors. Most patients note that migraine is improved by sleep, but occasionally the reverse is true. Sleep-related headache may be the presentation of raised intracranial pressure, exacerbated by the supine posture and episodic elevation in intracranial pressure during REM sleep. Morning headache is typical of sleep apnea syndrome and bruxism.

Associated with other medical disorders. Just as medical illness disrupts the quality of life during the day, it also affects the maintenance of sleep. A careful consideration of possible systemic disease is important in every patient with a sleep disorder. Almost every disease, at some point in its course, may disrupt sleep. Most painful disorders cause nocturnal arousal, especially arthritis and peptic ulcer disease. Insomnia may be the presenting complaint of congestive heart failure with nocturia, paroxysmal nocturnal dyspnea, or arousal secondary to Cheyne-Stokes respirations. Pulmonary dysfunction is exacerbated during sleep and predisposes patients to sleep-disordered breathing. Sleep disruption is particularly prominent in hyperthyroidism and uremia.

Proposed sleep disorders

"*Menstrual-associated sleep disorder* is a disorder of unknown cause, characterized by a complaint of either insomnia or excessive sleepiness, that is temporally related to the menses or menopause." Premenstrual excessive sleepiness is a sometimes dramatic disorder that appears within the first 2 years after the onset of menstruation. Periodic episodes of hypersomnolence tend to occur 6 to 10 days before the onset of menses. The disorder is treated successfully with birth control pills. Menopausal insomnia is characterized by recurrent awakenings, often associated with hot flashes or night sweats. Premenstrual insomnia is common, characterized by difficulty both initiating and maintaining sleep, and often associated with other symptoms attributed to the premenstrual syndrome.

"*Sleep-related laryngospasm* refers to episodes of abrupt awakenings from sleep with an intense sensation of inability to breathe, and stridor." The disorder is frightening but apparently benign. Otolaryngologic examination reveals no abnormality. The disorder usually recurs several times and then resolves. It is more common in smokers and patients with esophageal reflux. Sleep apnea and upper-airway abnormality need to be considered.

REFERENCES

Anch A et al: Sleep, a scientific perspective. Englewood Cliffs, NJ, 1988, Prentice-Hall.

Bootzin RR, Engle-Friedman M, and Hazelwood L: Insomnia. In Lewinsohn PM and Teri L, editors: Clinical geropsychology, new directions in assessment and treatment. New York, 1983, Pergamon Press.

Broughton RJ: Sleep disorders: disorders of arousal? Science 159:1070, 1968.

Guilleminault C et al: Sinus arrest during REM sleep in young adults. N Engl J Med 311:1006, 1984.

ICSD—International classification of sleep disorders: diagnostic and coding manual. Diagnostic Classification Steering Committee, Thorpy MJ, Chairman. Rochester, MN 1990, American Sleep Disorders Association.

Kryger MH et al, editors: Principles and practice of sleep medicine. Philadelphia, 1989, Saunders.

Lewy AJ et al: Antidepressant and circadian phase-shifting effects of light. Science 235:352, 1987.

Matsuki K et al: DQ (rather than DR) gene marks susceptibility to narcolepsy. Lancet 339:1052, 1992.

Moore-Ede MC et al: Medical progress: circadian timekeeping in health and disease. N Engl J Med 309:469, 530, 1983.

Schenck CH et al: Rapid eye movement behavior disorder. JAMA 57:1786, 1987.

Thorpy MJ, editor: Handbook of sleep disorders. New York, 1990, Marcel Dekker.

CHAPTER

111 Coma and Related Disorders

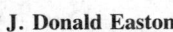

J. Donald Easton

COMA

Coma is a clinical state of total unresponsiveness to all external stimuli; only residual reflex activity remains. It represents the final stage of brain failure in the continuum of consciousness from alert, sentient awareness to inattentive drowsiness, obtundation, stupor, and finally coma. Since many of these terms have imprecise meanings, it is best to describe the patient's behavior in terms of spontaneous activity and response to spoken words or noxious stimulation.

A large number of structural and metabolic conditions may disrupt brain function and impair consciousness. However, the pathophysiology of coma can be divided into four basic mechanisms (see box, p. 1015) according to a classification modified from Plum and Posner. The first diagnostic objective of the physician confronted with a comatose patient is to determine which of the four fundamental types of coma is operant, as this will have implications for both diagnosis and treatment. By evaluating five important physical findings (state of consciousness, pupillary responses, oculocephalic responses, motor responses, and respiratory pattern), it is usually possible to determine which pathophysiologic type of coma the patient is experiencing (see box, p. 1015, and Table 111-1).

The state of consciousness is characterized best by describing the examiner's stimulus (e.g., a quiet question, a shout, a gentle shake, a painful compression of the sternum) and the patient's response (e.g., eye opening and meaningful speech, a semipurposeful attempt to remove the painful stimulus, decorticate posturing, no response). The

Pathophysiologic and etiologic classification of coma

I. Supratentorial mass lesions
  A. Intracranial hemorrhage
    1. Epidural
    2. Subdural
    3. Intracerebral
  B. Neoplasm
  C. Infarct plus edema
  D. Abscess
II. Subtentorial structural lesions
  A. Hemorrhage
    1. Pontine
    2. Cerebellar
  B. Infarction
    1. Brainstem
    2. Cerebellar plus edema
  C. Tumor
  D. Abscess, cerebellar
III. Metabolic (diffuse)
  A. Poisoning
  B. Hypoxia
  C. Hypoglycemia
  D. Diffuse ischemia
  E. Concussion-contusion
  F. Meningoencephalitis
  G. Primary organ failure
    1. Lung
    2. Kidney
    3. Liver
  H. Acid-base, electrolyte disorders
IV. Psychogenic

Evaluation of the comatose patient

Is the cause
  1. Supratentorial structural disease (mass)?
  2. Infratentorial structural disease?
  3. Diffuse brain disease (metabolic)?
  4. Psychogenic?

Physical examination emphasizing five key findings will determine the cause
  1. Five key physical findings*
    a. Level of consciousness
    b. Pupils
    c. Oculocephalic reflex
    d. Respiratory pattern
    e. Motor tone and responses
  2. Simplified brainstem schema (Table 111-1).

*See Table 111-1.

pupillary response is best elicited by a very bright light. Small constrictions are especially difficult to visualize when the pupils are small, and small reactive pupils are commonly mistaken for unreactive ones. Such a mistake may be very important.

The oculocephalic reflex (doll's eye response, doll's head eye phenomenon) is elicited by holding the patient's eyelids open and gently rocking the head briskly from side to side. If the reflex is intact, the eyes deviate conjugately to the side opposite that to which the head is rotated and then drift quickly back to the resting position. An intact reflex indicates that the tegmentum of the midbrain, pons, and medulla is largely intact structurally.

Motor responses may occur spontaneously (e.g., purposeless thrashing of the limbs on one or both sides of the body, decerebrate posturing) or only with voice or painful stimulation. Spontaneous respiratory patterns should be observed first before stimuli are applied by the examiner.

PATHOPHYSIOLOGY

Supratentorial mass lesions impair consciousness by compressing the diencephalic ascending reticular activating system. If the mass expands sufficiently, the brain may herniate downward through the tentorial notch. The rostral brainstem may be displaced caudally and be associated with hemorrhagic infarction of the central brainstem, which results in irreparable injury. Initially, the focal hemispheric lesion generally produces focal symptoms such as aphasia, hemiparesis, or homonymous hemianopia. As the mass grows, headache and altered consciousness often occur. If the hemispheric mass is located laterally rather than medially, the uncus of the temporal lobe may be squeezed over the notch of the tentorium; this compresses the ipsilateral

Table 111-1. Neurologic signs in central transtentorial herniation

Stage	Level of consciousness	Pupils	Oculocephalic reflex	Respiratory pattern	Motor tone and responses
Diencephalon	Lethargy to stupor	Small and reactive	Brisk	Sighs and yawns to C-S*	Semipurposeful to decorticate
Midbrain	Coma	MPF†	Decreased to absent	Tachypneic hyperpnea	Decerebrate
Pons	Coma	MPF	Absent	"Eupnea"‡	Decerebrate to flaccid
Medulla	Coma	MPF	Absent	Ataxic	Flaccid

Adapted from Plum F and Posner JB: The diagnosis of stupor and coma, ed 3. Philadelphia, 1980, Davis.
*Cheyne-Stokes respiration.
†Midposition and fixed: i.e., 4-5 mm in diameter and unresponsive to light.
‡Regular respiration, often shallow; rate of 25-40 per minute.

oculomotor nerve and cerebral peduncle and produces an ipsilateral dilated pupil and a contralateral hemiparesis (uncal, or lateral, herniation syndrome). Sometimes the contralateral cerebral peduncle is compressed against the opposite notch of the tentorium, causing a hemiparesis ipsilateral to the hemispheric mass. With more centrally placed masses, as the diencephalon becomes compressed, brain function is impaired just as though the diencephalon were functionally transected (central herniation syndrome). The patient becomes stuporous; pupils are small but reactive; the oculocephalic responses are brisk; generalized paratonia (also called *gegenhalten*) or decorticate posturing occurs; and Cheyne-Stokes respiration becomes apparent (see Table 111-1). It is imperative that this constellation of physical findings resulting from transtentorial herniation be recognized and that the patient be treated urgently for intracranial hypertension. Otherwise, hemorrhagic infarction of the brainstem results if further herniation occurs. As caudal deterioration to the midbrain level evolves, with both the uncal and central syndromes, coma supervenes; the pupils become 4 to 5 mm in diameter, without reaction to light; oculocephalic and oculovestibular (caloric) responses disappear; decorticate posturing becomes decerebrate; and transient hyperventilation appears. With further decompensation, the patient remains comatose, with unreactive midposition pupils and absent oculovestibular responses. Tone becomes flaccid, and respiration becomes eupnea-like at the pontine level. Ataxic respiration follows as the medullary level of function is reached. Hypotension and death typically follow. Except for the pupillary and motor asymmetry that occurs early in the herniation process with a laterally placed supratentorial mass (uncal herniation syndrome), neurologic function deteriorates symmetrically and in an orderly rostral-to-caudal sequence from diencephalon, to midbrain, to pons, and to medulla (central herniation syndrome).

In subtentorial structural disease, coma is commonly preceded by nausea, vomiting, vertigo, diplopia, nystagmus, ataxia, and occipital headache. The coma is produced by destruction or compression of the reticular formation. It is uncommon for the brainstem to be transected in a single plane as it is with transtentorial herniation, and asymmetric dysfunction is common (e.g., unilateral oculomotor, gag, pharynx, tongue or sympathetic palsies, hemiparesis, and hemianesthesia). Often the dysfunction is focal and can be localized to a specific area such as the right midbrain or left pons.

Metabolic encephalopathy is a diffuse disorder of cerebral function resulting from impaired neuronal metabolism. It is caused by (1) systemic disorders that result in inadequate delivery of nutrients to the brain, (2) endogenous or exogenous systemic poisons, (3) electrolyte disturbances, or (4) the products of intracranial infection or hemorrhage (see box at upper right). In its mildest form, it is manifested by inattention, indifference to the surroundings, and mild intellectual impairment. As confusion worsens, there may be irritability, agitation, hallucinations, aberrant perception, and other signs of delirium before brain function is more severely impaired and stupor and coma supervene.

Common causes of metabolic encephalopathy

- Substrate deprivation
  - Hypoxia
  - Diffuse ischemia
  - Hypoglycemia
  - Vitamin deficiency
- Systemic diseases
  - Respiratory failure (hypercapnia)
  - Kidney failure (uremia)
  - Liver failure
  - Endocrine dysfunction
    - Thyroid
    - Parathyroid
    - Adrenal
    - Pancreas
  - Hypertensive encephalopathy
  - Fever
  - Sepsis
  - Porphyria
- Poisoning
  - Alcohol
  - Prescribed drugs
  - Poisons
  - Drug withdrawal
- Meningitis
- Encephalitis
- Subarachnoid hemorrhage
- Electrolyte disorders
  - Water, sodium, calcium, magnesium, possibly aluminum
- Acid-base disorders
- Concussion-contusion
- Seizures plus postictal states
- Mixed metabolic encephalopathy
- Intensive care unit delirium

Asterixis, tremulousness, myoclonus, and convulsions may also occur. Although neurologic dysfunction is generally symmetric, multiple levels of brainstem function may be impaired simultaneously. For example, in opiate poisoning, the patient may be conscious and have "thalamic" (small, minimally reactive) pupils, purposeful movements, and near apnea. It is not known why certain functions are selectively vulnerable to the effects of specific metabolic disturbances, but the "liver flap" (asterixis), multifocal myoclonus of uremia, posthypoxic action myoclonus, and opiate-induced miosis-hypopnea are characteristic enough to suggest a specific cause for the encephalopathy. Unless the patient has ingested substances that directly affect the autonomic nervous system, the pupils are nearly always symmetric and reactive in metabolic brain disease, even in deep coma. Many of these metabolic disorders can be treated, and cerebral function may fully recover. However, some of them can produce irreparable brain injury. Consequently, the physician must proceed quickly, with an orderly and thorough consideration of the conditions known to produce this clinical syndrome, and should obtain appropriate laboratory confirmation (see box at upper right).

In psychogenic coma, the neurologic examination is nor-

High-yield laboratory studies

Blood glucose
Blood PO_2, PCO_2, pH, NH_3
Na^+, Ca^{2+}, Mg^{2+}, BUN
Liver function tests
Sedative drug screen
Lumbar puncture
Blood and CSF cultures
EEG

Diagnostic studies in coma patients

- Supratentorial mass lesions
  - Primary
    - CT scan
    - MR scan
  - Secondary
    - Angiography
- Subtentorial structural lesions
  - Primary
    - CT scan
    - MR scan
    - Angiography
- Metabolic diffuse*
- Psychogenic
  - Opticokinetic nystagmus
  - Calorics
  - EEG
  - Amobarbital (Amytal) interview

*See box on p. 1016.

mal except for the patient's unresponsiveness. Response to visual threat is normal, and the corneal, pharyngeal, abdominal, and other reflexes are also normal. Opticokinetic nystagmus, caloric-induced nystagmus, and the electroencephalogram (EEG) are normal. The fast phase of opticokinetic and caloric-induced nystagmus is absent in neurogenic coma. Covering the nose and mouth asphyxiates the patient and often induces immediate "awakening." This practice is discouraged, however, since some catatonic schizophrenic and hysterical patients have failed to arouse in this setting and have experienced hypoxic seizures and circulatory collapse. However, inhaled ammonia is a powerful noxious stimulus, and ammonia capsules often induce awakening.

The neurologic examination usually establishes the pathophysiology of the coma. When this information is coupled with the history of how the unresponsiveness came about, and in what setting, it is often possible to limit the diagnostic possibilities to just one or two. Selected laboratory studies then may provide definitive diagnostic information.

LABORATORY STUDIES

The box at upper right lists the most useful diagnostic studies. Computed tomography (CT) has contributed immeasurably in the evaluation of the comatose patient (see Chapter 108). It demonstrates intracranial mass effects and often provides specific information about the pathologic lesion and its precise location. Consequently, the CT scan is especially valuable in patients with suspected structural or mass lesions. MR scanning is extremely precise in the information its images provide but the technique is expensive, time consuming, and difficult to utilize in patients on ventilators. Cerebral angiography is more cumbersome and generally provides less precise information than does CT scanning. However, angiography may provide definitive information regarding aneurysms, arteriovenous malformations, vascular occlusions, and other lesions. In addition, angiography often provides information about abnormal vasculature that is important for the neurosurgeon in planning an operation. The EEG may demonstrate a focal or epileptic disturbance, but it is considerably less helpful than CT and MR scanning. The EEG can demonstrate diffuse physiologic disturbances and is helpful in diagnosing metabolic brain disease and brain death.

Lumbar puncture should be avoided in any patient suspected of having an intracranial mass lesion or noncommunicating hydrocephalus, because it may accentuate an intracranial pressure gradient and facilitate herniation of the intracranial contents from one compartment to another. Obtundation, focal signs, and papilledema are warning signs of a possible intracranial mass and suggest that other studies may be indicated before lumbar puncture. If treatable causes of meningitis (e.g., bacteria, fungi) are considerations, however, immediate examination of the spinal fluid may be mandatory, even if there is some risk of harm.

MANAGEMENT

The first step in managing the comatose patient is to protect the airway. Often, this simply requires gentle oropharyngeal suction and an oral airway, while at other times intubation and assisted ventilation are required. To prevent detrimental vasovagal effects of pharyngeal stimulation, atropine 1.0 mg I.V. should be given to any obtunded patient whose oropharynx will be stimulated by suctioning or by endotracheal or nasogastric intubation. The circulation must be maintained simultaneously. Hypotension in the coma patient is often caused by systemic acidosis, and correcting coexisting respiratory failure corrects the hypotension. Unless it is virtually certain that hypoglycemia is not playing a role in the patient's unresponsiveness, a sample of blood should be obtained for glucose determination, and 50 ml of 50% glucose should be given intravenously. Thiamin, 50 mg, can be given intravenously at the same time to any patient in whom Wernicke's encephalopathy is a consideration. If there is any possibility of a narcotic overdose, naloxone 0.4 mg, should be given intravenously one or more times. It must be used cautiously, however, in persons suspected to be physically dependent on opioids, because it may precipitate an acute abstinence syndrome. Once these supportive measures have been carried out to protect the patient from anoxia, ischemia, and hypoglycemia, one can obtain a history and examine the nervous system, paying particular attention to the aforementioned five physical findings.

HYPOXIC-ISCHEMIC ENCEPHALOPATHY AND PERSISTENT VEGETATIVE STATE

Hypoxic-ischemic encephalopathy after cardiopulmonary arrest is a frequent cause of prolonged coma. Survivors of cardiopulmonary arrest can experience a wide range of brain injury, varying from full recovery to brain death. In patients who have neurologic damage but whose brainstem functions are intact, management is often an ethical and medicolegal dilemma, especially since the extent of cortical damage may be severe, moderate, or mild.

Patients with prolonged survival who have intact brainstem function but virtually no cortical function are said to be in a *persistent vegetative state*. During hypoxia-ischemia, neocortical neurons are especially susceptible to anoxic injury and can be irreversibly damaged while the brainstem remains largely intact. After 1 to 2 weeks of sleeplike coma with brainstem reflexes present, patients in the persistent vegetative state resume periods of "wakefulness" in which the eyes are open and moving, but responsiveness is limited to primitive reflexes. The return of spontaneous eye opening often gives false hope to families because patients in a persistent vegetative state remain mindless, devoid of thought or emotion.

Predicting which survivors of cardiopulmonary arrest will remain in a permanent vegetative state is a frequent problem. Reliable clinical predictors of long-term neurologic outcome have been developed (Table 111-2), but none are absolute. Rare instances of remarkable recoveries belying these predictors have occurred, especially in young patients. The decision to either limit or terminate intensive supportive treatment in patients with severe neurologic deficits who have only a small chance of functional recovery is difficult for both physicians and families. Each clinical situation must be dealt with individually when considering limitation of care in this setting. However, several general principles apply to this ethical and medicolegal dilemma: (1) an adequate period of observation must occur, during which careful neurologic examinations should be recorded; (2) the prognosis, if maximal care if provided, should be clearly stated; (3) the wishes of the patient, if previously expressed, and of the patient's family, should be considered; and (4) a second neurologic consultation is often advisable. In cases deemed hopeless, withdrawal or limitation of supportive treatment is not mandatory but may be permissible, if the family agrees.

Other neurologic syndromes can follow less severe hypoxic-ischemic encephalopathy. In the "man-in-the-barrel" syndrome, patients recovering from hypoxic-ischemic brain injury can move their face and lower limbs

Table 111-2. Features predictive of neurologic recovery in hypoxic-ischemic coma patients in accordance with their best functional state within the first year*

	No recovery or vegetative state	Severe disability	Good recovery
Third-day examination			
No →	93%	7%	0%
↑			
Motor response: withdrawal or better			
↓ No →	61%	21%	18%
↑			
Yes → Spontaneous eye movements with fixation			
↓			
Yes →	8%	15%	77%
Seventh-day examination No →	100%	0%	0%
↑			
No → Spontaneous eye opening at 3 days			
↓			
Yes →	58%	42%	0%
No → Initial eye movements roving and conjugate			
↓			
Yes →	67%	17%	16%
Obeys commands			
↓	6%	22%	72%
Yes →			

Adapted from Levy DE et al: Predicting outcome from hypoxic-ischemic coma. JAMA 253:1420, 1985.

*Residual anesthetics, anticonvulsants, or metabolic derangements may be confounding.

spontaneously, or in response to pain, but not their upper limbs. Hypoperfusion of the distal branches of the middle cerebral artery causes selective damage to cortical motor neurons subserving the upper extremities. This syndrome is often transient and, when prolonged, is often associated with substantial cognitive impairment. Isolated cortical blindness caused by occipital lobe ischemia may also be seen following hypotension, presumably by a similar mechanism. Spinal cord ischemia, action myoclonus, and delayed, postanoxic leukoencephalopathy are uncommon neurologic sequelae of hypoxia-ischemia.

BRAIN DEATH

Since the late 1950s, it has been possible to keep patients alive who have irreversibly lost all brain function by using mechanical ventilation and vasopressors. In these patients who are brain dead, the heart and peripheral circulation continue to function in the absence of brain activity. *Brain death* implies irreversible damage to the entire brain, including the brainstem. This state is to be clearly distinguished from the persistent vegetative state, in which partial preservation of brainstem function occurs. The growing importance of organ donation for human transplantation has been a major impetus for the generation of reliable clinical criteria for brain death.

The medicolegal criteria for brain death vary widely, according to local laws and medical customs. The recommendations of the President's Commission (1981) are guidelines widely accepted in the United States for defining brain death in adults (see box at right). Criteria often differ for adults and children, the latter usually requiring more prolonged observation. The criteria may seem needlessly complex because no false-positive determinations are allowable. False-negative conclusions are more acceptable. The diagnosis of brain death should be made only by clinicians who are experienced in evaluating comatose patients, and documentation should be meticulously recorded in the medical record.

A patient with reactive pupils, a corneal or gag reflex, or any respiratory activity is not brain dead. Any type of decerebrate or decorticate posturing, even though nonpurposeful, reflects brainstem activity and also precludes the diagnosis of brain death. The pupils in brain death are usually midposition or dilated, and unreactive. Small pupils are uncommon and should be carefully checked for reactivity; they indicate possible drug intoxication. The preservation of purely spinal reflexes (e.g., tendon stretch reflexes, Babinski response) is consistent with brain death in most criteria. A general drug screen is usually required to exclude the occult presence of central nervous system depressants. Hypothermia and occult drug ingestion are the two conditions most often producing a reversible loss of brain function that is misdiagnosed as brain death. Neuromuscular blocking agents may also abolish motor and respiratory activity.

Apnea testing is an important measure of brainstem function. It should be carried out in a standardized manner to prevent hypoxemia and to ensure that the partial pressure of carbon dioxide (pCO_2) reaches the critical level to stimulate medullary respiratory centers. The patient is given 100% oxygen for 10 minutes; then oxygen is delivered at 6 liters per minute by a catheter placed in the trachea to maintain tissue oxygenation during apnea testing. Arterial blood gases are initially obtained and are then repeated after 8 to 10 minutes. The pCO_2 usually increases at a rate of 2.0 to 2.5 mm Hg per minute in immobile, comatose patients. If no respiratory activity is associated with a pCO_2 of more than 60 mm Hg, apnea compatible with brainstem death exists. This test is invalid in patients with severe pulmonary disease who are carbon dioxide retainers and who have hypoxemia as the driving mechanism for respiration.

Criteria for brain death in adults*

I. Cessation of all function of the entire brain
   - A. Unresponsive coma
   - B. Absent brainstem reflexes
     1. Pupillary light reflex
     2. Corneal reflex
     3. Cephalic (caloric) reflexes
     4. Oropharyngeal (gag) reflex
     5. Respiration (apnea testing)

II. Irreversibility
   - A. Coma of known cause without potential for reversibility
   - B. Exclusion of contributory, reversible conditions
     1. Drug intoxication
     2. Neuromuscular blockade
     3. Hypothermia (<32.2° C, 90°F)
     4. Shock
     5. Major metabolic disturbance
   - C. Persistence for an appropriate period of observation (6-24 hours, depending on cause of coma and local practice)

III. Confirmatory investigations (may be optional or required)
   - A. Electrocerebral silence (isoelectric EEG)
   - B. Absence of circulation to the brain

Adapted and abridged from Guidelines for the determination of death: report of the medical consultants on the diagnosis of death to the President's Commission for the Study of Ethical Problems in Medicine and Biomedical and Behavioral Research. JAMA 246:2184, 1981.

*Note: Local and institutional rules are superseding.

An isoelectric EEG is not synonymous with brain death, but only reflects electrical silence of the cerebral cortex. Drug intoxication, hypothermia, and viral encephalitis are well-known causes of an isoelectric EEG, and each is associated with a high probability of complete or partial neurologic recovery. An isoelectric EEG is a necessary but not sufficient requirement for brain death in many of the published criteria, although other criteria do not require EEG testing.

All reversible metabolic derangements that might contribute to central nervous system dysfunction must be absent to strictly meet most criteria of brain death, although the degree of allowable derangement is largely a matter of clinical judgment in individual patients. The potential importance of contributing metabolic derangements requires careful clinical consideration. In equivocal cases, confirmatory tests to document the absence of blood flow to the brain (e.g., angiography) may be considered.

Once brain death has been diagnosed according to local medical and legal standards, withdrawal of supportive treatment is legally and ethically justified. In the opinion of many experts, it is actually indicated. In patients with suspected brain death in whom the criteria are incompletely met, or in whom other uncertainties exist, observation with continued support is proper. Most patients who are brain dead experience somatic death from cardiovascular collapse within 48 to 72 hours despite supportive treatment, and prolonged somatic survival is rare, in contrast to patients in a persistent vegetative state.

Unusual movements of the extremities can occur for 15 to 30 minutes after ventilatory assistance is withdrawn in brain dead patients and are presumably a manifestation of terminal spinal cord ischemia. Families of patients should be discouraged from remaining at the bedside during this period.

REFERENCES

Council on Scientific Affairs and Council on Ethical and Judicial Affairs: persistent vegetative state and the decision to withdraw or withhold life support. JAMA 263:426, 1990.

Jennett B and Bond M: Assessment of outcome after severe brain damage: A practical scale. Lancet 1:480, 1975.

Levy DE et al: Predicting outcome from hypoxic-ischemic coma. JAMA 246:2184, 1981.

Medical Consultants on the Diagnosis of Death: Guidelines for the determination of death. JAMA 246:2184, 1981.

Plum F and Posner JP: The diagnosis of stupor and coma, ed 3. Philadelphia, 1980, Davis.

Spudis EV: The persistent vegetative state—1990. J Neurol Sci 102:128, 1991.

Teasdale G and Jennett B: Assessment of coma and impaired consciousness: a practical scale. Lancet 2:81, 1974.

CHAPTER

112 Faintness and Syncope

Robert A. O'Rourke
Richard A. Walsh
J. Donald Easton

Syncope (fainting) is a transient cessation of consciousness with spontaneous recovery caused by generalized cerebral ischemia. *Presyncope* (faintness) is the sensation of impending loss of consciousness that usually precedes full syncope. This symptom often is confused with the more general sensation of dizziness, which is often referred to by the patient as giddiness, lightheadedness, disequilibrium, imbalance, fuzziness in the head, a floating feeling, and so on (See Chapter 115).

Presyncope is manifested by lightheadedness, weakness, nausea, visual spots or vision dimming, ringing or roaring in the ears, diaphoresis, and skin pallor. It usually comes on over several seconds, although it may be sudden; except when it is caused by cardiac arrhythmias, the patient is usually in an upright position. If alteration of consciousness progresses to complete syncope, the person usually slumps, with minimal injury, and remains unconscious for a few seconds, sometimes for 1 to 2 minutes and, occasionally, for 5 to 10 minutes or longer. A few clonic jerks often occur and, occasionally, an intense, generalized tonic spasm results. Fecal and urinary incontinence are infrequent. Simple syncope rarely produces a rhythmic, clonic convulsion. The person usually awakens feeling weak but mentally clear, without headache or drowsiness. If he or she is prevented from falling to a recumbent position, the unconsciousness may be prolonged, and ischemic cerebral injury may occur. Presyncope often aborts before progressing to a full faint, but most faints are preceded by presyncope.

To diagnose syncope, the physician needs a detailed, chronologic account of precisely what the patient was doing, what his or her position or posture was, and the first thing that appeared to the patient to be wrong, in addition to other details, summarized in the box below.

Questions to ask the patient and observers in the evaluation of syncope

Questions for the patient

1. What were you doing during the hours and minutes preceding the blackout?
2. What was your situation regarding loss of sleep, ingestion of food and alcohol, and use of drugs or medications prior to the blackout?
3. What was your body position or posture?
4. What was the first thing you noticed to be wrong?
5. What symptoms did you experience next, in what order, and for how long?
6. Do you remember slumping or striking the floor?
7. What was the next thing you remember, and what position were you in when you regained awareness?
8. Did you hurt yourself in the fall?
   a. Did you injure your tongue or mouth?
   b. Did your back or muscles ache?
   c. Did you have a headache?
   d. Did you lose control of your bladder or bowels?
   e. How did you feel on awakening, and how long did it take for you to feel entirely normal again—seconds, minutes, or longer?

Questions for the observers

1. Ask the observers to answer the preceding questions when appropriate.
2. Was there any turning of the eyes or head?
3. Was there any twitching or jerking of the face or extremities?
4. Was the skin sweaty, pale, flushed, or blue?
5. Did the patient respond to observers in any way during the apparent unconsciousness?

The physician who can visualize the precise clinical picture at the completion of the history taking usually has considerable confidence in his or her diagnosis of syncope, or its exclusion; often, the setting provides major clues to the cause of the spells. The physician can then determine the specific cause of the syncope if it is not already clear (see the box below).

Pathophysiology

Cerebral blood flow is determined largely by arterial blood pressure and cerebrovascular resistance. *Cerebral blood flow autoregulation* is the phenomenon by which cerebral vessels automatically constrict or dilate in response to rising or falling systemic blood pressure. This intrinsic control mechanism maintains a virtually constant cerebral blood flow despite significant physiologic or pathologic fluctuations in arterial blood pressure. In healthy young adults in the upright position, the systolic blood pressure may fall to 60 to 70 mm Hg without significant cerebral ischemia. Below that, cerebral resistance vessels become maximally dilated, and further decreases in blood pressure result in progressive decreases in cerebral blood flow. Presyncopal symptoms result; if the blood pressure continues to fall, total loss of consciousness finally occurs. In older patients with diminished capacity for cerebral vasodilation in response to relative hypotension, there may be significant cerebral ischemia with much smaller reductions in arterial blood pressure.

Thus, whatever its specific cause, syncope results from a relatively sudden fall in cerebral blood flow to very low levels. A decrease in flow sufficient to cause presyncope can result from increased cerebrovascular resistance (e.g., hyperventilation, with its fall in arterial PCO_2, induces $[H^+]$ changes in the interstitial space around precapillary arterioles that mediate a vasoconstriction of these resistance vessels). However, syncope usually is caused by a fall in systemic blood pressure, either from a loss of peripheral or splanchnic vascular resistance or from a decrease in cardiac output. With most causes of syncope, blood pressure returns to the critical cerebral perfusion level as soon as the recumbent position is assumed.

Types of syncope

- I. Neurogenic syncope
  - A. Vasovagal (vasodepression)
  - B. Orthostatic hypotension
    1. Occasional normal individuals
    2. Peripheral neuropathy
    3. Medications
    4. Primary autonomic insufficiency
    5. Intravascular volume depletion
  - C. Reflex
    1. Cough
    2. Micturation
    3. Acute pain states
    4. Carotid sinus hypersensitivity
- II. Cardiogenic syncope
  - A. Mechanical
    1. Outflow tract obstruction
    2. Pulmonary hypertension
    3. Congenital heart disease
    4. Myocardial disease
  - B. Electrical
    1. Bradyarrhythmias
    2. Tachyarrhythmias

Neurogenic (circulatory) syncope

In each type of neurogenic syncope there are inadequate vasoconstrictor mechanisms.

Vasovagal (vasodepressor) and vasomotor syncope. Vasovagal syncope is the common faint and is the most common type of syncope. It occurs frequently in the young adult population but it may occur in any normal person. Situations that decrease central venous volume or increase cardiovascular adrenergic tone often aggravate vasodepressor syncope. It is often precipitated by emotional stress, or pain or threat of pain; it tends to be recurrent. For example, the sight of a shocking accident or of a hypodermic needle or blood withdrawal may evoke an attack. The primary event appears to be a decrease in splanchnic and extremity vascular resistance. At the same time, there is a sudden excess of vagal activity; this produces prompt bradycardia and a decrease in cardiac output; the combined result is a progressive fall in blood pressure until syncope occurs. Sometimes there is no evidence of excessive vagal activity, and it appears that peripheral vasodilation alone is causative *(vasomotor syncope)*. The common faint is aggravated by fasting, poor physical condition, warm environment, and excessive fatigue.

Orthostatic hypotension with syncope. Hypotension with syncope occurs in individuals who have either chronic or transient vasomotor instability, or intravascular volume depletion. Sudden rising from the recumbent or sitting position to a sitting or standing position or standing still for several minutes results in the pooling of blood in the lower extremities and viscera as a result of the loss of compensatory reflex peripheral vasoconstriction: blood pressure falls and syncope ensues.

Orthostatic hypotension results from: (1) impaired autonomic reflex control; (2) depletion of central or total blood volume, or both autonomic dysfunction and blood volume depletion; (3) circulating vasodilators (e.g., carcinoid syndrome); and (4) pharmacologic agents (e.g., nitrates and calcium blockers). Orthostatic hypotension occurs in otherwise normal people after physical deconditioning, especially with prolonged bed rest, fasting, and alcohol use. Varicose veins and normal pregnancy may also be implicated, and some patients also suffer orthostatic hypotension with faints after surgical sympathectomy.

Diabetic and other neuropathies affect the autonomic nervous system and cause sexual impotence, impaired sweating, and paralysis of vasomotor reflexes. Diminished ankle jerk reflexes and diminished sensation in the feet should be sought on examination as evidence of a peripheral neuropathy and should suggest the possibility of a concomitant autonomic neuropathy.

Antihypertensive, antidepressant, and some other medications commonly cause orthostatic hypotension by plasma volume depletion or sympatholytic vasomotor effects. Medications are probably the most common cause of neurogenic syncope in adults. Bleeding and persistent vomiting and diarrhea also may cause volume depletion.

Primary autonomic insufficiency may be caused by several degenerative diseases of the autonomic nervous system, and a common feature of these diseases is orthostatic hypotension with syncope.

Reflex syncope. *Cough syncope* usually occurs after a vigorous paroxysm of coughing in men with chronic obstructive lung disease. It may be caused by the sudden increase in intrathoracic and intra-abdominal pressure, which increases intracranial pressure and decreases cerebral blood flow. This Valsalva effect also may diminish cardiac output. A prolonged Valsalva maneuver in association with hyperventilation certainly appears to produce syncope in breath-holding spells of infancy, weight-lifter's blackout, and various blackout pranks indulged in by teenagers.

Micturition syncope is usually seen in elderly males who arise from sleep to urinate and faint while voiding. Orthostatic hypotension may be a significant part of the cause, but sudden decompression of the distended bladder may induce a reflex vasodilation of the peripheral vasculature.

Acute pain states occasionally produce syncope, probably by stimulating the dorsal motor nucleus of the vagus nerve, which then induces a prominent bradycardia and splanchnic vasodilation. Vagal and glossopharyngeal neuralgia, gallbladder colic, perforation of a viscus, and needling of body cavities are among the causes of reflex syncope. Intense vertigo and migraine headache occasionally induce syncope, presumably through this reflex vagal mechanism. Carotid sinus hypersensitivity also may cause syncope.

Cardiogenic syncope

Syncope of cardiac origin involves loss of consciousness produced by a sudden, marked reduction in effective cardiac output. Etiologic classification of these disorders may be divided broadly into mechanical and electrical (arrhythmic) causes.

Mechanical causes. Left ventricular outflow tract obstruction is the most frequently encountered cause of mechanical cardiac syncope in adults. Obstruction may occur at the valvular, subvalvular, or supravalvular level and may be fixed (e.g., aortic stenosis) or dynamic (e.g., hypertrophic cardiomyopathy). In these conditions, cardiac output may not increase sufficiently during skeletal muscle exercise to meet peripheral oxygen demands. Blood preferentially flows to the exercising muscle, and this results in systemic arterial hypotension, cerebral anoxia, and effort-related syncope. By a similar mechanism, primary pulmonary hypertension and severe pulmonic stenosis occasionally may be associated with effort syncope. Cyanotic congenital heart defects characterized by right-to-left shunting and either pulmonary hypertension or right ventricular outflow obstruction are associated occasionally with exertional syncope. Decreased peripheral resistance with exercise increases right-to-left shunting, which maintains cardiac output but results in further reduction of systemic arterial oxygen saturation and cerebral hypoxia, and occasionally produces faintness or syncope. Vagal reflexes, however, may be involved in these conditions as well as in the syncope that occurs with massive pulmonary embolism. Syncope at rest may occur in any of these disease states resulting from arrhythmias (see under Electrical Causes, below). Left atrial myxomas are an uncommon, but definite, cause of mechanical cardiac syncope (Chapter 24). The patient may have clinical findings suggestive of mitral stenosis but will complain of faintness or syncope, which occurs with change of position as the tumor mass suddenly obstructs the mitral orifice. Thrombosis or prosthetic valve malfunction also may produce sudden mechanical obstruction of the circulation and syncope. Cardiac syncope also may result from acute massive myocardial infarction on the basis of low cardiac output or transient severe arrhythmias.

Electrical causes. Electrical (arrhythmia) disorders are more frequent causes of cardiac syncope than are mechanical abnormalities. Cerebral blood flow is maintained in supine healthy individuals over a wide range of heart rates from approximately 40 to 185 beats per minute. Alterations in pulse rate outside these limits may reduce cerebral circulation and function. In addition, cerebrovascular disease, upright posture, and coronary artery, valvular, or myocardial dysfunction of any etiology may diminish tolerance to even more modest alterations in heart rate.

Advanced degrees of atrioventricular (A-V) block are the most frequent arrhythmic causes of faintness or syncope (the Stokes-Adams-Morgagni syndrome). Symptomatic chronic or acute forms of heart block usually involve the distal conduction system (His-Purkinje system), occur in the elderly or postinfarction patient, and may be persistent or episodic. The resting electrocardiogram may provide evidence of impaired conduction in one or any combination of the three fascicles through which the ventricles are normally activated (Chapter 9). Heart block involving the proximal conduction system (A-V node) is less often symptomatic and is most frequently congenital, drug-induced (e.g., digitalis, beta blockers, calcium blockers), or ischemic in origin.

Stokes-Adams syncope is characterized by its abrupt onset and lack of relation to posture, position, or effort. Like seizures, it may occur in the recumbent position. Sometimes, as a result of prolonged cardiac asystole and attendant severe cerebral anoxia, seizure like activity and sphincter incontinence may occur and be misdiagnosed as epilepsy. Self-limited, malignant ventricular arrhythmias (fibrillation or tachycardia) constitute another important cause of cardiac syncope. Ventricular fibrillation, occurring in patients with a prolonged Q-T interval, may result from sympathetic autonomic imbalance of ventricular innervation as a genetically determined cause of prolonged syncope and sudden death. This familial condition may occur alone (Romano-Ward syndrome) or may be associated with congenital deafness (Jervell-Lange-Nielsen syndrome). The most common supraventricular arrhythmia associated with cerebral symptoms is impaired sinoatrial impulse formation or conduction (sick sinus syndrome), a disorder that is recognized increasingly in the elderly and in the postoperative patient with congenital heart disease. Paroxysmal atrial tachyarrhythmias occasionally are associated with frank syncope, usually in the elderly patient with underlying cerebrovascular disease. Vagally mediated heart block or ventricular asystole has been observed in many disease states (carotid sinus or mediastinal tumors, esophageal diverticula, peritoneal or pleural irritation) and during a variety of diagnostic procedures (e.g., endoscopy and cardiac catheterization). Vagal and glossopharyngeal neuralgia may induce a similar reflex form of syncope. The diagnosis is suggested by the invariable sequence of severe pain in the posterior oropharynx or ear, followed by loss of consciousness caused by profound sinus bradycardia or asystole.

Ambulatory electrocardiogram (ECG) recordings, atrial pacing studies, and bundle of His recordings, alone or in combination, are often necessary to define the presence or absence of a responsible cardiac arrhythmia in patients with dizziness or syncope. In patients with arrhythmia-induced syncope, appropriate pacemaker or drug therapy depends on demonstrating the causative rhythm disturbance (Chapter 9).

Differential diagnosis

Although an accurate history points to a correct diagnosis, several disorders frequently are confused with syncope. These include (1) epilepsy, (2) hypoglycemia, (3) cerebrovascular disease, (4) "drop attacks," (5) hysterical faints, and (6) hyperventilation syndrome.

Epileptic seizures usually differ from syncope in that they are of immediate onset and occur day or night and while the patient is active or supine. They often result in injury and commonly are associated with urinary or fecal incontinence. Clonic convulsive activity commonly lasts for several minutes, and often there is postictal confusion, drowsiness, and headache. While no single aspect of a seizure differentiates it from syncope, the total sequence of events usually does. Partial complex (temporal lobe, psychomotor, limbic) seizures may be confused with presyncope or syncope because of autonomic symptoms and signs and because the patient loses awareness during the seizure (even though he or she may not have convulsions). Usually, there is an aura at the onset of the seizure. Although episodes may resemble the symptoms of presyncope, they commonly produce a "dreamy" or confused state; patients often experience hallucinations, illusions involving themselves or their environment, or unusual feelings of déjà vu. During the ictus, the patient frequently carries out automatic activity that is generally stereotypic for that patient. *Akinetic seizures* are brief attacks of unconsciousness with loss of muscle tone; they are uncommon, occur primarily in children and may be confused with syncope.

Hypoglycemia typically produces confusion or behavioral abnormalities and then hunger and salivation. This is followed by sympathetic hyperactivity manifested by sweating, tachycardia, and nervousness. Obtundation progressing to coma and seizures may ensue. It is unusual for hypoglycemia to produce a relatively abrupt and transient loss of consciousness; thus this condition generally is not confused with syncope.

Cerebrovascular disease rarely causes transient loss of consciousness. Subarachnoid hemorrhage may cause temporary unconsciousness, but it usually has an explosive onset, with severe headache; the patient is typically left with obtundation, often prominent neurologic deficits, and neck stiffness after several hours. A major cerebral embolism or thrombosis may produce transient unconsciousness, but residual neurologic deficits are present. Transient cerebral ischemic attacks involving the carotid artery distribution almost never produce transient unconsciousness. Whereas dizziness is one of the cardinal signs of brainstem ischemia, true syncope is uncommon. When dizziness results from brainstem ischemia, it usually is associated with tinnitus, deafness, diplopia, dysarthria, extremity paralysis or numbness, or other symptoms of brainstem ischemia. Therefore, cerebrovascular disease usually produces many associated symptoms of focal cerebral dysfunction that readily distinguish it from syncope.

The drop attack is a puzzling phenomenon. It usually occurs after the sixth decade and is characterized by a sudden drop to the ground with no apparent loss of consciousness. The patients may bruise their knees but usually are otherwise unhurt and able to stand immediately. While the cause of this disorder is unknown, it has been attributed to basilar artery insufficiency producing transient ischemia to the part of the reticular formation that regulates postural tone. Because these patients often have attacks for many years without other evidence of brainstem ischemia, many physicians believe that a diagnosis of vertebral-basilar insufficiency cannot be made with confidence.

Hysterical faints or swoons must be differentiated from syncope, particularly emotion-induced vasovagal syncope. Hysterical faints occur dramatically and in the presence of others; they are not associated with pallor, diaphoresis, or weakening or slowing of the pulse. They draw attention to the hysterical personality who may be seeking secondary gain through this and other physical complaints. There may be prolonged periods of "unresponsiveness" with resistance to passive opening of the eyelids, bizarre posturing, or resistance to movement of the limbs.

Hyperventilation rarely causes syncope. However, it does cause presyncope. This faintness, together with anxiety, dyspnea, palpitations, and paresthesias of the distal extremities and perioral area in a setting of overventilation, constitutes the hyperventilation syndrome. It is usually caused by acute anxiety. Sometimes, vasodepressor mechanisms are superimposed, and syncope results.

Evaluation of syncope

Most patients of middle age or older who have a syncopal episode without an easily identifiable benign cause probably should be hospitalized.

Emphasis is placed on a detailed history because it is the most important aspect of the evaluation (Fig. 112-1). In reflex syncope induced, for example, by cough, micturition, or acute pain states, the history is virtually diagnostic. The same can be said of vasodepressor syncope, although a search should be made for factors contributing to orthostatic hypotension. The physical examination and electrocardiogram (ECG) provide important information. Gentle massage of one and then the other carotid sinus, with monitoring of the pulse rate and rhythm and the blood pressure, is essential in evaluating possible carotid sinus hypersensitivity.

In orthostatic hypotension with syncope, the mechanism is proved by obtaining the blood pressure in the supine, sitting, and standing positions. In some patients, vasomotor tone will not fail immediately, so it is important to record the blood pressure immediately after standing and then at 1, 3, and 5 minutes or longer. Passive head-up tilt has been identified as a modality for detecting vasodepressor and orthostatic syncope. A positive response to sudden upright tilt of 10 to 60 minutes, with or without an isoproterenol challenge, is defined as syncope or near-syncope in association with hypotension, bradycardia, or birth. A careful examination of reflexes and sensory and motor function should be made to look for evidence of an associated peripheral neuropathy. If it is found, a specific cause should be sought. Screening drugs and alcohol level should be considered. Central venous pressure can be measured if volume depletion is a concern. Neurologic consultation would seem prudent in a patient with any of the widespread neurologic abnormalities suggesting one of the primary nervous system diseases associated with degeneration of the preganglionic or postganglionic autonomic nervous system (e.g., Parkinson's disease, Shy-Drager syndrome). An EEG and cerebral CAT scan often provide important information when neurologic syncope is suspected (see Fig. 112-1).

Two or three minutes of hyperventilation should be observed in any patient suspected of the hyperventilation syndrome. Normal people may become intensely dizzy with this maneuver, so it is important that the patient's spontaneous episodes be mimicked by deep breathing before one attributes etiologic significance to the hyperventilation.

A glucose tolerance test, prolonged fasting, or other provocative tests for hypoglycemia, and electroencephalography for epilepsy, should be reserved for patients in whom the diagnosis of syncope is uncertain. Aortic arch and cerebral angiography rarely need to be considered. Even if vascular abnormalities are found in elderly patients, they will not necessarily be diagnostically meaningful.

In the work-up of suspected cardiac syncope, inquiry should be made regarding the association of the syncope with exertion, dyspnea, palpitations, chest pain, or other symptoms of cardiac awareness. A history of rheumatic

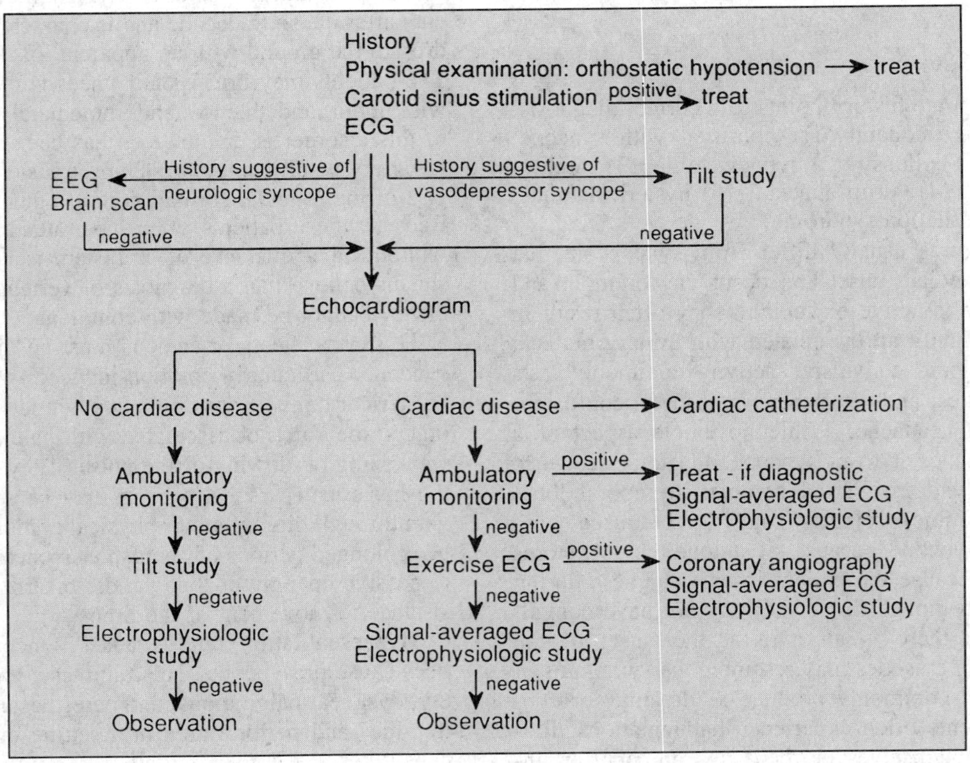

Fig. 112-1. Approach to evaluation of syncope, beginning with the history and physical examination. (From Schaal SF et al: Curr Probl Cardiol 4:211, 1992.)

heart disease, coronary artery disease or hypertension may be important. Although one rarely has the opportunity to examine the patient during an episode of syncope for the presence of an arrhythmia, one should examine for abnormalities of cardiac rhythm or rate, hypertension, signs of congestive heart failure, murmurs, or carotid sinus hypersensitivity. The echocardiogram is an important diagnostic test when cardiogenic syncope is probable. It often confirms the presence of heart disease and may point to the most likely cause for syncope (see the box on p. 1021 and Fig. 112-1). Depending on the history, ECG, and results of echocardiography, signal-averaged ECG (for "late potentials"), exercise electrocardiography (for arrhythmias and/or ischemia), and electrophysiologic studies are indicated in specific patients (Chapter 9, Fig. 112-1). Ambulatory ECG recordings are obtained in most patients in whom a noncardiac cause of syncope cannot be identified.

Treatment

The treatment of neurogenic syncope should be directed toward preventing or correcting the cause of the decreased cerebral perfusion. Vasovagal vasodepressor syncope is best treated by eliminating such precipitating factors as emotional excitement, fatigue, hunger, inactivity, or sedative drugs. These patients should be instructed to assume a sitting or recumbent position with the first presyncopal symptoms. The management of vasodepressor syncope often is very challenging. Therapeutic options include (1) volume expansion (support garments, flurocortisone acetate); (2) beta-adrenergic blockade; (3) anticholinergic agents; (4) methylxanthines (theophylline); (5) disopyramide, and (6) dual-chamber cardiac pacing. The last-mentioned is controversial and most useful in patients with bradycardia. Reflex syncope associated with micturition or coughing may be improved by having the patient avoid standing at the time of these activities.

Treatment of cardiogenic syncope depends on making the correct pathophysiologic diagnosis. Tachyarrhythmias may be treated in various ways, depending on the seriousness of the arrhythmias (Chapter 9). Maneuvers such as breath-holding or Valsalva or carotid sinus massage may abort supraventricular tachyarrhythmias. More serious arrhythmias may be controlled by the use of such drugs as quinidine, procainamide, digitalis, or propranolol. Electrocardioversion or insertion of a pacemaker may be necessary in other patients. Syncope caused by a valvular lesion may not be relieved without surgical correction.

REFERENCES

Almquist A et al: Provocation of bradycardia and hypotension by isoproterenol and upright posture in patients with unexplained syncope. New Engl J Med 320:346, 1989.

Kapoor WP: Diagnostic evaluation of syncope. Amer J Med 90:91, 1991.

Kenny RA et al: Head-up tilt: a useful test for investigating unexplained syncope. Lancet. 1:1352, 1986.

Klein RC and Machell C: Use of electrophysiologic testing in patients with non-sustained ventricular tachycardia: prognostic and therapeutic implications. J Amer Coll Cardiol 14:155, 1989.

Rubenstein LZ et al: The value of assessing falls in an elderly population. A randomized clinical trial. Ann Int Med 113:308, 1990.

Schaal SF et al: Syncope. Curr Probl Cardiol 17:211, 1992.

Silverstein MD et al: Patients with syncope admitted to medical intensive care units. JAMA 248:1185, 1985.

Teichman SL et al: The value of electrophysiologic studies in syncope of undetermined origin: report of 150 cases. Am Heart J 110:469, 1985.

CHAPTER

113 Headache and Facial Pain

John Edmeads

HEADACHE

Mechanisms of headache

The brain itself is not sensitive to pain. When lesions of the brain cause headache, they do so by involving pain-sensitive structures inside the skull, such as the arteries at the base of the brain, the dural venous sinuses, other portions of the dura, and cranial nerves that carry pain fibers (i.e., cranial nerves V, VII, IX, and X). The external structures of the head are all pain-sensitive and give rise to a variety of headaches (see Table 113-1).

The richly innervated superficial structures tend to localize the headache fairly precisely. For example, inflammation of the right temporal artery (temporal arteritis) produces right temporal headache, and purulent left frontal sinusitis causes left frontal headache. When a superficial structure is more diffusely affected, it produces a more diffuse headache (e.g., the generalized extracranial vasodilatation thought to underlie some attacks of migraine produces a generalized headache). Involvement of deeper structures leads to less precise localization (e.g., while sphenoidal sinusitis may cause pain between the eyes, it may also refer pain to the vertex of the skull). Intracranially, pain localization is quite imprecise, and headache often is felt in an area distant from the lesion. A right occipital lobe tumor may cause frontal headache because the structures of both the anterior and middle cranial fossae are innervated by the first division of the trigeminal nerve (V1). Stimulation of any of these structures produces pain referred to the superficial distribution of V1, which is the front half of the head. Posterior cranial fossa structures are innervated mostly by pain fibers from the second cervical cord segment. Disease of these structures generally causes pain that is referred to the back of the head or the neck. Thus, a left cerebellar abscess usually causes a left occipital headache. Lesions at the craniocervical junction or in the upper part of the neck may, however, produce pain felt in the front of the head. This occurs because the descending portion (nucleus caudalis) of the trigeminal nucleus extends down to the third or fourth cervical segments (C3-C4), becoming confluent there with the dorsal horn of the cervical cord, so that pain impulses from the upper cervical segments can

Table 113-1. Mechanism of headaches

Structure involved	Mechanism	Headache syndrome
Cranial blood vessels		
Intra- and extracranial	Neurogenic and humorally induced vasodilatation and inflammation	Migraine, cluster headache
	Immunogenic inflammation	Vasculitis, including temporal arteritis*
Intracranial	Chemically induced vasodilatation	Hunger, fever, medications, hangover, hypoxia, hyperthyroidism
	Pyogenic inflammation	Meningitis
	Chemical inflammation	Subarachnoid hemorrhage
	Mechanical dilatation	Severe hypertension, postpuncture headaches†
	Traction (displacement)	Postpuncture headaches, mass lesions (tumors, hydrocephalus, etc)
Mucosa of sinuses	Inflammation, pressure changes	Sinus headaches
Eyes	Inflammation, increased pressure	Iritis, glaucoma
Muscles		
Face and jaw	Mechanical strain, inflammation	Myofascial pain dysfunction syndrome ("TMJ headache")
Neck and scalp	Sustained contraction	Some tension-type headaches
Unknown	Unknown	Most tension-type headaches

*The headache of temporal arteritis comes mainly from extracranial arteries.
†Postpuncture headaches are caused by a combination of traction and vasodilatation.

gain access to the trigeminal system and be referred anteriorly.

Headache syndromes (see Tables 113-1, 113-2, and the box on p. 1028)

Though ideally headaches should be understood in terms of what structures they arise from, this information is not always clear (Table 113-1). Therefore the International Headache Society (IHS) has devised a classification of headaches and facial pains, with diagnostic criteria, based entirely on clinical attributes. Intended primarily to ensure uniformity of terminology for researchers, the IHS classification is quite lengthy and thus unwieldy for clinical use. The boxed material on p. 1028 is a simpler, much shorter classification. It incorporates some of the new IHS terminology (in italics) but is not entirely consistent with the groupings used by the IHS.

Table 113-2. Important headache syndromes

	Migraine			
	Without aura	**With aura**	**Cluster headache**	**Tension-type headache**
Incidence	Common	Uncommon	Uncommon	Very common
Age of onset	Childhood, adolescence, or young adulthood	Childhood, adolescence, or young adulthood	Young adulthood, middle age	Young adulthood, middle age
Sex bias	Female	Female	Male	No
Family history of headaches	Yes	Yes	No	Yes
Onset and evolution of headache	Slow to rapid	Slow to rapid	Rapid	Slow to rapid
Time course of headache	Episodic	Episodic	Clusters in time	Episodic, may become constant
Quality	Usually throbbing	Usually throbbing	Steady	Steady
Location	Variable, often unilateral	Variable, generally unilateral	Orbit, temple cheek	Variable
Exacerbators	Head-low position, exertion	Head-low position, exertion	None	Stress
Associated features	Prodrome, vomiting	Prodrome, aura, vomiting	Lacrimation, rhinorrhea, Horner's syndrome	None
Physical signs	No	No	Partial Horner's syndrome	No

Migraine. Migraine affects 10% to 20% of the population. It is the second most common headache syndrome, next to tension-type headache. Migraine is not a single entity but a group of disorders sharing the following characteristics: (1) a constitutional predisposition (about 70% of patients with migraine have a first-order relative with a history of migraine); (2) a pattern of repeated unilateral or bilateral headaches of a vascular type (see below), with freedom from pain between attacks; and (3) association of the headaches with autonomic and/or neurologic features that may vary in type and prominence from person to person and from attack to attack.

Most migraine sufferers have their first attack in childhood or adolescence. While migraine can begin at any age, its commencement after the age of 50 is uncommon, so another diagnosis should be sought in those who begin to have headaches for the first time after middle age. Women are affected more often than men, in a ratio of 3:2, possibly because hormonal factors such as menstruation may play a prominent role in precipitating attacks.

Migraine without aura (formerly called "common migraine") is the most frequently encountered form. Criteria for diagnoses are multiple attacks of headaches that last, untreated, for a few hours to a few days and that have at least two of the following characteristics: unilaterality, pulsatility, moderate to severe intensity, and aggravation by activity. The headaches should be accompanied by aversion to noise and light (phonophotophobia) and/or by nausea or vomiting.

Migraine with aura (formerly called "classic migraine") is much less frequent and is characterized by the occurrence of a neurologic aura before or in the early part of a headache that meets the above criteria. Typically the aura consists of bright shimmering visual manifestations of crude or well-formed configuration, beginning in one part of the visual field and slowly spreading and expanding to involve other portions of it. Various types of visual auras include fortification spectra, flickering photopsias, heatwavelike distortions, and less frequently, negative phenomena such as hemianopia. Occasionally the visual symptoms may be succeeded by transient paresthesias in the mouth or face, or in one upper limb. These neurologic features fade after 15 to 30 minutes to be replaced by a throbbing headache, often associated with nausea and vomiting.

Many attacks of migraine appear out of the blue, but some seem to be precipitated by stress, excitement, bright lights, menstruation, alcohol, or food such as chocolate or cheese. Oral contraceptive medication may increase the frequency of migraine attacks, and some evidence suggests that it increases the risk of permanent neurologic deficits such as hemianopia and hemiparesis occurring in the wake of attacks of migraine with aura.

Some people, a few hours to a day or so before the onset of headache, experience behavioral alterations such as depression, elation, hyperactivity, or craving for specific foods. These prodromal syndromes suggest hypothalamic or limbic complicity in the pathogenesis of migraine.

The pathophysiology of migraine is complex and obscure, with neurological, vascular, and chemical aspects. Most believe that the pain of migraine headache comes from dilatation and perhaps sterile inflammation of cranial arteries both inside and outside the skull. These vascular changes may be produced by various blood-borne substances such as serotonin (5HT), estrogens, and alcohol, among others. A purely vascular pathogenesis, however, is insufficient to account for all the phenomena of migraine, including the aura; the brain must be involved. The aura of migraine is associated with a wave of oligemia that begins

Temporal arteritis	Subarachnoid hemorrhage	Meningitis	Brain tumor
Uncommon Over 50	Uncommon Over 35	Uncommon Any age	Uncommon Any age
No No	No No	No No	No No
Slow	Abrupt	Rapid	Slow
Increasing, becoming constant	Persists for days	Persists for days	Duration steadily increases
Constant Localized	Steady Diffuse	Steady Diffuse	Steady Localized, then diffuse
None	None	None	Head-low position, exertion
Generally ill	Altered consciousness, sometimes vomiting	Altered consciousness, sometimes vomiting	Altered consciousness, sometimes vomiting
Arterial changes	Meningeal irritation, sometimes focal signs	Meningeal irritation, sometimes focal signs, fever	Focal signs common, sometimes papilledema

A classification of headaches and facial pain

I. Vascular headaches
  A. Migraine
    1. Migraine with headaches and inconspicuous neurologic features
      a. *Migraine without aura* ("common migraine")
    2. Migraine with headaches and conspicuous neurologic features
      a. With transient neurological symptoms
        (1) *Migraine with typical aura* ("classic migraine")
        (2) *Sensory, basilar,* and *hemiplegic migraine*
      b. With prolonged or permanent neurologic features ("complicated migraine")
        (1) *Ophthalmoplegic migraine*
        (2) *Migrainous infarction*
    3. Migraine without headaches but with conspicuous neurological features ("migraine equivalents")
      a. Abdominal migraine
      b. *Benign paroxysmal vertigo of childhood*
      c. *Migraine aura without headache* ("isolated auras," transient migrainous accompaniments)
  B. Cluster headaches
    1. *Episodic cluster headache* ("cyclic cluster headaches")
    2. *Chronic cluster headaches*
    3. *Chronic paroxysmal hemicrania*
  C. Other vascular headaches
    1. Headaches of reactive vasodilatation (fever, drug-induced, postictal, hypoglycemia, hypoxia, hypercarbia, hyperthyroidism).
    2. *Headaches associated with arterial hypertension*
      a. Chronic severe hypertension (diastolic > 120 mm Hg)
      b. Paroxysmal severe hypertension (pheochromocytoma, some coital headaches)
    3. Headaches caused by cranial arteritis
      a. *Giant cell arteritis* ("temporal arteritis")
      b. Other vasculitides

II. Headache associated with demonstrable muscle spasm
  A. Headaches caused by posturally induced or paralesional muscle spasm
    1. Headaches of sustained or impaired posture (e.g., prolonged close work, driving)
    2. Headaches associated with cervical spondylosis and other diseases of cervical spine
    3. Myofascial pain dysfunction syndrome (*headache or facial pain associated with disorders of teeth, jaws, and related structures, or "TMJ syndrome"*)
  B. Headaches caused by psychophysiologic muscular contraction ("muscle contraction headaches," or *tension-type headache associated with disorder of pericranial muscles*)

III. Headaches and facial pain without demonstrable physical substrate
  A. Headaches of uncertain etiology
    1. "Tension headaches" (*tension-type headache unassociated with disorder of pericranial muscles*)
    2. Some forms of posttraumatic headache
  B. Psychogenic headaches (e.g., hypochondriacal, conversional, delusional, malingered)
  C. Facial pain of uncertain etiology ("atypical facial pain")

IV. Combined tension-migraine headaches
  A. Episodic migraine superimposed on chronic tension headaches
  B. Chronic daily headaches
    1. Associated with analgesic and/or ergotamine overuse ("rebound headaches")
    2. Not associated with drug overuse

V. Headaches and head pains caused by diseases of eyes, ears, nose, sinuses, teeth, or skull

VI. Headaches caused by meningeal inflammation
  A. Subarachnoid hemorrhage
  B. Meningitis and meningoencephalitis
  C. Others (e.g., meningeal carcinomatosis)

VII. Headaches associated with altered intracranial pressure ("traction headaches")
  A. Increased intracranial pressure
    1. Intracranial mass lesions (neoplasm, hematoma, abscess, etc.)
    2. Hydrocephalus
    3. Benign intracranial hypertension
    4. Venous sinus thrombosis
  B. Decreased intracranial pressure
    1. Post-lumbar-puncture headaches
    2. Spontaneous hypoliquorrheic headaches

VIII. Headaches and head pains caused by cranial neuralgias
  A. Presumed irritation of superficial nerves
    1. Occipital neuralgia
    2. Supraorbital neuralgia
  B. Presumed irritation of intracranial nerves
    1. Trigeminal neuralgia ("tic douloureux")
    2. Glossopharyngeal neuralgia

at the occipital pole and spreads anteriorly across the cortex; this spreading oligemia is believed to result from primary alterations in cortical metabolism and function.

Moskowitz's work may provide the missing link between brain and blood vessel. He has emphasized that the trigeminal nerve in its relationship with cranial blood vessels is more than just a passive conductor of pain impulses from vessel to brainstem. Neural traffic in the trigeminal nerve may also be in the opposite direction, with impulses from the brainstem impinging on the blood vessels and, via release of substance P and other peptides, producing dilatation and inflammation of the vessels. These neurogenic changes in the vessel may themselves generate pain, which ascends the trigeminal nerve to the brainstem. The painful aspects of the migraine attack may thus originate in or be perpetuated by reverberations up and down this trigeminovascular system. Further linking the brain and the cranial blood vessels are studies on serotonin (5HT) in migraine. The concentration of this neurotransmitter declines during an attack, and restitution to normal levels by intravenous injection of serotonin aborts an attack. Moskowitz has demonstrated that substances that stimulate the 5HT-1 receptors located presynaptically on the terminals of the trigeminal nerve can inhibit the release of substance P from the terminals and prevent or reverse the dilatation and inflammation of the blood vessels. This effect has been demonstrated with the selective 5HT-1 agonist sumatriptan and the nonselective 5HT-1 agonist DHE (dihydroergotamine). Both these substances have clear efficacy in terminating acute attacks of migraine.

Cluster headache. Unlike migraine, with its predilection for young females, the much less common condition of cluster headache affects males almost exclusively. It usually begins in the third or fourth decades. Cluster headaches take their name from their tendency to cluster in time. An affected individual typically suffers up to eight headaches every day for a few weeks or months, and then the headaches cease, only to reappear in successive clusters months or years later (episodic cluster headache). Occasionally the headaches recur daily and the cluster never ends (chronic cluster headaches).

Each cluster headache lasts 0.25 to 3 hours, commonly 45 minutes. Typically they come on during sleep, rousing the patient and forcing him to pace the floor moaning—unlike the migraine sufferer, who prefers to lie quietly in bed. The headache is a deep, agonizing, nonthrobbing pain that involves the same part of the head or face in every headache. It usually involves one eye and the adjacent temple, cheek, or forehead. It is associated with watering and redness of the affected eye, drooping of the ipsilateral lid, sometimes miosis of that eye (i.e., a partial Horner's syndrome), and congestion or running of the ipsilateral nostril. Nausea is uncommon, and vomiting is rare. After the headache disappears the patient typically sinks into exhausted sleep, only to be awakened hours later by another headache. Although night is the time of predilection, some cluster headaches occur during the daylight hours, particularly if the patient drinks alcohol, which can be a powerful trigger. The pathophysiology of cluster headaches is unknown, but they may arise from periodic spasm, edema, or inflammation of the internal carotid artery near the skull base. Extremely little is known about the chemical concomitants of cluster headache.

Tension-type headache. Physicians once believed that these headaches, the most common type of headache, were caused by sustained, painful contraction of the muscles of the scalp and neck occurring as a somatic manifestation of psychic tension. The evidence for this is flimsy. Electromyography may show increased activity of these muscles during a so-called "muscle contraction headache," but equally often it does not. Sometimes more electromyographic activity is present in people with migraine headaches than in those believed to have tension-type headaches. All in all, the pathogenesis of tension-type headaches is obscure. Very likely some headaches, particularly those incurred during prolonged close work or associated with fatigue, are caused at least in part by painful neck or scalp muscle spasm. Other headaches, perhaps those more overtly connected with depression or other forms of emotional stress, may have no organic substrate but rather represent a referral of psychic pain to the soma. The IHS classification avoids controversy by coining a new term, "tension-type headache," which makes no statement about pathogenesis.

Tension-type headaches tend to be bilateral, dull, nonpulsatile, and from the point of view of the observer, not very intense. They may be bifrontal or nuchal-occipital and are often described as "like a weight on top of the head," "like a tight band around the head," or "like a feeling of expansion within the head." Nothing seems to aggravate these headaches except more stress or fatigue, and nothing seems to benefit them except removal of stress and, in the milder and less entrenched cases, analgesics and antidepressants.

Nausea is uncommon, unless it occurs as a side effect from medication, and vomiting is not seen. Neurologic accompaniments do not occur.

These headaches run a spectrum of seriousness. At one end is most of the normal population who have occasional mild to moderate headaches in response to easily recognized transient stress or fatigue. These headaches respond promptly to simple analgesics and to removal of stress. Further along the spectrum are patients who are habitually somewhat tense and worried or depressed, who have more frequently recurring headaches, but who are well most of the time. These people usually have some insight into the relationship between their symptoms and their life and feelings, and usually show some response to counseling, to antidepressant medication, and to analgesics.

At the far end of the spectrum are the patients with "chronic daily headaches." They have headaches all day, every day and have had them for months or years. It is in these patients that the admixture of migraine is most apparent. They often have, superimposed on their constant dull background headaches, recurrent severe hemicranial throbbing headaches associated with nausea and vomiting.

These patients often organize their entire lives, and those of their family, around their headaches and complain bitterly of the pain. Nevertheless, they do not appear to be in physical distress. Their headaches are "worsened by everything and helped by nothing." They have been unresponsive to, or have developed side effects from, a wide range of medications. Though adamant that analgesics are "useless," they frequently overuse them. Their insight is defective, and they are resistant to and resentful of any suggestion that their intractable headaches are related to serious psychologic disequilibrium. Convinced that organic disease is being missed, they demand and receive repeated investigations, all of which are normal.

Temporal arteritis. Unlike the foregoing headache syndromes, temporal arteritis (1) characteristically begins after the age of 50 years, (2) is caused by visible pathology, and (3) is dangerous.

This progressively obliterative giant-cell arteritis involves not only the arteries of the scalp, causing headache, but also other vessels, including those supplying the eyes and occasionally the brain. About half of those with the headache of temporal arteritis who are not treated go on to develop blindness. The syndrome of temporal arteritis is recognizable, and treatment is effective. The headaches are but part of a generalized arteritis. They occur in individuals who feel and look ill with malaise, fever, sweating, weight loss, arthralgias, and aching in the back and shoulders (polymyalgia rheumatica). Claudication of the jaw is uncommon but virtually pathognomonic. It is produced by narrowing of the arteries supplying the muscles of mastication. Typically the headache involves one temple, although any part of the scalp can be involved depending on which branches of the external carotid artery are inflamed. The headache is often described as head soreness rather than headache. It typically begins as an intermittent soreness or burning discomfort and steadily escalates over several weeks or months to become a constant, well-localized pain. Sometimes the affected scalp artery is prominent, tender, incompressible, and pulseless. Rarely there may be a red streak in the overlying skin.

The diagnosis is suspected with the occurrence of a localized, progressively worsening "sore" headache in an elderly individual. Suspicion is heightened by other complaints suggesting a more generalized illness, by the finding of an abnormal scalp artery, and by the demonstration of an elevated erythrocyte sedimentation rate present in about 90% of cases. The diagnosis is confirmed by biopsy of the affected artery.

Corticosteroids are effective in relieving the headache and preventing complications. They should be started in a dose of 80 to 100 mg per day (prednisone equivalent) and be continued at that dose until symptoms resolve and the erythrocyte sedimentation rate normalizes. The dose is then tapered to the smallest dose that keeps the patient asymptomatic and the erythrocyte sedimentation rate normal.

Subarachnoid hemorrhage. The headache of subarachnoid hemorrhage is one of the most dramatic events in clinical medicine. It is usually abrupt in onset and incapacitating in severity. The headache involves the entire head and often radiates into the neck and even into the back. It is often accompanied by some blunting of consciousness, and vomiting is common. The headache remains severe for several days and then gradually abates. On examination the patient is typically in severe pain. There are signs of meningeal irritation, such as nuchal rigidity and sometimes limitation of straight-leg raising, and occasionally subhyaloid hemorrhages in the optic fundus. Often there are no focal neurologic deficits; however, if the hemorrhage or associated infarction involves the brain parenchyma, hemiparesis, aphasia, or visual field abnormalities may occur. Subarachnoid hemorrhage is most often caused by rupture of a berry aneurysm, and the majority occur in middle age.

The initial pain of subarachnoid hemorrhage is probably produced by tearing and distortion of the blood vessel and its adjacent arachnoid membrane, with the pain perpetuated through chemical irritation by blood of the pain-sensitive vessels and perivascular meninges. Increased intracranial pressure may contribute to the headache.

A full-blown subarachnoid hemorrhage is difficult to misdiagnose. Sometimes, however, an aneurysm or arteriovenous malformation bleeds only a little, causing a moderate or severe headache of sudden onset but without signs of meningeal irritation or neurologic injury. These patients are worrisome. Is this headache a migraine or is it a "minibleed" that may precede by a few hours or days a massive subarachnoid hemorrhage? In general, young people who have a previous history of similar headaches, whose present headache is easing, who did not have the headache come on during exertion, who are alert and oriented, and who on repeated examinations have no neurologic abnormalities or neck stiffness, probably do not have a subarachnoid hemorrhage. All others are suspect for subarachnoid hemorrhage and need a CT scan to demonstrate or exclude a mass lesion or obvious subarachnoid blood. If the CT scan is normal, a lumbar puncture should be obtained to detect small amounts of blood in the CSF. A normal CT scan does not exclude a small subarachnoid hemorrhage. MRI is not useful for showing early hemorrhage.

Meningoencephalitis. The headache of meningoencephalitis is also caused by meningeal irritation and in many respects resembles a subarachnoid hemorrhage. The onset, instead of occurring instantaneously, takes place over several minutes to an hour or so. The headache of meningitis may ultimately become as intense as that of a subarachnoid hemorrhage and may similarly be associated with blunted consciousness and vomiting, especially in children. Like subarachnoid hemorrhage, meningitis is usually associated with signs of meningeal irritation. The very young, the very old, and the very sick may fail to exhibit nuchal rigidity despite overwhelming meningitis. The slower onset of meningitis pain and its association with symptoms and signs of infection usually distinguishes it from the pain of subarachnoid hemorrhage.

Headaches caused by meningeal irritation—subarachnoid hemorrhage and meningitis—are intense and serious.

Failure to recognize them and to institute immediate appropriate treatment is often fatal.

Brain tumor (increased intracranial pressure). In this syndrome a progressively enlarging mass, such as a neoplasm or subdural hematoma, causes progressive displacement of, or traction on, pain-sensitive intracranial structures, producing a progressively worsening headache. Initially the headache is mild and intermittent, but over a period of days, weeks, or months it becomes more persistent and more intense. It is aggravated by factors that increase intracranial pressure such as the head-low position (the headache is typically worse in the morning and improves as the patient gets up and about), coughing and straining, or by transient displacement of the intracranial contents such as with jarring the head. The headache is constant in location.

By the time an intracranial mass lesion is big enough to produce headaches, it generally produces other neurologic symptoms and signs that may be subtle. There may be vague dizziness, slight difficulty in thinking, or changes in the personality. There may be mild signs such as a droop of one corner of the mouth or a reflex abnormality.

The syndrome of a progressively worsening headache, always in the same location and perhaps associated with other neurologic symptoms and signs, should prompt immediate investigation for an intracranial mass lesion.

Hypertension. High blood pressure is an infrequent cause of headache. Most people with hypertension either have no headaches or have the same migraine or tension headaches experienced by the normotensive population. However, moderately severe hypertension (diastolic greater than 120 mm Hg) may produce headaches that appear in the morning, sometimes awakening the patient. This dull, sometimes throbbing ache, either diffuse or occipital, eases as the patient gets up and about. Paroxysmal very severe hypertension, as sometimes seen in pheochromocytoma, may also be associated with paroxysmal headaches.

Evaluation

The key to the diagnosis of headache is in the patient's history. Important factors include the duration of the complaint, the age at onset, the time course pursued by the headache, factors that exacerbate and relieve it, and the constancy and location of the headache. The physical examination is normal in most of the benign headache syndromes but gives crucial information regarding the serious ones (see Table 113-2).

Features of the history and examination suggesting that a particular headache may be ominous are shown in the box at upper right. When any of these danger signals are recognized, investigation is mandatory.

A contrast-enhanced CT scan is the single most productive test for identifying serious lesions causing headache. This scan detects most space-occupying lesions (e.g., brain tumors, subdural hematomas, abscesses), reveals hydrocephalus and cerebral edema, and shows some arteriovenous malformations. CT scanning can miss aneurysms.

Danger signals of an ominous headache

1. Failure to conform *readily* to an innocuous pattern such as migraine, tension headache, or cluster headache
2. Onset in or after middle age
3. Recent onset and progressive course
4. Association with other neurologic or systemic symptoms
5. The presence of abnormal physical signs

However, aneurysms seldom produce headaches unless they rupture or leak, and when they do, the blood in the brain parenchyma or in the CSF is commonly visible on the CT scan. If there is still suspicion of a subarachnoid hemorrhage in the presence of a normal CT scan or if there is suspicion of meningitis, a lumbar puncture should be done.

The erythrocyte sedimentation rate should be checked in all patients with new onset of headache after the age of 50, to help identify temporal arteritis.

Treatment

Migraine. A careful history may elicit dietary, environmental or behavioral triggers of the migraine attacks. These may include habitual overwork and fatigue, caffeine, monosodium glutamate (MSG), nitrates in smoked meats, alcohol, cheese, sleep deprivation or excess, oral contraceptives and other estrogenic hormones, and poorly handled anxiety. Sometimes the patient is unaware of these triggers until asked about them. Avoidance of the triggers, if feasible, may substantially improve the migraine and reduce the need for medication.

Most migraine sufferers for acute attacks simply take over-the-counter (OTC) analgesics such as aspirin or acetaminophen, usually with adequate results. The efficacy of these OTC analgesics can be improved by taking them in a large dose (1000 mg rather than the 650 mg usually advised) and, if possible, in a liquid or effervescent form to enhance absorption. Many physicians prescribe analgesics containing codeine and/or a barbiturate, and these can be quite effective *when taken properly*. However, they have a high potential for abuse; taking them too frequently (that is, on consecutive days or on more than 3 days in any one week) may establish a rebound headache cycle. In this cycle some hours after the last dose of analgesic, withdrawal symptoms including headache may occur; the patient takes more analgesic for the headache, raising the tissue level of the analgesic and lessening or abolishing the headache . . . until withdrawal from that dose occurs some hours later. In this fashion a patient can be sucked in to taking narcotic or barbiturate analgesics every day, often many times per day. Some authorities believe that these rebound headaches may occur from overuse of even the generally benign OTC analgesics. All agree that rebound headaches can result from the overuse of ergotamine.

Properly prescribed and taken, ergotamine tartrate in a

dose of 1-2 mg orally very early in an attack aborts about 50% of migraine episodes. In some of the remainder, poor absorption may be a factor; ergotamine can then be taken by other routes, such as 2 mg rectally or sublingually. Some patients can be taught to self-inject dihydroergotamine (DHE) subcutaneously or intramuscularly in a dose of 0.5 to 1.0 mg. To minimize the risk of habituation and of rebound headaches, ergotamine should not be given on consecutive days or more often than 2 days per week. Ergotamine is believed to exert its antimigraine effects by stimulating the 5HT-1 receptors in cranial vessels, producing vasoconstriction and reducing neurogenic inflammation. Because it combines with other receptors, including dopamine and adrenergic receptors, side effects such as nausea, vomiting, and peripheral vasoconstriction may occur; administration of an antinauseant before or with the ergotamine may be helpful.

Sumatriptan is believed to combine only with the 5HT-1 receptor and thus has a more specific action with fewer side effects. It can be given in a dose of 100 mg orally or 6 mg subcutaneously using a self-injector. So far, rebound cycles have not occurred from sumatriptan.

Status migrainosus occurs when, as a result of a severe prolonged (more than 72 hours) attack of migraine unresponsive to self-administered medications, the patient has decompensated emotionally and physically and has presented to a physician for emergency treatment. After ensuring through history, examination, and appropriate investigations (sometimes a CT scan and a lumbar puncture) that the diagnosis truly is status migrainosus and not a leaking aneurysm or early meningitis, treatment comprises intravenous rehydration of the patient followed by the use of *one* of the following regimens:

1. Antiemetic (e.g., promethazine 25 mg) by slow IV push followed by narcotic (e.g., meperidine 75–100 mg) by slow IV push.
2. Antiemetic (e.g., promethazine 25 mg or metoclopramide 10 mg) by slow IV push followed by DHE (0.5-1.0 mg) by slow IV push; DHE 0.5 mg may be repeated if necessary in 1 hour.
3. Double-check that the patient is adequately rehydrated and then give chlorpromazine by repeated miniboluses of 7.5 mg every 10 minutes until either the headache is relieved or a maximum of 30 mg have been given; watch for hypotension.
4. Sumatriptan 6 mg SC (note: sumatriptan should not be given within 24 hours of the last dose of ergotamine or DHE, and DHE should not be given within 6 hours of the last dose of sumatriptan).

Prevention of migraine attacks. Prophylactic medications are used when ergotamine, analgesics, or sumatriptan do not abort attacks or, if they do, are consumed so regularly as to risk habituation, abuse, or toxicity. Medications useful in the prophylaxis of migraine include propranolol, 80 to 240 mg per day (and other beta blockers—atenolol, metoprolol, nadolol, timolol); verapamil, 240 mg per day, or nifedipine, 60 mg per day; amitriptyline, 50 to 125 mg per day; and methysergide, 4 to 12 mg per day for no more than 5 consecutive months.

All medications mentioned should be started in low doses and gradually increased. Other agents occasionally useful in the prophylaxis of certain types of migraine include nonsteroidal anti-inflammatory drugs, lithium, platelet antiaggregation agents, phenothiazines, and monoamine oxidase inhibitors. Nonpharmacologic modalities such as biofeedback and hypnotherapy are occasionally useful.

Cluster headaches. Treatment of the acute attack with medication is often not feasible because of the sudden nocturnal onset. Inhaled ergotamine or self-injected dihydroergotamine may occasionally be helpful. Oxygen inhalation shortens attacks in about half of patients. Prophylaxis is preferable, using any of the following regimens for the expected duration of the headache cluster: (1) methysergide, 4 to 12 mg per day; (2) lithium carbonate, 600 to 1200 mg per day; (3) prednisone, 15 to 60 mg per day; (4) verapamil, 240 mg per day; or (5) valproic acid, 750 to 1500 mg per day. *Warning:* methysergide and prednisone must not be used long-term, as in *chronic* cluster headache.

Tension-type headaches. Occasional tension-type headaches respond well to over-the-counter analgesics and are seldom a medical problem. More frequent headaches may improve with explanation and reassurance, although, as a rule, the more frequent and prolonged the headaches, the less the patient's insight and the less likely their benefit from this brief, informal psychotherapy. Antidepressant medication (e.g., amitriptyline) alone or in combination with a phenothiazine or benzodiazepine can be useful in some cases of chronic recurrent tension-type headaches. If there is a vascular component, the addition of a migraine prophylactic agent can be helpful.

Chronic daily headaches. At least half of these patients have their headaches as the result of analgesic and/or ergotamine rebound cycles; in the others the chronic daily headaches are fueled by psychological disturbances or, very rarely, by undetected disease. If the headaches are drug-induced, the only treatment likely to work is to get the patient off all analgesics and ergotamine, a daunting task that usually requires hospitalization. Raskin, and Silberstein et al. have developed regimens for using DHE to assist in this (see references). Close, prolonged follow-up of these patients is essential; they have a tendency to slip back into overuse of medications and once again develop chronic daily headaches.

FACIAL PAIN

Facial pain frequently is caused by easily diagnosed local diseases, such as a tooth abscess, sinusitis, or parotitis. Diagnosis is a problem only with certain neuralgic, vascular, and psychogenic syndromes (Table 113-3). *Tic douloureux,* or trigeminal neuralgia, is the most common neuralgic facial pain. It typically affects the elderly and presents as recurrent 1- or 2-s jabs of sharp, severe, unilateral pain most often located in the V2 or combined V2-V3 distribution of the trigeminal nerve. Pathognomonic of tic douloureux is

Table 113-3. Facial pain

	Location	Nature	Timing	Associated physical findings
Tic douloureux	V2, then V2-V3; rarely V1	Triggered	Brief jabs	None
Geniculate neuralgia	Ear	Not often triggered	Brief jabs, or long duration	Vesicles in ear, VII palsy, ± VIII findings
Glossopharyngeal neuralgia	Tonsillar fossa, ear	Triggered	Brief jabs	Episodes of syncope
Postherpetic neuralgia	One or more adjacent cranial or cervical nerves	Burning	Constant	Healed skin lesions, sensory loss, or hyperpathia
Posttraumatic neuralgia	Usually one cranial or cervical nerve	Burning, aching	Constant	Sensory disturbances
Cluster headache	Retro-orbital, cheek, temple	Boring, deep, intense	Attacks of 30-120 min	Lacrimation, ptosis, rhinorrhea
"Lower-half headache"	Orbit, nose, cheek, mastoid; may spread to neck and arm	Boring, deep, intense	Attacks lasting one or more hours	Sometimes flushing, lacrimation, rhinorrhea
Carotidynia	One side of neck	Deep, aching	Several days	Tender carotid in neck
Atypical facial pain	Cheek, jaw, entire face	Aching, may be bizarre	Constant	Emotional disturbance

the ability of the patient to trigger the pains by stimulating the face or the buccal mucosa (e.g., washing the face, eating, or brushing the teeth). While the cause is unknown, some cases may be caused by irritation of the root of the trigeminal nerve by a pulsating loop of an elongated arteriosclerotic vessel. When typical tic douloureux appears in a young person, multiple sclerosis should be suspected. Carbamazepine, in a dose of 200 to 800 mg per day, is effective treatment in the majority of patients. When carbamazepine fails, a percutaneous radiofrequency lesion of the ipsilateral trigeminal ganglion or surgical decompression of the trigeminal root in the posterior fossa can be helpful.

Cluster headache is the most common vascular cause of facial pain. Diagnosis is rarely a problem, except for cases in which the pain is primarily in the cheek. Several other facial pain syndromes (e.g., Sluder's syndrome, lower-half headache, Vail's neuralgia) have been described, but they may be unusual variants of cluster headache.

Atypical facial pain is a poorly understood and uncommon syndrome in which constant deep aching pain affects one side of the face, rarely both sides. It affects patients who have no abnormal physical signs but who usually manifest prominent psychological disability. There is no evidence that the pain is neuralgic, and considerable evidence that it is psychogenic. Treatment is difficult, but psychotherapy and antidepressant medication may help.

REFERENCES

Headache Classification Committee of the International Headache Society: Classification and diagnostic criteria for headache disorders. Cranial neuralgias and facial pain. Cephalalgia 8(suppl. 7):1, 1988.
Moskowitz MA: The neurobiology of vascular head pain. Ann Neurol 16:157, 1984.
Moskowitz MA and Buzzi MG: Neuroeffector functions of sensory fibres: implications for headache mechanisms and drug actions. J Neurol 238:S18, 1991.
Raskin NH: Repetitive intravenous dihydroergotamine as therapy for intractable migraine. Neurology 36:995, 1986.
Raskin NH: Headache, ed 2. New York, 1988, Churchill Livingstone.
Silberstein SD, Schulman EA, Hopkins MM: Repetitive intravenous DHE in the treatment of refractory headache. Headache 30:334, 1990.

CHAPTER

114 Neck and Back Pain

Kenneth K. Nakano

In medicine, pain in the neck and back is a common clinical problem encountered by every physician. Pain in the neck and back is normally limited in its duration and is responsive to rest, local measures (ice, heat, massage), and nonnarcotic analgesics and muscle relaxants. The pathophysiologic basis for episodes of neck or back pain includes inflammatory, degenerative, and traumatic changes of the fascia, ligaments, apophyseal joints of the spine, and paraspinal muscles. Strain of the muscle or ligaments produces inflammation, edema, and spasm, resulting in pain and stiffness. Irritation of spinal nerve roots from a herniated disk (nucleus pulposus), an ostophytic spur, or, less likely, a malignancy may produce diffuse spasm and discomfort, as well as radicular pain, sensory loss, and weakness in the distribution of the affected nerve root (dermatome pattern). Disk herniation occurs when the anulus fibrosus encircling the soft nucleus pulposus becomes weakened or torn, allowing the central disk material to extrude into the spinal canal to compress nerve roots or the spinal cord. Degenerative changes in the disk and adjacent vertebrae (spondylosis) occur in older people, are seen on x-rays of the spine, and generally do not produce symptoms unless the spondylytic changes encroach on the intervertebral foramina (and produce symptoms of nerve root irritation). In patients with congenitally narrow spinal canals, degenerative disk changes compromise the spinal canal and intervertebral foramen and may produce symptomatic spinal stenosis, a condition now much more easily diagnosed with the use of magnetic resonance imaging.

Knowledge of the dermatome, sclerotome, and myotome distribution patterns for the cervical and lumbosacral nerves can aid in the diagnosis (Table 114-1). It is important to confirm the source of dysfunction in the neck and low back, understand the mechanism by which the symptoms occur, and recognize the tissues capable of eliciting clinical signs. A careful, thorough history and complete physical examination will reveal the problem clearly. Only after the clinician recognizes certain conditions and arrives at a diagnosis can he or she direct effective therapy.

Structures causing neck pain

Acromioclavicular joint
Heart and coronary artery disease
Apex of lung, Pancoast's tumor, bronchogenic cancer (C3, C4, C5 nerve roots in common)
Diaphragm muscle (C3, C4, C5 innervation)
Gallbladder
Spinal cord tumor
Temporomandibular joint
Fibrositis and fibromyositis syndromes (upper thoracic spine, proximal arm, and shoulder)
Aorta
Pancreas
Disorders of any somatic or visceral structure (produces cervical nerve root irritation)
Peripheral nerves
Central nervous system (posterior fossa lesions)
Hiatus hernia (C3, C4, C5)
Gastric ulcer

NECK PAIN

In clinical practice, neck pain occurs slightly less frequently than does low back pain; a major difference is that neck pain becomes less disabling, seldom compromising work capacity. Neck stiffness exists as a common disorder: for the age group 25 to 29 years in the U.S. working population, there is up to a 30% frequency of one or more attacks of stiff neck. For the work population over 45 years of age, this figure rises to 50%. Episodes of "simple" stiff neck last 1 to 4 days and seldom require medical care. Radicular pain to the shoulder and arm occurs later in life than does stiff neck: a frequency of up to 10% in the 25 to 29 age group, subsequently rising to 25% to 40% after age 45. Overall, 45% of working men experience at least one attack of stiff neck, 23% report at least one attack of radiculopathy, and 51% suffer both these symptoms at some time during their career.

Pain in the neck exists in all occupational groups. Stiffness of the neck appears first, followed by headache and shoulder-arm pain. The pain-sensitive structures of the neck include the ligaments, the nerve roots, the articular facets and capsules, the muscles, and the dura. Pain in the neck area can originate from several tissue sites and result from a number of mechanisms (see box at upper right).

Clinical examination

The essential means of diagnosis and management of neck pain include elicitation of the history and the physical examination. Neuroimaging procedures (x-rays, computed tomography [CT], magnetic resonance imaging [MRI], and electrodiagnostic procedures (electromyography—nerve conduction) help confirm the clinical formulation.

The most common symptom of cervical spine disorders is pain. Cervical nerve root irritation causes a well-localized area of pain, whereas poorly defined areas of pain arise from deep connective tissue structures, muscle, joint, bone, or disk. The patient's ability to describe the pain gives the physician essential clues to diagnosis. Stiffness with consequent limitation of motion of neck, shoulder, elbow, wrist, and even fingers may occur subsequent to prior injury response, articular involvement, nerve root irritation, or reflex sympathetic dystrophy. Tenosynovitis and tendinitis often accompany syndromes of the cervical spine and may involve the rotator cuff; tendons around the wrist or hand, with stenosis or fibrosis of tendon sheaths; and palmar fascia. Numbness and tingling follow the segmental distribution of the nerve roots in cervical spine disorders; however, this condition occurs frequently without demonstrable sensory change. Muscular weakness and fasciculation indicate a lower motor neuron disorder secondary to a radiculopathy. Pain and guarding produce functional weakness. Head pain is common and is characteristic of cervical spine disorders; it results from nerve root compression, vertebral artery pressure, compression of sympathetic nerves, and posterior occipital muscle spasm, as well as osteoarthritic changes of the apophyseal joints of the upper three cervical vertebrae. A lesion at C6 and C7 may produce neurologic or myalgic pain with tenderness in the precordium or scapular region, producing confusion with angina pectoris.

Systematic physical examination of patients with neck pain includes examination of the head, neck, upper thoracic spine, shoulders, arms, forearms, wrists, and hands with the patient fully undressed. The physician observes the patient's posture, movements, facial expression, gait, and various positions (sitting, standing, supine). As the patient walks into the office, the physician observes the head position and how naturally and rhythmically the head and neck move with body movement. There is a large range of motion of the cervical spine, which, in turn, provides a wide scope of vision and is essential to the sense of balance. The basic movements of the neck include flexion, extension, lateral flexion to the right and left, and rotation to the right and left. A decrease in specific motion may occur with blocking at a joint, pain, fibrous contractures, bony ankylosis, muscle spasm, mechanical alteration in joint and skeletal structures, or a tense and uncooperative patient. Other causes of muscle spasm include injury to muscle, involuntary splinting over painful joints or skeletal structure, and irritation or compression of nerve roots of the spinal cord. Reflexes indicate the state of the nervous system and its afferent pathways (Table 114-2). Certain abnormal reflexes appear only with spasticity and paralysis; these indicate injury to the corticospinal tract. The primary deep tendon re-

Table 114-1. Relation of reflexes to peripheral nerves and spinal cord segments

Reflex	Site and mode of elicitation	Response	Muscle(s)	Peripheral nerve(s)	Cord segment
Scapulohumeral reflex	Tap on lower end of medial border of scapula	Adduction and lateral rotation of dependent arm	Infraspinatus and teres minor	Suprascapular (axillary)	C4 to C6
Biceps jerk	Tap on tendon of biceps brachii	Flexion at elbow	Biceps brachii	Musculocutaneous	C5 and C6
Supinator jerk (also called *radial reflex*)	Tap on distal end of radius	Flexion at elbow	Brachioradialis (and biceps brachii and brachialis)	Radial (musculocutaneous)	C5 and C6
Triceps jerk	Tap on tendon of triceps brachii above olecranon, with elbow flexed	Extension at elbow	Triceps brachii	Radial	C7 and C8
Thumb reflex	Tap on tendon of flexor pollices longus in distal third of forearm	Flexion of terminal phalanx of thumb	Flexor pollices longus	Median	C6 to C8
Extensor finger and hand jerk	Tap on posterior aspect of wrist just proximal to radiocarpal joint	Extension of hand and fingers (inconstant)	Extensors of hand and fingers	Radial	C6 to C8
Flexor finger jerk	Tap on examiner's thumb placed on palm of hand; sharp tap on tips of flexed fingers (Tromner's sign)	Flexion of fingers	Flexor digitorum superficialis (and profundus)	Median	C7 and C8 (T1)
Epigastric reflex (exteroceptive)	Brisk stroking of skin downwards from nipple in mammillary line	Retraction of epigastrium	Transversus abdominis	Intercostal	T5 and T6
Abdominal skin reflex (exteroceptive)	Brisk stroking of skin of abdominal wall in lateromedial direction	Shift of skin of abdomen and displacement of umbilicus	Muscles of abdominal wall	Intercostal, hypogastric, and ilioinguinal	T6 and T12
Cremasteric reflex (exteroceptive)	Stroking skin on medial aspect of thigh (pinching adductor muscles)	Elevation of testis	Cremaster	Genital branch of genitofemoral	L2 and L3 (L1)
Adductor reflex	Tap on medial condyle of femur	Adduction of leg	Adductors of thigh	Obturator	L2, L3, and L4
Knee jerk	Tap on tendon of quadriceps femoris below patella	Extension at knee	Quadriceps femoris	Femoral	(L2), L3, and L4
Gluteal reflex (exteroceptive)	Stroking skin over gluteal region	Tightening of buttock (inconstant)	Gluteus medius and gluteus maximus	Superior and inferior gluteal	L4, L5, and S1
Posterior tibial reflex	Tap on tendon of tibialis posterior behind medial malleolus	Supination of foot (inconstant)	Tibialis posterior	Tibial	L5

From Nakano KK: Neck pain. In Kelley WN et al, editors: Textbook of rheumatology. Philadelphia, 1985, Saunders.

Continued.

Table 114-1. Relation of reflexes to peripheral nerves and spinal cord segments—cont'd

Reflex	Site and mode of elicitation	Response	Muscle(s)	Peripheral nerve(s)	Cord segment
Semimembranosus and semitendinosus reflex	Tap on medial hamstring tendons (patient prone and knee slightly flexed)	Contraction of semimembranosus and semitendinosus muscles	Semimembranosus and semitendinosus	Sciatic	S1
Biceps femoris reflex	Tap on lateral hamstring tendon (patient prone and knee slightly flexed)	Contraction of biceps femoris	Biceps femoris	Sciatic	S1 and S2
Ankle jerk	Tap on tendo calcaneus	Plantar flexion of foot	Triceps surae and other flexors of foot	Tibial	S1 and S2
Bulbocavernosus reflex (exteroceptive)	Gentle squeezing of glans penis or pinching of skin of dorsum of penis	Contraction of bulbocavernosus muscle, palpable at root of penis	Bulbocavernosus	Pundendal	S3 and S4
Anal reflex (exteroceptive)	Scratch or prick of perianal skin (patient lying on side)	Visible contraction of anus	Sphincter ani externus	Pudendal	S5

flexes and plantar responses should be routinely examined (Table 114-3).

Differential diagnosis

Several clinical conditions arising outside the cervical spine but perceived in or around the neck area mimic cervical nerve root irritation, muscle spasm, ligament strain, bone disease, and joint disorders (see box on p. 1038).

Peripheral neuropathy may produce pain, both proximal and distal to the irritative site. Muscle spasm is not associated with peripheral neuropathy. Spinal cord tumors produce a poorly localized and ill-defined neck pain, hyperreflexia, and spasticity; immobilization does not relieve the pain, and deep tenderness and local muscle spasms are absent. Cerebral or subarachnoid hemorrhage, meningitis, head and neck trauma, or a central tumor produce neck pain, mimicking cervical spine syndromes. In these instances, clinical examination, CT scan, MRI, and spinal fluid evaluation can be used to differentiate the various conditions.

An important clinical fact in the differential diagnosis of neck pain is that compression or irritation of cervical nerve roots with radiation of pain is associated with deep tenderness at the site of pain. Segmental areas of deep tenderness that are not painful until palpated indicate nerve root involvement. A 1% injection of lidocaine into the painful area results in transient reproduction of the radicular pain, followed by relief of pain for days or weeks in the patient with nerve root involvement. If local anesthetic injection fails to reproduce (and relieve) the pain, one then looks at potential visceral or somatic structures having the same segmental supply.

Neck pain occurs in malingerers, depressed people, persons seeking compensation, and hysterical and psychoneurotic individuals. These patients possess no concomitant nerve root irritation and derive no relief from local anesthetic injections. Furthermore, absence of muscle spasm, an antalgic position, and feigning of limitation of neck motion should arouse the clinician's suspicion. Skilled clinical elicitation of historic data and the physical examination constitute the principal reproducible means of making a differential diagnosis (Fig. 114-1).

Table 114-2. The six primary reflexes

Reflex	Nerve roots necessary for reflex	Muscle carrying out the reflex
Ankle jerk	S1	Gastrocnemius
Posterior tibial	L5	Posterior tibial
Knee	L2-L4	Quadriceps
Biceps	C5, C6	Biceps
Radial	C5, C6	Brachioradialis
Triceps	(C6), C7, C8	Triceps

Treatment

Cautious clinical, electrodiagnostic, and neuroimaging assessment must precede the planning of medical treatment, since it is important to exclude other causes of neck pain (see box on p. 1038). In the treatment regimen of neck pain,

Table 114-3. Neurologic findings in lumbosacral nerve root disorders

Nerve root	Pain distribution	Weakness	Sensory findings	Reflexes
L3	Anterior thigh	Paresis of quadriceps, psoas, and adductors	L3	Knee jerk reduced or absent
L4	Upper gluteal region to anterior and medial thigh and to knee	Mild paresis of adductor and quadriceps	L4	Knee jerk reduced or absent
L5	Lateral gluteal area to posterior, lateral thigh, lateral calf, lateral malleolus, dorsum of foot, and into big toe	Paresis of extensors of big toe; with severe weakness, toe and foot extensors weaken	L5	Posterior tibial reflex reduced or absent (significant if unaffected side is normal)
S1	Gluteus maximus to lateral posterior thigh, leg, and into heel and lateral foot	Paresis of plantar flexion muscles of foot	S1	Ankle jerk reduced or absent
S2	Gluteus maximus to posterior medial side of thigh and medial posterior calf; pelvic pain	Slight weakness plantar flexion; occasional bladder dysfunction	S2	Ankle jerk may be slightly reduced.

the physician considers the following: (1) severity of the symptoms; (2) the presence or absence of neurologic findings; and (3) the severity of the condition as seen by electrodiagnostic and radiographic procedures (when indicated) (see Fig. 114-1).

Bed rest should be reserved for severe acute cases, for chronic cases with an acute exacerbation of symptoms, and for patients in whom ambulatory treatment fails. For relief of pain, anti-inflammatory and muscle relaxant medications suffice. With the above medical regimen, most acute neck pains subside within 7 to 10 days. When the acute pain subsides, the patient may commence therapeutic exercises (anterior-neck mobilizing; shoulder raising; and muscle strengthening—active, passive, isotonic, isometric, and isokinetic) and appropriate postural training. Traction, either continuous or intermittent, should be considered when bed rest fails. Continuous cervical traction should be reserved for more severe cases with symptoms of nerve root compression. Cervical collars may be helpful, in part because they also help correct posture faults. These should fit well and maintain the neck in the most comfortable position. Collars should not be worn continuously for more than 2 months, to prevent weakness and wasting of neck muscles.

Physical therapy benefits most patients with neck pain; some persons are helped by cryotherapy; others benefit from heat (both superficial and deep). Mechanical therapy (whirlpool baths and/or massage) may also help relieve symptoms. In certain cases, electrotherapy and transcutaneous nerve stimulation may be beneficial. Still other patients may respond to biofeedback and relaxation techniques.

Two main groups of patients appear appropriate for surgical therapy. In the first group, symptoms relate primarily to the nerve roots emerging from the cervical spine, and the condition presents with either persistent neck pain or arm pain associated with anatomic weakness. In the second group, a slowly progressive spinal cord syndrome involves the legs first, then the arms.

LOW BACK PAIN

Low back pain is one of the most common of medical complaints encountered by physicians. Many disorders cause low back pain (see box on p. 1038); as a result, there are various modes of diagnosis and treatment. More than 50% of the population complains of low back pain at some time, and for at least one fourth of the people, the pain problem is ongoing. In the majority of cases of low back pain the problem is easy to treat; it responds well to therapy and surgical intervention rarely is needed. The majority of patients do not need consultation by a specialist, except when conservative care fails.

Clinical evaluation

Documentation of the history becomes the most important aspect of the examination. If the pain is localized to the low back alone, symptomatic care often suffices. When true sciatica is present, the patient can usually describe the course of the pain and trace the dermatome. Lumbar disk herniation with radiculopathy becomes unlikely if there is no sciatica. Most low back pain of musculoskeletal origin is worsened by activity and sitting and is relieved with rest. Trauma is overemphasized as a cause of low back and leg pain. In legal matters, however, it is important to document the events that brought on the pain.

The physical examination is aimed at determining if nerve root compression exists, whether there is instability, and if there is a hint of nonmusculoskeletal origin for the pain. In patients with acute lumbar pain, there is lumbar muscle spasm that straightens the normal lumbar lordosis (this can be both seen and palpated). Most often, the muscle in spasm is tender. When only one side is involved with low back pain, there is a compensatory scoliosis (scoliosis concave to that side; this shortens one leg by lifting the pelvis). Motor examination should test the strength of plantar flexion and dorsiflexion of the foot and toes. The ability of

Cervical spine syndromes

Localized neck disorders

Osteoarthritis (apophyseal joints, C1-C2-C3 levels most often)
Rheumatoid arthritis (atlantoaxial)
Juvenile rheumatoid arthritis
Sternocleidomastoid tendinitis
Acute posterior cervical strain
Pharyngeal infections
Cervical lymphadenitis
Osteomyelitis (staphylococcal, tuberculosis)
Meningitis
Ankylosing spondylitis
Paget's disease
Torticollis (congenital, spasmodic, hysterical)
Neoplasms (primary or metastatic)
Occipital neuralgia (greater and lesser occipital nerves)
Diffuse idiopathic skeletal hyperostosis
Rheumatic fever (infrequently)
Gout (infrequently)

Lesions producing neck and shoulder pain

Postural disorders
Rheumatoid arthritis
Fibrositis syndromes
Musculoligamentous injuries to neck and shoulder
Osteoarthritis (apophyseal and Luschka)
Cervical spondylosis
Intervertebral osteoarthritis
Thoracic outlet syndromes
Nerve injuries (serratus anterior, C3-C4 nerve root, long thoracic nerve)

Lesions producing predominantly shoulder pain

Rotator cuff tears and tendinitis
Calcareous tendinitis
Subacromial bursitis
Bicipital tendinitis
Adhesive capsulitis
Reflex sympathetic dystrophy
Frozen shoulder syndromes
Acromioclavicular secondary osteoarthritis
Glenohumeral arthritis
Septic arthritis
Tumors of the shoulder

Lesions producing neck and head pain with radiation

Cervical spondylosis
Rheumatoid arthritis
Intervertebral disk protrusion
Osteoarthritis (apophyseal and Luschka joints; intervertebra disk osteoarthritis)
Spinal cord tumors
Cervical neurovascular syndromes
Thoracic outlet and associated syndromes

Classification of disorders causing low back pain

- Lumbar disk syndromes
  - L4 nerve root compression
  - L5 nerve root compression
  - S1 nerve root compression
  - Large midline disk herniation
- Congenital abnormalities
  - Facet asymmetry
  - Transitional vertebral (Bertolloti's syndrome)
  - Spondylolisthesis-spondylolysis
  - Scheuermann's disease
  - Achondroplasia
- Arthritic conditions
  - Hypertrophic arthritis
  - Osteoarthritis
  - Ankylosing spondylitis
  - Rheumatoid arthritis
  - Osteitis condensans ilii
- Infections
  - Acute bacterial disk space infection
  - Tuberculous spondylitis
  - Sacroiliac infection
- Tumors
  - Benign
    - Meningioma or neurinoma
    - Osteoid osteoma
    - Osteoblastoma
  - Malignant
    - Metastatic cancer (breast, lung, prostate, etc.)
    - Primary neural tumors
    - Myelogenous diseases
      - Multiple myeloma
      - Hodgkin's disease
      - Lymphoma
      - Eosinophilic granuloma
      - Hand-Schüller-Christian syndrome
- Metabolic disease
  - Osteoporosis
  - Ochronosis
  - Paget's disease
  - Sickle cell disease
- Trauma
  - Lumbar strain
  - Compression fracture
  - Subluxation of facet joint
- Nonskeletal disorders
  - Myofascial pain
  - Pelvic disorders (pelvic inflammatory disease, uterine fibroids, tumors)
  - Ectopic pregnancy
  - Retroperitoneal tumors or hematoma
  - Prostatitis
  - Abdominal aortic aneurysm
  - Kidney stones
  - Pyelonephritis
  - Pancreatitis
  - Peptic ulcer
  - Large bowel obstruction

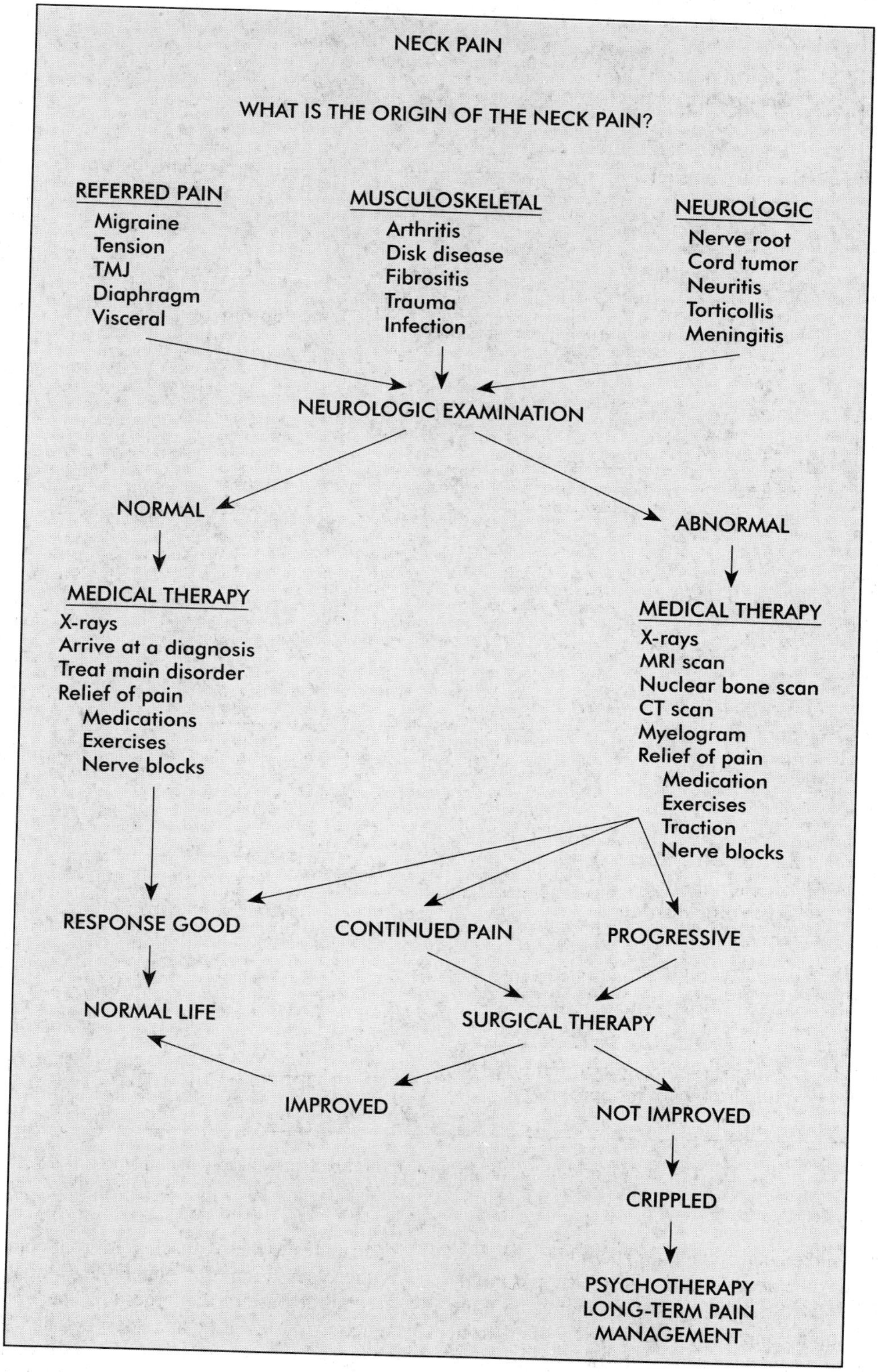

Fig. 114-1. Neck pain algorithm for diagnosis and therapy.

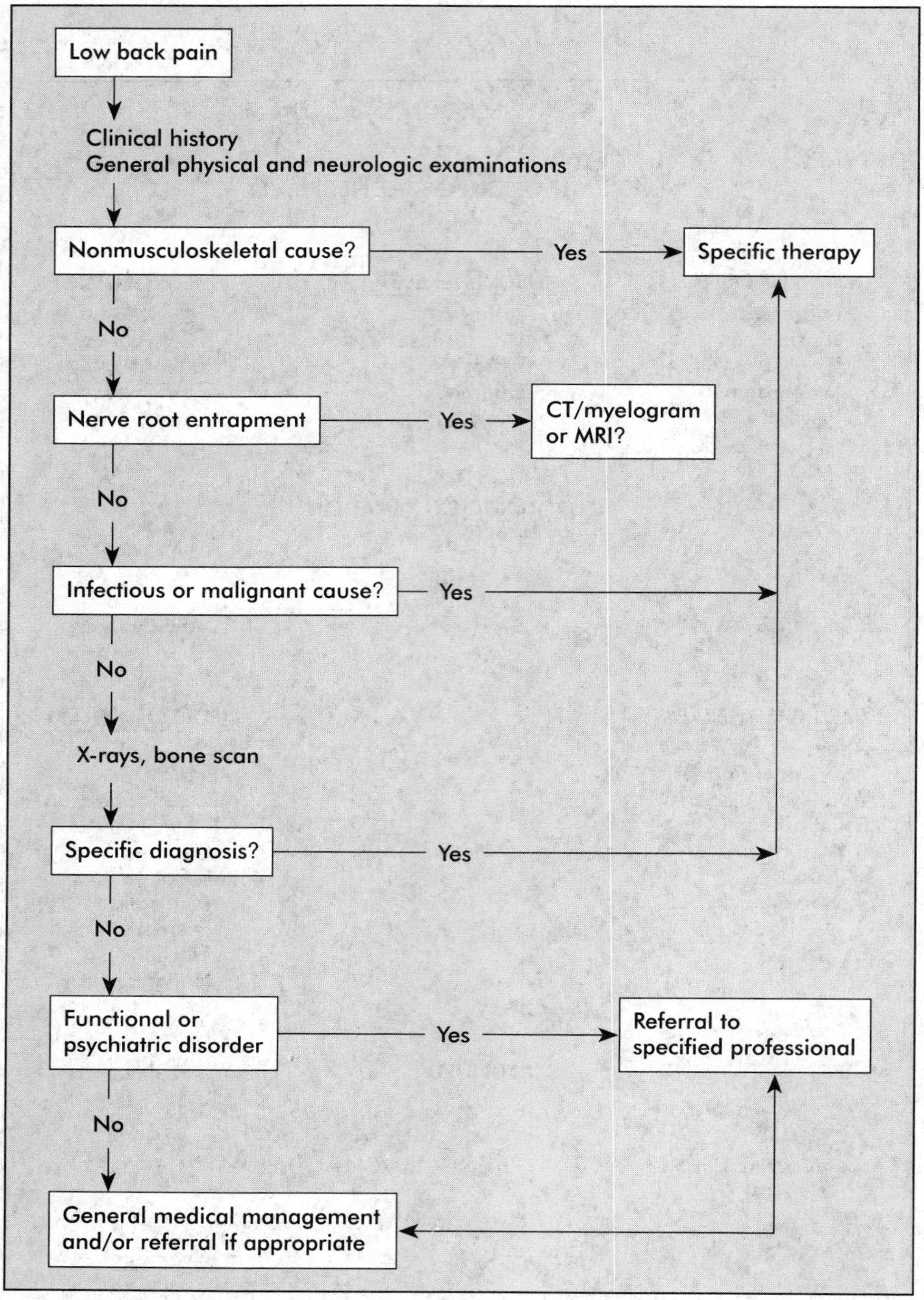

Fig. 114-2. Algorithm for the evaluation of a patient with low back pain.

the patient to flex and extend at the knee should be assessed, and the ankle and knee deep tendon reflexes should be recorded (Table 114-3). Straight-leg testing should be done with the patient supine and each extended leg lifted from the bed. If this produces sciatic pain in either leg, nerve root compression can be assumed. With L4 nerve root compression, there is diminution of the knee jerk and altered sensation of the medial side of the leg. There is some weakness of the quadriceps—but this is inconstant, since L3 also contributes to these muscles. L5 root compression produces reduced sensation of the lateral leg, dorsum of the foot, and around the base of the large toe. There is weakness of dorsiflexion of the foot and toes but no deep tendon reflex change. Root compression of S1 shows a loss or diminution of the ankle reflex and sensory loss on the lateral side of the foot and sole. Additionally, there will be weakness of plantar flexion (often brought out by the patient walking on the toes). With lumbar disk herniations, the great majority occur at L4-5 and L5-S1 and a small minority affect L3-4. Lumbar disk herniations at higher levels are unusual.

Lumbar facet degeneration or injury may cause both back pain and nonradicular leg pain. Leg pain may occur without nerve root compression. Referral of pain by facet syndromes will be diffuse: into the hip and coccyx from L5 to S1, down the back of the thigh from L4 to L5, and into the anterior thigh from L3 to L4.

Diagnostic evaluation

If the clinical history or physical examination raises the question of atypical low back pain or presentation, plain x-rays should be taken to screen for tumor, infection, fracture, congenital anomaly, or other serious medical problems mimicking the common acute musculoskeletal low back pain syndrome (Fig. 114-2). Spondylosis or a congenital anomaly produces an intractable low back pain syndrome that does not respond to an adequate conservative program.

Electrodiagnostic studies (EMG, etc.) have the greatest diagnostic value in atypical sciatic syndromes or in patients who have had prior lumbosacral surgery. The purpose of these studies is to define the nerve roots involved in the pain syndrome. With intractable sciatica or progressive pain/weakness, CT scan/myelography and MRI become the definitive tests and often dictate the need for surgical intervention.

Treatment

For the acute episode of low back pain, the fundamental conservative therapy is strict bed rest. Bed rest is indicated when the patient's pain becomes so severe that ambulation is impossible. As soon as the severe pain relents, the person should be allowed progressive ambulation and physical therapy.

Nonnarcotic anti-inflammatory medications often ease the pain, and muscle relaxants can curtail the spasm. In cases of severe acute low back pain, narcotic drugs may be necessary, although only on a short-term basis, to minimize the possibility of addiction.

Physical therapy measures include cryotherapy (ice packs) or heat, depending on the patient and the clinical setting; massage; and ultrasound. Lumbar traction may be applied below the knees or at the pelvis. Additionally, traction often assures bed rest.

Often, in both acute and chronic musculoskeletal disorders, the clinician finds trigger points. There are two approaches to the management of focal myositis. The traditional technique is to identify the area of local spasm and pain by palpation and then inject it with local anesthetic combined with steroids. An alternative method of eliminating the trigger point, especially in the acute phase, is the use of local electrical stimulation, which also provides local analgesia. Good results can be achieved with local electrical stimulation, which often speeds the resolution of the painful area. Injection into the trigger point is most useful in the chronic pain state in which a specific area of myositis is well established. Repeated injection of these areas often provides long-lasting pain relief. These techniques should provide more than temporary relief. Active physical therapy emphasizing range of motion and exercise must supplement trigger point injection or stimulation.

When the back pain problem becomes chronic or regularly recurrent, a lumbosacral brace may be beneficial. Bracing in the acute musculoskeletal pain syndrome is seldom indicated. It is best to begin with the lightest brace that is efficacious and then move to heavier braces if necessary. The brace must provide support from the rib cage to the pelvis and must limit motion. In most cases of back pain, bracing should be a temporary measure.

Neither bracing nor active physical therapy should be long-term modalities in the majority of cases of low back pain. The aim of physical therapy is to relieve muscle spasms, which usually last only a few weeks. Prolonged, repetitive physical therapy programs are not indicated.

The judicious use of an exercise program should eliminate the need for bracing relatively soon for most patients with back pain. As soon as the patient's acute pain and spasms are relieved, it becomes important to begin active therapy to restore range of motion and restoration of function. Long-term limitation of activities weakens muscles, stiffens ligaments, and may produce an unnecessary and prolonged disability. Exercises designed to increase range of motion, including stretching at the knees and hips and restoration of range of motion in all directions of bending for the lumbar spine, should be pursued. Leg strengthening is important, and back and abdominal muscles should be exercised regularly. One goal is to prevent recurrence of acute back pain syndromes and eventual alleviation of chronic symptoms. Isometric exercises in association with range-of-motion techniques are satisfactory and tolerated well by most patients in the course of rehabilitation.

Conservative regimens should not be used in the following conditions: (1) if the patient has loss of bowel and/or bladder function; and (2) if the patient has another major or progressive neurologic deficit, or such intractable pain that adequate analgesia becomes impossible. In the above clinical situations, prompt diagnosis and surgical treatment are imperative.

Most patients—even those with minor neurologic changes such as a reflex abnormality, radicular sensory change, or discernible but unimportant weakness—should be placed on a conservative, noninterventional medical regimen. In those populations complaining of low back and leg pain only 1% to 2% suffer from a significant disk herniation and require low back surgery.

REFERENCES

Bradley WG et al: Comparison of CT and MRI in 400 patients with suspected disease of the brain and spinal cord. Radiology 152:695, 1984.

Cailliet R: Neck and arm pain, ed 2. Philadelphia, 1980, Davis.

Cailliet R: Low back pain syndrome, ed 3. Philadelphia, 1981, Davis.

Frymoyer JW: Back pain and sciatica. N Engl J Med 318:291, 1988.

Murayama S, Numaguchi Y, and Robinson AE: The diagnosis of herniated intervertebral discs with MR imaging: a comparison of gradient-refocused-echo and spin-echo pulse sequences. AJNR 11:17, 1990.

Nakano KK: Neck pain. In Kelley WN et al, editors: Textbook of rheumatology. Philadelphia, 1989, Saunders.

CHAPTER

115 Otoneurology

Stephen W. Parker

ANATOMIC SUBSTRATE OF BALANCE

Balance is controlled by sensory systems in the central and peripheral nervous systems. These are organized so that an individual can still function after damage to one system; if more than one is damaged, the individual is unstable. Sensory receptors of the vestibular system reside in the inner ear. The semicircular canals respond to angular acceleration and the utricle and saccule to movements in relation to gravity (linear acceleration). These structures are connected to the vestibular nuclei in the brainstem via the eighth nerve. The midline cerebellar structures, including the flocculus, nodulus, and vermis, are integral parts of the vestibular system and have a powerful inhibitory effect on the vestibular nuclei. The cerebellar hemispheres are not part of the vestibular system, but they play an important role in balance by modulating motor activity and coordination. Vision also plays a major role in balance and in normal individuals often overrides other balance modalities. The final major sensory modality contributing to balance is proprioception mediated by peripheral nerves. Disease processes that impair one or more of these modalities impair the individual's ability to balance. If multiple systems are not functioning, balance is severely impaired. A syndrome of multiple sensory deficits may be seen in elderly patients with degenerative central nervous system or labyrinthine changes, plus neuropathy, retinopathy, or arthropathy.

DISEASES AND THEIR LOCI

Systemic

Systemic or distant causes of dizziness include postural hypotension, which is a frequent cause of a lightheaded type of dizziness that occurs on standing from a supine or sitting position, although there may be a delay in the onset of symptoms. Anemias often produce dizziness on standing. Pernicious anemia has been associated with episodes of spinning dizziness and positional dizziness. Cardiac arrhythmias can produce a lightheaded type of dizziness and episodes of spinning dizziness, which suggest ear rather than cardiac disease. Aortic stenosis may be associated with a lightheaded or faint feeling that occurs after limited exercise. Hypothyroid patients may have a Ménière's-like picture, with bilateral hearing loss and episodes of spinning dizziness. The dizziness usually resolves with treatment, but the hearing loss may not improve. Hyperthyroid patients rarely have hearing loss but may complain of tinnitus. They may have spinning dizziness, but more frequently they complain of a lightheaded, off-balance sensation. Hypoglycemia may produce a lightheaded type of dizziness and, less frequently, spinning.

Inner ear

Diseases affecting the inner ear are among the most common causes of dizziness but are relatively few in number. Labyrinthitis is an inflammation of the inner ear that most typically affects both auditory and vestibular portions of the inner ear. Symptoms are the sudden onset of hearing loss and dizziness. The hearing loss may resolve or persist. The dizziness may be quite intense at the onset but gradually resolves. The time course of resolution of symptoms may be hours, days, weeks, or months. This illness is a monophasic one with the possibility of some fluctuation. Labyrinthitis has been classified in three types. The most severe is bacterial labyrinthitis, which occurs in the setting of a meningitis. Often these patients are so sick that the initial dizziness and hearing loss are not clinically apparent, and instability and hearing loss are appreciated after the patient has recovered from the acute effects of the meningitis. Serous labyrinthitis is seen in patients with middle ear infections. Bacteria do not appear to enter the inner ear, but toxic substances appear to do so. Pathologically, one sees mononuclear cells in the inner ear and damage to the hair cells of the basal turn of the cochlea adjacent to the round window. There may be high-frequency hearing loss as well as dizziness. The most common type of labyrinthitis is viral, the prototypes of which are measles and mumps. The clinical entity of vestibular neuronitis is used to explain the sudden onset of dizziness associated with decrease in vestibular function on one side without auditory symptoms. Thus, it is characterized by the sudden onset of severe dizziness with no auditory symptoms. Examination reveals instability with a tendency to fall to one side. There may be spontaneous or gaze nystagmus with the fast-phase beating to the side opposite that to which the patient is falling. No other neurologic signs or symptoms are present. Testing reveals a reduced response to caloric stimulation on the side to which the patient is falling and the side opposite spontaneous and gaze nystagmus fast phase.

Ménière's syndrome is a multiphasic illness characterized by repeated episodes of spinning dizziness, fluctuating hearing with gradual deterioration, a feeling of pressure in the affected ear, and tinnitus in the affected ear. The etiology of this process is unclear, but the pathophysiology appears to be an overproduction of endolymph or a problem with absorption of endolymph that results in swelling of the endolymphatic space (endolymphatic hydrops) with episodes of dizziness and hearing loss, possibly occurring at the time of repeated rupture of membranes in the inner ear. The process has a variable course and may resolve spontaneously. Many forms of medical treatment have been tried without well-documented success. Sometimes, vestibular suppressant medication helps to decrease the severity of symptoms. If symptoms persist in a severe form, surgical treatment may be helpful. Operations to change the abnormal pathophysiology have had limited success in relieving symptoms (66% with improvement). Destructive procedures, such as labyrinthectomy or selective sectioning of the vestibular portion of the eighth nerve, have had a higher incidence of success if patients are carefully selected to include only those with documented unilateral inner ear dysfunction. Over a period of 5 years, 15% to 30% of patients may have involvement of both inner ears. There may be systemic causes of Ménière's-like symptoms, especially with bilateral involvement. This can be seen with hypothyroidism, lues, and vasculitis.

Positional vertigo and nystagmus are common symptoms that often come from the inner ear. The most common type is benign paroxysmal positional vertigo (BPPV), which is characterized by spinning dizziness on lying down as well as sitting up. There may be dizziness on turning the head from side to side or on flexing and extending the neck. The classic finding on examination is a burst of rotary nystagmus when the patient is rapidly placed in the right- or left-ear-down position. This nystagmus has a brief latency and a duration of less than 60 seconds, and it is associated with dizziness. The nystagmus and dizziness fatigue (decrease) on repeated movements into the provoking ear-down position. On sitting up from the provoking ear-down position, there are similar symptoms of nystagmus and dizziness, but the nystagmus reverses direction so that it has a downward rather than upward vertical component. Other features—latency, brief duration, dizziness, and fatiguing—are unchanged. BPPV comes from the posterior semicircular canal of the inner ear on the side from which the symptoms may be provoked. This is a self-limited process of unknown cause (although it can occur after trauma) that resolves spontaneously after weeks to months. Patients learn to deal with the symptoms or to avoid the provoking positions. Some physicians advocate exercises in which the patient repeatedly attempts to provoke the symptoms in an attempt to produce a central adaptation to them. This may be effective in selected groups of patients, but many cannot tolerate the repeated induction of symptoms over a short period of time. There are other forms of positional vertigo and nystagmus, some of which come from the inner ear and others of which originate in the central nervous system. Central nervous system lesions are characterized by purely vertical nystagmus, persistent nystagmus (lasting more than 60 seconds), and nystagmus occurring without dizziness. Head trauma frequently causes dizziness secondary to concussive effects on the labyrinth. This is frequently a positional dizziness that may be a variant of BPPV.

The most common causes of serious ototoxicity in the United States are aminoglycoside antibiotics, which may produce vestibular and auditory damage in the inner ear by damaging hair cells. The incidence of this damage may be decreased but not eliminated by careful attention to blood levels and renal function. The relative amount of auditory and vestibular dysfunction varies among the different members of this group. Neomycin and kanamycin have mainly auditory effects. Gentamicin and tobramycin affect vestibular function more than auditory function, and streptomycin affects vestibular function much more than auditory function. Damage to hearing occurs initially in the higher frequencies, and there is relative preservation of speech discrimination. Eventually a profound hearing loss may occur. The vestibular dysfunction may be insidious and often is initially not appreciated in critically ill patients. It becomes apparent as an instability on attempting to walk and as an instability of the environment when sitting in a bouncing car or wheelchair. The patient finds it difficult to read when the head is moving. Although there may be some improvement in the damage to the vestibular system, most of the functional improvement comes from central nervous system adaptation and the ability to use information from other sensory systems, such as the visual and the proprioceptive. Thus, patients with multiple sensory deficits may not be able to compensate for the loss of inner ear vestibular information and may remain unstable.

Perilymph fistulas between the inner and middle ear occur with erosive tumors and after barotrauma, such as explosions and rapid pressure changes in scuba diving. With classic barotrauma, there is sudden onset of hearing loss and dizziness. Over the past several years, the possibility of chronic perilymph fistulas being responsible for much of the unexplained dizziness and hearing loss has been raised. This issue is still a controversial one.

Eighth nerve

Abnormalities of the eighth nerve are less frequent than those of the inner ear. Acoustic neuromas constitute 2% of intracranial tumors and are the most common tumor of the cerebellopontine angle. These Schwann cell tumors of the vestibular portion of the eighth nerve originate in the internal auditory canal, because it is at this point that the eighth nerve changes its sheath from glial to Schwann cell. Symptoms are produced by compression of the neurovascular bundle in the internal auditory canal. The most common symptom is a slowly progressive unilateral hearing loss. Dizziness is less common and may be only a mild instability as the central nervous system adapts to the slow loss of peripheral vestibular function. Although the seventh nerve is compressed in the internal auditory canal, facial paralysis is relatively rare, because motor function is resistant to the compressive effects of this type of tumor. Other symptoms appear as the tumors grow out of the internal auditory canal and fill the cerebellopontine angle. The next most common finding is decreased facial sensation from compression of the fifth nerve or fifth-nerve nucleus, but tumors must be at least 2 cm in posterior fossa extension to symptomatically compress the fifth nerve. Other late symptoms from compression of the brainstem include limb ataxia, gait ataxia, headache, and memory loss from hydrocephalus. Approximately one fourth as common are cerebellopontine angle meningiomas. These tumors tend to be larger at the time of presentation, since they originate on the dura of the posterior fossa and often must fill the cerebellopontine angle before causing symptoms.

Brainstem

Although diseases of the brainstem that cause dizziness are less common than diseases of the inner ear, they are often more dangerous. These include strokes, tumors, and demyelinating and degenerative diseases. Strokes are the most worrisome, because they can progress to irreversible loss of function in a matter of hours. Two well-defined stroke syndromes are the lateral medullary stroke and the anterior inferior cerebellar artery (AICA) stroke. The presenting symptoms of the lateral medullary stroke are dizziness with veering toward the side of the lesion, nystagmus beating toward the side of the lesion, ipsilateral limb ataxia, loss of pin and temperature on the contralateral foot, and decreased sensation on the ipsilateral side of the face. In the AICA syndrome there is dizziness with severe ipsilateral hearing loss, ipsilateral peripheral-type facial paralysis, ipsilateral decreased facial sensation, contralateral decreased limb sensation, and, sometimes, ipsilateral limb ataxia. The AICA syndrome is much less common than the lateral medullary syndrome. Other basilar branch occlusions and lacunae may produce dizziness. Cerebellar hemorrhages may present with symptoms similar to those of vestibular neuronitis. There may be sudden onset of dizziness, which may be spinning and made worse by movement. Limb ataxia and headache are often absent, and unassisted walking is impossible. That there usually is no nystagmus is an important differential point, since patients with acute peripheral vestibular lesions who are unable to walk usually have nystagmus. The diagnosis of cerebellar hemorrhage can be made with a computed tomography (CT) scan without contrast enhancement. If cerebellar hemorrhage is suspected, it is imperative that a CT scan be performed without delay, because once these patients become obtunded from brainstem compression, the prognosis is poor. Cerebellar infarction in the distribution of the distal posterior inferior cerebellar artery (PICA) is important, because with intravenous free water these infarcts often swell and result in brainstem compression. Infarction in this distribution spares the brainstem and damages the inferior and medial ipsilateral cerebellar hemisphere. Patients are dizzy and unsteady; there is no limb ataxia. The clinical clue is nystagmus beating to the left on left lateral gaze and to the right on right lateral gaze, whereas in acute labyrinthine disease the nystagmus should beat only in one direction whatever the direction of gaze. Tumors involving the brainstem may affect both balance and hearing. Usually, there are other neurologic signs and symptoms suggestive of brainstem disease. Demyelinating disease may present with dizziness as the initial symptom; with time, other signs and symptoms suggestive of central nervous system abnormality appear. In many degenerative diseases of the central nervous system, dizziness and instability of gait and posture are prominent symptoms. These disorders include cerebellar and spinocerebellar degenerative diseases and progressive supranuclear palsy.

Cerebral cortex

The sensation of dizziness occasionally can come from the cerebral cortex. Penfield demonstrated that stimulation of the parietal cortex provoked sensations of dizziness. Vestibular epilepsy occurs with two types of presentation. In the more common type, spinning dizziness is an ictal phenomenon of a partial seizure disorder. The less common type is a generalized seizure disorder provoked by a vestibular stimulus such as rotation or caloric stimulation. Hydrocephalus may produce problems with balance and stability. Patients complain of unsteady gait and instability of balance. They have a shuffling, small-stepped gait and, often, difficulty initiating gait, called *apraxia of gait*. Memory loss and urinary urgency or incontinence are often part of this syndrome.

DIFFERENTIATION OF CENTRAL (BRAINSTEM) AND PERIPHERAL (EIGHTH NERVE AND INNER EAR) Dizziness

The sensation of motion alone does not permit a differentiation between ear and central nervous system disease. Spinning dizziness can come from the ear or the brain. Only the associated symptoms and signs enable one to make the differential diagnosis. Headache at the back of the head or between the ears can come from ear or brain disease. Pain perceived on the forehead, in the eye, or at the root of the nose is suggestive of disease in the posterior fossa. Facial or extremity numbness is consistent with disease in the brain, as is limb ataxia, focal weakness, double vision, trouble with speech, and trouble swallowing. In acute situations, close attention must be given to disturbances of consciousness. One must differentiate between the vertiginous patient who wants to lie still and the patient who is unable to maintain alertness. The combination of dizziness and impairment of consciousness suggests widespread involvement of the brainstem consistent with a tumor or basilar artery occlusion. It is important to recognize basilar artery disease, because relatively mild symptoms can rapidly progress to devastating and irreversible deficits. The clues to the identification of brainstem disease are the associated neurologic symptoms and signs; it is not possible to make the diagnosis of brainstem disease on the basis of dizziness alone. Although as many as 25% of patients who subsequently develop clear basilar transient ischemic attacks initially present with unaccompanied dizziness, the diagnosis cannot be made at that time. Fortunately, these patients usually demonstrate other signs and symptoms before a permanent deficit occurs. Hearing loss and positional dizziness are more common with inner ear disease but can be seen with diseases of the brainstem.

Spontaneous and gaze nystagmus

The characteristics of nystagmus can sometimes help localize an abnormality. The usual inner ear nystagmus is horizontal or rotary and beats in only one direction. The components of the nystagmus may vary as the eyes are moved in different positions. Thus, in one position the nystagmus may be mainly horizontal and in another position more vertical. After acute severe damage to one inner ear or eighth nerve, there may be nystagmus with the fast-phase beating to the side opposite the lesion in all directions of gaze. Nystagmus beating to the right on right lateral gaze and to the left on left lateral gaze is characteristic of nystagmus from the central nervous system. The most common cause of this type of nystagmus is drug effect. Nystagmus that is different in the two eyes (dissociated), pure vertical nystagmus, and direction-changing nystagmus all are from the central nervous system. If nystagmus is present for days or weeks without accompanying dizziness, it is from the central nervous system. Nystagmus that does not change its components as the eyes are moved around is consistent with a central nervous system lesion.

HEARING

Disorders of the auditory system are manifested by reduced ability to hear, distortion of the ability to hear, increased sensitivity to sound, and the production of sound or the perception of sound when it is not present (tinnitus). A conductive hearing loss occurs when sound is better conducted through the bone of the skull than through the air and the ossicles in the middle ear to the inner ear. Fluid, infection, tumor, and fixation of the ossicles (as in otosclerosis) result in a conductive hearing loss. Damage to the cochlea results in a sensory neural hearing loss characterized by a decrease in the ability to hear pure tones and a proportionate decrease in the ability to understand speech. There also may be distortion of perceived sounds. Lesions affecting the eighth nerve, such as acoustic neuromas, produce hearing losses that may vary. Typically, there is a high-frequency hearing loss, and speech discrimination is more severely affected than would be expected from the pure tone loss. Damage to the auditory pathways in the brainstem often does not produce hearing loss, because there is so much crossing of the auditory pathways that it requires large bilateral lesions to produce hearing loss. However, there may be difficulty with complicated or competing auditory stimuli or with localization of sound. Lesions in the temporal lobe may produce impairment of the ability to understand speech, with competing background words in the ear contralateral to the lesion.

Testing of hearing is precise and standardized in the audiogram. This test investigates behavioral hearing by presenting pure tones or words at different frequencies, by either air or bone conduction, to determine the thresholds for pure tone hearing at frequencies from 250 to 8000 Hz. The ability to understand speech is an important function of the auditory apparatus and can sometimes help localize the site of an auditory lesion. Speech discrimination is tested by giving phonetically balanced words at an intensity 40 Db above threshold and recording the percentage of correct responses. The audiogram is most helpful in documenting behavioral hearing and in identifying and localizing hearing loss from the middle and inner ear. At times, it can help differentiate inner ear from eighth nerve disease. A more sensitive test of abnormalities of the eighth nerve or brainstem is short-latency auditory-evoked potentials. These are submicrovolt potentials that can be recorded in the first 7 msec after an auditory stimulus such as a broad-band click with surface electrodes at the scalp and the ear lobe. A series of reproducible waves at constant interwave latencies is found in normals. With conductive or cochlear hearing loss, all waves are delayed. With damage to the auditory pathways in the eighth nerve or brainstem, there may be interwave latency prolongations, loss of waves, or distortion of waves. This test is extremely sensitive in the diagnosis of acoustic neuromas, with a false-negative rate of between 4% and 8%, and may show abnormalities in brainstem lesions when hearing is normal, as is often the case in multiple sclerosis.

CLINICAL EVALUATION

The clinical evaluation of patients with balance and hearing problems should begin with a thorough and careful history and a physical examination focused especially on hearing loss and dizziness, as well as possible associated neurologic symptoms and signs. The audiogram should often be the initial test for patients with hearing loss or auditory symptoms, and it should be performed on most patients with balance problems. If there is a unilateral hearing loss, the next test should be auditory-evoked potentials, to search for a possible retrocochlear locus of abnormality. If the evoked potentials are abnormal and consistent with an eighth-nerve lesion, an imaging study must be performed. The most sensitive technique for looking at the posterior fossa, and especially the internal auditory canal, is contrast-enhanced magnetic resonance imaging (MRI) scan. This imaging method permits the identification of intracanalicular acoustic neuromas and small brainstem lesions, as well as large cerebellopontine angle lesions. The CT scan is still a good way to look at the posterior fossa. It is superior to the MRI scan for acute hemorrhages, but it does not visualize intracanalicular acoustic neuromas or tumors extending less than 1 cm into the posterior fossa. It is necessary to use intravenous contrast enhancement to visualize acoustic neuromas on the CT scan.

If the symptom of concern is dizziness or imbalance, it is often helpful to obtain tests of vestibular and balance function. Among the battery of tests of balance that can help localize and characterize abnormalities are the electronystagmogram (ENG), sinusoidal vertical axis rotation, visual-vestibular interaction rotation testing, and posturography. The ENG is a battery of tests in which eye movements are recorded under conditions designed to demonstrate different functions of the vestibular system. Eye movements are recorded with eyes open in the light, eyes open in the dark, and eyes closed. Spontaneous, gaze, optokinetic, positional, and caloric nystagmus are recorded, as well as saccades and pursuit eye movements. These tests give information about the brainstem control of eye movements, the brainstem vestibular system, and the inner ear and eighth-nerve vestibular system. Sinusoidal vertical axis rotation is a sensitive computerized test of the vestibulo-ocular reflex of the horizontal semicircular canals that is complementary to caloric stimulation but more sensitive and more reliable. Visual-vestibular interaction testing gives information about the relationships among the inner ear vestibular system, the brainstem, the cerebellum, and the visual systems by rotating the patient with eyes open in the dark, with visual fixation, and with optokinetic stimulation. Dynamic posturography permits a different and more direct investigation of balance than has been previously available. Patients stand on a platform that can measure sway with strain gauges and computer control. The platform can be moved in different directions, as can a visual surround, to make the task more difficult and to selectively abolish or distort sensory inputs such as vision and proprioception. These tests permit an objective characterization of standing balance under a variety of conditions and may give functional information about an individual's difficulty with balance.

TREATMENT

Choice of treatment depends on the cause of symptoms and the type of symptoms. Acoustic neuromas are usually surgically resected. Dizziness associated with hypothyroidism often resolves upon treatment with thyroid, and dizziness from partial seizures resolves with anticonvulsant treatment. Episodes of spinning dizziness from inner ear dysfunction may be treated with vestibular suppressant medications such as meclizine, dimenhydrinate, and promethazine. The disadvantages of these medications are that they often cause drowsiness and that they may make some patient's balance worse by suppressing a damaged vestibular system. Diphenidol is an effective vestibular suppressant that does not cause drowsiness, but in a small percentage of patients it causes visual hallucinations. Some physicians advocate treatment with low-salt diets, diuretics, and the avoidance of caffeine. These treatments have not been proven to be effective. Lightheaded unsteady dizziness often decreases when patients are treated with small doses of benzodiazepines. There is evidence from animal experiments that diazepam suppresses vestibular nucleus firing rates and therefore acts as a vestibular suppressant as well as having a tranquilizing effect. This class of medication usually only partially suppresses symptoms and may be habituating, so stopping medication can exacerbate symptoms. Persistent episodes of spinning dizziness that do not stop with medication and can be proven to come from one ear can usually be stopped with a labyrinthectomy or selective vestibular nerve section. The nerve section is designed to preserve hearing. The labyinthectomy completely destroys hearing. Patients with positional dizziness or persistent (rather than episodic) dizziness or instability are often able to decrease their symptoms by performing exercises designed to produce central nervous system adaptation or compensation. These exercises (vestibular physical therapy) are most effective when they are tailored to the patient's deficit and modified by interaction between a trained therapist and the patient. Preliminary data from several groups suggest that vestibular physical therapy is very helpful in decreasing symptoms of dizziness and imbalance.

REFERENCES

Baloh RW: Dizziness, hearing loss, and tinnitus: the essentials of neurotology, Philadelphia, 1984, Davis.

Baloh RW and Honrubia V: Clinical neurophysiology of the vestibular system, ed 2. Philadelphia, 1990, Davis.

Honrubia V and Brazier MAB, editors. Nystagmus and vertigo: clinical approaches to the patient with dizziness. Orlando, Fla, 1982, Academic.

Rudge P: Clinical neuro-otology. New York, 1983, Churchill-Livingstone.

CHAPTER

116 Disorders of Speech and Language

Daniel B. Hier

Disordered speech and language are among the most important signs of neurologic disease. Careful evaluation of the speech-disordered patient gives clues to the etiology and anatomic site of neurologic illness. A disorder of language always implies disease of the cerebrum. A language disorder is a defect in the ability to understand linguistic symbols or a defect in the ability to express meaning using linguistic symbols. Language disorders can disrupt either oral language (aphasia) or written language (alexia or agraphia). These language disorders are usually caused by injury to language-related structures in the frontal, temporal, parietal, and occipital lobes of the dominant hemisphere or their underlying subcortical connections. In addition to aphasia, a variety of other speech disorders may result from injury elsewhere in the nervous system (the nondominant hemisphere, the frontal lobes, the cerebellum and its connections, the basal ganglia and their connections, the corticospinal tract and its connections, the peripheral nerves innervating respiratory and oropharyngeal muscles) or dysfunction outside the nervous system, including the respiratory apparatus, the oropharynx, and the tongue.

APHASIA

Testing for aphasia

Aphasia is tested at the bedside by examining the patient for defects in repetition of speech, impairment in comprehension, abnormalities in speech fluency, and difficulties in word retrieval.

Repetition. Repetition is tested by having the patient repeat short phrases (e.g., "I am here," "no ifs ands or buts," etc.). Repetition is normal or near-normal in anomic aphasia and the transcortical aphasias. Repetition is abnormal in conduction aphasia, Broca's aphasia, Wernicke's aphasia, and global aphasia.

Comprehension. Comprehension is tested by having the patient follow one-step, two-step, and three-step spoken commands. Patients who can follow simple two-step or three-step commands are considered to have grossly intact comprehension for the purposes of aphasia classification.

Although gross comprehension is generally impaired in Wernicke's aphasia, patients with milder degrees of aphasia show a less severe pattern of comprehension defects. Even aphasics without gross comprehension deficits have trouble comprehending complex logicogrammatical constructions (e.g., "Put the red chip in front of the white chip," "What relation to you is your mother's brother?" or "Does summer come before spring?").

Fluency. Fluency encompasses two somewhat different concepts: quantity of speech output and ease of speech output. Fluent aphasics produce utterances of longer length (usually five or more words) and produce more words per unit time than do nonfluent aphasics (normal speakers produce more than 100 words per minute). Furthermore, fluent aphasics speak easily and without effort. Nonfluent aphasics produce sparse speech that is hesitant, labored, and effortful. Problems in classification occur with aphasics who speak their utterances effortlessly, but generate little output because of severe word-retrieval problems. This often occurs in Wernicke's aphasia where speech output (quantity of words per minute) is reduced as a result of severe anomia. Since utterances are easily articulated these aphasics should still be classified as fluent despite sparse speech output. Wernicke's, conduction, anomic, and transcortical sensory aphasias are classified as fluent aphasias. Nonfluent aphasias include Broca's aphasia, transcortical motor aphasia, transcortical mixed aphasia, and global aphasia.

Word retrieval. Word retrieval problems can be elicited by asking the patient to name commonplace objects, or they may become apparent during spontaneous speech. Word retrieval deficits are called *anomia.* Anomia is a central feature of all aphasias but also occurs in dementia, encephalopathy, and delirium. Anomia may occur upon confrontation naming of objects or in running speech. Among aphasic and demented subjects, speech is altered in predictable ways by word-retrieval problems. Lexical access is generally more difficult for nouns than for verbs and adjectives. Prepositions and conjunctions are least affected. High-frequency nouns (e.g., *cat*) are easier to retrieve than low-frequency nouns (e.g., *gyroscope*). Picturable nouns are easier to retrieve than abstract nouns. Indicators of anomia are numerous. *Circumlocutions* are attempts by anomic patients to substitute a description of a word for the unretrievable word (e.g., a watch is called "something I tell time with"). Excessive use of circumlocutions makes the speech verbose. Empty words such as *thing, one, those,* etc. are used in place of more specific nouns. Pronouns are used in place of nouns, giving anomic speech an empty quality. Other manifestations of word retrieval difficulties include verbal paraphasia (substitution of one word for another, such as *clock* for *watch*) and neologisms (invented words).

Classification of aphasia

Controversy exists about the validity of aphasia syndromes. Although aphasics are routinely assigned a diagnostic category, one third of aphasics cannot be easily categorized. Discrepancies in classification of aphasics are commonplace even among experienced raters. Within a given aphasia category (e.g., Wernicke's aphasia), heterogeneity exists among aphasics. Furthermore, there is not an exact relationship between areas of cerebral injury and any given aphasia syndrome. Despite these problems, aphasia categorization is a routine and often useful exercise. The most widely accepted classification scheme is that of the Boston Diagnostic Aphasia Examination. Most aphasiologists recognize eight forms of aphasia: anomic, conduction, Broca's, Wernicke's, global, transcortical motor sensory, transcortical mixed, and transcortical sensory.

Wernicke's aphasia. The speech of patients with Wernicke's aphasia is well articulated with normal melody, rhythm, and inflection. Fluency (as measured by both ease of articulation and quantity of output) is often normal. Some Wernicke's aphasics are laconic with sparse output, reflecting severe word-retrieval problems. Other Wernicke's aphasics are verbose with sometimes uncontrollable verbal output (logorrhea). Although grammatical structure is often intact, the information conveyed is diminished. An excess of words is used to convey little meaning (circumlocution), reflecting the limited use of substantive words. Nonspecific or empty words (*it, thing, this,* etc.) are used excessively. In Wernicke's aphasia, verbal paraphasic errors (word substitutions) predominate over phonemic paraphasic errors (sound substitutions). Some word substitutions are invented words; these are termed *neologisms.* Frequent use of neologisms creates jargon. Reading comprehension, auditory comprehension, naming, and repetition of speech are impaired. Oral reading is occasionally relatively spared. Elementary neurologic findings such as hemiparesis and sensory loss are generally not present. A right superior quadrantanopia is present when the lesion injures optic radiations in the left temporal lobe. The responsible lesion is usually in the posterior superior temporal lobe.

Broca's aphasia. Broca's aphasia is a syndrome of nonfluent speech associated with relatively spared comprehension. Speech is laconic and hesitant, giving it a telegraphic quality. Speech is uttered effortfully and lacks normal melody *(dysprosody).* Repetition is severely impaired. Confrontation naming deficits are variable. Articulatory disturbances are often prominent, and a marked dysarthria is usually present. Although commonly associated with Broca's aphasia, these articulatory disturbances are not a true aphasic disorder. Phonemic paraphasias (sound substitution errors) abound in Broca's aphasia. Agrammatism is a further hallmark of Broca's aphasia. Agrammatic speech is characterized by an abundance of substantive words (nouns, verbs, etc.) and few functor words (prepositions, conjunctions, articles). The failure to utilize functors leads to speech that is economical but violates the rules of syntax. Broca's aphasia is usually associated with a dense right hemiparesis. However, rare instances of Broca's aphasia without hemiparesis have been reported. Visual fields and sensation are usually normal. Oral-buccal-lingual apraxia (inability to protrude tongue, pucker lips, whistle, etc.) frequently accompanies Broca's aphasia, reflecting injury to the prefrontal motor cortex. Ideomotor apraxia of the left upper extremity may also accompany Broca's aphasia. These patients pantomime the acts of waving good-bye, hammering, dealing cards, or saluting clumsily with their nonparetic left arm, reflecting interruption of crossing callosal fibers from the left premotor cortex. The ideomotor apraxia can be demonstrated only in the nonparetic left arm that has been disconnected from motor programs in the left parietal lobe (callosal apraxia). The lesion responsible for Broca's aphasia is a large left frontal lesion extending backward to the Rolandic fissure. Lesions limited anatomically to Broca's area produce a transient syndrome of muteness followed by effortful speech that rapidly resolves.

Conduction aphasia. Conduction aphasia is a less common aphasic disorder. Comprehension is well preserved. Spontaneous speech is usually fluent, although it may be contaminated by both phonemic (sound substitution) and verbal (word substitution) paraphasic errors. The hallmark of the disorder is repeated speech that is impaired compared to spontaneous speech. Writing and spelling are impaired. Anomia of varying degrees accompanies conduction aphasia, although the anomia may be mild. Anatomic site of injury in conduction aphasia may be the superior left temporal lobe, the inferior parietal lobe, or the insula and underlying arcuate fasciculus.

Global aphasia. Global aphasia is a common aphasic syndrome characterized by disruption of all language functions including spontaneous speech, naming, repetition, reading, writing, and comprehension. Patients are nonfluent, with little or no speech output. Marked deficits in repetition and comprehension of spoken language are present. Reading comprehension and writing are severely impaired. Global aphasia is often associated with a dense right hemiplegia, right hemisensory loss, and right hemianopia. Uncommon instances of global aphasia without hemiparesis have been reported. The responsible lesion is usually large and encompasses both Wernicke's area in the temporal lobe and Broca's area in the frontal lobe. Global aphasia may follow left carotid occlusion, embolism to the stem of the left middle cerebral artery, or large left basal ganglionic hemorrhages.

Anomic aphasia. Anomic aphasia or amnestic aphasia is a common form of aphasia but one with little localizing significance. In its purest form, it is characterized by normal comprehension and fluent speech complicated by word-finding difficulties. Repetition is normal. Speech may be circumlocutory with verbal paraphasic errors. Confrontation naming is impaired. In its less pure (and more common) form, anomic aphasia is associated with a mild reduction in comprehension of spoken and written language. Characteristically, articulation, prosody, oral reading, repetition, and writing from dictation are normal. Etiologies of anomic aphasia include raised intracranial pressure, brain tumors, toxic and metabolic disorders, head injury, and Alzheimer's disease. In cases of cerebral infarction, anomic aphasia is of little anatomical localizing value (lesions may be left frontal, occipital, parietal, temporal, or deep). Some cases of Wernicke's aphasia resolve into an anomic aphasia during recovery.

Transcortical aphasia. In transcortical aphasia repetition of speech is markedly superior to spontaneous speech. In a few transcortical aphasics, the tendency to indiscriminately repeat all heard speech constitutes *echolalia*. However, echolalia is not an essential feature of transcortical aphasia. Transcortical aphasia contrasts with conduction aphasia, which is characterized by spontaneous speech that is superior to repetition. The major forms of transcortical aphasia are transcortical motor aphasia, transcortical sensory aphasia, transcortical mixed aphasia, and isolation of the speech area. Transcortical motor aphasia resembles Broca's aphasia, but repetition is relatively intact. The lesion is often in the deep subcortical structures of the left frontal lobe. Transcortical sensory aphasia resembles Wernicke's aphasia except that repetition is intact. Transcortical sensory aphasia may occur after posterior temporal or parietal lobe lesions or subcortical lesions that undercut parietal or temporal cortex. Marked deficits in naming, comprehension, and spontaneous speech characterize transcortical mixed aphasia. Repetition is disproportionately spared. Some patients are echolalic and lack spontaneous speech. These severe instances of transcortical mixed aphasia have been termed *isolation of the speech area*.

Thalamic aphasia. The aphasia that follows left thalamic hemorrhage or infarction often has "transcortical" features. Repetition is usually spared. Voice volume is low. Variable word access and comprehension problems occur. When speech output is reduced, the aphasia of left thalamic infarction or hemorrhage resembles transcortical mixed aphasia. Echolalia may occur. When speech output is greater, the aphasia that follows left thalamic stroke resembles transcortical sensory aphasia.

Crossed aphasia. Since the left hemisphere is dominant for language in nearly all right-handers and as many as 60% of left-handers, aphasia after right hemisphere injury is unusual. Crossed aphasia is the combination of right hemisphere injury with aphasia in a right-handed patient. With regard to left-handers, the concept of crossed aphasia is moot since their hemispheric dominance for language is unpredictable. The frequency of crossed aphasia in right-handers after right hemisphere injury ranges from 0.4% to 1.8%. Crossed aphasia may be either fluent or nonfluent. The pattern of anatomical localization of aphasia in cases of crossed aphasia resembles the left hemisphere pattern. Anterior (frontal) lesions are associated with Broca's aphasia and posterior (temporal) lesions with Wernicke's aphasia.

Aphasia therapy

Since its inception, the issue of the efficacy of speech therapy for aphasia has been controversial. Evaluation of the efficacy of speech therapy requires controlling for many variables that influence recovery from aphasia, including age at onset (younger aphasics do better than older aphasics), size and site of lesion (patients with smaller lesions away from the central language zone do better than patients with larger lesions in the central language zone), etiology (those with hemorrhages tend to do better than those with infarctions), handedness (some studies have found that left-handers do better than right-handers), educational and socioeconomic backgrounds, neurobehavioral complications, motivation, insight into language deficits (patients with better insight into their deficits tend to do better), general health of the patient, quality of therapy available, and time elapsed before the onset of therapy. Within 1 to 2 weeks after a stroke or other brain injury, spontaneous recovery begins because of resolution of acute ischemia, hemorrhage, or mass effect. A concomitant improvement in language function also occurs spontaneously. However, the mechanisms governing improvement in aphasia over the long term (months to years) are not understood. Many approaches to therapy have been taken, including both traditional approaches based on principles of education (reteaching language) and techniques aimed at facilitating recovery for specific types of linguistic deficits. In addition to providing therapy, the therapist accurately assesses the speech status of the patient and the psychological support needed. Recent controlled studies have suggested that speech therapy may be efficacious in the recovery from aphasia, especially when motivation, insight, and comprehension are spared.

SPEECH DISORDERS

In addition to aphasia, a variety of speech disorders are frequently encountered, including impaired articulation (dysarthria), impaired melody of speech, impaired voice volume, mutism, and perseveration.

Hypophonia

Decreased voice volume *(hypophonia)* may reflect respiratory or airway difficulties, diseases of the basal ganglia such as Parkinson's disease, or psychiatric disease (hysteria, malingering, depression, or schizophrenia). *Aphonia* is a complete loss of voice. Aphonic patients may be unable to phonate for a variety of reasons, including respiratory difficulties; paralysis of respiratory muscles; abnormalities of the tongue, larynx, and oropharynx; bulbar paralysis; and pseudobulbar palsy.

Dysarthria

Dysarthria is a broad term that encompasses a variety of disorders of speech articulation. Dysarthria is a disorder of speech, not language. Dysarthric patients need not be aphasic, although many patients with aphasia (especially motor or Broca's aphasics) are dysarthric. Dysarthria can arise from structural lesions of the pharynx, tongue, palate, or lips, from dysfunction of muscles that control the vocal apparatus, or from neurologic dysfunction of the peripheral and cranial nerves, brainstem nuclei, or cortical centers and pathways controlling the vocal apparatus. Three major types of dysarthria are recognized.

Paretic dysarthria or *flaccid dysarthria* is characterized by weakness of the muscles of articulation. The responsible lesion disrupts the function of the lower motor neuron with paralysis of the lips, tongue, or soft palate. Paretic dysarthria may complicate bulbar poliomyelitis, progressive bulbar palsy, brainstem stroke, or idiopathic polyneuritis. The flaccid state of the musculature of both respiratory apparatus and oropharynx produces speech that is of low volume, hypernasal, and poorly articulated.

Spastic dysarthria or *rigid dysarthria* occurs with lesions of the upper motor neuron. The most common cause of spastic dysarthria is single or multiple strokes. Voice volume may be good but the voice has a harsh, sometimes strangled quality. Melody and rhythm of speech are choppy *(dysprosody)*. Articulation is impaired.

Ataxic dysarthria occurs with cerebellar disease. It is seen most commonly with cerebellar degeneration (hereditary or alcoholic) or multiple sclerosis. The speech of these patients is characterized by the inappropriate stress on unstressed syllables (scanning speech) that is one hallmark of cerebellar disease. Voice volume may vary excessively. Speaking rate is decreased. At times poorly controlled expirations of air betray the ataxic quality of the speech. Voice volume is generally good.

Hypokinetic dysarthria is typical of Parkinson's disease and multi-infarct dementia. Voice volume is low and there is marked hypoprosody.

Hyperkinetic dysarthrias occur with certain other basal ganglia diseases such as Huntington's chorea and torsion dystonia. The speech disorder tends to parallel the hyperkinetic movements found in the limbs. There may be excessive variations in speaking rate, voice tremor, excessive variation in voice volume, and impaired articulation.

Mutism

Mutism is failure to speak. Mutism may occur for a variety of reasons. *Pure word mutism* (also known as *cortical anarthria* or *aphemia*) is inability to speak caused by cerebral injury. Auditory and reading comprehension are intact. Written expression is usually normal. Recovery from initial mutism is the rule. The cerebral lesion is usually in the area of the left frontal lobe responsible for articulation. Loss of language (aphasia) is an important cause of mutism. Patients with global aphasia or severe Wernicke's aphasia may be mute because they cannot formulate any language. Similarly, mutism may complicate the late phases of the degenerative dementias (Pick's disease and Alzheimer's disease) when profound aphasia deprives the patient of spontaneous speech.

Mutism may be a complication of certain psychiatric conditions, including catatonic schizophrenia, severe depression, malingering, and conversion reaction. Mutism also occurs with akinetic mutism, chronic vegetative state, and "locked-in" state. In *akinetic mutism* there is a profound abulia (usually resulting from hydrocephalus or bifrontal damage). Patients fail to speak as a result of profound lack of motivation and mental inertia. Patients in a *chronic veg-*

etative state have sustained massive brain damage and are severely demented. Although these patients go through sleep-wake cycles, they show little evidence of intellectual activity. They may gaze purposively about the room, but never speak. Chronic vegetative state may follow severe anoxia, hypotension, hypoglycemia, or head trauma with diffuse brain injury. In chronic vegetative state the electroencephalogram is abnormal with severe slowing and low voltage. *Locked-in* patients are alert but are unable to move or speak as a result of a brainstem lesion, usually in the mid or low pons. The lesion is low enough in the pons to spare the reticular activating system in the upper pons and midbrain so alertness is preserved. "Locked-in" patients are quadriplegic and unable to move most oral-facial musculature. The electroencephalogram shows relatively normal activity, and the patient can understand speech and writing. Vertical eye movements and eyelid blinking (which are controlled by midbrain structures) are preserved as the only communication system available to the "locked-in" patient.

Perserverative speech disorders

Cortical stuttering. Although stuttering is a common developmental disorder of childhood, it also occurs in some adults after brain injury. *Stuttering* is characterized by the abnormal repetition of individual syllables. Most cases of cortical stuttering are associated with aphasia and left hemisphere damage.

Palilalia. *Palilalia* is abnormal repetition of syllables, words, or short phrases. It may be difficult to distinguish palilalia from cortical stuttering, which involves the involuntary repetition of an initial syllable. Palilalia occurs in Parkinson's disease and other diseases of the basal ganglia. Palilalia may also complicate aphasia or dementia.

Echolalia. *Echolalia* is the abnormal tendency to echo words and phrases. In striking cases the patient may fail to comprehend the request but accurately repeat it (e.g., when asked "Tell me your name?" the patient may simply reply "Tell me your name.") Echolalia may occur in a variety of disorders including advanced Alzheimer's disease, infantile autism, schizophrenia, and transcortical aphasia.

Disordered speech melody

Prosody is the musical quality of speech produced by variations in pitch, rhythm, and stress of pronunciation. In *hyperprosody,* normal prosodic variations are exaggerated. Hyperprosody sometimes occurs in manic psychiatric states. *Dysprosody* is the loss of normal melody of speech that occurs after left frontal lobe damage. The speech is halting, dysarthric, and lacks normal rhythm and melody. Dysprosody is a characteristic of Broca's aphasia and other motor aphasias. In hypoprosody, normal prosodic variations are lost. Speech has a dull and monotonous quality. Hypoprosody is characteristic of Parkinson's disease and is often accompanied by low voice volume. After right hemisphere damage, some patients are unable to intone affect into their speech. Their speech has a flat, unemotional quality. This deficit is known as *aprosody*. In practice, it is difficult to distinguish aprosody from hypoprosody. However, the term *aprosody* is usually reserved for the prosodic disturbance that follows right hemisphere damage, whereas *hypoprosody* is used to describe the prosodic disturbance of Parkinson's disease and other basal ganglionic disorders.

DISORDERS OF WRITTEN LANGUAGE

Agraphia

Agraphia is a disorder of written language caused by brain disease. Writing may be disrupted by several mechanisms: words may be misspelled (a disorder of language), letters may be malformed (dysmorphic letters suggest either constructional or ideomotor apraxia), or words may be misplaced on the page (a spatial disorder). *Pure agraphia* is the misspelling of words in the absence of gross aphasia, apraxia, or alexia. It is usually associated with focal left parietal lobe disease. It may occur in association with the other elements of Gerstmann's syndrome (dyscalculia, right-left confusion, and finger agnosia). *Aphasic agraphia* is impaired writing found in association with aphasia. Agraphia may occur with either fluent aphasia (e.g., Wernicke's) or nonfluent aphasia (e.g., Broca's). The writing deficit is at least as severe as the oral language deficit, although exceptions have been reported. *Apraxic agraphia* results from loss of the skilled motor programs necessary for writing. Handwriting is performed clumsily and the letters are poorly formed. Other signs of ideomotor apraxia are usually present. Apraxic agraphia may follow damage to the left parietal lobe. Spatial agraphia may occur after right hemisphere injury. There is no aphasic deficit and words are properly spelled. However, left unilateral spatial neglect interferes with the correct placement of letters and words on the page. Constructional apraxia is often present as well.

Alexia

Pure alexia or *alexia without agraphia* is an acquired disorder of reading with preserved writing. Pure alexia is also known as *occipital alexia, posterior alexia, pure word blindness, verbal alexia,* and *receptive* or *sensory alexia*. Gross aphasia is absent, although mild degrees of anomia may be present. A right homonymous hemianopia regularly accompanies pure alexia, although rare cases without hemianopia have been reported. Color agnosia (the inability to name colors present visually) frequently accompanies pure alexia. Typically the lesion responsible for pure alexia is in the left occipital lobe and is large enough to involve both the left visual cortex and fibers crossing the splenium of the corpus callosum from the right visual cortex. Pure alexia may also occur after deep lesions near the angular gyrus. These subangular lesions presumably disconnect the angular gyrus from visual input. *Alexia with agraphia* is most commonly associated with lesions in the angular gyrus region. It is also known as *parietal alexia* or *aphasic alexia*. Both reading and writing are disturbed. A mild fluent aphasia often accompanies alexia with agraphia. Anomia and verbal paraphasias are often present. Visual field disturbances (either a right homonymous hemianopia or a right inferior quadrantanopia) are variably present. Elements of Gerstmann's syndrome and constructional apraxia often accompany alexia with agraphia. *Frontal alexia* is the alexia that occurs with frontal lobe damage and Broca's aphasia. Oral reading and reading comprehension are often limited to single substantive words, with little ability to read paragraph-length material aloud or for comprehension.

REFERENCES

Albert ML and Helm-Estabrooks N: Diagnosis and treatment of aphasia. Parts I and II. JAMA 259:1043 and 259:1205, 1988.

Damasio AR: Aphasia. N Engl J Med 326:531, 1992.

Darby JK, editor: Speech and language evaluation in neurology: adult disorders. Orlando, Fla, 1985, Grune & Stratton.

Hier DB, Gorelick PB, and Shindler AG: Topics in behavioral neurology and neuropsychology. Stoneham, Mass, 1987, Butterworths.

II NEUROLOGIC DISEASES

CHAPTER

117 Epilepsy

John Davenport

PATHOPHYSIOLOGY

The term *epilepsy,* or *seizure disorder,* broadly denotes recurrent episodes of disturbed behavior caused by paroxysmal, uncontrolled, hypersynchronous discharges of cerebral neurons. Clinical seizure events are symptoms of intrinsic cerebral disease or of alteration of cerebral function by systemic conditions.

Epileptic hyperactivity arises in the complex circuitry of cerebral gray matter. The patterned, asynchronous activity of cortical neurons, which is the physiologic basis of normal integrative cerebral function, is replaced by an abnormal synchronous discharge of cortical cells. When restricted to only a small portion of cerebral gray matter, this pathologic electrical activity is termed an *epileptogenic focus.* Such asymptomatic localized disturbances may spread by physiologic mechanisms to recruit anatomically contiguous gray matter, to create a larger abnormality and cause focal cerebral symptoms. They may also involve more widely projecting connections within or between the hemispheres. When conditions are suitable, subcortical integrating mechanisms may become involved, resulting in a generalized discharge of the cerebral cortex and its downstream connections.

The great variety of clinical seizure manifestations is thus the result of the interaction of several possible disturbances: (1) local alterations of cerebral cortex structure, either congenital or acquired, resulting in a tendency to abnormal synchronization; (2) local and systemic biochemical and metabolic factors that alter a given cell's firing characteristics; (3) variations of the interconnections between cortical and subcortical regions that integrate normal cerebral function; and (4) the maturation and evolution of brain tissue during childhood, adolescence, and adulthood. Interactions among these multiple factors determine the effective threshold for seizure discharge, the route and speed of spread from a focal abnormality, the presence or absence of generalized convulsions, and the likelihood of recurrent attacks. The physiologic functions of the brain areas where the discharge begins and through which it spreads determine the form of the individual patient's seizures.

CLINICAL SEIZURE PATTERNS

The archetype of epileptic seizures, the generalized tonic-clonic convulsion (major motor, or grand mal, seizure), is an impressive and frightening experience for both patient and observer (see box below). The patient abruptly ceases ongoing behavior and falls. There is rigid stiffening of the muscles, including chest and abdomen, causing cyanosis, a garbled cry or groan, and often incontinence of urine. This tonic phase gives over shortly to rhythmic clonic muscular jerking that gradually decreases in frequency and dies away. The ictal convulsion rarely lasts more than 2 or 3 min and leaves the patient in a limp, unresponsive state. Progressive recovery occurs in a postictal phase characterized by confusion, lethargy, headache, and diffuse myalgia, which lasts several hours or, less often, up to several days, until full baseline function is restored. The patient has only vague or no recall of the onset and no memory of the ictal events or of a portion of the postictal period.

A second common pattern is the *absence seizure (petit mal seizure),* wherein the patient, almost always a child,

Classification of epileptic seizures

- Generalized (no detectable focus)
  - Tonic-clonic (grand mal)
  - Absence (petit mal)
  - Tonic
  - Myoclonic
  - Clonic
  - Akinetic
- Partial (focal onset)
  - Simple (consciousness intact)
    - Motor
    - Sensory
    - Autonomic
    - Psychic
  - Complex (consciousness impaired)
    - Simple onset, with later impairment of consciousness
    - Impaired consciousness at onset
- Partial evolving to secondarily generalized convulsion

abruptly stops activity and stares vacantly, perhaps with a fluttering of the eyelids or minor changes in muscle tone or posture. A motor convulsion does not occur, and after only 5 to 10 seconds the child quite abruptly recovers to a completely normal state, with partial or complete amnesia of the period of staring.

Other less common generalized seizure types also occur primarily in infants and children, including *tonic seizures,* a sudden stiffening of trunk or limb muscles with loss of consciousness lasting 10 to 60 seconds; *myoclonic seizures,* manifested by single or sequential sudden jerks of limb muscles without altered consciousness; *clonic seizures,* with impaired consciousness and jerking lasting for several minutes and demonstrating quite variable distribution and symmetry; and *akinetic seizures,* brief loss of tone with intact awareness, producing head nodding if involving only neck muscles but, with more diffuse distribution, leading to falling and possible injury.

All these generalized seizure types can be related to more or less complete involvement of both hemispheres. In many attacks, however, restricted electrical discharge leads to a wide range of focal or partial symptoms and signs.

Simple partial seizures may occur in the form of isolated, self-limited motor or sensory features. There can be rhythmic jerking of the hand or part of the face, turning of the head or eyes, speech arrest, or inarticulate vocalization when the precentral cortex is involved. Unpleasant paresthesias of limbs or face, clicking or buzzing sounds, flickering unformed light patterns, or foul smell or taste sensations may result from discharges in the various primary sensory cortical areas. More often, partial seizures are composed of a series of symptoms caused by a "march" of epileptic neuronal activity sequentially involving different cortical areas. *Jacksonian seizure* is the historic eponym applied to clonic movements gradually migrating from face to hand, or the reverse; but this is only one of many diverse patterns of involvement of multiple cortical functions.

Extremely varied and complicated experiences result from activation of temporal-parietal association areas, with psychic symptoms of inappropriate familiarity (deja vu) or unfamiliarity, detailed sensory distortions or hallucinations, intricate memory experiences, and "dreamy states." Emotions of anxiety, fear, or, less commonly, euphoria or ecstasy may be produced by activation of medial temporal areas. Any of these may be reported by the patient with intact consciousness and complete memory for the spell, an essential criterion for *simple partial seizures* (SPS).

Complex partial seizures (CPS), on the other hand, by definition have total or partial interruption of memory and consciousness, and patients usually have inappropriate responsiveness to the environment during the ictus. These deficits correlate with discharge within the limbic system circuits in the medial temporal and frontal lobes of one or both hemispheres, including cingulate gyrus, hippocampus, and septal area.

CPS attacks often begin with a motionless stare, abruptly interrupting previous behavior. After only a few seconds there is a second phase of stereotyped nonpurposeful movements, or *automatisms,* such as swallowing, lip-smacking, chewing, pacing, repetitive or fumbling hand movements, humming, or mumbling. This phase lasts a minute or so, during which the patient is amnestic and apparently unaware of the environment. After this there is a subtle transition to more environmental responsiveness, with more coordinated and purposeful activity, including intelligible verbalization, but with persistent amnesia. The return of memory, roughly defining the end of the ictal phase, occurs about 3 and rarely more than 5 minutes after onset. The stereotypic ictal automatisms have been related to discharge in the anteromedial temporal areas, near the amygdala nucleus, and are common and objective features of CPS attacks. Although CPS usually arise from lesions in the temporal lobe *(temporal lobe epilepsy, psychomotor seizures),* they may be manifestations of pathology in the frontal or parietal lobes.

An *aura* is a brief sensation remembered by the patient before loss of consciousness occurs in a complex partial or generalized seizure. An aura indicates that the seizure began focally and, by its specific quality, suggests the seizure's anatomic focus. An aura lasting more than a few seconds is classified as SPS; if proceeding to evolve to other stereotyped ictal signs without responsiveness or memory, it then would become CPS, especially if an automatism occurs. A common example of CPS would be a feeling of strange, fearful uneasiness, followed in a few seconds by an involuntary turning of the head to the side; then with lapse of memory, a smacking of lips, and staring lasting 2 minutes; and finally, a dazed and confused period of 20 minutes.

Attacks of amnesia or staring spells occurring with other simple or complex patterns but without convulsion are often erroneously called "petit mal." Particularly in adulthood, such attacks are usually CPS and imply a need for investigation of the responsible focal lesion. Similarly, seizures that appear to be classic nonfocal grand mal attacks may result from the rapid generalization of an initially focal discharge.

In childhood and early adolescence, approximately two thirds of patients with recurrent seizures have no detectable epileptic focus. In late adolescence and adulthood, the distribution inverts, and "late-onset" seizures are usually the result of acquired localized cerebral damage.

ETIOLOGY

Metabolic causes (see box at upper right)

Cerebral neuronal function is dependent on critical supplies of glucose and oxygen, on electrolyte distribution across cell membranes, and on the detoxifying processes of visceral organs. In general, the more rapid the metabolic change, either from normality or back toward normality during therapeutic procedures, the more likely a seizure is to occur. Seizures caused by metabolic disturbances are usually generalized motor convulsions, although partial seizures may result from hypoglycemia, and from hypocalcemia in neonates. Focal features appearing in these and other systemic derangements should be considered to have an underlying structural cause until it is reasonably demonstrated otherwise.

Single or even multiple seizures occurring in the con-

Common causes of seizure

- Metabolic factors, especially
  - Hypoglycemia
  - Hypoxia
  - Hyponatremia
  - Hypocalcemia
  - Acid-base disturbances
  - Organ failure: renal, hepatic
  - Drug withdrawal: alcohol, sedatives
  - Drug intoxication: aminophylline, lidocaine
- Focal cortex lesions, including
  - Infarction
  - Contusion
  - Tumor
  - Abscess
  - Meningitis
  - Encephalitis
- Congenital: hereditary or acquired
  - Idiopathic
    - Grand mal
    - Petit mal
  - Perinatal injury
  - Maldevelopment
  - Degenerations

text of an acute illness, with metabolic derangement, fever, and possible medication side effects, are not considered to be epilepsy. They are regarded as *provoked* or *symptomatic seizures*. With resolution of the illness the prognosis is usually good unless structural damage has occurred, and chronic antiepileptic drug treatment is unnecessary.

Focal cortex lesions

Any disease that results in damage to cortical tissue may cause a seizure and lead to a chronic epileptic disorder. Determining factors include the magnitude and acuteness of the derangement and the specific site of injury. The temporal and basal frontal lobes and the peri-Rolandic motor and sensory areas are more likely to support epileptic dysrhythmias than are the parietal and occipital lobes, in part because of their extensive limbic and thalamic connections. A partial or generalized seizure may occur at the time of an ischemic stroke, or brain hemorrhage. Some patients may first have seizures several months after the acute event, following evolution of the cortical scar. Seizures occur rarely in transient ischemic attacks (TIAs) or cerebral and brainstem lacunar strokes.

Head trauma may cause epileptogenic cortical scarring as a result of brain laceration by depressed fracture or penetrating wounds. More frequently, closed head injuries are associated with contusions of the frontal or temporal lobes. Again there is usually delayed onset of partial or secondarily generalized seizures, 6 months to a few years after the traumatic incident. The risk of late epilepsy is directly related to the duration of posttraumatic stupor and identifiable local brain contusion, hematoma, or direct penetration.

A partial or generalized seizure may be the first symptom of brain tumor, either primary or metastatic. Seizures occur in about one third of tumor patients sometime during the course of illness; low-grade primary neoplasms occasionally are discovered after many years of follow-up for "idiopathic" epilepsy. The highest incidence of neoplastic epilepsy occurs in middle-aged or elderly adults, particularly those with partial seizure patterns.

Acute bacterial and viral infections may be complicated by partial or generalized seizures precipitated by multiple pathophysiologic factors, including fever, dehydration, cerebritis, and abscess formation. The seizure may be one of the earliest clinical manifestations of the illness, but an infectious process can usually be determined easily by physical and cerebrospinal fluid (CSF) examination. A chronic seizure disorder may follow successful medical treatment of the infection.

Congenital causes

The importance of genetic factors has been demonstrated for certain childhood epilepsies. For example, the 3/s spike-wave electroencephalogram (EEG) abnormality of petit mal appears to be inherited as an autosomal dominant trait. A family history of seizures is statistically more likely to be obtained from patients with epilepsy beginning in childhood (7.5%) than in adulthood (1.5%) but still does not define the individual patient's condition as familial or "idiopathic." Rather, it indicates a possible contribution of lowered seizure threshold for physiologic stresses such as sleep deprivation, fever, hyperventilation, certain repetitive stimuli (e.g., light flashes), and psychic turmoil. Maturation of the infant brain that is congenitally maldeveloped or damaged in the perinatal period may produce seizures at any time during later life but most commonly in the first decade. Any of the rare hereditary cerebral degenerations may manifest seizures at some point in the clinical course.

Statistically, the most common seizure disorders are the idiopathic petit mal and grand mal types in which no structural lesion is apparent. It is common practice to describe patients with no EEG or CT lesion as having "idiopathic epilepsy." There is some danger in this description, in that an erroneous presumption arises that no focus ever will be found, and that a hereditary condition is present, which may be transmittable to offspring. It is preferable to maintain a more skeptical position and regard such cases as "cryptogenic"; only after many years may some neoplastic or degenerative process show other unmistakable signs of its presence.

DIAGNOSIS AND LABORATORY EVALUATION

The proper management of seizure disorders rests on a complete and accurate description of the patient's symptoms and confidence that they are epileptic events. Since the physician rarely sees the patient during the attack itself, the usual evaluation during the post- or interictal period depends on reports of other observers and on the patient's recollection, compromised as that may be by amnesia for ictal and postictal periods. Occasionally, the epileptic nature of the event may be obscured by the failure to elicit a description of a familiar seizure pattern. In dealing with such unusual and occasionally bizarre episodes, one should remember that diagnostic characteristics of seizure events include the following:

1. A sudden alteration of behavior. Typically, a seizure abruptly and unpredictably interrupts the normal flow of subjective and objective brain function. Only infrequently do patients have seizures precipitated by specific external events or stimuli or characterized by a slow crescendo of symptoms.
2. Stereotyped patterns. Although almost any human behavior can be produced by a seizure, the epileptic attacks of a given patient have only one or a few recurring patterns. The march of symptoms is predictable from one attack to the next. The characteristic headache, myalgia, sluggish mentation, lethargy and sleep craving, and gingival-labial contusions present after a brief unwitnessed amnestic period offer very strong circumstantial evidence of a tonic-clonic convulsion, nearly as reliable as an eyewitness account.
3. Alteration of consciousness. Loss of awareness, ranging from mild confusion to coma during the attack and various degrees of amnesia after it, should suggest epilepsy. If memory is preserved, the patient's recollected description should be consistent and clear.
4. Brief duration. The ictal period rarely lasts more than 4 or 5 minutes. The postictal period may be prolonged but has the characteristics of progressive normalization of function.

Careful history taking from the patient and all potential witnesses is of central importance in the diagnosis of seizures and deserves the utmost respect. Without this salient information, mistakes in evaluation and management are frequently made and are seldom adequately corrected by resort to laboratory testing. Even sophisticated computerized imaging and electrophysiologic technologies are limited in their diagnostic power by the context of the clinical problem at hand.

Table 117-1 lists other common disorders often considered in the differential diagnosis of epilepsy.

Once a seizure disorder is suspected or proved on clinical grounds, prompt medical evaluation is indicated to assess the clinical implication of the epileptic symptoms and to set a course of management. The neurologic examination is usually normal in patients with a seizure disorder, even in those with structural lesions. However, if focal neurologic abnormalities are present, they are often enhanced immediately after a seizure. The cortical anatomic correlation of the postictal focal signs is a clue to the site of the epileptogenic focus. Postictal focal abnormalities can be of any type (e.g., aphasia, hemianopsia, sensory deficit, conjugate gaze preference). Transient localized weakness that follows a convulsion is called *Todd's paralysis*.

The EEG holds special prominence in the diagnosis of epilepsy because of its exclusive ability to record and characterize the pathophysiologic electrical events. The EEG abnormalities that confirm a clinical diagnosis of epilepsy include sharp or spike discharges, spike-and-slow-wave patterns, and other paroxysmal rhythmic activity having anomalous location or form—all of which are evidence of pathologic hypersynchrony. In addition, the EEG may demonstrate a nonspecific localized slow-wave pattern that indicates a focal lesion is present, of which the seizure itself is a symptom. Since both slow and sharp abnormalities may be more prominent immediately after a seizure, *early post-*

Table 117-1. Differential diagnosis of epilepsy

Disorder	Unlike epilepsy	Like epilepsy
Syncope	Premonitory symptoms Precipitating factors Diffuse fading vision	Myoclonic jerks or tonic stiffening, on occasion
Transient ischemic attack	No "march" of symptoms No jerks, twitches No loss of consciousness, amnesia Brainstem symptoms	Focal EEG slowing Normal examination between attacks
Migraine	Prominent headache Preserved consciousness	Focal symptoms Focal EEG slowing
Hypoglycemia	Temporal relationship to fasting Initial sympathetic discharge	Focal symptoms and EEG slowing Loss of consciousness Postictal headache, confusion
Paroxysmal vertigo	Preserved consciousness Monosymptomatic spells Auditory, vestibular abnormalities	Severe temporary disability
Narcolepsy	Cataplexy Appropriate sleep behavior with attacks	Hallucinations Inappropriate, unpredictable timing of attacks
Psychogenic spells	Event-related Stressful context Lack of autonomic features Lack of incontinence	Dramatic convulsive behavior

ictal recording of the EEG is highly desirable. Finally, EEG abnormalities roughly parallel the frequency and severity of clinical manifestations. A repeatedly normal EEG in the presence of frequent clinical attacks should suggest another pathophysiologic diagnosis.

The diagnostic yield of epileptic EEG abnormalities may be increased with hyperventilation or photic stimulation, or by recording the EEG during sleep, as it may occur in a routine session, by induction with mild sedation, or by recording in the morning after overnight sleep deprivation. A potential pitfall is that an epileptic discharge on EEG may mislocalize a structural abnormality. Specific localization must be made with other clinical and imaging techniques.

Limitations of the EEG should be recognized. Because it is a short temporal sampling of relatively brief episodic events, a single interictal EEG recording may fail to disclose a significant abnormality in an epileptic patient. Consequently, *a normal EEG does not rule out epilepsy*. Of course, a specific EEG pattern is not at all required for diagnosis if epilepsy is undeniably present on clinical grounds. In this situation a normal study reduces the likelihood of serious pathology and can serve as documentation of cerebral electrical status for future comparison.

It should be emphasized that the diagnosis of epilepsy is primarily clinical, by the characterization of the attacks, supported by EEG evidence. One should therefore insist that EEG support be very convincing if the clinical information is incomplete, and be wary of overreading EEG studies that may be "compatible with epilepsy."

Although systemic metabolic derangements may be more or less obvious, specific investigation for occult abnormalities may substantially alter the diagnostic and therapeutic approach to the patient. Successful treatment of a significant systemic disturbance may result in control of seizures without specific antiepileptic drug therapy. Conversely, if metabolic disturbances are not corrected, attempts to suppress seizures with drugs will be unsatisfactory.

Evaluation of a partial seizure logically begins with clinical consideration of potential sources of cerebral pathology: a history of strokelike events, incidents of head trauma, or symptoms suggestive of progressing malignancy. Standard computed tomography (CT) scanning, with or without contrast enhancement, is recommended in every patient to identify treatable structural conditions—especially neoplasms. The great majority of these scans are normal or show nonspecific abnormalities, such as atrophy. Magnetic resonance imaging (MRI) (see Chapter 108) is more sensitive than CT in documenting epileptogenic lesions in temporal or frontal lobes, especially for the small atrophic scars resulting from cortical contusion and subtle white matter intensities after infection or concussion. The relatively high cost of MRI makes routine use inadvisable; rather, MRI should be considered in patients with suboptimal control from medical therapy, especially those being evaluated for epilepsy surgery.

Cerebral angiography is reserved for detailed evaluation of suspected vascular lesions, especially arteriovenous malformations, suspected embolic stroke in young patients, and some neoplasms. After a focal mass has been excluded by CT, lumbar puncture and CSF analysis may help resolve suspicions of bleeding, inflammation, and infection, in the pertinent setting. Routine CSF study is not advised.

The extent and urgency of the diagnostic evaluation depend greatly on the clinical status of the patient. In all cases, initial seizures must be investigated promptly and carefully. It is advisable to hospitalize the patient so that complete and perhaps repeated assessment can be made of the neurologic status. A careful search for a structural lesion—occult in the case of a generalized convulsion—should be completed soon after the first patient contact. This search should include a CT scan, a metabolic screen, and, in certain cases, a lumbar puncture (see box below). Additionally, the potential seriousness of the incident can be communicated to the patient, and intelligent and effective drug treatment can be started.

Two common types of metabolic seizures deserve special discussion. In febrile seizures, there is hereditary predisposition to experience brief generalized convulsions with sudden elevation of body temperature. This condition is essentially confined to children between 6 months and 5 years of age. With a relatively brief history of illness caused by a nonspecific viral infection, the child abruptly has a convulsion that lasts only a few minutes. There are no focal components, the neurologic examination discloses no sign of cerebral disease, and routine metabolic studies are normal. There is often a family history of epilepsy, including other febrile episodes. A lumbar puncture is usually advisable at the time of the first seizure, to be certain there is no CNS infection, and in other circumstances when the convulsion is prolonged beyond 10 minutes, focal or lateralized ictal or postictal features are present, or if there are other clues of suboptimal cerebral function. Although febrile seizures can recur, prophylactic antiepileptic drug therapy is usually not required unless the seizures are atypical or neurologic impairment is present.

Alcohol withdrawal seizures are encountered in chronic alcoholics. In the setting of an alcoholic debauch, often with nutritional impairment, the patient has a generalized convulsion and is brought to the hospital. There is a his-

Seizure diagnosis

- Detailed history: outside observers
- General and neurologic examinations
- EEG: waking, sleeping
- Metabolic evaluation
  - Electrolytes, calcium
  - Glucose
  - Acid-base status
  - BUN, liver function tests
  - Serum (or urine) drug screen
- Structural lesion evaluation
  - CT scan, MRI
  - Lumbar puncture
  - Angiography

tory of relative abstinence, although the blood alcohol level may still be elevated. The patient recovers from the convulsion rapidly, with normal neurologic function and early signs of the abstinence syndrome of mild anxiety, tachycardia, and tremulousness. Several brief seizures may occur while the patient is being evaluated, but the attacks are essentially self-limited. If focal signs are present during the attack or in the postictal period, CT scanning is recommended, as these patients often are self-neglectful and have poor memory, and they often sustain head injury. If the convulsions are prolonged, acute loading with phenobarbital is indicated. Hospitalization and treatment for the abstinence syndrome are advisable, since many patients proceed to develop delirium tremens. Chronic antiepileptic drug therapy is not indicated.

Table 117-3. Seizure types and preferred drug treatment

Seizure type	Preferred agents
Generalized tonic-clonic	Carbamazepine Phenytoin Valproate
Simple and complex partial	Carbamazepine Phenytoin
Absence	Ethosuximide Valproate
Myoclonic	Valproate Clonazepam
Status epilepticus (generalized)	Diazepam/phenytoin Phenobarbital Lorazepam

TREATMENT

Once systemic diseases, acute metabolic derangements, and progressive cerebral diseases have been excluded by appropriate testing, the patient can be assured that the attacks will probably be successfully suppressed with antiepileptic drugs (AEDs) (Tables 117-2 and 117-3). Three fourths of adults with recurring seizures have a major reduction of seizure frequency, and over half achieve complete control.

Primary generalized seizures, both grand mal and petit mal types, are most easily suppressed, and partial attacks less successfully, particularly complex partial seizures. Patients with multiple seizure types or progressive lesions usually experience more difficulty.

Effective AED treatment is promoted by attention to the following considerations.

1. Start with a single AED in an effective dose, increasing the dose until seizure control is achieved or clinical toxicity occurs. Most patients are successfully managed with single-drug therapy.
2. Use blood AED concentrations judiciously in assessing both under- and overtreatment. One or two samples in the first 2 months of therapy confirm compliance and allow early revision of the dose schedule. After any change of dose, four or five drug half-lives must elapse before stable blood concentrations are achieved. "Therapeutic range" should be considered as an initial target. Some patients require high doses and plasma levels for suppression of clinical seizures.
3. If the first-choice drug is inadequate or not tolerated, it should be stopped and another agent established. Some simultaneous treatment with both drugs may be appropriate temporarily, to avoid seizure relapse.
4. Treatment with a single AED (monotherapy) is the ideal strategy to maximize control with minimal side effects.
5. The sedative and cognitive side effects of phenobarbital and primidone are common and effectively limit these drugs to agents of second choice, in spite of their antiepileptic effectiveness.

Table 117-2. Antiepileptic drugs in common use

Generic name	Trade name	Typical adult dose range (mg/day)	Target plasma level (μg/ml)	Serum half-life (h)	Side effects: Dose-dependent	Side effects: Idiosyncratic
Carbamazepine	Tegretol	600-1200	4-12	15	Ataxia, diplopia, nystagmus	Hyponatremia, rash, aplastic anemia
Phenytoin	Dilantin	300-400	10-20	24	Ataxia, nystagmus, gingival hyperplasia	Rash, lymphadenopathy
Valproate	Depakote	1000-2500	50-100	12	Gastric distress, alopecia, weight gain	Tremor, hepatic failure, decreased platelets
Phenobarbital	Luminal	60-180	15-30	96	Sedation, ataxia, blurred vision	Hyperactivity
Primidone	Mysoline	500-1500	5-10	16	Sedation, ataxia, blurred vision	
Ethosuximide	Zarontin	750-1500	40-100	36	Ataxia, sedation, gastric distress, headache	Rash
Clonazepam	Klonopin	15-20	.01-.05	30	Sedation, ataxia	

Status epilepticus

Generalized tonic-clonic status epilepticus is characterized by continuous or frequent and repeated convulsions, without recovery of full consciousness. It requires prompt and vigorous treatment to prevent major morbidity and mortality from hypoxia, hyperthermia, hypoglycemia, and acidosis. The mortality of the condition increases proportionately with the duration of the convulsions. In the emergency room or intensive care setting, pathogenic mechanisms must be defined and treatment instituted simultaneously (see box below). The airway and ventilation must be ensured, intravenous lines established, and blood obtained for glucose, electrolytes, and antiepileptic and toxic drug determinations. Arterial blood gases and pH also should be measured. The patient then should be given 25 g glucose intravenously, as well as 50 mg thiamine. Acidosis should be treated with intravenous bicarbonate.

These maneuvers may be facilitated by temporarily suppressing active convulsions with diazepam, 5 to 10 mg given intravenously over 1 to 2 minutes.

The history of illness must be obtained simultaneously. Anticonvulsant drug withdrawal or noncompliance in treated epileptics is often at fault. Other common causes are brain trauma, neoplasms, infections, and major metabolic derangements.

In addition to terminating the seizures, it is important to prevent their recurrence. This is accomplished by treating the underlying pathogenic abnormality (an important point often neglected) and by administering antiepileptic drugs that rapidly penetrate brain tissue and also have long-lasting effects. The blood concentrations required in this situation may be considerably higher than the usual therapeutic range for ambulatory patients. Careful monitoring of the patient is required to avoid respiratory and circulatory failure and other complications of coma.

Management of generalized status epilepticus in adults

1. Observe seizures briefly while getting history: consider pseudoseizures.
2. Give diazepam, 10 mg I.V., to arrest convulsion.
3. Start I.V.s; intubate trachea; draw blood samples; give glucose 25 g, thiamine 50 mg, calcium gluconate 100 mg I.V.

Reexamine briefly.

4. Begin phenytoin infusion, 18 mg/kg, 50 mg/min maximum rate, with ECG and BP monitoring: expect convulsions to subside during or soon after phenytoin loading.
5. If seizures are uncontrolled, give phenobarbital 3-5 mg/kg I.V. over 5–10 min; expect prompt control.
6. If seizures are uncontrolled, assess plasma AED levels (phenytoin >30, phenobarbital >45), plasma glucose, oxygenation, and acidosis; give bicarbonate; get experienced neurologic advice.
7. If seizures are controlled, give maintenance AED.

Many methods of drug treatment have been recommended for status epilepticus. Occasionally, two or three 5- to 10-mg doses of diazepam given intravenously permanently terminate the seizures. More often, the rapid redistribution of diazepam to noncerebral tissue allows seizures to recur, and repeated doses lead to undesirable sedative toxicity without achieving lasting seizure control.

In most adults, intravenous phenytoin should be considered the drug of choice to suppress persisting seizure activity. The usual loading dose is 15 to 20 mg per kilogram body weight. It should be given no faster than 50 mg per minute, while respiration, blood pressure, and the electrocardiogram (ECG) are monitored. Attempts to give phenytoin more rapidly may cause hypotension or cardiac arrest, especially in the elderly. Phenytoin loading takes 30 to 60 minutes and seizures should come under lasting control within another 30 minutes. The plasma concentration can then be maintained either intravenously or orally. Phenobarbital likewise can be given intravenously rapidly enough to control seizures and also can provide long-term maintenance. It is limited primarily by its sedative side effects but is the drug of first choice in patients known to be intolerant of phenytoin and in children under age 15. Phenobarbital can be given secondarily to patients who have not been controlled by phenytoin as given above. The recommended loading dose is 3 to 5 mg per kilogram body weight for adults, given over 1 to 2 minutes. Up to 10 to 15 mg per kilogram may be given to children. Phenobarbital may interact with previously administered diazepam to cause respiratory arrest during the infusion. If seizures continue after another 30 minutes, a second dose of the same size may be administered, and maintenance doses are given after seizures are controlled.

Intravenous lorazepam (Ativan) is an alternative to diazepam for initial seizure control. Its longer duration of antiepileptic action—related to distribution kinetics—reduces the occurrence of early seizure relapse and is thus an advantage in the acute situation. It may avoid the complications of high-dose rapid PHT or PB loading. This use of lorazepam has not yet been approved for general application and is now undergoing controlled clinical study.

Status epilepticus refractory to both phenytoin and phenobarbital usually is caused by unresolved serious metabolic disturbances, drug toxicity, cerebral trauma, or infection. Experienced neurologic advice is recommended at that point, to help choose between several less-well-established and controversial treatments.

In general, status epilepticus is best controlled by adequate drug dosage given intravenously, so that effective brain concentrations are reached as rapidly as possible. Intramuscular or rectal administration may avoid some intravenous toxicity but, because of delayed absorption and low plasma levels, fail to attain the primary therapeutic goal. A leisurely approach is likely to fall short, and the physician should remain immediately available until seizure control is achieved.

Partial seizures may also be persistent, typically as focal motor status (continuous partial epilepsy, epilepsia partialis continua), most commonly with repetitive arm or face jerking, or psychomotor status, consisting of frequent behavioral automatisms with partial or complete amnesia. Although assessment and prompt AED management is desirable to avoid generalized status, these conditions are less hazardous to life and cerebral function and are often considerably more difficult to control. The aggressive protocol outlined above should be tempered to avoid AED overdosage, particularly when consciousness is minimally disturbed. If plasma levels of phenytoin are 25 to 30 μg per milliliter and of phenobarbital are 35 to 40 μg per milliliter, further increases are unlikely to improve the situation.

Relatively uncommon is the syndrome of nonconvulsive status epilepticus. A patient, usually with a seizure history, becomes stuporous or confused for hours or days but has had no obvious convulsion. Subtle nystagmoid conjugate ocular movements and random facial twitches or limb myoclonic jerks may indicate the true pathophysiology. An urgent bedside EEG shows a chaotic pattern with hypersynchrony or spike discharges, which can be suppressed easily with small quantities of diazepam, 1 to 2 mg intravenously, occasionally with prompt arousal of the subject as well.

Pseudoseizures

In some patients, episodes of convulsive or nonconvulsive seizurelike behavior can result from psychogenic influences. Pseudoseizure attacks have a superficial resemblance to true epilepsy but characteristically occur in a provocative or emotionally charged setting, have unusual convulsions consisting of alternating "thrashing" limb movements without bilateral symmetric features, and lack the autonomic discharge and pathologic reflex findings characteristic of organic epilepsy. Nonconvulsive, CPS-like attacks may present as episodes of amnesia, rage, or aggressive outbursts, staring spells, or any kind of "funny feeling" that may be misinterpreted by the patient as epileptic. The EEG is normal during the ictus—although often obscured and rendered unreliable by movement artifact—and normal waking EEG patterns are present immediately afterward, with no postictal slowing. Although in some instances the attacks may be under full voluntary control (malingering), it is more likely that the patient suffers from a personality disorder or some form of neuroticism, including classic hysteria or conversion disorder following the usually psychiatric criteria.

Many patients with pseudoseizures have an organic seizure disorder as well, and a confident differential diagnosis may be difficult even for an experienced observer—especially if the patient is medically sophisticated and the attacks take the form of CPS. Evaluation should include careful clinical observation of the attacks, including provocation of one or more spells by suggestion, possibly with the patient in the EEG laboratory.

An additional objective test is measurement of serum prolactin, which is temporarily elevated after GTC or CPS events. To use this test to identify true seizures, the blood sample must be obtained within 20 minutes of the spell and compared to a control sample drawn exactly 24 hours later, to account for normal diurnal variation of the hormone.

The occurrence of pseudoseizures in an epileptic patient demands a reassessment and a change in both AED and nondrug management. AEDs may have been increased in number or dosage in a vain attempt to stop the attacks, and reduction of dosage may be followed by improvement. It is essential to view pseudoseizures as psychiatric symptoms, requiring evaluation of the emotional and interpersonal stresses generating them. Although formal psychologic or psychiatric referral is usually helpful and sometimes necessary, the primary physician has a great advantage in defining the medical and epileptic context of the spells and in providing the patient with emotional support.

PSYCHOLOGIC ISSUES AND BEHAVIOR CHANGES

In some cases, the presence of epilepsy is associated with long-term changes in behavior and personality. This phenomenon is extremely variable among patients. It is at least multifactorial, the result of underlying personality traits, the effects of any structural lesions on cerebral function, the frequency and type of seizures, medication side effects, and ill-defined factors of self-perception and esteem. The relative contribution of these components is often difficult to resolve and considerable controversy has arisen regarding many practical and theoretic details, such as whether certain seizure foci lead to specific emotional reactions, or how much effect some medications have on cognition.

Prognosis

The natural history of seizure disorders is extremely varied and is influenced by heredity, age of onset, frequency of attacks and multiplicity of patterns, permanent brain injury, and perhaps promptness and adequacy of AED seizure control. The prolixity of salient determinants makes calculation of the future of a single patient unreliable. After a single unprovoked seizure (i.e., one not related to acute and transient metabolic stress), the risk of further attacks is a matter of some controversy, recurrence within 2 years being reported to vary in prevalence between 30% and 70%. Because of this uncertainty, many neurologists recommend no AED treatment until a second seizure occurs, unless a higher risk of recurrence can be presumed on the basis of clinical, EEG, or CT scan evidence that a structural lesion is present. This is especially true for children, in whom brain maturation may reduce future risks. After age 30, on the other hand, a structural lesion is highly probable even without independent evidence, and the social morbidity of even one more seizure may justify a more aggressive approach, with single-drug AED therapy given for 2 to 5 years.

After an appropriate—but admittedly arbitrary—seizure-free period, consideration may be given to AED withdrawal, accomplished by slow reduction of daily doses, changes being made at monthly intervals, or even longer. Rapid discontinuation may precipitate status epilepticus. The patient must be counseled about the possibility of future seizures even if the withdrawal period is uneventful—particularly with adults, who must decide whether the disruption of life attendant upon seizure recurrence is worth risking.

Intractable seizures

Some patients continue to have seizures in spite of therapeutic efforts—always a frustrating experience for both physician and patient. In this situation, several possibilities should be considered.

1. The patient is receiving inadequate drug treatment, because of either noncompliance, as assessed by blood levels, or the physician's failure to press dosages to clinical toxicity.
2. The specific seizure type has been incorrectly diagnosed and inappropriate AEDs prescribed (e.g., ethosuximide for petit mal, which is in fact a CPS atypical absence).
3. The patient is receiving multiple-drug therapy with sedative side effects that increase the tendency for seizures to occur.
4. Some or all of the attacks are pseudoseizures.
5. The epilepsy truly is medically refractory.

Intensive monitoring

Patients with uncontrolled seizures of any type should be referred to special inpatient units for intensive monitoring. The basic technology available is simultaneous recording of EEG and patient activity on videotape, continuously for many days up to 2 to 3 weeks. Both seizure events and interictal EEG patterns can be evaluated by a multidisciplinary team with neurologic, neurosurgical, pharmacologic, and psychologic expertise. Special procedures such as cerebral metabolic studies and intracranial electrode placements can be performed to document and critically define seizure types and their anatomic origins.

Epilepsy surgery—specific excision of cortex proven to be the source of the patient's typical seizures—can be considered for medically refractory patients with definitively localized seizure foci lying in anterior temporal lobes (the most common site) or in other locations where resection will not cause neurologic handicap. Other patient selection factors include lack of progressive pathology (e.g., tumor), relative youth, preserved intelligence, and psychologic stability. For patients without a defined focus or with diffuse or otherwise unresectable disease, enrollment in protocols investigating new AED agents may be an option. Intensive monitoring can also detect or provide proof of pseudoseizures. Subsequent psychologic evaluation and counselling may lead to improvement in social morbidity, even if all seizures are not completely controlled.

Chronic care

In spite of the statistically good prognosis for AED control of seizures, there is considerable need for the physician to maintain continuous and constructive contact with the patient with epilepsy. The unpredictability and dramatic appearance of the seizures often have serious consequences for the patient's personal and social life. Some occupations involving hazardous working conditions may no longer be possible, and the patient may require vocational rehabilitation. Life and health insurance policies may have to be renegotiated. Driving motor vehicles must be interdicted except for individuals with significant warning or restricted partial symptoms. The emotional stress of having such a potentially serious and often mysterious illness can have subtle or overt psychological effects that may be more difficult to manage than the seizures themselves. The need for conscientious daily drug treatment requires full understanding and acceptance of the condition by the patient. Supportive physician-patient interaction is the key to effective use of all available resources.

REFERENCES

Browne TR and Feldman RG: Epilepsy: diagnosis and management. Boston, 1983, Little, Brown.

Delgado-Escueta AV, Bascal FE, and Treiman DM: Complex partial seizures on closed-circuit television and EEG: a study of 691 attacks in 79 patients. Ann Neurol 11:292, 1982.

Delgado-Escueta AV et al: Management of status epilepticus. N Engl J Med 306:1337, 1982.

Engel J: Seizures and epilepsy. Philadelphia, 1989, FA Davis.

Penfield W and Jasper HH: Epilepsy and the functional anatomy of the human brain. Boston, 1954, Little, Brown.

Porter RJ: Epilepsy, 100 elementary principles, ed 2. Philadelphia, 1989, Saunders.

CHAPTER

118 Cognitive Failure Dementia

Thomas M. Walshe III

SYNDROMES OF MENTAL FAILURE

When a human being loses the traits that control behavior and fails to process information adequately, the cause is a failure in cerebral function. The general concept of cerebral failure is akin to that of heart failure, in that either can arise from many etiologies, can be transient or progressive, can be of several types, and can vary in exact localization. Cerebral failure causes the human being to deviate from his or her established character, personality, bearing, and intellect. Specific losses of language and praxis may also accompany the changes in behavior. In the most general sense, cerebral failure may produce disorders of thought and mood (psychiatric diseases) or disorders of memory and cognition (neurologic diseases). The mind, however, is not compartmentalized by medical specialty, so a person having a thought disorder (e.g., schizophrenia) may have signs of cognitive failure and a patient with dementia (e.g., Alzheimer's disease) may have signs of a mood disorder. The overlap of clinical signs is a pervasive theme in the description of disorders that alter mental function. By realizing that the different mental status changes are variations of a general cerebral failure, one is less disturbed by the overlap of the several types.

When the brain begins to fail in its mental function, the deficits may only disrupt the subtle relationships between spouses or interfere with the level of execution of complex tasks. Such changes are hardly measurable by clinical methods and are often reported not as failures in cognition, but as vague medical or emotional complaints. If the failure becomes worse, the patient fails at home, at work, and in other social interactions, making the source of the problem obvious. There are several signs of cognitive failure, each with its own neurologic features and underlying pathologies.

Dementia

The neurologic sign of dementia comprises failure of learning, loss of memory, and loss of analytical ability. Patients are alert (when not treated with drugs) and attentive to the given task but fail because of memory deficits. Dementia is almost always a chronic complaint. In some diseases, dementia coexists with other signs, such as aphasia (failure of language) and apraxia (failure to execute learned tasks). When memory alone is lost and other cognitive powers remain largely intact, the mental state is described as *amnesia*. Amnesia is a neurologic sign associated with specific brain lesions and may occur in neurotic patients who have no gross brain lesions. The causes of dementia are usually found to be diseases of the brain itself.

Confusional states

The neurologic sign of confusion combines inattention, apathy, and somnolence. Poor organization of information prevents a coherent sequence of thought. Specific memories may be preserved, although they appear out of context and so distorted that the patient cannot answer questions correctly. Language is preserved. Confusional states occur over short periods (hours or days). The causes of confusion are usually found outside the skull, and the cerebral failure often is reversible. Delirium is a confusional state in which hyperactivity replaces apathy. The archetype for delirium is the syndrome of acute alcohol withdrawal, delirium tremens. The quiet confusional state may lead to coma, whereas it is unusual for the delirious patient to progress to coma.

The neurologic signs dementia, amnesia, confusion, and delirium are caused by specific disorders. They may coexist, and because they are similar in many ways, they may not always be clearly separated. However, it is worth attempting to determine by the history and physical examination which sign is dominant in the case, so that one can focus on the most likely diagnostic possibilities. When the dominant sign is dementia, an organized approach often leads to the diagnosis.

APPROACH TO THE DEMENTED PATIENT

As with any clinical sign, dementia can be caused by many disorders. One can discover the etiology by noting the character of the dementia and its natural history. In discussion with the patient and the family one must determine the mode of onset, the speed of progression (if any), drug history, and associated illnesses or complaints. The examination reveals the severity of the cognitive failure, the presence of other neurologic signs, and clues to underlying medical illness. Armed with this data, one can isolate several groups of disease in which dementia is the primary sign, including dementia alone, dementia with medical signs, dementia with variable neurologic signs, and dementia as part of a neurologic syndrome. The most prevalent dementia, especially in the elderly, is Alzheimer's disease (AD); therefore, the diagnostic imperative is to separate other disorders, some of which can be cured, from AD.

DEMENTIA WITHOUT OTHER NEUROLOGIC OR MEDICAL SIGNS

Dementia is an age-related disorder. In a community study in East Boston, Massachusetts, the prevalence of dementia was found to be 10%. The prevalence rose steeply with age so that in persons older than 85 the rate was 47%. In that community 84% of the demented persons were diagnosed to have AD. In data reported from the Framingham study women were more often affected with dementia than men; in that population the rate for AD was 55% among all demented patients. Because it is so common, AD must enter into the differential diagnosis of any adult patient who is found to have dementia. By knowing the clinical features of AD and the disorders that resemble it, the clinician can usually make the diagnosis. AD occurs occasionally in patients as young as 40 but is extremely rare in younger patients.

AD occasionally passes through families as an autosomal-dominant trait. In such cases there is an age-specific risk of dementia among siblings and children. In the familial form of AD, there is an earlier onset, more severe dementia, and higher risk to the relatives. Two thirds of AD cases follow no set inheritance pattern, but the pedigrees of patients with AD show a higher incidence of degenerative diseases of all types.

In AD the cortical neurons degenerate along with their axons, so the white matter of the brain shrinks and the cerebral ventricles enlarge. The temporal, frontal, and parietal lobes bear the brunt of the disease. The occipital lobes show fewer changes, and the posterior fossa contents are usually not affected. Microscopic examination shows neuronal loss with neurofibrillary and granulovacuolar degeneration.

The pathogenesis of the underlying lesions in AD is a target of active research. The hallmarks of the disease are the beta amyloid plaques in the neuropil and the neurofibrillary tangles in the neurons. Beta amyloid deposition is of two types. In one type there is a diffuse noncompacted amyloid deposition, which is not associated with dystrophic neurites or neurofibrillary changes. This type of deposition occurs often in the brains of old persons without overt dementia. The other type of plaque is a compacted beta amyloid deposit with a dense core. The dense plaques are associated with neurofibrillary changes in the neurons, and they are numerous in patients with AD. The total number of amyloid plaques is not as important as the number of the dense plaques, which relates to the degree of dementia. The beta amyloid has been identified at least in tissue culture to be toxic to mature neurons. The exact mechanism of cell death remains unclear.

Exploration of the genetic factors in AD has led to chromosome 21, the site of abnormality in patients with Down syndrome, who as a group are at high risk to have AD by age 50. Genetic linkage studies in familial Alzheimer's disease (FAD) seemed to identify a locus of predisposition in the long arm of chromosome 21. In addition, the gene for the amyloid precursor protein from which the beta amyloid is formed was cloned and localized to chromosome 21. These lines of observation suggested that the genetic abnormality of FAD was located on chromosome 21. Further information substantially clouded the issue. Data reporting DNA recombination events between the locus of FAD and the amyloid precursor protein (APP) gene failed to confirm a correlation. Families with FAD did not show linkage to chromosome 21 markers. However, several kindreds of FAD have been shown to have a mutation in the gene located close to the beta amyloid sequence. The mutation, the conservative substitution of isoleucine for valine, does not appear in normals or late-onset AD. The underlying pathophysiology of AD remains unsolved although new information continues to provide clues.

Neurochemical studies show that the cholinergic system is affected more than other neurotransmitter systems in AD. Reduced acetylcholine and choline acetyltransferase in the cortex and deep nuclei such as the nucleus basalis suggest that the loss of cholinergic transmission plays a part in the syndrome. It has become increasingly clear that AD causes much more than cholinergic failure. The noradrenergic system is also affected, and there is cell loss in the locus coeruleus and decreased norepinephrine in many brain regions. Cell loss, nucleolar volume loss, and neurofibrillary tangles in the raphe nuclei implicate the serotonergic systems as a target of AD. Low serotonin levels in the caudate, hippocampus, and other nuclei are present and fit with the cellular losses.

The clinical syndrome of AD begins in midlife or late life and is usually unnoticed or ignored for several years. Patients change their habits and often lose interest in their usual pursuits before it becomes obvious what is happening. Some develop psychotic symptoms or appear depressed. Most patients present to the generalist with complaints not obviously associated with decreased mental functions. At that early stage the disease is clinically undiagnosable. Most patients with AD worsen over 6 to 12 months; the younger patients seem to progress more quickly than the older ones. By the time the patient is clearly demented, there is often a history of 2 or 3 years of gradually increasing dysfunction. Impairment of learning, loss of recent and remote memory, and failure to analyze information follow the initial behavioral symptoms. Language is almost always affected, so patients have a striking dysnomia. Losses in calculation, praxis, and other functions add to the global mental failure. The dementia is usually moderately severe by the time the patient appears at the neurologist's office. Patients with moderately severe AD sometimes have bradykinesia and gegenhalten. The disease progresses smoothly over 5 to 10 years, eventually leaving the patient bedridden, immobile, mute, and in a persistent vegetative state. Intermittent illness may cause transient worsening, but the dementia does not improve. Death intervenes from repeated aspiration pneumonia and recurrent infectious diseases. In the late stages, myoclonus or seizures occur in about 25% of cases. The gait is usually preserved until very late in the illness.

AD that begins late in life causes less severe aphasia, enabling the patient to maintain communication that reveals a rambling, incoherent stream of thought similar to that seen in acutely confused patients. Some elderly patients with AD become unable to walk but have no clear motor deficit to explain the gait failure.

Most patients with AD require chronic hospitalization in the last several years of their illness, because of uncontrolled aggressive behavior, wandering, urinary and fecal incontinence, and the need for constant supervision in all aspects of life.

There is no cure for AD. During the early stages the family can manage the patient's failure by reducing their expectations and simplifying the household routine. Sleep disorders can be treated with mild sedatives (diphenhydramine, chloral hydrate) at night. Incontinence can sometimes be reduced by toileting the patient on a time schedule and monitoring fluid intake. Wandering, incontinence, and general nuisance behaviors are rarely controlled with drugs unless the patient is heavily sedated.

Emphasis on the cholinergic deficit in AD has directed therapeutic trials of anticholinesterase drugs. A number of novel compounds are under study. Other strategies include attempts to slow the progress of the disorder or to interfere with the amyloid deposition. Drugs that treat the symptoms or the pathology of AD will become available in the future once the current trials are complete.

Aggressive and assaultive behavior responds in some cases to short-acting benzodiazepines (lorazepam, oxazepam) used only when the unwanted behavior is a problem. Continued use of sedatives sometimes reduces function in demented patients or may cause paradoxic agitation. Intermittent use of the drugs avoids oversedation and allows optimum function. If behavior is unacceptable and no other treatment works, neuroleptics (chlorpromazine, haloperidol) are useful in curtailing assaultiveness. Neuroleptics used in doses that control the unwanted behavior reduce function in demented patients and also cause tardive dyskinesia and parkinsonism. Drug-induced dysphagia and immobility increase the chances of aspiration pneumonia.

The chronic care of patients with progressive dementia depends on the understanding of the natural progression of the disease. The physician and family can agree on appropriate levels of care as the patient moves from stage to stage toward the inevitable end of the disease.

Other entities cause a clinical picture almost identical to that of AD. Lobar atrophy, or Pick's disease, is clinically indistinguishable from AD but has few neurofibrillary tangles or amyloid plaques. The neurons swell and contain cytoplasmic inclusions. The atrophy is particularly severe in the temporal and frontal lobes. Some patients with severe chronic dementia have a pathology unlike either Pick's or Alzheimer's disease yet have a similar clinical course. The course and management of the other progressive degenerative dementias is similar to that of AD. There are no diagnostic tests for AD, and the evaluation aims at excluding other causes of dementia. Treatable disorders almost never cause the isolated, chronic, severe, global dementia that is seen in advanced AD.

SYSTEMIC MEDICAL ILLNESS CAUSING DEMENTIA

Systemic illness affecting mental status usually causes a confusional state rather than dementia, but a few medical disorders cause a dementia that might be confused with early AD. Most of the time in systemic illness, the altered cognition is a secondary diagnostic clue rather than the major clinical feature. Elderly patients are more likely than young patients to present with dementia as the major sign of nonneurologic illness. The dementia is reversible when there is treatment for the underlying disease and the disease has not permanently damaged the brain.

The history of the dementia is usually short, decline almost always being reported in less than a year. The onset is rapid, with stabilization over a few months, and there is often a clear beginning, unlike in the progressive degenerative cases. The dementia is almost always mild or moderate, and language is often spared. The memory deficit is likely to fluctuate more widely than in AD. There may be elements of inattention and obtundation that make the separation between dementia and confusion difficult.

The major systemic medical causes of dementia are listed in Table 118-1. The details of their clinical profiles can be found elsewhere in this book. Many other medical disorders are associated with mental failure, but they usually cause delirium or confusional state and thus can be distinguished from AD. They are not listed.

As a rule, the reversible medical causes of dementia do not cause specific neuropathologic changes. There are, however, systemic disorders that attack the brain directly and create their own neuropathologic change. Patients with Whipple's disease have neuropathologic changes of the brain and may have neurologic signs other than the dementia. Likewise, a specific pathology is found in the AIDS dementia complex. The dementia in AIDS is not from an opportunistic infection or from the complications of lymphoma or immunosuppressive therapy—the neurons are infected with the HIV itself. Patients with dementia from AIDS lose the ability to perform complex sequencing tasks, develop a slowness of thinking, and become inattentive. The memory loss is mild at the beginning but becomes severe as the syndrome progresses. The dementia is usually accompanied by slowness of motor function, including the eye movements, and by hyperreflexia, Babinski signs, and ataxia. In addition to the motor findings, AIDS dementia can be distinguished from AD by the history of risk, the younger age of onset, and the less profound memory loss at the beginning.

Almost any systemic medical perturbation can cause an elderly patient, especially one with mild dementia, to decompensate and appear acutely confused. When the underlying dementia has gone unrecognized, there may be an illusion of an acute onset of the dementia that persists after the confusion abates. The progressive degenerative disorders do not begin acutely.

DEMENTIA IN DISORDERS WITH VARIABLE NEUROLOGIC FEATURES

Several neurologic disorders feature dementia that may be confused with AD but have neurologic signs or histories that help the clinician make the diagnosis. Table 118-2 enumerates the various diagnostic tests that help to distinguish the major disorders in which dementia is a key feature.

Subacute spongiform encephalopathy (Creutzfeldt-Jakob

Table 118-1. Nonneurologic diseases sometimes presenting as dementia

Disease	Diagnostic indicators
Thyroid disease	T_3, T_4, TRH
Adrenal disease	Serum cortisol
Hypoparathyroidism	Serum calcium (parathormone levels)
Chronic renal disease	History of renal disease, BUN, creatinine
Chronic liver disease, hepatocerebral degeneration	History of liver disease, ammonia, LFTs acquired
Chronic drug toxicity	History of drug use, screens
Thiamine deficiency	History of alcoholism or other cause of thiamine deprivation; purely amnestic dementia, Wernicke-Korsakoff syndrome
Pernicious anemia	CBC, vitamin B_{12} level, gastric analysis, dietary history, loss of vibratory sensation
Niacin deficiency	Dermatitis, history of malnutrition
Neurosyphilis	FTA-ABS of CSF, other neurologic signs
Acquired immunodeficiency syndrome (AIDS)	HIV antibodies, other neurologic signs
Paraneoplastic syndromes	Chest x-ray, signs and symptoms of cancer
Whipple's disease	Malabsorption, arthritis, gaze palsy, amnestic dementia
Chronic dehydration	Elderly patients, elevated serum and urine osmolality

Table 118-2. Neurologic tests that help to diagnose causes of dementia*

Cause	EEG	CT/MRI	LP
Trauma	Asymmetric waveforms, paroxysmal activity	Shows areas of damage	Normal
Tumor	Asymmetric waveforms, paroxysmal activity	Shows lesion	Abnormal
Chronic subdural hematoma	Normal or slow, low amplitude on side of lesion	Shows lesion	Normal in half
MS	Normal	MRI shows lesion	Elevated gamma globulin
Hydrocephalus	Generalized slowing	Enlarged ventricles	Pressure high "normal" or above
Progressive degenerative dementia	Nonspecific slowing or normal	Normal or general atrophy	Normal
Vascular dementia	Asymmetric changes, slowing, paroxysmal activity; may be normal	Shows lesions in many cases	Normal
Creutzfeldt-Jakob disease	"Burst suppression" late in disease	Atrophy	Normal
Medical causes	Nonspecific slowing or normal	Normal	Normal
Syphilis	Nonspecific slowing or normal	Normal or focal defects, atrophy	FTS-ABS+, cells in active cases
Depression	Normal	Normal	Normal

*A normal laboratory test almost never rules out the possibility of a disease.

disease) is a dementing disease caused by a transmissible agent thought to be a virus. It is an unusual cause of dementia, with an incidence of approximately one case per 1 million population. The disorder causes gliosis and cell loss in the cerebral and cerebellar cortices. A characteristic vacuolated (spongy) appearance of the tissues and the lack of inflammatory cells give it a distinct neuropathologic picture.

Creutzfeldt-Jakob disease usually affects patients beyond middle age and begins with altered behavior. Dementia develops rapidly and devastates the patient within a year in almost all cases. Ataxia, gait disorder, and other signs of cerebellar dysfunction are frequent and may precede the mental decline. Visual complaints occur in some patients. Myoclonus occurs in most cases. The EEG shows synchronous bursts of high-voltage sharp waves with intervals of low voltage.

The diagnosis can be suggested by brain biopsy, but for absolute certainty, diagnosis requires the transmission of the disorder by the inoculation of suspected tissue into brains of chimpanzees.

Creutzfeldt-Jakob disease is not contagious in the usual sense, but infected blood and other body fluids should be kept isolated. There is no treatment for the disease.

Patients with head trauma have residual abnormalities in mental function, often with failure of memory. The degree of the trauma determines the degree of dementia. Almost invariably, there are other signs and a clear history of trauma with a period of coma. Patients with repeated head trauma, such as professional boxers, exhibit a mental decline as they age that resembles AD. The dementia can be moderate or (sometimes) severe, but language is usually spared. Many head trauma patients are abulic and may have extrapyramidal features. Survivors of heat stroke also are sometimes left with a dementia, although the details of the syndrome are not well established.

A slowly growing brain tumor may present as dementia and be confused with progressive degenerative dementia. The onset is subacute, over weeks or months; there are almost always other signs of neurologic dysfunction, and in metastatic tumor a primary lesion may be identified. The dementia is mild or moderate. In many cases the patient suffers from increased intracranial pressure, causing somnolence and a confusional state instead of (or in addition to) dementia. Tumors of the diencephalon or the medial temporal lobe may cause an amnestic state. Frontal lobe tumors cause a failure of analytical thought, abulia, and increased intracranial pressure.

Chronic subdural hematoma (SDH) in elderly patients can cause an insidiously progressive dementia occurring over several days or weeks. The syndrome may mimic AD, except that most elderly patients with SDH are lethargic. Patients may not have other neurologic signs, but most have at least traces of motor dysfunction. Seizures and headache are also associated with chronic SDH. The CSF may be normal, but in one-half of patients there is xanthochromia, pleocytosis, and elevated opening pressure. The EEG is abnormally slow, with reduced amplitude on the side of the lesion. The hematoma is almost always identified by computed tomography (CT) or magnetic resonance imaging (MRI) scan. Subdural hematoma is a frequent cause of acute neurologic change in patients with AD.

Hydrocephalus causes lethargy and a variety of neurologic signs, along with changes in mental function. The CSF pressure in some cases may not be elevated but is almost always above 100 cm H_2O and usually at the upper normal limit. Normal pressure hydrocephalus is an unusual cause of dementia occurring as a late complication of intracerebral infection or subarachnoid hemorrhage. In a few patients no predisposing reason is identified. The syndrome develops subacutely over a few weeks, causing lethargy and mental failure accompanied by a gait disorder and incontinence. Frequent falls and failure in the pursuit of usual activity are the chief complaints. The dementia is moderate, and language is usually minimally affected. The patient is slow to respond (abulic) but when given time, often produces the right answer. The EEG is slow in most cases, and the CT or MRI shows dilated ventricles. Placement of a ventricular shunt to relieve the pressure improves the patient when hydrocephalus is the problem.

Dilated ventricles also occur in progressive degenerative dementia, in vascular dementia (vide infra), and in normal elderly persons. One must relate all the laboratory and clinical data to make the diagnosis of normal pressure hydrocephalus. Acute subdural hematoma is a complication of ventricular shunt in hydrocephalus.

VASCULAR DEMENTIA

Vascular dementia results from stroke and accounts for approximately 15% of patients who present with dementia as the primary complaint. Cerebrovascular disease, however, produces dementia in a larger number of patients who are not counted among those who present with dementia as the major complaint. One of the chief factors that prevents stroke patients from returning to their prestroke function is failure of mental function. Many patients have specific cerebral syndromes (aphasia, apraxia), but less obvious mental syndromes of inattention, failure of planning, poor memory, and other mental deficits also occur. The dementia occurs in most strokes along with other signs, but in some cases multiple recurrent strokes accumulate over years to cause a gradual decline in ability. There is often a clear history of at least one stroke in the past, and there is a stepwise deterioration in which the patient or family can mark plateaus and declines. The onset of the dementia can usually be dated within a few months. Risk factors for stroke (hypertension, atherosclerosis, family history) can also be found. Focal neurologic signs are the rule but may be only subtle reflex changes or changes in motor tone.

Multiple cerebral infarcts

Several vascular syndromes cause a progressive dementia that may mimic AD. Multiple cortical strokes occur in patients with cardiac arrhythmia, valvular disease, cardiomyopathy, and other sources for embolism. The CT scan shows medium-sized lesions in the distribution of the MCA involving the cortex. Thrombotic vascular disease of the carotid or cerebral arteries that causes multiple infarction can also produce dementia. Moya moya, a slowly progressive thrombosis of the large arteries at the base of the brain, may cause a dementia with few other neurologic signs.

Multiple lacunar strokes occur in the setting of chronic hypertension. The syndrome of multiple lacunar infarction from small vessel thrombosis sometimes is more indolent than multiple embolism, because the lesions are smaller and may go unnoticed longer. The CT scan shows enlarged ventricles and areas of damage in the deep white matter, basal ganglia, and brainstem. Dysarthria, dysphagia, and pseudobulbar palsy are frequently part of the picture. The dementia in these cases is not as severe as that seen in AD of equal duration, and there is usually no aphasia, apraxia, or hemianopia. Systemic lupus erythematosus (SLE) sometimes causes multiple cerebral infarctions. In SLE patients mental failure along with variable neurologic signs occur, but the finding is usually psychosis rather than dementia.

Single cerebral infarcts

Occlusion of the posterior cerebral artery is a single-stroke syndrome that causes amnesia. The deficit occurs with a hemianopia and may be transient. Anoxia and hypotension after cardiac arrest may leave the resuscitated patient with an amnestic dementia. Recurrent severe hypoglycemia may produce a dementia with abulia, memory loss, and other signs. Right middle cerebral artery occlusions are sometimes associated with depression and a chronic inattention, failure to form a coherent line of reasoning, and failure to analyze information properly. The syndrome resembles the confusional state except the patient is fully alert and the state is chronic. The vascular dementias do not progress unless strokes continue to accumulate.

NEUROLOGIC SYNDROMES WITH DEMENTIA

Several neurologic disorders combine dementia with specific neurologic findings. The dementia occurs as a part of a rather stereotyped syndrome. Huntington's disease, Parkinson's disease, and progressive supranuclear palsy are the best known. These disorders are discussed elsewhere in this book.

REFERENCES

Bachman DL et al: Prevalence of dementia and probable senile dementia of the Alzheimer type in the Framingham Study. Neurology 42:115, 1992.

Boller F, Lopez OL, and Moossy J: Diagnosis of dementia: clinicopathologic correlations. Neurology 39:76, 1989.

Evans DA et al: Prevalence of Alzheimer's disease and other dementing diseases in a community population of older persons higher than previously reported. JAMA 262:2551, 1989.

Joachim CL, Morris JH, and Selkoe D: Clinically diagnosed Alzheimer's disease: autopsy neuropathological results in 150 cases. Ann Neurol 24:50, 1988.

Sinder WD et al: Neurological complications of acquired immune deficiency syndrome: analysis of 50 patients. Ann Neurol 14:403, 1983.

Yankner BA and Mesulam M-M: β-amyloid and the pathogenesis of Alzheimer's disease. N Engl J Med 325:1849, 1991.

CHAPTER

119 Parkinsonism and Movement Disorders

Lewis R. Sudarsky

Disorders of motor control, once considered the exclusive province of the neurologic specialist, are seen with increasing frequency in general medical practice. The prevalence of Parkinson's disease exceeds 1% after age 65, affecting a growing segment of the population. Many more patients have essential tremor, and the sophistication of patients and physicians has increased available treatment options. Focal dystonias such as torticollis and writer's cramp are more often recognized. The deinstitutionalization of chronic psychiatric patients over the last decade has created important changes in Western societies. As these patients have hit the streets and shelters in growing numbers, phenothiazine-induced dyskinesias have become commonplace in office and hospital practice.

An established approach to the disorders of motor control is to divide manifestations into positive and negative symptoms: paucity of movement, and motor excess (Fig. 119-1). The positive manifestations can be divided further into excess tonic innervation (spasticity, dystonia) and abnormal involuntary movements (the dyskinesias). Positive and negative symptoms commonly coexist. Parkinson's disease features a manifestation from each category: bradykinesia, rigidity, and tremor. This approach nevertheless provides a descriptive framework for systematic review of a rather diverse group of disorders. In some cases, particularly with tremor, chorea, and myoclonus, the underlying physiology has been partially characterized. With Parkinson's disease, the pathophysiology is understood at the level of the synapse, and the cell biology is under active study.

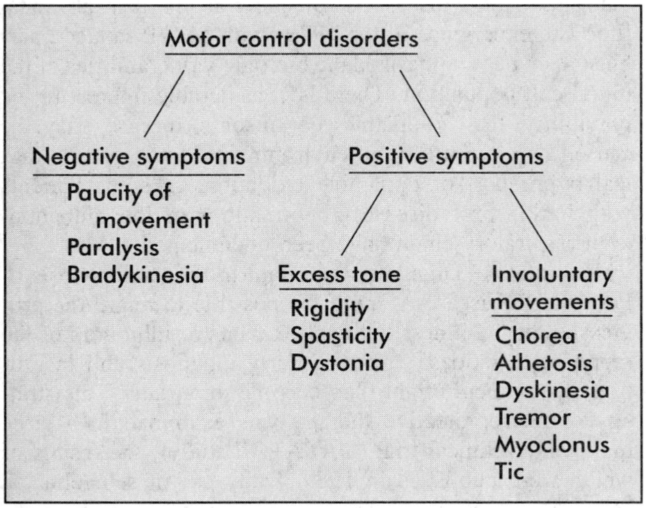

Fig. 119-1. Classification of motor control disorders.

PARKINSON'S DISEASE

Parkinson's disease was described by James Parkinson in 1817, though its full characterization and understanding have emerged with the modern neurochemical era. Incidence increases with age. Parkinson's disease is relatively uncommon under age 40; the prevalence approaches 2.5% at age 85. Familial cases are described, but the condition is generally not considered to be heritable.

Clinical features

The recognition of Parkinson's disease relies on four cardinal clinical features: bradykinesia, rigidity, tremor, and a characteristic disorder of posture and gait. Two or more features are usually present, though the diagnosis can sometimes be made from the tremor alone. Bradykinesia (slowness and difficulty in initiating movement) is the most disabling feature. It is commonly reported by patients as weakness or increased difficulty at daily activities, such as washing and dressing. Extrapyramidal rigidity with "cogwheeling" is most easily appreciated in passive movement of the neck and limbs. The resting tremor of 3-5/second subsides during limb movement. It is most evident in pronation/supination of the forearm and flexion of the fingers ("pill rolling"). The jaw and perioral area may be involved. A flexed posture is observed and the gait is shuffling, with a tendency to turn "en bloc." Patients may experience a tendency to accelerate (festination). Later in the illness, there is loss of postural stability and a tendency to fall. This is seldom an early feature in idiopathic Parkinson's disease, and early postural instability may be a clue to another akinetic/rigid disorder.

Associated features are also helpful in recognition and diagnosis. Facial expression is diminished; seborrhea and blepharospasm are often observed. There may be dysarthria (monotonous, hypophonic speech) or drooling. The patient's handwriting may degenerate into a micrographic scrawl. The differential diagnosis relies on distinguishing idiopathic Parkinson's disease from a long list of causes of secondary parkinsonism (see box, p. 1066). Associated pyramidal, autonomic, or cerebellar features are usually caused by a systems degeneration, a presentation sometimes referred to as *Parkinson's-plus*.

Parkinson's remains a clinical diagnosis, often based on impressions rather than formal criteria. No lab tests are used routinely. Of patients who present with an akinetic/rigid disorder, 10% to 20% ultimately turn out to have another illness, so MRI is sometimes used to screen patients with atypical parkinsonism. Parkinson's disease can be detected in a preclinical phase using positron emission tomography (PET) with fluoro-DOPA.

The natural history is one of gradual progression. In the pre-levodopa era, the median survival was on the order of 10 to 15 years. Death was from the complications of immobility: inanition and pneumonia. Patients today live longer. There is some suggestion that those who present with tremor have a more benign course. As levodopa has improved survival, it has also had an impact on the clinical

Differential diagnosis of parkinsonism

Idiopathic Parkinson's disease

Systems degeneration (Parkinson's-plus syndromes)
- Progressive supranuclear palsy
- Shy-Drager syndrome
- Olivopontocerebellar atrophy
- Striatonigral degeneration
- Cortical-basal ganglionic degeneration
- Huntington's disease (rigid variant)
- Wilson's disease
- Alzheimer's disease with extrapyramidal rigidity

Secondary parkinsonism
- Postencephalitic parkinsonism
  - Drug-induced parkinsonism
  - Cerebrovascular disease
    - Binswanger's disease
    - Basal ganglia lacunes
  - Normal pressure hydrocephalus
  - Trauma, midbrain injury
  - Tumor, vascular malformation (rare)
  - Toxic/metabolic
    - N-methyl-4-phenyl-tetrahydropyridine (MPTP)
    - Manganese
    - Carbon monoxide poisoning
    - Non-Wilsonian hepatocerebral degeneration
    - Hyperparathyroidism

spectrum of disease. More refractory late-stage patients are seen, and there is a greater awareness of mental status changes.

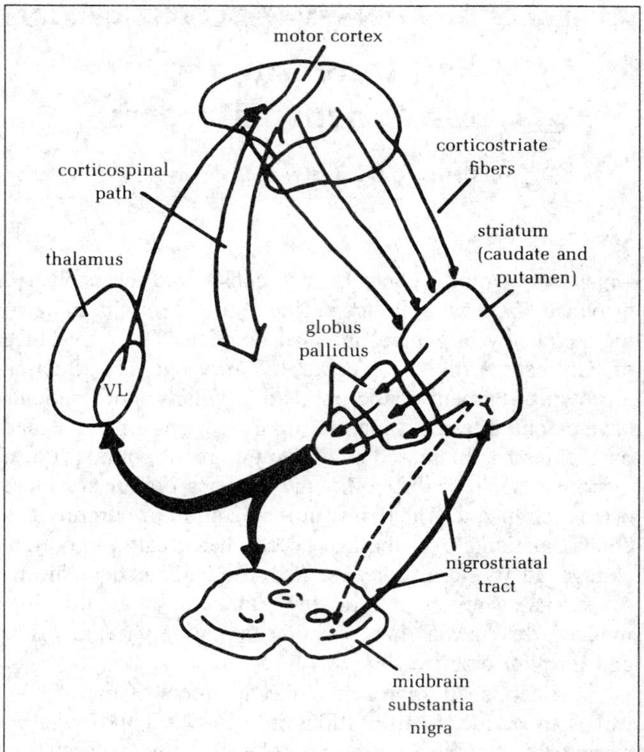

Fig. 119-2. The striatal loop is involved in the elaboration of voluntary movement. Cortical impulses are fed to the neostriatum (caudate and putamen). Output through the globus pallidus to the thalamus influences the execution of movement by the corticospinal tract. Midbrain substantia nigra neurons, via the nigrostriatal pathway, control the flow of process through the striatal loop. Dopamine is the principal neurotransmitter of nigral afferents to the striatum. (Redrawn from Sudarsky L: Parkinsonism, tremors, and gait disorders. In Branch WT, editor: Office practice of medicine, ed 2. Philadelphia, 1987, WB Saunders.)

Etiology and pathogenesis

There are approximately 500,000 specialized dopamine cells in the midbrain of the young adult, most of which lie in the pars compacta of the substantia nigra. These cells contain neuromelanin and manufacture neurotransmitter dopamine. Together with the pigmented cells in the adjacent ventral tegmental area, they supply virtually all of the dopamine innervation of the forebrain. The striatopallidal loop (Fig. 119-2) participates in the planning and automatic execution of learned movement. The dopamine pathway to the striatum is thought to have a modulatory role in this processing. The small population of substantia nigra neurons thus influences the motor production of the basal ganglia.

The substantia nigra is the principal site of pathology in Parkinson's disease. The large, pigmented cells in the midbrain degenerate, and pallor can be observed by gross inspection at postmortem. Intraneuronal inclusion bodies (Lewy bodies) are a biologic marker for the disease process. Symptoms and signs of parkinsonism emerge when 75%-80% of the dopamine innervation is gone. With steady progression past this point, the clinical disorder grows more severe.

The etiology of Parkinson's disease is still not understood. Incidence increases sharply with age, as noted above. Twin studies argue against inheritance and suggest that Parkinson's disease is somehow acquired in postnatal life. The experience in the 1970s with MPTP-induced parkinsonism has emphasized the biologic vulnerabilities of the nigral cell population. There is considerable interest in the possibility that idiopathic Parkinson's disease may be caused by exposure to an environmental toxin or free radical byproducts of dopamine oxidation. In some patients with Parkinson's disease, abnormalities of the mitochondrial respiratory chain have been documented.

If oxidative damage is important in the pathogenesis of Parkinson's disease, it might be possible to retard the progression of the illness with antioxidants or inhibitors of the monoamine oxidase enzyme. Early diagnosis and institution of treatment might then become important. This strategy of neuroprotective therapy was examined in a large multicenter clinical trial (DATATOP study), the results of which were published in 1989. Daily use of selegeline, a MAO B-isoenzyme inhibitor, significantly slowed the evolution of disability in treated patients. The study does not establish a neuroprotective mechanism for the drug effect, however, and its interpretation has been controversial.

Management

It is important for all patients with parkinsonism to remain physically active. Physical therapy and exercise are often as helpful as medication in the early stages. For consideration of drug treatment, we divide patients into three groups: early, moderate, and advanced disease. The patient with early disease, often newly diagnosed, is easily able to work and perform daily activities. Such patients primarily experience symptoms at a nuisance level, some social embarassment, and a great deal of anxiety about the outlook. Moderate parkinsonism begins to impinge on function as the patient shows a change in mobility. Daily activities require more time. Advanced disease is marked by limitations in daily activities despite drug treatment. Such patients may develop fluctuations, treatment-limiting side effects, and a loss of independence in activities of daily living.

While controversy persists about the interpretation of the DATATOP study, most movement disorder specialists would recommend the use of selegeline in all newly diagnosed patients. The drug is usually well tolerated; the standard dose is 5 mg morning and midday. At this dose, the MAO B-isoenzyme is selectively inhibited and no dietary restrictions are necessary. Five percent to 10% of patients experience insomnia or nausea. Selegeline can cause confusion in older, demented patients. It also aggravates postural hypotension when used with other antiparkinsonian medications. While not intended as symptomatic therapy, selegeline improves motor function (and mood) in some patients. Most new patients do well without requiring other medication for about a year. Patients need to understand the rationale for an expensive medication that is not dramatic in its effect on motor performance.

Table 119-1. Antiparkinsonian drugs

Preparation	Average daily dose
Levodopa	1.5-8.0 g
Levodopa/carbidopa (Sinemet)	300-1200 mg
Levodopa/benserazide (Madopa)	300-1200 mg
Amantadine (Symmetrel)	100-300 mg
Trihexyphenidyl (Artane)	2-15 mg
Benztropine (Cogentin)	1.0-6.0 mg
Ethopropazide (Parsidol)	100-400 mg
Bromocriptine (Parlodel)	7.5-30 mg (with DOPA)
Pergolide (Permax)	1.5-4.0 mg
Selegeline (Eldepryl)	5-10 mg

Moderate disease

Symptomatic therapy (some form of dopamine replacement) is added as soon as slowness or stiffness has begun to interfere with the patient's occupation or daily activities. Large studies have not demonstrated any advantage to withholding levodopa at this stage, though the best results are generally achieved in the first 5 or 6 years of its use. It is curious to think that one can influence the function of the brain by the oral loading (by feeding) of neurotransmitter precursors, yet this is precisely the mechanism of action of levodopa. Levodopa enters the nervous system by facilitated transport and is converted directly into neurotransmitter dopamine. The regulatory step in catecholamine synthesis is bypassed, so large quantities of neurotransmitter dopamine can be made and stored presynaptically. Peripheral inhibitors of dopa decarboxylase enhance the central accumulation of transmitter and diminish side effects caused by receptors in the periphery. For this reason, levodopa is usually given in combination with 75-150 mg/24 hrs of carbidopa (see Table 119-1). It is best to begin with a small dose (half a 25/100 Sinemet tablet, twice a day; or half a Sinemet CR). If nausea is a problem, options include reducing selegeline to 5 mg, adding extra carbidopa (available from the manufacturer), or adding an antiemetic. There is less nausea with Sinemet CR, which does not cause a rapid surge in the plasma levodopa level.

Authorities on the treatment of Parkinson's disease increasingly advocate early introduction of a dopamine receptor agonist drug, such as bromocriptine (10-15 mg) or pergolide (1.0-1.5 mg), together with levodopa. The principal advantage of this approach is that it allows the levodopa dose to remain in the low range (300-500 mg/day) for most patients. (For theoretical reasons, smaller doses of levodopa may be preferable.) In one commonly cited study, patients treated with bromocriptine from the outset had less difficulty in subsequent years with response fluctuations and dyskinesias.

One point against this strategy is the greater toxicity and expense of the dopamine agonists, which are generally less potent therapeutic agents that Sinemet. Synthetic dopamine agonists can cause nausea, dizziness, leg edema, orthostatic hypotension, confusion, and dyskinesias. In large doses, they can even produce symptoms of ergotism, including digital vasospasm and chest pain. Best results are obtained by starting with a small dose (1.25 mg bromocriptine, 0.05 mg pergolide) and gradually increasing over 2 to 3 weeks into the desired dose range. The agonist drugs have the advantage of a longer half-life, and used together with levodopa they provide a smoother response. Few patients succeed with these drugs alone as primary therapy.

Advanced disease

The transition to advanced Parkinson's disease is often marked by the development of response fluctuations. Patients have trouble maintaining an even response to levodopa after 5 or 6 years of therapy. The half-life of levodopa is short (90 to 120 minutes), and many late-stage patients experience "wearing off" of its effect 2 to 3 hours after a dose. At the same time, they may be more sensitive to CNS toxicity at the peak dose. Because of the narrow therapeutic window, replacement of neurotransmitter dopamine by interval administration of precursor is unphysiologic and unsatisfactory for these patients. The solution to the problem of end-of-dose "wearing off" is a greater reliance on long-acting medications. Dopamine agonists are a useful adjunct in this situation. Sinemet CR, a sustained-release preparation, provides delayed enteric absorbtion over 4 to 6 hours. Sinemet CR can be expected to last twice as long as regular Sinemet, though individuals differ with respect to their response to this medication. Selegeline has not been as successful for this indication, and we do not encourage its use in late-stage patients.

Other patterns of response fluctuation are more difficult to manage. Some patients describe transient freezing or episodes of "sudden off," which resolve over minutes without additional medication. Other patients develop a pattern of diphasic dyskinesia, in which involuntary movements accompany medication onset and wearing off. Greater reliance on dopamine agonist medications is often helpful, especially if the Sinemet dose can be reduced. Experimental treatment modalities such as fetal tissue transplantation are under investigation.

Patients with late-stage Parkinson's disease are quite often disabled by postural instability and falls. Postural reflexes are not responsive to medication, and such patients must be more cautious. They should be encouraged to use a cane or walker when ambulation is unstable. Symptoms of autonomic dysfunction such as postural hypotension and constipation require attention in some patients.

Mental status changes

Although James Parkinson described a motor disorder, it is now apparent that a subgroup of patients with Parkinson's disease suffer mental change (delirium, depression, dementia). Delirium is generally transient and reversible, related to medications. All the commonly used antiparkinsonian medications have the potential to cause delirium, even transient psychosis. Anticholinergic drugs are the worst offenders; it may be best to avoid them altogether in patients over 70. In the patient prone to confusion, the preferred strategy is to avoid polytherapy and focus on the single drug with the greatest therapeutic index (e.g., Sinemet).

Depression occurs in a substantial number of patients. It is generally mild to moderate, but can be a difficult management problem. Depression is not correlated with the magnitude of disability and is often a feature in early-stage Parkinson's disease. Selegeline elevates mood for some patients, but a tricyclic antidepressant may be required if depression is significant.

The natural history of Parkinson's disease has changed in the levodopa era. As more late-stage patients are alive and functioning, it is apparent that 10%-20% have a dementia syndrome as part of their illness. Episodic confusion (even off medication), slowness, and frontal behavioral features are most often observed. Neuropathologic examination of such cases at postmortem reveals cytoskeletal markers of Alzheimer's disease (cortical plaques and tangles) in about half. Some have only lesions of Parkinson's disease, with widespread involvement of subcortical structures (locus ceruleus, ventral tegmental area, basal nucleus of Meynert). It is best to avoid antipsychotic drugs, if possible, because their prolonged use inevitably worsens motor symptoms. Clozapine, an antagonist specific for the D4 dopamine receptor in the limbic system, has shown some promise for behavioral disturbance and hallucinations in Parkinson's disease.

SECONDARY PARKINSONISM

A number of diseases can present as an akinetic/rigid syndrome with features of parkinsonism. Drug-induced parkinsonism is particularly common in nursing homes and chronic care facilities, but is also seen among outpatients in the community. A systems degeneration is ultimately found in 4%-6% of patients who present with parkinsonism.

Systems degeneration (Parkinson's-plus syndromes)

Of patients initially thought to have Parkinson's disease, 3%-4% evolve the typical clinical picture of progressive supranuclear palsy (PSP, Steele-Richardson-Olszewski syndrome). It is distinguished clinically by axial dystonia (especially extension of the head), a characteristic facial expression (suggesting horror or astonishment), and supranuclear gaze palsy. Postural instability and mental change are prominent findings. Ocular signs may not be present initially, but the emergence of downward gaze palsy is pathognomonic. PSP is associated with nerve cell loss, gliosis, and globose neurofibrillary tangles in the substantia nigra, the subthalamic region, and the periaqueductal gray. Response is partial, at best, to antiparkinsonian medications.

A disorder known as cortical-basal ganglionic degeneration has poor response to levodopa, and additional motor signs not typical in idiopathic PD. Rigidity is often unilateral or highly asymmetric, and patients have apraxia or the "alien hand" phenomenon (in which the limb appears to wander without full volitional control). Dementia is often a feature of this disorder as well.

In the Shy-Drager syndrome, parkinsonism is associated with progressive autonomic failure. Sleep apnea and vocal cord paralysis are frequently associated. Mild orthostatic hypotension is not unusual in idiopathic Parkinson's disease, but hypotension is severe in these patients, and may be made worse by levodopa. Olivopontocerebellar atrophy (OPCA) is characterized by parkinsonism and cerebellar dysfunction, with gross atrophy of the pons and cerebellum on imaging studies. Dysarthria is a prominent feature. Some cases are familial, some sporadic. A wide range of heterogeneity is observed, even within an affected family. Bannister and Oppenheimer have suggested that OPCA, Shy-Drager syndrome, and striatonigral degeneration be lumped together under the heading *multiple system atrophy,* as the range of syndrome variability and overlap is so great.

Drug-induced parkinsonism

Chronic administration of drugs that depress dopamine synaptic function can cause a form of parkinsonism. Reserpine, which depletes catecholamines presynaptically, and the dopamine receptor antagonists (including haloperidol, prochlorperazine, and metaclopramide) have motor "neuroleptic" effects. Drug-induced parkinsonism is endemic in chronic psychiatric hospitals and common in nursing homes. It is difficult to distinguish clinically from idiopathic Parkinson's disease. Perioral tremor is somewhat more common, and gait impairment somewhat less. Coexistent tardive dyskinesia may be an important clue. The diagnosis is usually made after a review of the patient's medications. The disorder persists for 1-3 months (median 7 weeks) after discontinuation of neuroleptic drug treatment. Anticholinergic drugs are commonly employed to improve function pending recovery; most neurologists prefer not to use levodopa in this context.

Destructive lesions of the midbrain or corpus striatum

Strokes in the basal ganglia have long been recognized as the occasional cause of a parkinsonian syndrome. Such cases, often hypertensive patients with multiple subcortical infarcts, usually have pyramidal signs, frontal gait disorder ("gait apraxia"), and abnormal mental state. Rarely, late-life hydrocephalus presents a somewhat parkinsonian appearance. Other structural pathology in the midbrain or striatum is occasionally encountered in patients with parkinsonism. Trauma to the midbrain is a rare cause, as in patients with dementia pugalistica.

Postencephalitic parkinsonism

Encephalitis was once a common cause of parkinsonism. Most cases occurred in the wake of von Economo's encephalitis, an epidemic illness during the period 1916-1927. Today the condition is quite rare. Many of the patients are younger. An acute encephalitic illness progresses over days to akinetic mutism or coma. Features of the acute illness include external ophthalmoplegia, sleep, and respiratory disorder. A severe behavioral disturbance is often observed. Residua include chronic parkinsonism with dystonic features and oculogyric crises.

Toxic/metabolic etiology

A toxic parkinsonian syndrome was first recognized by Cotzias among workers in the manganese mines of South America. Carbon monoxide poisoning can produce a striking clinical picture, with necrosis in the globus pallidus, extrapyramidal rigidity, and dystonia. Such patients are rarely normal mentally. MPTP toxicity is a more recent phenomenon. Patients have an apparently normal mental state and a rather pure parkinsonism. The toxin was a by-product in the manufacture of "designer drugs" for recreational use. Asymptomatic patients known to be exposed should be followed closely for signs of emergent parkinsonism.

OTHER DISORDERS WITH INCREASED TONE

Spasticity

The term *spasticity* describes a range of phenomena associated with the upper motor neuron syndrome. The principal characteristics are (1) increased muscle tone, (2) velocity-dependent increase in tonic stretch reflexes, and (3) increased tendon jerks with clonus. The "clasp-knife" phenomenon is appreciated during passive movement. There is an initial resistance, followed by a collapse of tension, a response mediated by stretch receptors in the Golgi tendon organ. Clinically, spinal spasticity differs somewhat from spasticity seen with cerebral disorders.

The muscle spindle supports the tonic stretch reflex. Specialized receptors are found in the spindle within the intrafusal fibers for both static and dynamic stretch. Ia afferents convey this information to the gray matter of the spinal cord. Alpha and gamma efferents maintain contraction in the muscle. In spastic disorders, the spinal segment is released from inhibitory influences deriving from the upper motor neurons (the corticospinal tract). A cerebral lesion also facilitates excitatory influences from the vestibulospinal and pontine reticulospinal tracts. The end result is increased activation of both alpha and gamma efferents, an increase in tone and intrinsic spinal motor activity.

Baclofen, a $GABA_B$ agonist, promotes inhibition in multisynaptic spinal reflex pathways and is remarkably effective for painful flexor spasms in spinal patients. Diazepam promotes intrinsic inhibition but is sometimes sedating. These two medications are often used in combination. The benefits are sometimes disappointing in ambulatory patients, as the drugs cause some degree of weakness. Dantrolene acts primarily on skeletal muscle, decreasing excitation-contraction coupling. It is preferred by many patients with cerebral palsy. Cutaneous toxicity is common, and hepatotoxicity must be monitored. For severe spasticity refractory to oral agents, intrathecal administration of baclofen using a catheter and infusion pump has been quite successful. A variety of surgical procedures have been employed to reduce dysfunctional muscle contraction, ranging from nerve block to section of tendons or nerve roots.

Dystonia

The term *dystonia* means sustained abnormal fixed posture, and also refers to the spasms associated with dysfunctional posture. Dystonia may be generalized or restricted (focal or segmental). It is important to distinguish primary dystonia from secondary dystonia, for which a number of causes have been described (see box, p. 1070).

Primary generalized dystonia (idiopathic torsion dystonia, dystonia musculorum deformans) is a disorder with autosomal dominant inheritance; it is particularly prevalent

Causes of acquired (secondary) dystonia

- Cerebral palsy
  - Kernicterus
  - Asphyxia (hypoxic/ischemic encephalopathy)
- Posthemiplegic dystonia
- Dystonia resulting from encephalitis or trauma
- Acute drug-induced dystonia
- Chronic tardive dystonia
- Huntington's disease
- Progressive supranuclear palsy
- Wilson's disease
- Hallervorden-Spatz disease
- Neuronal ceroid lipofuscinosis
- GM_1, GM_2 gangliosidosis
- Lipidosis with sea-blue histiocytes
- Lesch-Nyhan syndrome
- Machado-Joseph disease
- Leigh's disease

among families of Ashkenazic Jewish extraction. The disorder has been localized to the long arm of chromosome 9. There are no consistent neuropathologic findings at the light microscope level, and the pathophysiology is not well understood. Albin, Young, and Penny have proposed a derangement of basal ganglia output. Changes in norepinephrine levels have been found in the hypothalamus, subthalamus, and locus ceruleus in postmortem brain, but the number of cases studied to date is small.

Dystonia musculoram deformans begins in childhood, usually with an inturned foot or torsion of the trunk. The mental state and deep tendon reflexes are normal. The postural distortions may be quite extreme, and distinguishing true dystonia from a hysterical disorder may be difficult. Periods of remission may occur, especially early. Successful treatment with high doses of anticholinergic drugs has been described. A disorder characterized by dystonia, young adult onset, and marked diurnal variation (fluctuations) responds to treatment with levodopa.

In patients with generalized dystonia, it is always necessary to exclude Wilson's disease and the other listed causes of secondary dystonia. Dystonic symptoms are very common in cerebral palsy patients and patients with neurodegenerative diseases involving the basal ganglia. Neuroleptic drugs can cause an acute dystonic reaction. Animal studies suggest that acute dystonic reactions to neuroleptic drugs result from a transient disorder of regulation at the dopamine synapse. They respond dramatically to anticholinergic drugs. A chronic, persistent dystonia sometimes occurs within the clinical spectrum of tardive dyskinesia (tardive dystonia).

Focal dystonias

The past decade has witnessed increasing recognition of focal dystonias, such as blepharospasm, torticollis, spastic dysphonia, and writer's cramp. Dystonias involving hand function are particularly common among certain occupational groups, such as keyboard operators and musicians. Focal dystonias involving the hand may be observed also in relation to peripheral nerve injury. Response to pharmacotherapy in these disorders has generally been disappointing, and botulinus toxin injection has rapidly become the treatment of choice. The pathophysiology of focal dystonia and the rationale for the therapeutic effect of botulinus toxin are not understood. The toxin produces a chemical denervation at the neuromuscular junction, which persists for 3 to 4 months. Patients require repeated treatments.

Idiopathic cervical dystonia (spasmodic torticollis) has its usual onset in middle adult life. There is sometimes a brief remission in the first year, after which the disorder tends to persist. Ten percent to 15% of patients have a positive family history. Head turning may be mixed with retrocollis or head tilt. In one large series, 75% of patients had neck pain. Attempts at treatment with anticholinergic drugs, carbamazepine, or baclofen rarely succeed for very long. Surgical procedures may weaken the support of the head, and the disorder usually recruits other muscles to express itself. Experience with botulinus toxin has been quite promising. Neck motion is substantially reduced in 60% to 80% of patients, and pain is relieved in up to 90%. Repeat injections using EMG to localize the posterior neck muscles are often required to achieve the best result.

Stiff-man syndrome

Originally described by Moersch and Woltman at the Mayo Clinic in 1956, stiff-man syndrome has re-emerged as a clinical entity with the discovery of associated autoantibodies to glutamic acid decarboxylase (GAD) in 85% of patients. Other immune-mediated disorders such as diabetes, vitiligo, and thyroiditis are frequently associated. Painful muscle spasms occur in the lower back and legs, with hyperlordosis of the spine and hypertrophy of the paraspinal muscles. This spinal deformity is the most characteristic feature of described cases. The disorder is quite uncommon. The spasms respond to benzodiazepines (often large doses are required). Plasmapheresis and corticosteroids are of unproved benefit.

ABNORMAL INVOLUNTARY MOVEMENTS

Tremor

The recognition of a tremor usually poses little problem. Technically, tremor is an oscillating involuntary movement about a joint. Contractions of reciprocally innervated antagonist muscles produce the movement. Tremor is divided into resting tremor and tremor with movement (action tremor). The latter category is subdivided into postural tremor, intention tremor, and task-specific tremor, such as primary writing tremor (Fig. 119-3). Essential tremor is sometimes mistaken for Parkinson's disease. Parkinsonian tremor subsides with activity. The topography of the tremor is also a clue. Involvement of the legs or jaw favors Parkinson's disease, while a whole-head tremor or vocal tremor is generally an essential tremor. Surface EMG or

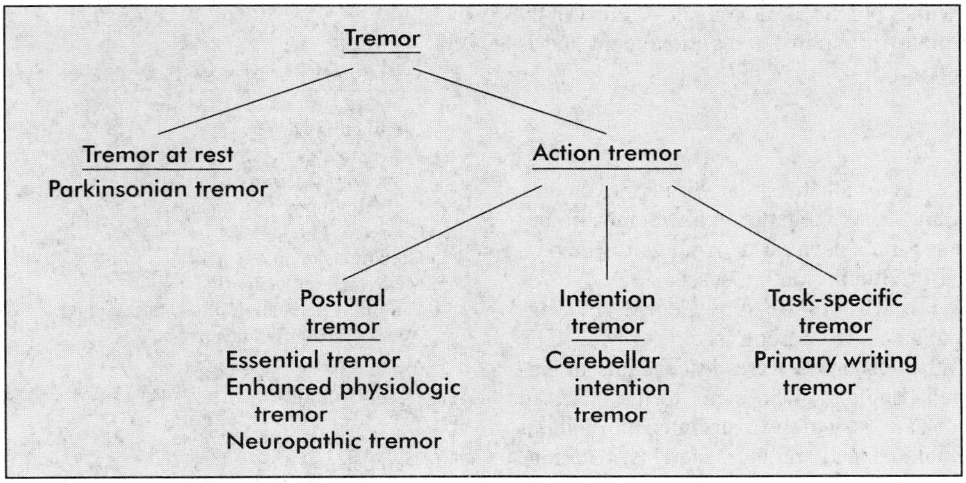

Fig. 119-3. Classification of tremor.

accelerometric recording can be used to resolve difficult cases. Distinguishing cerebellar intention tremor from the postural tremor group is often more difficult. In essential tremor, tremor amplitude and direction are more variable. Cerebellar intention tremor increases as the goal is approached, in a manner suggestive of a defective servomechanism.

Parkinsonian tremor is 3-7 Hz. EMG studies reveal an alternating pattern of activity in antagonist muscles. Resting tremor often responds to anticholinergic medications and usually improves with dopamine replacement therapy. In some stable patients with severe and refractory tremor, stereotactic neurosurgical ablations of the ventral-intermediate thalamic nucleus have been done with good result. For the vast majority of patients with longstanding PD, tremor is not the most limiting feature.

A low-amplitude, high-frequency tremor (8-12 Hz) is present among asymptomatic normal persons. It can be amplified by catecholamines, stress, fatigue, drug or alcohol withdrawal, thyroid hormone, caffeine, nicotine, or numerous other medications (see box at right). It is difficult to study physiologically because the tremor is buried in the normal interference pattern of the muscle. Young and Shahani suggest a peripheral mechanism, because intra-arterial injection of beta blockers can often quiet this tremor in a single limb. The use of small doses of beta blockers has become a common practice among performing artists. The preferred management of the symptomatic patient with enhanced physiologic tremor is treatment of the underlying disorder, commonly anxiety, thyroid disease, or substance abuse.

Essential tremor is a 4-12 Hz action tremor, often large enough in amplitude to interfere in activities of daily living. Physiological studies show cocontraction of agonist and antagonist muscles (a synchronous pattern) in 90% of cases. It may be familial, sporadic, or associated with other neurologic disease. In particular, Parkinson's disease and spasmodic torticollis are sometimes heralded by essential tremor. Many patients discover for themselves the beneficial effects of alcohol. Propranolol is the preferred treatment; a central mechanism has been proposed. Sustained trials of high doses (up to 320 mg/day) are sometimes required. Primadone in doses of 50-250 mg/day has also been employed. Tremors with lower frequency and head tremors in the elderly are notoriously difficult to treat.

Medications reported to induce tremor

Thyroid extract, synthroid
Epinephrine
Amphetamine, phenylephrine, and other sympathomimetics
Caffeine, theophyline, and other xanthenes
Nicotine, oxytremorine
Lithium
Phenothiazines
Methyl bromide
Monosodium glutamate
Corticosteroids (in high dose)
Insulin, oral hypoglycemic agents
Alcohol (withdrawal)
Metal intoxication (lead, arsenic, bismuth, mercury, manganese)
Tricyclic antidepressants

Intention tremor is a part of a cerebellar syndrome. It is characterized by rhythmic oscillation about the target of movement. Dysmetria, a tendency toward erratic movement, and gait ataxia are often more disabling to the patient than the tremor. Patients with cerebellar disease may have both intention tremor and a postural tremor. Limb weighting may be helpful; mechanical damping has been used to design assistive devices.

Patients with neuropathy may have a tremor, the mechanism for which is ill understood. Patients with motor neuron disease appear to have tremor caused by the irregular action of a small pool of giant motor units on the hand. Primary writing tremor is an example of a task-specific tremor associated with a practiced movement. It apparently resides within the motor program for the movement and is not otherwise expressed.

Huntington's disease

Chorea is a disorder in which irregular, brief movements occur in the limbs and trunk, together with facial grimacing, head movements, and a peculiar dancing gait. The prototype is the chorea of Huntington's disease.

Huntington's disease was described by George Huntington, an American physician from Long Island, in 1872. The cases he and his father observed were descendants of immigrants from Bures, England, who came to the states in 1649. Today the disease is widely distributed throughout northern Europe, South Africa, and the Americas. Huntington's disease is dominantly inherited, with onset in middle adult life. The cardinal clinical features are dementia, chorea, and a behavioral disorder. The prevalence is 7 to 10 per 100,000 population; patients enjoy a greater than normal "reproductive index." The genetics have been intensively studied and the defect localized to the short arm of chromosome 4. The gene product is presently not known, nor is the mechanism by which the gene produces premature loss of a selected neuronal population.

The disease has its usual onset in the 30s, though onset in childhood or late adult life is described. Behavioral disturbance usually occurs first, with depression the most common feature. Patients are often impulsive, erratic, or "hard to get along with." Chorea begins with piano-playing movements of the fingers or with facial grimace. Fast eye movements (saccades) are impaired. As the trunk becomes involved, there is a characteristic dancing gait, with relative preservation of balance. With further progression over a decade, rigidity and dystonia predominate and chorea may actually diminish. The patient with onset at age 35 is commonly bedridden in his 50s, with severe dysarthria, dysphagia, and dementia. There is dramatic weight loss caused by caloric expenditure from the movements. Childhood-onset cases are predominantly rigid, rather than choreic, and may have seizures.

Pathology reveals gross atrophy and neuronal loss in the caudate, with lesser changes in the putamen and globus pallidus, and mild change in the frontal cortex. Caudate atrophy can often be appreciated by the loss of the caudate impression on the lateral ventricle by CT or MRI. Microscopic examination reveals gliosis and loss of intrinsic neurons, especially the spiny cell population. Cell loss is selective, with marked depletion of GABA and enkephalin neurons and preservation of a class of aspiny stellate cells containing the diaphorase enzyme, somatostatin, and neuropeptide Y. The cell loss in the striatum results in excess inhibition of the subthalamic nucleus and disinhibition of thalamocortical afferents.

Definite diagnosis requires a pathologically confirmed case in the family. Initially the family history may be obscure. It is then important to rule out other causes of choreic movements (see box at upper right). There is presently no way to alter the progression of the disease. Haloperidol and diazepam are used in small doses by many patients to improve motor function. Presymptomatic diagnosis of relatives "at risk" is now feasible, though this application of genetic technology has been limited by patient preference.

Differential diagnosis of choreic disorders

Huntington's disease
Acute rheumatic chorea (Sydenham's)
Chorea gravidarum
Systemic lupus erythematosis
Chorea-acanthocytosis
Glutaric acidemia
Methylmalonic aciduria
Familial calcification of the basal ganglia
Acute vascular hemichorea
Senile chorea
Spontaneous oral dyskinesia in the edentulous patient
Drug-induced dyskinesias
- Levodopa, bromocriptine
- Anticholinergics
- Antihistamines
- Oral contraceptives
- Neuroleptics

Non-Huntington choreas

The box above provides a list of rather diverse disorders that have in common the tendency to cause choreic movements. These diseases all affect the basal ganglia and produce a disorder of striatopallidal output.

Sydenham's chorea is the neurologic manifestation of acute rheumatic fever. It is a self-limited condition, seen primarily in childhood. It is now uncommon in the United States. Chorea has been described with acanthocytosis in the peripheral blood, presumably a manifestation of an inherited membrane defect. CNS lupus (lupus cerebritis) may have chorea as a symptomatic manifestation when immunologic injury involves the basal ganglia. Transient chorea has been associated with pregnancy in some patients and with the use of oral contraceptives. It is unclear whether such patients have an underlying structural injury.

Stroke in the region of the subthalamic nucleus can cause severe flinging movements on the contralateral side. These violent movements (hemiballismus) improve over days, but may leave a residual hemichorea. Patients have been described with basal ganglia lacunes and generalized chorea, though it is striking how rarely small strokes in this region produce any involuntary movements. Spontaneous oral dyskinesias are found occasionally among older patients (senile chorea). Many of these cases occur among edentulous patients or are related to medications. Choreoathetosis (a slower, somewhat writhing movement disorder) is commonly caused by perinatal injury to the basal ganglia from ischemia or kernicterus. Athetosis has been described following hemiplegia when the injury occurs early in life.

Drug-induced dyskinesias

Dyskinesias related to medication can be acute or chronic. Unlike the chorea of Huntington's disease, movements are repetitive and stereotyped. Involvement of the perioral area (oral-buccal-lingual syndrome) is most typical, though not universally present. Acute dyskinesias have been reported with anticholinergics, dopaminergic agonists, antihistamines, and a variety of other drugs.

Chronic tardive dyskinesia is an array of dyskinetic and dystonic disorders, delayed in appearance, related to long-term administration of neuroleptic drugs. Three months exposure is probably the minimum necessary to produce a persistent dyskinesia. The problem is by no means universal in patients at risk. The prevalence of persistent dyskinesias in neuroleptic-treated patients (15%-40%) increases with age, and is greater among women. Tardive dyskinesia is thought to be a disorder of regulation at the postsynaptic dopamine receptor, caused by chronic exposure to neuroleptic drugs. Postsynaptic suprasensitivity to dopamine has been demonstrated in an animal model. Tardive dyskinesia and drug-induced parkinsonism may coexist in the same patient. The movements are not always permanent. If the offending agent is discontinued, spontaneous improvement may occur within 18 months, particularly in younger patients. Otherwise, treatment of tardive dyskinesia is not entirely satisfactory. The most successful approach has utilized drugs that deplete dopamine from the nerve terminal presynaptically (reserpine, tetrabenazine).

Myoclonus

Myoclonus is a brief muscle jerk originating from the central nervous system. It can be spontaneous, or it may be evoked by voluntary movement (action myoclonus), or triggered by sensory stimuli (reflex myoclonus). Myoclonus should be distinguished from asterixis, a brief lapse in tonic muscle activation. Both myoclonus and asterixis are seen together in certain metabolic encephalopathies. Sporadic myoclonus may be related to cortical epileptic activity. Long-duration jerks (50-300 ms) are sometimes caused by a disorder of the brainstem or spinal segmental mechanism. Spinal myoclonus is typically rhythmic. The physiology of myoclonus can be studied by recording the muscle jerk (using surface EMG), and by back-averaging the EEG to derive the related cerebral potential. The box at right adopts the etiologic classification proposed by Marsden, Hallett, and Fahn. Under some circumstances (transition to sleep, hiccup), myoclonus can be a physiologic phenomenon.

Etiologic classification of myoclonus (after Marsden, Hallett, and Fahn)

Physiologic

Sleep jerks
Hiccup

Essential

Familial essential myoclonus
Sporadic essential myoclonus
Startle syndromes

Epileptic myoclonus (fragments of epilepsy)

Partial continuous epilepsy
Photomyoclonic response
Primary generalized epileptic myoclonus
Juvenile atonic-myoclonic epilepsy (Lennox-Gastaut)
Infantile spasms
Benign myoclonus of infancy
Baltic myoclonus (Unverricht-Lundborg)

Symptomatic myoclonus

Storage disease with progressive myoclonus epilepsy
- Lafora body disease
- Neuronal ceroid lipofuscinosis
- Sialidosis
- Gaucher's disease
- GM_2 gangliosidosis
- Mitochondrial encephalomyopathy (MERRF)

Toxic/metabolic encephalopathy
Spinocerebellar, basal ganglia degenerations
- Friedreich's ataxia
- Wilson's disease
- Progressive supranuclear palsy
- Huntington's disease

Alzheimer's disease
Creutzfeldt-Jacob disease
Viral encephalitis
Posthypoxic (Lance-Adams)
Focal CNS damage
- Palatal myoclonus
- Spinal myoclonus

After Marsden CD, Hallett M, and Fahn S: In Marsden CD and Fahn S, editors: Movement disorders. London, 1982, Butterworth Scientific.

Essential myoclonus is often a familial disorder, with onset in the first or second decade, a benign course, and a normal EEG. Otherwise typical cases are commonly seen with no family history. Based on the success with posthypoxic myoclonus, 5-hydroxytryptophan has been used to treat other patients. Many respond as well to clonazepam, and some to valproate.

Quite frequently, myoclonus is observed as a fragment of an epileptic disorder. It may occur in relation to partial epilepsy or with some of the generalized epilepsies. In these cases, EEG is often diagnostic, and therapy is directed at the underlying seizure disorder. Valproate is preferred over phenytoin in predominately myoclonic generalized epilepsies.

Attention has recently been focused on the syndrome of progressive myoclonus epilepsy. Usually familial, these cases combine myoclonic seizures, tonic-clonic seizures, progressive ataxia, and dementia. The differential includes Lafora body disease, several of the storage diseases, and the recently characterized mitochondrial encephalopathies. The clinical syndrome known as MERRF (myoclonus epilepsy, ragged-red fibers) caused by a mitochondrial disorder may have onset in middle adult life.

In hospital practice, myoclonus is most often the marker of a metabolic encephalopathy caused by hepatic disease,

CO_2 retention, or chronic renal failure. Other causes of symptomatic myoclonus (myoclonus as a feature of a more generalized neurologic disorder) are listed. Myoclonus may be seen with late-stage Alzheimer's disease. Reflex myoclonus with periodic discharge on the EEG is characteristic of Creutzfeldt-Jakob disease. Segmental syndromes have been described that are restricted to the brainstem (palatal myoclonus) or the spinal cord. Spinal myoclonus has been described in association with tumor, infection, and rarely as a complication of spinal anesthesia or lumbar disc surgery.

Tics, Tourette's syndrome

A tic is a brief involuntary movement that is repetitive, often a caricature of a volitional movement that has taken on a life of its own. Patients describe a subjective aspect to the movement, an urge to tic. Tics may be suppressed for a time by act of will, unlike myoclonic movements, but reemerge when voluntary control is released.

Gilles de la Tourette's syndrome is a disorder characterized by multiple tics and vocalizations, which vary over time. Coprolalia (dirty talk) is present in most patients, but is not necessary for diagnosis. A pattern of autosomal-dominant inheritance has been demonstrated, though not everyone manifests the complete syndrome. Obsessive-compulsive disorder and childhood attention deficit disorder have been associated. Males are more commonly affected (3:1), though other family members may have obsessive compulsive disorder without motor manifestations. Onset of simple tics occurs between 5 and 10 years of age, while coprolalia emerges in adolescence. Compulsive behavior is a striking phenomenon in some patients. Cognitive function is usually normal. Haloperidol or pimozide have been used to suppress the movements, though many patients prefer not to take them. Small doses are best to reduce the risk of tardive dyskinesia. Clonazepam has also been used for tics, and fluoxitine can be helpful for obsessions and compulsions.

REFERENCES

Albin RL, Young AB, and Penny JB: The functional anatomy of basal ganglia disorders. Trends in neurosciences, 12:366, 1989.

Burke R: Tardive dyskinesia: current clinical issues. Neurology 34:1348, 1984.

Chan J, Brin MF, and Fahn S: Idiopathic cervical dystonia: clinical characteristics. Movement disorders 6:119, 1991.

Fahn S: Clinical variants of idiopathic torsion dystonia. J Neurol Neurosurg Psychiatry. 52(suppl):96, 1989.

Jankovic J and Brin M: Therapeutic uses of botulinum toxin. N Engl J Med, 324:1186, 1991.

Marsden CD: Parkinson's disease. Lancet, 335:948, 1990.

Marsden CD, Hallett M, and Fahn S: The nosology and pathophysiology of myoclonus. In Marsden CD and Fahn S, editors: Movement disorders. London, 1982, Butterworth Scientific.

Martin JB, Gusella JF: Huntington's disease: pathogenesis and management. N Engl J Med, 315:1267, 1986.

Parkinson Study Group, Effect of deprenyl on the progression of disability in early Parkinson's disease. N Engl J Med 321:1364, 1989.

Singer HS, Walkup JT: Tourette syndrome and other tic disorders: diagnosis, pathophysiology and treatment. Medicine, 70:15, 1991.

CHAPTER

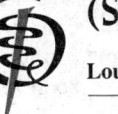

120 Cerebrovascular Disease (Stroke)

Louis R. Caplan

Stroke is a simple term, yet it describes a group of heterogeneous conditions that have in common death of brain tissue caused by disease of its vascular supply. The causes of stroke can be conveniently divided into two large categories: hemorrhage and ischemia. Bleeding and lack of blood are diametrically opposite conditions requiring quite different diagnostic and treatment strategies.

STROKE SUBTYPES

Hemorrhagic stroke

Hemorrhage injures tissues by exerting local pressure on brain structures, by interrupting and cutting vital brain pathways, and by increasing intracranial pressure, causing pressure shifts and herniations of brain tissue with brainstem compression. There are two large subcategories of hemorrhage: subarachnoid hemorrhage (SAH), in which bleeding is into the spaces surrounding the brain; and intracerebral hemorrhage (ICH), in which bleeding is directly into brain parenchyma. SAH and ICH are important to separate, since they have different causes, outcomes, and treatments.

SAH is most often caused by leakage of blood from abnormal blood vessels on the surface of the brain—aneurysms and vascular malformations. Aneurysms, often referred to as *berry* or *congenital,* are outpouchings on arteries probably caused by a combination of congenital defects in the vascular wall and degenerative changes. Aneurysms usually occur at branching sites on the large arteries of the circle of Willis at the base of the brain (Table 120-1). When an aneurysm ruptures, blood is released under arterial pres-

Table 120-1. Most common aneurysm sites and clinical signs

Location	Signs
ICA—posterior communicating artery junction	Ipsilateral third-nerve palsy
Anterior communicating artery	Bilateral leg weakness, numbness, and extensor plantar signs
MCA bifurcation	Contralateral face weakness, aphasia ([L] lesion) or visual neglect ([R] lesion)
Basilar bifurcation	Bilateral third-nerve palsies, extensor plantar reflexes, coma
Vert—PICA junction	Dizziness, lateral medullary infarct

MCA, middle cerebral artery; ICA, inferior cerebral artery; vert, vertebral; PICA, posterior inferior cerebellar artery.

sure into the subarachnoid space and quickly spreads through the cerebrospinal fluid around the brain and spinal cord. The sudden increase in intracranial pressure and meningeal irritation cause sudden headache, cessation of physical and intellectual activity, and, often, vomiting and alteration in the state of alertness. Drowsiness and restlessness with agitation are especially common. Most often, there is no associated bleeding into the brain, so severe focal neurologic signs such as hemiplegia and hemianopia are unusual. The expanding aneurysm or focal surrounding collections of blood within the cisterns and subarachnoid space can affect the cranial nerves and adjacent brain structures, causing characteristic focal features that depend on the location of the aneurysm (see Table 120-1). At times, the initial bleeding is so severe that death or irreversible brain damage occurs. If the bleeding is limited, the patient survives but is at risk of rebleeding in the days and weeks after the initial SAH. The arteries bathed by subarachnoid blood collections often become constricted, leading to delayed brain ischemia. Breakdown products of blood affect the vascular endothelia leading to transient, and later, fixed luminal narrowing. Aneurysms are less often caused by dissection (traumatic or spontaneous) through the adventitia of arterial walls, embolism of infected or myxomatous material to the vasa vasorum of distal cerebral arteries ("mycotic aneurysms"), or degenerative elongation and tortuosity of arteries ("dolichoectatic"). Vascular malformations (AVMs) contain abnormal capillary, venous, or arteriovenous channels. Bleeding from AVMs is mostly into the brain and/or into the subarachnoid space on the surface of the brain, and it is usually less vigorous and under less pressure than is hemorrhage from aneurysmal rupture. Less frequent causes of SAH include bleeding diatheses; trauma; amyloid angiopathy; bleeding into meningeal tumors; and the use of drugs that precipitously raise systemic blood pressure, such as methamphetamine and cocaine. Some patients who fall or hit their heads have concussions and so are amnestic for the trauma. Amyloid angiopathy is an important cause of SAH during the geriatric years.

Intracerebral hemorrhage (ICH) is most often caused by hypertension. Chronic hypertension causes degenerative changes in penetrating and subcortical arteries and arterioles with weakening of the arterial walls and small aneurysmal outpouchings (usually called *Charcot-Bouchard microaneurysms*). Acute increases in blood pressure and blood flow can also cause leakage from the same arteries. The affected penetrating arteries lie deep within the brain. Hypertensive ICH is most often located in the basal ganglia (putamen or caudate nucleus), thalamus, cerebral white matter, pons, and cerebellar white matter (Table 120-2). Bleeding is under arteriolar pressure and is cushioned by the resistance of tissue pressure in the surrounding brain structures. The initial release of blood into brain parenchyma causes pressure damage to local tissues and surrounding small vessels. The surrounding capillaries and arterioles break, leading to enlargement of the hematoma. The first signs of the hemorrhage are caused by dysfunction at the site of the bleeding: for example, in putamenal hemorrhage, weakness of the face, arm, or leg on the opposite side of the body; and in cerebellar hemorrhage, gait ataxia (see Table 120-2). If the hemorrhage is large, distortion of structures and increased intracranial pressure cause headache, vomiting, and decreased alertness. The cranial cavity is a closed system, and the bony skull and dura mater act as a fortress protecting the brain from outside injury. When swelling or hemorrhage arises inside the fortress, these structures may constitute a prison, restricting and strangulating their enclosed contents and forcing herniation of tissue from one compartment to another. Survival depends on the size and rapidity of development of the hematoma. ICHs are at first soft and dissect along white-matter fiber tracts. If the patient survives the initial pressure changes, blood is absorbed, and after macrophage clearing of the debris, a cavity or slit forms that may disconnect brain pathways. ICH can also be caused by bleeding from AVMs; trauma; bleeding diatheses, especially the prescription of anticoagulants; amyloid angiopathy; bleeding into brain tumors or granulomas; and sympatheticomi-

Table 120-2. Most common loci of hypertensive ICH and signs

Location (frequency)	Motor/sensory	Pupils	Eye movements
Putamen (40%)	Contralateral hemiparesia and hemisensory loss	Normal	Conjugate gaze paresis to opposite side
Caudate (8%)	Transient contralateral hemiparesis	Sometimes ipsilateral Horner's	Sometimes conjugate gaze paresis to opposite side
Lobar (15%)	Sometimes contralateral hemiparesis (aphasia, hemianopsia, etc., varying with lobe)	Normal	Sometimes conjugate gaze paresis to opposite side, depending on lobe
Thalamus (20%)	Contralateral sensory loss greater than motor	Small, poorly reactive, unilateral or bilateral	Eyes down and in, upgaze paralysis, sometimes ipsilateral conjugate gaze paresis
Pons (8%)	Quadraparesis	Small, reactive	Absent, horizontal gaze, ocular bobbing
Cerebellum (8%)	Ipsilateral ataxia, no paralysis	Sometimes ipsilateral pupil smaller	Ipsilateral sixth nerve or conjugate gaze paresis

metic drugs. Aneurysms rarely bleed only into the brain, causing a local hematoma near the brain surface.

Ischemic stroke

Deprivation of blood flow can be attributed to one of three different processes—thrombosis, local in-situ narrowing or occlusion of an artery obstructing or impeding distal blood flow; embolism, or blockage of an artery by material arising more proximally in the heart, venous system, or proximal arteries; and systemic hypoperfusion, which denotes a global decrease in brain blood flow caused by hypotension, cardiac pump failure, or hypovolemia. In thrombosis and embolism, ischemia exists in a local region of the brain fed by the affected artery, but in systemic hypoperfusion the decrease in blood flow and ischemia is more widespread.

Thrombosis implies obstruction of blood flow caused by a localized occlusive process within one or more blood vessels. The lumen of the vessel is narrowed or occluded by an alteration in the vessel wall or by superimposed clot formation (Fig. 120-1). The most common type of vascular pathology is atherosclerosis. Fibrous and muscular tissues overgrow in the subintima, and fatty materials form plaques that can encroach on the lumen. Platelets adhere to the crevices in the plaques and form clumps that serve as nidi for the deposition of fibrin, thrombin, and clot. Plaques and ulcers are associated with denudation of the endothelium and decreased release of endothelial relaxing factors (EDRF). Endothelins can promote platelet activation and thrombus formation. Intraluminal thrombi are of different types: so-called "white clots," which are comprised mostly of platelets and fibrin, and "red thrombi," which are red blood cells enmeshed in fibrin. White platelet clumps form most often in fast-moving streams, adhering to crevices and irregularities along the intimal surface. Fibrin-dependent red thrombi develop in slow-moving streams, for example, arteries with severe luminal narrowing. Atherosclerosis affects chiefly the large extracranial and intracranial arteries (Fig. 120-2), but there are important sex and racial differences in the distribution and incidence of lesions at these sites. White patients and men have more disease of the ex-

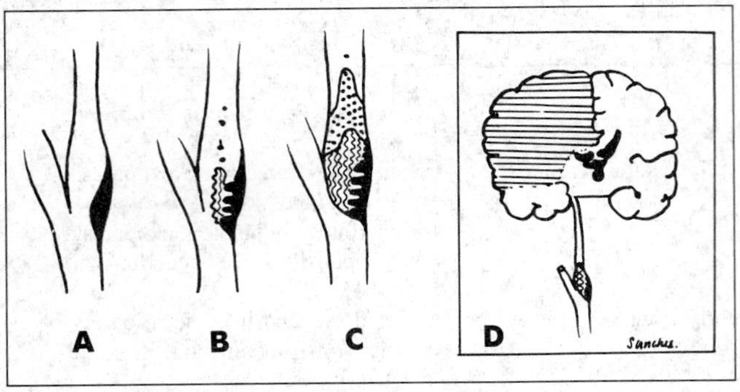

Fig. 120-1. Internal carotid artery atherosclerotic lesions. **A,** Flat plaque on the posterior wall. **B,** Plaque with platelet-fibrin emboli. **C,** Plaque with occlusive thrombus. **D,** Recent ischemic cerebral infarct in anterior and middle cerebral artery territories caused by internal carotid artery occlusion.

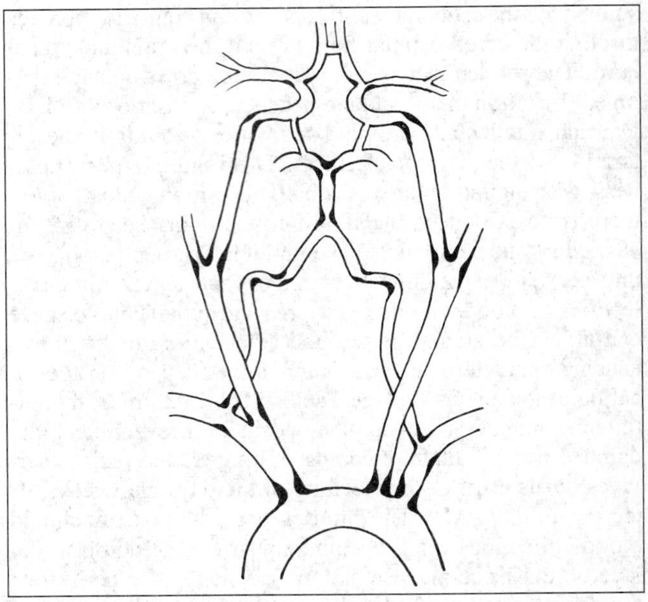

Fig. 120-2. Sites of predilection for atherosclerotic narrowing. Black areas represent plaques.

tracranial arteries, especially the internal carotid and vertebral artery origin; blacks, persons of Asian origin, and women have a predilection for narrowing of intracranial arteries, especially the middle and posterior cerebral arteries. Narrowing of arteries decreases blood flow, leading to stagnation of the blood column and activation of clotting factors. Clot and fibrin-platelet clumps form and break off, blocking distal arteries and further impeding flow in the parent affected artery. Less often, "thrombosis" is caused by a primary disorder of blood coagulation and not by a disease of the arterial wall. Deficiencies of natural coagulation-inhibiting factors (antithrombin III, protein C, protein S), abnormal fibrinolytic activity, acquired and inherited qualitative and quantitative abnormalities in serological coagulation factors, acquired immunologically mediated syndromes such as antiphospholipid antibodies, and systemic diseases such as cancer, inflammatory bowel diseases, and infections can all cause hypercoagulable states. Less common vascular pathologies leading to occlusive disease include fibromuscular dysplasia, an overgrowth of medial and intimal elements that compromise vessel contractility and the size of the luminal opening; "arteritis," especially caused by temporal arteritis; Takayasu's disease; injection of illicit drugs; and dissection of the arterial wall with luminal or extraluminal clot temporarily obstructing the lumen.

The small penetrating arteries deep within the brain substance are the sites of a different type of occlusive process from that of the larger extracranial and intracranial arteries. Variously called *lipohyalinosis* or *fibrinoid degeneration,* the changes in the penetrating arteries are mostly caused by hypertension. Subintimal lipid-laden foam cells and pink-staining fibrinoid material thicken the arterial walls, sometimes compressing the lumen. In places the areries are replaced by tangles and wisps of connective tissue that obliterate the usual vascular layers. The arteries affected are the lenticulostriate branches of the middle cerebral arteries (MCA), the thalamoperforating and thalamogeniculate branches of the posterior cerebral arteries (PCA), and the midline and paramedian penetrating branches of the vertebral and basilar arteries (Fig. 120-3). The small, deep infarcts that result from occlusion of these penetrating arteries are usually called *lacunes*.

Small, deep infarcts can also result from miniature atheromas (microatheromas) that form at the origin of penetrating arteries, and by plaques within the parent arteries that obstruct or extend into the branches.

Embolism is of two major types—cardiogenic and intra-arterial. Improved technology for evaluating cardiac disease has led to identification of previously unrecognized potential embolic sources and has documented that a higher proportion of ischemic strokes than previously suspected are emboli of cardiac origin. At least 30% of ischemic strokes are caused by embolism from the heart, a figure close to that derived from the Harvard Stroke Registry prior to sophisticated cardiac testing. Cardiac sources include endocardial and valve disease, myocardial infarcts and myocardopathies, arrhythmias, and intracardiac lesions such as tumors and clots (see box at right). Recently, transesophageal echocardiography has shown that protruding, often mobile and pedunculated atheromas and clots can be found in the thoracic aorta and are a relatively common source of embolism. Angiography and cardiac surgery with clamping of the aorta may promote embolism from aortic lesions. A less common form of cardiac embolism occurs when the heart serves as a conduit for emboli arising from clots in systemic veins; these clots pass through interatrial septal defects or patent foramen ovale to reach the brain and systemic circulation (so-called *paradoxical emboli*). Artery-to-artery emboli are composed most often of clot, platelet clumps, or fragments of plaques that break off from atherosclerotic lesions in proximal arteries. The most common sources of intra-arterial emboli are stenotic lesions in the carotid and vertebral arteries in the neck. Embolism is especially apt to occur just after a clot is formed, before it adheres to the arterial wall. Cholesterol crystals, fat, tumor, and foreign body material, particularly talc and cornstarch injected by drug abusers, are less frequent intra-arterial embolic materials. Embolic fragments, no matter what the source, tend to arrest in a recipient artery, depending on the location of branch points and the size of the embolic matter. Once lodged, the embolic matter often moves on within 48 hours, allowing reperfusion of the previously ischemic zone.

Blockage of arteries, whether caused by thrombi or emboli, sets in motion a series of events. Perfusion pressure distal to the occlusion drops, and the brain supplied by that artery is deprived of blood. Decreased blood flow in turn activates protective mechanisms that help restore blood flow to that ischemic region. Low pressure and release of lactic acid and other metabolites helps open collateral channels, bringing blood to the ischemic zone. At the same time, the process in the artery is not static; emboli pass, thrombolysis and fibrinolytic factors help lyse clots, and some clots propagate and embolize. These pathophysiologic events explain the clinical signature of thromboembolic stroke: that is, transient ischemic attacks and clinical fluctuations with progressive, stepwise, and fluctuating deficits.

Cardiogenic sources of emboli

- Myocardial ischemia
  - Mural thrombi
  - Hypokinetic zones
  - Ventricular aneurysms
- Arrhythmia
  - Atrial fibrillation (especially recent or paroxysmal)
  - Sick sinus syndrome
- Valvular
  - Bacterial or marantic endocarditis
  - Rheumatic mitral or aortic stenosis
  - Bicuspid aortic valve
  - Mitral valve prolapse
  - Calcific aortic stenosis
  - Mitral annulus calcification
- Cardiomyopathies
  - Endocardial fibroelactosis
  - Alcoholic cardiomyopathy
  - Myocarditis
  - Amyloid
- Intracardiac lesions
  - Myxomas
  - Primary or metastatic cardiac malignancies
  - Ball valve thrombi
- Intracardiac defects with paradoxic emboli
  - Atrial septal defects
  - Patent foramen ovale

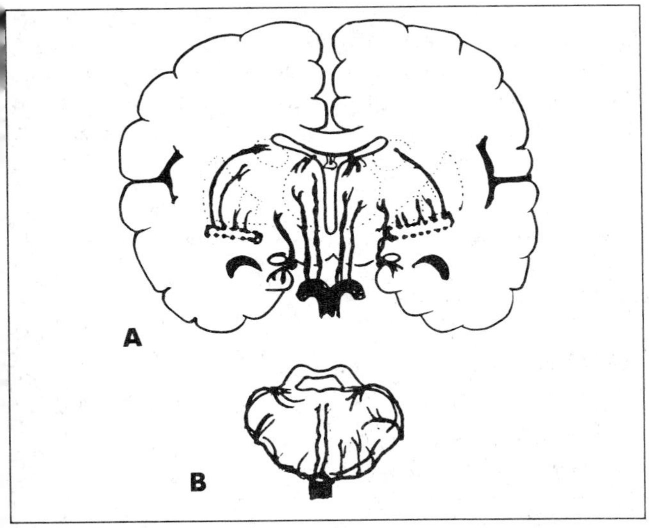

Fig. 120-3. Penetrating arteries prone to lipohyalinosis and microaneurysms: **A,** the lenticulostriate and thalmogeniculate arteries, and **B,** penetrating arteries to the pons. (From Caplan LR and Stein RW: Stroke: a clinical approach. Boston, 1986, Butterworth.)

Thrombosis is most frequent after sleep or a rest, the deficit being noticed on rising. Emboli come more often with activity, and the deficit often comes more abruptly than it does in thrombosis. Fluctuations, improvements, and stepwise and progressive changes in signs result from changes in the clot, emboli, and altered flow in collateral channels. During a period of 7 to 10 days the clot in the vessel and the collateral channels stabilize. The clinical signs depend on the part of the brain that is ischemic, but in thromboembolic stroke there are always prominent focal signs and not global neurologic dysfunction.

Systemic hypoperfusion is mainly caused by inadequate pumping of blood to the head. This occurs when there is too little blood in the system (shock, hypovolemia), when the pump itself fails (myocardial failure or severe arrhythmia), or when there is systemic hypotension. Faintness, pallor, dim vision, dim hearing and lightheadedness, dizziness, and lack of thought clarity are commonly noticed. The patient is worse when sitting or standing and the blood pressure is low. In contrast to thromboembolic stroke, hypoperfusion is global but favors the so-called border zone or watershed areas between the major regions of vascular supply (Fig. 120-4).

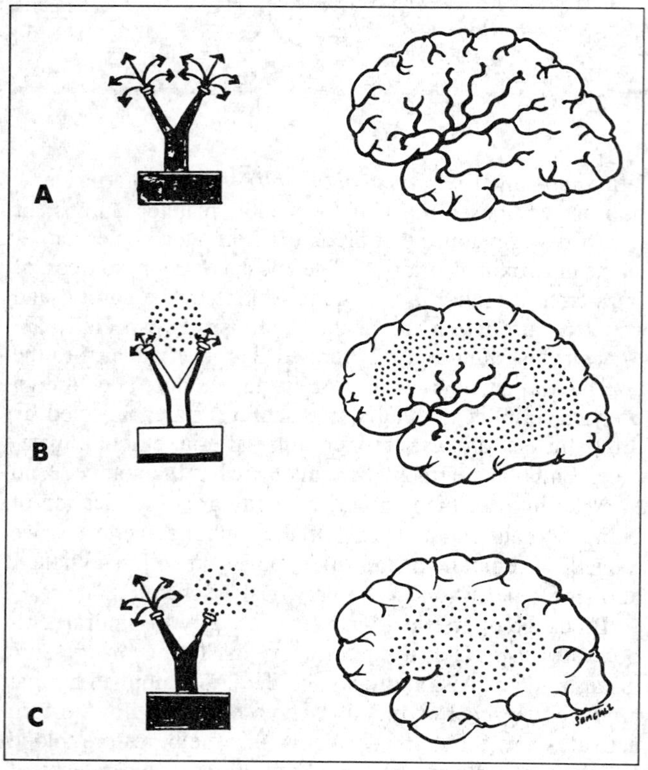

Fig. 120-4. Heart (pump) failure and watershed infarction. On the left is a diagrammatic schema of a water pump and two hoses. On the right are lateral surfaces of the brain. **A,** Normal pump and arterial circulation. **B,** Low pump pressure and border-zone ischemia: water goes to center of hoses (arteries); stippled areas are those of poor flow. **C,** "Blocked hose" and middle cerebral artery infarction. Water is deficient in center of supply *(stippled areas).* (From Caplan LR and Stein RW: Stroke: a clinical approach. Boston: 1986, Butterworth.)

CLINICAL SEPARATION OF STROKE SUBTYPES

The first question to ask is whether the patient has a stroke or a vascular lesion. Although most abrupt-onset focal neurologic disorders are caused by cerebrovascular disease, sometimes other disorders can mimic or be confused with stroke (see box below). These disorders should be considered. In patients with vascular disease, the next step is to place the patient in one of the stroke subtype categories discussed: that is, subarachnoid hemorrhage, intracerebral hemorrhage, thrombosis, embolism, or systemic hypoperfusion. Clinical data are often sufficient to arrive at a differential diagnosis in which some subtypes are seen as more likely than others and some are excluded. The use of probabilities is important, since a single diagnosis is seldom 100% certain. In a given patient, a single diagnosis—for example, thrombosis—usually is most likely (perhaps 70% probability), but embolic occlusion requires consideration (perhaps 20% probability), and ICH, although unlikely, is still possible (10% probability). SAH and systemic hypoperfusion can be excluded in this patient. Most of the data used to estimate probabilities come from the history of the development of the stroke. When the history is meager (for example, if the patient is stuporous, aphasic, or cannot recall what happened), the likelihood of an accurate clinical diagnosis diminishes. The clinical diagnosis can then be checked and amplified by laboratory data.

Demographics and past medical illnesses

The patient's age, sex, race, family history, and personal medical history strongly affect the probability of given stroke mechanisms. For example, if a young hypertensive black man without known heart disease had a stroke, ICH would be strongly suggested. In a 65-year-old diabetic man with coronary and peripheral vascular disease, there is a high probability of associated extracranial occlusive disease and thrombotic stroke or intra-arterial embolism. Of course, some diseases, such as hypertension, predispose to more than one stroke subtype. Hypertension can cause ICH, but

Important stroke mimics

- Migraine
- Syncope
- Hyperventilation
- Metabolic encephalopathy
- Drug overdose or intoxication
- Transient global amnesia
- Vestibular vertigo
- Seizures
- Hypoglycemia
- Hysterical conversion reaction

it also strongly increases the frequency of atherosclerosis of the extracranial arteries and thrombotic stroke. Patients with coronary artery disease have a predilection for associated extracranial vascular disease but also may have myocardial ischemic lesions that can lead to cardiogenic cerebral embolism. The racial and sex differences in the distribution of occlusive lesions have already been noted. Table 120-3 depicts relative weighting factors attributable to various risk factors.

Prior cerebrovascular events

Past strokes and transient ischemic attacks are especially important clues to stroke subtype. As an artery gradually becomes occluded, intermittent decreased distal flow or intra-arterial emboli, consisting of clot, fibrin platelet clumps, or plaque, are common. Approximately 50% of patients with infarcts caused by thrombosis of large extracranial or intracranial arteries have TIAs before their stroke, and 23% of patients with small-artery occlusion (lacunes) have premonitory TIAs. However, patients sometimes do not volunteer the occurrence of a prior attack, not recognizing the relationship. A patient with a left hemiparesis may not volunteer that 1 month ago he had a shade descend over his right eye for 2 minutes, because to him the eye has no relation to the weak limbs. A patient with arm weakness may not tell the physician about attacks of previous transient leg numbness, believing them to be unrelated. The physician must *repeatedly* ask about prior transient spells, specifically asking, Have you ever had temporary weakness, numbness, or shaking of a leg or a limp? Temporary weakness of an arm? Temporary speech trouble? A shade over your eye? and so forth. The presence of a transient ischemic attack in the same vascular territory as a stroke very heavily weights the probabilities to a thrombotic stroke. A past TIA or stroke in a different vascular territory makes cardiogenic embolism more likely.

Activity at stroke onset and early course of development of the signs

Thrombotic stroke often develops when the circulation is quiet—for example, during nocturnal sleep or a nap. Recent studies show that the hours between 8 to 12 in the morning are the most frequent time for ischemic stroke to develop. Embolism, ICH, and SAH more often develop during physical activity. Exceptions to this rule are common, and in practice most strokes begin during activities of daily living. The early course of the signs is very helpful in predicting stroke mechanism. Embolic strokes most often produce a neurologic deficit that develops abruptly and is maximal at onset (80%). Thrombotic strokes, in contrast, more often cause stuttering or stepwise signs (33%), gradual progression (13%), or signs that fluctuate from abnormal to normal (12%). Improvement or fluctuation early in the course of illness is virtually never found in ICH, which most often progresses gradually during minutes or hours (60%) or causes a deficit that appears to be maximal at onset (35%). Patients and family members are often not good at describing the progression of signs, but "walking through the events" near the time of the stroke can be very helpful. For example, a 63-year-old woman notes weakness of the left hand while fixing breakfast. Alarmed, she walks normally to her bed upstairs and lies down. Arising an hour later, she is happy to find her hand works well. Later in the morning she has a notable limp as she ascends the stairs. In the afternoon she cannot make the stairs, and her hand is weak. This course of illness with fluctuations and temporary improvement is characteristic of a thrombotic stroke.

Symptoms accompanying the neurologic deficit

Headache, loss of consciousness, vomiting, seizures, chest pain, and systemic symptoms such as fever are also important clues to the presence of stroke mechanism. All patients with SAH who are able to give a history have headache at

Table 120-3. Weighting of risk factors

	Thrombosis	Lacunae	Embolism	ICH	SAH
Hypertension	++	+++		++	+
Severe hypertension		+		++++	++
Coronary artery disease	+++		++		
Claudication	+++		+		
Atrial fibrillation			++++		
Sick sinus syndrome			++		
Valvular heart disease			+++		
Diabetes	+++	+	+		
Bleeding diathesis				++++	+
Hyperlipidemia	+++	+	+		
Cancer			++	+	+
Old age	+++	+		+	−
Black or Japanese origin	+	+		++	

Adapted from Caplan L and Stein R: Stroke: a clinical approach. Boston, 1986, Butterworth.

the onset of the stroke. The absence of headache virtually excludes the diagnosis of SAH. Seizures are most common in patients with ICH or embolism. Vomiting is most often caused by increased intracranial pressure caused by SAH or ICH or to ischemia within the posterior circulation. It is rare for a patient with thrombotic stroke other than basilar artery occlusion or embolism to lose consciousness at the onset of the stroke. Chest pain or arrhythmia before the stroke raises the possibility of cardiogenic embolism, and fever and malaise raise the possibility of bacterial endocarditis and temporal arteritis.

Findings from the neurologic and general examinations

Many nonneurologists, wary about the complexities of the neurologic exam, shy away from the stroke patient. The diagnosis of stroke subtype rests primarily on the items discussed so far—the background history and historical data about the stroke. The neurologic findings tell more about *where* the lesion is than *what* it is. At times the location of a lesion can heavily influence etiology: for example, a small deep lesion in the internal capsule or basal ganglia is likely to be a small ICH or a lacunar thrombotic infarct, whereas a superficial lesion in the left temporal lobe cortex is most likely an embolic infarct. Table 120-4 lists common localization patterns. Stroke localization heavily influences investigation of the vascular cause—posterior circulation ischemic events are not clarified by noninvasive or angiographic studies of the carotid artery.

Examination of the heart and arteries in the head, neck, and arms can also provide evidence of occlusive disease by the presence of delayed or absent pulses, collateral circulation, or bruits. The ocular fundus also gives important information about the arterial pressure and the carotid-ophthalmic circulation.

After acquiring the data items discussed, the physician, following the clinical encounter, should be able to construct a probability-oriented differential diagnosis of stroke mechanism and locale. These hypotheses can then be tested and amplified by eclectically chosen investigations.

LABORATORY DIAGNOSIS—AMPLIFICATION OF THE CLINICAL DIAGNOSIS

The choice of laboratory tests should depend on the question to be answered. Technology has vastly improved recently and is capable of determining where the brain lesion is, whether it is ischemic or hemorrhagic, how big it is, where lesion/s are within the vessels, how severe the vascular lesions are, whether there is a cardioembolic source, and whether there is a hematologic problem causing hypercoagability or excess bleeding. The box at right lists the various tests commonly available.

The most important first step is to determine whether the brain lesion is caused by hemorrhage or ischemia. In some patients, this will be obvious clinically: for example, a patient with a transient or rapidly improving neurologic deficit and no headache does not have a hemorrhagic process. The single best test to determine if a lesion is an ICH or an infarct is computed tomography (CT) scanning. CT or MRI should be used in every patient with a stroke or transient ischemic attack, because of the overwhelming amount of information gained and the safety of the procedure. Clinicians should not be swayed in this regard by those who, however appropriately, urge economy. Stroke is such an important, serious, and expensive disease that each case de-

Table 120-4. Common localization patterns

Brain locale or syndrome	Vessels	Findings
1. Left hemisphere anterior circulation	Left ICA, MCA, ACA	Aphasia, right-limb and -face weakness and/or sensory loss, right visual inattention
2. Right hemisphere anterior circulation	Right ICA, MCA, ACA	Left visual neglect, left-limb and -face weakness and/or numbness, poor drawing and copying, lack of recognition of deficit
3. Left occipitotemporal	Left PCA	Right hemianopsia, inability to read but not write and spell, no limb weakness, occasional right hemisensory loss
4. Right occipitotemporal	Right PCA	Left hemianopsia, occasional left hemisensory loss, occasional left neglect
5. Brainstem-cerebellum	Vertebral and basilar arteries	Vertigo, bilateral visual loss, quadraparesis, ataxia, crossed signs (cranial nerves on one side, limb weakness or sensory loss on other side), nystagmus
6. Pure motor stroke (internal capsule in pons)	Penetrating artery	Hemiparesis without cognitive, sensory, or visual loss
7. Pure sensory stroke (thalamus or postlimb internal capsule)	Penetrating artery	Hemisensory symptoms without motor, cognitive, or visual abnormalities

ICA, internal carotid artery; MCA, middle cerebral artery; ACA, anterior cerebral artery; PCA, posterior cerebral artery.

Laboratory procedures to evaluate cerebrovascular disease

- Brain imaging
  - Computed tomography (CT)
  - Magnetic resonance imaging (MRI)
  - Positron emission tomography (PET)
  - Single photon emission computed tomography (SPECT)
  - Xenon-enhanced CT
- Functional brain tests
  - Electroencephalography (EEG)
  - Topographic EEG
  - Evoked responses
  - PET
  - SPECT
  - Xenon cerebral blood flow (XeCBF)
  - Xenon-enhanced CT
- Vascular lesion
  - B-mode ultrasound
  - Continuous-wave (CW) or pulsed Doppler ultrasound
  - Oculoplethysmography (OPG)
  - Color-flow Doppler
  - Transcranial Doppler ultrasound (TCDU)
  - Magnetic resonance angiography
  - Catheter dye angiography
- Spinal fluid analysis
  - Lumbar puncture
- Hematologic tests
  - Hemoglobin
  - Platelet count
  - Prothrombin time
  - Partial thromboplastin time (PTT)
  - Antithrombin III
  - Protein C and S levels
  - Antiphospholipid antibodies
- Cardiac tests
  - Electrocardiography
  - Echocardiography
  - Ambulatory rhythm monitoring
  - Doppler
  - Multiple-gated acquisition scan (MUGA)

serves careful investigation aimed at minimizing deficits and logically treating the causative process. CT not only differentiates hemorrhages from infarcts—it also shows the extent of ICH and documents the size and location of the lesion, drainage into the CSF or surface, pressure effects on secondary structures, and the presence of edema surrounding the lesion. CT also accurately images the size and location of infarcts. In a highly significant number of patients, CT uncovers clinically unsuspected past vascular lesions and stroke mimics such as meningiomas, along with subdural hematomas.

Magnetic resonance imaging (MRI) is probably more sensitive but less specific than CT; it does not readily separate ischemia or edema or Wallerian degeneration from the primary infarct or hemorrhage. Casual inspection of an MRI scan usually does not allow easy distinction between ICH and infarction, but these two can be distinguished by analysis of the characteristics of different spin echo techniques: that is, the T1 and T2 weighting of images. MRI is more accurate in detecting posterior fossa lesions and lesions at the base of the brain. The MRI capability of imaging lesions in sagittal, horizontal, and coronal planes is a distinct advantage in localizing some lesions. When large and very recent (within 48 hours), subarachnoid hemorrhages are usually seen on CT but not imaged by MRI. Lumbar puncture with careful analysis of the CSF is a key diagnostic test for SAH.

The next question to settle is *the location of the brain dysfunction,* which not only helps in understanding and interpreting the symptoms, but is crucial for planning investigations of the vascular lesion. Most often, neurologic examination, CT, and/or MRI allow accurate definition of the brain localization and vascular territory involved. Some patients with transient or reversible neurologic deficits have normal examinations or findings that cannot be definitively localized to a brain region. For example, weakness of an arm could occur with lesions in the precentral cortex, cerebral white matter, or brainstem, whereas a patient with aphasia plus weakness and numbness of the right face and hand definitely has a left paracentral cortical lesion. Most patients with normal neurologic examinations have nondiagnostic imaging tests, and some patients with abnormal examinations also have normal images on CT and MRI. Brain tissue, although not functioning normally, has not been anatomically altered and so does not show abnormal findings on brain imaging. A number of "functional tests" can give evidence of abnormal brain functioning or abnormal blood flow. In some patients, EEG, evoked-response tests after visual, somatosensory, or auditory stimuli, and topographic EEG mapping can indicate the brain regions not functioning electrically normally. Positron emission tomography (PET) gives even more data about local brain metabolic and blood flow abnormalities. In practice, PET is seldom available clinically, and electrical testing is very infrequently of practical help. Some tests such as SPECT scanning, xenon cerebral blood flow (XeCBF), and xenon-enhanced CT provide functional information about blood flow, but these data tell more about the vascular lesions than about the brain lesion.

Once the localization and mechanism (ischemia or hemorrhage) have been determined, the clinician should turn to analysis of the *causative vascular lesion*. The investigations chosen differ depending on whether hemorrhage or ischemia is present. If SAH is present, CT with contrast occasionally images an aneurysm or AVM, but angiography is the method of choice for opacifying these causative vascular lesions. The blood should also be screened for a bleeding diathesis. If an ICH is present on CT in a common location for hypertensive hemorrhage (see Table 120-2) and the patient is hypertensive, no further evaluation usually is needed to diagnose a hypertensive ICH. If the location or morphology is atypical, contrast enhancement of CT or angiography sometimes is used to diagnose AVM, aneurysm, or tumor that could have precipitated bleeding. Blood screening for a bleeding diathesis is also important.

When an infarct is found on CT or when no hemorrhage is seen in a patient with stroke or TIA, an ischemic etiology is inferred. Tests chosen to document and define the vascular lesion depend on the location of the lesion (anterior or posterior circulation) and the patient's demographics and risk factors. B-mode ultrasound and Doppler examination of the carotid arteries are both excellent techniques for studying internal carotid artery occlusive lesions in the neck. Sometimes these two techniques are combined in a duplex system that improves the diagnostic yield of the examination. Oculoplethysmography can document important flow reduction in the ophthalmic artery branches of the internal carotid artery when occlusive carotid disease is suspected. Transcranial Doppler ultrasound is a good technique for quantifying intracranial occlusive disease of the internal carotid artery siphon, middle cerebral artery, and anterior cerebral artery, as well as the intracranial vertebral and basilar arteries. Doppler is also a good technique for diagnosing vertebral artery disease in the neck. Ultrasound and functional tests do not substitute for angiography, which shows the full extent of the major extracranial and intracranial arteries. Magnetic resonance imaging (MRI) is a promising new technique capable of showing most severe occlusive lesions and medium-sized aneurysms. Catheter angiography by femoral artery catheterization remains the most precise way of imaging the arterial tree, but it carries a small risk (1%-2% morbidity and mortality). All patients with ischemia should have at least screening studies of blood coagulation, to exclude a hypercoagulable state.

Cardiogenic embolism should be suspected strongly in patients with (1) infarcts in different vascular territories, (2) known cardiac disease, (3) sudden-onset neurologic deficits without premonitory transient ischemic attacks (TIAs), (4) relative youth (under 40 years old), (5) no occlusive vascular lesion found. Cardiac investigations usually include an electrocardiogram, echocardiogram, and ambulatory cardiac rhythm monitoring. Doppler study of the septum during echocardiography and after injection of a few bubbles of air helps detect septal defects and paradoxical embolism. Alternatively, monitoring of the intracranial arteries after intravenous injection of air bubbles also identifies passage of the bubbles across the septum. Large-vessel occlusive disease and cardiogenic embolism are especially likely if the lesion is superficial and affects the cerebral cortex. Small, deep lacunes are sometimes imaged by CT and MRI, thus defining the lesion and making further evaluation unnecessary if the risk factor profile and clinical picture are typical for lacunar disease. Border-zone bilateral infarction suggests cardiac disease or hypotension and should stimulate cardiac investigations. Tests of blood flow are useful only when the causative vascular lesions are known. PET, SPECT, xenon-enhanced CT, and xenon inhalation CBF studies all can show the regions of relatively decreased blood flow. When these regions of abnormal CBF are superimposed on the infarct, the physician can tell whether collateral flow is good or there are important or large areas of brain tissue that, although not yet infarcted, are tenuously supplied with blood. Knowing the causative vascular lesion, the state of the blood, and the extent of the brain damage, the clinician can logically tailor therapy to the patient.

THROMBOTIC STROKE

Treatment of patients with thrombotic lesions should be guided by (1) the severity and reversibility of the brain damage; (2) the nature, location, and severity of the vascular occlusive lesion; and (3) the state of the blood. In general, the more severe and irreversible the lesion, the more remote the possibility of effective reperfusion and restoration of function. Another aim of treatment is prevention of further damage. To judge the brain tissue still "at risk" for further ischemia, the physician must know the vascular lesion and mechanism of stroke. An example would be a patient with a small lesion in the white matter of the frontal lobe. If the damage is caused by a lacune, the entire territory of the lipohylanotic disorganized artery may be infarcted, so no further tissue is at immediate risk. If, however, the vascular process was occlusion of the internal carotid artery in the neck or in the siphon, then nearly the entire hemisphere is still at risk. In another patient with a large right-anterior cerebral and middle cerebral territory infarct, if the causative vascular lesion was occlusion of the internal carotid artery, then the entire territory of that vessel has been infarcted and little tissue is at further risk. If, however, the cause was an embolus from a cardiac mural thrombus, then the posterior circulation and entire opposite hemisphere are at risk. The less the cerebral damage, the higher the benefit/risk ratio. Especially likely to benefit from treatment are patients with TIAs but no brain damage.

In each series of ischemic stroke patients with a given vascular lesion—for example, stenosis of the internal carotid artery—the likelihood of stroke increases with increasing severity of stenosis. As stenosis becomes more severe, platelet fibrin deposits tend to form and embolize, and decreased flow through the stenotic vessel leads to the formation of fibrin-dependent "red clots." Red clots form in situations promoting stasis, such as leg veins and dilated cardiac atria, whereas "white platelet clumps" tend to form on rough areas in fast-moving arterial streams, such as the internal carotid artery. Theoretically, red clots would respond more to warfarin anticoagulants and heparin, and white clots would be prevented more with platelet antiaggregants, such as aspirin. Surgery (endarterectomy) or warfarin may be indicated for patients with tight stenotic lesions and important tissue at risk for further ischemia. The choice of warfarin or surgery depends on the accessibility of the lesions to the surgeons, the risk of surgery, the patient's wishes, the likelihood the patient will be compliant with anticoagulants, and any contraindication to the use of anticoagulants. Heparin should be used for 2 to 3 weeks when there is an acute occlusion of an artery, to prevent propagation and embolization of clot. Usually, long-term warfarin is not needed after the clot organizes and adheres to the vessel wall. Aspirin, 50 to 300 mg per day, can prevent platelet-fibrin emboli in patients with minor or moderate stenosis. Increasing the dose of aspirin (especially if an in-vitro aspirin effect is not shown at the lower dose) or use of ticlopidine should be tried if symptoms recur. Neither warfarin nor surgery is recommended in patients with slight to moderate stenosis. Obviously, if the patient has a primary coagulopathy, polycythemia, or thrombocytosis, these disorders should be treated more specifically.

Anterior circulation large-vessel occlusive disease

Internal carotid artery origin (ICAO). The distal common carotid artery (CCA) and first 3 cm of the ICA, especially along the posterior wall directly opposite the flow divider between the external carotid artery (ECA) and the internal carotid artery (ICA), is the most common site of plaque formation in the cerebrovascular system. Symptoms correlate with the severity of stenosis. The most common presentations are (1) TIA, (2) transient monocular blindness (TMB), and (3) sudden-onset stroke. TIAs are usually multiple. Temporary weakness and/or numbness of the limbs on the opposite side of the body is the most common symptom, and the hand and the arm are the most frequently affected body parts. Dysphasia is also common. Spells are often not stereotyped; a patient with right-ICA stenosis might have numbness of the left hand and foot in one spell, numbness and weakness of the left arm and hand in another, and sudden giving way of the left leg in a third spell. TMB is common and especially important to recognize, because it identifies the ICA-ophthalmic artery circuit as the location of the causative vascular lesion. The visual symptoms are usually described in terms of a dark shade or curtain descending over vision in the eye ipsilateral to the occlusive process. The shade may descend only halfway or, occasionally, may block vision from the side, like a stage curtain closing. The visual loss lasts seconds to minutes, then recedes, usually with no residual loss of vision. Attacks can be precipitated by bending, sudden rising, or straining. Some patients with chronic ocular ischemia note loss of vision in the ischemic eye when exposed to bright light, a kind of "visual claudication." Sudden-onset strokes are usually caused by embolism of plaque or clot from an occluded or tightly stenotic ICAO lesion. Less often, embolism can arise from a seemingly minor plaque, a clot loosely attached to the vessel wall, or carotid dissection.

Noninvasive tests are usually adequate to reflect the severity of ICA stenosis but not to predict ulceration. Duplex scans (B-mode and Doppler combined) give an accurate image of the CCA and its ICA and ECA branches. Oculoplethysmography (OPG), periorbital directional Doppler ultrasound (PDDU), and transcranial Doppler ultrasound (TCDU), by measuring flow or pressure in carotid artery tributaries, add information about the functional severity of the proximal lesion. When the ICAO lesion is severe (that is, greater than 70% stenosis), angiography, either by standard femoral artery catheterization or by digital intravenous or intra-arterial techniques, is usually needed to further define the ICA lesion and to opacify the important ICA intracranial branches.

Internal carotid artery siphon (ICAS). The tortuous S-shaped portion of the ICA from where it enters the bony skull to where it emerges from bone at the clinoid process to enter the cranial cavity, is usually called the *siphon*. When narrowing occurs before the ophthalmic artery branch, the symptoms are indistinguishable from those of ICAO disease except for the absence in ICAS disease of physical signs of disease in the neck, such as a bruit. When the occlusive lesion is above the ophthalmic artery branch, TMB does not occur, of course. ICAS disease causes TIAs or strokes with ischemia in the territories of the middle cerebral artery (MCA) and anterior cerebral artery (ACA). Weakness and/or numbness of the leg and face are most common. Because ICAS lesions have a much higher stroke-TIA ratio than ICAO disease, the former have a poorer prognosis.

Tests used to directly image the ICA in the neck, such as duplex scans and Doppler, are not helpful in ICAS disease. OPG can show reduced flow when the ICAS lesion is proximal to the ophthalmic artery. TCDU is effective in studying ICAS disease, but only an experienced technician can provide accurate interpretation. Angiography is the preferred method for showing the lesion. ICAS disease is not surgically accessible, so treatment is usually platelet antiaggregants or warfarin, depending on the degree of stenosis, the severity of the stroke, and the presence of still at-risk brain.

Middle cerebral artery. Intrinsic lesions of the MCA are less common than emboli to this vessel that arise from either the heart or the vascular system. In-situ narrowing usually affects the proximal portion of the artery before the lenticulostriate branches and is most common in blacks, individuals of Asian origin, and women. Strokes are caused by blockage of flow to the MCA territory or by embolization of material to MCA branches. Common symptoms are hemiparesis, aphasia, and neglect of the contralateral visual field. Weakness or numbness of one limb is less common than in ICAO disease. Compared with ICAO disease, strokes usually are more frequent but less severe. On CT scans, infarcts caused by MCA disease are usually deep, imaging as greater than 2-cm infarcts in the striatum and capsule (so-called striatocapsular infarcts) or wedge-shaped sylvian infarcts in the distribution of a branch of the MCA. TCDU can give accurate data about pressure and flow in the MCA, but other noninvasive tests are not useful. MRA and catheter angiography are the only procedures that provide an image of the lesions, but lack of distal flow in the MCA can sometimes be suspected on contrast-enhanced CT scans and MRI.

Anterior cerebral artery. This vessel supplies the paramedian frontal lobes. Symptoms of ischemia include weakness of the contralateral foot, leg, and thigh, incontinence, and abulia (lack of spontaneity and increased latency of responses). Embolism, especially from the ICA, is a more common cause of ACA occlusion than is intrinsic disease. Diagnosis usually depends on angiography.

Posterior circulation large artery occlusive disease

Subclavian artery and vertebral artery origin (VAO). Plaques most often occur within the subclavian artery before the vertebral artery origin; plaques can extend into the

VAO or originate within the first 2 to 3 cm of the proximal vertebral artery. When the subclavian artery is very stenotic or occluded, the most common symptoms relate to the ischemic arm—fatigue, coolness, and lack of power or endurance, along with a small, delayed pulse, cool hand, and asymmetrically reduced blood pressure are noted. Less often, patients report TIAs, with dizziness, staggering, or double vision occasionally precipitated by exercise of the ischemic arm. When the lesion is within the VAO and the subclavian artery is not narrowed, identical attacks of vertigo, imbalance, and transient double vision or visual blurring occur, but of course the arm is not symptomatic.

Diagnosis of subclavian stenosis is usually possible clinically by detection of a supraclavicular bruit, careful palpation of the wrist and arm pulses, and measurement of blood pressure in the two arms. Noninvasive tests of arm flow and Doppler studies of the vertebral arteries can usually identify obstruction of subclavian or vertebral flow and detect retrograde flow down the vertebral artery. Angiography with delayed films can identify the vascular lesion and the presence of retrograde flow ("subclavian steal"). Disease of the subclavian artery and vertebral artery origins is usually benign and occurs most often on the left. Usually, adequate collateral vessels develop to prevent serious arm or posterior circulation ischemia. When the proximal vertebral artery occludes, the clot can embolize to the intracranial posterior circulation; heparin should be used for 2 to 3 weeks in such a situation. Right-sided subclavian or innominate artery disease is more serious, since the clot can extend into or embolize to the right carotid artery. Occlusive disease of the remainder of the extracranial vertebral arteries is infrequent, but the distal extracranial vertebral artery, where the artery loops around the atlas, is a vulnerable place for injury or dissection during sudden movements or neck manipulation.

Vertebral artery intracranially (VAIC). The intracranial vertebral artery supplies the medulla oblongata and the inferior surface of the cerebellum. Stenosis or occlusion causes (1) lateral medullary infarction, for which symptoms and signs are noted in Table 120-5; (2) ischemia of the lateral and medial medulla, in which hemiparesis of the limbs opposite to the lesion is often found with symptoms of lateral medullary ischemia; and (3) cerebellar infarction, characterized by gait ataxia, dizziness, and vomiting. Sometimes, occlusion of the intracranial vertebral artery is detected asymptomatically when the patient is studied because of a sudden hemianopia caused by posterior cerebral artery territory infarction; the distal occlusion has been caused by intra-arterial embolization of clot from the VAIC. TCDU and continuous-wave Doppler can detect decreased flow in the VAICs. Bilateral occlusion or stenosis of the VAICs is particularly serious and can cause chronic medullary and cerebellar ischemia with posturally induced dizziness and visual blurring, as well as progressive weakness and ataxia of the limbs.

Basilar artery disease. The basilar artery supplies the pons. Occlusion develops because of in-situ atherosclerosis of the basilar artery or extension of clot from the distal VAIC. The most common symptoms are weakness of the limbs—often, both legs. At times, weakness is crossed (that is, one side of the face and opposite side of the body) or affects one side of the body, sometimes alternating sides in different attacks. Double vision, dysarthria, and dizziness are also common. The most severe risk of serious brainstem infarction occurs shortly after the basilar artery occludes. In some patients, collateral circulation develops quickly, and slight or no brain damage results despite basilar artery occlusion. Maintenance of blood volume and blood pressure during the crisis helps as collateral circulation develops, and heparin probably is useful in preventing clot extension and embolization. Long-term warfarin is probably not needed unless the basilar artery is tightly stenotic or harbors clot and is not yet occluded. Diagnosis is by angiography or TCDU. CT with contrast can identify tortuous dolichocetatic basilar artery aneurysms and can occasionally image a fresh basilar artery clot. MRI is the preferred technique for identifying brainstem and cerebellar infarction.

Occlusion of the rostral basilar artery is most often embolic, with clot arising from the heart or proximal verte-

Table 120-5. Signs and symptoms in lateral medullary infarction

Anatomic structure	Ipsilateral findings	Contralateral findings
Descending tract and nucleus of V	Jabs of pain in the face, loss of pain and temperature sensation in the face, loss of corneal reflex	
Vestibular nuclei	Whirling dizziness, nystagmus	
Restiform body and cerebellum	Clumsiness and inability to stand or walk; gait ataxia, leaning to the affected side; ataxia on finger-to-nose and toe-to-object testing	
Descending sympathetic fibers	Horner's syndrome	
Nucleus ambiguous	Dysphagia and hoarseness, decreased pharyngeal movement, paralysis of the vocal cord	
Spinothalamus tract		Loss of pain and temperature sensation on the body and limb, sometimes with a "level" on the trunk

bral basilar system. Symptoms include visual loss—hemianopia or bilateral visual loss—loss of memory, and various oculomotor signs. Ischemia is in the territories of the arteries penetrating from the basilar artery apex to the medial midbrain and thalamus and in the territories of the posterior cerebral arteries (PCAs).

Posterior cerebral arteries (PCA). These vessels supply the occipital lobes and the undersurfaces of the temporal lobes. Occlusion of a PCA is most often embolic, arising from the heart or proximal vertebral basilar system. When intrinsic stenosis of the PCA is present, the lesion almost always involves the proximal perimesencephalic or ambient segments. The most common symptom is loss of vision to one side. Patients describe a void or lack of ability to see to the side. Despite the hemianopia, and unlike visual loss in lesions of the middle cerebral artery territory, patients do not neglect or ignore the hemianopic side. Some patients with left PCA occlusion have alexia without agraphia: that is, they can write and spell but cannot read. They usually also cannot identify colors. Patients with right PCA territory infarction, especially if it is extensive and includes the temporal and parietal lobes, have left visual neglect. Hemisensory loss on the side contralateral to the lesion may accompany hemianopia, but paralysis is not common.

Penetrating artery disease

Treatment consists primarily of controlling the underlying causative process—hypertension. Hyperlipidemia and polycythemia may be contributory factors and should also be treated. During the acute phase, blood pressure should *not* be extensively lowered, since this decreases pressure in collateral channels and may extend the infarct. The patient should be kept supine and blood volume and flow maximized during the acute phase of the infarct; only during convalescence, 2 to 3 weeks later, should vigorous antihypertensive treatment be prescribed.

Neurologic deficit in patients with lacunar infarction can progress gradually or stepwise for 1 to 7 days. Evidence for a lacunar—that is, penetrating artery—etiology includes hypertension, past or present; short clinical history of TIAs or stroke progression; purely motor or purely sensory nature of clinical signs affecting face, arm, and leg; CT or MRI that images a small deep infarct or no lesion; and a normal or symmetric EEG.

EMBOLISM

The major treatment of cerebral embolism is prophylactic prevention of the next embolus. When the source is intraarterial, treatment depends on the nature of the arterial lesion and the severity of the resulting brain damage, and one should follow the guidelines given under thrombotic stroke. Heparin, then warfarin for 2 to 4 weeks should be used when an acute occlusion of a proximal artery has occurred. When the proximal arterial embolic source is a tightly stenotic artery, either surgery (if feasible) or longer-term warfarin is indicated. When the proximal source is plaque without severe stenosis, platelet antiaggregants, such as aspirin, should be used. Recent studies have shown that warfarin prophylaxis is very effective in preventing cardiogenic embolism in patients with atrial fibrillation. Treatment of other cardiac sources has not been as well studied. Some cardiac sources require direct treatment of the heart lesion, which may eliminate or reduce their embologenic potential—for example, surgery for valvular disease or a ventricular aneurysm or interatrial septal defect, and the use of cardioversion and antiarrhythmic drugs to convert atrial fibrillation to normal rhythm.

Because it has been demonstrated that warfarin anticoagulants decrease the incidence of embolism in patients with rheumatic mitral stenosis and atrial fibrillation and those with recent myocardial infarction, many physicians prophylactically use warfarin in any patient with cardiogenic embolism. When warfarin anticoagulation is used, it is advisable to keep the prothrombin time at approximately 1.5 times the control value (INR 2-3) and no higher. Many cardiac lesions occur in older patients in whom long-term anticoagulation poses important risks and problems. Some cardiac lesions known to be potential embolic sources probably have a relatively low frequency of embolism: for example, mitral valve prolapse and porcine valves. In elderly patients and in cases in which there is a low frequency of embolism, the risk-benefit ratio of anticoagulants is not known. Aspirin may also be effective prophylaxis in some patients with potential cardiac sources of embolism. Dipyridamole in high doses (400 mg a day) seems to add protection when used with warfarin in patients with prosthetic valves. Despite the lack of data, aspirin may be useful for prophylaxis in some patients with cardiac lesions of low embolic potential and in patients with absolute or relative contraindications to warfarin use.

The onset of neurologic signs in patients with cerebral embolism is usually abrupt, and most often the deficit is maximal at or near onset. Fluctuations or worsenings and sudden improvement are common during the first 24 to 48 hours, probably because of the passage of emboli distally. Angiography within the first 12 hours has a high yield of showing emboli, but after 48 hours most emboli are no longer detectable. The most common recipient arteries are the MCA and ACA in the anterior circulation and the vertebral, distal basilar artery, and PCA in the posterior circulation. The clinical signs and imaging findings are the same as those described in the discussion of these vessels in the section on thrombotic stroke.

HEMORRHAGIC STROKE

Treatment of patients with intracerebral hemorrhage (ICH) depends on the size and location of the hematoma, the severity of the clinical neurologic deficit, and the etiology of the bleeding. Bleeding diatheses, such as hypoprothrombinemia caused by warfarin prescription, hemophilia, or thrombocytopenia, should be reversed when possible, and hypertension should be controlled. Some have advocated surgical drainage of hematomas to relieve mass effect and accelerate recovery. Surgery can be life-saving in patients with increasing mass effect, but it should be remembered that surgical drainage does not remove the lesion—it merely replaces the hematoma with a hole or cavity more quickly than nature will. Small lesions (less than 1 cm) usually heal well by themselves and do not require drainage. Large lesions (greater than 4 to 5 cm) are invariably fatal, and usually the patient is devastated even before reaching a medical facility; drainage of these large lesions may allow survival in a very poor vegetative state. Surgery probably is most useful for moderate-size (greater than 2 cm) hematomas in surgically accessible sites, such as the cerebellum, cerebral lobes, and right putamen, in patients who are worsening while under observation, who are developing signs of increased intracranial pressure (e.g., increased stupor, headache, a dilated pupil), and in whom CT or MRI shows shifts of intracranial contents. Without surgery, the prognosis for such patients is poor.

In subarachnoid hemorrhage (SAH) the aim is to treat the source of the hemorrhage, usually an aneurysm or AVM, before it can bleed again. Most often, this involves surgical clipping or coating of an aneurysm and surgical removal of an AVM. In the acute stage after the bleed, brain swelling and the presence of blood make the surgery more difficult and the outcome of surgery more tenuous. Generally, the surgeon waits until the patient is in good clinical condition. Prevention of ischemia caused by vasoconstriction is also an important consideration while waiting for surgery and during the postoperative period. Calcium channel blockers such as nimodipine and nicardipine show promise and are being studied. Hypovolemia and hyponatremia are common after SAH, and volume depletion can augment ischemia caused by vasoconstriction. Volume replacement is an important treatment in patients with delayed cerebral ischemia after SAH.

STROKE PREVENTION, PREVENTION AND TREATMENT OF STROKE COMPLICATIONS, AND REHABILITATION

Prevention of cerebrovascular disease and stroke is clearly better than treatment after stroke has occurred. Several conditions—for example, hypertension, smoking, hyperlipidemia—are definite risk factors for stroke and heart disease. Others—such as birth control pills, excessive alcohol and coffee consumption, elevated hematocrit, obesity, chronic emotional stress, and lack of exercise—are possible risk factors, but the epidemiologic data are not definitive or sufficient. The earlier these risk factors are corrected or treated, the more likely is prevention or delay in the development of occlusive vascular disease. The presence of atherosclerosis (symptomatic coronary or peripheral vascular occlusive disease and extracranial carotid artery disease detected by noninvasive testing) carries a more immediate risk. The most immediate risk is the presence of a transient ischemic attack, which requires urgent evaluation, accurate diagnosis of mechanism, and treatment. Prevention is the job of every general physician who sees patients. Often forgotten is the duty of the specialist who cares for the patient during the acute stroke or ischemic attack. In the haste to deliver specific therapy to treat the lesion causing the present symptoms, specialists often overlook their responsibility to treat or moderate risk factors, in the hope of preventing further progression of any underlying atherosclerosis. If prevention is not begun early in treatment, it is often neglected.

Death, disability, and prolongation of hospitalization are most often caused by complications of stroke and its treatment, rather than by the stroke itself. Some of these complications are readily predictable and preventable with good medical and nursing care. Table 120-6 contains a brief list of these complications, the most important of which are pneumonia, phlebothrombosis, pulmonary embolism, nutritional deprivation, and depression.

In the United States, unfortunately, rehabilitation, prevention, and acute stroke care are generally managed at different sites and by different physicians. Yet all three form a continuum of care for patients with cerebrovascular disease. Rehabilitation, which emphasizes recovery and readaptation strategies, should begin very soon after the stroke, while the patient is in the acute care unit. Passive movement of weak limbs, use of ancillary devices to help maintain function, and education about specific neurologic deficits can be performed by the ward medical and nursing staff and should not be relegated solely to the therapist and physiatrist, who see the patient a small fraction of the day. If and when the patient is transferred to a rehabilitation unit, acute or preventive medical treatment begun in the acute unit should be vigorously pursued. All too often the patient is appropriately educated about treatment of hypertension, the need for avoidance of salt, and the value of a low-

Table 120-6. Common stroke complications and causes

Complication	Causes
Pneumonia	Aspiration and hypoventilation
Phlebothrombosis	Immobility of paretic lower extremities
Hypovolemia	Lack of fluid intake, often because of dysphagia
Hyponatremia	Inappropriate ADH, diuretics, poor intake
Seizures	Excitable partially injured cerebral tissue
Depression	Organic mental changes, discouragement
Shoulder dislocation	Lack of proper care of paralyzed arm
Peripheral nerve injuries	Improper positioning of paretic limbs
Decubiti	Immobility, lack of turning and movement, inanition
Urinary tract infection	Indwelling urinary catheter, bladder distention
Bleeding, brain or systemic	Excessive anticoagulation
Congestive heart failure	Fluid overload
Hypotension	Excessive use of antihypertensives

cholesterol, low-fat diet—only to be given free salt, butter, cream, and ice cream on the rehabilitation service.

Rehabilitation can also be overdone. The aim of rehabilitation is to allow readaptation to life's daily activities and full reintegration into home and the community life. During rehabilitation, however, therapy for specific deficits, such as weakness of the left arm and hand, may be emphasized. After returning home, patients may be so centered around exercising and improving left-arm strength and dexterity that they lose sight of the major aim—a return to full living. Most people's activities do not depend on having a "normal" left hand, normal gait, or normal visual fields. Despite a residual deficit, many patients are able to live full lives. Continued intense attention to deficits detracts from recovery instead of promoting it. Rehabilitation and acute care must be integrated. Each must come to appropriate closure.

REFERENCES

Albers G et al: Stroke prevention in nonvalvular atrial fibrillation: a review of prospective randomized trials. Ann Neurol 30:511, 1991.

Barnett HJ et al: Stroke: pathophysiology, diagnosis, and management. New York, 1985, Churchill Livingstone.

Caplan LR: Anticoagulation for cerebral ischemia. Clin Neuropharmacol 9:399, 1986.

Caplan LR: Diagnosis and treatment of ischemic stroke. JAMA 266:2413, 1991.

Caplan LR: Stroke: a clinical approach, ed 2. Boston, 1993, Butterworth.

Caplan LR et al: Race, sex, and occlusive vascular disease: a review. Stroke 17:648, 1986.

Caplan LR et al: Lumbar puncture and stroke. Stroke 18:540A, 1987.

Caplan LR et al: Transcranial doppler ultrasound: present status. Neurology 40:696, 1990.

Mohr JP: Lacunes. Stroke 13:3, 1982.

Mohr J et al: The Harvard Cooperative Stroke Registry: a prospective registry. Neurology 28:745, 1978.

Wolf P, Dyken M, and Barnett HJM: Risk factors in stroke. Stroke 15:1105, 1984.

CHAPTER

121 Demyelinating Diseases

David M. Dawson

The demyelinating diseases (see box above) are illnesses in which the primary site of histopathologic change is in the myelin sheath covering axons. By convention, the term is restricted to disorders of central nervous system myelin. Other illnesses, comparable in many respects, attack peripheral myelin, a product of the Schwann cell rather than the oligodendrogliocyte. These peripheral illnesses include acute Guillain-Barré syndrome and chronic inflammatory demyelinating polyneuropathy. *Dysmyelination,* or *leukodystrophy,* is a disease in which myelin degenerates, presumably because it is formed abnormally. A final category comprises illnesses involving subtotal necrosis of portions of the brain, involve primarily the white matter of the cerebral hemisphere, such as methotrexate leukoencephalopathy and subcortical arteriosclerotic encephalopathy.

Disorders of central nervous system myelin

- Demyelinating diseases
  - Unknown etiology, possible immune etiology
  - Multiple sclerosis
  - Transverse myelitis
  - Neuromyelitis optica (Devic's disease)
  - Acute disseminated encephalomyelitis
  - Acute hemorrhagic leukoencephalitis
  - Postviral, postvaccinial encephalomyelitis
- Viral etiology
  - Progressive multifocal leukoencephalopathy
  - Subacute sclerosing panencephalitis
  - Necrosis of white matter
- Systemic toxic, nutritional disorders
  - Anoxia
  - Nutritional deprivation
  - Vitamin B_{12} deficiency
  - Central pontine myelinolysis
  - Marchiafava-Bignami disease
  - Methotrexate
  - Cranial irradiation
  - Lead
  - Organic mercury
  - Triethyl tin
- Dysmyelinating diseases
  - Leukodystrophies
  - Lipidoses
  - Aminoacidurias
  - Congenital hypothyroidism

Although demyelinating diseases share certain histologic features, including infiltration by lymphocytes and plasma cells, some tendency for perivascular localization of cells, and a variable degree of infiltration by macrophages that remove the damaged myelin fragments, they are clinically quite distinct, and this discussion is based on the clinical features.

MULTIPLE SCLEROSIS

Multiple sclerosis (MS) is the most common demyelinating illness. It is far commoner in the temperate zones of the world, and particularly in the more highly developed countries, where in some instances the prevalence approaches 100 cases per 100,000 population. In Southeast Asia, in contrast, the illness is practically unknown in the native-born population. Population migration studies indicate that the risk of developing MS is carried with an individual if migration occurs after adolescence. All races are affected, but the illness is twice as common in whites as in blacks in the U.S. population. The ratio of female to male patients is approximately 3:2.

Course and prognosis

MS is a disease of middle life. It is common for the first symptoms to occur in the third or fourth decade of life, and onset of illness before adolescence is extremely rare. There are only a few documented cases of typical MS occurring in childhood. Onset after age 60 is rare. The illness is extremely variable in its course. About 20% of patients have benign illness, consisting of brief relapses of symptoms and signs (described below), with no accumulated deficit over the course of many years. Another 10% of patients have severe illness from the onset, with rapidly developing dementia, severe weakness, ataxia, and visual disorder within a few months. The majority of patients pursue an intermediate course, often beginning with attacks of illness (relapsing-remitting MS) and continuing with a chronic, progressive phase in later years. Some patients, particularly those with onset after age of 35, are in the progressive phase of the illness from the outset. Although there are no fully reliable guidelines as to the particular course an individual patient's illness will take, the pace of the disease is usually apparent within the first 5 years. MS has only a slight effect on overall life span, which is primarily attributable to those few patients who have highly aggressive forms of the illness.

Common clinical signs and symptoms

Although MS can attack almost any portion of the central nervous system, certain locations are especially characteristic (Table 121-1).

The first symptom often is acute optic neuritis, which presents as loss of central vision in one eye, impaired pupillary reflex, and pain on ocular movement. The symptoms often develop over the course of a few days to a week, then stabilize for a month or two, and then improve. In the majority of instances, optic neuritis resolves, leaving only some pallor of the disk and impaired appreciation of bright colors. About 40% of patients with acute optic neuritis go on to develop clinically apparent MS. Whether the others represent a *forme fruste* is not known.

An acute attack of MS affecting the brainstem or pons may produce double vision, dizziness, unsteady gait, numbness of one side of the face, and cerebellar ataxia. A highly characteristic finding is the internuclear ophthalmoplegia (INO) caused by a lesion of the medial longitudinal fasciculus. It consists of delay of adduction of one eye, with nystagmus of the abducting eye on lateral gaze.

An acute attack of MS affecting the cervical spinal cord may produce numbness of one or both hands; weakness of gait; brisk reflexes in the lower extremities, with extensor plantar responses; and the highly characteristic Lhermitte's phenomenon, in which flexion of the neck produces tingling and paresthesias into the legs.

MS may attack the most caudal portions of the spinal cord, in which case the patient may complain of atonic bladder, constipation, impotence, and loss of sensation in the saddle region. Lesions of the thoracic spinal cord often affect the sensory tracts or entering sensory fibers, so that patients complain of numbness of an area of skin or numbness from the waist or rib cage downward. A few patients present with primarily cerebral symptoms, such as depression, difficulty in concentration, defective memory, or speech disorder. Such symptoms are far more common in patients with well-advanced chronic, severe MS but in rare instances may occur at an early stage.

At all stages of the illness, fatigue is a recognizable and common symptom that may produce a specific type of disability over and above the disability produced by the neurologic deficit. All symptoms of MS, particularly the milder symptoms, tend to fluctuate with levels of fatigue, excitement, and body temperature. Patients report a change in visual acuity as the day progresses or report that they can walk a certain distance and then their legs tire. This day-to-day and hour-to-hour variability of symptoms is quite characteristic.

Etiology and pathogenesis

The cause of MS remains unknown. Recently accumulated evidence indicates an autoimmune attack on the central nervous system by activated lymphocytes, followed by macrophages. Why this attack occurs is unknown. Certain epidemiologic evidence suggests that MS is acquired, and that there is a long latency between exposure to an unknown agent and the development of clinically apparent symptoms. The incidence in close family members (parents and siblings) is at least five times what it is in the population at

Table 121-1. Differential diagnosis of common multiple sclerosis syndromes

Clinical syndrome	Alternate diagnoses	Distinctive findings	Laboratory examination
Optic neuritis	Ischemic optic neuropathy	Edema of disc margin, older age	Elevated ESR
	Serous retinopathy	Abnormal macula	
	Retro-orbital tumor	Slow progression	Visualization by CT or MRI scan
Brainstem disorder	Tumor	Slow progression	Visualization by CT or MRI scan
	Infarction	Older age, history of TIA	
Spinal cord syndrome	Cervical spondylosis	Neck pain, loss of some reflexes	Cervical x-ray
	Motor neuron disease (ALS)	No sensory loss	EMG
	Cervical tumor	Progressive course	Spinal MRI scan
Neurogenic bladder	Lumbosacral tumor	Pain, slow progression	Myelogram, spinal CT

large. It is not settled whether this represents a common exposure to a pathogenetic agent or an inherited disorder of immune regulation; the latter explanation seems more likely. If one identical twin has MS, in 50% of instances the other twin will have clinical or laboratory evidence of MS. Many unsuccessful efforts to isolate a virus from patients with MS have been made.

Unlike patients with other autoimmune diseases, such as lupus erythematosus and myasthenia gravis, patients with MS are singularly free of coexisting illness. Rare instances of chronic demyelinating neuropathy with MS are known. Bipolar manic-depressive illness is overrepresented among the MS population compared with other psychiatric illnesses.

The histopathologic lesions in the brain suggest a cell-mediated autoimmune disease. Studies of populations of lymphocytes in the brain have indicated that the lymphocytes show an overrepresentation of $T8^+$ (suppressor/cytotoxic) cells. Studies of the immunoglobulin G (IgG) that is present in the spinal fluid in patients with MS indicate a polyclonal response.

Many patients with chronic, active, progressive MS will show a reduction of $T8^+$ cells in the peripheral blood. Current efforts at many laboratories to define a regulatory defect in the immune system of MS patients, particularly a defect correlating with disease activity, have thus far proven unsuccessful.

Recent data indicate a role for circulating lymphocytes that are reactive to immunologically dominant peptides of myelin basic protein.

Diagnosis

Although several laboratory investigations are now available to assist in the diagnosis of MS, the diagnosis remains a clinical one. It must be based on the observation of a chronic recurring or chronic progressive disease of the central nervous system, affecting more than one location in the nervous system and dispersed over time. Mistakes in diagnosis usually can be traced to failure to observe these simple rules, or to overreliance on laboratory tests. There is commonly a delay of several years between the onset of the first symptoms and the confirmed diagnosis of MS.

Laboratory tests. Diagnostic aid from the laboratory allows earlier diagnosis in many instances. The five specific areas of laboratory investigation are discussed below.

Examination of the CSF. The cerebrospinal fluid (CSF) of a patient with MS commonly contains 5 to 100 lymphocytes per cubic millimeter, at any stage of the illness. The total protein is usually normal or mildly elevated. CSF protein over 100 mg% is distinctly unusual in MS and should immediately raise suspicion of some other process. Spinal fluid IgG is elevated, particularly in the middle or later stages of the illness. Elevation of CSF IgG can be measured as the total IgG in mg%, (normally less than 5 mg%), ratio of IgG to albumin (normally less than 12%), or as an index relating the ratio of CSF IgG synthesized within the nervous system to systemic IgG. All of these are satisfactory and give equivalent results, being positive in approximately 80% of patients with chronic relapsing or chronic progressive MS. Patients in the early phases of the illness are the most likely to have a normal CSF IgG.

If subjected to electrophoresis, the IgG is seen to form into one or more distinct bands (oligoclonal bands). This is characteristic of MS, although it is also observed in other illnesses in which IgG is synthesized within the nervous system, such as syphilis, subacute sclerosing panencephalitis, and, occasionally, lupus erythematosus.

Evoked-potential testing. These are electrophysiologic measurements in which a stimulus is delivered and its transit through the nervous system is timed. The commonly used tests include visual evoked response, brainstem auditory evoked response, and somatosensory evoked response. It is characteristic of demyelination of the central nervous system to produce electrophysiologic delay in these measurements. Evoked-response testing is abnormal in more than 80% of patients with chronic relapsing or chronic progressive MS. The visual evoked response is the most likely to be abnormal and is the most clinically relevant test. In patients who have only chronic progressive myelopathy on clinical examination, the discovery of delay, particularly an asymmetric delay, of visual evoked response is clear evidence of a second lesion of the nervous system and thus helps to confirm the diagnosis.

Computed tomography (CT) scanning. A minority of patients with MS show lesions on CT. Such lesions are often hypodense and may enhance with contrast, particularly when they are acute. Patients with chronic MS may show nonenhancing hypodense lesions as well as signs of cerebral atrophy. Diagnostic changes on CT scan occur in no more than 15% of all patients with MS.

Magnetic resonance imaging (MRI). MRI scans are usually positive in patients with MS. The lesions appear as high-intensity, bright lesions on scanning, particularly on late T1 or T2 weighted images (Figs. 121-1 and 121-2). Lesions may show as a diffuse periventricular plaque, as scattered round bright lesions in the central white matter, or, occasionally, as large confluent plaques in one or the other cerebral hemisphere. Many of the lesions visible on MRI scanning are clinically silent. The lesions may appear and disappear over the course of several months, but some may remain as permanent findings in patients scanned at intervals. It is not yet known whether the number of lesions or their apparent activity correlates well with clinical activity of the disease. Other conditions cause comparable MRI appearances, and a diagnosis of multiple sclerosis should never be based on the MRI appearance alone. In patients above the age of 50, small vascular lesions in the white matter are the most common confounding finding, but small, bright lesions may occur in any age group and are of unknown significance if a clinical history compatible with MS is absent.

Informing the patient. Under which circumstances a patient should be advised of the diagnosis of MS is often a difficult decision. The great majority of patients prefer to be told the diagnosis at the early stage. Only if there are

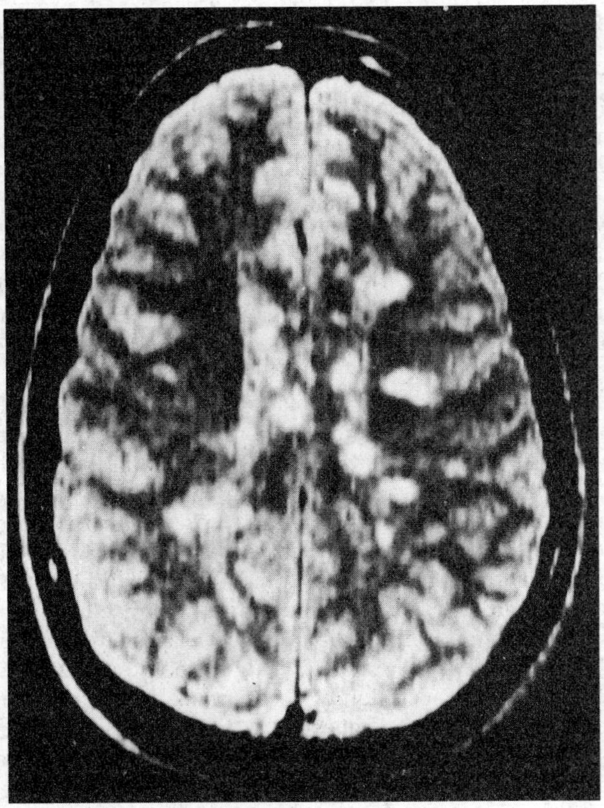

Fig. 121-1. MRI scan of cerebral hemispheres in a patient with early relapsing/remitting multiple sclerosis. The bright periventricular lesions are characteristic; in this patient they were asymptomatic.

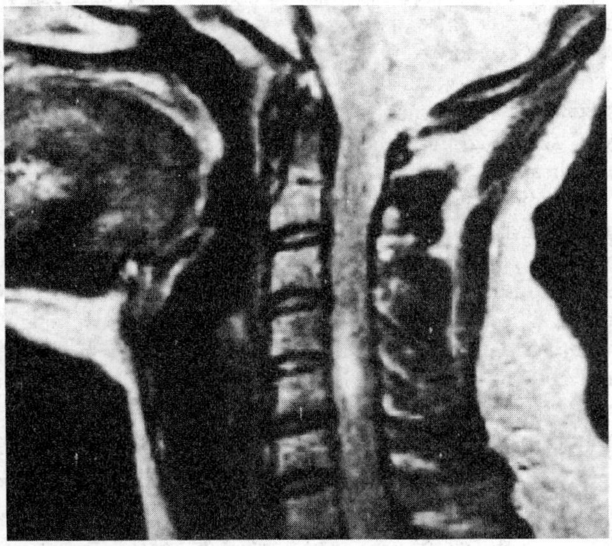

Fig. 121-2. MRI scan through the cervical region showing a lesion of multiple sclerosis in the C4-C5 region.

specific contraindications, such as emotional instability, depression, or turmoil within the family, should a diagnosis be withheld. Once a decision has been made to impart the diagnosis, the illness should be explained in a clear and easily comprehensible fashion, avoiding euphemisms and stressing the possibilities of treatment. At all stages of illness, alternate diagnoses should be considered. These possibilities are considered in Table 121-1.

TREATMENT

Myriad treatments have been proposed for this long-term, variable illness. The list of proposed treatments encompasses everything from diet to electrical stimulation to acupuncture, emotional support, and various forms of immunosuppressive therapy. Patients and families frequently seek guidance as to the veracity of such treatments. General supportive psychological and medical care is important. Specific symptoms can often be treated quite effectively, even when the overall course of the illness cannot be altered. Patients with significant degrees of depression may benefit from antidepressant medications, counseling, or formal psychotherapy. Flexor spasms of the limbs, spasticity when walking, and other symptoms of pyramidal tract dysfunction may respond to antispasticity medications such as baclofen, 20 to 60 mg per day. Benzodiazepines may be used for the same purpose but pose a significant risk of addiction. Patients with MS frequently have bladder dysfunction, either atonic bladder or neurogenic bladder with early urgency and rapid voiding, or various combinations of these two syndromes with dyssynergic contractions of the sphincter. Some patients may respond to anticholinergic medications such as oxybutynin, 5 mg once or twice per day, or to low doses of tricyclic antidepressants. Tonic spasms or trigeminal neuralgia may be treated by carbamazepine. For patients with specific types of motor disorders, particularly spasticity and weakness, physiotherapy may be very helpful in maintaining residual neurologic function.

For individual attacks of MS that occur in the setting of the relapsing/remitting disease, many neurologists use brief courses of corticosteroids. ACTH (adrenocorticotrophic hormone) has been demonstrated to have some slight but definite effect in shortening of the course of attacks of MS.

Intravenous steroids, in the form of 1000 mg per day of methylprednisolone given over 1-2 hours for 5-7 days, are now commonly used. Preliminary data indicates a better response in acute relapses than other forms of treatment. A recently completed trial of therapy for optic neuritis showed a better response for IV steroids than from placebo or oral prednisone, and demonstrated a higher subsequent relapse rate after oral steroids. This may serve to further limit the use of oral steroids for relapses of MS as well as for optic neuritis.

To influence the long-term course of the illness, many immunosuppressive regimens have been advocated. At present, this is a field of intense interest, and new protocols are being tried at many institutions. Long-term oral azathioprine accompanied by steroids and high-dose intravenous cyclophosphamide are the immunosuppressive therapies that have the best supporting data at present.

Limitations of azathioprine, as judged by meta-analysis of many trials, apparently derive from toxicity associated with its use. Limitations of effectiveness of cyclophosphamide seem to derive from lack of effect in patients aged 40 or older.

More specific treatments (anti-T-cell monoclonal antibodies, oral myelin desensitization, interferon-β)may be in the end be more useful but remain experimental.

It should be clear that the unpredictable course of MS requires great care in the choice of treatment. Patients should not begin ill-advised and dangerous treatments when it is possible that the overall nature of the illness may remain benign throughout. However, patients who enter an active progressive phase of the illness can expect that deterioration in all likelihood will continue, and such patients may be candidates for aggressive treatment.

ACUTE DISSEMINATED ENCEPHALOMYELITIS

This rare illness occurs in all age groups but is more commonly recognized in the pediatric age group and the young adult. It is a monophasic illness, consisting pathologically of a multitude of small perivenous demyelinating lesions throughout the nervous system. The symptoms frequently develop after a prior viral illness, such as the exanthems of childhood; they have also been reported following vaccinations, such as DPT, smallpox, and rabies. Unlike in MS, both the central and peripheral nervous systems characteristically are involved. Symptoms may consist of confusion, stupor, blindness, transverse myelitis, weakness of the extremities, ataxia, and incontinence—all occurring at approximately the same time.

Rarely, the CSF is normal; usually, it contains a mild-to-moderate elevation of total protein and several hundred lymphocytes per cubic millimeter.

ACUTE HEMORRHAGIC LEUKOENCEPHALOPATHY

This very rare illness presents as a large patch of demyelination affecting one hemisphere, frequently tracking down within the cerebral peduncles into the corresponding brainstem and cerebellum. The CSF may contain blood. It has a very high mortality rate. In all likelihood, this entity represents an acute and severe version of the preceding illness, although in a few cases that have been well studied, no prior exanthem or prior illness was recognized.

PROGRESSIVE MULTIFOCAL LEUKOENCEPHALOPATHY

Although still classified as a demyelinating illness, this rare disease is now known to be a chronic viral infection. It occurs in patients in whom the immune system is suppressed, particularly those with leukemia, lymphoma, or acquired immune deficiency syndrome, and also in rare patients receiving immunosuppressive drugs for renal transplantation or rheumatoid arthritis. The plaques of viral infection usually begin in one hemisphere and spread over the course of weeks or months throughout the nervous system. The plaques are normally visible by CT scan at a time when clinical symptoms appear. The CSF is characteristically normal. At biopsy or autopsy the lesions are shown to contain JC virus, a virus of the papova group. No effective therapy is known, and the disease is uniformly fatal.

TRANSVERSE MYELITIS

This term refers to a clinical syndrome in which a patient suffers a total or near total spinal cord lesion, usually over the course of a few days. Pathologically, the lesion not only is demyelinating, but also may include necrosis of neurons or axons as well. Thoracic and lumbar segments of the cord are usually those affected. Recovery is often incomplete, with significant residual disability. About 10% percent of patients with acute transverse myelitis are later found, on the basis of later-developing lesions, to have MS.

REFERENCES

Beck RW et al: A randomized, controlled trial of corticosteroids in the treatment of acute optic neuritis. N Eng J Med 326:581, 1992.

Hauser SL et al: Intensive immunosuppression in progressive multiple sclerosis. N Engl J Med 308:173, 1983.

Mackin GA et al: Treatment of multiple sclerosis with cyclophosphamide. In Rudick RA and Goodkin DE, editors: Treatment of multiple sclerosis. London, 1992, Springer-Verlag.

McDonald WI and Silberberg DH, editors: Multiple sclerosis. Stoneham, 1986, Butterworths.

McFarlin DE and McFarland HF: Multiple sclerosis. N Engl J Med 307:1183, 1982.

Paty DW et al: MRI in the diagnosis of MS. Neurol 38:180, 1988.

Poser CM, editor: The diagnosis of multiple sclerosis. New York, 1984, Thieme-Stratton.

Scheinberg L, editor: Multiple sclerosis: a guide for patients and their families. New York, 1983, Raven Press.

Weiner HL and Hafler DA: Multiple sclerosis. Current Neurology 6:123, 1986.

Yudkin PL et al: Overview of azathioprine treatment in multiple sclerosis. Lancet 338:1051, 1991.

CHAPTER

122 Myelopathies

Frisso A. Potts

Myelopathy is the term used to designate disease in the spinal cord. When there is evidence of inflammation, the term *myelitis* is preferred. The disease may involve one or many segments and may extend partially or completely across the transverse diameter of the cord. Lesions may arise within the cord *(intramedullary)* or be caused by pressure by an external mass *(extramedullary)*. The clinical presentation varies depending on the level and extent of the pathologic process. The box below lists a few of the more commonly encountered causes of myelopathy.

CLINICAL FEATURES

The spinal cord is composed of longitudinal tracts subserving motor and sensory functions. Motor tracts carry descending impulses from higher centers to the appropriate anterior horn cells, and from there, motor axons exit the cord by way of anterior roots into peripheral nerves, to innervate specific muscle groups. Conversely, sensory input carried by peripheral nerves enters the cord through posterior roots at discrete levels before forming ascending tracts. This segmental arrangement allows the clinician to localize precisely the rostral extent of a lesion. In addition, its anteroposterior and transverse extent can be inferred with some knowledge of the arrangement of these tracts. Fig. 122-1 diagrams the essential anatomy of the spinal cord.

Causes of myelopathy and myelitis

- Inflammatory
  - Infectious
    - Bacterial: spirochetal, tuberculous
    - Viral: poliomyelitis; herpes HTLV, HIV, zoster; rabies
    - Other: rickettsial, fungal, parasitic
  - Noninfectious
    - Idiopathic transverse myelitis, multiple sclerosis
- Toxic/metabolic
  - Arsenic
  - Pernicious anemia
  - Pellagra
  - Diabetes mellitus
  - Chronic liver disease
- Trauma
  - Spinal fracture/dislocation
  - Stab/bullet wound
  - Herniated nucleus pulposus
- Compression
  - Spinal neoplasm
  - Cervical spondylosis
  - Extramedullary hematopoiesis
  - Epidural abscess
  - Epidural hematoma
- Vascular
  - Arteriovenous malformation
  - Periarteritis nodosa
  - Lupus erythematosus
  - Dissecting aortic aneurysm
- Physical agents
  - Electrical injury
  - Irradiation
- Neoplastic
  - Spinal cord tumors
  - Paraneoplastic myelopathy

The most diagnostically useful tracts are the following:

1. *Corticospinal tract*. This tract carries motor input from the contralateral cerebral cortex to the anterior horn cells. It decussates in the medulla and remains ipsilateral (same side) to the point of exit of the motor roots. Fibers descending to sacral levels are laterally placed; those reaching the cervical segments are more medially placed.
2. *Dorsal columns*. These carry the sensations of discriminative touch, position, and vibration to the contralateral cerebral cortex. In the cord they remain ipsilateral to the side of entry of the posterior roots, since they do not decussate until they reach the medulla. The sacral segments are located medially; the cervical, laterally.
3. *Lateral spinothalamic tract*. This tract carries crude touch, pain, and temperature sensation from the contralateral side of the body. Fibers carrying these modalities from the periphery enter the spinal cord through posterior roots, synapse, and decussate within a segment or two. The resulting tract has sacral input outermost and cervical innermost.
4. *Autonomic fibers*. These run in the white matter of the cord near the central canal and carry sympathetic outflow to the thoracic cord, whence motor fibers exit to provide sympathetic innervation to various organs. These tracts also carry input to sacral centers concerned with voluntary bowel and bladder function, as well as erectile function in the male.

A few basic principles are helpful in defining the location and extent of cord disease.

1. Transverse spinal cord lesions give signs and symptoms below the level of the lesion.
2. Lesions in the region of the central canal affect primarily decussating pain and temperature fibers, giving signs and symptoms at the level of the lesion. However, if the transverse extent of the lesion is large, the longitudinal tracts and even the motor neurons in the anterior horn may be affected. When spinothalamic fibers are involved by an expanding central lesion, the sacral fibers tend to be spared.
3. Intrinsic cord lesions are usually painless and affect autonomic function early. Extrinsic compression is usually accompanied by focal pain in the affected segment of the spine, and autonomic involvement is late.

DIAGNOSIS

Once the lesion is localized clinically, plain x-rays of the spine may reveal bony abnormalities, such as fractures, bony spurs impinging on the spinal canal, or bone erosion by neoplasm. Abnormal uptake in bone scans also aids in identifying bony abnormalities and extramedullary masses. Myelography, particularly when combined with computerized tomography (CT) of the spine, is an excellent way of defining extra- and intramedullary lesions. However, the best method for defining spinal cord pathology is magnetic resonance imaging (MRI), which provides

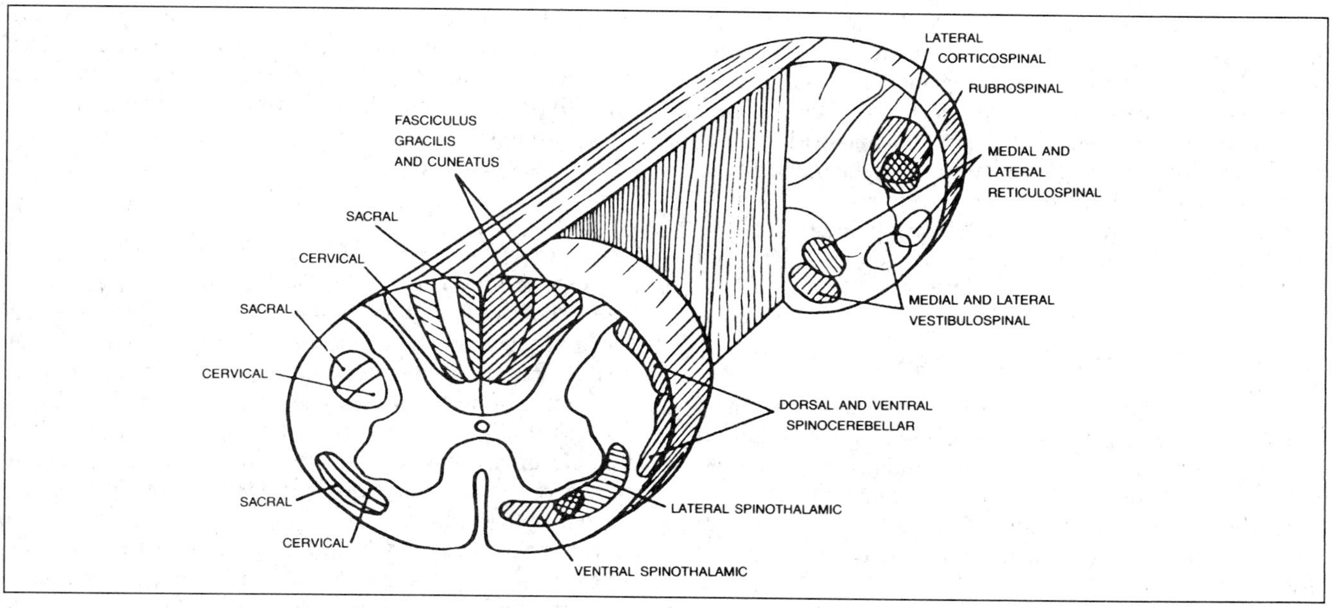

Fig. 122-1. Principal tracts of the spinal cord. Lamination in the posterior columns and corticospinal and spinothalamic tracts is shown in the left half of the diagram. The location of the sensory pathways is shown at the same level on the right, and the location of the motor pathways is shown at another level on the far right. (Adapted from Daube JR and Sandok BA: Medical neurosciences. Boston, 1978, Little, Brown.)

excellent resolution of intrinsic as well as extrinsic lesions (see Chapter 108). As an adjunct to these procedures, examination of cerebrospinal fluid (CSF) may demonstrate the presence of hemorrhage, of inflammatory or malignant cells, and of abnormal proteins, thus giving clues to etiology.

SPINAL CORD LESIONS AND THEIR CLINICAL SIGNS

Acute spinal cord compression or transection

This syndrome is most commonly the result of trauma, such as vertebral fracture or gunshot wound. Rarely, it may be seen as a result of intervertebral disk herniation or as a result of intramedullary spinal cord disease (hemorrhage or infarction). Complete spinal cord transections give rise to *spinal shock*. There is complete flaccid paralysis and sensory loss below the level of the lesion, and urinary and fecal retention occur. If the lesion is above the midthoracic level, interference with descending sympathetic tracts gives rise to failure of the sympathetic nervous system with attendant hypotension, and anhydrosis is evident below the level of the lesion. With high cervical lesions, severe respiratory embarrassment is the rule. If the patient does not succumb to respiratory failure or urinary tract infection, recovery from spinal shock starts in several days to weeks with return of stretch reflexes and the beginning of reflex micturition. As weeks and months progress, increasing spastic rigidity of previously flaccid muscles occurs, and patients usually experience involuntary muscle spasms (flexor spasms).

Subacute spinal cord compression

This syndrome is most likely to occur as a result of extrinsic cord lesions; tumors and degenerative joint disease of the spine are the leading causes. It is imperative for the physician to make an early diagnosis of spinal compression, since in many instances decompression is feasible and permanent loss of function may be avoided. Early signs of spinal compression include paresthesia and sensory loss below the level of the lesion. Stiffness and weakness of the legs are common. In more advanced cases, urinary frequency with urgency and flexor spasms of the lower extremities are seen.

Brown-Séquard syndrome

This syndrome of hemisection of the cord may be seen with intrinsic or extrinsic lesions and consists of motor weakness and spasticity in segments below and ipsilateral to the lesion. Loss of vibratory and position sense also occurs ipsilateral to the lesion (undecussated tracts), whereas loss of pain and temperature sensation (decussated tracts) is found contralateral to the lesion.

Central cord syndrome

This term is applied to myelopathies that affect the most central region of the cord. They give rise to deficits in pain and temperature sensation at the level of the lesion (since the incoming fibers decussate through the center of the cord) with sparing of vibratory and position sense—the so-called *dissociated sensory loss*. By the same token, stretch reflexes at the level of the lesion are impaired, and if the lesion is large enough to involve the more laterally placed tracts, there is spasticity and sensory loss to temperature and pain below the level of the lesion. Sacral sparing is the rule, as these segments are represented by laterally placed fibers. A classic example is the developmental anomaly known as *syringomyelia*. Hyperextension injuries of the neck have also been known to give rise to the central cord syndrome.

Syndrome of the anterior spinal artery

As its name implies, this myelopathy occurs as a result of ischemia in the territory of the anterior spinal artery. It causes a functional transection of the cord involving the spinothalamic and corticospinal tracts, as well as the anterior horn cells in the affected region. The posterior columns are spared, since they derive their blood supply from the posterior spinal artery.

CLINICAL CONDITIONS GIVING RISE TO MYELOPATHY

Cervical spondylosis

This is the most common cause of myelopathy. In its earliest or simplest form, it manifests itself with neck pain that may radiate into the arms. The sign of Babinski is usually present early in the course and may be the only sign of cord involvement. Indeed, it is thought that cervical spondylosis with asymptomatic cord compression is the underlying reason for the high incidence of extensor plantar responses in the elderly. The course is extremely variable, but in its progressive form it gives rise to the syndrome of subacute cord compression (see above). A coexistent radiculopathy may decrease or obliterate stretch reflexes in the upper extremities. In mild, slowly progressive cases, treatment consists of immobilization of the neck with a collar. If progression occurs, cervical laminectomy for cord decompression may be necessary. An anterior cervical approach with intervertebral disk removal and spinal fusion has also been used.

Transverse myelitis

This term is used to describe a rapidly progressive (hours or days) myelopathy characterized by necrosis of the spinal cord in one or several segments. The clinical picture is as described in acute spinal cord compression (see above). The CSF may show an inflammatory pleocytosis with or without evidence of a hemorrhagic component. Protein elevation is the rule. MRI may show a swollen cord at the involved level. The syndrome may be temporally related to a number of viral illnesses or to vaccinations (notably influenza and smallpox vaccines). In these cases, recovery does not often occur and no successful therapy is available, although treatment with steroids or ACTH may be palliative. When this condition is associated with multiple sclerosis (MS), there usually are signs of involvement elsewhere in the central nervous system and remissions and exacerbations are the rule. The presence of monoclonal bands on CSF protein electrophoresis would suggest that a transverse myelopathy is caused by MS, although it would not prove it unequivocally.

Epidural abscess

These abscesses usually occur in the lumbar region and are rarely the cause of spinal cord compression. When they occur in the thoracic or cervical cord, they give rise to subacute spinal cord compression (see above) with early involvement of posterior columns, since the usual site for the abscess is posterior to the cord. Frequently, there is pain at the site of involvement. In their more common location, they give rise to cauda equina syndrome, which is characterized by focal pain, development of hyporeflexia in the lower extremities, and in the most severe cases, progressive sensory loss, motor weakness, and, eventually sphincter paralysis. Although not every case develops in this inexorable, devastating fashion, a high index of suspicion is necessary to prevent worsening in mild cases. Radiologic studies easily demonstrate the abscess, and progression may be arrested with antibiotic therapy; surgical decompression is usually necessary, however.

Retrovirus infection

A slowly progressive, nonhemorrhagic, usually noninflammatory myelopathy has been associated with systemic infection by the HTLV-I and HIV (formerly known as HTLV-III) viruses. The former may occur in familial form and accounts for many cases of tropical spastic paraparesis. Spastic lower-extremity weakness with variable sensory loss develops over a period of months. The spinal level of the lesion may "ascend," originally starting in the thoracic cord but eventually involving the high cervical cord. Autonomic function may be spared. The CSF is usually acellular, with only mild protein elevations, and in most cases contains antibodies against the offending virus.

Metabolic myelopathies

The most notorious example of these disorders (although rarely seen today) is combined systems degeneration, the myelopathy associated with pernicious anemia (see Chapter 80) that consists of progressive lower-extremity spastic paraparesis with superimposed ataxia caused by posterior column involvement. There usually is a fairly well defined sensory cord level to vibratory sense. A peripheral neuropathy of vitamin B_{12} deficiency is invariably present. A similar myelopathy has been described with folate deficiency. Chronic liver failure is also associated with a myelopathy—a slowly progressive spastic paraparesis or quadriparesis with a poorly defined sensory level. Autonomic sparing is the rule. Its etiology is not clear, although it is thought that nutritional factors may play a role.

Paraneoplastic myelopathies

Spastic paraparesis or quadriparesis with a more or less well-defined sensory level may occur in the setting of systemic malignancy, such as lymphoma or various other tumors. When no evidence of concurrent retrovirus infection or direct involvement of the cord by tumor is evident, the term *paraneoplastic* may be applied. This is an uncommon manifestation of systemic malignancy and its pathophysiology and etiology are not clear.

Radiation-induced myelopathy

This complication of radiation treatment may occur in as many as 4% of patients who have received radiation for spinal or body cavity tumors. It occurs most often when the location makes incidental radiation of the cord possible, and its onset usually occurs between 12 and 15 months after completion of treatment, although it has been reported as early as 6 months and as late as 60 months. The process is a slowly progressive one involving the cord levels subjected to the radiation. Initial minor symptoms usually progress over a period of months to a full-blown spinal transection syndrome with severe motor, sensory, and autonomic impairment. No form of treatment has been successful, although steroids may have a transient beneficial effect. This complication is clearly related to radiation dose, and it is rarely seen when the cord has received less than 3300 rad.

Spinal tumors

About one-half of these tumors are metastatic to the extramedullary structures and invade locally to produce the subacute spinal cord compression outlined above. Bone involvement is usually heralded by focal pain and easily detected by plain films and bone scan. More subtly invasive tumors, such as the lymphomas and sarcomas, spread through the meninges and cause spinal compression with little bony evidence of their presence. Identification must rely on CT scanning or MRI. Once the tumor has been identified, irradiation and chemotherapy are the treatments of choice. The second most common spinal tumor is the meningioma that arises outside the cord but within the dural sac; these tumors are amenable to surgical excision. Primary intraspinal tumors are the rarest of the lot, and they consist mainly of gliomas. The myelopathies produced by primary intraspinal tumors (unlike those produced by metastatic tumors) generally are slowly progressive.

Complications of vascular surgery

Ischemic infarction of the spinal cord can complicate aortic surgery. The incidence of this complication is highest (28%) in procedures involving the thoracic and abdominal aorta. A much higher incidence of myelopathy (48%) has been reported in aneurysmal repair after dissection or rupture of the aneurysm. However, aortic surgery below the level of the renal arteries carries little or no danger of ischemic myelopathy. The clinical presentation in most cases is that of acute spinal transection at a mid or lower thoracic cord level. Hypotension, caused by spinal shock, may further complicate the clinical picture. Full recovery is the exception rather than the rule. Many procedures have been used in an attempt to prevent this surgical complication. Among these are artery-to-artery shunting, pretreatment with steroids, free-radical scavengers, thiopental, papaverine, and hypothermia. Of these only the last-mentioned seems to have a beneficial effect.

REFERENCES

Adams RD and Salam-Adams M: Chronic nontraumatic diseases of the spinal cord. Neurol Clin 9:605, 1991.

Danner RL and Hartman BJ: Update on spinal epidural abscess: 35 cases and a review of the literature. Rev Infect Dis 9:265, 1987.

Dawson DM and Potts FA: Acute nontraumatic myelopathies. Neurol Clin 9:585, 1991.

Helweg-Larsen SJ et al: Myelopathy in AIDS. A clinical, neuroradiological and electrophysiological study of 23 Danish patients. Acta Neurol Scand 77:64, 1988.

Johnson RT and McArthur JC: Myelopathies and retroviral infections. Ann Neurol 21:113, 1987.

Plum F and Olson ME: Myelitis and myelopathy. In Baker AB and Baker LH, editors: Clinical neurology, Hagerstown, MD, 1984, Harper & Row.

Salazar-Grueso EF et al: Familial spastic paraparesis syndrome associated with HTLV-I infection. N Engl J Med 323:732, 1990.

Yu YL et al: Cervical spondylotic myelopathy and radiculopathy. Acta Neurol Scand 75:367, 1987.

CHAPTER

123 Disease of Peripheral Nerve and Motor Neurons

Eric L. Logigian

Signs and symptoms of a peripheral nerve disorder depend on the fiber composition (sensory, motor, and autonomic) of the affected nerves, the selectivity of the disease process (which fiber types are affected), the part of the body they innervate, and the patient's sensitivity to dysfunction of the affected fibers. For example, mild entrapment of the median nerve at the wrist may spare motor and autonomic fibers and affect the sensory fibers alone, resulting in sensory symptoms, sometimes without signs, in the median nerve distribution of the hand. Such symptoms may be more disturbing to a musician than to someone whose livelihood is not so dependent on optimal hand function.

Disorders of peripheral nerve result in "negative" and "positive" symptoms and signs, many of which are listed in Table 123-1. Not listed are functional problems that the patient may notice, such as dropping things from the hand, which may signify finger weakness or sensory loss. Simi-

Table 123-1. Signs and symptoms of peripheral nerve disease

Fiber type	Negative	Positive
Motor	Weakness, atrophy, fatigability, clumsiness, areflexia, hypotonia, deformities (pes cavus, kyphoscoliosis)	Muscle twitches (fasciculations, myokymia), cramps
Sensory	Sensory loss, ataxia, clumsiness, areflexia, hypotonia	"Tingling," "pins and needles," "burning"
Autonomic	Postural hypotension, loss of sweating, impotence, bowel and bladder symptoms	Hyperhidrosis, gustatory sweating
Trophic		Foot ulceration, Charcot arthropathy

larly, falling or unsteadiness when walking may be caused by polyneuropathy affecting the sensory or motor fibers in the lower extremities. Inquiry about what the patient can and cannot do is often useful in characterizing muscle weakness. Oculobulbar weakness presents as ptosis, diplopia, swallowing or chewing trouble, nasal regurgitation of fluids, and drooling. Proximal limb weakness typically causes trouble reaching above the head, getting out of a chair, trouble going upstairs, or a waddling gait, whereas distal limb weakness results in trouble unscrewing jar lids, buttoning, zipping, holding a pen or eating utensils, or tripping.

Peripheral nerve disease not only may selectively affect motor, sensory, or autonomic fibers, but also may affect nerve fibers according to size. Table 123-2 lists the sensory symptoms and signs referable to nerve fibers of large and small diameter. Not listed is autonomic dysfunction, which if on a peripheral basis is evidence for small fiber neuropathy, whereas motor dysfunction from pathology of motoneuron axons represents a disorder of medium to large fibers. Since large fibers are more thickly myelinated than are thinly- or unmyelinated small axons, "large fiber" dysfunction may result from disorders predominantly affecting myelin (i.e., myelinopathy), or larger axons (i.e., axonopathy). The two can frequently be differentiated with electrophysiologic studies.

Table 123-2. Large- and small-fiber sensory symptoms and signs

	Large fiber	Small fiber
Symptoms	"Tingling," "pins and needles"	"Burning," "aching," "jabbing"
Signs	Loss of vibratory and joint position sense, areflexia, ataxia	Loss of sharp-dull or temperature discrimination

DIFFERENTIAL DIAGNOSIS

Peripheral nervous system (PNS) versus central nervous system (CNS)

Before ascribing weakness or sensory loss to the peripheral nervous system, the physician should be certain there are no central nervous system signs (Table 123-3). Ordinarily, hyporeflexia, hypotonia, and muscle wasting are indicative of peripheral nerve disease, although acute lesions of the CNS can result in hyporeflexia and hypotonia and a chronic lesion of the CNS can lead to "disuse" atrophy. In addition, several diseases affect both the CNS and PNS. Therefore, CNS signs in a patient with peripheral neuropathy are important clues.

Nerve versus muscle; neuromuscular junction (NMJ)

Muscle weakness without any sensory signs or symptoms is rarely caused by peripheral nerve disease and should suggest disease of motor neurons, neuromuscular junction (NMJ), or muscle. Muscle weakness caused by NMJ disorders, such as myasthenia gravis or Lambert-Eaton syndrome, diurnally fluctuate; the former may get worse with continuous repetitive muscle contraction, whereas the latter may improve. In contrast to most polyneuropathies, muscle disease more frequently affects proximal muscles and is associated with preserved tendon jerks, elevated muscle enzymes, and "myopathic" abnormalities on electromyography (EMG). However, proximal weakness is seen in some of the spinal muscular atrophies and in selected polyneuropathies, sometimes with minimal sensory involvement, such as acute or chronic inflammatory demyelinating polyradiculoneuropathy (AIDP, CIDP) and porphyric neuropathy.

Clinicopathologic syndromes of nerve disease

Disease of peripheral nerve results in several clinicopathologic syndromes (Table 123-4) that should be recognized as a first step in making an etiologic diagnosis. The following discussion is organized according to the clinical presentation, which usually allows the physician to predict the

Table 123-3. Central nervous system signs and possible implications

Sign	Possible implication
Extensor plantar response	Lesion of the upper motor neuron
Hyperreflexia, hypertonus	Lesion of the upper motor neuron
Sensory or motor level	Spinal cord lesion
Loss of sharp-dull discrimination contralateral to limb weakness	Spinal cord lesion

Table 123-4. Clinicopathologic syndromes in peripheral neuropathy and neuronopathy

Syndromes	Primary pathology of
Neuronopathy	
Motoneuronopathy	Lower motoneurons in spinal cord, brainstem, and/or upper motoneurons
Sensory neuronopathy	Dorsal root ganglia
Autonomic neuronopathy	Autonomic ganglia
Radiculopathy	Dorsal and/or ventral roots, or both
Polyradiculopathy, cranial neuropathy, meningitis	Roots, cranial nerves, meninges
Polyradiculoneuropathy	Roots, plexus, and nerves
Plexopathy	Plexus
Mononeuropathy	One nerve (sensory, motor, or mixed)
Mononeuropathy multiplex	Two or more nerves
Polyneuropathy	Many or all nerves
Myelinopathy	Myelin
Axonopathy	Axon
Polyneuropathy or mononeuritis multiplex with CNS involvement	Peripheral and central nervous system

site of pathology and, subsequently, the etiology, on which treatment is based. This is occasionally complicated because the same etiology can result in different clinicopathologic syndromes (Table 123-5), and vice versa (see Table 123-10).

CLINICAL SYNDROMES

Progressive lower motor neuron (LMN) deficit (muscle wasting, weakness, fasciculations), with or without upper motor neuron (UMN) deficit (brisk tendon jerks, increased muscle tone)

Progressive loss of lower or upper motoneurons with relative sparing of those innervating extraocular and sphincter muscles occurs in several forms throughout life; collectively, these disorders are referred to as the motor neuron diseases. Inherited or sporadic forms with relatively symmetric proximal or distal muscle weakness caused by loss of lower motor neurons are referred to as the spiral muscular atrophies (SMAs). With the exception of infantile Werdig-Hoffman disease type I and progressive bulbar palsy of childhood (Fazio-Londe disease), which lead to death within 18 months of onset, SMA is compatible with long survival. There are even sporadic cases limited to one extremity (benign focal amyotrophy). The workup in suspected SMA should exclude muscle disease, postpolio syndrome, hexosaminidase deficiency, CIDP, diabetic motor neuropathy, and neuropathy caused by porphyria, lead, dapsone, or nitrofurantoin.

In the adult, pure UMN (primary lateral sclerosis) and LMN (spinal muscular atrophy, benign focal amyotrophy) forms exist, but *amyotrophic lateral sclerosis (ALS)* is the most common form with both UMN and LMN involvement. The findings usually are asymmetric initially, resulting in progressive skeletal muscle wasting, weakness, fasciculations, and cramping, often beginning in one limb but then becoming generalized. Tendon jerks may remain brisk

Table 123-5. Diseases associated with different types of neuropathy

	AIDP	CIDP	Axonal SMP	MN	MNMP	Plex	Small
Metabolic							
Diabetes			+	+	+	+	+
Acromegaly*			+	+ (CTS)			
Hypothyroidism*		+	+	+ (CTS)			
Infectious							
AIDS*	+	+	+		+		
Leprosy			+		+		
Connective tissue							
SLE*	+		+		+		
Rheumatoid arthritis			+	+	+		
Sjögren's syndrome			+		+		
Periarteritis nodosa*			+		+		
Wegener's granulomatosis*			+		+		
Cranial arteritis*			+		+		
Churg-Strauss syndrome			+		+		
Cryoglobulinemia			+		+		
Hypersensitivity angiitis			+		+		
Lyme disease	+		+	+	+		
Idiopathic							
Sarcoidosis*			+		+		

AIDP, acute inflammatory demyelinating polyneuropathy; CIDP, chronic idiopathic demyelinating polyradiculoneuropathy; axonal SMP, axonal sensorimotor polyneuropathy; MN, mononeuropathy; MNMP, mononeuropathy multiplex; plex, plexopathy; small, small-fiber polyneuropathy; CTS, carpal tunnel syndrome; AIDS, acquired immune deficiency syndrome; SLE, systemic lupus erythematosus.

*Central nervous system manifestations may be present.

despite muscle atrophy. Some cases have predominant involvement of brainstem motoneurons (progressive bulbar palsy). Mean disease duration is 2.5 years, but survival in a given patient depends mainly on maintenance of bellows function (i.e., diaphragm and intercostal muscles) and airway protection (i.e., cough reflex and swallowing). Among the most important clinical signs in ALS are those originating from pathology above the foramen magnum (atrophy or fasciculation of the tongue, palate, face, and a brisk jaw jerk). If these signs are absent, the diagnostic workup must exclude disease of the spinal cord and roots, as in cervical spondylosis; such diseases can cause multiple root with LMN and spinal cord compression with UMN findings, and thereby simulate ALS.

Because of vaccination, poliomyelitis, resulting in a flulike illness followed by rapid asymmetric paralysis, is now rare. However, some polio survivors from the epidemics of 30 to 40 years ago are now beginning to experience pain, muscle fatigue, and weakness (postpolio syndrome). Some have progressive weakness and wasting in muscles that were not necessarily weak at the onset of polio (postpolio muscular atrophy). A reduced motoneuron pool resulting from the original illness, further depleted by progressive loss of anterior horn cells that occurs with aging and by the increased metabolic demand placed on the residual cells, may be the cause. The workup should exclude other causes of muscle weakness, such as radiculopathy or entrapment neuropathy.

Treatment of motor neuron and related diseases is largely supportive at this time. Decisions regarding respiratory support and hyperalimentation should be discussed early in the course. Rehabilitative techniques (discussed below) and individual or group psychiatric support for both the patient and the family are often helpful.

Proximal pain in one limb with sensory, motor, or reflex abnormalities

This constellation suggests radiculopathy, plexopathy, or proximal mononeuropathy (i.e., spinal accessory nerve palsy, femoral neuropathy; see Table 123-7) but can be simulated by a primary rheumatologic disorder affecting the shoulder or hip joint, as well as adjacent bursae or tendons. Although in the latter case patients may be weak from guarding or disuse atrophy, the correct diagnosis is suggested by limited range of motion, localized tenderness, and a normal EMG examination.

Cervical radiculopathy usually presents with sensory symptoms, which sometimes worsen with neck movement. These include a nonspecific neck, shoulder, or scapular pain, and, occasionally, a more "localizing" sensation that radiates into the dermatome of the specific nerve roots involved. Similarly, side-to-side asymmetries in muscle strength, sensation, or tendon jerks depend on the involved roots (Table 123-6). The most common causes of cervical radiculopathy are nerve root compression from intervertebral foraminal stenosis or disk herniation and, rarely, extra- or intramedullary tumors. Signs of cervical myelopathy (i.e., hyperactive tendon jerks, extensor plantar response), which can occur in addition to cervical root compression (i.e., cervical spondylosis), should be sought in the legs.

Lumbosacral radiculopathy presents with low-back, hip, or buttock pain, with occasional "dermatomal radiation" and sensory, motor, and reflex changes, depending on the involved root or roots (Table 123-6). The pain may begin after heavy lifting and is generally worse in the sitting position or when coughing, sneezing, or straining at stool. Pressure over the sciatic notch and straight-leg raising may reproduce the pain somewhat. Common causes are com-

Table 123-6. Spinal root signs and symptoms

Spinal root	Distribution of pain, paresthesias, or sensory loss	Weak muscles	Diminished reflexes
C5	Shoulder, anterolateral arm and forearm	Deltoids, infra- and supraspinatus, biceps	Pectoralis, biceps
C6	Shoulder, radial forearm, thumb	Biceps and brachioradialis, pronator teres	Biceps, brachioradialis
C7	Pectoral area, axilla, posterolateral forearm, 2nd and 3rd digits	Triceps, wrist extensors	Triceps
C8	Axilla, posteromedial arm, 4th and 5th digits	Hand interossei (ulnar nerve), abductor pollicis brevis (median nerve)	Finger flexors
L4	Hip, anterior thigh, anteromedial leg, great toe	Knee extensors, hip flexors	Knee
L5	Hip, posterolateral thigh, anterolateral leg, middle of foot	Foot extensors, great toe extensors, knee flexors	Medial hamstring
S1	Gluteal area, posterior thigh and leg, lateral foot	Foot flexors	Ankle
S2	Posterior thigh and leg	Toe flexors	—
S3-5	Sacral area	Sphincters	Bulbo cavernosus, anal wink

C, cervical; L, lumbar; S, sacral.

pression by a laterally herniated intervertebral disk (most commonly, L4-5 or L5-S1) followed by tumor and herpes zoster. A midline herniated disk, lumbar spondylosis, and arachnoiditis are other causes, but these usually produce bilateral lumbosacral polyradiculopathy.

The diagnosis of unilateral cervical or lumbar radiculopathy may be supported by spine films and EMG. Metrizamide myelogram, computed tomography (CT) scan, or magnetic resonance imaging (MRI) may be needed to determine the cause of root compression in cases without clear etiology and to visualize (1) the cervical cord in patients with myelopathy or (2) the cauda equina/conus medullaris in patients with bilateral lumbosacral radiculopathy with bladder dysfunction or symptoms of spinal claudication. Conservative treatment (cervical collar, traction in cervical radiculopathy, or bed rest in lumbosacral radiculopathy) is usually successful. Patients may benefit from a course of nonsteroidal anti-inflammatory drugs and, if necessary, a short course of narcotic analgesics. Some cases may require surgery to decompress roots, the spinal cord, or the cauda equina. Although comprehensive therapy of chronic low back pain in patients with lumbosacral radiculopathy is beyond the scope of this chapter, some of the simpler measures are discussed below.

Another form of radiculopathy occasionally seen is thoracic or thoracolumbar radiculopathy. It is most commonly caused by reactivation of herpes zoster and produces dermatomal pain and skin rash with little if any sensory loss; it can also be caused by diabetes and Lyme disease. Pain control is the main problem (discussed below).

The diagnosis of plexopathy is suggested when the sensorimotor deficit is not limited to or affects more than one nerve or two roots. Proximal limb or girdle pain is often present. In the arm, brachial plexopathy occurs as a result of traction injury from two-wheeled vehicle accidents, tumor infiltration, or radiation and immunologic causes (postinfectious or vaccination). A recurrent, autosomal dominantly inherited form has also been described. In the lower extremity, common causes of lumbosacral plexopathy are retroperitoneal tumor or hemorrhage and irradiation. In addition, elderly type II diabetics sometimes develop asymmetric, painful lower extremity weakness and wasting associated with weight loss, often with minimal sensory findings. Although presenting as plexopathies, such cases probably represent a localized lumbosacral radiculoneuropathy. They are sometimes referred to as *diabetic amyotrophy, diabetic motor neuropathy,* or *proximal diabetic neuropathy.*

EMG can be helpful in the diagnosis of plexopathy. CT or MRI scan of the plexi can be performed to rule out tumor infiltration or hemorrhage. The therapeutic aims are pain control and treatment of the underlying disease.

The mononeuropathies are among the simplest neurologic lesions, and each has its own clinical presentation (Table 123-7). Single-cranial-nerve palsies are occasionally seen in diseases that produce mononeuritis multiplex or in those that simultaneously infiltrate nerve and the leptomeninges (see below), but the most common cranial mononeuropathies are diabetic third- or sixth-nerve palsies, trigeminal neuropathy secondary to herpes zoster, and Bell's (seventh cranial nerve) palsy. Isolated seventh nerve palsy is usually idiopathic but can be caused by herpes zoster (with vesicles in ear, palate, or tongue), trauma, sarcoidosis, or Lyme disease. Patients present with acute onset of panfacial weakness of varying severity with prominent affection of the frontalis muscle, indicating that the facial weakness is lower rather than upper motor neuron. Hyperacusis and abnormalities of tearing, taste, and even sensation (pain, sensory loss) may also occur. In idiopathic cases, some recommend an early course of prednisone (1 mg per kilogram per day) for 5 to 16 days, depending on the severity of facial paresis, followed by a 5-day taper. In cases with incomplete eye closure, the eye should be protected with artificial tears during the day and an ointment during sleep. Mononeuropathies of the extremities (Table 123-7) are most often caused by chronic compression, stretch, or angulation as nerves pass through bony or ligamentous canals (i.e., carpal/tarsal tunnel syndrome, ulnar neuropathy at the elbow or wrist, meralgia paresthetica). Nerves that pass around bony or ligamentous structures are also vulnerable to acute compression from external pressure (i.e., peroneal, radial nerve palsy). Early on, the pathologic substrate of these so-called entrapment neuropathies is myelinopathy, but later, or in more severe cases, axonal injury occurs as well. EMG and nerve conduction studies confirm the diagnosis, rule out other causes for the clinical deficit, and determine the degree of axonal injury. In cases of acute compression, and in mild-to-moderate chronic nerve compression, treatment is usually conservative: splinting, pain control, and prevention of further injury. In refractory cases with severe pain or significant axonal degeneration, surgical therapy aimed at decompressing or transposing the nerve may be required.

Stepwise, asymmetric, neuropathic symptoms, signs, or EMG findings over days to weeks

This constellation suggests *mononeuropathy multiplex,* a term indicating discrete pathology of two or more named nerves in more than one limb. Nerve pathology usually is outside areas where entrapment commonly occurs—a feature that distinguishes mononeuritis multiplex from the more chronic condition of hereditary predisposition to pressure palsy. Most commonly, this syndrome is caused by systemic vasculitis with nerve infarction. It is important to remember that this syndrome can sometimes present as a symmetric polyneuropathy (see Table 123-5). Workup and therapy should be directed to the underlying illness. Biopsy of an involved nerve may be diagnostic.

Headache, back pain, multiple-cranial-nerve palsies, polyradiculopathy

Because the nerve roots and cranial nerves traverse the subarachnoid space, they are sometimes affected by disease processes that also affect the meninges. This syndrome can

Table 123-7. Common mononeuropathies

Nerve	Clinical presentation	Causes
Spinal accessory	Shoulder pain, droop and weakness of abduction, trapezius wasting	Nerve trauma
Long thoracic	"Winging" of scapula	Backpacking, idiopathic
Axillary	Deltoid weakness, sensory loss over lateral upper arm	Trauma
Radial at the spiral groove (Saturday-night palsy)	Wrist and finger drop, weakness and areflexia of brachioradialis, sensory loss over dorsum of first web space	Acute compression
Musculocutaneous	Weakness of elbow flexion, sensory loss over radial aspect of forearm	Trauma, elbow hyperextension
Ulnar at the elbow	Wasting, weakness of interossei; sensory loss over palmar and dorsal surface of the ulnar aspect of the hand	Chronic compression
Median in the forearm (pronator syndrome)	Forearm ache, weakness of intrinsic and extrinsic median muscles, sensory loss over the palmar, radial aspect of the hand	Chronic compression
Radial in the forearm (posterior interosseous palsy)	Forearm pain, finger drop, radial deviation of the extended wrist	Mass lesion, trauma, idiopathic
Median at the wrist (carpal tunnel syndrome)	Nocturnal hand "tingling"; weakness, wasting of abductor pollicis brevis; sensory loss over volar aspect of fingers 1-3	Chronic compression
Ulnar at the wrist	Weakness, wasting of interossei; variable sensory loss over 4th and 5th fingers	Occupational trauma
Femoral	Hip, groin pain; knee buckling; knee extensor weakness; absent knee jerk; sensory loss over anteromedial thigh and medial calf	Diabetes, retroperitoneal hemorrhage or tumor, postsurgical
Lateral femoral cutaneous at inguinal ligament	Thigh pain, sensory loss over lateral thigh, Tinel's sign lateral inguinal ligament	Chronic compression
Sciatic	Weakness of dorsiflexion plantar flexion, foot eversion and inversion, sensory loss over dorsum and sole of foot	Hip surgery, prolonged bed rest
Peroneal at the fibular head (peroneal palsy)	Tripping; foot drop; sensory loss over lateral calf and dorsum of foot; normal foot eversion and inversion	Acute compression (i.e., leg crossing)
Posterior tibial at ankle (tarsal tunnel syndrome)	Nocturnal foot pain and tingling, Tinel's sign posterior to medial malleolus	Chronic compression, trauma

be caused by tumor infiltration from carcinomatous meningitis, leptomeningeal inflammation from neurosarcoidosis, or infectious causes such as chronic meningitis (i.e., tuberculosis, cryptococcus, neurosyphilis, Lyme disease). CSF examination is crucial to the diagnosis.

Polyneuropathy

The first step in narrowing the differential diagnosis of polyneuropathy is to note its time course and tempo. Other important issues in the diagnosis and treatment of polyneuropathies are shown in the box below.

Important factors in the evaluation and therapy of polyneuropathy

1. Tempo
2. Symmetry of signs and symptoms
3. Physiology: axonal versus demyelinative
4. Clues to etiology: family history, drugs, occupational exposure, nutrition, systemic disease, vaccination
5. Functional impairment
6. Efficacy, risks, cost of treatment

Acute symmetric, generalized weakness with sensory complaints progressing over 1 to 4 weeks. Today, this presentation is almost always an acute inflammatory demyelinating polyradiculoneuropathy (AIDP), often referred to as the Guillain-Barré syndrome. However, other causes should be considered (see box at upper right). AIDP is usually preceded by an infectious illness, vaccination, or surgery. Ataxia of gait or limbs is often an early symptom, followed by weakness of proximal and then distal muscles; sometimes, facial, extraocular, and respiratory muscles are eventually involved. Sensory loss occurs but is generally exceeded by sensory symptoms. Autonomic abnormalities affecting the cardiac rhythm, thermoregulation, and the pupils or sphincters may develop, presumably as a result of involvement of the white rami communicantes. After several days, the cerebrospinal fluid (CSF) reveals an elevated protein with little or no cellular response, and electrical studies can often demonstrate a demyelinating neuropathy. ICU monitoring of respiratory function and cardiac rhythm is required for progressive cases, with timely intubation if necessary, prophylaxis of venous thrombosis, frequent turning to prevent decubiti, intermittent catheterization for urinary retention, pain control, and emotional support. Finally, early plasmapheresis has been shown to shorten the course in AIDP patients with significant weakness. Intravenous immunoglobulin (IVIg) also appears to be effective.

Acute neurologic diseases in the differential diagnosis of acute inflammatory demyelinating polyradiculopathy (AIDP)

Central nervous system
- Acute cervical myelopathy
- Basilar artery thrombosis

Anterior horn cell poliomyelitis

Nerve
- Acute inflammatory demyelinating polyradiculoneuropathy (AIDP)
- Porphyric neuropathy
- Diphtheritic neuropathy
- Drugs: dapsone, nitrofurantoin (occasionally)
- Toxins: organophosphate, arsenic (single exposure), thallium (single exposure)
- Tick paralysis

Neuromuscular junction
- Botulism
- Myasthenia gravis

Muscle membrane
- Hypo-, hyper-, and normokalemic periodic paralysis

Muscle
- Acute polymyositis

Causes of myelinopathy

I. Hereditary conditions
   A. Hereditary motor sensory neuropathy
      1. Type I (Charcot-Marie-Tooth disease)
      2. Type III (Dejerine-Sottas disease)
      3. Type IV (Refsum's disease)
   B. Hereditary predisposition to entrapment neuropathy
   C. Metachromatic leukodystrophy*
   D. Globoid cell leukodystrophy (Krabbe's disease)*
   E. Adrenoleukodystrophy or adrenomyeloneuropathy*
   F. Cockayne syndrome*

II. Acquired conditions
   A. CIDP
   B. "Benign" monoclonal gammopathies, particularly IgM
   C. Osteosclerotic myeloma
   D. Waldenström's macroglobulinemia
   E. Perhexiline therapy
   F. Acquired immune deficiency syndrome*

*Central nervous system manifestations.

Table 123-8. Small-fiber neuropathies

	Diagnosis made by
Amyloidosis Hereditary types I-IV Nonhereditary	Positive family history in some cases, mucous membrane, nerve biopsy
Diabetes (sometimes)	Fasting and postprandial blood sugar, Hgb AlC
Dimethylpropionitrile (DMAPN)	History of exposure
Fabry's disease* (alpha-galactosidase A deficiency)	Family history, high serum phytanic acid
Hereditary sensory neuropathy types I, III, IV	Family history, clinical presentation
Tangier's disease (hereditary high-density lipoprotein deficiency)	Reduced high-density alpha lipoproteins and cholesterol

*Central nervous system manifestations.

Stepwise, relapsing, or slowly progressive symmetric motor-sensory polyneuropathy with slow nerve conduction velocities. Most commonly, this presentation is caused by chronic inflammatory demyelinating polyradiculoneuropathy (CIDP), which has features in common with AIDP (proximal muscle weakness, motor greater than sensory deficit, elevated CSF protein, similar pathology) but has a different time course (onset to peak deficit longer than 8 weeks) and less autonomic involvement. The demyelinating forms of hereditary motor sensory polyneuropathy (HMSN), such as HMSN I, III, IV, should be considered in cases of childhood onset, along with other acquired disorders simulating CIDP, such as some of the paraproteinemias and AIDS (see box at upper right). Immunosuppressive agents, plasmapheresis, and IVIg are useful in treating idiopathic CIDP and the paraproteinemias. Plasmapheresis may be used to treat AIDS-related CIDP.

Chronic, symmetric, slowly progressive sensorimotor polyneuropathy affecting legs more than arms (onset to peak deficit, months to years). The majority of chronic polyneuropathies are axonopathies, predominantly affecting large or medium fibers and initially affecting the longest axons, which subsequently "die back" with progressive involvement of shorter axons. Hence, sensory dysfunction, weakness, and areflexia begin in the toes and, depending on the severity of the neuropathy, ascend, in order, to the lower legs, fingertips, upper legs, forearms, midline trunk, upper arms, and top of the head. Far less frequent are chronic small-fiber axonopathies (Table 123-8), whose signs and symptoms (discussed above) can often be recognized at the bedside, and the chronic myelinopathies (see box above), which can be distinguished from axonopathies by nerve conduction studies and electromyography.

Clues to the etiology of chronic axonopathy primarily affecting large and medium fibers are the presence of systemic illness, hereditary predisposition (Table 123-9), and exposure to drugs or toxins (Table 123-10). To elicit a family history of neuropathy, one should determine if family members have deformity of foot, spine, or hand or can walk only with the use of assistive devices. In cases without a known cause, examination of family members is necessary to rule out hereditary neuropathy.

The most common cause of polyneuropathy in Western civilization is diabetes, which in addition to chronic sym-

Table 123-9. Causes of chronic axonopathy

	Diagnosis confirmed by
I. Malnutrition or malabsorption	
A. Thiamine deficiency (beriberi)*	Erythrocyte transkelolase assay
B. Pyridoxine deficiency	Measurement of tryptophan metabolites after tryptophan loading
C. Pantothenic acid	Clinical presentation
D. Vitamin B_{12} deficiency*	Schilling test, vitamin B_{12} level
E. Pellagra* (deficiency of niacin and other B vitamins)	Clinical presentation
F. Vitamin E deficiency*	Clinical presentation, vitamin E levels
II. Metabolic disease	
A. Diabetes	Fasting and postprandial blood sugars
B. Renal failure	BUN, creatinine
C. Hypothyroidism, hyperthyroidism	Thyroid function tests
D. Acromegaly	Growth hormone studies
III. Infection	
A. Acquired immune deficiency syndrome	HIV titer, clinical presentation
B. Leprosy	Nerve biopsy
IV. Neuropathy associated with malignancy	
A. Para- or dysproteinemia	
1. "Benign" monoclonal gammopathy	Serum and urine protein and immunoelectrophoresis
2. Multiple myeloma	Bone films, bone marrow aspirate, serum and urine protein and immunoelectrophoresis
3. Cryoglobulinemia	Serum for cryoglobulins
B. Carcinoma	
1. Lung carcinoma	Thorough physical examination, chest x-ray, etc.
2. Gastrointestinal malignancy	Thorough physical examination, stool guaiacs, etc.
3. Breast cancer	Thorough breast examination, mammography
4. Genitourinary carcinoma	Pelvic examination, urinalysis, etc.
C. Lymphoma, Hodgkin's disease	Biopsy of lymph node, etc.
V. "Connective tissue" diseases (see Table 123-5)	ANA, RF, ESR, etc.
VI. Hereditary axonopathies	
A. Hereditary sensorimotor polyneuropathy—type II (Charcot-Marie-Tooth)	Clinical presentation, including skeletal deformities
B. Hereditary sensory neuropathy—type II	Clinical presentation, including nerve biopsy
C. Neuropathy associated with the hereditary ataxias*	Clinical presentation, including presence of ataxia
D. Ataxia telangiectasia*	Clinical presentation
E. Xeroderma pigmentosa	Genetic studies, clinical presentation
F. Abetalipoproteinemia* (Bassen-Kornzweig disease)	Diminished vitamin E level, cholesterol, and low-density lipoproteins
G. Porphyric neuropathy*	
1. Acute intermittent	Elevated urinary porphyrin precursors, erythrocyte assay of uroporphyrinogen synthetase I
2. Coproporphyria	Elevated fecal porphyrin
3. Variegate	Elevated fecal and urinary porphyrins and urinary porphyrin precursors
VII. Idiopathic	Absence of peripheral neuropathy in family members, negative workup

*Central nervous system involvement.

metric sensorimotor or small-fiber polyneuropathy also produces several asymmetric forms: cranial or limb mononeuropathy, thoracolumbar radiculopathy, lumbosacral plexopathy, and mononeuritis multiplex. Whereas the asymmetric forms are probably ischemic in origin, the symmetric forms may have either an ischemic or a metabolic cause (i.e., abnormalities of sorbitol metabolism). Treatment of diabetic neuropathy should include good glucose control, control of pain and autonomic symptoms, and good foot care (discussed below).

In U.S. society, neuropathy caused by vitamin deficiency occurs in malnourished, alcoholic patients; in patients treated with isoniazid or hydralazine; and, rarely, in malabsorption syndromes. In alcoholics, the neuropathy presents as a subacute or chronic, symmetric, painful sensorimotor axonopathy and represents the result of months to years of inadequate nutrition with deficiency of B vitamins, particularly thiamine. Treatment of alcoholic neuropathy consists of adequate nutrition, thiamine and other B vitamin supplementation, and pain control. Isoniazid (INH) and hydralazine appear to interfere with pyridoxine metabolism and can produce an axonal sensorimotor polyneuropathy. Administration of oral pyridoxine (50 mg two times a day) prevents INH neuropathy. (Note that higher doses—

Table 123-10. Sensorimotor neuropathy caused by drugs and toxins

Drugs	
Anesthetics/hypnotics	
Glutethimide	
Nitrous oxide	
Thalidomide	
Antibiotics	
Chloramphenicol, clioquinol,* dapsone,† ethambutol,* ethionamide, isoniazid, metronidazole,* nitrofurantoin†	
Anticonvulsants	
Phenytoin	
Cardiovascular medicines	
Amiodarone	
Hydralazine	
Perhexilene maleate	
Cancer chemotherapeutic agents	
Cisplatin, misonidazole,* vincristine	
Rheumatologic medicines	
Gold	
Toxins	Associations
Acrylamide	Used in production of grouting and flocculating agents
Arsenic†	Smelting, mining
Carbon disulfide	Used in production of rubber, rayon, or cellophane
Cyanide*	Consumption of stone fruits, cassava plants
Dichlorophenoxyacetic acid (2,4 D)	Used as a herbicide
Dimethylpropionitrile (DMAPN)	Used in production of polyurethane grouting agents
Ethylene oxide	Used in chemical sterilization
Hexacarbons (i.e., h-hexane methyl *n*-butyl ketone)	Industrial solvents, glue sniffing
Lead	Smelting, battery production, repair of automobile radiators, moonshine whiskey
Mercury*	Used in a number of industries, fungicide
Methyl bromide	Used as insecticide, fire extinguisher, refrigerant, fumigant
Organophosphorus esters* Leptophos, mipafax, trichlorfon, triorthocresyl phosphate	Used as insecticides and petroleum or plastic additives
Polychlorinated biphenyls	Used as plasticizers, electrical insulators, fungistatic agents
Thallium*†	Rodenticides, insecticides

*Central nervous system manifestations.
†Sometimes associated with acute polyneuropathy.

i.e., 500 mg per day—can result in a sensory neuronopathy.) Vitamin B_{12} deficiency is among the most important of the diseases that can affect both the peripheral and the central nervous systems (see diseases with asterisk in Tables 123-5, 123-8, 123-9, 123-10 and the box on p. 1101), because replacement therapy is curative if begun early. Although peripheral nerves are often mildly affected in vitamin B_{12} deficiency, the predominant pathology tends to be in the posterior and lateral columns of the spinal cord. Indeed, the initial symptoms and signs appear to be peripheral, but the distal limb paresthesias (i.e., tingling), followed by vibratory and joint position sense loss, sometimes loss of ankle jerks, and, subsequently, gait ataxia can all be caused by dorsal column rather than peripheral nerve pathology. Pyramidal signs eventually develop, too. The usual cause is pernicious anemia; rarely, other causes of malabsorption may be involved.

Peripheral neuropathy frequently results from cancer or its treatment. Direct invasion of spinal roots, cranial nerves, or plexi occurs, as does sensorimotor polyneuropathy, a "remote effect" of cancer. The latter, sometimes referred to as *paracarcinomatous neuropathy,* has several forms: AIDP, CIDP (see the box on p. 1101), motor or sensory neuronopathy, and, most commonly, sensorimotor axonopathy. Patients with significant polyneuropathy without obvious cause should be screened with a careful examination and judicious laboratory testing (see the box on p. 1101 and Table 123-9) to rule out an underlying malignancy. However, without some clue from the history, the examination, and screening lab studies, extensive evaluation for occult malignancy is generally fruitless and not recommended. Of the several chemotherapeutic drugs that produce sensorimotor polyneuropathy (Table 123-10), the most common is vincristine, and the neuropathy improves when the drug is stopped. Radiation therapy can result in plexopathy, which can usually be distinguished from tumor invasion of the plexus by slower progression, little or no pain, and a tendency to involve the upper or whole brachial or the lower or whole lumbosacral plexus. However, CT scanning or MRI, or even biopsy of the plexus, may be required to be certain of tumor invasion, since its treatment usually includes radiation.

THERAPY OF PERIPHERAL NERVE DISORDERS

Treatment of these disorders includes specific treatment of the underlying disease process and general supportive measures. The latter consists of preventive care, such as (1) good foot care for all with insensate feet, particularly for the diabetic (competent podiatry, proper-fitting shoes, prompt treatment of infection); and (2) avoidance of nerve trauma, as in leaning on elbows or crossing legs, since polyneuropathy predisposes to compressive mononeuropathy. Rehabilitative techniques are important: (1) range of motion to prevent contractures and subsequent disability in the event of nerve recovery; (2) strengthening exercises; and (3) proper selection of (a) orthoses, such as a lightweight plastic ankle foot orthosis to prevent foot drop while walking, (b) wrist splints for carpal tunnel syndrome or radial nerve palsy, and (c) assistive devices for ambulation, such as canes, crutches, and wheelchairs. Pain can sometimes be controlled with nonsteroidal anti-inflammatory medicines, but narcotics may be required in acute circumstances. In chronic neuropathy, anticonvulsants (carbamazepine, phenytoin) or tricyclic antidepressants (amitriptyline), sometimes in conjunction with phenothiazines (fluphenazine), may be required. Occasionally, pain results from altered biomechanics (i.e., knee or back hyperextension in postpolio patients) and may be amenable to rehabilitative therapy (i.e., bracing). Other spontaneous positive sensory symptoms, such as distal "tingling" or "pins and needles," may be ameliorated by the wearing of gloves or socks. Autonomic dysfunction, such as orthostatic hypotension, can be treated by (1) "dangling" the legs prior to standing up, (2) avoidance of prolonged bed rest and elevating the head of the bed, (3) the use of made-to-measure elastic stockings, and (4) fludrocortisone therapy. Cholinergic therapy may be useful in treating gastroparesis (metoclopramide) or cystopathy (bethanechol).

REFERENCES

Asbury AK and Gilliat RW, editors: Peripheral nerve disorders. London, 1984, Butterworths.

Dawson DM, Hallett M, and Millender LH: Entrapment neuropathies, ed 2. Boston, 1990, Little, Brown.

Dyck PJ et al, editors: Peripheral neuropathy, ed 2. Philadelphia, 1984, Saunders.

Schaumberg HH, Berger AR, and Thomas PK: Disorders of peripheral nerves, ed 2. Philadelphia, 1991, Davis.

CHAPTER

124 Diseases of the Neuromuscular Junction

Marjorie E. Seybold

MYASTHENIA GRAVIS

Myasthenia gravis (MG) is a disorder of neuromuscular transmission that affects approximately 1 in 20,000 persons. It has an autoimmune basis characterized by a 7 S gamma globulin antibody (AChR-ab) directed against the nicotinic acetylcholine receptor (AChR) of the neuromuscular junction. There is no racial or geographic predilection, and the disorder can occur at any age. It most commonly begins in young adulthood, and females are affected more often than males in this age group. In the elderly, males are affected at least as frequently as females. Familial cases are rare. HLA typing has revealed a frequent association of MG with HLA-A1, -B8, and -DR3 in patients without thymoma with onset of the disease in young adulthood, but these HLA types are inconsistently present, even in familial cases.

Two other disorders of neuromuscular transmission clinically similar to MG are recognized. Neonatal MG is the development of transient weakness in an infant born to a myasthenic mother. It occurs in only 15% of at-risk infants, despite the transplacental transfer of AChR-ab from the mother to her infant in almost all pregnancies involving a mother with MG. The possibility of brief autonomous infant production of AChR-ab in the affected cases has been suggested. There is no correlation between maternal disease severity and occurrence of MG symptoms in the neonate. Treatment with anticholinesterase medication is necessary if weakness is severe. Fortunately, spontaneous recovery occurs, usually within 3 to 4 weeks after birth. Reoccurrence of MG in later life is very unlikely.

Penicillamine-induced MG (PEN-MG) describes the development of MG symptoms in patients treated with the drug D-penicillamine. It occurs in patients with a variety of underlying disorders, including rheumatoid arthritis, Wilson's disease, biliary cirrhosis, and systemic sclerosis. Preliminary HLA studies have raised the possibility of association between B35/DR1 and the development of PEN-MG. This differs from the increased prevalence of B8/DR3 reported in spontaneous MG. PEN-MG appears to be clinically identical to spontaneous MG, and AChR-ab is characteristically present. The symptoms usually are predominantly ocular, but generalized weakness may occur. The disorder responds to treatment with anticholinesterase medications and usually remits spontaneously within 1 year of the discontinuation of penicillamine. Occasional cases of persistent MG have been reported, however.

Pathophysiology

The autoimmune form of MG is characterized by the presence of AChR-ab and a reduction in the number of AChRs on the postsynaptic portion of the neuromuscular junction. These changes result in reduction in postsynaptic response to ACh. Acetylcholine, although released in normal amounts from the nerve terminal, is at times unable to induce sufficient depolarization of the postsynaptic membrane to initiate muscle excitation. Muscle weakness and fatigability result.

The mechanisms responsible for AChR-ab induction of MG in humans are poorly understood. Some information regarding MG has been extrapolated from studies of experimental autoimmune myasthenia gravis (EAMG) in animals. This disease, induced by injecting animals with adjuvant and purified AChR, mimics MG pharmacologically, histologically, physiologically, and clinically. The animals develop AChR-ab and appear to represent a valid immunologic model for MG in humans.

Studies in EAMG have implicated humoral, cellular, and complement factors in the disease. The disease may be transferred from animal to animal or from MG patient to animal by antibodies. However, this passive transfer of disease is blocked in animals depleted of complement (C3). EAMG also may be transferred by lymph node cells from immunized animals. Production of AChR-ab and EAMG in animals treated with AChR and adjuvant can be prevented in animals depleted of T cells.

In MG, immunoglobulin G and complement have been identified on the postsynaptic folds of the neuromuscular junction, and a prominent reduction in AChR has been documented. The reduction in receptors is presumed to be induced by the AChR-ab, both by enhancing receptor degradation and by complement-mediated destruction of the end plate. AChR-ab enhances destruction of AChR by cross-linking receptors, which, in turn, accelerates internalization and degradation of AChR. Complement-mediated injury of the postsynaptic membrane reduces the numbers of receptors by direct destruction and probably also by interference with proper insertion of the new AChR into the membrane.

Almost 90% of MG patients with generalized weakness, but only 50% to 60% of those with purely ocular findings, have detectable AChR-ab in their sera. The concentration of antibody does not correlate well with clinical symptoms, although patients with only ocular symptoms usually have relatively low levels of AChR-ab. AChR-ab response in MG is polyclonal, being directed against the various subunits of the AChR. Unfortunately, no specific subunit antibodies appear to be linked to clinical severity or to the presence of thymoma. In most patients, the majority of the AChR-ab are directed against a specific region of the alpha subunit separate from the ACh binding site on that subunit.

Evidence of altered cellular immunity in MG has been reported, but no specific defect has been identified as yet. Peripheral blood lymphocytes (PBLs) undergo antigen-specific transformation when exposed to AChR. This increased PBL responsiveness appears to occur in helper T cells and, although proportional to disease severity in EAMG in rats, has not been correlated consistently with disease activity or patient age in MG.

Either hypo- or hyperthyroidism occurs in approximately 10% of MG patients. Other presumed autoimmune diseases, such as lupus erythematosus, rheumatoid arthritis, pernicious anemia, and polymyositis, occur in MG patients more often than expected by chance. Myasthenic patients, even those without overt symptoms of other disease, often produce antinuclear, antithyroid, and antistriated muscle antibodies. The latter are particularly common in MG patients who also have thymomas.

Pathology

The most striking pathologic change observed in MG is the "simplification" of the postsynaptic portion of the neuromuscular junction. AChR, which is concentrated at the tips of the postsynaptic membrane folds, is frequently reduced to less than half the normal amount, and much of the remaining AChR has antibody bound to its surface. Complement components C3 and C9 are localized to the AChR area, and fragments containing AChR, antibody, and complement are detected in the synaptic cleft. The cleft itself is wider than normal.

Pathologic changes in the muscle itself are not prominent. Local collections of lymphocytes ("lymphorrhages") are sometimes seen within the muscle, but the role and etiology of these cells are not clear.

Thymus gland abnormalities are usually present in MG patients. At least 10% have a thymoma, and most of these patients are 30 years of age or older at the time of MG onset. The distinction of malignant, as opposed to benign, thymoma is based on the presence or absence of tumor invasion of the surrounding tissue, rather than on cell type. Thymomas rarely metastasize outside the thoracic cavity.

Patients without thymoma frequently have germinal centers in the thymic medulla, often called *thymic hyperplasia*. Hyperplasia is common in young patients, whereas those over 60 years old often have little remaining thymic tissue. Thymic cells from MG patients often spontaneously produce AChR-ab in vitro and, after irradiation, stimulate peripheral blood lymphocytes to produce AChR-ab, suggesting the presence of both specific B cells and helper T cells in thymic tissue.

Clinical and laboratory findings

The hallmark of MG is weakness that is made worse with exercise and improved with rest. Other factors, such as heat, menses, emotional stress, and intercurrent illness, frequently exacerbate the weakness. The onset of symptoms may be gradual or abrupt. Any skeletal muscle can be affected, but ocular symptoms are the most frequent initial complaint. Ptosis, ocular muscle weakness, or both may occur. Dysarthria, chewing fatigue, and dysphagia are also common. Involvement of the muscles of respiration may be sufficiently severe to require assisted ventilation. The extremities are often weaker proximally than distally, but either or both muscle groups may be involved. Arm weakness may result in an inability to shave or comb the hair, and leg weakness may result in sudden falls. Fluctuations in severity usually occur during the day, and asymmetry is common. Pain may occur in a fatigued muscle and is common in weakened neck muscles after prolonged head support. Paresthesias and sensory loss do not occur.

Muscle examination may be normal in rested patients, but weakness usually can be brought out with exercise. Patients with more severe disease are weak even at rest. Muscle atrophy is uncommon, and tendon reflexes and sensory examination are normal.

Myasthenia gravis can be remitting, static, or progressive. Some patients have only ocular symptoms, although the majority develop generalized disease. Rapid development of severe symptoms refractory to anticholinesterase medications is called a *myasthenic crisis*.

Laboratory testing reveals an elevated level of AChR-ab in as many as 90% of patients, depending on the laboratory method used. Repetitive nerve stimulation shows a decrement of the compound motor action potential of muscle in approximately 90% of patients if three or more muscles, especially proximal ones, are studied. Individual motor units also show an abnormal fluctuation in amplitude from moment to moment on electromyographic needle examination and reflect the fatigue of individual muscle fibers. More-sophisticated electromyographic testing, such as single-fiber electromyography, can detect abnormalities when conventional repetitive stimulation is normal.

Because of the increased incidence of thyroid disease in MG patients, thyroid test results may be abnormal. Likewise, B_{12} levels may be low because of associated pernicious anemia. Autoantibodies such as antinuclear antibody, antithyroid, rheumatoid factor, antistriated muscle, and antiparietal cell antibody are often present.

Chest x-ray or computed tomography may demonstrate a thymoma or a prominent thymus gland.

Diagnosis

People with myasthenia gravis commonly see several doctors before the disease is recognized. The patient may be considered to be hysterical or malingering for a time before the correct diagnosis is suspected.

The clinical diagnosis is based on the history of fluctuating weakness and on the demonstration of skeletal muscle weakness. Confirmation is obtained by demonstrating improvement after injection of anticholinesterase medication, either in the short-acting (edrophonium) or long-acting (neostigmine) form. A decrementing response of the muscle potential to repetitive nerve stimulation and demonstration of AChR-ab in the serum are further confirmatory evidence of MG. Patients in clinical remission may still have AChR-ab present. The use of minimal doses of curare as a diagnostic test to bring out weakness should be discouraged, as respiratory failure may occur.

Other disorders of neuromuscular transmission, such as the Lambert-Eaton myasthenic syndrome (frequently associated with oat-cell carcinoma of the lung), botulism, organophosphate poisoning, and antibiotic-induced neuromuscular block, usually can be distinguished by their mode of clinical presentation, poor response to anticholinesterase drugs, differing electrical characteristics, and the absence of AChR-ab. Dysthyroid ocular disease, dystrophies of ocular muscles, and brainstem-induced eye movement abnormalities must be distinguished from MG in the patient with only ocular symptoms. Easy fatigue as the result of metabolic imbalance, drug abuse, depression, or systemic disease also must be considered in the differential diagnosis of generalized MG.

Treatment

Treatment usually begins with anticholinesterase medications. The dosage varies widely, depending on the patient's symptomatic response and sensitivity to side effects. The most commonly used drug, pyridostigmine, is given in divided doses as needed during the day. Its onset of effect is about 30 minutes and it lasts up to 4 hours. A long-acting form (Timespan) is available for bedtime use if bulbar or respiratory weakness occurs throughout the night or on awaking in the morning. The uneven Timespan release makes it less popular than the shorter-acting form for daytime use. Muscarinic side effects of the anticholinesterase medications may be reduced by the use of low doses of atropine. Excessive anticholinesterase medication can induce muscle weakness by depolarizing or desensitizing available AChR and may lead to severe distress, termed *cholinergic crisis*. This crisis is treated by withdrawal of all anticholinesterase drugs for 24 to 48 hours and provision of ventilatory support as needed. Supplementary medications such as ephedrine, potassium, and calcium are of uncertain value.

Additional therapy for MG includes thymectomy, adrenal corticosteroids, other immunosuppressant drugs, plasmapheresis, and gamma globulin, although each of these modalities is controversial.

Thymectomy is accepted treatment for thymoma. Radiation therapy also has been used, especially if a contraindication to surgery exists. Thymectomy in the absence of evidence for thymoma is more controversial. Some authorities propose thymectomy for all patients with generalized MG; others favor it only in patients not responding well to medical treatment. The likelihood of improvement or remission after thymectomy is thought by some to be greater in younger patients with recent onset of the disease. Sustained improvement, when it occurs, may begin months or up to several years after the surgery.

Steroid therapy is used frequently. Many different regimens have been suggested, although alternate-day prednisone is used most often. Exacerbations of weakness may occur when therapy is initiated, especially if large doses are given. Frequently, when alternate-day prednisone is used, more weakness is experienced on the steroid off-days during the early stages of therapy. The course usually becomes smoother with prolonged use of the drug. Most patients require steroids indefinitely. Cataracts, osteoporosis, aseptic necrosis of bone, and decreased resistance to infection are long-term side effects.

Immunosuppressant drug therapy with azathioprine is now being used more commonly, especially in patients with severe disease who are poorly responsive or refractory to corticosteroids. Azathioprine may be given in conjunction with steroids or as the only immunosuppressant therapy. Side effects such as bone marrow suppression and the late development of neoplasms must be considered.

Other immunosuppressant therapies, such as cyclophosphamide and cyclosporine, have been used in a small number of MG patients. The toxicity of these medications probably precludes their frequent use in this disease.

Plasmapheresis and leukoplasmapheresis have been used successfully in seriously ill patients. Their application to less severely involved patients is not widely accepted at present, but it may be in the future.

Intravenous gamma globulin has recently been reported to be effective in treating some patients with MG. Its efficacy, however, has not yet been established in controlled clinical trials, nor has its usefulness relative to other treatments been established.

CONGENITAL MYASTHENIA

Congenital myasthenia is a general term used to designate several different developmental defects in neuromuscular structure and function, including a presynaptic disorder characterized by impairment of acetylcholine resynthesis or storage (familial infantile myasthenia) and one associated with a paucity of synaptic vesicles and reduced quantal release. The several postsynaptic defects include impaired acetylcholine (ACh) breakdown (congenital endplate acetylcholinesterase [AChE] deficiency), slow acetylcholine receptor ion channel closure (slow channel syndrome), inadequate acetylcholine receptor (AChR) production (congenital endplate AChR deficiency), abnormal interaction of ACh and AChR, high AChR channel conductance and shorter-than-normal channel open time (high-conductance fast channel syndrome), and prolonged channel open time with mutation of the epsilon subunit of the AChR. Autosomal-recessive inheritance has been described in familial infantile myasthenia, congenital endplate AChR deficiency, AChE deficiency, and high-conductance fast-channel syndrome. Slow-channel syndrome is an autosomal-dominant or sporatic disorder. AChR-ab has not been detected in congenital myasthenia, and there is no evidence linking it with an abnormality in the immune system.

Ptosis, ocular movement abnormalities, poor suck and cry, weakness, and easy fatigue may all occur in congenital myasthenia and may be clinically indistinguishable from autoimmune myasthenia gravis. Symptoms are usually present at birth, but particularly with slow-channel syndrome, later onset may occur. All of the disorders are reported to display a decremental response to 2 Hz stimulation, at least in muscles that are clinically weak. A repetitive response to a single-nerve stimulus occurs with slow-channel syndrome and endplate AChE deficiency.

Familial infantile myasthenia, endplate AChR deficiency, abnormal ACh-ACh-R interaction syndrome, and the syndrome associated with a paucity of synaptic vesicles have all been reported to respond to anticholinesterase medication. Because there is no evidence of immune abnormality, thymectomy, corticosteroids, and other immune-suppressant drugs are not recommended.

LAMBERT-EATON MYASTHENIC SYNDROME

Lambert-Eaton myasthenic syndrome (LEMS) is a disorder of neuromuscular transmission resulting from defective release of ACh by the nerve terminal after nerve stimulation. It is frequently seen in association with malignancy and is presumed to be autoimmune in origin.

The disorder is most often seen in adults, usually over the age of 40. Males are affected more often than females, both those with cancer and those without a detected carcinoma. The association with underlying malignancy approaches 60%; the majority of tumors are oat cell carcinomas of the lung.

Pathophysiology

LEMS is presumed to be an autoimmune disorder directed against the presynaptic nerve terminal. Exocytosis of synaptic vesicles containing ACh is felt to occur at the active zones on the presynaptic membrane by a calcium-dependent process. Antibody-induced disruption of these active zones would hinder calcium uptake and thus impair ACh release.

In favor of an autoimmune etiology for LEMS is the observation that mice injected with immunoglobulin G from LEMS patients develop a loss of active zones and active zone particles and display electrophysiologic abnormalities characteristic of LEMS. Antibodies directed against voltage-gated calcium channels (VGCC) are detected in over 50% of LEMS patients in some series. The response of LEMS patients to plasmapheresis and immunosuppressant therapy also favors an autoimmune basis for the disease.

Pathology

In humans, morphologic studies show both pre- and postsynaptic abnormalities. Freeze fracture electron microscopy shows a decrease in and disorganization of the active zones. Postsynaptic studies reveal reduplication of endplate folds. Whether this change is caused by the disease process or is secondary to presynaptic events is not known.

Clinical and laboratory findings

Clinical signs of LEMS include weakness and fatigability. Proximal muscles, especially those of the pelvic girdle, are often affected, and gait difficulty is a frequent presenting complaint. Ptosis and diplopia are often present but bulbar weakness, common in myasthenia gravis, is infrequently present in LEMS. Autonomic nervous system involvement occurs in LEMS and complaints of dry mouth and impotence may result. Paresthesias are frequently reported but detectable sensory loss is rare. Despite patient complaints of severe disability, it is common to find only mild weakness on examination. Tendon reflexes are usually depressed or absent.

The only presently readily available laboratory test for LEMS is repetitive nerve stimulation. At low (2 to 3 Hz) rates of stimulation, a small motor response is detected that further diminishes between the first and fifth response. Brief exercise (10 to 20 seconds) results in an improvement in the amplitude of muscle response toward the normal range. Two minutes later, the defects seen in the rested muscle have recurred, and the amplitude of response is once again small. Repetitive stimulation of rested muscle at rapid (20 to 50 Hz) rates of stimulation produces an increasing amplitude of response that may reach 2 to 20 times the amplitude of the initial response.

Microelectrode studies of the neuromuscular function in LEMS patients show that the number of quanta of ACh released by a nerve impulse is small. Rapid repetitive stimulation or voluntary activation briefly facilitates the release of quanta, enhancing the depolarization of the postsynaptic membrane and improving neuromuscular transmission. VGCC antibody detection will probably soon be commercially available as a diagnostic aid.

Associated disorders

LEMS frequently occurs in association with tumors, usually oat cell carcinoma of the lung. In these cases, it is suspected that antibodies made to tumor determinants cross-react with the active sites on the nerve terminals. Symptoms usually precede recognition of the tumor, at times by as long as several years. Treatment of the underlying tumor sometimes results in improvement in LEMS symptoms as well.

Patients with LEMS may have evidence of other autoimmune disorders, especially those that are organ-specific.

Organ-specific autoantibodies, (thyroid, gastric, and/or skeletal) are seen in up to 45% of LEMS patients. Thyroid disease, vitiligo, and pernicious anemia have been clinically observed. Over 10% of LEMS patients also have detectable antibodies to acetylcholine receptors. In these cases differentiation between LEMS and myasthenia gravis must be based on clinical and electrophysiological markers.

Treatment

Anticholinesterase medications usually produce modest improvement. Drugs that enhance ACh release, such as guanidine hydrochloride, are more effective. However, side effects such as paresthesias and toxicity, including aplastic anemic and renal failure, often limit prolonged use. 3, 4, Diaminopyridine, a drug that promotes acetylcholine release from presynoptic vesicles, has shown some encouraging beneficial effects in patients with LEMS, but is not yet available for general use. Corticosteroids, azathioprine, and plasmapheresis have been used with success in LEMS.

Some centers favor postponement of immunosuppressive therapy in those patients without recognized tumors because of concern that such treatment might undermine natural control of any underlying malignancy.

REFERENCES

Myasthenia Gravis

Finley JC and Pascuzzi RM: Seminars in neurology 10:70, 1990.

Lindstrom J et al: Myasthenia gravis. Advances in immunology 42:233, 1988.

Penn AS et al, editors: Myasthenia gravis and related disorders: experimental and clinical aspects. Ann NY Acad Sci 1993 (in press).

Seybold ME: Myasthenia gravis. In Lichtenstein LM and Fauci AS, editors: Current therapy in allergy, immunology and rheumatology—3. Toronto, 1988, Decker.

Seybold ME: Update on myasthenia gravis. Hosp Med 27:71, 1991.

Congenital Myasthenia

Engel AG: Congenital disorders of neuromuscular transmission. Semin Neurol 10:122, 1990.

Engel AG et al: Newly recognized congenital myasthenic syndromes: I. Congenital paucity of synaptic vesicles and reduced quantal release. II. High-conductance fast-channel syndrome. III. Abnormal acetylcholine receptor (AChR) interaction with acetylcholine IV. AChR deficiency and short channel-open time. Prog Brain Res 84:125, 1990.

Penn AS et al, editors: Myasthenia gravis and related disorders: experimental and clinical aspects. Ann NY Acad Sci 1993 (in press).

Lambert-Eaton Myasthenic Syndrome

Chalk CH et al: Response of the Lambert-Eaton myasthenic syndrome to treatment of associated small-cell lung carcinoma. Neurology 40:1552, 1990.

Engel AG: Review of evidence for loss of motor nerve terminal calcium channels in Lambert-Eaton myasthenic syndrome. Ann NY Acad Sci 635:246, 1991.

Lennon VA et al: Autoimmunity in the Lambert-Eaton myasthenic syndrome. Muscle Nerve 5:S21, 1982.

Lennon VA and Lambert EH: Autoantibodies bind solubilized calcium channel—conotoxin complexes from small cell lung carcinoma: a diagnostic aid for Lambert-Eaton myasthenic syndrome. Mayo Clin Proc 64:1498, 1989.

Lundh H et al: Current therapy of the Lambert-Eaton myasthenic syndrome. Prog Brain Res 84:163, 1990.

O'Neill JH et al: The Lambert-Eaton myasthenic syndrome. A review of 50 cases. Brain 111:577, 1988.

Penn AS et al, editors: Myasthenia gravis and related disorders: experimental and clinical aspects. Ann NY Acad Sci 1993 (in press).

Vincent A et al: Autoimmunity to the voltage-gated calcium channel underlies the Lambert-Eaton myasthenic syndrome, a paraneoplastic disorder. Trends Neurosci 12:496, 1989.

CHAPTER

125 Muscle Disease

Robert H. Brown, Jr.

The cardinal symptom of muscle disease is weakness. A careful clinical analysis usually distinguishes the weakness of primary muscle disease from that caused by problems elsewhere in the motor unit or central nervous system. Distinguishing diagnostic features are outlined in Table 125-1. Most primary muscle diseases preferentially affect the proximal muscles. Thus there may be difficulty lifting the arms to comb the hair or rising from a low chair, while fine finger movements, removing a lid from a jar, and walking on tiptoes may be normal. Weakness is sometimes described as fatigue. In primary myopathies, weakness and fatigue symptoms usually significantly disrupt normal daily activities, while in systemic or psychiatric illnesses producing fatigue this may not be the case. By the same token, in the primary myopathies the actual signs of muscle dysfunction may be more severe than the symptoms. Patients with primary myopathies such as disorders of muscle metabolism may complain of muscle cramping and pains. Myalgias induced by brief bursts of intense activity such as sprinting may occur in disorders of glycogen utilization; such activity depends primarily on recruitment of anaerobic type II muscle fibers that are glycogen-dependent. Conversely, in disorders of lipid metabolism, muscle pain may be most severe after sustained, low-level activities such as hiking that recruit oxidative, lipid-dependent type I fibers. Indeed, the lipid myopathies may be associated with episodic dark urine after chronic muscle exercise, indicating frank muscle breakdown and myoglobinuria. Weakness in primary myopathies is generally constant from day to day, perhaps with some worsening with sustained exercise; this is in marked contrast to the weakness in neuromuscular junction disorders such as myasthenia gravis or Eaton-Lambert syndrome, which may be highly variable over the course of only a few hours. It is axiomatic that the primary myopathies, in contrast with peripheral neuropathies or central nervous system diseases, do not produce numbness or sensory loss.

It is useful to begin the muscle examination by observing the exposed torso and extremities. The hallmark of longstanding muscle disease is muscle wasting, which is often symmetrical and proximal. Myopathic weakness and wasting of the face and eyelids is prominent in facioscapulohumeral, myotonic, and oculopharyngeal dystrophies; in

Table 125-1. Differential diagnosis of disorders of the motor unit

Finding	Nerve	Neuromuscular junction	Muscle
Clinical			
Weakness, wasting	+	+/−	−
Fasciculations	+	−	−
Cramps	+	−	+
Sensory loss	+/−	−	−
Hyperreflexia	+/−	−	−
Laboratory			
Elevated CPK	−	−	+
Elevated myoglobin	−	−	+/−
High CSF protein	+/−	−	+/−
EMG-NCT			
Slowed conduction	+/−	−	−
EMG potential amplitude	Increased	Normal	Decreased
EMG potential duration	Increased	Normal	Decreased
Number EMG potential	Decreased	Normal	Increased
Fasciculations	+	−	−
Decremental response	−	+/−	−
Muscle biopsy	Grouped atrophy	Normal	Degeneration-regeneration

the latter two there may also be pharyngeal weakness. Focal atrophy may be evident after muscle trauma or focal denervation. There is generally little visible spontaneous twitching of myopathic muscles; by contrast, muscles atrophied by denervation often reveal fasciculations. In some disorders there is infiltration of muscle with connective tissue and fat, which increases muscle bulk. Such pseudohypertrophy is particularly prominent in the calves in Duchenne and Becker's dystrophies. Muscle swelling with tenderness may be evident in focal or diffuse inflammatory muscle diseases.

It is conventional to rate muscle strength on a scale of 0 to 5 as follows: 5—full power; 4—nearly full power against both resistance and gravity; 3—moves against gravity but not resistance; 2—moves but not against gravity or resistance; 1—trace of movement; 0—no movement. In practice, rating muscle strength numerically is less important than describing performance of standard tests of muscle function such as lifting the head from a position of hyperextension or flexion over the edge of a bed; doing a sit-up; holding the arms overhead; rising from a chair or a squat without using the arms; walking; stepping up onto a stool; hopping on either foot alone; or pursing the lips to blow.

LABORATORY EVALUATION

Several laboratory tests assist in the diagnosis of neuromuscular disorders. Particularly helpful are serum levels of muscle enzymes released with muscle injury such as aldolase or the MM isoform of creatine kinase CK. In fulminant myopathies such as Duchenne dystrophy, CK may be elevated as much as a hundredfold. By contrast, in slowly progressive disorders it may be normal or elevated no more than twofold to threefold. Increases in CK are not specific to primary myopathies; the enzyme may be mildly elevated in active denervating disease such as amyotrophic lateral sclerosis. Levels may also rise after incidental trauma or intramuscular injections. Like muscle enzyme levels, serum and urine creatine and myoglobin are elevated when there is active muscle breakdown. Myoglobin release does not necessarily correlate with CK elevations; indeed, myoglobinuria is rare in Duchenne dystrophy. Systemic and muscle-specific carnitine deficiencies produce lipid myopathies that may be diagnosed by assaying serum and muscle levels of this substance. Abnormalities in the major pathways of muscle energy production may be detected with two simple clinical tests. In the ischemic forearm lactate test, the forearm is exercised vigorously for 1 minute under ischemic conditions, which effectively disables mitochondria, rendering the muscle dependent on glycolysis for ATP production. Normally there is at least a twofold rise in serum lactate by about 6 minutes after the ischemic exercise. A flat lactate response is typical of glycolytic enzyme disorders such as myophosphorylase deficiency (McArdle's disease). By obtaining pyruvate and ammonia levels simultaneously, one may also screen for deficiencies of lactate dehydrogenase or myoadenylate deaminase. To test muscle for ATP generation from lipids, the patient is fasted until glycogen stores are depleted, usually more than 24 hours, while serum glucose and urinary ketone levels are monitored. In normal glycogen-depleted muscle, glucose levels are maintained by fatty acid metabolism, which secondarily produces urinary ketones. In disorders such as deficiencies of carnitine or carnitine palmityltransferase, blood glucose may fall precipitously without ketonuria. Fasting serum lactate and pyruvate levels may be elevated in mitochondrial disorders. Finally, it is increasingly possible to diagnosis specific muscle gene defects using small quantities of blood lymphocyte DNA and polymerase chain reaction methods; thus, blood-based diagnosis is now possible for most cases of Duchenne and Becker's dystrophy and the respective carrier states, myotonic dystrophy, hyperkalemic periodic paralysis, some mitochondrial muscle diseases, and some neuropathiies such as Charcot-Marie-Tooth disease and familial amyloidosis.

ELECTROMYOGRAPHY

Analysis of the electrophysiological properties of muscle by electromyography (EMG) helps distinguish primary myopathies from other disorders producing weakness. The first major diagnostic EMG parameter is *spontaneous activity*. When muscle undergoes active denervation, spontaneous twitches of single muscle cells or fibrillations occur, reflecting electrical irritability. Fasciculations, that is, spontaneous discharges of an intact motor unit, may be seen in normal or denervated muscle. The second major parameter is *amplitude and shape of the muscle compound action potential*. In primary myopathies the action potential is often brief and reduced in amplitude; in denervating diseases with chronic reinnervation and motor unit enlargement, the action potential may be enlarged and prolonged. *Electrical irritability of the muscle membrane* is the third parameter. In myotonic disorders, the muscle membrane or sarcolemma shows sustained high but variable frequency discharges after needle insertion and after volitional contraction of muscle fibers (the "dive-bomber" sound heard on audio analysis of the EMG). In contrast, the sustained muscle contraction caused by energy deficiency, as seen in McArdle's disease, is electrically silent. The final parameter is a *pattern of recruitment of fibers* with voluntary muscle contraction. In primary muscle disease, the number of recruitable motor units is normal; however, the number of fibers per unit may be decreased, resulting in a pattern of low amplitude on recruitment. In contrast, denervating diseases such as poliomyelitis or motor neuron disease may reduce the number of recruitable motor units although the actual recruited compound muscle action potentials may be of normal or increased amplitude. Nerve conduction studies should be normal in primary muscle disease.

PATHOLOGY

Muscle biopsy may distinguish myopathic from neurogenic disease and may lead to specific morphologic diagnoses. In primary myopathies, muscle is characterized by fiber size vaiation and evidence of degeneration (fiber necrosis and phagocytosis; possibly inflammation) and regeneration (basophilia; central nucleation; fiber splitting). In chronic myopathies there may be extensive connective tissue proliferation and fatty infiltration. By contrast, in denervating diseases there may be evidence of active (small, angulated fibers) and chronic (fiber type grouping and grouped atrophy) denervation. Other features may suggest specific diagnoses such as the presence of fibers with a ragged red appearance in mitochondrial myopathies; marked lymphocytic infiltration of interstitium in polymyositis; glycogen-rich vacuoles in some glycolytic enzyme deficiency states (e.g., Pompe's disease or acid maltase deficiency); or lipid inclusions in the lipid myopathies. Muscle from biopsies is also useful for direct muscle biochemical assay or protein analysis using Western immunoblotting or immunofluorescence.

SPECIFIC CATEGORIES OF MUSCLE DISORDERS

The box below lists the major categories of muscle diseases. The inflammatory myopathies are discussed in detail elsewhere. Several categories of myopathy are inherited, as outlined in Table 125-1; the largest is the muscular dystrophies, a diverse group of disorders whose common feature is a period of relatively normal muscle function early in life

Classification of primary myopathies

- I. Hereditary
  - A. Muscular dystrophies
  - B. Congenital myopathies
  - C. Metabolic myopathies
    - 1. Glycogenolysis and glycolysis
      - a. Myophosphorylase, phosphofructokinase deficiency
      - b. Distal glycolytic enzyme deficiencies
    - 2. Lipid
      - a. Carnitine-palmityl-transferase A or B deficiency
      - b. Systemic and muscle carnitine deficiency
      - c. Defective beta decarboxylation
    - 3. Purine
    - 4. Mitochondria
      - a. Defined biochemical defects
      - b. Mitochondrial DNA mutations (Table 125-3)
      - c. Mitochondrial DNA depletion (e.g., AZT therapy)
  - D. Membrane excitability disorders
    - 1. Myotonia
      - a. Myotonic dystrophy
      - b. Myotonia congenita
    - 2. Periodic paralysis
      - a. Sodium channel mutations
        - (i) Hyperkalemic periodic paralysis
        - (ii) Normokalemic periodic paralysis
        - (iii) Paramyotonia congenita
      - b. Hypokalemic periodic paralysis
- II. Inflammatory
  - A. Polymyositis (± dermatomyositis)
  - B. Polymyositis with vasculitis
  - C. Inclusion body myositis
  - D. Infectious
    - 1. Bacterial (e.g., clostridial)
    - 2. Viral and retroviral (e.g., Coxsackie, HIV)
    - 3. Parasitic (e.g., toxoplasmosis)
  - E. Drug-induced
  - F. Miscellaneous (e.g., sarcoidosis, paraneoplastic)
- III. Endocrine metabolic
  - A. Electrolyte disturbances (e.g., calcium, magnesium, potassium)
  - B. Endocrine disturbance
    - 1. Cushing's disease
    - 2. Hypo- and hyperthyroidism
    - 3. Hypo- and hyperparathyroidism
- IV. Toxic (e.g., alcohol, steroids, halothane, vincristine, chloroquine)
- V. Primary muscle tumors
- VI. Miscellaneous (e.g., malignant hyperthermia)

followed by deterioration in strength in selected muscle groups. Despite recent dramatic research progress, these disorders remain untreatable.

Duchenne muscular dystrophy (DMD)

This is the most common muscular dystrophy, affecting about 1 in 3000 boys. It is an X-linked disorder that frequently arises as a spontaneous mutation. Boys with DMD often have some delay in motor milestones and generally do not run normally. By the age of about 4 they may have difficulty walking upstairs and may fall easily. They are unable to rise from a squat unless they use the hands and arms to push off on the legs (Gowers' maneuver). Early in the course the calves show "pseudohypertrophy" or enlargment caused by fatty and connective infiltration. Before about the eighth year, most DMD boys experience heel cord tightening and tend to toe walk. Most use wheelchairs by about the twelfth year. The myocardium may be involved, as indicated by persistent tachycardia, ectopic rhythms, subtle conduction defects, and EKG abnormalities (tall R waves and deep Q waves respectively over the right and left precordium). Death is usually from pulmonary failure with recurrent pneumonias. Becker's muscular dystrophy (BMD) is a less severe variant of DMD; it is usually also characterized by calf pseudohypertrophy and progressive proximal muscle weakness; BMD and DMD do not occur within the same family. BMD patients remain ambulatory beyond the age of 15 and often well into adult life.

Recent studies have identified both the DMD/BMD gene on the X chromosome and its product dystrophin. This is a large, muscle-specific protein, which has a rodlike structure and is membrane-associated. It is almost uniformly absent in DMD biopsies; in BMD muscle it is usually present but abnormal in size. The laboratory diagnosis of BMD and DMD has conventionally relied on elevation of serum CK levels and the presence of myopathic findings on EMG and muscle biopsy. It is now possible to assay muscle directly for dystrophin with immunoblotting and immunofluorescence. One may also use polymerase chain reaction to diagnose deletions characteristic of DMD/BMD in blood DNA; this can assist in prenatal and preclinical diagnosis as well as carrier detection for genetic counselling.

Facioscapulohumeral dystrophy typically affects muscles of the face and proximal upper extremities; weakness of the peronei and anterior tibial muscles may produce footdrop as well. The disorder is usually autosomal-dominant; most cases of FSH dystrophy are genetically linked to the distal long arm of chromosome 4. There is considerable variation in the onset and severity of the illness. Most patients come to medical attention in the third decade, some never do, and some are diagnosed as children. In infants the earliest manifestation may be a tendency to get soap in the eyes while bathing. In children it may be an inability to purse the lips to whistle. In affected individuals there is prominent scapular winging. Abduction of the arms produces scapular elevation, which appears anteriorly as a step between the neck and shoulders. Weakness of the trapezeii and rhomboids may produce extreme shoulder sagging and even, in rare cases, brachial plexopathies.

Limb girdle dystrophy is an autosomal recessive disorder, linked in some families to a gene locus on chromosome 15, which is characterized by slowly progressive weakness of the proximal arms and legs but not the face. The age of onset is variable. In later stages pulmonary manifestations are common as a result of diaphragmatic weakness. In general, the disease is characterized by long-term survival. Muscle biopsy and electrophysiologic studies are essential to exclude polymyositis and spinal muscular atrophy of the Kugelberg-Welander type. Without EMG the latter may be clinically indistinguishable from limb girdle dystrophy. Indeed, in chronic denervating diseases biopsied muscle may acquire a "myopathic" histopathologic appearance, although fiber type grouping should point to denervating disorders.

Myotonic dystrophy is an autosomal-dominant, multisystem disorder whose muscle features include myotonia (prolongation of muscle contraction caused by sustained firing of the muscle membrane) and progressive wasting of the facial (eyelids, masseters, temporalis), neck, and distal limb muscles. The myotonia is painless; individuals first diagnosed in adulthood often describe lifelong difficulty letting go of a doorknob. Nonmuscle features include frontal balding, cataracts (posterior, subcapsular, stellate), testicular atrophy and infertility, diminished insulin sensitivity, cardiac disease (particularly conduction system defects), and mental retardation. Facial muscle involvement produces a pathognomonic "hatchet" face with ptosis, prominent temporal and masseter wasting, and jaw slackness. In adults the onset of the illness is insidious in the second or third decade. In babies of mothers with myotonic dystrophy, there may be severe hypotonia and floppiness with weak respiration and sucking but no myotonia. The most useful laboratory investigation of any myotonia is the EMG, which demonstrates the typical myotonic dive-bomber bursts as mentioned above. Muscle biopsy shows typically myopathic features and prominent type I fiber atrophy, increased central nucleation, chains of nuclei, and ring fibers. Phenytoin may improve the myotonia; other membrane-active medications such as quinine may be hazardous because of potential cardiac conduction defects. The genetic defect in myotonic dystrophy appears to be an expanded CTG trinucleotide repeat arising in a protein kinase encoded on chromosome 19.

In contrast to myotonic dystrophy, *myotonia congenita* (MC) is a muscle-specific disorder that begins in early childhood and produces profound, sometimes disabling muscle stiffness. Strictly speaking, this is not a dystrophy. Most MC patients have a "herculean" appearance with muscle hypertrophy and unusually distinct definition of muscle bulk; as a rule there is no muscle wasting. Paramyotonia congenita (PMC) is a related disorder in which there is cold-provoked muscle stiffness, particularly of the eyes and hands, and in severe instances, paralysis. PMC is caused by mutations in a skeletal muscle sodium channel, as are hyperkalemic periodic paralysis and some forms of MC. It is thus not surprising that the muscle stiffness in these diseases may respond to the sodium channel blocking agent mexiletine.

Oculopharyngeal dystrophy is a late-life, dominantly inherited disorder characterized by ptosis and difficulty swallowing leading to recurrent aspiration pneumonia and cachexia. In large kindreds from French Canada relative sparing of the extraocular muscles is reported. By contrast, in families of Italian origin external ophthalmoplegia may be profound.

The classification in Table 125-2 includes several other inherited myopathies; most are uncommon. The congenital dystrophies are somewhat arbitrarily grouped because they are clinically evident at birth or very early in life and because they lack distinguishing pathologic features. For example, in Fukuyama congenital muscular dystrophy, hypotonia and weakness of the face and proximal limbs occur with severe myopathy and developmental abnormalities in the central nervous system. By contrast, the congenital myopathies are characterized by distinctive myopathological features. They often produce hypotonic weakness at birth followed by a nonprogressive or even an improving course; patients may show skeletal abnormalities, minimal CK elevations, and only mildly myopathic findings on EMG. In central core disease, one additionally finds weakness of the eyelids and face. Muscle biopsy reveals long, centrally located cores lacking oxidative enzymes. In nemaline rod myopathy, clumps of bacilliform rods or threads are seen in the subsarcolemmal space predominantly in type I fibers. Ultrastructurally these are composed of enlarged Z bands. The majority of fibers in myotubular myopathy are of small diameter with centrally positioned nuclei and resemble embryonic myotubes. Patients with myotubular myopathy may have external ophthalmoplegia. In congenital fiber type disproportion, type I fibers are relatively smaller than type II fibers and there is a tendency toward type I fiber predominance.

Metabolic myopathies

Numerous inherited disorders alter muscle metabolism. It is convenient to group the familial metabolic myopathies into three categories: glycogen and glucose, lipid, and mitochondrial disorders (see Fig. 125-1). Defective glucose metabolism may arise from defects in enzymes either of glycogenolysis or glycolysis; not all of the enzyme disorders are muscle-specific. Deficiency of the lysosomal enzyme acid maltase results in abnormal glycogen accumulation in multiple tissues. In its infantile form, Pompe's disease, absence of acid maltase, is characterized by myopathy, dysfunction of CNS neurons, cardio- and hepatosplenomegaly, and macroglossia. Muscle weakness is a consequence both of myopathy and denervation. By contrast, in adult acid maltase disease, myopathy is the primary manifestation. Slowly progressive proximal weakness and in some instances respiratory failure occur with mild

Table 125-2. Inherited myopathies

Disease	Genetics/chromosome*	Onset (yrs)	Involvement: Heart	Involvement: Other	Course
Major muscular dystrophies					
Duchenne	R, X	3-5	+	± MR	Rapid
Becker's	R, X	5-10	±	−	Slow
Facioscapulohumeral	AD, 4	5-40	−	−	Slow
Limb girdle	AR, 15†	5-15	±	−	Slow
Myotonic dystrophy	AD, 19	15-25	±	+++	Slow
Myotonia congenita	AD, 17 AR	<10	−	−	Slow
Hyperkalemic paralysis	AD, 17	3-10	−	−	Slow
Hypokalemic paralysis	AD	>12	−	−	Slow
Oculopharyngeal dystrophy	AD	50-60	−	−	Slow
Related myopathies					
Congenital dystrophies					
Congenital muscular dystrophy		Birth			Slow
Fukuyama disease		Birth		+CNS	Slow
Rigid spine syndrome					
Congenital myopathies					
Central core disease	AD/AR, 19				
Nemaline rod disease	AD/AR, 1				
Myotubular myopathies	AD/AR; R, X				
Congenital fiber type disproportion					
Myoshi distal myopathy	AR	15-25	−	−	Slow
Scapuloperoneal dystrophy	AD;R, X	20-40	+	−	Slow

*In some disorders, the chromosomal assignments may differ in different families despite similar clinical phenotypes.
†It is likely that more than one disorder can mimic limb girdle dystrophy.
R = recessive; AR = autosomal recessive; AD = autosomal dominant R, X = X-linked recessive

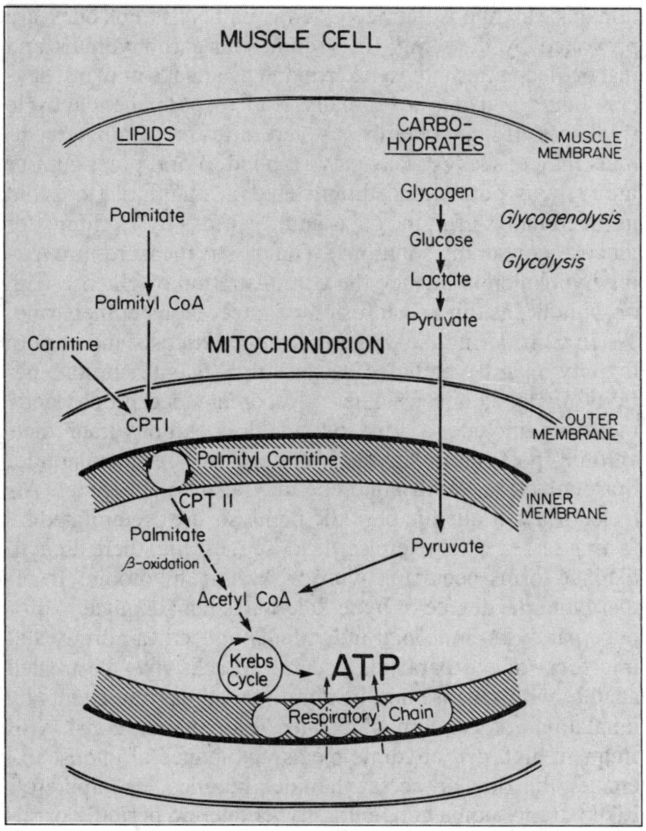

Fig. 125-1. Overview of energy production in muscle. CPT I and II respectively designate forms I and II of the enzyme carnitine-palmityl-transferase, located in the inner membrane of the mitochondrion. The major pathways in the generation of adenosine triphosphate (ATP) entail breakdown of either carbohydrates or lipids; the mitochondrion is the final common pathway in the process.

elevation of serum CK. The EMG is myopathic and may show high-frequency discharges. The enzyme deficiency may be measured in lysosomal preparations from fibroblasts and lymphoblasts as well as muscle.

Myophosphorylase deficiency (McArdle's disease) and *phosphofructokinase* deficiency impair glycolysis and cause painful muscle cramping after intense exercise, which preferentially uses glycogen-rich type II fibers. Patients may develop a "second wind" with sustained, submaximal exercise. Prolonged exertion may induce rhabdomyolysis, myoglobinuria, and even renal failure. Muscle microscopy demonstrates subsarcolemmal glycogen accumulation. As described above, the absence of a rise in lactate after ischemic forearm exercise is a useful screening test for these disorders. Because the enzymes are muscle-specific, definitive diagnosis requires enzyme assay of muscle tissue.

Deficiencies of distal glycolytic enzymes (phosphoglycerate kinase, phosphoglycerate mutase, and lactate dehydrogenase) are associated with exercise-induced muscle pain and myoglobinuria. In these diseases, lactate elevations after ischemic forearm exercise are subnormal. Muscle biopsy is required for definitive diagnosis.

Several disorders of muscle lipid metabolism have been defined. With sustained muscle exercise, muscle glycogen stores are depleted and lipid becomes essential for generation of energy in muscle. Carnitine, an essential factor in the breakdown of muscle lipids, may be deficient systemically or selectively in muscle. In the former case, a progressive myopathy develops early in life in association with recurrent hepatic encephalopathy and even coma; the systemic features are absent in selective muscle carnitine deficiency. Some patients in both categories respond to treatment with oral carnitine. Recurrent crises of rhabdomyolysis and myoglobinuria may occur when either form of the enzyme carnitine palmityl-transferase is deficient. Once palmitate enters the mitochondrion, it is degraded to acetyl-CoA by sequential steps of beta oxidation; defective beta oxidation may also be associated with aberrant muscle lipid metabolism. As described above, one may screen for defective lipid metabolism by fasting a patient and monitoring for maintenance of normal blood glucose by gluconeogenesis as indicated by production of urinary ketones. Confirmation of the diagnosis requires assay of levels of carnitive palmityl-transferase or beta-oxidation activity in muscle. Some patients may improve with increased intake of carbohydrates or medium-chain triglyceride diets.

A syndrome of diffuse, postexertional muscle pain has been ascribed to deficiency of the enzyme myoadenylate deaminase. However, inasmuch as the deficiency is common even in asymptomatic individuals the significance of this entity remains uncertain. The enzyme deficiency causes a subnormal rise in ammonia after ischemic forearm exercise; it must be confirmed by direct histochemical or enzymatic assay in muscle.

Mitochondrial abnormalities underlie a disparate group of myopathies whose most common feature is their multisystemic character. In many the muscle is characterized by peripheral, submembrane accumulations of mitochondria described as ragged red fibers because of their irregular, reddish appearance on trichrome staining. Ultrastructural examination of the mitochondria may reveal enlargement, crystalline inclusions, and morphologic abnormalities of cristae such as elongation, flattening, or concentric duplication. In many instances, specific biochemical defects or mutations in mitochondrial DNA (mtDNA) have been defined (Table 125-3). While some patients have isolated myopathies, in most there is additional involvement of other tissues. In many adults the major clinical manifestation is chronic progressive external ophthalmoplegia (PEO), which develops symmetrically and insidiously with ptosis and sometimes proximal muscle weakness. This may be inherited (below) but is often sporadic. Individuals with this disorder may eventually be afflicted with dementia, epilepsy, retinal pigmentary degeneration, pyramidal and extrapyramidal signs, cerebellar ataxia, cardiomyopathy and heart block, neuropathy, diabetes, and hypoparathyroidism. When these features develop sporadically in childhood or adolescence in individuals with abundant ragged red fibers, the term *Kearns-Sayre syndrome* may be applied. KSS is caused by large deletions in mtDNA; these are described as heteroplasmic because not all species of mtDNA in a

Table 125-3. Myopathic mitochondrial DNA (mtDNA) mutations

Mutation	Phenotype	Inheritance
Single deletions	PEO (OM, KSS)	Sporadic
Multiple deletions		
	PEO	Autosomal dominant
	Recurrent myoglobinuria	Autosomal dominant
	Encephalomyopathy	Autosomal dominant
	MNGIE	
Duplications	KSS	Sporadic
Point mutations		
Complex 1, ND4	LHON	Maternal
tRNA (lys)	MERRF	Maternal
tRNA (leu-UUR)	MELAS	Maternal
tRNA (leu-UUR)	PEO	Maternal
tRNA (leu-UUR)	MiMyCa	Maternal
ATPase 6	NARP	Maternal
ATPase 6	Infantile Leigh's	Maternal

Reviewed in Schon EA: In Schapira ANV and DiMauro S, editors: Mitochondrial disorders in neurology. London, 1992, Butterworth-Heinemann.
PEO = progressive external ophthalmoplegia
OM = ocular myopathy
KSS = Kearns-Sayre syndrome
MNGIE = myoneurogastrointestinal encephalomyopathy
LHON = Leber's hereditary optic neuropathy
MERRF = myoclonic epilepsy with ragged red fibers
MELAS = mitochondrial encephalopathy with lactic acidosis and stroke
MiMyCa = mitochondrial myopathy and cardiomyopathy
NARP = neuropathy, ataxia, retinitis pigmentosa

given tissue are mutated in KSS. Other categories of mitochondrial disorders include those with myoclonic epilepsy and ragged red fibers (or MERRF) and mitochondrial encephalopathy, lactic acidosis, and stroke (or MELAS). In MERRF, MELAS, and Leber's hereditary optic neuropathy (LHON), the primary defect appears to be a point mutation affecting regions of mitochondrial DNA encoding tRNAs or respiratory complex proteins (Table 125-3). As in LHON, many of the point mutations are homoplasmic; the mtDNA mutation is uniformly present in all mitochondria. In some cases, pedigree analysis indicates maternal inheritance of the disease trait; this pattern is expected for a mutation in mitochondrial DNA which at conception is transmitted to the fetus via the egg cytoplasm. Another recently defined category of mtDNA diseases is characterized by tissue-specific depletion of mtDNA. This may arise either as an inherited condition or secondary to exposure to drugs such as azidothymidine (AZT), which are nucleoside analogs used in HIV therapy.

Several inherited myopathies are characterized by abnormal electrical excitability of the muscle cell. The myotonias are mentioned above. A second important category is the periodic paralyses, disorders characterized by periodic weakness occurring with abnormal serum levels of potassium. These disorders are dominantly inherited, typically begin in adolesence, and affect males more commonly than females. In hypokalemic periodic paralysis, episodes are provoked by diets high in sodium and carbohydrates and rest or sleep after intense exertion. The attacks may last several hours and may eventually lead to permanent muscle weakness. If hypokalemia is severe, life-threatening arrythmias may ensue. Attacks may respond to oral potassium or intravenous potassium administered in mannitol (to avoid intracellular shifts in potassium caused by sodium- or glucose-containing solutions). Diagnostic measures provoking hypokalemia include the administration of glucose with or without insulin and infusion of intravenous epinephrine. When considering the diagnosis, thyrotoxicosis and barium toxicity must be excluded because they may precipitate periodic hypokalemic weakness. Recommended prophylactic measures include a low-sodium, low-carbohydrate diet, chronic potassium supplementation, and acetazolamide. Spironolactone and triamterene may also be beneficial. Attacks of hyperkalemic periodic paralysis are precipitated by fasting or rest after exercise. Data suggest that there are two distinct forms occurring with or without myotonia. In either type, the degree of hyperkalemia is not adequate to produce paralysis in normal individuals; indeed, a normokalemic form of the paralysis occurs. Attacks may be treated acutely with glucose and insulin, beta adrenergic agents by inhalation, or calcium gluconate. Prophylaxis consists of frequent high-carbohydrate meals, avoidance of intense exercise, thiazide or acetazolamide diuretics, or albuterol. Like paramyotonia congenita, hyperkalemic periodic paralysis is caused by mutations in the muscle-specific voltage-sensitive sodium channel. It is therefore of interest that some individuals with PMC may develop hyperkalemic periodic paralysis. As in paramyotonia congenita, the myotonia in hyperkalemic paralysis may respond to mexiletine.

Several endocrinologic and toxicologic disorders produce myopathy. Perhaps the best example is the myopathy associated with excess glucocorticoids or adrenocorticotropic hormone (ACTH). Whether secreted endogenously or administered in treatment of other disorders, these substances may produce severe proximal muscle weakness, usually with other manifestations of glucocorticoid excess. Hyperthyroidism may also produce a severe proximal myopathy, which may worsen subacutely and mimic polymyositis; unlike polymyositis, thyrotoxic myopathy does not elevate the serum CK. It should be recalled that thyrotoxicosis may be associated with a higher incidence of myasthenia gravis than normal and may in some individuals produce periodic weakness with hypokalemia closely resembling familial hypokalemic periodic paralysis. Thyrotoxic patients may also demonstrate selective dysfunction of the eye muscles occurring in association with exophthalmos, or thyrotoxic ophthalmopathy. Hypothyroidism may produce proximal weakness and fatigue with muscle stiffness and hyporeflexia; in these patients serum CK may be elevated as much as 10 to 100 times above normal. Pituitary disorders may impair muscle function. Proximal weakness may be evident in up to 50% of patients with acromegaly and may also result from pituitary failure. Disorders of calcium metabolism may mimic myopathies. A syndrome of proximal muscle wasting and easy fatiguability has been described with both primary and secondary hypoparathyroidism usually with a normal serum CK. Hypoparathyroidism may produce hyperexcitability of nerve and muscle and even frank tetany. In some patients this is latent, but may be provoked by metabolic or respiratory alkalosis or by percussing the facial nerve (Cvostek's sign). A chronic myopathy has been described with calcium deficiency, responding to calcium and vitamin D treatment. Pathologic evaluation of muscle is not specifically diagnostic in any of the endocrine myopathies; some may show selective type II fiber atrophy.

A variety of substances are directly or indirectly toxic to muscle. Alcohol may produce a skeletal and cardiac myopathy, although it remains unclear whether this is direct toxicity of ethanol or secondary to nutritional deficiencies. There is clearly an alcoholic, hypokalemic myopathy characterized by subacute evolution of profound muscle weakness in conjunction with elevated serum CK values and vacuolar changes on muscle biopsy. Several drugs cause rhabdomyolysis and myoglobinuria, including heroin, amphetamines, phenformin, phenfluoramine, clofibrate, phencyclidine, barbiturates, and azathioprine. There is evidence that myopathy without rhabdomyolysis may be caused by chloroquine, emetine, vincristine, colchicine, and the beta blockers labetalol and propranolol. Rarely, intramuscular injections of certain agents may cause local fibrosis and contracture; offending substances include pentazocine, meperidine, and the antibiotics penicillin, streptomycin, and chloramphenicol (Chloromycetin). Selected drugs such as cimetidine, d-penicillamine, and procainamide may produce muscle inflammation.

One other muscle disorder with which the general clinician should be familiar is malignant hyperthermia (MH), a clinical syndrome induced by certain anesthetic agents and characterized by acute development of severe, diffuse muscle rigidity, acidosis, tachycardia, and fulminant life-threatening fever. MH may be inherited as an autosomal-dominant trait caused by a mutation in the gene for the ryanodine receptor, a protein that triggers muscle contraction by releasing calcium from the sarcoplasmic reticulum. MH may be more common in individuals with certain myopathies such as Duchenne dystrophy and central core disease. Hyperthermic crises are triggered by multiple agents including depolarizing cholinergic agonists such as succinylcholine, volatile anesthetics such as halothane, or membrane active agents such as lidocaine. Fortunately, if recognized, the disorder may be treated specifically with dantrolene and symptomatic measures.

REFERENCES

Brooke M: A clinician's view of neuromuscular disease, ed 2. Baltimore, 1986, Williams and Wilkins.

Dubowitz V: Muscle biopsy, a practical approach. London, 1985, Bailliere Tindall.

Engel AG and Banker BQ: Myology. New York, 1986, McGraw-Hill.

Kakulas BA and Adams RD: Diseases of muscle: pathological foundations of clinical myology. Philadelphia, 1985, Harper & Row.

Schon EA: Mitochondrial DNA and the genetics of mitochondrial disease. In Schapira AHV and DiMauro S, editors: Mitochondrial disorders in Neurology. London, 1992, Butterworth-Heinemann.

Walton JN, editor: Disorders of voluntary muscle. Edinburgh, 1981, Churchill-Livingstone.

THE NEUROLOGY OF BEHAVIOR IV

CHAPTER

126 Behavioral Neurology

Roy Freeman

Cognition, language, personality, and the emotions, the traditional province of psychologists, psychiatrists, and philosophers, were for decades of only cursory interest to the neurologist. The past 30 years, however, has seen a movement, spearheaded by Dr. Norman Geschwind, built on the careful European clinicopathologic correlations of the nineteenth and early twentieth centuries and furthered by modern anatomic and neuroradiologic techniques, which has culminated in the legitimate establishment of the study of behavior within the realms of neurology.

The traditional approach to lesion localization, based on a careful examination of the patient's mental status, is as much a part of this dimension of clinical neurology as it is in examination of the cranial nerves, motor system, or sensory system.

This chapter discusses the most common derangements of cognition, emotion, and behavior seen in clinical practice. Knowledge of these behavioral syndromes is of more than theoretical importance. A detailed neurobehavioral evaluation in conjunction with the motor and sensory examination often enables the examiner to accurately localize the site of pathology or identify a clinical syndrome before any abnormality becomes evident on computed tomography (CT) or magnetic resonance imaging (MRI) scan. Furthermore, attention to this aspect of the neurological examination permits the early diagnosis of those neurobehavioral disorders that occur in the absence of any abnormality on the general neurological exam. Early recognition that the personality change occurring as a consequence of an occult frontal lobe tumor or the confusion presenting as a result of a right parietal lobe stroke is caused by neurologic disease is of obvious clinical importance.

THE ACUTE CONFUSIONAL STATE

The acute confusional state is unquestionably the most common cause of mental status change and probably the most frequent reason for neurologic consultation in any general hospital. The hallmark and salient deficit in this condition is the inability to maintain attention. Confused or inattentive patients have difficulty focusing their cognitive faculties on relevant environmental stimuli and, of equal importance, fail to exclude irrelevant stimuli from consciousness. The wide spectrum of mental states accompanying this inattention range from apathy and lethargy to agitation and hypervigilance. The confused patient may also display inappropriate jocularity and facetiousness. Confusion associated with agitation that is frequently accompanied by autonomic overactivity, such as mydriasis, tachycardia, diaphoresis, and tachypnea, is called *delirium*.

Disorientation is a frequent accompaniment to an acute confusional state, although it is not essential to the diagnosis. A peculiar form of disorientation known as *reduplicative paramnesia* is occasionally seen. In this case the patient places him- or herself appropriately in the hospital environment and simultaneously believes he or she is in a second environment, usually closer to home.

On mental status testing, the patient in a confusional state may be disoriented and has difficulty with tests of attention. Such tests include the digit span (most patients normally are able to repeat seven digits forward and five digits backward), continuous performance tests (such as the serial subtractions of 7s or the recitation of the months of the year backward), and tests of vigilance (such as the recognition of the letter *A* from a list of letters randomly recited by the examiner). Spontaneous speech may be mildly aphasic and the patient is typically agraphic. This agraphia is characterized by poor penmanship, as well as by spelling and grammatic errors. Further cognitive testing is usually limited by inattention.

On physical examination the patient may appear tremulous, with asterixis, myoclonus, and picking behavior. Autonomic overactivity as mentioned above is sometimes seen. The electroencephalogram (EEG) usually shows generalized slowing.

The acute confusional state is most frequently a result of a primary disorder outside the central nervous system. In the evaluation of the confused patient, careful attention should be paid to the possibility of metabolic dysfunction, drug and toxin ingestion or withdrawal, and infection both in and out of the central nervous system (see box at right).

Focal cerebral lesions at several sites—usually occurring as a consequence of a cerebrovascular event—can result in an acute confusional state. Nondominant parietal lobe lesions frequently produce this syndrome. In this case the neurologic examination may reveal denial of illness (anosognosia), a left homonymous hemianopsia or neglect, spatial or constructional difficulties, and contralateral cortical somatosensory loss or extinction.

Infarcts in the distribution of the posterior cerebral artery resulting in lesions affecting the fusiform and parahippocampal gyri (right or left) may also produce an agitated confusional state. Cortical blindness and short-term memory loss may be present, although a tendency to deny these deficits (Anton's syndrome) or amnestic confabulation sometimes confounds the examination.

Right frontal lobe lesions, particularly involving the medial orbital cortex, are another focal cause of an acute confusional state. Hemorrhage from a cerebral aneurysm or arteriovenous malformation is a frequent cause of such lesions.

Causes of acute confusional state

- Metabolic dysfunction
  - Electrolyte abnormalities
  - Hepatic failure
  - Renal failure
  - Hypoxia
  - Hypercarbia
  - Endocrinopathies (e.g., thyroid, parathyroid, and adrenal dysfunction)
  - Blood glucose abnormalities
  - Acidosis
  - Alkalosis
  - Porphyria
  - Vitamin deficiencies
- Drugs and toxins
  - Psychoactive medications
  - Alcohol
  - Toxic ingestions
  - Drug and alcohol withdrawal
- Infections
  - Systemic infections
  - CNS infections (meningitis, encephalitis)
- Seizures
  - Complex partial seizures
  - Psychomotor and absence status epilepticus
  - Postictal states
- Brain disease
  - Focal brain lesions
    - Right parietal lobe
    - Medial occipital lobes
    - Right frontal lobe
  - Generalized brain lesions
    - Head trauma
    - Hypertensive encephalopathy
    - Subdural hematoma
    - Space-occupying masses
    - Vasculitis
    - Petechial hemorrhages

THE AMNESIC SYNDROME

The salient feature of the amnesic syndrome is memory loss with grossly normal attention, language, motivation, and cognition. Typically, there are several aspects to this syndrome, including an anterograde memory loss (the inability to acquire new information since the onset of the responsible illness); a retrograde memory loss (the inability to recall information and events memorized prior to the onset of the illness); and confabulation (a tendency to fabricate, or "fill in," the memory hiatus). The latter, when present, occurs early in the course of an amnesic syndrome and is invariably accompanied by confusion.

Because a reciprocally connecting circuit of limbic structures involving medial temporal lobes, specific diencephalic structures, and the basal forebrain, is responsible for memory function, a variety of clinical conditions that produce lesions in diverse anatomic sites may cause an amnestic syndrome. Specific structures in this circuit include the hippocampus, the fornix, the mammillary bodies, the anterior and dorsomedial thalamic nuclei, the septal area, the cingulum, and the amygdala.

Researchers have delineated several phases in the process of memorization and recall. A useful clinical approach divides memory into registration (the reception of information), retention (the storage of information), and retrieval (the recall of stored information). Recent evidence suggests that different diseases that produce different neuroanatomic and neurochemical lesions cause specific patterns of memory loss. For example, disease processes affecting structures in the medial temporal, diencephalic, and basal frontal regions produce deficits in declarative memory (the recall and recognition of events and facts) while sparing procedural memory (skill learning). In contrast, diseases such as Huntington's disease that involve the basal ganglia produce procedural memory deficits.

Memory is best tested at the bedside by considering the somewhat artificial division of immediate, recent, and remote memory. Clinical tests for immediate memory are identical to those used to test attention and are described above. Recent memory is tested by asking the patient to recall events that took place in the preceding minutes, hours, or days. Alternatively, the patient can be asked to recount presented material (both visual and verbal) after a similar interval. Remote memory is tested by asking the patient to recall personal and historical events of the preceding years.

Several focal cerebrovascular lesions produce an amnestic syndrome. The best described syndrome occurs as a result of a medial temporal lobe infarct in the distribution of the posterior cerebral artery, resulting in hippocampal- and parahippocampal-region injury. Coincident neurologic findings include alexia with or without agraphia, color anomia, hemianopsia, and, less frequently, central achromatopsia and prosopagnosia. Bilateral lesions are probably necessary to produce a permanent amnestic syndrome.

Strokes in the distribution of the thalamoperforate and tuberothalamic arteries, supplying diencephalic structures, also produce an amnestic syndrome. The neurologic examination in this case may reveal apathy and akinesia, as well as supranuclear paralysis of vertical gaze and other motor deficits.

Vascular lesions (in particular, ruptured arteriovenous malformations and anterior communicating aneurysms) of the basal forebrain (septal area) also produce memory loss.

The term *transient global amnesia* is used to describe a syndrome of uncertain cause in which there is a sudden loss of recent and remote memory. This condition is sometimes preceded by an emotionally charged situation, exertion, pain, or sexual intercourse. Patients develop an anterograde amnesia that is characterized by bewilderment and mild agitation. They ask questions repeatedly and are not placated by appropriate replies. There is a retrograde amnesia of variable extent in which the patients have difficulty recalling events ranging from the preceding hours to past years. Intellectual function remains otherwise intact. The amnesia terminates abruptly and the entire episode usually lasts less than 24 hours. There remains, however, a permanent memory hiatus for the duration of the spell. Migraine, transient vertebrobasilar ischemia, epileptiform discharges, medication reactions, occult head trauma, and conversion hysteria have been reported as etiologies of this restricted disorder of registration and recall, but most cases remain unexplained.

Korsakoff's syndrome is another frequently encountered cause of the amnestic syndrome. Wernicke's encephalopathy, a clinical triad of confusion, ataxia, and ophthalmoplegia, frequently precedes the development of this chronic amnestic state. Thiamine deficiency associated with the malnutrition of alcoholism is the most common cause of the Wernicke-Korsakoff syndrome, but hemodialysis, hyperalimentation, hyperemesis gravidarum, gastric plication, and other causes of malnutrition may also produce this devastating clinical picture. Symmetric lesions are present at the base of the third and fourth ventricles and the aqueduct of Sylvius. Mammillary body and thalamic (in particular, the dorsomedial thalamic nuclei) lesions appear critical for the development of the amnestic syndrome.

Further causes of an amnestic syndrome are listed in the box below.

THE FRONTAL LOBE SYNDROME

The frontal lobes encompass over one third of the cerebral hemispheres and are divided into motor, premotor, and prefrontal regions. Injury to the prefrontal region, which comprises one half of the frontal lobe, produces the so-called frontal lobe syndrome. This syndrome manifests as a disorder of behavior and personality producing only subtle deficits in cognitive and intellectual function.

Patients with frontal lobe lesions do not adequately regulate or monitor their behavior, and thus language, conduct, and demeanor may be profane, childish, exhibitionistic, and

Causes of amnesia

- Cerebrovascular events
  - Hippocampal lesions
  - Thalamic lesions
  - Basal forebrain lesions
- Wernicke-Korsakoff syndrome
- Head trauma
- Hypoxia
- Hypoglycemia
- Herpes simplex encephalitis
- Degenerative diseases
  - Alzheimer's disease
  - Pick's disease
  - Huntington's disease
- Creutzfeldt-Jakob disease
- Transient global amnesia
- Neoplasms
- Limbic encephalitis
- Postsurgery
  - Bilateral temporal lobectomy
  - Bilateral fornix section
  - Mammillary body surgery
  - Cingulectomy

socially inappropriate. Such patients appear thoughtless, impulsive, and unable to delay gratification. Their behavior lacks reverence for prevailing environmental and social conventions, and their actions are poorly planned and executed with limited insight into possible consequences. It is as if frontal lobe injury allows previously latent thoughts and actions to become manifest.

Disorders of mood and affect also occur with frontal lobe injury. Patients can display depression (particularly with left frontal lobe damage), as well as euphoria or elation (perhaps more commonly with right frontal lobe damage). Anger and irritability also are commonly seen. Characteristically, these moods are shallow and superficial, with labile and easily elicited shifts from one emotional state to another.

Apathy, indifference, and diminished arousal with lack of spontaneity and motivation are known as *abulia* and may also be seen as a consequence of frontal lobe injury. An extreme form of this behavior, in which there is an absence of self-generated or stimulus-elicited speech or movement, is referred to as *akinetic mutism,* or *coma vigil*. The akinetic mute patient neither speaks nor moves spontaneously, is only minimally responsive to the environment, and yet appears alert and is able to track objects within his visual field.

Patients with frontal lobe lesions may also display reduced cognitive flexibility, diminished creativity and capacity for abstract thought, and disordered regulation of motor skills such as motor sequencing. These dysfunctions manifest as perseveration, impersistence, imitative behavior, and lack of personal autonomy, particularly in an unstructured environment.

These abnormalities of mental status are sometimes associated with gait disturbance, alterations in muscle tone, incontinence, and grasp or other primitive reflexes.

A similar constellation of symptoms and signs that includes deficits in planning, abulia, loss of initiative and drive, anxiety with agitation, and obsessive-compulsive behaviors occurs with lesions of the basal ganglia. This may reflect interruption of the circuits that link the striatum to the frontal cortex.

This clinical profile can be produced by head injury, brain tumors (including gliomas, meningiomas, and metastases), hydrocephalus, demyelinating disease, degenerative disease (such as Alzheimer's and Pick's diseases), and cerebrovascular lesions (such as strokes in the distribution of the anterior cerebral artery and rupture of arteriovenous malformations or anterior communicating artery aneurysms).

Researchers have attempted to correlate specific features of the frontal lobe syndrome with certain anatomic regions. In this regard, it has been suggested that lesions of the orbitofrontal surface of the frontal lobe result in behavioral and emotional abnormalities, medial frontal lesions result in disorders of arousal, and dorsolateral lesions result in disorders of cognitive and motor flexibility and abstract reasoning. The concurrence of various signs and symptoms, the close anatomic juxtaposition of the various anatomic regions, and the failure of the various clinical conditions to respect anatomic boundaries, has rendered such an approach merely a hypothetical model at this point.

VISUAL AND VISUOSPATIAL BEHAVIORAL DISTURBANCES

The visual system is arguably the most complex sensory network in the primate brain. Lesions within this system and its connections produce a variety of perceptual and behavioral disorders. The disorders of perception primarily reflect damage in the visual and visual association cortex, whereas the more complex neurobehavioral disorders associated with visual dysfunction are most commonly caused by the disconnection of visual cortex from other cerebral regions.

The most frequent disturbance of visuospatial behavior is the hemi-inattention or hemineglect syndrome. Such patients fail to report, respond to, or orientate to stimuli contralateral to a brain lesion. In the most severe form of this disorder the patient fails to respond to all contralateral sensory modalities; dresses, shaves, and grooms only one half of the body; eats only from one half of the plate; and visually and motorically ignores one half of the environment. In milder forms this abnormality can only be demonstrated by simultaneously providing a rival perceptual stimulus.

Several other behavioral disorders may accompany the syndrome of hemineglect. Patients may minimize the neurologic deficit (anosodiaphoria) or even refuse to acknowledge it (anosognosia). The patient may even deny ownership of a limb or express hatred of it.

Hemispatial neglect may be demonstrated by tests of line bisection (the patient divides the line closer to his intact hemifield), cancellation tests (the patient fails to cross out all letters or lines in the affected hemifield), and tests of drawing (the patient fails to complete the drawing of a clock or flower in the affected hemifield). Hemispatial neglect can result in a "paralexia." In this circumstance the patient neglects one half of a word: for example, a word such as *greenhouse* would be read as *house*.

Typical neglect syndromes have been described with lesions involving the frontal lobe, parietal lobe, basal ganglia, and reticular formation. The neglect syndrome occurs more commonly, is more severe, and is of greater duration with right hemisphere lesions. This observation, together with the proclivity of right hemisphere lesions to produce global disorders of inattention (see above), lends credence to the notion that the right hemisphere is dominant for attention.

Numerous disorders of perception have been associated with diseases within the visual system. These include illusions of size (micropsia and macropsia), shape (metamorphopsia), and number (monocular diplopia, triplopia, or polyopia). Patients have described a visual image shifting to another part of their visual fields (visual allesthesia) and even the persistence or recurrence of visual images after the removal of the visual stimulus (palinopsia).

Visual hallucinations may be simple (flashes of light, dots, colors, lines, and geometric forms) or complex (objects, animals, persons, and landscapes). Simple visual hallucinations are usually associated with local ocular disease, but occipital lobe lesions, occipital epilepsy, migraine, and, occasionally, toxic metabolic states can produce these phenomena.

Complex hallucinations are most frequently associated with a state of agitated confusion or delirium (see above). Other causes include the Charles-Bonnet syndrome, which is the appearance of hallucinations caused by eye disease in elderly individuals, as well as hemianopsias and seizure foci involving the temporoparietal cortex. Brainstem and diencephalic lesions have also been associated with characteristically vivid, often pleasant hallucinations, a condition known as *peduncular hallucinosis*.

The cortically blind patient is unable to perceive visual stimuli throughout the visual field while maintaining normal pupillary light reflexes and extraocular movements. This state is often accompanied by other disturbances of higher function, and the patient is frequently amnestic or confused. Such patients may fail to acknowledge their lack of vision and confabulate when asked to describe their visual world (Anton's syndrome). They typically rationalize their errors by attributing them to an environmental cause, such as dim light or the wrong pair of spectacles. Bilateral lesions of the geniculocalcarine tract are necessary to produce this syndrome and may occur as the result of a single embolus to the basilar artery bifurcation or a posterior circulation cerebrovascular accident in a patient with a preexisting contralateral hemianopsia, following vertebral angiography, with arrested transtentorial herniation, after hypoxic or ischemic events, and, rarely, with brain tumors and demyelinating disease.

Balint described a curious constellation of abnormal visuospatial behavior. In this syndrome the patient is unable to direct his or her gaze on command or in response to an orientating stimulus (apraxia of gaze), manual reaching under visual guidance is impaired (optic ataxia), and the patient cannot willfully direct his or her gaze appropriately (psychic paralysis of gaze). The patient is unable to perceive the visual field as a whole (simultanagnosia) and tends to focus on small, often irrelevant, peripheral aspects of the visual panorama. This syndrome is most frequently associated with bilateral occipitoparietal disease (i.e., dorsal cerebral regions) resulting in disconnection of the visual cortex from those cerebral areas mediating visuomotor exploration.

In contrast to this, visual agnosias—such as visual object agnosia, prosopagnosia (the failure to identify familiar faces), environmental agnosia, and color agnosia—have all been associated with bilateral inferotemporal and medial occipital damage (i.e., ventral cerebral regions). These disorders of recognition probably reflect the disconnection of the visual cortex from those regions of the brain subserving memory.

DISORDERS OF EMOTIONAL EXPRESSION

Disorders of affect, mood, and emotion associated with brain disease have been mentioned above. In this section, two commonly seen disturbances of emotional expression will be discussed—pseudobulbar affect and aprosodia.

Pseudobulbar affect refers to brief, inappropriate, uncontrollable outbursts of laughing and/or crying that occur spontaneously or with minimal provocation. The observation that the laughing or crying lacks congruence with the mood state of the patient has led to terms such as *forced, released,* or *inappropriate* laughter and crying. The laughter or crying fails to elicit a similar response among observers, and the patient usually becomes distraught and embarrassed at the lack of control over his or her demeanor.

Pseudobulbar affect is usually associated with other stigmata of pseudobulbar palsy, such as dysarthria, dysphagia, a brisk jaw jerk, and hyperactive gag reflex, as well as with bilateral motor and sensory findings. Bilateral lesions caused by vascular disease, trauma, and demyelinating and degenerative disease that involve cortical, subcortical, or upper brainstem structures are responsible. Although the exact mechanism for producing inappropriate laughter and crying is unknown, the phenomenon is thought to result from the release of brainstem regions from inhibitory hemispheric control.

Involuntary laughing and crying may also occur as an ictal manifestation, as in gelastic and dacrystic epilepsy, respectively. The emotional response is stereotyped, unprovoked, and usually unaccompanied by the appropriate mood state. This symptom is most frequently associated with epileptic foci in limbic regions and thus may be accompanied by other characteristic complex partial seizures and lead to secondary generalized seizures.

Another common disorder of emotional expression is the inability to impart emotion to spoken language. This disruption in the production of prosody—the pitch, tempo, rhythm, and melody of speech—is most frequently seen with lesions occurring in the right hemisphere. The loss of prosody, called *aprosodia,* results in monotonous, expressionless speech and may be mistaken for depression. This disturbance in the production of prosody may be accompanied by a disturbance in the interpretation of prosody. Aprosody, a disorder of the emotional aspects of language, should be seen in contrast to aphasia, which is a disruption in the semantic, syntactic, and grammatic components of language.

CONCLUSION

This chapter has covered the neurobehavioral syndromes most frequently encountered in the clinical environment. Our knowledge of the relationship between brain and behavior is rapidly expanding as a consequence of more sophisticated neuropsychological research methods, neurochemical techniques, and brain metabolic and blood-flow-imaging studies. The reader desiring a more detailed review of this rapidly growing area should consult the references listed below.

REFERENCES

Cummings JL, editor: Clinical neuropsychiatry. New York, 1985, Grune & Stratton.

Cummings JL, editor: Subcortical dementia. New York, 1990, Oxford University Press.
Freeman R, Bear D, and Greenberg MS: Behavioral disturbances in cerebrovascular disease. In Vinken PJ, Bruyn GW, and Klawans HL, editors: Handbook of clinical neurology, vol II (SS) 137.
Geschwind J: Disorders of attention: a frontier in neuropsychology. Philos Trans R Soc Lond (Biol) 298:173, 1982.
Heilman KM and Valenstein E, editors: Clinical neuropsychology, ed 2. New York, 1985, Oxford University Press.
Levin HS, Eisenberg HM, and Benton AL: Frontal lobe function and dysfunction. New York, 1991, Oxford University Press.
Mesulam MM, editor: Principles of behavioral neurology. Philadelphia, 1985, F.A. Davis.
Squire LR and Zola-Morgan S: The medial temporal lobe memory system. Science 253:1380, 1990.
Strub RL and Black WF, editors: The mental status examination in neurology, ed 2. Philadelphia, 1988, Davis.

CHAPTER

127 Anxiety

Barry S. Fogel

Anxiety may be a transient mood, a persistent or recurrent dysfunctional mood, or a rigorously defined psychiatric illness—an anxiety disorder. Anxiety disorders include panic disorder (recurrent stereotyped panic attacks), generalized anxiety disorder (persistent unrealistic or excessive worry for 6 months or more), phobias, obsessive-compulsive disorder, and posttraumatic stress disorder. These disorders are the most common psychiatric disorders in the United States, with a lifetime prevalence approaching 15%. They are even more prevalent in medical practice, because of the frequent presentation of anxiety with somatic symptoms. Panic disorder and generalized anxiety disorder usually present with multiple somatic symptoms, including dyspnea, dizziness, numbness and tingling, palpitations, trembling, sweating, choking, dysphagia, nausea, flushing, and chills. Panic attacks frequently include fears of dying or "going crazy," feelings of unreality, or chest discomfort. Chronically anxious people may complain of fatigue, tension, impaired concentration, irritability, or insomnia, the last-mentioned being experienced early in the night. Although each of the somatic symptoms of panic disorder and generalized anxiety disorder has a wide differential diagnosis, the simultaneous occurrence of multiple somatic symptoms of anxiety favors a psychiatric diagnosis, particularly if the onset occurs prior to age 35, symptoms have been long-standing, and the physical examination and laboratory screening are negative.

Patients with anxiety disorders often offer a chief complaint appropriate to the internist's subspecialty: chest pain to the cardiologist, dyspnea to the pulmonologist, numbness to the neurologist. If multiple additional symptoms are elicited, the diagnosis of an anxiety disorder is supported. If not, anxiety can still be the cause of the symptoms. It should remain in the differential diagnosis, and a trial of antianxiety treatment should be undertaken if the complaint is not explained sufficiently by other medical findings. In this situation, monosymptomatic anxiety with definite recurrent attacks would be treated as panic disorder, and monosymptomatic anxiety with continual symptoms would be treated as generalized anxiety disorder.

The differential diagnosis of anxiety includes medical disorders, drug-induced anxiety, and anxiety as a manifestation of depression. Severe anxiety beginning after age 40 usually implies one of these possibilities. Common medical conditions in which anxiety can be a prominent presenting feature include angina pectoris, cardiac arrhythmias, recurrent pulmonary emboli, asthma, congestive heart failure, hypoglycemia, limbic (temporal lobe) epilepsy, and hyperthyroidism. Rarer possibilities include parathyroid disease, pheochromocytoma, and carcinoid. Drugs frequently associated with anxiety include psychostimulants (including amphetamines and cocaine), sympathomimetic agents including barbituates and nonprescription decongestants, theophylline, and indomethacin. Withdrawal from sedative hypnotic drugs, benzodiazepines, opiates, tricyclic antidepressants, neuroleptics, or alcohol is an even more frequent precipitant of anxiety symptoms. Caffeine, at levels as low as 250 mg per day (two to three cups of brewed coffee) can produce or aggravate anxiety symptoms. Thus, the diagnostic workup of the anxious patient includes a careful cardiopulmonary and neurologic history and examination, an alcohol and drug history, and a detailed inquiry about the symptoms of depression. All anxious patients require tests of thyroid function, a calcium level, and laboratory screening appropriate to their age and epidemiologic setting, including an electrocardiogram for patients over 40. Those with prominent episodic neurologic symptoms or treatment-refractory panic attacks deserve an electroencephalogram (EEG).

The psychiatric history focuses on data especially relevant to treatment selection. Past history should include inquiry about prior psychiatric illness, treatment and response, prior substance abuse, and whether there have been major traumatic life events. Review of current symptoms should include inquiry about obsessions and compulsive rituals, phobic avoidance of particular situations, and "flashbacks" suggesting a posttraumatic stress disorder.

Patients with anxiety disorders usually require both psychological management and drug therapy. Regarding the former, patients definitely should not be given bland reassurance that they are "just anxious." Their physical complaints should be attributed to a benign disturbance of nervous system function that produces frightening physical symptoms. Patients should be advised to avoid caffeine and other stimulants and should be taught some formal method of relaxation. Drug therapy should be offered in all cases and strongly encouraged in cases in which the patient has begun to avoid work or usual life activities. Patients with specific interpersonal difficulties, posttraumatic stress disorders, or poor adjustment to a current life situation should be referred for formal psychotherapy.

Patients with significant phobic avoidance require systematic exposure to the situations they fear. In milder cases this can be accomplished with informal support from the physician and family or friends. In more severe cases, formal behavior therapy is necessary. Patients with compulsive rituals such as handwashing are best treated with serotonergic drugs (e.g., clomipramine or fluoxetine), but behavior therapy that prevents their rituals is a useful adjunct. Patients with posttraumatic stress disorder should be referred for formal psychotherapy, which usually involves reviewing the traumatic event in a therapeutic setting. Support groups are also helpful, particularly for homogeneous groups such as incest survivors or veterans with combat-related trauma.

Benzodiazepines are the most common treatment for anxiety in general medical practice. They are most valuable in the treatment of transient anxiety caused by life stresses or medical procedures. In these situations, they offer the advantages of rapid action and low toxicity.

Long-term use of benzodiazepines often leads to pharmacologic and psychologic dependence. Also, the drugs can be abused by patients with addictive tendencies. Thus, in the context of chronic anxiety disorders, the best strategy usually is to initiate treatment with a benzodiazepine and then start a more suitable longer-term pharmacologic or psychologic therapy, after benzodiazepines have provided quick relief and have promoted cooperation. While long-term benzodiazepine use is occasionally justified, psychiatric consultation usually should be obtained before large, refillable prescriptions for benzodiazepines are issued.

For generalized anxiety without panic, drugs of choice include the tricyclic antidepressants imipramine and nortriptyline, and buspirone. Tricyclics should be started at 10 mg per day and increased gradually until symptoms are relieved, side effects develop, or a full antidepressant dose is reached (see Chapter 128 on Mood Disorders for further details). Buspirone should be started at 5 mg t.i.d. and increased every few days as tolerated to a maximum of 20 mg t.i.d. if necessary for control of symptoms.

Patients with panic attacks respond best to tricyclic antidepressants or to the MAO inhibitor phenelzine given at a dose of 45-90 mg per day. While phenelzine involves the inconvenience of dietary restrictions, it may have specific benefits for patients whose anxiety is associated with social phobia and may more rapidly and completely relieve phobic avoidant behaviors.

Patients with obsessions and compulsions should be treated with either clomipramine, fluoxetine, sertraline, or puroxetine in full antidepressant dosages, building up gradually to minimize side effects. For posttraumatic stress disorder there is no specific pharmacologic treatment, but antidepressants are helpful in patients with prominent depressive symptoms, and lithium or carbamazepine may stabilize mood in patients with frequent and intense mood swings.

The prognosis of anxiety disorders is variable, both chronic and relapsing-remitting courses being common. Patients with milder disorders often discontinue treatment on their own. For those who have more severe symptoms that have remitted on medication, gradual withdrawal of medication should be attempted every 3 to 6 months, unless experience indicates a need for chronic maintenance therapy.

Rational benzodiazepine selection is based on the expected duration of treatment, the patient's hepatic status, and the specific indication and route of administration. The short-acting benzodiazepines oxazepam and lorazepam do not have persistent active metabolites that accumulate if hepatic function is decreased by age or disease. Longer-acting agents, such as diazepam and chlordiazepoxide, do have persistent active metabolites; however, these agents offer the advantage of once-a-day dosage and a milder withdrawal syndrome on abrupt discontinuation. Lorazepam is reliably absorbed with intramuscular injection and is the preferred agent when this route is to be used. Acute panic attacks respond to almost any benzodiazepine if the dosage is sufficient; alprazolam and clonazepam are more effective than other benzodiazepines for recurrent panic attacks.

In the elderly, shorter-acting benzodiazepines are preferable because of an increased risk of falls and fractures associated with longer-acting agents. When the latter are prescribed, the long half-life of active metabolites implies that the drug may not be in steady state for weeks following initiation or change in dosage. Thus, frequent monitoring for ataxia is necessary, and dosage increases must be spaced several weeks apart.

REFERENCES

Baldessarini RJ: Chemotherapy in psychiatry, principles and practice. Cambridge, Mass, 1985, Harvard University Press.

Diagnostic and Statistical Manual of Mental Disorders, ed 3. Washington DC, 1987, American Psychiatric Association.

Gorman JM and Papp LA, section editors: Anxiety disorders. In Tasman A and Riba B, editors: Review of psychiatry, vol 11. Washington DC, 1992, American Psychiatric Press.

Meltzer HY, editor: Psychopharmacology: the third generation of progress. New York, 1987, Raven Press.

Orne MT and Frankel FH: Anxiety disorders. In Karasu TB et al, editors: Treatment of psychiatric disorders. Washington DC, 1989, American Psychiatric Association.

CHAPTER

128 Mood Disorders

Barry S. Fogel

Mood disorders are widespread in the general population. The lifetime prevalence of major depression in the United States is approximately 10%. In patients who seek medical treatment, the prevalence is especially high, both because illness and trauma can precipitate depression and because major depression frequently presents with primarily physical symptoms.

The mood disorders comprise depression in its various

forms, and bipolar (manic-depressive) disorders. The term *depression* in common usage may refer to a transient mood, a persistent and dysfunctional mood, or a mood disorder with physical as well as mental symptoms of sufficient severity, multiplicity, and duration to warrant formal diagnosis as an illness. Patients with depressive symptoms seemingly explained by a life stress or a physical illness still qualify for a psychiatric diagnosis if the symptoms are persistent and cause dysfunction. An exception is made for bereavement: physical and mental symptoms of grief are not diagnosed as a mental disorder unless they exceed cultural norms for severity, duration, or degree of impairment.

Medical illness and mood disorder usually have a circular relationship. Medical illness is a stress that can precipitate or aggravate depression, and depression can produce or intensify physical symptoms and impair a patient's ability to participate fully in treatment and rehabilitation. Major depression impairs cognitive efficiency with potential consequences of memory impairment and poor judgment. It also can alter immune functions; this possibly influences prognosis in infectious, autoimmune, and neoplastic diseases.

The presentation of depressive disorders varies with the patient's age. Young and middle-aged adults complain primarily of sad, depressed, or irritable moods, and their emotional symptoms usually are prominent. Children and adolescents often present with changes in behavior, such as displaying a negative attitude toward, or withdrawal from, friends, school, and hobbies. Elderly patients often focus on the somatic or cognitive accompaniments of depression, such as insomnia, anorexia, constipation, memory loss, or difficulty concentrating. They may deny depressed mood altogether or may attribute their mood changes entirely to physical symptoms and steadfastly resist the diagnosis of a mental disorder. A common feature of major depression in all age groups is loss of pleasure or interest in activities that the patient usually enjoys.

Major depression is diagnosed when the entire syndrome lasts at least 2 weeks and a change of mood or interest is accompanied by four or more of the following symptoms: (1) changes in appetite or weight; (2) insomnia or hypersomnia; (3) fatigue and energy loss; (4) feelings of worthlessness or excessive guilt; (5) impaired concentration or indecisiveness; (6) recurrent thoughts of death, death wishes, or suicidal ideas, plans, or actions. Only three of the additional symptoms are needed if the patient has both a mood change and a loss of interest or pleasure in activities.

Physical signs of depression include a persistently sad or pained affect, slowed speech or movement (psychomotor retardation), and agitation. A severe depression may be accompanied by thought disorder, as discussed in Chapter 130.

Depressed mood with fewer associated symptoms and a close temporal association with a life stress is termed an *adjustment disorder with depressed mood;* a longstanding persistent depression with less than the full major depressive syndrome is called *dysthymia*.

At least 20% of patients with major depression also have some history of distinct periods of elevated, expansive, or irritable mood. These periods may be accompanied by (1) inflated self-esteem or grandiosity, (2) decreased need for sleep, (3) talkativeness, (4) racing thoughts, (5) distractibility, (6) increased goal-directed activity, or (7) excessive involvement in pleasurable activities with potentially painful consequences, such as sexual indiscretions or spending sprees. Hypomania would be diagnosed if an elevated or expansive mood were accompanied by at least three of these features or if an irritable mood were accompanied by four of these features. Mania is diagnosed when hypomania is accompanied by marked impairment in social or occupational function, or by psychiatric hospitalization.

Mania and hypomania usually present before age 40, unless the patient has had prior depressive episodes. The differential diagnosis of new-onset mania in a younger person always must include drug-induced mental disorders and brief reactive psychosis. If thought disorder is prominent, schizophreniform disorder must be considered, and if the patient is confused or disoriented, agitated delirium is a relevant consideration.

New onset of manic symptoms in a patient over 40 without a prior history of depression strongly suggests secondary mania caused by a specific organic disorder, such as hyperthyroidism or right hemisphere stroke. Other relatively common causes of secondary mania include multiple sclerosis, head injury, and medications, including stimulants, antidepressant drugs, dopamine-agonist antiparkinsonian drugs, corticosteroids, cimetidine, procarbazine, and baclofen.

Patients with a mood disorder who have had any episodes of mania or hypomania carry the diagnosis of *bipolar disorder;* major depression without mania is called *unipolar depression*.

ORGANIC FACTORS

Organic factors frequently precipitate or aggravate mood disorders; on occasion, they are causal. Removal of relevant organic factors is usually a necessary but not always a sufficient step in treating the mood disorder. Specific investigations for organic factors should be based on the medical history and epidemiologic setting. Comprehensive lists of medical disorders associated with depression can be found in the references by Cummings and by Lishman; some particularly common organic factors are discussed here.

Substance abuse can be associated with either major depressive or manic episodes. Major depression can occur in the context of alcohol abuse; most, but not all, patients' major depressions clear with 1 month of abstinence. The remainder require specific treatment for depression. Alcohol abuse can precipitate manic episodes in individuals with a previous history of bipolar disorder, but more commonly, excessive drinking is a symptom of hypomania, rather than its cause. Sympathomimetic drugs, including cocaine and amphetamines, can produce mania; after prolonged use, and especially after withdrawal, they may precipitate a major depression. Depression after stimulant withdrawal usually resolves spontaneously with abstinence but occasionally persists unless specifically treated.

Prescribed medications can provoke depression. Some well-known offenders are reserpine, methyldopa, propranolol, cimetidine, corticosteroids, and barbiturates. Even when a drug is not known to commonly provoke depression, the new onset of depression shortly after a new drug is started or its dosage is increased should raise the suspicion that the drug is an aggravating factor. The prescribed drugs that most commonly precipitate mania are stimulants, antidepressants, and corticosteroids.

Thyroid disorders commonly are associated with mood disorders. Hypothyroidism may present with depression, or depression may supervene later in the course of hypothyroidism. Depression caused by hypothyroidism can occur with a normal or low-normal T4; the thyroid-stimulating hormone (TSH) level is elevated and a thyrotropin-releasing hormone-stimulation test shows an exaggerated response. Hyperthyroidism can present as either depression or mania, but care should be taken not to overdiagnose hyperthyroidism, because T4 may be transiently elevated by the stress of acute mental illness. Cushing's disease usually produces depression. Adrenal insufficiency causes fatigue, which usually is not confused with depression, because physical signs normally are evident by the time mood symptoms develop.

Neurologic diseases associated with a high prevalence of depression include Parkinson's disease, multiple sclerosis, temporal lobe epilepsy, and stroke. All but the last can present with depression alone, the neurologic problem emerging on neurologic history and examination or, occasionally, with longitudinal follow-up. Tumors and infections of the CNS may present with depression before unequivocal neurologic signs are manifest. Therefore, neurodiagnostic tests are indicated when a patient in a high-risk group for CNS infection, malignancy, or stroke develops a new depressive illness. Both multiple sclerosis and stroke, particularly in the right hemisphere, can precipitate mania or hypomania.

Patients who reside in or have recently traveled to developing countries may be at risk for depression caused by parasitic disease. Parasitic diseases with central nervous system involvement (e.g., trypanosomiasis) or with hepatic involvement (e.g., schistosomiasis) are most likely to present with depression. Lyme disease and HIV disease can present with mood changes; serological tests are indicated in patients at risk.

Depression, but usually not mania, may be the manifestation of occult malignancy; cancer of the pancreas is particularly notorious for presenting with depression. New-onset depression in late life, particularly if accompanied by weight loss, anemia, elevated ESR, or other signs of internal disease, should trigger a thorough search for occult cancer.

TREATMENT

Treatment of mood disorders begins with establishing the diagnosis and treating relevant organic factors, including those related to substance abuse. Hospitalization is considered if the patient poses a significant threat to self or others because of suicidal, self-destructive, or violent behavior, or if outpatient treatment is not feasible. Common impediments to outpatient treatment include cognitive impairment, lack of insight into the illness, lack of informed, supportive family, and unstable medical conditions that raise the risk of psychotropic drug treatment.

Patients with severe thought disorders, and particularly those with delusions and hallucinations, initially are treated with neuroleptic drugs while specific treatment for their mood disorder is begun.

Major depression is treated with a combination of psychologic and pharmacologic modalities. Psychological treatment for depression can be either educational and supportive or more formally psychotherapeutic. Formal psychotherapeutic treatment is indicated when interpersonal conflicts, unresolved grief, or habitual self-defeating behavior and thinking contribute to the illness. Patients with fewer psychological symptoms and more physical symptoms often respond to informal supportive counseling, education about the disease, and reassurance that medical treatment is likely to be effective in relieving symptoms.

The principal drug therapies for depression are of the tricyclic antidepressants, the selective serotonin reuptake inhibitors (fluoxetine and sertraline), bupropion, trazodone, and the monoamine oxidase inhibitors (MAOIs). A list of antidepressant drugs with usual and extreme dosages is presented in Table 128-1. Different antidepressants are comparable in efficacy if given at appropriate dosages, so initial drug choice should aim at minimizing those side effects to which the patient would be especially vulnerable or would be unlikely to tolerate. A second consideration is whether the drug is sedating or stimulating. Fluoxetine, bupropion, and MAOIs are the most stimulating; trazodone and amitriptyline are the most sedating. Finally, drug choice can take into account additional features of the patient's mental illness. The serotonin reuptake inhibitors may be particularly useful for patients with long-standing chronic depression or depression with obsessive-compulsive symptoms. Imipramine, nortriptyline, and the MAOIs are simultaneously effective for depression, panic attacks, and phobias. Clomipramine and the MAOIs may help patients unresponsive to other drug treatments. Bipolar depressed patients may have a lower risk of drug-induced mania with bupropion.

Successful drug therapy for depression is based on several principles. First, the patient must understand the diagnosis and be aware that full antidepressant response to a drug may take several weeks. This sometimes requires bearing with side effects before the depression lifts. During this period, the physician must be available by telephone for the patient's questions and concerns, and frequent appointments should be scheduled if the patient is physically frail, anxious, or ambivalent about treatment. Patients with suicidal ideation insufficient to warrant hospitalization should be seen frequently also.

Second, initial dosages should be relatively low in all patients and very low in patients who are physically frail,

Table 128-1. Antidepressant drugs

Drug	Typical full dose	Dosage range	Notes
Tertiary amine tricyclic:			
Amitriptyline	100-200	10-300	1 2 3 4
Doxepin	100-200	10-300	1 2 3 4
Imipramine	100-200	10-300	1 2 3 4
Trimipramine	100-200	25-300	1 2 3 4
Clomipramine	100-200	25-250	1 2 3 4
Secondary amine tricyclic:			
Desipramine	100-200	10-300	3 4
Nortriptyline	50-100	10-150	4
Protriptyline	20-30	10-60	1 4 5
Amoxapine	100-200	25-300	3 4 5 6
Maprotiline	100-200	25-225	2 3 4 7
Trazodone	200-400	50-600	2 3
Bupropion	300-400	150-450	5 7
Serotonin reuptake inhibitors:			
Fluoxetine	20-60	5-80	5
Sertraline	50-150	25-200	8
Paroxetine	20-60	10-60	
MAO inhibitors:			
Phenelzine	45-60	30-90	3 5 9
Tranylcypromine	30-40	20-60	3 5 9

NOTES

1. Relatively high anticholinergic effects
2. Relatively high sedation
3. Relatively high rate of orthostatic hypotension
4. Quinidine-like effects on cardiac conduction
5. Prominent stimulating effect; may cause agitation early in treatment
6. Neuroleptic effects—risk of tardive dyskinesia and parkinsonism
7. Relatively high seizure risk; raise dosage slowly and avoid single doses >150 mg for bupropion
8. Frequent GI side effects
9. Special diet and drug interaction precautions needed

neurologically impaired, very anxious, or have a history of tolerating medications poorly. Dosage should be advanced every few days as tolerated until symptoms remit, a full therapeutic dose is reached, or treatment is limited by dose-related side effects. Further increases in dosage beyond the average range are justified if the patient has responded partially and side effects are not too severe. Patients receiving extreme dosages of tricyclics should have electrocardiograms to rule out conduction delay. Patients with unusually severe side effects on low doses or a lack of response to high doses should have antidepressant blood levels determined. Therapeutic ranges are best validated for nortriptyline, imipramine, and desipramine.

Third, side effects should be managed actively. Transient worsening of insomnia and anxiety on stimulating antidepressants responds to benzodiazepines. Constipation is helped by stool softeners. Orthostatic hypotension on tricyclics is helped by stopping diuretics, liberalizing fluids, elevating the head of the bed at night, and using fludrocortisone if necessary.

Fourth, difficulty in drug treatment of a disabling major depression should lead to psychiatric consultation rather than abandonment of treatment. Timely consultation is preferable to many months of unsuccessful drug trials that exhaust the patient while function and morale decline further.

Patients with major depression unresponsive to medications usually remit with electroconvulsive therapy (ECT). Approximately 60% of patients with delusional depression do not improve with antidepressant drugs alone, and either antidepressant-neuroleptic combinations or ECT are required to attain remission. Patients with bipolar depression may respond less well to tricyclics than patients with unipolar depression and may do better with MAOIs or ECT. Most require maintenance therapy with mood-stabilizing drugs such as lithium, carbamazepine, or valproate.

Patients with depression complicating severe medical illness or physical frailty usually cannot tolerate full doses of antidepressant drugs. Many respond to very low doses of antidepressants. Methylphenidate or dextroamphetamine, 5-10 mg once or twice a day, can be used in the short term to help mobilize a lethargic, depressed patient. Since stimulants have not been proved to be an effective treatment for major depression, patients who respond to stimulants should be switched to antidepressants if continued drug therapy appears necessary once the patient is mobilized.

Major depression remits with the first drug therapy chosen in about 70% of cases; ECT is effective in 80% to 90% of cases. Less than 10% of patients fail to respond eventually to some biological treatment. Regardless of what treatment is used to produce remission, continued treatment with antidepressant drugs for 6 to 12 months is advisable to reduce the risk of early relapse.

The primary treatment for mania and hypomania is therapy with a mood-stabilizing drug—lithium, carbamazepine, or valproate. Lithium has been the standard drug in the United States; direct comparison studies suggest that carbamazepine is equally effective. Valproate has also been proved effective in controlled clinical trials, but the evidence is less extensive. Patients unresponsive to lithium definitely should receive trials of carbamazepine and valproate before it is concluded that they are unresponsive to treatment and long-term neuroleptic therapy is instituted. Patients with very frequent cycling between highs and lows (more than four times a year) should be started on carbamazepine or valproate initially.

Patients with bipolar disorder usually require long-term, or even lifetime, treatment with mood-stabilizing drugs to minimize relapses. Psychological therapy begins with an educational and supportive approach to the patient and family; selected patients profit from formal psychotherapy once their mood has been stabilized.

REFERENCES

Amsterdam JD, editor: Refractory depression. New York, 1991, Raven Press.

Baldessarini RJ: Chemotherapy in psychiatry, principles and practice. Cambridge, Mass, 1985, Harvard University Press.

Clayton PJ: Bipolar illness. In Winokur G and Clayton P, editors: The medical basis of psychiatry. Philadelphia, 1986, Saunders.

Cohen-Cole SA, Brown FW, and McDaniel S: Diagnostic assessment of depression in the medically ill. In Stoudemire A and Fogel B, editors: Psychiatric care of the medical patient. New York, 1993, Oxford University Press.

Cummings JL: Clinical neuropsychiatry. Orlando, Fla, 1985, Grune & Stratton.

Fogel BS and Stone AB: Practical pathophysiology in neuropsychiatry: a clinical approach to depression and impulsive behavior in neurologic patients. In Yudofsky SC and Hales RE, editors: American psychiatric press textbook of neuropsychiatry, ed 2. Washington, DC, 1992, American Psychiatric Press.

Klerman GL, editor: Mood disorders in treatment of psychiatric disorders. Washington, DC, 1989, American Psychiatric Association.

Lishman WA: Organic psychiatry. The psychological consequences of cerebral disorders, ed 2. Oxford, 1987, Blackwell.

Stoudemire A et al: Psychopharmacology in the medically ill. In Stoudemire A and Fogel B, editors: Psychiatric care of the medical patient. New York, 1993, Oxford University Press.

CHAPTER

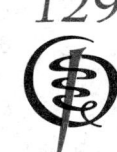

129 Personality Disorders, Maladaptive Illness Behavior, and Somatization

Barry S. Fogel

Physicians most often encounter disturbances of personality in the form of noncompliance with treatment, inappropriate behavior in medical settings, self-defeating health habits, litigiousness, doctor shopping, or apparent attachment to physical symptoms and the sick role. Personality traits are labeled *disorders* when they are inflexible and maladaptive and lead to functional impairment, subjective distress, or both. Personality traits and personality disorders form a continuum, as do most behavioral variables. However, certain constellations of maladaptive traits occur with sufficient frequency to be readily recognized; some of these have acquired the status of formally diagnosable mental disorders. The obsessive-compulsive personality and the antisocial personality are two well-known examples.

PERSONALITY DISORDERS

Personality disorders are not diagnosed unless the maladaptive traits persistently affect the patient's function. Thus, individuals who show inflexible, maladaptive behavior patterns only at times of acute stress, pain, or physical illness would not receive a personality disorder diagnosis. Such patients present more frequently in medical practice than do those with definite personality disorders. The same principles of assessment and management can be applied to both groups of patients, but definite diagnoses of personality disorders should be deferred until patients have recovered from acute physical illness.

The common personality disorders have been grouped into three clusters; within each cluster, the disorders have a common feature. Diagnostic assignment to a given cluster is much more reliable than is assignment to a particular disorder within the cluster. The three clusters of personality disorders are presented in the box on p. 1126.

The cluster of greatest interest to most nonpsychiatric physicians consists of the antisocial, borderline, histrionic, and narcissistic personality disorders. These disorders have the common feature of dramatic, erratic, or overly emotional behavior. The specific criteria for each disorder can be found in DSM-III-R, the standard reference on American psychiatric nosology. The disorders overlap, and it is not uncommon for patients to simultaneously meet criteria for two or three disorders within this cluster. Patients with these disorders come to their physicians' attention by displaying behavior that is overly dramatic, unstable, or unreasonable—such as threatening suicide, self-injury, or lit-

Personality disorder clusters

"Dramatic"
- Antisocial
- Borderline
- Histrionic
- Narcissistic

"Odd"
- Schizoid
- Schizotypal
- Paranoid

"Anxious"
- Avoidant
- Compulsive
- Dependent
- Passive-aggressive

igation; misusing medications; or abruptly terminating medical treatment, as by signing out of the hospital against medical advice. In addition, patients with antisocial personalities may engage in overtly criminal acts, such as stealing drugs or forging prescriptions, or may violate others' rights by assaultive or disruptive behavior in hospitals, clinics, or physicians' offices.

Another cluster consists of avoidant, dependent, obsessive-compulsive, and passive-aggressive personality disorders. Patients with these disorders have a common feature of anxiety or fearfulness, although these feelings may be more implicit in their behavior than directly expressed. Patients with these disorders come to their physicians' attention through noncompliance with treatment; difficulties engaging fully in self-care; and trouble making adjustments in their personal habits when required for medical treatment, rehabilitation, or disease prevention. Thus, dependent personalities may excessively request advice and reassurance from the physician, while simultaneously relishing a sick role that gives them a claim on their relatives' attention. Passive-aggressive personalities may forget appointments, miss doses of medications, and misunderstand instructions, while declining responsibility for their lack of success in medical treatment.

The third cluster consists of paranoid, schizoid, and schizotypal personality disorders. These disorders feature odd or eccentric behavior. Patients with these disorders have difficulties in all personal relationships, including the relationship between physician and patient. Patients may fail to confide in the physician or fail to accept medical advice because of mistrust, suspicion, or social discomfort; or they may have unusual and strongly held ideas that conflict with medical recommendations and are not open to reconsideration.

Personality disorders are diagnosed on the basis of a detailed personal and social history, ideally corroborated by a third party. A social history must show that the patient's maladaptive traits have been continually present since early adulthood. In the case of antisocial personality, a history of antisocial conduct must begin in childhood, with truancy, running away, cruelty to animals, lying, stealing, or other evidence of irresponsible or heedless behavior.

The social history usually accumulates over the course of medical diagnosis and treatment. Occupational and educational history, marital history, military history, and history of involvement in litigation, if explored systematically, usually permit a diagnosis. For example, a dishonorable discharge from military service raises a suspicion of antisocial personality; apparently frivolous lawsuits suggest a paranoid personality.

Antisocial and borderline personalities are common among drug addicts. Alcoholics are more likely than nonalcoholics to have some form of personality disorder, although there is no unique personality common to all alcoholics. Survivors of childhood abuse or incest have an increased prevalence of borderline personality, and the perpetrators of abuse and incest almost always have a personality disorder, often antisocial, borderline, or narcissistic.

MALADAPTIVE ILLNESS BEHAVIOR

Any maladaptive personality trait can be aggravated by anxiety, depression, pain, stress, or mild delirium. Thus, any patient who presents with maladaptive behavior in a medical setting deserves evaluation for anxiety, depression, and adequacy of pain relief, and a cognitive mental status examination specifically screening for a confusional state. The stress of illness and its treatment often can be reduced by careful explanation of the illness and its treatment and by informed-consent procedures tailored to the patient's intelligence and cognitive style. For example, obsessive-compulsive patients may benefit greatly from receiving reading material about their illness, whereas dependent patients may do better with less information and more reassurance. Further, all patients profit from careful explanation of what they can expect from their treatment and what the physician expects from them regarding cooperation with treatment.

Patients with more severe personality disorders, such as antisocial and borderline, may be manipulative, threatening, or dishonest, at times putting themselves or others at risk of physical harm. In these situations, the patient must be told firmly but without anger what limits must be respected if medical treatment is to continue. Violation of these limits should imply termination of the physician-patient relationship. If a patient is too physically ill to be released from treatment, psychiatric consultation should be obtained. If the patient has committed unlawful acts or is threatening them, law enforcement personnel may need to be involved.

Frequently, patients with severe personality disorders gain the favor of a particular physician or nurse and through charm, manipulation, or threats enlist the latter's support against other health professionals, with the objective of bending or violating accepted behavioral limits or rules of medical practice. A patient might request unreasonable quantities of narcotics and convince one physician that all other physicians and nurses are unfairly denying appropriate relief from pain. In such situations, the physician primarily responsible for the patient's medical treatment must bring together all involved health professionals, review the case, and promote a joint decision on a single, consistent policy; this decision usually should be put in writing.

When medical treatment is significantly compromised by a personality disorder or maladaptive personality traits, formal psychiatric consultation should be obtained. It is generally best not to wait for major behavioral excesses, such as suicide attempts, violence, or self-injury. The psychiatrist should be asked to help develop a viable management plan, or, when appropriate, to arrange referral to a different treatment setting. If the patient is not to be referred away, the primary physician should maintain the same frequency of patient contact after psychiatric consultation, to avoid evoking feelings of abandonment in the patient.

SOMATIZATION

Many patients consult physicians with multiple somatic complaints affecting several organ systems and interfering with function, the symptoms of which are out of proportion to physical findings and laboratory abnormalities. Others have single symptoms or signs with no demonstrable organic basis. These patients, whose behavior is called *somatization,* fall into several distinct groups:

1. Patients with a lifelong conviction that they are sickly, and multiple physical complaints beginning before age 30. These patients suffer from somatization disorder, a psychiatric condition of unknown etiology. They tend to have continual medical complaints that fluctuate in intensity throughout life, despite medical or psychiatric treatment. They often abuse prescribed medications and many also have a personality disorder of the dramatic cluster.
2. Patients with personality disorders, usually in the dramatic cluster, who somatize at times of stress, whether to dramatize their plight, to attract attention, to obtain compensation, or to avoid responsibility.
3. Patients with primary psychiatric disorders, such as panic disorder, major depression, or schizophrenia, in whom the multiple somatic complaints are symptoms of the psychiatric illness and remit with effective treatment of it.
4. Patients with chronic physical disorders that may present with multiple physical symptoms before unequivocal diagnostic signs are manifest, such as multiple sclerosis, Lyme disease, HIV disease, and systemic lupus erythematosus.
5. Patients with specific physical symptoms or signs without a demonstrable organic cause, that have an evident emotional significance of which the patient is unaware. For example, a patient may become blind after witnessing a gruesome scene or become paraplegic on the eve of an athletic contest he fears losing. These patients suffer from *conversion disorder,* or hysterical conversion. Their symptoms are not consciously feigned and the patients feel themselves to be ill.
6. Patients who consciously feign illness or deliberately cause themselves to be sick, for example, by covert injection of drugs or toxins. The former are malingerers, the latter have factitious illness. The former always have the motive of personal gain of some kind; the latter may be motivated either by external reward or by an emotional need to be ill, to receive care, or to deceive others. Most patients with factitious illness have personality disorders of the dramatic cluster.

Patients with somatization disorder should be managed by their primary physician, with a conservative approach to laboratory tests and invasive procedures and with regular visits not contingent on new or increased symptoms. Patients with somatic complaints caused by other psychiatric disorders or resulting from disordered personality benefit from psychiatric consultation and treatment appropriate to the diagnosis.

Physical disorders with multiple somatic complaints are most often misdiagnosed as psychiatric when the patient also shows dramatic or abnormal behavior. Simultaneous and comprehensive medical, neurologic, and psychiatric evaluation helps avoid error. When apparent somatization develops in middle age or later and without definite historical evidence of personality disorder or major mental illness, occult medical illness is the most likely possibility.

Conversion disorder usually has a good prognosis. It is treated either with formal psychotherapy or with support and reassurance by the primary physician regarding the excellent chance of recovery. Gross malingering is a legal and administrative issue, although its confrontation may precipitate behavior requiring psychiatric assessment. Factitious illness indicates psychiatric consultation because it is a form of self-injury. However, psychiatric treatment is of limited help.

MALADAPTIVE ILLNESS BEHAVIOR

Patients without psychiatric illness or personality disturbance may respond behaviorally to medical illness in ways that impede a good outcome. Two common forms of maladaptive illness behavior are amplification of pain or disability and denial phenomena.

Emotional factors that cause excess pain or disability can be internal, such as a need to suffer or identification with a loved one who had similar pain or disability, or interpersonal, such as receiving more attention from a spouse when in pain. These factors are best identified by structured psychosocial assessment, including a conjoint interview with the patient and his spouse or family. Treatment is by individual or family therapy, which may focus on either the emotions or the overt behavior, depending on the apparent reason for symptom amplification.

Denial phenomena include gross denial of illness ("There is nothing wrong with me") or denial of the implications of illness ("It's cancer, but I've got it licked"). They are common in acute myocardial infarction and when severe chronic or life-threatening illnesses are first diagnosed. They are maladaptive when they interfere with treatment or rehabilitation. Appropriate management consists of gradual and repeated confrontation in the context of support and empathy. Attempts to frighten the patient into compliance usually are unsuccessful.

REFERENCES

Diagnostic and statistical manual of mental disorders, ed 3, rev. Washington, DC, 1987, American Psychiatric Association Press.

Fogel BS: Personality disorders in the medical setting. In Stoudemire A and Fogel B editors: Psychiatric care of the medical patient. New York, 1993, Oxford University Press.

Fogel BS and Martin C: Personality disorders in the medical setting. In Stoudemire A and Fogel BS, editors: Principles of medical psychiatry. Orlando, Fla, 1987, Grune & Stratton.

Folks DG and Houck CA: Somatoform disorders, factitious disorder, and malingering. In Stoudemire A and Fogel B, editors: Psychiatric care of the medical patient. New York, 1993, Oxford University Press.

Frances AJ and Hales RE, editors: American Psychiatric Association annual review, vol 5. Washington, DC, 1986, American Psychiatric Association Press.

Glickman LS: Psychiatric consultation in the general hospital. New York, 1980, Dekker.

Kellner R: Somatoform and factitious disorders, In Karasu TB et al, editors: Treatment of psychiatric disorder. Washington, DC, 1989, American Psychiatric Association.

Sadavoy J and Fogel B: Personality disorders in old age. In Birren JE, Sloan RB, and Cohen G, editors: Handbook of mental health and aging, ed 2. Orlando, Fla, 1992, Academic Press.

Tyrer P, editor: Personality disorders: diagnosis, management and course. London, 1988, Wright.

Widiger TA and Gunderson JG: Severe personality disorders. In Tasman A and Riba MB, editors: Review of psychiatry, vol 11. Washington, DC, 1992, American Psychiatric Press.

CHAPTER

130 Thought Disorders

Barry S. Fogel

Disordered thinking may be either a disorder of thought content, such as false beliefs or hallucinated experiences, or a disorder of thought process, as reflected by incoherence of speech, illogical thinking, or disorganized behavior. Disordered thinking is remarkably common in medical patients. Delirium and dementia are the most common causes. Other causes of thought disorder are listed in the box at upper right and discussed further below.

Patients with impaired attention and orientation and with disorders of higher cortical function caused by metabolic disturbance or degenerative disease may misperceive their environment, have difficulty producing coherent speech, and produce logical inconsistencies of which they are unaware. Actual delusions, or specific false beliefs, can occur in delirious or demented patients, but they are rarely elaborate. General suspiciousness and hyperarousal are much more common in organic disorders than are specific and detailed delusions. Any patient showing a new onset of conspicuous suspiciousness in the context of medical illness deserves careful evaluation of cognitive mental status and screening for toxic, metabolic, and primary neurologic disorders if cognitive abnormalities suggest delirium.

Causes of thought disorders

- Gross brain dysfunction
  - Delirium
  - Dementia
  - Neurologic diseases, for example, Huntington's chorea
- Brief reactive psychosis
- Mood disorders
  - Depression with delusions
  - Mania
- Schizophrenic disorders
- Drug-induced

A second common cause of disordered thinking in medical settings is brief reactive psychosis. This disorder is diagnosed when a patient without a conspicuous prodrome develops florid psychotic symptoms after a major life stress, such as serious illness, physical trauma, or the loss of a significant person.

Personality disorders, particularly of the dramatic and odd clusters, are predisposing factors, as are mild organic cognitive disorders of insufficient severity or generality to warrant a diagnosis of delirium. A social history and a cognitive mental status examination therefore are necessary for accurate diagnosis. Drugs, both prescribed and self-administered, also can produce brief psychotic experiences of acute onset; an appropriately targeted drug history should be obtained from all psychotic patients, and toxic screens should be performed routinely.

Both delirium with thought disorder and brief reactive psychosis can be accompanied by agitation, uncooperativeness, insomnia, and paranoid thinking that can interfere significantly with medical diagnosis and treatment and can cause considerable suffering for the patient and family. Therefore, both disorders usually are treated with neuroleptic medication. High-potency neuroleptics generally are preferable, because of their lesser autonomic and anticholinergic side effects. The dose range used is wide; elderly, debilitated, or brain-damaged patients may need an order of magnitude less neuroleptic than young, large, physically healthy, and severely agitated men with histories of violent assault. The lower end of the dose range is 1 mg per day of haloperidol or 2 mg per day of thiothixene; at the upper end, 5 mg of haloperidol or 10 mg of thiothixene can be used every half-hour until the patient is calm. Combining haloperidol with lorazepam at the ratio of 5:1 controls agitated behavior more rapidly, and the lorazepam mitigates the side effects of muscle stiffness and motor restlessness that can be caused by haloperidol. The drugs can be mixed and given by intravenous or intramuscular route in patients unable or unwilling to take oral medication. The total dose needed for behavioral control can be repeated every 24 hours until the disorder causing the agitation has begun to resolve. When haloperidol is given alone, extrapyramidal side effects, such as dystonia, rigidity, and tremor, are not unusual. Antiparkinsonian medication should be given promptly if these side effects develop, and prophylactic antiparkinsonian medication should be strongly considered for older patients, brain-damaged patients, and patients with a past history of extrapyramidal reactions to neuroleptics. Typical antiparkinsonian drug dosages are amantadine, 100 mg two to three times a day, or benztropine, 2 mg two or three times a day. Lower doses are appropriate for elderly or debilitated patients and for individuals with impaired renal function.

In addition to drug therapy, patients with acute psychoses are aided by a calm, consistent environment and a minimum number of different caretakers, by frequent reorientation to place and situation, and by minimizing the use of medical drugs that have frequent psychotoxicity. Examples of the latter include pentazocine, meperidine, cimetidine, methyldopa, corticosteroids, indomethacin, and procainamide.

Thought disorder can accompany the more severe forms of depression and invariably accompanies mania. Severely depressed patients usually are preoccupied with negative ideas that may relate to guilt, physical illness or incapacity, persecution, poverty, or regret. These ideas can assume delusional proportions—a development that implies a poorer prognosis and a less satisfactory response to antidepressant drugs. Auditory hallucinations ("voices") may deprecate the patient or command the patient to commit suicide. Patients with mania overvalue themselves and their projects and frequently have delusions of grandeur and importance. Auditory hallucinations usually are in keeping with the patient's exalted ideas—he may hear the voice of God or take direct orders from powerful figures. Both in severe depression and in mania, thought process is also disturbed. Depressed patients experience a slowing of thought that at times produces the impression of dementia or an apathetic confusional state. Manic patients have a rapid stream of thought that can degenerate into a confusing flight of ideas or even into total incoherence and confusion suggesting an agitated confusional state.

Disordered thought content not compatible with the patient's mood can also occur. Such mood-incongruent delusions imply a worse long-term prognosis, even with appropriate treatment.

The treatment of thought disorder associated with mood disorder begins with neuroleptic medication and provision of a stable calm environment, as in the treatment of brief reactive psychosis. Once the patient is more cooperative and less agitated, specific treatment is directed toward the mood disorder. Lithium, carbamazepine, or valproate are used for mania, antidepressant drugs or electroconvulsive therapy for depression. Long-term use of neuroleptics usually is unnecessary in patients with mood disorders and should be avoided whenever possible because of the risk of tardive dyskinesia.

Chronic, persistent, or recurrent thought disorder not associated with a mood disorder usually is caused by one of the schizophrenic disorders. Schizophreniform disorder is diagnosed when the illness lasts less than 6 months; schizophrenia is diagnosed when the illness lasts 6 months or more. Both conditions involve active symptoms associated with overt behavioral changes and prodromal or residual symptoms that precede and follow episodes of active symptoms. The active symptoms include delusions, hallucinations, incoherence, markedly abnormal motor behavior (catatonia), and inappropriate or markedly unreactive affect. The delusions tend to be bizarre, such as the belief that one's thoughts are being controlled by occult forces or creatures from another planet. Hallucinations, usually auditory, can consist of a running commentary on the patient's actions, or of a dialogue between different voices. Visual hallucinations are not rare but occur less often than do auditory hallucinations; their presence should suggest delirium or drug intoxication.

The prodromal or residual symptoms include social isolation or withdrawal, impaired occupational function, impaired hygiene and grooming, inappropriate or flat affect, abnormal speech, odd beliefs, unusual perceptual experiences, and peculiar behavior such as talking to oneself in public. The abnormal speech may be vague or lacking in content, or, alternatively, overelaborate and circumstantial.

Schizophrenia is a chronic disease of multifactorial causation that affects 1% of the world's population. Genetic factors are known to be significant in its etiology, with monozygotic twins having a 65% concordance rate. People with schizoid or schizotypal personality disorders are more vulnerable to the disease. Hallucinogens or psychostimulants, such as amphetamines and cocaine, can precipitate psychoses clinically indistinguishable from schizophrenia, although most drug-induced psychoses are of relatively short duration. A chronic thought disorder resembling schizophrenia occurs in a minority of patients with limbic (temporal lobe) epilepsy.

Since schizophrenia is a subacute or chronic disease with blatant psychologic symptoms, the diagnosis of a major mental illness usually is obvious by the time a patient sees a physician. Alternate, less common presentations include obscure or bizarre somatic complaints representing somatic delusions, serious organic disease neglected because of apathy or delusional beliefs, or unexplained academic or occupational failure. Because patients with schizophrenia often avoid medical care or neglect physical problems, the newly presenting schizophrenic patient requires thorough physical evaluation, and laboratory screening appropriate to physical findings, nutritional status, the history of alcohol or drug use, and epidemiologic risks.

Treatment of schizophrenia combines drug treatment with psychosocial interventions. Drug treatment is based on the long-term use of neuroleptic drugs. Drug treatment is more effective for the positive symptoms of schizophrenia, such as delusions and hallucinations, than for its negative symptoms, such as flat affect or social withdrawal. A typical daily maintenance dose of a high-potency neuroleptic would be 5 to 10 mg of haloperidol or 10 to 20 mg of thiothixene. The range of doses used in practice is wide, because there is marked interindividual variation both in clinical response and in sensitivity to side effects. Antiparkinsonian drugs often are necessary when high-potency agents are used. Tardive dyskinesia, a persistent and often permanent movement disorder involving involuntary facial movements, choreoathetosis, and/or dystonia, is the most common complication of long-term neuroleptic treatment, occurring in approximately one quarter of patients treated long-term. Informing the patient about the risk of tardive dyskinesia is a medical/legal necessity if the patient is to be continued on long-term neuroleptic therapy.

Probably the most disturbing acute side effect of neuroleptics is akathisia. This is a motor disorder characterized by subjective restlessness and continual motor activity, such as rocking or pacing. Patients describe an almost unbearable discomfort if they attempt to hold still. Treatment begins with reducing the dosage of the neuroleptic and/or adding antiparkinson medication. Propranolol is the best specific treatment. The usual starting dose is 20 mg t.i.d.

Neuroleptics usually are classified by potency and route of administration. The high-potency drugs, such as haloperidol and fluphenazine, have the fewest anticholinergic and cardiovascular side effects but cause the most extrapyramidal reactions. The low-potency drugs, such as chlorpromazine and thioridazine, have the opposite profile and are substantially more sedating. Thioridazine and perphenazine have substantial antianxiety effects that sometimes are desirable. Two high-potency drugs, haloperidol and perphenazine, come in a depot intramuscular preparation that permits treatment by biweekly or even monthly injections in patients unable to comply with daily oral medication.

High-potency neuroleptics usually are seen as the initial treatment of choice. However, if patients cannot tolerate them because of extrapyramidal side effects, a low- or medium-potency agent should be substituted.

In patients on neuroleptics, adverse effects can be minimized by keeping the dose at the minimum level necessary to control major positive symptoms such as hallucinations and delusions. If additional mental symptoms require drug treatment, these should be handled with specific non-neuroleptic adjuncts. Depression should be treated with antidepressants, anxiety with benzodiazepines or buspirone, and fluctuating moods with lithium or carbamazepine. Adequate psychosocial treatment also should be provided.

When symptoms of schizophrenia fail to respond to two different standard neuroleptics at adequate dosage, the treatment of choice is clozapine. Clozapine can be dramatically effective in patients unresponsive to other neuroleptics and rarely causes extrapyramidal side effects. Its use is limited by a 1% to 2% risk of life-threatening agranulocytosis. Clozapine also causes seizures in 3% to 4% of patients, can cause drug fever up to 103 degrees Fahrenheit during the first 6 weeks of treatment, and can produce numerous other side effects including sedation, tachycardia, hypotension, EKG changes, and hypersalivation. Side effects require drug discontinuation in about 6% of cases. Clozapine should be started at a dosage of 25-50 mg per day and increased gradually to an average dosage of 300-500 mg/day. Weekly blood counts are mandatory for the full duration of therapy; the drug should be stopped immediately if neutropenia develops.

Psychosocial measures are directed at preserving and enhancing social function. Individual, group, and family psychotherapy all have a place, but the last-mentioned has the greatest proved benefit and is usually the treatment of choice for patients who live with their families. Formal training in social skills is valuable when those skills are lacking, as is vocational rehabilitation for the unemployed. Employment, when the patient is able to work, is particularly valuable in preserving social skills and function. With treatment, 60% of schizophrenics have social recovery within 5 years and about one third are able to work.

REFERENCES

Baldessarini RJ: Chemotherapy in psychiatry: principles and practice. Cambridge, Mass, 1985, Harvard University Press.

Bradley PB and Hirsch SR, editors: The psychopharmacology and treatment of schizophrenia. Oxford, 1986, Blackwell.

Canoro R: Schizophrenia. In Karasu TB et al, editors: Treatment of psychiatric disorders. Washington, DC, 1989, American Psychiatric Association.

Carpenter WT and Jauch DA: Treatment of brief reactive psychosis. In Karasu TB et al, editors: Treatment of psychiatric disorders. Washington, DC, 1989, American Psychiatric Association.

Coryell W: Schizoaffective and schizophrenic disorders. In Winokur G and Clayton P, editors: The medical basis of Psychiatry. Philadelphia, 1986, Saunders.

Fogel BS: Organic mental disorders. In Sederer LI, editor: Inpatient psychiatry: diagnosis and treatment, ed 3. Baltimore, 1991, Williams & Wilkins.

Lieberman JA, Kane JM, and Johns CA: Clozapine: guidelines for clinical management. J Clin Psychiat 50:329, 1989.

Lipowski ZJ: Delirium: acute confusional states. New York, 1990, Oxford University Press.

Meltzer HY, editor: Psychopharmacology: the third generation of progress. New York, 1987, Raven Press.

Nasrallah HA: The neuropsychiatry of schizophrenia. In Yudofsky SC and Hales RE, editors: The American Psychiatric Press textbook of neuropsychiatry, ed 2. Washington, DC, 1992, American Psychiatric Press.

Tsuang MT and Loyd DW: Schizophrenia. In Winokur G and Clayton P, editors: The medical basis of psychiatry. Philadelphia, 1986, Saunders.

Weinberger DR, section editor: Schizophrenia. In Tasman A and Goldfinger SM, editors: American Psychiatric Press review of psychiatry, vol 10. Washington, DC, 1991, American Psychiatric Press.

V Neurology in General Medicine and Surgery

CHAPTER

131 Head Trauma

Peter McL. Black

Head trauma is an important medical problem both in its acute management and its long-term sequelae. This chapter discusses the pathology, clinical presentation, differential diagnosis, management, and possible complications of patients with head injuries.

PATHOPHYSIOLOGY

The skull acts as a rigid container that does not allow expansion of masses within it. Intracranial pressure (ICP) rises exponentially as volume increases. Cerebral perfusion pressure (CPP), defined as mean arterial pressure minus mean intracranial pressure, is a measure of the effect of increasing brain pressure on cerebral blood flow: it should be kept at 40 mm Hg or higher to assure adequate brain perfusion.

Head injuries can be divided into three categories: skull fractures, which may be linear, basilar, or depressed; focal brain injuries, including contusions, intracranial hematomas, and missile wounds; and diffuse injuries, including concussion and diffuse axonal injury.

Skull fractures may be associated with underlying brain injury, such as epidural or subdural hematoma, or may be silent with respect to the brain.

Focal injuries include epidural, subdural, and intracerebral hematomas; and cerebral contusions. Epidural hematomas occur between dura and skull and separate the dura from the skull at the inner table of the bone; they have a characteristic lenticular shape and are associated with skull fractures in 75% to 90% of cases. Subdural hematomas occur between the surface of the brain and the dura. Hematomas of this type have major mass effect on the whole hemisphere because of the continuous nature of the subdural space. Intracerebral hematomas are surrounded by brain parenchyma: they may be difficult to separate from contusions. Brain contusions may occur adjacent to prominences such as the frontal or middle fossa or may occur in the brainstem. They are usually mottled in computed tomography (CT) appearance and contain pulped brain. They may be "coup," (under the impact site) or "contrecoup" (on the opposite side of the brain from impact). The coalescence of brain contusions after the initial injury is an important cause of delayed neurologic deterioration. Diffuse injuries include subarachnoid hemorrhage and shear lesions. Subarachnoid hemorrhage is the most common hemorrhage in head injury and may be responsible for delayed hydrocephalus as well as diffuse brain dysfunction. Shear lesions of white matter involve axonal tearing and may be devastating despite minimal CT evidence of injury.

Intracranial hemorrhage may precede rather than follow a head injury; an example is a middle cerebral aneurysm that ruptures and creates a subdural hematoma that results in loss of consciousness, leading to an automobile accident and subsequent head injury. This possibility should always be considered when evaluating unusually placed hematomas.

CLINICAL PRESENTATION

Head injury presentations can be classified as acute or chronic, and in the acute phase can be classified as severe, moderate, or mild. For the patient with acute head injury, the problem is appropriate management. For the patient with chronic head injury, it is often recognizing the diagnosis.

Acute head injury

The patient with a significant acute head injury may have findings ranging from full alertness to deep coma. The Glasgow Coma Scale is useful in classifying and following severity in the acute case (Table 131-1). A mild injury has a coma score of 13 to 16; a moderate injury, 8 to 15; and a severe injury, less than 8.

Evaluation of patients with severe head injury

The evaluation and management of patients with severe head injury should proceed together. In the evaluation, four important questions must be answered.

1. *How severe is the injury?* The most widely used mechanism for evaluating severity of injury is the Glasgow Coma Scale summarized in Table 131-1.

Table 131-1. Glasgow Coma Scale

Function tested	Response	Grade
1. Eye opening (E)	Spontaneously	E4
	To voice	3
	To pain	2
	None	1
C = eyes closed by swelling		
2. Best motor response	Obeys commands	M6
	Localizes pain	5
	Withdraws	4
	Decorticate to pain	3
	Decerebrate to pain	2
	None	1
3. Best verbal response	Oriented, appropriate	V5
	Confused conversation	4
	Inappropriate words	3
	Incomprehensible sounds	2
	None	1
T = intubated or tracheostomy		

Three features are examined: the best verbal response; best motor response, usually in the best limb; and what is required for eye opening. The coma score is important for initial grading and also for follow-up of the patient. Patients with a coma score of less than 8 have a 40% likelihood of requiring immediate surgery.

2. *What brain structures are affected?* This question has importance for the prognosis and for therapy. The major structures potentially affected are the cerebral hemispheres, brainstem, and cerebellum. Aphasia, cortical sensory loss, or visual field loss suggest focal cortical injury or mass. Ataxia is an important sign of a cerebellar mass. Pupillary or eye movement abnormality suggest a brainstem lesion. Most comatose states after head injury appear to result from shear injury to the white matter of the cerebral hemispheres rather than to brainstem injury, as was once believed.
3. *Is there evidence of a lateralizing mass?* Lateralization of signs is an important physical finding in head injury evaluation. The lateral tentorial herniation syndrome, discussed below, is especially important and should be recognized by every physician.
4. *Is the patient worsening?* This question is best answered by sequential examinations using the Glasgow Coma Scale.

Herniation syndromes

The most important syndromes to recognize after head injury are the lateral tentorial herniation syndrome, central herniation, and tonsillar herniation. These indicate imminent brainstem damage and death.

Lateral tentorial herniation is characterized by increasing restlessness or drowsiness, followed by weakness of the limb opposite the mass (pyramidal tract compression at the tentorial notch), pupillary dilation on the side of the lesion (oculomotor nerve and therefore parasympathetic compression), and, ultimately, central herniation.

Central tentorial herniation occurs with bilateral compression through the tentorial notch: small pupils, increasing obtundation, and decorticate or decerebrate posturing are its findings. It is usually caused by bilateral subdural hematoma, but acute hydrocephalus may also give this appearance.

Tonsillar herniation is heralded by headache and ataxia, with sudden subsequent respiratory arrest. It is the most treacherous form of herniation, because a patient may be well one moment and moribund the next; it is caused by an expanding cerebellar mass.

Radiologic diagnosis

The CT scan has made an enormous difference in the management of head injury. In the acute injury, four patterns should be recognized by the physician: epidural hematoma, subdural hematoma, intracerebral hematoma, and contusion. All are best evaluated in an unenhanced scan.

An epidural hematoma has a characteristic white lenticular shape adjacent to bone. An associated skull fracture may be seen on bone windows. A subdural hematoma tracks over the entire convexity. There is often greater shift associated with it than the hematoma itself would suggest; this is because of its distribution over the entire hemisphere. An intracerebral hematoma is characterized as a high-absorption mass within parenchyma. Mass effect may not be associated with this injury initially. A cerebral contusion is a mottled pattern of high and low absorption representing both axonal shearing and hemorrhage. Edema, characterized by diffuse absorption on CT, is also present after head injury in some patients. These patterns, especially in the acute phase, are much better seen on the CT than on the MRI, which may not demonstrate an acute hematoma.

On CT scans, three brain regions are particularly treacherous in the acute stage. The first is the temporal fossa, where bony artifact may obscure an epidural hematoma. The second is the vertex of the brain; because of the CT sections passing transversely through brain tissue, a high subdural hematoma may be missed, and coronal scans may be necessary to detect it. The third is the posterior fossa, where bony artifact may obscure a hematoma; 4-mm sections may be necessary to achieve good resolution.

Differential diagnosis

The diagnosis of acute head injury is usually straightforward. One problem is to establish whether a preexisting neurologic condition led to the head injury. Potential problems of this kind include aneurysm rupture with intracerebral hemorrhage, hypertensive intracerebral hemorrhage, and carotid occlusion or dissection.

Drug overdosage may make the head injury appear worse than it is. A toxic screen should be obtained if there is any question of drug usage.

Management of severe head injury

Evaluation and management of acute severe head injury proceed simultaneously. A history of the injury should be obtained as quickly as possible from ambulance drivers or other witnesses while initial neurologic evaluation is proceeding. This evaluation, as noted previously, should include the Glasgow Coma Scale, assessment of degree and level of injury, possible asymmetries in examination, and assessment of whether the patient is worsening.

In the initial management, three steps are of paramount importance: first, assuring that the airway and ventilation are adequate; second, assuring that there is no bleeding elsewhere that might lead to death during the neurologic evaluation; and finally, excluding cervical spine injury.

A good rule for head injury management is to intubate patients who will tolerate intubation, since considerable hypoxic brain damage may accompany an acute injury. Bleeding elsewhere can be excluded by chest film and physical examination, as well as by evaluation of the extremities. Cervical spine injury is best assessed by a lateral cervical spine film done portably in the emergency room.

In the triage of acute head injury, three levels can be distinguished: the first is the patient with a Glasgow Coma Scale of less than 8 who does not respond purposefully to commands. This patient requires immediate CT scanning. If this cannot be done expeditiously in the institution, the patient should be transferred to a larger center where CT scanning facilities and neurosurgical help are available. The second is the patient who is drowsy but is still following commands: this patient requires CT scanning to be performed within 4 to 6 hours; if the neurologic status is changing, immediate scanning is necessary. Finally, patients who have evidence of a significant injury by history or examination but are now clinically well require observation for 12 to 24 hours or CT scanning.

Nonoperative management of patients with severe head injury includes support of ventilation and blood pressure, limitation of intravenous fluids, use of phenytoin or another anticonvulsant if there is a discrete mass, and intensive-care neurologic monitoring. An ICP monitor may be used—usually a subarachnoid bolt or fiberoptic catheter—which allows maintenance of cerebral perfusion pressure above 40 torr. ICP itself should be maintained below 20 torr. Methods used to decrease ICP include mannitol intravenously to keep osmolarity at 300 to 310 mOsm per liter and hyperventilation to sustain PCO_2 at 30 to 35 mm Hg. Corticosteroids are of uncertain efficacy in posttraumatic edema, although they are used in many centers. The use of barbiturates has also diminished, as it may lead to increased incidence of a chronic vegetative state. However, pentobarbital in boluses, 50 mg intravenously, to maintain ICP less than 25 mm Hg, may be a useful adjunct to keep intracranial pressure under control.

Chronic sequelae of head injury

Several patterns should be recognized as sequelae of head injury. The first is global deterioration in an elderly patient, characterized by increasing memory loss, gait trouble, and slowing of activity. Even without an antecedent history of head injury, this presentation deserves CT scanning; chronic subdural hematoma and hydrocephalus are two head injury sequelae that may be found. A second pattern is loss of mental acuity and ambition in a young patient with a normal CT scan after mild head injury. This posttraumatic/postconcussive syndrome is very subtle but is increasingly being recognized. Seizure disorder and cerebrospinal fluid (CSF) leak may also be late sequelae of head injury.

For the patient with chronic head injury, management decisions are less emergent but are sometimes quite difficult. They include how long the patient should stay away from work or school and to what extent difficulties with work or school are a result of the head injury. There are few good guidelines for these decisions.

Management of minor head injury

A minor head injury can be defined as one with a Glasgow Coma Scale of 13 to 15. There are several recurring questions with such patients.

Should a patient with a mild head injury be admitted for observation? Patients who are feeling unwell following head injury require observation by a competent observer. Whether this is done in the hospital or in the home depends on the circumstances. Admission, in the author's opinion, is necessary if there is evidence of contusion on the CT scan or if the patient is drowsy or confused at the time of examination. Children under age 5 should also usually be admitted if they have been at all unresponsive. For other patients, observation at home may be adequate if another adult is continuously present and the patient has only signs of mild discomfort with a normal CT. A set of instructions should be given to each patient.

Should every patient with a head injury have skull films? Obtundation, CSF leak, asymmetric neurologic findings, and an obvious depressed fracture are accepted guidelines for skull films. In fact, skull films are being used less and less, as CT scanning becomes more prevalent. Any patient who had a loss of consciousness and who is not feeling perfectly well should be given a CT scan.

What should be done if a patient is deteriorating? In most institutions a CT can be obtained quickly enough that an emergency room burr hole is not indicated. Mannitol, 100 g, can be given intravenously during a brief sojourn at the CT scan for rapid sequence examination of the temporal fossa or any other area where there is a contusion. However, if the patient's status is changing rapidly, with evidence of increasing hemiparesis, obtundation, and pupillary dilatation, serious consideration must be given to emergency evacuation of a presumed epidural hematoma. This is best done in the operating room with a burr hole on the side with the dilating pupil, although in exceptional circumstances it may be necessary to proceed in the emergency room. Surgical help should be obtained for this.

Specific clinical entities

Epidural hematomas are the most reversible intracranial hematomas. They usually occur in the temporal fossa from middle cerebral artery tears or in the posterior fossa from transverse sinus tears. In 75% to 90% of cases there is an associated fracture. The clinical presentation is often of a transient loss of consciousness with recovery (the "lucid interval"), followed by increasing drowsiness, headache, weakness on the side of the body opposite the epidural hematoma, and pupillary dilation on the same side. Treatment is emergency evacuation of the clot; overall mortality is 15% to 43%.

Subdural hematomas are often associated with underlying brain contusions. They are more common after automobile injuries and may appear initially in patients with coma or as the herniation syndromes noted previously. Mortality is 35% to 50% despite CT scanning; younger patients have better outcomes, as do patients operated on within 3 hours of injury.

Intraparenchymal hematomas occur in 2% of severe injuries. They should be removed if there is more than a 1-cm associated CT shift or unless they are in an important area of brain, such as the speech or motor areas: mortality varies from 25% to 72%, depending primarily on the level of consciousness prior to surgery.

Missile wounds are generally treated by debridement of the missile track in the operating room. Deep fragments of bullet need not be removed.

Linear skull fractures require no treatment except observation for potential hematomas.

Depressed skull fractures should be elevated if the depression is deeper than the inner table of the skull; if there is an associated CSF leak; or if there is intracranial air on CT, which suggests a dural tear.

COMPLICATIONS

Acute head injury may be complicated by delayed intracerebral hematoma formation, increasing brain edema, and disseminated intravascular coagulation. Other complications include the following.

Posttraumatic epilepsy may be early (within 1 week) or delayed: early seizures occur in 2.5% to 7% of patients, delayed seizures in 7.1%. Prophylactic anticonvulsants may diminish the incidence of later seizures. Parenchymal hemorrhage or dural lacerations appear to be associated with a greater likelihood of these late seizures.

Posttraumatic hydrocephalus mainly results from subarachnoid hemorrhage at the time of injury but may also be contributed to by shearing of white matter fibers and subsequent dilation "ex vacuo." There is progressive enlargement of ventricles, and shunting may help. However, distinguishing those patients in which shunts are not helpful is sometimes quite difficult with this posttraumatic syndrome.

Chronic subdural hematoma is an important and sometimes overlooked sequela of even minor injury in the elderly. The hematoma increases in size by continued oozing of blood from subdural membranes and therefore increasing the size of the lesion. The treatment for this condition is still debated, but surgical evacuation of one kind or another is necessary.

Posttraumatic syndrome is a poorly characterized condition marked by loss of concentration, memory difficulty, headache, and difficulty with work. Over 50% of patients with minor head injury have one or more of these complications 3 months after injury. Psychometric tests may help in the evaluation. There is no specific treatment at present, but there is increasing recognition of this important problem.

REFERENCES

Becker DP et al: The outcome from severe head injury with early diagnosis and intensive management. J Neurosurg 47:491, 1977.

Black P McL and Swann K: Management of severe head injuries. In Burke JF, Boyd RJ, and McCabe CJ, editors: Trauma management. Chicago, 1988, Year Book.

Gennarelli TA and Timbault LE: Biomechanics of head injury. In Wilkins RH and Rengachary SS, editors: Neurosurgery. New York, 1985, McGraw-Hill.

Jamieson K and Yelland JDN: Traumatic intracerebral hematoma: report of 63 surgically treated cases. J Neurosurg 37:528, 1972.

Phonprasert C et al: Extradural hematoma: analysis of 18 cases. J Trauma 20:679, 1980.

Rimel RW et al: Disability caused by minor head injury. Neurosurgery 9:221, 1981.

Seeling JM et al: Traumatic acute subdural hematoma: major mortality reductions in comatose patients treated within 4 hours. N Engl J Med 304:1511, 1981.

CHAPTER

132 Spinal Cord Injury

Paul A. Gutierrez
Michael Vulpe
Robert R. Young

Until the middle of this century, spinal cord injury (SCI) was considered a malady with little hope for successful treatment. Ernest Bors and Sir Ludwig Guttman, leaders in the development of specialized centers dedicated to the care and rehabilitation of patients with spinal cord injuries, were instrumental in demonstrating that these patients could be successfully managed. The advent of antibiotic therapy and rational management of the neurogenic bladder has significantly decreased mortality from urosepsis, which was previously the major cause of death in these patients. It is now well established that an organized and comprehensive management plan can successfully return most spinal-cord-injured patients to a functional status as valuable and productive members of society. This plan must include rapid identification of the degree of neurologic impairment and protection of the spinal cord from further primary damage or from secondary damage. In addition, early treatment of associated injuries to other parts of the body should be a top priority. Once the patient has been stabilized from the initial injuries, a comprehensive rehabilitation program must be started to enhance the return of function and reduce the incidence of secondary complications.

An important concept to remember is that some or much of what follows in this chapter is applicable to the management of spinal cord impairment produced by nontraumatic disorders. These include cord infarction (caused by atherosclerosis, hypotensive episodes, dural arteriovenous malformations, or surgery for abdominal aortic aneurysm), cord compression from tumor or abscess, Foix-Alajouanine syndrome, multiple sclerosis, and the end-stage degenerative diseases and amyotrophic lateral sclerosis. The management of spinal cord injury or impairment constitutes a particularly well developed area within neurologic rehabilitation and provides us with paradigms for similar approaches to patients with other neurologic impairments.

EPIDEMIOLOGY

Spinal cord injury predominantly affects males, who make up 85% to 90% of the patients. Most are single and young, with 60% of injuries occurring in individuals between the ages of 16 and 30 years.

The incidence of spinal cord injuries in the United States is estimated at 8000-10,000 new cases annually. These are roughly equally distributed between incomplete tetraplegics, complete tetraplegics, incomplete paraplegics, and complete paraplegics. There is an increased incidence of SCI in the summer months, in the early hours of the morning, and on weekends; alcohol and drug use are frequently involved. Causes include motor vehicle accidents (50%), falls (20%), sports (15%), and violence (15%). Approximately two thirds of sports-related spinal cord injuries occur in diving accidents. Two particularly common causes are motor vehicle accidents in 16- to 30-year-olds and falls in 61- to 75-year-olds.

Most spine injuries occur at levels where there is relatively increased mobility. The midcervical region and the thoracolumbar junction are the sites in the spine with the greatest mobility, in contrast to the thoracic spine, which is stabilized by the rib cage. In the cervical region, movement of the relatively massive head produces large forces that are apt to cause fractures during rapid deceleration such as occurs with motor vehicle and diving accidents and falls. The pelvic girdle and legs inferiorly and the thorax superiorly act as large masses producing stress at the thoracolumbar junction during deceleration.

Spinal cord injuries rarely occur in isolation. Associated trauma includes head injuries, closed or open, in 15% of patients. Limb fractures are seen in approximately 10% of patients with acute spinal cord injuries, fractures of some portion of the trunk are seen in about 20%, and significant chest or thoracic injuries are seen in 15%. Associated operations after an acute spinal cord injury include spinal fusion in 35%, halo traction in 20%, open reduction of fractures in 20%, and tracheostomy in 10%.

CLASSIFICATION

Spinal cord injuries can be classified according to anatomic or functional schemes. The skeletal level of injury (SLI) is determined by radiologic examination. It is named after the vertebra with the greatest damage, or the two adjacent vertebrae with the greatest damage. This is often referred to as the *motion segment*.

The neurologic level of injury (NLI) is determined by the neurologic examination. The NLI is defined as the most caudal segment with good motor and sensory function. The motor level of injury should be determined independently from the sensory level of injury on each side of the body. Good motor function is defined by the most caudal myotome with at least enough power to overcome gravity, a grade of 3 out of 5: (0/5—no movement, 1/5—only trace movement, 2/5—movement through full range with gravity eliminated, 3/5—movement through full range against gravity, 4/5—movement through full range against some resistance, 5/5—normal power). Key muscles used to determine the motor level for classification are listed in the box below. Normal sensory function is determined according to dermatomal testing. Key sensory areas recommended for testing the dermatomes are listed in the second box below and shown in Fig. 132-1.

When the most caudal segments with good function are the same on both sides of the body, the NLI may be identified as one segment. When they are different, each side's NLI should be described independently. The zone of par-

Key muscles determining motor level

C1-4	Diaphragm
C5	Elbow flexors (biceps)
C6	Wrist extensors
C7	Elbow extensors (triceps)
C8	Finger flexors, distal phalanx
T1	Hand intrinsics (interossei)
T2-L1	Use sensory level and Beevor's sign
L2	Hip flexors (iliopsoas)
L3	Knee extensors (quadriceps)
L4	Ankle dorsiflexors (tibialis anterior)
L5	Long toe extensors (extensor hallucis longus)
S1	Ankle plantar flexors (gastrocnemius)
S2-5	Use sensory level and sphincter ani

Key areas determining sensory level

C2	Occipital protuberance
C3	Supraclavicular fossa
C4	Top of the acromioclavicular joint
C5	Lateral side of the antecubital fossa
C6	Thumb
C7	Middle finger
C8	Little finger
T1	Medial side of the antecubital fossa
T2	Apex of the axilla
T3	Third intercostal space
T4	Fourth intercostal space, nipple line
T5	Fifth intercostal space
T6	Sixth intercostal space, xiphisternum
T7-9	Intercostal spaces
T10	Umbilicus
T11	Intercostal space
T12	Inguinal ligament
L1	Upper anterior thigh
L2	Midanterior thigh
L3	Medial femoral condyle
L4	Medial malleolus
L5	Dorsum of the foot at the third MTP joint
S1	Lateral heel
S2	Popliteal fossa in the midline
S3	Ischial tuberosity
S4/5	Perianal area

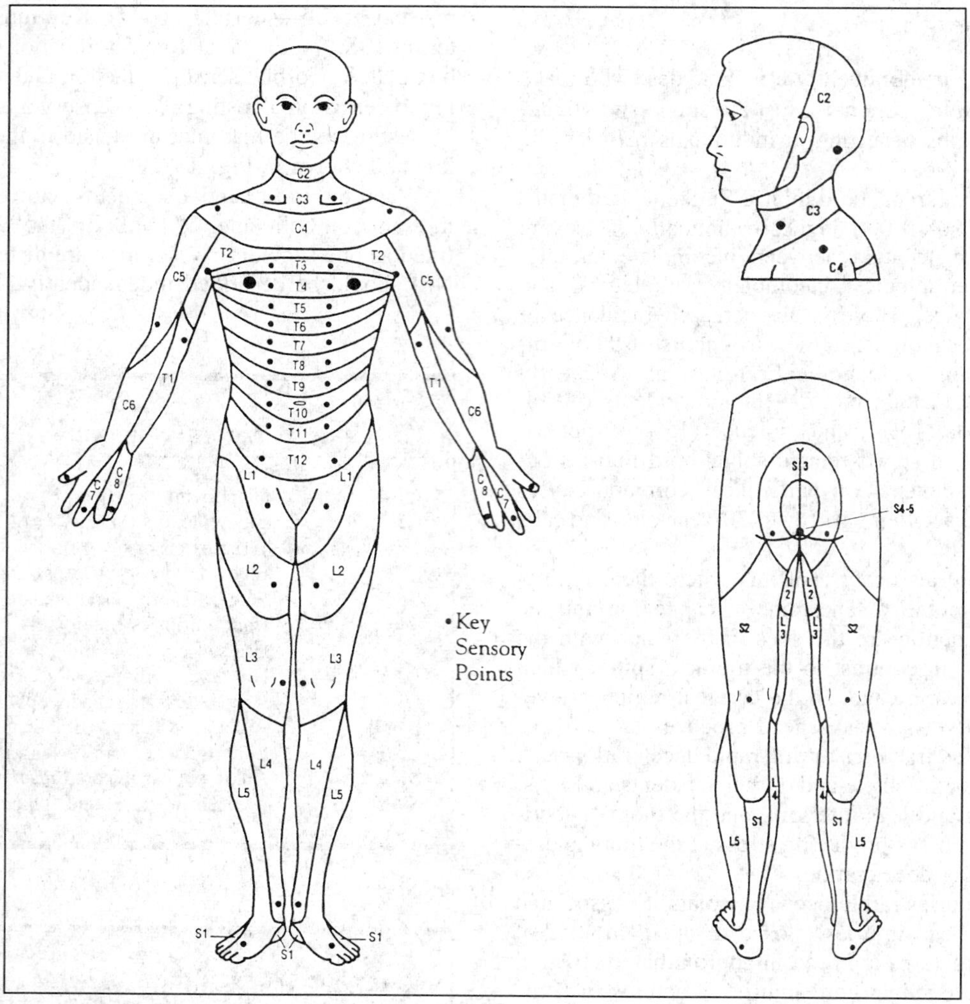

Fig. 132-1. Areas to test to determine sensory level of injury. (By permission from Dittunno JF, editor: Standards for neurologic and functional classification of spinal cord injury. Chicago, 1992, American Spinal Injury Association.)

tial preservation (ZPP) is the region of the cord immediately below the NLI with some remaining sensation or motor function. If it includes up to three consecutive segments caudal to the NLI, the injury is still considered complete. If any nonreflex neurologic function is found below the ZPP, the injury is considered incomplete.

The Frankel classification system describes the degree of preservation of function below the NLI. Frankel A lesions are complete, with no preservation of motor or sensory function below the ZPP. Frankel B lesions are incomplete, but with only preserved sensation below the ZPP. Frankel C lesions are those with preserved, but useless, voluntary motor function below the ZPP. Frankel D lesions are those with preserved, useful, voluntary motor function below the ZPP. This is defined as preserved voluntary motor ability below the NLI with most of the key muscles having at least grade 3 power. Frankel E denotes return of normal motor and sensory function, but reflexes may remain abnormal.

The Frankel classification system can be used as a prognostic indicator for functional recovery. This makes it imperative that a careful and complete neurologic evaluation be done as soon as possible after a spinal injury. Of all patients with spine fractures from C1-S5, 50% present to the hospital as Frankel A, 10% as Frankel B, 10% as Frankel C, and 30% as Frankel D. Of all patients presenting as Frankel A, 94% are still Frankel A (complete lesions) on discharge from the hospital despite all therapeutic efforts. The remaining 6% are Frankel B (50%) or Frankel C or D. None have complete recovery. Of patients presenting as Frankel B, 62% are unchanged at the time of discharge. Fifty percent of those presenting as Frankel C injuries and 94% of those presenting as Frankel D injuries are unchanged or improved at the time of discharge.

SPINAL CORD INJURY SYNDROMES

Central cord syndrome

Incomplete spinal cord injuries can be further classified into clinical syndromes based on the anatomic location of damage within the cord. The central cord syndrome is seen most commonly with hyperextension injuries of the cervical spine. This syndrome is particularly common in the elderly and in individuals with congenital or acquired cervical stenosis. As a result of the trauma, they develop hemorrhagic necrosis of the central gray matter and the more medial white matter. With the central cord syndrome, patients have greater weakness in the arms than the legs. Thus the term "upside-down quadriplegia" is used to describe the physical findings. Anatomically, this can be explained by the fact that the corticospinal and spinothalamic tracts are organized such that the sacral fibers are more lateral and the cervical fibers are more medial in location (Fig. 132-2). The more caudal fibers are protected from central cord necrosis and have a greater chance of surviving damage in this type of cervical cord injury. The significance of these facts is that many patients with the central cord syndrome are eventually able to ambulate, although they may still have significant weakness in their arms.

Brown-Séquard syndrome

The Brown-Séquard syndrome results from injury on one side of the cord that interrupts ascending and descending fiber tracts. It results in ipsilateral motor weakness, loss of fine touch and position sense, and contralateral sensory deficits in pain and temperature. At the neurologic level of injury, there is also ipsilateral flaccid weakness and anesthesia caused by damage to the nerve roots and motor and sensory neurons in that area. This syndrome can result from any spinal injury, but is more common with penetrating injuries and asymmetric herniations of the nucleus pulposus. A pure Brown-Séquard syndrome is rare; usually one finds the two major features to be predominantly ipsilateral spastic weakness and contralateral loss of pain and temperature sensation.

Anterior cord syndrome

The anterior cord syndrome is rare in its pure form. It may be seen with flexion injuries, acute central herniations of the nucleus pulposus, and some vascular insults to the spinal cord. The regions of the cord involved are those supplied by the anterior spinal artery. The areas spared include the posterior columns and dorsal horns. Thus, below the level of injury, there is weakness and loss of pain and temperature sensation.

Posterior column syndrome

The posterior column syndrome is the rarest syndrome in its pure form. It has been associated with hyperextension injuries. The clinical manifestations are those of loss of posterior column function: vibratory and fine touch sensations, and proprioception. Power and gross sensation are preserved, so these patients have a chance for useful functional recovery after rehabilitation.

Cauda equina/conus medullaris syndrome

The cauda equina syndrome results from low-level spine injuries, those at or below the thoracolumbar junction. This differs from the other syndromes mentioned above in that the damage does not leave any intact caudal spinal cord: the damage is primarily to spinal nerve roots and perhaps the conus. Loss of motor power results from lower motor neuron dysfunction, which produces flaccid rather than spastic weakness. Sensory loss is to all modalities in the

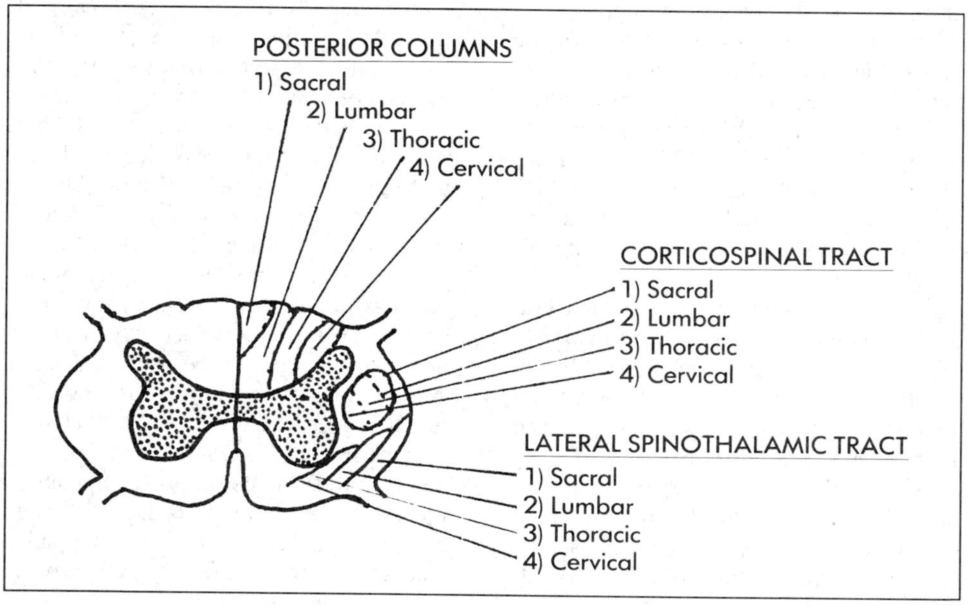

Fig. 132-2. Organization of fibers within tracts by level of origination or termination.

affected dermatomes, since all fibers run in close proximity in the spinal nerves. There is partial or complete loss of sacral reflexes leading to bladder and bowel dysfunction. Sphincter tone tends to be reduced in the bladder and bowel, and incontinence rather than retention of urine and feces is the rule.

Immediate management of spinal cord injury

In the last decade, the eventual outcome from spinal trauma has improved significantly. A major emphasis was placed on spine stabilization in the field to prevent further neurologic injury during transport to the trauma center. This has involved well-trained emergency medical technicians and paramedics and has resulted in a shift from the majority of injuries being complete (Frankel A) to incomplete (Frankel B-E) lesions. At the accident scene, the top priorities remain the ABCs (airway, breathing, circulation), but spinal column stabilization on a spine board or splint is the next greatest priority. More sophisticated stretchers have been developed, even some that can be used during x-ray and other imaging studies. Intravenous fluids should be administered, and transport in the Trendelenburg position may decrease the risk of shock and aspiration.

On arrival at the hospital, a reassessment of the patient should include a brief history, physical examination, and neurologic evaluation. Spinal column immobilization and cardiopulmonary stabilization must be maintained. The latter must emphasize prevention of hypoxia and hypotension. A Foley catheter should be inserted into the bladder and urinalysis performed to look for hematuria. Sources of internal bleeding in the abdomen, chest, and pelvis need to be identified and treated. The National Acute Spinal Cord Injury Study II (NASCI II) demonstrated that intravenous megadose methylprednisolone therapy, instituted within 8 hours of the initial injury, decreases the neurologic deficits resulting from spinal cord injury. The dose used in that study was an initial bolus of 30 mg/kg body weight, followed by a continuous intravenous infusion of 5.4 mg/kg/hr over the next 23 hours. Patients receiving that therapy had statistically significant improvement in recovery of motor and sensory function at 6-month follow-up compared to those given placebo or naloxone. It should be emphasized, however, that this treatment has not been shown to produce dramatic functional recovery and should not replace surgical decompression if that is indicated by radiologic examination.

Patients with cervical spinal cord injuries often have bradycardia caused by the unopposed action of the parasympathetic nervous system on the heart. Parasympathetic inputs to the heart are from the vagus nerve, which reaches this organ via an extraspinal pathway. It is rarely damaged in cervical spine trauma, whereas sympathetic function may be impaired. The vagal outflow can be increased by tracheal suction, which may lead to serious bradycardia or even asystole with sudden death. These patients should therefore be fully oxygenated before they are suctioned. Atropine should be readily available in the event of a sudden bradycardic episode or cardiac arrest. In addition, both patients with head injuries and those with spinal cord injuries can suffer loss of autoregulation of cerebral blood flow for weeks or several months after the initial trauma. In the early stages, this can lead to or extend ischemic injuries in the cord or cerebrum, should hypotension occur.

Once the patient's cardiovascular status is stable, radiographic evaluation should be performed. Continued caution is needed to prevent further neurologic injury. Fractures of the cervicothoracic junction, thoracic spine, and thoracolumbar junction can easily be missed unless roentgenograms, including CT, of these regions are obtained. The highest level of neurologic injury may clinically but not radiologically mask a second, lower level of injury. If there is no radiographic evidence of compression of neural elements or spinal column instability, the patient should be managed medically in the intensive care unit. When there is recognition of mechanical neural compression or stretch in patients with *incomplete* injuries, this should be relieved as soon as possible by restoring spinal alignment, removing bony or disc fragments or blood from the neural canal, or providing spinal stability by the appropriate technique. In patients presenting with *complete* injuries (Frankel A), emergency decompression or stabilization is not warranted since recovery of useful neurologic function in such patients is virtually nil, even with surgery. Spinal alignment in cervical spine fractures is best restored through spinal traction. This may require application of hardware such as Garner-Wells tongs by a surgical trauma team and placing the patient on a fracture bed or frame. Closed reduction can then be achieved by the application of weights. Careful monitoring of the neurologic exam and serial radiographs are essential to avoid overdistraction. Traction is generally not effective in lower-level fractures.

Surgical management of spinal cord injury may be necessary when closed reduction cannot be achieved (some fracture dislocations), when decompression of the spinal cord from bone fragments or blood is needed (some burst fractures), or for definitive stabilization of any unstable fracture of the spine. Many of the last-mentioned would eventually heal with bed rest, but surgical stabilization permits the patient to be out of bed sooner, thus accelerating the rehabilitation process. Again, it must be emphasized that timing of any surgical procedure depends on findings on the neurologic exam. Acute surgery is not indicated for patients with complete (Frankel A) spinal cord injuries. In patients with incomplete injuries, including sacral sparing, stabilization may be anterior, posterior, or both, depending on the site and type of fracture. Bone grafts, metal plates or rods, or wires can be used; a discussion of the type of surgery for a given injury is beyond the scope of this chapter. It is essential to remember that spinal fusion does not provide immediate, complete stabilization, and care should be taken to avoid destabilization when the patient is moved postoperatively. It may take 12-24 weeks for bony fusion to mature, and during this time the patient needs to be protected with external bracing such as a halo device, rigid collar, or thoracolumbar jacket.

SUBACUTE MANAGEMENT OF SPINAL CORD INJURY

Cardiovascular system

Homeostasis is interrupted by a spinal cord lesion, so once immediate stabilization of the patient is achieved, it is essential that the care-providing team address multiple other systems affected by the altered nervous system function. As previously mentioned, the cardiovascular system is compromised in its ability to regulate blood pressure. Hypotension may be particularly prominent after meals. This results from increased blood volume in the splanchnic bed, secretion of intestinal vasoactive peptides, and vasodilatation caused by insulin release. These patients should be sat up only slowly and may require ephedrine to maintain adequate blood pressure. Eventually, the renin/angiotensin system usually compensates for loss of autonomic nervous system control. Patients may maintain a greater intravascular volume and better orthostatic blood pressure if they do not lie absolutely horizontal; the bed may need to be tilted in the head-up position. Angiotensin-converting enzyme inhibitors are usually not well tolerated in the treatment of hypertension in chronic spinal cord injury patients.

Peripheral cardiovascular consequences of spinal cord injury include potentially life-threatening deep-venous thrombosis (DVT). In the first few weeks, SCI patients are especially susceptible to DVT as a result of immobilization, lack of muscle tone, and altered vascular tone. Subcutaneous heparin, pneumatic stockings, or almost continuous electrical stimulation of the calves can help prevent development of DVT and its most dangerous consequence, pulmonary embolism. Once an acutely injured patient is able to get out of bed into a wheelchair, the risk of DVT begins to diminish. In chronic SCI patients, arterial atrophy and distal ischemia, especially in the legs, may lead to the need for amputations. Quadriplegics have difficulty with thermoregulation because of their altered peripheral vascular control. They have lost normal mechanisms to prevent hypothermia (such as cutaneous vasoconstriction and shivering) or hyperthermia (vasodilatation and sweating).

Autonomic dysreflexia, a condition equivalent to "spasticity" of the sympathetic nervous system, should be treated as a life-threatening emergency. It is generally seen in patients with neurologic levels of injury at T6 and higher, because most of the spinal sympathetic system is below this level. It results from massive discharge of a relatively intact sympathetic nervous system triggered reflexly by a noxious stimulus below the level of injury. This is most commonly urinary bladder distention, but may be fecal impaction, skin lesions, or any noxious stimulus that would produce discomfort if its effects could reach the cerebrum. Because of the spinal cord injury, the sympathetic outflow, once begun, cannot be turned off by descending outflow from higher brain centers. Blood pressure rises dramatically, and bradycardia is commonly seen, in contrast to most other causes of hypertension. The patient experiences a pounding headache, piloerection and sweating below the NLI, nasal congestion, flushing, or even simple malaise (one cause of the "feel terrible syndrome"). While severe hypertension is the most dangerous of the consequences of dysreflexia (because of the risk of intracerebral hemorrhage), it can be missed if the patient is not examined early in the course of an episode. Sometimes reactive hypotension occurs if the noxious stimulus is removed before the blood pressure is taken.

The most important immediate management for autonomic dysreflexia involves removing the source of the noxious stimulus. The patient should be sat up in bed to help decrease intracerebral pressure, and the urinary bladder should be drained. Topical anesthetic jelly can be used for catheterization, and the bladder can be irrigated with topical anesthetic. If this does not relieve the symptoms or control the blood pressure, the rectum should be checked for fecal impaction after topical anesthetic jelly is applied. If these measures fail to bring the blood pressure down within a few minutes, nifedipine should be given. A 10 mg capsule should be bitten and swallowed by the patient. This dose of nifedipine can be repeated in 15 minutes if needed. Alternatively, hydralazine 0.25 cc (5 mg) can be given intravenously and repeated every 5 to 10 minutes as necessary, but the total dose should not exceed 1 cc (20 mg). Blood pressure should then be monitored every 5 minutes until it is back to normal, and then every 30 minutes for 4 hours. Should the hypertension prove to be refractory to the above measures, the patient should be transferred to an intensive care unit for more definitive treatment including intravenous hypotensive agents and, if all else fails, spinal anesthesia.

Respiratory system

The respiratory system is compromised to varying degrees in almost all SCI patients, depending on the neurologic level of injury. Injuries at or above C4 can paralyze the phrenic nerves and compromise function of the diaphragm and other muscles responsible for inhalation. This may result in ventilator dependence, although the patient may be able to compensate for short periods by using accessory muscles in the neck. The ventilator must be adjusted not only to produce physiologic levels of pO_2 and pCO_2, but also to avoid prolonged increased intrathoracic pressure, which would reduce venous return to the heart. Spinal cord injured patients also have compromise of their thoracic and abdominal muscles of exhalation, which results in a poor cough. This, plus the production of abnormally viscous mucous, makes spinal cord patients particularly susceptible to mucous plugging, atelectasis, and pneumonia. Patients with high-level lesions are also at great risk of aspiration.

Gastrointestinal system

Gastrointestinal manifestations of spinal cord injury are predominantly those of hypomotility. Gastric hypomotility can lead to nausea, dyspepsia, and reflux with eventual esophagitis and aspiration pneumonitis. Stress gastritis and upper gastrointestinal hemorrhage are additional problems, especially early after the injury. Gallstones develop frequently, even in young men, perhaps as a result of gallbladder hypomotility and hypercalcemia. Colonic hypomotility and anal sphincter spasticity lead to chronic constipation and megacolon. Patients need to be placed on a bowel training program where digital rectal stimulation is performed every other day to help promote regular evacuation of the bowel. Stool softeners and dietary fiber supplements can be helpful in avoiding fecal impaction. Suppositories and enemas should be avoided if possible. Hemorrhoids, anal fissures, and fistulas are complications that may further complicate the care of spinal-cord-injured patients.

Genitourinary system

Genitourinary complications of spinal cord injury were once a major factor in the early demise of these patients. While great advancements have been made in urologic management and antibiotic therapy, renal failure is still an important cause of their morbidity and mortality. The primary goal in management of the urinary system is to maintain renal function. Once the new patient has been stabilized, initiation of intermittent catheterization is a major priority. Prolonged management with an indwelling catheter can lead to refractory urinary tract infections, bladder stones, neoplasms, and in males, urethritis and epididymitis. Intermittent catheterization can be started at intervals of 4 to 6 hours, depending on fluid intake. The frequency of catheterization can then be adjusted to allow the accumulation of no more than 300-350 cc of urine at a time. The achievement of a "balanced bladder" is the goal, defined as a bladder with sufficient capacity to store urine reliably and the ability to empty sufficiently without excessively high pressure or vesicoureteral reflux.

Many patients develop spontaneous voiding after the initial period of spinal shock. Urodynamic studies to assess intravesicular pressures should be done on all patients. Those who are voiding should have a simultaneous uroflow and EMG of the external sphincter. The finding of increased EMG activity and excessive intravesicular pressure with decreased flow suggests that there is detrusor-sphincter dyssynergia. This occurs when there is simultaneous contraction of the detrusor muscle (which decreases the size of the bladder) and external sphincter (which obstructs outflow through the urethra). It is seen most commonly in patients with suprasacral injuries and is accompanied by bladder hyperreflexia. These patients tend to have urinary retention and can develop vesicoureteral reflux of varying degrees. If the bladder pressure is less than 60 to 70 cm H_2O and the residual urine less than 75 cc, spontaneous or stimulated voiding can be used. Otherwise, something must be done to lower bladder pressure and residual volume. In patients with outflow obstruction resulting from dyssynergia, the external sphincter can sometimes be successfully relaxed with alpha sympatholytics such as phentolamine, phenoxybenzamine, or prazosin. Transurethral external sphincterotomy can also be used to relieve the obstruction. Some patients, in addition, require transurethral resection of the prostate and bladder neck. An external urine collection device can be used to prevent incontinence in men, and high-absorbency pads can be used by women. Patients with hyperreflexia and high intravesicular pressures can sometimes be managed with detrusor-relaxing agents such as oxybutnin or propantheline and intermittent catheterization.

Patients with areflexic bladders who are unable to empty the bladder by abdominal straining should be managed with intermittent catheterization. Areflexic bladders are most commonly seen in low-level paraplegics or those with the cauda equina syndrome. They should be instructed in the methods of clean intermittent self-catheterization and urinary acidification. Fluid intake should be regulated to avoid rapid filling of the bladder so that a regular schedule of self-catheterization can be followed. Some patients are unable or unwilling to perform self-catheterization. In patients with hyperreflexic bladders, sometimes the bladder can be stimulated to empty reflexively by tapping the suprapubic region, stimulating the anal sphincter, or pulling the pubic hair. Every possible effort should be made to avoid using a chronic indwelling catheter because of the long-term complications mentioned previously.

Urinary tract infections are a common problem in spinal-cord-injured patients. In general, prophylactic antibiotics have not proven to be useful in either catheter-free or catheter-dependent individuals. Most patients have bacteriuria, but this should be considered only colonization of the urine and not a tissue infection. Bacteriuria should not be treated unless there is significant pyuria (at least 50 WBCs per high-power field) and/or other symptoms such as fever, bladder spasms, and malaise.

Bladder and renal calculi are another important long-term complication of spinal cord injury. Bladder calculi are usually infected and can cause severe irritation to the bladder. If detected early, they can sometimes be flushed out through a catheter. Larger stones can be crushed during cystoscopy or with transurethral electrohydraulic lithotripsy. Renal calculi are most common in the first year after injury. Calcified stones are common because impaired mobility leads to bone resorption, hypercalcemia, and hypercalciuria. Struvite stones are also much more frequent than in the general population. In fact, up to 98% of stones in SCI patients include struvite in their composition, whereas only 15% of stones in the general population have struvite. Struvite stones are frequently infected with urease-producing bacteria, which cause chronic urinary tract infections. Also, urease-producing bacteria release ammonia, which alkalinizes the urine and promotes stone formation in the kidneys and urinary tract.

Sexual dysfunction is another major source of concern for spinal-cord-injured patients. In males, approximately two thirds of patients regain some erectile function within 6 months of their injury, but only 10% ejaculate normally. Sexual function depends on the level and completeness of the neurologic injury. Patients with suprasacral lesions can have reflexively induced erections, but those with complete lesions cannot have psychologically induced erections. Patients with conus or cauda equina injuries are less likely to have any erections, but some with incomplete lesions may have only psychogenic erections. Electroejaculation, vacuum tumescence, injection of prostaglandins or other medications into the penis, and vibratory stimulation are methods that have been developed to aid in the generation of erection and ejaculation. Those with retrograde ejaculations who desire to have children can have the ejaculate retrieved from the bladder.

Musculoskeletal system

Bone demineralization occurs rapidly and irreversibly after spinal cord injury. The elimination of gravitational load/stress of bone caused by immobilization is probably the major cause of this. The resultant hypercalcemia and hyperphosphatemia may lead to nausea and vomiting in the first few weeks after spinal cord injury. Inactivity may also lead to rapid muscle atrophy below the neurologic level of injury, even if lower motor neurons remain intact. Eventually, demineralization leads to fragility and an increased tendency for fractures of long bones and compression fractures of vertebral bodies. Any fall or trauma should be considered a potential cause of fractures, and radiographs may be necessary despite lack of pain or immediate swelling. A more comprehensive review of this subject is provided in the references.

Heterotopic ossification (HO) is bone formation in abnormal locations, most commonly around the hips and knees after spinal cord injury. The clinical presentation varies and it can be asymptomatic. HO may present as swelling around the joint or decreased range of motion. It can also cause distal extremity swelling as a result of vascular compression, and in this presentation needs to be distinguished from deep venous thrombosis. Diagnosis is usually possible with plain radiographs but radionuclide triphasic bone scans may be necessary early in the development of HO. Etidronate disodium (Didronel) is the treatment of choice with an initial dose of 20 mg/kg/day for 2 weeks followed by 10 mg/kg/day for 10 weeks. If gastrointestinal side effects such as diarrhea occur, the dosage can be divided. For more severe cases, the treatment can be continued up to 6 months. Surgical removal of HO should not be undertaken until nuclide scans show it is no longer active (i.e., no longer being formed).

Integumentary system

Skin integrity can be difficult to maintain in any immobilized or paralyzed patient. A pressure sore is an area of skin that has become necrotic because unrelieved pressure causes ischemia and mechanical damage. This occurs most commonly over a bony prominence such as the ischium, greater trochanter, or heel, or in the sacrococcygeal region. Other factors that can contribute to the development of pressure sores include fecal and urinary incontinence, friction, shear forces, elevated body temperature, sepsis, accumulation of metabolic waste products, altered lymph drainage, hypoalbuminemia, advanced age of the patient, and fractures. Persons with normal sensation and mobility subconsciously detect prolonged pressure in tissues and periodically shift their position to relieve this pressure. Patients with impaired sensation and mobility must consciously move or rely on others to move them to relieve pressure on skin and subcutaneous structures.

Prevention of pressure sores should be given a high priority for spinal-cord-injured patients. The goal can best be met if the patient can be regularly turned in bed at least every 2 hours without generating excessive shear forces. In addition, many cushions and beds have been designed to spread out pressure over as great an area as possible. Flotation beds of various types (air, water, or silicon beads and air) have generally proven to be the most useful. Wheelchair cushions with cutouts to relieve pressure in one area must be carefully designed to avoid causing excessive shear forces in surrounding skin. Controlling flexor spasms with medications or nerve blocks can also help prevent sores resulting from friction. Additionally, patients can be trained in methods to provide pressure relief in their chairs every 20-30 minutes.

Treatment of pressure sores can involve surgery or more conservative approaches. In general, local therapy of wounds should include removal of pressure and regular debridement of necrotic tissue, control of infection, and promotion of epithelialization. Traditionally, gauze soaked with Dakin's solution, sterile saline, hydrogen peroxide, or silver nitrate has been used to pack the wound in a wet-to-dry manner. As the dried dressings are removed, debridement takes place. It is now generally accepted that drainage from wounds should be absorbed with hydroactive dressings and granules. Hyperbaric oxygen treatments have been used to promote wound healing and decrease recovery time. Promising new approaches such as the use of calcium alginate preparations are currently under study. Another innovative approach to the treatment of pressure sores has been the reintroduction of maggot-debridement therapy, which had previously fallen out of favor with those treating pressure sores in this country. It is promising in that sterile maggots can be used safely in debridement of dirty wounds in fragile patients to promote epithelialization of those wounds.

Surgical therapy can include split-thickness skin graft over a well-granulated superficial wound. Larger, deeper sores may need to be excised and underlying bony prominences reduced, with the wound then being closed with a myocutaneous flap, the muscles serving as padding. Postoperatively, pressure must be kept off the wound, so the patient should be placed in a flotation bed.

Nervous system

Initially after spinal cord trauma, there may be a period during which there appears to be no function in any portion of the caudal spinal cord. This period of areflexia and flaccid paralysis has been termed *spinal shock* and may last for a few weeks. Eventually, however, function begins to return to the areas of the cord not directly damaged in the trauma. First is the bulbocavernosus reflex, which returns almost immediately, followed by deep-tendon reflex activity. This is followed shortly by enhancement of sacral parasympathetics and the strengthening of anal and bladder sphincter reflexes. Primitive withdrawal responses from noxious stimuli such as an extensor plantar response or a triple flexion response in the leg may then soon appear. Exaggerated flexor spasms can be seen in response to tactile stimuli. An extreme "mass response" may involve bilateral flexion at the knee and flexion and adduction at the hip. Abdominal contractions may result in evacuation of the bowel and bladder. Reflex diaphoresis may also be seen.

Spasticity after spinal cord injury is a result of loss of descending inhibitory input from motor systems that normally control and coordinate movement and muscle activity. Below the neurologic level of injury, segmental reflex arcs remain intact so that sensory inputs can still trigger motor and autonomic outflow. Spasticity can interfere with functional activities, personal care, and positioning, and can cause discomfort for the patient. It can sometimes be controlled with range-of-motion exercises, which stretch muscles. It can be exacerbated by a noxious stimulus such as a urinary tract infection, pressure sore, fecal impaction, or other intra-abdominal process. It may improve when these conditions are treated.

Pharmacologic control of spasticity should be instituted with specific treatment goals defined; for example, paresis or inability to use the upper limb is rarely improved. These goals would include a noticeable increase in a few restricted functional abilities, a decrease in the need for intensive nursing care, or relief of pain and discomfort. Baclofen is generally considered the medication of choice because of its effectiveness and relatively low incidence of adverse reactions. It is thought to be an agonist of the inhibitory neurotransmitter gamma-amino butyric acid (GABA). Its primary site of action is believed to be in the spinal cord, where it presumably mimics some of the descending inhibitory actions lost after spinal cord injury. It apparently also has actions on higher centers, since it can cause sedation in some patients early in treatment. The treatment usually recommended is 15-80 mg per day in divided doses, starting at a minimum and increasing to the dose needed to achieve the desired response without intolerable adverse effects. Some have had better success with higher doses than those recommended by the manufacturer (e.g., 240-300 mg per day) without producing intolerable adverse reactions.

Diazepam is another medication that acts centrally to mimic the action of descending inhibitory motor systems. Diazepam is effective in the control of spasticity, but it has prominent actions on the limbic system, thalamus, and hypothalamus and can cause sedation and other cognitive adverse reactions that may limit its usefulness. Dosage should be started at 2 mg twice per day and titrated up to a maximum of 20 mg per day, although some patients can tolerate at least 10 mg four times per day. Clonazepam is another benzodiazepine that can be effective for the control of myoclonus. These are brief jerks of predominantly flexor groups and can interfere with functional abilities and annoy the patient. Sometimes as little as 1 mg per day can decrease these myoclonic jerks, but usually higher doses are needed. Clonidine is a centrally acting $alpha_2$-adrenergic agonist that has also been shown to be effective in the control of spinal spasticity. It may be given orally or through a transdermal patch at dosages of 0.1 to 0.5 mg per day. The limiting adverse reactions include hypotension (rare in patients with complete spinal cord injury) and sedation. Dry eyes and mouth generally are transient problems.

Dantrolene works peripherally to inhibit the release of calcium from the sarcoplasmic reticulum and thus decreases the contractility of skeletal muscle. Its use is limited by adverse reactions including drowsiness, lethargy, lightheadedness, and a potentially serious hepatotoxicity. Hepatotoxicity is more common in the elderly, women, and anyone receiving estrogen therapy. Liver enzymes must be checked regularly, especially in these groups. Dosage should start at 25 mg twice per day and be titrated up slowly to a maximum of 100 mg four times per day.

Medical therapy has varying effectiveness and some patients may require more aggressive therapy to control their spasticity. Motor point blocks with phenol may be used to selectively decrease spasticity in desired muscle groups. Surgical procedures, including tendon lengthening and peripheral neurectomy, should only be used as a last resort, and never in the first year after injury. Dorsal rhizotomies, either open surgical or percutaneous radiofrequency procedures, and myelotomies restricted to the dorsal root entry zone can be effective. Unfortunately, recurrence of spasticity has been seen even after these destructive procedures. The latest developments in the treatment of spasticity include the use of a small, implantable pump to deliver a continuous infusion of baclofen to the intrathecal space. This procedure has shown promising results. Botulinum toxin may be injected into spastic muscles to weaken them for periods of approximately 3 months.

Syringomyelia is a condition in which cavitation develops in the central region of the spinal cord. It is seen commonly as a posttraumatic phenomenon in SCI, but can be associated with Arnold-Chiari malformation and can be idiopathic. These cavitations may be single or multiloculated, and they may extend both caudal and rostral from the site of the initial trauma. Fluid with a composition similar to cerebrospinal fluid fills these cavities, although extensive analysis of the cyst contents has not yet been carried out. Clinical manifestations include loss of pain and temperature sensation (classically in a capelike distribution over the shoulders and neck), muscle atrophy and loss of motor power, respiratory insufficiency, pain, and changes in the degree of spasticity. The presentation is highly variable depending on the location and extent of the cyst, but increased pain and deterioration of function, especially above the original level, are serious complications of SCI. Diagnosis is best made with an MRI, but a delayed CT after myelography may show the water-soluble contrast collected in the cavity after it has cleared the subarachnoid space.

The exact etiology and pathogenesis of syringomyelia is not known. Tethering of the cord from adhesions is a commonly associated finding on MRI. Some speculate that increases in pressure within the cysts during Valsalva's maneuvers may lead to further breakdown of tissue and extension of the cyst. Another possible mechanism is that an as-yet-unknown substance in the cyst fluid acts as a destructive agent leading to further tissue breakdown. Treatments for syringomyelia include spine stabilization, release of the tethered cord, and shunting or fenestration of the cyst cavity to allow drainage of the fluid into the subarachnoid space. Results are variable and are generally limited to halting progression of the cystic degeneration of the spinal cord and maintaining function rather than restoring it.

SPINAL CORD INJURY REHABILITATION

Rehabilitation after spinal cord injury is best provided by an interdisciplinary team at a specialized facility. A comprehensive program encompassing therapies for both physical handicaps and psychological adjustments is essential and should include peers and other patients. It should encourage patient participation, which is vital to promote the resumption of meaningful integration into society.

Rehabilitation can and should begin even in the acute phase of the injury. Prevention of pressure sores should be an important part of care given from the onset of medical therapy. As previously discussed, frequent turning of the patient, flotation beds, and constant inspection of the skin are essential to protect the skin of the immobile patient. Prevention of joint contractures should include range-of-motion exercises and splinting as soon as the patient is medically stable. This is especially true if associated trauma has occurred to any limb or joint. These measures, applied early in the treatment of a spinal-cord-injured patient, can reduce the time needed for rehabilitation; if contractures are allowed to develop, they are difficult to overcome. As spasticity develops, the frequency of range-of-motion exercises needs to be increased. These can be performed by both therapists and nurses, and in some selected cases can be a way to involve family members in the rehabilitation and healing process.

Once the patient is medically and surgically stable, the neurorehabilitation team should be actively involved in primary care of the patient. The physician coordinates the activities of the team and manages the medical complications. He or she obtains the appropriate consultations from other physicians and surgeons for assistance in the complex care of the spinal-cord-injured patient.

The rehabilitation nurse in a center specializing in spinal cord injury or impairment has multiple responsibilities. These include basic nursing care, skin care, bowel and bladder care, patient and family education, and ensuring that skills learned in therapies are put to use on the nursing unit. The nursing team member is also most involved in the prevention and management of complications such as autonomic dysreflexia, deep venous thrombosis, and urinary tract infection.

The occupational therapist provides training in activities of daily living and works with the patient on improving upper extremity function. This includes training in dressing, feeding, grooming and personal hygiene, and homemaking. It also includes maintenance of range of motion, which may require the construction of splints for some patients. The occupational therapist may also be involved in providing environmental control devices and in electric wheelchair training with chin controls or sip-and-puff controls.

Physical therapists (and kinesiotherapists in VA hospitals) work with the patient to develop a reconditioning and strengthening program. Physical therapists are also highly involved in mobility skills such as training in safe wheelchair operation, sitting balance, and turning in bed. They are most involved with lower extremity function including range of motion and, if applicable, gait training with walkers, braces, canes, or crutches. They also are involved in training paraplegics and some low-level quadriplegics to do transfers from bed to wheelchair and back and into shower chairs or automobiles. Another function of these therapists is to help in the ordering of appropriate adaptive devices for the home and evaluation of the patient for an appropriate wheelchair. They also may assist with adaptive devices for an automobile and driver training, and may be involved in treating pain with physical modalities such as heat, cold, stretching, ethyl chloride sprays, and transcutaneous electrical nerve stimulation devices.

Social workers are important members of the rehabilitation team whose responsibilities involve coordination of discharge planning and reentry into the community. They provide important support to the patient and family members to help find means for financing the hospitalization and equipment or attendant care that may be needed after hospitalization. They help apply for government benefits that may be available for the physically disabled. They also coordinate linking the patient with peer support groups who may be able to provide additional assistance in coping with the challenges of life after a spinal cord injury. This "peer counseling" can be both formal and informal (i.e., newly injured patients talking with and watching other inpatients at the SCI center). Social workers work closely with clinical psychologists to anticipate and manage any psychosocial problems that may arise.

The clinical psychologist provides counseling services to both the patient and family members to assist in their adaptation to the physical and psychological stresses of a spinal cord injury. Depression and grieving for the loss of abilities are natural parts of the rehabilitation process. Many patients go through a period of denial before they are ready to begin active participation in rehabilitation. Neuropsychologic testing may also have to be performed to identify any subtle cognitive deficits that may have resulted from either traumatic or ischemic brain injuries. This can be crucial in planning for vocational rehabilitation and directing interventions that may be necessary for maximizing rehabilitation outcome.

Vocational rehabilitation counselors help patients return to work or obtain training or schooling so that they can find a new career. They work with representatives of the state offices of rehabilitation services and other community organizations to give the patient opportunities to re-enter the work force if at all possible. They may also be involved in evaluations of the patient's capabilities and aptitudes so that a wise career choice can be made.

Rehabilitation engineering is another important aspect of the team approach to treatment of the spinal-cord-injured patient. Rehabilitation engineers help design and construct various prosthetic and orthotic devices used to improve a patient's abilities. They modify wheelchairs to improve a patient's posture and prevent pressure sores. They may also supervise modifications to the patient's home or automobile and construct environmental control devices that allow the paralyzed patient to control telephones, lights, televisions, radios, heating and air-conditioning systems, and other appliances in the home.

Functional outcomes for patients after rehabilitation for spinal cord injury differ according to many factors, but the most important is the neurologic level of injury (NLI). If the NLI is C4 or higher, the patient requires assistance for virtually everything, including assisted coughing, feeding, grooming, dressing, bathing, bowel and bladder care, and ambulation. Patients with a C5 NLI are totally dependent for bowel and bladder care, lower extremity dressing, and bathing. They usually need an assisted cough and upper extremity dressing. With special adaptive devices, C5 quadriplegics can be independent after setup for electric wheelchair ambulation, feeding, and grooming. A C6 quadriplegic usually needs assistance for bladder management, coughing in the supine position, and lower-extremity dressing. They can be independent with adaptive equipment in their bowel care, bathing, upper extremity dressing, grooming, and feeding. Some of these patients can safely operate an adapted van, driving with specially designed hand controls.

The addition of elbow extension that comes with a C7 NLI is extremely important for enhancing transfer and mobility skills. These patients can be nearly independent if they are highly motivated and are provided proper adaptive equipment. Wheelchair propulsion may be strong enough to negotiate slopes and uneven terrain, but curbs and stairs remain a barrier. Feeding, grooming, bathing, bowel and bladder care, bed mobility, and pressure relief can all be managed with equipment without the assistance of an attendant. Driving can be independent with hand controls, and some may be able to transfer and then independently place their wheelchair into the car. Patients with C8/T1 NLI additionally are totally independent for all grooming, bathing, etc., and have significantly better control of fine movements with the hands.

Patients with NLI below T6 need no assistance with cough or pulmonary hygiene. Some can ambulate to a limited degree with a physical assist or guarding and orthoses and walkers. Those with injuries below T10 through L2 have the potential for independent functional ambulation for short distances with orthoses such as long leg braces, ankle/foot orthoses, and forearm crutches. Patients with hip extension, L3 NLI, have potential for community ambulation. The Vannini-Rizzoli boot is a custom-fitted device that patients with levels at or below T6 NLI can be trained to use for community ambulation. Current research is ongoing to develop elaborate systems of microprocessor-controlled electrodes (functional electrical stimulation [FES]), which can be used for stimulation of lower extremity muscles in a pattern that allows ambulation with walkers and braces. These systems are not yet practical because of their bulk and inefficiency and the difficulty of activating small, nonfatigable motor units. However, FES in the form of phrenic nerve pacemakers is very successful in providing respiration for quadriplegics with injuries above C4 that spare phrenic motor neurons. FES is also increasingly useful in restoring upper limb function in patients with good biceps function but paralysis of muscles controlling the hand.

SUMMARY

Spinal cord injury or impairment remains a devastating lesion of the nervous system. Current therapies have not proven to be particularly effective in preventing or reversing damage to the spinal cord. Still, every effort should be made to preserve remaining function and prevent complications. The care of these patients has been significantly improved with the development of specialized multidisciplinary centers. The emphasis in current treatment focuses on rehabilitation and adaptation to the disability and prevention of secondary disabilities. Ongoing research provides hope for further advancement in the care and treatment of spinal cord injury, but even when new developments become practically implemented, the neurorehabilitation team is essential in the care of these patients. It is important that ongoing efforts continue to be made to integrate people with disabilities into society so that they may lead full and productive lives.

REFERENCES

Bracken MB et al: A randomized controlled trial of methylprednisolone or naloxone in the treatment of acute spinal cord injury. N Engl J Med 322(20):1405, 1990.

Care and treatment of spinal cord injury patients. Washington, DC, IB 141-85, 1991, Department of Veterans Affairs. Also see J Am Paraplegia Soc 15:295, 1992.

Elias AN and Gwinup G: Immobilization osteoporosis in paraplegics. J Am Paraplegia Soc 15:163, 1992.

Lee BY et al, editors: The spinal cord injured patient: comprehensive management. Philadelphia, 1991, Saunders.

NIDRR consensus statement: The prevention and management of urinary tract infections among people with spinal cord injury. J Am Paraplegia Soc 15:194, 1992.

Woolsey RM and Young RR, editors: Disorders of the spinal cord, Neurologic clinics 9(3). Philadelphia, 1991, Saunders.

CHAPTER

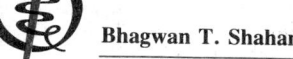

133 Principles of Neurorehabilitation

Bhagwan T. Shahani

NEUROLOGIC REHABILITATION

Neurologic rehabilitation is a relatively new area of specialization for neurologists and physiatrists. Prior to introduction of newer techniques for diagnosis of neurologic disease, especially neuroimaging and clinical neurophysiology, neurologists usually depended on meticulous history and detailed physical examination to localize a lesion in the central and/or peripheral nervous systems. It was sometimes necessary to wait a long time for the development of physical signs to make a proper diagnosis. Recent technologic advances in the diagnosis of neurologic disease have demphasized the traditional dependence on these age-old methods. In addition, development of new therapies and better medical management have resulted in greater survival of victims with disabling neurologic diseases and neurotrauma. It is therefore not surprising that increasing numbers of neurologists, who were formerly interested primarily in the intellectual exercise of making the diagnosis and pinpointing a lesion in the central nervous system, are now focusing their attention on long-term management using principles of rehabilitation medicine.

Rehabilitation medicine, as practiced today, uses a "team approach," drawing on the specialized skills of the physician, physical therapist, occupational therapist, social worker, psychologist, speech-and-hearing therapist, nurse, vocational counselor, and specialists in orthosis and prosthesis. In addition, a biomedical engineer can play an important role on the rehabilitation team. This interdisciplinary approach is usually available at specialized centers for rehabilitation. However, as Rusk points out:

> If patients are to benefit from present-day developments in rehabilitation, the concept of rehabilitation and the basic technics must be made a part of the medical programmes of all our hospitals. The concept of rehabilitation and the basic technics must also be made a part of the armamentarium of all physicians: for, regardless of the type of disability, the responsibility of the physician to his patient can not end when the acute injury or illness has been cared for. Medical care is not complete until the patient has been trained to live and work with what he has left.

In recent years new research techniques in cellular and molecular biology have resulted in awareness of the growth potential of neurons in the central nervous system (CNS) of human subjects. Studies are being performed to evaluate mechanisms responsible for the increasing or decreasing nerve fiber growth in the adult CNS. It has been documented that fetal neuronal transplants in adult mammalian brain result in synaptogenesis with beneficial functional effects. These findings, as well as experiments documenting CNS regeneration with evidence of plasticity, have brought new hope to the field of rehabilitation medicine.

Some important topics in neurorehabilitation are discussed below. The principles of rehabilitation of the patient with stroke can also be applied to other neurological disorders of the central nervous system.

Stroke rehabilitation

The estimated prevalence of stroke in the United States population is 1.4 million. Several studies have shown that comprehensive rehabilitation programs improve the functional outcome of stroke patients. Patients receiving comprehensive stroke rehabilitation do better in ambulation, ADL activities, and transfer function. Furthermore, rehabilitation methods help patients (and their families) to cope with their deficits much better.

After determining the etiology of the stroke, emphasis is placed on managing fluid and electrolyte balance, dysphagia, and during the acute phase, bowel and bladder control. In some instances where dysphagia is a prominent feature, a gastroenterologist and/or speech therapy consultant interested in dysphagia can be helpful in organizing the feeding program for the patient. It may be necessary to perform a modified barium swallow videofluoroscopy to evaluate the patient's ability to swallow liquids and solid foods. Many patients may find that a pureed diet of puddings or custards is easier to swallow than liquids. Patients with dysphagia can be trained to produce compensating head and neck movements and perform specific exercises with the help of the speech therapist. Dieticians are helpful in recommending foods with proper consistency that can provide sufficient caloric input. In severe cases of dysphagia it may be necessary to use nasogastric feeding or to perform gastrostomy to provide adequate nutrition for the patient.

To prevent pressure sores, the patient must be turned once every 2 hours and the limbs should be positioned properly. The two most vulnerable areas for development of pressure sores are the ankle and the lateral malleolus. The other areas where pressure sores may develop are over the greater trochanter of the femur, the sacrum, and the coccyx. Once the pressure sore develops, the treatment consists of removing pressure over the area where the sore has developed, high-protein diet, heat-lamp application, and cleansing the area with an antiseptic solution. The application of povidone-iodine is controversial. Plastic surgery with a skin-muscle flap is rarely needed if proper precautions are taken to prevent pressure sores.

Bowel and bladder management is of utmost importance in the acute phase after stroke. For proper bowel management, the patient must receive sufficient fiber or stool softener (e.g., docusate sodium [Colace] 100 mg three times a day). If spontaneous bowel movements do not take place, bisacodyl (Dulcolax) suppositories may be used every other day to regulate bowel evacuation. For proper bladder management it may be necessary to use intermittent catheterization if the residual urine is greater than 100 cc.

If preventive measures with anticoagulant agents are not taken, up to 75% of patients may show evidence of deep vein thrombosis. The risk of venous thrombosis persists as long as the patient is nonambulatory.

Physical and occupational therapy must be started immediately during the acute phase of stroke. Every joint must be given a full range of motion at least once a day. Active assistive exercises should be given whenever possible. If the patient is able to cooperate, an occupational therapist can train the patient to use the unaffected limb (as much as possible) for activities of daily living. Speech therapists are helpful for teaching proper methods for communication with the patient and management of dysphagia.

In the subacute phase the patient can be transported to physical therapy, occupational therapy, speech therapy, and cognitive rehabilitation therapy programs for the rehabilitation treatment. Starting with "mat exercises," physical therapists gradually use different forms of therapies based on established techniques (e.g., Bobath, Rood, Brunnstrum, Knott and Voss) either to increase or decrease tone in appropriate muscles or suppress and/or enhance associated movements. Although different proprioceptive neuromuscular techniques are used, no one particular method of treatment has been proved to be superior to others. A skilled physical therapist usually uses a combination of these techniques to develop the best possible motor performance in the hemiparetic limbs. Once the patient is able to develop good sitting balance and turn on the mat, it is usually possible to start ambulation training at the fixed hemibar or parallel bars. The patient progresses from periods of standing with the help of parallel bars or a hemibar to walking with the help of a cane. During this phase the patient is evaluated for bracing as necessary. By the time of discharge most patients need no more than a light polypropylene ankle brace. While the patient is progressing in ambulation it is important to teach the patient simple transfers. The patient should be allowed to go home on a day pass so that family members can adjust and participate in the patient's rehabilitation program.

In addition to receiving physical therapy, the patient is regularly sent to an occupational therapy clinic where he receives cognitive and ADL retraining and training in transfer techniques and wheelchair use, if indicated. Computer-based technology can be used for cognitive rehabilitation for higher-level patients. Dressing using clothing adaptations such as Velcro closure, feeding using special devices such as friction plates, and grooming are taught by occupational therapists. Wheelchair assessment and training can also be done in the occupational therapy department under supervision of a physiatrist. To prevent shoulder subluxation, occupational therapists provide shoulder support in the form of figure-eight support, a Bobath sling, a Brunnstrum support, or modifications of these. It is essential that the patient receive full range of motion of upper extremity joints during these sessions; this is provided by occupational therapists as well as members of the patient's family.

Although controlled scientific studies have produced uncertain results, every patient with dysarthria and dysphasia deserves to be evaluated and treated by a speech therapist. In addition to teaching patients to respond to simple questions, speech therapists can help train the family to cope with the patient's language deficit. As mentioned earlier, speech therapists also contribute significantly to management of dysphagia in patients with stroke.

Shoulder-hand syndrome

Shoulder-hand pain syndrome or reflex sympathetic dystrophy is common in patients with stroke. Many of these patients have proprioceptive sensory loss in the affected upper extremity. The main treatment aims to reduce pain and provide active range of motion to joints of the affected upper extremity. Initially, pain medication consists of nonsteroidal anti-inflammatory agents. Some patients respond to treatment with prednisone, 30-40 mg per day. It is usually not necessary to subject the patient to stellate ganglion blocks, which are recommended by some authors.

Brachial plexus and peripheral nerve injuries

Brachial plexus and peripheral nerve injuries are not uncommon in stroke patients. Detailed electrophysiological studies in the electrodiagnostic laboratory can provide useful information to document lower motor neuron involvement.

Biofeedback

In a controlled study we have found that biofeedback hastens recovery of function of dorsiflexion of the foot, significantly improving the strength, repetitive activity, and active range of motion. However, biofeedback does not affect the course of recovery of function in proximal muscles, such as quadriceps and hamstrings. Biofeedback has also not been useful for treating the control of distal musculature in the upper extremity.

Functional electrical stimulation

The results of functional electrical stimulation to improve strength and active range of motion are controversial. Further studies are needed to evaluate its role in managing spasticity in patients with stroke.

SPASTICITY

The strict physiological definition of spasticity describes it as a motor disorder characterized by a velocity-dependent increase in tonic stretch reflexes ("muscle tone") with exaggerated tendon joints, resulting from hyperexertability of the stretch reflex as one component of the upper-motor-neuron syndrome. This definition has many limitations. The vast majority of patients who have lesions in the spinal cord (e.g., multiple sclerosis) have abnormalities of polysynaptic reflexes resulting in spontaneous flexor spasms and flexor dystonia. This group of patients, who can be treated successfully with pharmacological agents, are excluded from the definition if spasticity is considered an abnormality *only* of the stretch reflex arc.

Baclofen has been found to be the drug of choice for the treatment of spontaneous flexor spasms. Sometimes a combination of lower doses of baclofen and diazepam (Valium) may be more effective than either drug alone. Dantrolene sodium (Dantrium) is reserved for some bedridden patients with severe spasticity, where the goal is to "weaken" the muscles to reduce spasticity and help in the nursing care.

Approximately 2 to 3 months after stroke, patients are ready to be discharged home. The social worker, who works with the family and the patient throughout the inpatient stroke rehabilitation, assesses the structure of family support and financial needs for proper care of the patient at home. During the transition period it is useful to arrange a visiting nurse to be with the patient three or four times a week. If indicated, the patient can be followed up in the outpatient rehabilitation clinic, where he can receive physical, occupational, and speech therapy. However, it must be recognized that the goal of stroke rehabilitation is to make the patient and his family fully responsible for the care of the patient.

MANAGEMENT OF PATIENTS WITH MULTIPLE SCLEROSIS (MS)

There are approximately 200,000 to 500,000 people suffering from MS in the United States; it is one of the commonest causes of severe disability during the young productive years of life. Since no pharmacological agent can cure MS, the best that can be done for these patients is symptomatic treatment with techniques used in rehabilitation medicine. The principles of rehabilitation are similar to those described for the stroke rehabilitation; the neurologist, physiatrist, physical therapist, occupational therapist, speech therapist, social worker, rehabilitation nurse, and neuropsychologist all play important parts in the team effort to rehabilitate the MS patient.

Most patients with MS complain of gait disturbance as a major primary symptom. Gait disturbance is produced by a variety of underlying causes, including weakness (usually upper-motor-neuron type), spasticity, cerebellar or sensory ataxia, or a combination of these factors. As mentioned earlier, spinal spasticity in MS patients responds well to treatment with baclofen. There is no specific treatment for weakness; patients are advised to exercise regularly within the limits of their tolerance to improve endurance. In some instances assistive devices are necessary to improve gait.

There are no pharmacological agents for the treatment of cerebellar ataxia. Some patients improve by performing specific exercises in front of mirrors to provide visual feedback. Some evidence suggests that attaching weights to different appropriate parts of the body may improve motor performance in patients with cerebellar ataxia. If none of these methods work, it may be necessary to train the patient to walk with a cane, crutch, or walker. Patients unable to ambulate safely may have to use a wheelchair.

One of the most disabling symptoms of MS patients is related to bladder dysfunction. The detailed diagnosis and management of the bladder dysfunction is beyond the scope of this chapter but has been well described in reviews of neurorehabilitation (see Scheinberg 1987). Not infrequently, urinary symptoms are accompanied by bowel dysfunction in these patients. Most patients complain of constipation as the primary symptom. Principles of management of bowel dysfunction are similar to those described for stroke rehabilitation.

In some patients with severe neurologic impairment, dysarthria and dysphagia may require treatment by a speech pathologist. Fortunately these symptoms are not frequently severe enough to cause a major disability for MS patients. Pressure sores develop in approximately 15% of the patients with MS, and every effort should be made to prevent their occurrence as described previously in this chapter.

BRAIN INJURY REHABILITATION

Whereas at one time physical restoration was the emphasis in brain injury rehabilitation, in recent years the focus has been on cognitive and behavioral aspects. However, it should be recognized that it is not possible to treat cognitive deficits without influencing the patient's behavioral, social, and motor functions. Cognitive remediation after brain injury, along with new pharmacological therapies, has become one of the most exciting areas in neurorehabilitation.

REFERENCES

DeLisa JA et al: Rehabilitation medicine: principles and practice. Philadelphia, 1988, Lippincott.

Scheinberg L and Shahani BT, editors: Neurologic clinics. Philadelphia, 1987, Saunders.

Shahani BT, editor: Electromyography in CNS disorders: central EMG. Boston, 1984, Butterworth.

CHAPTER

134 Ocular Manifestations of Neurologic Disorders

John E. Carter

ABNORMALITIES OF VISION

The neural networks involved in processing vision and eye movements are complex and involve multiple areas of the nervous system, including the retina, several cranial nerves and many regions of the cortex, hemispheric white matter, and brainstem. The basic anatomy and physiology of the visual and ocular motor system is clearly understood. Consequently, the physician who learns the anatomy and common diseases of these systems has invaluable knowledge for understanding many neurologic disease processes.

Many instances of visual loss are caused by local ocular disease. Other visual disturbances, some with visible funduscopic changes and some with normal-appearing eyes, are only one part of a larger neurologic condition. The temporal profile of the visual loss, the characteristics of the visual deficit, and the funduscopic appearance are all important in establishing a diagnosis.

Patient's history

The nature of a lesion causing visual loss is most likely to be indicated by an accurate history. What did the patient first notice: a film over the eye, dirty glasses, looking through a fog? An observant patient may report changes in the color of objects or difficulty with tuning a color television. Bumping into objects on one side may lead to awareness of a visual field defect. Is the disturbance throughout the visual field or in one specific area? Are the symptoms in one or both eyes? What happens when each eye is covered individually? Both formed and unformed visual hallucinations are common in patients with visual loss, but these patients may be reluctant to mention them unless specifically questioned.

The temporal profile of the visual loss is most important. When did the patient first become aware of the problem? Difficulty in establishing this point often means that a slowly progressive lesion is present. Sudden onset, on the other hand, suggests a vascular cause. It is important, however, to determine how the patient first noticed the visual loss. If the patient happened to cover one eye and suddenly became aware of visual loss in the other eye, the loss is often interpreted as an acute change by the patient when it may have been present for some time. How long did it take the deficit to become maximal? Is it improving, stable, or continuing to worsen? If the visual loss is intermittent, how often does it occur and are there any factors that seem to precipitate it? Fig. 134-1 provides a graphic representation of the temporal profile of the major processes causing visual loss.

Clinical evaluation

The patient's best acuity should be obtained with glasses on, and if not 20/20, the acuity may be further tested by having the patient look through a pinhole in a card. If there is no ocular pathology and the best corrected acuity is less than 20/20, a neurologic cause must be sought.

Color vision is tested with Ishihara or American Optical color plates and is most useful in diagnosing an optic neuropathy. With lesions of the optic nerve, color vision becomes abnormal before there is any loss of visual acuity or is abnormal out of proportion to the acuity loss.

The pupillary reaction to light may be abnormal as a result of a lesion of the efferent limb of the reflex in the third nerve, in which case the consensual reaction is still present and normal. An afferent limb pupillary defect indicates a lesion of the optic nerve; the response to light is smaller, less brisk, and often unsustained.

Confrontation visual field testing is performed with the examiner seated in front of the patient. The important areas to explore are the horizontal and vertical meridians (Fig.

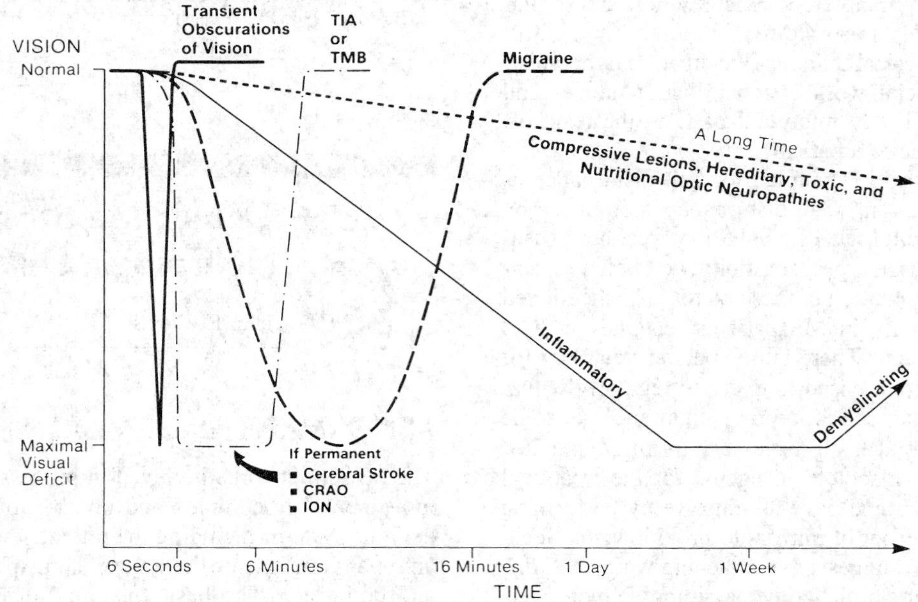

Fig. 134-1. Temporal profile of visual loss caused by different disease processes. *TIA*, transient ischemic attack; *TMB*, transient monocular blindness; *CRAO*, central retinal artery occlusion (retinal infarction); *ION*, ischemic optic neuropathy. Idiopathic demyelinating optic neuritis is the most common inflammatory optic neuropathy and has a good prognosis for recovery, whereas more specific inflammatory processes such as infections or systemic arteritis are less likely to be associated with good recovery. (From Carter JE: Visual field defects. In Taylor RB, editor: Difficult diagnosis. Philadelphia, 1985, Saunders. Reproduced with permission.)

134-2). The left and right sides of the vertical meridian are compared superiorly and inferiorly; then superior and inferior areas are compared along the horizontal meridian. These comparisons should allow the examiner to detect a qualitative difference in function in the two eyes (e.g., a central scotoma or optic nerve lesion), in the superior and inferior fields of an individual eye (altitudinal defect), or in the left and right hemifields of each eye (either bitemporal or homonymous hemianopia).

Examination of the fundus with the direct ophthalmoscope should be done after dilating the pupils. Tropicamide 1% provides good dilation for a short duration.

OCULAR VASCULAR DISEASE IN NEUROLOGY

Three syndromes reflecting ocular circulatory insufficiency have neurologic implications: amaurosis fugax (or transient monocular blindness), retinal artery occlusion, and ischemic optic neuropathy. Retinal arterial emboli may be found in association with any of these syndromes or may be an incidental finding.

Retinal arterial emboli occur in three common compositions: platelet-fibrin aggregates, cholesterol crystals (Hollenhorst plaques), and calcific emboli. Platelet-fibrin aggregates disintegrate within a few minutes or less and therefore are seen only when the patient has an episode of amaurosis fugax while being examined. A column of white material is seen in the retinal arterial tree, where it stops briefly at an arterial bifurcation, pulsating with the heart, and then breaks up into smaller columns and moves along the arteries to the next bifurcation. Shortly after this material disappears, the vision begins to return, and the retina and optic disc become hyperemic.

Cholesterol crystals are the most common arterial emboli observed in the eye (Fig. 134-3). They can occlude the artery and cause retinal infarction. However, they are flat crystals and typically lodge at arterial bifurcations that are too narrow for their width, but blood is able to flow over the top and bottom surfaces without causing symptoms. Cholesterol crystals are highly refractile and yellow in color. They often appear to be larger than the vessel in which they lie, reflecting the fact that the vessel walls themselves are not visible; rather, it is the column of blood that is observed during fundoscopy. Cholesterol emboli may lodge at one location permanently or may disappear between examinations; they are an important indicator of risk for future stroke and for future coronary artery disease and death.

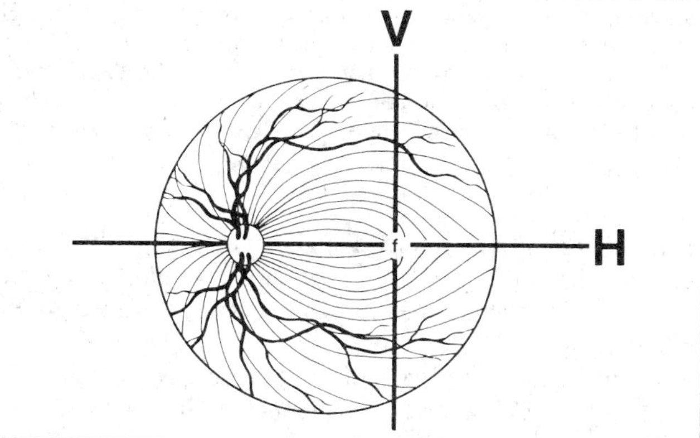

Fig. 134-2. The pattern of the retinal circulation and the relationship of the circulation, optic disc, and fovea *(f)* to the vertical *(V)* and horizontal *(H)* meridians of the visual field.

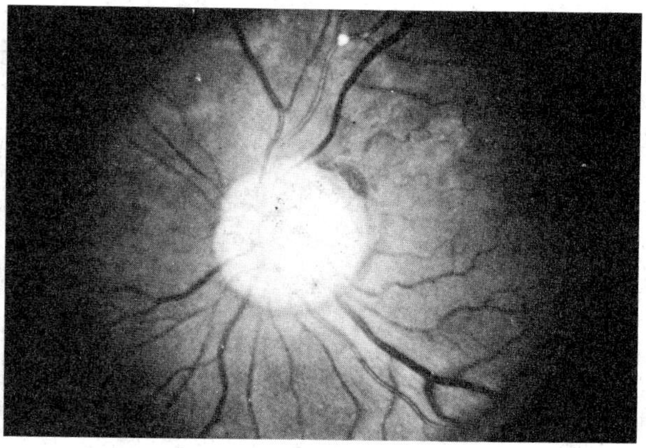

A

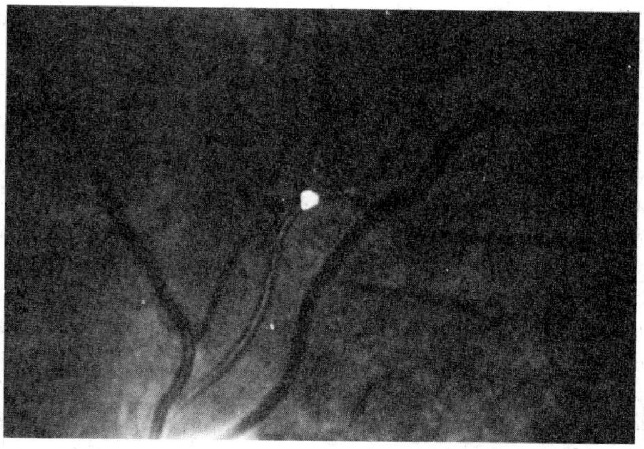

B

Fig. 134-3. A and **B**, A cholesterol crystal embolus lodged at an arterial bifurcation.

Calcific emboli are much less common and consist of whitish-gray clumps of material (Fig. 134-4) that usually lodge in the retinal arteries between bifurcations. They are often the product of calcific cardiac valvular disease, but may be seen associated with carotid atherosclerosis. All forms of retinal emboli are serious indicators of potential stroke.

Transient monocular blindness, or amaurosis fugax, consists of sudden loss of vision in one eye. Vision may simply fade out, or there may be the sensation of a shade being drawn across the eye, usually from top to bottom. The visual loss usually lasts for 2 to 10 minutes and either fades back in or resolves in a manner similar to a shade being

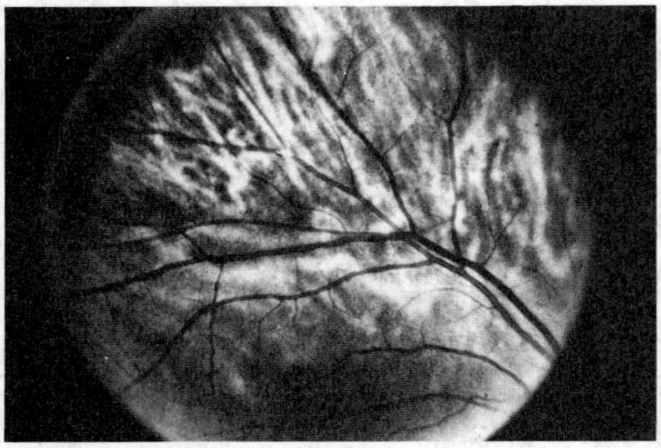

Fig. 134-4. An amorphous clump of calcific material that has lodged at an arterial bifurcation.

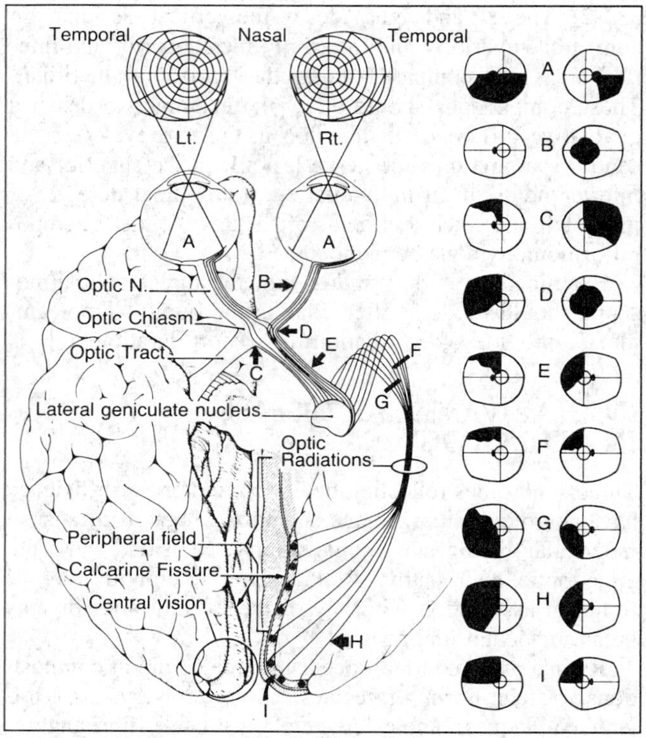

Fig. 134-5. A, Two examples of altitudinal visual field defects that could be caused either by occlusion of a superior branch of the central retinal artery or by an episode of ischemic optic neuropathy involving the superior optic disc. On the left is a large field defect involving both lower quadrants. On the right the injury is more limited and the defect involves only the temporal quadrant, but it connects with the blind spot and does not go to fixation or have a border at the vertical meridian. **B,** A central scotoma in the visual field of the right eye caused by a lesion of the right optic nerve. **C,** Bitemporal hemianopia caused by a lesion of the optic chiasm. The asymmetry is typical of chiasmal field defects until a late stage, when the hemianopia may be complete in both eyes. **D,** Junctional scotoma, that is, a central scotoma on the side of a lateral chiasmal lesion with a temporal hemianopia in the visual field of the opposite eye. **E,** Markedly incongruous homonymous hemianopia seen with a lesion of the optic tract. **F,** Homonymous superior quadrantanopia seen with lesions of the optic radiations in the temporal lobe. **G,** Homonymous inferior quadrantanopia seen with lesions of the superior optic radiations in the low parietal or parietotemporal lobe junction. **H,** Congruous homonymous hemianopia seen with lesions either of the optic radiations close to their termination or of the calcarine cortex itself. **I,** Precise inferior quadrantanopia seen if an occipital lobe lesion involves just the superior bank of the calcarine cortex.

pulled up. Transient monocular blindness is the ocular equivalent of transient ischemic attack. Identical symptoms have been described in migraine, with Raynaud's phenomenon, and in young patients with no known cause. Therefore, transient monocular blindness as an indicator of carotid system ischemia is limited to the stroke-aged population and conditions predisposing to stroke at a young age. Even in the stroke-aged population, about 40% of patients with transient monocular blindness have normal carotid angiograms. Since the fundus is usually normal between episodes, diagnosis of transient monocular blindness is made from history alone.

When ischemia is not transient and infarction with permanent visual loss occurs, the cause is either occlusion of the central retinal artery or one of its branches or ischemic optic neuropathy. In either case the characteristic pattern of visual loss is the result of damage to the retinal ganglion cell axons. Within the eye the ganglion cell axons must swing above and below the fovea to reach the optic nerve (see Fig. 134-2). This arcuate pattern of the ganglion cell axons effectively divides the retina and its respective visual field into superior and inferior halves. This division occurs along a horizontal line drawn through the point of visual fixation and the optic disc and is referred to as the *horizontal meridian*. The vascular supply of the retina is the central retinal artery and its branches, which also follow this arcuate pattern. The blood supply of the optic disc itself does not come from the central retinal artery but rather from short, penetrating arterioles derived from the posterior ciliary arteries. These arterioles supply individual segments of the optic disc, and vascular injury here produces a discrete visual field defect whose location is related to the group of nerve fiber bundles that have been damaged. This characteristic distribution of the nerve fibers and the blood supply within the eye provides localization of altitudinal visual field defects (i.e., visual field defects that lie in one vertical half of the visual field with a sharp border at the horizontal meridian [Fig. 134-5, *A*]) to the eye itself. The other disease that can destroy large numbers of nerve fibers at the optic disc is glaucoma, which may progress insidiously to produce a large altitudinal field defect. The intraocular pressure must be determined to exclude glaucoma.

Central retinal artery occlusion produces infarction of the entire retina. The arteries are attenuated, and the retina is a milky color. This complication may be caused by nonembolic occlusion of the central retinal artery as it enters the eye through the lamina cribrosa, or it may be associated with emboli from the carotid arteries or heart. When emboli are in the fundus, the likelihood of finding major occlusive disease in the carotid system is higher. Occlusion of a branch of the retinal artery (Fig. 134-6) is almost always caused by an embolus, even if the embolus is no longer present and visible. Retinal branch arterial occlusion has the same significance as a visible embolus.

Ischemic optic neuropathy consists of infarction of the optic nerve at the optic disc. The entire optic disc may be involved, producing monocular blindness, but more often only a segment of the disc is infarcted, producing an altitudinal visual field defect. The appearance funduscopically is that of a normal retina with a swollen optic disc. The swelling is characteristically pale, lacking the hyperemia seen with optic neuritis or papilledema (Fig. 134-7). However, the area of pale swelling may include only a segment of the disc while the remainder of the disc exhibits secondary hyperemic swelling (Fig. 134-8). Most ischemic optic neuropathy is idiopathic, but it may be caused by temporal arteritis.

Most patients with nonarteritic ischemic optic neuropathy are between 55 and 70 years old, but they may be as young as 40. These patients are generally healthy, although hypertension and diabetes are common findings. Ischemic optic neuropathy occasionally occurs in association either with occlusion of the internal carotid artery or with multiple cholesterol emboli in the retinal arterioles. Emphasis should be on control of hypertension. Idiopathic ischemic optic neuropathy seldom occurs a second time in the same eye, but 20% to 40% of patients have a subsequent episode in the other eye.

Temporal arteritis is commonly diagnosed because of an episode of ischemic optic neuropathy. Most patients are over 70 years old. Other symptoms of temporal arteritis, such as progressively worsening headaches, jaw claudication, polymyalgia rheumatica, night sweats, anemia, or fever of unknown etiology, may be relatively mild. As many as 40% of patients with temporal arteritis may experience visual loss. Sixty-five percent of patients who present with ischemic optic neuropathy caused by temporal arteritis in one eye experience visual loss in the other eye, often within 24 hours and usually within the first week, if they are not

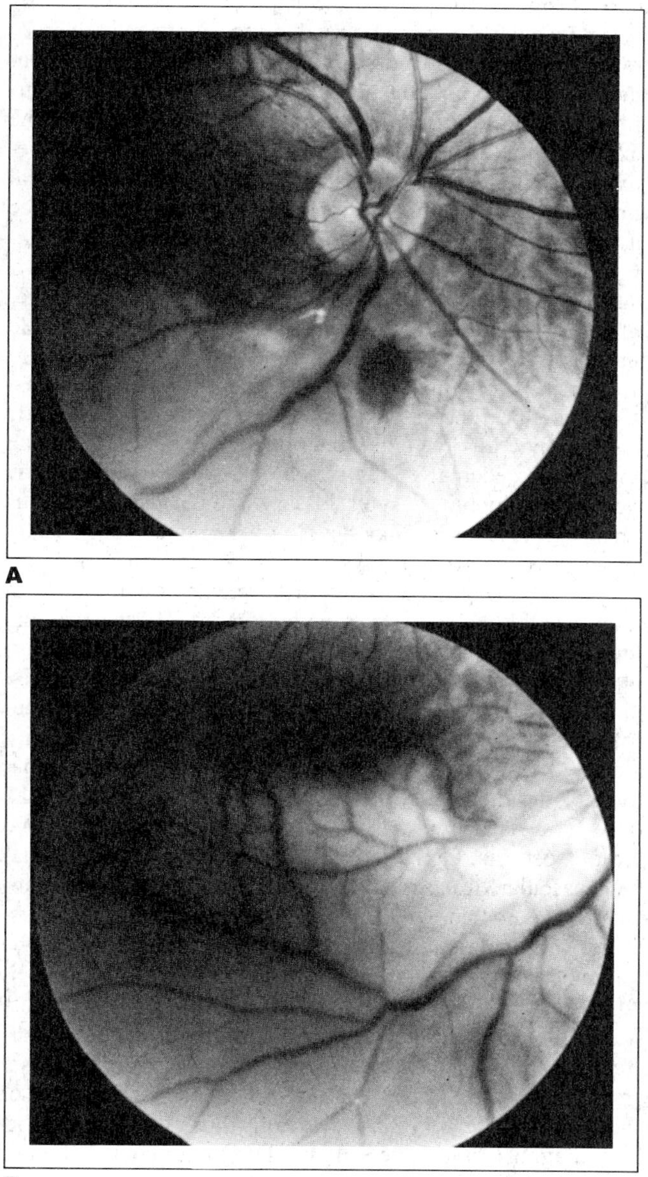

A

B

Fig. 134-6. A, An embolus at an arterial bifurcation. The resulting ischemia has produced an intraretinal hemorrhage below the optic disc and a pale, infarcted retina distal to the embolus and extending across the inferior retina below the fovea in **B.** (From Carter JE: Visual field defects. In Taylor RB, editor: Difficult diagnosis. Philadelphia, 1985, Saunders. Reproduced with permission.)

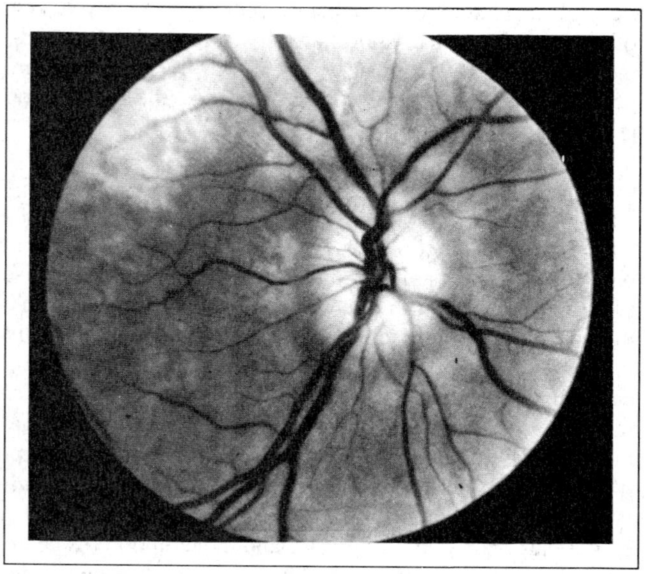

Fig. 134-7. Pallor and swelling of the entire optic disc in an elderly lady with sudden total visual loss and ischemic optic neuropathy caused by temporal arteritis. Compare the inner area of this optic disc with the hyperemic central area optic disc swelling caused by papilledema or optic neuritis in Fig. 134-9. (From Carter JE: Ophthalmic and neuro-ophthalmic aspects of headache. In Packard RC, editor: Neurologic clinics, vol 1. Philadelphia, 1983, Saunders. Reproduced with permission.)

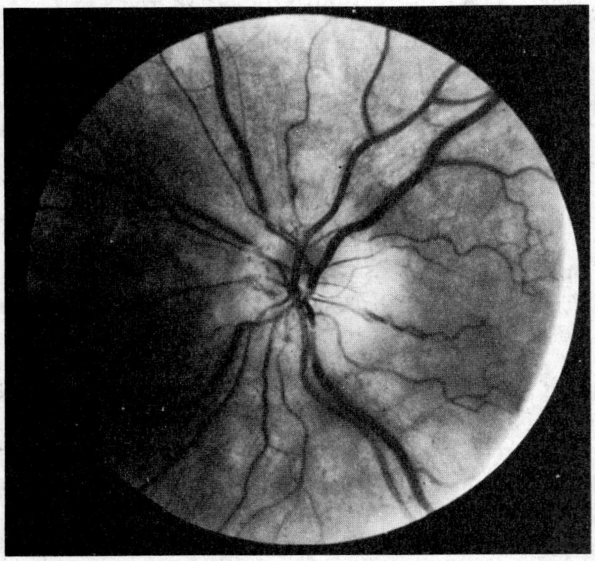

Fig. 134-8. Ischemic optic neuropathy with loss of the superior visual field. Note that the inferior aspect of the optic disc is pale, while superiorly the disc is also swollen but remains adequately perfused and does not exhibit pallor. (From Carter JE: Visual field defects. In Taylor RB, editor: Difficult diagnosis. Philadelphia, 1985, Saunders. Reproduced with permission.)

treated. A history suggestive of this disorder should prompt therapy with corticosteroids pending a temporal artery biopsy. In a patient with ischemic optic neuropathy but no other symptoms of temporal arteritis, the erythrocyte sedimentation rate should be determined. A value above 40 mm per hour justifies the use of corticosteroids until a temporal artery biopsy is performed.

Papilledema

An arbitrary distinction is made between disc edema from other causes and papilledema. Papilledema is passive disc swelling secondary to increased intracranial pressure transmitted to the optic discs by the cerebrospinal fluid (CSF) in the subarachnoid space surrounding the optic nerves. Except for transient obscurations of vision (i.e., episodes of monocular visual loss lasting a few seconds), visual function is normal until the late stages of chronic atrophic papilledema. Papilledema is often asymmetric but seldom unilateral. Elevation and blurring of the disc margins is seen earliest superiorly and inferiorly, and the temporal disc margin is the last to be affected. The optic disc is hyperemic. The veins are dilated and tortuous, and the vessels may be indistinct at the disc margin where they are obscured by the swollen nerve fiber layer of the retina. Venous pulsations are not seen, although they are also absent in 20% of normal individuals. If present, venous pulsations indicate a CSF pressure of 220 mm or less. Nerve fiber layer hemorrhages (splinter and flame-shaped hemorrhages), nerve fiber layer infarcts (cotton-wool spots), and exudates may all be present as the papilledema becomes more severe (Fig. 134-9).

Papilledema is usually the result of chronic elevation of intracranial pressure, although it may develop within a few hours after subarachnoid or intracerebral hemorrhage.

Benign intracranial hypertension typically causes papilledema (see Chapter 136).

Optic neuritis and optic neuropathies

Retinal ganglion cell axons enter the optic nerve in an orderly fashion. Those from the papillomacular bundle carrying macular or central visual information enter temporally, but assume a more uniform distribution throughout the optic nerve as they progress toward the brain. Axons from the papillomacular bundle make up the majority of the axons within the optic nerve. Clinically, the optic nerve behaves as though it were primarily carrying central visual information. Therefore, lesions of the optic nerve produce a combination of the following: loss of visual acuity, diminished color perception, diminished brightness of the visual environment (visual dimming), defective pupillary reaction to light, and a depression of the central visual field in a central scotoma (see Fig. 134-5, *B*).

When the findings indicate an optic neuropathy, the history is the best indicator of the nature of the process. Optic neuritis may involve either the optic nerve head, producing visible disc edema, or the retrobulbar portion of the optic nerve, producing visual loss without visible fundus changes. Visual loss may develop very rapidly but usually progresses for several days to a week, and an aching orbital pain exacerbated by eye movements is common. Vision usually begins to improve by the end of 2 weeks, and most patients experience good visual recovery. The majority of cases occur in patients 20 to 40 years old and are unilateral. In patients less than 20 years of age, optic neuritis is commonly bilateral. Optic neuritis is usually idiopathic, but is occasionally caused by contiguous inflammation of the meninges, orbit, or paranasal sinuses and may also be caused by syphilis, sarcoidosis, tuberculosis, and cryptococcosis. Optic neuritis is occasionally seen in collagen vascular diseases such as systemic lupus erythematosus. If there is no evidence of a systemic inflammatory disease or inflammation in structures along the course of the optic nerve, the patient may be followed expectantly. If visual recovery begins within 2 to 3 weeks, further diagnostic studies may be unnecessary. Corticosteroids do not affect the final outcome of idiopathic optic neuritis, but they may temporarily improve visual function in some cases of neoplastic optic nerve compression, thus delaying the correct diagnosis. Optic neuritis is a common manifestation of multiple sclerosis, but in a patient who has no past history of neurologic dysfunction the diagnosis of multiple sclerosis is not justified.

Optic nerve compression may be caused by neoplastic, aneurysmal, or cystic mass lesions and is usually unilateral. Diffuse infiltrative lesions such as sarcoidosis, lymphoma, or leukemia may affect one or both optic nerves in the or-

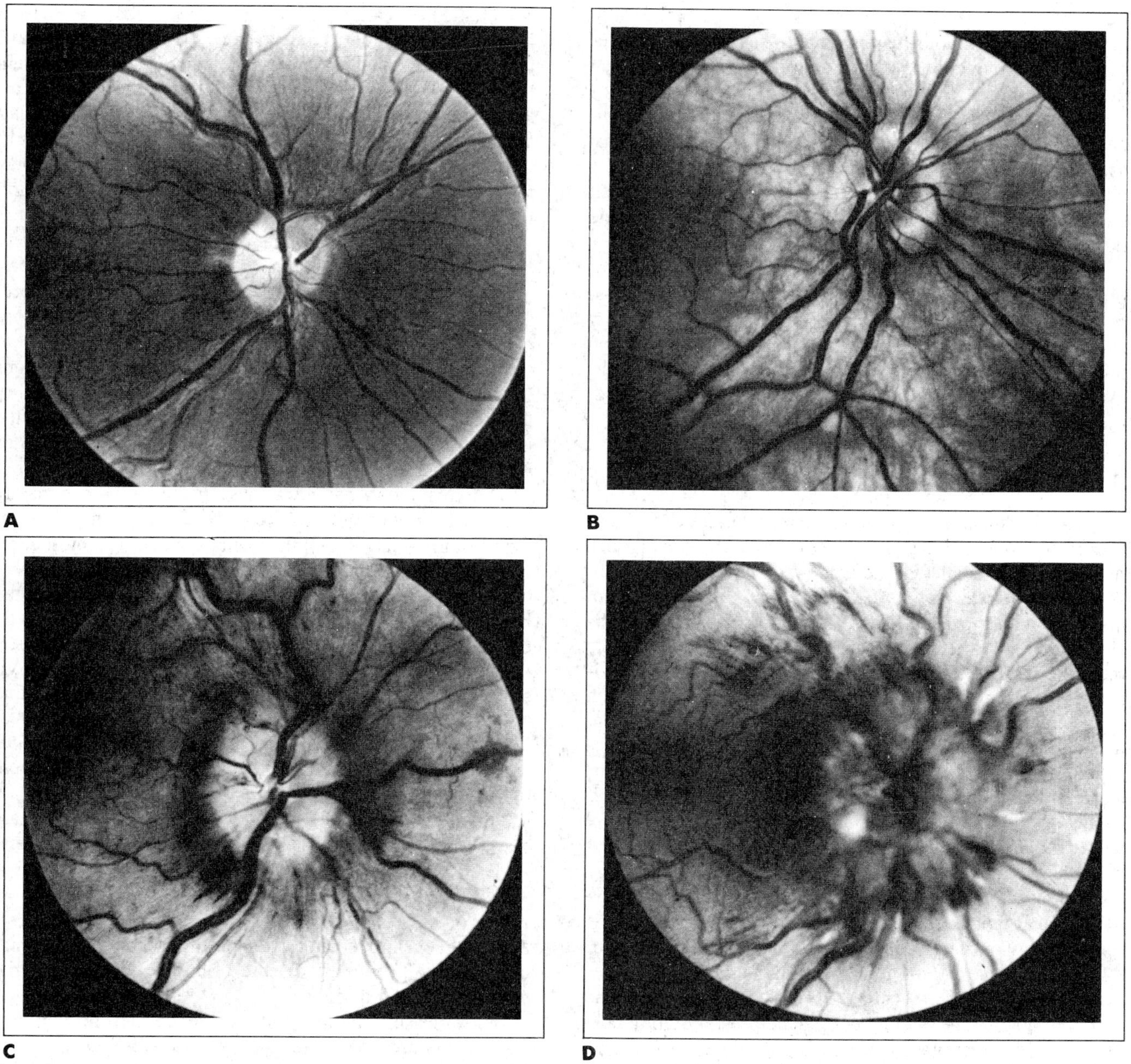

Fig. 134-9. A, A normal optic disc with the macula to the left of the disc. The arcuate fibers enter the disc superiorly and inferiorly and make the nerve fiber layer thicker and the disc margins less clearly visualized in these two quadrants. The earliest changes in papilledema will be seen in these quadrants. The nerve fiber layer at the nasal quadrant on the right in the picture is intermediate in thickness, and the disc margin is more clearly seen, but not as sharply as the temporal quadrant on the left where the nerve fiber layer is thinnest. **B,** Mild disc edema in a patient with pseudotumor cerebri. There is marked hyperemia and opacification of the peripapillary nerve fiber layer. **C** and **D** illustrate progressively more severe swelling of the optic disc, with splinter hemorrhages located in the nerve fiber layer and cotton-wool spots, which are microinfarctions of the nerve fiber layer. (From Carter JE: Ophthalmic and neuroophthalmic aspects of headache. In Packard RC, editor: Neurologic clinics, vol 1. Philadelphia, 1983, Saunders.)

bit or intracranially. Meningeal carcinomatosis frequently affects the optic nerves bilaterally. Insidious and slowly progressive bilateral loss of vision with central scotomas suggests a toxic or nutritional optic neuropathy or hereditary optic atrophy.

Chiasmal disease

At the optic chiasm all visual axons from the nasal half of each retina cross to the contralateral side. A unilateral visual system lesion posterior to the chiasm causes a visual field defect that affects one lateral half of the visual field in each eye (homonymous hemianopia). These visual field defects should not cross the vertical meridian that runs through the fixation point (see Fig. 134-2).

A lesion of the chiasm produces a bitemporal hemianopia that is often asymmetric (Fig. 134-5, *C*). The chiasm is not an isolated structure, however, and a laterally placed lesion may give a combination of optic nerve deficit on the ipsilateral side and a temporal hemianopia on the other (Fig. 134-5, *D*).

Most chiasmal visual disturbances are caused by compression and are usually the result of pituitary adenomas, craniopharyngiomas, and suprasellar meningiomas. Other neoplastic processes that can produce chiasmal dysfunction include optic glioma, teratoma, and metastases, as well as cysts, vascular malformations, demyelinating disease, trauma, infarction, and arachnoiditis.

Retrochiasmic disease

Behind the chiasm all visual information relates to the contralateral visual field. Lesions behind the chiasm produce homonymous visual field defects (Fig. 134-5, *E* to *I*). Incongruous field defects are homonymous but of different degree in the two eyes (Fig. 134-5, *E*). This defect indicates a lesion either of the optic tract or of anterior optic radiations where the axons from the same area of the visual field of the two eyes have not yet moved close to each other. Farther posteriorly, and in the occipital lobe where these fibers synapse in adjacent areas, a lesion creates a congruous visual field defect (Fig. 134-5, *H*). Since the vertical meridian splits the fixation point, and since either half of the fovea is capable of maximal visual resolution, visual acuity is normal even with a complete, unilateral homonymous hemianopia.

Lesions of the optic tract cause incongruous homonymous visual field defects. Since the optic tracts encircle the midbrain, associated brainstem abnormalities are expected. After leaving the lateral geniculate nucleus, the most inferior fibers of the optic radiations run forward around the temporal horn of the lateral ventricle before continuing posteriorly to the occipital lobe. Lesions here create a homonymous superior quadrantanopia (Fig. 134-5, *F*). The most superior fibers of the optic radiations run in the inferior parietal lobe, where lesions produce a homonymous inferior quadrantanopia (Fig. 134-5, *G*). A discrete lesion in the occipital lobe produces a homonymous visual field defect that is identical in the two eyes (Fig. 134-5, *H*). The optic radiations synapse in the calcarine cortex, which lies on the medial surface of the occipital lobe, is split into superior and inferior banks by the calcarine fissure. The superior bank receives all information originating in the inferior half of the visual field, and the inferior bank receives information from the superior field. A lesion limited to one of the banks is the only lesion likely to produce a visual field defect that occupies exactly one quadrant of the homonymous visual fields (Fig. 134-5, *I*).

The majority of patients with symptomatic homonymous visual field defects have vascular lesions, usually within the occipital lobe. Other patients may have substantial visual field defects without being aware of them and may have vascular or neoplastic lesions anywhere along the visual pathways. Because both left and right posterior cerebral arteries have a common origin from the basilar artery, bilateral infarction of the occipital lobes may occur. The resulting visual loss affecting both visual fields in both eyes may resemble bilateral optic nerve lesions. However, the pupil reactions to light are normal.

Lesions of the dominant hemisphere that disrupt projections from the occipital lobe to the parietal and temporal lobes may create an inability to read while writing is preserved (alexia without agraphia), or an inability to recognize objects visually despite the preserved ability to identify them by sound or feel (visual agnosia). Similar lesions of the nondominant hemisphere may produce an inability to recognize familiar faces despite the ability to identify the persons by their voices (prosopagnosia). These conditions are accompanied by a homonymous hemianopia.

Unlike auditory hallucinations, visual hallucinations are not usually indicative of psychiatric illness and can occur with lesions at any site in the visual system. The most common neurologic process causing visual hallucinations is classic migraine, which produces unformed hallucinations. Formed visual hallucinations, that is, recognizable objects, places, or people, occur only with lesions in the central nervous system, usually anterior to the calcarine cortex in visual association areas. Occasionally patients complain that an object or face they have just seen persists in the visual field (palinopia), or that when an object is seen it is reduplicated once or many times, creating a cerebral diplopia or polyopia. All of these "positive" visual phenomena are usually indicative of an ongoing pathologic process and are almost always accompanied by a homonymous hemianopia.

ABNORMALITIES OF EYE MOVEMENT

Abnormal eye movements often provide localizing information about both primary disease of the nervous system and various systemic diseases.

With the exception of convergence, all normal eye movements are conjugate: that is, the two eyes move an equal distance in the same direction. Most cases in which an abnormality of eye movement is the primary neurologic problem involve an acquired weakness of one of the extraocular muscles that results in diplopia. This paralytic strabismus is distinguished from nonparalytic strabismus, which is usually congenital and is caused by an inherent imbalance of tone in the extraocular muscles. During the developmental period the brain is capable of suppressing the visual image from one of the two eyes to prevent diplopia. If nonparalytic strabismus is not corrected early, this suppression may produce a permanent loss of visual acuity referred to as amblyopia ex anopia. In the adult with disconjugate eye position, the absence of diplopia and the presence of diminished visual acuity in one eye, without other signs of retinal or optic nerve disease, indicate the presence of a congenital rather than an acquired strabismus. Acquired disconjugate eye movements with associated diplopia are most likely to be caused by injury to one of the ocular motor nerves (i.e., cranial nerves III, IV, and VI), myasthenia gravis, skew deviation, or dysthyroid myopathy.

Ocular motor nerve disorders

An isolated palsy of one of the ocular motor nerves is the most common cause of acquired disconjugate eye movements and diplopia. Head trauma is a common cause of third-, fourth-, and sixth-nerve palsies, and it presents no diagnostic difficulty. Other identifiable causes are aneurysms; neoplasms; infections such as meningitis, encephalitis, otitis, ethmoiditis, or syphilis; postinfectious cases associated with a viral illness; collagen vascular diseases; multiple sclerosis; and complications of surgery. There is a large group in whom the injury is assumed to be ischemic secondary to atherosclerotic or diabetic vascular disease and another large group in whom the injury is idiopathic. The primary concern is to distinguish between patients in these latter two groups, who generally recover in 2 or 3 months, and those in whom ocular motor palsy is the presenting sign of a neoplasm or an intracranial aneurysm. Pain may be a prominent complaint in all of these conditions, but the pain should resolve within a few days in patients with benign etiologies. Table 134-1 shows the frequency of the various causes of ocular motor palsies.

Sixth-nerve palsy. A sixth-nerve palsy produces horizontal diplopia, most notable when the patient looks at distant objects. An esotropia is present on examination, and the diplopia worsens when the eyes are moved in the direction of the weak lateral rectus muscle. A lesion of the sixth-nerve nucleus or its axons in the brainstem is associated with other neurologic abnormalities. Table 134-1 details the most common causes of isolated sixth-nerve palsies. While the majority of sixth-nerve palsies are benign, the sixth nerve has a long course next to bony structures as it travels up the base of the skull, and involvement by metastatic tumor, especially by direct invasion from the nasopharynx, is common enough that patients with a sixth-nerve palsy should have computed tomography with attention to bony detail at the base of the skull. Increased intracranial pressure from any cause can produce a sixth-nerve palsy as a false localizing sign. Sixth-nerve palsies can occur as the result of a subarachnoid hemorrhage, but are rarely the presenting sign of an unruptured intracranial aneurysm.

Table 134-1. Frequency of causes of impaired function of the ocular motor nerves

Cause	Sixth cranial nerve (%)	Fourth cranial nerve (%)	Third cranial nerve (%)
Undetermined	24	31	24
Head trauma	14	31	14
Neoplasm	21	5	13
Ischemic	15	22	20
Intracranial aneurysm	3	1	17
Other	23	10	12

Fourth-nerve palsy. Fourth-nerve palsy produces vertical or oblique diplopia that is worse when looking down. The central nervous system attempts to compensate for this abnormality, and the resulting pattern of eye movements may be confusing. However, the diplopia of the fourth-nerve palsy should follow a "marching" pattern. The examiner must first determine which of the two eyes is the higher one. The diplopia worsens when the eyes are moved toward the opposite side, and also worsens when the head is tilted toward the side of the high eye. Thus, a right fourth-nerve palsy results in the right eye being higher than the left eye, worsening diplopia when the eyes move to the left side, and worsening diplopia when the patient tilts his or her head to the right side. A left-right-left pattern when the left eye is the higher of the two eyes indicates a left fourth-nerve palsy. Any other pattern in this three-step test indicates a weakness of one of the other vertically active extraocular muscles. If this is the case, and if there are no other signs of third-nerve dysfunction, such as impaired adduction, ptosis, or impaired pupillary reaction to light, the patient most probably has a skew deviation, myasthenia gravis, or dysthyroid myopathy (see below).

Fourth-nerve palsy is the least commonly encountered ocular motor nerve palsy and is the least likely to be associated with a serious disease process (see Table 134-1). Intracranial aneurysm is a very uncommon cause. Neoplasm is also not common, and most patients with a neoplasm have other neurologic signs early on. A limited laboratory evaluation may be undertaken, and the patient can be observed expectantly if the remainder of the neurologic history and examination is normal.

Third-nerve palsy. Third-nerve palsy is recognized by combinations of ptosis, impairment of ocular movements in medial, upward, or downward directions, and impairment of direct and consensual pupil reaction to light. Table 134-1 summarizes the causes of isolated third-nerve palsy. The third nerve is the only ocular motor nerve that is commonly affected by an expanding intracranial aneurysm prior to its rupture, so consideration must be given to performing cerebral arteriography even if computed tomography is normal. The pupillomotor fibers travel superficially in the third nerve and are susceptible to external compressive lesions. Ischemic damage to the third nerve tends to involve the substance of the nerve, sparing the most superficial fibers. Three fourths of patients with ischemic third-nerve palsy have a normal pupillary reaction to light, and less than 5% of patients with an aneurysmal third-nerve palsy have spared pupillary function. Therefore, a patient with diabetes or an older patient with hypertension or atherosclerotic disease and a pupil-sparing third-nerve palsy is unlikely to have an aneurysm. Even if such a patient has a third-nerve palsy with the pupil involved, the frequency of ischemic third-nerve palsy is high enough that the morbidity of cerebral arteriography justifies a period of observation if computed tomography of the head is normal and the spinal fluid is clear.

Combined injury to the ocular motor nerves. Dysfunction of a combination of the third, fourth, and sixth cranial nerves can occur. In general, this parasellar syndrome indicates pathology in the region of the cavernous sinus. Since the ophthalmic division of the trigeminal nerve also runs in the wall of the cavernous sinus, sensory disturbances of the upper face may be seen. Primary neoplasms sometimes occur in this region, but metastatic lesions are more common. Other processes producing the parasellar syndrome include cavernous sinus thrombosis, carotid-cavernous sinus fistula, and aneurysm of the intracavernous carotid artery. If a specific cause cannot be found, the diagnosis of Tolosa-Hunt syndrome may be considered. Tolosa-Hunt t syndrome is a nonspecific inflammation of the cavernous sinus and responds dramatically to corticosteroids.

Skew deviation. Skew deviation is an acquired, vertical strabismus caused by a disturbance of vertical eye movement pathways proximal to the ocular motor nerve nuclei. Patients complain of vertical diplopia, but examination demonstrates a pattern of extraocular muscle weakness that is not consistent with weakness of the superior oblique muscle (fourth cranial nerve), and the remaining function of the third nerve is intact, making a lesion of the third cranial nerve unlikely. Skew deviation always indicates a lesion in the posterior fossa and is almost always caused by pathology within the substance of the brainstem or cerebellum rather than by an external, compressive lesion. Skew deviation is frequently associated with an internuclear ophthalmoplegia. In younger patients a skew deviation is most commonly seen in multiple sclerosis, whereas in older patients it is probably caused by a stroke.

Myasthenia gravis. Myasthenia gravis may be the most commonly missed diagnosis in patients presenting with abnormal eye movements. Eighty percent of patients with myasthenia gravis present with symptoms and signs of ocular motor dysfunction. Myasthenia may mimic an internuclear ophthalmoplegia, a sixth-nerve palsy, or a fourth-nerve palsy, or it may present any of the features of a third-nerve palsy except a dilated pupil. The hallmark of myasthenia gravis is ocular ptosis or diplopia, which varies from hour to hour and day to day, typically being variable on successive examinations. Myasthenia gravis should be considered in any patient with disconjugate eye movements.

Dysthyroid ophthalmopathy. Thyroid eye disease, or dysthyroid ophthalmopathy, consists of an infiltration of the extraocular muscles and other orbital contents by inflammatory cells and a mucilaginous ground substance, followed later by fibrosis of orbital tissues. Patients often have diplopia caused by restriction of the extraocular muscles, most commonly the inferior rectus. Forced ductions in which the examiner attempts to manually rotate the eye show that the passive movement of the eye is limited by the involved muscle. Other findings include proptosis, vascular congestion seen over the insertion of the lateral or medial rectus muscle on the globe, lid retraction or lid lag, and edema of the eyelids. Dysthyroid ophthalmopathy can occur in a patient who is hyperthyroid but can also occur in patients who have been treated for hyperthyroidism and are euthyroid or even hypothyroid. It may even occur in patients who have not yet developed other evidence of thyroid disease. Therefore, it is a clinical diagnosis based on the findings of the eyes rather than on laboratory evidence of thyroid dysfunction. Dysthyroid ophthalmopathy is probably the leading cause of unilateral exophthalmos and is the leading cause of bilateral exophthalmos in adults.

Lid retraction, when seen with exophthalmos, is diagnostic of dysthyroid myopathy. Lid retraction by itself, without signs of parkinsonism or dorsal midbrain disease, is also probably caused by dysthyroid myopathy. Computed tomography is often used to demonstrate the enlarged extraocular muscles, but orbital echography is more sensitive. Even if these studies do not demonstrate muscle enlargement, they do not exclude the clinical diagnosis of dysthyroid myopathy.

DISTURBANCES OF CONJUGATE EYE MOVEMENTS

Patients with a disturbance of conjugate eye movements commonly do not experience symptoms, in contrast to patients with disconjugate eye movements that produce diplopia. Conjugate eye movement abnormalities are more often recognized by abnormal signs on examination.

There are three types of conjugate eye movement: saccadic, pursuit, and vestibular. Fast eye movements, or saccades, are refixation eye movements that shift the eyes from one object to another. Saccadic eye movements are modulated by a pathway arising in the frontal lobes anterior to the primary motor cortex. The pathway for rightward gaze arises in the left frontal lobe, descends through the internal capsule to the midbrain reticular formation, decussates in the caudal midbrain at the level of the fourth cranial nerve nucleus, and synapses in the right pontine paramedian reticular formation (PPRF). The PPRF is also known as the para-abducens nucleus or the pontine gaze center. The PPRF is the brainstem integrator or the final common pathway for all conjugate horizontal eye movements. From the right PPRF, the same eye movement output is delivered to the right sixth-nerve nucleus to move the right eye to the right, and, via the medial longitudinal fasciculus, to the medial rectus subnucleus of the left third-nerve nucleus to move the left eye to the right. Thus, impulses arising in the left frontal lobe ultimately move the eyes conjugately to the right. Lesions of the frontopontine pathway for saccadic eye movements are common and, in the acute phase, produce a gaze paresis in which the patient's gaze tends to be tonically deviated in the direction of normal gaze. That is, damage to the left frontal lobe causes a right gaze paresis. The patient cannot voluntarily look to the right, and the eyes spontaneously deviate to the left (toward the injured frontal lobe). Although the patient may be able to voluntarily return his gaze to the midline, he is unable to move his eyes past the midline into the paretic field of gaze. If a single, unilateral lesion is responsible, recovery occurs in a few days or weeks. Consequently, gaze paresis is seen predominantly with acute lesions. During recovery the patient's relaxed gaze returns to the primary position. The eyes can be moved voluntarily in the paretic direction, but this movement often cannot be sustained, and there may be a gaze-evoked nystagmus. Optokinetic nystagmus with the target moving toward the opposite side produces the slow component but no return fast phase. When associated with a hemiparesis, a gaze paresis may be either ipsilateral, indicating a hemispheric lesion, or contralateral, indicating a lesion in the brainstem where the pathway has crossed to the contralateral side.

Pursuit eye movements are modulated by a pathway descending from the occipital cortex close to the lateral ventricle into the midbrain reticular formation to the PPRF. This pathway appears to be uncrossed. A lesion in this pathway produces an absence of optokinetic nystagmus when the target is moving toward the side of the lesion. The lesion may or may not be associated with a homonymous hemianopia on the opposite side. When no homonymous hemianopia is present, the lesion is usually deep in the hemispheric white matter and is more likely to be neoplastic than ischemic.

Conjugate vertical eye movements are bilaterally modulated. They are not usually affected by hemispheric disease unless the disease is bilateral and fairly extensive. Lesions of the pretectum or rostral midbrain tectum produce Parinaud's syndrome (dorsal midbrain syndrome, or Sylvian aqueduct syndrome), consisting of impaired vertical gaze, lid retraction, light-near dissociation of the pupillary reaction, and convergence-retractory nystagmus. Upward gaze progressively diminishes with increasing age, but downward gaze is not affected. Impaired downgaze combined with features of Parkinson's disease is characteristic of progressive supranuclear palsy in which diffuse neuronal degeneration occurs in brainstem motor nuclei.

Impaired vertical movement of a single eye caused by a supranuclear lesion is very uncommon, because of the bilaterality of vertical gaze mechanisms and because of the close anatomic association of the vertical gaze centers in the pretectum and rostral midbrain and the third-nerve nuclei in the rostral midbrain.

Interruption of the medial longitudinal fasciculus between the sixth-nerve nucleus and the contralateral third-nerve nucleus produces an internuclear ophthalmoplegia. On attempted horizontal gaze the adducting eye remains in the primary position or adducts poorly, and the abducting eye exhibits horizontal nystagmus. Since the medial longitudinal fasciculus crosses just rostral to the sixth-nerve nucleus, the interruption is on the side of the eye that fails to adduct. Patients with internuclear ophthalmoplegia may have preserved convergence, demonstrating intact function of the third-nerve nucleus input to the medial rectus. The eyes are usually aligned normally in the primary position so that the patient does not complain of diplopia, although bilateral cases may manifest an exotropia in the acute stage. The absence of ptosis, with normal pupillary action and vertical eye movements, distinguishes these cases from medial rectus weakness caused by a third-nerve palsy. Unilateral or bilateral internuclear ophthalmoplegia in younger adults is a common manifestation of multiple sclerosis.

Nystagmus and other ocular oscillations (Table 134-2)

Nystagmus is a rhythmic, to-and-fro oscillation of the eyes. Jerk nystagmus has clearly defined slow and fast phases and is named for the fast phase. Pendular nystagmus appears to have equally rapid to-and-fro components. Most cases of pendular nystagmus are congenital. Congenital nystagmus is horizontal in the primary position, remains horizontal in vertical gaze positions, appears to convert to jerk nystagmus on lateral gaze, and is decreased by convergence. Congenital nystagmus produces some decrease in visual acuity but does not produce oscillopsia, the sensation of movement of the environment.

The most common nystagmus is gaze-evoked nystagmus. It is seen when the gaze is sustained in an eccentric position. The slow phase is back toward the primary posi-

Table 134-2. Types of nystagmus with localizing value and the common location and cause of the responsible lesions

Type of nystagmus	Common location of responsible lesion	Common causes of responsible lesion
Up-beat nystagmus		
Worse on upgaze	Brainstem or cerebellar vermis	Alcoholic cerebellar degeneration
Worse on downgaze	Medulla or pons	Multiple sclerosis, anticonvulsants, neoplasm
Down-beat nystagmus	Cervicomedullary junction	Cranial malformation, multiple sclerosis, infarction, anticonvulsants, alcoholic cerebellar degeneration, lithium toxicity
Periodic alternating nystagmus	Cervicomedullary junction	Multiple sclerosis, cranial malformation
Seesaw nystagmus	Anterior third ventricle	Neoplasm
Convergence-retractory nystagmus	Dorsal midbrain	Neoplasm, multiple sclerosis
Ocular myoclonus	Dentatorubro-olivary triangle	Infarction, multiple sclerosis
Ocular flutter and opsoclonus	Cerebellar pathways	Brainstem or cerebellar encephalitis, occult neuroblastoma
Ocular bobbing	Pons	Infarction, toxic or metabolic encephalopathy

tion, and the fast phase is in the direction of gaze. Gaze-evoked nystagmus may be present on lateral gaze only or also on upgaze. It is seldom present on downgaze. Gaze-evoked nystagmus is a physiologic nystagmus that is more likely to be seen when the patient is subjected to external factors such as fatigue, drugs, and head trauma. This type of nystagmus has no localizing significance unless it is markedly asymmetric, in which case a brainstem lesion may be suspected.

Vestibular nystagmus may be the result of injury to the peripheral vestibular apparatus or nerve, or injury to the central vestibular pathways. Vestibular nystagmus is present in the primary position and is increased in amplitude when the eyes are moved in the direction of the fast component. This nystagmus is usually horizontal but always has some torsional component, and it remains horizontal even on upgaze. If the lesion is peripheral, the direction of apparent environmental spin is the same as the fast phase of the nystagmus, while the patient past-points and falls toward the side of the slow component. These relationships may not be maintained when the lesion is in the brainstem. Peripheral lesions are more likely to be associated with tinnitus and hearing loss and are more likely to produce acute symptoms and associated nausea and vomiting.

Several varieties of nystagmus are less common but are more important, because they provide specific localizing information and are very likely to be associated with an active process producing acquired changes in the central nervous system. These varieties of nystagmus all exhibit nystagmus in the primary position and are often associated with oscillopsia. Although most of these cases occur with injury anywhere in the brainstem or cerebellum, each is most commonly associated with a lesion in one specific location.

Down-beat nystagmus is present in the primary position. It may be accentuated by downgaze but is most accentuated by moving the eyes to the side and down. Down-beat nystagmus is most commonly associated with a disturbance at the cervicomedullary junction: for example, Arnold-Chiari malformation.

Up-beat nystagmus occurs in two varieties. The first type is a relatively fine up-beating nystagmus in the primary position that increases on downgaze. Like down-beating nystagmus, it is most often associated with a lesion of the medulla. A more coarse up-beating nystagmus that increases on upgaze is seen in association with injury to the anterior vermis of the cerebellum and is commonly seen with alcoholic cerebellar degeneration.

Periodic alternating nystagmus is a horizontal jerk nystagmus that periodically changes direction. It begins with a brief period of no nystagmus lasting a few seconds. Then there is beating to one side, with increasing amplitude followed by decreasing amplitude, until the nystagmus ceases for a few seconds, followed by the same crescendo-decrescendo pattern beating in the other direction. The entire cycle typically lasts 3 to 4 minutes. Periodic alternating nystagmus is also most commonly associated with injury to the medulla.

Convergence-retractory nystagmus is a feature of the dorsal midbrain syndrome; thus, there is associated impaired upgaze. With attempts to look up, especially attempted saccadic upward eye movements, there is a cocontraction of all the extraocular muscles, producing convergence of the two eyes and retraction of the eyes into the orbit. This nystagmus is best elicited with an optokinetic nystagmus target moving downward, which induces downward pursuit movements and repetitive upward saccades that evoke convergence-retractory nystagmus.

Ocular myoclonus describes rhythmic, pendular vertical eye movements, which sometimes accompany palatal myoclonus. These findings indicate disruption of the pathway between the red nucleus, the ipsilateral inferior olivary nucleus, the contralateral dentate nucleus of the cerebellum, and the red nucleus again.

Ocular flutter and opsoclonus are saccadic intrusions during which saccades interrupt fixation. Ocular flutter is a brief flurry of horizontal saccades around fixation; opsoclonus is a burst of conjugate saccadic eye movements in random directions. Both findings are indicative of a lesion in the cerebellar pathways within the cerebellum or brainstem.

Ocular bobbing describes a rapid downward movement of the eyes, followed after a short variable delay by a slow drift of the eyes back to the primary position. This is most often seen in comatose patients with extensive pontine damage. Similar movements with different patterns have been called reverse bobbing when the eyes have a quick movement upward and a slow movement back to the primary position or inverse bobbing when the eyes drift downward followed by a quick movement upward. Inverse bobbing is associated with metabolic encephalopathy.

REFERENCES

Burde RM, Savino PJ, and Trobe JD: Clinical decisions in neuro-ophthalmology. St. Louis, 1985, Mosby.

Ellenberger C: Perimetry: principles, technique, and interpretation. New York, 1980, Raven Press.

Glaser JS: Neuro-ophthalmology, ed 2. Hagerstown, Md, 1990, Harper & Row.

Leigh RJ and Zee DS: The neurology of eye movement. Philadelphia, 1983, Davis.

Miller NR: Walsh and Hoyt's clinical neuro-ophthalmology, vol 1. Baltimore, 1982, Williams & Wilkins.

Miller NR: Walsh and Hoyt's clinical neuro-ophthalmology, vol 2. Baltimore, 1985, Williams & Wilkins.

Paton D, Hyman BN, and Justice J Jr: Introduction to ophthalmoscopy. Kalamazoo, Mich, 1976, The Upjohn Company.

CHAPTER

135 Neurology of the Lower Urinary Tract

Frances M. Dyro

INNERVATION OF THE LOWER URINARY TRACT

Bladder function depends on interaction among sacral parasympathetics, somatic micturition centers, and pontine micturition centers. Cortical regions 6 and 9 of the frontal lobes impose voluntary control over voiding reflexes. The peripheral innervation of the lower urinary tract consists of preganglionic parasympathetic fibers that travel with the pelvic nerves through the inferior hypogastric plexus, then synapse with postganglionic neurons distributed in ganglionic clumps in the adventitia of the detrusor and internal sphincter. Sympathetic fibers originating in the lower thoracic and upper lumbar segments descend along the aorta to form the superior hypogastric plexus. These act to contract the internal sphincter during ejaculation, preventing retrograde ejaculation. The pudendal nerve arises from the anterior primary rami of S2, S3, and S4, with pelvic floor efferents deriving mainly from the S3 and S4 motor roots. The nerve also carries afferents from the posterior urethra. Sensation of bladder fullness as well as painful impulses from the bladder dome and trigone travel along the pelvic nerve.

BLADDER ANATOMY

The bladder is composed of a meshwork of smooth-muscle fibers forming the detrusor and the trigone. The contractile properties of smooth muscle are similar to those of striated muscle, but the velocity of shortening and rate of relaxation are much slower in smooth muscles. The smooth-muscle cells form "tight junctions" representing low-resistance extrasynaptic pathways of excitation (electrical rather than pharmacologic). Distention and stretch of the smooth muscle lowers its transmembrane potential, rendering the muscle cells hyperexcitable as the bladder fills. There is also a nonneural component of bladder tonus attributable to the elastic properties of smooth muscle and collagen.

BLADDER FILLING

Urination is a phenomenon that can be considered in two phases. During the filling phase the detrusor muscle of the bladder is relaxed, and the internal and external sphincters are contracted. The detrusor is kept relaxed by inhibition by parasympathetic cholinergic nerve impulses and stimulation of sympathetic beta-adrenergic impulses. Sphincter and pelvic floor muscle contraction is a function of somatic nerves and sympathetic alpha-adrenergic receptors in the proximal urethra and bladder neck.

Filling of the bladder stimulates the stretch receptors in the detrusor muscle. Afferent information from the stretch receptors is conveyed to the central nervous system via pelvic nerves. This may produce increased efferent discharges in the preganglionic nerves of the thoracolumbar sympathetic outflow, which inhibits efferent transmission across pelvic ganglia. This promotes bladder filling by beta-adrenergically mediated relaxation of the detrusor. Alpha-adrenergic effects increase tone in the proximal urethra.

BLADDER EMPTYING

The normal emptying, or micturition, phase begins when the bladder neck smooth muscle and the striated external sphincter relax in response to inhibition of alpha-adrenergic impulses. Contraction of the detrusor smooth muscle then occurs in response to parasympathetic cholinergic stimulation. Failure of the sphincters to relax as the detrusor contracts is called *dyssynergia*. Continence has active and passive components. Passive continence is a result of resting tonus of the somatic innervated striated sphincters, alpha-adrenergic innervated smooth muscle, and the elastin and collagen of the urethra and pelvic floor. Active continence is the result of voluntary contraction of the sphincter and pelvic floor muscles. Key features and treatment of the major categories of bladder-emptying dysfunction are summarized in Table 135-1.

Reflexes

The baseline activity of muscles of the pelvic floor and the striated sphincter mechanism is increased during increases in intra-abdominal pressure (Valsalva or cough) with cutaneous stimulation of the perineum and with bladder filling. Voiding is initiated by silencing of sphincter activity followed by detrusor contraction. This coordinated or synergic voiding pattern is mediated by pontine nuclei. In lesions below the pons but above the sacral segments, there is dyssynergia or inappropriate contraction of the sphincter in response to detrusor contraction.

PHARMACOLOGY

Anticholinergic agents such as propantheline, imipramine, atropine, and hyoscyamine block muscarinic receptors and inhibit detrusor contractions. These may be used therapeutically to control the urgency and frequency resulting from uninhibited contractions of the bladder. Anticholinergic agents used in the treatment of Parkinson's disease may produce urinary retention by inhibiting detrusor contractions; cholinergics such as bethanecol stimulate muscarinic receptors, increasing detrusor tone and increasing force of contraction in cases in which poor detrusor contraction results in incomplete emptying.

Adrenergic agents such as levarterenol, ephedrine, and phenylephrine stimulate alpha- and beta-adrenergic receptors, causing relaxation of detrusor but tightening of the bladder neck.

Oxybutynin is a smooth-muscle relaxant with adrener-

Table 135-1. Key features and treatment of the major categories of bladder-emptying dysfunction

Dysfunction	Site of lesion	Voiding pattern	Treatment
Detrusor hyperactivity			
Coordinated sphincter	Cerebrum or basal ganglia, dementia, Parkinson's, CVA, multiple sclerosis	Urgency, urge incontinence voiding without awareness	Anticholinergics
External sphincter dyssynergia	Suprasacral spinal cord	Incomplete emptying, low volume, uninhibited contractions	Anticholinergics, intermittent catheterization
Internal sphincter dyssynergia	Cord lesion above T6-T12	Incomplete emptying, autonomic dysreflexia	Phenoxybenzamine, anticholinergics
Detrusor areflexia			
Coordinated sphincter	Sacral cord or cauda equina	Interrupted flow, voiding by straining	Bethanechol, intermittent catheterization, credé
External sphincter overactivity	Sacral cord	Decreased sensation of fullness, voiding by straining	Bethanechol, diazepam, intermittent catheterization
External sphincter denervation	Sacral cord, peripheral nerves, cauda equina	Incontinence, large residual urine	Intermittent catheterization
Poor relaxation of smooth-muscle sphincter	Sacral cord	High capacity	Phenoxybenzamine, bethanechol

gic properties that increases bladder capacity and decreases uninhibited contractions. Drugs used for other reasons may produce bladder dysfunction. Tricyclic antidepressants with anticholinergic properties and calcium channel blockers may produce urinary retention by decreasing detrusor contractibility. Some alpha-adrenergic antagonists, such as pseudoephedrine and phenylpropanolamine in cough remedies, can increase urethral resistance. Alpha-adrenergic antagonists may be used to lower urethral resistance in prostatic obstruction.

VOIDING DYSFUNCTION (Also see Chapters 361 and 370)

Aging

Voiding dysfunction, incontinence, or inability to empty the bladder may be a result of neurologic abnormality or physical or mechanical abnormality. Many structural changes occur with aging. Bladder capacity may be reduced below the lower limit of normal (400 ml). Uninhibited contractions may occur, giving a sense of urgency and uncontrollable loss of varying amounts of urine. This phenomenon is often accompanied by inefficient detrusor contractions, resulting in incomplete emptying and frequent urinary tract infections because of high residual urine volumes.

The outflow obstruction caused by benign prostatic hypertrophy in turn can produce supersensitivity to a range of different agonists of the smooth muscle, analogous to the denervation supersensitivity. The result is frequent contractions of the detrusor but reduced effectiveness of contractions. The patient reports a decreased stream and incomplete emptying.

Following prostatic surgery, incontinence may result from injury to striated or smooth-muscle sphincters. In elderly women, weakened pelvic musculature and damage to the striated sphincter during childbirth or tissue changes secondary to estrogen deficiency result in incontinence during any activity that increases intra-abdominal pressure.

Cortical disease

In cortical disease (cerebrovascular accident, Parkinson's disease, or loss of neural function from diffuse atherosclerotic disease), there may be loss of cortical inhibitory impulses to the bladder. The patient feels the desire to void but is unable to prevent voiding by inhibiting reflex contractions.

ABNORMALITIES OF INNERVATION

Neuropathic bladder

If sensory pathways are interrupted between sacral spinal neurons and cortical centers, there may be loss of sensation of bladder fullness. If the sphincters are functioning, overflow incontinence results when bladder pressure exceeds pressure generated by sphincter contraction. This results in chronic infection, because there is always a high residual urine volume. Intermittent catheterization usually results in a reduction in urinary tract infections and dryness.

Motor paralytic bladder

The atonic neurogenic bladder is often caused by the peripheral neuropathy of diabetes or alcoholism but may be the result of trauma or pelvic surgery. Sphincter weakness may be caused by damage to pudendal nerves or sacral roots, or by trauma to the sphincter during childbirth or with perineal injuries.

Dyssynergia

Outflow obstruction occurs when the detrusor contraction fails to inhibit sphincter contraction. This dyssynergia is seen in spinal cord and bilateral cortical lesions. The simultaneous contraction of the detrusor and sphincters gives rise to incomplete emptying and reflux. If it is not detected, hydroureter and hydronephrosis with renal damage may result.

Autonomic dysreflexia is seen in complete neurologic lesions above the T5 level and is usually a result of bladder overdistention or urethral instrumentation. The exaggerated sympathetic response gives a huge rise in diastolic and systolic blood pressure, producing headache and even intracranial bleeding. Minor symptoms of autonomic dysreflexia such as sweating in normally innervated areas may be helped by an adrenergic blockade.

Sophisticated techniques are available for the study of the voiding mechanism. The complete urodynamic study begins with uroflowmetry, in which the patient urinates into a commode fitted with a sensor that measures rate and volume of urine flow.

The bladder is then catheterized to measure the amount of residual urine. An electromyographic needle electrode is placed in the sphincter to give information about the amount of muscle activity and the presence or absence of denervation. The urethral catheter is slowly moved through the urethra while measurements of pressure are made. This procedure indicates the length of the active sphincter mechanism ("the continence zone") and the amount of maximum resistance. During filling of the bladder, pressure within the bladder is measured as sphincter activity is monitored. At capacity the sphincter should relax completely, the detrusor contracts, and the bladder empties smoothly and completely. Measurements may also be made of the sacral reflex arc. This is obtained by electrically stimulating the perineum and measuring a two-component response from the sphincter. This analog of the blink reflex is a measure of the integrity of the sacral cord and roots. Somatosensory evoked potentials may be obtained by stimulating the pudendal nerve and recording over the cortex or magnetic stimulation of the cortex while recording from the external sphincter if cord injury or demyelinating disease is suspected.

CONCLUSION

Function of the lower urinary tract is the result of a complex interplay between physical and neurologic parameters. Malfunction can occur at many levels. Treatment must be based on a clear understanding of the source of the problem.

REFERENCES

Dyro FM: Electrophysiology of the lower urinary tract. In Yalla SV et al, editors: Neurourology and urodynamics. New York, 1988, Macmillan.

Ertekin C et al: Examination of the descending pathway to the external anal sphincter and pelvic floor muscles by transcranial cortical stimulation. EEG and Clin Neurophys 75:500, 1990.

MacKeith RC, Meadow SR, and Turner RK: How children become dry. In Kolvin I et al, editors: Bladder control and enuresis. Philadelphia, 1973, Lippincott.

Percy JP et al: Electrophysiological study of motor nerve supply of pelvic floor. Lancet 1:16, 1980.

Resnick NM, Yalla SV, and Laurino E: The pathophysiology of urinary incontinence among institutionalized elderly persons. N Eng J Med 320:1, 1989.

Yeates WK: Bladder function in normal micturition. In Kolvin I et al, editors: Bladder control and enuresis. Philadelphia, 1973, Lippincott.

CHAPTER

136 Neuro-Oncology

Amy A. Pruitt

INTRACRANIAL NEOPLASMS

Incidence

Intracranial neoplasms are the second most common neurologic cause of death, next to stroke. In 1989, 13,000 new primary brain tumors were reported in the United States, along with approximately 80,000 metastatic brain neoplasms. Since a high percentage of primary brain tumors are malignant and since most metastatic tumors are unresectable, inexorable clinical deterioration is the course for most patients. Both neurologists and internists are asked to treat increasing numbers of patients with neurologic cancers because of more successful treatment of systemic malignancies. Recent advances in diagnostic techniques and in perioperative management of cerebral edema have resulted in valuable palliative therapy for these tumors.

Adequate clinical management of neurologic cancer requires (1) recognition of signs and symptoms suggesting intracranial neoplasm; (2) early use of appropriate diagnostic tests to distinguish tumor from other causes of progressive neurologic dysfunction, such as metabolic derangement, infection, and subdural hematoma; (3) efficient exclusion of systemic malignancy prior to directing the patient to a neurosurgeon for biopsy; (4) appropriate use of medication to control cerebral edema and seizures; and (5) recognition of the medical problems to which these patients are prone both from their tumor and from its treatment.

Pathophysiology

The symptoms and signs caused by brain tumors are determined by their size, location, invasiveness, and rate of growth. Brain tumors produce focal disturbances of function by infiltrating or compressing brain tissue. When the tumor becomes large enough, the mass and its associated edema may result in more generalized neurologic dysfunction from raised intracranial pressure. Symptoms of tumor masses reflect expansion within a fixed bony vault into space normally occupied by brain, blood, and cerebrospinal fluid (CSF). Although the brain can accommodate the presence of slow-growing tumors, both benign and malignant masses larger than 3 cm in diameter increase the intracranial pressure. The increased pressure in the subarachnoid space surrounding the optic nerves impairs venous and lymphatic drainage and causes papilledema. Vessels associated with a growing tumor contain gaps or fenestrations through which a plasma filtrate escapes, producing "vasogenic cerebral edema" and greatly increasing the effective tumor volume. If brainstem structures become distorted or if the pressure becomes high enough to impair cerebral blood flow, stupor and coma result.

As brain tissue is compressed, it may herniate under the falx cerebri or through the tentorium that forms immobile divisions between the various intracranial compartments. Decompression of the spinal subarachnoid space by lumbar puncture accentuates the pressure gradient and may precipitate brain herniation.

Clinical findings

Based on the mechanisms discussed above, brain tumors may produce both focal deficits and more generalized, or "nonlocalizing," disturbances in brain function. Headache, the initial symptom in 50% of patients with brain tumors, results from traction on pain-sensitive dura, blood vessels, or cranial nerves caused by edema, intracranial hypertension, hydrocephalus, or local compression. In most patients with supratentorial tumor, this pain radiates to the side of the tumor, while posterior fossa masses elicit retroorbital or nuchal pain. Tumors of the frontal and temporal lobes can grow very large before producing symptoms, and such symptoms may be quite nonspecific. Subtle, progressive disturbances of mentation and memory, or simply apathy and drowsiness, may be noted.

Seizures are the initial symptom in 20% of patients with brain tumors. Any adult with a first seizure that is not readily explainable on other grounds is a brain tumor suspect. Occasionally the first symptom is an event simulating a transient ischemic attack.

Tumors of the posterior fossa produce specific, progressive signs and symptoms. Rapidly growing tumors may cause obstructive hydrocephalus, resulting in headache, vomiting, lethargy, abducens nerve palsies, and papilledema. More slowly growing tumors give rise to a unilateral sixth-nerve deficit along with a combination of progressive unilateral hearing loss, facial weakness, and facial pain or numbness, a symptom complex suggestive of a lesion in the cerebellopontine angle. Gait ataxia results from cerebellar tumor, and nuchal or occipital head pain along with corticospinal signs develop with further tumor enlargement and encroachment on brainstem connections.

Tumors typically produce a gradual, progressive loss of function. Metastatic tumors are more likely to produce acute symptoms that evolve in days to weeks, or even in minutes as in the case of such hemorrhagic tumors as melanoma, hypernephroma, lung carcinoma, and choriocarcinoma. In contrast, a careful history in patients with primary brain tumors may disclose subtle personality changes or partial seizures that antedate the diagnosis by months or years.

Laboratory evaluation

Contrast-enhanced computed tomography (CT) and magnetic resonance imaging (MRI) have largely replaced the combination of skull radiograph, electroencephalogram, radionuclide brain scan, and arteriography as the principal diagnostic tests for the evaluation of patients with suspected brain tumor.

CT scan without contrast enhancement detects tumors whose density exceeds that of normal brain parenchyma, including meningioma, melanoma, and primary cerebral lymphoma; tumors with spontaneous hemorrhage; and hydrocephalus produced by masses obstructing the ventricular system. The use of iodinated contrast is essential in detecting intracranial neoplasms and outlines the tumors as homogeneous or ring-enhancing masses surrounded by variable amounts of edema. Ringlike enhancement can occur in conditions other than tumor such as abscesses, recent cerebral infarctions, the plaques of multiple sclerosis, and certain vascular malformations. An initially negative CT scan is sometimes found in patients with glial tumors, meningeal carcinomatosis, metastases, and primary brain lymphoma, but repetition of the scan 4 to 6 weeks later, when the clinical circumstances remain highly suspicious for tumor, usually detects the lesion. An MRI should be obtained as well.

MRI may be more sensitive but less specific than CT for evaluating central nervous system (CNS) neoplasms. In situations in which only nonspecific mass effect can be discerned on CT, MRI can more fully define the extent of infiltrating tumor. The ability of MRI to detect small amounts of increased brain water content allows assessment of the full extent of tumor and its surrounding edema. High-resolution, high-contrast images of the brain in axial, coronal, and sagittal planes allow for three-dimensional assessment of tumor volume and location for surgical and radiation therapy planning (Fig. 136-1). Administration of the paramagnetic contrast agent gadolinium diethylene-triamine pentaacetic acid (gadolinium DTPA) further defines tumor vascularity and the degree of blood-brain barrier breakdown, which often correlates with histologic malignancy (Fig. 136-2).

MRI specifically may be better than CT for the assessment of tumors at the skull base, pineal region, posterior fossa, and spinal cord. Large arteries and veins associated with the tumor may be well demonstrated, obviating arteriography in some cases. Subacute or remote hemorrhage has a characteristic MRI appearance (shortened T1 signal—see Chapter 108), allowing distinction between tumor and arteriovenous malformations and suggesting tumor histology in those tumors prone to hemorrhage, such as melanoma, choriocarcinoma, and metastases of lung and renal origin. Fat-containing tumors, such as epidermoids and lipomas, may be well outlined. Cysts can be evaluated to determine if their characteristics match those of CSF (arachnoid cyst, porencephalic region) or differ from those of CSF (cystic astrocytoma).

Arteriography provides selective visualization of intracranial arteries. Some malignant tumors are characterized

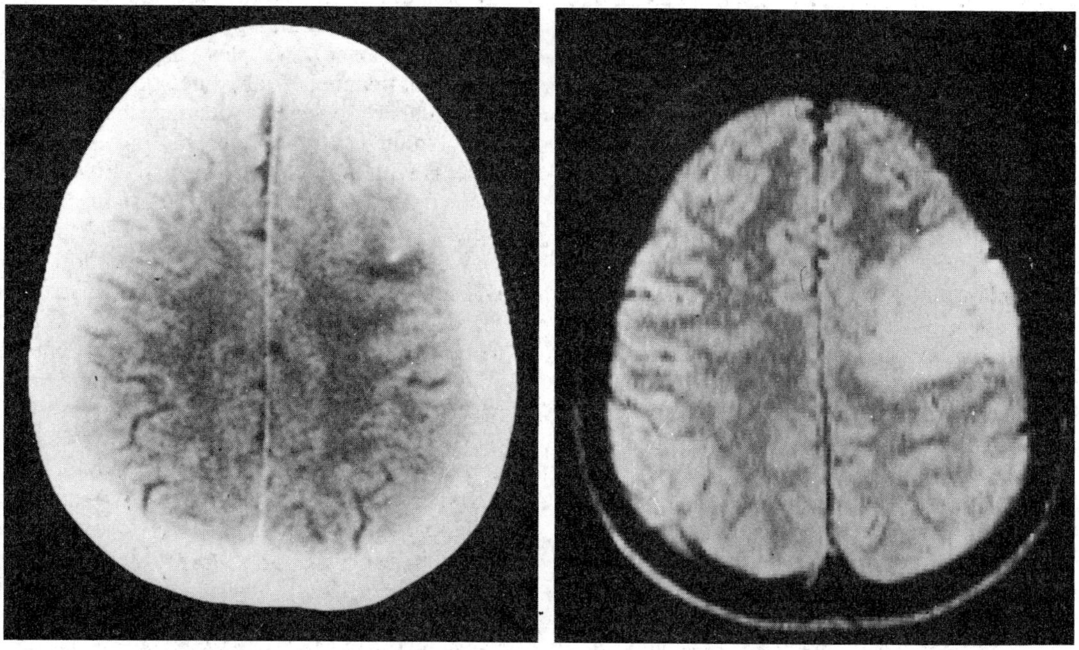

Fig. 136-1. This oligodendroglioma appears as a small area of hypodensity with calcium on CT *(left)* but as a much larger area of T_2 signal abnormality on MRI *(right)*. Contrast images (not shown) showed no enhancement on either CT or MRI consistent with the low-grade histology found on biopsy.

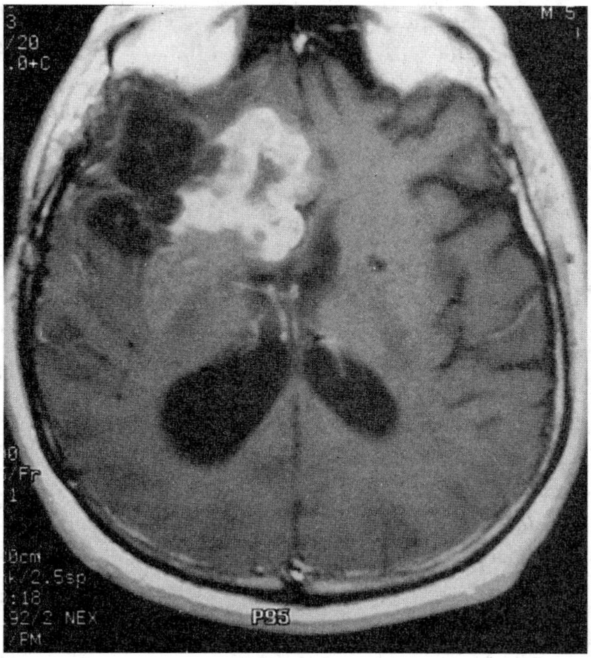

Fig. 136-2. MRI of a glioblastoma multiforme arising at a site of previously resected low-grade glial neoplasm shows pronounced enhancement of the tumor when gadolinium is administered. The tumor now extends into the corpus callosum.

by an angiographic "blush" with early draining veins. Demonstration of the vascular anatomy aids in neurosurgical planning, but the accuracy of MRI, and more recently magnetic resonance angiography (MRA), in defining tumor vascularity has reduced the use of arteriography for this purpose.

Surgery produces specific tissue diagnosis in patients with solitary or multiple intracranial masses. In general, brain masses should be biopsied even if they cannot be excised when the clinical diagnosis is in doubt. In the setting of multiple intracranial masses, a biopsy often follows an unrewarding systemic search for malignancy. This evaluation should include a hemogram, chest x-ray, CT scan of the chest, sputum cytology in a smoker, liver function studies, carcinoembryonic antigen (CEA), radionuclide bone scan, and perhaps intravenous pyelography. Biopsy is performed through an open craniotomy or by using CT- or MRI-guided stereotactic techniques. Resection may be curative for histologically benign tumors that are surgically accessible, including meningiomas, acoustic neuromas, ependymomas, oligodendrogliomas, pituitary adenomas, and some astrocytomas. Partial resection improves symptoms and seizure control and reduces dependence on corticosteroids.

Preoperative surgical management is based on the need to control cerebral edema and seizures. Corticosteroids may relieve symptoms dramatically within 48 hours of their initiation. Dexamethasone, 10 mg intravenously followed by

4 to 6 mg orally or intramuscularly every 6 hours, is the initial therapy usually recommended. Steroids may not suffice to control symptoms caused by tumors blocking the ventricular system, and emergency ventriculoperitoneal shunting may be required. Anticonvulsants are usually prescribed only for patients who have already had a seizure, but many physicians choose to treat prophylactically.

Pathology

Common intracranial tumors are listed in the box below. In all adult age groups, malignant astrocytoma or glioblastoma is the most common type of primary tumor. Metastases account for nearly two thirds of intracranial neoplasms treated in general hospitals in 1985 and are discussed under Systemic Cancer and the Nervous System, later in this chapter.

Anaplastic astrocytoma and *glioblastoma multiforme* represent three fourths of the glial tumors diagnosed yearly in adults in the United States. These highly invasive, rapidly growing tumors commonly occur in the corpus callosum; the frontal, parietal, and temporal lobes; and the thalamus. Peak age of tumor development is between 40 and 70, and the tumor is somewhat more common in males. The tumor may be vascular, and CT scan reveals a usually solitary, heterogeneously enhancing lesion. Clinical history may reveal symptomatic changes for several months; however, the clinical history is much shorter if seizures are the presenting feature. If untreated, patients survive only 17 weeks. Surgery is the first line of treatment with an extensive debulking of surgically accessible lesions and biopsy of critically located ones. Recent data suggest that biopsy alone may underestimate the grade of malignancy in glial tumors. Despite refinement in radiotherapeutic schedules, aggressive surgery, and recent chemotherapy, median survival after all available therapeutic modalities is only 62 weeks. Nineteen percent of patients are alive at 18 months from the time of diagnosis. Current chemotherapeutic programs include single-agent chemotherapy (BCNU, CCNU, and cisplatin) and multiagent programs (CCNU, vincristine, and procarbazine). Mahaley (1991) provides a compilation of current treatment trials. Interstitial implantation of tumor with radioactive seeds containing iodine or iridium is also being studied, but is applicable only to a small subset of patients with tumor volumes small enough for implantation and with a possibly better prognosis because of small size alone.

Well-differentiated astrocytomas (formerly grades I and II) occur throughout the brain and spinal cord and slowly infiltrate the white matter of these areas. Subcortical white matter of the hemispheres is the most common location in adults, while optic nerve, cerebellum, and brainstem are the usual locations in children. These tumors are avascular and on CT or MRI appear as indistinct masses with little or no contrast enhancement. The tumors may evolve over several years. Excision is curative for some cerebellar, optic nerve, and lobar astrocytomas. Biopsy is recommended for all suspected low-grade astrocytomas with surgical resection if the tumor is favorably located. Biopsy confirms diagnosis and identifies patients with anaplastic tumors that do not enhance on CT or MRI. Cyst drainage and partial resection are feasible for many supratentorial tumors. Median life expectancy is 67 months with tumors in supratentorial locations and 89 months when the growth is in the cerebellum. Chemotherapy has no established role. The timing of radiation therapy of low-grade astrocytomas remains controversial and is currently under investigation in a multicenter protocol.

Meningioma is the only brain tumor more common in women and represents 20% of intracranial masses. These tumors are generally benign histologically, although they can invade adjacent skull; since meningiomas may involve critical brain structures or blood vessels, they sometimes cannot be completely removed. The mass is frequently quite round and hyperdense with respect to surrounding brain tissue on the unenhanced CT scan with homogeneous enhancement after contrast administration. An arteriogram may reveal striking vascularity, with some of the blood supply coming from external carotid artery branches. Common sites are in the midline along the falx, the olfactory groove, the tuberculum sellae, the foramen magnum, the sphenoid ridge, and along the lateral cerebral convexity and tentorium of the cerebellum. Resection is both diagnostic and curative for subfrontal, intraventricular, and parasagittal tumors. Incompletely excised tumors and those with more invasive histologic features are sometimes irradiated.

Recent data suggest an increased incidence of *primary central nervous system lymphoma* (PCNSL), in part because of the increased frequency of PCNSL in patients with the acquired immune deficiency syndrome, but the incidence is also increased in apparently immunocompetent individuals. Patients with PCNSL may present with symptoms resulting from intracranial mass lesions, or with symptomatic uveal/vitreal deposits, diffuse meningeal seeding (lymphomatous meningitis), or intradural spinal masses.

PCNSL has a distinctive radiographic appearance with diffusely enhancing lesions, often in a periventricular loca-

Common intracranial tumors

- Metastatic carcinoma
  - Lung
  - Breast
  - Melanoma
  - Kidney
  - Gastrointestinal
- Glioblastoma
- Anaplastic astrocytoma
- Meningioma
- Astrocytoma (grades I and II)
- Ependymoma
- Oligodendroglioma
- Pituitary adenoma
- Cranial nerve neuromas
- Primary cerebral lymphoma
- Medulloblastoma

tion. In about one half of patients the lesions are multifocal. These lesions are highly sensitive to the administration of high-dose glucocorticoids and may disappear entirely. Since lysis of lesions by corticosteroid may result in nondiagnostic biopsy results and since other processes such as multiple sclerosis and sarcoidosis can be improved by steroid administration, steroid use should be deferred, if possible, until histologic confirmation of the diagnosis is obtained.

The surgical approach to PCNSL is different from that used for most primary brain tumors. Surgical resection does not contribute to overall survival with this disease, and patients should have a stereotactic biopsy. At times, the diagnosis can be established by CSF cytology or vitreous biopsy. Recent studies have strongly suggested improved survival in patients receiving chemotherapy in addition to cranial irradiation. The chemotherapy is usually administered prior to radiation therapy. Various combinations of methotrexate and high-dose cytosine arabinoside have been roughly comparable in extending median survival to 42 months, compared with 15- to 18-month survival in patients receiving radiation therapy alone.

Tumors of the pineal region include germ cell neoplasms, true tumors of the pineal body (pineocytoma and pineoblastoma), and uncommon presentations of metastatic, glial, and meningeal growths. Recent surgical advances allow more specific histologic diagnosis than previously was possible. Since the prognosis is quite variable and since treatment depends heavily on histology, every effort should be made to refer the patient to a surgeon experienced with surgery in this site. Germ cell tumors include germinomas, endodermal sinus tumors, teratoma, embryonal carcinoma, and choriocarcinoma. Symptoms of such tumors may involve diabetes insipidus, bitemporal visual field defects, headache caused by hydrocephalus, failure of upward gaze, and pupillary abnormalities. Germinomas may be very sensitive to relatively small amounts of radiation, but other histologic types have worse prognoses and may seed the cranial and spinal nerves. Pineocytoma and the more primitive pineoblastoma are treated with radical surgical excision. Both tend to recur, and some recent successes with chemotherapy have been reported.

Most previously discussed types of tumor can occur in the posterior fossa. However, several histologic types are specific to this region. *Medulloblastoma,* one type of primitive neuroectodermal tumor, is commonly located in the midline cerebellum and presents with headache and ataxia. Removal of the tumor is the first step in treatment, followed by lumbar puncture and gadolinium-enhanced MRI of the spinal cord to detect spinal seeding. Radiation is given to the posterior fossa and to the neuraxis. Chemotherapy has been somewhat successful in controlling recurrent tumors. Commonly used regimens include nitrogen mustard, vincristine, procarbazine, and prednisone (MOPP); and lomustine, vincristine, and methotrexate. *Ependymomas* are glial tumors occurring largely in childhood and young adulthood; their typical intracranial location is at the fourth ventricle. After resection of tumor, sampling of spinal fluid, and radiation to the cranium or whole neuraxis (depending on CSF results), 5-year survival is nearly 70%.

Acoustic neuroma is a benign tumor composed of the cells covering the acoustic nerve as it leaves the brain through the internal auditory meatus. When bilateral, these tumors suggest the central form of neurofibromatosis. Early detection is essential, as hearing may be spared when the tumor is removed while it is still confined to the canal. Brainstem auditory-evoked potentials, CT, MRI, and metrizamide or air cisternography have greatly accelerated diagnosis of such tumors. Patients with progressive unilateral hearing loss should be referred to a neurologist for further investigation.

Benign intracranial hypertension (pseudotumor cerebri)

Benign intracranial hypertension is an idiopathic syndrome of increased intracranial pressure manifested by headache, papilledema, sixth-nerve palsies, and progressive visual loss. The syndrome is most often seen in obese adolescent females. Although the majority of cases are of unknown cause, associated clinical settings include pregnancy, corticosteroid administration, sex hormone use, adrenal and parathyroid disorders, venous sinus thrombosis, and use of vitamin A, tetracycline, or nalidixic acid.

The CT or MRI scan commonly shows small, "slitlike" lateral ventricles, and the CSF is found to be under elevated pressure, often with a low spinal fluid protein. The syndrome may resolve spontaneously over several months, although it may take as long as 2 years. However, the pressure on the optic nerve can lead to permanent visual loss.

Repeated lumbar punctures, initially at daily intervals, to lower the pressure to less than 180 mm Hg are the appropriate treatment. This treatment provides symptomatic relief, although lumbar-peritoneal shunting may be required when vision is seriously threatened. Adrenal corticosteroids, acetazolamide, furosemide, and oral glycerol have all been advocated, but their efficacy has not been proved.

SYSTEMIC CANCER AND THE NERVOUS SYSTEM

Neurologic complications are common in patients with systemic cancer, largely because improved therapy has resulted in longer survival. Metastatic complications have increased along with adverse effects of the therapy itself. One third of cancer patients are found at autopsy to have metastatic, infectious, or vascular complications affecting the nervous system.

Clinical findings

Metastatic complications. The clinical findings arising from metastasis to various elements of the nervous system are outlined in Table 136-1 and have, in large part, been discussed earlier. The hallmarks of cerebral metastasis are headache, mental status changes, seizures, focal motor or sensory signs, and papilledema.

Table 136-1. Metastatic complications of cancer

	Intracranial	Spinal	Meningeal	Nerves, roots, plexus
Clinical findings	Headache Seizures Mental status changes Focal signs Papilledema	Back pain Weakness Bladder dysfunction Sensory loss Increased DTRs Babinski signs	Cranial nerve findings: diplopia, bulbar palsy Spinal root findings: weakness, areflexia, bladder dysfunction Hydrocephalus: headache, mental status changes	Pain Cranial nerve palsies Brachial plexus: C7, C8, T1 palsy; Horner's syndrome; extremity edema Lumbosacral plexus: extremity pain with weakness and sensory loss in multiple segmental pattern; unilateral
X-ray and laboratory findings	CT, MRI	Spine x-ray Bone scan Myelogram: block MRI: block	MRI, CT: hydrocephalus CSF: low glucose, elevated protein Cytology: malignant cells Myelogram: nodules	Skull x-ray: erosion Tomography: erosion MRI, CT: mass lesion
Differential diagnosis	Primary CNS tumor Cerebral hemorrhage Cerebral infarction Cerebral abscess	Primary cord tumor Radiation myelopathy Herniated disk Epidural hematoma	Peripheral neuropathy Myopathy Chronic fungal meningitis	Radiation effects Radiation-induced neoplasm Surgical trauma
Common primary tumors	Lung Breast Melanoma Genitourinary Leukemia Lymphoma Gastrointestinal	Breast Lung Prostate Kidney Lymphoma Myeloma Melanoma	Leukemia Breast Lymphoma Lung Melanoma	Breast Lung Lymphoma Prostate Head and neck

CT, computed tomogram; DTRs, deep tendon reflexes; MRI, magnetic resonance imaging.

Pathophysiology

The nervous system complications of cancer can be classified as metastatic or nonmetastatic (see box at right). Direct neoplastic invasion of the brain, meninges, spinal roots, or peripheral nerves causes most of the neurologic symptoms. Spinal epidural metastases are also common and are manifested as a myelopathy (see Chapter 122). Metabolic effects occur owing to the failure of other organs (e.g., liver, lungs). Increased susceptibility to nervous system infections results from altered host resistance as a consequence of either the tumor itself or its treatment. Cerebrovascular disorders are common in cancer patients. Multiple cerebral infarctions are the most common pathology and may result from septic embolization or nonbacterial thrombotic endocarditis. Disseminated intravascular coagulation (DIC) and intracerebral hemorrhage are more common in patients with leukemia or lymphoma than in those with solid tumors, coagulopathies being the major risk factor for these patients. Like DIC, multiple cerebral infarctions may present either in a focal, strokelike series of events or with diffuse, progressive encephalopathy. Moreover, direct toxic effects of chemotherapeutic agents and radiation therapy may cause persistent neurologic disability, even in the patient who has no residual tumor. Finally, occasional patients manifest one of the "remote" effects of cancer that are presumably caused by toxic or metabolic influences of the primary neoplasm (see box on p. 1169).

Neurologic complications of systemic cancer

- Metastatic
  - Intracranial
  - Intraspinal
  - Meningeal
  - Nerves, plexuses, roots
- Nonmetastatic
  - Metabolic encephalopathy
  - Infections
  - Vascular disorders
  - Complications of therapy
  - Remote effects of cancer

Sixty percent of cerebral metastases occur in the setting of previously diagnosed systemic cancer. Cancers of lung in men and breast in women account for the largest absolute number of metastases, although melanoma is the tumor with the highest likelihood of spread to the central nervous system. Twenty percent of patients with cerebral metastasis have neurologic symptoms predating the diagnosis of the primary malignancy, which is most often in the lung. Multiple metastases are present in one half of all cases.

Contrast-enhanced MRI is the procedure of choice for the diagnosis of cerebral metastases. MRI should be done as part of the initial or pretreatment evaluation for three groups of patients: (1) Patients with lung carcinoma for whom curative lobectomy is planned require a preoperative MRI. (2) Patients with small-cell lung carcinoma should be scanned prior to prophylactic cranial radiation. (3) Patients with widely disseminated melanoma, breast, or testicular tumors about to undertake an aggressive chemotherapy regimen should have MRI as part of their staging evaluation. Patients for whom MRI is contraindicated because of surgical clips or cardiac pacemakers should have a contrast-enhanced CT scan.

An apoplectic onset occurs 5% to 10% of the time and is often caused by hemorrhage into a metastatic lesion. Intracerebral hemorrhages are particularly common in metastasis of choriocarcinoma and melanoma. Occasionally, multiple small metastases to the cerebral hemispheres or a small metastasis to the brainstem reticular formation may present as an encephalopathy.

Metastasis to the base of the skull produces a number of "syndromes" depending on the area involved. The orbital syndrome presents as painful ophthalmoplegia or diplopia, with visual acuity preserved until late in the course of the disease. A CT scan typically identifies a metastasis to the orbit and adjacent bone. The parasellar syndrome results from metastasis to the petrous apex and sellar region, with compression of the structures within the cavernous sinus. The patient complains of a dull, aching, ipsilateral frontal or temporal headache accompanied by diplopia. Proptosis is not present, and there is impairment of the oculomotor, abducens, or trochlear nerves and the ophthalmic division of the trigeminal nerve. The middle fossa, or gasserian ganglion, syndrome is characterized by progressive facial numbness caused by metastasis to the gasserian ganglion. Occasionally the tumor may extend laterally to involve either the abducens or facial nerves. The tumor may be confined to the ganglion and therefore may not be readily seen by CT or plain radiographs. The jugular foramen syndrome is characterized by retroauricular pain, hoarseness, and dysphagia, which are manifestations of glossopharyngeal, vagus, and accessory nerve dysfunction. Bony erosion adjacent to the jugular foramen can usually be demonstrated by CT scan. The occipital condyle syndrome is characterized by severe, unremitting, ipsilateral occipital headache accompanied by dysphagia and dysarthria from a hypoglossal nerve paralysis.

Spinal cord compression from metastatic tumor is most commonly the result of vertebral body metastasis with extension into the adjacent epidural space causing compression of the spinal cord, roots, or cauda equina. Back pain is the first symptom in over 95% of these patients, often preceding other neurologic symptoms or signs by several weeks, and local spine tenderness is common. Spine x-rays, bone scan, and myelography are the most important methods for establishing the diagnosis. MRI has begun to play an increasing role in the emergency diagnosis of epidural spinal cord compression and is particularly valuable for those patients whose coexisting intracranial metastases preclude lumbar puncture.

Meningeal carcinomatosis is manifested clinically by cranial nerve and spinal root palsies that often are accompanied by localized pain. Communicating hydrocephalus may result from impaired CSF flow and cause increased intracranial pressure, with headache and mental status changes. CSF pleocytosis and hypoglycorrhachia are common. Repeat CSF cytologies may be necessary before malignant cells are identified and the diagnosis is established.

Computed tomography and MRI of the head may be of value in the diagnosis of carcinomatosis of the meninges. Some of the findings suggestive of this complication include ventricular enlargement, sulcal and/or cisternal obliteration, enhancing cortical nodules, and leptomeningeal enhancement. These changes may be seen before clinical evidence of meningeal metastasis; at other times changes may be noted only after serial scans are performed.

Metastatic involvement of peripheral nerves or plexuses may be difficult to differentiate from dysfunction resulting from prior surgical or radiation therapy. If weakness and sensory symptoms in the arm are the result of neoplastic infiltration of the cervical roots or brachial plexus, there is often pain in the shoulder, Horner's syndrome, and a pattern of weakness suggesting involvement of C7, C8, and T1 roots. Patients who have received previous radiation therapy to the area and have a radiation-induced brachial plexopathy less often have shoulder pain or Horner's syndrome, and their pattern of weakness suggests C5 and C6 root involvement.

Nonmetastatic complications

Vascular disorders. Certain cancer patients are predisposed to ischemic and hemorrhagic cerebrovascular complications. DIC and septic embolization are more common in patients with leukemia and lymphoma than in patients with solid tumors. Like DIC, nonbacterial thrombotic endocarditis with cerebral embolization may manifest itself either in a focal, strokelike event or in diffuse, progressive encephalopathy. Intracerebral hemorrhage may occur because of bleeding into a parenchymal metastasis; it is particularly common in melanoma and choriocarcinoma. Spontaneous intracerebral and subarachnoid hemorrhages are common in acute myelogenous leukemia and treatment-induced thrombocytopenia.

Complications of therapy. Unfortunately, the successful treatment of many tumors is accomplished at the cost of injury to normal tissue.

A therapy-related complication can mimic recurrent tumor, infection vascular disease, metabolic derangement, or paraneoplastic process, all of which must be excluded before ascribing the new problem to therapy. Familiarity with the more commonly occurring therapy complications and their temporal relationship to treatment spares the patient unnecessary diagnostic studies.

Chronic corticosteroid therapy may induce insulin-dependent diabetes in some patients. At doses of greater than 8 mg dexamethasone, or its equivalent, for more than a few weeks, myopathic changes are often seen. Painless symmetric weakness of the proximal arm and leg muscles responds to tapering of the steroids and to vigorous physical therapy. The combination of corticosteroids, relative immobility, and perhaps a hypercoagulable state caused by the underlying tumor leads to a high incidence of thrombophlebitis. Many physicians recommend insertion of a vena cava filter rather than anticoagulation with coumadin in patients with brain neoplasms.

The second most commonly used type of medication in these patients, anticonvulsants, is associated with rashes and altered steroid metabolism. Allergy to an anticonvulsant may be masked by the corticosteroid and revealed later when the patient is tapered off the steroid.

Many chemotherapeutic agents adversely affect several parts of the nervous system (Table 136-2). In addition, radiation therapy to the nervous system may be associated with acute (1 to 2 days), subacute (10 to 13 weeks), or chronic (4 to 30+ months) complications. Acute effects take the form of headache, nausea, lethargy, and transient worsening of focal symptoms and signs, apparently resulting from edema. These acute symptoms are more likely to occur with high initial radiation doses. The subacute injury occurs 10 to 13 weeks after radiation, at which time demyelination occurs, accompanied by attendant cerebral, cerebellar, or spinal cord findings that may resolve spontaneously in 6 to 8 weeks.

The late, chronic irradiation injury is accompanied by pathologic changes of small-vessel occlusion with infarction and glial proliferation in the white matter. These patients may present with either an insidiously progressive multifocal encephalopathy or a sudden strokelike onset. The CT scan shows single or multiple low-density lesions predominantly in the white matter. MRI reveals widespread areas of prolonged T2 signal both at the site of the original tumor and remote from it. MRI does not clearly differentiate radiation necrosis from recurrent tumor. The problem of mass effect may become significant enough to justify surgical removal both for diagnosis and for therapy if the lesion is located in an accessible area. This situation is more likely to arise after radiation therapy of primary tumors, in which the radiation doses used are usually larger than are those employed for metastatic tumors.

Late radiation injury to the spinal cord results in progressive weakness and sensory loss below the level of treatment, often with prominent painful paresthesias. MRI is useful for excluding recurrent tumor and demonstrates prolonged T2 signal in the radiation-injured cord. Unfortunately, spinal radiation injury does not respond to corticosteroids or any other form of treatment.

Radiation-induced brachial or lumbar plexopathies and peripheral neuropathies may develop months or years following radiation to these structures. Weakness and atrophy insidiously develop in the innervated muscles, with pain and sensory loss absent or late. If pain and sensory loss are early findings, the possibility of tumor infiltration of the nerve or plexus increases. Radiation-induced tumors of the plexus or peripheral nerves may develop many years after high-dose irradiation to the nerve. The typical clinical findings are painful, progressive, asymmetric motor and sensory dysfunction in regions innervated by the irradiated plexus or nerve, with enlargement of the nerve or plexus demonstrated on clinical examination, CT scan, or MRI.

In patients with cancer previously treated with radiation therapy to ports encompassing the brachial plexus, it may be difficult to differentiate tumor invasion of the plexus from radiation effects when shoulder and arm symptoms occur. Lung and breast cancer are the commonest neoplasms to invade the brachial plexus. Pain in the shoulder and arm is the major initial complaint in 90% of these patients. Weakness and atrophy are present in over two thirds and typically involve muscles innervated by the lower portions of the brachial plexus (C7, C8, T1). This portion of the plexus is in closest proximity to the lymphatic channels from the chest and breast. Horner's syndrome is present in

Table 136-2. Neurologic complications of chemotherapy

Neurologic problem	Drug	Route of administration
Encephalopathy (including cerebral edema and leukoencephalopathy)	Corticosteroids	Oral/intramuscular/intravenous
	L-Asparaginase	Intravenous
	Procarbazine	Oral/intravenous
	Nitrosoureas	Oral/intravenous/intra-arterial/high-dose intravenous
	Cytosine arabinoside	High-dose intravenous
Optic nerve damage	Nitrosoureas	Intra-arterial/high-dose intravenous
Cerebellar ataxia	5-Fluorouracil	Intravenous
	Cytosine arabinoside	Intrathecal
Cranial neuropathy	Vincristine	Intravenous
	Cisplatin	Intravenous/intra-arterial
Myelopathy/radiculopathy	Thiotepa	Intrathecal
	Methotrexate	High-dose intravenous/intrathecal
	Cytosine arabinoside	High-dose intravenous/intrathecal
Peripheral neuropathy	Vincristine	Intravenous
	Cisplatin	Intravenous
Myopathy	Corticosteroids	Oral/intramuscular/intravenous
	Vincristine	Intravenous

Modified from Young DF: Neurological complications of chemotherapy. In Silverstein A, editor: Neurological complications of therapy. Mt. Kisco, NY, 1982, Futura.

half of the patients with plexus metastasis and is especially useful in predicting those patients with brachial plexus metastasis who will have cervical epidural metastasis found at myelography. Arm symptoms caused by the effects of radiation to the brachial plexus typically have their onset 4 to 5 years after radiation therapy. Symptoms may, however, begin as soon as a few months after therapy. Surprisingly, the dose of radiation seems to correlate poorly with the likelihood of developing radiation-induced changes. Pain is not a prominent complaint but it does occur in 20% of patients. Compared with the patients who have brachial plexus metastasis, these patients more often have a swollen limb, weakness and atrophy occur in the upper plexus (C5, C6), and Horner's syndrome is uncommon.

At times it may be difficult to differentiate tumor infiltration of the lumbosacral plexus from the delayed effects of prior radiation to the pelvis. Tumor infiltration of the plexus is typically first manifested by an ever-increasing pain in the hip, back, and leg, which is often worse at night. A radiation-induced plexopathy normally presents with the slow progression over months or years of hip and leg weakness, and numbness. The symptoms frequently are bilateral. An electromyogram (EMG) may show myokymic discharges not generally present with metastasis. A CT or MRI scan of the pelvis is unremarkable in radiation damage but often confirms the presence of a tumor mass or adenopathy in the patient with recurrent tumor.

Vascular complications of remote radiation have been reported, particularly in patients who have received cervical and mediastinal irradiation for Hodgkin's disease or high-dose (6000 cGy) cervical radiation for head and neck primary tumors. The neurologic presentation of these problems mimics naturally occurring atheromatous stroke or transient ischemic attack. Angiographic findings in these patients include disproportionate involvement of the distal common carotid artery and unusually long carotid lesions. Surgical reconstruction of these vessels is difficult, and the vessels demonstrate destruction of the internal elastic lamina and replacement of the normal intima and media with fibrous tissue.

Neurologic paraneoplastic syndromes. Several neurologic syndromes associated with systemic cancer but not the result of direct invasion of the CNS by tumor are summarized in the box at upper right. General clinical characteristics of paraneoplastic processes involving the nervous system include acute or subacute onset, severe disability at peak, stereotypical syndromes irrespective of the type of underlying neoplasm, modest CSF pleocytosis, elevation of CSF protein, IgG elevation, oligoclonal bands, frequent involvement of more than one type of neural cell, and low incidence (less than 1%) in patients with cancer despite the relative frequency of cancers associated with paraneoplastic syndromes such as small cell lung cancer, lymphomas, and breast carcinoma/gynecologic malignancies.

Though rare, these syndromes assume an importance out of proportion to their incidence, for several reasons. From one half to two thirds of patients develop the paraneoplastic syndrome prior to the diagnosis of systemic neoplasm. Paraneoplastic syndromes may be mimicked by many other processes, leading to inappropriate diagnostic tests or treatments. Symptoms of the paraneoplastic disease, which is often acute or subacute in onset, are often more disabling than the symptoms of the tumor, and though usually unaffected by treatment directed at the tumor, occasionally can be ameliorated by treatment of the systemic neoplasm. Anecdotal evidence suggests that the cancer of patients with paraneoplastic syndromes often runs a more benign course.

The recent demonstration of circulating antibodies and antigens identified by these antibodies in both the nervous system and in the tumor tissue of some patients with paraneoplastic syndromes offers clues about the body's immunologic response to neoplasms. The identification of specific antibodies, summarized in Table 136-3 in a patient without known cancer, may focus the search on one or a few malignancies.

Neurologic paraneoplastic syndromes

- Brain/cranial nerves
  - Limbic encephalitis
  - Brainstem encephalitis
  - Retinal degeneration
  - Optic neuritis
- Cerebellum
  - Paraneoplastic cerebellar degeneration
  - Opsoclonus/myoclonus
- Spinal cord/dorsal root ganglia
  - Myelitis
  - Necrotizing myelopathy
  - Subacute motor neuropathy
  - Motor neuron disease
  - Subacute sensory neuropathy
- Peripheral nerve
  - Subacute or chronic peripheral neuropathy
  - Acute polyradiculopathy (Guillain-Barré)
  - Chronic inflammatory neuropathy
  - Mononeuritis multiplex
  - Brachial neuritis
  - Acute or subacute autonomic neuropathy
  - Peripheral neuropathy associated with paraproteinemia
- Neuromuscular junction and muscle
  - Lambert-Eaton myasthenic syndrome
  - Myasthenia gravis
  - Dermatomyositis/polymyositis

Treatment of metastatic cancer

The treatment of nervous system metastasis primarily involves radiation therapy, surgery, glucocorticoids, and chemotherapeutic agents. The therapeutic plan for a patient with cerebral metastasis is dictated by the clinical status. Patients with solitary, accessible lesions and little or no active systemic disease may be considered for surgery with postoperative radiation. Those with advanced, widespread systemic cancer may be treated with corticosteroids alone to maximize neurologic function and to reduce headache. Most patients with multiple metastases or unresectable sol-

Table 136-3. Autoantibodies in neurologic paraneoplastic syndromes

Syndrome	Tumor	Antibody	Specificity	Antigen (Western blot)
PCD	Ovary Breast	Anti-Yo	Purkinje cell cytoplasm	34 and 62 kd band from Purkinje cells and breast and ovary tumors
	Lung	One anti-Hu	Nuclei of CNS neurons	35-40 kd band from neurons and sclc
	Hodgkin's	No antibody		
SSN limbic encephalopathy	Sclc ? Prostate	Anti-Hu	Nuclei of CNS neurons	35-40 kd band from neurons and sclc tumors
Retinal degeneration	Sclc	Antiretinal	Ganglion cells	20-24, 65, 145, 205 kd band from retina
Opsoclonus/myoclonus	Breast	Anti-Ri	Neuronal nuclei	55 and 80 kd band from neurons
Lambert-Eaton myasthenic syndrome	Lung (sclc) No tumor	Antivoltage sensitive Ca^{++} channels	L-Ca^{++} channels (particles in presynaptic active zones)	VGCC

Modified from Posner JB: Paraneoplastic syndromes. Curr Neurol 9:245, 1989.
Sclc, sclerosing.

itary lesions are referred for radiation therapy. Three fourths of patients treated with any of the various radiation schedules in common use improve both clinically and by CT or MRI. Over one half are able to discontinue their steroid medication. While treatment failure for primary brain tumors is caused by local recurrence or to spinal dissemination of tumor, for two thirds of patients with cerebral metastases the cause of death is recurrent systemic tumor at a time of neurologic remission.

Upon demonstration of a block caused by spinal epidural cancer, high doses of corticosteroids (dexamethasone, 10 to 20 mg intravenously, followed by 16 to 24 mg per day in divided doses orally or parenterally) are administered, and radiation therapy is recommended. Recently, reconsideration has been given to surgical therapy as a primary mode of treatment for radioresistant malignancies such as prostate, lung, and colon cancers. The clinical condition of the patient at the time of treatment appears to be the most important factor in outcome. Only 3% of patients who are paraplegic at the time of diagnosis regain the ability to walk, regardless of type of therapy, while nearly 50% of those with only mild weakness are ambulatory after surgery or radiation therapy. Meningeal carcinomatosis is managed with combined irradiation and intrathecal chemotherapy (e.g., methotrexate or cytosine arabinoside, often instilled through an indwelling ventricular reservoir). Meningeal tumor caused by leukemia, lymphoma, or breast carcinoma is more likely to respond to treatment, whereas leptomeningeal metastases of lung or melanoma origin are resistant to currently available intrathecal chemotherapeutic agents.

REFERENCES

Black P McL: Brain tumors. N Engl J Med 324:1471, 1991.

Clouston PD: The spectrum of neurological disease in patients with systemic cancer. Ann Neurol 31:268, 1992.

DeAngelis LM: Primary CNS lymphoma: combined treatment with chemotherapy and radiotherapy. Neurology 40:80, 1990.

Florell RC: Selection bias, survival and brachytherapy for glioma. J Neurosurg 76:179, 1992.

Gilbert RW: Epidural spinal cord compression from metastatic tumor: diagnosis and treatment. Ann Neurol 3:40, 1978.

Glantz MJ: Influence of the type of surgery on the histologic diagnosis in patients with anaplastic gliomas. Neurology 41:1741, 1991.

Graus F: Cerebrovascular complications in patients with cancer. Medicine (Baltimore) 1:16, 1985.

Greenberg HS: Metastasis to the base of the skull: clinical findings in 43 patients. Neurology 31:530, 1981.

Helweg-Larsen S: Recovery of gait following radiation therapy in paralyzed patients with metastatic epidural spinal cord compression. Neurology 40:1234, 1990.

Horowitz MD: Central nervous system germinomas: a review. Arch Neurol 48:652, 1991.

Jaeckle KA: Evolution of computed tomographic abnormalities in leptomeningeal metastases. Ann Neurol 17:85, 1985.

Kori SH: Brachial plexus lesions in patients with cancer: 100 cases. Neurology 31:45, 1981.

Kornblith PL: Chemotherapy for malignant gliomas. J Neurosurg 68:1, 1991.

Laws ER: Neurosurgical management of low-grade astrocytomas of the cerebral hemispheres. J Neurosurg 61:665, 1984.

Leibel S: Radiation therapy for neoplasms of the brain. J Neurosurg 66:1, 1987.

Loeffler JS: The treatment of recurrent brain metastases with stereotactic radiosurgery. J Clin Oncol 8:576, 1990.

Mahaley MS: Neuro-oncology index and review: adult primary brain tumors. J Neuro-Oncol 11:85, 1991.

Olin JW: Treatment of deep vein thrombosis and pulmonary emboli in patients with primary and metastatic brain tumors. Arch Intern Med 147:2177, 1987.

Otter R: Solitary brain metastasis treatment: a randomized trial. Neurology 38:393, 1988.

Patchell R: A randomized trial of surgery in the treatment of single metastases to the brain. N Engl J Med 322:494, 1990.

Posner JB: Paraneoplastic syndromes. Curr Neurol 9:245, 1989.

Recht LD: Suspected low grade glioma: is deferring treatment safe? Ann Neurol 31:431, 1992.

Walker MD: Randomized comparison of radiation therapy and nitrosoureas for the treatment of malignant glioma of the brain. N Engl J Med 303:1323, 1980.

Wasserstrom WR: Diagnosis and treatment of leptomeningeal metastases from solid tumors. Cancer 49:759, 1982.

Weisberg LA: Benign intracranial hypertension. Medicine (Baltimore) 54:197, 1978.

CHAPTER

137 Neuroendocrinology

Steven E. Hyman

Neuroendocrinology is the field that deals with the relationship between the nervous system and the endocrine system. Because of its scope, this chapter serves only as an introduction. Interactions between the central nervous system (CNS) and endocrine glands are critical for homeostatic maintenance; for responses to environmental stimuli, such as danger; for control of reproductive function; and for many behaviors. In addition, the nervous system exerts control over such hormonally mediated developmental processes as growth and sexual maturation. Communication between the nervous system and the endocrine system travels in both directions; neurons of the hypothalamus and the autonomic nervous system transduce signals from the CNS to the endocrine system, whereas peripherally released hormones—especially steroids, which cross the blood-brain barrier easily—have many sites of action within the brain.

In recent years the purview of neuroendocrinology has been broadened to include all of neurosecretion, because of the realization that many of the classic distinctions between the nervous system and the endocrine system had been too simplistically drawn. In retrospect, it is not surprising that the two major systems responsible for intercellular communication share many physiologic mechanisms and even the molecules they use for signaling. For example, by definition endocrine glands secrete directly into the bloodstream; neurons, on the other hand, were initially thought to secrete their transmitters only at specialized structures called *synapses*. More recently, it has been found that the mechanisms of neurosecretion are quite varied. Within the nervous system, many transmitters appear to be released not at classic synapses, but into the intercellular space between neurons, and to diffuse over relatively large distances before reaching postsynaptic receptors. In addition, certain hypothalamic neurons secrete hormones directly into the blood; not only are these secreting cells morphologically neurons, but their secretion is caused by depolarization. This latter type of release, often called *neuroendocrine secretion,* is the mode of secretion of the hypophysiotropic-releasing hormones and the posterior pituitary hormones, oxytocin and vasopressin. Another initially unsuspected similarity between the nervous system and endocrine systems has been the discovery that peptides, many of which act as classical hormones, may also serve as transmitters within the CNS; indeed, almost all of the traditional peptide hormones of the endocrine system have now been found in the CNS.

NEUROENDOCRINE REGULATION (also see Chapter 147)

The major anatomic substrates of neuroendocrine regulation are the basal forebrain, limbic system, and midbrain, all of which have major inputs into the hypothalamus; the hypothalamus itself, with its median eminence-portal capillary system; and the anterior and posterior pituitary (see Chapters 160 and 161). Neurons from the higher centers projecting to the hypothalamus regulate hormone synthesis and release by the hypophysiotropic neurosecretory cells. The major inputs from higher centers probably utilize the excitatory neurotransmitter glutamate to evoke hormone release, but these effects are powerfully modulated by noradrenergic and serotonergic afferents from the brainstem, by dopaminergic and opioid peptide-containing afferents from within the hypothalamus, and by inputs from the circadian pacemaker located within the suprachiasmatic nucleus of the hypothalamus. In addition to these regulatory systems within the brain, there are inhibitory feedback loops mediated by peripheral hormones. What results are the complex patterns of hormone release required for the optimal end-organ effects of each hormone. These patterns include basal release; pulsatile release, as in the case of gonadotropin-releasing hormone (GnRH); circadian patterns of release, as with growth hormone–releasing hormone (GHRH) and corticotropin-releasing hormone (CRH); and evoked release, as occurs in stress (e.g., producing extra bursts of CRH). Loss of these patterns can lead to abnormalities of function: for example, continuous, as opposed to pulsatile, release of GnRH leads to desensitization of its receptors with resulting hypogonadism; loss of normal diurnal variation in corticotropin-releasing factor (CRF) release with excessive afternoon and evening secretion may produce signs of hypercortisolism, even if the absolute peak levels of cortisol are not elevated.

Neurotransmitter regulation of the releasing hormones may involve both single and multisynaptic pathways. The dopaminergic pathways involved in neuroendocrine regulation arise mainly in the arcuate nucleus of the hypothalamus and descend into the median eminence (the tuberohypophyseal system), where they are involved in the control of anterior pituitary secretion, most prominently the inhibition of prolactin release. The noradrenergic pathways that affect pituitary secretion ascend to the hypothalamus from their nuclei of origin in the pons, which are adjacent to the major noradrenergic nucleus of the brain, the locus coeruleus. Serotonergic projections to the hypothalamus ascend from the brainstem raphe nuclei.

An understanding of the neurotransmitter inputs into neuroendocrine regulation can lead to important clinical implications. Since hypophysiotropic-releasing hormones are under neuronal control, drugs that affect neurotransmitters or their receptors can alter endocrine function. For example, because dopamine has inhibitory effects on prolactin synthesis and release, dopamine receptor agonists, such as bromocriptine, have been used successfully in the treatment of prolactinomas. Drugs that affect neurotransmitters can also result in significant neuroendocrine side effects. For example, because the antipsychotic drugs are dopamine antagonists, they may result in hyperprolactinemia.

The fact that monoamine neurotransmitters have critical effects on neuroendocrine secretion means that hormone regulation can possibly serve as a window on the brain. For example, although the pathophysiology of major depressive disorders is unknown, it is believed to involve dysfunction of monoamine neuronal systems, including noradrenergic and possibly serotonergic projections, and it has been found that nearly 50% of patients with major depression have a strikingly abnormal pattern of cortisol secretion, with hypersecretion and loss of normal diurnal variation. Although tests of the hypothalamic-pituitary-adrenal axis are neither sensitive nor specific enough to provide a useful medical test for depression, study of neuroendocrine dysregulation in CNS disorders such as depression may eventually yield useful insights into the pathophysiology of depression and of stress-related disorders.

NEUROPEPTIDES

During recent years, a large number of peptides, many of them originally identified as hormones, have been found to act as transmitters in the nervous system. Although the occurrence of the same peptide both within and outside the CNS initially suggested that certain peptides might be involved in the regulation of related functions at different anatomic sites, there is little evidence to suggest that this is the case. The classification of brain peptides given in the box at right is therefore more a reflection of the history of their discovery than of their functions within the CNS, which remain largely unknown.

Although somewhat simplistic, it is possible to think of the brain's neurotransmitters as divided into three major groups: (1) the excitatory and inhibitory amino acids, (2) the biogenic amines, and (3) the neuropeptides. The amino acids have the highest concentration in brain (10^{-3} molar) and a uniform distribution, as would be expected of transmitters that probably subserve classical "fast" synaptic transmission among neurons. The biogenic amines, norepinephrine (NE), dopamine (DA), serotonin (5-HT), histamine, and acetylcholine (ACh), and all of the neuropeptides generally produce what have been called modulatomy effects on postsynaptic neurons. A full description of these effects is beyond the scope of this chapter, but they include relatively long-term changes in the behavior of the postsynaptic neuron's ion channels and thus modulation of the way it can subsequently process information. The biogenic amines have greater regional variability of concentration than do the amino acids, but in major brain areas they have a concentration of about 10^{-6} molar. Anatomically they are organized for the most part as diffusely projecting systems originating from a small number of cell bodies in the brainstem or basal forebrain, and they give the appearance of regulatory systems, perhaps setting the responsiveness of other circuits. Peptides, on the other hand, have an extremely irregular distribution in brain, with individual peptides being represented in some areas but not others. Where present, they often occur in very low concentrations in comparison to other transmitters (about 10^{-9} molar). Like the biogenic amines, they appear to function largely as modulators of other neural circuits but to act more locally.

Because of rapid progress in application of radioimmunoassay, immunohistochemistry, and molecular cloning techniques, the identification of peptide transmitters has proceeded rapidly. Understanding their particular functions, however, has remained a difficult problem. The functions of some peptides are known, at least in limited contexts:

Classification of CNS peptides by other tissues and functions in which they are prominent

- Neurohypophyseal hormones
  - Vasopressin
  - Oxytocin
  - Neurophysins
- Hypophysiotropic-releasing hormones
  - Thyrotropin-releasing hormone
  - Gonadotropin-releasing hormone
  - Somatostatin
  - Corticotropin-releasing hormone
  - Growth hormone–releasing hormone
  - Prolactin inhibitory factor
- Pituitary hormones
  - Corticotropin
  - Beta-LPH, beta-endorphin
  - Prolactin
  - Growth hormone
  - Luteinizing hormone
  - Thyrotropin
- Opioid peptides
  - Beta-endorphin
  - Methionine enkephalin
  - Leucine enkephalin
  - Dynorphin
- Gastrointestinal peptides
  - Vasoactive intestinal polypeptide
  - Cholecystokinin
  - Gastrin
  - Neurotensin
  - Insulin
  - Glucagon
  - Secretin
  - Motilin
  - Pancreatic polypeptide
- Tachykinins
  - Substance P
  - Substance K
- Invertebrate peptides
  - Hydra head activator
  - FMRF amide
- Other peptides
  - Angiotensin
  - Bradykinin
  - Calcitonin
  - Calcitonin gene–related peptide (CGRP)
  - Carnosine
  - Neuropeptide Y
  - Atrionatriuretic peptide
  - Bombesin

for example, substance P appears to be involved in transmitting pain messages from the periphery, and methionine enkephalin and leucine enkephalin are involved in suppression of incoming pain signals. But even for peptides with some known functions, many remain undiscovered, and the roles of most of the neuropeptides in physiology remain a challenge for the future.

REFERENCES

Gold PW et al: Responses to corticotropin-releasing hormone in the hypercortisolism of depression and Cushing's disease: pathophysiologic and diagnostic implications. N Engl J Med 314:1329, 1986.

Hokfelt T: Neuropeptides in perspective: the last ten years. Neuron 7:867, 1991.

Lindberg I: The new eukaryotic precursor processing proteinases. Mol Endocrinol 5:1361, 1991.

Sossin WS, Fisher JM, and Scheller RH: Cellular and molecular biology of neuropeptide processing and packaging. Neuron 2:1408, 1989.

van den Pol AA, Wuarin JP, and Dudek FE: Glutamate, the dominant excitatory transmitter in neuroendocrine regulation. Science 250:1276, 1990.

CHAPTER

138 Metabolic and Toxic Disorders

Stephen M. Sagar

METABOLIC ENCEPHALOPATHY

A wide variety of toxins and metabolic derangements depress CNS function and produce metabolic encephalopathy (see box at right). The clinical signs are relatively stereotypes and reflect a rostral-caudal gradient of sensitivity to metabolic and toxic insults. The cerebral cortex is most vulnerable and hence affected earliest. As the degree of abnormality progresses, there is successive involvement of basal ganglia, diencephalon, and brainstem.

Consequently, the earliest signs of metabolic encephalopathy are those of diffuse depression of cerebral cortical activity. There is impairment of attention and of higher intellectual function. The patient has difficulty with abstractions and constructional problems, such as drawing a clock, and may become dysarthric, have word-finding difficulty (anomia), and make paraphasic errors. As the encephalopathy progresses, the patient becomes confused and then delirious and progressively drowsy. Periodic (Cheyne-Stokes) respiration is common in the early stages of metabolic encephalopathy. Asterixis, a flapping tremor of the outstretched hands caused by brief lapses in postural muscle tone, is a nonspecific sign of metabolic encephalopathy that helps distinguish the condition from focal lesions.

As the patient becomes stuporous, a stage is reached where the patient is responsive only to noxious stimuli, but characteristically has no lateralizing neurologic signs (unless there is a pre-existing lesion, the manifestations of which can be brought out by diffuse encephalopathy). There may be extrapyramidal rigidity, or, unusually, posturing of the extremities. Importantly, however, the brainstem reflexes, including pupillary responses and extraocular movements, are intact.

It is important to distinguish this state from the syndrome of central herniation, in which the patient becomes stuporous and may not have lateralizing neurologic signs, but has sluggish or absent pupillary reflexes and decorticate or decerebrate posturing of the extremities. A more complex picture may be presented by overdoses of drugs that have direct autonomic actions (e.g., tricyclic antidepressants, neuroleptics, atropine-like drugs, and sympathetomimetic agents) that may impair pupillary light responses early in the course of encephalopathy.

Causes of acute metabolic encephalopathy

I. Substrate deficiency
   - Hypoxia/ischemia
   - Hypoglycemia
   - Carbon monoxide poisoning
   - Hypoxia

II. Cofactor deficiency
   - Thiamin
   - Vitamin B_{12}
   - Pyridoxine (isoniazid administration)

III. Electrolyte disorders
   - Hyponatremia
   - Hypercalcemia
   - CO_2 narcosis
   - Dialysis disequilibrium syndrome

IV. Endocrinopathies
   - Diabetes
     - Ketoacidosis
     - Nonketotic hyperglycemic hyperosmolar coma
   - Thyroid
   - Adrenal
   - Parathyroid

V. Endogenous toxins
   - Liver disease
     - Portal-systemic shunting
     - Liver failure
   - Uremia
   - Porphyria
   - Subarachnoid hemorrhage

VI. Exogenous toxins
   - Drug overdose
     - Sedative/hypnotics
     - Ethanol
     - Narcotics
     - Salicylates
     - Tricyclic antidepressants
   - Industrial toxins (e.g., organophosphorus insecticides, heavy metals)
   - Meningitis
   - Sepsis

VII. Heat stroke

VIII. Epilepsy (postictal)

IX. Drug withdrawal

With progressive involvement of more caudal areas of the brain, the patient becomes unresponsive to even noxious stimuli; decorticate or decerebrate posturing occurs. The extraocular movements become progressively more difficult to elicit, but pupillary light reflexes are typically maintained. Finally, medullary respiratory centers are affected, leading to respiratory arrest and death unless the patient is supported. This entire sequence of events may occur over minutes in the case of hypoglycemia, over about an hour if rapidly absorbed sedative-hypnotic drugs such as pentobarbital are ingested, or over weeks for slowly developing metabolic conditions.

With certain causes of metabolic encephalopathy, particularly hyponatremia, uremia, and porphyria, generalized major motor seizures may intervene. These may occur at any stage of the encephalopathy, but are usually seen at the point that the patient enters the delirious phase or later. In withdrawal syndromes from alcohol and short-acting barbiturates, seizures may occur before signs of encephalopathy appear.

Laboratory and radiographic data are helpful in defining the cause of encephalopathy and excluding structural causes of altered mental status. The electroencephalogram (EEG) is quite sensitive to metabolic derangements of the cortex and demonstrates symmetric slowing of background rhythms. The EEG is therefore helpful in excluding focal cortical pathology and in following the progression and resolution of encephalopathy. CT and MRI scans are normal in uncomplicated metabolic encephalopathy; in severe cases and cases complicated by global hypoxia or ischemia there may be diffuse brain swelling.

Other specific laboratory abnormalities relate to the etiology of individual cases. Endocrine and electrolyte abnormalities, abnormal liver or renal function, abnormalities of blood gases, and the presence of toxic levels of drugs may be diagnostic in cases of obscure etiology.

SPECIFIC DISEASES CAUSING METABOLIC ENCEPHALOPATHY

Hypoglycemia

Since glucose is the major fuel for brain metabolism and brain neurons contain only minimal glycogen stores, a rapid fall in blood glucose can produce severe impairment of CNS function. The level of blood glucose at which encephalopathy occurs is variable and depends on the rapidity with which the glucose falls. Diabetic patients whose glucose drops rapidly from hyperglycemic levels in response to an insulin injection may develop symptoms at levels of blood sugar that are well tolerated by a nondiabetic, starved person. With rapidly falling glucose, the encephalopathy may progress over minutes. Seizures may occur and are usually major motor in type. Unlike other causes of metabolic encephalopathy, hypoglycemia commonly causes focal neurologic signs, including aphasias and hemiparesis, in the absence of an underlying brain lesion.

These deficits are rapidly correctable with the administration of glucose. Because the administration of glucose to thiamin-deficient patients can precipitate Wernicke's encephalopathy, it is standard practice to administer thiamin along with the glucose if the patient's history is unknown or if there is a question of malnutrition or alcoholism. The routine administration of glucose in cases of acute encephalopathies of unknown cause is standard practice in the emergency ward setting.

Hyponatremia

Serum hypo-osmolality associated with hyponatremia causes water to enter cells, including cells of the central nervous system. This results in brain edema and disruption of neuronal physiology. Serum sodium levels below 125 mEq/L are frequently associated with seizures and encephalopathy. As in hypoglycemia, the level of serum sodium at which a given patient becomes symptomatic depends on the rapidity with which hyponatremia develops; chronic hyponatremia of modest degree is better tolerated than a rapid fall of serum sodium.

Hyponatremia is common in three settings (see Chapter 350): when dehydrated patients are given hypotonic fluids, particularly common postoperatively; with the syndrome of inappropriate ADH (vasopressin) secretion (SIADH) in association with pulmonary or CNS disease; and with the ectopic secretion of vasopressin-like substances by tumors, most commonly small cell carcinoma of the lung. A syndrome of cerebral salt wasting has also been described in association with subarachnoid hemorrhage. This condition produces hyponatremia and is associated with elevated circulating levels of both atrial natriuretic peptide and vasopressin, but it responds to salt repletion rather than fluid restriction.

The treatment of hyponatremia is detailed in Chapter 350. The rapidity with which symptomatic hyponatremia should be corrected is a matter of controversy. It is generally agreed that in severe hyponatremia the serum sodium should be raised rapidly to about 125 mEq/L to prevent seizures. The rate at which the serum sodium should be corrected from that point to normal depends on the underlying cause and the rate at which the hyponatremia developed. Rapidly developing hyponatremia, as in postoperative patients, is probably best corrected to nearly normal sodium levels over about 24 hours. Chronic hyponatremia should probably be more slowly corrected over several days to avoid central pontine myelinolysis (see p. 1176).

Acute hepatic encephalopathy

The clinical manifestations of acute hepatic encephalopathy caused by portal-systemic shunting are discussed in Chapter 56. Of interest neurologically is that tremor and other extrapyramidal movement disorders, including chorea and parkinsonian-like rigidity, are more common in hepatic encephalopathy than in other metabolic encephalopathies. Hyperventilation with respiratory alkalosis is also characteristic. The EEG may show triphasic waves, high-amplitude wave forms in the delta frequency range with characteristic appearance. These waves can occur in other encephalopathies, but are typical of hepatic disease. Laboratory confirmation of the diagnosis of hepatic encephalopathy may be difficult, as liver enzymes and bilirubin are not necessarily abnormal in portal-systemic shunting. Arterial ammonia concentration is difficult to measure in a standardized fashion and is highly variable in normal patients. Cerebrospinal fluid glutamine concentration is a more reliable indicator and is now readily available, but it requires a lumbar puncture, which is risky in the presence of clotting abnormalities.

The treatment of hepatic encephalopathy is based on reducing the ammonia levels in the brain, although ammonia is probably only one of several toxins responsible for the encephalopathy. Protein restriction, lactulose, and nonabsorbable antibiotics administered orally or by enema are the mainstays of treatment. There is evidence that overactivity of neuronal systems that employ γ-amino butyric acid (GABA) may play a role in hepatic encephalopathy; experimental trials are under way with benzodiazepine antagonists that inhibit GABAergic transmission. Fever of any cause may make hepatic encephalopathy suddenly worse and requires immediate treatment. Patients with portal-systemic shunting may have subclinical neuropsychiatric abnormalities without overt encephalopathy. It is possible that their daily functioning can be improved by dietary protein restriction and lactulose therapy.

The neurologic syndrome of acute liver failure is indistinguishable from that of portal-systemic shunting, but generally develops rapidly. The same treatment modalities are employed for both conditions.

ALCOHOL-RELATED DISORDERS

Acute intoxication

Ethanol intoxication produces a clinical syndrome familiar to everyone in its mild and moderate form; it is identical to intoxication with other sedative/hypnotics in its severe form. Ataxia is usually obvious at blood ethanol levels of 50-100 mg/dl, confusion at levels over 200 mg/dl, and stupor and coma at levels above 300 mg/dl. Chronic alcoholics demonstrate tolerance to the neurologic effects of ethanol; they show fewer signs of intoxication at a given blood alcohol concentration than do naive drinkers.

Unless ethanol intoxication is complicated by respiratory or cardiovascular failure, all of the manifestations of acute ethanol intoxication are reversible. The treatment, therefore, is medical support as necessitated by the level of intoxication. There is no benefit from the administration of caffeine or other CNS stimulants. Rare individuals exhibit pathological intoxication after ingestion of even small amounts of ethanol. They display bizarre and aggressive behavior and delusional thinking and are usually amnestic for the episode. The condition resolves after a few hours, but may require observation in a protected and supervised setting.

Ethanol withdrawal

The mildest manifestation of withdrawal from chronic ethanol ingestion is tremulousness, which appears several hours after the last drink and may persist for several days. The tremor responds to propanolol, benzodiazepines, and renewed ethanol ingestion, but is self-limited and does not require specific therapy.

Withdrawal seizures characteristically occur 18-48 hours after cessation of heavy drinking and are major motor in type. They are usually brief, few in number, and self-limited; but prolonged seizures and even status epilepticus can occur. It is unclear if alcohol withdrawal seizures can be prevented with anticonvulsants, but in many detoxification programs alcoholics being withdrawn from ethanol are treated with a brief course of phenytoin or carbamazepine.

Alcohol withdrawal may also precipitate seizures in patients with underlying epilepsy, but the occurrence of a generalized, uncomplicated major motor seizure during ethanol withdrawal does not imply the presence of epilepsy. Since alcoholics are susceptible to head trauma, infections, and other causes of epilepsy, it may be difficult to decide in an individual case if the patient's seizures are purely withdrawal seizures or whether chronic anticonvulsant therapy is indicated.

Delirium tremens is the most dramatic and potentially life-threatening result of acute ethanol withdrawal. The syndrome begins 1-5 days after the last drink and persists for 1-5 days, depending on severity. It is heralded by increasing tremulousness, agitation, and signs of sympathetic overactivity, including diaphoresis, tachycardia, hypertension, and hyperthermia. The patient becomes confused, then delirious. Visual hallucinations, characteristically vivid and disturbing, are a prominent feature. These agitated, delirious patients are challenging management problems. Cardiac arrhythmias, dehydration, and complications of intercurrent illnesses, such as pancreatitis, liver disease, and infection, may be life-threatening.

Treatment consists of careful hydration and electrolyte management, sedation with benzodiazepines, cardiac monitoring and treatment of arrhythmias, and fever reduction with antipyretics. Excess free water sufficient to produce hyponatremia should not be administered, but fluid losses from diaphoresis and hyperthermia must be replaced. Patients are frequently hypomagnesemic, but there is no evidence that replacement of magnesium ameliorates the syndrome. The patients are frequently hypokalemic; but because of sympathetic overactivity and resulting cardiac arrhythmias, particular care must be taken with the intravenous administration of potassium. If possible, oral potassium supplementation should be used.

Sedation is best carried out with benzodiazepines. Upon presentation, the patient may be given diazepam intravenously in increments of 5 mg every 10-20 min until the patient is sedate but still easily arousable. The patient must then be monitored frequently and supplemental doses given I.V. or I.M. as needed. It is important to recognize the long-acting nature of diazepam and not put the patient on a fixed schedule of doses, which frequently results in oversedation and can produce respiratory failure.

Alcoholic hallucinosis is a relatively benign withdrawal syndrome during which patients experience recurrent hallucinations, which are typically auditory and which may be threatening and disturbing. This syndrome usually lasts a few days and is self-limited, but rarely runs a prolonged course.

Nutritional deficiency

Chronic alcoholics may obtain much of their daily caloric intake as ethanol. Therefore, they are subject to nutritional deficiency, especially of folate and thiamin. The cardinal manifestation of folate deficiency is a macrocytic anemia, but it is possible that peripheral neuropathy may also result. The central nervous system bears the brunt of thiamin deficiency. Wernicke's encephalopathy is an acute neurologic emergency. The disease is most commonly seen in alcoholics, but occurs in other malnourished people as well. The neuropathology consists of focal hemorrhagic necrosis, especially in sites surrounding the third ventricle and aqueduct. The mammillary bodies are the most vulnerable regions, but thalamus, hypothalamus, the periaqueductal gray matter, the floor of the fourth ventricle, and the cerebellar cortex are affected as well.

The clinical syndrome has three cardinal manifestations: an acute confusional state with loss of ability to form new memories (from diencephalic lesions), ophthalmoplegia (from brainstem lesions), and ataxia (from brainstem and cerebellar involvement). Rarely, the patient may be stuporous or comatose. Immediate therapy with thiamin, 50 mg I.V. and 50 mg I.M. plus daily doses of 50 mg I.M. or P.O., is undertaken whenever the disease is suspected. The ophthalmoplegias respond best to therapy, ataxia less well. The loss of recent memory shows the slowest and least improvement.

Patients may be left with Korsakoff's psychosis, the chronic inability to form new memories. Typically, these patients confabulate; that is, they manufacture untruthful stories and experiences in response to questions. When presented with verbal material in memory testing, they register the information correctly but retain it for less than 1 minute.

Chronic ethanol toxicity

Chronic ethanol ingestion is directly toxic to the nervous system. It commonly produces a distal, symmetric sensory-motor peripheral neuropathy that can be painful. The neuropathy is primarily axonal and recovers slowly if ethanol ingestion ceases. Cerebellar degeneration also occurs, both in association with acute Wernicke's encephalopathy and as an isolated disease. The anterior vermis is the most vulnerable region, producing trunkal ataxia as the major manifestation. Focal cerebellar atrophy can frequently be seen on CT or MRI scans; pathologically there is loss of Purkinje cells in the regions affected.

Myopathy may result from chronic ethanol abuse and may be acute or chronic. Binge drinking may result in acute rhabdomyolysis, with generalized muscle weakness and soreness, serum CPK values in the thousands, and myoglobinuria. The myopathy is reversible. Hydration and medical management to prevent renal failure are required. The chronic form of alcoholic myopathy produces progressive proximal muscle weakness with only modest elevation of serum CPK. The muscles are not tender. The electromyogram and muscle biopsy show a myopathic picture, although peripheral neuropathy frequently coexists.

Two rare conditions associated with chronic alcoholism are optic neuropathy, a subacute demyelinating lesion of the optic nerves sometimes called alcohol-tobacco amblyopia, and Marchiafava-Bignami disease, a demyelinating disease beginning in the corpus callosum and spreading bilaterally into centrum semiovale. Mild, asymptomatic cases of this illness are being recognized by MRI scanning, but the disease can be devastating, with the subacute development of dementia, paralysis, and even coma and death. The pathophysiology of these uncommon demyelinating diseases is unknown.

CHRONIC EFFECTS OF METABOLIC DERANGEMENT

Chronic acquired hepatocerebral degeneration

Patients who undergo repeated bouts of hepatic encephalopathy develop a chronic and irreversible neurologic syndrome characterized by dysarthria, tremor, and ataxia. The patient may develop a rigid extrapyramidal movement disorder as well. There is no specific therapy for this condition except avoidance of acute hepatic encephalopathy.

Central pontine myelinolysis

Since the advent of intravenous fluid therapy, an apparently new disease has appeared marked by the acute development of quadraparesis, ataxia, and abnormalities of extraocular movements. The neuropathology consists of a focus of demyelination in the basis pontis, without inflammation, hemorrhage, or necrosis. More recently, the disease has been recognized to be associated with hyponatremia, although it is not known if the hyponatremia per se or its too-rapid correction produces the damage. Other factors, including liver disease and alcoholism, may also play an important role, as the condition occurs in liver transplant recipients, some of whom have no documented hyponatremia.

Posthypoxic leukoencephalopathy

A small minority of patients who suffer global brain hypoxia or ischemia (including survivors of cardiac arrest and carbon monoxide intoxication) develop, several days to 2 weeks after the insult, a subacutely progressive demyelinating disease affecting the white matter of the centrum semiovale and the internal capsules. Spastic quadraparesis, pseudobulbar palsy, and dementia are prominent manifestations. The pathophysiology of this delayed reaction to hypoxia/ischemia is unknown and no specific therapy is available.

REFERENCES

Charness ME, Simon RP, and Greenberg DA: Ethanol and the nervous system. N Engl J Med 321:442, 1989.

Estol CJ et al: Central pontine myelinolysis after liver transplantation. Ann Neurol 39:493, 1989.

Plum F and Posner JB: The diagnosis of stupor and coma. Philadelphia, 1980, F.A. Davis.

Record CO: Neurochemistry of hepatic encephalopathy. Gut 32:1261, 1991.

Sterns RH: The management of symptomatic hyponatremia. Sem Nephrol 10:503, 1990.

Victor M, Adams RD, and Collins GH: The Wernicke-Korsakoff syndrome and related neurological disorders due to alcoholism and malnutrition, ed 2. Philadelphia, 1989, F.A. Davis.

Wijdicks EFM, et al: Atrial natriuretic factor and salt wasting after aneurysmal subarachnoid hemorrhage. Stroke 22:1519, 1991.

CHAPTER

139 Principles of Neurologic Emergencies and Intensive Care

Allan H. Ropper

Certain neurologic problems cause catastrophic, usually abrupt, brain damage and coma. These intracranial diseases include trauma, subarachnoid hemorrhage, parenchymal cerebral hemorrhage, status epilepticus, encephalitis, severe meningitis, brain tumor, brain edema after large cerebral infarctions, and basilar artery occlusion. All except the last have in common an increase in the volume of the intracranial contents and associated rise in intracranial pressure (ICP). Other neurologic diseases require emergency or intensive care because they cause respiratory failure; foremost are the Guillain-Barré syndrome, myasthenia gravis, and upper cervical spinal cord injury. These specific problems, representing the extremes of otherwise less severe neurologic diseases, require immediate diagnosis and management, frequent nursing attention, and the ability to respond quickly to clinical and pathophysiologic changes.

The clinical principles of neurologic intensive care, therefore, have to do with raised intracranial pressure, respiratory failure, and general medical complications of critical illness. A parallel emerging field, cerebral resuscitation, is concerned with minimizing neuronal damage after cardiac arrest. Despite interesting scientific leads, cerebral resuscitation has not yet achieved great clinical depth. A major controlled study of the use of high-dose barbiturates after cardiac arrest, used for their property of reducing cerebral metabolic requirements, has shown no benefit. There has also recently been increased appreciation of the frequency and importance of the neurologic complications of severe systemic diseases in medical and surgical intensive care units. These include encephalopathy, polyneuropathy, and seizures. The next decade promises important further clinical testing in these related fields.

PATHOPHYSIOLOGY OF ACUTELY RAISED ICP

Intracranial masses generally produce brain death or brain ischemia by raising the pressure within the skull to levels near arterial pressure in the cranium. This reduces the difference between systemic blood pressure and ICP, called *cerebral perfusion pressure:* CPP = BP − ICP. Reduced CPP from systemic hypotension appears to cause more neural damage than an identical reduction in cerebral perfusion from raised ICP. In both circumstances, the length of time and rapidity of ischemia, as well as the absolute level of cerebral blood flow, determine the extent of brain damage. ICP is normally below 10 to 15 mm Hg, and persistent elevation indicates that the compensatory mechanisms for the addition of volume to the brain, such as shifting of cerebrospinal fluid (CSF) and brain tissue away from the mass, are failing. Despite the imprecise methods available for measuring ICP and the uncertainty of blood pressures within cerebral vessels, ICP above approximately 40 mm Hg, with normal systemic blood pressure, appears to cause direct ischemic damage to neurons. Although an ICP between 15 and 40 mm Hg is not itself harmful, these levels indicate that precipitous further rises are about to occur, thus reducing the margin of safety before brain death. The relationship between ICP and volume, termed *compliance,* approximates an exponential function (Fig. 139-1); the risk of deterioration of CPP increases greatly as ICP or intracranial volume increases. The aim of therapy is to keep the ICP below or near 15 to 20 mm Hg, to prevent sudden deterioration from critically low CPP.

Blood pressure has a complex relationship to ICP and cerebral perfusion. Undamaged areas of the brain are able to autoregulate a constant cerebral blood flow (CBF), as systemic systolic blood pressure varies from approximately 80 to 170 mm Hg. When mean blood pressure is less than approximately 60 mm Hg, perfusion pressure begins to drop in parallel with blood pressure (Fig. 139-2). Inadequate

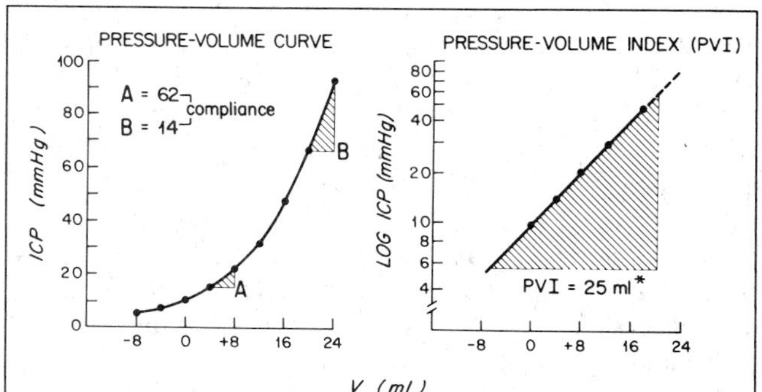

Fig. 139-1. Intracranial compliance curve showing the exponential relationship between ICP and increments of volume in the cranial cavity of a normal adult. The steepness of the curve changes with age, mannitol, and other factors. (* = calculated volume to raise ICP × 10.) (Reprinted with permission from Ropper AH: Neurological critical care. Semin Neurol 4:397, 1984.)

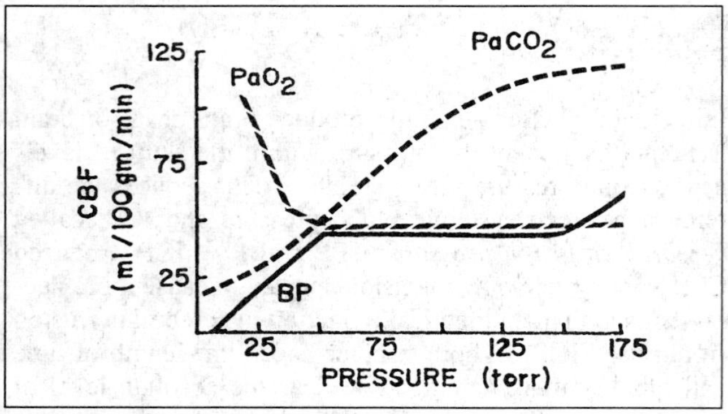

Fig. 139-2. Relationship between blood pressure, $PaCO_2$, and cerebral blood flow (CBF). The cerebral circulation autoregulates over a wide range of blood pressures. (From Shapiro HM: Anesthesia 43:445, 1975.)

blood flow may occur even earlier in regions subject to raised pressure from an adjacent mass. Simply elevating blood pressure to match raised ICP does not ensure adequate CPP, since elevated blood pressure worsens edema in damaged regions, eventually acting as an enlarging mass. The edema associated with trauma, hemorrhages, or infarctions—all associated with acute spontaneous hypertension—are particularly prone to enlarge with even moderate hypertension.

Patients with raised ICP have spontaneous or iatrogenically induced elevations in ICP caused by loss of autoregulation and by cerebrovascular dilation. These episodes, termed *plateau waves,* cause ICP to rise to extremely high levels for up to 30 minutes, often with clinical deterioration or brain death. Cerebral blood volume generally parallels CBF so that increases in flow result in elevated ICP, particularly if compliance is poor.

Normal regions of brain respond to changes in arterial CO_2 and oxygen tension in a predictable way (see Fig. 139-2). The reductions in CBF caused by lowering arterial CO_2 may be used as a therapeutic method of lowering ICP (see below); conversely, hypercarbia causes increased CBF and raised ICP. Arterial oxygen has less effect on CBF and ICP, but severe hypoxia causes cerebral vasodilation and increased ICP. All these relationships of systemic physiology to CBF and ICP occur in undamaged regions of brain, an effect quite different from ischemic, hemorrhagic, traumatized, or electrically discharging areas where blood flow has been uncoupled from the normal stimuli to vascular tone. Moreover, pressure dysautoregulation and CO_2-related flow changes are disrupted regionally in acute disease, resulting in exaggerated pressure gradients between brain compartments and signs of clinical deterioration.

Other derangements that exaggerate cerebral edema include serum hypo-osmolarity relative to brain that creates a gradient for water into brain tissue; increased cerebral venous pressures, as from sagittal sinus thrombosis, jugular vein compression, or congestive heart failure; and increased cerebral blood flow from fever or seizure.

CLINICAL SIGNS AND PATHOANATOMY OF INTRACRANIAL MASSES

The clinical features associated with an intracranial mass are the result of both direct damage in brain regions around lesion (hemiplegia is most common) and signs caused by secondary distortion of the lower thalamus and upper brainstem that lead to a diminished level of consciousness. The falx, a thick fold of dura separating the cerebral hemispheres, and the tentorium, the dural sheath separating the posterior fossa from the hemispheres, create natural limitations to tissue displacements as a hemispheric mass expands. The classic literature attributes the clinical signs caused by a mass lesion to movements of tissue downward through the tentorial opening or across the falx. These displacements, called *herniations,* are seen commonly in pathologic specimens and are associated with obvious compression and deformation of the upper midbrain, either laterally, from parahippocampal and uncal herniation, or more symmetrically, from downward transtentorial central herniation. Each of these distortions has been associated with a characteristic clinical syndrome that reflects dysfunction progressing from rostral to caudal regions of the brainstem. The central syndrome begins with drowsiness and bilaterally miotic, 1 to 2 mm diameter pupils that are light-reactive, and proceeds to stupor and enlarging 4 to 6 mm diameter pupils that eventually become unreactive to light. The uncal syndrome has as its main feature a unilaterally enlarging pupil (on the side of the mass in over 90% of cases, or paradoxically, on the other side in the remainder), followed by progressively diminished alertness. Both syndromes then converge with loss of horizontal eye movements (a sign of pontine damage), abnormalities of respiratory rhythmicity (a signal medullary dysfunction), and eventual loss of all clinically testable brain function. The central syndrome has been interpreted as the clinical result of symmetric downward compression of the upper midbrain as it is displaced centrally through the tentorial opening. The uncal syndrome is thought to represent compression of one third nerve by the uncal gyrus of the medial temporal lobe as it is pushed over the edge of the tentorium, or in some cases, by the downward movement of the posterior cerebral artery. Other well-described phenomena related to herniations in other regions are compressions of the posterior or anterior cerebral arteries against the dura causing infarction of the occipital lobe or frontal lobes; hemorrhages within the brainstem caused by distortion and rupture of small arteries (multiple small hemorrhages in the medulla, near the lower fourth ventricle are properly called *Duret hemorrhages,* although this term is in common use for all secondary brainstem hemorrhages); and damage to the pituitary stalk. Similar concepts connect downward impaction of the cerebellar tonsils (inferiorly and medially lying structures) into the foramen magnum as a cause of direct medullary compression, apnea, and death; upward herniation of the superior cerebellum through the tentorial opening, causing a syndrome that involves early pupillary abnormalities; and horizontal herniation of the medial cingulate gyrus of the frontal lobe under the falx, causing frontal lobe dysfunction. With the advent of computed tomography (CT) scanning and magnetic resonance imaging (MRI), other features of secondary tissue distortion from an acute hemispheric mass have been emphasized—most commonly, enlargement of all or of the posterior portion of the lateral ventricle on the side opposite a mass.

The relationship between a mass, herniation, and clinical signs depends on the size and location of the mass, the speed of evolution, and the shape and size of the tentorial opening. The brain tolerates large masses in the frontal and occipital lobes, distant from the tentorial aperture, better than central or parietal lesions, and tolerates slowly evolving masses, such as tumors, better than acute lesion, such as hemorrhages. The spaces surrounding the upper midbrain at the level of the tentorial opening vary greatly among individuals, which may account for some of the variation in clinical signs with herniation syndromes.

The fidelity of the various herniations to clinical signs varies, and complete classically described syndromes are uncommon in practice. They more often appear in fragmented fashion. There is a relatively consistent relationship between the horizontal displacement of the hemispheres by an acute unilateral mass and the level of consciousness; specifically, alertness is maintained with horizontal displacement of the pineal gland less than 3 mm from the midline, drowsiness occurs with 4 to 6 mm displacement, stupor with 6 to 8 mm displacement, and coma with greater than 8 mm displacement (Fig. 139-3). These may occur without evident downward herniation, although most displacements are invariably associated with so much tissue distortion that both vertical and horizontal herniations are seen. The pineal calcification serves only as an approximate but easily identifiable marker of midline displacement of the lower-thalamic and upper-midbrain region, where the important reticular nuclei reside. On occasion, substantial displacement of more anterior portions of the hemispheres—greater than a 12 mm horizontal shift of the septum pellucidum—is associated with stupor.

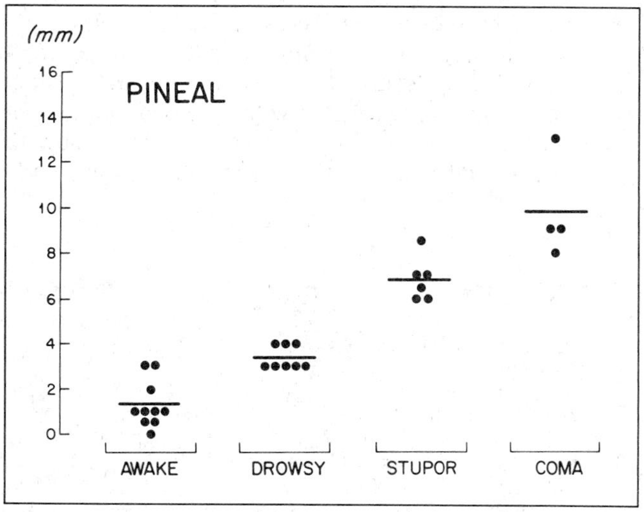

Fig. 139-3. Horizontal displacement of the pineal calcification from the midline, and the corresponding clinical state in patients with an acute hemispheric mass (hemorrhage, edema with middle cerebral artery infarction, or subdural hematoma). (Reprinted with permission from Ropper AH: N Engl J Med 314:953, 1986.)

The relation between clinical features of coma and raised ICP is complicated by drowsiness that commonly occurs in the several hours after a large hemispheric stroke, preceding any mass effect or horizontal displacement. Plum has suggested that acute large hemispheric lesions cause drowsiness or stupor by a mechanism of reticular activating system "shock." He has proposed that acute damage in the reticular system, at any level, disrupts the system temporarily and gives rise to a decreased level of consciousness. This view is corroborated by drowsiness acutely after large middle-cerebral-artery infarctions, at which time there is no mass effect (edema generally takes 24 to 72 hours to develop).

It is often not possible to separate the effects of herniations or large displacements from the damage caused by hypotension, hypoxia, or unseen traumatic damage at the time of many intracranial catastrophes. A clinical state worse than expected from horizontal shift is usually from one of these simultaneous injuries.

BRAIN DEATH

Brain death has become increasingly important as transplantation progress continues and public awareness increases. Most jurisdictions in the United States have determined that there is no legal difference between cessation of heart's activity and brain death. The pathologic state is characterized by progressive softening of the entire brain and the histologic changes of early cell death (respirator brain). This is reflected clinically by cessation of all function of the hemispheres and brainstem. Bedside testing to document brain death includes the observation of deep coma with absence of classical posturing (segmental spinal reflexes and unusual limb movements do occur); light-unreactive pupils that should be midposition or dilated, but not small; no spontaneous or caloric-induced eye movements; no facial movement or corneal reaction; and apnea when the ventilator is removed (see box on p. 1180). The latter has been defined in various ways, and some standardized tests have been suggested to demonstrate that the $PaCO_2$ has risen above 50 or 60 mm Hg without stimulating breathing. An isoelectric electroencephalogram (EEG) is often used as a confirmatory test to demonstrate massive cortical dysfunction but is not always necessary. In all circumstances, drug overdose must be excluded by history or laboratory testing. This clinical state is only an indirect reflection of the severe underlying brain damage of brain death, but it serves well as an operational definition. Another approach has been to equate brain death with cessation of cerebral blood flow that can be demonstrated with angiographic or radionuclide brain scan techniques. Some nuances of the clinical state, criteria for its demonstration, and the appropriate management

Clinical features of brain death

Hemisphere death
- Deep coma
- Absence of purposeful movement, well-defined posturing, or convulsions
- Can be corroborated by EEG, brain scan, or angiography*

Brainstem death
- Unreactive midposition or enlarged pupils
- Absent eye movements with oculocephalic ("doll's eyes") and oculovestibular (caloric) stimulation
- Absent corneal responses
- Absence of spontaneous breathing with apnea testing

Exclusions
- Sedative drugs
- Severe hypothermia
- Immediately preceding circulatory arrest

*Brain death is a clinical diagnosis; laboratory confirmation may be used in special circumstances.

of the family and approach to transplantation are usually established at the local hospital level.

RELATIONSHIP OF ICP TO OUTCOME

A number of studies have demonstrated a strong association between raised ICP and poor outcome in head trauma. The most important lesson learned from this work was that one half or more of hospital deaths in head-injured patients were caused by uncontrolled elevation in ICP that eventually led to global ischemia and brain death; the remainder were caused largely by sepsis and other medical complications. This work also suggested that aggressive therapy for raised ICP would improve clinical outcome. Skeptics have begun to question this premise, instead believing that uncontrollable ICP reflects severe and widespread damage that cannot be ameliorated. There is, however, a consensus that careful attention to ICP therapy avoids unnecessary deaths from raised ICP.

Several small series of nontraumatic intracranial lesions—including cerebral hemorrhage, large strokes that become edematous, encephalitis, and the few cases of massive brain swelling after cardiac arrest—suggest that there is also a relationship between raised ICP and poor outcome, particularly because of the absence of associated systemic injuries that cloud the issue in head trauma. Nevertheless, uncertainty exists about the beneficial effects of aggressive ICP therapy, and many neurologic practitioners currently favor an approach that usually stops short of monitoring ICP directly. In some experienced units, however, therapy is guided by ICP measurements, and there is the clinical impression that a few patients are salvaged who would otherwise have died from severe rises in ICP. The alternative to using ICP measurements to guide therapy is to treat all patients with moderate doses of mannitol and with hyperventilation, as well as to assume that those able to respond to therapy will do well and that those who cannot would have done poorly anyway.

MEDICAL TREATMENT OF RAISED ICP

Medical treatment of raised ICP reduces intracranial volume by (1) extracting extracellular water from brain tissue with osmotic agents, (2) reducing cerebral blood volume by constricting capacitance vessels with hypocarbia (hyperventilation) or barbiturates, and (3) preventing avoidable elevations of cerebral blood flow and edema caused by reversible entities such as fever, hypoxia, hypercarbia, inhaled anesthetics, and, especially, hypertension, or reductions in perfusion pressure from hypotension (see the box below).

Mannitol, given in bolus infusions, is currently the most commonly used hyperosmolar therapy for raised ICP, although glycerol is favored by some, and renal loop diuretics may produce a similar effect. The major effect of osmotic agents is thought to be the creation of an osmotic gradient between brain and blood in undamaged brain, extracting water that is subsequently excreted in a diuresis. There may also be a more acute effect from a brief but rapid cerebral vasoconstriction in response to extreme serum hyperosmolarity. Hyperosmolar therapy initially produces serum osmolarities of 290 to 325 mOsm per liter. Contributions to serum osmolarity from sodium or glucose alone are ineffective in reducing brain volume. Like hyperventilation, hyperosmolar therapy is effective mainly in undamaged regions of brain. Although free water administration is avoided by restricting fluids and giving only normal saline intravenously (all other standard intravenous fluids are hypoosmolar), intravascular hypovolemia from "fluid restriction" must be avoided in order to prevent hypotension. In other words, the ideal state is euvolemic hyperosmolarity. Intravascular volume support with crystalloid, colloid, or, least desirably, pressors, is necessary in some cases.

Hyperventilation, by reducing arterial PCO_2, causes a serum and CSF alkalosis that leads to cerebral vasoconstriction and begins to reduce ICP within 15 seconds. Hypocarbia continues to be effective for minutes to an hour or more in most cases. The CSF pH eventually returns to nor-

Therapies for raised intracranial pressure

Conventional
- Hyperventilation
- Hyperosmolar infusion and fluid restriction
- Blood pressure control

Unconventional or used in special circumstances
- High-dose barbiturates
- CSF drainage
- Craniectomy
- Surgical evacuation of clot or necrotic brain tissue
- Diuretics

mal (slightly lower than blood), and vasoconstriction ceases. The precise level of hypocarbia necessary to reduce ICP and its effective duration vary; little additional benefit occurs from $PaCO_2$ levels below approximately 24 mm Hg (there are exceptions in children, who continue to respond down to $PaCo_2$ 17 to 19 mm Hg). The theoretical possibility of creating ischemia by excessive hyperventilation seems to be rare or minimal in clinical practice. The benefits of hyperventilation have recently been questioned and a small group of head-injured patients may have better outcomes without hyperventilation. The problem of the limited duration of effect of hyperventilation is partially improved by the administration of buffers such as THAM that delay the equilibration of CSF pH. As with most other ICP therapies, hypocarbia is effective only in undamaged areas of brain where vessels remain reactive to physiological stimuli.

Hypertension may exaggerate edema more than almost any other physiologic abnormality in patients with raised ICP. Since most patients with intracranial masses become acutely hypertensive (especially those with hemorrhages or trauma), blood pressure control is a prime objective in ICP therapy. Normal areas of brain autoregulate to keep perfusion pressure approximately normal while damaged areas leak edema fluid that cannot be extracted. Raising blood pressure is, therefore, not a viable way of maintaining cerebral perfusion pressure. Conversely, excessive reduction in blood pressure creates a risk of hypoperfusing brain regions subject to raised ICP. Although the precise levels of desirable blood pressure in patients with acutely raised ICP have not been determined, a slow return toward normal seems desirable. Antihypertensive drugs that cause vasodilation, such as nitroglycerin and most calcium channel blockers, are generally avoided to avoid increased cerebral blood volume and raised ICP.

High-dose barbiturates dependably reduce raised ICP, but their use has gone through cycles of popularity and, more recently, decline. Although the addition of high-dose barbiturates does not improve outcome in head trauma, they remain useful adjuncts for controlling ICP, particularly by muting the blood pressure and ICP rises associated with endotracheal intubation or suctioning, chest physical therapy, and other ICU treatments. Some clinicians believe that the judicious use of barbiturates after conventional measures have failed to reduce ICP salvages a few patients who would otherwise become brain dead. The major risk in the use of high-dose barbiturates is hypotension, particularly when there is also dehydration and positive pressure ventilation—all of which conspire to reduce cardiac output. Should ICP fail to be controlled, barbiturates also confound the clinical diagnosis of brain death.

Surgical therapies, including ventricular CSF drainage, removal of blood clots or necrotic brain tissue, and hemicraniectomy, are dictated by the CT scan and the clinical state. There is currently no evidence that surgery improves the ultimate deficit caused by traumatic or hemorrhagic lesions, but removal of clot and drainage of hydrocephalus, by reducing intracranial volume, remain definitive ways to lower ICP. When hydrocephalus is thought to be the cause of stupor or coma, as it is after subarachnoid hemorrhage, ventricular drainage is the treatment of choice.

CEREBRAL BLOOD FLOW, METABOLISM, AND BRAIN RESUSCITATION

Normal function of neurons depends on the delivery of oxygen and glucose by adequate blood flow. Neurons have a very limited anaerobic capacity, so cortical electrical activity, as measured by EEG, stops several seconds after severe cerebral ischemia. Cerebral blood flow (CBF) in the hemisphere is approximately 60 ml per 100 g per minute (75 ml per 100 g per minute in gray matter, 45 ml per 100 g per minute in white matter, and 15 to 30 ml per 100 g per minute in the brainstem). Regional flow can change at least 50% in response to the metabolic demands of cortical neurons, especially if the motor strip is activated. As gauged by the EEG and evoked potentials, neurons become electrically dysfunctional when CBF falls below 20 to 30 ml per 100 g per minute, and spontaneous or evoked neuronal activity is reduced with CBF below 18 ml per 100 g per minute. Neurons are probably not irrevocably damaged until CBF is reduced below 12 to 15 ml per 100 g per minute; at that level, energy processes that maintain membrane and mitochondrial stability are disrupted. However, abrupt CBF reduction is less well tolerated than is subacute or chronic ischemia.

The observation that barbiturates can reduce the cerebral damage caused by experimental hypoxia or ischemia has led to clinical attempts at brain sparing, or "brain resuscitation," that aims to optimize substrate delivery and reduce neuronal metabolic demands during and after cardiac arrest. Despite success with barbiturates administered before or soon after cardiac arrest in animals, a large randomized trial has failed to show benefit in clinical circumstances of cardiac arrest. Modifications of CPR to improve CBF by increasing cerebral venous pressure, through increases in intrathoracic venous pressure, have also been suggested. Some work, still not fully corroborated, suggests that hyperglycemia may be harmful during ischemia. Control of hyperglycemia has therefore also become a part of some stroke and brain resuscitation therapy.

The most recent interest in brain resuscitation derives from the provocative observation that excitatory neurotransmitters in the cortex, especially glutamate in the hippocampus, are highly neurotoxic. Their release in large quantities after arrest of circulation may lead to ongoing but reversible neuronal damage after ischemia has been corrected. Glutamate may act as a neurotoxin by at least two mechanisms: by opening channels that allow calcium influx, causing mitochondrial and cell death; and by modifying sodium channels and causing cell swelling. Calcium-channel blockers and specific glutamate-binding antagonists are being studied as brain protectors as a result of these findings.

Generalized brain ischemia is associated with combinations of three types of anatomic distribution of injury. The classic ischemic-hypoxic injury causes loss of neurons predominantly in Sommer's sector of the hippocampus, with shrinkage and gliosis of the hippocampal gyri. This is manifested in some postcardiac arrest patients as a Korsakoff's-type memory loss with sparing of other mental performance. Disproportionate hypoxia compared to ischemia may be responsible for this type of injury. The dense distribution of glutamate receptors in the hippocampus may be a factor in the region's preferential susceptibility to ischemia-hypoxia. A more severe syndrome after cardiac arrest may result from widespread cortical neuronal damage. Virtually all regions of the cortex are affected, with most neuronal loss in layers 2 and 5 of the cortex, Purkinje cells of the cerebellum, and the hippocampus. The clinical state varies from severe dementia with apathy to virtually functionless hemispheres, manifest as "neocortical death" or the "apallic" state in which only brainstem function persists. More severe degrees of especially bad generalized ischemia can damage the basal ganglia as well. The third type of anatomic lesion results from a brief and purely ischemic insult that produces infarction in "watershed" or low flow border-zone regions of large arterial territories. These cause bilateral strokes in the high frontoparietal cortex between the middle and anterior cerebral artery blood supplies or in the posterior-inferior parietal cortex between the middle and posterior cerebral artery territories. In complete form the first watershed stroke produces shoulder and proximal arm weakness; the second, cortical blindness or related visual difficulties.

Status epilepticus represents a special type of intracranial derangement in which the metabolic demands of neurons are greatly increased and blood flow increases to match the metabolic needs of neurons. In the presence of an intracranial mass the increased flow may cause dangerous elevations of ICP. In addition to the risks associated with status epilepticus, including aspiration, hypoxia, cardiac stress, and self-injury, prolonged and continued electrocerebral seizures, even without convulsions, lead to cortical damage that simulates generalized ischemic injury.

NEUROLOGIC COMPLICATIONS OF CRITICAL ILLNESS (see box)

Approximately 20% of patients with acute illnesses in medical intensive care units have major neurologic complications, mainly encephalopathy from hepatic or renal failure or from the hypoxia of cardiac arrest, seizures, polyneuropathy, or stroke. The occurrence of any of these substantially worsens prognosis. A special syndrome of encephalopathy and polyneuropathy has been found to follow sepsis or multiorgan failure. The neuropathy (critical-illness polyneuropathy) is a major cause of inability to wean mechanical ventilation in critical care or postoperative settings. Seizures in critically ill medical patients are often not clinically evident and manifest only as periods of confusion or unresponsiveness. An EEG is required to detect this complication. Many neurologic conditions that lead to consultation in an ICU are the result of medication use, particularly the use of sedatives and neuromuscular blocking drugs.

Neurologic complications of critical medical illness

- Cerebral
  - Encephalopathy
    - Septic
    - Hepatic
    - Uremic
    - Anoxic
    - Hyponatremic
    - Hypo- or hyperglycemic
    - Medication induced
  - Seizures
    - From underlying brain lesion
    - From metabolic derangement
    - Medication induced
  - Stroke
- Polyneuropathy paralysis
  - Septic, multiorgan failure
  - Guillain-Barré syndrome
  - Uremic
  - Prolonged effect of neuromuscular blockers
  - Malnutrition
  - Profound hypokalemia or hypophosphatemia

RESPIRATORY FAILURE IN NEUROLOGIC DISEASES

Several important neurologic diseases cause diaphragmatic weakness and require intensive care, foremost among them Guillain-Barré syndrome, myasthenia gravis, critical-illness polyneuropathy, amyotrophic lateral sclerosis, and spinal cord injuries. A few of these illnesses can, rarely, present as primary respiratory failure. Coma from any source also creates a special situation of combined failure of airway protection and central respiratory failure. The neurologic aspects of these diseases are discussed elsewhere in the text, but the management of mechanical respiratory failure is common to all of them.

Diaphragmatic weakness is manifest first by reduced air flow rates through the airways that result in poor coughing and airway clearing. As weakness progresses, the maximum volume of breathing is diminished, resulting in atelectasis and mild hypoxemia. Because the diaphragm has special physiologic properties that cause it to fatigue and fail when muscle contraction exceeds narrow limits of rate and tension, respiratory arrest can occur rapidly and may not reflect weakness in other muscles. Most peripheral neurological diseases also affect oropharyngeal muscles and impair airway protection, compounding the risk of aspiration and poor airway clearing. Chest physical therapy and deep breathing are mainstays for assisting airway clearing. Once the diaphragm fatigues, air exchange is compromised and hypercarbia occurs. The complications of mechanical neuromuscular respiratory failure can be anticipated and are ultimately treated by endotracheal intubation and mechanical ventilation.

REFERENCES

Ivan B, editor: Coma: physiopathology, diagnosis and management. Springfield, 1982, Charles C. Thomas.

Plum F and Posner JB, editors: Diagnosis of stupor and coma, ed 3. Philadelphia, 1980, F.A. Davis.

Ropper AH: Acute increased intracranial pressure. In Asbury AK, McKhann GM, and McDonald WI, editors: Diseases of the nervous system, ed 2. Philadelphia, 1991, Saunders.

Ropper AH, editor: Neurological and neurosurgical intensive care, ed 3. New York, 1993, Raven Press.

CHAPTER

140 Neurocardiology

Martin A. Samuels

CARDIAC MANIFESTATIONS OF NEUROLOGIC DISEASE

Duchenne's muscular dystrophy

Boys with Duchenne's progressive fatal sex-linked dystrophy rarely have clinical evidence of myocardial dysfunction before the age of 10 years, but by age 18 all patients have clinically detectable cardiomyopathy. Congestive heart failure is a frequent terminal event, and autopsy invariably shows dystrophic myocardial involvement. Early dystrophy is characterized by tachycardia, large electrocardiogram (ECG) R/S wave ratios in V_1, diminished systolic function of the left ventricular posterior wall and septum, and decreased rate of relaxation of the posterior wall. With the development of a dilated cardiomyopathy in late dystrophy, additional cardiac abnormalities appear, including enlarged heart volume by x-ray; reduced left ventricular ejection fraction; diminished left ventricular diameter; and a decreased rate of circumferential fiber shortening, as detected in the echocardiogram (Chapter 5). The ECG in Duchenne's dystrophy characteristically indicates posterior wall fibrosis and is abnormal in nearly every case. It consists of tall, upright, precordial R waves with increased R/S amplitude ratios, often with deep limb lead and lateral precordial Q waves. Similar ECG abnormalities are regularly seen in affected siblings and even in female carriers. Sudden death may be more common in patients with Duchenne's dystrophy, but this has not been as well documented as it has been in the case of myotonic dystrophy.

The cardiac pathology is distinctive. It consists of dilation of both ventricles and patchy but fairly extensive scarring in both subendocardial and subepicardial locations within the posterolateral left-ventricular free wall, without narrowing of the extramural coronary arteries. The classic histologic changes seen in skeletal muscle are basically the same as those seen in cardiac muscle: that is, degeneration and subsequent loss of fibers, variation in fiber size, abnormal enlargement and atrophy of some fibers, concomitant proliferation of endomysial and perimysial connective tissue, and subsequent replacement with adipose tissue. The distinctive ECG pattern associated with Duchenne's dystrophy probably results from multifocal myocardial degenerative changes involving predominantly the posterobasal left ventricle and the posterior papillary muscle.

Facioscapulohumeral (Landozy-Dejerine) dystrophy

Facioscapulohumeral muscular dystrophy is consistent with a normal life expectancy and is usually transmitted as an autosomal-dominant trait. Most patients do not suffer from congestive heart failure during life, although rare cases have been reported in which cardiac involvement was predominant.

Limb-girdle (Erb's) muscular dystrophy

Little is known about the cardiac disease in limb-girdle dystrophy. It may be frequent pathologically but is rarely of clinical importance.

Myotonic dystrophy and myotonia congenita

Approximately two thirds of patients with myotonic dystrophy have cardiac involvement with conduction disturbances, including prolonged P-R and QRS intervals and left bundle block, frequent cardiomegaly, and congestive heart failure. Pathologically, there is fatty infiltration and replacement of myocardium, interstitial fibrosis, and destruction of muscle fibers. Many patients with myotonic dystrophy have symptomatic congestive heart failure and rhythm disturbances; sudden death is not at all unusual, probably as a result of cardiac arrhythmias. Even patients with congenital myotonic dystrophy have evidence of myocardial involvement as manifested by conduction defects and sometimes impaired systolic function.

Myotonia congenita (Thomsen's disease) is not a progressive disorder and may actually improve in adult life. Although there is often no cardiac involvement, cases have been reported with findings identical to those seen in myotonic dystrophy.

Other rare dystrophies

Cardiac involvement has been reported in isolated instances of nearly every type of the less common muscular dystrophies, including Becker's X-linked benign dystrophy and humeroperoneal dystrophy. Abnormalities in common include frequent atrial arrhythmia and conduction disturbances that range from P-R prolongation and abnormal P waves to sinus node arrest. Congestive heart failure is rare during life, but arrhythmias seem to be a common cause of death.

Metabolic myopathies

A myopathic illness caused by abnormal glucose metabolism is called a *metabolic myopathy*. Many of these illnesses result from abnormal mitochondrial function in various parts of the nervous system, and sometimes in other organs. These illnesses are unique because they are inherited in a non-Mendelian fashion—the mitochondrion is the only subcellular organelle that possesses its own DNA. These mitochondrial illnesses are divided into five types: (1) deficits of transport (e.g., carnitive deficiency); (2) defects in substrate utilization (e.g., pyruvate carboxylase deficiency, pyruvate dehydrogenase complex deficiency); (3) defects of the Krebs cycle (e.g., fumarase deficiency, alpha keto-glutamate deficiency); (4) defects of oxidation-phosphorylation coupling, and (5) defects in the respiratory chain (e.g., complex I, II, III, IV, or V deficiency). Clinically, many disorders in this group include a cardiomyopathy, the manifestations of which vary from asymptomatic cardiac enlargement to severe cardiac arrhythmias (e.g., complete heart block) and occasionally even overt heart failure. Two well-recognized clinical syndromes with cardiomyopathy are carnitive deficiency and the Kearns-Sayre syndrome. The former is characterized by attacks of hypoketotic hypoglycemia and progressive dilated cardiomyopathy resulting from a lipid storage myopathy, which is usually inherited as an autosomal recessive trait. The latter is a triad of progressive external ophthalmoplegia, retinal pigmentary degeneration, and heart block, apparently occurring as a sporadic condition. Most of the other mitochondrial myopathies, such as myoclonus epilepsy with ragged red fibers (MERRF), mitochondrial encephalomyopathy, lactic acidosis and strokelike episodes (MELAS), Leigh subacute necrotizing encophalomyelopathy, and Menke's trichopoliodystrophy, have little or no effect on cardiac muscle.

Polymyositis and dermatomyositis

This group of disorders is divided into several subgroups: polymyositis, dermatomyositis, childhood myositis, myositis with malignancy, and overlap syndromes.

Approximately one half of patients with polymyositis and dermatomyositis have ECG abnormalities. These changes are rare in patients with myositis with malignancy and in childhood myositis.

Approximately one third of patients with polymyositis have laboratory abnormalities indicating left ventricular dysfunction. Thus, subclinical cardiac dysfunction is a fairly common manifestation of polymyositis but rarely requires specific therapy.

Myasthenia gravis

Cardiac abnormalities clearly exist in myasthenia gravis. Prolonged Q-T intervals, sinus tachycardia, sinus arrhythmias, right bundle branch block, and nonspecific ST-T wave changes occur more frequently among myasthenic patients. The incidence of congestive heart failure is not greater among myasthenic patients, and these ECG changes probably do not represent myasthenic disease of cardiac neuromuscular junctions.

Neuropathic diseases

Neuropathies only affect the heart through the mechanism of autonomic neuropathy. The most common autonomic polyneuropathy is diabetes mellitus. The specific cellular mechanism is unknown, but diabetics are known to show significant orthostatic instability without the normal heart rate increase and maintenance of blood pressure on standing, to have abnormal sweating patterns, and, frequently, to complain of bowel, bladder, and sexual dysfunction. There is no specific therapy for this orthostatic instability except control of the diabetes and mechanical assistance, such as elastic stockings or body suits. Amyloidosis may produce a similar circumstance, but much more rarely.

In familial dysautonomia (Riley-Day syndrome), there is gross dysfunction of the autonomic nervous system with severe orthostatic hypotension.

Blood pressure control may be a major problem in patients with acute idiopathic polyradiculoneuritis (Guillain-Barré syndrome). Hypotension, labile hypertension, and persistent hypertension have all been seen in this disease. Several mechanisms have been considered. Some believe that the hypertensive episodes are caused by denervation hypersensitivity of vessels to circulating catecholamines because of an autonomic neuropathy. Denervation of baroreceptors could also theoretically produce hypertension, as has been proved experimentally. In most cases the clinically significant problem is orthostatic hypotension and labile blood pressure in the acute phase of the illness. Because of the extreme sensitivity of the blood pressure to posture, blood pressure control can usually be obtained merely by adjusting the head of the patient's bed. Antihypertensive agents and pressors should be avoided if possible, because of their probable excessive effect, probably from denervation hypersensitivity. It is rare for the problem to persist after the illness has reached its improvement phase.

ECG and myocardial abnormalities in neurologic disease

Many different ECG abnormalities have been seen in the setting of acute neurologic illness (see Chapter 4). The classic clinical setting is that of a subarachnoid hemorrhage, and the most characteristic ECG changes are tall, peaked, or inverted T waves, sometimes referred to as *cerebral T waves*. More worrisome are prolonged Q-T intervals and S-T segment changes suggestive of anterior wall myocardial ischemia. These and other, less dramatic abnormalities are seen in up to half of patients with subarachnoid hemorrhages and in as many as 90% of patients with ischemic strokes, many of whom have hypertension. Head injury and psychological stress have also been associated with arrhythmias.

Cardiac arrhythmias have been produced by electrical stimulation of several structures in the brains of experimental animals. Posterior hypothalamic stimulation is particularly effective, but subthalamic, hippocampal, and midbrain stimulation have also produced abnormalities. The most consistent and dramatic ECG abnormalities are produced by stimulation of the stellate ganglia in the neck. Lengthening of the Q-T interval (and thus, susceptibility to ventricular arrhythmias) is relatively easily effected by stimulation of the left stellate ganglion, but ablation of the right stellate ganglion can produce the same result.

The asymmetry of autonomic innervation of the heart is striking. Sympathetic fibers from the left stellate ganglion are dominant over the posterior aspect of the left ventricle, whereas the right stellate ganglion supplies the anterior wall. Similarly, the right vagus nerve supplies the sinoatrial (SA) nodes and has a dominant role in setting heart rate, whereas the left vagus nerve supplies the atrioventricular (AV) node, and its stimulation can lead to AV block.

For many years the ECG changes found in acute neurologic illness were thought to represent some noncardiac electrical disturbance, partly because autopsy studies showed no clear abnormalities in the myocardium. However, histopathologic abnormalities in heart muscle have been repeatedly demonstrated in cases of acute neurologic illness with ECG changes but no preexisting cardiac disease.

Endocardial hemorrhages have followed head trauma, seizures, and subarachnoid or other intracranial hemorrhages, particularly those involving the orbitalfrontal area, which appears to be part of the cortical representation of the autonomic nervous system. In acute neurologic illness with cardiac changes, the characteristic abnormality is myocardial contraction band necrosis (MCBN). This cardiac abnormality can also be seen with marked catecholamine excess, with reperfusion of the myocardium (such as after bypass surgery), and in sudden death attributed to stress. These cardiac changes are distinctly different from the coagulative necrosis seen in cases of coronary artery disease and myocardial infarction. Similar focal cardiac necrosis has been found in as many as one third of patients with raised intracranial pressure and in victims of sudden death.

It is clear that ECG abnormalities in the setting of acute neurologic illness are "cerebral" only in the sense of etiology. It is a threatened or damaged myocardium that produces the abnormal ECG. Of course, hypoxia and other metabolic stresses can be synergistic with the nervous system input in the induction of cardiac lesions. Experimentally, hypoxia and steroids potentiate catecholamines in the generation of cardiac lesions.

Experimentally, the subendocardial hemorrhages that follow hypothalamic stimulation can be prevented by section of the cervical spinal cord. Lack of a similar benefit from vagotomy again suggests that the cardiac lesions are mediated by the sympathetic nervous system. Prevention of CNS stimulation–induced arrhythmias by treatment with sympathetic antagonists or by reserpine also implicates the sympathetic nervous system. The effects of stellate ganglia stimulation and lesions suggest the same.

Several preventive therapies are possible. Sympathetic nervous system blockade by beta-adrenergic antagonists may provide protection against arrhythmias. More speculative treatment includes the use of calcium-channel blockers. Left stellate ganglion block has been employed successfully in cases of refractory cardiac arrhythmias after subarachnoid hemorrhage.

Specific neurocardiac syndromes

Friedreich's ataxia. Cardiac involvement has long been recognized in this familial neurologic disorder. Three of Friedreich's original six cases showed severe fatty degeneration of the heart. This incidence of 50% has remained constant, although ECG changes, not necessarily associated with cardiac symptoms, occur in over 90% of patients. In rare cases the cardiac disease may be much more severe than the neurologic disease and may even be the presenting symptom.

In the typical patient the cardiac symptoms are those of progressive congestive heart failure and angina pectoris. ECG changes include arrhythmias, heart block, and Q waves in I, II, V_1, V_5-V_6. Pathologically the heart is large, with fatty infiltration and fibrous replacement of myocardium. The fibers are hypertrophied, and the pathologic picture is often that of a hypertrophic cardiomyopathy.

The prognosis is poor, and most patients die of congestive heart failure. The importance of the cardiac aspect of the disease is clear, but, unfortunately, there is no evidence at this time that any treatment alters the course of this hypertrophic cardiomyopathy.

External ophthalmoplegia with cardiac conduction disorders (Kearn-Sayre's syndrome). One of the many "ophthalmoplegia plus" syndromes includes pigmentary degeneration of the retina and disorders of cardiac conduction. Most of these patients have severe disease of the conduction system with propensity to complete heart block. These patients are often young, and lifelong insertion of a permanent pacemaker is required to prevent sudden death.

NEUROLOGIC ASPECTS OF CARDIAC DISEASE

Arrhythmias

Atrial fibrillation (see Chapter 9). Atrial fibrillation greatly increases the risk of systemic embolism in patients with mitral valve disease, and it has been common practice to anticoagulate all such reliable patients for life to prevent systemic emboli, including cerebral emboli. In the past, however, patients with atrial fibrillation in the absence of mitral valve disease were not anticoagulated, since they were said not to have the same risk for systemic embolism as patients with mitral valve disease. It is now known that atrial fibrillation, regardless of its etiology, imparts a high risk for stroke. Although mitral disease plus atrial fibrillation does indeed produce the highest risk group, atrial fibrillation in other settings also produces a greatly increased risk, many times that of the control group.

Several large prospective studies have now shown conclusively that low-intensity anticoagulation with warfarin reduces the risk of stroke in patients with nonrheumatic atrial fibrillation. The lowest effective dose of warfarin thus far demonstrated in a well-done trial is an amount capable of prolonging the prothrombin time to 1.2-1.5 times the control.

A further dilemma arises when a patient with atrial fibrillation has an embolic stroke. Such infarctions often are hemorrhagic, presumably because of lysis of the embolic material and reflow of blood under arterial pressure into necrotic vessels. The amount of hemorrhage is usually small and insufficient to be seen on the CT scan, so the clinician is often faced with the problem of treating an embolic source with an anticoagulant that theoretically could convert a relatively benign hemorrhagic infarction into a full-blown intracerebral hemorrhage. Indeed, anecdotal cases have been reported in which a very atypical intracerebral hemorrhage was seen to develop after an embolic stroke in a patient on an anticoagulant. It is common practice to maintain anticoagulation in patients who suffer small embolic strokes and to temporarily discontinue anticoagulation in patients with large embolic strokes.

Ventricular arrhythmias and heart block (see Chapter 9). Ventricular arrhythmias (particularly ventricular tachycardia) and heart block with bradycardia may produce transient or permanent neurologic syndromes. Whether the deficit is transient or permanent is determined primarily by the length of time the arrhythmia persists, with the consequent decreased cerebral blood flow. Additional factors such as fixed arterial lesions in the carotid or vertebrobasilar arterial system, probably modulate the degree and distribution of deficit to some degree, but firm data are lacking.

Transient deficits from brief periods of generalized decreased cerebral blood flow are probably extremely common, particularly in the elderly. Often, these arrhythmias are sufficiently brief and infrequent to elude detection by routine ECG examination. Ambulatory ECG recording techniques have permitted the diagnosis of many brief arrhythmias and clarified their clinical correlates (see Chapter 4).

Cardiac arrest

Cardiac arrest refers to absent cardiac output for any cause, but its most common etiology is probably ventricular tachyarrhythmia (ventricular tachycardia and fibrillation). The patient loses consciousness promptly when cardiac output ceases, and the degree of recovery of neurologic function after resuscitation depends on the efficiency and speed with which cerebral circulation is restored. There is clearly a great deal of individual variation in the amount of time that must elapse before irreversible damage has occurred. In clinical practice it is extremely difficult to weigh the efficiency of a cardiac resuscitation. Its true effectiveness is, after all, reflected most accurately in the residual state of the patient's nervous system.

Until recently, the clinician had very little information on which to estimate the prognosis for useful life after cardiac arrest. Only the syndrome of brain death was clearly identified, defined as apnea, unresponsiveness, and absence of cranial reflexes with an isoelectric electroencephalogram. This circumstance is actually rare after a cardiac arrest. Most often, the physician is faced with a patient who is severely impaired but does not meet the full criteria for brain death. It is in this circumstance that additional guidelines are badly needed. Briefly stated, the absence of eye movements after cardiac arrest is a bad prognostic sign despite other intact brainstem functions, including respiratory and blood pressure control mechanisms. Few patients without eye movements after cardiac arrest recover to a level of useful neurologic function. In other words, these patients, although not meeting the strict definition of brain death, are left in a permanent vegetative state. It should be clearly understood, however, that these guidelines are purely medical and do not necessarily reflect the prevalent legal or social attitudes toward death and vegetative states.

Between the extremes of brain death and persistent vegetative state on the one hand and full recovery on the other is a wide spectrum of neurologic abnormalities consequent to cardiac arrest. These fall into two major categories: cases in which the return of blood flow occurs promptly but with a prolonged period of hypoxia (nonischemic anoxia) and cases in which the return of blood flow is delayed (ischemic anoxia).

In the former case, damage occurs in areas of the brain known to be particularly sensitive to hypoxemia despite adequate blood flow. These areas include layers three and five of the cerebral cortex (laminar necrosis), the Sommer sector of Ammon's horn, the basal ganglia (particularly the globus pallidus), and the Purkinje cells of the cerebellum. The dentate nucleus of the cerebellum and the inferior olivary nucleus of the medulla also are particularly vulnerable to anoxia. The prototypic form of nonischemic anoxia is carbon monoxide poisoning, in which cerebral blood flow is normal but with a very low oxygen content. From the distribution of cerebral damage described above, one might predict the types of syndromes that are commonly seen. These include epilepsy and myoclonus, particularly intention myoclonus (Lance-Adams syndrome); various degrees of cortical dysfunction, including aphasia, apraxia, visual disturbance, and behavioral and intellectual dysfunction; movement disorders, including dystonias, choreoathetosis, and tremors; memory loss; and cerebellar ataxia.

Ischemic anoxia entails both decreased blood flow and anoxia. The lesions of nonischemic anoxia are often seen but frequently are more severe and widespread. Furthermore, there may be additional lesions in the distribution of stenotic arterial circulations (e.g., a middle cerebral distribution infarction distal to a high-grade carotid stenosis) or in the border zones between major arterial circulations. The circumstance of cardiac arrest most resembles that of ischemic anoxia. When the underlying cerebral circulation is normal and the period of anoxia relatively brief, the syndrome more approaches the circumstance of nonischemic anoxia. The more prolonged the period of ischemia, the more the syndrome approaches that of ischemic anoxia.

Patients must be approached individually. Maximal recovery may take many months, but the majority of the improvement occurs within 72 hours of the insult. A few of the postanoxic syndromes can be treated with some success—for example, anticonvulsants, diazepam, clonazepam, or tryptophan for postanoxic myoclonus—but many are best managed with patience and physical rehabilitation.

Ischemic heart disease—acute myocardial infarction

It is logical to assume a relationship between myocardial (see Chapter 14) and cerebral infarction, since the underlying process in both conditions is atherosclerosis, a systemic disease. Obviously, if the acute myocardial infarction is attended by cardiogenic shock with severe systemic hypotension, the patient may show some or all of the manifestations of ischemic anoxia mentioned in the previous section.

Aside from the problem of systemic hypotension or cardiac arrhythmias, there is a definite correlation between cerebral infarction and recent myocardial infarction. Of all patients admitted to a hospital with stroke, about one in eight are found to have suffered recent myocardial infarctions, three quarters of which are asymptomatic. The 1-year mortality rate for patients with both heart and brain infarct is about 50%—twice that of patients with only stroke.

Several possible explanations for this association are possible. The first is that the myocardial infarction predated the cerebral infarction and led to the stroke by acting as a source for systemic emboli, perhaps arising from a mural thrombus on a dyskinetic ventricular wall. A second, less likely hypothesis is that an unknown source for embolus produced both cerebral and coronary emboli. The third possible explanation would be that the cerebral infarction predated and somehow caused the myocardial infarction. This may seem an unlikely sequence, but suggestive evidence was provided by Feibel and colleagues, who studied 27 patients with various types of stroke (14 with hemisphere infarction, 5 with brainstem infarction, and 8 with subarachnoid hemorrhage) with serial ECGs and systemic catecholamine determinations. Nine patients showed severe myocardial ischemia or infarction and had elevated catecholamine levels; of these, 5 who had myocardial infarction had the most elevated levels and the worst prognosis (4 died). Twelve patients showed mild or possible ischemia, had mild elevations of catecholamines, and survived; and 6 others with normal ECGs and cardiac enzymes had normal catecholamine levels and survived as well. The criteria for myocardial infarction were not only ECG changes, but also characteristic cardiac enzyme elevations. These data suggest that CNS disease may actually cause myocardial ischemia and infarction, possibly mediated via catecholamine release.

In general, it appears that there is a positive association between myocardial infarction and cerebral infarction. This population may contain some cases of myocardial infarction causing embolic stroke, some cases of cerebral infarction precipitating cardiac ischemia, and a few cases of concomitant cerebral and coronary ischemia, possibly from another embolic source or generalized hypotension.

Concomitant coronary and carotid occlusive disease

It is not surprising to find a high incidence of cerebral occlusive vascular disease in a population of patients with coronary occlusive vascular disease, since the underlying process is systemic. The frequent coexistence of these two disorders leads to a number of difficult problems in the management of patients who are to undergo coronary artery bypass surgery. In this circumstance, most vascular surgeons would recommend combined surgical management of the carotid and coronary disease, either simultaneously or in a staged procedure. In the circumstance of impending coronary artery bypass surgery, most neurologists would demand the occurrence of hemisphere transient ischemic attacks, with or without transient monocular blindness or submaximal cerebral hemisphere infarction in the distribution of a stenotic carotid artery, before recommending carotid endarterectomy.

Endocarditis

The modern spectrum of neurologic complications of infective endocarditis has been well analyzed in two large retrospective studies: one from the Massachusetts General Hospital, analyzing 218 patients between 1964 and 1973 and a second from the University of Texas at San Antonio affiliated hospitals, studying 166 patients between 1978 and 1986. The results of these two studies are remarkably similar and may be summarized as follows:

Neurologic complications are common (see Chapter 15), and they were recognized clinically in 35% to 39% of the patients. These neurologic complications were clinically important, in that 40% to 58% of these patients died, whereas only 20% without neurologic complications succumbed. The frequency of neurologic complications is clearly related to the infecting organism. The more virulent organisms, such as *Staphylococcus aureus, Streptococcus pneumonia,* anaerobic streptococci, or enterobacteriaceae, have a higher incidence (53% to 90%) whereas infection with a less virulent organism, such as *Streptococcus viridans,* shows a much lower incidence (28%). Furthermore, the major valve involved is related to the frequency of neurologic complications, with mitral valve disease carrying nearly twice the risk of either aortic or tricuspid valve involvement.

By far the most frequent neurologic complication seen in bacterial endocarditis is major cerebral embolic infarction, which occurred in 17% to 20% of the 218 patients. In the vast majority of cases, the middle cerebral artery or one of its branches was involved, with an appropriate clinical syndrome. The majority of these patients died, and postmortem examination showed a characteristic hemorrhagic infarction. An occluded vessel was sometimes found, but microorganisms were very rarely found in the brain parenchyma. Thus, most emboli arising from cardiac vegetations in this situation are bland and produce typical embolic hemorrhagic infarction of the brain. The very high mortality probably reflects merely the combined mortality of stroke plus infective endocarditis.

Microscopic (i.e., less than 1 cm^3) brain abscesses are seen rarely (8 of 218 MGH patients) and almost certainly result from miliary spread of infected emboli arising from cardiac vegetations (see Chapter 15). However, this is quite rare compared to the relatively common event of major bland cerebral emboli. Macroscopic brain abscess is practically unknown in pure bacterial endocarditis. The treatment of microscopic abscesses requires antibiotic therapy alone, and macroscopic abscess requires surgical drainage plus antibiotic therapy. The latter should not be considered a manifestation of pure bacterial endocarditis, regardless of the infecting organism.

Cerebral mycotic aneurysm, another rare complication of endocarditis, is presumably caused by infected emboli from cardiac vegetations. Most occur with *S. aureus* infection and are found in branches of the middle cerebral artery. The characteristic clinical picture is sudden onset of middle cerebral artery syndrome followed by an intracerebral hemorrhage.

The question of whether to use anticoagulant or antiplatelet therapy to prevent cerebral emboli in endocarditis patients is an extremely difficult one. The crucial issue is whether the increased risk of intracerebral hemorrhage produced by anticoagulants is greater or less than the decrement in cerebral emboli prevented by the anticoagulant. Unfortunately, most data remain anecdotal.

Seizures are seen in approximately 10% of patients with endocarditis. Focal seizures, which are seen in approximately one half of this 10%, usually represent cerebral infarction from embolus, whereas generalized seizures may belie numerous metabolic disturbances, including uremia, hypoxemia, electrolyte disturbances, and penicillin toxicity, but usually do not indicate focal neurologic disease.

Spinal fluid examination is not particularly useful clinically in the setting of endocarditis, and findings generally depend on the virulence of the infecting organism rather than on any specific neurologic complications.

Nonbacterial (marantic) thrombotic endocarditis (NBTE) is a paraneoplastic syndrome most often associated with adenocarcinoma. In about one fifth of the cases, there is evidence of some degree of disseminated intravascular coagulation (DIC), suggesting that at least in some cases, NBTE represents the abnormal coagulation of DIC. Arterial thrombosis and/or embolism may occur in many peripheral organs, including the brain, but much less is known about the detailed neurologic syndromes that occur in this entity than about those in bacterial endocarditis, primarily because of the former's relative rarity. In cancer patients, NBTE may be a more common cause of stroke than previously recognized. The treatment is that of the underlying tumor. Anticoagulants are contraindicated because of the fear of hemorrhagic complications from disseminated tumor.

REFERENCES

Boston Area Anticoagulation Trial for Atrial Fibrillation Investigators: The effect of low-dose warfarin on the risk of stroke in patients with nonrheumatic atrial fibrillation. N Engl J Med 323:1505, 1990.

DiMauro S et al: Mitochondrial encephalomyopathies. Neurol Clin 8:483, 1990.

Drislane FW et al: Myocardial contraction band lesions in patients with fatal asthma: possible neurocardiologic mechanisms. Am Rev Respir Dis 135:498, 1987.

Forsberg H, Ologsson B-O, and Eriksson A: Cardiac involvement in congenital myotonic dystrophy. Br Heart J 63:119, 1990.

Kanter Mc and Hart RG: Neurologic complications of infective endocarditis. Neurology 41:1015, 1991.

Karch SB and Billingham ME: Myocardial contraction bands revisited. Hum Pathol 17:9, 1986.

Levy DE et al: Predicting outcome from hypoxic-ischemic coma. JAMA 253:1420, 1985.

Nigro G, Comi LI, and Vain RJI: The incidence and evolution of cardiomyopathy in Duchenne muscular dystrophy. Int J Cardiol 26:271, 1990.

Pruit AA, Rubin RH, and Karchmer AW: Neurologic complications of bacterial endocarditis. Medicine (Baltimore) 57:329, 1978.

Rudehill A et al: ECG abnormalities in patients with subarachnoid haemorrhage and intracranial tumors. J Neurol Neurosurg Psychiat 50:1375, 1987.

Samuels MA: The heart and neurologic disorders. In Tyler HR and Dawson DM, editors: Current neurology. Boston, 1979, Houghton Mifflin.

Samuels MA: Neurogenic heart disease: a unifying hypothesis. Am J Cardiology 60:15J, 1987.

Samuels MA: Cardiopulmonary aspects of neurological catastrophes. In Ropper AH and Kennedy S, editors: Neurological and neurosurgical intensive care, ed 2. Rockville, Md, 1988, Aspen.

Samuels MA: Unexpected demise: sudden death in neurology. In Hachinski V, editor: Challenges in neurology. Philadelphia, 1992, F.A. Davis.

CHAPTER

141 Neurorheumatology

Kenneth K. Nakano

The neurologic manifestations of the rheumatologic disorders can be conveniently categorized (Table 141-1 and box, p. 1190). Approximately 75% of patients with rheumatoid arthritis (RA) who have had symptoms of the disease for less than 1 year improve, and approximately 15% to 20% show complete remission. However, when the disease becomes recurrent or is sustained over the years, increasingly serious and permanent disturbance in joint function develops. Neurologic complications manifest themselves in patients with moderate and severe forms of the disease. Ankylosing spondylitis (AS) and the diseases under the "collagen vascular" rubric (systemic lupus erythematosus [SLE], periarteritis nodosa, scleroderma, polymyositis [PM]–dermatomyositis [DM], Wegener's granulomatosis, temporal

Table 141-1. Neurologic manifestations of the collagen vascular diseases

Entity	Prevalence rate	Genetics	Age of onset	M:F	Clinical features	Pathology	Therapy
Systemic lupus erythematosus (SLE)	Rare in general population, CNS complications in 30%-75%	Sporadic	24 mos. after diagnosis	1:9	Seizures 54%, CNS 42%, mental change 33%, hemiparesis 12%, paraparesis 4%, movement disorder 4%, polyneuropathy 8%	Microinfarcts in the CNS; globulin in choroid plexus; fibrinoid degeneration	Probably steroids and/or immunosuppressive therapy
Temporal arteritis (TA)	Rare	Sporadic	60-80 years of age	M = F	Headache (temporal more than occipital), fever, weight loss, ESR >50 mm; prominent temporal artery; 30% can go blind; CNS involved	Giant-cell arteritis in media of vessels	Temporal artery biopsy, steroids for at least 6 mos
Polymyalgia rheumatica (PMR)	Rare	Sporadic	60-80 years of age	M = F	Malaise, weight loss, ESR >50 mm; brainstem strokes occasionally; normal enzymes, EMG; not much weakness	Can show similar pathology as TA or nothing	Steroids until ESR remains low
Granulomatous giant-cell arteritis (GGA) Wegener's (W)	Rare	Sporadic	30-60 years of age (but any age)	M < F	CNS: seizures, hemiparesis, SAH, infarcts, MS change. PNS: mononeuritis multiplex, neuropathy	Granulomatous lesions in resp. tract, kidneys; vasculitis in nerves and CNS	Steroids and/or immunosuppressives (especially cyclophosphamide)
Periarteritis (P)	Rare	Sporadic	30-40 years of age in 50%	M = F	Acute or insidious; fever, malaise, weakness, arthralgias, visceral involvement. PNS: neuropathies 50%. CNS: Sz, HA, psychosis	Inflammatory arteritis of medium-sized arteries, vasonervorum ischemia; progressive	Steroids
Polymyositis (PM)	$6.3/10^5$	Sporadic	40-70 years of age	5:1	Subacute girdle muscle weakness 98%; dysphagia 51%; muscle pain 58%; ESR, CPK, EMG abnormalities in the majority	?sensitized lymphocytes; ?virus; Degenerative and inflammatory changes in muscle with perivascular lymphs and plasma cells	Steroids; for severe, relapsing cases immunosuppressives may be of benefit
Dermatomyositis (DM)		Sporadic	Child, adult	M = F	Skin findings in DM; often associated with cancer	Skin DM involved	

CNS, central nervous system; ESR, erythrocyte sedimentation rate; EMG, electromyogram; SAH, subarachnoid hemorrhage; MS, mental status; PNS, peripheral nervous system; Sz, seizure; HA, headache; CPK, creatine phosphokinase.

Neurologic manifestations of rheumatoid arthritis

Articular-cervical spine disease
- Cervical subluxations (four types)
  1. C1 moves anteriorly on C2
  2. C1 moves posteriorly on C2
  3. Vertical subluxation of odontoid
  4. "Staircase" or multiple lower-level subluxations
- Radiologic findings often with clinical symptoms
  1. Double-crush syndrome
  2. Narrowed disk spaces above C5
- Radiologic findings without clinical symptoms
  1. Vertebral plate erosion
  2. Apophyseal joint erosion
  3. Basilar impression of the skull

Extra-articular
- Peripheral neuropathies
  1. Compression leading to entrapment
  2. Mild sensory neuropathy with a good prognosis
  3. Diffuse sensorimotor neuropathy
  4. Fulminant sensorimotor neuropathy
- Diffuse myopathy and focal myositis
- Polymyositis-dermatomyositis
- Vasculitis—often with other connective tissue disorders
  1. Mononeuritis complex
  2. "Cerebral vasculitis"—often with lupus and rheumatoid arthritis
- Dural rheumatoid nodules causing brain and spinal cord compression
- Progressive multifocal leukoencephalopathy

arteritis–giant cell arteritis, polymyalgia rheumatica, and related syndromes) infrequently produce neurologic complications.

RHEUMATOID ARTHRITIS (see Chapter 304)

The neurologic manifestations of RA can be divided into articular and extra-articular disorders (see the box above).

Articular involvement

The main synovial joints in the neck are the apophyseal joints. Several synovial bursae also lie around the odontoid and its associated ligaments. Chronic inflammation of these bursae may lead to erosion of bone and ligaments with subsequent loss of stability. Approximately 30% to 40% of all patients with chronic RA and severe peripheral joint disease who are hospitalized have radiologic evidence of cervical spine subluxation. Often, these radiologic findings are not associated with neurologic symptoms. However, in 2% to 5% of all patients with significant cervical subluxation, pyramidal tract signs or vague subjective sensory findings are evident on neurologic examination. Usually, RA affects the upper levels of the cervical spine and produces different clinical features at different ages. In children with RA, growth is deficient and apophyseal joints often fuse, with resultant limitation of neck movement. In adults, the main change in the cervical spine is subluxation, which can take four forms: (1) C1 moves anteriorly on C2 (this is the most common form and results from insufficiency of the transverse ligament or from erosion or fracture of the odontoid); (2) C1 moves posteriorly on C2 (this results from severe erosion or fracture of the odontoid); (3) vertical subluxation of the odontoid and body of C2 (a result of destruction of the lateral atlantoaxial joints or of the bone around the foramen magnum, the rarest form of cervical subluxation in RA); and (4) "staircase" subluxation, or subluxation of one vertebra on another, often multiple and below the C2 level (second most common cervical subluxation in RA; depends on destruction of the apophyseal joints rather than on loss of ligamentous connections).

Characteristic neuritic pain radiating up to the occiput is frequently present. Crepitation and instability of the cervical spine can cause alarm. Paresthesias can be caused by head or neck movement and Lhermitte's sign may be elicited by sudden flexion of the neck. Rarely, the complaints reflect transient ischemic attacks in the posterior cerebral circulation (transient visual disturbances, such as diplopia, vertigo, paresthesias, or paresis). Early spinal cord compression or ischemia may produce subtle spastic quadriparesis and hyperreflexia, which may be especially unwelcome when a patient is already debilitated. Pyramidal tract signs (increased reflexes and Babinski responses) or early proprioceptive loss in the hands represent early signs of impending spinal cord compression. The classic spinal cord compression picture, including an altered sensory level to all modalities, bladder and bowel dysfunction, and flaccid quadriplegia, is a late development. To make a clinical diagnosis of cervical subluxation in RA, radiologic confirmation becomes necessary. Lateral views of the cervical spine, in extension and flexion to open the gap between the odontoid and the arch of C1, are helpful. Tomography, computed tomography (CT), and magnetic resonance imaging (MRI) may become necessary for detailed anatomic study and precise measurement of the spinal canal and the cord.

Treatment for the less severe and neurologically asymptomatic cases of cervical subluxation includes firm cervical collars aimed at improving stability and easing pain. Neurosurgical and orthopedic surgical immobilization of the neck and halo traction should be considered in the patient with progressive spinal cord signs. Stabilization becomes most useful before permanent neurologic or vascular damage occurs to the spinal cord. If surgery is considered, it should be done before the patient has suffered permanent cord injury and at a center familiar with chronic RA and techniques of cervical and occipitocervical fusion.

Extra-articular manifestations

Peripheral neuropathies. Various types of neuropathies have been reported in RA: compression leading to entrapment (e.g., carpal tunnel syndrome, ulnar nerve at the elbow, posterior interosseous nerve syndrome, tarsal tunnel syndrome), mild sensory neuropathies with a good prognosis, diffuse sensorimotor polyneuropathy, and a fulminant sensorimotor disorder often related to a generalized vasculitis. Proposed causes of the neuropathy in RA include vascular disturbances, nutritional deficiencies, and demyelination. The neuropathy most commonly encountered, however, is a mild sensory one, primarily of the feet and legs. Patients often complain of varying degrees of paresthesias, dysesthesias, or "burning feet" for varying periods of time. Often when the RA stabilizes, the symptoms of the peripheral neuropathy subside over weeks. Optimal nutrition, additional vitamins, and carbamazepine have offered some relief of the subjective dysesthesias and burning feet.

A more severe sensorimotor polyneuropathy can be seen occasionally in patients with acute joint disease, in which the patient has some objective weakness in addition to the sensory symptoms. Vasculitis is not present clinically, and the patient may show symmetric distal weakness of the limbs as well as diminished vibration and touch sensations in the feet and legs, more than in the hands and arm. Often, the patients in this category have neglected their RA, or there has been an acute recurrence of the disease.

The aim of therapy should be to effect remission of the RA. One must rule out other possible causes of peripheral neuropathy (e.g., diabetes, toxins, alcohol excess, drugs). Subjective relief of pain can be achieved with phenytoin or carbamazepine. Generally, the patient recovers most of the neurologic function independent of therapy, and the neuropathy improves. A small number of patients may be left with a chronic neuropathy, as evidenced by neurologic examination and nerve conduction studies. In a small percentage of cases, malignant rheumatoid vasculitis presents with a fulminant sensorimotor disorder, often with a mononeuritic component. Often, these patients have been treated with steroids or their disease has followed an unremitting course. Evidence of vasculitis is seen on the skin, and the neurologic picture can be similar to that in periarteritis nodosa. These patients may have concomitant collagen vascular disease, or their symptoms may represent a spectrum of diseases (e.g., a patient can have RA and features of SLE). Medical therapy should be directed at control of the vasculitis and the RA. Even with optimal therapy, most of these patients are left with severe neuropathies.

Myopathy and focal myositis. Seventy percent to 80% of patients with chronic and recurrent RA have some muscle weakness, usually around the areas of joint involvement. These patients report diminished proximal strength and peripheral joint disability. RA myopathy is independent of steroid therapy, and these patients do not progress to diffuse and severe muscle necrosis if the RA remains controlled with medications and physical therapy. Although there is a combination of muscle and joint inflammation, the prognosis depends more on the joint disease than on the muscle involvement.

Vasculitis. Generalized RA vasculitis is rare. In a severe case of RA with multiple neurologic findings suggesting central nervous system (CNS) involvement or a mononeuritis complex, a complete neurologic evaluation includes electroencephalogram, CT, MRI, and spinal fluid examination. Short-term, high-dose steroid therapy and/or immunosuppressive drugs may be indicated in the acute condition.

Dural rheumatoid nodules. If the patient with RA has severe subcutaneous nodules, he or she may rarely go on to develop dural nodules, which can compress the brain or spinal cord. Dural nodules cannot be clinically separated from other disorders causing compression either of the brain or spinal cord (e.g., subdural hematoma, metastatic cancer, or neurofibroma). When a compressive syndrome within the CNS is suspected, CT scan of the brain and MRI scans of the spine should be performed to make the diagnosis.

Progressive multifocal leukoencephalopathy (PML). PML, a rare complication of RA, is an asymmetrically diffuse CNS disorder evidenced by multifocal areas of demyelination. It is an infection by the papova viruses that overwhelms an immunologically suppressed host. No known therapy exists, and the patient's course is rapidly fatal.

ANKYLOSING SPONDYLITIS
(see Chapter 312)

AS represents a chronic progressive form of arthritis involving the sacroiliac joints, the spinal apophyseal (synovial) joints, and the paravertebral soft tissues. Characteristically, this disease produces ossification of the annulus fibrosus of the intervertebral disks and of the connective tissue immediately adjacent to the annulus and changes in the intervertebral diarthrodial joints similar to those occurring in RA. Over a period of 10 to 20 years the patient with AS develops the poker-type deformity or the cervicodorsal kyphosis. Both atlantoaxial and atlantooccipital subluxations occur. External bracing may provide relief of bulbar symptoms from vascular ischemia in the latter situation. Other neurologic involvement in AS includes the cauda equina syndrome, vertebrobasilar insufficiency, and peripheral nerve lesions. Therapy should be directed at controlling the AS. In the event of the cauda equina syndrome, neurosurgical decompression of the lower spine may be necessary.

COLLAGEN VASCULAR DISEASES
(see Chapter 206)

The symptoms and signs resulting from these disorders (see Table 141-1) include those resulting from systemic reaction to the disease and involvement of the viscera.

Vasculitis can be defined as inflammation of blood vessels and is associated with necrosis causing compromise of vessel lumen and secondary ischemia in involved tissues. Consequently, vasculitis appears often in the differential diagnosis of nearly all neurologic disorders, because it can closely mimic most central nervous system (CNS) and peripheral nervous system (PNS) diseases. However, certain clinical symptoms and signs, alone or in combination, can be suggestive of a vasculitic disorder.

Three basic types of peripheral neuropathy appear when vasculitis affects the PNS: (1) mononeuritis multiplex (MM); (2) distal symmetric "stocking-glove" sensorimotor peripheral neuropathy (PN); and (3) overlapping, extensive MM. Regardless of the type of PN seen in the vasculitis syndromes the symptoms include a severe, burning paresthesia in the distribution of the involved nerve or nerves.

When skeletal muscle becomes involved with vasculitis, patients demonstrate symmetric proximal muscle weakness that appears clinically indistinguishable from that seen in polymyositis (PM) or dermatomyositis (DM). In patients with an underlying collagen vascular disease (viz., SLE, RA, Sjögren's syndrome, scleroderma), the skeletal muscle involvement is often caused by a primary inflammatory involvement of the muscle itself rather than to vasculitis.

Two primary patterns of clinical involvement occur for CNS vasculitis, depending on whether the vasculitis is predominantly diffuse or focal. With diffuse involvement the patient complains of acute or subacute headache, psychiatric impairment (personality, behavioral, and affective disturbances), and cognitive impairment (memory and mental status changes). Generalized seizures may occur in association with an encephalopathy. On the other hand, focal CNS vasculitis causes focal cerebral deficits. Any stroke-like event, especially in a young person without risk factors of stroke, should alert the clinician about a vasculitis. Furthermore, single or multiple cranial nerve palsies (visual loss, diplopia, facial paresthesias or weakness, vertigo, tinnitus, dysphagia) can be manifestations of focal CNS vasculitis. Less commonly, focal CNS vasculitis causes intracerebral or subarachnoid hemorrhage, movement disorders (e.g., chorea), and an isolated myelopathy (e.g., isolated granulomatous angiitis). Overlap in the symptoms of these two patterns occurs because all of the vasculitides can produce either diffuse or focal CNS disease.

It is important to note that most of the vasculitic syndromes can produce disease in both the CNS and PNS, often simultaneously (Table 141-1). Atypical cases that do not fit neatly into any of the diagnostic categories occur frequently and suggest that there is some overlap of clinical syndromes (e.g., SLE and RA). The institution of therapy (including immunosuppressive therapy) can alter the natural history of many forms of vasculitis that were previously untreatable and often fatal. Therefore, it becomes vital that the clinician arrive at an early diagnosis and classification to prevent the development or progression of CNS and PNS manifestations of the collagen vascular disorders, including the various vasculitides.

SUMMARY

Neurorheumatology encompasses the neurologic syndromes and complications seen in RA, AS, and the various collagen vascular disorders. Although the involvement of the peripheral and central nervous systems may be infrequent with the rheumatologic diseases, they represent well-defined clinical entities that require a keen clinical awareness and medical (and at times surgical) treatment.

REFERENCES

Hawke SHB et al: Vasculitic neuropathy. A clinical and pathological study. Brain 114:2175, 1991.

Kissel JT: Neurologic manifestations of vasculitis. Neurol Clin 7:655, 1989.

Nakano KK: Neurology of musculoskeletal and rheumatic disorders. Boston, 1979, Houghton-Mifflin.

Nakano KK: Entrapment neuropathies. In Kelley WN et al, editors: Textbook of rheumatology, ed 3. Philadelphia, 1989, Saunders.

Nakano KK: The neurological complications of rheumatoid arthritis. Orthop Clin North Am 6:861, 1975.

Sigal LH: The neurologic presentation of vasculitic and rheumatologic syndromes: a review. Medicine 66:157, 1987.

CHAPTER

142 Neuropulmonology

Frank W. Drislane
Martin A. Samuels

Respiratory abnormalities in patients with neurologic disease are found both in normally alert patients and in those with altered states of consciousness.

RESPIRATORY PATTERNS IN PATIENTS WITH ALTERED STATES OF CONSCIOUSNESS

In altered states of consciousness, the most common (but least specific) respiratory abnormality is periodic breathing, most often Cheyne-Stokes respiration (CSR): that is, a regular waxing and waning of respiratory rate and volume, with apneic periods at the low points. CSR represents an increased sensitivity of the respiratory drive in response to CO_2. This is usually the result of bilateral cerebral dysfunction, although other factors contributing to an aberrant modulation of respiratory rhythms (such as hypoxia, other metabolic derangements, or prolonged circulation time, as in congestive heart failure) can lead to CSR.

The pneumotaxic center in the upper pons modulates inspiratory and expiratory centers lower in the brainstem. Bilateral abnormalities anywhere above this center can disrupt descending influences from forebrain structures and lead to CSR.

Ventilation persists in CSR, and patients do not become hypoxic. While periodic breathing is of limited localizing value in neurologic illness, its appearance may be the only sign of deterioration in a patient with known disease—for example, a mass lesion.

CSR may also be the primary respiratory abnormality in sleep apnea syndrome (rather than the more sudden apneas usually associated with this syndrome). In this case, CSR, possibly through increased upper airway resistance, can lead to sleep fragmentation, increased arousals, and diminished oxygen saturation. In these patients (though not in sleep apnea in general), theophylline has been helpful in reversing the hypoxemia.

Posthyperventilation apnea (PHVA) also signifies an abnormal responsiveness to CO_2. An apnea of over 10 seconds after five deep breaths is considered abnormal and can be seen with bilateral hemispheric dysfunction (including those caused by metabolic abnormalities or drugs). Most individuals with CSR or PHVA have neurologic illness, although each is seen occasionally in normals, especially during sleep.

Central neurogenic hyperventilation (CNH) is often discussed but rarely seen. To be certain of the diagnosis of CNH, one should demonstrate a low arterial PCO_2 and a high PO_2 on room air; the hyperventilation should persist during sleep and in the absence of stimulant medications. Respirations are very large in volume, with equal phases of inspiration and expiration. CNH has been seen in a few cases of anterior and medial pontine lesions, sparing the lateral pontine regulatory centers. Even in comatose patients, however, CNH is far less frequent than is pulmonary disease (especially congestive failure), which should always be sought. It is most prudent to look for metabolic and pulmonary causes of deep regular respiration, even in stuporous and comatose patients. An elevated respiratory rate, if associated with actual hyperventilation, is a poor prognostic sign.

Apneustic breathing (or failure of normal expiration) is similarly rare but of much greater localizing value. These prolonged inspiratory cramps signify neurologic damage in the lower pons, often the result of a pontine stroke, though they can also be seen with hemorrhage and meningitis. Often, these strokes are extensive and produce near transection of the pons. An apneustic (inspiratory) center at the pontomedullary junction is presumably released from higher controls by these lesions.

Ataxic breathing is completely irregular respiration and is a clear marker of disease in the medulla. Respirations have no discernible pattern and consist of unpredictable gasps. This is most characteristically seen with compression of the medulla caused by mass lesions, such as cerebellar tumors and hemorrhages; less often, it is seen in demyelination and in strokes (less common because of the bilateral blood supply of the medulla). It may be seen in poliomyelitis as part of a spectrum of hyporesponsiveness of the respiratory centers to chemical stimuli such as hypoxia. This loss of rhythmicity in respiration denotes a failure of the most fundamental (and essential) respiratory centers, as opposed to an interruption of higher centers that modulate respiratory rhythms. It is in such cases that the basic inspiratory and expiratory centers in the medulla are most imperiled. Not surprisingly, when there is ataxic breathing, even the mildest sedation can lead to complete respiratory failure.

As a general rule, rapidity of respiration suggests pulmonary or metabolic disease, whereas loss of regularity is more suggestive of brainstem dysfunction.

RESPIRATORY PATTERN ABNORMALITIES IN AWARE PATIENTS

Respiratory failure can be caused by several neuromuscular diseases, usually long after the diagnosis is made, such as in muscular dystrophies (Chapter 125). Exacerbations of myasthenia gravis (Chapter 124) can do the same—again, usually after the diagnosis has been made, but myasthenic syndromes caused by aminoglycosides or rare cases of botulism may be less obvious. Early diagnosis is particularly important in Guillain-Barré syndrome (Chapter 123) because the diagnosis is often missed, because it can lead to respiratory failure in a substantial percentage of patients, and because supportive care and other treatments are effective in nearly all patients. In this section we will concentrate on respiratory abnormalities with a neurologic basis, without more widespread weakness.

Hypoventilation, presumably caused by medullary failure and insensitivity of medullary receptors to the usual chemical stimuli, can also be seen after encephalitis. A diminished responsiveness to CO_2 can also be demonstrated even years after recovery from acute poliomyelitis. Such chronic medullary failure appears to be irreversible. Attempts at treatment of primary hypoventilation have included the use of progesterone as a respiratory stimulant and the use of phrenic nerve pacers.

Failure of automatic breathing (Ondine's curse) is readily understood on consideration of the two independent systems of neural control of respiration. Conscious and voluntary breathing, used in speech, music, and other voluntary activities, is largely mediated by the corticospinal tracts and can be damaged in strokes and other lesions. For example, a stroke can diminish respiratory movements on the affected side of the body during wakefulness and leave automatic breathing symmetric during sleep. Bilateral damage can lead to "respiratory apraxias," sometimes in association with a pseudobulbar palsy.

Most respiration, however, is automatic and occurs in response to metabolic demands. Failure of automatic breathing is uncommon and is usually acquired rather than congenital. Its cause is a bilateral interruption of fibers from the medullary respiratory centers to the upper spinal cord, where the phrenic nerves and other nerves to respiratory muscles originate. These fibers are separate from the corticospinal tract and can be interrupted by bilateral infarctions in the medullary tegmentum—a rare situation, given the bilateral blood supply. Whereas cortical and other lesions above the pons can alter voluntary breathing without disturbing automatic respiration, medullary and cervical spinal cord lesions can interrupt automatic breathing, leaving voluntary respiration intact. Patients with a failure of automatic breathing breathe adequately while awake, but they may develop hypocapnia, hypoxia, and pulmonary hypertension caused by respiratory failure during sleep.

Ondine's curse has occurred in several cases of bilateral cervical cordotomy performed to sever the spinothalamic tracts for treatment of intractable pain. Nearby reticulospinal fibers can be damaged in this procedure, leading to a failure of automatic respiration while leaving voluntary respiration intact. A similar situation may occur after poliomyelitis. Failure of automatic respiration can also be seen after bilateral carotid endarterectomy caused by the loss of chemosensitivity in the carotid bodies.

Those rare patients with a history and symptoms suggestive of failure of automatic breathing usually need to be studied during sleep to reach a diagnosis. The far more common cases of sleep apnea syndromes are diagnosed in the same studies. Interestingly, REM sleep can lead to more precipitous apnea in cases of Ondine's curse, possibly because of the inhibition of muscular tone that REM produces. Failure of automatic respiration is a rare condition; phrenic pacers are a potential treatment. Seizures are a rare cause of respiratory dysrhythmias.

Tic syndromes, and especially Gilles de la Tourette syndrome (see Chapter 119), commonly present with respiratory symptoms and signs. They are often misdiagnosed for years and often mistaken for primarily respiratory ailments. In fact, repetitive throat clearing is the most frequent symptom in Tourette's syndrome (TS), and a tic in the form of a vocalization is necessary for the diagnosis of TS. Such involuntary respiratory movements can be extremely frequent and include such noises as barking, coughing, snoring, sniffing, shrieking, grunting, and sneezing. Often the diagnosis is not made until the patient displays involuntary shouting of obscenities (coprolalia), but this occurs only in a minority of TS patients and is often absent for several years after the initial symptoms. Eye blinking, facial grimacing, and tics of the limbs are common, and even sensory tics have been reported, but vocalizations are the most common presenting symptom. Tics must be differentiated from other causes of movement disorders, such as Wilson's disease, Huntington's disease, and late effects of neuroleptics.

Up to one fourth of all children may have tics at some time. Most, however, are transient and last weeks to months. The more persistent tics of TS appear at an average age of 7 years, but the diagnosis may be delayed up to decades. TS is not rare, occurring in perhaps up to 1% of the population. There is increasing evidence that TS is transmitted genetically in an autosomal dominant manner, though with variable penetrance and expression. Penetrance is higher in males, who make up over three fourths of the patients. TS is strongly associated with both obsessive-compulsive disorder (OCD) and attention-deficit–hyperactivity disorder.

Pharmacologic evidence argues for an abnormality in dopamine neurotransmitter function in TS. Amphetamines (often used in cases of attention-deficit disorder) and levodopa have led to the exacerbation or beginning of TS, and it has been seen after phenothiazine withdrawal. Dopamine receptor blockade with haloperidol or pimozide has been the mainstay of therapy and is effective in over three quarters of patients. Pimozide, which can lead to a prolonged QT cardiogram interval, has been thought to produce fewer movement disorder side effects than haloperidol, but one controlled trial found no difference in efficacy or side effects. Clonidine (thought to act on the norepinephrine system) appears helpful in a smaller percentage of patients, and possibly for a shorter duration, but it is often the first choice because of lessened concern about serious long-term side effects. It is important to tailor the treatment to a target symptom, and many patients require no medication. For some others, it is the associated OCD or attention-deficit disorder that is most troublesome. Fluoxetine has been helpful for OCD in Tourette's patients. Some patients benefit from a combination of haloperidol and stimulants to treat both the TS and attention-deficit disorder. A taper of medications is appropriate if tics have been under control for many months.

Diaphragmatic flutter can be caused by thoracoabdominal or neurologic disease. This rare condition may present with chest pain and is often caused by irritation of the phrenic nerve or abnormalities in the pleura, such as adhesions. On examination, it is readily realized that the diaphragmatic movement (often 100 to 150 times per minute) is independent of the heartbeat. It usually does not lead to hypo- or hyperventilation, because voluntary respiration continues to be superimposed, but it can be very distressing. Most cases improve with sleep and are intermittent. Individual episodes may last from seconds to months and may recur. Medications are usually of no help. Phrenic nerve section has been used as a treatment in some patients, but the disease is often bilateral.

In some patients, electromyographic studies have demonstrated synchronous contractions of the diaphragm and intercostal muscles, suggesting a central neurologic basis for the "respiratory myoclonus." Thus, the syndrome can be considered analogous to palatal myoclonus, seen with lesions in the lower brainstem caused by stroke, tumor, demyelination, or encephalitis. Some of these patients have responded to treatment with phenytoin.

Hiccups are extremely common, are almost always benign, and are usually caused by chest or abdominal causes. Their central component is shown by the simultaneous involvement of all inspiratory muscles. They are inhibited by breath holding and hypercarbia, whereas hyperventilation can lead to an exacerbation of bursts of hiccups. Rarely, they are manifestations of primary neurologic disease, such as syringomyelia, strokes, tumors, and medullary compression. Similarly, yawning may be a sign of medullary compression from a posterior fossa mass or a sign of raised intracranial pressure, and it may be a useful sign in comatose patients.

NEUROGENIC PULMONARY EDEMA

Neurogenic pulmonary edema (NPE) is seen in a wide variety of cerebral insults. It is characterized by the rapidity with which it may develop and by the high protein content of the pulmonary edema fluid. The most characteristic etiologies are head injury, prolonged seizures, and subarachnoid hemorrhage, although many causes have been described. In its most severe form, it is rare and has a grim prognosis, but a less severe, more gradual, and unrecognized form of NPE may be relatively common.

The pathophysiology of NPE is complex and controversial and is expertly summarized by Malik, from whose review much of this section derives.

Hypothalamic lesions provided some of the earliest experimental models of NPE. Bilateral preoptic lesions in rats have led to hemorrhagic and fatal pulmonary edema. The observation that prior midline lesions more caudal in the hypothalamus prevent this effect led to the concept of NPE as a "release phenomenon" caused by failure of inhibition of posterior hypothalamic structures, which produce an intense sympathetic nervous system discharge. Subsequent experiments have suggested that the preoptic lesions were actually irritative and that purer ablations give different results—thus putting into question the idea of a release phenomenon. The hypothalamus, however, is not *the* essential structure involved in NPE, since transection of the brain below the hypothalamus does not prevent the NPE produced by abnormalities in the brainstem below.

The medulla oblongata is the crucial brain structure involved in the genesis of NPE. Exquisite physiologic studies done by Chen and colleagues have detailed the interactions of the nucleus of the solitary tract (NTS), the dorsal motor nucleus of the vagus nerve, and the nucleus ambiguus, as well as their roles in mediating the autonomic dysfunction that leads to pulmonary and systemic hypertension and pulmonary edema. Cardiopulmonary abnormalities can be produced by ischemia in the medulla. More common than ischemia, however, is the presumed compression (or distortion) of the brainstem found in raised intracranial pressure (ICP), head injury, and hemorrhage. Medullary lesions may cause an interruption of the baroreceptor reflex arc, leading to an intense sympathetic vasomotor activation. This is mediated through circulating catecholamines and, more powerfully, through direct sympathetic innervation. That NPE produced by cerebral compression is prevented by spinal transection at the C7 level (but not by vagotomy, adrenalectomy, or decerebration) implicates the sympathetic outflow tracts in the generation of NPE. NPE produced by cerebral compression or by NTS lesions can be prevented by pretreatment with phentolamine, which demonstrates mediation by alpha-adrenergic receptors. Stellate ganglion stimulation can produce the same rise in pulmonary vascular resistance, also preventable with alpha-adrenergic blockade.

Vagotomy prevents some of the bradycardia and gastric erosions seen with CNS lesions but does not prevent the systemic and pulmonary hypertension and NPE produced by raised ICP and medullary lesions. The bradycardia seen in the Cushing response to raised ICP is effected through the vagus nerves, but this appears to be separable from the hypertension and NPE. (Vagotomy has produced pulmonary edema in some species, but it is unclear whether respiratory obstruction and airway constriction leads to some of this effect.)

Autonomic innervation of the lungs is extensive. Nerves to the lung enter through the anterior and posterior pulmonary plexus from the sympathetic trunks and vagus nerves. At the hila the nerves follow the airway and blood vessels to smaller branches. Sympathetic fibers extend to pulmonary vessels as small as 30 μm in diameter. Although innervation is less extensive than that in the systemic circulation, CNS insults can lead to a reduction in pulmonary vascular compliance and a dramatic rise in both systemic and pulmonary pressures.

Adrenal catecholamines may contribute to pulmonary vasoconstriction (catecholamine concentrations can increase by up to 1000 times their baseline value with raised ICP!), but adrenalectomy does not abolish the NPE that follows raised ICP. The local effect of splanchnic sympathetic innervation appears to be primary, as section of these splanchnic nerves prevents development of NPE.

Systemic hypertension is often found with raised ICP or other neurologic catastrophe. Some have postulated that systemic vasoconstriction causes a shift of blood volume toward the lower resistance pulmonary vasculature, thus causing NPE. At the same time, the sympathetic stimulation of vessels in the pulmonary circulation leads to elevated resistance. In the lung, alpha receptors (vasoconstricting) predominate over beta receptors (dilating), so vasoconstriction is the predominant sympathetic response. The effect of the adrenergic receptor appears to be greater in the pulmonary venous circulation than in the arterial, thus leading to a marked rise in the pulmonary capillary hydrostatic pressure.

Pulmonary vascular hypertension has been thought to be important in NPE, but it may be neither sufficient nor necessary. Experimentally, NPE can be produced by raised ICP even with control of the systemic blood pressure. Also, the pressure produced even with the most intense sympathetic vasoconstriction seems insufficient to lead to the pulmonary dysfunction seen in NPE. Finally, the high protein content of the pulmonary fluid in NPE clearly implies an alteration of vascular permeability.

This alteration in pulmonary vascular permeability appears necessary for the development of NPE, but its origin is unclear. Its rapid development and the frequent accompanying pulmonary hypertension have led to the theory that a pulse, or "blast," of hypertension leads to structural damage of the vascular endothelium. Other studies, however, have shown increased permeability with no alteration in vascular pressures whatsoever. Conversely, no alteration in permeability was seen when a rapid pulse of pulmonary hypertension was applied experimentally.

Direct changes in the vascular endothelium with loosening of tight junctions have been produced by CNS lesions. This may be even more damaging when superimposed upon vascular hypertension. The permeability changes seem to be mediated by the sympathetic nervous system, but additional "second messengers," such as histamines, opioids, or prostaglandins, could be involved locally. Increased permeability may be the result of a distortion in the contractility of the endothelial cells or pericytes by bradykinin or histamine. This may explain the mechanism of opiate-induced and other noncardiac forms of pulmonary edema.

In summary, despite the frequent occurrence of systemic and pulmonary vascular hypertension following CNS lesions, a direct, probably sympathetic-mediated, alteration in pulmonary vascular permeability appears to be essential in the production of NPE.

Treatment of NPE is dependent on recognition of the syndrome in the appropriate neurologic setting and differentiation of it from other illnesses, such as aspiration pneumonia, common in the same settings. Assurance of a good airway, oxygenation, and diuresis are appropriate, as in other forms of pulmonary edema. Especially when cerebral edema is involved, diuresis with osmotic agents such as mannitol may be helpful. The complications of beta-receptor blockade in such a situation would argue against its use in hypertension after neurologic catastrophe, even before NPE develops. Conversely, alpha-blocking agents such as phentolamine may be useful in treating NPE, assuming the systemic blood pressure tolerates this medication. Positive pressure breathing is a controversial treatment that might be helpful in the pulmonary edema, but it raises concern about diminution of cardiac output and elevation of ICP. When NPE is the result of status epilepticus, anticonvulsants are obviously indicated, and some have suggested that phenytoin may be useful in NPE even without overt seizures. Naloxone has been helpful in animal experiments in NPE, although its use in clinical settings has not yet been determined. Considering the physiology postulated above, some have suggested the use of antihistamines in treatment of NPE.

REFERENCES

Chen HI and Chai CY: Integration of the cardiovagal mechanism in the medulla oblongata of the cat. Am J Physiol 231:454, 1976.

Kamholz SL: Pulmonary aspects of neurological diseases. New York, 1987, PMA.

Malik AB: Mechanisms of neurogenic pulmonary edema. Circ Res 57:1, 1985.

Mitchell RA and Berger AJ: Neural regulation of respiration. Am Rev Resp Dis 111:206, 1975.

Plum F and Posner JB: The diagnosis of stupor and coma, ed 3. Philadelphia, 1980, Davis.

Singer HS and Walkup JT: Tourette syndrome and other tic disorders: diagnosis, pathophysiology, and treatment. Medicine 70:15, 1991.

CHAPTER

143 Neurogastroenterology

Martin A. Samuels

MALABSORPTION AND DEFICIENCY STATES (see Chapters 28, 42, and 49)

The neurology of gastrointestinal diseases is largely related to maldigestion, malabsorption, and malnutrition. It stands to reason that the developing nervous system is particularly sensitive to deprivation of protein, carbohydrate, fat, minerals, and vitamins. As a consequence, it is generally true that inherited defects that lead to a deficiency of one or more of these critical elements cause dramatic, often devastating neurologic disease. Acquired deficiencies, on the other hand, lead to more circumscribed, often reversible syndromes. In general, neuronal systems that utilize long axons are the most susceptible to defects that disable energy metabolism. Thus, polyneuropathy and focal encephalopathies (e.g., spastic paraparesis caused by dying back of corticospinal axons or blindness caused by dying back of retinal ganglion cell axons) are the most common manifestations of many of the dietary deficiency or malabsorption syndromes. For a detailed description of the neurologic consequences of the many deficiency states, the interested reader should refer to the excellent monograph by Pallis and Lewis.

Most substances of neurologic significance in adults are absorbed from the proximal and middle thirds of the small bowel. Vitamin B_{12}, the notable exception, is absorbed with its gastric-derived intrinsic factor in the terminal ileum. Deficiencies of nearly all of the water-soluble vitamins (i.e., thiamine, riboflavine, nicotinic acid, pyridoxine, pantothenic acid, vitamin B_{12}, folic acid, and ascorbic acid) are known to be associated with a polyneuropathy in which sensory symptoms (e.g., burning feet and paresthesias) overshadow motor difficulties. Since in real life, patients usually have multiple water-soluble vitamin deficiencies, it is difficult to know precisely which one causes a particular symptom.

For example, pure folate deficiency does not cause a neurologic syndrome in animals, whereas patients with folate deficiency almost invariably have a polyneuropathy, possibly as a result of the associated deficiency of other vitamins or other dietary substances.

Above and beyond the neuropathy, several of the water-soluble-vitamin deficiency states produce specific neurologic syndromes that deserve mention. Thiamine (vitamin B_1) deficiency causes Wernicke's encephalopathy, an acute syndrome characterized by a mental abnormality (usually confusion and amnesia), ataxia, and various oculomotor problems (e.g., nystagmus, bilateral abducens palsies). All of the clinical syndromes are caused by biochemical (and ultimately pathologic) lesions in central nervous system nuclei (paraventricular regions of the thalamus and hypothalamus mammillary bodies, periaqueductal gray, floor of the fourth ventricle, vestibular nuclei, and superior cerebellar vermis), which presumably are particularly dependent on thiamine-mediated reactions. Most severe thiamine deficiency is caused by malnutrition, often associated with alcoholism—although any cause of malnutrition (e.g., nausea and vomiting caused by chemotherapy) can result in enough thiamine deficiency to cause clinically evident Wernicke's encephalopathy. Multiple clinical or subclinical attacks of Wernicke's encephalopathy may result in a chronic state of amnestic dementia (Korsakoff's disease). Severe untreated Wernicke's encephalopathy may be fatal or result in irreversible amnestic dementia, so all suspected patients (e.g., alcoholics, severely malnourished people, comatose patients) should be treated with parenteral (intravenous or intramuscular) thiamine, 100 mg initially followed by 50 mg per day for 5 days or until a normal diet can be reestablished. Carbohydrates should never be given to severely malnourished patients until thiamine has been infused, because that results in thiamine-dependent cells becoming more acidotic as a result of anaerobic metabolism of the carbohydrate.

Nicotinic acid deficiency (pellagra) produces a dementia in addition to its classic effects on the skin and gastrointestinal tract (dermatitis and diarrhea). The dementia is characterized by memory loss and attentional defects similar to that seen in vitamin B_{12} deficiency and is therefore nonspecific in and of itself. Whether nicotinic acid deficiency can cause an acute encephalopathy progressing rapidly to coma (Jolliffe's disease) is unsettled, since most patients in this circumstance have unequivocal signs of Wernicke's encephalopathy as well. Pellagra is now rare, probably because bread is enriched with niacin (nicotinic acid); however, it can be seen in severely malnourished patients.

Pyridoxine (vitamin B_6) deficiency is known to result in seizures, particularly in infancy. Some infants require large nonphysiologic doses of pyridoxine (i.e., 50 to 100 mg per day) to terminate neonatal seizures. This disorder, which is inherited as an autosomal recessive trait, is known as pyridoxine dependency. Most pyridoxine deficiency in adults is caused by the use of pyridoxine antagonists, such as isonicotinic acid hydrazide (INH) for the treatment of tuberculosis. It is recommended that patients on INH be given pyridoxine, 50 mg daily, to prevent the polyneuropathy and seizures caused by vitamin B_6 deficiency. Patients with various malabsorption disorders, such as sprue and celiac disease, may also become pyridoxine-deficient.

Vitamin B_{12} deficiency also causes neurologic syndromes above and beyond neuropathy. This subject is covered in Chapter 88.

The fat-soluble vitamin-deficiency states do not produce polyneuropathies but have other characteristic neurologic manifestations.

Vitamin A (retinol) deficiency results in impaired dark adaptation (night blindness).

Vitamin D deficiency causes osteomalacia, which may be associated with a proximal myopathy similar clinically to that seen in thyroid disease.

Vitamin E deficiency is known to be associated with abetalipoproteinemia (Bassen-Kornzweig disease), a disorder characterized by retinitis pigmentosa, ataxia, pes cavus, areflexia, red blood cells with spikelike processes, and fat malabsorption. Beta lipoprotein and vitamin E are both totally absent from the blood, but the relationship of vitamin E deficiency to the pathogenesis of the Friedreich's ataxia-like neurologic illness remains obscure.

Vitamin K deficiency results in a bleeding diathesis that may result in hemorrhages in or around neurologic structures.

WHIPPLE'S DISEASE (see Chapter 42)

Whipple's disease is a multisystemic chronic disease that regularly affects both the nervous system and the gastrointestinal tract. It is characterized by weight loss with steatorrhea, arthralgias, and abdominal pain. The patients may be asymptomatic neurologically or may show visual disturbances, amnestic dementia, ophthalmoplegia, myoclonus, and a relatively specific movement disorder called *oculomasticatory myorhythmias,* in which rhythmic convergence or vertical pendular eye movements are combined with synchronous opening and closing of the jaw. Neuropathologically, the same PAS-positive macrophages can be found in the brain as are found in other tissues of the body. Although this PAS-positive material suggests a bacterium, no single organism has been proved to be the cause, though the best evidence supports a beta-hemolytic streptococcus. The diagnosis is usually made by intestinal biopsy but in pure central nervous system cases, brain biopsy may be required. If an organism can be cultured from the biopsy specimens, antimicrobial therapy is chosen based on its specific sensitivities. If no organism can be cultured, then empiric treatment with tetracycline, erythromycin, or trimethoprim-sulphamethoxazole is usually tried. Some patients respond well to therapy, stabilizing and even dramatically improving in some circumstances. The role of altered immunity is uncertain, but the condition has been seen in patients with AIDS.

PANCREATIC DISEASE (see Chapter 67)

Patients with pancreatic disease often suffer from episodes of hypoglycemia. It is unlikely that mild degrees of hypoglycemia (i.e., greater than 50 mg per deciliter) have any transient or lasting effect on neurologic function. However, severe hypoglycemia has clear neurologic and neuropathologic correlates. This is obvious when one considers how dependent the brain is on a constant supply of glucose, being virtually unable to use any other energy substrate. Acute hypoglycemia results in a massive effort by the autonomic nervous system to mobilize sugar from stored carbohydrate. This results in tachycardia and sweating. If this effort fails to maintain an adequate blood sugar, the level of consciousness rapidly falls, descending from confusion through drowsiness and stupor to coma. The cellular structures most susceptible to the ravages of hypoglycemia are similar to those that fail in circumstances of anoxia. These include the deep layers of the cerebral cortex, the basal ganglia (particularly the globus pallidus), the hippocampal formation (particularly the Sommer sector), and the cerebellar Purkinje cells. With repeated attacks of hypoglycemia, a clinical syndrome develops that probably relates to the cell loss in these and other regions of the brain—namely, an amnestic dementia (the hippocampal lesion); myoclonus, often worse on action or intention (the cortical lesions); various movement disorders, such as myoclonus, chorea, and dystonia (the basal ganglia lesion); and ataxia (the cerebellar lesion). This syndrome progresses if the episodes of hypoglycemia continue to occur, as frequently happens in severe insulin-dependent type I diabetics or in alcoholics with severe pancreatic insufficiency and liver disease.

Pancreatic encephalopathy refers to a vaguely characterized disorder seen in the course of acute pancreatitis and consisting of an abnormality in the level of consciousness ranging from confusion to coma, slowing of the electroencephalogram, and, sometimes, motor disorders such as tetraparesis and increased tendon reflexes. It is difficult to be certain that the neurologic disorder in such acutely ill patients is in fact caused by the pancreatic failure, rather than by commonly associated conditions such as shock, sepsis, alcohol withdrawal, Wernicke's encephalopathy, metabolic acidosis, hepatic failure, and electrolyte disturbances. It is clear that some of the pathologic reports of so-called pancreatic encephalopathy actually are examples of central pontine myelinolysis, a condition now thought to be associated with hyponatremia or its rapid correction.

PARASITIC INFESTATIONS

A number of intestinal parasitic diseases affect the nervous system. These include protozoan diseases (e.g., *Entamoeba histolitica* causes a meningoencephalitis) and platyhelminth-caused diseases, the most important and frequent of which is cysticercosis, the larval phase of the human tapeworm, *Taenia solium*. The life cycles and clinical manifestations of these parasitic diseases are covered in Chapters 280 and 282.

INFECTIOUS DIARRHEAS

The infectious diarrheas, such as shigellosis and salmonellosis, may cause profound neurologic disturbances, but these are almost certainly caused by the electrolyte disturbances, fever, and generalized illness produced by these pathogens rather than to any direct effect on the nervous system.

REFERENCES

Pallis CA and Lewis PD, editors: The neurology of gastrointestinal disease. London, 1974, Saunders.

Sharf B and Bental E: Pancreatic encephalopathy. J Neurol Neurosurg Psychiatry 34:357, 1971.

Victor M, Adams RD, and Collins GH: The Wernicke-Korsakoff syndrome, ed 2. Contemporary neurology series, vol 30. Philadelphia, 1989, Davis.

Wroe SJ et al: Whipple's disease confined to the CNS presenting with multiple intracerebral mass lesions. Neurol Neurosurg Psychiatry 54:989, 1991.

CHAPTER

144 Neurohepatology

Martin A. Samuels

The neurologic aspects of liver disease can be divided into two major categories: the reversible portosystemic encephalopathies (also known as hepatic encephalopathy) and irreversible portosystemic encephalopathies (i.e., Wilson's disease and acquired non-Wilsonian hepatocerebral degeneration).

Reversible means that the neurologic aspects of the illness will disappear, assuming the underlying process causing the liver failure can be treated successfully. Many patients with potentially reversible neurologic complications of liver disease die of the hepatic failure before the nervous system can recover. Upon pathologic examination of brains of patients who succumb to acute hepatic failure, one finds only cerebral edema and an increase in the size and number of the protoplasmic astrocytes. These so-called Alzheimer type II glia are pathognomonic of liver failure.

REVERSIBLE PORTOSYSTEMIC SYNDROMES

Reversible portosystemic encephalopathy (PSE) may be acute (e.g., acute yellow atrophy or Reye's syndrome), or chronic recurrent (episodes of acute PSE superimposed on stable liver disease, such as alcoholic cirrhosis).

When symptomatic, patients with reversible PSE show a mental disorder, ranging from slight inattention to coma, prominent motor abnormalities (e.g., tremor, asterixis, myoclonus, hyperreflexia), and fairly consistent laboratory abnormalities (e.g., hyperammonemia, mild hypoxemia, respiratory alkalosis, elevated CSF glutamine, and high-voltage sharp triphasic delta waves on the electroencephalogram). The neurotoxin is still not definitely known. False neurotransmitters, such as octapamine, and other potential toxins, such as fatty acids, mercaptans, and amino acids, have all had advocates. Probably, the original idea that ammonia is the toxin is as accurate as any hypothesis. It may be true that the glutamate-glutamine detoxification system for ammonia is compartmentalized to the glial cells and that the Alzheimer type II glia are a reflection of brain efforts to detoxify high levels of ammonia. When this system becomes saturated, the nervous system is no longer capable of removing ammonia, which then produces its toxic effects on neuronal function.

The other prevalent hypothesis is that liver disease somehow results in the elaboration of a substance that activates the gamma aminobutyric acid receptor, type A ($GABA_A$). This $GABA_A$ receptor is modulated allosterically by benzodiazepines, barbiturates, and the endogenous family of peptides derived from the precursor polypeptide, diazepam binding inhibitor (DBI). It is possible that endogenous benzodiazepine-like substances may be synthesized by animals or ingested from dietary sources and that these substances may reach the brain in larger than normal amounts when there is portosystemic shunting, thereby activating the inhibitory action of the $GABA_A$ receptor and producing coma. The major argument supporting this hypothesis is that the benzodiazepine antagonist, flumazenil, ameliorates portosystemic encephalopathy in animals and humans. However, the drug is not yet available in the United States.

Whatever the mechanism of the neurotoxic effects of liver failure, it can be treated by reducing the production and absorption of nitrogenous products from the gastrointestinal tract. This can be done using protein restriction, antibiotics, catharsis, and lactulose.

IRREVERSIBLE PORTOSYSTEMIC SYNDROMES

There are two major chronic, progressive, irreversible portosystemic encephalopathies: hepatolenticular degeneration (Wilson's disease) and acquired hepatocerebral degeneration. Wilson's disease is an autosomal dominantly inherited illness in which there is an inability to synthesize ceruloplasmin, the copper-carrying enzyme. Copper is deposited in many tissues, including the liver (leading to cirrhosis) and the cornea (the pathognomonic Kayser-Fleischer ring). The neuropathology shows cavitation of the lenticular nuclei (putamen and globus pallidus), laminar cortical necrosis, and widespread Alzheimer type II glial cells—findings that imply that the chronic liver disease produces many of the neurologic and neuropathologic features of the illness. The treatment is copper chelation with D-penicillamine (see Chapter 60).

In some patients with chronic liver disease, there develops a relentlessly progressive neurologic illness, similar neurologically in many ways to Wilson's disease. These patients show prominent dysarthria and akinesia, often with tremor. Tendon reflexes are increased and Babinski signs are present. In some patients there develops a pure motor spastic paraparesis that, rarely, can dominate the clinical picture (the so-called hepatic paraplegia). Superimposed on this degenerative process are often episodes of acute reversible PSE with worsening confusion and asterixis. Pathologic examination reveals laminar cortical necrosis and Alzheimer type II glial cells, reminiscent of those seen in acute PSE and in Wilson's disease. There is no abnormality in copper metabolism, no deposition of copper in the brain, and no Kayser-Fleischer rings. It appears that the sine qua non in the development of this syndrome in the context of liver disease is the existence of a portosystemic shunt. This shunt may be produced surgically (e.g., splenorenal shunt or portocaval shunt) in an effort to reduce portal pressures or may happen spontaneously within the liver itself (intrahepatic portosystemic shunts) in the course of hepatic cirrhosis. Some of these patients seem to respond transiently to levodopa or dopamine-receptor agonists (e.g., bromocriptine), implying that neurotransmitter failure is part of the pathogenesis of the illness (see Chapters 50 and 56).

Neurologic effects of liver transplantation

Orthotopic liver transplants are associated with a variety of neurologic complications, which fall into several major categories. About 10% of patients have seizures, 90% of which are single. The remaining 10% with recurrent seizures can usually be managed with phenobarbital. However, some of these patients have a prolonged period of unconsciousness followed by a persistent or slowly resolving cerebrocerebellar syndrome characterized by ataxia, dysarthria, and weakness. It is probable that this is caused by cyclosporine toxicity. About 2.5% of patients are clinically diagnosed as having a stroke. Infarctions are possible, but most are subarachnoid and/or intracerebral hemorrhages, probably related to the coagulopathy of the liver disease. In some cases hemorrhagic infarction is related to infection with an organism known to produce a vasculitis (e.g., *Aspergillus*). In the immediate postoperative period these patients are nearly all encephalopathic related to infections, metabolic imbalance, drug toxicity, and the effects of the graft's malfunction.

REFERENCES

Estol CJ, Pessin MS, and Martinez AJ: Cerebrovascular complications after orthotopic liver transplantation. Neurology 41:815, 1991.

Morgan MY et al: Successful use of bromocriptine in the treatment of chronic hepatic encephalopathy. Gastroenterology 78:663, 1980.

Mousseau R and Reynolds T: Hepatic paraplegia. Am J Gastroenterol 66:343, 1976.

Plum F and Hindfelt B: The neurological complications of liver disease. In Vinken PJ and Bruyn GW, editors: Handbook of clinical neurology, vol 27. Amsterdam, 1976, Elsevier.

Victor M, Adams RD, and Cole N: The acquired (non-Wilsonian) type of chronic hepatocerebral degeneration. Medicine (Baltimore) 44:345, 1965.

Victor M and Rothstein JD: Neurologic manifestations of hepatic and gastrointestinal disease. In Asbury AK, Mcdonald WI, and McKhann CM, editors: Diseases of the nervous system, ed 2. Philadelphia, 1992, Saunders.

Vogt DD et al: Neurologic complications of liver transplantation. Ann Neurol 31:644, 1992.

Wilson SAK: Progressive lenticular degeneration: a familial nervous system disease associated with cirrhosis of the liver. Brain 34:295, 1912.

CHAPTER

145 Neurohematology

Martin A. Samuels

ANEMIA (see Chapter 80)

Anemia in its own right rarely produces neurologic symptoms. When severe, it can result in a generalized dull headache, and, occasionally, retinal hemorrhages may occur. Iron-deficiency anemia is, for unknown reasons, associated with obsessive-compulsive behaviors that fall into two categories: compulsive eating (pica) and compulsive moving of the limbs, usually the legs (restless legs syndrome). Common pica behaviors include the eating of starch, paint chips, clay, earth (geophagia), or ice (pagophagia). It is clear that the pica does not represent replacement of iron since eating ice, the most common pica behavior, usually does nothing in this regard and many clays actually contain substances that chelate iron. The restless legs syndrome is a common cause of insomnia. It consists of an unpleasant creeping sensation deep in the legs (and occasionally in the arms) when the person is at rest. The person feels compelled to move the legs. Most frequently affected are women who pace the floors at night and complain of insomnia. The syndrome may progress to severe motor restlessness (akathisia), which in its severest form occurs throughout the day (Ekbom syndrome). Serum iron and total iron-binding capacity should be measured in all patients complaining of pica or restless legs syndrome. If iron replacements fail to relieve the symptoms, the patient may respond to low-dose benzodiazepines (particularly clonazepam) at bedtime, or dopamine agonists (e.g., Sinemet, bromocriptine). The megaloblastic anemias are associated with very specific neurologic syndromes. Vitamin B_{12} deficiency, once a common and dreaded illness, now is quite rare, although sporadic cases of pernicious anemia, dietary deficiency of vitamin B_{12}, malabsorption, and infestation with the fish tapeworm *(Diphyllobothrium latum)* are still seen (see Chapter 88). It is probably true that all forms of vitamin B_{12} deficiency produce the same array of neurologic complications, although most of the experience is with patients suffering from pernicious anemia. The neurologic manifestations of vitamin B_{12} deficiency span nearly the entire nervous system. There is a myelopathy (subacute combined degeneration of the spinal cord), an encephalopathy, and an optic neuropathy. The myelopathy produces a spastic weakness of the legs (and sometimes arms), a profound loss of vibration and joint position senses out of proportion to the severity of the neuropathy, and a positive Romberg sign. The encephalopathy produces a dementia best characterized in modern terms as a chronic confusional state with poor memory and a severe attentional deficit but little or no aphasia or apraxia—thus distinguishing it from typical Alzheimer's disease. The optic neuropathy may produce anything from red desaturation to severe loss of visual acuity with a deafferented pupil in one or both eyes.

Despite its once-high prevalence and intense interest by generations of physicians, the precise mechanism by which vitamin B_{12} deficiency produces neurologic problems remains a mystery. The fact that vitamin B_{12} is necessary for DNA synthesis may explain the megaloblastic anemia, leucopenia, and glossitis seen in patients with B_{12} deficiency, but this does not explain the effects on neurons of the adult nervous system, which do not divide. The role of vitamin B_{12} in other enzymatic reactions (i.e., the conversion of 1-methylmalonyl CoA to succinyl CoA and the methylation of homocystine to methionine) is well known, but the connection between these reactions and neuropathology is tentative at best.

Folate deficiency, another cause of megaloblastic anemia usually produced by malnutrition, is often part of a multiple vitamin deficiency syndrome. For this reason, it is not clear whether folate deficiency itself causes any neurologic disorder. Many patients with folate deficiency have a polyneuropathy, but this may be caused by deficiencies in other elements in the diet (see Chapter 123).

HEMOGLOBINOPATHIES AND THALASSEMIA (see Chapter 89)

The hemoglobinopathies and thalassemia often are associated with neurologic complications. Patients with sickle cell anemia have painful crises and may suffer small-vessel occlusions involving the brain or spinal cord. These small-vessel occlusions produce infarctions, hemorrhagic infarctions, and, occasionally, intracerebral hemorrhages. The supraclinoid carotid is a location that seems predisposed to occlude in patients with sickle cell anemia. The precise mechanism for this predisposition is not known, but it is possible to noninvasively predict an impending occlusion using transcranial Doppler technology. Seizures may also occur, probably as a result of small-vessel distribution infarcts of various ages. These patients are also subject to recurrent attacks of bacterial meningitis, possibly related to functional or surgical asplenism. Although the incidence of these neurologic problems is higher in the patients with homozygous sickle cell anemia, they may all be seen occasionally in patients with various heterozygous hemoglobinopathies, including SC, SD, SF, and S thalassemia syndromes. Patients with thalassemia may also suffer recurrent episodes of meningitis, particularly after surgical splenectomy. They also may have extramedullary hematopoiesis (see below) and an array of vaguely described neuromuscular disorders that may be coinherited with the thalassemia, rather than caused by the thalassemia per se.

EXTRAMEDULLARY HEMATOPOIESIS

Extramedullary hematopoiesis is the production of blood cells outside of the usual bone marrow compartments. This usually occurs in reticuloendothelial organs, such as liver and lymph nodes, but can occasionally be found near the nervous system—usually in the thoracic epidural space, rarely in the intracranial subdural space. These masses can compress the spinal cord or brain, producing a myelopathy or an encephalopathy. Approximately one half of the patients with dural extramedullary hematopoiesis have had thalassemia, and a quarter have had myelofibrosis. The other quarter comprises a potpourri of diagnoses, including polycythemia, sickle cell anemia, pyruvate-kinase deficiency, and Paget's disease of bone. Extramedullary hematopoiesis can be treated very effectively with radiation therapy.

HEMORRHAGIC DIATHESIS

Hematologic disorders associated with a hemorrhagic diathesis may produce neurologic complications resulting from bleeding into or around the brain, spinal cord, roots, plexuses, or nerves. Hemophiliacs until quite recently often succumbed to neurologic complications; however, modern replacement therapy has made these problems quite rare. Patients with hemophilia still are more prone than normal people to develop intramuscular or retroperitoneal hemorrhages, particularly when there is a history of trauma. Retroperitoneal hemorrhages may produce a compressive sacral plexopathy that usually recovers slowly with resolution of the blood. Intracranial and interspinal hemorrhages (epidural, subdural, subarachnoid, or parenchymal) are still more common in hemophiliacs than in normals, but only slightly so. Thrombocytopenia of any cause may result in intracranial or spinal hemorrhages. In conditions in which the remaining few platelets are presumed normal (e.g., immune-mediated idiopathic thrombocytopenic purpura), patients usually do not suffer serious neurologic hemorrhages until the platelet count approaches 10,000 per cubic millimeter. However, when platelets are both abnormal and reduced in number (e.g., in chemotherapy patients), one can expect neurologic hemorrhages when the platelet count reaches about 50,000 per cubic millimeter. Thrombotic thrombocytopenic purpura (TTP) is a particular neurohematologic syndrome consisting of thrombocytopenic purpura, hemolytic anemia, and various neurologic symptoms and signs (e.g., headache, confusion, aphasia, seizures, cranial neuropathies, weakness, sensory loss), which are now known to be caused by small-vessel occlusions in the brain and spinal cord. Renal failure and fever are also frequently seen. Various therapies (e.g., heparin, antiplatelet drugs, steroids) in the past had shown equivocal results. It now appears that plasma exchange provides the best chance for the patient, but despite this, the prognosis for this cryptogenic syndrome remains poor.

Disseminated intravascular coagulation (DIC) of any etiology rarely causes gross neurologic hemorrhage. In a few patients with DIC, multiple cerebral infarctions may occur, and autopsy may show multiple small petechial hemorrhages. It is likely that these findings would produce little persistent neurologic deficit should the patient survive the episode of DIC and not die of the underlying cause (e.g., sepsis). Hypoprothrombinemia is usually iatrogenic, caused by the various anticoagulant drugs used to prevent thromboembolism. It is now clear that anticoagulation to prothrombin times longer than 18 seconds carries an increased risk of nervous system hemorrhages. It is probable (but not yet proved) that antithrombotic therapy aiming for a prothrombin time of 15 to 18 seconds (coumadin light) can produce the same protection without the associated risk of hemorrhage.

HYPERCOAGULABLE STATES (see Chapters 76 and 83)

A patient is said to have a hypercoagulable state if he or she has laboratory or clinical conditions related to an increased risk for thrombosis. Hypercoagulable states are divided into a primary (usually inherited) type (e.g., antithrombin IV deficiency, protein C and protein S deficiencies) and a secondary (acquired) type (e.g., malignancy, pregnancy, use of oral contraceptives, anticardiolipin antibodies). In both types, cerebral vessels may suffer thrombosis in situ, with consequent infarction. Most standard hematologic tests do not reveal the presence of a hypercoagulative state, but specialized studies can be obtained if one suspects that such a state exists based on arterial or venous thrombosis in otherwise risk-free patients. Young women with stroke represent a group of patients in whom a hypercoagulable state should be sought. In one circumstance, a standard hematologic test, the partial thromboplastin time (PTT), may be found to be prolonged in a patient suffering a thrombotic event. This artifactual prolongation of the PTT is caused by the presence of an acquired immunoglobulin, usually directed against cardiolipin (the so-called lupus anticoagulant). The prolongation of the PTT results from the fact that the antibody inhibits the activity of phospholipid in the in vitro clotting reaction. It is not really an anticoagulant and is, in fact, a cause of a hypercoagulable state that can result in thrombosis of cerebral veins or arteries. The lupus anticoagulant is found in some patients with systemic lupus erythematosus, as well as in patients on neuroleptic drugs and patients with other autoimmune disorders. In the near future it will probably be possible to screen for the hypercoagulable state in stroke patients.

HYPERVISCOSITY

The hyperviscosity state is a clinical syndrome characterized by confusion, headache, blurred vision, and specific retinal funduscopic findings (i.e., venous engorgement [sausage veins] and retinal hemorrhages). It is caused by sludging of blood in brain vessels as a result of increased viscosity and is seen in polycythemia (particularly when associated with iron deficiency) and paraproteinemias. Among the paraproteinemias, macroglobulinemia has the greatest propensity for the production of hyperviscosity. The presence of cryoglobulins and cold agglutinins is also associated with hyperviscosity. The treatment for the hyperviscosity syndrome is plasma exchange.

PARAPROTEINEMIAS (see Chapters 75 and 95)

Paraproteinemias cause an array of neurologic complications above and beyond their tendency to produce hyperviscosity. This may be a result of the fact that immunoglobulins produced by the neoplastic clone of cells may be directed against components of the normal nervous system (e.g., myelin-associated globulin [MAG]) or to the production of amyloid that infiltrates nervous tissue. Thus, multiple myeloma is commonly associated with many different types of peripheral neuropathy (i.e., polyneuropathy and mononeuropathy multiplex). In addition, in some patients with paraproteinemias, plasma cells emanating from cerebral veins may actually infiltrate the brain, producing a clinical syndrome (the Bing-Neel syndrome) characterized by cerebrospinal fluid pleocytosis, multifocal neurologic signs with a downhill course, and sometimes the appearance of a histiocytic lymphoma in the brain. The disorder is unresponsive to plasma exchange and probably represents a widespread neoplastic infiltration of the nervous system.

Monoclonal gammopathy of undetermined significance (MGUS) is associated with various peripheral and sometimes central nervous system manifestations. It is probable that these paraproteins (particularly the IgM type) are directed against components of the peripheral and, rarely, central nervous system, thereby producing polyneuropathies, mononeuropathies, and possibly even multifocal central nervous system demyelination, which may clinically and by imaging techniques look like multiple sclerosis. There is some evidence that the neurologic manifestations of MGUS respond partially to plasmapheresis.

REFERENCES

Adams R et al: The use of transcranial ultrasonography to predict stroke in sickle cell disease. N Engl J Med 326:605, 1992.

Dyck PJ et al: Plasma exchange in polyneuropathy with monoclonal gammopathy of undetermined significance. N Engl J Med 325:1482, 1991.

Feldmann E, editor: The antiphospholipid antibody and stroke (APASS symposium. Stroke 23:I1, 1992.

Grotta JC et al: Red blood cell disorders and stroke. Stroke 17:811, 1985.

Petty GW et al: Complications of long term anticoagulation. Ann Neurol 23:578, 1988.

Samuels MA: Neurologic manifestations of hematologic diseases. In Asbury AK, McKhann GM, and Mcdonald WI, editors: Diseases of the nervous system: clinical neurology, ed 2. Philadelphia, 1992, Saunders.

Schafer AI: The hypercoagulable states. Ann Intern Med 102:814, 1985.

CHAPTER

146 Neuronephrology

Martin A. Samuels

Patients with renal failure are subject to several major classes of neurologic disease, caused by either the uremia itself or its treatment (e.g., dialysis).

NEUROLOGIC COMPLICATIONS OF UREMIA (see Chapters 347 and 348)

Uremic encephalopathy occurs in the course of renal failure when the glomerular filtration rate falls below 10% of normal and usually is dramatically relieved by dialysis or renal transplantation. Its neurologic characteristics are nonspecific, consisting of an abnormality in the level of consciousness ranging from inattention to coma, with variable numbers of motor signs, such as asterixis, myoclonus, tremor, and seizures. When a patient with uremia develops an encephalopathy, other contributing factors, such as drugs or concomitant hepatic failure, should be identified and treated. It is important to bear in mind the fact that drugs that are cleared by the kidney may reach toxic levels in uremic patients even when taken in normal doses.

There is no absolute relationship between the degree of renal failure, as measured by any of the usual blood chemistries, and the severity of the encephalopathy. The most consistent abnormality found in brains of animals and humans who have died of uremia is a dramatic increase in calcium content. Furthermore, some of the encephalopathy can be reversed with parathyroidectomy or medical suppression of parathyroid hormone (PTH). Since calcium is important in neurotransmitter release and action, it is possible that PTH-mediated changes in calcium metabolism may underlie some of the encephalopathy seen in uremic patients. In addition, there is evidence that PTH may itself be toxic to the nervous system, above and beyond its effect on calcium metabolism.

At the moment, the best treatment for uremic encephalopathy is improvement in the uremic state.

Uremic neuropathy is common in patients with chronic renal failure but is only a significant clinical problem in about 10% of those patients on chronic renal dialysis. Most of these patients also have diabetes mellitus (diabetics compose about one third of patients on chronic renal dialysis), which is well known to produce a similar neuropathy, so it is usually difficult in practice to separate the true uremic neuropathy from the diabetic neuropathy. However, it is clear that in a small number of nondiabetic patients, there is a neuropathy severe enough to become a significant clinical problem.

The most common uremic neuropathy is a symmetric sensorimotor polyneuropathy affecting the longest nerves first and then dying back toward the spinal cord. The clinical phenomena (i.e., burning feet, tender feet and calves, "restless legs," and, rarely, distal weakness) are indistinguishable from those in any other metabolic axonopathy (e.g., diabetes mellitus, alcohol abuse, vitamin deficiency, cancer). Electrophysiologic studies are rarely helpful, in that they invariably show mild slowing of the nerve conduction velocities and widespread denervation but nothing pathognomonic of the uremic neuropathy. The neurotoxic substance(s) in renal failure have not been convincingly identified.

Another neuropathy seen in uremic patients is the mononeuropathy syndrome, caused by compression of metabolically deranged nerves. Compression in bedridden patients of the ulnar, radial, femoral, or peroneal nerves can produce neuropathies in uremic patients more readily than in normal people.

Carpal tunnel syndrome is particularly common in uremic patients, and some of these patients have been shown to have secondary amyloidosis with accumulation of the amyloid in the carpal tunnel. The amyloid in this circumstance is made from a beta-2 microglobulin that normally is cleared by the kidney. Being a large molecule with a molecular weight of about 12,000 daltons, beta-2 microglobulin is not cleared by hemodialysis. It can therefore accumulate and be incorporated into a beta-pleated sheet (i.e., amyloid) and be deposited in soft tissue or the heart, producing clinical syndromes such as carpal tunnel syndrome.

NEUROLOGIC COMPLICATIONS OF THE TREATMENT OF UREMIA (see Chapter 348)

Hemodialysis is associated with two distinct neurologic conditions: the dialysis dysequilibrium syndrome (DDS) and dialysis dementia (also known as dialysis encephalopathy).

DDS consists of a spectrum of neurologic abnormalities ranging from headache and muscle cramps to coma. The severe form (i.e., severe encephalopathy, stupor, or coma) is very rare in modern practice, probably because patients are dialyzed at much higher levels of renal function than in prior eras. It may be inferred from this fact that severe DDS is caused by rapid correction of extreme hyperosmolarity. This probably explains the fact that patients on chronic dialysis or in whom the BUN is allowed to slowly drift down over many days or weeks rarely suffer severe DDS. Mild forms of DDS (i.e., headache, muscle cramps, and mild confusion) still are seen and usually respond favorably to infusions of hypertonic saline, glucose, or mannitol.

It was originally hypothesized that DDS was caused by the so-called reverse urea effect: urea was thought to be cleared less rapidly from the brain than from the blood during hemodialysis, thereby leading to a movement of water into the brain and resulting in cerebral edema, which was said to cause the symptoms. It has subsequently been shown that urea is cleared from the brain and blood at the same rate, making the reverse urea effect hypothesis untenable. Currently, it is theorized that a cerebral intracellular acidosis is caused by the production of organic acids (so-called idiogenic osmoles) by the brain and that this pH disturbance produces the neurologic symptoms. The precise stimulus for the production of these organic acids remains obscure.

Dialysis dementia (or dialysis encephalopathy) is a progressive, usually lethal disease characterized by dysarthria, with a rather characteristic stuttering quality, polymyoclonus, and rapidly progressive dementia. The electroencephalogram (EEG) is usually quite abnormal, often showing rhythmic bursts of high-voltage sharp activity. Early in the course of the disease, intravenous diazepam infusion often strikingly improves the EEG and the speech disorder. The brain pathology is usually unimpressive but may show a spongioform encephalopathy, reminiscent in many ways of the pathology of Jakob-Creutzfeld disease. This disease has not been transmitted to subhuman primates by intracerebral injection of brain material from affected patients. There is some evidence that high levels of aluminum in the dialysate are associated with this illness, and most dialysis units now employ routine deionization of water used to prepare dialysate. It is known that high levels of aluminum are neurotoxic and that aluminum can produce neurofibrillary tangles in animals; however, the pathology of the dialysis dementia syndrome is not reminiscent of Alzheimer's disease, and there is very little direct evidence that aluminum actually causes this disease in animal models.

It had been argued that elevated aluminum levels decrease the activity of an enzyme, dihydropteridine reductase, which in turn is involved in neurotransmitter synthesis. This neurotransmitter deficiency would then cause the dialysis encephalopathy. However, recent studies have failed to show any relationship between this enzyme's activity and either aluminum levels or cognitive function. Thus, the etiology of dialysis encephalopathy remains obscure.

REFERENCES

Bolla KI et al: Dihydropteridine reductase activity: lack of association with serum aluminum levels and cognitive functioning in patients with end stage renal disease. Neurology 41:1806, 1991.

Fraser CL and Arieff AI: Nervous system complications of uremia. Ann Intern Med 109:143, 1988.

Part Five

Endocrinology, Metabolism, and Genetics

I BASIC PHYSIOLOGY

CHAPTER

147 Principles of Endocrine Physiology

Richard M. Jordan
Peter O. Kohler

Traditionally *hormones* are defined as secretory products that travel through the blood to affect distant tissues and organs. It is now apparent that these concepts are too restrictive. Some hormones such as testosterone and estradiol have important local effects on their secretory organs in addition to the tissues they reach via the circulation. Such localized action, known as paracrine function, is also characteristic of several other classes of chemical mediators not usually considered hormones. These include mediators of the inflammatory response (histamine, bradykinin, slow-reacting substance) and a host of neurotransmitters. Overlap of function further blurs the distinction between neurotransmitters and hormones. Norepinephrine functions both as a neurotransmitter and as a hormone. Likewise, small peptides manufactured in the hypothalamus (thyrotropin-releasing hormone and somatostatin) appear to serve as neurotransmitters as well as hormones.

A single hormone can be manufactured in several different organs. For example, proopiomelanocortin, the precursor for corticotropin (ACTH) endorphins and beta-lipotropin, is synthesized not only in the anterior pituitary but also in the brain, placenta, gastrointestinal tract, and reproductive organs. Other small peptides have been found common to the brain and the gastrointestinal tract. Thus the identity of separate specific organs constituting an endocrine system is no longer adequate because organs not normally considered endocrine are now known to secrete hormones important for maintaining the body's homeostasis. This is true for the gastrointestinal tract, kidney, liver, and lungs, which are all sites of hormone synthesis.

CLASSES OF HORMONES

One scheme of categorizing hormones is based on their chemical structure. Four major classes are generally recognized: peptides, amines, iodothyronines, and steroids. Peptide hormones are the largest class and are divided into smaller peptides (thyrotropin-releasing hormone, gonadotrophin-releasing hormone, somatostatin, etc.), larger peptides (insulin, growth hormone, parathyroid hormone, etc.), and glycoproteins (luteinizing hormone, follicle stimulating hormone, chorionic gonadotropin, and thyroid stimulating hormone). Structurally glycoproteins are composed of alpha and beta chains. Glycosylation may be necessary for interaction of the alpha and beta subunits.

Iodothyronines (l-thyroxine [T_4], triiodothyronine [T_3]) are derivatives of a single aromatic amino acid, tyrosine. Two iodinated tyrosine molecules are attached to form the final hormone product. Catecholamines (norepinephrine, epinephrine, and dopamine) are enzymatic modifications of tyrosine. Similarly, melatonin is formed from tryptophan. Steroid hormones are derived from cholesterol, and all have a similar core known as the cyclopentanoperhydrophenanthrene nucleus. Variations in bond saturation and side chain modifications of this core give a unique biologic action to each steroid hormone.

HORMONE SYNTHESIS

Peptide hormones

Peptide hormone synthesis proceeds in the same manner as that of other proteins. This process is illustrated in Figs. 147-1 and 147-2. A typical gene (Fig. 147-1) responsible for hormone synthesis includes a strand of deoxyribonucleic acid (DNA) containing the base sequence responsible for transcription of the complementary nucleotide sequence of premessenger ribonucleic acid (RNA) (pre-mRNA). Interspersed in the transcription unit are base sequences that are not translated (introns). Their function, if any, is unknown. Exons are the base sequences that dictate the formation of a specific protein. The entire transcription is flanked by a promoter region at the 5′ end that determines where the transcription coding sequence begins and has regions that respond to regulatory influences such as steroid hormones. The 3′ end of the gene contains the signal sequence that terminates transcription.

The pre-mRNA formed contains the sequences derived from both introns and exons. The intron-derived sequences are removed during RNA processing, leaving mature mRNA. More than one mRNA can be formed from a single pre-mRNA. The mRNA is exported from the nucleus into the cytoplasm, where it becomes associated with ribosomes (Fig. 147-2). Ribosomes function as the machinery of protein synthesis and perform the process of elongating peptide chains (see later discussion). The ribosome-cytoplasmic mRNA complex is called the polyribosome. Amino acids from the cytoplasm are carried to this complex by transfer RNA (tRNA) and are attached to a growing peptide chain as the ribosome moves along the mRNA from the 5′ to the 3′ end. As the newly synthesized protein emerges from the ribosome, a sequence of 15 to 30 mostly hydrophobic amino acids (the signal peptide) is exposed to the cytoplasm. The signal peptide binds to a cytoplasmic molecule called signal recognition particle (SRP). This association blocks further translation until the SRP binds to a signal receptor on the endoplasmic reticulum. There is also a receptor on the endoplasmic reticulum for the ribosome. This binding process frees the signal peptide from the SRP, and the elongation of the protein resumes, thereby pushing it through the membrane to the interior of the endoplasmic reticulum. As long as the hormone precursor molecule has the signal peptide attached, it is called a preprohormone.

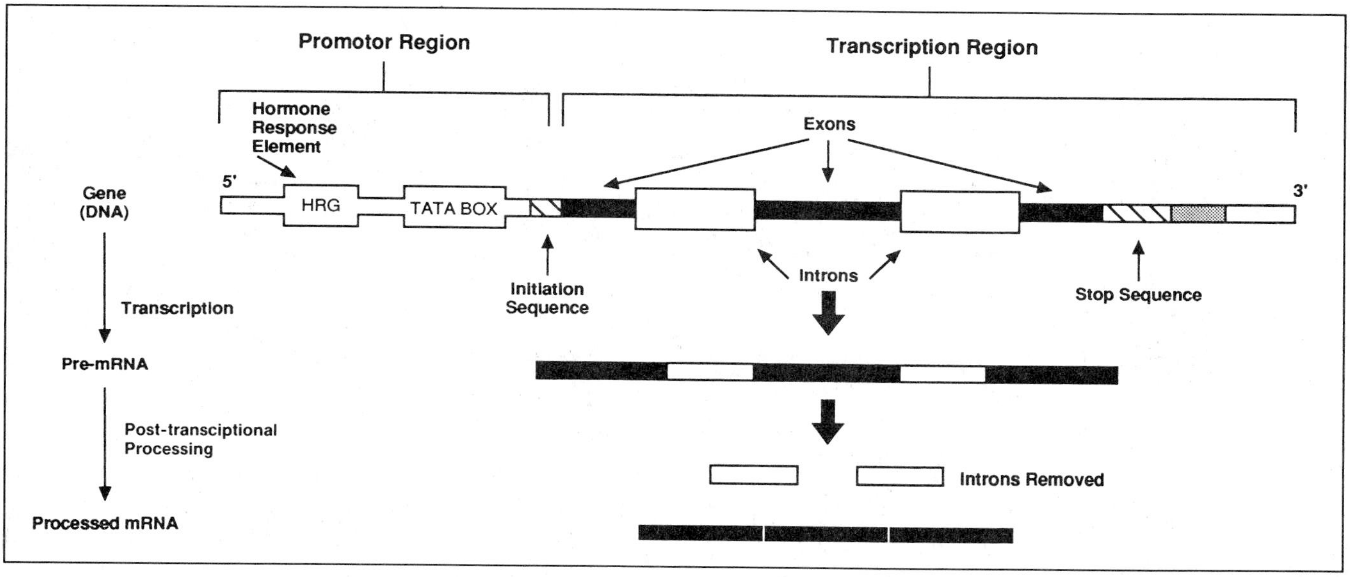

Fig. 147-1. Gene structure and the steps involved in encoding a polypeptide. Exons contain the complementary base sequence that forms the processed mRNA. Some base sequences (introns) are transcribed into pre-mRNA from the gene but are removed during posttranscriptional processing and do not contribute to the translated amino acid sequence of a protein. Hormone response elements interact with steroid hormone–receptor complexes to affect the transcription product. The TATA box is a base sequence that promotes the action of RNA polymerase, the enzyme responsible for polymerization of RNA into complementary base sequences from the DNA template. HRE, hormone response element; mRNA, messenger ribonucleic acid; DNA, deoxyribonucleic acid.

The signal peptide, however, is quickly cleaved by a trypsin-like enzyme residing in the membrane of the endoplasmic reticulum, changing the precursor to a prohormone. When a termination sequence on the mRNA is reached, translation stops and the peptide chain is released. The ribosome then dissociates into its two subunits and drifts off into the cytoplasm. The prohormone is transfered via transport vesicles to the Golgi apparatus, where further posttranslational modifications occur such as glycosylation and cleavage of amino terminal residues. In the Golgi apparatus, the peptide hormones are packaged into microvesicles or secretory granules and are either stored or immediately secreted into the extracellular fluid. The entire process from the beginning of synthesis to hormone secretion or storage can occur in less than 1 hour.

Steroid hormones

The various steroid hormones are derived from enzymatically induced alterations of a cholesterol core. In the adrenals and gonads, pituitary trophic hormones stimulate these changes. Unlike peptide-secreting cells, the precursor (cholesterol) is supplied by plasma lipoproteins or is synthesized directly by the cell. Inside the mitochondria, cholesterol is converted to pregnenolone. Further transformation of pregnenolone occurs after it leaves the mitochondria and enters the endoplasmic reticulum. It is here that side chain modifications occur. These biosynthetic processes occur in the adrenal cortex, testis, ovary, and, to some extent, fat.

The synthesis of the steroid vitamin D differs considerably from that of other steroid hormones in that transformation occurs in several different organs. Cholecalciferol (vitamin D) is either initially synthesized in the skin nonenzymatically by the action of ultraviolet radiation on 7-dehydrocholesterol or absorbed from the intestine. Vitamin D then is transported to the liver, where it is converted to a 25-hydroxylated product. This product is the major circulating form of the vitamin. Conversion to the most active vitamin D metabolite, 1,25-hydroxyvitamin D, occurs in the kidney.

Catecholamines

Catecholamines are synthesized from the amino acid tyrosine in nerves and in the adrenal medulla. The synthetic process involves hydroxylation and decarboxylation (removal of a COOH group) of tyrosine (Chapter 164). Tyrosine is first converted to dihydroxyphenylalanine by the rate-limiting enzyme tyrosine hydroxylase and then to dopamine by a decarboxylase. Dopamine enters granulated vesicles and is transformed to norepinephrine by dopamine beta-hydroxylase. Tissues that contain phenylethanolamine N-methyl transferase (adrenal medulla, organ of Zuckerkandl, and some central nervous system neurons) are capable of converting norepinephrine to epinephrine.

Thyroid hormone

Thyroglobulin is a large, 660,000 dalton protein produced by the thyroid follicular cell. This molecule contains more

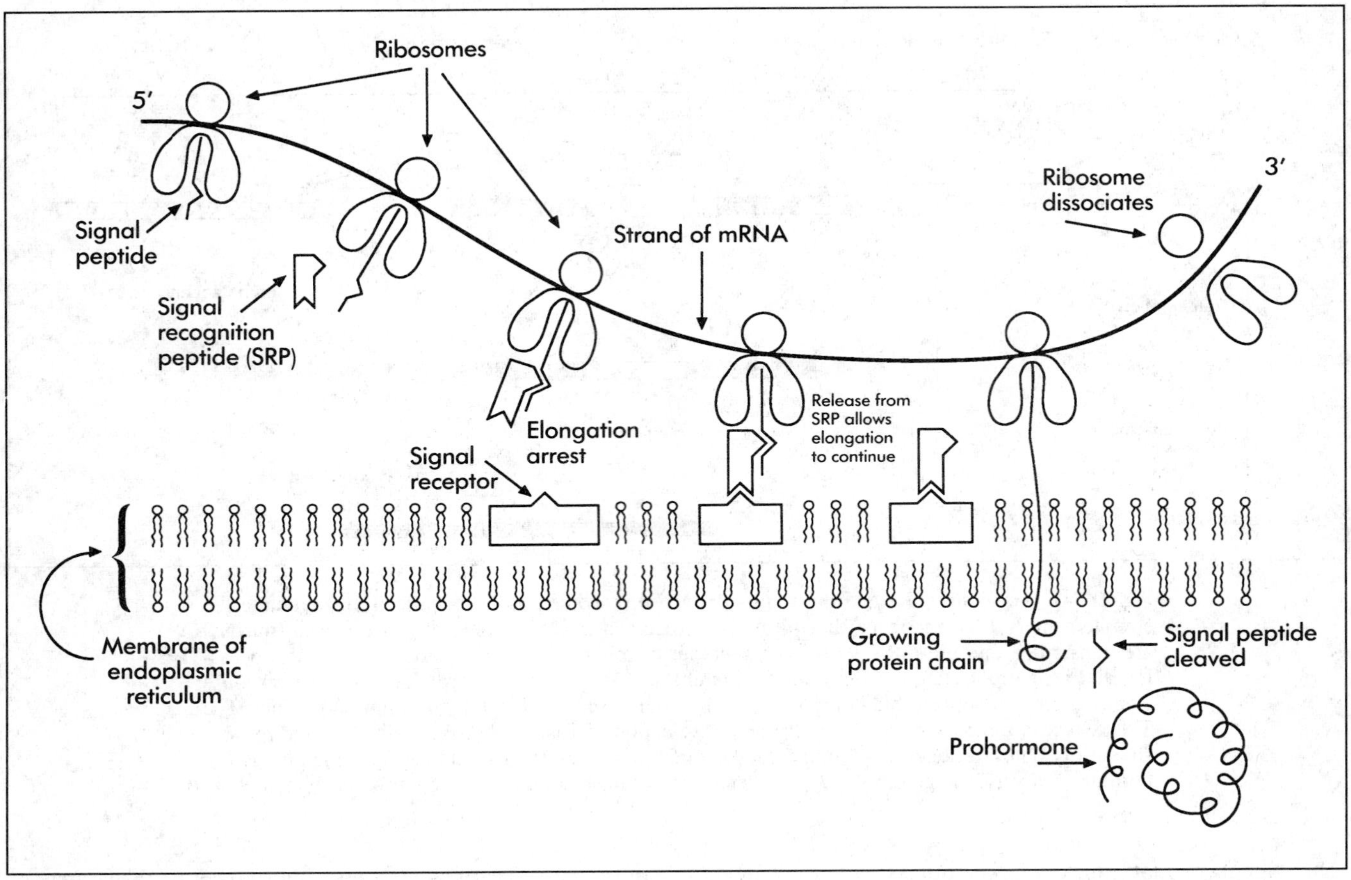

Fig. 147-2. Process of peptide hormone synthesis. The protein chain is extruded from the ribosome complex until signal peptide combines with signal recognition peptide. This stops further elongation until SRP binds to the signal receptor on the surface membrane of the endoplasmic reticulum. This frees the peptide chain, allowing it to resume elongation. Signal peptide leads the protein chain through the membrane, and once it reaches the interior of the endoplasmic reticulum, signal peptide is cleaved. SRP, signal recognition peptide.

than 100 tyrosine residues that have a spatial orientation that makes them susceptible to iodination. Iodide is actively trapped by the follicular cell, oxidized to iodine, and then attached to tyrosine residues *(organification).* Either monoiodotyrosine (MIT) or diiodotyrosine (DIT) is formed, depending on whether one or two molecules are added to the tyrosine moiety. While still incorporated in the thyroglobulin molecule, two DIT molecules are enzymatically coupled to form thyroxine (DIT + DIT $\rightarrow$ T_4), or MIT and DIT are joined to form triiodothyronine (DIT + MIT $\rightarrow$ T_3).

MECHANISMS OF HORMONE ACTION

Hormone action is intimately linked to the interaction between a hormone and a specific cellular receptor. The receptor serves two important functions: One is to allow the target cell to recognize the hormone from myriad other circulating substances. Second, the hormone-receptor interaction initiates the final pathway leading to hormone action. At present, two broad categories of hormone receptors are recognized: receptors that reside on the cell membrane surface and receptors found in the interior of the cell.

Membrane receptors

Recent evidence indicates that cell surface receptors are glycoproteins of two general classes (Fig. 147-3). The first class contains a large external portion that binds the hormone. The class of receptor also contains a small hydrophobic transmembrane component and an intracellular component that has intrinsic tyrosine kinase activity. Receptors for insulin and insulin-like growth factor 1 are examples. The second class is less well defined but in general reacts with G proteins (see later discussion). These receptors are often large and may span the cell membrane up to seven times. Many receptors appear to be highly mobile and "float" in the lipid bilayer of the plasma membrane. The hydrophilic portions of the protein are exposed at the surface, whereas the more lipid-soluble portions of the molecule are anchored in the hydrophobic portion of the membrane.

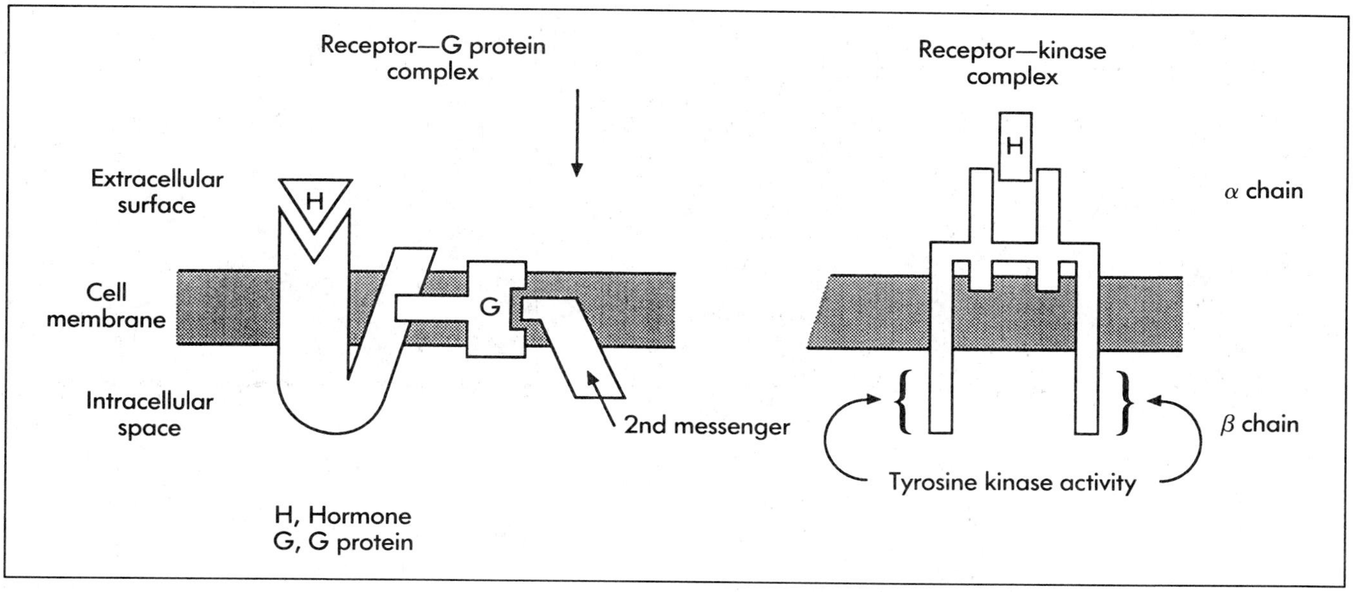

Fig. 147-3. Structure of cell surface receptors.

Membrane receptors bind water-soluble hormones that include all peptide hormones and catecholamines. These hormones travel freely in the circulation and are not bound to plasma proteins. Being water soluble, however, they do not readily cross the cell membrane. Thus membrane receptors allow the hormonal message to be internalized within the cell. Binding of the hormone to the receptor appears to involve both hydrophobic and electrostatic interactions. This process is reversible, so receptors may be recycled and used more than once. In some instances the receptor-hormone complex is internalized, and at that point it is subject to degradation by cytoplasmic proteases.

Activation of adenyl cyclase

The translation of hormone message involves a cascade of complex events illustrated in Fig. 147-4. The initial steps are hormone recognition by the receptor and formation of the hormone-receptor complex. This interaction increases the affinity of the hormone complex for a family of guanosine triphosphate (GTP) regulatory proteins called G proteins that bind and hydrolyze guanosine triphosphate (GTP). There are stimulatory (G_s) and inhibitory (G_i) G proteins. Both classes are heterotrimers composed of alpha, beta, and gamma subunits. The beta and gamma subunits are identical in the stimulatory and inhibitory systems, whereas the alpha subunits differ. In the absence of hormone being bound to the receptor, the G protein is kept inactive by the alpha subunit binding guanosine diphosphate (GDP). When the hormone occupies the receptor the alpha subunit binds GTP and dissociates from the beta-gamma complex. The alpha-GTP stimulatory subunit then activates adenyl cyclase (the second messenger). The beta-gamma subunit also may activate other second messengers.

Once adenyl cyclase is activated, it catalyzes the conversion of adenosine triphosphate (ATP) to cyclic 3′5′-adenosine monophosphate. In the cytoplasm of the cell, cyclic AMP combines with regulatory subunits of cyclic AMP–dependent protein kinases, causing the subunits to dissociate from the enzyme, thereby activating the protein kinase. Activated protein kinase in turn catalyzes the phosphorylation of other enzymes or proteins by ATP, and this leads to an alteration of cell function in a hormone-specific fashion. Cyclic AMP activity is in part regulated by the cytoplasmic enzyme phosphodiesterase, which deactivates cyclic AMP by converting it to 5′ adenosine monophosphate.

The G_i protein complex works in a parallel fashion and is activated by a separate hormone-receptor interaction. When the alpha inhibitory subunit dissociates from the G_i protein complex, however, it inhibits adenyl cyclase. This additional mechanism gives precise control over regulation of hormone action.

Calcium mediation of hormone action

Not all hormones use adenylate cyclase as their intracellular messenger. Influx of Ca^{2+} plays an important role as an effector of hormone action (Fig. 147-5). One means by which intracellular Ca^{2+} concentration increases is by the hormone-receptor complex opening Ca^{2+} channels of the plasma membrane and allowing influx of extracellular Ca^{2+} into the cell along an electrochemical gradient. It is also possible that intracellular calcium bound by organelles is released. The increase in intracellular Ca^{2+} activates protein kinases and causes subsequent phosphorylation of protein as described for cyclic AMP. This and numerous other effects of Ca^{2+} are mediated through a low-molecular-weight, ubiquitous, intracellular protein called *calmodulin*. Calmodulin is a single-chain peptide structure with four binding sites for Ca^{2+}. After Ca^{2+} is bound to calmodulin, the protein undergoes conformational changes and becomes activated. Activated calmodulin becomes associated with

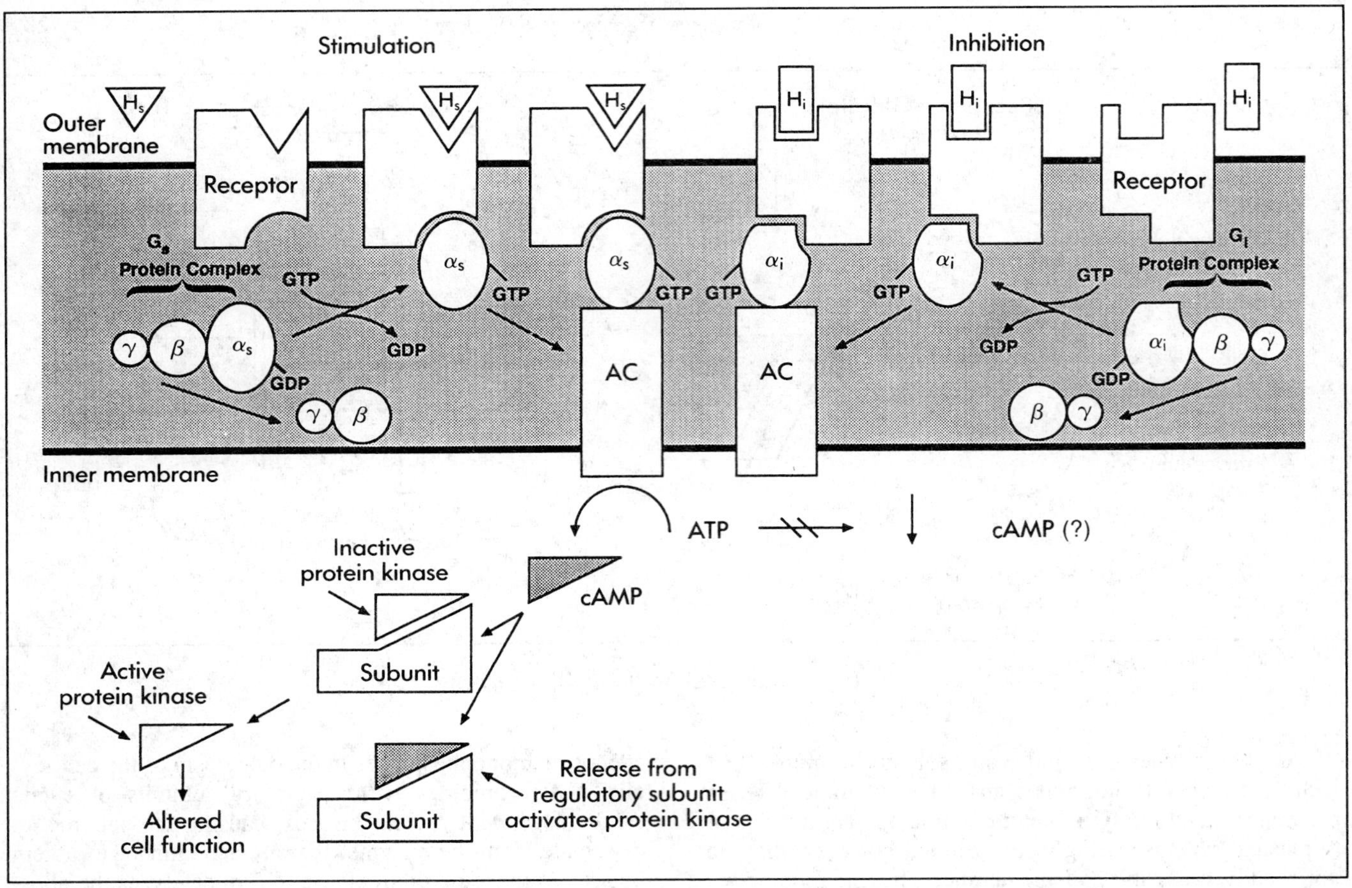

Fig. 147-4. The multiple steps leading to simulation and inhibition of adenylate cyclase and subsequent altered cell function *(see text for discussion)*. The alpha subunit of stimulatory G protein complex stimulates adenylate cyclase, whereas the alpha subunit of inhibitory G protein complex decreases cyclic AMP formation. H_s, stimulatory hormone; H_i, inhibitory hormone; G_s, stimulatory G protein; G_i, inhibitory G protein complex; AC, adenylate cyclase.

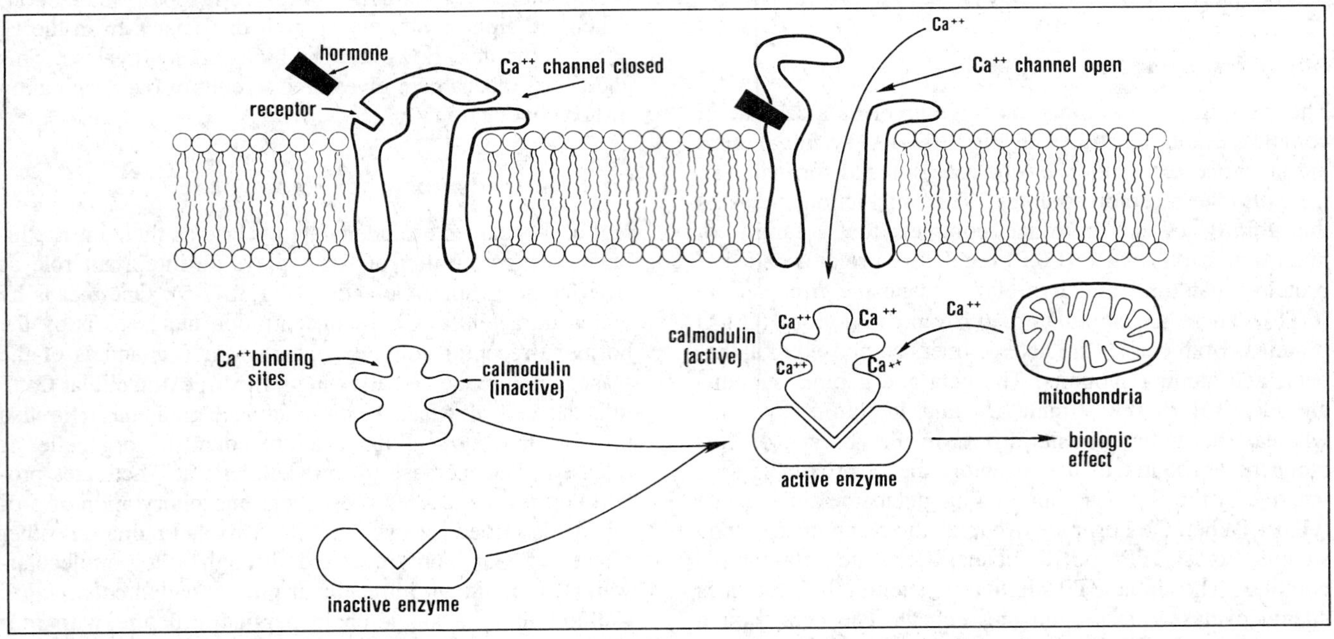

Fig. 147-5. Schematic diagram showing a hormone stimulating calcium entry into the cell. Once inside the cell calcium may bind to a ubiquitous regulatory protein, calmodulin, and activate it, which in turn activates protein kinase enzymes (see text for details). (From Kohler PO and Jordan RM, editors: Clinical endocrinology. New York, 1986, Wiley.)

calmodulin-sensitive enzymes such as protein kinases, and this interaction enhances the catalytic ability of the enzyme. Recent evidence suggests that many intracellular enzymes are regulated by calmodulin. After the calcium-dependent activity, intracellular Ca^{2+} levels are restored by the action of calcium-sodium ATPase pumps, which normally act to keep the intracellular Ca^{2+} concentration low.

Other intracellular messengers

Some hormone-receptor interactions activate a membrane phospholipase C via a unique G protein (Fig. 147-6). The active phospholipase C causes hydrolysis of membrane phosphoinositides yielding diacylglycerol (DAG) and inositol triphosphate (IP_3). IP_3 causes release of Ca^{2+} from intracellular organelles such as the mitochondria. The Ca^{2+} associates with calmodulin, which activates protein kinases (see earlier discussion). DAG remains in the membrane and, with Ca^{2+}, activates protein kinase C. Like other kinases, protein kinase C facilitates phosphorylation of proteins.

For insulin and epidermal growth factor the receptor itself has intrinsic kinase activity, which becomes active after the hormone binds to the receptor. Another intracellular messenger is guanylate cyclase. It catalyzes the conversion of cyclic guanosine triphosphate (GTP) to cyclic guanosine monophosphate in a way analogous to that which occurs for cyclic AMP from ATP. Presumably cyclic GMP–dependent kinases are activated.

Receptor regulation

Regulatory processes controlling the concentration of cell surface receptors are being elucidated. Receptors are proteins synthesized on the rough endoplasmic reticulum and processed in the Golgi apparatus and are transported via secretory vesicles to the plasma membrane. Because they are integral membrane proteins, receptors are subject to recycling processes and are continuously synthesized and degraded. The presence of agonist (hormone) appears to regulate receptor function and number. In the case of insulin, high hormone levels decrease the number of active receptors able to bind insulin, a process known as *down regulation*. In some cases hormones may actually increase receptors, an example of which is the action of estrogen and follicle-stimulating hormone (FSH) to increase granulosa cell luteinizing hormone (LH) receptors during ovarian follicular maturation.

A concept different from reduced receptor number is that of change in receptor affinity for hormone. Alterations of affinity involve true changes in the kinetics of association and dissociation between hormone and receptor ($H + R \sim HR$). With reduced affinity, the biologic response for a given concentration of hormone decreases. An example of this phenomenon is the effect of elevated blood insulin levels, which reduce the affinity of the receptor for insulin (negative cooperativity).

An interesting observation is that membrane receptors are often present in considerable excess of what is needed

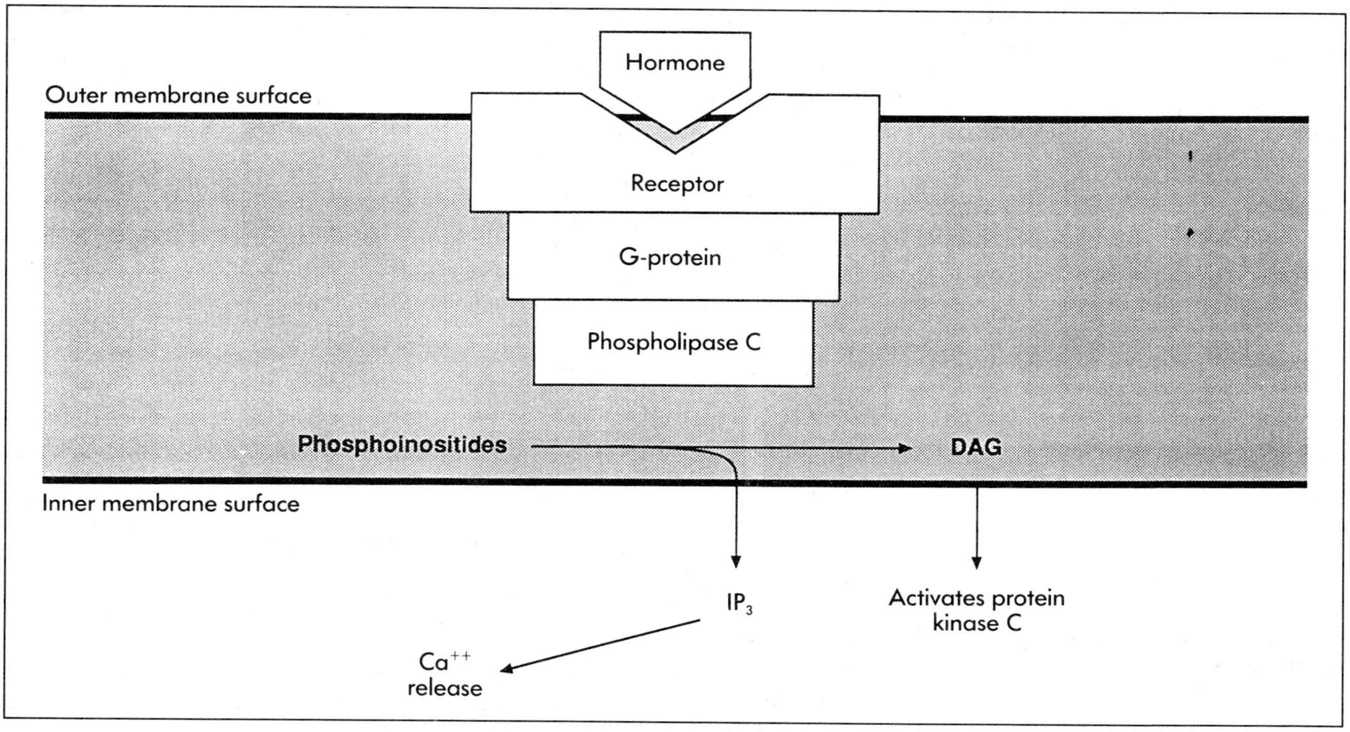

Fig. 147-6. Activation of inositol triphosphate and diacylglycerol from phosphoinositides. Both IP_3 and DAG act as second messengers. IP_3 inositol triphosphate; DAG, diacylglycerol.

for a maximal hormone response ("spare receptors"). Although the biologic significance of this is uncertain, it may allow for a maximum hormone response despite a reduced level of hormone.

Nuclear and cytoplasmic receptors

Thyroid hormones and steroid hormones are lipid soluble and can, therefore, penetrate the cell's plasma membrane. The classic model for steroid hormone action holds that, once inside the cell, steroid hormones bind to cytoplasmic receptors. These receptors are proteins that have a hormone binding area at the carboxy terminal and midmolecular region, rich in cystine residues, that forms loops. This folded area binds coordinately with zinc (zinc fingers) and attaches to nuclear chromatin. Interaction with the steroid changes the size, charge, and chemical properties of the protein, creating in the entire receptor-hormone complex a high affinity for nuclear chromatin. The movement of this complex to the nucleus is called *translocation*. The chromatin contains specific areas called hormone responsive elements (HREs) that binds the hormone-receptor complex. This interaction either enhances or reduces transcription of new mRNA and thus modifies the cell's activity. For some steroids the receptors reside in the nuclei of target cells rather than in the cytoplasm.

Thyroid hormone receptors are located on nuclear chromatin. They are acidic, nonhistone proteins that have high-affinity but low-capacity–binding properties and bind T_3 better than T_4. The hormone-receptor interaction induces changes in the chromatin that lead to transcription of new mRNA and new protein synthesis.

Our understanding of the regulatory processes governing nuclear and cytoplasmic receptors is even more rudimentary than that of membrane receptors. However, we know that progesterone is capable of reducing the concentration of its receptor. Progesterone also reduces the number of estrogen receptors. Estrogen, on the other hand, increases the synthesis of its own as well as progesterone receptors. Recycling and degradation mechanisms are poorly understood.

HORMONE SECRETION

Endocrine cells that store peptide or amine hormones in granules have a readily releasable pool of hormone. Granules are discharged in close temporal relationship with the appropriate stimulus *(stimulus-secretion coupling)* regardless of whether the stimulus is neural or hormonal. The process of secretion is dependent on an influx of calcium into the cell. In some cells the entry of ionic calcium causes contraction of a microfilament system that appears to be important in guiding hormone granules to the cell surface. At the surface the storage vesicle surrounding the granule fuses with the plasma membrane, and the granule is expelled at the cell-capillary interface (exocytosis). For a number of endocrine cells, the stimulus for secretion causes new hormone synthesis. This phenomenon results in a biphasic release, an early pulse of stored hormone followed by a more sustained release of newly synthesized hormone.

In contrast to peptide and amines, steroids are secreted by simple bulk transfer, down concentration gradients from the gland to the blood. Steroid-producing cells store very little of their final product, and therefore, the stimulus for hormone release is linked to the stimulus for accelerated hormone synthesis.

Thyroid hormone secretion is unique. Substantial amounts of thyroid hormone are stored within the thyroid follicles attached to the colloid protein. Follicular colloid-containing thyroglobulin is engulfed by the projections from the follicular cells. Thyroglobulin isolated in this fashion is subjected to proteolysis with release of thyroid hormone. The thyroid hormone then diffuses out of the cell. In this case, the secretory process does not respond rapidly to a stimulus, distinguishing it from the stimulation-release relationship seen with peptide and amine hormones.

Hormone secretion does not occur at a uniform rate. Peptide and catecholamines in particular are released episodically. Feeding, fasting, or nonspecific stress may have stimulatory or inhibitory effects on hormone secretion. Sleep-related hormone release occurs with many hormones, including growth hormone and prolactin. Circadian variation, which is a self-sustaining repetitive fluctuation with a period of approximately 24 hours, is characteristic of ACTH release. In many clinical situations a knowledge of these variations may be crucial for accurate interpretation of blood hormone concentration levels.

Transport

Most hormones are transported at least some distance to their target organs. Usually transport occurs in blood, but lymph and cerebrospinal fluid may also be important transport media. Peptide hormones and catecholamines are water soluble and travel freely in these fluids. Lipid-soluble hormones (thyroid hormone and all steroid hormones), however, are transported in association with plasma carrier proteins. Many carrier proteins such as cortisol-binding globulin, thyroid-binding globulin, sex hormone–binding globulin, and vitamin D–binding globulin have a high affinity for a single hormone. Nonspecific, low-affinity binding also occurs, because most of the lipid-soluble hormones bind to albumin. The physiologic function of carrier proteins is uncertain. Binding is not necessary for hormone action to occur. In fact, it is the free hormone that initiates hormone-mediated activity. Carrier proteins possibly act to buffer sudden increases in hormone availability or serve as a reservoir by preventing rapid hormone degradation. Despite such plausible theories of function, an absence or excess of carrier proteins does not cause any apparent clinical disease.

Regulatory mechanisms for hormone secretion

Regulation of hormone action occurs at all levels from the process of secretion to action at the target cell. Possible regulatory mechanisms by receptor activity, postreceptor phenomena, and transport proteins were mentioned in preceding sections.

Influences that directly stimulate hormone secretion can be divided into two broad categories: neural discharge and feedback regulation responding to changing blood levels of hormone or other chemical mediators. Although either variety of stimulus may occur independently of the other, more often they are coupled to control secretion.

Examples of neural-mediated hormone secretion are stress-induced release of pituitary hormones (ACTH, growth hormone, prolactin) via action of hypothalamic peptides, circadian release of ACTH, sleep patterns of growth hormone secretion, and nocturnal gonadotropin release during puberty. Vasopressin release after hypotension and oxytocin secretion after suckling are mediated by neural stimuli.

The most familiar example of a changing hormone level causing hormone secretion is that of feedback regulation (Fig. 147-7). In most instances, active secretion of a trophic hormone is inhibited by feedback suppression from the target hormone. There are numerous examples of this type of servomechanism in endocrinology including regulation of thyroid-stimulating hormone (TSH), ACTH, and the gonadotropins by their respective target cell hormones. A nonhormonal mediator of feedback inhibition is calcium. Small changes in extracellular ionic calcium are quickly followed by reciprocal changes in parathyroid hormone secretion.

A more complex example of feedback regulation is the relationship between glucose and insulin. Elevation of the blood glucose level causes insulin release, which acts to return the glucose level to normal. Conversely, hypoglycemia decreases insulin secretion. Hypoglycemia, however, also triggers the release of insulin counterregulatory hormones (glucagon, epinephrine, cortisol, and growth hormone), which stimulate either glycogenolysis or glyconeogenesis, or both, in an active effort to increase the blood glucose concentration.

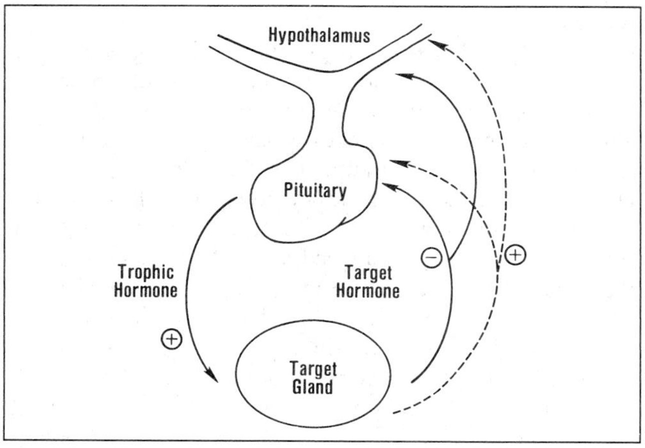

Fig. 147-7. General schematic drawing showing feedback relationships between the pituitary gland and the target organ. (From Kohler PO and Jordan RM, editors: Clinical endocrinology. New York, 1986, Wiley.)

Feedback may be positive as well as negative. An example of positive feedback is the effect of estradiol on gonadotropin secretion at a specific time during the follicular phase of the human menstrual cycle. At this point in the cycle, estradiol levels reach a critical level for a sustained period, causing the midcycle LH and FSH surge. At other times estradiol feedback is negative. The exact mechanism by which such a dual feedback occurs is not known.

Degradation of hormone

In order to make adaptive changes to the environment, the endocrine system must be able to dispose of hormone as well as secrete it. Several mechanisms for hormone degradation exist, some of which are rapid and others comparatively slow. The rate of hormone removal usually parallels the rapidity with which a hormone effects adaptive changes.

The half-life of peptide hormones is short, varying between 8 and 60 minutes. A percentage of intact hormone and fragments of hormone is filtered by the kidney and excreted in the urine. Peptides are also degraded by proteases and peptidases in plasma and at the target gland after internalization. Other organs such as the liver also metabolize peptides.

Steroid hormones are metabolized primarily in the liver through reductions, oxidations, hydroxylations, side chain cleavages, and conjugation to glucuronates and sulfates. These transformations not only render the compounds inactive but also increase their water solubility, thereby facilitating excretion in urine and bile. Catecholamines are cleared very rapidly from the circulation and are inactivated through methylation and oxidative deamination. These transformations occur either intraneuronally or extraneuronally. The degradation of thyroid hormone is accomplished by iodine removal via a deiodinase and also by conjugation with glucuronates and sulfates. Deiodinated metabolites are excreted in urine, whereas most of the conjugated metabolites are excreted in bile. Vitamin D metabolites also are eliminated in the bile.

Another mechanism of hormone metabolism is routing to pathways of either an active or an inactive product. The 25-hydroxylated derivative of vitamin D is converted by the kidney to a largely inactive 24,25-hydroxylated compound when the blood ionic calcium level is normal. If calcium conservation is needed, the kidney converts 25-hydroxyvitamin D to 1,25-hydroxyvitamin D. The 1,25-hydroxylate product is very active in promoting gastrointestinal absorption of calcium, and it also acts on bone to increase calcium resorption.

REFERENCES

Ascoli M and Segaloff DL: On the structure of the luteinizing hormone/chorionic gonadotropin receptor. Endocr Rev 10:27, 1989.

Berridge MJ: Inositol triphosphate and diacylglycerol: two interacting second messengers. Annu Rev Biochem 56:159, 1987.

Brown MS, Anderson RGW, and Goldstein JL: Recycling receptors: the round-trip itinerary of migrant membrane proteins. Cell 32:663, 1983.
Herbert E and Uhler M: Biosynthesis of polyprotein precursors to regulatory peptides. Cell 30:1, 1982.
Gilman AG: G proteins: transducers of receptor-generated signals. Annu Rev Biochem 56:615, 1987.
Means AR and Chafouleas JG: Calmodulin in endocrine cells. Annu Rev Physiol 44:667, 1982.
Neer EJ and Clapham DE: Roles of G protein subunits in transmembrane signaling. Nature 333:129, 1988.
O'Malley BW: Steroid hormone action in eukaryotic cells. J Clin Invest 74:307, 1984.
Rasmussen H: The calcium messenger system. N Engl J Med 314:1094, 1164, 1986.
Roth J and Taylor SI: Receptors for peptide hormones: alterations in disease of humans. Annu Rev Physiol 44:639, 1982.
Welshons WV, Lieberman ME, and Gorski J: Nuclear localization of unoccupied estrogen receptors. Nature 307:747, 1984.

CHAPTER

148 Physiology of Bone and Mineral Homeostasis

Gregory R. Mundy
Charles A. Reasner II

FUNCTIONS OF THE SKELETON

Bone is a unique mineralized connective tissue that comprises cortical or compact bone and trabecular or cancellous bone. Cortical bone makes up approximately 75% of the total skeleton and trabecular bone 20%. Cortical bone is present in the shafts of the long bones, whereas cancellous bone occurs in the vertebrae, ends of the long bones, and ribs. Bone not only provides structural support for the body but is the storehouse for 99% of the body's calcium, 80% of the phosphate, and substantial amounts of magnesium, sodium, and carbonate. Because the skeleton is a source of these ions, they are available when systemic deficiencies occur. When calcium deficiency occurs, bone resorption maintains the serum and tissue calcium supply but weakens the skeleton. Bone also provides a defense mechanism against systemic acidosis and assists renal and respiratory systems in maintaining acid-base balance. Bone resorption leads to release of additional phosphate and carbonate to buffer systemic acidosis.

NATURAL HISTORY OF THE SKELETON

Fig. 148-1 illustrates the changes that occur in bone with aging. Throughout life bone is continually being resorbed and reformed at discrete sites throughout the skeleton. This process is known as *bone turnover* or *bone remodeling*. The total bone mass depends on the closely associated processes of bone resorption and bone formation, which are under the control of specialized bone cells called *osteoclasts* (for bone resorption) and *osteoblasts* (for bone formation). During adolescence, bone formation exceeds bone resorption, and an increase in bone mass occurs. Bone mass reaches a maximum after linear growth stops, remains constant for approximately 10 years, and then begins to fall in the third or fourth decade. The bone mass declines to half its maximum value by age 80 or 90 (age-related bone loss). Women have less bone mass at maximum and show an accelerated phase of bone loss just after menopause. This loss involves predominantly endosteal resorption with loss of cancellous bone, particularly in the vertebrae, without adequate replacement by new bone. Cortical bone mass also declines rapidly after the menopause.

Bone remodeling and the balance between rates of bone formation and bone resorption determine bone volume. Because the remodeling of bone occurs asynchronously at local and discrete sites throughout the skeleton, the regulation of bone volume, particularly trabecular bone volume, is probably under the control of local rather than systemic factors. The factors that control bone volume have not yet been identified. Clearly, their characterization is vitally important for understanding normal bone turnover, age-related bone loss, and osteoporosis (see later discussion).

CELLULAR PHYSIOLOGY OF BONE

Osteoprogenitor cells, which are fibroblast-like and derived from local mesenchymal cells in the bone marrow, differentiate into *osteoblasts,* which synthesize collagen and other components of the bone matrix. Osteoblasts are also probably responsible for the orderly mineralization of the bone matrix, although the precise role of these cells in this process is unclear. When surrounded by new bone, osteoblasts become *osteocytes* and gradually stop synthesizing collagen. Osteoblasts and osteocytes are connected by cell processes that form a continuous "bone membrane," which establishes a functional boundary between blood and bone mineral.

Osteoclasts (bone-resorbing cells) are independent of the bone membrane. Their precursor cell is a circulating mononuclear cell that originates in the bone marrow and is probably a member of the monocyte-macrophage family. They are highly specialized multinucleated cells with a characteristic area of the cell membrane called a *ruffled border,* which is the site at which bone resorption occurs. Bone surfaces are covered by a flattened layer of spindle-shaped lining cells that probably represent cells in the osteoblast lineage. Osteoclasts lie above this layer and resorb bone by insinuating processes containing ruffled borders between the lining cells. Bone resorption occurs extracellularly as a two-step process. Initially, it involves calcium removal, possibly requiring H^+ secretion across the ruffled border. H^+ is generated within osteoclasts by an isoenzyme of carbonic anhydrase. The second part of this resorption process is the degradation of bone matrix by lysosomal enzymes and collagenase and occurs after the mineral has been re-

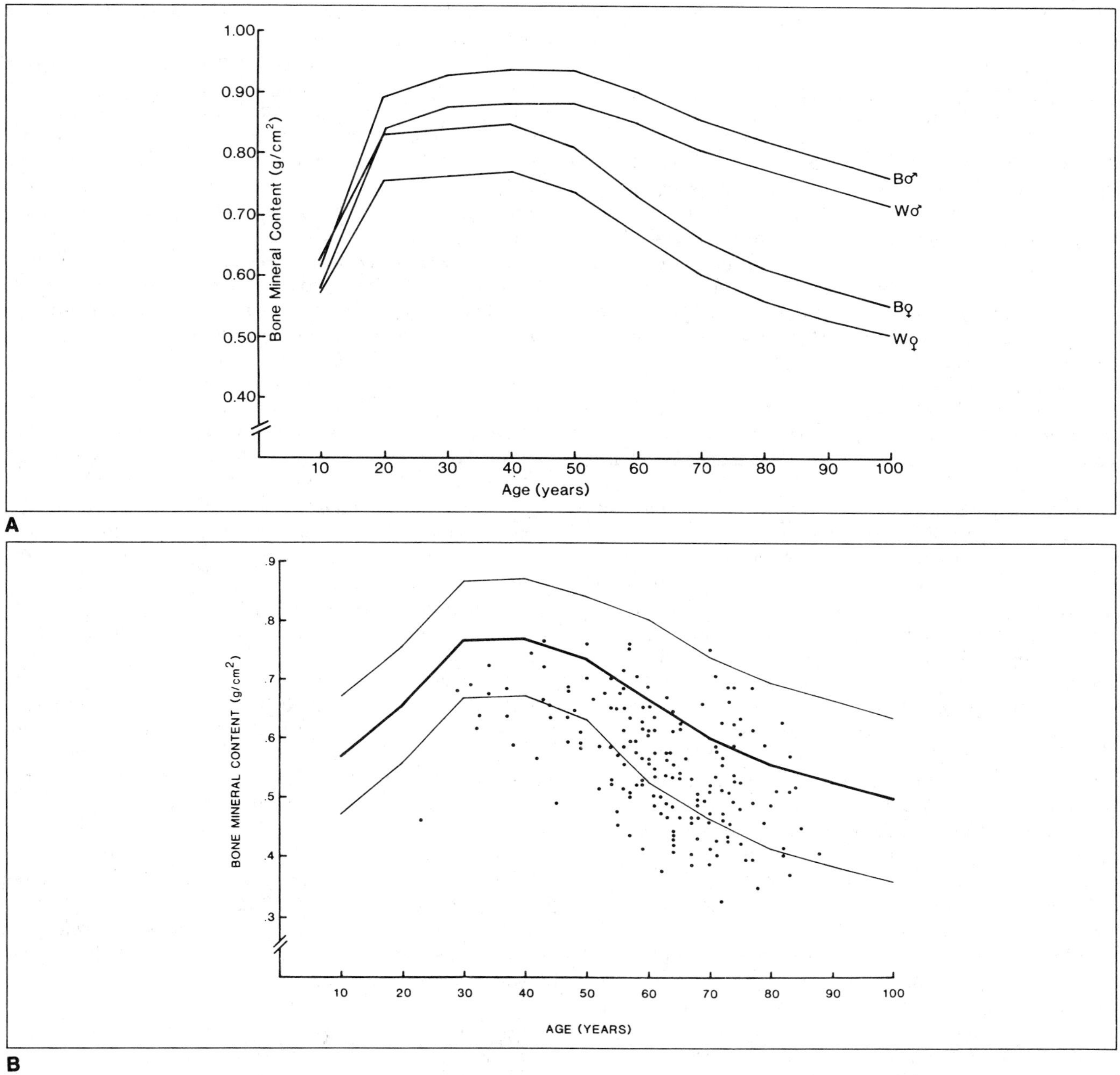

Fig. 148-1. A, Relationship between bone mineral content (radial midshaft) and age. Note that males have higher bone mineral content than females, blacks have higher bone mineral content than whites, and decline in bone mineral content is accelerated in females in the immediate postmenopausal years. **B,** Bone mineral content in osteoporotic white females plotted in relation to age. The solid center line is the mean value for normal white females, and the outer line marks the 95% confidence limits. Each point represents an individual patient. Note that there is considerable overlap between normal and osteoporotic patients, although the majority of patients have a value below the mean normal value.

moved. The number and activity of osteoclasts are under hormonal regulation. Osteoclasts are activated by parathyroid hormone (PTH); the vitamin D metabolites, prostaglandins E; cytokines, such as interleukin 1, and tumor necrosis factor; thyroid hormones, and growth factors such as epidermal growth factor and the transforming growth factors. Osteoclast activation involves an increase in size and number of ruffled borders. Osteoclast activity is inhibited by calcitonin transiently, glucocorticoids (depending on the stimulus), plicamycin, oral phosphate, and the bisphosphonates. Osteoclast-like cells also resorb calcified cartilage and dentin.

MATRIX FORMATION AND CALCIFICATION

Bone organic matrix consists predominantly of type I collagen (about 95%), but it also contains acidic glycoproteins, sulfated proteoglycans, and a calcium-binding protein that contains gamma-carboxyglutamic acid residues (called the *bone Gla protein* or *osteocalcin*). The function of the bone *Gla* protein is unknown, but its measurement is now being used as a marker of bone turnover (Chapter 151). It is synthesized by a cell in the osteoblast lineage, and it has been suggested that its function may be to inhibit and thereby regulate bone matrix mineralization. The bone *Gla* protein comprises about 20% of the noncollagen protein in bone. Other similar noncollagen proteins are *osteonectin,* osteopantin, and bone sialoprotein II. Their functions are also unknown.

The cellular mechanisms by which bone is formed differ in different parts of the skeleton. Intramembranous bone formation is the mechanism by which the flat bones of the calvarium and face are formed and by which the width of the long bones is determined. In this process, bone formation begins with a condensation of an island of mesenchymal cells that differentiate into osteoblasts and produce surrounding new bone that enlarges circumferentially and gradually mineralizes. As the osteoblasts become buried in the new bone matrix, they become osteocytes. The mechanism of bone formation is entirely different in the long bone shafts. In these bones, bone formation begins on an anlage of cartilage. A collar of bone develops around this cartilage anlage to form the midshaft of the bone *(diaphysis).* The cartilage is formed by chondroblasts. The cartilage anlage is eventually penetrated by blood vessels and is gradually resorbed by multinucleated cells to form the marrow cavity. Specialized areas of the anlage near each end of the long bone contain hypertrophic chondrocytes and are known as the *epiphyseal plates* or *growth plates*. This area is responsible for continued increase in length of the bone. As the resorption of cartilage by multinucleated cells occurs, bone forms on cartilaginous trabeculae and is remodeled by osteoclasts and replaced by osteoblasts. The origin of these osteoblasts is unclear. This entire process is known as *endochondral bone formation*. It is disturbed in states of vitamin D deficiency, so that the growth plate expands and matrix mineralization is impaired.

One of the unique qualities of bone that distinguishes it from other connective tissues is that its protein matrix is mineralized. Mineralization of bone occurs only after several days of *osteoid maturation,* a process that involves secretion of the collagen and noncollagen proteins of bone by active osteoblasts. The precise steps involved in mineralization of this matrix are unclear, but cell-free matrix vesicles that contain alkaline phosphatase and other enzymes that may be important in producing increased local concentrations of mineral may initiate this process. These matrix vesicles are probably derived from the cytoplasm of osteoblasts and chondroblasts and form nucleation sites for the precipitation of the mineral required for normal calcification of the matrix. The bone mineral is eventually deposited as hydroxyapatite $[Ca_{10}(PO_4)_6(OH)_2]$ crystals within the *hole zones* of collagen, which are the gaps between the ends of two collagen molecules. It is clear that these processes of bone formation and mineralization must be carefully regulated, but the precise manner in which this is achieved is not known. However, adequate supplies of calcium and phosphate are essential, as are the active metabolites of vitamin D. It is likely that the effect of the vitamin D metabolites is mediated by their providing a supply of calcium and phosphate at the mineralizing site rather than by affecting mineralization directly.

STRESS AND COUPLING

Rates of skeletal growth are influenced by stress, and in particular by weight bearing. This may be mediated through a piezoelectric effect, which can be generated by compression or tension on collagen. Bone growth is also dependent on a number of hormones including growth hormone, insulin-like growth factor I (also called *somatomedin C*), insulin-like growth factor II, transforming growth factor B, bone morphogenetic proteins, fibroblast growth factors, thyroid hormones, vitamin D metabolites, corticosteroids, and sex hormones.

Once the skeleton is formed, it is remodeled continuously by resorption of old bone in haversian canals and on the endosteal (trabecular) surfaces and by formation of new bone, which is deposited at these sites of resorption. The mechanism of this "coupling" of bone formation to bone resorption is unknown. This process of coupling of bone formation to bone resorption is the key event in bone that controls skeletal mass. Age-related bone loss is due to a relative increase in bone resorption over bone formation. When the factors and events that regulate this coupling are understood, it may be possible to understand the pathogenic events involved in age-related bone loss and other metabolic bone diseases.

CALCIUM METABOLISM

Distribution

Extracellular fluid calcium is a tightly controlled variable that has a number of vital functions. About 40% of the total calcium in the extracellular fluid is ionized or free and is closely regulated by homeostatic mechanisms. Of the total body calcium, 99% is distributed in bone, with the rest in soft tissue and the extracellular fluid. Ionized calcium in the extracellular fluid is regulated at the sites of calcium flux, which occur across the gastrointestinal tract, bone, and kidney. Precise regulation of extracellular ionized calcium concentration is necessary because ionized calcium influences a number of important metabolic processes including (1) cellular secretion of secretory proteins, hormones, and other products including neurotransmitters; (2) coupling between cell excitation and contraction, in the case of muscle cells, or secretion by secretory cells; (3) cell growth and division; (4) blood coagulation mechanisms, by acting as a cofactor for the enzymes involved in clotting; (5) maintenance of cell membrane stability and permeability; (6) regulation of enzyme activity including enzymes involved in glycogenolysis, gluconeogenesis, and protein kinases, which are calcium dependent; and (7) mineralization of newly formed bone. The mechanisms by which calcium influences these processes are unclear. However, movement of calcium ions into or out of the cytosol by regulated processes is clearly important.

The necessity for having a precise regulatory mechanism for maintaining the serum ionized calcium concentration between narrow limits is clear. When variations in the serum calcium concentration outside the normal range occur, disturbances in cell function result that can be anticipated from knowledge of the effects of ionized calcium on cell metabolic processes. For example, hypocalcemia is associated primarily with nerve conduction disturbances. Common symptoms include paresthesias, tetany, and convulsions. Hypercalcemia is also associated with disturbances in neuronal function. In severe hypercalcemia, patients may suffer from lethargy and impaired mental status; gastrointestinal disturbances including nausea, vomiting, and constipation; and disturbances in neuromuscular function characterized by muscle weakness and hypotonicity.

Intracellular calcium is distributed in subcellular compartments in a unique manner. Extracellular fluid calcium concentration is similar to the intramitochondrial calcium concentration (approximately 10^{-3}M). In contrast, the concentration of calcium in the cytosol is 1000 to 10,000 times less (10^{-6} to 10^{-7}M). It appears likely that there are separate active transport mechanisms responsible for pumping calcium from the cytosol into the extracellular fluid, into mitochondria, and possibly into microsomes. The mechanisms that are responsible for controlling fluxes of calcium across the plasma membrane and across the mitochondrial membrane are unclear but are clearly important for regulation of many important cellular events. Calcium is present in relatively high concentrations in the endoplasmic and sarcoplasmic reticula and is important for muscle contraction. During muscle excitation, the initial event is depolarization of the plasma membrane, which leads to release of calcium from the sarcoplasmic reticulum into the cytosol. Increases in cytosolic calcium in the muscle cell lead to conformational change in the protein troponin, which subsequently initiates the actin-myosin interaction, the basis of muscle contraction. Only small changes in cytosolic calcium concentration are required for excitation-response coupling in secretory cells. Excitation and depolarization of the plasma membrane are associated with entry of calcium from the exterior to the cytosol and with release of proteins stored within secretory granules. This may involve interactions with cyclic nucleotides and subsequent events, including facilitation of binding and fusion of secretory granules with the plasma membrane; activation of the tubulin-microtubule system, causing movement of secretory granules toward the cell exterior; and activation of specific adenosine triphosphatase (ATPase) enzymes involved in release of secretory granule contents to the exterior. In the gut and kidney and possibly in bone, calcium is transported across cells to the extracellular fluid. The molecular mechanisms involved in entry of calcium into the cell, transcellular calcium transport, and exit from the cell are not clear. Calmodulin is a ubiquitous calcium-binding protein with a molecular mass of 7000 daltons that is present in all cells. It is an intracellular receptor protein for calcium that may be responsible for delivering calcium to specific intracellular sites where calcium-regulated metabolic events occur. It is likely that the binding of calcium to calmodulin leads to specific conformational changes in the calmodulin molecule that in turn influence the way calmodulin interacts with specific target proteins, leading to changes in their activity.

Major systems controlling extracellular calcium homeostasis

Extracellular fluid calcium is a closely guarded variable that is regulated within 5% of mean by hormonal control of calcium fluxes that occur across the gut, renal tubules, and bone (Fig. 148-2).

Gastrointestinal tract. In the gastrointestinal tract, calcium is absorbed predominantly in the small bowel and excreted via the bile and pancreatic ducts. Calcium absorption from the gut occurs by two regulated processes, active calcium transport and facilitated diffusion. Secretion of calcium in the intestinal juices is probably unregulated but takes place mostly proximal to the sites of calcium absorption. The amount of calcium absorbed can vary from 20% to 70%, depending on the amount of calcium in the diet and vitamin D status. This adaptation of calcium transport to the available dietary calcium is probably mediated by 1,25-dihydroxyvitamin D. The variation in calcium absorp-

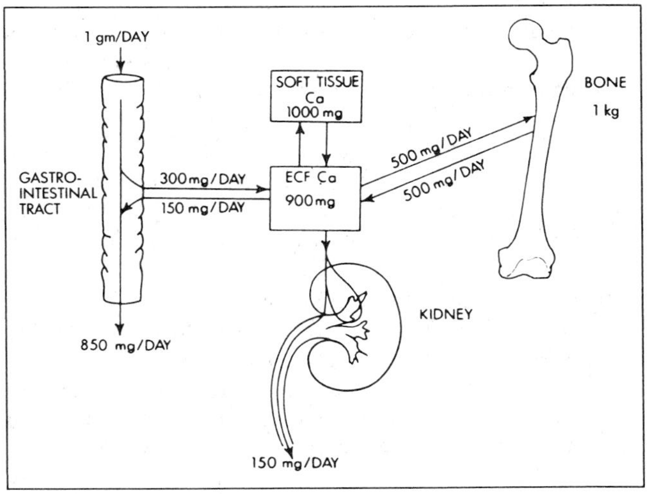

Fig. 148-2. Major sites of calcium regulation and control of calcium homeostasis. Values are for a normal adult at zero calcium balance. Younger growing individuals show a higher percentage of absorption from the gut and bone resorption with net positive calcium balance. (Mundy GR, Canalis EM, and Raisz LG: Conn Med 40:680, 1976.)

tion is less than the variation in dietary supply of calcium. The average American diet contains approximately 1000 mg calcium per day, although many elderly people ingest less. The highest rate of absorption of calcium occurs in the duodenum. However, calcium absorption also occurs in the ileum and jejunum, and because these segments of intestine are longer, the major part of calcium absorption takes place in these segments. Active calcium transport is associated with synthesis of a calcium-binding protein in intestinal cells whose activity is regulated by 1,25-dihydroxyvitamin D and that is probably important in the translocation of calcium across the gut wall. The active transport of calcium requires metabolic energy and is a saturable process. This indicates that a point can be reached when the addition of more calcium will yield no further increase in calcium transport. Calcium transport across the gut is inhibited by corticosteroids and by dietary components such as oxalate and phytate. It is decreased in patients with chronic renal failure and vitamin D deficiency. Parathyroid hormone (PTH) increases calcium absorption in the gut indirectly by increasing the synthesis of 1,25-dihydroxyvitamin D. Calcium absorption is increased in patients with vitamin D intoxication and the absorptive form of idiopathic hypercalciuria. Calcium absorption is also increased by dietary sugars such as lactose and fatty acids.

Kidney. The renal handling of calcium comprises two steps—namely, filtration across the glomerulus and reabsorption in the renal tubules. About 99% of the calcium filtered across the glomerulus is reabsorbed in the renal tubules. This occurs primarily in the proximal convoluted tubule but also in the ascending limb of the loop of Henle and the distal tubule. Only the distal tubular calcium reabsorption is finely regulated. The transport of calcium in the proximal tubule and the loop of Henle (which comprises about 90% of the total tubular calcium reabsorption) is linked to sodium chloride transport. When sodium transport is increased, calcium transport is also increased. Thus saline loading and loop diuretics that decrease sodium chloride reabsorption also promote calcium excretion in the urine. Calcium transport in the proximal tubule and loop of Henle is isotonic and is probably unaffected by PTH. In the distal convoluted tubule, calcium transport is not associated with sodium chloride transport, but is under the control of PTH, which promotes calcium reabsorption. It is not known whether PTH exerts its effects on calcium reabsorption by increasing cyclic AMP concentration in distal tubular cells. Vitamin D metabolites and calcitonin probably have only minor effects on the renal handling of calcium. Thiazide diuretics decrease calcium excretion, probably by direct effects on increasing calcium reabsorption in the loop of Henle and the distal segments.

Bone. Increases in osteoclast activity cause release of bone calcium into the extracellular fluid. This process is stimulated by PTH and 1,25-dihydroxyvitamin D and is inhibited by calcitonin. The effects of these three systemic hormones are regulated by negative feedback controls. There are other hormonal factors that stimulate or inhibit bone resorption, but the effects of these factors on bone do not appear to be regulated. The effects of bone resorption and bone formation on maintenance of extracellular fluid calcium concentration are considered in more detail later.

Parathyroid hormone

Synthesis and secretion. Parathyroid hormone is an 84 amino acid, single-chain polypeptide hormone that is secreted by the chief cells of the parathyroid glands. The PTH gene product is a larger precursor molecule called *pre pro-PTH* comprising 110 amino acids and having a molecular weight of about 13,000. This precursor is rapidly processed in the rough endoplasmic reticulum to a smaller molecule known as *pro-PTH,* which is a linear peptide of 90 amino acids with a molecular weight of approximately 10,000. Within the Golgi zone, pro-PTH is further processed to native PTH (1-84), which is stored in secretory granules in the parathyroid cells and released from the parathyroid cells in response to a fall in the ionized calcium concentration bathing the parathyroid glands. The hormone that is secreted by the glands is further cleaved in the periphery by the kidneys and liver into smaller fragments. The amino-terminal (or N-terminal) fragments comprise the biologically active moiety of the molecule. The first 34 amino acids of the molecule are required for biologic activity. The carboxyl-terminal (C-terminal) fragments are biologically inert.

Biosynthesis and release of PTH are regulated by the extracellular fluid calcium concentration. A fall in calcium concentration stimulates PTH secretion, and an increase inhibits it. PTH secretion is also stimulated by adrenergic agonists, prostaglandins of the E series, and, acutely, by falls in magnesium ion concentration. The physiologic significance of these latter stimuli is unknown. PTH secretion is inhibited by severe magnesium depletion of chronic duration and by active vitamin D metabolites.

Biologic effects. Parathyroid hormone affects calcium and phosphate fluxes in the bone, kidneys, and gastrointestinal tract. In *bone,* the major effect of PTH in vivo is to increase bone turnover, to stimulate osteoclastic bone resorption, and to increase new bone formation. In vitro, PTH inhibits bone collagen synthesis, so that the effects observed in vivo may be indirect and secondary to the effects on osteoclastic bone resorption. It is likely that the effects of PTH to increase bone resorption are not mediated directly by an action on the osteoclasts but through an intermediate cell. Although the effects of PTH on the osteoblast may be mediated by cyclic AMP, it is still not clear that PTH acts on osteoclastic bone resorption through this second messenger.

In the kidney, PTH increases renal tubular reabsorption of calcium and decreases urinary calcium excretion relative to the filtered load. It also decreases renal tubular reabsorption of phosphate, leading to renal phosphate wasting. Both of these effects are probably mediated by cyclic AMP. The major regulatory effect of PTH on calcium and phosphate handling by the renal tubules occurs at the distal tubule site. Parathyroid hormone has other effects on the kidneys including inhibition of renal tubular bicarbonate reabsorption in the proximal tubule and stimulation of the complex renal 1-hydroxylase enzyme, which leads to increased production of 1,25-dihydroxyvitamin D.

Parathyroid hormone's effects on the *gut* are indirect. PTH causes increased absorption of calcium from the gut indirectly through its effects on the kidney to increase synthesis of 1,25-dihydroxyvitamin D.

PTH mediates its effects on target organs via a receptor that has recently been identified and molecularly cloned. The receptor is a transmembrane protein that appears to be related to the calcitonin receptor structurally and activates both adenylate cyclase and the phosphoinositol pathway signaling mechanisms.

The overall effect of PTH therefore is to increase the serum calcium concentration and decrease the serum phosphorus level because of its combined effects on the gut, kidney, and bone.

Calcitonin

Synthesis and secretion. Calcitonin is a 32 amino acid peptide that is synthesized and secreted by the parafollicular cells of the thyroid. In birds, fish, and reptiles, these cells form a separate organ known as the *ultimobranchial gland*. The calcitonin gene encodes a larger molecular species than the secreted form known as *pro-calcitonin*. In humans, this molecule has a molecular weight of about 17,500. The calcitonin molecule has a proline-amide group at the carboxyl-terminal and a disulfide bridge linking amino acids 1 and 7 from the amino-terminal, which is necessary for biologic activity. The major circulating form is the calcitonin monomer or 32 amino acid molecule. It is metabolized predominantly in the kidney. The plasma half-life of calcitonin is approximately 5 minutes.

The calcitonin gene also encodes another recently described peptide known as *CGRP* (the *calcitonin gene-related peptide*), whose physiologic function at the present time is unknown, but that is secreted mole for mole with calcitonin. CGRP has potent effects on vascular smooth muscle. It also inhibits bone resorption but is much less potent than calcitonin. Cells other than the thyroid parafollicular cells can synthesize calcitonin. Biologically inert calcitonin may be synthesized by certain nonthyroid tumors, and there is some evidence for calcitonin secretion in the brain. The physiologic significance of extrathyroidal calcitonin production is unknown.

Calcitonin is released from the thyroid parafollicular cells in response to an increase in extracellular fluid calcium or by the action of gastrointestinal hormones including gastrin, glucagon, secretin, and cholecystokinin-pancreozymin. Gastrin is the most potent of these secretagogues. Calcitonin release from the parafollicular cells is inhibited by a fall in serum calcium concentration.

Biologic effects. The precise physiologic role of calcitonin is still unknown. Calcitonin's most prominent effect is to inhibit osteoclastic bone resorption, which it does rapidly and effectively. Calcitonin inhibits all stages of osteoclast differentiation from its precursors, decreases the activity of preformed osteoclasts, and causes the dissolution of osteoclasts into mononuclear cells. Calcitonin's effects on inhibiting osteoclastic bone resorption are transient, and this loss of responsiveness in the continued presence of calcitonin (known as the *escape phenomenon*) may be due to *down regulation* (decreased calcitonin receptor number or binding of calcitonin in the continued presence of calcitonin). Therefore, in patients with an absence of calcitonin-secreting cells (after thyroidectomy) and in patients with medullary thyroid carcinomas who have markedly increased circulating concentrations of calcitonin, there are no clear abnormalities in either bone cell function or in calcium homeostasis.

It has been postulated that calcitonin is required to protect the body against postprandial hypercalcemia and to protect the growing or maternal skeleton from continued bone resorption when calcium is being absorbed from the gut after a calcium-rich meal. Calcitonin has no major effects on bone formation, on vitamin D metabolism, or on absorption of calcium from the gut. Patients with medullary thyroid carcinoma and excess calcitonin secretion may have diarrhea caused by increased secretion of fluid and electrolytes in the small intestine. The precise mechanism is unclear.

The gene for the calcitonin receptor has also recently been molecularly cloned. The calcitonin receptor belongs to the same family of receptors as PTH; it is a transmembrane receptor protein that mediates its effects through adenylate cyclase.

Calcitonin receptors have been described on many cells outside bone including many tumor cells, lymphocytes, and neuronal cells. The physiologic or pathologic significance of these extraosseous receptors is entirely unknown. Calcitonin has been used as a therapeutic agent in diseases associated with increased bone resorption, including Paget's disease, hypercalcemia, and osteoporosis. It is a very useful agent in Paget's disease, is effective in hypercalcemia when used in association with glucocorticoids (which inhibit bone resorption), and may be of slight benefit in some patients with osteoporosis and increased rates of bone resorption. The form of calcitonin that has been most widely used in treatment is salmon calcitonin, which is biologically very potent. Eel and human calcitonin are also now used in different countries and have similar biologic effects.

Vitamin D

Synthesis and metabolism. The vitamin D metabolites are a group of steroid-like compounds known as *sterols* that are derived exogenously from plant ergosterol in the diet or endogenously from 7-dehydrocholesterol in the skin.

Vitamin D_3 is synthesized in the skin by the action of ultraviolet light on 7-dehydrocholesterol (previtamin D_3) in epidermal cells. This process occurs in several intermediate steps that are not enzyme controlled. Vitamin D_3 synthesized in the skin is absorbed in the small intestine and is transported in the plasma bound to a carrier protein known as the *vitamin D–binding protein*. An additional major source of vitamin D in humans is the diet. Plant ergocalciferol (previtamin D_2) is analogous to 7-dehydrocholesterol and is converted to vitamin D_2 by exposure to ultraviolet irradiation. The subsequent metabolism and biologic activity of the active forms of vitamin D_2 (from plant origins) and vitamin D_3 (from synthesis in the skin) are identical in humans. In the liver, vitamin D undergoes the first metabolic step that involves biologic activation. Here it is hydroxylated in the 25 position to 25-hydroxyvitamin D, which is the major circulating form of the sterol. 25-Hydroxyvitamin D is transported in the plasma bound to the vitamin D–binding protein to the kidney, where it undergoes a number of further hydroxylation steps. The major biologically active metabolite produced by the kidney is 1,25-dihydroxyvitamin D, which is the most potent and rapidly acting of all the vitamin D metabolites. The other major renal metabolite of vitamin D metabolism is 24,25-dihydroxyvitamin D. Whether or not it has any important biologic effects is still controversial.

Vitamin D metabolism is carefully regulated. Synthesis in the skin is influenced by sunlight exposure, and there are seasonal variations in the circulating concentrations of 25-hydroxyvitamin D. Synthesis in the skin is greatest in summer in persons exposed to the sun. However, it is not clear whether degree of skin pigmentation has a major effect on vitamin D_3 production. The 25-hydroxylation process in the liver is not well understood. This activation process does not appear to be tightly regulated. When availability of substrate vitamin D is high (excess sunlight exposure, excess vitamin D ingestion), there is increased production of 25-hydroxyvitamin D, and when substrate availability is low, production is decreased. Thus measurement of circulating 25-hydroxyvitamin D is a reliable index of vitamin D supply.

In contrast, 1-hydroxylation in the kidney is carefully controlled by ambient phosphate concentration and PTH. In addition, there possibly is regulation by sex hormones and prolactin. However, the major regulators of 1-hydroxylation are PTH and phosphate. Dietary phosphate deprivation causes increased activity of the 1-hydroxylase reaction by mechanisms that are unclear. Parathyroid hormone stimulates the 1-hydroxylation mechanism by a direct effect. Thus the effect of a decrease in dietary phosphate or serum phosphate concentration is to increase production of 1,25-dihydroxyvitamin D. The renal 1-hydroxylase is a complex mitochondrial p450 cytochrome enzyme system that is present in the proximal convoluted tubule of the kidney. Other extrarenal 1-hydroxylation enzyme systems have been described in the placenta, bone, and chronic inflammatory cells. The physiologic significance of extrarenal 1-hydroxylation is not clear, but this mechanism is probably important in diseases such as sarcoidosis in which 1-hydroxylation does occur outside the kidney and leads to hypercalcemia.

The 24-hydroxylase system is much less well described. It is present in the proximal convoluted tubule and is stimulated by 1,25-dihydroxyvitamin D. 25-Hydroxyvitamin D is metabolized in the kidney and possibly other sites to 24,25-dihydroxyvitamin D. Whether 24,25-dihydroxyvitamin D has a physiologic role remains unknown. It may merely represent an alternative inactivation pathway to the 1-hydroxylase pathway. Both 1,25-dihydroxyvitamin D and 24,25-dihydroxyvitamin D are converted to 1,24,25-trihydroxyvitamin D. 1,24,25-Tri-hydroxyvitamin D is further metabolized by removal of a side chain to form calcitroic acid. How these degradation pathways are controlled is presently unknown, but the overall process resembles the formation of bile acids from cholesterol.

The vitamin D metabolites are bound to serum proteins in the circulation, like other steroids and sterols. The major serum transport protein is an $alpha_2$ globulin known as the *vitamin D–binding protein,* the *group-specific component,* or *Gc protein.* 1,25-Dihydroxyvitamin D is also probably bound to glycoproteins in the circulation. The circulating forms of the sterols are more than 99% bound to transport proteins. The concentration of the metabolites of vitamin D_3 is higher than that of vitamin D_2 in human subjects. Vitamin D_3 and vitamin D_2 probably have identical biologic activity. Vitamin D_2 and vitamin D_3, 25-hydroxyvitamin D, 1,25-dihydroxyvitamin D, and 24,25-dihydroxyvitamin D are all conjugated in the liver to form glucuronides and sulfates that have enterohepatic circulation.

Biologic effects. 1,25-Dihydroxyvitamin D is the major active metabolite of vitamin D. 25-Hydroxyvitamin D is biologically active but has only one thousandth the activity of 1,25-dihydroxyvitamin D. Vitamin D itself is inactive biologically and can be regarded as a prohormone. The vitamin D metabolites increase the absorption of calcium and phosphate from the gut into the blood by active transport. They also increase bone resorption by stimulating osteoclast activity. The overall effect is to increase serum concentrations of calcium and phosphorus. In the absence of vitamin D or in conditions of impaired vitamin D metabolism, there is a failure of mineralization of newly formed bone with subsequent development of the metabolic bone disease known as *rickets* (children) or *osteomalacia* (adults). 1,25-Dihydroxyvitamin D corrects this failure to mineralize newly formed bone. It is still controversial whether it does this solely by providing a supply of calcium and phosphate that is available at the mineralizing site or whether the active metabolites of vitamin D are also required to stimulate the osteoblast to mineralize bone normally. However, recent data suggest that the former is the more likely mechanism.

1,25-Dihydroxyvitamin D also causes the kidney to stimulate calcium and phosphate reabsorption. It also increases 24-hydroxylase activity, which may be a major step in inactivation. The renal effects of 1,25-dihydroxyvitamin D are probably relatively unimportant compared with its bone and gut effects.

Recent studies have shown that 1,25-dihydroxyvitamin D affects osteoclast activation differently than other hormonal stimulators of bone resorption such as PTH or the prostaglandins. 1,25-Dihydroxyvitamin D seems to be an important factor in stimulating fusion and differentiation of osteoclast progenitors into mature osteoclasts, in addition to causing activation of preformed osteoclasts. It also has significant local effects in the bone marrow microenvironment on modulating immune responses and inhibiting lymphocyte activation. It inhibits lymphocyte mitogenesis and production of the lymphokine interleukin 2 but can stimulate production of the bone-resorbing monokine interleukin 1 in some systems. These local interactions between the vitamin D metabolites, immune cells, and osteoclasts and their progenitors may be very important factors in our understanding of normal bone cell metabolism and function and constitute an active area of current research.

The vitamin D receptor has recently been characterized and molecularly cloned. It belongs to the same family of receptors as all of those for the steroid hormones, as well as those for retinoic acid and thyroid hormones. Recent observations have shown that point mutations in the vitamin D receptor are responsible for some inherited forms of rickets associated with vitamin D resistance.

OTHER HORMONES AFFECTING CALCIUM HOMEOSTASIS AND THE SKELETON

1. *Growth hormone and somatomedin C*. Growth hormone accelerates skeletal growth, partly through somatomedin C (also called *insulin-like growth factor I*), which stimulates protein synthesis and sulfation in cartilage. Somatomedin C also stimulates bone collagen synthesis directly.
2. *Thyroxine and triiodothyronine*. The thyroid hormones stimulate bone turnover and are required for normal skeletal growth and bone remodeling. They have a direct effect on bone similar to that of PTH, which probably explains the osteopenia and hypercalcemia that occasionally occur in hyperthyroidism. Patients with hyperthyroidism have increased renal tubular phosphate reabsorption and may have hyperphosphatemia, increased serum alkaline phosphatase concentration, and increased urine hydroxyproline excretion.
3. *Glucocorticoids*. Glucocorticoids can inhibit both bone formation and bone resorption directly in pharmacologic doses; this characteristic may explain their causing osteoporosis when used chronically. Their inhibitory effect on osteoclastic bone resorption explains the lowering of the serum calcium level seen in some patients with hypercalcemia of malignancy treated with these agents. However, bone resorption may be increased in humans with prior normal calcium homeostasis who are treated with glucocorticoids because of (1) impaired calcium absorption in the gut, which leads to secondary hyperparathyroidism, and (2) direct stimulation of PTH secretion. The effect on the intestinal mucosa in inhibiting calcium absorption may be direct or may be due to impaired metabolism of vitamin D. The overall increase in bone resorption and decrease in bone formation cause decreased bone mass and osteoporosis.
4. *Estrogens and androgens*. The sex steroids, especially estrogens if they are given to females around the time of menopause, stimulate skeletal maturation and epiphyseal closure at puberty and can prevent loss of bone mass in adults. Inhibition of bone resorption by estrogens and androgens has been postulated but has never been demonstrated directly. Their effects on bone may be indirect and may be mediated by changing the concentrations of other hormones such as PTH or cytokines such as interleukin 1 and interleukin 6.
5. *Insulin*. Insulin stimulates bone collagen synthesis in vitro. In patients with diabetes mellitus osteopenia frequently develops and this may be due in part to insulin lack. It is likely that these effects of insulin are mediated through the insulin-like growth factor I receptor.
6. *Epidermal growth factor and related peptides*. Epidermal growth factor and a family of related peptides produced by tumors and some normal tissues have important effects on bone. The tumor-derived growth factors, platelet-derived growth factor (PDGF), and transforming growth factor alpha (TGF alpha) stimulate bone resorption in vitro and may play a role in bone destruction associated with some solid tumors. In addition, these factors are present in the normal embryo and may be important for skeletal modeling during growth and remodeling during wound and fracture repair.
7. Growth regulatory factors stored in bone. Recent observations have shown that the bone matrix is a repository for a number of powerful bone growth regulatory factors. These include transforming growth factor beta (TGF beta), insulin-like growth factors I and II, the fibroblast growth factors, and a newly described family of growth factors that are related to TGF beta called the bone morphogenetic proteins. These factors cause the formation of new bone when injected into subcutaneous tissue in vivo and may be important in endochondral bone formation, fracture repair, and repair of bone defects.
8. *Local hormones* (cytokines).
   a. *Prostaglandins* produced by chronic inflammatory cells stimulate bone resorption and may mediate localized bone loss in periodontal disease, rheumatoid arthritis, and certain neoplasms. These locally acting factors are produced by cells found at sites of chronic inflammation such as macrophages.
   b. *Osteoclast-activating factor (OAF)* is a potent stimulator of bone resorption that is produced by activated lymphocytes. OAF does not represent one molecule but is probably composed of the cytokines interleukin 1, interleukin 6, lymphotoxin, and tumor necrosis factor, which have recently been purified and molecularly cloned. These cytokines are potent bone-resorbing factors in vitro and in vivo. In multiple myeloma, which is usually associated with bone destruction and often with hypercalcemia, the malignant cells secrete these and related cytokines.

c. Other local factors in the bone cell microenvironment may play a role in osteoclast generation and activity. These include gamma-interferon and transforming growth factor beta (TGF beta), which inhibit osteoclast activity, and monocyte-colony-stimulating factor, which increases osteoclast differentiation. In this regard, it is possible that 1,25-dihydroxyvitamin D can also be considered a local hormone. There have been indications (not yet confirmed) that it could be produced by cells in the bone marrow microenvironment. If this turns out to be true, this sterol may also be important in controlling local osteoclast differentiation as well as in modulating immune function.

REFERENCES

Agus ZS, Goldfarb S, and Wasserstein A: Calcium transport in the kidney. Rev Physiol Biochem Pharmacol 90:155, 1981.

Eisman J: Vitamin D metabolism. In Mundy GR and Martin TJ, editors: Physiology and pharmacology of bone: Handbook of experimental pharmacology. Springer, (in press).

Garrett IR et al: Production of the bone resorbing cytokine lymphotoxin by cultured human myeloma cells. N Engl J Med 317:526, 1987.

Hauschka PV et al: Growth factors in bone matrix. J Biol Chem 261:12665, 1986.

Hirsch PF and Munson PL: Thyrocalcitonin. Physiol Rev 49:548, 1969.

Hughes MR et al: Point mutations in the human vitamin D receptor gene associated with hypocalcemic rickets. Science 242:1702, 1988.

Juppner H et al: A G-protein linked receptor for parathyroid hormone and parathyroid hormone related peptide. Science 254:1024, 1991.

Klahr S and Hruska K: Effects of parathyroid hormone on the renal reabsorption of phosphorus and divalent cations. In Peck WA, editor: Bone and mineral research: annual 2. Amsterdam, 1983, Excerpta Medica.

Kronenberg HM: Parathyroid hormone—molecular biology, chemistry and actions. In Mundy GR and Martin TJ, editors: Physiology and pharmacology of bone. Handbook of experimental pharmacology. Springer, (in press).

Lin HY et al: Expression cloning of an adenylate cyclase-coupled calcitonin receptor. Science 254:1022, 1991.

Moseley JM et al: Parathyroid hormone-related protein purified from a human lung cancer cell line. Proc Natl Acad Sci USA 84:5048, 1987.

Mundy GR: Bone resorption and turnover in health and disease. Bone 8:S9, 1987.

Mundy GR: The hypercalcemia of malignancy revisited. J Clin Invest 82:1, 1988.

Mundy GR and Martin TJ: Hypercalcemia of malignancy—pathogenesis and treatment. Metabolism 31:1247, 1982.

Mundy GR and Roodman GD: Osteoclast ontogeny and function. In Peck WA, editor: Bone and mineral research V. Amsterdam, 1987, Elsevier.

Nordin BEC: Plasma calcium and plasma magnesium homeostasis. In Nordin BEC, editor: Phosphate and magnesium metabolism. Edinburgh, 1976, Churchill-Livingstone.

Suva LJ et al: A parathyroid hormone-related protein implicated in malignant hypercalcemia: cloning and expression. Science 237:893, 1987.

Yates AJP et al: Effects of a synthetic peptide of a parathyroid hormone-related protein on calcium homeostasis, renal tubular calcium reabsorption and bone metabolism. J Clin Invest 81:932, 1988.

Wozney JM et al: Novel regulators of bone formation: molecular clones and activities. Science 242:1528, 1988.

CHAPTER

149 Principles of Genetic Disorders

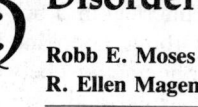

Robb E. Moses
R. Ellen Magenis

Medical genetics has been recognized as a medical field for some time but is only now beginning to serve as a distinct discipline. It is a cross-discipline specialty in which patient care may extend to other areas of medicine. The tools available for diagnosis and treatment in medical genetics apply not only to inherited disorders but also to diseases that reflect an alteration of the function or structure of the genome and its expression during the life of an individual. Recently available techniques indicate that gene therapy or modification of the expression of genes is part of future medical practice.

INTRODUCTION

An intuitive as well as a practical knowledge of genetics has been of long-standing benefit to medical practice. Traits such as polydactyly and color-blindness were described in the eighteenth century with regard to patterns of inheritance. In the nineteenth century, the characteristics of X-linked recessive inheritance for hemophilia were recognized by Otto in New England. Autosomal recessive inheritance was also described in the nineteenth century. The use of twins for separating environment and heredity in analysis of human disease was another nineteenth century development.

These observations were placed on a rational basis with the rediscovery in the early part of this century of the mid-nineteenth century work of Mendel. The core contribution of Mendel's work was to recognize that inheritance can be viewed as a unit or packet of information, passed from parent to offspring. The term *gene* refers to this unit of inheritance. The definition has changed through the years with increasing refinement of knowledge of what constitutes a gene. Mendel established the principle of *segregation,* that is, that genes encoding the same function (alleles) in diploid organisms pass through generations separately, and the effect of these genes can be monitored in subsequent generations. This observation led to the concepts of *dominance* and *recessiveness,* which refer to the expressed traits (phenotypes) and not to the genes themselves. The dominant phenotype is a trait that is expressed in the heterozygote; the recessive trait is not noted in heterozygotes. Today a phenotype may be analyzed at the molecular level. An individual may demonstrate the dominant trait with a variable *expressivity*. Indeed the appearance of the dominant trait may even be so low as to be absent, referred to as *nonpenetrant*.

Independent assortment refers to Mendel's observation that unrelated genes behave in an independent matter. Alleles segregate; nonalleles (independent genes) assort. Genes that assort completely independently are unlinked. *Linkage* refers to the observation that genes on the same chromosome may be close enough to travel together at meiosis. This linkage is a reflection of physical distance. A new combination of genes after meiosis is referred to as *recombination*. Because humans carry two copies of each gene, 50% recombination is equivalent to independent assortment and reflects that the two *loci* (physical locations of the gene) are either on different chromosomes or so far apart on one chromosome that recombination is frequent enough to produce independent assortment. Units of recombination are morgans; 1 centimorgan (cM) equals approximately one megabase of DNA.

DNA has been identified as the physical basis for inheritance. The symmetry of the double helix model gave a rationale for transmission of genes. The mesh between the two DNA strands implied that genetic information is encoded in a linear array that can be duplicated by template function. The linear array is composed of a variable sequence of only four basic repeating units.

Within the last 20 years the number of defined genetic syndromes that can be assigned to a single gene with characterized inheritance has gone from several dozen to more than 4000. Of even greater importance perhaps has been the recognition of *multifactorial* or *polygenic* traits, in which multiple genes interact with the environment to produce a disease. Patients in this category may state to the physician that "a disease such as hypertension runs in my family." An appreciation of the interaction of the genome of an individual and the environment will become increasingly important.

MOLECULAR GENETICS OF THE HUMAN GENOME

Genes are organized in the DNA double helix. This helix is composed of two chains of deoxynucleotides in antiparallel construction; the polarity of each strand follows the 5′ to 3′ phosphodiester linkage between the deoxyribose moieties. Deoxyribonucleic acid (DNA) and ribonucleic acid (RNA) are synthesized only in the 5′ to 3′ direction. One strand of DNA, in coding the gene, is recognized as the "sense" or coding strand. The gene is "read" or transcribed from the 3′ to 5′, so the messenger RNA can be synthesized in the permissible 5′ to 3′ direction. The initiation of transcription typically occurs at a significant distance before the start of the coding region of the gene. Coding regions of genes are frequently separated by long stretches or spacers of apparently noninformative DNA. The intervening stretches are termed *introns;* the coding regions, *exons*. The primary RNA message from the coding unit of the gene contains RNA complementary to both exons and introns in a continuous fashion. At the 3′ end of the RNA transcript, there is typically a polyadenylation signal. The initial RNA transcript is processed into mature RNA by the removal of introns by the RNA splicing process and addition of adenosine residues at the 3′ end. This process is dependent on ribozymes, catalytic RNA molecules. The processed messenger RNA is translated into the protein product (Fig. 149-1). There are several steps at which the expression of the gene product might be regulated: transcription, splicing, translation, and modification or activation of the protein product. In addition, the appropriate transport of the protein product to the appropriate site for

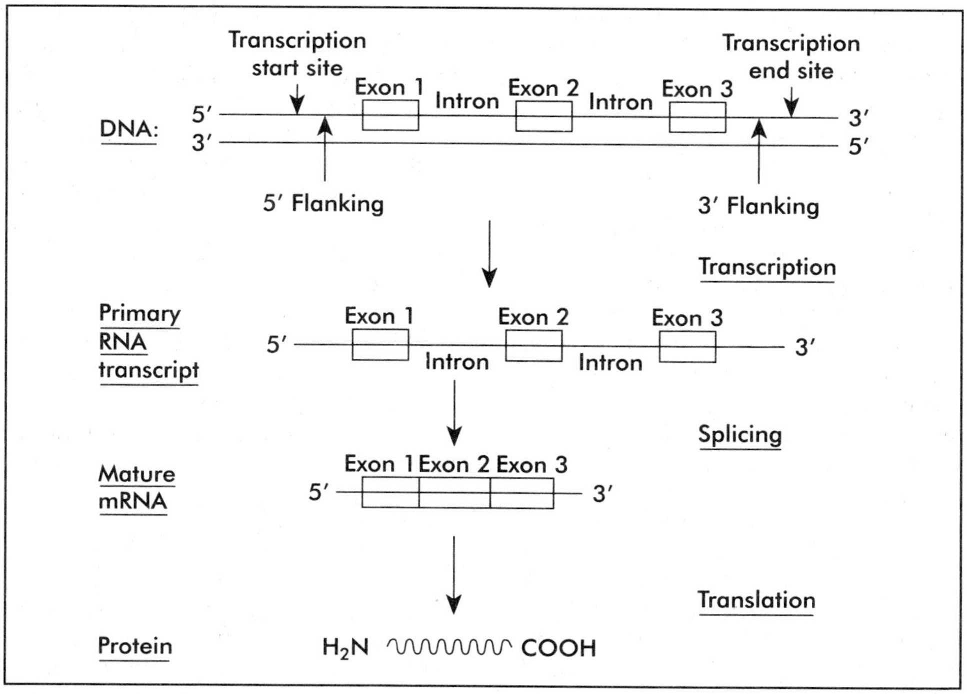

Fig. 149-1. Processing of genomic information.

action in the cell is required. If transport signals are not encoded and processed appropriately, failure of transportation of the protein to the proper location for activity may result.

DNA is notable for its chemical stability. It is a good repository for the genetic information of a cell. The replication of DNA is accomplished and monitored by accurate enzymes. The overall mistake level is approximately 1 in 10^{10} nucleotide addition events. The cellular processes responsible for this very low error rate include the accuracy of enzymes responsible for synthesis of the DNA. These enzymes appear to have an overall mistake frequency of about 1 in 10^5 to 10^6 incorporations. DNA polymerases in humans are associated with a "proofreading" or "editorial" 3′ exonuclease activity, which removes mismatched nucleotides preferentially and reduces the error rate an additional 100-fold. Finally, newly incorporated bases are screened for mismatches by an elaborate correction system. These systems have the ability to recognize the correct or parental strand of DNA that serves as template. Corrections are preferentially made in the newly synthesized DNA strand. Mismatch correction lowers the overall mistake frequency an additional 100-fold.

However, the genome is not a static entity. The very low mistake level resulting from DNA replication still provides a degree of variability in newly synthesized DNA. Mutations can also result from physical agents such as high energy radiation or from chemical agents. Cells have processes for recognition and repair of damage to the DNA. Damage or alteration to the DNA must be passed by the replication complex in the synthesis of new DNA in order to "fix" the mutation in the genome. A point mutation may be "silent" because of degeneracy in the code, in which case the alteration in the nucleotide still permits coding for the same amino acid that was previously encoded. Amino acid incorporation is encoded in a triplet code and the third position is particularly tolerant of change. Alternatively, a mutation may be silent because of a conservative substitution of an amino acid with similar physical characteristics to the original amino acid and no alteration in the properties of the resulting gene product. An additional reason for a silent mutation is a nonconservative amino acid change in a portion of the protein that is not required for function. Finally a silent mutation may occur in an intron and thus cause no alteration in the resulting protein product.

On the other hand, several types of mutations may significantly alter the function of the gene product. In one case, the mutation may alter the junction sites between introns and exons in such a way that splicing is altered. Such a mutation may result in the omission of an entire exon from the coding RNA. Another result that produces noticeable change in the gene product can be the substitution of a dissimilar amino acid in the portion of the gene encoding the active site of the protein or required for formation of required tertiary structure. A mutation may also produce a "stop" codon that is recognized by the cellular machinery as a signal to cease synthesis of protein. Occurrence of such a mutation early in the coding sequence for the protein can lead to the production of a truncated peptide without function. In addition to point mutations resulting from single base substitutions, large deletions and rearrangements may result from recombination. Indeed, such events may be large enough to be recognizable in chromosome analysis.

Multiple alleles existing at the same locus are the result of independent mutational events. If a given allele reaches a level of 1% in the population, it is a *polymorphism*. Sometimes polymorphisms can be recognized at the protein level, as in the case of a number of erythrocyte enzymes. However, variation at the nucleotide sequence level qualifies equally well as a polymorphism. Such polymorphisms are useful in DNA diagnostic procedures. In addition, nucleotide sequence variation may occur at sites outside the gene, but close enough to the gene to be tightly linked and therefore unlikely to be subject to recombination. If such a variance outside a gene is associated with an allele of the gene, the extragenic variation or polymorphism is said to be in *disequilibrium* with the mutated gene. The linkage of detectable nucleotide polymorphisms constitutes a *haplotype*. Through the use of *restriction endonucleases* that recognize and cleave DNA only at sites of specific sequence, diseases have been associated with recognized nucleotide polymorphisms either inside or outside the gene. Thus significant detectable molecular diversity is present in the human genome, and this diversity may serve as a signature for detection of an allele and tracking of that allele through a family with inherited disease.

The sexual process also provides for a rich genetic diversity. With independent assortment of genes on separate chromosomes and random reassociation of chromosomes during meiosis, there are 2^{23} combinations for the 46 chromosomes in each fertilized egg as a result of spermatogenesis and oogenesis and fertilization to form a diploid individual.

Variations in the nucleotide sequence that are detected as a result of the infrequent cutting by restriction endonucleases are termed *restriction fragment linked polymorphisms* (RFLPs). These reflect the variation in the size of the product after digestion of the DNA with a given restriction enzyme and detection with a "probe" of DNA, a labeled fragment known to lie within the region (Fig. 149-2). By the process of hybridization on a solid matrix, a variation in size can be detected. This process, the *Southern blot,* serves as a basis for detection of polymorphisms at the nucleotide level. This is the basic study for establishing linkage of a nucleotide polymorphism with an allele.

There has been a rapid accumulation of probes, assigned to each of the human chromosomes, which has allowed construction of a *restriction map* that on refinement will provide an overlapping linkage map for each human chromosome (Fig. 149-3). This is the first plateau for the Human Genome Project.

As analysis of the genome of higher organisms proceeded, it became clear that there were frequently occurring patterns of repeat sequences that took place as often as a million times in the genome. The size of the repeating unit is a continuum from two nucleotides to dozens of nucleotides. Such repeats are random in occurrence but are relatively stable in location. One of the frequently occur-

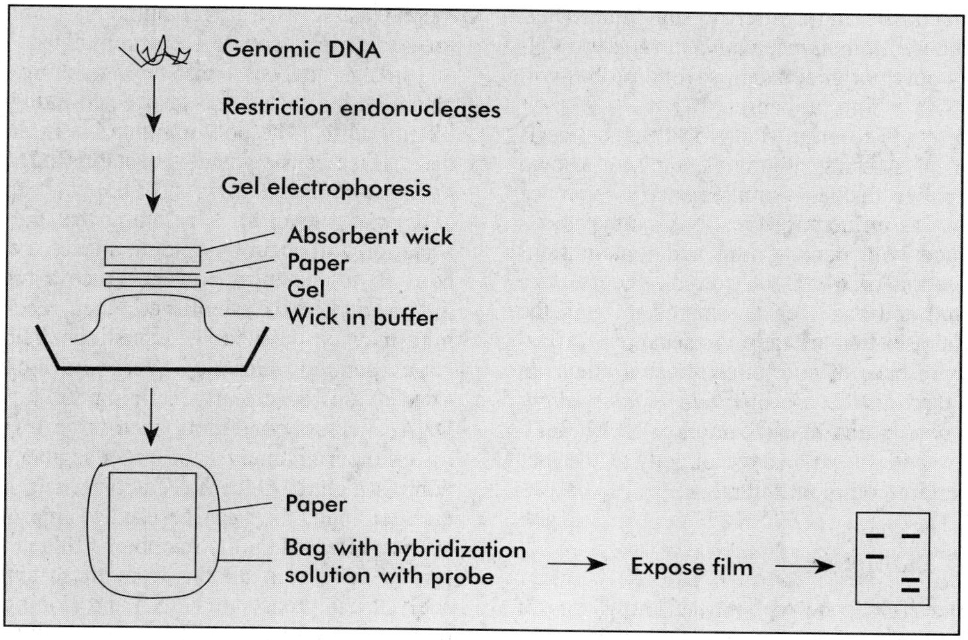

Fig. 149-2. Southern hybridization. Flow of method for detecting polymorphism at restriction sites.

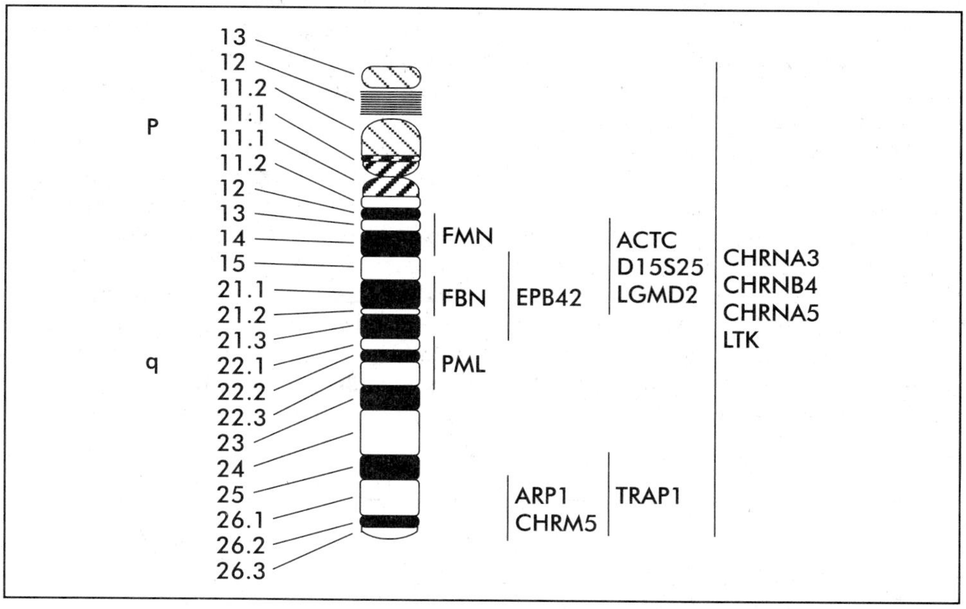

Fig. 149-3. Ideogram of chromosome 15. The abbreviations denote DNA fragments known to be on chromosome 15, and the vertical bars indicate localization of the markers.

ring repeated sequences in the human genome can be cleaved by the restriction endonuclease Alu I. These *Alu sites* may serve as convenient anchor points in the genome for molecular analysis. Because the sequence of such sites is known, DNA probes that will hybridize to these sequences are readily available. Additional repeating units have been described in a variety of subunit sizes. There is variation from individual to individual in the number of times the unit is repeated at a given site. Thus through cleavage by restriction enzymes, it is possible to detect variation between individuals. The repeat sites are polymorphic for such reiteration and therefore differ among individuals. This variation in length of the tandem repeat units forms the basis for DNA fingerprinting of individuals and is useful from both a diagnostic and a forensic standpoint (Fig. 149-4). Because the *variable number tandem repeats* (VNTRs) are extremely polymorphic, use of several probes will establish identity with a high probability.

The *polymerase chain* reaction (PCR) utilizes synthesis across a region of DNA using oligonucleotides of known sequence that hybridize to their complementary sequence in the genomic DNA as primers for the DNA synthesis. As the cycle is repeated with denaturation and renaturation, geometric amplification of the DNA strands occurs. The process is facilitated and has been automated through the use of DNA polymerases that are thermoresistant. It is possible to detect the presence of normal or mutated alleles in amplified regions through the use of *allele specific oligonucleotide* (ASO) *probes* and hybridization or RFLP analysis. Thus it is now possible to analyze directly at the molecular level for certain common mutations.

POSITIONAL CLONING

It is possible to identify a gene without the knowledge of the gene product or its function. The "classic" approach to isolation and cloning of a human gene involves purification of a gene product with generation of antibodies to that product, screening of an expression cDNA library, identification of clones expressing the epitopes from the gene product by screening with the antibody, and isolation of the cDNA and hybridization to a genomic library. In the absence of identification and purification of the gene product, it is still possible to clone the gene by positional cloning (Fig. 149-5). This approach has been used successfully for the cystic fibrosis and Duchenne muscular dystrophy genes.

A critical step in *positional cloning* is the identification of the region of the genome where the gene lies. This requires either good fortune in recognition of a patient with the genetic disorder carrying a recognizable deletion or rearrangement in the chromosomes, pinpointing an area of likely position of the gene, or family linkage studies in which several affected and unaffected family members are screened with unique DNA probes of known location. The latter technique requires many individuals but becomes more feasible as a larger number of unique DNA probes for the human genome are accumulated.

Linkage analysis consists of tracking a DNA polymorphism with affected and unaffected individuals until a high likelihood that the polymorphism is in disequilibrium with the disease-causing gene is established. The *logarithm of the odds of disequilibrium* (LOD) is accepted as being suggestive at a level of 3, meaning that the odds that the association will occur by random chance are only 1:1000 (the base 10 to the third power). Once a high LOD score to linked markers is established, then recombinational mapping may be pursued by screening of libraries containing large genomic inserts. Yeast artificial chromosomes (YACs) are capable of containing 800 kilobases or more of DNA. Vectors containing such large fragments of genetic material permit analysis of larger segments of the intact genome structure. Once YACs containing regions of interest are identified, they can be used to improve linkage analysis with affected family members further. As specific cDNA probes become available from these studies, the linkage analysis can proceed to cDNA and cloning in phage or plasmids and eventually to direct sequencing of the gene.

MECHANISMS OF MONOGENIC INHERITANCE

Single gene disorders are inherited defects traceable in a unit inheritance pattern. More than 4000 such disorders are recognized. Individually they tend to be rare, but overall they represent a significant health burden on the population (perhaps 1% or more of all birth defects).

If an individual has one defective allele, he or she is described as being *heterozygous* for that gene. An individual completely defective in both alleles at that locus or completely normal in both alleles at that locus is described as being *homozygous*. In reality, as a result of variability, individuals differ in alleles at any given locus. However, the concept of homozygous and heterozygous is useful. Dominance and recessiveness relate to the function of the gene product and not to the gene. *Dominance* refers to the observable trait seen in an individual who is heterozygous

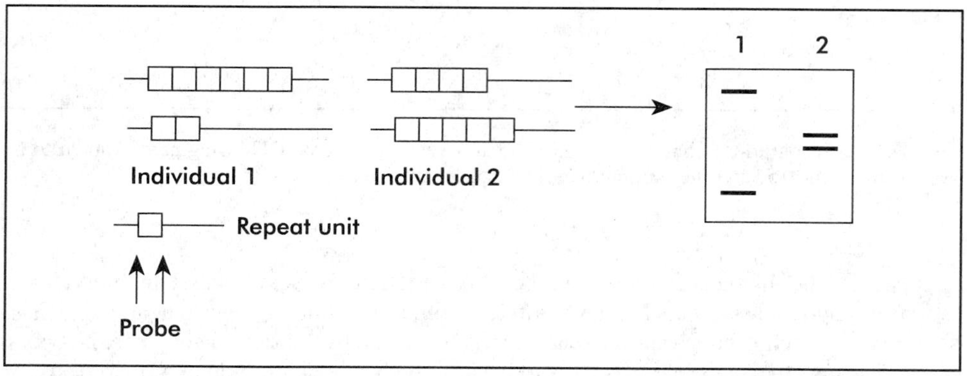

Fig. 149-4. VNTR analysis. Individuals 1 and 2 differ in the number of repeats of the basic unit detected by the probe. The Southern blot reflects the size difference of the fragments containing the repeat. VNTR, variable number tandem repeat.

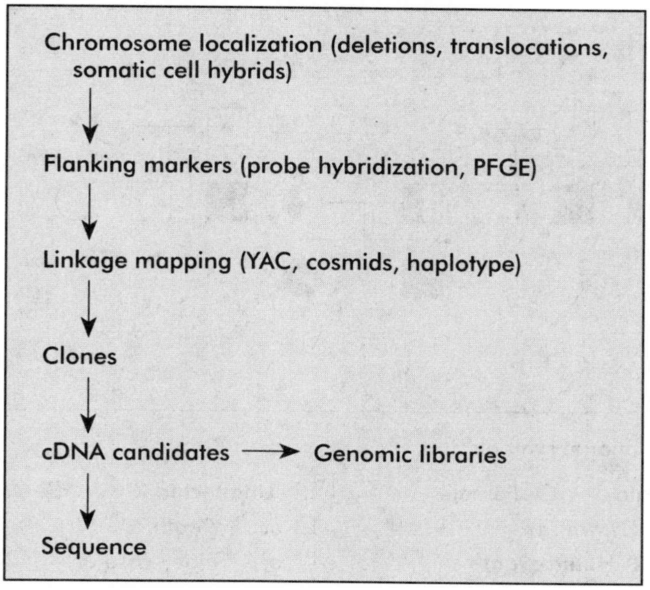

Fig. 149-5. Typical sequence of steps in positional cloning.

for a given gene function, and *recessiveness* refers to the trait observed in the individual who is completely defective in that gene function. Note that these terms refer to the function of the gene product and not to the gene itself. In many instances, the function of the gene product is not completely dominant or recessive, and therefore *codominant* and *incompletely dominant* refer, respectively, to traits that are simultaneously expressed or appear to be masked in the presence of the function of an additional gene product. In the case of most metabolic enzymes, a relatively modest level of activity is sufficient to supply the requirements. Individuals who are phenotypically normal may be demonstrated to be partially deficient in the enzymatic activity. In some instances it is possible to identify such individuals as genetically heterozygous biochemically.

Autosomal recessive inheritance

The pedigree of a typical autosomal recessive inheritance pattern is illustrated in Fig. 149-6 for the disease cystic fibrosis. This is one of the most common genetic diseases and has a carrier frequency of about 1 in 25 to 30 among the white population in North America.

In the case of cystic fibrosis, heterozygotes show no defect and are detectable only by detailed molecular analysis. Therefore the defective gene is not detected in the population at large. However, affected individuals carry a life-threatening burden with digestive problems, thick secretions, and impaired pulmonary function. The isolation and identification of the cystic fibrosis gene were triumphs of reverse genetics. The gene appears to be a membrane protein responsible for a "channel" function.

There are several characteristics of the pedigree analysis for a typical autosomal recessive disorder (Fig. 149-6):

- The pattern of inheritance is "horizontal." The hallmark is that several siblings are affected when neither parent is affected.
- Males and females are equally affected.
- The parents are carriers and may be demonstrated as such if testing is available. This is the notorious "silent" gene disease.
- Consanguinity of the parents becomes more common with increasing rarity of the disease.

The autosomal recessive inheritance pattern demonstrates the principles of segregation defined by Mendel. Each of the parents, who is normal, carries one normal and one defective allele and therefore has a 50% chance at meiosis of donating a defective allele to the gamete. It follows that the offspring will have genotypes in the ratio of 1:2:1 and a ratio of 3:1 for phenotype. That is, 75% of the offspring of such a mating will appear normal and 25% will show the recessive or disease phenotype. Note that "normal" offspring have a two thirds risk of being carriers for the defective gene. Think of each parent as (Ff), where F represents the normal gene and f represents the deficient gene encoding the cystic fibrosis gene product. With a 50% chance of F or f in germ cells for each parent, inspection shows that (FF) will occur in one fourth of the pregnancies, (Ff) will occur in half of the pregnancies, and (ff) will occur in one fourth of the pregnancies.

Diseases such as cystic fibrosis that are burdensome but not absolutely lethal before reproductive age are not "genetic lethal." Defective alleles may be inherited, as well as arise by new mutation. Variant alleles can be maintained stably in the population. The equilibrium for two alleles is described by the Hardy-Weinberg formula:

$$p^2 + 2pq + q^2 = 1$$

where p = frequency of one allele (A), q = frequency of other allele (a), and $p + q = 1$.

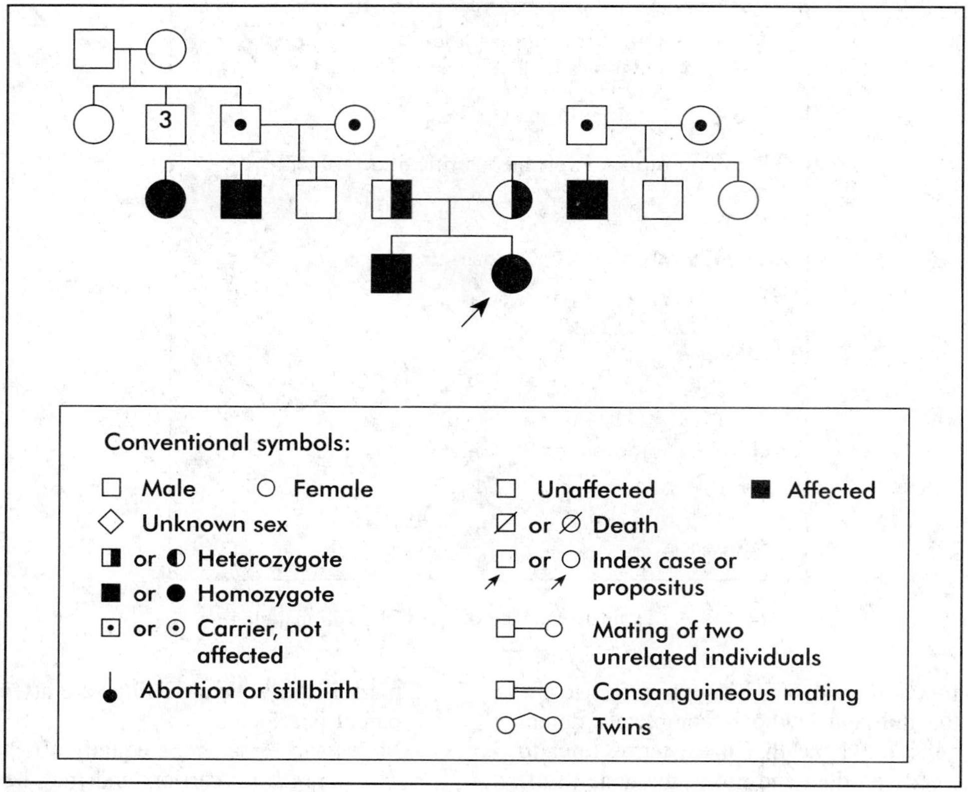

Fig. 149-6. Autosomal recessive pedigree.

Several deficient alleles exist in the population. Therefore the presence of a disease does not connote the presence of a specific allele. An autosomal recessive disease phenotype also may result from different deficiencies and not those attributable to a single gene. Several genes may be involved in a metabolic pathway, and a deficiency in any of the genes may produce the same "terminal phenotype." Good examples are the DNA repair diseases such as xeroderma pigmentosum, where more than one gene is involved, but the ultimate phenotype in the disease is the same. Thus in a sequential multigenic biochemical pathway, a deficiency in any one of the genes may produce the same disease.

In the case of autosomal recessive diseases, it is important for the clinician to consider the possibility of consanguinity, or incest. The likelihood increases as the rarity of the disease increases. Decreasing carrier frequency makes the likelihood of mating with a heterozygote less likely. Because decreasing gene frequency means that heterozygotes become increasingly rare in the population, then the likelihood of consanguinity or incest increases proportionately. In the case of cystic fibrosis, the likelihood that a carrier (heterozygote) will marry a carrier is about 1 in 900. However, in the case of a disease that is rarer and has a carrier frequency of, for example, 1 in 100, the chances of heterozygotes' marrying is 1 in 10,000. When such a disease appears in a family, it is important for the clinician to assess the possibility of consanguinity carefully.

Autosomal dominant inheritance

Autosomal dominant inheritance shows a somewhat different pattern from that of autosomal recessive inheritance (Fig. 149-7). The pedigree illustrated shows the inheritance pattern for neurofibromatosis. The hallmarks of autosomal dominant inheritance patterns are:

- A "vertical" transmission pattern.
- Males and females equally affected.
- A 50% risk for the disease in each child of an affected parent.

Particularly intriguing aspects of autosomal dominant disorders are *variable expressivity* and *penetrance*. Partial or complete effect of the genetic defect in individuals carrying a single mutated allele is the result of variable expressivity. Nonpenetrance is no observable phenotype in an individual known to have the defective allele. Individuals who bear the disease have one normal and one affected allele. Because an individual has a 50% chance of donating either allele to a gamete at meiosis, there should be a 50% probability that the offspring of an affected individual will demonstrate the genetic defect. For example, in the case of neurofibromatosis, expression is variable. It is not uncommon to inspect a patient who manifests a number of the findings of neurofibromatosis, including neurofibromas, multiple café-au-lait spots, altered pigmentation patterns, and intracranial tumors, but has "normal" parents. On inspection, one parent may manifest no more findings than

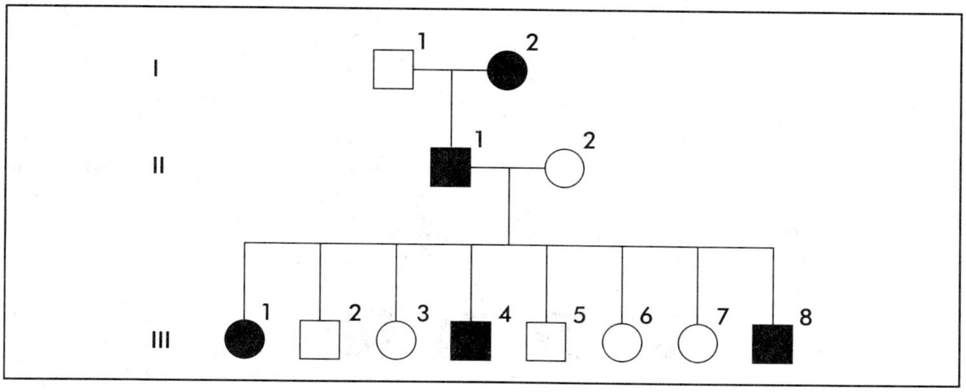

Fig. 149-7. Autosomal dominant pedigree. The symbols are as in Fig. 149-6.

axillary freckling, which is a hallmark of neurofibromatosis. Although the deficient allele is clearly present in the parent, it has not been noted to cause disease.

Autosomal dominant inheritance patterns may reflect new mutations. If two individuals who are normal have an affected child with an autosomal dominant disease, the offspring may well represent a new mutation. In such an instance, the likelihood that additional offspring will be affected is low for that couple, with established paternity. The certainty with which the clinician can make this prediction is linked to the likelihood of high penetrance and high expressivity for the defective gene; a disease with a high expressivity is achondroplasia. A secondary consideration is that the mutation rate may increase with the age of the parents, best demonstrated with paternal age. Thus if an older normal couple have an achondroplastic child, it is a relatively safe conclusion that the offspring represents a new mutation. In this case, the recurrence risk for subsequent children with achondroplasia is low.

As in the case of autosomal recessive diseases, more than one gene defect may be involved in producing the same terminal phenotype in autosomal dominant diseases. This is the case in neurofibromatosis, in which two individual genes apparently cause a very similar but not completely overlapping phenotype. It is recognized that one of the genes is located on chromosome 17 and one on chromosome 22.

Myotonic dystrophy, classified as autosomal dominant, is an example of a triplet (CTG) expansion mutation. The nucleotide triplet repeat causes the disease if the number of repeat units is sufficient. With succeeding generations the number of repeats tends to increase, causing earlier and more severe appearance of symptoms. This gives a molecular basis for the clinical phenomenon of *anticipation*.

X-linked inheritance

X-linked inheritance involves genes that are on the X chromosome and can be detected or cause disease when deficient. Several points are important in consideration of X-linked inheritance. First, in females two X chromosomes are present, but one is inactivated. The inactivation process is random. Thus females are mosaic for X chromosome alleles. Some genes on the X chromosome have been shown to escape inactivation. The inactivated X chromosome condenses as a sex chromatin or Barr body that can be observed as a dark spot on the edge of the nucleus. It is late in duplicating in the cell cycle. X inactivation occurs at an early stage in embryologic development, at about 16 days after fertilization. Once inactivated, a given X chromosome remains inactivated in that somatic cell line and all cells derived from that cell line. The random X inactivation process is referred to as *lyonization*. Random inactivation means that females carry a number of X chromosomes that contain deficient alleles but may or may not be inactivated, thus giving them partial activity for a number of enzymes. If a female has a gene for an X-linked recessive disorder on one of her X chromosomes, cells may express the deficient allele or the normal allele. Because X inactivation is random, females carry approximately equal numbers of active paternal and maternal X chromosomes. Should a number of X chromosomes bearing the normal gene be inactivated, the female may express or partially express the deficiency. On this basis the occasional female is a carrier of Duchenne muscular dystrophy, who shows some impairment of muscular function. Only rarely does one discover a female who is homozygously defective for an X-linked disorder. Presumably such an occasion arises from a nondisjunction event or in a situation in which mutant alleles are common in the population. The latter would produce a mixed homozygote defective for gene function. Alternatively, females may lack an X chromosome (45 XO, Turner's syndrome) and therefore manifest deficiencies in the X chromosome. An X-linked pedigree (Fig. 149-8) shows a different inheritance pattern from either recessive or dominant autosomal characteristics:

- No male-to-male transmission.
- All daughters of an affected male are carriers.

The X-linked disease Duchenne muscular dystrophy presents a good example of identification of the gene involved by reverse genetics. The identification and cloning of the Duchenne muscular dystrophy gene and recognition of its

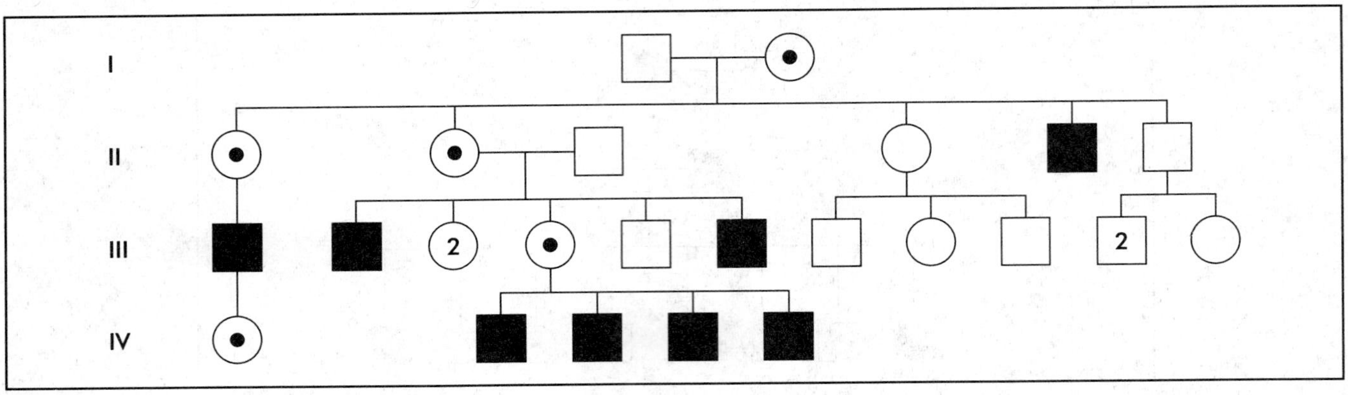

Fig. 149-8. X-linked pedigree. The symbols are as in Fig. 149-6.

product, dystrophin, rested on fortuitous observations of translocation/breakpoints or deletion of the X chromosome in affected males. This allowed identification of DNA sequences present in normal individuals but not in the affected male. This led to the identification of the region of the chromosome containing the affected gene and was followed by rapid cloning. The gene structure is unusually large, as is the size of the protein product.

The X-linked fragile-X syndrome is notable as an example of a disease caused by expansion of a triplet repeat sequence (CGG). An increase in the number of times the triplet is repeated in the maternal X chromosome predisposes sons to fragile-X syndrome. Expansion appears to occur in the mother. Depending on X inactivation daughters may be affected as well as sons, but only at half the frequency because of the randomness of X inactivation.

MULTIFACTORIAL INHERITANCE

Multifactorial inheritance is by far the most commonly observed influence in normal individuals. It is readily recognized that height, skin color, hair color, and intelligence are related to characteristics common to each parent. A number of frequently occurring diseases, such as diabetes mellitus, hypertension, coronary artery disease, schizophrenia, metabolic disorders, neural tube defects, and facial defects, are known to be polygenic or multifactorial disorders. These are the disorders that are recognized as "running in the family." A feature of multifactorial disorders is that the pattern of inheritance is not simple and cannot be demonstrated to fit a mendelian pattern. In all likelihood, the appearance of these disorders is dependent on the interaction of the environment and the genotype of the affected individual.

Association of multifactorial diseases with DNA polymorphic markers has been reported. The "anonymous" probes are not identified with any known gene function but can be associated statistically with the multifactorial disease. For example, there is evidence that certain DNA probes are associated with an increased risk for coronary heart disease. It is likely that an accumulation of probes will be used as a battery to test for increased risk for diseases that are commonly thought of as not being primarily genetic. Such an analysis may well establish an increased risk for an individual relative to the general population. Obviously, the application of such testing and the identification of such individuals involve questions of privacy and cost but may allow prophylactic treatment.

HUMAN CHROMOSOMES

At the beginning of cell division the apparently homogeneous nuclear material condenses into discrete elements, called chromosomes because of the color obtained with various stains. The distribution of chromosomes in germ cell division was noted by Sutton and Boveri in 1902 to be similar to the transmission of hereditary characteristics. They surmised that chromosomes are physical carriers of hereditary traits. Though it was known that the number and structure of these chromosomes were characteristic for each species examined, the chromosome number for humans was disputed until 1956, when Tjio and Levan established the number as 46.

The discipline of human cytogenetics has expanded rapidly since 1956 to include many areas, several of clinical relevance:

- The delineation of numerous congenital malformation syndromes caused by chromosome rearrangement.
- The detection of specific chromosome *aneuploidies* (incorrect number) and rearrangements associated with many specific leukemias and solid tumors.
- The investigation of the possibility that viruses, chemicals, radiation, drugs, and other environmental agents that have a direct effect on chromosomes may be responsible for some congenital anomalies and neoplasias.

The human karyotype

The human *karyotype* is a standardized way of arranging metaphase chromosomes that facilitates their classification and identification and aids in the detection of chromosome anomalies. The normal human karyotype has 23 pairs of chromosomes representing the *diploid* complement of 46 chromosomes. Twenty-two of these pairs are the *autosomes;* the remaining pair consists of the *sex chromosomes,* which are morphologically distinctive in males and females. A normal karyotype is noted as 46,XX (female) or 46,XY (male). The longer arm of the chromosome is termed *q,* the other *p*.

In females the sex chromosomes are identical in size and are called the "X's." Although the X's in females are genetically homologous chromosomes (as in the case of autosomes), in the normal diploid interphase cell, one of the X's forms a condensed *heterochromatic* body in interphase called the *Barr body*. The Lyon hypothesis states that (1) in each somatic cell there is inactivation of one of the X chromosomes, (2) this process occurs early in development and is random with respect to X chromosomes in different cells, and (3) once a particular X is inactive, it is inactive in all daughter cells. This process is important with regard to X chromosome *dosage compensation* (more genetic material in XX females than XY males).

In males, one of the sex chromosomes is smaller and is called the *Y;* it is not strictly homologous, except at the end of the short arm, to the X and there is no Barr body present in the nondividing cells of normal males. However, the Y chromosome has distinctive fluorescent staining properties that in most cases distinguish it from every other human chromosome.

Chromosome identification and chromosome banding techniques

Before the advent of chromosome banding in 1971, chromosomes generally could only be classified into groups based on size and position of the *centromere*. Chromosome banding techniques have provided the means of distinguishing each of the 22 pairs of autosomes and the X and Y chromosomes. A nomenclature that assigned a number for each band according to distance from the centromere and location on the long or short arm was devised. The occurrence of staining *heteromorphisms* (normal inherited variations) usually located at the centromere region allowed further distinction between homologues, and in some cases and their parental origin.

Cell culture and chromosome preparation

The most informative stage of the cell cycle for examination of chromosomes is early metaphase/late prophase. Because cells often are not dividing or not dividing synchronously (except for bone marrow), the method used to obtain sufficient numbers of cells in metaphase is tissue culture. Cells for tissue culture can be obtained from several sources, most commonly peripheral blood, skin biopsy specimens, amniotic fluid, chorionic villi, bone marrow, and solid tumors. Peripheral blood is the most convenient source of cells for chromosome analysis. The lymphocytes are normally in a resting stage but can be stimulated to transform into actively growing cells by addition of a mitogen such as phytohemagglutinin. During the last 1 to 2 hours of culture a mitotic arresting agent, colchicine, is added to the culture to prevent cell entry into metaphase.

There are now many techniques for staining human chromosomes. Some are useful for distinguishing pairs of chromosomes; others are useful for detecting heteromorphisms. Commonly employed techniques can display routine banding or reverse banding, centromeric regions, and heteromorphisms. Methods to increase the band number *(high-resolution chromosomes)* have been devised. Most commonly, cells are synchronized for division with the use of a methotrexate "block"; the block is released and the cells harvested at the times predicted to "catch" the chromosomes in late prophase or early metaphase, revealing more bands. These can be stained with any of the techniques described; G banding provides the best resolution (Figs. 149-9, 149-10).

CHROMOSOME ABNORMALITIES

Types of chromosome abnormalities

There are two major types of human chromosome abnormalities: numerical and structural. Numerical abnormalities may involve extra or missing entire chromosomes *(aneuploidy),* an extra set of chromosomes *(triploidy),* or extra sets of chromosomes *(polyploidy)*. Structural aberrations include partial loss of a chromosome or addition of chromosomal material on a chromosome (partial aneuploidy), such as terminal and interstitial deletions, duplications, rings, and isochromosomes. In addition, translocations or rearrangements of material within a chromosome or between chromosomes may occur. Each of the structural abnormalities may be familial or sporadic in origin.

Mechanism of formation and parental origin of abnormalities

Aneuploidy most often results from a meiotic segregation error *(nondisjunction)* in meiosis I or II. Such errors occur in both male and female meiosis, but more often in meiosis I in the female, and incidence increases with age. Postmeiotic or mitotic nondisjunction can also occur. The result is then *mosaicism* (e.g., 45,X/46,XX) and the individual has two distinct cell populations. The detection of the source of error can be either by molecular techniques or by chromosome heteromorphism.

In trisomy 21, the most common chromosome aneuploidy, a maternal age effect has been demonstrated. The cause is unknown. Because the errors appear to occur primarily in meiosis I, postulates have focused on (1) possible failure of pairing or lack of chiasma formation, (2) desynapsis or premature separation after pairing, or (3) actual nondisjunction.

Utilization of chromosome heteromorphisms has allowed parental origin to be determined in other types of chromosome aberrations. Origin studies have shown the majority of triploids to have two sets of chromosomes from the father, most often as a result of double fertilization. Certain structural abnormalities, such as the deletion of bands q11.2 to q13 of chromosome 15 in Prader-Willi syndrome,

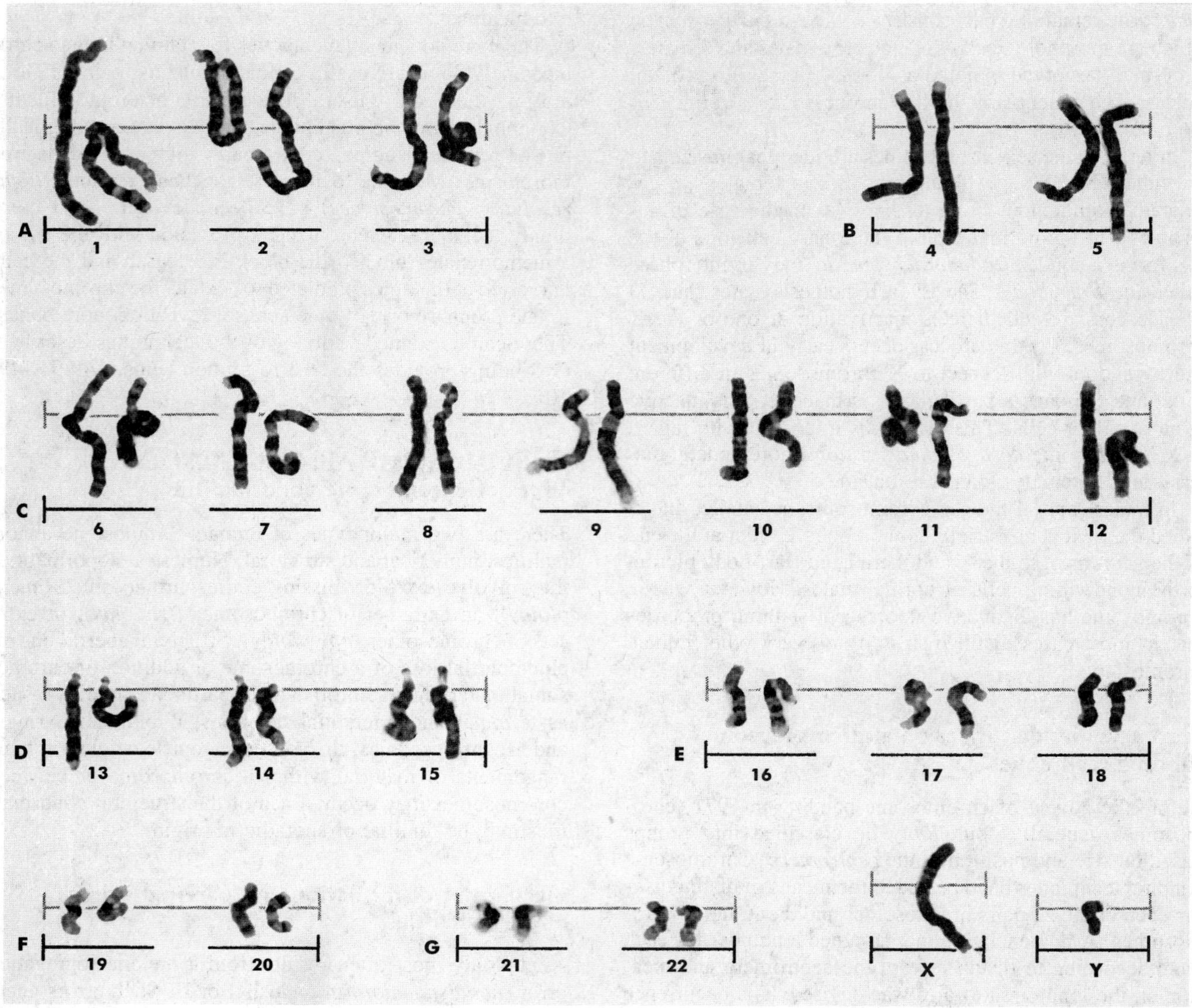

Fig. 149-9. G-banded male karyotype at the approximate 650 band stage according to the International System for Human Cytogentic Nomenclature (ISCN) (1985).

have appeared to be almost exclusively of paternal origin (Fig. 149-11). On the other hand, when the structural aberration is accompanied by *nondisjunction*, as in the case of the extra *bisatellited* (a terminal heteromorphism) 15 and the extra bisatellited 22 in cat eye syndrome, the origin has been almost exclusively maternal.

Xg^a blood group studies have been informative in a few cases of *Turner syndrome* with 45,X karyotypes (X0) and indicate that most often, the paternal sex chromosome is absent. This has been substantiated by molecular techniques. Y chromosome abnormalities are clearly of obligate paternal origin; the frequency of Y chromosome abnormalities is such that paternal errors must not be uncommon.

Partial deletions, duplications, or aneuploidy may result from *translocations* between chromosomes in a parent. By far the most frequent translocation is the robertsonian type, in which two acrocentric chromosomes fuse at their centromeres, thus reducing the number of chromosomes. Affected individuals, when balanced carriers, are themselves normal, but have a higher risk for abnormal offspring. Balanced reciprocal exchange between two chromosomes in a parent may result in unbalanced or balanced as well as normal products, but the chance of having chromosomally unbalanced offspring is relatively high. *Inversion* refers to the reorientation of a part of a chromosome within the chromosome. Inversions also may be balanced or unbalanced. When they are balanced, chromosome imbalance occurs only if there is an odd number of crossovers.

Somatic chromosome aberrations, including aneuploidy, deletion, duplication, and translocation, have also been associated with human disease. These abnormalities are presumably not inherited because they are localized only to

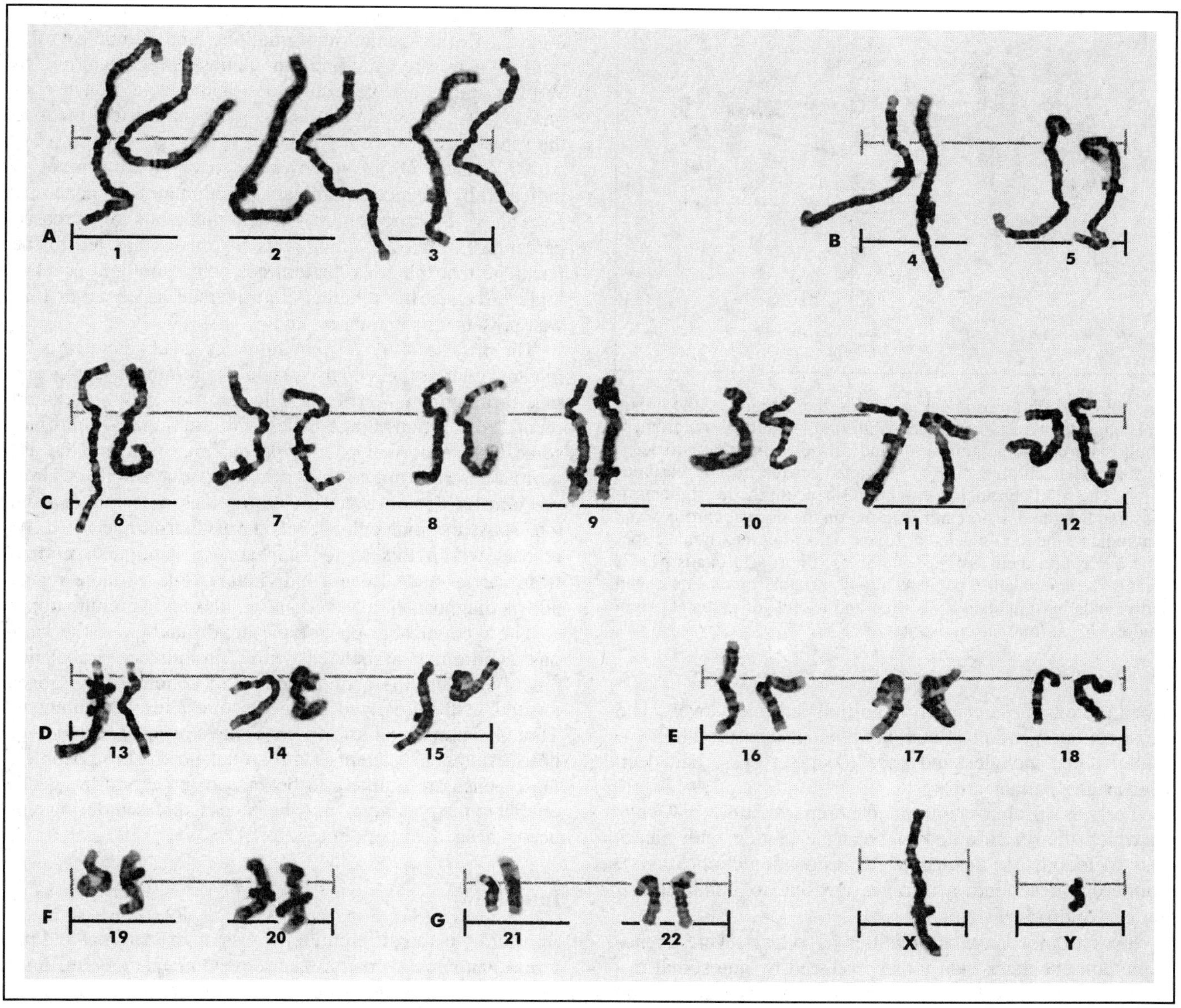

Fig. 149-10. High-resolution G-banded male karyotype at the 900 band stage. Note that there are bands present in this karyotype that are not visible in the karyotype in Fig. 149-9.

specific tissues. The molecular basis is known for some of these abnormalities, for example, the *Philadelphia chromosome* (a chromosome 9/22 translocation), which is usually present in chronic myelogenous leukemia. However, the precipitating event for the translocation is not known.

Chromosome syndromes

Approximately 50% of first trimester spontaneous abortions are chromosomally abnormal. Abnormalities in the early abortuses tend to differ from those found later in gestation and include trisomy for all the chromosomes except chromosome 1. The two most common abnormalities occurring in about 25% of the chromosomally abnormal abortuses are triploidy and 45,X Turner syndrome. Triploidy is characterized by cystic degeneration of the placenta, sometimes appearing as hydatidiform mole; there is usually an accompanying fetus. The fetus is small for gestational age and has low-set ears and syndactyly. A yet to be explained phenomenon is the markedly increased incidence of toxemia of pregnancy and eclampsia with triploidy. About 0.5% to 1% of all liveborns have chromosome abnormalities, and 7% to 10% of stillbirths and neonatal deaths are due to chromosome imbalance.

The infants with autosomal trisomies who survive to term include trisomies 13, 18, and 21. Of these, only trisomy 21 cases survive beyond infancy. These trisomies are also found in early spontaneous abortions. About 70% of trisomy 21 conceptuses are lost before term. Individuals who have a trisomy for other chromosomes may survive

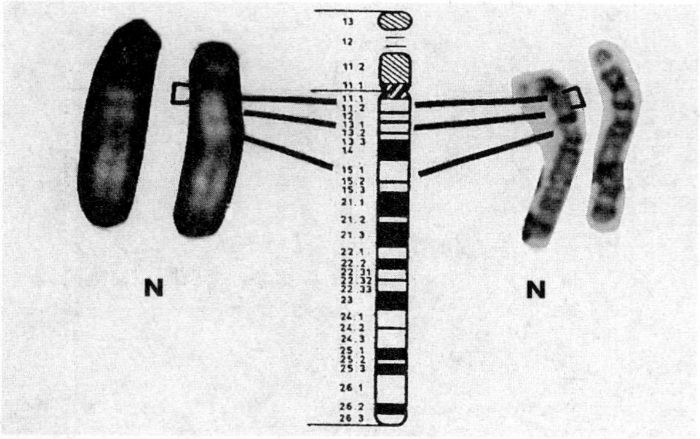

Fig. 149-11. Chromosome 15 showing the deletion of the proximal long arm typical of Prader-Willi and Angelman syndromes. The left chromosome pair is R-banded; the region that is deleted in the far-left chromosome is bracketed on the normal chromosome. The right chromosome pair is G-banded; the far right chromosome has the deletion and brackets on the normal chromosome that indicate the region deleted. Lines to the idiogram indicate specific bands and their assigned members. Short arm bands p11.2, stalk p12, and satellite p13 are highly variable among unrelated individuals but are stably inherited and useful for parental origin studies. N, normal chromosome.

when there is mosaicism for a normal cell line as well. The most common and characteristic is mosaic trisomy 8. Typical features include snub nose, deep-set eyes, and deep plantar and palmar grooves.

There is an almost unlimited number of different ways in which the 46 chromosomes can be broken with pieces lost (deletions) or reattached (translocation/duplications). Numerous described syndromes are due to imbalance of such chromosome segments.

Sex chromosome abnormalities have less severe phenotypic consequences than those produced by autosomal imbalance. This may be caused by lyonization (inactivation) of the excess X chromosomes, and paucity of genes affecting the brain or body structure on the Y. 45,X *Turner syndrome* individuals who survive to term are relatively undamaged. The patients are females, who are short and infertile and have variable somatic abnormalities. Typically the individual has a short, wide or webbed neck; downslanted eyes; shield chest; and short fourth metacarpals. Mosaicism is frequent; the other cell line may be normal XY or XX or an X long arm rearranged chromosome. Less often other structural rearrangements occur. 45,XO occurs in 1/2500 live female births.

Triple X females (47,XXX) occur in about 1/1000 births; they are phenotypically normal females with varying degrees of mental retardation and behavioral difficulties. XXY patients (Klinefelter syndrome), on the other hand, are tall and may be mildly mentally retarded. The occurrence is 1/800 male births. They are almost always infertile as a result of hypogonadism (Chapter 166).

Several *microdeletion* syndromes have recently been described. The deletions generally include only a single chromosome band. An example is the *WAGR syndrome* (Wilm's tumor, aniridia, genital abnormalities, and mental retardation). There are multiple anomalies, predisposition to Wilm's tumor, and generally loss of the lactic dehydrogenase A gene. A dominant disease gene for aniridia maps to the same region.

XYY males (1/500 in newborn surveys) are normal as indicated by physical examination, although they generally have above-average height. The fact that there are increased percentages of XYY individuals in prisons has led to the postulate that the XYY pattern has behavioral and psychologic effects. This remains controversial as observer bias was present in some early studies.

The *fragile X syndrome* in males is characterized by mental retardation, coarse facies, prominent ears, and macro-orchidism. Carrier females may or may not exhibit mental retardation. Some males with the fragile-X chromosome have a normal phenotype but may transmit the abnormal chromosome to their offspring. The fragile-X chromosome is demonstrated in culture, as a lesion at band Xq27. At the molecular level, a varying number of CGG repeats within this region appears to distinguish normal from carrier and affected individuals. The variable repeat allows diagnosis of affected individuals and "premutation."

The recognizable phenotypic abnormalities of the various syndromes associated with chromosome imbalance must be due to the actions or loss of actions of the genes located in the involved segments that alter development. Though a number of known genes have been shown to have dose effects in patients with unbalanced chromosomes, these genes are unlikely to be causative factors; the genes crucial to the phenotype may be genes expressed during embryogenesis and then "turned off."

Imprinting

Imprinting is the differential expression of maternal and paternal genomes in mammalian development. Several lines of evidence favor the occurrence of differential expression. For example, nuclear transplantation experiments in mice have shown that a parthenogenetically produced egg develops to birth only when a male-derived genome is introduced by fusion of karyoplasts. Thus a maternally and a paternally derived genome are necessary for mammalian development. The mechanisms of imprinting are not known but differential methylation is suspected.

In humans, the Prader-Willi and Angelman microdeletion syndromes seem to be examples of imprinting. A small deletion of the proximal long arm of chromosome 15 is found in approximately 85% of Prader-Willi patients, with normal chromosomes in the parents (Fig. 149-11). Parental origin studies show in all cases examined that the deletion occurred as a de novo event in the father. The Angelman syndrome includes characteristic minimally dysmorphic facies, small hands, but normal growth, delayed development, and frequent unprovoked laughter. Feeding problems provided by incoordination of suck and swallow, sleep difficulties, hyperactivity, tremulousness, and seizures generally develop in infancy. A deletion of the same region of chromosome 15 as in Prader-Willi syndrome is found in these patients, but chromosomes of the parents are normal. However, in all cases of Angelman syndrome in which parental origin studies were performed, the affected chromosome was from the mother.

Uniparental disomy, or two copies of a chromosome from one parent, has been noted in most of the Prader-Willi patients who do not have a cytogenetic or molecular deletion, providing further evidence for the role of imprinting in this region of chromosome 15. In these cases there are two copies of the maternal chromosomes (most frequently both of the mother's 15's, but occasionally two copies of the same chromosome 15) and no chromosome 15 from the father. Though uniparental disomy is unusual in the Angelman syndrome, there are the expected findings of two chromosome 15's from the father and no chromosome 15 from the mother.

DIAGNOSIS AND MANAGEMENT OF GENETIC DISORDERS

Approach to the patient

Medical genetics is a cross-discipline field with an interesting combination of tertiary and primary care. In evaluating patients, the clinical geneticist may interact with specialists in several areas of medicine and should work with the patient and the family as a unit. Counseling and ability to communicate, particularly with regard to accurate historical information, are requisites. Medical genetics is a family-oriented specialty. The physician should view the patient as a member of a group and not as an isolated case with a potentially important inherited problem. Consideration must be given to the carrier status of other family members, and whether or not appropriate tests are available to detect that status. Medical genetics is perhaps one of the most cost-effective specialties for preventive medical practice. Many times, the cost both psychologically and financially is extremely high for patients with inherited diseases. However, the recognition of a *proband* (index case) can alert the medical geneticist to effective screening measures for the remainder of the family, perhaps leading to a decrease in cost and suffering. Conversely, patients with inherited diseases frequently consult a clinician because of knowledge of a family member affected with the disease.

A careful history is the keystone to a successful medical genetics diagnosis. Particular attention should be paid to the onset of symptoms, whether or not milestones of development have been gained appropriately, whether or not such milestones have been lost, food intake and tolerance history, and whether or not other family members show similar findings or afflictions. Another important element in history taking is *pedigree analysis*. This is most conveniently done with forms that readily delineate the generations in the family and include adequate space for annotation with names. Two important points with regard to pedigree analysis are last names before marriage and ethnic and locale origins of families. Frequently, such information can be a clue to consanguinity. Attention should be given to individuals who die suddenly or in an unexplained manner or who manifest certain phenotypic features that may be associated with the disease of interest. A good example is Marfan syndrome, in which sudden death produced by aortic rupture is associated with numerous phenotype findings. The age at onset of symptoms should be noted. In history taking, it is important to obtain details of the obstetric history for any pregnancies involving affected individuals, with attention to intercurrent infections, unexplained fevers, and drug or teratogen exposures for the mother. It is also important to note a history of any spontaneous miscarriages. Medical records to substantiate the diagnosis and photographs of other affected family members, when they cannot be present, can be invaluable.

The physical examination in the practice of medical genetics should note the symmetry of the body and its parts as well as relative size and conformation compared to those of the normal population. A readily available set of tables of height, weight, head circumference, interocular distance, and other parameters is indispensable in evaluating dysmorphology and establishing a base for diagnosis. Diagnosis in medical genetics frequently begins with an orderly listing of abnormal physical findings followed by a systematic comparison to listings of associations of abnormalities in recognized syndromes. Such dysmorphology data bases are available in computer software packages.

Testing and diagnosis

After history taking and physical examination, the physician faces the decision of ordering additional tests to establish a diagnosis or to evaluate the relative severity of the disease in the individual. The decision is based on the physical findings and the suggestions from the history as well as information from the referring physician. During the evaluation of patients, psychometric testing to establish development and intelligence is appropriate. With infants, developmental testing and comparative evaluation in relation to normal milestones are as significant as in older children and adults. Where appropriate, psychologic evaluation can be very helpful.

The use of consultations is critical in medical genetic diagnosis. For example, an ophthalmologic consultation should be routinely used for patients who manifest mental retardation. Many inherited diseases have ocular features that are helpful, if not pathognomonic. For a number of inherited diseases, radiologic studies can be definitive—for example, vertebral films in the muccopolysaccaridoses, and three-dimensional radiologic techniques to evaluate central nervous system development as well as standard films. Ultrasonography both for diagnosis and for monitoring is appropriate in a number of inherited disorders. Establishing the diagnosis is the keystone to successful family counseling.

With regard to laboratory testing, it is helpful to divide the approach into three categories: metabolic, karyotype analysis, and DNA or molecular testing (Fig. 149-12). Metabolic testing is appropriate in the case of mental retardation as a screening test using the urine or serum. It is good practice to include evaluation of levels of organic acids and

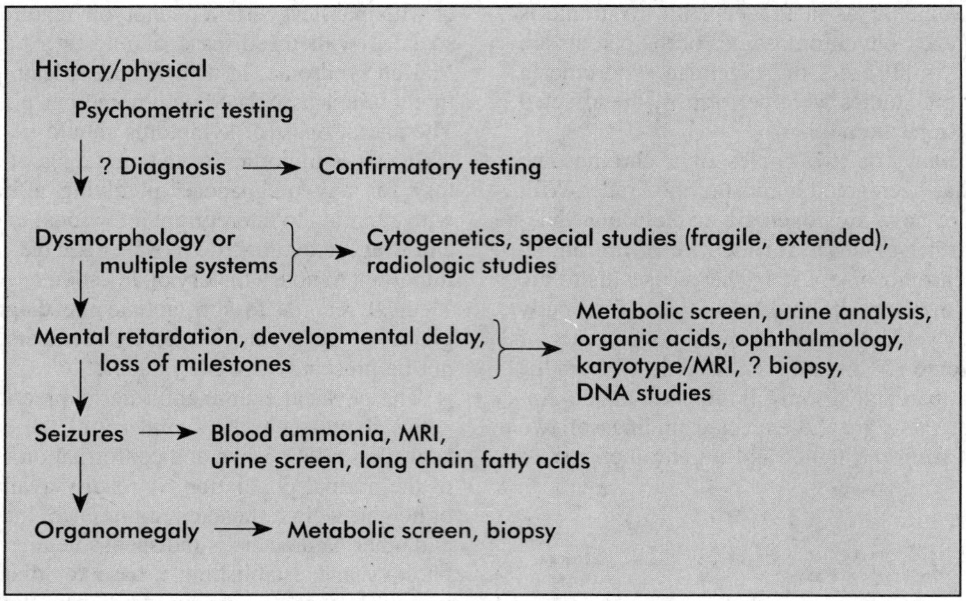

Fig. 149-12. Diagnostic testing. Flow chart for patient evaluation with regard to laboratory procedures.

amino acids, especially with the presence of seizures. If the patient in the perinatal period has seizures, evaluation of levels of organic acids and blood ammonia is appropriate. If symptoms appear to be related to dietary history, metabolic evaluation is also suggested. Loss of developmental milestones is a hallmark of storage disease and should alert the physician to that possibility.

Karyotype analysis is indicated when a patient exhibits dysmorphology, involvement of several organ systems, and/or mental retardation. In a number of situations it is appropriate to request a specialized karyotype analysis, such as a fragile site study in a patient who is suspected of having fragile-X syndrome. It is appropriate to look for "microdeletions" in some instances, such as chromosome 15q in Prader-Willi syndrome.

The number of tests to which DNA diagnosis can be advantageously applied is relatively small at the present time but is growing rapidly. This technique is most promising when a disease has a low new mutation frequency, no available metabolic test exists, but the defective gene has been identified. At the present time, the tests must be targeted to a given disease. None of the testing methods should be viewed as operating in isolation from the others. It is likely that tests that are now performed at the DNA level may be performed at the "metabolic" level once the gene product and its function have been further assessed.

COUNSELING AND PRENATAL DIAGNOSIS

Medical genetics is unusual in the extent of its requirement for and reliance on patient and family counseling. In this respect, the physician frequently uses the services of genetic counselors who are trained in gathering information and explaining heritable disorders to patients. Counseling is an integral part of diagnosis and treatment and must be adjusted to the needs of the patient: that is, does the patient require primarily recurrence risk data or outlook for his or her own disease? The salient points of genetic counseling are:

- Basis for and certainty of the diagnosis
- Burden of the disease
- Recurrence risk
- Treatment

The first step in genetic counseling is to inform the patient of the diagnosis, the basis of the conclusions regarding the diagnosis, and the level of certainty. It is important at this step to be thorough. It is also important not to attach a label to a patient if the diagnosis is uncertain. During this phase of the counseling, pictures are frequently helpful. For example, in chromosomal disorders, the basis for the diagnosis can be established more clearly if the clinician uses diagrams or actual pictures of chromosomes, if possible, of the disorder under discussion. Are any additional tests required? The level of certainty of the diagnosis justifies the administration of additional tests. The burden of the diagnosis is the physical, emotional, and financial load the diagnosis implies. Some diagnoses, such as malformations, have a relatively light impact in regard to viability of the patient but a significant psychologic impact, as well as its implications for reconstructive surgery. Other diagnoses bode ominous outlooks. Recurrence risk is important to establish with regard to future childbearing, risk for the offspring who already exist, and implications for other family members. Here the counselor must be circumspect.

Sensitivity to both the patient's and other family members' privacy must be considered. The physician is dependent on the goodwill of family members and the action of the patient or the patient's relatives for identifying additional affected family members, obtaining specimens for further diagnostic tests, and collecting additional historic information. Many times, information about other family members is helpful in forming a basis for diagnosis. For example, a history of family members' dying suddenly of aneurysms is compatible with a history of Marfan syndrome in the family and implies that the patient under consultation does not represent a new mutation.

Treatment options and outlooks are important considerations for the patient. Can the recurrence risk for a couple be lowered by prenatal diagnosis or by artificial insemination? Are these alternatives acceptable to the patient? In genetic counseling, the physician must provide information that the patient will use to make decisions within his or her ethical framework. Will termination after prenatal diagnosis be an acceptable alternative? If not, is the cost of the prenatal diagnostic procedures worthwhile? What is the level of certainty for prenatal diagnostic procedures? These are significant points that should be considered by the counselor in talking with the family.

Prenatal diagnosis and counseling are usually based on a couple's desire for prenatal diagnosis because of an empiric risk for disease or a patient's desire for prenatal diagnosis because of a familial history. In the first category, advanced maternal age, with increased risk of chromosomal aneuploidy, would be the most common reason for counseling. In the latter category, a typical reason for prenatal diagnosis would be screening tests that indicated that the couple were carriers for Tay Sachs disease, an autosomal recessive disease with a high burden. Other common reasons for prenatal diagnosis and counseling would be a family history of chromosomal disorders, multifactorial disorders, or a disease manifesting dysmorphology. In the case of dysmorphology, the diagnosis can occasionally be established in utero by ultrasound. For example, achondroplasia can be observed in utero in an ultrasound given on a routine basis. Amniocentesis with karyotype analysis can lower the risk of chromosomal disorders to well below 0.5% if the results are normal.

In counseling, it is useful to inform the patient of the general population risk of birth defects (approximately 3%), with the exact level depending on where one sets the boundaries for a "birth defect." This risk places the increasing chance of chromosomal abnormality with increasing maternal age in perspective. It is important to inform the patient of what prenatal diagnosis cannot rule out, and the physician should emphasize that a normal result in a given test does not represent a clean bill of health for the pregnancy. The statements of the counselor should be couched in terms of risk estimates and percentage of chances.

TREATMENT

Treatment of individuals with genetic disorders is not a new field. The psychologic and social support requirements of the patient, although not curative, are an integral part of treatment. For example, in Prader-Willi syndrome patients regularly require psychologic counseling and evaluation as well as considerable monitoring for eating disorders. Although not representing a cure, such elements can be effective in controlling the results of the abnormal gene. Phenylketonuria (PKU) offers an example of biochemical treatment, in which the dietary restriction of phenylalanine is critical to the patient's achieving normal or nearly normal intelligence. There seems little doubt that early institution of and strict adherence to the dietary regimen are required for normal function. In other instances, supplying a cofactor can be remarkably effective. For example, in biotinidase deficiency, pharmacologic doses of biotin prevent the appearance of disease.

Enzyme therapy has been an attractive goal in the treatment of inherited disorders. Important considerations in this regard still include the blood-brain barrier and the half-life or duration of the infused enzyme in the bloodstream. Several promising examples are the treatment of Gaucher's disease with sphingomyelinase and Fabry's disease with alpha-galactosidase. Enzyme replacement therapy is feasible when the metabolic defect can be corrected by circulating enzymes available in large amounts of high purity. Production of human enzymes in mammalian expression systems avoids antigenic stimulus and proper modification to permit "targeting" for uptake by specific tissues.

Therapy by substituting normal functional genes for deficient genes seems an attainable goal. It is useful to distinguish somatic cell gene therapy from germ cell gene therapy. In the former, the goal would be to cure the defect in a patient, and in the latter, an additional goal would be to prevent a defect in the offspring of the patient. The ethical implications are viewed by society as somewhat different: in the former, the net effect would be little different from that of treating a patient with a dietary supplement; in the latter, the result is that future generations may be affected in terms of permanent alteration. In either instance the question of adverse risk produced by derepression or repression of a gene product remains an open question. Is it possible, for example, to inactivate a tumor suppressor gene and increase the risk of cancer in a patient? Evidence seems to indicate that, in fact, such questions can be answered satisfactorily and that gene therapy can be undertaken in a safe manner.

One of the approaches to gene therapy, ex vivo, is to isolate the patient's cells, modify the genome in those cells, and then reintroduce those cells into the patient in such a way that an expansion of the cells would supply sufficient gene product to prevent the symptoms of the disease. For example, liver cells, muscle cells, and bone marrow cells can all be isolated, manipulated, and reintroduced into the body with a subsequent increase in number of the modified cells. In this approach, retroviruses have been the primary experimental model vector. Cloning vectors derived from retroviruses with the desired gene inserted in an expression cassette can be packaged in viral capsids to allow infection of human cells. Replication defective vectors are used to "force" integration into the host genome for stable expression, indexed by a selectable trait for cell marking. RNA retroviruses carrying a drug resistance marker are model systems. If adequate expression can be monitored and demonstrated in vitro, then the cell line that has been modified is reintroduced. Variables that must be controlled to assure successful gene therapy include adequate expression of the gene and its product, appropriate modification of the product to allow function, and delivery of the gene product in sufficient levels. With regard to these points, tissue-specific promoters and the tissue of production are important considerations. If the enzyme must be modified to allow proper transport and persistence, it must be ensured that the altered gene is being produced in tissues that will appropriately carry out such functions.

Adequate means of delivering and monitoring the expression of genes are therefore at hand. Other essential needs for routine application of gene therapy include a demonstration of safety, mechanisms for tissue targeting on a routine basis, vectors with promoter-enhancer systems active in a given tissue over a long time frame, possible controllable expression, and, most importantly, safety. Meeting each of these needs appears feasible.

The potential applications for gene therapy are much broader than in "genetic" diseases. It seems likely that gene therapy will not be limited to rare inherited disorders but may find use in other areas such as immune dysfunction and cancer. The cost-effectiveness and range of usefulness promise to make gene therapy the treatment of choice in a broad array of disorders. We may expect to see application of this technology in a variety of situations within the next decade.

REFERENCES

Collins FS: Positional cloning: let's not call it reverse anymore, Nature Genetics 1:3, 1992.

Desnick RJ: Treatment of genetic diseases. New York, 1991, Churchill Livingstone.

Emery AE and Rimoin DL, editors: Principles and practice of medical genetics, ed 2. New York, 1990, Churchill Livingstone.

Jones KC: Smith's recognizable patterns of human malformation, ed 4. Philadelphia, 1988, Saunders.

McKusick VA: Mendelian inheritance in man, ed 4. Baltimore, 1992, Johns Hopkins University Press.

Richards RI and Sutherland GR: Heritable unstable DNA sequences, Nature Genetics 1:7, 1992.

Schlessinger D: Yeast artificial chromosomes: tools for mapping and analysis of complex genomes, Trends Genetics 6:248, 1990.

Scriver CR et al: The metabolic basis of inherited disease, ed 6. New York, 1989, McGraw-Hill.

Thompson MS, McInnes RR, and Willard HP: Thompson and Thompson genetics in medicine, ed 5. Philadelphia, 1991, Saunders.

LABORATORY TESTS II

CHAPTER

150 Laboratory Diagnosis in Endocrinology

Richard M. Jordan
Peter O. Kohler

In no other area of internal medicine is the laboratory more crucial for diagnosis than in endocrinology. The physician, however, faces a difficult challenge in making effective use of laboratory technology. There are usually more tests available to evaluate a condition than are necessary to diagnose it, and the diagnostic procedures often involve complex and expensive manipulations. Thus the clinician needs a thorough understanding of endocrine pathophysiology, not only to interpret results but also to know which tests to order. Without this knowledge, it is inevitable that time and resources will be wasted.

GENERAL PRINCIPLES OF ENDOCRINE TESTING

General categories of endocrine tests

Endocrine evaluation can be divided into two broad categories—testing in the basal state and testing designed either to increase or to decrease hormone secretion (stimulation and suppression tests).

Basal tests. Basal testing should be done when the patient is resting and has fasted for a period of approximately 8 to 12 hours. Ideally, the patient should not be acutely ill, and medication should be withdrawn. The last stipulation is often difficult to meet.

Stimulation tests. Stimulation testing is used primarily to assess the adequacy of hormone reserve. Direct testing utilizes a specific trophic hormone or an agent known to induce a target gland hormone response. The patient's response is then compared with standards derived from normal individuals. Stimulation testing is also used to elicit an inappropriate secretory response. An example is the secretion of calcitonin after pentagastrin injection in patients with medullary carcinoma of the thyroid. A calcitonin response is not seen in normal individuals. Thus the anomalous response becomes a diagnostic marker for disease.

Another variety of stimulation testing involves tests that inhibit feedback suppression. There are two general mechanisms by which this can be accomplished. The testing agent can block target gland hormone secretion, which then results in increased trophic hormone release. This occurs as a result of diminished feedback inhibition caused by a lower concentration of target gland hormone. Metyrapone stimulation utilizes this physiologic principle. A testing agent can also inhibit feedback suppression by blocking the action of the target hormone at the site of trophic hormone secretion. In this instance, the agent employed usually occupies the receptors for the target hormone but has little or no ability to decrease trophic hormone release. Clomiphene stimulation is an example of this form of feedback inhibition.

Suppression tests. Suppression testing is commonly used in the evaluation of endocrine hypersecretory disorders. Usually these testing procedures inhibit physiologic hormone secretion. With autonomous hormone secretion there is loss of feedback to signals that normally suppress hormone secretion. Failure of appropriate suppression to occur offers strong evidence for loss of normal control mechanisms and associated glandular abnormality.

Measurement of hormone concentration in blood

Many hormones are released episodically. Fortuitous determination at either the height of a secretory burst or its nadir may therefore give misleading results. To obviate this problem, it is helpful to obtain three blood specimens at intervals of 15 minutes or more. Equal aliquots from the specimens are pooled into a single combined specimen. The value obtained should closely approximate the average hormone concentration, and the patient is charged for only a single hormone determination. It is especially important to obtain pooled specimens when measuring gonadotropins, estrogens, and testosterone; it is not necessary for most other hormones. The difficulty of collecting several blood specimens is greatly lessened by using an indwelling catheter kept patent with a heparin-saline solution.

Hormones also are subject to biologic variations and rhythms that reflect either influences from the environment or regular oscillations originating from within the patient *(endogenous rhythms)*. External stimuli causing a stress reaction may cause acute release of several hormones including adrenocorticotropic hormone (ACTH), cortisol, growth hormone, prolactin, and epinephrine. The endogenous rhythmic oscillations of hormone concentration may have a 24 hour periodicity *(circadian)* or exhibit cyclicity of more than 24 hours *(infradian)*. These factors must be considered when interpreting hormone concentrations in blood.

Many hormones are transported in plasma partly bound to binding proteins and partly unbound or free. It is only the free portion that is active; however, in some cases (i.e., thyroid hormone), the great majority exists in the bound form. Routine testing techniques are not capable of separating the bound from the free portions of the hormone and measure only the total hormone concentration. Thus conditions that greatly alter protein binding of hormones may lead to an inaccurate estimate of the active hormone level. When conditions exist that alter binding (discussed later), the clinician should request that the free hormone concentration be measured.

Measurement of hormone concentration in urine

The measurement of a hormone or its metabolites in urine theoretically corrects for fluctuating blood levels and integrates the concentration over a longer period (usually 24 hours). To assess whether a urine collection is complete, creatinine excretion in the urine should be measured. The creatinine content in an adult is usually 1 g or more per day. For testing procedures requiring multiple urine collections during a series of diagnostic manipulations, such as dexamethasone suppression for Cushing's syndrome, it is essential to save a small aliquot from each total volume until all testing is completed and results are returned to the physician. This will allow retrieval and retesting of specimens that are lost or improperly handled by laboratory personnel. Many hormones measured in the urine are metabolic products of conjugation. Their measurement commonly utilizes laborious extraction procedures or chromatography. Very large and dilute urine volumes make total extraction and accurate measurement of the products difficult.

Immunoassay

No single technologic development has advanced endocrinology further than the immunoassay. It allows investigators to understand the pathophysiology of many diseases and provides a powerful tool for diagnosing endocrine disorders. Despite its importance, the principles of immunoassay are relatively simple (Fig. 150-1). It consists of the following major components:

1. An antibody that is specific for the particular hormone being measured.
2. A fixed and specific amount of the hormone that is labeled with a radioactive marker.
3. A specimen that contains an unknown amount of hormone.

To perform the assay, the antibody and the labeled hormone are added to the specimen with the unknown amount of hormone. The endogenous hormone (the hormone originally present in the specimen) and the labeled hormone (the hormone added in the laboratory) compete for binding sites on the antibody. If there is a large concentration of endogenous hormone, most of the antibody will be bound to it and little antibody remain to bind the labeled hormone. Thus the antibody-hormone complex will contain only a small amount of labeled hormone and therefore little radioactivity. Conversely, if the concentration of endogenous hormone is small, the antibody will bind relatively more labeled hormone, and the antibody-hormone complex will contain considerable radioactivity. To measure the amount of radioactivity that is bound, the hormone bound to the antibody and the unbound hormone must be separated, and there are a variety of techniques for accomplishing this. One method commonly used employs a "second antibody," which binds the hormone-specific "first antibody" and facilitates the precipitation of the hormone-antibody complex. Determining the unknown hormone level is possible by comparing the amount of binding in the unknown specimen to a standard curve (Fig. 150-2). Standard curves are es-

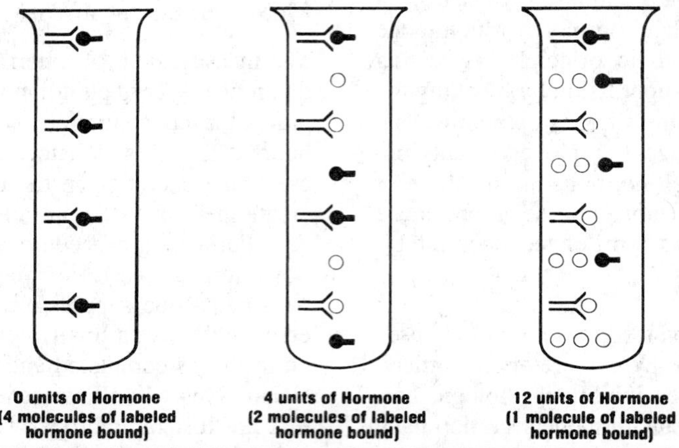

Fig. 150-1. The principles of radioimmunoassay *(see text)*. With no endogenous hormone, all of the labeled *(radioactive)* hormone is bound by antibody specific for the hormone. A precipitate of antibody and hormone would then show increased radioactivity. With very high levels of endogenous hormone, the great majority of antibody is bound by endogenous hormone. In this case, very little radioactivity would be detected in the hormone-antibody precipitate. ≺, antibody; ●, labeled hormone; ○, endogenous hormone.

tablished by adding known quantities of unlabeled hormone and determining the percentage of radiolabeled hormone bound.

The immunoassay is usually sensitive and reliable. Different antibodies to the same hormone, however, can vary in *specificity* (degree of binding to other proteins in addition to the one being measured) and *affinity* (concentration of antibody needed to bind a given amount of hormone). Therefore results of laboratories employing different assay systems often are not strictly comparable. It is also important to realize that an antibody may bind prohormones or hormone fragments (which often are not active), so the value determined is not necessarily a measurement of biologically active hormone.

Newer techniques offering a modification of the immunoassay are being utilized by commercial laboratories. Use of monoclonal antibodies (a single clone of antibody with affinity for only a single antigenic site on a hormone) improves the specificity of an assay and diminishes interlaboratory variation of results.

Chemiluminescence immunoassay may offer an alternative to immunoassay. It is similar to the classic immunoassay except that it employs the antigen labeled with a chemiluminescent compound (acridinium esters) as the tracer. When acridinium is oxidized, it emits photons at approximately 430 nm wavelength that are detected by a photonmultiplier. The photon strikes are counted and converted to counts in a way similar to that of a gamma counter that quantitates radioactivity.

Other methods of hormone measurement

Although immunoassay is presently the most widely used means of measuring hormone concentration, other methods are still occasionally employed. *Competitive protein binding* is a displacement assay in which a specific binding protein and a labeled tracer hormone are mixed with the substrate to be measured. Its principles are entirely analogous to those of the radioimmunoassay except that the binding protein is substituted for an antibody. Cortisol is sometimes measured with this technique by using a cortisol-binding globulin (transcortin) as the binding protein.

Radioenzymatic conversion is a technique that employs the addition of radiolabeled hormone to a specimen and then, with a fixed amount of an added enzyme, causes conversion of a portion of the hormone to metabolites that are radiolabeled. The quantity of labeled metabolites is then measured. If the endogenous concentration of hormone is large, the enzyme will convert relatively little labeled hormone to metabolite. If the endogenous hormone concentration is low, more of the added labeled hormone will be converted, thereby increasing the total labeled metabolites. This technique is helpful when the hormone metabolites are easier to measure than the hormone, as in the case of catecholamines.

Fluorometric methods to determine steroid or catecholamine concentration utilize a substance that absorbs light at one wavelength and then emits light at a characteristic longer wavelength of lower energy. This technique is relatively sensitive, but drugs and hormones other than the one being measured can also fluoresce, giving false-positive results.

Colorimetry utilizes a chemical reagent to cause the substance being measured to form a specific colored product. The intensity of the color is used to determine the concentration of the substance. Except for its use in enzyme-linked immunosorbent assays (ELISAs) and steroid hormone measurement, colorimetry is now employed less frequently because of its low sensitivity. The presence of many nonspecific chromogens (drugs, other hormones) may also make interpretation of results difficult.

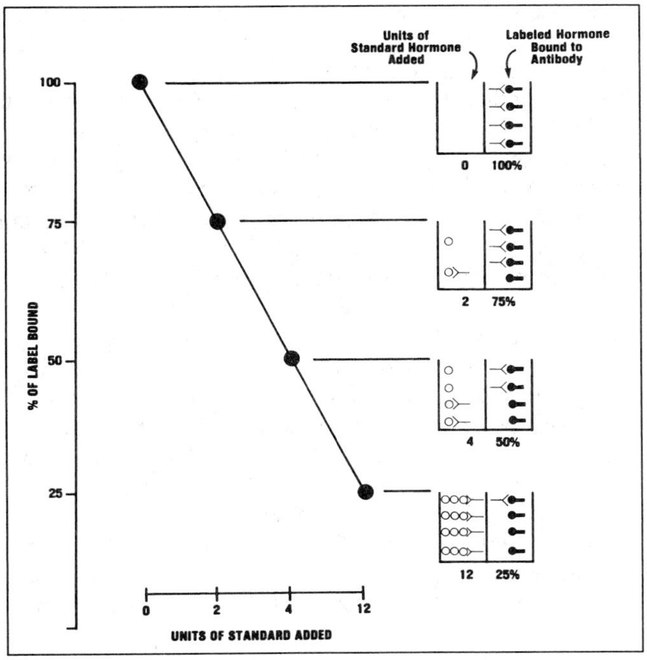

Fig. 150-2. Standard curve for radioimmunoassay. As the amount of standard *(unlabeled)* hormone is increased, less of the labeled hormone is bound by antibody specific to the hormone. Thus knowledge of the amount of radioactivity bound by antibody when a known amount of hormone is added allows determination of the amount of endogenous hormone in an unknown sample. For accurate measurement, the same quantity of antibody and label must be used in unknown samples as is used in plotting the standard curve. The standard curve illustrated here is linear and therefore is idealized. Most standard curves show considerable flattening and less sensitivity at the lower and upper limits of assay detectability. This is not a problem at the upper limits of detectability (high levels of endogenous hormone) because such samples can be diluted and reassayed. ≺, antibody; ●━, labeled hormone; ○, endogenous hormone.

Radiographic and isotopic studies in endocrinology

Computed tomography has had a great impact on the neuroradiologic evaluation of patients with suspected hypothalamic-pituitary disease. High-resolution scanners demonstrate abnormalities as small as 1.5 mm within the pituitary gland. Small hypothalamic tumors can be seen but may be hard to distinguish from normal tissues if the tumor is a well-differentiated neural cell neoplasm. Computed tomography is a very sensitive means of detecting suprasellar calcifications in patients with craniopharyngiomas. Adrenal tumors as small as 0.5 cm can be seen if they lie in the lateral wings of the adrenal gland. The adrenal gland, however, thickens considerably where the lateral wings join, and if a tumor is located there it must be larger than 1.5 cm to be identified consistently. Adrenal tumors may not be detected if there is little fat surrounding the adrenal glands. Fat outlines the adrenal borders, and its absence obscures abnormalities in adrenal gland contour.

Computed tomography of the pancreas is sometimes helpful in detecting insulinomas. However, the tumor must be larger than 2 cm to be identified. Another application of this technique includes evaluation for extraocular muscle enlargement or a retro-orbital mass in patients with unilateral exophthalmos. Less common uses of computed tomography are the evaluation of thyroid and parathyroid tumors and detection of early osteoporosis. The place of computed tomography in the evaluation of these disorders, however, is not yet established.

Ultrasonography is an increasingly important tool in endocrine evaluation. Thyroid nodules are often studied with ultrasonography to ascertain whether or not they are solid, mixed (solid and cystic components), or purely cystic. Predominantly cystic nodules are very unlikely to be malignant. In patients with exophthalmic Graves' disease, the orbital contents can be visualized by this technique and distinguished from tumors causing exophthalmos. Ultrasound is also valuable for evaluating ovarian structure in patients with hirsutism. Although it is a sensitive means of detecting polycystic ovaries, ultrasound does have some limitations in detecting ovarian tumors. In thin patients, tumors as small as 1 cm can be identified. Adipose tissue, however, is echogenic and makes interpretation of the study very difficult in obese patients, in whom tumors as large as 5 cm can be missed. This is unfortunate because physical examination of the ovaries is most likely to be inadequate in obese patients.

Radioisotope studies are particularly important in the evaluation of thyroid disease. An iodine-123 tracer is given to patients with suspected hyperthyroidism; if hyperthyroidism is present, the 24 hour thyroid uptake of this isotope is usually greater than 30%. The test is not useful for diagnosing hypothyroidism because iodine is present in ever-increasing quantities in our diet, effectively abolishing a lower normal limit to the uptake. Functional characteristics of thyroid nodules can also be studied with thyroid scans. Areas with autonomous function often show increased uptake, whereas hypofunctional areas show diminished uptake. Technetium-99, which delivers very little radioactivity to the thyroid, also can be used for this purpose. Technetium, however, is trapped but not organically bound to thyroglobulin and may make some nonfunctional nodules appear functional. This may inappropriately lower the suspicion of cancer because functioning nodules are very unlikely to be cancerous. Iodocholesterol scanning is sometimes used to image the adrenal glands; however, the study is tedious and in most centers has been replaced by computed tomography.

Magnetic resonance imaging (MRI) is not invasive and does not use ionizing radiation. It delivers anatomically detailed images of the pituitary and hypothalamus. Tumors to 0.3 cm in diameter can be seen. The neck and mediastinum can be visualized well in searching for metastatic thyroid cancer, substernal goiter, or parathyroid adenoma after an unsuccessful surgical exploration. It also holds promise for ovarian imaging because it delivers a negligible amount radiation.

Selective venous catheterization with hormone measurement in venous effluent can be a useful means of locating the source of hormone hypersecretion. The technique is most widely employed in the study of primary hyperaldosteronism after other localizing techniques have failed to determine whether a single adenoma is present or both glands are hyperplastic. The right adrenal vein cannot always be entered because of its small size and variable anatomic position. Venous catheterization is also used to locate a parathyroid adenoma in patients with a previously failed parathyroidectomy or in those with difficult-to-diagnose Cushing's syndrome in which selective catheterization of the inferior petrosal vein and measurement of ACTH concentration can establish the presence of pituitary-dependent Cushing's syndrome. Occasionally these studies are used to localize pheochromocytoma, insulinoma, and carcinoid.

SPECIFIC ENDOCRINE TESTS

Hypothalamic-pituitary testing

A large number of tests are available for evaluating the reserve of specific anterior pituitary hormones (Fig. 150-3) (Chapter 160). Stimulatory agents increase secretion either by hypothalamic pathways or by direct stimulation of the anterior pituitary. Some testing agents cause release of multiple hormones.

Thyrotropin-releasing hormone. In normal individuals thyrotropin-releasing hormone (TRH) causes the release of thyroid-stimulating hormone (TSH) and prolactin (PRL). Theoretically, the test can distinguish between hypothalamic and pituitary deficiency. Unfortunately, there is overlap between the responses observed in these two disease states in that some patients with pituitary disease have a normal TSH response (the expected response with hypothalamic disease), and patients with hypothalamic disease may demonstrate a subnormal TSH response (the expected response for pituitary disorders). These paradoxic responses and the fact that PRL reserve rarely needs to be tested limit the usefulness of TRH testing for pituitary disease. The test is used to evaluate patients for suspected hyperthyroidism because an even slightly excessive thyroid hormone concentration suppresses the TSH response to TRH. Thus an absent or blunted TSH response to TRH is supportive evidence for hyperthyroidism in patients with an equivocally elevated thyroid hormone level in blood. For evaluation of most cases of hyperthyroidism, however, a finding of a suppressed TSH level using the newer, sensitive assay has largely replaced the TRH test. TRH testing remains useful in the evaluation of hyperthyroidism with a normal or elevated TSH concentration. Patients with TSH-secreting pituitary tumors rarely show any TSH responsiveness to TRH, whereas those with pituitary resistance to thyroid hormone feedback do have a TSH response to TRH. To perform this test, 500 μ of TRH is administered intravenously, and blood for TSH is collected at 0, 15, 30, and 60 minutes. The TSH level should show increments of at least 5 μU per milliliter. Age blunts the TSH response, and the increase may be less than 2 μU per milliliter in normal men over 50 years old.

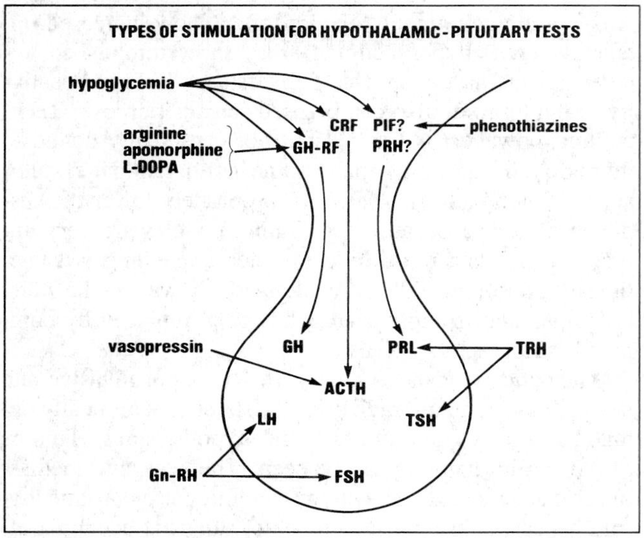

Fig. 150-3. Stimulatory agents cause increased anterior pituitary hormone secretion either by hypothalamic pathways or by direct stimulation of the anterior pituitary gland. The level at which these stimulatory agents exert their effects is shown. GH-RF, growth hormone–releasing factor; PIF, prolactin-inhibiting factor; PRH, prolactin-releasing hormone.

Gonadotropin-releasing hormone. Both luteinizing hormone (LH) and follicle-stimulating hormone (FSH) are released by gonadotropin-releasing hormone (GnRH). In adults, the LH response is greater than the FSH response. In children, the responses of LH and FSH are approximately equal except during puberty, when the FSH response exceeds that of LH. As with TRH, a single injection of GnRH may not distinguish between a hypothalamic origin and a pituitary origin of gonadotropin deficiency. However, with intermittent injections (over a period of at least 2 weeks), virtually all patients with a hypothalamic defect will respond to GnRH. Patients are given 100 μ of GnRH intravenously, and blood is collected at 0, 30, and 60 minutes. In adults the LH level increases by at least 20 mIU per milliliter. The FSH concentration is much less responsive, and an increase of less than 2 mIU per milliliter is seen in some normal individuals.

Corticotropin-releasing hormone. In identifying the cause of Cushing's syndrome corticotropin-releasing hormone (CRH) may be useful. Patients with pituitary-dependent Cushing's syndrome have an ACTH response to CRH. Those with ectopic ACTH syndrome do not show an ACTH increase. However, there is overlap of the ACTH response between these disorders and CRH does not always distinguish between them. Measurement of simultaneously obtained ACTH specimens from the inferior petrosal sinus and a peripheral vein is a more reliable means to separate pituitary-dependent Cushing's syndrome from ectopic ACTH secretion. CRH (1 μ/kg) is given by bolus, and blood samples for ACTH are obtained at 0, 15, 30, and 60 minutes. The maximum ACTH response occurs at 15 minutes and the cortisol peaks at 30 to 60 minutes.

Growth hormone–releasing hormone. Growth hormone–releasing hormone (GHRH) is not available for clinical use. When 3.3 μ per kilogram is given intravenously, a peak growth hormone response is seen between 30 and 90 minutes. Levels attained range from 5 to 50 ng per milliliter. An increase of growth hormone concentration occurs in patients with hypothalamic disease and in some with pituitary disease. This overlap limits its diagnostic utility.

Insulin-induced hypoglycemia. In response to the stress of hypoglycemia, ACTH, PRL, and GH are secreted. Stimulation occurs via activation of hypothalamic pathways; therefore a subnormal hormone response occurs with either hypothalamic or pituitary disease. Regular insulin is administered at a dose of 0.1 unit per kilogram. Obese patients or those with acromegaly need 0.15 to 0.2 unit per kilogram because they have relative insulin resistance. To be confident that the stress level is adequate, the blood glucose concentration should drop below 40 mg %. Blood specimens are obtained at 0, 30, 60, and 90 minutes. If symptoms of hypoglycemia are excessive, the patient can be given intravenous glucose without fear of compromising the test's accuracy because the hypoglycemic stress will have already occurred. In a normal response, GH exceeds 7 ng per milliliter, and cortisol exceeds 20 μ per deciliter. PRL usually increases to 30 ng per milliliter or more, but there is rarely a need to measure it during dynamic testing. The presence of seizure disorders or coronary artery disease is a contraindication for the test. The test also should be avoided in elderly people. Subnormal increments in GH without pituitary disease are seen in obese patients and in those with long-standing hypothyroidism and hypogonadism.

Other stimulation tests. GH is released by a number of pharmacologic agents including *levodopa, arginine,* and *apomorphine* (Table 150-1). All work through activation of hypothalamic pathways. Obesity blunts the GH response to hypoglycemia. *Chlorpromazine* and *metoclopramide* are antidopaminergic drugs that stimulate PRL secretion (Table 150-1). These PRL stimulatory tests do not aid in the diagnosis of PRL-secreting pituitary tumors. Lysine vasopressin directly stimulates the pituitary to release ACTH (Table 150-1). This agent directly tests the pituitary-adrenal axis while it bypasses the hypothalamus. It is best given by intravenous infusion but can also be given as an intramuscular injection. Side effects are abdominal pain, nausea, defecation, and occasional attacks of angina. Side effects have limited the clinical application of vasopressin stimulation, and the test is obviously contraindicated in patients with coronary artery disease or hypertension.

Tests utilizing feedback inhibition. *Metyrapone* inhibits the adrenal enzyme 11-beta-hydroxylase, thereby blocking the conversion of 11-deoxycortisol to cortisol (Fig. 150-4). Cortisol levels fall, and because 11-deoxycortisol is not an effective inhibitor of ACTH, ACTH levels increase. This stimulates the production of more 11-deoxycortisol, which is measured directly in the blood by radioimmunoassay or in the urine as a 17-hydroxycorticosteroid. The test should not be done in patients with suspected adrenal insufficiency because the reduced cortisol production can precipitate adrenal crisis. The test is very helpful in identifying patients with pituitary-dependent Cushing's syndrome because this is the only variety of Cushing's syndrome in which the urinary 17-hydroxycorticosteroid level increases after administration of metyrapone. There are two varieties of the metyrapone test, an overnight test and a 3 day test. To perform the overnight test, metyrapone, 30 mg per kilogram, is given orally at midnight. At 8:00 AM, blood is drawn for 11-deoxycortisol and cortisol level determinations. The 11-deoxycortisol level should increase to more than 8 μ per deciliter in patients with a normal pituitary-adrenal axis, and the cortisol concentration should be less than 5 μ per deciliter (a low cortisol level indicates that the block of 11-hydroxylase is adequate). The 3 day test is accomplished by measuring a baseline urinary 17-hydroxycorticosteroid value and then administering 750 mg of metyrapone every 4 hours for six doses. The urinary 17-hydroxycorticosteroid concentration should increase two to three times over the baseline value on day 2 or day 3. Several drugs (diphenylhydantoin, phenobarbital, primidone, and phenylbutazone)

Table 150-1. Pituitary stimulation tests

Agent	Protocol	Normal response
Levodopa	500 mg is given orally; blood specimens are obtained at 0, 30, and 60 min	GH level should exceed 7 ng/ml
Arginine infusion	Dose of 0.5 g/kg (30 g maximum) is infused over 30 min; blood is drawn at 0, 30, 60, 90, and 120 min	GH level should exceed 7 ng/ml
Apomorphine	750 μ is given subcutaneously. Blood is obtained at 0, 30, 60, and 90 min	GH level should exceed 7 ng/ml
Metoclopramide	10 mg is given intravenously; blood is collected at 0, 30, 60, and 90 min	PRL level exceeds 100 ng/ml
Chlorpromazine	25 mg is injected intramuscularly; blood is obtained at 0, 30, 60, and 90 min	PRL level increases 2 times baseline level or achieves an absolute value >20 ng/ml
Vasopressin	Infuse 2 U/h over 2 hours with blood specimens collected at 0, 30, 60, and 120 min	Plasma cortisol should exceed 20 μ/dl

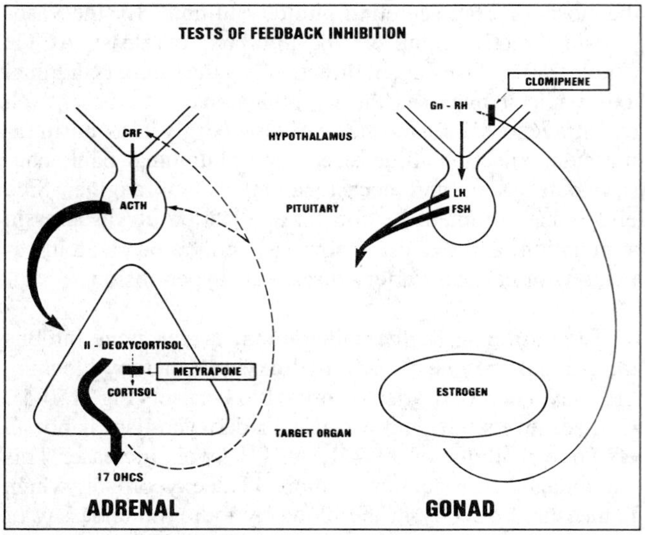

Fig. 150-4. Metyrapone and clomiphene cause increasing trophic hormone secretion by blocking feedback inhibition. Metyrapone blocks the conversion of 11-deoxycortisol to cortisol by inhibiting the enzyme 11-beta-hydroxylase. Cortisol levels fall, thereby diminishing feedback inhibition. This results in increased ACTH secretion. Clomiphene, a weak estrogen analog, binds to hypothalamic estrogen receptors and blocks estrogen feedback inhibition, resulting in increased gonadotropin secretion. ACTH, adrenocorticotropic hormone.

may accelerate the clearance of metyrapone and cause the urinary 17-hydroxycorticosteroid response to be blunted or absent.

Clomiphene citrate is an estrogen analog that blocks estrogen effect. Loss of estrogen feedback activity at the hypothalamus causes gonadotropin secretion to increase, allowing evaluation of the hypothalamic-pituitary axis (Fig. 150-4). To conduct the test, pooled specimens of LH and FSH are obtained on day 1, and then clomiphene is given orally, 50 mg twice daily, for 10 days. The maximum gonadotropin response is usually seen approximately 10 days after beginning the drug. FSH and LH should increase by at least 50% over baseline levels when measured at day 10. Depression is the only major side-effect. Ovulation may be induced in a previously infertile woman.

Suppression tests. The *dexamethasone suppression test* measures the intactness of glucocorticoid-ACTH feedback regulation. Patients with a higher setpoint of ACTH secretion or autonomous cortisol secretion are resistant to dexamethasone suppression. The test is used for the diagnosis of Cushing's syndrome. There are two types of dexamethasone suppression tests, an overnight screening test and a 6 day test used for definitive diagnosis. The overnight screening test is performed by giving 1 mg of dexamethasone at 11 P.M. and obtaining an 8 A.M. plasma cortisol level. This amount of glucocorticoid is sufficient to suppress ACTH (cortisol) secretion in normal individuals but not in patients with Cushing's syndrome regardless of type. Normal individuals suppress the cortisol level to less than 5 μ/dl. In patients with Cushing's syndrome the level remains greater than 5 μ/dl and is often above 10 μ/dl. The 6 day test, when coupled with an accurate 8 A.M. plasma ACTH level determination, allows the physician to distinguish between the different types of Cushing's syndrome. The 6 day test is divided into two parts. Initially, a "low dose" (0.5 mg q6h) and then a "high dose" (2 mg q6h) of dexamethasone are administered. The low dose suppresses ACTH secretion (and therefore cortisol level) in normal individuals but not in patients with Cushing's syndrome. Patients with pituitary-dependent Cushing's syndrome, however, show ACTH suppression when they are given sufficiently high doses of dexamethasone. This higher threshold of suppression occurs because of an altered feedback mechanism to glucocorticoids. Patients with other varieties of hypercortisolism such as ectopic ACTH secretion and adrenal tumors show no change in cortisol secretion regardless of the dosage of dexamethasone given. Thus the differential response to low-dose dexamethasone is used to separate normal individuals from patients with Cushing's syndrome, and the high-dose test separates patients with pituitary-dependent Cushing's syndrome from those with adrenal tumors or ectopic ACTH secretion. Adrenal tumors suppress ACTH concentration to undetectable levels, allowing them to be distinguished from the ectopic ACTH syndrome, which has a high ACTH concentration. False-positive results may result from accelerated metabolism of dexamethasone induced by certain drugs such as diphenylhydantoin, phenobarbital, primidone, and phenylbutazone. Thyrotoxicosis also increases the clearance of dexamethasone and may cause a false-positive result.

Glucose suppression of GH is used to evaluate autonomous GH secretion. In normal individuals GH secretion is suppressed to less than 2 ng per milliliter 60 to 120 minutes after 100 g of oral glucose is given. In contrast, acromegalic patients rarely show a decrease to less than 5 ng per milliliter, and in some instances a paradoxic increase of GH occurs. To perform this test, 100 g of glucose is given orally, and GH level is measured 90 minutes later. It is not helpful to obtain a baseline GH level.

Basal pituitary hormone measurements. A basal level of PRL is useful in the evaluation of hyperprolactinemia. A concentration of greater than 200 ng per milliliter almost always indicates a PRL-secreting pituitary tumor. Values less than this are not discriminatory because they may be due to tumors as well as to other causes of hyperprolactinemia (Chapter 160).

In patients with suspected hypothyroidism a basal *TSH* concentration should always be obtained with the initial battery of thyroid function studies. A low or normal TSH level in patients with established hypothyroidism indicates that hypothalamic or pituitary disease is responsible because with even mild primary hypothyroidism the TSH level is elevated. (Fig. 150-5 illustrates the principle of loss of feedback inhibition with increased secretion of trophic hormone.) A caveat is the "sick euthyroid syndrome" (Chapter 162), in which a low total thyroxine (T_4) level is seen

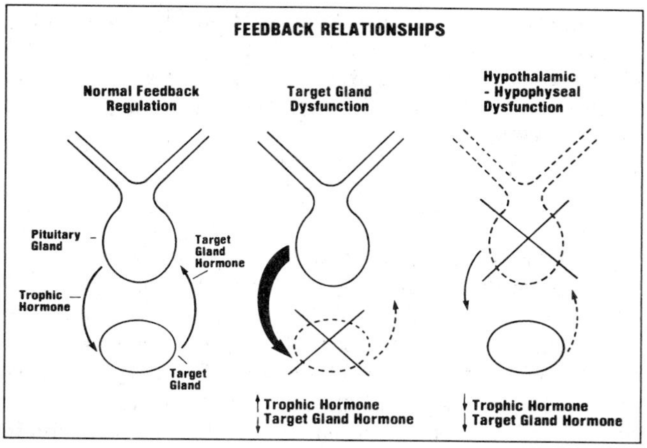

Fig. 150-5. Normally the endocrine target hormone causes feedback suppression of its anterior pituitary trophic hormone. With loss of target gland function, feedback inhibition decreases, causing increased trophic hormone secretion. Hypothalamic-hypophyseal dysfunction results in both decreased trophic hormone level and target hormone secretion.

Table 150-2. Gonadotropins

Clinical state	LH mIU/ml	FSH mIU/ml
Prepubertal	2-6	1-3
Adult	6-25*	4-20*
Menopausal, castrate	>25	>20

*Midcycle peak of LH is 2 to 3 times baseline value and for FSH is approximately 2 times baseline value.

with a normal TSH level. These patients are not clinically hypothyroid and have normal levels of free T_4.

The same principle applies to *LH* and *FSH* measurements as that described for TSH. A low or normal concentration in the presence of low gonadal steroid levels suggests hypothalamic or pituitary disease (Table 150-2). In women, such information must be interpreted in conjunction with the menstrual cycle because in the early follicular phase both gonadotropin and gonadal steroid levels may normally be low. As a rule, however, women with normal menstruation rarely need evaluation for hypogonadism.

Basal ACTH levels are helpful in the diagnosis and differentiation of Cushing's syndrome (Fig. 150-6). High levels are seen with ectopic ACTH syndrome, and undetectable levels are observed with adrenal tumors. It is not necessary to measure ACTH level to document that hypocortisolism is primary rather than secondary. Normal ACTH levels vary widely between 20 and 110 pg per milliliter. Higher concentrations are seen in normal individuals in response to stress.

Determination of a basal *GH* level is rarely helpful in evaluation of either GH deficiency or GH excess. In contrast, measurement of *somatomedin C* level by radioimmunoassay gives useful information about both of these conditions. Somatomedin C (insulin-like growth factor) is the mediator of GH action. In acromegaly, somatomedin C levels are usually greater than 4 units per milliliter. GH deficiency is suggested by values lower than the age-related lower limits listed in Table 150-3. One unit of somatomedin C is equal to 32.1 ng.

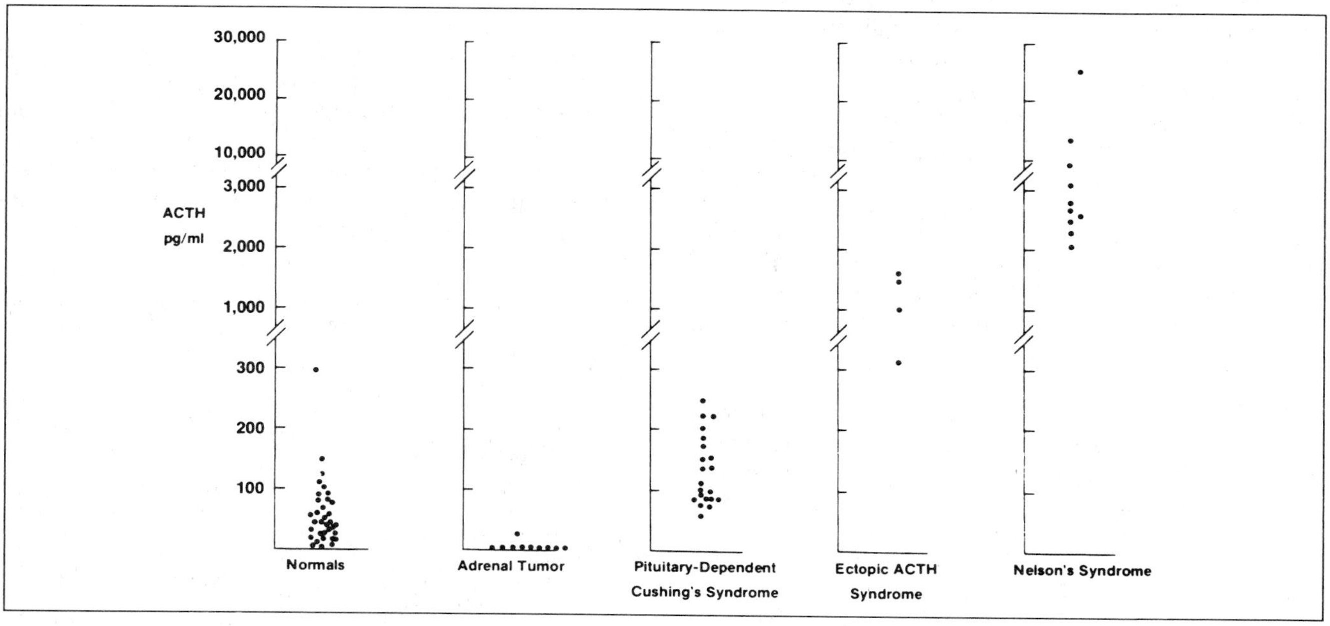

Fig. 150-6. Plasma ACTH concentration in patients with Cushing's syndrome. (From Cook et al: West J Med 132:111, 1980.)

Table 150-3. Normal age-related changes of somatomedin C

	Somatomedin C concentration (U/ml)	
Age in years	Male	Female
0-3	0.08-1.1	0.11-2.2
3-6	0.12-1.6	0.18-2.4
6-11	0.22-2.8	0.41-4.4
11-13	0.28-3.7	0.99-6.8
13-15	0.90-5.6	1.2-5.9
15-18	0.91-3.1	0.71-4.1
Adult	0.34-1.9	0.45-2.2

Posterior pituitary testing (Chapter 161)

Plasma vasopressin concentration. Measurement of the plasma vasopressin concentration with a simultaneously performed plasma osmolality evaluation is an accurate method of diagnosing diabetes insipidus. A low vasopressin concentration with elevated plasma osmolality is virtually diagnostic of central diabetes insipidus. Patients with elevated vasopressin concentration in the face of an elevated plasma osmolality and polyuria have nephrogenic diabetes insipidus, assuming that hypotension, diabetes mellitus, and salt-wasting nephropathy are excluded. Unfortunately few reliable assays are available to the clinician. There also is a delay of days to weeks before the results of the assay are available and a diagnosis established.

Water deprivation

The water deprivation test assesses the urine-concentrating ability of a patient and the effect of exogenously administered vasopressin on urine osmolality. In patients with diabetes insipidus urine is not concentrated during water deprivation despite developing hyperosmolality. Vasopressin is then given, to decrease free water clearance and allow the urine to become concentrated in patients with central diabetes insipidus. Patients with nephrogenic diabetes insipidus do not respond to vasopressin, and the urine remains dilute. In patients with primary polydipsia the urine is concentrated during water deprivation, although not always to normal values. They do not respond to vasopressin if water deprivation has been continued to the point of maximum urine osmolality. The testing procedure protocol is outlined in Chapter 161.

Water loading. Most cases of inappropriate vasopressin secretion (SIADH; inappropriate secretion of antidiuretic hormone) can be diagnosed on the basis of the history, physical examination, serum and urine electrolyte levels, and plasma and urine osmolality. Occasionally, however, it is necessary to subject a difficult-to-diagnose patient to water loading. Most individuals excrete 50% of an administered water load (20 ml/kg body weight of tap water given over 30 minutes) within 4 hours. Failure to do so is presumptive evidence of SIADH if hypocortisolism and hypothyroidism are excluded. Drugs such as chlorpropamide, clofibrate, diphenylhydantoin, and procainamide may decrease water clearance and cause false-positive results. As a precautionary measure, hourly serum osmolarity should be determined.

Tests of thyroid function (Chapter 162)

Radioimmunoassay of thyroid hormone. Thyroid hormone radioimmunoassays (RIAs) routinely measure the total thyroxine level (T_4-RIA) and the total triiodothyronine concentration (T_3-RIA). Because most of the circulating T_4 and T_3 is bound to thyroglobulin (99.95% and 99.5%, respectively), the assay results are greatly affected by drugs and clinical conditions that alter thyroid-binding globulin (TBG) concentration (Chapter 162). The normal T_4-RIA is 5.5 to 11.5 μ per deciliter. The normal T_3-RIA concentration is 80 to 195 ng per deciliter. A number of conditions decrease the conversion of T_4 to T_3 and subsequently cause low total levels without hypothyroidism (refer to the box below). For this reason and also because the T_3 level often remains normal despite mild hypothyroidism, the T_3-RIA is an unsuitable screening test for hypothyroidism.

Free thyroid hormone concentration. Measurement of the free thyroid hormone level is more difficult and expensive than assays that measure the total thyroid hormone concentration. Generally, the free T_4 or the free T_3 concentration is determined by equilibrium dialysis. Newer, less time-consuming methods have appeared, including kits that measure the free T_4 by radioimmunoassay. The reliability of these faster methods, however, is still in question. The advantage of determining the free thyroid level is that changes in TBG do not affect the result. The normal free T_4 concentration is 0.8 to 2.4 ng per milliliter, and the normal free T_3 level is less than 350 pg per milliliter.

Thyroid-stimulating hormone. The use of monoclonal antibodies has increased the sensitivity of the TSH assay to the degree that low TSH levels can be distinguished from normal. Conventional TSH assays are only capable of discriminating high levels from normal. The sensitive TSH assay is useful as a screening test for hyperthyroidism. Suppressed TSH levels coupled with borderline or elevated thy-

Conditions that decrease conversion of T_4 to T_3

- Caloric restriction
- Acute febrile illness
- Liver disease
- Renal insufficiency*
- Burns
- Drugs (propranolol, glucocorticoids, propylthiouracil, iodinated contrast agents)

*T_4 level also may be low.

roid hormone levels are indicative of primary hyperthyroidism. Not all commercially available assays are uniformly accurate, however, and some euthyroid patients have suppressed sensitive TSH levels. An elevated TSH level with high thyroid hormone levels suggests the rare disorder of secondary hyperthyroidism from a pituitary or hypothalamic source. High TSH levels, however, are usually indicative of primary hypothyroidism. A value of less than 0.4 μU per milliliter is low or suppressed, values 0.5 to 5 μU per milliliter are normal, and values greater than 7 μU per milliliter are elevated.

Thyroid hormone-binding globulin. TBG level is assessed indirectly by the T_3 resin uptake test (Fig. 150-7). This test measures the capacity of a resin to bind radioactive T_3 in the presence of TBG. The key to understanding the test is the realization that TBG binds radiolabeled T_3 preferentially compared with the resin. In hyperthyroidism excess thyroid hormone occupies the TBG, leaving few sites for the radiolabeled T_3 to be bound. Thus most of the added radiolabeled T_3 is bound by the resin, giving a high resin uptake. In hypothyroidism, there are many unoccupied thyroid hormone-binding sites on TBG; therefore most of the T_3 is bound by TBG and little is taken up by the resin, resulting in a low resin uptake. Confusing results may be obtained in the presence of conditions that either increase or decrease TBG level (Fig. 150-7). Estrogens, for example, increase TBG level and cause more thyroid hormone to be bound, thus increasing the total thyroid hormone concentration. A new equilibrium is reached, however, and the free thyroid hormone level remains normal. Because of excess TBG, more radiolabeled T_3 is bound, causing the resin uptake to be low. Thus a paradoxic situation results in which the total T_4 (or total T_3) level is elevated, but the T_3 resin uptake is low. Conversely, if TBG levels are reduced, the total thyroid hormone level is low, but the resin uptake is elevated. The normal T_3 resin uptake value varies among laboratories. A common normal range is 25% to 35%. TBG can be measured directly by radioimmunoassay. In most instances, however, this offers little advantage compared with the less expensive T_3 resin uptake test. The normal TBG concentration is 1 to 15 mg per deciliter.

Corrected thyroxine concentration. A simple calculation can be performed to correct for alterations in the total T_4 concentration induced by changes in TBG.

$$\text{Corrected total } T_4 = \text{patient's } T_4 \times \frac{\text{patient's } T_3 \text{ resin uptake}}{\text{average } T_3 \text{ resin uptake}}$$

For example, if the patient's T_4 concentration is elevated to 14 μ per deciliter but the T_3 resin uptake value is low at 20%, it is unclear whether or not hyperthyroidism is present. Using the equation, the corrected T_4 is 9.3 μ%.

$$14\ \mu \times \frac{20}{30} = 9.3\ \mu\%$$

The average T_3 resin uptake value is the midpoint between the upper and lower limits of the particular T_3 resin uptake assay being used. The normal range for the corrected T_4

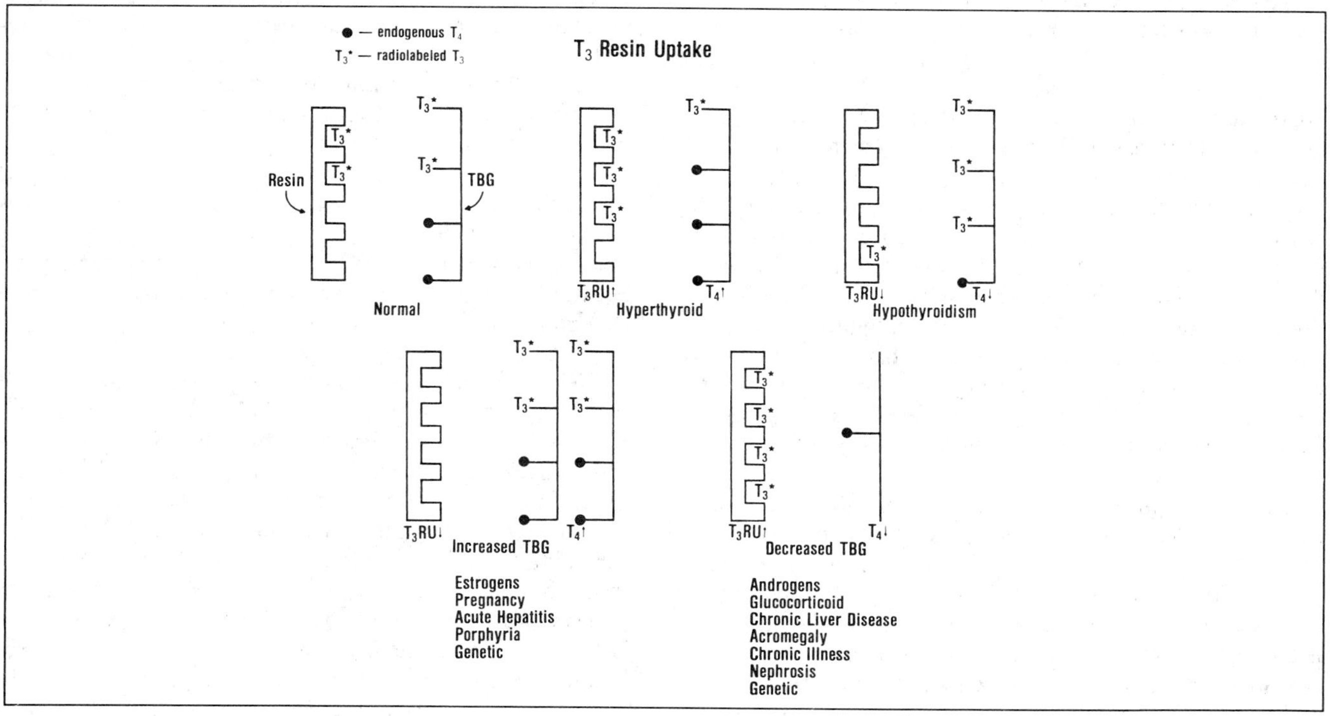

Fig. 150-7. The effects of hyperthyroidism, hypothyroidism, increased TBG, and decreased TBG on the T_3 resin uptake. Clinical states that either increase or decrease TBG concentrations are listed.

concentration is the same as that of total T_4. A similar calculation is used to determine a corrected total T_3 level.

Antithyroid microsomal antibodies and antithyroglobulin antibodies. Circulating antibodies to these antigens imply inflammation and destruction of thyroid tissue. High titers of either antibody strongly suggest autoimmune lymphocytic thyroiditis (Hashimoto's thyroiditis). It is unusual, however, for knowledge of these antibody titers to influence the management of a patient.

Serum thyroglobulin level. Normal individuals usually have low but readily detectable levels of thyroglobulin in serum. After a total thyroidectomy, however, thyroglobulin levels should be undetectable while taking replacement amounts of thyroid hormone. This relationship makes thyroglobulin level a useful index to follow in patients with thyroid cancer. Detectable levels after thyroidectomy for thyroid cancer or the subsequent development of titers usually indicates the presence of metastatic disease. Thyroglobulin is also helpful for differentiating between "painless" subacute thyroiditis and factitious hyperthyroidism (Chapter 162). Patients with subacute thyroiditis should have high levels reflecting thyroid gland damage and release of its products into the circulation, whereas patients taking thyroid hormone have low or undetectable thyroglobulin levels. In normal individuals thyroglobulin levels vary from 5 to 25 ng per milliliter.

T_3 suppression test. In normal individuals, exogenously administered T_3 suppresses TSH secretion, which in turn decreases the thyroid uptake of radioiodine. Resistance to suppression indicates either autonomous thyroid hormone secretion, as occurs in Graves' disease, or toxic multinodular goiter. The test is accomplished by performing a 24 hour radioiodine uptake determination and then administering 75 μ of T_3 for 10 days. On the tenth day the 24 hour uptake test is repeated (the tracer dose is given on the ninth day). Most normal persons suppress the uptake to less than 2%. Patients with autonomous thyroid hormone secretion show less than 50% suppression of the baseline radioiodine uptake. The test is helpful in patients who have symptoms that suggest hyperthyroidism but show equivocal results in thyroid function testing. Thyrotoxic symptoms may develop during the period of T_3 administration; therefore concurrent administration of a beta-blocking agent increases patient tolerance of the test. The test is contraindicated in individuals with coronary disease and in the elderly.

TSH stimulation test. The TSH stimulation test measures the ability of the thyroid gland to incorporate radioiodine in response to exogenously administered TSH. The test can determine whether or not primary hypothyroidism is present in a patient taking thyroid hormone, although it is a somewhat impractical means of accomplishing this end. A response to TSH does not exclude hypothyroidism secondary to hypothalamic or pituitary disease. Its major use is to distinguish silent subacute thyroiditis from factitious hyperthyroidism. The damaged gland in the former condition prevents uptake of iodine, whereas patients taking thyroid hormone, even to the point of hyperthyroidism, still have normal uptake (>10%) in response to TSH. Bovine TSH, 10 units daily, is administered for 3 days, and the radioiodine uptake test is performed on the third day. Occasionally, severe allergic reactions occur, so patients should be skin-tested with TSH before testing.

Thyroid-stimulating immunoglobulin. Thyroid-stimulating immunoglobulin (TSI) is an antibody to the TSH receptor. TSI is usually detectable in patients with Graves' hyperthyroidism. Its measurement, however, is rarely helpful in the diagnosis or treatment of thyroid disease.

Pentagastrin and calcium stimulation tests of calcitonin. Patients with medullary thyroid cancer secrete calcitonin after the administration of pentagastrin or calcium to a much greater extent than normal individuals. Pentagastrin is given at a dose of 0.5 μ per kilogram or 150 mg per kilogram of calcium chloride is infused over 10 minutes and blood is collected at 0, 2, 5, and 10 minutes. Basal levels are normally less than 20 pg per milliliter in women and less than 30 pg per milliliter in men. With a tumor, stimulated values almost always exceed 425 pg per milliliter. Normal individuals may show some increase, but it is considerably smaller.

Adrenal medullary hormones (Chapter 164)

Metanephrines. Metanephrine and normetanephrine are formed when epinephrine and norepinephrine, respectively, are methylated by the enzyme catechol-O-methyltransferase. Together, these urinary catecholamine metabolites are termed *metanephrines*. A 24 hour urine collection for metanephrines is an accurate, reliable, simple, and cost-effective screening test for the diagnosis of pheochromocytoma. Normal values are less than 1.3 mg per 24 hours.

Vanillylmandelic acid. Vanillymandelic acid (VMA) is a metabolic product formed by the action of monoamine oxidase on metanephrines. It is also a good screening test but is somewhat less sensitive than metanephrines. Normal excretion is less than 8 mg per 24 hours.

Urinary catecholamines. Normally, only about 1% of plasma catecholamines are excreted in the urine unchanged. In patients with pheochromocytoma, this figure may approach 10%. Unfortunately, the assay is affected by many interfering agents and is technically difficult to perform. Thus it is less valuable than metanephrines or VMA as a screening test. Fractionation of the total urinary catecholamines into epinephrine or norepinephrine may be useful in patients with multiple endocrine neoplasia types IIA and IIB. Patients with these disorders who also have a pheochromocytoma may have an elevation of only the epinephrine fraction of the total urinary catecholamines. Normal adults excrete 20 to 70 μ of norepinephrine and 0 to 15 μ of epinephrine during a 24 hour period.

Plasma catecholamines. A carefully collected and meticulously measured plasma catecholamine determination is a very sensitive method for diagnosing pheochromocytoma. At present, however, few commercially available assays can duplicate the sensitivity of the expensive and technically difficult research assays. We therefore reserve plasma catecholamine level measurement for cases in which clinical suspicion is very high but results of repeated urine studies are normal. The clinician should take special care to choose a laboratory that has an assay of proven reliability. When the measurement is made, the patient should be medication free. An indwelling, heparinized catheter should be inserted, and the patient should remain supine for 30 minutes before collection. This will reduce the chance of stress-induced plasma catecholamine elevation. Total catecholamine level is usually greater than 2000 pg per milliliter in patients with pheochromocytoma. Normal values are listed in Table 150-4.

Clonidine suppression. If results of urine and blood studies are equivocal for pheochromocytoma or if suspicion remains high despite normal testing results, clonidine suppression of plasma norepinephrine levels may be helpful. Clonidine is a central alpha-adrenergic stimulant that ultimately results in diminished sympathetic outflow and a fall in norepinephrine levels. If norepinephrine production is autonomous, as it is with a pheochromocytoma, norepinephrine levels remain elevated and unchanged 3 hours after 0.3 mg of oral clonidine. Norepinephrine levels generally fall into the normal range if another cause is generating the hypertension even if the basal level is elevated. However, false-negative and false-positive results occasionally occur.

Agents interfering with catecholamine assays. In general, interfering agents are most likely to cause spurious elevation of the urinary and plasma catecholamine levels. Metanephrines are least likely to be affected, although x-ray contrast media such as sodium diatrizoate (Renografin) depress values for as long as 1 week. VMA colorimetric assays that rely on a diazotized p-nitro-aniline reaction are sensitive to interference with numerous dietary substances such as coffee, tea, chocolate, bananas, cheese, and vanilla. This method is now used infrequently, and dietary restriction before VMA measurement is usually not necessary. Clinical conditions, including acute myocardial infarction, diabetic ketoacidosis, burns, and shock, all may cause elevations of catecholamine levels and those of their urine metabolites. Table 150-5 lists the drugs that may interfere with each of the assays.

Table 150-4. Plasma catecholamine concentration

	Epinephrine (pg/ml)	Norepinephrine (pg/ml)
Basal	25-70	150-400
Major stress*	100-500	200-2000
Hypertension	20-100	200-5000
Pheochromocytoma	50-2000	>2000

*Hypoglycemia, surgery, cardiac ischemia.

Adrenal cortex (glucocorticoids) (Chapter 163)

Plasma cortisol. Blood cortisol levels are measured by radioimmunoassay. Because it is released in a pulsatile fashion, random measurements are rarely diagnostic of either hypocortisolism or hypercortisolism. An exception, however, is the acutely ill patient with adrenal crisis. Major stress causes the cortisol level to exceed 20 μ per mil-

Table 150-5. Agents interfering with catecholamine assays

	Metanephrines	VMA	Catecholamines
Drugs that increase urine metabolites			
Methylxanthine	↑	↑	↑
Ephedrine	↑	↑	↑
Amphetamines	↑	↑	↑
Catecholamines	↑	↑	↑
Clonidine withdrawal	↑	↑	↑
Hydralazine	↑	↑	↑
Minoxidil	↑	↑	↑
Nitroglycerin	↑	↑	↑
Nifedipine	↑	↑	↑
Tricyclic antidepressants*	↑	↑	↑
Levodopa	↑	↑	↑
Nalidixic acid	—	↑	—
Bretylium	—	—	↑
Methylphenidate	—	—	↑
Glyceryl guaiacolate	—	↑	—
Quinidine	—	—	↑
Quinine	—	—	↑
Isoproterenol	—	—	↑
Drugs that decrease urine metabolites			
Alpha methylparatyrosine	↓	↓	↓
Clonidine	↓	↓	↓
Reserpine	↓	↓	↓
Guanethidine	↓	↓	↓
Clofibrate	—	↓	—
Disulfiram	—	↓	—
Sodium diatrizoate	↓	—	—
Drugs that have a mixed effect on urine metabolites			
Ethanol	↑	↓	↑
Methyldopa	↑	↓	↑
Methenamine mandelate	—	↓	↑
MAO inhibitors	↑	↓	↑
Chlorpromazine	—	↓	↑

*Acute effect.

liliter in normal persons. A concentration significantly less than this is strong evidence of adrenal insufficiency. Patients receiving estrogens may have extremely elevated plasma cortisol levels (>60 μ/ml) without Cushing's syndrome because of an estrogen-induced increased production of cortisol-binding globulin. Some clinicians measure morning and evening cortisol levels as a screening test for Cushing's syndrome because there is a loss of circadian cyclicity in this disorder. Normal 8:00 A.M. levels are 6 to 22 μ per milliliter. The P.M. cortisol level should be measured between 10:00 P.M. and midnight when the concentration is less than 5 μ per deciliter. Values obtained earlier than 10:00 P.M. may still approach morning levels and may therefore be misleading.

Urinary 17-hydroxycorticosteroids. The urinary 17-hydroxycorticosteroid test measures the 17,21-dihydroxy-20-keto metabolites of cortisol and cortisone and, when the formation of these compounds is inhibited by metyrapone testing, the metabolites of 11-deoxycortisol. Like plasma cortisol, 17-hydroxycorticosteroid levels are seldom helpful as an isolated measurement. The advantage of this measurement over a plasma cortisol measurement is that secretion is evaluated over a 24 hour period. Normal values are 3 to 10 mg per 24 hours (or 2.5 to 7.0 mg/g of creatinine).

Urinary free cortisol. Less than 1% of cortisol is excreted unchanged in the urine. Measurement of the free cortisol level is particularly valuable as a screening test for Cushing's syndrome because more than 90% of patients have elevated values. Urine free cortisol is not a reliable screening test for adrenal insufficiency. Acute illness and pregnancy may cause false elevations. Normal levels vary greatly from laboratory to laboratory depending on the extraction procedure used to remove cortisol. A common normal range is 20 to 90 μ in 24 hours. In some assays, however, the upper limit of normal is only 35 μ in 24 hours, whereas in others a value as high as 240 μ in 24 hours may be normal.

ACTH stimulation tests. ACTH directly stimulates the adrenal gland to secrete cortisol. The lack of an increase of cortisol or urinary 17-hydroxycorticosteroid level (if they are low at onset) demonstrates primary adrenal insufficiency. The test does not reliably detect secondary adrenal insufficiency. There are two varieties of tests, a rapid test and a prolonged test. Most cases of adrenal insufficiency are adequately demonstrated with the rapid test. To perform the rapid test, 250 μ of cosyntropin is administered either intramuscularly or intravenously. After 1 hour the injection is repeated. One hour after the second injection, blood is drawn for cortisol measurement. In normal individuals the cortisol level increases to an absolute value of greater than 20 μ per milliliter. Although a baseline cortisol value at 0 minute is often obtained, it rarely adds useful information to the patient's evaluation.

To demonstrate primary adrenal insufficiency definitively, the long ACTH stimulation test is used. This test is conducted by measuring baseline urinary 17-hydroxycorticosteroids on day 1 and day 2. On days 3, 4, and 5, 250 μ of cosyntropin is administered intravenously for 8 hours each day while urine collection for 17-hydroxycorticosteroids continues. By day 5, in normal individuals 17-hydroxycorticosteroid levels increase to greater than 25 mg in 24 hours. Patients with hypopituitarism have a stepwise increase of the urinary 17-hydroxycorticosteroid level even if the value on day 5 is less than 25 mg in 24 hours. Patients with primary adrenal insufficiency show little or no increase at any time during the test. Patients can be treated with dexamethasone 0.5 mg twice daily to prevent the development of symptomatic adrenal insufficiency during the 5 day test. Dexamethasone does not cross-react with assays for cortisol or 17-hydroxycorticosteroid level.

Adrenal cortex (androgens)

Urinary 17-ketosteroids. Androgens such as androstenedione, dehydroepiandrosterone, and androsterone are metabolized to 17-ketosteroids. All of these compounds have a keto group at C-17. Although measurement of the 17-ketosteroids provides an assessment of both adrenal and ovarian androgen production, testosterone normally forms less than 1% of this metabolite. Thus patients with testosterone-secreting tumors may have normal levels of urinary 17-ketosteroids. Very high 17-ketosteroid levels are seen in androgen-secreting adrenal tumors (especially adrenal carcinoma) and congenital adrenal hyperplasia. Women normally excrete 5 to 15 mg in 24 hours and men 5 to 17 mg in 24 hours. Because 24 hour urine collections can be cumbersome, a single determination of a blood dehydroepiandrosterone sulfate level (discussed later) has largely replaced measurement of 17-ketosteroids.

Plasma dehydroepiandrosterone and DHEA-sulfate. Approximately 80% of dehydroepiandrosterone (DHEA) is formed by the adrenal gland. DHEA-sulfate is a sulfated conjugate and is present in higher quantities than is DHEA. Also, a somewhat higher percentage of total DHEA-sulfate is of adrenal origin than is the total percentage of circulating DHEA. However, either can be used to evaluate adrenal androgen secretion, and in many laboratories measurement of one or the other hormone has replaced 17-ketosteroid values because of its ease of collection. Normal concentrations of DHEA and DHEA-sulfate in women are 3 to 6 ng per milliliter and 850 to 1350 ng per milliliter, respectively. DHEA in men ranges from 4 to 7.5 ng per milliliter and DHEA-sulfate from 1100 to 1600 ng per milliliter.

Plasma 17-hydroxyprogesterone. 17-Hydroxyprogesterone is the precursor of 11-deoxycortisol in the cortisol synthetic pathway. Its conversion to 11-deoxycortisol is dependent on the enzyme 21-hydroxylase. Thus patients with the 21-hydroxylase deficiency variety of congenital adrenal hyperplasia (the most common type) and 11-hydroxylase deficiency have elevated basal levels of 17-hydroxyprogesterone that may be 5- to 50-fold higher than normal.

Patients with mild deficiency of 21-hydroxylase may have elevated levels only after ACTH stimulation. Unstimulated levels in normal women are 25 to 85 ng per milliliter in the follicular phase, and 100 to 275 ng per milliliter in the luteal phase. In men, normal levels are less than 25 ng per milliliter. One hour after administration of 250 μ of cosyntropin, in normal individuals 17-hydroxyprogesterone levels rarely increase to greater than 300 ng per milliliter. In congenital adrenal hyperplasia, levels increase to greater than 1000 ng per milliliter even in mild deficiency states when the basal 17-hydroxyprogesterone concentration is normal.

Adrenal cortex (mineralocorticoids)

Plasma aldosterone. The concentration of aldosterone in blood is highly dependent on posture and salt intake. With normal salt intake (approximately 110 mEq/day), the supine plasma aldosterone level is 5 to 15 ng per deciliter, and the 2 hour upright level is 20 to 75 ng per deciliter. To diagnose primary hyperaldosteronism, it is necessary to demonstrate poor suppressibility of aldosterone with salt administration; this can be done with the *saline infusion test*. The test is performed by infusing 2 L of saline solution over a 4-hour period with the patient recumbent. In patients with an aldosterone-secreting tumor, the plasma aldosterone concentration is usually not suppressed to less than 10 ng per milliliter, although levels occasionally fall below this in patients with bilateral hyperplasia of the zona glomerulosa.

18-Hydroxycorticosterone. Measurement of this mineralocorticoid is useful to separate patients with an aldosterone-secreting adenoma from those with bilateral hyperplasia. The 18-hydroxycorticosterone concentration is less than 60 ng/dl in patients with hyperplasia, whereas patients with an adenoma have values greater than 100 ng/dl.

11-Deoxycorticosteroid. The level of 11-deoxycorticosteroid (DOC) is elevated in patients with congenital adrenal hyperplasia from 11- and 17-hydroxylase deficiency. It also is elevated in some patients with ectopic ACTH syndrome and adrenal carcinoma. The normal concentration is 4 to 12 ng per deciliter.

Plasma renin activity. Plasma renin activity (PRA) is not a direct measurement of plasma renin concentration. Rather, it is a determination of the ability of plasma to generate angiotensin I from renin substrate. Normal levels are highly dependent on volume status, posture, and salt intake (Table 150-6). Patients with primary mineralocorticoid excess almost invariably have subnormal PRA even under conditions that stimulate renin. One stimulating procedure is to maintain a low-salt diet for 4 days and then measure PRA. Another means of evaluating PRA is to institute a low-salt diet for 2 days and then administer 80 mg of furosemide, then for the patient to maintain upright posture for 4 hours (Table 150-6).

Table 150-6. Plasma renin activity

	ng/ml/hr
Normal diet (100 mEq/day)	
Supine	1.1 ± 0.8
Upright	1.9 ± 1.7
Low-salt diet (10 mEq/day)	
Supine	2.7 ± 1.8
Upright	6.6 ± 2.5
Diuretic and low-salt diet	10.0 ± 3.7

Urinary aldosterone excretion. As with plasma aldosterone, the urinary aldosterone level depends on volume status and salt intake. During high-normal sodium intake (greater than 120 mEq/day) aldosterone excretion ranges between 4 and 17 μ per 24 hours. Values higher than 17 μ per 24 hours during salt loading suggest a diagnosis of primary aldosteronism. After 4 days of salt restriction (10 mEq/day), the urinary aldosterone excretion should be 20 μ per 24 hours. Patients with isolated aldosterone deficiency generally have values of less than 15 μ per 24 hours during salt restriction.

Tests of male gonadal function (Chapter 166)

Testosterone. Testosterone level is measured by radioimmunoassay. Its determination should be accompanied by gonadotropin level measurement. Low testosterone levels with low gonadotropin values suggest pituitary-hypothalamic disease, whereas with primary testicular disease gonadotropin concentrations are high with a low testosterone level. Acute or chronic stress also may lower the testosterone level in the absence of gonadal disease. The normal adult male concentration is 350 to 1200 ng per deciliter.

Estradiol. Estradiol level should be measured in men with gynecomastia and other feminizing conditions. Elevated levels are seen with neoplasms, liver disease, and hyperthyroidism and in older men. In normal men, the estradiol level should not exceed 45 pg per milliliter.

Beta-subunit human chorionic gonadotropin. Beta-subunit human chorionic gonadotropin, placental hormone is produced by trophoblastic tumors, germinal cell neoplasms, and nongerminal cell cancers such as adenocarcinoma of the lung, gastric cancer, and islet cell tumors. The presence of beta-human chorionic gonadotropin in a man with gynecomastia or impotence of recent onset is an indicator of serious disease. Normally, levels should be undetectable or very low (less than 5 mIU/ml).

Chorionic gonadotropin stimulation. During the onset of puberty it may be necessary to assess the capacity of the testis to secrete testosterone because at this time low gonadotropin secretion may normally exist with low testosterone levels. A dose of 1500 units of human chorionic gonadotropin is injected intramuscularly, and testosterone level is measured 48 hours later. Values should be increased into the normal adult male range (300 to 1200 ng/dl), thereby indicating that the testosterone secretory capacity of the testis is normal.

Semen analysis. Semen analysis is an excellent test of gonadal function. Normal parameters indicate that gonadal function is normal without the need to perform hormonal analysis (which is generally more expensive). A normal sperm count is 20 to 50 million sperm per milliliter with 60% of the sperm demonstrating normal structure. Fertility, however, has been documented in men with counts of less than 10 million per milliliter. The normal volume of the ejaculate is between 2 and 6 ml. It is sometimes helpful to test for the presence of seminal fructose. Fructose is the product of the seminal vesicles, and its absence in azoospermic men implies blocked ejaculatory ducts or congenital absence of the vas deferens. Specimens for semen analysis should be collected by masturbation after at least 48 hours of sexual abstinence and should be examined within 1 hour of collection.

Tests of female gonadal function (Chapter 165)

Estradiol. Estradiol concentration varies widely during the normal human menstrual cycle (Table 150-7). In amenorrheic patients, estradiol levels may be needed to evaluate ovarian secretory capacity. Gonadotropins also should be obtained to allow separation of primary and secondary deficiency states.

Progesterone. In some women, progesterone secretion is inadequate to maintain the corpus luteum and may account for infertility. Normal levels are listed in Table 150-7.

Total testosterone. Testosterone level is often elevated in women with anovulation or hirsutism. Mild elevations are seen in polycystic ovarian disease and other nonneoplastic virilizing disorders. Patients with testosterone-secreting tumors generally have levels that are greater than 200 ng per deciliter. Normal values are 20 to 90 ng per deciliter.

Unbound testosterone. Approximately 99% of testosterone is bound in women. In some women with hirsutism, the total testosterone concentration is normal, but the unbound fraction is elevated. Normal unbound levels range from 0.09 to 1.2 ng per deciliter.

Table 150-7. Estrogen and progesterone concentration in women

Phase of cycle	Estradiol (pg/ml)	Progesterone (ng/dl)
Early follicular	10-30	—
Late follicular	30-70	2-90
Luteal	100-300*	600-3000
Menopausal	5-25	<30

*Midcycle estradiol peak may be up to 600 pg per milliliter.

Androstenedione. Androstenedione is a relatively weak androgen which originates from the ovary, adrenal glands, and by conversion in peripheral tissues. Although it has several sources, its level is commonly elevated in women with an ovarian cause (e.g., polycystic ovarian disease) of hyperandrogenization. Normal levels are 50 to 250 ng/dl.

Dihydrotestosterone. Testosterone is converted to the potent androgen dihydrotestosterone (DHT) by the enzyme 5-alpha-reductase. DHT is the major androgen that affects hair follicles. Elevated levels indicate increased 5 alpha reductase activity, although level of androstanediol glucuronide (discussed later) is probably a better measure of this activity. Normal DHT levels range from 5 to 30 ng/dl.

Androstanediol glucuronide. Androstanediol glucuronide is a tissue metabolite of DHT, and serum levels correlate well with 5 alpha reductase activity and androgen cellular activity. Absolute increases in level of this metabolite are often found in hirsuite women with normal levels of total and unbound testosterone. The finding of an elevated androstanediol level, however, does not often affect therapy and the test should not routinely be done for the diagnosis of hirsutism. Normal adult female levels are 60 to 800 ng/dl.

Progesterone withdrawal test. The progesterone withdrawal test evaluates whether there is sufficient estrogen secretion to cause endometrial development in women with amenorrhea. If estrogen effect is present, a normal menstrual period will occur after administration of progesterone. Withdrawal bleeding indicates that the hypothalamic-pituitary-gonadal-uterine axis is intact. Lack of bleeding gives no information about the level of the defect. To perform the test, 10 mg of oral medroxyprogesterone is administered for 5 days. Alternately, 100 mg of progesterone-in-oil as a single dose can be given intramuscularly. Vaginal bleeding should occur within the following 14 days.

Sequential estrogen-progesterone stimulation. Patients who do not have vaginal bleeding after progesterone withdrawal should be treated with sequential estrogen and progesterone to exclude a primary endometrial disorder as the cause of amenorrhea. If, despite adequate hormonal stimulus, there is no bleeding, an endometrial cause of the amenorrhea is likely. If bleeding occurs, the lesion is at a level higher than the endometrium. The test is completed by administering either 2.5 mg of conjugated estrogens or 0.2 mg of ethinyl estradiol for 21 days. On day 16, 10 mg of medroxyprogesterone is added and continued until day 21. In the following 10 days, menstrual bleeding should appear. For the test result to be conclusively abnormal, the cycle of medication should be repeated three times without the occurrence of vaginal bleeding.

Basal body temperature. Basal body temperature is measured to determine whether ovulation has occurred. The temperature is taken for 5 minutes before the woman gets out of bed in the morning. Normally, temperatures are stable during the follicular phase, but just before ovulation, a dip is seen. If ovulation occurs and progesterone secretion is sufficient to maintain the corpus luteum, the basal body temperature increases by at least 1° F.

Genetic studies

Buccal smear. Cells with more than one X chromosome have detectable chromatin (Barr body) on the nuclear membrane. Normal women have 20% to 40% of somatic cells with Barr bodies. In men the total is less than 5%. To obtain cells, the cheek is scraped with a metal spatula, and the cells are smeared on a glass slide and then placed in a fixative. The slide is then stained and read by a technician experienced in cytologic analysis.

Chromosomal analysis. Chromosomal analysis is very expensive and as a rule does not need to be done for confirmation of disorders such as Turner's syndrome, Klinefelter's syndrome, XX sex reversal syndrome, and XYY syndrome. Women with gonadal dysgenesis and virilization, however, should have a karyotype. In this case, the finding of a Y chromosome indicates that testicular elements are probably present in the gonad. This abnormality requires surgical intervention because such gonads are at increased risk for malignant degeneration.

Miscellaneous

Urinary 5-hydroxyindoleacetic acid. 5-Hydroxyindoleacetic acid (5-HIAA) is a product of serotonin metabolism. Its excretion is above normal in almost all patients with the carcinoid syndrome. Dietary products that contain serotonin must be excluded before measurement; these include walnuts, bananas, avocados, chocolate, and red plums. Cough preparations that contain glyceryl guaiacolate falsely elevate 5-HIAA level, and phenothiazines falsely depress 5-HIAA level. Reserpine releases serotonin and can cause a mild elevation. False elevations are also seen in nontropical sprue. Normal excretion is from 5 to 9 mg per 24 hours; however, most patients with carcinoid excrete more than 50 mg per 24 hours. Modest elevations of less than 25 mg per 24 hours are often due to one of the factors mentioned other than carcinoid.

Gastrointestinal hormones. A basal *gastrin* level of more than 500 pg per milliliter in a patient with acid hypersecretion is highly suggestive of a gastrinoma (Zollinger-Ellison syndrome). Gastrin values between 250 and 500 pg per milliliter are equivocal and require evaluation with the *secretin stimulation test*. It is performed by administering 2 IU/kg of secretin intravenously and collecting blood at 0, 2, 5, and 10 minutes. The gastrin level increases by at least 200 pg per milliliter in patients with a gastrinoma. Duodenal ulcer, gastric outlet obstruction, retained antrum, G cell hyperplasia or hypertrophy, and renal insufficiency may cause elevations of basal gastrin levels but do not show an increase after secretin. *Somatostatin* is produced by somatostatinomas and can be measured in blood. Patients with somatostatinomas have levels that range from 150 to 100,000 pg per milliliter. Normal individuals have levels of less than 80 pg per milliliter.

Insulin. Measurement of insulin is useful in evaluating a patient with fasting hypoglycemia. During a fast, when the plasma glucose concentration is less than 40 mg %, the plasma insulin level should be less than 5 to 10 μU per milliliter. Values higher than this are very suggestive of insulinoma if C-peptide is also elevated (discussed later). Higher fasting insulin levels are seen in obese patients without insulinoma as a result of insulin resistance. In thin and normal-weight persons, the insulin/glucose ratio should be less than 0.25 when the plasma glucose level is less than 40 mg %.

Connecting peptide. Connecting peptide (C-peptide) is formed when proinsulin is cleaved into insulin. It is therefore an indicator of endogenous insulin secretion. Hypoglycemic patients with inappropriately elevated insulin level but undetectable or low C-peptide concentration probably have factitious hypoglycemia from insulin injection because commercially prepared insulins do not contain C-peptide. Sulfonylurea agents, however, stimulate C-peptide secretion, and patients taking these drugs cannot be distinguished from insulinoma patients on the basis of a high C-peptide concentration. Normal fasting levels of C-peptide range from 1 to 2 ng per milliliter.

REFERENCES

Cryer PE: Diagnostic endocrinology. Oxford, 1979, Oxford University Press.

Dudley R: Chemiluminescence immunoassay: an alternative to RIA. Lab Med 21:216, 1990.

Goldzieher JW et al: Improving the diagnostic reliability of rapidly fluctuating plasma hormone levels by optimized multiple sampling techniques. J Clin Endocrinol Metab 43:824, 1976.

Kater CE et al: Stimulation and suppression of the mineralocorticoid hormones in normal subjects and adrenocortical disorders. Endocr Rev 10:149, 1989.

Nakamura T et al: The value of paramagnetic contrast agent gadolinium-DTPA in the diagnosis of pituitary adenomas. Neuroradiology 30:481, 1988.

Sheps SG et al: Recent developments in the diagnosis and treatment of pheochromocytoma. Mayo Clin Proc 65(1):88, 1990.

Spencer CA et al: Thyrotropin secretion in thyrotoxic and thyroxine-treated patients: assessment by a sensitive immunoenzymetric assay. J Clin Endocrinol Metab 63:349, 1986.

Vaitukaitis JL: Hormone assays. In Felig P et al, editors: Endocrinology and metabolism. New York, 1987, McGraw-Hill.

CHAPTER

151 Diagnostic Approach to Bone and Mineral Disorders

Gregory R. Mundy
Charles A. Reasner II

SERUM CALCIUM

The total serum calcium level has three components. About 45% is protein bound (predominantly to albumin) and is biologically inert, about 5% is complexed or chelated to citrate and is also biologically inert, and about 50% belongs to the ionized or free component, which is metabolically active. Measurements of the ionized calcium component are not generally available except in special laboratories and as a special procedure. The autoanalyzers used in most laboratories measure total serum calcium level accurately and reproducibly, although probably not as accurately as the atomic absorption spectrophotometer. The normal total serum calcium concentration is between 8.5 and 10.2 mg per deciliter of serum unless there are abnormalities in the serum proteins. The serum calcium level is a remarkably well guarded variable, but it should be appreciated that the only component of the total serum calcium level that is regulated by calciotropic hormones is the ionized calcium. Clinicians should not base decisions on the total serum calcium concentration without considering changes in concentrations of plasma proteins, particularly albumin. The ionized calcium component is more difficult to measure than the total serum calcium, and, provided the serum protein concentrations can be measured, measurements of ionized calcium are rarely necessary. One possible exception occurs in patients with myeloma in whom the total serum calcium concentration is occasionally increased as a result of excessive binding of calcium to the myeloma protein, while ionized calcium level may be normal. In these patients, the ionized calcium determination would be useful. The blood for serum calcium evaluation should be drawn without a tourniquet. It is also important to be aware of the changes that pH causes in the ionized calcium without changing the total calcium level. Alkalosis leads to a decrease in the ionized component, and acidosis leads to an increase in the ionized component of calcium.

As a general rule, one can correct for changes in the serum albumin by adding 0.8 mg per deciliter to the total serum calcium level for every gram of albumin that the serum albumin is less than 4.0 g per deciliter of serum. Expressed as a formula for a patient with suspected hypercalcemia or hypocalcemia, corrected total serum calcium level = observed total serum calcium − 0.8 (4.0 − measured serum albumin level in g/dl). The normal corrected total serum calcium concentration is 8.5 − 10.2 mg per deciliter. The serum calcium concentration at which symptoms result from hypocalcemia or hypercalcemia cannot be predicted with certainty. It depends on both the rapidity of change and the absolute serum calcium concentration. However, patients rarely experience symptoms caused by hypocalcemia if the corrected serum calcium level is greater than 8 mg per deciliter and rarely have symptoms produced by hypercalcemia if the corrected serum calcium level is less than 11 mg per deciliter.

URINE CALCIUM

Urine calcium excretion is useful in the differential diagnosis of recurrent renal calculi and in the diagnosis of familial hypocalciuric hypercalcemia, a condition readily confused with asymptomatic primary hyperparathyroidism. Urine should be collected for 24 hours in containers with an acid preservative, and creatinine should be determined on the same specimen to ensure adequacy of the collection. Urine calcium concentration is an important parameter to follow in patients with hypoparathyroidism who are being treated with vitamin D and calcium supplementation. The dose of vitamin D should be titrated against the urine calcium level so that urine calcium does not rise over 350 mg per day. This is usually accomplished with a serum calcium level that is below the normal range but still high enough to keep the patient asymptomatic because the effect of parathyroid hormone (PTH) of increasing calcium reabsorption is absent. In the differential diagnosis of idiopathic hypercalciuria, it is important to know the calcium intake because normal calcium excretion varies considerably with dietary calcium level. Although any absolute criterion for the diagnosis of hypercalciuria is arbitrary and is likely to include some normal individuals and overlook some patients with abnormal calcium homeostasis or abnormal renal tubular calcium handling, on an average daily intake of 600 to 1000 mg of elemental calcium, most normal men have urine calcium excretion of less than 300 mg per day, and women have less than 250 mg per day. In idiopathic hypercalciuria, values are higher. On a restricted calcium diet (400 mg/day), most normal men have urine calcium excretion of less than 250 mg per day, and normal women have less than 200 mg per day. In familial hypocalciuric hypercalcemia, urine calcium excretion is usually less than 100 mg per day despite hypercalcemia.

SERUM ALKALINE PHOSPHATASE

Alkaline phosphatase is an enzyme found in and released by active osteoblasts. Its precise physiologic role is still a mystery, although it is likely to be involved in bone mineralization. An increased serum alkaline phosphatase concentration is associated with increases in bone formation. The concentration of this enzyme in the serum reflects bone turnover and is usually elevated when bone resorption is increased, for example, during childhood and in hyperthyroidism, because bone formation and bone resorption are linked or coupled. The enzyme is secreted from cells into the blood and is measured routinely on small samples of serum in an autoanalyzer. The most striking increases in serum alkaline phosphatase concentration occur in Paget's disease and occasionally in osteoblastic metastases caused by metastatic carcinoma. Alkaline phosphatase level is also usually increased in patients with osteolytic metastases from metastatic solid tumors. However, it is often normal in patients with myeloma, reflecting the fact that bone formation is usually not increased in this disorder. The total serum alkaline phosphatase concentration is composed of a number of isoenzymes produced by both the liver and the bone. These may be distinguished by electrophoresis or by the relative heat lability of the bone fraction at 56° C for 15 minutes ("bone alkaline phosphatase burns"). In the near future, bone-specific alkaline phosphatase level is likely to be measured by using monoclonal antibodies. Liver alkaline phosphatase concentration is increased in biliary tract obstruction and in hepatocellular disease. Elevation of the concentration of alkaline phosphatase of liver origin is accompanied by increases in other serum enzymes of hepatic origin, including gamma glutamic pyruvic transaminase and 5′ nucleotidase.

SERUM BONE GLA PROTEIN

The bone Gla protein (also called osteocalcin) is a major protein constituent of the bone matrix whose function is unclear. It may function as an inhibitor of normal bone mineralization. It comprises 20% of the noncollagenous protein in bone. It can be measured in the serum by radioimmunoassay as a parameter of increased bone turnover, and in particular as a parameter of osteoblastic activity. Recently developed sandwich assays using monoclonal antibodies may improve the sensitivity and specificity. Circulating concentrations do not correlate perfectly with serum alkaline phosphatase concentration, and it is likely that these two proteins are the products of different cells in the osteoblast lineage. This measurement is primarily an investigative tool currently, and its clinical usefulness remains to be determined.

URINE HYDROXYPROLINE

Hydroxyproline is an amino acid that is almost unique to collagen and is a breakdown product of collagen degradation. Its urinary excretion can be measured, and it reflects increased collagen turnover from any source including bone. However, urinary hydroxyproline level varies with the diet. For accurate assessment of collagen turnover, the patient should be on a gelatin-free diet. This limits the usefulness of the test. Urinary hydroxyproline is increased in any condition associated with increased collagen turnover such as Paget's disease, thyrotoxicosis, or acromegaly. It has limited clinical use but has been a reasonable marker of response to therapy in patients with Paget's disease. In patients with Paget's disease who are being treated with bisphosphonates or calcitonin, the fall in urinary hydroxyproline level appears several weeks before the fall in alkaline phosphatase level, suggesting that the reduction in bone formation is due to the inhibition of osteoclastic bone resorption caused by the drug therapy.

URINARY EXCRETION OF COLLAGEN PYRIDINIUM AND DEOXYPYRIDINIUM CROSSLINKS

Pyridinoline (Pyr) and deoxypyridinoline (D-pyr) are two nondigestible pyridinium crosslinks present in the mature form of collagen. D-pyr is present only in significant amounts in the type 1 collagen of bone. Thus its measurement in the urine is a reflection of rates of bone resorption. Because its urinary excretion is not altered by diet, it has potential as a much more helpful measure of rates of bone resorption than urine hydroxyproline level. Preliminary information indicates that urinary D-pyr is increased in all states of increased bone resorption, including the postmenopausal period in women.

It should be remembered that the techniques of measurement of bone mineral density, bone histomorphologic characteristics, and biochemical markers of rates of bone resorption measure essentially different things. The biochemical markers reflect bone turnover in the whole skeleton but give no information about local or regional changes. In contrast, bone histomorphometry limits assessments to a localized area of the skeleton but does provide morphologic information on the nature of the abnormality. Bone mineral density provides a static measurement at one point in time but gives no information on structure or relative rates of bone resorption or bone formation. These techniques are thus complementary.

SERUM PHOSPHORUS

Serum phosphorus concentration is determined in most laboratories by autoanalyzer. It is not as tightly regulated as the serum calcium level and can vary by 50% in the normal individual with changes in diet, fasting, vomiting, or renal function. The serum phosphorus value may fall by 30% 2 hours after a carbohydrate-rich meal, and this should be considered when serum phosphorus level measurements are being assessed. It also varies with age and sex and is slightly higher in females than in males at any age but is clearly higher in childhood and adolescence when bone turnover is high. However, the serum phosphorus concentration is a helpful additional diagnostic parameter in measurement of the serum calcium level in patients with hypercalcemia and hypocalcemia. The measurement of phosphate excretion and its expression as the tubular reabsorption of phosphate (TRP), fractional excretion of phosphate, or tubular maximal reabsorption of phosphate as a fraction of the glomerular filtration rate (GFR [T*m*P/GFR]) is useful in patients with hypophosphatemia in whom renal phosphate loss is suspected; however, it is less useful in the differential diagnosis of hypercalcemia, because patients with primary hyperparathyroidism or malignancy may have increased urinary phosphate excretion.

IMMUNOREACTIVE PARATHYROID HORMONE

Parathyroid hormone (PTH) level is now readily measurable in the serum by radioimmunoassay. For many years this assay was beset with problems, but these problems have been resolved considerably during the last 5 years. Prior difficulties were caused by fragmentation of PTH that occurs in the circulation that yielded multiple circulating fragments varying both in biologic activity and in immunoreactivity. PTH measurements by the newer immunoradiometric assays (IRMAs) are valuable because they measure the complete intact molecule (Table 151-1).

The biologically active portion of the PTH molecule resides in the first 34 amino acids from the amino or N-terminal end. The carboxy terminal (C-terminal) end of the molecule is biologically inert. Unfortunately, the portions of the PTH molecule that have been most readily measured by immunoassay in the past are not biologically active. Most of the earlier assays used antibodies that cross reacted with fragments that included the carboxy terminus of the PTH molecule, called *C-terminal assays*. Results from these assays are difficult to interpret in patients with impaired renal function because the C-terminal fragments of PTH depend on the kidneys for clearance. Immunoreactive plasma PTH concentrations increase according to these assays when the serum creatinine level is greater than 2 mg per deciliter. The newer amino terminal or N-terminal assays more closely reflect minute-to-minute secretion by the parathyroid gland and measure the biologically active portion of the molecule. The amino-terminal assays were more useful in patients with renal failure or in those in whom it was necessary to localize abnormal parathyroid tissue using selective sampling of veins draining the neck and mediastinum.

Older intact or midregion assays have some of the advantages of both the C-terminal and N-terminal assays, although the fragments they detect also depend on the adequacy of renal function.

There is probably no point in measuring PTH unless the serum calcium level is abnormal. By and large, measurement of immunoreactive PTH is most useful in making the differential diagnosis of hypercalcemia and in particular in distinguishing patients with primary hyperparathyroidism from those with other causes of hypercalcemia. Patients who have a PTH concentration that is 30% greater than the top of the normal range in any assay can be confidently diagnosed as having primary hyperparathyroidism in the absence of renal failure. A PTH measurement in the normal range is difficult to distinguish from low values in most of the commonly available assays, and probably in all assays some patients with proven primary hyperparathyroidism have values in the normal range. Nomograms comparing serum PTH values with serum calcium values have been widely used but have often been overinterpreted. In the differential diagnosis of hypocalcemia, measurement of PTH should distinguish patients with pseudohypoparathyroidism from those with primary hypoparathyroidism. In the latter condition, secretion of PTH does not occur and the immunoreactive serum concentrations are low. In patients with pseudohypoparathyroidism (peripheral tissue resistance to PTH), the serum concentrations are increased secondary to hypocalcemia. Another use of the PTH assay is to follow patients with chronic renal failure and secondary hyperparathyroidism.

In using PTH assays it should be emphasized that only one assay should be used in following one patient, because assays are likely to vary in terms of the tracer, the standard, and the antisera. Several studies have been performed comparing the older assays from different laboratories and have shown considerable discrepancies.

Table 151-1. Disorders of calcium metabolism—use of circulating measurements of calcium, phosphorus, and PTH concentrations

Serum Ca	Serum P	Plasma PTH	Disorder
↑	↑	↓ or Nl	Increased gut absorption of calcium (vitamin D intoxication, sarcoidosis, milk-alkali syndrome)
↑	↑	↑	Hypercalcemia of any cause and renal failure
↑	↓	↑	Primary hyperparathyroidism
↑	↓	↓ or Nl	Humoral hypercalcemia of malignancy
↓	↓	↑	Vitamin D deficiency, hypomagnesemia*
↓	↑	↑	Pseudohypoparathyroidism, renal failure, acute pancreatitis
↓	↑	Nl or ↓	Primary hypoparathyroidism

*PTH release is stimulated by acute hypomagnesemia. In contrast, chronic hypomagnesemia is associated with low serum PTH. Nl, normal.

VITAMIN D METABOLITES

Two biologically active metabolites of vitamin D, 25-hydroxyvitamin D and 1,25-dihydroxyvitamin D, are frequently measured in the blood. The serum 25-hydroxyvitamin D measurements are more useful clinically. This metabolite is the major circulating form of the vitamin and reflects vitamin D intake. It is particularly valuable if the physician suspects either vitamin D intoxication or vitamin D lack caused by dietary deficiency or malabsorption. The 25-hydroxyvitamin D level is measured by competitive protein-binding assay, and normal values are in the range of 10 to 80 ng per milliliter. Levels are higher in patients living in sunny climates and during the spring and summer. Concentrations of less than 5 ng per milliliter are seen in vitamin D deficiency.

1,25-Dihydroxyvitamin D is the most active metabolite of vitamin D, but it is more difficult to measure, and knowledge of the serum concentration has limited clinical usefulness. This hormone is increased in patients with hypercalcemia produced by sarcoidosis and other granulomatous diseases, in those with primary hyperparathyroidism, and in some patients with lymphomas. However, the 1,25-dihydroxyvitamin D level provides only slightly more information than measurement of the serum calcium in these situations. Possibly one situation where it is clearly indicated is the rare patient with rickets caused by tissue resistance to 1,25-dihydroxyvitamin D (vitamin D–dependent rickets type II). In this syndrome, the serum 1,25-dihydroxyvitamin D concentrations are markedly increased.

SERUM CALCITONIN

Serum immunoreactive calcitonin concentration is easier to measure than PTH level, and there are better correlations from laboratory to laboratory in the results. Unfortunately, it has limited clinical usefulness. Calcitonin levels are increased in patients with medullary carcinoma of the thyroid and are used in such patients for making the diagnosis as well as for monitoring response to therapy or for recurrence. Calcitonin measurement can also be used for localizing the site of tumor by selective venous sampling. In patients with early disease or with familial medullary thyroid carcinoma when the disease is still occult, abnormal calcitonin level measurements may be recognized only after provocative testing with pentagastrin or calcium infusion. Both of these agents are calcitonin secretagogues, and patients with excess calcitonin-secreting cells usually show an exaggerated calcitonin response after their administration. Of these two secretagogues, pentagastrin is the more reliable. Serum calcitonin level is lower in women than in men at all ages, but recent data suggest that there is no age-related decrease, despite earlier reports to the contrary. Some patients with nonthyroid malignancies may have high circulating calcitonin levels produced by ectopic secretion. Ectopic calcitonin is usually biologically inert.

URINARY CYCLIC ADENOSINE MONOPHOSPHATE

The measurement of urinary cyclic adenosine monophosphate (AMP) level gives information similar to that yielded by PTH assays, and its concentration in urine depends mainly on biologically active PTH. As with the PTH immunoassay, measurements are difficult to interpret in the presence of renal failure. Urinary cyclic AMP values have been used in the differential diagnosis of the subtypes of idiopathic hypercalciuria, but the clinical usefulness in this situation is doubtful. In the differential diagnosis of hypercalcemia, many patients with hypercalcemia of malignancy also have an increase in urinary cyclic AMP level. Therefore the efficacy in distinguishing malignancy from primary hyperparathyroidism as the cause of hypercalcemia is limited. The major use of urinary cyclic AMP level in the past has been to distinguish pseudohypoparathyroidism from primary hypoparathyroidism. In the latter condition, there is a sharp rise in urinary cyclic AMP level after PTH infusion, whereas in the former condition there is tissue insensitivity to PTH. Nephrogenous cyclic AMP level has been measured by many workers in investigative studies but probably does not give more useful clinical information than the simpler measurement of urinary cyclic AMP level. The urine collection should be made in the same way as that for urinary calcium determination. Ideally, the measurement should be expressed in terms of the glomerular filtration rate, that is, as nanomoles per deciliter of glomerular filtrate.

BIOCHEMICAL MARKERS OF RATES OF BONE RESORPTION AND BONE FORMATION

Accurate measurements of overall rates of bone resorption and bone formation would be very helpful in clinical practice. For example, to assess efficacy of therapies that inhibit bone resorption, an inexpensive measurement of resorption rates such as a biochemical parameter that can be determined by noninvasive techniques would be very useful (see the box below). Biochemical markers are not useful for diagnosis, because they are not specific for the different disease states. An exception may be Paget's disease of bone, in which rates of bone resorption and bone formation may greatly exceed those of other conditions, and markers such as urine hydroxyproline or serum alkaline phosphatase level may be so markedly increased that the diagnosis is apparent.

BONE HISTOMORPHOMETRY

Quantitative bone histomorphometry data obtained from nondecalcified biopsy specimens from the iliac crest are now frequently used to make an accurate diagnosis of the nature of a metabolic bone disease. Bone biopsies are particularly useful in the differential diagnosis of osteopenia. The technique is to take a through-and-through section of bone from the iliac crest by percutaneous needle biopsy after the patient takes two short courses of tetracyline separated by a known number of days, usually 10. Tetracycline is laid down at the site of mineral deposition, and this technique allows measurement of rates of bone formation in terms of the mineral apposition rate. Tetracyclines can be identified in nondecalcified bone sections because these an-

Biochemical markers of bone turnover

Markers of bone formation

Serum total and bone specific alkaline phosphatase
Serum osteocalcin (bone Gla protein)
Serum procollagen 1 extension peptides

Markers of bone resorption

Total and dialyzable urine hydroxyproline
Urine pyridinoline and deoxypyridinoline (collagen cross-links)
Serum tartrate–resistant acid phosphatase

tibiotics have a characteristic fluorescence in ultraviolet light. A suitable labeling regimen is to give tetracycline hydrochloride (500 mg po bid) for 2 days, wait 10 days, and then give demethylchlortetracycline (demeclocycline 300 po bid) for 4 days. The biopsy is taken 2 to 4 days after cessation of the demeclocycline. Drugs that interfere with absorption of tetracyclines such as phosphate binders or antacids should be avoided while the tetracyclines are being administered.

The bone biopsy specimen must be nondecalcified so that evaluation of the amount of mineralized bone relative to unmineralized bone can be assessed. This is necessary for the diagnosis of osteomalacia. The bone biopsy also allows evaluation of the surfaces involved in osteoclast activity, but unlike bone formation, no measurement of the rate of bone resorption is possible. The biopsy needle must be of sufficient size and diameter to permit the core of bone to be removed without compression or distortion, which would make it impossible to assess the relative trabecular bone volume. The procedure is generally well tolerated and is associated with low morbidity. Bone histomorphometry is most useful clinically in the differential diagnosis of osteopenia, particularly in distinguishing osteomalacia from osteoporosis (see the box below). Bone biopsy is also useful in assessing bone abnormalities in patients with renal osteodystrophy.

Although this technique provides valuable information, there are problems with sampling, because cellular events occurring in the iliac crest may not be representative of those in the thoracic or lumbar vertebrae. It allows the diagnosis of osteomalacia to be excluded, but it does not give a precise measurement of total bone mass because of the imprecision of the technique and the potential sampling error between the iliac crest and the spine. For the same reasons, it is not a useful technique for monitoring therapy. The most important parameters that can be determined are trabecular bone volume, mineral apposition rate, and percentages of the total bone surfaces involved in osteoclastic bone resorption and bone formation. In osteoporosis, there is a decrease in bone volume but no increase in unmineralized bone (osteoid tissue). In osteomalacia, there is an increase in osteoid tissue with a decrease in the mineral apposition rate. The osteoid tissue is assessed by the percentage of total bone surfaces covered with osteoid tissue and the width of the osteoid seams. In states of high bone turnover such as primary hyperparathyroidism, hyperthyroidism, or Paget's disease, there is increased osteoid tissue, but this can be distinguished from osteomalacia because in these conditions the mineral apposition rate is increased.

Possible assessments with bone biopsy

Osteoporosis

Volume of trabecular bone relative to volume of tissue

Osteomalacia

- Area of bone surface covered by osteoid tissue
- Width of osteoid seams
- Volume of osteoid tissue
- Mineral appositional rate (requires serial biopsies and tetracycline markers)
- Calcification front (requires tetracycline marker or special stains)

Others

- Area of bone surface involved in resorption (scalloped margins with or without osteoclasts)
- Area of bone surface involved in formation (lined by osteoblasts)

STEROID SUPPRESSION TEST

The steroid suppression test has a limited but definite place in the differential diagnosis of hypercalcemia. In this test 100 mg of cortisone acetate or its equivalent is given per day for 10 days, and the serum calcium level is measured on alternate days. Patients with primary hyperparathyroidism essentially never show a decrease in serum calcium concentration in response to glucocorticoids. However, the serum calcium level in patients with sarcoidosis or other causes of hypercalcemia produced by increased calcium absorption from the gut is almost invariably suppressed. About 30% of patients in whom malignant disease is responsible for hypercalcemia show suppression of the serum calcium level during the steroid suppression test. These tests are most useful in the asymptomatic patient in whom the plasma PTH determination is not diagnostic, and the possibility that sarcoidosis or occult malignancy is responsible for the hypercalcemia needs to be excluded.

MEASUREMENT OF BONE MINERAL CONTENT

During the past 20 years, a number of techniques for measuring bone mineral density have been introduced. The technology for measurement of bone mineral density and evaluation of patients with osteoporosis is continuing to evolve. These techniques have improved because of the growing interest in osteoporosis and have now become part of routine medical practice. Moreover, the great demand for these instruments together with improvements in technical performance have made the measurements less expensive. These instruments now make it possible not only to evaluate the total skeleton but also to evaluate bone mineral density in specific regions of the skeleton separately and thus provide information on the independent status of cortical and cancellous bone. These measurements also allow estimation of bone strength and prediction of future fracture risk. However, it should be appreciated that they do not make a diagnosis of specific bone diseases and do not distinguish the nature of the bone disease responsible for a decline in bone mineral density. Four techniques are widely used currently: single-beam photon absorptiometry, dual-beam photon absorptiometry (DPA), dual-energy x-ray absorptiometry (DEXA), and quantitative computed tomography (QCT). Newer noninvasive techniques, ultrasound and magnetic resonance imaging (MRI), are also currently being investigated.

Single-beam photon absorptiometry

The single-beam photon absorptiometry technique uses ^{125}I and a scintillation detector to measure bone mineral content in the forearm bones. The reproducibility and precision of the determination (approximately 2% to 3%) are impaired because of the difficulty of repositioning the forearm precisely in successive measurements. It gives information only on bone mineral densities in the distal extremities and cannot determine the nature or extent of diseases of generalized bone loss. This technique measures cortical bone predominantly, and correlations between changes in the bone mineral content in the cortical bone of the forearm and the bone mineral content of the cancellous bone of the vertebrae are often poor. For example, about 30% of persons with clinical osteoporosis have normal forearm bone mineral density according to some investigators. However, in individual patients with abnormal findings, this method may be useful for monitoring changes in bone mineral densities during a long period of observation. This is more likely to be valuable in primary hyperparathyroidism, in which beneficial therapeutic intervention is possible, than in osteoporosis, in which treatment is difficult for established disease. Because many patients with vertebral body collapse produced by osteoporosis have normal forearm bone mineral density measurements according to this technique, it is obviously inadequate as a screening test to select patients at risk for the development of osteoporosis. The radiation exposure is minimal, and recent technical advances using rectilinear scanning have improved both precision and sensitivity.

Dual-beam photon absorptiometry

The dual-beam photon absorptiometry (DPA) technique utilizes a multienergy isotope, gradolinium-135. It allows measurement of bone mineral content in the lumbar spine. It measures all the bone (both cortical and trabecular) in the vertebral body, with a precision of 2% to 3%. An online computer image is used to assess results. Modifications in the technique also allow measurement of bone mineral content in the femoral neck. This technique is still very new, and variations in results are reported by different groups. It has the advantage of measuring bone mineral density in the bones that are primarily affected in osteoporosis and age-related bone loss. The radiation exposure is minimal, but DPA scanning is time-consuming.

Computed tomography

The computed tomography (CT) technique uses CT scanners operated in a quantitative rather than an imaging mode. It measures a defined amount of trabecular bone in the vertebrae and compares it with a known standard. Bone in the femoral neck can also be examined. The precision and sensitivity of the current measurements are greatly improved, although there is still controversy about how reproducible and how accurate they are. Many investigators feel that the current techniques are not precise enough to allow meaningful sequential measurements. A major problem is that intramedullary fat and subcutaneous tissue can make the results difficult to interpret. Patients with dorsal kyphosis may find this procedure less acceptable than the other techniques because of discomfort in positioning the patient during the performance of the test.

Dual-energy X-ray absorptiometry

In the dual-energy x-ray absorptiometry (DEXA) technique, a dual x-ray source replaces the isotope source used in DPA. This technique has the advantage of greater accuracy and precision than DPA and can be performed much more rapidly. Moreover, radiation exposure is even lower. It is used for the same measurements and in the same situations as DPA. This is the current state-of-the-art method. Newer applications such as lateral spine scanning (which may provide better measurements of cancellous bone) and body composition analysis are now possible with this technique.

Newer techniques

The potential of ultrasound for measurement of bone mineral density is currently under evaluation. Ultrasound is a simple noninvasive technique that is being used to assess bone mineral density in the patella, cortical bone of the femur and radius, and os calcis. Magnetic resonance imaging (MRI) provides indirect measurements of bone mineral density and is still in the early stages of investigation.

REFERENCES

Bijvoet OLM: Kidney function in calcium and phosphate metabolism. In Avioli LV and Krane SM, editors: Metabolic bone disease, vol 1. New York, 1977, Academic Press.

Delmas PD: Clinical use of biochemical markers of bone remodeling in osteoporosis. In Christiansen C and Overgaard K, editors: Osteoporosis 1990. Third International Symposium on Osteoporosis, Copenhagen, 1990, Osteopress.

Delmas PD, et al: Urinary excretion of pyridinoline crosslinks correlates with bone turnover measured on iliac crest biopsy in patients with vertebral therapy. J Bone Min Res 6:639, 1991.

Dent CE: Cortisone test for hyperparathyroidism. Br Med J 1:230, 1956.

Eastell R and Riggs BL: Diagnostic evaluation of osteoporosis. Endocrinol Metab Clin North Am 17:547, 1988.

Epstein S: Serum and urinary markers of bone remodeling: assessment of bone turnover. Endocr Rev 9:437, 1988.

Eyre D: Collagen crosslinking amino-acids. Methods Enzymol 144:115, 1987.

Genant HK et al: Non-invasive bone mineral analysis: recent advances and future directions. In Christiansen C and Overgaard K, editors: Osteoporosis 1990, Third International Symposium on Osteoporosis, Copenhagen, Denmark, 1990, Osteopress.

Meunier PJ: Histomorphometry of the skeleton. In Peck WA, editor: Bone and mineral research annual 1. Princeton, 1983, Excerpta Medica.

Mundy GR: Anatomy, physiology and function of bone: bone resorbing cells. In Favus MJ, editor: Primer on the metabolic bone disease and disorder of mineral metabolism. Kelseyville, Calif, 1990, American Society for Bone and Mineral Research.

Mundy GR: Differential diagnosis of osteopenia. Hosp Pract 11:65, 1978.

Parfitt AM, Oliver I, and Villaneuva AR: Bone histology in metabolic bone disease: the diagnostic value of bone biopsy. Orthop Clin North Am 10:329, 1979.

Robins SP et al: Measurement of the cross linking compound, pyridinoline, in urine as an index of collagen degradation in joint disease. Ann Rheum Dis 45:969, 1986.

Uebelhart D et al: Effect of menopause and hormone replacement therapy on the urinary excretion of pyridinium crosslinks. J Clin Endocrinol Metab 72:367, 1991.

Uebelhart D et al: Urinary excretion of pyridinium crosslinks: a new marker of bone resorption in metabolic bone disease. Bone Mineral 8:87, 1990.

Watson L, Moxham J, and Fraser P: Hydrocortisone suppression test and discriminant analysis in differential diagnosis of hypercalcemia. Lancet 1:1320, 1980.

III CLINICAL SYNDROMES

CHAPTER 152 Weight Loss

Richard M. Jordan
Peter O. Kohler

Severe loss of weight in the absence of intentional dietary restriction is virtually always a sign of serious systemic or psychiatric disease. In general, this problem can be separated into two broad categories (see the box on the right). The first group of patients have weight loss with normal or excessive food intake. Insulin-dependent diabetes mellitus, thyrotoxicosis, and malabsorption belong in this category. The second group of patients have weight loss with diminished food intake. Here, the etiologic agent is often cancer, a psychiatric disorder, chronic infection, or gastrointestinal disease in which eating is associated with distressful symptoms. Some patients in this category have disease processes that actually cause increased caloric needs despite decreased intake. The disease states most notable for causing weight loss and the mechanisms by which weight loss is produced are briefly discussed later (Chapters 37 and 49).

Causes of weight loss

I. Weight loss with normal to increased food intake associated with unimpaired appetite
   A. Insulin-dependent diabetes mellitus
   B. Thyrotoxicosis
   C. Pheochromocytoma
   D. Carcinoid
   E. Malabsorption and maldigestion
   F. Intestinal parasite infestation
   G. Diencephalic syndrome
   H. Malignancy (uncommon)
   I. Luft's syndrome
II. Weight loss with normal or decreased food intake
   A. Impaired appetite that in some cases may be coupled with an increased caloric requirement
      1. Malignancy
      2. Psychiatric disorders (including anorexia nervosa)
      3. AIDS
      4. Liver disease
      5. Addison's disease
      6. Uremia
      7. Chronic infection
      8. Chronic lung disease
      9. Chronic inflammatory disease
      10. Cardiac cachexia
      11. Diabetic neuropathic cachexia
      12. Hypothalamic tumor (very rare)
   B. Unimpaired appetite but decrease of food intake secondary to other factors
      1. Gastric ulcer
      2. Duodenal ulcer with outlet obstruction
      3. Postgastrectomy syndrome
      4. Regional enteritis
      5. Ulcerative colitis
      6. Food faddism

ENDOCRINE DISORDERS

Endocrine diseases are almost always a consideration in the differential diagnosis of weight loss. Although clearly important, these disorders are less frequently responsible for weight loss than are gastrointestinal disease, malignancy, and depression.

Insulin-dependent diabetes mellitus, especially in young persons, often causes weight loss. This is in part a consequence of fluid and calorie loss secondary to glycosuria. Although many patients manifest polyphagia and polydipsia, some are anorectic. In patients with long-standing diabetes mellitus, additional factors may contribute to weight loss. The chronic debilitating nature of the disease may cause depression and anorexia. A few patients have gastric atony with greatly delayed gastric emptying (gastroparesis diabetacorum), causing nausea, vomiting, and painful abdominal distention. These symptoms discourage regular or adequate food ingestion and lead to poor diabetic control and undernutrition. Many diabetic patients develop a diarrhea that is commonly accompanied by steatorrhea, although uncomplicated diabetic steatorrhea is usually not a primary cause of weight loss. True malabsorption from celiac disease or pancreatic exocrine insufficiency, however, occasionally is associated with diabetes mellitus and must be considered in the diabetic patient with weight loss. Rarely, in older diabetic male patients profound weight loss is combined with autonomic and peripheral neuropathy (diabetic neuropathic cachexia). The cachexia is so impressive that malignancy is usually suspected. The pathophysiologic features of the disorder are unknown, but patients usually recover spontaneously after approximately 1 year.

Thyrotoxicosis and pheochromocytoma cause hypermetabolism and produce weight loss. In both diseases weight loss may be prominent despite excessive caloric intake. Usually, neither disorder is difficult to recognize. In elderly patients, however, hyperthyroidism may occur with very few of the classic symptoms (apathetic thyrotoxicosis). Thus unexplained weight loss in an older patient should always prompt the physician to measure the thyroid hormone concentrations. Luft's syndrome is a rare disease of skeletal muscle mitochondria in which there are excessive respiration and uncoupling of oxidative phosphorylation. Although not actually an endocrine disorder, the hypermetabolism present suggests the diagnosis of hyperthyroidism. The carcinoid syndrome may increase the metabolic rate, and when this is coupled with diarrhea and malabsorption (features that are often present), considerable weight loss can occur. Almost 50% of patients with carcinoid suffer a significant loss of body weight.

When Addison's disease presents insidiously, weight loss is a prominent manifestation. Weakness, fatigue, nausea, and abdominal cramping are all additive factors that cause anorexia and weight loss. Dehydration may also contribute. Hypothalamic tumors, although more commonly associated with marked obesity, can interfere with appetite generation and cause cachexia. Such patients have been diagnosed mistakenly as having anorexia nervosa. In early childhood, an anterior hypothalamic tumor sometimes causes a poorly understood disorder in which cachexia occurs despite increased food intake (diencephalic syndrome).

GASTROINTESTINAL DISEASE

Gastrointestinal disease causes weight loss through anorexia, distressful symptoms that discourage eating, and malabsorption. Chronic liver disease—especially chronic active hepatitis or alcoholic liver disease with cirrhosis—may cause anorexia and weight loss (Chapters 57 and 59).

In esophageal disorders, gastric ulcers, duodenal ulcers with outlet obstruction, postgastrectomy syndromes, and chronic pancreatitis, the ingestion of food may cause such discomfort that patients severely limit oral intake. Abdominal pain and bloody diarrhea initiated by eating may cause patients with regional enteritis and ulcerative colitis to experience significant weight loss. The edentulous patient may be incapable of mastication and lose weight.

Malabsorption or maldigestion can result from many diseases (Chapter 42). Although malabsorption is usually symptomatic and clinically quite evident, it can occasionally be subtle in presentation. Protein-losing enteropathy may also cause weight loss. The edema and ascites resulting from hypoalbuminemia may overshadow any gastrointestinal symptoms present.

PSYCHIATRIC DISORDERS

Anorexia nervosa is always a consideration when a young woman has unexplained weight loss (Chapter 37). The disorder is rare in men. Although there are differing theories concerning the psychiatric aspects of the disorder, virtually all patients demonstrate some degree of psychologic abnormality. Pathologic interrelationships between mother and daughter are commonly present. The conflict in many cases is the parent's need to stay in control, opposing the child's desire for independence. In some patients depression is present. This disorder has several endocrine manifestations, and some evidence suggests that anorexia nervosa may be associated with a hypothalamic disorder. Many (if not all) of the endocrine abnormalities, however, are also seen in simple starvation without anorexia nervosa.

In moderate to severe depressive illness, 70% to 80% of patients experience diminished appetite and weight loss. Because depression is present in up to 4% of the U.S. population, it is probably the single most overlooked disease in a medical practice. Schizophrenia, manic-depressive disorders, and chronic anxiety states may also be associated with weight loss. Drug dependence, especially alcoholism and narcotic addiction, commonly results in weight loss. The mechanism is complex and involves primary effects of the drugs, decreased intake of food, associated chronic illnesses, and depression. Rarely, transient weight loss occurs in patients who surreptitiously ingest thyroid hormones and amphetamines. Weight loss results primarily from induced hypermetabolism and muscle wasting and, in the case of amphetamines, from anorexia. Weight usually stabilizes, however, in spite of continued ingestion of these agents. Extremely heavy tobacco abuse also is a cause of anorexia and weight loss.

CANCER

The possibility of cancer is always a major concern in any unexplained weight loss. The cause of weight loss is usually multifactorial. The basal metabolic rate is often elevated, with values of +35% to +74% being reported (+15% is the usual upper limit in normal persons). Patients with leukemia and lymphoma tend to have the highest metabolic rates. Rapid cell growth is in part responsible. The patient's nutrients are used by the tumor, and a considerable amount of energy is expended by the neoplastic cells in maintaining such functions as active transport, synthesis of new proteins, and other processes of cell growth. One specific metabolic abnormality that has been identified is excessive activity of the Cori cycle. The Cori cycle (which consumes considerable energy) involves the conversion of glucose to lactate by the liver and kidney and then the resynthesis of glucose from these substrates. Studies indicate that cancer patients with the greatest weight loss also have the highest activity of the Cori cycle. Alterations in taste and production of an anorexigenic substance are other likely contributing factors. Cachectin or tumor necrosis factor is a polypeptide produced by mononuclear macrophages. It is capable of producing both weight loss and fever and may be a cofactor causing weight loss in some cancer patients as well as in chronic infections. Depression on learning that cancer is present also contributes to anorexia. Local tumor factors such as mechanical obstruction can interfere with assimilation of nutrients, and malabsorption may be present in pancreatic cancer. The treatment to which many cancer patients are subjected (surgery and chemotherapy) may increase metabolic demands and cause anorexia.

INFECTIONS

Acquired immunodeficiency syndrome (AIDS) or AIDS-related complex is now an important consideration in any patient who experiences weight loss. Often other symptoms or signs (fatigue, fever, lymphadenopathy, night sweats, or diarrhea) are present to suggest this possibility. Tuberculosis and other insidious infections such as subacute bacterial endocarditis and brucellosis should be considered in patients with low-grade fever and weight loss. For each degree of fever (Fahrenheit), the patient's metabolic rate increases 7%. Besides anorexia and fever, there is evidence that acute and chronic infections have primary metabolic effects on the cell, contributing to the patient's negative nitrogen balance. Cachectin (see Cancer) may play a role in the pathogenesis of the weight loss.

All of these factors operating together have the potential to cause weight loss of significant proportion. Infestation with intestinal parasites that consume host nutrients is rare in Western countries but should be considered when weight loss occurs despite normal caloric intake.

MISCELLANEOUS DISORDERS

Uremia from any cause can be responsible for decreased appetite and weight loss. Chronic inflammatory disease, especially rheumatoid arthritis and lupus erythematosus, also should be considered, although usually the presence of either disease is obvious. Likewise, cardiac cachexia is rarely occult. Loss of weight in severe congestive heart failure results from anorexia coupled with increased metabolic demands of the hypertrophied myocardium and respiratory muscles. In advanced cases of chronic lung disease, the work of breathing increases caloric needs; however, the effort of eating may become so taxing that food intake actually decreases, thereby causing loss of weight. A cause of malnutrition and weight loss that recently appears to be increasing in frequency is food faddism. Occasionally distance-running enthusiasts who have greatly increased caloric requirements follow unusual diets that are calorically and nutritionally inadequate.

APPROACH TO THE PATIENT WITH WEIGHT LOSS

Several factors deserve emphasis when a patient with weight loss is evaluated. The starting weight, final weight, and period over which weight was lost are obviously important. The patient's weight should then be expressed as a percentage of the ideal body weight to quantify the degree of weight loss and malnutrition. Rapid loss of more than 10% of normal weight may compromise the patient, whereas the same loss over a prolonged period may have few deleterious effects. A weight loss of approximately 20% in the nonobese patient is indicative of moderate malnutrition. Loss of 35% to 50% of normal body weight represents severe malnutrition and is virtually always life-threatening.

A history of increased or depressed appetite suggests conditions in one of the two major categories listed in the box on p. 1260. Dietary composition also should be known because foods of low nutritive value (snack foods) or alcohol abuse may mask the presence of protein malnutrition. Symptoms of diarrhea, bulky malodorous stools, nausea, and vomiting suggest a gastrointestinal cause of the weight loss. The presence of anorexia may indicate depression or other psychiatric disturbance that may be revealed by a detailed social and personal history. Anorexia and associated symptoms of hemoptysis, fever, lymph node swelling, hematuria, change in bowel habits, or abdominal pain may provide evidence for the possibility of cancer or an infectious process.

In addition to the physical findings specific to the disease entities listed in the box on p. 1260, general physical manifestations that indicate severe malnutrition may occur with weight loss. Dermal changes of perifollicular hyperkeratotic papules, pellagrous dermatitis, petechiae, and ecchymoses may occur, although these changes are most common in children. Cheilosis, glossitis, and stomatitis with superficial ulcerations may be found. The presence of edema, either from malnutrition or secondary to a disease associated with weight loss, may camouflage the wasting and weight loss.

Usually the differential diagnosis is apparent at the conclusion of the history and physical examination. Laboratory and radiologic studies should be used to confirm the diagnosis. However, if weight loss remains unexplained, the patient must have thorough testing for cancer. This may require a full complement of gastrointestinal radiography, abdominal computed tomography scans, intravenous pyelography, ultrasonography, and bone marrow examination. Although virtually any neoplasm may cause weight loss, tumors that are especially associated with this sign are pancreatic cancer, gastrointestinal malignancies, renal cell cancer, lung cancer, lymphomas, and leukemias.

REFERENCES

Berkman B et al: Failure to thrive: paradigm for the frail elderly. Gerontologist 5:654, 1989.

Beutler B and Cerami A: Cachectin: more than a tumor necrosis factor. N Engl J Med 316:279, 1987.

Forse RA and Shizgal HM: The assessment of malnutrition. Surgery 88:17, 1900.

Grunfeld C and Feingold KR: Metabolic disturbances and wasting in the acquired immunodeficiency syndrome. N Engl J Med 327:329, 1992.

Holroyde CP et al: Altered glucose metabolism in metastatic carcinoma. Cancer Res 35:3710, 1975.

Hsu LKG: The treatment of anorexia nervosa. Am J Psychiatry 143:573, 1986.

Marton KI, Sox HC Jr, and Krupp JK: Involuntary weight loss: diagnostic and prognostic significance. Ann Intern Med 95:568, 1981.

Weiss RJ: Unexplained weight loss in an elderly patient: delayed diagnosis of thyrotoxicosis. Postgrad Med 86:177, 1989.

CHAPTER

153 Obesity

Edward S. Horton

Obesity is a condition in which there is an excess of body fat. It is usually, but not always, associated with being "overweight" when compared to population norms for body weight related to age, gender, height, and frame size. The increased fat mass may be due to an increase in the lipid content of individual fat cells, an increase in total fat cell number, or a combination of the two. The distribution of body fat may be generalized or localized to specific regions. Thus obesity is not a single disease entity but a syndrome with many causes, including combinations of genetic, nutritional, environmental, and sociologic factors. This results in a varied picture of obesity with regard to its natural history, complications, association with other diseases, and response to treatment.

No completely satisfactory classification of the various forms of obesity has been developed, although attempts have been made to categorize obesity according to the distribution of body fat (central vs. peripheral), proposed pathogenetic mechanisms (metabolic vs. regulatory), age of onset (childhood, early adulthood, gestational, middle age), cellular character of the adipose tissue (hypertrophic vs. hyperplastic), and cause (genetic, hypothalamic, dietary, physical inactivity, and endocrine disease). Recent studies have focused on the possibility that low resting metabolic rates and decreased spontaneous physical activity may be predisposing factors to the development of obesity in some individuals. Another area of active investigation is focused on understanding the several factors that regulate food intake, including central nervous system, gastrointestinal, and hormonal mechanisms. These investigations may lead to a better understanding of the cause and pathogenesis of the various forms of obesity and an improved classification system. Currently, however, the classification in the box on the right may be useful in developing an approach to the diagnosis and treatment of the obese patient.

Classification of obesity

- Familial
  - Onset usually in childhood
  - Prevalence in first-degree relatives
  - Genetic and cultural determinants
  - Potential association with other diseases such as non–insulin dependent diabetes mellitus, hyperlipidemias, hypertension, gout
- Isolated
  - Onset usually in adolescence or adulthood
  - Common contributing factors
    - Increased food intake
    - Decreased physical activity
    - Withdrawal from smoking
    - Estrogens
    - Drugs affecting energy intake or expenditure
      - Phenothiazines, serotonin antagonists tricyclic antidepressants, marijuana, sulfonylureas
  - Commonly associated diseases
- Hypothalamic disorders
  - Tumors—craniopharyngioma, glioma, cyst, etc.
  - Inflammation—sarcoidosis, tuberculosis, eosinophilic granuloma, encephalitis, leukemia
  - Trauma—after head injury
  - Benign intracranial hypertension
- Endocrine disorders
  - Cushing's syndrome
  - Insulinoma
  - Hypothyroidism
  - Hypogonadism
  - Polycystic ovary syndrome
  - Growth hormone deficiency
- Congenital disorders
  - Prader-Willi syndrome
  - Laurence-Moon-Biedl syndrome
  - Alstrom's syndrome
  - Familial partial lipodystrophy

DIAGNOSIS

Just as there has been difficulty in classifying obesity, there has also been a lack of uniformity in defining diagnostic criteria. This is due, in part, to the fact that methods for accurately measuring body fat content are not readily available in clinical practice. Often the diagnosis is obvious clinically. Examination of the patient may reveal large amounts of subcutaneous adipose tissue that can be demonstrated by the "pinch test" or measured as skinfold thickness by specially designed calipers. In general, approximately 50% of body fat is in subcutaneous tissue, so measurement of skinfold thickness at one or more sites can be used to estimate total body fat. The upper limit of normal for skinfold thickness over the triceps area is considered to be 23 mm in adult men and 30 mm in adult women with somewhat lower values in children. Others have correlated the sum of skinfold thickness measured at several sites (e.g., biceps, triceps, subscapular, and suprailiac) with measurements of total body fat content and from these data have developed predictive tables for adult men and women.

Perhaps the most common method for diagnosing obesity is by the use of tables of desirable weights for sex and height, such as those developed by the Metropolitan Life Insurance Company in 1959 and revised in 1985. The patient's weight compared to "desirable weight" is usually expressed as the "percent overweight" with the upper limit of normal considered to be 20% above the standard. What is actually determined by the use of these tables is the body weight of an individual relative to an arbitrary standard and not the degree of body fatness. Thus a person who has a large skeletal and muscle mass may be "overweight" by the tables but not obese.

Several other parameters of height and weight have been used to diagnose obesity, the most commonly used being the body mass index (BMI), which is the ratio of weight in kilograms to height in meters squared (kg/m^2). This is now the preferred method of expressing body size and correlates well with more precise measurements of body composition. The normal range for BMI is 20 to 25; 25 to 30 indicates mild obesity, 30 to 40 moderate obesity, and more than 40 severe obesity.

Where available, estimates of total body fat by body density measurements, isotope dilution, ^{40}K counting, or total body electrical conductivity, or electrical impedence methods can be used to diagnose obesity with greater accuracy. Current practice is to consider a fat content of greater than 20% in men and 28% in women to indicate obesity. However, such a definition is arbitrary and does not consider the anatomic character, distribution, or health consequences of the obesity.

Measurement of the waist to hip circumference ratio (WHR) as an index of upper body (abdominal) obesity versus lower body (buttocks and thighs) obesity is also useful, because an increase in intra-abdominal fat is associated with an increased risk for metabolic abnormalities and adverse health consequences. The WHR is determined by measuring the circumference at the navel and the maximum circumference of the hips and buttocks. It is normally greater in men than in women and tends to increase somewhat with increasing age in both sexes. Precise upper limits of normal have not been defined, but a WHR more than 1.0 in men and more than 0.85 in women is associated with an increased risk of metabolic abnormalities.

PATHOPHYSIOLOGY

Regardless of the underlying cause, the final common pathway for the development of obesity is an excess of energy intake over energy expenditure leading to deposition of body fat. In humans, very little de novo lipogenesis occurs in adipose cells. Lipids, either derived directly from the diet or synthesized in the liver from excess carbohydrates, are transported to adipose tissue as chylomicrons or very-low-density lipoproteins (VLDLs). The triglycerides in these particles are hydrolyzed by lipoprotein lipase located in capillary endothelium, taken up in adipose cells, and then re-esterified into cellular triglycerides. During periods of negative energy balance, stored triglycerides are released from adipose cells as glycerol and free fatty acids and metabolized for energy production. When energy intake exceeds energy expenditure over a long period, obesity results.

It is now clear that many factors regulate both energy intake and energy expenditure and that defects in one or more of these factors may play a significant role in the pathogenesis of obesity. Energy intake is regulated by internal factors governing hunger, satiety, and appetite; by the efficiency with which ingested food is digested, absorbed, and metabolized; and by external factors such as the availability of food, composition of the diet, social pressures, and environmental conditions. Energy expenditure is determined by factors that regulate the basal metabolic rate, thermic response to food ingestion, energy used during physical activity, and responses to environmental conditions such as exposure to cold temperatures. Changes in thyroid hormone metabolism, sympathetic nervous system activity, and insulin sensitivity all affect energy expenditure.

The concept that obesity is always associated with hyperphagia is no longer tenable. Daily energy intake may be the same or less than in lean subjects if energy expenditure is also reduced. This may occur if the resting metabolic rate is low or physical inactivity is present. However, in most patients, total daily energy expenditure correlates well with the fat-free mass when corrected for levels of physical activity.

DIFFERENTIAL DIAGNOSIS

By far the most common forms of obesity are those that occur in adolescence or adulthood in association with one or more contributing factors such as excessive food intake, decreased physical activity, withdrawal from smoking, use of oral contraceptives, or use of medications that affect the regulation of food intake or energy expenditure. Familial forms of obesity are also common, although onset is usually during childhood and a positive family history of lifelong obesity is present. To assess these patients a detailed history is required to determine the age of onset, rate of progression, prior treatments, and present status of the obesity. In addition, the presence or absence of associated diseases and any identifiable contributing factors, including medications, diet, physical activity, and psychologic, social, and environmental characteristics, should be determined. The physical examination should include an assessment of the severity of the obesity and the anatomic distribution of body fat. Both the BMI and the WHR should be calculated and recorded.

Hypothalamic disorders associated with obesity are characterized by hyperphagia and, in some cases, decreased physical activity. Other signs of hypothalamic dysfunction such as altered temperature regulation and fluid balance as well as signs of neurologic disease are often present. Endocrine disorders associated with obesity should be considered if other characteristic signs and symptoms are present.

The various congenital syndromes associated with obesity are rare but should be considered if the characteristic stigmata are present. Prader-Willi syndrome is suggested by a combination of muscle hypotonia in infancy, short stature, delayed bone maturation, cryptorchidism, and mental retardation. Other manifestations may include small hands and feet, strabismus, and dental enamel hypoplasia. The Laurence-Moon-Biedl syndrome is characterized by retinitis pigmentosa, polydactyly or syndactyly, mental retardation, and hypogonadism. Nerve deafness and abnormalities of the heart and kidneys may also occur. Alstrom's syndrome is similar to Laurence-Moon-Biedl syndrome and includes atypical retinitis pigmentosa, nerve deafness, hypogonadism, and diabetes mellitus. Familial lipodystrophy is a variable disorder characterized by a marked decrease in subcutaneous fat in one segment of the body and hypertrophy of fat in another. It is more frequent in women, and a familial pattern of fat distribution is common. For example, several members of one family may have a marked decrease in fat over the torso and upper extremities and a marked increase in the hips, buttocks, and legs, whereas another family may exhibit the opposite pattern.

ASSOCIATED DISEASES

Taken as a group, the obese have an increased overall mortality rate when compared to a normal weight population. The mortality ratio increases with increasing severity of obesity. At a BMI of 30, the relative risk is approximately 1.3, and with a BMI of 40 the risk is increased to 2.5, compared to that of a normal weight population. Obesity is also associated with several other diseases that may result in significant morbidity or may be the primary cause of death. These include a cluster of metabolic abnormalities commonly referred to as the syndrome of insulin resistance (SIR), which includes hyperinsulinemia, insulin resistance, non–insulin dependent diabetes mellitus (NIDDM), hyperlipidemia, hypertension, and gout. In women, hyperandrogenism may also be present. Other diseases associated with obesity include coronary artery disease, cerebral and peripheral vascular disease, biliary tract disease, osteoarthritis, and gout. In addition, menstrual irregularities and diseases of the reproductive tract, particularly endometrial carcinoma, are more common in obese women.

Many of these conditions are improved significantly by weight reduction, and treatment of obesity plays a major role in their prevention and management. It is particularly important in the management of NIDDM, hyperlipidemia, and hypertension. In these conditions, even modest degrees of weight reduction may result in marked improvements in blood glucose and VLDL concentrations, moderate decreases in cholesterol level, and significant fall in blood pressure.

Metabolic abnormalities that lead to the development of one or more of the associated diseases are not present in all obese individuals. A population of "healthy" obese exists and epidemiologic data suggest that in the older age groups life expectancy may actually be increased when a moderate degree of obesity is present. This may represent a "selected" population and re-emphasizes the fact that obesity is not a single entity but a group of conditions with various causes and prognoses.

Psychologic and social handicaps may be a major problem for the obese and should be considered in evaluating the patient. Discrimination against obese individuals in several sectors of society, including acceptance into universities and professional schools, job promotion, and fashion design, has been demonstrated in a variety of studies, and the obese are frequently treated as if they are lazy or lack will-power to control their weight. Depression, lack of self-confidence, and a sense of guilt are common in patients with obesity and may constitute barriers to successful treatment.

TREATMENT

The basic goal of treatment is to reduce the excess adipose tissue mass by creating a negative net energy balance. Ideally, this should be accomplished with the least possible loss of lean body mass and without impairment of vital organ functions. Once the desired body weight is achieved, a new steady state of energy balance should be maintained by balancing caloric intake with energy expenditure. Nutritional adequacy of the diet with regard to vitamins, minerals, and other essential nutrients should be maintained as much as possible during weight loss and is a major goal during weight maintenance. If the obesity is caused by another disease process, treatment of the underlying condition may be sufficient to improve or cure the condition without specific dietary interventions.

The vast majority of patients with obesity should be treated by a program combining reduction in energy intake, increased physical activity, and attention to correcting identified factors contributing to the obesity. Support systems to promote modifications in life-style are particularly important for long-term success of weight reduction and weight maintenance programs.

A negative energy balance of 500 kcal/day can usually be maintained over many weeks or months. This is safe and can be expected to result in an average rate of weight loss of 1 lb/wk. If more rapid weight loss is desired, diets ranging from 600 to 1000 kcal/day can be used but require careful monitoring and supplementation of essential nutrients. These very low calorie diets are not generally recommended for long-term use. Daily energy intakes of less than 600 kcal/day have been associated with sudden death, most likely caused by cardiac arrhythmias associated with electrolyte imbalance or myocardial degeneration. They also result in significant negative nitrogen balance and loss of lean body mass. For these reasons they should rarely be used.

Medications that suppress appetite or stimulate energy expenditure are commonly used to potentiate weight loss, but their effects are often transient. Many have undesirable side-effects and/or potential for habituation. New compounds are currently being developed that may be more effective and prevent these problems.

A number of surgical procedures have been developed for the treatment of severe, life-threatening obesity. Of these, the most common in current use are gastric bypass and gastroplasty procedures. Complications of these procedures, although fewer than those of some of the other surgical treatments, are still troublesome and include development of stomal ulcers, obstruction of the anastomosis, reflux esophagitis, recurrent vomiting, diarrhea, and dumping syndrome.

In general, patients seeking treatment for severe obesity for the first time should be considered for medical therapy including appropriate dietary, physical exercise, and behavior modification regimens and support. Gastric restrictive or bypass procedures could be considered for well-informed and motivated patients with acceptable operative risks, provided they are selected carefully after evaluation by a multidisciplinary team with medical, surgical, psychiatric, and nutritional expertise. Regardless of the therapeutic approach selected, obesity is a chronic disease and long-term management and surveillance are necessities.

REFERENCES

Bogardus C et al: Familial dependence of the resting metabolic rate. N Engl J Med 315:96, 1986.

Bray GA: Syndromes of hypothalamic obesity in man. Pediatrics 13:525, 1984.

Bray GA: Complications of obesity. Ann Intern Med 103:1052, 1985.

Bray GA: Obesity. Disease-a-Month 35:451, 1989.

Fujioka S et al: Contribution of intra-abdominal fat accumulation to the impairment of glucose and lipid metabolism in human obesity. Metabolism 36:154, 1987.

Gastrointestinal Surgery for Severe Obesity NIH Consensus Development Conference Concensus Statement. Volume 9(1) March 25–27, 1991.

King AC et al: Diet vs. exercise in weight maintenance: the effects of minimal intervention strategies on long-term outcomes in men. Arch Intern Med 149:2741, 1989.

Kissebah AH et al: Relation of body fat distribution to metabolic complications of obesity. J Clin Endocrinol Metab 54:254, 1982.

Landin K et al: Importance of obesity for the metabolic abnormalities associated with an abdominal fat distribution. Metabolism 38:572, 1989.

Ravussin E et al: Determinants of 24-hour energy expenditure in man: methods and results using a respiratory chamber. J Clin Invest 78:1568, 1986.

Ravussin E et al: Reduced rate of energy expenditure as a risk factor for body-weight gain. N Engl J Med 318:467, 1988.

Roberts SB et al: Energy expenditure and intake in infants born to lean and overweight mothers. N Engl J Med 318:461, 1988.

Sims EAHS and Danforth E Jr: Expenditure and storage in man. J Clin Invest 79:1019, 1987.

Stunkard AJ et al: The body-mass index of twins who have been reared apart. N Engl J Med 322:1483, 1990.

Williamson DF et al: The 10-year incidence of overweight and major weight gain in U.S. adults. Arch Intern Med 150:665, 1990.

Woo R, Kush-Daniels R, and Horton ES: Regulation of energy balance. Annu Rev Nutr 5:411, 1985.

CHAPTER

154 Weakness

David L. Vesely

Weakness, fatigue, and *loss of energy* are all terms used by patients to describe similar subjective symptoms. On closer questioning, *fatigue* usually refers to a loss of power or strength associated with exertion. *Loss of energy,* on the other hand, more often refers to a generalized feeling of inability to begin movement not associated with exertion. *Weakness* usually relates to a loss of strength in one or more muscle groups. Weakness becomes a more objective finding when decreased muscular power is demonstrated. Objective weakness may be divided into several groups based on where the majority of the patient's weakness is located anatomically (see the box on the right).

The mode of onset and progression of the weakness are helpful in distinguishing particular disorders in the differential diagnosis of weakness. Several disorders are associated with rapid onset of weakness, including the Guillain-Barré syndrome, botulism, organophosphate poisoning, se-

Causes of muscle weakness

I. Primary proximal weakness
  A. Muscle
    1. Endocrine: hyperthyroidism, hypothyroidism, subacute thyroiditis, hyperparathyroidism, acromegaly, Addison's disease (acute adrenal insufficiency), primary aldosteronism, steroid myopathy (Cushing's syndrome; iatrogenic), and male hypogonadism
    2. Metabolic: diabetes mellitus, insulin-induced hypoglycemia, glycogen storage diseases (acid maltase deficiency, muscle phosphorylase deficiency, muscle phosphofructokinase deficiency), lipid storage disease (carnitine deficiency), and alcoholic myopathy
    3. Muscular dystrophies: limb-girdle, Duchenne's, Becker's
    4. Inflammatory myopathies: polymyositis, dermatomyositis, other collagen vascular diseases including rheumatoid arthritis, sarcoidosis, human immunodeficiency virus
    5. Hypercalcemia, hypophosphatemia, hypokalemia, and hyperkalemia of any cause
    6. Drug induced: colchine, chloroquine, cimetidine, amidarone, beta blockers, D-penicillamine, cyclosporin
  B. Neuromuscular junction: myasthenia gravis, Eaton-Lambert, botulism, organophosphate poisoning
  C. Peripheral nerve: diabetic proximal neuropathy, Guillain-Barré syndrome, acute intermittent porphyria, tick paralysis, and arsenic poisoning
  D. Anterior horn cell: poliomyelitis, chronic spinal muscular atrophy
II. Primary distal weakness
  A. Muscle: myotonic dystrophy
  B. Peripheral nerve: beriberi, diphtheria, lead, porphyrins, carcinomatous neuropathy, chronic progressive demyelinating neuropathy, peroneal muscle atrophy (Charcot-Marie-Tooth), Guillain-Barré syndrome, Refsum's disease, compressive lesions (root, plexus, nerve)
  C. Anterior horn cell: poliomyelitis, motor neuron disease
III. Generalized weakness
  A. Decreased cardiac output (mitral stenosis, tricuspid stenosis, mitral regurgitation)
  B. Acute infectious diseases and chronic infectious diseases such as tuberculosis, brucellosis, and trichinosis
  C. Chronic glomerulonephritis and other causes of uremia, including generalized rhabdomyolysis
  D. Pernicious anemia (and other anemias)
  E. Hepatitis
  F. Neurosyphilis
  G. Psychiatric illnesses such as depression
  H. Multiple sclerosis
  I. Mitochondrial myopathy—genetic, zidovudine
  J. L-tryptophan (eosinophilia-myalgia)

vere electrolyte imbalance, diphtheria, and acute polymyositis. A history of relapses and remissions could suggest myasthenia gravis, a relapsing peripheral neuropathy, one of the periodic paralyses, exogenous potassium depletion, or a collagen-vascular disease. Other disorders are slow in onset, with a progressive deterioration of strength that should make one think of one of the muscular dystrophies. Any consideration of differential diagnosis must take into account associated signs such as atrophy or muscle wasting. It is important to note whether the muscle wasting follows the distribution of any particular nerve; this can provide a clue to the neurologic basis of the wasting. Careful note should be made of the way a patient walks into a room, sits down, or gets up from a chair. A patient who has no difficulty in removing a shirt over the head but gives way when formal muscle testing of the shoulders is attempted may not have organic weakness. The diagnosis of hysterical weakness or malingering depends chiefly on the discovery of inconsistencies when all the clinical signs are considered as a whole.

ENDOCRINE CAUSES

Of the various causes of muscle weakness, endocrine myopathies currently represent the most easily correctable of the neuromuscular disorders (Chapter 124). Weakness as a symptom of hyperthyroidism was reported by Graves as early as 1835 and is found on physical examination in approximately 80% of hyperthyroid patients. Usually the proximal limb muscles are involved, and the shoulder girdle muscles are involved more often than the muscles of the pelvic girdle. As with other types of proximal muscle involvement described later, these patients have difficulty in walking up stairs, getting up from a chair, and combing their hair without resting. With increasing severity of the thyrotoxic myopathy, the distal musculature often becomes involved, and occasionally bulbar weakness also occurs. After successful treatment of hyperthyroidism, the patient usually fully recovers muscular strength, as with other endocrine myopathies described later. With respect to weakness in hyperthyroid patients, it should be remembered that there is also a 30-fold increase in incidence of myasthenia gravis in Graves' disease patients compared with the incidence in the general population. Periodic paralysis is also associated with Graves' thyrotoxicosis but differs from familial hypokalemic periodic paralysis (which it closely resembles) in that 95% of thyrotoxic patients have no familial pattern and periodic paralysis attacks disappear without recurrence after the patient becomes euthyroid. Asians are especially prone to thyrotoxic periodic paralysis.

Weakness is also present in up to 40% of all hypothyroid patients but is generally less marked than in hyperthyroid patients. Weakness is likewise a presenting symptom of hyperparathyroidism, and 20% to 30% of these patients have objective signs of proximal muscle weakness in the lower extremities on neurologic testing. In addition to hyperparathyroidism, hypercalcemia and hypophosphatemia of any cause are also causes of proximal muscle weakness.

Weakness is a major symptom in approximately 40% of patients with acromegaly and is related to a combination of myopathy and neuropathy. A large percentage of patients with acromegaly are still clinically weak a year or more after treatment. Muscle weakness is a common symptom in Addison's disease. It appears to be closely related to the hyperkalemia because, when potassium levels are normalized, weakness usually disappears. Hyperkalemia or hypokalemia (e.g., primary aldosteronism) of any cause may produce proximal muscle weakness.

Cushing's syndrome typically becomes manifest with proximal muscle weakness in 80% to 90% of these patients. Steroid myopathy, including that produced by exogenous steroids, may be the most common endocrine cause of weakness. Noticeable muscle weakness resulting from corticosteroid administration usually occurs 3 to 20 months after starting the respective steroid. Male hypogonadism is sometimes associated with a generalized weakness.

METABOLIC CAUSES

Of the metabolic causes of weakness, poorly controlled diabetes mellitus is the most common. Severe hypophosphatemia in the diabetic or nondiabetic patient may cause weakness. Weakness is one of the symptoms of marked hyperglycemia as well as acute hypoglycemia of any cause. The glycogen storage and lipid storage diseases are relatively rare, but proximal muscle weakness is one of their prominent features. Proximal muscle atrophy and weakness, mainly of the lower limbs, occur in the chronic alcoholic patient.

MUSCULAR, NEUROMUSCULAR, AND NEURAL CAUSES

The progressive muscular dystrophies are among the genetic causes of marked proximal muscle weakness. Thus Duchenne's pseudohypertrophic pelvifemoral muscular dystrophy and Becker's pseudohypertrophic (milder course) muscular dystrophy are inherited as X-linked recessive diseases. Limb-girdle dystrophy is usually inherited as an autosomal recessive trait, but it occasionally follows an autosomal dominant pattern of inheritance.

The inflammatory myopathies are characterized by (1) the relatively common polymyositis, which is a symmetric, painless weakness of the proximal limb and trunk muscles without any clinically apparent skin lesions, and (2) dermatomyositis, which has a similar distribution of proximal muscle weakness accompanied by skin lesions, the most pathognomonic of which is the heliotrope (lilac-colored) rash over the eyelids, nose, forehead, and fingernails. All the collagen-vascular diseases as well as sarcoidosis can cause a myopathy that is similar to polymyositis.

Human immunodeficiency virus type 1 (HIV-1) may cause a proximal myopathy usually of the nemaline rod type or an inflammatory myopathy similar to polymyositis. A far more common myopathy in HIV-1 infected individuals is due to treatment with zidovudine (AZT). This myopathy usually presents after more than a year of therapy and is characterized by wasting of the buttock muscles with associated leg weakness, which is usually reversible with cessation of AZT treatment. Other drugs that induce myopathies are colchicine, chloroquine, D-penicillamine, cimetidine, amidarone, beta blockers, and cyclosporin. The newly described eosinophilia-myalgia syndrome is caused by the ingestation of L-tryptophan.

Myasthenia gravis in its advanced stages causes a weakness of the proximal muscles of the limbs. True myasthenia gravis rarely occurs without weakness of the muscles innervated by the cranial nerves. The weakness of myasthenia gravis is episodic and is characterized by partial recovery of strength after a period of rest and after administration of anticholinesterase drugs. Eaton-Lambert syndrome is a myasthenia-like condition associated with cancer, such as small-cell carcinoma of the lung. The weakness in this syndrome usually involves the pelvic, thigh, and shoulder muscles and spares the ocular and bulbar muscles.

With peripheral nerve involvement, weakness may advance during a period of days to involve the proximal and distal limb muscles, as in the Landry-Guillain-Barré syndrome, tick paralysis, and acute intermittent porphyria, or it may develop rather slowly, over a period of weeks, as in arsenic or lead poisoning or the diabetic neuropathies. Diabetic mononeuropathy may, however, develop rapidly. If proximal muscle weakness is asymmetric and is accompanied by atrophy, hyperreflexia, and fasciculations, one should think of diseases of the anterior horn cell.

Distal muscle weakness gives rise to difficulty with fine coordinating movements and with grip, causing problems with performing such daily activities as buttoning a shirt or tying a shoelace. Severe distal symmetric weakness that rapidly advances to the point where the patient is confined to a wheelchair is seen with the carcinomatous and uremic polyneuropathies. An exception to the general rule that muscle disease becomes manifest with proximal weakness is the profound distal weakness seen in patients with myotonic dystrophy, in which hand, facial, and neck muscles are usually affected. Genetic causes of distal weakness include Charcot-Marie-Tooth (peroneal muscle) atrophy and Refsum's disease (chronic polyneuropathy with ichthyosis, deafness, and retinitis pigmentosa). Compression of a nerve against the underlying bone also results in distal weakness; mild cases recover fairly rapidly (2 to 12 weeks). All of the polyneuropathies caused by diphtheria, diabetes, and lead intoxication also can lead to distal muscle weakness.

MISCELLANEOUS CAUSES

A general weakness is seen in disorders of decreased cardiac output such as mitral stenosis, tricuspid stenosis, and mitral regurgitation. Acute and chronic infectious diseases such as brucellosis, tuberculosis, and trichinosis may show weakness frequently accompanied by fever. All severe anemias, including acute blood loss and hepatitis, may cause a generalized feeling of fatigue. A generalized weakness is often associated with chronic glomerulonephritis. Uremia of any cause may lead to a generalized weakness in addition to the distal muscle weakness discussed above. If the patient has weakness in only one limb, and that is associated with optic neuritis and an alteration in emotional response, multiple sclerosis should be considered. A generalized weakness in an individual or family may be due to mitochondrial dysfunction, which has been reported in more than 100 cases. Finally, neurosyphilis and psychiatric illnesses that mimic many disease states should be considered in patients with a generalized weakness.

APPROACH TO DIAGNOSIS

Diagnostic aids for determining the cause of weakness include serum enzyme levels. Of the serum enzymes, creatine phosphokinase (CPK) shows the largest increase in neuromuscular disease, so this enzyme is routinely obtained. Other intramuscular enzymes whose levels are elevated in the serum in the conditions described earlier are aldolase, glutamic oxaloacetic transaminase, glutamic pyruvic transaminase, and lactic dehydrogenase. Another diagnostic aid is electromyography, which suggests denervation of muscle if fasciculations are seen, or anterior horn cell disease if fibrillations are present. With this technique, myasthenia gravis with a progressive decrement in muscle response to tetanic stimulation can be differentiated from the Eaton-Lambert syndrome, which has a terminal increase in response. At rest, patients with myopathies generally show no electrical activity. Muscle biopsies with ultrastructural studies are often helpful if the above studies plus the history and physical examination do not reveal the diagnosis. Thus muscle biopsies help make the diagnosis in denervation atrophy, in muscle dystrophies, and in the glycogen storage diseases. Lumbar puncture with examination of the spinal fluid is also helpful in diagnosing certain causes of weakness such as the Guillain-Barré syndrome and neurosyphilis.

REFERENCES

Brew BJ: Central and peripheral nervous system abnormalities. Med Clin North Am 76:63, 1992.

Espinoza R et al: Characteristics and pathogenesis of myositis in human immunodeficiency virus infection - distinction from azidothymidine-induced myopathy. Rheum Dis Clin North Am 17:117, 1991.

Tritschler HJ: Mitochondrial myopathy of childhood associated with depletion of mitochondrial DNA. Neurology 42:209, 1992.

Vesely DL: Recognition and managing acute adrenal insufficiency. J Crit Illness 3:101, 1988.

CHAPTER

155 Hirsutism

D. Lynn Loriaux

The human body, except the palms of the hands, the soles of the feet, and the lips, is covered with hair follicles. Two kinds of hair grow from these follicles: vellous hairs and terminal hairs. Terminal hairs are typified by the hairs of the scalp. Vellous hairs are typified by the facial hairs of children. The relative distribution of terminal and vellous hair differs between men and women. This results from the effect of androgens. Androgens change vellous hairs to terminal hairs in certain *androgen-sensitive* areas such as the face, upper back and shoulders, chest, and, to some extent, the arms and legs. *Androgen-dependent* hirsutism is a disorder of women in which the hair distribution acquires a male pattern. Hirsutism in any other pattern is referred to as *non–androgen* dependent hirsutism. It is most commonly an untoward side-effect of some medication. Examples of drugs that cause non–androgen dependent hirsutism include diazoxide, minoxidil, phenytoin, glucocorticoids, and cyclosporin A. The following discussion applies only to the androgen-dependent form of the disorder.

SYMPTOMS

Most patients with hirsutism complain of increased hair growth on the face. In particular, the need to remove the hair leads to a feeling of "defeminization." Many women with hirsutism complain of oligoamenorrhea and infertility. Symptoms of virilization are uncommon. When present, they include deepening of the voice, increasing muscle bulk, and qualitative changes in libido that can be characterized as masculine.

SIGNS

Terminal hairs in a masculine distribution define the condition. Less than 5% of normal women have terminal hairs on the cheeks, less than 3% have terminal hairs over the sternum, and, for practical purposes, normal women never have terminal hair over the shoulders, upper back, and upper abdomen. The quantity and quality of the hair distribution over the arms and legs are not in themselves useful in establishing the diagnosis. Signs of virilization include temporal balding, deepening of the voice, and clitoromegaly.

ETIOLOGY

The cause of androgen-dependent hirsutism is increased androgen effect. This can result from the overproduction of androgens or from increased sensitivity to their action. In women, androgens arise from two organs: the ovary and the adrenal. Thus most of the disorders that result in hirsutism are disorders of one or both of these organs (refer to the box on the right). When an abnormality of the ovary or adrenal gland cannot be identified, the disorder is called *idiopathic hirsutism*. The ovary is usually the source of increased androgen secretion in these cases.

The adrenal causes of hirsutism include adrenal cancer, virilizing adrenal adenoma, and the virilizing forms of congenital adrenal hyperplasia; 21-hydroxylase deficiency, 11-hydroxylase deficiency, and 3-hydroxysteroid dehydrogenase deficiency.

The ovarian causes of hirsutism include ovarian neoplasms, idiopathic hirsutism, polycystic ovary, insulin resistance, and persistent corpus luteum of pregnancy.

Iatrogenic and factitious forms exist. Synthetic *impeded androgens* currently are used to treat disorders such as endometriosis, fibrocystic breast disease, and hereditary angioneurotic edema. This treatment is usually accompanied by some degree of hirsutism. The attempt to improve athletic performance through the use of androgens has also led to many cases of hirsutism.

Causes of androgen-dependent hirsutism

- I. Ovarian
  - A. Neoplastic
    - 1. Tumors of gonadal stroma
      - a. Sertoli-Leydig tumors (arrhenoblastoma)
      - b. Granulosa-theca tumors
      - c. Sertoli cell tumor
      - d. Lipid cell tumor
      - e. Gynandroblastoma
    - 2. Germ cell tumors
      - a. Teratoma
    - 3. Mixed stroma and germ cell tumors
      - a. Gonadoblastoma
  - B. Nonneoplastic
    - 1. Idiopathic hirsutism
    - 2. Polycystic ovary syndrome
    - 3. Insulin resistance
- II. Adrenal
  - A. Neoplastic
    - 1. Adrenal carcinoma
    - 2. Virilizing adrenal adenoma
  - B. Nonneoplastic
    - 1. Congenital adrenal hyperplasia
      - a. 21-Hydroxylase deficiency
      - b. 11-Hydroxylase deficiency
      - c. 3-Beta-hydroxysteroid dehydrogenase deficiency
    - 2. Cushing's disease
- III. Iatrogenic or factitious
  - A. Androgens
    - a. Synthetic androgens
    - b. Parenteral testosterone esters
  - B. "19-nor" progestins

DIAGNOSIS

The physician evaluating a hirsute patient should have the possibility of serious underlying disease foremost in mind. Points that tend to separate the serious causes of hirsutism from the benign should be emphasized in the evaluation.

History

The benign forms of hirsutism usually have their onset in the peripubertal period. Hirsutism having its onset distinctly before or after puberty suggests a serious underlying disorder. Benign hirsutism usually develops over a course of 2 or 3 years and then becomes relatively stable. Hirsutism that is progressive is worrisome. Oligoamenorrhea and amenorrhea are found in both benign and malignant forms of hirsutism. Virilization, manifest by deepening of the voice, temporal balding, and changes in libido, is an ominous finding. A family history of hirsutism or a history of medication use that has hirsutism as an untoward side-effect suggests benign disease.

Physical examination

A careful quantitation of the distribution of terminal hair is of primary importance. This assessment will be used to evaluate the extent to which the patient deviates from the normal distribution of terminal hair growth in women and the rate of progression of hirsutism as well as its response to therapy if and when initiated. "Soft" findings of virilization include increased skin thickness, acne, increased muscle bulk, and a masculine pattern of fat distribution. A more objective measure of masculinization is clitoral size. This can be assessed conveniently by the method described by Tagatz and colleagues. A careful search should be made for pelvic and abdominal masses. Truncal skin creases, the axillae, and the wrinkles of the neck should be examined carefully for acanthosis nigricans. Signs of other diseases associated with hirsutism, including Cushing's syndrome and acromegaly, should be noted.

Laboratory evaluation

The measurement of plasma testosterone concentration plays a central role in the laboratory evaluation of the disorder because the process is androgen mediated. Ideally, the concentration of plasma testosterone should be measured at least three times to provide a more reliable estimate of the "true" concentration of the hormone. Testosterone concentrations greater than 200 ng per deciliter are rarely seen in the benign forms of hirsutism. Thus testosterone concentrations of this magnitude require a thorough evaluation for adrenal and ovarian neoplasms using pelvic ultrasound and imaging of the adrenal glands. On the other hand, testosterone concentrations in the normal range are rarely associated with serious abnormality.

Low testosterone concentrations in association with a "benign" history suggest the diagnosis of idiopathic hirsutism or the polycystic ovarian syndrome. These conditions have a benign course and a good outcome. Plasma testosterone values between the upper limit of normal and 200 ng per deciliter can have any cause. Patients with attenuated congenital adrenal hyperplasia usually fall into this range. This disorder should be excluded with the "short" adrenocorticotropic hormone (ACTH) stimulation test. After intravenous administration of synthetic ACTH, 250 μ over 1 minute, the plasma concentrations of several steroid biosynthetic intermediates are measured at 45 and 60 minutes. The most common form of congenital adrenal hyperplasia, the 21-hydroxylase deficient form, can be diagnosed by measuring the plasma concentration of 17-hydroxyprogesterone, the steroid intermediate just before the enzyme block. The concentration of 17-hydroxyprogesterone should not exceed 350 ng per deciliter in normal subjects after the administration of ACTH. The plasma concentration of 17-hydroxyprogesterone usually exceeds 2000 ng per deciliter in subjects with the disease. 11-Deoxycortisol and 17-hydroxypregnenolone are the appropriate steroid intermediates to measure for the diagnosis of the 11-hydroxylase and 3-beta-hydroxysteroid dehydrogenase forms of the disorder, respectively.

If congenital adrenal hyperplasia is excluded, the possibility of neoplasm remains. Pelvic ultrasound and adrenal computed tomography are the best tests for this evaluation.

TREATMENT

The treatment of adrenal and ovarian neoplasms is surgical extirpation. The treatment for the attenuated forms of congenital adrenal hyperplasia is administration of exogenous glucocorticoids. The preparation of choice is hydrocortisone at a dose of 12 to 15 $mg/m^2/day$ given once a day in the morning. The treatment of virilization associated with insulin resistance is gonadotropin suppression using either the gonadotropin-releasing hormone superagonists or a combination of estrogen and progesterone in a dose sufficient to suppress luteinizing and follicle-stimulating hormone secretion (the standard birth control pill is usually adequate for this purpose).

The choice of treatment for the benign forms of hirsutism, idiopathic hirsutism, and the polycystic ovary syndrome is less clear. Because the pathophysiology of these disorders is still in an imperfect stage of understanding, rational therapy remains elusive. The general guide should be to intervene, if necessary, in the least noxious way acceptable to both patient and physician.

The available therapeutic modalities for hirsutism are shown in the box below. Briefly, shaving is always effective. It is usually rejected because of feelings of defeminization. Wax depilatories and electrolysis are more acceptable; electrolysis is the more effective and expensive of the two. Birth control pills result in improvement in about 70% of treated subjects but expose the patient to the risks of systemic estrogen therapy. These risks become more frequent and severe with advancing age. Glucocorticoids improve symptoms in about 50% of subjects but expose the patient to the risk of adrenal suppression, a potentially lethal condition.

Treatment modalities for hirsutism

- Physical removal
  - Shaving
  - Wax depilatories
  - Electrolysis
- Suppression of androgen secretion
  - Ovary
    - Birth control pills
    - Gonadotropin-releasing hormone superagonists
  - Adrenal
    - Glucocorticoids
    - Synthesis inhibitors (ketoconazole)
- Androgen antagonists
  - Cyproterone acetate
  - Spironolactone

In the author's view, exogenous glucocorticoids are only indicated in the treatment of hirsutism when the diagnosis of attenuated congenital adrenal hyperplasia is unequivocal. Finally, antiandrogens such as cyproterone acetate and spironolactone have recently gained popularity for the treatment of idiopathic hirsutism and polycystic ovary syndrome. Most studies show success rate approaching 100%, but the long-term consequences of treatment with these agents remain unknown.

It should be noted that improvement in hirsutism is a slow process, and final judgment on the success or failure of a given intervention should not be made before at least 6 months has elapsed.

REFERENCES

Adashi EY: Insulin and related peptides in hyperandrogenism. Clin Obstet Gynecol 34:872, 1991.

Barbieri RL: Hyperandrogenic disorders. Clin Obstet Gynecol 33:640, 1990.

Barbieri RL: Hyperandrogenism: new insights into etiology, diagnosis, and therapy. Curr Opin Obstet Gynecol 4:372, 1992.

Bates GW and Cornwell CE: Iatrogenic causes of hirsutism. Clin Obstet Gynecol 34:848, 1991.

Ehrmann DA and Rosenfield RL: Clinical review 10: an endocrinologic approach to the patient with hirsutism. J Clin Endocrinol Metab 71:1, 1990.

Kessel B and Liu J: Clinical and laboratory evaluation of hirsutism. Clin Obstet Gynecol 34:805, 1991.

Lobo RA: Hirsutism in polycystic ovary syndrome: current concepts. Clin Obstet Gynecol 34:817, 1991.

Moghissi KS: Clinical applications of gonadotropin-releasing hormones in reproductive disorders. Endocrinol Metab Clin North Am 21:125, 1992.

Redmond GP and Bergfeld WF: Treatment of androgenic disorders in women: acne, hirsutism, and alopecia. Cleve Clin J Med 57:428, 1990.

Shelley DR and Dunaif A: Polycystic ovary syndrome. Compr Ther 16:26, 1990.

CHAPTER

156 Amenorrhea

William F. Crowley, Jr.

Amenorrhea is usually a distressing symptom. In adolescent women amenorrhea raises the possibility of reproductive inadequacy in adulthood. In women of reproductive years the absence of a menstrual period suggests the possibility of pregnancy, which may cause distress or joy, depending on life's situation. In older women, the possibility of the beginning of menopause and the end of the reproductive life span represents yet another of life's transitions with which the patient must deal. Thus the appearance of amenorrhea never fails to evoke strong feelings in the patient and frequently leads to an interaction with the physician.

When consulted by a patient with amenorrhea, the physician must use all resources at his or her command. In almost no other area of endocrinology does one use every aspect of the history and physical examination, especially the social and dietary history, the concurrent use of medications, the exercise history, a careful examination of body weight versus height, and a skin examination. Data from each of these lines of evidence are critical to the generation of a differential diagnosis, which, when combined with carefully targeted laboratory testing, can identify most of the organic causes of amenorrhea and permit a presumptive diagnosis of the functional causes. Thus in the evaluation of amenorrhea, there is no substitute for a detailed history and physical examination to focus one's laboratory testing and make the evaluation cost-effective and accurate.

Amenorrhea can be classified into four etiologic categories: disorders of the hypothalamus, the pituitary gland, the ovary, and/or the uterus. The initial evaluation of a patient with amenorrhea is aimed at localizing the defect to one of these four areas, and then, once the defect has been localized to a given anatomic level, generating a differential diagnosis that employs the previously gleaned historic and physical examination information. In this sense, the approach to a patient with amenorrhea is similar to that of a patient with a neurologic lesion in that the anatomic localization often precedes and focuses the subsequent generation of a differential diagnosis and the initiation of therapy.

HYPOTHALAMIC CAUSES

The hypothalamus, the site of the most common defect in a population of women with amenorrhea, secretes gonadotropin-releasing hormone (GnRH) in an episodic fashion. This hypothalamic secretion of GnRH is modulated by many factors. Suspension of GnRH secretion, for example, is a mechanism by which reproductive processes can be suppressed by environmental stresses such as malnutrition and/or weight loss. A residual of this normal feedback mechanism so necessary from an evolutionary view is commonly seen in women suffering from anorexia and/or bulimia. In both of these circumstances, the hypothalamic input to the reproduction system is suppressed, depending on the metabolic signals arriving at the hypothalamus from the periphery. Similarly, stress exerts its primary impact on hypothalamic GnRH secretion and is a frequent cause of amenorrhea in young women. When seen in this perspective, many of the circumstances that are viewed clinically as pathologic are really adaptive responses to environmental stress. Most of these challenges mediate their effect on the reproductive system primarily through extinction or alteration of the pattern of the GnRH secretion.

Because GnRH cannot be measured easily in the systemic circulation, clinicians must rely on gonadotropin measurements for inferential information about the hypothalamic secretion of GnRH. When extensive studies using frequent sampling of peripheral luteinizing hormone (LH) and follicle-stimulating hormone (FSH) measurements as an index of GnRH secretion are undertaken, it becomes clear that the vast majority of patients with a defect in the hypothalamic secretion of GnRH (termed *hypothalamic amen-*

orrhea) exhibit a spectrum of disorders of GnRH secretion. These vary from a totally apulsatile pattern of GnRH release to defects of its amplitude or frequency, as well as a persistently pubertal pattern termed a *developmental arrest* (Fig. 156-1). Because two thirds to three fourths of all patients with amenorrhea have hypothalamic amenorrhea, an understanding of the spectrum of the abnormalities of GnRH secretions and their various modes of clinical and biochemical presentation is essential to any systematic approach to the amenorrheic patient.

The clinical circumstances in which hypothalamic amenorrhea most frequently occurs are those of psychologic stress. These include recent loss of a loved one, change of residence or job, or affective disorders such as depression. Previously referred to as *stress-related* amenorrhea or *boarding-school* amenorrhea, these terms all describe the net impact of a series of psychologic stresses on the central nervous system, which are, in turn, played out in abnormalities of GnRH secretion. More often, however, the individual psychologic stresses are more subtle and frequently not manifest during the initial visits to the physician. As one comes to know the patient better, these individual stresses may reveal themselves during repeated interactions. Similarly, there is a wide degree of personal variability in the responsiveness to a given stress such that no two women may respond in a similar fashion.

One of the puzzling features of patients with hypothalamic amenorrhea is the wide spectrum of biochemical abnormalities of gonadotropin and sex steroid testing these patients may present. If the patients are completely deficient in endogenous GnRH secretion, as is often found in severe anorexia nervosa, the random levels of peripheral LH and FSH are very low, often with LH level much lower than that of FSH, for unclear reasons. Because a profound estrogen deficiency accompanies such a complete absence of GnRH-induced gonadotropin secretion, one explanation for the relative preservation of FSH secretion in these patients is the absence of estrogen-induced negative feedback. Alternatively, the possibility of a second releasing factor governing FSH secretion, which is not as severely affected in subjects with hypothalamic amenorrhea, is possible. Whichever explanation may obtain, the pattern of low-level LH with normal follicular phase levels of FSH is a frequent occurrence in the most profound type of hypothalamic amenorrhea. The attendant hypoestrogenemia is often apparent on physical examination as vaginal dryness and pallor. Such patients frequently have vaginal dryness and dyspareunia. Despite these manifestations of severe peripheral

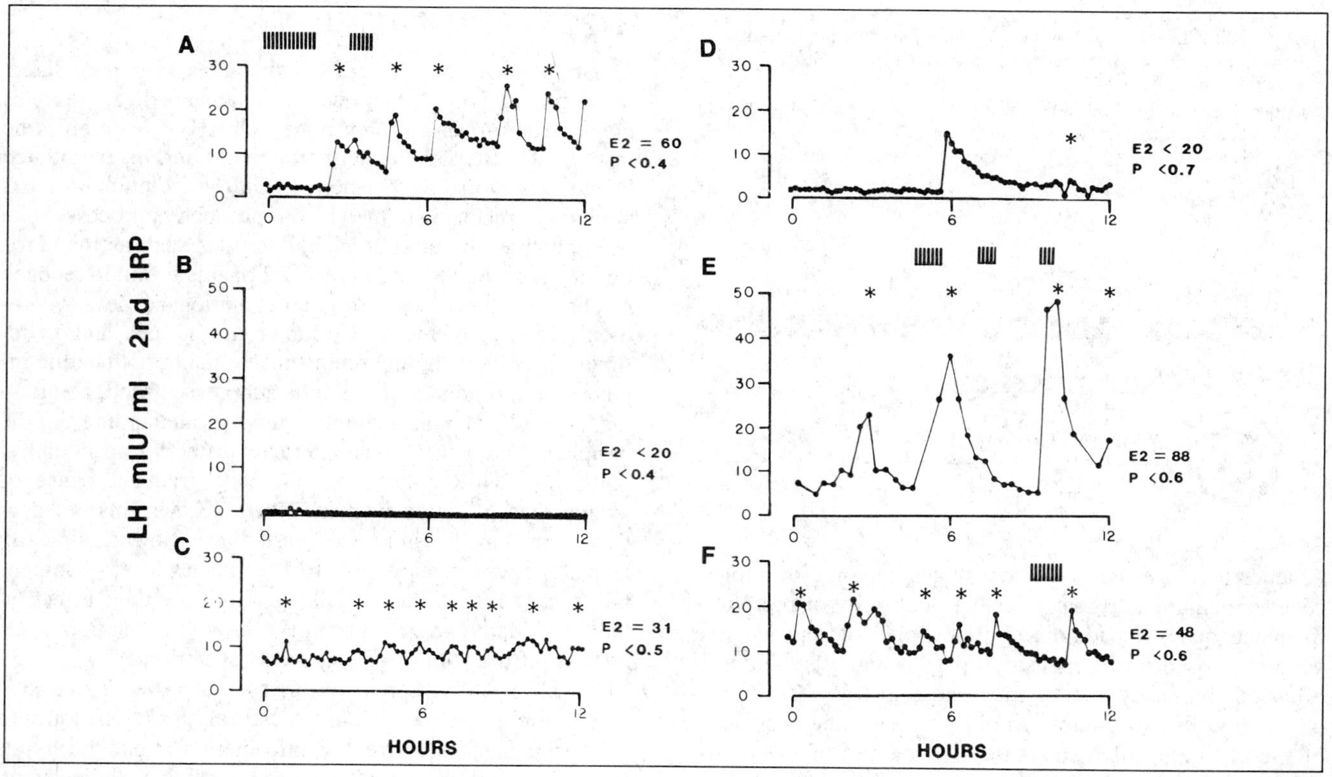

Fig. 156-1. GnRH secretion in women with hypothalamic amenorrhea. Luteinizing hormone secretion in normal women and women with hypothalamic amenorrhea, demonstrating the spectrum of GnRH-induced LH secretory patterns seen. **A,** Normal women. **B-F,** Women with hypothalamic amenorrhea. **B,** Apulsatile pattern. **C,** Disordered amplitudes. **D,** Disordered frequency. **E,** Sleep-entrained pattern *(developmental arrest)*. **F,** Unclassified pattern. LH, luteinizing hormone; GnRH, gonadotropin-releasing hormone.

estrogen deficiency, hot flashes are virtually absent in patients with hypothalamic amenorrhea as opposed to those patients with a primary ovarian defect who exhibit severe hot flashes, sometimes with less evidence of estrogen deficiency.

Although these clinical and biochemical findings suggest the complete form of total GnRH deficiency, more frequently patients with hypothalamic amenorrhea experience a partial defect in endogenous GnRH secretion such that the peripheral levels of gonadotropins vary, depending on the particular period of random sampling. Should the patient have recently experienced an isolated burst of GnRH-induced gonadotropin secretion, the plasma LH levels may exceed those of FSH (Fig. 156-1, *D*), producing a pattern that can suggest other disorders such as polycystic ovarian disease. However, on repeated testing during multiple office visits or during a prolonged period of sampling during an inpatient evaluation (generally reserved for a research setting), mean LH and FSH levels are generally documented to be in the normal, follicular phase range. Thus the total daily pattern of gonadotropin pulsations is aberrant and insufficient to initiate and sustain folliculogenesis and to mount an ovulatory LH surge in these patients. This combination of random levels of gonadotropins and sex steroids within the follicular phase ranges in an otherwise amenorrheic subject is often puzzling to the physician, if one does not keep in mind that the pattern of GnRH-induced gonadotropin secretion over longer periods is defective in such patients. Consequently, most diagnoses of hypothalamic amenorrhea are made on a presumptive basis in which the history and physical examination are compatible; the biochemical testing fails to reveal specific evidence of primary ovarian failure or hyperprolactinemia, and the elimination of other anatomic causes of amenorrhea has been made.

Given the presumptive diagnosis of hypothalamic amenorrhea, the therapeutic considerations must be tailored to individual circumstances. For example, if the environmental stress is soon to be removed, the disorder will be self-limited and may not require any therapy other than educating the patient. If prolonged amenorrhea is present, hypoestrogenemia, with attendant decreases in bone density, may prompt the institution of estrogen replacement therapy. It is important to remember that other specific causes of amenorrhea (such as a prolactin-secreting pituitary tumor) must be eliminated before undertaking estrogen replacement therapy because estrogen therapy can induce growth of such tumors in certain circumstances.

Should the patient wish to conceive, then institution of clomiphene citrate, an antiestrogen capable of blocking endogenous estrogen receptors and stimulating GnRH secretion, may be administered in increasing doses to induce ovulation and to attempt conception. It is important to reserve this form of therapy for women who have some evidence of endogenous GnRH secretion as witnessed clinically by estrogen effects on examination or direct measurement and who wish to conceive because the obvious attendant dangers of pregnancy must be prevented, unless specifically desired. Should clomiphene fail to induce ovulation or result in a conception, then administration of graded doses of menotropins (Pergonal) (human FSH and LH) or Menotropin (isolated human FSH) can be undertaken only under circumstances in which careful monitoring of both peripheral levels of estradiol and ovarian ultrasound evaluations, as well as prior experience with Pergonal, are available to the clinician.

More recently, the administration of pulsatile GnRH in a physiologic pattern using portable infusion pumps has been demonstrated to restore a normal pattern of gonadotropin secretion, induce the growth of a single follicle, and stimulate ovulation. The ability of pulsatile GnRH to limit attempts at ovulation to single folliculogenesis represents a significant achievement of a physiologic hypothalamic replacement schedule that has several advantages over the other regimens of clomiphene and menotropins, with their inherent risks of hyperstimulation and multiple gestation.

Finally, the literature has suggested that progestin-induced menstrual bleeding can be used either as a diagnostic test for patients with hypothalamic amenorrhea or, administered monthly, as an alternative therapy. However, this test is neither sensitive nor specific because the response to progestin administration ultimately depends on the degree of endogenous GnRH-induced gonadotropin secretion, which, in turn, is stimulating ovarian sex steroid production. Should the patients be completely deficient in GnRH, then progestin administration invariably results in the absence of any withdrawal bleeding. Conversely, should sufficient endogenous GnRH secretion be present, then a progestin-induced menstrual period occurs. However, the same patient, at various times during the natural history of recovery or relapse from hypothalamic amenorrhea, may exhibit differing responses to this intervention. Thus this test is not helpful diagnostically in this clinical setting.

PITUITARY CAUSES

Pituitary defects, particularly prolactinomas, comprise approximately 20% of cases of amenorrhea. Although patients with prolactin-secreting tumors may exhibit the more typical presentations of a pituitary tumor, including headache, visual field defects, and other hormonal deficiencies, such clinical presentations are increasingly rare (Chapter 160). In fact, amenorrhea is usually the earliest symptom of a prolactin-secreting microadenoma, which, before the ability to determine prolactin levels in the peripheral circulation, was classified as an example of hypothalamic amenorrhea. This historical misclassification attests to the similarity of biochemical presentation of some pituitary prolactinomas and hypothalamic amenorrhea. Although the anatomic defect in prolactinomas is at the pituitary gland, the cause and pathologic characteristics of the amenorrhea occurring in this clinical setting generally result from the ability of prolactin to disrupt endogenous GnRH secretion. Consequently, the biochemical and clinical presentations of prolactinomas are often indistinguishable from those of hypothalamic amenorrhea.

The fact that the defect in prolactinoma patients is not

in the pituitary is suggested by several observations. First, many prolactinomas are so small, they are undetectable by conventional radiographic techniques. Thus their mass effect cannot account for the associated disruption of the accompanying menstrual cyclicity. Second, institution of bromocryptine therapy promptly restores menstrual cyclicity in these patients, implying functional integrity of the residual gonadotroph population. Finally, when persons have examined prolactinoma patients with intensive sampling of their gonadotropin levels, they have been able to discern a spectrum of GnRH-induced pattern of gonadotropin release that is indistinguishable from that of subjects with hypothalamic amenorrhea.

Consequently, once the anatomic considerations of diagnosing a prolactinoma by computed tomography and/or nuclear magnetic resonance scanning in a patient demonstrating hyperprolactinemia have been addressed, these patients generally revert to a normal menstrual cyclicity with reinstitution of normal prolactin levels via administration of a long-acting dopamine agonist such as bromocryptine. Because dopamine serves as the natural prolactin-inhibiting factor, patients with prolactinoma may represent an example of endogenous catecholamine defect, giving rise to reduced dopaminergic inhibition of prolactin secretion. After surgery for removal of some of these tumors, a 30% to 50% recurrence rate has been noted despite apparent cure after initial tumor removal. This observation supports the notion that the basic defect is indigenous to the hypothalamus. Consequently, surgery is now generally reserved for those cases in which there is an anatomic defect secondary to the tumor size such as headaches, visual field compression, or extraocular movement paralysis. Radiotherapy has been used rarely in this circumstance and is generally reserved for those patients in whom tumor size rather than menstrual irregularity is the major symptom.

Finally, it is important to remember that other pituitary defects such as acromegaly, Cushing's syndrome, and gonadotropin-secreting tumors, as well as postpartum pituitary infarction, also can cause amenorrhea. These are rare causes and should be treated on an individual case basis, depending on tumor size and/or biochemical function. In most of these circumstances, the appearance of amenorrhea is but one of several symptoms heralding the onset of the process and therefore of secondary concern.

OVARIAN CAUSES

Ovarian causes of amenorrhea can be divided into two broad categories: those associated with hyperandrogenic dysfunction of ovarian secretion and those associated with premature failure of ovarian secretion.

Androgen-secreting defects of the ovary can be either benign (such as polycystic ovarian disease and/or hyperthecosis) or neoplastic (such as Sertoli-Leydig cell tumors, lipoid cell tumors, and other hormonally functioning ovarian tumors that secrete androgens, estrogens, or, more typically, a combination of both).

Polycystic ovarian disease and/or hyperthecosis is a condition that is part of a spectrum of benign hyperandrogenic lesions of the ovary, presenting with recurrent anovulation, oligoamenorrhea, signs and symptoms of hyperandrogenemia, ovarian enlargement in most cases, and an abnormally high LH/FSH ratio in the peripheral circulation. The presumed pathophysiologic characteristics of polycystic ovarian disease represent a vicious cycle in which ovarian androgen hypersecretion initiates an abnormally high LH/FSH ratio. This abnormal gonadotropin ratio thwarts adequate follicular growth and ovulation and results in an overstimulation of the thecal component of the ovary, which, in turn, begets further hyperandrogenemia. This cycle seems to be multifactorial, as suggested by the accompanying features in several subsets in patients with polycystic ovarian disease. These associations include insulin resistance, attenuated congenital adrenal hyperplasia, and acanthosis nigricans. Although these patients typically have irregular menstrual periods, they often experience amenorrhea. Physical examination often reveals hirsutism, acne, and excessive oiliness of the skin—all manifestations of hyperandrogenemia. The treatment of this condition depends on the wishes of the patient but generally requires ovarian suppression to ameliorate the hyperandrogenic symptoms. When fertility is desired, ovulation induction with clomiphene and/or menotropins is required. Hyperthecosis is generally viewed as a variant of the polycystic ovarian syndrome in which the number of follicles is reduced and the thecal component is increased. Both of these conditions must be differentiated from tumors of the ovary, and this differential can usually be made by a combination of the extreme levels of hyperandrogenemia present in tumors (i.e., plasma testosterone concentrations in excess of 200 ng/dl) and unilateral ovarian enlargement by ultrasound examination.

Premature ovarian failure represents the other group of ovarian disorders that are characterized by amenorrhea and symptoms typical of menopause. Thus hot flashes, vaginal dryness, elevated FSH and LH levels, and "castrate" ranges of estradiol are the typical biochemical findings of this condition. The causes of this group of conditions include a familial syndrome of unknown origin; karyotypic abnormalities, particularly those of the X chromosome; autoimmune variations of ovarian failure; the "resistant ovary" syndrome, in which the ovary is insensitive to gonadal stimulation but retains primordial follicles; and those following exposure to environmental toxins or chemotherapy. Treatment for premature ovarian failure includes sex steroid hormone replacement to alleviate the symptoms of estrogen deficiency and to prevent diminution of bone density with time. Pregnancy is now possible with fertilized donor egg insemination into the uterus.

UTERINE CAUSES

Uterine sources of amenorrhea, particularly Asherman's syndrome, in which severe endometrial scarring obliterates the endometrial lining, are the most frequently overlooked causes of amenorrhea by internists. The clinical history of these patients is usually preceded by an intrauterine infection, recent uterine manipulation such as dilation and curettage, and/or uterine packing after excessive hemorrhaging with abortion. Intrauterine devices can cause endometrial scarring, which, over time, can also lead to this condition. Usually, there is a history of antecedent, gradual decreases in menstrual flow, often with increasing cramping and abdominal pain produced by cervical stenosis. This diagnosis is best considered by a thoughtful history and examination of the basal body temperature charts, which demonstrate a biphasic pattern typical of ovulatory periods but are not accompanied by endometrial bleeding at the end of the menstrual period. In fact, cyclic monthly pain may replace normal endometrial withdrawal bleeding, indicating a hematocolpos. Transvaginal ultrasound examinations can be relied on to make this diagnosis. The use of estrogen followed by progesterone withdrawal bleeding also results in the lack of menstrual withdrawal bleeding, providing the patient takes an adequate dose of the sex steroid hormone replacement therapy.

SUMMARY

A careful history and physical examination can usually localize the cause of amenorrhea to one of four anatomic locations. Specific blood testing can then eliminate the anatomic causes of amenorrhea, focus the differential diagnosis to a given level, and often foreshadow rational therapy of that condition.

REFERENCES

Fries H et al: Epidemiology of secondary amenorrhea. II. A retrospective evaluation of etiology with special regard to psychogenic factors and weight loss. Am J Obstet Gynecol 118:473, 1974.

Kleinberg DL et al: Galactorrhea: a study of 235 cases, including 48 with pituitary tumors. N Engl J Med 296:589, 1977.

Santoro N et al: Hypogonadotropic disorders in men and women: diagnosis and therapy with pulsatile GnRH. Endocr Rev 7:11, 1986.

CHAPTER

157 Impotence and Altered Libido

John C. Marshall

Impotence is the inability to achieve or maintain a penile erection that is adequate to allow satisfactory sexual intercourse. Penile erection is due to vascular engorgement of the corpora cavernosa. This process is incompletely understood but results from complex mechanisms involving emotional, neurologic, vascular, and hormonal components. Abnormalities of any of these systems can result in impotence. Impotence is a common complaint in middle-aged men, and previous estimates suggested that psychogenic causes were responsible in 50% to 90% of cases. Recent evidence has indicated that this view may be incorrect, and the presence of defined pathologic abnormalities has been emphasized in several studies. Medications, psychogenic causes, and endocrine abnormalities each accounted for approximately 25% of cases in these studies, with diabetes, other neurologic diseases, urologic abnormalities, and miscellaneous causes accounting for the remaining 25% of patients. Thus psychogenic impotence is a diagnosis of exclusion, and impotence should be formally evaluated by history, clinical examination, and appropriate laboratory tests.

CLINICAL ASSESSMENT

Disorders commonly associated with impotence are shown in Table 157-1; specific endocrine causes are shown in Table 157-2.

History

The history should document the onset of impotence (acute or gradual) and establish whether impotence is complete or whether erections still occur at night or in response to a full bladder. Sexual desire or libido may be normal or reduced. A careful history of past and present medications and their relationship to the onset of symptoms should be established. Detailed questions should evaluate the presence of neurologic disease (both central and peripheral), and symptoms of vascular insufficiency such as angina or claudication should be assessed. In particular, the presence of polyuria and polydipsia may indicate diabetes mellitus, and a family history of non–insulin dependent (type 2) diabetes suggests the possibility of subclinical diabetes. Abdominal or pelvic surgery, particularly radical prostatectomy or rectal surgery, may be important. The patient's mental status should be evaluated, especially the presence of depression or emotional lability. A detailed history of the marital relationship is essential, and the attitudes of both partners to sexual relations established. A history relating to family stability, recent family bereavement, or evidence of alcohol or other substance abuse should be obtained.

Physical examination

Physical examination should emphasize the neurologic, vascular, and endocrine systems. Detailed examination of the external genitalia is essential. Examination of the vascular system should include auscultation and palpation of peripheral pulses, particularly in the lower limbs, and evidence of ischemia (cold feet, skin changes, ulceration) should be sought. Neurologic examination should include gait and coordination, and assessment of peripheral motor and sensory function in the legs is particularly important. Genital and perineal sensation should be assessed and the presence of a normal cremasteric reflex and anal sphincter tone determined. Autonomic nervous system function can be assessed by means of changes in heart rate and blood pressure during a Valsalva maneuver or isometric hand grip. Endocrine evaluation should include a careful search for the presence of hypogonadism with its associated skin changes (thin, pale skin) and diminished sexual hair

Table 157-1. Disorders associated with impotence

Disorder	Mechanisms and clinical features	Serum hormones
Medications/substance abuse Antihypertensives, diuretics, tranquilizers, antidepressives, phenothiazines, spironolactone, cimetidine, estrogens, chemotherapeutic agents, marijuana, opiates; alcohol	Medication history: Most antihypertensive agents can interfere with autonomic nervous function. Spironolactone and cimetidine act as peripheral androgen antagonists	LH, FSH, and testosterone concentrations usually normal LH, FSH, and testosterone concentrations suppressed by estrogens Prolactin concentration increased by phenothiazines, opiates, and some antidepressive agents
Psychogenic	Diagnosis of exclusion. Impotence with only one partner. Erections may occur at night or with a full bladder	Normal
Neurologic Depression, peripheral neuropathy, parkinsonism, syphilis, demyelinating diseases, spinal cord section, pelvic nerve section	Abnormalities of autonomic and/or somatic innervation. Detailed examination essential including peripheral and perineal sensation and anal sphincter tone. History of radical prostatectomy or pelvic surgery. Diabetic neuropathy is the most common problem and may precede marked elevation of blood glucose level	Normal
Vascular Atherosclerosis, sickle cell disease, thrombotic disorders	Impaired blood flow to the corpora cavernosa. Claudication and evidence of lower limb ischemia may be present	Normal Testosterone concentration may be low and LH and FSH concentrations elevated if severe testicular ischemia is present.
Endocrine* Hypothalamic-pituitary disorders, primary testicular disease	Usually caused by reduced testosterone secretion. Onset is gradual and associated with reduced libido. Clinical evidence of hypogonadism (pale soft skin, reduced beard growth) may be present. Testes may be slightly reduced in size and of soft consistency	Testosterone concentration low LH and FSH concentrations elevated in testicular disease and normal or low in hypothalamic-pituitary disorders Prolactin concentration may be elevated
Cirrhosis Alcoholic, hemochromatosis	Probably related to abnormal estrogen metabolism. Stigmata of liver disease (spider nevi). Gynecomastia is often present, and the testes are soft and reduced in size	Testosterone concentration low or low normal Estradiol concentration elevated or upper normal LH and FSH concentrations variable—normal or low
Uremia	Multifactorial causes, related to endocrine and other metabolic abnormalities. Anemia present and clinical evidence of renal failure	Testosterone concentration low LH and FSH concentrations normal or elevated Prolactin concentration elevated
Penile abnormalities Peyronie's disease, congenital vascular abnormalities	Impaired blood flow resulting from local causes. Erections may be painful in Peyronie's disease. Chordee or fibrous plaques may be present in the penis	Normal

*A detailed listing of endocrine disorders causing impotence is given in Table 157-2.

growth. The penis should be examined both for normal pubertal development and for presence of chordee or fibrous plaques in the corpora cavernosa. Testicular size and consistency should be documented together with the presence or absence of gynecomastia. Additionally, evidence of hypothyroidism or hyperthyroidism should be sought.

DIFFERENTIAL DIAGNOSIS

The differential diagnosis of impotence should focus on determining whether impotence is a manifestation of an underlying disease process or simply a functional disturbance. In some instances the temporal relationship of symptoms (i.e., to previous prostate surgery or to initiation of medications) points to the cause. Similarly, the occurrence of impotence only with a specific partner, or the presence of spontaneous erections at night or with a full bladder, suggests a psychological basis. Additionally, reduced libido together with impotence suggests an endocrine disorder, depression, or a systemic disease as opposed to vascular or peripheral neuropathic causes.

In many cases, the exact cause remains uncertain after clinical examination, and hormonal measurements are required to exclude endocrine disease. The usual hormonal changes are shown in Tables 157-1 and 157-2. Laboratory assessment of gonadal function is indicated in all patients

Table 157-2. Endocrine disorders causing impotence and decreased libido

Disorder	Mechanisms and clinical features	Hormonal and radiologic abnormalities
Hypothalamic—tumor or cyst, granuloma (sarcoid, tuberculosis, histiocytosis X), trauma, idiopathic	Reduced secretion of gonadotropin-releasing hormone (GnRH) or interrupted hypothalamic-portal blood flow. Clinical evidence of TSH or ACTH deficiency may be present as a result of failure of hypothalamic-releasing factors. Diabetes insipidus is often present. Prolactin may be elevated because of reduced dopamine secretion	Testosterone level low, LH and FSH levels low Prolactin level may be elevated but not above 150 ng/ml CSF cytologic and/or culture result abnormal in granulomatous disease Normal sellar radiographic result, but CT scan shows hypothalamic abnormality
Pituitary		
Tumors—chromophobe adenoma, prolactinoma, Cushing's disease, acromegaly	Hypopituitarism is due to a mass effect in chromophobe tumors. Hyperprolactinemia inhibits GnRH secretion, which is reversible. Glucocorticoids inhibit gonadotropin secretion. Clinical evidence of hypogonadism is usually present with soft testes. Signs of Cushing's syndrome or acromegaly may be present. Variable degrees of TSH and ACTH deficiency may be present, more commonly in chromophobe tumors	Testosterone level low, LH and FSH levels low or low normal Prolactin levels >200 ng/ml indicate a prolactinoma Variable degrees of hormone deficiency on pituitary reserve testing Sellar radiographic result often normal in Cushing's disease CT scan shows pituitary tumor in almost all cases
Carotid artery aneurysm	Compression of pituitary by the aneurysm with variable degrees of pituitary failure	Hormonal abnormalities similar to tumors. CT scan with contrast usually reveals diagnosis, but carotid angiography may be needed to distinguish from a chromophobe adenoma
Hemochromatosis	Deposition of iron in pituitary. Variable degrees of hypogonadism and hypopituitarism are seen clinically. May be associated with cirrhosis and diabetes mellitus	Testosterone level low, LH and FSH levels low or low normal Variable hormonal deficiencies revealed by pituitary reserve testing Radiographic and CT scan findings normal
Testicular		
Klinefelter's syndrome	Presence of extra X chromosome and 47,XXXY karyotype. Most men have partial pubertal development and eunuchoidal habitus. Testes are small (<2 cm) and firm. Mosaicism may occur, and some men have normal secondary sex characteristics with small testes. These patients usually are infertile	Testosterone level low, LH level elevated, FSH markedly elevated Testosterone and LH levels occasionally normal and only FSH level may be elevated 47, XXY karyotype
Tumors—Leydig's cell, embryonal cell, teratoma, choriocarcinoma	Leydig cell tumors secrete estradiol, which suppresses LH, FSH, and testosterone secretion. Embryonal cell tumors and teratomas may secrete hCG, which stimulates estradiol secretion. A testicular nodule is usually palpable, and gynecomastia is commonly present	Leydig cell—testosterone level low, LH and FSH levels low, and estradiol level elevated Teratomas—testosterone levels often normal, estradiol level elevated, LH and FSH levels low or low normal; hCG may cross-react in LH assays
Hemochromatosis	Iron deposition in the testes. Variable degrees of hypogonadism are seen, and the testes are usually small and soft	Testosterone level low. LH and FSH levels are variable because iron may also be deposited in the pituitary, producing gonadotropin deficiency
Orchitis—mumps, venereal disease, tuberculosis	Usually results in infertility caused by seminiferous tubule damage, but rarely Leydig's cell failure and hypogonadism also occur. Testes are small and soft and often asymmetrically affected	Testosterone level low, FSH level markedly elevated, LH level elevated
Radiation therapy or chemotherapy—alkylating agents	The germinal epithelium is damaged, but Leydig's cell involvement may occur. Seminiferous tubule damage may be reversible over months to years. Testes are usually small and soft	Testosterone level may be low, FSH level markedly elevated, LH level may be elevated

Continued

Table 157-2. Endocrine disorders causing impotence and decreased libido—cont'd

Disorder	Mechanisms and clinical features	Hormonal and radiologic abnormalities
Idiopathic	Testicular degeneration affecting both the seminiferous tubules and Leydig's cells. The patient is clinically hypogonad, and the testes are small and soft	Testosterone level low, LH and FSH levels elevated
Thyroid disease		
Hypothyroidism, hyperthyroidism	Mechanisms are uncertain. In hypothyroidism LH, FSH, and testosterone secretion may be reduced. Hyperthyroidism increases sex hormone–binding globulin levels, and increased amounts of testosterone are protein bound. Peripheral conversion of androgens to estrogens may also be increased. Gynecomastia may be present in hyperthyroidism	Hypothyroidism—testosterone level low or low normal. LH and FSH levels low or normal; prolactin level elevated in severe hypothyroidism Hyperthyroidism—testosterone level normal or elevated, estradiol level normal or elevated, LH and FSH levels normal or elevated
Other disorders—chronic disease, usually associated with weight loss (malignancy, infections, gastrointestinal granulomatous disorders)	Chronic weight loss is associated with reduced GnRH secretion, which is reversible if weight regain occurs	Testosterone level low, LH and FSH levels low

for two reasons. First, hypogonadism may coexist with other disorders such as diabetic neuropathy or vascular insufficiency. Second, the clinical manifestations of hypogonadism are subtle and develop slowly in adult men over months to years. In men who have undergone spontaneous puberty, diminished testosterone secretion may be manifest initially by reduced libido and impotence, and only months to years later will clear clinical evidence of hypogonadism be found. Postpubertally, penile size does not decrease in the absence of testosterone. Testicular size and consistency mainly reflect seminiferous tubule mass, and this only partly regresses with reduced secretion of pituitary follicle-stimulating hormone (FSH) and luteinizing hormone (LH). Thus diminished testosterone secretion may not be evident from clinical examination, and the serum testosterone level should be measured in all impotent men.

Clinical evidence can provide important clues to the diagnosis. The presence of gynecomastia (in the absence of medication use) suggests estrogen excess or testosterone lack. Testosterone-deficient men are more sensitive to the effects of estradiol, and gynecomastia may occur in the presence of a normal serum estradiol level. Estrogen excess can occur as a result of testicular tumors (Leydig's cell tumors; secretion of estradiol, choriocarcinoma or teratomas secreting human chorionic gonadotropin [hCG]), and rarely adrenal tumors. Testosterone insufficiency may be secondary to hypothalamic-pituitary disease or may result from primary testicular disorders (Table 157-2). In hypothalamic-pituitary disease, LH and FSH secretion is reduced, resulting in a low serum testosterone concentration. In primary testicular disease, a low serum testosterone level is accompanied by elevated levels of LH and FSH caused by the absence of testosterone-negative feedback. Evidence of hypothyroidism or adrenal insufficiency together with hypogonadism suggests a pituitary tumor as the underlying cause. Galactorrhea, rarely present in men, suggests the presence of a prolactinoma. Signs of Cushing's syndrome or acromegaly may indicate a pituitary tumor.

Small, soft testes may reflect prolonged reduction of gonadotropin secretion or primary testicular disease. The testes may be soft and small after mumps orchitis, but very small testes (less than 2 cm in length) of firm consistency suggest Klinefelter's syndrome. In this disorder, most men are clinically hypogonadal with low levels of testosterone, but 20% have a normal or low-normal testosterone level and infertility. Polyuria and polydipsia may be manifestations of diabetes insipidus resulting from hypothalamic disorders. More commonly, however, polyuria, especially when associated with weight loss, suggests diabetes mellitus. Diabetes mellitus is the most common endocrine disorder causing impotence, and in approximately 50% of diabetic men impotence develops. The underlying abnormality is usually a diabetic autonomic neuropathy, and this may be indicated by a history of nocturnal diarrhea, bladder dysfunction, postural hypotension, or abnormal pulse rate changes after a Valsalva maneuver. Less often, diabetic impotence is due to vascular insufficiency, which may be clinically evident as lower limb ischemia.

Thyroid disease, both hypothyroidism and hyperthyroidism, may be associated with impotence, although the mechanisms are not fully understood. In hyperthyroid men, serum estradiol and testosterone concentrations may both be increased as a result of elevated levels of sex hormone–binding globulin (TeBG). TeBG has a higher affinity for testosterone than estradiol, and more testosterone is bound to protein, which can reduce the concentration of biologically active "free" testosterone. In addition, peripheral conversion of androgens to estrogens is increased by thyroid hormone, which may result in increased serum estradiol concentration. In hypothyroidism, gonadotropin secretion may be impaired, and in severe hypothyroidism hyperprolactinemia may contribute to reduced gonadotropin and testosterone secretions. Hyperprolactinemia also occurs in chronic renal failure. Serum estradiol level may be elevated in cirrhosis of the liver caused by impaired metabolism of estrogen, and estradiol may inhibit gonadotropin secretion, resulting in soft testes and low testosterone secretion rates. Cirrhosis may be a manifestation of hemochromatosis, and iron deposition may also be present in the pituitary and in the gonad, leading to hypogonadism of pituitary and/or testicular origin. Impotence together with hypogonadism may be present in many chronic diseases, particularly those associated with marked weight loss such as malignancy or Crohn's disease. Severe weight loss results in reduced hypothalamic secretion of gonadotropin-releasing hormone (GnRH) and consequent reduced gonadotropin secretion from the pituitary.

LABORATORY INVESTIGATION

Laboratory screening should include a complete blood count, assessment of hepatic and renal function, and measurement of a fasting serum glucose level. A borderline fasting glucose level or family history of non–insulin–dependent diabetes (type 2) may occasionally need to be pursued by a glucose tolerance test. If thyroid disease is suspected, thyroxine and T_3-resin uptake should be measured, particularly in the elderly as clinical signs of hyperthyroidism may be absent. In view of the subtle clinical presentation of hypogonadism, serum testosterone level should always be measured and used as the basis on which to pursue further endocrine evaluation. The need for subsequent testing depends on the serum testosterone level and is summarized in the box on the right. Additional laboratory tests may be indicated by the clinical findings. The presence of gynecomastia indicates that serum estradiol level should be measured. Similarly, if a testicular tumor is suspected, measurement of beta-hCG and alpha-fetoprotein levels may reveal the presence of a teratoma. A normal serum testosterone value usually precludes the need for further endocrine evaluation, and other causes of impotence should be sought (Table 157-1). If serum testosterone level is normal and a psychogenic cause of impotence is suspected, measurement of nocturnal penile tumescence using a strain gauge may be indicated. The presence of nocturnal erections indicates normal function and helps to support the diagnosis of psychogenic impotence. If suspected, vascular insufficiency can be established by measurement of penile blood pressure by Doppler ultrasound. A penile/brachial blood pressure index of 0.6 or less suggests impairment of arterial blood flow.

Laboratory investigation of impotent men

1. Complete blood count; BUN, creatinine clearance; bilirubin, SGOT, SGPT, alkaline phosphatase; fasting glucose level (postprandial glucose or GTT if borderline). Serum thyroxine and T_3-resin uptake if clinically indicated
2. Serum testosterone
   If normal: no endocrine diseases (pursue other causes—see Table 157-1)
   If low or low normal*: Measure LH and FSH levels

If LH and FSH levels are low or low normal	*If LH and FSH levels are elevated*
Hypothalamic-pituitary disease, chronic illness or weight loss	Primary testicular failure
Serum prolactin	Pursue etiology (Table 157-2)
Thyroxine, T_3-resin uptake	Chromosome karyotype if hypogonad or small, firm testes
CT or MRI scan of pituitary	
Pituitary reserve function tests (insulin hypoglycemia and releasing hormones)	

*Serum testosterone level may be low in marked obesity as a result of decreased levels of sex hormone–binding globulin. LH, FSH, and prolactin levels are normal. BUN, blood urea nitrogen; SGOT, serum glutamic-oxaloacetic transaminase; SGPT, serum glutamic-pyruvic transaminase; GTT, glucose tolerance test; CT, computed tomography; MRI, magnetic resonance imaging.

MANAGEMENT

Wherever possible, management of impotence should be directed toward the underlying cause. If medications are suspected, the feasibility of stopping the drug or changing to an alternative form of therapy should be considered. This is particularly important in patients receiving treatment for hypertension. With the exception of prolactinomas, resection of pituitary tumors is not usually associated with a return of gonadotropin secretion, and replacement therapy with androgens is required. Treatment of prolactinomas, however, particularly medical therapy with bromocriptine, often results in a return of normal gonadal function, although this process is slow and occurs over several months. Removal of estrogen-secreting Leydig's cell tumors is usually followed by recovery of reproductive function. Primary testicular failure should be treated by replacement of testosterone, using intramuscular injections of a long-acting testosterone ester (testosterone enanthate or cypionate). A dose of 200 mg at 2 to 3 week intervals maintains serum testosterone level in the normal range. In patients with psychogenic impotence, marital or psychologic counseling of both partners may be helpful. When impotence is due to neuropathy, libido is often normal, and failure to achieve an erection may be a cause of considerable marital disharmony. In this situation, a penile prosthesis may be considered as a means of alleviating symptoms. Alternatives to a penile prosthesis include intracavernosal self-injection of papaverine or phentolamine. This results in a penile erection that persists for 30 to 40 minutes and allows intercourse. Complications include priapism and fibrosis of the corpora cavernosa, and the long-term safety and efficacy of this treatment remain to be established.

REFERENCES

Diagnostic and therapeutic technology assessment: vasoactive intracavernous pharmacotherapy for impotence: papaverine and phentolamine. JAMA 264:752, 1990 (editorial).

Kelly TM et al: Hypogonadism in hemochromatosis: reversal with iron depletion. Ann Intern Med 101:629, 1984.

Kursh ED et al: Injection therapy for impotence. Urol Clin North Am 15:625, 1988.

Nickel JC et al: Endocrine dysfunction in impotence: incidence, significance and cost-effective screening. J Urol 132:40, 1984.

Sidi AA et al: Intracavernous drug-induced erections in management of male erectile dysfunction—experience with 100 patients. J Urol 135:704, 1986.

Slag MF et al: Impotence in medical clinic outpatients. JAMA 249:1736, 1983.

Sparks RF, White RA, and Conolly PB: Impotence is not always psychogenic—new insights into hypothalamic pituitary gonadal dysfunction. JAMA 243:750, 1980.

Swerdloff RS et al: Infertility in the male. Ann Intern Med 103:906, 1985.

Whitehead ED et al: Diagnostic evaluation of impotence. Postgrad Med 88:123, 1990.

Whitehead ED et al: Treatment alternatives for impotence. Postgrad Med 88:139, 1990.

CHAPTER

158 Gynecomastia

John C. Marshall

Gynecomastia is an increase of breast tissue in males. True gynecomastia consists of proliferation of both ductal and stromal tissue and results from conditions that cause imbalance of levels of serum androgens and estrogens—either estrogen excess or testosterone deficiency. Estrogen excess occurs infrequently as a result of estrogen-secreting tumors. More commonly a relative excess of estrogens is present when serum testosterone concentration is reduced. In adult men, approximately 10% of serum estradiol level is from secretion by the testis; 40% is from peripheral conversion of testosterone to estradiol (aromatization), which occurs predominantly in fat cells; and 50% is derived from peripheral conversion of estrone to estradiol. Estrone itself is primarily derived from peripheral aromatization of adrenal androstenedione. The testes are the source of virtually all testosterone in plasma. Thus disorders that reduce testicular hormone secretion remove the major source of plasma testosterone but have much less effect on circulating estradiol, producing a situation of relative estrogen excess.

CLINICAL ASSESSMENT

Conditions commonly associated with gynecomastia and the mechanisms involved in it are shown in Table 158-1.

History and physical examination

In addition to documenting the onset and duration of gynecomastia, a careful history of pubertal maturation and a detailed medication history should be obtained. A family history of hypogonadism or infertility may be helpful, and the presence of infertility or anosmia in family members may point to a diagnosis of isolated gonadotropin deficiency. Gynecomastia is usually bilateral, but because marked asymmetry is often present, it may appear unilateral. True gynecomastia consists of concentric hypertrophy of breast tissue and is usually palpable as a discrete plaque of tissue beneath the areola. Commonly the plaque is 3 to 5 cm in diameter, but in severe cases it may be similar to a normal female breast. Gynecomastia should be distinguished from lipomastia, a diffuse increase in adipose tissue. Palpation of the breast over tensed pectoralis major muscles (by apposition of the hands) allows delineation of gynecomastia and differentiation from lipomastia. Evidence of cirrhosis, renal failure, or marked weight loss and presence or absence of a goiter should be sought on physical examination. Secondary sexual characteristics, including those of skin (thin, soft, and pale with reduced sebum secretion in testosterone deficiency), sexual hair and beard growth, and genital development, should be assessed. Examination of the genitalia is most important. The penis and testicles should be measured and the presence of developmental abnormalities noted. Hypospadias or partial scrotal fusion together with other evidence of incomplete masculinization suggests a partial form of an androgen-resistance syndrome. Testicular nodules or a marked inequality in testis size may indicate the presence of a testicular tumor.

DIFFERENTIAL DIAGNOSIS

Gynecomastia is present in the majority (up to 75%) of boys during pubertal maturation and is usually transient, lasting from 6 to 18 months. Breast enlargement may be associated with breast tenderness and reflects the initial transient stage of gonadotropin stimulation of an immature testis when estrogen secretion exceeds that of testosterone. Rarely, gynecomastia fails to regress during the later stages of normal puberty, but persistence of gynecomastia should initiate a search for other pathologic factors. Medications may be important, and the use of marijuana may be associated with persistence of gynecomastia. Gynecomastia occurs with increased frequency in elderly men, and its cause is probably multifactorial. Many elderly patients take medications for other disorders. Additionally, serum testosterone level tends to fall, and sex hormone–binding globulin level rises after the sixth decade, which may reduce biologically available testosterone and produce a relative estrogen excess.

Gynecomastia may be present in hypogonadism as a result of hypothalamic-pituitary or gonadal disorders, but it is more common in gonadal disorders, Klinefelter's syndrome is important in this regard, and 50% of men have gynecomastia in addition to small, firm testes. Abnormalities of the genitalia, partial masculinization, and development of gynecomastia at adolescence suggest an androgen-resistance syndrome. These men have a normal 46, XY karyotype, and genital abnormalities vary from small testes and hypospadias (Reifenstein's syndrome) to failure of scrotal fusion and abnormal descent of the testes (partial

Table 158-1. Causes of gynecomastia

Cause	Mechanisms and clinical features
Physiologic	
Puberty	Gonadotropin stimulation of the prepubertal testis initially produces estradiol secretion. Later, testosterone secretion is dominant and gynecomastia is consequently transient
Senescence	Uncertain mechanisms but probably related to decreased serum levels, testosterone and increased sex hormone-binding globulin (TeBG) resulting in a reduction in biologically available testosterone
Pathologic	
Hypogonadism	
Primary testicular disease or secondary to hypothalamic-pituitary disorders	Reduced testosterone secretion. Estrogens from the adrenal and from peripheral conversion of androstenedione produce a relative estrogen excess. Gynecomastia is usually present in Klinefelter's syndrome and less commonly in hypothalamic-pituitary disease
Androgen-resistance syndromes	
Testicular feminization, complete and partial forms; Reifenstein's syndrome	Abnormalities of the cytosolic androgen receptor, which is absent in testicular feminization and is reduced in number or has abnormal function in partial syndromes. Testosterone action is absent or reduced. Elevated LH and FSH levels stimulate testosterone and estradiol secretion, but only estradiol has peripheral effects. Gynecomastia is usually present. The phenotype may be female in testicular feminization, and varying degrees of abnormal scrotal fusion or hypospadias are present in partial forms
Tumors	
Testicular—Leydig's cell	Estradiol secreted by Leydig's cell tumors
Teratoma or choriocarcinoma	hCG secretion may be present
Adrenal	Some adrenal carcinomas secrete estradiol
Other—adenocarcinomas of lung and stomach, hepatoblastomas	Secretion of gonadotropins or hCG by tumors
Starvation and refeeding	Weight loss caused by starvation, malabsorption, or chronic illness is associated with gonadotropin-releasing hormone (GnRH) deficiency. With recovery, GnRH secretion increases, hormonal changes resemble those seen in normal puberty, and transient gynecomastia may occur
Hyperthyroidism	Mechanisms uncertain. Thyroid hormones increase TeBG synthesis, and testosterone binding is increased. Peripheral conversion of androgens to estrogen is increased and leads to a relative estrogen excess
Cirrhosis	Reduced estradiol metabolism. Increased serum estrogen concentrations suppress LH and FSH levels and also increase TeBG levels. Testosterone binding is increased, and a state of relative estrogen excess results
Renal failure	Mechanisms are uncertain, but serum testosterone level is reduced and levels of gonadotropins are usually elevated. Prolactin level is elevated but the significance is uncertain
Carcinoma of the male breast	Rare tumor. Gynecomastia is unilateral and may be very tender
Medications	
Spironolactone, cimetidine, cyproterone, flutamide	Compete for androgen receptors. Spironolactone also decreases testosterone secretion
Marijuana, digitalis	Weak intrinsic estrogen effects. Marijuana may also compete for androgen receptors
Chemotherapy (alkylating agents)	Predominant effect is on germinal epithelium, but Leydig's cells may be involved
Estrogens, testosterone, hCG	Testosterone treatment of hypogonadism is initially associated with transient gynecomastia produced by peripheral conversion to estradiol. hCG stimulates estradiol secretion in addition to testosterone secretion
Methyldopa, reserpine tricyclic antidepressants	Unknown mechanisms. Serum prolactin level may be elevated, but significance is uncertain

forms of testicular feminization). Serum hormone level measurements in these patients vary but usually include elevated levels of gonadotropins and estradiol. A similar clinical presentation may result from abnormalities of testosterone metabolism (deficiency of the 5-alpha-reductase enzyme that converts testosterone to dihydrotestosterone).

The presence of a testicular nodule indicates a possible testicular tumor, which may secrete estradiol (Leydig's cell tumor) or human chorionic gonadotropin (hCG) (teratoma, choriocarcinoma). The diagnosis of a Leydig cell tumor is suggested by an elevated serum estradiol concentration and low levels of luteinizing hormone (LH), follicle-stimulating hormone (FSH), and testosterone. hCG-secreting tumors may be associated with normal or elevated levels of estradiol and testosterone, but measurement of the beta subunit of hCG in serum confirms the diagnosis. Rarely, the source of hCG is an extratesticular tumor of the lungs, stomach, pancreas, or liver.

Gynecomastia occurred in many prisoners after World War II when food was made available. Starvation or severe weight loss from any cause results in reduced hypothalamic gonadotropin-releasing hormone (GnRH) secretion and consequent low serum levels of gonadotropins and testosterone. Weight gain is associated with a return of GnRH secretion, and the pattern of increased gonadotropin and sex steroid levels is similar to that seen during normal puberty. Thus gynecomastia results from the same mechanisms that occur during pubertal maturation.

Abnormalities of sex hormone—binding globulin (TeBG) concentrations may play a role in the gynecomastia associated with alcoholic cirrhosis and hyperthyroidism. In cirrhosis, impaired estrogen metabolism leads to upper normal or elevated serum estradiol levels, which inhibit gonadotropin secretion and increase TeBG production. Testosterone binding is increased, and as gonadotropin secretion is inhibited, levels of unbound biologically active testosterone fall. Similarly, excess thyroid hormone directly stimulates TeBG synthesis, which may explain the gynecomastia seen in some thyrotoxic men.

Medications that may cause gynecomastia are shown in Table 158-1 together with their presumed mechanism of action. Gynecomastia is common associated with use of drugs that increase serum estradiol levels (directly or indirectly) and drugs that interfere with testosterone binding to its intracellular receptor. Many medications have been associated with gynecomastia, but in most instances the exact mechanisms are unknown.

LABORATORY INVESTIGATION AND MANAGEMENT

In pubertal adolescents with normal genitalia, the presence of gynecomastia is assumed to be normal unless it is very severe or does not regress spontaneously. In some cases, however, severe gynecomastia may occur in the absence of demonstrable hormonal abnormalities and may require excision to spare the adolescent undue emotional trauma. In adult men, the appearance of gynecomastia should always be investigated unless it is clearly related to the use of a medication such as spironolactone. Initial investigation should include a complete blood count and assessment of hepatic and renal function. If thyroid disease is suspected, serum thyroxine and T_3-resin uptake measurements should be obtained, especially in elderly men as clinical manifestations of thyrotoxicosis may be absent. Hormonal measurements should include serum estradiol, testosterone, LH, and FSH levels. A low testosterone level with elevated LH and FSH values points to primary gonadal disease. A chromosome karyotype may be indicated, particularly if the testes are small and firm or if clinical evidence of abnormal penile and scrotal development is present. Low testosterone, LH, and FSH values indicate hypothalamic-pituitary disease. In these patients serum prolactin level should be measured and a computed tomography (CT) scan performed. Elevated serum estradiol levels may indicate a testicular tumor, and the level of the beta subunit of hCG should be measured. In the absence of a testicular nodule and beta hCG, an increased serum estradiol value may indicate an adrenal feminizing tumor. Urinary 17-ketosteroid or serum dehydroepiandrosterone sulfate level may be elevated, but a CT or magnetic resonance imaging (MRI) scan of the adrenals should be performed to exclude an adrenal tumor.

Management should be directed at the cause whenever possible. Medication-related gynecomastia usually regresses after the drug is stopped. Gynecomastia associated with the use of hCG or testosterone for treatment of hypogonadism is transient and should simply be observed. If tenderness is severe or the patient excessively embarrassed, tamoxifen given for 1 to 2 months may be effective. In most cases, removal of a testicular or adrenal tumor will result in regression of gynecomastia, but if gynecomastia is severe, complete regression may not occur. In such cases, or when the exact cause is not known, the breast tissue should be excised if the degree of gynecomastia is sufficient to cause the patient embarrassment.

REFERENCES

Bardin CW, Wright W: Androgen receptor deficiency: testicular feminization, its variants and differential diagnosis. Ann Clin Res 12:236, 1980.

Berkovitz GD et al: Familial gynecomastia with increased extraglandular aromatization of plasma C^{19} steroids. J Clin Invest 75:1763, 1985.

Carlson HE: Gynecomastia. N Engl J Med 303:795, 1980.

Casey RW, and Wilson JD: Antiestrogenic action of dihydrotestosterone in mouse breast; competition with estradiol for binding to the estrogen receptor. J Clin Invest 74:2272, 1984.

Kim I, Young RH, and Scully RE: Leydig cell tumors of the testis: a clinicopathological analysis of 40 cases and review of the literature. Am J Surg Pathol 9:177, 1985.

McDonald PC et al: Origin of estrogen in normal men and in women with testicular feminization. J Clin Endocrinol Metab 49:905, 1979.

Moore DC et al: Hormonal changes during puberty vs. transient pubertal gynecomastia and abnormal androgen/estrogen ratios. J Clin Endocrinol Metab 58:492, 1984.

Parker LN et al: Treatment of gynecomastia with tamoxifen: a double-blind cross-over study. Metabolism 35:705, 1986.

Webster DJT: Benign disorders of the male breast. World J Surg 13:726, 1989.

Wilson JD, Aiman J, and McDonald PC: The pathogenesis of gynecomastia. Adv Intern Med 25:1, 1980.

CHAPTER

159 Disorders of Adolescent Growth and Development

H. Verdain Barnes

Adolescence is characterized by dramatic physical, psychologic, and social growth and development. For the physician to provide optimal comprehensive medical care, each feature must be considered in evaluating, diagnosing, and treating the adolescent. This chapter discusses the normal physical growth and development characteristics of puberty, their assessment, and selected abnormalities of height, weight, and secondary sexual development.

PUBERTY

For clinical purposes, *puberty* can be defined as the interval from the earliest prepubertal changes in adrenal steroid secretion to the attainment of adult height, weight, and secondary sexual characteristics. Puberty is the concluding segment of normal physical growth. This continuum of growth begins in utero with sexual differentiation and the ontogeny of the adrenals, hypothalamus pituitary, and gonads. The result is a physically mature adult with the capacity to reproduce. Consequently human puberty is best viewed as a part of this continuum of maturation rather than an isolated event. The primum movens that initiates puberty remains unknown, although much is known about the process.

Hormone changes

The endocrine system provides the first measurable evidence that puberty has begun. The primary endocrine systems involved include the adrenals, hypothalamic-pituitary unit, and gonads. The first identifiable changes occur in the adrenal: adrenarche. Histologically the medullary capsule begins to disappear, and the zona reticularis develops. Accompanying these changes is a substantial increase in the microsomal enzymes, 17, 20-desmolase and 17-alpha hydroxylase, and sulfokinase activity appears. The result is a substantial increase in circulating dehydroepiandrosterone (DHEA) and its sulfate (DHEAS), and modest increases in delta-4-androstanedione and androsterone. In both sexes DHEA and DHEAS concentrations begin to rise between the ages of 7 and 9 years. Both hormones are produced almost entirely (> 90%) by the adrenal gland and rise progressively during puberty. The initiator of normal adrenarche is unknown.

The next identifiable event occurs within 1 to 2 years when both sexes appear to have a progressive decrease in the sensitivity of the hypothalamic-pituitary unit to the negative feedback supplied by the prepubertal levels of gonadal steroids. The result is an increase in the production and episodic release of gonadotropin-releasing hormone (GnRH) by the hypothalamus. Initially major pulsatile releases of GnRH occur only during non–rapid eye movement (REM) sleep. The resulting sleep-related increase in gonadotropin secretion is accompanied by a rise in circulating gonadal steroid levels.

Additional evidence of decreasing sensitivity of the hypothalamic-pituitary unit includes an increased luteinizing hormone (LH) response to a single intravenous bolus of GnRH. During the prepubertal period the LH response is small compared with the response seen at the onset of puberty. With the onset of puberty, there also appears to be a change in gonad sensitivity to stimulation by human chorionic gonadotropin (HCG). This change may in part be explained by an increased number of gonadotropin receptor sites on the gonad, a change that may be follicle-stimulating hormone (FSH) induced.

During puberty there is a progressive increase in DHEA, DHEAS, GnRH, LH, FSH, testosterone, dihydrotestosterone, and estradiol concentrations in both sexes. The progression correlates clinically with the Tanner stages of secondary sexual development.

As female puberty progresses, a positive hypothalamic-pituitary-gonad feedback system develops. Near the time of menarche, the hypothalamus and pituitary begin to respond to estrogen feedback with a pulsatile release of GnRH followed by LH when the critical level of circulating estradiol is reached. This monthly occurrence produces the LH peak that heralds ovulation. When this positive feedback mechanism is fully developed, regular ovulatory menstrual cycles occur (2 to 5 years post menarche).

Growth hormone (GH) and insulin-like growth factor I (IGF-I) (somatomedin C) appear to have significant roles in somatic growth during puberty. GH and IGF-I are needed for normal growth during puberty and the growth spurt. Higher levels of 24 hour integrated concentrations of GH and increased pulse amplitude of GH spikes are seen in adolescents as compared with prepubertal children and young adults. IGF-I level rises progressively through childhood and peaks at about the time of the maximum pubertal increase in lean body mass, height, and weight. This temporary rise in IGF-I level usually begins at about 10 years of age in the average female and 12 to 24 months later in the male. These changes in GH and IGF-I levels appear to be triggered by a progressive rise in growth hormone–releasing hormone (GHRH), which typically peaks during Tanner stage 3 and/or 4. The precise role of insulin in this process is not clear, but recent data suggest an increase in peripheral insulin resistance during puberty associated with a compensatory increase in insulin with which IGF-I has a strong correlation. In addition, appropriate gonadal steroids and nutrition, especially adequate protein, are required for normal IGF-I production and growth stimulation.

There is no convincing evidence that the concentrations of thyroxine, triiodothyronine, cortisol, glucagon, or parathyroid hormone change significantly during normal puberty. Prolactin level does not change in the male and changes only after menarche in the female. On the other hand, some and perhaps all of these hormones may have an important permissive or facilitating role in normal pubertal growth and development. For example, it is known that low or elevated levels of thyroid hormone and cortisol, low insulin and parathyroid hormone levels, and elevated prolactin levels can significantly alter growth and/or development. Level of inhibin, produced by Sertoli (testes) and granulosa (ovary) cells, also rises progressively during puberty. Current data suggest an important role for inhibin in the negative feedback control of FSH secretion. The level of antimüllerian hormone, also produced by the Sertoli and granulosa cells, is known to decrease during puberty, but a precise role in the normal physiologic processes of puberty has yet to be elucidated. The primary hypothalamic, pituitary, adrenal, and gonadal hormones of puberty, along with their primary actions in pubertal growth and development, are shown in Table 159-1.

GROWTH DURING PUBERTY

All body components except the thymus, tonsils, and adenoids normally increase in size during puberty. The most obvious changes occur in height, weight, and the sex organs.

Normal linear growth

The height increase that follows adrenarche usually accounts for 20% to 25% of the final adult height in the sexes. The majority of the growth occurs during a 36 month span within which the pubertal growth spurt, the peak height velocity (PHV) year, occurs. PHV occurs in the female 12 to 24 months before it does in the male. Although there is substantial normal variability in linear growth velocity in this age group, there is minimal variability for a given individual. Consequently the norm is for the adolescent to remain near his or her own percentile of linear growth velocity until he/she reaches adult height.

Normal weight growth

The adolescent's gain in weight after the onset of adrenarche accounts for about 50% of his or her optimum adult weight. More than half of this weight gain occurs during a 36 month period within which the peak weight velocity year (PWV) occurs. In general, the PWV year coincides with the PHV year. In the female, menarche usually occurs within 6 to 12 months after her peak weight velocity. Each individual normally remains near his or her established percentile for weight gain after about age 6 years.

The major contributors to adolescent weight gain are muscle, fat, and bone masses. The increase in lean body mass (for practical purposes, muscle mass) begins near the onset of adrenarche and peaks at the time of PHV and PWV. The total gain in lean body mass is quantitatively and qualitatively greater in males than in females with comparable stages of secondary sexual development. On the other hand, non–lean body mass (for practical purposes, fat) increases considerably in females and minimally in males during puberty. The percentage of body weight as fat in the male decreases to about 9% by the completion of the adolescent "growth spurt," whereas in the female it typically increases to about 20%.

Bone mass increases in parallel to muscle mass. Importantly, skeletal maturation or bone age can be assessed radiographically by evaluating the relative shape, position, and degree of epiphyseal fusion of the hand, wrist, and knee. Bone age has been pictorially defined in the standard Greulich and Pyle atlas. In general, the hand and wrist epiphyses are completely fused by the age of 17 years in the female and 19 years in the male. Once fusion has occurred, there is no significant increase in height.

Table 159-1. Actions of selected hormones during puberty

Hormone	Sex	Actions
Gonadotropin-releasing hormone (GnRH)	M/F	Stimulates pituitary secretion of LH and FSH
	F	Stimulates midmenstrual cycle LH surge
Growth hormone–releasing hormone (GHRH)	M/F	Stimulates pituitary secretion of GH
Growth hormone (GH)	M/F	Stimulates bone and lean body mass growth
Insulin-like growth factor I (IGF-I)	M/F	Is necessary for growth hormone action
Luteinizing hormone (LH)	M	Stimulates Leydig cell production and secretion of testosterone
	F	Stimulates theca cells to production and secretion of estrogens; induces ovulation by midcycle surge; initiates and maintains the corpus luteum and may stimulate the release of progesterone
Follicle-stimulating hormone (FSH)	M	Stimulates late stages of gametogenesis, maintains normal spermatogenesis, and may influence seminiferous tubule growth
	F	Stimulates cyclic growth and development of primary ovarian follicle, stimulates theca cell transformation
Testosterone	M	Stimulates phallus, scrotum, prostate, and seminal vesicle growth; accelerates linear growth; hastens epiphyseal fusion; increases pubic axillary and facial hair growth, skin oiliness, libido, red cell mass, muscle mass, and larynx size
	F	Accelerates linear growth; increases pubic and axillary hair
Estrogen	M	Hastens epiphyseal fusion; stimulates breast development
	F	Stimulates labia, uterus, vagina, and ductal breast development; increases areolar pigmentation; markedly hastens epiphyseal fusion; increases fat mass and distribution; triggers midcycle LH surge
Adrenal androgens (DHEA, DHEAS)	M/F	Initiates pubic hair and linear growth
Progesterone	F	Converts proliferative to secretory endometrium; stimulates lobuloalveolar breast growth

M, male; f, female.

Normal secondary sexual development

The development of adult secondary sexual characteristics is a major milestone for the body-conscious adolescent. During puberty the normal male experiences about a sevenfold increase in the size of the testes, epididymis, and prostate as well as about a twofold increase in phallus size. The normal female has a five- to sevenfold increase in the size of the uterus and ovaries as well as a substantial increase in the size of the vagina, fallopian tubes, labia, clitoris, and breasts. In both sexes, pubic hair and areola size progressively increase during puberty, axillary hair develops, and, in the male, the voice lowers and the beard growth appears.

SELECTED DISORDERS OF PUBERTAL GROWTH AND DEVELOPMENT

The most common concerns and problems of adolescent growth and development seen by the physician are constitutional delay of growth and/or development, idiopathic (familial) short stature, exogenous obesity, and gynecomastia. Less frequent but notable are familial tall stature, the chronic diseases associated with a delay in growth and/or development, and the gonadal dysgenesis syndromes. Of the chronic diseases, the most common are Crohn's disease and hypothyroidism, which in this group may have an occult presentation.

Constitutional delay of growth and/or development

Constitutional growth or developmental delay is estimated to occur in 1% to 2% of the adolescent population. Because a delay for the male tends to carry more cultural stigmata than for the female, they tend to seek help earlier and more frequently. Constitutional delay of growth and/or development, often referred to in the literature as constitutional delay of puberty, is the most common cause (90% to 95%) of growth and development concerns in adolescents. Consequently, the physician needs to be knowledgeable about its diagnosis and management. The cause of this normal variation in growth and development is unknown. These patients ultimately achieve full adult secondary sexual characteristics, ability to reproduce, and height compatible with their genetic background. A diagnosis of constitutional delay of growth and/or development must remain provisional until adult maturation is achieved, a process that may extend into the adolescent's middle 20s. Typically, however, the delay is about 3 years compared to peers of the same sex.

These patients usually seek medical attention between ages 14 and 16 years (mean = 14.9 years). In all published studies the number of females is small.

The typical male patient has an uneventful medical history including an uncomplicated birth and a normal birth length. At presentation, height is usually at or below the fifth percentile (15% to 25% above the fifth percentile) with an average yearly linear growth velocity of 4.0 to 5.5 cm. A history of constitutional delay of growth and/or development in one or more family members is obtained in more than 50%. When present, this can often be used to reassure the adolescent and his or her parents. Finally, these patients typically exhibit some degree of impaired self- and/or body image.

The physical examination findings are normal for a prepubertal male except for delayed development. In most studies the mean presenting height is about 145.0 cm and weight 39.7 kg, giving a derived height age of about 11.3 years and weight age of 12.0 years. The mean bone age is about 12.0 years, or a delay of about 2.7 years compared to chronologic age.

The subsequent growth and development pattern in these patients is variable. The most common is a relatively normal rate of progression to maturity once puberty begins. Next in frequency is a slow rate of progression with maturity attained in the early 20s. The remaining few patients have a very slow progression and reach maturity in the middle 20s.

In the differential diagnosis, idiopathic (familial) short stature and five other entities merit special consideration.

A confident provisional clinical diagnosis of constitutional delay of growth and/or development can be made by using the guidelines detailed in the box below. A variety of laboratory tests and procedures have been reported to distinguish hypogonadotropic hypogonadism from constitutional delay of puberty, but no single test has proved highly

Guidelines for a provisional diagnosis of constitutional delay of pubertal growth and development

Required features

1. Detailed negative review of the endocrine, neurologic, cardiorespiratory, gastrointestinal, renal, and musculoskeletal systems
2. Evidence of appropriate nutrition and eating habits
3. Linear growth rate of at least 4.0 cm/yr (average about 5 cm/yr)
4. Normal physical examination result, including genital anatomy, smell, and body proportions
5. Normal hemogram, erythrocyte sedimentation rate, chemistry profile, urinalysis, thyroid profile including TSH (third generation) findings; negative stool for blood, and noncastrate level of urinary or serum LH (IRMA) and FSH
6. Normal sella turcica on CT or MRI
7. 1.5 to 4.0 yr Delay in bone age compared to chronologic age

Supportive features

1. Family history of constitutional delay of growth and development
2. Height near fifth percentile for chronologic age

TSH, thyroid stimulating hormone; LH, luteinizing hormone; FSH, follicle-stimulating hormone; CT, computed tomography; MRI, magnetic resonance imaging.

sensitive or specific and easily and reliably reproducible. Presently the use of a highly sensitive bioassay and immunofluorometric assay for LH appears to be most promising. For the moment the confirmation of the onset of puberty by the presence of testes greater than 2.5 cm in diameter, serum testosterone level above 50 mg/dl, increase in LH (IRMA) to intravenous GNRH stimulation by more than 7.6 IU/L, or pubertal pattern of nocturnal LH (IRMA) pulsatility correlates well with a final diagnosis of constitutional delay.

Crohn's disease

In about 30% of Crohn's disease patients there is a delay in secondary sexual development and/or growth (Chapter 43). In up to 20% of adolescents with Crohn's disease, abdominal and bowel complaints may be subtle with no history of diarrhea. In most, one or more of the following laboratory abnormalities is identified: elevated erythrocyte sedimentation rate in 84%, decreased serum albumin level in 64%, or iron deficiency anemia in 50%.

Hypothyroidism

In the adolescent, thyroid hormone deficiency is often occult and usually insidious in onset. A delay in secondary sexual development may be less pronounced than linear growth retardation. Of the author's last 36 hypothyroid adolescents, less than 50% had such common manifestations as lethargy, excess weight gain, dry or coarse skin, constipation, cold intolerance, bradycardia, weakness, or facial edema, and one third did not have an obvious goiter. The most common cause is chronic lymphocytic thyroiditis (Hashimoto's) (Chapter 162). The laboratory test of choice is a third-generation TSH.

Turner's syndrome

Gonadal dysgenesis is the most common cause of hypergonadrotrophic hypogonadism in phenotypic females. The classic 45, XO chromatin pattern is found in roughly half of these patients and a mosaic pattern (XX/XO) in the remainder (Chapter 149). The mosaic patient may have few and occasionally no somatic stigmata other than short stature (i.e., well below the first percentile for chronologic age) to suggest Turner's syndrome.

In males with very short stature for chronologic age and delayed secondary sexual development, Noonan's syndrome is a consideration. This syndrome can occur in both sexes.

Klinefelter's syndrome

Klinefelter's syndrome is the most common form of male primary hypogonadism. Adolescent males with normal or tall stature who have an abnormal delay in the onset or progression of secondary sexual development should be evaluated for this diagnosis, particularly if the testes are relatively small and firm, fat distribution is eunuchoid, and/or gynecomastia is present (Chapter 166).

The second most common cause of eunuchoidism is a classic or variant form of Kallmann's syndrome. This type of hypogonadotrophic hypogonadism is usually a X-linked recessive or autosomal dominant disorder. The syndrome typically manifests as delayed puberty. In the classic form, the patient has eunuchoid features with anosmia or hyposmia (Chapter 166).

Idiopathic (familial) short stature

Second in frequency to constitutional delay in growth and/or development among adolescents with growth concerns is idiopathic (familial) short stature. Shortness is often a major concern to an adolescent and his or her parents and may be a concern regardless of whether the adolescent is lagging behind peers in secondary sexual development. These adolescents usually have a benign medical history and normal physical examination findings including body habitus and proportions. Secondary sexual development is typically not abnormally delayed. The family history of short stature is often impressive.

Growth hormone deficiency

The neuroregulation of GH production and secretion is complex because the neurohormones (GHRH and somatostatin), neurotransmitters (e.g., adrenergic, cholinergic, dopaminergic), and neuropeptides (e.g., corticotropin-releasing hormone, thyrotropin-releasing hormone) are all involved. Currently many GH-related causes of short stature with and without pubertal delay are controversial.

The classic form of pituitary GH deficiency is usually diagnosed in childhood. The congenital causes are a deletion of the GH gene, idiopathic GHRH deficiency, or developmental anomalies such as pituitary aplasia/hypoplasia or midline brain abnormality. These patients have low basal levels of GH, an abnormal response to standard GH provocative tests (exercise, levodopa, arginine, and/or insulin), a low basal level of IGF-I/somatomedin C, a decreased 24 hour integrated GH concentration, and a low nocturnal GH peak. In gene deletion or a developmental anomaly, there is an abnormal response to GHRH, whereas in idiopathic GHRH deficiency there is a near-normal response to the intravenous administration of GHRH. The former patients respond to GH therapy and the latter to GH or GHRH therapy. These congenital causes occur in only a small number of the patients with GH-related short stature.

A larger, less clearly defined, and more controversial group of patients appear to have GHRH, GH, and/or IGF-I problems, which may occur during puberty with short stature for chronologic age with or without pubertal delay. The spectrum of laboratory features in these patients ranges from a normal response to provocative GH stimulation tests, low basal IGF-I levels for chronologic age, low 24 hour integrated GH concentration, and low nocturnal GH peak (i.e., GH neurosecretory dysfunction), to normal basal

IGF-I levels and an apparent target cell resistance to IGF-I; to excess level of somatostatin, which inhibits GH release; to normal GH test results and low IGF-I levels with an apparently abnormal GH molecule or perhaps increased GH degradation. Growth hormone neurosecretory dysfunction (GHND) is by far the most common. Patients with the first two types of laboratory characteristics respond in varying degrees to GH therapy.

Familial tall stature

Normal adolescents who are above the 95th percentile for height for their chronologic age may seek medical attention. Most often the patient is a tall female with a tall mother and/or father. These adolescents have a normal health history and physical examination findings including body habitus. The predicted adult height can be estimated on the basis of midparental height (discussed later) and/or bone age. If the predicted adult height is more than 5 cm above the midparental height, or the parents and family are not tall, constitutional early normal maturation, acromegaly, giantism (cerebral or lipodystrophic), hyperthyroidism, Marfan's syndrome, tumor of the ovary (granulosa cell) or testicle (interstitial cell), and homocystinuria enter the differential diagnosis. In males, an XYY chromosome abnormality and Klinefelter's syndrome are also a consideration. For those with constitutional early normal maturation, the adult height is usually within 5 cm of the midparental height.

Weight abnormalities

The desire to control body weight and its distribution is a fanatic concern of many adolescents in the developed countries of the Western world. The most common weight problems (eating disorders) encountered by the physicians are obesity and anorexia nervosa.

Among overweight adolescents, exogenous obesity is the primary type (~95%). An accentuation of long-standing obesity or the onset of excessive weight gain during puberty is relatively common. The former is usually familial, as there are several obese first-order relatives, often including one or both parents. The problem begins in childhood, and the distribution of fat tends to follow that of obese family members. Hyperplasia of the adipose tissue is a common finding. A rare patient in this age group may have associated type II diabetes mellitus or hyperlipidemia.

Those in whom the onset of obesity occurs during puberty often do tend to have a family history of obesity. Their dietary history typically demonstrates an excess in calorie intake, often accentuated by stress, depression, and/or boredom.

In both groups caloric intake typically exceeds expenditure. No definite metabolic or endocrine dysfunction has yet been proved to be the cause of these conditions. The other possible causes of obesity in adolescents are rare; however, the possibility of an identifiable hypothalamic, adrenal, thyroid, pancreatic, or gonadal cause should not be overlooked. When one of these rare causes is present, there is usually ample evidence in the history and physical examination to suggest the diagnosis.

Anorexia nervosa should be considered, in females (female/male ratio ~ 19:1) who are underweight and have delayed or normal secondary sexual development associated with primary amenorrhea, particularly if they are rapidly losing weight. Most are white, middle- to upper-class, intelligent teenagers. Virtually all have a fear of being fat and a distinctly distorted perception of their body. Without these latter two characteristics, some other diagnosis is likely. Most also have a history of physical hyperactivity, usually including a preoccupation with exercise, a strong appetite, constipation, cold intolerance, depression, and/or anxiety. They are typically obsessive-compulsive and perfectionistic and have frequent and at times dramatic mood swings. On physical examination bradycardia, systolic hypotension, hypothermia, dry carotenemic skin, and lanugo hair are common findings (Chapter 37).

Adolescent breast growth abnormalities

The most common breast abnormality called to the physician's attention is gynecomastia. In a third to a half of adolescent males 1 to 3 cm of breast tissue below the areola, *benign adolescent gynecomastia,* develops. It is typically bilateral and nontender but may be unilateral and/or sporadically tender. The age of onset is usually between 12.5 and 14 years of age during gonad stage 3 before the PHV year. This gynecomastia tends to develop over a 1 to 6 month period, and in the majority it resolves spontaneously over the ensuing 6 to 18 months. When it persists longer than 2 years, spontaneous regression is rare. Gynecomastia should be suspected when an adolescent male refuses to be seen at home or at school without his upper body covered, refuses to attend or shower in physical education classes, or voices a concern about his masculinity (Chapter 158).

In the adolescent female a variety of breast growth problems may occur. In descending order of frequency they are breast asymmetry, polythelia, areolar overgrowth, inverted nipple, massiveness of breasts, breast hypoplasia, virginal hypertrophy, and amastia. The most common concern called to the attention of the physician is breast asymmetry. This is a normal finding and usually is minimal by breast stage 5. About 5%, however, continue to have a noticeable difference. Polythelia is a normal variant seen in about 2% of adolescent females. Areolar overgrowth usually occurs in early puberty but typically resolves or becomes far less prominent as the breasts develop. The failure of the nipple to extend beyond the surface of the areola may be often a concern to the adolescent; this normal variant rarely has medical significance in this age group.

The development of massive breasts that produce physical discomfort because of their weight is rare, as is virginal hypertrophy. The former condition is usually symmetric and develops progressively over the duration of pubertal breast growth, whereas the latter is typically rapid in onset and progression and may be unilateral. The presence of large, heavy, pendulous breasts in this age group may result in a negative self- and body image leading to a withdrawal from social and sports activities.

EVALUATING PUBERTAL GROWTH AND DEVELOPMENT

Virtually all adolescents have some degree of concern about the appropriateness of their personal growth and secondary sexual development. Their questions in these areas are often indirectly stated or not verbalized at all. Consequently the physician should be aware that such concerns are normal. Any adolescent's growth and development concern should be seriously and carefully considered by the physician, whether or not it meets the criteria for a medical concern.

A complete medical history is crucial, including an assessment of the adolescent's diet and exercise. Inadequate nutrition, especially protein, can adversely affect growth. Unusual or bizarre eating habits may signal the presence of an eating disorder such as anorexia nervosa, bulimia, or obesity. Excess, little, or no exercise may also adversely affect weight growth.

The adolescent's psychosocial function at home, with peers, and in school should be carefully assessed, because a real or perceived abnormality in growth and development may arrest or impede function in one or more of these areas. For example, an underdeveloped adolescent may refuse to attend or shower after physical education class. A detailed review of systems for subtle as well as overt endocrine, neurologic, cardiorespiratory, gastrointestinal, renal, or musculoskeletal signs and symptoms is essential because chronic diseases that affect growth and/or development (hypothyroidism, Crohn's disease, etc.) may have an occult presentation.

A complete physical examination is mandatory, including an accurate assessment of height, weight, and secondary sexual development. Such an examination cannot be adequately performed when clothing is covering the area to be examined. If there is a possibility of inflammatory bowel disease, a rectal examination and stool sample for occult blood are required. A pelvic examination in the adolescent female is necessary if delayed secondary sexual development and/or primary amenorrhea is being evaluated. Finally, adolescents are almost invariably apprehensive about the examination; therefore, a brief explanation of the specific components of the examination before beginning, preferably with the patient still clothed, often allays anxiety and makes both the patient and the physician more comfortable with the process, thus maximizing the benefits of the examination.

Assessing height and weight

Because height is genetically determined, the adolescent's height and linear growth velocity must be considered in the context of the mother's and father's individual as well as family heights. An accurate measurement of height without shoes using a stable measuring scale that has a right-angle device to extend from the crown of the head to the scale is important for the evaluation and follow-up observation of growing adolescents, particularly those suspected of having a growth problem.

Weight and its distribution as well as body composition appear to be polygenetically determined, although significantly modified in some instances by the environment. From current data it is not possible to predict an "ideal" body weight for age confidently. Likewise, it is not possible to state a precise weight at which medically significant undernutrition or unhealthy overnutrition begins.

The adolescent's current height and weight as well as all known previous values should be plotted by chronologic age on a longitudinal growth chart (Tanner and Whitehouse, or 1976 National Center for Health Statistics) and/or a growth velocity chart (Tanner and Whitehouse). These graphs provide a simple and useful method of (1) following the patient's growth rate, (2) establishing his or her own growth percentile, and (3) determining his or her height age and weight age. The latter are derived by drawing on a longitudinal growth chart a line from the patient's current height or weight to the 50th percentile and a perpendicular line to the age axis. For practical purposes, the 5th and 95th percentiles represent two standard deviations from the mean for a given chronologic age, thus providing clinically acceptable limits of normal variability. For an adolescent in a tall (adult male heights greater than 188 cm or female > 174 cm) or short (adult male height <166 cm for female <149 cm) family, his or her established linear growth velocity can be used as the basis for assessing growth during the pre-PHV years. Distinct deviations from a patient's own growth percentile merit evaluation. If the patient's weight percentile is well below his or her linear growth percentile, a careful search for an underlying chronic disease such as Crohn's disease or anorexia nervosa is needed.

Although no absolute criteria for recognizing abnormal linear growth and weight gain can be applied to all adolescents, the following guidelines have proved clinically useful. The guidelines for abnormal height are (1) a linear growth rate that is less than 4.5 cm or more than 9.0 cm in the years before the PHV year, (2) an acceleration of linear growth velocity that is equivalent to the individual's velocity for his or her PHV year before age 11.5 years in males and 9.5 years in females, (3) no PHV year by age 16 years, or (4) a distinct plateau or deceleration from the individual's established linear growth velocity. The latter is best assessed by using a linear growth velocity chart because longitudinal growth curves are based on cross-sectional height for chronologic age data. The guidelines for abnormal weight are (1) a distinct acceleration (>7 kg/yr) before the PWV year or deceleration (<1kg/yr) in weight gain, or (2) an unexplained weight loss of more than 2 kg during the peripubertal years.

Those adolescents identified as potentially abnormal by these guidelines should, at a minimum, have a careful and complete history and physical examination to search for those disorders known to affect pubertal growth and development adversely (Table 159-2).

Table 159-2. Selected disorders associated with growth and/or development problems in the adolescent

Causes	Pubertal delay alone	Pubertal delay and short stature	Short stature alone
Normal variants*			
Constitutional delay of puberty	X	X	—
Idiopathic short stature	—	X	X
Growth hormone deficiency disorders			
Classic isolated pituitary GH	—	X	X
Idiopathic GHRH/GH	—	—	X
Neurosecretory dysfunction	—	X	X
Panhypopituitarism	—	X	—
Gonadotropin deficiency disorders			
Idiopathic isolated LH and/or FSH	X	X	—
Idiopathic GnRH	X	X	—
Acquired LH and/or FSH	X	X	—
Acquired GnRH	X	X	—
Gonad deficiency disorders			
Idiopathic gonadal steroid	X	X	—
Acquired gonadal steroid	X	X	—
Congenital syndromes			
Klinefelter's	X	—	—
Kallmann's	X	—	—
Turner's	—	X	X†
Noonan's	—	X	X
Pure or mixed gonadal dysgenesis	—	X	—
Chronic diseases‡			
Diabetes mellitus	X	X	X
Crohn's disease	X	X	X
Ulcerative colitis	X	X	X
Renal tubular acidosis	—	X	X
Hypothyroidism	X	X	X
Hyperthyroidism	X	—	—
Anorexia nervosa	X	X	X
Malnutrition	—	X	X
Sickle cell disease	X	X	X

X, reported; —, not reported, GH, growth hormone; GHRH, growth hormone–releasing hormone; LH, luteinizing hormone; FSH, follicle-stimulating hormone; GnRH, gonadotropin-releasing hormone.
*Most common.
†Mosaic.
‡Variable incidence of linear growth retardation and/or pubertal delay.

Assessing secondary sexual development

The changes in the adolescent male's gonads, phallus, and scrotum and in the female's breast (areola and papilla) along with pubic hair growth in both sexes provide an important index of secondary sexual development. A descriptive staging system developed by Tanner and colleagues is the current standard for assessment. A clinically useful modification of their system is shown in Table 159-3. Such staging affords the physician objective parameters by which to assess the onset, status, and progression of an adolescent's sexual maturation.

Because the correlation between gonad or breast and pubic hair is variable, each should be assessed independently. The use of a Prader orchidometer improves accuracy and reproducibility in quantitating testicular volume. There are no standards for female breast size; therefore size per se is not evaluated in staging.

The age of onset for secondary sexual development and the duration of intervals between stages vary considerably within as well as between the sexes. Although there are no absolute criteria for recognizing abnormal secondary sexual development that apply to all adolescents, clinically useful guidelines can be stated by using the mean ±2 standard deviations or an approximation (5th and 95th percentiles). Guidelines for the age of onset and rate of progression are shown in Table 159-4. Those adolescents who vary beyond these limits should be carefully evaluated (Table 159-2) for hypothalamic, pituitary, or gonadal disorders and the chronic diseases known to affect pubertal growth and development.

For adolescents with short or tall stature and/or a delay in secondary sexual development, a hand or wrist radiograph for bone age should be obtained. For those being evaluated for constitutional delay in growth and development, a bone age delayed by more than 4.5 years suggests another diagnosis, such as an underlying chronic disease, or, if delayed less than 1.5 years, familial short stature. The

Table 159-3. Staging guidelines for secondary sexual development

MALE			
Genital stage	**Size of testes**	**Scrotum**	**Phallus (length)**
G1	<2 cm	Prepubertal	Prepubertal (4-8 cm)
G2	2-6 cm	Becomes reddened and thinner	Minimal or no enlargement (4-10 cm)
G3	6-12 cm	Greater thinning and enlargement	Increased length (6-14 cm)
G4	12-18 cm	Color darkens and further enlargement	Increased length, circumference, and gland size (8-15 cm)
G5	>18 cm	Adult	Adult (10-18 cm)

FEMALE		
Breast stage	**Breast**	**Areola and papilla (nipple diameter)**
B1	Prepubertal	Prepubertal (1.3-4.5 mm)
B2	Budding-elevation above chest wall by mound of subareolar breast tissue	Areola widens Papilla erect
B3	Larger and more elevation	Further widening of areola (1.5-6.7 mm)
B4*	Larger and more elevation	Areola and papilla form a mound projecting from the breast contour (4.50-10.9 mm)
B5	Adult (size variable)	No mound; areola and breast in same plane (7.1-12.7 mm)

MALE AND FEMALE			
Pubic hair stage	**Area**	**Amount**	**Type**
PH1	Male	0	
	Female	0	
PH2	Male—base of phallus and/or scrotum	+	Long (straight or curly), slightly pigmented, and downy
	Female—labia majora and/or mons veneris	+	
PH3	Male—spread to mons veneris	++	Increased curl, coarseness, and pigmentation
	Female—increased area of mons veneris		
PH4	Male—greater areas of mons veneris	+++	Greater curl and coarseness
	Female—almost entire mons veneris	+++	
PH5	Male and Female—entire mons veneris and medical aspect of the thighs	++++	Adult

Modified from Barnes HV. In Moss AJ, editor: Pediatrics update. New York, 1979, Elsevier.
*Does not occur in all individuals.

Greulich and Pyle bone age tables for height and chronologic age can also be used to make a reasonable prediction of the anticipated adult height. Patients with short stature and/or pubertal delay also merit computed tomography (CT) of the skull to assess the size and structure of the sella turcica.

A hemogram, erythrocyte sedimentation rate, chemistry profile, urinalysis, thyroid profile including a third generation measurement of thyroid-stimulating hormone (TSH), and blood or urine LH (IRMA) and FSH evaluation should be determined. If the patient's erythrocyte sedimentation rate is elevated and he or she has anemia, hypoalbuminemia, or stool positive for blood, Crohn's disease should be sought. If only anemia and/or hypoalbuminemia is present, anorexia nervosa should also be considered.

When familial short stature is considered the likely diagnosis, a helpful adjunct in assessment is a calculation of the adolescent's expected adult height based on midparent height. The determination of midparent height using Tanner and colleagues' method for calculation can provide a final adult height range for the adolescent. The value is calculated for males by plotting the father's and mother's height on the right coordinate of a standard growth chart, adding 13 cm to the mother's height to correct for the difference in the mean heights of adult men and women, then calculating the mean of the father's and mother's (corrected) heights. This midparent height is then used as the midpoint for the target adult height for the adolescent. A clinically useful approximation of the 3rd and 97th percentiles is obtained by subtracting or adding 10 cm, respectively, to the midparent height. The midparent height for females is similarly derived, but her 13 cm is subtracted from the father's height with no adjustment to the mother's height. The respective percentiles for females are approximated by subtracting or adding 9 cm to the midparent height. These values are useful in adolescent and parent

Table 159-4. Mean age of onset and interval between pubertal events

Event	Mean age of onset*	Stage and interval between stages (yr)†	
Males			
G2	11.9 ± 2.2		
PH2	12.3 ± 1.6	G2-3	0.4-2.2
G3	13.2 ± 1.6	PH2-3	0.1-1.0
PHV	13.8 ± 2.2	G3-4	0.2-1.6
PWV	13.9 ± 1.8	PH3-4	0.3-0.5
PH3	13.9 ± 1.8	G4-5	0.4-1.9
AH	14.0 ± 2.2	PH4-5	0.2-1.5
VC	14.1 ± 1.8		
G4	14.3 ± 1.6	G2-5	1.9-4.7
PH4	14.7 ± 1.8		
FH	14.9 ± 2.2		
G5	15.1 ± 2.2		
PH5	15.3 ± 1.6		
Females			
B2	11.2 ± 3.2		
PH2	11.9 ± 3.0	B2-3	0.2-1.0
PHV	12.5 ± 3.0	PH2-3	0.2-1.3
PWV	12.4 ± 2.8	B3-4	0.1-2.2
B3	12.4 ± 2.4	PH3-4	0.2-0.9
PH3	12.7 ± 1.0	B4-5	0.1-6.8
AH	13.1 ± 1.6	PH4-5	0.6-2.4
B4	13.1 ± 1.4		
Menarche	13.3 ± 2.6	B2-5	1.5-9.0
PH4	13.4 ± 2.4		
B5	14.5 ± 3.2		
PH5	14.6 ± 2.2		

*Data derived from Lee PA: J Adolesc Health Care 1:26–1980; mean ± 2 standard deviations.

†Data from Marshall WA et al: J Arch Dis Child 44:291–1969; 45:13, 1970; and Tanner JM et al: Arch Dis Child 51:170, 1976, 5th to 95th percentiles.

G, genital stage; PH, pubic hair stage; AH, axillary hair; VC, voice change; FH, facial hair; B, breast stage; SD, standard deviation.

counseling and assist in assessing the need for therapy. If the extrapolated height of the adolescent is more than 5 cm below the midparental height, a comprehensive evaluation for possible endocrine dysfunction or occult chronic disease is warranted.

When the diagnosis is questionable or the adolescent requests further evaluation, the patient's GH status should be evaluated. A basal GH, IGF-I/somatomedin C, and GH provocative test (exercise, levodopa, and/or insulin) or a nocturnal GH evaluation is commonly used for initial assessment. However, this battery of tests may not identify a substantial number of patients with GHND who might benefit from GH therapy. For GHND, a 24 hour integrated GH concentration is probably the most reliable test, although recent studies suggest that a 12 hour nocturnal integrated GH concentration may be equally reliable. Patients with a height at or below the first percentile for chronologic age, a linear growth velocity equal to or less than 4 cm per year, a bone age delayed by 2 years or more for chronologic age, a normal GH provocative test response, and a low-normal or low basal IGF-I level for chronologic age should be evaluated for this disorder.

When Turner's syndrome is suspected, a chromosome analysis with banding should be performed. If anorexia nervosa is suspected, the patient should have a psychiatric evaluation. Patients who are overweight but otherwise healthy as indicated by history and physical examination need not have an extensive evaluation for the rare causes of obesity.

THERAPY

Therapeutic intervention may be aggressively sought by a distraught adolescent and/or his or her parents. Consequently the physician must be prepared to provide a measured discussion of the diagnosis as well as effective patient and parent counseling if optimum patient care and satisfaction are to be achieved.

In the past, patients with normal habitus and no known chronic disease have been classified as having constitutional or familial short stature or a combination of the two. Adolescents with constitutional short stature were characterized by a delayed bone age without pubertal delay and familial short stature patients by a normal bone age and short parents; in addition, neither met the standard criteria for growth hormone deficiency. Several studies have now demonstrated that many of these patients as children or adolescents have a significantly increased rate of linear growth when treated with biosynthetic growth hormone without inappropriate acceleration of their bone age or interference with the daily pulsatile secretion of endogenous growth hormone. In current terminology, such patients have *idiopathic short stature*. More longitudinal studies to establish the precise indications for therapy and to identify better methods for predicting clinical outcomes are needed before routine clinical use can be recommended.

The vast majority (80% to 90%) of patients who have constitutional delay in growth and development require only supportive counseling, which stresses that the patient is normal but slow in developing to his/her full adult maturation and reproductive capability. Follow-up observation is needed about every 6 months. Some males, however, experience a profound arrest in psychosocial maturation or are so psychologically distraught that pharmacologic intervention is an appropriate consideration. In such cases, the patient and parents should be made aware of the pros and cons of hormone therapy. The adolescent, in conjunction with the parents, should make the decision to have or not to have hormone therapy. If such therapy is warranted and chosen, 200 mg of testosterone enanthate in oil administered intramuscularly once a month for a maximum of 4 to 6 months produce a progression of pubic hair and phallus development by a mean of 1.6 stages and 3.4 cm, respectively, plus an acceleration of linear growth by a mean of 9.8 cm. For most, these changes have a dramatic positive effect on body perception and psychosocial maturation. This regimen, according to several studies, does not compromise final adult height. Similar results can also be achieved with oral testosterone or oxandrolone administration, but a problem with intentional overdosing by the adolescent often makes oral therapy less desirable. Currently no accepted hormone therapy can be recommended for females with constitutional delay of growth and development.

Patients with secondary hypothyroidism should be treated with L-thyroxine in doses sufficient to maintain the third-generation TSH level in the normal range. For most adolescents, the dose ranges from 0.125 to 0.175 mg daily.

Turner's syndrome patients should have hormone therapy designed and initiated by a physician with expertise in managing both the psychosocial and the hormonal components of therapy for these patients. Patients with Klinefelter's syndrome can be treated with an oral or intramuscular testosterone preparation (Chapter 166).

Benign pubertal gynecomastia often resolves spontaneously and requires no therapy. When there is major psychologic dysfunction regardless of the amount of breast tissue present or the amount of breast growth is considerable, surgical therapy is indicated. Simple mastectomy is immediately successful and continues to be the only mode of therapy when the amount of breast tissue is large or the gynecomastia has persisted 2 years or longer. When treated within 6 to 12 months of onset, about 70% of adolescents with small to moderate gynecomastia appear to respond to 200 to 300 mg of danazol a day for 4 to 6 months.

Adolescents with a chronic disease that retards linear growth may or may not have a delay in the onset of sexual development. Controlling the disease process as quickly and completely as possible is important to ensure maximum linear growth. Once secondary sexual development is complete, catch-up growth cannot occur. If the disease requires the use of a growth-retarding medication such as glucocorticoids, it is critical to use the smallest possible dose to control the disease so that appropriate linear growth can be attained. In general, alternate-day doses of 30 mg of prednisone or its equivalent among the intermediate-acting steroids allow greater linear growth than a 5 to 10 mg daily dose. For example, most Crohn's disease patients with growth retardation grow about 2.0 to 3.0 cm per year. If secondary sexual development and epiphyseal closure occur at the expected time, such a patient may lose close to 21.0 cm (8.4 in) in height. When the disease is controlled with 15 mg of prednisone a day, growth is similar, whereas twice that dose every other day allows 70% to 80% of expected normal linear growth. Chronic disease patients with growth and development retardation should be managed jointly with a physician knowledgeable about adolescent growth and development.

REFERENCES

Barnes HV: Recognizing normal and abnormal growth and development during puberty. In Moss AJ, editor: Pediatrics update. New York, 1979, Elsevier.

Bercu BB et al: Growth hormone neurosecretory dysfunction. Clin Endocrinol Metab 15:537, 1986.

Genentech Collaborative Study Group: Idiopathic short stature: Results of a one-year controlled study of human growth hormone treatment. J Pediatr 115:713, 1989.

Goldstein S et al: The physiology of puberty. In Moss AJ, editor: Pediatrics update. New York, 1984, Elsevier.

Hamill PV et al: Physical growth: National Center for Health Statistics percentiles. Am J Clin Nutr 32:602, 1979.

Lee PA: Normal ages of pubertal events among American males and females. J Adolesc Health Care 1:26, 1980.

Rosenfeld RG et al: A prospective, randomized study of testosterone treatment of constitutional delay in growth and development in male adolescents. Pediatrics 69:681, 1982.

Rosenfeld RL: Diagnosis and management of delayed puberty. J Clin Endocrinol Metab 70:559, 1990.

Schuh R et al: Breast disorders of adolescence. In Kreutner AK and Reycroft-Hollingsworth D, editors: Adolescent obstetrics and gynecology. Chicago, 1978, Year Book.

Smith CP et al: Relationship between insulin, insulin-like growth factor I, and dehydroepiandrosterone sulfate concentrations during childhood, puberty and adult life. J Endocrinol Metab 68:932, 1989.

Tanner JM et al: Clinical longitudinal standards for height and velocity for North American children. J Pediatr 107:317, 1985.

Wu FCW et al: Patterns of pulsatile luteinizing hormone secretion before and during the onset of puberty in boys: a study using an immunoradiometric assay. J Clin Endocrinol Metab 70:629, 1990.

SPECIFIC ENDOCRINE, METABOLIC, AND GENETIC DISORDERS

IV DISORDERS OF THE ENDOCRINE GLANDS

CHAPTER

160 Disorders of the Hypothalamus and Anterior Pituitary

Shlomo Melmed
Glenn D. Braunstein

ANATOMY AND PHYSIOLOGY OF HYPOTHALAMIC-PITUITARY AXIS

Anatomy of the pituitary gland

The pituitary gland, weighing between 500 and 1000 mg, lies in the sella turcica within the sphenoid bone. The roof of the sphenoid sinus forms the floor of the sella, allowing direct surgical approach to the anterior pituitary gland via the transsphenoidal route. The cavernous sinus, containing the carotid arteries and third, fourth, and sixth cranial nerves, bounds the pituitary gland laterally; the optic chiasm lies over the superior aspect of the pituitary fossa. The diaphragma sella, the dural roof of the pituitary, separates the pituitary gland from the optic chiasm and cerebrospinal fluid. The soft tissue structures surrounding the pituitary gland may be compressed by superior or lateral extension of sellar or parasellar space-occupying lesions, resulting in cranial nerve palsies or visual field defects. The bone surrounding the pituitary gland may also be eroded by an expanding pituitary mass, resulting in the thinning and erosion of bony structures such as the clinoids.

The hypothalamus, extending from the margin of the optic chiasm to the mammillary bodies posteriorly, contains cell bodies that synthesize the specific hypothalamic-releasing and -inhibiting hormones, as well as the neurohypophyseal hormones.

Blood is supplied to the anterior pituitary primarily through the hypothalamus from the internal carotid arteries and superior hypophyseal arteries. The hypothalamic-pituitary-portal circulation consists of a rich venous connection between the hypothalamus and the pituitary, constituting the major blood supply of the anterior lobe. A secondary and less important blood supply to the anterior lobe is derived directly from the superior hypophyseal artery, whereas the inferior hypophyseal artery directly supplies the posterior pituitary gland. The primary blood supply to the pituitary therefore facilitates the transport of hypothalamic peptides to the anterior pituitary lobe (Fig. 160-1).

The hypothalamus synthesizes and secretes releasing or inhibiting hormones into the hypophyseal-portal blood supply. These hormones impinge directly on the anterior pituitary gland and regulate synthesis and secretion of the pituitary trophic hormones from specific cells that exhibit distinctive immunohistochemical and specific morphologic characteristics (Table 160-1). Somatotroph cells secrete growth hormone (GH); prolactin (PRL) is secreted by lactotrophs; corticotrophs secrete adrenocorticotropic hormone (ACTH) as well as opiate derivatives of its precursor, proopiomelanocortin (POMC); gonadotrophs secrete follicle-stimulating hormone (FSH) as well as luteinizing hormone (LH). Thyrotropin is secreted by thyrotrophs.

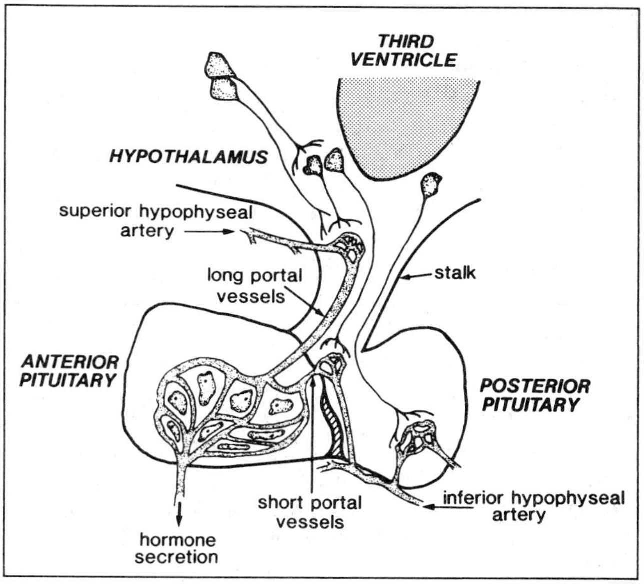

Fig. 160-1. Hypothalamic-pituitary axis. Diagram showing sites of hypothalamic nuclei that synthesize releasing and inhibiting hormones and hypothalamic closed portal system impinging on specific target cell types in the anterior pituitary gland. The anterior pituitary hormones, GH, PRL, ACTH, TSH, FSH, and LH, are secreted into the systemic circulation through the pituitary veins and inferior petrosal sinuses into the internal jugular vein. The posterior pituitary *(neurohypophysis)* derives hypothalamic signaling by direct neural extension of the nuclei synthesizing antidiuretic hormone and oxytocin. GH, growth hormone; PRL, prolactin; ACTH, adrenocorticotropic hormone; TSH, thyroid-stimulating hormone; FSH, follicle-stimulating hormone; LH, luteinizing hormone.

Table 160-1. Hypothalamic-pituitary axis

		Hormone expression	
Hypothalmic hormone	**Pituitary target cell**	**Trophic**	**Peripheral**
Stimulatory			
Growth hormone–releasing hormone	Somatotroph	Growth hormone	Insulin-like growth factor I
Corticotropin–releasing hormone	Corticotroph	ACTH and related peptides	Cortisol
Thyrotropin–releasing hormone	Thyrotroph	Thyrotropin	Thyroid hormones
Gonadotropin–releasing hormone	Gonadotroph	Luteinizing hormone	Gonadal steroids
		Follicle-stimulating hormone	Inhibin
Inhibitory			
Somatostatin	Somatotroph	Growth hormone	
Dopamine	Lactotroph	Prolactin	

Modified from Melmed S et al: Ann Intern Med 105:238, 1986.

HYPOTHALAMIC-PITUITARY TARGET HORMONE SYSTEMS

Hypothalamic-pituitary thyroid system

Thyrotropin-releasing hormone. Thyrotropin-releasing hormone (TRH), a tripeptide (pyroglutamyl histidylprolinamide), interacts with receptors on the thyrotroph, where it stimulates thyroid-stimulating hormone (TSH) secretion. In addition, TRH also stimulates the lactroph cell to secrete PRL.

Thyroid-stimulating hormone. Thyroid-stimulating hormone (TSH) is a glycoprotein hormone synthesized in the thyrotroph cell of the anterior pituitary. The alpha subunit of TSH is common to each of the glycoprotein hormones including TSH, FSH, LH, and human chorionic gonadotropin (hCG). The biologic specificity of these hormones is conferred by their unique beta subunits. Thyroid-stimulating hormone stimulates the thyroid gland to synthesize and secrete thyroid hormones. The secretion of TSH is stimulated by hypothalamic TRH and is inhibited by a potent negative feedback system mediated by peripheral thyroid hormones. Hypothalamic somatostatin (SRIF) and dopamine also inhibit TSH secretion. Nevertheless the negative feedback inhibition of TSH secretion by thyroid hormone overrides positive input from the hypothalamus. For example, hyperthyroid patients with mildly elevated T_4 levels do not respond by releasing TSH after an injection of TRH.

Testing of thyroid-stimulating hormone reserve. To test for pituitary TSH reserve, TRH (200 μ) is administered intravenously. Normal response is a two- to threefold increase in TSH levels occurring within 30 minutes after injection. Hypothyroidism caused by thyroid failure results in an exaggerated TSH response to TRH. Thyroid-stimulating hormone response is blunted in hyperthyroidism, exogenously administered thyroid hormone, and pituitary failure. Pituitary hypothyroidism is also characterized by low basal TSH levels in the face of thyroid failure, whereas hypothalamic hypothyroidism may have normal, low, or slightly elevated TSH level with low serum thyroxine level. In the latter situation, the TSH may have reduced biologic activity.

Hypothalamic-pituitary adrenal system

Corticotropin-releasing factor. Corticotropin-releasing factor (CRF) is a 41 amino acid hypothalamic peptide that stimulates the release of ACTH from the corticotrophs of the anterior pituitary. Corticotropin-releasing hormone is synthesized in the paraventricular nucleus of the hypothalamus as well as in higher brain regions.

Adrenocorticotropic hormone. The corticotroph cell of the anterior pituitary contains a large polypeptide molecule, POMC, which is the precursor for beta lipotropin, beta endorphin, and ACTH. Adrenocorticotropic hormone, a 39 amino acid single-chain polypeptide, stimulates adrenal steroidogenesis. Adrenal cortisol participates in the negative feedback regulation of both pituitary ACTH and hypothalamic CRF release. Loss of cortisol inhibition in patients with primary adrenal failure results in extremely high ACTH levels. The circadian rhythm of ACTH secretion results in peak levels in the early morning; the lowest levels are attained in the late evening. Stress overrides both the negative feedback regulation of cortisol and the circadian rhythm of ACTH secretion.

Testing for adrenocorticotropic hormone reserve. Testing for ACTH reserve is potentially hazardous in patients with compromised adrenal function and should be performed under careful supervision.

Insulin hypoglycemia. Regular insulin should be administered intravenously, 0.05 to 0.1 units per kilogram. The blood sugar level should fall to 50% of baseline within 30 minutes. Normal ACTH reserve is confirmed by a plasma cortisol response of 7 μ per deciliter above the baseline, a doubling of the baseline cortisol level, and a peak value of at least 20 μ per deciliter. The peak cortisol response occurs approximately 30 to 45 minutes after hypoglycemia develops. Insulin hypoglycemia is contraindicated in patients who have primary adrenal insufficiency or who are elderly, suffer from heart disease, or are susceptible to seizures.

Metyrapone. 3 g Metyrapone is given orally at 11 P.M. with a snack. Serum compound S (11-deoxycortisol) and cortisol levels are measured at 8 A.M. the following morning. The metyrapone causes a block in the conversion of

11-deoxycortisol to cortisol, blocking the major negative feedback inhibitor of ACTH secretion. The resultant surge in ACTH secretion stimulates production of compound S, which should be at a level greater than 8 μ per deciliter in individuals with a normal pituitary adrenal axis. Plasma cortisol levels must fall to less than 5 μ per deciliter for the result of this test to be valid.

Cortrosyn stimulation test. As an indirect test of pituitary ACTH reserve, adrenal cortisol reserve may be evaluated. Injection of synthetic ACTH 1 to 24 (cortrosyn 250 μ) intravenously or intramuscularly is followed by measuring serum cortisol levels after 30 and 60 minutes. Normally cortisol levels should double, rise at least 7μ per deciliter, or have peak levels of more than 20 μ per deciliter. A blunted response indicates either impaired pituitary ACTH level reserve or primary adrenal failure.

Corticotropin-releasing hormone test. As a direct test of corticotroph function, corticotropin-releasing hormone, 1 μ per kilogram, is administered intravenously. Plasma and/or serum cortisol responses are measured frequently during the next 60 minutes. Hypopituitary patients show a blunted response to CRF. Interestingly, patients harboring a corticotroph cell adenoma causing Cushing's disease often have an exaggerated ACTH response to CRF. Patients with ectopic ACTH-secreting tumors do not demonstrate a further rise in ACTH levels in response to CRF.

Test for adrenocorticotropic hormone hypersecretion. Dexamethasone suppression test should be performed to rule out a corticotroph-secreting adenoma resulting in Cushing's disease. Details of this test are provided in Chapter 163.

Hypothalamic-pituitary gonadal system

Gonadotropin-releasing hormone (GnRH). Hypothalamic gonadotropin-releasing hormone (GnRH), a 10 amino acid peptide, is synthesized in the preoptic region of the hypothalamus and regulates the secretion of both LH and FSH by pituitary gonadotrophs. The synthesis of this decapeptide appears to be under positive feedback control by peripheral estrogens. It is secreted in a pulsatile fashion every 60 to 120 minutes.

Gonadotropins. The two gonadotrophic hormones, LH and FSH, are glycoprotein hormones produced by the gonadotroph cell. Like TSH, the specific beta subunit confers biologic specificity on each of these hormones. In women, LH appears to mediate ovulation and maintenance of the corpus luteum; in men, LH controls testosterone synthesis and secretion by the Leydig cell. In women, FSH regulates the development and maturation of the ovarian follicle and stimulates the secretion of ovarian estrogen. In men, FSH is responsible for the development of seminiferous tubules and stimulates spermatogenesis. Feedback regulation of gonadotropin secretion is complex with both positive and negative components mediated by levels of gonadal steroids, especially estradiol, and gonadal polypeptide inhibitory (inhibins) or stimulatory (activins) hormones.

Testing for luteinizing hormone and follicle-stimulating hormone reserve

Gonadotropins. The best diagnostic test of gonadotropin deficiency is the concurrent measurement of peripheral serum gonadotropin and gonadal steroid concentrations. Circulating testosterone or estradiol levels are low in patients with pituitary gonadotropin deficiency. Three pooled serum samples drawn 20 minutes apart are used to measure serum LH and FSH levels to compensate for the neurosecretory pulses of gonadotropin release. The normal values are 4 to 20 mIU per milliliter for the gonadotropin hormones. Normal testosterone levels are above 280 ng per deciliter. Normal estradiol levels vary with the menstrual cycle but should be greater than 30 pg per milliliter in postpubertal premenopausal women.

Gonadotropin-releasing hormone test. To stimulate the gonadotrophs to secrete gonadotropins directly, 100 μ GnRH is administered intravenously. Luteinizing hormone levels usually peak within 30 minutes, whereas FSH levels plateau after 1 hour. Normal responses vary according to the menstrual cycle, age, and sex of the patient. Generally, LH levels increase about threefold; the FSH increase is somewhat more blunted. A normal response does not exclude the presence of pituitary hypogonadism, just as an absent response cannot reliably distinguish pituitary from hypothalamic causes of hypogonadism.

Hypothalamic-pituitary growth hormone system

Growth hormone–releasing hormone. Growth hormone–releasing hormone (GHRH), a 44 amino acid peptide, is synthesized in the hypothalamus and stimulates the release of GH from the somatotrophs. It was originally characterized from an ectopic pancreatic tumor and has potent GH-releasing activity when administered intravenously.

Somatostatin. Somatotropin release–inhibiting factor (SRIF) is synthesized in the medial preoptic area of the hypothalamus. This hypothalamic hormone inhibits the secretion of pituitary GH. It participates together with GHRH in a dual control system for the regulation of GH secretion. Interestingly, SRIF is also found in many extrahypothalamic tissues, including the central nervous system, gastrointestinal system, and pancreas.

Growth hormone. Growth hormone, quantitatively the main hormone secreted by the pituitary, is composed of 191 amino acids and has a molecular weight of 22,000 daltons. This polypeptide mediates linear growth together with other hormones and growth factors. Hypothalamic stimulatory and inhibitory peptides regulate GH secretion. Secretion is stimulated by GHRH and inhibited by SRIF. The pulsatile secretion of GH appears to involve a tonic balance between GHRH and SRIF. The secretion of these two peptides appears to be out of phase, which results in sequential peaks and troughs of GH secretion. Peak secretory bursts occur between 11 PM and 1 AM. Physical exercise, emotional stress, and nutritional status all appear to regulate GH secretion at the level of the hypothalamus.

Growth hormone binds to receptors in the liver and induces insulin-like growth factor I (IGF-I) production, which has been shown to mediate most of the growth-promoting actions of GH. Acting by way of a negative feedback loop, IGF-I suppresses GH secretion. Insulin-like growth factor I is also produced by extrahepatic tissues and may play a role in local tissue growth.

In the circulation, IGF is bound to a family of structurally homologous binding proteins (IGFBPs). Six distinct IGFBPs have been identified. IGFBP-3 acts as the main reservoir of circulating IGF, and its molar concentration corresponds to the concentration of total IGF peptide. IGFBP levels are low in states of growth hormone deficiency, liver disease, and malnutrition. In fact, measurements of serum IGFBP-3 concentrations may be useful as reflections of growth hormone deficiency. Smaller IGF binding proteins may also act to regulate the accessibility of IGF-I to target tissues.

Testing for growth hormone reserve. Tests of GH reserve have classically involved the indirect stimulation of the somatotroph to secrete GH.

Insulin hypoglycemia. Insulin hypoglycemia is administered 0.05 to 0.1 unit per kilogram intravenously. Blood glucose concentration should be reduced to at least 40 mg per deciliter or to at least 50% of the patient's initial blood glucose levels. Serial blood samples are drawn for measurement of GH and glucose levels. Peak response of GH occurs between 60 and 90 minutes and should be at least 7 ng per milliliter in 90% of normal patients.

Arginine infusion. Arginine infusion, 0.5 g per kilogram administered intravenously over 30 minutes, normally results in peak GH response to 60 to 90 minutes of at least 7 ng per milliliter.

L-Dopa and clonidine. L-Dopa (500 mg) or clonidine (0.025 mg), administered orally, may also be used to stimulate GH secretion. These oral tests are far safer than insulin tests and are preferred for elderly patients. Blood is drawn every 30 minutes and peak GH levels are found between 60 and 90 minutes.

Growth hormone–releasing hormone test. To test somatotroph secretory capacity directly, GHRH (1 μ/kg) is administered intravenously and serial blood samples drawn. Growth hormone levels usually peak within the first hour after injection. Patients with GH deficiency caused by hypopituitarism do not respond to GHRH. A GH response after repeated GHRH stimulation may indicate the presence of a hypothalamic disorder and defective synthesis or release of endogenous GHRH. Obesity and type II diabetes also cause a flattened GH response to GHRH.

Testing for growth hormone hypersecretion. After the oral administration of 75 g of glucose, GH normally is suppressed to less than 5 ng per milliliter within 60 minutes. Paradoxic GH responses to glucose are seen in about 75% of patients with acromegaly. A similar paradoxic decline may be found with L-dopa. Furthermore, a GH response to TRH may be seen in about 50% of patients with acromegaly.

Basal IGF-I levels are useful for the screening of GH excess because IGF-I levels do not fluctuate rapidly and they reflect the integrated secretion of GH over time. Levels above 2.2 units per milliliter are usually found in patients with acromegaly or gigantism. However, IGF-I levels are not as useful for screening for hypopituitarism, because the levels in hypopituitary patients may overlap with those of normal individuals.

Hypothalamic-pituitary prolactin system

Prolactin-inhibiting factor. The primary hypothalamic prolactin inhibitory factor is dopamine, which is a potent inhibitor of pituitary lactotroph prolactin synthesis and release. This tonic inhibition of prolactin by dopamine can be blocked by dopamine antagonists. Administration of potent dopamine antagonist drugs such as metoclopramide which do not cross the blood-brain barrier and which impinge directly on the anterior pituitary gland, result in enhanced basal prolactin secretion. Furthermore, depletion of hypothalamic dopamine by drugs, including the phenothiazines, causes hyperprolactinemia and even galactorrhea. This observation of the dopaminergic inhibition of prolactin secretion has allowed the design of therapeutic agents such as bromocriptine to suppress excessive secretion of prolactin.

Although no hypothalamic prolactin-releasing factor has been proved conclusively, vasoactive intestinal polypeptide (VIP) appears to be an important stimulator of prolactin synthesis and secretion by the pituitary.

Prolactin. Prolactin has a molecular weight of 21,500 daltons, contains 199 amino acids, and has a high degree of homology with GH and placental lactogen concentrations. Prolactin secretion is directed by inhibitory hypothalamic control. Dopamine inhibits whereas TRH and VIP stimulate PRL secretion. However, the physiologic role of TRH is unclear, because the level of TSH, which is released by TRH, does not rise during lactation when PRL levels are high. Prolactin secretion is also stimulated by estrogen, which may be the most important peripheral regulator of PRL secretion. Prolactin levels are often elevated in hyperestrogenemic states.

Testing for prolactin reserve. Thyrotropin-releasing hormone (200 μ intravenously by bolus) is administered. The peak PRL response after 10 to 20 minutes should be three- to fivefold above the baseline. Normal basal PRL levels are less than 20 ng per milliliter. Metoclopromide, 10 mg intramuscularly, may also be used as a stimulator of PRL release. The normal response is a doubling of PRL levels after 1 hour.

Testing for prolactin hypersecretion. A basal PRL level greater than 200 ng per milliliter strongly suggests the presence of a PRL-secreting adenoma. Although responses to TRH, metoclopromide, and L-dopa may be variable in patients harboring PRL-secreting adenoma, these tests are of limited utility in diagnosing the presence of such adenomas.

Quadruple-bolus testing. To provide an efficient and sensitive method for comprehensive testing of anterior pituitary reserve function, all four hypothalamic-releasing hormones may be administered simultaneously (Table 160-2) (Fig. 160-2).

Table 160-2. Administration of hypothalamic-releasing hormones as a combined anterior pituitary function test*

Hypothalamic hormone	Radioimmunoassay of pituitary hormone	Venous sampling time after infusion (min)
TRH 200 μ	TSH	15, 30
	PRL	10, 15
CRF 1 μ/kg	ACTH	10, 45, 60
GHRH 1 μ/kg	GH	45, 60
GnRH 100 μ	FSH	45, 60, 90
	LH	15, 30

Modified from Sheldon WR et al: J Clin Endocrinol Metab 60:623, 1985.
*Basal (zero time) samples are initially drawn for each hormone measurement. All four hypothalamic-releasing hormones are administered intravenously sequentially over 60 seconds, then followed by venous sampling for specific hormone radioimmunoassay at the indicated times.

CLINICAL SYNDROMES

Hypothalamic dysfunction

The hypothalamic nuclei surrounding the third ventricle are essential for the normal physiologic regulation of water metabolism, temperature control, appetite and food intake, the sleep-wake cycle, visceral (autonomic) functions, and control of anterior pituitary function. In addition, emotional expression, behavior, and short-term memory are influenced by this region. Small lesions in the hypothalamus therefore may give rise to several clinical abnormalities.

Several disease processes may involve the hypothalamus, including primary intracranial tumors, infiltrative disorders, trauma, vascular abnormalities, and developmental malformations. Over half of these patients have neuro-ophthalmologic abnormalities, pyramidal tract or sensory nerve involvement, headaches, and extrapyramidal cerebellar signs. Approximately one third exhibit recurrent vomiting, diabetes insipidus, somnolence, dysthermia, appetite dysfunction, and hypogonadism or precocious puberty.

Specific signs and symptoms of hypothalamic clinical syndromes have been localized to nuclear lesions (Fig. 160-3). Slow-growing lesions generally remain asymptomatic

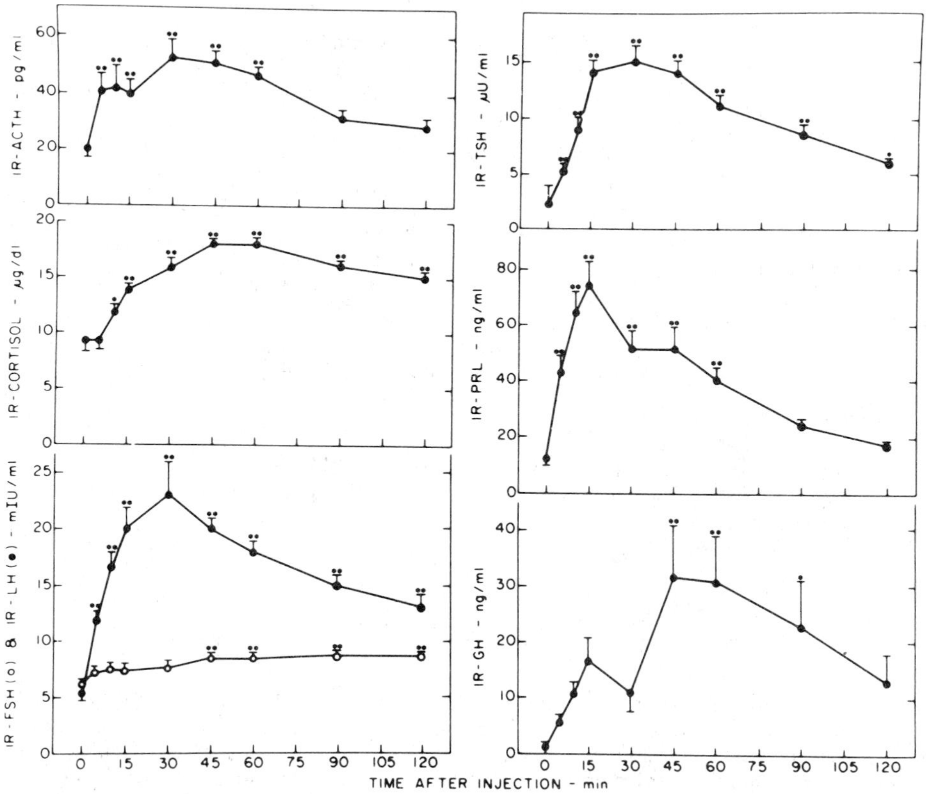

Fig. 160-2. Quadruple bolus test of anterior pituitary hormone reserve. Mean plasma or serum (± SEM) levels of hormones at intervals after administration of all four hypothalamic-releasing hormones in 26 normal subjects. $P < 0.05$; ** $P < 0.01$ (compared to baseline value). All four hypothalamic-releasing hormones are administered as depicted in Table 160-2. SEM, standard error of the mean. (From Sheldon WR et al: J Clin Endocrinol Metab 60:623, 1985.)

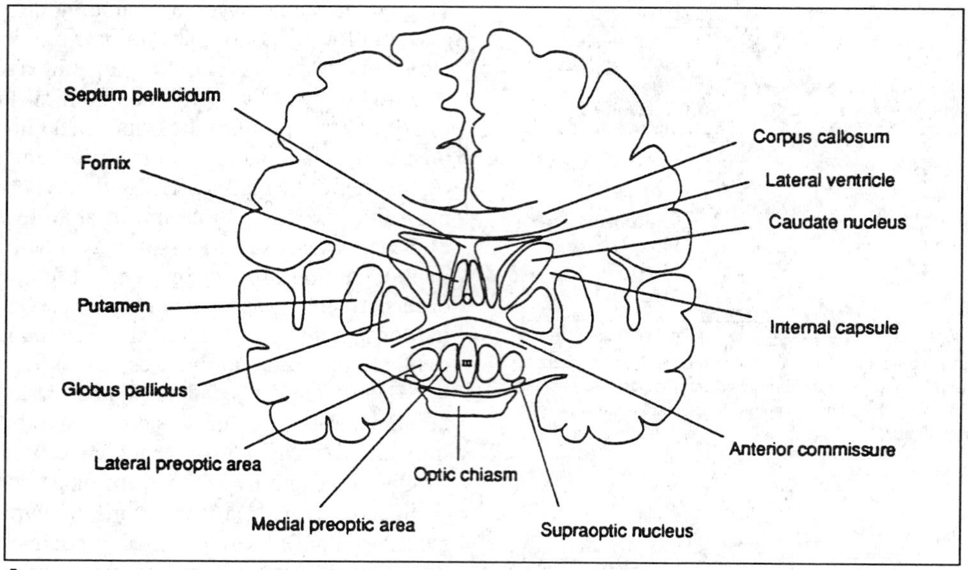

A

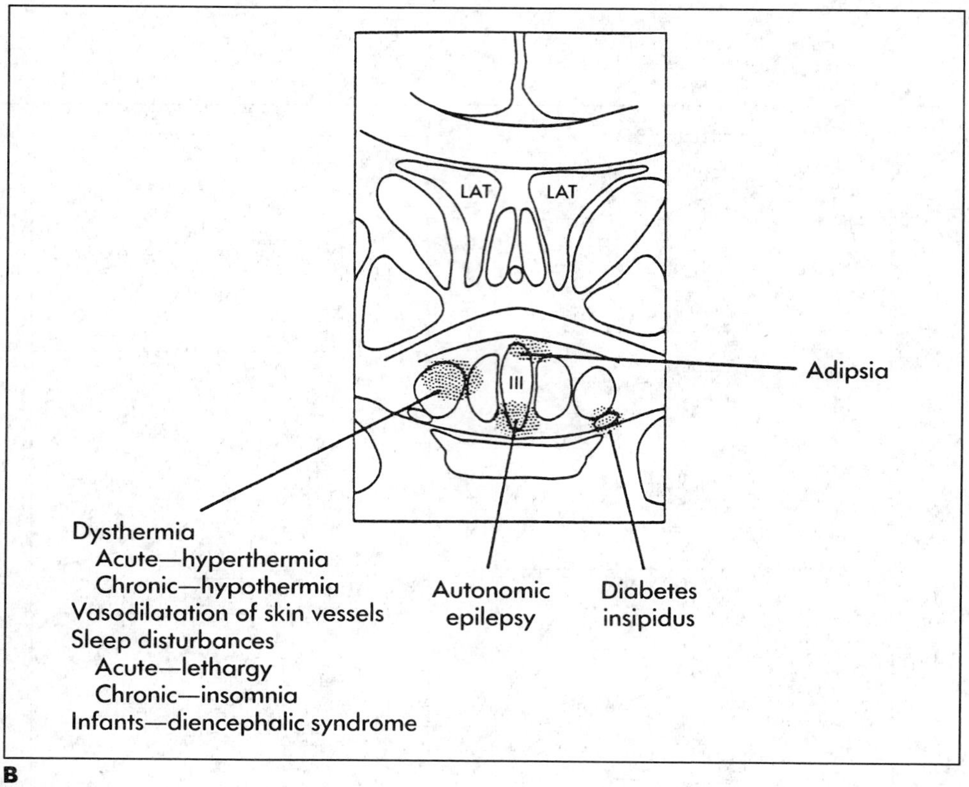

B

Fig. 160-3. A, Frontal section of the preoptic region of the hypothalamus. **B,** Clinical findings associated with lesions affecting the preoptic region. **C,** Frontal section of the supraoptic region of the hypothalamus. **D,** Clinical findings associated with lesions in the supraoptic region. **E,** Frontal section of the mammillary region of the hypothalamus. **F,** Clinical findings associated with lesions involving the mammillary region. III, third ventricle; LAT, lateral ventricle. (From Braunstein GD: In Melmed S, editor: The pituitary. Cambridge, MA: 1993, Blackwell Scientific.

Continued.

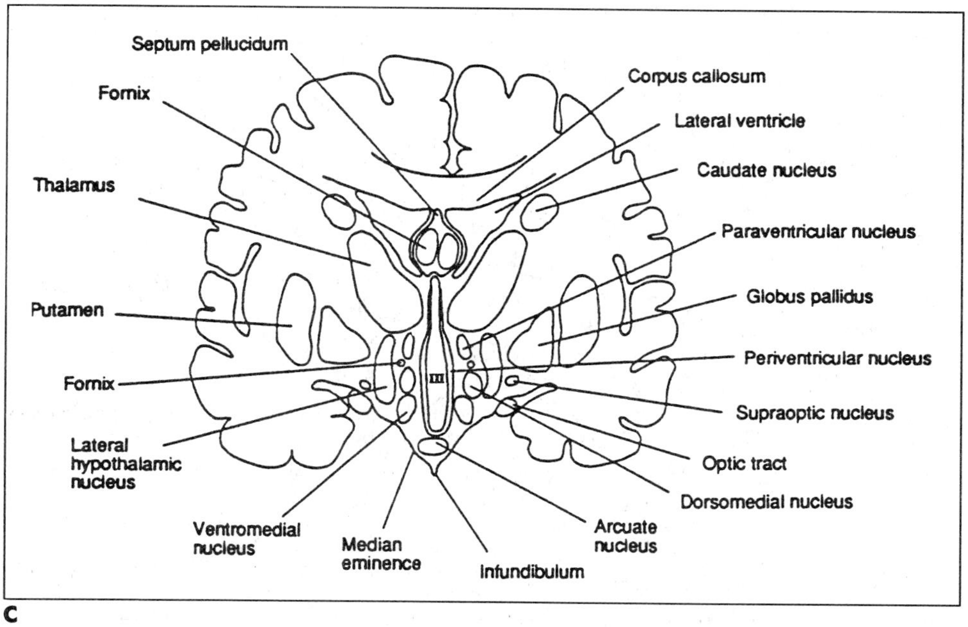

C

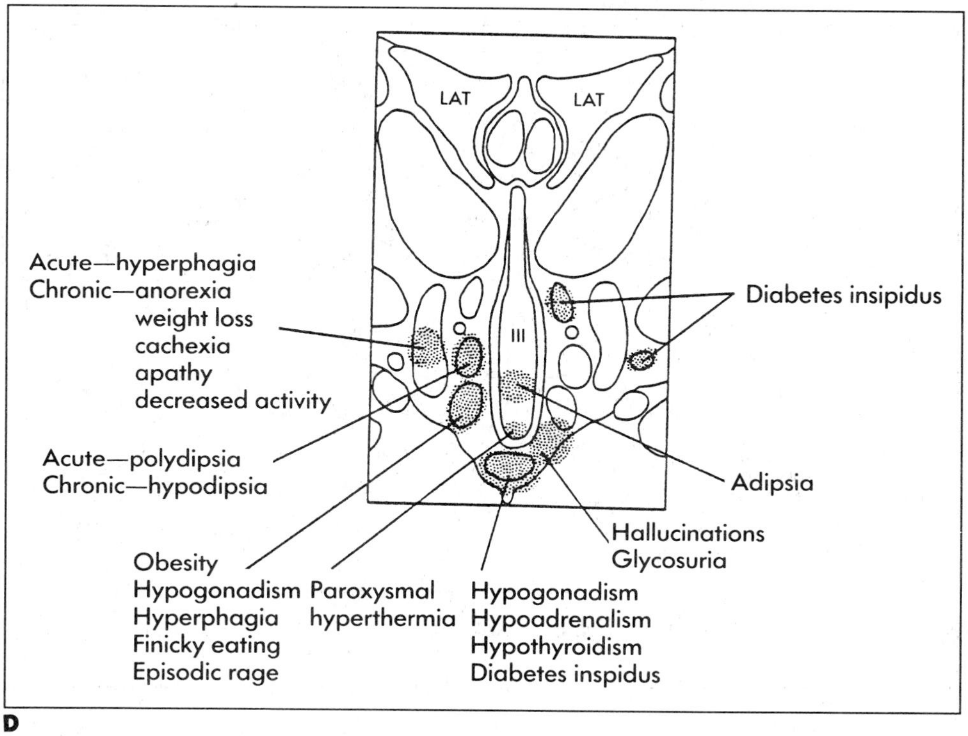

D

Fig. 160-3, cont'd.
For legend, see opposite page.

Continued.

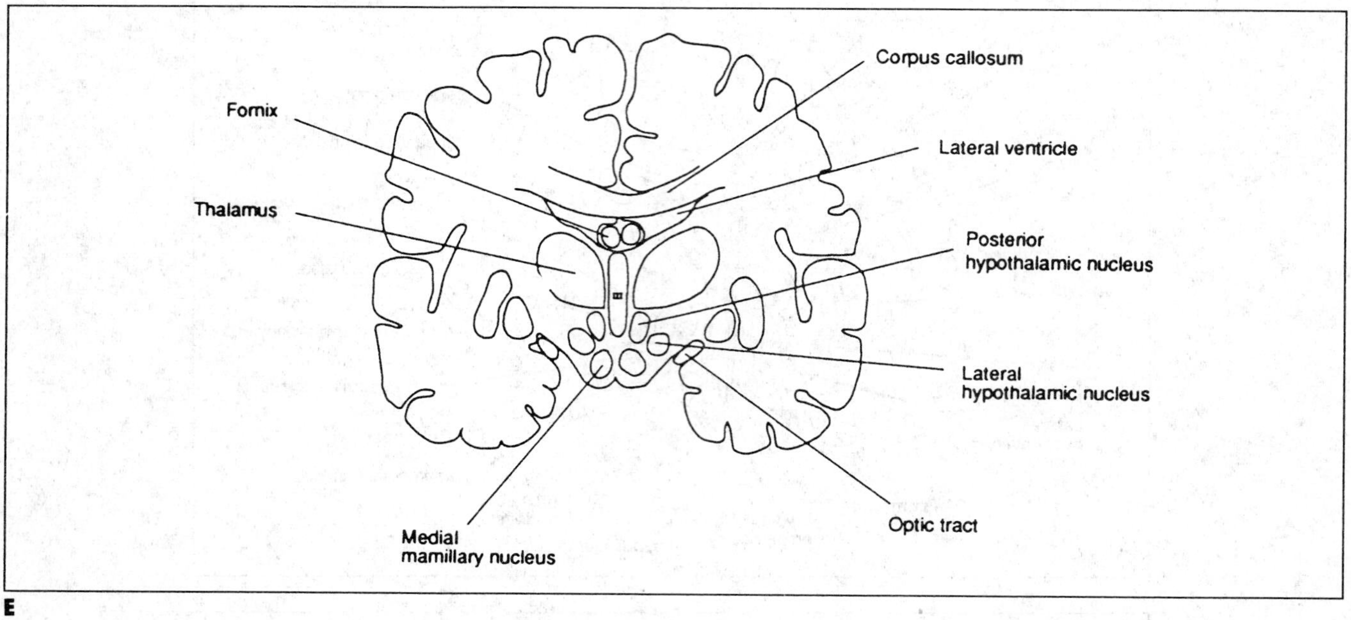

E

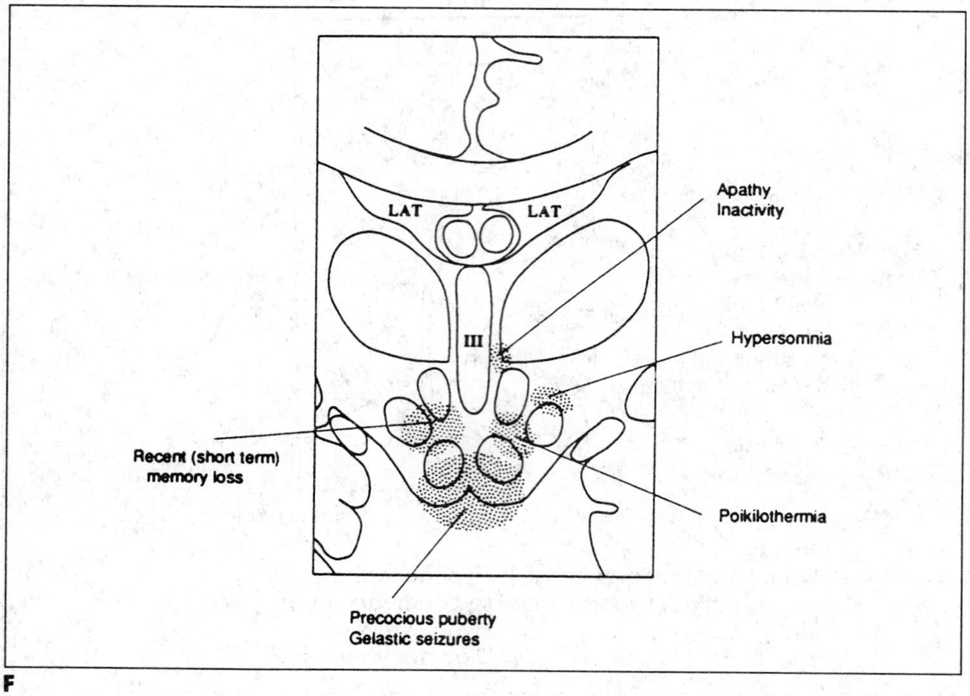

F

Fig. 160-3, cont'd.
For legend, see page 1298.

for substantially longer periods than acute insults. Destruction of a single unilateral nucleus usually does not result in a clinical syndrome as the remaining intact contralateral nucleus is sufficient to maintain appropriate physiologic homeostasis. Lesions arising from the third ventricle or basal hypothalamus or diffuse infiltrative conditions are most likely to lead to symptoms resulting from involvement of both homologous nuclei. Clinical manifestations also depend on whether a lesion involving a nucleus is stimulatory or destructive. For example, a tumor invading and destroying the tuberal area may result in hypogonadism, whereas a hamartoma in the same region may lead to precocious puberty. Systemic diseases such as sarcoidosis or histiocytosis that involve the hypothalamus usually have extrahypothalamic manifestations that may provide a clue to the underlying cause of the hypothalamic disorder.

Hypopituitarism

The clinical manifestations of hypopituitarism depend on the degree of pituitary hormone deficiency. The deficiency of anterior pituitary hormones may be isolated or may result from a combination of several hormone deficiencies. Generally, the pattern of hormone loss in a destructive pituitary lesion results in initial loss of GH, followed by gonadotropin, TSH, and finally ACTH secretion.

Causes. The causes of hypopituitarism are outlined in the box at right. Congenital conditions such as septo-optic dysplasia, Prader-Willi syndrome, and Laurence-Moon-Biedl syndrome usually are apparent in childhood. Isolated GH deficiency is an important cause of short stature. Recently, a neurosecretory GH deficiency has been described. These patients usually have short stature and an absence of normal nocturnal peaks of GH secretion. This may be diagnosed by performing serial GH testing every 20 minutes. The integrated GH secretion over 24 hours is low in these patients because of a presumed deficit of hypothalamic GHRH. Cysts of the base of the brain impinging on the hypothalamus may also cause pituitary failure. The vascular causes of hypopituitarism include pituitary apoplexy, Sheehan's syndrome, carotid aneurysm, as well as connective tissue disease and arteritides including systemic lupus erythematosus.

Causes of hypopituitarism

- Congenital or acquired
  - Septo-optic dysplasia
  - Hypogonadotrophic hypogonadism
  - Prader-Willi syndrome
  - Laurence-Moon-Biedl syndrome
  - Isolated GH deficiency
  - Neurosecretory GH deficiency
  - Basal encephalocele
- Vascular
  - Pituitary apoplexy
  - Sheehan's syndrome
  - Arteritides
  - Carotid aneurysm
- Inflammatory
  - Autoimmune lymphocytic hypophysitis
  - Histiocytosis
  - Sarcoidosis
  - Tuberculosis
  - Syphilis
  - Mycoses
- Physical agents
  - Cranial trauma and hemorrhage
  - Ionizing radiation
  - Stalk section
  - Surgery
- Infiltrations
  - Hemochromatosis
  - Metastatic carcinoma (breast and bronchus)
  - Amyloidosis
- Tumors
  - Hypothalamic
    - Craniopharyngioma
    - Glioma
    - Germinoma
    - Meningioma (sphenoidal ridge)
    - Hamartoma
    - Leukemia and lymphoma
  - Pituitary
    - Functioning macroadenomas
    - Nonfunctioning macroadenomas
- Idiopathic
  - Empty sella
  - Diabetes insipidus

Autoimmune lymphocytic hypophysitis is a recently recognized cause of pituitary failure. This condition has been described in association with pregnancy. The pituitary failure usually involves all the trophic hormones. The magnetic resonance image (MRI) of this condition may be difficult to differentiate from that of a pituitary tumor. Although the treatment of patients with this disorder does not require surgery, the diagnosis may be difficult and may only become evident on histologic examination of a surgical specimen. Other inflammatory causes of pituitary failure include histiocytosis, sarcoidosis, and chronic infection giving rise to granulomatous disease of the hypothalamus or pituitary including tuberculosis, syphilis, and various mycoses.

Damage to the hypothalamus or hypothalamic-pituitary unit cause pituitary failure. Trauma to the base of the brain may result in a stalk section and hemorrhage in the pituitary fossa. Ionizing radiation, especially with doses above 4000 rad, and surgery are iatrogenic causes of pituitary damage. Hemochromatosis, amyloidosis, and metastatic carcinoma are important lesions that may infiltrate the hypothalamus, and sometimes the pituitary itself, and cause pituitary failure. Interestingly, metastatic carcinoma is relatively rare in the anterior pituitary and is more commonly found in the posterior pituitary. This may be explained by the blood supply of the anterior pituitary, which comes primarily from the hypothalamic portal system, whereas the posterior pituitary has a direct blood supply from the internal carotid and the inferior hypophyseal arteries. The important tumors that metastasize to the pituitary are breast and bronchial carcinomas.

Tumors of the hypothalamus and pituitary are important causes of destruction and compression of the anterior pituitary, frequently resulting in its failure. The most common hypothalamic tumors are craniopharyngioma; this nonfunctioning mass may damage the hypothalamic neurons responsible for releasing factor production or may disrupt the vascular or neural connections between the hypothalamus and pituitary, resulting in growth failure and other features of hypopituitarism. Hypothalamic gliomas, germinomas, and hamartomas may impinge on the normal hypothalamic function through their mass effects, and there may also be functional and elaborate excessive amounts of hypothalamic-releasing hormones. Both functioning and nonfunctioning pituitary adenomas may compress normal surrounding pituitary tissue, resulting in pituitary failure. Usually the destruction of local pituitary tissue has to be fairly significant for pituitary failure to occur. Finally, idiopathic pituitary failure is occasionally seen in patients with primary empty sella and with idiopathic diabetes insipidus.

Pituitary apoplexy

Acute massive infarction of the pituitary gland (apoplexy) is a rare, life-threatening disorder that requires prompt diagnosis and treatment.

Causes. Predisposing factors that may lead to occlusion or severe spasm of the arteries supplying the anterior lobe and pituitary stalk include pregnancy, pituitary tumor, acquired or hereditary bleeding or clotting disorders, trauma, carotid angiography, radiation therapy of pituitary tumors, artificial respiration, increased intracranial pressure, diabetes, and atherosclerosis. Pathogenesis of this condition results from total ischemia associated with initial acute arterial spasm. This is followed by vascular congestion and thrombosis.

Signs and symptoms. The clinical presentation of pituitary apoplexy includes a wide range of symptoms and signs including sudden death. Retro-orbital or frontal headache occurs most commonly and is usually severe in nature and of very sudden onset. This may be accompanied by diplopia caused by compression of the cranial nerves (especially III and VI) supplying the extraocular muscles as a result of increased cavernous sinus pressure. Impaired visual acuity, photophobia, and visual blurring may precede the other clinical manifestations of apoplexy. Neurologic features of apoplexy commonly include alteration in consciousness, drowsiness, coma, and death. These signs may be accompanied by hemiparesis, hemianesthesias, signs of meningial irritation, nausea, vomiting, and diabetes insipidus. Hyperpyrexia is also commonly seen. Less common physical findings include seizures, aphasia, dementia, and lower cranial nerve palsies. Systemic alterations in temperature, respiratory rates, and blood pressure may occur if hypothalamic compression is significant. The clinical manifestations of apoplexy usually reflect the anatomic focus of the lesion. Accompanying adrenal insufficiency caused by pituitary failure may also contribute to the clinical picture.

Examination of the cerebrospinal fluid (CSF) usually reveals xanthochromia or fresh blood. Cerebrospinal fluid pressure and protein levels are usually elevated, and peripheral blood may show a leukocytosis. Computed tomography (CT) scan or MRI of the pituitary may identify a pituitary mass with or without suprasellar extension and associated perisellar bleeding.

Differential diagnosis. Differential diagnosis of this condition must be made quickly to ensure lifesaving intervention. The conditions to be considered in the differential diagnosis include ruptured intracranial aneurysm, acute meningitis, infarction of the base of brain, degenerative encephalopathy, and supratentorial herniation.

Signs and symptoms of pituitary failure. Any combination of single or multiple hormone loss may occur in lesions of the pituitary gland. Isolated deficiency of a single hormone may also occur.

Growth hormone deficiency. Growth retardation, short stature, and fasting hypoglycemia are the clinical hallmarks of GH deficiency during infancy and childhood. Delayed puberty may also be present. Children with this deficiency, which may be isolated, are usually round faced with a chubby appearance and lack good muscular development. Adults may not have any manifestations of GH deficiency, unless combined with ACTH deficiency, which may result in fasting hypoglycemia.

Gonadotropin deficiency. Central hypogonadism during childhood results in failure to enter normal puberty. Breast development is delayed, and pubic and axillary hair do not develop normally, although some sexual hair growth takes place if ACTH secretion is intact and stimulates adrenal androgen production. In females, primary amenorrhea is also present. In boys, small testes and phallus and sparse body hair are evident. If the gonadotropin deficiency is isolated, growth may be delayed but continues as a result of failure of long-bone epiphyseal closure. Therefore isolated hypogonadism causes adolescents to be tall and have eunuchoidal proportions. In these individuals, the upper/lower segment ratio is less than 1. Their arm span is usually greater than their height by 5 cm or more. In postpubertal women, hypogonadism is manifested as secondary amenorrhea, breast atrophy, and loss of pubic and axillary hair. In men, testicular atrophy, decrease in body hair growth, decrease in libido, impotence, and infertility are present.

Thyroid-stimulating hormone secretion deficiency. Deficiency of TSH secretion causes failure of thyroid function. The thyroid gland becomes involuted, and clinical features of hypothyroidism including lethargy, cold intolerance, constipation, bradycardia, delayed reflex relaxation time, and hoarseness become apparent. These patients may be differentiated from those who have primary hypothyroidism by a low circulating level of TSH in the presence of low thyroid hormone levels. The low TSH levels do not respond to exogenously administered TRH because of the pituitary lesion.

Adrenocorticotropic hormone deficiency. Deficiency in ACTH results in adrenal failure with a spectrum of presentations including orthostatic hypotension, weakness, hypothermia, nausea, vomiting, dehydration, lethargy, coma, and even death. Hypokalemia is usually not seen because of the maintenance of mineralocorticoid secretion through the renin-angiotensin-aldosterone system.

Vasopressin deficiency. Vasopressin (ADH) deficiency occurs when lesions involve the posterior pituitary. Damage to the hypothalamic nuclei or the posterior pituitary extensions of their axons results in diminished release of ADH. The symptoms of diabetes insipidus include polyuria, polydypsia, and nocturia.

Treatment of hypopituitarism

Adrenocorticotropic hormone replacement. The usual adult replacement dose of hydrocortisone is 20 mg in the morning and 10 mg at night. Alternatively, 25 mg cortisone acetate can be administered in the morning and 12.5 mg at night. Patients should be advised to increase the amount of medication to two to three times the normal replacement level before minor stresses such as dental procedures and to carry a Medi-Alert (Turlock, California) identification explaining the necessity to administer cortisol during any accident or other stress.

Thyroid-stimulating hormone replacement. The usual recommended replacement of thyroid hormone is in the form of synthetic L-thyroxine. This should be given in doses ranging from 0.1 to 0.15 mg once daily. Peripheral conversion of T_4 to T_3 provides physiologic amounts of T_3, as the majority of circulating T_3 is normally derived from peripheral hepatic conversion from T_4.

Gonadotropin replacement. In males, replacement of testosterone should be in the form of testosterone enanthate or cyprionate injections, 200 mg intramuscularly every 2 weeks. In females, estrogens can be replaced by administering ethinyl estradiol 0.02 to 0.05 mg, or conjugated equine estrogens, 0.65 to 1.25 mg daily for the first 25 days of each month. Alternatively, estradiol skin patches containing 4 or 8 mg of estrogen may be administered twice weekly for 3 weeks of every month. It is recommended that progesterone be added to facilitate cyclical uterine shedding. Medroxyprogesterone acetate 5 to 10 mg on day 16 through 25 of each month may be administered, and withdrawal bleeding generally begins between days 24 and 28 of the month. In both sexes, if fertility is desired, then gonadotropin therapy with menopausal gonadotropins and hCG should be instituted to induce ovulation or spermatogenesis. Alternatively, synthetic GnRH may be given in a pulsatile fashion via an infusion pump.

Growth hormone replacement. Children with short stature caused by GH deficiency or GH neurosecretory defect are treated with synthetic human GH derived from molecular recombinant techniques. The hormone is administered intramuscularly or subcutaneously at a dose of 0.1 mg per kilogram three times a week until fusion of the long-bone epiphyses takes place. Growth hormone therapy is currently being evaluated in adults who are in catabolic states including those who have burns, respiratory insufficiency, and postoperative recovery. The hormone is also being tested for use in the management of osteopenia and loss of lean body mass associated with aging.

Vasopressin replacement. ADH is provided by intranasal desmopressin (DDAVP). Recommended dose is 0.05 to 0.1 ml twice daily but must be titrated in each patient.

Treatment of pituitary apoplexy. The treatment of pituitary apoplexy is a medical emergency. Intravenous fluid and oxygen should be administered immediately with intravenous hydrocortisone (200 mg). Intravenous hydrocortisone boluses should be repeated as required during the initial phase of recovery. Intravenous thyroxine should not be administered until the hydrocortisone has been given. The increased metabolic demands of the administered thyroid hormone may precipitate adrenal crisis if the patient has not had adequate cortisone replacement. The dose of intravenous thyroxine is usually 500 μ administered as an intravenous bolus. Thereafter up to 100 μ intravenously daily is continued, as required. Blood glucose level should also be carefully monitored during the acute phase of apoplexy as these patients may be acutely hypersensitive to insulin because of the absence of the pituitary hormones that usually antagonize insulin action (e.g., GH, ACTH). These patients may therefore require intravenous glucose administration in addition to their initial acute hormonal replacement.

Pituitary tumors

Sensitive and specific immunotechniques have provided insight into the cellular pathophysiology of the anterior pituitary tumors. Each of the anterior pituitary cells as well as their putative primitive stem cell precursors, either singly or in combination, may give rise to pituitary adenomas that express functional hormones. Prolactin, GH, and POMC-expressing adenomas account for the vast majority of adenomas removed surgically. Prolactin-secreting adenomas account for at least one third of all pituitary adenomas. Gonadotropin- and TSH-secreting tumors account for less than 5% of all pituitary tumors. Recent studies have shown that some "nonfunctioning" tumors that do not secrete biologically active hormones may contain and/or secrete the common glycoprotein hormone alpha subunit.

Diagnosis. The mass effects or hormonal aberrations induced by pituitary tumors lead to the signs and symptoms that alert the patient and clinician. These manifestations may appear initially as a result of compression of adjacent neurologic structures while causing systemic effects by way of excess peripheral hormonal action. Depending on its structure, a tumor may cause hyposecretion of one hormone and hypersecretion of another. Hypersecretion of a pituitary trophic hormone can cause acromegaly, amenorrhea-galactorrhea, impotence, or Cushing's disease. Hyposecretion may result in hypogonadism, hypothyroidism, or hypoadrenalism.

Diagnosis of pituitary adenomas has been aided by the advent of sophisticated imaging techniques: CT and MRI (Fig. 160-4). These noninvasive procedures have many advantages over multidirectional polytomograms, pneumoencephalograms, angiograms, and venograms because they

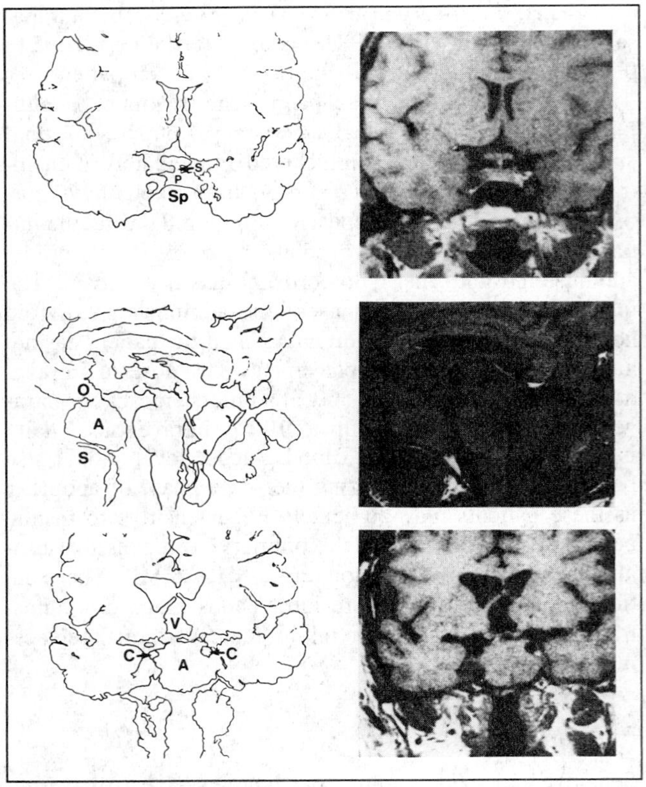

Fig. 160-4. MRI scans of head showing the normal anatomic relations of the pituitary gland *(top panel)* and a large GH-cell pituitary macroadenoma enlarging the sella and extending ventrally *(lower panels)*. Bony and soft tissue structures are clearly identified. *A*, adenoma; *C*, internal carotid arteries; *O*, optic tract; *P*, normal pituitary; *Sp*, sphenoid sinus; *S*, pituitary stalk; *V*, fourth ventricle. MRI, magnetic resonance imaging.

eliminate morbidity, decrease the cost of preoperative evaluation, and lessen the length of hospital stay. In addition, MRIs have the ability to detect microadenoma masses smaller than 3 mm that might otherwise be missed by less advanced techniques and also provide the best visualization of the hypothalamus.

Local neurologic effects. Nearly one half of all patients with pituitary tumors larger than 1 cm experience severe headache. Although the cause of the headache is unknown, it may result from pressure on the diaphragma sella by the tumor mass.

The optic chiasm, which lies above the sella turcica of the pituitary, is frequently impinged on by the encroaching tumor, causing visual field defects, initially beginning with loss of red perception. Approximately one half of patients with pituitary tumors before 1972 had evidence of a bitemporal hemianopsia or a superior bitemporal defect. Today, because of the ready availability of hormone assays and sensitive sellar and parasellar imaging techniques, pituitary masses can be diagnosed much earlier, and the incidence of ophthalmologic lesions has declined.

Hypothalamic involvement by pituitary tumors can result in diabetes insipidus, as well as sleep or appetite disorders. In addition, changes in autonomic nervous system function, fluid output, temperature regulation, and behavior can occur.

When macroadenomas invade the cavernous sinus, the third, fourth, and sixth cranial nerves, as well as the ophthalmic and maxillary divisions of the fifth cranial nerve, can be affected. These neurologic changes may result in ptosis, ophthalmoplegia, or diplopia; they may also cause decreased facial sensation. Hemorrhage into the tumor may result in pituitary apoplexy or acute necrosis. When this occurs, severe headache, visual impairment, paralysis, lethargy, coma, or evidence of meningeal irritation or increased intracranial pressure may follow.

Growth hormone-secreting pituitary tumors

Hypersomatotropism may be caused by pituitary or extrapituitary tumors (see the box below). Hypersecretion of GH can manifest itself in different ways, depending on the age of the patient. In children or adolescents whose epiphyseal growth centers have yet to fuse in the long bones, hypersomatotropism can cause gigantism. In adults, this excessive secretion results in acromegaly.

Acromegaly

Clinical manifestations. The clinical features of acromegaly occur slowly and are often only noticed after many years of gradual change (Fig. 160-5). Tumor size tends to be larger in younger acromegalic patients. The clinical presentation reflects the response to local tumor growth, the effects of peripheral tissue changes, and the indirect and direct effects of continuous GH hypersecretion (refer to the box on p. 1306).

Clinical manifestations of acromegaly include viscero-

Causes of hypersomatotropism

- Pituitary
  - Eutopic
    - Densely or sparsely granulated GH cell adenoma
    - Mixed GH cell and PRL cell adenoma
    - Mammosomatotroph cell adenoma
    - Acidophil stem cell adenoma
    - Plurihormonal adenoma
  - Ectopic
    - Sphenoid sinus or parapharyngeal GH cell adenoma
- Extrapituitary
  - Ectopic GH-secreting tumor
    - Pancreas, breast, lung
  - Excess GHRH secretion
    - Eutopic
      - Hypothalamic hamartoma
    - Ectopic
      - Bronchial and intestinal carcinoid tumors
      - Pancreatic islet-cell tumors
  - Acromegaloidism

Modified from S Melmed et al: Endocr Rev 4:271, 1983.

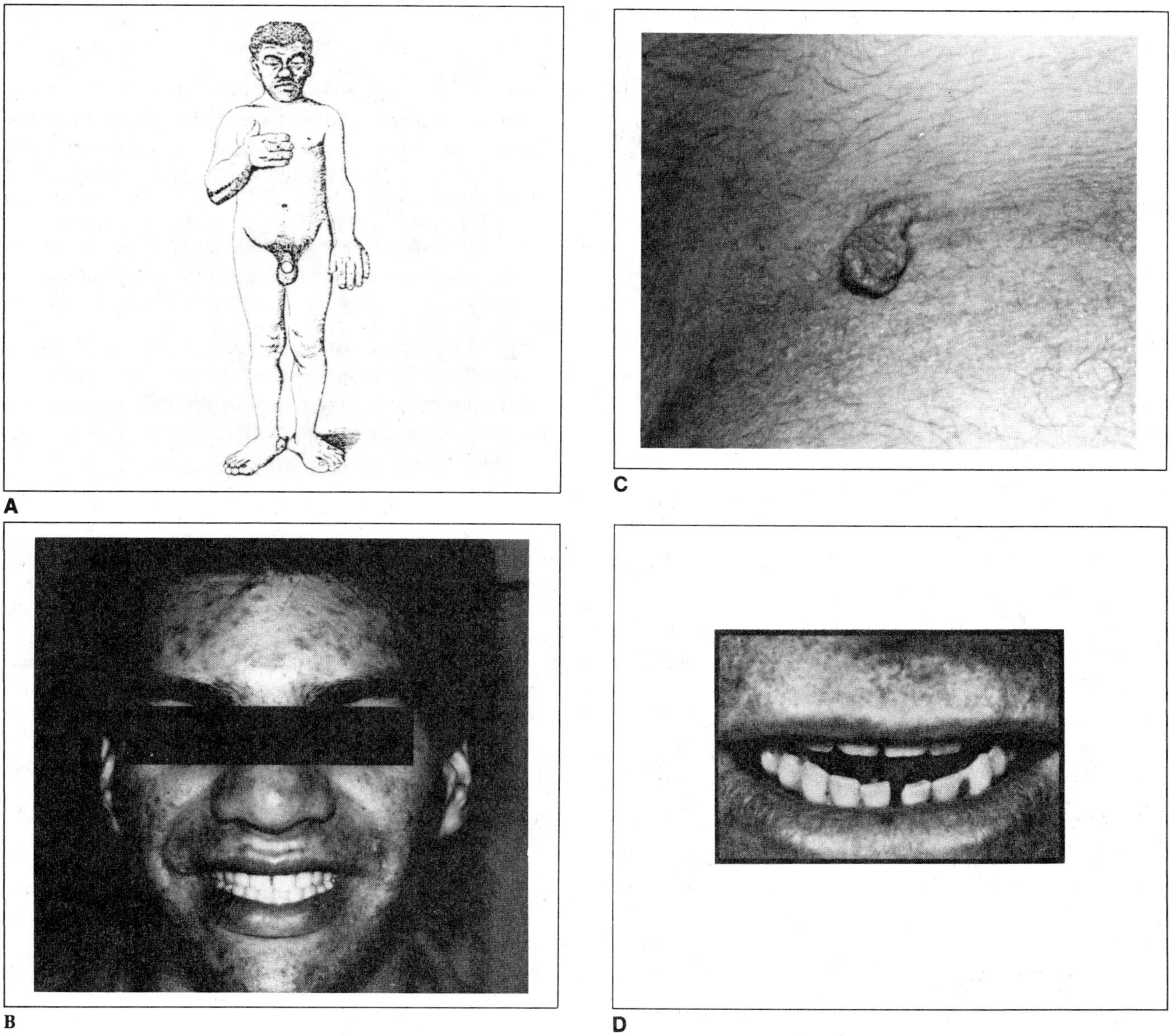

Fig. 160-5. Clinical signs of hypersomatotrophism seen in acromegaly. **A,** Original figure depicting earliest illustration of clinical features of acromegaly by Minkowski in 1887. Note acromegalic facies, fleshy fingers and toes, and frontal bossing. **B,** Young male acromegalic with active perspiration, oily skin, acne, and widened tooth gap. **C,** Prominent skin tags are important signs of acromegaly and may be associated with the presence of colon polyps. **D,** Increased overbite and widening of spaces between incisors caused by mandibular growth in acromegaly. (A from Minkowski: Berliner Klinische Wochenschrift, May, 1887.)

megaly of the kidney, heart, and, rarely, liver, and spleen. Cardiac abnormalities such as asymmetric septal hypertrophy and left ventricular hypertrophy also result from acromegaly. The excessive growth of soft tissues results in the characteristic coarsening of the facial features. In addition, the hands, feet, and tongue become larger, and excess skin develops around the neck and axillae; skin tags are prominent. The changes in bone, cartilage, and skin can result in prognathism, frontal bossing, kyphosis, and dental malocclusion. A further complication of acromegaly occurs when the median nerve becomes entrapped in the carpal tunnel; this leads to acroparesthesia. Hypertension may develop, as well as colonic polyps, which may become carcinomatous.

Insulin-like growth factor I, which is secreted under the influence of GH rather than the presence of the GH itself, is responsible for the acral enlargement seen in acromegaly. On the other hand, GH has direct anti-insulin effects, which can lead to insulin resistance and hyperinsulinism.

Clinical features of acromegaly

- Local tumor effects
  - Pituitary enlargement
  - Visual field defects
  - Cranial nerve palsy
  - Headache
- Somatic
  - Acral enlargement
    - Thickening of soft tissue of hands and feet
  - Musculoskeletal
    - Prognathism
    - Malocclusion
    - Arthralgias
    - Carpal tunnel syndrome
    - Acroparesthesia
    - Proximal myopathy
    - Hypertrophy of frontal bones
  - Skin
    - Hyperhydrosis
    - Oily
    - Skin tags
  - Colon
    - Polyps
    - Carcinoma
  - Cardiovascular
    - Left ventricular hypertrophy
    - Asymmetric septal hypertrophy
    - Hypertension
    - Congestive heart failure
  - Sleep disturbances
    - Sleep apnea
    - Narcolepsy
  - Visceromegaly
    - Tongue
    - Thyroid
    - Salivary gland
    - Liver
    - Spleen
    - Kidney
- Endocrine-metabolic
  - Reproduction
    - Menstrual abnormalities
    - Galactorrhea
    - Decreased libido, impotence, low sex hormone–binding globulin
  - Multiple endocrine neoplasia (I)
    - Hyperparathyroidism
    - Pancreatic islet-cell tumors
  - Carbohydrate
    - Impaired glucose tolerance
    - Insulin resistance and hyperinsulinemia
    - Diabetes mellitus
  - Lipids
    - Hypertriglyceridemia
  - Mineral
    - Hypercalciuria, increased 1,25 $(OH)_2D_3$
    - Urinary hydroxyproline
  - Electrolyte
    - Low renin
    - Increased aldosterone
  - Thyroid
    - Low thyroxine-binding globulin

Modified from Melmed S and Fagin J: West J Med 146:328, 1985.

However, although glucose intolerance is common at presentation, clinical diabetes mellitus is present in only approximately 15% of cases.

Menstrual disturbances are common in women with acromegaly. Similarly, males frequently have hypogonadism. The gonadotrophs can be destroyed by macroadenomas, which may cause hypogonadotropic hypogonadism. When tumors secrete both GH and PRL, hyperprolactinemia can result. This may also occur when a macroadenoma compresses the pituitary stalk, resulting in the disruption of dopamine transmission from the hypothalamus to the adenohypophysis. In both instances, hypersecretion of PRL can inhibit the normal cyclic discharge of GnRH, which in turn inhibits gonadotropin release and gonadal steroid secretion, resulting in hypogonadism.

Recently extrapituitary causes of acromegaly have been documented (see the box on p. 1304). Immunoreactive GH has been found in lung adenocarcinoma, breast cancer, and ovarian tissue extracts in vitro, and ectopic GH production has been documented in a patient with intramesenteric islet-cell tumor. Hypothalamic tumors, including hamartomas, choristomas, gliomas, and gangliocytomas, may be associated with acromegaly, resulting from the somatotroph hyperplasia or adenomas with excessive pituitary GH secretion stimulated by the GHRH elaborated by these tumors. Ectopic GHRH secretion has also been documented in pancreatic islet-cell, lung, and intestinal carcinoid tumors. Regardless of the tumor's location, patients with acromegaly have the classic clinical features of acromegaly, along with elevated circulating levels of GH and GHRH. The structure of GHRH was originally derived from extracts of pancreatic islet-cell tumors.

In contrast to classic acromegaly, acromegaloidism is a rare abnormality in which the clinical features of acromegaly are present in the absence of a pituitary or extra-adenohypophyseal tumor. In fact, acral enlargement can occur in the absence of elevated GH levels. It has been speculated that in such cases, the patient has a unique growth factor distinct from the known growth factors that promote in vitro erythroid growth.

Diagnosis. Although elevated GH levels are the hallmark of acromegaly, evidence of these increased levels does not necessarily mean an exclusive diagnosis of the disease. Elevated GH levels of more than 10 ng per milliliter, although found in more than 95% of all acromegalics, can also occur in patients with anorexia nervosa, malnutrition, diabetes, renal failure, porphyria, cirrhosis, or stress. For a conclusive diagnosis of acromegaly, an oral glucose tolerance test must be administered. This test usually demonstrates a failure to suppress GH. Nearly one third of patients who have acromegaly exhibit no change in their GH levels after a glucose tolerance load. Twenty to forty percent experience a paradoxic increase of GH secretion, and 5% to 7% show normal suppression. Abnormalities of GH secretion may also occur in response to other stimuli (e.g., dopamine agonists, TRH, GnRH, and VIP).

As mentioned previously, increased IGF-I levels are responsible for the classic acral enlargement that clinically defines acromegaly. Biochemical evidence of IGF-I hypersecretion correlates well with a diagnosis of active acromegaly, perhaps even better than do fasting or glucose-suppressed GH levels. Thus the first step in screening for acromegaly should entail measuring the patient's serum concentration of IGF-I; there is virtually no overlap in these levels between patients with acromegaly and normal individuals. When an elevated IGF-I level is detected, the patient should be evaluated further with an MRI or CT scan of the anterior pituitary and a postglucose GH determination. If no pituitary mass is detected, then further imaging should be performed to establish the location of an ectopically secreting GHRH or GH tumor. Measurements of immunoreactive serum GHRH levels may help to distinguish between these latter entities.

Therapy of acromegaly. Management of patients harboring pituitary tumors is aimed at reducing or ablating the tumor mass, correcting visual and neurologic defects, preserving anterior pituitary function, and preventing progression or recurrence of the condition. Pituitary secretion of GH should be totally suppressed to stop the progression of physical signs caused by hypersomatotropinemia. In addition, any other pituitary trophic hormone disorders should also be corrected. Criteria for absolute cure of acromegaly include GH suppressibility after administration of oral glucose, (<2 ng/ml), reappearance of normal circadian rhythm of GH secretion, normal GH increase after provocative stimulation, normal circulating IGF-I levels, and, finally, disappearance of paradoxic GH responses. By these criteria, no single therapeutic option (see the box below) really offers a 100% successful, long-term cure of acromegaly. Surgery is the primary therapy, and medical or radiation therapy is often required as an adjuvant. The development of newer pharmacologic agents, especially SRIF analogs combined with bromocriptine, holds much future promise.

Transsphenoidal surgery. The recommended primary therapy for acromegaly is transsphenoidal pituitary adenomectomy performed by a skilled and experienced neurosurgeon. Growth hormone levels fall rapidly to normal within 1 hour of selective excision of GH cell adenomas, and the amelioration of soft tissue and metabolic effects caused by elevated GH levels begins almost immediately.

Several clinical and biochemical features usually predict the success of surgery. Almost 90% of patients with preoperative random serum GH levels less than 40 ng per milliliter and harboring an adenoma totally confined within the pituitary fossa have an initial reduction in serum GH levels to less than 5 ng per milliliter after surgery. Normal postoperative pituitary function is expected if the tumor is well encapsulated. Long-term follow-up results (5 years and later) in these patients, however, are less favorable. Tumor recurrence with or without clinical features of acromegaly and evidence of failure to suppress GH levels after oral glucose has been observed in patients who had initially met the criteria of cure. Incomplete surgical resection of tumor tissue may result in postoperative recurrence of acromegaly. Although GH cell adenomas are usually well encapsulated, functioning tumor cells may be seeded in the dura and escape visualization and resection. The most important endocrine side-effects of surgery are damage to the remainder of the normal pituitary gland, resultant pituitary failure, and necessity for lifelong hormone replacement. Cerebrospinal fluid leaks, sinusitis, central nervous system damage, hemorrhage, transient or permanent (infrequent) diabetes insipidus, meningitis, and arachnoiditis occur in about 5% of patients. The frequency of these complications is related to the size of the tumor. Postoperatively, an empty sella may rarely lead to impingement of the optic chiasm. A mortality rate of about 1% is seen, especially with large invasive tumors.

Radiation therapy. Irradiation is recommended as an adjuvant form of therapy in acromegaly. A total dose of 5000 rad is administered over 4 to 6 weeks. The time required to lower GH levels effectively by 50% is usually at least 2 years. After 10 years, GH levels are normalized in about 75% of acromegalics. The arrest of tumor growth is almost universal, and most GH cell adenomas eventually shrink after irradiation.

Radiation damage to the surrounding tissues may occur, especially if more than 5000 rad is administered. Some degree of hypopituitarism develops in approximately one half of all patients after 10 years. Hypocortisolism and hypogonadism are the usual hormone deficits; isolated hypothyroidism occurs in about 20% of these patients. Proton beam therapy has the advantage over conventional radiotherapy that the patient can receive the total radiation dosage in only one or two visits without resulting skin damage. Radiation damage to cranial nerves and other surrounding structures, however, is a significant side-effect of this form of radiation. Radiation therapy is an inappropriate option for young patients because of the slow decrease in GH concentration.

Medical treatment of acromegaly

Bromocriptine. Bromocriptine (bromo-alpha-ergocryptine), a lysergic acid ergot derivative with dopamine agonist properties, may be used to treat acromegaly. Because neoplastic somatotrophs respond inappropriately to dopamine agonists by suppression of GH secretion in more than 50% of acromegalics, bromocriptine is useful as both primary and adjuvant medication for acromegaly. The doses of bromocriptine used in acromegaly are usually higher than those required to suppress PRL secretion. If a beneficial effect of bromocriptine is observed, it is usually seen with

Acromegaly: treatment options

Surgical
- Transsphenoidal pituitary adenomectomy or extrapituitary tumor resection

Medical
- Bromocriptine
- Somatostatin analog

Radiation
- Conventional or proton beam

up to 30 mg of bromocriptine daily. Basal serum GH levels are decreased to less than 10 ng per milliliter in about 50% of cases. A GH level of less than 5 ng per milliliter has been observed in 20% of reported cases; shrinkage of tumor size probably only occurs in about 10% to 20% of cases. Most patients report a significant improvement in clinical symptoms, including reduction of perspiration, decreased soft tissue swelling, and decreased ring size. Bromocriptine therefore causes clinical improvement in many patients despite persistently raised GH and/or IGF-I levels.

Because bromocriptine is a dopamine agonist and possesses ergot-like properties, side-effects involving the cardiovascular, nervous, and digestive systems are anticipated. Although the incidence of adverse reactions to bromocriptine is quite high, these are usually transient in nature and mild or moderate in degree. Nausea, headache, dizziness, fatigue, lightheadedness, vomiting, abdominal cramps, nasal congestion, constipation, diarrhea, and drowsiness have been reported. Furthermore a mild hypotensive effect may result in postural orthostasis when therapy is initiated. Tolerance to these effects generally develops within 2 to 3 weeks of continued usage. Less frequent reactions include gastrointestinal bleeding, dizziness, exacerbation of Raynaud's syndrome, hair loss, alcohol potentiation, and visual hallucinations. These side-effects may be ameliorated by temporarily reducing the dosage of the medication and by increasing the dose by intervals no more frequent than every 3 days or longer. Gastrointestinal side-effects may be eased by prescribing the medication with meals. Nevertheless, the drug is remarkably free of major side-effects and has been used successfully for many years in patients with hyperprolactinemia, acromegaly, and Parkinson's disease.

Somatostatin analog. The physiologic inhibitor of GH secretion, SRIF, was a natural candidate as a pharmacologic agent in acromegaly. An octapeptide SRIF analog (octreotide, D-Phe-Cys-Phe-D-Tryp-Cys-Thr-[OH]) with high potency and prolonged inhibition of GH secretion has been used successfully to lower GH levels in most acromegalic patients and to shrink some GH cell adenomas.

The octapeptide SRIF analog (Octreotide) because of its prolonged half-life inhibits growth hormone secretion for 6 to 8 hours after a subcutaneous injection. Octreotide (100 μ every 8 hours subcutaneously) lowers growth hormone levels in most acromegalic patients and suppresses integrated growth hormone secretion over 6 hours to less than 5 ng/ml in about two thirds of patients. Similarly, IGF-I levels are normalized in about two thirds of the patients. The drug shrinks about 30% of growth hormone cell adenomas and also alleviates soft tissue swelling, excessive perspiration, joint pains, and headache. Side-effects include transient gastrointestinal upset and loose stools during the first 2 weeks of treatment. Intestinal malabsorption and asymptomatic gallstones occur in up to a third of patients receiving the medication long term. This promising new drug awaits further evaluation for safety and efficacy as a primary therapy of acromegaly, as a presurgical drug to shrink tumors, or in postoperative treatment of recurrent acromegaly.

Hyperprolactinemia

Causes. Among the various physiologic states that influence PRL secretion are exercise, pregnancy, lactation, nipple stimulation, diet, and female orgasm (refer to the box below). Serum PRL levels are elevated by 60% within 2 hours of sleep onset, resulting in a circadian diurnal variation in PRL levels. Stress such as surgery or acute myocardial infarction can also result in hyperprolactinemia. Various pharmacologic agents have the ability to influence PRL secretion. These include dopamine receptor antagonists (e.g., metoclopromide), tricyclic antidepressants, reserpine, estrogens, opiates, and cimetidine. Hypothalamic and pituitary disorders are among the pathologic causes of hyperprolactinemia; diseases of the hypothalamus may lead to a reduction in dopamine secretion, resulting in disinhibition of PRL secretion. Lactotroph microadenomas or macroadenomas directly secrete PRL; pathologic processes directly involving the pituitary stalk may disrupt the hypothalamohypophyseal portal system and prevent dopamine from reaching the lactotrophs. Primary hypothyroidism may be associated with hyperprolactinemia, especially in chil-

Causes of hyperprolactinemia

- Physiologic
  - Pregnancy and lactation
  - Sleep
  - Stress
  - Exercise
  - Chest wall stimulation or trauma
  - Coitus
- Pathologic
  - Hypothalamic
    - Inflammation
    - Tumor
  - Pituitary
    - Lactotroph microadenoma or macroadenoma
    - Acromegaly
    - Stalk section caused by pituitary or parasellar mass
    - Empty sella syndrome
  - Peripheral
    - Hypothyroidism
    - Chronic renal failure
- Pharmacologic
  - Psychotropic agents
    - Phenothiazines
    - Tricyclic antidepressants
    - Opiate alkaloids
  - Antiemetics and antihistamines
    - Metoclopramide
    - Sulpiride
    - Cimetidine
  - Antihypertensives
    - Methyldopa
    - Reserpine
  - Hormones
    - Estrogens
    - Thyrotropin-releasing hormone

Modified from Melmed S et al: Ann Intern Med 105:238, 1986.

dren, presumably through enhanced TRH stimulation of the lactotroph.

Thus hypersecretion of PRL may be accounted for by a factor that impedes dopamine synthesis or release, or by an increase in the release of a putative PRL-releasing factor. Similarly, factors that antagonize dopamine receptors may also account for elevated serum PRL levels.

Prolactin-secreting pituitary tumors

Clinical presentation. Prolactinomas are the most common pituitary tumors. Although the tumorigenesis of prolactinomas is incompletely understood, the high rate of postsurgical recurrence implies that hypothalamic dysfunction is an important pathophysiologic factor. These tumors are diagnosed more often in women than men, possibly as a result of the difference in clinical manifestations between women and men (Table 160-3). Microadenomas are more common in women, and macroadenomas are more frequent in men. This may reflect a different natural history for these tumors in men and women. Only a small percentage of microadenomas in women appear to become macroadenomas. Furthermore, prolactinomas frequently cause menstrual disturbances, and thus tumors in women are generally discovered earlier than are the analogous tumors found in men. The presenting symptoms in men include decreased libido and impotence; these problems tend to become clinically manifest 10 to 15 years later than the presenting symptoms in women. By the time of diagnosis, the macroadenomas found in men may also have caused visual field abnormalities, secondary hypogonadism, hypothyroidism, and adrenal insufficiency.

The frequency of hyperprolactinemia correlates well with reproductive abnormalities in women. Approximately 15% of women with amenorrhea have elevated levels of serum PRL. In addition, 28% of women with galactorrhea without amenorrhea have hyperprolactinemia. Of women who have both problems, more than three fourths have increased PRL levels. Infertility is found in many women with PRL-secreting tumors and is the result of anovulation or an insufficient luteal phase.

Table 160-3. Clinical features of patients with prolactin-secreting pituitary adenomas

	Women (%)	Men (%)	P value
Mean age, yr	28.4	43.3	<0.001
Amenorrhea	83	—	—
Primary amenorrhea	6	—	—
Oligomenorrhea	10	—	—
Galactorrhea	81	6	<0.001
Headaches	38	36	NS*
Weight gain	25	22	NS
Visual abnormalities	10	38	<0.001
Decreased libido or impotence	14	71	<0.001
Fatigue	12	12	NS
Acne or hirsutism	8	—	—
Gynecomastia	—	21	—
Delayed sexual development	—	14	—
Macroadenoma	36	91	<0.001
Microadenoma	64	9	<0.001

Modified from Melmed S et al: Ann Intern Med 105:238, 1986.
*NS, nonsignificant.

Elevated PRL levels have the potential to impede the cyclic release of gonadotropins. In addition, they may interrupt the peripheral activity of gonadotropins on the gonads. Thus women frequently suffer from estrogen deficiency, which in turn may lead to decreased vaginal secretions causing dyspareunia and to osteopenia. Hyperprolactinemia can also cause elevated androgen levels. In women, this can lead to hirsutism and acne. In men, however, serum testosterone levels are depressed in at least two thirds of patients with prolactinomas. When the tumor is detected and treated early, testosterone levels may ultimately increase back to normal. In other instances, irreversible damage to the pituitary gonadotrophs may prevent the normalization of testosterone levels. Furthermore elevated PRL levels may impede the peripheral action of testosterone, perhaps by interfering with the conversion of testosterone to dehydrotestosterone. Clinically, this condition can manifest as impotence.

Diagnosis. The first stage of diagnosis of PRL-secreting pituitary tumors involves measuring basal serum PRL concentrations. When levels exceed 200 ng per milliliter (upper limit of normal is 20 to 25 ng per milliliter), a pituitary tumor is very likely. Prolactinomas are invariably present when levels surpass 300 ng per milliliter. Levels below 200 ng per milliliter might be caused by a variety of conditions, including drug-induced hyperprolactinemia, renal failure, and thyroid or hypothalamic disorders. To confirm the presence of a tumor, CT or MRI scanning of the pituitary-hypothalamic region should be performed when several serum samples show persistent hyperprolactinemia.

Unfortunately, no definitive test determines whether elevated PRL levels result from pituitary tumors or from other causes. Nevertheless, TRH stimulation tests are commonly administered. In controls, serum PRL concentrations more than double during this test; most patients with PRL-secreting tumors exhibit no, or very little, change; however, this lack of response occurs despite the source of elevated PRL.

Medical management of hyperprolactinemia. Bromocriptine is the treatment of choice for hyperprolactinemia associated with amenorrhea, galactorrhea, and infertility. The initial dose of bromocriptine is 2.5 mg daily. An additional 2.5 mg tablet should be added every week until therapeutic response is achieved. The therapeutic dosage required to suppress PRL level and to reverse the signs and symptoms of hypogonadism ranges from 2.5 to 15.0 mg per day. Women should be counseled to use a mechanical contraceptive device to prevent unwanted pregnancy during bromocriptine treatment, because ovulatory menstrual cycles generally resume within 2 to 3 months. If menstruation does not occur within 3 days of the expected period once ovulatory cycles are established, treatment with bromocriptine should be discontinued and a pregnancy test performed.

Bromocriptine is used for initial therapy in patients with PRL-secreting macroadenomas or persistent postsurgical hyperprolactinemia. The drug is also indicated to attempt shrinkage of large tumors before surgery. A number of studies have demonstrated the efficacy of bromocriptine as primary therapy for macroadenomas in treating visual and neurologic impairments as well as normalizing PRL levels. In a multicenter prospective study, tumor size was reduced by 50% or more in two thirds of patients harboring a PRL-secreting macroadenoma. In about a third of patients, tumor size was reduced by 10% to 25%. Even with dramatic reductions in PRL secretion and tumor size, pituitary function generally remains intact. Long-term postsurgical treatment prevents tumor regrowth and hyperprolactinemia. Bromocriptine treatment extending over 4 to 6 years has been continued with sustained benefits and few adverse effects. The drug lowers PRL levels, restores reproductive function in males and females, shrinks tumor size, and restores visual field deficits. Bromocriptine therefore offers safe and effective long-term therapy for prolactinomas. If, however, the bromocriptine is discontinued, the tumor may rapidly return to its original size.

Cushing's disease

The clinical presentation of hypercortisolism is discussed elsewhere (Chapter 163). The primary therapy of Cushing's disease is surgical removal of the ACTH-secreting corticotroph cell adenoma. Because this tumor may be very small, in some patients no pituitary tumor is visualized even by current imaging techniques. In others, postsurgical recurrence of the excessive ACTH secretion occurs. The major causes of patient morbidity and mortality resulting from Cushing's disease include arteriosclerosis, infection, and depression leading to suicide. Because of these deleterious effects on patient morbidity and a 5 year mortality rate of 50%, aggressive therapeutic intervention is warranted.

Medical management

Neuropharmacologic. As several brain and hypothalamic neurotransmitters that regulate POMC secretion have now been recognized, several neuropharmacologic agents have been used to control excessive ACTH secretion.

Serotonin is a potent stimulator of ACTH release. Cyproheptadine, an antiserotoninergic agent that acts to block ACTH release at the level of the hypothalamus, has been used to treat recurrent or primary Cushing's disease when surgery is contraindicated. Clinical and biochemical remission occurs in a small percentage of patients after about 3 months of medication. The drug has also been used as an adjuvant to pituitary irradiation. The initial dose of 4 mg three times a day is increased gradually to 4 mg every 4 hours. Side-effects of cyproheptadine include hyperphagia and somnolence. Excessive ACTH secretion invariably recurs after the drug is discontinued.

Although bromocriptine is not primarily indicated for treating corticotroph cell adenomas, it may acutely suppress ACTH secretion in some patients. Bromocriptine nonresponders often harbor relatively easily excisable ACTH-secreting adenomas. Patients who suppress ACTH levels with bromocriptine appear to have a less favorable response to surgical resection of the adenoma.

Steroidogenesis inhibitors. The biosynthesis of adrenal steroids is a complex posttranslational event, involving several key enzymes. *Ketoconozole,* an antifungal agent, inhibits steroidogenesis and has been used successfully to suppress urinary cortisol excretion during long-term treatment with 400 to 800 mg daily. Because gonadal steroidogenesis may also be blocked, some patients may require sex steroid replacement. Limited evidence suggests that ketoconozole inhibits ACTH secretion at the pituitary or hypothalamic level. *Metyrapone,* an inhibitor of 11-beta-hydroxylase as well as of pregnenolone production, suppresses cortisol synthesis and secretion within a week of starting treatment. The side-effects of the drug include exacerbation of hirsutism, nausea, and gastrointestinal discomfort. Although long-term treatment effectively inhibits steroidogenesis, hypertension and hypokalemia may result from the accumulation of mineralocorticoids above the enzymatic block. *Aminoglutethimide* blocks the conversion of cholesterol to pregnenolone. Within 3 to 5 days of administration (up to 1.5 g/day), adrenal steroidogenesis is suppressed, but the resultant increased release of ACTH may override the enzyme block and continue to stimulate cortisol production. Side-effects include skin rash and lethargy. Combination therapy with metyrapone may allow lower doses of aminoglutethimide to be used. Mitotane is a potent inhibitor of adrenal steroidogenesis, and its long-term use results in a "medical" adrenalectomy. The doses used in Cushing's disease (5 to 12 g daily) are lower than those usually used for adrenal carcinoma. Significant lowering of cortisol levels occurs in approximately 50% of patients within 6 months. Side-effects of o,p DDD include hypotension and secondary hypercholesterolemia. Mifepristone (RU-486), a peripheral glucocorticoid antagonist, acutely lowers cortisol levels, but its long-term efficacy is not proved.

Gonadotropin-secreting pituitary tumors

Clinical presentation. Gonadotropin-secreting pituitary tumors are rare pituitary tumors that occur mainly in male patients. They usually appear as a result of local pressure signs, for example, visual impairment. The patient also may have hypogonadism caused by down regulation of the pituitary gonadal axis by the high levels of secreted gonadotropins, although some patients may actually have long-standing primary hypogonadism resulting in gonadotroph hyperplasia and adenoma formation.

The majority of these patients have increased circulating levels of FSH and LH with respective discordant increases of the beta LH and beta FSH subunits, as compared to the alpha subunit. Most patients respond to GnRH by enhanced secretion of gonadotropins. Some patients may retain a degree of normal feedback regulation by showing suppression of gonadotropin levels with administration of sex steroids.

Gonadal function is usually suppressed in these patients

with low or normal testosterone levels, or low or normal sperm counts. Rarely, excessive production of LH alone by a tumor may result in increased levels of testosterone.

Differential diagnosis. The diagnosis is difficult to make in females because of the associated high gonadotropin levels of postmenopausal women. Primary gonadal failure or menopausal failure may result in secondary pituitary enlargement, further confounding the differential diagnosis.

Treatment. Treatment of these tumors is primarily surgical. The large pituitary mass should be resected. Adjuvant treatment with bromocriptine has been successful in several patients who have shown suppression of the elevated gonadotropin levels. The drug is especially useful for recurrences of the excess gonadotropin secretion after surgery.

Thyroid-stimulating hormone-secreting tumors

The thyroid-stimulating hormone-secreting tumors are extremely rare and are often plurihormonal and secrete GH, PRL, and alpha glycoprotein subunits as well as TSH. Approximately one half of the patients with these tumors have associated acromegaly or hyperprolactinemia. Thyroid-stimulating hormone-secreting tumors exhibit the signs and symptoms of hyperthyroidism. The cardinal features include inappropriately elevated TSH levels in the presence of elevated thyroid hormone levels. Interestingly, about a third of patients treated for TSH-secreting pituitary tumors have TSH levels less than 10 μU per milliliter. New ultrasensitive TSH radioimmunoassay should therefore be used to discriminate between low and inappropriately "normal" circulating TSH levels in patients with hyperthyroidism.

Treatment. The treatment of these tumors is primarily surgical excision. Bromocriptine and SRIF analog may be used as adjuncts to surgical management. Octreotide also effectively controls the hypersecretion of TSH and the associated hyperthyroidism in several patients as well as shrinking tumor size.

Empty sella syndrome

Acquired or congenital anatomic defects in the diaphragma sella may allow arachnoid herniation into the pituitary fossa, leading to formation of an empty sella. The sella becomes partially filled by arachnoid membrane, CSF, and the compressed pituitary gland. The empty sella syndrome is fairly common and accounts for about one third of radiologically demonstrable pituitary sella abnormalities.

Causes. A primary empty sella probably results from a congenital weakness in the diaphragma sella. This has been associated with obesity in females, increased intracranial pressure, multiparity, and hypertension. Other primary causes include intracranial tumors, pseudotumor cerebri, hydrocephalus, and hypoventilation with or without associated congestive heart failure. Several conditions may lead to a secondary empty sella. These include damage to the pituitary gland after pituitary surgery, radiation, hemorrhage, and infarction. The infarction may occur spontaneously in a normal pituitary gland (e.g., Sheehan's syndrome) or in a pituitary adenoma.

Clinical presentation. The empty sella is usually asymptomatic and is detected on routine imaging of the head. Approximately 10% of patients with the empty sella syndrome, however, have a history of chronic headaches. Visual field disturbances are rare and may result from herniation of the optic chiasm into the CSF compartment within the sella.

Endocrine function in such patients is usually normal, although partial hypopituitarism may be present in a minority. A blunting of the GH or cortisol response to insulin-induced hypoglycemia may be a subtle indication of pituitary failure in patients primarily affected by empty sella syndrome. The presence of isolated or multiple trophic pituitary hormone deficiencies in association with the empty sella suggests that the lesion may have been caused by infarction of a pituitary adenoma. Acromegaly, hyperprolactinemia, and Cushing's disease have also been described in the presence of an empty sella.

Differential diagnosis. The primary diagnosis of empty sella is made by sensitive imaging techniques including MRI and CT scanning. The classic radiologic picture is the infundibulum "sign," in which the pituitary stalk is clearly identified with the flattened pituitary tissue. The density of the CSF occupying the sella is also clearly distinguishable from normal pituitary density by MRI. Finally, herniation of the optic chiasm may be noted in the sella. It is important to distinguish intrasellar pituitary lesions from empty sella syndrome. The MRI and CT imaging may usually help make this distinction. Nevertheless, the presence of a microadenoma in the remnant pituitary tissue may pose a difficult radiologic diagnostic dilemma.

Treatment. Corrective surgery may be required for persistent CSF rhinorrhea, visual field defects, or prolapse of the optic chiasm. Endocrine deficits should be treated by replacement with specific hormones, and endocrine hyperfunction should be treated in relation to the specific hormone being hypersecreted by the concurrent adenoma.

REFERENCES

Frohman LA and Jansson J: Growth hormone releasing hormone. Endocr Rev 7:223, 1986.

Herman VS and Braunstein GD: Gonadotropin secretory abnormalities. Endocr Metab Clin 20:519, 1991.

Jorgensen JOL: Human growth hormone replacement therapy: pharmacologic and clinical aspects. Endocr Rev 12:189, 1991.

Karpf D and Braunstein GD: Current concepts in acromegaly: etiology, diagnosis and treatment. Compr Ther 12:22, 1986.

Kohler PO: Treatment of pituitary adenomas. N Engl J Med 317:45, 1987.

Lamberts SWJ et al: Long-term treatment of acromegaly with the somatostatin analogue SMS 201-995. N Engl J Med 313:1576, 1985.

Loriaux L: Treatment of Cushing's syndrome and adrenal cancer. Endocr Metab Clin 20:767, 1991.

Melmed S: Acromegaly. N Engl J Med 322:966, 1990.

Melmed S et al: Pituitary tumors secreting growth hormone and prolactin. Ann Intern Med 105:238, 1986.
Molitch M: Pituitary tumors: diagnosis and management. Clin Endocrinol Metab 16(3), 1987.
Molitch ME et al: Bromocriptine as primary therapy for prolactin-secreting macroadenomas: results of a prospective multicenter study. J Clin Endocrinol Metab 60:698, 1985.
Sheldon WR et al: Rapid sequential intravenous administration of four hypothalamic releasing hormones as a combined anterior pituitary function test in normal subjects. J Clin Endocrinol Metab 60:623, 1985.
Vance ML, Evans WS, and Thorner MO: Bromocriptine. Ann Intern Med 100:78, 1984.

CHAPTER

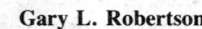

161 Disorders of the Posterior Pituitary

Gary L. Robertson

BASIC PRINCIPLES

Anatomy

The *posterior pituitary,* or *neurohypophysis,* is an extension of the ventral hypothalamus that penetrates the diaphragma sellae and attaches to the dorsal and caudal surfaces of the adenohypophysis. The part above the diaphragm is variously referred to as the *infundibulum* or *median eminence,* and that below as the *infundibular process* or *pars nervosa*. The posterior pituitary is supplied with blood by the superior and inferior hypophyseal arteries, which arise from the posterior communicating and intracavernous portion of the internal carotid. The arterioles divide in the pars nervosa into localized capillary networks that drain directly into the jugular vein via the sellar, cavernous, and lateral venous sinuses. In the infundibulum, the capillary networks coalesce into the portal veins, which supply blood to the adenohypophysis.

On histologic examination, the neurohypophysis appears as a network of capillaries, pituicytes, and nonmyelinated nerve fibers containing numerous electron-dense neurosecretory granules. The neurons terminate as bulbous enlargements juxtaposed to capillary networks scattered throughout all levels of the neurohypophysis. Those that reach the pars nervosa appear to originate primarily in nuclei of the supraoptic and, to a lesser extent, the paraventricular regions of the hypothalamus. Those neurons that terminate more proximally, particularly in the median eminence, probably arise in other hypothalamic areas, primarily the paraventricular nucleus (Fig. 161-1). Neurosecretory neurons from this nucleus also project to other parts of the brain, most notably the nucleus tractus solitarius and/or vasomotor center in the medulla.

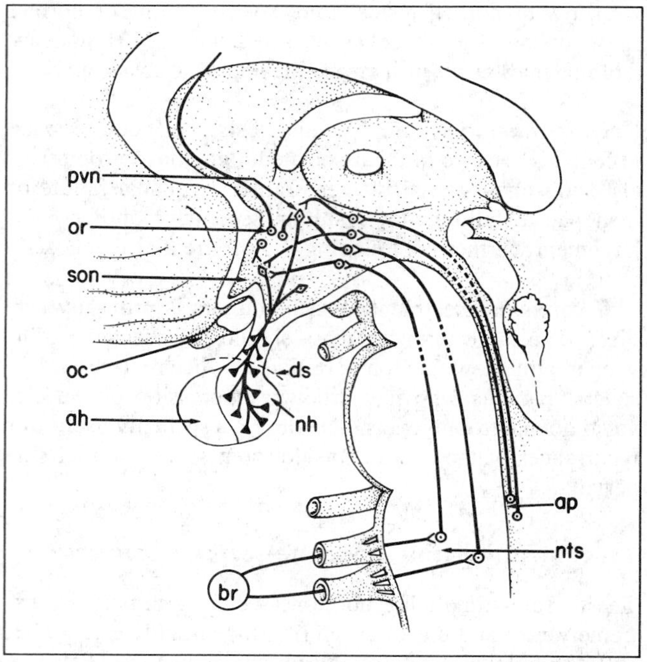

Fig. 161-1. The neurohypophysis and its principal regulatory afferents. *nh*, neurohypophysis; *ah*, adenohypophysis; *ds*, diaphragma sellae; *oc*, optic chiasm; *son*, supraoptic nucleus; *pvn*, paraventricular nucleus; *or*, osmoreceptor; *br*, volume and baroreceptor; *nts*, nucleus tractus solitarius; *ap*, area postrema (emetic center). (Modified from Robertson GL: In Ingbar SH, editor: The year of endocrinology 1977. New York, 1978, Plenum.)

Biochemistry

Chemistry. Vasopressin and oxytocin are the major if not the only hormones secreted by the neurohypophysis in adult humans. Both hormones are nonapeptides composed of a six membered disulfide ring and a three membered tail, on which the terminal carboxyl group is amidated (Fig. 161-2). Vasopressin differs from oxytocin in that phenylalanine is substituted for isoleucine in the ring, and arginine for leucine in the tail. These two changes confer markedly different biologic properties on the peptides.

Both vasopressin and oxytocin are stored in the posterior pituitary as insoluble complexes with specific proteins known as *neurophysins*. Two distinct types of neurophysin have been identified in humans. One is found exclusively in granules containing oxytocin, the other in association with vasopressin. Both neurophysins appear to be single-chain polypeptides of approximately 10,000 molecular weight (MW). Each neurophysin binds oxytocin and vasopressin equally well, indicating that the specific hormonal associations found in vivo are a function of cellular compartmentalization as well as a common biosynthesis.

Synthesis and hormone release. Vasopressin and oxytocin are synthesized in the supraoptic and paraventricular nuclei, packaged in granules with neurophysins, and transported down the axons to terminal dilatations, where they

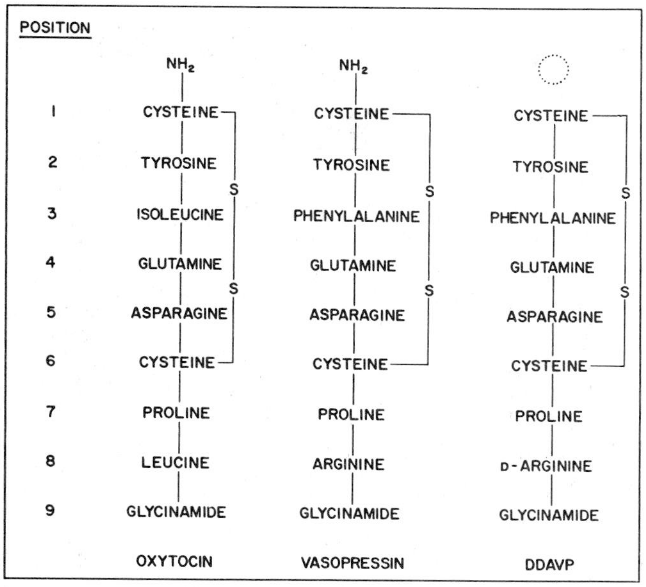

Fig. 161-2. The structure of oxytocin, vasopressin, and a synthetic analog, 1-desamino-8-D-arginine vasopressin (DDAVP).

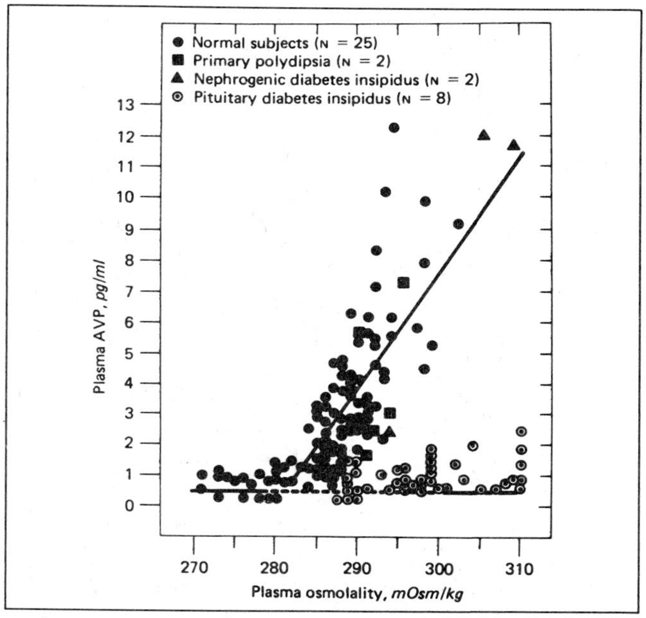

Fig. 161-3. The relationship of plasma vasopressin (AVP) to plasma osmolality in healthy adults and patients with polyuria of diverse causes. AVP, plasma vasopressin. (From Robertson GL et al: J Clin Invest 52:2340, 1973.)

are stored until release. Each hormone is produced by a different population of neurons. However, the biosynthetic mechanisms appear to be similar. Synthesis of vasopressin occurs via a macromolecular precursor that also contains the sequence for neurophysin and a glycoprotein. The gene that codes for this precursor is located on chromosome 20 and is composed of three exons. The precursor is cleaved during transport to yield the active hormone, neurophysin, and other still unidentified peptides. Stimuli, such as dehydration, increase synthesis as well as secretion of the hormone. Mutations in the gene that codes for the vasopressin precursor recently have been linked to the inherited form of neurogenic diabetes insipidus (discussed later).

Vasopressin secretion, together with that of its associated neurophysin, probably occurs through a calcium-dependent process of exocytosis similar to those described for other neurosecretory systems. In plasma, the neurophysin-hormone complex dissociates completely, and most if not all plasma vasopressin circulates in the free or unbound state. However, platelets contain relatively large amounts of vasopressin that is taken up from plasma and released or metabolized very slowly.

Physiology

Control of secretion. Vasopressin secretion is influenced by a number of different factors. Probably the most important influence under physiologic conditions is the osmotic pressure of body water. This effect is mediated by osmosensitive neurons located in the anterior hypothalamus near the supraoptic and paraventricular nuclei (Fig. 161-1). The osmoregulatory system can be examined by measuring plasma vasopressin level in healthy adults during various states of hydration (Fig. 161-3). At plasma osmolalities below a certain minimum or "threshold" value, plasma vasopressin is uniformly suppressed to low or undetectable levels. Above the threshold, plasma vasopressin level rises in direct proportion to osmolality. A plasma osmolality change of only 1% is sufficient to cause a measurable change in plasma vasopressin level. This extreme sensitivity enables the osmoregulatory system to play a dominant role in mediating the vasopressin response to changes in water balance.

The response of this osmoregulatory system is also remarkably precise. Although there is a relatively large scatter in the relationship between plasma vasopressin level and plasma osmolality in the normal adult population (Fig. 161-3), this variation is due principally to large individual differences in the set and sensitivity of the system. The basis for these individual differences in osmoregulatory function is not completely known. Aging is associated with some increase in sensitivity but cannot be the only cause, because even among young adults, sensitivity may differ by more than 10 times. Recent studies indicate that these individual differences are relatively constant and are determined to a great extent by heredity. The function of the osmoregulatory system is similar in males and females, although the threshold or set of the system is reduced during pregnancy and the luteal phase of the menstrual cycle.

The sensitivity of the osmoreactor is not the same for all plasma solutes (Fig. 161-4). Sodium and associated anions, which normally constitute more than 95% of the total osmotic pressure in plasma, are the most effective solutes in stimulating vasopressin secretion. Sugars, such as mannitol and sucrose, are also very potent when given intrave-

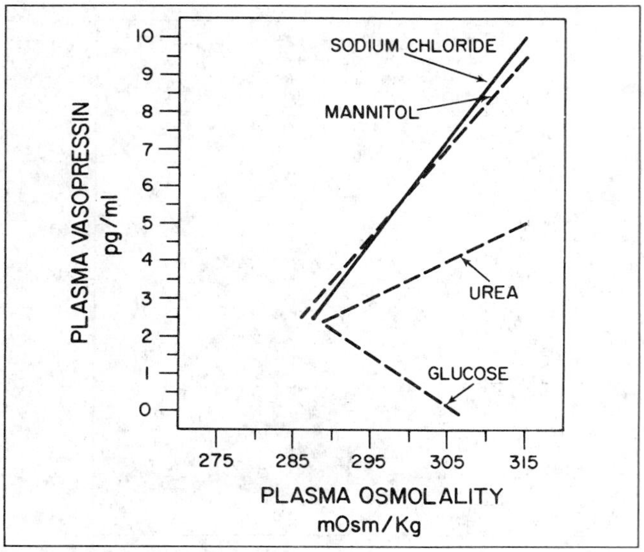

Fig. 161-4. The relationship of plasma vasopressin to plasma osmolality in healthy adults during the infusion of hypertonic solutions of various solutes.

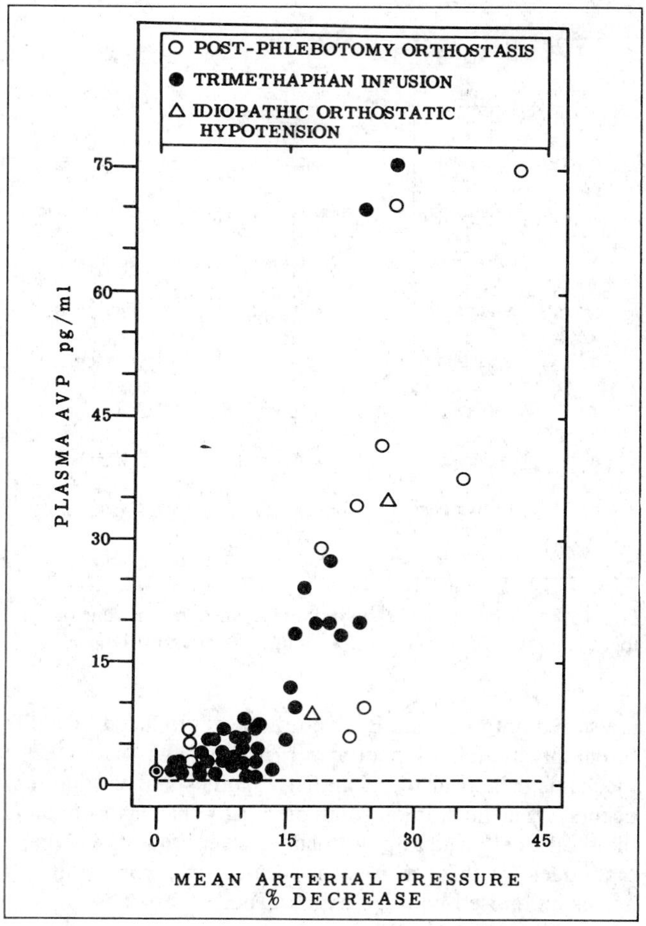

Fig. 161-5. The relationship of plasma vasopressin to percentage fall in blood pressure in healthy adults and patients with idiopathic postural hypotension. (From Robertson GL: In Felig P et al, editors: Endocrinology and metabolism. New York, 1981, McGraw-Hill.)

nously. In contrast, an increase in plasma osmolality produced by urea or glucose causes minimal or no stimulation of vasopressin secretion in healthy persons. In patients with insulin-deficient diabetes mellitus, however, hyperglycemia is moderately stimulatory. The mechanism by which the osmoreceptor discriminates between different solutes or the same solute under different conditions is not known with certainty, but it is thought to be based on the differences in cellular permeability.

Vasopressin secretion also can be influenced by alterations in blood volume or pressure. These effects are mediated primarily by afferent fibers that arise in baroreceptors in the heart, aortic arch, and carotid sinus and reach the brainstem through the vagal and glossopharyngeal nerves (Fig. 161-1). The pathways over which these signals are transmitted to the neurohypophysis are uncertain but probably involve a primary synapse in the nucleus tractus solitarius of the medulla.

The characteristics of this baroregulatory system are demonstrated by the relationship between plasma vasopressin and changes in arterial pressure (Fig. 161-5). In normal adults, an acute fall in blood pressure increases plasma vasopressin level by an amount that is roughly proportional to the degree of hypotension. However, because this relationship is exponential or curvilinear, a fall in blood pressure of as much as 10% may have little or no effect on vasopressin level, even though severe hypotension almost always evokes a very large response. The volume control of vasopressin secretion in humans appears to respond in an exponential or curvilinear fashion in a manner quite similar to that of the baroregulatory system. Thus upright posture, which lowers central or effective blood volume by 8% to 15%, usually has minimum effects on vasopressin in healthy adults. The relative insensitivity of vasopressin secretion to small changes in blood volume is considerably different from the extreme potency of osmotic stimuli. This difference in sensitivity is important for understanding both the physiologic processes of water balance and the mechanism of action of certain commonly used diagnostic tests for vasopressin activity.

Blood volume or pressure changes sufficient to affect vasopressin secretion do not necessarily disrupt the control of the osmoreceptor. In fact, they appear to shift the set of the system in such a way as to increase or decrease the effect of a given osmotic stimulus (Fig. 161-6). Therefore even during significant hypovolemia and/or hypotension, plasma vasopressin level can still be suppressed or stimulated appropriately by changes in plasma osmolality. This type of interaction indicates that osmotic and hemodynamic stimuli ultimately converge and act on the same population of neurosecretory neurons. Recognition of this interaction is essential to a proper understanding of many clinical disorders of vasopressin function.

Vasopressin secretion also may be stimulated by nonosmotic and nonhemodynamic factors. In humans one potent stimulus is nausea. The pathway mediating this response has not been defined but appears to involve the chemore-

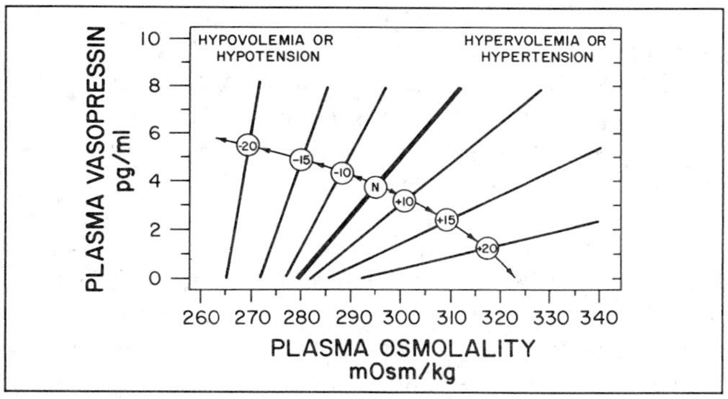

Fig. 161-6. The relationship between plasma vasopressin and plasma osmolality in the presence of differing states of blood volume and/or pressure. The line labeled *N* represents normovolemic, normotensive conditions. Minus numbers to the left indicate percentage fall; positive numbers to the right, percent rise in blood volume or pressure. (Modified from Robertson GL, Shelton RL, and Athar S: Kidney Int 10:25, 1976.)

ceptor trigger zone in the area postrema of the medulla (Fig. 161-1). Drugs and procedures, including apomorphine, morphine, nicotine, and alcohol and chemotherapy, can activate this pathway. The effect on vasopressin secretion is potent and immediate. Vasopressin levels elevations up to 100 to 1000 times basal levels may occur even when the nausea is transient and no vomiting or blood pressure changes are noted. Fluphenazine, haloperidol, or promethazine in doses sufficient to prevent nausea prevents the vasopressin response.

Acute insulin-induced hypoglycemia is a less potent stimulus for vasopressin release. The receptor and pathway mediating this effect are unknown but appear to be different from those for osmotic, hemodynamic, and emetic stimuli. The degree of hypoglycemia required to evoke vasopressin release has not been defined precisely but appears to be similar to that for other hormones responding to hypoglycemia. A 50% fall in plasma glucose level induced by insulin increases plasma vasopressin two- to fourfold. Whether other forms of hypoglycemia have similar effects on vasopressin level is unknown, but 2-deoxyglucose, which produces intracellular glucopenia, is also stimulatory.

Angiotensin II also has been implicated in the control of vasopressin secretion. Its mode of action is uncertain but appears to involve one or more sites in the central nervous system. The levels of plasma renin and/or angiotensin required to stimulate vasopressin release are probably quite high. Most of the studies have reported infusion of angiotensin in pressor doses with two- to fourfold increases in plasma vasopressin level. Whether the endogenous renin-angiotensin system plays an important role in the pathophysiology of vasopressin secretion has not been established.

Acute hypoxia or hypercapnia also stimulates vasopressin release. The pathways that mediate these effects have not been well defined but appear to involve peripheral as well as central chemoreceptors. The "thresholds" for these stimuli in humans are also uncertain, but, in the case of acute hypoxia, a fall in PaO_2 to less than 40 torr appears to be necessary. This mechanism probably is responsible for the osmotically inappropriate secretion of vasopressin that occurs in many patients with acute respiratory failure.

Pain, emotion, physical exercise, or other forms of nonspecific stress have long been thought to cause the release of vasopressin. However, it is unknown whether the response to stress is specific or due simply to some secondary stimulus such as the hypotension and/or nausea that often accompanies a vasovagal reaction to pain or intense emotion. In humans as well as rats, pain or other noxious stimuli of an intensity sufficient to activate the pituitary adrenal axis and sympathetic nervous system do not stimulate vasopressin secretion unless they also produce nausea and/or hypotension. Elevations in temperature are also reported to stimulate vasopressin release, but again, it is unclear whether the effect is primary or secondary to changes in blood volume and pressure. Resolution of these issues is necessary for understanding the pathogenesis of the inappropriate secretion of the hormone that occurs in a variety of clinical conditions (Chapter 350).

Many drugs and hormones also influence the secretion of vasopressin (Table 161-1). Stimulants, such as isoproterenol, nicotine, and apomorphine, probably act, at least in part, by producing nausea or lowering blood pressure. Agents such as histamine, bradykinin, the prostaglandins, beta-endorphin, morphine, and cyclophosphamide may act by the same mechanisms. Vincristine and lithium may stimulate by a direct effect on the neurohypophysis. The increase of vasopressin caused by chlorpropamide, clofibrate, and carbamazepine is still controversial, and a mechanism of action has not been proposed.

Pressor agents such as norepinephrine inhibit vasopressin release indirectly by raising arterial pressure. Dopam-

Table 161-1. Drugs and hormones that effect vasopressin secretion

Stimulatory	Inhibitory
Acetylcholine	Norephinephrine
Nicotine	Fluphenazine
Apomorphine	Haloperidol
Morphine (high doses)	Promethazine
Epinephrine	Oxilorphan
Isoproterenol	Butorphanol
Histamine	Morphine (low doses)
Bradykinin	Alcohol
Prostaglandins	Carbamazepine
Beta-endorphin	Glucocorticoids
Cyclophosphamide (iv)	? Phenytoin
Vincristine	Clonidine
Insulin	Muscimol
2-Deoxyglucose	
Angiotensin	
Lithium	
? Chlorpropamide	
? Clofibrate	

inergic antagonists, including fluphenazine, haloperidol, and promethazine, appear to act through suppression of the chemoreceptor trigger zone because they inhibit vasopressin release to emetic but not to osmotic or hemodynamic stimuli. Glucocorticoids appear to inhibit vasopressin secretion in healthy adults as well as in patients with adrenal insufficiency. However, it is still unclear whether these steroids act centrally or by raising blood volume and pressure. Intravenous phenytoin may inhibit vasopressin release, but the effect is inconsistent and the mechanism has not been defined. Opiates, including oxilorphan, butorphanol, and low doses of morphine, inhibit vasopressin secretion by raising the osmotic threshold. Carbamazepine inhibits vasopressin by decreasing the sensitivity of the osmostat.

The regulation of oxytocin secretion is understood less well because assays with the requisite sensitivity and specificity were not developed until very recently. However, secretion is known to be stimulated by breast-feeding. In humans, it is not stimulated by hyperosmolality or nausea but may be increased slightly by acute hypoglycemia.

Distribution and clearance. After release into the systemic circulation, vasopressin is rapidly distributed throughout the extracellular fluid. Equilibration between the intravascular and extravascular compartments occurs within 15 minutes. This rate is consistent with the molecular size and absence of binding to macromolecular components of plasma. After achieving equilibrium, vasopressin is cleared more slowly from the plasma. This slower disappearance probably reflects irreversible or metabolic clearance. The rate of this clearance varies considerably from person to person; average half-time is about 16 minutes.

Most of the vasopressin clearance in vivo appears to take place in the liver and kidney. These organs appear to inactivate vasopressin through reduction of the disulfide bridge followed by cleavage of the bond between residues 1 and 2. In pregnant women, the metabolism of vasopressin is increased slightly by a proteolytic enzyme known as *vasopressinase,* which appears in plasma by the second trimester and does not disappear until the second to fourth postpartum week. Because the activity of the enzyme is increased by contact with plastic or glass, reliable measurement of vasopressin level in pregnancy plasma requires the use of special proteolytic inhibitors during collection and processing of the samples.

Some undegraded vasopressin is excreted intact in urine. The amount varies considerably, but in normally hydrated healthy adults, it is rarely more than about 1% to 5% of the total metabolic clearance rate. Although the mechanisms involved in vasopressin excretion are not known, it probably is filtered at the glomerulus and reabsorbed to varying degrees by the tubules. This readsorption seems to be linked in some way to the renal clearance of sodium, because the urinary clearance of vasopressin varies markedly in close association with changes in solute clearance. Therefore measurements of urinary vasopressin do not always provide a reliable guide to changes in plasma vasopressin, particularly when there are changes in glomerular filtration and/or solute excretion.

Oxytocin distribution and clearance appear to be similar to those of vasopressin. Almost nothing is known about the metabolism or clearance of neurophysin except that it too can be recovered from urine.

Action. The major function of vasopressin is conservation of body water by reduction of urine output. This antidiuretic effect is achieved by promoting the reabsorption of solute-free water in the distal and/or collecting tubules of the nephron (Chapters 338 and 350). The degree of urinary concentration varies as a function of the plasma vasopressin level (Fig. 161-7). In healthy adults, this relationship is quite sensitive, because maximum urinary concentration occurs at a plasma vasopressin level of only about 5 pg per milliliter. At similar concentrations, vasopressin also reduces the rate of extrarenal water loss.

In addition to its effects on water output, vasopressin also causes contraction of smooth muscle in blood vessels and the gastrointestinal tract, secretion of ACTH by the anterior pituitary, hepatic glycogenolysis, platelet aggregation, release of factor VIII by endothelium, and alterations in firing by a variety of brain neurons. The concentrations of vasopressin required to affect these systems is not known, but it appears to be many times greater than those found in systemic plasma under physiologic conditions. It is conceivable, however, that the marked increases in vasopressin secretion produced by such stimuli as hypotension or nausea reach levels sufficient to affect vascular tone, gastrointestinal motility, portal blood flow, or clotting. The cellular mechanisms involved in the extrarenal actions of vasopressin are still undefined. It has been found, however, that the vascular, pituitary, and renal tubular effects of the hormone are mediated by different receptors (V1A, V1B, and V_2) with affinities for different parts of the vasopressin molecule. Structural modifications that abolish pressor activity do not decrease, and may even enhance, its antidiuretic activity. Analogs capable of antagonizing selectively the pressor and antidiuretic actions of vasopressin have been developed but, to date, they have been effective only in animals.

A major biologic action of oxytocin is to facilitate breastfeeding by causing the ejection of milk. This effect occurs through stimulation of contractile epithelial cells in the lactating mammary gland. Oxytocin appears to stimulate contraction of the uterus at parturition. Whether the hormone has any significant effect in males is unknown. Recently it has been shown that oxytocin has significant antidiuretic effects in some patients with neurogenic diabetes insipidus, suggesting that a chronic deficiency of vasopressin alters the V_2 receptor to enhance its receptivity and/or responsiveness to oxytocin.

The neurophysins have no recognized biologic action apart from complexing oxytocin and vasopressin in neurosecretory granules. Although present in plasma, they do not serve as binding or transport proteins because, in blood, the higher pH and lower concentration of the reactants favor complete dissociation.

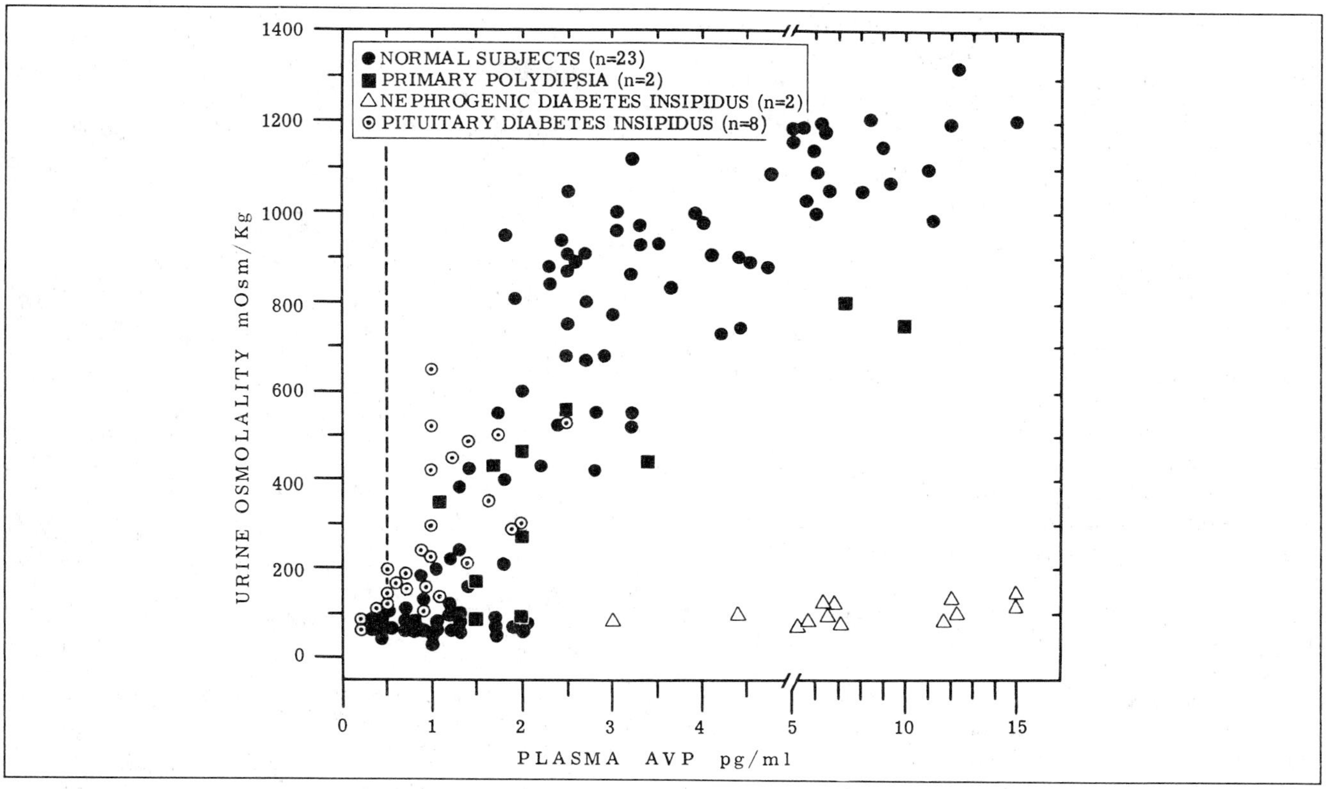

Fig. 161-7. The relationship of urine osmolality to plasma vasopressin concentration in healthy adults in various states of hydration and in patients with polyuria of diverse causes. (From Robertson GL et al: J Clin Invest 52:2340, 1973.)

Extrarenal water output. The volume of water lost by evaporation from skin and lungs varies markedly, depending on such factors as dress, humidity, environmental temperature, activity, and vasopressin secretion. Under conditions typical of modern, sedentary urban life, insensible water loss in a healthy 70 kg man or woman approximates urine output (1 L/day). However, if vasopressin is absent or activity or temperature increases, the rate of insensible water loss also rises and, under extreme conditions, may approach the maximum rate of water excretion by the kidney (20 L/day). Hence, in quantitative terms, insensible water loss and the factors that influence it are just as important to the economy of water balance as are the factors that regulate urine output.

Water intake. The thirst mechanism provides an indispensable adjunct to the antidiuretic mechanism in controlling water balance. In physiologic usage, *thirst* is defined as a consciously perceived need for water. This drive must be distinguished from dietary, social, psychogenic, and other environmental causes of drinking. Thirst is stimulated by many of the factors that cause vasopressin release. Hypertonicity of the plasma appears to be the most potent stimulus. Normally, an increase in plasma osmolality of only 2% to 3% above basal levels results in a strong desire to drink. The absolute level of plasma osmolality at which thirst develops varies somewhat from person to person but averages about 295 mOsm per kilogram. This level is considerably above the osmotic threshold for vasopressin release and closely approximates that at which maximum concentration of the urine normally occurs. Water intake can also be osmotically inhibited. This inhibitory control manifests as a sense of satiation and a reduction in the basal rate discretionary fluid intake when healthy adults are treated with saturating doses of antidiuretic hormone. It occurs with reductions in plasma osmolality and sodium of only 1% to 3% and is normally sufficient to prevent water intoxication even if antidiuresis is fixed at maximum levels.

Although the neuronal pathways that mediate thirst and satiation have not been totally defined, they appear to involve osmoreceptors located in the anterolateral hypothalamus near, but not totally coincident with, the osmoreceptors that regulate vasopressin release. The specificities of the two systems appear to be similar. Thus plasma solutes such as sodium or mannitol are potent dipsogens, whereas plasma urea or glucose has little or no effect on thirst.

A decrease in blood volume or pressure is also dipsogenic. The degree of hypovolemia and/or hypotension required to produce thirst is not well defined for humans but again appears to be greater than that needed to effect vasopressin release. Therefore it appears unlikely that hemodynamic variables have an important influence on water intake, except under pathologic conditions. The mechanism by which hypovolemia and/or hypotension produces thirst is unknown but may involve a resetting of the osmoregulatory system via the same or similar pathways as vasopressin release. Recent evidence suggests that thirst may also be influenced by receptors in the oropharynx, but their role in water intake regulation has not yet been clarified.

VASOPRESSIN DEFICIENCY: DIABETES INSIPIDUS (See also Chapter 350)

Clinical features

Neurogenic diabetes insipidus is a disorder characterized by the excretion of large amounts of dilute urine. The polyuria varies considerably from patient to patient, ranging from as little as 3 to as much as 20 L/day. It must be distinguished from simple *urinary frequency,* a disorder in which total output may be normal. Thirst and polydipsia are also prominent features of diabetes insipidus. In correlation with the polyuria, they also vary in severity from patient to patient.

Apart from polyuria and increased thirst, diabetes insipidus is associated with few other symptoms or complaints. Fatigue and irritability are sometimes mentioned, but these symptoms are mild and rarely, if ever, prompt the patient to seek medical care. Even the polyuria and polydipsia are remarkably well tolerated and often are not even mentioned to a physician until they become severe. As often as not, they come to light only during a careful examination for some other complaint such as headache, loss of vision, or symptoms referable to a deficiency of some other pituitary hormone. The scant attention paid to symptoms of polyuria and polydipsia is unfortunate because they can be treated quite easily and are often the harbinger of a more serious disorder.

Diabetes insipidus also is associated with relatively few physical signs. Except in unusual cases associated with damage to the thirst mechanism, dehydration is not sufficiently severe to be evident on physical examination. The only other physical signs are those caused either by the underlying disease itself (see the box at right) or by concurrent damage to other pituitary hormones or neighboring neuronal systems. The latter may be manifested as visual field defects, obesity, hypogonadism, hypothyroidism, secondary adrenal insufficiency, and, in children, retarded growth or delayed pubescence.

Except for hyposthenuria, results of routine laboratory tests are usually normal in uncomplicated neurogenic diabetes insipidus. As with symptoms and physical signs, all other laboratory abnormalities are due to the underlying disease itself or to concurrent damage to neighboring hormonal and/or neuronal systems. Plasma osmolality and/or sodium concentration is not appreciably elevated unless the patient's thirst mechanism is also damaged or the ability to drink is otherwise impaired.

Causes of diabetes insipidus

- I. Vasopressin deficiency (neurogenic or central diabetes insipidus)
  - A. Decreased secretion
    - 1. Idiopathic
      - a. Sporadic (? autoimmune)
      - b. Familial (autosomal dominant inheritance)
    - 2. Traumatic (accidental or surgical)
    - 3. Malignancy
      - a. Primary (craniopharyngioma, germinoma, meningioma, pituitary adenoma with suprasellar extension)
      - b. Metastatic (lung, breast, leukemia)
    - 4. Granuloma (sarcoid, histiocytosis, xanthoma dissemination)
    - 5. Infectious (meningitis, encephalitis, syphilis)
    - 6. Vascular (aneurysm, Sheehan's syndrome, cardiac arrest, vasculitis)
    - 7. Psychobiologic (anorexia nervosa)
    - 8. Toxic (carbon monoxide)
    - 9. Congenital malformations
  - B. Increased metabolism
    - 1. Pregnancy
- II. Vasopressin resistance (nephrogenic diabetes insipidus)
  - A. Idiopathic
    - 1. Sporadic
    - 2. Familial (X-linked recessive inheritance)
  - B. Post obstructive
  - C. Malignancy (retroperitoneal fibrosarcoma)
  - D. Granuloma (sarcoid)
  - E. Infectious (pyelonephritis)
  - F. Vascular (sickle cell disease or trait)
  - G. Metabolic (hypokalemia, hypercalciuria)
  - H. Toxic (lithium, demeclocycline, methoxyflurane, methicillin)
  - I. Malformations (polycystic disease)
  - J. Pregnancy
- III. Excessive water intake (primary polydipsia)
  - A. Psychogenic (schizophrenia, affective disorders)
  - B. Dipsogenic
    - 1. Idiopathic
    - 2. Traumatic
    - 3. Granuloma (neurosarcoidosis)
    - 4. Infectious (meningitis)
    - 5. Other (multiple sclerosis)

Differential diagnosis

Neurogenic diabetes insipidus must be differentiated from other causes of polyuria and polydipsia (see the box at right). The most common is the *solute diuresis* that accompanies severe uncontrolled diabetes mellitus or other conditions associated with deficient reabsorption of salt and water in the proximal nephron. It is characterized by a greatly increased rate of total solute excretion, an abnormality that is useful in distinguishing it from other causes of polyuria and polydipsia. Besides neurogenic diabetes insipidus, the latter include *nephrogenic diabetes insipidus* (resulting from an impaired response to the antidiuretic effect of vasopressin) and *primary polydipsia* (caused by excessive ingestion of water); see Chapters 350 and 360.

Pathogenesis and pathophysiology

Neurogenic diabetes insipidus is caused by insufficient amounts of plasma vasopressin. This deficiency results in a decrease in the hydroosmotic permeability of the distal and collecting tubules of the kidney. As a consequence, dilute urine formed in more proximal parts of the nephron is excreted essentially unchanged. The resultant loss of solute-free water causes mild dehydration, a rise in plasma osmolality, and the stimulation of thirst. The net effect is that water intake rises to a level sufficient to balance output, and the osmotic pressure of body fluid is stabilized at a new level, slightly above normal.

The magnitude of the polyuria and polydipsia depends on several variables, including the severity of vasopressin deficiency, the integrity of the thirst mechanism, the solute load, and the state of renal function. As a general rule, clinically significant polyuria does not occur until the secretory capacity of the neurohypophysis has been reduced by more than 50%. Because many patients with neurogenic diabetes insipidus retain some capacity to release vasopressin in response to osmotic stimulation, the concentration of hormone that circulates under basal conditions is determined by the level of plasma osmolality at which thirst occurs. If this limit is raised or abolished (e.g., by damage to the osmoreceptor or by externally imposed water deprivation), plasma osmolality may rise sufficiently to stimulate the release of vasopressin in amounts adequate to produce urinary concentration. This interplay between the factors that determine water intake and output explains the seeming paradox that many patients with neurogenic diabetes insipidus exhibit concentrated urine during a standard dehydration test. Vasopressin release also can be effected by nonosmotic stimuli. Because they are so potent, nausea or orthostatic hypotension may evoke significant increases in plasma vasopressin level even in patients who fail to respond to hypertonicity. In some patients, smoking has a similar effect. Hence these and other variables known to influence vasopressin level must always be kept in mind when interpreting the antidiuretic response to diagnostic or therapeutic procedures.

Changes in renal function also influence the severity of polyuria in patients with neurogenic diabetes insipidus. For any given level of plasma vasopressin, a rise or fall in solute excretion results in a proportionate increase or decrease in the volume of filtrate delivered to the collecting tubules. Hence the volume of urine excreted is influenced appreciably by changes in salt intake or other factors that alter solute load. In addition, neurogenic diabetes insipidus often results in two changes in the antidiuretic response to vasopressin. First, many such patients appear to be supersensitive to the antidiuretic effect of very low plasma concentrations of the hormone. The mechanism of this change is unknown, but it may involve increased affinity and/or number of renal vasopressin receptors, as occur with chronic deficiency of certain other hormones. Second, the hypersensitivity to very low concentrations of vasopressin is usually accompanied by a reduction in maximum urinary concentrating capacity. As a result, raising plasma vasopressin to normal or even supranormal levels increases urine osmolality less in patients with neurogenic diabetes insipidus than it does in healthy adults. This diminution in maximum concentrating response is thought to be due to "washout" of the medullary concentration gradient caused by chronic polyuria. It is not sufficiently severe to interfere with treatment of the polyuria and quickly resolves when antidiuresis is re-established; however, in conjunction with the changes in receptor affinity noted, it complicates the interpretation of certain commonly used diagnostic procedures (discussed later).

Nephrogenic diabetes insipidus is caused by deficient renal response to the antidiuretic actions of vasopressin (see the box on the left). Vasopressin secretion is normal. In other respects, the pathophysiology of nephrogenic and neurogenic diabetes insipidus is similar. Increased excretion of solute-free water results in mild hypertonic dehydration and stimulation of thirst. The degree of polyuria also depends to a great extent on the rate of solute excretion. Two distinct forms of nephrogenic diabetes insipidus have now been recognized. In one, the renal resistance is complete, and urine remains dilute even when there are marked increases in plasma vasopressin (type I). In the second, the renal resistance is partial or relative and urinary concentration does occur if plasma vasopressin level is elevated to more than 20 times normal (type II). As might be expected, there are important differences in the clinical behavior of these two forms of disorder. Unlike those with type I, patients with type II nephrogenic diabetes insipidus have concentrated urine in response to marked elevations in plasma vasopressin level produced either by prolonged water deprivation or by administration of vasopressin in standard diagnostic doses (0.05 to 0.1 U/kg). Hence in conventional indirect tests, they behave like patients with neurogenic diabetes insipidus yet respond inadequately to the standard therapeutic doses of the hormone.

Primary polydipsia is caused by excessive water intake. It results in a slight fall in plasma osmolality and an appropriate decrease in vasopressin secretion and urine concentration. As a result, water excretion rises to balance intake, and plasma osmolality stabilizes at a new level, only slightly below normal. In some cases, the polydipsia is associated with inappropriate vasopressin secretion, which, by retarding water excretion, leads to a marked reduction in plasma osmolality and/or sodium concentration. In some patients, the excessive intake of water appears to be due to an abnormality in the osmoregulation of thirst (dipsogenic). In many others, however, thirst is denied, and the excessive drinking appears to be due to more generalized cognitive dysfunction caused by serious mental illness (psychogenic). Like other forms of chronic polyuria, primary polydipsia results in a reduction in maximum urinary concentrating capacity. Whether primary polydipsia also causes supersensitivity to the antidiuretic action of small amounts of vasopressin is unclear.

Solute diuresis causes polyuria by overwhelming the distal diluting and concentrating mechanisms. As a consequence, large volumes of nearly isotonic urine are excreted, regardless of the plasma vasopressin level. Because water is lost in excess of sodium, the effective osmotic pressure of plasma tends to rise, and thirst is stimulated. The severity of the polyuria depends primarily on the rate of solute excretion. At high flow, it is largely independent of vasopressin secretion, water intake, or type of solute present.

Thus increased excretion of sodium, mannitol, urea, or glucose has essentially the same diuretic effect.

Diagnosis

Evaluation of the patient with polyuria and polydipsia should begin with a check for solute diuresis. In most cases, testing the urine for glucose suffices. If the test result is negative, other forms of solute diuresis can be ruled out simply by calculating the osmolar excretion rate. Depending on diet, healthy adults normally excrete somewhere between 500 and 1000 mOsm per day. If the product of urine volume in liters per day and urine osmolality in milliosmoles per kilogram exceeds 1500, solute diuresis is likely, and efforts to identify and correct it should be undertaken before proceeding with the testing. If the product is less than 1500 mOsm per day, solute diuresis is unlikely, and further tests to differentiate among the other three causes of polyuria are indicated (see the box on the right).

The next step is to assess the state of hydration by measuring plasma osmolality during ad libitum intake of fluids. To be meaningful, this measurement must be made on fresh plasma with the use of a carefully calibrated osmometer. Serum should not be used for this purpose because its use sometimes results in relatively large artifacts. If these requirements cannot be met or if plasma glucose or urea level is abnormal, it may be preferable to rely on measurements of plasma sodium. If hypertonicity and/or hypernatremia is present under basal conditions, the polyuria almost certainly is not due to primary polydipsia, and the testing can proceed directly to the vasopressin (Pitressin) test to differentiate between neurogenic and nephrogenic diabetes insipidus. To prevent misdiagnosis of patients with partial nephrogenic diabetes insipidus, the dose of hormone administered should be no greater than 10 mU per kilogram of aqueous vasopressin. The drug should be given parenterally, and urine osmolality measured before administration and at half-hour intervals for 2 hours after injection. Under these conditions, a maximum rise in urine osmolality of 50% or more is almost invariably diagnostic of neurogenic diabetes insipidus. A smaller increase or no change indicates nephrogenic diabetes insipidus. The complete and incomplete forms of the latter disorder can be further differentiated by repeating the test using larger doses of aqueous vasopressin (50 mU/kg).

In most patients plasma osmolality and sodium level are within normal limits under basal conditions (Fig. 161-8). In this case, a dehydration test should be performed. All liquids are withheld, and body weight as well as plasma and urine osmolality are measured hourly as dehydration develops. If urinary concentration does not occur before body weight falls by 5% or plasma osmolality and sodium level rise to 295 mOsm per kilogram and 143 mEq per liter, respectively, primary polydipsia is excluded, and the vasopressin test described previously can be used to differentiate between neurogenic and nephrogenic diabetes insipidus.

However, if fluid deprivation leads to urinary concentration, this indirect test does not distinguish reliably among primary polydipsia, "partial" neurogenic diabetes insipidus, and "partial" nephrogenic diabetes insipidus because all three conditions can manifest identical changes in urine osmolality (Fig. 161-9). Hence some other diagnostic approach must be used. The simplest, safest, and most reliable method is to measure plasma vasopressin level as well as plasma and urine osmolality at the end of the dehydration test (see the box above). By plotting urine osmolality as a function of the concurrent plasma vasopressin level on a suitable nomogram, almost all patients with type I or II nephrogenic diabetes insipidus can be identified (Fig. 161-7). A similar plot of plasma vasopressin level as a function of plasma osmolality serves to differentiate patients with

Evaluation of suspected diabetes insipidus

1. Measure plasma osmolality and/or sodium concentration under conditions of ad libitum fluid intake. If they are above 295 mOsm/kg and 143 mEq/L, the diagnosis of primary polydipsia is excluded, and the testing should proceed directly to step 3 to distinguish between neurogenic and nephrogenic diabetes insipidus
2. If basal plasma osmolality and/or sodium is not elevated, perform a dehydration test. If urinary concentration does not occur before plasma osmolality and/or sodium reaches 295 mOsm/kg or 143 mEq/L, the diagnosis of primary polydipsia is again excluded, and the evaluation should proceed to step 3
3. Inject aqueous vasopressin (Pitressin) in a dose of 10 mU/kg body weight and collect urine every 30 minutes for the next 2 hours. If urine osmolality rises more than 50% above the value obtained at the end of the dehydration test, neurogenic diabetes insipidus is established. If not, administer a larger dose of vasopressin (50 mU/kg) to distinguish partial from complete nephrogenic diabetes insipidus
4. If dehydration results in urinary concentration, measure plasma vasopressin level and relate it to concurrent plasma level and to urine osmolality level by using suitable nomograms (e.g., Figs. 161-3 and 161-3). If the level of plasma osmolality achieved is insufficient to permit a clear distinction between normal and subnormal vasopressin response (>292 mOsm/kg), infuse 3% saline solution at a rate of 0.1 ml/kg/min for 2 hours, and repeat the measurements of plasma osmolality and vasopressin level
5. If vasopressin level measurements are not available, admit the patient and perform a closely monitored therapeutic trial with intranasal desmopressin, 25 μ every 12 hours. If the trial corrects polydipsia as well as polyuria, and hyponatremia does not occur, the diagnosis of neurogenic diabetes insipidus is established. If the trial reduces polyuria, but not polydipsia, or produces other evidence of water intoxication, primary polydipsia is likely, and therapy should be discontinued until definitive diagnosis can be made by vasopressin assay. If desopressin does not reduce either polyuria or polydipsia, the diagnosis of nephrogenic diabetes insipidus is established. In some patients, repeat tests with higher doses of the drug may be indicated to distinguish between the complete and incomplete forms of the disorder

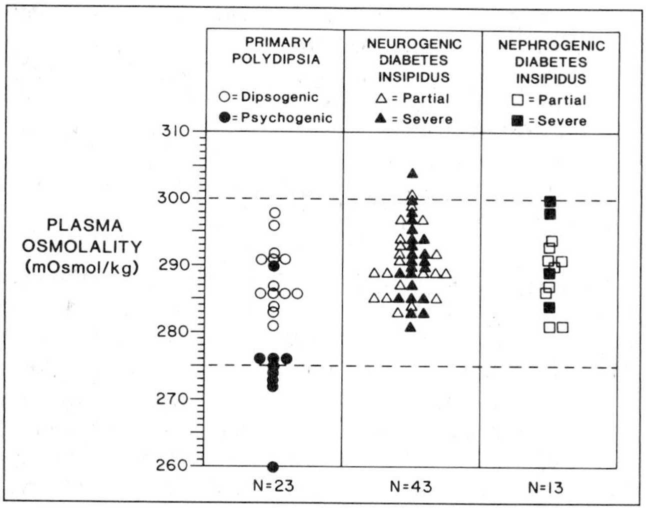

Fig. 161-8. Basal plasma osmolality in patients with polyuria of diverse causes.

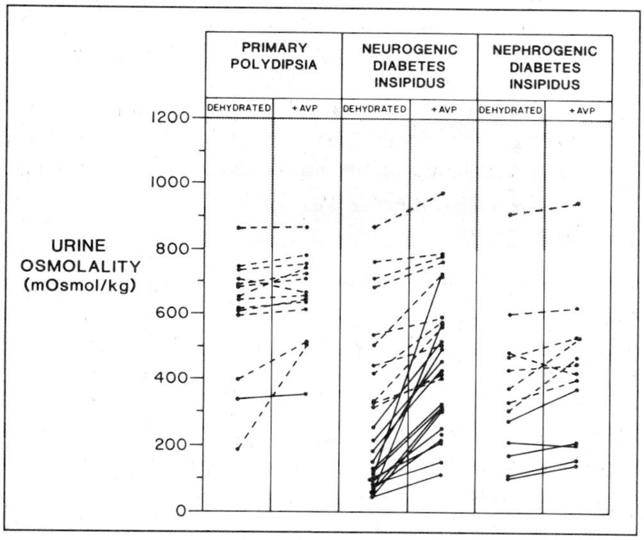

Fig. 161-9. Urine osmolality after a standard dehydration test and administration of vasopressin in patients with polyuria of diverse causes. In the category of primary polydipsia, the solid line indicates the values obtained in a patient with severe psychogenic polydipsia. The broken lines indicate the values obtained in 13 patients with dipsogenic polydipsia. In the categories of neurogenic and nephrogenic diabetes insipidus, the solid and broken lines indicate the values obtained in patients with severe or partial defects, respectively. AVP, vasopressin.

neurogenic diabetes insipidus from those with primary polydipsia (Fig. 161-3). In a few cases in which the level of plasma osmolality achieved is insufficient to permit unambiguous interpretation of the vasopressin concentration values, repeat assay after infusion of hypertonic (3%) saline solution (0.1 ml/kg/min for 2 hours) almost always clarifies whether secretion of the hormone is normal or subnormal.

If a vasopressin assay suitable for diagnosing diabetes insipidus is not available, the best alternative is to perform a closely monitored therapeutic trial with standard doses of desmopressin. If treatment for 1 or 2 days has no effect, the patient probably has nephrogenic diabetes insipidus. On the other hand, if the polyuria and polydipsia are abolished without producing significant hyponatremia, the diagnosis of neurogenic diabetes insipidus is indicated. If treatment reduces polyuria but not polydipsia, or produces other signs of water intoxication, the diagnosis of primary polydipsia should be strongly suspected. In such a case, however, other evidence should be sought because an occasional patient with unequivocal neurogenic diabetes insipidus also responds in this way.

Recent studies suggest that magnetic resonance imaging (MRI) may also permit diagnosis of neurogenic diabetes insipidus. On T_1-weighted images, the normal posterior pituitary displays a high signal indistinguishable from that of fatty tissue. In patients with neurogenic diabetes insipidus, this high-intensity signal is absent. However, the sensitivity and reliability of this approach as a means for diagnosis have not yet been established.

Because of possible involvement of neighboring structures, other diagnostic studies are indicated in patients with neurogenic diabetes insipidus. Besides radiographic evaluation by computed tomography or MRI of the sella and hypothalamus, visual fields and anterior pituitary function should also be thoroughly tested. In addition, other studies to determine the underlying disease process may be indicated.

SPECIFIC DISEASE ENTITIES

Deficiency of vasopressin secretion results from destruction of the neurohypophysis by any of several different pathologic processes. The most common cause before the advent of transsphenoidal approaches was surgical removal of pituitary tumors. Because the neurohypophyseal neurons originate in the hypothalamus and have many fibers that terminate above the sella turcica, pituitary adenomas that are confined to the sella turcica usually do not destroy enough of the gland to cause clinically apparent diabetes insipidus. However, tumors such as craniopharyngioma or germinoma that arise in the hypothalamus often manifest first as diabetes insipidus. Metastases from cancer of the lung or breast, leukemic infiltrates, and extramedullary hematopoiesis can also cause the syndrome. Certain granulomatomas or lipid storage diseases, such as sarcoidosis, histiocytosis, or, more rarely, xanthoma disseminatum, cause diabetes insipidus by infiltrating the pituitary or meninges at the base of the brain. These diseases are usually systemic, and, by the time they cause diabetes insipidus, usually have manifested themselves elsewhere (e.g., in lung, bone, or skin). Acute infections occasionally involve the neurohypophysis. Perhaps because the neurohypophysis has such a large secretory reserve and a bilateral blood supply, vascular disease is an unusual cause of diabetes insipidus. For reasons not altogether clear, some patients with anorexia nervosa have a mild form of neurogenic diabetes insipidus that disappears when the malnutrition is corrected.

Much, if not most, of the neurogenic diabetes insipidus now seen in an office practice is idiopathic in nature. The few histologic studies done in such patients reveal extensive loss of neurosecretory neurons in the supraoptic and, to a lesser extent, paraventricular nuclei. Idiopathic neurogenic diabetes insipidus can occur in sporadic or familial patterns. The familial form begins in childhood and is inherited in an autosomal dominant mode. It is due to a missense mutation in the part of the vasopressin precursor gene that codes for the signal peptide (exon 1) or the central, highly conserved structure of the neurophysin moiety (exon 2). By some as yet to be determined mechanism, these mutations cause postnatal degeneration of the neurons that express the gene, leading to severe deficiency of vasopressin.

Primary polydipsia is often associated with schizophrenia or other psychiatric illnesses. The pathogenic link is unknown, but, in many cases, the polydipsia seems to be prompted not so much by true thirst as by other motives, such as a desire to cleanse the body of poisons or other harmful substances. Primary polydipsia can also be due to an abnormality in the osmoregulation of thirst. Most of these cases are idiopathic, but the syndrome also is associated frequently with neurosarcoid and has been observed with trauma, tuberculous meningitis, and multiple sclerosis.

Renal resistance to the antidiuretic action of vasopressin can also result from a variety of diseases and drugs (see the box on p. 1318). Nephrogenic diabetes insipidus is discussed in Chapters 350 and 360.

Treatment

Vasopressins. For many years, the only practical therapy for neurogenic diabetes insipidus was injection of Pitressin tannate in oil. Intramuscular injection of 5 to 10 units every 48 to 72 hours gives satisfactory relief of the polyuria and polydipsia in most patients but could also result in inadequate or erratic response caused by failure to emulsify the mixture adequately by shaking and warming the vial before use. Recently, this preparation of vasopressin was withdrawn from the market. Because its duration of action is only a few hours, aqueous vasopressin is not suitable for long-term treatment of diabetes insipidus and therefore is used primarily for diagnostic purposes.

Desmopressin or DDAVP (Fig. 161-2) is a synthetic analog of vasopressin. This preparation possesses many advantages in the treatment of diabetes insipidus. Modifications in positions 1 and 8 of the molecule double its antidiuretic potency, eliminate its pressor actions, and increase the resistance to metabolic degradation. Desmopressin has much longer antidiuretic action than does native vasopressin. Administration of 10 to 25 μ by nasal insufflation twice daily affords complete relief of polyuria in most adults. Rhinitis and/or sinusitis may interfere with its absorption, but resistance caused by antibody production has not been reported. DDAVP is also available in a form suitable for parenteral use. A dose of 1 to 4 μ administered once daily by intramuscular injection usually provides complete relief of polyuria and polydipsia in patients with neurogenic diabetes insipidus. DDAVP has few side-effects. Excess water retention may occur, but the effect is usually transient even if therapy is continued. Sustained hyponatremia almost always indicates an abnormality in the thirst mechanism and is a reason to discontinue treatment and repeat the diagnostic studies. The only significant disadvantage of DDAVP is its cost, which is approximately 6 to 10 times that of other forms of antidiuretic therapy.

Oral agents. Chlorpropamide (Diabinese), a sulfonylurea drug more commonly used to treat hyperglycemia in diabetes mellitus, is also effective in diabetes insipidus. When given in conventional doses of 250 to 500 mg a day, it reduces urine output by 30% to 70% in patients with neurogenic diabetes insipidus. This decrease in urine volume is accompanied by a proportionate rise in urine osmolality and a reduction in polydipsia similar to that caused by small doses of vasopressin. Like vasopressin or DDAVP, chlorpropamide is ineffective in the treatment of nephrogenic diabetes insipidus. Unlike the hormones, however, chlorpropamide has little or no antidiuretic effect in normal persons or patients with primary polydipsia. Its antidiuretic effect in neurogenic diabetes insipidus may also be attenuated by concomitant or recent treatment with vasopressin or DDAVP. These seemingly paradoxic observations suggest that chlorpropamide acts via a mechanism similar to that of vasopressin itself but does so only if there has been a prolonged deficiency of the hormone. Studies in the toad bladder and rats suggest that chlorpropamide acts by potentiating the renal tubular effects of small, subthreshold amounts of vasopressin. Other mechanisms may also be involved because, in contrast to earlier impressions, the antidiuretic effect of the drug is as great in patients with severe deficiency as in those with partial deficiencies of vasopressin. The side-effects of chlorpropamide therapy include hypoglycemia and alcohol-induced flushing. The former is rare and usually can be prevented by avoidance of prolonged fasting or exercise. The latter is more common but is usually mild and may subside with repeated exposure. Other sulfonylurea drugs do not have a significant antidiuretic effect in patients with diabetes insipidus and, in some cases, may even have a mild diuretic action.

Clofibrate (Atromid-S), which is commonly used to treat hyperlipidemia, also may reduce polyuria and polydipsia in patients with diabetes insipidus. At conventional doses of 0.5 to 1.0 g three times daily, its antidiuretic effect is usually less than that of chlorpropamide, although in some patients clofibrate is more effective. The mechanism of action is not known. Clofibrate is also ineffective in nephrogenic diabetes insipidus and has only minimal antidiuretic action in normal subjects and patients with primary polydipsia. Clofibrate has not been shown to potentiate the renal actions of vasopressin. Major side-effects include myalgia, increased transaminase level, and gastroenteritis. These abnormalities often subside with continued treatment but in some cases may necessitate discontinuation of the drug.

Carbamazepine (Tegretol) also reduces or eliminates polyuria and polydipsia in patients with neurogenic diabetes insipidus. Its mechanism of action is also unclear but probably does not involve increased secretion of vasopressin. Its use in the treatment of diabetes insipidus is limited by the seriousness of some of its side-effects.

Thiazide diuretics also reduce polyuria in patients with diabetes insipidus. Unlike chlorpropamide and clofibrate, the thiazides are equally effective in patients with nephrogenic diabetes insipidus, indicating that they work by a different mechanism. By inhibiting sodium reabsorption in the ascending limb of Henle's loop, the thiazides interfere with maximum urinary dilution. At the same time, they contract the extracellular fluid volume and increase salt and water reabsorption in the proximal tubule. The net effect is a slight rise in urine osmolality and a proportionately larger reduction in urine volume. At conventional doses, thiazide diuretics significantly potentiate the antidiuretic effect of chlorpropamide in neurogenic diabetes insipidus and are most useful in conjunction with one of the other oral agents. Other than occasional hypokalemia, serious side-effects are rare. Because thiazides reduce the ability to excrete a water load in all persons, they may produce water intoxication in patients with primary polydipsia.

The appropriate role of the oral drugs in the management of diabetes insipidus is not clear. Used alone or in combination with thiazide diuretics, chlorpropamide or clofibrate can reduce polyuria to asymptomatic levels in most patients. Oral drugs have the advantage of convenience and relatively lower cost. This form of treatment is associated, however, with a greater incidence of undesirable side-effects, and there are unresolved questions about their long-term safety. Moreover, oral drugs probably should not be used in pregnancy, because of possible teratogenic effects. These medications also are potentially hazardous to young children. In these situations, desmopressin appears to provide the safest and most effective form of therapy.

Several other measures may be helpful in reducing polyuria in either nephrogenic or neurogenic diabetes insipidus. Salt restriction reduces urine output by increasing the volume of filtrate reabsorbed isosmotically in the proximal nephron. Caffeine and other methylated xanthines have exaggerated diuretic effects in patients with diabetes insipidus. Often elimination of coffee or tea from the diet substantially improves control of polyuria.

REFERENCES

Anderson B: Regulation of water intake. Physiol Rev 58(3):582, 1978.

Barron WM: Water metabolism and vasopressin secretion during pregnancy. In Lindheimer MD and Dawson JM, editors: Baillier's clinical obstetrics and gynecology. 1. Renal disease in pregnancy. Philadelphia, 1987, Lea & Febiger.

Goldman M, Luchios D, and Robertson GL: Mechanisms of altered water metabolism in polydipsic, hyponatremic, psychotic patients. N Engl J Med 318(7):397, 1988.

Richardson DW, and Robinson AG: Desmopressin. Ann Intern Med 103:228, 1985.

Robertson GL: Dipsogenic diabetes insipidus: a newly recognized syndrome caused by a selective defect in the osmoregulation of thirst. Trans Assoc Am Physicians 1(C):241, 1988.

Robertson GL: Thirst and vasopressin function in normal and disordered states of water balance. J Lab Clin Med 101(3):351, 1983.

Robertson GL: Differential diagnosis of polyurias. Annu Rev Med 39:425, 1988.

Robertson GL, Aycinena P: Neurogenic disorders of osmoregulation. Am J Med 72:339, 1982.

Robertson GL and Berl T: Water metabolism. In Brenner BM and Rector FC, editors: The kidney. ed 3. Philadelphia, 1986, Saunders.

Schmale H, Fehr S, and Richter D: Vasopressin synthesis—from gene to peptide hormone. Kidney Int [suppl S] 8-S:13, 1987.

Schrier RW, Berl T, and Anderson RJ: Osmotic and nonosmotic control of vasopressin release. Am J Physiol 236(4):F321, 1979.

Vokes TJ et al: Osmoregulation of thirst and vasopressin during normal menstrual cycle. Am J Physiol 254:R641-47, 1988.

CHAPTER

162 Disorders of the Thyroid

Gerald S. Levey
Irwin Klein

THYROID GLAND ANATOMY

The thyroid gland arises from embryonic endoderm and migrates caudad during development to its adult position at the base of the neck. Occasionally accessory thyroid tissue can be found along this path of descent either at the base of the tongue or along the thyroglossal duct. By the 12th week of gestation the thyroid gland is morphologically and functionally intact and the thyroid epithelial cells have formed small, intact colloid-containing follicles. The thyroid also contains C cells known to secrete calcitonin.

The normal thyroid gland weighs approximately 25 g and is composed of two lateral lobes and an isthmus. The isthmus lies just below the cricoid cartilage anterior to the trachea, and the lateral lobes extend superiorly and somewhat laterally in the jugular groove for approximately 4 to 5 cm (Fig. 162-1). Inspection and palpation of the thyroid allow identification of symmetric or asymmetric enlargement of the lateral lobes (goiter), discrete nodules, thyroid tenderness, or changes in consistency of the normally fleshy gland. Various methods have been recommended for the proper palpation of the thyroid, but no single technique is necessarily superior and each examiner should employ the approach that best suits the individual case.

THYROID HORMONE FORMATION AND METABOLISM

The formation of the thyroid hormones thyroxine (T_4) and triiodothyronine (T_3) depicted in Fig. 162-2 requires an adequate supply of exogenous iodine. Iodine is usually provided by the ingestion of food, water, or dietary supplements. Once absorbed, the iodine is converted to inorganic iodide and then concentrated by the thyroid gland by a trapping process that requires an intact membrane, sodium-potassium-adenosinetriphosphatase (Na^+-K^+ATPase), ade-

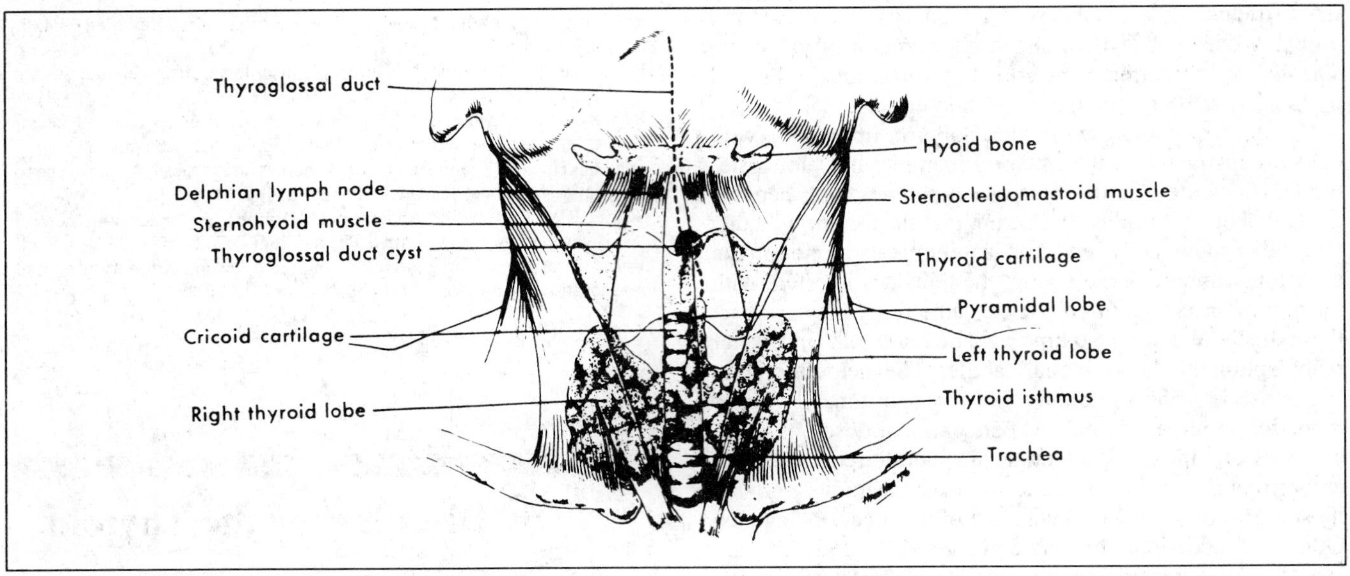

Fig. 162-1. Normal thyroid gland anatomy. (From Prior JA and Silberstein JS: Physical diagnosis: The history and examination of the patient, ed 7. St. Louis, 1981, Mosby.)

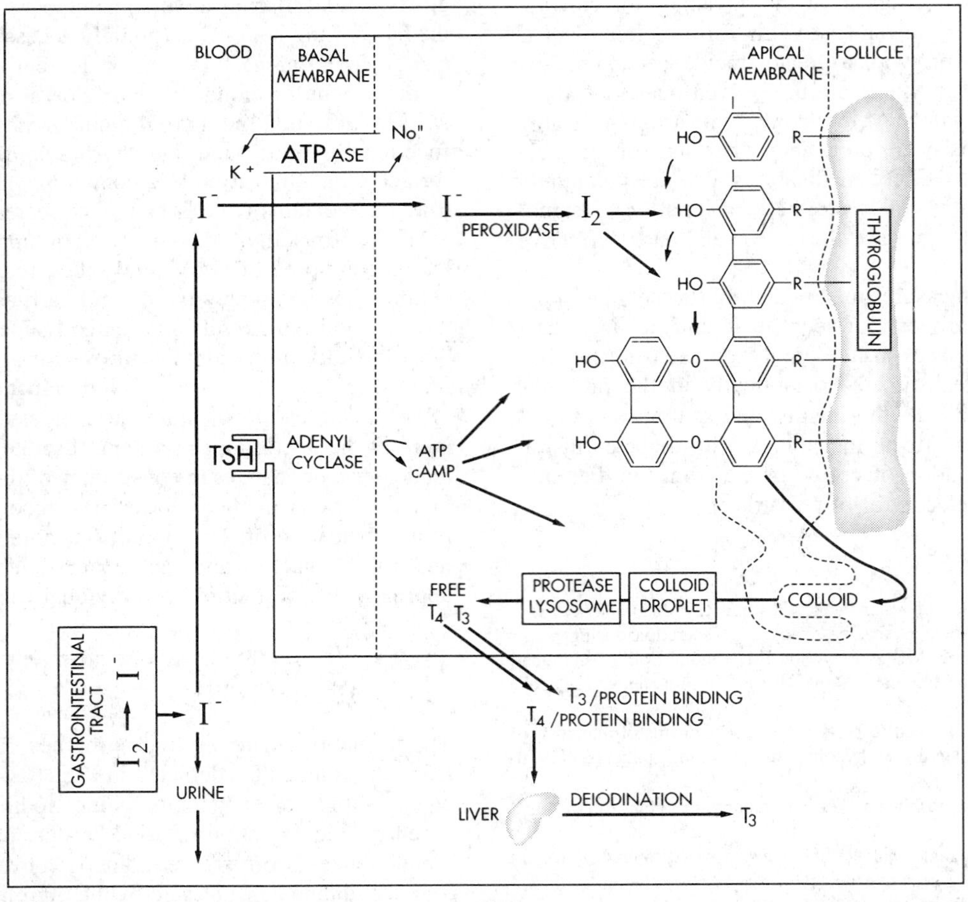

Fig. 162-2. Formation of thyroid hormone within the thyroid epithelial cell. (Modified from Berkow R, editor: The Merck manual of diagnosis and therapy, ed 16. Merck, 1992.)

nylate cyclase, and specific membrane lipids. Inorganic iodide is converted to organic iodine by a membrane bound peroxidase enzyme, which in the presence of hydrogen peroxide incorporates the newly organified iodine into tyrosine molecules in thyroglobulin, a glycoprotein in the colloid within the thyroid follicle. The iodination of the tyrosines occurs at either one (monoiodotyrosine [MIT]) or two (diiodotyrosine [DIT]) sites. MIT and DIT are in turn coupled, probably by an enzymatic reaction, in which two molecules of DIT would yield T_4 and one molecule each of MIT and DIT would yield T_3. The reaction producing T_4 is the major one, because the T_4/T_3 ratio in thyroglobulin is about 13:1. Most T_3 is produced by deiodination of T_4 in peripheral tissues. After the coupling reaction, the nascent thyroid hormones are still bound to thyroglobulin in the colloid follicle.

In order to make thyroid hormone available for transport to the bloodstream, pieces of thyroglobulin are removed from the follicle by endocytosis, resulting in the formation of vesicles known as colloid droplets. Within the cell, lysosomes containing proteases fuse with the colloid droplets and hydrolyze thyroglobulin, causing the release of free T_3 and T_4. Although some of the free thyroidal T_3 and T_4 is deiodinated in the thyroid gland with the iodine re-entering the thyroid iodine pool, most of the T_3 and T_4 diffuses into the bloodstream, where it is bound to specific serum transport proteins.

The major thyroid transport protein for T_4 is thyroxine binding globulin (TBG), a glycoprotein that normally accounts for about 80% of the bound serum thyroid hormone. T_4 is also bound by transthyretin (TTR, formerly known as thyroxine binding prealbumin [TBPA]) and to a much more limited extent by albumin. T_3 is mostly bound by TBG and to a minor degree by albumin. TBG has about a 10-fold higher affinity for T_4 than T_3; therefore approximately *0.05%* of the total serum T_4 and *0.5%* of the total serum T_3 are in an unbound (free) state, although in reversible equilibrium with the bound hormone. The concentration of free hormone is a function of this equilibrium and the number of occupied and unoccupied binding sites on TBG. This characteristic assumes particular importance in interpreting the laboratory tests (described later) measuring the concentrations of thyroid hormone in serum.

Thyroid-stimulating hormone (TSH) is the major regulator of thyroid gland growth and function. All of the reactions necessary for the intrathyroidal formation of T_4 and T_3 are under the influence and control of TSH, a glycoprotein formed and secreted by the thyrotroph cells of the anterior pituitary. TSH is composed of two distinct subunits; the alpha subunit is common to three other glycoprotein hormones including follicle-stimulating hormone, luteinizing hormone, and human chorionic gonadotropin and is responsible for adenylate cyclase activation in the thyroid cell membrane. The beta subunit confers binding specificity to the hormone for its cell surface receptor. Once the TSH binds to its thyroid plasma membrane receptor on the external cell surface, it activates the enzyme adenylate cyclase, increasing the formation of cyclic adenosine monophosphate (AMP), the nucleotide that serves as an intracellular messenger to mediate the effects of TSH on the thyroid cell. The control of TSH secretion and synthesis is complex and involves local mechanisms within the pituitary as well as the hypothalamus. Within the pituitary regulation is primarily modulated by the intrapituitary T_3 concentration derived from both circulating free T_3 and intrapituitary conversion of T_4 to T_3. Elevation of the circulating levels of free thyroid hormones inhibits TSH secretion from the pituitary, and more sustained elevation of the levels of free thyroid hormone decreases the biosynthesis of TSH in the thyrotroph cell. Conversely, decreased circulating levels of free thyroid hormone result in increased synthesis and release of TSH from the pituitary and subsequent rise in the circulating TSH.

TSH secretion from the pituitary is also influenced by thyrotropin-releasing hormone (TRH), a 3 amino acid peptide (pyro-Glu-His-Pro-NH) synthesized in the supraoptic and paraventricular nuclei in the hypothalamus and stored in the median eminence (Fig. 162-3). TRH is released into the portal venous system between the hypothalamus and pituitary, binds to the thyrotroph cells of the anterior pituitary, increases the entry of extracellular calcium into the thyrotroph cells, and results in both synthesis and release of TSH. The precise regulation of TRH has not been completely elucidated, although it appears to be a classic endocrine feedback mechanism with excess thyroid hormone depressing and deficient thyroid hormone stimulating its production and release.

It is now clear that thyroidal production of T_3 accounts for only about 15% to 20% of the circulating T_3. The remainder (80% to 85%) is produced by monodeiodination of the outer ring of T_4 by the membrane-bound enzyme 5′-deiodinase (Fig. 162-4). It is also clear that T_3 is at least 3 and perhaps as much as 10 times more potent than T_4 in its biologic activity and that T_4 may in this sense be regarded as a prohormone serving mainly as a substrate for the all-important peripheral conversion to T_3 in the liver, pituitary,

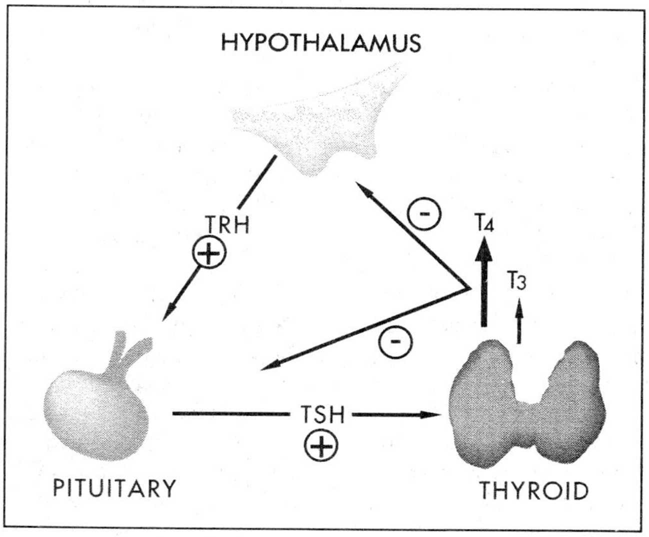

Fig. 162-3. Schematic representation of the regulation of thyroid gland function by the hypothalamus and the pituitary gland.

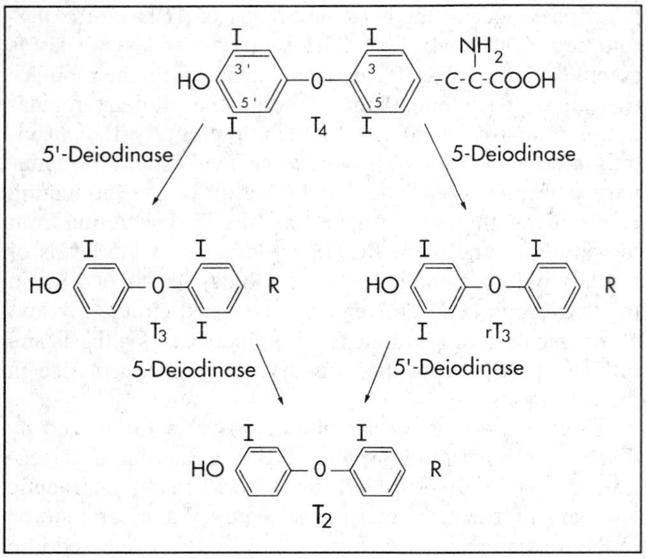

Fig. 162-4. Enzymatic metabolism of thyroxine.

kidney, and other organs. Monodeiodination of the inner ring of T_4 yields a metabolite known as reverse T_3 (rT_3), which has no significant metabolic activity. rT_3 is present in normal human serum, and, in trace amounts, in thyroglobulin. From 15 to 40 weeks of fetal life, amniotic fluid concentrations of T_3 are low and rT_3 levels are much higher than the corresponding values in maternal serum. The rT_3 in amniotic fluid is derived primarily from the fetus via the action of the 5-deiodinase enzyme. At delivery, the deiodination pattern is switched to the normal adult pattern and rT_3 levels fall rapidly and T_3 levels rise. Subsequent deiodinations of T_3 and rT_3 shown in Fig. 162-4 result in a series of metabolites probably having no biologic activity.

In recent years, an increasing amount of research has been directed at understanding the fundamental biochemistry and cellular biology of the deiodinases. The 5′-deiodinase has two distinct forms: 5′-deiodinase type I and 5′-deiodinase type II. Type I is located predominantly in liver and kidney; its activity is decreased in the fasted state and hypothyroidism and increased in hyperthyroidism; is inhibited by propylthiouracil, amiodarone, and the contrast agents iopanoic acid (Telepaque) and ipodate (Oragrafin); and has a substrate preference for rT_3. The 5′-deiodinase II is located predominantly in pituitary and brain; its activity is increased in hypothyroidism, unchanged by fasting, and decreased in hyperthyroidism; is inhibited by amiodarone, iopanoic acid, and ipodate but not by propylthiouracil; and has a substrate preference for T_4, which enables the pituitary thyrotroph cell to metabolize T_4 independently.

About 80 to 90 μ of T_4 is produced each day and deiodination is the major pathway by which it is metabolized. Approximately 80% of T_4 secreted by the thyroid is deiodinated in the periphery, half to T_3 and half to rT_3, and eventually to the other metabolites shown in Fig. 162-4. T_4 that is not deiodinated is eliminated by fecal excretion.

LABORATORY TESTS TO ASSESS THYROID FUNCTIONAL STATUS AND ANATOMY

There are a number of readily available laboratory tests to assess a patient's thyroid functional status and anatomy. Numerous complexities and pitfalls pose a distinct challenge to the clinician who must interpret the results and employ the findings to arrive at a diagnostic conclusion. Each of the commonly used tests is discussed and the inherent problems in interpretation noted.

Serum total T_4 and T_3

Serum total T_4 and T_3 levels have been classically measured by radioimmunoassays and more recently by nonisotopic enzyme linked immunoassay (ELISA). The tests are highly sensitive, specific, and reasonably inexpensive and accurately measure the total concentrations of T_4 and T_3. T_4 is generally the determination used routinely to assess thyroid functional status. Normal serum levels in most laboratories are about 5 to 11 μ/dl for T_4 and 80 to 160 ng/dl for T_3. Measurement of total T_4 is unaffected by contaminating non-T_4 iodine. In most cases changes in thyroid gland function result in a corresponding change in T_4 and T_3 levels. It must be remembered that over 99% of the T_4 and T_3 are protein-bound and that the free hormone, which is biologically active, is only a fraction of the total T_4 and T_3 levels. Therefore changes in serum binding protein (most commonly TBG, but occasionally TTR or albumin) levels produce elevations or depressions of total T_4 level. Thus a patient with an increase or decrease in the concentration of TBG may have normal thyroid gland function despite serum total T_4 and total T_3 levels equivalent to what is found in hyperthyroidism or hypothyroidism. In hyperthyroidism or hypothyroidism, the concentration of the free hormone changes, whereas isolated changes in TBG, TTR, or albumin leave the free T_4 or free T_3 at normal levels (changes in thyroid binding proteins in euthyroid patients are discussed later).

T_3 resin uptake and thyroid hormone binding ratio

The T_3 resin uptake is used to circumvent the problem of alterations in amount of serum TBG and is only useful in conjunction with a simultaneous measure of total T_4 or T_3. The T_3 resin uptake reflects the unsaturated thyroid hormone binding sites on TBG (Fig. 162-5) and is not a measure of circulating T_3. In the normal subject 25% to 35% of the TBG binding sites are occupied by thyroid hormone. When $^{125}I\text{-}T_3$ is added to the patient's serum, in vitro, a portion binds to the unoccupied TBG sites; a resin is then added that binds the remaining unbound $^{125}I\text{-}T_3$, and the result is expressed as a function of the resin uptake. In hypothyroidism, characterized by decreased levels of circulating thyroid hormone, there are decreased numbers of occupied and increased numbers of unoccupied TBG binding sites. Increased amounts of the $^{125}I\text{-}T_3$ are bound to TBG, resulting in a decreased uptake of $^{125}I\text{-}T_3$ by the resin. In hyperthyroidism, the converse pertains.

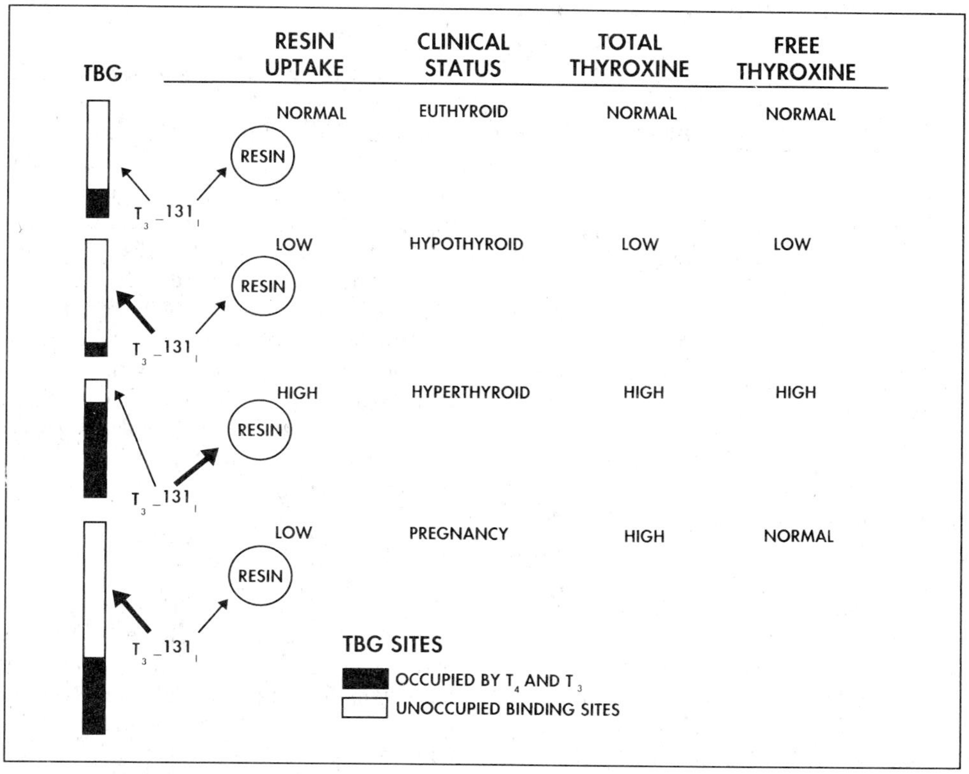

Fig. 162-5. Schematic representation of the T_3 resin uptake test. (Modified from Berkow R, editor: The Merck manual of diagnosis and therapy, ed 16. Merck, 1992.)

The T_3 resin uptake is most useful for interpreting alterations of serum total T_4 when there is an increase or decrease in the amount of TBG without any actual change in thyroid gland function. For example, when TBG is increased in hyperestrogenemic states, there are increased numbers of both occupied and unoccupied binding sites on TBG (see *lower panel,* Fig. 162-5). The total T_4 is increased because the actual number of TBG sites binding T_4 or T_3 is increased. However, as in the euthyroid state with normal free T_4 levels, only about 25% to 35% of the total sites are occupied, leaving an increase in unoccupied sites to bind $^{125}I-T_3$, resulting in a decreased resin uptake. In settings where the TBG is decreased, the opposite is found; there is a decrease in total serum T_4 level and unoccupied binding sites, and an increased amount of $^{125}I-T_3$ is available for resin uptake.

To avoid the use of percentages and to help standardize this test some laboratories now report a thyroid hormone binding ratio (THBR) instead of a T_3 resin uptake. This ratio is a normalization of the T_3 binding capacity of the patient's serum compared to a control from a euthyroid person with normal amounts of binding protein. Results are expressed as a ratio; the normal range is 0.85 to 1.10 in most laboratories. Many laboratories also report additional results known as the free thyroxine index (FTI), or T_7, which are simply mathematically derived figures based on the values for T_4 and T_3 resin uptake that although theoretically correct have only modest accuracy.

Free T_4 and free T_3

Theoretically free T_4 and free T_3 determinations would be the ideal test because they most accurately reflect thyroid status. However, the concentrations of free T_4 and free T_3 are low and difficult to measure. The methods used, including radioimmunoassay and equilibrium dialysis, are fraught with technical pitfalls and expensive. Equilibrium dialysis gives the most reliable results.

Serum TSH

The measurement of serum TSH concentration is the single best test for demonstrating hypothyroidism produced by thyroid gland failure (primary hypothyroidism). In primary hypothyroidism TSH level is elevated; however, in the unusual setting of secondary hypothyroidism caused by pituitary or hypothalamic failure the TSH level may be normal or low (Table 162-1).

Until recently, TSH was measured by a radioimmunoassay that lacked sensitivity at and below the lower range of normal. Its limited sensitivity prevented the use of TSH as a measurement for the investigation of hyperthyroidism when levels would be expected to be suppressed (nonmeasurable). Using the standard radioimmunoassay for measurement of TSH, a proportion of euthyroid patients had undetectable levels of TSH indistinguishable from levels found in hyperthyroidism. This limitation led to the devel-

Table 162-1. Serum TSH concentrations in various thyroid disease states

	Serum TSH (μU/ml) range
Normal*	0.1-5.0
Hyperthyroid	<0.1
Hypothyroid	
Subclinical	6-16
Overt primary	20-200
Secondary	0.1-5.0
Euthyroid sick syndrome	0.1-5.0
Recovery phase	0.1-15

*Varies with the specific assay employed.

opment of methods with greater sensitivity. The introduction of ELISA and chemiluminescent methods has provided a major advance in the sensitivity, specificity, and speed of TSH assays. At present, the basal serum TSH level measured by a highly sensitive and specific method can reliably discriminate hyperthyroid from euthyroid patients. The basal serum TSH level measured by such an assay is now the preferred alternative to the TRH stimulation test in assessing hyperthyroidism. The normal range in most assays is 0.1 to 5.0 μU/ml. A detectable serum TSH level has the same significance as a normal response to TRH and excludes hyperthyroidism except in rare cases of TSH-producing thyrotroph tumors of the pituitary. An undetectable basal TSH level has the same significance as a subnormal response to TRH and indicates either subclinical or overt hyperthyroidism. As a result the measurement of basal serum TSH level now provides a reliable index of thyrotroph activity across the entire spectrum of thyroid disease from primary hypothyroidism to hyperthyroidism.

Thyrotropin-releasing hormone test

The sensitive thyrotropin-releasing hormone (TSH) test has decreased the usefulness of the TRH stimulation test. The TRH test measures serum TSH levels after synthetic TRH is injected intravenously or intramuscularly. Normally, there is a rapid rise in TSH level of 5 to 25 μU/ml, reaching a peak in 30 minutes. In males older than 40 years of age, the release of TSH in response to TRH declines. The release of TSH in response to TRH is exaggerated in primary hypothyroidism: maximal stimulated values of TSH exceed 30 μU/ml. In hyperthyroidism TSH release is suppressed in response to injected TRH by the inhibitory effects of elevated intrapituitary free T_3 and T_4 levels on the pituitary thyrotroph cell.

The TRH test is useful in distinguishing thyroid dysfunction caused by pituitary disease that results from failure to release TSH in response to TRH in the clinical setting of hypothyroidism. Patients who are hypothyroid secondary to hypothalamic failure (a rare entity) and deficient TRH level have either normal or delayed release of TSH.

Antithyroid antibodies

The most common determinations of antithyroid antibodies are antimicrosomal and antithyroglobulin. Both tests are highly organ specific and sensitive; however, the antimicrosomal antibodies are most useful because they most frequently yield positive findings in the two thyroid autoimmune diseases of major concern to the clinician, Hashimoto's thyroiditis and Graves' disease.

Antimicrosomal antibodies are directed primarily against the membrane bound thyroid peroxidase. The antibody levels are elevated often in very high titers in the majority of patients with Hashimoto's thyroiditis and frequently in patients with Graves' disease. In contrast, antithyroglobulin antibodies are present in a smaller percentage of patients with Hashimoto's thyroiditis and less than half of those with Graves' disease.

TSH receptor antibodies

The thyroid goiter and autonomous hyperfunctioning of the thyroid characteristic of Graves' disease is due to an antibody directed against the thyroid TSH receptor. The antibody, which is an immunoglobulin G, (IgG) can be detected in about 90% of patients with Graves' disease. Because Graves' disease has characteristic clinical manifestations and diagnosis is usually not difficult, TSH receptor antibody (TRAb) determination is unnecessary in most cases. Measurement is most useful in women who are pregnant because high titers are associated with a greater risk of development of thyrotoxicosis in the neonate—key information for the obstetrician and pediatrician. Measurement of TRAb is also of some value in establishing the diagnosis of euthyroid Graves' disease in patients with ophthalmopathy and normal thyroid function.

Serum thyroglobulin

Thyroglobulin is present in low serum concentrations in the normal population. Concentrations are elevated in pregnancy (normal finding) and in a number of thyroid disorders including nontoxic goiter, hyperthyroidism, subacute thyroiditis, thyroid adenoma, and differentiated (usually metastatic) thyroid cancer of the papillary and follicular types. Determination of serum thyroglobulin is of greatest use in follow-up care of patients who have been treated for differentiated thyroid cancer. After successful treatment and institution of thyroid hormone in suppressive doses, serum thyroglobulin level is usually well within the normal range (<5 ng/ml). Elevations of serum thyroglobulin level in this setting indicate the presence of residual or recurrent thyroid cancer.

THYROID IMAGING TECHNIQUES

Radioisotopic scintiscanning

Scintiscanning has been used as an important tool for the evaluation of thyroid function and the noninvasive assessment of thyroid anatomy for many years. Originally the isotope used for scanning was ^{131}I. More recently, ^{123}I has superseded ^{131}I as the isotope of choice. Technetium (^{99m}Tc) pertechnetate, an anion concentrated by the thyroid, is also used to assess thyroid anatomy. In scintiscanning studies, the radiation emitted by the isotopes is recorded by a scanner and scintillation detectors on x-ray film or on a fluorescent screen that can be directly viewed and photographed. In addition, the use of ^{131}I or ^{123}I permits the quantitation of the thyroidal uptake of iodine over a fixed period and can be selectively used to assess the functional state of the thyroid gland.

At the present time, ^{123}I is the isotope of choice for scanning procedures. It has a much shorter half-life than ^{131}I and because of the absence of beta radiation gives a significantly smaller radiation dose to the thyroid. ^{99m}Tc has a short half-life and delivers a low dose of radiation to the thyroid but does not readily permit the calculation of a functional uptake and is not organically bound, thus creating its own technical and interpretive problems.

There are a number of indications for thyroid imaging studies. One is the assessment of thyroid nodules to define whether they are functional (hot or warm nodules) or nonfunctional (cold nodules). Warm or hot nodules are rarely malignant, and almost all thyroid cancers are cold on scintiscanning. Specificity is not ideal, because most benign thyroid nodules are also cold on scintiscan. A second indication for scanning techniques is to permit localization of the thyroid, which is of particular importance in patients with substernal goiters. A third is the localization of metastatic deposits of differentiated thyroid cancer or of residual normal thyroid tissue after surgery. A fourth indication is the anatomic evaluation of the thyroid, important in differentiating agenesis of one lobe of the thyroid versus a hyperfunctioning nodule that has suppressed the opposite lobe of the thyroid. Finally, scintiscanning helps in distinguishing a multinodular goiter from other goitrous enlargements of the thyroid.

For functional assessment, the uptake of ^{123}I or ^{131}I is measured at two time intervals, 6 and 24 hours. Normal individuals vary somewhat from laboratory to laboratory but in general, normal 24 hour uptake ranges from 2% to 35%. Because of the high iodine content of the diet in the United States, the lower limit of ^{123}I or ^{131}I uptake in normal individuals has declined and therefore the radioiodine uptake is no longer useful in the assessment of hypothyroidism. The 24 hour uptake is most useful in diagnosing hyperthyroidism of the Graves' disease type in which it is uniformly elevated and therefore can serve in distinguishing some of the various types of hyperthyroidism described late.

In addition to radiation exposure, the use of these tests has disadvantages in terms of high cost and time inconvenience for the patient. In addition, myriad factors increase or decrease the uptake. Therefore scintiscanning should only be used in a cost-effective and discriminating approach to medical care.

Ultrasound

The ultrasound technique provides a sensitive assessment of thyroid anatomy including a reasonably accurate estimation of size. It has the advantage of not requiring radioactive isotopes so there is no radiation exposure to the patient. The main use of ultrasound is to determine whether a nodule is solid, cystic, or a mixture of the two. A purely cystic nodule has a greatly reduced chance of being malignant. The main disadvantages of ultrasound are that it does not allow discrimination of benign and malignant nodules solely on the basis of solid or cystic characteristics and is costly.

INVASIVE TECHNIQUES

Thyroid biopsy provides the most useful and specific tool for deciding whether or not a thyroid nodule is benign or malignant and therefore is the routine procedure of choice for the evaluation of a solitary thyroid nodule. There are two basic biopsy techniques. The more commonly employed is fine-needle (22 to 27 gauge) aspiration. It is simple and safe, requiring only local anesthesia. The needle is inserted into the nodule, suction is applied at various angles, cells are drawn into the barrel of the needle, and the aspirate is placed on a microscopic slide for cytologic examination. Closed percutaneous biopsy using a Vim-Silverman needle is highly effective as a diagnostic tool but is more difficult to perform and occasionally associated with serious complications such as hemorrhage.

Fine needle aspiration is highly sensitive and specific and has decreased the need for surgical removal of thyroid nodules by at least 50%. As a result of biopsy technology, the prevalence of thyroid cancer in a surgically removed nodule has risen from about 5% to 15% to 35% to 50%.

Thyroid biopsy is not reliable for diagnosing follicular cancer, because histologic evidence of capsular or blood vessel invasion must be demonstrated to establish the diagnosis. Biopsy can confirm the clinical and/or serologic evidence for Hashimoto's thyroiditis; however, if lymphoma of the thyroid is a consideration, cutting needle (core) or open biopsy may be required. The problem of the management of nodules whose aspirates are interpreted as suspicious or indeterminate has not been resolved. Depending on the clinical setting, surgical removal or observation during suppression therapy with thyroxine is the usual course of action.

ALTERATIONS OF THYROID FUNCTION TESTS IN EUTHYROID PATIENTS

Euthyroid sick syndrome

The occurrence of both elevated and low concentrations of total T_4 and total T_3 in clinically euthyroid patients is well established. Patients with a variety of acute or chronic nonthyroidal illnesses, other stresses, or abnormal nutritional states may have abnormal thyroid function test results. Although serum total T_4 levels may vary, the hallmark of the euthyroid sick syndrome is a low serum T_3 level. In large part, the decreased serum total T_3 level is secondary to decreased peripheral conversion of T_4 to T_3, secondary to a decrease in the activity of the 5′-deiodinase. This leads in turn to decreased metabolism (outer ring deiodination) of rT_3 with consequent rise in serum rT_3 level. In severe stress there is decreased binding of thyroid hormones to TBG, lowering the total T_4 level while the serum free T_4 level remains normal. The serum TSH level is usually normal although in the recovery period from the euthyroid sick syndrome, the TSH level may be moderately elevated. The box below shows the wide variety of conditions and diseases commonly associated with this syndrome, including fasting, starvation, protein-calorie malnutrition, general surgical trauma, myocardial infarction, chronic renal failure, diabetic ketoacidosis, anorexia nervosa, cirrhosis, thermal injury, and sepsis.

The interpretation of thyroid function test result abnormalities observed in the euthyroid sick syndrome may be further complicated by the effects of a variety of drugs frequently used in acute and chronic illness that impair the peripheral conversion of T_4 to T_3 in liver and kidney (propranolol, dexamethasone) and in liver, kidney, and pituitary (amiodarone, iodinated contrast agents).

The diagnostic dilemma usually confronting the clinician in euthyroid sick syndrome is whether the patient is hypothyroid or euthyroid. The most sensitive indicator of hypothyroidism caused by primary thyroid gland failure is a marked elevation of serum TSH level; patients with the euthyroid sick syndrome have normal levels of serum TSH. In some cases of cirrhosis and in the recovery phase of euthyroid sick syndrome modest increases in TSH level may be found. However, corticosteroids and dopamine, which are frequently used in seriously ill patients, may lower TSH levels and can complicate the interpretation of the thyroid tests. Hypothyroidism in the patient with a coexistent acute or chronic systemic illness is suggested by a low or low normal serum rT_3 level because rT_3 level should otherwise be increased in the euthyroid sick syndrome.

The laboratory diagnosis of hyperthyroidism may also be obscured in the euthyroid sick syndrome by the often dramatic lowering of the serum total T_3 concentration. In this situation, clinical signs of hyperthyroidism, presence of a goiter and/or exophthalmos, blunted TRH-stimulation test result, and elevated radioiodine uptake serve as key determinants establishing the underlying presence of thyrotoxicosis.

Because of the many pitfalls in the interpretation of thyroid function test results in the euthyroid sick syndrome, there is no substitute for sound clinical judgment based on a meticulous history and physical examination when attempting to interpret thyroid function test result abnormalities in the acutely or chronically ill patient.

Euthyroid sick syndrome (nonthyroidal illness)

Fasting	Thermal injury
Starvation	Heart failure
Protein-calorie malnutrition	Hypothermia
Sepsis	Myocardial infarction
Trauma	Chronic renal failure
Cardiopulmonary bypass	Diabetic ketoacidosis
Widespread malignancy	Cirrhosis

Euthyroid hyperthyroxinemia

Since the advent of the routine assays of serum T_4 level, a number of conditions have been recognized to increase the level in euthyroid patients (refer to the box below), producing a state called euthyroid hyperthyroxinemia. Elevation in the concentration of TBG is recognized as the most common cause of elevation of the serum total T_4 level in the euthyroid patient. TBG level is most commonly increased by pregnancy and use of oral contraceptives; in the acute phase of infectious hepatitis; and on a genetic or idiopathic basis (see the box at bottom). It is occasionally increased in hypothyroidism, acute intermittent porphyria, and prolonged therapy with perphenazine. Hyperestrogenemic states, such as those produced by pregnancy and oral contraceptive therapy, are the most common cause of increased TBG levels, and treatment with the antiestrogen tamoxifen can also increase TBG. Because hyperthyroidism and hypothyroidism are commonly found in women between the ages of 20 to 50, it is important that the clinician

Euthyroid hyperthyroxinemia

Elevated thyroxine binding globulin level
Thyroid hormone resistance state
Iodine and iodine-containing drugs (amiodarone, ipodate)
High-dose propranolol
Acute psychiatric illness
Familial dysalbuminemic hyperthyroxinemia
Hyperemesis gravidarum

Alterations in thyroxine-binding globulin levels

Increased	Decreased
Estrogens	Androgens
Pregnancy	Glucocorticoids
Oral contraceptives	L-Asparaginase
Tamoxifen	Nephrotic syndrome
Perphenazine	Acromegaly
Clofibrate	Severe illness
Acute hepatitis	Starvation
Acute intermittent porphyria	Chronic hepatitis
Genetic	Genetic

be aware of the effects of estrogens on TBG level. Recently it has been shown that estrogens do not increase TBG level by increasing its synthesis, but rather prolong its half-life by increasing the sialic acid content of TBG.

Other causes of an elevated T_4 level in the euthyroid state in addition to TBG elevation include abnormalities of the other binding proteins, TTR and albumin; autoantibodies that bind T_4; generalized thyroid hormone resistance; drugs such as amiodarone and the contrast agents ipodate and iopanoic acid; acute psychiatric illness; acute nonthyroidal medical illness; and ingestion of synthetic thyroxine.

Abnormalities in T_4 binding to albumin and TTR, although rare, provide useful insights into these binding proteins. A recently described condition known as familial dysalbuminemic hyperthyroxinemia (FDH) is associated with serum total T_4 levels two to three times normal. FDH is an inherited disease transmitted as an autosomal dominant trait and appears to be more common in Hispanic populations. In the affected patients, the defect results from the presence of an abnormal binding site for T_4 on one quarter to one half of the circulating albumin molecules, which have an affinity for T_4 about 50 times normal. T_3 levels are normal because albumin binds T_3 only weakly. The T_3 resin uptake is usually normal, free thyroxine index is elevated, and serum free T_4 level, serum TSH level, and TSH response to TRH are normal, confirming the euthyroid state despite the marked elevation of T_4 level.

Euthyroid hyperthyroxinemia is also found in two rare syndromes characterized by increased binding of T_4 to TTR. One syndrome was described in a family in which the TTR was characterized by an abnormally high binding affinity of prealbumin for T_4. The other syndrome was described in two patients with a glucagonoma in which an increased amount of TTR was synthesized by the alpha cells of the pancreatic tumor. Serum T_3 level, T_3 resin uptake, TSH level, and TSH response to TRH are normal in these syndromes.

Rarely hyperthyroxinemia may be the result of anti-T_4 antibodies. These autoantibodies may cause an assay artifact or an actual increase in bound circulating T_4 level. Other thyroid function test findings are normal.

In recent years, the sporadic or familial occurrence of generalized resistance to thyroid hormones has been described; it is characterized by elevated total and free T_4 and T_3 levels and inappropriately elevated levels of TSH for the measured levels of T_4 and T_3. Some patients have a goiter, and selected young patients show signs of thyroid hormone deficiency such as growth retardation, delayed bone maturation, and deaf-mutism. Patients with generalized thyroid hormone resistance are most often clinically euthyroid. The generalized defect in cellular thyroid hormone action appears to reside in either the c-erbA family of T_3 nuclear receptors or a postreceptor step.

A few patients have selective pituitary resistance to thyroid hormone and usually exhibit the symptoms and signs of hyperthyroidism, increased serum total and free T_4 and T_3 levels, increased TSH level, and a normal TSH response to TRH. The defect may reside in a decreased intrapituitary conversion of T_4 to T_3, but this relationship has not been definitively established. Pituitary resistance to thyroid hormone can be distinguished from hyperthyroidism secondary to a TSH-producing pituitary adenoma by the finding that TSH produced by the adenoma is unresponsive to TRH stimulation and the serum level of the alpha subunit of TSH is increased. Amiodarone and the radiographic contrast agents iopanoic acid (Telepaque) and ipodate (Oragrafin) inhibit 5′-deiodination in liver and kidney and therefore impair the peripheral conversion of T_4 to T_3, resulting in a decrease in serum T_3 levels and increase in rT_3 levels (Fig. 162-4). In addition, these drugs inhibit the 5′-deiodinase II found in the pituitary, decreasing intrapituitary T_4 to T_3 conversion and causing a rise in TSH. Serum T_4 levels may be elevated, either secondary to the TSH elevation or as a result of decreases in the T_4 clearance rate. It should be noted that these drugs contain high concentrations of iodine and may also result in either iodide-induced hypothyroidism or, rarely, iodide-induced hyperthyroidism.

The beta-adrenergic blocking drug propranolol, when given in high doses, occasionally is associated with elevated T_4 levels. The mechanism appears to be secondary to the membrane stabilizing effect of propranolol in liver and kidney (but not in pituitary), which results in inhibition of T_4 to T_3 conversion and decrease in the disposal rate of T_4. Other beta-adrenergic blockers do not exert this effect.

Acute psychiatric illness

Acute psychiatric illness is associated with an increased incidence of T_4 level elevation, especially in patients having unipolar or bipolar depression, hyperemesis gravidarum, or paranoid schizophrenia. Although the patients are invariably euthyroid clinically, they frequently have a blunted to absent TSH response to TRH. The T_4 values and TRH responsiveness usually return to normal with treatment or resolution of the underlying condition. The mechanism of the abnormality is unknown.

L-thyroxine therapy

Patients treated with oral L-thyroxine may have elevated T_4 levels despite being clinically euthyroid and having normal T_3 levels. The mechanism of the increase is unclear; however, it seems to be greater 2 to 4 hours after ingestion of the dose. Thus it is probably best to obtain the blood sample for testing before the daily dose is administered. The serum T_3 level is normal if the patient is euthyroid. The supersensitive TSH appears to be the preferred test to assess the patient's metabolic state and to guide thyroxine replacement dosing.

Euthyroid hypothyroxinemia

A decrease in serum total T_4 level in euthyroid patients is known as euthyroid hypothyroxinemia. It is most commonly due to a decrease in the major binding protein, TBG. A decrease in TBG level is seen in a number of conditions (refer to the box on p. 1332). Pharmacologic doses of glucocorticoids and testosterone, high levels of growth hor-

Euthyroid hypothyroxinemia

Nonthyroidal illness
Decreased thyroxine-binding globulin level
Drugs
- Phenytoin
- Salicylates
- Tegretol
- Triiodothyronine

Genetic

Causes of thyrotoxicosis

Common	Uncommon
Graves' disease	Pituitary adenoma
Subacute thyroiditis	Struma ovarii
Silent	Metastatic thyroid cancer
Painful	Embryonal carcinoma of the testes
Toxic adenoma	Choriocarcinoma
Toxic multinodular goiter	Hyperemesis gravidarum
Excessive thyroxine hormone replacement	Isolated pituitary resistance to thyroid hormone
Iodide (Jodbasedow)	

mone as found in active acromegaly, and loss of large amounts of protein in the urine of patients with the nephrotic syndrome are among the more common causes of TBG deficiency and euthyroid hypothyroxinemia. A decrease in TBG level may also occur on a genetic basis and is X-linked; males are more severely affected than females. The deficiency of TBG on a genetic basis may be found in as many as 1 in 2000 people and is much more common than the genetic condition producing an increase in TBG. Because transthyretin and albumin are minor binding proteins for T_4, decreases in these proteins alone do not lower T_4 to below normal levels.

Two types of drugs, phenytoin and salicylates, cause euthyroid hypothyroxinemia. Phenytoin appears to decrease the binding of T_4 to TBG and, most importantly, accelerates T_4 degradation and disposal. Salicylates inhibit the binding of T_4 and T_3 to TBG.

Severe systemic illness in a euthyroid patient may be associated with a decreased serum total T_4 level secondary to endogenous inhibitors of T_4 binding to TBG.

THYROTOXICOSIS

Thyrotoxicosis is a complex pathophysiologic state secondary to excessive concentrations of free, biologically active thyroid hormone (T_4/T_3) in the blood and tissues. The term *thyrotoxicosis* is frequently used interchangeably with *hyperthyroidism*. However, in the strictest sense, *hyperthyroidism* comprises conditions in which the excessive amounts of thyroid hormone are derived from an overactive, hyperfunctional thyroid gland; *thyrotoxicosis* applies more broadly and includes all causes of excess thyroid hormone whether or not they are intrinsic or extrinsic to the thyroid gland.

Causes of thyrotoxicosis

There are many causes of thyrotoxicosis (see the box at upper right). The most common are Graves' disease, toxic multinodular goiter, toxic adenoma, thyrotoxicosis factitia, subacute thyroiditis, silent thyroiditis, excessive thyroid hormone replacement therapy, and iodide (Jodbasedow). Uncommon causes include TSH-producing tumor of the pituitary, metastatic embryonal carcinoma of the testis, choriocarcinoma, struma ovarii, metastatic follicular thyroid cancer, and isolated pituitary resistance to thyroid hormone.

Signs and symptoms

The general signs and symptoms of thyrotoxicosis may be among the most dramatic found in clinical medicine or conversely may be subtle. The more overt signs and symptoms tend to occur most frequently in the young, whereas in elderly patients, many of the typical findings may be masked and are more likely to be misdiagnosed. The general clinical features of thyrotoxicosis are extraordinarily diverse because thyroid hormone affects virtually every organ system in the body. Some of the signs and symptoms are associated with all forms of thyrotoxicosis and some are found only in specific types. The expression of the various signs and symptoms is also influenced by the duration of the thyrotoxicosis. The most frequent signs and symptoms associated with thyrotoxicosis are shown in the box below. The signs and symptoms are common to all forms of thyrotoxicosis with notable exceptions such as ophthalmopathy and infiltrative dermopathy, which are specific representatives of the immunologic aspects of Graves' disease (discussed later). Goiter is present in most, but not all, types of thy-

Common symptoms and signs of thyrotoxicosis

Tachycardia	Goiter
Anxiety	Tachycardia
Tremulousness	Widened pulse pressure
Increased appetite	Tremor
Weight loss	Warm smooth skin
Heat intolerance	Lid lag
Excessive sweating	Stare
Proximal muscle weakness	Exophthalmos*
Emotional lability	Infiltrative dermopathy*
Increased defecation	Hyperreflexia
Decreased sleep time	

*Specific for Graves' disease.

rotoxicosis. Symptoms and signs referable to the cardiovascular system are regularly present in all cases and include sinus tachycardia, palpitations, widened pulse pressure with an elevated systolic blood pressure, hyperdynamic precordium, and brisk carotid upstrokes. Patients may have supraventricular arrhythmias, classically atrial fibrillation. Elderly patients may exhibit this arrhythmia as the only clue to the presence of otherwise apathetic thyrotoxicosis.

The skin is usually smooth, warm, and moist with increased sweating. The hair is fine and grows faster than normal. Areas of depigmentation (vitiligo) or increased pigmentation are characteristic of Graves' disease. Patients complain of hypersensitivity to heat and may feel uncomfortably warm even in winter. Appetite is often dramatically increased and classically associated with a significant weight loss because of the increased metabolic rate. Patients complain of excessive nervousness and anxiety and many describe it as feeling as though they've had "too much caffeine." A tremor of the hands, which may interfere with fine movements such as writing or using utensils, is regularly found and is most easily demonstrated with the hands outstretched. Patients usually have excessive energy and frequently complain of decreased sleep time although fatigue and proximal muscle weakness are associated with longer-duration disease. Complaints suggesting proximal muscle weakness include exercise intolerance and difficulty in lifting or carrying heavy objects, combing hair, climbing stairs, or arising from a chair. Gastrointestinal complaints include an increased number of bowel movements and occasionally frank diarrhea. Women may notice a decrease in frequency of menstrual periods; men may note mild gynecomastia. Eye signs common to all types of thyrotoxicosis include stare, lid lag, and lid retraction. Exophthalmos and extraocular muscle palsies are potentially more serious developments and are specific for Graves' disease.

Many of the symptoms and signs of thyrotoxicosis are secondary to excessive adrenergic hormone stimulation. Although the hyperadrenergic state characteristic of thyrotoxicosis has been recognized for most of the 20th century and subjected to numerous investigations, the precise mechanism of increase in adrenergic tone is unclear. Direct measurements of serum catecholamine levels yield normal or low findings. Despite the lack of understanding of this clinical finding, drugs that counteract adrenergic hormones such as beta blockers are highly effective, improving a number of the signs and symptoms of thyrotoxicosis.

The role of the adrenergic nervous system is further emphasized when considering the differential diagnosis of thyrotoxicosis. Anxiety states and pheochromocytoma can produce many of the same clinical findings. Meticulous history and physical examination are usually sufficient to rule out these diagnoses. Patients with anxiety states have cool skin, cool and moist palms of the hands, normal sleeping pulses, and, unless fortuitously present, no goiter. Patients with pheochromocytoma have paroxysmal symptoms and usually manifest diastolic hypertension. Goiter is absent. If history and physical examination are insufficient to establish the diagnosis, routine thyroid function tests including a supersensitive TSH assay should be used to rule out thyrotoxicosis.

Graves' disease

Graves' disease, also known as diffuse toxic goiter, Basedow's disease, or Parry's disease, is an immunologic disorder characterized by the presence of one or more of the following: goiter, hyperthyroidism, ophthalmopathy, and infiltrative dermopathy. The typical patient has goiter and hyperthyroidism and usually has either overt or subtle ophthalmopathy. Infiltrative dermopathy is much less common. Graves' disease occurs more commonly in women in a ratio of about 8:1 and has a prevalence as high as 2% of the female population. There is a strong genetic component with an increased frequency of HLA-B8 and HLA-DR3 in Europeans, HLA-BW35 in Japanese, and HLA-BW46 in Chinese. Families may have some members with Graves' disease and some with Hashimoto's thyroiditis. Graves' disease occurs at all ages and is the most common form of hyperthyroidism, particularly in patients less than 50 years of age; hyperthyroidism secondary to nodular goiter assumes increasing importance in older patients, although some of these may have Graves' disease variants.

Graves' disease is an autoimmune disease. Patients and their families have an increased frequency of other autoimmune diseases such as myasthenia gravis, lupus erythematosus, insulin-dependent diabetes mellitus, pernicious anemia, Sjögren's syndrome, Addison's disease, and autoimmune thrombocytopenic purpura. There is a high frequency of thyroid-antimicrosomal antibodies. In some patients with Hashimoto's thyroiditis Graves' disease may ultimately develop and in some patients with Graves' disease Hashimoto's thyroiditis and later hypothyroidism evolve.

Graves' disease is well established as one of several diseases secondary to antibodies to a cell surface receptor. The antibody in Graves' disease is directed at the TSH receptor (TRAb). The antibody may be a family of antibodies directed against different domains of the TSH receptor, one being stimulatory of all the thyroid hormone biosynthetic processes within the thyroid, one predominantly an inhibitor of TSH binding, and another perhaps a stimulator of thyroid cell growth. TRAbs are present in approximately 90% of all patients with Graves' disease. They are G immunoglobulins that may arise secondary to a defect in suppressor T-lymphocyte function, which permits helper T lymphocytes to interact with thyroid specific antigens, proliferate, and ultimately interact with lymphocytes, producing the TRAb. The observation that the thyroid cell expresses human leukocyte antigen (HLA) class II antigens may further our understanding of how the autoimmune process of Graves' disease is initiated.

The clinical picture of a patient with Graves' disease serves as the prototype for all patients with thyrotoxicosis with notable exceptions unique to Graves' disease. The plethora of symptoms and signs can be categorized into three basic components. The first are those produced by adrenergic stimulation, including tachycardia, palpitations, nervousness, anxiety, depression, irritability, tremor, ocular stare, lid lag, increased systolic blood pressure, widened pulse pressure, increased cardiac contractility and output. These are characteristically dependent on the continuing presence of adrenergic stimulation and are amenable to acute therapeutic intervention with antiadrenergic agents and relatively easily reversed. A second component are those signs caused by excess thyroid hormone, including increased oxygen consumption, hyperphagia, increased synthesis of a variety of structural and enzymatic proteins, myopathy, some psychologic disturbances, and possibly some component of the tachycardia, arrhythmias, and cardiac hypertrophy. Because thyroid hormone effects are mediated at the nuclear level by changes in specific protein synthesis, the alterations produced by thyroid hormone excess tend to be prolonged and therefore slower to reverse with therapy, which must be directed first at achieving normal levels of thyroid hormone.

The third or immunologic component is unique to patients with Graves' disease and is not part of the symptoms and signs found with the other causes of thyrotoxicosis. The most constant sign in this component is a diffuse goiter that is secondary to the growth stimulation of the thyroid provided by TRAb. The goiters of Graves' disease are of variable size, ranging from the minimum enlargement so common in elderly patients to the massive enlargement characteristic of younger patients. Lymphadenopathy, splenomegaly, and vitiligo are present in a small but significant percentage of patients.

Two prominent manifestations of the immunologic component deserve special mention. Ophthalmopathy (Fig. 162-6), including exophthalmos and extraocular muscle inflammation, results from a complex, apparently antigen- and organ-specific immunologic reaction. The immunologic process is characterized by proliferation of retro-orbital tissue, producing exophthalmos, lymphocytic infiltration, edema, inflammation, and later fibrosis of the extraocular muscles. Conjunctival irritation, injection, edema, lacrimation, and photophobia are also observed. The exophthalmos can occasionally be so pronounced and progressive that corneal irritation and visual loss are threatened, requiring orbital decompression. Extraocular muscle paralysis can arise secondary to myositis and produce disabling double vision; most commonly patients manifest difficulty in convergence, upward, and/or superolateral gaze.

The ophthalmopathy may occur before the onset of signs, symptoms, and laboratory abnormalities characteristic of hyperthyroidism, a condition known as euthyroid Graves' disease. Ophthalmopathy may worsen or improve during the treatment of Graves' disease; it may make its appearance many years after the treatment of the disease.

Infiltrative dermopathy, also known as pretibial myxedema, occurs in less than 5% of patients. It is characterized by nonpitting swelling and induration over the pretibial area and dorsa of the feet. The swelling and induration may be localized to plaques or be more generalized and is usually violaceous and often intensely pruritic. Most commonly arising contemporaneously with the symptoms of hyperthyroidism, the lesions may also appear years after successful treatment.

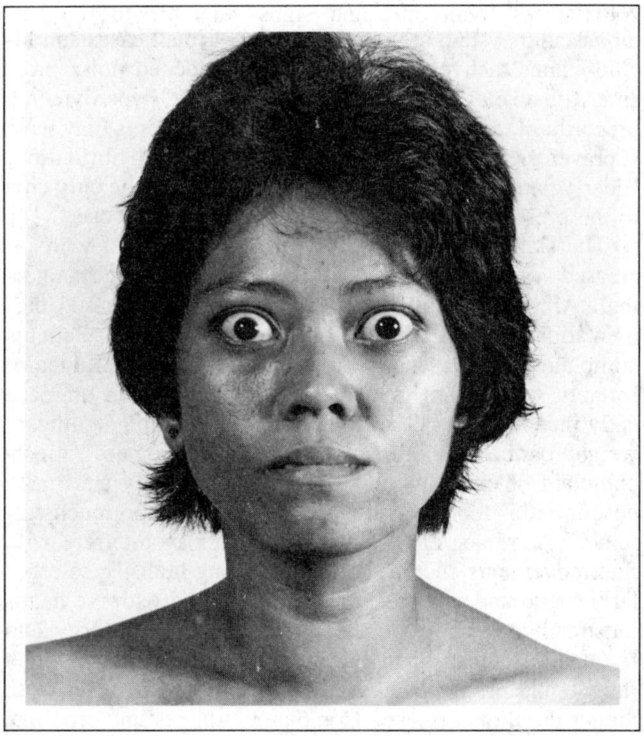

Fig. 162-6. Graves' disease manifesting as hyperthyroidism and ocular involvement with significant proptosis and stare.

Diagnosis. The diagnosis of Graves' hyperthyroidism is usually quite straightforward and depends on a careful clinical history and physical examination, a high index of suspicion, and routine determinations of blood levels of the thyroid hormones. A combination of serum total T_4 level, THBR, or free thyroxine index are appropriate initial tests because together they are highly accurate for assessing the presence of thyroid hyperfunction. A new useful and cost-effective alternative is a sensitive TSH evaluation to determine whether or not the level is suppressed. The sensitive TSH determination is also very useful when the diagnosis of hyperthyroidism remains unclear after the initial T_4 and THBR evaluations. Such a circumstance occurs in selected cases of Graves' hyperthyroidism, in which the serum total T_3 level is elevated, and the T_4 level normal (T_3 toxicosis). The suppressed TSH level confirms the thyroid overactivity.

Radioiodine scanning should not be considered a routine test in Graves' disease and should generally be used to discriminate among the various forms of thyrotoxicosis when this distinction may guide therapy (e.g., Graves' disease versus toxic multinodular goiter). Radioiodine uptake is useful in the diagnosis and plays a particularly helpful role in distinguishing Graves' disease from silent thyroiditis and in the calculation of the dose of ^{131}I when the latter is selected as the treatment modality. Radioiodine scanning and uptake should not be performed in women in the childbearing years until pregnancy has been ruled out. TRAb levels may be determined in women who are pregnant in order to define a potential risk of neonatal thyrotoxicosis.

Treatment. A number of highly effective therapeutic agents and approaches are used for the treatment of Graves' disease, including propylthiouracil and methimazole, ^{131}I, surgery, adrenergic blocking drugs, and iodide. The selection is determined primarily by the clinical setting and the preference of the physician.

Propylthiouracil and methimazole are thionamides that inhibit thyroid hormone biosynthesis and are most commonly used in younger patients. They act to decrease organification and impair the coupling reaction in a dose-dependent manner. At high doses (>600 mg/day) propylthiouracil, but not methimazole, inhibits the peripheral conversion of T_4 to T_3. Both drugs may exert some of their effects via the immune system. There is clinical evidence that they decrease activated helper T cells and increase activated suppressor T cells as well as lower TRAb levels. Recent reports suggest that this latter effect may be potentiated by simultaneous thyroxine administration.

The usual starting dose for propylthiouracil is 100 to 150 mg orally every 8 hours and for methimazole 30 to 45 mg orally in one daily dose. When the patient becomes euthyroid, the dose is decreased to the lowest possible total daily dose to maintain normal thyroid function. Complications of these agents include nausea, loss of taste, and, in less than 0.5% of patients, agranulocytosis. After treatment with these drugs for periods up to 1 to 2 years, a variable number of patients (15% to 40%) with Graves' disease enter remission. Evidence that a patient with Graves' disease is undergoing remission is provided by a marked decrease in size of the goiter, a fall in TRAb levels, and the return of a normal TRH stimulation test result. Relapses are frequent and unpredictable.

In comparing these two drugs both have relative advantages in different situations. Methimazole has a long duration of action, enabling it to be given in one daily dose enhancing patient compliance. Propylthiouracil crosses the placenta and crosses into breast milk much less than methimazole and is the preferred drug, if antithyroid drug therapy must be used in pregnancy or during breast-feeding. It also decreases T_4 to T_3 conversion, which is of theoretic advantage in emergency situations such as the treatment of thyroid storm.

Radioiodine. (^{131}I) has received widespread acceptance as the treatment of choice for Graves' disease, especially in older patients. It is safe, is economical over the long range, and effectively ablates functioning thyroid tissue. Its limitation in treatment of younger patients stems from the persistent concern about its potential effect on the progeny of patients treated with this isotope. Thus far there is no evidence of any increased genetic damage in the offspring. There has been no proven increased incidence of leukemia, carcinoma of the thyroid, or other tumors in the patients or their progeny. Hypothyroidism is the major undesired effect of ^{131}I therapy. It is difficult to gauge the dose even after measurements of iodine uptake and thyroid size, and there is no way to predict the response of the gland. One year after ^{131}I therapy, at least one fourth of the patients are hypothyroid, and this percentage further increases with time. On the other hand, if smaller doses are used, there is a higher incidence of recurrence of hyperthyroidism.

Surgery. Subtotal thyroidectomy is no longer a preferred treatment for patients with Graves' disease. It is reserved for young patients with the disease who do not enter remission with propylthiouracil or methimazole and who are not candidates for radioiodine therapy. Surgery may be used for patients who have a clinically palpable, cold nodule in the Graves' disease goiter.

Iodide. Iodide is mainly used for the emergency management of thyroid storm and for thyrotoxic patients about to undergo surgery because of its rapid effect and ability to decrease the vascularity of the thyroid gland. In pharmacologic doses (>5 mg per day), iodide rapidly inhibits the release of T_3 and T_4 from the thyroid gland. It also inhibits the organification of iodine, a transitory effect in almost all patients, lasting a few days to a week. Iodide is not used for routine treatment of hyperthyroidism and frequently complicates treatment because it greatly expands glandular iodide stores, making it more difficult to treat with antithyroid drugs and subsequent ^{131}I administration.

Complications of iodide therapy include inflammation of the salivary glands, conjunctivitis, and skin rashes. Rarely, administration of iodide to a euthyroid patient may precipitate hyperthyroidism (discussed later).

Beta-adrenergic blockade. Beta-adrenergic blocking agents are very effective in the short-term treatment of many of the most acute and prominent symptoms of hyperthyroidism. Propranolol is the beta-adrenergic blocking drug used most frequently. Within hours it improves palpitations, tachycardia, anxiety, and tremor. Associated depression may improve within 2 weeks, and proximal myopathy occasionally improves significantly. Beta-blocking drugs do not affect the nonadrenergically mediated symptoms or signs of hyperthyroidism such as goiter, heat intolerance, or ophthalmopathy.

Beta blockers are indicated in the following settings: (1) the short-term management of tachycardia or other debilitating cardiovascular symptoms, especially in older patients with no history of congestive heart failure; (2) symptomatic relief of severe anxiety or tremor; (3) with self-limited hyperthyroidism such as that found in subacute and silent thyroiditis; and (4) in thyroid storm, in which they produce a very rapid decrease in heart rate (in 2 to 3 hours when given orally; in minutes when given intravenously) that may be critical in management. The usual daily dose of propranolol taken orally is 40 to 160 mg in four divided doses.

Contraindications to the use of propranolol and other beta blockers include chronic lung disease (asthma, emphysema, bronchospasm) wherein abolition of the beta-adrenergic mechanisms responsible for bronchodilatation may lead to severe bronchospasm and respiratory failure, sinus bradycardia or greater than second-degree heart block, in treatment of patients receiving other myocardial depressants such as quinidine or procainamide, and in congestive heart failure. If a patient has heart failure that is heart rate–

related, in conjunction with proper monitoring, propranolol may be given with other cardiotropic drugs cautiously by intravenous (IV) titration to decrease the heart rate; shorter-acting beta blockers such as esmolol may be preferable. Propranolol is also contraindicated in patients receiving monoamine oxidase inhibitors and in those prone to spontaneous hypoglycemia, such as insulin-dependent diabetics.

Toxic nodular goiter (Plummer's disease)

Autonomous, hyperfunctioning nodules may develop in a setting of a single-nodule or multinodule goiter. The reason for the hyperfunction is unknown, but there seems to be a clear progression from a nontoxic to a toxic state with time. In a single nodule the excess levels of T_4 and T_3 suppress the remainder of the thyroid gland. Multinodular goiters may have one or more hyperfunctioning nodules. Toxic nodular goiters are more common in older patients. The symptoms and signs are typical of hyperthyroidism, are usually milder than those seen in Graves' disease, and have no immunologic component. The diagnosis is established by routine thyroid blood tests. There is a high frequency of T_3 toxicosis. Radioiodine scanning is necessary to define the anatomy of the thyroid. Radioactive iodine (^{131}I) and surgery are the usual treatment options. Many toxic nodular glands are relatively resistant to ^{131}I therapy and require high doses for successful treatment.

Thyrotoxicosis factitia

The syndrome of thyrotoxicosis factitia usually results from deliberate, surrepitious administration of thyroid hormone or inadvertent overdose during thyroid hormone treatment. The physician should have a high index of suspicion for this diagnosis in thyrotoxic patients who do not manifest a goiter. If T_4 is ingested in excess, the laboratory findings consist of high total T_4 and T_3 levels, high THBR a low radioiodine uptake, and absent goiter. If T_3 is ingested in excess, the laboratory findings consist of a low total T_4 level, high total T_3 level, low normal to normal THBR, low radioiodine uptake, and absent goiter (see the box below).

Subacute (DeQuervain's) thyroiditis

Subacute, or DeQuervain's, thyroiditis, or inflammatory disease of the thyroid characterized by a tender goiter, is discussed in more detail in the section Thyroiditis. During the acute inflammatory stage of several weeks' duration preformed stores of thyroid hormone within thyroglobulin are released into the bloodstream and the thyroid hormone is made available to the tissues after hydrolysis of the thyroglobulin. The thyrotoxicosis is self-limited, lasting only as long as the preformed stores of hormone are released by the inflammatory process. Serum total T_4 and T_3 levels are elevated, TSH level is suppressed, and classically the radioiodine uptake is 0% or only 1% to 2%.

> **Causes of thyrotoxicosis with a low radioiodine uptake**
>
> Thyrotoxicosis factitia
> Subacute thyroiditis
> Iodine
> Struma ovarii

Silent thyroiditis

Silent thyroiditis, an autoimmune disorder, is discussed in more detail in the section Thyroiditis. Although silent thyroiditis occurs in both women and men, it is more common in women, particularly in the postpartum period. The thyrotoxic stage of this thyroiditis is usually quite mild, generally seen in the first few weeks to months after delivery, and self-limited. There is only a mild degree of thyroid enlargement and the gland is nontender. Serum total T_4 and T_3 levels are elevated, TSH level is suppressed, and radioiodine uptake is normal or low. Thyroid antimicrosomal antibodies are present in many patients.

Thyroid hormone therapy

In the course of thyroid hormone replacement therapy, patients may be euthyroid clinically and have normal or high normal total T4 and T3 concentrations but suppressed TSH concentration indicated by sensitive assay. These patients have subclinical hyperthyroidism. It is important to adjust the replacement dose downward because patients such as these are at risk for increased bone turnover and a loss of bone mass if allowed to remain hyperthyroid.

Iodide-induced (Jodbasedow)

Iodine-induced thyrotoxicosis (Jodbasedow syndrome) usually occurs when large doses of iodine are administered to patients with underlying thyroid disease such as nontoxic multinodular goiter or iodine deficient goiter and was originally described in patients with a diffuse goiter. The source of excess iodine is frequently provided in the course of a diagnostic test using iodinated-contrast agents but occasionally is derived from dietary supplements or from drugs such as amiodarone that are 30% (by weight) iodine. The hyperthyroidism is generally of short duration, lasting several days to several weeks. Total T_4 and/or T_3 level is elevated and radioiodine uptake is low. Definitive therapy may be required, depending on the underlying thyroid abnormality.

Rare causes of thyrotoxicosis

The hyperthyroidism secondary to a TSH-producing tumor of the pituitary is due to direct overproduction of T_4 and T_3 after sustained stimulation of the thyroid by TSH. The goiter is usually small and the condition may not be suspected unless a TSH level is obtained and found to be inappropriately elevated. Hyperthyroidism secondary to choriocarcinoma is due to the ability of human chorionic gonadotropin (HCG) to bind to thyroid TSH receptors weakly and stimulate the gland. Struma ovarii is an ovarian teratoma containing functioning thyroid tissue; radioiodine scanning reveals uptake in the ovarian tumor and suppression of thyroid uptake of radioiodine. Widely metastatic follicular thyroid cancer of substantial mass may have enough functional thyroid tissue to produce either T_4 or T_3 toxicosis. Treatment of all these causes is surgical removal of the tumor, appropriate chemotherapy, or, in the case of metastatic follicular cancer, administration of ^{131}I.

Special problems

Thyrotoxic storm. Thyrotoxic storm is a dreaded complication of Graves' disease characterized by abrupt onset of florid symptoms of thyrotoxicosis, with some additional symptoms and signs not typical of uncomplicated Graves' disease including fever, hypotension, marked weakness, extreme restlessness, confusion, psychosis or even coma, cardiovascular collapse, and shock. These signs and symptoms are a manifestation of the loss of the normal ability to regulate heat dissipation, maintain circulatory hemodynamics, and control oxygen consumption in a severely hypermetabolic state. Thyroid storm occurs in untreated or inadequately treated Graves' disease and may be precipitated by infection, trauma, surgery, diabetic acidosis, stress, toxemia of pregnancy, labor and delivery, or discontinuance of antithyroid medication.

The patients have obvious signs of Graves' disease and almost always have large goiters. The presence of fever is a sine qua non for the diagnosis, which is made by the usual tests. Radioiodine uptake is particularly useful because 2 hour uptake of ^{123}I or ^{131} I is markedly elevated, helping to establish the diagnosis very quickly. Total T_4 and T_3 levels are elevated to the same degree observed in uncomplicated Graves' disease.

Acute treatment of thyroid storm consists of administration of propranolol orally or intravenously, intravenous sodium iodide, and an antithyroid drug such as propylthiouracil (900 to 1200 mg daily) (refer to the box at upper right). Supporting measures including administration of intravenous fluids, oxygen, a cooling blanket, and glucocorticoids are usually required. Plasmapheresis may be required to lower T_4 and T_3 levels rapidly. Histologic mortality in thyroid storm is about 20%; however, prompt recognition and treatment should lead to a satisfactory result. Improvement should be expected within 24 hours and recovery within a few days to a week. Ultimate definitive therapy after recovery should consist of ablation of the thyroid gland with ^{131}I.

Treatment of thyroid storm

Propranolol—160 mg/day orally in 4 divided doses; or 1 mg *slowly* IV q 4 h under careful monitoring
IV glucose solutions
Correction of dehydration and electrolyte imbalance
Iodide-30 drops Lugol's solution daily orally in 3 or 4 divided doses; or 1 to 2 g sodium iodine slowly by IV drip
Propylthiouracil—900 to 1200 mg/day orally or by gastric tube
Cooling blanket for hyperthermia
Plasmapheresis to lower T_4 and T_3 levels (in selected cases)
Digitalis if necessary
Treatment of underlying disease (e.g., infection)
Corticosteroid—100 mg hydrocortisone IV q 8 hr
Definitive therapy after control of the crisis—ablation of the thyroid gland with ^{131}I or surgery.

T_3 toxicosis. In general, T_3 and T_4 concentrations are regularly increased in patients with hyperthyroidism. In Graves' disease, increases in serum T_3 concentrations are usually somewhat greater on a proportional basis compared to T_4 concentrations, probably as a result of both increased thyroidal secretion of T_3 and increased peripheral conversion of T_4 to T_3. Occasional patients early in the course of Graves' disease may demonstrate all or most of the signs and symptoms of hyperthyroidism but normal values for serum total T_4 level, THBR, and radioiodine uptake. When measurement of serum total T_3 level is shown to be elevated, the condition is called T_3 toxicosis. In these patients eventually the classic laboratory abnormalities of hyperthyroidism develop when the state of T_3 toxicosis continues untreated for several weeks to months. In addition to Graves' disease, the incidence of T_3 toxicosis appears to be increased in areas where dietary intake of iodide is lowest and in patients with nodular goiter or a toxic adenoma. Because T_3 toxicosis is merely an early manifestation of thyrotoxicosis when it is discovered, it should be treated by the usual means.

Thyrotoxicosis in pregnancy. Graves' disease may arise de novo during pregnancy or the patient may have Graves' disease, treated or untreated, and become pregnant. In any case, thyrotoxicosis in pregnancy is often a significant diagnostic and management challenge. Diagnosis is difficult because in pregnant women a small degree of thyroid enlargement and symptoms and signs of hypermetabolism such as anxiety, irritability, polyphagia, heat intolerance, increased sweating, and warm, moist skin develop. By the fourth to fifth month of pregnancy, total T_4 and T_3 levels are normally elevated about twofold and T_3 resin uptake or THBR is low secondary to TBG level elevation. Therefore the presence of a normal or high normal T_3 resin uptake or THBR is suggestive of hyperthyroidism. Discovery of suppressed TSH level by the supersensitive TSH assay is diagnostic. Serum TRAb level should be determined to alert the pediatrician to the possibility of neonatal thyrotoxicosis. Radioiodine uptake and scanning are absolutely contraindicated because radioiodine crosses the placenta and can destroy the fetal thyroid gland, which is formed and functioning by the 12th week of pregnancy.

Treatment should be initiated with propylthiouracil in the usual starting dosage; methimazole is relatively contraindicated because it crosses the placenta to a greater extent than propylthiouracil. Propylthiouracil should be decreased to the lowest effective dose necessary to control the hyperthyroidism as soon as possible to minimize the risk of fetal goiter and/or hypothyroidism. If necessary, surgical treatment of the hyperthyroidism can be performed in the second trimester, but it is best to avoid surgery and the attendant risks of anesthesia and operative complications to the fetus. Surgery is contraindicated in the first and third trimesters because of a high risk of induction of premature labor and miscarriage. The fact that Graves' disease is difficult to manage adds a compelling reason to treat the disease definitively in any woman in the childbearing years to prevent potential complications of hyperthyroidism and its therapy in pregnancy.

Thyrotoxicosis in adolescence. The most common cause of thyrotoxicosis in adolescence is Graves' disease. Its general clinical features in adolescence are similar to those in adulthood. Additional considerations arise in selection of therapy. Treatment options include antithyroid drugs, radioiodine, and surgery. Posttreatment hypothyroidism should be promptly treated to prevent the disruptive effects of hypothyroidism on growth and development.

HYPOTHYROIDISM

Deficiency in the amount of biologically active thyroid hormone at the tissue level is called hypothyroidism. Hypothyroidism is generally classified into two major groups: (1) primary hypothyroidism caused by thyroid gland failure and (2) secondary or central hypothyroidism produced by failure of the pituitary or hypothalamus in which the defect is a deficiency of TSH. Hypothyroidism caused by hypothalamic failure is also referred to as tertiary hypothyroidism because TRH deficiency causes inadequate TSH secretion from an otherwise functional thyrotroph cell of the anterior pituitary.

Causes

The most common type of hypothyroidism is that due to primary thyroid gland failure. Within this group are five basic causes of primary hypothyroidism (see the box below): autoimmune (atrophic), which includes chronic lymphocytic thyroiditis (Hashimoto's thyroiditis) and silent thyroiditis, postablative (^{131}I, thyroidectomy, head and neck irradiation), goitrous, athyreotic, and nonautoimmune thyroiditis (such as Riedel's thyroiditis), and subacute thyroiditis. The hypothyroidism of silent thyroiditis and subacute thyroiditis is usually but not always transient.

Causes of hypothyroidism

Autoimmune (atrophic)
Postablative
Goitrous (iodine or synthetic defect)
Athyreotic
Nonautoimmune thyroiditis

The most common cause is the atrophic autoimmune type, which is most likely a late stage of Hashimoto's (autoimmune) thyroiditis because the majority of the cases have significant elevations of thyroid antimicrosomal antibody levels. It is more common in women than men and is often associated with other autoimmune diseases of the endocrine system, including autoimmune hypoparathyroidism, adrenal failure, hypogonadism, and insulin-dependent diabetes mellitus. Recent studies have identified the presence of TSH receptor blocking antibodies as an important and potentially reversible cause of hypothyroidism. Postablative primary thyroid gland failure is quite common and is usually found after ^{131}I treatment of thyrotoxicosis or subtotal or near-total thyroidectomy for thyroid cancer, Graves' disease, or toxic multinodular goiter. External mantle irradiation for Hodgkins' disease may also lead to thyroid gland failure; this generally evolves over a period of 5 to 10 years.

In goitrous hypothyroidism, goiter ensues because of decreased ability of the thyroid gland to synthesize thyroid hormone, leading to increased TSH secretion, which results in an increase in the size of the thyroid gland. Among the causes of goitrous hypothyroidism are endemic goiter, which occurs in regions of iodide deficiency such as the mountainous areas of Europe and South America. Children born of parents having an endemic goiter may be born with goitrous hypothyroidism (endemic cretinism). Drugs can produce goitrous hypothyroidism. The chronic administration of large doses of iodides as in expectorants sometimes results in goiter and hypothyroidism because of an inhibition of the organification step within the thyroid and an absence of the normal escape mechanism. Propylthiouracil and methimazole used for the treatment of hyperthyroidism may produce hypothyroidism. When used in pregnant women, they cross the placenta, occasionally causing goitrous hypothyroidism in the fetus. Lithium, which inhibits thyroid hormone synthesis and release, commonly produces a goiter and in a small subset of patients (primarily those with antimicrosomal antibodies) can induce hypothyroidism. Some vegetables, such as cassava, rutabaga, and white turnips, contain natural goitrogens. Drugs and natural goitrogen-induced causes are completely reversible when the offending agent is removed. Finally, a variety of genetic defects affecting thyroid hormone biosynthesis cause goitrous hypothyroidism. These genetic defects can affect transport of iodide, organification of iodide (with sensory nerve deafness and Pendred's syndrome), coupling of iodinated tyrosines, and intrathyroidal deiodination of thyroid hormone.

Athyreotic cretinism is found in children born with an absence of the thyroid gland. The various forms of thyroiditis which can result in atrophic or goitrous hypothyroidism are described in the section Thyroiditis. Hashimoto's thyroiditis may be the most common form of hypothyroidism if it is in fact the cause of end-stage, atrophic thyroid gland failure. In the early stages of Hashimoto's thyroiditis, the thyroid gland is typically enlarged, firm and rubbery in consistency, and infiltrated with lymphocytes. Although the production of thyroid hormone may remain normal, a subset of patients develop an inability to synthesize thyroid hormone. Defects in iodide organification with maintenance of iodide trapping are characteristic of Hashimoto's thyroiditis.

Riedel's thyroiditis is characterized by a dense fibrosis of the thyroid gland. Silent thyroiditis and subacute thyroiditis usually evolve through a hyperthyroid stage before the hypothyroid stage, and the hypothyroidism is usually transient.

Secondary forms of hypothyroidism are unusual and the tertiary subgroup (hypothalamic) are rare in ordinary practice. Secondary and tertiary forms include pituitary tumors, vascular anomalies, infections, and other causes.

Symptoms and signs

The symptoms and signs of primary thyroid gland failure are extraordinarily varied as a result of the multiple physiologic and biochemical effects of thyroid hormone on virtually every organ system. The symptoms and signs stand in stark contrast to those found in thyrotoxicosis and may be equally dramatic in their clinical presentation, which comprises the syndrome known as myxedema. On the other hand, they may be so subtle and insidious that the diagnosis may be overlooked for many months or even years unless the physician has a high index of suspicion and the patient or family is alert to the changes. The most common and characteristic symptoms and signs of hypothyroidism (myxedema) are listed in the box below. The patients complain of weakness, fatigue, and general lack of energy. The voice is hoarse and speech is dysarthric and slow. The facial expression is dull, and puffiness and periorbital swelling are caused by infiltration with the mucopolysaccharides hyaluronic acid and chondroitin sulfate. Patients frequently complain of cold intolerance and constipation.

Eyelids droop because of decreased adrenergic drive; hair is sparse and coarse; the skin is dry, scaly, and thick, and has a definite pallor. There is often carotenemia, which is particularly notable on the palms and soles because of deposition of carotene in the lipid-rich epidermal layers. Patients are forgetful and show other evidence of intellectual impairment, with a gradual change in personality. There may be frank psychosis ("myxedema madness").

Deposition of a proteinaceous material as well as an increase in muscle fibers in the tongue may produce macroglossia, thick speech, and snoring. Bradycardia is regularly found, and diastolic hypertension occurs in approximately 20% of patients. The heart may appear to be enlarged, usually as a result of the accumulation of a serous effusion of high protein content in the pericardial sac. There may also be pleural or abdominal effusions. The pericardial and pleural effusions develop slowly and only infrequently cause respiratory or hemodynamic distress. Paresthesias of the hands and feet are common, produced by carpal-tarsal tunnel syndromes caused by deposition of proteinaceous fluid in the ligaments around the wrist and ankle, producing nerve compression. Neuromuscular manifestations are varied, ranging from reflexes that are characterized by a slow relaxation to muscle hypertrophy, percussion myoedema, and myotonia. There is often menorrhagia, in contrast to the hypomenorrhea of hyperthyroidism. Hypothermia is commonly noted if the temperature is measured rectally.

It is important to differentiate secondary or central hypothyroidism from primary. There are a number of clinical clues, which usually result from secondary involvement of other endocrine organs when the pituitary and/or hypothalamus fails. These clues include amenorrhea rather than menorrhagia in a woman with known hypothyroidism; atrophic breasts; skin and hair that are thin and not coarse; skin depigmentation, diastolic hypotension, and a small heart without pericardial effusion.

Common symptoms and signs of hypothyroidism

Weakness	Eyelid droop
Fatigue	Facial puffiness
Cold intolerance	Periorbital edema
Constipation	Hoarse voice
Weight gain	Dry skin and hair
Snoring	Bradycardia
Menorrhagia	Diastolic hypertension
Muscle cramps and stiffness	Delayed deep tendon reflex
Paresthesias in hands and feet	Hypothermia

Laboratory diagnosis

The laboratory diagnosis of primary hypothyroidism is reasonably straightforward. Serum total T_4 and T_3 levels and THBR are low and the sine qua non is an elevated serum TSH level, usually to values above 20 μU/ml. The TSH level is the single best test for the diagnosis of primary thyroid gland failure for several reasons. The serum concentration of TSH rises early in the disease when serum concentrations of T_4 and/or T_3 may still be in the low normal range. The TSH allows primary and secondary hypothyroidism to be distinguished, is normal in cases of euthyroid hypothyroxinemia, and plays the key role in the complex differentiation of hypothyroidism from the euthyroid sick syndrome.

Thyroid antimicrosomal antibodies can be useful in the laboratory assessment of hypothyroidism because they are present in most cases of hypothyroidism caused by Hashimoto's thyroiditis and also in the atrophic form of primary hypothyroidism. Radioiodine uptake is of no value in the diagnosis of primary thyroid gland failure.

Other laboratory abnormalities present in primary hypothyroidism may occasionally be the precipitating reason to diagnose hypothyroidism. These include elevation of serum cholesterol level and unexplained anemia, which may be normochromic-normocytic, hypochromic-microcytic, or occasionally macrocytic; increased serum levels of creatine kinase with a normal percentage of the CK-MB isoenzyme; elevation of other muscle enzymes, including aldolase, lactic dehydrogenase, and serum glutamic–oxaloacetic acid (SGOT); and hyperuricemia and hyponatremia. The electrocardiogram (ECG) classically shows a sinus bradycardia with low voltage in the precordial leads. Chest radiograph may show an enlarged heart, which on echocardiogram is usually noted to be secondary to a pericardial effusion.

The laboratory assessment of secondary hypothyroidism reveals several important differences from primary hypothyroidism. Most significantly serum TSH levels are low or normal despite low serum total T_4 and T_3 levels. The TRH test is useful in confirming the diagnosis of secondary versus primary hypothyroidism and pivotal in distinguishing between pituitary failure and hypothyroidism resulting from hypothalamic failure. In the former, TSH is not released in response to the injection of TRH, whereas in the latter it is released, albeit usually more slowly and with a delayed peak. Cholesterol levels are not increased by secondary or tertiary hypothyroidism. Other abnormalities noted are consistent with the associated failure of other pituitary hormones such as growth hormone (GH), luteinizing hormone (LH), follicle-stimulating hormone (FSH), and adrenocorticotropic hormone (ACTH).

Differential diagnosis

The fully expressed picture of hypothyroidism (myxedema) is classic, and the diagnosis usually obvious to the clinician. Many of the clinical features can be suggestive of chronic renal failure, nephrotic syndrome, or severe anemia. Patients who have euthyroid sick syndrome can pose a significant diagnostic challenge because of the degree of illness and the complexity of changes in the thyroid function tests. The euthyroid hypothyroxinemias require an understanding of thyroid function tests to prevent misdiagnosis as hypothyroidism. More subtle or subclinical presentations of hypothyroidism require a high index of suspicion based on the clinical setting such as age, sex, family history, postpartum history, associated autoimmune disease, or the finding of the other laboratory changes noted.

Treatment

The treatment of hypothyroidism is usually relatively simple and begins to produce highly satisfactory relief of symptoms within several days to several weeks. A variety of thyroid hormone preparations are available for replacement therapy, including synthetic preparations of T_4 and T_3, combinations of the two in purified thyroglobulin, and desiccated animal thyroid. Synthetic preparations of pure T_4 (L-thyroxine) are preferred and should be used for the routine treatment of all cases of hypothyroidism. Synthetic L-thyroxine is given once per day, generally in the morning. The average maintenance dose is 100 to 125 μ/day orally. In general, the maintenance dose decreases in the elderly and may increase in pregnant women. A wide variety of incremental dosages are available to accommodate those requiring maintenance doses significantly above or below the average. Absorption is fairly constant at about 75% of the administered dose. T_3 is generated by peripheral conversion of T_4, preventing the chemical and clinical T_3 toxicosis found in the administration of T_3 or T_3-T_4 combinations. The dose used should be the minimum that restores TSH levels to normal. The induction of subclinical hyperthyroidism as demonstrated by a suppressed TSH level by the sensitive assay should be prevented in the replacement therapy for hypothyroidism. This is important from a long-term perspective to prevent cardiac complications such as supraventricular arrhythmias, tachycardia, angina pectoris, and calcium loss from bone with possible worsening of osteoporosis.

Most patients under the age of 50 tolerate the initiation of full thyroid hormone replacement therapy without any difficulty. However, in older patients and in hypothyroid patients with known coronary artery disease the initiation of thyroid hormone therapy with full replacement doses may precipitate angina pectoris caused by the increase in myocardial oxygen consumption and heart rate and the demand this places on the coronary artery blood supply. Therefore in older patients with or without known coronary artery disease it is prudent to begin replacement therapy with a low dose. A reasonable scheme would be to begin with 25 μ T_4/day orally and increase by 25 μ T_4/day orally every 4 weeks, the time required for thyroid hormone to exert its maximum effects. Serum TSH level should be determined before each additional increase, until the desired replacement dose is attained. Smaller increments in dose may be required in some patients.

Patients with hypothyroidism and coexistent adrenal insufficiency caused by either primary adrenal gland or secondary pituitary (ACTH) failure should receive replacement therapy with corticosteroids before or at the time of replacement with thyroid hormone to prevent the potential induction of acute adrenal insufficiency by the increase in cortisol metabolism imposed by thyroid hormone therapy.

T_3 should not be used alone for long-term replacement because its rapid turnover usually requires that it be taken at least twice daily. Some clinicians occasionally use T_3 as starting therapy because of the potential for more rapid onset of action. With the exception of myxedema coma, the chronic nature of hypothyroidism does not require rapid reversal of the metabolic and clinical changes. In addition, administering standard replacement amounts of T_3 (25 to 75 μ/day) results in rapidly increasing serum T_3 concentrations to potentially supranormal levels that return to normal or below normal by 24 hours. Therefore patients who receive T_3 are subject to varying therapeutic effects as a result of the short half-life (24 hours) of this preparation. Similar patterns of serum T_3 concentrations are seen when mixtures of T_3 and T_4 are taken orally. As noted, replacement regimens with synthetic preparations of T_4 reflect a different pattern of serum T_3 response with increases in serum T_3 to normal levels that occur gradually over 4 to 6 weeks.

Desiccated animal thyroid preparations are too variable in potency to be reliable and should not be used.

Special problems

Myxedema coma. Myxedema coma is a life-threatening but uncommon complication of hypothyroidism. It occurs most commonly but not exclusively in colder weather. Myxedema characteristically is found in patients with longstanding untreated primary hypothyroidism. Patients have a combination of altered mental status or coma, extreme hypothermia (temperatures 24° to 32.2° C [75.2° to 90° F]) hypo- or areflexia, seizures, CO_2 retention, bradycardia, hypoxemia, and respiratory depression caused by decreased cerebral blood flow. Severe hypothermia may be overlooked unless special low-reading thermometers are used. Precipitating factors include exposure to cold, infection, trauma, and drugs such as sedatives that suppress the central nervous system (CNS). Rapid diagnosis based on clinical judgment, history, and physical examination is imperative because early death is likely if the diagnosis is overlooked. Once the diagnosis is seriously considered, treatment needs to be instituted before the return of the laboratory test results because the usual delay in the reporting of these tests is too long under these circumstances. It is preferable to initiate therapy and terminate if thyroid function test results rule out the diagnosis rather than not start therapy and discover too late that the patient had myxedema with coma.

The treatment of myxedema coma is outlined in the box below. The cornerstone is the administration of an intravenous bolus of thyroxine (300 to 500 μ) to saturate the unoccupied binding sites on TBG, making free hormone available for response, followed by daily intravenous doses of 50 to 100 μ of synthetic L-thyroxine. Because triiodothyronine is now commercially available for parenteral use, this may provide more rapid metabolic responses in the treatment of myxedema coma. Supporting measures consisting of gentle warming and administration of intravenous fluids, glucocorticoids, and antibiotics as necessary are lifesaving. The patient should not be rewarmed rapidly because it may precipitate cardiac arrhythmias. If alveolar ventilation is compromised, mechanical ventilation should be instituted.

Treatment of myxedema coma

Thyroid hormone administration
  I-thyroxine 300 to 500 μ IV then 100 μ daily
or
  Triiodothyronine 25 to 50 μ IV then 25 μ q 8 h
Intravenous fluids
Gentle warming
Glucocorticoid 50-100 mg hydrocortisone q 8 h
Antibiotics for suspected infection
Respiratory support

Subclinical hypothyroidism. The entity of subclinical hypothyroidism is characterized by normal serum total T_4 and T_3 concentrations and modest elevations of serum TSH level to between 6 and 15 μU/ml in patients who either are clinically euthyroid or have only subtle signs of hypothyroidism. The disorder is more common in women: overall prevalence estimates range from 5% to as high as 20% of women over the age of 60. Subclinical hypothyroidism appears to be part of the spectrum of autoimmune thyroiditis because of the frequent association of increased levels of thyroid antimicrosomal antibodies. The diagnosis is usually made in the course of general screening of patients, particularly elderly patients, for nonspecific complaints such as mild fatigue, lack of energy, mild depression, and constipation.

The decision as to whether or not to treat a patient with normal serum T_4 and T_3 levels and modest elevations of serum TSH level is a difficult one. In younger patients the tendency is to treat any reproducible TSH level elevation, especially in the setting of autoimmune thyroiditis (positive antibodies). In elderly patients the issue is less clear, and in the absence of information from randomized clinical trials, therapy should be reserved for patients with both elevated TSH and thyroid antimicrosomal antibody concentrations (>1:1600). In the absence of these antibodies the rate of progression to overt hypothyroidism is low. The metabolic complications of the milder, subclinical forms of hypothyroidism remain unresolved.

Once therapy has been initiated, it is important to ensure that the TSH concentration is normalized and not suppressed. Otherwise subclinical hypothyroidism is exchanged for subclinical hyperthyroidism with its attendant risks.

THYROIDITIS

Hashimoto's thyroiditis (chronic lymphocytic thyroiditis, autoimmune thyroiditis)

Hashimoto's thyroiditis is characterized by a modest-sized goiter, lymphocytic infiltration of the thyroid, presence of organ-specific autoantibodies in a majority of patients, and hypothyroidism. It is one of the three major causes of primary thyroid gland failure. Hashimoto's thyroiditis is more common in women (8:1), is most frequent between the ages of 30 to 50, is frequently familial, and tends to be chronic and progressive.

Substantial evidence suggests that Hashimoto's thyroiditis is an autoimmune disease. Thyroid antimicrosomal and antithyroglobulin antibodies are commonly present; however, the thyroid inflammation is a cellular mediated immune response. Occasionally the hypothyroidism is due to the presence of thyrotropin-blocking antibodies that block the binding of TSH to its receptor. In some patients Hashimoto's thyroiditis may evolve into the classic thyrotoxicosis of Graves' disease, and Graves' disease may have certain features in common with Hashimoto's thyroiditis, such as the presence of antimicrosomal and antithyroglobulin antibodies. Hashimoto's thyroiditis frequently coexists with other autoimmune diseases such as Sjögren's syndrome, pernicious anemia, rheumatoid arthritis, lupus erythematosus, progressive systemic sclerosis, myasthenia gravis, autoimmune hepatitis, primary biliary cirrhosis, Addison's disease (adrenal insufficiency), hypoparathyroidism, and insulin-dependent diabetes mellitus.

The incidence of Hashimoto's thyroiditis is increased in patients with chromosomal disorders including Turner's, Down's, and Klinefelter's syndromes. There may be an increased incidence of papillary cancer of the thyroid, and there is a high concordance with thyroid lymphoma (see the section Thyroid Cancer). The early stages of the disease, which may last months to several years, are characterized by a nontender goiter of variable size that is firm and rubbery in consistency. Other features are lymphocytic infiltration of the thyroid, elevated levels of antithyroid antibodies (antimicrosomal and antithyroglobulin), normal or decreased serum T_4 level, and increased serum TSH level. Thyroid radioiodine uptake is increased with a patchy distribution caused by abnormalities within the thyroid epithelial cell that permit trapping of iodide but disrupt normal organification. About 20% of patients are frankly hypothyroid in the early stages.

The late stage of Hashimoto's thyroiditis is most likely represented in part by the typical adult atrophic, thyroid gland failure. The thyroid gland at this stage is fibrotic in addition to being atrophic and may no longer be palpable. However, many patients have an enlarged, irregular, firm thyroid gland. Elevated levels of antithyroid antibodies may decline with time. Serum T_4 and T_3 levels are generally below normal and serum TSH level is markedly elevated in the late stages of the disease, although some patients maintain normal thyroid function throughout. The hypothyroidism of classic Hashimoto's thyroiditis is almost always permanent; however, hypothyroidism associated with the presence of thyrotropin-blocking antibodies may be transient and remit.

Histopathologic examination of the gland reveals diffuse infiltration with lymphocytes, disruption of follicle architecture, and some degree of fibrosis. Epithelial cells demonstrating oxyphilic changes in the cytoplasm, called Askanazy cells, are pathognomonic of Hashimoto's thyroiditis.

The differential diagnosis is quite limited and the laboratory abnormalities usually clearly distinguish Hashimoto's thyroiditis from nontoxic, euthyroid goiter. The most difficult differential is between Hashimoto's thyroiditis and thyroid lymphoma, which may also be associated with markedly elevated levels of thyroid antimicrosomal antibodies. Open biopsy may be required to obtain enough tissue to establish the diagnosis.

Thyroid hormone is provided to correct hypothyroidism and to attempt to decrease the size of the goiter or prevent its further growth. Surgical resection of the thyroid is reserved for large, cosmetically unattractive glands or in the unusual circumstance when compressive symptoms of the trachea or esophagus develop. Thyroid hormone replacement is given after surgery.

Subacute thyroiditis (granulomatous, giant-cell, or DeQuervain's thyroiditis)

Subacute thyroiditis is an inflammatory disease of the thyroid that may be caused by a virus. Mumps and viruses associated with upper respiratory infections are suspected etiologic agents. The clinical features are characteristic and the diagnosis straightforward. Patients usually experience sudden onset of "sore throat" (neck pain) with progressive tenderness in the neck and low-grade fever (37.8° to 38.3° C). The neck pain shifts characteristically from side to side and finally settles in one area, frequently radiating to the jaw and ears. It is often confused with dental problems, pharyngitis, or otitis and is aggravated by swallowing or turning the head. There are profound lassitude and fatigue not seen in other thyroid disorders. Symptoms and signs of thyrotoxicosis regularly occur in the first few weeks of the disease because of preformed hormone release from the markedly inflamed gland. Physical examination reveals a thyroid that is asymmetrically enlarged, very firm to hard in consistency, and exquisitely tender.

Histologic studies show destruction of follicles, a characteristic giant cell infiltration surrounding a central core of colloid, inflammation, and mild fibrosis. Laboratory findings early in the disease include an increase in T_4 level, a suppressed TSH level, a decrease in radioiodine uptake (often to 0%), leukocytosis, and a markedly elevated sedimentation rate. After several weeks, the T_4 level is decreased, the TSH level remains suppressed, and the radioiodine uptake remains low. At this stage symptoms of hypothyroidism may develop. Once the TSH level begins to rise and inflammation disappears, thyroid function test results normalize. Subacute thyroiditis is self-limiting, generally subsiding in a few months, and full recovery is the rule. Occasionally the thyroiditis recurs, and rarely it results in permanent hypothyroidism. Because the disease is self-limited, treatment should be conservative, consisting of administration of beta blockers for disturbing symptoms of thyrotoxicosis, aspirin 650 mg every 4 hours, and, only as a last resort, glucocorticoids such as prednisone 5 mg orally every 6 hours. On discontinuance of the latter, there is often a severe rebound in symptoms.

Subacute thyroiditis most frequently must be differentiated from hemorrhage into a nodule or cyst. This is best accomplished by the normal sedimentation rate and thyroid function test results associated with hemorrhage into a nodule or cyst. Pyogenic thyroiditis, although rare, also must be differentiated. The thyroid in this case is reddened, fever and leukocytosis are very high, and a specific septic site extrinsic to the thyroid is evident. *Pneumocystis carinii* can cause painful nodular thyroiditis in patients with acquired immunodeficiency syndrome (AIDS).

Silent thyroiditis

Silent thyroiditis is an autoimmune disorder more common in women, often in the postpartum period. It is characterized by a variable but mild degree of thyroid enlargement and absence of thyroid tenderness. There is a self-limited hyperthyroid phase of several weeks to several months, often followed by a period of hypothyroidism (postpartum hypothyroidism) lasting weeks to months.

Many of the patients have elevated antimicrosomal antibody levels. This disease may be an autoimmune variant of Hashimoto's thyroiditis because biopsy results show lymphocytic infiltration. Diagnosis requires a high index of suspicion based on the clinical setting and generally mild symptoms. Total T_4 and T_3 levels are elevated and the radioiodine uptake normal or low. The white blood cell count and sedimentation rate are normal.

Because silent thyroiditis is a self-limited transient disorder that lasts 1 to 6 months, treatment is conservative. The thyrotoxic stage usually requires only adrenergic blockade with propranolol. Surgery and radioactive iodine therapy are contraindicated and thionamides ineffective. The transient phase of hypothyroidism may require thyroid hormone replacement therapy if the patient is symptomatic. Most patients recover normal thyroid function; however, in some permanent hypothyroidism develops. Relapses may occur, particularly in those cases of postpartum thyroiditis in which subsequent pregnancies may be followed by additional attacks. Some evidence suggests that thyroid hormone treatment before pregnancy can prevent these relapses.

Riedel's thyroiditis

Riedel's thyroiditis, a rare form, is most common in women above age 50 and is characterized by an intense fibrosis of the thyroid gland and surrounding tissues in the neck. The thyroid is enlarged, nontender, and fixed in position and feels woody-hard on palpation. The thyroiditis may progress to clinical hypothyroidism. Frequently, Riedel's thyroiditis results in compression of adjacent structures producing respiratory distress and/or dysphagia. Surgical resection of the thyroid gland may be required to preserve and restore tracheal and esophageal function. A cine esophagram or flow volume loop can give objective confirmation of clinical symptoms of dysphagia or dyspnea. The administration of synthetic L-thyroxine corrects any hypothyroidism but does not result in regression of the goiter.

EUTHYROID GOITER

Euthyroid (nontoxic) goiter is a common endocrine disease that may be defined as an enlargement of the thyroid gland without clinical hypothyroidism or hyperthyroidism. There are two general classes of euthyroid goiter: endemic and sporadic.

Endemic goiter is for all intents and purposes synonymous with iodine deficiency. The optimum intake of iodine for adults is about 100 to 150 μ daily. About 800 million people live in iodine-deficient areas of the world, including the mountainous regions of Central Europe, Asia, and South America, as well as lowland regions of Greece, the Netherlands, and Finland. In these population groups, endemic goiter occurs in at least 10% of the population, and there may be as many as 200 million endemic goiters worldwide. There are no iodine-deficient areas in the United States although in the early part of the 20th century there were several areas, most notably the Great Lakes region. Iodine prophylaxis achieved by the supplementation of table salt and foods such as bread and cereal eliminated the problem of iodine-deficient goiter.

Sporadic goiter occurs in less than 10% of any population group. Its prevalence is about 4% in the United States. It is more common in women than men (8:1), and onset is frequently noted at the time of puberty, pregnancy, and menopause. Euthyroid goiters may be subclassified as either diffuse or nodular, and nodular goiters may be characterized by either single or multiple nodules. Nodular goiters are more frequent in women than men (4:1), and the prevalence increases with age. The nodular goiters pose specific and significant diagnostic and therapeutic challenges for the clinician. Decisions must frequently be made as to whether a nodule is benign or malignant or whether a patient with a multinodular goiter having areas of autonomous function is hyperthyroid.

Pathogenesis

Endemic goiter is clearly related to iodine deficiency, which leads to a sequence of events characterized by impaired production of thyroid hormone, increased TSH secretion, enlargement of the thyroid to a clinically evident goiter, and increased ability of the hyperplastic thyroid gland to trap iodide, permitting synthesis of adequate amounts of thyroid hormone to maintain the euthyroid state. Failure to trap enough iodide results in inability to maintain the euthyroid state and ultimately in the endemic form of goitrous hypothyroidism.

The pathogenesis of either the diffuse or nodular type of sporadic goiter is not completely understood. In some cases there may be an inherent enzymatic defect in thyroid hormone biosynthesis that impairs the production of thyroid hormone, leading to increased TSH secretion and thyroid gland size. Defects at any of the biosynthetic steps such as trapping, organification, or coupling presumably may be congenital or acquired. Obvious congenital defects are rare; sporadic, acquired defects are largely unproved. If they exist, they theoretically should be associated with demonstrable increases in serum TSH concentrations. However, most if not all patients with nontoxic goiter have normal serum TSH concentrations, raising serious questions as to the validity of this theory. Over the past decade immunologic growth factors that may play a role in the development of sporadic goiter have been identified. These factors, called thyroid growth immunoglobulins (TGIs), in contrast to TRAb found in Graves' disease, stimulate growth but not biosynthesis of thyroid hormone and probably bind to a different domain of the TSH receptor.

The evolution of a nontoxic, diffuse goiter to a multinodular goiter remains unexplained. Neither TSH nor TGI stimulation seems to explain the heterogeneity of the multinodular goiter, characterized by areas of autonomous function and hypofunction and areas of hyperplasia and involution.

Histopathology

Endemic goiters are hyperplastic and show a significant reduction in the amount of intrafollicular colloid and a decrease in size of columnar epithelial cells. Microscopic areas of papillary cancer may be found in long-standing endemic goiter. Sporadic goiter has a normal histologic appearance except for slight hyperplasia. Multinodular goiters have areas of hyperplasia, involution, cystic degeneration, fibrosis, hemorrhage, and, late in the disease, areas of calcification. Hyperplastic areas are presumably functionally autonomous and may be hyperfunctional, leading to clinical or subclinical hyperthyroidism.

Clinical presentation

Endemic or sporadic goiters are of variable size, are diffusely enlarged, and may be quite firm on palpation. Nodular goiters are irregular on palpation; nodules may be soft, firm, and even stony hand. Patients are generally asymptomatic and the goiter incidentally detected by the patient, a family member, or the physician on routine physical examination. Patients may note a tightness, tickling, or irritation in the throat, precipitating frequent dry cough or clearing of the throat. Large goiters may produce tracheal and/or esophageal compression, leading to respiratory distress and/or dysphagia. Infrequently, these large benign goiters may result in superior vena cava obstruction. Narrowing of the thoracic inlet produces obstruction of venous return from the head, neck, and arms, which is accentuated by raising the arms; this may cause lightheadedness or dizziness. The goiters may also be of sufficient size to compress the recurrent laryngeal nerve, producing hoarseness. Hemorrhage into one of the nodules of a multinodular goiter produces exquisite tenderness and enlargement of a nodule that may be confused with subacute thyroiditis.

Laboratory assessment

Thyroid function testing in patients with endemic goiter usually reveals a low or low normal serum total T_4 level, normal serum total T_3 level, and mildly elevated TSH levels. The 24 hour radioiodine uptake is elevated, reflecting the avidity of the iodine-deficient thyroid gland for iodide. Scanning reveals a homogeneous distribution of iodide. Serum total T_4, T_3, and TSH levels and 24 hour radioiodine uptake are generally normal in sporadic diffuse and multinodular goiter. Radioiodine scanning of multinodular goiters reveals a patchy distribution of the isotope with areas of hyperfunction and hypofunction corresponding to the various autonomously functioning macronodules and micronodules. The picture of the multinodular goiter provided by the scintiscan and the irregularity of the gland on palpation can be confused with Hashimoto's thyroiditis. Determination of serum thyroid antimicrosomal and antithyroglobulin antibody levels should differentiate the two conditions, because uncomplicated multinodular goiter is not associated with the presence of these antibodies.

Treatment

The cornerstone of treatment of endemic goiter is the provision of supplementary dietary iodine. Most, but not all, long-standing goiters regress in size. Prevention is the ideal treatment, and population groups in iodine-deficient areas should receive iodide supplementation in their diet. Therapeutic amounts of iodide given to a patient with iodine deficiency may in selected cases precipitate thyrotoxicosis. The iodine-deprived thyroid gland has developed a highly efficient trapping and biosynthetic pathway that is sufficiently autonomous that it may transiently overproduce thyroid hormone when provided with excess iodide. This mechanism is similar to what may occur when excess iodide is provided to patients with sporadic or multinodular goiters when receiving iodinated contrast agents or expectorants containing iodide (see Jodbasedow Thyrotoxicosis).

The treatment of sporadic goiter is straightforward. Drugs or natural goitrogens should be removed and the goiter will regress. Because TSH may be responsible for the thyroid cell growth in some patients with sporadic goiter, synthetic L-thyroxine should be given in adequate dosage to decrease the serum TSH concentration, to prevent induction of subclinical or clinical thyrotoxicosis. The dose of synthetic L-thyroxine required varies from patient to patient over a range of 0.05 to 0.15 mg daily and cannot be predicted in any given case. It is best to begin with the lower dose. Many nontoxic diffuse goiters shrink rapidly within several weeks to several months, others regress in size slowly, and some remain unchanged, providing the insight that TSH may be only partly or not at all responsible for the goitrous enlargement of the thyroid in some patients. Multinodular goiters usually do not decrease in size in response to synthetic L-thyroxine administration because of the functional autonomy of many areas of the thyroid gland. The existence of autonomously functional areas frequently results in the induction of thyrotoxicosis when exogenous thyroid hormone is provided because it is in effect additive to the autonomous endogenous production. Therefore when using synthetic L-thyroxine therapy in patients with a multinodular goiter the physician must be careful to initiate therapy with lower doses, 25 to 50 μ daily. A baseline sensitive TSH determination should be obtained to determine whether or not the patient already has a suppressed TSH level from the autonomously functioning areas of the goiter.

Surgical therapy should be reserved for diffuse or nodular goiters that cause objectively confirmed significant obstructive symptoms and signs that do not respond to exogenous thyroid hormone. Thyroid hormone replacement is provided after surgery.

THYROID NEOPLASMS

Benign neoplasms

Benign neoplasms of the thyroid are classified as adenomas. Most adenomas are seen to be nonfunctional (cold nodule) on scintiscan of the thyroid (Fig. 162-7), although occasionally they may demonstrate normal function (warm nodule) or hyperfunction (hot nodule), thereby suppressing the remainder of the thyroid tissue and causing thyrotoxicosis.

Thyroid adenomas are of greatest concern clinically because they must be differentiated from follicular thyroid cancer, which can be a significant diagnostic challenge. History and physical examination provide useful but generally inconclusive insights as to whether a nodule is malignant. Fig. 162-8 shows a suggested schema to differentiate benign from malignant nodules. Certain factors increase clinical suspicion of malignancy. A history of radiation exposure to head, neck, or upper chest during childhood is perhaps the single most important historical finding (see Special Problem, in the section Thyroid Cancer). Nodules developing in young (< age 20) or older patients (> age 60) or in males (any age) are more likely to be malignant. Rapid growth of the nodule, fixation to local structures in the neck, stony-hard consistency, and associated lymphadenopathy all suggest thyroid cancer. Occasional patients with differentiated thyroid cancer may have anterior cervical adenopathy in the absence of a palpable thyroid nodule. Family history is usually not contributory except in cases of medullary thyroid cancer occurring as part of the multiple endocrine neoplasia (MEN) syndrome types 2A and 2B.

The traditional laboratory evaluation procedures for a thyroid nodule fail to discriminate between benign and malignant lesions. A malignant thyroid nodule is almost always cold on radioiodine scan and most adenomas are cold nodules. However, a nodule that is clearly functional (warm or hot) is rarely a cancer; therefore, scintiscanning has a selective role in diagnostic testing. Ultrasonography provides good information about size and cystic elements but cannot reliably identify a malignancy and should not be used routinely.

Fine needle aspiration (FNA) thyroid biopsy is the most reliable and useful diagnostic technique for assessing whether a nodule is benign or malignant. Fine needle aspiration has excellent sensitivity and specificity, thereby significantly decreasing the indiscriminant removal of thyroid nodules. Nodules read as benign after aspiration biopsy have only a very small chance (range <1% to as high as 5%) of being malignant in actuality. Fine needle aspiration also assists in discriminating solid from cystic nodules. When the fine needle aspirate reveals a cyst, the fluid should be examined cytologically because a small percentage of cysts are associated with thyroid cancer. Unfortunately, the technique does not distinguish follicular adenoma from follicular carcinoma because the diagnosis of follicular carcinoma is largely based on capsular or vascular invasion, which cannot be discerned on a cytologic preparation from an aspiration biopsy. Biopsy findings of nodules that are interpreted to be malignant should prompt surgical removal. Biopsy results read as suspicious, significantly atypical, or indeterminate present a further problem. The nodule can be evaluated by radioiodine scanning and functioning nodules observed over time or, if cold, surgically removed.

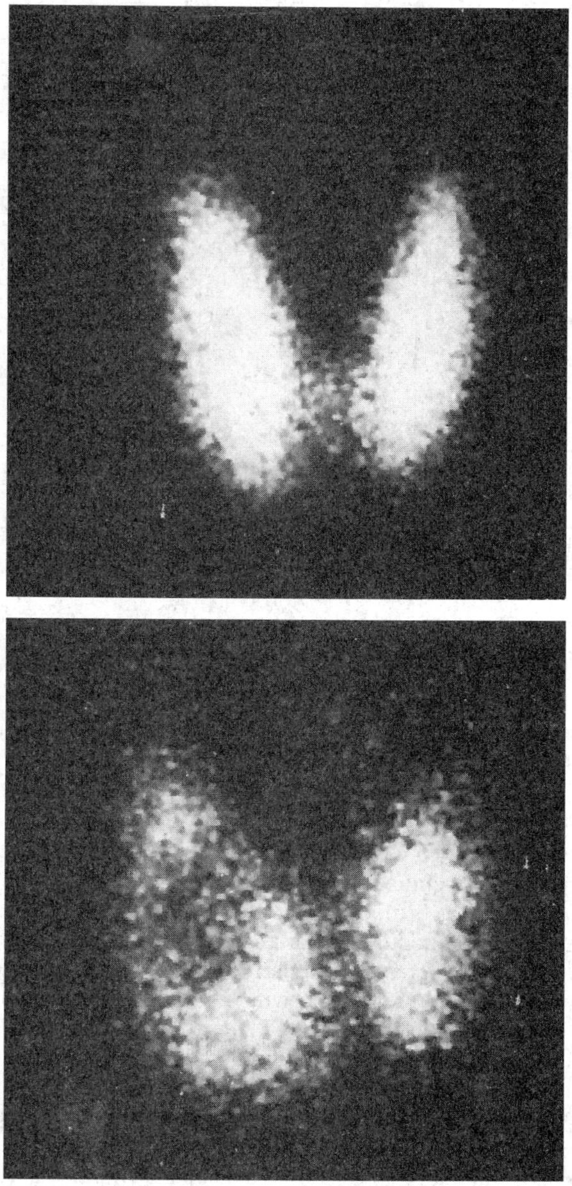

Fig. 162-7. Radioactive iodine scanning of the thyroid gland. The upper figure is that of a normal thyroid. The lower demonstrates a cold (nonfunctional) area in the right lobe.

Treatment. The medical treatment of a benign thyroid nodule is currently controversial. Historically such nodules are treated with suppression by synthetic L-thyroxine to de-

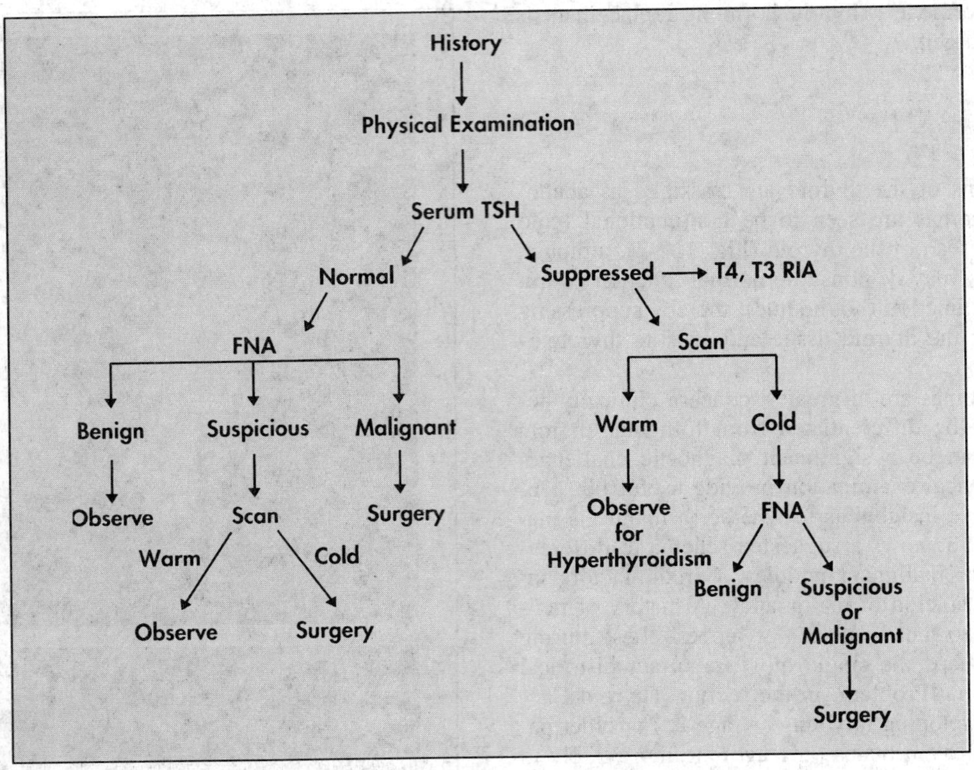

Fig. 162-8. Evaluation of a patient with a palpable thyroid nodule.

crease TSH level. A serum TSH level should be determined to prevent subclinical hyperthyroidism. Patients should be re-examined at 6 month intervals to determine changes in the size of the nodule. A variable percentage of warm and cold nodules regresses; similarly a variable percentage of thyroid nodules regresses without L-thyroxine therapy. Therefore the decision to use L-thyroxine must take into account this diversity of information, and perhaps pending updated clinical trials. Hyperfunctioning benign nodules may be treated with ^{131}I or surgery. Usually ^{131}I therapy is preferred because it is simple, safe, noninvasive, and less expensive than surgery and does not entail significant complications. Hypothyroidism usually does not ensue, in contrast to ^{131}I treatment of Graves' disease, because the hyperfunctioning nodule has suppressed TSH and the rest of the gland does not incorporate ^{131}I and is not destroyed.

Malignant neoplasms

Thyroid cancer is the most common endocrine cancer; however, among all types of cancers in the general population it is distinctly uncommon: there are about 10,000 to 12,000 new cases and about 1100 deaths per year. In its occult form thyroid cancer is much more common because routine autopsy studies reveal that as many as 5% to 20% of normal thyroid glands may have foci of malignant thyroid tissue, the clinical significance of which is unclear. The general term *thyroid cancer* incorporates different types of cancer ranging from well-differentiated, slow-growing tumors having an excellent prognosis to aggressive, poorly differentiated cancer with a poor prognosis. The facts that thyroid cancer represents less than 1% of all deaths of cancer and less than 10% of patients with thyroid cancer represents less than 1% of all deaths of cancer and less than 10% of patients with thyroid cancer die of the disease have promoted the reputation of thyroid cancer as a relatively benign malignancy. Because many patients who have the common thyroid malignancies are disease-free 20 to 30 years after diagnosis, various surgical and medical approaches may claim a certain success. Accepted therapies for the various thyroid cancers are discussed in the section devoted to each tumor.

The various types of primary thyroid cancers are listed in the box below. Three of the types are derived from follicular epithelium: papillary, follicular, and anaplastic. The other primary cancers of the thyroid are thyroid lymphoma and medullary cancer. The latter arises from the parafollicular or C cells and has distinctive biochemical manifestations.

Types of primary thyroid cancer

Papillary
Follicular
Anaplastic
Medullary
Lymphoma

Papillary carcinoma. Papillary carcinoma is the most common of the primary thyroid cancers, accounting for about 60% to 70% of all thyroid cancer in adults. It is more common in women than men (2:1 to 3:1), has a peak incidence in the third and fourth decades of life, may occur at any age, and is more aggressive in older patients. Most patients have an asymptomatic neck mass, occasionally several nodules are palpable, and in about one third of patients palpable cervical lymph nodes are present. Patients with papillary cancer may have a history of irradiation of the head, neck, or upper chest during childhood.

Papillary carcinoma is the slowest growing thyroid cancer. The tumor is unencapsulated and may infiltrate surrounding tissue, spreading by lymphatics to the cervical lymph nodes. In as many as 5% of patients an isolated cervical metastasis (formerly known as a lateral aberrant thyroid) may be the dominant finding and the thyroid gland may have only a microscopic focus of papillary cancer. Vascular invasion is rare. Distant metastases occur in about 10% of adults and are most frequent in lung, bone, and brain.

The tumor has a characteristic histopathologic picture consisting of folds of columnar epithelium, papillary projections (fronds), and scattered concentrically layered deposits of calcium called psammoma bodies. Most tumors are mixtures of papillary and follicular tumor elements. This characteristic has important therapeutic implications because follicular tumor tissue concentrates radioiodine whereas papillary does not.

Several factors are associated with a poorer prognosis for patients with papillary carcinoma, including age greater than 50, male sex, local tumor invasion at the time of surgery, and presence of distant metastases. Unlike that in primary cancers found in other organs, the presence of local lymph node metastases does not adversely affect the prognosis. The overall mortality rate of papillary carcinoma is quite low: survival rates of 90% or more at 20 or 30 years are the rule influenced by the risk factors noted earlier. The cause of death produced by this tumor is usually local tumor invasion involving the trachea and/or esophagus. In some patients, the tumor undergoes an anaplastic change, becoming more virulent and metastasizing widely.

Follicular carcinoma. Follicular carcinoma is a primary thyroid cancer that accounts for about 15% of all thyroid carcinoma. It is more common in women than men (2:1 to 3:1) and more common in patients over the age of 40. Many patients have a history of irradiation of the head, neck, or upper chest. There are a number of important differences between well-differentiated follicular and papillary carcinomas. Follicular carcinomas are encapsulated and usually spread by vascular invasion and not to regional lymph nodes. Patients with follicular cancer tend to have smaller thyroid tumors and may have distant metastasis. Bone metastases may occur early, are very destructive, and respond poorly to radioiodine therapy. Liver and lung are other common sites of distant metastases. Follicular tumor tissue has the ability to concentrate radioiodine, albeit less efficiently than normal thyroid tissue, and to synthesize thyroid hormone in minor amounts. Therefore widespread metastatic follicular carcinoma of substantial mass can occasionally produce enough thyroid hormone to induce thyrotoxicosis, most commonly T_3 toxicosis.

Follicular carcinoma, like papillary carcinoma, is a slow growing tumor; however, follicular carcinoma has a less favorable prognosis. The age of the patient and the degrees of capsular and vascular invasion influence the prognosis. Patients with lesser degrees of invasion have survival rates of 85% to 90% at 10 years, and greater degrees of invasion are associated with 50% or lower 10 year survival rates.

An uncommon variant of follicular carcinoma is the Hurthle cell carcinoma. This tumor is characterized by increased amounts of acidophilic cytoplasm, which on electron microscopy is shown to contain an abundance of mitochondria. These tumors may also metastasize widely. However, unlike follicular carcinoma, they rarely concentrate radioiodine.

Treatment. The surgical treatment of well-differentiated papillary and follicular carcinomas remains controversial; however, certain generalities can be stated. A papillary carcinoma less than 1.0 cm (micro carcinoma) in size is usually treated by lobectomy and isthmusectomy and examination of ipsilateral lymph nodes with removal of grossly involved nodes. Cure rates are high and postoperative radioiodine treatment unnecessary. Synthetic L-thyroxine should be given postoperatively in doses that lower TSH, but at the same time prevent subclinical thyrotoxicosis. TSH suppression is important because papillary (and follicular) cancers are to some degree TSH dependent.

Papillary carcinoma greater than 1.0 cm in size or infiltrative into surrounding tissues requires an operation that safely removes all thyroid tissue without associated complications of hypoparathyroidism or nerve paralysis. Surgery may be either a total thyroidectomy or a lobectomy on the involved side and near-total lobectomy on the contralateral side. In the higher risk patient thyroid hormone is withheld postoperatively until the patient has become hypothyroid, at which time radioiodine scanning is performed. Residual normal thyroid and tumor tissue is destroyed using high doses of ^{131}I. One week after this treatment a whole body scan is performed in an attempt to determine the presence of any distant, functional metastases. On completion of the postoperative diagnostic and therapeutic maneuvers synthetic L-thyroxine therapy is begun in doses adequate to suppress TSH as described. After surgery and adjunctive treatment yearly follow-up evaluation is required; this entails careful neck examination and serum thyroglobulin level determinations that provide a sensitive indicator for residual or recurrent tumor tissue, because normal tissue has been destroyed by the ^{131}I. Selected patients require radioiodine scanning.

Follicular cancer regardless of size is treated by total thyroidectomy or a procedure modified to perform a total lobectomy on the involved side and near-total lobectomy on the contralateral side. Unlike in papillary carcinoma there is no relationship of size to the aggressive behavior of the tumor. ^{131}I is administered and follow-up evaluation is conducted as described.

Anaplastic carcinoma. About 5% of thyroid cancers are anaplastic. The tumor is slightly more common in women than men and may arise from pre-existing papillary carcinoma or multinodular goiter. It has a peak incidence in the sixth and seventh decades of life, although it has been reported in patients less than 40 years old, including some children. The clinical picture is usually that of a rapidly growing thyroid mass that may be associated with dysphagia, hoarseness, hemoptysis, and respiratory distress. The mass is very firm to stony-hard on palpation and is fixed to surrounding structures. This aggressive clinical course must be differentiated from that of thyroid lymphoma (discussed later), which is treatable and generally has a more favorable prognosis. Most patients with anaplastic carcinoma die within months after the diagnosis is made, and few survive more than 1 year.

Histopathologic examination of needle biopsy specimens reveals anaplastic spindle and multinucleated giant cells with many mitoses; areas of necrosis and inflammation are prominent. Islands of papillary and/or follicular carcinoma may be present, supporting the likelihood of a precursor role for these tumors in some cases.

Treatment is palliative. Surgery is best used to relieve tracheal and esophageal obstruction. Chemotherapy and radioiodine therapy are usually ineffective; radiotherapy can in some cases slow disease progression.

Lymphoma. Thyroid lymphoma accounts for only a small percentage of thyroid cancer cases. It is more common in women than men (3:1) and has a peak incidence in the seventh or eight decade of life but may occur as early as the third decade. The history is usually one of a rapidly enlarging mass in the thyroid associated with varying degrees of pain and tenderness. There may be hoarseness and respiratory distress. The tumor is very firm to stony-hard on palpation.

Findings of histopathologic examination are most often consistent with a diffuse histiocytic lymphoma. Importantly, there is almost always histologic evidence of Hashimoto's thyroiditis and many patients are hypothyroid. Most thyroid lymphoma patients have markedly elevated levels of thyroid antimicrosomal and antithyroglobulin antibodies. The relation of Hashimoto's thyroiditis to thyroid lymphoma appears to be more than coincidental. Although the actual number of cases of thyroid lymphoma arising in patients with Hashimoto's thyroiditis is small, the risk of development of thyroid lymphoma is higher in patients with Hashimoto's thyroiditis, as is the risk of development of other lymphoproliferactive or myeloproliferative syndromes.

The diagnosis of thyroid lymphoma is usually made by fine needle aspiration, large (core) needle biopsy, and occasionally open biopsy. Large needle biopsy or open biopsy results may be more reliable because the specimens obtained provide an opportunity to assess intact histologic features that are critical to distinguishing lymphoma from Hashimoto's thyroiditis. Evidence for associated Hashimoto's thyroiditis and the biopsy results serve to distinguish thyroid lymphoma from anaplastic carcinoma, which has similar clinical features.

The prognosis is improved by early diagnosis. When lymphoma is confined to the thyroid gland, 5 year survival rates are as high as 75% to 85%; extension into the neck has a 5 year survival rate of about 35% to 40% and widely disseminated lymphoma a 5 year survival rate of only about 5%. Patients below the age of 65 and men have significantly longer median survival rates.

The treatment of thyroid lymphoma usually consists of radiotherapy and chemotherapy alone or in combination. Surgery is only performed to relieve tracheal obstruction or occasionally to stage for more extensive disease.

Medullary carcinoma. Approximately 5% to 10% of all new cases of thyroid cancer are medullary carcinomas. The tumor arises from the parafollicular C cells, which produce the polypeptide hormone calcitonin. It is slightly more common in women than men and has a peak incidence in the fifth and sixth decades of life. There are three forms of medullary thyroid cancer: sporadic, that associated with multiple endocrine neoplasia (MEN) type 2A (Sipple's syndrome), and that associated with MEN type 2B. Patients usually have a clinically apparent thyroid mass that is cold on scintiscan. When associated with MEN type 2A there may be a history of pheochromocytoma or hyperparathyroidism; with type 2B there may be a history of pheochromocytoma and a clinical picture of marfanoid habitus and diffuse ganglioneuromas most evident on the tongue.

The sporadic form is more common (about 4:1), occurs in older age groups (above age 40), and is usually unilateral. The familial forms are inherited as an autosomal dominant trait, are usually bilateral, and occur at a younger age. Medullary carcinoma associated with MEN 2A has the overall best prognosis, that associated with MEN 2B the worst; the prognosis for the sporadic form is intermediate. Disease prognosis is directly related to the degree of tumor calcitonin as measured by immunohistochemistry. Medullary carcinoma spreads via lymphatics to lymph nodes in the neck and mediastinum. It also regularly metastasizes to distant sites, most commonly lung, bone, and liver.

Medullary thyroid carcinoma has demonstrable biochemical markers and may be associated with several paraneoplastic syndromes. Calcitonin level is the biologic marker for this tumor and is elevated in the basal state or with stimulation by pentagastrin or calcium infusion in most cases. Calcitonin level provides a unique marker to detect early stages of medullary cancer in patients having the familial forms because basal and/or stimulated calcitonin levels are elevated when C-cell hyperplasia, the precursor lesion of medullary carcinoma, is present. Serum calcitonin levels provide the most useful tool for detecting the existence of residual tumor tissue postoperatively. Despite its role in downward regulation of serum calcium, the elevated level of calcitonin associated with this tumor only rarely results in hypocalcemia.

Medullary thyroid carcinoma is also associated with

classic Cushing's syndrome or carcinoid syndrome caused by the ectopic production of ACTH or serotonin by the tumor. Ectopic production of prostaglandins, kinins, and vasoactive intestinal peptide leads to watery diarrhea in certain patients. The tumor also produces histaminase, which is a useful marker for metastatic disease, and carcinoembryonic antigen, another potential tumor marker.

Diagnosis of medullary carcinoma of the thyroid is usually made by the determination of basal and/or stimulated levels of calcitonin. In the familial forms a diagnostic evaluation for pheochromocytoma is imperative before any surgical intervention. Patients with MEN type 2A should also have determinations of serum calcium and parathyroid hormone levels.

Tissue diagnosis is readily made by large needle or open biopsy, most commonly at the time of surgery. The tumor consists of large aggregates of C cells, epithelial cells, fibrous tissue, and deposits of amyloid. Deposits of calcium salts account for the occasional observation of dense, homogeneous conglomerate calcifications on routine radiographs of the primary or metastatic tumor.

Treatment of medullary carcinoma of the thyroid consists of total thyroidectomy with prophylactic central lymph node dissection. Lateral cervical lymph nodes are sampled, and if the result is positive, lymphadenectomy is performed. Normal-appearing nodes are usually not removed. Most surgeons do not perform aggressive, radical neck dissection as its utility in producing longer survival rates and cures is uncertain. Radiotherapy, radioiodine therapy, and chemotherapy are generally ineffective. In the familial forms determination of basal and stimulated calcitonin levels is essential to detect the precursor of medullary carcinoma, C-cell hyperplasia, because thyroidectomy at this stage is curative.

Risk factors associated with poor prognosis include male sex, lymph node involvement, extrathyroidal extension, and association with MEN type 2B. Five to ten year survival rates of 67% to 80% are not uncommon in the various reported series with sporadic tumors and tumors associated with MEN type 2A.

Special problem: external irradiation of the head, neck, and upper thorax in infancy and childhood. External irradiation of the head, neck, or upper thorax was administered in the past to treat a variety of conditions, including recurrent tonsillitis, adenoiditis, acne, tinea capitis, and thymic enlargement. The thyroid was incidentally irradiated by these procedures. Although not appreciated at the time, relatively small doses of radiation during infancy and childhood increase the risk of developing benign and malignant thyroid neoplasms. Another unfortunate demonstration of the effects of external irradiation has been a consequence of the atomic bomb blasts (Japan and Marshall Islands), which resulted in an increased incidence of both benign and malignant thyroid nodules.

It requires a latency of approximately 5 years after exposure to develop a thyroid tumor, but the patient remains at increased risk for at least 30 to 40 years after exposure and possibly for life. Probably a thyroid neoplasm develops in no more than half of those irradiated and most are benign. However, in about 5% of the irradiated group differentiated thyroid carcinoma develops. The tumors are generally slow-growing, relatively nonaggressive, and frequently multicentric, and thyroid scintiscanning does not always reflect areas of involvement. Microscopic foci of cancer have been observed in areas indicated to be normal by scintiscanning.

The initial evaluation of all patients who have received external irradiation to the thyroid gland should include examination of the thyroid gland for any palpable abnormality. In the absence of any abnormality, some physicians recommend physiologic replacement therapy with thyroid hormone, with the aim of suppressing TSH secretion to decrease the chance of developing a thyroid neoplasm. Whether this desirable goal can be accomplished is uncertain. Any palpable thyroid nodule is a candidate for open surgical biopsy, but perhaps fine needle aspiration cytologic evaluation can be used to guide therapy. All patients should have a determination of thyroid autoantibody levels in the initial evaluation, because a scan abnormality or a diffuse or irregular enlargement of the thyroid gland may be due to Hashimoto's thyroiditis. Physical examination of the neck should be performed yearly.

Total or near-total thyroidectomy is the treatment of choice for thyroid cancer in this setting followed by ablation of residual thyroid tissue with radioiodine. The overall prognosis is no different from that described for differentiated thyroid cancer.

REFERENCES

DeGroot LJ: Diagnostic approach and management of patients exposed to irradiation to the thyroid. J Clin Endocrinol Metab 69:925, 1989.

Demeure MJ and Clark OH: Surgery in the treatment of thyroid cancer. Endocrinol Metab North Am 19(3):663, 1990.

Gharib H et al: Suppressive therapy with levothyroxine for solitary thyroid nodules. N Engl J Med 317:70, 1987.

Goodwin TM et al: The role of chorionic gonadotropin in transient hyperthyroidism of hyperemesis gravidarum. J Clin Endocrinol Metab 75:1333, 1992.

Hamburger JI: The various presentations of thyroiditis: diagnostic considerations. Ann Intern Med 104:219, 1986.

Hashizume K et al: Administration of thyroxine in treated Graves' disease: effect on the level of antibodies to thyroid-stimulating hormone receptors and on the risk of recurrence of hyperthyroidism. N Engl J Med 324:947, 1991.

Helfand M and Crapo LM: Monitoring therapy in patients taking levothyroxine. Ann Intern Med 113:450, 1990.

Klein I and Ojamaa I: Cardiovascular manifestations of endocrine disease. J Clin Endocrinol Metab 75:339, 1992.

Levey GS and Klein I: Catecholamine-thyroid hormone interactions and the cardiovascular manifestations of hyperthyroidism. Am J Med 88:642, 1990.

Mazzaferri EL: Thyroid cancer in thyroid nodules: finding a needle in the haystack. Am J Med 93:359, 1992.

Spencer CA: Clinical utility and cost-effectiveness of sensitive thyrotropin assays in ambulatory and hospitalized patients. Mayo Clin Proc 63:1214, 1988.

Utiger R: Vanishing hypothyroidism. N Engl J Med 326:562, 1992.

VanHerle AJ et al: The thyroid nodule. Ann Intern Med 96:221, 1982.

CHAPTER

163 Disorders of the Adrenal Cortex

John Kendall
D. Lynn Loriaux

STRUCTURE AND FUNCTION OF THE ADRENAL GLANDS

The adrenal cortex, like the steroid-producing cells of the gonads, arises from the splanchnic mesoderm during the second month of fetal life. The adrenal medulla is derived from the neuroectoderm and joins the cortical cells during the sixth week of fetal life. The adrenal glands are in the retroperitoneal space adjacent to the upper pole of the kidney and derive their blood supply from small arteries arising from the aorta, the inferior phrenic, and the renal arteries. The venous drainage of the left adrenal gland is into the left renal vein, whereas the right adrenal gland empties directly into the inferior vena cava. The glands are conical in shape and have a combined weight of 6 to 10 g. The cortical portion of the gland is divided into three zones, each having special functional properties. The outermost zone, *zona glomerulosa,* is composed of clusters of lipid-poor cells that primarily synthesize aldosterone and 18-hydroxy-corticosterone. The intermediate layer, *zona fasciculata,* is thicker and primarily synthesizes cortisol and its precursors. The innermost zone, *zona reticularis,* primarily synthesizes the weak adrenal androgens, dehydroepiandrosterone and androstenedione. Both of these inner zones are lipid-rich.

The adrenal medulla occupies the central core of the gland and is composed of chromaffin cells that synthesize and secrete norepinephrine and epinephrine. The conversion of norepinephrine to epinephrine is a cortisol-dependent reaction, and the location of the adrenal medulla inside the cortisol-producing adrenal cortex facilitates this reaction.

Biosynthesis of adrenocortical hormones

The core structure of all adrenal steroids is the four-ring cyclopentanoperhydrophenanthrene nucleus. It is composed of 17 carbon atoms. Modifications, primarily at positions 11, 17, and 18, lead to a series of compounds with glucocorticoid, mineralocorticoid, androgenic, and estrogenic activities (Fig. 163-1). Adrenal steroid biosynthesis begins with cholesterol. Cholesterol can be synthesized in the adrenal gland de novo, or taken up from the circulating plasma. The first step in steroid biosynthesis occurs in the mitochondria, where the cholesterol desmolase enzyme system removes six carbons of the cholesterol side chain, yielding pregnenolone. Most of the remaining biosynthetic steps occur in the microsomes. Certain enzymatic modifications are specific to the different zones of the adrenal cortex. For example, in the zona glomerulosa, pregnenolone is converted to progesterone and then to a series of aldosterone precursors. In the zona fasciculata and reticularis, pregnenolone and progesterone are hydroxylated at the 17-position to form precursors of all other adrenal steroids. Cortisol accounts for about 50% of the total adrenal steroid secretion. The "adrenal androgens," dehydroepiandrosterone (DHEA) and androstenedione, account for most of the remainder. Small amounts of estrogen and testosterone are derived from the adrenal androgens.

Regulation of adrenocortical secretion

The adrenal cortex is under the control of two stimulatory peptides: ACTH and angiotensin II. Other factors such as serum sodium and potassium can modulate aldosterone secretion. The principal modulator of adrenocortical steroid biosynthesis, however, is ACTH. ACTH is a 39 amino acid polypeptide. A synthetic derivative, cosyntropin contains the first 24 amino acids of the native molecule and is commercially available for the clinical evaluation of adrenocortical function.

ACTH binds to cell surface receptors and stimulates cell growth and biosynthesis of steroid hormones. ACTH increases the adrenal cellular uptake of cholesterol and stimulates the first rate-limiting step in steroid biosynthesis, the conversion of cholesterol to pregnenolone. ACTH is secreted by pituitary corticotrophs that are regulated, in turn, by two hypothalamic hormones: corticotropin-releasing hormone (CRH) and vasopressin. ACTH secretion is episodic. There are about 10 secretory "bursts" during each day, the majority clustered between 6 and 10 A.M. The nadir of ACTH secretion occurs during the early hours of sleep. Cortisol secretion is entrained to ACTH secretion, leading to the familiar diurnal pattern of plasma cortisol concentration: high cortisol levels in the early morning, low cortisol levels in the evening.

Stresses such as trauma, infection, fear, and volume depletion lead to increased cortisol secretion. This increase in secretion usually is sustained for the duration of the stress. With the termination of stress, it subsides in a matter of hours. Circulating concentrations of cortisol are maintained in the "normal" range by a negative feedback system. Cortisol restrains its own secretion by inhibiting corticotropin-releasing hormone (CRH) secretion and by inhibiting the ability of CRH to stimulate ACTH secretion from the anterior pituitary gland. This effect of cortisol is blunted by stress and is absent in some diseases such as Cushing's disease. As expected, glucocorticoid administration can suppress ACTH secretion. If glucocorticoids are administered in supraphysiologic amounts for a prolonged period, pituitary-adrenal axis suppression can be clinically significant. Gradual recovery of the pituitary-adrenal axis follows withdrawal of corticosteroids. It can require more than a year if the duration of treatment is prolonged.

Aldosterone secretion is regulated primarily by the renin-angiotensin system. Renin is secreted by the juxtaglomerular cells in response to decreased "effective" blood pressure in the afferent arterioles of the kidney. Renin, in turn,

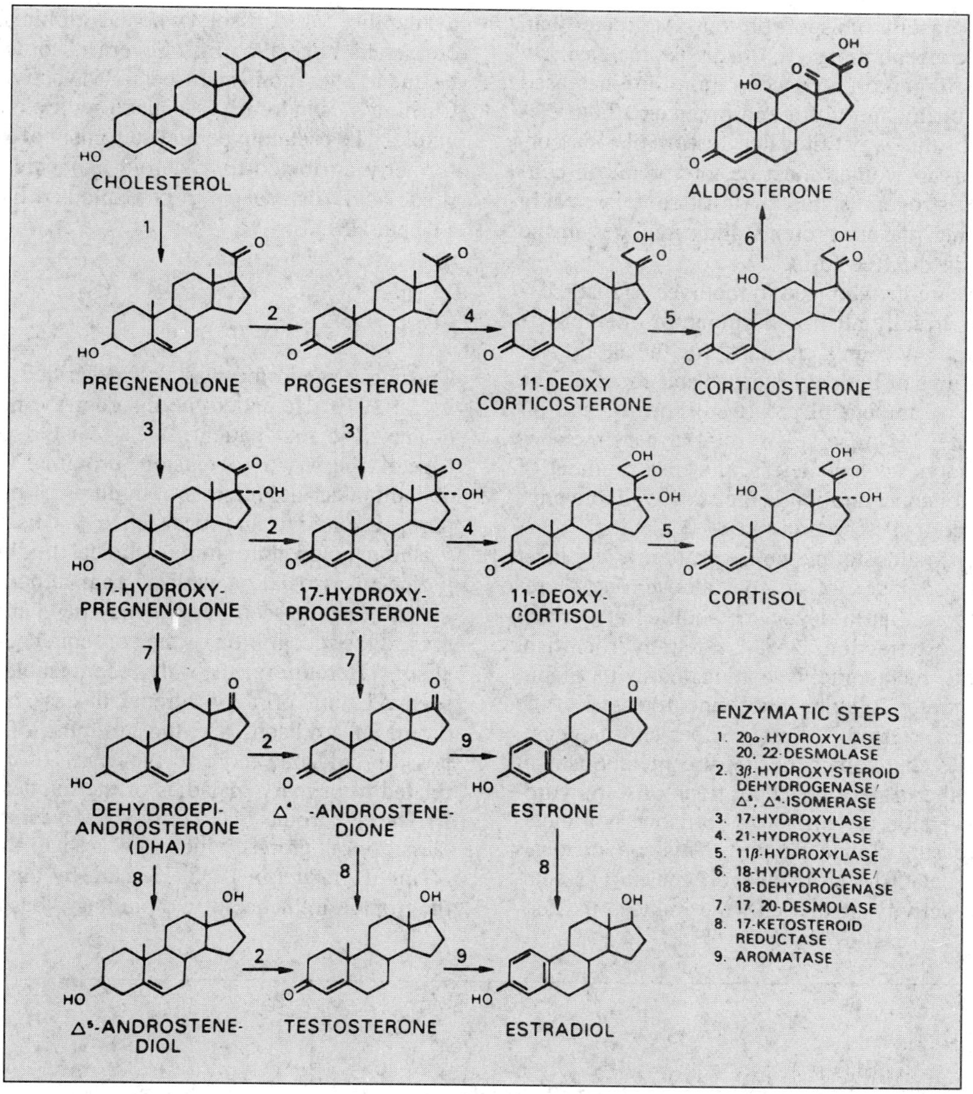

Fig. 163-1. The steroid biosynthetic cascade from cholesterol to the four classes of steroid hormones of adrenal origin: glucocorticoids, mineralocorticoids, androgens, and estrogens.

converts angiotensinogen, a polypeptide prohormone of hepatic origin, to angiotensin I, a decapeptide. Angiotensin I in turn is converted to angiotensin II, the bioactive octapeptide, by angiotensin converting enzyme (ACE) in vascular endothelial cells. Angiotensin II acts directly on the zona glomerulosa to stimulate aldosterone biosynthesis and secretion. Like that of ACTH, its primary action is on the rate-limiting biosynthetic step that converts cholesterol to pregnenolone. Aldosterone and the less potent mineralocorticoid precursors, desoxycorticosterone, corticosterone, and 18-hydroxycorticosterone, act principally on the kidneys to retain sodium and expand extracellular fluid volume. As volume expands, the stimulus for renin secretion is reduced, angiotensin II production is diminished, and mineralocorticoid secretion slows. In addition to the important role in regulating aldosterone secretion, angiotensin II has several effects on normal circulating fluid volume and blood pressure. It stimulates vascular smooth muscle contraction, renal tubular sodium reabsorption, and decreases free water clearance.

Potassium and sodium also can modulate aldosterone secretion. Potassium and angiotensin II both increase free calcium level in zona gomerulosa cells. It has been proposed that the final common pathway for both of these effects, and perhaps for that of ACTH as well, is through a calcium mediated "second messenger" transduction system. Sodium also affects zona glomerulosa function, but its regulatory effects appear to be mediated through changes in vascular volume. Other suggested modulators of aldosterone production include dopamine (inhibitory), proopiomelanocortin derivatives (stimulatory), and atrial natriuretic hormone (stimulatory).

Circulating cortisol is bound to plasma proteins. At normal plasma cortisol concentrations, only 10% is free. The protein bound fraction is divided between transcortin, a high-affinity low-capacity alpha globulin, and albumin, a low-affinity high-capacity transport protein. At greater than normal plasma concentrations, cortisol is increasingly bound to albumin. Transcortin concentrations are increased by estrogen. The birth control pill and pregnancy both elevate transcortins in this way. Elevated resting plasma cortisol concentrations in women must be interpreted in conjunction with the estrogen "status." Aldosterone is weakly bound to circulating plasma proteins and circulates in the plasma primarily in the free form.

Both hormones are metabolized in the liver. Hepatic extraction removes virtually all free hormone in one "pass." This rapid clearance accounts, in part, for the lability of plasma concentrations of both aldosterone and cortisol. The urinary excretion of unmetabolized (free) cortisol and aldosterone constitutes less than 1% of total urinary metabolites of these hormones. Nonetheless, the measurement of urinary free cortisol concentration is the best available clinical index of the cortisol secretion rate.

Urinary tetrahydroaldosterone concentration is the most commonly employed index of adrenal aldosterone secretion. There are more than a dozen metabolites of cortisol in urine. The largest fraction, 25%, is tetrahydrocortisol (Fig. 163-2). This metabolite is conjugated with glucuronide, making it water-soluble. It accounts for most of the urinary "17- hydroxysteroids" (Porter-Silber chromogens). Drugs and diseases that affect the hepatic metabolism of cortisol can alter the urinary concentrations of tetrahydrocortisol. The conversion of cortisol to cortisone is a metabolic step of increasing clinical interest. This conversion is dependent on 11-betaOH-steroid dehydrogenase (11-beta-HSD). Enhanced activity of this enzyme reduces the bioavailability of cortisol, whereas diminished activity increases its bioavailability. Several disorders are thought to be due to alterations in 11-beta-HSD activity. The "pseudo-Cushing's" syndrome associated with alcoholism is an example. The pseudohyperaldosteronism of licorice ingestion, formerly attributed to a steroid agonistic effect of glycyrrhizic acid, also seems to be explained by an inhibition of 11-beta-HSD.

ADRENAL HYPERFUNCTION

Cushing's syndrome

Cushing's syndrome was first described by Harvey Cushing in 1910. He called the disorder the polyglandular syndrome. The first patient, a 23-year-old woman, had centripetal obesity, hypertension, proximal muscle weakness, abdominal striae, hirsutism, thinning of the scalp hair, purpura, insomnia, and backache. In discussing the case, Cushing noted that similar clinical findings had been reported in association with adrenal tumors and concluded, "It will thus be seen that we may perchance be on the way toward the recognition of the consequences of "hyperadrenalism." Heretofore, the only recognizable clinical state associated with primary adrenal disease has been the syndrome of Addison, and the grouping of these cases may possibly add one more to the series of clinical conditions related to primary maladies of the ductless glands."

The syndrome was codified 20 years later in his now classic monograph, which appeared in the *Johns Hopkins Medical Journal* in 1932. He had, by this time, recognized the trophic influence of the pituitary "basophils" on the ad-

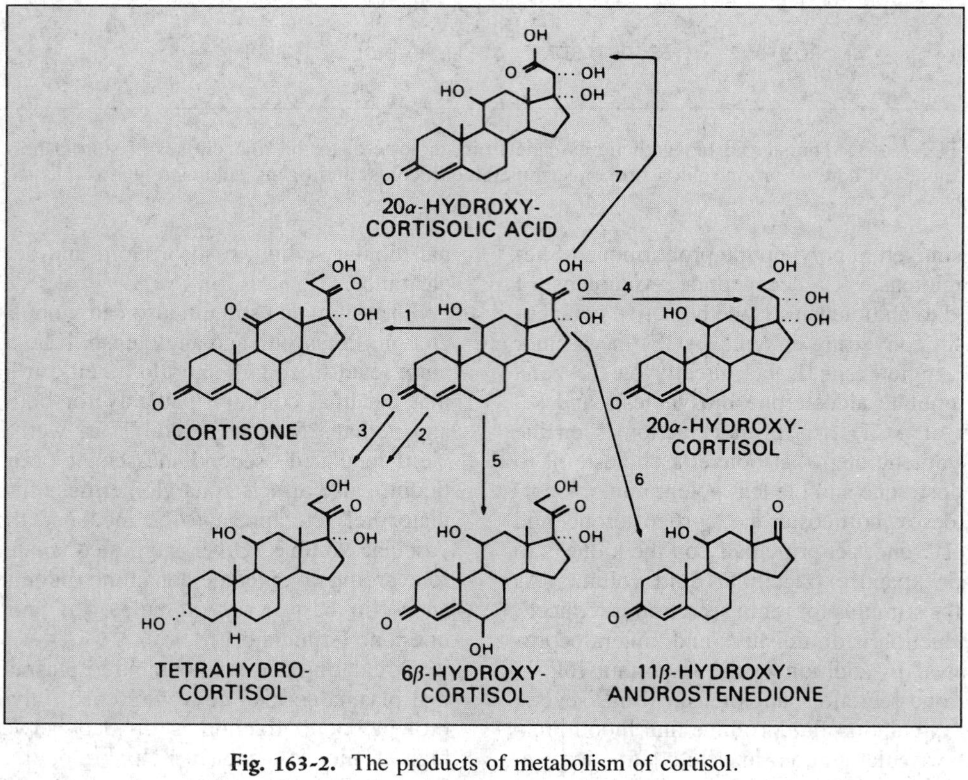

Fig. 163-2. The products of metabolism of cortisol.

renal glands and shown that basophilic tumors of the pituitary gland can cause the same clinical syndrome as tumors of the adrenal gland. The stage was thus set for the current classification of Cushing's syndrome into ACTH dependent and ACTH independent forms.

Clinical manifestations. The adrenal cortex produces three classes of steroid hormones: glucocorticoids, mineralocorticoids, and sex steroid (androgen and estrogen) precursors. Hyperfunction of the gland can produce clinical signs of increased activity of one or all of these steroid hormone types. Cushing's syndrome is the clinical expression of the overproduction of glucocorticoid.

Increased glucocorticoid action can be thought of as "antianabolic." The biochemical mechanism can be conceptualized as energy deprivation resulting from a glucocorticoid mediated antagonism of insulin action. The concept, even though an oversimplification, explains why so many cell types diminish "specialized" activity as a consequence of glucocorticoid excess. As a prime manifestation, protein wasting occurs, with the result that muscles become weak, bones become thin, and skin is rendered unable to sustain the stresses of normal activity, leading to striae and poor wound healing. The vasculature becomes fragile and ecchymosis results. The immune system is less efficient, encouraging opportunistic infection. Insulin resistance leads to glucose intolerance.

Most patients with Cushing's syndrome gain weight; some lose it. As expected, the difference appears to depend on food intake. A good appetite in the presence of hypercortisolism leads to truncal obesity with a characteristic accentuation of fat deposition in a yoke-like distribution over the clavicles and around the neck. Failure of appetite prevents this. Thus cancer and other wasting illnesses, when associated with hypercortisolism, can manifest only the "antianabolic" features of the illness.

To the extent that sex steroid precursors are produced, women manifest some degree of masculinization and men manifest some degree of feminization. To the extent that mineralocorticoids are produced, arterial hypertension and hypokalemic alkalosis occur. Laboratory findings associated with hypercortisolism are confined mainly to the complete blood count, in which erythrocytosis, granulocytosis, and lymphocytopenia are prominent manifestations.

Causes of Cushing's syndrome

There are six recognized causes of Cushing's syndrome. They can be divided into ACTH dependent and ACTH independent types (Table 163-1). ACTH dependent Cushing's syndrome has two causes, the ACTH secreting pituitary adenoma and the nonpituitary ACTH secreting tumor. ACTH secreting pituitary tumors are referred to as Cushing's disease, the most common cause of Cushing's syndrome. For reasons yet unknown, the small tumors that cause this disorder are resistant, to varying degrees, to the "feedback" effects of cortisol. Thus they maintain plasma cortisol "homeostasis" in a range that is too high for all tissues but the microadenoma itself. Like the normal gland, these tumors secrete ACTH in a pulsatile fashion. Unlike in the normal gland, the diurnal pattern of cortisol secretion is lost. These tumors are usually small and rarely alter the bony architecture of the sella turcica.

The ectopic production of ACTH is most commonly caused by neoplasms of the lung. Other tumors include endocrine tumors of foregut origin and the pheochromocytoma (Table 163-2). These tumors often process the proopiomelanocortin parent protein differently than pituitary tissue. Hence ACTH from these tumors frequently can be distinguished from that of pituitary origin.

The hallmark of the ACTH dependent forms of Cushing's syndrome is the presence of a measurable plasma ACTH level in a patient with clinical and biochemical "hypercortisolism."

The ACTH independent forms of Cushing's syndrome are adrenal in origin. (This excludes factitious or iatrogenic causes of Cushing's syndrome, which are becoming more common.) Adrenal cancers are usually large when Cushing's syndrome becomes manifest. As many as half of these tumors can be palpated through the abdominal wall at the first visit to a physician. The average size of these tumors is about 6 cm in diameter, making them easily detectable

Table 163-1. Causes of Cushing's syndrome

Cause	Relative incidence
ACTH dependent	75%
Cushing's disease	60%
Ectopic ACTH secretion	15%
Ectopic CRH secretion	<1%
ACTH independent	25%
Endogenous	
Adrenal cancer	15%
Adrenal adenoma	10%
Micronodular adrenal disease	<1%
Exogenous	
Factitious	<1%
Iatrogenic	Very common

Table 163-2. Tumors associated with the ectopic ACTH syndrome

Tumor	Frequency (%)
Oat cell carcinoma	50
Tumors of foregut origin	35
Thymic carcinoma	
Islet cell tumor	
Medullary carcinoma of thyroid	
Bronchial carcinoid	
Pheochromocytoma	5
Other	10
Gonadal	
Prostate and cervical carcinoma	
Tumors of unknown origin	

by computed tomographic (CT)-scan. Adrenal cancers can produce steroids other than cortisol. Thus when Cushing's syndrome is accompanied by virilization, feminization, or mineralocorticoid excess, the likelihood of adrenal cancer increases.

Adrenal adenomas average 3 cm in diameter. These tumors are not commonly associated with other steroid mediated syndromes and usually produce only cortisol.

Micronodular adrenal disease is a disorder of children, adolescents, and young adults. The adrenal glands contain numerous small (<3 mm) pigmented nodules that secrete cortisol in sufficient quantity to suppress pituitary ACTH secretion. The cortex between the micronodules is atrophic, in contrast to the ACTH mediated processes. The biochemical pathogenesis of this disorder is unknown. It can occur in sporadic or familial form. Several pigmented lentigines, cardiac myxomas, and other neoplasms can be associated with it.

The most common cause of ACTH independent of Cushing's syndrome is iatrogenic. Glucocorticoids in pharmacologic quantities are used to treat many diseases with an inflammatory component. Given enough time, this leads to Cushing's syndrome with all its attendant untoward sequelae. Rarely glucocorticoids are taken surreptitiously, posing a difficult diagnostic challenge for the clinician.

Diagnosis and differential diagnosis. The diagnosis of Cushing's syndrome requires the clinical picture of the disorder in association with supporting biochemical evidence of glucocorticoid excess. The biochemical abnormalities of Cushing's syndrome are two: an increased secretion rate of cortisol and a disordered circadian pattern of cortisol secretion. There are two important caveats. First, these abnormalities can have a periodic variation in intensity or can even be intermittent. Second, they are not found in most cases of factitious or iatrogenic Cushing's syndrome.

The most useful clinical test for assessing the cortisol production rate is the urinary free cortisol excretion rate. Values consistently in excess of 250 μg/day are virtually diagnostic of Cushing's syndrome. Depression, alcoholism, hypoglycemia, and psychic or physical stress can produce urinary free cortisol excretion rates above normal, but these values are rarely greater than 250 μg/day. Thus in the "gray" zone between normal (<100 μg/day) and 250 μg/day are many patients with "pseudo-Cushing's" syndrome and a few with "true" Cushing's syndrome.

Characteristic of the pseudo-Cushing's disorders, however, is a "normal" diurnal pattern of cortisol secretion. This contrasts with Cushing's syndrome, in which that rhythm is lost. Thus a clear demonstration of the loss of normal diurnal variation is strong evidence for the diagnosis of Cushing's syndrome. Because cortisol is secreted in a pulsatile fashion in normal and abnormal states, single morning and evening values are inadequate for this demonstration. We recommend sampling blood at 30 minute intervals between 6:00 and 8:00 A.M., and 10:00 and 12:00 P.M. for the measurement of cortisol. The rule of thumb is that the mean evening value should be less than half of the mean morning value, assuming a "normal" sleep-wake cycle. This approach allows the diagnosis of Cushing's syndrome in some patients who are excreting urinary free cortisol in amounts less than 250 μg/day.

Once the diagnosis of Cushing's syndrome has been established, effective therapy depends on an accurate differential diagnosis of the underlying cause. The traditional approach to this problem employs the dexamethasone suppression test. Administration of exogenous dexamethasone, at a dose of 2 mg/day for 2 days, suppresses the urinary excretion of Porter-Silber chromogens to less than 2 mg/day in virtually all normal people. The same qualitative phenomenon occurs in patients with Cushing's disease, but the necessary dose is greater. In 80% to 90% of patients with Cushing's disease the excretion of Porter-Silber chromogens is reduced by more than 50% of "baseline" at a dose of dexamethasone 8 mg/day. In patients with other causes of Cushing's syndrome this dose of dexamethasone usually fails to suppress the excretion of Porter-Silber chromogens. Because Cushing's disease accounts for 70% of patients with Cushing's syndrome, the majority of patients can be classified in this way. Failure to suppress the excretion of Porter-Silber chromogens with dexamethasone should lead to a careful search for primary adrenal disease with adrenal CT scan and, if it is absent, a thorough search for an ectopic source of ACTH secretion. This search should concentrate on the chest, where more than 90% of these lesions are found. Full lung CT and magnetic resonance imaging (MRI) scanning is the procedure of choice.

This approach to the differential diagnosis of Cushing's syndrome, however, misclassifies as many as 15% of patients with Cushing's disease. In addition, certain ACTH secreting tumors, notably the bronchial carcinoid, can meet the criteria in up to 40% of cases. Finally patients with "periodic" Cushing's syndrome are easily misclassified by this traditional approach.

Recent improvements in ACTH measurement technique have allowed a new approach to the differential diagnosis of Cushing's syndrome based on the measurement of plasma ACTH concentration and the response of ACTH to CRF.

The concept underlying this approach is that if ACTH is measurable in the plasma of a "hypercortisolemic" patient, the process is ACTH dependent. This categorizes patients into ACTH dependent and ACTH independent forms of Cushing's syndrome. The precise localization of the site of ACTH production can be accomplished with the technique of inferior petrosal sinus sampling for plasma ACTH.

Inferior petrosal sinus sampling allows the measurement of ACTH concentrations in blood immediately draining the pituitary gland. The average gradient of ACTH concentration, central to peripheral blood, is 20. The lower limit of this range in patients with a pituitary ACTH source is a ratio of 2. If the gradient is measured 3 to 5 minutes after CRF administration, the lower bound is 3. The maximum gradient seen in subjects with an ectopic source of ACTH is 2 in either circumstance. Thus the test has immense power for localizing disease "to" or "away from" the pituitary gland.

The test has the added benefit of allowing the preoperative localization of the ACTH secreting microadenoma to the right or left hemisphere of the anterior pituitary gland. A right to left gradient greater than 1.5 has been associated with correct localization in 85% of surgically confirmed cases. The gradient can be attributed to the almost complete lateralization of the venous drainage from the right to left halves of the pituitary gland into the right or left inferior petrosal sinuses.

This information allows the surgeon, in the absence of an identifiable tumor, to remove the "hemipituitary" suspected of harboring the lesion. It should be noted that the interpretation of apparent lateralization in samples obtained by inferior petrosal sinus sampling is reliable only if the sella turcica has not been surgically explored previously. Once operated on, the venous drainage of the pituitary gland is so altered that interpretation of relative ACTH concentrations, right to left, has no diagnostic value.

When ACTH cannot be measured in the plasma, the search for primary adrenal disease or a factitious cause of Cushing's syndrome should proceed as outlined under the traditional approach to differential diagnosis.

If either the traditional approach or the contemporary "ACTH directed" approach discloses contradictory or inconsistent results, periodic or intermittent hypersecretion of cortisol should be suspected. This can be verified only by serial urine collections for the measurement of urinary free cortisol or Porter-Silber chromogens. Once it is established, however, inferior petrosal sinus sampling during a "hypersecretory" period is a powerful approach to differentialed diagnosis.

Treatment

Cushing's disease. The rediscovery of the transsphenoidal approach to the pituitary fossa, coupled with modern optics and image intensification, has moved neurosurgical treatment of Cushing's disease into the forefront of the treatment options for this disorder. In the hands of a skilled surgeon, the success of this approach exceeds 90% on the first attempt. If the first attempt fails, and it can be documented that there is still a central gradient of ACTH, a second surgical attempt has a success rate of about 50%. The advent of inferior petrosal sinus sampling for ACTH has provided the surgeon with a rational procedure in the event that a pituitary tumor cannot be found; hemihypophysectomy. The current estimate of the recurrence rate of Cushing's disease is about 5%. Transsphenoidal microadenectomy is not without occasional complications. The mortality rate is about 1%. Infection in these immunocompromised patients is a common cause of death. Morbidity such as cerebrospinal fluid (CSF) leak, sinusitis, and diabetes insipidus (usually transient) occurs in about 5% of patients.

When surgery is not a viable therapeutic option, x-irradiation coupled with op'DDD should be considered. Conventional irradiation, 4500 rad over a 6 week period, is given in association with op'DDD at a dose of 3 g/day. In most patients the disorder can be controlled with this regimen. When "control" has been maintained for 1 year, op'DDD should be discontinued. If the disorder recurs, op'DDD is reinstated for another year. Most patients, with time, can discontinue op'DDD permanently as the effects of irradiation become established. This approach has no known mortality and a high rate of success. Morbidity includes the nonspecific effects of sella turcica irradiation: hypopituitarism in varying degree and nonspecific cognitive changes. In addition, the long-term consequences of op'DDD therapy are unknown.

Bilateral adrenalectomy is the final option for patients who refuse treatment or when the first two approaches fail. Although almost always curative, bilateral adrenalectomy is associated with a high mortality rate, approaching 5% in some series. The requirement for lifelong treatment with glucocorticoid and mineralocorticoid should also be taken into consideration. Finally, patients with Cushing's disease run the risk of subsequent pituitary tumor enlargement and pigmentation, Nelson's syndrome. The extent of this risk has been estimated at 5% to 10%.

Ectopic ACTH secretion. Surgical ablation of the ectopic ACTH source is the preferred treatment of this disorder. When the source of ACTH cannot be localized, or is too advanced or widespread for an effective surgical approach, blockade of adrenal steroidogenesis is the treatment of choice. The availability of ketoconazole for this purpose has considerably facilitated this therapeutic option. Ketoconazole blocks adrenal steroidogenesis at several levels, the most important being the 20-22 desmolase step that catalyzes the conversion of cholesterol to pregnenolone. Because this is the earliest step in the steroid biosynthetic cascade, the accumulation of troublesome intermediates such as 11-deoxycorticosterone, which can worsen hypertension, is prevented. Patients with a "fixed" ACTH secretion rate (i.e., without an intact feedback axis) usually respond well to this agent at doses ranging between 400 and 1200 mg/day. Effective blockade in patients with an occult source of ACTH often can be maintained for years. In this setting, regular re-evaluation in search of the responsible neoplasm can successfully identify the source and allow definitive surgical treatment. The primary toxicity of ketoconazole is hepatocellular. Rising plasma liver enzyme concentrations necessitate cessation of the drug. This is an uncommon occurrence; when it does occur, other blocking agents are available and can be used singly or in combination. These include metyrapone, aminoglutethimide, and trilostane.

Adrenal adenoma and carcinoma. The primary treatment of the disorders of adrenal adenoma and carcinoma is surgical. The prognosis for malignant behavior based on gross and microscopic pathologic examination is unreliable. Clinically, lesions greater than 6 cm tend to have malignant behavior. Failure to image with iodocholesterol also has bad prognostic implication.

Small tumors can be removed through a unilateral flank incision. Large tumors must be removed via the transabdominal approach to allow careful examination of the liver, the pararenal structures, and the great veins.

Benign lesions are cured by surgery. Hence with continued absence of local spread or metastases, watchful waiting should be emphasized. Evidence of malignancy, be it local recurrence or distant spread, calls for the addition of chemotherapy.

Chemotherapy for adrenal cancer is little changed from the early 1960s, when op′DDD was introduced. A congener of chlorophenothane (DDT), this drug is an adrenolytic agent that has variable efficacy against adrenal cancer. Because the drug is very fat-soluble, changes in dose are reflected slowly in changes in the circulating concentrations of the compound. The urinary excretion of op′DDD continues for months after cessation of its administration. When used to treat adrenal cancer, the drug traditionally has been pushed to toxicity. Recent findings support this practice and suggest that success may relate to dose and plasma levels of op′DDD achieved. The common toxic effects of the drug are nausea, somnolence, ataxia, and reduced attention span. When they are encountered, reduction of the dose by increments of 20% usually halts the progression of side-effects. Liver and bone marrow toxicity are not problems with this drug.

Treated this way, about 25% of patients have an objective remission manifested by shrinkage of a measurable lesion. The average duration of these remissions is 7 months. Throughout the course, surgically negotiable tumors should be removed even though it is clear that the operation will not be curative. The rationale behind this approach is that hemorrhagic or septic episodes associated with large tumor masses are a common and serious complication in this disease and, theoretically, can be prevented by early surgical intervention. With this approach, these patients follow a survival curve with a half-time of about 4 years.

Finally, op′DDD alters the pathway of adrenal metabolism so that, in the absence of significant tumor effect, the excretion of Porter-Silber chromogens or 17-ketosteroids is reduced. This does not constitute "true" remission and should not be confused with it. Urinary free cortisol is free of this artifact, and, if a chemical parameter of progress is deemed essential, this should be the chosen one.

Micronodular adrenal disease. The treatment for this disorder is bilateral adrenalectomy.

Recovery. A final word about the treatment of Cushing's syndrome: Successful intervention invariably makes patients feel worse, leading to an occasional "credibility gap." This should be anticipated: recovery to a usual state of good health can require a year or more. Foreknowledge of this can prevent anxiety and depression and work as a positive force in the rehabilitation process.

MINERALOCORTICOID EXCESS

In humans aldosterone is the major mineralocorticoid. It is a product of the zona glomerulosa of the adrenal gland. Aldosterone exchanges sodium ions for potassium and hydrogen ions in the proximal tubule of the kidney. Because sodium is primarily an extracellular ion, its balance is reflected in vascular volume. Vascular volume in turn regulates the secretion of aldosterone via the renin-angiotensin system. Thus the metabolic picture of mineralocorticoid excess is hypokalemic metabolic alkalosis associated with suppressed plasma renin activity. When aldosterone is the offending mineralocorticoid, plasma aldosterone concentrations are normal or high. When some other mineralocorticoid is the offending agent, aldosterone concentrations are suppressed.

Causes of mineralocorticoid excess

The mineralocorticoid excess syndromes can be thought of as primary or secondary. The primary causes are those in which the secretion of excess mineralocorticoid is the fundamental lesion. The secondary causes are those in which the excess secretion of mineralocorticoid is a response to another fundamental lesion. Examples of primary disease are aldosterone secreting adenoma and adrenal cancer; examples of secondary mineralocorticoid excess are cirrhosis of the liver and congestive heart failure. The primary syndromes of mineralocorticoid excess are usually associated with hypertension and require treatment. The secondary syndromes of mineralocorticoid excess are usually associated with normotension or hypotension and usually do not require specific therapy other than that directed to the underlying lesion. The common causes of mineralocorticoid excess are listed in the box below.

Diagnosis and differential diagnosis

The symptoms most frequently reported by patients with primary mineralocorticoid excess are headache, easy fatigu-

Common causes of mineralocorticoid excess

- With hypertension (primary mineralocorticoid excess)
  - Produced by aldosterone
    - Aldosterone secretion the *primary* lesion
      - Aldosterone secreting adenoma
      - Idiopathic hyperaldosteronism
      - Dexamethasone suppressible hyperaldosteronism
      - Adrenocortical carcinoma
    - Aldosterone secretion *secondary* to another lesion
      - Renal artery stenosis
      - Renin secreting tumor
      - Malignant hypertension
      - Chronic renal disease
  - Produced by some other mineralocorticoid
    - Adrenal cancer
    - 11-Beta hydroxylase deficiency
    - 17-Hydroxylase deficiency
    - Liddle's syndrome
    - 11-Beta hydroxysteroid dehydrogenase deficiency
    - Licorice ingestion
- With normal blood pressure
  - Chronic renal disease
  - Hepatic cirrhosis
  - Cardiac failure
  - Vomiting
  - Diuretic abuse
  - Laxative abuse
  - Familial chloride diarrhea

ability, and weakness. Hypertension is the most common sign. The finding of hypokalemia and metabolic alkalosis in a hypertensive patient should lead to further evaluation. The first step in this evaluation is to measure *stimulated* (4 hours of upright posture) plasma renin activity. Values less than 2 ng/ml/hr strongly indicate the presence of mineralocorticoid excess. A plasma aldosterone level measured at the same time categorizes the mineralocorticoid excess syndrome as that caused by aldosterone versus that caused by some other mineralocorticoid. A plasma aldosterone concentration greater than 14 ng/dl is virtually diagnostic of primary hyperaldosteronism. Lower levels are compatible with the diagnosis but must be shown to be "nonsuppressible" with an infusion of 2 L of normal saline solution over 4 hours to confirm the diagnosis. At the conclusion of the infusion, the plasma aldosterone concentration should be greater than 5 ng/dl and usually exceeds 10 ng/dl in proven cases of primary aldosterone excess.

Patients with aldosterone excess require localization of the source of aldosterone secretion before definitive therapy can be planned. This boils down to determining whether aldosterone is being secreted by one or by both adrenal glands. Unilateral aldosterone secretion is almost always produced by an aldosterone secreting adenoma and can be cured by adrenalectomy on that side. Bilateral secretion of aldosterone is the result of bilateral hyperplasia of the zona glomerulosa and this condition responds poorly to adrenalectomy.

The most reliable way to localize the source of excess aldosterone secretion is by bilateral adrenal vein catheterization. Thirty minutes after the intravenous injection of 250 μg cosyntropin, aldosterone and cortisol concentrations are measured in blood samples drawn simultaneously from both adrenal veins. In patients with bilateral disease, the aldosterone/cortisol ratio is the same; in those with unilateral disease, there is marked asymmetry in the ratios, the larger of the two identifying the gland harboring the adenoma. Treatment can be planned on the basis of these findings.

Patients with hypertension and mineralocorticoid excess produced by a mineralocorticoid other than aldosterone should be suspected of having adrenal cancer. The single best test for identifying this cause of mineralocorticoid excess is the adrenal CT scan. Because adrenal cancers are nearly always large at the time of discovery, usually greater than 6 cm in diameter, the CT scan can be counted on to identify nearly all such lesions. Identification of the remaining causes of nonaldosterone mineralocorticoid excess, aside from licorice ingestion, requires the measurement of steroid biosynthetic intermediates that are not widely available. This evaluation should be pursued in a specialty center.

Treatment

Aldosterone-mediated mineralocorticoid excess syndromes usually require treatment. Aldosterone secreting adenomas usually can be managed successfully with surgery. An ongoing puzzle in the management of these disorders is the well-established observation that bilateral adrenal secretion of aldosterone does not respond well to surgery. The metabolic changes can be reversed, but the associated hypertension is rarely improved.

The mineralocorticoid excess syndromes associated with normal blood pressure, the "secondary" syndromes, are treated with therapy directed at the underlying disorder. These patients are best treated by a combination of an aldosterone antagonist, spironolactone, to control hypokalemia, and a standard drug regimen for the associated hypertension.

The therapy for adrenal cancer is primarily surgical, with the addition of op'DDD in cases of metastatic disease. The enzyme deficiency disorders, 11-beta hydroxylase deficiency and 17-hydroxylase deficiency, are treated with exogenous glucocorticoid, and 11-beta hydroxysteroid dehydrogenase deficiency is treated with spironolactone.

ADRENAL HYPOFUNCTION

Adrenal hypofunction results from destruction of the adrenal cortex (primary adrenal insufficiency) or from ACTH deficiency (secondary adrenal insufficiency). In both instances, lack of glucocorticoid and mineralocorticoid accounts for the major clinical manifestations.

The clinical manifestations of chronic adrenal insufficiency include weakness, fatigue, weight loss, hypotension, anorexia, and, occasionally, diarrhea. Cutaneous hyperpigmentation is characteristic of primary adrenal insufficiency and is a useful differential diagnostic sign. The hyperpigmentation is typically located over the elbows and knuckles, in axillary folds, and in the buccal mucosa. Areas of existing pigmentation such as the palmar creases, the areolae, and the lip margins can become strikingly hyperpigmented. It is useful to inquire about recent injuries or surgical procedures because healing tissues can exhibit transient hyperpigmentation. Hyperpigmentation can be difficult to assess in dark-skinned people and in "weathered" individuals. In these instances, examination of the oral mucosa, especially the buccal mucosa, tongue, and gingival margins, is important because these are frequently hyperpigmented in primary adrenal insufficiency and only rarely so otherwise.

Pubic and axillary hair in women are dependent on weak adrenal androgens and can be absent or sparse in women with chronic adrenal insufficiency. Diminished or absent axillary hair is a frequent finding in men with hypopituitarism and reflects diminished secretion of adrenal and gonadal androgens. Sexual hair is present in men with primary adrenal insufficiency because the gonadal secretion of androgens is not materially affected by hypocortisolism.

Acute adrenal insufficiency often is first recognized during a stressful event such as surgery or infection. The hallmark of this disorder is hypotension resistant to correction with "volume" and pressor agents. Common laboratory tests often provide the first clues of adrenocortical hypofunction. The combination of hyponatremia, hyperkalemia, mild metabolic acidosis, and slight elevation of the blood urea nitrogen concentration and hematocrit are classic findings.

Causes of adrenal insufficiency

Primary adrenal insufficiency (Addison's disease) is most commonly due to autoimmune destruction of the adrenal cortex (refer to the box below). This accounts for 80% of cases. Tuberculosis is cited as the second leading cause, accounting for about 10% of cases. The balance is made up by fungal infections (blastomycosis, histoplasmosis), hemorrhage into the gland (coagulopathies, iatrogenic anticoagulation, surgery), metastatic neoplasms, sarcoidosis, amyloidosis, acquired immunodeficiency syndrome (AIDS), adrenal leukodystrophy, and congenital adrenal hypoplasia. Autoimmune adrenocortical destruction spares the adrenal medulla, whereas all other destructive causes can involve both the adrenal cortex and the adrenal medulla.

Autoimmune adrenalitis is associated with several other endocrine autoimmune glandular disorders. Most notable among these are thyroiditis and diabetes mellitus. The triad of adrenalitis, thyroiditis, and diabetes mellitus is also known as Schmidt's syndrome. Other less common autoimmune associations include pernicious anemia, vitiligo, hypoparathyroidism, and mucocutaneous candidiasis. The autoimmune disorders of the endocrine system do not always manifest themselves simultaneously.

Secondary adrenal insufficiency is more common than primary adrenal insufficiency. Secondary adrenal insufficiency is caused by a lack of ACTH stimulation of the gland and most commonly follows prolonged glucocorticoid therapy. Intrinsic or metastatic hypothalamic and pituitary disease, the second most common cause, is uncommon.

Causes of adrenocortical insufficiency

- Primary adrenocortical insufficiency
  - Acquired disorders (Addison's disease)
    - Idiopathic autoimmunity
    - Infectious causes (tuberculosis, AIDS, fungal infections, sepsis)
    - Metastic or invasive disorder (tumors, sarcoidosis, amyloidosis)
    - Adrenal hemorrhage (trauma, shock, coagulopathies)
    - Iatrogenic (surgery, adrenal inhibitors, anticoagulation)
  - Congenital and familial
    - Congenital adrenal hyperplasia (enzymatic deficiencies)
    - Congenital adrenal hypoplasia
    - Congenital unresponsiveness to ACTH
    - Adrenoleukodystrophy
    - Adrenomyeloneuropathy
- Secondary adrenocortical insufficiency
  - Hypothalamopituitary suppression by glucocorticoids
    - Exogenous glucocorticoid or ACTH administration
    - Endogenous suppression by adrenal or pituitary hyperfunction (Cushing's syndrome)
  - Hypothalamopituitary disease
    - Invasive neoplasms (pituitary tumor, craniopharyngioma, eosinophilic granuloma, lymphoma, leukemia)
    - Infections (tuberculosis, fungal)
    - Surgery and trauma

Diagnosis

The diagnosis of adrenal insufficiency can be confirmed definitively by demonstrating an impaired adrenal response to exogenously administered ACTH. A single injection of 250 μg of the synthetic ACTH (cosyntropin) should produce a plasma cortisol concentration of at least 20 μg/dl 45 minutes after administration in normal individuals. A diminished or absent response usually establishes the diagnosis of adrenal insufficiency but does not distinguish primary from secondary causes of the disorder. The exception would be a patient currently taking or having recently stopped high-dose steroids. In primary adrenal insufficiency, plasma ACTH values are elevated, and the combination of an impaired cortisol response to cosyntropin challenge and a high plasma ACTH level is strong evidence for the diagnosis of primary adrenal insufficiency.

Treatment

The therapy of adrenal insufficiency is straightforward: replace the deficient hormones, cortisol and aldosterone. The cortisol replacement dose is 12 to 15 mg cortisol/m^2 body surface/day. The total dose ranges between 20 and 30 mg/day for most adults. Traditionally, cortisol is given as a divided dose, two thirds in the morning, and one third in the afternoon. In the authors' opinion, a single daily dose in the morning is sufficient. Compliance is enhanced by this regimen. Patients with primary adrenal insufficiency require both cortisol and fludrocostisone. Orally administered aldosterone is not readily absorbed from the gastrointestinal tract. A synthetic analog of aldosterone, fludrocortisone (Florinef), is orally active and is given in doses ranging from 0.05 to 0.2 mg daily. Generally an oral dose of 0.1 mg daily suffices. Measurable indices of therapeutic efficacy include changes in body weight and postural blood pressure. Laboratory measures of adrenal function such as serum electrolyte, plasma ACTH, renin, and urinary cortisol levels can be reserved for resolving issues such as questions of compliance or lack of response to traditional maintenance therapy. Of particular note, the plasma ACTH concentration is not a useful tool for monitoring primary adrenal insufficiency because it remains high with adequate treatment.

Acute adrenal insufficiency is usually manifested as shock, poorly responsive to volume and pressor therapy. This condition requires emergency treatment. Infusion of isotonic saline solution should be started immediately. Intravenous cortisol, 100 mg as a bolus injection, should be given immediately after blood is taken for the measurement of cortisol and ACTH concentrations. This should be repeated every 6 hours thereafter for the first 48 hours. When the crisis is past, a return to the usual oral replacement dose can be accomplished over 48 hours. This diagnosis is often suspected in seriously ill patients. Therapy should be initiated without waiting for laboratory confirmation with the decision to continue dependent on the results of pretherapy tests.

Patients treated chronically with systemic corticosteroids may require replacement therapy if the treatment is terminated abruptly or tapered too quickly. Withdrawal from chronic therapy can be associated with fatigue, weakness, arthralgia, and occasional desquamation, mimicking, in part, the symptoms of chronic adrenal insufficiency. Suppression of the pituitary-adrenal axis rarely occurs in patients treated with corticosteroids for less than 2 or 3 weeks. If the suppression has been prolonged, however, recovery can require up to 1 year. Patients receiving chronic corticosteroid therapy are thought to require an increase in cortisol dose during periods of acute stress. It is traditional to cover such periods of stress by doubling the cortisol dose on the day of and the day after the stressful event. Some experts recommend tapering the dose back to maintenance levels over several days. In the authors' opinion, tapering can be omitted and the patient returned to maintenance doses as soon as the stress is over.

Isolated mineralocorticoid deficiency causes urinary retention of potassium, resulting in hyperkalemia, retention of hydrogen ions, and urinary sodium wasting. Hyperkalemia, although usually asymptomatic, can cause muscle weakness and life-threatening cardiac arrhythmias. Sodium wasting classically presents as orthostatic hypotension. However, in the most common presenting form of hypoaldosteronism, the sodium wasting can be offset by the sodium retention associated with severe renal disease. Hyporeninemic hypoaldosteronism is the most common form of isolated mineralocorticoid deficiency. The disorder is frequently associated with diabetes mellitus and usually appears late in the course of that disease.

The hyporeninemic hypoaldosteronism of diabetes is usually accompanied by asymptomatic hyperkalemia and mild acidosis. The renal complications of diabetes, including glomerulopathy and nephropathy, can predominate and result in seemingly paradoxic sodium retention and absence of orthostatic hypotension. In other circumstances, however, the sodium depleting effect of hypoaldosteronism predominates and leads to the expected orthostatic hypotension. This form of hypoaldosteronism is most likely the result of impaired renin secretion caused by the complications of diabetes in the afferent arterioles of the kidney. Although the resultant hyperkalemia of hypoaldosteronism would be expected to stimulate aldosterone synthesis, the stimulus is not sufficient to overcome the absence of renin.

Other causes of isolated mineralocorticoid deficiency are intrinsic nondiabetic renal disease and, more rarely, congenital adrenal hyperplasia.

The objectives of treatment of isolated mineralocorticoid deficiency are to reduce hyperkalemia and, if sodium wasting predominates, to expand effective blood volume. Fludrocortisone can be used to replace deficient mineralocorticoids. Serum potassium concentration falls and fluid volume expands as sodium is retained. In hyporeninemic hypoaldosteronism, the effective blood volume may be increased as a result of advanced diabetic renal disease. In this instance, a combination of dietary potassium restriction and administration of potassium binding agents and diuretics may be required to maintain appropriate potassium levels and an effective blood volume. It should be noted that asymptomatic mild elevations of serum potassium concentration may require only close clinical observation rather than therapy.

CONGENITAL ADRENAL HYPERPLASIA

Categories of congenital adrenal hyperplasia

There are five enzymatic steps between cholesterol and cortisol that, when attenuated, lead to specific syndromes of congenital adrenal hyperplasia (CAH). All are transmitted as autosomal recessive traits. The affected enzymes, in order from cholesterol to cortisol, are 20-22 desmolase, 3-beta-hydroxy-steroid dehydrogenase, 17-hydroxylase, 21-hydroxylase, and 11-hydroxylase (Fig. 163-3). The most common of these, 21-hydroxylase deficiency, accounts for 85% of cases. 11-Hydroxylase deficiency and 3-beta-HSD deficiency constitute most of the remainder.

A convenient way to categorize these disorders is into virilizing and feminizing forms. 21-Hydroxylase deficiency and 11-hydroxylase deficiency are virilizing forms; 20-22 desmolase deficiency and 17-hydroxylase deficiency are feminizing forms. 3-Beta HSD is virilizing in females and feminizing in males. All forms of CAH can adversely affect reproductive competence by altering sex-steroid synthesis and secretion. The most common form of CAH to do this, by far, is the 21-hydroxylase deficient form of the disease.

21-Hydroxylase deficiency occurs in two major clinical forms: classic and attenuated. The classic form is usually manifested in neonatal life or early childhood. It has two clinical presentations, roughly equal in prevalence: the simple virilizing form and the salt wasting form. The simple virilizing form is the most common cause of heterosexual precocious puberty in girls, and isosexual sexual precocity in boys. It usually is manifested after the neonatal period. The salt wasting form of the disorder occurs when the synthesis and secretion of both cortisol and aldosterone are impaired. These children are usually discovered in the neonatal period because of failure to thrive. Female infants with both forms of the disease may have ambiguous genitalia.

Several different mutations of the 21-hydroxylase gene have been associated with the classic form of 21-hydroxylase deficiency. These include gene deletions, gene conversion events, and point mutations. The attenuated form of the disorder is usually detected in the peripubertal period of life. The usual manifestations are those of idiopathic hirsutism and polycystic ovary syndrome. Hirsutism, oligomenorrhea, and infertility dominate the clinical picture.

There is only one clinical form of this variety, 21-hydroxylase deficiency, although there is great variability in severity. "Salt loss" is not a feature, but mild impairment of mineralocorticoid secretion can be demonstrated in most cases. There is an association with the human leukocyte antigen HLA-B14 and HLA-DR1 haplotypes. In these

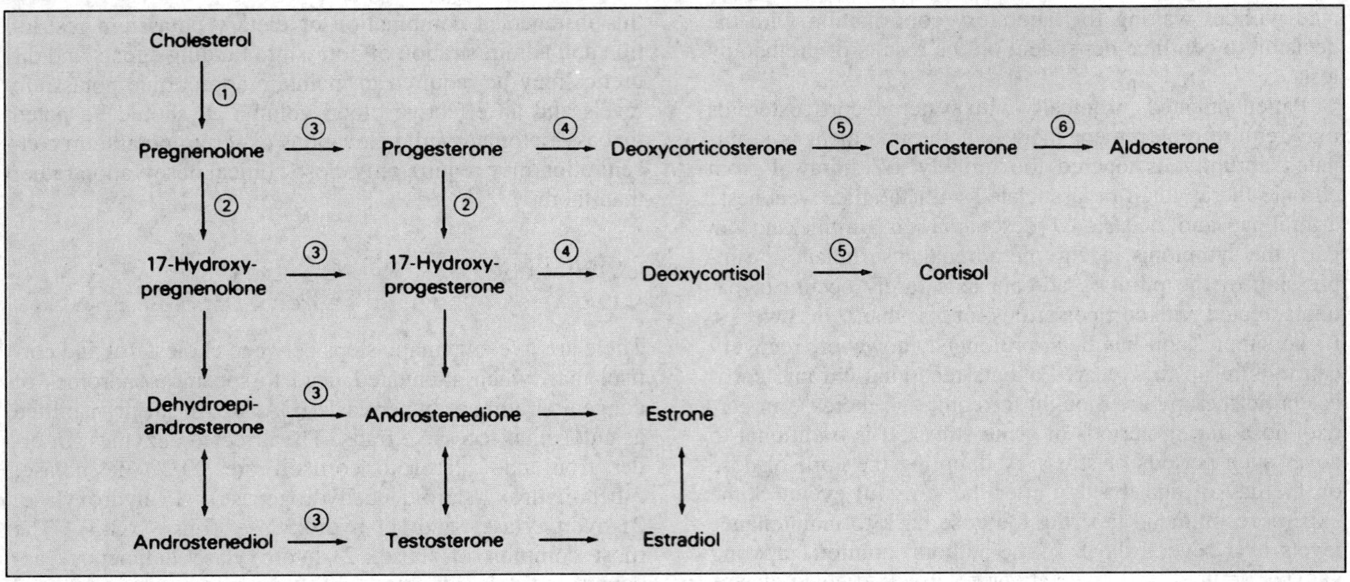

Fig. 163-3. The sites of the five enzyme blocks leading to the various syndromes of congenital adrenal hyperplasia. 1, 20-22 desmolase; 2, 17-hydroxylase; 3, 3-beta hydroxysteroid dehydrogenase; 4, 21 hydroxylase; 5, 11-hydroxylase.

cases, a single base change occurs in the 21-hydroxylase gene.

The incidence of the attenuated form of the disease varies widely, depending on the specific population under study. For example, it occurs in 1 in 27 Ashkenazic Jews, 1 in 53 Hispanics, 1 in 63 Yugoslavs, and 1 in 333 Italians. Other studies show "carrier" rates ranging between 1% and 6%. The disorder can vary in severity from hirsutism, oligomenorrhea, and infertility at one extreme, to normal phenotype at the other extreme with no abnormality other than the characteristic biochemical markers of the disease.

Diagnosis

The disorder should be considered in all cases of hirsutism, oligomenorrhea, or unexplained infertility. If plasma testosterone concentrations are in the normal range, attenuated CAH is unlikely. At the other extreme, plasma testosterone levels above 200 ng/dl are rarely, if ever, associated with the attenuated forms of CAH. Plasma testosterone levels between 65 and 150 ng/dl, however, are characteristic of attenuated CAH. The appropriate diagnostic test is a plasma 17 hydroxy-progesterone measurement 45 minutes after the administration of 250 μg cosyntropin. In normal subjects, 17-hydroxyprogesterone levels do not exceed 350 ng/dl after an ACTH challenge. The 17-hydroxyprogesterone value after cosyntropin administration virtually always exceeds 1000 ng/dl in attenuated CAH.

Treatment

Because the basic lesion is an inefficient production of cortisol caused by an altered 21-hydroxylase enzyme, the process can be reversed by supplying cortisol from an exogenous source. The production rate of cortisol ranges between 12 and 15 mg/m^2/day, and supplying this amount by mouth, once a day, effectively reduces the increased testosterone production rate. In most instances, hirsutism improves and cyclic menses resumes.

ADRENAL TUMORS

Adrenal tumors are being discovered with increasing frequency as a by-product of improved radiologic imaging of the abdomen. The current best estimate is that an adrenal mass is identified in 4% of abdominal CT scans. Because an adrenal mass is found in about 15% of autopsy specimens, it can be predicted that the incidence of previously unsuspected adrenal masses will approach this figure as imaging modalities continue to improve. Because these tumors are found by diagnostic procedures carried out for another purpose, they have been termed the *incidental adrenal mass*. The primary concern surrounding the incidental mass is that it might represent an adrenal carcinoma for which the appropriate treatment is early surgical intervention. In fact, the only chance of cure of an adrenal carcinoma is successful surgery. Balanced against this is the rarity of the lesion. Adrenal cancers account for only 0.2% of cancer deaths and have an estimated incidence of two per million population per year. It is estimated that the mean duration of disease before discovery is about 6 years. If all people with adrenal cancer are assumed to have an adrenal mass, about 1 in every 4000 adrenal masses will represent an adrenal carcinoma. More than half are discovered in the context of a clinical presentation of Cushing's syndrome. The other half are "silent" and thus usually discovered when large (5 cm or greater in diameter) and after distant metastases are established. Thus the incidental adrenal mass presents a diagnostic and therapeutic dilemma: the compelling need to identify accurately which incidental adrenal masses represent an adrenal cancer versus the extremely expensive and cost-ineffective testing necessary to do so.

The differential diagnoses of unilateral and bilateral incidental adrenal masses are listed in the boxes below.

All lesions must be evaluated for function. The history and physical features are important guides in this determination. Features of glucocorticoid excess are those of Cushing's syndrome. Hypertension associated with an adrenal mass suggests Cushing's syndrome, hyperaldosteronism, or pheochromocytoma. Hirsutism of recent onset, particularly if associated with signs of virilization such as temporal balding, deepening of the voice, and clitoromegaly, suggests androgen secretion.

The syndrome of adrenal insufficiency has already been mentioned. Unilateral disease, of course, is not associated with adrenal insufficiency. Said another way, the diagnosis of primary adrenal insufficiency implies bilateral disease. When bilateral masses are present, the differential diagnosis includes infection and neoplastic infiltration. The most common infections are tuberculous and fungal. The most common tumors are of the breast and lung.

The laboratory evaluation of the incidentally discovered adrenal mass should concentrate on the best screening tests for disorders of hormone excess or deficiency. The best screening test for Cushing's syndrome is the 24 hour urinary free cortisol excretion rate; for primary aldosteronism, the upright plasma renin activity; for pheochromocytoma, plasma catecholamines concentration after Clonidine; and for sex steroid secreting adenomas, plasma testosterone concentration in women, and estrone concentration in men. In bilateral disease, congenital adrenal hyperplasia should be excluded by measuring plasma 17-hydroxy-progesterone concentration and 11-deoxycortisol concentration 45 minutes after administration of 250 μg of intravenous synthetic ACTH. Adrenal insufficiency can be identified by an attenuated response of plasma cortisol to the standard 250 μg intravenous injection of synthetic ACTH. A single plasma ACTH measurement differentiates primary from secondary adrenal insufficiency in those patients who "fail" the screening test.

Functional lesions other than congenital adrenal hyperplasia must be treated surgically. Congenital adrenal hyperplasia is treated with exogenous glucocorticoid and, when indicated, mineralocorticoid. Current recommendations for nonfunctional lesions range from fine needle aspiration for all to expectant observation for all. Adrenal lesions found to represent disease metastatic to the adrenal gland should be treated as part of the therapy for the underlying neoplasm. Incidental masses of adrenal origin should be excised if greater than 3 cm in diameter. Masses of adrenal origin that are less than 3 cm in diameter are rarely malignant and can be safely managed conservatively. Unequivocal growth, however, is generally considered an indication for surgical intervention.

Although surgical treatment is palliative when the cancer is metastatic, surgery can be helpful in "debulking" the mass to reduce symptoms of hormone excess. The only effective medical treatment for adrenocortical carcinoma is op'DDD. It is not curative. The side-effects of this drug are serious, and the disadvantages of its use can outweigh the symptomatic benefits to the patient.

Bilateral adrenal masses

A. Functional Lesions
   1. ACTH dependent Cushing's syndrome
   2. Congenital adrenal hyperplasia
   3. Pheochromocytoma
   4. Conn's syndrome, hyperplastic variety
   5. Micronodular adrenal disease
   6. Idiopathic bilateral adrenal hypertrophy

B. Nonfunctional lesions
   1. Infection (tuberculosis, fungi)
   2. Infiltration (leukemia, lymphoma)
   3. Replacement (amyloidosis)
   4. Hemorrhage
   5. Bilateral metastases

Unilateral adrenal masses

Functional lesions
- Adrenal adenoma
- Adrenal carcinoma
- Pheochromocytoma
- Primary aldosteronism, adenomatous type

Nonfunctional lesions
- Adrenal adenoma
- Adrenal carcinoma
- Ganglioneuroma
- Myelolipoma
- Hematoma
- Adrenolipoma
- Metastasis

REFERENCES

Cushing H: The pituitary body and its disorders. Philadelphia and London, 1912, Lippincott.

Loriaux DL: The treatment of Cushing's syndrome and adrenal cancer. Endocrinol Metab Clin North Am 20:767, 1991.

Miller WL: Congenital adrenal hyperplasias. Endocrinol Metab Clin North Am 20:721, 1991.

Moore CC and Miller WL. The role of transcriptional regulation in steroid hormone biosynthesis. J Steroid Biochem Mol Biol 40:517, 1991.

Vallotton MB: Endocrine emergencies: disorders of the adrenal cortex. Baillieres Clin Endocrinol Metab 6:41, 1992.

Young WF, Jr et al: Primary aldosteronism: diagnosis and treatment. Mayo Clin Proc 65:96, 1990.

CHAPTER

164 Disorders of the Adrenal Medulla

Alan Goldfien

The human adrenal medulla is composed of cells derived from the sympathogonia of the primitive neural crest. During the fifth week of gestation, groups of these cells collect around the central vein of the fetal adrenal cortex to form the adrenal medulla. During the third month of gestation, the cells mature into pheochromacytes (chromaffin cells) arranged in nests and cords surrounding blood vessels. They contain typical catecholamine storage granules by the twelfth week.

The cells of the adrenal medulla are richly supplied by capillaries and sinusoids arising in the adrenal cortex and therefore are exposed to high levels of adrenal cortical steroids. The cells are innervated by the preganglionic fibers of the sympathetic nervous system, which synapse to form a plexus in the capsule on the posterior surface of the gland. The nerves enter the gland along with the blood vessels.

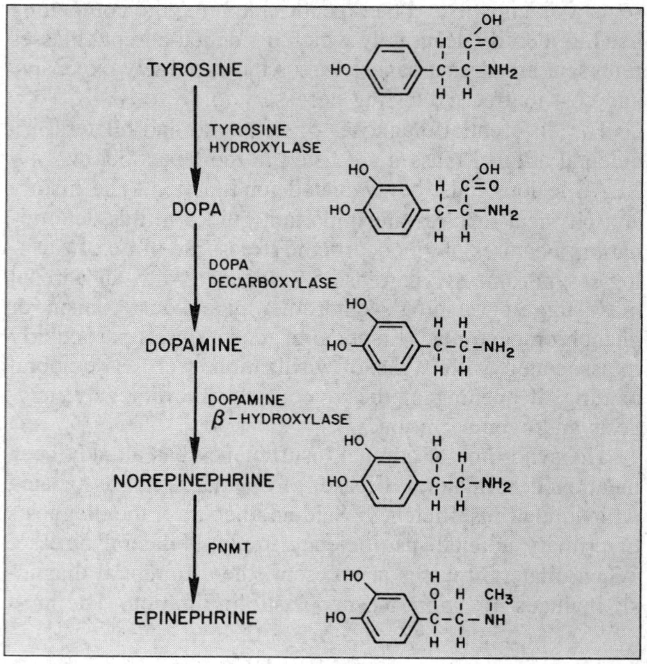

Fig. 164-1. Biosynthesis of the catecholamines.

HORMONES OF THE ADRENAL MEDULLA

The adrenal medulla synthesizes and secretes catecholamines as well as enkephalins. Special techniques indicate that other active peptides such as dynorphins, vasoactive intestinal peptide, somatostatin, and substance P can be found in chromaffin cells of various species. The physiologic significance of these findings is unknown.

Catecholamines: biosynthesis and metabolism

The catecholamines, epinephrine and norepinephrine, are normally produced in the adrenal medulla, brain, and sympathetic neurons. In peripheral adrenergic neurons, L-tyrosine entering the cell from the circulation is converted to dihydroxyphenylalanine (dopa) by the mitochondrial enzyme tyrosine hydroxylase. Dopa decarboxylase converts dopa to dopamine, which is taken up by specific storage granules. Dopamine in the granule is converted to norepinephrine by dopamine beta-hydroxylase. In the adrenal medulla, in some neurons in the brain, and in tumors producing epinephrine, norepinephrine is converted to epinephrine by the action of the enzyme phenylethanolamine N-methyltransferase. This process is summarized in Fig. 164-1. In the adrenal medulla and sympathetic nerve endings, catecholamines are stored in granules that appear to contain and release a number of active peptides including adrenocorticotrophic hormone (ACTH), vasoactive intestinal peptide (VIP), and the enkephalins. Recent studies indicate that peptides derived from the chromogranins are physiologically active and may modulate catecholamine release.

In the basal ganglia, in some hypothalamic nuclei, and in other central and peripheral neurons, dopamine is the final product and neurotransmitter. Dopamine is also secreted by some tumors.

When norepinephrine is released at nerve endings, 85% to 90% is taken up by the neuron and reutilized or metabolized there by monoamine oxidase (MAO). Amines not taken up by the neuron or bound to the adrenergic receptor are taken up at other sites on the effector cell and metabolized by catechol-O-methyltransferase (CMT). A small amount of the norepinephrine enters the circulation. The catecholamines released by tumors enter the circulation and are metabolized in the same manner as those released by the adrenal medulla. They circulate bound to albumin or a closely associated protein and act by binding to the adrenergic receptors in the membranes of cells. Catecholamines not bound to the receptor are metabolized by CMT or MAO. A single passage through the liver or kidney removes two thirds of the free amine. Normally, only a few percent of these amines appear in the urine unchanged or conjugated to glucuronic or sulfuric acid. About half of the catecholamine released is acted on by both enzymes and excreted in the urine as vanillylmandelic acid (VMA). These pathways of metabolism are summarized in Fig. 164-2. The plasma concentration of epinephrine and norepinephrine and the amounts of catecholamines and metabolite excreted daily are shown in Table 164-1.

Release of these hormones at synaptic clefts and into the circulation regulates many important cellular functions and organ responses. These responses are mediated by specific adrenergic receptors in the cell membrane.

There are two classes of adrenergic receptors, alpha and beta, each of which has several subtypes. These receptors were classified by the relative potencies of a series of ad-

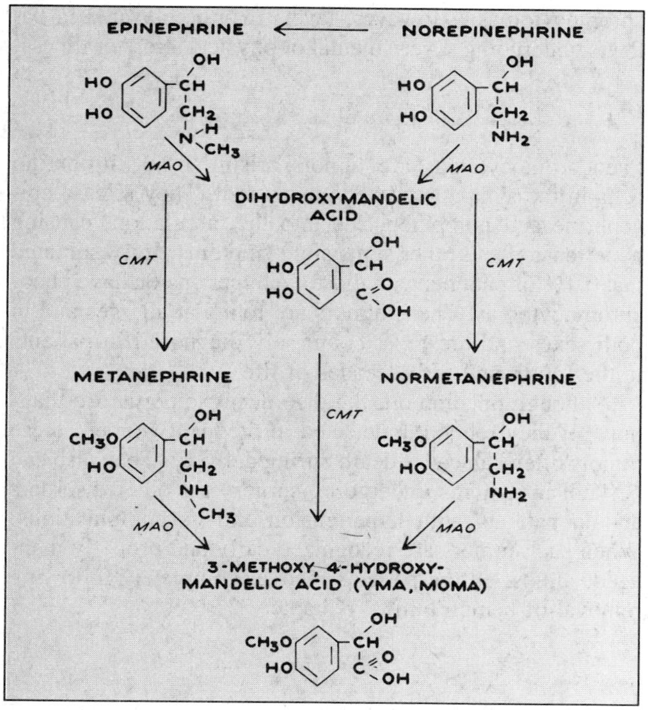

Fig. 164-2. Metabolism of epinephrine and norepinephrine by monoamine oxidase (MAO) and catechol-O-methyltransferase (CMT).

renergic agonists and antagonists. Each of the subtypes is now known to be coded by one or more separate genes.

The $alpha_1$ subtype are postsynaptic receptors that typically mediate vascular and other smooth muscle contraction. When agonist binds to this receptor, the alpha subunit of the guanyl nucleotide-binding protein G_q activates phospholipase C, which acts on phosphatidylinositol bis phosphonate to produce 1,4,5-inositol trisphosphate and diacylglycerol. These second messengers mediate intracellular effects of the agonist. Epinephrine and norepinephrine are potent agonists for this receptor, whereas isoproterenol is weakly active. The $alpha_2$ subtype is found on sympathetic nerve terminals, where it acts to inhibit the release of norepinephrine. It is also found in platelets and at many postsynaptic sites. The binding of agonist to $alpha_2$ receptors releases G_i alpha, which inhibits the enzyme adenylyl cyclase and reduces the formation of cyclic adenosine monophosphate (cAMP). Prazosin is a selective antagonist at the $alpha_1$ receptor and yohimbine is selective for the $alpha_2$ receptor, whereas phentolamine and dibenzyline act at both.

There are several beta-receptor subtypes. Agonist binding to these receptors activates adenylyl cyclase via the G_s alpha subunit to increase the production of cAMP, which in turn converts protein kinase A to its active form. The $beta_1$ receptor, which mediates the direct cardiac effects, is more responsive to isoproterenol than to epinephrine or norepinephrine whose potencies are similar. At the $beta_2$ receptor, which mediates vascular, bronchial, and uterine smooth muscle relaxation, isoproterenol is also most potent; but epinephrine is much more potent than norepinephrine. Some of the physiologic effects of the catecholamines are listed in Table 164-2.

Table 164-1. Normal plasma levels of catecholamines, their urinary excretion rates, and their major metabolites

Catecholamine or metabolite	Normal subjects: At rest	Normal subjects: Marked activity or stress
Plasma		
Epinephrine	20-50 pg/ml	150 pg/ml
Norepinephrine	100-400 pg/ml	1000 pg/ml
Urine		
Epinephrine	5-20 μg/24 hr	100 μg/24 hr
Norepinephrine	20-60 μg/24 hr	200 μg/24 hr
Metanephrines	<1.3 mg/24 hr	
VMA	<7.0 mg/24 hr	

HYPOFUNCTION OF THE ADRENAL MEDULLA

Hypofunction of the adrenal medulla is most often the consequence of bilateral adrenalectomy. In these patients, when adrenal corticoid replacement therapy is instituted, careful studies show only minor delays in recovery from insulin-induced hypoglycemia. The loss of this response is of no clinical significance, except in patients with diabetes mellitus in whom the glucagon response is also deficient,

Table 164-2. Adrenergic responses of selected tissues

Organ or tissue	Receptor	Effect
Heart (myocardium)	β_1	↑ Force of contraction ↑ Rate of contraction
Blood vessels	α	Vasoconstriction
	β_2	Vasodilatation
Kidney	β	Renin release
Gut	α, β	↓ Motility ↑ Sphincter tone
Pancreas	α	↓ Insulin release ↓ Glucagon release
	β	↑ Insulin release ↑ Glucagon release
Liver	β	↑ Glycogenolysis
	α	
Adipose tissue	β	↑ Lipolysis
Most tissues	β	↑ Calorigenesis
Skin (apocrine glands on hands, underarms, etc.)	α	Sweating
Bronchioles	β_2	Dilatation
Uterus	α	Contraction
	β_2	Relaxation

↑ = increased; ↓ = decreased

leaving them more susceptible to severe bouts of hypoglycemia. Adrenal medullary deficiency occurring as part of a more generalized autonomic insufficiency is associated with severe orthostatic hypotension; however, the role of the adrenal medulla is difficult to assess. Causes of orthostatic hypotension are shown in Table 164-3.

Autonomic insufficiency is associated with disorders of nervous system function (Table 164-3). In normal individuals, assuming that the upright position allows pooling of blood in the lower extremities. The initial fall in blood pressure stimulates baroreceptor activity, which activates central reflex mechanisms causing arterial and venous constriction, increased cardiac output, and release of renin and vasopressin. In patients with autonomic insufficiency, however, the interruption of afferent, central, or efferent components of this reflex results in failure to compensate for the fall in blood pressure and blood supply to the brain. This result leads to lightheadedness, syncope, and/or convulsions.

The most effective treatment of these symptoms is volume expansion using fludrocortisone. However, simple measures such as raising the head of the bed at night and using support garments may be sufficient to control the symptoms in some patients. Chronic constriction of the vascular bed using sympathomimetic agents has also been used but is not as effective as volume expansion.

HYPERFUNCTION OF THE ADRENAL MEDULLA

Increased production of catecholamines occurs during severe stress. The physiologic role of the adrenal medulla differs from that of the remainder of the peripheral sympathetic nervous system. Whereas the sympathetic nerves provide fine regulation of cellular function, the medulla secretes large amounts of catecholamines when deviations from homeostasis are extreme. Abnormal increases in circulating catecholamines are most commonly seen in patients with tumors derived from chromaffin tissue (pheochromocytomas). However, levels may be elevated in patients undergoing severe mental or physical stress or illness.

PHEOCHROMOCYTOMAS

Pheochromocytomas are tumors arising from chromaffin cells in the sympathetic nervous system. They release epinephrine and norepinephrine into the circulation, causing hypertension and other signs and symptoms. It is estimated that 0.1% of patients with diastolic hypertension have pheochromocytomas. These tumors are found at all ages and in both sexes and are most commonly diagnosed in patients in the fourth and fifth decades of life.

Although uncommon, the disorder is important to diagnose. If they remain undetected in pregnant women, these tumors often can cause death during delivery. They also can be fatal in patients undergoing surgery for other disorders and in patients with hypertension and its complications. When such tumors are recognized early and properly managed, almost all the patients recover completely following removal of benign tumors (Chapter 23).

Clinical manifestations

Although the majority of patients with functioning tumors have symptoms most of the time, they vary in intensity and are perceived to be mainly episodic or paroxysmal in about half the patients. Most patients with persistent hypertension also have superimposed paroxysms. A small number of patients are entirely free of symptoms and hypertension between attacks and may give no evidence of excessive catecholamine release during these intervals.

In patients with paroxysmal release of catecholamines, the symptoms resemble those produced by the injection of epinephrine or norepinephrine, and the symptom complex is far more consistent than is suggested by the variability of patients' complaints (see the accompanying box). An episode usually begins with a sensation of "something hap-

Table 164-3. Causes of orthostatic hypotension

Functional	Neurogenic (autonomic insufficiency)
Reduction in effective blood volume	Familial dysautonomia
Hemorrhage	Shy-Drager syndrome
Prolonged bed rest	Parkinson's disease
Adrenal insufficiency	Tabes dorsalis
Pregnancy	Syringomyelia
Drugs altering vascular reactivity or nervous system function	Cerebrovascular disease
Antihypertensives	Peripheral neuropathy due in diabetes
Adrenergic antagonists	Idiopathic orthostatic hypotension
Ca^{2+} channel blockers	Sympathectomy
Antidepressants	
Alcohol and depressants	

Common symptoms in patients with hypertension due to pheochromocytoma

Symptoms during or following a paroxysm
- Headache
- Sweating
- Forceful heartbeat ± tachycardia
- Anxiety or fear of impending death
- Tremor
- Fatigue or exhaustion
- Nausea and vomiting
- Abdominal or chest pain
- Visual disturbance

Symptoms noted between paroxysms
- Increased sweating
- Cold hands and feet
- Weight loss
- Constipation

pening" deep inside the chest, and a stimulus to deeper breathing is noted. The patient then becomes aware of a pounding or forceful heartbeat caused by the $beta_1$ receptor-mediated increase in cardiac output. This throbbing spreads to the rest of the trunk and head, causing a headache. The intense alpha receptor-mediated peripheral vasoconstriction causes cool hands and feet and pallor in the face. The combination of increased cardiac output and vasoconstriction causes marked elevation of the blood pressure when large amounts of catecholamines are released. The decreased heat loss and increased metabolism may cause a rise in temperature. These factors also cause reflex sweating. This sweating may be profuse and usually follows the cardiovascular effects, which begin in the first few seconds of the attack. The increased glycolysis and alpha receptor-mediated inhibition of insulin release cause an increase in blood sugar levels. Patients experience marked anxiety with all but the mildest attacks, and when episodes are prolonged, severe nausea, vomiting, visual disturbances, chest or abdominal pain, and paresthesias or seizures can occur. A feeling of fatigue or exhaustion usually follows.

In patients with paroxysmal symptoms, attacks may occur at intervals of months or as frequently as 25 times daily and may last from minutes to days. Usually, they occur several times weekly or more often, and last for 15 minutes or less. As time passes, the attacks usually increase in frequency but do not change much in character. They often are precipitated by activities that compress the tumor, such as changes in position, exercise, lifting, defecation, or eating, and by emotional distress or anxiety.

Patients with persistently secreting tumors also may experience the symptom complex described earlier when transient increases in the release of catecholamines are provoked by the same stimuli. In addition, the increased metabolic rate usually causes weight loss or, in children, a lack of weight gain, as well as heat intolerance and increased sweating. The effects on glycogenolysis and insulin release can produce hyperglycemia and glucose intolerance.

Chronic constriction of the arterial and venous bed leads to a reduction in plasma volume in most of these patients. The inability to further constrict this bed on arising and the down regulation of receptors and desensitization cause the postural hypotension that is characteristically observed. Chronic exposure to increased levels of circulating catecholamines produces a diffuse myocarditis in some patients. Unfortunately, specific electrocardiographic changes may be absent or may be attributable to left ventricular hypertrophy, and heart failure under cardiovascular stress may be the first clinical manifestation. Retinal and renal vascular lesions commonly associated with hypertension may be found.

A few patients with tumors secreting large amounts of dopamine rather than epinephrine or norepinephrine have been described and found to be normotensive.

In addition to the catecholamines, pheochromocytomas produce a wide variety of active peptides. These include somatostatin, substance P, adrenocorticotropin, beta-endorphin, lipotropin, vasoactive intestinal peptide, interleukin 6, parathyroid hormone-related protein, neuropeptide Y, calcitonin, calcitonin gene-related peptide, met-enkephalin, serotonin, gastrin, neurotensin, pancreastatin, galanin, and IGF-II. Secretion of large amounts of these substances may result in atypical clinical presentations.

Familial syndromes and other tumors

These tumors occur sporadically or as a heritable disorder, either alone or, more commonly, in association with other endocrine tumors. In multiple endocrine neoplasia (MEN) type II or type IIa, or Sipple's syndrome, the patient may also have a calcitonin-producing adenoma of the parathyroid. In MEN type IIb or III, pheochromocytomas occur in association with mucosal neuromas, which are numerous and small and are found around the mouth. The transmission of these disorders follows the pattern of an autosomal dominant gene with incomplete penetrance. In these syndromes there appears to be a genetic defect on chromosome 10 that can lead to a general stimulus to tumor formation in selected glands. These tumors may be preceded or accompanied by hyperplastic changes in the adrenal medulla, thyroid, and parathyroid glands and are multicentric in origin. Pheochromocytomas in these patients are bilateral, and additional tumors may be found outside the adrenal glands, and bilateral adrenalectomy may be advisable. It is necessary to screen the families of these patients for evidence of tumors. The diagnosis of medullary carcinoma of the thyroid and tumors of the parathyroid glands is discussed in Chapters 162 and 187, respectively.

Pathology

Pheochromocytomas occur wherever chromaffin tissue is found. The adrenal medulla contains the largest collection of chromaffin cells. In the fetus, the organ of Zuckerkandl is also very large, but it is gradually replaced by fibrous tissue after birth and is small in the adult. Chromaffin cells also are found in association with sympathetic ganglia, nerve plexuses, and nerves.

More than 95% of pheochromocytomas are found in the abdomen and 85% are in or near the adrenal. Common extra-adrenal sites are near the kidney and in the organ of Zuckerkandl. Those in the chest are in the posterior mediastinum. The intracranial lesions reported are thought to be metastatic in origin. The tumors may be multicentric in origin, particularly when familial. Although fewer than 10% of adults have multiple tumors, they are found in about one third of children with pheochromocytomas.

Pheochromocytomas vary in weight from under 1 g to several kilograms; however, they are usually small, most weighing well under 100 g. They are vascular tumors and commonly contain cystic or hemorrhagic areas. The cells tend to be large and contain typical catecholamine storage granules like those in the adrenal medulla. Multinucleated cells, pleomorphic nuclei, mitoses, and extension into the capsule and vessels are sometimes seen but do not indicate that the tumor is malignant.

Adrenal medullary hyperplasia also has been described

as the cause of an indistinguishable clinical picture and has been suggested to be a precursor of the tumors seen in the MEN syndrome, as well as occurring sporadically.

Diagnosis

Although the pattern of the manifestations described earlier can be elicited in almost all patients with functioning tumors who are capable of clear communication, the variability of presenting complaints may be confusing and is sometimes misleading. Women whose episodes are first noted around the time of the menopause may be thought to be experiencing "hot flashes." The diagnosis may be made only when hormonal therapy has failed to alleviate the symptoms or the episode is observed and the blood pressure taken during the attack. When a pheochromocytoma causes hypertension late in pregnancy, it may be confused with pre-eclampsia. Other causes of increased sympathetic activity that must be distinguished from pheochromocytomas are listed in the box below.

On physical examination, hypertension is usually present. Wide fluctuations of blood pressure are characteristic, and marked increases may be followed by hypotension and syncope. When pressure is elevated, postural hypotension is present. Typically, the hypertension does not respond to commonly used antihypertensive regimens, and such drugs as guanethidine and ganglionic blockers can induce paradoxical pressor responses. These patients, usually thin, have a forceful heartbeat, which is often visible and easily palpable. They feel warm, may have pallor of the face and chest, perspire, have cool and moist hands and feet, and prefer a cool room. Patients with long-standing and persistent symptoms and hypertension may have retinopathy. A mass may be palpable in the abdomen or neck, and deep palpation of the abdomen may produce a typical paroxysm.

The diagnosis of pheochromocytoma should be considered in all patients with paroxysmal symptoms; in children with hypertension; in adults with severe hypertension that does not respond to therapy; in hypertensive patients with diabetes and/or hypermetabolism; in patients with hypertension in whom symptoms resemble those described earlier or can be evoked by exercise, position change, emotional distress, or antihypertensive drugs such as guanethidine and ganglionic blockers; and in patients who become severely hypertensive or go into shock during anesthesia, surgery, or delivery. Patients who have disorders sometimes associated with pheochromocytomas (neurofibromatosis, mucosal adenomas, von Hippel's disease, or medullary carcinoma of the thyroid) or first-order relatives with a pheochromocytoma should be investigated.

Ganglioneuromas (which are usually small, well-differentiated tumors arising from ganglion cells) and neuroblastomas (highly malignant tumors arising from more primitive sympathoblastic cells) can produce catecholamines and present a similar clinical picture. Dopamine is usually the major active catecholamine produced and leads to elevation of homovanillic acid levels in the urine.

Differential diagnosis of hypertension secondary to other etiologies

- Severe anxiety attacks
- Paroxysmal tachycardias
- Coronary insufficiency
- Hypertensive crises associated with paraplegia
- Acute porphyria
- Autonomic epilepsy
- Monoamine oxidase inhibitors
- Tyramine in patients on monoamine oxidase inhibitors
- Menopausal "hot flashes"
- Hyperdynamic beta-adrenergic states

Diagnostic tests and procedures. The assay of catecholamines and their metabolites has markedly simplified the diagnosis of this disorder. Surgical exploration of a patient for this disorder should not be undertaken without chemical confirmation of the diagnosis.

In patients with continuous hypertension and/or symptoms, levels of plasma or urine catecholamines and their metabolites usually are clearly increased. A reliable assay of the catecholamines, metanephrines, or vanillylmandelic acid (VMA), is usually sufficient to confirm the diagnosis. Patients with large tumors may excrete disproportionately greater amounts of catecholamine metabolites because the amines can be metabolized by enzymes in the tumor cells before their release. Malignant tumors may release large amounts of dopamine, leading to the excretion of large amounts of homovanillic acid in the urine. It is important to eliminate drugs and dietary substances that interfere with these assays or to choose an appropriate assay procedure so that results are not misleading.

In patients having brief and infrequent paroxysms with symptom-free intervals, confirmation of the diagnosis may be more difficult. Although large amounts of catecholamines are produced during the brief episode, the total amount excreted during a 24-hour urine-collection period may not be clearly abnormal; this is in contrast to values in patients whose tumors secrete continuously. The latter group will accumulate larger amounts of catecholamines and metabolites even though secretion rates are lower and symptoms are less severe. Therefore sampling of blood or timed urine collections during a carefully observed episode may be necessary to confirm the diagnosis.

In patients with typical symptoms, provocative tests with glucagon or histamine are rarely needed; however, the possibility of a pheochromocytoma may be strong enough, or its presence dangerous enough (e.g., in pregnancy or before surgery), to require the use of these testing procedures to rule out the presence of such a tumor.

Assays for catecholamines and their metabolites are used to screen patients at high risk. Indications for screening patients are listed in the accompanying box. When blood cannot be obtained from patients at rest, the administration 0.3 mg of clonidine given 2 to 3 hours before sampling will

Patients to be screened for pheochromocytoma

Hypertensive patients with symptoms in the box on p. 1364
Young hypertensives, particularly with:
- Weight loss
- Seizures
- Orthostatic hypotension
- Unexplained shock

Family history of pheochromocytoma or medullary carcinoma of thyroid
Hypertension associated with:
- Neurofibromatosis and other neurocutaneous syndromes
- Mucosal neuromas
- Hyperglycemia
- Severe uncontrollable hypertension

Shock or severe pressor responses to:
- Induction of anesthesia
- Delivery
- Antihypertensive drugs

Incidentally discovered adrenal tumors

reduce the neurogenic contribution to norepinephrine levels.

In the occasional patient in whom the chemical tests are inconclusive, it may be useful or more convenient to institute therapy with phenoxybenzamine over 1 to 2 months to observe effects both on the nature and frequency of attacks and on the blood pressure. A salutary effect will sometimes be observed for a few weeks but seldom lasts longer in the absence of a pheochromocytoma. A good response indicates the need for reappraisal of the patient.

Localization of tumors. When the diagnosis has been established, the tumor must be located. Computed tomography (CT) and magnetic resonance imaging (MRI) are of great value in localizing these tumors (Fig. 164-3). MRI is somewhat more successful in locating extra-adrenal tumors and has the advantage of producing brighter images with T_2-weighting in contrast to most other adrenal tumors. Sonography also has proved to be safe and useful. Central venous sampling of blood for catecholamine assay via percutaneous venous catheter has been of great value in cases in which radiographic procedures fail, in which multiple tumors or metastases are suspected, or in which previous exploration has not disclosed all the tumor tissue. An example of the catecholamine levels in a patient with an intrarenal tumor is shown in Fig. 164-4; this procedure is rarely required.

Although not as widely available, scintograms following the injection of ^{131}I-labeled meta-iodobenzylguanidine (MIBG) are quite specific for identifying masses producing catecholamines, including neuroblastomas and pheochromocytomas. Administration of MIBG in these patients results in detectable images in 48 to 72 hours. It is particularly useful in identifying extra-adrenal tumors and metastases. It has also been used in the treatment of malignant tumors not amenable to surgical removal (see later).

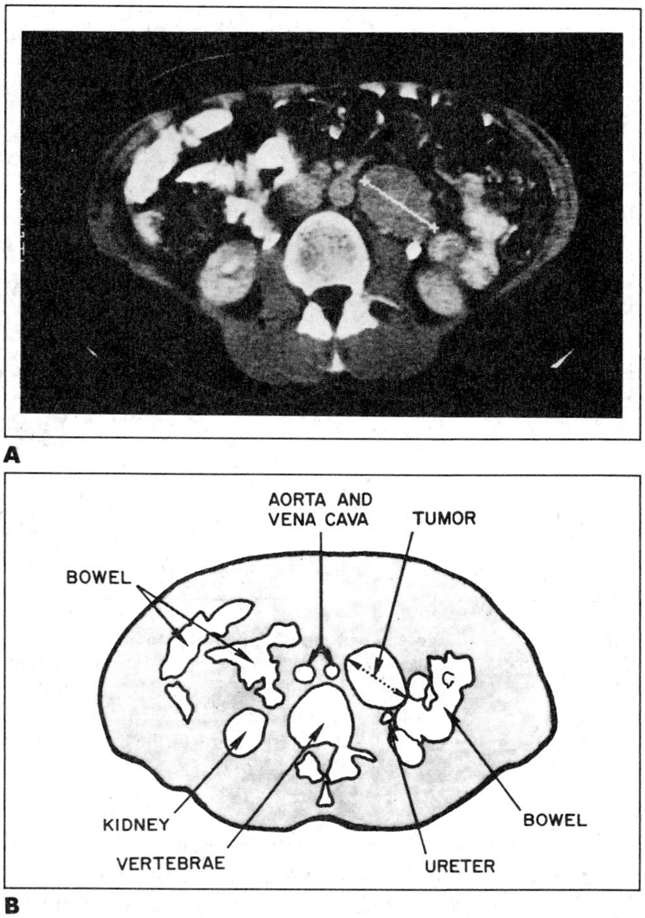

Fig. 164-3. **A,** An extra-adrenal pheochromocytoma localized to the left infrarenal area of the sympathetic chain by computed axial tomography. **B,** Identification of the important features of the scan. (From Goldfien A: Diseases of the adrenal medulla. In Basic and clinical endocrinology, Los Altos, Calif, 1982, Lange.)

Incidentally discovered tumors. As noted earlier, the use of CT and MRI to localize these tumors is indicated only after the diagnosis has been confirmed. Because these procedures are frequently used diagnostic tools, tumors in the region of the adrenal gland, are found in 2% to 5% of patients having CT or MRI scans. These patients should be screened for pheochromocytomas clinically and chemically as part of their workup.

Management

Optimal management of patients with pheochromocytomas requires an understanding of the pathophysiology produced by excessive catecholamines and an acquaintance with the action of adrenergic antagonists and other drugs used in the treatment of these patients (Chapter 23).

As soon as the diagnosis has been confirmed, therapy with adrenergic antagonists should be instituted. Appropri-

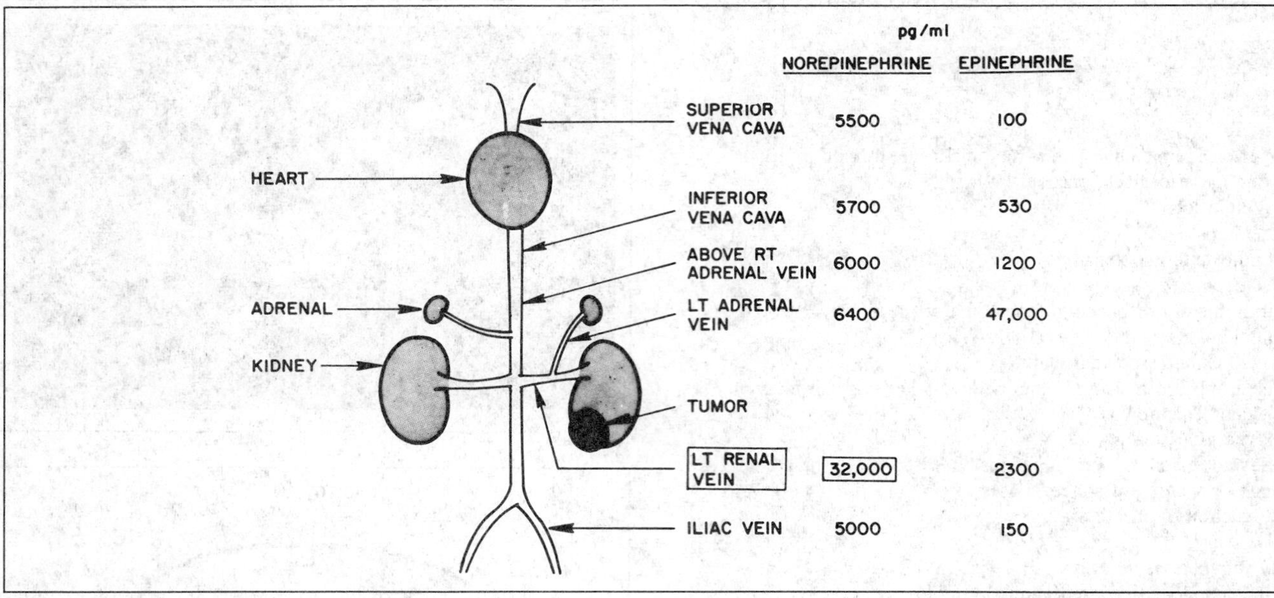

Fig 164-4. Catecholamine levels in blood obtained by percutaneous catheterization of the vena cava. The epinephrine concentration in the left adrenal vein is elevated as expected. However, the high concentration of norepinephrine in the left renal vein predicted that the tumor blood supply drained into that vessel and that the tumor would be found in the vicinity of the left kidney. (From Goldfien A: Diseases of the adrenal medulla. In Basic and clinical endocrinology, Los Altos, Calif, 1982, Lange.)

ate treatment is directed toward reducing the patient's symptoms, lowering of blood pressure, and amelioration of the paroxysms that either occur spontaneously or are induced by studies undertaken to localize the tumor or tumors. Such treatment will allow expansion of the vascular bed and plasma volume and will reduce the amount of transfused blood required for the maintenance of blood pressure after surgical removal of the tumor.

Although only a few days of this therapy are required for the preoperative study and preparation of these patients for surgery, prolonged medical therapy is advantageous in patients who have had recent myocardial infarctions, who have clinical evidence of catecholamine cardiomyopathy, or who are in their last trimester of pregnancy. They can be maintained on medical therapy until surgical removal of the tumor is undertaken.

Agents that commonly have been used in therapy include phentolamine and phenoxybenzamine. In patients with persistent paroxysms, phenoxybenzamine, a noncompetitive alpha-adrenergic antagonist with a prolonged effect, is indicated. Treatment is begun with doses of 20 to 40 mg/day and can be increased by 10 to 20 mg every 1 to 2 days until the desired effect is achieved. Completely normal blood pressure (lower than 140/90) may not be achieved and is not required. A dose of 60 to 80 mg daily is usually adequate, but two to three times as much may be necessary. When marked tachycardia or dysrhythmias occur, small doses of propranolol may be required but should only be given after alpha-receptor blockade is established.

Patients with infrequent paroxysms and an absence of interval manifestations can be treated similarly. Rapid titration of the dose may be difficult using phenoxybenzamine, however, because of its long half-life (36 hours). Prazosin, an alpha-antagonist, has also been found to be effective in these patients.

Preparation of the patient in this manner minimizes the hazards of anesthesia and surgery. The patient's blood pressure and cardiogram should be monitored continuously, and phentolamine and/or nitroprusside, propranolol, and other antiarrhythmic agents should be available. When multiple intra-abdominal tumors are suspected, they should be approached through a transabdominal incision to allow exploration of the adrenals, sympathetic ganglia, bladder, and other pelvic structures. When bilateral adrenal tumors are found and the adrenals removed, adrenocortical steroid replacement is required (Chapter 163).

When the tumor is removed, the blood pressure usually falls to levels of about 90/60 mmHg. A lower pressure or poor peripheral perfusion may indicate the need for blood volume expansion with whole blood, plasma, or other fluids. Pressor therapy is not usually required and should not be substituted for volume expansion.

The lack of a fall in pressure at the time of tumor removal (even in the presence of adrenergic blockade) suggests the presence of additional tumor tissue.

In patients with tumors producing persistent hypertension, the initial fall in blood pressure may be followed by an elevation of blood pressure postoperatively. The accompanying symptoms of sympathetic stimulation disappear, however, and the blood pressure and catecholamine levels return to normal over the next few weeks. If the blood pressure remains elevated, but the patient is otherwise asymptomatic, another cause for the elevated blood pressure should be considered. The presence of a renal vascular lesion or other coexistent causes of hypertension have been reported in several patients with pheochromocytomas. These tumors may be silent, secreting only small amounts of hormone. When these tumors are resected, the patient may show little change, and hypertension, if present, may persist.

Patients with nonresectable malignant tumors, metastases, or those who for other reasons are not amenable to successful surgical treatment can be managed medically for prolonged periods. Phenoxybenzamine can be used chronically as described. Patients with malignant tumors have also benefited symptomatically from treatment with alpha-methyl metatyrosine, an inhibitor of tyrosine hydroxylase, the rate-limiting enzyme in the biosynthetic process.

The incidence of malignant tumors in reported studies varies from less than 5% to more than 10%. These tumors can be recognized during surgery when there is significant local infiltration or metastases are identified. About 5% to 10% of patients thought to have been cured later experience recurrence of the tumor. Patients with extra-adrenal tumors and those whose tumors cells contain increased amounts of nuclear DNA are at higher risk of recurrence and should be screened at regular intervals after surgery. Although some patients with malignant pheochromocytomas die early because of disseminated disease, there are long-term survivors. The most common site of metastases is the skeleton, and these lesions may respond well to radiation therapy. The use of combination chemotherapy, alone or in combination with radiation, for soft tissue lesions has been successful in reducing the size and activity of metastases in some patients. The therapeutic use of ^{131}I-metaiodobenzylguanidine is being explored. Preliminary reports indicate that half of the patients treated experience partial remissions.

REFERENCES

Averbuch SD et al: Malignant pheochromocytoma: effective treatment with a combination of cyclophosphamide, vincristine, and dacarbazine, Ann Intern Med 109:267, 1988.

Clutter WE et al: Epinephrine plasma metabolic clearance rates and physiologic thresholds for metabolic and hemodynamic actions in man, Clin Invest 66:94, 1980.

Cryer PE: Physiology and pathophysiology of the human sympathoadrenal neuroendocrine system, N Engl J Med 303:436, 1980.

Gagel RF et al: The clinical outcome of prospective screening for multiple endocrine neoplasia type 2a. An 18-year experience, N Engl J Med 318:478, 1988.

Goldfien A: The adrenal medulla. In Greenspan FA and Forsham PH, editors: Basic and clinical endocrinology, Norwalk, Conn, 1989, Appleton & Lange.

Hollister AS: Orthostatic hypotension: causes, evaluation, and management, West J Med 157:662, 1992.

Krempf M et al: Use of m-[^{131}I]Iodobenzylguanidine in the treatment of malignant pheochromocytoma, J Clin Endocrinol Metab 72:455, 1991.

Manger WM and Gifford RW: Pheochromocytoma, New York, 1977, Springer.

Ponder BAJ and Jackson CE, editors: The Second International Workshop on Multiple Endocrine Neoplasia Type 2 Syndromes, Henry Ford Hosp Med J 335:2,3, 1987.

Ross NS and Aron DC: Hormonal evaluation of the patient with an incidentally discovered adrenal mass, N Engl J Med 323:1401, 1990.

Schatz IJ: Orthostatic hypotension, Arch Intern Med 144:733, 1984.

Sheps SG et al: Recent development in the diagnosis and treatment of pheochromocytoma, Mayo Clin Proc 65:88, 1990.

CHAPTER

165 Disorders of the Ovary

William F. Crowley, Jr.

BASIC PHYSIOLOGY

The human ovary is divided functionally and morphologically into two separate compartments. The first, composed of the granulosa and thecal cells, is responsible for steroidogenesis. The cells of this compartment secrete the steroids that initiate the appearance of secondary sexual characteristics at puberty, sustain cyclic estrogen and progesterone secretion throughout the reproductive years, and finally maintain low-level estrogen and androgen secretion after the menopause. These steroidogenic cells additionally secrete numerous peptides into the follicular milieu to sustain the maturing oocyte.

The second ovarian compartment, which is responsible for gametogenesis, consists of the germinal epithelium, or the oocyte population. The steroidogenic constituents of the ovary support the final stages of development of these oocytes and ensure their timely preparation for ovulation and possible fertilization (Fig. 165-1).

Ovarian function then can be viewed developmentally in four distinct periods: the neonatal period, puberty, the reproductive years, and the menopause.

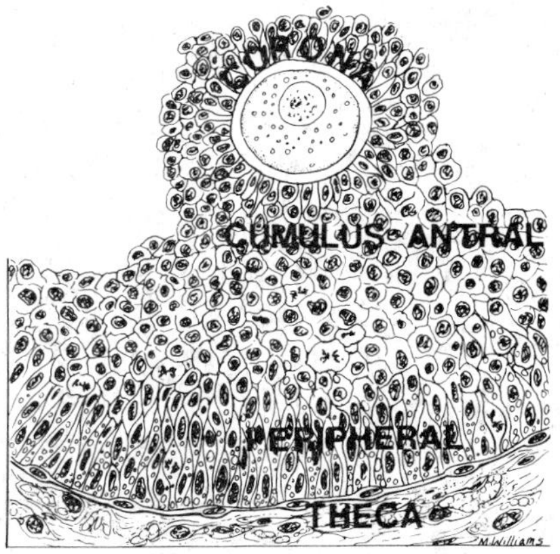

Fig. 165-1. A section through a graafian follicle. Granulosa cells surround the oocyte and secrete estradiol. (Courtesy of Dr L Zoller, Department of Anatomy, Boston University School of Medicine.)

Neonatal period

Throughout early development, the ovary is undergoing a continual attrition of its germ cell population. The peak population of 7 million oocytes is attained by the fifth month of embryonic development, whereas only 2 million remain at birth. Thus fetal development is associated with a progressive loss of germ cells. The steroidogenic compartment is also generally inactive until the final trimester of pregnancy.

At the time of delivery, pulsatile gonadotropin secretion occurs with a predominance of follicle-stimulating hormone (FSH) over luteinizing hormone (LH) secretion. This gonadotropin secretion initiates steroidogenesis and early folliculogenesis, both of which are maintained during the neonatal period. After this brief developmental window of hypothalamic-pituitary-ovarian activity, the ovary undergoes a quiescence that is accompanied by a decrease in steroidogenesis during the ovarian latency of childhood; however, follicular attrition continues. Of the remaining 2 million oocytes present at birth, only 300,000 are left by puberty.

Puberty

At puberty, sleep-entrained gonadotropin secretion (Fig. 165-2) becomes manifest, initially with a marked predominance of FSH secretion in the female. The gonadotropins secreted with a high FSH/LH ratio reinitiate ovarian function with subsequent steroidogenic secretion from the granulosa cells and secondary sexual maturation. Numerous ovarian follicles also develop, but the vast majority of these early follicles do not ovulate. This early anovulation is primarily related to the failure of estradiol-induced positive feedback and consequent lack of an LH surge in response to estradiol.

By late puberty, the sleep-entrained pattern of gonadotropin secretion gives way to a sleep-suspended state of gonadotropin-releasing hormone (GnRH) release in the early follicular phase of the menstrual cycle, the development of estradiol-induced LH surge and ovulation. These earliest ovulatory cycles of the adolescent period, however, are frequently characterized by inadequate length or insufficient progesterone secretion during the luteal phase, that is, an inadequate luteal phase. Only with progressive gynecologic maturity does a fully normal ovarian cycle occur.

Reproductive years

During the reproductive years, cyclic folliculogenesis occurs in a regular 28-day cycle (Fig. 165-3). During the earliest part of the follicular phase there is an increase in the frequency of GnRH secretion, which begins during the late luteal phase of one cycle and progresses across the early follicular phase of the next. This abrupt change in GnRH frequency occurs during the nadir of sex steroids and inhibin, which are reached at the luteal-follicular transition. Such an increase in hypothalamic-pituitary activity causes a temporary predominance of FSH secretion, which subsequently recruits a new wave of folliculogenesis in the ovaries. By days 5 to 7 of the menstrual cycle, the dominant

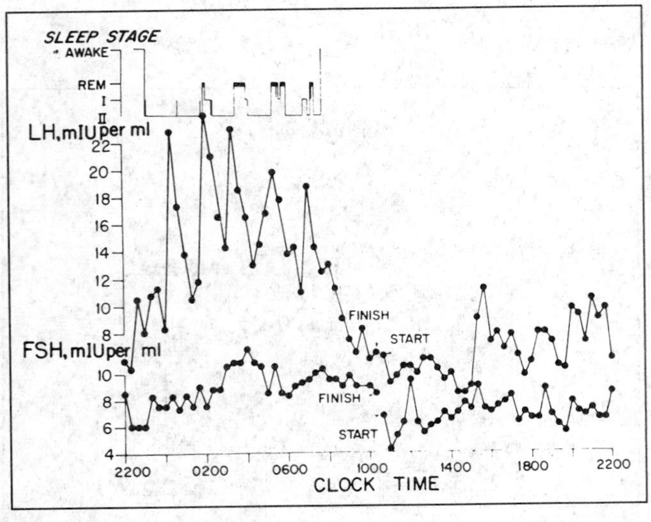

Fig. 165-2. Serial blood LH and FSH concentrations obtained every 20 minutes during sleep and wakefulness in a 13-year-old pubertal girl. (From Boyar RM et al: N Engl J Med 289:282-286, 1973.)

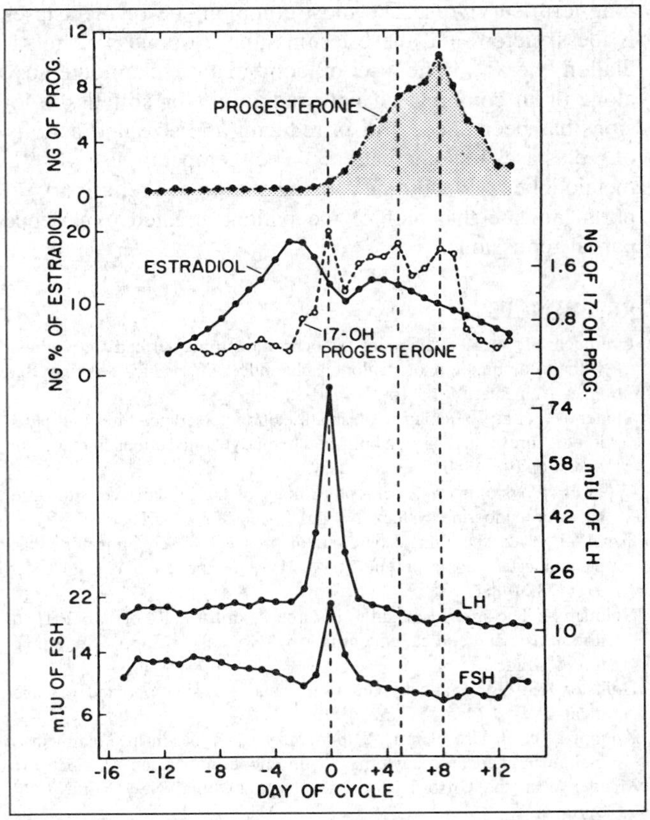

Fig. 165-3. Mean plasma LH, FSH, and steroid concentrations in apparently normally cycling young women. Levels are synchronized about the midcycle or periovulatory surge of LH. (From Vaitukaitis JL and Ross GT: Pharmacol Ther 1:317-329, 1976.)

follicle is manifest. Enhanced estradiol secretion from this follicle can be documented by ovarian vein sampling. Soon thereafter, the dominant follicle becomes visible ultrasonographically, eventually reaching a diameter of approximately 1.5 to 2.5 cm by midcycle.

During the follicular phase of the menstrual cycle, the development of the dominant follicle is associated with a coordinated atresia of the remaining cohort of recruited follicles. Eventually, the rising tide of estradiol secreted from the emerging dominant follicle evokes an LH surge from the pituitary. This LH secretion causes rupture of the follicle, permitting release of the mature oocyte. Thereafter, the corpus luteum secretes progesterone, estradiol, and inhibin, which act in concert to slow GnRH secretion and suppress pituitary function. This combination of biochemical events results in a nadir of circulating gonadotropin levels by the midluteal phase, a marked slowing of the GnRH pulse generator, and eventually, luteolysis. After dissolution of the corpus luteum, the frequency of GnRH secretion increases abruptly once again, with FSH levels rising more rapidly than LH, and the next wave of folliculogenesis ensues. Should fertilization have occurred in the cycle, the corpus luteum of pregnancy is sustained by human chorionic gonadotropin (hCG) and other, as yet undescribed, factors that support the corpus luteum of pregnancy until the time of placentation.

Menopause

Commencing in the fifth decade of life, the ovarian complement of oocytes approaches exhaustion. As this loss of germ cells occurs, there is an initial rise of FSH followed by LH levels (Fig. 165-4). After the complete disappearance of oocytes, a marked atrophy of the ovaries ensues with a consequent rise of both gonadotropins to castrate levels. However, there remains a persistent secretion of androstenedione and low levels of estrogen from the menopausal ovary. Although insufficient to sustain menstrual cyclicity and prohibit symptoms of estrogen deficiency, these hormone levels are significant in that symptoms occur if the postmenopausal ovary is removed. At menopause, symptoms of estrogen deficiency such as hot flashes, vaginal dryness, atrophy of the secondary sexual characteristics, and decreased bone density may appear after the decrease in steroidogenesis is complete.

Summary

The ovary undergoes a series of specific developmental and physiologic changes over the life span of the female that reflect a delicate balance of steroidogenesis and gametogenesis. Sex steroid secretion from the ovary initiates sexual maturation, maintains the sex steroid-dependent target organs in a state of readiness for implantation, and eventually decreases at the menopause. Gametogenesis occurs in the milieu of this carefully coordinated sex steroid environment, permits fertility, and ensures the reproductive capability of the individual as well as the propagation of the species.

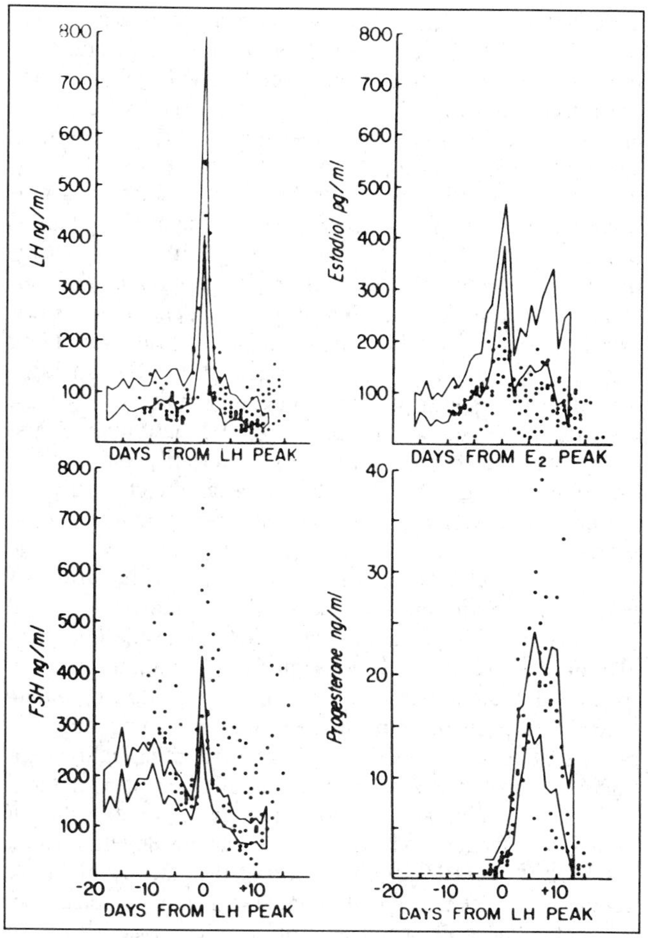

Fig. 165-4. Circulating levels of LH, FSH, estradiol, and progesterone among perimenopausal women. The 95% competence limits for gonadotropin and sex steroid levels among women during their earlier years of reproduction are encompassed by the connected line. (From Sherman BM, West JH, and Korenman SG: J Clin Endocrinol Metab 42:629-636, 1976.)

MODULATION OF GONADOTROPIN SECRETION

General

Ovarian function is principally determined by the timing, relative ratios and pattern of gonadotropin secretion from the anterior pituitary gland. These are, in turn, modulated by both hypothalamic GnRH secretion and ovarian sex steroid and peptide secretion. The relative influences of these predominantly positive (hypothalamic input) and negative (ovarian feedback) inputs to the gonadotroph then determine the milieu to which the ovary respond, and the changes in these inputs vary dynamically across development and the menstrual cycle.

Hypothalamic secretion of the gonadotropin-releasing hormone

GnRH is secreted into the hypophyseal-portal blood supply from the nerve terminals of the parvocellular neurons predominantly in the anterior hypothalamus. Release of GnRH secretion into the hypophyseal-portal circulation, and consequently on the gonadotropin-secreting cells of the anterior pituitary, is episodic in nature. Classic studies by Knobil and his colleagues have determined that this intermittency of GnRH stimulation is of critical importance for maintenance of physiologic levels of gonadotropin secretion. Continuous stimulation of the pituitary by GnRH and/or its long-acting agonistic analogs produces a paradoxic and selective desensitization and suppresses gonadotropin secretion. In fact, this resulting biochemical castration has been the basis of treatment for a wide variety of reproductive disorders by long-acting GnRH analogs. Therefore the input to the hypothalamic-pituitary axis must be pulsatile in nature for physiologic functioning of the ovary. This intermittent mode of secretion offers several different methods of modulating ovarian function by differences in patterns, ratios, and intervals of gonadotropin secretion.

GnRH secretion is also modulated by a wide variety of hormonal, environmental, metabolic, and developmental inputs (Fig. 165-5). These factors determine the ontogeny of GnRH secretion and, consequently, gonadotropin, and ovarian output. Several of these influences that modulate GnRH secretion have been identified, including biogenic amines (adrenergic, serotonergic and dopamanergic), peptidergic (substance P. endorphins), and sex steroid feedback. Other modulating factors such as the relationship of GnRH secretion to body weight and various developmental inhibitors of GnRH secretion during the latency of childhood are not yet elucidated. Together, however, these various modulators determine the quiescence or activation of gonadotropin secretion and ovarian function.

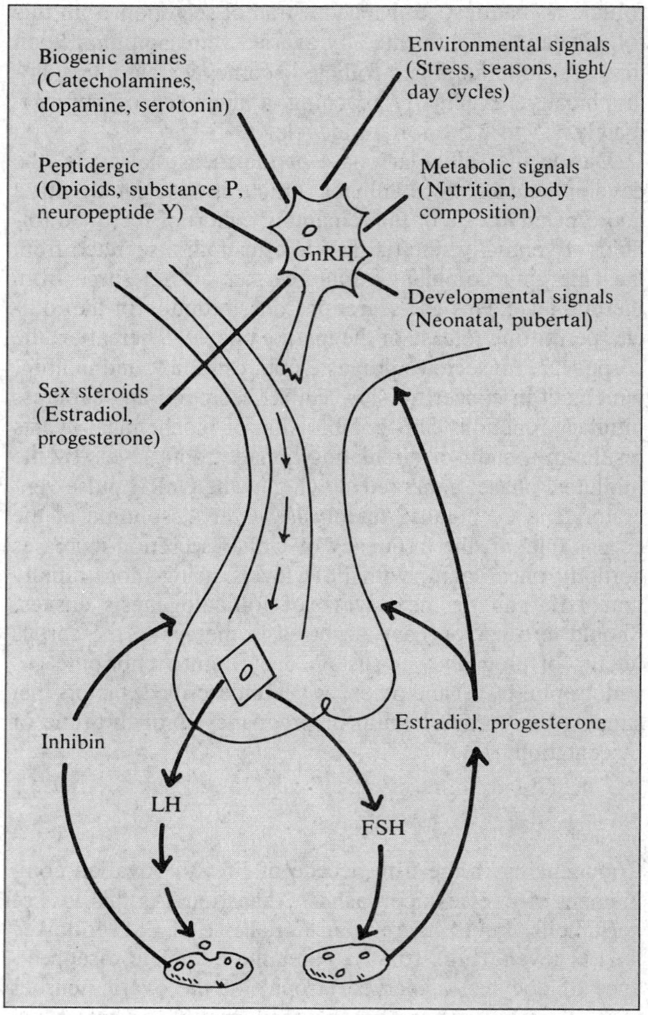

Fig. 165-5. Overview of the hypothalamic-pituitary-ovarian axis. GnRH is secreted episodically from the hypothalamus and causes pulsatile release of LH and FSH.

Pituitary gonadotropin secretion

The pituitary gonadotropins LH and FSH, are glycoproteins comprising common alpha-subunit and a unique beta-subunit (Chapter 160). The frequency of secretion of these gonadotropins depends solely on the frequency of antecedent GnRH secretion from the hypothalamus. The amplitude of their secretion, however, is determined by the quantity of GnRH secreted within a given episode of hypothalamic firing as well as by negative feedback of sex steroids and other ovarian products. Thus by a combination of varying the amount and frequency of GnRH secretion from the hypothalamus, as well as the sex steroid and peptide secretion from the ovarian follicle, the anterior pituitary gonadotroph is essential in determining both the paracrine hormonal milieu within the ovary and the intensity of gonadotropin secretion to the ovary. The combined feedback mechanism modulates the level of FSH secretion, such that only a single dominant follicle will develop each month.

Ovarian feedback mechanisms

The major sex steroids that exert feedback effects on gonadotroph are estradiol and progesterone. Estradiol, secreted by the granulosa cells of the growing follicle, initially exerts a negative feedback effect on LH and FSH secretion by two different mechanisms. The initial feedback effects of estradiol on the pituitary gonadotroph are to decrease FSH secretion and increase GnRH pulse frequency across the follicular phase of the cycle. However, the negative feedback exerted by estradiol on FSH secretion is the predominant effect. This limits the quantity and, possibly, the bioactivity of the FSH available to the growing follicle in such a manner that only a single follicle is cultivated. The hormonal support for other, nondominant follicles of the cohort is insufficient, and they become atretic. The dominant follicle has an increased number of FSH receptors, and therefore is relatively protected from the effects of a decline in circulating FSH. The dominant follicle thus is capable of surviving the progressively lower amounts of FSH occurring across the mid-to-late follicular phase of the cycle from the negative feedback effects of increasing estradiol levels. Atretic follicles do not have this capability and therefore involute during this period.

In addition to its early negative feedback on gonadotropin secretion, estradiol has a later, positive feedback effect on GnRH frequency. This feedback combined with the positive effects of estradiol on the pituitary ultimately culminates in the midcycle LH and FSH surge. These ovarian feedback effects, taken in combination, determine the declining FSH levels across the follicular phase with progressive increases in LH levels, culminating in the midcycle surge of both gonadotropins, which ruptures the dominant follicle and releases the egg.

At the uterine level, estradiol secretion across the follicular phase induces growth in the glandular elements, a consequent increase in the width of the endometrium, and initiation of a number of secretory events designed to result in successful implantation of the subsequently fertilized ovum.

Commencing at the time of ovulation, progesterone becomes the dominant ovarian sex steroid. Progesterone has a marked feedback effect on the hypothalamus, resulting in progressive and near total slowing of GnRH secretion over the ensuing 14 days of the luteal phase. Progesterone also halts the progressive proliferation of the endometrium that occurred during the estrogen-dominant follicular phase of the cycle and causes differentiation of the glandular epithelium into a secretory pattern with the appearance of glycogen at the base of the endometrial cells. With declining levels of progesterone across the last half of the luteal phase, there is a gradual withdrawal of steroid support, resulting in a series of microinfarctions of the glandular element and culminating in sloughing of the endometrium at the time of the menstrual period.

The granulosa and thecal cells of the ovarian follicle also produce inhibin, a dimeric protein comprising an alpha-subunit covalently linked with a beta-subunit to form a biologically active dimer. This glycoprotein has been isolated, sequenced, and cloned. When the alpha- and beta-subunits are combined, they exert a potent and relatively selective inhibition of FSH secretion, both basally and in response to GnRH, at the level of the anterior pituitary gland. This selective inhibition of FSH secretion is particularly evident in the midluteal phase of the cycle, during which inhibin combines with the midluteal peaks of estradiol and progesterone to achieve a maximal suppression of FSH secretion. Inhibin levels subsequently decline by the late luteal phase, thus permitting a rise in FSH to occur, which reinitiates the next wave of folliculogenesis. Ovarian cells also appear capable of making a beta/beta homodimer termed *activin,* which has opposing actions to those of inhibin. Thus whereas inhibin suppresses basal FSH and GnRH-stimulated FSH secretion from the anterior pituitary, activin produces a stimulation of FSH secretion.

In addition to the ability to secrete these modulatory peptides, developing granulosa cells of the follicle contain both estrogen and androgen receptors, which permit a local response to secreted sex steroids. Moreover, the mechanisms of action of these sex steroids are often in opposition, thus providing a local set of modulators of follicular growth. Estrogen increases the number of FSH receptors on the follicle and thus contributes to the emerging dominance of one follicle. In contrast, androgens binding to their receptors inhibit this process in the soon-to-be-atretic follicle. Estrogens also increase the number of LH receptors on the granulosa cells and thus further prepare the dominant follicle for responding to the ensuing LH surge. Androgens oppose this mechanism of action.

Thus it is clear that there are several active autocrine and paracrine systems at work within the ovary. These ensure the achievement of dominance and ovulation of that dominant follicle at the time of the midcycle while opposing forces induce atresia of the competing follicles.

LABORATORY TESTS AND DIAGNOSTIC PROCEDURES

Gonadotropin levels (Chapter 160)

Because the secretion of gonadotropins is intermittent in nature, randomly obtained gonadotropin levels are of somewhat limited value in assisting with the diagnosis of various conditions likely to affect the ovary. Given these limitations, the diagnosis of certain ovarian dysfunctions can be greatly facilitated by random gonadotropin determinations. For example, premature ovarian failure is uniformly characterized by a striking elevation of the serum FSH levels into the menopausal ranges (see Table 165-1). In this circumstance, FSH levels are often the first gonadotropins to be elevated, in addition to being elevated to a greater degree than LH levels, thereby becoming a sine qua non for this diagnosis. Similarly, patients with polycystic ovarian disease (Fig. 165-6) have a remarkable elevation of their LH/FSH ratio due to an increased frequency and amplitude of gonadotropin pulsations when compared with normal levels. Consequently, random samples of gonadotropins are often useful in assisting with this diagnosis because they demonstrate consistently high LH/FSH ratios.

All gonadotropin determinations must be interpreted in view of the patient's menstrual history, including both the preceding as well as the subsequent menstrual period, because dramatic changes occurring across the menstrual cycle can often mimic the changes seen in various disease states. Additionally, any gonadotropin determinations have to be viewed in the perspective of accompanying sex steroid levels. For example, if LH and FSH levels are elevated in a random sample, one needs to know whether the patient is cycling, and therefore was possibly at midcycle at the time of the determination, or amenorrheic with hot flashes and low estradiol levels, in which case a diagnosis of premature ovarian failure is more appropriate. Therefore a good menstrual cycle history and accompanying sex steroid levels are critical for the interpretation of random gonadotropin levels.

Most gonadotropin assays are increasingly specific for the beta-subunit of each of the gonadotropins. Because no pure standard exists for gonadotropin determinations, however, these levels are by necessity referenced to an international reference preparation, most often the *Second International Reference Preparation of Human Menopausal Gonadotropin (hMG).* Perhaps more important than the indi-

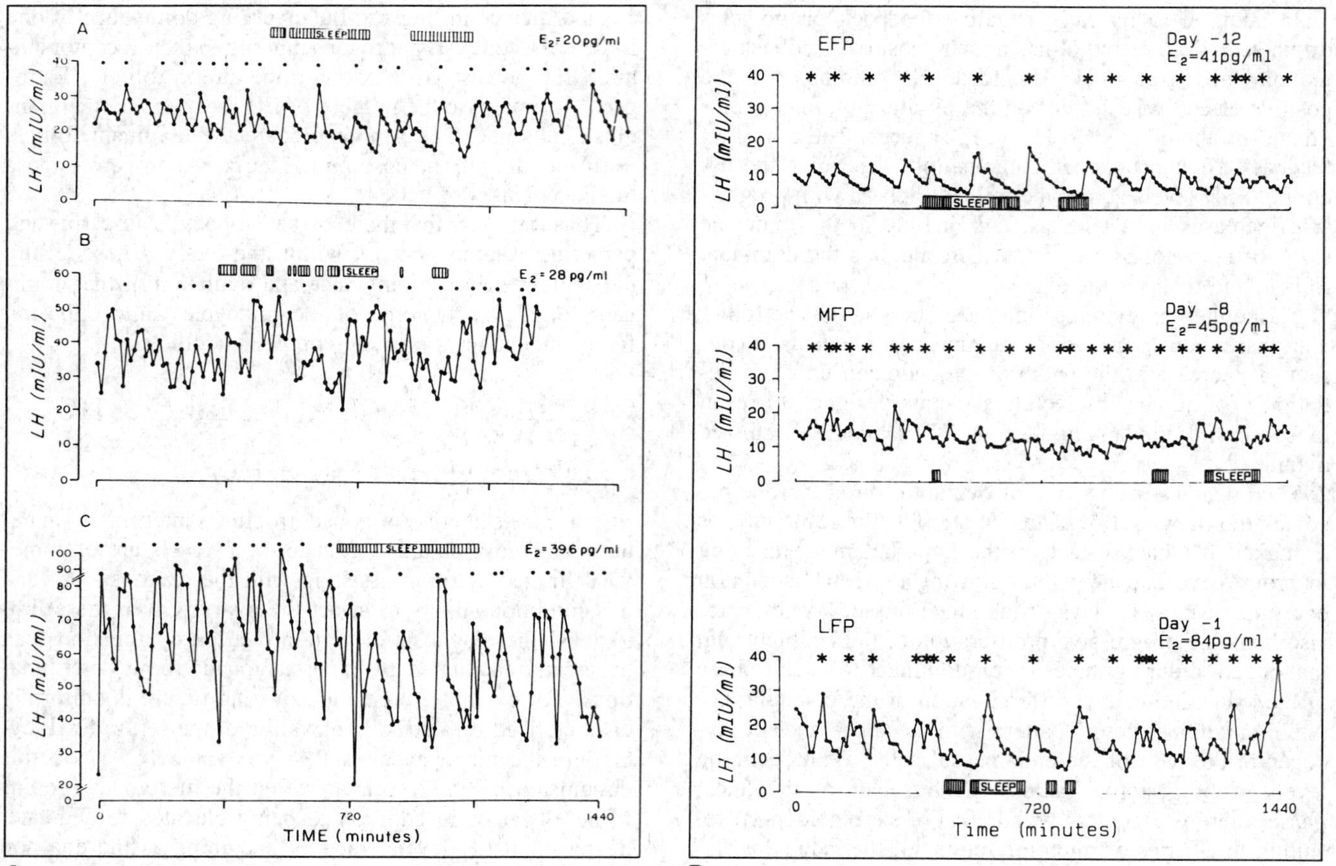

Fig. 165-6. Gonadotropic pulsations in three women with polycystic ovarian disease on the left, as compared with three normal women from early follicular *(upper right),* midfollicular *(middle right)* and late follicular *(lower right)* phase of a normal ovulatory cycle. The increase in both the frequency and amplitude of GnRH-induced gonadotropin pulsations in PCOD women is apparen (From Waldstreicher et al: J Clin Endocrinol Metab 66:165-172, 1988.)

vidual reference standard used is the need for the clinician to be familiar with the laboratory and its normal ranges. To achieve this goal, the physician must communicate with the laboratory to determine the confidence in the normative ranges. Table 165-1 demonstrates normal gonadotropin and sex steroid levels performed on the basis of daily bloods across 80 ovulatory cycles, and thus the levels are reasonably precise determinations of the normal range for this particular reference laboratory.

With the recent availability of recombinant gonadotropins and monoclonal antibodies, it will soon become possible to make more precise and universally applicable determinations of gonadotropins based on molar equivalents. In addition, the specific epitopes recognized by these antibodies will be determined, and thus the combination of improved measurements and pure standards will address many of the previous methodologic problems inherent in gonadotropin determinations.

Sex steroid levels

Estradiol and progesterone levels are usually measured by radioimmunoassay following organic solvent extraction of plasma to eliminate sex steroid binding to testosterone-estrogen binding globulin (TEBG) and cortisol-binding globulin (CBG), which bind estradiol and progesterone, respectively. These binding globulins obscure direct plasma measurements and therefore necessitate a preassay extraction step. Normative values for each of these levels are listed in Table 165-1 and do not vary as much from laboratory to laboratory as do gonadotropins because pure standards and relatively specific antisera are now widely available.

Inhibin/activin levels

At present, there are no widely validated assays for inhibin and activin. However, it is expected that specific assays for both will become widely available in the near future and for use in diagnosing various infertility states.

Ultrasonographic studies

With the advent of transvaginal ultrasound, it has now become clear that fine anatomic details of the ovary can be visualized by this noninvasive method, including total ovar-

Table 165-1. Normative data: female reproductive hormones

	Prepuberty	Menstrual cycle* EF	Midcycle	LF	Menopause
Estradiol (pg/ml)	<10	23-56	115-500	68-180	<20
Progesterone (ng/ml)	<0.2	0.2-0.6	0.3-3.5	6.5-32	<0.2
LH (mIU/ml)	<0.8-5.0	5-26	43-187	2-35	30-150
FSH (mIU/ml)	1-10	5-28	13-41	5-15	30-170
Testosterone (ng/dl)	<50	—	<90	—	<70

*Based on 80 ovulatory cycles.

ian size, number and size of developing ovarian follicles, and the stroma/theca ratio. Thus it is relatively easy to distinguish a neonatal ovary from one that is inactive during the latency of childhood. The pubertal ovary also has been identified to have a distinct morphologic appearance, with numerous, large cysts, very similar to some patients with polycystic ovarian disease. However, pubertal patients show a change in this morphology over time, whereas patients with polycystic ovarian disease show an increasing tendency to subcortical cysts, nonovulatory follicles, increase of stromal/cortex ratio, and an increased ovarian size over time. Similarly, the postmenopausal ovary reveals the absence of follicular structure and small-sized ovaries, although this is very difficult to distinguish from a relatively inactive ovary in an amenorrheic patient. Serum gonadotropin levels, however, are helpful in distinguishing primary gonadal failure from that secondary to a hypogonadotropic state. Thus ultrasound will serve as an increasing alternative for laparoscopic visualization of ovarian size and morphology in the future.

PATHOPHYSIOLOGIC DISORDERS

Ovarian disorders may be differentiated into two broad classes. The first includes disorders whose pathophysiology stems from inappropriate input to the ovary by the hypothalamic-pituitary axis. These include primary amenorrhea due to GnRH deficiency, "hypothalamic amenorrhea" due to an inappropriate secretion of GnRH, and polycystic ovarian disease. In the second group of ovarian disorders, there is an intrinsic disorder within the ovary itself. Typical examples include Turner's syndrome, in which the gametogenic portion of the ovary is exhausted before menarche, and premature ovarian failure. In both disorders there are elevated gonadotropins secondary to an intrinsic ovarian abnormality.

Ovarian disorders associated with abnormal hypothalamic-pituitary input

Hypothalamic amenorrhea. As described in detail in Chapter 156, the clinical presentation of subjects with hypothalamic amenorrhea can occur before puberty (primary amenorrhea) or after menarche (secondary amenorrhea). The usual clinical associations with this form of amenorrhea include stress, recent medical illness, exercise, severe weight loss (anorexia nervosa), bulimia, or other medical disorders that are usually accompanied by an alteration of body weight or other metabolic stress.

The central pathophysiologic abnormality of hypothalamic amenorrhea relates to disordered endogenous secretion of GnRH from the hypothalamus. These abnormal patterns of GnRH secretion (see Fig. 156-1) include a spectrum of abnormalities of GnRH secretion, varying from the total absence of GnRH secretion to disorders of its frequency or amplitude. Correction of this condition often results from mere removal of the stress to the hypothalamic-pituitary-gonadal axis. For example, in the vast majority of cases, instituting nutritional rehabilitation, decreasing exercise, removal of stress, etc. results in a restoration of menstrual cycles. If menses do not resume spontaneously and fertility is the goal of the patient, then a variety of agents can be used to induce ovulation, including clomiphene citrate, pulsatile GnRH, or exogenous gonadotropin administration. It should be recalled that hypothalamic amenorrhea is always a diagnosis of association and exclusion. Therefore anatomic defects of the hypothalamic-pituitary axis, prolactin-secreting tumors, and polycystic ovarian disease must be excluded on the basis of history, physical examination, appropriate anatomic studies, and measurement of serum prolactin and androgen levels.

Polycystic ovarian disease and hyperthecosis. Polycystic ovarian disease (PCOD) can have a myriad of presentations, including oligoamenorrhea, hirsutism, amenorrhea, or, rarely, frank virilization. The most typical presentation is severe oligoamenorrhea in association with a slowly progressive hirsutism having its onset in the peripubertal period. These clinical features are often combined with variable elevations of androgen secretion, abnormally high LH/FSH ratios, and recurrent anovulation. More recently, sensitive ultrasonographic visualizations of the ovary have revealed enlarged ovaries, a very high stroma/follicle ratio, and a peripheral array of numerous small follicles underlying a thickened capsule. These changes are in sharp distinction to the typical changes in the ovary in the peripubertal period, in which a lesser degree of ovarian enlargement occurs. A consistent array of large follicles are interspersed throughout the ovary, and there is a lack of consistent demonstration of a thecal hyperplasia to the ovaries. Pathologic examination confirms what is seen by ultrasound, that is, a number of peripherally arrayed and luteinized follicles without evidence of recent ovulation and marked thecal as well as interstitial hyperplasia of the ovary itself.

Hyperthecosis is believed to be a variant of PCOD in which the number of follicles is even more dramatically reduced, with a corresponding increase in the hyperplastic theca associated with normal-sized ovaries. This dense thecal involvement is also accompanied by higher degrees of hyperandrogenemia.

Undoubtedly, the polycystic ovary can be produced by several pathophysiologic mechanisms. In this regard, it is much akin to an end-stage kidney. Most certainly one of the pathophysiologic schemas involves an increase in the amplitude and frequency of endogenous GnRH secretion, resulting in an abnormally high LH/FSH ratio. This abnormal ratio results, in turn, in an overstimulation of the thecal components of the ovary by LH, insufficient stimulation of folliculogenesis by FSH, and a recurrent anovulatory state associated with thecal hyperplasia and hyperandrogenemia from the ovary. It is unclear whether this abnormality of hypothalamic-pituitary secretion is primary or merely secondary to hyperandrogenemia elsewhere. However, pituitary suppression by oral contraceptive agents or GnRH analogs results in a complete reversion of the biochemical abnormalities and the reduction in size of the ovaries during serial follow-up studies.

Yet another mechanism of production of polycystic ovarian disease syndrome seems to occur in its association with insulin resistance. The clinical marker of this pathophysiologic subset of PCOD patients is acanthosis nigricans, which serves as the dermatologic marker of severe insulin resistance. It appears that the theca of the ovary has receptors for somatomedin-C that are stimulated by the high circulating insulin levels, which, in conjunction with the high LH levels, results in an overresponsiveness of the ovary with androgen secretion. Undoubtedly, further pathophysiologic pathways to the production of PCOD will be uncovered.

Treatment of this condition depends on the patient's complaint. For patients merely requiring regular menstrual periods and/or relief of their hirsutism, suppression of the pituitary-ovarian axis with birth control pills or GnRH analogs results in an orderly shedding of the endometrium, reduction of endometrial hyperplasia, institution of regular menses, and a decrease of ovarian production of androgens with their attendant hirsutism. For those subjects desiring fertility, induction of ovulation with clomiphene citrate, pulsatile GnRH, or exogenous gonadotropin administration can be undertaken. Special care should be given to patients with PCOD, as they are particularly prone to ovarian hyperstimulation and multiple gestation by each of these methods of ovulation induction. Finally, for the rare subset of patients with PCOD in association with congenital hyperplasia or mild hyperprolactinemia, correction of the underlying defect results in restoration of normal menstrual cycles and fertility. In vitro fertilization is playing an increasing role in the fertility wishes of patients with PCOD.

Disorders of the ovary with intrinsic ovarian pathology

Turner's syndrome. Patients with Turner's syndrome demonstrate a complete deletion of their second X chromosome, and thus most commonly have a karyotype of XO. Usually, this is a lethal defect and approximately 99% of Turner's karyotypes are associated with early fetal loss. Approximately 1% of patients with the Turner's karyotype survive; this number is even greater when one considers subtle mosaicism of the X chromosome with more variable clinical abnormalities that resemble Turner's syndrome. Typical children with Turner's syndrome present with various dysmorphic features such as hypertelorism, widely spaced nipples, increased carrying angles of the elbow, cardiac abnormalities, and, most commonly in early childhood, lymphedema. By mid-childhood, their growth deficiency becomes manifest, multiple cutaneous nevi appear, and many of the other skeletal features such as increased carrying angles of the elbows become more apparent. For those subjects with mosaicism, all of these manifestations are attenuated.

The ovarian morphology in Turner's syndrome consists of an ovary that is generally similar to that of a postmenopausal ovary. Although the disease may be recognized at birth or during early childhood, most typically Turner's patients present at menarche with primary amenorrhea in association with short stature. Some patients with retention of a portion of the second X chromosome and consequent mosaicism can retain sufficient numbers of ovarian follicles to have a normal puberty, secondary amenorrhea, and even conception if their presentation is sufficiently attenuated. The mechanism by which this accelerated atresia of ovarian follicles in childhood occurs in patients with the absence of an X chromosome is unknown. It is quite clear, however, that the presence of a second X chromosome is protective against this rapid depletion of the follicles in early childhood that produces menopause before the age of menarche in the XO patients.

Therapy is generally supportive in childhood, although the combination of growth hormone plus nonaromatizable androgens now appears to offer promise for increasing mid-childhood growth velocities and, perhaps, adult stature. During puberty, estrogen administration promotes secondary sexual characteristics at the appropriate time. Should fertility become a request, in vitro fertilization with donor eggs can be explored.

Gonadal dysgenesis in phenotypically and karyotypically normal women. A small subset of women have hypergonadotropic amenorrhea, with a normal karyotype presenting at puberty. Whereas some of these women may have subtle deletions of the X chromosome not demonstrable by usual karyotypic methods, others may also have had in utero or neonatal viral infections such as mumps that may have destroyed the germinal cell epithelium before puberty. Generally, these patients present with primary amenorrhea with elevated gonadotropins quite similar to patients with Turner's syndrome, but lack the other dysmorphic features suggestive of deletion of the other X chromosome. In general, these patients grow normally during childhood, but lack a pubertal growth spurt. Because they do not exhibit sex steroid secretion from the gonads at puberty, however, their epiphyses do not fuse until early in adult life, and thus they may have eunucoidal body proportions, their span exceeding their height by several inches. The upper/lower segment ratio is also increased in these subjects, depending on the time of diagnosis.

Premature ovarian failure. Approximately 10% of patients presenting at a reproductive clinic with secondary amenorrhea will demonstrate a hypergonadotropic condition, termed *premature ovarian failure,* if it occurs before age 35. This syndrome has many etiologies and typically presents with a history of a waxing and waning course characterized by periods of hot flashes, elevated gonadotropins and amenorrhea alternating with periods of breast tenderness, remission of hot flashes, and ovulation with spontaneous pregnancy. Such a course is quite similar to that occurring during the normal perimenopausal period in women aged 40 to 45 immediately before the completion of the menopausal process.

Conditions associated with this process, suggesting an autoimmune basis in a subset of patients, include autoimmune thyroiditis and adrenal failure, in conjunction with premature menopause (Schmidt's syndrome). In other women onset follows chemotherapy in early life for childhood malignancies, abdominal irradiation, or toxic exposures such as mumps or oophoritis. Other subsets have a familial pattern and have been determined to have subtle deletions of an otherwise normal X chromosome so that only premature ovarian failure is manifest. Finally, other subjects with premature ovarian failure have been demonstrated to have "resistant" ovaries, in which follicles are histologically evident in their ovaries despite hypergonadotropic hypogonadism. In this subset, an antibody to the FSH receptor, suggesting an autoimmune etiology, has been demonstrated in several cases.

The waxing and waning nature of this condition makes interpretation of any treatments particularly problematic. Thus pregnancies have been reported with low-dose estrogen, high-dose glucocorticoid, oral contraceptive, and GnRH analog suppression of this condition. Whether any of these are truly effective or are merely temporarily associated with a natural remission of the process remains unclear. From a practical viewpoint, in vitro fertilization with donor egg insemination is an alternative for patients seeking fertility.

Swyer's syndrome. A rare form of XY gonadal dysgenesis, Swyer's syndrome, is an uncommon disorder in which patients are usually phenotypically normal females who present with amenorrhea and streak ovaries bilaterally. They may exhibit some sign of Turner's syndrome such as wide carrying angles of their elbows and short stature. However, they differ from Turner's patients in that they have some signs of androgen excess that typically only appear at the time of pubertal activation of gonadotropin secretion.

Because the gonads of these patients are quite dysgenetic and have a high incidence of neoplastic transformation beginning in the second decade of life, their gonads should be removed as soon as the diagnosis is made. These tumors are often malignant, and gonadoblastoma or dysgerminoma can present in adolescence. Therefore prompt attention to this aspect of their care is mandatory.

Ovarian tumors. Most tumors of the ovary, including follicular cysts, corpus luteum and theca lutean cysts, and endometrial cysts, are benign. Functional ovarian tumors account for only 1% to 3% of all ovarian tumors. The granulosa cell tumors are usually small and unilateral in nature and secrete estrogens. They may present in childhood as isosexual precocity or as postmenopausal bleeding in older women. During the reproductive years, their most common endocrine presentation is prolonged and irregular bleeding. However, it is the ovarian enlargement that is most generally manifest in the reproductive years.

Androgen-secreting tumors of the ovaries include Sertoli-Leydig cell tumors, which are often small, but can reach 8 to 10 cm. These rare tumors secrete androgen, which usually calls attention to them with varying degrees of hirsutism and virilization from their elevated serum testosterone levels, which may achieve adult male ranges. This diagnosis is suspected on the basis of an unusually high serum testosterone concentration, which exceeds levels seen in patients with PCOD (generally < 150 ng/dl in patients with PCOD). The weaker androgens may or may not be elevated, depending on the individual tumor. Urinary 17-ketosteroids, which measure the metabolites of these weak androgens, however, are almost always elevated and should always be determined in the presence of an ovarian mass with hirsutism. Tumors secreting either estrogens or androgens may be very small and difficult to identify by most imaging procedures, although transvaginal ultrasound has recently been quite helpful in identifying even small tumors.

The treatment for all of these ovarian tumors is surgical removal. Ultrasound evaluation is quite useful when followed by laparotomy for removal and determination of cell type.

REFERENCES

Auletta F and Flint A: Mechanisms controlling corpus luteum function in sheep, cows, nonhuman primates, and women especially in relation to the time of luteolysis, Endocr Rev 9:88, 1988.

Channing CP et al: The role of nonsteroidal regulators in control of oocyte and follicular maturation. Recent Prog Horm Res 38:331-408, 1982.

DiZerega GS and Hodgen GD: Folliculogenesis in the primate ovarian cycle, Endocr Rev 2:27, 1981.

Engel E and Forbes AP: Cytogenetic and clinical findings in 48 patients with congenitally defective or absent ovaries, Medicine 44:139, 1965.

Hodgen G: The dominant ovarian follicle, Fertil Steril 38:281-300, 1982.

McKenna TJ: Pathogenesis and treatment of polycystic ovary syndrome, N Engl J Med 318:558-562, 1988.

Morris JL and Scully RE: Endocrine pathology of the ovary, St. Louis, 1958, Mosby–Year Book.

Richards JS: Maturation of ovarian follicles: actions and interactions of pituitary and ovarian hormone on follicular cell differentiation, Physiol Rev 60:51-89, 1980.

Stouffer RL, editor: The primate ovary, New York, 1987, Plenum.

CHAPTER

166 Disorders of the Testis

Richard J. Santen

ANDROGEN METABOLISM

The testes contain Leydig or interstitial cells, typical of active steroid secretory tissue. These cells contain high-affinity G protein coupled receptors for luteinizing hormone (LH). Binding of LH to these receptors induces an increase in Leydig cell steroidogenesis and ultimately an increase in testosterone production. The testes secrete approximately 7000 μg testosterone/day into the peripheral circulation. A diurnal rhythm of testosterone with peak levels at 4 to 8 AM and nadir concentrations 20% to 30% lower at 4 to 8 PM occurs in younger men and less so in the elderly. A small percentage of testosterone, approximately 2%, circulates in a nonbound state in plasma, whereas the remainder is bound either to testosterone-estrogen-binding globulin (TEBG) or to albumin (Fig. 166-1). Only TEBG binds testosterone with sufficiently high affinity to retard entry into tissues. Several clinicopathologic events alter the absolute levels of TEBG in plasma (Fig. 166-1).

Testosterone serves as a prehormone and undergoes conversion to more potent metabolites through two activation pathways. In the first pathway, testosterone is converted to estradiol, a compound with 200-fold greater gonadotropin-suppressive potency than testosterone on a mass basis. In the second pathway, testosterone is converted via the enzyme 5α-reductase to dihydrotestosterone, the androgen bound to nuclear receptors in most androgen-responsive tissues. Two 5α-reductase enzymes, coded by separate genes, are present in variable proportions in prostate and in seminal vesicles, sebaceous glands, kidney, skin, hair, and other tissues. Degradative androgen metabolism takes place in liver (50% to 70%) as well as in peripheral tissues (30% to 50%) where inactive metabolites and glucuronide or sulfate derivatives are formed.

Androgens induce their hormonal effects (see the box on the right) through binding to an androgen receptor. The gene for this receptor, which binds dihydrotestosterone with 1.2-fold greater affinity than testosterone, has recently been cloned.

GERM CELL PRODUCTION

Seminiferous tubules, which are tightly coiled and up to 70 cm long, provide a continuous pathway for delivery of sperm from the testes to the rete testis, caput epididymis, and vas deferens. The seminiferous tubule is lined by a basal laminar layer and by myoid cells, which impart the ability for propulsion of fluids within the lumen (Fig. 166-2). Immature stem cells called *spermatogonia* lie along the basal lamina, interspersed between the supporting cells called Sertoli cells (Fig. 166-2). Follicle-stimulating hor-

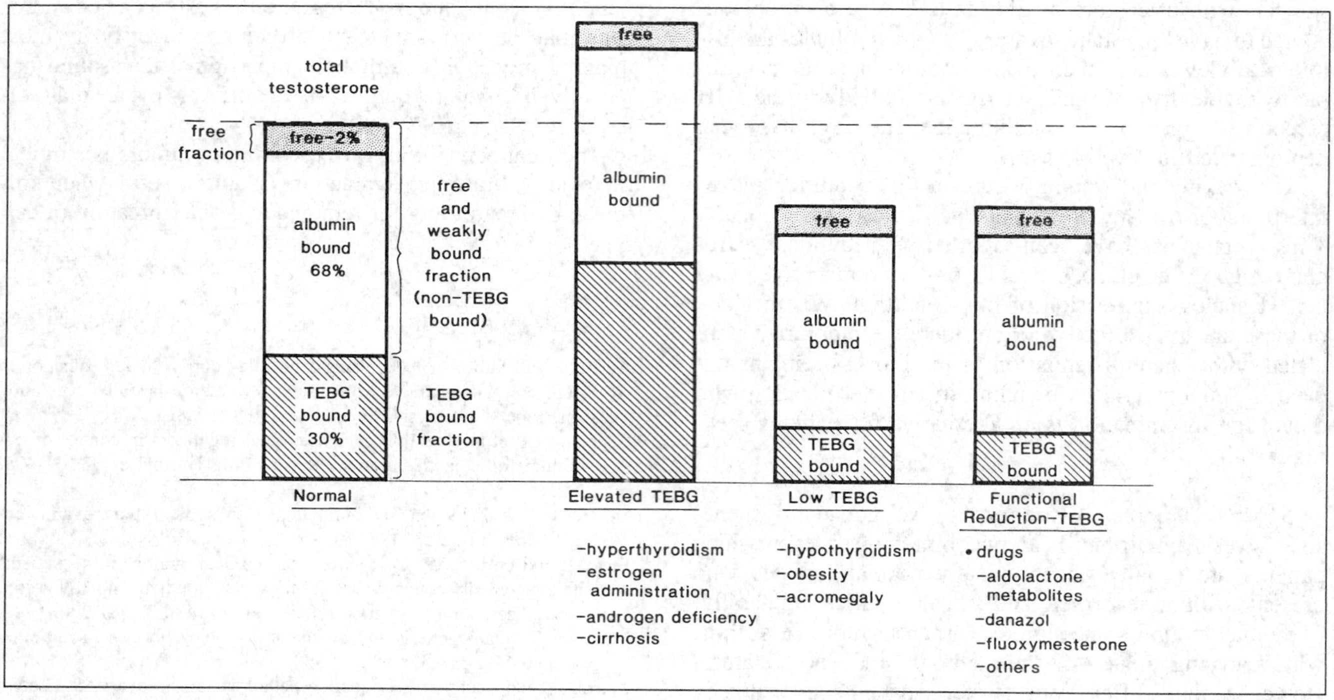

Fig. 166-1. Fractions of bound, weakly bound, and free testosterone in normal men and in women with disorders producing high or low levels of the sex hormone-binding protein also known as *testosterone-estrogen-binding globulin* (TeBG).

Clinical actions of androgen

In utero
- External genitalia development
- Wolffian duct development

Prepubertal
- Possible male behavioral effects

Pubertal
- External genitalia
  - Penis and scrotum increase in size and become pigmented, and rugal folds appear in scrotal skin
- Hair growth
  - Mustache and beard develop, and scalp line undergoes recession. Pubic hair develops. Axillary, body, extremity, and perianal hair appears
- Linear growth
  - Pubertal growth spurt appears. Androgens interact with growth hormones to increase somatomedin C levels
- Accessory sex organs
  - Prostate and seminal vesicles enlarge and secretion begins
- Voice
  - The pitch is lowered because of enlargement of larynx and thickening of vocal cords
- Psyche
  - More aggressive attitudes are manifest, and sexual potential develops
- Muscle mass
  - Muscle bulk increases and positive nitrogen balance is demonstrable

Adult
- Hair growth
  - Androgenic patterns are maintained. Male baldness may be initiated
- Psyche
  - Behavioral attitudes and sexual potency are maintained
- Bone
  - Prevention of bone loss and osteoporosis
- Spermatogenesis
  - Interaction with FSH to modulate Sertoli cell function and to stimulate spermatogenesis
- Hematopoiesis
  - Stimulation of erythropoietin and direct marrow effect on erythropoiesis

Modified from Bardin CW and Paulsen CA: The testis. In Williams RH, editor: Textbook of endocrinology, ed 6, Philadelphia, 1981, WB Saunders.

mone (FSH) binds to specific receptors in the Sertoli cell and modulates the process of spermatogenesis. Testosterone, whose concentrations in the testis are 100 times those in peripheral plasma, acts in concert with FSH. Testosterone stimulates the spermatogonia and primary spermatocytes to complete meiotic divisions, and FSH facilitates maturation of spermatids to spermatozoa during the process of spermiogenesis. The human testis manufactures $123 \pm 18 \times 10^6$ sperm daily. The full process of spermatogenesis requires 74 ± 5 days, whereas transport through the epididymis and further maturation there takes another 12 days.

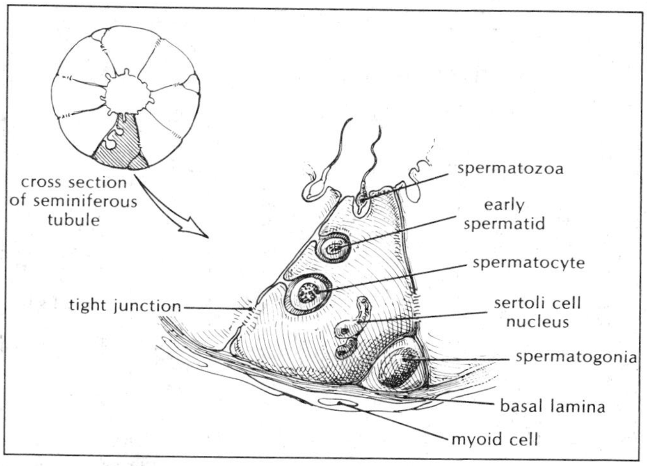

Fig. 166-2. Diagrammatic representation of a seminiferous tubule to illustrate the relationship between the lining membrane structures (i.e., basal lamina and myoepithelial cells), Sertoli cell cytoplasm, and germinal cells. Specialized tight junctions between Sertoli cells form a blood testis barrier and create the outer or basal compartment and the inner or adluminal compartment.

HYPOTHALAMUS-PITUITARY

Complementary servomechanisms control LH and FSH secretion precisely in men (Fig. 166-3, A, B). Both of these gonadotropins are secreted in a pulsatile fashion. Two steroids, testosterone (T) and estradiol (E_2), independently control gonadotropin secretion at two separate anatomic sites: the hypothalamus and pituitary. Negative feedback, the primary mechanism of this control, can be mediated either by an alteration in LH pulse frequency or by modulation of pulse amplitude. Testosterone inhibits LH secretion predominantly at the hypothalamic level through a reduction in pulse frequency (Fig. 166-3, *A*). Estradiol acts both at hypothalamic and pituitary levels to lower GnRH secretion as well as pituitary responsiveness to GnRH.

The control of FSH secretion is more complex. Testosterone and estradiol both inhibit FSH through a reduction in gonadotropin-releasing hormone (GnRH) secretion. In addition, a polypeptide heterodimer with alpha and beta subunits, a product of the testes (Fig. 166-3, B) called *inhibin,* exerts suppressive effects on FSH exclusively, acting primarily at the level of the pituitary. FSH (and also LH) stimulates increments in plasma inhibin, thus providing an ancillary negative feedback control system for FSH. Interestingly, beta-beta subunit homodimers of inhibin, called *activin,* paradoxically stimulate FSH and provide another potential means of FSH regulation.

AGE-DEPENDENT PHYSIOLOGIC CHANGES IN TESTICULAR FUNCTION

During the first 2 months of life, LH and testosterone levels approach those of adult life. After this brief period, the hypothalamic-pituitary-testicular axis becomes quiescent, and LH and testosterone levels are low (i.e., < 1 mIU/ml and < 20 ng/dl, respectively) during childhood. Testicular

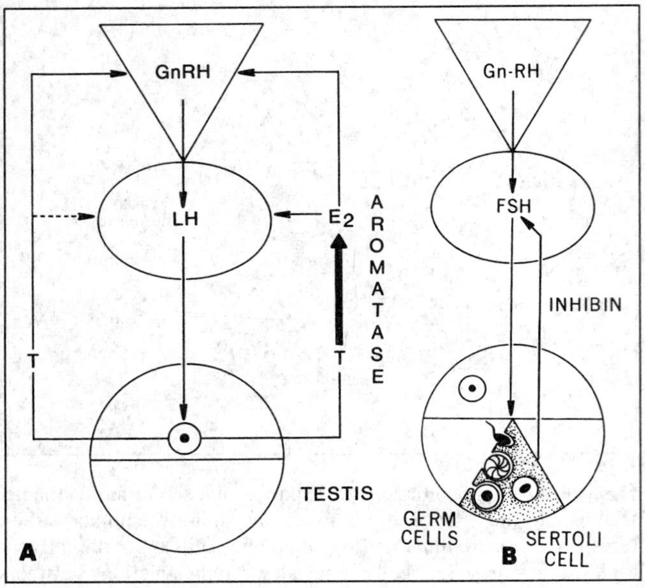

Fig. 166-3. Diagrammatic representation of the feedback interactions between the hypothalamus *(triangle)*, pituitary *(ovoid)*, and testis *(circle)*. **A,** The Leydig's cells of the testis secrete testosterone *(T)*, which exerts negative feedback effects on LH secretion at the hypothalamic level and through conversion to estradiol on the pituitary. Testosterone is converted into estradiol, E_2, by the enzyme, aromatase, which is present in fat, muscle, and liver. Estradiol exerts negative feedback effects at both hypothalamic and pituitary levels. Because estradiol and testosterone both lower GnRH levels, sex steroids also inhibit FSH secretion (not shown). **B,** An additional control mechanism exists for FSH whereby the Sertoli cells of the testis secrete inhibin. This protein product is thought to act at the pituitary to inhibit FSH secretion.

size is stable from birth until age 6 years when the testes gradually enlarge in proportion to somatic growth. The pubertal process begins on an average at age 11 in boys (95% confidence limits 9 to 13), when an increase in LH, FSH, and testosterone secretion occurs. The first physical evidence of puberty, rapid testicular enlargement, appears approximately 6 months later when the testes increase to greater than 2.9 cm on the long axis or 6 ml in volume. Once the process begins, pubertal testosterone increments occur rapidly over a 10- to 12-month period and reach levels 20-fold higher than those observed in the prepubertal period. During puberty, the major testosterone increase occurs during sleep when concomitant nocturnal LH and testosterone secretory pulses are observed. With progression into late puberty, the diurnal testosterone rhythm persists but that for LH is dampened.

After puberty, the hypothalamic-pituitary-testicular axis remains stable until approximately the fourth decade. Thereafter, the efficiency of Leydig cell steroidogenesis declines variably as a function of aging and of illness. The number of Leydig cells falls from 432 ± 45 million per testis to 243 ± 27 million in men older than 50, and each Leydig cell decreases in size. The decrease is progressive as Leydig cell number correlates negatively with age from ages 50 to 90 ($r = -.51$). As a function of this reduction in steroidogenic capacity, LH levels gradually rise and responsiveness to human chorionic gonadotropin (hCG), as a test of Leydig cell reserve function, diminishes. In spite of this process, free testosterone levels may be maintained in certain healthy men, but most experience a fall with aging. Total testosterone declines to a lesser extent than free levels because TEBG concentrations increase with age. The diurnal rise in testosterone that is easily observed in younger men becomes less pronounced.

ASSESSMENT OF CLINICAL STATUS

Assessment of patients is based on an understanding of the normal actions of androgens in utero, during puberty, and in adulthood (refer to the box on p. 1379). Patients with congenital hypogonadism have sexual infantilism and retarded growth for age. The history and physical examination focus on external genitalia, hair growth, linear growth, accessory sex organs, voice, psyche, and muscle mass. Acquired hypogonadism results in a loss of maintenance of normal androgen-mediated effects (see the box on p. 1379). Evaluation in these men is directed toward patterns of hair growth, testis size, sexual potentia, behavioral patterns, maintenance of bone density, spermatogenesis, and hematopoiesis.

ASSESSMENT OF HORMONAL STATUS

Basal levels

GnRH circulates in plasma in concentrations too low for practical measurement. The gonadotropins are detectable in plasma, but pulsatile secretion introduces an error in estimates from single samples that approximate ± 60% for LH and ± 20% for FSH. Measurements of LH or FSH in pools of plasma obtained at 20-minute intervals or in timed 3-hour (or longer) urine collections allow integration of secretory pulses. Recently developed ultrasensitive plasma gonadotropin assays or radioimmunoassay of urinary concentrates provide sensitivity in measuring the gonadotropins in states of markedly reduced secretion. Practical recommendations for gonadotropin assessment based on cost and precision include either of two approaches: (1) Obtain a single measurement of LH and FSH in plasma and confirm by repeat measurements in a pool of four samples taken at 20-minute intervals if the initial level is borderline high or low; or (2) measure LH and FSH in a precisely timed 3-hour urine collection.

Quantitation of gonadal steroid levels for clinical purposes presents fewer inherent problems than gonadotropin measurements. The lower amplitude of secretory pulses attenuates the error introduced by single-sample measurements to approximately half that for LH. Single samples are usually adequate for clinical assessment of testosterone and dihydrotestosterone levels. The diurnal rhythm of testosterone, however, necessitates obtaining early morning (i.e., 8 AM to 10 AM) samples and using normative values for that time of day. When abnormal values for total testosterone are detected, attention should be directed toward the possibility of TEBG abnormalities (see Fig. 166-1), and

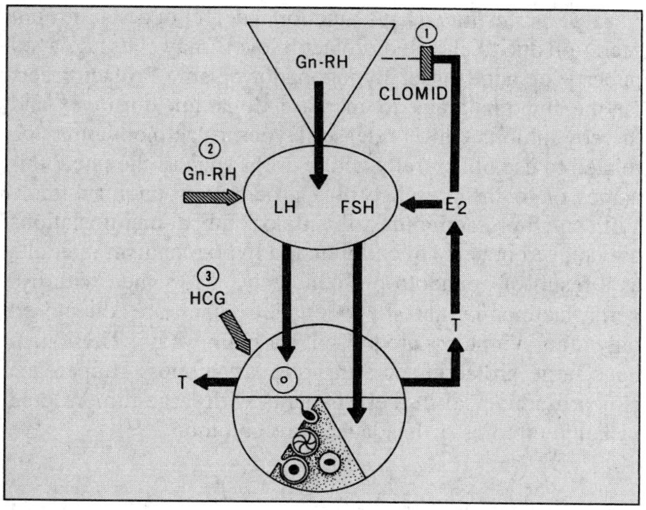

Fig. 166-4. Diagrammatic representation of sites of action of stimulation tests of the testis. Hypothalamus *(triangle)*, pituitary *(ovoid)*, Leydig and germ cell compartments of the testis *(circle)*.

non-TEBG-bound testosterone should be specifically requested.

Dynamic tests

Interruption of the estrogen-negative feedback axis with the antiestrogen, clomiphene citrate (Figs. 166-4 and 166-5; Table 166-1), stimulates both LH and FSH and secondarily testosterone and estradiol. Exogenous GnRH administration releases LH and FSH from the pituitary. Direct provocative testing of the testes requires administration of hCG and assessment of plasma testosterone increments at various time intervals (Figs. 166-4, 166-5).

Karyotype analysis provides a direct method for assessing chromosomal abnormalities and is determined on blood lymphocytes, skin fibroblasts, or gonadal tissues. Special banding stains allow identification of individual chromosomes and portions of these chromosomes. The DNA sequence on the Y chromosome, which controls testicular development (SRY gene), can now be probed by cDNA hybridization to determine the presence of this portion of the Y chromosome.

Table 166-1. Normal basal and stimulated hormone levels

		Stimulated		
		Mean % increase (range)		
	Basal	**Clomiphene**	**GnRH**	**hCG**
Plasma				
LH	4-20 mIU/ml	100 (30-400)	450 (50-1200)	—
FSH	4-20 mIU/ml	50 (20-200)	70 (9-176)	—
Testosterone	300-1200 ng/dl	25 (0-65)	No rise	100 (50-200)
Urine				
LH	500-2500 mIU/h	100 (0-200)	100 (15-200)	—
FSH	200-3300 mIU/h	100 (20-180)	63 (30-100)	—

Test protocols
Clomiphene test: 100 mg clomiphene citrate (clomid) daily by mouth for 7 d, draw blood sample or collect timed 3-hour urine before and on day 8
GnRH test
Plasma: 25 μg GnRH i.v. with collection of blood before and at 30, 60, 90, 120 minutes later
Urine: 100 μg GnRH i.v. with collection on timed 3-hour urine before and after injection
hCG test: 4000 IU hCG on day 1; draw blood sample before and on day 5

DISORDERS AFFECTING ANDROGEN PRODUCTION

The physician requires a logical framework on which to base an approach to patients with complaints referable to reproductive dysfunction. A useful classification scheme is based on the functional status of gonadotropin secretion and focuses on hypogonadotropic, hypergonadotropic, and eu-

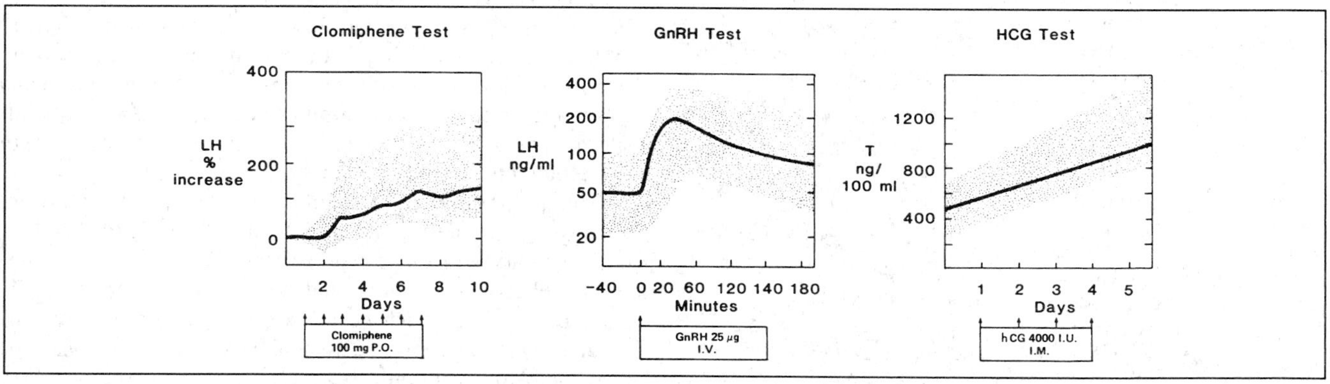

Fig. 166-5. Mean *(solid lines)* and ranges *(shaded areas)* of LH and testosterone increments during clomiphene, GnRH, and hCG tests.

gonadotropic syndromes. This approach provides a starting point on which to initiate a rational evaluation and allows Leydig cell and germinal cell dysfunction to be considered separately.

HYPOGONADOTROPIC SYNDROMES
(see the box below)

Organic hypogonadotropism

Multiple. Prepubertal patients with multiple tropic hormone deficiencies (see the accompanying box) commonly present with severe growth retardation, whereas older boys present with delayed adolescence. Adults reach attention because of impotence, headaches, or visual disturbance. Testosterone, LH, and FSH levels are low in patients with each of these disorders; and response to the clomiphene test is absent. Use of the exogenous GnRH test to distinguish hypothalamic from pituitary lesions is problematic. GnRH elicits a variable release of LH and FSH depending on the degree of pituitary gonadotropin reserve but also on preexposure of the pituitary to endogenous GnRH from the hypothalamus.

Classification of hypogonadotropic hypogonadism

I. Organic causes
  A. Multiple tropic hormone deficiencies
    1. Idiopathic
    2. Secondary to tumor
    3. Miscellaneous causes
      a. Histiocytosis X
      b. Tuberculosis
      c. Sarcoidosis
      d. Collagen vascular diseases
      e. Hypophysitis
  B. Secondary to hyperprolactinemia
  C. Isolated gonadotropin deficiency
    1. Hypogonadotropic eunuchoidism (Kallmann's syndrome)
      a. Complete
      b. Partial (predominant LH deficiency—"fertile eunuch syndrome")
      c. Variant form (isolated FSH deficiency)
    2. Specific genetic syndromes
      a. Prader-Labhart-Willi
      b. Laurence-Moon-Biedl
      c. Möbius
      d. Other rarer disorders
  D. Acute and chronic illness
    1. Malnutrition
    2. Miscellaneous acute illnesses
    3. Emotional disorders
    4. Liver disease (one subgroup)
    5. Renal disease (one component)
    6. Hemochromatosis
    7. Human immunodeficiency virus infection
II. Functional cause
  A. Physiologic delayed puberty

Hyperprolactinemia. A functional defect in gonadotropin secretion due to elevated prolactin levels may cause delayed puberty or adult-onset hypogonadotropism. Prolactin acts on the hypothalamus to increase dopamine turnover and thereby inhibits GnRH release. Hyperprolactinemia may be related to use of centrally active drugs such as the phenothiazines or to the presence of a prolactin-producing tumor. With small prolactinomas, the major clinical manifestations are delayed puberty in children and hypogonadism in adults as a result of gonadotropin deficiency. Most men with hyperprolactinemia and hypogonadotropism are diagnosed only after symptoms are present for many years. These men have large prolactin-secreting pituitary tumors. Impotence is nearly universal in these patients with large tumors, and visual symptoms or headaches are common.

Isolated gonadotropin deficiency

Gonadotropin deficiency without loss of other anterior pituitary hormones results from a number of genetic disorders (see the box at left). Subjects with these conditions present with sexual infantilism or incomplete sexual development. The specific diagnosis may be made easily if a family history is elicited or if characteristic physical findings are demonstrated. The specific disorders and their associated anomalies are discussed later.

Kallmann's syndrome. Hypogonadotropic eunuchoidism, or Kallmann's syndrome, is the most common cause of isolated gonadotropin deficiency and is inherited either as an autosomal dominant syndrome with relative sex limitation to males or with X-linked autosomal recessive inheritance in other kindreds. This disorder results from a reduction in the secretion of GnRH by the hypothalamus. GnRH-containing neurons fail to migrate into the hypothalamus from olfactory tissue anlage during embryologic development. Abnormalities observed with this condition in addition to the hypogonadism include hyposmia or anosmia, cryptorchidism, cleft lip or cleft palate, and congenital deafness. When anosmia is present, atrophy or absence of the olfactory sulcus can be demonstrated on magnetic resonance imaging (MRI) studies.

The degree of gonadotropin deficiency in patients with Kallmann's syndrome may vary. In the complete form, both FSH and LH levels are very low and no evidence of sexual maturation is apparent. With partial deficits, incomplete sexual development results and gonadotropin measurements can range up to the lower limit of adult normal values. Full spermatogenesis and normal testicular size may occur in some patients (fertile eunuch syndrome).

The major problem in diagnosis of isolated gonadotropin deficiency in patients under 18 years of age is to differentiate patients with an organic defect from those with delayed puberty on a functional basis. No definitive test is available to distinguish between these two groups of individuals. Demonstration of associated somatic abnormalities (e.g., anosmia with an abnormal olfactory sulcus on MRI, cleft lip or palate, etc.) provides the best means of confirming the diagnosis of Kallmann's syndrome. Approximately

80% of boys with hypogonadotropic hypogonadism exhibit either anosmia or hyposmia; therefore this clinical finding is useful. If no associated congenital anomalies or positive family history is present, the only definitive means of making the diagnosis of hypogonadotropic eunuchoidism may be to restudy the patient at 18 to 20 years of age when most boys with physiologic delay will have undergone pubertal changes. Intermittent androgen therapy is usually warranted until the patient reaches 18 to 20 years of age (see Treatment).

Patients with Kallmann's syndrome have low levels of LH, FSH, and testosterone under basal conditions. Provocative testing of pituitary reserve function with GnRH is not helpful diagnostically because this test elicits a spectrum of responses from complete absence to near normality. Stimulation of the hypothalamic pituitary axis with clomiphene has been suggested as a means to differentiate organic from physiologic disorders of sexual maturation. However, boys with delayed puberty, as well as those with hypogonadotropic eunuchoidism, respond to clomiphene similarly with a paradoxic suppression of LH and FSH. The fall in gonadotropin levels reflects their sensitivity to the minimally estrogenic properties of clomiphene. Measurement of growth hormone, thyroxine, prolactin, and adrenal hormones and assessment of the size of the sella turcica are usually necessary to rule out multiple trophic hormone deficiencies.

Specific genetic syndromes with predominant hypogonadotropism

The Prader-Labhart-Willi syndrome is an inherited disorder characterized by hypotonia (especially in infancy), obesity, mental retardation, short stature, and adult-onset diabetes mellitus. Other distinguishing features include acromicria, micrognathia, strabismus, fishlike or Cupid's bow mouth, clinodactyly, and absence of auricular cartilage. The degree of hypogonadotropism in this disorder is variable and ranges from partial to severe. Recently, a defect in chromosome 15 has been described in nearly half the cases studied.

The Laurence-Moon-Biedl syndrome is characterized by retinitis pigmentosa, obesity, mental retardation, and polydactyly and is associated with hypogonadism in 50% of affected patients and delayed adolescence in another 30%. In prepubertal boys, microphallus, hypospadias, and undescended testes are common. Retinal degeneration occurs between 4 and 10 years of age and obesity somewhat earlier.

Chronic illnesses

A variety of systemic illnesses with associated malnutrition may cause depressed testosterone levels or frank hypogonadism. Intestinal disease with malabsorption, recurrent infections, neoplastic disease, or primary malnutrition may lower testosterone levels in adults or cause poor growth and delayed pubertal progression in adolescents.

Acute illnesses

Patients with severe burns, coma, acute myocardial infarction, elective surgery, and critical illness may experience a reduction of LH and testosterone. These changes are usually multifactorial and represent the effects of stress, malnutrition, drugs, and other factors.

Emotional disorders

Adult men with anorexia nervosa present with gonadotropin deficiency and hypogonadism in association with weight loss. In adolescents, psychiatric illness or emotional stress may cause inhibition of gonadotropin secretion and delay the pubertal process. It has been suggested recently that stress increases corticotropin-releasing factor (CRF), which, in turn, activates the opiatergic neurons, which then lower GnRH secretion. This pathway could provide the mechanism for low LH levels in association with stress.

Obesity

Massive obesity is associated with low testosterone levels and low to low-normal LH levels. Reductions in TEBG levels are partially responsible for the lowering of total testosterone, but free or weakly bound testosterone levels are often low as well. Increased aromatization of testosterone to estradiol is present, but the testosterone levels can be returned to normal with weight loss of insufficient degree to lower estradiol levels.

Liver disease

Hypogonadism, gynecomastia, and testicular atrophy are commonly observed in men with hepatic cirrhosis and two subgroups of patients are described. In the hypogonadotropic subgroup, LH and FSH levels are suppressed because of associated malnutrition or because of enhanced aromatization of testosterone to estradiol and increased estrogen-negative feedback. The hypergonadotropic subgroup has a form of primary gonadal disease characterized by high LH levels and a diminished testosterone response to exogenous hCG. Direct effects of alcohol on the testes to inhibit steroidogenesis may partially explain this abnormality. Additional effects of alcohol on the liver to increase testosterone metabolic clearance rate may also lower circulating androgen concentrations.

Other chronic diseases

Chronic renal failure is associated with hypogonadism and hyperprolactinemia. Gonadotropin levels, although normal to slightly elevated, are reduced relative to the level of circulating testosterone. Hemochromatosis may also involve the pituitary and produce gonadotropin deficiency with hypogonadism. Isolated gonadotropin deficiency and fractional panhypopituitarism may be caused by lymphocytic hypophysitis. Nearly 50% of men with acquired immunodeficiency syndrome (AIDS) and some with AIDS-related complex (ARC) have low plasma testosterone levels. In the majority (75%), gonadotropin levels are inappropriately low. Narcotic analgesics reduce the secretion of LH and testosterone resulting in a reversible form of hypogonadotropin hypogonadism.

PHYSIOLOGIC DELAYED PUBERTY (CONSTITUTIONAL DELAY)

From an early age, boys with this disorder lag 1 to 3 years behind their peers in statural growth and bone age and may fall as low as the first percentile on growth charts. The diagnosis is suspected in a short, adolescent-aged boy of 14 years or older, with testes of prepubertal size whose father, brothers, or cousins initiated puberty between the ages of 14 and 18. The absence of hyposmia, anosmia, cryptorchidism, or other congenital anomalies supports the diagnosis of physiologic delay rather than other causes. Retardation in bone age and/or height of more than 3.5 standard deviations below the mean raises the question of an organic cause for delayed puberty. Additionally, clinical evidence of growth hormone, thyroxine, or cortisol deficiency by history or physical examination points to organic rather than physiologic causes of delayed sexual maturation.

The major problem in diagnosis is the differentiation of boys with physiologic delayed puberty from those with complete or incomplete forms of hypogonadotropic eunuchoidism. There is no definitive means of establishing the diagnosis of delayed puberty other than careful, prolonged observation. Measurement of urinary gonadotropin levels at six monthly intervals over 1 to 2 years provides reassurance if levels rise appreciably during the period of observation.

HYPERGONADOTROPIC HYPOGONADISM

Primary disorders of testicular function result in incomplete sexual maturation and hypogonadism (see the accompanying box). Demonstration of elevated LH and FSH levels (hypergonadotropism) allows this group of patients to be differentiated from those with hypothalamic-pituitary disorders in whom gonadotropin secretion is diminished. The clinical presentation differs based on the patient's age. In boys, the defect in testosterone secretion is often partial, and androgen-related somatic changes occur at puberty but are incomplete. Testicular growth is diminished because of the dysgenetic nature of the gonad. The gynecomastia that frequently develops during puberty is more severe than that observed in normal boys. In adults, testicular failure produces impotence as an early symptom and loss of secondary sex characteristics as a late finding, often taking 5 to 10 years to develop.

Hypergonadotropic hypogonadism

I. Gonadal defects
  - A. Genetic
    1. Klinefelter's syndrome
    2. Myotonic dystrophy
    3. Syndrome of webbed neck, ptosis, hypogonadism, congenital heart disease, short stature
    4. XYY syndrome
    5. Down syndrome
    6. Miscellaneous
  - B. Anatomic
    1. Functional prepubertal castrate
  - C. Gonadal toxins
    1. Drugs
    2. Ionizing irradiation
  - D. Enzyme defects
    1. 17α-hydroxylase deficiency
    2. 17-ketoreductase deficiency
  - E. Viral
    1. Mumps orchitis
  - F. Diabetes mellitus
  - G. Associated with aging

II. Hormone resistance
  - A. Androgen insensitivity
  - B. 5α-reductase deficiency

Genetic disorders

Klinefelter's syndrome is a type of testicular dysgenesis characterized by the presence of one or more supernumerary X chromosomes (Table 166-2). Classic and variant forms are described. The classic (XXY) form occurs in approximately 1 in 500 males (0.21% infants, 0.15 to 0.24% adults). Clinical features, laboratory findings, and testicular biopsy appearance are listed in Table 166-2. This disorder is highly suspect in an adult with firm testes of less than 2 cm long who has clinical signs of androgen deficiency of variable degree. Gynecomastia occurs in 85% of patients. These patients are of normal stature or tall. Large prospective surveys indicate a decrease in mean intelligence test scores and educational level achieved in men with Klinefelter's syndrome compared with controls of similar age. A slightly increased proportion may have frankly subnormal intelligence. Personality disorders are reported to occur more commonly in men with Klinefelter's syndrome than in the normal population.

The degree of Leydig cell dysfunction in Klinefelter's syndrome is variable. Mean testosterone concentrations in patients as a group are approximately one half (i.e., 300 ng/dl) those in normal men (600 ng/dl); however, 40% of patients have total testosterone levels in the normal, albeit low-normal range. Plasma estradiol on the other hand, is twofold higher in patients with Klinefelter's syndrome because of an increased conversion of testosterone into estradiol in peripheral tissues. In response to elevated estradiol, plasma TEBG levels are increased, and the fraction of non-TEBG-bound testosterone is reduced. Consequently, some patients with normal total testosterone levels will exhibit low "free and weakly bound" testosterone concentrations (see Fig. 166-1). The diagnosis of Klinefelter's syndrome of any type is confirmed by karyotype analysis of blood lymphocytes. Elevation of plasma FSH is uniform and of

Table 166-2. Clinical features of Klinefelter's syndrome

Parameter	Classic form	Variant forms*: XX	Mosaic forms*	Poly X + Y
Incidence	1/500	1/9000	Unknown	Unknown
Clinical features	Testes <2 cm and firm Eunuchoidal proportions Gynecomastia Personality disorder Androgen deficiency of variable degree	Shorter in stature Hypospadias	Testis may be normal sized	Increased incidence of cryptorchidism Radioulnar synostosis
Laboratory determinations	LH elevated FSH extremely elevated Testosterone lowered (in 50%) Barr body present			
Karyotype	47,XXY	46,XX	XXY/XY; XXY/XX	XXXY,XXXXY,XXXXXY
Spermatogenesis	Azoospermia		Impairment less severe	
Testis biopsy	Hyalinized tubules Relative Leydig cell hyperplasia		Less severe damage	

*Only divergent features are listed.
Modified from Bardin CW and Paulsen CA: The testes. In Williams RH, editor: Textbook of endocrinology, ed 6. Philadelphia, 1981, Saunders.

LH nearly uniform. Response to exogenous hCG is blunted, indicating decreased testicular reserve function.

Other syndromes. Myotonic dystrophy is a familial disorder characterized by cataracts, baldness, muscle weakness, and hypogonadism in 80% of affected males. The syndrome of webbed neck, ptosis, hypogonadism, congenital heart disease, and short stature is also called Noonan's syndrome or male Turner's syndrome. Clinical findings include facies typical of Turner's syndrome in girls, a webbed neck, short stature, low-set ears, ptosis, shieldlike chest, cryptorchidism, diminished spermatogenesis, decreased Leydig cell function, cubitus valgus, and cardiovascular anomalies (especially pulmonic stenosis). Also present may be mental retardation, low hairline, small penis, and lymphedema of the hands and feet, particularly at birth. The XXY syndrome, Down syndrome, sickle cell disease, and autoimmune disorders may also be associated with testicular failure and other endocrine deficiency states.

Functional prepubertal castrate syndrome (anorchia)

Individuals with this disorder present with signs and symptoms of severe androgen deficiency; they lack anatomically demonstrable or functioning testes, but exhibit normal external genitalia. Bilateral testicular torsion, which occurs sometime after embryologic development is completed, likely explains the loss of testes in these patients. Patients with complete anorchia present before puberty because bilateral cryptorchidism is suspected. Elevated gonadotropin levels for age suggest this diagnosis. A substantial rise in testosterone levels during administration of hCG practically excludes anorchia and supports the diagnosis of bilateral cryptorchidism. In the teenage or adult years, patients present because of sexual infantilism and lack of palpable testes. The combination of castrate levels of gonadotropins and low testosterone confirms the diagnosis and obviates the need for anatomic studies to localize testicular tissue.

Gonadal toxins

Cytotoxic drugs used as treatment of the nephrotic syndrome or of neoplastic diseases commonly produce testicular damage. The alkylating agents are particularly common offenders. Nearly 100% of patients receiving MOPP (mechlorethamine, vincristine, procarbazine, prednisone) chemotherapy develop azoospermia and compromised androgen production. Radiation therapy that includes the gonads also results in testicular failure. Spermatogenic elements are more sensitive to these effects than are Leydig cells. Polychlorinated insecticides, dibromochloropropane, and marijuana may also cause a reduction in sperm count and motility.

Enzyme defects

Genetic males with complete 17α-hydroxylase and 17-ketosteroid reductase deficiencies present as phenotypic females with partial virilization at puberty. Incomplete defects result in lack of full pubertal development, hypospadias, and gynecomastia in phenotypic males.

Mumps orchitis

In 15% to 25% of pubertal or postpubertal subjects, mumps involves the testes and produces a highly painful, inflammatory disorder. After the acute illness subsides, the germ cells gradually degenerate over a period of several years and Leydig cell dysfunction develops. In later years, patients present with symptoms of androgen deficiency or infertility and relate a past history of painful orchitis. Gynecomastia and testicular atrophy may be present as well as clinical evidence of androgen deficiency or infertility.

Diabetes mellitus

Impotence, which occurs in 50% of diabetic men, is usually multifactorial, with evidence of vascular, neurologic, or psychogenic factors. A subgroup of men with organic impotence without vascular disease has diminished testosterone but elevated LH levels, suggesting a primary gonadal defect. Impotence improves with testosterone therapy if candidates for therapy are carefully selected.

Male climacteric

The hormonal changes associated with aging include both gonadal and pituitary components. Free testosterone levels diminish gradually and gonadotropins increase as a function of age. Decreased sexual function may correlate with these changes. A decreased capacity for testosterone production by the Leydig cell is the main defect, but abnormalities of the hypothalamic-pituitary axis may also be present (i.e., abnormal LH pulse frequency, heightened negative feedback responsiveness to androgen). Replacement of testosterone may be warranted as a therapeutic trial in highly selected patients after a clear demonstration of low androgen levels. Further study is required to develop clear guidelines in the evaluation and treatment of such patients.

Hormone resistance

Syndromes of androgen insensitivity may be complete or incomplete. In the complete form, affected men present as phenotypic females with primary amenorrhea and breast development, the so-called testicular feminization syndrome. With incomplete insensitivity, the defect ranges from mild to severe and patients may exhibit diminished body hair, gynecomastia, hypospadias, bifid scrotum, cryptorchidism, or only azoospermia. Puberty is initiated at an appropriate age. Elevated LH levels in such patients reflect resistance to androgens at the hypothalamic-pituitary level. FSH titers are usually normal. Testis biopsy reveals a variable picture, with complete tubular sclerosis and peritubular hyalinization on one extreme and immature germ cells without sclerosis on the other. Genetic mutations of the androgen receptor gene and absent or abnormal receptor function have been described in individual patients with androgen resistance.

Another type of partial androgen resistance results from deficiency of the enzyme 5α-reductase, which converts testosterone to dihydrotestosterone. These patients exhibit ambiguous genitalia at birth and are usually reared as females. At puberty, partial virilization with penile growth and increase in muscle mass ensue. Facial hair, acne, and frontal balding are lacking, whereas spermatogenesis is normal. In primitive cultures these individuals take on a male role at puberty.

TREATMENT

Approaches to treatment differ depending on the clinical circumstances and desires of the patient (Table 166-3).

Table 166-3. Treatment of testis disorders

Group	Goal of treatment	Treatment modality	Dosage
Delayed adolescence	Short-term maintenance of plasma testosterone at 100-300 ng/dl	hCG	1000-4000 IU i.m. 1-3 times/wk
		Testosterone enanthate or cypionate	50-100 mg i.m. q3-4 wk
Adult hypogonadotropic hypogonadism	Long-term maintenance of testosterone levels at 300-1200 ng/dl	GnRH*	2-20 μg s.c. q2-3 h
		hCG	1000-4000 IU i.m. 1-3 times/wk
		Testosterone enanthate or cypionate	300 mg q14-21 d 200 mg q10-17 d 100 mg q5-10 d
Adult hypergonadotropic hypogonadism	Long-term maintenance of testosterone levels at 300-1200 ng/dl	Testosterone enanthate or cypionate	300 mg q14-21 d 200 mg q10-17 d 100 mg q5-10 d
	Provide subreplacement doses of androgen	Fluoxymesterone	5-10 mg p.o. daily
		Methyltestosterone	25 mg daily by linquet
		Testosterone† undecanoate	200 mg p.o. 4 times daily

*Experimental, requires programmed pump.
†Not available in the United States.

Delayed adolescence

Major psychologic effects may result from a delay in adolescent sexual development. Precise differentiation of physiologically delayed adolescence from isolated gonadotropin deficiency may not always be possible in boys of pubertal age. These considerations favor treatment empirically in patients over 14 years of age when clinical circumstances warrant. The usual goal of therapy is to initiate androgenic effects with intermittent, subreplacement doses of testosterone (i.e., maintenance of testosterone levels of 100 to 300 ng/dl) while observing for spontaneous maturational changes during periods off medication. Two therapeutic modalities, hCG or synthetic androgen replacement, are practically available but testosterone is preferred (Table 166-3). To initiate pubertal changes, 50 to 100 mg is administered intramuscularly every 3 to 4 weeks for 3 to 4 months with cessation for an equal time period. The goal is to promote secondary sex characteristics and normal linear growth. Evidence of spontaneous pubertal development such as testicular enlargement and spontaneous increments of gonadotropins and testosterone should be sought during the 3 to 4 months off therapy. If no significant progression is noted, several intermittent courses of low-dose testosterone can be administered until spontaneous puberty is initiated or the need for long-term exogenous therapy is confirmed.

Adult hypogonadotropic hypogonadism

The treatment goal is to maintain plasma testosterone levels in the adult normal range (300 to 1200 ng/dl) over a prolonged period. Injectable testosterone (Table 166-3) is preferred unless fertility is an immediate goal. In that instance, hCG is given until testosterone levels are normal for at least 6 months and then FSH preparations such as menotropins (Pergonal) are added.

Adult hypergonadotropic hypogonadism

Direct replacement of androgen provides the only effective therapy in adults with hypergonadotropic hypogonadism and also can be used in hypogonadotropic patients not immediately desiring to father children. The goal of therapy is to maintain plasma testosterone in the adult male range, that is, 300 to 1200 ng/dl. Injectable testosterone esters are required for full androgen maintenance, as oral androgens are insufficiently potent.

DISORDERS AFFECTING SPERMATOGENESIS

Germinal cell dysfunction occurs in 3% to 5% of the male population and produces infertility. Initial evaluation of the infertile man involves documentation of low sperm counts in at least three semen analyses obtained at monthly intervals. If quantitative counts are consistently below 20 million/cm^3 or 50 million total count, germinal cell dysfunction is highly suspect. A work-up is then initiated to identify possible etiologic causes. Disorders of germinal cell function can be classified as hypogonadotropic, hypergonadotropic, and eugonadotropic.

When germinal cell mass or Sertoli cell function is sufficiently reduced, plasma or urinary FSH levels increase, often without a concomitant rise in LH. A current hypothesis attributes this monotropic FSH rise to a reduction in testicular inhibin with partial interruption of FSH-negative feedback, although other explanations are possible. The degree of plasma FSH elevation can be used as a marker for the severity of germinal cell dysfunction. The availability of this measurement has largely obviated the need for testicular biopsy, as the specific histologic pattern seen does not usually influence patient management decisions.

Many therapies including exogenous gonadotropin administration, endogenous gonadotropin stimulation with clomiphene or tamoxifen, testosterone rebound, and kallikrein therapy have been proposed to enhance sperm production in men with germinal cell failure. Although uncontrolled studies report benefit, carefully randomized, placebo-controlled trials do not demonstrate the efficacy of these approaches.

Hypergonadotropic disorders

The Sertoli-cell-only syndrome is a disorder in which all germinal cell elements in the testis except Sertoli cells are lost, but Leydig cell function is relatively preserved. Clinical examination reveals normal pubic and axillary hair but small soft testes averaging 2 to 4 cm on their long axes (10 to 20 ml). FSH levels are uniformly elevated, and azoospermia is found on semen analysis. One half of the patients exhibit subclinical Leydig cell dysfunction, characterized by elevated LH levels with normal or slightly reduced testosterone concentrations and blunted responses to hCG.

Idiopathic seminiferous tubular failure with hyalinization is diagnosed on testicular biopsy in men with oligospermia or azoospermia whose FSH levels are elevated. Testis size may be reduced to below adult normal limits of 3.5 cm on the long axis or 20 ml.

Eugonadotropic disorders

Patients with oligospermia but normal FSH levels are considered to have eugonadotropic germinal cell failure. Two subtypes are described: arrest of germinal cell maturation at a specific step and generalized hypospermatogenesis affecting all germ cell elements. Clinical examination reveals no abnormality, and testis size is usually normal. On testis biopsy, only minimal peritubular hyalinization or normal peritubular elements are present.

Incompetence of the left or less commonly the right, testicular vein, results in the formation of dilated veins in the scrotum, a condition called *varicocele*. Empirical observations suggest an etiologic association between varicocele and infertility, but the precise mechanism is only speculative. Varicocele can be palpated during a Valsalva maneuver in approximately 40% of men with oligospermia or azoospermia. Reduced motility and a stress pattern of sperm morphology with increased numbers of immature or tapered forms are commonly found. The majority of reports indicate improved semen quality in 60% to 70% and fertility in 30% to 40% of men after high venous ligation to correct the varicocele; however, no definitive study including a control group conclusively establishes the validity of this treatment.

A thorough search for infectious agents has identified a variety of organisms in the seminal fluid of men with oligospermia or with decreased sperm motility. Mycoplasma infection, and particularly *Ureaplasma urealyticum,* has been suggested as a causative agent in infertility, but this theory remains controversial. The presence of an excess number of leukocytes in the seminal fluid suggests the possibility of infection. A cause and effect relationship between the documented infection and the associated infertility has not yet been established. Most large infertility clinics, however, routinely recommend antibiotics such as doxycycline when infection is suspected by the presence of pus cells on several seminal fluid examinations or when cultures are positive.

The sinopulmonary-infertility syndrome is diagnosed in patients with recurrent sinopulmonary infections, defective sperm motility, and dysfunction of cilia in the respiratory tract and on the spermatozoa. Cystic fibrosis and Young's syndrome (azoospermia in association with inspissated secretions in the vas deferens) represent two well-defined subtypes.

Genetic syndromes

Fifteen percent of men with azoospermia have genetic abnormalities, including XXY and XYY karyotypes, reciprocal autosomal and other translocations, and a variety of other abnormalities. The frequency of these disorders in oligospermic men with counts of 1 to 20 million/cm^3 is 1.65%.

Autoimmunity

Infertility and oligospermia occur in association with certain autoimmune disorders such as Addison's disease and the familial autoimmune endocrine deficiency syndrome. The presence of autoantibodies against the testis has been demonstrated in these subjects as well as in other patients with oligospermia or azoospermia.

Heat

Exposure to heat reproducibly reduces sperm production temporarily in a number of animal species. Although this effect has been incompletely documented in men, studies suggest that the heat encountered in a sauna may be sufficient to temporarily reduce sperm production.

Hypogonadotropic syndromes

These disorders are uniformly associated with androgen deficiency and are described under disorders of androgen production.

REFERENCES

Baker HWG et al: Relative incidence of etiologic disorders in male infertility. In Santen RJ and Swerdloff RS, editors: Male sexual dysfunction: diagnosis and management of hypogonadism, infertility and impotence, New York, 1986, Marcel Dekker.

Blackman MR et al: Comparison of the effects of lung cancer, benign lung disease, and normal aging on pituitary-gonadal function in men, J Clin Endocrinol Metab 66:88, 1988.

Brown-Woodman PD et al: The effect of a single sauna exposure on spermatozoa, Arch Androl 12:9, 1984.

David G et al: Sperm characteristics and fertility in previously cryptorchid adults. In Job JC, editor: Cryptorchidism, Basel/New York, 1979, Karger.

Dean JCS, Johnston AW, and Klopper AI: Isolated hypogonadotrophic hypogonadism: a family with autosomal dominant inheritance, Clin Endocrinol (Oxf) 32:341, 1990.

Dobs AS et al: Endocrine disorders in men infected with human immunodeficiency virus, Am J Med 84:611, 1988.

Fauser BCJM et al: Bioactive and immunoreactive FSH in serum of normal and oligospermic men, Clin Endocrinol (Oxf) 32:433, 1990.

Franchimont P, Demoulin A, and Bourguignon JP: Regulation of gonadotropin secretion. In Santen RJ and Swerdloff RS, editors: Male sexual dysfunction: diagnosis and management of hypogonadism, infertility and impotence, New York, 1986, Marcel Dekker.

French FS et al: Molecular basis of androgen insensitivity, Recent Prog Horm Res 46:1, 1990.

Green JS et al: The cardinal manifestations of Bardet-Biedl syndrome, a form of Laurence-Moon-Biedl syndrome, N Engl J Med 321:1002, 1989.

Griffin JE and Wilson JD: Disorders of the testes and the male reproductive tract. In Wilson JD and Foster DW, editors: Textbook of endocrinology, ed 8, Philadelphia, 1992, WB Saunders.

Grumbach MM and Conte FA: Disorders of sexual differentiation. In Wilson JD and Foster DW, editors: Textbook of endocrinology, ed 8, Philadelphia, 1992, WB Saunders.

Knuth UA et al: Treatment of severe oligospermia with human chorionic gonadotropin/human menopausal gonadotropin: a placebo-controlled, double-blind trial, J Clin Endocrinol Metab 65:1081, 1987.

Mendel CM: The free hormone hypothesis: distinction from the free hormone transport hypothesis, J Androl 13:107-116, 1992.

Murray FT et al: Gonadal dysfunction in diabetic men with organic impotence, J Clin Endocrinol Metab 65:127, 1987.

Rimoin DL and Schimke RN, editors: The gonads. In Genetic disorders of the endocrine glands. St. Louis: Mosby, 1971.

Rivier C, Vale W, and Rivier J: Studies of the inhibin family of hormones: a review, Horm Res 28:104, 1987.

Rosenfield RL: Diagnosis and management of delayed puberty, J Clin Endocrinol Metab 70:559-562, 1990.

Santen RJ: The testis. In Felig P, editors: Endocrinology and metabolism, ed 3, New York, McGraw-Hill, in press.

Snyder PJ: Clinical use of androgens, Annu Rev Med 35:207, 1984.

Spratt DI et al: The spectrum of abnormal patterns of gonadotropin-releasing hormone secretion in men with idiopathic hypogonadotropic hypogonadism: clinical and laboratory correlations, J Clin Endocrinol Metab 64:283, 1987.

Veldhuis J: The hypothalamic-pituitary-testicular axis. In Yen SSC and Jaffe RB, editors: Reproductive endocrinology, ed 3, Philadelphia, 1991, WB Saunders.

Whitcomb RW: The approach to the oligoazoospermic male, The Endocrinologist 1:125-130, 1991.

CHAPTER

167 Benign Disorders of the Breast

David L. Page

ANATOMY AND PHYSIOLOGY

The adult female breast is composed of 15 to 20 separate lobes of glandular tissue radiating out from individual openings at the nipple. A branching system of ducts end in lobular units, which are made up of branching alveolar elements. Most of the glandular tissue is present beneath the region of the areola and within the upper outer quadrant extending into the axilla. In most nonlactating women, the majority of breast tissue is made up of connective tissue and fat. The structural connective tissue of the breast suspends the glandular units between the fascia of the pectoral muscles and the overlying dermis. Menopause is followed by senile involution of the breast, with patchy and finally complete disappearance of the glandular units.

Several hormones affect the breast. Estrogen is required for both ductal and alveolar growth, but progesterone activity is also necessary for alveolar differentiation. Glucocorticoids and insulin support lactational development, and growth hormone is important for ductal and lobular growth. Placental lactogen stimulates alveolar growth and lactogenesis, and prolactin stimulates lactogenesis and maintenance of lactation. Oxytocin causes contraction of the myoepithelial cells, expelling milk into the ducts.

GENERAL FEATURES

The conditions presented here are often collectively referred to as *benign breast disease,* a general term recognizing only the absence of cancer. Although some histologic and radiographic findings indicate varying magnitudes of increased cancer risk, none of these has a known link to the clinical presentations of lumpiness or pain. It is important to remember that benign breast disorders may be clinically, histologically, or radiographically defined and that any relationship between these variously defined elements is tenuous despite the common use of similar terms. See also Chapter 159 for benign breast disorders of adolescents.

PAIN

Pain, lumps, and/or nipple discharge dominate the presentation of benign disease. The evaluation and perception of pain are intertwined with psychological factors; however, neuroticism is not a common cause of breast pain. Rarely, pain is a presenting sign of carcinoma. A detailed history will separate physiologic causes (thelarche, pregnancy) from secondary causes of pain such as infection and exogenous estrogen from primary breast pain. Breast pain must also be distinguished from referred pain secondary to gallbladder disease, lung disease, costochondral pain of Tietze's disease, or trauma as well as cervical disk disease.

The most frequent presentations of primary breast pain have no evident physical or pathologic basis and are often related to the menstrual cycle, with discomfort in the premenstrual or midcycle days being the most common. Mild symptoms are frequent enough to be considered normal. Assurance that these symptoms are not related to malignancy is important because with fears allayed, many women tolerate the discomfort better. Pain may be focal or diffuse, with or without associated nodularity.

The distinction between cyclic and noncyclic pain is useful because the former is likely to respond to hormonal therapy. The cyclic type of pain has its onset usually in the late twenties with increasing incidence with age until menopause, when pain often disappears. Breast pain may be recognized as cyclic even when constant, with increases in intensity related to the menstrual cycle.

Pregnancy as well as oral contraceptives may reduce or eliminate this pattern of breast pain. Progestins used to correct a supposed luteal insufficiency in patients with breast pain have no proved value. Bromocriptine, a dopamine agonist that lowers prolactin levels, is an effective drug in some patients with cyclic mastalgia. The physiologic basis for this therapeutic effectiveness is unknown, but is not related to basal prolactin levels. A dose of 2.5 mg twice daily causes nausea and dizziness in some patients and may be avoided in many patients by gradually increasing dosage from low levels. Symptoms of pain should be severe and steady over several months before considering this medication because of side effects.

Danazol, a weak androgen that suppresses gonadotropin secretion, is useful in cyclic mastalgia. Although side effects of amenorrhea, weight gain, and acne from weak androgenic effects are common at higher doses (200 to 400 mg/day), they are rare with 100-mg doses daily. The lower dose may be as effective as the higher one in cyclic pain. Prolonged therapy over several months should be avoided to limit long-term suppression of the pituitary-ovarian axis and to allow detection of spontaneous cessation of symptoms, which is common. Other therapeutic approaches are unproved despite popularity. Reduction or elimination of caffeine and related methylxanthines in the diet or treatment with pyridoxine, B vitamins, or vitamin E have been reported to benefit some patients; but all are still of unproved effectiveness. Increased intake of various essential fatty acids as a possibly effective measure is being studied. The establishment of treatment efficacy with any regimen is difficult because both pain and benign nodularity are notoriously inconsistent with time.

Noncyclic pain is much more difficult to manage because hormonal therapy has little effectiveness. The average age of onset for this pain pattern is over the age of 40, and the pain may not disappear with menopause. Noncyclic pain is usually unilateral and localized. The local injection of corticosteroids or local anesthetics may help in local pain. Surgical excision will often cure the pain of duct ectasia, a condition often associated with nipple discharge and acquired nipple inversion. Spontaneous resolution is unusual.

LUMPS

Palpable irregularity of breast tissue may vary from diffuse, fine irregularities to poorly defined lumps to discrete or dominant masses. Less well-defined nodularity is very common, particularly in thin women. Clinical nodularity is often decreased with oral contraceptive medication. The clinical evaluation of lumps requires documentation of duration, size, and location within the breast as well as examination of the breast contour and careful palpation of the axillae. Previous diagnostic examinations should be documented. The clinical importance of lumps and lumpiness in the breast rests largely on the mimicry of breast carcinoma; however, no degree of clinical nodularity or pain has known linkage to increased breast cancer risk.

Discovery of a dominant or discrete mass within the breast requires tissue definition by needle biopsy or surgical means. Because masses other than cancer may vary with the menstrual cycle, re-evaluation of less than completely discrete masses within a month's time is appropriate. Menstrual cycle-related changes are usually most prominent in the week or so preceding menses and least prominent immediately after menses. Thus a dominant mass that remains stable through a menstrual period should be histologically or cytologically evaluated. Mammography is recommended, but this technique is not sufficient to rule out cancer. False-negative mammograms are seen in at least 10% of cases with palpable breast cancer. Small and deep masses within the breast are more difficult to detect and evaluate by physical examination; however, limitations of size and depth do not apply to mammograms. Therefore mammography is indicated for deeper masses because it is more sensitive and specific than physical examination. Mammography excels in its ability to detect very small malignant processes, especially in the very large, fatty breast in which physical examination is difficult.

The lumpiness produced by benign alterations within the breast is most evident in the perimenopausal age group, producing the greatest number of benign breast biopsies (done to rule out the presence of cancer). After menopause, lumps with a clear definition to physical examination represent a higher likelihood of cancer. This development reflects both increasing age as a major cancer risk factor and decrease in background benign lumpiness. Other factors are associated with an increased incidence of breast cancer, but the great majority have increased risk to 1.5 or less times that of the general population. These factors include nulliparity, late first childbirth, and early onset or late cessation of menses. Strong evidence exists that oral contraceptive and current estrogen replacement medications (low dose, conjugated estrogen) have no effect on breast cancer risk, although there remains at least a possibility that some young groups (as yet inadequately studied) may have enhanced tumor development with estrogen. Generally, a single factor should double the risk of breast cancer before increased concern should be transformed to clinical action, including even relaying concern to the patient (which is currently translated into following regular mammographic surveillance).

Family history of breast cancer, particularly in a first-order relative (mother, daughter, or sister) is an important indicator of cancer risk. This level of risk is reliably known to be approximately double that of all women. Risk of carcinoma increases with increasing evidence of close relatives with breast cancer, particularly if the carcinoma in relatives appeared before menopause.

FIBROCYSTIC CHANGE OF THE BREAST

The relative incidence of fibrocystic change and cancer is shown in Fig. 167-1. Varying clinical presentations of local or diffuse lumps and pain are imprecisely linked to histopathologic patterns of fibrosis, cyst formation, epithelial hyperplasia (increased cell number), and adenosis (increased glandular units). This constellation of tissue alterations is often enclosed within terms of convenience such as *fibrocystic change*. These terms have little utility except to imply that biopsy was indicated and to document that cancer is absent. Biopsies may have changes that reliably indicate an increased subsequent breast cancer risk. Various hyperplastic or proliferative lesions are found in about 30% of such biopsies. About 4% of these benign biopsies contain hyperplastic changes approximating the histologic appearance of carcinoma in situ and are properly termed *atypical hyperplasia*. Their increased risk of carcinoma development is about four times that of the general population in the 15 years after biopsy, justifying effort in surveillance by mammography. The remaining 26% of women who have had a biopsy showing hyperplasia without atypia

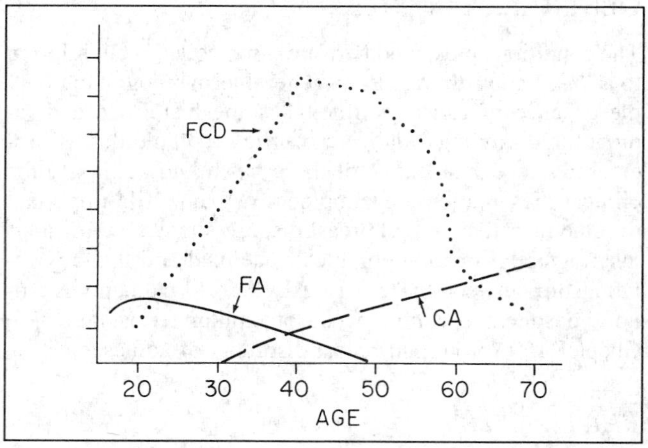

Fig. 167-1. Relative incidence of fibrocystic change (or disease, *FCD*), fibroadenoma *(FA)*, and carcinoma *(CA)* of the breast related to age at biopsy. Absolute numbers are not given because they depend on the frequency of breast biopsy and the ratio of benign to malignant rises when suspicion of cancer in poorly defined lumps is high and incidence of biopsy is high. This graph demonstrates the age dependency of these diagnostic possibilities. Other benign conditions, with papilloma predominating, are about half as frequent as FA and have an age distribution intermediate between FA and FCD.

have a risk approximately twice that of all women. Thus, 70% of biopsied women without these changes have no elevation of breast cancer risk beyond that of the general population.

MISCELLANEOUS SPECIFIC CONDITIONS

Bilateral nipple discharge of material resembling milk and containing fat globules is known as *galactorrhea*. Most cases are idiopathic, are found after cessation of oral contraceptive medication, or represent continuing discharge after pregnancy. The evaluation of this condition is discussed in Chapter 160. Nipple discharge other than a milky liquid is usually confined to a single breast and often to a single duct opening. The discharge is usually somewhat blue or brown and usually indicates benign alterations within the breast. If the discharge is bloody, particularly if it exists from a single opening at nipple, surgical exploration is warranted for what is usually a benign intraductal papilloma.

Cysts may present as dominant masses. Small cysts are present in a majority of perimenopausal women. Their occurrence decreases rapidly after age 50. The pathogenesis of cysts is unknown, and their linkage to carcinoma is unproved. The identification of a mass as possibly cystic makes an attempt at needle aspiration appropriate. If the mass persists or reappears, surgical removal is indicated.

Fibroadenomas are benign tumors usually occurring in young women (Fig. 167-1). They are regularly round, firm, sharply circumscribed, and nontender and appear movable within the mammary substance. These tumors are more common in Blacks and may be multiple. A rich stroma is an integral part of these lesions, closely associated with evenly distributed glandular elements. They may appear rapidly and can vary in size with the menstrual cycle. Surgical removal remains the standard therapy, although the tumors are benign, and avoidance of surgery in some cases is supportable after aspiration cytology, particularly in women younger than 25 years. A probable variant of fibroadenoma is the phyllodes tumor, which may attain large size and is occasionally malignant. Any soft tissue neoplasm may also appear in the breast, and a variety of other benign mass lesions may occur in the breast. The most common is the ductal papilloma.

Radial scars are uncommon lesions that have been widely recognized only in the last few years and have no known association with increased cancer risk. Larger examples are known as *complex sclerosing lesions or sclerosing papillary proliferations*. The clinical importance of these lesions lies in their simulation of invasive carcinoma on both physical and mammographic examination.

Fat necrosis is an unusual cause of a dominant mass in the breast and is probably caused by trauma. The condition often produces a firm, spiculated mass that can even dimple the skin and thus may closely mimic carcinoma.

Infections of the breast other than lactational abscesses are rare. They usually are caused by staphylococci and should be treated like any other local infection. Acid-fast and fungal organisms may involve the breast. Many parasitic and spirochetal organisms have also produced local infection in the breast.

REFERENCES

Deckers PJ and Ricci A Jr: Pain and lumps in the female breasts, Hosp Pract 27:67-68, 1992.

Dupont WD and Page DL: Menopausal estrogen replacement therapy and breast cancer, Arch Intern Med 151:67-72, 1991.

Dupont WD and Page DL: Risk factors for breast cancer in women with proliferative breast disease, N Engl J Med 312:146, 1985.

Gateley CA and Mansel RE: Management of the painful and nodular breast, Br Med Bull 47:284-294, 1991.

Goodwin PJ, Neelam M, and Boyd NF: Cyclical mastopathy: a critical review of therapy, Br J Surg 75:837-844, 1988.

Hendler FJ: Breast diseases and the internist, Am J Med Sci 293:331, 1987.

Hughes LE, Mansel RE, and Webster DJT: Benign disorders and diseases of the breast, London, 1989, Bailliere Tindall.

Page DJ and Anderson TJ: Diagnostic histopathology of the breast, Edinburgh, 1987, Churchill Livingstone.

Rohan TE and McMichael AJ: Methylxanthines and breast cancer, Int J Cancer 41:390, 1988.

Wisbey JR et al: Natural history of breast pain, Lancet 2:672, 1983.

CHAPTER 168 Diabetes Mellitus

Alan J. Garber

Diabetes mellitus is a disease complex characterized primarily by relative or absolute insufficiency of insulin secretion and concomitant insensitivity or resistance to the metabolic action of insulin on target tissues. Hyperglycemia results as a consequence of the defects in insulin secretion and action. Ultimately, in the diabetic process, there may be widespread involvement of virtually every organ system. This involvement is characterized by microvascular disease with capillary basement membrane thickening, macrovascular disease with accelerated atherosclerosis, neuropathy involving both the somatic and autonomic nervous systems, neuromuscular dysfunction with muscle wasting, embryopathy, and decreased resistance to infection. Hyperglycemia may be undetected before the development of such chronic complications of diabetes mellitus as nephropathy, retinopathy, myocardial infarction, or gangrene of the lower extremities.

Although diabetes mellitus was recognized as a clinical entity 2000 to 3000 years ago, clearly effective long-term treatment was unavailable until insulin was extracted from pancreatic tissues in 1921 by Banting and Best. Since the development of crystalline insulin, refinements in therapy have sought to make use of the improvements in insulin pharmacology that have resulted from complexing insulin with other proteins such as protamine or from producing crystalline zinc precipitates of insulin. Research based on the hypoglycemic effects of sulfonamide antibiotic derivatives has resulted in a class of orally administered hypoglycemic agents, the sulfonylureas. These drugs are useful in the treatment of diabetic patients who secrete inadequate amounts of endogenous insulin. Despite the clinical availability of insulin since the mid-1920s, patients have continued to die of diabetes mellitus and its complications. In contrast to the situation in the preinsulin era, patients may now easily survive multiple episodes of diabetic ketoacidosis or hyperosmolar nonketotic coma only to succumb slowly to the chronic complications of diabetes mellitus.

Diabetes mellitus is now the third leading cause of mortality in the United States and the leading cause of irreversible blindness and chronic renal failure. The estimated prevalence ranges from 3% to 6% of the population, and it is increasing at a rapid rate within the United States. Accelerated atherosclerosis produces 80% of all diabetic mortality, three fourths of it owing to coronary disease. The socioeconomic impact of diabetes is devastating to individual patients and society as a whole. Although inheritance and obesity are major risk factors for the development of diabetes mellitus, particularly the type II non-insulin-dependent form, the disease is found throughout the world and is seemingly independent of the carbohydrate content of the local diet.

PHYSIOLOGY

Regulation of human carbohydrate and fuel metabolism

In the resting or postprandial state, normal humans have an absolute requirement for approximately 180 g of carbohydrate per day to meet the energy requirements of the central nervous system and other tissues, such as erythrocytes, which are devoid of mitochondrial oxidative metabolism. This daily requirement is usually met by the ingestion of foodstuffs containing at least this quantity of carbohydrate. Increased glucose concentrations after eating stimulate pancreatic beta-cell insulin secretion while simultaneously reducing pancreatic alpha-cell glucagon secretion. These changes are amplified by the simultaneous secretion of enteric hormones that augment the insulin response to orally ingested glucose. The ingested carbohydrate is taken up by the liver and is also passed through to peripheral tissues for subsequent utilization. Initially, glucose is phosphorylated and stored in the form of hepatic glycogen, which may contain as much as 125 g of glucose (Fig. 168-1). Glycogen synthesis in the liver is stimulated by insulin activation of hepatic glycogen synthetase activity as well as by a possible inhibition of phosphorylase activity. This activity is reinforced by the declining glucagon level. The increased insulin and decreased glucagon concentrations also combine to increase the rate of flux in the pathway of anaerobic glycolysis in the liver by activating key enzymes of glycolysis. By these mechanisms, glucose, once phosphorylated as glucose 6-phosphate, may be stored as glycogen and also may be catabolized to the important three-carbon pyruvate within the liver.

When the sites available for further glycogen synthesis have been saturated, excess carbohydrate in the liver can then be transformed and subsequently stored in the form of fatty acids. The increased insulin and decreased glucagon concentrations provide an activation of pyruvate dehydrogenase. This substance, combined with pyruvate carboxylation to form oxalacetate, supplies both substrates required for net citrate formation. The large quantities of reducing equivalents generated by glycolysis at the level of glyceraldehyde-3-phosphate dehydrogenase are transported within the inner mitochondrial membrane and tend to shift the oxidation reduction potential of the mitochondria to a more reduced state.

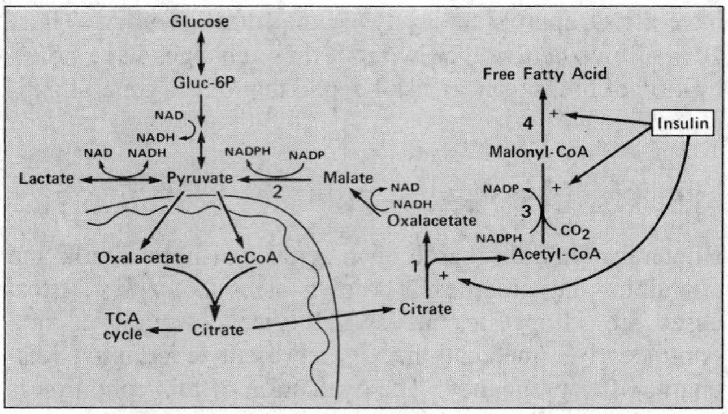

Fig. 168-1. Mitochondrial-cytosolic interactions for lipogenesis and gluconeogenesis. **1,** citrate cleavage enzyme; **2,** malic enzyme; **3,** acetyl coenzyme A carboxylase; **4,** fatty acid synthetase.

In the absence of substantial energy demands, adenosine triphosphate (ATP) levels remain high, and reduced nicotinamide-adenine dinucleotide (NADH) levels relative to NAD levels are also elevated. For these reasons, citrate oxidation and forward flow of the citric acid cycle are inhibited, most notably at isocitrate dehydrogenase (Fig. 168-1). Citrate efflux from the mitochondria occurs, and hydrolytic cleavage catalyzed by citric cleavage enzyme produces acetyl coenzyme A (acetyl CoA) and oxalacetate. Insulin induces fatty acid synthetase and acetyl CoA carboxylase activities. Acetyl CoA is carboxylated to form malonyl-coenzyme A (malonyl CoA), which is the first committed substrate for fatty acid synthesis and is also a key intermediate that inhibits fatty acid oxidation in liver. This regulation of fatty acid oxidation results from the potent inhibition by malonyl CoA of carnitine acetyltransferase I activity in the liver mitochondrial membrane. As a result, synthesized fatty acids cannot re-enter the mitochondria for subsequent degradation via the beta oxidation sequence. By these mechanisms, fatty acid accumulation follows the ingestion of large quantities of carbohydrate. These fatty acids are esterified to form triglycerides and are subsequently exported from the liver as very-low-density lipoprotein (VLDL) particles. Owing to the activation by insulin of peripheral lipoprotein lipase activity in the capillary vasculature surrounding adipose tissue, the secreted VLDL particles are hydrolyzed. The fatty acids are taken up by human adipose tissue and subsequently re-esterified and stored as triglycerides. Insulin facilitates the latter process (1) by increasing glucose transport and glycolysis in the adipocyte, thereby increasing alpha-glycerolphosphate availability for triglyceride synthesis, and (2) by an antagonism of cyclic adenosine monophosphate (cAMP)-mediated processes of triglyceride hydrolysis.

Metabolic fate of ingested protein

Ingestion of a pure protein meal produces an amino acidemia that stimulates the secretion of both glucagon and insulin. The increased glucagon concentration stimulates amino acid utilization by the liver, primarily to supply substrate for hepatic gluconeogenesis. Many amino acids are catabolized wholly or in part to compounds that ultimately form oxalacetate, aspartate, or malate. Oxalacetate is the substrate for phosphoenolpyruvate carboxykinase, a key gluconeogenic enzyme (Fig. 168-2). Amino acid carbon skeletons forming pyruvate require the enzymatic action of pyruvate carboxylase to synthesize oxalacetate. Glucagon induces the synthesis of phosphoenolpyruvate carboxykinase messenger RNA. Glucagon also stimulates the gluconeogenic enzyme fructose-1,6-diphosphatase activity.

After protein feeding, insulin also stimulates amino acid uptake and protein synthesis in peripheral tissues. Amino acids taken up by the liver are used for hepatic protein synthesis as well as for hepatic gluconeogenesis. The latter is critical in the absence of adequate carbohydrate intake.

Glucose homeostasis during fasting

Because the liver stores only about 100 to 125 g of glucose as glycogen, maintenance of circulating glucose concentrations, even after an overnight fast, must depend on gluconeogenesis (Fig. 168-3). Lactate is the principal precursor for hepatic gluconeogenesis in humans, generating approximately 50 g/day of glucose. Lactic acid must be recycled to glucose within the liver, or lactic acidosis will ensue. This cyclic pathway is called the *Cori cycle*.

To meet the continuing loss of glucose carbon during fasting or in periods of carbohydrate deprivation, which is oxidized to carbon dioxide in the central nervous system, large quantities of carbon from nonglucose sources must be mobilized and converted to glucose. Some of this requirement may be supplied by recycling of glucose-derived glycerol, which is liberated by triglyceride hydrolysis in adipose tissue. However, only amino acids derived from protein may provide the bulk of the precursor requirement for hepatic glucose production because a net synthesis of carbohydrate cannot be supported by fat oxidation. Of all amino acids studied, only alanine is taken up significantly by the liver. Indeed, the utilization of alanine is second only to the uptake and utilization of lactate by the liver. The source of this alanine is muscle. Alanine and glutamine synthesized largely from other amino acids account for the bulk of amino acid carbon released from skeletal muscle (Fig. 168-3). The amino acid precursors are liberated by the degradation of skeletal muscle proteins. Muscle protein homeostasis is modulated in part by insulin, which facilitates muscle protein synthesis and retards muscle protein degradation. Glutamine released from skeletal muscle is oxidized in the small intestinal mucosa leading in part to a net formation of alanine and lactate. Both these compounds are released into the portal venous circulation as fuels for subsequent hepatic glucose production. Muscle protein mass may be preferentially mobilized and delivered as gluconeogenic precursors to the liver for maintenance of hepatic glucose production in the fasting state (Fig. 168-3).

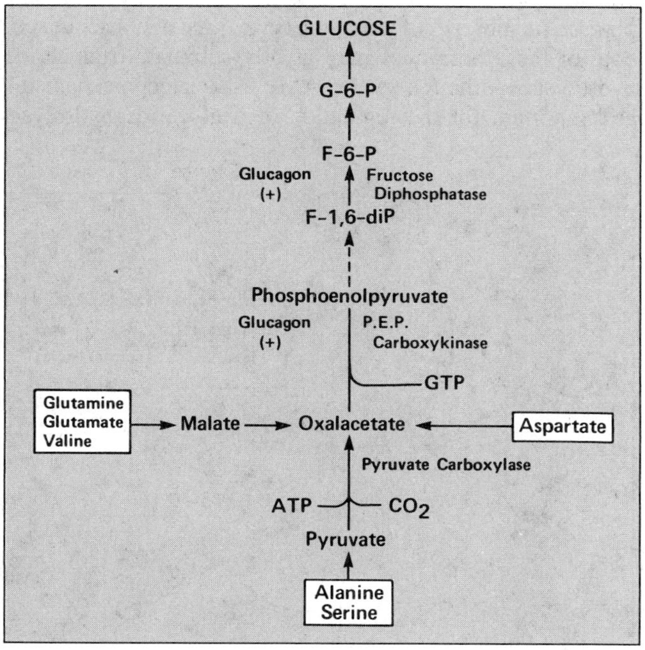

Fig. 168-2. Hepatic gluconeogenesis in humans.

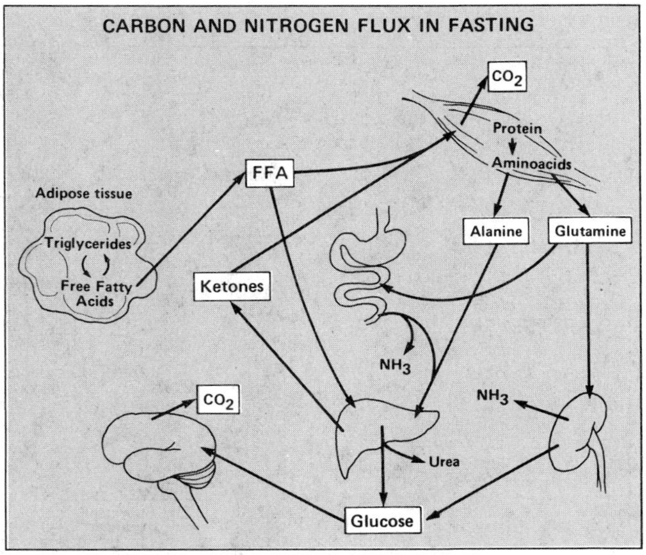

Fig. 168-3. Organ-organ interactions for glucose homeostasis during fasting.

Regulation of hepatic ketogenesis

Despite the availability of relatively large quantities of muscle protein, the obligate glucose need would require that more than 1 kg of muscle/day be degraded to meet the glucose requirement of fasting. Because the skeletal muscle mass accounts for 40% to 50% of body weight, it is apparent that no more than 10 days of starvation could be endured before substantial impairment of muscle function would occur from muscle wastage (Fig. 168-3). To meet the energy requirements of the central nervous system during starvation without impaired muscle function, alternative fuels are utilized. Because the bulk of excess ingested calories are stored as triglycerides, fatty acids become a primary source of energy for most tissues under conditions of starvation. Thus skeletal muscle, heart, liver, and most other tissues sharply increase their metabolism of fatty acids for energy production. The central nervous system, however, is unable to oxidize large quantities of free fatty acids. Instead, keto acids are used.

During fasting, rapid rates of hepatic fatty acid oxidation are accompanied by high glucagon and low insulin levels, which increase hepatic mitochondrial carnitine acyltransferase activity owing to a marked diminution of malonyl-CoA concentrations in the fasted state (Fig. 168-4). At the same time, mitochondrial oxalacetate also may be depleted by hepatic gluconeogenesis (removal by phosphoenolpyruvate carboxykinase) (Fig. 168-2). Acetyl-CoA accumulation occurs because the compound cannot be cleared by condensation with oxalacetate to form citrate. Disposal of the accumulated, excess hepatic acetyl-CoA occurs via condensation to form beta-hydroxy beta-methylglutaryl CoA, which is subsequently cleaved to form acetoacetate and acetyl CoA (Fig. 168-4). Acetoacetate is secondarily reduced by β-hydroxybutyrate dehydrogenase to form its hydroxy analog, β-hydroxybutyrate. These two compounds are referred to jointly as *ketone bodies* or *keto acids*.

During fasting, rates of hepatic ketogenesis increase rapidly, and keto acids accumulate in blood, to concentrations of 3 to 5 mM. Because of this, ketonuria develops within 48 hours in females and 72 hours in males. At concentrations of 3 mM or greater, circulating keto acids become an important and competitive substrate for central nervous system oxidative metabolism. Keto acids are utilized in the brain, heart, and skeletal muscle. Through this use of keto acids, central nervous system glucose consumption may be reduced dramatically. Thus in prolonged starvation, total glucose requirements can be decreased to between 50 and 80 g/day; muscle wastage is thereby reduced to less than 0.2 kg/day. This prevents significant muscle dysfunction during fasting.

Fatty acid metabolism during fasting

Triglyceride turnover in adipose tissue is controlled by a variety of hormones and cyclic nucleotides. Storage of triglycerides is promoted by insulin, which induces lipoprotein lipase. This enzyme is necessary for triglyceride hydrolysis and to clear circulating chylomicrons and VLDL of free fatty acids, for subsequent uptake by adipose tissue. Esterification of these free fatty acids requires insulin together with availability of intracellular glucose. The adipocyte is dependent on insulin for glucose transport. Glucose-derived alpha-glycerophosphate is the essential substrate for fatty acid esterification (Fig. 168-5). Because of the absence of glycerol kinase in adipose tissue, reutilization of glycerol liberated by triglyceride hydrolysis does not occur.

Triglyceride hydrolysis to fatty acids is regulated by both cyclic adenosine monophosphate-dependent and -independent mechanisms. Catecholamines and, to a lesser extent, glucagon stimulate adenylyl cyclases on the plasma membrane of the adipocyte. As a consequence, both of these hormones may greatly stimulate triglyceride hydrolysis. Although cyclic AMP-associated mechanisms are important for the regulation of triglyceride hydrolysis

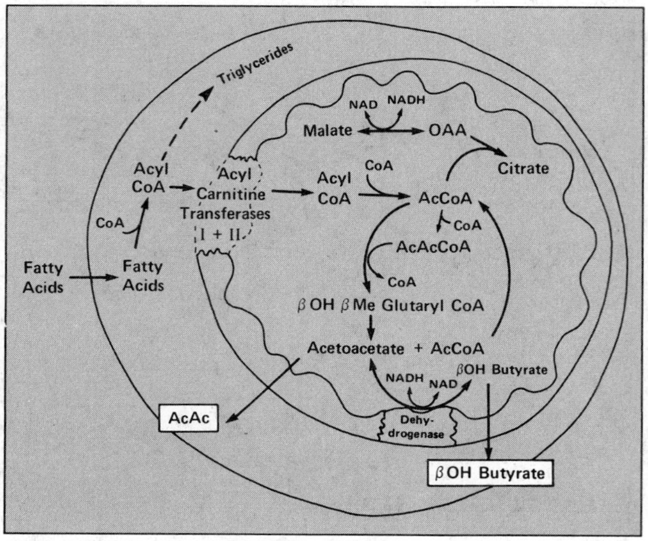

Fig. 168-4. Hepatic ketogenesis.

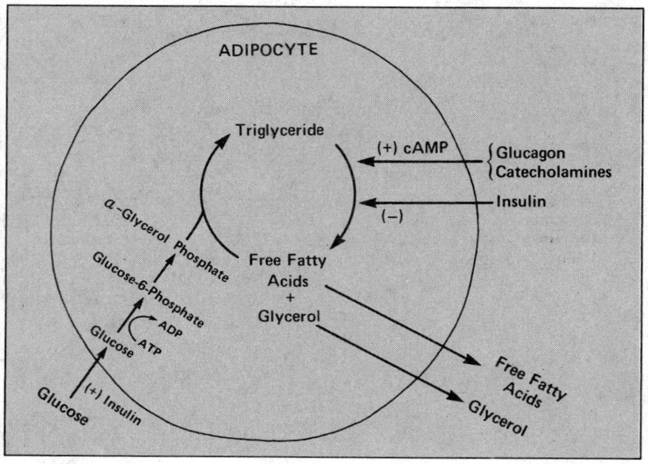

Fig. 168-5. Triglyceride turnover in the adipocyte.

in adipose tissue, growth hormone and cortisol also influence triglyceride breakdown in adipose tissue via noncyclic nucleotide-dependent mechanisms. Most of the anti-insulin hormones increase net free fatty acid delivery from adipose tissue so that oxidative fuel can be made available for all tissues of the body during physical or metabolic stress. In diabetes mellitus, increased triglyceride turnover and increased net triglyceride hydrolysis produce high levels of free fatty acids in blood, and these tend to accelerate rates of hepatic ketogenesis. Because blood levels of free fatty acids can increase by 10- to 20-fold during periods of maximal glucagon and catecholamine stimulation, they are oxidative fuels for energy generation in peripheral tissues. Indeed, free fatty acids are so well utilized that they effectively compete with keto acids for oxidation in the citric acid cycle and thereby block the disposal of keto acids when their concentration would have otherwise been sufficient to induce rapid rates of keto acid utilization. By this competition, free fatty acids contribute significantly to the development of ketoacidosis in patients with diabetes mellitus.

Integrated fuel homeostasis

From the preceding discussion it can be seen that the blood glucose level is a closely regulated, finely controlled parameter. Because of the obligate requirement for glucose maintained by the central nervous system, numerous metabolic systems have been evolved and organized to maintain blood glucose levels in all circumstances.

Insulin is the major anabolic hormone regulating the metabolism of virtually all body fuels and substrates. It promotes the storage of carbohydrate, initially in the form of hepatic glycogen, as well as skeletal muscle glycogen. The latter is available primarily as an emergency fuel for skeletal muscle contraction during periods of severe hypoxia or anoxia. Insulin is also strongly anabolic for the long-term storage of fuels in the form of triglycerides, the most efficient form of fuel storage available to humans. Insulin also promotes the net synthesis of free fatty acids in liver. The free fatty acids formed from excess carbohydrate ingestion are then stored in peripheral adipose tissue. Insulin plays a primary anabolic role in skeletal muscle, as it facilitates amino acid uptake as well as protein synthesis by independent mechanisms, and it retards the degradation of skeletal muscle proteins.

Glucagon, cortisol, and catecholamines are the major catabolic hormones in humans. The importance of glucagon is focused primarily on maintenance of blood glucose concentrations during fasting or periods of inadequate carbohydrate intake. To reduce the total body requirement for glucose, glucagon facilitates hepatic ketogenesis so that an alternative fuel, namely keto acids, may be produced for central nervous system energy requirements. Glucagon does not play a major role in the mobilization of substrates from peripheral tissue for subsequent metabolism in the liver. Glucagon is without effect on the mobilization of skeletal muscle proteins, which provide the ultimate carbon source for the bulk of glucose formed from amino acids during short-term starvation. Furthermore, glucagon plays only a secondary role in the regulation of triglyceride hydrolysis and free fatty acid mobilization from adipose tissue. In these peripheral tissues, a combination of high glucagon and especially low insulin levels appears to make available the amino acid and free fatty acid substrates for hepatic metabolism. Reinforcement of these effects of glucagon by catecholamines occurs in adipose tissue and by cortisol in both skeletal muscle and adipose tissue.

CLASSIFICATION

Over the years, a variety of classifications and diagnostic criteria for diabetes mellitus have been proposed. Although diabetes mellitus is primarily a disease of inadequate insulin secretion and action, measurements of abnormal insulin action in terms of serum or blood glucose are used almost exclusively to diagnose diabetes mellitus. In most formulations, basal euglycemia in the fasting state and an unimpaired ability to dispose of a carbohydrate load have been most widely used to assess the presence or absence of diabetes. Conditions other than diabetes mellitus also are associated with abnormal carbohydrate metabolism, carbohydrate intolerance, and even fasting hyperglycemia. A recent attempt has been made to resolve these differences and to organize the available clinical data to provide a scientific basis for interpretations of fasting serum or plasma glucose concentrations and also of serum glucose responses during glucose tolerance tests. Three major types of patients with diabetes mellitus are now recognized.

Type I insulin-dependent diabetes mellitus

Patients with type I diabetes mellitus have little or no endogenous insulin secretion. The onset of the disease is usually clinically abrupt, with marked polyuria, polydipsia, polyphagia, weight loss, and fatigue. These patients are highly prone to ketosis and frequently may present themselves for treatment in an initial episode of diabetic ketoacidosis. In other classifications, this form was termed *juvenile-onset diabetes mellitus,* or *ketosis-prone diabetes mellitus*. These patients generally have lost weight and are frequently at or below ideal body weight. As a result, there is marked sensitivity or brittleness to exogenous insulin administration, particularly with regular insulin.

This form of diabetes mellitus can occur at any age. Incidence most commonly peaks in the middle of the first decade and again at the time of the growth acceleration of adolescence. A prodromal phase of polyuria, polydipsia, and weight loss may precede the development of ketoacidosis by a period of days to months, but it most commonly is noted for only 2 to 4 weeks before onset of ketoacidosis. As with all other forms of primary diabetes mellitus, a genetic predisposition appears to underlie the pathogenesis of type I diabetes mellitus, although the family history is less strongly associated than in type II. Patients with type I disease have in common one of several human leukocyte antigen histocompatibility antigens (e.g., B8, B15, DW3, DW4), and islet cell antibodies frequently are observed at the time of diagnosis. A viral etiology involving one of several enteroviruses such as coxsackievirus B_4 and mumps has been proposed in these patients. Recently, evidence has been developed to suggest that an ongoing, autoimmune destruction of pancreatic beta cells may underlie type I diabetes mellitus. Clinical trials with immunosuppressive medications such as cyclosporine have demonstrated efficacy in prolonging the honeymoon phase of type I diabetes and in arresting the loss of residual insulin secretion in newly diagnosed patients. The toxicity of such therapy presently outweighs the benefits derived. Recent evidence, however, suggests that a brief period of early, aggressive glucose control, as with a biostator, may prolong residual, endogenous insulin secretory capacity and improve long-term glucose control.

Type II non-insulin-dependent diabetes mellitus

Patients with type II diabetes mellitus maintain some endogenous insulin secretory capability despite the overt abnormalities of glucose homeostasis, including fasting hyperglycemia and/or carbohydrate intolerance. Unlike type I patients, patients with type II diabetes mellitus are relatively resistant to the development of ketosis in the basal state because of the retention of endogenous insulin secretory capabilities. These patients generally demonstrate marked resistance or insensitivity to the metabolic actions of endogenous as well as exogenous insulin, in part as the result of decreased insulin receptors. A failure of postreceptor coupling and of intracellular insulin action is a more important cause of insulin resistance. In offspring of type II patients, insulin resistance appears inherited and is present at maturity. This resistance may also be the best predictor of a future diabetic state. A syndrome of insulin resistance (syndrome X) has been proposed to explain the frequent association of hypertension, carbohydrate intolerance, abdominal obesity, dyslipidemia, and accelerated atherosclerosis. Mild to marked obesity is present in approximately 80% of type II diabetic patients at the time of diagnosis. Obesity is a major risk factor for the development of this type of diabetes mellitus, owing in part to the associated insulin resistance. Nevertheless, it is clear that a primary insufficiency of insulin secretion is the pathologic essential for the clinical development of type II diabetes mellitus.

Although there can be limitations on insulin secretory capacity in type II diabetes, together with the presence of insulin insensitivity, these patients do not have an absolute dependence on injectable insulin for their survival. The clinical presentation of patients with type II disease varies greatly. These patients may manifest diabetes only after the development of complications such as retinopathy or nephropathy. On the other hand, type II patients may also seek treatment because of significant polyuria, polydipsia, easy fatigability, and irritability. In patients having one or more of the chronic complications of diabetes, marked abnormalities of carbohydrate metabolism are generally not observed, and these patients may even have normal fasting glucose levels. The frequency of vascular complications in diabetes is also amplified synergistically by common comorbid illnesses such as hypertension and dyslipidemia.

Most patients with type II diabetes mellitus are diagnosed after the age of 40 years. This form of diabetes often is called *adult-onset* or *ketosis-resistant diabetes mellitus*. Nevertheless, the onset of type II diabetes mellitus, including the so-called maturity-onset diabetes mellitus of the young (MODY), can occur at any age. Most forms of type II disease show strong heritable influences in their transmission. In MODY, an autosomal dominant inheritance has been established. In other forms of type II diabetes mellitus, the mode of transmission is less clear; however, a dominant inheritance is suspected. Nevertheless, because of the relationship between pre-existing obesity and the development of type II disease, environmental influences clearly play a strong role in the development of the disease.

Secondary diabetes mellitus

Secondary diabetes mellitus is a category that constitutes a heterogeneous grouping of patients for whom a designation of either of the traditional forms of diabetes mellitus appears inappropriate. Although abnormal glucose metabolism may be demonstrated by fasting hyperglycemia or an impaired ability to dispose of a carbohydrate load, genetically determined inadequacies of insulin secretion or action are not the primary pathogenic abnormality in secondary diabetes. The age of onset and clinical presentation may vary according to the etiology of the secondary diabetes. In general, any disease producing an impairment of insulin secretion or resulting in antagonism to insulin action can be associated with secondary diabetes mellitus. These primary diseases may include endocrine pancreatic insufficiency following chronic recurrent pancreatitis or cystic fibrosis. Other diseases, such as acanthosis nigricans, may be associated with antibodies to the insulin receptor. These may block the metabolic actions of insulin and therefore produce marked insulin resistance and secondary diabetes mellitus (see the box on the right).

A large number of diseases may interfere with the metabolic actions of insulin at the post-insulin-receptor level. These diseases include endocrinopathies such as acromegaly, glucagonoma, Cushing's syndrome, pheochromocytoma, and thyrotoxicosis. In addition, carbohydrate intolerance and fasting hyperglycemia have been observed in a variety of metabolic disorders, such as the muscular dystrophies, glycogen storage disease (type I), lipoatrophic diabetes mellitus, and in several chromosomal diseases such as Klinefelter's and Down syndromes. A variety of drugs also have been associated with carbohydrate intolerance and secondary diabetes mellitus. Some diuretics and antihypertensives such as diazoxide have direct antagonistic effects on endogenous insulin secretion, whereas others produce hypokalemia, which reduces insulin output. Neuroactive agents such as phenytoin, lithium carbonate, and tricyclic antidepressants also can impair glucose tolerance. A more complete listing of drugs that induce secondary diabetes mellitus is provided in the box at far right.

Pathologic processes producing secondary diabetes

I. Processes causing reduced insulin secretion
   A. Pancreatitis or pancreatectomy
   B. Cystic fibrosis
   C. Hemochromatosis
   D. Pheochromocytoma
   E. Somatostatinoma
   F. Aldosteronoma
   G. Hypokalemia
II. Processes producing impairment of insulin action
   A. Insulin receptor defects
      1. With acanthosis nigricans
      2. Insulin receptor antibodies
   B. Anti-insulin antibodies
   C. Diseases producing excess anti-insulin hormones
      1. Pheochromocytoma
      2. Cushing's syndrome
      3. Acromegaly
      4. Glucagonoma
      5. Thyrotoxicosis
III. Diseases producing secondary diabetes by unknown mechanisms
   A. Muscular dystrophies
   B. Myotonic dystrophy
   C. Acute intermittent porphyria
   D. Glycogen storage disease, type I
   E. Hyperlipidemia
   F. Friedreich's ataxia
   G. Laurence-Moon-Biedl syndrome
   H. Syndrome of progeria
   I. Prader-Willi syndrome
   J. Chromosomal aberrations
      1. Klinefelter's syndrome
      2. Turner's syndrome
      3. Down syndrome
   K. Sexual ateliotic dwarfism

Drugs producing impaired glucose tolerance and/or hyperglycemia

Diuretics and antihypertensive agents
- Thiazide diuretics
- Clonidine
- Furosemide

Agents with hormonal activity
- Glucocorticoids
- Oral contraceptives
- Thyroid hormone
- Progestins

Neuroactive agents
- Haloperidol
- Lithium carbonate
- Phenothiazines
- Tricyclics
- Adrenergic agonists

Anti-inflammatory agents
- Indomethacin

Miscellaneous
- Isoniazid
- Nicotinic acid
- Cimetidine
- Heparin

Diagnostic criteria for diabetes mellitus

In most normal subjects mean fasting serum glucose concentrations of approximately 80 mg/dl with a maximal increase in the postprandial state to approximately 140 mg/dl are routinely observed. However, considerable variability among individuals has been observed in large-scale patient population studies. There also may be considerable variation in group mean data for fasting circulating glucose concentrations between ethnic groups such as the Pima Indians as compared to white Americans. Individual variations may reflect the influence of age and metabolic and hormonal states, which can profoundly influence fasting glucose concentrations in otherwise normal subjects. Physical or emotional stress, infection, undernutrition, bed rest, and trauma are some of the more common causes of transient carbohydrate intolerance. Marked variation among multiple glucose tolerance tests on the same individual has been observed without subsequent deterioration of fasting glucose levels. For this reason, fasting hyperglycemia or abnormal carbohydrate tolerance should be reproducible on two or more occasions before the diagnosis of diabetes mellitus or impaired carbohydrate metabolism is made.

Because of the complexity of glucose tolerance testing and the variability encountered among tests, glucose tolerance testing is not advisable as a routine screening measure for diabetes mellitus unless there is a reason to establish this diagnosis. Standardization of glucose tolerance tests seems essential for their interpretation. In an otherwise healthy, unstressed ambulatory patient, at least 3 days of a relatively high carbohydrate diet (a minimum of 150 g of carbohydrate per day) are required for study of normal insulin secretory dynamics. The glucose tolerance test should always be performed in the morning, after 10 to 12 hours of overnight fasting, and the patient should refrain from significant caffeine or nicotine use during this period. A load of 75 g of glucose or of rapidly absorbed dextrins (e.g., Glucola) should be ingested and plasma glucoses determined at 0, 0.5, 1.0, 1.5, 2.0, and 3.0 hours after initiation of the test.

There are two major reasons to perform glucose tolerance tests. First, patients with multiple borderline fasting serum glucose levels (115 to 139 mg/dl) should be evaluated further with glucose tolerance tests to establish the degree of hyperglycemia. Second, patients with symptoms that may be clearly related to diabetes mellitus, or those with overt pathology that may be a complication of diabetes mellitus (e.g., an otherwise unexplainable neuropathy) must have the possible diagnosis of abnormal carbohydrate metabolism clearly established or refuted. In the latter group, a complete workup for other causes of symptoms or pathology consistent with diabetes mellitus also should be initiated. A second glucose tolerance test may be necessary to establish firmly the diagnosis of diabetes mellitus in these patients.

The 2-hour postprandial glucose level is of questionable value as a screening test for diabetes mellitus. The quantity of carbohydrate ingested, the other constituents of the meal, and the prior nutritional state of the patient may all combine to produce a false-negative, as well as false-positive, result. Such an outcome usually is not acceptable for any screening test. For these reasons, glucose tolerance screening is better performed by measuring a 2-hour sample after proper preparation and a defined glucose load.

Specific diagnostic criteria. The diagnosis of diabetes mellitus is made by a reproducible demonstration of fasting hyperglycemia. Fasting serum glucose levels of 140 mg/dl or greater on two or more occasions are diagnostic of diabetes mellitus in the adult, and this finding obviates the need for a glucose tolerance test in the absence of other causes of hyperglycemia. Increased certainty in the diagnosis is produced by such concomitant symptoms of classic diabetes mellitus as polyuria, polydipsia, polyphagia, weight loss, fatigue, and ketonuria. When one is testing glucose tolerance for diagnosis, a 2-hour venous plasma or serum glucose and one other sample (either the 30-, 60-, or 90-minute sample) must both exceed 200 mg/dl. Other criteria have been used to evaluate and diagnose diabetes by glucose tolerance testing. However, because of the relative absence of retinal and renal microvascular complications in those patients having a 2-hour plasma glucose less than 200 mg/dl the less stringent criteria indicated earlier are more appropriate for the diagnosis of type II diabetes mellitus. Otherwise, a large group of patients with only abnormal carbohydrate tolerance (peak $\geq$ 200 mg/dl; 2-hour $>$140 and $\leq$199 mg/dl) may be misdiagnosed as having diabetes mellitus, and they may thereby experience unnecessary difficulties with employment and insurability. Based on large population surveys, it seems that only patients with marked hyperglycemia (fasting $\geq$140 mg/dl; postglucose peak $\geq$200 mg/dl, and 2-hour postglucose $\geq$200 mg/dl) are subject to the development of diabetic macrovascular and microvascular complications such as retinopathy and nephropathy. On the other hand, patients with less marked hyperglycemia (fasting 115 to 139 mg/dl; postglucose peak $\geq$200 and 2-hour postglucose between 140 and 199 mg/dl) although not subject to the development of microvascular complications do have accelerated macrovascular disease.

Impaired glucose tolerance is a functional diagnosis that is likely an intermediary diagnosis in the evolution of clinical diabetes mellitus. A proportion of patients with abnormal glucose tolerance tests will progress to overt diabetes mellitus if a sufficient period of time elapses (5%/year or 30% after 10 years) or if endogenous or exogenous stress factors develop. A diagnosis of impaired or abnormal glucose tolerance assumes a fasting plasma glucose concentration of 139 mg/dl or less. If, on glucose tolerance testing, a patient has a 30-, 60-, or 90-minute plasma or serum glucose concentration greater than 200 mg per deciliter and a 2-hour serum or plasma glucose level ranging between 140 and 200 mg/dl, the diagnosis of probable impaired glucose tolerance may be entertained. From these criteria, it can be seen that the diagnosis of diabetes mellitus and that of impaired glucose tolerance is somewhat similar, in that the 30-, 60-, or 90-minute plasma or serum glucose sample must exceed 200 mg/dl. The only difference between these two diagnoses lies in the result obtained for the 2-hour sample, which ranges between 140 and 199 mg/dl for a diagnosis of impaired glucose tolerance, whereas values of 200 mg/dl or greater are diagnostic of diabetes mellitus. Of course, these results must be reproducible if either diagnosis is to be established by glucose tolerance testing alone.

Gestational diabetes

Pregnant women with no previous history of abnormal carbohydrate metabolism may develop impaired glucose tolerance or overt diabetes mellitus during pregnancy, particularly during the third trimester of the pregnancy when substantial resistance to the metabolic actions of insulin becomes apparent. A diagnosis of gestational diabetes implies that carbohydrate metabolism was normal before pregnancy. Most patients will return to normal glucose tolerance or impaired glucose tolerance in the postpartum state. Less commonly, such patients may maintain an overt diabetic state and therefore must be reclassified as type II diabetes mellitus. Because of the increased risk of perinatal fetal morbidity and mortality, it is essential to establish a diagnosis of gestational diabetes as early as possible. Because approximately one third to one half of patients with gestational diabetes will develop most commonly, type II diabetes mellitus after 5 to 10 years, careful characterization of the diagnosis again is essential.

The incidence of gestational diabetes is approximately 1% to 2% of all pregnancies. It must be suspected in any patient having glycosuria, a positive family history of diabetes mellitus, a history of unexplained stillbirth or prior abortion, a previous history of possible diabetic embryopathy, or previous congenital abnormalities. Because of the metabolic stress of pregnancy, independent values for interpretations of glucose tolerance tests are essential for the diagnosis of gestational diabetes (Table 168-1). All women should be screened with either a 2-hour glucose after a 50-g

Table 168-1. Criteria for diagnosis of gestational diabetes*

Sample time	Venous plasma (mg/dl)	Venous whole blood (mg/dl)
Fasting	105	90
1 h	190	170
2 h	165	145
3 h	145	125

*Values obtained from glucose tolerance testing must be equal to or greater than at least two of the values above.

glucose load or a 100-g oral glucose tolerance test (OGTT). Considerably lower fasting and 2-hour values must be exceeded for a diagnosis of gestational compared to type II diabetes mellitus. Additionally, the criteria of O'Sullivan and Mahan require only that two or more of the values be met or exceeded out of the fasting and 1-, 2-, and 3-hour samples drawn after a 100-g oral glucose challenge. Because other criteria for the diagnosis of gestational diabetes are presently unavailable for evaluation, the dissimilarity between those of O'Sullivan and Mahan and the diagnostic criteria presented for nonpregnant adults must remain. Because of the improved fetal viability in mothers adequately treated for gestational diabetes, the diagnostic criteria shown previously must be applied carefully. A high index of suspicion must be maintained for patients with any major risk factor that may lead to a deterioration of carbohydrate tolerance in the third trimester. To avoid fetal loss, proper therapy must be established during this period.

MANAGEMENT

The two basic forms of diabetes mellitus (type I, insulin-dependent, and type II, non-insulin-dependent) both require intensive patient education and management by the physician; however, the patient must also assume a major proportion of responsibility for management of the disease. The physician should assume the posture of a counselor or advisor who can best outline treatment modalities or options and counsel the patient regarding therapeutic decisions. It is essential that the patient actively participate in these therapeutic decisions, particularly because successful implementation of such decisions frequently is determined by the patient's sense of responsibility for treatment.

Motivational and behavioral approaches to management are especially important in adolescent diabetic patients, who may experience enormous adjustment difficulties owing to disturbances of their self-image produced by diabetes mellitus. Rebellious, defiant, and self-destructive behavior; manipulative maneuvers for secondary gain; and depressive episodes are common in the adolescent patient newly diagnosed with diabetes mellitus. However, similar psychologic disturbances may occur in any patient who has been diagnosed as having insulin-dependent diabetes mellitus. In obese adults with type II diabetes mellitus, equally difficult, but far more subtle, problems relating to weight reduction are frequently encountered. Habitual overeating, together with a lack of appropriate physical activity, results in obesity, which the patient maintains despite strong societal and peer pressures. Therefore considerable effort must be initiated and maintained to negate the secondary gain that these patients obtain from continuing their excessive food intake. A third major area requiring a thoughtful, motivational approach is the introduction of insulin therapy to patients who object to self-injection. This problem with the acceptance of insulin therapy is compounded by the relative dietary rigidity imposed by pharmacologic preparations of insulin. Total deletion of meals or a complete revamping of dietary intake on impulse can produce disastrous acute hypoglycemic episodes or periods of profound hyperglycemia. The induction of guilt in the patient by an admonishing physician can produce counterproductive behavior that ultimately results in a vicious circle of even greater difficulty in management. As patients become increasingly frustrated and made guilty by their maladaptive behavior, they may become depressed and self-destructive. As a consequence, a further deterioration in diabetic control results. An agreed on consensus for standards of diabetic control and the degree of control are shown in Table 168-2.

Other medical approaches to diet therapy, including behavioral modification, insight psychotherapy, and supportive psychotherapy, may be required to supplement the counseling and advice provided by the physician caring for the patient with diabetes mellitus. A supportive and conciliatory role on the part of the practitioner will usually prove far more rewarding than admonitions in the long-term management of the patient's diabetes.

Dietary management

The first and essential treatment for all patients with diabetes mellitus is diet management. Diet therapy is aimed at achieving four major goals:

1. Maintenance or establishment of ideal body weight
2. Distribution of the caloric intake into many small loads taken through the widest possible interval during the day
3. Avoidance of rapidly absorbed carbohydrate loads
4. Maintenance of proper, long-term nutritional balance

In prescribing a diet, the prescription must be arrived at rationally and with the patient's understanding. Capricious estimations of patients' caloric requirements to lose or gain weight can become punitive and therefore are unlikely to produce desirable outcomes. For the vast majority of patients with type II diabetes mellitus, weight reduction is necessary. On the other hand, a minority of patients with type II and a majority of patients with type I diabetes are already at or near ideal body weight, and weight maintenance is all that is required. A minority of patients with type I diabetes may be substantially underweight. Such individuals show extreme sensitivity to pharmacologic injec-

Table 168-2. Recommended standards of glucose control for patients with diabetes mellitus*

Index	Good	Acceptable	Fair	Poor
Fasting-serum (capillary)†	≤115(100)	≤140(120)	≤200(170)	>200
2-hour postprandial-serum (capillary)†	≤140(120)	≤175(150)	≤235(200)	>235
Glycosylated hemoglobin	≤6%	≤8%	≤10%	>10%

*Standards set by the American Diabetes Association and the US Department of Public Health Service, 1986.

†Each value expressed as mg/dl.

tions of insulin, and this sensitivity considerably complicates the induction and maintenance of good control of blood glucose concentrations. To calculate the caloric prescription required for patients with diabetes mellitus, the patient's present body weight and an estimation of his or her customary degree of physical activity are required. Most of the calories are consumed by the basal metabolic rate, and only about 25% to 40% more calories are required in any sedentary life-style (Table 168-3).

Thus the 70-kg sedentary subject (e.g., office worker) consumes approximately 2100 calories per day to maintain that weight. At most, a 20% variance can be attached to this number. For this patient, a caloric prescription ranging between 1700 and 2500 calories per day should be adequate. To prevent weight gain, particularly during the initial phases of insulin administration, a diet containing slightly fewer than the calculated required number of calories is advisable. It is particularly important to emphasize to the patient the need to determine carefully the portion size during the initial phase of therapy. Most patients consistently underestimate the sizes and quantities of the foods they consume.

A more frequent consideration in the dietary prescription is the need to adjust the patient's present weight to the estimated ideal body weight. Most commonly, this requires weight reduction. Behavioral modification approaches that attempt to elucidate the underlying causes of compulsive overeating in each patient may provide good long-term results. A successful weight-reducing diet must provide a sufficiently attractive and pleasant food experience for the patients so that they can follow modified diets for the rest of their lives. This requirement cannot be met by unbalanced, markedly hypocaloric, semistarvation diets, which produce excessive ketosis and wastage of lean body mass. A weight reduction greater than 1.0 to 1.5 kg per week is usually inadvisable. An even slower rate of weight reduction is advisable for the older patient.

Because a pound of fat represents approximately 3500 calories, a 1-kg weight loss per week amounts to a caloric deficit of 1000 calories per day. Thus a 100-kg obese, active woman who eats approximately 2500 to 3000 calories per day to maintain her weight should receive a caloric prescription for not more than 1500 to 2000 calories if she is to lose 1 kg per week. Some adjustment for individual metabolic differences and overestimations of portion size may be necessary, thereby justifying an initial prescription of 1200 to 1800 calories per day. As the patient's weight and caloric expenditure decline, downward readjustment of the caloric prescription will be necessary to reflect the decreased caloric needs. For example, when the patient has reduced to 90 kg, the diet must be reduced by 250 to 300 calories to maintain the same rate of weight loss. Periodic re-evaluation requires periodic downward adjustments of the caloric intake. At 70 kg, this same active woman would need to consume about 1750 to 2100 calories per day to maintain that weight. A continuing weight loss of 1 kg per week would require a caloric prescription of about 1000 calories to maintain constant weight loss. As the diet progresses, the patient becomes both more familiar with and accepting of the diet. An initial prescription of 1000 calories will not be as well tolerated by the patient because of inadequate secondary gain from food ingestion. The slower approach substitutes secondary gain from weight reduction and the resultant improved body image for that derived from food intake. This dietary approach requires periodic supervision and monitoring by the physician and, perhaps, by a nutritionist, of calories ingested, with considerable advice regarding the pitfalls of portion size, food tasting while preparing the family meals, and unprescribed snacks. If increased physical activity is also a component of the weight-reducing regimen, appropriate increases in caloric intake have to be considered (see also Chapter 49).

Table 168-3. Approximate caloric requirements to maintain body weight in adults

Activity level	Calories/kg/day
Basal (bed rest)	20-25
Sedentary (desk work)	30
Vigorous (postal worker)	35
Extraordinarily active (lumberjack)	40-50

Exchange lists. The most commonly used dietary prescriptions are obtained from the exchange lists developed by the American Diabetes Association. Although considerable variation can be produced in the caloric content per day, diets derived from these lists distribute daily calorie intake as about 20% for breakfast, 30% for lunch, 40% for dinner, and about 10% for a snack (usually given at bedtime). The diet contains approximately 15% to 20% protein, 30% to 35% fat, and 50% to 60% carbohydrate. Most of the carbohydrate is in the form of complex starches that do not produce accentuated peaks of hyperglycemia similar to those produced by equal quantities of refined sugars such as sucrose. Modifications of these diets may be made easily by moving bread, fruit, or meat exchanges from one meal to another or by substituting exchanges, as each exchange contains a known amount of calories in the form of protein, fat, or carbohydrate. A diet high in fiber should be prescribed to further reduce postprandial hyperglycemia. Although detailed dietary instruction regarding the implementation of an exchange list diet usually requires counseling from a dietitian, the physician should be familiar with the prescribed diet to counsel patients properly. Allowances should be made for ethnic food preferences and occasional off-diet food consumption.

Considerable care and forethought are required in using exchange lists. The use of these lists may not be practical for some patients because of financial, occupational, or uncommon dietary preferences. For such patients, a constant carbohydrate diet is frequently prescribed in which the amount of carbohydrate, particularly that in the form of rapidly absorbed carbohydrate, is controlled, and less attention is paid to the distribution of protein and fat. It also should be noted that for patients with hyperlipidemias secondary to poorly controlled diabetes mellitus, the American Diabetes Association diet is usually sufficient for control of types IV and V hyperlipidemia. However, modifications of the American Diabetes Association diet must be made for the less frequently occurring type IIB hyperlipidemia (Chapter 171). Lastly, it must be emphasized that food consumption must be modified in accordance with gross changes in physical activity, especially for type I diabetic patients in whom, if hypoglycemic reactions are to be avoided, ingestion of concentrated carbohydrates such as candy and sweetened beverages may be needed before, during, and sometimes after, strenuous exercise.

Oral hypoglycemic agents

Two major classes of oral hypoglycemic agents are currently available for use in patients with type II diabetes mellitus. The largest and only class available in the United States is the sulfonylureas. During the initial phase of treatment, sulfonylureas increase the quantity of insulin secreted in response to a given glucose concentration. With prolonged use, however, additional effects of the sulfonylureas tend to maintain lower blood sugars. These effects may be at the level of tissue insulin-receptor density or of the coupling of insulin receptors to metabolic processes in target cells. Sulfonylureas diminish hepatic glucose production and gluconeogenesis from alanine. Sulfonylureas also diminish or abolish the delayed insulin release in response to glucose noted in patients with type II diabetes. For this reason, sulfonylureas may be particularly useful in the treatment of that form of reactive hypoglycemia caused by early diabetes mellitus.

The other major class of oral antidiabetic agents are the biguanides, such as metformin and phenformin. Although not available in the United States, they are nonetheless widely used worldwide. They produce their hypoglycemic action by retarding glucose absorption from the gut and by direct effects on mitochondrial oxidative phosphorylation. The latter effect may be important, however, only at toxic levels of the drug. Biguanides improve insulin resistance in obese type II patients, but may cause toxic reactions including acute lactic acidosis, particularly in patients with renal disease in whom these agents may accumulate to toxic levels.

Six major sulfonylureas are presently available in the United States for the treatment of diabetes mellitus. Of these, tolbutamide, acetohexamide, tolazamide, and chlorpropamide are so-called first-generation agents, whereas glyburide and glipizide are more recently available second-generation agents (Table 168-4). The principal differences among these sulfonylureas lie in their ability to induce hypoglycemia, in their adverse effects profile, and in their duration of action. Tolbutamide (Orinase) has a relatively low potency/weight ratio and a short biologic effect. For these reasons, tolbutamide is the mildest hypoglycemic sulfonylurea available, and more than one daily dose generally is needed. It must be given either one-half hour before each meal or two to three times daily. Chlorpropamide (Diabinese) has a considerably prolonged biologic action and increased potency/weight ratio, so a dose need be taken only once daily. The more potent sulfonylureas have the disadvantage of producing hypoglycemia if a meal is delayed or omitted, or if the drug is taken in an excessive dose.

Differences among these agents result from variations in their means of metabolism and disposal. For example, chlorpropamide is cleared almost entirely by glomerular filtration. Thus its use is ill advised in patients with compensated renal insufficiency or with significant fluctuations in renal filtration, as with congestive heart failure. On the other hand, acetohexamide (Dymelor) must be metabolized in the liver to an active metabolite to obtain maximal biologic effect. The active metabolite is excreted in the urine. Coexisting liver or kidney disease may determine the sulfonylurea to be used. A serious complication of the use of chlorpropamide lies in its tendency to potentiate the action of antidiuretic hormone on renal water excretion and hence to produce hyponatremia and potential water intoxication. This problem may be an untoward complication in patients with chronic congestive heart failure. Instances of spontaneous hypoglycemia induced by glyburide as well as the other agents have been reported. Both second-generation agents—glipizide and glyburide—have the highest poten-

Table 168-4. Characteristics of oral hypoglycemic agents (sulfonylureas)

Generic name	Brand name	Strength (mg)	Onset of action (hr)	Duration of action (hr)	Dosage range (mg)	Major toxicity
Tolbutamide	Orinase	500	0.5	6-12	500-3000	Photosensitivity after alcohol ingestion; occasionally hypoglycemia
Chlorpropamide	Diabinese	100, 250	1	60-90	100-500	Hypersensitivity, jaundice, skin rash, pancytopenia; occasionally edema, hyponatremia
Acetohexamide	Dymelor	250, 500	0.5	12-24	250-1500	Hypoglycemia, gastrointestinal disturbances, headache; occasionally allergic skin manifestations, photosensitivity, jaundice
Tolazamide	Tolinase	100, 250, 500	4-6	10-18	100-1000	Rare gastrointestinal disturbances
Glyburide	Micronase	1.25, 2.5, 5	1	18-24	2.5-20.0	Hypoglycemia
Glipizide	Glucotrol	5, 10	0.5	12-24	5-40	Hypoglycemia

tial and efficacy of all sulfonylureas. Neither agent potentiates antidiuretic hormone action, increases water retention, potentiates congestive heart failure, nor results in hyponatremia as does chlorpropamide. Indeed, both second-generation agents have a mild diuretic property. Glipizide appears primarily to increase the quantity and rapidity of insulin secretion and secondarily to potentiate insulin action. It is therefore most useful in normal weight to moderately obese patients with type II diabetes mellitus, as these patients may be relatively insulopenic. On the other hand, glyburide primarily potentiates insulin action and receptor coupling on target tissues and secondarily increases insulin secretion. Thus glyburide is most efficacious in severely obese patients with diabetes, as they have relative hyperinsulinism and marked insulin resistance.

It seems evident that sulfonylureas are well suited for patients with type II diabetes who have persistent mild to moderate fasting hyperglycemia after an adequate trial of dietary therapy. Ideally, these patients should not have complications of diabetes mellitus that would be more responsive to insulin therapy. When combined with a vigorous dietary regimen, fasting glucose levels of 200 to 300 mg/dl often can be normalized by using one or another of the sulfonylureas. In general, the higher the initial fasting glucose level, the less likely the sulfonylureas are to produce primary control of the patient's hyperglycemia. In all subjects, lowering the fasting plasma or serum glucose concentration to a value below 115 mg/dl and the 2-hour postprandial glucose concentration to a value below 140 mg/dl is essential for good control of diabetes and to avoid the increased risk of vascular complications.

Although the oral sulfonylureas are appropriate therapy for patients with type II diabetes mellitus, they are not appropriate for patients with type I diabetes mellitus, as the latter group has markedly reduced or wholly absent endogenous insulin secretory capabilities. Because type I diabetes is associated with episodic ketosis, any patient in whom significant weight loss or ketosis has occurred is generally not a candidate for oral sulfonylurea therapy. The incidence of secondary failure with oral antidiabetic agents appears to correlate with failure to maintain ideal weight or with prolonged inability to reverse a moderately to morbidly obese state. In instances of secondary failure, alterations of the dose of sulfonylurea administered, emphasis on reevaluation of diet therapy, and institution of higher-potency second-generation sulfonylureas should be tried; however, in no event should the patient be maintained on oral antidiabetic agents in the presence of substantial fasting hyperglycemia with osmotic diuresis or ketosis. In these patients, insulin should be administered. Only in the most extreme cases of patient refractoriness to insulin or of inability to tolerate the concept of insulin therapy should oral antidiabetic agents be continued. In selected cases of secondary failure, combination insulin-sulfonylurea therapy may be of value. The most successful applications rely on bedtime neutral protamine hagedorn (NPH) insulin together with daytime sulfonylureas, generally second-generation agents such as glipizide and occasionally glyburide. In rare instances, rapid-acting insulin may be given before meals in severely insulin-resistant patients already taking glyburide. In that formulation, bedtime NPH insulin is omitted.

Insulin therapy

Insulin preparations have varying quantities of immunoassayable glucagon, pancreatic polypeptide, vasoactive intestinal peptide, somatostatin, and proinsulin. In general, the insulin preparations developed over the past 10 years are relatively pure, containing less than 50 contaminating protein molecules per million (ppm). More highly purified preparations are available for the unusual patient with adverse reactions to the more commonly used preparations. In addition to the ordinary commercial preparations of insulins derived from mixtures of beef and pork insulin, purified monospecies insulins isolated from pork or beef are also available. In addition, two forms of human insulin are commercially available. The first uses standard techniques of genetic engineering to produce authentic, pure human insulin of recombinant DNA origin by way of human proinsulin biosynthesis from transformed *Escherichia coli;* the second generates human insulin directly in genetically engineered yeast cells. In general, the use of purified monospecies human insulin is preferred for new patients and for all patients who have localized or systemic reactions or allergies to subcutaneous insulin of animal origin.

There is a wide variety of pharmacologic insulin preparations including relatively rapid-acting and intermediate-acting insulin; specially marketed mixtures of NPH (isophane insulin USP) and regular insulins; intermediate-acting insulins such as NPH and lente insulin, and prolonged-acting insulins such as ultralente and protamine zinc insulin (Table 168-5). Despite this variety of preparations, their use either alone or in combination, even with multiple daily injections, does not in any way reproduce the exquisite physiologic regulation of the blood glucose level observed in nondiabetic patients. This no doubt reflects the absence of finely regulated endogenous insulin secretion. Greater than normal levels of circulating insulin are required to suppress the gluconeogenic, glycogenolytic, and ketogenic potential of the pathologic hyperglucagonemia in patients with diabetes, perhaps as the result of systemic rather than portal insulin delivery.

Subcutaneous injections of insulin commit the patient to an organized and predictable life-style with respect to both food ingestion and exercise patterns. Continuous subcutaneous insulin infusion by a portable pump has shown promise in selected patients, particularly those who are pregnant. These pumps infuse a relatively small hourly dose of insulin, with much greater increments administered immediately before and during each meal. Although better, near-normal control of blood glucose levels has been demonstrated in these patients, there is some question as to whether this route of insulin delivery is routinely applicable to all patients with insulin-dependent (type I) diabetes mellitus. As an alternative to infusion pump usage, intensive, multidose regular insulin therapies have been proposed. These rely on the use of subcutaneous regular insulin before meals together with one or two small daily doses

Table 168-5. Selected clinical characteristics of insulin preparations

Onset of action	Insulin	Duration of action (h)		Peak effect (h)		Compatible mixed with
		Initial	Chronic use	Initial	Chronic use	
Rapid	Crystalline zinc (CZI, regular crystalline soluble actrapid)	6	16	2-3	5-6	All insulin preparations
	Semilente	12		3-6		Lente preparations
Intermediate	Neutral protamine (Isophane, NPH)	14-24	24	6-12	10-12	Regular insulin
	Globin	18		6-8		
	Lente	18-24	24	8-14	10-12	Regular insulin and semilente preparations
Long	Protamine zinc (PZI)	36		16-24		
	Ultralene	36		20-30		Regular insulin and semilente preparations

of ultralente to suppress ketogenesis. Glycemic control with this paradigm is fundamentally identical to that produced by continuous pump infusion. Either technique allows more variability in meal timing than does the use of one or two doses of intermediate-acting insulin. Intensive research work is also presently ongoing regarding nasal insulin administration, glucose sensors to be used with automated insulin pump systems, as well as islet cell transplantation. Routine clinical application of the latter would appear to be years in the future if ever. Segmental pancreas transplantation, performed simultaneously with transplantation of a kidney in patients with renal failure, offers promise of improved glycemic control and may require little or no exogenous insulin.

Types of insulin therapy. A number of approaches to the use of insulin therapy are presently used. In one, multiple small doses of regular insulin are administered before meals together with a small evening dose of intermediate-acting (NPH or lente) or long-acting (ultralente) insulin to prevent nocturnal glycosuria and early morning hyperglycemia and ketosis. This method of insulin administration tends to produce good to excellent control of the blood glucose concentrations, but it has several major disadvantages. First, patients must be willing to accept three or four injections of insulin per day and must be prepared to give these injections before meals. Second, patient self-reliance in judging meal size and regular insulin requirements is necessary, as type I patients tend to be sensitive to small changes in the dose of regular insulin administered. Further, these dose schedules depend on knowing the premeal glucose level by self-monitoring before each meal. The patient must therefore be willing and able largely to self-regulate therapy. Many physicians believe that this method of insulin administration produces the best control of blood glucose concentrations and the lowest incidence of the development of the chronic complications of diabetes mellitus. However, adequate studies comparing this method of insulin administration to the use of intermediate-acting insulin, alone or in combination with regular insulin, are presently unavailable. A consensus also has developed that the attainment of true euglycemia with insulin administration is a difficult, if not impossible, goal using presently available means of insulin administration. Nevertheless, normalization of the glucose level to the degree possible without inducing multiple episodes of serious hypoglycemia is the most prudent long-term management goal for patients with diabetes mellitus. Combination oral agent insulin therapy may also produce superior glycemic control. One or two doses of intermediate or long-acting insulin coupled with glipizide may produce excellent preprandial and postprandial control in mild to moderately obese type II patients. Rapid-acting insulin before each meal together with one to two doses of glyburide is preferable in morbidly obese patients.

Evaluation of hypoglycemic therapy. Available means of evaluating the extent of diabetic control include multiple fasting and spot serum glucose determinations and hemoglobin A_{1c} determinations.

The development of assays for determining the extent of glycosylation of hemoglobin resulting in the formation of hemoglobin A_{1c} in red blood cells permits a general assessment of the overall extent of hyperglycemia experienced by patients with diabetes mellitus. The nonenzymatic addition of glucose to hemoglobin A appears to occur in approximate proportion to the extent of hyperglycemia. In normal subjects only about 5% of hemoglobin A is glycosylated, whereas in patients with diabetes, it may be as great as 20%. It should be noted, however, that the rate of formation of hemoglobin A_{1c} is considerably faster than its rate of disappearance. Thus hemoglobin A_{1c} may be useful in monitoring diabetic outpatients during periods of stable and rapidly deteriorating control but is not suitable to detect rapid metabolic improvement. Because of the relatively long half-life of hemoglobin in the circulation, glycosylation of other proteins may be more useful for assessments of improving or deteriorating control. One such protein is serum albumin, which is also glycosylated but has a much shorter life span in blood. The fructosamine reaction is a crude assessment of primarily glycosylated albumin levels and therefore reflects diabetes control in the prior 2-week period. Another shortcoming of hemoglobin A_{1c} measurements is the many technical difficulties only recently recognized by the most sophisticated research laboratories.

Home monitoring of blood glucose by using glucose oxidase-based strip technology with or without electronic monitoring devices has virtually revolutionized diabetes management. Aside from the ability to assess blood glucose directly at any time desired, home glucose monitoring has generally produced vastly improved patient compliance. This improvement may be the result of the relative obscurity of urine test results to the average patient who never fully grasped correlations between an abstract number of urine glucose "pulses" or percentage of glucose excretion and the blood glucose level. Home glucose monitoring provides an instantaneous, direct assessment of the blood glucose concentration, which has far greater immediacy and impact on the patient's awareness. Correlation of medication or dietary errors follows as the natural consequence. Home monitoring should be used for all patients on insulin and has even proved quite useful for diet- or diet- and sulfonylurea-controlled patients. In the latter instances, negative feedback of dietary indiscretions tends to reduce or eliminate maladaptive behavior. In patients on weight reduction programs, the early and rapid fall in glucose levels, which is disproportionate to the extent of weight loss, tends to reinforce the beneficial effects of diet and to compensate for the reduced secondary gain to the patient resulting from reduced food intake. In general, capillary glucoses preprandially and postprandially for an entire day provide a pattern of glucose control that otherwise would represent unavailable data for patient and physician alike.

Insulin dosage. Therapy is begun by administering a comparatively small dose of intermediate insulin such as NPH or lente insulin. This dose should be approximately 40% of the estimated daily insulin requirement for the patient. At ideal body weight, most patients require 30 to 50 units per day of exogenously administered highly purified insulin, whether given as a single preparation or in combination with another insulin preparation. With increasing weight, however, higher insulin dosage is required. In general, the greater the body weight of the patient, the greater the insulin requirement. Thus in an average-sized adult, an initial dose of 15 to 20 units of intermediate insulin is usually given; this is raised over the next several days to weeks by 4- to 6-unit increments until a good therapeutic effect is attained. Administered insulin behaves somewhat differently from patient to patient, and the time of occurrence of peak action must be determined for each person. Some patients will experience a relatively rapid onset of peak effects of NPH or lente insulin, occurring 4 to 6 hours after injection, whereas most patients will have peak effects from a morning injection of NPH or lente insulin coincident with, or immediately before, the evening meal. A third group of patients will have peak biologic effects of insulin at considerably later periods, perhaps many hours after the evening meal. If the patient is not easily controlled, the approximate time of the biologic peak should be determined. In subjects having a peak action of NPH or lente insulin occurring at the time of the evening meal, blood glucose concentrations should be reduced to approximately 80 to 100 mg/dl immediately before the meal, so that the resulting caloric surge may be well controlled.

A minority of patients will be well controlled throughout the day and night on one dose of intermediate-acting insulin. Even though excellent control can be obtained before the evening meal, noticeable hyperglycemia may persist before breakfast or in the late morning hours after breakfast. In most instances, a second dose of NPH insulin may be necessary to normalize fasting glucose levels in these subjects. This second dose of insulin should be considerably less than the morning dose and should be administered immediately before the evening meal or occasionally at bedtime. When the second dose of insulin is begun, it is usually necessary to continue the same total insulin dosage to prevent hypoglycemia before the evening meal.

Changes in the amounts of insulin administered should be made no more frequently than every other day in outpatients and should usually not be more than 10% to 20% of the total insulin dose. If marked hyperglycemia is observed after breakfast and before lunch, a mixture of regular together with NPH (or lente) insulin may be necessary, instead of solely NPH insulin in the morning. The addition of regular insulin in the morning usually requires a proportional reduction of the intermediate-acting insulin dosage. Mixtures of rapid- and intermediate-acting insulins will broaden the duration of peak actions of NPH and lente insulins and will tend to make peak biologic effects of insulin injections coincident with postprandial hyperglycemia after the evening meal. This approach is recommended for patients with an idiosyncratic late peak action of NPH or lente insulin. The mixed-insulin morning dose plus a second evening dose produces improved control of difficult to manage diabetic hyperglycemia. Aside from idiosyncratic biologic responses to insulin, most patients tend to show progressive lengthening of the interval between the time of insulin injection and the appearance of peak hyperglycemic action as the dosage of intermediate-acting insulin is increased, particularly for doses of NPH or lente insulin greater than 40 units per day. Thus in patients with obesity or other reasons for insensitivity to pharmacologic preparations of insulin, dosages in excess of 40 to 60 units per day may show peak biologic activity occurring considerably later than the evening meal, and, in many circumstances, in the early morning hours. Such patients must either be treated with mixtures of rapid- and intermediate-acting insulin or, alternatively, switched to human insulin of recombinant DNA origin. The latter tends to produce more rapidly appearing and more pronounced peak biologic effects regardless of the pharmacologic nature of the preparations. This effect may result from the lower antigenicity of human insulin and its reduced antibody binding. As a consequence, human insulin is preferred in most clinical settings in which large insulin doses are used and in which delayed insulin responsiveness is noted.

The pattern of delayed responsiveness toward large dosages ($>$ 40 U/day) is a consequence of the depot nature of subcutaneous insulin injection. Diminishing the morning dose of NPH or lente insulin by approximately 10 units and adding equal amounts of regular or semilente insulin produces a faster onset of activity, assuming that human insulin is already being used. It may also be necessary to split the total dose of insulin into a morning dose containing two thirds to three fourths of the total and a smaller evening dose containing one fourth to one third of the total when the single morning dose is in excess of 40 to 60 units per day. Splitting the total dose of intermediate-acting insulin results in significantly greater overall hypoglycemic action for the total dose of insulin administered, and therefore it should not be accompanied by a large increase in the total dose prescribed. Indeed, a small reduction in total insulin administered per day may be wise if dose splitting is considered on an outpatient basis. Evening doses of insulin of between 8 and 20 units of NPH or lente given with the evening meal or at bedtime are usually adequate to produce fasting euglycemia in these subjects. Rarely, a "dawn phenomenon," characterized by insulin hypersensitivity from midnight through 4 AM followed by rising insulin resistance from 4 AM onward, may complicate insulin therapy in adolescents and young adults. Administration of the evening insulin dosage at bedtime is usually effective treatment, as the peak insulin action is then shifted to the point of rising relative insulin resistance, without producing antecedent hypoglycemia during the phase of insulin hypersensitivity. If residual hyperglycemia remains at the time of the noon meal, larger morning doses of regular or semilente insulin should be used. These approaches may be summarized into the following sequential guidelines:

1. Control blood glucose before the evening meal (single dose of intermediate-acting insulin or a mixed dose of rapid plus intermediate insulin for late peak action).
2. Control residual fasting hyperglycemia (split dose of intermediate-acting insulin).
3. Control late-morning hyperglycemia (mix rapid-acting with morning intermediate-acting insulin).
4. Control bedtime hyperglycemia (mix rapid-acting with evening intermediate-acting insulin).
5. Use enough insulin in appropriate mixtures to maintain near normal fasting venous glucose concentrations (< 115 mg/dl) and postprandial venous blood glucose concentrations below values that appear to be associated with microangiopathies (< 140 to 200 mg/dl).

Insulin allergy and the so-called honeymoon effect are two relatively common complications noted soon after starting insulin therapy. In type I subjects having severe hyperglycemia or ketoacidosis, insulin requirements may decrease dramatically, and the patient may no longer appear to require insulin, as hyperglycemia is no longer present. This honeymoon period may last from days to months and is invariably accompanied by a subsequent deterioration in metabolic control, after which the patient is usually left insulin dependent. Despite this seeming lack of need for insulin, these injections should never be totally discontinued, but the dose should be reduced to the smallest amount not producing hypoglycemia. Even if one unit per day is given, this dose should be sufficient to prevent an anamnestic response in which increased doses are required later.

Approximately 5% to 20% of patients begun on insulin will show some manifestation of local or systemic insulin allergy. Most commonly, local reactions include erythema and dysesthesias at the injection site. Continued insulin together with antihistamine therapy should be efficacious, and most cases clear spontaneously within 6 to 12 months. More serious, but less common, generalized and systemic reactions to insulin may also occur, including local and generalized urticaria, angioneurotic edema, and anaphylaxis. Changing insulin preparations to highly purified monocomponent, monospecies insulin, particularly human insulin, is generally helpful. Desensitization may be necessary, but it is not always permanent and may therefore need to be repeated if symptoms recur. Angioneurotic edema and anaphylaxis must be treated immediately with glucocorticoids, antihistamines, and epinephrine if necessary.

Somogyi and dawn phenomena. Episodic hypoglycemia, usually nocturnal, followed by rebound hyperglycemia, with or without mild ketosis, may occur in patients receiving excessive quantities of insulin. In most instances, this Somogyi phenomenon develops in response to excess insulin administration. The pathogenesis of this effect has been attributed to the adrenergic and glucagon response and, to a lesser extent, cortisol and growth hormone hypersecretion caused by hypoglycemia. These hormones increase glycogenolysis and gluconeogenesis, and epinephrine diminishes glucose uptake by peripheral tissues. Collectively, these events cause hyperglycemia. These hormones also increase free fatty acid mobilization from adipose tissue and favor hepatic ketogenesis, thereby causing ketosis.

Most commonly, the hypoglycemic episode occurs in the early morning hours and may be attributed to an evening dose of insulin that is in excess of the patient's needs or to a late peak hypoglycemic action of the morning dose of insulin. As a consequence, such patients have bedtime urinary glucose and ketone body spillages that are usually absent, yet awaken the next morning with substantial glycosuria, and perhaps ketonuria, before breakfast. The presence of ketonuria is a helpful point for the differential diagnosis in this setting, as the patient must be clearly and substantially underinsulinized or substantially overinsulinized for ketosis to develop in the morning. If the total dose of insulin administered to the patient is in excess of what might be expected, then the Somogyi effect should be suspected. Confirmation of these suspicions can be obtained by hospitalizing the patient and sampling blood for glucose concentrations at frequent (1- to 4-hour) intervals during a 24-hour period. The Somogyi phenomenon is documented by wide fluctuations in blood glucose concentrations (40 to 400 mg/dl) despite a lack of food intake. Alternative evidence for this effect can be obtained by determinations of blood glucose at 3 AM and 5 AM; however, this requires accurate home glucose monitoring technique for the outpatient management of diabetes. Treatment of the Somogyi effect is straightforward once the diagnosis is made. The offending insulin injection should be reduced until the rebound hyperglycemia clears. Modification of a morning intermediate-acting insulin dose with rapid-acting insulin or a complete change to a shorter-acting insulin such as semilente may be necessary. The dawn phenomenon is morning hyperglycemia and insulin resistance, not as the result of antecedent hypoglycemia, but instead owing to predawn surges in growth hormone and, to a lesser extent, other counterregulatory hormones. This phenomenon occurs primarily in younger, generally type I patients and requires 3 AM glucose monitoring for verification. Treatment consists of moving evening intermediate insulin shots to bedtime (10 PM), thereby producing peak morning hyperinsulinism at 6 AM, the peak time of insulin resistance.

Insulin resistance. Insulin resistance was traditionally defined as the requirement for more than 200 units of insulin per day to control hyperglycemia. By definition, this requirement must be exceeded in the absence of diabetic ketoacidosis, sepsis, and other causes of acute and transient insensitivity to the metabolic actions of insulin. In view of the more recently noted lower need for exogenous insulin in completely depancreatized patients, however, definitions of insulin resistance have been reconsidered, and it is now thought to be present when the exogenous insulin requirement exceeds 100 units per day. Clinically, insulin resistance was recognized in patients with overt hyperglycemia who responded inappropriately to conventional insulin doses and were found to have neutralizing antibodies to circulating insulin, but both the spectrum and subsequent recognition of insulin-resistant states have undergone a major expansion in recent years. It is now known that insulin resistance may occur independently of overt glucose intolerance with hyperglycemia. Thus insulin resistance may be present despite a euglycemic status, provided that supranormal concentrations of insulin are present. On the other hand, persistent hyperglycemia may be present even though pharmacologic quantities of exogenous insulin are administered.

In the majority of patients with true insulin resistance, resistance is the result of obesity, anti-insulin antibodies, malignancies, associated endocrinopathies, lipodystrophy, an immune dysfunction characterized by antireceptor antibodies (type B) or a reduction in receptor concentration (type A), acanthosis nigricans, a variety of autoimmune disorders, primary ovarian abnormalities with and without features of lipodystrophy, pregnancy, or the secretion of endogenous abnormal insulins. To discern the cause of insulin resistance, it is important to recognize that the first step in the action of insulin is its binding to insulin-receptor molecules on the external surface of the target cell plasma membrane. Therefore for simple convenience, it is easy to categorize insulin resistance as resulting from events occurring before, at, or after the point of hormone-receptor interaction.

The presence of substantial quantities of anti-insulin antibodies to animal (or human) insulin preparations can produce considerable wastage of insulin and also successfully compete with the insulin receptor for available circulating insulin. Practically all insulin-treated patients develop low concentrations of IgG anti-insulin antibodies, but in less than one patient per thousand do the anti-insulin antibody titer and affinity become sufficient to cause clinically apparent insulin resistance. Most commonly, antibody-mediated insulin resistance develops in a patient previously exposed for a period of time to exogenous insulin that is then discontinued and subsequently readministered. The repeated challenge with insulin induces an immunologic reaction similar to the anamnestic responses observed to other antigens.

Substantial antibody titers to insulin can be detected by modifications of the radioimmunoassay techniques for measuring insulin in serum or plasma. The titer of anti-insulin antibody present and the degree of clinical insulin resistance, however, are not closely correlated. Beef insulin has three amino acid residues that differ from those of human insulin; pork insulin has only one such differing amino acid residue. Thus most antibodies to pharmacologic preparations of insulin have higher affinities for beef than for pork or human insulin. As a consequence, switching the patient to a purified pork or human regular insulin generally proves effective in reducing the quantities of insulin required for controlling acute hyperglycemia. As much as 100,000 units of regular insulin have been administered to overcome the insulin-antagonistic action of antibodies in patients having diabetic ketoacidosis. If purified human regular or lente insulin does not reduce the high insulin requirements of patients with antibody-mediated insulin resistance, prednisone therapy as an immunosuppressive measure often will be efficacious, despite its relative antagonism to insulin action.

The lowest possible steroid dose producing acceptable and predictable insulin requirements should be given. Prednisone should be started at doses of 60 to 100 mg/day and continued until the insulin dosage decreases, usually within several days. A daily tapering of the prednisone should then be initiated. Maintenance prednisone dosage is generally 10 to 30 mg/day. The natural history of antibody-mediated insulin resistance is characterized by a spontaneous remission of this phenomenon 6 to 18 months after its presentation. As a consequence, marked hypoglycemia can result at the time of remission if the patient is maintained on large quantities of subcutaneous insulin.

A relatively rare cause for prereceptor insulin resistance results from the secretion of an abnormal insulin molecule that binds with less affinity to insulin receptors and has a diminished biologic activity. Another nonimmune form of insulin resistance noted very rarely in insulin-dependent diabetic patients (type I) derives from a reduced bioavailability of insulin after subcutaneous, but not intravenous, injections. This phenomenon is thought to be the result of local destruction or sequestration of insulin in its subcutaneous depot. Some investigators believe that this syndrome results from compliance failures or from occult infection and is not a unique pathologic entity.

Obesity is associated with the most common and best studied form of insulin resistance. This resistance is a heterogeneous disorder that is not directly proportional to the degree of obesity. In mildly hyperinsulinemic but resistant obese patients, the density of insulin receptors is reduced, and the resistance is primarily the result of the decreased receptor density. A postreceptor defect in coupling to metabolic processes may also be present. Weight reduction is the only effective therapy for the insulin resistance of obesity because the loss of receptors is reversible with weight reduction, and insulin responsiveness usually reverts toward normal.

Insulin resistance syndromes. Other forms of insulin resistance occur in three recently recognized syndromes. One syndrome, *type A,* occurs in females and is usually characterized by hyperglycemia, acanthosis nigricans, and polycystic ovaries. Various degrees of virilization have been observed, and serum testosterone concentrations may be increased slightly. The concentration of insulin receptors on circulating monocytes is reduced, and the receptor defect is not improved by dietary restriction as it is in obesity. In addition, some of these patients seem to have a postreceptor defect in coupling to insulin-responsive metabolic pathways.

Another of these syndromes, *type B,* is an autoimmune disease characterized by hyperglycemia, acanthosis nigricans, and diminished binding of insulin to its cellular receptor owing to the presence of circulating antireceptor antibodies. This syndrome may be associated with several accompanying disorders such as lupus erythematosus, Sjögren's syndrome, and ataxia telangiectasia. Anti-insulin-receptor antibody titers may fall after immunosuppressive therapy.

The *type C* syndrome of insulin resistance is characterized by the familial occurrence of insulin resistance coupled with acanthosis nigricans, acral hypertrophy, and muscle cramps. Ovarian dysfunction may occur in females, although testicular function may be normal in males. Fasting euglycemia or hyperglycemia may be present, but patients are resistant to the hypoglycemic effects of intravenous insulin injection at customary doses. Endogenous hyperinsulinemia is present, and insulin-receptor density on circulating monocytes is reduced.

Endocrinopathies such as Cushing's syndrome, pheochromocytoma, acromegaly, thyrotoxicosis, and profound hyperlipidemias are all associated with increased insulin requirements for diabetic control. Glucocorticoid excess is associated with reduced affinity of insulin receptors, but insulin requirements are usually not increased in patients taking less than the equivalent of 20 mg of prednisone daily. Epinephrine induces peripheral and hepatic insulin insensitivity through beta-adrenergic receptor mediation. As a result, peripheral tissues are insensitive to incremental changes in plasma insulin concentrations. The mechanism of this catecholamine effect is unclear. Medical or surgical management for hyperthyroidism, Cushing's disease, and acromegaly is indicated before good control of carbohydrate disturbances can be obtained.

The *syndrome of insulin resistance* or *syndrome X,* as it is also termed, describes the frequent association as comorbid illnesses of carbohydrate intolerance, essential hypertension, dyslipidemia, abdominal obesity, and accelerated atherosclerosis. Hyperuricemia may also occur. The hyperinsulinemia and dyslipidemia may account, at least in part, for the accelerated atherosclerosis of these disease entities. Both insulin resistance and dyslipidemia tend to antedate the subsequent appearance of diabetes or hypertension by years or decades. The precise etiologic significance of these associations is unclear at present and may not occur in all racial and ethnic groups equally. Nevertheless, the postulation of insulin resistance as a unifying mechanism linking many associated atherogenic illnesses has proved extremely attractive to many investigators concerned with macrovascular disease in patients with diabetes.

Lipoatrophic diabetes mellitus is an insulin-resistant state characterized by the lack of subcutaneous fat and by hyperlipidemia and an elevated metabolic rate. In some patients, lipoatrophy is associated with acanthosis nigricans and a variety of autoimmune disorders. This rare and complex disease appears to consist of a spectrum of disorders that at one extreme is associated with circulating anti-insulin-receptor antibodies or with altered insulin binding to receptors and at the other extreme with reversible hyperlipidemia with normal insulin-receptor number. There may be a primary disturbance of receptor coupling that produces rapid insulin desensitization. Therapy is limited primarily to dietary manipulations, including a low-carbohydrate diet and exogenous insulin administration.

ACUTE METABOLIC COMPLICATIONS OF DIABETES MELLITUS

Among the acute metabolic consequences of diabetes mellitus or its treatment are four distinctly different forms of coma. These are (1) diabetic ketoacidosis, (2) hyperosmolar nonketotic coma, (3) lactic acidosis, and (4) hypoglycemia. Diabetic patients are also subject to the other causes of coma found in the nondiabetic patient population including alcohol-induced ketosis. Certain features of the history and physical examination, as well as selected laboratory determinations, are extremely useful for the rapid differentiation of the forms of diabetic coma. For example, insulin hypoglycemia is a fulminant disorder generally precipitated by vigorous exercise, omission of food intake, or overdosage with either insulin or sulfonylureas. In addition, the patient is usually profusely diaphoretic, tachycardic, tremulous, and hypothermic. The specific clinical presentations and the diagnostic and therapeutic maneuvers pertaining to each of these comas are discussed in the following pages.

Diabetic ketoacidosis

Diabetic ketoacidosis is a life-threatening metabolic disorder characterized by accelerated rates of hepatic glycogenolysis, gluconeogenesis, ketogenesis, and impaired glucose and ketoacid utilization, all of which result in elevated concentrations of glucose and keto acids in blood. These disturbances, coupled with increased fatty acid mobilization from adipose tissue and increased muscle proteolysis, flood the bloodstream with an overabundance of fuels for hepatic glucose and ketone overproduction (Fig. 168-6).

The major hormonal abnormalities are an insufficient

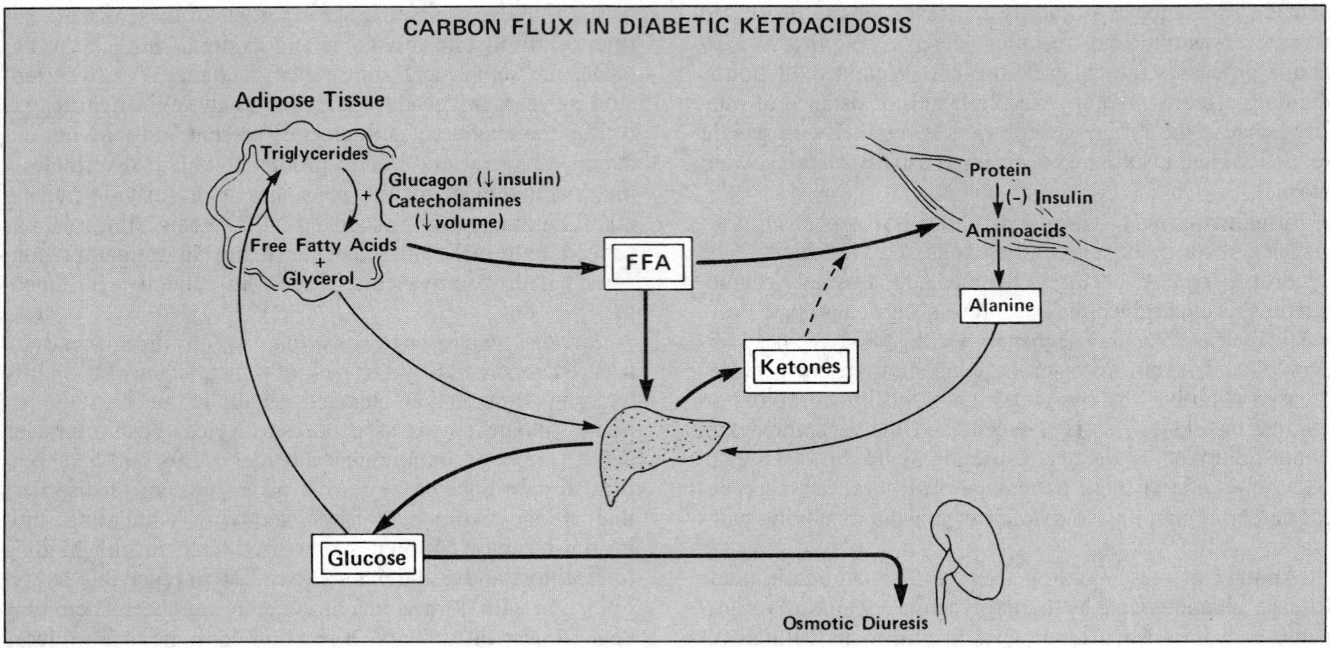

Fig. 168-6. Metabolic alterations in diabetic ketoacidosis.

quantity of circulating insulin to restrain catabolism and profound hyperglucagonemia. Hyperglycemia produces an osmotic diuresis and thereby causes intravascular volume depletion, which in turn stimulates sympathetic outflow and catecholamine release. The increased catecholamines dramatically increase free fatty acid mobilization from adipose tissue. Increased levels of epinephrine and glucagon in the blood augment hepatic gluconeogenesis, glycogenolysis, and ketogenesis. In addition, epinephrine diminishes any residual endogenous insulin secretion. The hypoinsulinemia and hyperglucagonemia decrease hepatic malonyl CoA concentrations and may increase hepatic carnitine concentrations. Both effects facilitate fatty acylcarnitine translocation across the liver inner mitochondrial membrane so that increased free fatty acid oxidation results in accelerated hepatic ketogenesis. The markedly increased free fatty acid levels also diminish ketone-body oxidation in peripheral tissues, thereby producing a marked hyperketonemia and massive ketonuria. The release of other stress hormones such as cortisol and growth hormone reinforces these pathogenic developments in diabetic ketoacidosis, as these hormones generally exhibit anti-insulin activity. Even though glucose and ketone bodies have no maximal renal tubular reabsorption rates, glycosuria and ketonuria during diabetic ketoacidosis occur because less than 100% of these filtered compounds are reabsorbed by the renal tubules. Massive renal glucose and keto acid excretion with the resultant osmotic diuresis produces large losses of sodium, potassium, calcium, phosphate, ammonium, and other ions in the urine. These severe losses of water and electrolytes, combined with the marked acidemia, may ultimately produce cardiovascular failure and death.

Diabetic ketoacidosis is usually accompanied by a history of several days of polyuria and polydipsia, but can appear as a fulminant disorder within a few hours, especially in cases of insulin pump failure. It occurs in lean or obese patients and may be found in younger, as well as older, patients. Contrary to popular opinion, there are more new cases of diabetes presenting with ketoacidosis in adults than in children. Morbid cardiovascular events, infections, trauma, pregnancy, emotional stress, excessive alcohol ingestion, and omission of prescribed insulin are frequent precipitating causes of diabetic ketoacidosis. On occasion, there may be no obvious precipitating cause. The physical findings of tachypnea, dehydration, and some degree of acetone halitosis (a fruity odor to the breath) are usually present. Abdominal pain with or without findings consistent with pancreatitis also may occur. Kussmaul respirations are usually present when the arterial pH is less than 7.3, but these finally may disappear owing to patient exhaustion. The central nervous system may no longer respond to severe acidosis when the arterial pH values are less than 6.9. These patients may have marked hyperlipidemia in serum or blood since type IV and type V hyperlipidemias are common in ketoacidosis. Lipemia retinalis is present when the plasma triglyceride concentration is greater than 2000 to 5000 mg/dl.

Laboratory confirmation of diabetic ketoacidosis should be made rapidly. Criteria for the diagnosis—hyperglycemia, hyperketonemia, and metabolic acidosis—may be present to varying degrees. For example, in a young, pregnant, insulin-dependent diabetic patient with a propensity for excreting urinary glucose, severe hyperketonemia and metabolic acidosis may be present despite a plasma glucose concentration of 200 mg/dl or less. On the other hand, in an insulin-dependent diabetic patient with prerenal azotemia, plasma glucose concentrations can be greater than 1000 mg/dl, and arterial pH less than 7.2, with only modest hyperketonemia; however, patients with advanced renal failure are generally resistant to the development of ketoacidosis. The finding of metabolic acidosis in these patients may be the result, instead, of lactic acidosis. Rarely, an insulin-dependent diabetic patient with protracted vomiting may manifest severe hyperglycemia, hyperketonemia and yet have a paradoxical metabolic alkalosis, owing to the marked gastric loss of hydrochloric acid in vomitus.

Patients with diabetic ketoacidosis usually urinate profusely, and thus urine demonstrating 4+ glycosuria and intense ketonuria can be obtained readily. In patients with neurogenic bladder atony, catheterization may be necessary. An adequate intravenous route for administering saline should be established; simultaneously, blood should be drawn for determinations of glucose, urea, creatinine, and electrolytes (Na^+, K^+, Cl^-, and HCO_3^-). If available, Dextrostix or Chemstrips can be used to determine rapidly the presence of hyperglycemia while awaiting the more accurate plasma glucose concentration from the clinical laboratory. Arterial blood gases should be obtained if possible. Additional plasma or serum should be obtained for semiquantitative determinations of circulating ketone bodies. The routinely used reagent for ketoacid detection in blood and urine is nitroprusside (Ketostix, Acetest).

Nitroprusside reacts with acetoacetate, the ketone body with the lowest concentration in blood, and with acetone only to a slight extent. Nitroprusside does not react with beta-hydroxybutyrate, the ketone body in greatest concentration in blood and urine. In general, beta-hydroxybutyrate concentrations are threefold to tenfold greater than acetoacetate concentrations in uncomplicated ketoacidosis. Because nitroprusside reacts only with acetoacetate, diagnostic difficulties may rarely be encountered. Changes in total keto acid load may not be reflected by changes in acetoacetate concentrations. For example, concomitant lactic acidosis, alcoholic ketoacidosis, or hypoxia may depress acetoacetate concentrations and increase beta-hydroxybutyrate concentrations. On the other hand, insulin therapy for ketoacidosis may decrease beta-hydroxybutyrate concentrations rapidly but also may cause transient increases in acetoacetate concentrations, tending to produce the false impression of a worsening state. Therefore severe diabetic ketoacidosis may be present irrespective of the results of nitroprusside testing of ketone reactivity in serum or plasma. Nonetheless, patients in severe diabetic ketoacidosis usually have great reactivity of serum or plasma to nitroprusside test reagents. Since ketones are unmeasured anions, a positive nitroprusside test together with an increased anion gap ($Na^+ - [Cl^- + HCO_3^-]$ in excess of 15) confirms hyperketonemia. Lactic acidosis also may be present.

Treatment. After the presence of hyperglycemia, hyperketonemia, and metabolic acidemia has been rapidly established, therapy should be initiated immediately. The treatment of diabetic ketoacidosis must be tailored to the individual patient. Five general areas of treatment can be broadly differentiated: (1) constant patient monitoring and re-evaluation, (2) fluid and electrolyte replacement, (3) rapid-acting insulin administration, (4) glucose supplementation as necessary, and (5) therapy for the precipitating cause. The patient should be weighed and the degree of dehydration assessed. The patient's state of consciousness, respiratory and heart rates, blood pressure, and temperature should be recorded at frequent intervals on a clinical flow sheet. This record also should contain notations of all fluid, electrolytes, and insulin administered as well as the laboratory data (including serial glucose, electrolytes, urea, creatinine, arterial or venous gases and pH, and urinary glucose and acetoacetate reactivities). Because hypothermia is an occasional finding, the presence of even a mild temperature elevation suggests an underlying infection. Parenteral and oral intake and urinary output should be recorded hourly on the flow sheet. In the unconscious patient with a history of vomiting or apparent gastric dilatation, nasogastric aspiration should be performed.

Having established the diagnosis, one should begin fluid and electrolyte replacement immediately. Intravascular volume depletion and a diminished glomerular filtration rate usually will be present. To expand the contracted intravascular volume rapidly and thereby improve tissue perfusion, normal saline should be first administered. Such expansion will also reduce adrenergic outflow and thereby diminish free fatty acid mobilization. Rates of saline administration should approximate 1 L/hr, and at least 1 to 2 liters of normal saline should be administered, except to patients with marked cardiovascular disease in whom slower rates of fluid administration may be necessary.

For patients with arterial pH levels less than 6.9 or in whom Kussmaul's respiration has ceased because of physical exhaustion, bicarbonate administration is advisable. Otherwise, for pH values greater than 7.0, sodium bicarbonate in itself is usually not necessary or even desirable. Diabetic ketoacidosis tends to be a self-correcting acidosis because complete oxidation of the accumulated strong organic acids (acetoacetate and beta-hydroxybutyrate) will restore arterial pH to normal. If excess quantities of bicarbonate are administered, rebound peripheral alkalosis with paradoxical central nervous system acidosis may occur because of differential transport of carbon dioxide, but not bicarbonate, across the blood-brain barrier. These changes can then produce obtundation and the appearance of secondary relapse or coma in patients seemingly cured of diabetic ketoacidosis. Lastly, excessive sodium bicarbonate administration to patients increases the sodium load dramatically and therefore may lead to hypernatremia and the subsequent development of a hyperchloremic metabolic acidosis (normal anion gap). This development is of particular consequence in patients with known cardiovascular disease, a major complication of long-standing diabetes mellitus.

An estimate of the total quantities of fluid and electrolytes to be replaced for patients with diabetic ketoacidosis is best made at the initiation of therapy so that clear treatment goals can be defined in advance and progress during treatment can be assessed periodically. As shown in Table 168-6, one should calculate the total fluid requirement for the patient on the basis of body weight and the extent of

Table 168-6. Fluid and electrolyte replacement per kilogram in diabetic ketoacidosis and hyperosmolar nonketotic diabetic coma

Replacement substances	Diabetic ketoacidosis (per kg)	Hyperosmolar nonketotic diabetic coma (per kg)
Water	100-150 ml	150-200 ml
Sodium	7 mEq	7mEq
Potassium	5 mEq	2-4mEq
Phosphate	1 mmol	1 mmol

dehydration and administer this over an approximate 8- to 12-hour interval in otherwise healthy subjects with no known cardiovascular disease. In patients with cardiovascular or renal complications of diabetes mellitus, in whom fluid loading at a rapid rate would be inadvisable, a more prolonged period of fluid replacement, averaging 16- to 24-hour may be preferred. During fluid replacement therapy, insulin administration will reduce the hyperglycemia, but not to levels sufficient to prevent the continuation of some degree of osmotic diuresis. Thus during the initial period of fluid replacement, one fourth to one half of fluids administered are usually excreted in the urine. Replacement of urinary losses by 0.5 N saline should be performed for a second 8- to 12-hour period after the initial 1 to 2 liters of saline are administered for rapid expansion of intravascular volume, fluid and sodium replacement should consist exclusively of 0.5 N saline until the blood sugar falls to 250 to 300 mg/dl.

Patients having ketoacidosis are frequently oliguric as a result of the markedly diminished glomerular filtration rate caused by hypovolemia. Despite the marked potassium losses observed in these patients, they are usually normokalemic or hyperkalemic at the time of presentation. For this reason, an admitting electrocardiogram is frequently useful. In patients without signs of hyperkalemia and in whom reasonable urine output can be observed, potassium administration should be initiated early in the course of fluid therapy for diabetic ketoacidosis. Otherwise, profound hypokalemia will be observed 4 to 8 hours after initiation of therapy for ketoacidosis. This development is a result of H^+-K^+ shifts that occur with rising blood pH and with transport of potassium intracellularly during glucose uptake by cells. After the development of a satisfactory urinary output, approximately 20 to 40 mEq/L of potassium should be added to replacement solutions of half normal saline as they are administered to patients, generally at a rate of 0.50 to 1.0 L/hr. Potassium administration in patients with diabetic ketoacidosis should be continued as long as fluid replacement is ongoing.

Hypophosphatemia often develops in patients with severe diabetic ketoacidosis and marked dehydration. This hypophosphatemia initially may not be apparent because of phosphate shifts from intracellular to extracellular compartments. Phosphate is primarily an intracellular anion, and levels of phosphate in blood may not provide an adequate assessment of the extent of intracellular phosphate depletion. In general, phosphate must be given judiciously to patients with renal failure because of the potential for intravenous phosphate to produce marked hypocalcemia and hypomagnesemia. Although phosphate losses may be as high as potassium losses in patients with diabetic ketoacidosis, phosphate replacement by continuous intravenous infusion should deliver approximately 20 mmol of phosphate per liter of 0.5 N saline. Intravenous phosphate should be given to markedly dehydrated, severely hyperglycemic patients or to those with serum phosphate levels less than 1.5 mmol/L. Serious hypophosphatemia ($<$ 1 mmol/L) may produce late-developing complications of diabetic ketoacidosis, most notably rhabdomyolysis. As a secondary result of the destruction of skeletal muscle, oliguric renal failure may be produced. Other complications of hypophosphatemia include hemolysis and cardiac conduction abnormalities. Mild hypophosphatemia may be repleted by oral ingestion of foodstuffs after reversal of ketosis.

Insulin administration must be initiated early in the management of diabetic ketoacidosis. It may be given by four major therapeutic modes, including intermittent intravenous boluses, intermittent split-dose subcutaneous and intravenous injection, intermittent intramuscular injection, and continued intravenous infusion. Each method of administration possesses its own unique advantages and disadvantages, and no single method is appropriate for all patients with diabetic ketoacidosis.

The route of administration should be chosen with a prior knowledge of insulin pharmacokinetics. Several major guiding principles for insulin therapy can be outlined. First, intravenous administration alone should be considered for all patients in whom marked hypotension or hypovolemia is observed. Absorption of subcutaneous insulin may be impaired as a result of poor tissue perfusion in these patients. Second, if intermittent bolus intravenous administration is chosen, the frequency of boluses should be sufficient to maintain adequate serum insulin levels of at least 200 to 400 μU/ml throughout the course of treatment of diabetic ketoacidosis. Because the half-life of intravenous insulin is approximately 4 minutes, boluses of insulin should be administered at 30- to 60-minute intervals to maintain adequate peripheral levels of insulin. Intermittent intravenous boluses of insulin in usual dosages of 0.5 to 2.0 units/kg produce hypoglycemia more frequently than any other method of insulin administration. Continuous intravenous insulin administration has the advantage of producing a predictable rate of decline in blood glucose levels and a satisfactory response in most patients with diabetic ketoacidosis. The recognition and management of insulin-antibody-mediated diabetic ketoacidosis, however, is considerably more complicated in patients receiving continuous intravenous insulin infusions. In general, infusion rates that would be sufficient to saturate the insulin-antibody-binding capacities are far greater than the customary rates of infusion used to treat uncomplicated ketoacidosis.

For continuous intravenous administration, a priming dose of approximately 0.1 unit/kg should be administered, followed by a continuous infusion of 0.1 unit/kg/hr. This dose may be given by infusion pump or by an independent intravenous drip system. Higher rates of infusion may be necessary for markedly obese patients or for patients in whom extraordinarily high levels of anti-insulin hormones might be encountered, such as patients with sepsis. Doses for bolus intravenous insulin administration should approximate 0.5 unit per kilogram administered at half-hour intervals.

At any time that urine glucose spillage becomes less than 4+ and blood glucose levels fall below 250 mg/dl, a change in fluid administration to include 5% dextrose will be necessary. This dose will prevent symptomatic hypoglycemia and facilitate the reversal of ketosis, because glucose is essential for free fatty acid re-esterification in adipose tissue. Doses of 25 to 100 units of regular insulin administered both subcutaneously and intravenously at 2-hour intervals are also appropriate therapy for most patients with diabetic ketoacidosis. Higher doses may be necessary in patients with insensitivity to insulin action, as might be expected in obese or septic subjects. Regardless of the route of insulin administration, only regular insulin should be administered to patients in diabetic ketoacidosis.

Each patient must be re-evaluated at 1- to 2-hour intervals to ensure improved metabolic status. A failure of improvement can be inferred from a lack of arterial or venous pH changes or from the lack of reduction of glucose levels. Initially, hemodilution produced by administration of normal saline will result in a falling blood glucose level because of renal glucose excretion. Increases in arterial pH, however, generally are not produced by rehydration to any significant extent; and pH thus may be the best guide to treatment in patients with diabetic ketoacidosis. This guideline is particularly important as it is the acidosis itself that is generally the most life-threatening component of the syndrome of diabetic ketoacidosis.

In general, patients presenting with diabetic acidosis in the late afternoon or early evening may be started on intermediate insulin the next morning because this interval should be sufficient to change arterial pH to values greater than 7.35 and to improve bicarbonate levels to normal. If the patient is capable of maintaining adequate food intake, the usual and customary dose of intermediate-acting insulin should be given. For patients in whom severe metabolic stress secondary to infection has precipitated the episode of diabetic ketoacidosis, additional insulin, in the form of small doses of regular insulin, may be necessary to prevent recurrent ketosis. This dose may be administered on the basis of a supplementary sliding scale based on double voided urines at 4- to 6-hour intervals or by the judicious use of regular insulin using serum glucose determinations before meals and bedtime. Although sliding scales that give 10 to 25 units for 4+ glucosuria are in common use, routine coverage for acetonuria should be avoided. The latter requires physician re-evaluation. In patients never previously managed on insulin, a starting dose of 20 to 25 units of intermediate-acting insulin may be given and supplemented with small quantities of regular insulin, as indicated earlier. These doses should be adjusted on a daily basis so that the patient is ultimately discharged on one or two doses of intermediate insulin, alone or in combination with short-acting insulin.

During the initial phase of management for patients with diabetic ketoacidosis, the precipitating cause of the ketoacidosis must be identified. Thus urinary tract infections or other (occult as well as more obvious) bacterial or viral illnesses must be identified and treated appropriately to successfully manage the ketoacidosis. Lumbar puncture should be considered in all patients with evidence of serious, unexplained infection or with disturbances in their level of consciousness, particularly if there are other neurologic findings. Antecedent or intercurrent myocardial infarction and cerebrovascular accident also must be considered in the evaluation of potential precipitating causes of diabetic ketoacidosis. Because diabetic subjects tend to evolve asymptomatic or atypical angina and myocardial infarction, electrocardiographic evaluation at the time of admission and after reversal of diabetic ketoacidosis seems essential. One must deal with such antecedent or intercurrent conditions appropriately in addition to giving treatments designed to reverse ketoacidosis.

Alcoholic ketosis

Ketoacidosis may be noted in clinical circumstances other than diabetes mellitus, (e.g., acute ethanol intoxication in a fasted patient). These patients are generally suffering from chronic hypocaloric malnutrition and chronic ethanol abuse. Pertinent clinical features of alcoholic ketoacidosis include dehydration, vomiting, and the presence of associated manifestations of alcoholism, particularly pancreatitis, gastrointestinal bleeding, hepatitis, cirrhosis, and delirium tremens. At the time of presentation, serum glucose concentrations may vary greatly but are usually less than 200 mg/dl. Nitroprusside reactivity in serum varies from "trace" to "strong," but there is usually a moderate reactivity even though a fulminant hyperketonemia and a large anion gap are present. This discordance occurs because of the high beta-hydroxybutyrate/acetoacetate ratio produced by high rates of ethanol oxidation to acetate in the liver. The arterial pH may reveal either an acidemia or alkalemia, the latter occurring because these patients tend to lose hydrogen ions during vomiting. Concentrations of lactate, uric acid, bilirubin, urea, triglycerides, transaminases, alkaline phosphatase, and amylase are generally elevated. In most instances, rehydration with normal saline and parenteral nutrition with glucose is the only treatment necessary. Only occasionally will insulin be required because of underlying diabetes or because of the impaired insulin release of starvation. Potassium and phosphate supplements are needed. Rarely, bicarbonate therapy may also be necessary. When treating alcoholic ketosis, it should be recognized that diabetic patients also may suffer from alcoholism. Thus a patient in alcoholic ketoacidosis with a low blood glucose concentration, a high blood beta-hydroxybutyrate concentration, and moderate acidemia can become overtly diabetic in hyperglycemic coma if glucose is infused intravenously unaccompanied by adequate amounts of insulin. Therefore the same degree of cautious clinical monitoring and repeated examinations of blood glucose, electrolytes, gases, and pH are required for these critically ill patients as for patients in diabetic ketoacidosis (Chapter 353).

Hyperosmolar nonketotic coma

This form of diabetic coma occurs less frequently than diabetic ketoacidosis. It is most common in the elderly diabetic person and is only rarely observed in younger patients. Hyperosmolar nonketotic diabetic coma is characterized by marked hyperglycemia, which is usually greater than that accompanying diabetic ketoacidosis. Initial serum glucose concentration ranges from 600 to 2400 mg/dl. The greater hyperglycemia in hyperosmolar nonketotic coma as compared to ketoacidosis is the result, in part, of more severe dehydration. In the past, it has been associated with a mortality of 30% to 80%. Hyperosmolar coma is defined by values of serum osmolality greater than 325 mosm/L. (Osmolality may be determined directly or may be approximated by mathematical formulas such as $2[Na^+ + K^+] + glucose/18 + BUN/2.8$.) These patients are, most typically, nonacidotic at the time of presentation; but mild to moderate metabolic acidosis may be observed, with arterial pH levels as low as 7.2. This acidosis may result in part from a concurrent element of lactic acidosis from the impaired tissue perfusion due to marked hypovolemia. Frequently, a small degree of ketosis is found in undiluted sera in patients whose primary disorders are hyperglycemia and hyperosmolality.

Factors precipitating hyperosmolar nonketotic coma are generally similar to those precipitating diabetic ketoacidosis. Often this disorder develops in a patient not previously known to have diabetes mellitus. Precipitating causes include administration of fluids high in glucose content either intravenously or during peritoneal dialysis or hemodialysis. Other causes are administration of glucocorticoids, diuretics, and phenytoin. The hyperosmolar state, in contrast to diabetic ketoacidosis, is preceded by a more prolonged period of polyuria, polydipsia, and increasing progressive dehydration. This period may range from 5 to 21 days and is often accompanied by a history of increasing enfeeblement, mental confusion, somnolence, and, ultimately, coma. The early phases of the hyperosmolar coma also may be marked by urinary incontinence secondary to a profound osmotic diuresis, which combined with the mental symptoms, may be confused with primary cerebrovascular disease by friends and relatives. This comparatively slow and progressive deterioration of the patient, together with a high mortality rate, stands in marked contrast to the dramatic presentation and relatively low morbidity and mortality of diabetic ketoacidosis.

Because of the relative absence of ketosis in patients with hyperosmolar nonketotic coma, it has been postulated that there must be more circulating insulin activity in this condition than in diabetic ketoacidosis. Clinical studies, however, have failed to discern any significant difference in insulin levels between these two forms of diabetic coma. The essential biochemical difference between the two syndromes is that free fatty acid levels in hyperosmolar nonketotic coma are normal in contrast to the tenfold or greater elevation of free fatty acid levels in diabetic ketoacidosis. This difference may be the result of a relative failure of adrenergic nervous system adaptation to hypovolemia. In the elderly, the lack of a volume-dependent augmentation of free fatty acid mobilization from adipose tissue because of a diminished catecholamine output could thus explain the absence of ketosis in these persons.

Thrombotic events are the principal cause of death in patients with hyperosmolar nonketotic coma. These may be the result of increased platelet coagulability combined with the more extensive atherosclerotic vascular disease in the elderly. Patients initially may appear with antecedent myocardial infarctions, cerebrovascular accidents, or acute renal failure. Any or all of these also may develop during the course of treatment for hyperosmolar nonketotic coma. Because the fluid deficit in these patients is extremely severe (ranging from 10% to 20% of body weight), extreme care must be taken to avoid precipitating congestive heart failure or pulmonary edema after rapid rehydration in patients already having compromised myocardial function.

Treatment of the hyperosmolar state. Treatment of the hyperosmolar nonketotic state should be directed first to fluid and electrolyte replacement, as this is undoubtedly the most dangerous element of the syndrome. An average net fluid deficit of 150 ml/kg has been observed, but with extremely severe hyperglycemia, greater fluid losses (up to 200 ml/kg body weight) can be expected. The estimated fluid loss should be replaced in the first 18 to 24 hours of therapy, and rates of intravenous infusion should be adjusted every 2 to 4 hours, with frequent reassessments of the patient's cardiovascular status and electrolyte balance. As in diabetic ketoacidosis, water is lost in excess of sodium. Saline 0.5 N will generally adequately replace the salt and water deficit in these patients.

Early in the course of treatment, a more rapid expansion of intravascular volume and correction of prerenal azotemia is accomplished by the use of normal saline rather than 0.5 N saline. Furthermore, normal saline is hypotonic compared to the marked hypertonicity of the hyperosmolar state. Thus extracellular tonicity can be reduced and free water obtained even using normal saline. Lastly, normal saline has the additional advantage of producing smaller volume or fluid shifts in tissue compartments such as the central nervous system, which have maintained intracellular volume status by the creation of intracellular idiogenic osmols. These osmotically active equivalents may be generated by the uncovering of charge groups on intracellular proteins, and they must be allowed to be recovered during the period of fluid replacement so as to avoid marked brain edema. For these reasons, 1 to 2 liters of normal saline given at a rate of 0.5 to 1.0 L/hr should be used as early fluid therapy. After initiation of a urinary output or other clinical improvement in tissue perfusion, 0.5 N saline should be utilized for the remainder of volume replacement.

Potassium replacement should also be initiated after urinary output is ensured since hypokalemia will occur during insulin treatment of the hyperglycemia. The extent of the hypokalemia in untreated patients is, however, somewhat less than that observed in patients with diabetic ketoacidosis, as no hydrogen-potassium ion exchange secondary to acidosis has usually occurred. Because acute oliguric renal failure is a common concomitant of hyperosmolar nonketotic coma, intravenous potassium therapy must be given judiciously and with monitoring of serum potassium concentrations. It may also be advisable in the presence of anuria to maintain electrocardiographic surveillance of T-wave configuration in such patients. Phosphate depletion also may be observed in patients with hyperosmolar nonketotic coma, particularly during successful rehydration and normalization of serum glucose concentrations. Therapy with intravenous phosphate should be undertaken under the same circumstances as outlined for diabetic ketoacidosis.

Insulin therapy of the hyperglycemia in patients with the hyperosmolar nonketotic coma also must be approached carefully and with frequent monitoring of blood glucose concentrations. Choices regarding the route and manner of insulin delivery in the hyperosmolar nonketotic coma are similar to those for insulin delivery in diabetic ketoacidosis. A relatively high proportion of patients, however, demonstrates poor tissue perfusion secondary to the marked hypovolemia. Therefore subcutaneous, and even intramuscular, insulin may be inappropriate in these persons. Intermittent boluses of 5 to 10 units of rapid-acting insulin at 30- to 60-minute intervals should be sufficient to produce steady decreases in blood glucose concentrations in these patients. Alternatively, a priming injection of 0.1 unit/kg followed by continuous intravenous infusion of 0.05 to 0.10 unit/kg/hr of rapid-acting insulin will produce a sufficiently rapid decline in circulating glucose concentrations.

Rapid correction of the hyperglycemia is ill advised in these patients because such a rapid glucose reduction may be accompanied by unwarranted shifts of water from extracellular to intracellular compartments, including the brain. Throughout the course of therapy for hyperosmolar nonketotic coma, appropriate treatment for any underlying precipitating cause, such as infection, sepsis, or myocardial infarction, must be undertaken. Unlike the case in ketoacidosis, glucose or insulin infusion after reduction of hyperglycemia to concentrations below 200 mg/dl may not be necessary. Adequate fluid replacement, however, may not have been achieved by this time in the course of therapy. If such is the case, then small doses of intermediate-acting or rapid-acting insulin, followed by surveillance of blood glucose concentrations, may be necessary while rehydration continues. After resolutions of the acute disorder, maintenance therapy for diabetes mellitus obviously is needed.

Lactic acidosis

In normal humans at rest, lactate is produced as the end product of glycolysis, primarily by tissues devoid of mitochondrial oxidative metabolism. However, under anaerobic conditions, virtually all tissues can produce lactate, including the central nervous system, muscle, and skin. Of these tissues, skeletal muscle may be the major site of lactic acid production, particularly during vigorous or hypoxic exercise. On the other hand, the liver is the major organ extracting lactic acid from the blood, although in certain states lactate is utilized by the kidney, the heart, and even skeletal muscle. Indeed, lactate is the predominant substrate for hepatic gluconeogenesis. When rates of peripheral lactic acid production and hepatic lactate extraction are balanced and equal, acid-base balance is unchanged. Lactic acidosis develops only when lactic acid production exceeds lactate utilization (Chapter 353).

Both accelerated production and diminished utilization occur as consequences of decreased tissue oxygenation. This may result from tissue hypoperfusion secondary to occlusive vascular disease or congestive cardiomyopathy. Hyperglycemia and dehydration are also important mechanisms predisposing patients to the development of lactic acidosis. For these reasons, it is not surprising that about one half of the patients who develop lactic acidosis are diabetic. Sepsis, hemorrhage, overdose with ethanol, methanol, salicylates, or biguanides may also cause lactic acidosis. Neoplastic tissue that depends on anaerobic glycolysis for energy may greatly increase lactate production but will not produce lactic acidosis unless lactate extraction by the liver is diminished, perhaps as the result of hepatic metastases. A variety of enzymatic defects—such as a depressed pyruvate dehydrogenase activity (which can develop in diabetes mellitus or in thiamine deficient states) or congenital enzyme defects in glucose-6-phosphatase, fructose-1,6-diphosphatase, pyruvate carboxylase, or pyruvate dehydrogenase—can also result in lactic acidosis. A relatively large proportion of patients, however, develop acute lactic acidosis with no discernible cause; these must be termed *idiopathic*.

Patients with lactic acidosis generally are acutely ill; they may be stuporous or obtunded, tachypneic, or hypotensive. The diagnosis of lactic acidosis should be suspected in patients with a metabolic acidosis that is not accounted for by drug ingestion, uremia, or ketoacidosis. The finding of an increased anion gap should arouse suspicion. The diagnosis may be confirmed by the demonstration of an arterial pH of less than 7.3 and a blood lactate concentration of greater than 5 to 10 mmol/L. In practice, however, the diagnosis is usually made on clinical grounds by exclusion of all other causes of metabolic acidosis. Confirmation of the diagnosis of lactic acidosis is difficult because lactate is not easily or rapidly measured in most laboratories. Specific enzymatic assays for lactate are available, but these are time-consuming and not routinely offered in most hospitals.

The initial therapy for lactic acidosis should include intravenous sodium bicarbonate in sufficient amounts to buffer the acidemia. One half of the measured bicarbonate deficit in total body water should be replaced in the first hour of treatment. Arterial pH should then be measured, and further bicarbonate administered if necessary. Unless the specific precipitating cause of the lactic acidosis is identified and treated, continued bicarbonate infusions will be necessary. Intravenous regular insulin should be infused to reverse hyperglycemia and to activate pyruvate dehydrogenase in the diabetic patients. Glucose infusion should be initiated concurrently with insulin once the hyperglycemia is corrected. Identifying and treating the initiating or predisposing cause of the lactic acidosis are essential. Hemorrhagic hypovolemia requires fluid and/or blood replacement. Sepsis requires appropriate antibiotic therapy, pharmacologic doses of glucocorticoids, and fluids. Myocardial infarction and congestive heart failure require inotropic agents and diuretics. Peritoneal dialysis may rarely be needed in renal failure to treat salt overload after sodium bicarbonate administration or to remove drugs. Serial arterial blood gases and pH values are needed in monitoring the patient's responses. Vasoconstrictive drugs increase lactate concentrations and should be avoided.

Hypoglycemic coma

There are two major forms of hypoglycemic symptoms. The first group is adrenergic-mediated events including profuse sweating, tachycardia, tremulousness, and nervousness. The second group of symptoms is attributable to central nervous system fuel deprivation and includes slurred speech, diplopia, headache, confusion, somnolence, coma, and seizures. Although sensitivity to hypoglycemia among patients varies greatly, adrenergic reactions and mechanisms usually become apparent with acute falls of blood glucose levels to less than 40 mg/dl. The most notable exception is in patients on beta-blocking drugs or with long-standing diabetes mellitus and central or peripheral adrenergic autonomic neuropathy. Cerebral symptoms also begin at blood glucose levels less than 50 mg/dl, with initial symptoms generally consisting of headache. Disorientation frequently is observed at blood glucose levels less than 30 mg/dl; seizures and coma generally appear at blood glucose levels less than 25 mg/dl.

Hypoglycemia always should be considered in any patient brought to the emergency room in coma. In known diabetics on insulin or sulfonylurea therapy, hypoglycemia is an even more likely cause of coma. The absence of Kussmaul's respiration and dehydration and a significant lack of acetone in the breath should increase the suspicion of hypoglycemia. The presence or recent history of grand mal seizures or of focal seizures in elderly persons having underlying cerebrovascular disease should further increase the suspicion of hypoglycemic coma. A history of a missed meal or of unusually vigorous exercise also may be obtained. Confirmation of this diagnosis can be obtained rapidly by Chemstrip analysis of blood glucose levels. Values less than 50 mg/dl should be considered as representing hypoglycemic coma until it is proved otherwise.

Therapy with 50% glucose solution should be initiated at once. Of this solution, 50 to 100 ml may have to be given to revive patients in hypoglycemic coma. Patients with longstanding hypoglycemia may not respond to this amount of glucose. Factors such as body weight and the amount of insulin or hypoglycemic agent ingested will determine the quantity of dextrose required for normalization of blood glucose concentrations. Many patients will awaken immediately when adequate circulating glucose concentrations are achieved. A significant proportion of these patients will show temporary or persistent features of residual neurologic deficit.

In small children or in subjects with veins difficult to access for 50% glucose administration, glucagon (0.5 mg) may be given intramuscularly, followed by a second dose within 15 minutes. Failure to respond to this dose of glucagon can be observed in patients with pre-existing depletion of hepatic glycogen stores, as might occur in a patient after severe and prolonged exercise. In no instance should the patient be regarded as cured simply because an improved state of consciousness is produced. If an overdose of large quantities of insulin or of sulfonylureas has occurred, relapse into hypoglycemia can be anticipated if no effort is made to ensure a continued intake of carbohydrate. The latter may be achieved by having the patient ingest orange juice or tea with added sucrose or glucose. Intravenous glucose administration using 10% glucose and water may be necessary. This is of some consequence in patients with sulfonylurea overdosage in whom a vigorous insulin secretory response to 50% glucose infusion will be observed. In these subjects, a prolonged course of therapy using a progressive reduction in the rate of infusion of 10% glucose and water is necessary to prevent relapse into hypoglycemia. Rarely, patients may require glucocorticoids to raise the blood glucose concentration to acceptable levels. This therapy should extend generally over two and preferably three half-lives for the ingested sulfonylurea (Table 168-4). Focal seizures or residual neurologic deficit that does not clear in a conscious patient after hypoglycemia should prompt the physician to investigate potential abnormalities of cerebrovascular supply or central nervous system structure.

Re-evaluation of diabetes management should be initiated in patients having serious hypoglycemic episodes. In particular, attention must be focused on the manner in which hypoglycemic agents are being self-administered and on the nature of diet regulation in these subjects. Other potential problems causing a marked increase in insulin sensitivity, such as that produced by adrenal insufficiency, renal insufficiency, liver disease, and pituitary dysfunction, also should be considered.

Prevention of diabetic comas

In addition to control of blood glucose, other aspects of diabetic care are important in the prevention of acute complications. Control of infections is particularly important. Hyperglycemia in patients with diabetes mellitus impairs a number of aspects of leukocyte function. These include leukocyte chemotactic response, phagocytosis, and bacterial killing. These impairments, together with the predilection of diabetic patients to microvascular and macrovascular disease, which impairs regional blood flow, tend to increase both the frequency and severity of acquired infectious processes. Staphylococcal pyoderma, gram-negative and anaerobic infections of the extremities, and pyelonephritis with papillary necrosis all occur more commonly in patients with diabetes mellitus. Mucormycosis of the paranasal sinuses is a rare infection, found almost only in patients with diabetes. Often, patients with severe bacterial infections develop bacterial sepsis. Such a state leads to a marked deterioration in the degree of diabetic control and may even precipitate diabetic ketoacidosis or hyperosmolar nonketotic coma. The worsening hyperglycemia tends in turn to facilitate a more severe bacterial infection because of further impairment in white cell function owing to hypovolemia with impaired tissue perfusion. For these reasons, serious infections in patients with diabetes mellitus must be treated vigorously and early in their course. Therapy with bactericidal antibiotics, preferably with combinations of therapeutic agents having synergistic interactions, should be instituted immediately after cultures are obtained. Control of the blood glucose level cannot be achieved in this setting by using routine or pre-existing dosage of insulin or of oral sulfonylureas. Under these circumstances, particularly with sepsis, continuous intravenous infusion of insulin in relatively low doses (0.05 to 0.4 unit/kg/hr) should be considered as an initial treatment. For patients with marked obtundation or inability to ingest food, intravenous glucose may be administered concurrently with insulin. At least 150 to 200 g/day of carbohydrate should be given in the form of glucose in order to suppress starvation ketosis. This method is generally preferable to the use of intermittent sliding-scale urinary glycosuria coverage, which allows intervals of 6 hours or more to pass before supplementary insulin is administered. The disadvantages of sliding-scale coverage include failures to obtain a urine specimen so that coverage can be given, potential variance between urinary glucose spillage and blood glucose concentrations, and interfering agents that can yield either false-positive or false-negative tests. In patients with severe sepsis, more frequent intervals for the administration of relatively small doses of insulin by sliding scale may yield acceptable results. In most instances, the blood glucose levels should be monitored at 1- to 4-hour intervals. The glucose levels should be held to 100 to 150 mg/dl in patients with severe infection.

CHRONIC COMPLICATIONS OF DIABETES MELLITUS

Chronic complications of diabetes mellitus are divided into three major categories: macrovascular disease, microvascular disease, and the neuropathies. Treatment of these disorders is not satisfactory. Prevention or at least a retardation of the progression of these complications is the goal of the physician. Although the mechanisms accounting for the development of diabetic complications are probably multifactorial, most authorities accept a correlation between the degree and duration of hyperglycemia and the frequency of complications. These relationships are probably valid for the macrovascular lesions as well as the microvascular and neuropathic lesions. Unfortunately, the precise pathogenic mechanisms for the development of diabetic complications are still poorly understood.

Macrovascular disease

Occlusive coronary artery disease and concomitant congestive heart failure account for more than 70% of mortality in all patients with diabetes. Although this phenomenon is generally noted after 15 or more years of diabetes, it may be the initial finding in some patients with diabetes mellitus. Atherosclerosis occurs at a frequency nearly twofold to fourfold greater in males and females, respectively, than that in the nondiabetic population. At least three major elements of the diabetic process together accelerate the complex mechanism(s) of atherosclerosis. First, the insulin-resistant state, which appears years to decades before clinical hyperglycemia, produces hyperinsulinemia; the latter is an important growth factor for vascular smooth muscle and fibroblast proliferation in the arterial wall. Second, a dyslipidemia in patients with diabetes and in the prediabetic, insulin-resistant state is frequently apparent. Such a dyslipidemia is characterized by elevated concentrations of triglyceride as VLDL and depressed levels of high-density lipoprotein (HDL)-cholesterol; this is seen in patients either with type I insulin-dependent disease or type II non-insulin-dependent disease, whether in males or females. Indeed, the depression of HDL-cholesterol levels in females with diabetes mellitus is greater than that seen in males and accounts, in part, for the differentially greater acceleration of atherosclerosis in diabetic females, particularly premenopausal females, as compared to diabetic males of the same age. Depressed HDL-cholesterol levels are a clear and well-characterized risk factor for coronary atherosclerosis. The hypertriglyceridemia may itself be atherogenic or may lead to the formation of atherogenic precursors such as modified LDL-cholesterol particles known as LDL subclass B, or small, dense LDL. The latter appears in most insulin-resistant states and has been shown to be three times more atherogenic than ordinary, unmodified LDL. The latter is generally replaced by smaller, denser LDL when triglyceride concentrations are well in excess of 150 mg/dl. Third, hyperglycemia accelerates atherogenesis by way of protein glycation. Such glycation modifies endothelial-basement membrane permeability and function, so as to allow greater rates of lipoprotein deposition in the arterial wall. The glycation simulates the production of a macrophage chemotaxis factor, thereby recruiting cells responsible for the early foam cell phase of atherosclerosis.

Glycation also generates growth factors capable of accelerating the cellular proliferation characteristic of the fibrous plaque. These factors include platelet-derived growth factors and other advanced glycosylation product growth factors. Glycation modifies the function of a number of lipoprotein particles, including LDL particles. When glycated, ApoB 100, the receptor-binding protein on LDL, shows greater cellular uptake of LDL particles. Glycation also modifies the tendency towards oxidation of LDL lipids. Oxidized LDL is more readily taken up by macrophages in the so-called scavenger pathway. Glycation of HDL is also observed. When glycated, HDL binds less well to its cellular and tissue receptors and catalyzes processes related to reverse cholesterol transport at rates only about half those seen with the unglycated lipoprotein. Other aspects of the diabetic state contribute to accelerated atherosclerosis, including potential modifications of VLDL particles themselves in such a fashion as to produce smaller, denser VLDL. These modified particles appear to interact with vascular endothelium to produce increased levels of thromboxane and reduced PGF_1a, thereby explaining, in part, an increased tendency toward thrombosis in patients with diabetes. Atherosclerotic macrovascular disease appears to be histologically similar in both diabetic and nondiabetic subjects, despite the rapid and occasionally fulminant progression of the disorder in diabetics. Thus patients in their late teens and early 20s may begin to be symptomatic from severe atherosclerosis, particularly in type I (insulin-dependent) diabetes.

The precise pathogenesis of the accelerated atherosclerosis is unclear. Although qualitatively similar in diabetic and nondiabetic patients, atherosclerosis in diabetes mellitus has several unique aspects. Coronary atherosclerosis in diabetic patients can involve the whole of the right and left coronary circulation and may not be limited primarily to proximal lesions as noted in nondiabetic patients. Such diffuse coronary artery disease frequently is accompanied by marked left ventricular dysfunction, which is frequently out of proportion to the degree of reduction in coronary blood flow. In the absence of previous myocardial infarction, a hypokinetic left ventricle in patients with diabetes has been interpreted to suggest a diabetic cardiomyopathy. Whether such cardiomyopathy exists independent of either macrovascular or microvascular disease is somewhat open to question, although it should be suspected in all poorly controlled diabetic patients with marked protein wasting.

Treatment for diabetic cardiomyopathy is similar to that of other forms of congestive cardiomyopathy. If there is impaired runoff in the distal coronary circulation of a patient, coronary artery bypass surgery may be more hazardous and less satisfactory in its overall outcome. Nevertheless, patients having high risk for myocardial infarction or demonstrating moderate to severe left ventricular impairment to exercise are still good candidates for coronary artery revascularization procedures.

Atypical angina as well as atypical symptomatology of myocardial infarction occur in diabetic persons. Some patients will not experience the usual degrees of pain during episodes of myocardial ischemia or infarction. The absence of severe chest pain or pressure in postoperative subjects must therefore be compensated for by a higher index of suspicion in the attending physician. Diabetic patients may have a greater tendency to manifest atypical symptoms of coronary insufficiency such as epigastric distress or heartburn. Neck pain or pain radiation to both shoulders is also more common. Lastly, patients with diabetes mellitus also tend to manifest coronary artery insufficiency by the episodic development of painless congestive heart failure with exercise or stress.

Medical management of coronary artery disease, as well as peripheral vascular disease, should aim at normalizing the hyperglycemia and eliminating obesity and dyslipidemias. Exercise and weight loss, with reduced fat intake and avoidance of alcohol consumption, is the preferred form of therapy for type II diabetes mellitus in patients with mild to moderate dyslipidemia or hyperlipidemia. Insulin is required in hypoinsulinemic patients. With insulin lack, the lipid disturbances are characterized by an excess accumulation of VLDL triglyceride-rich particles in blood and by an increase of substrate delivered to the liver for VLDL synthesis. This process leads to an acquired type IV hyperlipidemia. In more severe cases, a type V hyperlipidemia characterized by the presence of chylomicrons in addition to VLDL particles also may be observed. In general, these patients have triglyceride levels greater than 1500 mg/dl and manifest lipemia retinalis at triglyceride levels of 2000 or greater. Virtually all types of hyperlipidemia, with the possible exception of type IIa hypercholesterolemia alone, may occur in uncontrolled diabetes mellitus.

The treatment of the acquired hyperlipidemia of diabetes mellitus should be directed initially toward control of the blood glucose concentration by using exercise and diet therapy, and insulin if necessary. Patients with hyperlipidemia and hyperglycemia require greater than normal quantities of insulin. Insulin requirements of 100 to 200 units per day may be encountered, and these may not necessarily decrease as the hyperlipidemia is improved. Appropriate diet therapy such as an American Diabetes Association or American Heart Association diet for hyperlipidemia must be instituted. Caloric restriction to achieve ideal weight is essential. For most patients, these therapies will not completely control hypertriglyceridemia. Additional therapies using gemfibrozil may also be indicated, but only after attempts to control the hyperglycemia have been made. Nicotinic acid tends to worsen diabetic control and therefore should only be instituted in selected patients with careful monitoring of the patient (Chapter 171). An overall approach to the management of hyperglycemia and dyslipidemia in diabetic patients is provided in Fig. 168-7. For patients with familial combined or mixed dyslipidemias characterized by high LDL-cholesterol, high VLDL-triglyceride and low HDL-cholesterol levels, a combination of lipid-lowering agents may be necessary. Ideally, double therapy should use gemfibrozil plus a bile salt resin or an HMG-CoA reductase inhibitor with reduced skeletal muscle toxicity such as pravastatin. Furthermore, two or three agents may be useful in patients with advanced coronary disease in whom regression of atherosclerosis may be possible, particularly if a low-fat diet can be followed.

As with coronary artery disease, peripheral vascular disease in diabetic patients tends to be qualitatively similar, but quantitatively greater, than that observed in nondiabetic patients. However, the frequency of distal involvement, particularly of the lower limb, is far higher in diabetic subjects, especially in those who smoke. As a consequence of the impaired distal runoff in the circulation below the popliteal fossa, peripheral vascular bypass surgery for distal lower extremity ischemia is often less rewarding in diabetic than nondiabetic patients. If relatively isolated aneurysms or occlusions of the distal aorta or the common iliac or femoral artery can be demonstrated, then resection and graft or

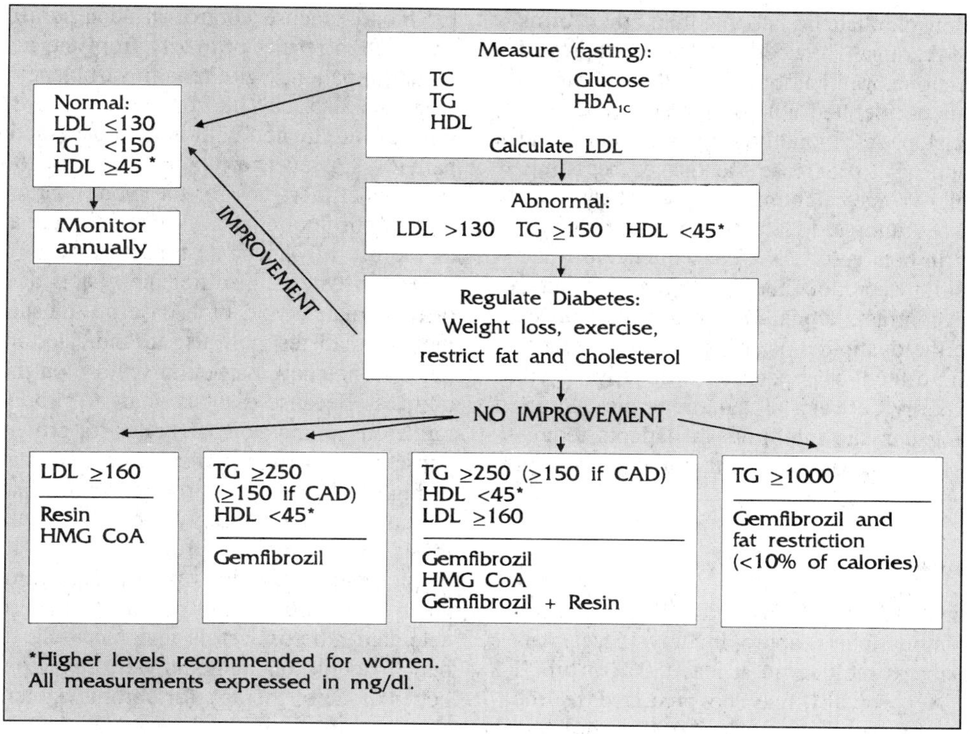

Fig. 168-7. Management of dyslipidemia in patients with diabetes. (Reprinted with permission from Diabetes Care 15:1068, 1992. Copyright © 1992 by the American Diabetes Association, Inc.)

bypass surgery may prove helpful in ameliorating symptoms such as claudication and in improving the muscle dysfunction of diabetic patients with severe peripheral vascular disease. In the more common syndromes of peripheral vascular insufficiency such as the Leriche syndrome, bypass surgery has proved helpful, although not totally satisfactory, in diabetic subjects. Lumbar sympathectomy is sometimes helpful in relieving mild rest pain but probably does not alter the long-term course of atherosclerosis. Little evidence, however, suggests that sympathectomy produces a lasting improvement in peripheral vascular blood flow; sympathectomy does not appear to reverse gangrenous complications or prevent amputations in patients with severely impaired circulation either. Attempts aimed at reducing risk factors such as obesity, cigarette smoking, and a lack of exercise should be encouraged.

Microvascular disease

Capillary basement membrane thickening or the accumulation of periodic acid Schiff-positive material within the microvasculature of diabetic subjects is a characteristic lesion of diabetes (Chapter 355). In the kidney, the formation of nodular areas of intercapillary glomerulosclerosis (Kimmelstiel-Wilson's disease) tends to be pathognomonic, but it is less common in diabetic subjects than is the more frequent diffuse glomerulosclerosis.

In almost all forms of diabetic microangiopathy, hypertension appears to be an important co-morbid risk factor requiring more aggressive attention to control than previously afforded. Recent studies have clearly indicated that so-called "high normal" blood pressures are clear, independent risk factors, particularly in the later phase of both proliferative retinopathy as well as diabetic nephropathy. To this end, therapy with antihypertensive agents to a diastolic pressure of 80 mm Hg or less is a general goal for the prevention, or at least amelioration, of the progression of diabetic microangiopathy. Some antihypertensive agents are more effective in this regard than others. For example, angiotensin-converting enzyme inhibitors, particularly short-acting inhibitors, may have unique nephroprotective properties with regard to diabetic kidney disease. In part, as the result of preferential action on efferent as compared to afferent arterials, intraglomerular hypertension may be reduced, thereby improving hyperfiltration, an initial lesion of diabetic nephropathy. As a consequence, proteinuria is also improved. Although blood pressure reduction in hypertensive patients has some beneficial effect on intrarenal hemodynamics and protein excretion rates in all patients with diabetic nephropathy, converting enzyme inhibitors appear to have unique, additional advantages independent of the elimination of hypertension per se.

On the other hand, a number of antihypertensive agents have untoward side effects in patients with diabetes. These agents magnify the potential for atherosclerosis, thereby vitiating potential benefits on atherosclerosis accruing from the reduction of hypertension by worsening such concomitant abnormalities as the insulin resistance and hyperglycemia of diabetes or the dyslipidemia of diabetes. Thiazide diuretics may more likely be associated with an increased mortality in hypertensive diabetic patients than other forms of antihypertensive therapy. They certainly have not proved satisfactory, either alone or in combination with beta blockers, in reducing the accelerated atherosclerosis of patients treated for hypertension. Additionally, each agent alone and in combination, appears to increase the risk of becoming diabetic substantially. Some calcium slow channel entry antagonists also have untoward effects on the calcium-potassium channel in beta cells. As a consequence of their use, impaired insulin secretion and hyperglycemia have been reported. In contrast, $alpha_1$-adrenergic antagonists appear to improve the dyslipidemia in patients with diabetes while producing effective, hypertensive therapy. There is evidence for synergy between alpha-adrenergic antagonists and converting enzyme inhibitors in patients requiring multiple drug therapies or for step therapy protocol in patients with diabetes.

Diabetic nephropathy

Diabetic nephropathy (Chapter 355) becomes clinically apparent (initially as albuminuria) approximately 15 years after the onset of diabetes mellitus in at least 50% of type I diabetic patients. Nephropathy may be predicted by the early development of microalbuminuria ($>$ 30 mg/min) in patients years before clinical macroproteinuria is seen. The disease has a slowly progressive course over a 10-year interval, at which point azotemia generally becomes apparent. A small fraction of diabetic patients with proteinuria develop an overt nephrotic syndrome. The appearance of obvious proteinuria often is correlated with the appearance of overt diabetic retinopathy, although the two do not necessarily appear simultaneously. Impairment of urinary bladder emptying because of diabetic autonomic neuropathy may aggravate advancing renal insufficiency.

Management of diabetic nephropathy focuses on preventing further deterioration by using low-protein diets, angiotensin-converting enzyme (ACE) inhibitors, as well as vigorous glucose and hypertension control. A reduction of glomerular hyperfiltration by decreased protein intake and especially by ACE inhibition with captopril, in particular, will tend to arrest the long-term decline in glomerular filtration rates. Hypertension must be normalized in all diabetic patients, as it increases the incidence, severity, and progression of all microvascular and macrovascular complications.

The management of diabetic patients with renal insufficiency is often complicated considerably by increased insulin sensitivity. This increase may result in part from an impaired glomerular clearance of insulin because renal disposal of insulin can account for the removal of up to one third of subcutaneously administered insulin. There is a tendency toward developing a progressively greater interval between the time of insulin injection and the time of peak biologic action of the drug. As a consequence, intermediate insulins such as NPH or lente may have peak biologic activity in diabetic patients with renal insufficiency at 18 to 30 hours after injection. Shorter-acting insulins, such as semilente on a twice-daily basis, may prove more effective for blood glucose control in such subjects. The delay in peak action results primarily from the delayed rates of removal in patients with renal insufficiency. Rebound hyperglycemia also may be frequently observed in patients with renal failure treated with intermediate-acting insulin. These patients, however, are highly resistant to ketosis.

Adjunct therapies for the more characteristic abnormalities of chronic renal insufficiency must also be used, such as the use of phosphate binders to control the hyperphosphatemia of renal insufficiency. Diets of 2000 to 3000 calories, which would otherwise be unusual in the management of diabetes mellitus, are indicated in patients with renal insufficiency, particularly those on maintenance hemodialysis. Because dialysis tends to produce a clearance of numerous amino acid substrates for protein synthesis, compensatory increases in dietary protein intake to 80 or 110 g of high biologic value protein per day and rigorous insulin therapy to maintain euglycemia and stimulate protein synthesis while inhibiting protein breakdown may be essential in such patients. However, low-protein diets are preferred when only mild renal impairment exists. In view of the accelerated atherosclerosis and metabolic instability of diabetic patients on hemodialysis, renal transplantation is a better mode of therapy for chronic azotemia.

Diabetic retinopathy

Diabetic retinopathy is a progressive deterioration in the microcirculation to the retina observed in patients with diabetes mellitus. Deterioration in intimal integrity, as evidenced by fluorescein leakage from retinal capillaries, can be observed within weeks of the development of flagrant hyperglycemia. After approximately 10 years of poorly controlled diabetes mellitus, microaneurysms are present in at least 50% of patients. Retinal microaneurysms, saclike excrescences of intimal basement membrane from the extended walls of the capillaries, are best seen by using fluorescein angiography. Evidence has been presented that vigorous control of glucose concentrations is associated with a diminished rate of microaneurysm formation in type I diabetic patients compared to patients having relatively less well-controlled hyperglycemia. Retinopathy is present in 90% of patients with diabetes for over 30 years.

After the appearance of microaneurysms, the course of diabetic retinopathy may progress to the development of punctate hemorrhages together with hard waxy-appearing exudates. The triad of hemorrhages, exudates, and microaneurysms is frequently called *background retinopathy* (Plate IV-1). This type can be accompanied by fluffy, so-called cotton wool exudates over the retina, which result from microinfarcts and retinal scarring. Hard exudates are the extravasation of proteinaceous and lipid-rich intravascular fluid that appear because of the increased permeability of retinal capillaries and are analogous to the proteinuria of the glomerular disease of diabetes mellitus (Plate IV-2).

In most patients, background retinopathy tends to remain relatively stable, although slowly progressive. In a minority of patients, retinal hemorrhages on a much larger scale develop from the weakened membranes of the dilated and tortuous retinal vessels. After resorption of much of the blood-containing material, progressive scarring develops. New retinal vessels that form in the scar area (a process termed *neovascularization*) appear to penetrate into the vitreous. In later stages, the vascular tufts contract toward the vitreous, producing a secondary retinal detachment. This process of proliferative retinopathy causes the profound loss of vision and ultimate blindness in patients with diabetes mellitus (Plate IV-3). Recent well-controlled studies have demonstrated that photocoagulation with argon laser light or retinal coagulation with a xenon lamp may prevent retinal detachment and preserve sight. Laser therapy may be used to accurately photocoagulate the contents of a dilated and tortuous vessel. Much of the stimulus to neovascular proliferation is the apparent result of the production of an angiogenesis factor by an ischemic retina. A decreased production of this factor by the destruction of portions of the retina using peripheral retinal photocoagulation ameliorates this proliferation by reducing angiogenesis. In patients with advanced vitreous involvement, surgical vitrectomy and vitreous replacement may offer some restoration of vision. For these reasons, ophthalmologic consultation and follow-up of all patients having moderate to advanced background retinopathy should be obtained at least annually.

Other parts of the eye also may be involved by diabetes mellitus. Chronic hyperglycemia may lead to temporary changes in lens shape that may result in marked fluctuations of visual acuity. Approximately 6 to 8 weeks of glucose control is required to re-establish lenticular curvature. Cataracts develop in patients with diabetes mellitus more frequently than in the normal population. In patients with galactosemia, the role of polyol formation has been clearly demonstrated in the hydration cataract. Similar mechanisms also have been postulated to explain the excessive rate of cataract formation in diabetic subjects. Chronic hyperglycemia may lead to excess sorbitol formation in the diabetic lens, thereby causing an osmotic gradient along which extracellular waste may flow into the lens. As a consequence, lens protein architecture may be disrupted, thereby generating a cataract. There is no evidence to demonstrate that good control of the blood glucose level prevents the development of cataracts in diabetic subjects. Once developed, reversal of cataract formation by nonsurgical means appears to be futile. Glaucoma also occurs with increased frequency in diabetic subjects. Presumably, the mechanisms of glaucoma development in such patients relates to posthemorrhagic fibrosis and scarring of the outflow tract for fluids (the canal of Schlemm) as the result of stimulated anterior chamber angiogenesis by the same factor(s) produced by the ischemic retina.

Diabetic neuropathy

Diabetic neuropathy is a troublesome consequence of diabetes mellitus. Unlike many of the other chronic consequences of diabetes, the neuropathy may occur early in the disease. Nevertheless, the frequency and severity of diabetic neuropathy increase proportionately with the duration and severity of the hyperglycemia in diabetes mellitus. In some patients, an acute loss of diabetic control may be accompanied by abrupt manifestations of diabetic neuropathy, most commonly distal paresthesias and dysesthesias.

Although diabetic neuropathy does not contribute substantially to mortality in patients with diabetes mellitus, it does contribute to high morbidity and impairment of lifestyle. Of all the chronic complications of diabetes, neuropathy appears to be the most responsive to therapies that normalize circulating glucose concentrations.

Virtually every aspect of the peripheral nervous system can be involved in diabetic neuropathy. Such neuropathy may be classified according to the area of peripheral nervous system involvement. For example, the most commonly encountered form of diabetic neuropathy is that of the symmetric distal polyneuropathy, usually affecting the lower extremity more commonly than the upper extremity. Diabetic neuropathy also may present as a radiculopathy or as a mononeuropathy of either a single nerve or multiple nerve trunks. Spinal cord and visceral involvement also may be evidenced in syndromes such as the tabetic-like neuropathy mimicking tertiary syphilis. In this neuropathy, lancinating pains of the abdomen or distal lower extremity may be excruciating. Charcot's joints also may be observed in patients with diabetes mellitus and usually involves the foot, although, rarely, involvement of the knee and upper extremity has been observed.

Virtually any cranial nerve, alone or in combination, may be involved in an acute presentation of diabetic neuropathy. Cranial nerves III, IV, and VI are most frequently affected. Other cranial nerves, however, such as VII, VIII, and XII may also be involved by the diabetic neuropathic process. Finally, almost every aspect of autonomic nervous system function may be seriously impaired by diabetic neuropathy. Such neuropathy may be patchy and incomplete in nature and may involve either a single aspect of autonomic function or a broad spectrum of functions.

The pathogenesis of diabetic neuropathy is unclear. Multiple mechanisms may be involved. Acute mononeuropathies alone (simplex), or in combinations (multiplex) in which nearly total dysfunction of whole nerve trunks can be observed, may result from a relatively sudden infarction of one or more branches of the vasa nervorum (the penetrating arteries delivering and maintaining circulation to nerve trunks). On the other hand, the slowly progressive deterioration of peripheral nervous system function seen in the systematic distal polyneuropathies may not be attributed to an infarction process. With progressive deterioration, axonal and nerve cell death may occur, accounting for the sensory anesthesia observed in these patients. Chronic hyperglycemia may lead to excess sorbitol formation in Schwann cells of nerve trunks. The enzyme responsible for sorbitol formation, aldose reductase, has a relatively low affinity for glucose, the concentration of which is the primary rate-controlling event for sorbitol formation. Clearance of osmotically active sorbitol depends on diffusion of the hexatol to the axon, where reoxidation to fructose may occur via sorbitol dehydrogenase. In diabetic nerve, sorbitol content is increased. Consequently, the increased osmotically active substances in the Schwann cell may produce an extracellular-to-intracellular fluid shift resulting in Schwann cell swelling and disruption. Because these cells are responsible for the maintenance of axonal integrity, axonal dysfunction and death may be observed.

Distal polyneuropathies. These complications are the most commonly encountered complaints of diabetic patients related to diabetic neuropathy. The distal paresthesias and dysesthesias may occur insidiously or may be acute during loss of diabetic control secondary to infection or other forms of severe stress. In the lower extremities, the involvement is usually bilateral, symmetric, and accompanied by severe pain. In individual subjects the pain may be perceived differently, e.g., as cramping, burning, or lancinating. The painful polyneuropathies of diabetes are often experienced with increased intensity at night. Paresthesias are most commonly expressed as numbness, tingling, or pins-and-needles sensations. The physical examination is generally unremarkable because neurologic functioning, including vibratory sensation, may be preserved. However, the sensational pain and light touch, particularly differentiation of sharp from dull objects, may be impaired. The most common concomitant of symmetric polyneuropathy in diabetic subjects is the bilateral absence of ankle and/or knee jerks. Indeed, diabetes mellitus is the most common explanation for bilaterally absent ankle jerks. Other explanations must be sought for unilaterally absent reflexes in the lower extremity, even in diabetic patients.

Unfortunately, treatment of diabetic polyneuropathy is usually unsatisfactory. Initial therapy should be directed toward establishing good control of the serum glucose concentrations in patients with diabetes mellitus. Treatment of residual symptoms has been attempted by using a combination of vitamin B therapies including thiamine (100 mg three times a day), folic acid (3 mg daily), vitamin B_{12} (1000 μg intramuscularly daily for 5 days), and a broad spectrum of other vitamins.

Initial expectations of this type of therapy were somewhat more enthusiastic and positive than subsequent results have warranted; however, there is increased protein and B-vitamin catabolism in diabetic subjects, and such patients do have lower serum vitamin concentrations than comparable diabetic patients without diabetic neuropathy. Additional therapy with either phenytoin or carbamazepine may be tried. Both agents have been reported to improve diabetic paresthesias in one third to one half of subjects studied. These pharmacologic agents may act by stabilizing axonal transmembrane potentials, thereby blocking pain and paresthesias. Carbamazepine is associated with a higher incidence of side effects than is phenytoin. The latter should be tried initially at full anticonvulsant doses. These agents are most effective for pseudotabetic symptoms. Amitriptyline and fluphenazine are also useful in the treatment of diabetic neuropathy. The effectiveness of aldose reductase inhibitors is presently being assessed.

Advanced sensory loss producing peripheral anesthesia in the lower extremity results in the development of a Charcot's joint. Destruction of the cartilaginous joint lining occurs from repeated trauma incurred as a result of loss of sensation. Abnormalities of chondrocyte metabolism and function also have been suggested as being involved in the pathogenesis. With continued use of the joint, destruction of the normal architecture and the attendant appearance of loose bodies within the joint may be observed on radiographic examination. Ultimately, a total destruction of the normal joint architecture and a loss of normal function occurs. Treatment of Charcot's joints of the lower extremity requires combined orthopedic, podiatric, and rehabilitative efforts.

A more frequent concomitant of distal anesthesia is the development of neurotropic ulceration, particularly on the plantar aspect of the foot. Anesthesia leads to a worsening of any minor injury because of the absence of protective painful stimuli. This problem in addition to pre-existing microvascular and macrovascular circulatory impairments characterizes the underlying mechanisms that may lead to rapid gangrene after foot injury.

All patients with diabetes mellitus should perform careful self-examination of their feet. Foot hygiene should be maintained with particular attention to the care and trimming of toenails and calluses. Extreme care should be taken in selecting footwear. Because diabetic patients have an early tendency toward hyperhidrosis and subsequent anhidrosis, the use of all-leather shoes is advised, as leather maintains an adequate rate of evaporation of perspiration. Absorbent socks also should be worn at all times. In the diabetic patient, shortening of the flexor tendons may occur, leading to hammer-toe deformities. This problem produces maldistribution of the weight on the foot and causes callosities. Therefore correction of maldistributed weight to prevent pressure on ulcerated lesions is important. Vigorous treatment of any form of ulceration of the diabetic foot is essential in preventing gangrene and ultimate amputation of the extremity. Prevention of infection in moderate- to large-sized ulceration initially should be attempted by topical antibiotic therapy. Advanced infected ulcerations require large doses of bactericidal antibiotic, generally given intravenously. Frequent debridement of the ulcerated area, particularly to prevent undermining of the ulcer margin by the spreading necrotic process, is also essential. Rest and elevation of the foot and frequent soaks in warm, but not hot, Betadine-water mixtures are also useful.

In diabetic patients with advanced microvascular and macrovascular impairments to nutrient flow and waste-product removal in the foot, amputation may be required if progressive unremitting infection or gangrene occurs. An obvious line of demarcation should develop. In all instances, amputation should be performed well above this line. Transtarsal amputation for infected ulcerations of the diabetic metatarsal area usually is not successful. To provide maximum rehabilitation of these patients, however, amputation below major joints such as the ankle or knee is more advisable than amputation above these joints. In particular, below-the-knee amputations almost always provide greater patient mobility and rehabilitation than do above-the-knee amputations. In the acutely infected patient, surgical therapies, such as vascular bypass procedures, aimed at increasing regional blood flow rarely prevent the need for amputation. In all instances, osteomyelitis should be considered in cases of persistent, nonhealing diabetic foot ulceration with consistent evidence of bacterial infection.

Diabetic neuromuscular disease

Diabetic neuromuscular disease can be differentiated into several different syndromes. In the upper extremity, painless atrophy of the intrinsic muscles of the hand can be observed. This is most obvious for the thenar and hypothenar eminences as well as the interosseous spaces. The atrophy may progress to a point of nearly total loss of intrinsic musculature. This process is always accompanied by a loss of motor power in the upper extremity, particularly the distal muscles. This form of peripheral neuropathy may or may not be accompanied by sensory anesthesia in the upper extremity. Upper extremity diabetic neuromuscular disease appears to be more common in the elderly and in males. Many of these patients have mild to moderate hypertriglyceridemia. Control of hyperglycemia and hypertriglyceridemia may be accompanied by improvement of the neuromuscular disease after a period of 6 to 12 months.

Diabetic neuromuscular disease of the lower extremity, more commonly referred to as *diabetic amyotrophy,* resembles a progressive weakness and wasting of proximal lower extremity muscles involving the pelvic girdle and anterior thigh compartments, most commonly the quadriceps femoris. This condition is usually accompanied by severe pain, although anesthesia may be observed. Unlike upper extremity diabetic neuromuscular disease, lower extremity disease may be asymmetric in distribution and generally heals spontaneously in 2 to 4 months from time of diagnosis. A similar, but less painful, variant of diabetic amyotrophy occurs in the upper extremity and is associated with progressive wasting of the intrinsic musculature of the shoulder girdle. In many patients, a combined defect involving the proximal musculature of both upper and lower extremities may also be observed. In these subjects, vigorous control of the blood glucose level by insulin therapy may provide the only beneficial form of therapy.

Acute mononeuropathies

Acute mononeuropathies may manifest themselves in virtually any single nerve trunk. Most commonly encountered are acute mononeuropathies of the cranial nerves, although other mononeuropathies such as acute foot drop also may be observed. Diabetic mononeuropathies may manifest themselves as acute, painful extraocular muscle palsies. In general, pain precedes the development of palsy by 5 to 10 days. Although the pain may be trigeminal in distribution, the diplopia and subsequent clinical involvement of the cranial nerves III, IV, or VI alone or in combination soon provide the basis for a diagnosis. When the third cranial nerve is involved, there is characteristic sparing of the pupillary fibers in more than 80% of cases, which provides a point of important differential significance because aneurysms or intracranial mass lesions generally involve both the pupillary fibers and the myelinated fibers to the extraocular muscles.

Specific therapies for diabetic extraocular palsy do not exist. Rest and local supportive measures generally will suffice until there is regression of the self-limited condition. Approximately 2 to 3 months is required for relatively complete healing. Other cranial nerves may be involved, producing considerable concern regarding the underlying diagnosis. Most commonly, extraocular involvement affects the seventh and eight cranial nerves and may manifest itself initially with a Bell's palsylike syndrome together with equilibrium or hearing impairment. On occasion, patients with diabetes mellitus may also have isolated primary pupillary abnormalities such as anisocoria with diminished reactivity to light but generally not accommodation. This may resemble an Argyll Robertson pupil.

Diabetic autonomic neuropathy

The autonomic neuropathies of diabetes may be manifested as a heterogeneous and complex combination of disorders involving virtually every organ system. The autonomic neuropathies are discussed here in terms of the organ system involved.

Gastrointestinal neuropathies. Virtually every aspect of gastrointestinal dysfunction may be produced by diabetic neuropathy. This may range from disordered esophageal motility to diabetic gastroparesis with impaired gastric emptying and may even include impaired peristalsis with diabetic diarrhea. Most common and distressing of the neuropathies affecting gastrointestinal function is that of diabetic diarrhea. The patient complains of explosive diarrhea, seemingly worse at night, although daytime hyperactivity is fairly common. The diarrhea is not preceded by cramps and may be sufficiently severe and sudden in nature as to produce the appearance of fecal incontinence. Characteristic roentgenographic patterns of disordered small bowel motility are sometimes observed in patients with diabetic diarrhea. Control of diabetic hyperglycemia is effective in improving the diarrhea in a small proportion of patients. Anticholinergics such as diphenoxylate (Lomotil) and stool-bulking agents have limited utility. Therapies using oral antibiotics such as tetracycline for relative bacterial overgrowth in the small intestinal lumen may be efficacious. Clonidine (0.2 to 0.3 mg/day) appears to be the most successful treatment to date.

Diabetic gastroparesis leads to early satiety and unpredictable gastric emptying accompanied by nausea and vomiting. This is a relatively distressing concomitant of diabetic visceral autonomic neuropathy. Gastroparesis tends to produce unpredictable losses in diabetic control owing to the inconstancy of food absorption. Multiple small feedings of a predominantly liquid, low-fat diet may be effective in maintaining nutrition. Approximately 1 to 3 months of rigorous euglycemia are essential before the symptoms of this disorder will disappear. Metoclopramide may be very useful in facilitating gastric emptying; cholinergic agonists in general have limited utility.

Genitourinary neuropathies. Mild to severe urinary bladder dysfunction occurs in more than 50% of patients with diabetes mellitus of more than 20 years' duration. Decreased bladder propulsive power and increased residual volume may be observed on voiding cystometrogram studies. As a consequence of the increasing residual volume, there is a deterioration in the utility of double-voided urines as indices of diabetic control. Therapy with cholinergic agonists is only partially effective. Because of the impairment of the sensation of the need for micturition, a reasonably successful strategy has been to urge patients with this complication to perform timed voidings regardless of the perceived need to void. As increasing paresis of the detrusor muscle occurs, increasing residual volume develops. Proportional to the degree of residual volume, there is early asymptomatic bacteriuria and, ultimately, overt cystitis. In more advanced cases, bladder neck resection may be attempted to reduce the amount of detrusor power required for bladder emptying. Urinary diversion may become necessary in a few patients.

Impotence and impairment of sexual function occur in more than 50% of men with long-standing diabetes and may be the first manifestation of the disease. Psychogenic causes for impotence should be excluded because diabetes does not preclude the relatively more common, psychologic etiology of impotence. A characteristic history of progressive loss of penile tumescence, diminution of morning erection, and inability to masturbate despite preservation of libido is highly suggestive of diabetic impotence. Serum testosterone concentrations are usually normal. Cystometrograms should be performed to establish whether bladder neuropathy coexists in these patients. Sleep laboratories that determine organic penile dysfunction may be helpful in establishing the diagnosis.

If mild to moderate impotence has occurred for only a brief time, rigorous control of the blood glucose concentrations may occasionally re-establish penile function. Hormone replacement therapy with testosterone, vitamins, or other medications is largely unsuccessful. In advanced cases, surgical implantation of penile prostheses may be the only available treatment. Sexual dysfunction in women with diabetes mellitus is rarely observed.

Cardiovascular neuropathy. Autonomic neuropathy manifested by orthostatic hypotension is relatively common in patients with diabetes mellitus and may be disabling. These patients may not be able to rise from a supine position without a period of 10 to 30 minutes of adaptation to an increasingly upright posture. The diagnosis is made by demonstrating a decrease of approximately 25 mm Hg in systolic or 10 mm Hg in diastolic pressure after 2 minutes of upright posture without a compensatory increase of the heart rate. Other entities to be considered are adrenal insufficiency, Shy-Drager syndrome, and primary autonomic dysfunction. In the Shy-Drager syndrome central nervous system dysfunction, particularly extrapyramidal and cerebellar dysfunction, should be demonstrable. Irregularity of sweating may also accompany diabetic autonomic dysfunction. Partial or total anhidrosis may be observed. A patchy distribution of sweating may be particularly evident in the face. An unusual variant of autonomic instability may be manifested by the profuse, drenching perspiration observed in certain diabetic patients after meal ingestion (gustatory sweating).

Treatment of orthostatic hypotension can be difficult. A high-salt diet will increase intravascular volume and thereby tend to maintain central nervous system perfusion despite excessive pooling of venous blood in the legs on standing. Expansion of intravascular volume using fludrocortisone (Florinef) in doses of 0.1 to 0.5 mg/day may also be used. Both of these therapies must be used judiciously in patients with concomitant cardiovascular disease, as volume overload and supine hypertension may result. Jobst stockings or even antigravity suits may be useful in reducing the severity of venous pooling of blood. The use of adrenergic pressors such as ephedrine may be hazardous and should be avoided as an initial therapy.

Diabetic dermopathy

A variety of complex and poorly understood lesions of the skin have been reported in patients with diabetes mellitus. Most common of these is the change in color and consistency of the skin, particularly over the anterior pretibial area in both type I and type II diabetic patients. The skin becomes mildly atrophic, waxy in consistency, and has a pale, almost translucent appearance. This is accompanied by hair loss, to a level at least as high or higher than the change in skin consistency. These changes begin in the dorsum of the foot and ascend slowly with time. Treatment generally yields less than encouraging results, with the principal effort directed at good diabetic control. Necrobiosis lipoidica diabeticorum (Plate VI-19) is a far more dramatic lesion but is observed in less than 5% of patients with diabetes mellitus. It may occur before or coincident with the diagnosis of diabetes. Necrobiosis produces a focal area of atrophic scarring in the anterior pretibial area bordered by a painful margin of erythematous, maculopapular, almost xanthomatous-like eruptions. Subsidence of the inflammatory process is accompanied by enlargement of the atrophic scarring, which itself is painless. There may be areas of telangiectasia at the margin. Therapy is nonspecific, focusing on control of diabetic hyperglycemia. Corticosteroids have been advocated for necrobiosis but do not appear to stop the progression of this self-limited disease. Less dramatic than necrobiosis diabeticorum are the more darkly pigmented shin spots seen in diabetic subjects. These macular areas of hyperpigmentation are painless and proliferate slowly with increasing duration of diabetes mellitus.

The patient with diabetes may have lipoatrophy or lipohypertrophy at insulin injection sites. The pathogenesis of these phenomena is unclear. Lipohypertrophy may be up to 5 to 10 cm in diameter. Highly purified preparations of insulin, such as single-component insulin, cause the disorders less commonly. Treatment of a pre-existing lipoatrophy by injection of the purer insulin into the margin of the lesion appears to be one reasonably successful therapeutic approach. In patients not responding to these maneuvers, insulin administration should be restricted to areas of less cosmetic importance.

Diabetes and pregnancy

Pregnancy considerably accelerates several of the chronic complications of diabetes mellitus and is accompanied by a high incidence of fetal wastage. Therefore pregnancy is not advisable for diabetic patients with microvascular disease. With considerable patient effort and attention to self-management, successful pregnancies can be achieved in patients with advanced, noncardiac complications. To reduce the fourfold incidence of fetal malformation in the infants of diabetic mothers, a period of 6 to 12 months of excellent control of the hyperglycemia before pregnancy seems indicated. Based on the experience of a number of investigators, multiple insulin doses containing primary regular or at least two doses of intermediate-acting insulin with rapid-acting insulin as needed will be essential for excellent diabetic control. Alternatively, mechanical insulin delivery systems such as the insulin infusion pump may improve diabetic control. Regardless of the mode of insulin administration, frequent home monitoring by using Dextrostix with a reflectance meter or Chemstrip BG will greatly improve diabetic control, especially during the last half of pregnancy.

During pregnancy, an early decreased insulin requirement is followed by later insulin resistance and insensitivity. In the first trimester, insulin requirements may be observed to decrease concomitantly with the growth of the fetal-placental unit, which acts to consume glucose and other nutrients. It should be remembered that the central nervous system consumes the largest portion of the obligate daily glucose requirement in the healthy adult. In the pregnant patient, the growth of a second central nervous system increases the carbohydrate demand dramatically. This development is particularly important during the third trimester, when an unusual form of ketosis may develop without striking hyperglycemia. It may be that the fetal-placental unit accounts for rapid glucose utilization but still allows for ketosis owing to insulin insufficiency.

Because of the antagonism to insulin action produced primarily by placental hormones (human placental lactogen, estrogen, and progesterone), insulin insensitivity develops during the second half of pregnancy. These patients therefore may precipitously develop diabetic ketoacidosis with glucose levels unusually low for that condition. Excessive fetal wastage is produced either by extreme hypoglycemia or by an episode of ketoacidosis. The necessary reduction of insulin requirements in the first trimester can be easily accomplished if multiple serum glucose determinations and double-voided urine glucose assessments are made routinely. By the second trimester the increasing antagonism to insulin action becomes apparent, necessitating a return to approximately that dose of insulin used in the antegravid period. By the beginning of the third trimester, insulin requirements rise. Immediately after delivery the insulin requirement may again drop precipitously. During the third trimester there is an increased glomerular filtration rate in the mother, with a resulting decrease in the renal tubular reabsorption of glucose. At this point, glycosuria may also contribute to a significant reduction of serum glucose levels disproportionate to the degree of insulinization of the patient.

Although the patient in the third trimester is extremely prone to develop ketoacidosis, monitoring of urinary glucose levels may provide an overestimation of insulin requirements. For these reasons, early admission to the hospital of third-trimester patients may markedly increase fetal survival in infants of type I diabetic mothers. Excellent control of the blood glucose concentration must be maintained up to week 34 to 36 of the pregnancy. At this point, determinations of the fetal lung maturity become a paramount guide to the course of the pregnancy. If difficulties are encountered in maintaining diabetic control or if toxemia in the mother or macrosomia in the fetus develops, elective cesarean section should be considered when fetal lung maturity has occurred. The goals of management of the pregnant diabetic patient should be (1) rigid control of fasting glucose to between 80 and 100 mg/dl, (2) avoidance of glucosuria, and (3) adherence to weight schedules. Although multiple injections of mixed insulins or of regular insulin generally are adequate therapy, better results may be obtained from continuous subcutaneous insulin infusion pumps (see also Chapter 369).

REFERENCES

Adrogue HJ et al: Plasma acid-base patterns in diabetic ketoacidosis. N Engl J Med 307:1603, 1982.

American Diabetes Association: The physician's guide to type II diabetes. Alexandria, 1984, American Diabetes Association.

Bantle JP et al: Postprandial glucose and insulin responses to meals containing different carbohydrates in normal and diabetic subjects. N Engl J Med 309:7, 1983.

Bolli GB and Gerich JE: The "dawn phenomenon"—a common occurrence in both non-insulin-dependent and insulin-dependent diabetes mellitus. N Engl J Med 310:746, 1984.

Bolli GB et al: Glucose counterregulation and waning of insulin in the Somogyi phenomenon (posthypoglycemic hyperglycemia). N Engl J Med 311:1214, 1984.

Camerini-Davalos RA et al: Drug-induced reversal of early diabetic microangiopathy. N Engl J Med 309:1551, 1983.

Campbell PJ et al: Pathogenesis of the dawn phenomenon in patients with insulin-dependent diabetes mellitus. Accelerated glucose production and impaired glucose utilization due to nocturnal surges in growth hormone secretion. N Engl J Med 312:1473, 1985.

DeFronzo RA: Lilly Lecture 1987: The triumvirate: b-cell, muscle, liver. Diabetes 37(6):667-687, 1988.

Flier JS, Kahn CR, and Roth J: Receptors, antireceptor antibodies, and mechanisms of insulin resistance. N Engl J Med 300:413, 1979.

Galloway JA: Insulin treatment for the early 80s. Facts and questions about old and new insulins and their usage. Diabetes Care 3:615, 1980.

Ganda OP: Pathogenesis of macrovascular disease in the human diabetic. Diabetes 29:931, 1980.

Garber AJ, Vinik A, and Crespin SR: Detection and management of lipid disorders in diabetic patients: a commentary for clinicians. Diabetes Care 15:1068, 1992.

Hermann LS: Metformin, a review of its pharmacological properties and therapeutic use (Review). Diabete Metab 5(3):233-245, 1979.

Kreisberg RA: Diabetic ketoacidosis: new concepts and trends in pathogenesis and treatment. Ann Intern Med 88:681, 1978.

Liang JC and Goldberg MF: Treatment of diabetic retinopathy. Diabetes 29:841, 1980.

Miles JM et al: Effects of acute insulin deficiency on glucose and ketone

body turnover in man: evidence for the primacy of overproduction of glucose and ketone bodies in the genesis of diabetic ketoacidosis. Diabetes 29:926, 1980.
Owen OE, Boden G, and Shuman CR: Managing insulin-dependent diabetic patients. Postgrad Med 59:127, 1976.
Owen OE et al: Effects of therapy on the nature and quantity of fuels oxidized during diabetic ketoacidosis. Diabetes 29:365, 1980.
Polonsky K et al: Relation of counterregulatory responses to hypoglycemia in type 1 diabetes. N Engl J Med 307:1106, 1982.
Raskin P et al: The effect of diabetic control on the width of skeletal-muscle capillary basement membrane in patients with type I diabetes mellitus. N Engl J Med 309:1546, 1983.
Roy N, Chou MCY, and Field JB: Time-action characteristics of regular and NPH insulins in insulin-treated diabetics. J Clin Endocrinol Metab 50:475, 1980.
Skyler JS: Complications of diabetes mellitus: relationship to metabolic dysfunction. Diabetes Care 2:499, 1979.

CHAPTER

169 Hypoglycemia

William E. Clutter
Philip E. Cryer

PHYSIOLOGY

Certain human tissues have an obligate requirement for glucose. For example, the adult brain metabolizes approximately 150 g of glucose in a 24-hour period; even brief glucose deprivation causes severe cerebral dysfunction. Other tissues, such as muscle, fat, and liver, utilize glucose when it is plentiful (e.g., after a carbohydrate-containing meal) but can utilize other metabolic fuels. The glucose taken up by these tissues may be metabolized or stored in the form of glycogen.

In view of the obligate glucose requirements of the central nervous system, prevention of a low plasma glucose concentration (hypoglycemia) is critical to survival. Normally, the plasma glucose concentration is maintained within narrow limits by a tightly regulated balance between glucose efflux from, and influx into, the circulation. Moreover, entry of glucose from ingested carbohydrate normally is intermittent; the postprandial period is a state of enhanced glucose metabolism and storage and suppressed endogenous glucose production. In contrast, the postabsorptive period is a state of partially suppressed glucose utilization and enhanced glucose production. The latter is the result of the breakdown of glycogen (glycogenolysis) and the formation of new glucose (gluconeogenesis). Under most circumstances, endogenous glucose production can be assumed to be from the liver; the kidneys become a major source of glucose only during prolonged fasting. After an overnight fast, approximately 75% of endogenous glucose production is from glycogenolysis; the remaining 25%, from gluconeogenesis. After approximately 24 hours of fasting, virtually all the glucose produced is by gluconeogenesis (Chapter 168).

The prevention of hypoglycemia between meals requires (1) a structurally and enzymatically intact liver; (2) adequate hepatic glycogen stores and an adequate supply of gluconeogenic precursors (lactate and pyruvate, glycerol, and gluconeogenic amino acids such as alanine); and (3) appropriate regulatory signals.

The major regulatory signals involved in the transitions between the fed and the fasted state appear to be insulin and glucagon. Insulin, secreted from pancreatic beta cells into the portal circulation in response to a meal, suppresses hepatic glucose production and stimulates glucose utilization by insulin-sensitive tissues. Glucagon stimulates hepatic glucose production by both glycogenolysis and gluconeogenesis. Its secretion from pancreatic alpha cells is suppressed after a carbohydrate meal, which favors glucose conservation. In the postabsorptive state, insulin secretion is suppressed and glucagon secretion increases. This combination of low insulin and high glucagon hormonal signals results in accelerated hepatic glucose production and diminished glucose utilization.

In addition to glucagon, the adrenomedullary hormone epinephrine, the adrenocortical hormone cortisol, and the adenohypophyseal hormone growth hormone tend to promote glucose production and limit glucose utilization. Glucagon, epinephrine, cortisol, and growth hormone are often referred to as glucose counterregulatory hormones (insulin being the glucose regulatory hormone).

The mechanisms of glucose counterregulation, which prevent or correct hypoglycemia, have been clarified by recent physiologic studies of a variety of models. Recovery from hypoglycemia caused by intravenous insulin injection is not due solely to return of insulin levels to normal, but requires secretion of glucose counterregulatory hormones. Glucagon plays a primary counterregulatory role. Epinephrine, although not normally critical to correction of hypoglycemia, compensates and becomes critical when glucagon is deficient. Growth hormone and cortisol are not necessary for recovery from acute insulin-induced hypoglycemia, but play roles in defense against prolonged hypoglycemia.

The transition from exogenous glucose delivery to endogenous glucose production after glucose ingestion is the result of coordinated diminution of insulin secretion and resumption of initially suppressed glucagon secretion. The plasma level of epinephrine normally rises several hours after glucose ingestion, but this increase is not critical for prevention of hypoglycemia. When glucagon secretion is deficient, however, enhanced epinephrine secretion prevents hypoglycemia.

To prevent hypoglycemia in the postabsorptive (overnight fasted) state, or after a 3-day fast, insulin secretion must decrease appropriately, and secretion of glucagon or epinephrine, or both, must be intact. Physiologic studies have not shown an important role for growth hormone or cortisol in preventing hypoglycemia. Nevertheless, patients with chronic deficiencies of these hormones occasionally develop fasting hypoglycemia.

Thus, the following principles (summarized in Fig. 169-1) govern glucose counterregulation:

1. Glucose counterregulation is not due solely to dissipation of insulin but rather to the coordinated dissipation of insulin and activation of counterregulatory systems.
2. Glucagon plays a primary counterregulatory role.
3. Epinephrine is not normally required for glucose counterregulation but compensates to a large degree when glucagon secretion is deficient (e.g., during insulin-induced hypoglycemia in type I diabetes mellitus). Hypoglycemia occurs or progresses only when both glucagon and epinephrine are deficient and insulin is present, or when insulin action is excessive.
4. Although other hormones, neural mechanisms, or glucose autoregulation may be involved in counterregulation, they are not sufficiently potent to prevent or correct hypoglycemia when both glucagon and epinephrine are deficient and insulin is present.

In keeping with their role in prevention as well as correction of hypoglycemia, the glycemic thresholds for release of epinephrine, glucagon, and growth hormone in response to a decline in plasma glucose lie within or just below the physiologic plasma glucose range and well above the threshold for symptoms of hypoglycemia.

Prolonged fasting is the only state in which obligate glucose utilization by the brain has been shown to decrease. During prolonged fasting, the central nervous system utilizes ketone bodies as well as glucose as fuels.

CLINICAL SYNDROMES

Clinical manifestations of hypoglycemia

The symptoms caused by hypoglycemia can be divided into two categories: (1) neurogenic (autonomic) symptoms due to the sympathoadrenal discharge triggered by a falling plasma glucose level and (2) neuroglycopenic symptoms due to cerebral glucose deprivation.

Typical neurogenic manifestations include tachycardia, palpitations, anxiety, and sweating. The magnitude of the sympathoadrenal response to decrements in plasma glucose is inversely related to the glucose nadir, so in general, the lower the plasma glucose concentration, the more intense the neurogenic symptoms. Very gradual declines in plasma glucose, however, appear to elicit a less vigorous sympathoadrenal response, and neurogenic manifestations may be subtle or imperceptible if moderate hypoglycemia develops insidiously. The recent finding that one episode of hypoglycemia diminishes symptomatic and counterregulatory responses to subsequent hypoglycemia may explain some instances of minimally symptomatic hypoglycemia.

Neuroglycopenic manifestations range from subtle mental impairment to coma and death. Between these extremes, symptoms may include headache, lethargy, hunger, visual symptoms, confusion, behavioral changes, incoordination, seizures, and impairment of motor and sensory functions. Both hypothermia during hypoglycemia and posthypoglycemic fever have been described. Although neuroglycopenic symptoms generally correlate with the degree of hypoglycemia, some patients appear to tolerate low plasma glucose concentrations relatively well. This ability presumably reflects adaptation of the brain to hypoglycemia, perhaps by altered transport of glucose across the blood-brain barrier.

Hypoglycemic symptoms typically clear rapidly after the plasma glucose concentration is restored to normal. More gradual clearing of neuroglycopenic symptoms over hours, or even days, sometimes follows profound hypoglycemia. Prolonged, severe hypoglycemia can cause permanent cerebral damage.

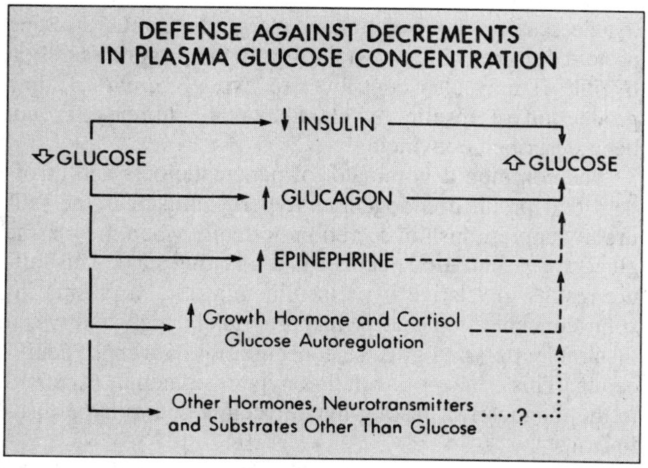

Fig. 169-1. Normal glucose counterregulation. The hierarchy of the redundant glucoregulatory factors involved in prevention or correction of hypoglycemia during decrements in plasma glucose counterregulation in normal humans. (From Cryer PE and Gerich JE: Hypoglycemia in insulin dependent diabetes mellitus: insulin excess and defective glucose counterregulation. In Rifkin H and Porte D, editors: *Ellenberg and Rifkin's Diabetes Mellitus,* ed 4, New York, 1989, Elsevier.

Classification of hypoglycemia

It is clinically convenient to divide patients with hypoglycemia into two broad categories: (1) those with fasting (or postabsorptive) hypoglycemia and (2) those with reactive (or postprandial) hypoglycemia. Fasting hypoglycemia is generally due to serious, potentially life-threatening disorders and requires aggressive diagnostic and therapeutic intervention. In contrast, reactive hypoglycemia (in the absence of fasting hypoglycemia) is usually due to a nonprogressive disorder that, although bothersome, is rarely life-threatening.

Pathophysiology of fasting hypoglycemia

The major causes of fasting hypoglycemia are outlined in the accompanying box. Hypoglycemia occurs when glucose use exceeds glucose production. Fasting hypoglycemia in patients with the various forms of hyperinsulinism and in those with tumors secreting insulin-like hormones is best attributed to suppressed hepatic glucose production coupled with inappropriately high rates of glucose utilization. Impaired hepatic glucose production with ongoing obligate

Causes of fasting hypoglycemia

- Drugs
  - Insulin
  - Sulfonylureas
  - Ethanol
  - Salicylates
  - Pentamidine
  - Quinine
- Critical organ failure
  - Renal failure
  - Hepatic failure
  - Cardiac failure
  - Sepsis
  - Malnutrition
- Hormonal deficiencies
  - Cortisol
  - Growth hormone
  - Glucagon plus epinephrine
- Extrapancreatic tumors
- Endogenous hyperinsulinism
  - Pancreatic beta-cell disorders: neoplastic (insulinoma), hyperplastic, or functional
  - Insulin secretagogues (e.g., sulfonylureas)
  - Autoimmune hypoglycemias: antibodies to insulin, antibodies to insulin receptors
- Hypoglycemias of infancy and childhood
  - Neonatal hypoglycemias
  - Congenital deficiencies of glucogenic enzymes
  - Ketotic hypoglycemia of childhood

glucose utilization (e.g., by the brain) is believed to be the predominant mechanism of fasting hypoglycemia due to drugs, hormonal deficits, hepatic dysfunction, chronic renal failure, and the childhood hypoglycemic disorders. Clearly, conditions characterized by accelerated glucose utilization, such as vigorous exercise and pregnancy, could exacerbate fasting hypoglycemia due to any of the disorders listed. Accelerated glucose utilization alone, however, seldom results in fasting hypoglycemia because of the normal capacity to increase glucose production.

By far the most common cause of hypoglycemia is therapy of diabetes mellitus with insulin or sulfonylureas. Although hypoglycemia is a major therapeutic limitation in diabetes, it seldom presents a diagnostic problem. These drugs may also be used to produce factitious hypoglycemia, however, especially among medical personnel and others with knowledge of diabetes. Ethanol inhibits gluconeogenesis but not glycogenolysis. Thus it causes hypoglycemia only when hepatic glycogen is depleted, in fasting or malnourished individuals. Salicylates cause hypoglycemia in children by an unknown mechanism. Pentamidine and quinine stimulate insulin release and presumably cause hypoglycemia by this means. A number of other drugs have been associated with hypoglycemia, but in most cases, other potential causes of hypoglycemia were present and a clear causal relationship was not established.

Renal insufficiency is a major factor associated with hypoglycemia in hospitalized patients. The mechanisms are not known, although the majority of patients who develop hypoglycemia are malnourished. The development of renal failure in diabetes mellitus often reduces insulin requirements and increases the risk of hypoglycemia.

Hepatic disease can cause hypoglycemia due to inadequate glucose production. Because the liver is normally able to increase glucose output severalfold, hepatic dysfunction must be rather severe to cause hypoglycemia.

Hypoglycemia in patients with cardiac failure or sepsis is probably secondary to impairment of hepatic and renal function. Hypoglycemia has rarely been attributed to malnutrition without other disorders.

Adrenocortical insufficiency commonly leads to anorexia and weight loss. Further, cortisol is required to maintain normal levels of hepatic gluconeogenic enzymes and to mobilize gluconeogenic precursors; it also antagonizes the effects of insulin. Deficiency of growth hormone produces enhanced insulin sensitivity. Despite these effects, most adults with cortisol or growth hormone deficiency, or both, do not develop hypoglycemia. On the other hand, hypoglycemia is an important manifestation of these disorders in children. Combined deficiency of glucagon and epinephrine occurs in some patients with insulin-dependent diabetes mellitus and greatly increases the risk of insulin-induced hypoglycemia. Deficiency of either glucagon or epinephrine alone, however, would not be expected to produce hypoglycemia, and indeed, hypoglycemia due to deficiency of either or both has not been shown convincingly in nondiabetic patients.

Fasting hypoglycemia occurs in some patients with large extrapancreatic tumors, especially mesenchymal tumors such as mesotheliomas and retroperitoneal sarcomas, and hepatic and adrenal carcinomas. In many cases, hypoglycemia appears to be caused by a combination of tumor production of insulin-like growth factor II (IGF-II) or its precursor and increased access of IGF-II to target tissues due to a decrease in sequestration by a large plasma IGF-binding protein complex. Suppression of growth hormone secretion by IGF-II may also contribute to hypoglycemia. Ectopic production of insulin by extrapancreatic tumors has not been described convincingly.

The common denominator of pancreatic beta-cell disorders that produce endogenous hyperinsulinism is the failure to suppress insulin secretion normally when the plasma glucose concentration declines in the fasting state. This failure results in relative hyperinsulinemia, i.e., a plasma insulin concentration that is inappropriately high relative to the ambient plasma glucose concentration, during hypoglycemia. This concept of relative hyperinsulinemia is central to the diagnosis of fasting hypoglycemia due to hyperinsulinism.

Intermittent hypoglycemia with inappropriately high serum free insulin concentrations has been recognized in a few patients found to have serum antibodies to insulin. It is presumed that insulin periodically dissociates from these antibodies, causing hyperinsulinism and hypoglycemia. In the absence of a history of insulin injection, these antibodies are considered to be autoantibodies to insulin. Autoantibodies to the insulin receptor usually produce insulin resistance, but in some patients they may cause hypoglycemia, presumably by mimicking the effects of insulin.

A number of hypoglycemic disorders are unique to, or typically present in, infancy or childhood. Transient neonatal hypoglycemia in infants of diabetic mothers is thought to be due to chronic fetal hyperglycemia with resultant fetal hypersecretion of insulin that persists for a time after birth. Many neonates who are small for gestational age suffer from transient hypoglycemia, which appears to be due to delayed induction of one or more gluconeogenic enzymes.

Ketotic hypoglycemia of childhood is a poorly understood syndrome that presents between the ages of 1 and 5 years, remits before the age of 10 years, and is characterized by fasting hypoglycemia with normal suppression of insulin secretion. Because normal children develop hypoglycemia with somewhat longer fasts, these patients may simply represent one extreme of the normal distribution of glucose production during fasting.

Pathophysiology of reactive hypoglycemia

Several disorders are known to cause reactive hypoglycemia. Alimentary hypoglycemia in patients who have undergone gastrectomy or gastric bypass is due to rapid entry of ingested carbohydrate into the small intestine, with a rapid rise in plasma glucose during the first hour. This early hyperglycemia, and perhaps enhanced secretion of insulinotropic gut factors, stimulates marked hyperinsulinemia. Hypoglycemia occurs during the second hour, due to persistent effects of the marked insulin response concomitant with cessation of intestinal glucose absorption.

Postprandial hypoglycemia can also occur in patients with the rare enzymatic defects, galactosemia and hereditary fructose intolerance, which are apparent in childhood.

Based on oral glucose tolerance testing, the diagnosis of idiopathic or functional reactive hypoglycemia has been made in patients without these known causes. Very few, if any, of these patients have hypoglycemia during daily life (after ordinary meals or during spontaneous symptoms), and most have evidence of psychiatric disorders. Thus hypoglycemia during a glucose tolerance test does not establish the cause of symptoms in daily life. Similarly, although reactive hypoglycemia has been attributed to early type II diabetes, it has never been shown that these patients have symptoms due to hypoglycemia.

CLINICAL AND LABORATORY DIAGNOSIS

Documentation and classification of hypoglycemia

The presence of hypoglycemia is often suspected on the basis of a history compatible with neurogenic or neuroglycopenic symptoms. Although sometimes compelling, the history is more often only suggestive, as such symptoms are commonly due to a variety of other disorders. Thus the diagnosis of hypoglycemia is suspected much more often than it is confirmed. Occasionally, a hypoglycemic disorder is first suspected because of a low glucose level in a plasma sample obtained for other reasons.

Once suspected, the diagnosis of hypoglycemia is most convincingly established when it is based on Whipple's triad: symptoms consistent with hypoglycemia, a concomitant low plasma glucose concentration, and relief of symptoms after the glucose level is raised to normal. The diagnosis of a hypoglycemic disorder is seldom tenable in the absence of consistent symptoms.

Symptoms that occur more than several hours after meals, often after exercise, raise the possibility of fasting hypoglycemia. Symptoms that occur shortly after meals raise the possibility of reactive hypoglycemia, but these symptoms can also occur at this time in patients with fasting hypoglycemia; the differential diagnosis in such patients is that of fasting hypoglycemia.

Fasting hypoglycemia

Patients with fasting hypoglycemia may have plasma glucose levels below 45 mg/dl (2.5 mmol/L) after a 10- to 12-hour overnight fast, especially with repeated measurements. Thus the first diagnostic step in suspected fasting hypoglycemia is to measure the plasma glucose concentration after an overnight fast, on several days if necessary. A value less than 45 mg/dl documents the presence of fasting hypoglycemia. If plasma glucose is greater than 45 mg/dl after an overnight fast, the fast should be prolonged until symptomatic hypoglycemia with a plasma glucose less than 45 mg/dl occurs, or for a maximum of 72 hours. Plasma glucose should be measured at least every 4 hours (more frequently as plasma glucose falls) and when symptoms occur. Bedside glucose monitoring devices may be used for rapid estimation, but are not accurate enough for definitive diagnosis; laboratory measurements should be performed. Symptomatic hypoglycemia usually occurs within the first 24 hours of a diagnostic fast in affected patients. A period of exercise at the end of a prolonged fast may precipitate hypoglycemia in an affected patient, in contrast to the normal stability of plasma glucose during exercise.

When symptomatic hypoglycemia with a plasma glucose less than 45 mg/dl occurs, certain tests should be performed to distinguish among possible causes. Plasma insulin and C-peptide should be measured, preferably on several samples, before the fast is ended, and a plasma or urine assay for sulfonylureas should be performed.

Failure of the plasma glucose concentration to fall below 50 mg/dl during a prolonged fast, particularly if a period of exercise is included, excludes the diagnosis of fasting hypoglycemia. In men, fasting plasma glucose values below 50 mg/dl document the presence of fasting hypoglycemia. The same statement cannot be made for women or children, in whom plasma glucose concentrations commonly fall below 50 mg/dl in the absence of symptoms during a prolonged fast. If values below 50 mg/dl are associated with unequivocal symptoms in a woman or a child, fasting hypoglycemia has been documented. If not, convincing biochemical evidence is required for diagnosis of a fasting hypoglycemic disorder (see below).

The differential diagnosis of fasting hypoglycemia can be narrowed rapidly with standard clinical data. A history of the use of insulin or other offending drugs may be obtained. Surreptitious use of hypoglycemic drugs, however, may be difficult to detect and requires screening of urine or plasma for such agents. Sulfonylureas may be inadvertently substituted for another drug, so the identity of each of the patient's medications should be confirmed by inspection. Critical organ dysfunction severe enough to cause hypoglycemia will be apparent clinically and with routine laboratory tests. Extrapancreatic tumors associated with hypoglycemia generally are large and clinically evident. The hypoglycemias of childhood are self-limited, except in patients with congenital enzymatic defects in whom associated findings suggest the diagnosis. In the absence of these causes, the differential diagnosis is limited to excessive insulin secretion or deficient glucose counterregulatory hormone secretion.

Hypoglycemia stimulates the secretion of cortisol, growth hormone, glucagon, and epinephrine. Thus the finding of elevated plasma concentrations of these hormones during spontaneous (or insulin-induced) hypoglycemia excludes deficiencies. It is conventional to assess the adequacy of growth hormone and cortisol secretion in patients with fasting hypoglycemia (Chapter 150). Because deficiencies of glucagon or epinephrine rarely if ever cause hypoglycemia except in patients with insulin-dependent diabetes, these hormones usually are not measured.

Diagnosis of hyperinsulinism requires the demonstration of an inappropriately elevated plasma insulin level during hypoglycemia. Plasma insulin concentrations are often not elevated above the fasting reference range. Because normal insulin secretion nearly ceases when the plasma glucose concentration falls to less than 45 mg/dl, plasma insulin concentrations should be measured when the fasting plasma glucose falls below this level. In such samples, a plasma insulin concentration greater than 10 μU/ml (60 pmol/L) is diagnostic of hyperinsulinism, and a concentration greater than 5 μU/ml is suspect and warrants further investigation.

Measurement of plasma C-peptide (the connecting peptide cleaved from proinsulin during conversion to insulin) can distinguish endogenous hyperinsulinism from surreptitious insulin administration. When plasma glucose is less than 45 mg/dl, a plasma C-peptide level greater than 1.5 ng/ml (0.5 nmol/L) confirms that hyperinsulinism is of endogenous origin, and a level greater than 1.0 ng/ml indicates probable endogenous origin. C-peptide levels are suppressed below these values in patients with exogenous hyperinsulinism (except in the presence of insulin antibodies—see below). In factitious hypoglycemia due to sulfonylureas, C-peptide levels are elevated, and tests for these drugs in plasma or urine are indicated, especially if the patient has access to these drugs.

Most patients with pancreatic beta-cell neoplasms have increased plasma levels of proinsulin. Although currently available only in research laboratories, specific proinsulin radioimmunoassays have a high degree of sensitivity for insulinomas and may be useful in confirming the results of a diagnostic fast. Other conditions, however, produce elevated proinsulin levels, so the diagnosis cannot be made on this basis alone.

The presence of circulating antibodies to insulin in patients with no history of insulin use suggests surreptitious insulin injection or autoimmune hypoglycemia. Such antibodies produce artifactually high values for plasma insulin in double-antibody immunoassays, and by binding endogenous proinsulin, which contains the C-peptide sequence, they also elevate plasma total C-peptide immunoreactivity. Methods are available for measuring free insulin and C-peptide levels in the presence of insulin antibodies. Injection of human insulin produces a much smaller immune response than animal insulins. Therefore surreptitious use of human insulin may produce hypoglycemia in the absence of detectable antibodies to insulin. This diagnosis will still be evident, however, from the combination of elevated plasma insulin and suppressed plasma C-peptide levels.

In summary, evaluation of a patient with fasting hypoglycemia should include a diagnostic fast, with measurement of plasma insulin and C-peptide when the plasma glucose is less than 45 mg/dl (and preferably several such measurements), along with assay for sulfonylureas and antibodies to insulin. If the diagnosis remains unexplained, assays for antibodies to the insulin receptor, for proinsulin, and for insulin-like growth factors may be of value and can be obtained from research laboratories. The differential diagnosis of hyperinsulinism is summarized in Table 169-1.

The preceding discussion assumes accurate measurement of the plasma glucose concentration. Artifactual lowering of the measured glucose level (pseudohypoglycemia) can occur if separation of the plasma from the formed elements of the blood is delayed for several hours, especially if glucose utilization by the formed elements is excessive (e.g., marked leukocytosis). This can be avoided by prompt centrifugation of the blood sample or by the use of special sampling tubes containing an inhibitor of glycolysis.

Reactive hypoglycemia

The prevalence of reactive hypoglycemia is unknown, largely because there are no widely accepted criteria for its diagnosis. There is strong evidence, however, that it is a very uncommon disorder that is erroneously diagnosed all too often.

Reactive hypoglycemia cannot be diagnosed on the basis of an oral glucose tolerance test, as plasma glucose concentrations reach nadirs less than 50 mg/dl after glucose ingestion in 10% of normal asymptomatic persons. Our diagnostic approach is to perform a 5-hour glucose tolerance test (with plasma glucose measurements at 30-minute intervals) and to ask the patient to record all symptoms and their time of occurrence. Unless typical symptoms occur, and both coincide with low plasma glucose values and abate as plasma glucose levels rise (Whipple's triad), the diagnosis of reactive hypoglycemia can be confidently excluded. The diagnosis can only be established, however, by frequent measurements of plasma glucose (along with a record of symptoms) after ordinary mixed meals, and if symptoms coincide with low plasma glucose levels after in-

Table 169-1. Differential diagnosis of hyperinsulinism

	Postabsorptive venous plasma glucose <45 mg/dl			
	Insulin	C peptide	Insulin antibodies	Other
Exogenous hyperinsulinism	↑	↓†	+	
Endogenous hyperinsulinism				
Insulinoma	↑	↑	—	↑ Proinsulin
Sulfonylurea	↑	↑	—	Positive sulfonylurea assay
Autoimmune hypoglycemia				
Antibodies to insulin	↑↑↑*	↓†	+	
Antibodies to insulin receptor	↑	?	—	Insulin receptor antibodies present; associated autoimmune disorder

*Insulin antibodies artifactually increase insulin levels measured by double-antibody radioimmunoassay.
†Free C-peptide levels are low, but total C-peptide levels may not be because of cross reactivity with antibody-bound proinsulin.

gestion of normal meals, and if fasting hypoglycemia has been carefully excluded.

SPECIFIC DISEASE ENTITIES

Only pancreatic beta-cell abnormalities causing endogenous hyperinsulinism are discussed here. The other disorders that may cause hypoglycemia are discussed elsewhere in this book.

Endogenous hyperinsulinism in adults is almost always due to pancreatic beta-cell tumors or insulinomas, which can occur anywhere in the pancreas. In about 80% of cases there is a single benign adenoma, whereas about 10% of cases are due to multiple benign adenomas, and 5% to 10% are due to carcinomas. Insulinomas occur in all age groups, although two thirds are diagnosed between the ages of 30 and 60 years. Approximately 60% of reported cases have been in women.

Most children with hyperinsulinism do not have insulinomas or other currently detectable pathologic lesions. Nesidioblastosis islet cells interspersed among pancreatic exocrine cells), once believed to be the basis for hyperinsulinism, is a normal finding in infants and is not associated with hypoglycemia.

Islet cell tumors, often multiple and including beta-cell tumors, are one component of the multiple endocrine neoplasia type I syndrome, along with hyperparathyroidism and pituitary tumors. This familial disorder is inherited as an autosomal dominant trait.

Ectopic secretion of insulin from extrapancreatic tumors has not been convincingly documented. Thus in an adult, fasting hypoglycemia due to hyperinsulinism implies the presence of an insulinoma, if factitious hypoglycemia has been excluded. Fasting hypoglycemia without hyperinsulinism can occur in many kinds of extrapancreatic neoplasms.

TREATMENT

Fasting hypoglycemia

Management of fasting hypoglycemia requires urgent treatment, diagnosis, and long-term prevention. The short-term treatment of hypoglycemia is the oral or intravenous administration of glucose. Glucagon (1.0 mg intramuscularly), which promotes hepatic glucose release, can be used when immediate glucose administration is impractical. The effect of glucagon is transient, however, and may not be great. Thus exogenous glucose administration should be started as soon as possible. It is common practice to give 25 to 50 g of glucose (in the form of a 50% glucose solution) by rapid intravenous injection immediately after drawing a sample for glucose determination and a sample to be saved for additional diagnostic studies. The plasma glucose concentration is then followed to ensure that hypoglycemia does not recur; continuous glucose infusions may be required to prevent recurrent hypoglycemia in some disorders.

After initial control of the hypoglycemia, attention can be turned to determining the hypoglycemic mechanism. Drug-induced hypoglycemia can be treated with glucose infusion (and drug withdrawal) alone. Documented hormonal deficits can be treated by hormone replacement. Hypoglycemia associated with extrapancreatic tumors may improve with reduction in tumor size achieved through surgery, chemotherapy, or radiotherapy. Hepatic dysfunction extensive enough to cause hypoglycemia is generally incompatible with survival, if it is not reversible. Recurrent fasting hypoglycemia associated with inanition, as in chronic renal failure, may respond to a high-caloric intake with frequent feedings.

The primary treatment of fasting hypoglycemia due to endogenous hyperinsulinism is surgical excision of the beta-cell abnormality. Computed tomography of the abdomen should be performed before surgery, although only a minority of beta-cell tumors can be detected. Some physicians also recommend angiography, which visualizes some tumors. Because insulinomas are usually small (median diameter 1 to 2 cm), negative examinations do not exclude their presence. In patients with fasting hypoglycemia clearly due to endogenous hyperinsulinism, many physicians recommend laparotomy, even in the absence of radiographic evidence of a pancreatic mass. In this setting, palpation by an experienced surgeon combined with intraoperative ultrasound examination of the pancreas allows successful removal of an insulinoma in the great majority of patients. At some centers, percutaneous pancreatic venous sampling is performed in an attempt to determine the region of the pancreas in which the tumor lies, but the benefits of this procedure have not been shown to outweigh its risks.

Solitary pancreatic tumors can be enucleated. Multiple tumors should be resected as much as possible, and sufficient pancreatic tissue to preserve function should be left. Because reduction of total tumor mass, even without cure, may render the patient euglycemic, total pancreatectomy should not be the primary procedure.

If a pancreatic tumor cannot be located at laparotomy, the optimal management is not clearly defined. Progressive pancreatic resection beginning with the tail is often recommended, but it may be preferable to forego resection and pursue further localizing studies.

In a collected series, 95% of patients with benign insulinomas were euglycemic after surgery. Complications include pancreatitis, pancreatic fistulae, and infections. Permanent diabetes may follow extensive pancreatic resection.

Medical palliation of hyperinsulinism that is not surgically correctable includes frequent oral feedings. Diazoxide, a drug that suppresses insulin secretion, may ameliorate hypoglycemia. Side effects include edema, nausea, and hypertrichosis, among others. The somatostatin analog octreotide ameliorates hypoglycemia in some patients, but is ineffective or worsens hypoglycemia in others. Chemotherapy may palliate symptoms in some patients with metastatic islet cell carcinomas; a combination of streptozocin and doxorubicin appears most effective.

Reactive hypoglycemia

No therapy has been shown to be effective, but a diet that includes frequent meals and avoidance of simple sugars is reasonable.

REFERENCES

Boyle PJ and Cryer PE: Growth hormone, cortisol, or both are involved in defense against, but are not critical to recovery from, hypoglycemia, Am J Physiol 260:E395-E402, 1991.

Cryer PE: Glucose homeostasis and hypoglycemia. In Foster DW and Wilson JD, editors: Williams textbook of endocrinology, ed 8, Philadelphia, 1992, WB Saunders.

Daughaday WH and Deuel TF: Tumor secretion of growth factors, Endocrinol Metab Clin North Am 20:539-63, 1991.

Doherty GM et al: Results of a prospective strategy to diagnose, localize, and resect insulinomas, Surgery 110:989-997, 1991.

Grunberger G et al: Factitious hypoglycemia due to surreptitious administration of insulin: diagnosis, treatment and long-term follow-up, Ann Intern Med 108:252-57, 1988.

Haymond MW: Hypoglycemia in infants and children, Endocrinol Metab Clin North Am 18:211-252, 1989.

Heller SR, Cryer PE: Reduced neuroendocrine and symptomatic responses to subsequent hypoglycemia after one episode of hypoglycemia in nondiabetic humans, Diabetes 40:223-226, 1991.

Hogan MJ et al: Oral glucose tolerance test compared with a mixed meal in the diagnosis of reactive hypoglycemia: a caveat on stimulation, Mayo Clin Proc 58:491-496, 1983.

Maton PN: The use of the long-acting somatostatin analogue, octreotide acetate, in patients with islet cell tumors, Gastroenterol Clin North Am 18:897-922, 1989.

Moertel CG et al: Streptozocin-doxorubicin, streptozocin-fluorouracil, or chlorozotocin in the treatment of advanced islet-cell carcinoma, N Engl J Med 326:519-523, 1992.

Rothmund M et al: Surgery for benign insulinoma: an international review, World J Surg 14:393-99, 1990.

Service FJ: Hypoglycemias, West J Med 154:442-454, 1991.

Service FJ et al: Functioning insulinoma—incidence, recurrence and long-term survival of patients: a 60 year study, Mayo Clin Proc 66:711-719, 1991.

Snorgaard O, Binder C: Monitoring of blood glucose concentration in subjects with hypoglycemic symptoms during everyday life, Br Med J 300:16-18, 1990.

CHAPTER

170 Heritable Disorders of Carbohydrate Metabolism

Alan J. Garber

NONDIABETIC MELLITURIAS

The nondiabetic melliturias comprise a heterogeneous group of disorders united solely by the presence of a reducing sugar in the urine. False-positive urine tests that can result from drug administration must be excluded. A variety of pharmacologic preparations such as levodopa, excessive quantities of salicylates, ascorbic acid, chloral hydrate, and x-ray contrast media can produce false-positive urine sugar testing using the Clinitest copper reduction method for reducing substances in urine. On the other hand, these same agents are capable of producing false-negative results in the presence of glucose when glucose oxidase enzyme strips are used, as they interfere with the coupling of the peroxide generated by glucose oxidase to the color-developing system in the enzyme strips. False-positive results with glucose oxidase testing generally result from oxidizing agents such as hypochlorite and peroxides. In all instances, the finding of glucosuria or glycosuria requires a careful evaluation to firmly exclude the diagnosis of diabetes mellitus.

Renal glucosuria

See Chapter 360.

Pentosuria

Pentosuria originally was described more than 80 years ago; since then, over 200 cases of patients with pentosuria have been reported in the literature. In all instances, the pentose excreted appears to be xylulose, although small amounts of L-arbitol have been isolated from the urine in some patients. In all patients thus far examined, the excretion of L-xylulose ranges between 1 and 4 g/day. This amount is virtually constant on a daily basis within the same patient and is largely unaffected by dietary pentose intake. The inheritance pattern of this autosomal recessive disease is largely confined to patients of Eastern European Jewish extraction and to a lesser number of Lebanese origin.

A diagnosis of pentosuria should be suspected in all patients having positive reducing substances in their urine that are consistently negative for glucose using glucose oxidase enzymatic strips. Diabetes mellitus also should be excluded in these patients. Further chemical testing of the reducing substance in the urine must demonstrate substantial quantities of L-xylulose. Pentosuria was originally classified as an inborn error of metabolism by Garrod in 1908. Subsequent studies have demonstrated that the metabolic defect arises from a deficiency of L-xylitol dehydrogenase ($NADP^+$). This enzyme catalyzes the reduction of xylulose to xylitol, an important step in the metabolism of glucuronic acid. Heterozygous states may be detected by using glucuronic acid loading with subsequent assessments of serum xylulose levels. Alternatively, the activity of the NADP-L-xylulose dehydrogenase may be assayed directly in red cells of the patient suspected of having this metabolic defect. Because this abnormality is harmless and individuals manifest no symptomatology, no treatment is necessary.

Essential fructosuria

In addition to pentoses such as L-xylulose, nonglucose reducing sugars such as fructose also may be found in the urine of otherwise asymptomatic patients. Patients having essential fructosuria excrete variable amounts of fructose, depending on the dietary intake of that sugar. Fructosuria is a relatively rare, genetically transmitted, inborn error of metabolism and is most probably an autosomal recessive disorder in patients having the fully developed expression of the defect. Although fructosuria is somewhat more common in patients of Jewish ancestry, the proportion of Jewish subjects to the total number of cases reported is lower than that with pentosuria. Fructosuria should be suspected in all nondiabetics having a nonglucose-reducing substance in the urine. However, specific enzymatic or chromatographic techniques are necessary for further elucidation of the reducing sugar present in the urine.

Fructosuria is believed to result from a relative or absolute deficiency in the activity of the first enzyme of hepatic fructose metabolism, fructokinase (Fig. 170-1). This enzyme, which rapidly phosphorylates fructose to form fructose 1-phosphate, is absent in essential fructosuria. Fructose excretion depends largely on the amount of fructose ingested. Renal disposal of ingested fructose may account for the clearance of 20% to 25% of the total ingested fructose. Fructosuria is an entirely benign condition. Unlike the more serious inborn error of fructose metabolism (hereditary fructose intolerance), benign fructosuria does not produce any other disturbance of intermediary metabolism. For this reason, no treatment is necessary.

Other forms of nondiabetic mellituria

A variety of other monosaccharides and disaccharides may appear in the urine of patients because of impaired or absent enzymatic function necessary for the disposal of these

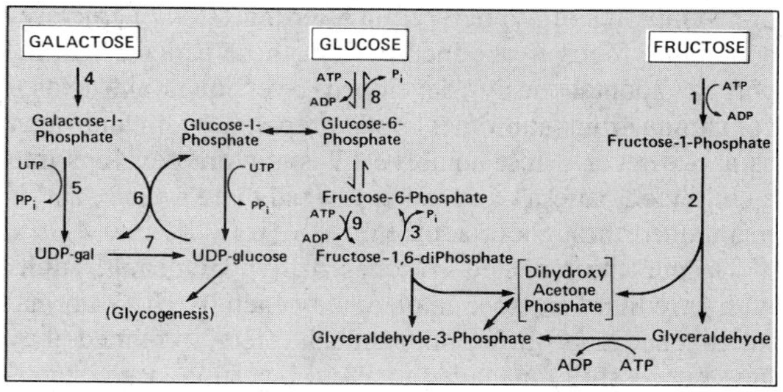

Fig. 170-1. Pathways of hexose metabolism in humans.

Enzyme	Deficiency state
1 Fructokinase	Essential fructosuria
2 Fructose-1-phosphate aldolase	Hereditary fructose intolerance
3 Fructose-1,6-diphosphatase	Fructose-1,6-diphosphatase deficiency
4 Galactokinase	Galactosemia
5 UDP galactose pyrophosphorylase	Galactosemia
6 Gal-1-phosphate uridyltransferase	Galactosemia
7 UDP glucose epimerase	Galactosemia
8 Glucose-6-phosphatase	Glycogen storage disease (GSD) type I (hepatorenal)
9 Phosphofructokinase	GSD type VII

sugars or because of a vast dietary intake that exceeds the capacity of normal enzyme activities to dispose rapidly of these sugars. In almost all instances, these forms of nondiabetic mellituria are not of clinical significance. Galactosuria may be noted occasionally in normal subjects ingesting large quantities of this monosaccharide. More commonly, galactosuria is seen in concert with galactosemia.

Mannoheptulose is a seven-carbon monosaccharide found in relatively large quantities in avocados. Accordingly, mannoheptulosuria may be observed in normal individuals after the ingestion of large amounts of this fruit. This condition is of no clinical consequence. Lactose may appear occasionally in the urine of women late in the third trimester of pregnancy. It also may be seen in patients with severe intestinal disease without lactase deficiency. In no event is lactosuria of major clinical consequence. Ingestion of large quantities of cane sugar may be followed occasionally by sucrosuria in otherwise normal individuals. In certain instances, patients with cystic fibrosis have also been described with sucrosuria after ingestion of sucrose.

Hereditary fructose intolerance

Although this autosomal recessive trait generally makes its appearance clinically at an early age, hereditary fructose intolerance was first diagnosed in an adult patient.

Hereditary fructose intolerance has two major clinical manifestations. In previously undiagnosed adults, a relatively characteristic history of nausea, vomiting, and cerebral symptoms of hypoglycemia after ingestion of fructose-containing foods is obtained. Often, these patients will report a spontaneously developed aversion to fructose-containing fruits and other foods prepared with cane sugar as a sweetener. Most notably, this symptom develops into a childhood pattern of aversion to candy and sweets, and is maintained throughout adult life.

Despite the repeated episodes of hypoglycemia, adults with hereditary fructose intolerance generally show normal intelligence and suffer no residual effect, provided they have successfully managed to avoid ingesting large quantities of fructose. In marked contradistinction to this relatively benign presentation in adults, children with hereditary fructose intolerance frequently manifest nausea, vomiting, cerebral dysfunction, and generalized failure to thrive. On occasion, the attacks of hypoglycemia can be so severe that they produce unconsciousness and tonic seizures. Physical examination may show hepatosplenomegaly and perhaps icterus. There may be ascites and marked liver dysfunction. Initial screening laboratory data in children with hereditary fructose intolerance may be markedly abnormal, with moderately severe elevations of serum glutamic-oxalacetic transaminase and serum pyruvate-oxalacetic transaminase. There may be hyperbilirubinemia and other findings of liver dysfunction as well as phosphaturia, glycosuria, bicarbonate wasting, and aminoaciduria. In contrast, adults may manifest few, if any, detectable biochemical abnormalities under routine screening procedures. In all instances, fasting blood sugars and serum phosphate levels are normal.

The key biochemical defect in hereditary fructose intolerance is the virtual absence of fructose 1-phosphate aldolase (aldolase B) activity owing to nonsense, missense, or splice site mutations. This second enzyme of fructose metabolism catalyzes the cleavage of fructose 1-phosphate into dihydroxyacetone phosphate and glyceraldehyde. The latter two compounds are subsequently degraded within the glycolytic pathway, ultimately to form pyruvic acid. Thus an absence of fructose 1-phosphate aldolase results in the accumulation of substantial quantities of fructose 1-phosphate in liver and in other tissues having a significant activity of fructokinase. After fructose ingestion, fructose 1-phosphate levels rise rapidly in the hepatocyte, thereby serving as a sink for inorganic phosphate and ultimately resulting in a relative depletion of adenosine triphosphate (ATP) in the hepatocyte. Because inorganic phosphate is a major determinant of the rate of oxidative phosphorylation by mitochondria, its depletion, together with a resulting loss of ATP, results in hypoglycemia, owing to a failure of hepatic glycogenolysis and gluconeogenesis. Additional direct effects of the accumulated excess fructose 1-phosphate on hepatic phosphorylase also may account for the lack of responsiveness of patients to exogenous glucagon during a hypoglycemic episode. The defect in fructose 1-phosphate aldolase appears to be an autosomal recessive trait. Asymptomatic carrier states having approximately one-half of normal enzymatic activities have been identified. In these carriers, recent studies using phosphorous NMR have shown abnormal hepatic energy metabolism on fructose loading and a clear tendency to hyperuricemia.

A diagnosis of hereditary fructose intolerance can be made by the demonstration of characteristic hypoglycemia and hypophosphatemia after fructose administration. Fructose may be given orally or, preferably, intravenously at a dose of 0.5 g/kg of body weight. This dose may be excessive for a relatively malnourished child or infant, but it is appropriate for adults or well-nourished children. Hypoglycemia in adults is observed 60 to 90 minutes after fructose ingestion, whereas in children the hypoglycemia occurs somewhat earlier, generally by 45 minutes after fructose administration. Concurrent with hypoglycemia or shortly preceding it, serum phosphate levels fall dramatically, generally to levels 60% or less of the initial serum phosphate level. Symptoms of hypoglycemia that may occur 15 to 30 minutes after fructose administration are largely due to the initial phases of hypoglycemia and reflect, initially, adrenergic responses, and, later, central nervous system responses to the hypoglycemia. A careful examination of the urine during a fructose tolerance test will demonstrate the presence of aminoaciduria; rising serum levels of hepatic enzymes also may be observed before the conclusion of the test. Treatment for hereditary fructose intolerance, elimination of fructose from the diet, is highly effective.

GLYCOGEN STORAGE DISEASES

The glycogen storage diseases are a heterogeneous group of metabolic disorders affecting many different tissues. Their common characteristic is the excessive accumulation of glycogen, usually with organ dysfunction. They are logically considered as defects at several points in the cycle of glycogen synthesis and breakdown.

Glycogen synthesis begins with phosphorylation of glucose to form glucose 6-phosphate, which is subsequently rearranged by the action of phosphoglucomutase to form glucose 1-phosphate (Fig. 170-2). This glucose 1-phosphate condenses with uridine triphosphate (UTP) to generate an active form of glucose, uridine diphosphate-glucose (UDP-glucose). This activated form of glucose is subsequently condensed with priming chains of pre-existing glycogen to produce chain lengthening by alpha-1,4-glucosyl linkage formation. The enzyme catalyzing this condensation, glycogen synthase or UDP-glucose-glycogen-alpha,1,4-glucosyltransferase, is the first major control point for the regulation of glycogen formation in mammalian liver. The enzyme exists in two forms. The independent, or dephosphorylated, form of the enzyme is fully active with respect to glycogen formation. Agents increasing muscle cyclic adenosine monophosphate (cyclic 3′,5′,AMP) levels, such as epinephrine and glucagon, accelerate glycogen degradation. Increased cyclic AMP levels also stimulate that kinase which phosphorylates glycogen synthase to form the D, or relatively inactive, form of the enzyme. The enzyme glycogen-synthase kinase, which phosphorylates glycogen synthase, is found in close association with the synthase as part of the glycogen particulate complex of mammalian liver and muscle. Glucose, vagal stimulation, and insulin tend to increase the activity of glycogen synthase, most probably by dephosphorylating the enzyme.

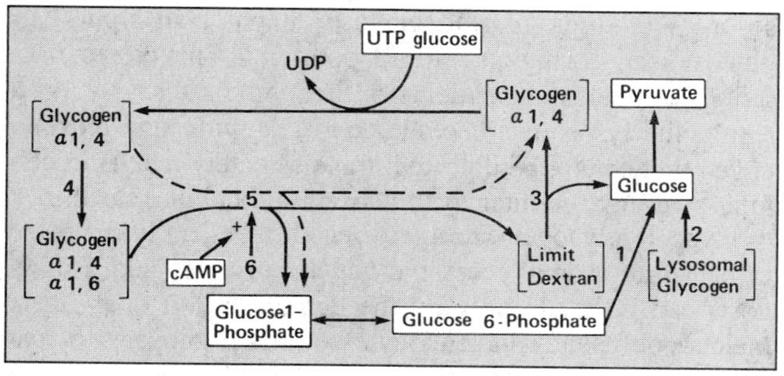

Fig. 170-2. Pathways of hepatic glycogen synthesis and degradation.

Enzyme	Deficiency state
1 Glucose 6-phosphatase	Glycogen storage disease (GSD) type I (hepatorenal)
2 Acid maltase	GSD type II (Pompe's disease)
3 Debranching enzyme	GSD type III
4 Branching enzyme	GSD type IV
5 Phosphorylase	Muscle: GSD type V (McArdle's disease) Liver: GSD type VI (Hers' disease)
6 Phosphorylase kinase	GSD type VIII

To maintain efficient storage of glucose as glycogen, long chains of alpha-1,4-glucosyl linkages must be modified so that alpha-1,6 branch points interrupt the linear array of glucose residues. The branching enzyme (alpha-1,4-glucan:alpha-1,4-glucan-6-glucosyltransferase) is responsible for rearranging alpha-1,4 linkages so that the linear array spans no more than six to ten glucose residues before a branch point occurs. This multibranched nature of glycogen structure results in a more rapid acceleration of glucose liberation by phosphorolysis than would otherwise occur using a much smaller number of linear alpha-1,4 sequences.

The second major point of hormonal regulation of glycogen metabolism is exerted on the enzyme catalyzing the primary step of glycogen degradation, phosphorylase. As is the case with glycogen synthase, glycogen phosphorylase exists in two forms—a phosphorylated form, which is active, and a dephosphorylated form, which is inactive. Phosphorylation of the inactive phosphorylase is catalyzed by the enzyme phosphorylase b kinase. This kinase itself exists in both active and inactive forms, which are phosphorylated and dephosphorylated, respectively. Regulation of phosphorylase b kinase by phosphorylation is catalyzed by cyclic AMP modifications of cyclic AMP-dependent protein kinase. Dissociation of the regulatory subunit from the catalytic subunit of cyclic AMP-dependent protein kinase rapidly accelerates the ATP-dependent phosphorylation of phosphorylase b kinase. Phosphorylase b kinase in turn phosphorylates the subunits of phosphorylase b, using ATP as substrate. Phosphorylase alone is not sufficient to maintain maximal rates of glycogenolysis in mammalian liver or muscle. Although phosphorylase cleaves alpha-1,4-glucosyl linkages to form glucose 1-phosphate, phosphorylase is without substantial activity on alpha-1,6-glucosyl linkages. Without further enzymatic activity, phosphorolysis of glycogen results in the formation of a limit dextran composed of peripheral alpha-1,6 linkages with interior, and a few exterior, alpha-1,4 linkages. Continuation of glycogenolysis then requires the action of debrancher enzyme (amylo-1,6-glucosidase), which hydrolyzes these linkages to form free glucose rather than glucose 1-phosphate. An intermediary enzyme responsible for continuing glycogenolysis is the oligo-1,4→1,4-glucan transferase, which rearranges the initial two or three alpha-1,4 linkages before the alpha-1,6 branch point to another locale in the glycogen molecule in such a way that the alpha-1,6 linkage is exposed to the catalytic site of the debrancher enzyme. Regulation of glycogenolysis by factors altering debrancher enzyme or the alpha-1,4-glucantransferase has not been described.

Finally, the glucose 6-phosphate formed by the action of phosphoglucomutase on the resulting glucose 1-phosphate is hydrolytically cleaved by the action of microsomal glucose 6-phosphatase in kidney and liver. Cleavage of the glucose ester results in the formation of free inorganic phosphate. The activity of the enzyme shows some hormonal regulation by agonists such as glucocorticoids. Direct effects of glucagon and of falling insulin levels, as during fasting, also have been postulated, although the precise biochemical mechanism for these effects has not as yet been defined.

Type I glycogen storage disease

Glucose-6-phosphatase deficiency is an inborn error of metabolism, known originally as *von Gierke's disease*. It results from a lack of hepatic and renal glucose-6-phosphatase activity. As a consequence, these patients have a characteristic history of hypoglycemia from infancy onward. Massive hepatomegaly is usually present. Splenomegaly is rare. Enlargement of the kidneys is also described. Characteristic symmetric, yellowish paramacular lesions are found in the retina in about half of the patients with von Gierke's disease. Osteoporosis is common, as are tendinous xanthomas on the extensor surfaces of the extremities. Many subjects have tophi because hyperuricemia accompanies this condition. Generalized platelet dysfunction, with a tendency to persistent bleeding after trauma or surgery, is described, as is inflammatory bowel disease. Hypoglycemia is present to a highly variable extent. The disorder is more common and much more serious in infants than in older children and adults. Metabolic acidosis often is found because lactic acidemia occurs, presumably as a consequence of impaired hepatic lactate clearance that is due to a failure of hepatic gluconeogenesis. Ketosis frequently occurs in patients with this disease, although careful study has not substantiated this as a central element. On the contrary, infants and children with hypoglycemia and ketosis should be investigated more carefully for the presence of other disorders such as fructose diphosphatase deficiency. A Fanconi-like syndrome is rare in patients with type I glycogen storage disease. These patients also have marked hyperlipidemia, most probably due to the inability to store glucose as glycogen; this causes an increased flux of ingested carbohydrate toward hepatic triglyceride and cholesterol metabolism. There is, in addition, a reduction in the activity of lipoprotein lipase in these patients. The hyperuricemia described in patients with type I glycogen storage disease was initially attributed to chronic metabolic acidosis with a resulting diminution in urinary uric acid clearance, but more recent study has shown that uric acid formation is increased. The precise biochemical mechanism producing the increased biosynthesis is not understood.

A diagnosis of type I glycogen storage disease should be suspected when hypoglycemia is unresponsive to epinephrine or glucagon administration. In the absence of glucose-6-phosphatase activity, significant amounts of free glucose cannot be released to the circulation after phosphorolysis of liver or kidney glycogen. The enzymatic assays of glucose-6-phosphatase activity in kidney or liver biopsies are an essential requisite for the diagnosis. The disease is inherited as an autosomal recessive trait, and carriers may have a reduced activity of the enzyme in liver, kidney, or intestinal mucosal biopsies. Carriers are asymptomatic.

Treatment of glycogen storage disease type I is relatively straightforward. The hypoglycemia requires frequent feedings. Treatment of the nocturnal hypoglycemia by continuous infusion via nasogastric tube has been effective. Approximately 10 mg/kg/min of carbohydrate must be administered. Recently, oral feedings of uncooked cornstarch at 6-hour intervals have been equally effective and better tolerated in children and adults but not in infants. Diminished insulin release may be produced by the use of diazoxide, which thereby reduces the tendency of the liver to store large quantities of glucose in the form of glycogen. Further amelioration of the hepatomegaly may be achieved by the somewhat more drastic use of portal diversionary procedures so that less glucose is stored as glycogen. Orthotopic liver transplantation may provide the best long-term therapy.

Type II glycogen storage disease

Alpha-1,4-glucosidase deficiency, also known as *Pompe's disease,* results in a glycogenosis most commonly noted in infancy. It primarily affects the heart, although other forms of the disease affecting primarily skeletal muscle also have been described. Pompe's disease manifests itself as generalized cardiac dysfunction with cardiomegaly, congestive heart failure, cyanosis, and ultimately death within the first year of life. The skeletal muscle form of the disease presents later in childhood or in adult life, tends to resemble a lysosomal storage disease or generalized myopathy, and must be differentiated carefully from such. The glycogenosis results from a failure of lysosomal hydrolysis of glycogen particles. In most mammalian tissues, cells are in a constant state of turnover in which older constituents are degraded and replaced by newly synthesized protein, lipid, and carbohydrate components of the cell. This remodeling process depends largely on lysosomal degradation of cellular constituents and organelles. Glycogen degradation in lysosomes requires an acid maltase enzyme, an alpha-1,4-glucosidase, having an acid pH optimum. This enzyme activity is deficient in patients with Pompe's disease. As a result, the lysosomes become engorged with ingested glycogen that cannot be digested; this ultimately results in cellular swelling, cellular dysfunction, and cellular death.

Type II glycogen storage disease is generally accepted to be an autosomal recessive genetic disease, and a diagnosis can be made only by the demonstration of the acid maltase deficiency in leukocytes or tissue biopsies of patients suspected of the diagnosis. Other biochemical tests generally are normal in these patients, except those resulting from the organ dysfunction produced. No treatment for this condition exists, and its inexorable course cannot be modified.

Type III glycogen storage disease

In *amylo-1,6-glucosidase deficiency,* also known as *debrancher enzyme deficiency,* a limit dextran glycogenosis results from the ongoing action of phosphorylase, but not of debrancher, activity. Thus as in type I glycogen storage disease, the patient has hepatomegaly (but less kidney enlargement) and, more commonly, splenomegaly. Although severe hypoglycemia and convulsions may occur in this condition, these tend to be generally milder than in patients with type I glycogen storage disease. Skeletal muscle and cardiac enlargement has also been described, but kidney enlargement is not common. Mild hyperlipidemia, but not hyperuricemia, may be anticipated, and biochemical abnormalities characteristic of liver dysfunction are observed frequently. The disease appears to be inherited as an autosomal recessive trait, and the treatment is similar to that of type I glycogen storage disease. Multiple small feedings may be used to ameliorate the hypoglycemia, and portal diversionary procedures may be necessary for the hepatomegaly and glycogenosis. Unlike the situation in type I glycogen storage disease, patients with type III glycogenosis frequently have a long and relatively asymptomatic life.

Type IV glycogen storage disease or branching enzyme deficiency

This relatively rare form of glycogen storage disease is also known as *amylopectinosis* or *Anderson's disease*. As with other forms of glycogen storage disease, growth retardation and failure to thrive are common in the early childhood period. Hepatomegaly, hypotonia, and splenomegaly also may be observed. The disease follows an inexorable course that is associated with cirrhosis, hepatic failure, and death within the first few years of life. Although the liver contains normal concentrations of glycogen, the biochemical nature of this glycogen is abnormal. Relatively long chains of alpha-1,4-amyloselike glycogen particles are synthesized. Because of the enzymatic deficiency, there is a markedly reduced number of branch points in each glycogen molecule. Consequently, glycogen solubility is reduced and phosphorylase activity becomes insufficient. An autosomal recessive inheritance has been described. No treatment for this condition is available.

Type V glycogen storage disease or muscle phosphorylase deficiency

In this disorder, originally described by McCardle, there is a prominent and unusual history of severe muscle cramps and a limitation of muscle function during exercise. The metabolic defect, which is the absence of glycogen phosphorylase in skeletal muscle, is undoubtedly present from birth but produces few if any symptoms during childhood. The disease becomes prominent in early adulthood, when severe muscle cramps and secondary myoglobinuria develop. Later, muscle wasting and weakness become increasingly severe as the myoglobinuria diminishes. Physical examination of these patients is generally unremarkable as are most routine biochemical determinations. The normal postexercise rise in venous lactate levels does not occur in patients with this glycogen storage disease owing to a failure of muscle glycogenolysis. This block in glucose mobilization during anoxic exercise thereby limits muscle ATP formation by anaerobic glycolysis. As a result of the diminished availability of high-energy phosphate, gross muscle dysfunction and cell leakage become apparent, causing myoglobinuria. Continued injury results in cell death and gross signs of muscle wasting. Muscle energy metabolism during aerobic states is otherwise intact owing to mitochondrial preservation and function. Phosphorous NMR studies clearly show normal work capacity provided that muscle atrophy has not occurred. This disorder is inherited as an autosomal recessive trait; the diagnosis is proved only by muscle biopsy and direct assays of the enzymes. Treatment with a variety of agents such as glucose, fructose, and isoproterenol to raise free fatty acid levels has been advocated. None of these provide consistent or long-lasting benefits. In all instances, strenuous exercise should be avoided.

Type VI glycogen storage disease

Recently, patients with increased hepatic glycogen levels and a 75% to 80% reduction of hepatic phosphorylase activity have been noted. Clinically, these patients resemble those with mild forms of type I glycogen storage disease. Owing to the intrinsic difficulties in the assay of liver phosphorylase activity, the precise biochemical defect, as well as its existence as a separate clinical entity, remains open to question.

Type VII glycogen storage disease or muscle phosphofructokinase deficiency

Phosphofructokinase is the key regulatory enzyme of the glycolytic pathway. The deficiency of this enzyme results in a diminished glycolytic clearance of glucose taken up by cells having an insulin-facilitated or insulin-requiring mechanism for glucose uptake. The glycogen storage in this condition results from the overaccumulation of fructose 6-phosphate and glucose 6-phosphate, which cannot be cleared by the usual pathways of anaerobic glycolysis. As a consequence, glucose 6-phosphate is converted to increased amounts of glycogen. An autosomal recessive inheritance seems apparent for this condition. Treatment is generally unavailable, although a low-carbohydrate diet with frequent small feedings may ameliorate the overaccumulation of glucose in the form of stored glycogen in skeletal muscle.

Type VIII glycogen storage disease or hepatic phosphorylase b kinase deficiency

As discussed earlier, phosphorylase activation requires at least two other enzymatic activities. Thus the findings of a low phosphorylase activity may suggest a diminished phosphorylase mass or a diminished activation mechanism regulating phosphorylase activity. In patients with a diminished phosphorylase b kinase activity, hepatomegaly and glycogenosis have been reported. Phosphorylase activation (conversion of phosphorylase b to phosphorylase a) is markedly slowed compared to that in normal persons. There is normal responsiveness to glucagon, however, and chronic glucagon administration produces a diminution of the hepatomegaly. This disease appears to follow an X-linked inheritance pattern. The patients have only mild symptoms, which are generally linked to the hepatomegaly, and they exhibit mild hypoglycemia on exertion. Treatment is not fully satisfactory at the present time.

GALACTOSEMIA

As is the case with the metabolism of most other hexoses in mammalian tissues, galactose is initially phosphorylated by a relatively specific galactokinase found in mammalian liver and, to a lesser extent, in other tissues. Galactokinase phosphorylates galactose in the presence of ATP to form galactose 1-phosphate and ADP (Fig. 170-1). Subsequently, the galactose 1-phosphate must be activated by transfer to a uridylyl group catalyzed by the galactose-1-phosphate-uridylyltransferase. In this reaction, galactose 1-phosphate condenses with UDP-glucose to form UDP-galactose + glucose 1-phosphate. The resulting UDP-galactose is converted to UDP-glucose by the action of UDP-galactose-4′-epimerase. Subsequently, the UDP-glucose is hydrolyzed by a pyrophosphorylation reaction such that UTP + glucose 1-phosphate is subsequently generated. The glucose 1-phosphate formed from galactose metabolism may be utilized directly for glycogen biosynthesis or, alternatively, may be converted to glucose 6-phosphate by the action of phosphoglucomutase and subsequently metabolized by anaerobic glycolysis or released as free glucose, depending on the fuel and energy requirements of the organism. Reduction of galactose to galactitol (a hexitol) is an alternative means of galactose disposal.

Two relatively specific and different presentations of galactosemia have been described. In the first and more serious of these inborn errors of metabolism, there is a near absence of the UDP-glucose-galactose-1-phosphate-uridylyltransferase. This absence most commonly manifests itself as a failure to thrive in infancy. Vomiting, diarrhea, and abnormal liver function with jaundice or hepatomegaly are generally present within the first week of life or at any time after milk ingestion. Because the predominant sugar of milk is lactose, a disaccharide composed of glucose and galactose, the infant is exposed to large quantities of galactose early in life. Severe hemolysis, ascites, and cataracts within a few days of birth have all been reported in a large proportion of patients who have the transferase form of galactosemia. If the disorder is left untreated, severe mental retardation and a failure of neurologic development will become apparent after the first few months of life. On occasion, failure to thrive and vomiting may be relatively less in some patients, and, after 3 to 6 months, these patients may manifest motor retardation, neurologic deficits, hepatic enlargement, and cataracts. In rare instances this presentation may not occur until the second to fourth year of life.

Routine laboratory testing usually will reveal a hyperchloremic metabolic acidosis, albuminuria, aminoaciduria reminiscent of Fanconi's syndrome, and, occasionally, lower-than-normal fasting glucose levels. The specific tests for galactose in blood will reveal substantial elevations in all patients studied. A diagnosis of galactosemia may be suspected on the basis of the appearance of a nonglucose reducing sugar in the urine.

Because the toxicity resulting from galactosemia is produced by accumulations of large quantities of intracellular galactose 1-phosphate or galactitol, therapy for this state must be directed toward producing a galactose-free diet for these patients. Initially, this means an elimination of milk and milk products from the diet. More commonly, Nutramigen and soy bean milks are used. Because of the difficulties of dietary adherence, this therapy is not always successful. Nevertheless, rapid relief of all symptoms will be observed in patients ingesting minimal quantities of galactose. Even the cataracts will regress, although they may not clear completely in most circumstances. Reversal of the mental retardation or, indeed, its prevention depends on an early initiation of a diet free of galactose. Mothers known to have produced galactosemic infants in the past should be kept on a galactose-free diet throughout subsequent pregnancies. This appears to be most helpful in preventing mental retardation and leads to early diagnosis in subsequent offspring with galactosemia. The diagnosis may be suspected in patients having galactose in blood or urine, but confirmation is required by direct assay of the activity of the uridylyltransferase in leukocytes, skin fibroblasts, or liver biopsies of these patients.

More recently, a second form of galactosemia has been described in which the biochemical defect appears to be an absence or deficiency of galactokinase. This condition was initially described in a 44-year-old adult. In general, these persons have milder involvement of the liver and spleen. Cataracts are considerably smaller in size, although they occur at remarkably young ages in galactosemic, as compared to nongalactosemic, patients. Most commonly, these findings should make the clinician suspicious of galactosemia. Screening tests for nonglucose-reducing sugars in the urine should be performed. Specific enzymatic assays should be used to confirm the diagnosis. In general, toxicity produced by the galactokinase deficit results primarily from the reduction of excessive quantities of galactose to galactitol in tissues such as the lens. The resulting hexitol produces premature cataracts by osmotic swelling and disruption of lens architecture. Similar mechanisms may occur in neuronal tissue, and it is possible that part of the central nervous system toxicity associated with more severe deficiency of the uridylyltransferase may result from galactitol formation. Treatment, as with the other form of galactosemia, rests primarily on the institution and maintenance of a galactose-free diet. Symptoms may resolve and cataracts may improve, although they do not disappear completely.

REFERENCES

Bondy PK and Rosenberg LE, editors: Diseases of metabolism, ed 8. Philadelphia, 1980, WB Saunders.

Buiman D, Holton JB, and Pennock CA, editors: Inherited disorders of carbohydrate metabolism. Baltimore, 1980, University Park Press.

Burmeister LA, Valdivia T, and Nuttall FQ: Adult hereditary fructose intolerance, Arch Intern Med 151:773, 1991.

Chen YT, Cornblath M, and Sidbury JB: Cornstarch therapy in type I glycogen-storage disease, N Engl J Med 310:171, 1984.

Couper R, Kapelushnik J, and Griffiths AM: Neutrophil dysfunction in glycogen storage disease Ib: association with Crohn's-like colitis, Gastroenterology 100:549, 1991.

Greene HC et al: Continuous nocturnal intragastric feeding for management of type I glycogen-storage disease, N Engl J Med 294:423, 1976.

Kirschner BS, Baker AL, and Thorp FK: Growth in adulthood after liver transplantation for glycogen storage disease type I, Gastroenterology 101:238, 1991.

Schwenk WF and Haymond MW: Optimal rate of enteral glucose administration in children with GSD-I, N Engl J Med 314(11):682-685, 1986.

Seegmiller JE et al: Fructose-induced aberration of metabolism in familial gout identified by 31P magnetic resonance spectroscopy, Proc Natl Acad Sci USA 87:8326, 1990.

Stanbury JB, Wyngaarden JB, and Fredrickson DS, editors: The metabolic basis of inherited disease, ed 5, New York, 1983, McGraw-Hill.

CHAPTER

171 Disorders of Lipids and Lipoproteins

Scott M. Grundy

This chapter describes the more common disorders of lipid metabolism, particularly those leading to accelerated coronary atherosclerosis. Certain rarer abnormalities of lipid metabolism also will be considered because their recognition is essential and because they provide insights into key steps of lipid regulation. Before considering abnormal states, however, lipid metabolism under normal circumstances is reviewed.

LIPID METABOLISM

The major lipids of the body are triglycerides, cholesterol, and phospholipids. The predominant phospholipid is lecithin, but others—sphingomyelin and cephalins—also are important for cellular function and transport of lipids. The chemical structures of the major lipids, including representative fatty acids, are presented in Fig. 171-1.

Triglycerides consist of three fatty acid molecules esterified to glycerol. Fatty acids vary in chain length and degree of saturation. The most common fatty acids of the saturated series are palmitic acid (16:0) and stearic acid (18:0); they are the primary constituents of most hard fats, whether of animal or plant origin. The major monounsaturated fatty acid is oleic acid (18:1ω9); it is the most prevalent fatty acid consumed in most diets. Oleic acid can be synthesized by both animals and plants.

Plants, but not animals, can synthesize two types of polyunsaturated fatty acids: they are ω6 and ω3 fatty acids. The major ω6 fatty acid, linoleic acid (18:2ω6), has 18 carbon atoms with two double bonds, the second being six carbons removed from the terminal methyl group. Linoleic acid occurs mainly in plant oils; it comprises 77% and 56% of the fatty acids of safflower oil and soybean oil, respectively. Linoleic acid is an essential dietary fatty acid for humans because it cannot be made by the body but is required for normal metabolism. It is an important constituent of cell membranes and it is a precursor for longer-chain fatty acids that are transformed into prostaglandins, thromboxanes, and prostacyclins of the one and two series (Fig. 171-2).

The parent ω3 fatty acid is linolenic acid (18:3ω3), and it too cannot be synthesized by the body. A deficiency of linolenic acid uniquely induces abnormalities in retinal function; thus it appears to be an essential fatty acid. It can be converted to fatty acids of longer-chain length and

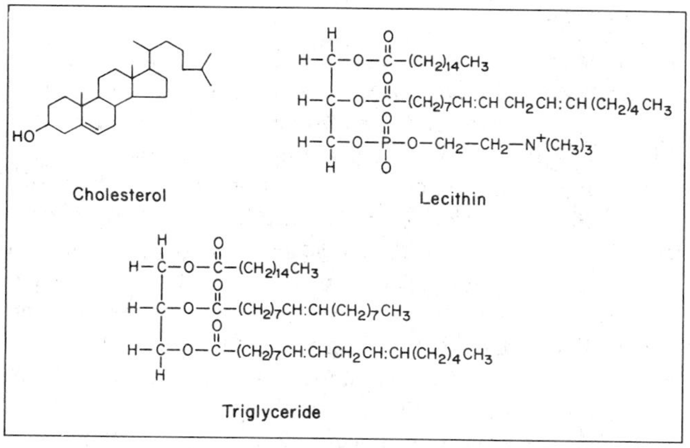

Fig. 171-1. The major lipids of plasma: cholesterol, lecithin, and triglyceride. Typical fatty acids are shown esterified to the latter two lipids.

greater unsaturation, which become precursors to prostaglandins, thromboxanes, and prostacyclin of the three series. Linolenic acid occurs in substantial amounts in soybean oil and rapeseed oil. Humans apparently have a limited capacity to convert linoleic acid to longer-chain, ω3 polyunsaturates. The latter must be obtained from other sources, of which the richest are fish oils. The ω3 fatty acids of fish oils may have therapeutic uses. They inhibit aggregation of platelets and thereby may prevent coronary thrombosis and also lower plasma triglycerides in patients with hypertriglyceridemia.

The triglycerides are stored mainly in adipose tissue and serve as a reservoir of energy and essential fatty acids. Triglycerides in adipocytes undergo lipolysis to free fatty acids (FFA). Adipose tissue lipolysis is inhibited by insulin and stimulated by catecholamines, glucagon, and adrenal corticoids. The FFA, which are released into the circulation, bind to albumin and are transported to various tissues—the liver, muscle, and heart. The liver extracts a portion of circulation FFA and either oxidizes them or incorporates them into triglycerides. Muscle and heart derive a substantial portion of their energy from circulating FFA.

Cholesterol is another important lipid but is not an essential nutrient. It plays a key role in maintaining the integrity of cellular membranes and is the sole source of steroid hormones and bile acids. Cholesterol is made in most tissues but mainly in the liver and intestinal mucosa. It is synthesized from acetate by a series of about 20 reactions (Fig. 171-3). In the sequence, acetate is condensed to acetoacetate, which takes another acetate residue to form hydroxymethylglutaryl coenzyme A (HMG CoA). The conversion of HMG CoA to mevalonic acid, catalyzed by the enzyme HMG CoA reductase, is the rate-limiting step in the synthesis of cholesterol. Mevalonic acid undergoes a series of condensation reactions, resulting in a straight-chain hydrocarbon, squalene, and squalene cyclizes to a sterol, lanosterol; the latter is converted to cholesterol. The rate of synthesis of cholesterol is influenced by the concentration of cholesterol within cells. For example, a rise in cellular concentration of cholesterol suppresses the activity of HMG CoA reductase. Thus feedback control maintains cellular cholesterol at optimum levels. As cells accumulate excessive amounts of cholesterol, a portion is esterified with a fatty acid, a reaction is catalyzed by the enzyme acylcholesterol acyltransferase (ACAT), and the product is stored temporarily as cholesterol ester until needed by the cell.

The liver promotes the excretion of cholesterol in two ways. First, a portion of hepatic cholesterol is converted into the "primary" bile acids, cholic acid and chenodeoxycholic acid; and second, cholesterol is secreted directly into bile. Direct secretion is made possible by the solubilizing power of bile acids. Both cholesterol and bile acids enter the intestine through the biliary tract. About 40% to 60% of intestinal cholesterol is reabsorbed, and the remainder is excreted into feces. Cholesterol is absorbed almost exclusively in the upper small intestine. Normally, almost all of the bile acids (approximately 98%) are reabsorbed, mainly in the distal small intestine. Only a very small fraction of

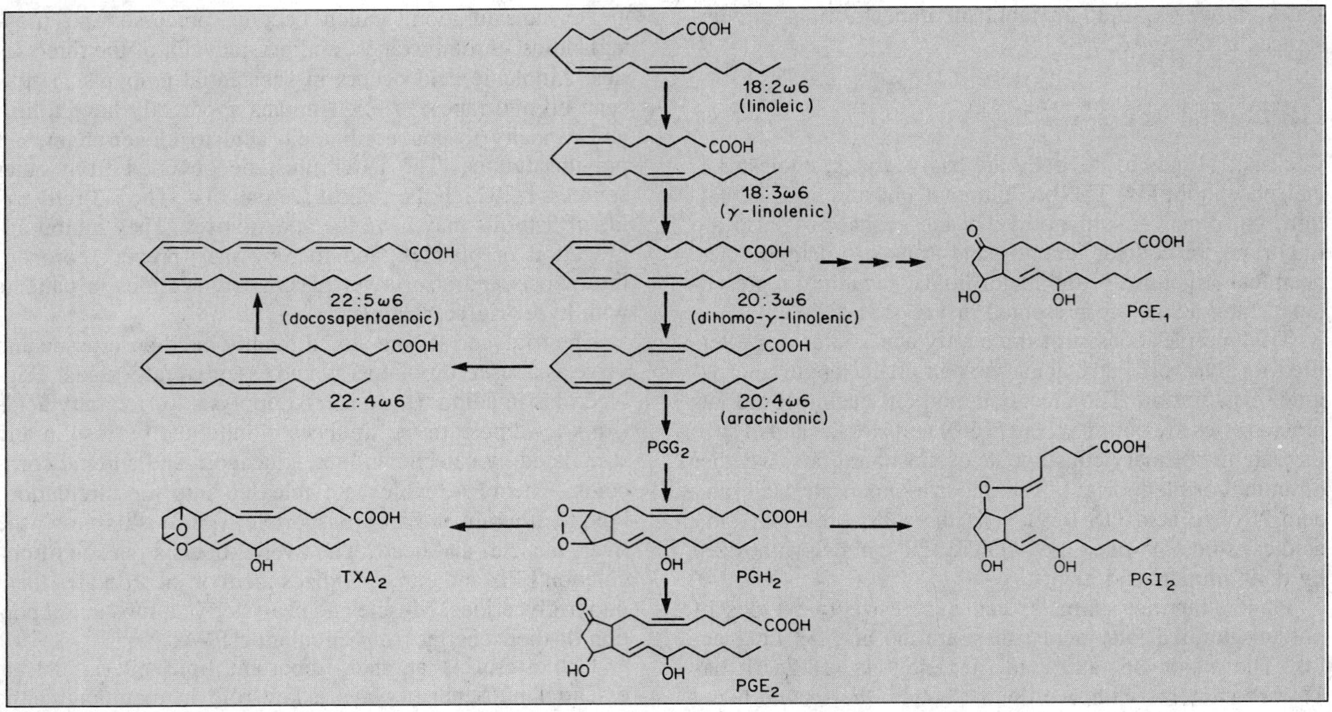

Fig. 171-2. Synthesis of prostaglandin of the 1 series (PGE_1) and prostanoids of the 2 series, prostaglandin (PGE_2), thromboxane (TXA_2), and prostacyclin (PGI_2). Also, docosapentaenoic acid is synthesized from the key intermediate, arachidonic acid.

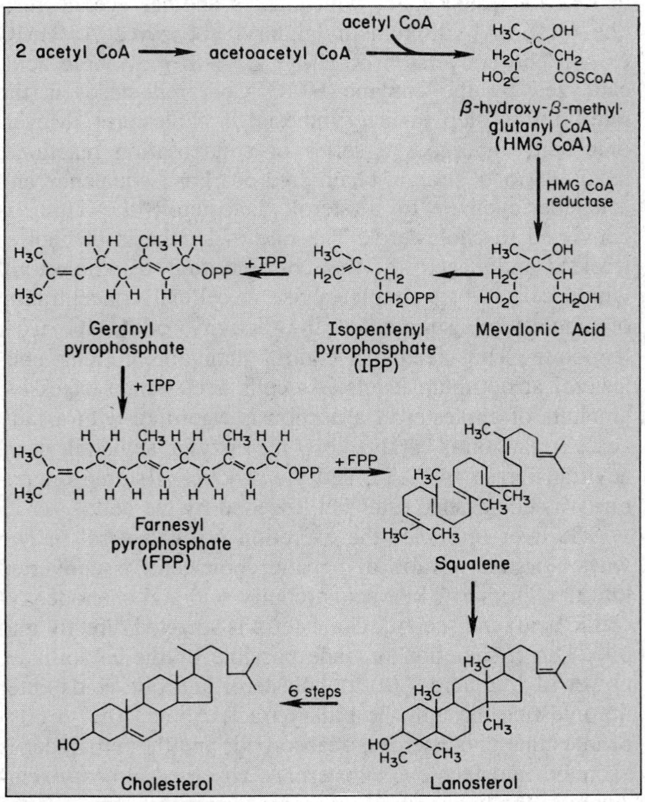

Fig. 171-3. Key steps in synthesis of cholesterol.

bile acids entering the intestine reaches the colon and is excreted in feces.

The bile acids return to the liver in portal blood and are extracted almost completely in their first pass. They are resecreted rapidly into bile to complete the enterohepatic circulation. In the liver, the bile acids inhibit the conversion of cholesterol into bile acids by suppressing the rate-limiting reaction in bile acid synthesis, the 7-alpha-hydroxylation of cholesterol. The rate of flux of bile acids through the liver thus regulates cholesterol catabolism and indirectly influences hepatic concentrations of cholesterol.

LIPOPROTEIN METABOLISM

Lipids are insoluble in aqueous solutions, and they cannot circulate freely in plasma. Instead, they are complexed with specialized proteins called *apolipoproteins,* or *apoproteins.* Lipid-apoprotein complexes are named lipoproteins, and they have a central core of nonpolar lipids (cholesterol ester and triglycerides) and a surface coat of more polar constituents—unesterified cholesterol, phospholipids, and apoproteins. Lipoproteins are produced by the gut and liver but are modified extensively in plasma. The major function of lipoproteins is to transport lipids (i.e., triglycerides, cholesterol, and lipid-soluble vitamins) from one site to another. They also help to stabilize the plasma membranes of cells that are bathed by plasma and lymph. The major lipoproteins of plasma and their constituents are listed in Table 171-1.

Table 171-1. The plasma lipoproteins

Lipoprotein	Origin	Major lipid constituent(s)	Major apolipoproteins
Chylomicrons	Gut	Triglycerides	B-48, E, C-II, C-III, A-I, A-II, A-IV
Very-low-density lipoproteins (VLDL)	Liver	Triglycerides	B-100, C-II, C-III, E
Intermediate-density lipoproteins (IDL)	VLDL catabolism Liver (?)*	Triglycerides Cholesterol	B-100, C-11, C-III, E
Low-density lipoproteins (LDL)	IDL catabolism Liver(?)*	Cholesterol	B-100
High-density lipoproteins (HDL)	Liver Gut Other lipoproteins†	Cholesterol Phospholipids	A-I, A-II, Others‡

*Several reports suggest that IDL and LDL can be secreted directly by the liver, although this has not been proved.
†Various constituents of HDL are acquired as these lipoproteins circulate in plasma. HDL may obtain phospholipids and apoproteins C-II, C-II, and E during lipolysis of triglyceride-rich lipoproteins. Cholesterol can be derived from the plasma membranes of cells.
‡Several other apoproteins—apo Cs, apo E, apo A-IV, and apo D—have been reported in HDL.

Apolipoproteins

The apoproteins of lipoproteins possess unique sequences of amino acids that allow them to bind to lipids and yet be dissolved in aqueous plasma. Each apoprotein has one or more specific functions, including (1) solubilizing lipids for secretion from cells, (2) transporting lipids in plasma, (3) activating enzymes responsible for hydrolysis of lipids, (4) accepting lipids through exchange reactions, and (5) binding to specific cell-surface receptors that provide a mechanism for cellular uptake and degradation of lipoproteins. The major apoproteins, along with their sites of origins, molecular weights, and general functions, are listed in Table 171-2.

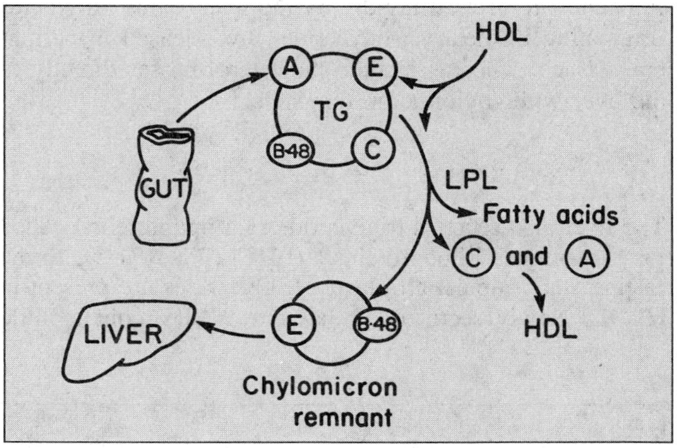

Fig. 171-4. Formation and catabolism of chylomicrons. The chylomicrons are produced by the intestine and contain mainly triglycerides (TG) in their lipid core. The surface coat contains apoprotein As (A-I, A-II, A-IV), Es, Cs, and B-48. The apo Es and Cs are derived in part from HDL. Triglycerides undergo lipolysis by lipoprotein lipase (LPL) to release fatty acids. Simultaneously, apo Cs and apo As are released and enter HDL. The residual lipoproteins, chylomicron remnants, retain apo E and apo B-48, and are taken up by the liver.

Chylomicrons

After dietary lipids are digested and absorbed, they are transported away from the intestinal tract by lipoproteins called chylomicrons (Fig. 171-4). The triglycerides are the major class of lipids in the diet, and as they enter the upper small intestine, they undergo lipolysis by pancreatic lipase, being degraded to fatty acids and monoglycerides; the latter then are taken up by the intestinal mucosa and resynthesized into triglycerides. Simultaneously, unesterified cholesterol of dietary and biliary origin enters mucosal cells and is esterified. Newly formed triglycerides and cholesterol esters are incorporated into chylomicrons, which are secreted into chyle. Chylomicrons are the largest of the plasma lipoproteins. More than 95% of their weight is triglyceride, and only 1% is cholesterol ester. Apoproteins also constitute only about 1% by weight. The major apoprotein of chylomicrons is apoprotein B-48 (apo B-48), a highly insoluble protein with a molecular weight of approximately 250,000. Other apoproteins—the apo Cs, apo Es, and apo As—also are present; they are either secreted with chylomicrons or are transferred from high-density lipoproteins (HDL).

Chylomicrons enter the bloodstream through the thoracic duct and pass into peripheral capillary beds. At the surface of capillary endothelial cells, they come in contact with an enzyme, lipoprotein lipase (LPL). This enzyme is activated by one of the C apoproteins, apo C-II. The triglycerides of chylomicrons are hydrolyzed to fatty acids and glycerol. The rate of lipolysis may be modulated by apo C-III, an apoprotein that apparently inhibits LPL. During lipolysis, the soluble apoproteins (apo Cs and apo As) are released into the circulation and loosely attach to HDL; here they are held in reserve for reutilization by VLDL.

When lipolysis of chylomicrons is almost complete, smaller lipoproteins, called *chylomicron remnants,* return to the circulation. These partially degraded lipoproteins contain only small amounts of triglyceride but retain almost

Table 171-2. Major apolipoproteins of plasma lipoproteins

Apolipoprotein	Origin	Lipoprotein source(s)	Molecular weight	Function
B-48	Gut	Chylomicrons	260,000	Chylomicron transport
B-100	Liver	VLDL, IDL, LDL	550,000	Transport of VLDL, IDL, LDL
A-I	Gut, liver	Chylomicrons, HDL	28,300	Activator of LCAT
A-II	Gut, liver	Chylomicrons, HDL	17,000	Transport of HDL
C-I	Liver	VLDL, IDL, HDL	6,500	Activation of LCAT*
C-II	Liver	VLDL, IDL, HDL	8,800	Activator of LPL*
C-III	Liver	VLDL, IDL, HDL	8,750	Unknown
E	Liver	VLDL, IDL, HDL	35-39,000	Receptor-mediated clearance of remnant lipoproteins

*LCAT, lecithin-cholesterol acyltransferase; LPL, lipoprotein lipase.

all of the newly absorbed cholesterol esters. Chylomicron remnants are cleared rapidly by the liver. Thus fatty acids originating in dietary triglycerides are released in peripheral tissues, whereas dietary cholesterol passes directly to the liver with chylomicron remnants.

Very-low-density lipoproteins

The liver also secretes triglyceride-rich lipoproteins, called very-low-density lipoproteins (VLDL) (Fig. 171-5). In the fasting state, almost all plasma triglycerides are present in VLDL. Newly secreted, or nascent, VLDL contain little cholesterol ester. The major apoprotein of VLDL is apo B-100, which is a very large molecule (molecular weight about 550,000) and is highly insoluble. Nascent VLDL also contain apo E, and as they circulate, they acquire apo Cs and more apo E from HDL. VLDL also accept cholesterol esters from HDL. In contrast to chylomicrons, VLDL have no apo A-I or apo A-II. Circulating VLDL are smaller than chylomicrons and have less triglycerides but more cholesterol esters.

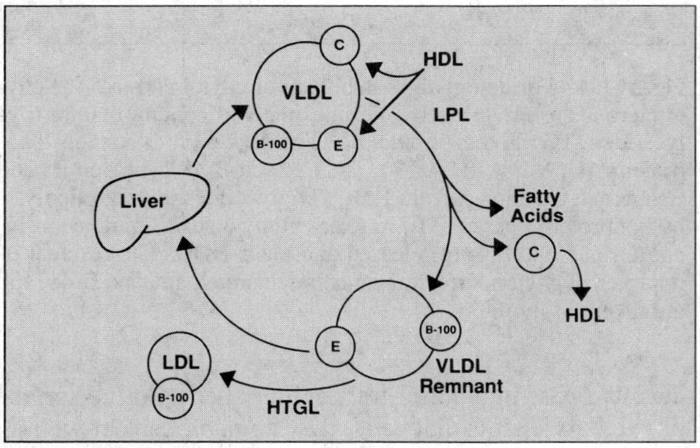

Fig. 171-5. Metabolism of VLDL. The liver secretes VLDL, which contain triglycerides as its major core lipid. Nascent VLDL contain apo B-100 and some apo E, and as these lipoproteins circulate they acquire apo Cs, possibly more apo Es, and cholesterol esters from HDL. The VLDL are degraded by lipoprotein lipase (LPL) with release of fatty acids and apo Cs, the latter returning HDL. The product of lipolysis, VLDL remnants, contain both cholesterol esters and smaller amounts of triglycerides as core lipids, and mainly apo-100 and apo Es as surface apoproteins. VLDL remnants can be taken up by the liver, or they can be degraded to LDL. The latter may be mediated in part by hepatic triglyceride lipase (HTGL). Normally, about 60% of VLDL remnants are removed by the liver, whereas the remainder are converted to LDL.

As VLDL enter the peripheral circulation, they too come in contact with LPL, and their triglycerides undergo lipolysis. The soluble apo Cs are released, but apo B-100 and much of apo E remain attached to the residual lipoproteins, which are called VLDL remnants. The latter have been largely depleted of triglyceride but remain enriched in cholesterol ester. VLDL remnants can have two fates. In normal persons, at least 60% of circulating VLDL remnants is removed by the liver, and their uptake is mediated by receptors that recognize apo E. More than one receptor may be involved in this process. VLDL remnants not removed by the liver are converted to low-density lipoproteins (LDL). The precise mechanisms by which conversion to LDL occurs are unknown, although the liver may be involved. A hepatic enzyme, *hepatic triglyceride lipase,* located on the surface of liver cells, may hydrolyze the remaining triglycerides of VLDL remnants, which results in loss of essentially all apoproteins except apo B.

Low-density lipoproteins

The LDL normally transport most of the cholesterol in plasma; they originate from catabolism of VLDL through intermediate-density lipoproteins (IDL) or VLDL remnants (Fig. 171-6). LDL contain mostly cholesterol esters in their nonpolar cores and carry very little triglyceride. Each particle of LDL has approximately 17,000 molecules of cholesterol ester. The only apoprotein of LDL is apo B-100, which is retained after catabolism of VLDL. Most LDL are cleared from the circulation by LDL receptors. These receptors are the same as those that remove VLDL remnants. Both the liver and many extrahepatic tissues express LDL

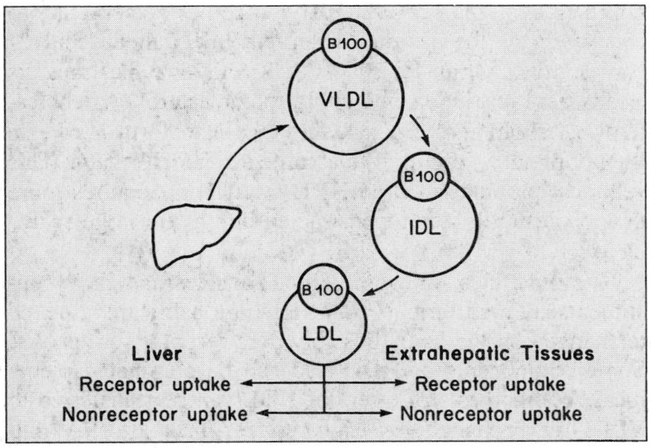

Fig. 171-6. Metabolism of LDL. The sole apoprotein of LDL is apo B-100. LDL contain mainly cholesterol esters in their lipid core. LDL are derived from the catabolism of VLDL and IDL. LDL can have several fates. About 70% of LDL are removed by the liver, and the remainder by extrahepatic tissues. About 50% to 75% of LDL are cleared by LDL receptors (receptor uptake), either in the liver or in extrahepatic tissues. The remaining LDL are removed by nonreceptor pathways, either in liver or extrahepatic tissues. Thus the major pathway of clearance of LDL is receptor uptake in the liver, but other pathways are involved.

receptors, but LDL are removed principally by the liver. Most LDL are cleared by LDL receptors, but smaller amounts leave by nonreceptor pathways, either in the liver or extrahepatic tissues. Normally, 10% to 15% of the circulating pool of LDL is taken up each day by nonreceptor pathways. Another 15% to 30% of the pool is eliminated daily by LDL receptors. In total, 30% to 45% of the plasma pool of LDL is cleared from the circulation every day.

A cell commonly used for study of LDL receptors is the fibroblast (Fig. 171-7). In tissue culture, each fibroblast expresses 20,000 to 50,000 receptors. The LDL receptor is a protein molecule that resides on the surface of cells in specialized regions of the plasma membrane called coated pits. The latter are indentations in the membrane. These pits are covered by a protein, *clathrin,* which gives the pits a fuzzy-coated appearance. These "coated" pits cover only about 2% of the cell surface, but they contain almost all LDL receptors. When LDL (or VLDL remnants) bind to the receptor, the resulting complexes of receptor and lipoprotein are internalized. This process occurs by invagination of the coated pit to form endocytic vesicles. These vesicles, containing the coated surface, pass through the cytoplasm until they fuse with lysosomes. In lysosomes, the components of LDL undergo hydrolytic degradation. Apo B is degraded to amino acids, and cholesterol esters to unesterified cholesterol. Cholesterol passes out of the lysosome, where it inserts into membranes or remains in cytoplasm to regulate the cell's synthesis of cholesterol.

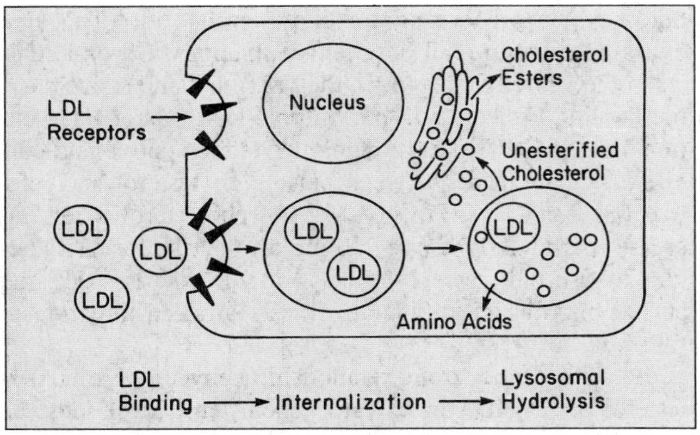

Fig. 171-7. Cellular metabolism of LDL. The plasma LDL bind to LDL receptors located in coated pits of cells. The LDL are then internalized, and the components undergo hydrolysis in lysosomes. The protein moiety of LDL is degraded to amino acids, and unesterified cholesterol is released to the cell cytoplasm. In the cytoplasm it can inhibit the cell's own synthesis of cholesterol, or it can be stored as cholesterol ester.

The number of LDL receptors synthesized by cells is adjusted by feedback regulation, and when intracellular concentrations of unesterified cholesterol rise, synthesis of receptors diminishes; on the contrary, when the concentration of cholesterol drops, synthesis of receptors escalates. Thus cellular concentrations of cholesterol couples inversely with the quantity of LDL receptors fabricated by the cell.

Small numbers of LDL particles are dispatched by other varieties of receptors. The macrophage, for example, maintains only few receptors for normal LDL, but it has numerous receptors for chemically modified LDL. Derivatives of LDL can be created in vitro that bestow recognition by these other macrophage receptors. One such derivative is acetyl LDL. Each macrophage has 20,000 to 40,000 receptors that bind to acetyl LDL, whereas these same receptors do not recognize native LDL. One attribute of the acetyl LDL receptor is that it is not under feedback regulation by intracellular cholesterol. Macrophages can acquire large amounts of cholesterol via modified LDL receptors, yet the number of receptors per cell remains constant. Macrophages also express receptors for another lipoprotein called beta-VLDL, a variant of the VLDL remnant. If VLDL remnants are delayed in their clearance from plasma, they become enriched in cholesterol esters, and the product, beta-VLDL, is recognized by the macrophage. Macrophage uptake of lipoproteins could be important in atherogenesis because once LDL enter the arterial wall, they may become chemically modified, and uptake of this modified LDL could transform macrophages into foam cells.

Recent evidence suggests that oxidation of LDL within the arterial wall may be one of the critical modifications leading to uptake by macrophages. Oxidized LDL not only is susceptible to macrophage uptake, but also may promote atherosclerosis in other ways (e.g., as a chemoattractant for macrophages and a cytotoxin).

High-density lipoproteins

Cholesterol can enter extrahepatic tissues either by uptake of LDL cholesterol or by new synthesis within these cells.

Because cholesterol cannot be degraded in extrahepatic tissues, it must be returned to the liver for excretion, a process called *reverse cholesterol transport*. Although the mechanisms for reverse cholesterol transport are not fully understood, another lipoprotein, HDL, may play an important role. The metabolism of HDL is complex and remains to be elucidated fully, but a general outline has emerged and can be reviewed.

The core lipids of HDL are mainly cholesterol esters. The HDL are relatively small particles, and their surface-coat constituents—apoproteins, phospholipids, unesterified cholesterol—predominate over core lipids. Several apoproteins (A-I, A-II, Cs, and Es) reside in HDL. The major apoproteins are A-I and A-II. Apo A-I is a single polypeptide chain of 243 amino acid residues. Apo A-II is a dimer of two identical chains, each chain having 77 amino acids; the chains are linked by a disulfide bond. Lesser amounts of other apoproteins—apo Cs and apo Es—are sequestered in HDL for transfer later to triglyceride-rich lipoproteins. HDL consist of relatively small particles, ranging in diameter from 40 to 100. More particles of HDL are in circulation than any other type of lipoprotein. HDL can be divided into two major subfractions, HDL_3 and HDL_2, the former being more dense than the latter.

The components of HDL have multiple origins. The apoproteins stem from both liver and gut. The liver apparently secretes apo A-I and apo A-II complexed with phospholipids. These complexes are called nascent HDL (Fig. 171-8). The intestine also secretes nascent HDL containing apo As. As nascent HDL circulate, they undergo transformation into mature HDL. Additional phospholipid is acquired by transfer from the surface coats of both chylomicrons and VLDL. Unesterified cholesterol also is transferred to HDL from the surfaces of cells or from other lipoproteins. This cholesterol undergoes esterification, catalyzed by the action of an enzyme called lecithin-cholesterol acyltransferase (LCAT); this enzyme transfers a fatty acid residue from lecithin to cholesterol. As cholesterol esters are synthesized, they begin to form a core in the lipoprotein, forcing it to assume a spherical shape. This spherical particle is called HDL_3; as HDL_3 acquires more new cholesterol, it is reconstructed into a still larger particle, HDL_2.

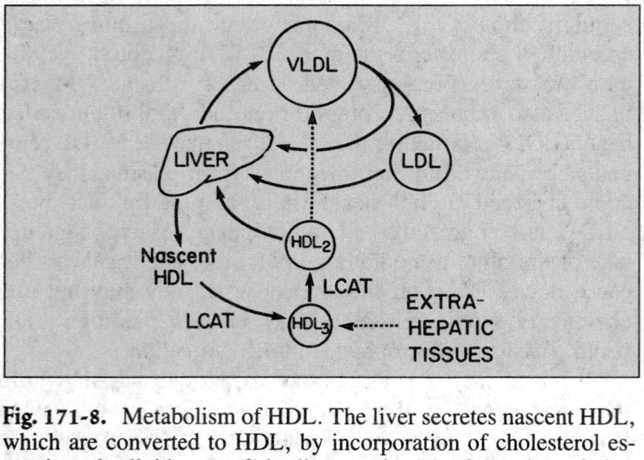

Fig. 171-8. Metabolism of HDL. The liver secretes nascent HDL, which are converted to HDL, by incorporation of cholesterol esters into the lipid core of the lipoprotein. The formation of cholesterol esters is catalyzed by the enzyme LCAT. Unesterified cholesterol for incorporation into HDL can be derived from extrahepatic tissues. The dashed lines indicate the flow of cholesterol molecules. HDL_3 is converted to HDL_2 by further incorporation of cholesterol esters. HDL_2 may be removed intact by the liver, but HDL_2 also can transfer some of its cholesterol ester to VLDL. This cholesterol can return to the liver with either VLDL remnants or LDL.

The outcomes for whole HDL particles and their constituents are multifarious. Some HDL probably are removed unchanged by the liver, possibly by a receptor for apo As. Some components of HDL also can be eliminated piecemeal. The cholesterol esters of HDL can be transferred to VLDL in exchange for triglycerides. Thereafter, VLDL cholesterol esters can reach the liver via hepatic uptake of the products of VLDL catabolism, namely, VLDL remnants and LDL. Further, some of the phospholipids of HDL may be lost on the surface of liver cells during interaction with hepatic triglyceride lipase; this reaction may convert HDL_2 back into HDL_3. Thus return of cholesterol from peripheral tissues to the liver seemingly does not occur by a single mechanism but probably follows a variety of pathways.

LIPOPROTEINS AND ATHEROSCLEROSIS

A major component of atherosclerotic plaques is cholesterol, and multiple lines of evidence implicate elevated levels of plasma cholesterol as a cause of atherosclerosis. For example, in several species of animals, feeding of cholesterol induced marked hypercholesterolemia and in turn atherosclerosis. In addition, patients with severe genetic hypercholesterolemia frequently develop premature atherosclerotic disease. According to many studies in both animals and humans, most of the excess cholesterol in atheromatous plaques is derived from plasma cholesterol.

The level of plasma cholesterol is positively correlated with the risk for coronary heart disease (CHD). Many epidemiologic surveys have demonstrated that this correlation holds over a broad range of cholesterol levels. This link exists both within and between populations. Several studies in the United States (e.g., the Framingham Heart Study, the Pooling Project, and the Multiple Risk Factor Intervention Trial [MRFIT]) have demonstrated a positive and curvilinear relationship between plasma cholesterol and relative risk for CHD (Fig. 171-9). As cholesterol levels increase, particularly above 200 mg/dl, the risk for CHD begins to rise more steeply. At 240 mg/dl, risk is twice that at 200 mg/dl, and at 300 mg/dl risk is raised threefold to fourfold.

Because of the strong relationship between plasma cholesterol and CHD, an elevated cholesterol level must be considered a major risk factor for CHD; however, it is only one of several other proved risk factors, the latter including hypertension, diabetes mellitus, cigarette smoking, and low levels of plasma HDL. The Framingham Heart Study has shown that coronary risk at any given level of cholesterol is compounded when several risk factors exist concurrently (Fig. 171-10). Even in the absence of other risk

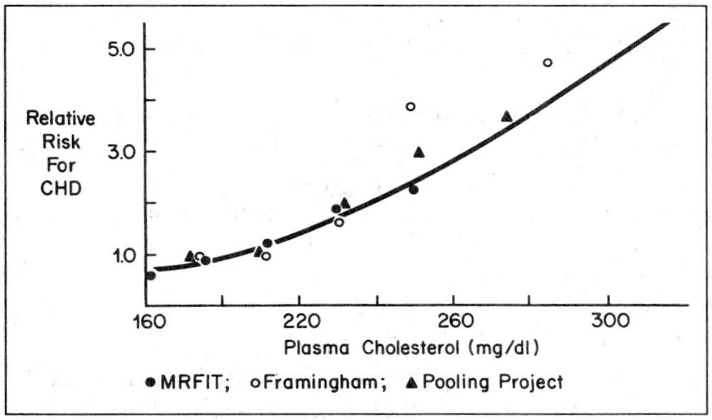

Fig. 171-9. Relative risk for CHD at various levels of plasma cholesterol. Data are shown for the Multiple Risk Factor Intervention Trial, the Framingham Heart Study, and the Pooling Project.

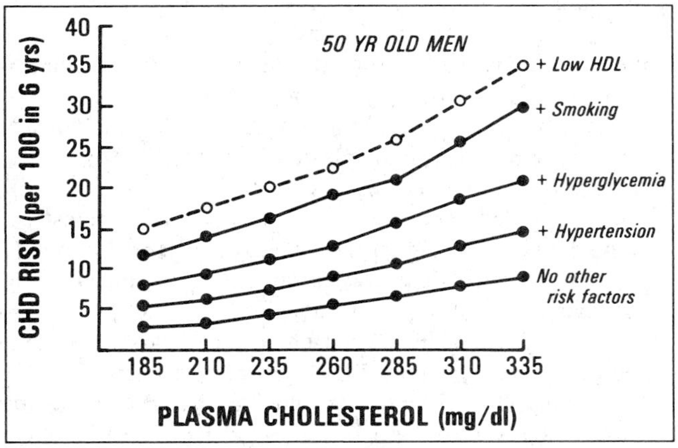

Fig. 171-10. Risk for CHD at various levels of plasma cholesterol in the presence or absence of other risk factors. Risk is expressed as number of new cases of CHD per 100 men at age 50 over a 6-year period. Data were obtained from the Framingham Heart Study. The addition of risk factors progressively increases risk for CHD at any level of cholesterol.

factors, the risk for CHD rises with increasing cholesterol levels, but for any given concentration of cholesterol, the likelihood of CHD is magnified by the joining of these other risk factors.

A link between high plasma triglycerides and CHD risk is not as firmly established as that for cholesterol. Nonetheless, several epidemiologic studies indicate that hypertriglyceridemia is associated with increased risk for CHD. Without question, a large proportion of patients with CHD have high plasma triglyceride levels, but in prospective studies, when other major risk factors (e.g., high total cholesterol and low HDL cholesterol) are factored out, triglyceride levels appear to lose their power to predict CHD. This finding has led some investigators to claim that hypertriglyceridemia is not an independent risk factor for CHD. In truth, however, both cholesterol and triglycerides merely reflect lipoproteins that carry them, and the lipoproteins are the agents that convey lipids into and out of the arterial wall. To describe the role of lipids in atherogenesis, therefore, the atherogenic potential of the different species of lipoproteins must be reviewed.

Chylomicrons

These lipoproteins in their native form may not be atherogenic. Their major constituent, triglycerides, contributes little to the lipid component of atherosclerotic plaques. Chylomicrons are large particles and seemingly filter poorly through the endothelium and into subintimal spaces; this lack of penetration probably minimizes their atherogenic capability. This fact could explain why severe hyperchylomicronemia, due to a deficiency of LPL, does not induce premature atherosclerosis. Nevertheless, some investigators believe that chylomicrons are indirectly atherogenic. When these particles interact with endothelial-surface LPL, cholesterol may be released, which then passes through the intima and into the arterial wall. If so, more cholesterol may infiltrate the arterial wall when high cholesterol intakes enrich chylomicrons with cholesterol.

Chylomicron remnants

Lipolysis of triglycerides of chylomicrons spawns smaller, cholesterol-enriched particles, chylomicron remnants. Chylomicron remnants thus presumably are more atherogenic than native chylomicrons. However, plasma concentrations of chylomicron remnants generally are low even after a fatty meal because they are cleared rapidly by the liver. Consequently, it is not known whether chylomicron remnants contribute to atherosclerosis under normal circumstances.

Very-low-density-lipoproteins

The atherogenic potential of VLDL likewise is uncertain. Elevated levels of VLDL often are found in patients having premature CHD, but VLDL nonetheless are relatively large particles, contain mainly triglycerides, and probably filter poorly through the endothelial lining of the arterial wall. Furthermore, some patients with high VLDL levels seem remarkably free of atherosclerosis. In spite of these factors, under some circumstances VLDL may deliver cholesterol into the arterial wall. If the protective endothelium becomes disrupted, VLDL could penetrate the intima and thus be atherogenic. One cause of endothelial injury may be smoking, and our clinical experience suggests that most hypertriglyceridemic patients with CHD are smokers. In addition, there are growing signs that the hypertriglyceridemic state may predispose to coronary thrombosis; several elements of the clotting system have been reported to be abnormal in patients with elevated triglycerides.

VLDL remnants

These lipoproteins are probably the most atherogenic of the various forms of VLDL. They are the smallest particles in the VLDL fraction, have the least triglycerides, and are relatively enriched in cholesterol esters. Indeed, patients displaying high concentrations of VLDL remnants seem at risk for premature CHD. Some types of remnants, specifically beta-VLDL, are particularly susceptible to uptake by macrophage receptors and appear to be highly atherogenic.

Low-density lipoproteins

The LDL are thought to be the most atherogenic of all lipoproteins. Elevated concentrations of LDL definitely accelerate atherosclerosis, and when their levels are very high, CHD often occurs prematurely. LDL are relatively small particles, are rich in cholesterol ester, and readily penetrate the arterial intima. LDL contain the highly insoluble apo B-100, which may be responsible for entrapment of LDL in the subintimal space. Indeed, intact particles of LDL can be identified in most atherosclerotic plaques. The passage of an excess of LDL into the arterial wall is considered by many to be the major factor responsible for atherosclerosis. The lack of CHD in countries where levels of LDL are low, despite a relatively high prevalence of other risk factors (e.g., smoking, hypertension, diabetes mellitus), supports the concept that excessive filtration of LDL into the artery is a necessary condition for atherogenesis.

High-density lipoproteins

Although HDL contain a high percentage of cholesterol, they are not atherogenic; indeed high plasma levels of HDL may protect against atherosclerosis. This protection could be due to HDL's role in reverse cholesterol transport; that is, HDL may remove excess cholesterol from the arterial wall. This function may occur maximally when circulating levels of HDL are high, and reverse cholesterol transport may be retarded by low levels. This concept agrees with the inverse correlation between HDL levels and CHD risk. Limited studies suggest that HDL_2 is more protective against CHD than is HDL_3. Recent data suggest that the most protective form of HDL is that in which apo A-I is the exclusive apoprotein of the HDL particle. It has been shown that the HDL_2 fraction is enriched with this type of particle.

There is not universal agreement that reverse cholesterol transport explains the inverse correlation between HDL levels and CHD risk. High HDL concentrations may merely reflect a "healthy" transport system for plasma lipids; for instance, when plasma total cholesterol and triglycerides are high, HDL levels frequently are low. Thus increased atherogenicity might reside more in an elevation of apo B-containing lipoproteins than in HDL per se. In addition, low HDL levels frequently occur in the presence of other CHD risk factors (e.g., smoking, obesity, and lack of exercise). Thus the low HDL-CHD link may be the result of several factors beyond the action of HDL to promote reverse cholesterol transport. In recent years, a lipoprotein Lp(a) has come into prominence as a definite risk factor for coronary heart disease.

EFFECTS OF DIETARY FACTORS ON LIPOPROTEIN METABOLISM

Several dietary factors influence the plasma lipoproteins. Because the diet has been implicated in atherogenesis, a review of dietary effects on lipoprotein metabolism seems appropriate. Each of the major dietary constituents is considered separately.

Saturated fatty acids

The American diet typically is rich in saturated fatty acids. These acids come from animal meats (beef and pork), dairy products (milk, butter, and cheese), eggs, tropical oils (coconut oil, palm oil, cocoa butter, and hard margarines), and baked goods. Many Americans consume from 15% to 18% of their total calories as saturated fatty acids. Three types of saturated fatty acids—lauric acid, myristic acid, and palmitic acid—raise the plasma total cholesterol; a fourth, stearic acid, does not. For every 1% of total calories consumed as cholesterol-raising saturated acids, the plasma total cholesterol increases by about 2.7 mg/dl. This response is relative to a baseline of carbohydrate, which is considered to have no effect on cholesterol levels; in other words, when the diet contains 18% of its calories as cholesterol-raising saturated fatty acids, the plasma total cholesterol will be 45 mg per/d higher than when the diet is completely free of saturated acids, and carbohydrate is consumed in their place.

Most of the rise in plasma cholesterol caused by saturated fatty acids occurs in LDL, but the cholesterol level in VLDL and HDL may rise slightly. The major action of the saturated acids is to impair the clearance of LDL, most likely by suppressing the synthesis of LDL receptors. They probably free up increased amounts of unesterified cholesterol in the liver to inhibit LDL-receptor synthesis.

Polyunsaturated fatty acids

The polyunsaturate, linoleic acid, lowers the plasma cholesterol when substituted for saturated fatty acids. Every 1% of calories of linoleic acid, when exchanged for carbohydrate, reduces the plasma cholesterol levels by about 1 mg/dl. The major reduction occurs partly in LDL, but levels of VLDL and HDL also fall. Whether linoleic acid has an inherent plasma LDL-lowering property has not been determined.

In the past, relatively high intakes of linoleic acid were recommended. In recent years, however, concern has been mounting about possible harmful effects of excessive intakes of linoleic acid. No large population has ever consumed high amounts of linoleic acid for prolonged periods, and consequently their safety has not been proved. Moreover, several additional adverse effects for polyunsaturates have been postulated. High intakes of linoleic acid may increase the risk of gallstones, potentiate chemical carcinogenesis, or suppress the immune system. Beyond these effects they can alter the composition of membrane phospholipids, the consequences of which are unknown. Thus it is now recommended that intakes of linoleic not exceed the current intake of 7% of total calories.

Monounsaturated fatty acids

The major monounsaturated fatty acid of the diet is oleic acid. When oleic acid replaces dietary saturated acids, plasma total cholesterol level falls. The percentage reduction in LDL levels with oleic acid is similar to that for linoleic acid. Oleic acid, however, does not reduce the HDL as much as does linoleic acid. A major advantage of oleic acid is that large amounts of olive oil, containing mainly oleic acid, have been consumed in the Mediterranean region for many years without evidence of side effects. Nor does it produce the adverse effects in animals that have been noted for linoleic acid. Furthermore, populations consuming large amounts of olive oil have a low prevalence of CHD. Thus oleic acid-rich diets appear preferable to those high in linoleic acid in preventing coronary disease.

Carbohydrates

Dietary carbohydrates can be considered neutral in their effect on total cholesterol and LDL levels. When they are substituted for dietary saturated fatty acids, therefore, the plasma cholesterol levels fall. The degree of fall in LDL levels may be slightly less than when linoleic acid or oleic acid is substituted for saturates, but in practical terms the differences are small. However, a sudden increase in carbohydrate intake may raise plasma triglyceride levels and lower HDL concentrations. If the carbohydrate intake is gradually increased and is in the form of fiber-containing foods, such induced hypertriglyceridemia may be avoided. Thus the neutrality of carbohydrates extends only to LDL levels.

High-carbohydrate diets by definition are low in fat. Low-fat diets are consumed in many regions, particularly in developing countries where prevalence of CHD is low. No adverse effects of low-fat diets are known, provided intakes of protein and other essential nutrients are adequate. Both simple and complex carbohydrates (i.e., starch) have similar effects on lipoprotein metabolism, although complex carbohydrates are thought to be preferable for a variety of other reasons. They cause fewer dental caries and they contain more fiber and usually are consumed with fruits and vegetables that contain various vitamins and minerals.

Cholesterol

American adults typically consume 350 to 500 mg of cholesterol per day, about half of which is absorbed. The influence of dietary cholesterol on plasma lipoproteins is variable. Cholesterol in the diet can raise concentrations of cholesterol in all lipoprotein fractions—VLDL, LDL, and HDL. The dietary cholesterol effect on LDL is enhanced when saturated fatty acids are present. Dietary cholesterol raises LDL levels by suppressing synthesis of LDL in the liver.

Protein

In some species, the type of protein in the diet can influence levels of plasma lipids. In rabbits, for example, casein raises the cholesterol level, and vegetable proteins lower it. In humans, even if serum cholesterol responses to different types of proteins are not identical, differences are relatively small. In general, animal proteins do not raise cholesterol levels relative to vegetable proteins.

Alcohol

Alcohol stimulates the synthesis of hepatic triglycerides, promoting secretion of VLDL triglycerides. The latter raises serum triglycerides, especially in obese people or in those having a lipolytic defect. In the latter, ingestion of alcohol, even in moderate quantities, can cause a striking hypertriglyceridemia. Alcohol also raises HDL-cholesterol concentrations leading some to postulate benefit. In truth, however, the consequences of this change, as they pertain to coronary risk, are not known. In contrast, alcohol ingestion has almost no effect on the metabolism of LDL.

Caloric restriction and weight loss

The obese state, characterized by a high caloric intake, has several effects on lipoprotein metabolism, most notably, increasing synthesis of VLDL and raising serum triglycerides. Even in obese patients who do not develop frank hypertriglyceridemia, secretion rates of VLDL are high; they are protected from elevated VLDL concentrations only by enhanced efficiency of their lipolytic system. Overproduction of VLDL, in turn, increases conversion of VLDL to LDL, and consequently, LDL levels often rise. Again, however, concentrations of LDL are not invariably boosted in obese people, suggesting that some people compensate by increasing their clearance of LDL. Obesity, in general, is associated with low HDL levels, and, as might be expected, weight reduction tends to restore levels to normal. Weight reduction furthermore lowers plasma triglycerides. In contrast, changes in LDL levels consequent to weight result are less constant; in some patients, levels of LDL fall; in others there is no change, and in a few there is even an increase in LDL.

EFFECTS OF DRUGS ON LIPOPROTEIN METABOLISM

Several drugs can be used to treat abnormalities in lipoprotein metabolism. They differ in their actions and are classified here according to their major mechanisms.

Drugs that enhance the clearance of LDL

Levels of LDL can be reduced by promoting the clearance of LDL from plasma. This process is usually accomplished by stimulating the activity of LDL receptors. The liver is the major site of clearance of LDL. As indicated before, the expression of LDL receptors on liver cells depends in part on hepatic cholesterol content. Of most importance for drug therapy, a fall in cholesterol content in the liver enhances the synthesis of LDL receptors. The potential for drug action to effect this change exists at several sites of metabolic control: synthesis of cholesterol, secretion of cholesterol into bile, intestinal reabsorption of cholesterol, secretion of cholesterol into bile, intestinal reabsorption of cholesterol, and conversion of cholesterol into bile acids (Fig. 171-11, *A*). Therapeutic modification of these key pathways affects hepatic cholesterol concentration, thereby modifying LDL-receptor synthesis (Fig. 171-11, *B*). Thus receptor synthesis can be amplified by hindering reabsorption of cholesterol, restricting synthesis, or upgrading conversion of cholesterol into bile acids; the latter response is customarily achieved by barring the reabsorption of bile acids.

The reabsorption of bile acids can be constrained by bile-acid binding resins, called *sequestrants;* these agents include cholestyramine and colestipol. These nonabsorbable resins have quaternary amine groups that secure to the acidic group of bile acids, lessening the backtracking of bile acids to the liver. Consequently, feedback repression on transformation of cholesterol into bile acids is disengaged; secondarily, hepatic concentration of cholesterol is reduced, LDL-receptor synthesis is augmented, and plasma levels of LDL and VLDL remnants fall. For reasons yet to be discerned, the bile acid sequestrants also spur the synthesis of VLDL triglycerides, leading to mild hypertriglyceridemia in some patients.

Actually, bile acid sequestrants are not highly proficient for binding of bile acids in the intestine, and large doses (e.g., 16 to 30 g/day) are required for a maximal reduction of LDL level. Many patients cannot abide such high doses. In these individuals lower doses can be tried and may yield a sufficient response. The sequestrants constipate many patients because they prevent the normal laxative action of bile acids. They can cause other gastrointestinal symptoms—heartburn, abdominal pain, bloating, belching, and nausea; however, these usually dissipate after several weeks of therapy. The sequestrants have no untoward effect outside the gastrointestinal tract, other than raising triglycerides in some patients, nor have they been shown to be carcinogenic.

Blocking the absorption of cholesterol also lowers hepatic cholesterol content and increases LDL-receptor synthesis. The ideal drug for blocking the reabsorption of cholesterol has yet to be discovered and developed. The most potent agent currently available is neomycin. At 2 g/day, it effectively blocks the absorption of cholesterol. Unfortunately, the drug has potential side effects. It alters the flora of the bowel, which theoretically can induce a resistant infection. It also has a toxic potential, and prolonged usage might impair hearing, although this response has not been proved for low oral doses. The Food and Drug Administration (FDA) has not approved neomycin for treatment of hypercholesterolemia, and its use for routine management of high LDL levels cannot be recommended. Other drugs that interfere with absorption of cholesterol are beta-sitosterol and sucrose polyester. Beta-sitosterol is not available at present as a therapeutic agent in the United States, and sucrose polyester, a synthetic nonabsorbable fat, has not yet been approved for use.

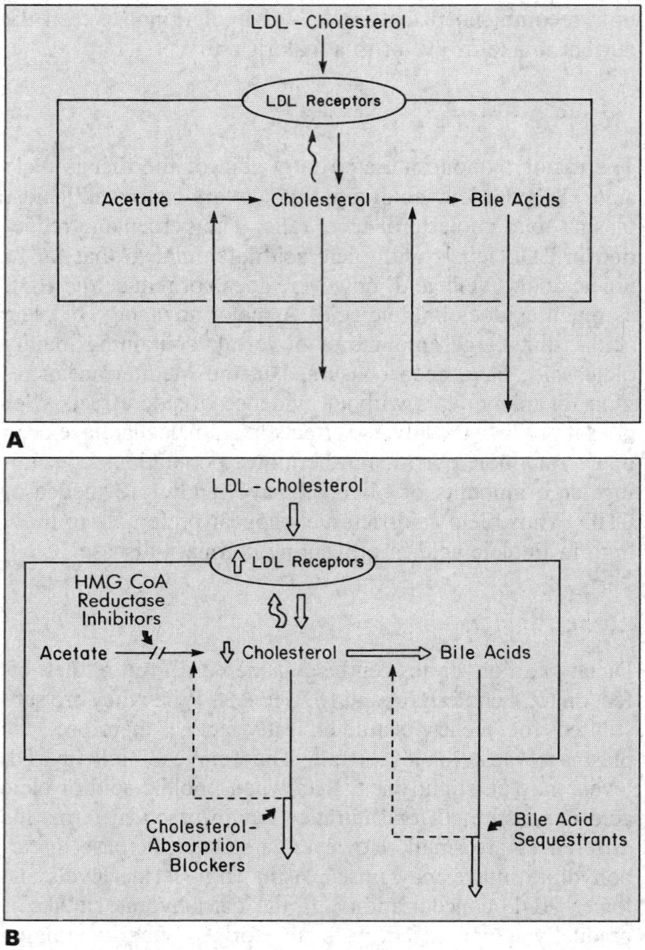

Fig. 171-11. Relationship between LDL receptors and the enterohepatic circulation (EHC) of cholesterol and bile acids. **A,** In the liver cell, cholesterol is formed from acetate and is partially converted to bile acids. Both cholesterol and bile acids are secreted into the intestine and are partially reabsorbed to complete the enterohepatic circulation. The return of cholesterol to the liver causes feedback inhibition on cholesterol synthesis, and the return of bile acids inhibits the conversion of cholesterol into bile acids. Both processes regulate the amount of cholesterol in the liver cell. This quantity of hepatic cholesterol determines the number of LDL receptors synthesized, which in turn regulates the uptake of LDL cholesterol. Thus the EHC plays an important role in modulating the activity of LDL receptors. **B,** Effects of induced alterations in the enterohepatic circulation on the activity of LDL receptors. The quantity of cholesterol in the liver cell can be reduced in three ways: (1) by blocking the reabsorption of bile acids, (2) by blocking the reabsorption of cholesterol, and (3) by inhibiting the synthesis of cholesterol (with HMG CoA reductase inhibitors). The fall in hepatic cholesterol due to any of these mechanisms stimulates the synthesis of LDL receptors, which in turn causes increased hepatic uptake of LDL and a fall in plasma LDL levels.

A third category of drugs that enhance the activity of LDL receptors is the group of inhibitors of cholesterol synthesis. The most promising are drugs that competitively inhibit HMG CoA reductase, the rate-limiting step in cholesterol synthesis. Three agents in this class have been approved by the FDA: lovastatin, pravastatin, and simvastatin. All drugs have the same mechanism of action and similar side effects. The standard doses of lovastatin and pravastatin are 20 to 40 mg/day, whereas simvastatin, which is approximately twice as potent for cholesterol levels, is administered in half these doses. At the usual doses, these drugs lower LDL cholesterol by about 20% to 30%. Side effects include myopathy (myalgia, muscle weakness, elevations of serum creatine kinases, and in severe cases, hemoglobinuria) and mild hepatotoxicity. These are reversible by discontinuation of the drug.

The thyroid hormones also enhance clearance of circulating LDL. This effect explains the low level of plasma cholesterol in hyperthyroidism and the opposite in hypothyroidism. These hormones apparently enhance LDL-receptor activity. In the past, D-thyroxine was used to treat hypercholesterolemia, but because of cardiac side effects, it was abandoned.

Finally, another drug, probucol, promotes the clearance of LDL. Probucol either enhances the affinity of LDL for LDL receptors or promotes removal of LDL by nonreceptor pathways. Probucol apparently does not alter hepatic metabolism of cholesterol, and apparently does not increase LDL receptor activity. It nonetheless lowers levels of LDL by 10% to 20%; unfortunately, probucol also lowers HDL levels. Whether this fall in HDL negates the beneficial effect of LDL lowering is not known. Other significant side effects for probucol have not been reported.

Drugs that inhibit the synthesis of lipoproteins

Nicotinic acid seemingly inhibits hepatic secretion of VLDL particles and thereby lowers both VLDL and LDL. It effectively reduces plasma lipids in several types of hyperlipidemia. Unfortunately, for many patients, its side effects make it impossible to take nicotinic acid for long periods or in adequate doses. Side effects that may occur with this drug include gastrointestinal distress, flushing and itching of the skin, elevation of plasma glucose, rise in uric acid level, hepatic dysfunction, and skin rash. Peptic ulcer disease may be exacerbated or reactivated. For maximum lipid lowering, nicotinic acid must be given in relatively large doses—3.0 to 6.0 g/day. To minimize side effects, it should be started in small doses (i.e., 100 mg three times daily with meals) and increased gradually as tolerated. Its flushing effect may be mitigated by low-dose aspirin.

Drugs that potentiate lipoprotein lipase

The fibric acids enhance the activity of LPL. Two such agents, clofibrate and gemfibrozil, are currently available in the United States; and two others, bezafibrate and fenofibrate, are used in Europe. By enhancing the activity of LPL, these agents promote the catabolism of triglyceride-rich lipoproteins—chylomicrons, VLDL, and VLDL remnants.

The fibric acids appear to influence the metabolism of lipoproteins in ways other than increasing the activity of LPL. Some of these changes, however, such as a rise in HDL-cholesterol levels, may be secondary to enhanced lipase activity. In most hypertriglyceridemic patients, the chemical composition of LDL is abnormal, and this abnormality is corrected by fibric acid therapy. The fibric acids may reduce the hepatic secretion of VLDL to a modest extent, which may enhance the triglyceride lowering. In patients with hypercholesterolemia, the fibric acids have a moderate LDL-lowering action. The fibric acids may cause abdominal discomfort, cholesterol gallstones, or myalgias, the latter being accompanied by a high creatine kinase level. Muscular side effects are particularly common in patients with renal impairment. The fibric acids increase risk for gallstones by causing supersaturated bile due to increased output of biliary cholesterol and by inhibited synthesis of bile acids. The fibric acids must be given in low doses to patients with renal insufficiency, and they are contraindicated in patients with liver disease. One clinical trial suggested that clofibrate may raise the risk of gastrointestinal cancer, although convincing proof is lacking. In another trial, gemfibrozil reduced the risk for CHD in hypercholesterolemic patients without inducing serious side effects. In the latter study, the major benefit for CHD prevention was observed in patients who had elevated plasma triglycerides accompanying hypercholesterolemia.

HYPERLIPIDEMIA

Hyperlipidemia can be defined as an increase in either plasma cholesterol or plasma triglycerides. Although there are multiple causes of hyperlipidemia, in general they fall into three categories: dietary, genetic, and secondary to other conditions. Dietary hyperlipidemias tend to be mild, whereas genetic disorders often are severe. Secondary hyperlipidemias result from various metabolic disorders or certain drugs. Hyperlipidemias commonly accelerate atherosclerosis, but they also can have other clinical consequences.

Hyperlipidemia is synonymous with hyperlipoproteinemia (HLP), an increase in plasma lipoproteins. HLP results from defects at any of several regulatory steps in lipoprotein metabolism (Fig. 171-12), including (1) production of VLDL, (2) lipolysis of VLDL (or chylomicrons), (3) removal of VLDL remnants, (4) conversion of VLDL remnants to LDL, and (5) clearance of LDL. Hyperlipoproteinemia has been categorized into *phenotypes*, or patterns of elevations of the different lipoproteins (Table 171-3). This classification is merely a shorthand notation for the types of lipoproteins present in excess. The phenotype alone does not reveal the underlying metabolic defect, and several different abnormalities can produce the same phenotype. For clinical purposes, HLP can be divided into hypercholesterolemia or hypertriglyceridemia.

Hypercholesterolemia

The term *hypercholesterolemia,* high plasma cholesterol, has undergone an evolution in meaning over the past de-

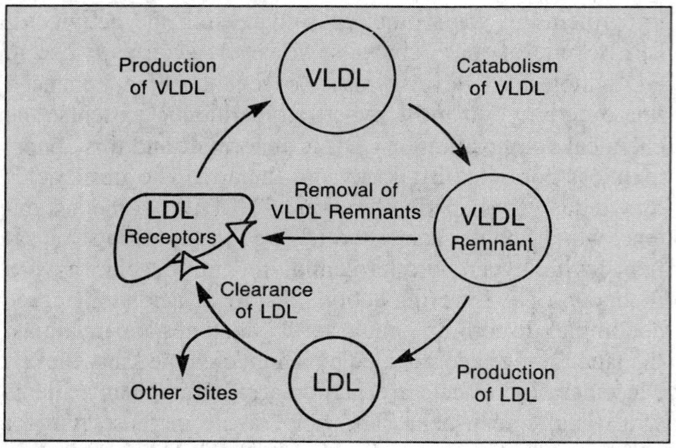

Fig. 171-12. Key steps in the metabolism of lipoproteins containing apo B-100: (1) production of VLDL by the liver, (2) catabolism of VLDL to VLDL remnants, (3) hepatic removal of VLDL remnants, (4) conversion of VLDL remnants to LDL (production of LDL), and (5) clearance of LDL by the liver or extrahepatic sites.

Table 171-3. Phenotypic classification of hyperlipoproteinemia

Phenotype	Lipoprotein present in excess
I	Chylomicrons
IIa	LDL
IIb	LDL + VLDL
III	Beta-VLDL
IV	VLDL
V	Chylomicrons + VLDL

cade. Previously, the term was defined as a plasma cholesterol level above the 95th percentile cut point for the population distribution. More recently, hypercholesterolemia has been defined according to its relation to CHD risk. For example, the National Cholesterol Education Program has classified the serum total cholesterol into three categories: desirable cholesterol level (< 200 mg/dl), borderline-high cholesterol (200 to 239 mg/dl), and high cholesterol (> 240 mg/dl). The current distribution of total cholesterol levels in the American population is presented in Table 171-4. For all adults (ages 20 to 74), approximately 25% have cholesterol levels exceeding 240 mg/dl. For many persons, the total cholesterol level is a fairly good indicator of the LDL-cholesterol level, but for some it is not. Therefore measurement of LDL cholesterol can be helpful. The distributions of LDL-cholesterol levels for American men and women are given in Table 171-5. In the present discussion, hypercholesterolemia will be classified as mild, moderate, or severe. The approach outlined for management of these grades of hypercholesterolemia is consistent with that recommended by the National Cholesterol Education Program.

Mild hypercholesterolemia (borderline-high cholesterol) can be defined as a total cholesterol in the range of 200 to 239 mg/dl. Epidemiologic studies indicate that risk for CHD at a level of 240 mg/dl is about twofold above that for levels below 200 mg/dl, and within the borderline zone (200 to 239 mg/dl), coronary risk rises progressively (see Fig. 171-9). Other risk factors compound the risk imparted by mild hypercholesterolemia (see Fig. 171-10). Therefore patients with cholesterol levels in the range of 200 to 239 mg/dl should be evaluated carefully for the risk factors shown in Fig. 171-10. A man who exceeds age 45 can be considered to be at increased risk through the combination of aging and male sex. Postmenopausal women also can be regarded at increased risk. If a patient with mild hypercholesterolemia has two CHD risk factors, but not established CHD, an attempt should be made to lower LDL-cholesterol levels to below 130 mg/dl. If CHD is present, the goal of LDL lowering should be less than 100 mg/dl. Recent clinical trial evidence indicates LDL lowering in patients with established CHD reduces risk for subsequent cardiovascular death.

The predominant cause of mild hypercholesterolemia (and borderline-high risk LDL cholesterol) is an excessive intake of saturated fatty acids, cholesterol, and total calories, the latter leading to obesity. A sedentary lifestyle also may raise the cholesterol level. Current eating habits and lifestyles of American adults probably increase the plasma cholesterol by 40 to 50 mg/dl above those that would occur on a diet low in saturated fatty acids and cholesterol combined with desirable body weight and a habit of vigorous exercise. Therefore the primary therapy of mild hypercholesterolemia is dietary modification, and when appropriate, weight reduction and increased exercise. The patient should be urged to reduce intake of saturated fatty acids and cholesterol to cut calories if overweight and to begin an exercise program. An acceptable dietary regimen is the Step I diet of the American Heart Association and the National Cholesterol Education Program; this diet restricts intake of fat to about 30% of total calories, saturated fatty acids to less than 10% of calories, and dietary cholesterol to less than 300 mg/day (see the box at far right).

Moderate hypercholesterolemia is defined as a plasma cholesterol in the range of 240 to 300 mg/dl. This definition includes an LDL-cholesterol level in the range of 160 to 210 mg/dl. Over this range, the risk for CHD increases from approximately twofold to fourfold above baseline. Although dietary excesses contribute to moderate hypercholesterolemia, genetic influences also are at play. In fact, genetic factors may render an individual unusually sensitive to dietary excesses, such that the latter produce an accentuated rise in LDL-cholesterol levels. The nature of these genetic factors is poorly understood, but a common abnormality seemingly is a reduced activity of LDL receptors, which may be the result of a metabolic suppression in synthesis of LDL receptors. Hepatic metabolism of cholesterol may be defective, interfering with the normal feedback regulation of receptor synthesis. Effects of a deficiency of LDL receptors on lipoprotein metabolism are shown in Fig. 171-13. Occasionally, suppression of LDL receptor synthesis is caused by hypothyroidism, and reduced thyroid function

Table 171-4. Population distribution of plasma total cholesterol (mg/dl)*

	White men				White women				
	Percentiles				Percentiles				
Age (yr)	5	50	75	95	5	50	75	90	95
20-24	118	159	179	212	121	165	186	220	237
25-29	130	176	199	234	130	178	198	217	231
30-34	142	190	213	258	133	178	199	215	228
35-39	147	195	222	267	139	186	209	233	249
40-44	150	204	229	260	146	193	220	241	259
45-49	163	210	235	275	148	204	231	256	268
50-54	157	211	237	274	163	214	240	267	281
55-59	161	214	236	280	167	229	251	278	294
60-64	163	215	237	287	172	226	251	282	300
65-69	166	213	250	288	167	233	259	282	291
70 +	144	214	236	265	173	226	249	268	280

*Modified from the Lipid Research Clinics Population Studies Data Book. The Prevalence Study. Bethesda, Md, 1979, National Institutes of Health Publication No. 79-1527.

should be sought in any hypercholesterolemic patient. An appreciable number of hypercholesterolemic patients apparently have an abnormality in LDL apolipoprotein B-100—an abnormality that interferes with the normal binding between LDL and LDL receptors. Still another cause for elevated LDL levels is an abnormally high conversion of VLDL to LDL.

Because LDL cholesterol levels in the range of 160 to 210 mg/dl impart a distinct increase in coronary risk, an effort to lower the LDL level is fully justified. Diet should be modified first, and again, intake of saturated fatty acids, cholesterol and total calories (if obesity is present) should be reduced. The Step I diet should be instituted by the physician and immediate staff (see the box on the right). A lipoprotein profile should be checked at 6 weeks and 3 months, and if the LDL cholesterol has not fallen to 160 mg/dl (in the absence of two other risk factors), or to below 130 mg/dl (in the presence of two other risk factors), saturated fatty acids and cholesterol in the diet should be further curtailed. A registered dietitian can help modify the diet to achieve this goal. Dietary therapy should then be continued for another 3 months before considering use of cholesterol-lowering drugs.

If the therapeutic goals for LDL lowering are not achieved by dietary modification alone, the use of drugs can be considered. The decision to use drugs depends on a va-

Table 171-5. Population distribution of plasma LDL cholesterol (mg/dl)*

	White men				White women			
	Percentiles				Percentiles			
Age (yr)	5	50	75	95	5	50	75	95
20-24	66	101	118	147	57	102	118	159
25-29	70	116	138	165	71	108	126	164
30-34	78	124	144	185	70	109	128	156
35-39	81	131	154	189	75	116	139	172
40-44	87	135	157	186	74	122	146	174
45-49	98	141	163	202	79	127	150	186
50-54	89	143	162	197	88	134	160	201
55-59	88	145	168	203	89	145	168	210
60-64	83	143	165	210	100	149	168	224
65-69	98	146	170	210	92	151	184	221
70 +	88	142	164	186	96	147	170	206

*Modified from the Lipid Research Clinics Population Data Book. The Prevalence Study. Bethesda, Md, 1979, National Institutes of Health Publication No. 79-1527.

American Heart Association Recommended Diet (Step I)

Composition
- Limit intakes of total fat to 30%, saturated and polyunsaturated fatty acids to 10%, and monounsaturated fatty acids to 15% of total calories; limit dietary cholesterol to 300 mg/day.

General description
- Limit meat to no more than 7 oz/day
  - Include only chicken and turkey with skin removed, and use lean cuts of fish, veal, beef, pork, or lamb.
- Restrict eggs to two per week, including those used in cooking.
- Restrict milk products to 1% fat milk, ice milk, sherbert, low-fat frozen yogurt, low-fat cheese, and low-fat cottage cheese.
- Avoid hard fats; use only vegetable oils, olive oil, or margarines.
- All vegetables and fruits are allowed except for coconut.
- Bread, cereals, pasta, potatoes, and rice are allowed except when made with eggs; limit starchy foods to prevent weight gain.
- Avoid whole-milk products, marbled meats, fish eggs, organ meats, bakery goods made with hard fats and eggs, and rich desserts.

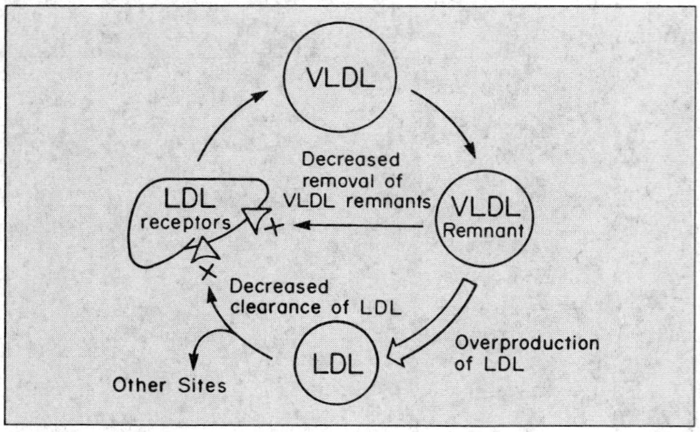

Fig. 171-13. Effects of a deficiency (or reduction) of LDL receptors on lipoprotein metabolism. First, hepatic clearance of VLDL remnants is reduced, and consequently, more VLDL remnants are converted to LDL; second, clearance of LDL is reduced. The net result of both changes is an increase in LDL concentrations.

riety of factors, including an estimate of the patient's overall risk status, age, motivation, and general health. The preferable drug for moderate hypercholesterolemia is a bile acid sequestrant. Its use is supported by the Lipid Research Clinics Coronary Primary Prevention Trial; in this trial, therapy with cholestyramine safely and effectively reduced the risk for CHD in patients with hypercholesterolemia. Some patients, however, cannot tolerate bile acid sequestrants, and alternative drugs must be considered. Nicotinic acid also is a potent cholesterol-lowering drug, and it has proved effective for reduction of coronary mortality. Unfortunately, nicotinic acid is accompanied by side effects in some patients that prevent its use. HMG CoA reductase inhibitors are highly effective for reducing LDL levels in patients with moderate hypercholesterolemia. Because their long-term safety has not been proved, they probably should not be used in the absence of CHD or other risk factors, but if these conditions are present, HMG CoA reductase inhibitors can be justified for many cases. Fibric acids generally are not effective LDL-lowering drugs, and they have little place for treatment of moderate hypercholesterolemia. Finally, probucol decreases LDL concentrations similarly to the fibric acids, but it unfortunately reduces HDL cholesterol levels. The latter effect theoretically could be deleterious, although probucol was shown recently to retard development of atherosclerosis in rabbits with genetic hypercholesterolemia. This finding is promising, and probucol deserves more investigation for its role in prevention of CHD.

If a patient with moderate hypercholesterolemia has established CHD, the goal of therapy is to reduce the LDL level to below 100 mg/dl. Often, this level cannot be achieved by dietary therapy alone, and it is necessary to resort to drug therapy. In such patients, dietary therapy need not be tried for 6 months before initiating to drug therapy. After a short period of dietary training, drug therapy can be instituted. HMG CoA reductase inhibitors are particularly attractive for treatment of moderate hypercholesterolemia in patients with established CHD, but often LDL-cholesterol levels will not be reduced to below 100 mg/dl. In these cases, the addition of bile acid sequestrants to the treatment regimen is highly effective for most patients and can be recommended for patients with established CHD in whom a maximal lowering of LDL levels is desirable.

A special case is the postmenopausal woman with moderate hypercholesterolemia (and elevated LDL cholesterol). LDL levels rise after the menopause because of loss of estrogens. This effect appears to be due to a reduction in LDL receptor activity, because estrogens are known to stimulate the synthesis of LDL receptors. The risk for CHD rises strikingly in postmenopausal women, and increased risk may be due in part to the increment in LDL levels. Concomitantly high HDL levels may afford an element of protection in some postmenopausal women, but elevated LDL concentrations probably still impart increased risk. One approach to postmenopausal hypercholesterolemia is to institute estrogen replacement therapy. A reduction of LDL levels of 10% to 15% occurs in many patients. If LDL lowering is not sufficient by estrogen replacement therapy alone, or if the woman has established CHD or other CHD risk factors, the use of HMG CoA reductase inhibitors can be considered.

Severe hypercholesterolemia consists of plasma cholesterol level over 300 mg/dl (LDL cholesterol over 210 mg/dl). Risk for CHD above this level exceeds that at baseline by at least four times. The most severe elevations of plasma cholesterol occur in patients with hereditary defects in the gene encoding the LDL receptor. Several different genetic defects in the primary structures of the receptor have been delineated, ranging from complete absence to aberrant receptor protein. These defects collectively cause the syndrome called *familial hypercholesterolemia*. Their effects on LDL metabolism are shown in Fig. 171-13. Because one gene for the LDL receptor is inherited from each parent, the disease usually occurs in the heterozygous form. One in 500 persons have heterozygous familial hypercholesterolemia; the homozygous form is much rarer (1 per 1,000,000). Heterozygous familial hypercholesterol is manifest as plasma total cholesterol in the range of 300 to 500 mg/dl, tendon xanthomas, and premature CHD. Men frequently develop CHD in their thirties or forties, or even earlier, whereas women often develop CHD in their fifties and sixties.

About 1% of adult Americans have cholesterol levels that consistently exceed 300 mg/dl. Some of these patients will have undetected familial hypercholesterolemia, but in most a monogenic inheritance cannot be demonstrated. Even so, most of them appear to have a reduced activity of LDL receptors, possibly due to a metabolic suppression of LDL receptor synthesis. Such patients rarely have tendon xanthomas, and CHD generally does not occur as early as in patients with familial hypercholesterolemia; nevertheless they are at high risk for CHD and should be treated appropriately. First, however, secondary forms of elevated LDL cholesterol should be ruled out. Hypothyroidism can cause severe hypercholesterolemia, as can biliary obstruction. In the latter condition, the excess plasma cholesterol is mainly unesterified, and the increased serum cholesterol is not found in LDL per se but in an abnormal lipoprotein called *lipoprotein X*. The nephrotic syndrome also causes severe hypercholesterolemia, and it may or may not be accompanied by hypertriglyceridemia.

Because primary severe hypercholesterolemia imparts a high risk for CHD, LDL levels should be lowered. Maximal dietary therapy should be initiated; for most patients, this means a diet very low in saturated fatty acids (less than 7% of calories) and cholesterol (less than 200 mg/day). Although dietary therapy helps in management, cholesterol-lowering drugs may be needed to bring the LDL cholesterol to acceptably low levels. Bile acid sequestrant generally should be the first drug prescribed. Nicotinic acid is a satisfactory second drug, but for most patients, HMG CoA reductase inhibitors are preferred in combination with sequestrants because of their potency and relative lack of side effects.

Hypertriglyceridemia

Hypertriglyceridemia is defined here as a plasma triglyceride level that exceeds 250 mg/dl. In its pure form, the plasma total cholesterol is less than 240 mg/dl. Most patients with pure hypertriglyceridemia have an increase in VLDL triglycerides, hence the term *endogenous hypertriglyceridemia,* also called type IV HLP. Serum triglycerides generally are in the range of 250 to 500 mg/dl. An elevation of endogenous triglycerides can be due either to an hepatic overproduction or to a defective lipolysis of VLDL triglycerides (Fig. 171-14). Either defect produces several metabolic consequences for the metabolism of other lipoproteins: an increased concentration of VLDL cholesterol, abnormalities in the composition of VLDL particles, increased concentrations of VLDL remnants and IDL, increased conversion of VLDL to LDL, enhanced catabolism of LDL, reduction in particles of reduced size, and decreased concentrations of HDL cholesterol. Any or all of these metabolic consequences of hypertriglyceridemia may be responsible for an increased rate of atherogenesis accompanying the hypertriglyceridemic state. The more common forms of hypertriglyceridemia are considered here.

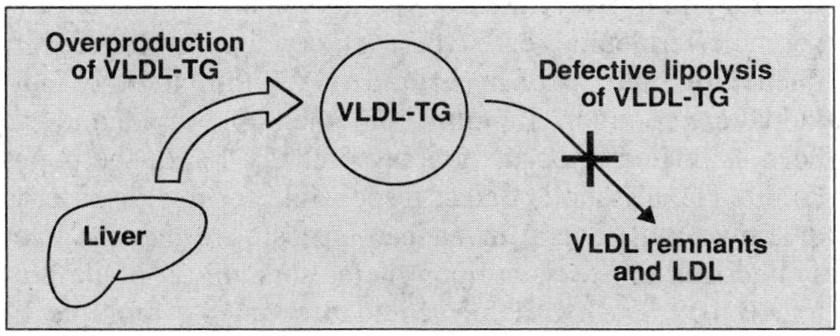

Fig. 171-14. Mechanisms of primary hypertriglyceridemia. An increase in VLDL triglyceride concentrations can be the result of either of two mechanisms: (1) hepatic overproduction of VLDL triglycerides (VLDL-TG) or (2) defective lipolysis of VLDL triglycerides.

Diet-induced endogenous hypertriglyceridemia. Certain dietary factors (e.g., excessive intakes of total calories, carbohydrates, and ethanol) stimulate the production of VLDL triglycerides. In some persons, high outputs of VLDL triglycerides do not induce hypertriglyceridemia because of a concomitant high activity of LPL. In other patients, however, LPL fails to compensate adequately, and overproduction of VLDL triglycerides causes mild hypertriglyceridemia. When this condition occurs, triglyceride levels rise to between 250 and 400 mg/dl. In obese patients, the number of VLDL particles entering the plasma is increased; consequently, more VLDL particles are converted to LDL. Regardless of whether lipoprotein concentrations are elevated in obese patients, the transport of an excessive number of lipoproteins through the plasma compartment may contribute to the increased risk for CHD associated with obesity. In contrast, high-carbohydrate diets and high intakes of ethanol increase the triglyceride content of each VLDL particle, but they do not raise the number of VLDL particles secreted into plasma. A higher flux of VLDL triglycerides, due to an excess of dietary carbohydrates or alcohol, may not be atherogenic.

Primary endogenous hypertriglyceridemia. This disorder can result from either overproduction of VLDL triglyceride or defective lipolysis of VLDL triglycerides (Fig. 171-14). When several members of a single family have elevated serum triglycerides, the condition is called *familial hypertriglyceridemia*. Primary overproduction of VLDL triglycerides is analogous to the high secretion of VLDL triglycerides induced by dietary carbohydrates or alcohol. The number of VLDL particles secreted into plasma is not increased, and only the quantity of triglycerides per particle is raised. The cause of primary overproduction of VLDL triglycerides is not known, but in some cases it may be due to resistance to the peripheral action of insulin. The causes of defective lipolysis of VLDL triglycerides are poorly understood. Most patients probably have a mild deficiency of LPL, but some may have defects in the chemical composition of VLDL, making the lipoprotein a poor substrate for LPL. Defective lipolysis of VLDL triglycerides is difficult to distinguish from overproduction of VLDL triglycerides, and for clinical purposes, it is sufficient to recognize the presence of primary endogenous hypertriglyceridemia. Either cause of hypertriglyceridemia can give rise to the metabolic consequences mentioned previously. Increasing evidence suggests that elevated triglyceride levels raise the risk for CHD, possibly because of these secondary metabolic changes in lipoprotein metabolism.

For patients with primary endogenous hypertriglyceridemia, changes in life-style (control of weight, increased physical activity, and restriction of excess carbohydrates [especially sucrose], and alcohol) are the first modes of therapy. If dietary therapy is not successful for normalizing triglyceride levels, drug therapy can be considered, especially if the patient has CHD or other coronary risk factors outlined in Fig. 171-10. Nicotinic acid is the drug of choice, but if it is not tolerated, gemfibrozil is a good alternative. If the patient does not have CHD or other risk factors, it may be prudent to withhold drug therapy and to attempt to control elevated triglycerides by diet modification and exercise.

Secondary hypertriglyceridemia. An increase in VLDL triglycerides, without a concomitant increase in cholesterol levels, can be produced by certain diseases or drugs: (1) poorly controlled diabetes mellitus, (2) chronic renal failure, (3) rare dyslipoproteinemias, (4) oral contraceptives, and (5) beta-adrenergic blocking agents. Commonly, these secondary causes will accentuate a latent primary hypertriglyceridemia.

A common cause of secondary hypertriglyceridemia is non-insulin-dependent diabetes mellitus (NIDDM). This condition induces both overproduction of VLDL triglycerides and reduced lipolysis of triglyceride-rich lipoproteins. The high output of VLDL triglycerides may be caused by two factors: increased serum FFA and hyperglycemia; it also can be accentuated by obesity. Reduced lipolysis of plasma triglycerides may be the result of a decrease of LPL activity, secondary to an impaired action of insulin. Hypertriglyceridemia may be one factor responsible for the increased risk for CHD associated with NIDDM. Treatment should be directed first toward improving glycemic control, reducing weight in obese patients, and increasing exercise. Lipid-lowering drugs have not been investigated extensively in NIDDM. Nicotinic acid unfortunately can worsen hyperglycemia and raise uric acid levels in diabetics. Gemfibrozil will lower triglycerides but may increase the LDL-cholesterol level. HMG CoA reductase inhibitors show promise for serum cholesterol-lowering diabetic patients, but their benefit in hypertriglyceridemic diabetes has not been established.

Mixed hyperlipidemias

Mixed hyperlipidemias are defined as an increase in plasma, total cholesterol (< 240 mg/dl), and plasma triglycerides (> 250 mg/dl). Mixed hyperlipidemia is identified when a lipoprotein profile is determined on a patient found to have high plasma cholesterol. It can be the result of several primary and secondary disorders in lipoprotein metabolism, and not uncommonly, primary and secondary disorders are present in the same individual. The major forms of mixed hyperlipidemia can be considered.

Marked hypertriglyceridemia with elevated cholesterol levels. When triglyceride levels exceed 500 mg/dl, increases in both VLDL and chylomicrons typically are present (type V HLP). Cholesterol levels usually exceed 240 mg/dl. Raised concentrations of cholesterol usually are limited to triglyceride-rich lipoproteins, and LDL cholesterol levels typically are normal or even reduced. Type V HLP usually results from combined overproduction of VLDL and reduced lipolysis of triglyceride-rich lipoproteins (Fig. 171-15). These two abnormalities together can result from any combination of dietary, primary, or secondary hypertriglyceridemia, as discussed in the previous section. The most immediate danger of severe type V HLP is acute pancreatitis. Many, but not all, older patients with type V HLP also

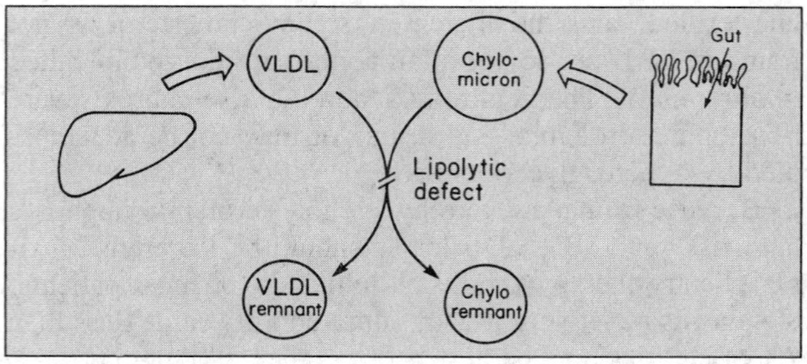

Fig. 171-15. Mechanism of type V HLP. An elevation of both VLDL and chylomicrons in type V HLP is the result of two metabolic defects: (1) overproduction of VLDL, and (2) a lipolytic defect for triglyceride-rich lipoproteins including both VLDL and chylomicrons.

have premature atherosclerotic disease; the latter is more likely to occur when other risk factors, such as smoking or diabetes mellitus, are present.

When triglyceride levels are in the range of 500 to 1000 mg/dl, the principles of therapy are similar to those described previously for endogenous hypertriglyceridemia. For severe type V HLP, treatment frequently requires a combination of diet and drugs. The intake of fat should be curtailed to reduce the formation of chylomicrons. Clearance of chylomicrons can be promoted in some patients by a fibric acid, such as gemfibrozil. If the fibric acid does not clear chylomicronemia, elevated triglycerides may respond to nicotinic acid, a drug that inhibits the synthesis of VLDL. Recent reports indicate that high intakes of fish oil also inhibit synthesis of VLDL, and fish oils may be used as an adjunct to therapy in some patients with type V HLP. If a patient has a dietary component to overproduction of VLDL (e.g., obesity or excessive alcohol intake), emphasis should be on dietary modification; if a second disorder is the major factor, treatment should be aimed at eliminating this disorder.

Familial combined hyperlipidemia. A more common form of mixed hyperlipidemia is familial combined hyperlipidemia. This disorder was first defined as a monogenic hyperlipidemia characterized by multiple lipoprotein phenotypes (types IV, V, III, IIA, and/or IIB) in a single family. Some family members may have elevations in both cholesterol and triglyceride levels; others manifest isolated hypercholesterolemia or hypertriglyceridemia. Moreover, fluctuating patterns of hyperlipidemia within a single individual are common. Familial combined hyperlipidemia has been estimated to occur in approximately 1% of the population. The metabolic defect responsible for this disorder is unknown, but several investigators postulate that the liver synthesizes an excess of lipoproteins containing apolipoprotein B-100. Such a defect could account for multiple lipoprotein abnormalities in a single individual or family. Regardless of which lipoprotein phenotype is present, the risk for CHD appears to increase.

An alternate explanation for multiple lipoprotein phenotypes within a single family might be that several lipoprotein defects are inherited simultaneously (Fig. 171-16).

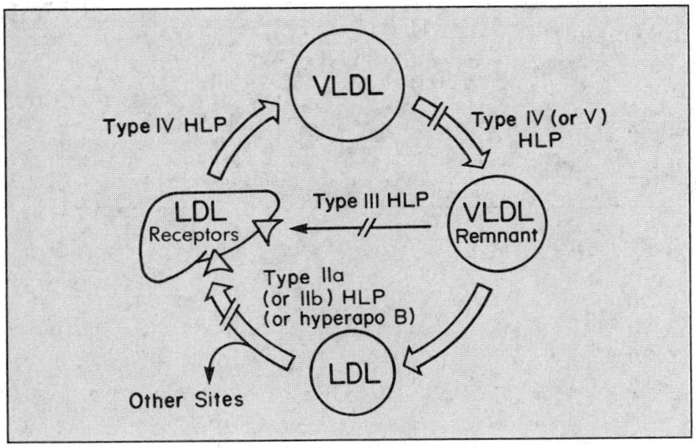

Fig. 171-16. Factors contributing to multiple lipoprotein phenotypes. Type IV HLP can result from either overproduction or defective clearance of VLDL. When both defects are present, the patient may have type V HLP. The E-2/2 genotype delays clearance of VLDL remnants, and when combined with another defect in triglyceride metabolism, results in type III HLP. Finally, a defective clearance of LDL, in association with other defects, can produce either hyperapobetalipoproteinemia (hyperapo B) or type II HLP (IIa or IIb).

Such defects could include overproduction of lipoproteins, defective lipolysis of triglyceride-rich lipoproteins, defective clearance of remnant lipoproteins, and/or reduced activity of LDL receptors. Considering the relatively high prevalence of all of these abnormalities among American adults, coinheritance of metabolic defects should be relatively common.

Treatment of mixed elevations of cholesterol and triglycerides, manifest by various combinations of increased VLDL and LDL, requires attention to both types of lipids. Elevated serum cholesterol and triglycerides can be treated together or separately. Weight reduction, increased exercise, and reduced intakes of saturated fatty acids may lower both serum cholesterol and triglyceride levels. If drug therapy seems appropriate, either because of inadequate response to dietary therapy or the presence of CHD or other risk factors, nicotinic acid is the drug of choice because it acts to reduce levels of all lipoproteins. If nicotinic acid is not effective or tolerated, various combinations of drugs can be tried. The combination of fibric acid and a HMG CoA reductase inhibitor can be highly effective but is associated with an increased risk for drug-induced myopathy. A fibric acid and bile acid sequestrant is another effective and relatively safe combination.

Primary mixed hyperlipidemia. Most patients with mixed hyperlipidemia cannot be shown to have multiple lipoprotein phenotypes. Some patients belong to the category of undetected familial combined hyperlipidemia, whereas others will have two or more concomitant defects in lipoprotein metabolism (Fig. 171-16). Primary mixed hyperlipidemia is a relative common abnormality in patients with premature CHD. Treatment is basically the same as that described for familial combined hyperlipidemia.

Secondary mixed hyperlipidemia. A common cause of mixed hyperlipidemia is NIDDM. In most NIDDM patients, weight reduction and better control of hyperglycemia will reduce both cholesterol and triglyceride levels, but the lipid-lowering response can be enhanced by use of HMG CoA reductase inhibitors. In the nephrotic syndrome, hypercholesterolemia and increased serum triglycerides often coexist; one abnormality responsible for the mixed hyperlipidemia appears to be an overproduction of lipoproteins by the liver, although the hypertriglyceridemia may be due in part to a defective lipolysis VLDL triglycerides. The hyperlipidemia of the nephrotic syndrome has proved difficult to treat successfully, but the HMG CoA reductase inhibitors appear to hold promise.

HYPOALPHALIPOPROTEINEMIA (LOW HDL)

The well-recognized inverse correlation between concentrations of HDL cholesterol and the risk of CHD justifies measurement of HDL cholesterol when plasma cholesterol exceeds 200 mg/dl. This measurement especially should be made if other risk factors are present. The distributions of HDL cholesterol levels in Americans are given in Table 171-6. For patients with high-normal or elevated LDL cholesterol, an HDL cholesterol level of below 35 mg/dl definitely is a cause for concern. A reduced HDL can be caused by one or more factors, many of which are reversible (see the box on p. 1454).

Whether raising HDL cholesterol by therapy will decrease coronary risk is unknown, but modification of several causes of a low HDL can be justified because of other benefits. For example, HDL cholesterol can be increased by weight reduction in obese persons, by cessation of smoking, by frequent and vigorous exercise, and by correction of elevated cholesterol or triglyceride levels. These regimens can be recommended for most patients with a low HDL. More controversial is whether regular consumption of alcohol for the purpose of raising the HDL level is advisable; its utility in preventing CHD has not been proved, and the serious social and physical consequences of excess intake of alcohol cannot be ignored.

Some regimens that reduce LDL (or total cholesterol) also may lower the HDL level. For example, diets high in polyunsaturated fatty acids or carbohydrates reduce the plasma HDL, as does the cholesterol-lowering drug probucol. The argument has been made that the decrease in the plasma LDL accompanying these regimens more than offsets any reduction in HDL because in populations in which levels of LDL and rates of CHD are low, the HDL cholesterol level may be low as well. The concept thus has arisen that the total cholesterol/HDL cholesterol ratio may be a better indicator of coronary risk than either the total cholesterol or HDL cholesterol level alone. The risk ratios for varying total cholesterol/HDL cholesterol ratios for American men are listed in Table 171-7, and these ratios can be used to predict coronary risk. It should be kept in mind, however, that a high level of HDL does not completely negate the risk imparted by an elevated LDL.

Table 171-6. Population distribution of plasma HDL cholesterol (mg/dl)*

	White men						White women					
	Percentiles						Percentiles					
Age (yr)	**5**	**10**	**25**	**50**	**75**	**95**	**5**	**10**	**25**	**50**	**75**	**95**
0-4												
5-9	38	42	49	54	63	74	36	38	47	52	61	73
10-14	37	40	46	55	61	74	37	40	45	52	58	70
15-19	30	34	39	46	52	63	35	38	43	51	61	74
20-24	30	32	38	45	51	63	33	37	44	51	62	79
25-29	31	32	37	44	50	63	37	39	47	55	63	83
30-34	28	32	38	45	52	63	36	40	46	55	64	77
35-39	29	31	36	43	49	62	34	38	44	53	64	82
40-44	27	31	36	43	51	67	34	39	48	56	65	88
45-49	30	33	38	45	52	64	34	41	47	58	68	87
50-54	28	31	36	44	51	63	37	41	50	62	73	91
55-59	28	31	38	46	55	71	37	41	50	60	73	91
60-64	30	34	41	49	61	74	38	44	51	61	75	92
65-69	30	33	39	49	62	78	35	38	49	62	73	98
70 +	31	33	40	48	56	75	33	38	48	60	71	92

*Modified from the Lipid Research Clinics Population Studies Data Book: The prevalence study. Bethesda, Md, 1979, National Institutes of Health Publication No. 79-1527.

RARE DISORDERS OF LIPID METABOLISM

Because the metabolism of lipids and lipoproteins is complex, defects can occur at multiple sites. Most defects result from abnormalities in the synthesis of a key protein or lipid. Some defects can produce hyperlipidemia, but other abnormalities cause low levels of lipoproteins or bizarre defects in lipoprotein metabolism. Although these disorders are rare, they can be devastating to the affected patient.

Abnormalities in the synthesis of apolipoproteins

Apolipoprotein B. A failure to synthesize lipoproteins containing apo B is responsible for the disorder called abetalipoproteinemia. In the most common form of this disorder, both apo B-100 and apo B-48 are absent, but one patient has been reported who had apo B-48 but no apo B-100. Classic abetalipoproteinemia is characterized by a lack of chylomicrons, VLDL, and LDL. A failure to synthesize chylomicrons causes malabsorption of fat, and absence of VLDL and LDL results in severe reductions in plasma triglycerides and cholesterol. Low levels of plasma cholesterol induce deformities of red blood cells (acanthocytosis), and after several years, patients develop progressive neurologic involvement—retinitis pigmentosa and ataxic neuropathy. Failure to transport vitamin E in LDL probably is responsible for neurologic signs, and their progression apparently can be retarded by parenteral administration of large doses of vitamin E.

A congenital reduction in synthesis of apo B-containing lipoproteins causes hypobetalipoproteinemia, or a very low level of LDL. Synthesis of defective forms of the apo B

Causes of reduced plasma HDL cholesterol

- Obesity
- Tobacco use
- Lack of exercise
- Hypertriglyceridemia
- Hypercholesterolemia
- Genetic factors (poorly defined)
- Drugs
  - Progestational agents
  - Anabolic steroids and androgens
  - Beta-adrenergic blocking agents
  - Thiazide diuretics
- Some cholesterol-lowering regimens
  - Diets (low-fat, low-cholesterol, high-polyunsaturated fat diets)
  - Drugs (probucol)

Table 171-7. Relation of total cholesterol/HDL cholesterol ratio to risk for coronary heart disease (men aged 50-70)

Total cholesterol/HDL cholesterol ratio	Coronary heart disease risk ratio
3.0	0.5
4.4	1.0
6.2	2.0
7.7	3.0
9.5	4.0

Castelli WP, Abbott RD, and McNamara PM: Summary estimates of cholesterol used to predict coronary heart disease, Circulation 67:730, 1983.

molecules produces a similar clinical picture. Although the LDL concentration is markedly reduced in these disorders, it is not absent. Patients with hypobetalipoproteinemia generally are spared the severe sequelae of abetalipoproteinemia, although occasionally these may occur when LDL reduction is severe.

Recently, a familial defective form of apo B-100 has been reported. The defect prevents the binding of LDL apo B to LDL receptors and results in hypercholesterolemia.

Apolipoprotein A. A rare disorder secondary to a defect in metabolism of apo A is Tangier disease. This disorder appears to be the result of enhanced catabolism of HDL. Both apo A-I and apo A-II in plasma are greatly reduced, but neither apoprotein has been shown to be structurally abnormal. Patients with Tangier disease accumulate large amounts of cholesterol esters in reticuloendothelial tissues, most notably in the tonsils; they commonly have a relapsing neuropathy and corneal opacities. Tangier disease follows autosomal recessive inheritance, and consanguinity is common. The disease apparently does not accelerate atherosclerosis despite the marked reduction in HDL levels.

Another disorder in metabolism of apo A is characterized by a familial deficiency of both apo A-I and apo C-III and severe coronary atherosclerosis. In this disorder, xanthoma of skin and tendons and corneal clouding are present. The reason for the presence of premature atherosclerosis with combined deficiency of apo a-I and apo C-III but not in Tangier disease is unclear. Finally, certain abnormal forms of apo a-I, such as one called A-I Milano, cause relatively low levels of HDL but not premature atherosclerosis.

Apolipoprotein E. A point mutation in the synthesis of apo E produces an abnormal isoform of this apo E. Two normal isoforms of apo E, apo E-3 and apo E-4, bind tightly to hepatic receptors for chylomicron remnants and LDL. In so doing, they promote hepatic uptake of chylomicron remnants and VLDL remnants. The abnormal isoform of apo E is called apo E-2, and it binds poorly to receptors. Every person inherits two genes encoding for apo E. Six genotypes thus are possible: E-3/3, E-3/4, E-3/2, E-4/4, E-4/2, and E-2/2. The E-2/2 genotype occurs in about 1 in 100 Europeans and Americans, and its presence in the absence of other defects of lipoprotein metabolism causes hyperlipidemia. The E-2/2 pattern, however, occasionally contributes to a unique form of hyperlipidemia called familial dysbetalipoproteinemia or type III HLP. This disorder is characterized by accumulation of remnantlike lipoproteins called beta-VLDL. Affected patients frequently have tuberous or tuberoeruptive xanthoma; yellow discolorations of palmar and digital creases; and premature atherosclerosis of coronary arteries, internal carotids, and abdominal aorta. Beta-VLDL are VLDL remnants enriched in cholesterol esters; they are identified by a cholesterol/triglyceride ratio in VLDL exceeding 0.3. Most patients with dysbetalipoproteinemia have the E-2/2 genotype combined with overproduction of VLDL (Fig. 171-16). The overproduction of VLDL may be primary or secondary to diabetes mellitus and/or obesity. Recently, a new kindred of patients has been described who have no plasma apo E. This disorder, which also may be characterized by dysbetalipoproteinemia, presumably represents a complete failure to synthesize apo E.

Apolipoprotein C. As indicated previously, a deficiency of apo C-III can occur with a lack of apo A-I; low levels of HDL but not hyperlipidemia result. In another rare condition, apo C-II, the apoprotein required for activation of LPL, is genetically absent. Its absence causes severe hypertriglyceridemia and chylomicronemia. Affected patients are prone to repeated bouts of acute pancreatitis and sometimes chronic pancreatitis. Premature atherosclerosis accompanying deficiency of apo C-II has not been reported.

Abnormalities in enzymes affecting lipoprotein metabolism

Lipoprotein lipase. A familial deficiency of LPL is a rare autosomal recessive condition. It results in a severe lipolytic defect for chylomicrons and consequently severe chylomicronemia (type I HLP). Levels of VLDL are relatively normal, and apparently atherosclerosis is not accelerated. Severe chylomicronemia is present from birth, and skin xanthomas and pancreatitis may occur in infancy or childhood. The plasma creams with chylomicrons, but the infranatant remains relatively clear because VLDL are only mildly elevated. Treatment requires a marked reduction of dietary fat, if possible to less than 10% of total calories. Medium-chain triglycerides can provide a partial replacement of dietary fat, but because these cause ketosis when given in large doses, their intake must be limited. Lipid-lowering drugs are of no value in treatment of type I HLP.

Lecithin-cholesterol acyltransferase. A genetic deficiency of LCAT occurs rarely as an autosomal recessive disease. It is characterized by failure to form cholesterol esters in plasma. Clinical manifestations include multiple defects in metabolism of lipoproteins, corneal opacities, anemia, renal failure, and premature atherosclerosis. The absence of cholesterol esters in plasma results in an array of abnormalities in lipoproteins. The LDL are unusually large and disk-shaped. HDL also are abnormal in size and shape, and various abnormalities are present in VLDL.

Abnormalities in enzymes affecting sterol metabolism

Lysosomal acid lipase. This enzyme hydrolyzes both the triglycerides and cholesterol esters that enter lysosomes with LDL. The absence of this lipase causes either a severe disease or a more benign one. The former, called Wolman's disease, is usually fatal before the age of 1 year. Features of Wolman's disease include massive accumulation of lipids in liver and spleen and a generalized failure to thrive. In the less severe form, cholesterol ester storage disease, patients often live to adulthood. They nonetheless have hepatomegaly because of accumulation of cholesterol esters in the liver. These patients frequently have hypercholesterolemia and premature atherosclerosis.

Defective bile acid synthesis. A defect in the side chain oxidation of cholesterol in its conversion to bile acids causes a disease called cerebrotendinous xanthomatosis. The primary defect in this disease appears to reside in mitochondrial 26-hydroxylation, a key reaction in the conversion. Consequently, the synthesis of the primary bile acids, cholic acid and chenodeoxycholic acid, is reduced. The resulting deficiency of bile acids causes a loss in the feedback regulation of bile acid synthesis, and increased amounts of cholesterol begin to be converted into bile acids. Because of the block in this conversion, however, intermediate steroids are shunted into other products including complex bile alcohols and cholestanol (dehydrocholesterol). Cholestanol becomes incorporated into plasma lipoproteins and, because of its unique physicochemical properties, promotes deposition of both cholesterol and cholestanol into tendons, brain tissue, and the arterial wall. The result is tendinous xanthomatosis, progressive neurologic dysfunction including dementia, spinal cord paresis and cerebellar ataxia, and premature atherosclerosis. A recent report indicates that the neurologic components of cerebrotendinous xanthomatosis can be reversed by oral administration of chenodeoxycholic acid, which inhibits the rapid catabolism of cholesterol, reduces the formation of cholestanol, and apparently reverses tissue deposition of sterols.

REFERENCES

Brown MS, and Goldstein JL: A receptor-mediated pathway for cholesterol homeostasis, Science 232:34-47, 1986.

Consensus Development Conference: Lowering blood cholesterol to prevent heart disease, JAMA 253:2080-2086, 1985.

Frick MH et al: Helsinki Heart Study: Primary-prevention trial with gemfibrozil in middle-aged men with dyslipidemia: safety of treatment, changes in risk factors, and incidence of coronary heart disease, N Engl J Med 317:1237-1245, 1987.

Grundy SM: Cholesterol and coronary heart disease: a new era, JAMA 256:2849-2858, 1986.

Grundy SM:-HMG CoA reductase inhibitors for treatment of hypercholesterolemia, N Engl J Med 319:24-32, 1988.

Grundy SM and Denke MA: Dietary influences on serum lipids and lipoproteins, J Lipid Res 31:1149-1172, 1990.

Lipid Research Clinics Coronary Primary Prevention Trial Results: I. Reduction in incidence of coronary heart disease, JAMA 251:531-564, 1984. II. The relation of reduction in incidence of coronary heart disease to cholesterol lowering, JAMA 251:365, 1984.

National Institutes of Health Consensus Conference: Treatment of hypertriglyceridemia, JAMA 251:1196, 1984.

Report of the Expert Panel on Population Strategies for Blood Cholesterol Reduction: National Cholesterol Education Program, Circulation 83:2154-2232, 1991.

Report of the Expert Panel on Blood Cholesterol Levels In Children and Adolescents: National Cholesterol Education Program, Pediatrics 89:525-583, 1992.

Report of the National Cholesterol Education Program Expert Panel on Detection, Evaluation, and Treatment of High Blood Cholesterol in Adults, Arch Intern Med 148:36-69, 1988.

Ross R: The pathogenesis of atherosclerosis—an update, N Engl J Med 314:488-500, 1986.

The cholesterol facts: A summary of the evidence relating dietary fats, serum cholesterol, and coronary heart disease. A joint statement by the American Heart Association and the National Heart, Lung, and Blood Institute, Circulation 81:1721-1733, 1990.

CHAPTER

172 Lipodystrophies

M. Joycelyn Elders

The lipodystrophies are a group of rare metabolic disorders characterized by abnormalities in adipose tissue, generalized or partial loss of body fat, abnormalities of carbohydrate and lipid metabolism, severe resistance to endogenous and exogenous insulin, and immunologic dysfunction. These disorders differ in the anatomic distribution of the dystrophic tissue and are associated with variable degrees of multiple system involvement. The lipodystrophies may be divided into three major categories: total, partial, and localized, based on the anatomic distribution of the lipodystrophic change.

Total lipodystrophy consists of congenital or acquired complete loss of adipose tissue, usually associated with hepatomegaly, hyperglycemia, hyperlipidemia, and hypermetabolism. Other associations include acanthosis nigricans, acromegalic gigantism, generalized hyperpigmentation, renal disease, central nervous system disorders, cardiomegaly, hypertrichosis, hypertrophy of external genitalia, and advanced bone age. Partial lipodystrophy is usually manifest as symmetric or asymmetric loss of adipose tissue with or without facial involvement and with or without atrophy of the extremities or the trunk. This syndrome has also been associated with renal disease, diabetes, hyperpigmentation, hirsutism, hepatomegaly, and hyperlipemia. Localized lipodystrophy is usually manifest as well-demarcated, multifocal atrophic lesions with or without other associated diseases. In each of these categories there are several syndromes that have distinguishable physical, genetic, immunologic, or biochemical characteristics.

A classification of this heterogeneous group of disorders is shown in the accompanying box. Whether each of these disorders is a distinct entity or whether they together represent a spectrum of disease has not been completely determined. The specific pathophysiology is not clear; however, the clinical syndromes are fairly distinct.

LEPRECHAUNISM

Leprechaunism is a rare inherited syndrome that includes characteristic facial features, intrauterine growth retardation, phallic enlargement, marked deficiency of subcutaneous fat stores, and striking cutaneous abnormalities (Figs.

Classification of the major lipodystrophic syndromes

I. Total lipodystrophy
   A. Leprechaunism
   B. Congenital
   C. Acquired
II. Partial lipodystrophy
   A. Acquired
   B. Familial
   C. Lipoatrophic diabetes mellitus
III. Localized lipodystrophy
   A. Mesenteric
   B. Membranous
   C. Centrifugal

172-1 and 172-2). Biochemical alterations have included postprandial hyperglycemia, hyperinsulinism, insulin resistance, abnormalities of the insulin receptor, and fasting hypoglycemia.

The high frequency of consanguinity and familial occurrence suggests that leprechaunism is transmitted by an autosomal recessive mode of inheritance. There is a 2:1 female/male ratio, and most of the infants manifest severe failure to thrive and early death.

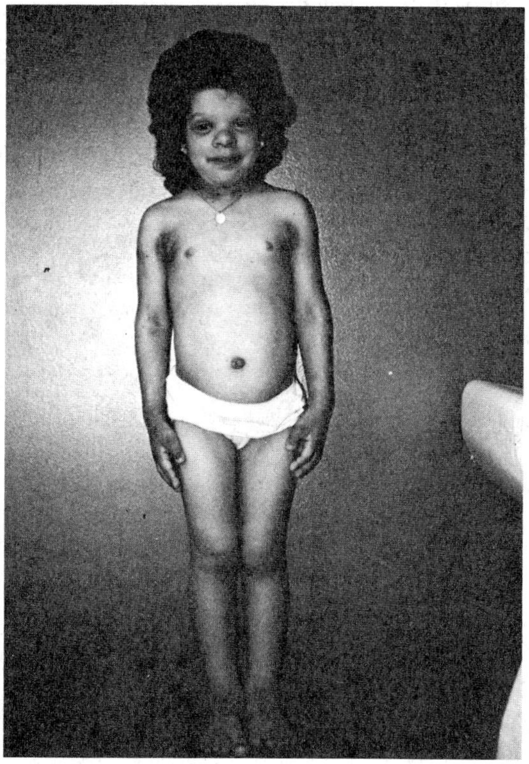

Fig. 172-1. Patient with leprechaunism. Note characteristic facies, absence of subcutaneous tissue, acanthosis nigricans, and hypertrichosis.

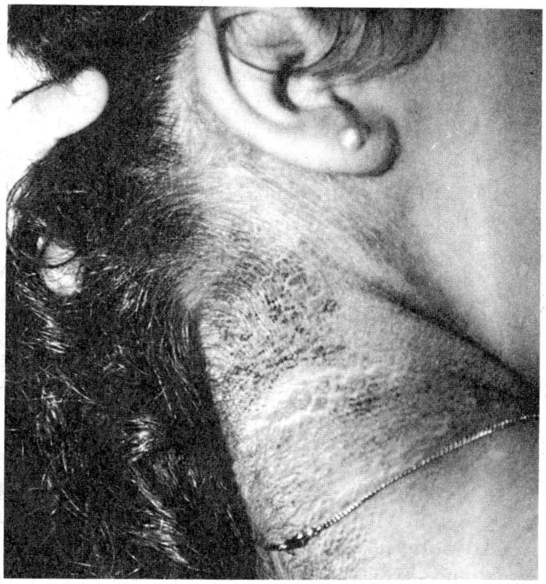

Fig. 172-2. Same patient as shown in Fig. 172-1.

Carbohydrate metabolism and insulin-receptor abnormalities in leprechaunism

All patients with leprechaunism studied thus far have shown evidence of abnormal glucose homeostasis. Fasting hypoglycemia has been a frequent finding and is thought to be secondary to an accelerated response to fasting or to decreased glycogen synthesis during feeding with decreased glycogen stores. Excessive elevations of the blood glucose level are frequent in association with elevated blood insulin levels and pancreatic islet cell hyperplasia. Pathologic findings have included enlarged kidneys, ovaries, and testes; increased iron deposition in the liver; calcific deposits in the kidneys; decreased lymphoid tissue; marked ductal hyperplasia of the breast; severe acanthosis nigricans; and marked hyperkeratosis of the skin. Recently, one of these patients exhibited increased excretion of epidermal growth factor (EGF) in the urine, suggesting one possible mechanism for the skin changes (Chapter 168).

Pathophysiology

The severe insulin resistance seen in leprechaunism is due to abnormalities of the insulin receptor rather than an abnormal insulin molecule. Recent studies have shown a correlation between point mutations of a single amino acid in the insulin receptor and severe insulin resistance. In some patients a homozygous leucine-proline mutation at amino acid position 233 in the alpha chain of the insulin receptor is found. In others an arginine for glycine substitution at amino acid position 31 has been found in the alpha-beta proreceptor. In both instances the mutation blocks cleavage of the proreceptor and transport from intracellular sites to the cell surfaces.

DNA amplification techniques have demonstrated that patients with leprechaunism were homozygous for these amino acid substitutions, whereas the parents and grandparents studied were heterozygous for these amino acid substitutions. Heterozygous family members had mild to moderate in vitro binding defects, but no clinical manifestations. Both the leucine to proline mutation at amino acid 233 in the alpha chain of the insulin receptor and the glycine to arginine at amino acid 31 in the proinsulin receptor alters conformation of the receptor such that transport to the Golgi compartment where proteolytic processing occurs is inhibited.

These mutant insulin receptors are associated with the following: (1) decreased insulin binding to the receptor, (2) decreased insulin stimulated 2-deoxy glucose uptake, (3) decreased autophosphorylation of the beta subunit of the insulin receptor, and (4) decreased half-life and a lack of recognition of the receptor by monoclonal antibodies directed against conformation-dependent epitopes. Further study will likely detect other amino acid mutations that will explain the similarities between leprechaunism, congenital lipodystrophies, other lipodystrophies, and insulin-resistant syndromes.

CONGENITAL TOTAL LIPODYSTROPHY

Congenital total lipodystrophy is a rare disorder of carbohydrate and lipid metabolism. In the majority of cases, it has an autosomal recessive inheritance pattern. The disease is characterized anatomically by a generalized and extreme lack of fat in subcutaneous tissue, clinically by extreme insulin resistance and diabetes mellitus, and biochemically by hyperglycemia and triglyceride hyperlipidemia. In addition to the lack of adipose tissue, a number of clinical features are observed from birth or early infancy.

Clinical manifestations

Congenital total lipodystrophy is a very rare syndrome (Table 172-1) that affects twice as many females as males. The onset is usually about the time of birth. The most striking feature of this condition is total lipodystrophy. There is virtual absence of fat from all subcutaneous tissue, including the distal portions of the body. The musculature is prominent, giving the patient a herculean appearance (Fig. 172-3). It is thought that these patients have an actual increase in muscle mass; however, some data suggest that the muscles are not truly hypertrophic but only appear to be so because of the lack of subcutaneous tissue.

The facies are very distinct. The masseters are prominent. The cheeks appear sunken owing to the lack of buccal fat pads, and the forehead is wrinkled, giving the patient an appearance of senility. The bony prominences and muscles are clearly outlined, and most patients have a very prominent abdomen.

Skeletal growth and maturation appear to be accelerated. There is mild to moderate hypertension, and the liver is always enlarged but not enough to account for the very prominent abdomen. These patients frequently develop acanthosis nigricans, which may be observed at any age but is most prominent in pubertal patients. It most frequently involves the neck, axillary, and inguinal areas; but it can have a generalized distribution. Other dermatologic features include

Table 172-1. Clinical comparison of the major lipodystrophic syndromes

	Total lipodystrophies			Partial lipodystrophies	
Clinical findings	**Leprechaunism**	**Congenital**	**Acquired**	**Acquired**	**Familial**
Inheritance	Autosomal recessive	Autosomal recessive	Sporadic	Usually sporadic	Always familial More than one generation affected Autosomal dominant
Age at recognition	Infancy	Infancy	Childhood-adult	Childhood-adult	Puberty
Sex incidence	Female/male (2:1)	Female/male (2:1)	Female predominance	Female predominance	Female predominance
Sites of lipoatrophy	Generalized	Face, trunk, limbs	Face, trunk, limbs	Face, upper trunk, upper limbs	Trunk and limbs
Prominence of muscles	Absent	+	Absent	Absent	Absent
Genital enlargement	+++	+	+	Absent	Common
Hepatomegaly/cirrhosis	±	Common	Common	Usually absent	Absent
Acanthosis nigricans	+++	++	+	Rare	+
Hypertension	Absent	Absent	+	Absent	Common
Associated abnormalities	Absent	Hepatic, renal, neurologic, cardiac	None	Renal, neurologic	None

+, mild; ++, moderate; +++, severe.

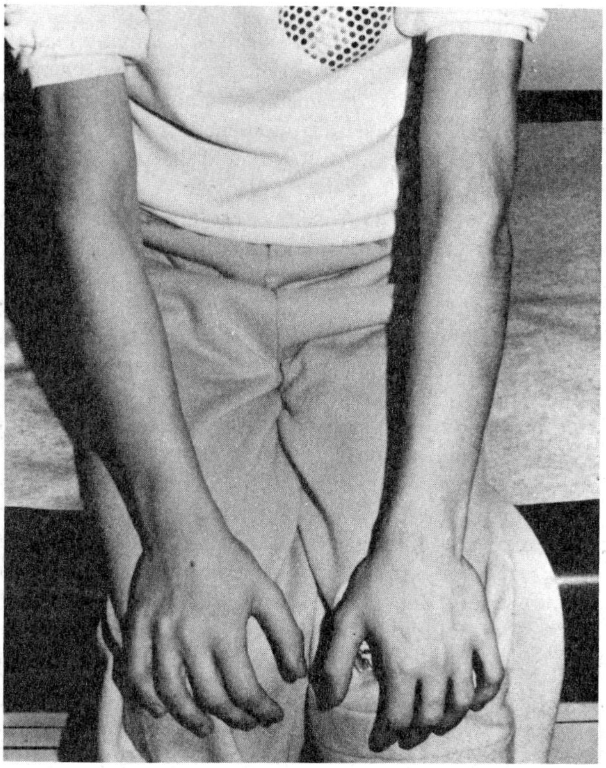

Fig. 172-3. Patient with acquired total lipodystrophy. Note prominent triceps muscles and absence of subcutaneous tissue.

hirsutism, eruptive xanthomas, and marked thickening of the skin. Genital hypertrophy is frequently observed.

Developmental milestones in children are usually normal, but mental retardation has been associated with total lipodystrophy in some instances. There are usually a very few symptoms until the onset of diabetes, which usually appears during the pubertal years. Ketosis is rare despite the lack of dietary therapy or insulin treatment. Renal disease may occur. The most common cause of death at any time from infancy to the fourth decade is hepatic failure.

Laboratory findings

The laboratory findings in generalized lipodystrophy are dominated by marked disturbance in fat and carbohydrate metabolism and, in most patients, by an increased basal metabolic rate (Table 172-2). The glucose tolerance and fasting insulin levels are normal early but may be slightly elevated. Early in the disease the insulin response to glucose is exaggerated and prolonged, with mild insulin resistance. From the ages of 8 to 10 years, glucose tolerance decreases rapidly, with grossly elevated insulin levels. The insulin responses to oral and intravenous glucose and to tolbutamide are exaggerated. Insulin resistance is marked and increases with age. After 12 years, there is a cessation of growth and onset of frank diabetes, with fasting hyperglycemia and diabetic glucose tolerance curves. A decreased insulin response to glucose stimulation occurs, suggesting the partial exhaustion of the beta cells. Hyperlipidemia, present in a majority of patients, is a constant feature in older patients, but the younger child may have normal lipid fractions.

An increased metabolic rate has been encountered in some patients with total lipodystrophy; however, thyroid, adrenal, and gonadal function studies have been normal. There is an exaggerated luteinizing hormone (LH), follicle-stimulating hormone (FSH), thyroid-stimulating hormone (TSH), and prolactin response to exogenously administered releasing hormones, suggesting lesions in the target organs. Although rapid growth is observed and the bone age is advanced in children, growth hormone and somatomedin levels are normal.

Liver function tests may be normal, especially in the late stages of the disease, when liver fibrosis occurs. All of the liver enzymes are frequently elevated. Alkaline phosphatase may demonstrate transient increases secondary to the increase in triglyceride levels. Renal function is usually nor-

Table 172-2. Laboratory comparison of the major lipodystrophic syndromes

	Total lipodystrophies			Partial lipodystrophies	
	Leprechaunism	**Congenital**	**Acquired**	**Acquired**	**Familial**
Hypertriglyceridemia	—	+++	++	±	++
Hypoglycemia	+++	—	—	—	—
Ketosis	Absent	Absent	Absent	Absent	Absent
Insulin resistance	+++	+++	++	+	+
Hyperinsulinemia	+++	+++	++	—	—
Insulin receptor abnormal	++	Affinity	—	—	—
Glucose intolerance	+++	++	++	++	++
Liver dysfunction	—	++	++	—	—
Hypothalamic-pituitary function	Normal	Normal	Normal	Normal	Normal
Bone age	Retarded	Accelerated	Normal	Normal	Normal

—, absent; ±, mild; ++, moderate; +++, severe.

mal in children; however, there is a progressive decline with increasing age of the patient. The intravenous pyelogram may reveal kidney enlargement. The ventriculogram and pneumoencephalogram frequently reveal ventricular dilatation. Pathologic findings are related to the complete lack of fat in the subcutaneous tissues and to hepatomegaly. This histology of the liver is that of marked fatty changes, congestion, and fibrosis, with abundant glycogen. Microscopic study of the muscle demonstrates hypertrophy associated with areas of degenerative fibrosis or infiltration with adipose tissue. The heart and kidneys are usually enlarged.

Pathophysiology

The etiology of this disorder is unknown. Insulin-receptor binding in a patient with total lipodystrophy is decreased. When these patients fast for 48 to 72 hours, however, insulin-receptor binding improves. Other studies have suggested a reversible loss of coupling of normal insulin receptors to metabolic pathways. The receptor loss is thought to be tissue specific, involving only adipose tissue and liver.

The mechanism of insulin resistance in total lipodystrophy is unknown. Previous studies that have attempted to determine whether there is an abnormality in receptor function have produced varying results. In some patients there is a quantitative receptor defect, in which there is a decrease in the number of receptors, but the residual receptors appear to be normal in all respects. The quantitative defect in receptor number persists in cell culture in vitro, suggesting that this defect is genetic. In other patients there appears to be a qualitative defect in the insulin receptor, in which insulin may bind to its receptor with a different affinity, or there may be a lack of insulin binding to the high-affinity receptor component. In still other patients, receptors are abnormally insensitive to changes in temperature and pH.

Along with qualitative and quantitative receptor defects, some patients are considered to have postreceptor defects or an abnormality in the insulin receptor that interferes with the coupling of insulin binding to insulin action. The biochemical defect resides at a step distal to the hormone receptor. No insulin antibodies or insulin receptor antibodies have been found. Some patient have entirely normal insulin binding to erythrocytes, monocytes, and cultured fibroblasts. Heterogeneity of insulin receptor interaction has been reported even in the same family of patients with lipodystrophy.

The mechanism of the lipemia is not understood but has been postulated to be related to (1) excessive secretion of "adipokinin," (2) somatotropin action, (3) intact lipogenesis from carbohydrate, owing to lack of an unknown enzyme necessary for the deposition of subcutaneous fat, or (4) absence of functional adipose tissue and saturation of other storage sites (e.g., liver). None of these postulates has been substantiated.

Differential diagnosis

Total lipodystrophy can usually be differentiated from other disorders by the generalized absence of fat tissue and the "athletic" appearance and prominent abdomen of affected children.

Congenital generalized lipodystrophy has many features of leprechaunism, including genital hypertrophy, acanthosis nigricans, and hypertrichosis (see Table 172-1). However, the disease differs from leprechaunism because it is associated with increased growth and muscle mass and hepatosplenomegaly. Acanthosis nigricans with insulin resistance type B has anti-insulin-receptor antibodies, not found in leprechaunism, whereas acanthosis nigricans and insulin resistance type A have defective insulin receptors and are associated with accelerated growth and virilization (Chapter 168). The typical triglyceride hyperlipidemia and insulin-resistant diabetes further substantiate the diagnosis.

Partial lipodystrophy has many features in common with total lipodystrophy (e.g., the facial appearance and well-outlined musculature of the involved areas). The muscles in partial lipodystrophy, however, are not hypertrophied, and the fat tissue remains intact in distal portions of the extremities. Some patients with hypothalamic lesions may present a clinical picture resembling that of total lipodystrophy. For example, patients with diencephalic syndrome of early infancy experience neither complete loss of adipose tissue nor accelerated growth. They usually have markedly increased appetites, increased motor activity, abnormal cerebrospinal fluid findings, skin pallor with normal hemoglobin concentrations, decreased pituitary reserve, and inadequate thyroid function.

The masculine appearance, advanced growth, clitoral or penile enlargement, and hirsutism seen in lipodystrophy may be confused with the appearance of patients with congenital adrenal hyperplasia. Adrenal function in patients with total lipodystrophy, however, is normal.

Treatment

There is no known specific drug treatment for the lipodystrophies. Pimozide, a dopamine-receptor blocker, has been reported to be useful, but long-term clinical trials have shown no effect.

Fenfluramine, another dopamine-receptor blocker, blocks the synthesis of triglycerides, reduces intestinal absorption of triglycerides, increases carbohydrate utilization in vivo, and decreases brain serotonin, suggesting a possible defect in serotonin metabolism in the central nervous system. Despite reports of its usefulness, long-term use of this drug has also been ineffective.

Diet therapy is of some value in the control of hyperglycemia and hyperlipidemia. The use of small, frequent feedings and partial substitution of medium-chain triglycerides for polyunsaturated fats appears beneficial.

Plastic surgery with implants of monolithic silicon rubber for correction of the deficient soft tissue of the face is an effective therapy. Dental prostheses may be useful in some instances. Long-term management is usually related to therapy for the renal and endocrine dysfunctions that occur.

PARTIAL LIPODYSTROPHY

The partial lipodystrophies, like the total lipodystrophies, may be inherited or acquired and may have a symmetric or asymmetric distribution. The etiology of partial lipodystrophy is unknown. Postulated etiologies include familial or genetic disease, infections, immunologic disorders, or neurogenic dysfunctions. Partial lipodystrophy has been documented to occur in successive generations and to be associated with a genetically determined hypocomplementemia.

Hypocomplementemia and C3 nephritic factor are known to occur in partial lipodystrophy. Abnormalities of the complement system are thought to precede the development of the dystrophy. However, the occurrence of partial lipodystrophy without complement and C3 nephritic factor has been documented. Partial lipodystrophy is also known to be associated with other autoimmune disorders, such as systemic lupus erythematosus, Sjögren's syndrome, idiopathic thrombocytopenic purpura, thyrotoxicosis, and myasthenia gravis.

In addition to the genetic, infectious, and immunologic hypotheses proposed as etiologic in partial lipodystrophy, a neurogenic etiology has also been postulated. This postulate is based on the (1) anatomic distribution of the atrophic adipose tissue, (2) autonomic dysfunction, (3) fatty tissue transplant studies showing atrophy of normal graft when transplanted into dystrophic areas and normal development of dystrophic tissue when implanted into a normal field, (4) abnormalities of hypothalamic-pituitary function, and (5) headache as a common manifestation.

ACQUIRED PARTIAL LIPODYSTROPHY

Acquired partial lipodystrophy is the most common of the lipodystrophies and occurs predominantly in females. There is a loss of fat from the face and trunk, with normal or excessive deposition in the pelvic girdle or lower limbs. This disorder is usually progressive and has been called cephalothoracic progressive lipodystrophy. Occasionally, only one side is affected, although some authors have suggested that unilateral partial lipodystrophy is a separate disorder.

Partial lipodystrophy has its onset from age 2 to 40 years, but the majority of patients are younger than 16 years. Clinical manifestations associated with this disease include a sensation of coldness of involved areas, vague abdominal complaints or vomiting, frequent defecation, headache, nervousness, and fatigue. Some of the signs are tachycardia, Raynaud's phenomenon, and excessive sweating. Various pathologic conditions have been associated with partial lipodystrophy, including central nervous system dysfunction, hyperthyroidism, diabetes mellitus, menstrual disorders, ovarian abnormalities, and hypogonadism. Hepatomegaly has been observed in some patients, but the most serious pathologic association is renal dysfunction. Proteinuria is much more frequent in partial lipodystrophy than in the other syndromes. The complement system is abnormal, with decreased levels of C3. Treatment of this condition is symptomatic.

LIPOATROPHIC DIABETES

Classically, this disease has been divided into congenital and acquired forms. The congenital forms of lipoatrophic diabetes are rare. The lipodystrophies may be generalized (transmitted as an autosomal recessive trait) or partial (transmitted as an autosomal dominant trait). The acquired form may develop in children or adults and may be generalized or partial. It often develops after an acute illness but may have an insidious onset. Both congenital and acquired lipoatrophic diabetes are associated with abnormalities in carbohydrate metabolism, manifested by hypoglycemia, glucosuria, increased plasma insulin levels, and insulin resistance. Patients usually do not develop ketoacidosis, but it has been known to occur. Familial lipoatrophic diabetes is a syndrome that appears to have a dominant mode of inheritance and is characterized by fat atrophy of the limb and trunk with sparing of the face, which may actually be rounded. The neck may also be spared. The disease usually begins at puberty but may not appear until middle age. It primarily involves females; males are rarely affected. Insulin resistance and hyperglycemia are usual, with severe hypertriglyceridemia and eruptive xanthomas. The vaginal labia are hypertrophied, and polycystic ovaries may be seen. Acanthosis nigricans is usually present. Liver and renal disease usually do not occur. The pattern of inheritance is consistent with an autosomal dominant transmission with variable expression.

Laboratory findings reveal a mild type V hyperlipidemia, chemical diabetes, and high plasma insulin levels. This disease has to be distinguished from the partial or total absence of subcutaneous fat as well as from the congenital lipodystrophies.

Acquired lipoatrophic diabetes usually begins in adolescence or early adult life. It shares certain features with congenital lipodystrophy such as acanthosis nigricans, hyperlipidemia, and hepatosplenomegaly, leading in some cases to frank cirrhosis. Insulin-resistant diabetes mellitus is almost invariably present; but neurologic, cardiac, and renal abnormalities are usually absent.

PARTIAL LIPODYSTROPHY ASSOCIATED WITH OTHER ANOMALIES

This autosomal dominant form of partial lipodystrophy involves the face and buttocks and is nonprogressive. It has its onset in infancy or early childhood and is associated with Rieger's anomaly, short stature, midface hypoplasia, hypotrichosis, and insulinopenic diabetes. Rieger's anomaly is a nonspecific defect associated with variable eye and tooth abnormalities. Eye anomalies include hypoplasia of iris stroma, prominent Schwalbe's ring, iridocorneal synechiae, microcornea or megalocornea, strabismus, and a predisposition to glaucoma. Tooth abnormalities include hypodontia, microdontia, enamel hypoplasia, atypically shaped teeth, and malocclusion. This condition differs from familial autosomal lipodystrophy in that onset occurs in infancy, other anomalies are associated, and the face is involved.

LOCALIZED LIPODYSTROPHY

The localized lipodystrophies have well-demarcated, multifocal lesions and often are associated early with a lymphocytic panniculitis, suggestive of an inflammatory mechanism.

MESENTERIC LIPODYSTROPHY

This isolated lipodystrophy of the fatty tissue surrounding the small intestine has also been called mesenteric panniculitis, lipogranuloma of the mesentery, and other names. Whatever the terminology, histologic findings are uniform in all cases: abundant adipose tissue interspersed with fibrous tissue. Forty-two percent of patients develop mesenteric thickening, 32% show a large single tumor, and 26% have multiple tumors. Clinical symptoms vary from an acute condition of the abdomen to vague nonspecific abdominal pain. Displacement of the gastrointestinal tract, a frequent finding on on x-ray film, is believed to be caused by enlarged mesenteric fat arising from the celiac axis.

MEMBRANOUS LIPODYSTROPHY

This condition is a rare inherited disease characterized by symmetric multiple cystic bone lesions and progressive neuropsychiatric symptoms including progressive dementia, seizures, ataxia, tremors, and loss of consciousness. The neuropsychiatric symptoms are considered to be related to a sclerosing leukoencephalopathy of the cerebrum. These patients may also have ischemic necrosis of the lens.

CENTRIFUGAL LIPODYSTROPHY

This rare discrete condition is characterized by a localized cutaneous depression enlarging in a centrifugal distribution. The depression is due to a marked dystrophic change of the subcutaneous adipose tissue.

REFERENCES

Aarskog D et al: Autosomal dominant partial lipodystrophy associated with Rieger anomaly, short stature, and insulinopenic diabetes, Am J Med Genet 51:29, 1983.

Bier DM et al: Glucose kinetics in leprechaunism: accelerated fasting due to insulin resistance, J Clin Endocrinol Metab 51:988, 1980.

Grunberger G et al: Insulin receptors in normal and disease states, Clin Endocrinol Metab 12:191, 1983.

Keenan BS et al: The effect of diet upon carbohydrate metabolism, insulin resistance, and blood pressure in congenital total lipoatrophic diabetes, Metabolism 29:1214, 1980.

Oseid S et al: Decreased binding of insulin to its receptor in patients with congenital generalized lipodystrophy, N Engl J Med 296:245, 1977.

Rosenberg AM et al: A case of leprechaunism with severe hyperinsulinemia, Am J Dis Child 134:170, 1980.

Rossini AA et al: Metabolic and endocrine studies in a case of lipoatrophic diabetes, Metabolism 26:637, 1977.

Van der Vorn ER et al: An Arg for Gly substitution at position 31 in the insulin receptor, linked to insulin resistance, inhibits receptor processing and transport, J Biol Chem 267:66, 1992.

Wachslicht-Rodbard H et al: Heterogeneity of the insulin-receptor interaction in lipoatrophic diabetes, J Clin Endocrinol Metab 52:416, 1981.

METABOLIC DISORDERS IN ADULTS V

CHAPTER

173 Disorders of Amino Acid Metabolism

Jess G. Thoene

Disorders of amino acid metabolism, transport, and storage constitute a heterogeneous group of conditions whose clinical impact ranges from mild (e.g., cystathioninuria) to severe (e.g., propionic acidemia) with death occurring during infancy or childhood. Most disorders of amino acid metabolism are associated with mental retardation and decreased life span. Those resulting from disorders of amino acid transport or storage (cystinosis, Hartnup's disease, iminoglycinuria, cystinuria, Lowe's syndrome) have a varied clinical presentation. Though each disease is rare in the general population, with incidences ranging from 1:10,000 to 1:200,000 live births, collectively they impose a substantial disease burden. They are inherited, with a few exceptions, as autosomal recessive conditions. In the diseases that manifest themselves in infancy, rapid and accurate diagnosis is essential because, in some instances, therapy is highly effective if instituted early. In all cases, genetic counseling can be offered. Until recently, most patients with disorders of amino acid metabolism have not survived to young adulthood; however, the development of effective therapies for some previously lethal disorders (see Disorders of the Urea Cycle and Disorders of Branched-Chain Amino Acid Metabolism) has permitted greatly improved life expectancy. In the near future, therefore, these conditions will assume a practical significance for internists as they previously have for pediatricians. A list of some disorders of amino acid metabolism that may be encountered in the adult population is given in Table 173-1.

The amino acids known to be associated with human disease and the availability of therapy are listed in Table 173-2. The listing is not exhaustive, and the reader is referred to the general references at the end of the chapter for more detailed discussions. Although the structures of the 20 amino acids required for protein synthesis and the urea-cycle intermediates have been known for approximately 50 years, new amino acids continue to be discovered (e.g., gamma-carboxyglutamic acid, beta-carboxyaspartic acid). It is reasonable to assume that new inborn errors of amino acid metabolism will continue to be described as knowledge concerning normal amino acid metabolism and genetic regulation accumulates.

The diagnosis of disorders of amino acid metabolism can be difficult due to the nonspecific modes of presentation, the nature of the analytic instruments required in establish-

Table 173-1. Disorders of amino acid metabolism that may be encountered in adults

Condition	Age of presentation	Major symptoms
PKU*	Infancy	Seizures, retardation (untreated)
Cystinuria	Adolescence—young adult	Kidney stones
Citrullinemia (adult form)	Childhood	Mental retardation
Vitamin-responsive organic acidemias	Infancy	Variable
Homocystinuria	Childhood	Thromboses
Cystathioninuria	Variable	Variable
Cystinosis (benign form)	Childhood	Keratopathy
Hartnup's disease	Childhood	Dermatitis, neurologic abnormalities
Alkaptonuria	Adult	Arthritis, pigmentary changes
Gyrate retinal atrophy	Adolescence	Visual loss
Partial OTC* deficiency	Intrapartum Postpartum	Hyperammonemic coma

*PKU, phenylketonuria; OTC, ornithine transcarbamylase.

ing the diagnosis, and the relative scarcity of these diseases in the general population. Accumulation of significant clinical experience in this field requires a wide referral area and sufficient laboratory resources to permit rapid and reliable diagnosis. The National Organization for Rare Disorders (NORD) maintains a current database on diagnostic and therapeutic services for these and other rare disorders.*

Because the alpha-amino group of amino acids reacts with ninhydrin to form colored compounds, the diagnosis of amino acidopathies has relied on detection through the use of this reagent. Indeed, the number of known inborn errors of amino acid metabolism increased dramatically during the 20 years after the introduction of the automatic amino acid analyzer. Amino acids in plasma and urine also may be estimated qualitatively via one- or two-dimensional chromatography and also by high-voltage electrophoresis. Interpretation of these patterns requires familiarity with normal variants and artifacts; newborn and premature infants may show a physiologic aminoaciduria due to relative immaturity of the tubular reabsorption mechanism for amino acids. Certain antibiotics also stain with ninhydrin and cause false-positive tests.

After transamination, amino acids become "invisible" to methods that rely on the ninhydrin reaction for visualization and quantitation. Thus those inborn errors resulting from defects after transamination generally require means other than the amino acid analyzer for identification. This group, known collectively as *organic acidemias,* has been delineated by a variety of techniques, the most universal of which is gas chromatography-mass spectrometry (GC-MS).

*NORD. New Fairfield, CT. 06812. 1-800-447-NORD.

Table 173-2. Amino acids of clinical interest and some related diseases

Amino acid	Related diseases	Available therapy*
Glycine	Nonketotic hyperglycinemia	−
	Ketotic hyperglycinemia	+
Alanine	Lactic acidoses	+
Valine	Hypervalinemia	+
	MSUD*	+
	Methylmalonic aciduria	+
Isoleucine	Propionic acidemia	+
	MSUD	+
Leucine	Isovaleric acidemia	+
	MSUD	
Methionine	Hypermethioninemia	NI
Cysteine	—	NI
Cystine	Cystinosis	+
	Cystinuria	+
Serine	Hyperoxaluria II	−
Threonine	Hyperthreoninemia	−
Phenylalanine	PKU*	+
	Atypical PKU and variants	
Tyrosine	Hereditary tyrosinemia	+
Asparagine	—	NI
Glutamine	—	NI
Tryptophan	Tryptophanuria	−
Proline	Hyperprolinemia I and II	NI
Aspartic acid	—	NI
Glutamic acid	Pyroglutamic acidemia	−
Histidine	Histidinemia	+
Arginine	Hyperargininemia	+
Lysine	Hyperlysinemia	+
Arginisuccinic acid	Argininosuccinic aciduria	+
Ornithine	Hyperornithinemia	+
	Ornithine aminotransferase deficiency	+
Citrulline	Citrullinemia	+
Homocystine	Homocystinuria	−
Cystathionine	Cystathioninuria	NI
Pipecolic acid	Hyperpipecolatemia	−
	Zellweger's syndrome	
Beta-alanine	Beta-alaninemia	−

*+, potential or proved therapy; −, no effective therapy; NI, therapy not indicated; MSUD, maple syrup urine disease; PKU, phenylketonuria.

GC-MS instrumentation can provide unambiguous identification of nanogram amounts of all volatile metabolites present in a given sample. Commercially available computerized data systems have greatly facilitated the reduction of the enormous amount of information each plasma or urine sample analyzed produces. GC-MS analysis, however, has some drawbacks. It requires relatively extensive sample preparation, and the instruments are expensive and not generally available in clinical laboratories.

Because of the severity of presentation of many inborn errors of metabolism and lack of pharmacotherapy, patients are likely to be candidates for the initial trials of gene therapy. The objectives for gene therapy, in addition to successfully isolating the working gene for the disease in question, include developing a delivery system directed at the tissue(s) of interest and generating expression of sufficient activity to produce clinical improvement. Some diseases (ornithine transcarbamylase deficiency, see later discussion) are known to be clinically asymptomatic when only a few percent residual activity are present. Achievement of this level of activity by exogenous gene therapy appears possible.

HYPERPHENYLALANINEMIA

Classic phenylketonuria (PKU) was described in 1937 and is perhaps the most widely studied aminoacidopathy. The incidence of PKU in the North American population is 1:14,000. A number of other conditions producing hyperphenylalaninemia have since been described (Table 173-3), reinforcing the need for precise diagnosis in this as in other amino acidopathies.

Classic PKU is an autosomal recessive condition resulting from deficiency of hepatic phenylalanine hydroxylase, which converts phenylalanine to tyrosine. It requires tetrahydrobiopterin as a co-factor. Untreated classic PKU produces clinical symptomatology that includes severe mental retardation, hypopigmentation of skin and hair, eczematoid rash, seizures, microcephaly, and electroencephalographic (EEG) abnormalities. The plasma phenylalanine concentration is sustained at greater than 20 mg/dl. Urinary excretion of alternative metabolites of phenylalanine (phenylpyruvic, phenylacetic, and phenyllactic acids) is responsible both for the musty odor associated with these patients and also for the characteristic green color produced in the urinary ferric chloride test.

The specific mechanism responsible for mental retardation in these patients has not yet been identified, although direct cerebral toxicity from elevated phenylalanine and its keto analogs has been postulated. Deficits resulting from decreased production of neurotransmitters derived from tyrosine are also possible. Artificially produced hyperphenylalaninemia in experimental animals has led to disruption of cerebral polyribosomes, defective cerebral protein synthesis, decreased brain cerebroside and sulfatide content, and decreased DNA content of cerebrum and cerebellum. Additionally, depletion of certain amino acids from the brain has been proposed as a result of sustained hyperphenylalaninemia.

Dietary treatment of classic PKU has proved to be one of the most effective means of ameliorating the inborn errors of metabolism. Diets low in phenylalanine were first used to treat PKU in the 1950s. It has since been demonstrated that, if the diet is begun early in life (ideally less than 1 month of age), the mean IQ of the treated PKU patients is very close to 100. This is in marked contrast to the IQ of untreated PKU patients, which is always less than 50 and is generally around 20. Because of the need for early intervention, most states have initiated mandatory infant PKU screening during the nursery stay to ensure rapid detection and early treatment. The diet consists of a semisynthetic formula low in phenylalanine, and it is supplemented with natural foods low in phenylalanine. The amount of dietary phenylalanine is adjusted on an individual basis to maintain the plasma phenylalanine level between 2 and 12 mg/dl. This is usually achieved at an average daily intake of 250 to 500 mg of phenylalanine throughout childhood. The question of when to terminate the diet is currently unresolved. However, most workers in the field agree that maintenance of a low-phenylalanine diet is desirable through at least 8 years of age.

A number of children have been born to mothers with PKU. These offspring have had abnormalities thought to result from intrauterine hyperphenylalaninemia. They include a variety of congenital anomalies, growth retardation, and mental retardation (over 90%). These findings clearly indicate a need for effective management of maternal PKU, including maintenance of the mother on a low-phenylalanine

Table 173-3. Hyperphenylalaninemias

Condition	Clinical aspects	Presumed defect	Blood phenylalanine
PKU	Mental retardation, hypopigmentation	Phe* hydroxylase absent	>20 mg/dl on regular diet
Persistent hyperphenylalaninemia	Normal	Decreased Phe hydroxylase	May be same as PKU early; later 4-20 mg/dl on regular diet
Transient mild hyperphenylalaninemia	Normal	Maturational delay of hydroxylase	May be same as PKU early; progressively declines toward normal
Transaminase deficiency	Normal	Phe transaminase deficiency	Varies with dietary protein intake
Dihydropteridine reductase deficiency	Initially normal; seizures, abnormal development evident within first year of life	Deficiency of dihydropteridine reductase	Variable—may be as in type I
Abnormal dihydropteridine reductase function	Myoclonus, uncontrolled movements, tetraplegia, greasy skin, recurrent hyperthermia	Unknown; functional abnormality of dihydropteridine reductase	May be >20 mg/dl

*Phe, phenylalanine.
Modified from Stanbury J, Wyngaarden JB, and Fredrickson DS, editors: The metabolic basis of inherited disease, ed 5, New York, 1983, McGraw-Hill.

diet throughout pregnancy. Available data are too limited at present to judge the effectiveness of this therapy.

TYROSINEMIA

Plasma tyrosine is elevated in several conditions, including hereditary tyrosinemia, transient tyrosinemia, tyrosine aminotransferase deficiency, "tyrosinosis," and generalized liver dysfunction, as well as in other unrelated conditions. In all instances, significant tyrosinemia leads to excessive urinary excretion of phenolic metabolites, producing a positive urinary nitrosonaphthol test.

Hereditary tyrosinemia is an autosomal recessive condition that is very rare in the general population; however, it is concentrated in a certain French-Canadian community where the carrier frequency is approximately 1 in 30 individuals. The genetic defect is now known to be deficiency of hepatic fumarylacetoacetate lyase. The primary clinical manifestations of this condition are hepatocellular dysfunction progressing to nodular cirrhosis, associated with a renal tubular nephropathy producing the renal Fanconi syndrome and hypophosphatemic rickets. Deficiency of p-hydroxyphenylpyruvic acid oxidase produces elevated urinary excretion of the phenolic compounds p-hydroxyphenylacetic acid, p-hydroxyphenyllactic acid, and p-hydroxyphenylpyruvic acid. Detection of succinylacetone in the urine is virtually diagnostic of this condition. Treatment with a diet low in tyrosine is reported to improve renal function. Lasting improvement in the hepatocellular dysfunction and avoidance of cirrhosis have not yet been substantiated. Liver transplantation is effective and required frequently in this disorder.

Transient tyrosinemia of the newborn is the most commonly encountered defect of tyrosine metabolism and has been found in up to 30% of premature infants. It is characterized by marked elevation in plasma tyrosine (up to 36 mg/dl, normal less than 1.3 mg/dl), tyrosyluria, no consistent abnormal clinical findings, and rapid response to both protein restriction and vitamin C supplementation. It is thought to result from delayed maturation of p-hydroxyphenylpyruvic acid oxidase, which requires vitamin C as a co-factor. It appears not to be a hereditary disorder and is important chiefly in distinguishing this benign condition from other, more serious, disorders of tyrosine metabolism that are heritable.

Tyrosine aminotransferase deficiency has been reported in a small number of patients characterized by striking elevations in plasma tyrosine (30 to 50 mg/dl) and tyrosyluria accompanied by a constellation of clinical findings, including mental retardation, palmar-plantar keratosis, microcephaly, seizures, and corneal clouding. In contrast to patients with hereditary tyrosinemia, liver and kidney diseases are absent in these patients. A defect in hepatic cytosol tyrosine aminotransferase has been reported in one such patient. Amelioration of the skin lesions has been reported to result from a diet low in phenylalanine and tyrosine.

Generalized hepatic dysfunction is known to lead to aberrations in tyrosine metabolism, including elevation in plasma tyrosine and tyrosyluria. Associated pathologic conditions reported to induce tyrosinemia include viral hepatitis, cirrhosis, neonatal giant-cell hepatitis, and cytomegalovirus infection. Other illnesses that have been associated with tyrosinemia include fructose-1,6-diphosphatase deficiency, galactosemia, cystic fibrosis, and hypothyroidism.

HISTIDINEMIA

Histidinemia results from a deficiency of the enzyme histidine-alpha-deaminase, which converts histidine to urocanic acid. It is inherited as an autosomal recessive trait. Elevated histidine in plasma is associated with excessive urinary excretion of alternative histidine metabolites, primarily imidazole pyruvic acid, which produces a green color on reaction with ferric chloride. The clinical features of this condition include mental retardation (50%) and speech defects. Diets low in histidine are effective in lowering plasma histidine in this condition; however, clinical improvement has not been documented. Because mental retardation is an inconstant finding in this condition, neonatal screening for histidinemia has not been adopted widely.

DISORDERS OF THE UREA CYCLE

The urea cycle is the primary mechanism in mammalian tissues for the disposal of nitrogen waste generated primarily from protein metabolism. The urea cycle intermediates and their interrelationships are shown in Fig. 173-1. For each "turn" of the cycle, 2 moles of ammonia are excreted in the form of 1 mole of urea. Ammonia enters the cycle, both as free ammonium in the first reaction in the cycle, and as aspartic acid in the third reaction. Both carbamylphosphate synthetase (CPS) and ornithine transcarbamylase (OTC) are located within mitichondria; the remaining three enzymes, argininosuccinate synthetase (AS), argininosuccinate lyase (AL), and arginase (ARG), occur in the cytosol. Citrulline and ornithine shuttle between the mitochondrial interior and the cytosol. Understanding of the regulation of urea cycle activity has recently been advanced with the description of N-acetylglutamate as a positive modulator of CPS activity. N-acetylglutamate is formed via the action of N-acetylglutamate synthetase which is itself positively modulated by arginine. Thus conditions leading to elevated arginine, such as dietary protein load, also enhance activity of the urea cycle, tending to preserve homeostasis.

Interruption of the urea cycle due to an enzymatic deficiency impairs the organism's ability to excrete waste nitrogen and leads to a common complex of clinical findings, which usually include marked hyperammonemia, mental retardation, protein intolerance, seizures, coma, and death in infancy if untreated. All known genetic disorders of the urea cycle are inherited as autosomal recessive conditions, except OTC deficiency, which is X-linked.

The approaches to short-term therapy of ammonia intoxication due to a urea cycle defect are similar, regardless of the particular defect involved. Ammonia removal may be accomplished by exchange transfusion, peritoneal dialysis,

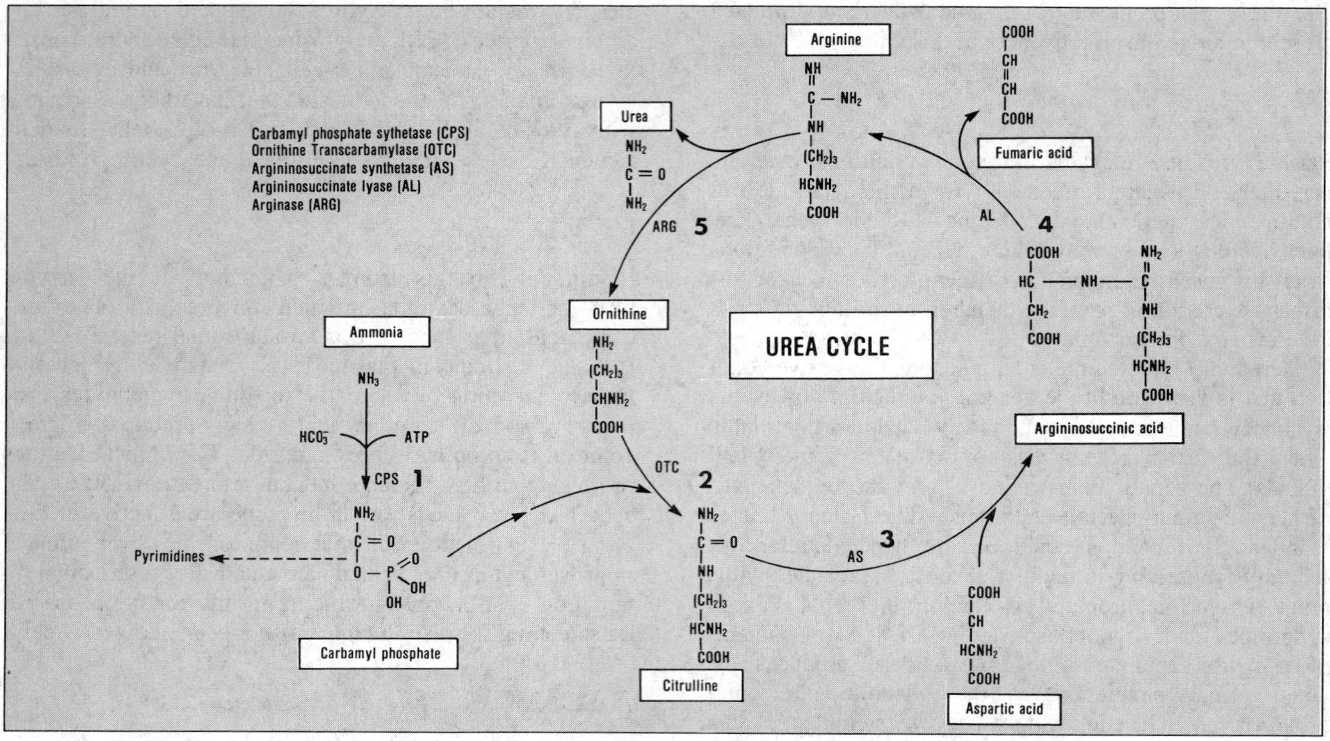

Fig. 173-1. The urea cycle. Enzymes: **1,** carbamylphosphate synthetase *(CPS)*; **2,** ornithine transcarbamylase *(OTC)*; **3,** argininosuccinate synthetase *(AS)*; **4,** argininosuccinate lyase *(AL)*; **5,** arginase *(ARG)*.

or hemodialysis. Hemodialysis appears to be the most effective short-term means of ammonia removal. In addition to general supportive care, which usually requires circulatory and respiratory support, patients with urea cycle disorders require protein-restricted diets to reduce the total nitrogen load. This diet can be accomplished by diluting a standard infant formula in such a way that appropriate fluid and caloric needs are supplied together with a total daily protein intake of approximately 1 g/kg of body weight. Long-term measures to assist in nitrogen removal have included administration of keto acid analogs of essential amino acids, arginine supplementation, and sodium benzoate. A drug comprising sodium benzoate and sodium phenylacetate (Ucephan, Kendall McGaw) has received Food and Drug Administration approval for the treatment of urea cycle disorders.

Differential diagnosis of hyperammonemia requires knowledge of the patient's blood ammonia concentration, plasma amino acid and volatile fatty acid pattern, and urinary orotic acid concentration (Table 173-4). Utilization of these data to specify the site of interruption of the urea cycle will be described under each condition.

Carbamylphosphate synthetase deficiency interrupts the first step in the classic urea cycle and leads to hyperammonemia, vomiting, protein intolerance, lethargy, and seizures. Patients with this condition have manifested symptoms from as early as 1 day of age to as late as several weeks. Hyperammonemia may be moderate (300 to 600 μg/dl; normal is less than 120 μg/dl). Because no other urea cycle intermediates are formed, no specific pattern of metabolites is found on analysis of plasma or urine. Lysine, glutamine, and alanine may be elevated as a nonspecific response to hyperammonemia. Urinary orotic acid level is normal or low. Because N-acetylglutamate synthetase activity is inhibited by propionylcoenzyme A (propionyl-CoA), a similar pattern may be seen in propionic acidemia; hence plasma volatile fatty acid determination should be made to rule out this and related conditions. The enzymatic defect should be confirmed in liver.

Ornithine transcarbamylase deficiency is manifested in a manner similar to that of CPS deficiency, except that only males are usually severely affected, owing to the X-linked nature of the disorder. Clinically affected females with a milder course, characterized primarily by protein intolerance, have been described and are thought to represent instances of unfavorable lyonization (inactivation of the normal X chromosome) and may demonstrate only minimal (1% to 5%) residual activity for OTC. Recent studies have shown that some heterozygote females develop hyperammonemic coma during the intrapartum period. One death and several catastrophic episodes of hyperammonemia have been reported from this previously unrecognized condition.

Carbamylphosphate is shunted into the pyrimidine pathway and results in a markedly elevated urinary excretion of orotic acid, distinguishing this condition biochemically from CPS deficiency. Pronounced hyperammonemia (>1000 μg/dl) occurs, accompanied by elevations in plasma alanine, glutamine, and lysine, with a reduced con-

Table 173-4. Laboratory aids in the differential diagnosis of hyperammonemia

Condition	Metabolic abnormality					
	Ammonia	Urinary orotic acid	Citrulline	Argininosuccinate	Arginine	Other
CPS deficiency	↑↑↑	N to ↓	Absent to low	N	N	↑ Glutamine and alanine
OTC deficiency	↑↑↑	↑↑	Absent to low	N	N	↑ Glutamine and alanine
Citrullinemia	↑↑↑	↑	↑↑↑	N	N	—
Argininosuccinic aciduria	↑↑	N	↑	↑↑↑	↑	—
Hyperargininemia	↑ to N	↑	N	Absent to low	↑↑	—
Transient hyperammonemia	↑↑↑	N	N	N	N	—
Organic acidemias	↑↑	N	N	N	N	Abnormal organic acid excretion

↑↑↑, marked elevation; ↑↑, moderate elevation; ↑, mild elevation; N, normal; CPS, carbamylphosphate synthetase; OTC, ornithine transcarbamylase.

centration of plasma citrulline. Confirmation should be made of the enzymatic deficiency in the liver.

Citrullinemia results from deficiency of argininosuccinic acid synthetase and is inherited as an autosomal recessive disorder. It is characterized by high blood levels of ammonia (1000 to 3000 μg/dl) and citrulline. Urinary orotic acid excretion is also elevated. Clinical symptomatology in the neonatal type of citrullinemia is very similar to the previously described urea cycle disorders with protein intolerance (characterized primarily by vomiting of protein meals) and obtundation occurring early in life. Genetic heterogeneity has been described, including variants with reduced ammonia concentrations and mild or intermediate symptomatology.

Argininosuccinic aciduria results from deficiency of argininosuccinase. It occurs in approximately 1:60,000 live births and presents clinically with seizures, coma, mental retardation, and hyperammonemia. A large proportion of affected patients do not survive infancy. There is marked elevation of argininosuccinic acid in plasma, cerebrospinal fluid, and urine. Fifty percent of patients have demonstrated a characteristic friability of the hair called *trichorrhexis nodosa*. As in citrullinemia, there is heterogeneity in the clinical expression of this condition. Subacute and late-onset variants have been described, as well as the classic neonatal type that is lethal if untreated. The condition is inherited as an autosomal recessive trait. Biochemical explanation for the variable clinical severity is lacking.

Hyperargininemia results from arginase deficiency and is distinguished from the preceding diseases in that it results in mental retardation but appears not to share the lethal neonatal expression characteristic of the other disorders. It is characterized by marked elevations of arginine in the blood, spinal fluid, and urine, whereas hyperammonemia is variable. The available data are consistent with an autosomal recessive mode of inheritance.

Organic acidemias may cause severe hyperammonemia as a result of inhibition of N-acetylglutamate synthetase by acylcoenzyme A (acyl-CoA) esters. Acyl-CoA esters are elevated in various disorders of branched-chain amino acid metabolism. Any infant with hyperammonemia should have plasma fatty acids measured early in the diagnostic work-up to avert use of inappropriate therapy designed for urea cycle disorders.

DISORDERS OF LYSINE METABOLISM

A variety of conditions characterized by elevations in the concentration of lysine in the plasma are known.

Periodic hyperlysinemia associated with hyperammonemia has been described, in which the ammonia level approaches 600 μg/dl. In this condition, oral lysine loading leads to a pronounced elevation in the concentration of ammonia in the blood. A reduced level of hepatic lysine dehydrogenase has been found.

Persistent hyperlysinemia is clinically different from the preceding disorder in that ammonia is not elevated. Mental retardation has been an inconstant finding.

Hyperpipecolatemia has been described in a small number of patients characterized clinically by hypotonia, hepatomegaly, and mental retardation. All known patients with this disorder are males, suggesting an X-linked inheritance pattern. Pipecolic acid is an alternative degradation product of lysine; however, lysine-loading tests in these patients have not produced elevation in the plasma pipecolic acid concentration. The biochemical defect is unknown, and effective therapy for this condition is lacking. Some, but not all, patients with Zellweger's syndrome also have manifested elevation in plasma pipecolate concentration. Patients with Zellweger's syndrome have hypotonia, mental retardation, hepatomegaly, renal cortical cysts, and early death.

DISORDERS OF BRANCHED-CHAIN AMINO ACID METABOLISM

Disorders of the branched-chain amino acids (leucine, isoleucine, and valine) account for the bulk of the organic acidemias, as the majority of defects in the metabolic pathways are located distal to an irreversible decarboxylation that occurs after transamination and thus all subsequent metabolites lack amino groups. Much of the clinical symptomatology is similar within this group of disorders. In the newborn period, symptoms may include protein intolerance and vomiting, lethargy, seizures, profound metabolic acidosis, coma, and death. Some of the disorders may also be manifested with hyperammonemia, unusual odors, and hypoglycemia. Survival of the initial episode may be followed by failure to thrive, mental retardation, recurrent attacks of severe ketoacidosis, thrombocytopenia, and neutropenia. All known disorders are inherited as autosomal recessive conditions. Because of the common clinical presentation, identification of the specific defect requires laboratory measurement of the abnormal metabolites that accumulate in blood and urine. This process entails analysis by gas chromatography, GC-MS, and/or high-performance liquid chromatography. Precise identification is essential, as some of these disorders are completely reversible with appropriate dietary therapy and/or vitamin supplementation. The metabolism of these three amino acids proceeds in a series of analogous reactions such that, in one instance, they share a common enzyme (branched-chain keto acid-decarboxylase) and, in others, they feed into a common metabolite (e.g., both valine and isoleucine are metabolized via propionyl-CoA). The disorders associated with each amino acid are given in Table 173-5. The following discussion is limited to the more widely characterized disorders. Many of those disorders lead to a secondary carnitine deficiency due to renal excretion of acyl-carnitine esters. Therapy with 100 to 300 mg/kg/day of L-carnitine can dramatically reduce the episodes of metabolic acidosis.

Maple syrup urine disease (MSUD) is due to a deficiency of the enzyme branched-chain keto acid-decarboxylase, which is common to all three degradation pathways. The disease has a frequency of about 1:220,000 live births and is characterized by a peculiar sweet smell to the urine, which gives this condition its name. This enzymatic deficiency gives rise to accumulation of the branched-chain amino acids and the corresponding keto acids. Leucine is grossly elevated and may reach concentrations 50-fold above normal. As in other inborn errors, the disease has variable clinical expression. The neonatal form manifests itself in the first week of life with vomiting, lethargy, hypertonicity, seizures, and, without appropriate therapy, death in the newborn period. These patients require a special diet low in branched-chain amino acids. Because of its severity and its responsiveness to early treatment, some states have included this condition in newborn screening programs. Milder variants have been described that have later onset of symptoms and intermittent acute episodes that correlate with the stress of infections or protein excess. A thiamine-responsive variant has also been described. This condition shows marked resolution of amino acid and keto acid elevations as well as clinical improvement on doses of thiamine of 10 to 150 mg/day.

Isovaleric acidemia results from a deficiency of isovaleryl-CoA dehydrogenase. It is characterized clinically by overwhelming neonatal illness, with vomiting, ketoacidosis, lethargy, coma, seizures, and a characteristic odor of "sweaty feet." These patients also may demonstrate thrombocytopenia and leukopenia. Isovaleric acid is elevated in plasma several hundredfold during acute episodes but may be only 10- to 50-fold elevated during stable intervals. Urinary isovalerylglycine excretion is relatively constant and provides a helpful diagnostic aid. Short- and long-term management is similar to that for the other disorders in this pathway. Oral glycine therapy also has been advocated to assist in clearance of isovaleric acid via enhanced excretion of isovalerylglycine. Glycine (100 to 200 mg/kg/day) appears to be an effective treatment.

Propionic acidemia results from deficiency of propionyl-CoA carboxylase, the enzyme that catalyzes conversion of propionate to D-methylmalonate. The enzyme requires biotin as a cofactor. Clinically, these patients manifest overwhelming illness in the neonatal period that may resemble neonatal sepsis. They are lethargic, with metabolic acidosis, ketosis, and hypotonia. Coma and seizures may supervene, with early death occurring in the majority of the untreated patients. Because of inhibition of synthesis of N-acetylglutamate by propionyl-CoA, these patients may have marked hyperammonemia and resemble patients with urea cycle defects. Propionic acid is markedly elevated in plasma as well as urine. Other elevated urinary metabolites include methylcitrate, beta-hydroxypropionate, and propionylglycine. Glycine is characteristically elevated in plasma and urine as well, a finding that led to the original term, *hyperglycinemia,* for this condition as well as methylmalonic aciduria. The glycine elevation may be due to inhibition of the glycine cleavage enzyme system by the accumulation of branched-chain amino acid metabolites proximal to propionyl-CoA. Short-term care requires cardiorespiratory support, correction of the severe metabolic acidosis, and removal of the excess accumulation of propionic acid and ammonia. This approach is usually accomplished by either peritoneal dialysis or exchange transfusions. Because some patients have been described who re-

Table 173-5. Disorders of branched-chain amino acid metabolism

Leucine	Isoleucine	Valine
Hyperleucine-isoleucinemia	Hyperleucine-isoleucinemia	Hypervalinemia
Maple syrup urine disease (MSUD)	MSUD	MSUD
Isovaleric acidemia	Beta-ketothiolase deficiency	Propionic acidemia
Beta-methylcrotonylglycinuria	Propionic acidemia	Methylmalonic aciduria
Beta-hydroxy-beta-methylglutaric aciduria	Methylmalonic aciduria	Multiple carboxylase deficiency
Multiple carboxylase deficiency	Multiple carboxylase deficiency	—

sponded to biotin, a therapeutic trial of 1 to 5 mg/day of biotin should be performed. Long-term care involves maintenance of a diet low in protein or use of special formulas low in the branched-chain amino acids. These patients can exhibit good metabolic control and acceptable growth and development on diets supplying 1.0 to 1.5 g/kg/day of protein.

Methylmalonic aciduria results from an enzymatic defect in the conversion of D-methylmalonic acid to succinic acid, or from a defect in the pathway for vitamin B_{12} transport and activation. These patients are clinically similar to patients with propionic acidemia, but they also may demonstrate hypoglycemia, neutropenia, thrombocytopenia, perammonemia, and hyperglycinemia. The diagnosis rests on demonstration of methylmalonic acid in plasma or urine. Because methylmalonic acid can decarboxylate to propionic acid during gas chromatographic analysis, it is important to assay each supposed propionic (acidemic) directly for methylmalonic acid by a colorimetric or other assay. Several variants of this condition are known, some of which are vitamin B_{12}-responsive. Again, an early therapeutic trial to determine vitamin responsiveness is indicated. Other disorders of branched-chain amino acid metabolism are listed in Table 173-5. They generally are rare in the newborn population and require extensive diagnostic evaluation.

Biotinidase deficiency deserves discussion because of the gratifying response biotin produces in these patients (Figs. 173-2 and 173-3). This disorder is not truly a defect in branched-chain amino acid metabolism per se; rather, it results from an inability to properly metabolize the vitamin biotin. Because four carboxylases require biotin as a cofactor (propionyl-CoA, acetyl-CoA, beta-methylcrotonyl-CoA, and pyruvate carboxylase), many metabolic ramifications result from this defect. Patients demonstrate ketosis, lactic acidosis, alopecia, ataxia, and developmental delay. The condition results from a defect in biotinidase, which releases biotin from the lysine moieties of dietary protein. A striking clinical response to 1 to 10 mg/day oral biotin is found. Some states have now instituted newborn screening programs for biotinidase deficiency.

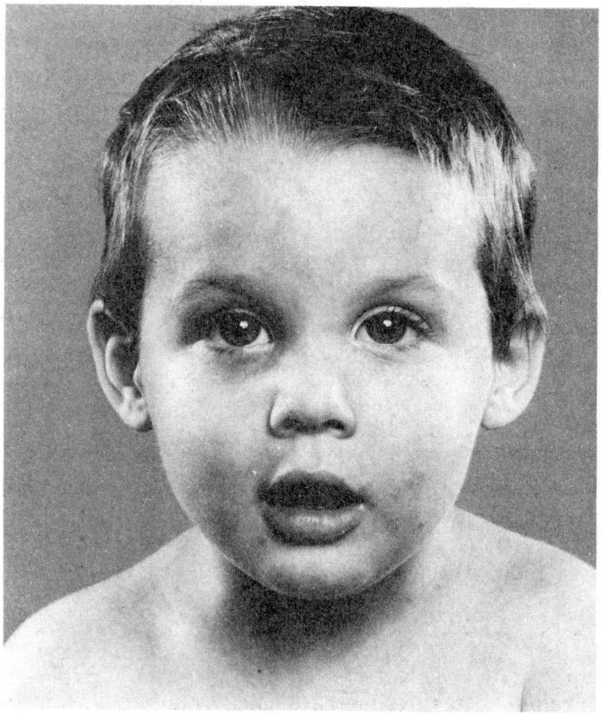

Fig. 173-3. The same patient as in Fig. 173-2 after 4 months of oral biotin, 10 mg/day.

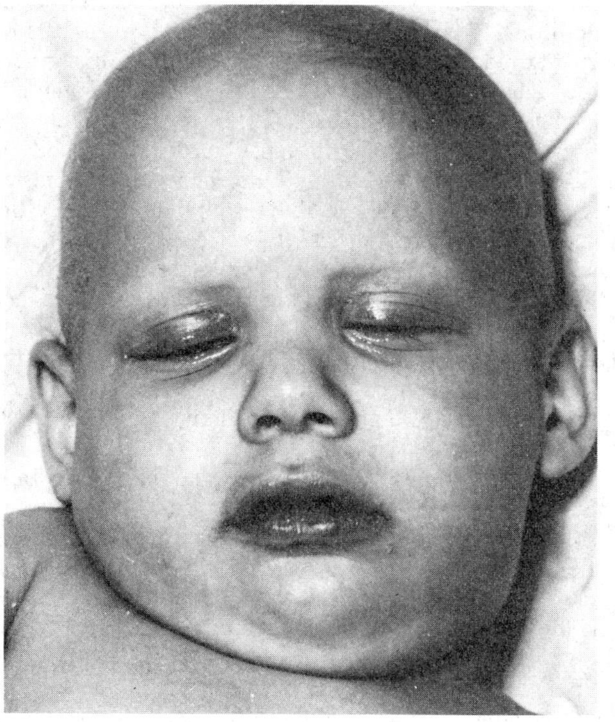

Fig. 173-2. A girl (2 years, 9 months old) with juvenile multiple carboxylase deficiency at the time of diagnosis.

DISORDERS OF METABOLISM OF SULFUR-CONTAINING AMINO ACIDS

Homocystinuria may result from the following causes: a deficiency of cystathionine synthetase (which catalyzes the conversion of methionine to cystathionine), from a block in the metabolism of N^5-methyltetrahydrofolate (the methyl donor in the above reaction) or from deranged vitamin B_{12} metabolism. Classic homocystinuria resulting from cystathionine synthetase deficiency is characterized by elevations in plasma homocystine and methionine up to 100 times normal. This enzymatic deficiency shows autosomal recessive inheritance, and the clinical phenotype includes failure to thrive, light complexion, and mental retardation. Patients also may demonstrate marfanoid habitus, and ectopia lentis develops by 3 years of age. The primary clinical disabilities are life-threatening venous and arterial thromboses, the biochemical explanation for which has not been elucidated. Therapeutic measures advocated include diets low in methionine and supplemented with cystine to avert the abnormal biochemical consequences of this block. Proof of effectiveness of this therapy is still accumulating. Some patients respond to large doses of vitamin B_6.

Cystathioninuria results from deficiency of cystathionase, which catalyzes the conversion of cystathionine to cysteine; the disorder appears to be the result of an autosomal recessive trait. A consistent clinical pattern in this condition has not been observed. Some patients are retarded, whereas others have normal intelligence.

Other disorders of sulfur-containing amino acid metabolism include sulfite oxidase deficiency, beta-mercaptolactate-cysteine disulfiduria, glutathionuria, and taurinuria. These patients generally are discovered as a result either of mass screening programs in retarded populations or a specific metabolic evaluation in a retarded patient.

MISCELLANEOUS DISORDERS OF AMINO ACID METABOLISM

Nonketotic hyperglycinemia results from a defect in the glycine cleavage enzyme system. It appears to be transmitted as an autosomal recessive trait and is manifested either as overwhelming disease in the newborn period, with coma, seizures, and death, or more gradually as failure to thrive and mental retardation. It is characterized clinically by massive elevation in the concentration of glycine in plasma, cerebral spinal fluid, and urine, without other abnormal metabolic findings. These signs distinguish the condition from the hyperglycinemia that accompanies propionic acidemia and methylmalonic aciduria. Effective therapy for this condition has not been devised, although some beneficial results have been reported from the use of strychnine, which acts as a specific antagonist of glycine at postsynaptic membrane receptors in the central nervous system.

Retinal gyrate atrophy is the result of ornithine-delta-aminotransferase deficiency. It produces a characteristic atrophic degeneration of retina and choroid and results initially in night blindness, followed by loss of peripheral vision leading to blindness during the fifth decade. The patients have a characteristic hyperornithinemia that responds to a diet low in arginine. Stabilization of visual function has been achieved on a low-protein diet.

DISORDERS OF AMINO ACID STORAGE

Cystinosis

The term *cystinosis* refers to disorders whose major biochemical characteristic is intralysosomal storage of the disulfide amino acid cystine in most body tissues. Cystine crystals may be seen in the cornea by slit-lamp examination as an aid to diagnosis. These crystals also are found in bone marrow aspirates and biopsies of rectal mucosa. There is marked heterogeneity of clinical expression, but all forms appear to be inherited as autosomal recessive traits. The clinical categories that have been distinguished are termed *infantile nephropathic, juvenile,* and *benign*.

Infantile nephropathic cystinosis is characterized by the onset within the first year of life of the renal Fanconi syndrome (aminoaciduria, glycosuria, proteinuria, phosphaturia, polyuria); failure to thrive; and photophobia, retinopathy, and keratopathy. Children with this condition have fair skin and blond hair if they are white. Non-whites generally appear to have lighter skin coloration than other family members. At about the fourth or fifth year of life, failure of glomerular filtration occurs, progressing to end-stage renal disease by the end of the first decade of life. Renal rickets also occurs concomitantly with the renal failure. Many patients also develop hypothyroidism by 10 years of age (Chapter 360).

The cause of cystine accumulation within cystinotic lysosomes is now known to be a defective lysosomal transport system for cystine. In normal lysosomes, the transport system removes cystine residues form the lysosomal compartment. The relationship between lysosomal cystine storage and clinical symptomatology has not been established.

Therapy for this disorder has traditionally included salt and water replacement, treatment with vitamin D for the vitamin D-resistant rickets, and ultimately, renal transplantation when end-stage renal disease has been reached. The transplanted kidney parenchymal cells do not accumulate cystine, and the transplantation experience in patients with cystinosis is parallel to that in patients of similar age who have received transplanted kidneys for other causes. Attempts at specific therapy for cystinosis have included a cystine-free diet, which has been demonstrated to be unhelpful and perhaps harmful, and a variety of agents directed at reducing intralysosomal cystine. The first among these agents to be tried extensively was dithiothreitol, which has been demonstrated to lower circulating leukocyte cystine concentrations. Unfortunately, the compound has considerable toxicity and is unpleasant to administer. Ascorbic acid has been tried because it reduces the cystine content of cystinotic fibroblasts in culture; however, a double-blind clinical trial revealed no beneficial effect from this agent. Subsequently, a clinical trial of cysteamine therapy was undertaken in cystinosis, because it is the most efficient compound known for reducing intracellular cystine in tissue culture. This study demonstrated improved linear growth and preserved renal function in patients treated with cysteamine.

Juvenile cystinosis is an intermediate variety in which the onset of renal disease occurs later, and end-stage renal disease may not be reached until the end of the second decade of life. Because few patients with this condition are known, few clinical investigations have been carried out and the biochemical reason for its milder presentation is unknown.

Benign cystinosis is a perplexing variant characterized by eye findings similar to those of the other forms, but no other clinical signs or symptoms. These patients are usually discovered during routine ophthalmologic examinations. The inheritance pattern is autosomal recessive, and the biochemical abnormality that permits heterogeneity in this condition has not yet been determined.

Alkaptonuria

Alkaptonuria was described in 1908 by Garrod. Inherited as an autosomal recessive condition, it is due to inability to further metabolize homogentisic acid, a tyrosine metabolite, to maleylacetoacetic acid. Homogentisic acid in urine oxidizes spontaneously to dark pigmentary material, drawing its presence to medical attention. The condition is usually asymptomatic until the fourth decade of life, when accumulation of homogentisic acid leads to ochronosis with pigmentary deposits in the sclera, ears, and other exposed cartilage. Ultimately, the joints and tendons become generally involved and degenerative arthritis occurs (Chapter 321). No effective treatment for the degenerative changes has been described.

DISORDERS OF AMINO ACID TRANSPORT

Cystinuria

Cystinuria is an autosomal recessive condition characterized by marked hyperexcretion of the amino acids cystine, lysine, ornithine, and arginine (Chapter 349). These amino acids share the structural characteristics of two amino groups separated by four to six intervening atoms and also share a common epithelial transport mechanism. Cystinuria results from a disorder of epithelial transport for these compounds, both in the intestinal mucosa and in the renal tubule. The clinical symptomatology, however, results solely from the hyperexcretion of cystine, the least-soluble amino acid. Precipitation of cystine in situ leads to the formation of renal and bladder calculi, which produce the potential for obstruction and infection and lead patients to seek medical attention. Pure cystine calculi are visible on x-ray films because of high sulfur content but are more radiolucent than calcium-containing stones. The diagnosis may be suspected by the nitroprusside test, which gives a pink color reaction in urine containing more than approximately 100 μg of cystine per milligram of urinary creatinine. The diagnosis is confirmed by qualitative or quantitative assessment of the other amino acids in urine. In the United States, the incidence is estimated at approximately 1 in 7000, making this one of the most common inborn errors. Therapy is directed toward maintaining cystine in solution, a goal that can be accomplished by maintaining a neutral or basic urinary pH and increasing urine flow. A usual regimen requires treatment with alkalinizing agents and maintaining fluid intake between 4 and 8 liters per day. Additionally, penicillamine has been proposed for enhancing the solubility of cystine because penicillamine forms a mixed disulfide with cystine that is markedly more soluble than cystine itself. Treatment with 1 to 3 g D-penicillamine per day has been demonstrated to enhance cystine excretion and to prevent renal calculi formation. Existing calculi also may be dissolved. However, penicillamine therapy may produce adverse side effects, primarily in the form of fever, erythematous skin rash, and arthralgias. These side effects usually reverse when therapy is stopped, and, in many instances, penicillamine may then be reintroduced at a slower rate of administration without recurrence of adverse reactions.

Other amino acid transport disorders

Hyperdibasic aminoaciduria results from an apparently isolated defect in renal and intestinal transport of lysine, arginine, and ornithine. Its existence indicates that there is an alternative transport system for these three amino acids that is not shared by cystine, and absence of increased cystine excretion distinguishes this disorder from cystinuria. Clinically, the disease is characterized by diarrhea, intestinal malabsorption, and growth retardation with, in a few instances, mental retardation. The disease appears to respond to treatment with a low-protein diet.

Familial iminoglycinuria results in the excretion of increased quantities of glycine and hydroxyproline. This observation gave rise to the hypothesis, since confirmed, that these two amino acids share a common transport system in the kidney. No clinical abnormalities have been reported, and it appears to be inherited as an autosomal recessive trait.

Hartnup's disease results from a defect in transport of

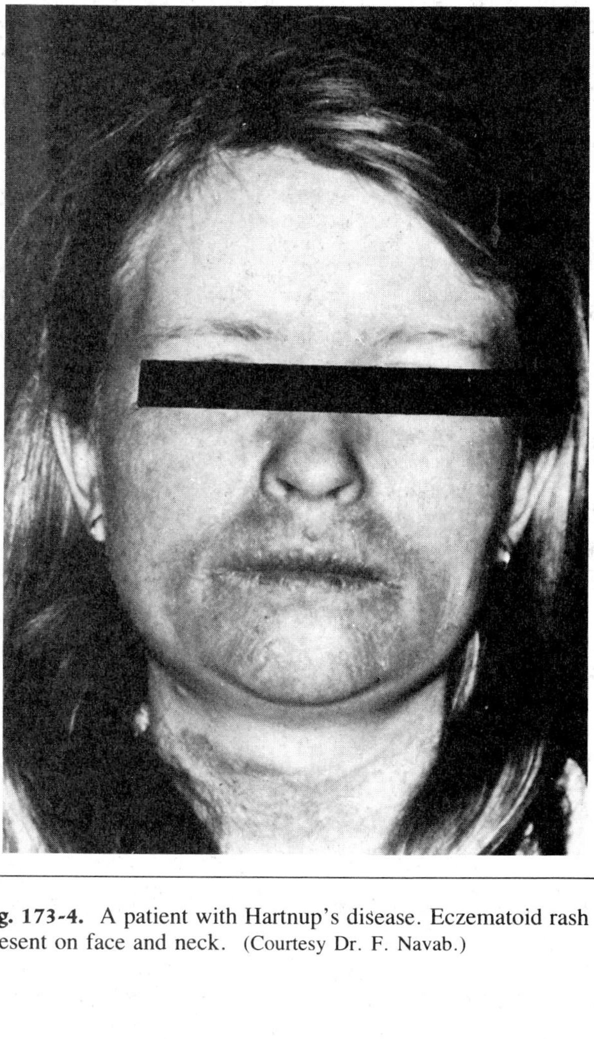

Fig. 173-4. A patient with Hartnup's disease. Eczematoid rash is present on face and neck. (Courtesy Dr. F. Navab.)

the "neutral" amino acids, which include alanine, serine, threonine, valine, leucine, isoleucine, phenylalanine, tyrosine, tryptamine, and histidine. These compounds are elevated fivefold to tenfold above normal in the urine of these patients. The condition is inherited as an autosomal recessive trait. Clinical features include a pellagra-like eczematoid, photosensitive rash of the extremities and face (Fig. 173-4); some inconstant neurologic symptoms including nystagmus, ataxia, tremor, and diplopia; and psychiatric disturbances ranging from emotional lability to frank hallucinations. Mental retardation is also an inconstant finding. The clinical features appear episodically and have been precipitated by sulfonamide therapy, exposure to sunlight, fever, or other stress. There is considerable similarity between this condition and pellagra, which results from dietary nicotinamide deficiency. Therapy with nicotinamide has resulted in improvement in both the skin and neurologic abnormalities.

Lowe's syndrome results in the renal Fanconi syndrome and is accompanied by X-linked inheritance, congenital cataracts, buphthalmos, failure to thrive, severe mental retardation, and hypotonia. The biochemical defect in this condition has not been identified.

REFERENCES

Brusilow S et al: Treatment of episodic hyperammonemia in children with inborn errors of urea synthesis, N Engl J Med 310:1630, 1984.

Buchanan D and Thoene J: Dual-column high-performance liquid chromatographic urinary organic acid profiling, Anal Biochem 124:108, 1982.

Chalmers R and Lawson A: Organic acids in man, London: Chapman & Hall, 1982.

Christensen H: Hypothesis: where the depleted plasma amino acids go in PKU, and why, Perspect Biol Med 30:186-196, 1987.

Gahl W et al: Cysteamine therapy for children with nephropathic cystinosis, N Engl J Med 316:971-977, 1987.

Msall M et al: Neurologic outcome in children with inborn errors of urea synthesis, N Engl J Med 310:1500, 1984.

Nyhan W: Abnormalities in amino acid metabolism in clinical medicine, Norwalk, Conn, 1984, Appleton-Century-Crofts.

Sassa S and Kappas A: Hereditary tyrosinemia and the heme biosynthetic pathway, J Clin Invest 71:625, 1983.

Scriver C et al, editors: The metabolic basis of inherited disease, ed 6, New York, 1989, McGraw-Hill.

Thoene J, editor: Physician's guide to rare diseases, Montvale, NJ, 1992, Dowden Publishing Co.

Thoene J and Wolf B: Biotinidase deficiency in juvenile multiple carboxylase deficiency, Lancet 1:398, 1983.

Wellner D and Meister A: A survey of inborn errors of amino acid metabolism and transport in man, Annu Rev Biochem 50:911, 1981.

CHAPTER

174 Lysosomal Storage Diseases

Alan J. Garber

Cellular composition is determined by the balance of degradation and resynthesis of intracellular components. Cells must adapt to changing internal and external demands by altering their structural and functional composition. The process of component turnover not only salvages damaged or degraded components but is essential to redirect ongoing processes toward new needs. For example, protein degradation rates are increased in both regenerating liver and hypertrophying muscle. Although in these states there is overall net synthesis, substantial redirection and adaptation are required. Lysosomes, cytoplasmic organelles containing hydrolytic enzymes, are the major site for the degradation of structural and functional cellular components; therefore, defects in lysosomal function impair cellular adaptive change and ultimately induce a loss of cellular function.

LYSOSOMAL PHYSIOLOGY

Lysosomes contain a host of degradative enzymes that are maximally active at an acid pH. The interior of the lysosome is maintained at about pH 4.5 by an adenosine triphosphate-dependent proton pump. Lysosomal enzymes are synthesized on the rough endoplasmic reticulum and processed as they pass through the endoplasmic reticula. A crucial step in this pathway is the addition of mannose 6-phosphate residues. This addition is generated by a two-step process. N-acetylglucosamine-1-phosphate is transferred to mannose residues, generating a phosphodiester. N-acetylglucosamine is then removed, leaving the mannose 6-phosphate residue as a lysosomal enzyme recognition marker. Receptors for mannose 6-phosphate reside on the specialized areas of the smooth endoplasmic reticulum that are destined to become the lysosome. These receptors bind the mannose 6-phosphate-labeled enzymes. As the new organelle is formed, it thereby incorporates lysosomal enzymes within it. Lysosomes internalize and subsequently degrade endogenous or exogenous materials. In addition to the ongoing degradation of endogenous cellular constituents, lysosomes are important to metabolize low-density lipoproteins (LDL) and some hormones via endocytosis and subsequent incorporation.

The concept of a lysosomal storage disease was first formulated by Hers to explain the pathogenesis of Pompe's disease, in which the histologic appearance of intracellular organelles filled with amorphous material results from a deficiency in lysosomal acid maltase. These findings correlate with progressive muscular dysfunction as described in Chapter 170. Lysosomal storage diseases were originally defined as a deficiency of a single lysosomal enzyme activity that causes undegraded material to accumulate within the lysosomes, leading to progressive disease. Subsequently, other lysosomal storage diseases were identified in which defects of lysosomal physiology cause multiple enzymatic defects (see ML II).

GENERAL CONSIDERATIONS

Dozens of lysosomal storage diseases have been identified. The most common have been grouped according to similarities in their clinical presentation, the biochemistry of the accumulated materials, and the enzymatic deficiencies involved. The schema in Fig. 174-1 attempts to guide the clinician toward a discrete group of diagnostic possibilities from among the many diseases described.

First, a reasonable index of suspicion is necessary. In infants and children, the classic findings of coarse facies with organomegaly, immobile joints, skeletal changes, and mental retardation suggest a mucopolysaccharide storage disease or mucolipidosis. Neurologic signs such as loss of developmental milestones, hypotonia or spasticity, exaggerated startle reflexes, or seizures are also indicative of lysosomal storage diseases, particularly the lipidoses. Clinical findings may be more subtle in adults, but progressive organomegaly, skeletal anomalies, mental retardation, affective disorders, and visual or auditory deficits all suggest a lysosomal disorder. The hallmark of lysosomal storage disease is the engorged lysosome. Circulating leukocytes, conjunctival biopsies, and cultured cells may all show cytoplasmic inclusions. The inclusions may display distinct morphology in light and electron microscopy and thus lead to a specific diagnosis. The biochemical demonstration of a specific enzyme deficiency is required for definitive diagnosis. Most lysosomal diseases may be diagnosed by assay of enzymes in circulating leukocytes, biopsy material, or cultured fibroblasts. The latter is often used for prenatal diagnosis by amniocentesis.

The great clinical heterogeneity seen within these diseases may occur for many reasons. Different isoenzyme deficiencies may produce different functional losses with the same observed total activity. Different mutations within the same structural gene may produce total or partial defects in enzymolysis; partial blocks produce lower activity but may also produce different substrate affinities. The loss of an activating factor may also impair enzymatic activity, without a mutation in the enzyme itself.

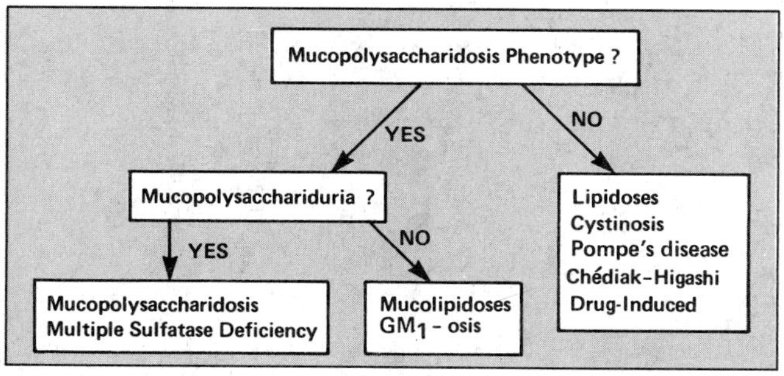

Fig. 174-1. Approach to the diagnosis of lysosomal storage diseases.

The impact of the loss of enzymatic activity will be serious when the enzymatic activity is crucial for cellular function. Disorders of mucopolysaccharides affect virtually all tissues. Gangliosidoses primarily affect the brain, and cystinosis affects the kidney, in which sulfhydryl exchange is active. Additionally, these diseases affect the young, in whom turnover and remodeling are great. Diseases mild enough to spare the patient until adulthood manifest more subtle lesions and are perhaps the greatest diagnostic challenges among the lysosomal storage diseases.

MUCOPOLYSACCHARIDOSES

The mucopolysaccharidoses (MPS) constitute a class of diseases characterized by an inability to completely degrade mucopolysaccharides. Mucopolysaccharides are nitrogenous polysaccharides that, when conjugated to core proteins, form the glycosaminoglycans. Enzymatic defects lead to the accumulation of mucopolysaccharides and chemically similar substrates within the lysosome. Because mucopolysaccharides are found throughout the body, it is understandable that most organ systems are affected by these diseases.

The organ systems most commonly affected include bone, viscera, connective tissue, and brain. Dysostosis multiplex denotes the characteristic bony abnormalities of widening of the medial clavicle, widening and shortening of the long bones, flattening of the ribs, beaking of the vertebrae with lumbar kyphosis, and enlargement of the sella turcica. Dysostosis multiplex is fully expressed in Hurler's disease and is present to some degree in most of the mucopolysaccharidoses. Hepatosplenomegaly is a frequent finding, as is asymptomatic carpal tunnel syndrome. Coarse facies, a depressed nasal bridge, corneal clouding, retinal disease, optic nerve swelling, and later atrophy, joint stiffness, deafness, cardiovascular anomalies, and neurologic abnormalities may all be present to a variable extent (Fig. 174-2). In particular, the degree of skeletal dysplasia and the presence or absence of corneal clouding or mental retardation may be useful in the differential diagnosis (Table 174-1). All mucopolysaccharidoses follow an autosomal recessive inheritance except for the X-linked MPS II (Hunter's disease) and may be diagnosed in utero by enzyme assay of cultured amniotic fibroblasts or through chorionic villus sampling. The detection of the carrier state of MPS types I, III, IV, and VI has not been reliable, owing to the overlapping of enzymatic activity values with those from normal individuals. MPS II heterozygotes may be diagnosed by the assay of cloned fibroblasts. Roughly half of the clones will be enzyme deficient by virtue of the random deactivation of X chromosomes in the carrier female.

MPS IH (Hurler syndrome)

MPS IH is the prototypic mucopolysaccharidosis. After the first few months of life, physical and mental abnormalities become obvious and usually prove fatal within

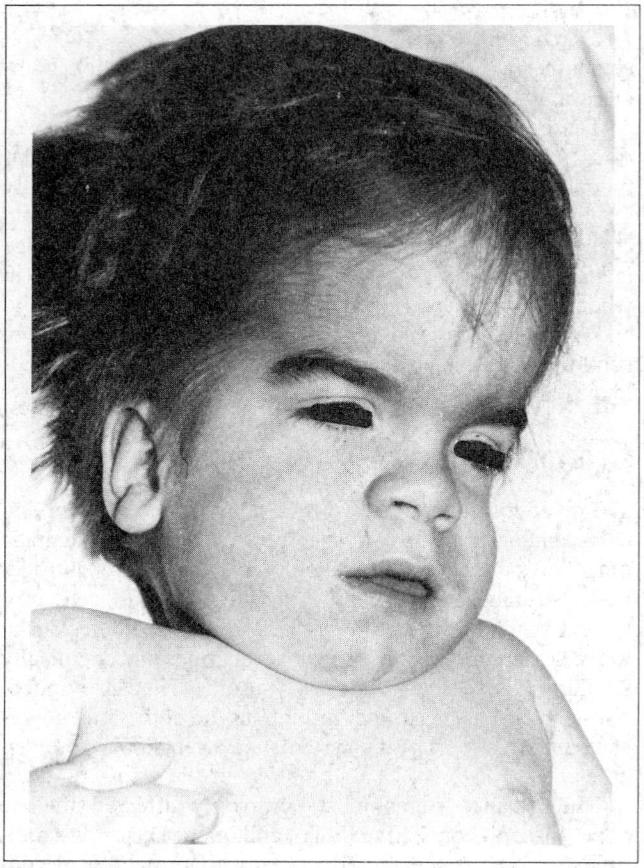

A

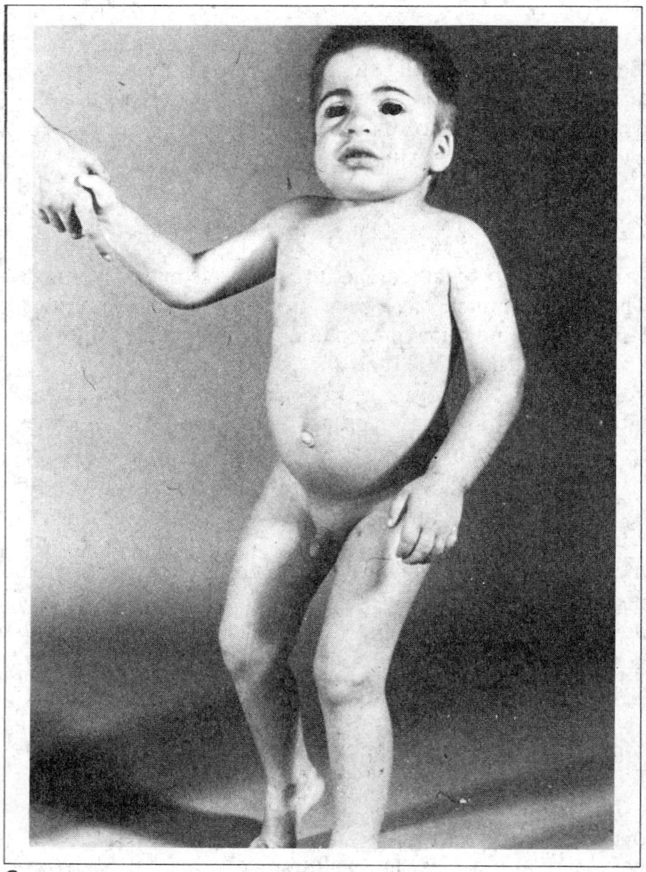

C

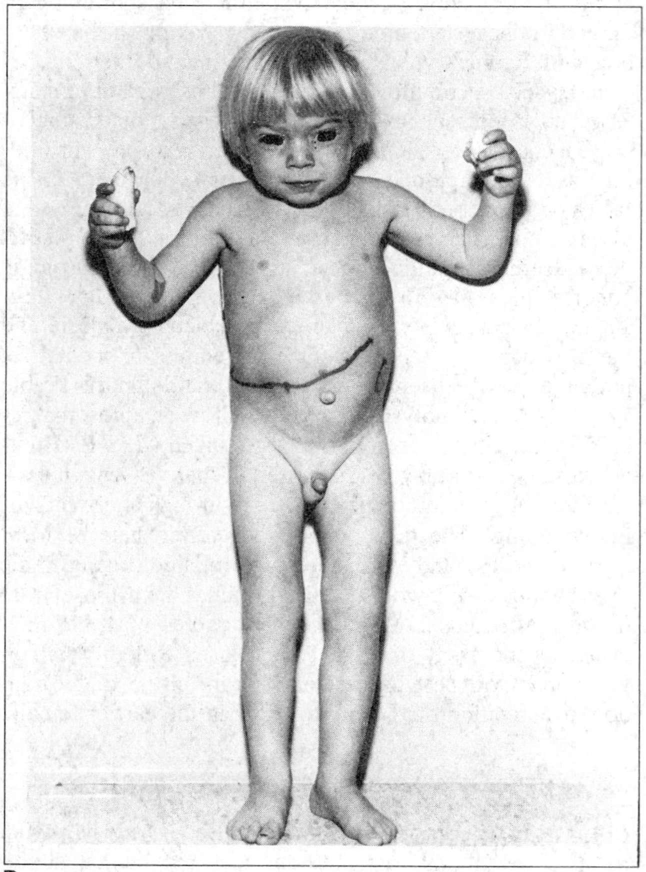

B

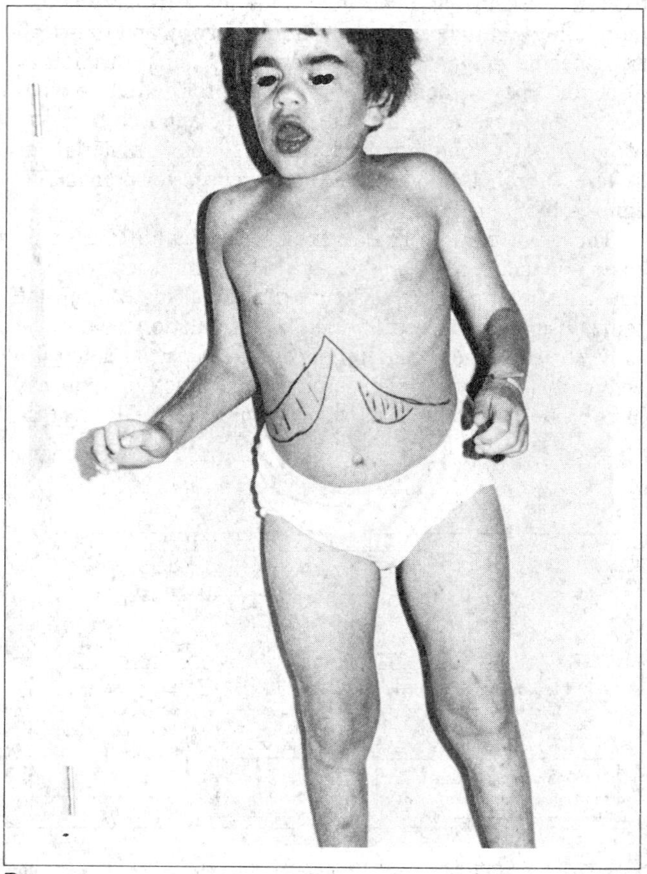

D

For legend see opposite page.

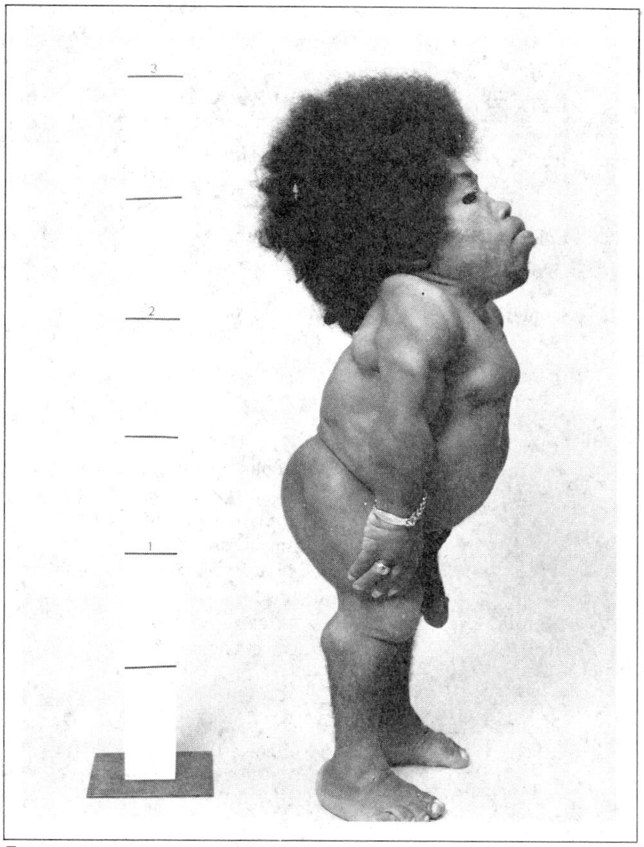

E

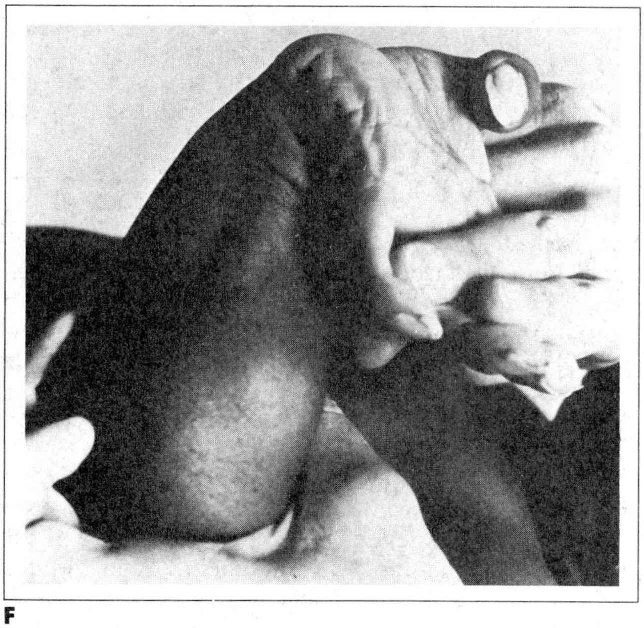

F

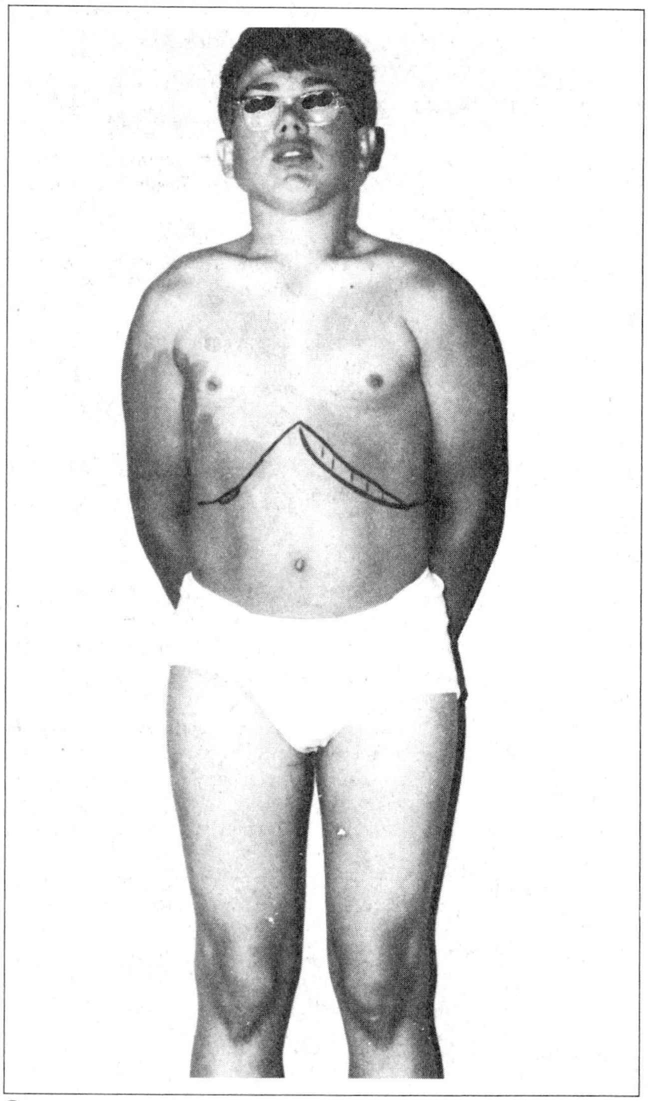

G

Fig. 174-2. Physical characteristics of patients with mucopolysaccharidosis. **A,** MPS IH (Hurler's disease). **B,** MPS IS (Scheie's syndrome). **C,** MPS II (Hunter's syndrome). **D,** MPS III (Sanfilippo's syndrome). **E, F,** MPS IV (Morquio syndrome). **G,** MPS VI (Maroteaux-Lamy syndrome). (Courtesy Dr. Nicola Diferrante,)

the first decade. Physical changes include dysostosis multiplex; hepatosplenomegaly; joint stiffness with claw hands; and a large head with coarse, thickened features (Fig. 174-2, *A*). Corneal clouding is a constant feature in this disease. Mental development slows and regresses after the first year. Cardiovascular abnormalities with valvular heart disease, pulmonary hypertension, and pulmonary insufficiency all lead to early mortality. The specific defect in alpha-L-iduronidase prevents normal catabolism of dermatan sulfate and heparan sulfate. Urinary mucopolysaccharides contain dermatan sulfate and heparan sulfate in a ratio of about 7:3.

Table 174-1. The mucopolysaccharidoses

Designation	Distinguishing characteristics	Urinary MPS	Eponym	Enzyme deficiency
MPS IH	Severe MPS phenotype, mental retardation, corneal clouding, early death (first decade)	Dermatan sulfate Heparan sulfate	Hurler	Alpha-L-iduronidase
MPS IS	Mild MPS involvement with nearly normal intelligence and stature, corneal clouding, normal life span	Dermatan sulfate Heparan sulfate	Scheie's	Alpha-L-iduronidase
MPS II	Mild: Mild MPS, short stature, mental retardation with nearly normal life span, X-linked, clear corneas Severe: Moderate MPS with mental retardation, deteriorating in second decade, X-linked, clear corneas	Dermatan sulfate Heparan sulfate	Hunter's	Iduronate sulfatase
MPS III	Mild MPS with clear corneas, severe mental retardation with neurologic decay	Heparan sulfate	Sanfilippo's	Type A: heparan-N-sulfatase Type B: N-acetylglucosaminidase Type C: acetyl-CoA glucosamide-N-acetyltransferase Type D: N-acetyl-alpha-D-glucosamine-6-sulfatase
MPS IV, A, B	Severe skeletal involvement with odontoid hypoplasia, lax joints, corneal clouding, normal intelligence	Keratan	Morquio	A: N-acetylgalactose sulfatase B: Beta-galactosidase
MPS V	Vacant			
MPS VI	Mild: Mild MPS phenotype, short stature, normal intelligence, corneal clouding, striking metachromatic inclusions Severe: Moderate MPS phenotype with mortality in second decade, odontoid hypoplasia, normal intelligence, corneal clouding, striking metachromatic inclusions	Dermatan sulfate	Maroteaux-Lamy	N-acetylhexosamine-4-sulfate sulfatase (arylsulfatase B)
MPS VII	MPS phenotype with odontoid hypoplasia and corneal clouding, mild to moderate retardation (very heterogeneous)	Dermatan sulfate	Sly	Beta-glucuronidase

MPS IS (Scheie's syndrome)

MPS IS is also caused by a defect in alpha-L-iduronidase, the same enzyme activity lacking in MPS IH. Although it seems likely that MPS IH and MPS IS are allelic mutations at the same locus, it remains to be explained how MPS IS also can have no demonstrable enzyme activity but display much less clinical severity than MPS IH. These patients enjoy a nearly normal life span and intelligence. Physical findings include corneal clouding, cardiovascular disease, and normal stature despite stiff joints and genu valgum (Fig. 174-2, *B*). The face is coarse, with a broad mouth. Retinitis pigmentosa may develop. Diagnosis rests with the demonstration of alpha-L-iduronidase deficiency in the presence of only moderate physical abnormalities. Urinary mucopolysaccharides contain dermatan sulfate and heparan sulfate in a ratio of about 3:2.

MPS I (Iduronidase deficiency)

A third MPS I, alpha-L-iduronidase-deficient phenotype has been reported. These patients present with physical features intermediate between MPS IH and MPS IS, with fair preservation of intelligence. This phenotype, termed *Hurler-Scheie syndrome* (MPS IH/IS), has been considered a compound of Hurler and Scheie alleles. However, reports of several patients from consanguineous parentage suggest the existence of a third independent allele.

MPS II (Hunter's syndrome)

MPS II is an X-linked disorder that produces a phenotype similar to, but less severe than, MPS IH. The lack of corneal clouding is a useful feature for differentiation. MPS II derives from a deficiency in iduronate sulfatase that causes urinary excretion of equal proportions of dermatan sulfate and keratan sulfate. The occurrence of enzymatically proved MPS II in females may be due to rare homozygosity, co-dominance, or an autosomal variant. Heterozygous females may be detected by enzyme assay of cloned fibroblasts. Two clinically distinct subtypes may be distinguished within this syndrome: severe and mild. Both subtypes segregate as an X-linked disorder.

The severe form of MPS II is distinguished by the development between the second and sixth year of life of physical defects including deafness, stiff joints, coarse facies, and skeletal abnormalities (Fig. 174-2, *C*). Mental deterioration follows. Death from respiratory and cardiovascular disease usually occurs in the second decade. The mild form of MPS II causes only mild physical abnormalities, which may include joint stiffness, carpal tunnel syndrome, short stature, deafness, and retinal dystrophy. Mental status may be normal or mildly retarded. Most patients survive between three and six decades.

MPS III (Sanfilippo's syndrome)

MPS III includes at least four phenocopies, which derive from different enzymatic defects. The clinical presentation begins between 2 and 4 years of age. First, there is loss of neurologic milestones, and this is followed by facial coarsening (Fig. 174-2, *D*), joint stiffness, and mild organomegaly reminiscent of mild MPS I. Corneal clouding, however, is notably absent. There is relatively slow progression of the disease, with severe neurologic deficits, severe mental retardation, spasticity, and seizures. Death is most common in the second and third decades. MPS III is currently divided into subtypes A, B, C, and D, each with a unique enzyme deficiency. All types show mild to moderate mucopolysacchariduria, with a predominance of heparan sulfate. Type A results from a deficiency of heparan-N-sulfatase; type B, from N-acetyl-alpha-glucosaminidase deficiency; type C, from a deficiency of acetyl-CoA-alpha-glucosamide-N-acetyltransferase; and type D from N-acetyl-alpha-D-glucosamine-6-sulfatase. Diagnosis depends on the clinical presentation of characteristic physical changes, severe mental degeneration, urinary excretion of heparan sulfate, and the identification of a specific enzyme deficiency.

MPS IV (Morquio's syndrome)

Morquio's syndrome displays unique physical findings among the MPSs. Skeletal abnormalities predominate (Fig. 174-2, *E*), with prominence of the lower ribs after the first year of life, spatulate ribs, flattening of the vertebra with kyphosis, and later osteoporosis. A constant and striking feature is hypoplasia of the odontoid process. This anomaly often leads to cervical compression and myelopathy, which may be a major source of morbidity. Corneal clouding and aortic valve disease are frequent findings. In contradistinction to MPS types I to III, the joints are lax with notable wrist instability (Fig. 174-2, *F*). Intellectual development is normal in MPS IV. The major sources of morbidity and mortality are respiratory insufficiency, cord compression, and cardiovascular disease. Two enzyme defects have been associated with the Morquio phenotype. Morquio A (MPS IVA) was originally described with deficiency of N-acetylgalactose sulfatase activity. A more recently described phenocopy, denoted Morquio B (MPS IVB), reveals a deficiency in beta-galactoside in which some residual activity toward GM_1 ganglioside avoids the presentation of frank GM_1 gangliosidosis.

MPS V

This classification, formerly held by Scheie's syndrome, is vacant since the discovery that Scheie's and Hurler's syndromes result from defects at the same gene locus.

MPS VI (Maroteaux-Lamy syndrome)

The clinical picture of MPS VI shows great heterogeneity. The severe form manifests in the second or third year of life and resembles MPS I, with kyphosis, anterior sternal protrusion, restricted joints, corneal clouding, and coarse facies (Fig. 174-2, *G*). Hydrocephalus and cervical cord compression may also develop owing to odontoid hypoplasia. Mortality often occurs in the second decade. A mild form characterized by corneal clouding, short stature, and inguinal hernia has been identified. This form seems compatible with a normal life span and may be distinguished from MPS IS by the inevitable short stature that it engenders. A normal intelligence seems to be preserved in all forms. Diagnosis relies on the clinical presentation, urinary excretion of dermatan sulfate, and the demonstration of a deficiency of N-acetyl-hexosamine-4-sulfate sulfatase activity.

MPS VII

First described as a separate disease in 1973, MPS VII is associated with characteristic mucopolysaccharidotic facies, dysostosis multiplex, and psychomotor retardation within the first year of life. Hypoplasia of the odontoid process and gibbous deformity are also present. The limited number of patients described thus far show significant heterogeneity in the severity of physical and mental abnormalities. Beta-glucuronidase activity is deficient in this disease, which leads to urinary excretion of heparan sulfate and dermatan sulfate.

MUCOLIPIDOSES

The mucolipidoses (ML) are grouped together on the basis of clinical similarities, but recent work has shown wide divergence in their pathogeneses. The key finding in this group of diseases is an MPS-type phenotype despite normal urinary mucopolysaccharides. ML types I and VI, mannosidosis, fucosidosis, and aspartylglucosaminuria result from classic single-enzyme defects that lead to the accumulation of glycosylated proteins. ML II and III result from the abnormal packaging of lysosomal enzymes in the organelle (Table 174-2). Chorionic villus sampling may be used in fetal diagnosis; however, care must be exercised to avoid contamination by maternal tissue.

ML I (Sialidosis I)

These patients develop a mucopolysaccharidosis-like phenotype during the first year of life and progress to mild somatic involvement with moderate mental retardation. There is considerable heterogeneity within this syndrome, and

Table 174-2. The mucolipidoses

Designation	Defect	Distinguishing features
ML I	Alpha-N-acetylneuraminidase	Moderate MPS phenotype, moderate retardation, neural degeneration in later years
ML II	N-acetylglucosamine-phosphotransferase	Severe MPS phenotype and retardation, clear corneas, neural decay by first decade
ML III	N-acetylglucosamine-phosphotransferase	Moderate MPS phenotype, mild retardation, corneal clouding
ML IV	Ganglioside sialidase	No MPS phenotype except corneal clouding, hypotonia, and hyperflexia; mild retardation
Mannosidosis	Alpha-mannosidase + packaging defect	Moderate MPS phenotype, severe retardation, clear corneas
Fucosidosis	Fucosidase	Type I: Moderate MPS phenotype, retardation with progressive decay to death in first decade Type II: Slight MPS phenotype with moderate retardation and slow neural deterioration, angiokeratoma corporis diffusum
Aspartylglucosaminuria	N-aspartyl-beta-glucosaminidase	Mild MPS phenotype; usually Finnish ancestry; pigmentation abnormalities with acne; severe retardation with affective disorders

there are reports of cherry-red spots and corneal opacities. The findings of a mild MPS phenotype, mental retardation, normal urinary mucopolysaccharides, and leukocyte inclusions point toward ML I and suggest further enzymatic analysis. This syndrome is associated with a deficiency in alpha-N-acetylneuraminidase. Two subtypes have been identified, and these have different clinical courses. The fusion of cells from these subtypes reconstitutes enzyme activity. Thus at least two alpha-N-acetylneuraminidase deficiency diseases seem to reside within ML I.

ML II (I cell disease)

Striking skeletal involvement coupled with respiratory difficulties brings these patients to attention within the first month of life. Progressive mental deterioration, heart disease, and respiratory failure occur within the first decade. Fibroblasts from ML II display numerous coarse inclusions, hence the denotation of "I"-cell disease. A number of lysosomal enzyme activities are lacking in ML II cells; however, culture medium from such cells contains high enzyme activities. This disease, and probably ML III as well, derives from defects in the packaging of certain lysosomal enzymes. Instead of clustering within primary lysosomes, the enzymes are secreted from the cell. The biochemical defect resides in the labeling of lysosomal enzymes with mannose 6-phosphate. ML II and ML III are now known to be deficient in N-acetylglucosamine-phosphate transferase, producing a defect in mannose 6-phosphate labeling of lysosomal enzymes. Without this marker, receptors in the endoplasmic reticulum membrane are unable to accumulate the enzymes for packaging into primary lysosomes. Thus in distinction to defects in lysosomal enzyme catalysis, these diseases stem from the disruption of general lysosomal physiology.

The diagnosis of ML II rests with the severe clinical presentation described above, the absence of mucopolysacchariduria, and a deficiency of N-acetylglucosamine-1-phosphotransferase. Plasma lysosomal enzyme activities are elevated, whereas cultured fibroblasts are deficient in several enzyme activities.

ML III (Pseudo-Hurler dystrophy)

Although this syndrome is biochemically similar to type II mucolipidosis, the clinical manifestations are less severe. Physical abnormalities begin during the first few years of life with the development of stiff joints that progress to claw-hand deformities. There are slightly coarsened facies, corneal clouding, and mild mental retardation. Although these findings suggest a mucopolysaccharidosis, urinary mucopolysaccharides are normal. Plasma lysosomal enzymes are elevated and cultured fibroblasts show multiple lysosomal enzyme deficiencies. The molecular defect in ML III leads to aberrant packaging of lysosomal enzymes. Current studies implicate considerable genetic heterogeneity in ML II and ML III, suggesting that multiple loci may reside within these clinical syndromes. Diagnosis depends on clinical presentation, the presence of normal urinary mucopolysaccharides, disproportionate changes in plasma and cellular lysosomal enzyme levels, and a deficiency in N-acetylglucosamine-1-transferase.

ML IV

A recently recognized syndrome, ML IV includes the clinical findings of corneal clouding, hypotonia, and developmental delay. Histologic studies show lysosomal inclusions; tissue analysis has indicated an increase in gangliosides GM_3 and GD_3. Recent reports implicate ganglioside sialidase as the deficient enzyme activity in this disorder.

Alpha-mannosidosis

This syndrome is typified by the early development of a mildly Hurler-like physical appearance. A broad skull with prominent jaw and forehead development is a nearly constant finding. These patients may die within the first decade of life, but studies also report that some survive into adulthood. Mental retardation is usually severe. Fibroblast studies show that large quantities of alpha-mannosidase are secreted into the culture medium. Coculture with ML II cells causes restoration of intracellular alpha-mannosidase activities. Thus it appears that this disease may be caused by improper incorporation of alpha-mannosidase into the primary lysosome. The diagnosis depends on an MPS-like phenotype without mucopolysacchariduria and is confirmed by finding a deficiency of lysosomal alpha-mannosidase activity.

Fucosidosis

Patients with fucosidosis display a wide diversity of clinical presentations, ranging from rapid progression and death in the first years of life to slow deterioration with survival into adulthood. In the type I infantile form, the first year of life brings muscular hypotonia, excessive sweating, Hurler-like disease phenotype, mental retardation, and death between 4 and 6 years of age. In the juvenile type II form, there is a slower progression, with a high incidence of angiokeratoma corporis diffusum, which formerly was thought unique to Fabry's disease. Diagnosis may be difficult in this heterogeneous disease. If there is a suspicion of this mucolipidosis, the presence of high sweat electrolytes and angiokeratoma corporis diffusum may suggest type II. Definite diagnosis requires a determination of fucosidase activity in leukocytes or cultured fibroblasts. Thus far, no relationship between the severity of disease and residual enzyme activity has been established.

Aspartylglucosaminuria (N-aspartyl-beta-glucosaminidase deficiency)

This disease is considered with the mucolipidoses because of its mucopolysaccharidosis-like phenotype in the absence of mucopolysacchariduria. Aspartylglucosaminidase cleaves carbohydrate-protein linkages from many glycolipids; its deficiency allows the accumulation of mucopolysaccharide-like materials within the lysosomes. These patients, almost exclusively of Finnish ancestry, come to attention because they miss developmental milestones and remain severely retarded. Most show no gross neurologic deficits but display aggressive or affective psychologic disorders. Coarse facies, broad nose, moderate dysostosis multiplex, and dermatologic abnormalities may suggest a mucopolysaccharidosis. Respiratory and gastrointestinal disorders also are reported. Circulating leukocytes have prominent inclusions. Urinalysis shows overexcretion of 2-acetamido-1-(beta-1-L-aspartamido)-1,2, dideoxy-beta-D-glucose in the urine. Definitive diagnosis depends on enzymatic assays in plasma leukocytes or circulating fibroblasts.

LIPID STORAGE DISEASES

Lipid storage diseases are associated with the finding of high levels of lipid compounds in the tissues of affected patients. Most of these patients lack the striking skeletal and soft-tissue abnormalities common to mucopolysaccharidoses and mucolipidoses. They do, however, commonly manifest severe derangements in central nervous system development (Table 174-3). Except for the X-linked Fabry's disease, these diseases are inherited in an autosomal recessive manner (Chapter 92).

Chemistry

Aside from acid lipase deficiency, the lipid storage diseases involve defects in sphingolipid metabolism. The sphingolipids are derived from sphingosine—fatty acid conjugates termed *ceramides* (Fig. 174-3). Ceramide may be conjugated with phosphocholine to form sphingomyelin, a widespread membrane component. Ceramide also may be sulfated to form sulfatides, glycosylated to form ceramide-n-hexoses, or further conjugated with sialic acid to form the gangliosides.

Farber lipogranulomatosis (acid ceramidase deficiency)

This disease presents a characteristic clinical syndrome. Although clinically normal at birth, within 2 to 4 months infants with Farber disease develop joint swelling and stiffness in their extremities. Superficial nodules and thickenings appear on the joints, which become painful. Flexure contractures result. Laryngeal swelling, stridor, and pulmonary consolidation lead to significant morbidity and mortality within the first 2 years. In a milder form of this disease, patients survive into their second decade. These patients accumulate subcutaneous nodules on extensor sur-

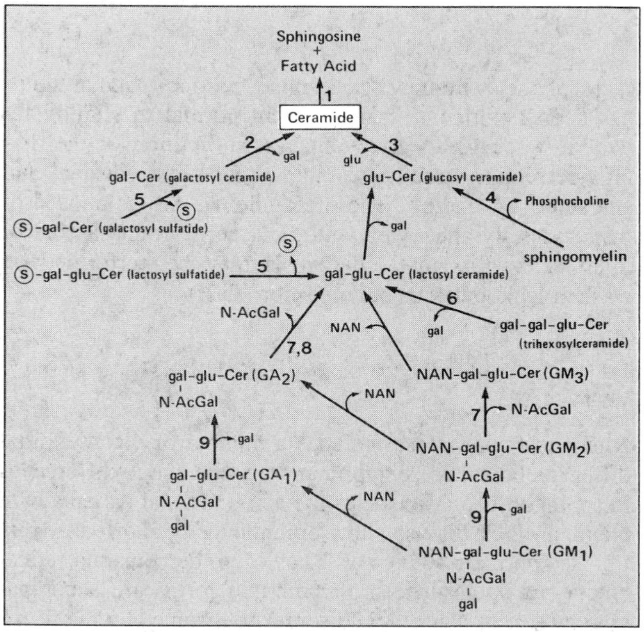

Fig. 174-3. Pathways of sphingolipid catabolism and disorders produced by enzyme deficiencies. *NAN,* N-acetyl neuraminic acid; *N-AcGal,* N-acetyl galactose; *gal,* galactose; *glu,* glucose.

Table 174-3. The lipidoses

Syndrome	Distinguishing features	Defect
Farber lipogranulomatosis	Joint swelling, stiffness, and pain in first year; widespread granuloma in dermis and pulmonary tree	Ceramidase
Niemann-Pick	Acute: failure to thrive, cachexia, neurologic signs, and cherry-red spots in the macula	Sphingomyelinase
	Juvenile: gait changes and ataxia in first year	
	Chronic: adult hepatosplenomegaly and respiratory disease with normal intellect	
Gaucher's	Infantile: failure to thrive, hypertonia, and neurologic signs with death in first 2 years; Gaucher's cells	Glucocerebrosidase
	Juvenile: as in infantile, with slower progression and survival into first decade; Gaucher cells	
	Chronic: adult hepatosplenomegaly, osteoporosis; Gaucher cells	
Krabbe's	Increased startle reflex, progressing to hyperreflexia and opisthotonos to vegetative state in first year; globoid cells	Galactocerebrosidase
Metachromatic leukodystrophy (MLD)	Infantile: gait changes progress to weakness and psychomotor disability and blindness in first years	Arylsulfatase A
Multiple sulfatase deficiency	MLD-like presentation in presence of MPS phenotype with urinary mucopolysaccharides	Arylsulfatase A,B,C
Fabry's	Angiectasis corporis diffusum, renal pain, renal and cardiac failure	Alpha-galactosidase
GM_1 gangliosidosis	Infantile: MPS-like phenotype with failure to thrive progressing to decerebrate rigidity and respiratory failure	Beta-galactosidase
	Juvenile: mild or no MPS features, psychomotor retardation in first decade	
	Adult: ataxia and seizures	
GM_2 gangliosidosis	Infantile (Tay-Sachs, Sandhoff): cherry-red retinal spots, exaggerated startle reflex progressing to hyperactivity, psychomotor retardation, and a vegetative state with death in first years	Tay-Sachs: hexosaminidase A
	Juvenile (Tay-Sachs): delayed progression of infantile form through first and second decades	Sandhoff's: hexosaminidase A and B.
	Adult (Tay-Sachs): dystonia and spinocerebellar degeneration	

faces of the extremities and spinal column. Mental status has been reported as ranging from normal to slightly retarded. Widespread granulomatous infiltration of the dermis, respiratory tract, and other organs is a constant and characteristic finding. These granulomas are composed of histiocytes, lymphocytes, and giant cells around a core of foam cells. Enzymatic diagnosis may be performed on washed leukocytes or cultured fibroblasts.

Niemann-Pick disease (sphingomyelinase deficiency)

Niemann-Pick disease includes a number of disorders that differ in clinical presentation and may be due to differences in sphingomyelinase isoenzyme activities. All patients with Niemann-Pick disease show organomegaly and foamy histiocytes on marrow biopsy. They often demonstrate retinal cherry-red spots. The most common forms are accompanied by severe neurologic disorder, but some chronic forms have mild or unappreciable neuropathology.

Acute infantile form (type A). This most common subtype manifests itself within the first months of life. Infants feed poorly, fail to thrive, and show slow neurologic development and hepatosplenomegaly. Retinal cherry-red spots occur in half of all patients. Cachexia, central neurologic decay, and death occur within the first few years of life.

Juvenile or subacute form (types C and D). The juvenile form is differentiated by a later onset of neurologic deterioration. These patients appear normal during the first few years of life and subsequently manifest gait disturbances and mild ataxia. Foam cells in the marrow and mild hepatosplenomegaly are present. Neurologic involvement becomes increasingly widespread and severe, leading to ataxia, spasticity, seizures, and ultimately to a vegetative state. These patients belong to type C, except for patients of Nova Scotian ancestry, for whom type D is reserved.

Chronic forms (types B and E). Types B (juvenile nonneuropathic) and E (adult nonneuropathic) probably represent a continuum of sphingomyelinase deficiencies without severe neurologic involvement. Mild hepatosplenomegaly, pulmonary infiltration, and occasional retinal cherry-red spots are the most common clinical findings. Some adult patients may have mild ataxia but are otherwise neurologically intact.

In addition to the aforementioned clinical and histologic findings, the diagnosis of Niemann-Pick disease requires a demonstration of a deficiency in one or all of the sphingomyelinase isoenzyme activities in circulating leukocytes or cultured fibroblasts. Recent evidence suggests that type C is due to an activating-factor deficiency. Types A and B show loss of sphingomyelinase enzyme.

Gaucher's disease (beta-glucocerebrosidase deficiency)

Most common of the sphingolipidoses, Gaucher's disease manifests itself in three distinct subtypes. The infantile neuropathic form (type II) becomes clinically apparent within the first months of life. Hepatosplenomegaly, failure to thrive, feeding difficulties, respiratory disease, and neurologic damage generally are found. Neurologic involvement proceeds to hypertonia, spasticity, and laryngeal stridor. Death occurs during the first year of life, usually owing to pulmonary failure. The infrequent juvenile neuropathic form (type III) displays many of the type II characteristics in a delayed form. In the first decade, hepatosplenomegaly, with easy bruisability, bone pain, abdominal pain, hyperreflexia, and spasticity, all develop. These patients often die in the second decade.

The most common form, chronic nonneuropathic (type I), may manifest itself in adulthood with hepatosplenomegaly, easy bruisability, anemia, and bone pain. No neurologic abnormalities are evident. Major findings include osteoporosis or necrosis of the vertebrae and proximal femur, hepatosplenomegaly, and an increased serum acid phosphatase level. All patients have diagnostic "Gaucher" cells on marrow biopsy. By phase microscopy, there is wrinkled cytoplasm with fibrillar inclusions. The nucleus is acentric; inclusions are periodic acid Schiff (PAS)-positive. The definitive diagnosis rests with increased tissue glucosylceramide levels and a deficiency of beta-glucocerebrosidase in circulating leukocytes or cultured fibroblasts.

Krabbe's disease (beta-galactocerebrosidase deficiency

This rare sphingolipidosis presents with acute central nervous system degeneration in the first few months of life; mortality usually occurs within the first year. Clinically, there are the findings of irritability, exaggerated startle reflex, and limb stiffening. Rapid deterioration follows, with the development of hypertonicity, opisthotonos, and blindness within months. The antemortem phase consists of a decerebrate vegetative state. Several late-onset cases have been described. Conjunctival biopsy reveals characteristically ballooned Schwann cells. The cerebral white matter shows a complete loss of myelin and a proliferation of globoid cells (histiocytes with PAS-positive inclusions). Animal models as well as human material show the accumulation of galactosylsphingosine, a potentially cytotoxic metabolite. Definitive diagnosis is made by the demonstration of beta-galactocerebrosidase deficiency in circulating leukocytes or cultured fibroblasts.

The sulfatidoses

Metachromatic leukodystrophy (sulfatide lipidosis). This disease also may be divided into subtypes according to the time of onset and progression of disease. The most common infantile form is manifested within the first few years of life in behavioral abnormalities, gait disturbances, weakness, and hypotonia. Hypertonia may then follow, together with cerebellar signs, quadriplegia, and blindness. These severely disabled patients may live for a decade or more. A less frequent juvenile form begins within the first decade of life and is manifested in behavioral or visual problems. These problems may be subtle initially but gradually progress to major deficits. This form may progress for decades, only to be terminated by a fatal infection.

The adult form is protean in presentation; initial symptoms suggest a psychiatric disorder. Beginning in the second to fourth decades, these patients exhibit thought disorders, disorientation, and bizarre behavior; they frequently are misdiagnosed as schizophrenic. A subsequent loss of intellectual function, with the appearance of ataxia, paresis, and seizures, indicates the true nature of this disorder. The diagnosis requires an assay of leukocyte or cultured fibroblasts for arylsulfatase A activity. Conjunctival biopsy shows dense metachromatic inclusions within Schwann cells. Brain histology shows demyelination with metachromatic staining of intracellular inclusions. Sulfatide levels are greatly increased in brain, kidneys, and liver.

Multiple sulfatase deficiency. This rare disease has clinical findings similar to those of late infantile metachromatic leukodystrophy; however, some findings are identical to those of the mucopolysaccharidoses, such as hepatosplenomegaly, flared ribs, and a J-shaped sella turcica. Urinary mucopolysaccharides show increased levels of dermatan sulfate and heparan sulfate. Cultured fibroblasts and peripheral leukocytes show deficiencies in arylsulfatases A, B, and C and in steroid sulfatase as well. This differentiates the disease from Maroteaux-Lamy and metachromatic leukodystrophies in which only arylsulfatases B and A, respectively, are deficient.

Fabry's disease (ceramide trihexoside lipidosis)

An X-linked disorder, Fabry's disease becomes apparent in the first decade of life with the onset of a characteristic skin lesion and pain. Female carriers manifest a full spectrum of involvement, from mild to severe. Angiokeratoma corporis diffusum begins as clusters of dark red, punctate angiectases grouping symmetrically over the hips, buttocks, thighs, lower abdomen, and lumbar region. Only fucosidosis type II exhibits this same lesion. Attacks of excruciating pain affect the digits and may radiate proximally to include the abdomen. These attacks are accompanied by fever and an increased erythrocyte sedimentation rate. Paresthesias or nagging pain in the extremities also may develop. Dysfunction of cardiovascular tissue leads to significant cardiovascular disability, with coronary artery disease and congestive failure. Renal failure leads to uremia and hypertension in the third to fifth decade. Cerebrovascular involvement may be evidenced by seizures and sensory or motor dysfunction. Whorl-like opacities in the superficial layers of the cornea provide a distinctive finding. This disease is diagnosed by the characteristic clinical presentation and the finding of alpha-galactosidase deficiency.

The gangliosidoses

GM_1 gangliosidoses (beta-galactosidase deficiency). This disease is divided into two forms: infantile (type I) and juvenile (type II). However, there is likely to be a spectrum from infantile to adult forms. Beta-galactosidase deficiencies lead to the accumulation of GM_1 and glycosaminoglycans. This leads to a mucopolysaccharidosis-like appearance in the acute infantile form without mucopolysacchariduria. The infantile form manifests itself at birth in peripheral edema, hypotonia, poor appetite, respiratory insufficiency, frontal bossing, and depressed nasal bridge. These patients commonly develop hepatosplenomegaly and dysostosis multiplex. A retinal cherry-red spot is often present. Retardation and hyperreactivity progress to decerebrate rigidity, blindness, and death from respiratory failure by the age of 2 years. The juvenile form shows intellectual and motor decline by 1 year of age. Hepatosplenomegaly and dysostosis multiplex are mild or absent. An adult form has been reported, which entails the development of ataxia and seizures in early adulthood. Coarse features, skeletal anomalies, and mild retardation are variable findings in this group. A diagnosis depends on the demonstration of an accumulation of GM_1 ganglioside in the brain or on the lack of beta-galactosidase activity.

GM_2 gangliosidoses. Tay-Sachs disease (hexosaminidase A deficiency) and Sandhoff disease (hexosaminidase A and B deficiencies) produce nearly identical clinical courses. The patients are notable for their doll-like features and pink, translucent skin. At 3 to 6 months of age, feeding difficulties, listlessness, motor weakness, and exaggerated startle reflex are noted. Retinal cherry red spots in the macula are almost always present. Later, progressive motor weakness, macrocephaly, deafness, blindness, and convulsions ensue. Death from pneumonia is usual by age 2 years. Much rarer juvenile forms of these diseases involve deterioration of intellectual and motor functions in the first decade, which progresses to retardation and decerebrate rigidity by the second decade. An adult form has been reported, with slow deterioration from childhood. Muscle atrophy, dystonia, and dysarthria suggest spinocerebellar degeneration, whereas visual and intellectual capacities remain intact.

Tay-Sachs disease is carried in high frequency by Ashkenazi Jews (0.033 carrier rate). Definitive diagnosis is by assay of hexosaminidase isoenzyme activities; heterozygotes show a 50% diminution of activity, whereas some patients with late-onset disease show an apparently less severe defect. In Tay-Sachs disease, GM_2 gangliosides accumulate in brain; in Sandhoff disease, GM_2 gangliosides accumulate in other viscera as well.

Acid lipase deficiencies

Two diseases stem from an inability to hydrolyze lysosomal triglycerides and cholesteryl esters. Wolman disease manifests itself within the first month of life in forceful vomiting, diarrhea, anemia, and thrombocytopenia. Massive hepatosplenomegaly and adrenal calcifications are characteristic findings. Neurologic development appears normal. The ensuing cachexia leads to death by 6 months of age. Cholesteryl ester storage disease is a more benign chronic condition, characterized by hepatosplenomegaly, accelerated cardiovascular disease, cholesteryl ester and triglyceride accumulation, and elevated levels of circulating LDL. This causes a pattern similar to Fredrickson's class II hyperlipidemia. These diseases stem from deficiencies in the same enzyme activity and are best diagnosed by the demonstration of low levels of acid lipase in circulating leukocytes or cultured fibroblasts.

OTHER LYSOSOMAL STORAGE DISEASES

Chédiak-Higashi syndrome

This childhood disease is manifested in photophobia and hypopigmentation of skin, hair, and eyes. Repeated severe bouts of infection precede the later onset of central and peripheral neuropathy, mental retardation, and seizures. Many patients survive into their teens, only to develop a lymphoreticular malignancy. The hallmark of this disease is giant peroxidase-positive granules in circulating leukocytes. Lysosomal inclusions also are found in Schwann cells, liver, and spleen. Abnormally large melanosomes are found in areas of cutaneous depigmentation.

Cystinosis

The acute nephropathic form of cystinosis (see Chapter 360) is manifested in the first year of life with failure to thrive, polyuria, and polydipsia. Metabolic acidosis, Fanconi-like syndrome, and vitamin D-resistant rickets ensue. These eventually result in dwarfism. Characteristic eye changes include patchy retinal hypopigmentation and fine corneal crystalline deposits demonstrable by slit lamp. Most patients have a light complexion and blond hair. Less acute forms have been reported, in which the patients have little or no nephropathy. Crystalline inclusions occur in conjunctiva, cornea, and leukocytes. A diagnosis depends on the clinical presentation, the histology, and the demonstration of high cystine content in leukocytes or cultured fibroblasts.

Drug-induced lysosomopathies

Chlorpromazine, tricyclic antidepressants, chloroquine, and the aminoglycoside antibiotics all interfere with lysosome function in cultured cells. Clinically, chloroquine and the aminoglycosides demonstrate toxicities that may result from an inhibition of lysosomal action. Chloroquine in moderate to high doses produces corneal opacities and myopathy characterized by intracellular lamellar inclusion bodies containing acid phosphatase. Retinal dysfunction also may be linked to chloroquine, which, in animal studies, produces lamellar inclusion bodies in retinal ganglion cells. Since chloroquine is an amphiphilic cationic drug, it concentrates in lysosomes, is protonated, and may then interfere with acidification or with enzyme-substrate interactions. The aminoglycosides concentrate in renal tubular lysosomes, where they may interfere with component turnover by inhibiting phospholipases, and thus produce phospholipid accumulation in lamellar inclusion bodies and subsequent cell toxicity. No histologic findings currently support a similar mechanism in aminoglycoside-mediated ototoxicity.

TREATMENT

The lysosomal storage diseases are presently incurable. The only area of therapy currently practicable consists of medical support and intervention when complications occur. Prevention rests with contraception or prenatal diagnosis and therapeutic abortion.

Several experimental therapies have attempted to restore the deficient enzyme activities within the affected organ systems. The most commonly used technique has been enzyme infusion. Since the liver accumulates and degrades infused enzymes, additional techniques have attempted to direct enzymes into other affected organs. Acid maltase has been linked to LDL to promote muscle uptake in patients with Pompe's disease. Enzymes have been encapsulated in liposomes, red cell ghosts, and synthetic polymers in order to maintain their circulating levels. Liposomes incorporating glycoproteins may serve to direct the liposomal contents to tissues with specific glycoprotein receptors. Intrathecal administration has been attempted in Tay-Sachs disease. These types of therapy have often shown short-term beneficial effects in reducing organomegaly and increasing peripheral substrate clearance.

Transplantation affords an indwelling source of circulating enzyme activity and may provide a site of peripheral substrate clearance. Fibroblast and amniotic membrane transplantation in mucopolysaccharidosis, kidney transplantation in Fabry's disease, and spleen or kidney transplantation in Gaucher's disease have all been attempted. Again, short-term improvement has been noted in tissue levels and plasma clearance of accumulated substrate.

Bone marrow transplantation has now been used in many of the lysosomal storage diseases. Because of host-versus-graft disease and because the host may produce antibodies to the new lysosomal enzymes, displacement bone marrow transplants have been used with ablation of the host marrow before transplantation. With the significant morbidity and mortality attendant to this strategy, transplantation has been used primarily in fatal diseases. Significant improvement in soft tissue involvement has been seen, particularly in the mucopolysaccharidoses and Gaucher's disease. Although some patients with MPS I have exhibited slowed mental decay with transplantation, little CNS improvement is seen in the lipid storage diseases. Skeletal abnormalities appear fixed in these patients by the time of transplant. Current work in this area involves decreasing the risk of transplantation and of modulating blood-brain barriers to enzyme passage.

With the cloning of many lysosomal enzymes, gene-specific reconstitution has become a realistic endeavor. Human gene replacement will be used first in tissue-specific diseases, such as severe combined immunodeficiency. Later, however, gene insertion may be used in fibroblasts or perhaps in other tissues with wider distribution. Successful implantation of human beta-glucoronidase in animal systems has been observed. Gene therapy of the lipid storage disorders will be most difficult because of central nervous system involvement. Retroviral targeting techniques or transplantation of fetal tissues will likely be used in this setting.

REFERENCES

Adinolfi M and Brown S: Strategies for the correction of enzyme deficiencies in patients with mucopolysaccharidosis, Dev Med Child Neurol 26(3):404, 1984.

Ben-Yoseph Y, Mitchell DA, and Nadler HL: First trimester prenatal evaluation for I-cell disease by N-acetylglucosamine 1-phosphotransferase assay, Clin Genet 33:38, 1988.

Durand P: Recent progress in lysosomal diseases, Enzyme 38:256, 1987.

Fortuin JJH and Kleijer WJ: Hybridization studies of fibroblasts from Hurler, Scheie, and Hurler/Scheie compound patients: support for the hypothesis of allelic mutants, Hum Genet 53:155, 1980.

Gijsbertus TJH et al: Morquio B syndrome: a primary defect in β-galactosidase, Am J Med Genet 16:261, 1983.

Glew RH et al: Mammalian glucocerebrosidase: implications for Gaucher's disease, Lab Invest 58(1):5, 1988.

Hobbs JR: Experience with bone marrow transplantation for inborn errors of metabolism, Enzyme 38:194, 1987.

Holton JB, editor: The inherited metabolic diseases, New York, 1987, Churchill Livingstone.

Igisu H and Suzuki K: Progressive accumulation of toxic metabolite in a genetic leukodystrophy, Science 224(4650):753, 1984.

Kolodny EH: Early detection of lysosomal storage diseases, Ann NY Acad Sci 477:312, 1986.

Libert J: Diagnosis of lysosomal storage diseases by the ultrastructural study of conjunctival biopsies, Pathol Annu 1:37, 1980.

Lüllman-Rauch R: Lysosomes in applied biology and therapeutics, Front Biol 48:49, 1979.

Muenzer J: Mucopolysaccaridoses, Adv Pediatr 33:269, 1981.

Stanbury JB, Wyngaarden JB, and Fredrickson DS, editors: The metabolic basis of inherited disease, ed 5, New York, 1983, McGraw Hill.

CHAPTER

175 Phakomatoses

Thomas D. Gelehrter

NEUROFIBROMATOSIS

Neurofibromatosis 1 (NF1), or von Recklinghausen neurofibromatosis, is a relatively common inherited hamartomatous disorder characterized by pigmented skin lesions, multiple cutaneous and subcutaneous tumors, and a variety of other manifestations affecting multiple organ systems. The severity of the disease varies widely among affected persons even within the same family. Because of its frequency (approximately 1 in 3000) and protean manifestations, NF1 is seen by every physician.

Clinical features

The clinical features of neurofibromatosis are extremely varied and are different by patient age. The most characteristic findings are café-au-lait spots and multiple neurofibromas, but neither finding alone is diagnostic of neurofibromatosis.

Café-au-lait spots are hyperpigmented macules that are distributed randomly on the body, though relatively few appear on the face. They are often present at birth or very early in life and tend to increase in number, size, and pigmentation over time. Approximately 10% of normal adults have one to five café-au-lait spots, usually less than 1.5 cm in greatest diameter; more than six spots greater than 1.5 cm in diameter are considered a diagnostic sign of neurofibromatosis and are found in 75% to 85% of affected patients. Less than 1% of normal children have more than two such spots; more than five spots greater than 0.5 cm in diameter are considered diagnostic in children. Axillary freckling is a characteristic though less frequently observed sign. Freckles are also found in other flexural, intertriginous areas, including the groin, antecubital, and inframammary regions. Such freckling is virtually never seen in unaffected individuals. Other forms of hyperpigmentation may be observed; occasionally large dark macules may overlie plexiform neurofibromas.

Multiple neurofibromas affect the skin of most patients, but may also be found in deeper tissues and internal organs innervated by the autonomic nervous system. Pedunculated dermal neurofibromas are rare in childhood, but increase in number at puberty and frequently increase during pregnancy in females. These benign multiclonal lesions contain a mixture of cells including fibroblasts, Schwann cells, and often mast cells. Although these skin neurofibromas virtually never undergo malignant transformation, they may be cosmetically disfiguring when present in large numbers and may cause pruritus. Subcutaneous neurofibromas frequently develop along the course of peripheral nerves. When present in the spinal canal or its foramina, they can produce significant neurologic symptoms because of compression. The most serious type of neurofibroma is the highly vascular, infiltrating plexiform neurofibroma, which is responsible for major disfigurements such as localized gigantism and overgrowth of extremities or the face.

The most characteristic ocular findings in neurofibromatosis are Lisch nodules, which are smooth, dome-shaped, tan nodules on the iris surface. These hamartomatous lesions are not neurofibromas and can be distinguished on slitlamp examination from the common flat iris freckles or nevi. Lisch spots are found in more than 90% of adult patients but appear to be less frequent in childhood. Whether they are seen in unaffected individuals is disputed. Other eye findings include choroidal hamartomas, myelinated corneal nerves, optic nerve tumors, and characteristic lesions of the eyelid caused by plexiform neurofibromas.

The central nervous system is also prominently affected in neurofibromatosis. Learning disabilities, common in children with this disease, are a significant problem in this age group. A variety of central nervous system tumors are found more frequently in neurofibromatosis than in the general population. Optic gliomas are a characteristic finding in NF1. It is now recognized that 15% to 20% of patients have such tumors detectable by computed tomography (CT); however, only about 1% of these patients are symptomatic. Therefore it is not recommended that patients with NF1 undergo routine CT or magnetic resonance imaging (MRI) scanning. If the patient's vision is not compromised, these tumors should simply be watched; therapy is indicated only if vision deteriorates. Radiation therapy is preferred because of the dangers of surgery and may help to arrest progression of the tumor. In a young child with NF1, decreased visual acuity or disconjugate gaze should suggest further evaluation for optic glioma. Acoustic neuromas do not occur with increased frequency in NF1; bilateral acoustic neuromas should suggest a separate and distinct entity, neurofibromatosis 2 (see later discussion). Other tumors such as astrocytomas and meningiomas are pathologically like those seen in patients without neurofibromatosis, but appear to occur more frequently in patients with neurofibromatosis. Approximately half of patients complain of headaches. Most headaches respond similarly to those in patients without NF1, and, if stable, need not raise concern. If the headaches are new or have changed in pattern, however, they should be carefully evaluated. Seizures and frank mental retardation are found only in a minority (<10%) of patients with neurofibromatosis.

Musculoskeletal involvement is common in neurofibromatosis, indicating an important mesodermal component of this disease. Mild short stature is usual and macrocephaly is very frequent, especially in the second decade of life. Macrocephaly does not correlate with intellectual impairment or other central nervous system abnormalities. The most common orthopedic problem is kyphoscoliosis. In addition to the usual form of scoliosis found in about one third of children with neurofibromatosis, there is an uncommon but characteristic acute anterior angulation of the lower cervical and upper thoracic spine. Congenital bowing of the tibia and/or fibula, and less frequently of the radius and/or ulna, is a characteristic lesion in neurofibromatosis and a difficult one to manage orthopedically. Although the bowing may remain static, it can progress to pathologic fractures and pseudarthrosis. Growth abnormalities including asymmetry and localized gigantism secondary to infiltrating plexiform neurofibromas may be a major source of morbidity, particularly in children.

Malignancy is generally considered a part of the clinical picture of neurofibromatosis. There does not appear to be an increase in the frequency of common cancers in patients with this disease; however, there is clearly a higher frequency of certain rare malignancies such as neurofibrosarcoma, malignant schwannoma, and pheochromocytoma, and probably of Wilms' tumor, rhabdomyosarcoma, and Ph^1 negative leukemia. The risk of sarcomatous degeneration of pre-existing neurofibromas is unknown. It is unlikely that pedunculated skin neurofibromas ever undergo malignant transformation; however, internal plexiform neurofibromas and schwannomas, especially those in the posterior mediastinum, apparently can undergo such change.

Hypertension is common in neurofibromatosis and is usually of the essential variety. Pheochromocytomas occur in less than 5% of patients with neurofibromatosis, far more frequently than in the general population. Rarely does this tumor occur before the age of 20 years in neurofibromatosis patients. Children with neurofibromatosis have a higher than usual frequency of renal artery stenosis. The lesions are usually located at the origin of the artery, are frequently bilateral, and are the result of vascular dysplasia rather than compression by neurofibromas.

Constipation occurs commonly, reflecting involvement of Auerbach's plexus of the colon. Gastrointestinal and genitourinary bleeding may be encountered because of neurofibromas in the lumen of the colon or bladder. Finally, disorders of sexual development including precocious puberty may also occur more frequently in neurofibromatosis than in the general population.

Genetics

Neurofibromatosis is inherited as a simple autosomal dominant trait that affects both sexes with equal frequency and severity. The gene appears to have a high penetrance; that is, an individual carrying the gene virtually always shows some manifestation of the disease by adulthood. However, the nature and severity of the pathologic manifestations vary widely, even within families. The causes of this variability are unknown. Neurofibromatosis occurs in approximately 1 in 3000 individuals and affects all races. Approximately one half of cases are sporadic and presumably represent new mutations. Estimates of the mutation rate for the neurofibromatosis gene are approximately 10^{-4} per gamete per generation, 100 times higher than those calculated for other human genes.

The gene for NF1 has been mapped to the centromeric region of chromosome 17 (17q11.2), and has been cloned. The gene for NF1 spans approximately 300 kb of genomic DNA and encodes a 13 kb mRNA that is ubiquitously expressed. There is no evidence of locus heterogeneity; that is, all cases of NF1 can be mapped to this single genetic locus.

All patients with neurofibromatosis and their families should be offered accurate and sensitive genetic counseling. The risk for each offspring of a patient with neurofibromatosis is 50% regardless of sex. This risk is the same whether the proband represents a familial or a sporadic case. Nevertheless, it is important to determine whether the patient represents a sporadic or familial case because in the latter circumstance other family members (e.g., siblings) are at risk. Therefore parents and siblings of a patient with neurofibromatosis should be evaluated through a careful history and physical examination. A postpubertal individual at risk of neurofibromatosis who has no signs of the disease is very unlikely to be carrying this gene, and the risk for his or her offspring should be no higher than that in the general population. Genetic counseling must also include a detailed explanation of the clinical spectrum of the disease, possible complications, and available therapy. The extremely variable expression of the disease should be clearly discussed. Because the disease can be very mild and benign in some patients and disfiguring and incapacitating in others, the genetic counselor must attempt to balance creating undue anxiety about the future with an unrealistically optimistic forecast for the patient and offspring.

PATHOGENESIS

The NF1 gene product is a cytoplasmic protein called neurofibromin, which is co-localized by immunofluorescence techniques with microtubules, suggesting that it is intimately associated with cytoskeletal elements. A small portion of the NF1 gene (approximately 10% of the coding region) shares sequence similarity with GTP activating proteins (GAP). GAP proteins accelerate the hydrolysis of *ras*-guanosine triphosphate to *ras*-guanosine diphosphate, converting the proto-oncogene protein *ras* from the active to the inactive form. Therefore it is tempting to speculate that neurofibromin acts as a tumor suppressor by regulating an intracellular protein, such as *ras,* essential for cell growth and proliferation.

Diagnosis, treatment, and natural history

The diagnosis of NF1 rests on clinical observations. Because none of the clinical features is found in every patient with the disease, no single clinical feature is absolutely diagnostic. The National Institutes of Health consensus diagnostic criteria for NF1 include the presence of two or more of the following: (1) six café-au-lait spots over 1.5 cm in greatest diameter in postpubertal individuals or 0.5 cm in children, (2) two or more neurofibromas of any type or one plexiform neurofibroma, (3) axillary or inguinal freckling, (4) optic glioma, (5) two or more Lisch nodules, (6) a distinctive bony lesion or thinning of long-bone cortex with or without pseudoarthrosis, and (7) a first-degree relative with NF1. There are no specific laboratory tests for this condition, and molecular diagnostic tests are not yet available. Thus far, only about 20 mutations have been described in the NF1 gene, and there is no clear correlation between the site of the NF1 mutation and the clinical phenotype. Given the great variability in clinical phenotype among affected individuals in a family with NF1, analysis of DNA mutations will most likely not be very helpful in predicting the patient's phenotype.

In the neonatal and early childhood period, most affected patients will be asymptomatic and have only café-au-lait spots. A minority will have severe involvement, including deforming plexiform neurofibromas of the face, limb overgrowth, or congenital pseudoarthrosis. Later in childhood, learning and behavioral problems, scoliosis, or central nervous system tumors such as optic glioma may bring the patient to medical attention. Cutaneous neurofibromas begin to appear at puberty. Although the majority of patients will not have severe problems resulting from this disease, patients cannot be reassured with any certainty. There appears to be no difference in the severity of manifestations between sporadic and familial cases.

Treatment of this condition is largely palliative. Dermal

neurofibromas can be removed by surgery, dermabrasion, or carbon dioxide laser treatment. Patients should be seen on at least a yearly basis, and evidence of complications should be sought. Particular attention should be paid to blood pressure and possible neurologic, ophthalmologic, and orthopedic problems, with appropriate specialized evaluations as needed.

Because the protean manifestations of neurofibromatosis require the services of multiple medical and surgical specialties, there is considerable risk that the patient's care can become fragmented. Patients with neurofibromatosis require considerable supportive care and should be provided with accurate and understanding genetic counseling. A network of specialized neurofibromatosis treatment centers around the country have been established for the care of patients with this condition. The National Neurofibromatosis Foundation* provides information and support for patients, families, and physicians dealing with this disease.

NF2

In addition to NF1, a separate and distinct entity known as bilateral acoustic neurofibromatosis, or neurofibromatosis 2 (NF2), is also an autosomal dominant trait, occurring in approximately 1 per 1,000,000 individuals. It is characterized by bilateral acoustic neuromas with onset of symptoms in the second and third decade, other central nervous system tumors, and, in 50% of patients, by cataracts. Multiple café-au-lait spots, multiple neurofibromas, Lisch nodules, and other manifestations of NF1 are uncommon. The gene for NF2 has been mapped to the center of the long arm of chromosome 22. Relatives at risk of NF2 who are more than 15 years old should be followed by regular MRI, ophthalmologic examination, and audiologic evaluation, including brainstem auditory evoked response (BAER).

TUBEROUS SCLEROSIS

Tuberous sclerosis is a dominantly inherited hamartomatous disorder characterized by seizures, mental retardation, and skin and eye lesions. The name reflects the characteristic subependymal hamartomas and cortical tubers that are the pathologic hallmark of the disease. Like neurofibromatosis, tuberous sclerosis is extremely variable in its manifestations and severity. Similarly, there is limited information on the natural history of this disease and on the frequency with which affected individuals manifest different clinical features of this condition.

Clinical features

The classic picture of tuberous sclerosis (TS) consists of the triad of mental retardation, seizures, and adenoma sebaceum. The seizures, found in 90% of patients, include characteristic myoclonic jerks and infantile spasms (hypsarrhythmia). Mental retardation is frequent but by no means universal, and when present it can be moderate to severe. Cranial CT scans reveal periventricular calcification and/or tubers in 60% to 90% of patients. The best known skin findings are adenoma sebaceum, which are actually facial angiofibromas, commonly occurring in the nasolabial region and over the cheeks. These lesions usually do not appear until the age of 3 to 5 years and blossom at about puberty, when they may be mistaken for acne. Facial angiofibromas are considered pathognomonic of TS, as are subungual and periungual fibromas. Hypomelanotic skin macules, often oval in shape (hence the name "ash leaf spots"), may be an even more frequent, though less often recognized, skin manifestation, but are not diagnostic. They are best seen with a Wood's lamp, and may be apparent in the newborn period. Other skin lesions include shagreen patches, and café-au-lait spots. Retinal astrocytic hamartomas or phakomas (including both white plaques and mulberry lesions) are seen in approximately half of patients with tuberous sclerosis and are diagnostic of this disease.

Other characteristic lesions include gingival fibromas, renal angiomyolipomas and cortical cysts (best detected by CT scans or ultrasound), cystic bone lesions in the phalanges, cardiac rhabdomyomas, and rarely pulmonary cystic lesions that may be associated with spontaneous pneumothorax. The renal angiomyolipomas and cysts usually do not cause functional impairment, but hemorrhage and progressive renal failure have been reported. Treatment of tuberous sclerosis is generally limited to the treatment of seizures when they occur.

Genetics

Tuberous sclerosis is inherited as an autosomal dominant trait with high penetrance and markedly variable expressivity. In some families, the genetic locus for tuberous sclerosis has been mapped to the long arm of chromosome 9 (9q34). In other families, there appears to be linkage to chromosomes 11 and 12, indicating locus heterogeneity for this condition.

A significant percentage of cases is sporadic and may represent new mutations. Because a parent may be very mildly affected, however, it is necessary to evaluate carefully parents and other first-degree relatives of diagnosed cases of tuberous sclerosis to distinguish new mutations from familial cases. If a parent of an affected child is not a gene carrier, the risk of having another affected child would be no greater than that in the general population, but it would be 50% if the parent is a gene carrier with mild manifestations.

Diagnosis of tuberous sclerosis is straightforward in severe cases with classic manifestations on the basis of history, examination of the skin and eyes, and confirmatory studies such as electroencephalography and CT. Diagnosis in mildly affected individuals, especially in adults who have neither retardation nor seizures, can be difficult. Parents and other first-degree relatives of an affected child should have a careful examination of the nailbeds and skin, including Wood's lamp examination, and examination of the retina through a dilated pupil. CT or MRI scans, renal ultrasound,

*141 Fifth Ave, Suite 7-S, New York, NY 10010.

and radiographs of the hands and feet may also be necessary to detect mildly affected individuals.

There are no specific laboratory tests for this disease, and prenatal diagnosis is not available, although fetuses have been diagnosed by echocardiographic demonstration of a rhabdomyoma. Genetic counseling should be offered to families with affected members. It is clear that a mildly affected parent may have a severely affected child, and there is considerable variation in severity even within families. Thus it is impossible to predict whether an affected child will have severe or mild manifestations. On the other hand, a mildly affected young adult is unlikely to develop more serious complications later in life. The National Tuberous Sclerosis Association* is available to help affected patients and families.

VON HIPPEL-LINDAU DISEASE

Von Hippel-Lindau disease is a relatively rare, dominantly inherited tumor disorder characterized by retinal angiomatosis and cerebellar hemangioblastoma. Retinal angiomas usually appear by the third decade of life. Angiomatous tumors, characteristically found in the cerebellum but also in other parts of the brain, spinal cord, adrenals, lungs, and liver, tend to develop later in life. Renal cell carcinoma is a particularly frequent cause of death. Polycythemia, pheochromocytoma, and pancreatic carcinoma are additional features of the disease, as are cysts of the pancreas, kidneys, and epididymis. von Hippel-Lindau disease is inherited as an autosomal dominant trait with considerable intrafamilial variation in age of onset and expression. No specific laboratory tests exist for its diagnosis. The gene has been mapped to the short arm of chromosome 3. Because von Hippel-Lindau disease is a precancerous disorder and some of the manifestations are amenable to treatment and cure when detected early, genetic counseling and careful screening and follow-up of relatives at risk are mandatory.

REFERENCES

Gomez MR, editor: Tuberous sclerosis, New York, ed 2, New York, 1988, Raven Press.

Gutmann DH and Collins FS: Recent progress towards understanding the molecular biology of von Recklinghausen neurofibromatosis, Ann Neurol 31:555-561, 1992.

Lamiell JM et al: von Hippel-Lindau disease affecting 43 members of a single kindred, Medicine (Baltimore) 68:1-29, 1989.

Martuza RL and Eldridge R: Neurofibromatosis 2 (bilateral acoustic neurofibromatosis), N Engl J Med 318:684, 1988.

Riccardi VM: Neurofibromatosis: phenotype, history, and pathogenesis, ed 2, Baltimore, 1992, Johns Hopkins University Press.

Seizinger BR: Toward the isolation of the primary genetic defect in von Hippel-Lindau disease, Ann NY Acad Sci 615:332-337, 1991.

Stumpf DA et al: Neurofibromatosis. NIH Consensus Development Conference Statement, Arch Neurol 45:575, 1988.

*800 Corporate Drive, Suite 120, Landover, MD 20785.

CHAPTER

176 Disorders of Porphyrin Metabolism

Joseph R. Bloomer
James G. Straka

The porphyrias are metabolic disorders in which excess accumulation and excretion of porphyrins and porphyrin precursors occur. The principal clinical manifestations are cutaneous lesions, neurologic dysfunction, and hepatic disease.

PATHOGENESIS OF BIOCHEMICAL ABNORMALITIES

Since the biochemical abnormalities in each of the porphyrias reflect an enzyme abnormality in the pathway of heme biosynthesis (Fig. 176-1 and Table 176-1), a knowledge of the pathway is necessary to understand the chemical findings.

Heme is synthesized by eight enzymatically controlled steps. The first and last steps take place within the mitochondria; the intervening steps occur in the cytosol or at the mitochondrial membrane.

The first step is catalyzed by the enzyme δ-aminolevulinic acid (ALA) synthase. The reaction involves the condensation of glycine with succinyl coenzyme A. The product is a β-keto acid (2-amino-3-oxoadipate), which spontaneously decarboxylates to form ALA. The enzyme requires pyridoxal phosphate, which "activates" the glycine molecule toward attack by the succinyl coenzyme A. As a branch point enzyme, ALA synthase is predictably the primary control point for the pathway. In liver its synthesis is repressed by the end product of the pathway, heme; its transport into the mitochondrion is inhibited by heme; and heme is an allosteric inhibitor of the enzyme reaction. The forms of porphyria that cause attacks of neurologic dysfunction have increased production of ALA due to induction of hepatic ALA synthase activity.

The second step of heme biosynthesis results in the condensation of two molecules of ALA with the elimination of two molecules of water, forming the monopyrrole porphobilinogen (PBG). The reaction occurs in the cytosol and is catalyzed by the enzyme ALA dehydrase.

The next two steps in the reaction series are catalyzed in concert by the enzymes PBG deaminase (or hydroxymethylbilane synthase) and uroporphyrinogen III synthase (formerly cosynthase). The first of these catalyzes the head-to-tail condensation of four PBG molecules (eliminating four molecules of ammonia) to produce a noncyclized tetrapyrrole called *hydroxymethylbilane*. Because of the structure of PBG, this intermediate has alternating acetate and propionate substituents on the pyrrole units. Uroporphyrinogen III synthase catalyzes a cyclization reaction with the concomitant "inversion" of the fourth pyrrole unit, result-

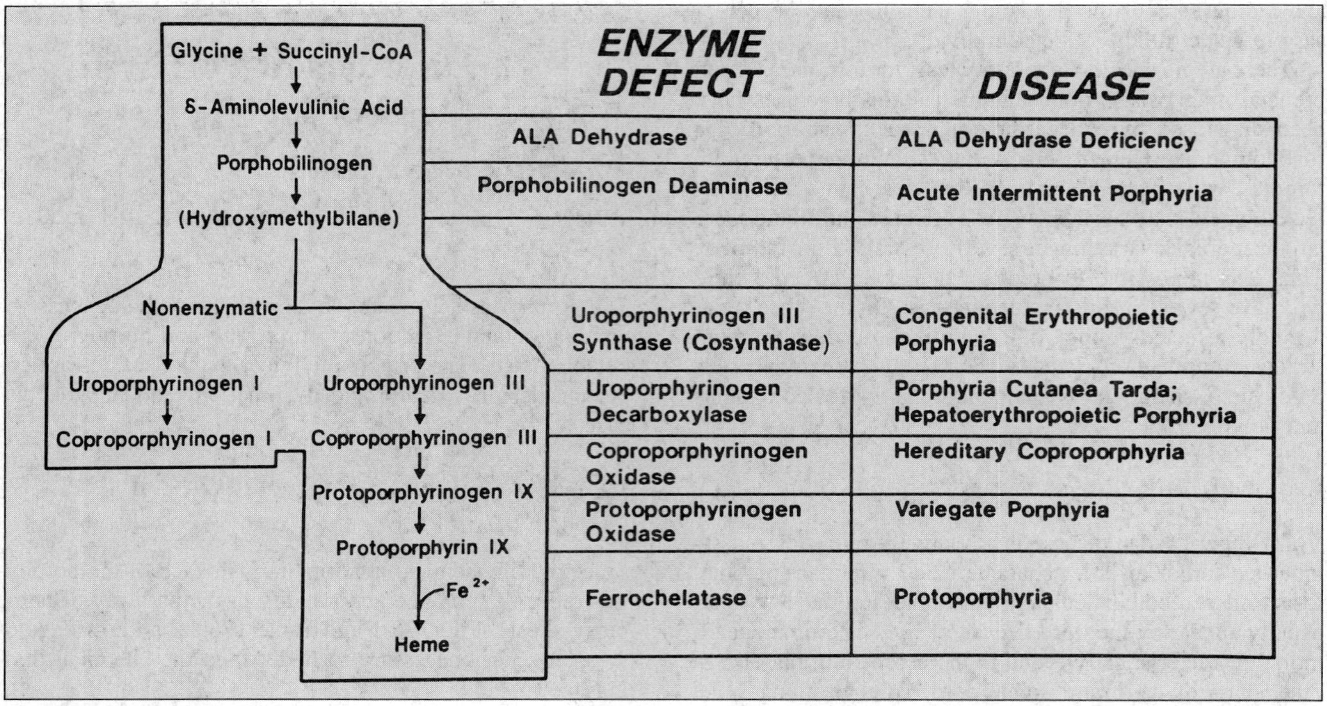

Fig. 176-1. Heme biosynthesis, showing the sites of enzyme defects in the different porphyrias. As a consequence of the enzyme defects, porphyrins and porphyrin precursors are accumulated and excreted in excessive amounts. (Reproduced from Bloomer JR and Bonkovsky HL: The porphyrias. Dis Mon XXXV:1-54, Jan 1989. With permission.)

ing in the formation of the asymmetric uroporphyrinogen III. In the absence of uroporphyrinogen III synthase, hydroxymethylbilane spontaneously cyclizes to form the symmetric, but biologically inactive, uroporphyrinogen I.

The fifth step in the pathway is catalyzed by uroporphyrinogen decarboxylase. The cytosolic enzyme sequentially removes the carboxylate groups of the four acetate substituents of uroporphyrinogen, leaving behind methyl substituents and producing coproporphyrinogen III. This enzyme also decarboxylates uroporphyrinogen I to form coproporphyrinogen I.

The next step converts two of the four propionate substituents of coproporphyrinogen III into vinyl groups by way of oxidative decarboxylation. The product is protoporphyrinogen IX. The enzyme responsible for this is coproporphyrinogen oxidase.

The penultimate step of heme biosynthesis results in the controlled six-electron oxidation of protoporphyrinogen to form protoporphyrin. The enzyme, protoporphyrinogen oxidase, is located within the inner mitochondrial membrane. The fate of the six electrons is unknown.

The final step of heme biosynthesis, catalyzed by ferrochelatase, results in the insertion of divalent iron into the center of the porphyrin nucleus with the displacement of two protons, forming heme. The reaction occurs at the inner face of the inner mitochondrial membrane.

All tetrapyrrole intermediates prior to protoporphyrin are at the oxidation state of a porphyrinogen, which consists of four pyrrole units separated by methylene groups. Porphyrinogens are nonplanar, nonaromatic colorless compounds. In vitro, they are susceptible to spontaneous oxidation, resulting in the conversion of the porphyrinogen to the porphyrin. The latter results from the formal loss of six hydrogen atoms, four from the methylene bridge carbons and two from pyrrole nitrogens. The resulting porphyrin, a cyclic compound composed of four pyrroles separated by methene bridges, is a planar aromatic compound that is deeply colored and fluorescent.

Defects in these enzymatic steps underlie the biochemical abnormalities that characterize the different porphyrias. In keeping with the importance of heme biosynthesis to aerobic cells, any inborn error of the pathway must cause only a partial reduction in the synthesis of heme. Thus, it is not surprising that most of the porphyrias are autosomal dominant traits (i.e., one normal and one mutant gene). The porphyrias that are autosomal recessive traits (congenital erythropoietic porphyria, ALA dehydrase deficiency, and hepatoerythropoietic porphyria) result in the production of enzymes with greatly reduced but not totally absent activities.

Whereas the enzyme defects may be expressed in any heme-forming tissue of a patient with porphyria, only the bone marrow and liver are quantitatively important in the overproduction of porphyrins and porphyrin precursors (Table 176-1). This formed the basis for the classification of the porphyrias as either erythropoietic or hepatic, depending on which tissue is the major site of expression of the biochemical abnormality.

Table 176-1. Principal clinical and biochemical manifestations in the porphyrias

Disorder	Cutaneous lesions	Neurologic dysfunction	Hepatic disease	Major site of porphyrin overproduction	Erythrocytes	Urine	Feces
Congenital erythropoietic porphyria	+	0	0	Bone marrow	↑ Uroporphyrin	↑ Uroporphyrin	↑ Uroporphyrin and coproporphyrin
Protoporphyria	+	0	+	Bone marrow and liver	↑ Protoporphyrin	—	↑ Protoporphyrin
Porphyria cutanea tarda	+	0	+	Liver	—	↑ Uroporphyrin	Isocoproporphyrin
Hepatoerythropoietic porphyria	+	0	+	Bone marrow and liver	↑ Zn-protoporphyrin	↑ Uroporphyrin	Isocoproporphyrin
Acute intermittent porphyria	0	+	0	Liver	—	↑ ALA and PBG	—
Variegate porphyria	+	+	0	Liver	—	↑ ALA, PBG, and coproporphyrin	↑ Protoporphyrin
Hereditary coproporphyria	+	+	0	Liver	—	↑ ALA, PBG, and coproporphyrin	↑ Coproporphyrin
ALA dehydrase deficiency	0	+	0	Liver	—	↑ ALA	—

ALA, δ-aminolevulinic acid; PBG, porphobilinogen.
This table does not list all of the biochemical abnormalities and only serves as a guide to indicate which measurements are most critical in the evaluation of the porphyrias.

Reduction in the activity of an enzyme may result from decreased synthesis of the enzyme protein, a structural defect leading to an unstable protein, or a structural defect resulting in altered enzyme function. The first two mechanisms reduce the amount of protein, which when evaluated using an antibody against the protein cause a reduction in cross-reactive immunologic material (CRIM) and are said to be *CRIM-negative*. The latter mechanism may also cause CRIM-negative mutations if the structural alterations are major or at the sites of immunologic determinants. However, the amount of CRIM may be unaffected. This is called *CRIM-positive*.

Both CRIM-positive and CRIM-negative mutations occur in specific types of porphyria, indicating that genetic heterogeneity exists for these disorders (i.e., more than one class of gene mutation causes the phenotype of the disease). For example, in acute intermittent porphyria, in which there is a deficiency of PBG deaminase activity, four classes of mutations have been identified by comparing the amount of CRIM to enzyme activity. Two of these mutations are CRIM-negative and two CRIM-positive. Similarly, both CRIM-positive and CRIM-negative mutations have been described in hepatoerythropoietic porphyria and in protoporphyria.

Recent studies using molecular techniques have clarified the reasons for the different CRIM mutations and have substantiated that genetic heterogeneity exists in the porphyrias. In one family with a CRIM-negative mutation in acute intermittent porphyria, a point mutation in exon 9 of the gene caused conversion of a glutamine codon to a stop codon, resulting in a truncated peptide that had neither enzyme activity nor immunoreactivity. In the CRIM-positive form of the disorder, three different mutations in the coding region of the gene have been identified. These mutations resulted in the formation of a protein that had markedly decreased enzyme activity but that was stable and immunologically crossreactive. Several more mutations are expected. Similar studies are being carried out in the other types of porphyria to categorize the different gene defects that cause the disease.

PATHOGENESIS OF MAJOR CLINICAL MANIFESTATIONS

The signs and symptoms most commonly seen in the porphyrias are cutaneous and neurologic (Table 176-1). In some both manifestations occur, whereas in others only one feature is present.

Cutaneous lesions result from the photosensitizing effects of porphyrins, which are deposited in the skin or are circulating in dermal blood vessels. Light with a wavelength of approximately 400 nm excites electrons of the porphyrins to elevated energy levels, causing the formation of compounds that react with molecular oxygen to form reactive oxygen species. The reactive oxygen may then damage tissue through peroxidation of membrane lipids and cross linking of membrane proteins.

Neurologic dysfunction occurs in those types of porphyria that are termed *acute* or *inducible* and may cause life-threatening complications such as respiratory paralysis. The pathogenesis of neurologic dysfunction has not been precisely determined, but one consideration is that ALA, which is overproduced in the liver as a consequence of the induction of hepatic ALA synthase activity, acts as a neurotoxin. A second possibility is a heme deficiency state. Experimental studies support both possibilities, and neurologic dysfunction may be caused by a combination of these factors.

Hepatic disease is also an important feature of some types of porphyria. The descriptions and pathogenesis of the hepatic disease are covered in the individual sections that follow.

TYPES OF PORPHYRIA

Congenital erythropoietic porphyria (Günther's disease)

This very rare disease is transmitted in an autosomal recessive manner. It results from a deficiency of uroporphyrinogen III synthase (cosynthase) activity. In the absence of uroporphyrinogen III synthase, PBG is converted to uroporphyrinogen I, which cannot be used and is excreted mainly in the urine.

The clinical manifestations involve the skin and erythron. Photosensitivity may begin in infancy. Vesicles or bullae occur on exposed portions of the body and, through the process of ulceration and healing, lead to scarring. Repeated episodes of ulceration and scarring cause severe deformity of the fingers, ears, and nose. Conjunctivitis, keratitis, changes in pigmentation, alopecia, and hypertrichosis of the face and limbs are other complications.

The excess uroporphyrin originates in developing erythrocytes in the bone marrow. Hematologic findings include a shortened red-cell life span, reticulocytosis, and circulating normoblasts. Splenomegaly is often present. Although slight elevation of serum bilirubin may be present, clinically evident jaundice is rare. In addition to hemolysis, ineffective erythropoiesis may play a role in causing anemia. In some patients, increased red cell production is sufficient to prevent anemia.

Pathologic findings include normoblastic hyperplasia in the marrow, fluorescence of a variable fraction of marrow normoblasts and circulating erythrocytes, increase of the pulp and follicular hyperplasia in the spleen, increased melanin in the epidermis, and fibroblast proliferation in the skin. The liver may be enlarged with an increase of hemosiderin, but histologic changes are nonspecific.

The diagnosis is indicated by severe cutaneous photosensitivity beginning in infancy or childhood, dark ("port wine") urine, erythrodontia, and hemolytic anemia. Confirmation comes from measurement of urinary uroporphyrin and demonstration of fluorescence of circulating erythrocytes and marrow normoblasts. Cells exhibit characteristic red fluorescence when irradiated with light of 400 nm wavelength (Soret band). Fluorescence of the teeth may also be found.

Treatment is directed to prevent skin lesions and manage the hemolytic anemia. Protection from sunlight is important. The creams and lotions used for standard sunburn protection are of no value because they do not absorb the long wavelengths that cause skin damage. Beta-carotene (Solatene) may be administered but has less efficacy than in protoporphyria (further details are presented under the treatment of protoporphyria). Secondary skin infections are treated with antibiotics.

Since excessive porphyrin production is augmented by the stimulation of erythropoiesis that results from hemolytic anemia, splenectomy has been used in treatment. In some cases, hemolysis has been reduced, and this has been associated with lessening of photosensitivity. Urinary and fecal porphyrin excretion often decrease after splenectomy. Transfusions inhibit erythropoiesis and decrease porphyrin excretion. Intravenous administration of hematin has also been shown to decrease erythrocyte and urinary uroporphyrin levels in a few patients.

Patients with congenital erythropoietic porphyria rarely survive beyond middle age. Although the cause of death has not always been clearly defined, renal failure or hepatic failure has sometimes been the terminal event.

Protoporphyria (erythrohepatic porphyria, erythropoietic protoporphyria)

This disease is transmitted as an autosomal dominant disorder with variable expression. It perhaps occurs in 10 to 20 individuals per 100,000 population. A deficiency of ferrochelatase activity has been demonstrated. As a consequence of the ferrochelatase defect, protoporphyrin accumulates in excessive amounts. This causes high levels of protoporphyrin in erythrocytes, bile, and feces. There is no increase of porphyrins in the urine. The absence of abnormalities in the urine is probably the reason the disease was not recognized as a type of porphyria until 1961.

Cutaneous symptoms usually begin in childhood. Burning or itching of the skin occurs after a variable period of exposure to sunlight (sometimes within a few minutes). Light that has passed through window glass may evoke symptoms. Burning is often accompanied by erythema and edema of exposed areas. The latter may persist for weeks. Chronic lesions cause thickening and scarring of the skin of the nose, cheeks, back of the hands, and fingers. An amorphous periodic acid Schiff-positive material is often demonstrable in and around capillary walls in skin that is exposed to light. This has also been found in variegate porphyria and porphyria cutanea tarda.

The other major clinical manifestation in protoporphyria is hepatobiliary disease. Protoporphyrin-rich gallstones are present in some patients. Liver biopsy specimens from patients frequently show mild abnormalities in the form of portal inflammation and fibrosis, along with deposition of brown pigment. A few individuals (less than 10% of patients) develop severe liver disease that can lead to death from hepatic failure. The livers of these patients have been black and cirrhotic. The black appearance is caused by massive deposits of pigment in hepatocytes, Kupffer's cells, portal macrophages, and bile canaliculi and small bile ducts. When examined by polarization microscopy, the pigment deposits are birefringent and by electron microscopy are shown to contain crystals. Isolation and characterization of the pigment crystals indicate they are composed of protoporphyrin, and it is currently thought that hepatic protoporphyrin deposition is the cause of the liver disease.

Approximately 20% to 30% of patients have mild anemia with hypochromic microcytic indices. A variable fraction of marrow erythroid cells and circulating erythrocytes have red fluorescence. The bone marrow morphology is normal.

Acute photosensitivity reactions, with or without objective skin changes, suggest the diagnosis. Confirmation requires the demonstration of increased erythrocyte protoporphyrin. In contrast to lead poisoning and iron deficiency anemia, the increased protoporphyrin in erythrocytes occurs as free protoporphyrin and not the zinc chelate.

Oral administration of beta-carotene (Solatene) is of value in increasing tolerance to light. This benefit may not be evident for 1 to 3 months after starting therapy. A yellowish discoloration of skin appears to be the only side effect. Methods to prevent and reverse hepatic protoporphyrin accumulation in patients with liver disease include attempts to suppress excess protoporphyrin production through red blood cell transfusions and intravenous administration of hematin, and interruption of the enterohepatic circulation of protoporphyrin by oral administration of cholestyramine or activated charcoal.

The prognosis depends on whether liver disease develops. Other manifestations probably do not affect life span.

Acute intermittent porphyria

This autosomal dominant disorder has an estimated prevalence of 5 to 10 cases per 100,000 population. Many cases exist in latent form. The manifest disease is more frequent in women. The fundamental defect is a deficiency of PBG deaminase activity.

The defect in PBG deaminase causes increased excretion of ALA and PBG in urine. When an acute attack of neurologic dysfunction occurs, excretion of these compounds increases because of induction of hepatic ALA synthase activity. Recovery is associated with a decline in their excretion, but values almost always remain above normal.

The disease may exist in latent form indefinitely, but several factors precipitate acute attacks. These include drugs (barbiturates and sulfonamides most commonly), starvation or excessive dieting, female sex hormones, and infections. Patients should not have pentobarbital for dental extractions or surgery.

The acute attack can involve any portion of the nervous system. The abdominal pain that frequently occurs during acute attacks is thought to result from imbalance in the autonomic innervation of the gut. Other manifestations of autonomic neuropathy are sinus tachycardia, labile hypertension, sweating, and vascular spasm (retina, skin, etc.). When peripheral neuropathy occurs, it is usually preceded by abdominal pain. The peripheral neuropathy may be sensory or motor. There may be pain in the back and legs or paresthesias. Motor neuropathy can involve any peripheral nerve and may be symmetric or asymmetric with a variable rate of progression. Complete flaccid paralysis can develop over a period of days. Respiratory paralysis sufficient to require assisted ventilation is a grave prognostic sign. In severe attacks, some patients are unable to speak, breathe, or swallow. Central nervous system manifestations include seizures, hallucinations, coma, hypothalamic dysfunction, cerebellar and basal ganglion manifestations, and bulbar paralysis. Depression and organic brain syndrome are the two most characteristic psychiatric problems.

The profound hyponatremia that develops in some patients results from gastrointestinal loss of sodium, inappropriate release of antidiuretic hormone, and, possibly, primary renal sodium loss. Hypercholesterolemia, hyperamylasemia, and increased serum thyroxin-binding globulin occur in some patients.

During the acute attack, the diagnosis is made by demonstrating increased PBG in the urine. Positive screening tests for PBG, such as the Watson-Schwartz or Hoesch test, should be confirmed by quantitative measurement of PBG. Since increased urinary PBG also occurs during acute attacks of variegate porphyria and hereditary coproporphyria, specific diagnosis is made by demonstration of decreased erythrocyte PBG deaminase activity.

Treatment involves prophylaxis, symptomatic management, and reversal of the fundamental disease process. All patients should be instructed to avoid the known precipitating factors. The abdominal pain often can be controlled with phenothiazines, but meperidine may be necessary. Propranolol has been used to control autonomic manifestations such as tachycardia and hypertension. A high-carbohydrate intake (400 g/day, or more if possible) causes a decrease of porphyrin precursor excretion and produce clinical improvement in some patients. The reason for the spectrum of responsiveness (from spectacular recovery to little or no effect) is unknown. Since this therapy has virtually no risk, it should be instituted in all acute attacks. Although the value of intravenous hematin administration has not been proved by double-blind studies, it does lower porphyrin precursor excretion, and is useful in the treatment of acute attacks, particularly if started early. Hematin therapy has little effect on established neuropathy, in which nerve regeneration is the rate-limiting factor in recovery. Since hematin affects blood clotting, caution should be exercised in patients with coagulopathies or in those receiving anticoagulants.

In previous studies, the mortality rate for serious paralytic attacks was 40% to 60%. Modern management of critically ill patients has reduced this rate, but mortality still occurs.

Variegate porphyria

The prevalence of this autosomal dominant disorder is unknown in the United States, but it is undoubtedly lower than that of acute intermittent porphyria. A deficiency of protoporphyrinogen oxidase activity is the fundamental defect. During acute attacks, the excretion in the urine of ALA and PBG is increased. During asymptomatic periods porphyrin precursor excretion is often normal, but urinary uroporphyrin and coproporphyrin may be increased, the latter usually exceeding the former. Fecal protoporphyrin is increased during both symptomatic and asymptomatic periods.

Cutaneous or neurologic manifestations (or both) occur. Increased skin fragility with formation of bullae, erosions, scarring, and pigmentation occur in skin exposed to sunlight. Facial hypertrichosis and chronic thickening of skin also occur. The acute attacks of neurologic dysfunction can be precipitated by the same factors as in acute intermittent porphyria, and the manifestations are the same.

The diagnosis during the acute attack is suggested by demonstration of increased ALA and PBG in the urine. Since this finding also occurs in attacks of acute intermittent porphyria and hereditary coproporphyria, it is not specific for variegate porphyria. So far as prophylaxis and treatment of the acute attack are concerned, however, distinction among these three disorders is academic. During asymptomatic periods or the presence of cutaneous symptoms alone, an increase of urinary uroporphyrin and coproporphyrin may be demonstrable, but these findings may be confused with those of porphyria cutanea tarda. The increase of fecal protoporphyrin that occurs in variegate porphyria allows the differentiation of these disorders.

Therapy of the acute attack of neurologic dysfunction is the same as for acute intermittent porphyria. Treatment of cutaneous manifestations is difficult. Beta-carotene therapy, as described for protoporphyria, has not been of value.

Hereditary coproporphyria

Like the other two acute types of porphyria, this dominantly transmitted disease can remain latent indefinitely, or attacks can be precipitated by the same factors that activate acute intermittent porphyria. Decreased coproporphyrinogen oxidase activity causes increased excretion of fecal coproporphyrin. Urine coproporphyrin may or may not be increased. An increase of urinary coproporphyrin without other urine findings is not specific for porphyria, since secondary coproporphyrinuria is seen in a number of hepatic, hematologic, malignant, and toxic diseases. During acute attacks, urinary excretion of ALA and PBG is increased, but it may be normal during asymptomatic periods.

Hereditary coproporphyria can cause both neurologic dysfunction and cutaneous manifestations. Treatment is the same as for acute intermittent porphyria and variegate porphyria.

Porphyria cutanea tarda

This disease can occur sporadically, as a familial disease, and also as a toxic disorder caused by exposure to hexachlorobenzene and related compounds. The disease is the most common of the porphyrias.

A deficiency of uroporphyrinogen decarboxylase activity is the basic defect. In the familial form of the disorder, this deficiency is found in all tissues, whereas in the toxic and sporadic forms, enzyme deficiency appears to be restricted to the liver.

Uroporphyrin and coproporphyrin are increased in the urine, with the former exceeding the latter. Urinary ALA may be minimally increased, but PBG is not. A group of tetracarboxyl porphyrins known as *isocoproporphyrins* are excreted in the feces.

Three factors that may activate the disease are increased ingestion of iron, alcoholism, and estrogen use. There are no neurologic manifestations. Minor trauma to skin causes vesicles or bullae that develop on sun-exposed areas, but acute photosensitivity reactions are not frequent. Vesicles and bullae rupture and are followed by erosions and scarring. Over a period of time, hirsutism, milia, areas of pigmentation and depigmentation, and sclerodermoid changes develop. Iron overload is present, and serum iron levels are often increased. Liver biopsy usually shows hepatocellular injury, along with fatty infiltration and hemosiderosis, and patients with long-standing untreated disease may develop cirrhosis and hepatocellular carcinoma. In the United States less than 10% of patients develop cirrhosis. Although alcoholism may be in part responsible for the hepatic damage, experimental studies indicate the porphyrin abnormality is possibly the most important factor.

The diagnosis should be considered when vesicles or bullae appear on exposed areas of skin. The disease is more frequent in men and usually appears after age 35. Young women have developed the cutaneous lesions while taking oral contraceptives, particularly when this has accompanied significant alcohol intake. During cutaneous symptoms, urinary uroporphyrin excretion usually exceeds that of coproporphyrin in porphyria cutanea tarda, whereas the opposite is generally seen in variegate porphyria. The high fecal protoporphyrin seen in variegate porphyria is also useful in distinguishing the two diseases. Decreased erythrocyte uroporphyrinogen decarboxylase activity can be used to diagnose porphyria cutanea tarda in its familial form.

Removal of body iron by repeated phlebotomy causes a decrease of urinary porphyrin excretion and clinical remission. Removal of 5 to 10 liters is usually required. Therapy is monitored by urinary uroporphyrin excretion. Chloroquine in low doses (125 to 250 mg three times a week) may also be used in treatment, particularly if the patient is intolerant of phlebotomy.

Hepatoerythropoietic porphyria

Hepatoerythropoietic porphyria is a rare form of porphyria, having been described in only about 20 patients. The disease is manifest within the first year of life as a skin disease resembling porphyria cutanea tarda. Patients are severely affected and develop excess facial hair, scarring of the hands and face, sclerodermoid changes, and acrosclerosis. The cutaneous symptoms improve somewhat as patients grow older, but hepatic disease supervenes. There are often slight to modest increases in serum transaminase and γ-glutamyl transpeptidase levels. The liver shows red fluorescence and a nonspecific hepatitis or portal inflammation. This may progress to cirrhosis. Adults usually have mild normochromic anemia, and fluorescent normoblasts are found in the bone marrow.

The abnormalities in porphyrin metabolism resemble those of porphyria cutanea tarda, with the additional feature that zinc protoporphyrin levels in erythrocytes are increased.

Hepatoerythropoietic porphyria is caused by a severe deficiency in the activity of uroporphyrinogen decarboxylase (5% to 10% of normal). The parents of such patients have approximately a 50% decrease in activity. Thus, hepatoerythropoietic porphyria is the homozygous form of decarboxylase deficiency, whereas familial porphyria cutanea tarda is the heterozygous form.

There have been few reports of therapy. The methods outlined for porphyria cutanea tarda seem rational, although iron removal is not likely to be of benefit. Administration of hematin and/or hypertransfusion may be considered when the bone marrow appears to be an important source of porphyrin overproduction.

ALA dehydrase deficiency

Patients who experienced acute porphyria-type symptoms were shown to have a 98% to 99% deficiency of enzyme activity. Their parents had 50% of normal activity. These findings suggest that rare instances of homozygous deficiency of ALA dehydrase activity produce acute attacks of porphyria.

Management is the same as that for the other acute types of porphyria.

REFERENCES

Bloomer JR and Bonkovsky HL: The porphyrias. DM 35:7, 1989.

Bloomer JR and Straka JG: Porphyrin metabolism. In Arais IM et al, editors: The liver. Biology and patholobiology. New York, 1988, Raven Press.

Bonkovsky HL: Porphyrin and heme metabolism and the porphyrias. In Zakim D and Boyer TD, editors: Hepatology. A textbook of liver disease. Philadelphia, 1990, Saunders.

Kappas A et al: The porphyrias. In Scriver CR et al, editors: The metabolic basis of inherited disease. New York, 1989, McGraw-Hill.

Lamon JM et al: Hematin therapy for acute porphyria. Medicine (Baltimore) 58:252, 1979.

Schmid R, editor: The hepatic porphyrias. Semin Liver Dis 2:87, 1982.

Schmid R, Schwartz S, and Watson CJ: Porphyrin content of bone marrow and liver in the various forms of porphyria. AMA Arch Intern Med 93:167, 1954.

With TK: A short history of porphyrins and the porphyrias. Int J Biochem 11:189, 1980.

CHAPTER

177 Hypercalcemia

John P. Bilezikian

CAUSES AND DIFFERENTIAL DIAGNOSIS

The causes of hypercalcemia are listed in the box below. Primary hyperparathyroidism and malignant neoplasms, the most common causes of hypercalcemia, are covered separately in Chapters 187 and 188. Despite the fact that in the great majority of patients with hypercalcemia (approximately 90%), one of these two etiologies is responsible, it is important to consider other causes of hypercalcemia in the course of a diagnostic evaluation.

The differential diagnosis of hypercalcemia depends on the history, the physical examination, and appropriate laboratory tests. If a malignancy is present, it is usually readily discovered. The malignant disorders most frequently associated with hypercalcemia are multiple myeloma; carcinoma of the lung, breast, esophagus, kidneys, ovary, or bladder; and lymphoma. The mechanisms for the elevated serum calcium in malignant disease are covered in Chapter 188. Primary hyperparathyroidism is distinguished from hypercalcemia of malignancy on clinical grounds and by obtaining a parathyroid hormone level (see Chapter 188). The concurrence of hypercalcemia and an elevated parathyroid hormone level, in the absence of renal failure, establishes the diagnosis of primary hyperparathyroidism. It is very rare for a malignant disorder, regardless of the mechanism of the hypercalcemia, to be associated with an elevated level of parathyroid hormone. In the syndrome of humoral hypercalcemia of malignancy, the parathyroid hormone-like protein (PTHRP) elaborated by the tumor does not cross-react in any of the commercially available radioimmunoassays or immunoradiometric assays for parathyroid hormone. Thus even when PTHRP is responsible for the hypercalcemia, the parathyroid hormone level is not elevated (see Chapter 187). Somewhat more difficult is the situation in which the concentration of parathyroid hormone is low and the diagnosis of malignancy cannot be made. The less common causes of malignancy must then be considered.

Causes of hypercalcemia

- Primary hyperparathyroidism
- Cancer
  - Parathyroid hormone-related protein
  - Ectopic production of 1,25-dihydroxyvitamin D
  - Other factors produced ectopically
  - Lytic bone metastases
- Nonparathyroid endocrine disorders
  - Thyrotoxicosis
  - Pheochromocytoma
  - Adrenal insufficiency
  - Vasoactive intestinal polypeptide hormone–producing tumor
- Granulomatous diseases (1,25-dihydroxyvitamin D excess)
  - Sarcoidosis
  - Tuberculosis
  - Histoplasmosis
  - Coccidioidomycosis
  - Leprosy
- Medications
  - Thiazide diuretics
  - Lithium
  - Estrogens and antiestrogens
- Milk-alkali syndrome
- Vitamin A intoxication
- Vitamin D intoxication
- Familial hypocalciuric hypercalcemia
- Immobilization
- Parenteral nutrition
- Acute and chronic renal insufficiency

Nonparathyroid endocrine disorders

Hypercalcemia occurs in approximately 5% to 10% of patients with hyperthyroidism, caused presumably by rapid bone turnover. The calcium is usually less than 11.5 mg per deciliter and is readily reversible after successful therapy for the hyperthyroid state. Hypercalcemia associated with pheochromocytoma may occur in the syndrome of multiple endocrine neoplasia type II, in which case primary hyperparathyroidism is concurrent. Alternatively, and analogous to humoral hypercalcemia of malignancy, some pheochromocytomas may elaborate a hypercalcemic factor. The proper approach to the patient with a pheochromocytoma and hypercalcemia is to remove the adrenal tumor first. Pancreatic islet cell tumors that secrete vasoactive intestinal polypeptide (VIP) can be associated with severe hypercalcemia. Similar to the situation with pheochromocytoma, the VIPoma may coexist with hyperparathyroidism as part of a multiple endocrine neoplasia syndrome (in this case, type I), but there are other patients in whom the hypercalcemia remits after removal of the pancreatic tumor. Addison's disease is another rare endocrine cause of hypercalcemia. The mechanism may be due to loss of the antagonistic properties of glucocorticoids on calcium absorption. Several decades ago, tuberculosis used to be the most common cause of adrenal insufficiency. In view of the presence of hypercalcemia in some patients with tuberculosis (see below), this possible etiology of the adrenal insufficiency should be borne in mind when hypercalcemia and adrenal insufficiency are seen together.

Vitamin D

Vitamin D toxicity can induce hypercalcemia among patients being treated for chronic hypoparathyroid states. When the parent compound, vitamin D, is responsible, hypercalcemia can persist for months because of the large potential storage depots for the vitamin in fat tissue. The serum calcium and phosphate are both elevated as is the 25-hydroxyvitamin D level. The active metabolite, 1,25-

dihydroxyvitamin D, is not usually elevated unless ingestion of this active metabolite is responsible for the hypercalcemia. The list of granulomatous diseases associated with hypercalcemia is long; the hypercalcemia in these diseases is caused, in many instances, by the granulomatous tissue producing 1,25-dihydroxyvitamin D. Sarcoidosis is the best example of a granulomatous disease that can induce hypercalcemia, but other noteworthy examples are tuberculosis, histoplasmosis, coccidioidomycosis, leprosy, berylliosis, candidiasis, eosinophilic granuloma, and silicone implantation. Ectopic production of 1,25-dihydroxyvitamin D by malignant lymphomas also occurs. Causes of hypercalcemia in acquired immunodeficiency syndrome (AIDS) may relate to malignant lymphomatous processes to which these patients are predisposed.

Medication-induced hypercalcemia

Thiazide diuretics may be responsible for hypercalcemia in the absence of any intrinsic abnormality in calcium metabolism. Thiazide-induced hypercalcemia is one of those situations in which the parathyroid hormone level may be elevated as a result of a nonparathyroid etiology. The hypercalcemia remits after withdrawal of the thiazide in a substantial number of patients, although it is also possible that primary hyperparathyroidism will be unmasked. The etiology of hypercalcemia, when it surfaces during thiazide therapy, cannot be made with confidence until 2 or 3 months after the diuretic is discontinued. Patients receiving lithium carbonate may develop hypercalcemia. Here again, the medication should be discontinued, if possible, to determine whether the lithium is responsible for the altered parathyroid sensitivity to calcium or whether primary hyperparathyroidism is present. Estrogens and antiestrogens (tamoxifen) have been reported to result in hypercalcemia in a significant number of patients with breast carcinoma. Usually these patients have known, extensive bone metastases. Very unusual examples of medication-induced hypercalcemia are milk-alkali syndrome and vitamin A toxicity.

Unusual causes

Familial hypocalciuric hypercalcemia (FHH) is an important consideration in the differential diagnosis of hypercalcemia because it can easily be mistaken for primary hyperparathyroidism. The distinction between FHH and primary hyperparathyroidism rests on several features: genetics (autosomal dominance) with early penetrance in childhood; normal parathyroid hormone level; low urinary calcium excretion (Ca/Cr clearance <0.01); and lack of typical clinical features of primary hyperparathyroidism (see Chapter 187). Immobilization hypercalcemia does not usually occur, despite the negative calcium balance to which all immobilized individuals are subject, unless there is an underlying abnormality in calcium metabolism such as Paget's disease or malignancy. Hypercalcemia, however, may regularly occur in growing children who have been immobilized because of a fracture or some other reason. Hypercalcemia in patients receiving parenteral nutrition may develop when administered calcium is greater than 300 mg per day and when renal function is impaired. Hypercalcemia after long-term parenteral nutrition also occurs but its mechanism is obscure. It is likely to be related to the osteomalacia that frequently develops in these individuals. Finally, hypercalcemia may occur in the setting of acute or chronic renal failure.

CLINICAL FEATURES

Hypercalcemia is associated with signs and symptoms that are independent of its etiology. When therapy for hypercalcemia per se is considered, these particular features should be assessed and not confused with signs and symptoms that may be caused more specifically by the patient's underlying disorder. Measures to reduce the serum calcium concentration do not ameliorate aspects of the patient's symptoms that are not a result of hypercalcemia. Admittedly, when rather general (e.g., weakness, lethargy), symptoms may be exceedingly difficult to pinpoint as to specific cause. In such cases, empiric but judicious therapy for the hypercalcemia may be warranted. The reported value for the serum calcium should always be interpreted with knowledge of the serum albumin, the major circulating calcium-binding protein. When the serum albumin is normal, approximately 50% of the total calcium value reflects the physiologically active, free ionized form. If the serum albumin is low, as is often the case in sick patients, the ionized calcium level is greater than 50% of the measured value, and the hypercalcemia is actually greater than that indicated by the total serum calcium. For every gram per deciliter reduction in the serum albumin, the measured total serum calcium concentration should be adjusted upward by 0.8 mg per deciliter to appreciate more accurately the degree of true hypercalcemia (see Chapter 151).

If the serum calcium is only mildly elevated (<11.5 mg/dl), there are few if any signs or symptoms of hypercalcemia. If the serum calcium is between 11.5 and 13.5 mg per deciliter, patients may or may not be symptomatic. Invariably, symptoms are present if the serum calcium is greater than 13.5 mg per deciliter. The rate at which the serum calcium rises is also a factor that helps to determine the degree of symptomatology. For a given calcium level, the patient who experiences the more rapid rise is the more symptomatic. A list of signs and symptoms of hypercalcemia is presented in the box on p. 1496. Included in the list is a set of problems that can make relatively mild hypercalcemia a medical emergency. Polyuria not accompanied by adequate oral fluid replacement can lead to decreased intravascular volume, thus increasing the severity of hypercalcemia. Worsening hypercalcemia in turn can lead to decreased fluid intake, because of anorexia, and more marked polyuria. Ensuing diminished renal function, because of dehydration, eventually leads to reduced clearance of the serum calcium. This cycle can rapidly lead to a hypercalcemic emergency. Such patients are invariably symptomatic both because of the level of the serum calcium and the rapidity of its rise. This pathophysiologic mechanism can be

Clinical features of hypercalcemia

General
- Weakness
- Dehydration
- Metastatic calcification

Central nervous system
- Impaired concentration
- Increased sleep requirement
- Altered states of consciousness (confusion, lethargy, stupor, coma)

Gastrointestinal tract
- Polydipsia
- Anorexia
- Nausea
- Vomiting
- Constipation
- Pancreatitis
- Peptic ulcer

Renal
- Polyuria
- Decreased function
- Decreased concentrating ability
- Nephrolithiasis
- Nephrocalcinosis

Cardiovascular
- Hypertension
- Electrocardiographic changes (shortened QT interval)
- Increased sensitivity to digitalis

operative in virtually any underlying cause of hypercalcemia.

TREATMENT

Therapeutic agents for hypercalcemia can lower the serum calcium in virtually all cases. The range of therapeutic options provides the opportunity to tailor treatment to the patient's condition. If the serum calcium is mildly elevated and not accompanied by any of the clinical features described above, therapy should be tempered accordingly. On the other hand, life-threatening hypercalcemia requires a much more aggressive approach. An important principle of therapy is to take into account the underlying cause of the hypercalcemia. In patients with mild, asymptomatic primary hyperparathyroidism, the approach is much different from the patient who presents in parathyroid crisis. In thyrotoxicosis, the hypercalcemia is best approached by treating the hyperthyroidism. In familial hypocalciuric hypercalcemia, patients are not treated. In hypercalcemia that develops late in the course of an incurable malignancy, the physician must consider the stark reality of the patient's prognosis. Severe hypercalcemia in the patient with terminal malignancy is sometimes best left untreated.

General measures to treat hypercalcemia are applicable to all hypercalcemic states, independent of their underlying etiology (see Table 177-1). Hydration is a key approach because the pathophysiologic events induced by the hypercalcemia lead invariably to dehydration. The serum calcium

Table 177-1. Management of hypercalcemia

General	Specific
Rehydration	Bisphosphonates
Saline administration	Plicamycin
Diuresis with furosemide	Calcitonin
	Gallium nitrate
Dialysis	Phosphate
Mobilization	Glucocorticoids
	Therapy of underlying etiology

declines simply by restoration of intravascular volume and improved renal glomerular filtration. Rehydration with intravenous saline has an additional advantage in that the saluresis so induced is associated with an obligatory increase in renal excretion of calcium. The use of a loop diuretic such as furosemide facilitates the loss of sodium and calcium and may be particularly valuable in patients whose cardiovascular tolerance to saline administration is limited. Diuresis with furosemide should be employed only after fluid therapy has first restored intravascular volume. Depending on the patient's capacity to handle the volume load, it is reasonable to administer judicious doses of furosemide (10 to 20 mg intravenously every 6 to 12 hours). If fluid tolerance is not viewed with concern, furosemide should not be used but rather reserved for signs of fluid overload, should they become evident. Thiazide diuretics should never be used because they may actually worsen the hypercalcemia. Peritoneal or hemodialysis should be considered if the hypercalcemia is severe and associated with renal failure. Although the patient with hypercalcemia may not be ambulatory at the time of admission to the hospital, every effort should be made to mobilize the patient as soon as possible. Mobilization helps to reduce the negative calcium balance associated with loss of weight bearing.

Specific measures to reduce severe hypercalcemia are often indicated. Most pathophysiologic mechanisms responsible for severe hypercalcemia lead to accelerated calcium mobilization from bone caused by activation of the osteoclast, the bone cell responsible for bone resorption. Specific therapies inhibit this process by impairing osteoclast-mediated bone resorption.

The bisphosphonates are pyrophosphate analogues that effectively inhibit osteoclast-mediated bone resorption. Three bisphosphonates are available worldwide: ethane hydroxy 1,1-diphosphonic acid (etidronate), dichloromethylene diphosphonate, and aminohydroxypropylidene diphosphonate (pamidronate). Etidronate and pamidronate are available at this time in the United States. Parenteral etidronate reduces the serum calcium effectively. An oral form may help to maintain reduced calcium levels. Concerns about a potential adverse side effect of etidronate, impaired bone formation, are not important when the drug is used acutely and in a limited way.

Pamidronate is a more potent bisphosphonate than etidronate but it has a similar time course of action, the serum calcium declining within 48 hours after the first dose. Adverse effects of parenteral pamidronate are limited to a transient temperature elevation (less than 2 degrees C), transient leukopenia, and a small reduction in serum phosphate concentration.

Plicamycin (mithramycin) is a specific osteoclast inhibitor and thus is effective in any hypercalcemic condition associated with accelerated osteoclast-mediated bone resorption. Potential side effects of plicamycin include nephrotoxicity, hepatotoxicity, and platelet dysfunction. These adverse effects and the need for parenteral administration limit the use of plicamycin to the acute therapy of hypercalcemia. It has no role as a chronic therapy.

Calcitonin should theoretically be an ideal therapy for hypercalcemia because it not only inhibits osteoclast function but also increases urinary calcium excretion. Although calcitonin is not as potent as the bisphosphonates or plicamycin, it nevertheless reduces the calcium transiently and may be of use as adjunctive therapy when the serum calcium is extremely high. Combinations of calcitonin and other agents have been employed to amplify and prolong the hypocalcemic effects of calcitonin. Combination therapy with glucocorticoids or bisphosphonates does not appear to be more effective than the additive effects of each agent alone. Calcitonin occasionally causes mild, transient nausea, abdominal cramps, and flushing.

Gallium nitrate, another inhibitor of bone resorption, reduces the serum calcium with a time course similar to that of the bisphosphonates. It should not be used when the serum creatinine is elevated or with other potential nephrotoxic agents. Clinical experience with gallium nitrate is still quite limited.

Glucocorticoid administration may be efficacious in certain malignant disorders such as multiple myeloma, lymphoma, and breast cancer, where it may decrease bone resorption. In other disorders characterized by excessive absorption of calcium from the gastrointestinal tract (vitamin D intoxication, sarcoidosis, milk-alkali syndrome), glucocorticoids can also be useful. In these settings, glucocorticoids act directly on gut epithelial cells to inhibit calcium transport. It is evident that these forms of hypercalcemia are also ameliorated by limiting the amount of calcium in the diet.

Phosphate inhibits bone resorption, limits gastrointestinal absorption of calcium, and complexes circulating calcium. Unfortunately, this last mechanism may lead to an adverse side effect, ectopic deposition of calcium phosphate salts in soft tissues. Because of this concern, parenteral phosphate is not used except in the most dire situations. Oral phosphate has no useful role in the therapy of life-threatening hypercalcemia because it is relatively weak and may not be tolerated by the patient who is likely to be suffering from the gastrointestinal manifestations of hypercalcemia.

An important consideration in the hypercalcemic patient is the underlying etiology. Specific therapy, if available, for the cause of the hypercalcemia may be as effective in lowering the serum calcium as the approaches outlined above.

REFERENCES

Bilezikian JP: Clinical utility of assays for parathyroid hormone-related protein. Clin Chem 38:179, 1992.

Bilezikian JP: Hypercalcemic states. In Coe FL and Favus MJ, editors. Disorders of bone and mineral metabolism. New York, 1992, Raven Press.

Bilezikian JP: Management of acute hypercalcemia. N Engl J Med 326:1196, 1992.

Broadus AE et al: Humoral hypercalcemia of cancer: identification of a novel parathyroid hormone-like peptide. N Engl J Med 319:556, 1988.

Mundy GR: Pathophysiology of cancer-associated hypercalcemia. Semin Oncol 17(suppl 5):10, 1990.

Ng KW and Martin TJ: Humoral hypercalcemia of malignancy. Clin Biochem 23:11, 1990.

Nussbaum SR et al: Highly sensitive two-site immunoradiometric assay of parathyrin, and its clinical utility in evaluating patients with hypercalcemia. Clin Chem 33:1364, 1987.

Singer FR et al: Treatment of hypercalcemia of malignancy with intravenous etidronate: a controlled, multicenter center study. Arch Intern Med 151:471, 1991.

Strewler GJ and Nissenson RA: Peptide mediators of hypercalcemia of malignancy. Ann Rev Med 41:35, 1991.

Warrell RP Jr and Bockman RS: Gallium in the treatment of hypercalcemia and bone metastases. In Freeman JS, editor: Important advances in oncology. Philadelphia, 1989, Lippincott.

CHAPTER

178 Hypocalcemia

John P. Bilezikian

Disorders associated with hypocalcemia include a long list of causes as noted in the box on p. 1498. The first consideration in any individual whose total serum calcium is below normal is to ascertain that hypocalcemia is actually present. The total serum calcium reflects the contribution of calcium bound to albumin (about 50%) as well as the physiologically active free calcium concentration. When the serum albumin is below normal, a relatively common feature in the very ill patient, the total serum calcium is low. If the serum ionized calcium were measured in patients with hypoalbuminemia, it would be normal. Because a direct determination of ionized calcium is not always available, the same correction factor indicated previously in consideration of hypercalcemia (Chapter 177) is made for hypocalcemia. The acid-base status of the patient is another factor that may influence the degree to which a patient may be symptomatic from hypocalcemia. In alkalosis, more calcium is bound to albumin. The change in equilibrium, favoring calcium in its inactive, bound form, gives rise to more symptoms for a given level of the total serum calcium when alkalosis is present. On the other hand, acidosis leads to a greater amount of free calcium and thus favors fewer symptoms for a given level of total serum calcium. Another factor that has only recently been recognized as potentially im-

Differential diagnosis of hypocalcemia

- Situational
  - Hypoalbuminemia
  - Alkalosis
  - Elevated concentrations of free fatty acids
  - Intensive care unit–associated
- Hypoparathyroidism
  - Postsurgical hypoparathyroidism
  - Idiopathic hypoparathyroidism
    - Isolated
    - Multiple glandular failure
  - Magnesium deficiency, severe
  - Hypermagnesemia
  - Infiltrative diseases of parathyroid glands
    - Hemochromatosis
    - Thalassemia
    - Wilson's disease
    - Metastatic carcinoma
    - Amyloidosis
  - Ionizing radiation or chemotherapy
  - Congenital disorders (DiGeorge's syndrome, Kearns-Sayre syndrome)
  - Neonatal hypocalcemia
- Relative hypoparathyroidism
  - Acute pancreatitis
  - Acute release of cellular phosphate
    - Rhabdomyolysis
    - Chemotherapy
    - Toxic shock syndrome
  - Osteoblastic metastases
  - Multiple, citrated blood transfusions
  - States of 1,25-dihydroxyvitamin D deficiency
  - Some vitamin D resistant states
- Resistance to parathyroid hormone
  - Pseudohypoparathyroidism
    - Type Ia and type Ib
    - Type II
    - Split target organ sensitivity

portant in shifting the partition ratio between bound and free calcium is circulating free fatty acids. Free fatty acids can permit more calcium binding to albumin and thus may lead to a reduced ionized calcium concentration. Despite these considerations and the underlying medical disorder, the presence of hypocalcemia in an acutely ill patient is not always easily explained. It is often obscure and not clearly related to abnormalities in parathyroid hormone or to 1,25-dihydroxyvitamin D.

DIFFERENTIAL DIAGNOSIS

Hypoparathyroidism

Hypoparathyroidism is defined as a state of hypocalcemia that occurs in association with deficient parathyroid glandular function. In all true hypoparathyroid states, the parathyroid hormone concentration is low. The coexistence of hypocalcemia and abnormally low parathyroid hormone levels differentiates the hypoparathyroid states from those hypocalcemic disorders caused by nonparathyroid abnormalities in which there is a compensatory increase in parathyroid hormone levels. The widespread availability of sensitive, reliable assays for parathyroid hormone permits one to rely on this assay for establishing the diagnosis of hypoparathyroidism. The serum phosphate tends to be in the upper range of normal, perhaps because of the loss of the phosphaturic actions of parathyroid hormone. The 1,25-dihydroxyvitamin D concentration may be low both because parathyroid hormone, a major stimulus to the formation of 1,25-dihydroxyvitamin D, is low and because elevated phosphate suppresses formation of the active vitamin D metabolite.

Postsurgical hypoparathyroidism. Hypoparathyroidism develops in a small percentage of patients who have undergone neck surgery. Following the removal of parathyroid tissue for hyperparathyroidism, a transient hypoparathyroid state may develop owing to several possible factors. These factors include interference with the vasculature of the remaining parathyroid tissue, a brief period required for the suppressed normal glands to recover function, or to rapid remineralization of bone in patients with hyperparathyroid bone disease (hungry bone syndrome). Management of the hypocalcemia in these patients is designed to cover the period before normal mineral homeostasis is reestablished, usually a matter of days. Some patients, however, develop permanent hypoparathyroidism following neck surgery. This condition is more likely to occur if the operation has been associated with major local anatomic dissection. Occasionally, all normal parathyroid tissue is inadvertantly removed or, in patients who have already undergone previous parathyroid surgery, normal parathyroid tissue may have been removed at an earlier time. Postsurgical hypoparathyroidism does not always occur in the days to weeks after surgery but rather may develop years later. In this situation, it is believed that functional parathyroid tissue, left with a marginal blood supply at the time of surgery, is rendered hypofunctional with further compromise of vascular integrity over the years. Postsurgical hypoparathyroidism can develop after any neck surgery, not just following parathyroid surgery.

Idiopathic hypoparathyroidism. *Idiopathic hypoparathyroidism* is a descriptive term encompassing a rather heterogeneous group of disorders characterized by deficient secretion of parathyroid hormone. The most common form is isolated, idiopathic hypoparathyroidism, unassociated with a family history or other glandular deficiencies. This form of hypoparathyroidism can occur at any age although it becomes apparent most commonly in children. Females are affected twice as often as males. Parathyroid antibodies are usually present in isolated, idiopathic hypoparathyroidism. These antibodies may be directed against the secretion of parathyroid hormone itself or against parathyroid tissue. In other cases of isolated, idiopathic hypoparathyroidism, the parathyroid glands are infiltrated with fat and replaced by fibrosis. Isolated, idiopathic hypoparathyroidism can occur, although much more rarely, as a familial syndrome. In this form of the disorder, parathyroid antibodies are absent. Genetic linkage studies have shown that the structural gene for parathyroid hormone is present in these individuals. Deficient parathyroid hormone secretion thus would appear to result from elements related to transcriptional, translation, or perhaps even secretory control of parathyroid hormone in the parathyroid cell.

Idiopathic hypoparathyroidism also occurs as a component of the multiple end-organ endocrine deficiency syndrome. When familial, the transmission pattern is most compatible with autosomal recessive inheritance. It may also be seen sporadically without a familial background. The most classic combination of endocrine glands involved is the parathyroids and the adrenals. Mucocutaneous candidiasis is usually also present. Gonadal failure, hypothyroidism, and diabetes mellitus may also be seen. Nonendocrine abnormalities, besides mucocutaneous candidiasis, such as pernicious anemia, chronic active hepatitis, alopecia, vitiligo, or malabsorption, may be present or develop over time. The clinical presentation of this form of idiopathic hypoparathyroidism varies with respect to the sequence of glandular involvement and also to the number of different glands affected in the course of the patient's life. Virtually every combination of end-organ deficiencies with or without the aforementioned nonendocrine manifestations of the syndrome has been described. Antibodies directed against specific endocrine tissues and T cell abnormalities suggest an autoimmune etiology. The multiple end-organ endocrine deficiency syndrome has also been described in connection with a constellation of developmental abnormalities.

Magnesium. Severe hypomagnesemia is associated with hypocalcemia caused in part by impaired secretion of parathyroid hormone. The functional hypoparathyroidism in severe magnesium deficiency is discussed in detail elsewhere (Chapter 180). Hypermagnesemia can also be associated with functional hypoparathyroidism and hypocalcemia. In this case, the parathyroid glands are inhibited in a normal physiologic way by the elevated magnesium level. Clinically, the setting in which this is most likely to occur is when magnesium is used to control premature labor. In most obstetric patients, however, the reduction in serum calcium is mild and usually not associated with symptoms.

Rare causes of hypoparathyroidism. Infiltration of the parathyroids by heavy metals such as iron (hemochromatosis, thalassemia) or copper (Wilson's disease) can lead, in rare instances, to hypoparathyroidism. Infiltration of the parathyroid glands can also occur, but very rarely, in metastatic carcinoma, in sarcoidosis, and in amyloidosis. Even more uncommon are reported examples of hypoparathyroidism in patients who have received previous irradiation to the head and neck. Similarly, parathyroid gland function has unusually been reported to be compromised following therapy with cytotoxic chemotherapeutic agents such as doxorubicin, cytosine arabinoside, asparaginase, and WR2721.

Neonatal and congenital disorders. A transient period of mild hypocalcemia is normal during the first 3 weeks of life, a normal consequence of immature parathyroid glands that are unable to compensate for the expected decline in the neonatal calcium concentration. Transient neonatal hypoparathyroidism may be more severe in the offspring of hyperparathyroid mothers. After feedings have begun, during the fourth through sixth week of life, neonatal hypocalcemia may be caused by the high phosphate content of foods, especially cow's milk. A milk mixture with a high calcium/phosphate ratio (4:1) is helpful until the parathyroid glands develop adequate maturity.

Hypoparathyroidism occurs as a component of anomalies associated with maldevelopment of the branchial pouches. The best known of these congenital causes of hypoparathyroidism is DiGeorge's syndrome, in which the absence of the third and fourth branchial pouches leads to absence of the parathyroid and thymus glands. Deficient T cell–mediated immunity caused by agenesis of the thymus is the most devastating part of this disorder, leading to death from severe viral and fungal infections within the first few years of life. When the first and fifth branchial pouches do not develop, hypoparathyroidism may be seen in association with a host of physical anomalies such as hypertelorism, antimongoloid slant, micrognathia, and aortic arch abnormalities. Hypoparathyroidism is also associated with other rare developmental abnormalities such as familial nephrosis, nerve deafness, lymphedema, prolapsing mitral valve, brachydactyly, and the Kearns-Sayre syndrome.

Relative hypoparathyroidism

Hypocalcemia can develop in patients who have normal parathyroid gland responsiveness. In this setting, the parathyroid glands react to the hypocalcemia, associated with a host of different primary disorders (see box, p. 1498), by secreting more hormone. The secondary hyperparathyroidism is an attempt to overcome the hypocalcemia induced by the pathophysiologic mechanisms involved in these various disorders. It is important to recognize the difference between primary hyperparathyroidism, a hypercalcemic disorder due to excessive secretion of parathyroid hormone (Chapter 187) and secondary hyperparathyroidism, an appropriate compensatory response to hypocalcemia. Primary hyperparathyroidism is virtually always associated with hypercalcemia whereas secondary hyperparathyroidism is associated with hypocalcemia, if compensatory secretion of parathyroid hormone is inadequate (i.e., relative hypoparathyroidism). If compensatory secretion of parathyroid hormone is adequate, the patient's calcium concentration may be in the low-normal range, at the expense of deleterious effects of elevated parathyroid hormone levels on bone and other target tissues.

Vitamin D deficiency or resistance. A major category of hypocalcemia associated with secondary increases in parathyroid hormone is deficiency of 1,25-dihydroxyvitamin D. A long list of gastrointestinal and renal diseases account for the majority of patients with 1,25-dihydroxyvitamin D deficiency. Defective mineralization of bones in adults gives rise to a clinical hallmark of vitamin D deficiency: osteomalacia. In these patients, the four parathyroid glands are hyperplastic. With appropriate management of the underlying disease, normal parathyroid function can sometimes be reestablished. Certain forms of vitamin D resistance may also be associated with a secondary hyperparathyroidism. These disorders are all considered in detail elsewhere (Chapter 181).

Pseudohypoparathyroidism. This classic disorder of calcium metabolism has an unmistakable physical appearance characterized by short stature, round facies, short neck, and foreshortened metacarpal and metatarsal bones (Albright's hereditary osteodystrophy or pseudohypoparathyroidism type Ia; Fig. 178-1). It is a genetic disease with several different transmission patterns: sex-linked dominant, autosomal recessive, and autosomal dominant. Patients usually have low-normal to frankly retarded intelligence. There may be a history of childhood seizures. Radiologically evident calcifications in the basal ganglia and cataracts are common. The serum calcium is low and the serum phosphate is elevated. In contrast to true hypoparathyroidism, the parathyroid hormone level is elevated, hence the designation *pseudohypoparathyroidism*. The salient biochemical feature of pseudohypoparathyroidism is resistance to the actions of parathyroid hormone. There is neither a phosphaturic nor a cyclic AMP response to parathyroid hormone in the classic (type Ia) syndrome (Fig. 178-2). The typical patient with pseudohypoparathyroidism type Ia may show resistance to the actions of other hormones besides parathyroid hormone. Hypothyroidism, hypogonadism, glucagon resistance, defective olfaction, and prolactin deficiency have all been reported in pseudohypoparathyroidism. Pseudohypoparathyroidism type Ib is identical to type Ia except for the fact that Albright's hereditary osteodystrophy is not present and other hormone resistant states are not seen. Patients do have the biochemical abnormalities. In

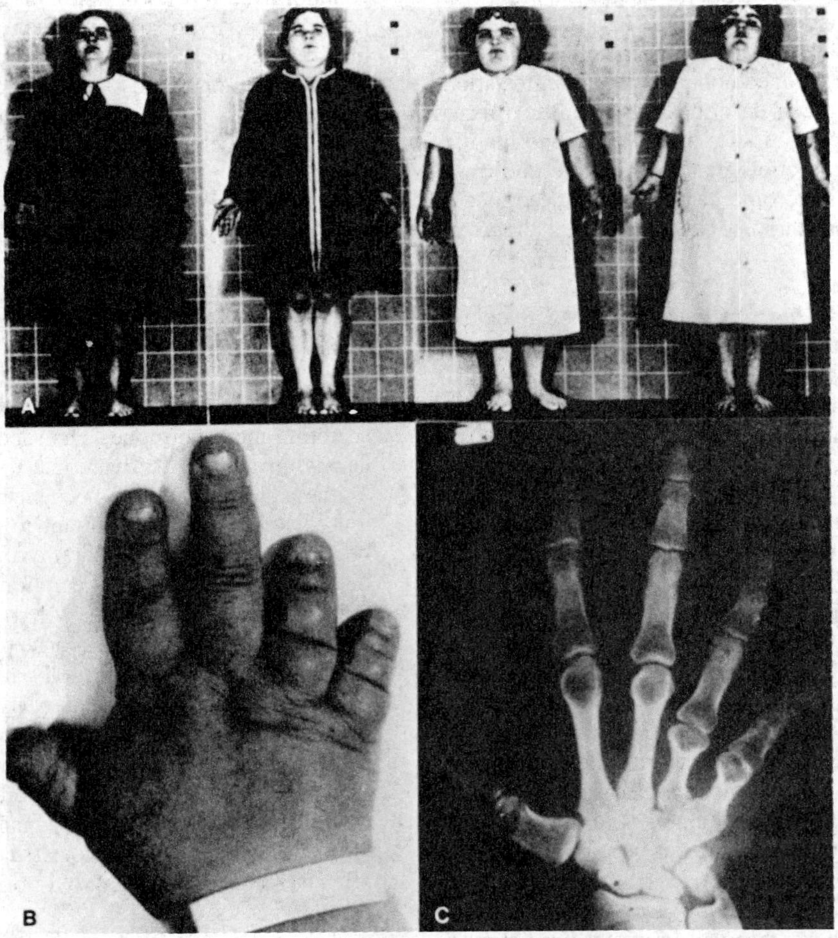

Fig. 178-1. The physical features of four sisters with pseudohypoparathyroidism. **A,** Note the short stature, round facies, and shortened neck. **B,** The metacarpal bones of the fourth and fifth digits are foreshortened, giving this characteristic appearance to the knuckles. **C,** Radiograph, demonstrating the shortened metacarpal bones. (**A** from Kinard RE et al: Arch Intern Med 139:204, 1979; **B** and **C** from Levine MA et al: Johns Hopkins Med J 151:137, 1982).

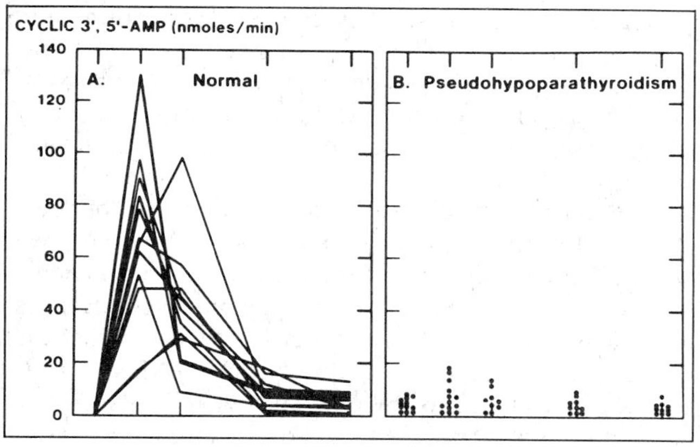

Fig. 178-2. Parathyroid hormone resistance in pseudohypoparathyroidism. **A,** Normal patients respond to an infusion of parathyroid hormone with a rapid and marked increase in the urinary excretion of cyclic AMP. **B,** In pseudohypoparathyroidism, this response to parathyroid hormone is markedly blunted. (Redrawn from Chase LW et al: J Clin Invest 48:1832, 1969.)

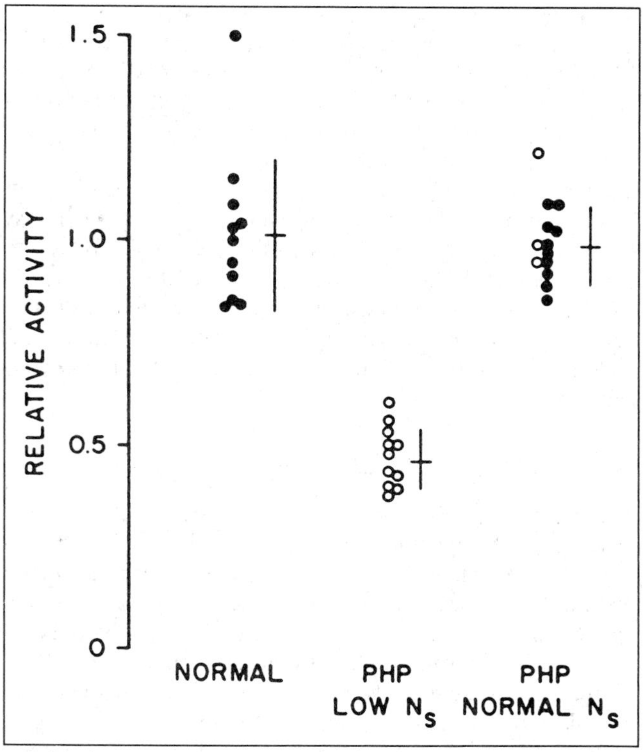

Fig. 178-3. Activity of the stimulatory guanine nucleotide–binding protein in pseudohypoparathyroidism. The data are expressed as activity relative to a standard, pooled erythrocyte membrane preparation from normal individuals. For each group, the mean ± standard deviation is shown. Open circles: patients with the complete phenotypic and biochemical defect, Albright's hereditary osteodystrophy (AHO). Closed circles: patients with normal body habitus but parathyroid hormone resistance (type Ib). Normal subjects are also shown as closed circles in the left-hand lane. Note three patients with classic AHO have normal G(N) protein levels. All patients with type Ib pseudohypoparathyroidism have normal levels of G(N). (Reprinted from Downs RW et al: J Clin Endocrinol Metab 61:351, 1985.)

contrast, after Albright described pseudohypoparathyroidism, he observed a patient with the typical body habitus but without evidence for hypocalcemia or target organ resistance. In his attempt to distinguish this variant from classic pseudohypoparathyroidism, Albright dubbed it *pseudopseudohypoparathyroidism*. Pseudo- and pseudopseudohypoparathyroidism clearly belong to the same genetic family as evidenced by family trees that contain both forms of the disorder, by selected patients whose biochemical profile has been known to cross over to the other, and by the molecular basis of the disorder (see below). Even other variants of pseudohypoparathyroidism exist such as those characterized by resistance to the renal actions of parathyroid hormone but sensitivity to its skeleton actions. Equally uncommon, some patients demonstrate a normal cyclic AMP response to parathyroid hormone but no phosphaturia (type II).

Important clues to the defect in pseudohypoparathyroidism were gained by observations related to the fact that the constellation of hormone resistance that is included in the syndrome involves the adenylate cyclase messenger system. A site common to all hormones that use adenylate cyclase is the guanine nucleotide binding protein, G_s, that links their different receptors to the catalytic unit of adenylate cyclase. Patients with Albright's hereditary osteodystrophy (pseudohypoparathyroidism type Ia) demonstrate a 50% reduction in G_s (Fig. 178-3). Levels of the inhibitory guanine nucleotide–binding protein, G_i, are normal. Despite the enthusiasm generated by this observation, reduced G_s levels do not entirely account for the syndrome. Patients with pseudopseudohypoparathyroidism in which the typical physiognomy is not accompanied by hormone resistance, nevertheless, do have reduced G_s levels. Only patients with the classic disorder, but not all, have the reduction in G_s. Patients with type Ib and parathyroid resistance in the absence of any other hormone resistance have normal levels of G_s, implying that this isolated hormone-resistant state might be caused by a defect in the parathyroid hormone receptor per se. There is even evidence for a circulating parathyroid hormone–like inhibitor in pseudohypoparathyroidism. These points suggest that reduced levels of G_s are not necessarily causally related to hormone resistance in pseudohypoparathyroidism and also that the underlying mechanisms for the various forms of pseudohypoparathyroidism are likely to be heterogeneous.

Acute pancreatitis. When acute pancreatitis is severe, it is associated with hypocalcemia, a very poor prognostic sign. It is still not known why patients may become so markedly hypocalcemic, but current evidence continues to focus on deposition of calcium soaps in conjunction with fatty acid lipolysis in pancreatitis. Although most patients have a secondary elevation of parathyroid hormone, there is debate about whether the parathyroid hormone response is sufficiently vigorous with respect to the extent of the hypocalcemia.

Other causes. Other causes of relative hypoparathyroidism may be caused by rapid release of phosphate from cells. Chemotherapy for acute leukemia or Burkitt's lymphoma, acute rhabdomyolysis, and toxic shock syndrome may all be associated with massive release of cellular phosphate into the circulation. Another mechanism is operative in the hypocalcemia associated with osteoblastic metastases in breast and prostatic carcinoma. The extremely rapid influx of calcium from blood to bone in these examples of osteoblastic metastatic bone disease is believed to be responsible for the hypocalcemia. Multiple, citrated blood transfusions can lead to complexing of free ionized calcium with citrate sufficiently great to reduce the ionized calcium concentration.

CLINICAL FEATURES

The presence of signs and symptoms of hypocalcemia is a function of the absolute level of the calcium concentration as well as the rate of its fall. Chronic hypocalcemia is much less likely to be associated with classic clinical features than acute hypocalcemia in which the serum calcium is reduced rapidly. The neuromuscular system is affected most often, giving rise to latent or frank excitability. The patient may complain of paresthesias of the extremities or a feeling of numbness, especially if the extremity is left in a resting position. Chvostek's sign is elicited by gently tapping the facial nerve anterior to the ear. Twitching of the proximate facial muscles indicates latent neuromuscular excitability. Mere contraction at the lip is a less reliable sign because it may be found in as many as 10% of normal subjects. Another classic sign of latent tetany is Trousseau's sign, elicited by carpal spasm after inflation of the blood pressure cuff to just above systolic blood pressure for 2 minutes. Carpal spasm consists of flexed elbow, flexed wrist, adducted thumb, flexed metacarpophalangeal joints, and extended interphalangeal joints. In acute hypocalcemia, spontaneous carpal-pedal spasm may be present. The QT interval on the electrocardiogram may be prolonged. Laryngospasm is a rare but life-threatening manifestation of hypocalcemia. Frank convulsions may be observed, especially in individuals with an underlying seizure disorder. A few examples of reversible congestive heart failure due to hypocalcemia have been reported.

In chronic hypocalcemia associated with hypoparathyroid states, long-term complications include ectopic calcium deposition in soft tissues, cataracts, and basal ganglia calcifications. Rarely, extrapyramidal signs suggestive of parkinsonism are observed. Papilledema and intestinal malabsorption with steatorrhea are also seen occasionally.

TREATMENT

The major aim of therapy is to alleviate signs and symptoms of hypocalcemia or, if possible, to prevent their appearance. There is no urgent need to treat the patient with mild hypocalcemia who is asymptomatic. Patients with marked hypocalcemia (less than 6.5 mg/dl) are a greater problem because symptoms can develop rapidly. Acute hypocalcemia is treated by the intravenous administration of calcium. As is true for infusion of any electrolyte solution, administration should be slow and deliberate. The goal of acute therapy is to control the signs and symptoms of hypocalcemia, not necessarily to normalize the serum calcium.

The chronic hypoparathyroid states require long-term therapy. Vitamin D and calcium are the mainstays of treatment. Theoretically, any of the preparations of vitamin D can be used to treat any of the chronic hypocalcemias. Knowledge of the state of vitamin D metabolism helps to adapt the treatment more specifically. Simple vitamin D deficiency is easily treated by providing enough vitamin D in the diet (400 to 1000 IU daily). For diseases of the gastrointestinal tract, larger amounts (50,000 IU twice weekly) are required. 25-Hydroxyvitamin D (25 to 50 μg daily) overcomes the initial hydroxylation defect in severe liver disease. The disorders associated with impaired conversion of 25-hydroxyvitamin D to 1,25-dihydroxyvitamin D (hypoparathyroidism, pseudohypoparathyroidism, renal disease, vitamin D–dependent rickets type I) can be treated with near physiologic doses of 1,25-dihydroxyvitamin (0.25 to 0.5 μg daily). If the parent form of vitamin D is used in these disorders associated with defective 1-hydroxylation of 25-hydroxyvitamin D, much larger amounts are required (50,000 to 100,000 units daily). The advantages of therapy with 1,25-dihydroxyvitamin D are the smaller required dose, its shorter half-life, and the fact that it does not appear to be stored in fat tissue. Thus, the unwanted complications of hypercalcemia and hypercalciuria are more readily reversible when 1,25-dihydroxyvitamin D is used.

If the diet does not contain at least 1 g of elemental calcium, patients require supplemental calcium in addition to vitamin D. The exact form of calcium salt is more a matter of convenience than effectiveness. Any preparation can provide enough supplemental calcium. The most convenient preparation to use is calcium carbonate because it contains a greater percentage of calcium (40%) than the citrate (21%), lactate (13%), gluconate (9%), or the glubionate (6.6%) forms. In older individuals, calcium citrate may be advantageous because it does not require gastric acid for efficient absorption. If achlorhydria or hypochlorhydria is present, calcium citrate should be considered.

REFERENCES

Albright F et al: Pseudohypoparathyroidism—an example of Seabright-Bantam syndrome. Endocrinology 3:922, 1942.

Aurbach GD et al: Parathyroid hormone, calcitonin, and the calciferols. In Wilson JD and Foster DW, editors: Williams textbook of endocrinology. Philadelphia, 1992, Saunders.

Chase LW, Melson GL, and Aurbach GD: Pseudohypoparathyroidism: defective excretion of 3′,5′-AMP in response to parathyroid hormone. J Clin Invest 48:1832, 1969.

Downs RW Jr: Hypocalcemia and hypoparathyroidism. In Bardin CW, editor: Current therapy in endocrinology and metabolism, ed 4. Philadelphia, 1990, BC Decker.

Downs RW and Levine MA: Hypoparathyroidism and other causes of hypocalcemia. In Becker KL, editor: Principles and practice of endocrinology and metabolism. Philadelphia, 1990, Lippincott.

Eastell R and Heath H III: The hypocalcemic states: their differential diagnosis and management. In Coe FL and Favus MJ, editors: Disorders of bone and mineral metabolism. New York, 1992, Raven Press.

Eisenbarth GS and Jackson RA: The immunoendocrinopathy syndromes. In Wilson JD and Foster DW, editors: Williams textbook of endocrinology. Philadelphia, 1992, Saunders.

Rude RK and Oldham SB: Magnesium metabolism. In Becker KL, editor: Principles and practice of endocrinology and metabolism. Philadelphia, 1990, Lippincott.

Stewart AF et al: Hypocalcemia due to calcium soap formation in a patient with a pancreatic fistula. N Engl J Med 315:496, 1986.

Tohme JF and Bilezikian JP: Hypocalcemic emergencies. Endocrinol Metab Clin North Am 1993 (in press).

CHAPTER

179 Disorders of Phosphate Homeostasis

Fuad N. Ziyadeh
Stanley Goldfarb

Phosphorus is among the most abundant constituents of all tissues and a major mineral component of bone. Almost all metabolic processes are critically dependent on phosphorus, particularly the provision of cellular energy in the form of adenosine triphosphate (ATP) and the phosphorylation of various enzymes such as protein kinases that express hormone action. In addition, phosphorus may influence the oxygen-carrying capacity of hemoglobin through regulation of 2,3-diphosphoglycerate (2,3-DPG) synthesis. Phosphorus is also an important constituent of membrane phospholipids that play an essential role in cell membrane integrity and in regulation of the phosphoinositide system, a critical regulatory system in cell homeostasis.

The total body content of phosphorus is about 1000 g, of which approximately 85% is in bone and most of the remainder is intracellular. Of the total plasma inorganic phosphorus, about 10% is protein-bound and about 5% is complexed. The remainder is in the form of orthophosphates. It has been customary to express concentrations in terms of elemental phosphorus but to refer to it as phosphate. The normal fasting serum phosphate in adults is 3.0 to 4.5 mg per deciliter. This value is higher in children and postmenopausal women. There is a diurnal variation of serum phosphate with a morning nadir. In addition, ingestion of carbohydrate lowers phosphate concentration by enhancing cellular uptake; ingestion of phosphate-rich food results in elevation of serum phosphate. Thus, it is important for the interpretation of serum and urinary levels that samples be obtained in the fasting state.

The average daily intake of phosphorus in the United States is about 1000 mg, mostly provided by dairy products, meats, eggs, and to a lesser extent, vegetables and grains. The mechanism of small intestinal absorption is complex, but the largest component is absorbed by passive diffusion. A smaller but significant component is absorbed actively under the influence of 1,25-hydroxycholecalciferol (1,25-DHCC). The net amount of phosphate that is absorbed from the gastrointestinal tract is approximately 600 to 700 mg per day. The gastrointestinal tract also secretes a relatively fixed amount of phosphate of about 200 mg per day. At steady state, adults must excrete in the urine an amount equal to net intestinal absorption every day to maintain normal external balance. This underscores the role of the kidney as the most important regulatory organ of serum phosphate and total body content of phosphorus.

Phosphate is freely filtered at the glomerulus. Approximately 80% of the filtered load is reabsorbed along the proximal tubule, 10% in the distal nephron, and the remainder appears in the final urine. Tubular phosphate transport is a result of a membrane carrier activated by cell sodium entry (sodium-phosphate cotransport) as well as the cellular use of phosphate in metabolic pathways. Parathyroid hormone (PTH) and dietary phosphate intake are the two most important regulators of urinary phosphate excretion. A rise in serum PTH depresses tubular reabsorption of phosphate by a process involving stimulation of proximal tubular cyclic AMP and phosphoinositide production, and leads to phosphaturia. Renal phosphate transport is also directly influenced by dietary intake of phosphate. If the diet is deficient in phosphate, normal individuals demonstrate an immediate and profound reduction in urinary phosphate excretion. The mechanism of this enhanced renal phosphate retention is unclear, but suppression of PTH secretion is not the primary factor. In experimental animals, the same acute response to reduction of dietary phosphate is observed despite PTH infusion or parathyroidectomy. Urinary phosphate excretion is also a function of the filtered load of phosphate, the product of serum phosphate, and the glomerular filtration rate (GFR). As the filtered load increases, the capacity to reabsorb phosphate increases until a maximum rate of transport for phosphate is reached. If the filtered phosphate load is above the maximum rate of transport for phosphate, urinary phosphate excretion is augmented; if the filtered load is below the maximum rate of transport, virtually no phosphate appears in the urine.

Movement of phosphorus between the extracellular and intracellular compartments (internal balance) occurs continuously, and enhanced shifts of phosphate between these compartments may produce marked changes in the serum phosphate concentration, which is discussed later.

HYPOPHOSPHATEMIA

Hypophosphatemia (see box, p. 1504) is defined as a low concentration of phosphate in the serum. Whether hypophosphatemia results in symptomatic and clinically important cellular phosphate depletion or not is a complex function of the level of cellular phosphate stores and the metabolic activity of the tissue, as discussed below. Hypophosphatemia may occur with or without a reduction in total body phosphate content, that is, phosphate depletion. Three major mechanisms may underlie hypophosphatemia: decreased intestinal absorption, enhanced urinary excretion,

Causes of hypophosphatemia

I. Decreased gastrointestinal absorption of phosphate
  - A. Starvation, malnutrition
  - B. Malabsorption
  - C. Phosphate-binding antacids

II. Increased renal excretion of phosphate
  - A. Primary hyperparathyroidism
  - B. Secondary hyperparathyroidism
  - C. Fanconi's syndrome
  - D. Familial hypophosphatemia
  - E. Oncogenic osteomalacia
  - F. Diuretic phase of acute tubular necrosis
  - G. Postrenal transplantation
  - H. Idiopathic hypercalciuria
  - I. Glycosuria
  - J. Acute volume expansion
  - K. Acetazolamide therapy

III. Enhanced cellular uptake
  - A. Glucose-insulin infusions
  - B. Catecholamine infusions
  - C. Respiratory alkalosis
  - D. Treatment of ketoacidosis
  - E. Recovery phase of malnutrition
  - F. Total parenteral nutrition
  - G. Hungry bone syndrome
  - H. Alcohol withdrawal
  - I. Fructose intolerance
  - J. Theophylline overdose
  - K. Severe hyperthermia

IV. Abnormalities in vitamin D metabolism*

*The predominant mechanism is secondary hyperparathyroidism but decreased intestinal absorption also contributes to hypophosphatemia.

and enhanced uptake of phosphate from the extracellular to the intracellular compartment or bone. At times, more than one mechanism may be involved in causing hypophosphatemia.

Etiology

Gastrointestinal causes. Since phosphate is ubiquitous in foods, hypophosphatemia secondary to a selective decrease in phosphate intake is unusual. The kidney responds to dietary restriction of phosphate almost immediately in such a way that urinary phosphate excretion falls within the first 24 hours (and probably within the first few hours) and negative phosphate balance is prevented. (The signal for this acute response is likely to be the acute fall in serum phosphate that results from dietary phosphate restriction.) However, since obligate intestinal secretion of phosphate persists, prolonged dietary phosphate deficiency may lead to phosphate depletion and a negative phosphate balance. Prolonged starvation can also lead to a negative phosphate balance, but the catabolic effects of a calorie-protein malnutrition result in increased breakdown of cells and release of large amounts of intracellular phosphate. This process may lead to normalization of serum phosphate and occasionally even to frank hyperphosphatemia despite severe total body phosphate depletion. An important cause of hypophosphatemia is the intake of large amounts of aluminum-, magnesium-, or calcium-containing antacids. In the intestinal lumen, these antacids bind both dietary and secreted phosphates and render them unabsorbable. Most syndromes of general intestinal fat malabsorption are also associated with hypophosphatemia. Although increased fecal excretion of phosphate does contribute to the negative phosphate balance, the predominant mechanism is the enhanced phosphaturia that develops as a result of secondary hyperparathyroidism (secondary to concomitant calcium and vitamin D malabsorption). Defects in gastrointestinal absorption of phosphate have also been noted in some patients with familial hypophosphatemic rickets and a subgroup of patients on maintenance hemodialysis.

Renal causes. Decreased renal tubular phosphate reabsorption is generally caused either by an intrinsic defect in tubular transport or, more commonly, by extrinsic factors that inhibit phosphate reabsorption. In all these disorders, the urine contains significant amounts of phosphate despite hypophosphatemia. Intrinsic tubular defects of phosphate transport may be a component of Fanconi's syndrome (glycosuria, generalized aminoaciduria, bicarbonaturia, uricosuria, and phosphaturia). Decreased renal tubular phosphate reabsorption is responsible for hypophosphatemia in familial hypophosphatemic rickets and oncogenic osteomalacia (see Chapter 182).

The most common cause of renal phosphate wasting is primary or secondary hyperparathyroidism (see Chapter 187). Other conditions associated with increased renal wasting of phosphate include the diuretic phase of acute tubular necrosis, postrenal transplantation, and idiopathic hypercalciuria. Hyperglycemia with glycosuria may promote renal phosphate excretion and contribute to phosphate depletion in uncontrolled diabetes. This effect may result from competition between glucose and phosphate for transport across the brush border of the proximal tubule. Acute volume expansion with saline, high-dose glucocorticoids, acetazolamide therapy, hyperthermia, and chronic metabolic acidosis are also known to promote urinary phosphate excretion.

Redistribution of phosphate. Increased cellular phosphate uptake may lead to various degrees of hypophosphatemia. In hospitalized patients, glucose infusions are the most common cause of hypophosphatemia. It is thought that glucose-induced insulin release promotes phosphate entry from the extracellular space into the cellular pool. Therapy of diabetic ketoacidosis can precipitate varying degrees of hypophosphatemia. Prior to therapy, patients with diabetic ketoacidosis may already be in marked negative phosphate balance because of glycosuria, metabolic acidosis, and poor intake of phosphate. However, serum phosphate is often normal, presumably as a result of the enhanced catabolic rate. On administration of large amounts of insulin, the serum phosphate level may rapidly fall, reaching between 1 and 2 mg per deciliter in the majority of patients within the first 24 to 48 hours. If insulin is administered at more physiologic rates, only mild reductions of serum phosphate are seen. During this time, urinary phosphate becomes very low, reflecting enhanced anabolism and insulin-stimulated tubular reabsorption of phosphate.

Acute respiratory alkalosis has been frequently associated with hypophosphatemia. However, experimental studies of this phenomenon were complicated by concurrent glucose infusions to the subjects; only mild hypophosphatemia develops in uncomplicated respiratory alkalosis in the absence of concomitant glucose infusions. The hypophosphatemia that develops in gram-negative septicemia and liver disease is presumably caused in part by respiratory alkalosis, but other factors may also be operative.

Stimulation of the beta-adrenergic system or catecholamine infusions may also be responsible for redistribution of phosphate from the extracellular to the intracellular compartment similar to the effects of insulin and respiratory alkalosis. Regimens of total parenteral nutrition that do not include phosphate may lead to profound hypophosphatemia. This effect may be caused in part by absence of phosphate supplementation, but the major cause of hypophosphatemia is the rapid cellular uptake of phosphate during refeeding. Rapid mineralization of bone after parathyroidectomy for primary hyperparathyroidism, after treatment of renal osteodystrophy by parathyroidectomy, or after renal transplantation may all be associated with severe hypophosphatemia, a situation often termed the *hungry bone syndrome*. Osteoblastic metastases, particularly in prostatic cancer, may have a similar effect whereby phosphate is taken up by bone from the extracellular space. Patients with rapidly growing malignancies such as Burkitt's lymphoma have recently been described in whom tumor uptake of phosphate has led to persistent hypophosphatemia. Eventual hyperphosphatemia occurred when tumor breakdown was induced by chemotherapy.

Several of the aforementioned mechanisms may be simultaneously present in the individual patient presenting with severe hypophosphatemia and phosphate depletion. Perhaps the most common clinical conditions are chronic alcoholism and alcohol withdrawal. Serum phosphate may be normal when patients are first admitted to the hospital but subsequently decline when withdrawal ensues and therapy is administered. Poor intake, malabsorption from concomitant pancreatic insufficiency, and increased urinary losses from the generalized catabolic state may all contribute to chronic phosphate depletion in alcoholic patients. On alcohol withdrawal, serum phosphate falls precipitously because of respiratory alkalosis, intravenous glucose infusions, refeeding, and therapy with oral antacids.

Patients with burn injury often develop hypophosphatemia, the lowest levels being reported on the fifth hospital day. Multiple causes are identified such as respiratory alkalosis, catecholamine release, total parenteral nutrition with rapid tissue deposition, and administration of large doses of antacids. Recent studies also suggest that hyperthermia-associated hypophosphatemia may be severe (serum PO_4 less than 1.0 mg/dl) and clinically important. Renewed interest in hyperthermia as an adjunctive therapy for treatment of malignancy makes this an important observation.

Clinical manifestations

Hypophosphatemia is commonly encountered in clinical practice. Approximately 2% of all patients admitted to a general hospital may have a serum phosphate level of less than 2 mg per deciliter. The incidence rises sharply in patients suffering from various debilitating illnesses such as malnutrition, malabsorption, alcoholism, burns, and sepsis. Glucose infusions and antacid ingestion, especially in the postsurgical patient, often result in further lowering of serum phosphate concentration.

Hypophosphatemia may or may not be associated with the syndrome of symptomatic phosphate depletion. Clinical manifestations may be totally absent in mild hypophosphatemia but may be life-threatening in prolonged severe hypophosphatemia (serum phosphate concentration less than 1 mg/dl). Significant complications of hypophosphatemia and phosphate depletion may involve many organic functions.

Two fundamental biochemical abnormalities may underlie the manifestations of hypophosphatemia: depletion of intracellular ATP and decreased levels of erythrocyte 2,3-DPG. These abnormalities may lead to organ dysfunction and tissue hypoxia. Typically, acute hypophosphatemia in a previously normal individual is not associated with any specific symptoms, since cellular stores are adequate to prevent critically low concentrations. If long-standing negative external phosphate balance has occurred and cell glycolysis and glycogen formation are then stimulated, for example by insulin, then critical cell phosphate deficits occur. ATP formation falls while use rises, and 2,3-DPG production falls. Enzymatic production of ATP and 2,3-DPG requires adequate cell inorganic phosphate.

Common symptoms of persistent hypophosphatemia include anorexia, dizziness, bone pain, paresthesias, proximal muscle weakness, and waddling gait. In general, neuromuscular symptoms predominate in acute hypophosphatemia, and skeletal symptoms in chronic hypophosphatemia. With extreme hypophosphatemia (serum phosphate level less than 0.5 mg/dl), an encephalopathy may develop with irritability, nervousness, dysarthria, confusion, stupor, seizures, and coma. In the alcoholic patient, these manifestations may mimic delirium tremens. Hallucinations, however, do not occur in hypophosphatemia. Skeletal muscle may be acutely affected by hypophosphatemia with resultant rhabdomyolysis. This entity is recognized by an abnormal elevation of creatinine phosphokinase and aldolase in serum. Alcoholics may be most vulnerable to development of rhabdomyolysis, especially during the first few days of hospitalization, when acute hypophosphatemia is superimposed on underlying chronic phosphate deficits.

Chronic hypophosphatemia is usually associated with musculoskeletal manifestations. Proximal muscle weakness and damage can develop, but the most serious consequence of this myopathy is respiratory muscle failure. Cardiac muscle may also be involved in severe hypophosphatemia, but frank congestive heart failure is rarely observed unless significant underlying myocardial disease is also present. A recent study has documented that acute, glucose-induced hypophosphatemia produces no detrimental effects on myocardial function in patients with no underlying heart disease.

Abnormalities in mineral metabolism are often noted in long-standing chronic hypophosphatemia. Rickets and osteomalacia develop as a result of impairment of osteoid mineralization. Bone pain, pathologic fractures, rheumatic complaints, and proximal muscle weakness are common features in adults with osteomalacia. Correction of phosphate deficiency results in striking bony healing.

Hypercalciuria is often associated with even mild degrees of hypophosphatemia and phosphate depletion. The major cause of hypercalciuria is a specific defect in calcium reabsorption in the distal nephron. Other mechanisms involved in the genesis of hypercalciuria include the direct stimulation of bone resorption by hypophosphatemia and the effect of hypophosphatemia to increase 1,25-DHCC. This compound stimulates both intestinal calcium absorption and bone resorption. All these effects tend to increase serum calcium and promote urinary losses of calcium. Interestingly, the syndrome of idiopathic hypercalciuria seen in approximately 50% of patients with calcium urolithiasis is often associated with a mild chronic hypophosphatemia and renal phosphate wasting.

Hematologic manifestations of hypophosphatemia involve disturbances in erythrocyte, leukocyte, and platelet functions. Since phosphate is a substrate for the generation of the high-energy phosphate bonds in ATP that are necessary for the initial phases of glycolysis, hypophosphatemia causes a reduction in red cell 2,3-DPG and a shift of the dissociation curve for oxyhemoglobin to the left. This results in decreased tissue delivery of oxygen and tissue hypoxia. In addition, hemolytic anemias may also be present because ATP deficiency produces enhanced membrane fragility and decreased erythrocyte survival. Hemolysis is rare unless profound degrees of hypophosphatemia develop (serum phosphate level less than 0.2 mg/dl). Depressed leukocyte phagocytic activity and migration may be observed in severe hypophosphatemia. This has been implicated as a contributory factor in the increased susceptibility to infection in critically ill patients. Defective aggregation and shortened survival of platelets have been observed in severe hypophosphatemia induced in laboratory animals. These defects were also implicated in specific bleeding abnormalities in a few patients.

Diagnostic approach

In the majority of patients with hypophosphatemia, the underlying cause is usually apparent from the history (Fig. 179-1). The most common causes of acute hypophosphatemia in hospitalized patients are glucose infusions and respiratory alkalosis. In other patients, additional diagnostic work-up may be required. The measurement of urinary phosphate can be helpful in many situations. Hypophosphatemia caused by deficient intake or antacid use leads to a marked decrease in urinary phosphate excretion (less than 100 mg/day). Inappropriately increased urinary phosphate excretion in the face of hypophosphatemia is usually caused by hyperparathyroidism or primary renal tubular defects. Measurement of serum calcium is very helpful in this setting. If serum calcium is high, primary hyperparathyroidism is the most likely diagnosis. If serum calcium is low, a form of secondary hyperparathyroidism is often present. Most patients with hypophosphatemia, hypocalcemia, and secondary hyperparathyroidism have a disorder in vitamin D metabolism such as occurs with poor nutritional intake, malabsorption, or postgastrectomy. When serum calcium and PTH are normal, hypophosphatemia associated with increased renal phosphate wasting denotes a defect in renal tubular function. The concomitant findings of bicarbonaturia, glycosuria, or aminoaciduria establish the diagnosis of Fanconi's syndrome. In the absence of these associated findings, however, the diagnosis is either familial hypophosphatemic rickets or oncogenic osteomalacia. The latter requires a careful search for an underlying neoplasm.

Prevention and treatment

In patients receiving total parenteral nutrition, prevention of hypophosphatemia can be achieved by supplementation with 10 to 15 mmol of potassium phosphate for every 1000 calories provided. Early resumption of oral feeding in the hospitalized patient and judicious use of antacids may decrease the incidence and severity of hypophosphatemia. In general, therapy for hypophosphatemia depends on its severity and acuteness, underlying causes, and the presence or absence of significant clinical symptoms of phosphate depletion. In most cases of mild to moderate acute hypophosphatemia (serum phosphate level of 1.5 to 2.5 mg/dl), especially in the absence of significant symptoms, parenteral therapy is not indicated. In fact, such therapy may be complicated by secondary hypocalcemia. Correction of the underlying disorder (e.g., glucose infusions, respiratory alkalosis, sepsis) and restoration of an adequate diet may be sufficient. Most patients with severe hypophosphatemia (serum phosphate level of less than 1 mg/dl) should be treated with adequate phosphate replacement therapy. Occasionally, such patients may be asymptomatic; hence, oral therapy is the preferred route of administration. Provision of milk (33 mmol PO_4/liter) or a balanced oral phosphate solution such as Fleet's Phospho-Soda (15 to 30 ml three to four times daily) or Neutra-Phos capsules (two capsules three times daily) is usually well tolerated. Higher doses may be associated with diarrhea. In the presence of severe symptoms or significant metabolic derangements, intravenous administration of phosphate salts at a dose of 0.08 to 0.16 mmol per kilogram over 6 hours is an effective and safe regimen. Frequent monitoring of serum phosphate and calcium to avoid hyperphosphatemia and hypocalcemia is necessary. The infusion should be stopped when serum phosphate rises above 1.5 mg per deciliter. Severe deficits may require larger doses in some patients, but this requirement cannot be predicted in any individual patient. In the presence of renal insufficiency, parenteral phosphate therapy should be used with extreme caution and with frequent monitoring of serum phosphate to avoid the rapid develop-

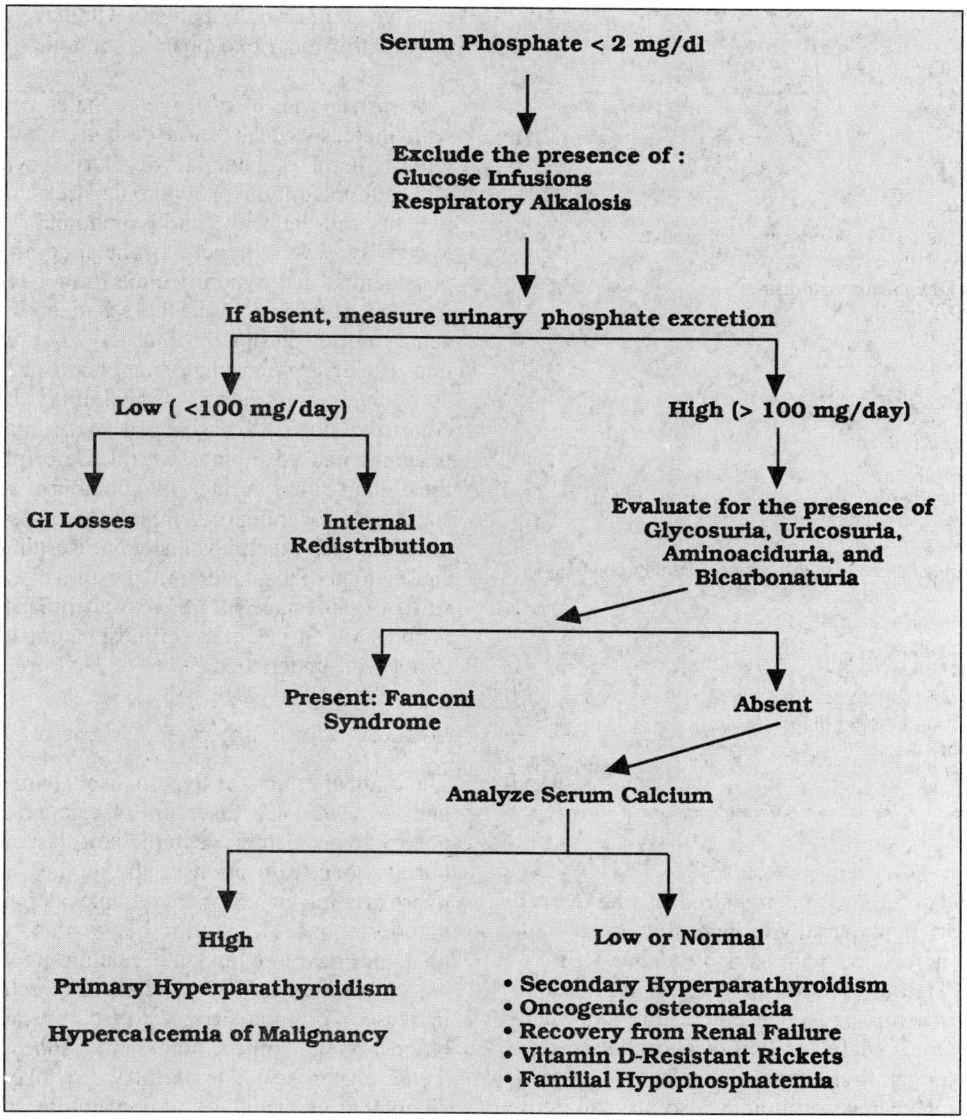

Fig. 179-1. Diagnostic work-up of hypophosphatemia.

ment of severe hyperphosphatemia. Treatment of hypophosphatemia in diabetic ketoacidosis has become popular, but its usefulness remains controversial. Hypophosphatemia may contribute to glucose intolerance and insulin resistance as well as to tissue hypoxia owing to decreases in erythrocyte 2,3-DPG. Recent clinical trials, however, did not show any evidence of significant clinical benefit from routine supplementation with phosphate, and many patients showed significant reduction in serum ionized calcium levels. Rarely, serum phosphate levels may fall below 1 mg per deciliter in patients treated for diabetic ketoacidosis; however, previous studies have not specifically addressed the benefits of phosphate treatment in this subgroup of patients. Chronic hypophosphatemia associated with renal phosphate wasting should be corrected by concomitant supplementation of oral phosphates (30 to 90 mmol/day) and a vitamin D metabolite to treat rickets or osteomalacia. In oncogenic osteomalacia, adequate excision of the underlying tumor (which is often a benign mesenchymal tumor) is curative. Hypophosphatemia of vitamin D deficiency may not require phosphate therapy; provision of adequate amounts of calcium and vitamin D is sufficient.

HYPERPHOSPHATEMIA

Hyperphosphatemia is frequently seen in clinical medicine practice. Three general mechanisms are responsible: massive intake of phosphate, impaired renal excretion resulting from renal failure or impaired PTH action on renal tubules, or enhanced release of phosphate from the intracellular to the extracellular compartment (see box, p. 1508).

Etiology

Renal causes. Renal failure is the most common form of hyperphosphatemia. With reduction of GFR below 30 ml

Causes of hyperphosphatemia

I. Renal causes
  A. Renal failure
    1. Acute
    2. Chronic
  B. Increased tubular reabsorption of phosphate
    1. Hypoparathyroidism
    2. Pseudohypoparathyroidism
    3. PTH suppression
    4. Acromegaly
    5. Thyrotoxicosis
    6. Bisphosphonate therapy
    7. Tumoral calcinosis
    8. Sickle cell anemia
II. Gastrointestinal causes
  A. Acute phosphate load
    1. Intravenous therapy
    2. Excess oral intake
  B. Surreptitious abuse of phosphate-containing laxatives
  C. Vitamin D overdose
III. Increased cellular release
  A. Rhabdomyolysis
  B. Tumor lysis syndrome
  C. Malignant hyperthermia
  D. Transfusion of stored blood
  E. Respiratory acidosis
  F. Lactic acidosis (?)

per minute, phosphate excretion is impaired despite marked degrees of secondary hyperparathyroidism. Acute renal failure is commonly associated with variable degrees of hyperphosphatemia. Trauma and rhabdomyolysis often lead to further elevations in serum phosphate concentration in acute renal failure. Impaired renal excretion of phosphate is uniformly seen in hypoparathyroidism and related disorders. Excess renal phosphate reabsorption is also seen in acromegaly and thyrotoxicosis because growth hormone, through increased insulin-like growth factor-1 (IGF-1) production, and thyroid hormone also elevate the maximum rate of transport for phosphate. Renal tubular phosphate reabsorption is also increased in sickle cell anemia, tumoral calcinosis, and treatment with some bisphosphonates. Tumoral calcinosis is a rare congenital disorder characterized by hyperphosphatemia, normocalcemia, normal PTH levels, and large calcified masses around large joints. The primary defect is an elevation in the maximum rate of transport/GFR for phosphate manifesting as increased tubular phosphate reabsorption (Chapter 360).

Gastrointestinal causes. Excess intake of phosphate may lead to transient hyperphosphatemia. Rapid increases in urinary phosphate excretion often normalize the serum phosphate level unless significant reductions in GFR are also present. Administration of phosphate-containing laxatives or enemas may lead to acute elevations in serum phosphate concentration in otherwise normal individuals, but this effect is more marked in patients with an atonic colon or ulcerative colitis, and in patients who have a concomitant impairment of renal phosphate excretion.

Redistribution of phosphate. States of rapid catabolism with increased destruction of body tissues are associated with hyperphosphatemia. Similarly, cytolysis associated with administration of cytotoxic drugs or radiotherapy to patients with leukemia and lymphomas is occasionally followed by severe hyperphosphatemia, hyperkalemia, hypocalcemia, and hyperuricemia (tumor-lysis syndrome).

Renal insufficiency in these patients is often caused by acute urate nephropathy, but may also result from deposition of calcium phosphate complexes in the kidney. Rhabdomyolysis after trauma, thermal injury, heat stroke, or narcotic overdose is associated with marked hyperphosphatemia caused by massive release of phosphate from intracellular sites. Acute myoglobinuric renal failure may supervene and impair renal phosphate excretion, further aggravating the hyperphosphatemia. Respiratory acidosis may cause hyperphosphatemia, presumably through cellular shifts of phosphate into the extracellular fluid. The mechanism involved in the hyperphosphatemia of lactic acidosis is not well understood.

Clinical manifestations

The clinical effects of hyperphosphatemia are primarily related to associated disorders of calcium metabolism. Secondary hypocalcemia, ectopic soft tissue calcifications, reduced bone resorption, and suppression of renal 1α-hydroxylation of 25-hydroxycholecalciferol are prominent manifestations. It seems likely that when hyperphosphatemia develops and the calcium-phosphate product in the serum exceeds 70, the chances of ectopic calcifications increase. Common sites of soft tissue calcification include blood vessels, cornea, lung, skin, kidney, and periarticular areas. Hyperphosphatemia may also play a role in the development of secondary hyperparathyroidism of renal failure. Moreover, the severity of renal osteodystrophy correlates well with the severity of hyperphosphatemia in chronic renal failure. It is also possible that uncontrolled calcium-phosphate deposition in the kidney may contribute to the inexorable progression of renal injury in chronic renal failure.

Diagnostic approach

In most situations, the cause of hyperphosphatemia is easily identified from examining the clinical situation. A reduction in the GFR below 30 ml per minute is the most common cause. The serum level of phosphate rarely exceeds 12 mg per deciliter even if severe renal failure supervenes, unless excessive amounts of phosphate are added to the circulation. Surreptitious abuse of phosphate-containing laxatives may pose some difficulty in diagnosis. In other conditions associated with hyperphosphatemia, measurements of urinary excretion of phosphate are helpful in making a diagnosis. Twenty-four-hour urinary excretion of phosphate is elevated (above 1000 mg/day) in association with excess phosphate loads and is depressed and reflects intake if the individual is in external balance (often below 1000 mg/day) in situations characterized by enhanced renal tubular reabsorption. In the latter disorders, determinations of serum calcium and PTH offer helpful clues to the underlying process. Serum PTH is low in idiopathic or postsurgical hypoparathyroidism but is elevated in pseudohypoparathyroidism or in secondary hyperparathyroidism, whereas serum calcium is often low in these conditions.

Treatment

Acute severe hyperphosphatemia with symptomatic hypocalcemia requires prompt treatment. If renal failure is not present, urinary phosphate excretion can be increased with the use of isotonic saline or sodium bicarbonate, 1 to 2 liters over 2 hours, and acetazolamide, 500 mg every 6 hours. When renal failure is present, institution of hemodialysis can promptly remove substantial amounts of phosphate and correct the hyperphosphatemia and the hypocalcemia. When very rapid control is required, glucose and insulin infusions promote cell phosphate uptake and may ameliorate hyperphosphatemia until dialysis is begun. The chronic hyperphosphatemia seen in chronic renal failure, hypoparathyroidism, or tumoral calcinosis is treated primarily by a low-phosphate diet and calcium-containing antacids.

REFERENCES

Agus ZS: Oncogenic hypophosphatemic osteomalacia. Kidney Int 24:113, 1983.

Agus ZS, Goldfarb S, and Wasserstein A: Disorders of calcium and phosphate balance. In Brenner BM and Rector FC, editors: The kidney, ed 2. Philadelphia, 1981, Saunders.

Delmez JA and Slatopolsky E: Hyperphosphatemia: its consequences and treatment in patients with chronic renal failure. Kidney Int 29:303, 1992.

Fisher NJ and Kitabachi AE: A randomized study of phosphate therapy in the treatment of diabetic ketoacidosis. J Clin Endocrinol Metab 57:177, 1983.

Gravelyn TR et al: Hypophosphatemia-associated respiratory muscle weakness in a general inpatient population. Am J Med 84:870, 1988.

Halevy I and Bulvik S: Severe hypophosphatemia in hospitalized patients. Arch Intern Med 148:153, 1988.

Knochel JP: Hypophosphatemia in the alcoholic. Arch Intern Med 140:613, 1980.

Lentz RD, Brown DM, and Kjellstrand CMM: Treatment of severe hypophosphatemia. Ann Intern Med 82:941, 1978.

Ritz E: Acute hypophosphatemia. Kidney Int 22:84, 1982.

Rubin M and Narins RG: Hypophosphatemia: pathophysiological and practical aspects of therapy. Semin Nephrol 10:536, 1990.

Ryan EA and Reiss E: Oncogenous osteomalacia. Review of the world literature of 42 cases and report of two new cases. Am J Med 77:501, 1984.

Shilo S, Werner P, and Hershko G: Acute hemolytic anemia caused by severe hypophosphatemia in diabetic ketoacidosis. Acta Haematol (Basel) 73:s5, 1985.

Wilson HK et al: Phosphate therapy in diabetic ketoacidosis. Arch Intern Med 142:517, 1982.

CHAPTER

180 Disorders of Magnesium Homeostasis

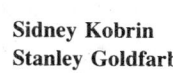

Sidney Kobrin
Stanley Goldfarb

The total body magnesium content is approximately 25 mEq per kilogram. (One mmol of magnesium is synonymous with 2 mEq and 24 mg.) Of this only about 1% is extracellular, giving a normal plasma magnesium concentration of between 0.75 and 1.0 mmol per liter. Magnesium is the second most abundant intracellular ion. About 20% to 30% of plasma magnesium is protein-bound, mainly to albumin. The rest exists in free ionized form or in complexes. In clinical practice, corrections of plasma magnesium concentrations are not made for alterations in protein (albumin) concentration, and no routine method exists for determining ionized magnesium concentration.

The bulk of total body magnesium is distributed between bone (approximately two thirds) and the intracellular compartment (approximately one third), primarily muscle. Bone magnesium is not readily available for defense against hypomagnesemia. In chronic magnesium depletion states, it is the skeletal pool that is most consistently diminished and is the most useful guide to total body magnesium stores.

NORMAL MAGNESIUM METABOLISM

Intestinal magnesium handling

The Food and Nutrition Board of the National Academy of Sciences recommends a daily dietary intake of 12 to 14 mmol of magnesium. This requirement may increase during pregnancy, lactation, and adolescence. The average American diet contains approximately 10 to 15 mmol/day, which is very close to the recommended amount. This suggests that magnesium deficiency may develop if dietary intake or intestinal absorption is modestly decreased or magnesium losses are slightly greater than normal. Gastrointestinal absorption of magnesium varies depending on the amount ingested. When dietary magnesium intake is typical (12 mmol/day), 30% to 40% of ingested magnesium is absorbed (Fig. 180-1). Under conditions of low magnesium intake (1 mmol/day), approximately 80% is absorbed, while only 25% is absorbed when magnesium intake is high (25 mmol/day). Presumably, only ionized magnesium is available for transport. Increased luminal phosphate or fat may precipitate with magnesium, decrease the amount of available ionized magnesium, and reduce intestinal magnesium absorption.

Although somewhat controversial, the majority of evidence suggests that two additional factors may play a role in the regulation of intestinal magnesium absorption. Vitamin D ($1,25[OH]_2D_3$) directly increases intestinal magnesium absorption, while parathyroid hormone probably in-

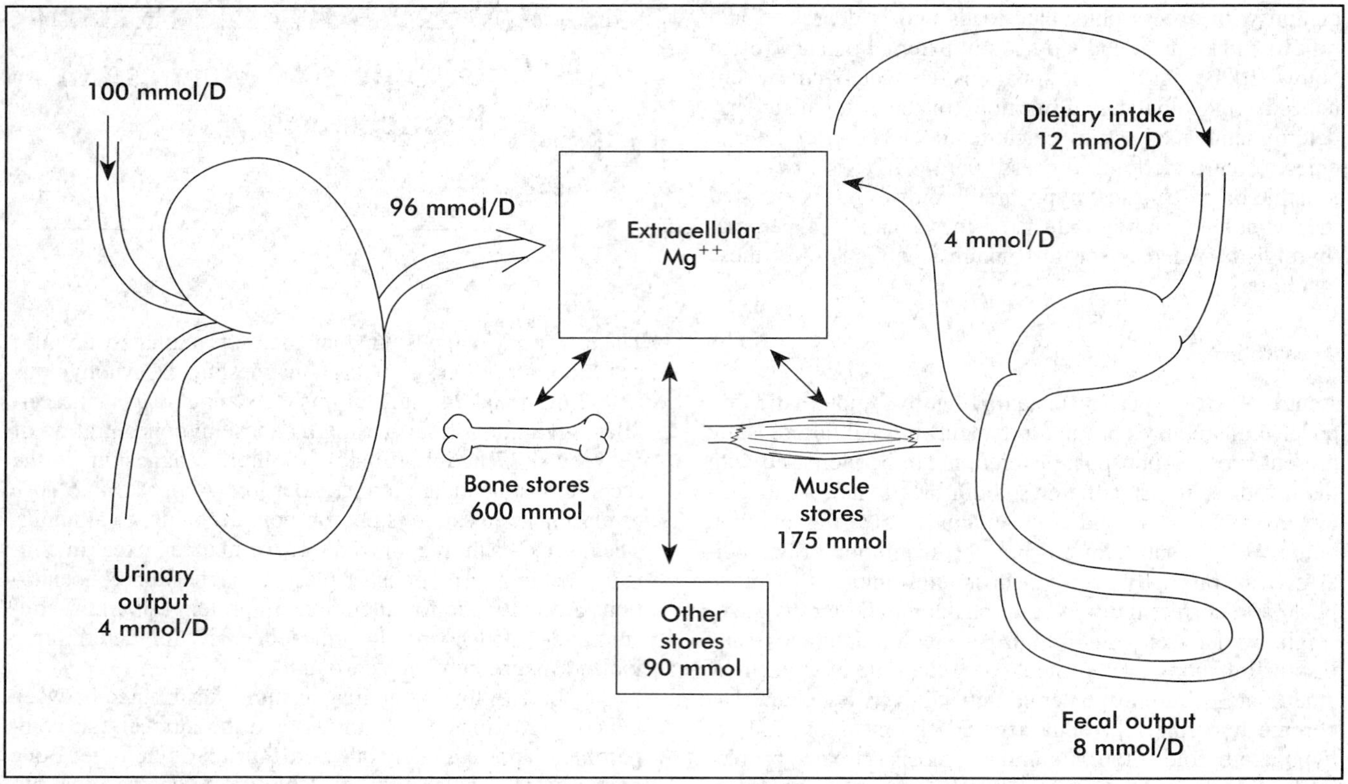

Fig. 180-1. Distribution of magnesium in the body and daily fluxes of magnesium between diet, GI tract, kidney, and various body pools.

creases magnesium absorption indirectly by increasing $1,25(OH)_2D_3$ synthesis.

Since magnesium absorption and secretion by the gastrointestinal tract are largely unregulated and little shift occurs in the various pools of magnesium on a day-to-day basis, the kidney serves as the major regulator of magnesium balance. Under normal conditions the non-protein-bound plasma magnesium is freely filtered at the glomerulus. About 20% to 30% of filtered magnesium is reabsorbed in the proximal tubule, and the major portion (60% to 65% of filtered load) is absorbed in Henle's loop. The distal nephron absorbs about 5% of magnesium, leaving about 5% of filtered load to be excreted in the urine. Both sodium loading and calcium loading decrease magnesium reabsorption in Henle's loop, thereby enhancing magnesium excretion. Parathyroid hormone may directly increase magnesium reabsorption in Henle's loop, opposing the indirect decrease in reabsorption as a result of hypercalcemia. An important factor regulating renal magnesium excretion is plasma magnesium level. Magnesium infusions and/or hypermagnesemia lead to prompt increases in urinary magnesium excretion, even in patients previously magnesium-depleted.

MAGNESIUM DEFICIENCY AND HYPOMAGNESEMIA

The plasma magnesium level may not be a reliable indicator of total body magnesium stores. However, except in a few clinical situations, persistent hypomagnesemia represents total body magnesium deficiency. Isolated primary magnesium deficiency as a result of dietary deficiency is extremely uncommon because of the ubiquity of magnesium in all foods and renal magnesium conservation. Therefore, magnesium deficiency usually occurs in the setting of large losses from the gastrointestinal tract or the kidney. The causes of hypomagnesemia are listed in the box on the right.

Etiology

Internal redistribution. Acute decreases in serum magnesium may occur with normal total body levels. Such redistribution may be seen with large infusions of intravenous glucose and during refeeding in children with protein-calorie malnutrition. Redistribution has also been reported with insulin therapy of diabetic ketoacidosis, during acute alcohol withdrawal, and in association with acute respiratory alkalosis. In acute pancreatitis, formation of magnesium-soap complexes has been postulated as contributing to hypomagnesemia. After parathyroidectomy for hyperparathyroidism, a significant decrease in serum magnesium may be seen in association with hypocalcemia and hypophosphatemia as part of the "hungry bone syndrome."

Gastrointestinal causes. During prolonged starvation, magnesium depletion may be seen as a consequence of de-

Causes of magnesium deficiency

Redistribution
Insulin administration
Hungry bone syndrome
Catecholamine excess states
(?) Acute respiratory alkalosis
Acute pancreatitis
Miscellaneous
  Excessive lactation and sweating

Gastrointestinal causes
Reduced intake
  Starvation
  Postoperative
Reduced absorption
  Specific magnesium malabsorption
  Generalized malabsorption syndrome
  Extensive bowel resections
  Diffuse bowel disease or injury
  Chronic diarrhea, laxative abuse

Renal causes
Primary tubular disorders
  Primary renal magnesium wasting
  Welt's syndrome
  Bartter's syndrome
  Renal tubular acidosis
  Diuretic phase of acute tubular necrosis
  Postobstructive diuresis
  Post–renal transplantation status
Extrarenal factors that increase magnesuria
  Drug-induced losses
    Diuretics, aminoglycosides, digoxin, *cis*-platinum, and cyclosporine
  Hormone-induced magnesuria
    Aldosteronism, hypoparathyroidism, hyperthyroidism
  Ion- or nutrient-induced tubular losses
    Hypercalcemia
    Extracellular fluid volume expansion
    Glucose, urea, mannitol diuresis
  Phosphate depletion
  Alcohol ingestion

Complex causes
Alcoholism
Diabetic ketoacidosis

creased intake and persistent renal losses caused by associated ketoacidosis. Magnesium deficiency is more readily seen in a variety of intestinal conditions associated with markedly diminished absorption and/or enhanced secretion. These include inflammatory bowel diseases such as ulcerative colitis and regional enteritis, extensive resections of small bowel, particularly involving the terminal ileum, and other conditions associated with generalized malabsorption. Formation of poorly soluble magnesium complexes with fat diminishes intestinal magnesium absorption. A rare syndrome of primary intestinal malabsorption of magnesium exists and is usually seen in association with hypocalcemia and seizures early in infancy. Large losses of magnesium may be associated with prolonged upper or lower intestinal fluid losses. The concentrations of magnesium in upper gastrointestinal (bile, gastric, pancreatic) fluid range between 0.2 and 0.5 mmol per liter. In the lower gastrointestinal tract, the magnesium concentration may be as high as 7 mmol per liter.

Renal losses. Urinary losses are usually reduced to less than 1 mEq per day shortly after institution of a magnesium-deficient diet. This efficient conservation may be diminished in the presence of various intrinsic or extrinsic renal disorders. These include the recovery phase of acute tubular necrosis, postobstructive diuresis, and postrenal transplantation. Renal tubular acidosis and Bartter's syndrome may also be associated with renal magnesium wasting. The associated potassium depletion and/or hyperaldosteronism in several of these states may contribute to impaired tubular reabsorption of magnesium. A primary renal magnesium-wasting syndrome exists in association with hypokalemia and nephrocalcinosis.

Use of drugs, particularly loop diuretics (furosemide, bumetanide, and ethacrynic acid), constitutes the largest single cause of renal magnesium wasting. These diuretics cause a greater fractional inhibition of magnesium than of sodium reabsorption in Henle's loop. Thiazides cause a much smaller increase in magnesium excretion. Multiple courses of high-dose aminoglycoside therapy have resulted in a tubulopathy characterized by hypomagnesemia, increased urinary potassium losses, hypokalemia, and hypocalcemia. *Cis*-platinum treatment for malignancy has been associated with a high frequency of hypermagnesuria and hypomagnesemia. The mechanism of the renal magnesium wasting has not been elucidated, although it probably results from damage to the ascending limb of Henle's loop.

Plasma volume expansion and osmotic diuresis induced with glucose, mannitol, or urea cause large renal losses of magnesium. Phosphate depletion has been associated with diminished tubular reabsorption of magnesium. Calcium loading and a variety of causes of hypercalcemia are associated with renal magnesium wasting and hypomagnesemia. The mechanism in each of these conditions is related to an inhibitory action on magnesium reabsorption in Henle's loop. The effect of alcohol is discussed below. Organic acidoses (lactic and ketoacids) are associated with increased renal magnesium losses.

The major effects of hormones on magnesium balance may be indirect. Thus, although parathyroid hormone enhances renal magnesium absorption, hyperparathyroidism may be associated with magnesuria because of the more potent counteracting effect of hypercalcemia on magnesium transport in the ascending limb of Henle's loop. Hypomagnesemia in hyperaldosteronism may be related to volume expansion and/or potassium depletion, although the possibility of a direct alteration of aldosterone on magnesium absorption has not been eliminated.

Complex causes

Alcoholism. Alcoholism is the clinical condition in which hypomagnesemia is seen most frequently. Multiple factors may contribute to the magnesium deficiency with or without hypomagnesemia in alcoholic patients. Poor nutrient intake in combination with increased losses from bouts of diarrhea produce external losses. Renal conservation may be impaired by associated starvation ketoacidosis. Acute ethanol administration also increases urinary magnesium excretion by a direct tubular effect. During acute illness, acute withdrawal from alcohol, acute respiratory alkalosis, and intravenous glucose administration may all cause intracellular shifts of magnesium with hypomagnesemia. Lastly, acute pancreatitis may cause further internal redistribution and hypomagnesemia. Other associated electrolyte disorders, for example, hypocalcemia and hypokalemia, may contribute to significant neuromuscular symptoms in the alcoholic patient.

Diabetic ketoacidosis. Hypomagnesemia develops in 7% of patients presenting with severe diabetic ketoacidosis. Renal magnesium wasting occurs because of the osmotic diuresis induced by hyperglycemia, ketoaciduria, and the catabolic effect of insulin deficiency, which leads to breakdown of intracellular organic compounds and release of magnesium from cells. During therapy, the anabolic effects of insulin drive magnesium back into cells and 50% to 60% of patients become transiently hypomagnesemic after 12 hours of treatment.

CLINICAL CONSEQUENCES OF MAGNESIUM DEFICIENCY

Whether the clinical effects of hypomagnesemia reflect total body deficiency or the low serum level is not well established. Clinical effects have been seen in acute hypomagnesemic states presumably not associated with total body magnesium deficiency, and magnesium administration may improve some clinical neuromuscular symptoms even in the absence of hypomagnesemia. Clinical interpretation of these effects is usually confounded by other coexisting electrolyte disturbances, mainly hypocalcemia and hypokalemia. The clinical spectrum of the consequences of magnesium deficiency are listed in the box on the right.

Clinical manifestations of magnesium deficiency

Definitely associated with magnesium deficiency

Metabolic

Refractory hypocalcemia responsive only to magnesium therapy

Refractory hypokalemia responsive only to magnesium therapy

Cardiovascular

Increased susceptibility to digoxin-related arrhythmias

Peripheral nervous system

Tremor of extremities and tongue

Myoclonic jerks

Chvostek's sign (common)

Trousseau's sign (rarely)

Tetany (rarely unless concomitant hypocalcemia)

General muscular weakness (particularly respiratory muscles)

Paresthesias

Central nervous system

Apathy, depression

Some or all facets of delirium, seizures

Coma, vertigo, nystagmus, and (rarely) movement disorders

Probably associated with magnesium deficiency

Cardiovascular

Ventricular arrhythmias: premature ventricular contractions, ventricular tachycardia, torsades de pointes

Ventricular fibrillation

Atrial arrhythmias (rare): atrial fibrillation and atrial tachycardia

Hypertension

Coronary artery spasm

Sudden death

Miscellaneous

Increased urolithiasis

Hemolysis

Gastrointestinal: esophageal spasm, anorexia, nausea, and adynamic ileus

Osteomalacia

Biochemical effects

Various plasma and total body electrolyte abnormalities are seen frequently with magnesium deficiency states. In experimental magnesium deficiency, hypokalemia and increased urinary potassium excretion occur. When hypokalemia coexists with hypomagnesemia, it is relatively refractory to potassium infusion unless the magnesium deficiency state is corrected. It is unclear whether the defect reflects primary renal tubular losses or alterations at the cellular membrane level leading to net cellular losses of potassium.

Hypocalcemia is also frequently seen in hypomagnesemic states. This may be related to decreased parathyroid hormone levels through a direct failure of secretion in the parathyroid gland or diminished bone response to the hormone in the presence of hypomagnesemia. Vitamin D fails to correct the hypocalcemia. Associated hypocalciuria and positive calcium balance suggest that decreased skeletal release is the predominant cause of the hypocalcemia.

Neuromuscular effects

The neuromuscular effects of hypomagnesemia occur commonly in association with hypocalcemia and/or hypokalemia. However, the symptoms and signs may be seen in the absence of any other electrolyte abnormalities. Moreover, when hypomagnesemia and hypocalcemia coexist in the face of neuromuscular symptoms, infusion of magnesium, but not calcium alone, may reverse the effects.

Cardiac effects

Arrhythmias are the most serious complications of magnesium deficiency. They frequently occur in association with digitalis therapy and/or hypokalemia. Even in the absence of other associated conditions, hypomagnesemia may predispose to arrhythmias. Atrial premature contractions and sinus or nodal tachycardia may occur. The PR and QT intervals may be prolonged, and flattening of T waves may be seen. Ventricular premature contractions and, in extreme cases, ventricular tachycardia and fibrillation may be caused by magnesium deficiency. Treatment with antiarrhythmic drugs may be ineffective unless magnesium deficiency is corrected. In some situations, magnesium infusions alone have abolished ventricular premature contractions.

Magnesium deficiency and cardiac glycosides interact to maximize cardiac toxicity. Magnesium deficiency increases the uptake of digoxin by myocardial cells, and both magnesium deficiency and cardiac glycosides decrease the activity of the sodium-potassium ATPase pump and may cause a reduction in intracellular potassium content.

ASSESSMENT OF MAGNESIUM STATUS

The majority of patients with clinical manifestations of magnesium deficiency have hypomagnesemia. Measurement of the serum magnesium concentration is relatively easy and has become the method of choice for estimating body magnesium content, although there are limitations on its use in evaluating total body magnesium stores. The normal serum magnesium concentration in humans is 0.9 ± 0.07 mmol/L. Symptoms of magnesium deficiency are generally not seen unless serum values are 0.25 to 0.35 mmol below the normal value.

There are two caveats to be considered when serum magnesium is used to diagnose magnesium deficiency. First, most methods of serum magnesium determination measure total magnesium concentration, while only free magnesium is biologically active. Because 25% to 30% of serum magnesium is bound to albumin and therefore inactive, measuring total serum magnesium may provide a spuriously low value in hypoalbuminemic states. Knoll et al have reported a formula to correct serum magnesium for hypoalbuminemia:

$$\text{Corrected serum } Mg^{++} \text{ (mmol/L)} = \text{measured total serum } Mg^{++} \text{ (mmol/L)} + .005\ (40 - \text{albumin g/L})$$

Serum contains only 0.3% of total body magnesium and may not always accurately reflect the intracellular magnesium status. It is possible for patients to be normomagnesemic but be depleted of intracellular magnesium and exhibit clinical manifestations of magnesium deficiency. Unfortunately, there is no quick, simple, and accurate test to measure intracellular magnesium concentration.

A surrogate for direct intracellular magnesium concentration is the measurement of magnesium retention after acute magnesium loading. Patients undergoing this test should not be receiving medication that affects renal excretion of magnesium. This method is useful only when there is a strong clinical suspicion of magnesium deficiency in the setting of normomagnesemia (e.g., unexplained electrocardiographic and neuromuscular disorders). Individuals with a deficit of magnesium retain a significant fraction of the injected magnesium. The method described by Bohmer et al is widely used in this regard.

The first step is to collect a 24-hour urine specimen and measure the magnesium content. If the content is less than 1 mmol/day, the magnesium load is administered. Thirty millimoles of magnesium sulfate are infused intravenously in 0.5 liters of 5% dextrose water over 8 to 12 hours. Once this infusion is initiated, a second 24-hour urine specimen should be collected and the magnesium content determined. Patients excreting less than 50% of the administered load are total body magnesium–deficient, while those with normal total body magnesium stores excrete more than 60% of the administered load. This test should be performed with great caution in patients with renal failure and cardiac conduction disturbances.

TREATMENT

Therapy depends on the severity of the hypomagnesemia and the associated clinical conditions. With mild hypomagnesemia and in the absence of severe clinical symptoms or signs, no specific treatment other than institution of a normal diet is required. When malabsorption is present, decrease in dietary fat intake may improve magnesium absorption. With severe deficits, supplemental oral and parenteral magnesium are needed. Renal reabsorption is complete only when hypomagnesemia is present; acute infusions transiently raise serum magnesium, and up to 50% of the replacement dose. The presence of renal insufficiency requires a reduction in the replacement dose as well as very close observation of serum levels and deep tendon reflexes. Several different oral salts are available. At high doses they induce catharsis. In general, the replacement dose should be less than that needed to induce diarrhea. Magnesium gluconate is well tolerated, but it provides less elemental magnesium per gram consumed than other salts. Magnesium oxide is also well tolerated and may be given in doses of 250 to 500 mg (6.25 to 12.5 mmol magnesium) four times daily, with up to 25% to 50% absorption.

In the presence of severe deficits (usually equal to 37.5 to 50 mmol), major neuromuscular or cardiac findings, or large gastrointestinal losses, parenteral administration is required. Magnesium sulfate is available in a 50% solution in 2-ml ampules (4.06 mmol). Twelve milliliters (24.5 mmol) may be diluted in a liter of 5% dextrose solution and infused over a 3 hour period. Another 40 mmol may be infused in 2 liters for the remainder of the first 24 hour period, and thereafter 24.5 mmol per day is given over the next 3 to 4 days. In patients who cannot tolerate the excess volume, the 50% magnesium sulfate solution may be given intramuscularly in divided doses. The intramuscular injection is usually painful. It is to be stressed that the presence of renal insufficiency of any degree requires significant reduction in dose. Serum level should be kept between 1.0 and 1.25 mmol per liter during replacement. When hypokalemia or hypocalcemia coexists with hypomagnesemia, the magnesium deficits must be corrected before adequate potassium or calcium replacement can be achieved.

HYPERMAGNESEMIA

Hypermagnesemia is an uncommon clinical disorder in the absence of renal insufficiency. In a normal individual up to 80% of an exogenous load is excreted by the kidney. As glomerular filtration falls, the fractional excretion of magnesium per nephron rises. Normal magnesium balance may be maintained until the glomerular filtration rate falls below about 30 ml per minute.

The causes of hypermagnesemia are listed in the box below. They may be subdivided into endogenous and exogenous sources and appear almost invariably in association with acute or chronic impairment in renal function. Decreased renal excretion may be seen with hyperparathyroidism, hypothyroidism, adrenal insufficiency, and lithium intoxication. In hyperparathyroidism the direct tubular effect of parathyroid hormone is usually counteracted by the magnesuric effect of hypercalcemia. Familial hypocalciuric hypercalcemia is characterized by a high serum magnesium level, in contrast to primary hyperparathyroidism.

Causes

Exogenous loads. Magnesium-containing antacids and enemas given in the presence of moderate to severe impairment in renal function represent the typical setting for hypermagnesemia. Large amounts of magnesium may be absorbed from colonic enemas. Though vitamin D normally plays no major role in magnesium metabolism, large doses of the active metabolites given in chronic renal failure may increase absorption of magnesium. Not infrequently, mild to moderate or even severe hypermagnesemia may be seen during therapy of toxemia of pregnancy, when large doses of intravenous magnesium sulfate are used. Neonatal as well as maternal hypermagnesemia may occur.

Clinical consequences

Clinical effects are usually not seen until the serum magnesium level exceeds 4 mEq per liter. The major effects are inhibition of neuromuscular transmission and cardiac electrical conduction. With a serum magnesium level of more than 4 mEq per liter, deep tendon reflexes are abolished. Lethargy is seen at levels approaching 7 mEq per liter. Paralysis of voluntary muscles and respiratory failure may occur at levels of 10 mEq per liter. Cardiovascular effects include hypotension and prolongation of the PR and QT intervals as well as QRS duration at levels of 5 to 10 mEq per liter. At levels of 15 mEq per liter, complete heart block or asystole may occur.

Moderate acute hypermagnesemia after parenteral infusions may cause hypocalcemia. The mechanism of this has recently been investigated in pregnant women receiving magnesium and is the result of direct suppression of parathyroid hormone secretion. Renal phosphate excretion may be reduced, and mild hyperphosphatemia may be seen, probably as a consequence of decreased parathyroid hormone levels.

Causes of hypermagnesemia

- I. Decreased renal excretion
  - A. Renal failure—glomerular filtration rate less than 30 ml/min
  - B. Hyperparathyroidism
  - C. Hypothyroidism
  - D. Addison's disease
  - E. Lithium intoxication
  - F. Familial hypocalciuric hypercalcemia
- II. Other causes: usually in association with decrease in glomerular filtration rate
  - A. Endogenous loads
    - 1. Diabetic ketoacidosis
    - 2. Severe tissue injury—burns
  - B. Exogenous loads
    - 1. Gastrointestinal
      - a. Magnesium-containing laxatives and antacids
      - b. High-dose vitamin D analogs
    - 2. Parenteral: management of toxemia of pregnancy

Treatment

Mild hypermagnesemia without major neuromuscular or cardiac disturbance requires no specific therapy other than withdrawal of magnesium-containing salts. During treatment with large doses of magnesium-containing salts, deep tendon reflexes should be monitored closely. If they are absent, magnesium administration should be withheld. Magnesium-containing antacids and enemas should be avoided in patients with chronic renal failure.

When severe hypermagnesemia exists with neuromuscular and/or cardiac depression, ventilatory assistance and cardiac electrical pacing may be required. Intravenous calcium acutely antagonizes the inhibitory effects of magnesium. Calcium gluconate or calcium chloride may be infused over a 5 minute period in a dose calculated to give 100 to 200 mg of elemental calcium. Intravenous glucose and insulin may be given to shift magnesium transiently into cells. Definitive therapy with hemodialysis is necessary.

REFERENCES

Agus ZS, Wasserstein A, and Goldfarb S: Disorders of calcium and magnesium homeostasis. Am J Med 72:473, 1982.

Aikawa JK: Biochemistry and physiology of magnesium. World Rev Nutr Diet 28:112, 1978.

Aurbach GD, Marx SJ, and Spiegel AM: Calcium homeostasis. In Wilson JD and Foster DW, editors: Textbook of endocrinology. Philadelphia, 1985, Saunders.

Bar RS, Wilson HE, and Mazzaferri EL: Hypomagnesemic hypocalcemia secondary to renal magnesium wasting: a possible consequence of high-dose gentamicin therapy. Ann Intern Med 82:646, 1975.

Cohen LF et al: Acute tumor lysis syndrome: a review of 37 patients with Burkitt's lymphoma. Am J Med 68:486, 1980.

Elin RJ: Magnesium metabolism in health and disease. DM 34:161, 1988.

Gonin RE and Knochel JP: Magnesium deficiency. Adv Intern Med 28:509, 1983.

Iseri LT, Freed J, and Barres AR: Magnesium deficiency and cardiac disorders. Am J Med 58:837, 1975.

Kobrin S and Goldfarb S: Magnesium deficiency. Semin Nephrol 10:525, 1990.

Massry SG: Pharmacology of magnesium. Ann Rev Pharmacol Toxicol 17:67, 1977.

Parfitt AM and Kleerekoper M: Clinical disorders of calcium, phosphorus, and magnesium metabolism. In Maxwell MH and Kleeman CR, editors: Clinical disorders of fluid and electrolyte metabolism, ed 3. New York, 1980, McGraw-Hill.

Rude RK and Singer FR: Magnesium deficiency and excess. Annu Rev Med 32:245, 1981.
Seller RH et al: Digitalis toxicity and hypomagnesemia. Am Heart J 79:57, 1970.
Shils ME: Experimental human magnesium depletion. Medicine (Baltimore) 48:61, 1969.

CHAPTER

181 Osteoporosis

Lawrence G. Raisz

Osteoporosis is by far the most common metabolic disorder of bone but is probably the least well understood. *Osteoporosis* can be defined as a disorder in which decreased bone mass and strength lead to an increased incidence of fractures with minimal or no trauma. The bone may show disordered architecture, but it is fully mineralized. Thus osteoporosis is distinguished from osteomalacia, in which mineralization is impaired. There is considerable disagreement as to whether osteoporosis should be diagnosed in individuals who clearly have decreased bone mass but have not yet developed a fracture. The term *osteopenia* has been used for these individuals as well as *asymptomatic osteoporosis*. *Osteopenia* has also been used as a nonspecific term for patients with functionally decreased bone mass before a diagnosis has been made to emphasize the need for differential diagnosis. Although age-related osteoporosis is by far the most common form of the disease, it is important to recognize atypical and secondary forms as well as diseases that can mimic or aggravate osteoporosis because there is specific and effective treatment for many of these disorders (see box on the right).

Classification of osteoporosis and related disorders

- Primary osteoporosis
  - Postmenopausal osteoporosis (type I)
    - Vertebral crush fracture syndrome
  - Senile osteoporosis (type II)
    - Fracture of the proximal femur
  - Idiopathic osteoporosis
  - Juvenile osteoporosis
- Endocrine osteoporosis
  - Hyperparathyroidism
  - Cushing's syndrome
  - Hyperthyroidism
  - Hypogonadism
  - Diabetes mellitus
- Nutritional osteoporosis
  - Scurvy
  - Malnutrition
  - Calcium deficiency
  - Malabsorption
- Secondary osteoporosis
  - Alcoholism
  - Liver disease
  - Renal disease
- Hematopoietic osteoporosis
  - Myeloma
  - Lymphoma
  - Leukemia
  - Mast cell disease
  - Thalassemia
- Congenital osteoporosis
  - Osteogenesis imperfecta
  - Homocystinuria
- Osteomalacia
  - Nutritional
  - Malabsorptive
  - Renal
  - Vitamin D-resistant
  - Anticonvulsant

CLINICAL DESCRIPTION

Clinically, osteoporosis is usually recognized because of symptoms related to fracture. Although there is considerable overlap, it is convenient to divide osteoporosis into two syndromes, type I and type II.

Type I osteoporosis, or the vertebral crush fracture syndrome, generally begins about 10 years after menopause and reaches its peak incidence in the sixties and early seventies. This syndrome is also termed *postmenopausal osteoporosis* because vertebral crush fractures caused by primary osteoporosis are rare in any group other than postmenopausal women; however, they can occur in younger women with amenorrhea or estrogen deficiency from other causes and in older men. Trauma is often absent; if present, it is minimal. Loss of trabecular bone in the vertebrae is the major underlying pathologic change. Trabecular bone loss in the wrist may also be important in the pathogenesis of Colles' fractures, which occur with increasing frequency after falls in women over the age of 45 and hence are part of type I osteoporosis.

Patients with type I osteoporosis differ from age-matched controls in that they have less trabecular bone. It is not clear, however, whether this occurs because their peak bone mass was lower earlier in life or because of rapid loss, particularly at the menopause. On the other hand, decreased lumbar bone density could be the result rather than the cause of vertebral fractures, since immobilization is likely to be substantial in these patients, and this can reduce lumbar bone mass.

Clinically, the diagnosis of type I osteoporosis is usually made because the patient complains of the acute onset of back pain and is found to have radiologic evidence of a vertebral compression fracture (Fig. 181-1). Some patients have chronic back pain and are found to have one or more compressed vertebrae; occasional patients show height loss and deformity without pain. The most frequently compressed vertebrae are those from T6 to L3. It is common to

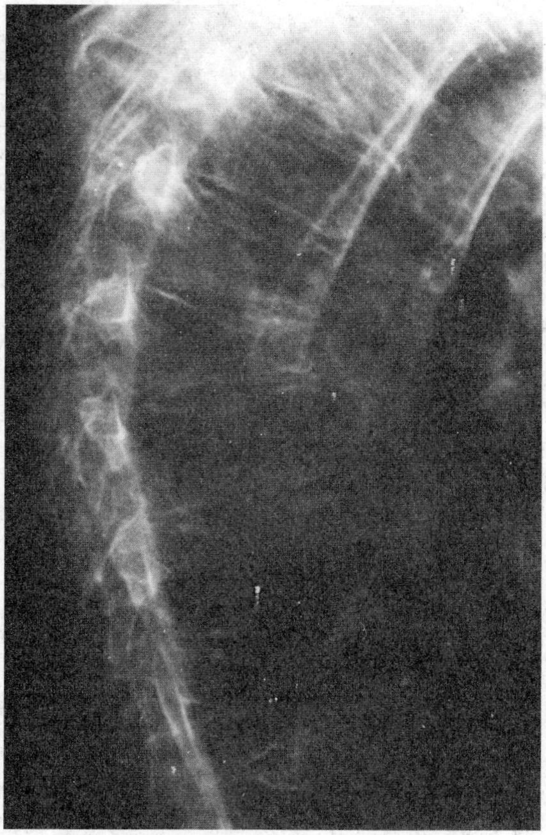

Fig. 181-1. Vertebral crush fractures. This radiograph of the lateral spine shows multiple compression and wedge fractures of the thoracic vertebrae that occurred without trauma between the ages of 60 and 70 in patient with severe postmenopausal (type I) osteoporosis.

find a loss of height of many vertebrae, with one or more markedly compressed. Anterior wedging, without loss of posterior height, is not as characteristic of type I osteoporosis. The disease has a remarkably variable course. Patients may have one or two fractures and no further episodes for many years. More often, the disorder is progressive, and additional vertebrae become involved. Using loss of 15% or more of posterior height of one or more vertebrae as a criterion, many patients show progression during the first year after diagnosis. This high incidence may decrease in subsequent years. Some patients show episodic disease with a cluster of fractures followed by a long period of remission before the second cluster of fractures occurs. Because of the extreme variability of the course, it is difficult to give a prognosis or to assess the effects of treatment in individual patients.

Type II osteoporosis is a term recently applied to older patients with fractures of the proximal femur. *Senile* and *involutional osteoporosis* are terms used to describe the same syndrome. Loss of both trabecular and cortical bone is probably involved, and there is some evidence suggesting that intertrochanteric fractures are more closely associated with trabecular bone loss, whereas fractures of the neck of the femur are associated with cortical bone loss. The incidence of these hip fractures begins to increase in women as early as the forties, but the major increase does not occur until after 65 in women and after 75 in men, and the fracture rate remains twice as high for women as for men. These fractures are usually traumatic, and there may be an inverse relationship between trauma and bone loss such that patients with marked bone loss suffer fractures after minimal or no trauma.

Patients with hip fracture or type II osteoporosis do not show substantially lower lumbar bone density than age-matched controls. This could be because both patients and controls are older and have already lost substantial amounts of bone or because their major abnormality is at a different site.

OTHER FORMS OF PRIMARY OSTEOPOROSIS

Juvenile osteoporosis is a relatively rare disorder that develops at the time of the pubertal growth spurt. In these patients there may be a dissociation between linear growth and the ability to consolidate and strengthen the skeleton. Thus vertebral or other fractures may occur. The disorder appears to be self-limited, and treatment is conservative, consisting of minimizing trauma, maintaining nutrition, and using a physiotherapy program that stimulates muscle and bone without injury. Calcitonin has been used in these patients, but no controlled studies have been done.

Idiopathic osteoporosis is a term applied to premenopausal women or relatively young men with osteoporosis for which there does not appear to be a secondary cause such as hypogonadism or alcoholism. The disorder is rare, ill defined, and probably heterogeneous. Biopsy may show increased bone turnover with accelerated resorption, and in such cases calcitonin therapy may be useful.

SECONDARY OSTEOPOROSIS

There are a large number of disorders associated with decreased bone mass in which the clinical picture may resemble primary osteoporosis. In some, the histologic appearance is different. For example, in primary and secondary hyperparathyroidism and in hyperthyroidism, the histologic picture is that of osteitis fibrosa cystica; in osteogenesis imperfecta there are abnormal collagen patterns; and in myeloma and mastocytoma characteristic abnormal cells are found. In Cushing's syndrome there is an unusual combination of increased bone resorption, impaired mineralization, and absence of wide osteoid seams because of inhibition of osteoblastic function. In patients with gastrointestinal, liver, and renal disease, osteoporosis may be seen, but there may also be osteomalacia. Presumably the development of osteomalacia depends on the relative severity of abnormalities in vitamin D metabolism or calcium and phosphate absorption, but the histologic picture is difficult to predict from clinical data. The separation between these disorders and primary osteoporosis may be indistinct, and they may coexist. For these reasons it is important to consider secondary forms of osteoporosis, not only in patients whose presentation is atypical, but also in patients who appear to have type I or type II osteoporosis, since identification of a specific cause or aggravating factor may result in much more effective treatment.

PATHOGENETIC FACTORS

The pathogenesis of primary osteoporosis is largely unknown. However, we can describe a number of factors that appear to contribute to this disorder and may be important in assessing risk and planning prevention or treatment.

Age-related bone loss

The pattern of gain and loss of skeletal mass in men and women is illustrated in Fig. 181-2. An important part of skeletal growth occurs during and after puberty when there is a substantial increase in bone mass. This involves endosteal apposition in the long bones and an increased amount of trabecular bone. Once peak bone mass has been reached, there is presumably a period during which skeletal remodeling is tightly coupled and rates of resorption and formation are essentially equal. However, this is a relatively short interval, and age-related bone loss begins in the thirties and forties, particularly in women. The loss of trabecular bone, which turns over more rapidly, is probably greater than that of cortical bone, but cortical thickness certainly decreases. In addition to loss of mass, aging may result in changes that affect mechanical properties. Changes in the size of osteons and haversian canals, death of osteocytes, and hypermineralization of lacunae, changes in collagen cross-linking, and decreased content of water in bone might result in increased brittleness and a propensity to fracture.

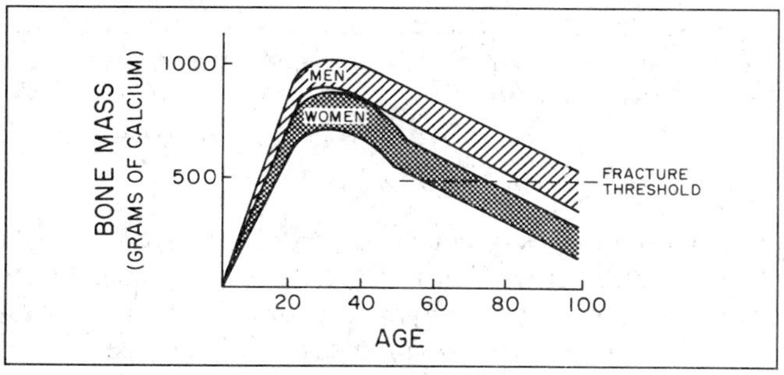

Fig. 181-2. Changes in bone mass with age. Note that bone mass is higher in men than in women and that age-related loss occurs in both sexes but is accelerated in women at the menopause. The concept of a fracture threshold is indicated by the dashed line. With age, increasing numbers of patients have a sufficient decrease in bone mass so that there is a higher likelihood of fracture with little or no trauma.

Genetic and constitutional factors

Certain populations, such as Northern European and Asian women, are at high risk for the development of osteoporosis. The lower prevalence of osteoporosis in blacks may be related to their greater bone and muscle mass, which appears to be associated with decreased bone turnover. Osteoporotic patients often have a positive family history, and first-degree relatives of these patients are likely to have a decreased bone mass. Patients with osteoporosis tend to be thinner and have a lighter frame with narrower bones than patients with osteoarthritis who are overweight. However, crush fractures do occur in women who have osteoarthritis. In these patients, the presence of vertebral spurs complicates the measurement of lumbar bone density.

Menopause

Accelerated bone loss associated with withdrawal of ovarian hormones is clearly a major pathogenetic factor (Fig. 181-3). Although there is extensive evidence that it is estrogen withdrawal that results in accelerated bone loss and that estrogen replacement can prevent it, the precise mechanism is not clear. One hypothesis is that estrogen increases the synthesis of or sensitivity to 1,25-dihydroxyvitamin D and this results in enhanced intestinal calcium absorption. In the presence of postmenopausal or other estrogen deficiency, a decreased calcium load might then increase parathyroid hormone and decrease calcitonin secretion. Alternatively, estrogen lack might have direct effects on calcitonin or parathyroid hormone secretion. However, the data supporting these possibilities are limited, and it seems more likely that estrogen has more direct effects on bone metab-

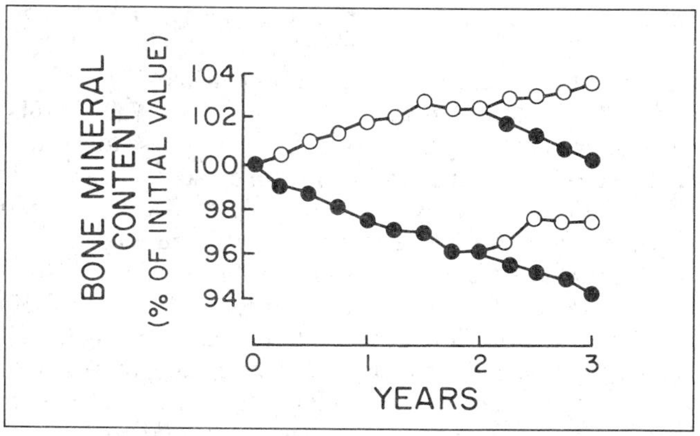

Fig. 181-3. Bone loss at the menopause. Bone mineral content of the distal radius was measured serially in women beginning with 3 years after the menopause. Untreated women showed progressive bone loss *(closed circles);* women treated with estrogen showed maintained or increased bone mass *(open circles).* If estrogen was begun in previously untreated women, at the end of 2 years there was a positive effect on bone mass, and if estrogen was discontinued at this time, bone loss occurred. However, the gains achieved during the prior 2 years of treatment were maintained. (Modified from Christiansen C et al: Lancet 1:459, 1981.)

olism by altering cellular function or the production of local bone-derived factors.

In addition to menopause, either natural and artificial following oophorectomy, other forms of estrogen deficiency such as Turner's syndrome and amenorrhea associated with anorexia nervosa or intense athletic training may result in decreased bone mass. Androgen deficiency in the male is also associated with bone loss. The mechanisms by which sex hormone deficiency produces bone loss are not fully understood. There is an increase in the rate of bone resorption when sex hormones are withdrawn, followed by a delayed increase in bone formation, probably as a result of the increased number of resorption sites. Since bone loss is progressive, the amount of bone formed must always be less than that required to replace the bone resorbed. This could be caused by loss of template for new bone formation because of perforations and discontinuities, particularly in trabecular bone, or could indicate that sex hormones are required not only to inhibit osteoclasts, but also to stimulate osteoblasts.

Calcium-regulating hormones

Despite many studies, there is no agreement about the role of calcium-regulating hormones in the pathogenesis of osteoporosis. To establish such a role, there should be a substantial difference in the level of or response to a particular hormone in osteoporotic patients compared to age-matched controls. Of course, some overlap is to be expected since some control patients may have asymptomatic osteoporosis. In type I osteoporosis parathyroid hormone levels are not elevated, and some data suggest a decrease. A small decrease in 1,25-dihydroxyvitamin D has also been reported, but measurement of both hormones shows that there is a substantial overlap of osteoporotic patients with normals. Most studies do not show a difference in calcitonin levels. The role of these hormones in the pathogenesis of hip fracture is even more difficult to evaluate. There is an age-related increase in parathyroid hormone levels, but the increase of 1,25-dihydroxyvitamin D in response to calcium deprivation or parathyroid hormone administration is blunted. There may also be an age-related decrease in calcitonin levels. All of these changes could be secondary to the decreases in renal mass and intestinal transport associated with aging. These may combine to impair 1,25-dihydroxyvitamin D synthesis and response, leading to secondary hyperparathyroidism and a decreased stimulation of parafollicular cells, which might result in a decrease in both resting and calcium-stimulated calcitonin secretion.

One difficulty with assigning a role for calcium-regulating hormones in osteoporosis is uncertainty concerning their long-term effects on bone formation. Parathyroid hormone and 1,25-dihydroxyvitamin D inhibit collagen synthesis acutely. However, in prolonged experiments, particularly those using intermittent administration, parathyroid hormone can increase trabecular bone mass. The vitamin D metabolites may have a similar effect, but this is not as well documented.

Other humoral factors

In addition to the calcium-regulating hormones, other factors influence bone resorption and formation and may be involved in the pathogenesis of osteoporosis. Somatomedins or insulin-like growth factors and insulin stimulate bone growth, whereas glucocorticoids inhibit it. There is little evidence that the systemic levels of these hormones are altered in osteoporosis, but cellular responses or local production could be altered. Bone turnover depends on local mechanisms that initiate resorption at particular sites and regulate the coupled formation response. Prostaglandins are produced by bone and have complex effects on bone formation and resorption. Increased prostaglandin production has been implicated in inflammatory bone loss. Prostaglandins may also be involved in the response to estrogen withdrawal since bones from oophorectomized rats produce an increased amount of prostaglandin E_2. Interleukin 1 and tumor necrosis factor are cytokines that could be produced in the marrow or possibly by bone cells. These "osteoclast-activating factors" stimulate bone resorption and inhibit bone formation. There is evidence that interleukin 1 production may be increased in some osteoporotic patients.

Bone cells also produce macromolecular factors that stimulate formation, termed *bone-derived growth factors, coupling factors,* or *bone morphogenetic proteins*. Unfortunately, until we can measure the local concentrations of these factors in patients, we cannot determine their potential pathogenetic role in osteoporosis.

Nutritional factors

Much remains to be learned about the role of calcium in the prevention and treatment of osteoporosis. There is evidence that a low calcium intake throughout life can result in a decrease in peak bone mass and that this could lead to an increased incidence of fractures. Age-related bone loss cannot be abrogated by calcium supplements but can be slowed. Although excessive intakes of protein and phosphate can produce negative calcium balance, it is not clear that these are important in the pathogenesis of osteoporosis. Ascorbic acid deficiency and excessive intakes of vitamins A and D can probably cause bone loss but are rarely encountered clinically.

Life-style

Immobilization results in rapid bone loss associated with both increased resorption and decreased formation. Moreover, moderate exercise can reverse bone loss in postmenopausal women. The effects of intense exercise appear to depend on whether sex hormone function is altered. In women who exercise intensely and have amenorrhea, particularly if this begins early after puberty, bone mass is lower than in age-matched controls.

Other aspects of life-style that may reduce bone mass are cigarette smoking, which appears to be associated with reduced estrogen levels, high alcohol intake, and possibly high caffeine intake. The mechanism of decreased bone mass in alcoholics is not known, but poor nutrition and direct effects of alcohol on bone have been implicated.

DIAGNOSIS

Type I osteoporosis is diagnosed by exclusion. In a postmenopausal woman with a crush fracture, a careful history and physical examination and a few laboratory studies are usually sufficient to rule out diseases that mimic or aggravate primary osteoporosis. The most important of these are primary hyperparathyroidism, osteomalacia, hyperthyroidism, multiple myeloma or lymphoma, and Cushing's syndrome. Gastrointestinal and renal disease may predispose to osteomalacia or secondary hyperparathyroidism as well as osteoporosis.

Patients with osteoporotic fractures should have routine laboratory studies to rule out secondary causes, including serum calcium, phosphate, creatinine, alkaline phosphatase, and protein electrophoresis. Levels of 25-hydroxyvitamin D can be used to assess vitamin D status.

There is some controversy concerning the use of bone density measurements in assessing osteoporosis. Measurement of bone mass is particularly useful in making decisions about prevention in postmenopausal women who have not yet fractured. Bone density measurements can also be used to follow the response to therapy, but the changes seen are often within the range of error of the method. Biochemical measurements of bone turnover have been advocated on the basis that patients with high turnover are likely to show more rapid bone loss and to respond best to inhibitors of bone resorption, such as calcitonin and bisphosphonates. Bone resorption can be assessed by measuring the excretion of hydroxyproline or pyridinoline cross-links in the urine. Measurements of osteocalcin, the bone gamma-carboxyglutamic acid—containing protein, and bone alkaline phosphatase can be used as indicators of bone formation. Bone biopsies, obtained after double tetracycline labeling, can be used to assess bone formation and mineralization. Biopsies are indicated in atypical or severe cases of osteoporosis, particularly when data suggest osteomalacia, which can only be diagnosed definitely by biopsy, or clinical findings that point to an unusual form of osteopenia, such as mastocytosis or a lymphoproliferative disorder.

Prevention

Once fractures have occurred, osteoporosis is often progressive despite therapy. At best, treatment can only reduce the incidence of further fractures. Because of this, there has been considerable emphasis on developing prevention programs for high-risk individuals before fractures occur. Efforts at prevention should probably begin in childhood and be reinforced in young adults. An adequate calcium intake of approximately 1200 mg/day in adolescents and 1000 mg/day in adults, combined with a program of physical activity that maintains muscle strength and bone mass, might reverse the current trend toward an increasing incidence of osteoporotic fractures in industrialized countries.

The most important time for establishing additional preventive measures is at the menopause. Hormone replacement has been shown to decrease the frequency of both vertebral and hip fractures. While the advantages and disadvantages of hormone replacement therapy have been much debated, the benefits are likely to outweigh the risks in patients who have low bone mass and are likely to develop osteoporotic fractures. For this reason, measurement of bone mass in perimenopausal women may be cost-effective. However, there are some contraindications to hormone replacement. Patients who have had breast cancer or serious thromboembolic complications from prior estrogen therapy should not be treated. There are relative contraindications including a family history of breast or endometrial carcinoma, fibrocystic breast disease, and gallbladder disease. Unopposed estrogen therapy increases the risk of endometrial carcinoma, but this is abrogated when a progestin is added to the regimen. The minimal effective dose of estrogen is probably 0.625 mg/day of conjugated estrogen or its equivalent. Estrogen can be given transdermally as well as orally. When the uterus is present, medroxyprogesterone or its equivalent can be given either for 10 to 14 days of each month in doses of 5 to 10 mg/day or continuously at doses of 2.5 to 5 mg/day. The former regimen results in regular menses, which many patients find difficult to accept. With continuous combined therapy, patients may have a few initial episodes of bleeding that then stop. Patients should have a mammogram before being placed on hormone therapy and yearly thereafter. Endometrial biopsy should be performed yearly if unopposed estrogen is used or whenever there is atypical bleeding. When estrogen is contraindicated in high-risk patients, other antiresorptive therapy can be considered (see below).

The preventive regimen should not be limited to hormone replacement therapy. Calcium supplementation and an exercise program that includes 3 to 4 hours of weight-bearing exercise weekly should be part of the program. Patients should be advised to discontinue smoking, reduce their intakes of alcohol and caffeine, and avoid excessive intake of protein and vitamins A and D. However, an adequate vitamin D intake of 400 units/day or its equivalent in sun exposure should be maintained. Compliance with a prevention program depends on patient motivation. Monitoring the patients with bone density measurements at 1- to 3-year intervals and maintaining exercise programs through group activities can help achieve good compliance.

Treatment

Patients who have had an osteoporotic fracture of the vertebrae, distal radius, proximal femur, or any other site should be put on the same conservative regimen used for prevention. Because most patients have limited mobility after fracture, the exercise regimen must be carefully tailored to their capacity and carried out under supervision. While many patients improve on this regimen, some show progressive bone loss and continue to fracture. In these individuals, additional therapy is indicated. Calcitonin can be used to inhibit bone resorption and increases bone mass, particularly in patients with high turnover. It currently must be given by subcutaneous injection and can produce anorexia and nausea, but a nasal preparation with fewer side effects is being tested. Bisphosphonates can also be used to decrease bone resorption and have been shown to increase bone mass in osteoporotic patients. A number of other agents are being tested, including calcitriol and other vitamin D metabolites as well as parathyroid hormone given intermittently. Sodium fluoride has been used extensively in patients with vertebral crush fracture, but high doses can cause side effects and may not decrease the incidence of fractures. Although treatment is limited, most patients improve given a comprehensive regimen, adequate encouragement, and appropriate follow-up.

REFERENCES

Cummings SR, Black DM, and Rubin SM: Lifetime risks of hip, Colles' or vertebral fracture and coronary heart disease among white postmenopausal women. Arch Intern Med 149:2445, 1989.

Delmas P: Biochemical markers of bone turnover for the clinical assessment of metabolic bone disease. Endocrinol Metab Clin North Am 19:1, 1990.

Eriksen EF et al: Cancellous bone remodeling in type I (postmenopausal) osteoporosis: quantitative assessment of rates of formation, resorption and bone loss at tissue and cellular levels. J Bone Miner Res 5:311, 1990.

Grisso JA et al: Risk factors for falls as a cause of hip fracture in women. N Engl J Med 324:1326, 1991.

Lindsay R, Hart DM, and Clark DM: The minimum effective dose of estrogen for prevention of postmenopausal bone loss. Obstet Gynecol 63:759, 1984.

Ott SM: Attainment of peak bone mass (editorial). J Clin Endocrinol Metab 71:A1082, 1990.

Raisz LG: Local and systemic factors in the pathogenesis of osteoporosis. N Engl J Med 318:818, 1988.

Riggs BL and Melton LG: Involutional osteoporosis. N Engl J Med 314:1676, 1984.

Silverberg SJ et al: Abnormalities in parathyroid hormone secretion and 1,25-dihydroxyvitamin D_3 formation in women with osteoporosis. N Engl J Med 320:277, 1989.

Tosteson ANA et al: Cost effectiveness of screening postmenopausal white women for osteoporosis—bone densitometry and hormone replacement therapy. Ann Intern Med 113:594, 1990.

CHAPTER

182 Osteomalacia and Disorders of Vitamin D Metabolism

L. Lyndon Key, Jr.
Norman H. Bell

Osteomalacia is a skeletal disorder in which mineralization of the newly formed osteoid or organic matrix of bone is defective. In children, the disease is rickets. In this condition, defective mineralization of cartilage that affects the epiphyseal growth plate leads to alteration in the maturation and pattern of cellular growth and development of epiphyseal plates, widening of the ends of long bones, retardation of growth, and the skeletal deformities described below.

PHYSIOLOGY OF BONE FORMATION

The normal sequence of bone formation first requires the production of an organic matrix or osteoid, which is then mineralized. The process of calcification is complex and still not well understood. Calcium and phosphate in the extracellular fluid are supersaturated, and metastatic calcification is prevented by pyrophosphate and possibly other substances, including peptides. Initially, bone mineral is deposited as amorphous calcium phosphate that is later converted to hydroxyapatite $[Ca_{10}(PO_4)_6(OH)_2]$ (see Chapter 148).

The rate of bone formation and calcification can be measured by histomorphometric techniques that employ tetracycline labeling. Tetracycline antibiotics have the fortuitous property of being deposited in a fluorescent, bandlike pattern at the mineralization front. As a consequence, they are readily visualized on histologic sections under a fluorescent microscope. Short-term administration of tetracycline in two series of doses with an intervening timed interval allows the appositional growth of the skeleton to be estimated by measuring the distance between the two fluorescent bands. In normal adult subjects, this distance averages approximately one μm per day. In osteomalacia and rickets, the distance is reduced. In severe cases of rickets and osteomalacia, the mineralization defect may be so marked that it is possible to discern only a single band of fluorescence (Plate IV-4). When the newly formed matrix mineralizes either poorly or not at all, it appears as a wide osteoid seam. The two distinguishing diagnostic features of osteomalacia on bone biopsy are wide osteoid seams and diminished mineralization. Both findings are essential to establish the diagnosis with certainty because an increase in width of osteoid seams is found in states of high bone turnover such as primary hyperparathyroidism, hyperthyroidism, and Paget's disease.

CLINICAL FEATURES

In children with rickets, growth is retarded and the skeleton is subject to deformities and fractures regardless of pathogenesis. Defective mineralization of cartilage and the skeleton produces the greatest abnormalities in the bones with the most rapid growth. Just as the rate of growth of different parts of the skeleton varies with age, the clinical findings of rickets also vary with age and often provide an indication of the age of onset of the disease. At birth and during the first year of life, softening of the cranium or craniotabes commonly occurs as a consequence of rapid growth of the skull. This results in widening of the cranial sutures, frontal bossing, and posterior flattening of the skull. In infancy and early childhood, thickening of the forearm at the wrist and of the costochondral junctions (the rachitic rosary), are the consequence of rapid growth of the arms and rib cage, respectively. The lower ribs at the site of attachment of the diaphragm, Harrison's groove, may be indented. Dental eruption is frequently delayed and abnormalities in dentition as well as an increased frequency of caries occur. In later childhood and adolescence, bowing of the lower extremities, especially around the knees, may result from rapid growth of the legs.

In infants and children, listlessness and irritability are common. In infants, myopathy is indicated by generalized hypotonia, whereas in older children, proximal muscles weakness is observed.

In adults, the clinical manifestations of osteomalacia are frequently subtle and may be overlooked, and the patients may be asymptomatic. When present, symptoms include diffuse skeletal pain and proximal muscular weakness. The pain is characteristically dull and aching, present in the lower back or hips or at sites where fractures have taken place; the pain is worsened by activity. Bone tenderness may be present on palpation. Fractures of the vertebrae, ribs, and long bones may occur, often with little trauma. Muscular weakness may be severe and is frequently associated with wasting. Since weakness usually involves the proximal muscle group, particularly the lower extremities, it may contribute to the waddling gait, a characteristic finding.

Hypocalcemia is sometimes found in patients with rickets and osteomalacia. As a result, lethargy, diarrhea, laryngeal stridor, grand mal seizures, cataracts, and increased intracranial pressure may ensue. Headaches and papilledema occur as a result of the increased intracranial pressure. In children, mental retardation sometimes results from chronic hypocalcemia.

LABORATORY FINDINGS

In osteomalacia, the serum calcium is normal or low, and serum phosphorus is normal or low depending on the absence or presence of secondary hyperparathyroidism and defects in phosphate handling. An elevation of the serum alkaline phosphatase is the most consistent abnormality. Serum immunoreactive parathyroid hormone is often increased. Reduction of the filtered load of calcium and increased circulating parathyroid hormone combine to produce a low urinary calcium. Increases in urinary cyclic AMP and hydroxyproline occur and are related to increased secretion of parathyroid hormone and enhanced bone resorption, respectively. Serum 25-hydroxyvitamin D and 1,25-dihydroxyvitamin D are normal, reduced, or elevated depending on the etiology of the underlying disease.

RADIOGRAPHIC AND NUCLEAR MEDICINE FINDINGS

The radiographic findings in rickets and osteomalacia are manifestations of the histopathologic abnormalities. In rickets, there is a widening of the epiphyseal growth plate, and the ends of the growing metaphyses are irregular or cupped. Loss of the trabecular pattern of the metaphyses, thinning of the cortices of the diaphyses, and bowing of the long bones may be present.

The most common radiographic finding in osteomalacia is a reduction in skeletal density, a nonspecific change that is of little value diagnostically since it is seen in other conditions, such as osteoporosis. More helpful in this regard are the less frequently occurring coarsening of the trabecular pattern and pseudofractures. The pseudofractures, or Looser's zones, are narrow lines of radiolucency that usually transect and lie either at right angles or obliquely to the cortical margins of bones (Fig. 182-1). They are often bilateral and symmetrical, and they commonly occur where major arteries cross bones. Sites include the axillary margins of the scapula, lower ribs, superior and inferior pubic rami, inner margins at the neck of the proximal femora, and posterior margins of the proximal ulna. Multiple bilateral and symmetrical pseudofractures in a patient with osteomalacia is called Milkman's syndrome.

The pathogenesis of Looser's zone is thought by some to represent a stress fracture that is repaired by laying down of osteoid that is inadequately mineralized. Since pseudofractures often lie adjacent to arteries, others attribute the lesion to mechanical erosion caused by arterial pulsations. This possibility is strengthened by arteriographic demonstrations that arteries frequently overlie sites of pseudofractures. Further, true fractures can occur at these weakened areas.

Another distinctive radiographic finding in osteomalacia is the "rugger jersey" appearance of the spine. This results from changes in advanced disease such that the vertebral bodies become concave as a result of softening of the bone. In contrast, the vertebral disks are large and biconvex. In osteomalacia, the incidence of compression fractures of the spine is lower than in osteoporosis.

In rickets and osteomalacia, skeletal changes sometimes result from secondary hyperparathyroidism. These include subperiosteal reabsorption of the phalanges and resorption of the distal ends of the long bones such as the clavicle and humerus. In some instances, radiographic features of excess parathyroid hormone may be more prominent than those of rickets or osteomalacia.

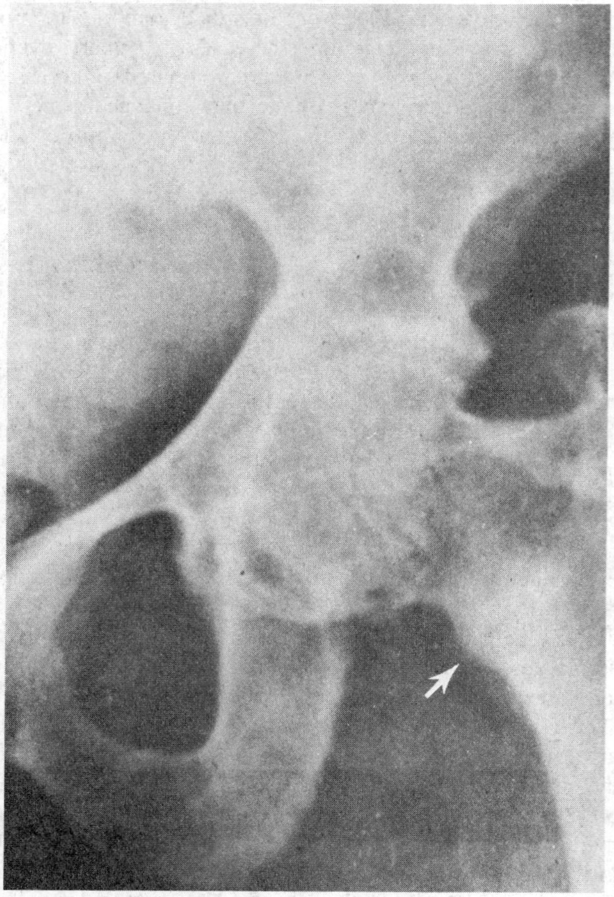

Fig. 182-1. Radiograph showing a pseudofracture of the femoral neck in a patient with osteomalacia. (Kindly provided by Dr. Robert Weinstein.)

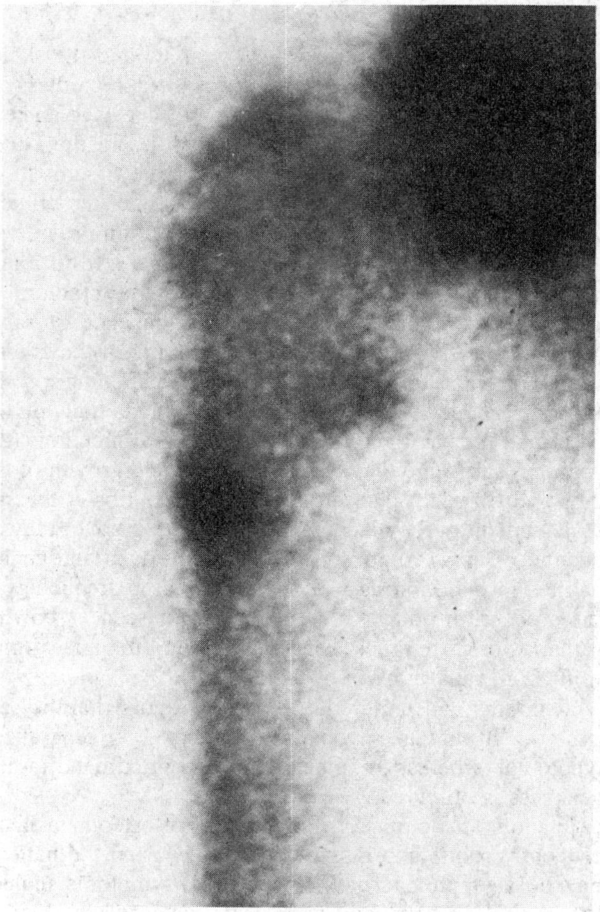

Fig. 182-2. Technetium-99 pyrophosphate bone scan of a femur showing a hot spot at the site of a pseudofracture in a patient with osteomalacia. (Kindly provided by Dr. Robert Weinstein.)

In patients with osteomalacia, bone scans show increased uptake of technetium-99 pyrophosphate by long bones and wrists and prominence of the calvarium and mandible. Less evident are beading of the costochondral junctions and marked uptake of the tracer by the sternum and its margins, the so-called "tie sternum." In addition, pseudofractures appear as hot spots (Fig. 182-2). In some instances, pseudofractures may be evident only on radiographs and in other instances, only on bone scan. Hot spots can be diagnosed erroneously as metastatic lesions.

In osteomalacia, bone mineral density as determined by single- and dual-photon absorptiometry may be diminished.

DIFFERENTIAL DIAGNOSIS

Mineralization is impaired by deficiencies of calcium, phosphate, or alkaline phosphatase. Rickets and osteoporosis can result from a number of causes, including abnormalities in the metabolism of vitamin D, deficiencies of calcium or phosphate, deficiencies of alkaline phosphatase, and defects in mineralization (see box at upper right). The pathogenesis of and clinical laboratory findings in selected individual diseases are described below.

NUTRITIONAL DEFICIENCIES

In children in the United States, rickets and osteomalacia resulting from deficiency of vitamin D are uncommon. When they do occur, they are usually caused by lack of sunlight and the resultant diminished dermal synthesis of vitamin D_3. Lack of dietary intake is an infrequent factor since milk and dairy products are fortified with vitamin D. Rickets may be an indication of child abuse and neglect. Rickets and osteomalacia are more common in other parts of the world, particularly in Third World countries. Rickets sometimes results from dietary deficiencies of vitamin D and calcium, even in tropical climates. In the United Kingdom, rickets occurs in immigrant Indians and Pakistanis. Several factors are contributory. Endogenous production of vitamin D is limited in women who remain indoors and wear traditional clothing because of diminished exposure to sunlight. Dietary practices such as the use of

Etiology of osteomalacia and rickets

I. Abnormalities in vitamin D metabolism
   A. Vitamin D deficiency
      1. Nutritional deficiency
      2. Lack of exposure to sunlight
      3. Malabsorption syndromes
         a. Postgastrectomy, partial or total
         b. Small bowel disease
         c. Pancreatic insufficiency
   B. Defective dermal production of vitamin D_3
      1. Chronic renal disease
      2. Aging
   C. Defective hepatic 25-hydroxylation of vitamin D
      1. Primary biliary cirrhosis
      2. Biliary atresia
      3. Biliary fistula
   D. Defective renal 1α-hydroxylation of 25-hydroxyvitamin D
      1. Hypoparathyroidism
      2. Pseudohypoparathyroidism
      3. Chronic renal insufficiency
      4. Vitamin D–dependent rickets type I
      5. Hypophosphatemic rickets
      6. Tumor-induced osteomalacia
      7. Age-related osteomalacia
   E. Defective target-organ response to 1,25-dihydroxyvitamin D
      1. Vitamin D–dependent rickets type II
      2. Anticonvulsant therapy
   F. Renal loss of vitamin D–binding protein
      1. Nephrotic syndrome

II. Phosphate deficiency
   A. Diminished intake
      1. Neonatal rickets
      2. Excess aluminum hydroxide ingestion
   B. Impaired renal tubular phosphate reabsorption
      1. Primary renal tubular defects
         a. X-linked hypophosphatemic osteomalacia
         b. Adult-onset hypophosphatemic osteomalacia
         c. Sporadic acquired hypophosphatemic osteomalacia
         d. Fanconi's syndromes
            (i) Wilson's disease
            (ii) Lowe's disease
            (iii) Tyrosinemia
            (iv) Glycogen storage disease
            (v) Cystinosis
            (vi) Ifosfamide therapy
      2. Secondary renal tubular "defects"
         a. Primary hyperparathyroidism
         b. Secondary hyperparathyroidism
         c. Renal tubular acidosis
         d. Tumor-induced osteomalacia

III. Mineralization defects
   A. Enzyme deficiency
      1. Hypophosphatasia
   B. Circulating inhibitor(s) of calcification
      1. Chronic renal failure
      2. Hypophosphatasia (increased pyrophosphate)
   C. Drugs and ions
      1. Diphosphonates
      2. Fluoride
      3. Aluminum intoxication
   D. Abnormal bone collagen or matrix
      1. Chronic renal failure
      2. Osteogenesis imperfecta
      3. Fibrogenesis imperfecta ossium

IV. States of rapid bone formation
   A. Postoperative primary hyperparathyroidism with osteitis fibrosa cystica
   B. Osteopetrosis

V. Miscellaneous
   A. Parenteral alimentation

chupputti flour is also a factor. This flour is derived from wheat with a high content of phytate that binds calcium, resulting in increased fecal excretion of the ion. Lignin, a component of wheat flour, binds to bile acids and prevents their absorption. Vitamin D, which normally forms micelles with bile acids, a requirement for its absorption by the intestine, is bound by the lignin-bile acid complex instead and is not absorbed. Removal of chupputti flour from the diet corrects abnormal vitamin D and mineral metabolism. Deficiency of vitamin D can be prevented by fortification of the diet with the vitamin. In women, dietary deficiency of the vitamin is often so profound that it causes rickets and hypocalcemia in their nursing infants.

In developed countries, the elderly are at greatest risk for developing osteomalacia. The reason is multifactorial. There is an age-related decline in the dermal synthesis of 7-dehydrocholesterol so that the production of vitamin D declines. In addition, impaired production of 25-hydroxyvitamin D in the liver, diminished synthesis of 1,25-dihydroxyvitamin D in the kidneys, and a decline in the transport of calcium in response to 1,25-dihydroxyvitamin D occur in aging individuals. These abnormalities in vitamin D metabolism and function, coupled with inadequate exposure to UV light in individuals who are housebound and chronically institutionalized as well as inadequate dietary intakes of vitamin D and calcium, provide the background for the development of osteomalacia.

GASTROINTESTINAL AND HEPATIC DISORDERS

Since vitamin D is absorbed in the proximal small intestine, a process that requires bile acids, and since vitamin D and its metabolism undergo an enterohepatic circulation, deficiency of the vitamin can result from gastrointestinal diseases that impair the intestinal absorption or interfere with the enterohepatic circulation of vitamin D. Diseases associated with osteomalacia include nontropical sprue, regional enteritis, scleroderma, blind loop syndrome, multiple jejunal diverticulae, and idiopathic steatorrhea. Osteomalacia is also a complication of a number of surgical procedures, including subtotal gastric resection with gastroenterostomy, small bowel resection, and intestinal bypass for the treatment of morbid obesity. The incidence of osteomalacia in these various conditions differs. For example, bone disease is common in patients with the Billroth II procedure that is used to treat peptic ulcer, but it is uncommon in patients with sprue. Impaired intestinal absorption of calcium as well as vitamin D contribute to the development of osteomalacia.

Osteomalacia and rickets also occur as a complication of hepatocellular, biliary, and pancreatic disorders. Biliary obstruction, which produces parenchymal disease of the liver, can diminish the synthesis of 25-hydroxyvitamin D and interfere with the intestinal absorption of vitamin D and calcium. Some patients can be improved by increasing their exposure to sunlight and the subsequent endogenous production of vitamin D. In others, a defect in synthesis of 25-hydroxyvitamin D is so severe that vitamin D is ineffective and 25-hydroxyvitamin D or 1,25-dihydroxyvitamin D_3 must be administered. In a patient with a defect in bile acid synthesis, replacement of the bile acid, chenodeoxycholic acid (125 mg twice a day), corrected abnormal absorption of vitamin D and healed the rickets. Thus, bile acid administration could be an alternative or supplemental means of treatment in patients with liver disease.

HYPOPARATHYROIDISM AND PSEUDOHYPOPARATHYROIDISM

Two diseases that infrequently result in osteomalacia are hypoparathyroidism and pseudohyperparathyroidism. Patients may present with complaints of bone pain, and the diagnosis of osteomalacia is made definitively by histomorphometric analysis of a bone biopsy. X-rays of the skeleton are sometimes unremarkable and therefore may not be helpful diagnostically.

In hypoparathyroidism, hypocalcemia and low or low normal serum 1,25-dihydroxyvitamin D are usually present and are important in the pathogenesis of the bone disease. Since parathyroid hormone is the major regulator of the renal synthesis of 1,25-dihydroxyvitamin D, low serum 1,25-dihydroxyvitamin D and hypocalcemia in hypoparathyroidism result from deficiency of the hormone. Patients with hypoparathyroidism often can be treated effectively with vitamin D, but some require more specific treatment with 1,25-dihydroxyvitamin D_3.

Pseudohypoparathyroidism is a disorder in which resistance to parathyroid hormone leads to hypocalcemia, retention of phosphate, and low serum 1,25-dihydroxyvitamin D. Impaired production of 1,25-dihydroxyvitamin D results from defective synthesis of cyclic adenosine 3′,5′-monophosphate since values are increased by administration of dibutyryl cyclic adenosine 3′,5′-monophosphate. In addition, patients with pseudohypoparathyroidism can develop skeletal manifestations of secondary hyperparathyroidism because of hypocalcemia and increased circulating parathyroid hormone. Some patients can be effectively treated with vitamin D and others may require 1,25-dihydroxyvitamin D_3.

VITAMIN D–DEPENDENT RICKETS TYPE I

Vitamin D–dependent rickets is an inborn error of vitamin D metabolism that is genetically transmitted as an autosomal recessive. Typically infants with this disorder appear normal at birth and develop the characteristic clinical and biochemical features of rickets during the first year of life. Biochemical features include hypocalcemia, normal or low serum phosphate, elevation of serum alkaline phosphatase, and increased serum immunoreactive parathyroid hormone. The disease results from an absence or inactive form of renal 25-hydroxyvitamin D-1-α-hydroxylase. As a result, serum 25-hydroxyvitamin D is normal and serum 1,25-dihydroxyvitamin D is markedly reduced. Patients sometimes can be treated successfully with large doses of vitamin D or 25-hydroxyvitamin D_3 but readily respond to physiologic doses of 1,25-dihydroxyvitamin D_3.

HYPOPHOSPHATEMIC OSTEOMALACIA

Hypophosphatemic rickets is usually an x-linked dominant familial disorder but is occasionally sporadic. The onset is between 1 and 1½ years of age and is associated with delayed or abnormal dentition. Screening studies in families indicate that fasting hypophosphatemia is the most common manifestation of the disorder. Serum immunoreactive parathyroid hormone and serum calcium are usually normal. There is a broad clinical spectrum of disease that varies from individuals who have hypophosphatemia and no apparent bone disease, usually females, to subjects who are symptomatic and have severe bone disease. The degree of hypophosphatemia and severity of bone disease are not correlated, although the diminished growth rate in these individuals is attributed to hypophosphatemia.

Hypophosphatemia in this condition is secondary to impaired reabsorption of filtered phosphate by the proximal renal tubule. Available evidence indicates that two separate mechanisms exist for phosphate transport in the renal tubule, a parathyroid hormone–dependent component that is responsible for two thirds of the tubular reabsorption of phosphate and a parathyroid hormone–independent component that is regulated by the serum calcium and is responsible for the remaining third net tubular reabsorption of the ion. The parathyroid hormone-dependent component is completely lacking in men with hypophosphatemia and is partially deficient in women with hypophosphatemia. Defective phosphate transport is also present in the intestinal mucosa, indicating that the deficit is generalized and not restricted to the kidney.

Renal production of 1,25-dihydroxyvitamin D is impaired in some patients and serum values are inappropriately low for the degree of hypophosphatemia. In addition, circulating 1,25-hydroxyvitamin D responds poorly to exogenously administered parathyroid hormone. The defect appears to be coupled to the abnormality in renal phosphate transport. As shown in Fig. 182-3, plasma 1,25-dihydroxyvitamin D varies directly with the tubular reabsorption of phosphate (TmP/GFR) in patients with X-linked hypophosphatemia, normal subjects, and patients with other defects in phosphate transport, including tumor-induced osteomalacia. Although it is quite likely that the renal production of 1,25-dihydroxyvitamin D and renal tubular reabsorption of phosphate are linked, treatment with 1,25-dihydroxyvitamin D_3 does not reverse the renal phosphate wasting and restoring serum phosphate to normal does not enhance the renal production of 1,25-dihydroxyvitamin D.

Of interest is the fact that tumoral calcinosis appears to be the mirror image of X-linked hypophosphatemia and tumor-induced osteomalacia (Fig. 182-3). In this disease, the renal tubular reabsorption of phosphate and plasma 1,25-dihydroxyvitamin D are both abnormally increased.

A type of hypophosphatemic rickets has been described, hereditary hypophosphatemic rickets with hypercalciuria, that is characterized by an elevation in circulating 1,25-dihydroxyvitamin D and hypophosphatemia. In this disorder, phosphate repletion alone results in healing of osteomalacia. In other forms of hypophosphatemic rickets and osteomalacia, treatment requires both phosphate and 1,25-dihydroxyvitamin D_3, which must be administered lifelong. If therapy is adequate, the bone disease can be almost completely reversed. Occasional complications of therapy include hypercalcemia and soft tissue calcification, including nephrocalcinosis, calcification at tendon attachments to bone, and cardiac valves. While soft tissue calcifications are widely believed to be secondary to increased calcium absorption and the resultant hypercalciuria in response to 1,25-dihydroxyvitamin D_3, there is evidence that complications correlate more strongly with the amount of phosphate administered.

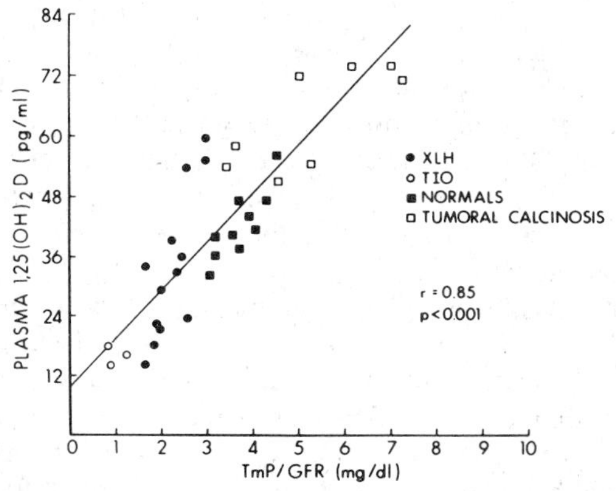

Fig. 182-3. Relationship between plasma 1,25-dihydroxyvitamin D and tubular reabsorption of phosphate (TmP/GFR) in normal subjects, patients with hypophosphatemic rickets (XLH), tumor-induced osteomalacia (TIO), and tumoral calcinosis. (With permission from Drezner MK: Understanding the pathogenesis of rickets. A requisite for successful therapy. In Zackson DA, editor: A CPC series: cases in metabolic bone disease. New York, 1987, Triclinica Communications.)

Early treatment of children with hereditary hypophosphatemic rickets results in an improved growth velocity and a more normal final stature. However, frequently the rate of growth is still below the expectations of the parents. Recently, treatment with growth hormone in combination with the standard therapy of phosphate and 1,25-dihydroxyvitamin D_3 has resulted in further improvement in growth velocity and more complete healing of rachitic changes. The beneficial effect of growth hormone appears to result from enhanced renal tubular reabsorption of phosphate, although its growth-promoting activity may contribute to the improved growth velocity.

TUMOR-INDUCED OSTEOMALACIA

Tumor-induced osteomalacia is a disorder similar to hypophosphatemic rickets in that the osteomalacia is associated with renal phosphate wasting and an inappropriately low serum 1,25-dihydroxyvitamin D. It is seen with a variety of benign or malignant neoplasms, such as sarcomas, hemangiomas, giant cell tumors of the colon, and carcinoma of the breast and prostate. Complete remission occurs with removal or irradiation of the tumor.

The clinical and biochemical features are typical of osteomalacia. Patients often present with generalized muscle weakness and bone pain. Serum calcium is usually normal to slightly reduced. Serum phosphate is low, and serum alkaline phosphatase and urinary calcium are elevated.

It is likely that the hypophosphatemia results from one or more factors produced by the tumors that alter the renal tubular reabsorption of phosphate in the proximal tubule and interfere with the renal production of 1,25-dihydroxyvitamin D. Treatment of the disorder is resection or irradiation of the lesion. If this is not possible, treatment with phosphates and vitamin D or 1,25-dihydroxyvitamin D_3 may be used.

VITAMIN D-DEPENDENT RICKETS II

Vitamin D-dependent rickets type II results from end-organ resistance to 1,25-dihydroxyvitamin D. The clinical, biochemical, and skeletal findings of the disorder may appear during infancy, childhood, or adolescence. The disease is sporadic or familial and is transmitted as an autosomal recessive trait. Infants with the familial disease may have permanent alopecia, usually a sign of severe disease. Studies with cultured skin fibroblasts from patients with the disorder demonstrate a wide variety of abnormalities in the uptake and nuclear binding of radiolabelled 1,25-dihydroxyvitamin D_3, indicating genetic heterogeneity in the disorder. More recent studies show mutations in the vitamin D receptor gene. Children with the most profound defects are difficult to treat and sometimes die of pneumonia. Patients with severe disease often respond poorly even to large doses of 1,25-dihydroxyvitamin D_3 but respond favorably to long-term infusions of calcium.

ANTICONVULSANT-INDUCED OSTEOMALACIA

Osteomalacia can be seen in patients with epilepsy who are receiving anticonvulsant therapy, especially phenobarbital and phenytoin (dilantin). The clinical spectrum ranges from asymptomatic individuals with a reduction in bone mass to patients with hypocalcemia, clinically apparent bone disease, fractures, and pseudofractures. The incidence of bone disease is higher in patients who receive more than one anticonvulsant drug.

Anticonvulsant drugs induce hepatic microsomal mixed-function oxidase activity. This results in increased hepatic conversion of vitamin D and 25-hydroxyvitamin D to more polar, biologically inactive metabolites. As a consequence, serum 25-hydroxyvitamin D is reduced. Since serum 1,25-dihydroxyvitamin D is normal, however, the bone disease may not be caused by abnormal vitamin D metabolism. In experimental animals, phenytoin inhibits the intestinal absorption of calcium and both phenytoin and phenobarbital inhibit mobilization of calcium from bone in vitro. Inhibition of the peripheral actions of 1,25-dihydroxyvitamin D is apparently responsible for the bone disease.

Administration of vitamin D corrects and prevents biochemical and radiographic abnormalities of osteomalacia and decreases the incidence of fractures in patients who are being treated with anticonvulsants.

RENAL DISEASE

Patients with renal disease develop rickets and osteomalacia based on all three mechanisms cited in the box on p. 1523, diminished renal production of 1,25-dihydroxyvitamin D and abnormal mineralization caused by aluminum toxicity and formation of abnormal collagen or matrix. Metabolic bone disease encountered in uremic patients includes osteitis fibrosa, osteomalacia, and a combination of the two disorders. With progressive renal failure, there is an inability to rapidly excrete phosphate, leading to a reciprocal reduction in serum calcium and increases in the secretion of parathyroid hormone. Phosphate retention, however, suppresses the renal production of 1,25-dihydroxyvitamin D, and the reduction is reversed or prevented by phosphate restriction. With advancing renal insufficiency, the kidney loses its capability to synthesize 1,25-dihydroxyvitamin D and rickets and osteomalacia may occur. Osteomalacia may also develop as a result of phosphate depletion induced by dialysis or secondary to renal phosphate wasting after kidney transplantation.

Aluminum is implicated in the defective mineralization seen in renal osteodystrophy. Evidence for this stems from several epidemiologic and experimental observations. First, a high prevalence of dialysis-dependent bone diseases was noted in patients undergoing hemodialysis with a water of high aluminum content. There was also a decreased incidence of these diseases after removal of aluminum. In addition, patients with dialysis-dependent osteodystrophy seem to manifest higher plasma aluminum levels, which correlate with bone aluminum content. Histomorphometric examination of bone reveals that aluminum is deposited along the mineralization front. Use of desferrioxamine in affected patients has resulted in clinical improvement of bone disease as well as decreased levels of plasma and bone aluminum concentrations. Animal studies demonstrate that aluminum loading in rats and dogs is associated with the development of osteomalacia. The severity of impairment in mineralization was increased in uremic animals. Inappropriately low or decreased serum parathyroid hormone secondary to parathyroidectomy seems to put patients at risk for the development of this entity.

On the other hand, several theoretical and experimental observations question the pathogenic role of aluminum in this disorder. It is not clear that aluminum is the only metal contaminating dialysis fluid that was removed with water purification. It is also noted that aluminum deposition at the mineralization front does not imply causality and may instead represent an epiphenomenon. Animals made osteomalacic by vitamin D depletion and given aluminum demonstrated aluminum deposits at the mineralization site in a pattern and to an extent that was identical to that found in the dialysis-dependent patients with osteomalacia. In addition, vitamin D repletion resulted in normal calcification even in the face of continued aluminum administration. Staining of the normally mineralized bone indicated that calcification had occurred at sites where aluminum had previously been deposited.

Chronic acidosis associated with renal disease, such as renal tubular acidosis without renal insufficiency, has also been associated with the development of osteomalacia. Treatment with alkali may suffice in these patients and avoid the possible complications of vitamin D therapy.

MINERALIZATION DEFECTS

Diphosphonates are protein-seeking agents that have the structure -P-C-P, are derivatives of pyrophosphate, and can impair mineralization. One of them, disodium etidronate, is effective in producing remission of Paget's disease. In high doses, 20 mg/kg of body weight, however, etidronate produces osteomalacia and fractures. At lower doses, 5 to 7.5 mg/kg of body weight, it corrects the biochemical and skeletal abnormalities of Paget's disease without impairing mineralization.

Fluoride, when ingested chronically in large doses, more than 20 mg of fluoride I.M. per day, produces skeletal fluorinosis. This syndrome is characterized by periosteal new bone formation, osteophyte formation, arthralgias, and abnormal hardening of the bone. Total osteoid surface area and width are increased. New periosteal bone formation may be abnormal and demonstrates a disordered lamellar structure.

Aluminum was implicated in the pathogenesis of osteomalacia and fractures that occur in patients on total parenteral nutrition who receive amino acids in the form of casein hydrolysate. High concentrations of aluminum were found in the casein hydrolysate and in skeletal tissue. In individuals who develop osteomalacia while on treatment with total parenteral nutrition, serum immunoreactive parathyroid hormone was either abnormally low or in the lower range of normal. The pathogenesis is thought to be similar to that of aluminum-related osteomalacia that occurs in patients with renal insufficiency.

HYPOPHOSPHATASIA

Hypophosphatasia is a rare disease characterized by low activity of serum and bone alkaline phosphatase. Abnormal mineralization of the skeleton resulting in rickets and osteomalacia are found together with premature loss of deciduous teeth and increased phosphoethanolamine and pyrophosphate in blood and urine. The disease is transmitted as an autosomal recessive and is prevalent in inbred populations.

Three types of hypophosphatasia are recognized based on the age of onset and clinical severity: infantile, childhood, and adult. Infantile hypophosphatasia usually develops before 6 months of age and can be diagnosed in utero. It is the most common form of this disorder and is associated with severe rickets and failure to thrive. Increased intracranial pressure, hypercalcemia, hypercalciuria, and nephrocalcinosis are found. The skeletal disease is so severe that less than 50% of infants survive. Childhood hypophosphatasia presents after 6 months of age and is characterized by premature loss of deciduous teeth, increased susceptibility to infection, and retarded growth. Radiographic findings include deossification with a coarse trabecular pattern, bowing deformities, and fractures. Irregular epiphyses and islands of radiolucency are present in the shafts of long bones. Spontaneous healing of rachitic skeletal changes occurs, but permanent teeth are lost early.

Adult hypophosphatasia is quite rare. Patients often have a history of rickets, loss of deciduous teeth in childhood, and early loss or extraction of permanent teeth. Radiographs may show a coarse trabecular pattern, Looser's zones, and subperiosteal bone formation.

The diagnosis is established by findings of low serum alkaline phosphatase and elevated serum and urine phosphoethanolamine. There is no effective form of treatment, although vitamin D has produced some improvement in a few patients. A number of patients have developed vitamin D intoxication. Treatment with phosphate improved mineralization of the skeleton in some instances when given in doses of 1.25 to 3.0 grams of neutral phosphate. Some clinical improvement has been observed when purified alkaline phosphatase is infused intravenously into patients with hypophosphatasia, but experience is limited.

TREATMENT

The goals of treatment of rickets or osteomalacia are to correct hypocalcemia if it is present; to prevent symptoms and sequelae of hypocalcemia including seizures and cataracts; to prevent or correct the skeletal deformities of rickets and osteomalacia and those of secondary hyperparathyroidism; to prevent hypercalcemia, hypercalcuria, and their consequences; and to produce normal growth and development of the skeleton in children. Vitamin D and a number of its derivatives are available in the United States. Vitamin D is available as 50,000 I.U. (1.25 mg) capsules for oral administration, in sesame oil (500,000 I.U. or 12.5 mg/ml) for injection, and in propylene glycol (200 I.U. or 6.25 μg per drop) for oral administration. The advantages of vitamin D are that the cost is modest and that it is often effective, even in patients with abnormal vitamin D metabolism. The disadvantages of vitamin D are that several weeks may be required to achieve optimal therapeutic effectiveness, the therapeutic dose is near the toxic dose, and biological activity persists after its administration is stopped.

25-hydroxyvitamin D_3 is available in capsules of 20 μg and 50 μg. The drug may be particularly useful in patients with hepatic disease and impaired synthesis of 25-hydroxyvitamin D. The onset of action of the drug is more rapid than that of vitamin D. The disadvantages are much the same as those of vitamin D. However, the half-life of the drug, 2 to 3 weeks, may be shorter than that of vitamin D, which is stored in fat so that in the event of toxicity, the biologic effects after cessation of administration may not be as long-lasting as those of vitamin D.

1,25-dihydroxyvitamin D_3 is marketed as capsules of 0.25 μg and 0.50 μg and an intravenous preparation containing 1 μg or 2 μg per ml. The advantages of the drug are its rapid onset of action and the rapid disappearance of its biological effect after discontinuation. The half-life of the drug is less than 6 hours. One disadvantage is that hypercalcemia may occur after long-term treatment during which the abnormal calcium metabolism is stabilized. Hypercalcemia can be treated by stopping the drug and prevented by decreasing the dose. Hypercalcemia occurs fairly frequently, so patients must be closely followed. 1,25-dihydroxyvitamin D_3 is most useful in diseases in which its synthesis by the kidney is impaired. It is sometimes of value in disorders in which resistance at the cellular level to its effects occurs. In the latter instance, higher doses are required.

Dihydrotachysterol is available as tablets of 0.125, 0.2, and 0.4 mg. The drug has a rapid onset of action and a relatively short duration of biological action after cessation of administration. The 180° rotation of the A ring permits the hydroxyl group in the free position to act as a pseudo–hydroxyl group. The drug becomes biologically active after it undergoes 25-hydroxylation in the liver. Since it does not need to be hydroxylated in the 1α position, the drug is of potential value in treating the same diseases as those for which 1,25-dihydroxyvitamin D_3 is indicated.

Calcium supplements should be administered in divided doses since calcium absorption is abnormally low in most patients with osteomalacia. Administration of calcium decreases the amount of vitamin D or its analogs required for treatment. The content of elemental calcium varies among preparations, so the amount that provides 1 gram of elemental calcium also varies. From 1 to 2 grams per day of elemental calcium should be administered to adults in divided doses. Children should receive 30 to 60 mg/kg body weight per day. The dose should be modified depending on the severity of the disease.

Deficiency of vitamin D in adults is treated by the daily administration of 5000 I.U. (125 μg) to 10,000 I.U. (250 μg) of vitamin D_2 until healing of bone disease occurs. Children should be treated with 1000 I.U. (25 μg) per day. This low dose does not mask vitamin D–resistant syndromes and rarely results in the hypocalcemia seen in the "hungry bone" syndrome associated with the initiation of vitamin D therapy. In noncompliant patients, a single high dose (500,000 IU, 12.5 mg) of vitamin D ("the stoss treatment"), delivered either as an intramuscular injection or by mouth, is frequently effective. After the bone disease is healed, 400 I.U. (10 μg) per day, the recommended requirement, prevents recurrence. Larger doses of 50,000 I.U. (1.25 mg) to 100,000 I.U. (2.5 mg) may be required in patients with gastrointestinal, renal, or hepatic disease. As already noted, treatment with 25-hydroxyvitamin D_3 is indicated when there is marked impairment of hepatic vitamin D-25-hydroxylase.

Vitamin D, 50,000 I.U. (1.25 mg) to 100,000 I.U. (2.5 mg) per day or more, is often effective in treating osteomalacia resulting from diseases associated with renal insufficiency, hypoparathyroidism, and pseudohypoparathyroidism but may not be effective in treating bone diseases associated with vitamin D–dependent rickets type I, hypophosphatemic rickets, and tumor-induced osteomalacia. In these disorders, 1,25-dihydroxyvitamin D_3, 0.5 to 3 μg per day, is usually effective. The dose of vitamin D, 25-hydroxyvitamin D_3, and 1,25-dihydroxyvitamin D_3 varies from patient to patient and in a given individual must be determined by trial and error for the treatment of hypophosphatemic rickets. Phosphate supplements of 2 to 4 grams per day in divided oral doses and as much as 4 μg per day of 1,25-dihydroxyvitamin D_3 are essential to heal the bone disease. Lifelong treatment is required. Removal or radiation of tumor is required to treat tumor-induced osteomalacia.

Osteomalacia associated with vitamin D–dependent rickets type II sometimes responds to treatment with vitamin D. However, in instances of a more profound target-organ defect, 1,25-dihydroxyvitamin D_3 is necessary. Doses as high as 15 to 20 μg per day are sometimes required and even so may not be effective. Under these circumstances, long-term parenteral administration of calcium can be used to heal the bone disease.

Osteomalacia associated with renal tubular acidosis is treated initially with 5000 I.U. (1250 μg) to 10,000 I.U. (2500 μg) of vitamin D. The acidosis is corrected by treatment with sodium bicarbonate. Once the bone disease heals, however, vitamin D is not required.

Hypercalcemia and hypercalciuria sometimes occur during treatment with vitamin D and its metabolites. Individuals may be asymptomatic or have anorexia, nausea, vomiting, weight loss, headache, constipation, polyuria, polydipsia, and altered mental status. The abnormal calcium metabolism is characterized by increased intestinal absorption and enhanced release of calcium from skeletal tissue. Decline of renal function, nephrocalcinosis, nephrolithiasis, urinary tract infections, and even death may ensue. Patients who are on long-term treatment with vitamin D and its analogs require careful follow-up at intervals of 4 to 6 weeks with measurement of serum and urinary calcium and serum creatinine. Careful evaluation of patients is important since there is no way to predict when or in whom vitamin D intoxication will develop. Of interest, vitamin D intoxication is almost never seen when the "stoss treatment" is used in children. The most effective means of treatment of side effects and complications is prevention. When intoxication does occur, the drug and calcium supplements should be stopped and fluids, 3 to 4 liters per day, should be given. Either the dose of vitamin D or its derivatives should be reduced, or another drug should be substituted. When intoxication is severe, treatment with prednisone or salmon calcitonin may be required.

REFERENCES

Balsan S and Tieder M: Linear growth in patients with hypophosphatemic vitamin D–resistant rickets: influence of treatment regimen and parental height. J Pediatr 116:365, 1991.

Drezner MK: Understanding the pathogenesis of X-linked hypophosphatemic rickets, a requisite for successful therapy. In Zackson DA, editor: A CPC series: cases in metabolic bone disease. New York, 1987, Triclinica Communications.

Epstein S et al: 1α,25-dihydroxyvitamin D_3 corrects osteomalacia in hypoparathyroidism and pseudohypoparathyroidism. Acta Endocrinol 103:241, 1983.

Gazit D et al: Osteomalacia in hereditary hypophosphatemic rickets with hypercalciuria: a correlative clinical-histomorphometric study. J Clin Endocrinol Metab 72:229, 1991.

Hodsman AB et al: Bone aluminum and histomorphometric features of renal osteodystrophy. J Clin Endocrinol Metab 54:539, 1982.

Hutchinson FN and Bell NH: Osteomalacia and rickets. Semin Nephrol 12:127, 1992.

Kumar R and Riggs BL: Vitamin D in the therapy of disorders of calcium and phosphorus metabolism. Mayo Clin Proc 56:327, 1981.

Lobaugh B, Burch WM Jr, and Drezner MK: Abnormalities of vitamin D metabolism and action in the vitamin D resistant rachitic and osteomalacia disease. In Kumar R, editor: Vitamin D, basic and clinical aspects. Boston, 1984, Martinas Nijhoff.

Okonofua F et al: Rickets in Nigerian children: a consequence of calcium malnutrition. Metabolism (U.S.) 40:209, 1991.

Ott SM et al: Aluminum is associated with low bone formation in patients receiving chronic parenteral nutrition. Ann Intern Med 98:910, 1983.

Pratt CB et al: Ifosfamide, Fanconi's syndrome, and rickets. J Clin Oncol 9:1495, 1991.

Verge CF et al: Effects of therapy in X-linked hypophosphatemic rickets. N Engl J Med 325:1843, 1991.

Wilson DM et al: Growth hormone therapy in hypophosphatemic rickets. Am J Dis Child 145:1165, 1991.

CHAPTER

183 Paget's Disease of Bone

Frederick R. Singer

In 1876, Sir James Paget, a remarkable English surgeon, described a focal disorder of bone that produced slowly progressive enlargement and deformity of the skeleton. He believed this was a rare disorder but in the ensuing years the application of biochemical testing and x-rays to clinical medicine made it apparent that this disease was not uncommon.

Paget's disease has been estimated to be present in 2% to 3% of the population over 50 years of age in countries where it is commonly found. Perhaps the population most affected by this condition is the Lancashire region of England, where the prevalence is estimated to be more than 8%. The disease follows patterns of English migration to Australia, New Zealand, South Africa, and the United States, and is relatively common on the continent of Europe and in cities in South America with heavy European immigration. Paget's disease is strikingly uncommon in Scandinavia, China, Japan, and India. The disease shows no clear predilection for either sex. Up to 25% of patients have at least one other family member affected by the disease. Examination of familial patterns of the disease suggests an autosomal dominant pattern of inheritance with incomplete penetrance. Studies in England have suggested that exposure to dogs may be a risk factor but this has not proven a universal finding.

PATHOLOGY

Generally, Paget's disease affects one or several bones, most often the skull, vertebrae, pelvis, femur, and tibia. It is believed that a focal increase in osteoclasts initiates an osteolytic process, which must evolve over decades before a bone such as the femur is totally involved. The osteoclasts in Paget's disease are sometimes quite large and may be found to have many more nuclei than normal. Behind the advancing front of osteoclasts into normal bone, there is evidence of great cellular activity. Osteoblasts have proliferated and line bony trabeculae that have undergone partial resorption by the osteoclasts. Fibroblasts, connective tissue, and blood vessels have replaced most of the hematopoietic cells of the marrow. The bone matrix has assumed a "mosaic" pattern with irregular cement lines instead of the normal symmetry of the collagen fibers in parallel. Sometimes a "burned-out" stage of Paget's disease is found in which cellular activity is reduced or absent but the abnormal matrix persists.

The ultrastructure of the osteoclast in Paget's disease is characterized by the presence of abnormal nuclear and cytoplasmic inclusions, which closely resemble the nucleocapsids of viruses of the Paramyxoviridae family. Immunocytochemical studies have demonstrated that the osteoclasts harbor measles virus and/or respiratory syncytial virus nucleocapsid antigens.

Attempts to identify specific viral mRNA transcripts have produced conflicting data. The identity of the osteoclast inclusions remains to be clarified.

CLINICAL COURSE

Paget's disease is not usually discovered until middle age. It is not known precisely what percentage of patients with Paget's disease are symptomatic. In a study in Germany it was estimated that less than 1% of affected individuals had symptoms. While this may be an underestimate of symptomatic patients, it is clear that many individuals are discovered to have this disease only when an abnormal x-ray or laboratory test is encountered during the course of a routine examination or while another disorder is being evaluated. In symptomatic patients, the most common complaints are skeletal deformity and musculoskeletal pain.

On physical examination, the skull, the clavicles, or the long bones of the lower extremities may be seen to be abnormal in an asymmetric distribution. Gross enlargement of these bones may be obvious and deformity of weight-bearing bones is also quite prominent. If the skull is involved, hearing loss is quite common in the later stages. Vertigo, tinnitus, and less commonly, headaches, may also be present. Basilar impression may be associated with neurologic syndromes related to compression of the spinal cord, the brainstem, the cerebellum, and the basilar and vertebral arteries. A common site of involvement is the spine, the thoracic and lumbar vertebrae most often being affected. Multiple vertebrae or a solitary vertebra may be abnormal.

Back pain is a common complaint and may be caused by Paget's disease, but degenerative arthritis of the spine is quite common. Less often, spinal stenosis may result in severe pain. Vertebrae affected by Paget's disease are also susceptible to compression fractures. A common site of involvement is the pelvis and femurs. When disease is present in these areas, degenerative arthritis of the hip is a major problem, leading to pain and impaired mobility. Bowing of the femur or tibia is also a cause of difficult ambulation. Degenerative arthritis in the knees and ankles may be associated with lower-extremity deformities.

Pathologic fractures sometimes occur in the femur and tibia of patients with Paget's disease. Nonunion is relatively infrequent but more likely to occur if the femur is fractured. A useful physical finding suggesting Paget's disease in the lower extremities is the observation of increased skin temperature over an affected bone. This is a consequence of increased blood flow not only to the bone but to the surrounding cutaneous region.

Examination of the fundus may reveal angioid streaks in about 10% of patients. This finding reflects defects in Bruch's membrane of the retina. This finding is seldom associated with impaired vision. Patients in whom more than 15% of the skeleton is affected by Paget's disease have increased cardiac output. This could predispose an individual to congestive heart failure, but high-output cardiac failure is not a common feature even in patients with very extensive disease.

The most deadly complication of Paget's disease is the development of a sarcoma in a preexisting lesion of Paget's disease. The prognosis in such patients is quite poor, probably because of the difficulties in early diagnosis. A relatively rapid increase in skeletal deformity or sudden worsening of bone pain suggests an underlying tumor. Fortunately, sarcomas occur in fewer than 1% of patients. Even less common are benign giant cell tumors, which can also arise in the pagetic bone.

RADIOLOGY

The diagnosis of Paget's disease is primarily made by x-ray since its features are so characteristic that a bone biopsy is seldom necessary. The early phases of the disease are most readily recognized in the skull and long bones. The initial lesion is a radiolucent area, which, in the skull, has been termed *osteoporosis circumscripta* (Fig. 183-1). In a long bone, the radiolucent lesion usually begins at either end of the bone and progresses with a sharply defined V shape either proximally or distally. The average rate of progress of such lesions has been measured to be approximately 1 cm per year. Uncommonly, this osteolytic phase may result in an expansile lesion resembling a cyst at the end of a long bone such as the tibia.

After many years, the osteolytic phase is transformed into an osteoblastic or osteosclerotic phase. Chaotic new bone formation leads to striking enlargement of the calvarium, which has a "cotton-wool" appearance (Fig. 183-2). It is likely that patients with severe enlargement of the skull have had their disease since childhood. The osteolytic lesions in the long bones evolve into lesions with thickened bone and irregular trabeculations. In the pelvis, a classical sign of Paget's disease is thickening of the iliopectineal line, the so-called "brim sign." The vertebral bodies are generally noted to be sclerotic at the time of diagnosis rather than radiolucent (Fig. 183-3). At times, a sclerotic vertebrae from Paget's disease may be difficult to distinguish from a malignant lesion. However, in Paget's disease the vertebral body is often larger than adjacent normal vertebrae (Fig. 183-3). In patients with back pain, computed tomography and magnetic resonance imaging of the spine are useful techniques to help evaluate the cause of the pain.

The most sensitive means of detecting Paget's disease is by utilizing radioactive tracers that localize in bone. Occasionally, lesions that are difficult to visualize on x-ray may be strongly positive on a bone scan.

BIOCHEMISTRY

Routine biochemical screening in patients with Paget's disease usually results in an isolated abnormality, elevation of serum alkaline phosphatase activity. The level of this index of osteoblastic activity correlates quite well with the extent and activity of the disease. Another index of osteoblastic activity, the blood level of the vitamin K–dependent protein osteocalcin, inexplicably is less useful. Indices of bone matrix resorption such as urinary hydroxypro-

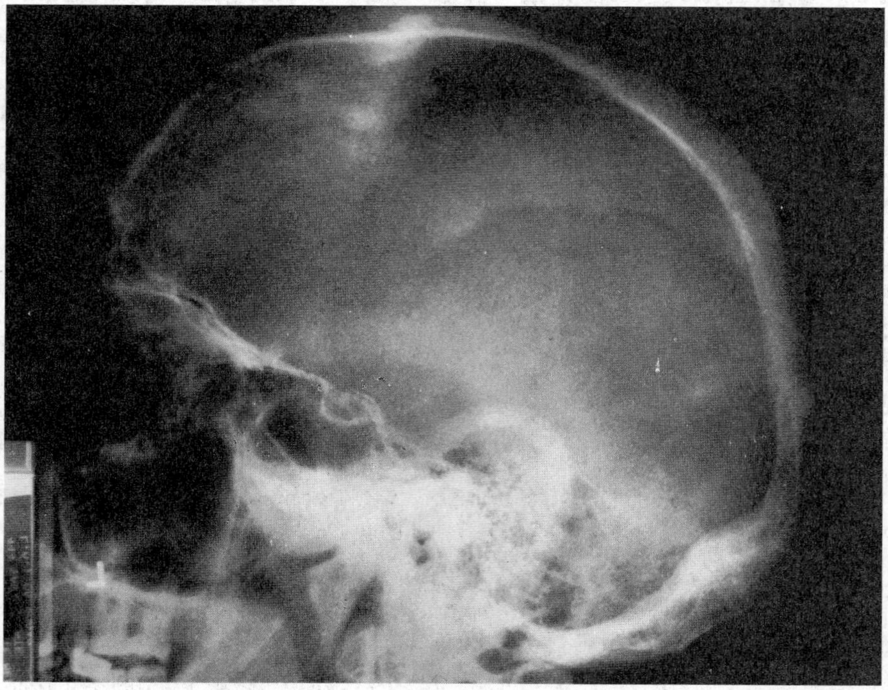

Fig. 183-1. Lateral x-ray of the skull demonstrating large radiolucent areas termed *osteoporosis circumscripta*. Early sclerotic lesions are also apparent.

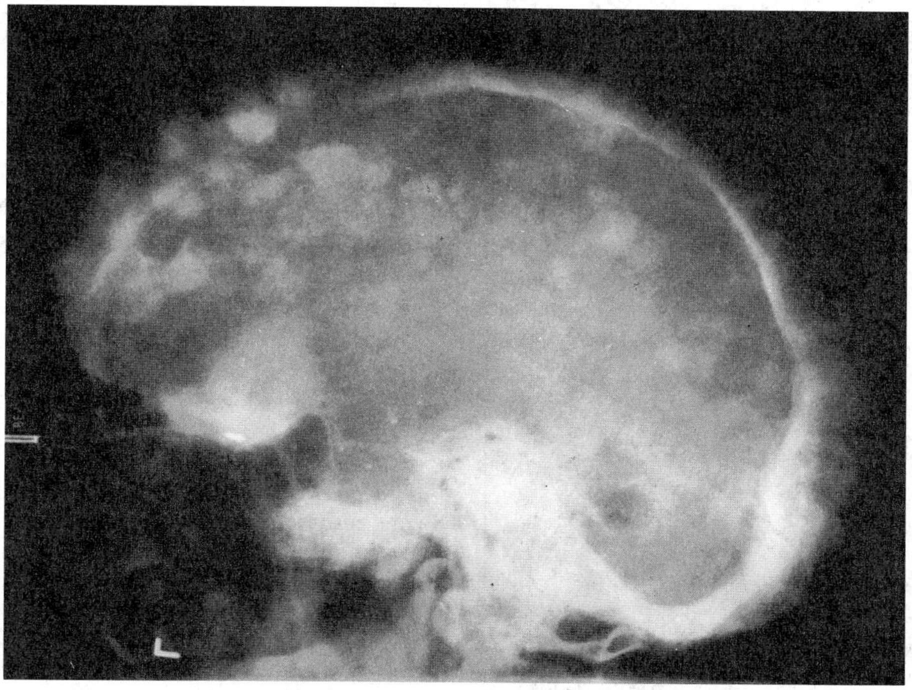

Fig. 183-2. Lateral x-ray of the skull of a patient with advanced Paget's disease. There is generalized thickening of the calvarium with patchy sclerosis exhibiting a "cotton-wool" appearance.

line or pyridinoline cross-links excretion are usually not needed for clinical evaluation unless liver disease or pregnancy complicates the clinical course. Hypercalcemia may occur if patients are immobilized or if primary hyperparathyroidism or a malignancy develops. Hyperuricemia, in the presence or absence of gout, may be found and perhaps reflect high turnover of nucleic acids.

TREATMENT

Until the etiology of Paget's disease is determined, definitive therapy is not possible. Nevertheless, during the past 20 years, it has become possible to deal effectively with many of the manifestations of the disease utilizing appropriate medical and surgical treatment.

Many patients require no treatment as they are asymptomatic and do not have disease in weight-bearing bones. The main indications for drug treatment are relief of bone pain, preparation for orthopaedic surgery, prevention of progression of osteolytic lesions in weight-bearing bones, and prevention or stabilization of hearing loss.

Calcitonin

Salmon and human calcitonin are inhibitors of osteoclast activity that reduce both bone resorption and, secondarily, bone formation when given chronically by subcutaneous injection. A nasal spray form of salmon calcitonin is available in some countries. Treatment results in relief of bone pain, resolution of osteolytic lesions, reduction of increased cardiac output, stabilization of hearing, and reversal of neurologic deficits in some patients. Subcutaneous treatment with 50 units of salmon calcitonin or 0.5 mg human calcitonin daily or on alternate days usually decreases serum alkaline phosphatase activity by 50%. Side effects include nausea and facial flushing, which usually is tolerable. Antibodies develop in about 50% of patients treated with the salmon hormone and may produce clinical resistance. These patients respond well to human calcitonin. If calcitonin treatment is discontinued, the disease becomes more active within months.

Bisphosphonates

The bisphosphonates, analogues of pyrophosphoric acid, are agents that localize to the surface of bone and inhibit bone resorption. The most widely available analogue, disodium etidronate, is administered orally at a dose of 5 mg/kg body weight daily for 6-month courses. It produces clinical benefits quite similar to those of the calcitonins. The main differences are that it is not effective in healing osteolytic lesions and doses greater than 5 mg/kg may induce osteomalacia. Much more potent bisphosphonates, which do not cause osteomalacia, are under study. Intravenous pamidronate, which is FDA-approved for malignant hypercalcemia only, is highly effective in suppressing disease activity. Even a single infusion can produce long-term improvement.

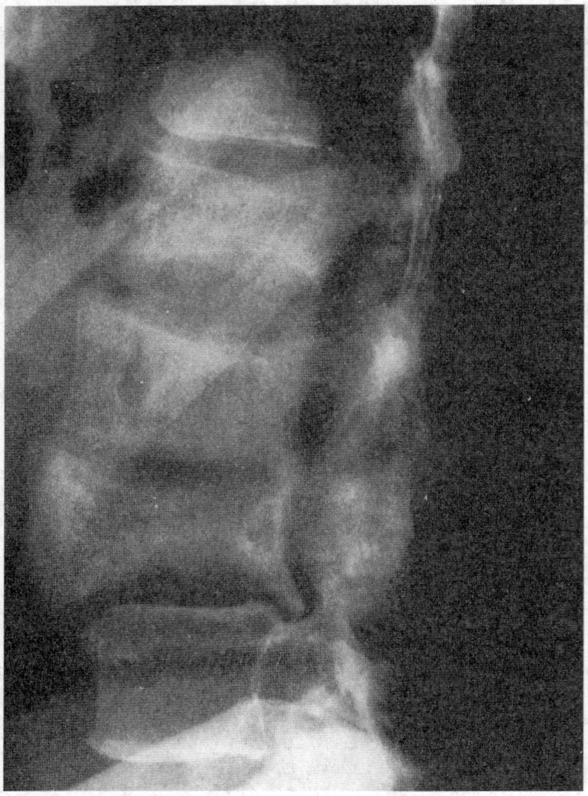

Fig. 183-3. Lateral x-ray of the lumbar spine demonstrating three enlarged vertebral bodies. The distal vertebral body is compressed and encroaching on the spinal canal.

Surgery

Drug therapy cannot reverse the structural abnormalities found to produce significant morbidity in some patients with advanced Paget's disease. Patients with neurological problems secondary to basilar impression require occipital decompression, and patients with spinal stenosis may need surgical intervention. The severe pain and impaired ambulation caused by degenerative arthritis of the hip can be effectively relieved by a total hip replacement. Impaired ambulation and knee or ankle pain caused by severe tibial bowing usually respond well to a high tibial osteotomy. Prior to elective surgery, it is wise to administer medical therapy for up to 3 months to minimize intraoperative and postoperative bleeding and prevent hypercalcemia caused by immobilization.

REFERENCES

Kanis JA: Pathophysiology and treatment of Paget's disease of bone. Durham, 1991, Carolina Academic Press.

McDonald DJ and Sim FH: Total hip arthroplasty in Paget's disease. J Bone Joint Surg 69 [Am]:766, 1987.

Meyers M and Singer F: Osteotomy for tibia vara in Paget's disease under cover of calcitonin. J Bone Joint Surg 60 [Am]:810, 1978.

Singer FR and Krane SM: Paget's disease of bone. In Avioli LV and Krane SM, editors: Metabolic bone disease and clinically related disorders, ed 2. Philadelphia, 1990, Saunders.

Singer FR and Wallach S, editors: Paget's disease: clinical assessment, present and future therapy. New York, 1991, Elsevier.

CHAPTER

184 Osteopetrosis

Gregory R. Mundy
Charles A. Reasner II

Osteopetrosis is the name given to a number of inherited bone disorders characterized by an increase in bone mass that impairs normal medullary hematopoiesis and obstructs osseous foramina. These disorders are characterized by a generalized increase in radiodensity and have been called *marble bone disease*. They are rare congenital disorders caused primarily by defective bone resorption. There is impaired remodeling of bone and a subsequent increase in trabecular and cortical bone matrix, usually with disorganized architecture and incomplete mineralization. The excess bone may obliterate the marrow cavity and encroach on nerve foramina. The bones are usually fragile despite their increased radiodensity and fracture easily. It has been suggested that *chalk bone disease* would be a more appropriate name than *marble bone disease*.

PATHOPHYSIOLOGY

There are several different types of osteopetrosis, but the primary underlying mechanism is the same—a failure of normal osteoclastic bone resorption. A particularly malignant childhood form, inherited as an autosomal recessive trait, is characterized by severe bone marrow failure and usually a poor prognosis. The more benign form that presents during adult life is inherited as an autosomal dominant trait. In this adult variety, bone marrow failure does not occur, but the patient may have an increased susceptibility to fracture, increased radiodensity, and encroachment on cranial nerves at the base of the skull. There is a third form in humans, a rare autosomal recessive disorder characterized by cerebral calcification, renal tubular acidosis, and osteopetrosis. This form has been called *marble brain disease*. In this variant, there appears to be a defect in an isoenzyme of carbonic anhydrase (carbonic anhydrase II), which is apparently necessary for normal osteoclastic bone resorption. This enzyme is present in the osteoclast and is probably essential for the normal osteoclast to generate an acid environment under its ruffled border, which is required in bone resorption.

There are a number of animal models of osteopetrosis in the mouse, rat, and rabbit. Much has been learned about normal bone resorption from studies of these models. Some variants can be cured by inoculation of normal mononuclear cells from the bone marrow or spleen of a littermate that presumably contain osteoclast precursors. In some variants osteoclast numbers are increased and in others they are decreased. Recent observations have shed considerable light on two murine models of osteopetrosis. These are the op/op variant, in which it has been shown that osteopetrosis is caused by impaired formation of osteoclasts. This occurs because stromal cells in this condition are unable to produce biologically active monocyte-macrophage-colony-stimulating factor (M-CSF). The disease in this case can be reversed by treatment with M-CSF. In another recently described variant of murine osteopetrosis, there is deficiency in expression of the src proto-oncogene. This proto-oncogene encodes an intracellular tyrosine kinase. Unlike op/op osteopetrosis, in src-deficient osteopetrosis the osteoclasts are formed but ineffective. This disorder can be cured by transplantation with normal osteoclast precursors. Thus, osteopetrosis is caused primarily by incompetent osteoclasts that are nonresponsive to hormones and other factors that normally regulate their activity, with subsequent impairment of normal bone resorption and bone remodeling. The different types of osteopetrosis are caused by a spectrum of abnormalities in the osteoclast, its precursor cells, or the factors necessary for normal osteoclast formation.

CLINICAL FEATURES

The common childhood form of the disease is severe and usually results in death during the first two years of life. In contrast, the adult form is mild and does not usually impair life expectancy. The rare childhood form of the disorder associated with carbonic anhydrase II deficiency is not characterized by bone marrow failure, and although it is compatible with long survival, renal tubular acidosis may shorten life expectancy.

Bone marrow failure is the critical feature of the childhood form; it is characterized by persistence of bony trabeculae, which almost completely fill the marrow cavity (Fig. 184-1). The consequences are anemia, leukopenia, and thrombocytopenia. As a result, extramedullary hematopoiesis may occur, but the children frequently die during infancy from the consequences of bone marrow failure such as infection or bleeding. If patients with this form of the disease survive into adult life, they suffer from anemia, recurrent fractures, and hepatosplenomegaly. Some have symptoms caused by encroachment of bone on cranial nerves, such as deafness or blindness, and most who survive have growth retardation. In the more benign adult form of the disease, sufficient marrow cavity is present for normal hematopoiesis, and the major symptomatology in these patients comes from their increased susceptibility to fracture. Many of these patients are asymptomatic, however, and the disease may be recognized accidentally when an x-ray is taken for some reason unrelated to the disease.

Despite their increased radiologic density, the bones are more likely to fracture because of poor organization of the bony architecture and the relative increase in woven bone. There is a failure of both primary modeling and subsequent haversian and trabecular remodeling. Although the bones are more susceptible to fracture, healing appears to proceed normally.

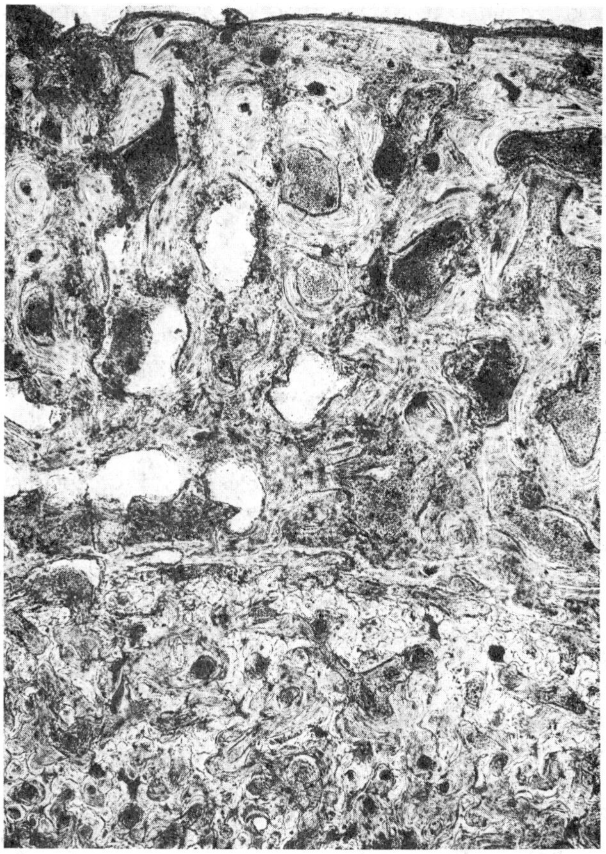

Fig. 184-1. Osteopetrosis. This illustration at low magnification reveals a densely calcified bone producing a pattern called *helter-skelter arrangement*. There is no peculiar pattern.

Despite the changes in bone histology and the propensity to fracture, deformity is usually not prominent. When it does occur, it is characterized by thickening of the shafts of the long bones so that the bones develop broad or club-shaped ends. The disease may be patchy in some bones, with some segments of bone appearing normal and some sections sclerotic on x-rays. This occurs most frequently in the vertebral bodies and the metacarpals. The skull and pelvis show a uniform increase in bone density, and the long bones show obliteration of the marrow cavity by dense compact bone.

Failure of resorption of cortical bone may result in obliteration of osseous foramina and entrapment of nerves, particularly the cranial nerves. As indicated above, this is characteristic of the severe childhood variant.

DIFFERENTIAL DIAGNOSIS

A number of other diseases may be associated with an increase in bone density. This is usually more localized than it is in most patients with osteopetrosis, and it does not date back to childhood. Some tumors are associated with focal osteoblastic metastases, which occur around metastatic tumor deposits. This is most common in patients with carcinoma of the prostate or breast, but it also occurs occasionally in patients with hematologic neoplasms such as Hodgkin's disease or myeloma. Most patients with myeloma have discrete osteolytic lesions. Bones affected by osteoblastic metastases are also more fragile and susceptible to fracture than normal bones, despite the increase in radiologic density. Pycnodysostosis is a very rare autosomal recessive disorder in which, although there is increased remodeling of the trabecular bone, cortical bone may be of increased density. There is frequently hypoplasia of the mandible and clavicle and resorption of the terminal phalanges of the fingers. The patients are usually very short, and the bones are susceptible to fracture. The x-ray appearance of many of the bones resembles that of osteopetrosis. van Buchem's disease, or hyperostosis corticalis generalisata, is characterized by thickening of cortical bone and is probably caused by increased bone formation rather than impairment of bone resorption. This condition is also inherited, although the mode of transmission is unclear. The skull is primarily involved. Engelmann's disease, or progressive diaphyseal dysplasia, is characterized by localized cortical thickening and is a rare autosomal dominant disorder.

Excess fluoride ingestion for many years causes generalized osteosclerosis, the formation of osteophytes, and calcification of ligaments. Endemic fluorosis is seen in some parts of the world where the drinking water contains enormous amounts of fluoride, such as India and South Africa. It does not occur with the much smaller amounts that are added to drinking water to prevent dental caries in many communities in the United States. It occurs occasionally in patients with osteoporosis who are treated with fluoride therapy. Fluorotic bone is radiologically dense but is poorly mineralized and characterized radiologically by excess osteoid. Fluoride stimulates osteoblast activity, but the mineral phase of bone is defective, and the bone is brittle.

TREATMENT

The benign adult form of osteopetrosis requires no treatment. Autosomal recessive infantile osteopetrosis has been treated recently with bone marrow transplantation, which has resulted in good responses in the short term in a few patients. The mortality caused by transplant complications is high, but in some of those who do survive there is evidence, at least for a few years, of normal osteoclastic bone resorption. This procedure was first tried only a few years ago, so the long-term results are not yet known.

Recently, several children with severe osteopetrosis have been treated with 1,25-dihydroxyvitamin D in an effort to provoke the nonresorbing osteoclast to resorb bone or to cause differentiation of mononuclear cell precursors to mature normal osteoclasts. Although there has been no improvement clinically, in one patient there was evidence in a bone biopsy of increased osteoclastic bone resorption. This therapy is also experimental at the present time.

REFERENCES

Coccia PF: Cells that resorb bone. N Engl J Med 310:456, 1984.

Coccia PF et al: Successful bone marrow transplantation for infantile malignant osteopetrosis. N Engl J Med 302:701, 1980.

Felix R, Cecchini MG, and Fleisch H: Macrophage colony stimulating factor restores in vivo bone resorption in the op/op osteopetrotic mouse. Endocrinology 127:2592, 1990.

Fischer A et al: Bone-marrow transplantation for immunodeficiencies and osteopetrosis: European survey, 1968–1985. Lancet 2:1080, 1986.

Key L et al: Treatment of congenital osteopetrosis with high dose calcitriol. N Engl J Med 310:409, 1984.

Kodama H et al: Congenital osteoclast deficiency in osteopetrotic (op/op) mice is cured by injections of macrophage colony stimulating factor. J Exp Med 173:269, 1991.

Mundy GR and Raisz LG: Disorders of bone resorption. In Bronner F and Coburn JW, editors: Disorders of mineral metabolism. New York, 1981, Academic.

Nordin BEC: Metabolic bone and stone disease. Baltimore, 1973, Williams & Wilkins.

Raisz LG et al: Studies on congenital osteopetrosis in microphthalmic mice using organ culture. Impairment of bone resorption and response to physiologic stimulators. J Exp Med 145:857, 1977.

Sly WS et al: Carbonic anhydrase II deficiency in 12 families with the autosomal recessive syndrome of osteopetrosis with renal tubular acidosis and cerebral calcification. N Engl J Med 313:139, 1985.

Sorell M et al: Marrow transplantation for juvenile osteopetrosis. Am J Med 70:1280, 1981.

Soriano P et al: Targeted disruption of the c-src proto-oncogene leads to osteopetrosis in mice. Cell 64:693, 1991.

van Buchem FSP: Hyperostosis corticalis generalisata. Acta Med Scand 189:257, 1971.

van Buchem FSP, Hadders HN, and Hansen W: Hyperostosis corticalis generalisata. Report of 7 cases. Am J Med 33:387, 1962.

Walker DG: Bone resorption restored in osteopetrotic mice by transplants of normal bone marrow and spleen cells. Science 90:784, 1975a.

CHAPTER

185 Fibrous Dysplasia

Gregory R. Mundy

Fibrous dysplasia is a disorder of expanding benign lesions occurring in either one or multiple sites in the skeleton. The condition is unusual but not rare. Occasionally multiple bone lesions may be associated with cutaneous pigmented macules and endocrine dysfunction. This triad of physical signs is also known as the *McCune-Albright syndrome*. Approximately one half of all patients have the classic triad, and most of the rest have two of the physical signs. The pattern of bones involved, the age of onset, and the natural history vary enormously from patient to patient. The bone disorder represents a developmental abnormality of bone-forming mesenchyma. The bone lesions are present in early childhood, but the diagnosis may not be apparent until later in life. Recently, it has been shown that in all affected tissues there is an activating mutation of the alpha subunit of the G protein ($G_s\alpha$) that couples hormone receptors to adenylate cyclase, resulting in constitutive activation of adenylate cyclase in those tissues. The condition is recognized at least three times as commonly in females as it is in males.

The McCune-Albright syndrome usually presents in childhood with spontaneous fracture or fracture after trivial injury, or premature vaginal bleeding in girls. The bone lesions may be monostotic or polyostotic. Fibrous tissue in the marrow proliferates and the adjacent cortical bone is eroded. The bones most frequently affected are the femur and tibia, skull, facial bones, and ribs. The clinical features are pain, deformity, pathologic fracture, and epiphyseal growth changes. Frequent deformities include leg-length discrepancies and bowing of the lower extremities. The characteristic deformity of the femur results in the "shepherd's crook," which causes a lateral or outward bowing of the femoral neck and shaft (Fig. 185-1). The tibia tends to bow inwards. The bone lesions may be multiple, but they are focal and discrete. The facial lesions may cause facial asymmetry, with severe distortions. The maxillary bones are frequently involved. The bone lesions are usually multifocal but unilateral, and on the same side of the body as the skin lesions. The natural history of the bone lesions varies enormously. In most patients the frequency of fractures is greatly increased during childhood but decreases after puberty.

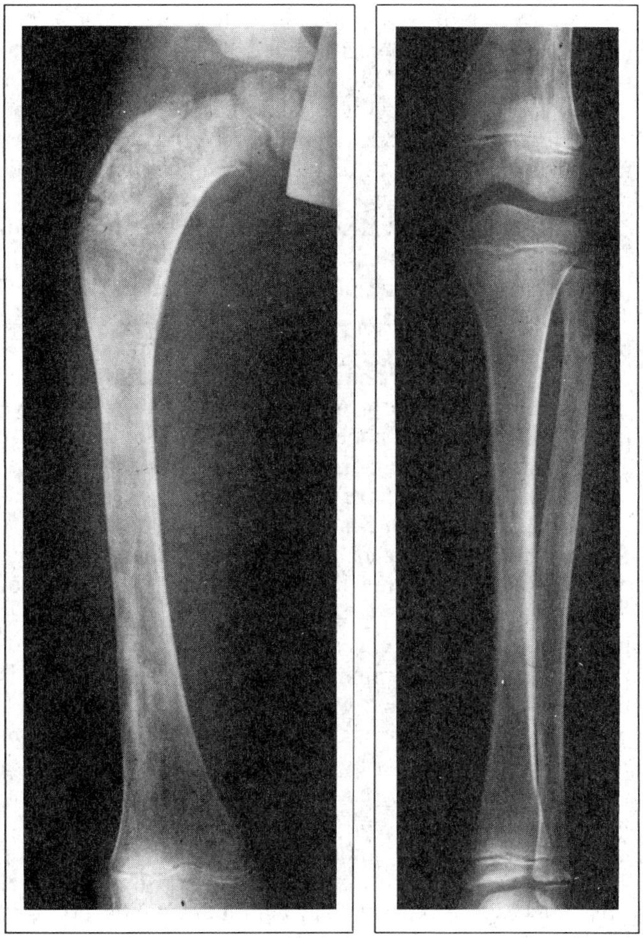

Fig. 185-1. Deformity of femur caused by fibrous dysplasia.

Skin lesions are the most common extraskeletal manifestations. The lesions occur most frequently on the sacrum, buttocks, and upper spine. They are hairless, flat, melanotic areas that do not cross the midline and have serrated margins. Because they may be confused with the lesions of neurofibromatosis, Albright claimed that their margins were like the coast of Maine whereas the margins of neurofibromatosis were more like the coast of California. However, dermatologists have been unable to distinguish the lesions on these grounds and there are no characteristic differences in the histology of the lesions in the two conditions. These pigmented macules may be present at birth.

A number of abnormalities of endocrine function have been described in Albright's syndrome. The most common has been precocious puberty, which may cause vaginal bleeding in infants or in young girls. Precocious puberty in girls can lead to rapid bone maturation, early epiphyseal closure, and subsequent short stature. The cause of precocious puberty is unknown. This feature of the condition is characterized by autonomous ovarian function and undetectable levels of circulating gonadotropins. Other endocrine conditions have been associated with Albright's syndrome including acromegaly, primary hyperparathyroidism, hyperthyroidism, Cushing's syndrome, and hypophosphatemia associated with vitamin D–resistant rickets. The relationship between these conditions and the bone lesions is unknown.

The x-ray appearance of the bone lesions of fibrous dysplasia is frequently diagnostic. In the long bones there is characteristically thinning of the cortical bone caused by endosteal erosion (Fig. 185-1). This thinning produces the appearance of a cyst, but in fact the lesions contain solid masses of fibroosseous tissue. The lesion may be radiolucent or have a ground-glass appearance if osseous trabecular bone is present. X-rays of the skull frequently show increased density at the base with thickening of the occiput (this is the most common radiologic sign) and lateral displacement of the orbital cavity. The lesions may be confused with those of Paget's disease, but the thinning of the cortical bone, absence of marked evidence of new bone formation in the long bones, and the younger age of the patient help to make the diagnosis of fibrous dysplasia.

The serum alkaline phosphatase level is usually normal in patients with fibrous dysplasia, but it may be slightly elevated, particularly after a pathologic fracture. The serum calcium is not increased unless the patient has coexistent primary hyperparathyroidism.

Treatment of this condition is primarily surgical. No medical therapy has been found to be valuable. Calcitonin has been tried and has been unsuccessful. Radiation therapy has also been used but has not produced any benefit and has been associated with later development of malignant transformation. When this rare complication occurs, it may be in the form of osteosarcoma, fibrosarcoma, chondrosarcoma, or mixed mesenchymal tumors. Treatment of the bone lesions of fibrous dysplasia is usually limited to correction of deformity or treatment of fracture. Curettage and grafting of the lesions do not necessarily lead to improvement.

REFERENCES

Albright F et al: Syndrome characterized by osteitis fibrosa disseminata, areas of pigmentation and endocrine dysfunction, with precocious puberty in females. N Engl J Med 216:727, 1937.
Dockerty MB et al: Albright's syndrome. Arch Intern Med 75:357, 1945.
Falconer MA and Cope CL: Fibrous dysplasia of bone with endocrine disorders and cutaneous pigmentation (Albright's disease). Q J Med 11:121, 1942.
Fibrous dysplasia of bone (editorial): Br Med J 1:685, 1971.
Gibson MJ and Middlemiss JH: Fibrous dysplasia of bone. Br J Radiol 44:1, 1971.
Harris WH, Dudley HR, and Barry RJ: The natural history of fibrous dysplasia. J Bone Joint Surg 44 [Am]:207, 1962.
Hunter D and Turnbull HM: Hyperparathyroidism: generalized osteitis fibrosa. Br J Surg 19:203, 1931.
Lee PA, Van Dop C, and Migeon CJ: McCune-Albright syndrome. JAMA 256:2980, 1986.
Lichtenstein L: Polyostotic fibrous dysplasia. Arch Surg 36:874, 1938.
Nordin BEC: Metabolic bone and stone disease. Baltimore, 1973, Williams & Wilkins.
Schwindinger WF, Francomano CA, and Levine MA: Identification of a mutation in the gene encoding the alpha subunit of the stimulatory G protein of adenylyl cyclase in the McCune-Albright syndrome. Proc Natl Acad Sci USA 89:5152, 1992.

CHAPTER

186 Renal Bone Disease

Hartmut H. Malluche
Marie-Claude Faugere

Bone changes are associated with various diseases of the kidney. They are seen mainly in patients suffering from kidney diseases resulting in impaired glomerular filtration. However, they also occur after kidney transplantation, with normal glomerular filtration rate and defects in tubular function, with renal stone disease, with nephrotic syndrome with or without loss of glomerular filtration, and with oxalosis.

The most prominent bone disease occurs in patients with partial or complete loss of glomerular filtration, and will be discussed in detail here (see also Chapter 348).

PREVALENCE

Histologic abnormalities of bone are found in virtually all patients with reduction in kidney function requiring chronic maintenance dialysis. The earliest histologic changes are seen after a relatively mild reduction in glomerular filtration rate (creatinine clearances between 70 and 40 ml/min). The histologic abnormalities at these early stages are usually not associated with clinical symptoms. They include mild to moderate secondary hyperparathyroid bone disease with or without defective mineralization. In patients with end-stage renal failure, a combination of both occurs, but one or the other lesion may predominate.

PATHOGENETIC FACTORS (see also Chapter 348)

Several interrelated and independent factors have been recognized in the pathogenesis of renal osteodystrophy. These factors include alterations in phosphate and calcium homeostasis, vitamin D metabolism, and parathyroid gland activity, accumulation of aluminum in bone and other organs, and dialysis-related factors. There is still considerable controversy about the sequence of pathogenetic events in the early stages of renal osteodystrophy.

Despite progressive loss of nephrons, serum phosphorus levels do not rise before the glomerular filtration rate is reduced to levels of less than 25% of normal. This is accomplished by an augmented excretion of phosphate through the remaining functioning nephrons, which may result in reduced activity of the renal C_1-α-hydroxylase and consequently in relative or absolute deficiency of the active vitamin D metabolite 1,25-dihydroxyvitamin D_3. This leads to secondary hyperparathyroidism. If the compensatory capacity of the kidney can no longer increase the excretion of phosphate through the remaining nephrons to compensate for advanced nephron loss, frank hyperphosphatemia ensues, which is usually associated with hypocalcemia. Thus, advanced renal osteodystrophy presents with hyperparathyroid bone disease and abnormal bone mineralization.

During the last decade, aluminum has been identified as an additional factor contributing to the severity of renal bone disease. Accumulation of aluminum in bone and other organs such as parathyroid glands has been observed in more than 50% of patients on dialysis and in 5% of patients before initiation of dialysis. Accumulation of aluminum in parathyroid glands results in decreased secretion of parathyroid hormone and suppression of bone turnover. In addition, aluminum inhibits renal and intestinal C_1-α-hydroxylase activity and may thus further reduce levels of 1,25-dihydroxyvitamin D_3. Aluminum accumulation in bone is associated with abnormal mineralization and reduction in bone formation and resorption with a disproportionately greater effect on formation, which leads to negative bone balance. These bone abnormalities may ultimately cause florid osteomalacia and/or osteopenia. Several sources of aluminum have been identified in dialyzed patients and include high concentrations of aluminum in water used for dialysis and aluminum-containing phosphate binders. The use of reverse osmosis and substitution of aluminum-containing phosphate binders by calcium salts have greatly reduced exposure of dialysis patients to aluminum. However, aluminum is ubiquitous in nature and is often present in drinking water, other drinking fluids, processed food, and medications. Also, its intestinal absorption may be aggravated by oral citrate intake. Recently, it has been observed that end-stage renal patients newly enrolled in a dialysis program and never exposed to aluminum-containing phosphate binders may develop aluminum-related bone disease. This worrisome observation emphasizes the fact that aluminum intoxication will continue to affect dialyzed patients.

The contribution of acidosis to the pathogenesis of renal bone disease in patients with reduced kidney function has not been fully elucidated and awaits further studies.

Institution of chronic maintenance dialysis may alter the course of renal bone disease. Dialysate calcium concentrations should be sufficient to counteract a negative calcium balance. Patients on peritoneal dialysis may have episodes of peritonitis, which may result in losses of vitamin D–binding protein. Neither exogenous nor endogenous calcitonin protects against development of hyperparathyroid bone disease in patients with renal failure.

HISTOLOGIC PATTERN

Renal bone disease in patients with reduced kidney function can be subdivided into three major histologic groups—predominant hyperparathyroid bone disease, low-turnover renal bone disease including osteomalacia and adynamic bone disease, and mixed uremic osteodystrophy of mild to moderate hyperparathyroid bone disease and defective mineralization. The histologic pattern is determined by the major pathogenetic factor responsible, namely, secondary hyperparathyroidism, deficiency of the active vitamin D metabolite, or accumulation of aluminum in bone. Even though these groups do not represent fully separate entities, it is worthwhile to distinguish them because therapy can be tailored according to the predominant histologic findings. Transformation from one form to another can occur. The prevalence of the different forms may vary depending on geographic factors, aluminum exposure, therapy with vitamin D metabolites, dietary intake, and dialysis-related factors. Approximately 45 to 90 percent of unselected patients with end-stage renal failure have mixed uremic osteodystrophy, 5 to 30 percent predominant hyperparathyroid bone disease, and 5 to 35 percent low-turnover renal bone disease. Over the past few years, the incidence of adynamic bone disease has increased gradually. The factors associated with the growing occurrence of adynamic bone disease include (1) the persistence of aluminum accumulation, (2) the increasing age of the patients, (3) the increased number of diabetics undergoing dialysis, and (4) chronic ambulatory peritoneal dialysis. The clinical relevance of adynamic bone disease is not yet fully known; however, preliminary observations point to a tendency toward hypercalcemia and a greater fragility of the skeleton in patients afflicted by this histological entity. Virtually all patients with mild to moderate renal failure present with mild hyperparathyroidism or mixed renal osteodystrophy.

Predominant hyperparathyroid bone disease (Fig. 186-1, Plate IV-5)

Histologic changes represent the effects of excess parathyroid hormone on the skeleton. There is an abundance of osteoclasts, osteoblasts, and osteocytes.

Disturbed osteoblastic activity results in disorderly production of collagen, which is deposited not only toward the trabecular surface but also into the marrow cavity, causing peritrabecular and marrow fibrosis. The nonmineralized

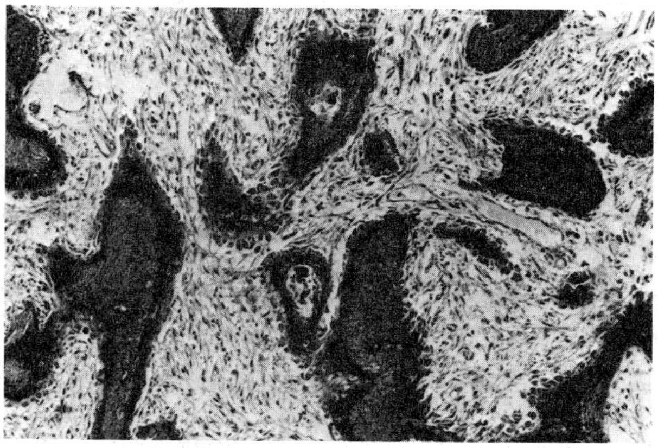

Fig. 186-1. (See Plate IV-5.) Predominant hyperparathyroid bone disease. Undecalcified 3-μm thick section of anterior iliac bone from chronically dialyzed patient. Abundance of osteoclasts, osteoblasts, and osteocytes. Marrow fibrosis. Irregular trabecular surface and tunneling resorption of mineralized bone underneath osteoid. Modified Masson-Goldner stain. Original magnification × 8. (Reprinted with permission from Malluche HH and Faugere MC: Atlas of mineralized bone histology. New York, 1986, Karger.)

component of bone, that is, osteoid, is increased, and the normal three-dimensional architecture of osteoid is frequently lost—that is, osteoid seams no longer exhibit their usual birefringence under polarized light; instead, a disorderly arrangement of "woven osteoid" and "woven bone" with a typical criss-cross pattern under polarized light is seen. The mineral apposition rate and number of actively mineralizing appositional sites are increased, as documented under fluorescent light after administration of time-spaced tetracycline markers. There is a tendency for cancellous bone mass to rise with increasing levels of parathyroid hormone. Approximately 35% of patients with predominant hyperparathyroid bone disease do have stainable bone aluminum.

Mixed uremic osteodystrophy (Fig. 186-2, Plate IV-6)

This form of renal osteodystrophy presents with two major abnormalities: hyperparathyroid bone disease and defective mineralization. Both histologic features may coexist at varying degrees in different patients. Cancellous bone volume is usually within the normal range. Factors that cause bone mass to decrease in dialyzed patients with mixed uremic osteodystrophy include accumulation of aluminum in bone, prolonged immobilization, and malnutrition. The major histologic abnormalities consist of accumulation of lamellar and woven osteoid with normal or increased thickness of osteoid, high-normal or increased number of osteoclasts and osteoblasts, and mild to moderate peritrabecular fibrosis. Evaluation of bone under fluorescent light after time-spaced tetracycline administration reveals a decrease in doubly labeled lamellar osteoid seams.

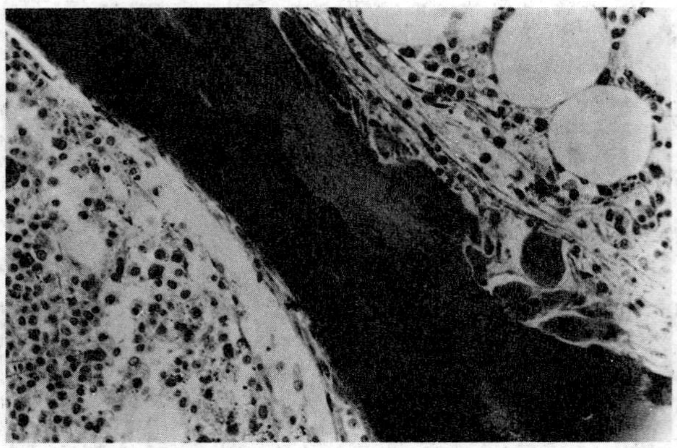

Fig. 186-2. (See Plate IV-6.) Mixed uremic osteodystrophy. Undecalcified 3-μm thick section of anterior iliac bone from chronically dialyzed patient. Presence of multinucleated osteoclasts resorbing bone and new bone apposition at the opposite side of the trabeculum. Increased osteoid seam thickness. Mild peritrabecular fibrosis. Modified Masson-Goldner stain. Original magnification × 20. (Reprinted with permission from Malluche HH and Faugere MC: Atlas of mineralized bone histology. New York, 1986, Karger.)

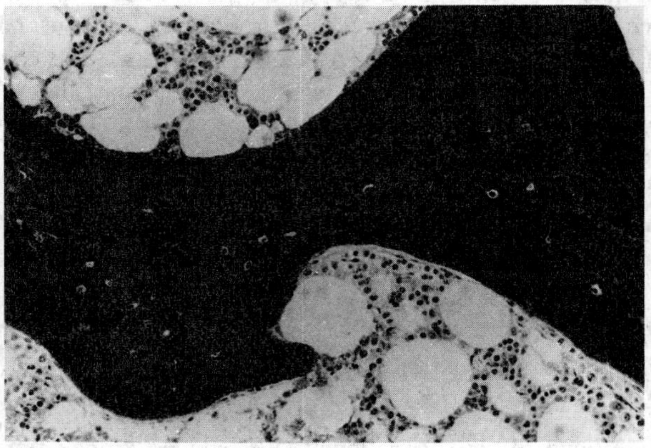

Fig. 186-3. (See Plate IV-7.) Low-turnover osteomalacia. Undecalcified 3-μm thick section of anterior iliac bone from chronically dialyzed patient. High osteoid volume caused by increased fraction of trabecular surface covered by osteoid seams and increased osteoid seam width. Irregular interface between osteoid and mineralized bone, reflecting previously enhanced resorptive activity. Absence of peritrabecular and marrow fibrosis. Paucity of bone-forming and bone-resorbing cells. Modified Masson-Goldner stain. Original magnification × 12.5. (Reprinted with permission from Malluche HH and Faugere MC: Atlas of mineralized bone histology. New York, 1986, Karger.)

Approximately 50% to 70% of patients with mixed uremic osteodystrophy present with stainable bone aluminum at the mineralization front. Aluminum in this location is associated with reduced osteoblastic activity, resulting in a decrease in bone formation and mineralizing activity.

Low-turnover renal bone disease
(Fig. 186-3, Plate IV-7)

The histologic hallmark of low-turnover osteomalacia is a dramatic reduction in the number of bone-forming and bone-resorbing cells associated with an accumulation of lamellar osteoid that occupies most of the trabecular surface and represents a considerable fraction of the trabecular bone volume. Total cancellous bone volume may be increased, mainly as a result of the excessive accumulation of osteoid. This is not infrequently accompanied by a reduction in mineralized trabecular bone mass. The smooth contour of the osteoid-marrow interface is in striking contrast to the irregular interface between osteoid and mineralized bone, which reflects past resorbing activity. More than 90% of patients with low-turnover osteomalacia have histologically stainable aluminum deposits at the bone-osteoid interface. When signs of low bone turnover are found with paucity of bone-forming and bone-resorbing cells, and osteoblastic dysfunction without accumulation of osteoid the histologic abnormality is *adynamic renal bone disease*.

CLINICAL FEATURES

Patients with mild or moderate renal insufficiency are rarely clinically symptomatic. Patients with end-stage renal disease requiring dialysis are liable to develop (1) mechanical insufficiency of the skeleton such as fractures of tubular bones, crush fractures of the vertebrae, rib fractures and epiphysiolysis in children (slipping of the epiphyses due to impaired transformation of growth cartilage into regular metaphyseal spongiosa), and (2) soft tissue and vascular calcifications.

Approximately 20% of dialyzed patients have bone pain and pseudogout and/or palpable extraosseous calcifications. Periarticular calcifications and soft tissue calcifications are preferentially seen in patients with predominant hyperparathyroid bone disease, whereas loss of height and spontaneous fractures occur mainly in patients with low-turnover osteomalacia. Clinical problems caused by soft tissue and vascular calcifications are seen earlier in the course of the disease, whereas orthopedic skeletal problems arise with increasing duration of dialysis. The "red eye syndrome" resulting from inflammatory reactions and irritation caused by conjunctival calcifications is seen in approximately 10% of dialyzed patients. If calcifications occur in the cornea, band keratopathy can be demonstrated by slit-lamp examination. Soft tissue calcifications—that is, tumoral calcifications, pseudogout, and skin calcifications in adult dialysis patients—are clearly related to the magnitude of the calcium-phosphate product and are responsive to its lowering. In contrast, vascular calcifications are unrelated to the calcium phosphorus product and do not respond to its normalization. In long-term dialysis patients, carpal tunnel syndrome and arthralgias are often associated with β2-microglobulin amyloid deposition in articular and periarticular structures. No specific therapy is known for this abnormality.

Renal osteodystrophy in children and growing individuals may present with a different clinical picture. Although bone pain, pseudogout, soft tissue calcifications, conjunctival calcifications, and serum biochemical changes are generally not strikingly different from those seen in adults, vascular calcifications are quite infrequent in children on chronic maintenance dialysis.

Encephalopathy is usually seen in association with low-turnover renal bone disease and is related to aluminum intoxication. The encephalopathy might evolve as the typical "dialysis dementia" with waxing and waning or as acute psychosis-like clinical presentation.

Morbidity and mortality are related to the severity of renal osteodystrophy. Severe hyperparathyroid bone disease as well as low-turnover renal bone disease are associated with a high degree of morbidity and mortality. Toxic effects of parathyroid hormone on the peripheral and central nervous system have been implicated in clinical complications such as pruritus, muscle weakness, and electroencephalographic disturbances. Morbidity, disability, and mortality are clearly increased when aluminum accumulation in bone is found. In unselected dialyzed patients, less than 20% of those with stainable aluminum in bone are asymptomatic, whereas 80% of those without aluminum are asymptomatic. Mortality is high in patients with more than 70% of the trabecular surface exhibiting aluminum if no specific therapy is instituted.

DIAGNOSIS

The diagnostic value of serum biochemical parameters is limited. Serum calcium is poorly related to histologic parameters of osteoclastic bone resorption. Spontaneous hypercalcemia or development of hypercalcemic episodes with vitamin D therapy is more frequently seen in patients with predominant hyperparathyroid bone disease and in patients with low-turnover renal bone disease (particularly with aluminum accumulation). Serum alkaline phosphatase is directly related to the amount of osteoid in the skeleton (regardless of the type). Therefore, alkaline phosphatase indicates the severity but not the quality of the bone disease. Serum parathyroid hormone levels are higher in the group of patients with predominant hyperparathyroid bone disease and lower in those with low-turnover renal bone disease, but there is a considerable overlap. Serum levels of 1,25-dihydroxyvitamin D_3 are decreased or low in most patients with renal osteodystrophy. Serum levels of the bone Gla protein reflect bone turnover and particularly bone formation, but further studies are needed to establish the place of this measurement. Measurements of serum concentrations of aluminum do not have a predictive value for aluminum accumulation in bone. Measurements of serum aluminum before and 5 to 48 hours after a single intravenous infusion of deferoxamine (Desferal, 20 mg/kg body weight infused at a rate not to exceed 15 mg/kg body weight per hour) can be used as a screening test; however, this test has limited sensitivity and specificity.

Information obtained from skeletal x-rays has to be interpreted with an understanding of the underlying histologic changes. In nondialyzed patients there is a notable discrepancy between cancellous and cortical bone, that is, cancellous bone mass may be increased and cortical bone may be normal or decreased. In dialyzed patients, normal, decreased, or increased cancellous bone mass may be found. The erosion of cortical bone by osteoclastic resorption accounts for the roentgenologic finding of subperiosteal resorption, periosteal and endosteal resorption cavities, cortical striation, and cortical thinning. These changes may be represented radiologically by erosive cortical defects in the skull ("pepper pot skull"), acro-osteolysis of the clavicula, and erosion of the terminal finger phalanges. A "rugger jersey" appearance of the spine, and a ground-glass appearance of the skull, ribs, pelvis, and metaphysis of tubular bones reflect cancellous changes. In advanced hyperparathyroid stages, "pseudocysts" or "brown tumors" may be observed. Looser's zones that are straight bands of radiolucency abutting onto the cortex and running perpendicular to the long axis of bone are of relatively low sensitivity and low specificity for the diagnosis of osteomalacia. The combination of hyperparathyroid bone disease and defective mineralization renders interpretation of the x-ray findings particularly difficult, since signs of increased bone resorption may be seen on x-rays reflecting past resorbing activity, which may have been succeeded by accumulation of osteoid. Since osteoid is radiolucent, the superimposed osteomalacia is missed by x-ray examination. Similar limitations apply to the measurement of bone mineral content by dual photon absorptiometry techniques.

Currently, the only unequivocal tool for diagnosis of renal osteodystrophy is histologic examination of nondecalcified bone biopsy specimens after in vivo administration of time-spaced tetracycline markers. The latter allows evaluation of bone dynamics such as mineralization rate and bone turnover. The bone specimens should also be stained for aluminum, because histochemically stainable deposits of aluminum at the bone-osteoid interface correlate better with histologic abnormalities in bone than concentrations of aluminum measured by atomic absorption spectrophotometry. Further specific histochemical stains may be necessary if other substances such as iron, lead, or amyloid are suspected.

PREVENTION AND THERAPY

Therapeutic intervention should begin before the patient develops far-advanced bone disease, that is, not later than at the time of institution of dialysis. Secondary hyperparathyroidism can be prevented by avoiding deviations of serum calcium and phosphorus levels from normal. An imbalance between dietary phosphate intake and renal phosphate excretion or phosphate removal through dialysis can be avoided by reducing dietary phosphate intake and intestinal phosphate absorption.

Even though prescription of phosphate-restricted diet appears logical in patients with reduced kidney function, it is often difficult to obtain full compliance. Therefore, phosphate binders are customarily prescribed to reduce intestinal absorption of phosphate. Unfortunately, most available potent intestinal phosphate binders contain aluminum. Calcium salts such as calcium acetate and calcium carbonate are at this time the preferred first-line preventative or therapeutic approach to hyperphosphatemia. The clinical efficacy and safety of other phosphate binders such as seraconium oxide and polyuronic acid await further study.

Persistent hyperphosphatemia despite therapy using phosphate binders may not always be related to lack of compliance. Excess circulating levels of parathyroid hormone may enhance release of phosphate from bone, thus maintaining hyperphosphatemia that is unresponsive to oral phosphate binders.

Serum calcium levels can be kept in the normal range by avoiding hyperphosphatemia, by oral administration of calcium salts such as calcium carbonate (0.5 to 1.5 g/day), or by therapy using the active vitamin D metabolite 1,25-dihydroxyvitamin D_3 (0.25 to 2.0 μg/day, Rocaltrol). It is advisable to start with low doses, increasing the daily dose in steps of 0.25 μg if serum calcium levels do not increase (at least 0.5 mg/dl) after 2 weeks of therapy.

More recently, intravenous administration of 1,25-dihydroxyvitamin D_3 (1-2.5 μm three times per week Calcijex) is used as therapy for hypocalcemia and elevated parathyroid hormone in dialysis patients. The intravenous administration has been shown to be associated with less-frequent episodes of hypercalcemia; this is apparently related to the relatively higher concentrations reached in the target organ parathyroid gland compared to the intestine.

Prospective clinical studies show that early administration of 1,25-dihydroxyvitamin D_3 can reverse the histologic bone abnormalities, and administration of pharmacologic doses of the drug is beneficial in patients with mixed uremic osteodystrophy. However, doses less than 0.5 μg per day should be used in early to moderate renal failure to avoid overcorrection, that is, suppression of bone turnover. Also, the positive response to 1,25-dihydroxyvitamin D_3 is reduced if there are deposits of stainable aluminum in bone.

In patients with predominant hyperparathyroid bone disease and those with low-turnover renal bone disease, vitamin D therapy frequently leads to hypercalcemia. Concomitantly elevated serum phosphorus levels may raise the calcium phosphorus product to critical levels (more than 70 mg/dl) associated with deposition of calcium salts in soft tissues. The hypercalcemia seen in patients with predominant hyperparathyroid bone disease receiving vitamin D therapy is caused in part by the effect of the active vitamin D metabolite on bone. In contrast, hypercalcemia in patients with low-turnover osteomalacia receiving vitamin D therapy results most probably from the positive effect of vitamin D on intestinal calcium absorption while the capacity of bone to incorporate calcium is reduced owing to low bone turnover and lack of excretory kidney function.

Since approximately 95% of patients with low-turnover renal bone disease do have severe aluminum accumulation in bone, intravenous therapy with deferoxamine should be beneficial for these patients. Deferoxamine is a potent drug for removal of aluminum from bone. However, it should be borne in mind that removal of aluminum from bone may transform the histologic findings of low-turnover osteomalacia to those of mixed uremic osteodystrophy and those of mixed uremic osteodystrophy to predominant hyperparathyroid bone disease. Deferoxamine should be given intravenously three times per week, preferably during dialysis, at a dose of 15-25 mg per kilogram body weight and at a rate not to exceed 15 mg/kg/hour. Considering the dialysance of the deferoxamine-aluminum complex and the total amount of aluminum that may accumulate in bone and other organs, long-term therapy is required for most patients.*

Predominant hyperparathyroid bone disease without aluminum accumulation in bone requires surgical reduction of parathyroid gland mass if administration of intravenous 1,25-dihydroxyvitamin D_3 results in hypercalcemia. The exact threshold at which intravenous 1,25-dihydroxyvitamin D_3 is no longer able to suppress parathyroid gland overactivity and when surgery remains the only tool awaits further study. Total parathyroidectomy with transplantation of parathyroid tissue to the forearm is the preferred choice for patients who need surgery. However, recurrent severe gland hyperplasia and invasive cell growth have been described. Thus, some authors advocate total parathyroidectomy. Other clinical indications for surgical reduction of parathyroid gland mass include spontaneous hypercalcemia, hyperphosphatemia, pruritus, and progressive extraosseous calcifications. Treatment with orally administered 1,25-dihydroxyvitamin D_3 should be considered postoperatively to avoid further hyperplasia of the transplanted gland. Withholding 1,25-dihydroxyvitamin D_3 replacement after surgery for days or a few weeks allows the transplanted gland to assume its function more rapidly at the new site and to mobilize soft tissue calcifications.

The occurrence of severe osteomalacia after parathyroidectomy in patients with bone aluminum and the finding of enhanced aluminum uptake by bone after parathyroidectomy call for careful documentation of the absence of stainable aluminum by bone histology before parathyroidectomy is contemplated. Lowering the serum parathyroid hormone levels is usually an effective therapy for pruritus. Before surgery, antipruritic medications such as diphenylhydramine (Benadryl) and/or activated charcoal may be helpful. Periarticular and soft tissue calcifications as well as symptoms of periarthritis respond to the lowering of the calcium-phosphorus product by parathyroidectomy.

REFERENCES

Baker LRI et al: $1,25(OH)_2D_3$ administration in moderate renal failure: a prospective double-blind trial. Kidney Int 35:661, 1989.

Coburn JW and Alfrey AC editors: Conference on aluminum related diseases. Kidney Int 29:S18, 1986.

Faugere MC and Malluche HH: Stainable aluminum and not aluminum content reflect histologic changes in bone of dialyzed patients. Kidney Int 30:717, 1986.

Faugere MC et al: Loss of bone resulting from accumulation of aluminum in bone of patients undergoing dialysis. J Lab Clin Med 107:481, 1986.

Malluche HH and Faugere MC: Atlas of mineralized bone histology. New York, 1986, Karger.

*Note: Approval by the Food and Drug Administration for the use of 1,25-dihydroxyvitamin D_3 and deferoxamine in the management of bone abnormalities of patients with renal osteodystrophy is pending.

Malluche HH and Faugere MC: Renal bone disease 1990: an unmet challenge for the nephrologist. Kidney Int 38:193, 1990.

Malluche HH and Faugere MC: Uremic bone disease: current knowledge, controversial issues and new horizons. Miner Electrolyte Metab 17:281, 1991.

Malluche HH et al: Bone histology in incipient and advanced renal failure. Kidney Int 9:355, 1976.

Malluche HH et al: The use of deferoxamine in the management of aluminum accumulation in bone in patients with renal failure. N Engl J Med 311:140, 1984.

Ott SM et al: Prevalence of bone aluminum deposition in renal osteodystrophy and its relation to the response to calcitriol therapy. N Engl J Med 307:709, 1982.

Smith AJ et al: Aluminum-related bone disease in mild and advanced renal failure: evidence for high prevalence and morbidity and studies on etiology and diagnosis. Am J Nephrol 6:392, 1986.

Teitelbaum SL. Renal osteodystrophy. Hum Pathol 15:306, 1984.

CHAPTER

187 Primary Hyperparathyroidism

John P. Bilezikian

Primary hyperparathyroidism is a common endocrine disorder caused by the excessive secretion of parathyroid hormone from one or more parathyroid glands. The major actions of parathyroid hormone—to mobilize calcium from bone and to conserve calcium in the kidney—account for hypercalcemia, a hallmark of the disease. In some cases, an additional action of parathyroid hormone, to facilitate the conversion of 25-hydroxyvitamin D to the active metabolite, 1,25-dihydroxyvitamin D, leads to increased absorption of calcium from the gastrointestinal tract. Despite the remarkable variability in clinical and biochemical features of primary hyperparathyroidism, the serum calcium level is virtually always elevated. As noted in Chapter 177, primary hyperparathyroidism, along with hypercalcemia of malignancy, is the cause of hypercalcemia in the vast majority of cases. It should always be seriously considered as a potential cause of hypercalcemia.

PREVALENCE

Estimates of prevalence of primary hyperparathyroidism range from 1 in 500 to 1 in 1000. This prevalence is markedly higher than estimates in the 1930s and 1940s when primary hyperparathyroidism was considered uncommon. The dramatic increase in recognized cases coincides with the widespread introduction of the multichannel autoanalyzer in clinical medicine in the 1970s. Primary hyperparathyroidism is now most often discovered incidentally when the patient is being evaluated by the physician for a set of complaints that are completely unrelated to hypercalcemia. Primary hyperparathyroidism occurs at all ages with a peak incidence in the sixth decade of life; women are affected more commonly than men by a ratio of 3:2. The disorder is relatively unusual in children.

PATHOLOGY AND ETIOLOGY

The vast majority of patients with primary hyperparathyroidism, 80% to 85%, have a single adenoma that varies in size from relatively small (less than 0.5 g) to very large (over 10 g). Even the modest parathyroid adenoma is much larger than the normal gland, which is only approximately 25 mg. Most adenomas are less than 1 g in size. They appear histologically as a confluence of encapsulated chief cells with a rim of normal tissue at the margin. It is unusual for a patient to harbor more than one adenoma. Cystic elements in an adenomatous gland may call attention to a rare familial variant, cystic parathyroid adenomatosis. Although the parathyroid adenoma is most commonly found at one of the usual locations of parathyroid tissue (the four poles of the thyroid gland), the tumor may be found at unusual locations in up to 10% of patients with adenomatous disease. Ectopic sites include the lateral neck, the retroesophagus, within the thyroid gland itself, and the mediastinum.

Approximately 20% of patients with primary hyperparathyroidism have a pathologic process involving all four glands with hyperplasia. Four-gland hyperplasia may occur sporadically but is seen also in conjunction with multiple endocrine neoplasia (MEN) type I or II. The extent to which each gland is involved varies in that some hyperplastic parathyroids appear to be abnormal only because of diminished fat content, whereas others are grossly enlarged. Involvement of all parathyroid glands in hyperplastic disease contrasts markedly with the normal appearance of three parathyroid glands when the pathology is adenoma. This distinction is important because the surgical approach to the patient is defined in part by the pathology of primary hyperparathyroidism.

The rarest presentation of primary hyperparathyroidism is parathyroid carcinoma, occurring in well under 1% of patients. As is the case for many endocrine neoplasms, it is difficult to distinguish on pathologic grounds benign from malignant disease. Several histologic features such as mitoses, vascular invasion, and fibrous trabeculae are important clues. In addition, metastases to contiguous (thyroid, neck muscles, esophagus) or more distant sites (cervical lymph nodes, lung, liver) help to establish the diagnosis of parathyroid malignancy.

The underlying cause of primary hyperparathyroidism is not known. Most patients develop the disease in the absence of a family history or possible predisposing factors such as childhood neck irradiation. Molecular analysis of adenomatous parathyroid tissue indicates that the disease is most likely monoclonal in origin. Several patients with primary hyperparathyroidism have been described in which the parathyroid hormone gene is rearranged and under the influence of a different, more active promoter. This observation has not been generally made in primary hyperparathyroidism, suggesting that it may not constitute the genetic basis for primary hyperparathyroidism in most patients.

SYMPTOMS AND SIGNS

The manifestations of primary hyperparathyroidism include potential involvement of many organ systems. They are caused either by the effects of excess parathyroid hormone on its target tissues or by the major biochemical consequences of hypercalcemia. Certainly, hypercalcemia may give rise to its own set of signs and symptoms such as shortened QT interval on the electrocardiogram, polyuria, polydipsia, anorexia, constipation, and depressed central nervous system function (see Chapter 177). These features are specific for hypercalcemia; they are not specific for primary hyperparathyroidism. The extent to which manifestations of hypercalcemia are present is related to the level of the elevated serum calcium, the rate of its rise, and the chronicity of the problem. In addition to hypercalcemia, primary hyperparathyroidism causes systemic abnormalities, some of which are classic manifestations of the disease. The designation *disorder of bones and stones* illustrates two specific organ systems at risk for damage or dysfunction from primary hyperparathyroidism.

Bone disease

The classic bone disease of primary hyperparathyroidism is *osteitis fibrosa cystica*. Clinically, patients develop bone pain and occasional pathologic fractures. Resorption of bone caused by excessive secretion of parathyroid hormone is associated with several typical radiologic signs. Subperiosteal resorption of the distal phalanges is the most specific sign of primary hyperparathyroidism. It is appreciated best on the radial side of the middle phalanges. Similar radiologic changes may be present in the skull, where a moth-eaten or salt-and-pepper pattern is evident. The distal third of the clavicles may demonstrate tapering of bone density. Locally destructive lesions appearing as bone cysts or "brown tumors" in the long bones and pelvis constitute another skeletal manifestation of primary hyperparathyroidism (Fig. 187-1). Brown tumors are collections

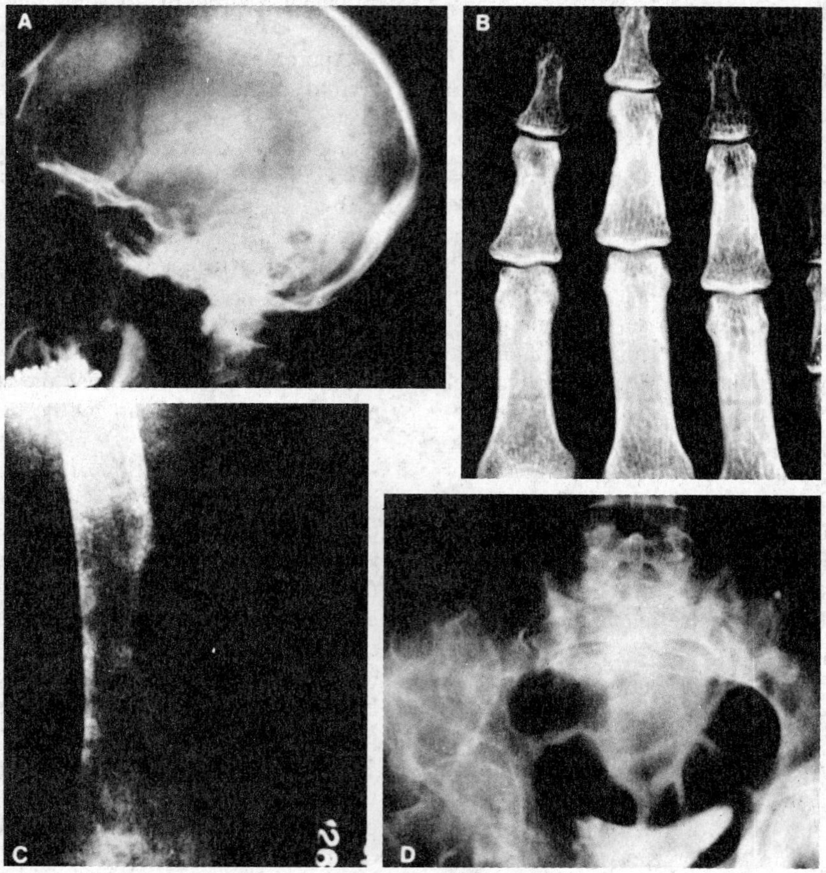

Fig. 187-1. Osteitis fibrosa cystica in primary hyperparathyroidism. **A,** Note the salt-and-pepper appearance of the skull. **B,** Subperiosteal bone resorption can be appreciated along the radial margins of the distal phalanges. **C,** The lytic lesion on the lateral border of the femur is a brown tumor that subsequently healed after successful parathyroidectomy. **D,** Confluent cystic bone disease in the pelvis of a woman with severe primary hyperparathyroidism.

of osteoclasts intermixed with poorly mineralized woven bone. Nonspecific generalized demineralization is sometimes evident in the absence of obvious hyperparathyroid bone disease. Osteitis fibrosa cystica was always uncommon in primary hyperparathyroidism, never composing more than 10% of the hyperparathyroid population. It is even more uncommon now. However, in populations without ready access to medical care, overt parathyroid bone disease is still seen.

Although the milder form of primary hyperparathyroidism seen today suggests that patients are discovered before radiologic signs develop, this does not mean that most patients are spared skeletal involvement. Approaches more sensitive than conventional radiography demonstrate the presence of bone involvement in a greater percentage of patients. Noninvasive densitometry of the skeleton, in fact, shows that many patients without overt radiologic hyperparathyroid bone disease have evidence of demineralization. The particular distribution of reduced bone mineral density in primary hyperparathyroidism appears to be preferential to cortical bone (long bones) as compared with cancellous bone (spine). Involvement of cortical bone with preservation of cancellous bone is compatible with the physiologic actions of parathyroid hormone. Subclinical involvement of cortical bone in primary hyperparathyroidism is confirmed with even greater sensitivity by histomorphometric analysis of the percutaneous bone biopsy. Among many asymptomatic patients, cortical width, formation, and resorption surfaces, as well as bone formation rates, are affected. Consistent with data obtained from bone densitometry, cancellous bone volume does not appear to be reduced in primary hyperparathyroidism. Scanning electron microscopy of bone biopsy specimens illustrates this point well (Fig. 187-2). It is not yet clear whether this information is going to be helpful in predicting or selecting those patients who are destined to experience important skeletal complications of primary hyperparathyroidism.

Renal disease (also see Chapter 349)

Kidney stones are one of the classic complications of primary hyperparathyroidism. Before the clinical profile of primary hyperparathyroidism began to change approximately 20 years ago, nephrolithiasis occurred in approximately one third of all patients with the disorder. The incidence of nephrolithiasis is now closer to 15% to 20%. In the occasional patient, a symptomatic kidney stone is the first manifestation of primary hyperparathyroidism. It is thus still strongly advisable to investigate the possibility of primary hyperparathyroidism in any patient who presents with a kidney stone, although fewer than 1 in 20 is ultimately shown to have the disease. Besides stones, the kidney may be affected in other ways, such as deposition of calcium-phosphate crystals throughout the renal parenchyma. This process, nephrocalcinosis, may or may not be associated with diminished renal function. Some patients with primary hyperparathyroidism demonstrate a decreased creatinine clearance without nephrocalcinosis or other obvious etiology. Perhaps the most common association between primary hyperparathyroidism and the kidney is hypercalciuria. Urinary calcium excretion over 250 mg daily is seen in 20% to 25% of patients with primary hyperparathyroidism. The hypercalciuria is caused by the greater load of filtered calcium which exceeds the capacity of the kidney to conserve it despite the conserving actions of parathyroid hormone. It is not clear whether hypercalciuria in this setting predisposes patients to nephrolithiasis and/or nephrocalcinosis.

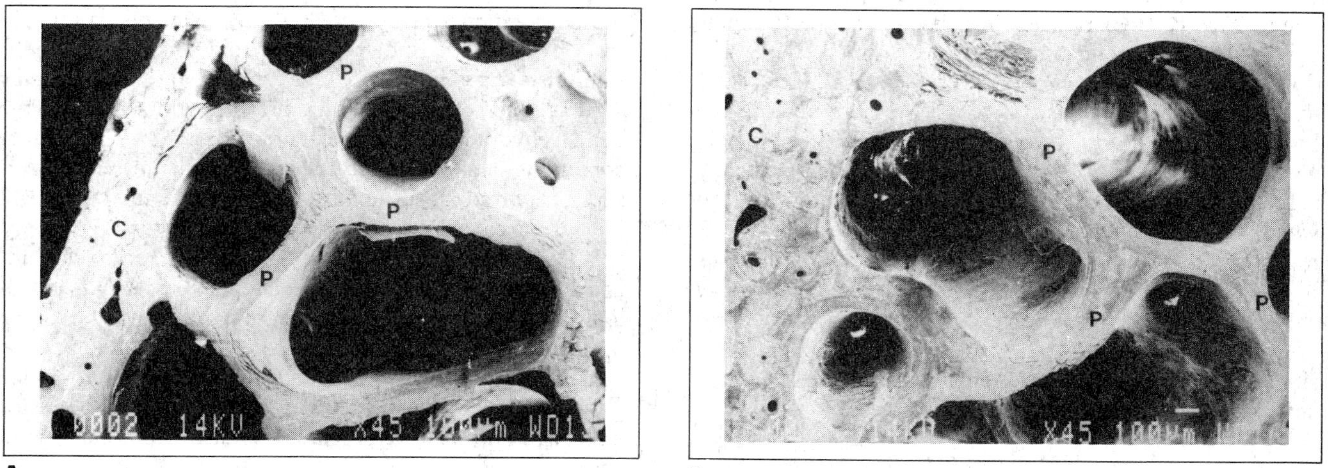

A B

Fig. 187-2. Primary hyperparathyroidism as seen by scanning electron microscopy. A 45-year-old man with primary hyperparathyroidism, **A,** is compared to an age- and sex-matched normal subject, **B.** Note that the trabecular plates *(P)* are conserved in hyperparathyroidism, but that the cortex *(C)* is considerably thinner. The field width is 2.4 mm in each case, and the magnification is the same for normal and hyperparathyroid bone. (Courtesy of Dr. David Dempster. Helen Hayes Hospital.)

Other organ involvement

The hyperparathyroid syndrome includes the potential for involvement of organ systems besides the skeleton and the kidneys. The common complaints of weakness and easy fatigability may be associated with a particular neuromuscular syndrome characterized by atrophy of type II muscle fibers. More recent experience suggests that the neuromuscular component of primary hyperparathyroidism is more likely to consist of a less specific set of neurologic manifestations. In fact, the weakness and easy fatigability of primary hyperparathyroidism is typically not associated now with any clinical neurological findings. However, muscle biopsy and electromyography testing are not routinely performed in the evaluation of the hyperparathyroid patient; thus it is not known whether patients with this complaint have any degree of neuromuscular dysfunction.

The gastrointestinal tract may also appear to be a target of the hyperparathyroid state. Historically, peptic ulcer disease was regarded as a frequent complication. It is now seen predominantly with MEN syndrome type I in which primary hyperparathyroidism and peptic ulcer may coexist. Otherwise, there is debate over whether there is a pathophysiologic association between these relatively common disorders. Similarly, the association between primary hyperparathyroidism and acute pancreatitis remains to be established on pathophysiologic grounds.

The articular system is affected in primary hyperparathyroidism, with gout and pseudogout both being seen. In the absence of symptoms, older patients with chondrocalcinosis of the knees and wrists may be at risk for the development of pseudogout. A well-known anemia of primary hyperparathyroidism is characterized by normocytic and normochromic indices. It is an unusual finding, occurring only when other systemic manifestations of primary hyperparathyroidism are present. The anemia is completely reversible after successful removal of the parathyroid adenoma. Finally, hypertension has been thought for many years to be a complicating feature of primary hyperparathyroidism. However, in only a very small minority of patients (less than 10%) is the blood pressure significantly lowered after surgery. As with the association with peptic ulcer disease, it is unclear whether hypertension and hyperparathyroidism are linked pathophysiologically or whether the incidence of both disorders together more likely reflects the expected coincidence of two common diseases. In yet another nonspecific association, a host of neuropsychiatric syndromes have been described in patients with primary hyperparathyroidism, the most common being depression. More subtle features include lack of concentrating ability and a sense of intellectual weariness.

DIAGNOSIS

Forms of clinical presentation

Given the extremely wide range of potential organ involvement in primary hyperparathyroidism, it is not surprising that the disease may present with one or more of the above complications (see box above). Isolated stone or bone disease or virtually any other potential target organ can be a focus of concern that accompanies the diagnosis. The most common presentation of primary hyperparathyroidism, however, is asymptomatic primary hyperparathyroidism, in which hypercalcemia is present in the absence of any specific signs or symptoms commonly or clearly attributed to the disease. Most often, patients have serum calcium values not more than 1 mg per deciliter above the upper limits of normal. Asymptomatic primary hyperparathyroidism dominates the modern clinical presentation of the disease. In this large cohort of asymptomatic patients, management decisions are imprecise and therapeutic guidelines are uncertain.

Clinical presentations of primary hyperparathyroidism

- Asymptomatic hypercalcemia
- Bone or stone disease
- Other recognized complications (neuromuscular, gastrointestinal, articular, hematologic, central nervous system)
- Acute primary hyperparathyroidism
- Parathyroid carcinoma
- Familial primary hyperparathyroidism
- Primary hyperparathyroidism in pregnancy
- Neonatal hyperparathyroidism
- Multiple endocrine neoplasia type I or II

In marked contrast to the most common presentation of primary hyperparathyroidism as an asymptomatic disorder, primary hyperparathyroidism presents rarely as life-threatening hypercalcemia with very high calcium values. Some of the highest serum calcium levels, up to 25 mg per deciliter, have been reported in patients with primary hyperparathyroidism. A history of mild hypercalcemia is present in approximately 25% of these patients. Acute primary hyperparathyroidism (parathyroid poisoning, parathyroid crisis) usually develops in patients who have an intercurrent illness for which they are immobilized or bedridden. Dehydration is another etiologic factor. Under these conditions, a state of further negative calcium balance ensues, parathyroid hormone levels increase markedly, and the serum calcium rises accordingly. Anorexia and polyuria lead to further dehydration and higher serum calcium, and a worsening cycle of escalating hypercalcemia is established. Acute primary hyperparathyroidism is an important consideration in acutely hypercalcemic individuals because it is curable and readily reversible. On clinical grounds, it may be difficult, if not impossible, to distinguish acute primary hyperparathyroidism from parathyroid carcinoma.

On the extreme other hand, there are occasional patients with normal serum calcium values who are suspected of having primary hyperparathyroidism because of nephrolithiasis or other well-known complications. The term *normocalcemic hyperparathyroidism* has been applied to these patients. It is a misnomer because the calcium can be shown to become abnormal in these patients at periodic intervals.

Primary hyperparathyroidism may be associated with MEN type I (parathyroid, pituitary, pancreas) or type II (medullary thyroid cancer, pheochromocytoma; see Chapter 164). Primary hyperparathyroidism can also occur rarely as an isolated familial disease involving only the parathyroids. A pathologic variant of familial primary hyperparathyroidism is cystic parathyroid adenomatosis, characterized by recurrent parathyroid disease over years as glands become sequentially involved.

Primary hyperparathyroidism can develop during pregnancy. The diagnosis may be suspected in retrospect after delivery when neonatal hypocalcemia and tetany occur in the offspring. The neonatal hypocalcemia is believed to be caused by suppression of neonatal parathyroid function by the maternal hypercalcemia. Finally, primary hyperparathyroidism can present as life-threatening hypercalcemia discovered soon after birth. These children display a characteristic hypotonia and can be managed only by emergency parathyroidectomy. At operation, all four glands are involved in a hyperplastic process. Of great interest is the fact that kindreds of families with neonatal primary hyperparathyroidism have been described in which familial cystic adenomatosis and/or familial hypocalciuric hypercalcemia are also present.

Physical findings

The most noteworthy aspect of the physical examination in primary hyperparathyroidism is that the examination is not noteworthy. There are usually no abnormal physical findings specifically related to the disease. By ophthalmologic slit-lamp examination, calcium phosphate deposition in the medial and lateral limbic margins of the cornea (band keratopathy) is seen rarely. Enlarged parathyroid tissue is rarely palpable except when parathyroid carcinoma is present.

Laboratory findings and differential diagnosis

Hypercalcemia is a *sine qua non* of the disease. The serum phosphorus is usually in the lower range of normal but in approximately one third of patients, it may be frankly low. If the serum alkaline phosphatase (bone-derived) is elevated, it usually reflects active bone disease and is accompanied by elevations in serum osteocalcin (a marker of osteoblast activity) and urinary hydroxyproline or collagen cross-links (markers of osteoclast activity). 1,25-Dihydroxyvitamin D levels may be elevated although this is not specific for primary hyperparathyroidism. 1,25-Dihydroxyvitamin D levels are elevated in a number of other conditions associated with hypercalcemia such as sarcoidosis, other granulomatous diseases, certain lymphomas, and vitamin D toxicity (see Chapter 177). The actions of parathyroid hormone to alter acid-base handling in the kidney lead sometimes to mild hyperchloremia and metabolic acidosis. Urinary calcium excretion is elevated in approximately one fourth of all patients. Phosphaturia, a major physiologic action of parathyroid hormone, may also be demonstrated.

The most useful test for the diagnosis of primary hyperparathyroidism is the parathyroid hormone measurement per se. The most useful assays are those that measure intact hormone or fragments with specificity for mid- or carboxy-terminal regions of parathyroid hormone. These assays show frank elevations in parathyroid hormone in well over 90% of patients with surgically proved primary hyperparathyroidism (Fig. 187-3). The urinary cyclic AMP level, another marker of parathyroid hormone activity, does not usually add much to the diagnostic evaluation in view of the utility of the assays for parathyroid hormone. The diagnosis of primary hyperparathyroidism is made by the simultaneous presence of hypercalcemia and an elevated level of parathyroid hormone (see Chapter 177). The only exceptions to this general rule are the hypercalcemias associated with the use of thiazide diuretics and lithium. The history usually points out these two possibilities fairly readily. In these situations, the only way to determine the etiology of the hypercalcemia is to withdraw the suspected medication, if possible, and to repeat the tests in 2 to 3 months.

Another important reason why the immunoassays for parathyroid hormone have become so useful in establishing the diagnosis of primary hyperparathyroidism relates to our better understanding of some of the other etiologies of hypercalcemia. In malignant disease, parathyroid hormone

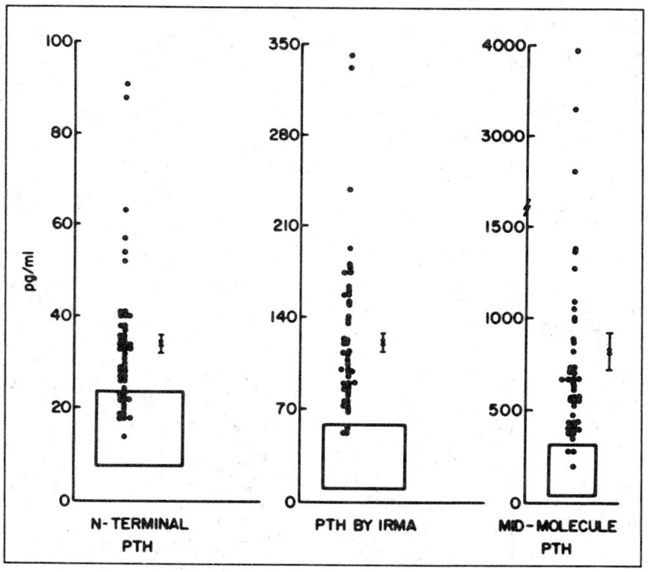

Fig. 187-3. Usefulness of radioimmunoassays and immunoradiometric assays for parathyroid hormone in establishing the diagnosis of primary hyperparathyroidism. The panels show levels of parathyroid hormone as determined by assays with specificities for *N*-terminal PTH *(left panel)*, intact PTH *(middle panel)*, and midmolecule PTH *(right panel)*. For intact PTH (immunoradiometric) and midmolecule PTH (radioimmunoassay), virtually all patients with established primary hyperparathyroidism have frankly elevated levels. In this series, the *N*-terminal radioimmunoassay shows frank elevations in a smaller number. The data represent individual blood samples determined by all three assays. (Reprinted from Silverberg SJ et al: J Bone Mineral Res 4:283, 1989.)

levels are not elevated. The parathyroid hormone–like protein, implicated in the syndrome of humoral hypercalcemia of malignancy, does not cross-react in the available immunoassays for parathyroid hormone (Fig. 187-4). Thus, virtually all malignant disorders, except for parathyroid carcinoma and the exceedingly rare example of ectopic production of authentic parathyroid hormone by a malignant tumor, show suppressed levels of parathyroid hormone. Similarly, in those malignancies and granulomatous disorders associated with hypercalcemia and elevated 1,25-dihydroxyvitamin D, the parathyroid hormone level is suppressed. Where multiple, local factors in bone are responsible for malignancy, here too, the parathyroid hormone level is not elevated.

Familial hypocalciuric hypercalcemia (FHH) should be considered in patients who appear to have primary hyperparathyroidism. FHH is a disorder characterized by mild hypercalcemia, very low urinary calcium excretion (calcium/creatinine less than 0.01), and mild hypermagnesemia. Parathyroid hormone levels are not elevated. Although the high penetrance of the disorder causes hypercalcemia in childhood, it may not be recognized until early adulthood. Patients with FHH are remarkably free from complications associated with primary hyperparathyroidism, an observation that has given rise to the description *benign familial hypercalcemia*. Adults with FHH need no treatment. Subtotal parathyroidectomy does not cure the disease. The possibility that FHH bears some relationship to primary hyperparathyroidism comes from observations in several families in which FHH and neonatal primary hyperparathyroidism were both present.

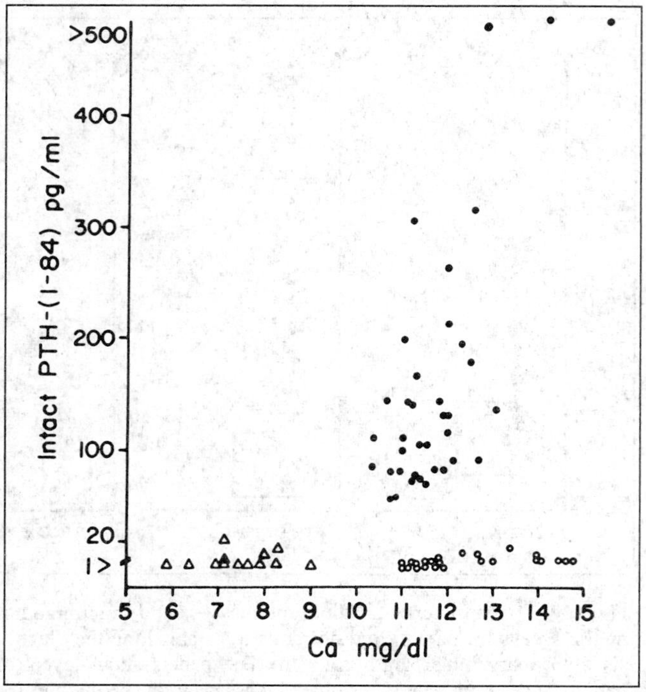

Fig. 187-4. Usefulness of the immunoradiometric assay for parathyroid hormone in the differential diagnosis of hypercalcemia. Patients with surgically proved primary hyperparathyroidism show elevations (greater than 65 pg/ml) in virtually all cases. Patients with malignancy show levels that are below or at the lower limit of normal (12 pg/ml). (Reprinted from Nussbaum SR et al: Highly sensitive two-site immunoradiometric assay of parathyrin and its clinical utility in evaluating patients with hypercalcemia. Clin Chem 33:1364, 1987. With permission.)

TREATMENT

Surgery

The definitive treatment for primary hyperparathyroidism is surgical removal of the abnormal gland(s). In the days when primary hyperparathyroidism was often accompanied by signs and symptoms, the case for parathyroid surgery was relatively straightforward. Now, however, the typical patient is asymptomatic. Complicating the consideration of surgery are additional points. We do not know and cannot yet predict who among the asymptomatic patients will develop complications of parathyroid disease. We do not even know who among the asymptomatic is truly asymptomatic. As newer methods to detect parathyroid bone disease become more widely used (bone densitometry, percutaneous bone biopsy), it is distinctly possible that our definition of *asymptomatic* will change and we will have a more certain basis for knowing whether a given patient is at risk for developing complications.

Current surgical guidelines include patients with any of the following six features: (1) a serum calcium level greater than 1 mg per deciliter above the upper limits of normal; (2) signs or symptoms of primary hyperparathyroidism, regardless of the actual serum calcium value; (3) markedly reduced cortical bone density; (4) age, under 50; (5) an episode of acute primary hyperparathyroidism; and (6) hypercalciuria. These groups are believed to present a long-term risk for the development of complications of primary hyperparathyroidism.

Parathyroidectomy should be performed by an expert neck surgeon who is intimately familiar with the difficult aspects of the procedure. Parathyroid surgery tends to be difficult because abnormal glands are still rather small. In addition, they do not always have the characteristic red-brown color and oval cigarlike configuration and may look very much like a fat globule. Moreover, they are occasionally found in ectopic sites. If an adenoma is discovered, an attempt is usually made to locate all other parathyroid glands to ascertain that they are normal. Pathology is checked during the operation by examination of frozen sections of tissue. Some surgeons will not explore the other side of the neck if the adenoma and a normal gland are discovered on the same side because the possibility of finding a second adenoma on the other side is small. If parathyroid hyperplasia is discovered, removal of 3½ glands is performed, leaving sufficient residual parathyroid tissue to maintain normal parathyroid function. Some surgeons remove all four hyperplastic glands and transplant remnants of parathyroid tissue into the forearm. Tissue from an adenomatous gland is not transplanted as a rule. When parathyroid surgery is successful, which should occur approximately 90% to 95% of the time, patients usually experience a transient 1- to 2-day period of mild hypocalcemia followed by a return of the serum calcium to normal as the suppressed normal glands regain function. In patients with overt skeletal disease, there may be a prolonged period of hypocalcemia caused by rapid reversal of the negative state of calcium balance and deposition of calcium into bone (hungry bone syndrome). A more permanent complication of parathyroid surgery is hypoparathyroidism. In the patient who has had previous neck surgery and removal of some parathyroid tissue already, postoperative hypoparathyroidism may be evident soon after surgery and documented by monitoring the lack of return of parathyroid function. However, hypoparathyroidism does not develop sometimes until months to years after surgery. In this situation, it is possible that the remaining parathyroid tissue is left with marginal vasculature and that with age, there is further reduction in vascular integrity. Another permanent complication of parathyroid surgery is recurrent laryngeal nerve damage with resultant hoarseness and loss of voice volume.

In patients who have had previous neck surgery, localization techniques are usually indicated. Among the noninvasive approaches to localization, interest centers around ultrasonography, computed tomography, magnetic resonance imaging, and scintigraphy. For all procedures, limitations include their resolving power, making adenomas smaller than 200 mg difficult to delineate, and an appreciable incidence of false-positive localization. These approaches nevertheless are destined to improve with advancing technology (Fig. 187-5). The invasive techniques of arteriography and selective venous catheterization can provide definitive anatomic and functional identification of parathyroid tissue, but they are time-consuming, operator-dependent, and expensive procedures. Nevertheless, they should be used in those patients with previous neck surgery for whom it is vitally important to identify the location of the adenoma preoperatively. Most medical centers do not routinely perform these procedures. Patients in need should therefore be referred to those few hospitals in the United States that have the requisite expertise to conduct these tests successfully.

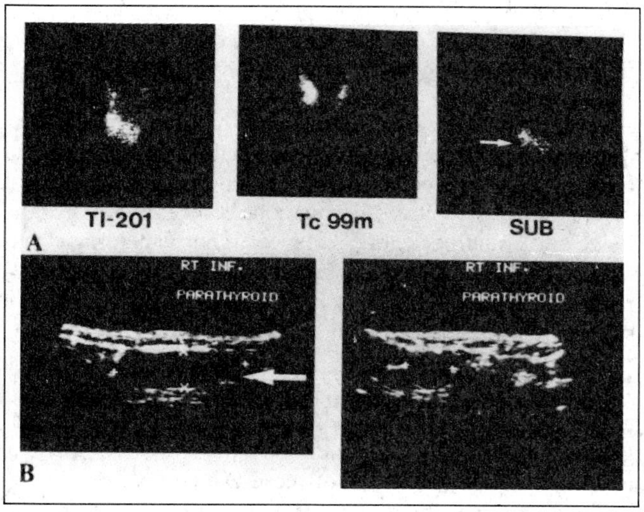

Fig. 187-5. Localization of parathyroid tissue by scintigraphy and ultrasound. Thallium-201-technetium-99m parathyroid scans in a patient with primary hyperparathyroidism. **A,** Increased thallium uptake is seen in the inferior aspect of the right lobe of the thyroid, which is confirmed by subtraction (sub) image *(arrow)*. **B,** In the two lower panels, high-resolution parathyroid sonogram in the same patient. Sagittal *(left)* and transverse *(right)* planes illustrate the adenoma. (Reprinted from Winzelberg GG: Parathyroid imaging. Ann Intern Med 107:64, 1987. With permission.)

Medical therapy

There are several groups of patients with primary hyperparathyroidism in whom surgery is not a clear option. The large cohort of patients with asymptomatic primary hyperparathyroidism illustrates the problem faced by the physician. It is not known which patients will eventually develop complications of the disease and which will remain asymptomatic. There are no clinical or laboratory criteria by which risks or probabilities of complications can be established. The variable natural history of primary hyperparathyroidism often leaves the clinician undecided between a surgical approach and a more conservative medical one. Many clinicians, however, do not recommend surgery unless the patient meets one of the surgical guidelines. Approximately 50% of patients will meet one or more surgical guidelines. In addition to the asymptomatic hyperparathyroid patient who does not meet surgical guidelines, medical management is often reserved for patients who refuse surgery and for patients who are no longer surgical candidates because of coexisting medical problems. Also included in this group are patients with persistent hyperparathyroidism who had unsuccessful previous neck operations and failed attempts at preoperative localization.

General guidelines for the patient with primary hyperparathyroidism follow from a consideration of the hypercalcemia per se. The management of acute hypercalcemia associated with primary hyperparathyroidism follows the same guidelines as those presented in Chapter 177. For routine primary hyperparathyroidism in which calcium levels are only mildly elevated, adequate hydration and ambulation are always to be encouraged as well as avoidance of diuretics such as thiazides that may actually worsen the hypercalcemia. Dietary recommendations for calcium intake should be moderate. A rationale to recommend high dietary calcium intake in order to suppress parathyroid glandular activity might be associated with worsening hypercalcemia, especially if the 1,25-dihydroxyvitamin D level is elevated. On the other hand, low dietary calcium intake could theoretically lead to further stimulation of parathyroid hormone secretion. Oral phosphate therapy may lower the serum calcium and is a reasonable mode of therapy. Chronic administration could conceivably predispose patients to ectopic calcium phosphate deposition and further elevation of parathyroid hormone levels. Postmenopausal women may be helped by estrogen therapy although parathyroid hormone levels do not decline and phosphate levels may be further reduced. Finally, a newer generation of pyrophosphate analogues known as *bisphosphonates* might be shown in the next several years to be useful in primary hyperparathyroidism.

REFERENCES

Arnold A et al: Monoclonality and abnormal parathyroid hormone genes in parathyroid adenomas. N Engl J Med 318:658, 1988.

Bilezikian JP et al: Characterization and evaluation of asymptomatic primary hyperparathyroidism. J Bone Min Res 6(suppl 2):S85, 1991.

Fitzpatrick LA and Bilezikian JP: Acute primary hyperparathyroidism. Am J Med 82:275, 1987.

Heath H III, Hodgson SF, and Kennedy MA: Primary hyperparathyroidism: incidence, morbidity, and potential economic impact in a community. N Engl J Med 302:189, 1980.

Law WM Jr and Heath H III: Familial benign hypercalcemia (hypocalciuric hypercalcemia)—clinical and pathogenetic studies in 21 families. Ann Intern Med 102:511, 1985.

Mallette LE et al: Familial cystic parathyroid adenomatosis. Ann Intern Med 107:54, 1987.

Nussbaum SR et al: Highly sensitive two-site immunoradiometric assay of parathyrin and its clinical utility in evaluating patients with hypercalcemia. Clin Chem 33:1364, 1987.

Potts JT Jr: Management of asymptomatic hyperparathyroidism. J Clin Endocrinol Metab 70:1489, 1990.

Proceedings of the NIH Consensus Development Conference on Diagnosis and Management of Asymptomatic Primary Hyperparathyroidism. In Potts JT Jr, editor: J Bone Min Res 6(suppl 2):S1, 1991.

Rao DS et al: Lack of biochemical progression or continuation of accelerated bone loss in mild asymptomatic primary hyperparathyroidism; evidence for a biphasic disease course. J Clin Endocrinol Metab 109:959, 1988.

Shane E and Bilezikian JP: Parathyroid carcinoma. In Williams CJ et al, editors: Textbook of uncommon cancer. New York, 1988, Wiley.

Silverberg SJ et al: Skeletal disease in primary hyperparathyroidism. J Bone Mineral Res 4:283, 1989.

Winzelberg GG: Parathyroid imaging. Ann Intern Med 107:64, 1987.

CHAPTER

188 Malignant Disease and the Skeleton

Gregory R. Mundy
Charles A. Reasner II

BONE METASTASES

Tumors frequently involve the skeleton. They may metastasize to bone to form either lytic (destructive) or blastic (formative) lesions (Fig. 188-1). Lytic metastases are much more common than blastic metastases, although most tumors that metastasize to bone have both lytic and blastic elements. The cellular and molecular mechanisms responsible for causing these increases in bone resorption and bone formation are undergoing intense investigation. As described in Chapter 148, bone that is resorbed is usually replaced by newly formed bone. However, in some tumors, the increase in bone formation is too pronounced to be accounted for simply by the physiologic coupling mechanism that normally links bone formation to bone resorption. It seems likely in these tumors that the tumor cells are producing a bone growth factor that stimulates adjacent osteoblasts to form new bone. The tumors that are most frequently associated with osteoblastic metastases are carcinomas of the prostate and breast, which also may be associated with osteoblastic lesions. Metastatic prostatic cancer frequently shows osteoblastic bone formation around metastatic deposits in bone.

Most tumors that metastasize to bone cause osteolytic bone destruction. These metastases may or may not be associated with hypercalcemia. The molecular mechanisms responsible for osteolytic metastases and bone destruction are unclear but comprise both the migration of tumor cells toward bone surfaces and then local destruction of bone tumor when cells are housed within the bone marrow cavity adjacent to endosteal bone margins. The destruction of bone is primarily mediated by osteoclasts, although there is evidence of direct involvement of tumor cells themselves. Local mediators of osteoclastic bone resorption that may be produced by a tumor within the bone marrow cavity include prostaglandins and the osteoclast-activating factors. Tumor cells may reach endosteal bone surfaces by chemotaxis or chemoattraction by fragments of type I collagen released during the normal bone remodeling process.

CLINICAL CONSEQUENCES OF MALIGNANT INVOLVEMENT OF THE SKELETON

The clinical consequences of malignant involvement in the skeleton include bone pain, fracture, and hypercalcemia (to be discussed later). Once tumors involve the skeleton, they are usually incurable, and only palliative therapy is possible. Bone metastases are frequently complicated by severe pain and occasionally by fracture after trivial injury. The most effective current form of therapy for localized tumor involvement of the skeleton is radiation therapy.

Hypercalcemia of malignancy

Although hypercalcemia is a frequent complication of malignant disease, there is a clear association between certain tumors and hypercalcemia. Hypercalcemia occurs most commonly in patients with squamous cell carcinomas of the lung, head, and neck, breast cancer, and hematologic malignancies such as myeloma and T cell lymphomas. The tumors most frequently associated with hypercalcemia are shown in Table 188-1.

Pathogenesis. For convenience we can classify hypercalcemia into three clinical categories, since a different pathogenetic mechanism is likely to be responsible in each case, and therapy differs in each of these categories.

Solid tumors without bone metastases. This group probably accounts for 30% to 40% of patients with hypercalcemia of malignancy. It has been designated *humoral hypercalcemia of malignancy,* since it appears likely that a humoral factor (or factors) released by the tumor cells is responsible for stimulating bone resorption and renal tubular calcium reabsorption, thereby causing hypercalcemia. Humoral hypercalcemia of malignancy is also often (but not

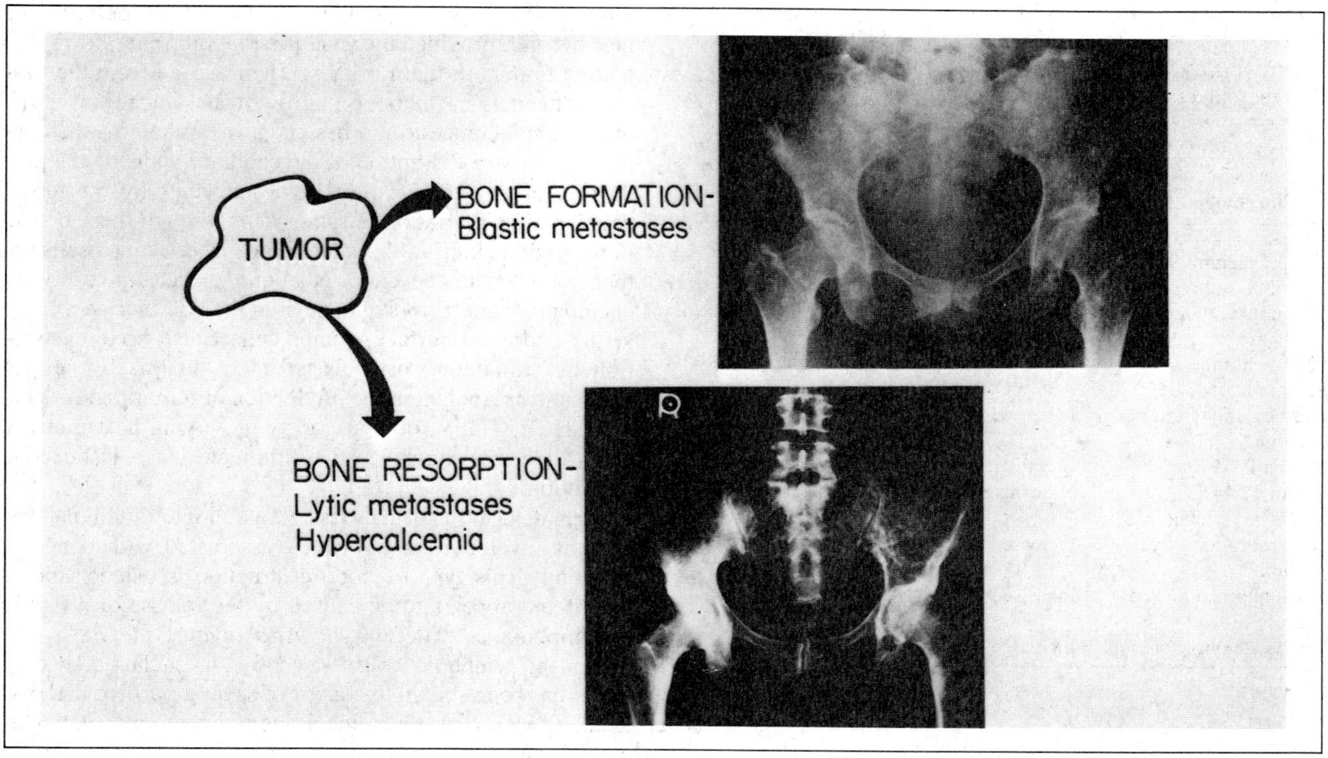

Fig. 188-1. Tumor products may cause increases in osteoblast activity (blastic metastases) or increases in osteoclast activity (lytic metastases and/or hypercalcemia).

Table 188-1. Malignancies associated with hypercalcemia

Types of malignancy	Percentage of total
Lung	35
Breast	25
Hematologic (myeloma, lymphoma)	14
Head and neck	6
Renal	3
Prostate	3
Unknown primary	7
Others	8

Modified from Mundy GR and Martin TJ: Hypercalcemia of malignancy—pathogenesis and treatment. Metabolism 31:1247, 1982.

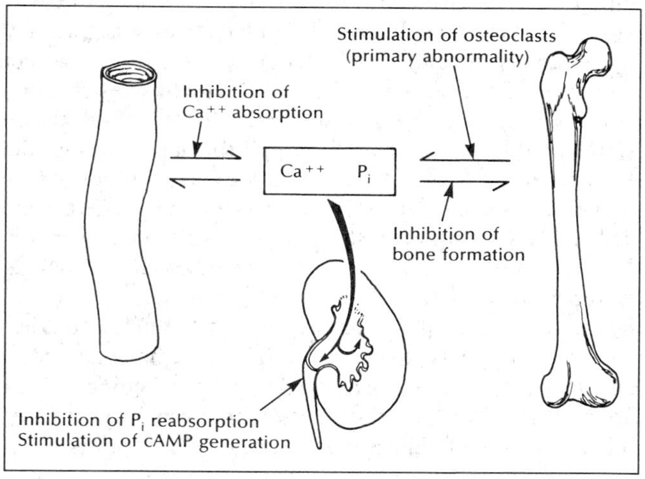

Fig. 188-2. Tumor products cause the syndrome of humoral hypercalcemia of malignancy by causing these effects on calcium and phosphate homeostasis.

always) associated with renal phosphate wasting and hypophosphatemia, increased nephrogenous cyclic AMP generation, and increased immunoreactive parathyroid hormone–related peptide (PTH-rP). (Table 188-2). Immunoreactive parathyroid hormone concentrations are suppressed. These features are depicted in Fig. 188-2. The condition occurs most frequently in patients with squamous cell carcinomas of the lung, head, and neck, carcinoma of the ovary, carcinoma of the pancreas, and carcinoma of the kidney.

The mechanisms by which tumor cells cause an increase in serum calcium have been clarified recently. Hypercalcemia occurs because of an increase in osteoclastic bone resorption and an increase in the reabsorption of calcium in the renal tubules. Most but not all patients with this syndrome of humoral hypercalcemia of malignancy (HHM) have increased circulating concentrations of the tumor peptide parathyroid hormone–related peptide (PTH-rP). This factor has homology with parathyroid hormone (PTH) at the

Table 188-2. Comparison of clinical features in primary hyperparathyroidism and humoral hypercalcemia of malignancy

Clinical feature	Primary hyperparathyroidism	Humoral hypercalcemia of malignancy
Serum calcium	Increased	Increased
Serum phosphorus	Decreased	Decreased
Serum alkaline phosphatase	N or increased	N or increased
Serum chloride	>103 mEq/liter	<98 mEq/liter
Serum bicarbonate	<25 mEq/liter	>25 mEq/liter
Plasma parathyroid hormone	Increased	N or decreased
Plasma PTH-rP	N or increased	Increased
Serum 1,25-dihydroxyvitamin D	N or increased	N or decreased
Gut absorption of calcium	Increased	Decreased
Urine phosphate excretion	Increased	Increased
Urine calcium excretion	Increased	Increased

N, normal.

N-terminal end, binds tightly to the PTH receptor, and shares with PTH the capacity to increase osteoclastic bone resorption, increase calcium reabsorption in the renal tubules, and increase the plasma calcium. Whether it has additional effects distinct from those of PTH is still not clear. However, the clinical syndromes of PTH excess (primary hyperparathyroidism) and PTH-rP excess (HHM) are not identical. The reasons may be that PTH-rP has effects distinct from those of PTH, or that other factors produced in HHM modify the effects of PTH-rP mediated through the PTH receptor. Since other factors are indeed produced by tumors associated with HHM that profoundly affect bone cells and calcium homeostasis in patients with cancer, the latter explanation seems likely. These other factors include tumor necrosis factor (TNF), which is produced by normal host cells stimulated by the presence of the tumor and has been shown to cause hypercalcemia in some human tumors, and interleukin-1α and transforming growth factor α, which are powerful bone resorbing factors that cause hypercalcemia and that are frequently produced by solid tumors in association with PTH-rP by solid tumors.

Solid tumors with metastasis. The most common tumor in this group is carcinoma of the breast. This group accounts for about 40% of all patients with hypercalcemia of malignancy. The mechanism of hypercalcemia is presumably related to the excessive osteolytic bone destruction that accompanies the metastatic process. The cellular events involved in the development of an osteolytic metastasis have been examined using in vitro techniques.

Liotta has described a multistep process by which tumor cells metastasize to different organs. The initial event is shedding of tumor cells from the primary tumor site followed by their entry into the bloodstream. After this, the tumor cells spread to vascular organs such as the red bone marrow and, provided the situation is appropriate, form secondary tumors in these organs. Their escape from the vascular channels in the bone marrow to the interstitial tissue involves adherence to the basement membrane of the capillary walls, the disruption of the capillary walls by the production of degradative proteolytic enzymes by the tumor cells, and the migration of tumor cells through these breaks in the endothelium to the interstitial space. Tumor cells are then attracted to the endosteal bone surface, possibly by chemoattractant factors in bone or at the bone surface. Once at the endosteal surface, tumor cells cause bone destruction by stimulating osteoclasts. They do this by several mechanisms, including the production of tumor factors such as PTH-rP, TGFα, or IL-1, or by provoking host immune cells to release cytokines that stimulate osteoclastic bone resorption.

Hematologic malignancies. Hematologic malignancies such as myeloma are frequently associated with bone destruction. This type of bone destruction is osteoclastic in nature and appears to be caused by the release of a family of lymphokines called *osteoclast-activating factors* by the malignant lymphoid cells. Recently, osteoclast-activating factor has been shown to consist of several purified and molecularly cloned proteins, including lymphotoxin, tumor necrosis factor, interleukin-6, and interleukin-1. In myeloma, lymphotoxin, interleukin-1, and interleukin-6 have all been implicated. Myeloma is almost invariably associated with osteoclastic bone resorption, and 20% of patients also develop hypercalcemia. Hypercalcemic patients with myeloma usually have impaired renal function.

A human type C retrovirus (human T cell lymphotrophic virus type I or HTLV-I) has been a consistent finding in a particular form of T-cell lymphoma. The patients universally have a paraneoplastic syndrome characterized by increased bone turnover, abnormal bone scans, and hypercalcemia. In several patients, the neoplastic cells have been shown to produce an osteoclast-activating factor–like peptide in vitro. It has also been found that some patients with T cell lymphomas and hypercalcemia have high circulating 1,25-dihydroxycholecalciferol concentrations. This is a result of metabolism of 25-hydroxyvitamin D to 1,25-dihydroxyvitamin D stimulated by the HTLV-infected cells.

Clinical features. The clinical features of patients with hypercalcemia of malignancy may be confused with the terminal features of malignant disease. Thus many of the symptoms of hypercalcemia such as nausea, vomiting, weight loss, confusion, and lethargy could be ascribed to the malignant disease itself, to the chemotherapy or irradiation therapy that many of these patients receive, or to hypercalcemia. It is important to distinguish these because hypercalcemia is potentially reversible.

There is a rough relationship between the absolute concentration of the serum calcium and symptoms caused by hypercalcemia. In patients with malignant disease, hypercalcemia usually develops fairly rapidly, so symptoms may become apparent at relatively lower serum calcium levels than in primary hyperparathyroidism, in which the patient may become adjusted to a high level of serum calcium and be relatively asymptomatic with much higher serum calcium concentrations. The symptoms depend on the rapidity of the rise in serum calcium as well as the absolute serum calcium concentration.

Differential diagnosis. In considering the differential diagnosis of hypercalcemia, one must consider all the other causes of hypercalcemia and their relative frequencies. Malignant disease and primary hyperparathyroidism are responsible for almost 90% of all causes of hypercalcemia, so that in any patient with hypercalcemia the cause is likely to be one of these two conditions. It is also important to note that primary hyperparathyroidism is a very common disease and may occur coincidentally in a patient with malignant disease. There are many case reports of the coexistence of these two conditions. It is particularly important to consider this possibility in patients with tumors that are rarely associated with hypercalcemia, such as carcinoma of the uterine cervix, or with cancers that may be frequently associated with hypercalcemia but not in the particular clinical situation in which it is being observed, for example, in early carcinoma of the breast without evidence of bone metastasis. In general, occult malignancy is an unusual cause of hypercalcemia. Since primary hyperparathyroidism is so common in the elderly female population, when an elderly woman presents with asymptomatic hypercalcemia without obvious malignant disease, the most likely diagnosis is primary hyperparathyroidism.

As indicated earlier, a number of diagnostic tests can be used to distinguish the hypercalcemia of malignancy from other causes of hypercalcemia. Of course, it is important initially to determine whether the patient has malignant disease or metastatic bone disease by a careful history and physical examination and possibly by the use of bone scans and skeletal x-rays. The other tests that may be used to separate hypercalcemia of malignancy from primary hyperparathyroidism and other causes of hypercalcemia include measurement of the serum chloride (usually less than 100 mEq/liter in patients with malignant disease but greater than 103 mEq/liter in patients with primary hyperparathyroidism); the serum phosphorus (usually less than 3.5 mg/dl in patients with primary hyperparathyroidism, but it may be less or more in patients with malignant disease); the parathyroid hormone radioimmunoassay, which is usually but not always increased in patients with primary hyperparathyroidism and is usually but not always in the normal range or suppressed in patients with malignant disease; measurement of urinary or nephrogenous cyclic AMP (which is increased in patients with primary hyperparathyroidism and may be increased, normal, or suppressed in patients with malignant disease); and the steroid suppression test, which essentially never decreases the serum calcium in patients with primary hyperparathyroidism but does suppress the serum calcium in about one third of patients with hypercalcemia or malignancy and in all patients with hypercalcemia caused by increased absorption of calcium from the gastrointestinal tract.

Sometimes the cause of hypercalcemia can be determined from a careful clinical history. For example, progressive increase in the serum calcium usually occurs fairly rapidly in patients with malignant disease, whereas in patients with primary hyperparathyroidism careful review of the patient's records may indicate that mild hypercalcemia has been present for many years. It is also important to appreciate that hypercalcemia may worsen very rapidly in patients with malignant disease after treatment with estrogen or antiestrogen therapy if the patient has metastatic breast cancer; after volume depletion caused by diuretic therapy; or after vomiting subsequent to treatment with cytotoxic drugs or radiation therapy.

The differential diagnosis of hypercalcemia is also considered in Chapter 177.

Treatment. The indication for treatment of patients with malignant disease is an increased serum calcium level in the symptomatic patient. Although it is controversial whether or not to treat patients who are asymptomatic, a reasonable approach is to treat all patients with definite hypercalcemia of malignancy. Even if patients are asymptomatic, the serum calcium may increase very rapidly, which could lead to the patient's rapid demise.

The treatment of hypercalcemia has been discussed elsewhere (Chapter 177). The agents available for urgent treatment include saline to correct dehydration and promote a calcium diuresis; calcitonin and glucocorticoids, which rapidly reverse increased bone resorption; and furosemide, which may promote a calcium diuresis when used in large doses in fully rehydrated patients. For the less urgent treatment of hypercalcemia, the currently available agents in the United States are pamidronate, etidronate, gallium nitrate, and plicamycin (mithramycin). Pamidronate and etidronate are bisphosphonates. Both should be given parenterally. Pamidronate is more effective than etidronate and is now the preferred agent. Both of these bisphosphonates are relatively slow acting, with maximal effects unlikely to be observed before 4 days of treatment. There is less experience with gallium nitrate, but initial response rates appear to be encouraging and possibly similar to those observed with pamidronate. Gallium nitrate is probably more effective than etidronate. Unlike these other agents, plicamycin has been available for many years. It is probably more toxic and should now be used only in situations where the other agents are ineffective. It is particularly dangerous to use in patients with renal failure because it has direct renal toxicity, and the kidney is responsible for its clearance.

REFERENCES

Case Records of the Massachusetts General Hospital: Case 15-1971. N Engl J Med 284:839, 1971.

Garrett IR et al: Production of the bone resorbing cytokine lymphotoxin by cultured human myeloma cells. N Engl J Med 317:562, 1987.

Liotta LA: Tumor invasion: role of the extracellular matrix. Cancer Res 46:1, 1986.

Moseley JM et al: Parathyroid hormone-related protein purified from a human lung cancer cell line. Proc Natl Acad Sci 84:5048, 1987.

Mundy GR: The hypercalcemia of malignancy revisited. J Clin Invest 82:1, 1988.

Mundy GR and Martin TJ: Hypercalcemia of malignancy—pathogenesis and treatment. Metabolism 31:1247, 1982.

Mundy GR et al: The hypercalcemia of malignancy: clinical implications and pathogenic mechanisms. N Engl J Med 310:1718, 1984.

Mundy GR et al: Tumor products and the hypercalcemia of malignancy. J Clin Invest 76:391, 1985.

Mundy GR: Pathophysiology of skeletal complications of cancer. In Mundy GR and Martin TJ, editors: Physiology and pharmacology of bone. Handbook of experimental pharmacology. Springer, (in press).

Myers WPL: Hypercalcemia in neoplastic disease. Arch Surg 80:308, 1960.

Powell D et al: Non-parathyroid humoral hypercalcemia in patients with neoplastic disease. N Engl J Med 289:176, 1973.

Sporn MB and Todaro GJ: Autocrine secretion and malignant transformation of cells. N Engl J Med 303:878, 1980.

Suva LJ et al: A parathyroid hormone-related protein implicated in malignant hypercalcemia: cloning and expression. Science 237:893, 1987.

Yates AJP et al: Effects of a synthetic peptide of a parathyroid hormone-related protein on calcium homeostasis, renal tubular calcium reabsorption and bone metabolism. J Clin Invest 81:9232, 1988.

Part Six

Pulmonary and Critical Care Medicine

I BASIC PHYSIOLOGY

CHAPTER

189 Respiratory Pathophysiology

Walter J. Daly
Jacob S. O. Loke

The respiratory system consists of (1) a gas exchanger, (2) a bellows to move gas in and out of contact with the exchanger, (3) a neural control mechanism, and (4) a transport fluid to move gases between the exchanger and the rest of the body. Disorders of respiration can affect any or all of these components. Many respiratory symptoms arise from failure of a system component resulting from increased work required to perform some component function or from pain or irritation arising from some component motion. The whole system is balanced to achieve the best possible aeration of the blood with the greatest economy of effort. In fact, in some instances, the control mechanism accepts compromise in blood gas levels rather than driving ventilation to achieve better results when the improvement would require uncomfortable effort.

NONRESPIRATORY FUNCTIONS OF THE LUNG

Filtering

The lung serves a vital filtering function. It protects the systemic circulation against constant threat of focal ischemia and even infarction by filtering embolic material of various types, that is, fibrin clumps, clots, and other material that may be endogenous or exogenous in origin.

Metabolic functions

The lung has an important set of metabolic functions. Since the entire cardiac output flows through the lung during a single circulation, a large fraction of the circulating blood is in contact with respiratory endothelial cells two or more times each minute. This finding suggests that the lung is uniquely situated to perform metabolic changes on the blood. In some instances, the lung seems to act like a metabolic filter, removing certain locally important vasoactive substances such as serotonin, bradykinin, norepinephrine, and certain prostaglandins (PGs). Substances important to systemic regulation such as epinephrine, prostacycline, and PGI_2 pass unaffected. Angiotensin I is specifically converted to angiotensin II by angiotensin-converting enzyme (ACE). These important activities are performed by the pulmonary endothelial cells. Disorders that impair endothelial cell function also affect amine-processing efficiency. Best studied of these disorders is oxygen toxicity.

Lung defenses (see Chapter 193)

Microvascular fluid exchanges

The principal forces active in transcapillary fluid movement in the lung are the capillary hydrostatic pressure and the plasma oncotic pressure. The balance of these pressures favors reabsorption of fluid from the interstitium and thus provides for a "dry" alveolocapillary membrane and unimpeded gas exchange. Fig. 189-1 depicts an electron microscopic view of the alveolocapillary relationship. Fig. 189-2 diagrams the forces of the capillary membrane. In everyday life, transient increases in capillary pressure during exercise must exceed the oncotic pressure; fluid transudation occurs particularly at the lung bases. Fluid is readily drained from the interstitium into the lymphatics, and lung water increases only a little. As long as interstitial oncotic pressure remains low and plasma protein concentration remains relatively normal, capillary hydrostatic pressure is usually not sufficiently high to cause edema. Factors that increase hydrostatic pressure or lower plasma oncotic pressure can be expected to produce interstitial edema. If the draining capacity of the lymphatics is exceeded, water accumulates in the interstitium, the lung stiffens, and alveolar flooding may occur. Fluid leaving the capillary bed under these circumstances is characteristically low in protein concentration.

If capillary pressure exceeds about 25 mm Hg, protein leakage occurs and edema formation is enhanced by decreasing the transendothelial oncotic gradient. At high capillary pressures the distinction between pressure (hemodynamic, hydrostatic) edema and permeability edema is lost as protein leaks through injured alveolocapillary membrane at high pressure.

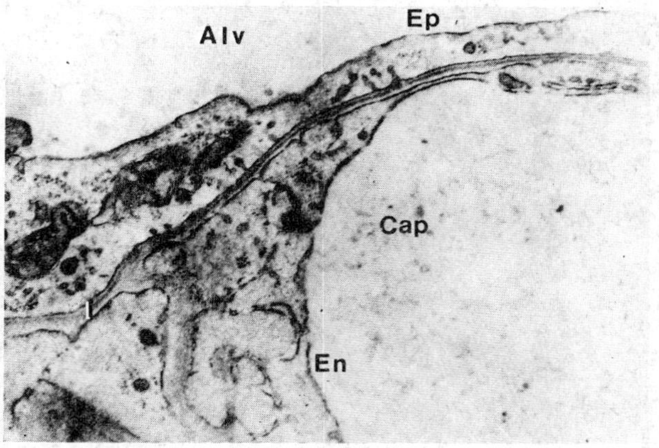

Fig. 189-1. Electron microscopic view of alveolocapillary membrane. Alv, alveolus; Cap, capillary; En, capillary endothelium; I, interstitium; Ep, alveolar epithelium.

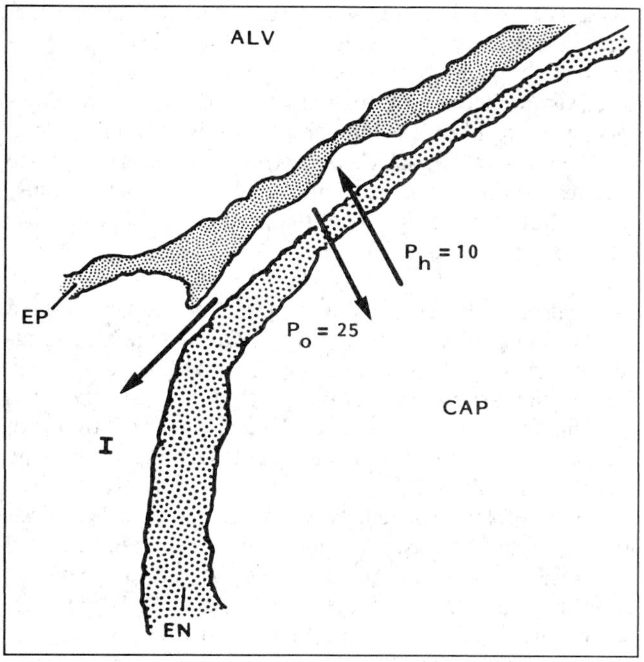

Fig. 189-2. Diagram of forces acting at alveolocapillary membrane. Alv, alveolus; Cap, capillary; Ep, alveolar epithelium; En, capillary endothelium; P_h, hydrostatic pressure; P_o, plasma oncotic pressure; I, interstitium.

Other conditions may increase the permeability of the capillary membrane directly, leading to a permeability edema. In this event, the membrane leaks protein as well as water at lower capillary pressures, the osmotic gradient is lessened, and fluid movement may occur at less elevated or even normal capillary pressures. When permeability is increased, lymph protein concentration increases. This change in lymph protein clearly differentiates lung fluid accumulation caused by permeability from that caused by hydrostatic pressures, except when pressure is very high and effective pore size increases.

As fluid accumulates in the interstitium, it finds its way to the lymphatics, which first appear at the level of the respiratory bronchioles. When the interstitium is fluid-filled and the draining capacity of the lymphatics has been exceeded, alveolar flooding occurs and clinical pulmonary edema is evident. Dyspnea, hypoxemia, and early radiographic changes may appear prior to alveolar flooding.

RESPIRATORY FUNCTION

As a gas exchanger, the lung is sufficiently effective so that up to 6 liters of oxygen can move into the blood each minute as comparable quantities of carbon dioxide leave. Thus, about 7×10^{23} molecules of oxygen individually diffuse across a surface of 90 m^2 into an instantaneous capillary volume of about 100 ml, which is changed 400 times each minute during extremes of exercise. During rest, transfer is appropriately reduced to the level of 200 to 400 ml of oxygen each minute.

The forces driving this remarkable movement of gas between alveolus and capillary are entirely those that drive diffusion of gas from places of higher to lower partial pressures. No active processes requiring metabolic energy are required.

Simply, the function of the lung as a gas exchanger has three components: delivery of gas to and from the alveolus, diffusion across the membrane, and movement of blood to and from contact with the membrane.

Mechanical properties

Briefly stated, the mechanical properties of the lung important to understanding clinical disorders are compliance and airway resistance. The forces applied to the surface of the lung are transmitted by the chest wall and diaphragm acting as a bellows.

Chest bellows. The forces driving the lung during ventilation are the muscles of the chest wall and diaphragm. These muscles are coordinated and cycled in response to metabolic and neurologic needs. The lung is ventilated as a passive response to movement of the bellows, modified by compliance and resistance factors. With muscle weakness or paralysis caused by a variety of disorders, for example, poliomyelitis, muscular dystrophy, paraplegia, or phrenic nerve palsy, hypoventilation may occur. Also, decreased deformability of the thorax (for example, kyphoscoliosis, obesity, or ascites) may impair bellows function. In any case, the volume of air moved during a tidal volume depends on the force of bellows activity and the mechanical impediments to movement. The force with which the diaphragm contracts must also affect the volume of air moved, especially when the work of breathing is increased. Diaphragmatic fatigue contributes to ventilatory failure and respiratory acidosis and weakens diaphragmatic contractions; theophylline increases the force of contraction.

Compliance. Compliance is an expression of the elastic properties of the lung. It is measured as the force required to hold an added air volume in the lung in the midvolume range, after all motion has ceased. Compliance (C_L) is expressed as liters per centimeter of water. Customarily, the transpulmonary pressure is measured as the difference between airway and esophageal pressure at one lung volume compared with similar pressure differential at another lung volume, when no air is flowing. In actual practice, static compliance is measured as the slope of a curve relating lung volume and transpulmonary pressure—measured during periods of no air flow. This relationship is outlined in Fig. 189-3. The normal lung compliance is about 0.2 liter per centimeter of water. The fibrotic lung and the congested lung are stiffer; that is, they have lower compliance. In emphysema, the lung contains less tissue per unit volume of air and has a higher compliance.

Total compliance (C_T) is the compliance of lung and chest measured together. If C_C = compliance of the chest, $1/C_T = 1/C_L + 1/C_C$. Normal C_T = 0.1 liter per centimeter of water. The compliance usually measured in patients

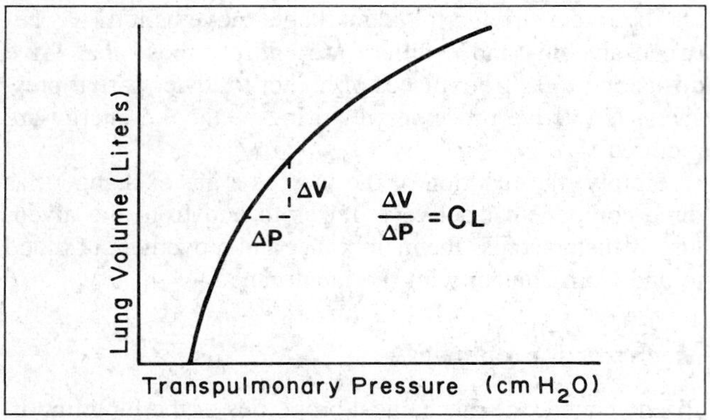

Fig. 189-3. Measurement of the static compliance (CL) of the lung. The change in lung volume (ΔV) is plotted against the change in transpulmonary pressure (ΔP) (the pressure required for lung inflation) during periods of no airflow.

connected to ventilators is total compliance. In such measurements, the condition of no airflow must be met, but chest wall relaxation or paralysis is crucial.

Since CL is a measure of the force required to stretch the lung, the lower the CL, the greater the force required for a given tidal volume. Thus, when CL is low, breathing tends to be with low tidal volumes at greater frequency.

Dynamic compliance. The pressure-volume relationship measured without allowing for complete cessation of airflow is called *dynamic compliance*. In normal individuals, static compliance and dynamic compliance approximate each other. If the internal mechanical properties of the lung are unevenly distributed, each breath is also unevenly distributed, and without the time that a period of no airflow allows for redistribution, volumes are unevenly distributed and each part of the lung may be on a different portion of its pressure-volume curve. Thus, when mechanical unevenness exists, dynamic compliance is less than static compliance and becomes still less as breathing frequency increases.

Airway resistance. Airway resistance expresses the force required to move air from alveolus to mouth. Normally the resistance of the upper airway is about 50% of the total. Resistance of airways less than 2 mm in diameter is only about 20%. Changes in resistance in small airways therefore have little effect on overall resistance or on clinical measurements such as FEV_1 until obstructive disease is far advanced. These earlier resistance changes, however, may have an important impact on distribution of ventilation, ventilation-perfusion matching, and arterial PO_2.

Since resistance measurements are made during airflow and really measure the force required to move the lung and to move air through the resistance of the airway, the force required is highly dependent on the rate of flow. For a given resistance (RL), rapid breathing requires more effort than slow, deeper breathing.

Work. The overall resistance (RL) and compliance (CL) account for the work required to ventilate the lung. Normally the process is so efficient that little added effort is necessary to increase ventilation within useful ranges. However, when resistance is high or the lung is very stiff, added ventilation is accomplished only with vigorous effort by the muscles driving the chest bellows. When the added muscular effort is inappropriate to the motion induced, the sensation of dyspnea is evoked.

Surfactant. Type II alveolar epithelial cells produce a unique phospholipid, dipalmitoyl-lecithin, which lines alveolar surfaces. This material is capable of changing its surface tension so that the surface tension of small alveoli is less than that of large alveoli. If such material were not present, small alveoli would be expected to empty into large alveoli and collapse.

Long before surfactant was demonstrated, its presence was suspected because of theoretical considerations of the hysteresis of pressure-volume curves of the lung and the difference between air-filled and fluid-filled pressure-volume curves. Surfactant has been extracted from the lung, its surface-active properties have been measured, its composition has been analyzed, and its presence at the alveolar surface has been demonstrated by special electron microscopic techniques. Surfactant is an "antiatelectasis" factor that tends to prevent alveolar closure at small volumes. In vivo or excised lungs seem to decrease their surfactant activity and compliance as their volume of expansion decreases. In other words, both compliance and surfactant activity are affected by the volume history of the lung. This change is partially explained by alveolar closure at small volumes, but may also be caused by extracellular changes in surfactant molecules; that is, surfactant molecules may aggregate or disaggregate as volume changes. Large-volume sighs at 4- to 5-minute intervals seem sufficient to maintain surfactant activity and prevent alveolar collapse.

Since it develops late in prenatal life, deficient or absent surfactant generation characterizes the immature lung of premature infants and contributes to the alveolar collapse, stiff lung, and faulty oxygenation of the neonatal respiratory distress syndrome. In adults, surfactant may be inactivated or displaced by edema, contributing to alveolar collapse in pulmonary edema.

Membrane functions

The alveolocapillary membrane has three layers: alveolar epithelium, interstitium, and capillary endothelium. Fig. 189-1 illustrates their relationship. The total thickness approximates 0.3 μm, but the thickness is unevenly distributed over the capillary surface. For gas to diffuse easily, a very thin and consequently fragile membrane is required. Membrane forces (e.g., hydrostatic pressure) and injurious substances (e.g., hyperoxia or bacterial or endogenous proteases) readily cause membrane leakage. Thus, reparative processes are important and probably active under many circumstances.

The process of gas transfer is so rapid that red cells are normally completely saturated with oxygen before they have traversed half the length of the alveolar capillary. If alveolar oxygen tension is reduced or circulation time quickened, the process may become time-limited, as during exercise at altitude. At rest (under normal conditions), with reasonably normal inspired oxygen partial pressure, it may be correctly assumed that hemoglobin is saturated with oxygen, and both carbon dioxide and oxygen in a given alveolus are in equilibrium with gas concentrations in the adjacent capillary by the time alveolar capillary transit is completed. Calculations show and physiologic observations confirm that oxygen transfer across the membrane is not limited by membrane thickness; that is, oxygenation is not diffusion-limited except during exercise while breathing hypoxic oxygen concentrations or at altitude. Although gas transfer is conceptualized as occurring from a single alveolus, across a single alveolocapillary membrane to a single capillary containing a single red cell, it is readily apparent that these processes take place in several million sets of alveoli and capillaries simultaneously. As shown in Fig. 189-4, each alveolus is liberally supplied with a network of capillaries.

It is possible to measure this aggregate transfer of oxygen as an oxygen-diffusing capacity (DLCO), but the measurement is too cumbersome for clinical use. Rather, trace carbon monoxide concentrations are used as a test gas, and the calculations become simpler because hemoglobin removes carbon monoxide from the plasma so rapidly that plasma PCO opposing diffusion across the membrane can be assumed to be zero. Low DLCO is characteristic of a number of lung diseases (e.g., fibrosis, sarcoidosis, emphysema), but the transfer is reduced not because of resistance at the membrane but because of a reduced overall alveolar gas–capillary blood contact as capillary bed is destroyed and/or blood-gas contact deranged. DLCO may be decreased in anemia as the capillary mass of hemoglobin available to bind carbon monoxide is decreased.

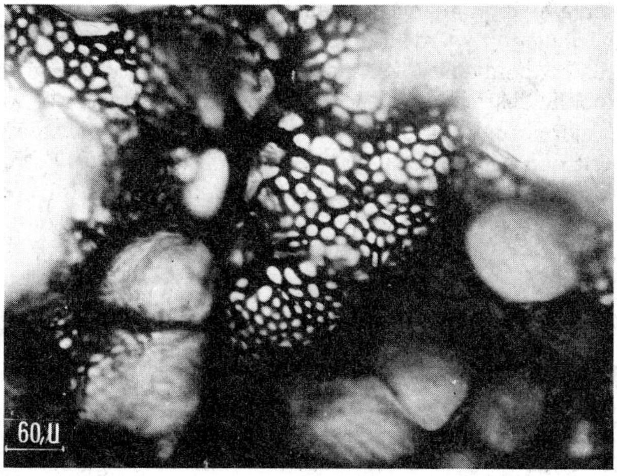

Fig. 189-4. Microscopic view of the capillary network at the alveolar surface viewed en face. This preparation was from a thick cut of an India ink–perfused, fume-fixed lung.

Alveolar gas and dead space

As the lung inspires, air enters, and as it expires, gas leaves, but the lung is not empty even at end-expiration.

At the end of an expiration, conducting airways are filled with expired gas. As inspiration begins, this gas is the first to reenter the alveoli. At the end of inspiration, those same nonexchanging parts are filled with inspired air that never reaches the alveoli. This space is called the *dead space*. Furthermore, regions of alveoli that are not perfused or are "underperfused" function as dead space because they do not contribute to oxygen absorption or carbon dioxide release. The gas contained in this dead space is called the *dead space volume* (V_D). The overall ventilation of the lung is greater than the alveolar ventilation by the amount of ventilation that never reaches perfused alveoli and is moved in and out of the dead space.

The volume of gas remaining in the lung at the end of a normal expiration is the functional residual capacity (FRC). Thus, functioning alveoli are not empty at end-expiration but contain a volume of gas that is diluted as inspiration occurs. This residual gas serves to buffer against wide swings in gas tension as respiration cycles.

The forces acting on the lung to drive ventilation are not directly applied to each alveolus, so given alveoli are ventilated according to the ease with which air flows into them; the inspired air flows to alveoli that are most easily opened, through bronchi with the least resistance. Since normally there is uneven distribution of ventilation, some unevenness of alveolar ventilation and of individual alveolar gas tensions occurs. However, in any single alveolus, given reasonable inspired oxygen concentrations and circulation time that is not excessively rapid, PO_2 and PCO_2 in the alveolus and end-capillary blood may be assumed to be nearly identical.

Selection of reasonable values of PO_2 and PCO_2 to represent the sum of all alveolar PO_2s and PCO_2s is a more complex consideration. The rapidity of carbon dioxide movement and the shape of the blood-carbon dioxide dissociation curve (Fig. 189-5) have led to the theoretical demonstration that arterial PCO_2 ($PaCO_2$) can be taken as equal to alveolar PCO_2 (P_ACO_2). The different dissociation relationship for blood and oxygen does not permit a similar assumption, and P_AO_2 must be calculated. A simplified calculation is

$$P_AO_2 = P_IO_2 - 1.25\ (PaCO_2)$$

P_IO_2 is the partial pressure of oxygen inspired. A respiratory quotient (RQ) of 0.8 is assumed.

Unevenness of ventilation

Since the forces applied to the surface of the lung by the chest bellows are not evenly distributed and since the indi-

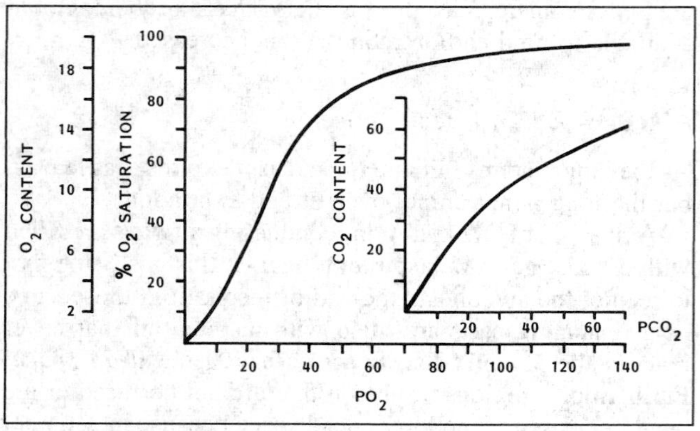

Fig. 189-5. Dissociation curves of O_2 and CO_2 with blood. These curves are represented as normal curves. Hemoglobin concentration = 15 g/dl. Content = ml gas per dl blood.

vidual resistances and compliances within the lung are not evenly distributed, some alveoli are normally better ventilated than others. Unevenness may be diffusely distributed as in the diffuse diseases of the lung, regionally distributed as with a local partial bronchial obstruction, or distributed according to top-to-bottom gradients. Unevenness of ventilation may be exaggerated by irregular stiffening of the lung with scattered foci of edema, inflammation, or fibrosis, or with irregularly scattered areas of increased airway resistance arising with diffuse obstructive pulmonary diseases. Furthermore, resistances are constantly changing with clearing of mucous plugs, coughing, deep breathing, or even local perfusion changes. It is well established that local bronchial constriction occurs in response to local decreases in alveolar PCO_2 caused by redistribution of perfusion to other areas. Local factors also cause frequency-dependent unevenness. Given irregularly scattered areas difficult to ventilate, increasing respiratory frequency causes redistribution of ventilation away from the difficult areas to the areas of easier access, thus exaggerating unevenness. With diseases such as asthma, chronic obstructive pulmonary disease (COPD), or fibrosis, that unevenness is exaggerated.

In normal individuals, regionally determined gradients of ventilation are more important than differences caused by local resistance changes. Such gradients are dependent on the structure of the chest and of the lung and on regional pressure-volume relationships. The net result is a gradient of ventilation such that the lower zones of the vertical lung receive the largest fraction of ventilation. At low lung volumes, there is even a tendency for lower zone airway closure, which accounts for some hypoxemia found at low lung volumes. Obesity may exaggerate airway closure in mechanically difficult lower lung zones.

Capillary blood gas

Once oxygen enters the plasma, it rapidly diffuses along concentration gradients into the red cell and loosely associates with hemoglobin according to the relationship known as the *oxygen-hemoglobin dissociation curve*. The shape of this curve (Fig. 189-5) and the factors affecting it are of great importance. Carbon dioxide leaves the blood, even more rapidly than oxygen enters, and diffuses freely into the alveolus. The carbon dioxide dissociation curve describes the carbon dioxide partial pressure–volume relationship (Fig. 189-5).

In normal gas environments, the principal alveolar gases are oxygen, carbon dioxide, nitrogen, and water. Water vapor remains as a constant pH_2O, dependent on body temperature and barometric pressure. Oxygen enters the alveolus as alveolar gas is partially exchanged during ventilation, and, with each breath, carbon dioxide is removed. Carbon dioxide diffuses into the alveolus from the capillary blood, having been delivered to the lung from peripheral production sites. Thus, there is a reciprocal relationship between $PACO_2$ and PAO_2. In fact, if PAN_2 remained constant, the sum of $PACO_2$ and PAO_2 would be a constant fraction of barometric pressure during air breathing.

It is evident that decreased ventilation of a given alveolus decreases end-capillary PO_2 and increases PCO_2 with resultant change in capillary blood oxygen and carbon dioxide content. When ventilation is increased above normal, however, alveolar PO_2 and end-capillary PO_2 move toward the level of inspired PO_2 and alveolar end-capillary PCO_2 decreases. Only blood carbon dioxide content changes appreciably since PO_2 increases above 80 mm Hg add little oxygen to hemoglobin, and increases above 100 mm Hg add almost none.

Perfusion

Just as alveolar ventilation is unevenly distributed, so is capillary perfusion. Unevenness of perfusion is dependent on gravity, local structural change, and local alveolar PO_2. In the normally low-pressure pulmonary circulation, the effect of gravity is large, increasing the perfusion of dependent areas and leaving uppermost parts unperfused. With increases in pulmonary vascular pressure, perfusion is "redistributed" toward the apices, a radiographic sign of increased pulmonary venous pressure. With local fibrosis, embolic obstruction of the pulmonary artery, or loss of vasculature caused by emphysema, foci of absent or decreased perfusion occur. Perfusion distribution is singularly sensitive to local alveolar PO_2, so that areas of focal alveolar hypoxia cause local arterial constriction and perfusion unevenness.

Relationship of ventilation to perfusion

When, for whatever reason, local ventilation and perfusion are not ideally matched, blood gas abnormalities occur in end-capillary blood. Arterial blood sampled peripherally for PCO_2 and PO_2 measurement represents the aggregate of end-capillary contributions together with admixture from venous blood totally bypassing alveolar exchange. When foci of alveolar underventilation with respect to perfusion occur (low $\dot{V}/\dot{Q}$), end-capillary blood has low PO_2 and high PCO_2. When such blood is mixed with blood from areas

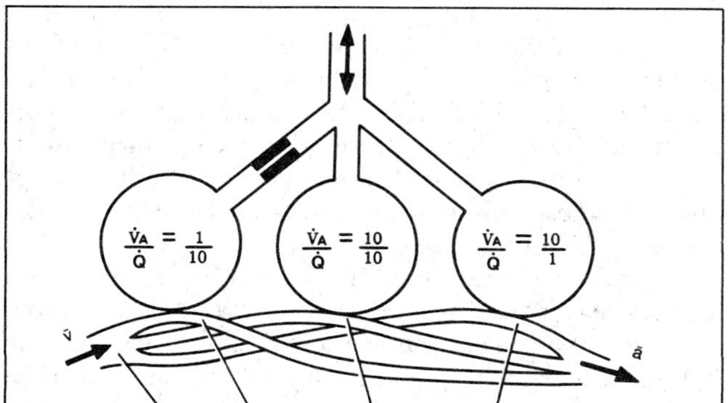

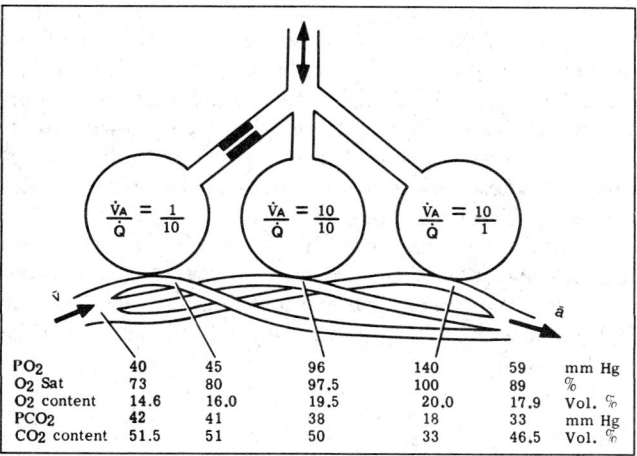

PO_2	40	45	96	140	59	mm Hg
O_2 Sat	73	80	97.5	100	89	%
O_2 content	14.6	16.0	19.5	20.0	17.9	Vol. %
PCO_2	42	41	38	18	33	mm Hg
CO_2 content	51.5	51	50	33	46.5	Vol. %

Fig. 189-6. Ventilation-perfusion mismatching. Three alveoli (A) with different $\dot{V}/\dot{Q}$ are illustrated. V, ventilation (volume/time); Q, blood flow (volume/time). Mixed venous ($\bar{v}$) values are tabulated in the first column. Values have been calculated and listed for each end capillary. Mixed arterial values ($\bar{a}$) are listed in the last column. Hemoglobin concentration = 15 g per dl.

Causes of hypoxemia

Anatomic shunting of venous to arterial shunt
- Pulmonary arteriovenous fistula
- Patent ductus arteriosus with reversal flow
- Intracardiac septal defect with severe pulmonary hypertension, pulmonic stenosis, tricuspid atresia, single ventricle

Physiologic derangements
- Hypoventilation
- Ventilation-perfusion mismatching

Altitude
- Low P_IO_2

of normal $\dot{V}/\dot{Q}$, the consequence is reduced arterial PO_2 and increased PCO_2. Increased PCO_2 stimulates increased ventilation, which is chiefly distributed to the areas of normal or high $\dot{V}/\dot{Q}$ ratios, reducing the PCO_2 and increasing the PO_2 in the blood from those areas. But the result of mixing this blood with blood from areas of low $\dot{V}/\dot{Q}$ is only correction of the PCO_2 levels, not PO_2. The slope of oxygen- and carbon dioxide–blood dissociation curves determines this difference. Thus, hyperventilation of some areas may remove sufficient carbon dioxide to compensate for carbon dioxide retained in foci of underventilation, whereas the hyperventilated areas do not add sufficient oxygen to correct for the hypoxemia generated from foci of underventilation. This important phenomenon is illustrated in Fig. 189-6. In this example, hyperventilation sufficient to reduce $PaCO_2$ to 33 mm Hg failed to raise PaO_2 above 59 mm Hg.

Mismatching of ventilation and perfusion is the most common cause of hypoxemia. A representative list of other causes of hypoxemia is presented in the box.

Hyperventilation and hypoventilation

Overall increases or decreases in alveolar ventilation have profound effects on alveolar and arterial blood gas levels. These effects are predictable from consideration of the oxygen- and carbon dioxide–blood dissociation curves (see Fig. 189-5). The rate of carbon dioxide production is also an important determinant of P_ACO_2. The relationship is expressed as

$$P_ACO_2 = 0.863\ (\dot{V}CO_2/\dot{V}_A)$$

0.863 being a conversion constant; $\dot{V}CO_2$, an expression of CO_2 production; and $\dot{V}_A$, alveolar ventilation. In other words, increases in carbon dioxide production require increases in alveolar ventilation if P_ACO_2 is not to rise.

As total alveolar ventilation increases without a change in carbon dioxide production, alveolar PCO_2 is reduced and alveolar PO_2 approaches inspired PO_2. Examination of the dissociation curves shows that this change profoundly affects blood carbon dioxide content with little change in oxygen content. Conversely, decreases in overall alveolar ventilation increase alveolar PCO_2 and decrease alveolar PO_2, affecting both arterial PO_2 and oxygen content as well as arterial PCO_2 and carbon dioxide content.

Since $PaCO_2$ is taken as a measure of overall P_ACO_2, increased $PaCO_2$ occurs when alveolar ventilation is decreased, and decreased $PaCO_2$ reflects increased alveolar ventilation. In clinical practice, increases in $PaCO_2$ do not occur unless there is alveolar hypoventilation. If the lungs are normal and central hypoventilation occurs, $PaCO_2$ rises. If the lungs are abnormal and ventilation-perfusion mismatching is present, $PaCO_2$ does not rise unless the neural control does not respond appropriately to increased $PaCO_2$, restoring it to normal. Thus, for clinical purposes, even with mismatching, $PaCO_2$ does not rise without absolute or relative "hypoventilation."

Oxygen transport

Oxygen transport is the volume of oxygen moved through the circulation in a unit of time. Thus, O_2 transport (ml/min) = O_2 content (ml/dl) × blood flow (dl/min). Cardiac output or blood flow to a specific site is important to oxygen transport and tissue delivery. Blood oxygen content depends on the pulmonary capillary PO_2 produced by gas exchange, the amount of hemoglobin present, and the slope of the oxygen-hemoglobin dissociation curve (see Fig. 189-5). If the curve is normal, PaO_2 above 80 mm Hg adds little more than dissolved oxygen to the blood. Since only 0.003 ml of oxygen/mm Hg PO_2/ml blood is carried as dissolved oxygen, oxygen in solution is not important to oxygen transport except during hyperbaric conditions. Given the shape of the dissociation curve, when PaO_2 is less than 60 mm Hg, the availability of oxygen changes greatly with small changes in PaO_2. Thus, addition of small concentrations of inspired oxygen adds substantial amounts of oxygen when PaO_2 is less than 60 mm Hg. Often attention is focused only at the upper end of the curve where the relationships determining loading of oxygen in the lung are described. The unloading of oxygen in the systemic capillaries also has great importance and is described by the same curve. Systemic capillary PO_2 varies widely from time to time and from place to place, depending on metabolic activity and local blood flow. The oxygen-hemoglobin relationship is sensitive to a number of factors that "shift the curve" to right or left, reflecting changing hemoglobin affinity for oxygen. These shifts have important implications for oxygen unloading.

DISORDERS OF OXYGEN TRANSPORT

Oxygen-hemoglobin curve

The right or left placement of the oxygen-hemoglobin dissociation curve expresses a relationship that is an important determinant of oxygen transport. Fig. 189-7 illustrates abnormal variations in the curve. If the lungs are producing reasonably normal PaO_2, the changes in the curve chiefly affect the unloading of oxygen since the curve is steeper in the unloading region. This effect can be readily appreciated with the use of Fig. 189-7 by determining the percent saturation of each curve for a given PO_2 in the 20- to 40-mm Hg range. The position of the curve can be expressed as P_{50}, the PO_2 at which hemoglobin is 50% saturated. Table 189-1 lists conditions that are characterized by changes in P_{50}. When P_{50} is greater than normal, the curve is shifted to the right; when P_{50} is less than normal, it is shifted to the left. If one supposes that unloading oxygen in the systemic capillary to the 30% saturated level is needed for oxygen delivery, a left shift or low P_{50} requires greater reduction in tissue PO_2 to accomplish the same oxygen unloading. In regional circulations, where flow is limited by partial vascular obstruction or fixed cardiac output, difficulty with oxygen unloading may aggravate tissue hypoxia. These patients are particularly troubled if PaO_2 is decreased, which should be avoided.

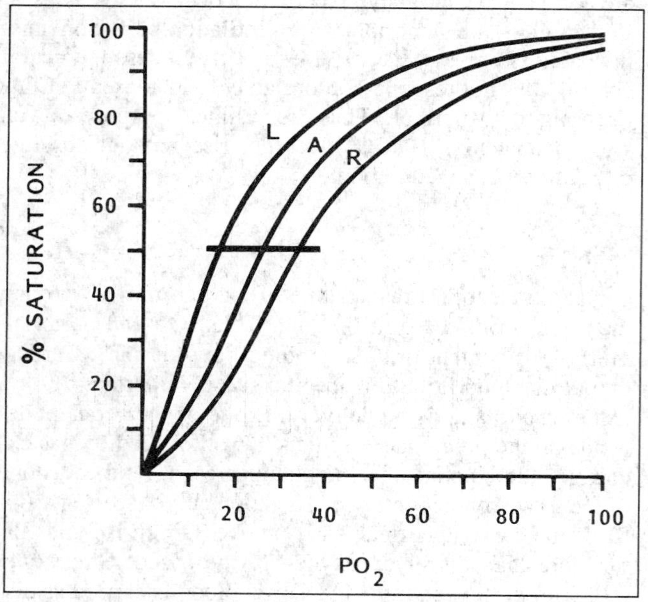

Fig. 189-7. Shifts in oxygen-hemoglobin affinity curve. Curve *A* depicts the normal relationship. *L* represents a left-shifted curve (increased affinity). *R* represents a right-shifted curve (decreased affinity). Curve L: P_{50} = 17 mm Hg. Curve A: P_{50} = 26 mm Hg. Curve R: P_{50} = 34 mm Hg.

Anemia may impede oxygen transport, but unless hemoglobin levels are severely reduced, increased flow satisfactorily accommodates. Furthermore, through increases in 2,3-diphosphoglycerate levels, oxygen unloading may be facilitated.

Carbon monoxide

Carbon monoxide poisoning produces important derangements in oxygen transport, mainly by occupying the oxygen-binding sites in the hemoglobin molecule. Since the carbon monoxide–hemoglobin affinity is 200 times greater than the oxygen-hemoglobin affinity, small concentrations of carbon monoxide can convert large quantities of hemoglobin to carboxyhemoglobin. The carbon monoxide–hemoglobin affinity further complicates oxygen transport by causing a left shift in the oxygen-hemoglobin curve (low P_{50}). Thus, what oxygen is transported is released with difficulty at the capillary level, driving tissue PO_2 even lower. Moreover, because carbon monoxide binds to myoglobin avidly, intracellular oxygen transport in active muscles—both skeletal and myocardial—is further impaired. The effect on oxygen transport of small quantities of carbon monoxide is greater than the loss of comparable quantities of oxygen capacity through anemia.

Abnormal hemoglobins

Rarely, congenital hemoglobinopathies (e.g., Kansas, Beth Israel) occur with oxygen-hemoglobin curves so far right-shifted that hemoglobin is barely saturated with the PO_2

Table 189-1. Factors affecting oxygen-hemoglobin affinity

Low P_{50}* Left shift of curve (increased affinity)	High P_{50} Right shift of curve (decreased affinity)
High pH (alkalosis)	Low pH (acidosis)
Low temperature	High temperature
Low 2,3-DPG	High 2,3-DPG
Stored blood	Anemia
Phosphorus deficiency	Altitude acclimatization
Carbon monoxide poisoning	Rare hemoglobinopathies (Kansas, Beth Israel)
Hemoglobinopathies (e.g., Kempsey, Yakima)	

2,3-DPG, 2,3-diphosphoglycerate.
*Normal P_{50} = 27 mm Hg.

available during air breathing. If oxygen-hemoglobin affinity is reduced far enough, oxygen unloading occurs so readily that sufficient amounts of reduced hemoglobin may be present in peripheral vessels to produce cyanosis without low tissue PO_2 or difficulty with oxygen transport. Conversely, other hemoglobinopathies have such increased oxygen-hemoglobin affinity that tissue PO_2 may be lowered to the point that erythropoietin is increased and erythrocytosis occurs. Often patients in this situation are detected through evaluation of polycythemia and demonstration of P_{50} that is abnormally low.

Other abnormalities of oxygen-hemoglobin affinity include sulfhemoglobinemia and methemoglobinemia. Sulfhemoglobin occurs as the consequence of binding of hydrogen sulfide to hemoglobin and, like carboxyhemoglobin, loses sites in the molecule usually available for oxygen binding. Sulfhemoglobin occurs after industrial or accidental exposure to hydrogen sulfide, in users of certain medications, and even as a consequence of environmental exposure to polluted air. In contrast to the left shift of the oxygen dissociation curve found in carboxyhemoglobin, the curve is right-shifted when sulfhemoglobin is present. Thus, the sulfhemoglobin effect on oxygen transport seems less than that predicted by estimating the fraction of sulfhemoglobin present, while the carbon monoxide effect is greater than predicted by carbon monoxide–hemoglobin levels.

Methemoglobinemia occurs as a congenital defect in hemoglobin metabolism or as a result of exposure to various toxic or medicinal substances such as nitrites, sulfonamides, and primaquine. The basic defect is conversion of the ferrous iron to the ferric form in the hemoglobin molecule, destroying its oxygen-carrying capacity. Methemoglobinemia, when present in sufficient concentrations (1.5 to 2.0 g/dl), produces brown discoloration of the skin. In acute situations, intravenous methylene blue (1 to 2 mg/kg) ordinarily causes rapid reversal. As with carbon monoxide–hemoglobin, methemoglobin causes a left shift of the dissociation curve, increasing oxygen affinity for hemoglobin and impeding oxygen unloading.

Acid-base regulation by the lung

The prime determinant of acid-base balance and arterial pH is the buffer ratio of carbon dioxide to bicarbonate. The concentration of gaseous carbon dioxide is rapidly changed by ventilation, whereas bicarbonate is more slowly regulated by the renal tubule. Abrupt changes in alveolar ventilation increase or decrease $PaCO_2$ and produce a set of pH levels dependent on the bicarbonate concentration. Chronic deviations in $PaCO_2$ are accommodated partially by tubular retention of bicarbonate or excretion to produce a different set of carbon dioxide–bicarbonate relationships. Thus, it is important to recognize both acute and chronic PCO_2-pH curves. Ordinarily, renal compensation for a given acute PCO_2 change is not complete for many hours. When carbon dioxide retention is produced, $PaCO_2$ increases, but respiratory acidemia may be severe or slight, depending on whether it is acute or chronic.

Given this relationship, it is possible to construct a series of curves to fit PCO_2-pH pairs characterizing acute or chronic respiratory acidemia or alkalemia (Fig. 189-8). Understanding of this difference between acute and chronic PCO_2-pH curves is important (1) to the diagnosis and management of respiratory acidosis and differentiation from metabolic acidosis, and (2) to the recognition of mixed states (i.e., combined respiratory and metabolic acidosis).

Alveolar-arterial difference—oxygen

It can be assumed that blood leaving alveolar capillaries has nearly the same PO_2 as the alveoli they perfused, providing reasonably slow circulation time and normal or high alveolar PO_2 (P_AO_2). Furthermore, if ventilation to all alveoli is equal, P_AO_2 is uniform throughout the lung. The ideal lung should have only such perfectly matched ventilation and perfusion relationships. If the ideal lung existed, there would be virtually no alveolar-arterial oxygen gradient.

The aggregate of individual alveolar PO_2s cannot be measured but is calculated as follows:

$$P_AO_2 = P_IO_2 - 1.25\ P_ACO_2$$

where $P_ACO_2 = PaCO_2$ (alveolar PCO_2 = arterial PCO_2).

Even in normal lungs, a small alveolar-arterial oxygen difference exists because of ventilation-perfusion mismatch. This difference, $P(A\text{-}a)O_2$, is normally about 6 mm Hg at ages less than 30 and about 15 mm Hg in normal persons older than 60 years of age. The effect of age on $P(A\text{-}a)O_2$ is depicted in Fig. 189-9. The $P(A\text{-}a)O_2$ is a rather sensitive index of the lung's performance and is easily calculated. Arterial PO_2 (PaO_2) is a less sensitive measure; it provides some information about the state of oxygenation but incomplete information about the lung. For example, a young asthmatic may have a PaO_2 of 80 mm Hg, indicating satisfactory oxygenation, but if $PaCO_2$ is 20 mm Hg

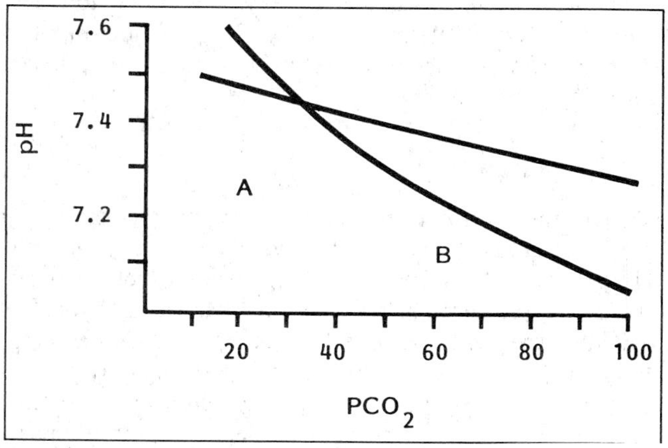

Fig. 189-8. PCO_2-pH curve. The steep curve outlines the PCO_2-pH relationship during acute changes in PCO_2. The flat curve represents changes during chronic PCO_2 deviations. Zone A is the area containing the PCO_2-pH pairs found during metabolic acidosis. Zone B contains a mixed area observed with combined respiratory and metabolic acidosis.

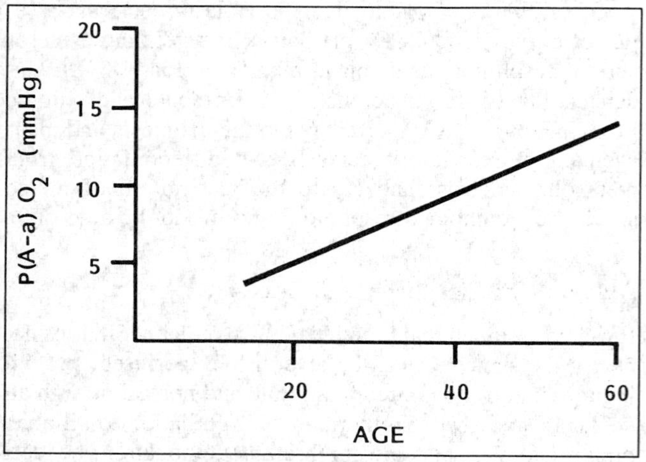

Fig. 189-9. Effect of age on alveolar-arterial oxygen difference.

during air breathing ($FiO_2 = 0.21$), it follows that $P(A\text{-}a)O_2$ is 42 mm Hg, a highly abnormal value, suggesting substantial ventilation-perfusion mismatch.

Calculations: Barometric pressure = 747 mm Hg
Water vapor pressure = 47 mm Hg
700 mm Hg

$$
\begin{aligned}
FiO_2 \times (P_B - 47) &= PiO_2 \\
0.21 \times (747 - 47) &= 147 \text{ mm Hg} \\
PAO_2 &= PiO_2 - 1.25\, PaCO_2 \\
&= 147 - 1.25\,(20) \\
&= 122 \\
P(A\text{-}a)O_2 &= PAO_2 - PaO_2 \\
&= 122 - 80 \\
&= 42 \text{ mm Hg}
\end{aligned}
$$

If alveolar ventilation is depressed in a patient with normal lungs (e.g., a patient taking narcotics), PaO_2 decreases and $PaCO_2$ increases without changing $P(A\text{-}a)O_2$. If, however, a patient has increased $PaCO_2$, it is useful to calculate $P(A\text{-}a)O_2$ to determine whether PaO_2 is appropriately decreased or whether concomitant ventilation-perfusion mismatch has occurred.

Venous admixture

Though the most common cause of hypoxemia during air breathing at rest (at sea level) is ventilation-perfusion mismatch, some "nonventilated" blood enters the left heart, having passed through thebesian cardiac veins, bronchial veins, or anatomic arteriovenous (A-V) shunts in the lung. In clinical situations, large right-to-left shunts may exist in pulmonary A-V fistulas or right-to-left intracardiac shunts. Furthermore, perfused but nonventilated or grossly underventilated alveoli contribute to this nonventilated circulation, which is collectively called *venous admixture*. Venous admixture is usually expressed as percentage of cardiac output ($\dot{Q}S/\dot{Q}T$). In general, $\dot{Q}S/\dot{Q}T$ is greater than 20% if PaO_2 is less than 100 mm Hg during 100% oxygen breathing.

Effects of oxygen breathing on blood gases

Air is 21% oxygen. If one assumes barometric pressure to be 747 mm Hg, the combined gas pressure at the alveolus is 747 mm Hg. At body temperature, water vapor has a pressure of 47 mm Hg, so this pressure contributes to the 747 mm Hg, leaving 700 mm Hg for the sum of PN_2, PO_2, and PCO_2. The highest that PO_2 could be if no CO_2 were present would be $0.21 \times 700 = 147$ mm Hg. If all metabolism converted oxygen only to CO_2 and all CO_2 were excreted, $PCO_2 + PO_2$ could then not exceed this ideal value of 147 mm Hg. If the lung were "ideal," $PaCO_2 + PaO_2$ would also equal 147 mm Hg, but this situation never occurs because $P(A\text{-}a)O_2$ always exists. The degree to which $PaCO_2 + PaO_2$ departs from 147 mm Hg (during air breathing) is another measure of the extent of ventilation-perfusion mismatch, venous admixture, and/or diffusion defect.

In clinical settings, $PaCO_2 + PaO_2$ often exceeds 147 mm Hg. This excess can happen only if there has been oxygen breathing or if the blood gas determinations are in error.

Each 1% of oxygen added to the inspired mixture adds 7 mm Hg PO_2 at the alveolar level. Given the shape of the oxygen-hemoglobin dissociation curve (see Fig. 189-5), it is evident that small increases in inspired oxygen concentration have large effects on oxygen transport unless substantial fractions of blood totally bypass alveoli and enter the arterial circulation as unoxygenated venous blood (venous admixture).

In patients who have advanced COPD or other disorders with profound hypoxemia and carbon dioxide retention, ventilation may be partially suppressed by hypercarbia but maintained only by hypoxic stimulation of the arterial chemoreceptors. Hypoxemia is dangerous and should be corrected with oxygen breathing, but excessive rises in PO_2 may remove the stimulus to continued ventilation and cause deepening respiratory acidosis, while small increases in

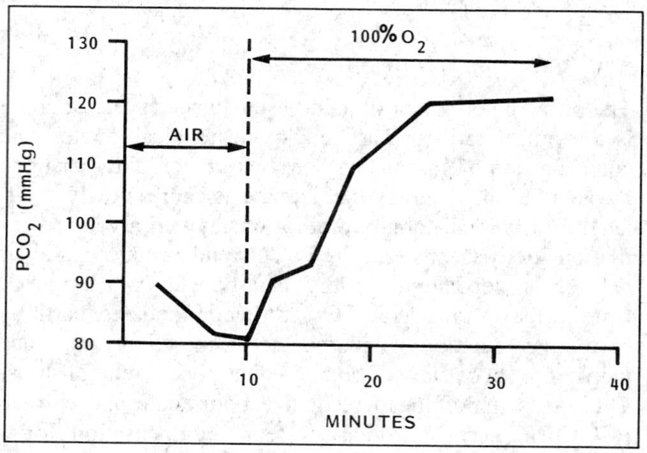

Fig. 189-10. Illustration of 100% oxygen breathing producing hypoventilation. Large increase in PCO_2 occurred within 25 minutes during O_2 breathing in a patient with advanced chronic obstructive pulmonary disease with ventilatory failure.

PO_2 may provide safer oxygenation levels with little effect on acidosis. The ability of uncontrolled oxygen breathing to produce carbon dioxide narcosis and acidosis in a patient with COPD is shown in Fig. 189-10. Since PO_2 and PCO_2 are closely linked during air breathing, the level to which PCO_2 can rise is limited by individual tolerance for hypoxemia during air breathing. During oxygen breathing, the limiting factor is tolerance for the narcotic effect of carbon dioxide and respiratory acidosis.

REFERENCES

Bates DV: Respiratory function in diseases, ed 3. Philadelphia, 1989, WB Saunders.

Forster RE II et al: The lung, physiologic basis of pulmonary function tests, ed 3. Chicago, 1986, Mosby–Year Book.

Handbook of physiology: the respiratory system. vol 1, Circulation and non-respiratory functions. Bethesda, Md, 1985, American Physiological Society.

Massaro D: The cellular and molecular basis of alveolar stability. J Lab Clin Med 98:155, 1981.

Said SI: Metabolic functions of the pulmonary circulation. Circ Res 50:325, 1982.

Weibel ER: How does lung function affect gas exchange? Chest 83:657, 1983.

West JB: Pulmonary pathophysiology: the essentials. Baltimore, 1982, Williams & Wilkins.

CHAPTER

190 Abnormalities of the Control of Breathing

Neil S. Cherniack

The constancy of blood gases (arterial PCO_2, PO_2, and pH) seen in healthy persons is accomplished by a complex interplay of control systems that rely on signals from chemo- and mechanoreceptors in the body. These control systems govern the rate and depth of breathing so that blood gases are maintained within a narrow range despite a variety of conditions that might otherwise cause unfavorable variations.

When respiratory function is severely impaired, these control systems may be unable to maintain arterial blood gases at normal levels. Indeed pulmonary disorders are the usual cause of persistent hypoxemia, hypercapnia, or hypocapnia, but frequently abnormalities are caused by a combination of impaired pulmonary performance and control system inadequacies. More rarely defects in the control system alone cause abnormal blood gases.

The respiratory control system itself is subject to two broad classes of disorder. The first affects the regularity of breathing and causes fluctuations in blood gas tensions. Acutely these fluctuations can be sufficiently great so as to be life-threatening. The second kind of abnormality affects the mean level of alveolar ventilation so that arterial PCO_2 is excessively low or high but breathing remains regular.

CHEMICAL CONTROL

Changes in blood gas tensions or in blood or brain pH cause compensatory changes in ventilation that tend to restore gas tension and pH toward their usual levels. Fig. 190-1 schematically diagrams the system responsible.

A reduction in ventilation, for example, usually decreases arterial PO_2, exciting chemoreceptors in the carotid bifurcation and aortic arch (the carotid and aortic bodies) that sample the level of PO_2 and increase their signal to respiratory neurons in the medulla according to the degree of the hypoxemia. This increased signal in turn augments the activity of respiratory neurons and the motor discharge to the inspiratory muscles. This is a feedback control system because information concerning the effect of ventilation on arterial blood gases (in this case arterial PO_2) is transferred (fed back) to the respiratory neurons through the chemoreceptors so that corrective action can be taken.

These are the only known receptors that increase ventilation in response to hypoxia. Changes in PO_2 rather than oxygen content are their stimulus. With a progressive reduction in arterial PO_2, chemoreceptor discharge increases hyperbolically. A decrease in arterial PO_2 from 50 to 40 mm Hg produces a greater change in chemoreceptor activity and ventilation than a change from 100 to 90 mm Hg, as shown in Fig. 190-2. Unlike its effects on the peripheral

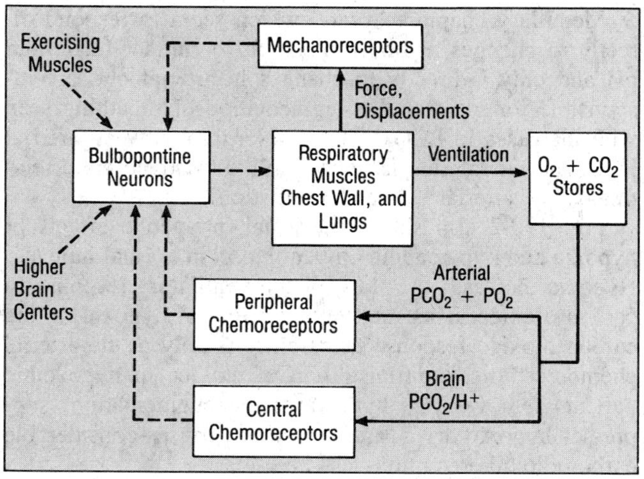

Fig. 190-1. Block diagram of respiratory control system. Dotted lines indicate actions of controller. Solid lines indicate information transfer through the controlled system. The bulbopontine neurons receive input from peripheral and central chemoreceptors, exercising muscles, and higher brain centers. They increase the activity of the respiratory muscles to augment ventilation. Ventilation changes the amount of O_2 and CO_2 stored in chemical combination and physically dissolved in the tissues, alters the PCO_2, PO_2, and H^+ concentrations in the arterial blood and brain, and thus affects chemoreceptor activity. Movements of the chest wall, lungs, and respiratory muscles alter mechanoreceptor activity.

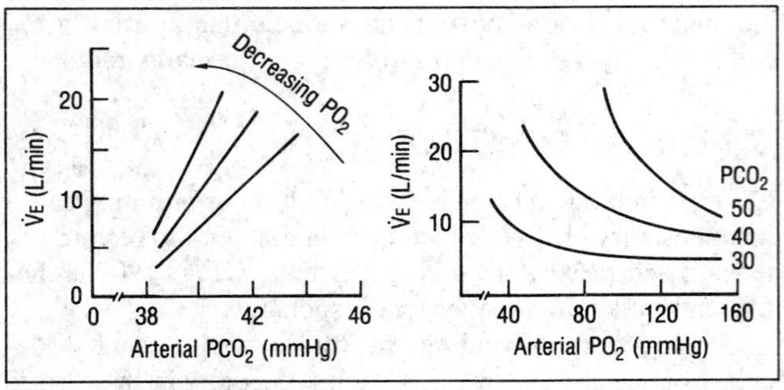

Fig. 190-2. Left panel: Ventilatory response to CO_2; the slope of the response line increases with hypoxia. Right panel: Ventilatory response to hypoxia. Note how hypercapnia increases the curvature of the ventilatory response to hypoxia.

chemoreceptors, hypoxia is believed to have a depressant effect on brain respiratory neurons. This seems to be caused by the release by brain cells of depressant neurotransmitters and neuromodulators such as gamma-aminobutyric acid (GABA), enkephalins, and adenosine. The exact level of arterial PO_2 at which depression of central respiratory neurons occurs probably depends on the rate of oxygen delivery by the cerebral circulation and ultimately on the ability of the cerebral blood vessels to dilate and brain blood flow to increase with hypoxia. An increase in arterial PCO_2 also stimulates peripheral chemoreceptors. But in normal individuals, the increase accounts for only 15% to 30% of the total ventilatory response to carbon dioxide.

Medullary chemoreceptors, which seem to respond directly to changes in brain interstitial or intracellular fluid pH and only indirectly to changes in arterial pH, are responsible for most of the augmentation of breathing seen with increases in PCO_2. The relationship between arterial PCO_2 and ventilation is linear, unlike the hyperbolic relationship of arterial PO_2 and ventilation.

Fig. 190-2 also shows the usual interactive effects of hypoxia and hypercapnia on ventilation in normal humans. Hypoxia increases the slope of the ventilatory response to carbon dioxide. This multiplying effect of hypoxia on the carbon dioxide response takes place mainly at the arterial chemoreceptors. Administration of oxygen to hypoxemic patients removes this hypoxia-driven augmentation, suppresses hypoxic drive, and sometimes causes considerable carbon dioxide retention.

Changes in arterial pH caused by metabolic disorders shift the position of the carbon dioxide response line. Metabolic alkalosis shifts the response line to the right so that resting PCO_2 is increased and ventilation is decreased, whereas acidosis causes a leftward shift so that resting PCO_2 is decreased and ventilation is greater. In addition, severe alkalosis seems to depress the effect of PCO_2 changes on ventilation, decreasing the slope of the ventilatory-carbon dioxide response line; acidosis has the opposite effect.

NEURAL FACTORS IN THE CONTROL OF VENTILATION

The rhythmic cycle of inspiration and expiration depends on the interaction among groups of neurons located in the medulla. The time spent in each phase of respiration is modified by signals from mechanoreceptors in the lungs and muscles of the chest wall. The mechanoreceptors in the lung are supplied to the vagus and can be classified into three broad categories: (1) receptors in the airways, which respond to stretch of the airways as the lungs expand and are responsible for the classic Hering-Breuer reflexes in which lung inflation inhibits inspiratory and excites expiratory activity; (2) irritant receptors located in the epithelial layer of the airways, which are excited by dust, noxious gases, and mechanical stimuli; and (3) J receptors located in the alveolar wall, which are activated by congestion of the lung interstitium.

Irritant receptors like the stretch receptors are innervated by myelinated fibers; unmyelinated fibers supply the J receptors. Both irritant and J receptors are rapidly adapting and have discharge patterns that bear little relationship to inspiration and expiration. Although neither receptor has an important influence in determining the usual pattern of breathing, stimulation of the receptors may be an important factor in the hyperventilation seen in asthmatic attacks. In addition, mechanical stimulation of the airways or the inhalation of potentially noxious agents, such as particulate matter, NO_2, SO_2, NH_3, or antigens, seems to excite irritant receptors producing airway constriction and rapid, shallow breathing. Irritant receptors in large airways are responsible for the cough reflex.

J receptors are excited by alterations in the lung interstitium produced, for example, by edema. They also can be activated by various chemical agents such as histamine, halothane, substance P, and phenyl diguanide. Excitation of the J receptors causes laryngeal closure and apnea, followed by rapid, shallow breathing. J receptors contribute to the tachypnea seen in persons with pulmonary edema and pneumonia.

Three types of receptors in the chest wall innervated by spinal nerves—joint, tendon, and spindle—signal changes in the force exerted by the respiratory muscles and movement of the chest wall. Although these receptors are not believed to be important in normal breathing, they affect breathing patterns in diseases of the lung and chest wall and seem to act to facilitate compensation to impediments for breathing. Adjustment of the relationships among tidal volume, inspiratory time, and expiratory time by chest wall and pulmonary mechanoreceptors may be important in minimizing the work of breathing and the energy expenditure of the respiratory muscles and so can affect the endurance characteristics of the respiratory muscles. Fatigue of these muscles occurs more quickly when the ratio of inspiratory time to total breath duration is greater; endurance is prolonged by smaller ratios.

Higher brain centers also affect breathing. In awake subjects, voluntary hyperventilation with oxygen even to extremely low levels of PCO_2 is rarely followed by apnea. This is not true in anesthetized or in sleeping subjects who stop breathing when overhyperventilated. This difference in the effect of hyperventilation in conscious and unconscious humans has been attributed to a "wakefulness drive" arising in the reticular formation of the brain, which preserves ventilation even in the absence of chemical stimulation. This drive may be caused by the impingement of random stimuli from the external environment on the brain, which maintains respiratory neuron activity.

Ventilation can be controlled consciously as well as involuntarily, that is, automatically influenced. Indeed, separate neural pathways for the voluntary and automatic control of the respiratory muscles have been described. Multiple inputs also allow the respiratory muscles to be sufficiently versatile so that ventilation can be adjusted to satisfy needs for chemical homeostasis and also to be used in communication and emotional expression. Higher brain centers may also play a key role in breathing, allowing adequate ventilation to be achieved with a minimum expenditure of work and with least discomfort.

IRREGULAR BREATHING

It has been known for many years that patients with congestive heart failure (particularly those with arteriosclerotic cardiac disease) as well as patients with brain disorders, such as tumors or cerebrovascular disease, sometimes breathe with a crescendo-decrescendo pattern of ventilation, each swing of ventilation terminating in apnea. This kind of breathing, called *Cheyne-Stokes respiration,* has been considered an ominous prognostic sign. However, a similar breathing pattern has been observed in apparently normal individuals during sleep and even during wakefulness in sojourners at altitude. A Cheyne-Stokes–like pattern of breathing is also common in metabolic alkalosis, in premature infants, and in adults with the sleep apnea syndrome (see box below).

Oscillations in several physiologic systems can be observed during Cheyne-Stokes breathing. Together with swings in ventilation, cyclic changes occur in blood pressure, heart rate, and cerebral blood flow. Upper airway resistance decreases during the periods of increased ventilation. There may also be striking fluctuations in alertness. Signs of depression occur during the apneic phase: the pupils are often constricted, and the patient may be motionless. With hyperventilation, the pupils dilate; there may be thrashing of the extremities and electroencephalogram (EEG) evidence of arousal.

When measured simultaneously, arterial blood and alveolar gas tension swings have been shown to be out of phase. During hyperventilation, alveolar PCO_2 tends to be low and alveolar PO_2 high; the reverse occurs during the apneic phase (Fig. 190-3). These alveolar changes are the expected effects of ventilation changes on lung gas tensions. On the other hand, arterial gas tensions seem to change in the opposite way so that arterial PO_2 is lower and arterial PCO_2 higher during hyperventilation than during apnea. This difference between arterial and alveolar gas tensions is believed to reflect the time required (circulation time) to transport blood from pulmonary capillaries to the systemic arteries. In general, the cycle length of Cheyne-Stokes respiration (the time required for a complete cycle of hyperventilation and apnea) is proportional to the circulation time; the time of hyperventilation and apnea increases as circulation time is prolonged.

It was previously thought that during the period of apparent apnea (as indicated by the absence of discernible airflow), all respiratory movements ceased, but in some patients respiratory activity seems to continue, and airflow is absent because of upper airway obstruction.

Many believe that Cheyne-Stokes respiration is a manifestation of instability in the feedback control of breathing similar to instabilities observed in manmade control systems

Causes of irregular breathing

- Congestive heart failure (particularly arteriosclerotic disease)
- Disease of the central nervous system (particularly cerebrovascular disease, meningitis, encephalitis, and brain tumors)
- Sleep-disordered breathing (central and obstructive apneas)
- Metabolic alkalosis
- Prematurity

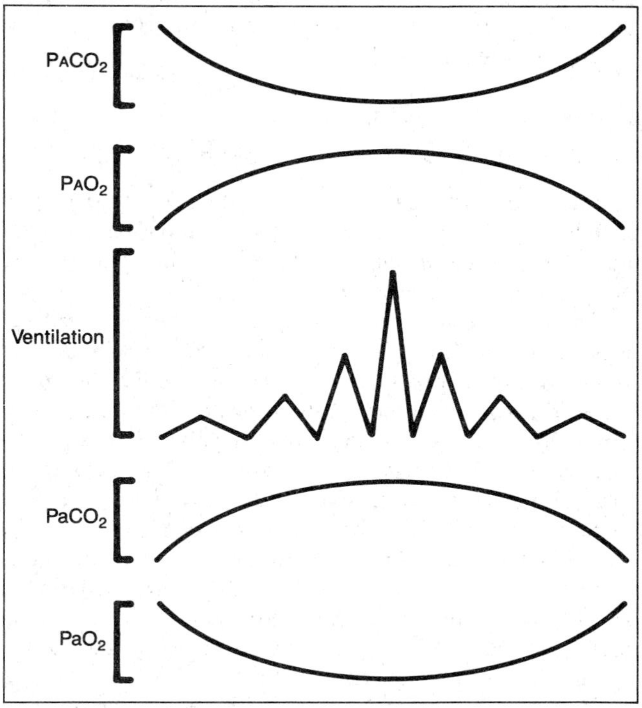

Fig. 190-3. Changes in alveolar and arterial blood gas tensions during Cheyne-Stokes breathing. Arterial PO_2 is lowest and arterial PCO_2 is highest during the hyperventilation phase.

that regulate temperature or the output of machines. In these physical control systems, delays in information transfer from the controller to the controlled system (corresponding to increases in circulation time in the respiratory system), increases in controller gain (analogous to heightened ventilatory responses to changes in PCO_2 and PO_2), or changes in set point (corresponding to increases in the level of PCO_2 and PO_2 needed to initiate breathing) cause the output of these systems to be oscillatory. Whether these analogies are correct is still controversial, but animal experiments suggest that Cheyne-Stokes respiration can be produced by interventions that cause change in physiologic function that would be expected to cause control system instability, such as artificial lengthening of circulation, controller gains, and changes in set point. Also, Cheyne-Stokes breathing seems to be more frequent at altitude in individuals with increased responses to hypoxia (heightened controller gain) and can be induced by breathing low oxygen in some individuals while they are asleep.

In patients with Cheyne-Stokes breathing and heart disease or some brain abnormality, treatment ought to be directed at reversing cardiac failure, increasing cerebral blood flow, or alleviating the central nervous system dysfunction. Occasionally the intermittent decreases in PO_2 that occur during apnea are sufficiently great as to be life-threatening. Oxygen inhalation is helpful in those patients and may abolish the breathing irregularity. Sometimes Cheyne-Stokes breathing can be made to disappear by theophylline administration. Breathing carbon dioxide–enriched gas mixtures also frequently eliminates Cheyne-Stokes respiration. Respiratory depressants, which increase resting PCO_2 levels and cause hypoxemia, frequently produce Cheyne-Stokes breathing in predisposed patients.

BREATHING DURING SLEEP AND THE SLEEP APNEA SYNDROME

Normally during sleep, ventilation decreases along with metabolic rate, but because the fall in ventilation is greater than the decrease in metabolism, PCO_2 rises slightly and arterial PO_2 decreases a bit.

The changes in blood gas tension probably reflect the loss of stimuli from the surroundings, such as light and sound, which normally excite breathing. Even though in most normals these blood gas changes are minimal, sometimes changes in arterial PO_2 are clinically significant, particularly in patients with lung disease or neuromuscular disorders if hypoxemia is present during wakefulness. Because of the shape of the oxyhemoglobin dissociation curve, the oxygen saturation of arterial blood can fall to dangerous levels even with small PO_2 changes once patients are on the steep slope of the curve. The hypoxia and hypercapnia occurring during sleep in these patients can contribute to the cardiovascular consequences of lung disease and may accelerate bicarbonate retention, leading to even more pronounced alveolar hypoventilation when awake. The changes in gas tensions resulting from altered controller properties during sleep are probably aggravated by other changes that accompany sleep, such as the fall in functional residual capacity (FRC), which may increase ventilation-perfusion mismatching, and the increase in upper airway resistance, which tends to reduce ventilation.

In addition to changes in blood gas tensions, normal subjects may experience brief periods of apnea during sleep. Usually these apneas are less than 10 seconds and occur sporadically less than ten times a night, especially in early slow-wave sleep (stages I and II) and in rapid eye movement (REM) sleep.

In individuals with the sleep apnea syndrome, there are longer repetitive pauses in which airflow is absent. During these pauses, there may be dramatic decreases in oxygen saturation accompanied by a variety of cardiac arrhythmias. These arrhythmias may take the form of premature beats, but more frequently there are episodes of bradycardia or asystole. Sleep apnea is more frequent in those who snore, in the obese, in the elderly, and in males. It is currently felt that sleep apnea accounts for most of the cases formerly termed the *obesity-hypoventilation* or *pickwickian syndrome*.

The apneas that occur during sleep are of two types: central, in which there is little evidence of respiratory activity, and obstructive, in which airflow is absent despite obvious respiratory activity; airflow fails to occur because of occlusion of the upper airway passages (Fig. 190-4). Usually obstructive apneas are more frequent than central ones, last longer, and hence are of greater clinical significance. Sometimes apneas occur irregularly, but frequently both central and obstructive apneas and EEG evidence of arousal during the hyperventilation phase are associated with a Cheyne-Stokes pattern of breathing.

The same mechanisms that have been used to explain Cheyne-Stokes respiration may also account for central apneas during sleep. On the one hand, shifts in the operating point of the control system (elevated PCO_2 during sleep) may cause unstable respiratory control, or it is possible de-

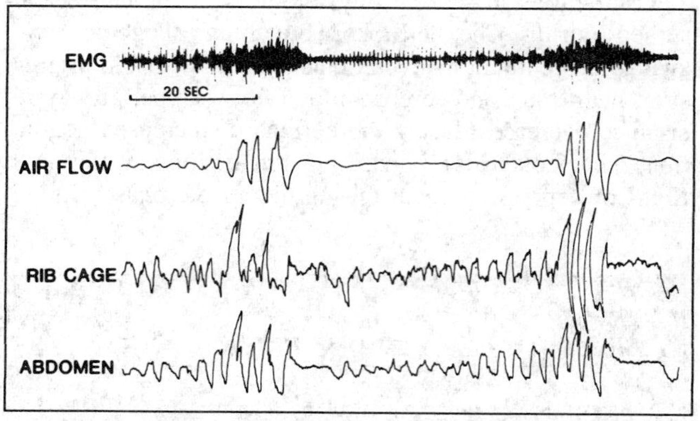

Fig. 190-4. Tracing of electromyogram (EMG) measured from a chin surface electrode, airflow, and rib cage and abdominal movement in a patient with sleep apnea. Note that the airflow pattern resembles that seen in Cheyne-Stokes respiration. Associated with the waxing and waning of airflow are swings in the chin EMG (reflecting change in the activity of upper airway muscles). Note that chest wall movements persist even in the absence of airflow so that the apnea is obstructive in type.

pressed drives to breathing caused by inherently low chemosensitivity or large reductions in metabolic rate during sleep may be instrumental.

Cephalometric measurements and computed axial tomography (CAT) scans reveal anatomic narrowing of the upper airway in some patients with obstructive sleep apnea. Nasal obstruction, for example, has been found to increase the number of sleep apneas. Many obese patients with obstructive sleep apnea seem to have narrower upper airway passages, which increase resistance to airflow.

The upper airway passages are formed by semirigid structures. The cross section of the upper airway can be actively narrowed or dilated by contraction of muscles in the nasal and oral cavities, the hypopharynx, and the larynx. During inspiration when the chest wall muscles contract, a negative pressure is produced in the pharynx that not only draws in air to inflate the lungs but also tends to collapse the upper airway. This can cause occlusion unless the muscles that dilate the upper airway can respond appropriately to withstand this collapsing force. It is believed that abnormalities in the control and coordination of the upper airway muscles may contribute to episodes of obstructive apnea during sleep.

The cranial nerves that innervate the upper airway muscles frequently display respiratory-related changes in their activity. In the case of the muscles that help widen the upper airway, such as the alae nasi (nostril flarer), the genioglossus (which protrudes the tongue), and the posterior cricoarytenoid (which abducts the vocal cords), activity is greater during inspiration than expiration. In addition, this respiratory-related activity increases with many of the same stimuli that excite breathing, for example, hypercapnia, hypoxia, and low blood pressure. The upper airway muscles may respond differently in patients with obstructive apnea than in normal patients. Arousal induced by hypoxia and hypercapnia occurs in association with the termination of apnea in many patients.

Negative pressure in the upper airways has been shown to stimulate activity of the upper airway muscles. The large intrapharyngeal negative pressures that develop during obstructive breathing during sleep may also help terminate the episodes of obstruction.

HYPOCAPNIA AND HYPERVENTILATION

The box above lists some causes of persistent hyperventilation. Diseases that decrease lung compliance, such as fibrosis or pulmonary edema, are often associated with constant and regular hyperventilation. Although these patients frequently have mild to moderate hypoxemia, the hyperventilation is disproportionate to the severity of the hypoxemia and persists even when hypoxemia is relieved by the administration of 100% oxygen. It has been postulated that increased activity of vagally mediated reflexes contributes to the hyperventilation. It was thought that increased stretch receptor discharge was responsible for the heightened reflex, but recent studies in animals suggest that stimulation of J receptors may be even more important.

Acidosis of the arterial blood or the brain extracellular fluid is sometimes the explanation for hyperventilation. Diabetes may produce a severe metabolic acidosis associated with hyperventilation (Kussmaul's breathing). In subjects returning to sea level after a stay at altitude, hyperventilation often occurs and continues for several days even though arterial pH is normal or even alkaline. In some, persistent acidity of the cerebrospinal fluid is associated with the phenomenon. A reduction in brain extracellular fluid bicarbonate usually occurs during a sojourn at altitude, which is only gradually restored to normal levels with return to sea level. Hyperventilation may be maintained until cerebrospinal fluid acidity is also reversed. Acidosis also seems to account for the hyperventilation observed in uremia. This hyperventilation, which remains for a time even after dialysis restores arterial pH to normal levels, may also be caused by a persistent acidosis of brain extracellular fluid.

Causes of persistent hyperventilation

Fibrotic lung disease
Metabolic acidosis (e.g., diabetes, uremia)
CNS disorders (midbrain and pontine lesions)
Hepatic coma
Salicylate intoxication
Fever
Psychogenic (e.g., anxiety)

The cause of the hyperventilation seen in hepatic failure is still not clear. The hypoxia sometimes seen in patients with this disease caused by venous to arterial shunting seems insufficient to explain the hyperventilation that may be caused by elevated levels of brain ammonia.

The most severe instances of respiratory alkalosis occur in the presence of central nervous system disorders such as meningitis. Pontine lesions are a well-known cause of hyperventilation. At times, though, pontine hemorrhage produces the prolonged inspiratory pauses of apneustic breathing rather than increased breathing.

Fever is known to produce a shortening of inspiratory time and an increase in respiratory frequency in humans and even in vagotomized animals. The increase in frequency seems to be a direct effect of temperature on the discharge of bulbopontine neurons.

Hyperventilation is a common sign of salicylate intoxication. Salicylates increase metabolic rate but also seem to have a direct respiratory-stimulating effect on the brain.

Occasionally, hyperventilation is intermittent and associated with changes in position. The tachypnea associated with orthopnea probably arises from pulmonary congestion and airway closure in the supine position, which produces hypoxia and J receptor stimulation. Rarely, tachypnea and hyperventilation are observed only when patients are placed in an upright position (so-called platypnea). The explanation for this is uncertain but may be caused by poor perfusion of the lung when the patient is in the upright position, which improves when pulmonary artery pressure is increased by making the patient supine.

Anxiety in psychoneurotic patients sometimes produces persistent hyperventilation associated with syncope, numbness, and tingling of the extremities. Sometimes arrhythmia and chest pain occur, which may mimic the occurrence of organic heart diseases. Training in controlled breathing techniques may reduce hyperventilation in these patients.

The deleterious effects of hyperventilation alkalosis are primarily cardiovascular (e.g., arrhythmias, reductions in cardiac output, hypotension) and nervous (e.g., decreases in cerebral blood flow, obtundation, tetany, seizures).

Treatment of acute hyperventilation should aim at reversal of the process inciting the disturbance (e.g., treatment of meningitis, sepsis). However, when the pH rises to 7.55 or above, special measures ought to be considered to raise the arterial PCO_2 and lower the pH. In subjects in whom an airway is in place, this can most easily be achieved by artificially increasing respiratory dead space. Sedative drugs, which may be tried only if hypoxemia is not present, are usually ineffective since the doses required to depress the medullary respiratory neurons also depress the vasomotor center and produce hypotension. Disturbances refractory to the above measures require controlled mechanical ventilation.

HYPOVENTILATION AND HYPERCAPNIA IN SUBJECTS WITH NORMAL LUNGS

Increased levels of arterial PCO_2 are generally a consequence of obstructive pulmonary disease but can also occur in patients with normal lungs in certain circumstances, as shown in the box below. Hypercapnia in patients without lung or chest wall disease sometimes results from an abnormality in the medullary respiratory neurons caused either by infection or cerebrovascular disease. Both the response to hypercapnia and hypoxia may be depressed, and minute ventilation is decreased. The rate and depth of breathing tend to be less regular than in normals, and breath-holding time is frequently prolonged. Although hypoxia as well as hypercapnia is present at rest, the hypoxia can be explained entirely by the hypoventilation, and the gradient between alveolar and arterial PO_2 is within normal limits. Arterial blood gases can be restored to normal limits by voluntary hyperventilation.

Causes of persistent hypercapnia

1. With normal lungs:
   a. CNS disturbances (e.g., cerebrovascular disease, Parkinson's disease, encephalitis)
   b. Metabolic alkalosis
   c. Myxedema
   d. Primary alveolar hypoventilation (Ondine's curse)
   e. Spinal cord lesions
2. Diseases of the chest wall (e.g., kyphoscoliosis, ankylosing spondylitis)
3. Neuromuscular disorders (e.g., myasthenia gravis, Guillain-Barré syndrome, amyotrophic lateral sclerosis, acid maltase disease, muscular dystrophy, poliomyelitis)
4. Chronic obstructive pulmonary disease

Progesterone stimulates respiration in some of these patients, and oral administration of this drug may produce a significant reduction in the $PaCO_2$. Phrenic nerve stimulation has been used successfully in these patients to restore normal blood gas tensions and pH.

Occasionally, extreme elevations in $PaCO_2$, hypoxia, and cor pulmonale occur in patients with severe metabolic alkalosis. In contrast, other patients with equally great blood bicarbonate elevations show little if any carbon dioxide retention. This discrepancy is not explained by differences in brain interstitial fluid pH but may reflect altered intracellular pH.

In part, the hypoventilation observed in myxedema is a direct effect of the disease on the lung and respiratory muscles. The vital capacity may be reduced by muscular weakness, and a decrease in diffusing capacity has been observed. Myxedema may also produce an abnormal EEG, and it has been suspected that respiratory neuron depression contributes to the hypoventilation, which is relieved by thyroid hormone replacement. Hyperventilation is not observed in hyperthyroid patients, and carbon dioxide sensitivity is within normal limits.

It should also be noted that patients with sleep apnea may also have persistent hypercapnia while awake.

Although depression of hypercapnic and hypoxic sensitivity usually occur together, in some subjects a selective blunting of hypoxic drive occurs. For example, hypoxic response is depressed, but the response to hypercapnia may be normal in patients with surgically resected carotid bodies in a now-discarded treatment for asthma or in whom inadvertent injury to the carotid body was produced (by carotid endarterectomy, for example).

Birth at altitude or long-term exposure to altitude depresses hypoxic response but has little effect on the response to hypercapnia. Children with congenital cyanotic heart disease who in effect also have had prolonged exposure to hypoxia, such as altitude dwellers, also display a blunted hypoxic response.

These patients with isolated defects in hypoxic response are able to maintain normal blood gas tensions during rest and exercise. However, anesthesia and the resulting depression of carbon dioxide sensitivity may produce hypoventilation and a progressive and life-endangering hypoxia.

Diseases that severely restrict movements of the chest wall, such as kyphoscoliosis and ankylosing spondylitis, may cause hypoventilation and retention of carbon dioxide.

Neuromuscular disorders, such as myasthenia gravis, the Guillain-Barré syndrome, amyotrophic lateral sclerosis, acid maltase disease, or muscular dystrophy, often terminate in respiratory failure with carbon dioxide elevation and depressed oxygen saturation. Bilateral paralysis of the diaphragm, the major muscle of inspiration, may cause carbon dioxide retention particularly when the patient is supine. This is associated with inward movement of the diaphragm during inspiration and outward movement of the rib cage. As in the patients with primary alveolar hypoventilation, in these patients, carbon dioxide retention occurs mainly because minute ventilation is reduced.

HYPERCAPNIA IN PATIENTS WITH OBSTRUCTIVE LUNG DISEASE

Chronic obstructive pulmonary disease (emphysema and bronchitis) is the most common cause of hypercapnia. An inborn decrease in chemosensitivity may contribute to the hypoventilation in some patients. In others, metabolic alkalosis or the use of sedatives or opiate drugs causes a depressed response to carbon dioxide and to hypoxia and further reduces ventilation. Some patients have a decreased minute ventilation, but in many patients with chronic obstructive pulmonary disease, the level of minute ventilation is even greater than normal. In these patients hypercapnia is associated with shallow, rapid breathing in which each breath has a reduced inspiratory time. The hypercapnia is caused by an increase in physiologic dead space ventilated with each breath. One explanation for this kind of respiratory pattern is reflex stimulation of breathing by inflamed airways. But some patients may adopt this pattern of breathing to avoid respiratory muscle fatigue. Since hyperinflation characteristically occurs in obstructive lung disease, the respiratory muscles are shortened and may be unable to produce normal amounts of force when stimulated. In addition, because airway resistance is increased, the respiratory muscles may become chronically fatigued. In a small group of patients the lungs are so damaged and the respiratory muscles are so inefficient that increased ventilation raises the carbon dioxide production of the respiratory muscles to a greater extent than it removes carbon dioxide from the body. It has been shown that respiratory muscle fatigue occurs when the tension time index of the respiratory muscles (defined as the product of the pressure produced as a fraction of maximum pressure and the inspiratory time as a fraction of time spent in inspiration and expiration) exceeds a critical value. Endurance can be prolonged by breathing shallowly with a small tidal volume so that muscle tension is reduced while shortening inspiratory time increases the opportunity for muscle recovery.

Normal subjects respond to acute airway obstruction with increased inspiratory effort. This response remains intact in asthmatic patients but is reduced in some patients with chronic obstructive pulmonary disease and may contribute to the development of hypercapnia. Aging and the sleep deprivation that occurs in the sleep apnea syndrome are other factors that decrease the respiratory response to obstruction.

BEHAVIORAL CONTROL OF BREATHING AND ITS RELATION TO DYSPNEA

In addition to being regulated automatically (through chemoreceptor and mechanoreceptor reflexes), breathing can be altered volitionally. Obvious examples of this are voluntary breath holding and the mild hyperventilation that occurs with speech. Anxiety and depression may have more long-lasting effects on ventilatory patterns. Emotional factors may also explain the irregular breathing observed at times in normal individuals.

Volitional factors may be more important clinically when dyspnea (a sensation of difficult or labored breathing) is present. Although normal breathing occurs effortlessly without conscious awareness, the dyspneic patient is cognizant of every breath. Dyspnea is one of the more common presenting symptoms in patients with lung disease. Sometimes dyspnea is the major cause of disability and appears to be out of proportion to the severity of the lung disease.

To study dyspnea, standard psychophysical methods that relate the physical intensity of a stimulus to the sensation experienced have been used. These studies show that the sensations produced by changes in tidal volume increase as they do to other stimuli (e.g., light and sound) as a power function of the physical intensity of the stimulus. It is of interest that this power relationship also applies to the sensations produced by changes in respiratory muscle contraction. The sensory effects that occur with respiratory muscle contraction and the degree of dyspnea experienced increase with the pressure produced and length of time the pressure is maintained. Of the two effects, pressure changes seem more potent than time changes. Some evidence shows that some patients breathe more shallowly and rapidly to relieve dyspnea. Although this would decrease the sensation produced by breathing, it worsens gas exchange.

Hypercapnia and hypoxia are respiratory stimulants that increase the force generated by the respiratory muscles. Relief of hypoxia and hypercapnia is an effective way of diminishing dyspnea. Nonetheless, a clear relationship between respiratory sensitivity to hypoxia or hypercapnia and the dyspnea experienced by patients with lung disease has not yet been demonstrated. Sedative drugs have been used to diminish sensitivity to hypoxia and hypercapnia with the expectation that this would also reduce dyspnea. Although lifestyle has been improved in a few patients by this kind of treatment, in many patients significant adverse effects on gas exchange have been demonstrated.

ASSESSMENT OF RESPIRATORY CONTROL

Usually chemosensitivity has been evaluated by plotting the relationship between ventilation and arterial PCO_2 and PO_2 after steady state inhalation of different inspired gas mixtures. These tests were long and tedious for both the patient and the examiner. Recently much more rapid single-breath and rebreathing methods of assessing ventilatory responses to hypoxia and hypercapnia have been developed.

Ventilation may not be an adequate measure of the response to chemical stimuli in patients with disease of the lungs or chest wall who have impaired respiratory mechanics. Methods of assessing efferent activity, which measures inspiratory pressures generated during airway occlusion or diaphragm electrical activity, have allowed respiratory regulation to be studied, even in the presence of significant lung disease.

Difficulties still remain; for example, methods of assessing the neural control of breathing are still in the developmental stage. However, there is now sufficient experience so that most patients with suspected abnormalities in respiratory control can be assessed and a diagnosis made.

Evaluation begins with the history, physical examination, and chest roentgenogram, which determine whether symptoms or signs of pulmonary or neuromuscular diseases are present. Tests that measure airway caliber and the strength of the respiratory muscles are particularly useful since obstructive lung disease and respiratory muscle weakness are the functional abnormalities most often associated with carbon dioxide retention.

Patients with obstructive lung disease rarely develop carbon dioxide retention if the forced expiratory volume at 1 second (FEV_1) is greater than 1.5 liters, although the ventilatory response to carbon dioxide will be reduced in patients with even modest reductions in FEV_1. Significant carbon dioxide retention with less reduction in FEV_1 should lead one to suspect concomitant respiratory controller dysfunction. If carbon dioxide retention is caused entirely by respiratory controller dysfunction, the A-a gradient is normal or nearly so, and breath-holding time will be unaffected by changes in PCO_2. Also, voluntary hyperventilation will return the arterial PCO_2 to normal values.

When lung function tests are normal, controller performance can be more directly evaluated by determining the ventilatory response to hypoxia and hypercapnia. When lung function is abnormal, measurements of occlusion pressure or the EMG of the diaphragm can be used to evaluate whether there is any response to chemical stimuli. Polysomnography during sleep is essential in determining whether carbon dioxide retention is caused by disordered breathing during sleep.

REFERENCES

Berger AT, Mitchell RA, and Severinghaus JW: Regulation of respiration. N Engl J Med 297:93, 1977.

Cherniack NS: Sleep apnea and its causes. J Clin Invest 73:1501, 1984.

Cherniack NS, Nochomovitz ML, and Altose MD: Disorders of respiratory control. In Simmons DH, editor: Pulmonology, vol 4. New York, 1982, Wiley.

Dowell AR et al: Cheyne-Stokes respiration: a review of clinical manifestations and critique of physiological mechanisms. Arch Intern Med 127:712, 1971.

Longobardo GS and Cherniack NS: Abnormalities in respiratory rhythm. In Cherniack NS and Widdicombe JG, editors: The handbook of physiology, sect. 3, vol 2, Washington, DC, 1986, American Physiological Society.

Sorli J et al: Control of breathing in patients with chronic obstructive lung disease. Clin Sci Mol Med 54:295, 1978.

Strohl KP, Cherniack NS, and Gothe B: Physiologic basis of therapy for sleep apnea. Am Rev Respir Dis 134:791, 1986.

van Lunteren E and Strohl KP: The muscles of the upper airways. Clin Chest Med 7:171, 1986.

CHAPTER

191 Respiratory Muscles and Respiratory Muscle Failure

Dudley F. Rochester

The respiratory muscles are striated skeletal muscles under both voluntary and automatic neural control. Their vital function is to generate the inspired breath or tidal volume at a size and rate appropriate to the prevailing metabolic needs. In effect, the respiratory muscles represent the "air pump" of the body, just as the heart is the blood pump.

The principal inspiratory muscles are the diaphragm, the parasternal intercostal muscles, and the scalene muscles in the neck. The principal expiratory muscles are the external and internal oblique and transversus abdominis muscles of the abdomen and the triangularis sterni muscles in the thorax. The lateral intercostal and sternocleidomastoid muscles also contribute to breathing.

RESPIRATORY MUSCLE CONTRACTILE PROPERTIES

The force produced by muscle contraction varies with (1) the degree of electrical or neural excitation, (2) the resting length of the muscle, and (3) the velocity at which it shortens during contraction. These considerations apply to the respiratory muscles, in vitro and in situ.

The physiologic range of phrenic nerve discharge rates lies between 5 and 40 impulses per second. Diaphragmatic contractile force and shortening vary approximately fivefold over this range, so increasing stimulation frequency is an important mechanism for regulating respiratory muscle force output and the size of the tidal volume.

Diaphragm muscle length changes with lung volume. At the normal breathing position (functional residual capacity, FRC) the diaphragm is at or near its optimal resting length, whereas at full inspiration (total lung capacity, TLC) the diaphragm is 40% shorter. Diaphragmatic force and volume displacing capacity are best near FRC, but are reduced by half at TLC.

During quiet breathing the diaphragm shortens by 5% to 10% per breath, but during maximal voluntary or exercise ventilation it shortens by approximately 20% per breath. The velocity or shortening increases almost tenfold from quiet breathing to maximal ventilation. Because of this, the dynamic diaphragmatic force during maximal ventilation is only half the maximal static force.

RESPIRATORY MUSCLE NEURAL CONTROL AND INTERACTIONS

Quiet breathing in the supine position is accomplished by the diaphragm and the parasternal muscles, and expiration is passive. Merely assuming an upright position causes inspiratory recruitment of the scalene muscles as well as tonic and phasic expiratory recruitment of the abdominal muscles.

At higher levels of ventilatory effort, recruitment extends to the sternocleidomastoid, intercostal, abdominal, and triangularis sterni muscles. This is a normal response to an increase in ventilatory load, for example, with physical exercise, when airway resistance increases, or when breathing at a higher than normal lung volume.

The abdominal muscles can assist inspiration, because their expiratory contraction increases abdominal pressure and pushes the diaphragm to a more cranial position. This lengthens the diaphragm and improves its mechanical advantage. In addition, the sudden relaxation of the abdominal muscles at the end of expiration facilitates the onset of inspiratory airflow.

Diaphragmatic contraction causes the dome of the diaphragm to descend, thereby displacing the abdominal wall outward and increasing abdominal pressure. This exerts a lateral force on the lower rib cage through the area where the diaphragm is apposed to the inner aspect of the rib cage. The diaphragm also lifts and flares the lower rib cage. All three of these actions expand the lungs, especially the lower lobes.

Because diaphragmatic contraction lowers the pressure inside the thorax, it tends to cave in the upper chest. Contraction of inspiratory muscles in the upper rib cage and neck not only prevents chest distortion, but also contributes to the inspired volume, especially in the upper lobes.

At a very high lung volume, diaphragmatic shortening capacity is impaired, and the diaphragm becomes flattened so it cannot effectively convert its contractile force into the pressure needed to inflate the lungs. The diaphragm no longer expands the lower rib cage, and the flat diaphragm may even draw the lower rib cage inward during inspiration (Hoover's sign).

RESPIRATORY MUSCLE STRENGTH

The strength of the respiratory muscles can be assessed by measuring the pressure generated by maximal inspiratory and expiratory efforts against a closed airway (PImax, PEmax). PImax is highest at RV and PEmax is highest at TLC. Typically, PImax and PEmax in young adult males are −120 and +250 cm H_2O, respectively. Values in young women are about 70% of those in men, and in both sexes over the age of 50, PImax and PEmax are about 10% to 15% lower than in young adults.

Alternatively, one can measure esophageal pressure (Pes) and gastric pressure (Pga) as reflections of pleural and abdominal pressures, respectively. The difference between Pga and Pes is referred to as *transdiaphragmatic pressure* (Pdi). During maximal inspiratory efforts against a closed airway, Pdi is similar in magnitude to Pes and PImax, but Pdi is twice as high during respiratory maneuvers that also increase abdominal pressure. The Pes during a sniff is similar to PImax, and Pes during a cough is similar to PEmax. Because sniffing and coughing are natural actions, they are useful to test patients who have trouble performing the PImax and PEmax maneuvers correctly, or in case of suspected malingering.

RESPIRATORY MUSCLE ENDURANCE AND FATIGUE

Breathing is an endurance activity that requires repetitive contraction of the respiratory muscles for life. Normal breathing requires very little energy expenditure, and the perceived effort of breathing is also small. Perhaps the most remarkable aspect of the respiratory muscle and neuromotor control system is its versatility. The respiratory muscles can support speech and singing, swimming the crawl and chopping wood, walking, cycling, and a host of other activities, all largely hidden from consciousness.

Two factors that bear on endurance are muscle fiber type and blood supply. About 75% of the fibers in respiratory muscles have good to excellent intrinsic endurance characteristics, and respiratory muscle blood supply is bountiful. Respiratory muscle endurance also depends on respiratory muscle strength and the force and duration of contraction with each breath.

The force and duration of inspiratory muscle contraction are assessed from the pressure required to inspire the tidal volume (Pbreath), and the duration of inspiration (Ti). Both Pbreath and Ti are expressed as fractions of their maximal values, PImax and Ttot (Ttot is the duration of one whole breath). Combining these variables yields a pressure-time index (PTI): PTI = (Pbreath/PImax) × (Ti/Ttot).

In normal subjects breathing quietly, Pbreath/PImax is typically 0.05, Ti/Ttot is 0.4, and PTI is 0.02. Any combination of Pbreath/PImax or Ti/Ttot that causes Pbreath/PImax to exceed 0.5 or PTI to exceed 0.15 leads to fatigue. The time to onset of overt fatigue is 90 minutes when PTI is 0.15, but only 3 minutes when PTI is 0.40. Thus, the respiratory muscles may be in a fatiguing pattern of contraction without having developed overt contractile failure.

There are at least three mechanisms of respiratory muscle fatigue. Central fatigue represents inhibition of neural drive, perhaps owing to inhibitory influences from the overstressed muscle. Transmission fatigue is failure at the level of the nerve or neuromuscular junction. Muscle cell fatigue is caused by impairment of the excitation-contraction coupling mechanism.

The best test for respiratory muscle fatigue is to detect a reduction in the Pdi response to stimulation of the phrenic nerves, while the amplitude of the electromyogram (EMG) is preserved. An increase in Pbreath/PImax or inspiratory PTI, slowing of relaxation rate, and a shift in the power in the electromyogram (EMG) from higher to lower frequency (fall in the high/low ratio) all indicate that the respiratory muscles are in a fatiguing pattern of contraction, but are not evidence of overt fatigue.

Several clinical signs indicate that the inspiratory muscles are severely stressed, including increasing dyspnea, tachypnea, and flaring of the alae nasi. Contraction of neck inspiratory and abdominal muscles can be assessed by palpation. The smooth outward inspiratory excursion of the chest and abdomen is replaced by abrupt, jerky movements in which the chest and abdomen are out of phase with each other (chest-abdomen asynchrony).

RESPIRATORY MUSCLE WEAKNESS

A leading cause of inspiratory muscle weakness is mechanical disadvantage to the diaphragm consequent to hyperinflation of the lung in obstructive lung diseases such as asthma, chronic bronchitis, and emphysema. Conversely, in severe obesity and ascites, the diaphragm may lose force because it is overstretched, especially when the patient is supine.

Severe global respiratory muscle weakness occurs in circulatory or septic shock, with hypokalemia, hypophosphatemia, acidosis, and from cachexia from infection, neoplasm, or malnutrition. Hypoxia limits respiratory muscle endurance, whereas hypercapnia exerts an immediate depressant effect on muscle contractility.

The clinical manifestations of respiratory muscle involvement in neuromuscular diseases depend on the nature of the underlying disease and the site of the lesion. In spinal cord injury, expiratory muscle paralysis exceeds inspiratory paralysis because most of the inspiratory muscles are innervated about the C5 level. Diseases such as myasthenia gravis, dystrophies, and myopathies tend to involve inspiratory and expiratory muscles about equally.

Paralysis of the diaphragm often occurs without other respiratory muscle weakness. Diaphragmatic paralysis is a complication of open-heart surgery, as a result either of cold injury to the phrenic nerves or damage to phrenic nerve blood supply. Diaphragmatic contractility is reflexly inhibited for about a week after upper abdominal surgery, and expiratory strength is reduced for approximately a week after thoracic surgery.

The consequences of respiratory muscle weakness are impaired coughing and sighing, atelectasis, pneumonia, limitation of exercise capacity, and ventilatory failure. A definitive diagnosis of respiratory muscle weakness is made by measuring PImax and PEmax. Other valuable clues are unexplained reductions in vital capacity and maximal voluntary ventilation, or unexplained increases in RV and $PaCO_2$. One should suspect respiratory muscle weakness in any patient with ventilatory failure, especially when the severity of underlying lung disease does not appear to account for CO_2 retention.

Significant ventilatory failure ($PaCO_2$ greater than 50 mm Hg) does not occur with muscle weakness alone until inspiratory muscle strength (PImax) falls below approximately 25% of normal. However, in obstructive lung disease and other conditions where the work of breathing is increased, ventilatory failure occurs when PImax falls below 50% of normal.

RESPIRATORY MUSCLE FAILURE, DYSPNEA, AND VENTILATORY FAILURE

In diseases that predispose to ventilatory failure, mechanical abnormalities of lungs, airways, and chest wall increase Pbreath, and respiratory muscle weakness reduces PImax. With a high Pbreath and a low PImax, as for example in COPD, Pbreath/PImax and PTI approach the fatigue threshold. More importantly, the increase in Pbreath/PImax leads to dyspnea and respiratory distress.

The link between respiratory muscle failure and ventilatory failure is rapid, shallow breathing. This breathing pattern is associated with an increase in the neural drive to breathe. It also reflects the respiratory center response to the respiratory distress associated with the increase in Pbreath/PImax. That is, with increasing severity of disease, both tidal volume and Ti/Ttot fall.

Smaller, shorter breaths reduce Pbreath and minimize dyspnea. The increase in respiratory rate maintains minute ventilation at normal levels, but the small tidal volume leads to CO_2 retention. This is especially true when the efficiency of gas exchange is severely compromised, as in COPD and other severe lung disease.

Respiratory muscle fatigue can lead to ventilatory failure, but in most cases it appears that ventilatory failure results from adopting the rapid, shallow breathing pattern. Evidently this strategy reduces Pbreath and Ti/Ttot enough that overt fatigue is avoided.

TREATMENT OF RESPIRATORY MUSCLE FAILURE

The immediate treatment of respiratory muscle failure is the treatment of acute ventilatory failure, that is, provide oxygen and initiate mechanical ventilation to normalize blood gas composition. The next step is to remove adverse influences on the muscles by correcting electrolyte balance and fluid volume status, controlling infection, and relieving bronchospasm.

When patients in ventilatory failure receive adequate levels of mechanical ventilation, their spontaneous breathing efforts cease and they lose their dyspnea. Dyspnea and tachypnea also occur with inflammation of the airways, pneumonia, pulmonary embolism, pulmonary edema, atelectasis, pleural effusion, and pneumothorax. If any of these complications are present in the mechanically ventilated patient, dyspnea and tachypnea persist despite adequate oxygenation and ventilation. During trials of weaning from mechanical ventilation, dyspnea, tachypnea, and chest-abdomen asynchrony signify that significant respiratory muscle failure persists and that the trial is likely to fail.

Patients with severely limited ventilatory endurance may need mechanical ventilator support several hours per day. Although this improves blood gas composition and respiratory muscle function, its mechanism of action is not clear. Relief of nocturnal hypoventilation and of dyspnea may be as important as rest to relieve muscle fatigue.

Methylxanthines (theophylline, caffeine), beta-adrenergic agonists, and digitalis glycosides enhance diaphragmatic contractility in vitro. For the most part, however, use of pharmacologic agents in treatment of respiratory muscle failure has been disappointing.

Nutritional repletion restores respiratory muscle strength

and endurance, provided caloric intake is approximately 1.5 times resting energy expenditure. The limitations are (1) it does not work unless underlying catabolic processes can be controlled, (2) excessive repletion of critically ill patients may lead to difficulty in weaning owing to excessive CO_2 production, and (3) patients with COPD find it hard to manage the diet.

Inspiratory muscles can be trained to enhance ventilatory endurance or to increase respiratory muscle strength and endurance. Inspiratory muscle training has only modest effects on dyspnea and almost none on capacity for activities of daily living. However, regimens that combine inspiratory muscle and walking training appear to be much better in this regard.

SUMMARY

Normal respiratory muscles have excellent endurance and use little energy. The extraordinary versatility of the respiratory musculature stems from a sophisticated control mechanism that can adapt the pattern of breathing to a wide variety of physical activities.

Respiratory muscle dysfunction is a significant component of diseases that predispose to ventilatory failure. Causes include mechanical disadvantage, malnutrition, metabolic disarray, hypoxemia, and respiratory acidosis. Respiratory muscle failure contributes to the development of ventilatory failure through a perception of dyspnea and the resultant rapid, shallow pattern of breathing.

Respiratory muscle function can be restored by relief of adverse influences, reducing the work of breathing, and treating the underlying disease to the extent possible. Improvement of respiratory muscle contractility by nutritional repletion and training is often the key to reversing ventilatory failure.

REFERENCES

Begin P and Grassino A: Inspiratory muscle dysfunction and chronic hypercapnia in chronic obstructive pulmonary disease. Am Rev Respir Dis 143:905, 1991.

Dekhuijzen PN, Folgering HT, and van Herwaarden CL: Target-flow inspiratory muscle training during pulmonary rehabilitation in patients with COPD. Chest 99:128, 1991.

Efthimiou J et al: The effect of supplementary oral nutrition in poorly nourished patients with chronic obstructive pulmonary disease. Am Rev Respir Dis 137:1075, 1988.

Leblanc P et al: Breathlessness and exercise in patients with cardiorespiratory disease. Am Rev Respir Dis 133:21, 1986.

Rochester DF: Ventilatory failure: an overview. In Marini JJ and Roussos C, editors: Update in intensive care and emergency medicine 15, ventilatory failure. New York, 1991, Springer-Verlag.

Rochester DF, editor: Respiratory muscle failure, parts one and two. Seminars in respiratory medicine, vols 12#6 Nov-Dec 1991 and 13#1 Jan-Feb 1992.

Rochester DF and Braun NMT: Determinants of maximal inspiratory pressure in chronic obstructive pulmonary disease. Am Rev Respir Dis 132:42, 1985.

Tobin MJ et al: Konno-Mead analysis of ribcage-abdominal action during successful and unsuccessful trials of weaning from mechanical ventilation. Am Rev Respir Dis 135:1320, 1987.

CHAPTER

192 Pulmonary Blood Flow

J. T. Sylvester
Roy G. Brower

The major function of the pulmonary vasculature is to bring blood into sufficiently intimate contact with ventilated air to allow adequate uptake of oxygen and elimination of carbon dioxide. In addition, this circuit provides the reservoir that fills the left ventricle during diastole and the mechanical filter that prevents air, thrombi, and other particulate material from reaching the systemic circulation, where embolic infarction or ischemia could have disastrous consequences. Finally, the pulmonary endothelium, with a large surface area of about 130 m^2, performs important metabolic functions, such as production and inactivation of certain vasoactive hormones.

STRUCTURE

The pulmonary arteries accompany the airways in bronchovascular bundles and branch asymmetrically as they travel peripherally. Arterial diameters, which approximate those of the accompanying airways, decrease from about 20 mm in the main pulmonary artery to about 20 to 50 μm in precapillary arterioles. Despite this, the increased number of branches causes the total cross-sectional area of the arterial vasculature to increase peripherally. At the central part of the acinus, the arterial end branches connect to a dense alveolar capillary network. This network is interconnected throughout the acinus, providing numerous pathways for blood to flow from the center of the acinus to the postcapillary venules at its periphery. The venules converge to form progressively larger veins, which follow an independent course toward the left atrium approximately midway between pairs of bronchovascular bundles.

Vascular smooth muscle allows active control of the flow through pulmonary vessels. The larger extraparenchymal pulmonary arteries contain several elastic lamini and a paucity of smooth muscle. Intraparenchymally, muscularity progressively increases until arteries about 2 mm in diameter are reached and then decreases so that virtually no arteries less than 30 μm in diameter have smooth muscle. At any given external diameter, pulmonary veins have thinner walls than arteries. In addition, the transitions from nonmuscular to muscular veins occur in larger vessels. Although they have no smooth muscle themselves, capillaries may nevertheless be subject to active control by interstitial myofibroblasts extending from the endothelial to the epithelial basement membrane. Contraction of these cells may cause capillary compression.

RESISTANCE

Although the entire cardiac output (CO) flows through the lung, the pressure gradient from the main pulmonary artery to the left atrium is usually no greater than 10 mm Hg, whereas about 100 mm Hg is normally required to drive the same CO through the systemic vasculature. Thus, in comparison to the systemic vasculature, the pulmonary vasculature is a low-resistance circuit. Under normal conditions, resistance in the pulmonary vasculature is approximately equally divided among arteries, capillaries, and veins. This contrasts with the systemic circulation, where most of the resistance is found in arterial vessels.

The flow-resistive properties of the pulmonary circuit are described by the relationship between mean pulmonary artery pressure (Ppa) and CO (Fig. 192-1). Two features of this pressure-flow relationship are noteworthy. First, the pressure axis intercept is the backpressure to flow, or the pressure that pulmonary artery pressure must exceed before blood can flow through the lung. The backpressure may vary in different parts of the lung because of gravity. This variation serves as the basis for dividing the lung into three zones. In zone 3, normally found in the basilar, dependent parts of the lung, both pulmonary arterial and left atrial pressures exceed alveolar pressure, and left atrial pressure is the backpressure to flow. In zone 2, normally found in the middle regions of the lung, gravity causes left atrial pressure to become less than alveolar pressure, but pulmonary artery pressure remains greater than alveolar pressure. The thin-walled capillaries are surrounded by alveolar pressure and do not resist collapse when left atrial pressure (and therefore intravascular capillary pressure) falls below alveolar pressure. For blood to flow through this region, pulmonary artery pressure must exceed alveolar pressure, which therefore acts as the backpressure. In zone 1, normally found at the apices of the lung, gravity causes both pulmonary arterial and left atrial pressure to become less than alveolar pressure. Thus, in this lung region, no blood flows through the collapsed alveolar capillaries.

The second noteworthy feature of this pressure-flow relationship is its curvilinearity: as Ppa increases, the change in pressure required to generate a given change in flow decreases. This occurs because at higher pressures perfused vessels distend and nonperfused vessels, such as those in zone 1, open and become perfused. The latter is termed *recruitment*. Both distention and recruitment increase the cross-sectional area of the vasculature and thereby lower its resistance.

Resistance can be measured as the inverse of the slope of the pressure-flow relationship ($\Delta Ppa/\Delta CO$); but, this is impractical in patients because the pressure-flow curve is unknown and difficult to determine. In patients with thermodilution pulmonary artery catheters, resistance can be quantified as the difference between mean pulmonary artery and wedge pressures divided by CO. This ratio, known as *pulmonary vascular resistance* (PVR), has a normal value of less than or equal to 4 mm $Hg \cdot L^{-1} \cdot min$.

Increases in PVR are usually interpreted to indicate an increase in the flow-resistive properties of the vasculature, and vice versa. This interpretation is unambiguous if the change in PVR occurs with either Ppa or CO remaining con-

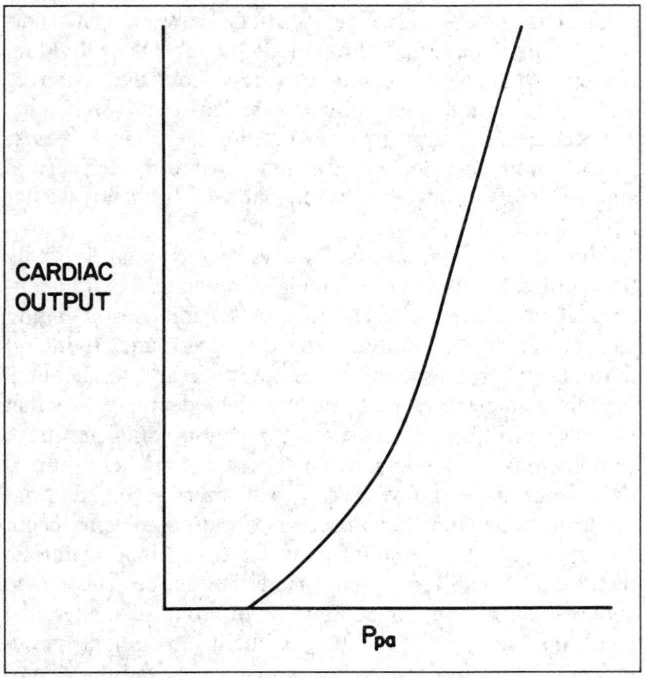

Fig. 192-1. Pulmonary artery pressure-flow relationship. Ppa, mean pulmonary arterial pressure.

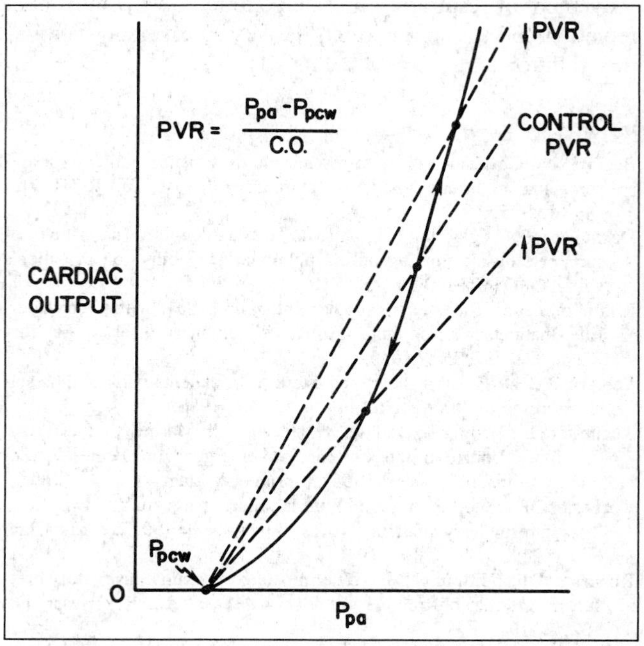

Fig. 192-2. Change in pulmonary vascular resistance (PVR), calculated as the difference between mean pulmonary arterial (Ppa) and capillary wedge pressures (Ppcw) divided by cardiac output (CO), can occur without a change in the pulmonary artery pressure-flow curve.

stant or with Ppa and CO changing in opposite directions; however, if Ppa and CO change in the same direction, changes in PVR can occur without any change in the pulmonary artery pressure–flow relationship, as shown in Fig. 192-2. Pulmonary vascular resistance is the inverse of the chord slope connecting two points on the pressure-flow relationship: mean Ppa at the measured CO and pulmonary capillary wedge pressure (Ppcw) at a CO of zero. Increases in CO along an unchanged pressure-flow relationship decrease PVR, and decreases in CO increase PVR because of the curvilinearity of the relationship. Furthermore, as illustrated in Fig. 192-3, changes in the pressure-flow relationship can occur without any change in PVR. If the pressure-flow curve were shifted to higher pressures, as would occur with vasoconstriction, and CO increased appropriately, the new Ppa-CO point could lie on the old PVR line. The result would be no change in PVR despite the vasoconstriction-induced change in the pressure-flow relationship. The same result could be obtained if the Ppa-CO relationship were shifted to lower pressures (vasodilation) and CO were appropriately decreased.

One way to deal with these ambiguities is illustrated in Fig. 192-4. Draw a straight line through the control Ppcw and Ppa-CO points on a set of pressure-flow coordinates. Draw a second straight line parallel to the flow axis through the control Ppa-CO point. Shade the area between the two lines. If a new Ppa-CO point falls to the right or left of the shaded area, then pulmonary vasoconstriction or vasodilation has occurred, respectively. If the new Ppa-CO point falls within the shaded area, it is not possible to conclude that the flow-resistive properties of the vasculature have changed.

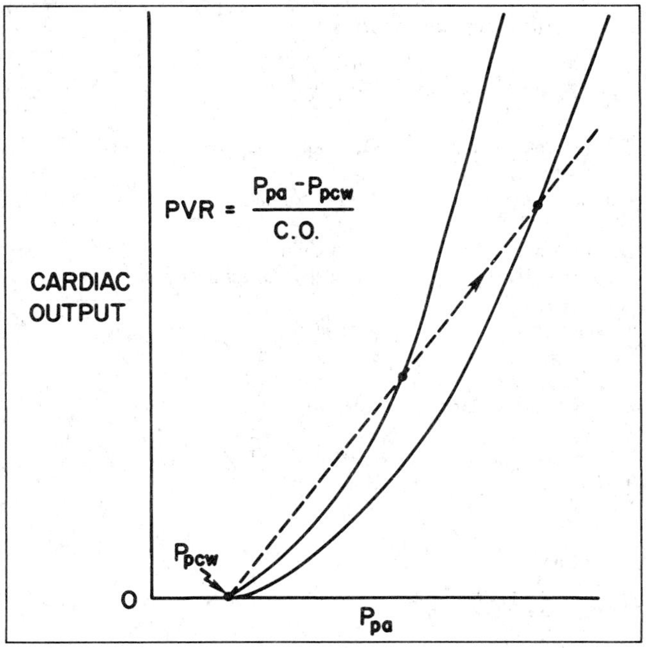

Fig. 192-3. A change in the pulmonary artery pressure–flow curve can occur without a change in pulmonary vascular resistance (PVR). Ppa, mean pulmonary arterial pressure; Ppcw, capillary wedge pressure; CO, cardiac output.

COMPLIANCE

Compliance is the property of the vasculature that allows it to change volume in response to a change in distending pressure. This property has not received as much attention as resistance but is nonetheless essential to normal circulatory function. For example, during diastole, the aortic and pulmonary valves are closed, and the left ventricle must be filled from the pulmonary vasculature. This could not occur if the pulmonary circulation had no compliance.

Like resistance, the compliance of the pulmonary circulation is less than that of the systemic circulation. For example, in animals pulmonary vascular compliance is about 0.25 ml•mm Hg^{-1}•kg^{-1}, whereas systemic vascular compliance is about 2.5 ml•mm Hg^{-1}•kg^{-1}. Because of its low compliance and intravascular pressure, the pulmonary circuit contains only about 10% of the total vascular volume. The distribution of this volume within the pulmonary circuit is not known with certainty, but recent studies suggest that the majority of pulmonary vascular compliance is located in the capillaries. This contrasts with the systemic circulation, where most of the compliance is thought to reside in small veins.

EFFECTS OF LUNG INFLATION

The lungs undergo cyclic changes in gas volume during the respiratory cycle, subjecting the pulmonary blood vessels to unique stresses. The effects of these stresses can be best understood by dividing the lung vessels into two functional categories. Alveolar vessels are surrounded by alveolar pressure, which rises relative to the pressure on the surface

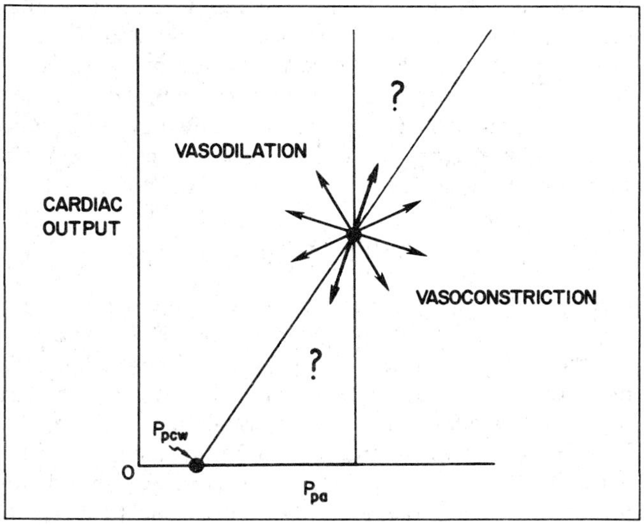

Fig. 192-4. Graphical method for assessing changes in the flow-resistive properties of the pulmonary circulation clinically. For explanation, see text. Ppcw, capillary wedge pressure; Ppa, mean pulmonary arterial pressure.

of the lung (pleural pressure) when the lung inflates. Thus, alveolar vessels tend to be compressed by inflation. Alveolar vessels include not only capillaries but also arteries and veins, which lack effective attachments to the pulmonary parenchyma. Extra-alveolar vessels are surrounded by the sum of inward-acting alveolar pressure and outward-acting tissue pressure exerted by connections between the vessel and lung parenchyma. The distending effect of the tissue connections is predominant, causing extra-alveolar vessels to expand as the lung inflates. Extra-alveolar vessels include most arteries and veins and also the capillaries located at the junctions of alveolar septae, the so-called corner vessels. Thus, the effect of inflation on the lung vasculature can be viewed as the net result of its opposing effects on alveolar and extra-alveolar vessels.

At residual lung volume, there is little tension in the parenchymal tissue, and extra-alveolar vessels may be narrowed, folded, or kinked. As lung volume increases, tissue tension increases, and the extra-alveolar vessels lengthen, expand, and unfold, decreasing their resistance. At low lung volumes, this decrease in extra-alveolar vessel resistance exceeds the simultaneous increase in alveolar vessel resistance caused by compression. Thus, total pulmonary vascular resistance falls. With further increases in lung volume, however, the increase in alveolar vessel resistance continues, while extra-alveolar vessels approach the limit of their distensibility. Thus, total pulmonary vascular resistance rises. Normally, pulmonary vascular resistance is minimal when lung volume is near functional residual capacity (FRC). Changes in lung volume in either direction elicit increased resistance, but the potential magnitude of the increase is much greater with inflation than with deflation.

The effects of inflation on pulmonary blood volume depend on the initial zonal conditions. If left atrial pressure is high and acting as the backpressure to flow (zone 3), the compliant alveolar vessels are distended and decrease their volume when subjected to the compressive effects of inflation. In contrast, if alveolar pressure is high and acting as the backpressure to flow (zone 2), the alveolar vessels are compressed, and little or no further compression occurs with lung inflation. These effects of inflation on alveolar vessel volume therefore variably oppose the increase in extra-alveolar vessel volume elicited by inflation.

EFFECTS OF VASOMOTOR TONE

Increased vasomotor tone shifts the pulmonary artery pressure-flow relationship to higher pressures, whereas decreased tone shifts it to lower pressures. These alterations in overall resistance can be accompanied by redistribution of blood flow among the parallel vascular channels, particularly if the change in tone is not uniform among the channels. In addition, the distribution of resistance, and therefore pressure and volume, within the channels can be altered. The consequences of vasomotion depend on both the site and magnitude of the response. For example, constriction anywhere along a channel can decrease its flow; however, if the constriction occurs in the venous part of the channel rather than the arterial, the volume of the channel and the amount of fluid filtered into the interstitium from its permeable region increases. Such effects could cause edema and deterioration of gas exchange.

A large number of substances are capable of changing pulmonary vasomotor tone (Table 192-1). Several substances can cause either constriction or dilation, depending on the initial state of tone, the presence of different receptor types, and other factors. Stimulation of the sympathetic nervous system and hypoxia cause pulmonary vasoconstriction. With the exception of hypoxia, the significance of these responses is not well understood.

When ventilation to a region of lung is impaired, as by a bronchial mucus plug or bronchoconstriction, the carbon dioxide tension of the region rises and the oxygen tension falls. If PO_2 falls below about 75 mm Hg, vasoconstriction occurs, resulting in a decrease in regional perfusion and readjustment of PCO_2 and PO_2 toward normal values. Thus, the pulmonary vasoconstrictor response to hypoxia adjusts local perfusion to match local ventilation, thereby ameliorating the detrimental effects of regional hypoventilation on systemic arterial oxygen tension. The ability of the hypoxic response to maintain appropriate regional ventilation-perfusion relationships becomes limited as the size of the hypoxic region increases. If, for example, the entire lung were hypoxic, vasoconstriction would occur in all regions and no redistribution of perfusion would occur. This occurs in normal subjects at high altitude, in patients with weak respiratory muscles or depressed ventilatory drive, and in patients with diffuse parenchymal lung disease se-

Table 192-1. Substances with vasoactive effects on the pulmonary circulation

Vasoconstriction	Vasodilation
Catecholamines (alpha-adrenergic)	Catecholamines (beta-adrenergic)
Acetylcholine	Acetylcholine
Histamine	Histamine
Bradykinin	Bradykinin
Serotonin	Vasoactive intestinal polypeptide
Angiotensin II	
Vasopressin	Substance P
Leu-enkephalin	Prostaglandin I_2
Prostaglandin H_2	Prostaglandin E_1
Prostaglandin F_2 alpha	Adenosine
Prostaglandin D_2	Adenosine triphosphate
Prostaglandin E_2	Carbon dioxide
Thromboxane A_2	Hydrogen ion
Leukotriene C_4	
Leukotriene D_4	
Leukotriene E_4	
Platelet activating factor	
Adenosine triphosphate	
Carbon dioxide	
Hydrogen ion	
Potassium ion	

From McMurtry I: Humoral control. In Bergofsky EH, editor: Abnormal pulmonary circulation. New York, 1986, Churchill-Livingstone.

vere enough to cause generalized alveolar hypoxia. Under these conditions, hypoxic pulmonary vasoconstriction usually increases right ventricular afterload but does little to optimize gas exchange.

Administration of pulmonary vasodilators such as isoproterenol can cause hypoxemia, presumably as a result of abrogation of hypoxic vasoconstriction and secondary deterioration of ventilation-perfusion matching. In some cases, hypoxemia does not occur despite deterioration of ventilation-perfusion relationships because the vasodilator simultaneously increases CO through reduction of right and left ventricular afterload. The result is an increase in mixed venous oxygen tension, which nullifies the deleterious effects of poor ventilation-perfusion matching on arterial oxygen tension.

The mechanism of hypoxic pulmonary vasoconstriction remains unknown despite intensive investigation. Much of this work has focused on the identification of a unique humoral mediator released from hypoxic lung tissue, such as catecholamines, serotonin, histamine, prostaglandins, and leukotrienes. Alternatively, hypoxia may act directly on vascular smooth muscle. The trigger to contraction could be a change in smooth muscle energy state, but evidence in favor of this theory remains circumstantial. A similar degree of confusion exists with respect to the mechanism of local hypoxic responses in systemic vessels, which dilate rather than constrict. Whatever the mechanisms, these opposite responses both act to maintain oxygen transport under conditions of hypoxic stress. Pulmonary vasoconstriction preserves systemic arterial oxygen content by matching pulmonary perfusion to ventilation. Systemic vasodilatation promotes distribution of oxygen-rich arterial blood to where it is most needed.

PATHOPHYSIOLOGY OF PULMONARY HYPERTENSION (see Chapters 20 and 216)

Pulmonary hypertension can occur by three mechanisms: an increase in pulmonary vascular resistance, an increase in the backpressure to pulmonary blood flow, or an increase in flow.

Pulmonary vascular resistance can be increased by removal, obstruction, or obliteration of vascular channels. For example, with lung resection or pulmonary embolism, the number of patent parallel channels is reduced. Normally, the remaining vessels can distend and be recruited sufficiently to accommodate all of the CO without a large increase in pressure. If, however, the remaining vasculature is not capable of recruitment or distention, the increase in pulmonary artery pressure after obstruction or obliteration of vascular channels is more severe. Pulmonary vascular resistance also increases if individual channels become narrowed by vasospasm or by medial and endothelial hypertrophy, as occurs with chronic hypoxia and primary pulmonary hypertension. Again, this decreases the total cross-sectional area of the vasculature, necessitating an increase in pulmonary artery pressure to maintain a normal flow of blood.

If the backpressure to flow rises, pulmonary artery pressure must also rise to maintain an adequate pressure gradient for blood flow. This occurs when left atrial pressure is increased to high levels by mitral stenosis. With high levels of positive end-expiratory pressure (PEEP), alveolar pressure can be increased sufficiently to compress alveolar vessels and become the backpressure to flow. Further increases in PEEP then necessitate increases in pulmonary artery pressure to maintain cardiac output. Hyperinflation caused by asthma has the same effect. In this case, contraction of inspiratory muscles decreases pleural pressure to very negative values while alveolar pressure remains close to zero. Since pleural pressure surrounds the heart as well as the lungs, the decrease in pleural pressure causes left atrial pressure to decrease relative to alveolar pressure, and thus alveolar pressure becomes the backpressure to flow. Pulmonary artery pressure is also lowered by the reduction in pleural pressure, resulting in a decrease in the pressure gradient (pulmonary artery pressure–alveolar pressure) for flow. To restore this gradient, the right ventricle must raise pulmonary artery pressure relative to pleural pressure. This form of pulmonary hypertension would not be detected by the usual measurement of pulmonary artery pressure, which uses atmospheric pressure as a reference. It becomes apparent only if pulmonary artery pressure is referenced to pleural pressure. Thus, from its perspective in the chest the right ventricle sees an increase in pulmonary artery pressure during hyperinflation whether the hyperinflation is produced by raising alveolar pressure relative to atmospheric pressure (PEEP) or lowering pleural pressure relative to atmospheric pressure (asthma).

Increased CO can also lead to pulmonary hypertension. In patients with atrial or ventricular septal defects or with a patent ductus arteriosus, there is left-to-right shunting and an increase in pulmonary blood flow at rest. At first, the resulting increase in pulmonary artery pressure is mild because of the distensibility and recruitability of the pulmonary vessels. With time, however, anatomic changes occur in the vasculature that decrease its cross-sectional area, causing pulmonary hypertension. The mechanisms by which these anatomic changes occur are not well understood.

To understand the effects of pulmonary hypertension on the heart, it is useful to consider the relationship between right atrial pressure and CO (the Frank-Starling, or CO curve) and the relationship between right atrial pressure and venous return (the venous return curve). The CO curve demonstrates that the output of the heart progressively increases to a plateau as its filling pressure is increased. The curve is shifted downward (lower right ventricular output at a given right atrial pressure) by a decrease in cardiac contractility or an increase in afterload. The venous return curve demonstrates that the flow of blood to the right heart form the peripheral circulation is progressively decreased as the backpressure to venous return (the right atrial pressure) is increased. The venous return curve is shifted upward (higher venous return at a given right atrial pressure) by an increase in blood volume, a decrease in systemic vascular compliance, or a decrease in the resistance to venous return. In the steady state, venous return must equal CO.

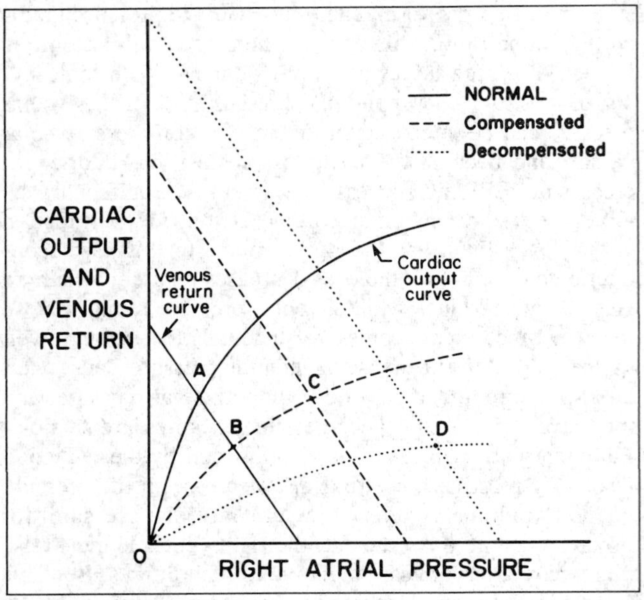

Fig. 192-5. Graphical analysis of the regulation of cardiac output and right atrial pressure under normal conditions and compensated and decompensated pulmonary hypertension. **A,** Normal; **B,** pulmonary hypertension without peripheral vascular compensation; **C,** pulmonary hypertension with peripheral vascular compensation; **D,** decompensated pulmonary hypertension. For details, see text.

The intersection of the curves (Fig. 192-5) indicates what the steady state CO and right atrial pressure must be (point A).

If pulmonary artery pressure and therefore right ventricular afterload are increased, the CO curve shifts downward, intersecting the venous return curve at a lower CO and higher right atrial pressure (point B). Compensatory mechanisms such as constriction of peripheral vessels and renal retention of sodium and water are activated, shifting the venous return curve upward. The new intersection (point C) indicates a restoration of CO, albeit at an even higher right atrial pressure. If this situation persists, the right ventricle may hypertrophy, causing an upward shift of the CO curve and perhaps some return of the right atrial pressure toward normal. If, however, the pulmonary hypertension progresses, as is frequently the case, further increases in right atrial pressure as well as peripheral vascular pressure and volume occur. At some point, the increase in peripheral vascular pressure results in edema. With time, the hypertrophied, dilated right ventricle weakens, particularly if hypoxemia and acidosis are present. This causes a further downward shift of the CO curve, leading eventually to lowered CO in the face of a markedly enlarged blood volume and massive peripheral edema (point D). This sequence of events can vary with the acuity of the insult. Under some circumstances, as in chronic bronchitis, the process may occur over a period of years and may be punctuated by numerous remissions and exacerbations. In contrast, when pulmonary hypertension is severe and occurs abruptly, as with pulmonary embolism, compensatory mechanisms may be inadequate or have insufficient time to develop fully. Under these conditions, CO may fall to severely low levels, resulting in shock and death.

The treatment and clinical causes of pulmonary hypertension are discussed in Chapters 20 and 216.

REFERENCES

Dawson CA: The role of pulmonary vasomotion in the physiology of the lung. Physiol Rev 4:2, 1984.

Fishman AP: Pulmonary circulation. In Fishman AP et al, editors: The respiratory system: circulation and non-respiratory function. Bethesda, Md, 1985, American Physiological Society.

Grover RF et al: Pulmonary circulation. In Shepherd JT and Abbored FM, editors: The cardiovascular system: peripheral circulation and organ blood flow part 1. Bethesda, Md, 1983, American Physiological Society.

Guyton AC, Jones CE, and Coleman TG: Circulatory physiology: cardiac output and its regulation. Philadelphia, 1973, Saunders.

McMurtry IF: Humoral control. In Bergofsky EH, editor: Abnormal pulmonary circulation. New York, 1986, Churchill-Livingstone.

Mitzner W: Resistance of the pulmonary circulation. Clin Chest Med 4:2, 1983.

Sylvester JT et al: Acute hypoxic responses. In Bergofsky EH, editor: Abnormal pulmonary circulation. New York, 1988, Churchill-Livingstone.

Weibel ER: The pathway for oxygen. Cambridge, Mass, 1984, Harvard University Press.

CHAPTER

193 Host Defense Mechanisms in the Respiratory Tract

Herbert Y. Reynolds

An elaborate network of mechanical barriers and of immunologic and cellular mechanisms situated in the naso-oropharynx and along the trachea and conducting airways clears the respiratory mucosa of particles and microorganisms that are inhaled with ambient air or aspirated with oropharyngeal secretions. This local defense system also impedes the attachment and growth of microbes that inhabit the nose, throat, and central airways. The peripheral airways generally protect the alveolar surfaces, which are devoid of microbes. However, particles of small size (less than 3.0 μm in diameter or with special aerodynamic properties such as fragments of asbestos fibers) can be carried to the alveolar surface where mucociliary clearance and coughing mechanisms are no longer effective. Thus, the air exchange surface has developed additional mechanisms to cleanse itself. These include the scavenger activity of mobile alveolar macrophages, aided by nonimmune (surfactant and fibronectin) and immune (immunoglobulin [Ig] antibody) opsonins, and the ability to generate an inflammatory reaction, which mobilizes polymorphonuclear (PMN) cells from adjacent capillaries plus other forms of systemic defense (complement components) to the alveoli.

This chapter reviews normal components of the defense apparatus in the conducting airways and on the air exchange surface. Impairment of one or several of these host defenses can predispose to sinopulmonary infection or chronic lung disease; overactivity or a smoldering inflammatory response can cause bronchitis or alveolitis, stimulating fibroblasts to make collagen, which leads to interstitial fibrosis.

CONDUCTING AIRWAYS

A mucosal surface covers the airways. In the nares and oropharynx, the surface is squamous epithelium, but, over the nasal turbinates and from the upper trachea down to the respiratory bronchioles, it consists of a pseudostratified, columnar, ciliated, mucus-secreting epithelium. A turnover of mucosal cells occurs approximately every 7 days. This ciliated epithelium (Fig. 193-1) is interspersed with goblet cells and orifices leading from the submucosal bronchial glands. A tuft of possibly 100 to 200 cilia on each epithelial cell beats with amazing speed, approaching 300 times per minute, and waves of coordinated ciliary motion move over the airways surface. Lymphocytes and plasma cells are distributed in the submucosa and lamina propria areas of the larger conducting airways and nasal passages. Some surface lymphocytes are found, perhaps extruded from bronchial-associated lymphoid aggregates. A few surface macrophages exist, either coming up from the alveoli, or perhaps they are dendritic macrophages, which have a special ability to process antigens that have been inhaled and impacted on the surface. These cells might initiate immune responses in the airways.

Autonomic nervous control regulates humidification of air and heat exchange on the mucosal surface, conserving fluid, especially in the nose and trachea. Attention is usually placed on the secretory potential of the mucosa, that is, mucus produced by bronchial glands and goblet cells, serous and Clara cell secretion, local immunoglobulin production, and transudation of proteins from the vascular space; however, absorption of fluid from the mucosa and across the alveolar epithelial surface can be equally impor-

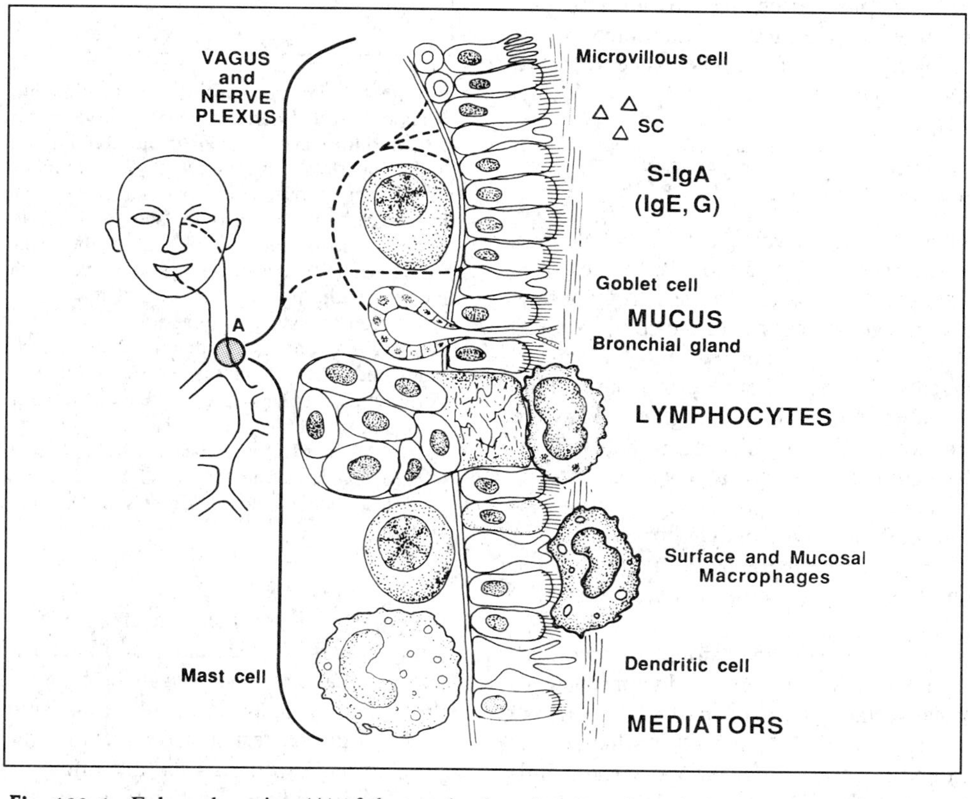

Fig. 193-1. Enlarged portion *(A)* of the conducting airway surface depicting the mucosa and the major submucosal structures. The pseudostratified ciliated epithelium has a covering layer of mucus (produced by goblet cells and bronchial glands) that contains various proteins, including immunoglobulins and secretory component *(SC)*, and surface cells such as lymphocytes (from bronchial-associated lymphoid aggregates) and macrophages. In submucosal areas plasma cells and mast cells reside that can secrete immunoglobulins or mediators such as histamine. Joining all of these glandular and cellular networks together are nerves, perhaps regulating their control through neuropeptides, and by adrenergic and cholinergic nerve fibers. A rich vascular supply exists also. In addition, the epithelial cell can produce arachidonic acid metabolites that control mucosal swelling and permeability. *S-IgA*, serum immunoglobulin A; *IgE, G*, immunoglobulin E and G. (Modified from Reynolds HY: Pulmonary host defenses—state of the art. Chest 95:223S, 1989.)

tant and must be considered. Lymphatic routes to clear fluid, removal of senescent cells and phospholipids by macrophages, and activity of brush cells with apical border microvilli submerged in the periciliary sol fluid are all operant. The integrity of tight apical junctions joining epithelial cells is also crucial in overall fluid balance or in preventing submucosal deposition of antigens, as these junctions can be affected by irritation from airborne pollutants and by immediate allergic injury, which can occur with antigen-antibody reactions. Selective sampling of respiratory lining secretions that permits accurate quantification of various components has just begun to be done in humans. General fluid balance along the airways and the status of local irritation on the mucosal surface are important variables in obtaining accurate values. As for local secretion of proteins, the thickness of the stratified epithelial surface separating the lamina propria and basement membrane from the luminal surface of the airway might be a significant factor, too. As an example, to facilitate secretion of dimeric IgA, epithelial cells have developed a receptor for secretory component. Mast cell or macrophage cytokines, perhaps leukotrienes, may alter local mucosal permeability. Bradykinin and neuropetides can change this also, so values for immune components measured on the mucosal surface can fluctuate along the surface; allowance must be made for this dynamic interplay.

DEFENSE MECHANISMS OF THE AIR EXCHANGE OR ALVEOLAR SURFACE

Toward the periphery of the airways, the epithelial layer gradually becomes thinner and less stratified; the cells become cuboidal in shape, and cilia are shorter. In the terminal air sacs and over the alveolar surface, the cell layer flattens and blends to a single layer of epithelium (type 1 pneumocytes) interspersed with type 2 pneumocytes found in the corners of alveoli. Goblet cells and mucous glands that were present in the conducting airways disappear (below level of respiratory bronchioles) as the alveolar surface is reached. This epithelial layer supports freely moving, detachable phagocytic cells and lymphocytes present on the alveolar surface. In the transitional zone at the level of the respiratory bronchioles, other secretory cells (Clara cells) are present.

Particles or microbes of small dimensions in inspired air can elude trapping mechanisms in the conducting airways and reach the alveolar surface. As an example, bacteria may have the critical size, between 0.5 and 3 μm diameter in an envelope of moisture, so they may escape aerodynamic filtration in the proximal airways (Fig. 193-2) and must be dealt with in the alveoli. As mentioned, mucociliary clearance and coughing are not effective in removing particles from the alveolar surface, so other mechanisms have been developed. Based on experiments in rabbits and rodents exposed to aerosolized bacteria, bacteria deposited on the alveolar surface are rapidly captured by alveolar macrophages and ingested within a half hour or so. As approximately one macrophage services three alveoli, these mobile cells can move quickly to cover a large area; shortcuts through

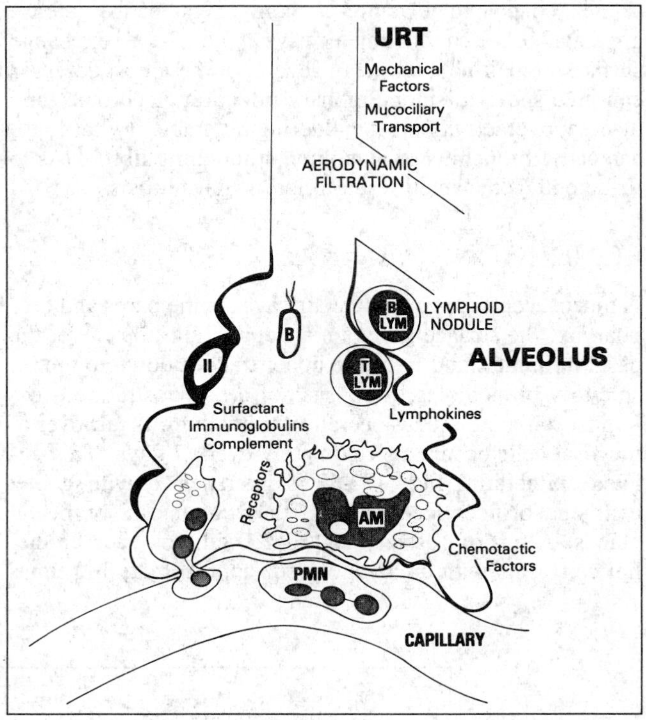

Fig. 193-2. Enlargement of the alveolar unit illustrating components of the host defense system active on the alveolar surface. If a bacterium *(B)* has escaped the aerodynamic filtration defenses in the upper respiratory tract *(URT)*, a number of adversaries await it. After being pushed against the alveolar wall where components in the epithelial lining fluid, such as surfactant, secreted by type II cells, and opsonins may coat it, the bacterium is left as prey for a roving alveolar macrophage. Several options can then be exercised. If the macrophage cannot inactivate and contain the microbe after ingesting it, lymphokines produced by lymphocytes in the lung may energize and activate the macrophage. These monokines and other mediators are described in Fig. 193-3. In addition, the macrophage may secrete chemotactic factors that can attract additional phagocytic cells, especially polymorphonuclear neutrophils (PMN) into the alveolar space. AM, alveolar macrophage. (Modified from Reynolds HY: Respiratory infections may reflect deficiencies in host defense mechanisms. Dis Mon 31:1, 1985. With permission.)

the pores of Kohn facilitate this rapid coverage. What actually occurs between entry of a bacterium into an alveolus and its phagocytosis by a macrophage is speculation, but the following scenario could be envisioned.

After the bacterium is free within the alveolus, the expansion and closure of the alveolus, a product of inspiration and expiration, probably forces the bacterium against the alveolar wall where it becomes mixed or coated with several constituents of the alveolar lining material. These could be surfactant and other glycoproteins (fibronectin) and humoral immune factors (IgG) and complement factor B. Two of these substances can be considered as nonimmune opsonins, surfactant, and fragments of fibronectin; immunoglobulin with antibody specificity would be an immune opsonin. Complement, particularly C_3b, can promote receptor-mediator attachment to a macrophage or interact with antibody to augment receptor binding. Also, a microbe might trigger activation of the alternate complement pathway and create directly a lytic situation for itself. Complement activation is not usual or easily done. Only minimal concentrations of complement factors are measured in normal bronchoalveolar lavage fluids (BAL), and inhibitors of complement that would be needed to modulate complement activity and prevent indiscriminate tissue injury by this lytic system seem to be absent, also.

Immunoglobulin G is the principal opsonic antibody available in BAL fluid. Immunoglobulin A is available in limited amounts and has much less opsonic activity than IgG. Immunoglobulin M occurs in minimal amount in normals. As IgM does not have prominent specific mu chain receptors on alveolar macrophages, its role is minor. Whatever the mixture of opsonins, a bacterium so coated is more easily phagocytosed by the macrophage. Macrophages can ingest inanimate particles (polystyrene balls) without prior opsonization, but they will not ingest many viable bacteria, especially gram-negative species, without an opsonic coating. Certainly, a specific opsonin increases the effectiveness of phagocytosis appreciably.

Once inside the macrophage, the fate of the microbe is in part its own device and in part reflects the condition of the macrophage. A large inoculum of microbes could overwhelm the defense system, or an unusually virulent species or an initial exposure to a new species not encountered before (hence no prior chance for the host to have mounted any cellular or humoral immunity) could allow a microbial species to take hold and create infection (pneumonia). Reactivity of the macrophage becomes another variable, and this requires coordination with lymphocytes in the lung. A number of cellular mediators generated from T lymphocytes can energize and activate macrophages, thus improving phagocytic and intracellular bactericidal capabilities. Examples are migration inhibitory factor and gamma interferon. These cellular interactions will be examined later.

Once the macrophage has encountered a microbe and ingested it, the phagocyte may be able to kill or contain it, and the problem is resolved; cell-mediated immune stimulation may be necessary to complete the action. Alternatively, conditions that favor proliferation of the microbe, that is, large inoculum, virulence, or virgin exposure of the host, may require that the macrophage recruit additional phagocytic help. One mechanism for doing this is elaboration of chemotactic factors that attract PMNs into the alveoli. There is a plentiful supply of PMNs marginated in capillaries adjacent to alveoli and readily available. In normal, uninflamed alveoli, few PMNs are present. About 1% of airway cells recovered in BAL fluid (Table 193-1) are PMNs. Human alveolar macrophages can produce several substances that initiate and direct the motion of granulocytes. These include a complex protein interleukin 8, and leukotriene B_4 of the lipoxygenase pathway of arachidonic acid metabolism. Although PMNs are the prominent inflammatory cells responding to bacterial infection, other cells such as eosinophils, lymphocytes, and monocytes may be under control of chemotactic factors important for other inflammatory responses as are found in granulomatous and eosinophilic lung diseases.

IMMUNOGLOBULINS

In the analysis of protein in BAL fluid recovered from normal subjects, albumin represents approximately one third of the total protein and accounts for the largest share. The percentage of albumin is not significantly different for smokers and nonsmokers (31% versus 35%, respectively).

A group of proteins found in high concentration and easily detected in lavage fluid are the immunoglobulins. Immunoglobulin A constitutes approximately 5% of the total protein in BAL fluid. Serum IgA is principally a monomer, and little exists in polymeric form. In contrast, IgA in BAL fluid is a typical secretory IgA, as found in breast secretions (colostrum), parotid fluid, and gastrointestinal fluid in that it contains bound secretory component glycoprotein as well as joining chain (J chain). Compared with values of about 2 mg per milliliter in serum, concentrated BAL fluid (about 25-fold concentration) contained about 150 μg per milliliter; differences between smokers and nonsmokers were not significant. Precipitin analysis of purified secretory IgA fractionated from BAL fluid has identified both alpha heavy chain subtypes. Delacroix and colleagues measured the relative proportions of IgA_1 and IgA_2 in serum and a variety of external secretions. In general, excretory fluids contain mostly A_1 but relatively more A_2 than in comparison with serum. In bronchial secretions about 33% of the IgA was the A_2 variety.

Although IgA accounts for a sizable percentage of the total protein in BAL fluid, IgG is more abundant. Immunoglobulin G, expressed as a ratio of albumin, is present in concentrated BAL fluid from nonsmokers in the same proportion as it is in serum (ratio about 0.25 to 0.3); for smokers, the lavage fluid contains slightly more IgG in proportion than does serum (ratio about 0.4), based on the finding that some 20% of normal smokers have elevated IgG

Table 193-1. Profile of respiratory cells recovery in BAL fluid (for nonsmoker normals following 100- to 300-ml lavage)

Cell number total	Viability	Differential count (%)			Cytocentrifuge cell stain (%)		
		Macrophages	PMN	Eosinophil/basophil	Lymphocytes	Ciliated cells	Erythrocytes
15×10^6	<90%	85	1-2	<1	7-12	1-5	<5

in their lavage fluid. As IgG approximates the serum value, this leads to the conclusion that most of it arrives in airspace secretions by transudation from the plasma compartment. In addition, intraluminal secretion of IgG and IgA is possible by alveolar space plasma cells or by release of cell membrane–bound immunoglobulin from lymphocytes and possibly macrophages.

Immunoglobulin G in BAL fluid is composed of the four heavy chain subclasses of IgG, and these are quantitative in almost the same proportions as found in serum. In BAL fluid, IgG_1 is most abundant (66%), IgG_2 is next (27%), and IgG_3 and IgG_4 are in small amounts accounting for 3% to 4% each of the total IgG. Immunoglobulin G_4 seems to be higher in BAL fluid than in serum.

Immunoglobulin E has been considered by some to be a secretory immunoglobulin that belongs to the mucosal secretory immune system because IgE plasma cells can be identified in the airway submucosa. It is present in BAL fluid obtained from normal humans, but its concentration of about 10 ng per milliliter of concentrated BAL is very low in the nonallergic subject. However, such measurements may not fairly represent the actual presence of IgE in the lungs because IgE is in part tissue bound, especially to submucosal mast cells and intraluminal mast cells. Immunoglobulin E–secreting plasma cells are not plentiful in normal nonatopic subjects.

Immunoglobulin M, an approximately 900,000 dalton molecular weight protein, may be detected in very low concentrations, but even so the values are minuscule compared with those for IgA and IgG. Lactoferrin is present in BAL fluid. As it is quite similar in size to secretory IgA, it is a difficult contaminant to remove when purifying IgA from BAL fluid for biochemical analysis. Transport of these two proteins into the airways has been considered to be linked. Lactoferrin and transferrin, which can also be identified in alveolar fluid, have antimicrobial activity because of iron required for microbial growth.

Several proteins collected with the lavage technique have more relevance for the conducting airways than the alveolar spaces. Secretory component (SC) is a glycoprotein selectively produced by serous epithelial cells along various mucosal surfaces of the body and is of special interest in the airways because it is added to respiratory secretions selectively without an additional source from the intravascular fluid. Much of the SC supply is bound to secretory IgA, but a surprisingly large amount exists in pulmonary lavage fluid in a free or unattached state.

RESPIRATORY CELLS

Bronchoalveolar lavage fluid provides a sample of cells that are present on the surface of the terminal conducting airways and alveoli. As BAL requires successive aliquots of saline to be infused and aspirated from a sublobar segment of a lung, cells are detached and recovered in serial aspirates. If serial BAL fluid samples are assessed for their content of cells, some variation can be found in that PMN cells may be disproportionately high in the first aspirate and more lymphocytes appear in later ones; macrophages are plentiful in all samples. A representative population of intraluminal cells in BAL fluid is given in Table 193-1. From cigarette smokers without overt bronchitis or other respiratory disease, the recovery of cells in lavage is usually three- to fivefold greater, reflecting primarily more alveolar macrophages. The population of alveolar macrophages is not homogeneous, and the variable size and morphology of these cells reinforce this. When alveolar macrophages are separated into subpopulations by cell surface markers or by size and density, different functions are evident. Moreover, macrophages should not be considered as just scavenger phagocytes for they have significant immune effector activities and secretory function as well and are important in modulating immune responses on the alveolar surface. As macrophages undergo a transition from blood monocytes into differentiated alveolar macrophages in the interstitial compartment of the lung tissue, intermediate stages, or so-called interstitial macrophages, may have a special role in forms of chronic lung injury and fibrosis.

As shown in Table 193-1, the usual cell recovery from a healthy nonsmoking volunteer is about 15 million cells, depending on the volume of lavage fluid used and recovered. The viability of the cells is about 95% and on a differential cell count (prepared from cytocentrifuged cell specimen and stained with Wright-Giemsa), most of the cells are macrophages. Polymorphonuclear cells are rare, as are erythrocytes; the amount of coughing induced by the bronchoscopy influences the number of ciliated epithelial cells found. These cells are often viable in a wet preparation mount of the BAL cells, and ciliary motion is visible.

Considerable interest has focused on the identification of lymphocytes, which may account for 10% or so of the total cells (Table 193-2). Aided by the use of T cell–specific monoclonal antibody staining, most of the lymphocytes are T cells, and with further T cell subset identification, about half of these are helper/inducer cells, and a

Table 193-2. Lymphocyte subsets (%)

T cells (% of total)	T helper/ inducer*,†	T suppressor/ cytotoxic*	T killer*,§ lymphocytes	B lymphocytes (plasma cells)‡	Untypeable lymphocytes
70	50	30	7	5-10	5

*As percent of T cells. The T_H/T_S ratio is approximately 1.5:1.8.
†The T helper subset contains approximately 7% of cells with HLA DR^+ antigen, and these can preferentially produce interleukin-2.
‡Among plasma cells are immunoglobulin-releasing cells with the following frequency: IgG = IgA > IgE.
§Killer lymphocytes seem inactive when retrieved from a normal lung.

lesser percentage are of the suppressor/cytotoxic variety. The ratio of T helper/suppressor cells is about 1.5 in the normal airways, and this is approximately the same ratio obtained for peripheral blood lymphocytes. Among the T helper cells, a small percentage (about 7% in normals) have an HLA-DR antigen; this subpopulation may increase when a lymphocytic alveolitis develops as in active sarcoidosis and is responsible for most of the interleukin-2 (IL-2) produced. Approximately 7% of the airway T cells are killer cells, but these seem dormant in normal subjects. In addition, about 5% of the lymphocytes are B cells or plasma cells. These cells can release various class-specific immunoglobulins from their surface as already mentioned. Finally, a small percentage of lymphocytes are not typeable with the usual immunologic reagents used and may in fact be "null" cells. The disordered interaction between lymphocytes and macrophages is important in the cause of several lung diseases; the complexity of this based on potential cell contact and action of soluble mediators is illustrated in Fig. 193-3. Although the interaction between activated lung macrophages and lymphocytes, subtype T helper/inducer (T_H) and T suppressor/cytotoxic (T_S), is emphasized, there are ramifications for other immune cells, such as killer lymphocytes, immunoglobulin-producing plasma cells, and B lymphocytes also.

Alveolar macrophages develop from circulating blood monocytes, which undergo further maturation or differentiation in the interstitial spaces before emerging on the al-

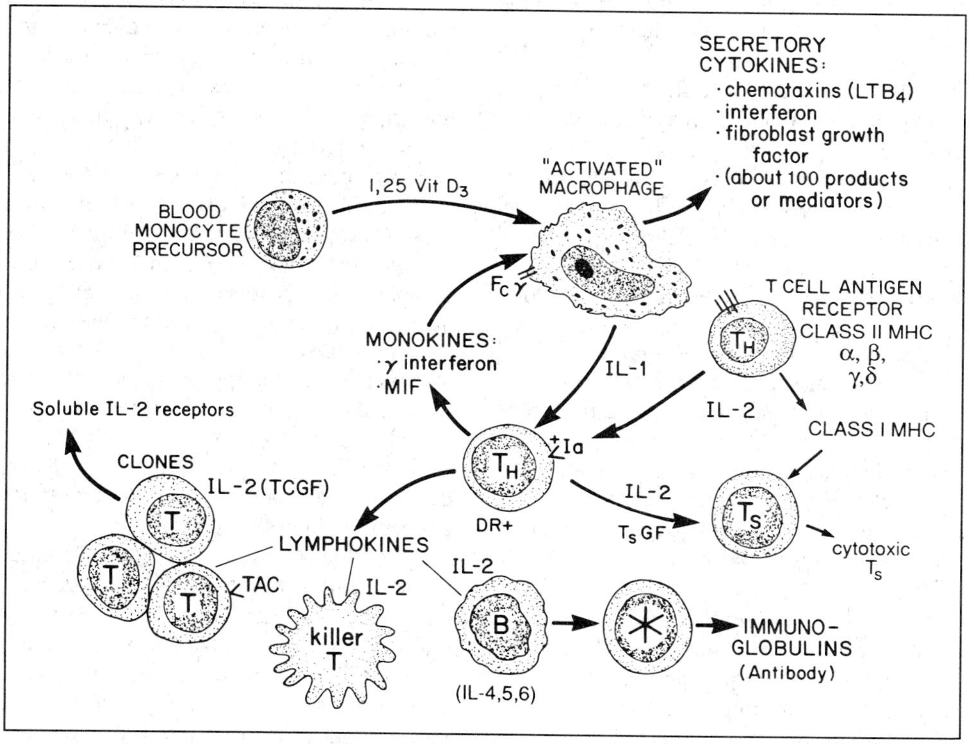

Fig. 193-3. Immunologic interactions on the alveolar surface illustrated by various secretory functions of alveolar macrophages and lymphocytes. Monocyte precursors from the blood differentiate into mature macrophages under the influence of vitamin D metabolites and other unknown stimuli to become long-living, aerobically metabolizing phagocytes. Their most important activity is to scavenge the alveolar surface, ingesting accumulated debris and aerosolized or aspirated microbes. However, macrophages have the potential to become "activated" cells capable of producing and secreting an enormous array of enzyme and cellular mediators. These "cytokines" can affect the function of other cells such as lymphocytes. Chemotactic factors can also attract polymorphonuclear neutrophils into the alveoli. One substance, interleukin-1 (IL-1), when secreted by activated macrophages, may be a chemoattractant for T lymphocytes to enter the alveoli. Activated T helper (T_H) cells are capable of producing lymphokines and monokines, which are important in modulating the function of other immune cells. Among the lymphokines interleukin-2 (IL-2) can stimulate other T cells to proliferate and thereby expand clones of lymphocytes. Interleukin-2 can activate killer T cells and may stimulate B-lymphocytes to become plasma cells capable of synthesizing various classes of immunoglobulins. Activated T helper cells can produce several monokines that affect macrophage function, such as migration inhibition factor (*MIF*) and gamma (γ) interferon. *LTB_4*, leukotriene B_4; *MHC*, major histocompatibility; *T_3*, subclass T suppressor cell; *TCGF*, T cell growth factor; *T_H*, subclass T helper cell. (Modified from Reynolds HY: Lung immunology and its contribution to the immunopathogenesis of certain respiratory diseases. J Allergy Clin Immunol 78:833, 1986.)

veolar surface. Vitamin D metabolites seem to be important in this process. The alveolar macrophage's first responsibility is to be a roving scavenger and phagocyte to clean debris from the alveolar surface. However, it is apparent that the macrophage, especially when activated, can secrete a large array of cellular substances and mediators that affect the function of other cells (cytokines). As an example, macrophage chemotactic factors, including leukotriene B_4, can attract other inflammatory cells to the alveoli, or fibroblast growth factors, such as platelet-derived growth factor and fibronectin, can influence fibroblast replication. Activated macrophages can secrete interleukin-1 (IL-1), which may attract lymphocytes. Such molecules as tumor necrosis factor and plasminogen activator can have local alveolar effects but may diffuse into the systemic circulation as well. The list of enzymes, regulatory proteins, and inhibitors produced by macrophages continues to lengthen as over 100 substances have been attributed to this heterogenous cell population.

The macrophage also serves as an antigen-presenting cell, which can process an antigen and display it on its cell membrane, where it is taken up by an appropriate T_H lymphocyte and matched with respect to class II histocompatibility antigens. Antigen is received on the lymphocyte's membrane by a T cell antigen receptor, which has an intricate structure composed of two beta and alpha chains.

Within the lumen of the alveolar spaces, the majority of lymphocytes are T cells with the proportion of T helper cells greater than suppressor cells; this ratio is approximately 1.5. The activated T_H cells can secrete a variety of monokines, such as gamma interferon and migration inhibition factor (MIF), that modulate macrophage activity in turn. Gamma interferon in particular can energize or activate the macrophage. Also T_H cells secrete lymphokines that affect other lymphocytes. Interleukin-2 appears to be an important mediator in this respect, produced by a subset of T_H cells identified as DR-positive lymphocytes. It can stimulate T cells to replicate, thus expanding the clone and number of cells in the alveoli (formerly known as T cell growth factor [TCGF]), or it can activate natural killer lymphocytes that usually are dormant in normal lung. Importantly, IL-2 in concert with other interleukins can stimulate B lymphocytes to secrete immunoglobulin and may promote their differentiation into plasma cells. The effect of T suppressor cells is less well defined in terms of special mediators produced, but T cells may produce T suppressor growth factors. Natural inhibitors exist that may neutralize the effect of lymphokines, or inhibition of IL-2 can be caused by such immunosuppressive drugs as corticosteroids and cyclosporin A. Thus, the potential for cellular interaction within the air spaces is multiple and complicated.

POTENTIAL DEFECTS OR DYSFUNCTION IN HOST DEFENSES THAT COULD LEAD TO RESPIRATORY ILLNESS

The naso-oropharynx and major conducting airways have an intricate network of barriers and moveable mechanisms that prevent particles or microbes from adhering and penetrating the mucosal surface and then sweeps them off. As reviewed, these include mucus coating of the surface, tight apical junctions between epithelial cells, beating cilia, angulation of the airways, and the cough reflex. Also present are immunologic components: secretory IgA and IgG, a few lymphocytes and macrophages that may initiate immune responses, and various mediators, such as histamine, produced by mast cells or macrophages. There is a very dynamic airway mucosal surface equipped to react breath to breath with the many toxic substances inhaled with ambient air. At the level of the respiratory bronchioles where the airways change from serving as conduits for airflow to adapting for air exchange, host defenses are different. On the alveolar surface, clearance of particles and microbes is a combined function of phagocytic cells and various lipids, glycoprotein, and immunoglobulins that serve as opsonins (Fig. 193-2). Individual components or a combination of them may malfunction or be defective from a hereditary deficiency in structure and predispose the host to illness. Usually the result is respiratory infections, often recurrent ones that involve the upper airways and sinuses and the lungs. More subtle defects, such as deficient antiprotease inactivation of proteolytic enzymes, may take longer to manifest and require additive effects of other injury, for example, cigarette smoking, to accelerate illness such as emphysema. Several key times in a patient's medical presentation would be appropriate points to consider at least whether a defect, hereditary or acquired, in pulmonary host defense was contributory. In some situations an accurate diagnosis can lead to replacement therapy of the absent component, or awareness of the specific problem can help put the illnesses into overall perspective for the patient and his or her family. Early on in infancy or childhood when recurrent infections occur, pediatricians are alerted quickly to the possibility of congenital illnesses such as cystic fibrosis. However, because children with acute respiratory infections are so well treated with antibiotics, the appearance of cystic fibrosis and related problems may be delayed and not recognized until later in life—as a teenager or young adult. Therefore, the internist may be confronted with a patient who has recurrent otitis media, sinusitis, and bronchitis, seemingly as independent problems; infertility concerns may be present also. At this juncture a differential diagnosis that includes cystic fibrosis, structural defects in cilia leading to dyskinetic ciliary action, and immunoglobulin deficiencies particularly of IgG subclasses IgG_2 and/or IgG_4 is appropriate to consider.

A second situation in which an acquired defect in pulmonary defenses could be the cause of respiratory infection(s) in a patient is the new onset of bacterial infections (at any age) or particular opportunistic microorganisms. Several components of the alveolar milieu could be indicated and are illustrated with these examples. As the macrophage is centrally positioned in the defense of the alveolar surface, it must be responsive to a number of things. This scavenger phagocyte first intercepts the microbe and either can kill or contain it or must call in some other phagocytic cell or inflammatory mediator(s) for assistance. Opsonic antibodies (IgG) and other nonimmune opsonins (complement and surfactant or fibronectin fragments) facilitate phagocytosis, but an absence of antibody may permit infection to develop with encapsulated bacteria such as *Streptococcus pneumoniae*. Insufficient bone marrow reserve of PMNs, reflecting antineoplastic chemotherapy, or a paucity of chemotactic factors to attract them into the alveoli is a situation that may permit gram-negative bacilli and fungal organisms to flourish. Inability of immune T lymphocytes to energize macrophages, through soluble cellular mediators that provide cell-mediated immunity and activation, makes containment of certain intracellular microbes impossible for these phagocytes (*Legionella* or mycobacteria). Similarly, concomitant infection of macrophages with viruses (human immunodeficiency virus, and cytomegalovirus or herpes viruses) plus an excessive T lymphocyte suppressor cell influence may make *Pneumocystis carinii* and common bacterial and fungal organisms difficult to contain in the lungs of acquired immunodeficiency syndrome (AIDS) patients.

Consideration about what the lung host deficiency might be can make therapy more specific through immunization to develop special antibodies, replacement of certain immunoglobulins (IgG subclasses), or selective administration of cell mediators (gamma interferon or interleukins). These ideas are expanded in several chapters (see Chapters 222, 243, 260, 272, and 297) that examine the specific diseases or infections cited above.

REFERENCES

Delacroix DL et al: IgA subclasses in various secretions and in serum. Immunology 44:383, 1982.

Merrill WW et al: Immunoglobulin G subclass proteins in serum and lavage fluid of normal subjects: quantitation and comparison with immunoglobulins A and E. Am Rev Respir Dis 131:584, 1985.

Reynolds HY: Respiratory infections may reflect deficiencies in host defense mechanism. Dis Mon 31:1, 1985.

Reynolds HY: Lung immunology and its contribution to the immunopathogenesis of certain respiratory diseases. J Allergy Clin Immunol 78:833, 1986.

Reynolds HY: Immunologic system in the respiratory tract. Physiol Rev 71:1117, 1991.

Reynolds HY: Immunoglobulin G and its function in the human respiratory tract. Mayo Clin Proc 63:161, 1988.

Reynolds HY: Pulmonary host defenses—state of the art. Chest 95:223S, 1989.

CHAPTER

194 Mechanisms of Lung Injury and Repair

Jamson S. Lwebuga-Mukasa

The lung has stereotypic responses to acute injury. The exact molecular mechanisms of acute lung damage and factors that control normal repair are poorly understood. Damage to the alveolar-capillary barrier is followed by exudation of serum components into the interstitium and ultimately into the alveolar space. Inflammatory cells, components of fibrinolytic or complement systems, cytokines, and leukotrienes amplify injury. All cellular and extracellular matrix (ECM) components of the alveolar wall may participate in amplification of the inflammatory reaction. They are also important in tissue repair. Injury to type I alveolar epithelial cells results in exposure of the underlying basement membrane. Type II cells, the precursor cells for type I pneumocytes, proliferate and migrate to cover the denuded basement membrane. They subsequently differentiate into type I cells, thus regenerating a continuous epithelial cell lining.

Although common mechanisms may be involved in the initial injury and inflammatory response, the course of lung repair is more complex. It is influenced by (1) the nature and severity of the initial insult and inflammatory response, (2) superimposition of a second insult during the recovery period or chronicity of injury, (3) cell-to-cell and cell-to-extracellular matrix interactions, (4) effects of soluble growth factors from alveolar macrophages (AMs) and lymphocytes, (5) growth factors and cytokines bound to lung extracellular matrix, which may be released during inflammatory reactions, and (6) secretion of autocrine and paracrine factors by lung parenchymal cells. Growth factors secreted by lung parenchymal cells may also influence macrophage and lymphocyte functions. The variety of factors released during an inflammatory reaction and the ensuing repair probably reflects the interaction among the different factors and the target cells.

Cell-to-cell adhesion is required for normal development, repair, and maintenance of continuous polarized alveolar, epithelial, and endothelial cell layers. Tight epithelial junctions are essential to maintain fluid-free alveoli. Cell-to-cell interactions may be mediated by homologous cell adhesion molecules (CAMs), which are involved in cell recognition and tight-junction formation. Cell adhesion molecules permit sorting, migration, and reestablishment of continuous epithelial layers consequent to lung damage. A number of cell-cell adhesion molecules have been isolated and characterized. They include the cadherins, members of the integrin superfamily, and the platelet-endothelial cell adhesion molecule-1 (PECAM-1). They localize at sites of cell-cell contact. E-cadherins are a subfamily of epithelial cell CAMs that are found on lung epithelial cells. They are integral membrane glycoproteins that mediate Ca^{2+}-dependent homophilic cell-to-cell adhesion.

Cell interaction with extracellular matrix (ECM) is a dynamic process. The major constituents of ECM are collagens, proteoglycans, and adhesive glycoproteins. Some proteoglycans have the capacity to bind other ECM molecules and growth factors. The cells synthesize ECM components, which assemble into complex three-dimensional structures. Both spacial organization and composition may be important for tissue-specific properties of the ECM. When ECM is damaged or modified, for example, after proteolysis during inflammatory reactions, solubilized fragments of ECM components may mediate many important biologic functions, such as chemotaxis and proliferation. The ECM, through cell-to-extracellular matrix receptors, is in turn capable of regulating cellular functions.

Integrins are a superfamily of cell surface receptors that allow cells to bind ECM molecules. Integrins are heterodimeric glycoproteins that consist of an α(130-200 kDa) subunit and a β(90-130 kDa) subunit. Both subunits span the plasma membrane. While the integrin family is determined by the β subunit, it is the structure of the α polypeptides that determines the substrate specificity of the receptor. When integrins bind to ECM ligands, the interaction is relayed into the cytoplasmic domains of the receptors, which results in activation of genes that in turn control diverse cellular functions such as migration, proliferation, adhesion, cell shape changes, and cell differentiation. Two complementary mechanisms are believed to be important for the signal transduction caused by integrins. In one mechanism the signal is transduced through the cytoplasmic domains to the cytoskeleton, which regulates cell shape. In another mechanism, the binding of the ligand to its integrin results in activation of phospholipase C and the tyrosine kinase cascade of the *src* family of oncogenes, which results in specific gene activation. The receptor levels may be regulated by the levels of their expression at the cell surface, as a consequence of posttranslational modification, or by differential splicing of ligands such as fibronectin or laminin. The expression of the integrins is controlled by the ECM, growth factors, and the cytokine network. All known integrin functions require divalent cations. Eight β, twelve α integrins, and at least nineteen α/β combinations have thus far been identified. In general, β_1 and β_3 integrins function as adhesive receptors for ECM while β_2 integrins mediate cell-to-cell interactions of leukocytes and the immune system. A β_4 integrin is involved in lymphocyte adhesion. α_v can associate with several different β subunits: α_v β_5, which binds vitronectin; α_v β_6, which is a fibronectin receptor; and α_v β_8, whose ligand has not yet been identified. α_4 can associate with β_1 and β_7 and functions as a receptor for fibronectin or for VCAM-1.

First, we review the structural and cellular components of the alveolar wall, using the adult respiratory distress syndrome (ARDS) to illustrate mechanisms of acute injury and the lung's defenses against them. Next, we discuss repair processes after acute lung injury.

COMPONENTS OF THE ALVEOLAR WALL

The alveolar wall consists of cellular and ECM components. Structural components of the alveolar wall provide a thin barrier across which gas exchange occurs. They also control the permeability of water solutes. In addition, cellular components of the lung perform many biochemical functions that are important for normal organ function and repair.

Cells of the alveolar epithelium

The alveolar epithelium is a mosaic consisting of type I and type II pneumocytes. Type I cells are extremely thin, flat cells that cover about 95% of the respiratory surface. They are the major barrier to diffusion of fluid and electrolytes into the alveoli. Because of their large surface area and their capacity for pinocytosis, they may contribute to the bulk transport of fluids across the alveolar septum. They may be capable of limited repair and of phagocytosis of particulate matter from the alveolar space. Little is known about their biosynthetic and metabolic functions.

Type II pneumocytes are cuboidal cells that are usually located at alveolar corners. They synthesize, store, secrete, and recycle surfactant. Type II cells synthesize, deposit, and remodel epithelial basement membrane. They regulate fluid and electrolyte transport. They are the precursors for adult type I cells during regeneration of the epithelium. In chronic hyperoxic states, type II cells adapt to oxygen injury by increasing cellular content of antioxidant enzymes. Along with Clara cells, type II cells are the major stem cells of the distal air spaces.

Cells of the interstitial space

The alveolar interstitial space contains fibroblasts, smooth muscle cells, and pericytes. Fibroblasts, of which there are several subpopulations, are the most commonly encountered cell type. They synthesize and secrete collagen, glycosaminoglycans, elastin, adhesive glycoproteins, and other components. Fibroblasts play important roles in pathologic conditions associated with abnormal deposition of extracellular matrix components. Their interactions with type II cells may be important for the maintenance of the type II pneumocyte–differentiated state. They also release enzymes that degrade the extracellular matrix such as collagenase and plasminogen activator (PA). The interstitial space at alveolar junctions contains lymphatics, which are important for removal of interstitial fluid and other metabolic products.

Capillary endothelium

The capillary endothelium provides a nonthrombogenic surface for gas exchange and accounts for 30% to 40% of the barrier to fluid efflux into the alveolus. Capillary cells are involved in receptor and bulk transport of macromolecules, metabolism of biogenic amines, and vasoactive peptides.

Capillary endothelial cells also function as endocrine cells and participate in immunologic reactions. It is not known whether endothelial cells secrete factors that regulate alveolar epithelial cell functions. Endothelial cells are active participants in initiation and amplification of inflammatory reactions of the lung. The endothelial surface nearest injury becomes more adhesive to leukocytes. In vitro interleukin-1 (IL-1), gamma interferon (IFN-γ), and tumor necrosis factor (TNF), all of which are macrophage products, induce expression of leukocyte adhesion molecules on cultured endothelial cells. IL-1 and TNF also induce endothelial cell production of IL-8, a potent chemoattractant of PMNs. Endothelial cells also synthesize platelet-activating factor (PAF), prostaglandins, platelet-derived growth factor (PDGF), and class II major histocompatibility (MHC) antigens. Gamma interferon causes organizational changes of endothelial cells, producing gaps between cells. Its effects are synergistic with those of TNF and IL-1. Finally, endothelial cells may release enzymes that degrade the ECM.

Lung extracellular matrix

Current knowledge of the composition of the lung ECM is incomplete. The lung ECM is made of at least 50 different protein components. Four broad classes of structural macromolecules exist: (1) collagen types I, II, III, IV, V, and VI, (2) noncollagenous adhesive glycoproteins—laminin, fibronectin, cytotactin, entactin, and osteonectin (SPARC), (3) elastin, and (4) glycosaminoglycans. Review of this area is beyond the scope of this chapter.

The ECM constitutes the three-dimensional mechanical framework that accounts for a significant component of the physical properties of the lung. Basement membranes separate the alveolar epithelium from the interstitium and thus provide boundaries along which orderly repair of the epithelium can occur. During repair the ECM provides a scaffold for attachment, proper orientation, support, shape determination, and migration of the cellular components of the alveolus. The ECM may function as a permissive substratum on which cells are responsive to soluble factors or as an inducer for the expression of new cellular functions in adherent cells during lung development and repair. Because of the net negative charge of alveolar epithelial basement membrane, the ECM may play an important role in the retention of cations. Intact or cleaved components of ECM may be important in chemoattraction of inflammatory cells into the alveolar space. Finally, ECM may function as a reservoir of growth factors such as fibroblast growth factor (FGF) and transforming growth factor β (TGFβ), which are released during lung remodeling.

MECHANISMS OF LUNG INJURY

Because of the large gaps in our understanding of the mechanisms of lung injury and repair, we borrow from observations made on nonpulmonary systems or on in vitro model systems and attempt to corroborate the observations with those in a clinical setting.

Acute lung injury resulting in ARDS may be direct, as occurs with inhalation lung injury, or it may be secondary such as occurs in settings of sepsis, massive trauma, or massive blood transfusions. The initiating injury mechanisms probably differ, depending on the clinical settings. However, once initiated, lung damage may be amplified by recruitment and activation of polymorphonuclear leukocytes (PMNs), complement, fibrinolytic and lipoxygenase products, and local tissue factors. Generalized damage to the alveolar septum leads to leakage of fluid and protein into the interstitium. When the capacity of lung lymphatics to clear the fluid is overwhelmed, fluid exudes to the alveolar space, resulting in pulmonary edema. As a result, there is reduced lung compliance and functional residual capacity (FRC), a large right-to-left intrapulmonary shunt, and impaired gas transport. Decrease or dysfunction of surfactant occurs and may be caused in part by influx of inhibitory plasma factors. Some of the postulated mechanisms of acute lung injury are detailed below.

Alveolar macrophages are the principal cells involved in the recruitment of PMN in the air space; however, other cellular constituents of the alveolar wall participate in this process. Epithelial cells, fibroblasts, and endothelial cells have been shown to produce IL-8 in response to TNF and IL-1. During inflammatory reactions, pulmonary endothelial cells express on their surfaces inducible adhesion molecules such as endothelial-leukocyte adhesion molecule-1 (ELAM-1), granulocyte-associated membrane protein 140 (GMP140), intracellular adhesion molecule-1 (ICAM-1), and vascular cell adhesion molecule-1 (VCAM-1). The adhesion molecules are important for PMN and platelet adhesion and thus serve to localize the PMN and platelet adhesion to sites of inflammation. Components of the lung extracellular matrix such as type IV collagen, fibronectin, and laminin in their mature state or cleaved state are PMN chemoattractants. Finally, arachidonic acid produced by pulmonary epithelial cells is metabolized to a potent chemoattractant, leukotriene B_4 (LTB_4), by pulmonary alveolar macrophages.

Inflammatory cell hypothesis

Both AMs and PMNs, which contain mechanisms for protease and oxidant lung injury, are believed to mediate lung damage. Macrophages contain lysosomal enzymes and neutral proteases that may damage the ECM. Activated AMs release substances that are chemotactic to PMNs. The latter are frequently found at sites of alveolar and endothelial damage. Polymorphonuclear leukocytes and products of leukocytes are observed in bronchoalveolar lavage fluid (BALF) of patients at risk of ARDS and those with ARDS. Polymorphonuclear leukocytes release oxygen radicals (superoxide anion $O_2^{\dot{-}}$ and the hydroxyl radical [•OH]) as well as hydrogen peroxide (H_2O_2). Finally, substances capable of activating both PMNs and AMs are present in pulmonary microvasculature and BALF.

Polymorphonuclear leukocytes are normally absent from lung parenchyma. However, activated PMNs adhere to the surface of the pulmonary endothelium at the site of alveolar injury. They migrate through the endothelium, between cell junctions, and penetrate the basement membrane into the interstitium and finally into alveolar spaces. Polymorphonuclear leukocytes may degranulate at any stage of their migration, releasing factors that may amplify the initial damage to cellular and ECM components. However, PMNs are not the sole source of lung injury since neutropenia does not completely protect the lung from prolonged hyperoxia.

Oxidant injury hypothesis

Both PMNs and AMs have mechanisms for release of toxic oxygen radicals, which damage cell membrane components and extracellular matrix. Superoxide dismutase, catalase, and ceruloplasmin are important protective mechanisms against oxidative damage to lungs. Oxygen radical scavengers, such as dimethyl thiourea (DMTU), protect alveolar cells from hyperoxic injury and resultant ARDS after phorbol myristate acetate–induced lung damage. Oxygen radicals may mediate their toxic effects by increasing pulmonary perfusion pressures and peroxidative damage to cell membranes and ECM. Thus, papaverine, an inhibitor of smooth muscle contraction, prevents increased lung damage in isolated lung preparations.

Cell-free systems consisting of xanthine and xanthine oxidase mixtures have been used to generate O_2^- (superoxide) and hydrogen peroxide (H_2O_2). In the presence of iron, they react to form hydroxyl radical (•OH). Hydroxyl radicals can be converted to water and oxygen by catalase. Superoxide anion $O_2^{\dot{-}}$ is converted to H_2O_2 by superoxide dismutase. The H_2O_2 or its derived product such as •OH probably causes the lung damage since superoxide dismutase does not protect from lung damage.

Protease hypothesis

According to this hypothesis, inflammatory cells release proteases, elastases, collagenases, trypsin/chymotrypsin, and plasminogen activator–plasmin system, which damage both cells and ECM. In all cases the enzyme system has a corresponding inhibitor for regulation of its activity. The degree of proteolysis is determined by the granule content of PMNs, timing, location of proteases, substrates, and corresponding enzyme inhibitors.

Elastases. Leukocyte elastase is a serine protease that is released from PMN granules. It is bound by AM membrane and is secreted when the macrophage is activated. This enzyme can degrade a wide range of substrates including elastin, collagen types III and IV, fibronectin, fibrinogen, factors VIII and XII, fibrin split products, and glycosaminoglycans. Alpha 1-antiprotease is the primary inhibitor of leukocyte elastase. This elastase is present in BALF of patients with ARDS. Cathepsin L is a cysteine protease with elastolytic properties and an acid pH optimum that is also found in the leukocyte granule and macrophages.

Collagenases. The PMN granule also contains leukocyte collagenase, which is a metalloenzyme capable of degrading all collagen types and fibronectin.

Trypsin/chymotrypsin. The trypsin activity can degrade type III collagen and cell surface glycoproteins. Leukocyte granules also contain chymotryptic activity, another serine protease, which degrades fibronectin and other glycoproteins.

Plasmin-plasminogen activator-inhibitor system. Plasminogen activators are involved in many cellular degradative processes and are distributed on many cell types. Plasminogen activators convert plasminogen to plasmin. Plasmin degrades fibrin and other proteins. There are two principal plasminogen activators: urokinase and tissue plasminogen activators.

Plasminogen activator is secreted as a 50,000-dalton proenzyme. Many cell types possess surface receptors for proPA. Cells also synthesize several PA inhibitors: type 1, which is secreted by placenta, macrophages, and monocytes. Type 3 PA inhibitor is produced by fibroblasts. Types 1 and 2 are specific for PA. Type 3 also inhibits plasmin, thrombin, and trypsinlike proteases. It is believed that secreted PA binds to a plasma membrane receptor. After activation, PA triggers localized proteolysis of ECM, thus facilitating cell migration and lung remodeling. PA's binding receptor may protect the enzyme from its inhibitors. The AM contains a PA that is identical to urokinase and enhances elastolytic activity of AMs.

Complement by-products hypothesis

Complement activation may play an important role in sepsis-induced lung damage. In septic shock and in an experimental model of sepsis, lung injury depends on complement activation and release of C5a, which is a chemotactic fragment. The C5a complement fragment may bind on surfaces of endothelial cells or on exposed endothelial cytoskeletal components, leading to further cellular and endothelial cell damage. The C5, 6-9 complexes cause irreversible target cell membrane damage. Protective mechanisms against complement-mediated cell damage include C_1 inhibitors (C1-INH), (C4Bp)-C4 binding protein, and factor 1 (C4b-C3b inhibitors), which are regulators of the classic pathway. The C4a, 3a, and 5a anaphylatoxins cause smooth muscle contraction and increased production of factors H (B-H), P (properdin), and factor 1, which are regulators of the alternate pathway. The S protein and antithrombin III are modulators of the common pathway.

Products of the fibrinolytic system

Diffuse intravascular coagulation with fibrinolysis often occurs during ARDS associated with trauma. It is associated with excessive formation of thrombin and plasmin in circulation. Platelet thrombi and microaggregates develop within lung microcirculation. Also during endotoxin-associated ARDS, activation of PMNs, AMs, and complement results in PMNs aggregation with release of PAF, endothelial cell injury, activation of blood-coagulating system and platelet microaggregation, and impaired clearance of activated blood products by the reticuloendothelial (RE) system. Purified fibrinogen fragment D causes progressive complement depletion and pulmonary dysfunction, presumably via endothelial cell damage. Release of tissue factor at the site of injury may trigger the blood coagulation system in this form of ARDS.

Factor XII is activated at the site of injury, and kallikrein is formed. Simultaneously, plasminogen is converted to plasmin, presumably by endothelial cell–derived PA. Alpha$_2$-macroglobulin and alpha$_2$-antiplasmin, which inhibit plasmin, are the protective mechanisms. When both inhibitors are overwhelmed, plasmin digests fibrinogen, fibrin, factor V, and factor VIII:C. Plasmin absorbed on fibrin surface is protected from both plasma inhibitors. Experimental data support possible toxic roles in the lung for fibrin (ogen) fragment D, fibrin peptide 6A, elastase or its fibrin (ogen) derivatives, kallikrein and the platelet derivatives (thromboxane A_2 and lipoxygenase derivatives), and leukocyte-produced mediators (leukotrienes such as LTC_4 and LTD_4).

Kininogen

Kinins cause marked permeability changes of the alveolar microvasculature. Proteases from human PMNs can generate kinins from kininogens. However, the exact enzyme responsible has not been established.

REPAIR MECHANISMS

Factors that determine the path of the repair process are only beginning to be elucidated. They include (1) severity and nature of the initial insult, (2) chronicity of the insult or superimposition of a second insult during the period of recovery from the initial injury, (3) cell-to-cell and cell-to-ECM interactions, (4) local effects caused by growth factors bound to ECM, (5) contributions of soluble growth factors secreted by inflammatory and parenchymal cells, (6) serum-derived growth factors, and (7) formation of cross-links of newly synthesized extracellular matrix components.

Normal recovery from acute alveolar injury

Repair of the lung epithelium requires remodeling of damaged basal lamina on which reorganization of cellular components and transformation of type II into type I cells occurs. Alveolar fluid is cleared by type II cells. Lung ECM provides a three-dimensional scaffold and boundaries along which re-epithelialization occurs. Its constituents (e.g., glycosaminoglycans, collagens, laminin, fibronectin, and entactin) influence many cellular functions. Newly synthesized ECM components undergo normal cross-linking, thus forming stable structures. Structural microdomains, which exist beneath type I and II pneumocytes, are probably reestablished at this stage and may play a role in transformation of type II into type I cells.

Mesenchymal-epithelial interactions are important for normal lung development; their role during repair is speculative at present. Type II cells have basal processes with which they interact with interstitial cells. The processes are most frequent during periods of lung remodeling and rapid growth. Their role during repair is speculative at the present time.

Alveolar macrophages phagocytize and break down cellular debris from sloughed epithelium. They synthesize and secrete numerous soluble growth factors, chemotactic factors, and cytokines that regulate cell proliferation and metabolic biosynthetic functions of lung cells. Responsiveness of the lung cells to the soluble factors is, in turn, regulated by the nature of the ECM that the cells are in contact with.

Pathologic reparative response to lung injury

Abnormal repair may occur when the lung's three-dimensional architecture is severely altered in the initial injury or ensuing response. Thus, after oleic acid injury when lung basement membranes are preserved, normal healing occurs. However, when the basement membranes are damaged, lung repair results in scar formation. In bleomycin-induced lung injury, the intensity of chronic inflammation and fibrosis has been found to be directly related to the severity of acute lung injury.

The nature of injury is important. For example, intratracheal instillation of elastase results in emphysematous response, whereas instillation of collagenase does not heal with emphysema. Chronicity of the insult is thought to be important. Thus, while the same inflammatory mechanisms are believed to be involved in lung damage in ARDS that may not progress to fibrosis, chronic inflammatory responses are thought to result in the fibrotic reactions of idiopathic pulmonary fibrosis.

A second insult superimposed during the recovery phase may result in a fibrotic response. For example, after radiation-induced lung damage, administration of oxygen exacerbates the injury and may result in a fibrotic response. Similarly, patients with bleomycin-induced lung damage may worsen when they are concomitantly treated with oxygen, which presumably enhances oxidant damage.

Formation of cross-links of newly synthesized ECM is an important determinant of the course of repair. For example, intratracheal administration of cadmium chloride ($CdCl_2$) to Golden Syrian hamsters causes acute lung injury that results in fibrosis. However, when beta-aminopropionitrile (BAPN), an inhibitor of lysyl oxidase, is simultaneously administered, bullous emphysema results. Lysyl oxidase is required for cross-linking of collagens and elastin during lung remodeling. Penicillamine similarly interferes with cross-linking of collagens and may prevent fibrotic lung reactions.

The exact molecular mechanisms that tip the balance toward normal, fibrotic, or emphysematous reparative responses in clinical settings are unknown at present; however, the general patterns tend to be (1) an initial inflammatory response; and (2) a proliferative, migratory, and biosynthetic phase under influence of ECM and soluble factors and cell-to-cell interactions. The transformation of the thickened alveolar epithelium into a normal respiratory surface occurs by differentiation of cuboidal type II cells into type I pneumocytes.

One of the mechanisms by which the inflammatory response and damage to ECM may influence repair is by recruitment of fibroblasts into the alveolar space. Fibroblast chemotaxis may be mediated by proteolytic products of ECM components such as collagens, tropoelastin, elastin, and fibronectin; peptides secreted by AMs, lymphocytes, and platelets; and LTB_4. Macrophages play key roles in repair processes of acute lung injury since they are capable of secreting factors that stimulate or inhibit proliferation of lung parenchymal cells (PDGF, TGFβ, PAF, IL_1, and prostaglandin E_2 [PGE_2]). Macrophages may also regulate procoagulant activity of alveolar fluid and thus promote fibrin deposition in alveolar spaces. In chronic inflammatory states, the lymphocyte may produce factors that directly regulate lung parenchymal functions. Lung parenchymal cells may also produce factors that regulate immune responses or macrophage functions. For example, endothelial cells can secrete IL_1, granulocyte monocyte colony—stimulating factor (GMCSF), and express MHC antigens.

The alveolar epithelial surface lining fluid is known to contain tissue factor and factor VII complexes and promotes coagulation of plasma. Thus, exudation of plasma into the alveolar space, as occurs in ARDS, results in fibrin clot deposition in alveolar spaces. Cross-linking reactions mediated by factor XIIIa may also cross-link serum growth factors into fibrin clots, providing for their subsequent slow release during repair phases of the injury. For example, serum fibronectin can be cross-linked to fibrin by factor XIIIa and is a component of the "fibrin" clot. Fibronectin is an adhesive, chemoattractant, and proliferative factor for lung fibroblasts. It may stimulate fibroblasts to migrate from the lung interstitium through breaks in damaged alveolar basement membranes and enter into the alveolar spaces. The fibroblasts adhere and proliferate in the fibrin clots and may, in severe cases, obliterate the respiratory spaces. Thrombin, an enzyme that mediates conversion of fibrinogen to fibrin, is also a known mitogen. Potentially, thrombin may stimulate type II and other parenchymal cells to proliferate.

Although the initial response to acute lung injury is the same regardless of the nature of insult, the outcome of the repair process may be either restoration of normal architecture, fibrotic reaction, or emphysema. Studies examining mechanisms of lung injury and repair may in future permit targeting of therapy to minimize further lung damage and promote restoration of normal lung architecture and function.

REFERENCES

Albelda SM: Endothelial and epithelial cell adhesion molecules. Am J Respir Cell Mol Biol 4:195, 1991.

Blasi F, Vassalli JD, and Dan K: Urokinase-type plasminogen activator: proenzyme, receptor and inhibitor. J Cell Biol 104:801, 1987.

Bone RC et al: Adult respiratory distress syndrome: sequence and importance of development of multiple organ failure. Chest 101:320, 1992.

Brody JS: Cell-to-cell interactions in lung development. Pediatr Pulmonol 1(3 suppl):PS42, 1985.

Fantone JL and Ward PA: Role of oxygen-derived free radicals and metabolites in leukocyte-dependent inflammatory reactions. Am J Pathol 107:397, 1982.

Hemler M: VLA proteins in the integrin family: structures, functions and their role in leukocytes. Ann Rev Immunol 8:365, 1990.

Lwebuga-Mukasa JS: Matrix-driven pneumocyte differentiation. Am Rev Respir Dis 133:452, 1991.

Osborn L: Leukocyte adhesion to endothelium in inflammation. Cell 62:3, 1990.

Paralka VM, Vukicevic S, and Reddi AH: Transforming growth factor β type I binds to collagen IV of basement membrane matrix: implications for development. Dev Biol 143:303, 1991.

Salvador RA, Fiedler-Nagy CA, and Coffey JW: Biochemical basis for drug therapy to prevent fibrosis in ARDS. In Zapol WM and Falke KJ, editors: Acute respiratory failure. New York, 1985, Dekker.

Standiford TJ et al: Interleukin-8 gene expression by a pulmonary epithelial cell line. A model for cytokine network in the lung. J Clin Invest 86:1946, 1990.

LABORATORY AND DIAGNOSTIC TESTS II

CHAPTER

195 Pulmonary Function Testing

Jacob S. O. Loke

In the clinical evaluation of patients with cardiopulmonary disorders, pulmonary function tests can be used to separate patients with pulmonary abnormalities from those with cardiac diseases, noting that both cardiac and pulmonary diseases may coexist. The respiratory system consists of the respiratory center, the lung with its conducting system of the upper airway and the tracheobronchial tree (the gas-exchanging portion), and a ventilatory pump composed of the chest cage and the respiratory muscles. Malfunction of any part of the respiratory system can lead to pulmonary disease, and specific tests may be needed to detect these abnormalities.

Pulmonary function tests are used to objectively evaluate the patient with respiratory symptoms such as dyspnea. The patient can present with psychosomatic complaints of dyspnea at rest and/or on exertion, and lung function tests are helpful in assessing whether the patient has obstructive or restrictive lung disease, or both, or normal lung function. This distinction is important because reassurance or antianxiety medication may be needed in those with a psychogenic respiratory disorder, whereas patients with a condition such as asthma may need bronchodilator therapy. In the latter, lung function tests are able to detect physiologic and abnormal changes in the respiratory system. In patients who use amiodarone for control of ventricular tachycardia or bleomycin for chemotherapy, lung function tests are able to detect pulmonary lung toxicity caused by these agents. Also, pulmonary function forms an integral part of the preoperative and functional assessment of the patient going for surgery. This is especially important in patients with significant bullous obstructive lung disease who will be undergoing bullectomy or lobectomy, or pneumonectomy for lung cancer. In occupational lung disease and lung disability evaluation, lung function tests are useful for assessing decreased function and impairment. Finally, lung function tests have been used to evaluate the success of therapy, be it bronchodilator therapy in asthmatic patients or corticosteroid therapy in patients with sarcoidosis. It is important to note that the pulmonary abnormalities may not be present at rest but may be evident when lung function tests are performed during exercise and sleep. Patients may present with dyspnea on exertion, and using the exercise test, exercise-induced asthma can be diagnosed. Similarly, in a patient who presents with hypersomnolence, sleep apnea, and cor pulmonale, obstructive or central sleep apnea may be demonstrated during the performance of a sleep study. Pulmonary function tests that are available in a complete pulmonary function laboratory include the measurement of (1) nasal airway resistance—to evaluate the patency of the nasal passages; (2) lung volumes—to assess hyperinflation, air trapping, and restrictive ventilatory defect; (3) spirometry—for assessing obstructive or restrictive processes; (4) single-breath diffusing capacity—for obstructive and restrictive defects; (5) pulmonary mechanics (airway resistance, compliance—dynamic and static, maximal elastic recoil pressures, and pressure-volume curves)—for obstructive and restrictive diseases; (6) maximal respiratory mouth pressures during expiration (PE_{max}), inspiration (PI_{max}), and transdiaphragmatic pressures (P_{di})—for assessing respiratory muscle function including the diaphragm; (7) spirometry before and after inhaled bronchodilator—to assess reversibility of airway obstruction in patients with obstructive airway disease; (8) bronchoprovocation inhalation tests with nonspecific or specific agents—to determine airway hyperreactivity and occupational asthma; (9) exercise testing—to evaluate cardiopulmonary integrity and function; (10) arterial blood gases—to assess the gas exchange properties of the lung (i.e., to detect hypoxia and/or hypoventilation and acid-base disturbances); (11) ventilatory control studies such as ventilatory responses to hypoxia and hypercapnia—to assess the respiratory control centers in patients with the pickwickian syndrome or Ondine's curse; and (12) sleep studies—to detect central or obstructive sleep apnea or sleep disturbance and to evaluate nocturnal oxygen therapy in patients with lung diseases.

SPIROMETRY

The lung has certain intrinsic properties, which include volume, elasticity, ventilatory ability, and gas exchange. Spirometry has been used to assess ventilatory ability. Also, one of the ways to detect airway obstruction is by measuring the forced expiratory volume in 1 second (FEV_1), the forced vital capacity (FVC), and the FEV_1/FVC ratio.

The FEV_1 and FVC can be determined with the patient exhaling into a water-sealed spirometer in which volume is measured against time (Fig. 195-1) or into a flow-volume device in which a pneumotachygraph with its associated circuits integrates flow into volume, and a flow-volume curve is generated (Fig. 195-2). The spirometer test requires a maximal effort during exhalation from total lung capacity. In obstructive airway disease, the FEV_1 is decreased more than the FVC so that the FEV_1/FVC ratio is less than 70%. The normal FEV_1/FVC ratio increases in children and young adults and decreases with age. Various criteria have been used to quantitate the severity of airway obstruction based on the predicted formula for FEV_1. When the FEV_1 is 65% to 79% of the predicted FEV_1, the airway obstruction is classified as mild; when it is 50% to 64% of predicted FEV_1, the airway obstruction is moderate, and when the FEV_1 is below 50% of predicted FEV_1, severe obstructive airway disease is present. The above criteria are used when the FEV_1/FVC ratio is decreased and obstructive in nature. However, it should be noted that in patients with asthma or lung disease who have significant coughing on exhalation, the FVC is underestimated or abruptly cut off because of coughing. Although the FEV_1 is decreased, the FEV_1/FVC may still be above 70%. A slow vital capacity (VC) maneuver should be performed, which may show an increase in slow VC compared to the FVC, thus showing an abnormal FEV_1/FVC ratio. In addition, clinical correlation should be done together with pulmonary function tests after inhaled bronchodilator therapy. Serial lung function tests may show an obstructive pattern later when the coughing episodes are resolved or diminished. The shape of the flow-volume curve is of value in assessing airway obstruction. The pattern of the airway obstruction can be caused by pressure limitation (Fig. 195-3, *A*) or volume-dependent limitation (Fig. 195-3, *B*). Expiratory wheeze caused by dy-

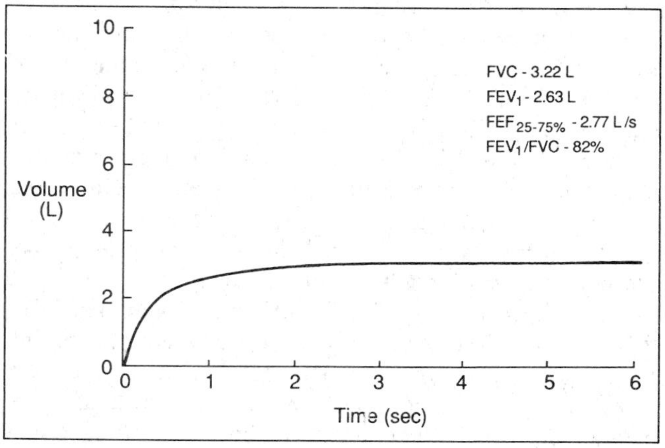

Fig. 195-1. Normal spirogram in a 59-year-old white female (154 cm in height). FEF_{25-75}, forced midexpiratory flow (L/s) between 25% and 75% of the forced vital capacity (FVC). FEV_1, forced expiratory volume in 1 second.

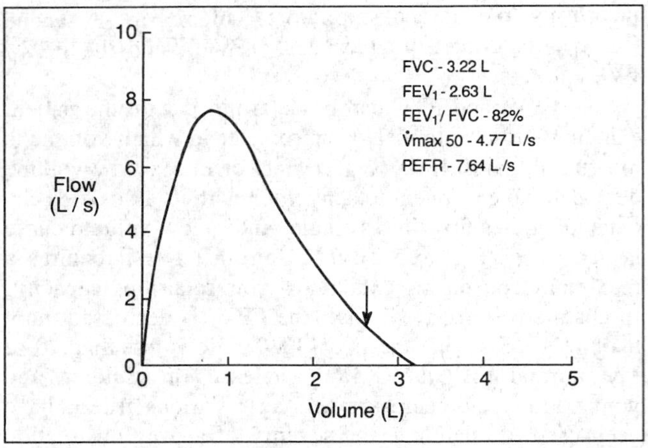

Fig. 195-2. Normal maximal expiratory flow-volume curve study in a 59-year-old white female (154 cm in height). *Small arrow* is the forced expiratory volume in 1 second (FEV_1) time marker. V_{MAX} 50, rate of air flow (L/s) at 50% of forced vital capacity (FVC). PEFR, peak expiratory flow rate in liters per second.

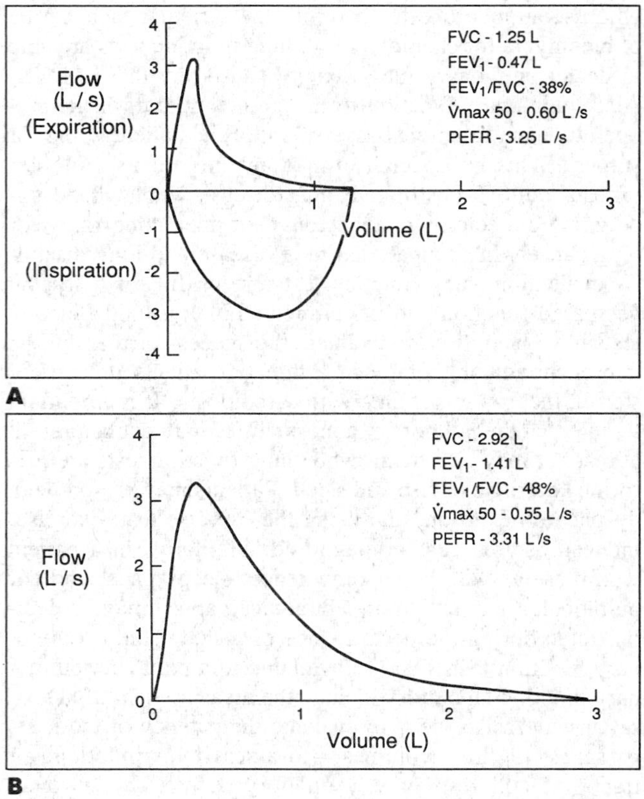

Fig. 195-3. A, Pressure limitation maximal expiratory and inspiratory flow-volume curve study in a 65-year-old white male (173 cm in height) with severe obstructive airway disease. V_{MAX} 50, rate of air flow (L/s) at 50% of forced vital capacity (FVC); PEFR, peak expiratory flow rate in liters per second; FEV_1, forced expiratory volume in 1 second. **B,** Volume-dependent limitation maximal expiratory flow-volume curve study in a 62-year-old white male (161 cm in height) with moderate obstructive airway disease. V_{MAX} 50, rate of air flow (L/s) at 50% of forced vital capacity (FVC); PEFR, peak expiratory flow rate in liters per second; FEV_1, forced expiratory volume in 1 second.

namic air compression can be heard during quiet or forced expiration on auscultation of the chest. For restrictive disease, FEV_1 and FVC decrease proportionally, but more so with the FVC such that the FEV_1/FVC is normal or increased.

From the spirometric studies, one can measure the flow rates at 25% to 75% ($FEF_{25\%-75\%}$) of the FVC. When the FEV_1, FVC, and FEV_1/FVC ratio are normal, a decrease in forced expiratory flow at 25% to 75% of FVC (below 70% of predicted) indicates small airway disease, which is the earliest obstructive lung disease pattern seen in cigarette smokers. With the computer system available in most pulmonary function laboratories, the computer can digitize the flow at 50% of FVC from the spirometric tracing, enabling the flow rate at 50% of FVC ($\dot{V}_{max}$ 50) to be calculated without performing flow-volume curve studies. The decrease in $\dot{V}_{max}$ 50 below 70% of predicted in the presence of a normal FVC, FEV_1, and FEV_1/FVC ratio indicates mild obstructive lung disease of the small airways.

Other studies that have been used to assess small airway function include the closing volume, and breathing air and an 80% helium–20% oxygen mixture for the flow-volume curve studies. These tests are generally investigational or research studies. The normal predictive range for pulmonary function test results, that is, spirometry, subdivisions of lung volume, single-breath diffusing capacity, are based on normal population studies. Generally, when the values are below 80% of predicted or above 120% of predicted (for total lung capacity [TLC] and residual volume [RV]), the values are abnormal. However, the 95% confidence limits of a normal reference population may be a better way of assessing the normal range. When one is evaluating results of pulmonary function tests, the predicted equations used in different pulmonary function laboratories should be taken into consideration. Also, predicted equations should be corrected for age, sex, and height and for race as well, since blacks and Asians have spirometry and lung volumes 15% lower than those of whites.

The maximal expiratory and inspiratory flow-volume curves are especially useful in detecting upper airway obstruction. Various types of upper airway obstruction can be elicited depending on the configuration of the flow-volume curves (Fig. 195-4, *A, B, C*). In fixed upper airway obstruction, the flow-volume curve shows a plateau in both the inspiratory and expiratory limb (Fig. 195-4, *A*). These upper airway obstructive lesions are caused by circumferential narrowings that are not influenced by intratracheal or extratracheal pressure changes. The constricted narrowed areas can be localized from the history or physical examination or by performing a fiberoptic bronchoscopic examination. At times, the patient may present with stridor, and the flow-volume curve is still normal in configuration. A critical narrowing of the trachea has to be attained in some cases before the plateau pattern is evident on flow-volume curve.

Variable extrathoracic upper airway obstruction

The suprasternal notch is used to separate extrathoracic upper airway obstruction from intrathoracic upper airway ob-

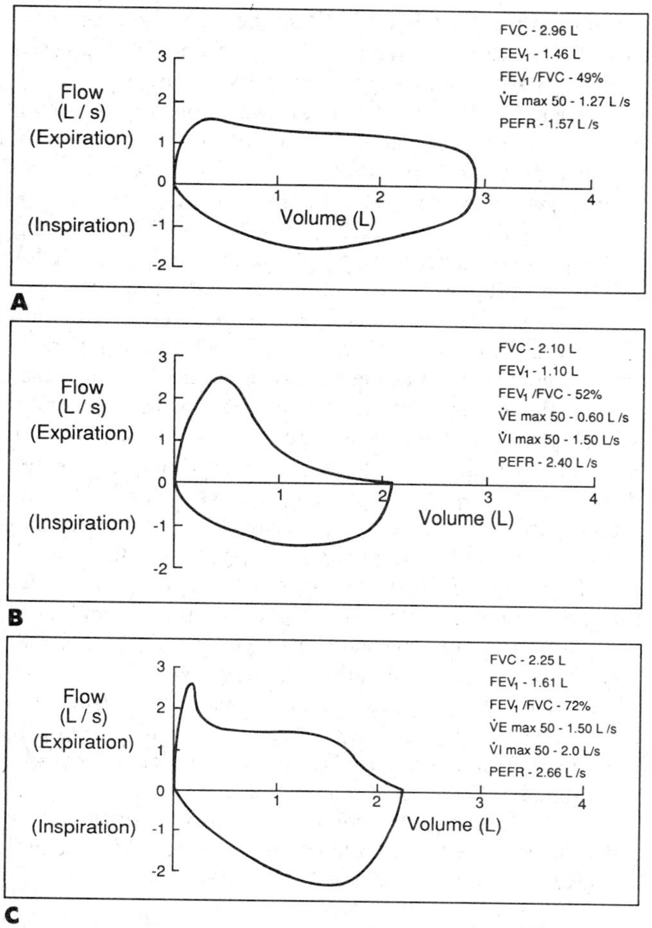

Fig. 195-4. **A,** Maximal expiratory and inspiratory flow-volume curve study in a 52-year-old black male who has obstructive airway disease in addition to fixed upper airway obstruction. VE_{max} 50, rate of air flow (L/s) at 50% of forced vital capacity (FVC) during expiration; PEFR, peak expiratory flow rate in liters per second; FEV_1, forced expiratory volume in 1 second. **B,** Maximal expiratory and inspiratory flow-volume curve study in a 77-year-old white male who has obstructive airway disease in addition to a variable extrathoracic upper airway obstruction caused by a thyroid carcinoma with tracheal compression. VE_{max} 50, air flow rate at 50% of forced vital capacity (FVC) during expiration; VI_{max} 50, air flow rate at 50% of FVC during inspiration; PEFR, peak expiratory flow rate in liters per second; FEV_1, forced expiratory volume in 1 second. **C,** Maximal expiratory and inspiratory flow-volume curve study in a 69-year-old black female who has a retrosternal goiter and a variable intrathoracic upper airway obstruction. VE_{max} 50 rate of air flow (L/s) at 50% of forced vital capacity (FVC) during expiration; VI_{max} 50 rate of air flow (L/s) at 50% of FVC during inspiration; PEFR, peak expiratory flow rate in liters per second; FEV_1 forced expiratory volume in 1 second.

struction. Any lesion (enlarged tonsils, goiter) that occurs in the upper airway and trachea above the suprasternal notch is extrathoracic in origin and may produce a plateau pattern on the inspiratory loop (Fig. 195-4, *B*). During inspiration the intratracheal pressure is less than the atmospheric pressure around the neck and leads to compression of the upper airway obstruction. During exhalation, the intratracheal pressures are greater than the atmospheric pressure, and, therefore, there is no limitation of airflow. The ratio of flow at 50% FVC during expiration ($\dot{V}E_{max}50$) and flow at 50% FVC during inspiration ($\dot{V}I_{max}50$), that is, $\dot{V}E_{max}$ 50/$\dot{V}I_{max}$ 50 is greater than 1.

Variable intrathoracic upper airway obstruction

Obstructive lesions in the tracheobronchial tree that are below the suprasternal notch give rise to a plateau pattern during expiration. During inspiration, the intrapleural pressure is negative relative to the tracheal lumen, and the caliber of the tracheal lumen increases; during forced exhalation, the positive intrapleural pressure is greater than the intratracheal pressure, leading to tracheal narrowing. The ratio of $\dot{V}E_{max}$ 50/$\dot{V}I_{max}$ 50 is less than 1. During a routine spirometric test, variable intrathoracic upper airway obstruction or fixed upper airway obstruction can be suspected when the FEV_1, FVC, midflow rates, and FEV_1/FVC ratio are normal but there is a significant decrement in peak flow rate such that the FEV_1(ml)/peak flow (liters per minute) is greater than 10 (normal, less than 10). A flow-volume curve study during inspiration and expiration is requested to further document the variable or fixed pattern of upper airway obstruction.

INHALED BRONCHODILATOR STUDIES

Bronchial asthma, asthmatic bronchitis, viral upper respiratory tract infection, chronic obstructive pulmonary disease (COPD), occupational asthma, and psychogenic vocal cord dysfunction are some of the causes of reversible airway disease. To evaluate the reversibility of airway obstruction, one gives an inhaled bronchodilator—isoproterenol or metaproterenol (two puffs)—and assesses again the spirometric findings of FEV_1, FVC, and $\dot{V}_{max}$ 50 or $FEF_{25\%-75\%}$. The most reliable parameter for the response to inhaled bronchodilator is the FEV_1. A 15% increase in FEV_1 from the baseline value after an inhaled bronchodilator is a significant improvement. Normal individuals do not usually increase the FEV_1 by more than 5% after inhaled bronchodilator, whereas an asthmatic subject can increase the FEV_1 by more than 15% after an inhaled bronchodilator. When the FEV_1 and FVC are normal, but the midflow rates are decreased, any increase in $\dot{V}_{max}$ 50 or $FEF_{25\%-75\%}$ by more than 15% is also considered significant improvement provided the FVCs before and after inhaled bronchodilator were comparable, that is, similar in values. If the FVC after an inhaled bronchodilator is much lower than the prebronchodilator FVC, the $\dot{V}_{max}$ 50 could be artificially high by calculation, as the $\dot{V}_{max}$ 50 is the midpoint of the FVC and may not represent a response to inhaled bronchodilator. Similarly, when the FVC after inhaled bronchodilator is higher than the prebronchodilator value, the $\dot{V}_{max}$ 50 may be artificially lower than the prebronchodilator value. Therefore, for the assessment of response to inhaled bronchodilator for the midflow rates, isovolume measurement of flow rates from the TLC on the flow-volume curve should be used to calculate pre- and postbronchodilator response. When the FEV_1 is below 1 liter, and especially if it is below 0.5 liter, any small change in FEV_1 can lead to significant response by the usual criteria of 15% increase from baseline. For example, an FEV_1 increase from 0.3 to 0.4 liter after inhaled bronchodilator indicates a 33% increase, but the changes are so small, and the patient will continue to have dyspnea. Although the response to inhaled bronchodilator is a significant one by the definition of response to inhaled bronchodilator, clinically it is not a significant one.

LUNG VOLUME DETERMINATION

The subdivisions of lung volume can be determined with the nitrogen washout–helium dilution technique or body plethysmography. The helium dilution technique accurately measures the lung volumes when there is no evidence of significant airway obstruction. In patients with obstructive lung disease, the helium dilution technique may underestimate lung volume because of poor mixing or inhomogeneity of gases in the lungs. However, the body plethysmograph determines intrathoracic lung volume whether or not the airways or alveoli are in communication with the other airways, and this is a more accurate way of determining the functional residual capacity. In patients with emphysema, there is usually hyperinflation and air trapping manifested by an increase (above 120% of predicted) in functional residual capacity (FRC) and RV, respectively. In contrast, for patients with restrictive ventilatory defect, TLC decreases and is classified as mild when TLC is between 66% to 81% of predicted, moderate when 51% to 65% of predicted, and severe when less than 51% of predicted value. In restrictive disease when the FEV_1/FVC is normal or increased, the increase in RV may be caused by muscle weakness and not to air trapping per se. In the presence of a normal TLC, FRC, RV, and FEV_1/FVC ratio, a decrease in FVC suggests also a restrictive process. The flow-volume curve shows a characteristic curve for restrictive process. Initially, the flow rates are increased with an increase in FEV_1/FVC ratio caused by an increase in elastic recoil in patients with interstitial lung disease or pulmonary fibrosis. Subsequently, with progressive increase in the restrictive process, the FEV_1, peak flow, and midflow rates are also decreased significantly but the FEV_1/FVC ratio is normal or increased. When the TLC is decreased significantly together with a decrease in the FEV_1/FVC ratio, then both a restrictive and obstructive disease process exists.

It has also been shown that an isolated decrease in RV in the subdivisions of lung volume may indicate a restrictive intrathoracic process whether it is caused by lymphoma, cardiomegaly, or pleural disease.

SINGLE-BREATH DIFFUSING CAPACITY

The single-breath diffusing capacity is useful to assess occupational and interstitial lung disease, pulmonary vascular disease, and the effects of certain drugs (such as amiodarone and bleomycin) or after chemotherapeutic agents that can affect the interstitial portion of the lung. Also it is of value in emphysema with destruction of the pulmonary parenchyma and loss of the pulmonary capillary bed. Since diffusing capacity is related to the capillary blood volume, any loss of the pulmonary capillary bed leads to a decrease in diffusing capacity. The diffusing capacity is increased in patients with asthma and pulmonary hemorrhage.

The test involves the patient inhaling a mixture of known concentration of air, carbon monoxide (CO), and an inert gas such as helium (He) or neon (Ne). After certain respiratory maneuvers, the patient exhales to RV and then inhales the mixture of 21.5% oxygen, 68.3% nitrogen, 0.295% carbon monoxide, 9.9% helium, and breath holds for 10 seconds. A portion of the exhalation is collected, and concentrations of the carbon monoxide and the helium exhaled are measured. During the breath-holding period, the concentration of carbon monoxide in the lung decreases as it "diffuses" into the blood in the pulmonary capillaries. A diffusion defect was originally considered to assess an increase in thickness of the alveolar capillary membrane, which would lead to a decrease in oxygen tension in the blood. Diffusion defect is not considered to be a major factor in causing arterial hypoxemia. Other factors that can affect the values of diffusing capacity include the hemoglobin concentration, capillary blood volume, ventilation-perfusion mismatch, the ratio of alveolar volume to capillary blood volume, and carboxyhemoglobin.

An increase in diffusing capacity is seen in patients with an increase in hemoglobin concentration or an increase in pulmonary blood volume. The hemoglobin level should be determined with the test since anemia leads to a decrease in diffusing capacity. Before assuming that the diffusing capacity is abnormal, it should be corrected for the hemoglobin level given by the formula:

$$\text{Corrected diffusing capacity} = \text{uncorrected diffusing capacity}/0.06965 \times \text{hemoglobin}$$

Smokers have higher carboxyhemoglobin levels in the blood than nonsmokers, and the single-breath diffusing capacity assumes that the carbon monoxide tension in pulmonary capillaries is zero. Therefore, without correcting for carboxyhemoglobin, the diffusing capacity may still be normal when it is above 70% of predicted in contrast to the above 80% of predicted for nonsmokers. Our normal predicted equations for single-breath diffusing capacity include smokers and nonsmokers.

The diffusing capacity in patients with restrictive lung disease such as interstitial fibrosis is decreased. This decrease is associated with a decrease in TLC and vital capacity (VC) and a normal or increased FEV_1/FVC. In contrast, patients with restrictive disease caused by chest cage or weakness of the respiratory muscles may have a decrease in TLC and VC and a normal or increased FEV_1/FVC ratio, but the diffusing capacity is normal.

The typical patterns of lung function tests in patients with restrictive or obstructive disease or both are shown in Table 195-1.

SPECIAL PULMONARY STUDIES

Ventilatory control studies

In a patient who presents with pulmonary hypertension and heart failure or alveolar hypoventilation in the absence of lung disease, abnormalities in the respiratory control cen-

Table 195-1. Patterns of pulmonary function abnormalities in various pulmonary diseases

Patterns of abnormalities	VC	RV	TLC	FEV_1/FVC	D_LCO
Obstructive					
Asthma	N or ↓	N or ↑	N or ↑	↓	N or ↑
Chronic bronchitis	N or ↓	N or ↑	N	↓	N
Emphysema	N or ↓	↑	↑	↓	↓
Restrictive					
Pulmonary parenchyma	↓	↓	↓	N or ↑	↓
Extrapulmonary	↓	↓	↓	N	N
Restrictive and obstructive diseases	↓	N or ↓	↓	↓	N or ↓

VC, vital capacity; RV, residual volume; TLC, total lung capacity; FEV_1, forced expiratory volume in 1 second; FVC, forced vital capacity; D_LCO, diffusing capacity of carbon monoxide; N, normal; ↓, decreased; ↑, increased.

ter should be suspected. Patients with primary alveolar hypoventilation (Ondine's curse) have no abnormalities in their lungs. Spirometry determinations of lung volumes and diffusing capacity in these patients are normal. However, one can detect the alveolar hypoventilation by performing an arterial blood gas analysis, which shows alveolar hypoventilation with a normal alveolar-arterial oxygen difference. Also, when one asks the patient to hyperventilate voluntarily, an increase in arterial oxygen tension (PaO_2) and a decrease in arterial carbon dioxide tension ($PaCO_2$) occurs. Also, arterial oxygen saturation determined noninvasively with the pulse oximeter increases when the patient hyperventilates. When the patient inhales a 5% carbon dioxide and 95% oxygen mixture using a rebreathing technique for the ventilatory response to hypercapnia, the response of ventilation is blunted or absent with progressive increase in end-tidal PCO_2. In normal individuals, there is a 2- to 3-liter increase in minute ventilation per 1 mm Hg change in end-tidal PCO_2. With regard to the ventilatory response to hypoxia, the patient breathes ambient air in a spirometer using the rebreathing technique. The rise in end-tidal PCO_2 is maintained at an isocapnic level of approximately 40 mm Hg by a carbon dioxide absorber. A pulse oximeter is used to assess oxygen saturation with progressive depletion of oxygen in the system as a result of the rebreathing maneuvers. When the ventilatory response is plotted against oxygen saturation, a linear relationship is found. Normally a 0.6-liter increase in minute ventilation occurs per 1% change in oxygen saturation. In patients with respiratory center abnormalities, the ventilatory response to hypoxia is blunted or absent. Subjects who have had removal of carotid bodies for treatment of asthma can also have a blunted ventilatory response to hypoxia.

The ventilatory response of breathing when there is a progressive decrease in arterial oxygen tension or hypoxia is a curvilinear one, but when oxygen saturation is plotted against ventilation, a linear relationship results. In patients with severe obstructive lung disease, the ventilatory response to hypercapnia and hypoxia may not be determined because of the mechanical abnormalities of the lung, which can produce a limitation in the ventilatory response. The occlusion pressure during the first 100 ms of inspiration has been used to assess the respiratory center output in these patients with lung disease.

Bronchoprovocation inhalation tests

The indications for bronchoprovocation inhalation tests are a clinical suspicion of hyperreactive airways, atypical presentation of asthma, and occupational asthma. Patients may have cough, dyspnea, and chest tightness and yet have normal pulmonary function tests at rest. Although abnormal lung function tests can be documented in the work place, normal lung function tests may be found away from the working environment. The two types of bronchoprovocation inhalation tests are specific antigen challenge tests and nonspecific bronchial challenge tests. For the former, the particular agent that is producing the occupational asthma is given to the patient to inhale. With the specific challenge tests, the patient should be observed in a hospital environment for 24 hours since there may be an immediate reaction followed by a delayed reaction in the decrement of pulmonary function tests being monitored. The provocation dose is the dose of the agent that produces a decrease in FEV_1 by 20% or more from baseline. It is also known as $PD_{20}(FEV_1)$.

In the nonspecific bronchial inhalation tests, methacholine or histamine is inhaled periodically at increasing concentrations, and the FEV_1 and FVC are monitored. In normal individuals, there is no decrease in FEV_1 below 20% of baseline values with the inhalation of the highest concentration of methacholine. In contrast, those patients with occupational asthma (symptomatic) or asthma usually react at a low concentration of methacholine. Since methacholine is a nonspecific bronchoprovocation test used to detect hyperreactivity of the airways, a negative test does not rule out a positive test with a specific antigen or agent to which the patient is allergic in the work place.

Bronchodilator therapy, coffee or tea, and beta blockers should not be taken prior to the nonspecific bronchoprovocation tests to avoid false-negative or false-positive tests.

Clinical exercise tests

Exercise testing is useful in the evaluation of patients with dyspnea with or without cardiopulmonary disease. Because of somatic complaints of dyspnea on exertion in an individual with a normal lung function test, an exercise test can be used to evaluate the cardiorespiratory responses to exercise. If one uses either a treadmill or bicycle ergometer for the exercise test, the blood pressure, heart rate (HR), electrocardiogram (ECG), ventilation, tidal volume, respiratory rate, carbon dioxide production, oxygen consumption, and oxygen saturation can be measured. The normal response of the cardiovascular system to progressive incremental exercise is an appropriate increase in HR and blood pressure reaching a targeted HR of close to 90% of the predicted maximal HR given by the formula ($210 - 0.65 \times$ age). There should be no exertional hypotension or significant increase in diastolic blood pressure above 90 mm Hg or ECG changes suggestive of S-T segment depression or ischemia. The oxygen consumption at maximal exercise ($\dot{V}O_{2max}$) should be normal, and the slope of the $\dot{V}O_2$/HR should be normal. $\dot{V}O_2$/HR is also known as oxygen pulse. The $\dot{V}O_{2max}$ is increased in athletes and in fit individuals. It is decreased in unfit persons and decreased markedly in patients with significant cardiovascular disease or congestive heart failure. Also, the $\dot{V}O_{2max}$ is decreased in subjects with pulmonary disease. In a normal individual, the cardiovascular system and not the pulmonary system is the main limiting factor of exercise performance.

Associated with the gradual increase in HR during exercise in a normal individual is an appropriate increase in minute ventilation (i.e., tidal volume × respiratory rate). The maximal minute ventilation that can be achieved with maximal exercise is about 60% of the estimated maximal voluntary ventilation (MVV) (based on the $FEV_1 \times 35$). Therefore, for a person with an FEV_1 of 3 liters, the estimated MVV is approximately 105 liters. There should be no oxygen desaturation with exercise, and if the subject achieves a maximal minute ventilation, which is approximately 60% of the estimated MVV, then some ventilatory reserve for exercise exists. In an individual with normal lung function test, an abnormal exercise test (in the absence of exercise-induced bronchospasm) may indicate cardiovascular abnormalities, especially if the $\dot{V}O_2$ is significantly decreased and associated with ischemic changes in ECG or exertional hypotension, and the ventilatory limitation was not reached.

In patients with obstructive lung disease, exercise tests may show that the targeted maximal HR is not attained, but that the patient may reach maximal ventilation as shown by the maximal ventilation ($\dot{V}E_{max}$)–estimated MVV ratio, that is $\dot{V}E_{max}/MVV \times 100\%$ approaching or greater than 100%, and thus indicates ventilatory limitation. In patients with obstructive lung disease, the estimated MVV is given by the formula $FEV_1 \times 40$. In COPD patients the anaerobic threshold is usually not reached, the $\dot{V}O_2$ is described as peak $\dot{V}O_2$ and not $\dot{V}O_{2max}$, and the peak $\dot{V}O_2$ is low. Also, oxygen desaturation can be seen if there is significant oxygen desaturation (below 90%) at a low exercise workload. This type of patient may need to receive supplemental nasal oxygen therapy with exercise.

In restrictive interstitial lung disease, exercise tests are useful to determine the work capacity and degree of oxygen desaturation. The patient can be ventilatory limited or may show significant oxygen desaturation before reaching ventilatory limitation. There is a decrease in the tidal volume response with the exercise because of the restrictive process, and this is associated with an inappropriate increase in respiratory rate to compensate for the blunted tidal volume response. Oxygen therapy is valuable in interstitial lung disease patients with significant oxygen desaturation to prevent the complications of pulmonary hypertension associated with hypoxia. Assessment of therapy can be done with serial exercise tests to determine the effect of corticosteroid or cyclophosphamide therapy.

The majority of patients with end-stage chronic obstructive lung disease may not be able to tolerate an exercise test on the treadmill or bicycle ergometer. Instead a walking test of 2-, 6-, and 12-minute duration can be performed with monitoring of oxygen saturation with a portable pulse oximeter. If the patient shows significant oxygen desaturation below 85% while ambulating on a level surface for short distances, oxygen therapy is warranted, and the amount of oxygen therapy can be assessed by repeating the walking test to ensure an adequate oxygen saturation with the required nasal oxygen concentration.

Sleep studies

Patients with chronic obstructive pulmonary disease may have relatively normal PO_2 and PCO_2 at rest when the arterial blood gases are performed. However, during sleep, they may show significant oxygen desaturation. The oxygen desaturation is associated with pulmonary hypertension and can aggravate their COPD, leading them to seek medical help for their dyspnea. Thus, sleep studies with monitoring of oxygen saturation provide us with the oxygenation status of patients with COPD. The use of oxygen therapy for prevention of oxygen desaturation or hypoxia has been shown in the nocturnal oxygen therapy trial studies in the United States and in the Medical Research Council studies in England to increase the survival of COPD patients with hypoxia.

The other major disease category for which sleep studies are indicated is the sleep apnea syndrome, whether it is central or obstructive sleep apnea (see Chapter 190).

A sleep study includes monitoring of stages of sleep, oral and nasal airflow, and ECG. By assessing the oral and nasal airflow and the rib cage and abdominal movements, obstructive or central types of sleep apnea syndrome can be diagnosed. Significant oxygen desaturation can occur with obstructive or central sleep apnea. Therapy can be directed at obstructive sleep apnea by using nasal continuous positive airway pressure, thus improving the oxygen saturation as well as their sleep pattern or stages of sleep. Sleep studies can also be used to evaluate narcolepsy and myoclonus. (see Chapters 142 and 190).

REFERENCES

American Thoracic Society: Evaluation of impairment/disability secondary to respiratory disorder. Am Rev Respir Dis 133:1205, 1986.

Bates DV: Respiratory function in disease, ed 3. Philadelphia, 1989, Saunders.

Clausen JL, editor: Pulmonary function testing. Guidelines and controversies. Orlando, 1984, Grune & Stratton.

Forster II RE et al: The lung. Physiologic basis of pulmonary function tests, ed 3. Chicago, 1986, Year Book.
Jones NL: Clinical exercise testing, ed 3. Philadelphia, 1988, Saunders.
Kryger MH, Roth T, and Dement WC: Principles and practice of sleep medicine. Philadelphia, 1989, Saunders.
Miller A, editor: Pulmonary function tests. A guide for the student and house officer. Orlando, 1987, Grune & Stratton.
Morris AH et al: Clinical pulmonary function testing. A manual of uniform laboratory procedures. Salt Lake City, 1984, Intermountain Thoracic Society.
Wilson AF, editor: Pulmonary function testing. Indications and interpretations. Orlando, 1985, Grune & Stratton.

CHAPTER

196 Invasive Diagnostic Techniques

John A. Rankin

SPUTUM EXAMINATION

Examination of an expectorated sputum sample is one of the easiest and most cost-effective analyses to perform in evaluating suspected pulmonary disease. Either direct wet-mount examination of unstained sputum or the examination of Gram- or Wright-Giemsa–stained specimens can yield valuable and occasionally diagnostic information. Use of the thick, purulent yellow or green matter and avoidance of obvious salivary components increases the reliability of the results. A thin layer of fresh sputum is smeared on a glass slide. For wet-mount examination, a cover slip is then placed over the slide. When a Gram stain is performed, the sample should be heat-fixed to the slide over a flame. When a Wright-Giemsa stain is made, the sample should be air dried. The specimen in all cases should be examined first under low power (100×) to assess if it is a sample from the lower respiratory tract. Confirmation is reflected by the presence of either alveolar macrophages or ciliated epithelial cells. An optimal sample contains one or both of these cells. Neutrophils present in sputum may arise from the gums, especially in patients with poor dentition, and therefore, their presence is not necessarily indicative of a lower respiratory tract source of the sample. The use of oil is necessary for the assessment of leukocytes and bacteria. A differential cell count is performed most easily on the Wright-Giemsa–stained specimen. The presence of large numbers of eosinophils (more than 20% to 30%) suggests atopic or parasitic disease. Additional findings supportive of asthma include the presence of Charcot-Leyden crystals, which are formed by the crystalization of eosinophil lysophospholipase; of Curschmann's spirals, which are bronchiolar casts; and of Creola bodies, which are composed of exfoliated epithelial cells.

The diagnosis of a specific bacterial pneumonia based on the presence or absence of bacteria and neutrophils in a Gram stain of a sputum specimen is subject to many pitfalls and consequently must be made with caution. The reliability of a sputum Gram stain can be maximized when the predominant organism is identified in an area with greater than 25 neutrophils and less than 10 squamous epithelial cells per low-power field. Even in these circumstances, however, false-positive and false-negative results occur frequently. One of the primary problems is that oral flora contaminate sputum as it is expectorated; thus differentiating contaminants from the etiologic agent(s) may be impossible. Other factors, such as the thickness of the smeared specimen, understaining or overstaining the slide, and the expertise of the reader, affect the reliability of the results. These problems are compounded in patients with chronic bronchitis because bacteria and neutrophils are present chronically in their lower respiratory tracts. Furthermore, severely neutropenic patients may not generate neutrophils in their sputum despite the presence of a bacterial pneumonia. For all of these reasons, the diagnosis of pneumonia caused by a specific etiologic agent can be made with certainty from a sputum sample only when the organism present in sputum is not part of the normal host oral flora and is not known to colonize the upper or lower respiratory tracts of subjects without pneumonia.

In some instances the induction of a sputum sample is helpful in establishing the etiology of suspected pulmonary pathology. This is especially true for patients who may have *Pneumocystis carinii* pneumonia complicating the acquired immunodeficiency syndrome (Chapters 242 and 281). A careful protocol has been worked out that has a sensitivity as high as 70%. Patients are allowed nothing by mouth for several hours and then prepped by brushing their teeth and gums and by washing their mouth several times with sterile saline or water. An ultrasonically generated mist of 3% saline is inhaled for approximately 10 to 15 minutes to induce cough and sputum production. The expectorated specimen then is liquefied using dithiothreitol and concentrated prior to making a slide to stain for the presence of *Pneumocystis* organisms.

Sputum also may be examined for the presence of malignant cells. If a sample cannot be delivered immediately for cytologic examination, it should be expectorated directly into a fixative solution. This procedure permits optimal preservation of cell morphology and helps maximize the positivity rate. Both outpatient and inpatient samples should be processed in this manner. As a general rule, the volume of sputum should not exceed the volume of fixative. If a patient is not spontaneously producing sputum, inhalation of an ultrasonically generated mist may induce cough and sputum production and thereby enhance the yield. It is important to note that the finding of malignant cells in sputum is not necessarily diagnostic of lung carcinoma as their presence may be caused by malignancy in respiratory passages above the vocal cords. In general, sputum cytologic examination has a sensitivity of approximately 30% to 50% in patients with centrally located tumors. The yield of sputum examination from patients with lung lesions located in the peripheral airways is significantly less. Examination of three to five specimens appears to maximize the yield in all instances. In view of the ease with which sputum may be obtained and the relatively low cost, cytologic examination is still regarded as the first step in the evaluation of a patient with suspected lung malignancy.

Alveolar macrophages with large cytoplasmic vacuoles can be seen in patients with lipoid pneumonia. These patients usually present with chronic infiltrates or masslike lesions on radiographic examination and result from aspirating oily substances such as mineral oil or oil-based nose drops. Industrial exposure to oil mists or aerosols might lead to more diffuse interstitial infiltrates. The presence of fat in the alveolar macrophage vacuoles can be confirmed by using a Sudan stain. A positive Sudan stain, however, is not pathognomonic of lipoid pneumonia or of fat embolism, since sudanophilic cytoplasmic inclusions may be of endogenous origin.

SKIN TESTING

Skin testing can be useful clinically in evaluating a patient with suspected tuberculous or mycotic infection and in identifying persons who have been infected previously. The skin test reactivity depends on the cell-mediated (type IV) immune reaction described in Chapter 286. This test relies on developing an area of induration at the site of injection. The peak of induration occurs at 24 to 72 hours after the intradermal injection of the antigen into the skin. With an especially strong immune reaction, skin necrosis can occur in the area of cellular infiltration, and regional lymphadenopathy can develop. Areas of vesiculation or necrosis of the skin are commonly treated with topical 0.1% hydrocortisone ointment.

A variety of both technical and host factors may be responsible for a false-negative reaction. The most common problem encountered is poor technique of administration. Any host factor that interferes with delayed hypersensitivity has the potential to interfere with a positive test. Recent viral infections or recent vaccination with a live virus may suppress, temporarily, delayed hypersensitivity. Patients with lymphomas, lymphoproliferative disorders, and sarcoidosis frequently fail to respond to skin testing. Therapeutic agents such as cyclophosphamide, nitrogen mustard, and corticosteroids depress delayed hypersensitivity. Reactivity may not return for several weeks after corticosteroid therapy has been discontinued. Elderly individuals and critically ill patients, including those with disseminated mycobacterial or fungal disease, also may demonstrate false-negative responses. It is always important to apply a control skin test reagent of mumps or trichophytin antigens to which most of the population should react, simultaneously with the specific test antigens.

Tuberculosis (Also see Chapter 276)

The tuberculin skin test becomes positive in most persons 6 to 8 weeks after infection. The standard preparation is a purified protein derivative (PPD) of the organism developed by Siebert in 1940. Three concentrations are commercially available that contain 1, 5, or 250 tuberculin units. The standard test dose used to screen for infection with tuberculosis is the intermediate strength (5 TU). The first- or second-strength concentrations have little clinical use. Second strength is so concentrated that many persons get a nonspecific inflammatory response whether or not they have been previously infected with *Mycobacterium tuberculosis* or other mycobacteria. As many as 8% of patients with culture-proven tuberculosis have been reported to have negative PPD skin tests when tested initially. These patients include the acutely ill whose skin tests become positive as they respond to antituberculous therapy and improve clinically. Many series report that 1% or 2% of patients with proved tuberculosis and no known reason for anergy fail to react to PPD. A negative tuberculin test, therefore, does not exclude the possibility of active tuberculosis.

Mantoux test. Intermediate PPD, 0.1 ml, is injected intradermally in the volar surface of the forearm with a 1 ml tuberculin syringe. If it is properly administered, a pale, raised wheal is immediately visible at the injection site. To interpret, measure the transverse diameter of induration, a firm raised area, 48 to 72 hours after injection. Erythema may or may not be present. Ten mm or greater of induration is a positive reaction in non-HIV-infected patients. In HIV-infected persons 5 mm of induration is considered a positive reaction because of a reduction in delayed-type hypersensitivity responses.

A positive test indicates past infection with *M. tuberculosis* and does not necessarily signify current active disease. Once a positive PPD has been determined and recorded, there is rarely any need to repeat the test since specific sensitivity for *M. tuberculosis* persists almost indefinitely after exposure. The size of the reaction may wane in the elderly. Four mm of induration or less is a negative reaction; 5 through 9 mm is a doubtful reaction. If the clinical picture or history of exposure warrants, the test should be repeated at a different site within 1 week. An indeterminate reaction can be seen in patients infected with nontuberculous mycobacteria that cross-reacts with PPD. Cross-reactivity to PPD does not occur with mycotic infections. In patients with an indeterminate reaction secondary to atypical mycobacterial infection or with a waning response to PPD, a repeat PPD applied within several weeks may yield an area of induration greater than 10 mm. This is referred to as a booster response and does not reflect true conversion from a negative to a positive response. The second test, therefore, may be a false positive but usually reverts to the indeterminate category if retesting is performed 6 to 12 months later. In most circumstances, a change of at least 6 mm from less than 10 mm to greater than 10 mm of induration can be considered indicative of new infection.

Various rapid multiple-puncture techniques are available for large-scale screening. Patients with positive reactions (palpable induration) must be rechecked with the quantitative intradermal Mantoux test because of a high incidence of cross-reaction to other mycobacteria seen with these rapid screening procedures.

Histoplasmosis (See Chapter 277)

Histoplasmin skin test reagent is primarily of value in epidemiologic studies. It is of little diagnostic or prognostic value in an individual patient. Moreover, its use can so interfere with interpretation of potentially more useful serologic tests for histoplasmosis infection that histoplasmin skin testing is inappropriate in clinical diagnosis.

Coccidioidomycosis (See Chapter 277)

The skin test can be useful diagnostically and prognostically in coccidioidomycosis. Unlike the histoplasmosis test, the coccidioidomycosis skin test does not influence serologies, and cross-reactivity of the standard concentrations is much less of a clinical problem. Two skin test materials are available.

Coccidioidin. Coccidioidin is a preparation from the mycelial phase of the yeast that has been used for more than 40 years. One tenth of a ml of a 1:100 dilution is injected intradermally. Induration of 5 mm or more at 24 to 48 hours is positive. The induration in some reactors may fade after 36 hours and might be missed if the skin site is checked only at 48 hours. The vast majority of patients with primary pulmonary infection with coccidioidomycosis have a positive skin test within 3 weeks of infection. The skin test reactivity persists for many years but eventually wanes and becomes negative.

In patients with erythema nodosum who have symptoms suggestive of coccidioidomycosis, skin testing with the 1:100 dilution can cause local skin necrosis and exacerbate the systemic disease. Initial testing should be done with a 1:1000 or even 1:10,000 dilution.

With disseminated coccidioidomycosis, anergy often develops. As patients begin to respond to therapy, initially negative skin tests become positive. If the skin test with the 1:100 dilution of coccidioidin is negative in a patient with disseminated coccidioidomycosis, a 1:10 dilution should be applied. Lack of skin reactivity to this higher concentration is a particularly bad prognostic sign.

Spherulin. Spherulin is prepared from the spherule phase of the organism and has been in use for about 10 years. Like coccidioidin, it is available commercially in a 1:100 (usual dose) and 1:10 (high) concentration. Its indications, application, precautions, and interpretation are the same as for coccidioidin. Epidemiologic studies show that 25% to 35% more persons in endemic areas have a positive skin test to the spherulin form, indicating that it is more sensitive than coccidioidin. The prognostic role of spherulin in patients with disseminated disease is not clear, and in this situation the coccidioidin form is currently more valuable.

Blastomycosis (See Chapter 277)

The skin test for blastomycosis yields many false-positive and false-negative results and therefore is of little or no value.

SEROLOGY

The detection of serum antibodies to a number of pathogenic organisms has diagnostic usefulness. Often a significant rise in titer occurs after an acute infection. There can be a subsequent fall with maintenance of persistent low levels for months to years. The documentation of the acute rise generally has the greatest clinical value. The peak rise occurring 3 to 4 weeks after the initial infection may allow serologic tests to be of diagnostic value only in retrospect.

Histoplasmosis (See Chapter 277)

Complement-fixation titers for both the mycelial and yeast phases of histoplasmosis are usually but not always high in patients with acute primary pulmonary disease (95%) or disseminated disease (65%). Only 35% of patients with chronic cavitary histoplasmosis have titers as high as 1:32, but 70% of patients with acute histoplasmosis have titers of 1:32 or greater. An initial histoplasmin complement-fixation titer of 1:64 or a serial fourfold rise in titer is generally considered diagnostic. Fewer than 5% of persons living in an endemic area have complement-fixation titers of 1:8 or 1:16 with no evidence of current disease. In patients with chronic cavitary histoplasmosis, a sudden rise in titer may presage clinical relapse. Prior application of a histoplasmin skin test can "artificially" elevate complement-fixation titers. The mycelial phase titers are most likely to show an acute elevation that lasts for several months after the skin test is applied. Also, cross-reactivity to multiple fungal agents has been demonstrated with the complement-fixation studies.

A gel diffusion test of sera for antibodies against concentrated histoplasmin can produce two significant bands in the patient with *Histoplasma* infection. The *M band* develops early in infection and can persist for long periods. It can be induced or increased by a histoplasmin skin test. The *H band* is usually found in patients with active disease only and is not influenced by skin testing. It disappears more rapidly than the M band but often can still be detected in a patient's serum several months after pulmonary involvement when the disease appears stable. A positive gel diffusion test can be used to rule out cross-reactivity as a cause of a positive histoplasmosis complement-fixation test.

Recently, evidence suggests that diverse forms of histoplasmosis can be diagnosed using techniques to detect antigen in serum and urine. These techniques are not widely available at this time.

Coccidioidomycosis (See Chapter 277)

Acute infection with coccidioidomycosis causes an early (1-3 weeks) but very transient rise in specific immunoglobulin M (IgM) antibodies. This increase can be detected by a tube precipitin test, immunodiffusion, or a latex particle agglutination test in serum. Ninety percent of symptomatic patients are positive for the tube precipitin test within 3 weeks of infection. The latex particle agglutination test is even more sensitive in detecting the early IgM levels but is less specific. There is a 10% false-positive rate. These tests have no prognostic value.

IgG levels increase later in infection but can remain elevated for years. This antibody is detected with complement-fixation or immunodiffusion tests. High titers, greater than 1:32, are seen often in patients with disseminated disease and portend a poorer prognosis. The titer falls with response to therapy. Serial studies, therefore, have prognostic value. Approximately 75% of patients with coccidioidomycosis meningitis have positive complement-fixation titers in the cerebrospinal fluid. An exoantigen test also is available to identify putative cultures of *C. immitis*.

Blastomycosis

A complement-fixation test is available for blastomycosis but is of little use, as it lacks sensitivity and specificity.

Aspergillosis (See Chapter 277)

Serologic tests are helpful in the diagnosis of patients with allergic bronchopulmonary aspergillosis (ABPA). Precipitating antibodies against *Aspergillus fumigatus* are found in the serum of almost all patients with ABPA but also in about 25% of patients with other forms of extrinsic asthma. Total serum IgE levels are high in both groups, and although they are highest in patients with ABPA, overlap occurs. Specific IgE and IgG levels against *A. fumigatus* determined by radioimmunoassay frequently are higher in patients with ABPA than with other forms of asthma, although overlap occurs.

Once a diagnosis of ABPA has been made by standard criteria, a total serum IgE level can be followed to monitor the response to therapy and clinical course.

Antibody titers are not helpful in the diagnosis of invasive aspergillosis. However, the determination of serum antigen titers is a promising diagnostic tool that is not yet widely available.

Cryptococcosis

Although cryptococcal antigen and antibody studies are most useful in patients with cryptococcal meningitis, they may have some value in patients with cryptococcal lung diseases (see Chapter 279).

Mycoplasma pneumoniae (See Chapter 255)

Mycoplasma pneumoniae can cause upper and lower respiratory tract infections. The pneumonic form can be confirmed, at least during the convalescent phase, by serologic testing. The *M. pneumoniae* complement-fixation titer assay is used most commonly. The complement-fixation titers start to rise about 1 week after onset of infection and reach a peak in another 3 weeks. High levels persist for approximately half a year and then taper to low levels, less than 1:16, over the next several years. A fourfold rise in titers between an acute and convalescent serum is considered diagnostic. If an acute serum was not obtained, a titer of at least 1:64 in the convalescent sera can be considered presumptive evidence of *M. pneumoniae* infection in an appropriate clinical setting. A promising and now commercially available test examines specimens for the organism's ribosomal RNA using a complementary radiolabeled DNA probe. The test appears to have a sensitivity and specificity approaching 90%. More clinical experience with this test is needed, however.

Cold agglutinin, a nonspecific IgM autoantibody directed at the I antigen on red blood cells, also rises in titer and reaches a peak in 2 to 3 weeks in most patients with pulmonary involvement with *M. pneumoniae*. Titers greater than 1:64 usually are seen. Very high titers can be associated with hemolysis. Cold agglutinin titer elevation is observed also with psittacosis, infectious mononucleosis, many viral infections, and lymphoproliferative diseases, and therefore, is nonspecific.

Legionnaires' disease (See Chapter 272)

Legionella pneumophila and other *Legionella* species cause the pneumonia known as *legionnaires' disease*. Three serologic methods are currently used to establish the diagnosis: (1) a direct fluorescent antibody test can be performed on sputum, pleural fluid, transtracheal aspirate secretions, bronchial washings, or lavage specimens, and on lung tissue. When performed by a skilled individual, this test is rapid and more than 90% specific, but only 50% sensitive. Each *Legionella* species requires a separate and specific fluorescent antibody. (2) An indirect fluorescent antibody technique and an enzyme-linked immunoabsorbent assay (ELISA) currently are used to detect specific serum antibodies. Most patients demonstrate a fourfold rise in titer within weeks of their illness. A single titer more than 1:256 suggests but does not prove recent infection. (3) Recently, a radioimmunoassay for antigen in urine has been developed and is commercially available. Positive results are 90% specific and about 80% sensitive. The test at this time is available only for *L. pneumophila* of serogroup 1. The concomitant culture of the organism along with serologic evidence of infection firmly establishes the diagnosis.

THORACENTESIS

The space separating the visceral pleura and the parietal pleura normally contains several ml of fluid. The parietal pleura is perfused by systemic arterial vessels with a mean capillary pressure of 30 cm H_2O. The visceral pleura is perfused by vessels of the pulmonary circulation with a mean capillary pressure of 11 cm H_2O. The 19 cm difference in hydrostatic pressure normally causes fluid to enter the pleural space from the parietal pleura and to be reabsorbed by the visceral pleura. Cells and macromolecules return to the circulation via the lymphatics. A variety of disorders can disrupt the normal equilibrium of transudation and reabsorption and lead to accumulation of a pleural effusion. Alterations in hydrostatic pressures, obstruction of lymphatic drainage, reduction in osmotic pressure, or changes in capillary permeability from inflammation or tumor invasion can result in fluid accumulation. Thus, pleural effusion can be a sign of either intrathoracic or extrathoracic disease. Thoracentesis, aspiration of pleural fluid for symptomatic relief and/or analysis, sometimes yields a specific diagnosis but often just narrows the diagnostic possibilities.

Conditions that alter the vascular and osmotic pressures without directly involving the pleura itself, such as heart failure, nephrotic syndrome, myxedema, and cirrhosis, cause a transudative fluid to accumulate.

Conditions associated with inflammation of the pleura such as tumor, connective tissue disease, trauma, and infection cause the accumulation of an exudative fluid. Criteria based on the pleural fluid protein concentration and pleural fluid lactic dehydrogenase concentration allow the differentiation of exudates and transudates (Table 196-1). In exudates the pleural fluid protein/serum protein concentration ratio is greater than 0.5. The pleural fluid lactic dehydrogenase concentration serum lactic dehydrogenase concentration ratio is greater than 0.6 and the absolute pleural fluid lactic dehydrogenase concentration is greater than two thirds of the upper limit of normal. Pleural fluid meeting any one of these three criteria qualifies as an exudate. WBC, RBC, and glucose determinations tend to be as shown in Table 196-1 but are not included in the separation of transudative and exudative effusions. Thoracentesis should be performed in any patient with a pleural effusion of unknown cause. The only major exception is a patient with clinical findings of congestive heart failure whose effusion decreases with appropriate therapy. With the initial diagnostic aspiration, no more than 1 liter should be removed. Acute pulmonary edema and hypotension have been reported after removal of larger quantities.

Information useful in the diagnosis of a pleural effusion is summarized in the box on the right. Two findings on analysis of the effusion can yield a specific etiologic diagnosis. A positive smear and/or culture for bacteria, fungi, or mycobacteria has clinical importance since the pleural space is normally sterile. In a patient with a pneumonic process and a pleural effusion, culture of the effusion provides a reliable means of identifying the pathogen. Only one third of patients with a tuberculous pleural effusion have a positive culture of the fluid. Pleural biopsy for microscopic examination and culture increases the diagnostic yield to almost 70%.

Table 196-1. Pleural fluid classification

	Transudate	Exudate
Pleural TP/Serum TP	<0.5	>0.5
LDH	<2/3 upper normal limit	>2/3 upper normal limit
Pleural LDH/Serum LDH	<0.6	>0.6
WBC	<1000	>1000
RBC	<1000	>100,000
Glucose	=blood	<blood

TP, total protein; LDH, lactic dehydrogenase; WBC, white blood count; RBC, red blood count.

Information useful for the diagnosis of pleural effusions

I. Specific diagnostic aids
   A. Positive smear and/or culture for bacteria, mycobacteria, or fungi
   B. Positive cytology for primary or metastatic neoplasm or for lymphoma
   C. "True" chylous effusion-disruption or invasion of thoracic ducts
II. Potentially useful characteristics in differential diagnosis
   A. Elevated pleural fluid amylase/serum amylase ratio suggests
      1. Pancreatitis
      2. Pancreatic pseudocyst
      3. Ruptured esophagus (salivary amylase)
      4. Neoplasm
   B. Pleural fluid/serum glucose ratio <0.5 suggests tuberculosis, tumor, parapneumonic effusion, rheumatoid arthritis, or systemic lupus erythematosus
   C. Red blood count >100,000/mm^3 associated most often with tumors, trauma, and embolus with infarction
   D. Lymphocytosis in exudate (>50% lymphocytes) seen in chronic effusions
   E. Pleural fluid eosinophilia rare in malignant and tuberculous effusions unless there is a coincident pneumothorax
   F. Greater than 1% mesothelial cells rare in tuberculous effusion
   G. Pseudochylous effusions (cholesterol crystals) seen with chronic effusion of rheumatoid disease, tuberculosis, and trapped lung
   H. Elevated acid mucopolysaccharide and hyaluronic acid levels usually associated with mesothelioma
   I. Lupus erythematosus cells: presence diagnostic of lupus pleuritis
   J. pH <7.1 in parapneumonic effusion suggests, but alone does not mandate, need for closed-tube thoracostomy
   K. Foul-smelling odor characteristic of anaerobic infection

A positive cytology is a second specific diagnostic aid from pleural fluid examination. For patients with malignant effusions, one third to two thirds have positive cytologic findings in their initial pleural fluid examination. The incidence of a positive cytology increases with the volume of fluid analyzed. Thus, up to 90% of malignant effusions can be confirmed cytologically if three separate pleural fluid specimens are analyzed. Inflammation can cause bizarre mesothelial cell changes that can be confused with neoplastic changes. Also, in patients with large, long-standing neoplastic effusions, the free malignant cells in the effusion can degenerate in vivo with time and prevent definitive cytologic diagnosis. A second or third thoracentesis specimen containing freshly shed cells might allow a more specific diagnosis.

A milky or creamy appearance to pleural effusion suggests chylothorax, which can be confirmed by Sudan III stain, by measuring triglyceride levels, and by the presence of a chylomicron band on lipoprotein electrophoresis. Chylous effusion is caused by disruption of the thoracic duct resulting from trauma, lymphoma, tumor invasion, or, less commonly, granulomatous involvement of the mediastinum. A pseudochylous appearance can occur in chronic effusion (e.g., in rheumatoid disease). Pseudochylous effusions are recognized by the presence of rhomboid cholesterol crystals, the absence of the lymphocytosis seen in association with true chylous effusion, and a high cholesterol but low triglyceride level.

An extremely low pleural fluid glucose level (0 to 20 mg/dl) suggests a rheumatoid effusion. A pleural fluid glucose level of 20 to 40 mg per deciliter is commonly noted with large intrathoracic tumors, the presence of free malignant cells in the pleural space, or empyema.

Approximately 10% of patients with pancreatitis have a pleural effusion in the left hemithorax. A pancreatic pseudocyst under the right side of the diaphragm can cause an effusion in that hemithorax. The pleural fluid amylase levels in these two conditions can be higher than the serum amylase concentration. With esophageal rupture, amylase of salivary origin can be found on thoracentesis. The source of this amylase can be differentiated by electrophoresis. Slight elevation in pleural fluid amylase, usually less than 1000 units, can be seen in patients with primary bronchogenic carcinoma or metastatic carcinoma of gastrointestinal or breast origin.

A complete cell count on pleural fluid is of relatively little diagnostic value. A red cell count greater than 100,000 per milliliter is usually found in association with trauma. About one fifth of patients with malignant effusions also have very high red cell counts. A smaller percentage of patients with pulmonary infarction have a pleural fluid red cell count greater than 100,000, though over half have a bloody appearance to their effusions. The finding of over 50% lymphocytes in an exudate is consistent with many chronic effusions and is not particularly suggestive of tuberculosis or malignancy. A predominance of eosinophils in pleural fluid does not have the specificity for allergic or noninfectious inflammatory disease that it does in sputum. A high pleural fluid eosinophil count, however, is reputedly rare in tuberculous or malignant effusions unless there is a concurrent pneumothorax. Several entities, such as hemothorax, pneumothorax, previous thoracentesis, fungal disease, and parasitic disease, predispose to pleural fluid eosinophilia. The presence of more than 1% mesothelial cells is also rare in a tuberculous effusion.

In some patients with pleural tumors such as mesothelioma, acid mucopolysaccharide and hyaluronic acid concentrations are increased. However, tests for these substances are not standardized, and normal values may vary markedly among laboratories. Hence, the reliability of these test results is difficult to determine. The specific cause of a pleural effusion usually is not determined from pleural fluid analysis alone, but from integration of the patient's history, physical findings, radiographic studies, and other laboratory data with pleural fluid characteristics. The various biochemical assays should be ordered selectively for each patient. In spite of appropriate analyses, 20% of patients may not have a specific etiology determined at the time of their initial examination.

PLEURAL BIOPSY

Percutaneous pleural biopsy can increase the diagnostic yield over thoracentesis alone when an exudate is documented and the etiology remains unclear. The complications of pleural biopsies should be little more than those of thoracentesis alone, if there is an adequate amount of pleural effusion. The procedure should not be uncomfortable for the patient if the skin, periosteum of the upper surface of the rib at the biopsy site, and parietal pleura are adequately anesthetized. Care must be taken to keep the biopsy needle on the superior surface of the rib to avoid the neurovascular bundles running along the inferior surfaces of the rib. Collection of four to six samples from separate sites increases the diagnostic yield. Pleural biopsies are particularly helpful in diagnosing pleural effusions secondary to tuberculosis or malignancy. A recent review of over 400 patients who had both thoracentesis and pleural biopsy showed that thoracentesis established a diagnosis of malignancy in 58% and pleural biopsy in 43%. The pleural biopsy was positive in 7% of patients with a tumor when thoracentesis cytology was negative.

Typical granulomas may be seen on microscopic visualization, and occasionally organisms are revealed by special stain. Culture of the pleural tissue may grow mycobacteria even if the histologic study does not show specific changes.

Primary pleural tumors, such as mesotheliomas, may be difficult to diagnose with certainty on the relatively small samples obtained from pleural biopsies. A variety of inflammatory processes can lead to bizarre changes in the mesothelial lining cells, which the pathologist may have difficulty in differentiating from neoplastic changes. The definitive diagnosis of mesothelioma often requires an open biopsy.

BRONCHOSCOPY AND BIOPSIES

Table 196-2 summarizes the invasive techniques used to evaluate potential pulmonary disease. The introduction of the flexible fiberoptic bronchoscope in the late 1960s added a powerful tool for the diagnostic workup of many patients with bronchial or pulmonary parenchymal abnormalities. It has largely, though not completely, replaced the older rigid bronchoscope for examination of the tracheobronchial tree. The typical diagnostic fiberoptic bronchoscope has a 4 mm to 6 mm external diameter and contains a 2 mm biopsy and suction channel. Biopsy forceps, cytology brushes, and saline for lavage and washings can be introduced through the channel. The distal end can be flexed at least at an angle of 120° for insertion into segmental and subsegmental bronchi. By contrast, the rigid bronchoscope can visualize directly only the trachea, the major bronchi, and the openings to some of the segmental bronchi. The fiberoptic bronchoscope, therefore, offers greatly increased visual and biopsy range with greater patient comfort.

Table 196-2. Summary of diagnostic techniques

Biopsy technique	Appropriate application	Potential complications
Thoracentesis	Pleural effusion Diagnostic and therapeutic reasons	Pneumothorax-R Hemothorax-R Infection-R
Pleural biopsy	Pleural fluid Exudate of uncertain etiology Increases diagnostic yield with malignancy and granulomatous disease	Pneumothorax-R Hemothorax-R
Fiberoptic bronchoscopy with brush and biopsy	Central endobronchial lesion	Hypoxemia Hemoptysis-R
	Peripheral nodules or infiltrates—moderate yield; drops to low yield with lesion <2 cm	Pneumothorax Hemoptysis
	Diffuse interstitial disease—moderate yield	Pneumothorax Hemoptysis
	Search for bleeding with mild to moderate hemoptysis	Worsens hemoptysis-R
	Preoperative staging for thoracotomy with neoplastic disease	
Rigid bronchoscopy	Massive hemoptysis	Worsens hemoptysis
	Biopsy of upper airway obstructive lesion	Further compromises upper airway
	Foreign body removal	
Needle aspiration	Peripheral nodules—high yield Pneumonic infiltrates (particularly in immunocompromised patients)—moderate yield	Pneumothorax-C Hemoptysis Air embolus-R
Bronchoalveolar lavage	Infiltrates (particularly in immunocompromised host)—high yield and very low morbidity. Particularly safe in patient at high risk for bleeding	Worsens hypoxia
Open biopsy	In patient in whom other techniques have not yielded a specific diagnosis and clinical condition warrants surgery; in patient who is critically ill and does not have time to try serial procedures prior to starting therapy Bleeding diathesis or pulmonary hypertension	Pneumothorax-C
Thoracoscopy	Pleural disease, peripheral lung mass, or interstitial lung disease	Pneumothorax-C
Mediastinoscopy	Right paratracheal masses	Pneumothorax-R

R, rare; C, common.

Fiberoptic bronchoscopy is useful (1) for diagnosing lung masses or infiltrates of uncertain etiology, (2) to evaluate hemoptysis or abnormal cytologic findings with normal chest radiograph, and (3) in preoperative evaluation of a patient with known chest malignancy. It is possible to perform biopsies or obtain aspirates for culture. In addition to having diagnostic functions, the fiberoptic bronchoscope is used therapeutically to remove retained secretions and to remove foreign bodies beyond the reach of the rigid bronchoscope.

The fiberoptic bronchoscope is used generally with only topical anesthesia while the patient is awake or slightly sedated. It can be introduced through either the nose or mouth, with or without an endotracheal tube. Diagnostic fiberoptic bronchoscopy is a very safe procedure. Fluoroscopic guidance is helpful when pulmonary parenchymal biopsies are to be obtained or when peripheral masses or nodules are to be sampled. About half of the primary chest neoplasms presenting as radiographic abnormalities can be visualized directly through the fiberoptic bronchoscope. Better than a 90% diagnostic yield is obtained for central endobronchial lesions. A greater than 70% diagnostic yield can be obtained from peripheral lesions when cytology brushes and biopsy forceps are guided into the lesion under fluoroscopic control. Carcinoma metastatic to the lung also can be diagnosed by biopsy through the fiberoptic bronchoscope. With the exception of tumors of genitourinary tract origin, metastatic lesions to the lung tend to be peripheral and need to be subjected to biopsy under fluoroscopic control. The diagnostic yield for fiberoptic bronchoscopy decreases to about 20% for lesions less than 2 cm in diameter and for those located in the outer periphery of the lung field.

In addition to establishing the cell type of primary or metastatic carcinomas of the lung, fiberoptic bronchoscopy is useful in preoperative staging. Blind biopsy of a normal-appearing main carina in patients with bronchogenic carcinoma has uncovered microscopic neoplastic invasion in as many as 10% of patients. This finding alters the therapeutic approach. In patients with positive cytologic findings and an abnormal chest radiograph, the tumor site has been localized to lobes other than the site of the apparent radiographic abnormality. In other patients tumors have been found bilaterally by bronchoscopy, although the involvement of only one side was apparent radiographically. In patients with hemoptysis or abnormal sputum cytologies but normal chest radiographs, the fiberoptic bronchoscope is the best diagnostic tool for locating the site of disease. Occult bronchogenic neoplasms can be found in a significant percentage of adult smokers presenting with hemoptysis and normal chest films. By including a thorough examination of the nasal and oral pharynx with the fiberoptic scope, one can uncover additional occult neoplasms. With the use of a transbronchial needle, subcarinal, right paratracheal, and, to a limited extent, left paratracheal nodes can be aspirated through the fiberoptic bronchoscope to aid in staging and diagnosis of carcinoma of the lung.

In patients with diffuse interstitial disease, transbronchial biopsy through the fiberoptic bronchoscope may provide adequate histologic material for specific diagnosis. Complications include a low (less than 5%) incidence of pneumothorax, fever, and hemoptysis of more than 10 ml of blood. Fluoroscopic control may be helpful in obtaining tissue. Multiple samples (six to eight) can be taken but are obtained generally from only one lung, since pneumothorax remains a risk even when the biopsy is done under fluoroscopic control.

Not all patients are candidates for fiberoptic bronchoscopy. As the procedure is performed under local anesthesia in awake patients with the instrument passed through either the nose or mouth, patient cooperation is important. Two relative contraindications are severe hypoxemia that cannot be readily corrected with supplemental oxygen and acute hypercapnia. Bleeding diatheses, recent myocardial infarction, and untreated pulmonary tuberculosis are additional relative contraindications. Patients at increased risk include those with bronchospastic disease such as asthma, pulmonary hypertension, superior vena cava obstruction, massive hemoptysis, and uremia. Patients at risk for a serious complication or with one or more relative contraindications can be sedated and intubated. The procedure then can be performed with or without mechanical ventilation. With careful preprocedure evaluation, proper technique, and monitoring during the procedure, the incidence of complications is low. However, bleeding, pneumothorax, adverse reaction to an anesthetic agent, blood gas deterioration with associated arrhythmias, and death are all potential complications. The procedure should be carried out only by well-trained physicians with adequate support personnel and in facilities that can handle emergencies.

The rigid bronchoscope still has a clinical role. It is of value in pediatric patients and in patients with partial upper airway obstruction in which the solid fiberoptic bronchoscope would completely obstruct the upper airway. The rigid scope is also useful in patients with massive hemoptysis and for internal drainage of lung abscesses in which the small suction channel of the fiberoptic scope would be overwhelmed by large volumes of fluid, blood, or pus. The rigid scope generally is used in an operating suite with the patient under general anesthesia.

BRONCHOALVEOLAR LAVAGE

Bronchoalveolar lavage (BAL) is a relatively new tool for the clinician. This procedure is performed through a fiberoptic bronchoscope that is wedged in a segmental bronchus. Usually 20 to 50 ml of a physiologic solution are infused sequentially with aspiration after each instillate. Instilled volumes totaling 100 to 300 ml are used most commonly. Swan-Ganz–like catheters now exist that can be inserted through the bronchoscope's channel. The balloon is inflated to sequester a portion of the lung and a smaller volume lavage is performed through the catheter's tip. Bronchoalveolar lavage fluid can be analyzed for total cells, differential cell count, and the presence of parasites. It can also be stained and cultured for bacteria, viruses, and fungi. The isolation of almost any organism that does not normally colonize the upper or lower respiratory tract, such as *Legionella, Histoplasma, P. carinii,* or *M. tuberculosis,* is diagnostic of infection. Recent data suggest that the isolation of commonly encountered gram-positive or gram-negative bacteria at greater than 10^5 colony-forming units/ml in a semiquantitative culture is very suggestive of pneumonia caused by the isolated organism(s). A few relatively uncommon diseases such as eosinophilic pneumonia, alveolar proteinosis, and eosinophilic granuloma also can be diagnosed by findings in BAL fluid from patients with a clinical syndrome that is consistent with the above diseases. Additional diagnoses that can be made with the assistance of BAL include lung carcinoma, berylliosis, and pulmonary hemorrhage (see box below).

Lung lavage initially was used as a method for the removal of inspissated airway secretions; later BAL was used to investigate immunopathogenic mechanisms relevant to numerous interstitial lung diseases or lung defense mechanisms in normal hosts. Some data suggest BAL cell differentials are useful in the initial evaluation of patients with undiagnosed interstitial lung disease. Likewise, BAL cell differentials also may be helpful in the assessment of the activity of various lung diseases such as idiopathic pulmonary fibrosis. However, most pulmonologists agree that its

Diagnostic applications of bronchoalveolar lavage

- Infectious pneumonias
  - *Pneumocystis carinii*
  - Cytomegalovirus
  - Legionellosis
  - Cryptococcosis
  - Histoplasmosis
  - Tuberculosis
  - Aspergillosis
- Other pulmonary disorders
  - Malignancy
  - Hemorrhage
  - Alveolar proteinosis
  - Eosinophilic granuloma
  - Chronic eosinophilic pneumonia
  - Drug-induced lung disease
  - Berylliosis
  - Hypersensitivity pneumonitis

usefulness as a clinical tool resides with the ease, safety, and sensitivity with which BAL can assist in the diagnosis of lung infections. A major advantage to BAL is that it can be performed with relative safety in patients with significant disturbances of their coagulation systems and on patients requiring mechanical ventilation. Potential major complications are similar to those for fiberoptic bronchoscopy except that pneumothorax and hemorrhage rarely occur. BAL should be distinguished from whole lung lavage, which is used only occasionally in the treatment of alveolar proteinosis.

PROTECTED BRUSH CATHETER

Samples of lower respiratory tract secretions can be retrieved with minimal contamination by upper respiratory tract organisms through the use of a protected brush catheter. This catheter has a brush within a double sheath that is sealed at the distal end with a soluble plug. After introduction through the fiberoptic bronchoscope and into the airway to be sampled, the plug is extruded, the sample is obtained, and the brush is withdrawn within its sheath. Data on the value of this technique in the diagnosis of pneumonia are variable, but it appears promising, particularly when meticulous attention is paid to details of the procedure. The isolation of organisms at greater than 10^4 colony-forming units/ml suggests bacterial pneumonia.

TRANSTRACHEAL ASPIRATION

Transtracheal aspiration is another technique used to obtain lower respiratory tract secretions relatively free from contamination by upper respiratory tract flora. The procedure is performed under local anesthesia using a needle with an indwelling catheter that is advanced through the cricothyroid membrane. Aspirated secretions can be stained and cultured for pathogenic organisms. As with the protected brush catheter, data on the value of this technique vary. Interpretation of results is particularly difficult for patients with chronic bronchitis, many of whom have tracheal colonization with bacteria. When the procedure is performed by an experienced individual, the incidence of significant complications is low, and the results are helpful in diagnosing infectious pneumonias.

TRANSTHORACIC NEEDLE ASPIRATION

An alternative approach to the fiberoptic bronchoscope is transthoracic needle aspiration. A small-gauge spinal needle or a thin-walled 23- or 25-gauge needle made specifically for needle aspiration can be introduced under local anesthesia into lung nodules percutaneously with the assistance of computed axial tomography or fluoroscopy. The operator can often determine when the lesion has been entered by seeing it move and feeling a sense of resistance at the end of the needle. If attempts to aspirate fluid and cells from the lesion are unsuccessful initially, a few cm^3 of saline can be injected into the lesion and the aspiration repeated. Material can be obtained for cytologic evaluation and culture. With malignant lesions, a greater than 90% diagnostic yield has been reported in some series.

The incidence of pneumothorax has been 20% to 30% although only a small percentage of the patients have required a chest tube to reexpand the lung. A 10% to 20% incidence of hemoptysis has been reported, but this side effect is usually self-limited. In addition to evaluating solitary pulmonary nodules, needle aspiration can sample parenchymal or pleural masses and mediastinal or hilar lymph nodes.

Contraindications to needle aspiration are a bleeding diathesis, the presence of blebs or bullae in the immediate vicinity of the potential biopsy site, pulmonary hypertension, suspected vascular lesions such as arteriovenous malformations, and the inability of the patient to cooperate or to hold his or her breath for short periods. Aspiration with a thin, flexible needle also can prove useful in diagnosing pneumonia, particularly in the complex setting of the host who has undergone immunosuppression. Thus, needle aspiration provides an alternative to BAL or brushing with a protected brush catheter.

THORACOSCOPY

Thoracoscopy (also referred to as *pleuroscopy*) is a procedure in which a fiberoptic thoracoscope is introduced into the pleural space through a small intercostal incision with the patient under general anesthesia. The pleura can be inspected visually and biopsied under direct observation. In addition, it is also possible to biopsy peripheral lung parenchyma. Thus, it can spare the patient the more invasive thoracotomy. Thoracoscopy has been used extensively in Europe and now is being used with an increasing frequency in the United States.

OPEN LUNG BIOPSY

The decision to proceed to open lung biopsy is predicated upon several points, such as the diagnostic success or failure of less invasive tests and the speed with which a diagnosis is needed. This procedure requires general anesthesia and is the most invasive of diagnostic tests used to diagnose thoracic disease. A significant advantage of open lung biopsy is that through a large chest wall incision, the surgeon gains access to one entire chest cavity. Consequently, masses deep within the lung can be biopsied. In addition, larger quantities of lung parenchyma can be removed than by other, less invasive techniques. Furthermore, hilar and mediastinal lymph nodes can be sampled, which permits an assessment of the spread of a disease.

MEDIASTINOSCOPY AND MEDIASTINOTOMY

For mediastinoscopy a small incision is made at the suprasternal notch under general anesthesia. A mediastinoscope is inserted and advanced as tissue planes are dissected along the right side of the trachea. Right paratracheal lymph nodes or masses can be biopsied as far down as the main carina. A similar procedure cannot be performed on the left side of the trachea because of the presence of the great vessels. When it is necessary to biopsy selectively anterior left-sided masses or nodes situated near the aorta and pulmonary artery, a mediastinotomy is performed in which a small incision is made in the area of the second or third costal cartilages near the sternum with the patient under general anesthesia. This permits an extrapleural approach to left-sided lesions and can be performed quickly.

REFERENCES

Sputum Examination

Epstein RL: Constituents of sputum: a simple method. Ann Intern Med 77:259, 1972.

Skin Tests and Serologies

Snider DE Jr: The tuberculin skin test. Am Rev Respir Dis 125(suppl):108, 1982.

Barnes PF et al: Tuberculosis in patients with human immunodeficiency virus infection. N Engl J Med 324:1644, 1991.

Wheat J et al: The diagnostic laboratory tests for histoplasmosis: analysis of experience in a large urban outbreak. Ann Intern Med 97:680, 1982.

Thoracentesis and Pleural Biopsy

Prakash UBS and Reiman HM: Comparison of needle biopsy with cytologic analysis for the evaluation of pleural effusion. Mayo Clin Proc 60:158, 1985.

Sahn SA: The pleura. Am Rev Respir Dis 138:184, 1988.

Bronchoscopy, Needle Aspiration, and Bronchoalveolar Lavage

Goldstein RA et al: Clinical role of bronchoalveolar lavage in adults with pulmonary disease. Am Rev Respir Dis 142:481, 1990.

Reynolds HY: Bronchoalveolar lavage. Am Rev Respir Dis 135:250, 1987.

Westcott JL: Percutaneous transthoracic needle biopsy. Radiology 169:593, 1988.

CHAPTER

197 Pulmonary Diagnostic Imaging

Vernon A. Vix
Dewey J. Conces, Jr.
Robert D. Tarver

Pulmonary imaging methods vary from noninvasive to invasive. They are associated with varying degrees of discomfort, risk, and expense. In approximately 90% of instances, the plain chest radiograph is the only imaging study needed. Unfortunately, it can be normal or nonspecific in the presence of significant disease.

To make the plain radiograph and other modes of imaging most useful, the clinician should:

1. View all films independently.
2. Review all films with a radiologist. Do not depend solely on the written report.
3. Know that previous or old chest radiographs can be invaluable. Most adults have had one. Take the trouble to obtain it.
4. Be aware that anatomic abnormalities may reflect physiologic changes, for example, elevated diaphragms in noncompliant lungs and large upper lobe vessels in pulmonary venous hypertension.
5. Use the radiologist as a consultant in planning the patient's investigation.

The variety of specialized pulmonary imaging modalities presented in the discussion that follows has not lessened the importance of a competent clinician.

COMPUTED TOMOGRAPHY

Computed tomography makes use of a collimated x-ray beam of variable width (1.5 to 10.0 mm) to obtain information limited to that slice thickness. The anatomy is studied and displayed in cross section. The area of interest is studied with successive slices of predetermined thickness and spacing. Information for each slice is obtained in approximately 2 seconds. Density discrimination on CT is ten times that of conventional radiographs. Soft-tissue pulmonary nodules as small as 1 mm can be detected. Density graduations called Hounsfield units (HU) are based on a scale of −1000 for air to 0 for water. The ability to discriminate density differences allows the detection of tissue interphases such as fluid in cysts or lymph nodes surrounded by fat in the mediastinum. Fat can be recognized by its low density (−70 to −130 HU).

Contrast agents may be given intravenously to identify normal or abnormal vascular structures. The information can be displayed at different window widths of density and at different levels of density, allowing optimal demonstration of abnormalities.

CT is not a routine screening procedure. It should be used to help clarify specific problems and should always be preceded by a recent chest radiograph.

Computed tomography is indicated in the presence of a known extrapulmonary malignancy, for example, renal cell carcinoma, osteosarcoma, and melanoma, when the detection of pulmonary metastasis alters therapy. A significant number of nodules of less than 5 mm are benign, so the problem of a false-positive diagnosis of metastasis is always present.

The solitary pulmonary nodule is a common problem. No change in growth over 2 years and the unequivocal presence of central calcification are the only two reliable signs of benignancy. CT is able to identify calcium not visible on plain films. Phantoms that simulate specific anatomic locations and appropriate test objects are available to avoid the technical variables that are inherent in density determinations. In our department CT density determination using this phantom has been found to be very useful in evaluating the solitary nodule that does not contain calcium on a low-kV radiograph. Density measurements done without the phantom require special care. Accuracy of the equipment cannot be presumed but requires frequent calibration. Emphasis is placed on previous films, history of a prior malignancy, smoking history, associated disease, and age factors that might indicate the need for needle aspiration biopsy or other more definitive studies.

CT is also useful to establish or exclude a questionable lesion seen on the chest radiograph and to detect the presence of cavitation.

Evaluation of lung nodules with CT is not without its difficulties. Since information is obtained during suspended respiration, it is essential that each slice be obtained with the same lung volume, otherwise the nodule may move out of the field of interest. A cooperative, instructed patient is required.

Hila and mediastinum

CT is useful in identifying hila adenopathy. When done with intravenous contrast (contrast enhancement), small nodes can be separated from confusing vessels. Magnetic resonance imaging (MRI) can also be used.

Computed tomography is clearly the superior method for examining the mediastinum, whether one is evaluating disease seen on the chest radiograph, looking for suspected abnormalities such as a thymoma in myesthesia gravis, or staging a known lung malignancy (Fig. 197-1). The low density of the normal fat of the mediastinum makes it possible to detect nodes as small as 5 mm regularly. Complete evaluation requires histologic study of these nodes. Location on CT determines the approach best for biopsy (mediastinoscopy, transbronchial aspiration, percutaneous aspiration, parasternal thoracotomy).

Not only can the extent of mediastinal disease be evaluated with CT, but the appearance of certain lesions is relatively specific. Lipomas are low density, and cysts usually have a denser rim than their center. Contrast enhancement identifies normal vessels and vessel variants and demonstrates aneurysms.

Chest wall and pleura

The demonstration of anatomy in cross section makes CT an excellent method for evaluating the pleura and chest wall. Empyemas can be differentiated from lung abscesses. Lipomas are readily apparent. The localization and extent of pleural implants from metastasis or mesothelioma are well shown. The best site for biopsy is apparent, and follow-up comparison studies are easily carried out. Unless there is obvious rib destruction or tumor bulging externally, suspected chest wall invasion requires histologic verification. When confusion exists, CT may be used to distinguish benign pleural plaques from extrapleural fat.

High-resolution CT

Compared to plain film radiography, CT has increased sensitivity for parenchymal disease. This is a result of the elimination of superimposition of structures and the increased ability of CT to discriminate parenchymal structures. Recently the technique of high-resolution CT (HRCT) has been developed. In this technique the slice thickness of 1.5 mm is used, which results in the images having much greater detail than conventional CT images.

HRCT has been found to be very useful in evaluating diffuse lung disease. It is useful in identifying parenchymal disease in patients who are symptomatic or with abnormal pulmonary function tests, but who have normal chest radiographs. Similarly, in febrile immune-compromised patients, infiltrates can be identified that are not visible on chest films. The HRCT findings can be used to characterize diffuse lung disease. The HRCT findings for sarcoidosis, lymphangitic spread of carcinoma, and bronchiectasis are fairly characteristic (Fig. 197-2). The activity of the lung disease can be assessed with HRCT since the presence of "ground glass densities" indicates active alveolitis. The response of the lung disease to therapy can be assessed with serial examinations. Finally, if biopsy is needed for diagnosis, HRCT can identify the best site for obtaining the biopsy.

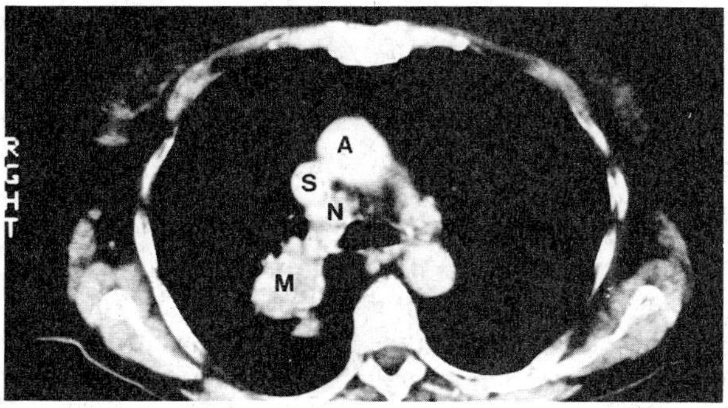

Fig. 197-1. Transverse CT image with intravenous contrast at the level of the tracheal bifurcation. Biopsy of nodes by mediastinoscopy showed poorly differentiated adenocarcinoma. M, right upper lobe mass; S, superior vena cava; A, ascending aorta; N, right paratracheal and retrocaval lymph nodes.

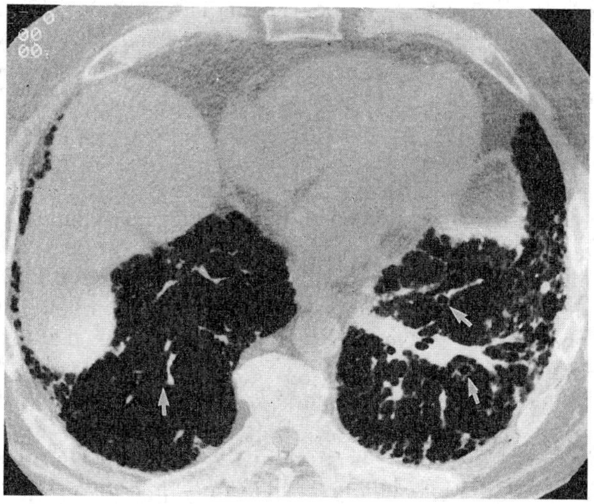

Fig. 197-2. HRCT scan through the lung base of a patient with idiopathic pulmonary fibrosis. Subpleural reticular opacities and traction bronchiectasis *(arrows)* are demonstrated bilaterally.

LUNG SCANS

The major use of scintiscanning studies of the lung is in the diagnosis of pulmonary thromboembolism (PE). Small particles introduced intravenously distribute themselves in the pulmonary capillaries according to blood flow. If these particles are tagged with radioactive material, their distribution can be recorded with a gamma camera. At the present time the most frequently used particles are macroaggregated albumin (10 to 60 μ in diameter) labeled with technetium 99m. These particles are biodegradable and their number is small in comparison to the total number of pulmonary arterioles providing a large margin of safety. Soon after perfusion (P) lung scans became an accepted clinical examination in the 1960s, it became apparent that although the study was highly sensitive in detecting abnormalities, it lacked specificity for thromboembolic disease. Almost any lung abnormality affects lung perfusion.

To improve specificity, ventilation (V) studies done with xenon-133 or xenon-127 were introduced. Their use was based on the fact that an area of diminished perfusion that maintains normal ventilation is most characteristic of vascular occlusion. Krypton-81m gas or DTPA technetium 99m as an aerosol may also be used. This is true in the absence of bronchoconstriction, congestive atelectasis, edema, hemorrhage, or infarction that may be produced by PE.

A normal V scan in an area of a P defect is a mismatch characteristic of vascular occlusion. The matched defect that is present when the V-P scans are both abnormal in the same area occurs in a wide spectrum of primary pulmonary diseases as well as in the parenchymal changes that may occur secondary to a vascular occlusion. Not only can pulmonary emboli show matched defects but less often other diseases can produce a V-P mismatch characteristic of an acute PE.

The evaluation of a patient with a suspected PE should include a chest x-ray to detect pulmonary infiltrates, pneumothorax, atelectasis, or other pulmonary diseases. Unless a contraindication exists, heparin may be started while the diagnostic evaluation is extended. Lung scans are then done within 12 to 24 hours; later scans are less diagnostic. For technical reasons related to photon energy, xenon-133 V scans are done before P scans. Both wash-in and wash-out ventilation should be evaluated, preferably both anteriorly and posteriorly. The labeled macroaggregated albumin for the P scan may be injected as a split dose in the vein of each foot to evaluate thrombi above the knees. The P scan should be imaged in multiple views. Ventilation done with xenon-127 is less available but has the advantage that it can be done after the P scan.

Abnormalities of ventilation are shown by failure of areas to fill during the wash-in phase and/or delayed clearing of xenon from areas during the wash-out phase. Perfusion is normal if radioactivity is uniformly present in all expected areas. An area of diminished or absent radioactivity indicates a perfusion abnormality.

Because V-P scans done for thromboembolism are an indirect demonstration of disease they are interpreted as "normal," "high probability," or "indeterminate." This is based on the appearance of the chest radiograph together with the presence and size of perfusion abnormalities and whether associated ventilation abnormalities exist. The larger the area of V-P mismatch or the larger the P defect compared to the density on the chest radiograph, the more likely is the presence of PE. Nonthromboembolic occlusion of vessels produces similar findings.

A normal P scan excludes the diagnosis of a PE. Over 80% of V-P scans done for suspected PE show some abnormality. A high-probability scan, which is 85%-90% accurate for a positive diagnosis, is present in fewer than half (41%) of patients who have a PE. The large number of nonspecific abnormal scans is where the major problems and controversies exist. Clinical evaluation is useful in deciding which abnormal scans should be further investigated with an angiogram. The patient with an indeterminate scan can be expected to have a PE more often than those with low-probability scans (33% vs 16%). In one series, however, 31% of patients with a low probability scan had angiographic PE. Most clinicians would agree that the majority of indeterminate scans should be evaluated with an angiogram. Since indeterminate scans are seen in at least 33% of patients with a suspected PE this would result in a relatively large number of pulmonary angiograms—more than are now being done. It might be useful to think of V-P scans as "normal," "high probability," or "nondiagnostic."

Most PEs have their origin in the large veins of the lower extremities. When thrombi are present in these large veins they are associated with a high incidence (50%) of PE. Impedance plethysmography and compression sonography are accurate methods for detecting and excluding large vein thrombi. Although the absence of vein clots does *not* exclude a PE, their presence would greatly facilitate the decision to use anticoagulants in patients with nondiagnostic lung scans. The role of these peripheral vein studies in patients with suspected PE is being evaluated.

V-P scintiscans can separate pulmonary hypertension secondary to old or recurrent PE from primary pulmonary hypertension. Unresolved emboli produce a high-probability scan; primary hypertension shows a low-probability or normal scintiscan.

V-P scans are useful in evaluating regional lung function. They may be especially helpful to evaluate the amount of lung resection that can be tolerated in a patient with lung cancer and in the evaluation of a patient with bullae being considered for resection.

Gallium-67 citrate has an affinity for inflammatory and neoplastic tissue. Scans done with this substance should be delayed at least 48 hours after the injection. The greatest value of gallium scans in the thorax is in evaluating the activity of diffuse pulmonary disease. Such applications include idiopathic fibrosis, sarcoidosis, and in patients receiving drugs with potential pulmonary toxicity such as amiodarone. Not only is the activity evaluated, but also the sensitivity of detecting diffuse abnormalities is often greater on gallium scans than on the chest radiograph.

PULMONARY ANGIOGRAM

Most pulmonary angiograms (PAs) are done to evaluate patients for suspected thromboemboli. A few angiograms are done to evaluate arteriovenous (AV) fistulas.

The decision to do a PA in a patient with a suspected PE is based on clinical circumstances and the findings of a prior V-P lung scan. A normal P lung scan excludes a significant pulmonary embolus and makes an angiogram unnecessary. Since the PA is the most definitive way of making the correct diagnosis, it should be used whenever the scan findings are inconclusive or at variance with the clinical evaluation. It is especially important to do a PA when the risk of therapy is so great as to make a correct diagnosis mandatory or when interventive therapy such as inferior vena cava occlusion or, more rarely, an embolectomy is considered. At most institutions 10% to 20% of patients with abnormal perfusion scans are evaluated with a PA. As with all imaging studies for pulmonary thromboemboli, the sooner an angiogram is done, the more reliable it is. Emboli begin to resolve within 24 hours and complete resolution may occur within 7 days. At times emboli do not resolve but organize and cause chronic pulmonary hypertension.

With few exceptions a PA done for suspected thromboembolic disease should be preceded by a V-P scan. An abnormal perfusion scan delineates those areas that must be well visualized on the angiogram. Using the lung scan and chest radiograph as a road map, the most probable areas of embolus can be studied first to shorten the study, decrease the contrast load, and allow more selective, detailed evaluation of abnormal areas.

Pulmonary angiograms are not easy studies. Considerable experience is required to ensure that examinations are satisfactory in patients whose ability to cooperate is often compromised by severe illness. The study is expensive and requires specialized equipment and an experienced team. Therefore, the indications should be carefully considered and do vary among medical centers. The procedure is safely accomplished by experienced operators. Serious complications are more frequent in the presence of pulmonary hypertension and/or a failing right ventricle. Even in such circumstances the mortality has been 0.5% or less. In the evaluation of chronic thromboembolism and pulmonary hypertension for possible surgery, a PA is essential and should not be avoided. The use of supplemental oxygen and nonionic contrast agents, which alter physiology less than the older contrast agents, should make the procedure safer. In the presence of left bundle branch block, facilities for pacing must be immediately available since complete heart block may occur. Major arrhythmias, though uncommon (about 1%), need to be recognized and appropriately treated. Contrast reactions, usually minor, occur in about 1% of patients. The currently used catheters have eliminated perforation as a complication.

To diagnose a PE, the actual clot must be visualized as a filling defect or an abrupt termination of a vessel (Fig. 197-3). If these criteria are followed, a falsely positive diagnosis is rare. A normal PA reliably indicates that therapy of pulmonary embolism is not needed. Follow-up of 311 such patients for periods up to 30 months showed no deaths from pulmonary embolism.

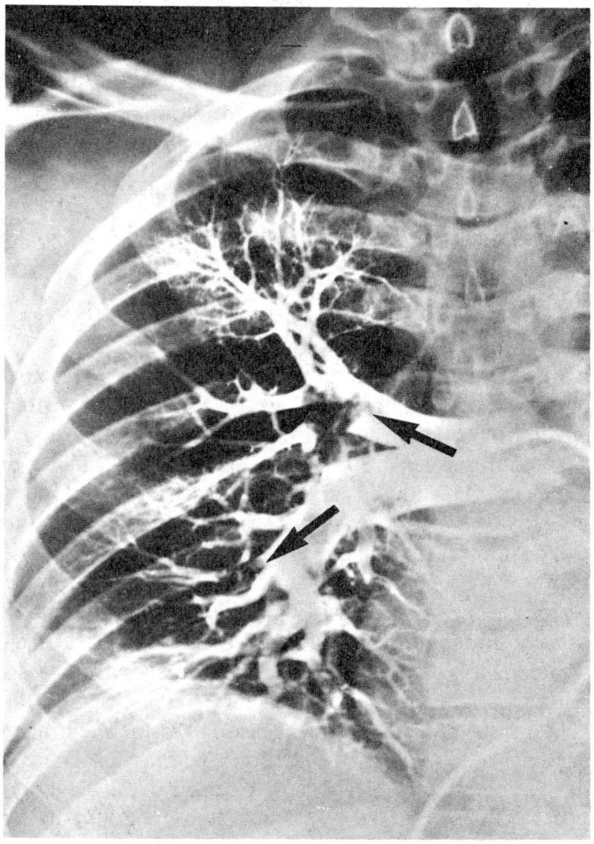

Fig. 197-3. Right pulmonary angiogram. Clots are located within arteries *(arrows)*.

The actual diagnosis of a pulmonary AV fistula requires demonstrating an extracardiac right-to-left shunt with blood gas studies in the absence of pulmonary parenchymal disease. The number and location of these fistulas are best determined by PA. Treatment of these pulmonary AV fistulas can usually be accomplished with some form of transcatheter embolization.

Bronchial artery angiograms as a preliminary to embolization may be useful in hemoptysis. Massive (500 to 600 ml per day), life-threatening hemoptysis is the most clear indication, but chronic episodic hemoptysis in a patient with poor pulmonary drainage and function impairment (e.g., cystic fibrosis) are possible candidates as well. The bleeding site is best localized endoscopically first. In some patients with recurrent hemoptysis, however, it may be necessary to rely on the degree of hypervascularization seen to decide which vessel to embolize. Gelfoam or more permanent Ivalon particles are usually used. A skilled and experienced operator is essential because the anatomy of the feeding arteries is variable, and care must be taken to avoid injecting the vascular supply to the spinal cord. Paraplegia is the most feared complication. Some operators monitor somatosensory-evoked potentials during test injections into the vessel prior to embolization.

Bleeding stops immediately about 70% of the time. Recurrence of bleeding is seen in 20% of cases. The most frequent causes of hemoptysis that lend themselves to this form of therapy are cystic fibrosis with bronchiectasis, aspergillosis (fungus ball), and occasionally tuberculosis, lung abscess, or lung cancer. The vast majority are high-risk patients for surgery.

PULMONARY ULTRASONOGRAPHY

Diagnostic ultrasonography depends on the reflections of sound waves from the interphase of tissues with different acoustic properties. These differences in acoustical impedance for soft tissues are relatively small. Much greater differences occur with air and bone, which do not permit enough sound to penetrate to evaluate deeper structures. Only those disease processes that can be approached without intervening air or bone can be studied. Therefore, except for the heart (echocardiography), ultrasound plays a relatively minor role in evaluating thoracic disease. Imaging is done through the intercostal spaces or from a subchondral or superasternal approach.

The most valuable use of ultrasound is to detect and/or accurately localize fluid collections within the thorax or about the diaphragm. Fluid is recognized by an absence of internal echoes (Fig. 197-4). Each study contains its own acoustically determined ruler so that once fluid is localized, its depth can be accurately measured. This measurement allows a needle tip for aspiration to be precisely placed, avoiding penetration of lung, diaphragm, liver, or spleen. On occasion, a fluid-containing cavity may contain some internal echoes from blood clots or tissue debris, and at times solid structures such as lymphomas and neurofibromas may be so uniform acoustically as to appear cystic: since the needle tip can be so accurately placed, no harm comes from attempts at aspiration in either situation. In the case of solid tumors, aspirated cells for cytology may be diagnostic.

Most pleural effusions are readily diagnosed from chest radiographs, including lateral decubitus and oblique views. Ultrasound is used when small effusions are to be aspirated to obtain material for diagnostic purposes, when densities adjacent to the chest wall cannot be differentiated from fluid collections, or when there has been a prior unsuccessful attempt at fluid aspiration.

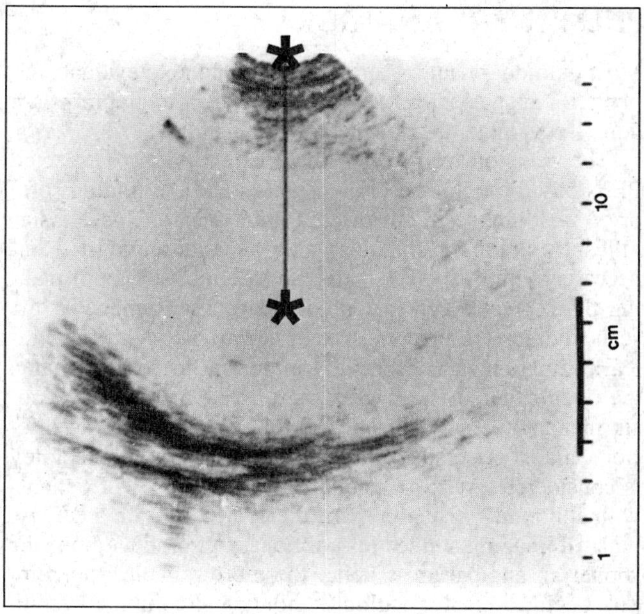

Fig. 197-4. Ultrasound of a left lower posterior thoracic density. Upper * on skin surface, lower * within echo-free fluid. Depth indicated by 1 cm gradation marker on right. Needle aspiration at 6 cm depth revealed an empyema.

MAGNETIC RESONANCE IMAGING

The nuclei of atoms that have an odd number of neutrons plus protons have a magnetic moment. When these nuclei are placed in a magnetic field, they attempt to align themselves to this field. In doing so they rotate (precess) about the direction of the magnetic field at a specific frequency for a given nucleus. These precessing nuclei can absorb energy if they are exposed to a radio wave of the same frequency (resonance). After such a pulse, the nuclei release energy as they return to their ground state (relaxation). Longitudinal (T_1) and transverse (T_2) relaxation times may be measured and are thought to be specific for each substance. The recording of this energy release is the basis of magnetic resonance imaging (MRI). Hydrogen nuclei are magnetic and, because of their abundance in living tissue, are the nuclei involved in imaging by most present-day devices.

All studies that use x-rays are limited in recording the differences in tissue based on photon absorption alone. Magnetic resonance imaging, however, can make use of a large variety of pulse sequences to enhance tissue discrimination. A further characteristic of MRI is that flowing blood usually gives no signal, allowing easy recognition of vascular structures from surrounding tissue. MRI has no known adverse biologic effects.

Tesla is the unit of strength of the magnet. Most newer scanners are 1.5 T, although excellent images can be obtained on lower field strengths of 0.3 T to 1.0 T. Cardiac gating is needed to image the chest and requires 4-6 minutes to scan 10 slices. Respiratory compensation, a form of respiratory gating, is also needed. MRI is not a routine study but should be used to solve specific problems.

MRI has a number of advantages over CT scanning in evaluating the heart and mediastinum. Moving blood can be made to have no signal or to have a bright signal without the addition of contrast material. This capability aids in the identification of masses and nodes in the hili or mediastinum and offers an alternative modality to CT in patients who are allergic to contrast. The ability to image the chest in saggital, coronal, and oblique planes is a significant advantage over CT. Cardiac gating allows improved visualization of intracardiac anatomy and pathology.

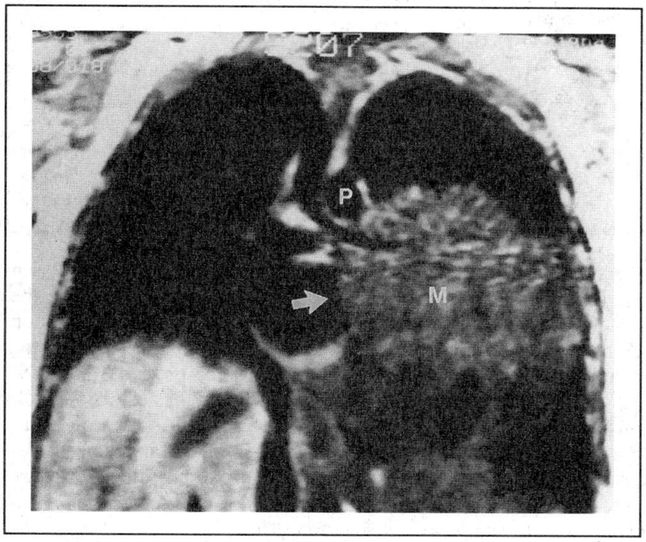

Fig. 197-5. Coronal plane magnetic resonance image in a patient with a lung mass (M) that has invaded the left atrium *(arrow)*. P, pulmonary artery lateral to the trachea and superior to the left bronchus.

In the evaluation of lung cancer and mediastinal masses CT and MRI offer similar results. However, MRI is better at evaluating invasion of the chest wall, brachial plexus and subclavian vessels such as in superior sulcus tumors. Coronal imaging improves detection of subcarinal and AP window adenopathy. MRI is the imaging method of choice for evaluating posterior mediastinal neurogenic tumors that may involve the spinal canal. MRI cannot detect calcification, which is often important in chest imaging. MRI of the aorta is very good at evaluating acquired diseases such as aneurysms and dissections as well as congenital lesions such as vascular rings and coarctations. The ability to image the entire aorta on one oblique scan is a distinct advantage. MRI is the imaging modality of choice for imaging intracardiac tumors and masses and for evaluating the extent of cardiac involvement by paracardiac lesions (Fig. 197-5). MRI is also useful in evaluating obstruction, compression, or thrombosis of the mediastinal veins.

Cardiac pacemakers, ferromagnetic vascular clips, implants or foreign bodies in critical areas (e.g., intracerebral, eye, cochlea), and the very early Starr-Edwards or other loosened heart valves are contraindications to MRI studies.

MRI of the chest is evolving rapidly as new imaging techniques are discovered. Imaging of the lung parenchyma and pulmonary arteries and more detailed cardiac imaging will be available in the near future.

REFERENCES

Kelley MA et al: Diagnosing pulmonary embolism: new facts and strategies. Ann Int Med 114:300, 1991.

Naidich DP, Zerhouni EA, and Siegelman SS: Computed tomography and magnetic resonance of the thorax, ed 2. New York, 1991, Raven.

Pinet F et al: Embolization of the systemic arteries of the lung. J Thorac Imag 2:11, 1987.

Webb WR, Muller NL, Naidich DP: High-resolution CT of the lung. New York, 1992, Raven.

Webb WR and Sostman HD: MR imaging of thoracic disease: Clinical uses. Radiol 182:621, 1992.

CHAPTER

198 Intensive Care Monitoring and Mechanical Ventilation

Herbert P. Wiedemann

Critically ill hospitalized patients are treated almost exclusively within specialized intensive care units. Two major developments during the last 25 years provided the impetus behind the flourishing of intensive care units. In the late 1960s, the value of volume-cycled ventilators and of delivering assisted ventilation in special centralized units was documented. The other major advance was the emergence of technologies that allowed the monitoring of important hemodynamic parameters. Most notable in this regard was the introduction of bedside pulmonary artery catheterization in the early 1970s.

In the intensive care unit, physicians are challenged to provide skillful and timely application of monitoring and support devices. Furthermore, the resulting data must be interpreted correctly, avoiding the pitfalls that might result in clinical mismanagement. In this chapter, the major procedures and techniques of hemodynamic monitoring and mechanical ventilation are discussed.

INVASIVE MONITORING OF HEMODYNAMICS AND GAS EXCHANGE

Peripheral artery catheterization

Cannulation of a peripheral artery is frequently performed in the intensive care unit, allowing (1) continuous monitoring and graphic display of the systemic arterial blood pressure, and (2) repeated analysis of arterial blood gases. Because of the low risk of serious complications, peripheral artery cannulation is warranted in all patients with hemodynamic instability in whom continuous monitoring of arterial pressures is important. Arterial catheters also improve accuracy in this setting, since sphygmomanometry usually underestimates the actual intra-arterial pressure in patients with increased peripheral vascular resistance caused by hypovolemia or overt shock. In addition, the need for frequent arterial blood gas analyses in patients with respiratory failure is a relative indication for the use of an indwelling catheter to avoid the inconvenience and discomfort of frequent "single-stick" arterial samples. However, the advent of noninvasive techniques for monitoring arterial oxygen satura-

Recommended technique for inserting and maintaining systemic artery lines

1. Do an Allen test prior to radial artery cannulation. Ischemic complications are lowest if ulnar artery refill time is less than 5 seconds.
2. Use sterile technique for insertion (antiseptic preparation, gloves, drapes).
3. Percutaneous insertion is preferred over surgical cutdown.
4. Use 20-gauge catheter if wrist circumference is small.
5. Use continuous flush system with a nondextrose solution (normal saline) containing heparin.
6. Transducer should have disposable dome.
7. Assess daily
   a. Catheter site for evidence of inflammation
   b. Distal extremity for evidence of ischemia
8. Limit cannulation to 4 to 5 days at one site
9. Remove catheter for
   a. Distal ischemia
   b. Local infection
   c. Persistently damped pressure tracing
   d. Difficulty with blood withdrawal

Modified with permission from Matthay MA: Invasive hemodynamic monitoring in critically ill patients. Clin Chest Med 4:233, 1983.

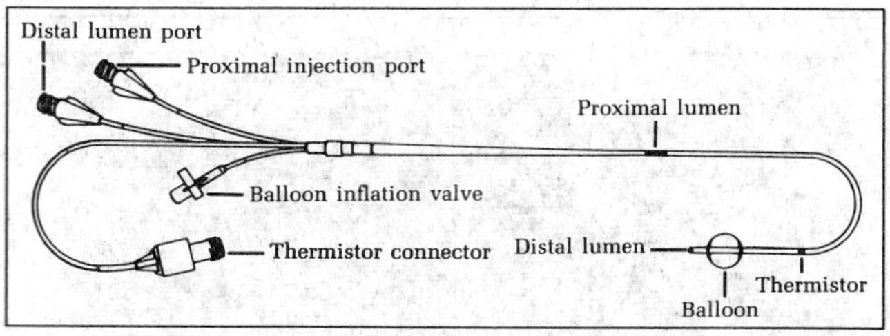

Fig 198-1. Typical triple-lumen pulmonary artery catheter. When the catheter is properly positioned and the balloon is deflated, the distal lumen records pulmonary artery pressure. When the balloon is inflated enough to occlude the segmental pulmonary artery, the distal lumen measures "wedge" pressure. The proximal lumen is 30 cm from the catheter tip and lies in the right atrium. A thermistor located just proximal to the balloon is used for cardiac output studies; the thermistor senses a temperature change shortly after a cold bolus of fluid exits from the proximal lumen. (Reproduced with permission from Matthay MA: Invasive hemodynamic monitoring in acute respiratory failure. J Resp Dis 2:40, 1981.)

tion (e.g., oximetry) and $PaCO_2$ (e.g., capnography) is reducing the need for indwelling arterial catheters in hemodynamically stable patients being monitored solely for respiratory failure.

Usually, the radial artery is chosen because of convenience and generally good collateral circulation. Prior to using this site, the patency of the ulnar circulation should be evaluated with an Allen test; ischemic complications are minimized if ulnar artery refill time is less than 5 seconds. Other common insertion sites include the brachial, femoral, and dorsalis pedis arteries. Cannulation is usually performed with an 18- or 20-gauge catheter inserted percutaneously or via surgical cutdown.

With proper technique (see box above) peripheral artery cannulation is generally safe. The major complications are ischemia distal to the insertion site and infection. Ischemia may be secondary to either local thrombosis or distal embolization. Subclinical and reversible arterial occlusion are common, with up to one fourth of arteries remaining angiographically occluded 1 week after catheter removal. However, clinically significant ischemia (e.g., necrosis of fingers or toes) is rare (less than 0.2%). Hypotension, severe peripheral vascular disease, and the use of vasopressor drugs increase the risk of serious ischemic complications. The incidence of catheter-related septicemia can be reduced to less than 1% with proper precautions. Risk factors favoring infection include cannulation exceeding 4 days at one site and insertion by surgical cutdown rather than percutaneously.

Pulmonary artery catheterization

Routine bedside catheterization of the pulmonary artery became feasible with the introduction of the balloon-tipped catheter by Swan and colleagues in 1970. Since the inflatable balloon at the tip allows the catheter to be directed by blood flow, fluoroscopy usually is not necessary for proper placement. Several versions of the pulmonary artery catheter, commonly referred to as the *Swan-Ganz catheter,* are now available. One important modification of the original design is the placement of a thermistor near the distal tip, which allows for measurement of cardiac output by the thermodilution technique. Fig. 198-1 depicts the most frequently used pulmonary artery catheter.

Pulmonary artery catheterization rapidly became an integral aspect in the management of many intensive care unit patients since the properly positioned catheter allows the direct acquisition of three important physiologic variables (see box below): (1) cardiac output, (2) intravascular pressures (right heart chambers, pulmonary artery, and pulmonary artery occlusion or "wedge" pressure), and (3) mixed venous oxygenation. Additionally, a large number of calculated physiologic parameters can be derived from these primary measurements (Table 198-1).

Insertion and normal wave forms. Venous access can be achieved via percutaneous insertion of the catheter through the subclavian, internal jugular, external jugular, femoral, or antecubital vein; cutdown may be necessary with the an-

Directly measured physiologic variables obtained with pulmonary artery catheterization

Cardiac output
Intravascular pressures
  Right atrial pressure
  Right ventricular pressure
  Pulmonary artery pressure
  Pulmonary artery "wedge" pressure
Mixed venous oxygenation

Table 198-1. Physiologic data derived from invasive monitoring

	Normal range
Cardiac index (L/min/m^2)	2.4-4.4
$CI = \frac{CO}{BSA}$	
Systemic vascular resistance (dynes • sec • cm^{-5})	900-1400
$SVR = \frac{MAP = CVP}{CO} \times 79.9$	
Pulmonary vascular resistance (dynes • sec • cm^{-5})	150-250
$PVR = \frac{MPAP = PAWP}{CO} \times 79.9$	
Stroke volume (ml)	
$SV = \frac{CO}{HR}$	
Stroke volume index (ml/m^2)	30-65
$SVI = \frac{SV}{BSA} = \frac{CI}{HR}$	
Left ventricular stroke work index (g • m/m^2)	43-61
$LVSWI = SVI \times (MAP - PAOP) \times 0.0136$	
Right ventricular stroke work index (g • m/m^2)	7-12
$RVSWI = SVI \times (MPAP - CVP) \times 0.0136$	
Oxygen content (ml/dl blood)	About 19.5
$CaO_2 = Hgb \times$ arterial O_2 saturation $\times 1.36 + (PO_2 \times 0.003)$	
Arteriovenous oxygen content difference (ml/dl)	3-5
$avDO_2 = CaO_2 - CvO_2$	
Oxygen delivery (ml/min)	800-1200
O_2 delivery $= CO \times CaO_2 \times 10$	
Oxygen consumption (ml/min)	180-280
$VO_2 = CO \times (CaO_2 - CvO_2) \times 10$	
Pulmonary shunt (venoarterial admixture) (%)	<3-5%
$\frac{QS}{Qt} = \frac{CcO_2 - CaO_2}{CcO_2 - CvO_2}$	

Modified from Sprung CL, editor: The pulmonary artery catheter: methodology and clinical applications. Baltimore, 1983, University Park.
BSA, body surface area; CaO_2, arterial oxygen content; CcO_2, pulmonary capillary oxygen content (assumed equal to alveolar PO_2); CI, cardiac index; CO, cardiac output; CvO_2, mixed venous oxygen content; CVP, central venous pressure; Hgb, hemoglobin concentration; HR, heart rate; LVSWI, left ventricular stroke work index; MAP, mean arterial pressure; MPAP, mean pulmonary artery pressure; PAWP, pulmonary artery wedge pressure; PVR, pulmonary vascular resistance; Qs/Qt, pulmonary shunt; RVSWI, right ventricular stroke work index; SV, stroke volume; SVI, stroke volume index; SVR, systemic vascular resistance.

tecubital route. In intensive care units and operating rooms, the internal jugular route is usually selected as offering the best compromise between ease of insertion and avoidance of major complications. The subclavian approach is rapid, and the site is immobile, but complications can be serious, including pneumothorax and inadvertent subclavian artery puncture. Because subclavian artery bleeding cannot be controlled by local pressure, abnormal clotting parameters constitute a strong contraindication to this approach. The antecubital vein is a safe insertion site, but it is sometimes difficult to maneuver the catheter into the central venous circulation from this site, and movement of the arm may cause difficulty in maintaining correct catheter position.

The catheter is advanced with continuous monitoring of the electrocardiogram (ECG) (for arrhythmia detection) and venous pressures recorded from the distal orifice. A sudden increase in the respiratory fluctuation of recorded pressures signals that the catheter tip has reached a central intrathoracic vein. The balloon is then inflated with air to the full recommended volume (1.5 ml for the 7 French catheter; 0.8 ml for the 5 French catheter) for flow-directed passage through the right atrium, right ventricle, and into the pulmonary artery. As a general guide, the right atrium should be reached about 10 cm from the subclavian vein, 10 to 15 cm from the jugular vein, 30 cm from a femoral vein insertion site, 40 cm from the right antecubital fossa, and 50 cm from the left antecubital fossa. Representative normal pressure tracings seen during passage of the catheter are shown in Fig. 198-2. The catheter is advanced until a pulmonary artery "wedge" tracing is obtained. This occurs when the balloon occludes the pulmonary artery segment; with absent flow, the pressure tracing from the distal orifice of the catheter reflects left atrial pressure. During flotation of the catheter, it is important to have the balloon fully inflated to prevent the catheter tip from protruding (Fig. 198-3). A catheter tip that is too distal and located in a small pulmonary artery may cause falsely high measurements of cardiac output and mixed venous PO_2.

Since measurement of the pulmonary artery wedge pressure (PAWP) is a major use of the pulmonary artery catheter and provides the basis for important diagnostic and

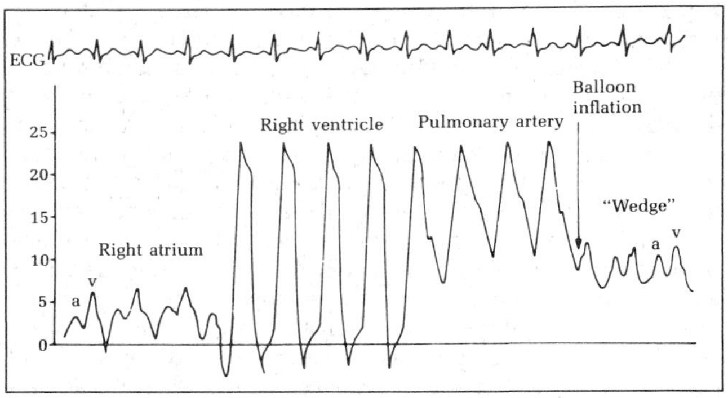

Fig. 198-2. Representative recording of normal pressures and wave forms as a Swan-Ganz catheter is passed through the right side of the heart into the pulmonary artery. The first waveform is a right atrial tracing with characteristic a and v waves. The right ventricular, pulmonary artery, and pulmonary artery wedge tracings follow in sequence. Note that the wedge tracing shows a and v waves transmitted from the left atrium. In addition, the wedge pressure (mean) is less than pulmonary artery diastolic pressure. The wedge tracing is not always this distinct, but a very damped tracing or a mean wedge pressure greater than pulmonary artery diastolic pressure usually indicates some mechanical problem in the system (e.g., air bubble in the connecting tubing, catheter tip "overwedged," balloon inflated over distal orifice, or catheter tip in zone 1 or zone 2). In severe mitral regurgitation, the large transmitted left atrial v waves occasionally may cause the wedge tracing to resemble a pulmonary artery tracing. In such a case, careful analysis of the waveforms and attention to where the peak pressure occurs in relation to the ECG complex (top tracing) usually will avoid misinterpretation. (Reproduced with permission from Matthay MA: Invasive hemodynamic monitoring in critically ill patients. Clin Chest Med 4:233, 1983.)

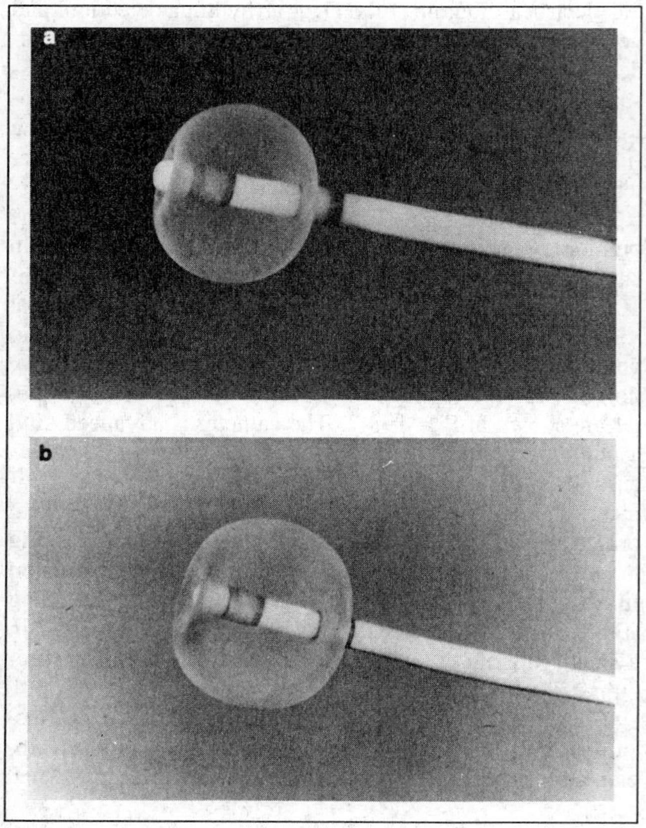

Fig. 198-3. Photographs of a 7 French Swan-Ganz catheter balloon inflated with either 1.0 ml *(a)* or 1.5 ml *(b)* of air. Notice that the catheter tip protrudes beyond the inflated balloon if less than the full recommended volume is used. The exposed catheter tip may cause endocardial damage, induce ventricular arrhythmias, or damage the pulmonary artery. Also, using the recommended volume helps ensure a relatively proximal wedge position, which is important to lessen the risk of pulmonary infarction and to help maintain accuracy of thermodilution cardiac output and mixed venous PO_2 determinations. A catheter tip that is too distal and located in a small pulmonary artery may cause falsely high measurements of cardiac output and mixed venous PO_2. (Reproduced with permission from Sprung CL: Complications of pulmonary artery catheterization. In Sprung CL, editor: The pulmonary artery catheter: methodology and clinical applications. Baltimore, 1983, University Park.)

therapeutic decisions, it is essential that a valid PAWP be obtained. Adherence to the following criteria help ensure a valid PAWP: (1) a tracing characteristic of a left atrial wave form should be seen; a highly "damped" tracing devoid of oscillations except those resulting from ventilation-induced pressure changes is not acceptable. The PAWP wave form should disappear promptly with balloon deflation, yielding a pulmonary artery tracing, and return rapidly after balloon reinflation. (2) The mean PAWP should be lower than or equal to the pulmonary artery diastolic pressure (the PAWP may transiently exceed pulmonary artery diastolic pressure in severe mitral regurgitation). (3) Catheter obstruction is ruled out by the ability of a saline flush solution to flow through the distal lumen. (4) Blood gas analysis of blood withdrawn from the distal port should reflect systemic arterial PO_2 and PCO_2 rather than that of mixed venous blood. Although this last criterion is usually not routinely tested, it may be of help in confusing situations. The validity of this criterion is supported by information that highly oxygenated blood is usually withdrawn from a true wedge position even in areas of radiographic infiltrates or in patients with large intrapulmonic shunts.

Although flow-directed passage of the catheter into the pulmonary artery usually presents little difficulty, a problem may occur in the presence of low cardiac output, tricuspid valve regurgitation, right ventricular dilatation, or severe pulmonary hypertension. In such circumstances, a left-sided venous access route is advantageous, since the catheter has to loop in only one direction in going from the left subclavian vein to the right ventricular outflow. In some instances it may be necessary to advance the catheter with fluoroscopy to provide a direct visual assessment of catheter position.

Inability to obtain a valid PAWP tracing could be caused by a catheter tip that is not located in zone 3 of the lung (Fig. 198-4). If the catheter tip is located outside zone 3, the pulmonary artery tracing may appear normal until the balloon is inflated. Since alveolar pressure exceeds pulmonary capillary pressure in zone 2, the vessel distal to the inflated balloon then collapses, causing PAWP to reflect al-

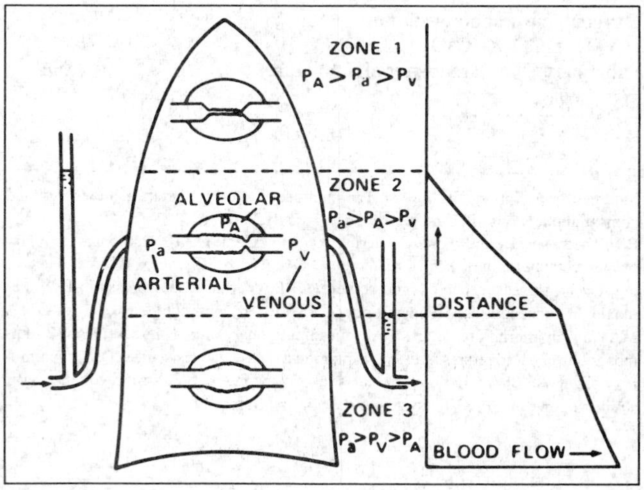

Fig. 198-4. Zones of the lung, based on the relationship among pulmonary artery (P_a) pressure, alveolar pressure (P_A), and pulmonary venous pressure (P_v). The zones are not constant. For instance, a decrease in P_v (e.g., diuresis) or an increase in P_A (e.g., PEEP therapy) converts some zone 3 area into zone 2 or zone 1. The pulmonary wedge pressure reflects P_v (and thus left atrial pressure) only if the tip of the Swan-Ganz catheter lies in zone 3 before balloon inflation. If the balloon is inflated in zone 2, the occluded vessel collapses since P_A is greater than P_v. Without a continuous column of the blood between the catheter tip and the left atrium, the wedge pressure cannot reflect left atrial pressure. (Reproduced with permission from West JB, Dollery CT, and Naimark A: Distribution of blood flow in isolated lung: relation to vascular and alveolar pressures. J Appl Physiol 19:713, 1964.)

veolar pressure rather than left atrial pressure. Because the vast majority of pulmonary blood flows through zone 3, the flow-directed catheter usually migrates into this region during initial insertion. However, the size of the lung zones may change in response to physiologic alterations. For instance, diuresis or ventilation with high levels of positive end-expiratory pressure (PEEP) reduces the size of zone 3 because of a decrease in pulmonary venous pressure or an increase in alveolar pressure, respectively. Thus, a catheter tip originally correctly positioned in zone 3 may subsequently be in zone 2. To obtain a valid wedge position, it may be necessary to refloat the catheter under these new physiologic conditions.

If a proper wedge tracing cannot be obtained, pulmonary artery diastolic pressure is sometimes used to estimate PAWP. In individuals with a normal heart rate and a normal pulmonary vascular bed, the relationship between these values is close. However, with tachycardia (especially heart rates above 120 per minute) or pulmonary hypertension, pulmonary artery diastolic pressure exceeds PAWP by large amounts. Thus, in many situations requiring monitoring (e.g., adult respiratory distress syndrome, pulmonary embolism), estimation of PAWP from the pulmonary artery diastolic pressure is unreliable.

The normal waveforms depicted in Fig. 198-2 may be altered significantly by pathophysiologic conditions. For example, infarction of the right ventricle may reduce the pressure generated by this chamber to such a degree that right atrial, right ventricular, and pulmonary artery wave forms and pressures are nearly identical. Severe mitral valve insufficiency leads to a wedge tracing with a large left atrial "v" wave that may mimic the pulmonary artery waveform. These and other situations may cause significant confusion unless the clinician anticipates the possibility of aberrant waveforms through an understanding of the clinical setting.

Since intravascular pressure readings such as PAWP are calibrated relative to atmosphere, these measurements reflect transmural vascular pressures (pressure difference across the wall of the vessel or heart chamber) only if the pleural and atmospheric pressures are equal. (The importance of correctly assessing transmural pressure and the interpretation of PAWP during PEEP therapy are addressed more fully in the subsequent discussion of the relationship between PAWP and left ventricular preload.) Since pleural pressure most closely approximates atmospheric pressure at end expiration, vascular pressure readings should be obtained at this time. In patients with rapid, labored breathing, this may present a problem because of the large deflection in vascular pressures and the short expiratory time. In such instances, a printout of the actual pressure tracing on a strip chart recorder, as shown in Fig. 198-5, may be required; end expiration can be identified visually, and the vascular pressure during the brief end-expiratory phase can be directly measured. In contrast, reliance on most currently available electronic digital displays could provide misleading information, since the displayed pressure represents an average value obtained during a scanning period that exceeds the end-expiratory phase.

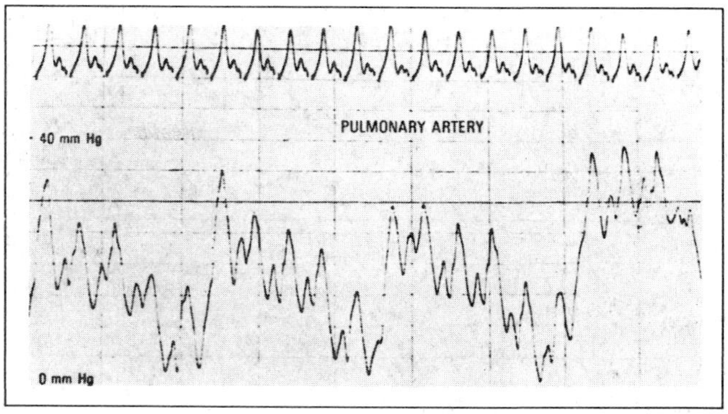

Fig. 198-5. Example of how rapid, labored respirations can result in marked fluctuations of the pulmonary artery pressure tracing *(lower tracing)*. The upper tracing is the ECG. The patient's respiratory rate was 40, and the peak pulmonary artery pressure varied from 35 to 40 to 18 mm Hg. Since the pressures are recorded on calibrated strip chart paper, the pressures corresponding to the brief period of end expiration can be easily identified. A digital readout could be very misleading, since this value would be an electronic average of a 3- to 4-second scanning period. (Reproduced with permission from Matthay MA: Invasive hemodynamic monitoring in critically ill patients. Clin Chest Med 4:233, 1983.)

Thermodilution cardiac output. (Also see Chapter 6.) With a thermistor-tipped pulmonary artery catheter and a commercially available bedside microprocessor, the measurement of cardiac output is an easy and rapid procedure that can be performed many times in a single day if necessary. Thermodilution measurements correlate well with the Fick or dye dilution techniques, which are much more difficult to perform. To obtain thermodilution cardiac output measurements, 10 ml of room temperature or iced saline solution is injected as rapidly as possible (ideally, less than 4 seconds) into the proximal injection port. The bolus exits the catheter in the right atrium and travels into the pulmonary artery where the thermistor detects the change in temperature over time. The bedside microprocessor quickly calculates and displays the cardiac output. The use of 0° C injectate solution (ice water temperature) carries a theoretical advantage over room temperature solution (22° C), since the contrast with core body temperature is greater with the former (better signal/background ratio). However, room temperature injectate is entirely acceptable except in severely hypothermic patients; if core body temperature is 6° to 11° C (10° to 20° F) below normal, ice temperature solution is mandatory.

Phasic changes in intrathoracic pressure and venous return induced by spontaneous or mechanical ventilation may cause significant variability in single measurements (Fig. 198-6). To reduce this problem, as well as other causes of variability, it is standard practice to average three consecutive measurements (about 1 minute apart), which are all obtained at end expiration, to constitute a single determination. Cardiac output determinations performed in this manner have an accuracy and reproducibility that are usually very acceptable for clinical use. However, the ther-

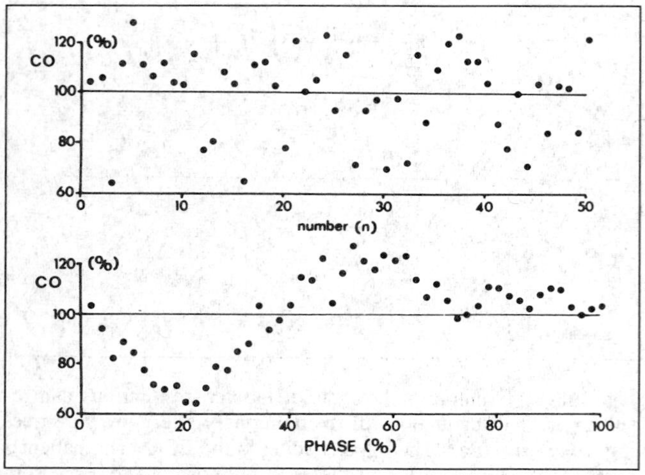

Fig. 198-6. Effects of respiratory phase during mechanical ventilation on thermodilution right-sided cardiac output (CO) determinations. Top panel shows a series of 50 random measurements. Bottom panel shows the same 50 injections plotted according to the respiratory cycle phase with the initial downward deflection occurring during ventilation-delivered inspiration. (Reproduced with permission from Jansen JRC et al: Thermodilution technique for measurement of cardiac output during artificial ventilation. J Appl Physiol 51:584, 1981.)

modilution technique may not be accurate in the presence of significant tricuspid valve regurgitation (which causes a falsely low measurement), intracardiac shunts, or a too distally placed catheter (may be suspected when less than 1.0 ml of air in the balloon produces a wedge pressure).

Mixed venous oxygen saturation. Mixed venous blood is sampled through the distal orifice of the pulmonary artery catheter with the balloon deflated. (The 7 French catheter has a 2.5 ml dead space that must first be eliminated by discarding the initial sample.) In patients receiving mechanical ventilation and very high inspired oxygen concentration, a fast rate of blood withdrawal may lead to a falsely elevated mixed venous oxygen saturation caused by contamination of the sample with pulmonary capillary blood. A slow rate of blood withdrawal (less than 3 ml per minute) eliminates this possibility. Severe mitral valve regurgitation may also cause a falsely elevated mixed venous oxygen saturation as a result of retrograde pulmonary capillary blood flow.

Clinically, mixed venous oxygenation is used to monitor changes in cardiac output and assess tissue oxygenation. In normal individuals and many patients, as oxygen delivery (cardiac output × arterial oxygen content) decreases, increased extraction of oxygen from circulating blood allows tissue oxygen consumption to remain stable (oxygen consumption is independent of oxygen delivery until a critically low level of delivery) but causes the mixed venous oxygen content to decrease. Thus, a decrease in cardiac output is reflected by a corresponding decline in mixed venous oxygen. Furthermore, as mixed venous PO_2 approaches 27 to 30 mm Hg (normal, 39 mm Hg), blood lactate levels usually increase, indicating that tissue oxygenation is reaching a critically low level. These interpretations of mixed venous oxygenation are most valid in patients with "simple" hemodynamic problems, such as isolated myocardial dysfunction. In more complex illnesses, including sepsis and the adult respiratory distress syndrome (ARDS), the interpretation of mixed venous oxygenation is much more complex. In sepsis, peripheral "shunting" of arterial blood past tissue beds may lead to maintenance of a high mixed venous oxygen level despite tissue oxygen deprivation indicated by high blood lactate levels. Furthermore, in some ARDS patients, oxygen consumption varies with oxygen delivery, even at normal or high cardiac outputs, suggesting an abnormal "supply dependency" of oxygen consumption. This phenomenon may be related in part to abnormalities in the systemic capillary circulation, which prevent normal tissue oxygen extraction. The result is that mixed venous oxygenation may remain high and relatively stable despite large, and presumably clinically important, decreases in cardiac output, oxygen delivery, and oxygen consumption. It is clear that solely monitoring mixed venous oxygenation in patients with sepsis or ARDS is inadequate. The clinician needs to monitor several other parameters, including cardiac output, arterial oxygen saturation, and lactate levels to be informed about changes in hemodynamic states of these patients.

Pulmonary artery catheters that provide a continuous measurement of the mixed oxygen saturation through use of fiberoptic reflectance oximetry are currently available. Although the continuous monitoring of mixed venous oxygenation may provide a helpful "early warning system" for detecting adverse hemodynamic trends, its value in this regard is limited by the factors outlined in the preceding discussion. Reliance on stable mixed venous oxygenation may provide a false sense of security in patients with illnesses such as ARDS or sepsis.

Left-to-right intracardiac shunts cause an elevated mixed venous oxygenation. This fact may be helpful in diagnosing atrial or ventricular septal defects; during passage of the catheter, blood samples show an abnormal "step-up" in oxygen saturation as the tip is passed into the right atrium or right ventricle. An example of how this maneuver may provide important diagnostic information is a patient with myocardial infarction who develops sudden hemodynamic instability and a systolic murmur. The major diagnoses to be considered are acute ventricular septal defect or acute mitral valve insufficiency. These possibilities can be easily distinguished through an assessment of oxygen saturation in the chambers of the right heart.

It is important to remember that mixed venous oxygenation has an important influence on arterial oxygenation saturation when there is a high degree of shunt through the lungs (e.g., ARDS) (Fig. 198-7). Although clinicians often reflexively attribute a decrease in PaO_2 to a worsening of lung function, such a decrease may in fact result from nonrespiratory factors that cause a reduction in mixed venous oxygenation (e.g., anemia, increased oxygen consumption, low cardiac output). If such factors are corrected, arterial oxygen saturation may improve even if lung disease does not improve.

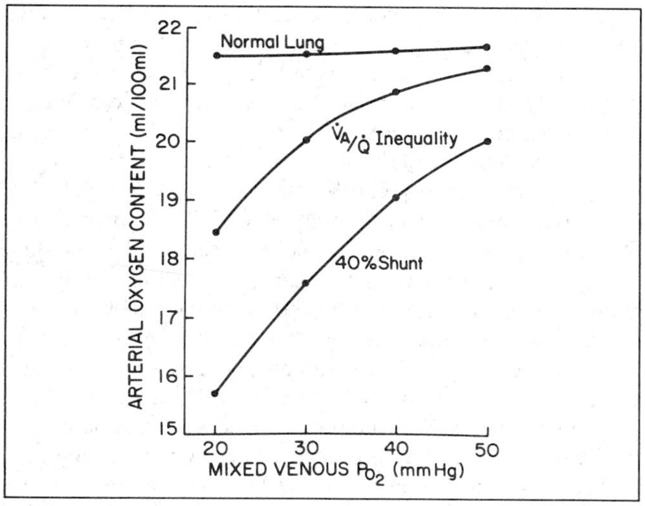

Fig. 198-7. The effect of changing the mixed venous PO_2 on the arterial oxygen content in a patient with normal lungs, one with marked ventilation-perfusion inequality, and one with a large shunt. Each theoretical patient was assumed to be breathing 50% oxygen, and cardiac output and minute ventilation were held constant. (Reproduced with permission from Dantzker DR: Gas exchange in the adult respiratory distress syndrome. Clin Chest Med 3:57, 1982.)

Pulmonary artery wedge pressure. The measurement of the PAWP is a major use of the pulmonary artery catheter. The PAWP allows the clinician to make important assumptions regarding left ventricular preload and pulmonary capillary hydrostatic pressure.

Balloon occlusion of a branch of the pulmonary artery causes flow to cease between the catheter tip and the "junction point" at which pulmonary venous radicles served by the occluded artery join other radicles in which blood is still flowing toward the left atrium. Pulmonary artery wedge pressure reflects venous pressure at this junction point, which appears to be located in a pulmonary vein of about the same size as the occluded pulmonary artery. Thus, the usual wedge pressure produced by balloon occlusion of a lobar artery correlates well with venous pressure at or near the left atrium. Because little pressure difference normally exists among the large pulmonary veins, left atrium, and left ventricle during end diastole, PAWP usually is a good approximation of intracavitary left ventricular end diastolic pressure (LVEDP). Under certain circumstances, however, normal pressure equilibration is prevented, and this relationship does not hold. For instance, obstruction of the large pulmonary veins (e.g., atrial myxoma, thoracic tumors, mediastinal fibrosis) may cause PAWP to exceed left atrial pressure. Similarly, mitral valve stenosis or insufficiency causes PAWP and left atrial pressure to exceed LVEDP. If left ventricular compliance is very reduced, left atrial contraction causes an increase in LVEDP such that it may exceed PAWP by 5 mm Hg or more. Although the clinician needs to be alert to these and related exceptions, PAWP usually provides a good estimate of LVEDP.

Relationship of PAWP to left ventricular preload. (See Chapter 6.) According to the Frank-Starling principle, left ventricular preload determines the force of cardiac contraction for any given level of myocardial contractility. Therefore, a measurement of left ventricular function (e.g., cardiac output) taken in conjunction with an assessment of left ventricular preload allows the clinician to make important conclusions regarding left ventricular contractility. Since PAWP is frequently used to assess left ventricular preload, it is important to understand the relationship between the two, which are sometimes incorrectly assumed to be identical.

Preload refers to stretch of myocardial fibers, and therefore is best assessed by left ventricular end diastolic *volume* (LVEDV). The LVEDV is determined by the transmural ventricular distending pressure (intracavitary pressure, or PAWP, minus juxtacardiac pressure) and ventricular compliance (pressure − volume relationship). The relationship between PAWP and left ventricular preload is shown in Fig. 198-8, which illustrates how a given PAWP may be associated with varying degrees of left ventricular filling in critically ill patients with altered juxtacardiac pressure (e.g., mechanical ventilation and PEEP) or ventricular compliance (e.g., myocardial ischemia, pericardial effusion).

Failure to understand the PAWP-LVEDV relationship

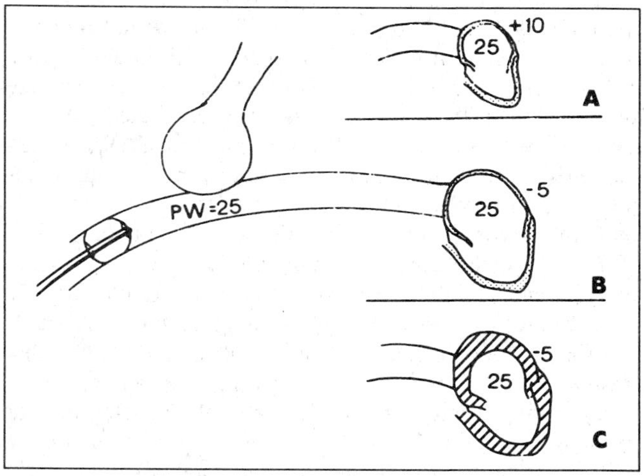

Fig. 198-8. Relationship of pulmonary artery wedge pressure (PW) to left ventricular preload (left ventricular volume or "stretch") in three situations, illustrating the importance of considering pleural (juxtacardiac) pressure and ventricular compliance, along with PW, when making assumptions about left ventricular preload. The PW is elevated in each example and reflects the intracavitary left ventricular end diastolic pressure. **A,** The pleural pressure is increased, as might occur with PEEP therapy. Transmural left ventricular pressure is approximately normal, as is the preload. **B,** The pleural pressure is normal. Transmural left ventricular pressure is elevated, and preload is increased. **C,** The ventricle is stiff, as might occur with myocardial ischemia. Although PW and pleural pressure are identical to example **B,** the preload in this instance is normal. (Reproduced with permission from O'Quin R and Marini JJ: Pulmonary artery occlusion pressure: clinical physiology, measurement, and interpretation. Am Rev Respir Dis 128:319, 1983.)

may lead to misdiagnosis and institution of inappropriate therapy. For instance, a hypotensive patient on high PEEP levels may have a relatively normal PAWP that erroneously may be interpreted to reflect adequate left ventricular preload. Assuming therefore that intrinsic cardiac dysfunction exists, the physician may begin treatment with inotropic or vasopressor agents. However, in this example, left ventricular filling volume may in fact be low since PAWP overestimates left ventricular transmural distending pressure when pleural pressure is elevated (e.g., Fig. 198-8, *A*); perhaps a volume infusion trial is the most appropriate initial therapy for this patient.

How can the clinician adjust for the effect of PEEP on PAWP measurements? For most purposes, it is sufficient to be cognizant of the influence of PEEP and to make the necessary mental adjustment in interpretation of PAWP, as outlined in the preceding paragraph. Most important, serial changes in PAWP that occur with therapeutic interventions should be correlated with other hemodynamic and clinical parameters (e.g., blood pressure, cardiac output, urine output) to determine empirically the optimum PAWP for a given patient. This approach is necessary since it is difficult to directly measure or calculate juxtacardiac pressure in patients. Pleural pressure at end-expiration cannot be assumed to be equal to PEEP, since lung and chest wall compliance affect the relationship between these pressures. In patients with poor lung compliance (e.g., ARDS), the change in pleural pressure is usually less than one half of the applied PEEP. Direct measurement of pleural pressure with an esophageal balloon is impractical in intensive care patients; furthermore, this measurement may underestimate the immediate juxtacardiac pressure in ventilated patients. Temporarily disconnecting PEEP to measure PAWP is discouraged. The resulting new measurement is of questionable value since hemodynamics are altered (e.g., an acute increase in venous return). In addition, abrupt removal of PEEP may cause dangerous hypoxemia, and this may not be fully and rapidly reversible with reinstitution of PEEP.

Relationship of PAWP to pulmonary capillary hydrostatic pressure. The other major clinical utility of PAWP is that it provides a means of assessing pulmonary capillary pressure, or the filtration pressure favoring the development of pulmonary edema. This information often allows for the distinction between cardiogenic ("hydrostatic") and noncardiogenic ("leaky capillary") origins of lung edema fluid. Thus, the presence of pulmonary edema with a normal PAWP suggests capillary injury (e.g., ARDS), whereas pulmonary edema with a high PAWP supports a cardiogenic cause such as congestive heart failure (but does not rule out coexisting lung injury). In most clinical settings, PAWP provides a reasonable assessment of pulmonary capillary pressure. However, these values are not equivalent, and the common practice of referring to PAWP as "pulmonary capillary wedge pressure" should be discouraged.

In fact, PAWP is less than true capillary pressure by a variable amount that depends on pulmonary venous resistance. Remembering that PAWP estimates pressure in the large veins near the left atrium, it is apparent that PAWP must be less than capillary pressure to maintain forward blood flow. The difference between these pressures depends on the magnitude of flow resistance between the pulmonary capillaries and left atrium. Usually about 40% of the total pressure drop from pulmonary artery to left atrium occurs on the pulmonary venous side of the capillaries. Since PAWP approximates left atrial pressure, pulmonary capillary pressure normally can be estimated as PAWP + 0.4 (mean pulmonary artery pressure − PAWP). However, influences such as hypoxia, sympathetic nervous system discharge, and vasoactive medications may significantly increase pulmonary venous resistance with the result that pulmonary capillary pressure may far exceed PAWP. A rare but prototypic example is pulmonary veno-occlusive disease, in which the PAWP is frequently normal but the chest roentgenogram exhibits pulmonary edema. Increased pulmonary venous resistance probably also sometimes contributes to pulmonary edema in more common problems such as central nervous system injury (neurogenic pulmonary edema), myocardial infarction, and ARDS. Further research is necessary, but it does appear that reliance on PAWP causes the physician to underestimate the role of hydrostatic forces in the development of pulmonary edema under some clinical circumstances. However, until more direct measurements of pulmonary capillary pressure become available, PAWP remains an extremely valuable, and often essential, measurement for the assessment and management of pulmonary edema.

Complications of pulmonary artery catheterization. The potential adverse effects of pulmonary artery catheterization are now well understood from over a decade of experience (see box below).

Complications of balloon flotation right heart catheterization

1. Arrhythmias
   a. Transient premature ventricular contractions (PVCs)
   b. Sustained ventricular tachycardia
   c. Ventricular fibrillation
   d. Atrial fibrillation
   e. Atrial flutter
2. Right bundle branch block
3. Pulmonary infarction
4. Pulmonary artery rupture
5. Catheter-related infections
6. Balloon rupture
7. Catheter knotting
8. Endocardial damage
   a. Valve cusps
   b. Chordae tendineae
   c. Papillary muscles
9. Complications at insertion site
   a. Pneumothorax
   b. Arterial puncture
   c. Venous thrombosis or phlebitis
   d. Air embolism

Ventricular arrhythmias occur frequently during insertion of the catheter but are usually self-limited. In critically ill patients, the incidence of ventricular tachycardia (three or more consecutive premature ventricular contractions [PVCs]) is reported to be 20% to 50%. However, sustained ventricular tachycardia requiring therapy occurs in only 1% to 2% of such patients. Risk factors for ventricular tachycardia include hypocalcemia, myocardial infarction or ischemia, hypotension, and hypokalemia. However, the two most significant risk factors are hypoxemia (PO_2 less than 60 mm Hg) and acidosis (pH less than 7.2). In such high-risk patients, the use of prophylactic lidocaine during catheter insertion should be considered.

During the initial years of Swan-Ganz catheter use, pulmonary infarction was one of the most common serious complications. The incidence of pulmonary infarction was found to be greater than 7% in the mid-1970s. However, more recent experience suggests that the incidence of pulmonary infarction is now at most 1%. The difference may result from better understanding of techniques that minimize this complication. For instance, the risk of thrombus developing on the catheter tip is now reduced by the use of continuous flush with heparin solutions. Equally important is the avoidance of persistent wedging of the catheter tip. Distal migration of the catheter can be prevented by maintaining it in a position where nearly the full recommended balloon inflation volume is required to produce a wedge tracing. Furthermore, the balloon should never be inflated for longer than is necessary to obtain a wedge pressure reading (15 to 20 seconds).

The incidence of pulmonary artery rupture is about 0.2%. This is a serious complication with approximately a 50% mortality. The major risk factor for pulmonary artery rupture is pulmonary artery hypertension. Proper technique can minimize the risk of this serious complication. The balloon should always be inflated slowly and with continuous pressure monitoring; inflation should cease as soon as a wedge tracing is obtained. Hand flushing of the catheter while it is in a wedge position should be avoided.

Some indications for pulmonary artery catheterization

1. Distinguish noncardiogenic and cardiogenic pulmonary edema
2. Adult respiratory distress syndrome: manage PEEP and volume therapy
3. Myocardial infarction complicated by
   a. hypotension unresponsive to volume challenge
   b. hemodynamic instability requiring vasoactive drugs or mechanical assist devices
   c. suspected cardiac tamponade (equalization of end diastolic pressures)
   d. suspected mitral regurgitation (giant "v" waves)
   e. suspected ruptured interventricular septum (step-up in right heart oxygen saturation)
4. Unresponsive congestive heart failure
5. Resolving doubts about volume and cardiovascular status in complex illnesses (e.g., sepsis, pulmonary embolism)
6. Diagnosis and monitoring of pulmonary hypertension
7. Major cardiac surgery

Modified with permission from Goldenheim PD and Kazemi H: Cardiopulmonary monitoring of critically ill patients. N Engl J Med 331:717, 1984.

Indications for pulmonary artery catheterization. Use of the pulmonary artery catheter should be reserved for those patients in whom the diagnosis or reasonable initial therapeutic plan remains unclear after a careful clinical and noninvasive assessment, or in patients who are so unstable that the proposed treatment requires invasive monitoring. Clinical settings in which pulmonary artery catheters are frequently used include complicated myocardial infarction or congestive heart failure, ARDS (especially if PEEP greater than 10 cm H_2O is required), septic shock, pulmonary embolism with hypotension, and during major cardiac or vascular surgery (see box at lower left).

The physician should maintain respect for the possibility of a serious complication, albeit uncommon, from the pulmonary artery catheter and avoid the overzealous use in patients in whom the information obtained is unlikely to change the diagnosis or therapy.

NONINVASIVE MONITORING OF GAS EXCHANGE

Pulse oximetry

Pulse oximetry provides a simple, accurate, and noninvasive technique for the continuous monitoring of arterial oxygen saturation. This technology is gaining widespread application in intensive care units. Pulse oximetry operates on a spectrophotometric principle that exploits the different absorptive properties of oxygenated and deoxygenated hemoglobin. A small lightweight device attaches to the finger (Fig. 198-9) or toe and directs through the nailbed usually two wavelengths of light; a photodetector measures absorption. Arterial pulsation is used to gate the signal to the arterial component of blood contained within the nailbed.

Loss of adequate finger pulsation interferes with the instrument's ability to calculate arterial saturation. Inadequate finger pulsation may occur with (1) infusion of vasoconstrictive drugs, (2) hypotension (mean blood pressure less than 50 mm Hg), and (3) hypothermia. With most instruments, inadequate pulsation triggers a "low-perfusion" alarm, which should prevent the clinical application of inaccurate data. Dark skin pigmentation and jaundice do not significantly affect accuracy. However, many units have a tendency to overestimate true arterial saturation at very low values. Furthermore, the presence of elevated carboxyhemoglobin or methemoglobin produces falsely high oxyhemoglobin saturation measurements. This could have serious clinical consequences since the physician may not recognize important decreases in arterial oxygen content. Direct measurement of an arterial blood sample with the traditional four-wavelength co-oximeter (arterial blood gases) distinguishes oxyhemoglobin from carboxyhemoglobin and methemoglobin.

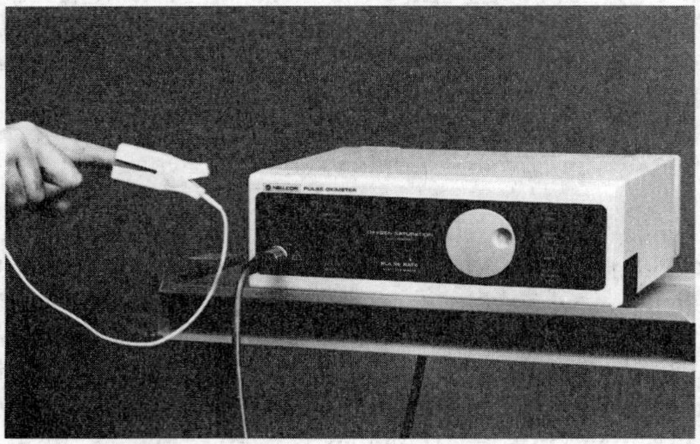

Fig. 198-9. Pulse oximeter. Pulse rate and oxygen saturation are displayed continuously.

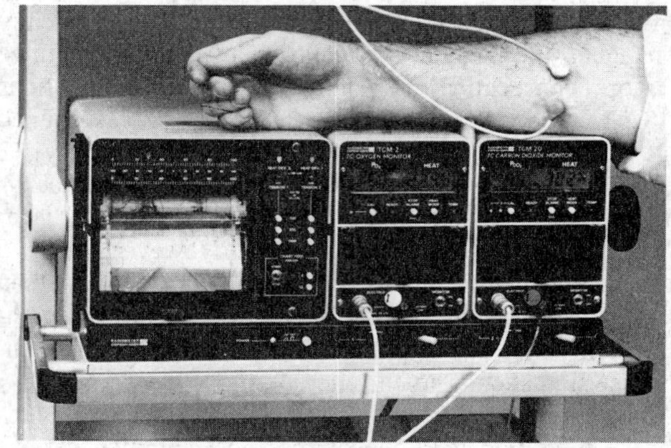

Fig. 198-10. Transcutaneous PO_2 and PCO_2 probes attached to forearm. Measurements are displayed continuously on digital monitors *(right)* and recorded on strip chart *(left)*. (For this photograph, probes were not calibrated or equilibrated.)

Transcutaneous oxygen and carbon dioxide

Heated skin probes are able to measure the concentration of oxygen or carbon dioxide that diffuses from the capillaries through the skin (Fig. 198-10). At relatively normal cardiac outputs, the transcutaneous PO_2 ($PtcO_2$) is a reliable trend monitor of the PaO_2, although the $PtcO_2$ averages only about 80% of the PaO_2 (a $PtcO_2$ value of 80 mm Hg corresponds to a PaO_2 of 100 mm Hg). However, at moderate levels of hypoperfusion (cardiac index between 1.5 and 2.2 L/min/m^2), even when not associated with frank hypotension, the $PtcO_2$ averages only about 50% of the PaO_2. This represents an important limitation of transcutaneous monitoring since such patients may not be easily distinguished without invasive monitoring of the cardiac output. And finally, in cardiogenic shock (cardiac index less than 1.5 L/min/m^2), changes in $PtcO_2$ actually reflect changes in the cardiac output (or tissue oxygen delivery), rather than the PaO_2. The physiologic interpretation of the $PtcO_2$ value therefore is complex but relatively well established. In patients with normal cardiac output and cutaneous blood flow, the $PtcO_2$ reflects PaO_2. However, in low-flow states, the $PtcO_2$ diverges from PaO_2 and reflects tissue oxygen delivery instead. This represents both a problem and an opportunity. The problem is that monitoring of the $PtcO_2$ alone may be inadequate in many clinical situations since a decreasing $PtcO_2$ may reflect either pulmonary decompensation (decreasing PaO_2) or hemodynamic failure (decreasing cardiac output). A separate, independent measurement of respiratory or cardiac function may be necessary to properly interpret the change in $PtcO_2$. On the other hand, $PtcO_2$ can detect overall decreases in tissue oxygen delivery that are otherwise difficult to assess noninvasively.

Several practical considerations affect the use of transcutaneous monitors. The heated electrodes may produce mild erythema, need to be moved frequently, have a fairly long initial equilibration time (about 5 minutes), and take time to fully respond to subsequent changes (about 1 minute). Conjunctival monitors are available, which have much shorter equilibration and response times.

The transcutaneous PCO_2 is usually about 5 to 20 mm Hg higher than $PaCO_2$. The transcutaneous PCO_2 measurement is less sensitive to changes in hemodynamic status than $PtcO_2$ and responds faster to changes in arterial gas tension.

Because of the practical and theoretical considerations, transcutaneous monitoring has not achieved widespread use as a noninvasive technique to monitor arterial blood gases in adult intensive care unit patients. However, as discussed, this technology does have immediate potential application in the noninvasive assessment of tissue oxygenation in patients with hypoperfusion.

End-tidal carbon dioxide monitoring

The carbon dioxide concentration of expired gas can be continuously monitored by mass spectroscopy or infrared absorption spectrophotometry. After anatomic dead space is cleared, the exhaled carbon dioxide tension tracks the mean alveolar value, which in turn closely approximates arterial carbon dioxide tension if pulmonary ventilation and perfusion are evenly distributed. However, in most critically ill patients, end-tidal carbon dioxide monitoring does not provide a reliable approximation of absolute arterial PCO_2 since ventilation and perfusion are usually not optimally matched. Nevertheless, capnography has several potential roles in the intensive care setting, including the monitoring of patients after attempted intubation, during cardiopulmonary resuscitation, and during weaning from mechanical ventilation. Quick confirmation of appropriate endotracheal intubation is sometimes difficult. Capnography is a rapid and practical technique for detecting inadvertent esophageal intubation, which causes the CO_2 tension of the "expired" gas to quickly fall to very low levels. Cardiac arrest is associated with a marked drop in the end-trial CO_2, and the return of adequate cardiac output during successful cardiopulmonary resuscitation is associated with a dramatic rise in expired CO_2. Capnography is therefore one of the earliest and most reliable indicators of adequate resuscitation. During weaning from mechanical ventilation, capnography allows easy visualization of low total volume breaths or apneic periods.

MECHANICAL VENTILATION

In the 1950s, positive pressure ventilation supplanted negative pressure ventilation (e.g., iron lung) as the method of choice for providing respiratory support to critically ill patients. The major advantages of positive pressure ventilators include (1) the ability to ventilate adequately despite the presence of increased airway resistance or decreased pulmonary compliance, (2) better "control" of the airway through endotracheal intubation (e.g., suctioning of secretions), and (3) significantly improved access to the patient since the ventilator does not encase the patient.

The major adverse consequences of positive pressure ventilation (see box below) are chiefly related to the altered physiology of inspiration. Instead of the normal bellows function of the chest wall and diaphragm, which creates negative pleural and airway pressure during spontaneous inspiration, positive pressure ventilation increases tracheal and pleural pressure during inspiration, altering normal interactions among lung, chest wall, and diaphragm. As a result, positive pressure ventilation may worsen ventilation-perfusion matching within the lung, leading to increased dead space ventilation and physiologic shunting. Usually, such inefficiency can be overcome by the increased ventilatory and oxygenation capacity of mechanical ventilation itself. Another physiologic consequence of positive pressure ventilation, decreased cardiac output, may present more of a clinical problem. This may be especially true when PEEP is also applied.

Initiating mechanical ventilation

Indications. The gas exchange function of the lung is twofold: (1) to provide oxygenation of arterial blood, and (2) to eliminate carbon dioxide and help regulate normal arterial acid-base balance. Inadequacy of either process such that there exists an immediate threat to life constitutes acute respiratory failure, which is the major indication for mechanical ventilation.

Hypoxemia severe enough to require mechanical ventilation is usually caused by disorders of the lung parenchyma that produce marked ventilation-perfusion mismatch or intrapulmonary shunting, and such hypoxemia remains relatively unaffected by increases in minute ventilation. Hypoxemia is therefore often referred to as "gas exchange" failure. In contrast, hypercapnia requiring mechanical support of respiration is usually the result of inadequate alveolar ventilation, or "ventilatory" failure. The box below lists some disorders that may require mechanical ventilation for treatment of gas exchange or ventilatory failure.

Acute respiratory failure is assessed by measurement of the arterial blood gases, but there are no absolute threshold values of arterial PO_2, PCO_2, or pH at which mechanical ventilation should be instituted. Rather, it is necessary also to consider the underlying disease process, the patient's course and response to therapy, and other factors within the overall clinical context. As a general guide, acute hypercapnia resulting in a pH less than 7.30 should lead to consideration of beginning mechanical ventilation. Hypoxemia frequently can be initially treated with supplemental oxygen via nasal prongs or face mask without resorting to mechanical ventilation. If the arterial PO_2 cannot be maintained above about 60 mm Hg with such external devices, intubation and mechanical ventilation are necessary. In addition to ensuring controlled delivery of a high oxygen concentration to the lungs, mechanical ventilation may reduce the oxygen requirement in some patients by lessening shunt through the recruitment of previously collapsed alveolar units.

Initial ventilator settings. After intubation, most patients are initially placed on a conventional positive pressure–volume-controlled ventilator. The settings typically selected at the start of mechanical ventilation include a tidal volume of 10 to 15 ml per kilogram, a respiratory frequency of 12 machine-delivered breaths per minute, an oxygen concentration of 100%, and an inspiratory flow rate of 40 to 60 liters per minute (80 to 100 liters per minute in patients with chronic obstructive lung disease to allow more expiratory time and improve ventilation-perfusion matching). The high-pressure alarm should be set at about 10 cm above the peak airway pressure observed on these settings.

Complications of mechanical ventilation

Barotrauma (e.g., pneumothorax, pneumomediastinum, subcutaneous emphysema)
Decreased cardiac output
Nosocomial pneumonia
Complications of endotracheal or tracheostomy tubes

Some indications for mechanical ventilation

Gas exchange (oxygenation) failure
- Pneumonia
- Adult respiratory distress syndrome
- Pulmonary edema

Ventilatory failure
- Neuromuscular disease (e.g., Guillain-Barré syndrome, myasthenia gravis, poliomyelitis)
- Drug overdose
- Respiratory muscle fatigue or dysfunction
- Restrictive defects of the chest wall
- Depressed respiratory center drive
- Severe asthma
- Exacerbation of chronic obstructive pulmonary disease

Within 20 minutes of initiating mechanical ventilation, arterial blood gases should be obtained to document the adequacy of the initial ventilator settings and to guide subsequent adjustments. If possible, the inspired oxygen concentration should be lowered to nontoxic levels (less than 40% to 50%), while maintaining an adequate arterial concentration (PO_2 more than 60 mm Hg). The minute ventilation (tidal volume and respiratory rate) is adjusted to achieve an appropriate arterial PCO_2 and pH.

Modes of mechanical ventilation

Mechanical ventilation can be delivered via different modes and modifications thereof (see box below). Although few data exist to support the overall superiority of one form of mechanical ventilation over the others, the purported advantages of certain modes have fostered their selective application in particular clinical circumstances.

Controlled mechanical ventilation. With this mode, a preset tidal volume is delivered at a predetermined frequency. The patient is unable to trigger additional ventilator breaths, frequently leading to patient discomfort. This mode of ventilation is now seldom used and is appropriate only for unconscious and apneic patients.

Assist/control ventilation. The assist/control mode, or assisted mechanical ventilation (AMV), allows the patient to trigger a ventilator-delivered breath (at the preselected tidal volume) by initiating a minimal inspiratory effort. If the patient does not make inspiratory efforts, the ventilator ensures a minimal minute ventilation at a frequency and tidal volume preselected by the physician. The major advantage of this system is that the patient is able to interact with the ventilator, thereby minimizing discomfort and allowing for an increase in minute ventilation in response to changes in physiologic demands. For these benefits to be realized, the sensitivity of the patient-triggering mechanism needs to be adjusted to avoid unintentional machine ventilation (leading to respiratory alkalosis) but should allow for patient-initiated breaths without excessive effort. Assist/control is the mode usually chosen for the initiation of mechanical ventilation.

Intermittent mandatory ventilation. Intermittent mandatory ventilation (IMV) delivers a preset tidal volume at a specified frequency, thereby guaranteeing a minimum ventilator-delivered minute ventilation, but additionally allows the patient to breathe spontaneously without triggering the ventilator. Respiration by the patient during IMV ventilation therefore mimics the physiology of normal spontaneous ventilation (e.g., full respiratory muscle effort throughout inspiration, negative pleural pressure during inspiration).

When compared to AMV, the putative advantages of IMV include (1) better patient synchrony with ventilator, (2) less tendency toward respiratory alkalosis, (3) maintenance of respiratory muscle function, (4) usefulness as a weaning technique, and (5) less reduction in cardiac output. Some evidence is available to support the contention that IMV is indeed helpful in patients who are "fighting" the ventilator in the assist/control mode or in patients whose cardiac output is depressed during positive pressure ventilation as a result of hypovolemia or the use of PEEP. A trial of IMV is warranted for these purposes. In contrast, no appropriately controlled studies indicate the superiority of IMV for enhancing respiratory muscle function or for expediting weaning. Two prospective investigations failed to find any clinically significant difference in pH among patients ventilated with IMV or AMV. Although there was a slight trend toward a reduction in alkalosis with IMV, this occurred because of an increase in carbon dioxide production rather than a reduction in minute ventilation. This suggests that the small improvement in alkalosis occurs at the expense of increased breathing work.

The consequences of IMV are most appropriately discussed in the context of the frequency of ventilator-delivered breaths. If the IMV rate is low, the patient is receiving only partial ventilatory support since the ventilator does not provide an adequate minute ventilation. In such a case, the patient is required to supplement the difference. For unstable patients or patients with respiratory muscle fatigue, a low IMV rate clearly is inappropriate. In contrast, a low IMV setting may be of benefit in weaning a stable patient from mechanical ventilation. A high IMV rate provides full ventilatory support to the patient and obviates the need for additional spontaneous breaths. Used in this manner, IMV differs little from the traditional use of AMV.

Positive end-expiratory pressure. Positive end-expiratory pressure can be used with any of the modes of ventilation. It generally improves arterial oxygenation when applied to patients with diffuse lung edema and refractory hypoxemia caused by intrapulmonary shunting (e.g., ARDS). This is accomplished by preventing atelectasis in fluid-filled alveoli and terminal bronchioles, thereby improving ventilation-perfusion relationships. Frequently, the improvement in arterial PO_2 allows reduction of the inspired oxygen concentration to less toxic levels. Most evidence suggests that PEEP does not reduce total lung water, prevent ARDS when applied early to patients at risk, or hasten lung repair. Most clinicians therefore advocate the use of PEEP only when necessary to support oxygenation and only at the minimal level necessary to achieve this goal. Ideally, the arterial PO_2 should be maintained greater than or equal to

Some modes of mechanical ventilation

Controlled mechanical ventilation (CMV)
Assist/control ventilation (AMV)
Intermittent mandatory ventilation (IMV)
Positive end-expiratory pressure (PEEP)
Pressure support ventilation (PSV)
High-frequency ventilation (HFV)
Inverse-ratio ventilation (IRV)

60 mm Hg (oxygen saturation greater than 90%) with an inspired oxygen concentration less than or equal to 50%.

The major adverse effect of PEEP is a depression of cardiac output. This is attributable chiefly to an increase in mean intrathoracic pressure and a consequent decrease in venous return to the thorax. No evidence shows that PEEP has a direct effect on myocardial contractility. A decrease in cardiac output is usually seen with PEEP levels greater than 10 cm H_2O, but this may occur at lower levels in patients with hypovolemia or cardiac disease. When cardiac output decreases significantly in a patient receiving PEEP, this may result in a net decrease in systemic oxygen delivery despite the improvement in PaO_2 and arterial oxygen saturation.

An empirical trial is necessary to determine the optimum level of PEEP under any given clinical circumstances. This usually involves gradually increasing the PEEP (e.g., 0, 5, 10 cm H_2O and so on) while monitoring arterial PO_2, lung compliance (compliance usually improves until excessive PEEP levels are reached), and the hemodynamic status. A pulmonary artery catheter should be placed to monitor hemodynamic variables if it is apparent that PEEP greater than 10 cm H_2O is required or if hemodynamic instability occurs at lower levels.

If PEEP is applied inappropriately to patients with *focal* lung consolidation (e.g., unilateral pneumonia), a paradoxical decrease in arterial PO_2 may occur. Alveolar expansion caused by PEEP preferentially occurs in the more compliant normal lung, increasing pulmonary vascular resistance in this area and thereby directing more pulmonary blood flow through the consolidated lung, aggravating the shunt.

Inverse ratio ventilation. Recent evidence suggests that conventional ventilatory support of ARDS patients with volume-cycled ventilation and PEEP (see above) may perpetuate lung injury by overinflating. A strategy termed *inverse ratio ventilation* (IRV) may maintain or improve gas exchange at lower levels of PEEP and lower peak airway pressures, thereby theoretically reducing lung damage caused by mechanical ventilation. IRV can be achieved by two methods: (1) with volume-cycled inspiratory flow rate, or (2) with pressure-controlled ventilation, by utilizing a long inspiratory time. A limitation of IRV is the need to heavily sedate or paralyze most patients during its use. Clinicians appear to be using IRV with increasing frequency, although no clinical trials have as yet compared the outcome in ARDS patients treated with IRV versus conventional ventilation.

Pressure support ventilation. A recent development in mechanical ventilation is pressure support ventilation (PSV), the augmentation of inspiratory efforts by a set amount of positive airway pressure. This pressure is sustained at a plateau level as long as a minimal inspiratory flow is occurring, providing the patient with significant control over the volume and duration of inspiration. Among different ventilators there is as yet no standard algorithm for maintaining and terminating pressure support during each breath; such pressure-flow specifications are dependent on the particular model used.

More clinical experience is necessary before conclusions about the role of PSV can be made. Pressure support ventilation may improve patient comfort and reduce pressure work during mechanical ventilation (e.g., spontaneous breaths during IMV) and may also be a valuable adjunct to weaning patients from mechanical ventilation.

High-frequency ventilation. High-frequency ventilation (HFV) is a generic term for mechanical ventilation with a frequency of greater than 60 cycles per minute. Three major types of ventilators are available: high-frequency positive pressure ventilators (HFPPV), high-frequency jet ventilators (HFJV), and high-frequency oscillators (HFO). Although each uses different mechanics and produces gas displacement in different ways, each is characterized by small tidal volumes that are less than or approximate to the anatomic dead space volume. Among other potential benefits, HFV provides adequate gas exchange at lower peak airway pressure than conventional positive pressure ventilation.

The HFPPV and HFJV are open systems that are effective without the use of a tight-fitting endotracheal tube. These systems are therefore useful when ventilatory support is required during upper airway surgery, laryngoscopy, or bronchoscopy. Except for these situations, HFV has not been documented to offer consistent benefits over conventional ventilation. A large prospective and randomized study comparing HFJV and conventional ventilation in intensive care unit patients with respiratory failure from a variety of causes (e.g., ARDS, pneumonia, aspiration) found no superiority for either technique. Conventional ventilation provided a higher PaO_2 at equivalent PEEP levels than HFJV, but alveolar ventilation was slightly better on HFJV. On HFJV, oxygenation and ventilation were maintained with lower peak inspiratory pressures than those with conventional volume-cycled ventilation. These differences were all small and not likely to be clinically significant. Similarly, no data are available indicating a reduction in the incidence of barotrauma with HFV or showing improved survival in patients with bronchopleural fistula, despite anecdotal reports that HFJV might be effective in ventilating patients with bronchopleural fistula.

Further clinical experience and investigation are necessary to define the role of HFV in the intensive care unit.

Monitoring ventilatory mechanics

Total thoracic (lung and chest wall) compliance characteristics can be assessed in the ventilated patient. The pressure dial on the ventilator indicates, for any given tidal volume, both peak pressure and a static pressure (assessed when there is no air flow just prior to the start of exhalation) (Fig. 198-11). Momentarily occluding the expiratory tubing immediately prior to exhalation may be necessary to reveal the brief plateau of the static pressure. Dividing the tidal volume by either peak or static pressure gives a measure of the thoracic dynamic characteristic or the thoracic static compliance, respectively. Static compliance re-

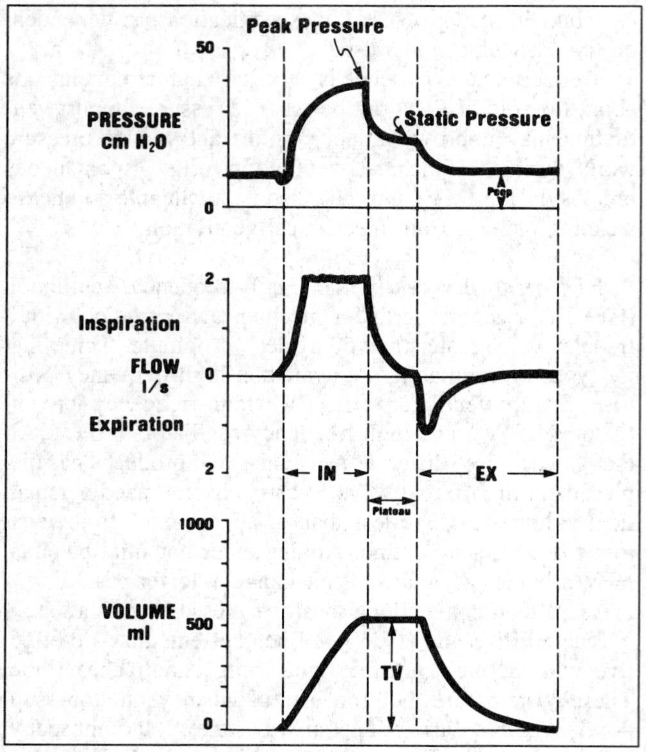

Fig. 198-11. Relationship of tidal volume (TV), air flow rates, and ventilator dial reading in a patient receiving mechanical ventilation with 10 cm H_2O of PEEP. The static pressure is more apparent if expiratory retard or inspiratory hold is used, or if the expiratory tubing is momentarily occluded or pinched.

$$\text{Static compliance} = \frac{\text{tidal volume}}{\text{static pressure} - \text{PEEP}}$$

In this example, static compliance equals 500 ÷ (20-10) = 50 ml/cm H_2O. The normal static compliance of the lung and chest wall in a mechanically ventilated patient is about 50 to 70 ml/cm H_2O. If lung and chest wall compliance is reduced (less than 25 ml/cm H_2O), the increased work of breathing will hinder weaning. If flow is also measured (requires a pneumotachograph), then airway resistance (Raw) can be calculated:

$$\text{Raw} = \frac{\text{peak pressure} - \text{static pressure}}{\text{flow}}$$

In this example (40-20) ÷ 2 = 10 cm H_2O/liters per second (l/s). Normal Raw is between 2 and 3 cm H_2O/liters per second. Increased airway resistance might be due to bronchospasm or secretions, for instance. (Reproduced with permission from Bone RC: Monitoring ventilatory mechanics in acute respiratory failure. *Respir Care* 28:597-604, 1983.)

flects changes in the lung parenchyma, whereas the dynamic characteristic additionally reflects changes in airways resistance. It is valuable to evaluate respiratory compliance characteristics when taking care of the critically ill. Such monitoring provides means of assessing therapeutic interventions such as PEEP (static compliance usually increases during initial application of PEEP and may begin to decrease if the optimal PEEP level is exceeded) or assessing disease trends (a decreasing compliance signals worsening of lung parenchymal disease). Furthermore, an acute increase in peak airway pressure may be a valuable early indicator of problems such as pneumothorax, endotracheal tube sliding into the right mainstem bronchus, or endotracheal tube (or airways) becoming plugged with blood or secretions.

Endotracheal intubation and tracheotomy

Mechanical ventilation requires intubation of the trachea with either an endotracheal or a tracheotomy tube. In a patient with acute respiratory failure, endotracheal intubation can be performed much quicker and with fewer complications than tracheotomy, which requires surgical expertise and is associated with a twofold to fivefold increase in complication rate when performed on an emergency rather than elective basis. With current respiratory care techniques and soft-cuff endotracheal tubes, endotracheal intubation can usually be maintained for several days or even a few weeks without excessive complications. Nevertheless, the requirement for "prolonged" mechanical ventilation is an indication for elective tracheotomy. However, the timing of elective tracheotomy in mechanically ventilated patients remains a controversial topic.

Proponents of delayed tracheotomy cite studies demonstrating that the complications from tracheotomy are greater than those of 2 or 3 weeks of endotracheal intubation. However, these nonrandomized investigations (in which the tracheotomy groups were exposed to the tracheotomy procedure only after fairly prolonged translaryngeal intubation) may be biased against tracheotomy since prolonged translaryngeal intubation increases the risk for airway injury from a subsequent tracheotomy. Advocates of early tracheotomy also point to studies suggesting that laryngeal injuries from endotracheal intubation may be more severe and difficult to repair than tracheal injuries from tracheotomy.

A reasonable approach is to continue translaryngeal intubation in most mechanically ventilated patients for a week to 10 days and consider tracheotomy if weaning and extubation are not likely within the next week. Clinical judgment and individual patient factors may provide grounds for altering this approach. Specifically, the risks and advantages of each technique need to be considered in the particular clinical context.

Problems encountered with endotracheal intubation may include patient discomfort, difficulty in suctioning tracheobronchial secretions, patient self-extubation, and with nasotracheal intubation, sinusitis or otitis. Problems with tracheotomy include stomal infection, stomal hemorrhage, and subcutaneous emphysema.

A major advantage of tracheotomy is less interference with the pharyngeal area, allowing possibilities for speech and eating. Tracheotomy tubes also are more easily changed when necessary and have less resistance to air flow as compared with endotracheal tubes. These considerations account for the need for tracheotomy in virtually all patients undergoing a prolonged weaning process.

Weaning from mechanical ventilation

The process of returning a mechanically ventilated patient to normal spontaneous breathing is termed *weaning*. The clinician faces two major issues in the weaning process.

First is the decision regarding when the patient is ready to begin the weaning process. Once the patient is deemed ready for weaning, an appropriate plan for accomplishing this goal must be devised. Prediction of weaning success and the weaning process itself are considerably more straightforward in the patient who has received short-term mechanical ventilation (less than 7 days). In contrast, patients who have received mechanical ventilation for longer than 1 month often require a fairly prolonged and complex weaning process.

Initiation of weaning should be considered when the patient has sufficiently recovered from the underlying processes that necessitated mechanical ventilation. The patient should also be hemodynamically stable, alert, cooperative, and without physical distress. At this point, gas exchange and spontaneous ventilatory parameters should be assessed. The criteria indicated in the box below are highly predictive of weaning success after short-term ventilatory support. In many of these patients, it is reasonable to allow the patient to breathe spontaneously on a T-piece circuit with an inspired oxygen concentration of approximately 40%. Provided that the arterial blood gases obtained after 30 to 60 minutes are adequate, and the patient does not exhibit tachypnea, tachycardia, cardiac arrhythmias, or hemodynamic instability, the patient can usually be extubated.

Patients who have received long-term mechanical ventilation or who have significant unresolved underlying lung disease or other medical complications are usually not appropriate for the rapid T-piece weaning technique. In such patients, fulfilling the criteria of the box below does not necessarily predict quick success, and the weaning process is frequently prolonged over several days or even weeks. Two methods that have traditionally been used in this setting are the use of intermittent T-piece and IMV weaning. The intermittent T-piece technique involves the use of progressively longer and more frequent periods of full spontaneous ventilation through the T-piece circuit, followed by periods of complete rest with full ventilatory support. The IMV method involves a gradual decrease in the IMV rate. In this method, the patient receives partial ventilatory support in a progressively decreasing manner, rather than intermittent periods of no ventilatory support as with the T-piece technique. In both methods, it is customary to return the patient to full ventilatory support during the night until the final stages of weaning are approached.

Criteria predictive of successful weaning from short-term mechanical ventilation

- Arterial oxygen tension >60 mm Hg with inspired oxygen concentration ≤40%
- Tidal volume >5 ml per kilogram
- Vital capacity >10 ml per kilogram
- Maximum inspiratory force <−25 cm H_2O
- Spontaneous minute ventilation ≤10 liters per minute (and maintains acceptable $PaCO_2$)
- Able to double spontaneous minute ventilation with maximal voluntary effort
- Respiratory frequency/tidal volume ratio <100 breaths per minute/liter

Nonpulmonary factors to consider in the difficult-to-wean patient

- Medications (e.g., sedatives, analgesics)
- Malnutrition
- Hypophosphatemia, hypomagnesemia, hypokalemia
- Small-bore endotracheal tube (8 mm tube or larger is preferred)
- Respiratory muscle dysfunction (e.g., diaphragm paralysis following open heart surgery)
- Metabolic alkalosis (depresses respiratory drive)
- Unstable medical status (e.g., uncontrolled infection)
- Interference with chest wall (e.g., casts, bandages, chest tube, restraints)
- Hypothyroidism

No conclusive data exist that indicate the superiority of either the T-piece or IMV technique. Some advocates of the T-piece method claim support from the physiology of muscle training, in which the usual approach is to work a muscle to the point of fatigue and then allow complete rest. If weaning the ventilator-dependent patient is analogous to the athlete in training, the T-piece method would appear to have an advantage (although IMV is not in conflict with this concept). Although further studies are necessary to define the relative merits of T-piece and IMV weaning, it is clear that each technique, when used appropriately, has been successfully used as a weaning method.

Pressure support ventilation is attracting attention as a possible new weaning technique. Experience with this method is limited, but there are some theoretical advantages to this approach. Pressure support may provide a more physiologic workload to the ventilatory muscles than does IMV (with pressure support, the pressure-volume load on the muscles is more normal and the work is applied more regularly). In addition, since the patient has more control over the flow and volume of each breath, patient comfort might be expected to be improved with pressure support ventilation. At the start of weaning, levels of pressure support that produce tidal breaths equivalent to that supplied by conventional ventilation are provided. Subsequently, the level of pressure support is gradually reduced as tolerated.

In the difficult-to-wean patient, it is worthwhile considering a number of nonrespiratory factors that may be contributing to the problem (see box above), such as medications, metabolic alkalosis, or hypothyroidism.

REFERENCES

Carlon GC et al: High-frequency jet ventilation: a prospective randomized evaluation. Chest 84:551, 1983.

Clark JS et al: Noninvasive assessment of blood gases. Am Rev Respir Dis 145:220, 1992.

Falk JL, Rackow EC, and Weil MH: End-tidal carbon dioxide concentration during cardiopulmonary resuscitation. N Engl J Med 318:607, 1988.

Heffner JE: Tracheal intubation in mechanically ventilated patients. Clin Chest Med 9:23, 1988.

Heffner JE: Timing of tracheotomy in ventilation-dependent patients. Clin Chest Med 12:611, 1991.

Higgins TL and Stoller JK: Discontinuing ventilatory support. In Pierson DJ and Kacmarek RM, editors: Foundations of respiratory care. New York, 1992, Churchill-Livingstone.

Hudson LD et al: Does intermittent mandatory ventilation correct respiratory alkalosis in patients receiving assisted mechanical ventilation? Am Rev Respir Dis 132:1071, 1985.

Marcy TW and Marini JJ: Intensive ratio ventilation in ARDS: rationale and implementation. Chest 100:494, 1991.

Marini JJ: Monitoring during mechanical ventilation. Clin Chest Med 9:73, 1988.

Morley TF: Capnography in the intensive care unit. J Intensive Care Med 5:209, 1990.

Pierson DJ: Weaning from mechanical ventilation in acute respiratory failure: concepts, indications, and techniques. Respir Care 28:646, 1983.

Sassoon CSH: Positive pressure ventilation: alternative modes. Chest 100:1421, 1991.

Weisman IM et al: State of the art: intermittent mandatory ventilation. Am Rev Respir Dis 127:641, 1983.

Wiedemann HP, Matthay MA, and Matthay RA: Cardiovascular-pulmonary monitoring in the intensive care unit (parts 1 & 2). Chest 85:537, 656, 1984.

Wiedemann HP and McCarthy K: Noninvasive monitoring of oxygen and carbon dioxide. Clin Chest Med 10:239, 1989.

Yang KL and Tobin MJ: A prospective study of indexes predicting the outcome of trials of weaning from mechanical ventilation. N Engl J Med 324:1445, 1991.

III Clinical Syndromes and Therapeutic Modalities

CHAPTER

199 Approach to the Patient with Respiratory Disease: History, Physical Examination, and Assessment of Major Symptoms*

Herbert Y. Reynolds

The diagnosis of pulmonary disease has changed remarkably over the past 20 years because of technology (i.e., computed tomography [CT], fiberoptic bronchoscopy, CT-guided needle aspiration, and nuclear magnetic resonance imaging) that allows a more direct view of lung tissue. Moreover, the spectrum of pulmonary disease is changing. Cancer of the lung, especially in females, continues to increase. The "white plague" of tuberculosis is on the rise again, especially in patients with acquired immunodeficiency syndrome (AIDS) who are at risk for many kinds of infection to common encapsulated bacteria, *Pneumocystis carinii,* and fungal organisms. Chronic obstructive pulmonary disease is increasing in the aging populations, and disorders of sleeping and obstructive apnea are recognized more often. Increasingly, lung transplantation is a reality for selected patients with pulmonary hypertension, interstitial fibrosis, and cystic fibrosis. Low-grade graft versus host disease causing mucositis and bronchiolitis obliterans is encountered in recipients of bone marrow transplants.

Advances and new forms of pulmonary illness notwithstanding, no speciality in medicine today depends more on the basic tools that have been in use for decades for the diagnosis of disease. The medical history alone may establish the diagnosis in many instances. Skillful interpretation of routine radiographs and pulmonary function tests is required. Identification of bacteria in the sputum Gram stain still determines initial or empirical antibiotic choices. The lung biopsy with light microscopy is the mainstay of tissue diagnosis.

The purpose of this chapter is to remind the reader of the usefulness of what is old but tested, and to present an approach to the respiratory patient by reviewing the history, the performance of the physical examination, and the main symptoms of some pulmonary diseases.

CONSIDERATION OF THE HISTORY

A thorough review of the patient's medical and social history, coupled with the presenting symptoms or circumstances of the acute illness, provides the background for the physician's initial diagnosis. These elements dictate how extensive a physical examination is needed and suggest what ancillary laboratory studies are necessary to confirm or identify the disease process. Acute situations created by trauma or catastrophic illness obviously curtail history taking and by necessity direct medical attention to emergency care. It is possible that a rushed and busy house staff physician or hurried practitioner may not take the time to question and listen to the patient or may quickly scan a checklist history sheet and go straight for objective laboratory data and a chest radiograph. The physician may plan to fill in the details of the history later but, as can happen, may not get back to this as originally planned. Thus, part of the patient's data base may not be evaluated adequately. Sometimes only in retrospect do possible omissions of history become important.

Many unrelated things may have to be asked of the patient before a composite history is formed: the patient's occupational history is an example. Inhalation exposure to chemical fumes or organic dusts can cause asthmalike symptoms; the breathing of airborne particles from the grinding or cutting of heavy metal, or inhaling of sand or asbestos fibers can initiate forms of diffuse interstitial pulmonary fibrosis that produce chronic dyspnea. Usually,

*Author appreciates the prior contributions of Dr. Richard E. Brashear.

many years must elapse between the initial exposure to such materials and the development of respiratory symptoms, so that dating the exposure(s) or correctly identifying the work-related circumstances may be difficult. A detailed account of each job, including summer work during youth and assignments in military service, may be necessary to pinpoint a casual exposure to asbestos, for example, which might explain parietal pleural plaques. Exposure can be insidious to inhaled mold spores and organic antigens that can cause hypersensitivity pneumonitis, so unsuspected avocations or unusual hobbies need to be probed. Sometimes a visit to the patient's work place or home is required to assess the environmental milieu.

Symptoms referable to asthma or bronchospasm can be confusing. Coughing instead of wheezing can be a presentation of asthma. Wheezing and shortness of breath occurring at night and awakening the patient might denote esophageal reflux and regurgitation from a hiatus hernia. This can cause glottic dysfunction, producing hoarseness and cough. Also, while recumbent, peripheral edema from congestive heart failure can be redistributed to the pulmonary tissue, causing wheezing and cough—so-called cardiac asthma.

An accurate history of cigarette smoking is usually obtained, but some attempt to quantify the exposure by calculating pack-years and noting if filtered or unfiltered cigarettes were smoked are of interest. A history of marijuana smoking may not be volunteered by the patient, since many erroneously think it is not as harmful or as much of a risk factor as tobacco. Abrupt cessation by a heavy smoker is often an ominous sign that lung cancer is feared, usually because some hemoptysis has occurred or because a persistent cough prompts the patient to seek medical help. Many patients with bronchitis and chronic obstructive pulmonary disease (COPD) continue to smoke despite very disabling symptoms. In contrast, patients with true asthma and adults with cystic fibrosis rarely smoke. Fractured ribs and a hemothorax sustained in a long-past motor vehicle accident could account for costophrenic blunting and pleural thickening noted on a chest radiograph. A question directed to the patient's spouse about the latter's perception of the patient's respiratory symptoms could evoke the complaint of fitful sleeping and snoring by the patient that directs attention to an upper airway obstruction or a sleep disorder syndrome. Particulars in a patient's travel history might raise alternate causes for a chest mass or mediastinal calcification and redirect the diagnostic evaluation. Likewise, recurrent bacterial respiratory infections, perhaps also with sinus involvement in a young adult, could prompt the physician to consider pursuing one of several congenital diseases that affect the respiratory system, such as impaired ciliary movement (syndromes associated with an intrinsic structural defect in the dynein arms or radial spokes of cilia that alters rhythmic beating), acquired hypogammaglobulinemia, selective immunoglobulin G (IgG) subclass deficiency, or a subtle presentation of cystic fibrosis. A family history revealing affected siblings is of obvious importance. An association between recurrent sinopulmonary infections and infertility problems could be a clue for cystic fibrosis or a ciliary defect. Increasingly, drugs are implicated as a cause of hypersensitivity and interstitial pulmonary fibrosis, and a complete inventory of drug taking must be recorded. Antineoplastic chemotherapy agents and immunosuppressant drugs are usually obvious, but gold or penicillamine therapy used for the patient with rheumatoid arthritis, an antibiotic prescribed for chronic suppression of a bladder infection or, rarely, a thiazide diuretic or some other very common medication can all be culprits.

PHYSICAL EXAMINATION OF THE RESPIRATORY SYSTEM

Some of the most helpful information about breathing mechanics can be obtained by simply observing the patient. The careful eye will note whether accessory muscles of respiration are used, nasal flaring is present, rib retractions occur, diaphragm-abdominal muscle incoordination exists, or splinting of the thorax is done. The manner in which the patient breathes is almost as helpful as auscultation of the lungs. Pursed-lip breathing, fixing the hands on the thighs to stabilize the shoulder girdle, sitting or leaning forward in bed, and conversing in short phrases or words instead of normal sentences all betray dyspnea. Anxiety, restlessness, sallow complexion or frank cyanosis, audible wheezing, and paroxysms of coughing can add to the appearance of respiratory difficulty. The depth and frequency of breathing should be recorded, as well as some judgment about the amount of air movement. For example, with severe asthma, a patient may have few wheezes because of poor air movement, or crackles may not be heard even in pulmonary edema if the patient is fatigued and respirations are shallow.

Tachypnea is obvious, but other patterns of abnormal breathing often relate to neurologic diseases that affect central respiratory centers in the brain and brainstem. Distinct breathing patterns accompany forms of sleep apnea or reflect upper airway obstruction. Sleep monitoring and polysomnography are needed to document the derangement precisely, and neurophysiologic study is required to confirm hypoglossal muscle or laryngeal dysfunction. In some cases, however, casual observation of the sleeping patient may reveal salient features of the obstructive process. A history of snoring, fitful sleep, daytime somnolence, and deteriorating mentation or violent, abusive behavior in a history, usually supplied by the spouse or a relative, are invaluable parts of the diagnostic workup in sleep disorders. The shape of the mandible and face (micrognathia) or a large tongue and small retropharyngeal area may give physical clues.

Careful inspection of the nose and throat is necessary. Evidence of nasal obstruction from polyps or a deviated septum can explain postnasal secretions and coughing. Polyps can be associated with asthma, allergic rhinitis, and other diseases such as aspirin-induced asthma and cystic fibrosis. Nasal ulceration and sinusitis may suggest a vasculitis of the respiratory tract (Wegener's granulomatosis). Parotid gland swelling can be found in sarcoidosis and with collagen vascular diseases.

Before auscultating the chest, it is worth observing the

patient take a few deep breaths and watching for asymmetrical expansion of the thorax; also assess the shape of the thoracic cage and note the presence of scoliosis or pectus excavatum. Barrel-chest development, overdevelopment or hypertrophy of pectoralis and strap muscles used as accessory muscles for respiration, gynecomastia, and any incoordination of chest and abdominal musculature should be noted. Next, cursory palpation at least of bony structures of the thorax and inspection for external signs of trauma and prior surgical scars are indicated. Conscientious palpation of nodal areas in the neck, axillary, and retroclavicular areas is required; breast examination in males and in females and careful palpation of the thyroid gland are also necessary. Percussion of the chest to ascertain diaphragm movement, to localize pleural effusion(s), or to elicit dullness over pneumonic areas is an age-old diagnostic technique that can yield helpful clues. Unfortunately, such clues seem less important for the accuracy of diagnosis, since radiographic and scanning procedures provide more objective data; however, auscultation of the lung fields remains useful because it provides unique information that the chest radiograph or CT scans cannot capture and helps the physician to immediately assess important disorders affecting the airways. Wet crackles from alveolar edema, wheezes, rhonchi, and diminished breath sounds can be distinguished. Merely listening at the posterior bases of the lungs, however, may not be sufficient, for axillary and frontal projections of the lungs to the chest wall may yield pleural rubs or important clues to infection. Patients with a variety of diffuse interstitial pulmonary diseases that lead to fibrosis usually have dry, inspiratory crackles throughout much of the lung fields. Descriptive adjectives, such as "cellophane" and "Velcro" rales, have been given to these adventitious lung sounds. Examination of the heart must be considered as an extension of the lung examination, and a thorough assessment of left and right ventricular function must be made. Evidence of right heart failure and/or pulmonary hypertension must be sought.

Obviously, an entire physical examination is required, and other sites, removed from the chest, can give important clues about lung function and the type of lung disease present. Needle puncture marks in the skin may identify an unsuspected intravenous drug user and provide a clue for the cause of multiple pulmonary abscesses and endocarditis. Acral cyanosis can reflect hypoxemia. Most collagen vascular diseases, particularly progressive systemic sclerosis, dermatomyositis, lupus erythematosus, and rheumatoid arthritis, involve the skin, as well as having an appreciable incidence of interstitial pulmonary fibrosis. Clubbing of the digits always provokes an interesting differential diagnosis. Evidence of primary tumor in other organs can explain pulmonary metastases, and a tumor-associated hypercoagulable state may cause deep-vein thrombosis and result in pulmonary emboli. Because so many interrelationships exist among systemic diseases and pulmonary dysfunction, it is useless to catalogue even the most frequent associations; the point for emphasis, however, is that a clear understanding of medical pulmonary disease requires a global view of the patient, and this requires a thorough physical examination.

RESPIRATORY SYMPTOMS

Certain respiratory symptoms are quite important, especially if volunteered by the patient. The cardinal ones include dyspnea or breathlessness, wheezing, coughing, expectoration of secretions, chest pain, and hemoptysis; each will be addressed.

Dyspnea

Dyspnea may be an insidious symptom that is difficult for the patient to define or to pinpoint with regard to onset. *Dyspnea* means difficult or uncomfortable breathing and in aggregate is more than just an abnormal breathing pattern, for example, tachypnea, hyperventilation, and irregular or nonsynchronous breathing. Dyspnea can be quantitated. It is a subjective sensation that often is described as breathlessness and an awareness of not being able to catch one's breath or having insufficient breath to perform a simple or mundane task (toweling off after bathing or stopping midway climbing a flight of stairs). Labored breathing is expected with exertion and exercise, but the point at which one becomes aware of an unusual breathing pattern or perceives an excessive effort to breathe or to recover the breath is quite subjective. Breathlessness, which is an approximate synonym for dyspnea, can be quantitatively quite different for various persons, and, as a symptom of respiratory illness, it must be verified for each patient. For a conditioned athlete or jogger, breathlessness is associated only with vigorous exertion, whereas an active parent, supervising children and a household, may find breathlessness in the course of accustomed activity very debilitating. At times, dyspnea may not be a specific symptom of respiratory disease, but a derivative symptom indicating mild left ventricular heart failure, anemia, thyrotoxicosis, or myositis and weak-muscle syndromes. Breathlessness commonly heralds a variety of interstitial lung diseases that produce less compliant lungs and restrictive patterns of pulmonary function. Because of its subjective nature, dyspnea may not correlate with various physiologic measurements; thus attempts have been made to quantitate it with various indices and scales. One such indexing method couples the patient's measured functional impairment with the magnitude of the task, the effort required, and the psychological factors contributing. Thus, a clinical rating of dyspnea may provide quantitative information that complements measurement of lung function.

Dyspnea is a respiratory symptom that needs to be evaluated, and its cause can stem from a myriad of pathologic processes in the lungs. As mentioned, it can reflect defective respiratory drive, impaired respiratory muscles, or be a secondary symptom of cardiac or hematologic dysfunction. Finally, emotional illness (e.g., depression, hysteria) can produce various forms of dyspnea that are manifested as sighing, hyperventilation, rapid shallow breathing, or throat clearing and frequent coughing. In evaluating dyspnea, it must be judged in the context of the history and physical examination, appropriate laboratory data, chest imaging studies, and pulmonary function testing. Determining whether dyspnea has developed acutely or is of a chronic nature is important. For patients with COPD, dyspnea seems to correlate reasonably well with the forced expiratory volume (FEV_1), maximum voluntary ventilation (MVV), and residual lung volume (RV). For patients with forms of interstitial lung disease, the fall in arterial oxygen desaturation with exertion and the carbon monoxide diffusion capacity (DLCO) are good parameters to monitor in assessing dyspnea or breathlessness. However, some patients with sarcoidosis may have normal lung spirometry yet have dyspnea, possibly reflecting endobronchial granulomatous disease and irritation. Finally, dyspnea may be a criterion used to determine disability in a legal or administrative sense that implies an inability to work or perform certain tasks; in other words, to define limitation. As dyspnea is a subjective feeling and can be coupled with many kinds of illness, it must not only be recognized but also judged with objectivity that requires a thorough history, examination, and substantiating pulmonary function studies. Its treatment should be appropriate for the underlying systemic or lung disease and for the patient's psychological situation.

Wheezing

Wheezing certainly contributes to dyspnea and is often interpreted as the same symptom by some patients. Wheezing, which can be considered a valid physical sign as well as a symptom, gives the sensation of inhaled air sticking in the airways and limiting a deep inspiration. It may terminate with a cough. Wheezing can be felt by the subject as tightness with breathing and is often audible; this sound has to be distinguished from stridor, which emanates from the larynx and oropharynx. Both sounds can evoke a feeling of panic and air hunger in the patient, but stridor can be easily heard and identified as coming from upper airway obstruction or choking. Wheezing is most commonly associated with asthma; however, the adage that "all that wheezes in the chest is not caused by asthma" must be remembered. Bronchospasm can be an aftermath of viral or bacterial infection and is ascribed to hyperactive, irritated airways; this can be intrinsic asthma associated with smoking and microbial infections and is not caused by an IgE antibody–mediated hypersensitivity reaction to an extrinsic allergen. Peribronchial fluid that accumulates from left heart failure can cause bronchospasm (cardiac asthma) as well. Showers of small pulmonary emboli may cause diffuse wheezing, but usually of a transient nature. Isolated areas of unilateral wheezing in the chest carry a different connotation and may reflect localized obstruction by an endobronchial lesion or an aspirated particle. Many patients with asthma are never wheeze-free, and diffuse expiratory phase wheezing can be felt and also heard even when the subject is asymptomatic and under good medication control. Wheezing heard in both the inspiratory and expiratory phases of breathing denotes a more advanced stage of bronchospasm and often an acute attack. The silent chest in an asthmatic when little air is moving is a signal that airway obstruction is severe and vigorous therapy is needed.

Cough

Coughing is a normal mechanism for forcefully expelling secretions or inhaled particles from the airways and it complements the mucociliary clearance system of the epithelial cell lining surface. Cough can be initiated voluntarily; however, it is most important as a protective reflex. Normal coughing is infrequent and develops little force. With deep, frequent coughing, it becomes more than a symptom or nuisance but an obvious sign of respiratory illness that demands attention and explanation.

The cough mechanism represents an interesting network of neurosensory-muscular coordination. The sensory arm of the cough reflex originates from afferent receptors in the epithelium of the airways. Excitation of the receptors by mechanical or chemical factors initiates impulses upward along the vagus nerve to integrative areas in the medulla oblongata and pons. Efferent impulses are transmitted to the diaphragm, the intercostal and abdominal muscles, and to the larynx.

Coughing has three phases. During the first, or inspiratory phase, the glottis opens wide and an initial inspiration increases static elastic recoil and lung volume. The compressive phase is initiated with closure of the glottis, continues with active contraction of the expiratory muscles, and ends with the sudden opening of the glottis. The expulsive phase begins with opening of glottis and the explosive release of the pressurized intrapulmonary gas. Rapid expiratory flow is maintained by continued contraction of the expiratory muscles. These three phases of cough are necessary to create the high flow and decreased cross-sectional area needed to produce the high linear velocity of air required for an effective cough.

Evaluation. Many diseases can have coughing as a symptom. Not only is the anatomic location or the organ system involved helpful in determining why coughing is present, for example, postnasal secretions irritating the glottis, or an enlarged thyroid gland, an aortic aneurysm, or another mediastinal structure compressing the trachea, but the kind of cough can be informative, too—its frequency, depth, sound, and what is expectorated, if anything. With airway irritation from inhaled fumes or infection and subsequent excessive formation of airway secretions, coughing usually becomes frequent and is an obvious sign of abnormal lung function. A raspy, wet cough productive of mucoid or discolored sputum (yellow, grey, green, or brown) characterizes patients with chronic bronchitis or bronchiectasis, whereas patients with asthma may have a cough that produces scant, tenacious whitish phlegm, and mucous plugs. As postnasal drip that consists of viscid secretions can trigger coughing, a thorough nose and laryngeal examination should be part of the evaluation of a patient with a chronic cough. A cough alone, without wheezing, can be the principal manifestation of asthma in some patients. In nonsmokers with a chronic persistent (more than 2 months) cough who have a normal chest radiograph, 25% or more may have unrecognized asthma—so-called cough variant asthma, in which coughing instead of wheezing is the main symptom. A cough can also herald the development of more obvious heart failure and pulmonary edema. A nonproductive, short, shallow cough is a usual manifestation of diffuse interstitial fibrotic lung disease, because stiff, noncompliant airways do not distend readily with inspiration, and stretching them seems to precipitate reflex coughing. With airway irritation after infection, even shallow breaths may evoke coughing by stimulating abnormally sensitive irritant receptors in the bronchial walls. Coughing and clearing the throat can also be anxiety responses, and some patients with a history of chronic cough may actually not have airway disease but may just be manifesting self-consciousness and nervousness. In the wake of respiratory viral or *Mycoplasma* infection, a persistent cough may linger for weeks. Such pathogens directly injure ciliated epithelial cells and can decrease the effectiveness of mucociliary clearance; thus, coughing may be a compensating or adaptive host mechanism to ensure adequate clearance of stagnant secretions. Thus, a cough is a symptom that usually needs evaluation and a reasonable explanation for its appearance.

For a cough of new onset to be worrisome enough to demand a thorough assessment, it should have been present for at least 6 to 8 weeks and not be just a residual from a prior mild respiratory infection. The cigarette smoking status of the patient is important, and an attempt to decrease smoking should be stressed. If the cough is productive, a sputum analysis of cells, a microbial culture, and a cytology should be obtained initially. Thereafter, the evaluation is largely dictated by the patient's history, which provides the clues for the origin of the coughing. As mentioned, an ear-nose-throat examination with sinus radiographs or CT scan and perhaps an allergy workup, if upper airway infection or rhinitis is likely, may be required. Nocturnal "asthma" or glottic dysfunction from regurgitation would suggest the need for a barium swallow and esophageal studies to document reflux from a hiatus hernia or esophageal dysmotility.

Coughing of an episodic nature or induced by exercise or athletics would warrant a methacholine inhalational challenge test to document hyperactive airways. Endobronchial obstruction can occur from either a benign cause resulting from aspiration of a particle or a piece of vegetable matter into the airways, or ominously suggest a tumor in patients of all ages, whether cigarette smokers or not. Therefore, a diagnostic bronchoscopy may be required. The appearance of a normal chest film may not obviate the need for bronchoscopy in assessing early manifestations of obstruction or endobronchial disease. If coughing is part of a diffuse interstitial lung process, an etiologic evaluation often requires tissue biopsy.

In systematically working through the differential diagnosis of a chronic, persistent cough and in deciding what tests and invasive procedures may be indicated, the problem of a habit or psychogenic cough should be placed purposely at the bottom of the differential list. Since this is a frequent cause of cough in children and in young, self-conscious adults, this form of coughing or throat clearing may be dismissed as something benign and often treated empirically. However, it must be a diagnosis of exclusion only after other diseases have been rigorously considered and eliminated. As mentioned, a habit cough or a psychogenic cough tic occurs primarily in older children and adolescents. School phobia is a frequent contributing cause. The cough is nonproductive, brassy, and repetitive, having an explosive barklike or "honking" quality. It characteristically does not occur during sleep, and these patients do not respond to cough suppressants or antibiotics. Treatment usually requires appropriate psychotherapy. After an upper respiratory infection, albeit mild, some adults continue for months or years to have a barking, nonproductive cough. This cough may be psychosomatic and provides some secondary gain from family, friends, or associates.

Treatment. Treatment of coughing requires therapy for the underlying problem that caused the cough. Cessation of cigarette smoking produces significant decreases in coughing. Within 4 to 6 weeks after stopping, a noticeable decrease in coughing may have occurred; however, the cough may linger and can persist for several years. A persistent cough in a smoker or exsmoker raises the possibility of neoplasm, and, therefore, the need for close observation.

Therapy includes aerosolized bronchodilators for asthma, cessation of smoking for chronic bronchitis, elevation of the head of the bed and no food or fluid before retiring for gastroesophageal reflux, and antibiotics and decongestants for sinusitis. Symptomatic (nonspecific) treatment is indicated only when the cause of the cough consistently eludes diagnosis so that specific or definitive therapy cannot be given. Cough suppressants are usually given for symptomatic relief rather than cure. Antitussive drugs act either on the afferent pathway of the reflex (peripherally) or centrally where the cough is coordinated. The drugs that appear to act on the afferent side of the cough reflex arc are local anesthetics. Central cough suppression is probably achieved by depressing the medullary integrative areas. The central cough suppressants include both narcotic and nonnarcotic agents. All narcotics are reasonably effective cough suppressants. The most commonly used is codeine phosphate. It is usually effective in oral doses of 8 to 15 mg, but as much as 30 mg is occasionally required. As an antitussive agent, dextromethorphan may be as effective as codeine. Clinical studies comparing 60 mg of dextromethorphan and 30 mg of codeine phosphate demonstrated similar antitussive effects. Expectorants and mucolytics do not function as cough suppressants. Guaifenesin (glycerol guaiacolate) has been demonstrated to have no antitussive effect in patients with the common cold.

Complications. *Cough syncope,* defined as a loss of consciousness preceded by a paroxysm of coughing, most often occurs in males. The patients are usually obese, well-muscled cigarette smokers, with underlying chronic obstructive disease. The more violent the cough, the more likely syncope is to occur. The duration of unconsciousness is brief, often only several seconds; rarely, a convulsion may occur. Many mechanisms have been postulated for cough syncope. After the buildup of intrathoracic pressure, several things might occur, including arterial hypotension, cerebral ischemia, inhibition of reticular areas in the midbrain, and a concussion-like effect from rapid rises in cerebrospinal fluid pressure.

Vigorous coughing may promote loss of urine and sometimes fecal material. This incontinence, usually occurring in women, may require use of an absorbent pad. Coughing is a frequent prelude to hemoptysis, which has many causes and will be discussed. Rib fractures caused by cough are common. In patients with infections of the respiratory tract, the incidence of cough fractures is 5% or less. Cough fractures commonly involve the lateral aspect of one of the fifth through the tenth ribs. Pain is a usual but not an invariable symptom of a cough fracture. Tenderness is usually found over the area of the fracture. Since the initial line of fracture is quite delicate, an early rib fracture may be invisible on radiographs. It is important to obtain oblique radiographs taken for rib detail when looking for rib fractures. After several weeks, callus formation occurs, and rib fractures may be more easily recognized.

Pneumothorax, pneumomediastinum, splenic rupture, rupture of the rectus abdominis muscle, heart block, inguinal hernia, and rupture of anal, nasal, and subconjunctival veins are some of the more unusual complications of coughing.

Expectoration

To eject phlegm or sputum from the throat or lungs by hawking and spitting or coughing is a common event. It may be an unconscious act, if secretions are minimal, or it may be an unpleasant habit, characterized by frequent snuffing and clearing of the throat that can be a manifestation of postnasal secretions. Usually, nasal and sinus drainage is unnoticed unless cold air, irritants, spicy foods, or a viral upper respiratory tract infection stimulates the mucosa; allergic rhinitis and sulfite food preservative sensitivity reactions are often recognized as causes. Clearing the throat can be a nervous habit of an anxious, self-conscious person. It is uncertain how much fluid is produced along the tracheobronchial surface normally because the humidification of inspired air and recovery of water from air during expiration are efficient mechanisms. The normal mucosal surface, viewed at bronchoscopy in normals, appears rather dry. Mucus does not uniformly cover the ciliated surface but is seen in patches. The pH of the mucosal surface of the trachea is 6.7. Ciliary clearance sweeps the surface secretions up the airways to the larynx where they are swallowed. Regular coughing and production of phlegm or sputum are not usual but when present are indicative of airway irritation, which can be from many causes and may require medical investigation.

The patient's description or physician's inspection of an expectorated specimen has always had value in deciding what the abnormal process is—discoloration suggesting an exacerbation of infection in a person with chronic bronchitis, mucous plugs in a decompensating asthmatic, or blood mixed with sputum versus pure hemoptysis. Smelling the specimen (anaerobes give a sweetish odor), looking at the layering of sputum in a container, and quantitating the amount are recommended. How accurate these parameters are in judging the nature or severity of the lung process is debatable. Blood streaking and hemoptysis become ominous signs of illness and will be given special description later. Assessing sputum purulence as a gauge of infection is an imprecise measurement. Purulence usually relates to a change in the color and consistency of baseline mucoid or whitish phlegm that is expectorated routinely by a person with underlying airway irritation and hyperreactivity, for example, a cigarette smoker with bronchitis or a symptomatic asthmatic. When the phlegm becomes grayish or greenish, perhaps sticky and more copious, an intercurrent microbial infection is suspected. Unfortunately, an analysis of inflammatory cells in sputum, ribonucleic acid value for polymorphonuclear content, and quantitative bacterial cultures do not correlate well with objective evidence of infection.

The origin of the secretions can be confusing. Postnasal secretions running down the retropharynx may not be perceived until they accumulate and cause clearing of the throat or trigger a cough. The patient may not realize that the phlegm is coming down from the throat and not up from the trachea. The texture of the sputum is often described by patients. Sticky phlegm in the trachea can be felt or perceived as a fullness and tickle when breathing and coughing, yet it might not be cleared; it remains adherent and does not come up and frustrates the subject. Hard flecks or strings of mucus can be interspersed in the sputum. Asthmatics often expectorate plugs of mucus variously described to be like rice particles, worms (bronchial casts), or pieces of spaghetti. Episodes of hard coughing that produce gelatinous, blood-colored plugs, perhaps as large as the tip of a small fifth finger, may be the clue for bronchiectasis and an allergic bronchopulmonary mycosis complicating asthma. The volume of expectorated fluid can be appreciable, roughly quantitated in quaint terms of tablespoons or portions of a cupful. A person with active bronchitis or with bronchiectasis as found with cystic fibrosis can produce several ounces a day or more of secretions. The purulent solid material may float on the watery secretions causing the specimen to layer, which is taken as evidence of bronchorrhea from bronchiectatic, infected airways or rarely of drainage from a lung abscess.

Chest pain

Chest pain(s) (see Chapter 7) is a symptom that is readily communicated by the patient; however, identifying its cause or origin may require considerable effort and thought. Pain, like hemoptysis, is not likely to be ignored by the patient unless it has a familiar and recurrent pattern, as in the case of the pain associated with angina or with esophageal irritation; even under these circumstances its appearance may cause considerable anxiety because of what it portends. Pain originating in the biliary tract and in epigastric structures may radiate to the chest and cause dyspnea, and it may mimic the pain arising from mediastinal organs or the parietal pleura; hence, the origin of chest pains may be confusing. Likewise, acute bacterial lobar pneumonia in a lower lung lobe may produce epigastric tenderness, directing attention to the abdomen as well as the lung. Atypical anginal chest pains can be difficult to differentiate from esophageal and gastric causes, especially if the patient has a known hiatus hernia or acid-peptic dysfunction. As postprandial heartburn can represent angina, exercise stress testing and often cardiac angiography may be needed to distinguish the cause. A rib injury or costochondritis can sometimes be a confusing cause of acute, severe chest wall pain, but the relationship of the pain to position or movement, and point tenderness elicited with examination, usually resolve the issue. The complex description of pain is subjective but is likely to contain at least six ingredients: intensity, sequence, duration, physical location, associated physiologic aspects, and the subject's behavior related to the pain. Pain has psychological and social connotations as well. Pain related to cardiac, pericardial, aortic, or pulmonary vascular problems is discussed in Chapters 7, 18, 20, and 24.

Pleural pain. *Pleuritis,* defined as rhythmic, sharp chest pain related to breathing, usually has an obvious relation to a respiratory infection, pulmonary infarction, or pleural tumor; pain emanates from irritation of the parietal pleura containing the afferent nerve fibers that convey pain sensation. The visceral pleura and lung parenchyma are insensitive and contain no pain fibers. Pain fibers that originate in the parietal pleura course through the chest wall as fine twigs of the intercostal nerves, and irritation of pain receptors in these nerve fibers produces pain in the chest wall that feels superficial, sharp, and lancinating and is aggravated by laughing, coughing, and deep inspiration. The presence of a pleural friction rub establishes that the cause of a pleuritic-type pain involves the pleura and is not some other chest wall pain syndrome with respiratory variation in the intensity of the pain.

The causes of pleural disease are discussed in Chapter 218.

Chest wall pain. All structures in the thoracic wall, including the skin and subcutaneous tissues, are potential sources for chest pain. The muscles, ligaments, cartilage, and bone, which are the most common sources of chest wall pain, can be involved with strain, inflammation, or malposition. The pain is most often a dull, aching soreness that varies in response to movement or local touch.

The "chest wall syndrome" is a catch-all occasionally applied to anterior chest pain that arises from multiple causes, including cervicothoracic nerve root irritation, inflamed tissues in the chest wall, or rib fracture. In this syndrome, chest tenderness can be evoked when firm, steady pressure is applied to the region of the chest where the spontaneous episodes of pain originate. Treatment is directed to the underlying abnormality.

Tumors of the ribs and soft tissues of the chest wall are not very common but are usually obvious when present. Traumatic intercostal neuritis, one of the more common painful afflictions of the intercostal nerves, can be produced by hypermobile costal cartilages (slipping rib syndrome) that pinch the intercostal nerve between the costal cartilages. Rib fractures are frequently unrecognized as the cause of chest pain. Strenuous coughing can be the culprit. Fractures may not be detected on roentgenograms until sufficient callus has formed. The deep, aching discomfort of herpes zoster may precede the skin eruption. Myogenic chest pain (myodynia or fibromyositis) is represented by local areas of hyperirritability and tenderness located deep in various muscles, particularly the pectoralis muscles. Mondor's disease, superficial thrombophlebitis of the chest wall and breast, is a relatively uncommon cause of chest pain. The chief complaint is sudden pain in or near the breast, followed by the appearance of the thrombosed, tender, cordlike vein and its branches. The hypersensitive xiphoid syndrome (xiphoidalgia) may cause confusing chest pain. The main diagnostic feature of xiphoidalgia is to reproduce the pain the patient has complained about by very moderate fingertip pressure on the tender portion of the xiphoid.

Tietze's syndrome (Tietze's disease, costal chondritis) is an unusual cause of chest pain in young adults and older children. On examination, a firm, fusiform or spindle-shaped swelling is confined to one or more of the upper four costal cartilages, usually the second. Tenderness is usually present, but heat and erythema are absent. The rare biopsies that have been done showed normal costal cartilage and no inflammation. The chief complaint is pain that is generally localized to the involved cartilage and is of mild to severe intensity. The pain is variously described as aching, gripping, sharp, dull, or neuralgic and may mimic that of angina pectoris, pleurisy, and intercostal neuritis. The pain tends to subside after several weeks or months, but the palpable swellings may persist. Treatment is essentially supportive with rest, reassurance, local heat, and analgesics.

Hemoptysis

Hemoptysis is the coughing or expectoration of gross blood or even blood-tinged sputum. It is a sign more than a symptom of respiratory illness, but its psychological impact is so strong that the anxiety and fear caused make hemoptysis a symptom too. If sputum is usually swallowed, hemoptysis is often not detected. The source of blood in true hemoptysis may be from the pulmonary parenchyma, larynx, or tracheobronchial tree. Bleeding from the mouth, throat, or nasopharynx must be carefully excluded. Blood from the gastrointestinal tract can create diagnostic confusion. Except when blood loss is extremely rapid, vomited blood is dark red, not frothy, and the pH is acidic. In contrast, hemoptysis is associated with coughing (not vomiting); a portion is often frothy since it is mixed with air and sputum. The color is usually (but not always) bright red. Hemoptysis may be followed by several days of blood-streaked sputum.

Clinical evaluation. Hemoptysis is a frightening occurrence and has to be investigated thoroughly with a careful history to ascertain the frequency and volume of blood expectorated and by physical examination to localize the source (see box below). Blood-tinged sputum from a patient with mitral stenosis and heart failure is of less concern than bright red blood coughed up by a patient with bronchiectasis or with an *Aspergillus* fungus ball in a residual lung cavity of sarcoidosis. Frothy sputum suggests pulmonary edema. An endobronchial neoplasm in the cigarette-smoking, middle-aged person is always a worrisome possibility, and fiberoptic bronchoscopy may be needed to inspect the various airways and obtain histologic tissue for diagnosis. Bleeding can originate in the posterior nasopharynx and actually drip into the back of the throat, or it can be aspirated into the airways without the patient being aware. A careful examination of the nose and throat is thus very important for excluding this possible site of bleeding that can be mistaken as the source for hemoptysis. Telangiectasis on the lips or buccal mucosa may indicate Rendu-Osler-Weber disease.

Aspiration of blood may also occur with brisk gastrointestinal bleeding and regurgitation of blood. Frank, bloody sputum is unusual with pulmonary embolus or infarction and with most forms of bacterial pneumonia, whereas gross bleeding is common from sarcoid or tuberculous lung cavities. Rusty-colored sputum may signal bacterial pneumonia. Recurrent hemoptysis strongly suggests a lung tumor, if tuberculosis, sarcoidosis, and bronchiectasis are not the cause. Radiation-induced pneumonitis can cause brisk and recurrent hemoptysis that can be difficult to control and can be a distressing complication for the patient; in this case the cause is known, and in time the bleeding subsides. Rarely, hemoptysis concurrent with menstrual flow may suggest a focus of endometrial tissue in the bronchial wall. Bloody sputum mixed with white gritty material suggests broncholithiasis.

Causes of hemoptysis in adults

- Infections
  - Chronic bronchitis
  - Bronchiectasis
  - Lung abscess
  - Bacterial pneumonias
  - Fungal infections
  - Tuberculosis
- Neoplasms
  - Bronchogenic carcinoma
  - Bronchial adenoma
  - Carcinoma metastatic to the lung
- Cardiovascular disorders
  - Mitral stenosis
  - Pulmonary infarction
  - Congenital heart disease, especially cyanotic heart disease
- Pulmonary arteriovenous fistula
- Parasitic diseases
- Pulmonary-renal diseases (Goodpasture's disease)
- Miscellaneous
  - Cystic fibrosis
  - Broncholith
  - Cysts and bullae
  - Endometriosis (catamenia)
  - Idiopathic (in 10%-15% cases no demonstrable cause is found)
  - Malingering and/or Münchausen's syndrome

Diagnostic studies. A careful history, physical examination, and chest radiographs (posteroanterior and lateral) are done first. A normal chest radiograph does not exclude serious disease and should rarely be the final study, for half the patients have a normal chest radiograph. Caution should also be exercised in attributing the site of bleeding to an obvious abnormality on a chest radiograph since bronchoscopy may reveal that the bleeding site is different from this area seen on the radiograph. A blood count, clotting evaluation, and urinalysis are necessary. Sputum should be examined for malignant cells, tuberculosis organisms, and fungi. A tuberculosis skin test plus anergy controls should be applied.

Fiberoptic bronchoscopy is essential in the evaluation of a patient with hemoptysis, even if the chest radiograph is normal. There are a few exceptions, for example, a young person with acute bronchitis, a few days of blood-streaked sputum associated with paroxysmal coughing, and complete clearing of the sputum when the bronchitis subsides. Fiberoptic bronchoscopy is diagnostic for the cause of hemoptysis in about 80% of lung cancer patients and in 60% of patients with a nonmalignant cause of hemoptysis. Early bronchoscopy (during hemoptysis or during the 48 hours after hemoptysis has ceased) is more likely to demonstrate active bleeding or localize the bleeding.

Thoracic CT can be valuable. Thoracic CT should be part of the evaluation of hemoptysis if a chest radiograph is negative and fiberoptic bronchoscopy is not revealing. Thoracic CT may demonstrate an area of bronchiectasis, inapparent lung cavity, or broncholithiasis causing hemoptysis when these were not detected on the conventional chest radiograph. Ultrathin-section "slices" of 1.5 mm, instead of 1.0 cm, may be required to see bronchiectatic areas (high-resolution scan or HRCT).

Other studies that are used in the appropriate situation include bronchograms (particularly for upper lobe bronchiectasis), ventilation-perfusion lung scans, pulmonary angiograms, and selective bronchial artery angiography.

Treatment. The objectives of therapy for significant and ongoing hemoptysis are to stop bleeding, prevent airway obstruction, and support the patient's vital functions. Adequate suctioning apparatus and equipment for endotracheal intubation should be immediately available (a double-lumen tube should be included). If the bleeding site is known, it is best to place that side in a dependent position to reduce blood spilling over into the uninvolved lung. Drugs that significantly depress cough or respiration should be avoided since failure to clear the bronchi of blood may lead to airway plugging by blood clots. Antibiotics may be necessary to treat an underlying infection that may be causing hemoptysis. Oxygen may be indicated if hypoxemia is present, and transfusions should be considered to maintain the hematocrit above 30%.

"Massive" or life-threatening hemoptysis has a significant mortality. *Massive hemoptysis* is variously defined as 100 to 600 ml per 24 hours or 600 ml per 48 hours. With pulmonary hemorrhage, asphyxia is a greater hazard than exsanguination. Bronchoscopy, preferably with a rigid bronchoscope, should probably be done as soon as possible to localize the site of bleeding. Patients with "massive" hemoptysis usually demonstrate a steady decrease of bleeding, with cessation of hemoptysis after 4 days. Most patients with serious hemoptysis can be successfully treated conservatively. However, in some situations, a pulmonary resection may be indicated. Selective embolization of bronchial arteries has also been found beneficial for treating life-threatening hemoptysis.

REFERENCES

Cooper A, White D, and Matthay RA: Drug-associated pulmonary disease. Am Rev Respir Dis 133:321, 1986.

Irwin RS et al: Chronic cough as the sole presenting manifestation of gastroesophageal reflux. Am Rev Respir Dis 140:1294, 1989.

Irwin RS, Curley FJ, and French CL: Chronic cough. Am Rev Respir Dis 141:640, 1990.

Mahler DA and Wells CK: Evaluation of clinical methods for rating dyspnea. Chest 93:580, 1988.

Maxwell SL and Reynolds HY: Variations of asthma: unusual presentations and causes. Consultant 32:48, 1992.

Palmer LP et al: Bacterial adherence to respiratory tract cells: relationships between in vivo and in vitro pH and bacterial attachment. Am Rev Respir Dis 133:784, 1986.

Simon PM et al: Distinguishable types of dyspnea in patients with shortness of breath. Am Rev Respir Dis 142:1009, 1990.

CHAPTER

200 Acute Respiratory Failure

Leonard D. Hudson

Acute respiratory failure (ARF) can be defined as the relatively sudden onset of failure of the respiratory system to carry out its major functions (i.e., the adequate delivery of oxygen into and adequate removal of carbon dioxide from the arterial blood) to a degree that causes a threat to life. Thus, ARF is not a disease but rather a syndrome marked by abnormal physiologic functions that can be caused by a variety of disease processes. The process causing failure of function is not necessarily limited to the lungs themselves, but may involve any part of the respiratory system: the ventilatory control system, the lungs (including the airways and the lung parenchyma), the lung vasculature, and the chest wall and muscles of respiration.

ARF can be more specifically defined by abnormalities of arterial blood gas values. It should be recognized that any specific definition is somewhat arbitrary and varies according to the clinical situation. A commonly used definition of ARF is an arterial PO_2 (PaO_2) less than 55 mm Hg and/or an arterial PCO_2 ($PaCO_2$) greater than 50 mm Hg with an accompanying acidemia. The defined limit of PaO_2 for ARF ranges from less than 50 to less than 60 mm Hg; a PaO_2 less than 55 is most commonly used. This range is chosen because of its position on the oxyhemoglobin dissociation curve (Fig. 200-1). If the PaO_2 falls below 50-55 mm Hg, the oxygen saturation, and thus the oxygen content of the arterial blood, falls sharply. Therefore, a PaO_2 below this level may be life-threatening. Above a PaO_2 of 60 mm Hg there is nearly complete saturation of the hemoglobin by oxygen. Raising the PaO_2 to higher values results in relatively little increase in arterial oxygen content.

A $PaCO_2$ greater than 50 mm Hg is used as a limit because a sudden change from a baseline normal $PaCO_2$ (40 mm Hg) with a normal serum bicarbonate (24 mEq/liter) causes significant respiratory acidosis. The life-threatening aspects of hypercapnia are related to the associated acidosis. Thus, chronic hypercapnia compensated by increased serum bicarbonate is not necessarily dangerous in itself. Since some patients with chronic pulmonary disease may constantly have PaO_2 and $PaCO_2$ values that fit these arbitrary definitions, the clinician must determine whether the observed abnormal blood gas values are chronic and stable or associated with an acute clinical worsening.

The syndrome of ARF is analogous to acute functional failure in any other organ system, for example, cardiac, renal, or hepatic. The syndrome represents a severe functional abnormality that is life-threatening and requires immediate attention. Identification of the syndrome allows the clini-

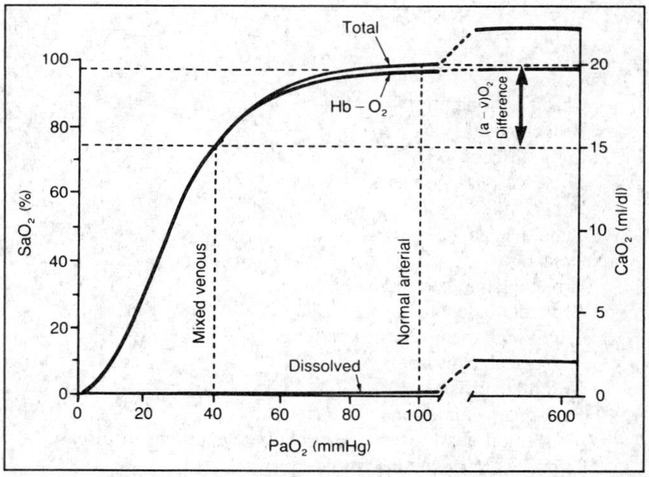

Fig. 200-1. The oxygen-hemoglobin dissociation curve, relating the partial pressure of oxygen in arterial blood (PaO_2) to arterial O_2 saturation (SaO_2) and to the O_2 content of arterial blood (CaO_2). A normal hemoglobin concentration in milliliters per deciliter is assumed. The curve descends steeply below PaO_2 values of 50 mm Hg, indicating severely reduced O_2-carrying capacity by hemoglobin below this PaO_2. The lower line represents O_2 in solution in the blood; the middle line depicts O_2 bound to hemoglobin at that PaO_2; the upper line shows O_2 bound to hemoglobin plus O_2 dissolved. Note that dissolved O_2 contributes little to CaO_2 at a PaO_2 in the normal range. (From Luce JM, Tyler ML, and Pierson DJ: Intensive respiratory care. Philadelphia, 1984, Saunders.)

cian to consider a particular approach to diagnosis and management. Indeed, the principles of management are similar once a diagnosis of ARF has been established, despite the variety of diseases that may lead to this functional abnormality. Certain therapeutic measures can be initiated once ARF has been diagnosed. On the other hand, optimal management usually depends on establishing a more specific diagnosis of the disease or diseases that cause or precipitate the organ failure.

PATHOPHYSIOLOGIC CAUSES OF ACUTE RESPIRATORY FAILURE

Four pathophysiologic mechanisms can lead to ARF: hypoventilation, ventilation/perfusion mismatch, shunt, and diffusion limitation. Only the first three mechanisms are important clinically, since diffusion limitation is uncommon as a cause of significant hypoxemia. Thinking of ARF in terms of these mechanisms is useful in establishing the differential diagnosis of the cause of failure and facilitating management.

Hypoventilation

Alveolar hypoventilation is characterized by an elevation in $PaCO_2$. Thus, hypoventilation is present when alveolar ventilation is inadequate to meet the body's requirements for removal of carbon dioxide, and the $PaCO_2$ level begins to rise. The total minute ventilation and even the alveolar ventilation may be increased above normal if this increase is not adequate for the level of carbon dioxide production. The resultant hypercapnia not only causes respiratory acidosis, but is also associated with hypoxemia. With hypoventilation, hypoxemia is a result of a decreased alveolar partial pressure of oxygen (P_AO_2). The level of alveolar ventilation is not adequate to remove the carbon dioxide produced, and the amount of atmospheric air containing oxygen brought in to the alveolus is also reduced. Since P_AO_2 is reduced, the PaO_2 must necessarily be reduced as well. If arterial hypoxemia is caused by hypoventilation alone, the difference between the alveolar oxygen and the arterial oxygen [$P(A\text{-}a)O_2$] is normal. All other mechanisms resulting in hypoxemia are associated with an increased $P(A\text{-}a)O_2$ (Chapter 189).

The hypoxemia associated with hypoventilation can be corrected by administering supplemental oxygen. However, this oxygen has no direct effect on respiratory acidosis. The more physiologic way to correct both respiratory acidosis and hypoxemia is to improve alveolar ventilation. How this is best accomplished depends on the cause of the alveolar hypoventilation. When air-flow obstruction is the cause of hypoventilation, bronchodilators and secretion removal are appropriate. However, when an overdose of sedatives has caused respiratory center depression, temporary mechanical ventilation allows time for drug metabolism or removal.

Ventilation/perfusion mismatching

Ventilation-perfusion ($\dot{V}/\dot{Q}$) mismatch is the most common explanation for hypoxemia. For hypoxemia to result, the mismatch must include lung regions where ventilation is decreased out of proportion to perfusion; this results in areas of increased $PaCO_2$ and reduced PaO_2. Blood passing by these alveoli reflects the reduced oxygen tension. Also, less carbon dioxide is removed from these regions, and end-capillary blood has an increased PCO_2. However, an increase in ventilation to the areas of lung where ventilation and perfusion are relatively normally matched provides enough carbon dioxide removal to compensate for the elevated PCO_2 from areas of mismatch. This effect is a consequence of the relatively linear shape of the carbon dioxide dissociation curve; an increase in ventilation in any local lung area strikingly lowers the carbon dioxide content of local pulmonary venous blood. However, increased ventilation of the relatively normally matched regions does not result in a significant increase in oxygen saturation or content because of the sigmoid shape of the oxygen-hemoglobin dissociation curve (see Fig. 200-1). Thus, increased ventilation does not compensate for the low $\dot{V}/\dot{Q}$ areas that result in hypoxemia.

Hypoxemia caused by $\dot{V}/\dot{Q}$ mismatching can be corrected by a relatively small increase in the inspired fraction of oxygen (F_IO_2). This correction occurs because airways to poorly ventilated alveoli remain open, and, if the gas mixture is administered for a long enough period, the increased pressure of inspired oxygen is eventually reflected in an increased PaO_2. Definitive therapy depends on reversal of the specific cause of the regional reductions in ventilation (e.g., bronchospasm).

Shunt

Intrapulmonary shunt can be thought of as one extreme of $\dot{V}/\dot{Q}$ mismatch. With shunt, however, there is no ventilation but perfusion continues, which, as with $\dot{V}/\dot{Q}$ mismatching, results in an increased $P(A\text{-}a)O_2$. Again, adequate carbon dioxide removal can usually be accomplished by increasing ventilation to areas of more normal $\dot{V}/\dot{Q}$ matching. The resulting normal $PaCO_2$ does not mean that carbon dioxide removal is entirely normal, since a very high minute ventilation is often required to achieve a normal or low $PaCO_2$. Shunt is distinguished from $\dot{V}/\dot{Q}$ mismatch by the magnitude of the increase in F_IO_2 required to provide adequate arterial oxygenation. In an area of shunt, added oxygen cannot reach the alveoli since there is no ventilation. Thus, blood flowing past these areas of filled or collapsed alveoli has oxygen tensions that are equal to those of mixed venous blood. Administration of a high F_IO_2 is still associated with hypoxemia and a greatly increased $P(A\text{-}a)O_2$.

Since processes that cause shunt must result in either alveolar filling or collapse, these areas are usually recognizable on chest x-ray because they are airless.

Diffusion limitation

Diffusion limitation is an uncommon cause of clinically significant hypoxemia. In normal circumstances blood flowing through the pulmonary capillary bed reaches nearly complete oxygen saturation of the hemoglobin in approximately one third of the total time available for exposure to the alveolar surface. Even when a limitation in diffusion of the oxygen is present there is usually ample time for the hemoglobin to be saturated with oxygen. Exceptions can occur with exercise, with markedly increased cardiac output and associated markedly reduced capillary transit time, or at high altitudes. Diffusion limitation of oxygenation should not be confused with the pulmonary function test of diffusing capacity. The diffusing capacity is measured by using trace amounts of carbon monoxide and is chiefly influenced by the matching of alveolar blood and gas surfaces. Thus, even a markedly abnormal diffusing capacity for carbon monoxide may not significantly affect oxygen transfer. Associated hypoxemia is more probably caused by $\dot{V}/\dot{Q}$ mismatch. For practical purposes, diffusion limitation is not a primary cause of ARF, although it could be a contributing factor in the critically ill patient with very high cardiac output. When diffusion limitation of oxygenation does exist, hypoxemia can be easily corrected by administering an enriched oxygen mixture (increased F_{IO_2}).

CLASSIFICATION OF ACUTE RESPIRATORY FAILURE

There are several possible classifications for ARF. None of these is entirely satisfactory for clinical purposes because none encompasses all the possible causes or types of ARF. Two of the commonly used classifications, taken together, can assist the clinician in planning a management approach to the patient with ARF. These classifications are based on (1) whether there is previous respiratory disease and (2) whether hypoxemia is associated with (a) normocapnia or hypocapnia or (b) hypercapnia (Table 200-1). Appropriate classification of a patient with ARF aids in diagnosis and also helps in application of treatment principles. It is very important to determine a specific etiology so that treatment can be optimally designed.

DIAGNOSIS

The diagnosis of ARF can be considered in three stages: (1) clinical suspicion that ARF might be present, (2) confirmation that ARF is present, and (3) identification of a specific etiology.

Clinical suspicion that ARF might be present should develop from the clinical situation. Two particular settings are important to recognize. The first involves the patient with preexisting lung disease in whom there has been some relatively sudden clinical deterioration. Examples include a patient with chronic obstructive pulmonary disease with clinical worsening and a patient with neuromuscular disease with a superimposed respiratory or metabolic complication and overall clinical worsening. The second setting involves patients who may or may not have preexisting lung disease, but have an acute injury or illness known to be associated with a high incidence of ARF, for example, the patient with septic shock, a circumstance known to be associated with a high incidence of acute diffuse lung injury (adult respiratory distress syndrome [ARDS]).

Compatible symptoms and signs may also suggest ARF and fall into two categories: (1) those reflecting the acute disease process, and (2) those reflecting hypoxemia and/or acidosis. Symptoms and signs reflecting the precipitating disease usually suggest some acute lung disease or disorder. These symptoms include increased cough and sputum production and/or increased shortness of breath. Since these symptoms usually are related to the respiratory system, the

Table 200-1. Classification of acute respiratory failure

Category	Example	Mechanism of hypoxemia	Chest x-ray
↓ PaO_2 with normal or ↓ $PaCO_2$			
Preexisting lung disease	Restrictive lung disease (pulmonary fibrosis)	$\dot{V}/\dot{Q}$ mismatch ± shunt	Diffuse interstitial infiltrate
	Asthma (until very severe)	$\dot{V}/\dot{Q}$ mismatch	Clear
No preexisting lung disease required (but could be superimposed on chronic disease)	Adult respiratory distress syndrome	Shunt	Diffuse alveolar-filling infiltrate
	Cardiogenic pulmonary edema	Shunt	Diffuse alveolar-filling infiltrate
	Pulmonary emboli	$\dot{V}/\dot{Q}$ mismatch and shunt	Clear (or localized infiltrate)
	Pneumonia	Shunt	Localized or diffuse alveolar-filling infiltrate
↓ PaO_2 with ↑ $PaCO_2$			
Previous lung disease	COPD	Hypoventilation and $\dot{V}/\dot{Q}$ mismatch	Clear
	Asthma (very severe)	Hypoventilation and $\dot{V}/\dot{Q}$ mismatch	Clear
Normal lungs	Sedative drug overdose	Hypoventilation	Clear
	Neuromuscular disease (e.g., myasthenia gravis, Guillain-Barré syndrome)	Hypoventilation	Clear

possibility of ARF is usually considered and the diagnosis sought. Perhaps more important are the symptoms and signs reflecting hypoxemia and acidosis. These symptoms may be more subtle and difficult to relate to ARF since they usually involve the central nervous system (CNS) and/or the cardiovascular system. CNS symptoms reflecting these physiologic abnormalities range from restlessness and irritability to confusion and coma. They may be as subtle as personality change in a patient with COPD, a change recognized by the family, but not necessarily by a stranger. Both hypoxemia and acidosis can cause CNS dysfunction. The CNS effects of respiratory acidosis are in part related to the vasodilatory effects of carbon dioxide, with accompanying central acidosis evident in the cerebrospinal fluid (CSF). Physical findings include papilledema and asterixis. Cardiovascular signs or symptoms can reflect either compensatory mechanisms to increase cardiac output and delivery of oxygen to the tissues or complications of hypoxemia and acidosis such as cardiac arrhythmia.

The clinical situation and symptoms and signs that provoke suspicion of ARF are obtained from appropriate history and physical examination. Diagnosis of this clinical syndrome is confirmed by arterial blood gas analysis. Since the syndrome is defined by abnormal arterial blood gases, measurement of arterial blood gases not only confirms the diagnosis but also provides information regarding the type of physiologic abnormality that causes the hypoxemia. Repeat arterial blood gas measurements following oxygen administration help separate $\dot{V}/\dot{Q}$ mismatch from shunt as possible mechanisms.

After the diagnosis has been established by arterial blood gas measurement, additional information can be obtained from a chest roentgenogram. The findings on the chest x-ray can help both with understanding the probable cause of hypoxemia and with diagnosis of the particular disease present. The chest roentgenogram can help determine the appropriate level of initial oxygen therapy by suggesting whether shunt or $\dot{V}/\dot{Q}$ mismatching is likely to be predominant. If shunt is present, usually there is evidence of alveolar filling or collapse; a density or infiltrate is caused by airless or edematous lung or lung filled with purulent secretions. If the chest x-ray is relatively normal, hypoventilation and $\dot{V}/\dot{Q}$ mismatching are more likely causes. Then the diagnoses to be considered include COPD with bronchitis, drug overdose, or neuromuscular diseases. If there is a diffuse alveolar-filling process involving most lung fields, ARDS or cardiogenic pulmonary edema must be considered, and shunt is likely to be an important mechanism contributing to hypoxemia. If there is a localized abnormality that involves alveolar filling, shunt is still the probable mechanism, but pneumonia must be considered. These examples are simplistic but are meant to illustrate only a few of the possible ways in which the chest roentgenogram is helpful in diagnosis (see Table 200-1).

PRINCIPLES OF MANAGEMENT

Establishing the diagnosis of ARF allows the application of general principles of management. These management principles apply to any type of ARF, although their specific application is greatly influenced by the type and specific cause of ARF. These principles are as follows.

Correction of inadequate oxygenation

The most life-threatening physiologic abnormalities should be corrected first. Hypoxemia does not have to be totally corrected to normal; the goal is improvement such that the acute threat to life is removed or greatly diminished. Since hypoxemia usually is the most life-threatening abnormality, correction should be started immediately with supplemental oxygen administration.

Correction of respiratory acidosis

The importance of the level of carbon dioxide is related primarily to its effect on pH; thus, treatment should be directed toward normalization of pH, not PCO_2. If possible, treatment should be aimed at correction of the process that resulted in hypercapnia. The decision to use mechanical ventilation is based on clinical findings and is discussed later.

Maintenance of cardiac output and tissue oxygen transport

Although ARF is defined by abnormal arterial blood oxygen tension, a goal of therapy is to maintain oxygen delivery to the tissue and cellular level. The other important determinant of tissue oxygen transport (in addition to the arterial content of oxygen) is cardiac output. Some therapies used in ARF can decrease cardiac output. Thus, even if there is an improvement in arterial oxygen content, the total amount of oxygen transported to the tissues might be adversely affected. Since hemoglobin concentration is an important determinant of arterial oxygen content, correction of anemia should be considered when planning therapy.

Treatment of the underlying disease

The first three principles of management are only supportive and temporizing. Definitive management depends on treatment of the processes that resulted in the initial physiologic abnormality. Table 200-2 outlines conditions that may precipitate ARF.

Avoidance of preventable complications

It is unusual for a patient with ARF to die of acute hypoxemia or respiratory acidosis with current methods of respiratory support. Death often occurs from other complicating factors such as infection or thromboembolism. For each clinical situation, the common complications should be known and measures taken to avoid them. Some complications of management are outlined in the box on p. 1638.

Since ARF is by definition a life-threatening process and since therapy can be complicated and carries potential risk, any patient with ARF is best managed initially in an intensive care unit. The typical COPD patient with ARF

Table 200-2. Factors that may precipitate acute respiratory failure

Category	Precipitating factor
I. Normal lungs	Central
	Head injury
	Stroke
	Drug overdose
	Bellows
	Guillain-Barré
	Rib fractures (flail chest)
	Airway
	Tracheal obstruction
II. Acute pulmonary disease (lungs previously normal)	Sepsis
	Shock
	Aspiration
	Pneumonia
	Edema
	Asthma
III. Acute pulmonary disease (lungs previously abnormal)	Pneumothorax
	Pneumonia
	Pulmonary embolism
	Factors in group II

Complications of management of acute respiratory failure

Infection (hospital-acquired)
Pneumothorax
Respiratory alkalosis
Cardiac arrhythmia
Thromboembolism
Tracheal injury
Sinusitis
Pulmonary oxygen toxicity
Decreased cardiac output

may require only overnight management in such a unit if there is a relatively rapid response to therapy, or may be managed in an acute care ward if personnel are experienced in the care of these patients and the patient is relatively stable. In other situations (e.g., ARDS), critical care facilities may be required until the lung lesion has resolved.

MEASURES TO IMPROVE OXYGENATION

The goal of measures to improve oxygenation is to increase the arterial oxygen saturation (SaO_2) and thus arterial oxygen content. If possible, this increase should be accomplished while avoiding the risk of oxygen toxicity. Certainly it should be accomplished without producing meaningful decreases in cardiac output. A PaO_2 in the range of 60 mm Hg or above usually provides adequate oxygen saturation. However, if this level is achieved by administration of a high FIO_2, oxygen toxicity may damage the lung. Unfortunately, the exact level of FIO_2 that represents a toxic threat is not known. It is known that oxygen toxicity is a time-dose relationship; that is, the higher the FIO_2 and the longer the time administered, the greater the risk. Data suggest that levels above 0.7 or 0.8 can be associated with parenchymal lung injury (similar to that seen with other causes of ARDS) after only a few days. Therefore, the use of FIO_2 0.8 or higher for more than 1 day should be avoided *if possible*. It must be kept in mind, however, that the primary goal of therapy is to oxygenate the arterial blood adequately, and a dangerously high FIO_2 may be necessary. Evidence exists for other types of less severe oxygen toxicity at lower FIO_2. Ciliary action may be reduced, and bacterial killing by alveolar macrophages may be impaired. The clinical importance of these possible toxic effects has not been established.

Measures usually available to improve oxygenation include administration of supplemental oxygen, use of positive end-expiratory pressure (PEEP) or continuous positive airway pressure (CPAP), improved ventilation or use of enhanced tidal volumes, and definitive therapy of the underlying pulmonary abnormality.

If positive airway pressure is required, it is important that cardiac output be maintained at satisfactory levels so that oxygen delivery is not impaired by decreased blood flow.

Supplemental oxygen

The clinician must decide initially whether a high or a low amount of supplemental oxygen is likely to be required. This estimate is based on knowledge of the clinical abnormality and the likely pathophysiologic mechanism involved, that is, whether the major mechanism of hypoxemia is shunt (requiring a high FIO_2) or hypoventilation and/or $\dot{V}/\dot{Q}$ mismatch (requiring only a small increment in FIO_2).

A low level of supplemental oxygen can be administered through nasal prongs. Nasal prongs are well tolerated by patients since they are relatively comfortable and allow the patient to cough out secretions and to eat or drink while receiving supplemental oxygen. If the nasal passages are open, nasal administration is effective even when a patient breathes through his or her mouth, as oxygen is entrained from the posterior nasopharynx during inspiration. The flow rate can be adjusted upward from 0.5 liter per minute to achieve the desired increase in PaO_2. Once a flow greater than 6 liters per minute is used, there is slight further augmentation of the actual FIO_2. High flows of nasal oxygen have a drying and irritating effect on the upper respiratory tract. Oxygen masks using the Venturi principle allow regulation of the FIO_2 at a given level and are particularly useful in transport or emergency situations in which it is important to maintain a known, relatively stable FIO_2 with a small amount of oxygen supplementation.

A higher FIO_2 can be provided with an appropriate oxygen mask, particularly one that has an oxygen reservoir so that all the oxygen inspired does not have to be provided by the flow rate delivered from the oxygen source. With such a mask, the reservoir fills from the oxygen source during expiration and is available to provide an additional volume of oxygen during inhalation. It is difficult to ensure that masks stay in place; if a patient is unstable and requires a high FIO_2 for more than several hours, it is safer to place an endotracheal tube and administer oxygen through a closed system.

PEEP/CPAP

PEEP and CPAP are ventilatory maneuvers used to improve arterial oxygenation when specific indications are present. *PEEP* refers to the maintenance of positive pressure throughout the expiratory cycle when applied together with mechanical ventilation. *CPAP* refers to the maintenance of positive pressure throughout respiration during spontaneous breathing. The mechanism of improvement in oxygenation is the same with both PEEP and CPAP; they both increase the functional residual capacity (FRC, the amount of air in the lungs at the end of a resting exhalation). This increase in FRC improves oxygenation when lung volumes are low as a result of widespread lung injury associated with intrapulmonary shunt. PEEP either opens areas of microatelectasis, previously not ventilated but still perfused, or holds an edematous lung at a higher volume so that the fluid that previously totally filled alveolar sacs now occupies only a portion of the alveolus, allowing some ventilation. With both of these possible mechanisms, areas of shunt are converted to low or normal $\dot{V}/\dot{Q}$ regions and oxygenation is improved.

PEEP may not improve oxygenation if the abnormality is limited to one area of the lung. In this circumstance, PEEP preferentially increases lung volume in the normal and more compliant areas of lung and may have little effect on focal abnormalities. A detrimental effect on oxygenation may even result since high alveolar pressure in areas of normal lung (with an associated increase in lung volume and resistance to blood flow) can divert blood from the normal areas of lung to the diseased portions and actually increase the shunt effect. Thus, a major indication for the use of PEEP/CPAP is ARDS, in which there is diffuse acute lung injury resulting in widespread areas of microatelectasis and pulmonary edema. In this clinical situation, the goals of the use of PEEP are to increase the PaO_2 to provide adequate oxygen saturation of hemoglobin and to allow a reduction in the FIO_2 below the potentially toxic range. There is little or no evidence that PEEP has other therapeutic effects on the lung or otherwise modifies the course of the disease.

Potential problems with PEEP include reduction in cardiac output, primarily through a decrease in venous return. This effect occurs as alveolar pressure is transmitted in part to the pleural space and mediastinum, impeding venous return. There is also a potential risk of barotrauma with resultant pneumothorax; this risk is increased by the concomitant use of mechanical ventilation with high tidal volumes. In general, airway pressure should be the least required to achieve the oxygenation required.

Increased tidal volume

The primary beneficial effects of mechanical ventilation are improvement of respiratory acidosis and reduced work of breathing, but *judicious use* can also improve oxygenation in selected patients. Although PEEP and CPAP are the primary methods to open areas of microatelectasis, the same effect can be achieved at times by use of mechanical ventilation with larger tidal volumes than the patient can generate spontaneously. To improve oxygenation in some animal models of lung injury (e.g., near drowning in fresh water), it is necessary to apply both mechanical ventilation and PEEP.

Definitive therapy

Efforts directed at improving oxygenation are only supportive and temporizing. A permanent improvement in oxygenation requires definitive therapy for the underlying disease. If no definitive therapy is available, the normal healing or repair process must be given time to occur. In either case, it is important to recognize which forms of treatment are merely supportive and which represent specific therapy directed at the cause of the oxygenation abnormality.

MEASURES TO CORRECT RESPIRATORY ACIDOSIS

Respiratory acidosis in the ARF patient can be life-threatening. The urgency for correction of acidosis and the type of therapy required depend on several factors, including the degree of acidosis, the time over which the acidosis has developed, and the specific cause of the respiratory acidosis. Each of these factors affects the risk/benefit relationship of the various types of treatment. Acidosis does not have to be totally corrected. Often partial correction suffices to remove the life-threatening aspects of respiratory acidosis, including impaired tissue functioning, impairment of enzyme systems, and presence or threat of severe cardiac arrhythmias.

Pharmacologic compensation

Administration of bicarbonate partially corrects respiratory acidosis. If acidosis is severe and an acute threat to life, bicarbonate administration can provide rapid improvement and has the additional benefit of allowing other medications (such as bronchodilators) to act in a more optimal pH range. The major drawback of bicarbonate administration is the alkalosis and sodium overload that may follow correction of the underlying cause of the respiratory acidosis. Therefore, bicarbonate administration is generally reserved for severe abnormalities, and then relatively small amounts are given as a temporizing measure.

Attempts at pharmacologic stimulation of respiration generally are not useful.

Mechanical ventilation

Mechanical ventilation usually corrects respiratory acidosis rapidly. Again the risk/benefit must be carefully considered (see below).

Treatment of the underlying disease

Treatment of the process that led to respiratory acidosis is obviously the most physiologic way to correct this abnormality. Once again, as with correction of oxygenation, administration of bicarbonate and mechanical ventilation are only temporizing supportive measures. In correction of respiratory acidosis, however, therapy aimed at correction of the underlying disease process may be the primary or only means of improving respiratory acidosis. This is particularly true in COPD and asthma patients in whom aggressive administration of bronchodilators and help with secretion removal can result in sufficient improvement in both airflow and respiratory acidosis. Within a few hours, the threat to life can be substantially reduced. In a patient with a sedative overdose, metabolism of the medication (or removal with dialysis when appropriate) requires more time, and correction of the acidosis with mechanical ventilation is a more prudent approach.

THE DECISION TO USE MECHANICAL VENTILATION

Whether or not mechanical ventilation is indicated is a major management decision in patients with ARF. Although there are some guidelines to follow, generally the decision is based on the specific clinical situation. The general indications for mechanical ventilation are (1) to improve respiratory acidosis, (2) to reduce excessive work of breathing, and (3) to improve hypoxemia.

One primary goal is improvement of respiratory acidosis, but not all patients with respiratory acidosis require mechanical ventilation. There is no particular PCO_2 or pH value that warrants ventilation in all cases of respiratory acidosis. The decision to ventilate is based on an evaluation of anticipated benefits and possible risks. This evaluation, in turn, depends on the underlying disease causing the respiratory acidosis and the associated dangers of mechanical ventilation in the particular patient. For example, mechanical ventilation should be used readily for a patient with CNS depression caused by sedative overdose since the benefits are substantial, the ventilation time is relatively short (until the sedative can be metabolized), and there are relatively few complications of intubation and mechanical ventilation in such a patient. On the other hand, mechanical ventilation should be reserved for the minority of COPD patients with ARF since endotracheal intubation and mechanical ventilation are associated with higher risks in patients with COPD.

Even in the absence of respiratory acidosis, mechanical ventilation may be useful in the patient with very high work of breathing and high minute ventilation, particularly if a patient has not responded to other therapy and may continue breathing with a high minute ventilation for some time. Unfortunately, there is no easy clinical way to measure work of breathing other than subjective clinical assessment.

In the patient with rapid shallow breathing, hypoxemia may respond to increasing the tidal volume with mechanical ventilation. This improvement in hypoxemia is presumably caused by reopening atelectatic areas of lung and either reducing shunt or improving low $\dot{V}/\dot{Q}$ lung regions.

ESTABLISHMENT OF AN ARTIFICIAL AIRWAY

One of the important decisions in the management of ARF is to determine whether an artificial airway is necessary. The indications for placing an artificial airway include (1) to protect the airway (especially from massive aspiration of gastric contents), (2) to close the system for delivery of an increased FIO_2, (3) to facilitate mechanical ventilation, and (4) to aid in control of secretions. It is rare that a patient requires establishment of an airway for secretion control alone. When suctioning is carried out through an artificial airway, only the trachea or one mainstem bronchus is usually accessible. Therefore, the patient must be able to bring secretions up into the major airways, but intubation impairs cough and makes it difficult to clear secretions from the lower airways. Often, clearance can be facilitated by stimulation of cough during suctioning.

When an indication for an artificial airway exists, an endotracheal tube is placed. Placement of the tube should be done under the most controlled circumstances and by the most experienced person available. Whether an oral or nasal tube is placed is largely a matter of individual preference, although one of the disadvantages of the nasotracheal tube is the increased risk of blocking drainage from paranasal sinuses and precipitating sinusitis. In fact, sinusitis should be considered as a possible source of infection in any patient with a nasotracheal tube and fever. Once the tube has been placed, physical examination should be performed to check for possible esophageal placement or placement in the right mainstem bronchus. Finally, proper tube placement should be confirmed by a chest roentgenogram.

Currently available endotracheal tubes have low-pressure, high-volume cuffs, which have reduced the rate of complication at the cuff site. However, these cuffs do not prevent aspiration of small amounts of secretions or fluid. On the other hand, they should allow protection against massive aspiration of gastric contents, at least until the patient can be appropriately positioned so that aspiration of a large amount of material does not occur.

Whether a tracheostomy should be performed rather than continuing use of the endotracheal tube is decided by weighing the risks and benefits of each type of airway in the specific clinical situation. The cuff complications of both endotracheal and tracheotomy tubes are similar. The use of endotracheal tubes is associated with laryngeal complications and upper airway complications, including sinusitis. Tracheostomy has a low but definite mortality and is associated with late development of tracheal stenosis at the tracheostomy stoma site. Use of modern materials and improved respiratory therapy techniques to reduce the movement of the endotracheal tube in the larynx have reduced trauma and laryngeal complications. Currently, it is common practice to leave an endotracheal tube in place for several weeks. The exact period of intubation associated with a rising incidence of laryngeal complications is not known. However, as a general guide, if a tracheal tube is to be in place for much longer than a month, tracheostomy is preferable. If this decision can be made early in the course of illness, tracheostomy should be done as soon as possible. If it is felt that a patient can be extubated prior to a month, the endotracheal tube can be left in place and this decision reassessed on a weekly basis or as indicated.

MANAGEMENT OF SPECIFIC ACUTE RESPIRATORY FAILURE SYNDROMES

The principles of management remain the same for any ARF patient regardless of the underlying etiology. However, the specific application of these principles differs considerably depending on the etiology.

COPD with ARF

Most patients with COPD and ARF require only a small increase in supplemental oxygen to correct the oxygenation abnormality. This increase can be achieved by administering 1 to 2 liters per minute of oxygen by nasal prongs, and then adjusting the flow rate according to the resulting arterial blood gases. An alternative method of administration is a 24% or 28% Venturi mask. In some patients with COPD, oxygen administration can be associated with worsening hypoventilation and respiratory acidosis. Previously, this association was thought to be secondary to removal of the hypoxic drive to breathe in patients with already diminished carbon dioxide ventilatory drive. Recent studies suggest that increased $PaCO_2$ related to the administration of oxygen results from changes in ventilation/perfusion with increased dead space ventilation.

Whatever the mechanism, an increased PaO_2 (usually greater than that necessary to achieve adequate SaO_2) can be associated with worsening respiratory acidosis in a minority of patients. Three aspects of this phenomenon must be emphasized: (1) it occurs only in a minority of COPD patients with ARF; (2) the primary objective in any ARF patient is still to oxygenate the arterial blood adequately; the potential of increasing $PaCO_2$ does not justify allowing a patient to remain significantly hypoxemic; and (3) a significant improvement in oxygenation (since the PaO_2 is usually in the steep portion of the oxygen-hemoglobin dissociation curve) can be achieved without a clinically important reduction in pH in nearly all patients by careful administration of oxygen and close monitoring together with other forms of therapy aimed at the precipitating causes of ARF.

Some COPD patients require a greater increase in FIO_2 than can be achieved with 2 liters per minute of nasal oxygen. In these patients there is usually an element of increased shunt, a result, for example, of pneumonia or congestive heart failure as the precipitating cause of respiratory failure.

Many COPD patients with ARF have significant respiratory acidosis. Experience with management of these patients has shown improved results if unnecessary application of mechanical ventilation is avoided and other means of improvement in acidosis are used. Coughing is extremely important for secretion removal in COPD patients with ARF. Effective mechanical ventilation requires placement of an endotracheal tube, which results in impairment of cough by preventing glottic closure. Also, mechanical ventilation often impairs mobilization of the patient. Although this impairment can be avoided with a great deal of effort, it is often an undesired side effect.

Other risks of endotracheal intubation and mechanical ventilation are higher in the COPD patient than in other patients with ARF. The COPD patient has increased lung compliance, which results in an increased risk of reduced cardiac output and barotrauma. In addition, the risk of infection in these patients is high. Therefore, unnecessary mechanical ventilation should be avoided.

When does mechanical ventilation become necessary in the COPD patient with ARF? This question can be answered in the negative sense as follows. If a patient is awake, can cough, and can cooperate with therapy (by taking inhaled bronchodilators and cooperating with measures to remove secretions), it is rarely necessary to use mechanical ventilation. Patients who meet these criteria should be given a trial of aggressive therapy before proceeding to mechanical ventilation. In these patients, mechanical ventilation should be employed only if a patient is not improving or is clearly tiring. On the other hand, if a patient initially is obtunded and difficult to arouse, intubation and mechanical ventilation should be carried out even before knowing the degree of acidosis. Thus, the decision to ventilate a COPD patient is primarily based on clinical findings. Mental status is of prime importance. In most medical centers, less than 10% of COPD patients with ARF require mechanical ventilation.

How should respiratory acidosis be treated in COPD patients? Therapy of respiratory acidosis is essentially the same as treatment of the underlying chronic disease. Worsening hypoventilation is usually associated with worsening airflow; potentially reversible elements of air-flow obstruction are bronchospasm and increased secretions. Therefore, treatment should be aimed at improving airflow with bronchodilators and aiding secretion removal. Aggressive bronchodilator therapy is indicated for potential improvement in airflow obstruction, even when a patient has not been previously shown to respond to bronchodilators in an outpatient setting. In most patients, simultaneous treatment with inhaled β-adrenergic and/or anticholinergic agents and intravenous or oral corticosteroids is warranted. β-adrenergic agents should be given by inhalation, using metered dose inhalers (MDI) or a nebulized solution. The bronchodilator effect of ipratropium bromide, an anticholinergic agent available by MDI, is equivalent to that of β-adrenergic agents in COPD patients. Although most studies in stable outpatients have failed to show added benefit if either agent is administered after a maximal dose of the other, a trial of administering both agents may be warranted in ARF.

In a study of patients receiving β-adrenergic agents and intravenous corticosteroids, addition of intravenous aminophylline had no beneficial effect on pulmonary function when compared to placebo. However, theophylline may have other beneficial effects including enhancement of recovery from respiratory muscle fatigue and stimulation of ventilatory drive; thus, the current role of theophylline administration in patients with COPD and an acute exacerbation is unclear. If theophylline is given, it is usually first administered in the form of intravenous aminophylline, with an intravenous loading dose, depending on whether the patient has been receiving chronic theophylline therapy. If the history indicates compliance with a reasonable outpatient theophylline regimen, the maintenance dose should be continued until therapy can be guided by actual measurement of the serum theophylline level. Since theophylline is well absorbed from the gastrointestinal tract, a change to an oral form can be carried out relatively early in the hospital course, after initial clinical improvement has occurred.

A well-controlled study of COPD patients with ARF caused by exacerbation by acute bronchitis demonstrated significant improvement in airflow when corticosteroids were administered during the first 3 days of therapy. Corticosteroids were administered as methylprednisolone sodium succinate, 0.5 mg per kilogram body weight every 6 hours.

Promotion of secretion removal should be encouraged. Patients should be stimulated to cough, especially after inhalation of a bronchodilator. A trial of chest percussion and postural drainage may be warranted, with evaluation of results compared with those with cough alone. Hypoxemia may worsen in the lateral postural drainage positions and may require a temporary further increase in F_{IO_2} to counteract this change.

A randomized controlled trial of antibiotic administration during an acute exacerbation in patients with COPD resulted in a slight but statistically significant improvement in the rate of successful outcomes in patients treated with antibiotics. Antibiotic use was not associated with increased side effects when compared to placebo. Although the clinical importance of these results could be debated, it seems prudent to err on the side of using antibiotics in a patient whose exacerbation is severe enough to precipitate ARF. In the absence of evidence for a specific bacterial etiology, any antibiotic that is effective against *Streptococcus pneumoniae* and *Haemophilus influenzae* is appropriate (Chapter 224).

Proper treatment of the underlying disease requires another diagnosis in addition to COPD—that of the cause precipitating ARF. Although the treatment described remains the same for the other aspects of COPD, specific therapy varies according to whether the acute illness is viral bronchitis, bacterial pneumonia, pulmonary embolism, congestive heart failure, and so on.

Respiratory muscle fatigue may contribute significantly to the development of ARF. Clinical findings suggesting respiratory muscle fatigue include rapid shallow respirations, paradoxical abdominal breathing, and respiratory alternans. The latter two are relatively specific for respiratory muscle fatigue. Paradoxical abdominal breathing is diagnosed by observing the abdomen move in as the chest moves outward. Usually, the abdomen and chest wall move out together during inspiration. Respiratory alternans is a more unusual finding. It consists of periods during which inspiratory muscle activity consists entirely of use of the chest wall muscles, alternating with periods of diaphragmatic breathing. At present, treatment of inspiratory muscle fatigue remains unclear; there is evidence that theophylline facilitates recovery, but the clinical importance of this observation is not yet known. It appears that rest is important in allowing recovery of the fatigued respiratory muscles; therefore, mechanical ventilation allowing respiratory muscle rest may assume increasing importance in selected patients with evidence of recent onset of respiratory muscle fatigue as a major component of their ARF.

ARF occurring with ARDS

ARDS usually occurs in clinical situations involving severe underlying illness or injury and therefore is associated with a variety of causes. The exact mechanism is not known but is generally believed to represent acute lung injury, either as a direct insult (e.g., from aspiration of gastric contents) or, more commonly, indirectly through activation of humoral or cellular mediators (such as with sepsis and severe multiple trauma). Treatment, other than specific therapy aimed at the underlying causes, is supportive.

Correction of the oxygenation abnormality in the ARDS patient requires a high F_{IO_2}. The initial F_{IO_2} should be high to ensure adequate oxygenation, and then should be adjusted downward as tolerated, monitoring blood gases. PEEP and CPAP are employed either to provide an adequate Pa_{O_2}, if this has not already been achieved, or to lower the F_{IO_2} to reduce the risk of oxygen toxicity. Depending on the initial blood gases and the initial F_{IO_2}, the clinician must decide on a reasonable goal, but at least reducing the F_{IO_2} to 0.7 and preferably to 0.5 seems important. The F_{IO_2} is reduced further as the Pa_{O_2} improves, until the F_{IO_2} is down to 0.4 or 0.5. Then the PEEP can be progressively decreased by 5 cm H_2O decrements. Once the initial level of PEEP that gives the desired improvement in oxygenation without a significant reduction in cardiac output has been established, the tidal volume should be adjusted if the patient is receiving mechanical ventilation. Usually, the tidal volume can be adjusted downward if the FRC has improved with PEEP. Selection of the appropriate tidal volume can be aided by measuring the total static compliance at various tidal volumes. The compliance usually decreases at both low and high tidal volumes. The lowest value with a stable plateau level of compliance should provide adequate lung expansion while reducing the risk of lung rupture and pneumothorax.

ARDS is rarely associated with respiratory acidosis. However, this does not mean that carbon dioxide removal is normal in these patients. Minute ventilation ($\dot{V}_E$) usually is very high, producing a normal or often somewhat reduced $PaCO_2$. Mechanical ventilation may be indicated to reduce the work of breathing and, in some instances, to help improve oxygenation. Estimation of the work of breathing requires subjective clinical evaluation.

Treatment of the underlying disease is mainly supportive. The one major exception is the treatment of sepsis. If a patient is thought to have sepsis, appropriate cultures and a thorough search for the source of possible infection should be made. Broad-spectrum antibiotics should be given until culture results are available. It is especially important to search for infections that may require surgical drainage, such as intra-abdominal abscesses.

Infection represents the most important complication in the ARDS patient because it frequently leads to a clinical sepsis syndrome with hypotension and multiple organ failure and is associated with a very high mortality. In managing these patients, careful infection control measures, including compulsive hand washing between patient contacts, are mandatory.

ARF without lung disease

Two categories of patients with ARF but no pulmonary abnormalities are (1) those with suppressed central drive—most common are patients who have taken an overdose of sedative or tranquilizing drugs; and (2) those with neuromuscular abnormalities leading to respiratory failure. Initial management of an overdose patient includes gastric lavage to remove any drug still in the stomach. If a patient is not awake, the airway should be protected during gastric lavage by endotracheal intubation. The decision to institute mechanical ventilation is based on both the patient's mental status and the presence of respiratory acidosis. If a patient is obtunded and respiratory acidosis is present, mechanical ventilation should be used until he or she is consistently awake. Aspiration of oropharyngeal or gastric contents is relatively common in the obtunded overdose patient. Antibiotic treatment of aspiration pneumonia is indicated only if evidence of a bacterial pneumonia develops, including purulent sputum with pathogenic organisms seen on Gram stain. Prophylactic corticosteroids or prophylactic antibiotics are not warranted.

Patients with progressive neuromuscular disease should be followed with serial measurements of vital capacity. As a general rule, ventilatory support should be considered when the vital capacity falls below 15 ml per kilogram body weight. Mechanical ventilatory support should be continued until muscle strength and spontaneous vital capacity improve and are adequate to sustain spontaneous ventilation without muscle fatigue.

DECISIONS IN VENTILATORY SUPPORT

Once it has been decided that mechanical ventilation is warranted, several other decisions need to be made: the type of ventilator, the FIO_2, the mode of ventilation, the tidal volume and respiratory frequency, whether to use PEEP or CPAP, and finally, what kind of monitoring should be performed. The FIO_2 should be the lowest necessary to achieve adequate arterial oxygenation; this level must be decided for each patient. It is best initially to use a high FIO_2 and then rapidly decrease it to the lowest level necessary as judged by arterial blood gas studies.

The modes of ventilation include controlled mechanical ventilation (CMV), assisted mechanical ventilation (AMV, also called *assist/control mode*), intermittent mandatory ventilation (IMV), and pressure support ventilation (PSV). With CMV the respiratory rate is set and the patient cannot adjust it by breathing spontaneously or by triggering additional breaths from the ventilator. Consequently, the patient on controlled ventilation usually has to be sedated, given a muscle-paralyzing agent, or ventilated with a frequency sufficiently high that respiratory alkalosis is produced. Both muscle paralysis and respiratory alkalosis have significant drawbacks; therefore, CMV should be limited to specific clinical indications.

Most patients can be ventilated with either AMV (assist/control) or IMV. With AMV the ventilator rate is set slightly below the patient's intrinsic respiratory rate, and the patient is able to trigger some or all of the ventilator breaths. With IMV some breaths are given by the ventilator at a predetermined rate, and the patient is allowed to breathe spontaneously from a pressurized high-airflow circuit to meet the rest of the ventilatory requirements.

There is considerable debate regarding the relative advantages and disadvantages of AMV versus IMV. It is clear that the majority of patients requiring mechanical ventilation can be effectively ventilated by either ventilatory mode. Perhaps it is more important to be aware of specific clinical situations in which one of these modes may have particular advantages over the other. IMV can be useful in a patient who is "fighting the ventilator" on CMV or AMV and in whom other causes for this so-called fighting (e.g., inadequate oxygenation, acidosis, or pain) have been ruled out. A change to IMV sometimes allows the patient to adjust to mechanical ventilation in a more comfortable fashion; each patient should be evaluated individually. A patient with severe airflow obstruction can develop progressive air trapping and "auto-PEEP" (positive alveolar pressure throughout exhalation) on AMV. This phenomenon can be associated with significant reductions in cardiac output as positive alveolar pressure is transmitted to the pleural space and to the great veins, thus impeding venous return. Changing to IMV might allow dissipation of the positive alveolar pressure and air trapping during the periods of spontaneous breathing. IMV has a theoretical advantage in patients with marginal cardiac output because mean alveolar pressure tends to be lower since some of the breaths are spontaneous; this lower pressure reduces the risk of impaired cardiac output. On the other hand, with the AMV mode, in the unstable critically ill patient with an already high minute ventilation requirement, further increased ventilatory demand could be met relatively easily by triggering the machine at a more rapid rate. With IMV in this situation, the patient may not be able to meet this increased ventilatory demand by increasing spontaneous ventilation. In patients with high ventilatory demands, the potential advantages of IMV may no longer exist if a high mandatory rate on IMV is used. AMV is associated with a lower work of breathing than IMV (because of the component of spontaneous breathing with IMV). Recent studies have shown that some patients on AMV continue to actively inspire after they initiate the ventilator breath and continue to perform inspiratory muscle work. Thus, the advantage of reducing work of breathing is not as great as it might seem. This phenomenon is particularly likely to occur if the inspiratory flow is relatively slow and unable to meet the patient's desired demands for inspiratory flow. There are no data to confirm that one mode has a clear advantage over the other in enhancing the process of weaning from mechanical ventilation.

PSV augments the patient's spontaneous breathing effort. As the patient triggers each breath, the airway pressure increases rapidly to the desired pressure setting and remains there until the flow rate decreases to a predetermined minimal flow or percentage of the peak flow, at which time the inspiratory flow of gas from the ventilator ceases. Thus part of the work of each breath is carried out by the patient and part by the ventilator. The amount of work contributed by the ventilator is determined by the set pressure and resulting tidal volume. PSV mainly has been recommended for weaning but can also be employed as a primary ventilatory mode. The patient has some control over the inspiratory pressure wave form, which appears to be associated with an improvement in patient comfort over other ventilatory modes in some patients. Use of PSV requires that a patient's ventilatory drive be intact.

The tidal volume and respiratory rate should be set so that the minute ventilation (their product) results in a normal pH (unless there are specific reasons for a different pH, for example, a temporary respiratory alkalosis in management of cerebral edema). The tidal volume should be large enough to prevent progressive microatelectasis; however, this usually occurs only at low tidal volumes, less than 5 ml per kilogram body weight.

A tidal volume in the range of 6 to 10 ml per kilogram body weight is recommended initially. High tidal volumes have been associated with increased risk of pneumothorax. This risk can be reduced by using measurements of total static compliance at various tidal volumes to choose the lowest tidal volume with the highest compliance. Choosing this tidal volume helps prevent relative overdistention of the more compliant alveolar units, an occurrence associated with a decrease in overall compliance.

It has been shown in patients with chronic air-flow obstruction that rapid inspiratory flow rates shorten the inspiratory time and allow a longer exhalation time for any given respiratory rate. This reduces air trapping and is associated with improved oxygenation and a decrease in the dead space to tidal volume ratio (V_D/V_T). Therefore, it is recommended that high inspiratory flow rates be used in COPD patients and that the inspiratory flow rate be adjusted to a level that is comfortable for patients without COPD.

PEEP (with AMV or CMV) or CPAP (with IMV) should be applied if specific needs to improve oxygenation are present in patients with acute diffuse alveolar disease. Some investigators feel that a certain amount of PEEP or CPAP is "physiologic" in that lung volume and arterial blood gas measurements made on a low level of PEEP are similar to those made after extubation and slightly greater than measurements made with a patient breathing without PEEP or CPAP with the endotracheal tube still in place. However, these differences are small and of doubtful clinical importance in most patients. It is not recommended that PEEP or CPAP be routinely applied to all patients. For example, PEEP or CPAP should not be applied in patients with possible increased intracranial pressure or in patients with increased risk for lung rupture, unless specific indications outweigh these risks.

Finally, it should be determined what monitoring is necessary for the patient receiving ventilatory support (see Chapters 198 and 203). In addition to general monitoring considerations, the patient receiving mechanical ventilation should have regular monitoring of the exhaled tidal volume, minute ventilation, peak and inflation hold pressures, and the volume and pressure in the tracheal tube cuff required to occlude the airway. Occasional measurements of carbon dioxide production and dead space (V_D/V_T) can be useful, particularly in patients requiring prolonged ventilation with high minute ventilation requirements.

REMOVAL FROM MECHANICAL VENTILATION AND WEANING

In removing ventilatory support, cessation of mechanical ventilation should be considered as a separate step from removal of the endotracheal tube. Some patients are able to breathe spontaneously with adequate maintenance of arterial blood gases but continue to require endotracheal intubation for airway protection.

In most patients the term *weaning from mechanical ventilation* is applied incorrectly. Weaning implies gradual removal from mechanical ventilation. Most patients receiving ventilatory support can be readily removed from mechanical ventilation once their underlying problem has been corrected. In these patients a gradual process is not necessary. In determining which patients can be removed from mechanical ventilation, two separate questions should be asked. First, can the patient maintain adequate arterial oxygenation on the FIO_2 that can be achieved by nasal prongs or face mask oxygen delivery? And second, can the patient maintain adequate ventilation spontaneously? A decision regarding the first question is made by interpretation of the PaO_2 in relation to the FIO_2. If the PaO_2 is adequate on an FIO_2 of 0.4, adequate oxygenation should be accomplished with an FIO_2 readily achievable after removal of the endotracheal tube. The second question is approached by measuring so-called ventilatory parameters during spontaneous breathing. These parameters should be used only as a guide to determining removal from mechanical ventilation because some patients, when breathing spontaneously in their chronic outpatient state, never meet the recommended criteria for removal from mechanical ventilation. However, if the ventilatory parameter criteria *are* met and the patient is otherwise stable, successful removal from mechanical ventilation can be virtually ensured.

Usual variables measured and guidelines for successful discontinuation of mechanical support include tidal volume (V_T) greater than 5 ml per kilogram body weight, vital capacity (VC) greater than 10 ml per kilogram body weight, inspiratory force less than (more negative than) −30 cm H_2O, and minute ventilation ($\dot{V}_E$) less than 10 liters per minute. Other measurements, including V_D/V_T, have been suggested but are used less frequently and are generally not necessary. Most of these criteria have not been subjected to critical study in a controlled trial. Established criteria include $\dot{V}_E$ less than 10 liters per minute and the ability to double this V_E value with a maximum voluntary ventilation (MVV) maneuver. All patients who met these criteria were able to be successfully removed from mechanical ventilation and subsequently extubated. Of patients who did not meet these criteria, some were successfully removed, while others had to be returned to ventilatory support. Of those who did not meet the criteria but could be successfully removed, several observations were helpful. Most of these patients had borderline values for the above criteria. However, they had a greater mean inspiratory force than the patients who had to be returned to mechanical ventilation, with an absolute cutoff between the two groups of −24 cm H_2O. Once the endotracheal tube was removed, many of these patients who previously could not double their $\dot{V}_E$ value with an MVV maneuver could now double or even triple this value. Thus, it is apparent that in some of these measurements, the endotracheal tube can add to airflow resistance, and these values might be improved once the tube has been removed. Tube sizes with an internal diameter less than 7.5 mm are particularly associated with increased resistance to airflow.

The resting $\dot{V}_E$ must be interpreted in view of the patient's body size, muscle mass, and physical state prior to the onset of ARF. For example, attempts at stopping mechanical ventilation might not be warranted in a small elderly woman with COPD and possible muscle fatigue until the $\dot{V}_E$ is less than 10 liters per minute, but a young, relatively large man in good health prior to the onset of ARDS might be removed when the $\dot{V}_E$ drops to 15 liters per minute. Once a patient is considered to be a candidate for removal from a ventilator, a trial of spontaneous breathing through a T piece usually is warranted. This trial should be relatively short (approximately 30 minutes) since ventilation will most likely be easier once the tube is removed. At the end of 30 minutes, arterial blood gases are obtained. If these values are judged to be adequate, mechanical ventilation can be discontinued and a decision made regarding removal of the endotracheal tube.

In a patient who cannot be readily removed from the ventilator, a program of weaning must be started. The major methods of gradual withdrawal are (1) IMV with a progressively lowered mandatory rate until the patient is breathing entirely spontaneously; (2) PSV with a progressively lowered pressure until only the pressure required to overcome airway resistance of the endotracheal tube is reached, or (3) short T-piece trials that are progressively lengthened until the patient essentially is breathing spontaneously. No data are available to prove the superiority of any given method over another. If the IMV method is used, it is important to continue to attempt to lower the mandatory rate progressively. Otherwise, the patient might actually be kept on mechanical ventilation longer by very slowly lowering the mandatory rate, a misuse of the method rather than a true failure of it. Recently, muscle physiologists have given theoretical support to the conventional intermittent T-piece method. Their hypothesis is that respiratory muscle training requires periods of working the muscles to a point of fatigue, with intermittent rest provided by total ventilatory support to allow the muscles to recover from this fatigue. Whether this theory is borne out in practice requires controlled studies comparing the two methods of withdrawal in appropriate patients.

Medical stability, appropriate nutritional status, and appropriate psychological preparation are extremely important when removing patients from mechanical ventilation. These aspects are probably more important than the specific method of weaning used.

OTHER ASPECTS OF MANAGEMENT OF THE ACUTE RESPIRATORY FAILURE PATIENT

If it is anticipated that the period of ARF might be prolonged, early attention should be directed at the nutritional state of the patient. Critical studies have not yet demonstrated at what point in the course of ARF feeding should be started to produce the best outcome. However, most clinicians suspect that early administration of adequate nutritional support is important, especially in a catabolic patient.

The ARF patient should not be limited to a supine position in bed, if at all possible. Moving from the supine to the sitting position improves lung volume. Moving to various positions is important in maintaining expansion of all areas of the lung and in enhancing secretion removal. In addition, sitting in a chair or walking helps maintain musculoskeletal function.

Attention to the psychological aspects of the patient with ARF is also important. These patients are often depressed. A patient with chronic underlying lung disease may be exhausted at hospital admission and irritable because of impaired sleep, in addition to any hypoxemia that might be present. Psychosocial support can be critical in influencing outcome.

All of these aspects of care are even more important if a patient requires mechanical ventilation. Institution of mechanical ventilation often results in a patient being kept in bed rather than getting up to walk or sit in a chair, prevents feeding by mouth, and impairs communication. Thus, these patients require more effort from the health care team.

REFERENCES

Derenne JP, Fleury B, and Pariente R: Acute respiratory failure of chronic obstructive pulmonary disease. Am Rev Respir Dis 138:1006, 1988.

Marini JJ: Lung mechanics in ARDS. Clin Chest Med 11:673, 1990.

Matthay MA: The adult respiratory distress syndrome: definition and prognosis. Clin Chest Med 11:575, 1990.

Pingleton SK: Complications of acute respiratory failure. Am Rev Respir Dis 137:1463, 1988.

Rosen RL and Bone RC: Treatment of acute exacerbations of chronic obstructive pulmonary disease. Med Clin N Amer 74:691, 1990.

Schmidt GA and Hall JB: Acute on chronic respiratory failure: assessment and management of patients with COPD in the emergent setting. JAMA 261:3444, 1989.

Stoller JK and Kacmarek RM: Ventilatory strategies in the management of ARDS. Clin Chest Med 11:755, 1990.

CHAPTER

201 Multiple Organ Dysfunction Syndrome (MODS) in the Context of ARDS

Jean E. Rinaldo

ARDS AND THE EVOLVING MODS CONCEPT

The Adult Respiratory Distress Syndrome (ARDS) has been evolving since the initial descriptions of the disorder in 1967. At first, the syndrome was defined by pulmonary physiologic parameters. Abnormal pulmonary microvascular permeability coefficients resulting in lung edema and abnormal regulation of ventilation-perfusion matching resulting in hypoxemia in the lung were considered necessary and sufficient physiologic hallmarks. Several factors led to the realization that this concept was oversimplified. Inflammation and cell biology began to be emphasized when neutrophils were implicated in causing permeability lung edema and when pulmonary histology from lungs of ARDS patients showed dramatic changes in the structure of lung parenchyma, including proliferation lung fibrosis and microvascular obliteration. These findings suggested an inflammatory basis of injury and intercellular miscommunication during healing, leading to a fibrotic response. Then concurrent extrapulmonary abnormalities that accompanied pulmonary dysfunction during ARDS were recognized. As supportive care improved, retrospective clinical studies showed that progressive physiologic failure of several interdependent organ systems often occurred concurrent with respiratory failure and ultimately was responsible for deaths. These extrapulmonary components of ARDS include, but are not limited to, hepatic dysfunction, renal dysfunction, altered mental status, coagulopathies, gastrointestinal bleeding and dysmotility, and a propensity for superinfection. Presence of infection and of extrapulmonary multisystem organ failure (MSOF) emerged as the most important predictors of mortality in ARDS patients. Accordingly, respiratory failure caused by ARDS is now commonly viewed as a part of a multisystem disorder.

Nomenclature is imprecise; because systemic infection is so intimately related to the syndrome, *sepsis syndrome, sepsis, multiple organ dysfunction syndrome (MODS), systemic inflammatory response syndrome (SIRS),* and *multisystem organ system failure* (MSOF) have been used almost interchangeably by different investigators to define the systemic response to infection or noninfectious inflammation with its associated organ dysfunctions. There have been attempts at standardization of nomenclature but these are not universally accepted. We use the term *multiple organ dysfunction syndrome* (MODS) here.

MECHANISMS OF MODS

By definition, MODS is a pansystemic process. For conceptual purposes, we may subdivide the underlying mechanisms into three subsets: (1) panvascular effects that cause tissue ischemia, (2) intracellular nonischemic metabolic or cytotoxic effects, and (3) signalled changes in cell function induced by cytokines. In the first category are vascular occlusive events that cause disturbances in regional blood flow. These may arise as a result of perturbations in vasomotor responsiveness or luminal plugging by leukocyte and platelet aggregates. Important vaso-occlusive mediators that have been implicated include thromboxane, a cyclooxygenase metabolite of arachidonic acid released by platelets, and endothelin, a peptide released by endothelial cells. Alternatively, synthesis of vasodilating mediator substances such as prostacyclin may be inhibited, producing a net vasoconstrictor effect. Many of the vaso-occlusive mechanisms that have long been thought to be involved in the pathogenesis of ARDS may work similarly in other organs. One example is sepsis-induced acute renal failure. Normal human glomeruli synthesize predominantly prostaglandin E_2 and prostaglandin F_2, but during sepsis there appears to be a shift in prostaglandin metabolism resulting in enhanced release of thromboxane, which acts as a potent vasoconstrictor. Presumably, related sequences occur in other tissues. In the second category are cytotoxic assaults and disturbances in intracellular metabolism that are not a direct result of vascular occlusion. These include generation of reactive oxygen species by intracellular enzyme systems or by the respiratory burst of contiguous phagocytes, as well as putative but poorly documented metabolic aberrations such as the uncoupling of oxidative phosphorylation. In the third category are specifically signalled changes in cell function induced by cytokines, which act as "hormones" of inflammation. The cytokines are protein molecules that are synthesized and released by cells, bind specifically to cell surface receptors on target cells, and thereby induce a functional change in the target cells. These functional changes include leukocyte priming and activation, activation of transcription factors that regulate gene expression, chemotaxis, and other effects that amplify a systemic inflammatory response. As "hormones," these blood-borne peptides can induce signalled changes in cells throughout the body that possess the requisite surface receptors, making them potential effectors of a pansystemic syndrome.

Autocrine, paracrine, and endocrine responses to cytokines have been particularly emphasized in MODS arising during sepsis. Gram-negative infections are a common predisposition to MODS. It has been estimated that 120,000 cases of gram-negative bacteremia occur yearly with a fatality rate ranging from about 20% to about 60%. The MODS syndrome commonly occurs and causes death. Bacterial endotoxin (lipopolysaccharide, LPS) is thought to be involved in triggering inflammatory cascades that cause organ system injury. In experimental studies, LPS causes a constellation of symptoms that may be termed the "sepsis syndrome": fever or hypothermia, leukocytosis or leukopenia, hyperventilation and hypoxemia, and hypotension. Also, LPS causes the release of cytokines into the circulation. It has been postulated that the cytokines serve important host defense and homeostatic roles in limited infection, but that during overwhelming or sustained infection they cause a cascade of unopposed physiologic reactions that threaten the host. The principal cytokines implicated in sepsis to date are tumor necrosis factor, interleukin-1, interleukin-2, interleukin-6, interleukin-8, and interferon-gamma. Evidence that LPS and these cytokines are major factors in sepsis syndrome and MSOF is as follows: the cytokines appear in the blood of infected patients and experimental animals given LPS, and the levels are higher in patients with septic shock. When infused, the physiologic effects of the LPS and of cytokines mimic those of septic shock, and antibodies to the cytokines block many of these physiologic effects. The cytokines circulate in blood and their molecular weights are generally small enough to permit them to cross the capillary endothelial barrier relatively freely. In vitro, the agents affect the functions of a wide variety of cultured cell types from different organs providing the potential for multisystem effects. This evidence for cytokine cascades being involved in the evolution of the sepsis syndrome has recently been reviewed in detail.

RECOGNITION OF MODS AND DIAGNOSTIC STRATEGY

MODS is diagnosed by demonstrating concurrent onset of otherwise unexplained pulmonary, CNS, renal, hepatic, and hematologic functional abnormalities in an appropriate clinical setting, usually one involving either infection or noninfectious inflammation or tissue injury. Respiratory abnormalities are often recognized first, prompting a clinical diagnosis of ARDS. Evidence of extrapulmonary involvement may be much more subtle than pulmonary dysfunction because injury to the lung microvasculature has immediate life-threatening clinical manifestations arising from pulmonary edema. In contrast, other organs may maintain functional integrity despite extravasation of fluid and protein. Thus ARDS often appears to precede MODS. The earliest signs of extrapulmonary dysfunction are confusion, glucose intolerance, unexplained volume requirement, diminished urine output, mild thrombocytopenia, slight prolongation of the prothrombin time, and heme-positive stools or gastric aspirates. If the underlying predisposition is self-limited or effectively treated, the extrapulmonary organ dysfunctions may resolve before becoming clinically significant and the multisystem nature of the illness may not attract attention. Inability to reverse the inciting event permits MODS to progress until elevations in creatinine, abnormal liver function studies, gastrointestinal hemorrhage, or other overt extrapulmonary manifestations occur. This sequence seems more common in immunosuppressed or chronically debilitated patients in whom an inciting infectious event is less easily controlled.

Other multiorgan dysfunctions and interactions may mimic MODS. Concurrently, a combination of primary organ system injuries may be present, for example, aminoglycoside-induced renal failure, cholestatic drugs, and volume overload contributing to pulmonary edema. Such patients may be incorrectly labelled as having MODS. It is important to recognize the possibility that concurrent primary dysfunctions may be present, because many of the causes are iatrogenic and potentially reversible. Another variation on the MODS theme is the deleterious interaction of dysfunctional organ systems that are causally unrelated. An example is the concurrence of ARDS with preexisting severe liver disease. The liver and lung are arranged in series and blood from the hepatic vein first encounters the lung microvasculature. The failing liver may contribute to pulmonary dysfunction by failing to synthesize proteins critical to host defense, by failing to metabolize mediators of ARDS or clear bacteria or cell remnants from the circulation, and by the active "export" of mediators such as tumor necrosis factor (and other cytokines) and xanthine oxidase, which injure the lung endothelium. Renal failure and ARDS of unrelated etiologies also may interact detrimentally. Renal failure itself is mildly immunosuppressive, but other logistical factors probably are just as important, including difficulty removing edema fluid from the lung, prolonging the need for invasive respiratory support, and the need for invasive central vascular access for dialysis and transfusions.

When faced with evidence of MODS, the diagnostic strategy is to uncover and treat the underlying etiology; to prevent, identify, and treat superinfection; and to exclude other etiologies for organ system dysfunction. Medications should be reviewed to uncover nephrotoxic, hepatotoxic, or marrow-suppressing drugs administered singly or in combination. In the case of renal dysfunction, diagnostic work-up should be undertaken to exclude prerenal and postrenal abnormalities such as intravascular hypovolemia, low cardiac output, and urinary obstruction. Evaluations for occult sources of infection usually include cultures of blood, sputum, urine, pleural fluid, and ascites if present; computerized tomography of the sinuses; abdominal ultrasound and/or computerized tomography; lumbar puncture; and evaluation of all invasive lines as a potential nidus of infection.

SUPPORTIVE THERAPY FOR MODS

Prevention and therapy of MODS are nonspecific. The overall goals are to identify and reverse the underlying cause of the systemic inflammatory response; to maintain tissue oxygenation; to provide nutritional support; to avoid iatrogenic complications; to prevent, diagnose, and treat infection; and to support or replace critically impaired functions of individual organs with mechanical ventilation, dialysis, transfusions of blood products, and cardiotropic and/or vasoactive pharmacologic agents.

The first goal is identification of the underlying etiology. MODS is most commonly associated with systemic infections. Noninfectious events may also cause MODS, including pancreatitis, extensive cutaneous burns, ischemia-reperfusion events, skeletal fractures and crush injuries, and hypovolemic or cardiogenic shock, but these should be considered diagnoses of exclusion and the patients should be evaluated for occult infection. In the case of burns and crush injuries, devitalized tissue should be aggressively debrided as early as possible. There is a growing population of immunosuppressed patients with profound impairments of host defense that predispose them to recurrent and/or ineradicable infections. This group includes patients with human immunodeficiency virus, patients with end-stage organ failure awaiting transplantation, organ transplantation recipients, patients who have received marrow ablative chemotherapeutic agents for hematologic malignancies, and debilitated, alcoholic, and/or malnourished patients. In these patients MODS may appear to result from occult infection even though the source of infection is difficult to identify, and empiric antibiotic therapy is usually employed.

A second major goal is to maintain tissue oxygenation. Regional blood flow, hemoglobin concentration, and hemoglobin saturation are the principal determinants of tissue oxygenation. It is important that *flow* rather than *blood pressure* be emphasized. Blood pressure may be maintained by sympathetic reflexes or supported artificially with vasopressor agents even though flow is greatly reduced. In such cases the normalization of the blood pressure by vasoconstriction may promote MODS by enhancing tissue ischemia, especially in the kidney. Reduced cardiac output measured by thermodilution, mixed venous oxygen desaturation, and/or arterial blood lactate levels may provide evidence that tissue oxygen delivery is inadequate. Skin capillary refilling and urine output are useful clinical indices of regional flow in these tissues, but currently no available technology reliably assesses regional tissue oxygenation. Restoration of intravascular volume should be the initial therapeutic approach. After fluid resuscitation is complete, careful titration of peripheral vasoconstrictors may increase cerebral, renal, and coronary perfusion, but should be employed only if there is a persistent and significant reduction in systemic vascular resistance that results in refractory hypotension despite euvolemia. Low-dose dopamine (2-5 μg/kg/min) may provide renal vascular dilatation, preserving renal blood flow. It should be emphasized that significant volume infusions may be needed initially to restore intravascular volume, which is lost to increased venous capacitance and ongoing loss of fluid into tissues resulting from increased microvascular permeability. However, it has been shown that persistent positive fluid balance in such patients is a poor prognostic factor; in the later stages of therapy, (usually several days after the septic event is treated), diuresis must be induced to mobilize and excrete this fluid and permit weaning from mechanical ventilation.

Substantial improvements in oxygen delivery can often be achieved by transfusion, especially in patients unable to augment cardiac output sufficiently to compensate for anemia. Hemoglobin concentration should be maintained at >12 g/dl in such patients, especially if arterial hypoxemia is enough of a problem to necessitate use of potentially toxic FIO_2. Transfusions of red blood cells may permit the FIO_2 to be lowered by increasing oxygen delivery and elevating mixed venous oxygen content. In contrast to substantial benefits achievable by transfusion of erythrocytes, little improvement in oxygen delivery can be achieved by using more oxygen to boost arterial pO_2 above 60 mm Hg, which provides 90% saturation in patients with a normal hemoglobin dissociation curve. Use of higher FIO_2 to elevate the arterial pO_2 to higher levels provides no benefit and increases the risk of pulmonary oxygen toxicity.

After initial stabilization, nutrition should be instituted. A major advance in supportive care of critically ill patients in recent years has been the emphasis on early adequate nutritional support. Such therapy has three major goals: to provide adequate caloric support; to provide adequate protein to maintain positive nitrogen balance wherever possible or to minimize proteolysis even when positive nitrogen balance cannot be achieved; and to maintain integrity of the gastrointestinal mucosa through enteral feeding. Total enteral nutrition has been shown to reduce the incidence of septic complications in trauma patients. Some but not all studies show superiority of enteral versus parenteral nutrition. It has been proposed that enteral nutrition provides substrate that helps maintain gastrointestinal mucosal villous morphology and prevents mucosal breakdown. It is further argued that mucosal breakdown plays a part in translocation of intestinal flora and endotoxin into the systemic circulation, which sustains sepsis syndrome leading to MODS. Although this hypothesis remains controversial, it seems prudent to provide as much enteral nutrition as can be tolerated, supplementing this with parenteral nutrition to fulfill caloric and protein requirements. Currently it is recommended to provide 25 to 35 kcal/kg/day (3-5 g/kg/day of glucose and 0.5-1 g/kg/day of fat, and 1.5 to 2.0 g/kg/day of protein). Some recommended assessment of caloric needs by indirect calorimetry and monitoring urinary nitrogen excretion to assess nitrogen balance.

Aggressive support in an ICU setting is usually required for days or weeks. During the period of chronic ICU supportive care, it is important to avoid iatrogenic complications, as these may be a major determinant of outcome. Some of the common preventable iatrogenic events are oxygen toxicity, barotrauma, and catheter-related sepsis. The toxic threshold for oxygen in man is unknown, but animal models indicate that use for 72 hours of an FIO_2 of 0.5 may cause the injured lung to develop fibrosis during the repair phase of injury. Thus an important aspect of care is to expeditiously and assiduously decrease the FiO_2 to the lowest level that provides a hemoglobin oxygen saturation of 87% to 90%. The routine use of bedside pulse oximetry has greatly simplified this task. PEEP is routinely employed to permit the FiO_2 to be lowered to <50%. When so doing, it is important to verify that cardiac output has not been inadvertently decreased by the preload reducing effect of positive intrathoracic pressure such that oxygen delivery is actually lower even though the pO_2 is higher. Barotrauma is common during PEEP administration, so as little PEEP should be employed as is needed to minimize the exposure to toxic oxygen concentrations. Balancing the complications of hyperoxia and PEEP requires careful titration to achieve a moderate level of both. Catheter-related sepsis is a continuous threat because of the need for ongoing vascular access for delivery of drugs and for monitoring. Strict aseptic technique should always be employed. Lines placed during emergency conditions should be replaced promptly. Lines should be changed every 72 hours, during febrile episodes, or if signs of inflammation are visible at the entry site. Every effort should be made to discontinue indwelling vascular catheters as soon as they are no longer needed.

Superinfection is a common cause of mortality in ARDS and is the usual factor associated with the development of MODS. The importance of continuous diagnostic vigilance in the evaluation of possible primary and secondary infections has already been emphasized. Pulmonary infections are the most common and least treatable secondary infections. Endotracheal intubation predisposes patients to such infections because mucociliary clearance is impaired. Weaning and extubation should be accomplished as expeditiously as possible to minimize the risk of nosocomial pneumonia as a sustaining factor for MODS.

PROPOSED FUTURE THERAPY: IMMUNOTHERAPY AND CYTOKINE-SPECIFIC AGENTS

Presently there is no specific pharmacologic therapy for MODS. Corticosteroids were used commonly in the past but have been shown in controlled trials not to be of value. The emphasis on cytokines as specific signalling molecules in the systemic inflammatory response, and on molecular technologies for cloning these cytokines and their receptors, has generated enthusiasm for potential future therapies aimed at interrupting the LPS-cytokine-cell signalling cascade. Clinical trials have been reported that test the efficacy of monoclonal antibodies against LPS, but to date the results are inconsistent. Trials are underway testing three classes of agents directed toward cytokines: cytokine-specific antibodies, soluble inhibitors of the cytokines, and receptor antagonists. The inhibitors are usually soluble molecules that resemble the cell surface receptors; they bind the cytokine so it cannot interact with receptors on cells. The receptor antagonists are usually analogs of the cytokine; they bind to the specific cytokine cell surface receptors of target cells but do not signal the functional response. Molecular cloning has made possible the identification, cloning, and recombinant synthesis of the cytokines and the inhibitors and receptor antagonists, but their clinical efficacy remains to be demonstrated.

REFERENCES

Asbaugh DG et al: Respiratory distress in adults. Lancet 2:319, 1967.

Bone RC et al: Definitions for sepsis and organ failure and guidelines for the use of innovative therapies in sepsis. Chest 101:1644, 1992.

Christman JW: Potential treatment of sepsis syndrome with cytokine-specific agents. Chest 102:613, 1992.

Christman JW and Bernard GR: Cytokines and sepsis: what are the therapeutic implications? J Crit Care 6:172, 1991.

Heard SO and Fink MP: Multiple organ failure syndrome. J Int Care Med, vol 6, December 1991.

Heyman SJ and Rinaldo JE: Multiple system organ failure in the adult respiratory distress syndrome. J Int Care Med 4:192, 1989.

Matuschak GM and Rinaldo JE: Organ interactions in the adult respiratory distress syndrome during sepsis: role of the liver in host defense. Chest 94:400, 1988.

Rinaldo JE and Christman JW: Mechanisms and mediators of the adult respiratory distress syndrome. Clin Chest Med 11:621, 1990.

Rinaldo JE and Rogers RM: Adult respiratory distress syndrome: changing concepts of lung injury and repair. N Engl J Med 306:900, 1982.

CHAPTER

202 Pulmonary Edema

Gordon R. Bernard
Kenneth L. Brigham

Heart failure remains the most common cause of pulmonary edema, that is, excess fluid in the lungs. Edema secondary to lung microvascular injury without heart failure (noncardiogenic edema or primary pulmonary edema) has become a more prominent clinical problem in the past 20 years, probably because of increased sensitivity to the diagnosis and improved emergency care with longer survival of patients at risk for lung injury. In its most severe form, noncardiogenic pulmonary edema is generally referred to as the *acute respiratory distress syndrome* (ARDS).

The functional consequences of pulmonary edema are partly caused by the physical presence of excess fluid in the lungs, but, especially in ARDS, other abnormalities of airway and vascular function contribute to the failure of gas exchange. Bronchoconstriction and pulmonary vasoconstriction are both important functional abnormalities that may not be direct results of the edema. In fact, in some forms of pulmonary edema, the amount of water in the lungs may not be the critical issue.

Pulmonary edema caused by heart failure is pathogenetically different from that caused by lung injury, but there are many similarities in diagnosis and treatment (Chapter 10). Understanding the clinical problem requires understanding the pathophysiology such that an otherwise bewildering list of etiologies can be comprehended by lumping pathophysiologically similar clinical problems together.

DEFINITION

Strictly defined, *pulmonary edema* is excess fluid in the lungs outside of the circulation. Increased intravascular volume (congestion) is commonly present, especially when edema is caused by heart failure, but congestion and edema are at least different phases of the process.

In the lungs extravascular fluid may accumulate in two major compartments. The interstitial compartment includes the thin interstitium of the alveoli but also the potential spaces around larger airways and blood vessels. This interstitial compartment is the initial site of fluid accumulation, resulting in cuffs of fluid around vessels and airways, which cause increased prominence of the bronchovascular shadows on chest radiographs (interstitial edema). Edema fluid may accumulate in this compartment without flooding of alveoli or significant interference with gas exchange at rest, but these cuffs of fluid may affect the lung volume at which small airways collapse and may also affect the distribution of blood flow in the lungs.

Airspaces in the lungs are an enormous potential space for fluid accumulation. Alveolar flooding usually occurs only after the interstitial compartment is filled and, when it occurs, results in significant deterioration of ventilation and oxygenation. In some forms of edema, the epithelial barrier lining alveoli appears to be injured. Normally, this epithelial layer is very tight and prevents movement of fluid into airspaces. When this barrier is breached, filling of alveoli can occur without filling of the interstitial compartment since fluid filtered from capillaries could enter directly into alveoli. Although this sequence is likely under some conditions, it has not been proved to actually occur.

A pathophysiologic classification of pulmonary edemas by etiology

I. Alterations in Starling forces
- A. Increased hydrostatic pressure (heart failure, mitral stenosis, ?neurogenic pulmonary edema)
- B. Decreased plasma oncotic pressure (malnutrition, hepatic failure, massive crystalloid infusion)

II. Altered pulmonary microvascular membrane permeability
- A. Shock (septic, ?hemorrhagic, ?neurogenic, ?cardiogenic)
- B. Infections (viral, fungal, tuberculosis, rickettsial)
- C. Multiple trauma (fat embolism, head trauma)
- D. Inhalation injury
  1. Gastric aspiration
  2. Near-drowning
  3. Hydrocarbons
  4. Irritant and poisonous gases (nitrogen dioxide, ammonia, phosgene, chlorine, cadmium, ozone), smoke
  5. Oxygen toxicity
  6. Hypersensitivity pneumonitis
- E. Drug-related (heroin, aspirin, paraquat)
- F. Hematologic disorders (disseminated intravascular coagulation, transfusion, cardiopulmonary bypass, pulmonary embolism)
- G. Metabolic disorder (pancreatitis, ketoacidosis)
- H. Immunologic (systemic lupus erythematosus, Wegener's granulomatosis, Goodpasture's syndrome)

III. Miscellaneous and poorly understood conditions
- A. Uremia
- B. Eclampsia
- C. Radiation pneumonitis
- D. High-altitude pulmonary edema
- E. Reexpansion of unilateral collapsed lung
- F. Idiopathic

PATHOPHYSIOLOGIC CLASSIFICATION OF PULMONARY EDEMAS

The outline in the box on the right is an attempt to place many of the causes of pulmonary edema into pathophysiologically similar groups (see Chapter 10). As a practical matter, understanding the etiologies responsible for the edema is not terribly useful in that treatment is dictated more by the pathophysiology than by the etiology.

Alterations in Starling forces

The physical forces determining the rate of fluid filtration across capillaries are usually called *Starling forces*. The four Starling forces are hydrostatic pressure inside and outside exchange vessels (capillary pressure and interstitial pressure, respectively) and the oncotic (protein osmotic) pressure inside and outside exchange vessels. The sum of these forces adjusted by the filtration coefficient ("leakiness" of the capillary membranes) determines the rate of fluid filtration into the pulmonary interstitium.

Any abnormality that interferes with blood flow distal to the lung capillaries can result in increased capillary pressure. The most common such abnormality is failure of the left ventricle. Left heart failure results in elevated left ventricular diastolic pressure, elevated left atrial pressure, and thus elevated pressure in pulmonary veins and capillaries.

Abnormalities proximal to the left ventricle, which may increase pulmonary downstream pressures, include obstruction to flow at the mitral valve (mitral stenosis) and occlusion of pulmonary veins. It is also possible that diffuse constriction of pulmonary veins can occur to a degree sufficient to elevate pulmonary capillary pressure enough to cause edema. This mechanism may be operative in pulmonary edema occurring with injury to the central nervous system (neurogenic pulmonary edema) where endogenous release of large amounts of catecholamines may cause dramatic pulmonary vasoconstriction as well as pulmonary edema occurring with sepsis syndrome.

It is clear that decreases in plasma oncotic pressure resulting from hypoproteinemia can predispose to pulmonary edema (see box above). Whether it is possible for edema to result from hypoproteinemia in the absence of elevated capillary pressure in human disease is not clear because elevated pulmonary vascular pressures are commonly present also in these situations.

Increased microvascular permeability

When capillary endothelium is injured, permeability is increased and excess fluid filters into the interstitium, resulting in edema without any derangement in the Starling forces.

As indicated in the box (p. 1650), increased permeability pulmonary edema occurs in a large and diverse group of clinical disorders. How microvascular injury occurs is not completely clear for any of these disorders, but some evidence shows that a common pathogenetic sequence is shared by many of them. In practice, the diagnosis usually depends on demonstration of edema by chest radiograph with a normal pulmonary arterial wedge pressure (PAWP) (see below). Increased permeability also results in edema fluid with higher protein concentration than in cardiogenic edema. Measurements of protein concentration in edema fluid suctioned have been used to distinguish between high-pressure and high-permeability edema.

Gram-negative sepsis and aspiration are the most common causes of increased permeability edema (ARDS), accounting for greater than half of the cases. Experimental work has clearly implicated prostanoids as mediators of some of the abnormalities in lung function. Marked alterations in lung mechanics and pulmonary hypertension after gram-negative endotoxemia appear to be mediated by increased endogenous production of cyclo-oxygenase products of arachidonic acid, and, at least experimentally, these changes are inhibited by nonsteroidal anti-inflammatory agents.

Mixed forms of pulmonary edema

Although the diagnosis of noncardiogenic pulmonary edema usually requires demonstration of normal left heart pressures, there is no a priori reason why increased permeability cannot occur in the presence of heart failure. In the absence of some specific measurement of pulmonary vascular permeability, diagnosis of this abnormality in the presence of increased left heart pressures is difficult. Several investigational techniques for measuring capillary endothelial or airway epithelial permeability are available that are potentially useful in critically ill humans, but none of these techniques is available for routine clinical use. Until such methods are available, the diagnosis of mixed forms of edema rests on the history and clinical course (see below).

DIAGNOSIS

The presence of pulmonary edema is suggested when a patient acutely develops cough, dyspnea, anxiety, pallor, and cyanosis. The physical examination and clinical setting are important in differentiating the many possible etiologies. Cardiac edema is usually associated with valvular or myocardial heart disease and may be heralded by such physical signs as drenching sweat, nausea, distended neck veins, hepatojugular reflux, tachycardia, a third heart sound (S_3) gallop, and often the murmur of mitral regurgitation. The pulmonary examination reveals diffuse rales usually more pronounced in the dependent portions of the lung. The extremities may be cold, clammy, and sometimes cyanotic (low cardiac output state).

The patient with ARDS, on the other hand, does not typically display signs of heart failure and may have a negative chest examination or only very fine rales and no orthopnea. The patient, however, is anxious, dyspneic, and cyanotic (but not cold) and usually has evidence of an underlying entity associated with ARDS. Cardiac output is usually normal or increased.

Given a typical clinical setting and a preponderance of differentiating clinical signs, distinguishing cardiac from noncardiac pulmonary edema can be relatively simple. However, the two entities often overlap sufficiently to make diagnosis difficult, and the two processes can occur simultaneously in the same patient. Since the diagnosis is not clear in most cases, additional data are required for optimal patient management.

Data supporting a diagnosis of cardiac edema include electrocardiographic evidence of myocardial ischemia or infarction, elevated cardiac enzymes, relatively small calculated pulmonary shunt, and an aspirated bronchial fluid protein concentration less than 50% of plasma protein concentration. Data supporting a diagnosis of ARDS include a very large pulmonary shunt and edema fluid protein concentration greater than 70% of plasma protein concentration. Finally, a critical measurement for differentiating cardiac from noncardiac edema is the PAWP. A high PAWP (more than 18 mm Hg) indicates heart failure or volume overload as the etiology of the edema until proved otherwise. A PAWP less than 18 mm Hg in the face of progressive pulmonary edema suggests ARDS. There are pitfalls in this logic because during left ventricular failure, the PAWP can be reduced rapidly with nitrates, diuretics, digoxin, and oxygen such that by the time the PAWP can be measured, it may have returned to the normal range. Usually if this is the case, the pulmonary edema and hypoxemia rapidly subside. In ARDS, the edema generally persists even up to several weeks.

Thus, any evidence of pulmonary edema (usually by chest radiograph) accompanied by an elevated PAWP is consistent with cardiogenic pulmonary edema. With ARDS, several other criteria must be met. There must be evidence of pulmonary edema by chest radiograph, and typically the pattern is of diffuse interstitial and alveolar infiltrates. However, the characteristics of the x-ray pattern may be diverse, as in the case of viral pneumonia (diffuse pattern), lung contusion (patchy), and unilateral pulmonary edema. There is no uniformly accepted description of what the chest radiograph should look like in ARDS.

Abnormal oxygenation is the hallmark of ARDS, but again there is no well-accepted level of hypoxemia required to make the diagnosis, and any attempt to establish such a level would certainly be arbitrary. For the purpose of defining populations for ARDS research, some of the criteria used include (1) PaO_2 less than 70 on fraction of inspired oxygen (FIO_2) of 0.40, (2) arterial/alveolar oxygen ratio of less than 0.3, (3) PaO_2 less than 60 mm Hg with FIO_2 of 0.60, and many others. Regardless of the oxygenation criteria, the patient populations defined are remarkably similar clinically.

Finally, the last criterion considered useful in the diagnosis of ARDS is lung compliance. In the acute care setting, static compliance is usually measured by dividing tidal volume (ml) by plateau airway pressure (obtained by occluding the exhalation port of the ventilator after delivery of a tidal breath) minus whatever level of positive and expiatory pressure may be present at the time. This is stated as *total thoracic compliance,* and values less than 50 ml per cm H_2O are common in ARDS.

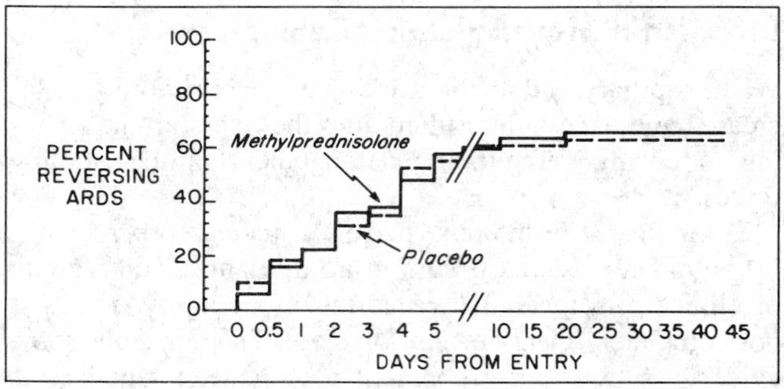

Fig. 202-1. Trends in arterial blood gas reversal in ARDS patients randomized to receive either methylprednisolone (30 mg/kg × four doses 6 hours apart) (N = 50) (- - - - -) or placebo (N = 49) (— —). No difference occurred in the mortality rate by treatment group, p more than 0.05. (Reprinted with permission from Bernard GR et al: High-dose corticosteroids in patients with the adult respiratory distress syndrome. N Engl J Med 317:1565, 1987.)

CLINICAL PRESENTATION

The box on p.1650 lists many, although by no means all, of the clinical settings in which pulmonary edema occurs. Table 202-1 lists some of the risk factors along with the percentage of patients at risk who develop ARDS. Patients with sepsis have the highest risk of developing ARDS of all groups studied (38%). In addition, in most hospitals, sepsis is one of the most common risk factors encountered.

Once the primary insult occurs there is a latent period before ARDS develops during which lung function may be normal. This time period can vary from 0 to more than 72 hours, but more than 80% of the cases manifest in the first 24 hours. It is important to recognize that a latent period occurs so that precautions such as intensive care observation can be instituted. Also, development of the syndrome remote from the primary insult can be confusing and lead to inappropriate treatment. Finally, if and when specific therapy for ARDS is available, the latent period may be the best time to intervene.

MANAGEMENT

The management of cardiac pulmonary edema is essentially the management of heart failure, a subject discussed elsewhere in this text (Chapter 10). Cardiac pulmonary edema can cause severe respiratory embarrassment requiring mechanical ventilation; in such cases, the management is similar to that for noncardiac pulmonary edema. Therefore, the discussion here concentrates on the therapy of noncardiac edema.

Oxygen is usually the first form of therapy offered the patient with pulmonary edema. Oxygen therapy should be initiated with the highest percentages of oxygen practical (such as can be delivered with a nonrebreathing 100% oxygen mask) in patients who are severely ill. Once arterial blood gases have been obtained, appropriate adjustments can then be made. Oxygen percentages of 100% are generally considered safe if used for less than 24 hours and it is probably safer to err on the side of too much oxygen briefly than to risk an extended period of severe hypoxemia. If oxygen therapy is essential to the patient's survival, endotracheal intubation should be considered. An endotracheal tube permits precise, consistent oxygen delivery, easy suctioning of airway secretions when necessary, and maintenance of a reliable airway for the institution of mechanical ventilation, if, and more likely, when the need arises. Fig. 202-1 depicts the rate of improvement in arterial blood gases in a large group of ARDS patients randomized to receive corticosteroids early in their illness.

Mechanical ventilation is usually required in the management of severe pulmonary edema. The ventilator is often used to control oxygen delivery and to maintain positive end-expiratory pressure (PEEP), but these functions can be performed by other means. The most important function of the ventilator is to provide adequate ventilation without requiring large energy expenditure by the patient. Work of breathing in patients with severe edema is increased for

Table 202-1. Clinical predictors of ARDS

	Total number of patients at risk	Number of patients developing ARDS	(%)
Sepsis syndrome	13	5	38
Aspiration of gastric contents	23	7	30
Pulmonary contusion	29	5	17
Multiple emergency transfusions	17	4	24
All patients at risk (includes other etiologic categories besides those listed above)	88	29	33

Adapted from Pepe P et al: Clinical predictors of the adult respiratory distress syndrome. Am J Surg 144:124, 1982.

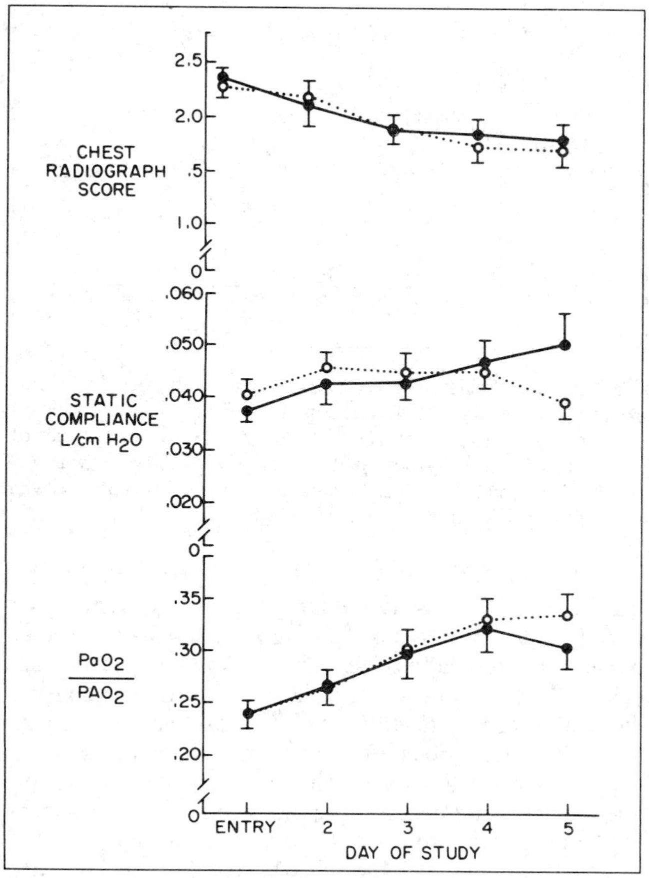

Fig. 202-2. Chest radiograph score (0 denotes normal, 1 mild, 2 moderate, 3 severe pulmonary edema), total thoracic static compliance, and arterial to alveolar PaO_2 ratio (PaO_2/PAO_2) in 99 patients randomized to receive either methylprednisolone 30 mg per kilogram q6h for 24 hours (- - - - -) (N = 50) or placebo (— —) (N = 49). There were no significant differences according to treatment group either at time of entry or at any point in the 5 days of close follow-up, p more than 0.05. (Reprinted with permission from Bernard GR et al: High-dose corticosteroids in patients with the adult respiratory distress syndrome. N Engl J Med 317:1565, 1987.)

three reasons. First, the lungs are stiff (decreased compliance) because of accumulated edema fluid and later in the course, fibrosis (Fig. 202-2). Second, the airways may be obstructed by edema fluid, mucus, debris, or bronchospasm. Third, severe mismatch of ventilation and perfusion produces large increases in physiologic dead space, which may require very large increases in minute ventilation to maintain alveolar ventilation. Mechanical ventilation is generally indicated when respiratory rates exceed 35 to 40 breaths per minute in a resting patient because this level of respiration exhausts ventilatory reserve and even slight complications (such as a lobar mucous plug or mild aspiration of secretions) may result in respiratory arrest.

Once intubated and mechanically ventilated, a patient with ARDS may survive with severely abnormal gas exchange for weeks, though significant improvement may occur in just a few days. Methods of assessing the course of such patients include chest radiographs, arterial blood gases, and hemodynamic measurements. To follow the efficiency of gas exchange, measurement of a derived variable that takes into account both alveolar oxygen tension (PAO_2, calculated from the alveolar gas equation) and arterial oxygen tension (PaO_2) is useful. The gold standard for the assessment of the efficiency of oxygenation is the calculation of pulmonary shunt. The shunt calculation requires knowledge of the FIO_2, PaO_2, mixed venous oxygen tension ($P\bar{v}O_2$) and saturation ($S\bar{v}O_2$), arterial PaO_2 and saturation (SaO_2), and $PaCO_2$. Because these values are not always readily obtainable, several substitutes for this determination have been derived. Examples include PaO_2/PAO_2 ratio, PaO_2/FIO_2 ratio, A-aDO_2 (alveolar to arterial oxygen difference), and others. Each has its limitations, but in terms of ease of calculation, the PaO_2/FIO_2 ratio is simplest. Fig. 202-2 shows the trends in oxygenation, chest radiograph score, and static lung compliance in a large group of patients with ARDS.

Although brief periods of exposure (less than 24 hours) to high oxygen concentrations (100%) are relatively safe, longer periods may not be. Therefore, when inspired oxygen concentrations must exceed 50% (a level generally accepted as safe for long periods), efforts must be made to allow for a lower FIO_2. Positive end-expiratory pressure is often used for this purpose after the institution of mechanical ventilation and is discussed below. Attention must also be paid to maintaining a clear airway by frequent suctioning and to minimizing oxygen demand whenever possible.

Even in the normal state, stress or exercise results in reduced mixed venous hemoglobin saturation. But, since normal individuals have very little shunt, the low mixed venous oxygen levels produced through increased oxygen demand have very little effect on arterial oxygen levels. In the case of patients with severe pulmonary edema, shunt can increase to extremely high levels (levels of 25% to 35% are common). This amount of shunt allows a significant volume of desaturated mixed venous blood to enter the arterial circulation, thus lowering the PaO_2 in systemic arterial blood. Treatable causes of increased oxygen demand include thyrotoxicosis, fever, and agitation; the latter two are very common in patients with ARDS. Fever should be treated with antipyretics rather than a cooling blanket because the shivering induced by cooling may increase oxygen demand. Agitation should be treated with narcotics or benzodiazepines, adding a paralyzing agent such as pancuronium only if necessary. If the latter is used, the sedating agents must also be maintained and possibly increased to offset the adverse psychological effects of paralysis.

Once oxygen consumption is minimized, attention should be given to maximizing oxygen delivery. The box on p.1654 lists medically attainable means of optimizing oxygen transport.

Corticosteroids

Based on animal studies and the inflammatory nature of ARDS seen in lung biopsy specimens, there has been a long-held belief that corticosteroids in high doses might be useful in this disorder. However, recent studies have shown

Methods for optimizing oxygen transport

Improve cardiac output
Maintain normal hemoglobin
Rightward shift of oxygen-hemoglobin curve
- Prevent hypothermia
- Increased 2,3-diphosphoglycerate
- Avoid alkalosis
- Avoid low PCO_2

Reduce oxygen consumption

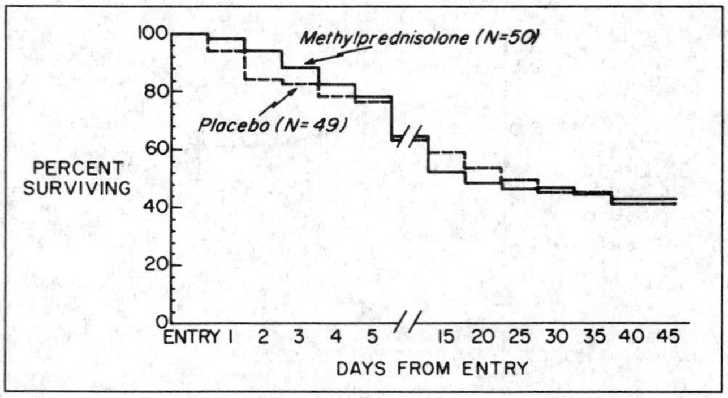

Fig. 202-3. Cumulative survival of patients with ARDS randomized to receive either methylprednisolone (30 mg/kg × four doses 6 hours apart) or placebo. No difference occurred in the rate of reversal by treatment group, p more than 0.05. (Reprinted with permission from Bernard GR et al: High-dose corticosteroids in patients with the adult respiratory distress syndrome. N Engl J Med 317:1565, 1987.)

that steroids neither prevent septic patients from developing ARDS nor affect the course of gas exchange, chest radiograph, and lung compliance abnormalities in patients with established ARDS (see Figs. 201-1 and 202-2). Finally, corticosteroids do not seem to affect overall mortality in patients with established ARDS even when treated early (Fig. 202-3).

Positive end-expiratory pressure (PEEP)

Venous admixture or shunt can be reduced dramatically with PEEP in some but not all patients with pulmonary edema. Adverse effects of PEEP include hypotension, decreased cardiac output, and the risk of barotrauma. Whether PEEP is of benefit depends on its effect on PaO_2 and cardiac output. For example, if PEEP increases PaO_2 from 60 to 80 mm Hg but reduces cardiac output by 30%, then oxygen delivery has been severely reduced. In practice one should obtain measurements of both PaO_2 and cardiac output before and after each PEEP level change so that oxygen delivery can be calculated. As a general rule, PEEP should be increased in a stepwise fashion in increments of 3 to 5 cm H_2O until the desired goal of reducing the FiO_2 into the nontoxic range is reached without significant reduction in cardiac output. There are little data to suggest that PEEP levels higher than the 20 to 25 cm H_2O range are more effective than levels less than 20 cm H_2O.

Fluid management

In both cardiac and noncardiac pulmonary edema, a balance must be sought between the positive effect of relatively high PAWPs on cardiac output and the negative effect on lung fluid balance. It is generally agreed that left ventricular filling pressure cannot be reliably estimated by physical examination or by direct measurement of central venous pressure. For these reasons, the flow-directed pulmonary artery catheter, which has been shown to give reliable estimates of left ventricular filling pressure, has become commonplace in the management of pulmonary edema. Measurement of PAWP and serum protein allows for the estimation of intravascular Starling forces, thus providing objective evidence of effects of therapy without having to wait for the more slowly evolving blood gas and chest radiograph changes (see Fig. 202-2). It is generally accepted that PAWP should be in the range of 15 to 18 mm Hg or slightly higher in patients with normal pulmonary vascular permeability and failing left ventricles to maximize cardiac output. It is prudent to keep patients with noncardiogenic pulmonary edema relatively volume restricted as long as there is no deleterious effect on cardiac output and hence oxygen delivery. Measurements of cardiac output and oxygen delivery are necessary to assess effects of fluid therapy in all patients with severe pulmonary edema.

If intravascular volume must be reduced, the primary therapy should be volume restriction and diuretics. Central vasodilators such as nitroglycerin and nitroprusside may decrease pulmonary vascular pressures more rapidly than volume reduction, but these drugs can increase pulmonary shunt by paralyzing hypoxic vasoconstriction, the autoregulatory process that maintains ventilation-perfusion matching.

For patients requiring intravenous fluids, controversy remains over the relative benefits of crystalloid versus colloid solutions. In cardiac pulmonary edema, infusions of albumin (especially if the serum albumin is low) can have a pronounced effect in mobilizing interstitial fluid from the lungs and from the rest of the body. This beneficial effect is most useful when left ventricular filling pressures are low, an uncommon circumstance in cardiac pulmonary edema. However, when pulmonary vascular permeability is increased, albumin readily crosses the microvascular barrier and therefore fails its intended purpose of increasing the oncotic gradient in favor of interstitial fluid resorption. Some studies suggest that crystalloid solutions may be superior to colloid solutions in the management of noncardiac pulmonary edema, but this area of management remains controversial.

Substantial controversy continues with regard to the value of volume restriction/diuresis in ARDS. Although numerous references in the medical literature suggest a benefit to volume reduction in ARDS, well-designed studies are lacking. The correct balance between risk of increasing lung water and decreasing oxygen balance has not been struck.

A proper clinical trial examining this important clinical question is needed.

REFERENCES

Ashbaugh DG et al: Acute respiratory distress in adults. Lancet 2:319, 1967.

Ashbaugh DG et al: Continuous positive-pressure breathing (CPPB) in adult respiratory distress syndrome. J Thorac Cardiovasc Surg 57:31, 1969.

Bernard GR et al: High-dose corticosteroids in patients with the adult respiratory distress syndrome. N Engl J Med 317:1565, 1987.

Bone RC et al: A controlled clinical trial of high-dose methylprednisolone in the treatment of severe sepsis and septic shock. N Engl J Med 317:653, 1987.

Brigham K, editor: Pulmonary edema. Semin Respir Med 4:267, 1983.

Pepe P et al: Clinical predictors of the adult respiratory distress syndrome. Am J Surg 144:124, 1982.

Rinaldo JE and Rogers RM: Adult respiratory distress syndrome: changing concepts of lung injury and repair. N Engl J Med 306:900, 1982.

Staub N: Pulmonary edema. Physiol Rev 54:678, 1974.

Sznajder JI and Wood LDH: Beneficial effects of reducing pulmonary edema in patients with acute hypoxic respiratory failure. Chest 100:890, 1991.

CHAPTER

203 Respiratory Therapy and Monitoring

David H. Ingbar
Theodore W. Marcy

Respiratory therapy is a useful adjunct in treating many pulmonary disorders. The spectrum of respiratory care is broad, encompassing normobaric and hyperbaric oxygen therapy, postural drainage, chest percussion, delivery of medications by nebulization or aerosols, ventilator care, and noninvasive respiratory monitoring. Unfortunately, respiratory therapy is quite labor-intensive and therefore costly. In only a small number of situations have respiratory treatments been scientifically proven to be of benefit, although few have been rigorously tested. Consequently the practitioner must be aware of the indications and contraindications for each modality of treatment and must work closely with the therapist to continually reevaluate the patient's response to therapy.

RESPIRATORY CARE TREATMENT MODALITIES

Oxygen therapy

Many hospitalized patients are administered supplemental oxygen either as treatment for documented hypoxemia (measured arterial oxygen pressure (PaO_2) < 60 mm Hg or oxygen saturation SaO_2 < 92%), or prophylactically to prevent hypoxemia in patients who have symptoms of myocardial ischemia or who are undergoing certain procedures (e.g., bronchoscopy). Prior to initiating oxygen therapy, an arterial blood gas (ABG) sample should be obtained to determine the baseline values of $PaCO_2$ and PaO_2 unless the patient is in severe respiratory distress. Hypoxemia is regarded as life-threatening when the PaO_2 is below 55 mm Hg or the SaO_2 is below 85%, because in this range the steep hemoglobin-oxygen dissociation curve results in a large decrease in hemoglobin saturation with any further small decrement of PaO_2.

Oxygen delivery devices. The choice of an oxygen delivery device for a specific patient depends, in part, on how high and how constant an inspired fraction of oxygen (FIO_2) is necessary. In the hospital, the maximal FIO_2 that can be delivered to the trachea is limited by the maximal flow rate from the wall outlet (usually 15-20 liters per minute). As the patient's inspiratory flow rate increases above that from the oxygen delivery device, a relatively larger fraction of the inspired gas consists of entrained room air. During respiratory distress or tachypnea, the inspiratory flow rate increases markedly from the normal resting value of 20 liters per minute, often exceeding the rate of oxygen supply and decreasing the delivered FIO_2.

Nasal prongs. Nasal prongs are used to deliver 0.5 to 6 liters of oxygen per minute. Higher flow rates are not used because they dry the nasal mucosa and may lead to epistaxis. Even the patient who appears to be breathing through the mouth entrains oxygen through the nasopharynx. The FIO_2 varies with the patient's inspiratory flow rate, but usually is between 0.22 and 0.40. This delivery method is useful for patients with hypoxemia caused by ventilation-perfusion mismatching, such as those with COPD and asthma, since their hypoxemia is responsive to small increases in FIO_2. In COPD patients with carbon dioxide retention, supplemental oxygen may lead to worsening respiratory acidosis because it either suppresses hypoxic respiratory drive or alters the dead-space-to-tidal-volume ratio. In these patients it is important to limit the increase in FIO_2 to the minimum that achieves an adequate SaO_2. Some authorities strongly advocate that nasal prongs should not be used in patients with CO_2 retention because the FIO_2 achieved varies with the patient's inspiratory flow rate. Other authorities are skeptical that these fluctuations of FIO_2 are clinically important and believe that this relative disadvantage may be outweighed by many patients' reluctance to wear face masks continuously.

Nasal prongs usually are the delivery device of choice for long-term oxygen therapy. Several oxygen-conserving devices are available that provide either a reservoir of oxygen or inflow only during inspiration. An alternative method of long-term oxygen delivery is via a transtracheal oxygen catheter. This silastic catheter is placed through the cricothyroid membrane directly into the trachea. It can be used to deliver higher FIO_2 levels and greater flow rates. Thus it may be beneficial for selected patients with hypoxemia that is resistant to therapy with 2-3 liters per minute of oxygen by nasal cannulae. In addition, some patients prefer this method since it avoids the stigma of wearing easily visible nasal prongs.

Aerosol face masks. Masks that cover the nose and mouth deliver a humidified mixture of oxygen and room air with a wide range of possible FiO_2s. Since the mask has side air holes and is not tightly fitted, a variable amount of room air is inhaled around or through the mask. As the set FiO_2 is increased, the flow rate provided from the mixing jet nebulizer falls since the mixed gas is more oxygen-rich. The patient may then need to entrain more room air to meet their inspiratory flow demand. Consequently, a setting of "100% oxygen" usually only achieves a tracheal FiO_2 of 50%-70% oxygen.

A very high FiO_2 sometimes is required for patients with hypoxemia from shunt physiology, as in multilobar pneumonia, pulmonary edema, or severe atelectasis. Three strategies have been used to increase the maximum FiO_2 delivered without intubating the patient. First, the mask's side holes can be covered with flaps that close the holes during inspiration but permit exhalation. Second, a bag can be attached to the mask to provide a reservoir of oxygen-rich gas. A one-way valve makes this bag fill with pure oxygen while the patient exhales. When the patient inhales at a rate greater than the rate at which gas is delivered into the mask, this valve opens and the oxygen from the reservoir bag is inhaled instead of entraining room air. This mask is called a nonrebreather reservoir mask because the patient's exhaled gas does not enter the reservoir bag. The combination of these two methods achieves FiO_2s in the range of 0.7-0.9, depending on how well the mask fits the patient. A less useful variant is the partial rebreather mask in which the bag is partially filled by the first portion of the exhaled gas. This gas is oxygen-rich because it comes from the patient's dead space. Third, the oxygen from two wall outlets can be yoked together into one mask to provide a total flow of 30 liters per minute of pure oxygen. This system provides an FiO_2 in the trachea of up to 80%-90%.

In the air-entrainment or "Venturi" face mask, a jet of oxygen is directed through an orifice engineered to entrain a fixed proportion of room air. By changing the orifice size, this mask can deliver a high flow of gas with a fairly precise FiO_2 of 24%, 28%, 32%, 36%, or 40% depending on the orifice selected. It often is used instead of nasal prongs for COPD patients with CO_2 retention to provide a controlled amount of FiO_2. Its disadvantages are that the inspired gas is not completely humidified and it must fit the face snugly.

Prescription of oxygen. Oxygen may be prescribed for continuous use, for use during exertion, or for nocturnal use, depending upon when the patient is hypoxemic. It never should be given to patients for prophylactic or as-needed use at home. Some patients recuperating from an acute illness may be given short-term home oxygen to treat hypoxemia while their underlying disease improves. The need for long-term oxygen should be determined after the patient is at baseline and on maximal medical therapy. Medicare requirements for long-term oxygen are that patients breathing ambient air either (1) have a $PaO_2 < 55$ mm Hg or $SaO_2 < 88\%$ or (2) have a PaO_2 56-59 mm Hg *and* either cor pulmonale on electrocardiogram or an hematocrit > 55%. In patients with COPD and hypoxemia at rest despite optimal therapy, continuous oxygen (24 hr/day) is more effective than shorter daily durations of treatment at improving survival and neuropsychologic function. Oxygen should be prescribed for use during sleep or with exertion to patients with hypoxemia while asleep or with exercise, respectively, but not at rest. Nocturnal hypoxemia commonly occurs in patients with COPD, restrictive lung diseases, and asthma, even in the absence of sleep apnea. Exertional oxygen also is indicated in patients who are able to be more active when using oxygen, but this improvement should be documented by a 6-minute walk test or exercise oximetry.

Third party payors, including Medicare, have very stringent guidelines for reimbursement of long-term oxygen therapy because of its high cost. The prescribing physician must document the need for oxygen, determine the appropriate flow rate and frequency, and specify the oxygen delivery system. For Medicare reimbursement, a specific form (HCFA-484) must be completed by the physician. Documentation of continued need for home oxygen in spite of maximal medical therapy is required at frequent intervals.

Home oxygen can be supplied from liquid oxygen tanks, compressed gas tanks, or oxygen concentrators. Home care companies are reimbursed a fixed amount based on the oxygen flow rate, and therefore have a disincentive to provide the more expensive oxygen systems that may be of maximum benefit to the patient. The physician must clearly specify and insist on the delivery system that is best for the patient. Although all supply methods are costly, the tanks are more expensive and require frequent replacement. However, small portable "walking tanks" can be filled from the main tank, allowing the patient to leave home and be active. Despite the added cost, liquid oxygen systems are preferred for ambulatory patients to allow these patients to fill portable oxygen units at home from stationary reservoirs. Justification for a portable oxygen system requires that the therapeutic purpose be specified and that some benefit be documented. Concentrators are electrically driven devices that concentrate oxygen from the air, but they can provide low-flow oxygen (<2-3 Lpm) only. For patients who are primarily homebound or bedbound, an oxygen concentrator with extension tubing is adequate and generally less expensive. The nonreimbursable added cost of electricity to power these units is significant and sometimes must be considered. Small oxygen cylinders that can be used for short excursions out of the home or in case of a mechanical or electrical failure of the concentrator usually should be provided along with a concentrator.

Secretion clearance and lung expansion

Atelectasis—the loss of lung volume—impairs gas exchange, increases the work of breathing, and probably leads to a higher incidence of pneumonia. A variety of therapeutic modalities attempt to reverse atelectasis by enhancing secretion clearance and by increasing and sustaining inspiratory lung volume. In addition to coughing, simple treatments include deep breathing, mobilizing the patient, incentive spirometry, humidification, and tracheal suctioning. Increasing the tidal volume of breaths by sighs, intentional deep breathing, or incentive spirometry recruits atelectatic alveoli. Dependent regions of the lung are especially prone to atelectasis since they are partially compressed, less well ventilated, and do not spontaneously drain their secretions with gravity. Frequent changes of position distribute the tidal breaths to these previously dependent portions of the lung and assist in clearing secretions. Sitting the patient upright in a chair significantly increases both tidal volume and vital capacity relative to the supine position.

Cough. Cough is probably the most effective way to clear excess secretions from the airway. Aggressive encouragement of coughing by nursing, medical, and respiratory therapy staff is more important than most of the treatment techniques discussed below. Special cough techniques such as quadriplegic coughing or "huff coughing" may be helpful to teach some patients to improve their cough efficacy.

In the past, ultrasonic nebulization of small particles of water or saline commonly was used to induce cough because the particles stimulate tracheal irritant receptors. Verbal encouragement, however, is preferred because most patients are capable of coughing, and ultrasonic particulates may trigger bronchospasm. Many hospitals have discontinued offering this treatment because it is not very effective, is expensive, and has significant side effects. On the other hand, ultrasonic nebulization of hypertonic saline increases the diagnostic yield of sputum induction for *Pneumocytis carinii* and *M. tuberculosis*. It also may be worth an empiric trial of ultrasonic saline nebulization to induce cough in comatose patients.

Tracheal suction. Suctioning of the trachea through the nose or mouth may help patients who cannot cough effectively by both stimulating cough and removing excess secretions within reach of the catheter. Harmful side effects include (1) tracheal damage that may result in bleeding or predispose to infection, (2) hypoxemia, (3) arrhythmias resulting from autonomic reflexes, (4) apnea, and (5) contamination of the lower respiratory tract. Unless special catheters or positioning are used, the right mainstem bronchus is more frequently entered than the left. By turning the patient's head to the right and/or using a special angled suction catheter, the left mainstem bronchus can be entered more often.

Humidification. Usually the upper airway provides very efficient humidification of gases reaching the lower airway, preventing mucosal drying and inspissation of mucus. For intubated or tracheotomized patients, inspired gas must be fully saturated with molecular (nonparticulate) water. For nonintubated patients, systemic hydration is probably the best way to avoid dessication of secretions. Bronchospastic patients may benefit from using heated jet nebulizers to humidify their supplemental oxygen because of the higher water vapor pressure and content in the warm gas. Inadequately humidified air may trigger airway hyperreactivity. Nebulized saline, a suspended particulate, does not thin secretions or aid in their clearance. Nebulized water, hypotonic saline, or hypertonic saline have not been demonstrated to thin secretions, and all can precipitate bronchospasm.

Incentive spirometry. Incentive spirometers of all types permit the patient to visually judge their inspiratory effort. The patient is encouraged to inhale as rapidly as possible for as long as possible, thereby achieving a maximal inspiratory volume. This is one of the best ways to reverse or prevent atelectasis. A major advantage is that once taught properly, the motivated patient can use it with little supervision. In the motivated patient, it is as effective at preventing postoperative pulmonary complications as other more complicated and time-consuming measures. A recent adaptation is to place a one-way valve on the device that blocks expiration. This allows the patient to make several "stacked" inspiratory efforts, leading to a higher cumulative lung volume—a strategy that may be particularly useful in patients with respiratory muscle weakness.

Intermittent positive-pressure breathing (IPPB). This modality assists the patient's inspiration by having a pressure-limited ventilator deliver a rapid inflow of gas into the mouth until the preset pressure limit is reached. In contrast to volume ventilation, the volume of gas administered is not regulated. IPPB once was widely used for patients with COPD and atelectasis, especially to nebulize aerosol medications. Many controlled studies demonstrated little or no objective benefit either of IPPB alone or as a method of medication delivery. Consequently it should be used only for the cooperative patient who is too weak to inspire effectively and who has a documented increase of tidal volume during and/or after treatment. With an increased tidal volume, it can help reverse atelectasis, rest the respiratory muscles, or transiently prevent the need for intubation. Contraindications to IPPB include pneumothorax, bullous lung disease, asthma, recent esophageal or gastric surgery, cardiac dysfunction, and an uncooperative patient.

Recently, devices besides mouthpieces, such as nasal or face CPAP masks, have been used to deliver several new types of IPPB. Nasal continuous positive airway pressure (CPAP) applied through a nasal mask often is used to treat sleep apnea. Tight-fitting CPAP face masks have been connected to mechanical ventilators and have provided positive pressure ventilation for 24-48 hours to treat nonintubated patients with rapidly reversible respiratory failure. Most recently, compact pressure ventilators are available that can provide different levels of inspiratory and expiratory pressure (bilevel positive airway pressure or Bi-PAP) applied to either nasal or face masks. These Bi-PAP machines can provide nocturnal ventilation for patients with respiratory muscle fatigue or chronic respiratory failure, thereby avoiding tracheotomy. They also may obviate the need for intubation of some patients with acute respiratory failure.

Postural drainage (PD). This technique involves lying the patient down in positions that encourage passive gravity drainage of secretions from either the segmental or lobar bronchi. Frequently this is combined with chest percussion or vibration, but this is not required. Sometimes PD is applied selectively to drain secretions from a region that has pneumonia, atelectasis, or a lung abscess. At other times it is applied to all of the lung segments in sequence.

Postural drainage is reasonable to use for patients with (1) COPD and who produce more than 30 ml of sputum per day; (2) bronchiectasis; (3) cystic fibrosis; (4) pneumonia and who cannot cough or spontaneously clear their secretions, especially as a result of neuromuscular disorders or a depressed level of consciousness; (5) atelectasis not reversed by incentive spirometry and other simple measures; and (6) lung abscess. If these conditions are chronic, then these patients and their families should be taught these techniques for regular outpatient use. Prophylactic treatment of intubated patients with PD to compensate for their diminished ability to cough is sometimes done, but this has not been rigorously demonstrated to be helpful. For hospitalized patients with one or more of the above indications, PD should be given as an empiric trial and discontinued if there is no beneficial response. There is no clear benefit of PD beyond incentive spirometry, deep breathing, and coughing for most patients with COPD, pneumonia, or routine postoperative care.

Some patients do not tolerate the positions required to achieve effective PD and may become very dyspneic or hypoxemic, especially with addition of percussion or vibration. Increased intracranial pressure is another contraindication to PD.

Chest percussion and vibration. These techniques frequently are used in conjunction with PD. They can increase the velocity of tracheal mucus movement up the tracheobronchial tree. However, they also may worsen hypoxemia, especially in patients with hemodynamic instability, low cardiac output, or arrhythmias. Their clinical benefit, beyond that from PD, has not been established. Rib fractures or recent hymoptysis are additional contraindications. Rarely, patients with a bacterial lung abscess suddenly drain abscess fluid or blood during PD. If this material spills throughout the tracheobronchial tree, respiratory failure may result.

Mucolytic agents. Several agents, such as N-acetyl cysteine, disperse mucus plugs in vitro. Direct instillation of this agent through a bronchoscope onto a visible plug may disrupt it. However, N-acetyl cysteine may injure epithelial tissue, especially the cilia, and often stimulates tracheal irritant receptors, causing bronchospasm. Nebulization of these agents has not been effective in several randomized studies of patients with COPD. Consequently it should be used cautiously, if at all, in patients with asthma or COPD. If used, treatment should be limited to only a few doses and should be accompanied by bronchodilators. It often is used chronically for patients with cystic fibrosis, but the evidence supporting this practice is not strong.

Iodinated glycerol is an oral agent that increases expectoration of respiratory tract secretions and that may aid liquification of mucus in patients with chronic bronchitis. It improved symptoms of cough frequency, severity, and the ease of clearing secretions in a randomized, double-blind controlled study, although there were no improvements in objective measures of pulmonary function. The lack of improvement in pulmonary function may be related to concomitant stimulation of mucus secretion by this drug. Other expectorants, such as guaifenesin and supersaturated solutions of potassium iodide (SSKI), stimulate sputum clearance, but also increase bronchial gland mucus production and secretion. Their overall clinical efficacy, however, has not yet been defined with careful clinical studies.

Nebulized and aerosolized medications

Aerosolized medications are being utilized increasingly for therapy of asthma and other forms of obstructive airways disease. In addition, aerosolized medications are indicated for some parenchymal lung diseases. Nebulized ribavirin is used for treatment of respiratory syncytial virus, pentamidine is used as prophylaxis against *Pneumocystis* pneumonia in HIV-infected patients, and aerosolized surfactant compounds are being investigated for use in patients with the adult respiratory distress syndrome.

Delivery methods. Three different delivery systems are available: nebulizers (jets and ultrasonics); metered dose inhalers (MDI); and dry-powder inhalers (DPI). There are advantages and disadvantages to each of these methods, and the choice of the delivery system must be individualized for the specific patient and medication.

The deposition of aerosolized medications in the lung is affected by the characteristics of the particle generated, the ventilatory pattern, and the airway geometry. Aerosol particles with a mass median aerodynamic diameter (MMAD) between 2-5 μm are optimal to deliver drugs to the airways, while particles with an MMAD of between 0.8-3 μm are optimal for drug delivery to the alveoli. Particles larger than 5 μm are filtered by the upper airway. Inspiratory flow rates of approximately 0.5 L/s appear to be best for aerosols generated by MDIs and nebulizers, while higher flow rates are required for DPIs. Aerosol deposition is adversely affected by the decreased airway diameter present in patients with airflow obstruction. Endotracheal tubes also significantly decrease the delivery of aerosolized medications to the lower respiratory tract.

MDIs have the advantage of convenience, relatively high lung deposition (10%-15%), and low cost. Oropharyngeal deposition can be reduced with the use of a holding chamber or spacer device. For example, spacers limit the systemic absorption of inhaled corticosteroids and decrease the incidence of steroid-induced oral candidiasis and dysphonia. MDIs are the delivery system of choice for most outpatients. Some studies suggest that they may be as effective as nebulizers in cooperative hospitalized patients with acute airflow obstruction. The major disadvantage of MDIs is that they require the patient to coordinate actuation of the device while initiating inspiration and then to perform a 4-second to 10-second breath hold. Holding chambers and spacer devices may improve drug delivery in patients who are unable to coordinate MDI inhalation. Other limitations include the limited number of available medications, the inconvenience associated with higher dosage regimens, and the dependence on chlorofluorocarbons as propellants.

Nebulizers can deliver larger volumes and higher doses of medication than MDIs or DPIs and can be used in patients who are too ill or who otherwise are unable to effectively use an MDI. A larger number of medications are available for nebulization, and medications intended for parenchymal deposition (pentamidine and ribaviran) must be delivered by a nebulizer. However, the fractional lung deposition is low (2%-10%), requiring longer administration time, more medication, and therefore, increased cost. There is also the risk of microbial contamination of the aerosol or aerosol generator.

DPIs, such as "spinhalers," are actuated as the patient initiates inspiration, improving the ease of administration, but they require a higher inspiratory flow rate than some patients can generate. Deposition appears to be equivalent to a properly used MDI. The disadvantages of DPIs are (1) limited numbers of medications are available for use with this system, (2) heavy oropharyngeal deposition may occur, and (3) high-humidity environments may cause clumping of the particles, preventing the use of DPIs in humidified ventilator circuits.

Both MDIs and nebulizers can be used in intubated patients, but dose adjustments are probably necessary to compensate for the deposition of drug in the circuit and on the endotracheal tube.

RESPIRATORY MONITORING

Noninvasive respiratory monitoring has increased markedly in the last 5 years. New methods monitor the pattern of breathing, including respiratory rate, tidal volume, and activity and synchrony of chest wall and abdominal muscles. Most useful are noninvasive determinations of the arterial blood percentage saturation with oxygen and the end-tidal CO_2 level ($P_{et}CO_2$).

Oximetry

This technique uses the different absorption spectra of oxy- and deoxyhemoglobin to determine the percentage of heme sites occupied with oxygen. Light of several wavelengths is passed through thin tissues of the ear lobe, finger, toe, or nasal bridge to obtain this ratio. Pulse oximetry uses plethysmographic techniques to eliminate the absorption contributed by nonpulsatile blood in the tissue. This direct measurement of hemoglobin SaO_2 avoids the problems encountered in using calculated saturations from ABG results. However, special situations may result in erroneous oximetric SaO_2 measurements. Poor tissue perfusion, strenuous exertion, the presence of other pigments in the skin or blood, and pulsatile venous blood flow all may cause inaccurate readings. Abnormal hemoglobins also may affect the accuracy of the saturation measurement.

Measurements may be made continuously or at a single point in time as a substitute for an ABG. Since oximetry does not accurately distinguish PaO_2 levels above 60 torr, its utility is restricted to (1) ensuring that a patient does not have life-threatening hypoxemia, or (2) titrating the FiO_2 in a patient with a low SaO_2. It is useful for monitoring patients during anesthesia or procedures and for detecting nocturnal hypoxemia during sleep. It is not appropriate, however, as a replacement for an ABG in the initial assessment of dyspneic patients with lung or heart disease or of patients with significant metabolic derangements because it does not provide information about the pH or $PaCO_2$. Large changes in PaO_2 above 70 torr are not detected because hemoglobin is fully saturated in this range. Finally, in monitoring the patient who is difficult to wean from a ventilator or who has recently been extubated, oximetry alone is not sufficient since it will not detect CO_2 retention. Nonetheless, oximetry is extremely useful and decreases the need for arterial blood gas measurements, as long as it is used appropriately.

Capnography or end-tidal CO_2 measurement

Methods to continuously measure the exhaled CO_2 pressure using either mass spectrometry or absorption of infrared light are becoming widespread, especially for intubated patients. The $P_{et}CO_2$ closely approximates the arterial PCO_2 if (1) there is complete equilibration of CO_2 across the alveolar capillary unit; (2) there is little physiologic right-to-left shunt; (3) there is uniform mixing of the exhaled gas; and (4) alveolar dead space is not significantly increased. A tracing of the exhaled wave form of PCO_2 over time should have a late expiratory plateau, indicating complete mixing. In the presence of severe lung disease or sepsis, there may be incomplete equilibration, resulting in an arterial to end-tidal CO_2 gradient. The CO_2 wave form may be altered in characteristic ways in different types of lung disease that suggest, for example, the presence of physiologic dead space caused by pulmonary embolism. Capnography is a useful adjunct to oximetry in monitoring intubated patients during ventilator changes, weaning, procedures, or anesthesia. Better methods for obtaining reliable measurements of $P_{et}CO_2$ in nonintubated patients will be very useful in caring for patients with COPD or neuromuscular disorders.

Other monitoring techniques

The evaluation of respiratory muscle strength and endurance is important in assessing the risk of respiratory failure in patients with neuromuscular disease such as the Guillain-Barré syndrome, polymyositis, and muscular dystrophy. Maximal inspiratory airway pressure (MIP) and vital capacity (VC) are global measures of respiratory muscle strength that can be repeatedly measured at the bedside of these patients. Significant reductions in VC (< 600 ml) and MIP (<20 cm H_2O) indicate severe impairment of respiratory muscle function and may be more sensitive indicators of the need for intubation than ABGs in these patients. However, these measurements require standardized techniques and full patient cooperation.

Abnormal respiratory patterns may also predict impending respiratory failure. Respiratory inductive plethysmography (Respitrace) provides a noninvasive method of continuously monitoring the respiratory pattern in spontaneously breathing patients. The simultaneous recording of movements of both the rib cage and abdominal compartments can detect abnormal patterns such as paradoxic motion (abdomen and rib cage moving in opposite directions) or asynchrony (time lag between motion of the rib cage and the abdomen). Indices that quantitate the degree of abnormal breathing may be useful in monitoring patients with respiratory impairment, but the equipment is expensive, and the bands placed around the rib cage and abdomen are easily dislodged.

REFERENCES

Aerosol Consensus Statement. Chest 100:1106, 1991.

Burton GG, Hodgkin JE, and Ward JJ, editors: Respiratory care: a guide to clinical practice, ed 3. Philadelphia, 1991, Lippincott.

Eid N et al: Chest physiotherapy in review. Respir Care 36:270, 1991.

Marini JJ, Pierson DJ, and Hudson LD: Acute lobar atelectasis: a prospective comparison of fiberoptic bronchoscopy and respiratory therapy. Amer Rev Respir Dis 119:971, 1979.

O'Donohue WT: Prescribing home oxygen therapy. Arch Intern Med 152:746, 1992.

Pierson DJ and Kacmarek RM, editors: Foundations of respiratory care. New York, 1992, Churchill Livingstone.

Sugarloaf Conference on the Scientific Basis of Respiratory Therapy. Amer Rev Respir Dis 22(S):1, 1980.

Tobin MJ: Respiratory monitoring in the intensive care unit. Am Rev Respir Dis 138:1625, 1988.

CHAPTER

204 Pulmonary Rehabilitation

Daniel M. Goodenberger
Barry J. Make

Pulmonary rehabilitation has been defined as "an art of medical practice wherein an individually tailored, multidisciplinary program is formulated which through accurate diagnosis, therapy, emotional support, and education, stabilizes or reverses both the physio- and psychopathology of pulmonary diseases and attempts to return the patient to the highest possible functional capacity allowed by his pulmonary handicap and overall life situation." Implicit in this definition is the recognition that the treatment of each patient as unique, the rehabilitation program being tailored to each individual. The practice of pulmonary rehabilitation requires that success be defined for each individual; goals desirable for one person may be unattainable or undesirable for another. A third corollary is that the whole patient is treated, and as a result, improvement may occur in several spheres simultaneously, making it difficult to attribute increased functional capacity to any single rehabilitation component (Fig. 204-1).

Broad goals for pulmonary rehabilitation may be defined. In general, attention is directed toward achieving maximum reversibility of obstruction, preventing and treating complications of the patient's underlying disease, and improving quality of life, a somewhat nebulous goal subject to individual value judgments and conditioned by patient expectations. An argument can be made that these goals are in fact the goals of any internist treating lung disease, and that formal rehabilitation programs are therefore unnecessary. Indeed, the principles of pulmonary rehabilitation should be considered in the management of all patients with respiratory disease. Although many of the medical and educational aspects of pulmonary rehabilitation may be applied by any well-trained internist, a formal program may involve input from a large number of highly specialized personnel who devote a significant portion of their time and effort to pulmonary rehabilitation. For a single practitioner to duplicate that input is enormously time-consuming on a per patient basis and may not represent optimal use of his time. Moreover, formal programs usually have concentrated patient educational resources and have developed efficient teaching techniques based on their experiences. Such programs are most often under the direction of a pulmonary internist whose major interest lies in this area and who devotes significant amounts of time to patients undergoing rehabilitation. Clearly, decisions regarding when and whether to refer are colored by multiple factors. Among these factors are availability of such programs in the area, patient financial resources, patient willingness to participate in a program, and desire of the individual practitioner to take advantage of a formal program instead of providing similar services himself.

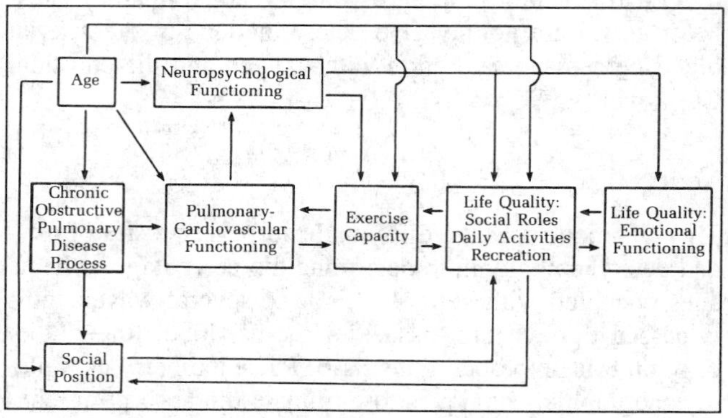

Fig 204-1. Heuristic model for interrelating chronic obstructive pulmonary disease and other variables that affect quality of life. (From McSweeney AJ et al: Life quality of patients with chronic obstructive pulmonary disease. Arch Intern Med 142:473, 1982. With permission.)

Who should be considered for referral? Although data are emerging that patients with other forms of respiratory impairment can benefit substantially from an organized rehabilitation program, the primary patient group is comprised of those who have chronic obstructive pulmonary disease (COPD). Although not firmly established, it seems reasonable to expect better outcome over a longer period for those with COPD who receive intervention earlier in the course of their illness. However, it has clearly been shown that rehabilitation benefits even those with very severe disease (FEV_1 less than 500 cc and/or severe hypercapnea). Benefits that may be expected from a rehabilitation program include symptomatic relief, with reduction of dyspnea as well as the subjective distress occasioned by dyspnea. In addition, quality of life may be improved with increased ability to perform activities of daily life, increased exercise tolerance, and a reduction in the anxiety and/or depression that may be associated with a chronic disease. Although it is clear that oxygen therapy reduces mortality in hypoxic patients with chronic lung disease, uncertainty remains as to any reduction in mortality associated with general pulmonary rehabilitation. However, little doubt exists that formal rehabilitation programs are associated with reduced morbidity in terms of acute hospitalizations, which may be reduced up to 60%. Similarly, data suggest that costs of medical care may be reduced substantially. Last, pulmonary rehabilitation may improve the capacity of the patient with COPD to remain gainfully employed, further reducing both social and psychological morbidity and societal cost.

PROGRAM STRUCTURE

Pulmonary rehabilitation may be conducted on either an inpatient or outpatient basis. The latter is less expensive, yields results similar to inpatient programs, and is more cost-effective in most circumstances. Inpatient programs allow multiple resources to be applied in a way that is convenient to both the patient and the multiple specialists participating and may be most beneficial for those with severely decreased functional ability. It is more expensive and gives results that are not significantly different from outpatient programs. Pulmonary rehabilitation programs should not be thought to be the exclusive province of tertiary care referral hospitals; community-based programs have clearly demonstrated and reported their success.

A typical pulmonary rehabilitation team in a formal program includes a variety of health care professionals. The director is most often a physician respiratory specialist with a particular interest in pulmonary rehabilitation. The day-to-day management of the program may appropriately reside in the hands of a clinical nurse specialist with expertise in respiratory care. A physical therapist may be in charge of a general conditioning program, breathing retraining, chest physical therapy, and an exercise program that may emphasize upper extremity and accessory respiratory musculature as well as standard walking or cycling. Occupational therapists bring special expertise to vocational counseling, and techniques and devices for energy conservation in daily activities. A respiratory therapist with particular interest in the area may be very effective in teaching the use and management of oxygen, inhaled medications, and ancillary equipment. Nutritional expertise may be appropriate not only for patients who are malnourished, but also for those who are affected by postprandial dyspnea. The complexities of medical reimbursement, home assistance, and available community resources may best be managed by a medical social worker. Last, the problems of anxiety, depression, and appropriate use of psychoactive medication may be greatly expedited by consultation with a psychiatrist.

When physician, hospital, and/or community resources are insufficient to support such a personnel-intensive approach, yet a need for pulmonary rehabilitation exists without conveniently available referral, it may be possible for two to three individuals to assume the multiple roles described above. There is no a priori reason that this cannot be successful; however, the advantages of scale will be lost, and the nonspecialist will necessarily have a smaller proportion of time to devote to such a program.

MEDICAL INTERVENTION

Baseline evaluation

Each patient should undergo a thorough baseline evaluation on entry. A careful history and physical examination, chest x-ray, laboratory tests indicated by the history and physical, and pulmonary function tests before and after bronchodilator administration constitute an acceptable minimum.

Smoking cessation

Smoking cessation is of paramount importance. Beneficial effects include a diminished rate of decline of pulmonary function over time and occasional outright improvement; diminished respiratory symptoms, particularly cough; diminished risk of influenza and other viral respiratory infections; and reduced carboxyhemoglobin concentration with subsequent improved oxygen saturation and reduced oxygen requirements in the hypoxemic. Many programs exclude from participation and refer for smoking cessation therapy those who continue to smoke. The ability to end nicotine addiction may be a barometer of motivation and implies greater motivation and compliance with the rehabilitation process. Attempts at smoking cessation may be tailored to the individual's desires and personality. At one extreme, unsupervised efforts may be augmented by written self-help materials such as those available from the American Lung Association. Supervised programs may be medical, with physician advice and monitoring and prescription of medication to reduce symptoms leading to relapse, or primarily psychotherapeutic with group or individual emphasis and adjunctive use of biofeedback, hypnosis, aversive conditioning, and group support. All approaches have reasonable short-term success in motivated individuals, but the recidivism rate is high, and no clear advantage of one approach over another has emerged. Nicotine-containing gum improves short-term quit rates, with an advantage over placebo that may be sustained for 2 years or more. Transdermal nicotine delivery systems also appear to increase abstinence at 1 year. As expected, a higher dosage of transdermal nicotine is more successful than a lower dosage. Clonidine also appears to reduce nicotine withdrawal symptoms and leads to increased abstinence rates for at least 6 months.

Although debate continues about the mechanism of action of theophylline and its place in the management of COPD, experience shows that it clearly benefits many patients. Several controlled trials show benefits that include decreased airflow obstruction, increased respiratory muscle strength, and a variable improvement in dyspnea. Multiple preparations are available; in general, compliance is improved with less frequent administration and minimization of side effects. The former can best be achieved with the use of long-acting preparations, and the latter by cautious dosing, aiming for levels somewhat lower (10 to 15 mg/dl) than those traditionally recommended for asthma. Although specific long-acting preparations may call for twice or once-daily dosing, a smoother serum theophylline level curve with fewer toxic peak and subtherapeutic through levels may be achieved with more frequent administration of smaller doses of sustained release products.

Corticosteroids

Patients for whom corticosteroids are prescribed indiscriminately long-term may experience one or more of the many adverse effects—Cushing's syndrome, myopathy, hyperglycemia, cataracts, and osteoporosis—without significant benefit. However, 10% to 20% of patients with stable non-asthmatic COPD show objective benefit from corticosteroids. Since it is difficult to predict which individuals will respond, a clinical trial remains the most useful way to select those who should receive steroids. The patient should receive 0.5 mg/kg/day of prednisone for a predetermined length of time, usually 2 to 4 weeks. If no objective pulmonary function benefit occurs, the prednisone should be tapered and discontinued. If, however, clear improvement results, the dose should be gradually reduced to the lowest effective level.

Infectious complications

Prevention of infection may help to reduce exacerbation of disease. Influenza vaccination given each fall is indicated for this high-risk group of patients; concern regarding elevation of serum theophylline levels postimmunization appears to be unnecessary. For the high-risk patient during an epidemic, amantadine prophylaxis is warranted, particularly in a closed community of the predominately elderly.

Although a large placebo-controlled trial demonstrated that antibiotics were worthwhile in the treatment of acute infectious exacerbations of COPD, not all studies have demonstrated such success. While these infectious exacerbations are most often viral, empiric antibiotic therapy directed at the pneumococcius, *Haemophilus influenza,* and *Branhamella catarrhalis* (moraxella) is justifiable from a cost-effectiveness point-of-view at the onset of respiratory symptoms and purulent sputum. Choice of antibiotics may be guided by community resistance patterns, but reasonable choices would include ampicillin, tetracycline, doxycycline, and cotrimoxazole. The practice of prescribing antibiotics chronically, or for an arbitrary fraction of time such as 2 weeks out of every 4, is not demonstrably useful in the majority of patients. Chronic antibiotics are most useful in the setting of bronchiectasis and in selected patients with common variable immunodeficiency or other humoral deficiencies.

Oxygen therapy

Oxygen therapy in the hypoxemic is associated with prolongation of life and improvement of its quality. The reason for this remains unclear but may be related to reduction in fatal dysrhythmias. Other beneficial effects include reduction of nonfixed pulmonary hypertension, improvement in right ventricular failure, reduction of polycythemia and associated viscosity, improvement of neuropsychiatric function, and provision of a margin of safety against further dangerous desaturation in those positioned on the steep portion of the oxygen-hemoglobin dissociation curve. Current indications include a persistent PaO_2 less than or equal to 55 mm Hg (or an oxygen saturation [SaO_2] less than or equal to 88%) in chronic stable patients on an optimal medical regimen. Oxygen may be prescribed for a PaO_2 less than 60 mm Hg or an SaO_2 of 89% in those with edema or other physical findings consistent with cor pulmonale, P pulmonale on ECG (P wave greater than 3 mm in leads II, III, and AVF), mental dysfunction, or polycythemia (hematocrit greater than or equal to 57%). Patients with exercise-related desaturation to a PaO_2 less than or equal to 55 mm Hg or an SaO_2 less than or equal to 88% are also eligible for chronic oxygen therapy during activity. Individuals who have desaturation to a similar level during sleep and have the end-organ dysfunction listed above may be candidates for nocturnal oxygen supplementation. A typical oxygen prescription is written for oxygen by nasal cannula at a flow rate sufficient to produce a PaO_2 greater than or equal to 65 mm Hg. Since nocturnal desaturation is common, the flow rate is arbitrarily increased by 1 L/min at night unless recording sleep oximetry demonstrates a different requirement.

Home oxygen use is widespread and expensive. As many as 800,000 individuals in the United States may be recipients. Medicare supports approximately 60% of home oxygen use, and as a result, increasing government regulation has been the rule. In 1989, the Health Care Financing Administration created extensive new requirements for prescription and justification of home oxygen. Reimbursement is fixed regardless of method of delivery, and this has had a profound effect on the delivery systems and availability of oxygen. This so-called "Six-Point Plan" provides reimbursement for a stationery system of approximately $295 monthly at this writing, of which Medicare pays 80%. Reimbursement is diminished by 50% for flow of less than 1

L/min and increased by 50% for flow rates greater than 4 L/min. In addition, a small supplement (approximately $40 monthly) is provided for portable oxygen, which is clearly necessary for individuals undergoing an active rehabilitation program.

Because of these considerations, many durable medical equipment vendors prefer to provide the least costly system possible (Table 204-1). An oxygen concentrator is least costly for the homebound patient requiring low flow rates, and home oxygen delivery is never required. However, because the concentrator is dependent on electricity, a back-up system or home generator may be required in rural areas, and a separate portable system is required to enhance mobility. Additionally, electricity cost is not covered by insurance. Compressed gas is widely available and is moderately expensive at low flow rates. Small portable cylinders are available that can provide up to 11 hours of oxygen when low flow rates are used. It is the most expensive method at higher flow rates and requires frequent home deliveries (a large H cylinder lasts about 4½ days at 1 L/min, and correspondingly less at higher flow rates). Liquid oxygen has the advantage of providing a longer-lasting supply (a reservoir may last 2 weeks at 1 L/min). The associated portable system is the lightest, longest-lasting, and thus most compatible with the goals of pulmonary rehabilitation. While the small "stroller" compressed gas tanks are "portable," they are much less compatible with ambulation than the over-the-shoulder liquid oxygen containers. However, liquid oxygen is expensive, and as a result, in many rural areas liquid oxygen is not available. Moreover, many durable medical equipment vendors tell prescribing physicians that Medicare no longer pays for liquid oxygen. While this is not true, carriers can review a prescription for liquid oxygen with their own physician staff and determine that a less costly system would be adequate despite documentation by the prescribing physician. An additional problem with the liquid oxygen system is that refilling the portable supply from the main reservoir may be difficult for the relatively infirm.

Patient compliance with continuous oxygen therapy is often limited, in part because of the high cost and symptoms related to mucous membrane drying. For these reasons methods to conserve oxygen have been developed. The most common are nasal cannulae with oxygen reservoirs, which collect the continuously flowing oxygen during patient exhalation and make it available during inhalation, allowing lower flow rates as well as less drying of the nose. Devices that pulse oxygen delivery only during inspiration also reduce oxygen needs, thereby allowing greater patient mobility. Patient compliance may be related to self-consciousness about visibility of oxygen tubing; in such cases systems that conceal or camouflage the reservoir and delivery system are best accepted. In the hands of some investigators, transtracheal catheter oxygen delivery has very high acceptance because of enhanced appearance as well as reduction in oxygen needs and lack of mucous membrane drying. Minute ventilation and work of breathing are clearly reduced by transtracheal administration of oxygen. This method has the disadvantage of requiring a minor surgical procedure, and long-term follow-up from multiple centers is lacking. In addition, because a large proportion of individuals receiving transtracheal oxygen may be able to be adequately oxygenated with flow rates less than 1 liter per minute, a significant financial disincentive may be created because of the reimbursement issues mentioned above. This needs to be taken into consideration when the oxygen prescription is written.

EDUCATION

The goal of the education process is to improve the patient's health. Objectives include increasing the patient's understanding of the disease process, its natural history, and the rationale for treatment of the pathophysiologic process as well as for measures designed to control symptoms. Anticipated effects of mastery of this knowledge include an improved ability to cope with daily life with this chronic illness, increased ability to perform self-care, clearer communication between care giver and patient, increased compliance with the medical and rehabilitative regimen, and a more realistic set of expectations regarding both short- and long-term outcome. The curriculum should include appropriate instruction about the disease process; rationale and importance of appropriate use of medications, and specific information about their dose and timing; instruction in the use of medication administration devices; oxygen use when appropriate; and physical measures when indicated. The various components are best taught by the individual specialists functioning as part of a well-coordinated team. Such coordination can be enhanced by regular meetings of all team members with patient-by-patient review of progress. Repetitive instruction is mandatory, and patients should demonstrate mastery of their new skills and knowledge repeatedly over the course of the program to reinforce the learning. Instructional aids may include pamphlets from national sources such as the American Lung Association, locally produced self-instruction materials, anatomic models, and audiovisual materials including slide-tape programs and videotapes. Family members must be included in the process, as their participation in the patient's rehabilitation and subsequent care is crucial both to success and to perception of success.

EXERCISE CONDITIONING

An exercise program is important in rehabilitation as it can clearly increase exercise capacity and reduce dyspnea at a given activity level in COPD (Fig. 204-2). The mechanism(s) for this improvement is somewhat unclear, as improvement occurs at levels of exercise not ordinarily associated with a training effect in individuals without lung disease. Traditional programs concentrate on lower extremity exercise, in various combinations of free walking, treadmill walking, and stationary cycling. Each has advantages and disadvantages (Table 204-2). Improvement in one form of exercise may transfer poorly to other forms, and thus the advantage of free walking is that it is a useful activity in daily life with improved capacity resulting in concrete

Table 204-1. Forms of oxygen supply for outpatient therapy

Form of oxygen	Reservoir duration, if used at 1 L/min	Associated portable system	Portable supply duration if used at 1 L/min	Portable supply weight (lb)
Compressed gas	4.8 d per large cylindrical "H" tank	Small tanks with wheels or shoulder strap		
		"E" cylinder	11 hours	17
		"D" cylinder	7 hours	10
		"C" cylinder	4 hours	8
		Mada cylinder	2 hours	5
Liquid oxygen	13-14 d per 70-75 lb of liquid O_2 in canister	Canisters with shoulder strap or wheels		
		Small canister	7 hours	6.5-7.5
		Large canister	13 hours	10-12
Oxygen concentrator	No limit; machine extracts O_2 from air	Small compressed gas tanks (see above)	Small compressed gas tanks (see above)	

Modified from Make BJ: Medical management of emphysema. Clin Chest Med 4:465, 1983. With permission.
*Medicare pays 80%; patient is responsible for remainder. Data provided by Glasrock Home Health Care for St. Louis area, 1992.

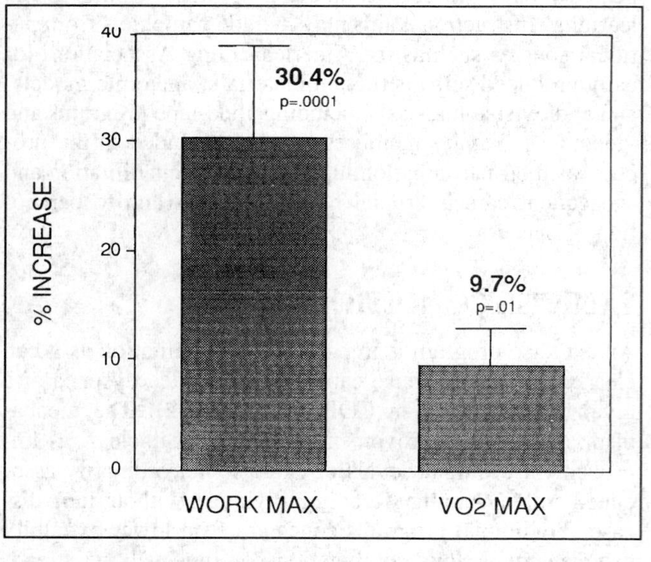

Fig. 204-2. Improvement in exercise capacity following pulmonary rehabilitation. There was a 30.4% increase in maximum work and 9.7% increase in maximum oxygen consumption on bicycle ergometry testing in 26 COPD patients completing a 3-week rehabilitation program at the National Jewish Center for Immunology and Respiratory Medicine.

benefits. Walking also requires no special equipment, and improvement is easy to measure in the distance achieved in either 6 or 12 minutes of continuous walking. The prescription should be formulated after a baseline exercise study that includes maximum oxygen uptake, minute ventilation, maximum heart rate, electrocardiographic monitoring, energy expenditure, and oximetry for detection of exercise oxygen desaturation. A typical training schedule should involve performance of the selected exercise repetitively to the level of dyspnea, for at least 20 minutes four times weekly. Three weeks or more should be allowed for improvement and a maintenance exercise regimen followed thereafter. Fig. 204-2 depicts the results of the National Jewish Center's rehabilitation program.

Increasing interest has focused on the benefits of upper extremity exercise. It has long been noted that activities of daily life involving elevation of the upper extremities produce dyspnea in patients with COPD out of proportion to energy expenditure. Recent work suggests that this results from interference with or fatigue of the upper extremity–related accessory muscles of respiration, and experience is accumulating to suggest that an exercise program involving upper extremity muscles improves arm activity endurance time and reduces dyspnea. Moreover, such a program

Approximate charge per month if used 24 hours a day				
1 L/min	**3 L/min**	**Medicare reimbursement***	**Advantages**	**Disadvantages**
Stationary $450 *Portable (additional)* $170	 $1180 $320	*Stationary* <1 L/min; $137.35 1-4 L/min; $274.70 >4 L/min; $412.05 *Portable* $46.76 (any system)	Widely available Moderate expense for use at home if used at low flow rates or for brief periods	Heavy and large, hard to move Portable system rather bulky Frequent tank deliveries may be needed
$460	$1025 (portable included)	Same as above	Portable system easiest to carry and longest lasting Most convenient and least expensive for extended or high flows	Expensive except for patients on high flow rates (>3 L/min) and those who spend long periods on portable use Oxygen evaporates slowly (2%/d) Some patients have trouble refilling some models of portable canisters
Stationary $360 for any amount of usage, plus cost of electricity		Same as above	Most economical for many patients who use O_2 24 hours a day and stay home	Dependent on electricity, so back-up system needed Alternate system needed for portable use
Portable (additional) $170	$320		Not dependent on deliveries of O_2 from supplier Attractive cabinetlike appearance of machine	Can deliver up to 4 L/min of >90% O_2 Cost of electricity ($25/mo) not covered by insurance

may be included as part of a rehabilitation group meeting, and has had considerable success when set to music. We use a graded upper extremity program consisting of multiple repetitions of arm lifts with very light weights and unloaded arm cycle ergometry.

Table 204-2. Advantages and disadvantages of exercise training methods

Method	Advantages	Disadvantages
Treadmill	Effective Easy to learn Direct supervision required	Expensive Labor intensive Equipment is physically large
Bicycle	Effective Cheaper than treadmill May be used at home	Moderately expensive Moderately labor intensive
12-minute walk	Effective Simple Inexpensive No equipment required Home or hospital based	Less supervision required Requires more patient self-motivation

From Make BJ and O'Brien R: Pulmonary rehabilitation: an adjunct to the management of patients with chronic obstructive pulmonary disease. In Brody JS and Snider GL, editors: Current topics in the management of respiratory diseases. New York, 1985, Churchill-Livingstone. With permission.

The role of specific inspiratory muscle training in respiratory rehabilitation remains unclear. Several studies have suggested that ventilatory muscle endurance may be enhanced and respiratory muscle strength improved by targeted inspiratory muscle training; however, improvement in exercise capability, sense of well-being, and increase in activities of daily living have not been reproducibly demonstrated.

The perception that the respiratory muscles of patients with severe COPD are chronically fatigued has led to several trials of respiratory muscle rest using external negative pressure ventilators ("iron lungs" or smaller equivalents) or nasal positive-pressure ventilation. Recent controlled studies do not show that elective ventilatory assistance adds anything to pulmonary rehabilitation in normocapnic COPD patients. Moreover, negative-pressure ventilation is poorly tolerated. Some studies report decreased $PaCO_2$ in hypercapnic COPD patients; this effect may be related to resetting of the chemoceptors and increased hypercapnic drive.

PHYSICAL THERAPY

Three general categories of physical therapy are available for the patient with COPD. The first includes measures to clear airway secretions. Removing excess poorly cleared sputum is theoretically attractive as it may reduce airway resistance, decrease ventilation-perfusion mismatch, improve oxygenation, and perhaps prevent infection. The most frequent methods are postural drainage alone or with chest percussion and/or vibration. Available evidence does not demonstrate fewer hospitalizations, diminished morbidity, or lesser mortality in those receiving chest physical therapy and is supportive of its use only in those producing more than 30 ml of sputum daily, a situation uncommon in COPD. These techniques may be aided by reduction of viscosity with adequate hydration and perhaps mucolytics, reduction of airway irritation by elimination of tobacco and other inhalant exposure, and improving mucociliary clearance with theophylline and inhaled $beta_2$ agonists.

A second category of physical therapy is breathing retraining. Although exercises aimed at emphasizing "diaphragmatic" breathing have been used for more than 40 years, little objective evidence shows improved function. A variety of postures and exercises have been described but appear to be useful chiefly in giving the patient a sense of control over dyspnea. Pursed-lip breathing is likewise standard. It diminishes minute ventilation with a larger tidal volume but lower respiratory rate and may be useful in allowing exhalation to a lower functional residual capacity by diminishing airway collapse, with resultant more advantageous respiratory muscle position and reduced work of breathing. Objective evidence of its effectiveness is, however, scanty.

Last, relaxation techniques such as internal visualization of a pleasant setting may be useful in giving patients another tool to control episodic nonexertional dyspnea.

OCCUPATIONAL THERAPY

Energy conservation techniques allow the COPD patient to accomplish more with less energy expenditure. Occupational therapists are experts in teaching patients how to plan tasks to eliminate unnecessary or duplicative effort, to work in the most efficient posture, and to proceed at a realistic pace. Evaluation of the patient's activities at work or at home may allow the use of work-reducing assistive devices. For example, kitchen work may be performed using a high chair with the opportunity to support the upper extremities on either the counter or the chair arms, rather than standing. Power kitchen appliances such as an electric can opener may reduce dyspnea-producing upper extremity work. The shelf storage may be rearranged to reduce walking and reaching, and long-handled gripping devices may be substituted for climbing. Similar principles may be applied to many other forms of work and activities of daily living, such as showering, shaving, toileting, and eating.

NUTRITIONAL EVALUATION AND THERAPY

More than 30% of patients with severe COPD have evidence of significant protein-calorie malnutrition. The causes for this malnutrition are poorly understood and probably multiple. Patients with severe hyperinflation commonly have increased dyspnea after a meal, and the resultant decrease in intake may contribute to poor nutrition. Although no data show nutritional repletion reduces mortality in COPD, it is clear that malnutrition has multiple negative effects on pulmonary function. Diaphragmatic and other respiratory muscle function is impaired, immune competence is compromised, and overall mortality is increased in COPD patients with weight loss. Additionally, surfactant production, ventilatory control, and lung repair after injury may all be less than optimal. Even though evaluation of nutritional status may include standard anthropometric measurements (arm circumference, triceps skin fold thickness), serum albumin and transferrin, lymphocyte count, and routine chemistries, actual versus ideal body weight (assuming freedom from edema) provides a simple, reasonably sensitive screen for long-term nutritional status. Patients whose actual weight is less than 90% of ideal need more thorough investigation. Those patients who become dyspneic during meals should have oximetry to detect the occasional patient who becomes hypoxemic with eating. Nutritional therapy should ideally be guided by nutritional consultation. Smaller, more frequent meals and snacks may reduce mealtime dyspnea. High-caloric dietary supplements (commercial or home-made frappes) may enable greater calorie intake. Relatively low-carbohydrate, high-fat supplements may reduce the respiratory quotient and carbon dioxide production. Although theoretically attractive, no evidence currently available clearly shows long-term benefit. Last, optimization of the underlying medical condition and minimization of drug side effects on the gastrointestinal tract may allow improved appetite and nutritional status.

PSYCHOSOCIAL MANAGEMENT

A vicious cycle of dyspnea evoking anxiety, which provokes further dyspnea, is familiar to most clinicians. Strong emotions increase adrenergic output, which increases minute ventilation. In the setting of COPD, this diminishes expiratory time, increases hyperinflation, and increases dyspnea. As a result, patients with severe COPD learn to avoid provocative activities and strong emotion, a condition that has been described as living in an emotional straitjacket. The patient's lifestyle becomes increasingly reclusive, and his or her social circle becomes progressively restricted. Diminished self-esteem is frequent and is made worse if employment is no longer possible. Reactive depression is thus very common (42% in the Nocturnal Oxygen Therapy Trial). Life-threatening depression is uncommon and is best approached by formal psychiatric evaluation and therapy. The much more common anxiety and reactive depression are more usefully managed by specific rehabilitation measures and support. However, an experienced liaison psychiatric consultant often provides great help in separating the two groups, guiding psychopharmacotherapy, and identifying psychosocial obstacles to rehabilitation. Rehabilitation, as described above, and breathing retraining may help the patient regain a sense of control, reducing anxiety. Both education and exercise training may result in desensitization to symptoms. Meditation as an approach to relaxation training may be useful. Group meetings allow the sympathetic support of the rehabilitation staff as well as the opportunity to share experiences, problems, solutions, and often friendship with similarly afflicted peers.

SPECIALIZED PULMONARY REHABILITATION

Patients with problems other than simple COPD may benefit from the services of specialized pulmonary rehabilitation units. Those with early respiratory failure from skeletal and chest wall deformities (e.g., kyphoscoliosis and thoracoplasty) and neuromuscular disease (e.g., postpolio syndrome, muscular dystrophy, and high spinal cord injury), may be helped to remain at home with partial ventilatory support. While negative pressure ventilation retains a role in this regard, its use is complicated by difficulties of application, particularly in the neuromuscularly impaired, and by its proclivity for inducing upper airway obstruction during sleep. A growing body of literature demonstrates that noninvasive positive-pressure ventilation, most often delivered via nasal mask, may be a reasonable nocturnal substitute for a significant number of these patients. Nocturnal hypoventilation is prevented and respiratory muscles are rested. Patients may become demonstrably stronger during the daytime, and gas exchange often returns toward normal during waking hours. Moreover, quality of life may be significantly improved. A smaller proportion of these patients may benefit from nocturnal ventilation via tracheostomy. Lastly, as respiratory failure progresses, these patients may have very productive lives with complete, tracheostomy-delivered positive-pressure ventilation. Portable ventilators and motorized wheelchairs allow considerable mobility, and many patients may have normal speech during mechanical ventilation through the use of a variety of techniques.

A real but more limited role exists for home management of partially or completely ventilator-dependent patients with COPD. Medical intensive care has resulted in an increasing number of these chronically ventilator-dependent patients; as they become otherwise medically stable, options for continued care include an acute care hospital, a chronic care hospital, a skilled nursing facility, or their own home. It is estimated that there are over 11,400 ventilator-dependent patients in United States hospitals. The care and maintenance of such individuals in the home is a labor-intensive effort that requires the coordinated skills of many of the individuals mentioned earlier in this chapter, with overall care directed by a skilled and motivated pulmonary subspecialist.

FOLLOW-UP CARE

Patients who have completed the formal rehabilitation program need continued follow-up. Those with relatively stable COPD may be seen regularly in the outpatient setting by a physician and/or nurse clinician. In addition to standard management of the lung disease, each visit should be used to reinforce the teachings of the formal program. Retention of knowledge and skills should be gently tested and emphasis given where needed. Those requiring home oxygen and home respiratory devices require periodic visits and assessment by the responsible home care company, and their reports should be examined by the physician. Patients who need physical therapy, or whose status is more tenuous, benefit from regular assessment and care from the personnel of the local visiting nurse association. Their services may allow the patient to remain in the home, and thoughtful attention to their reports and calls facilitates this.

REFERENCES

Anthonisen NR et al: Antibiotic therapy in exacerbations of chronic obstructive pulmonary disease. Ann Int Med 106:196, 1987.

Bach JR and Alba AS: Management of chronic alveolar hypoventilation by nasal ventilation. Chest 97:52, 1990.

Celli B et al: Controlled trial of external negative pressure ventilation in patients with severe chronic airflow obstruction. Am Rev Respir Dis 140:1251, 1989.

Corsello PR and Make BJ: Which oxygen conserving device is best for your patient? J Respir Dis 13:27, 1992.

Couser JI and Make BJ: Transtracheal oxygen decreases inspired minute ventilation. Am Rev Respir Dis 139:627, 1989.

Fernandez E et al: Sustained improvement in gas exchange after negative pressure ventilation for 8 hours per day on two successive days in chronic airflow limitation. Am Rev Respir Dis 144:390, 1991.

Foster S and Thompson HM: Pulmonary rehabilitation in lung disease other than chronic obstructive pulmonary disease. Am Rev Respir Dis 141:601, 1990.

Glassman AH et al: Heavy smokers, smoking cessation, and clonidine. Results of a double-blind, randomized trial. JAMA 259:2863, 1988.

Harver A et al: Targeted inspiratory muscle training improves respiratory muscle function and reduces dyspnea in patients with chronic obstructive pulmonary disease. Ann Int Med 111:117, 1989.

Hodgkin JE, Zorn EG, and Connors G, editors: Pulmonary rehabilitation—guidelines to success. Boston, 1984, Butterworth.

Make BJ, editor: Pulmonary rehabilitation. Clin Chest Med 7:519, 1986.

Make BJ and Gilmartin ME: Rehabilitation and home care for ventilator-assisted individuals. Clin Chest Med 7:679, 1986.

Murciano D et al: A randomized, controlled trial of theophylline in patients with severe chronic obstructive pulmonary disease. N Engl J Med 320:1521, 1989.

Niederman MS et al: Benefits of a multidisciplinary pulmonary rehabilitation program. Improvements are independent of lung function. Chest 99:798, 1991.

Nocturnal Oxygen Therapy Trial Group: Continuous or nocturnal oxygen therapy in hypoxemic chronic obstructive lung disease. Ann Intern Med 93:391, 1980.

Shigeoka JW and Stults BM: Home oxygen therapy under Medicare: a primer. West J Med 156:39, 1992.

Spessert C and Goodenberger D: Chairobics (an exercise and pulmonary rehabilitation educational videotape). Tucson, Ariz, 1991, Glasrock.

Strumpf DA et al: Nocturnal positive pressure ventilation via nasal mask in patients with severe chronic obstructive pulmonary disease. Am Rev Respir Dis 144:1234, 1991.

Transdermal Nicotine Study Group: Transdermal nicotine for smoking cessation. Six-month results from two multicenter controlled clinical trials. JAMA 266:3133, 1991.

IV Specific Disease Entities

CHAPTER

205 Chronic Obstructive Pulmonary Disease

Gordon L. Snider

DEFINITION

No generally accepted definition of chronic obstructive pulmonary disease (COPD) exists. This chapter defines COPD as a process characterized by the presence of chronic bronchitis or emphysema that may lead to the development of airways obstruction. The airways obstruction may be partially reversible, is often accompanied by airways hyperreactivity (Chapter 300), and thus may have features similar to asthma. Patients should be appropriately characterized by clinical, radiographic, physiologic, and other laboratory studies. The term *COPD,* or its frequently used synonym, *chronic obstructive lung disease,* permits a clinician to record a diagnosis that does not imply an indefensible degree of precision.

Chronic bronchitis

Chronic bronchitis is defined as the presence of chronic productive cough that does not result from a medically discernible cause (e.g., tuberculosis, lung cancer) and that has been present for an extended period. For clinical purposes, "extended period" is defined as the presence of symptoms in the patient half of the time for 2 years. This definition is based on symptoms. No known specific basis should exist for the sputum production that is the defining characteristic of chronic bronchitis.

Emphysema

Emphysema is defined as abnormal permanent enlargement of the air spaces distal to the terminal bronchioles accompanied by destruction of their walls and without obvious fibrosis. *Destruction* is defined as nonuniformity in the pattern of respiratory air space enlargement; the orderly appearance of the acinus is disturbed and may be lost.

AIRWAYS OBSTRUCTION

As its definition makes clear, COPD and its two major components, chronic bronchitis and emphysema, may occur with or without airways obstruction. However, it is airways obstruction that causes impairment of lung function, disability, and death. Asthma, by definition (Chapter 300), is always associated with airways obstruction. Remission of the airways obstruction, either spontaneously or in response to treatment, is the hallmark of asthma. On the contrary, the airways obstruction of COPD tends to be nonremitting once it develops. Therefore it may not be possible to differentiate between the patient with nonremitting asthma and the patient with COPD who has airways obstruction and hyperreactivity. These complex interrelations are shown in Fig. 205-1.

Note that the patient with asthma whose airways obstruction is completely reversible is diagnosed as having asthma. On the other hand, nonremitting asthma is included within the context of COPD. Patients whose airways obstruction results from a specific cause (e.g., bronchiectasis, cystic fibrosis, obliterative bronchiolitis) are not included under the umbrella of COPD. Preventive efforts are best directed at patients who have COPD with no or mild airways obstruction; therapeutic measures are directed at those with the more severe degrees of airways obstruction.

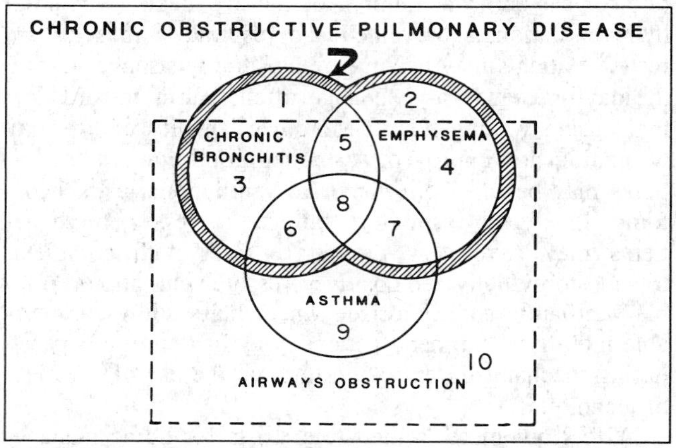

Fig. 205-1. Schema of chronic obstructive pulmonary disease (COPD). A nonproportional Venn diagram shows subsets of patients with chronic bronchitis, emphysema, and asthma in three overlapping circles. Subsets of patients within the rectangle have airways obstruction. Patients with asthma, subset 9, are defined as having completely reversible airways obstruction and lie entirely within the rectangle. Patients in subsets 6, 7, and 8 have reversible airways obstruction with chronic productive cough or emphysema; it may be difficult to be certain whether patients in these subsets have underlying asthma or have developed bronchial hyperreactivity as a complication of chronic bronchitis or emphysema. Patients in subset 3 have chronic productive cough with airways obstruction but no emphysema; the size of this subset is not known. Patients with emphysema alone fall into subset 4. Most patients who require medical care for their disease fall into subsets 5 and 8. Patients in subsets 1 and 2 do not have airways obstruction, as determined by the forced expiratory volume for 1 second (FEV_1), but have clinical or radiographic features of chronic bronchitis or emphysema, respectively. Since COPD does not have airways obstruction as a defining characteristic, and since pure asthma is not included in the term *COPD,* patient subsets 1 to 8 are included within the area outlined by the shaded band that denotes COPD. (Reprinted with permission from Snider GL, Faling LJ, and Rennard SI: Chronic bronchitis and emphysema. In Murray JF and Nadel JA, editors: Textbook of respiratory medicine, ed 2. Philadelphia, 1993, Saunders.)

EPIDEMIOLOGY

Prevalence and mortality

The National Health Interview Survey estimated that about 13 million persons in the United States had COPD in 1989. The Tecumseh, Mich., Community Health Study of more than 9000 males and females of all ages showed that about 14% of adult males and 8% of adult females have chronic bronchitis, obstructive airways disease, or both. In 1988 more than 80,000 deaths resulted from COPD and allied conditions, representing about 3.5% of all deaths and the fifth leading cause of death in the United States. COPD is cited as a contributing cause of death about 2.5 times more frequently than as an underlying cause. Between 1960 and 1986, the age-adjusted mortality rate for COPD rose 71%, during which time the death rate for cardiovascular disease declined by more than 40%. These data reflect the effects of cigarette smoking on persons now reaching an advanced age. They also reflect that, in contrast to cardiovascular mortality rates, COPD mortality rates are relatively insensitive to smoking cessation.

Prevalence, incidence, and mortality rates for COPD increase with age and are higher in males than females and are higher in whites than nonwhites. Incidence and mortality are generally higher in blue-collar workers than white-collar workers and in those with fewer years of formal education. Some evidence suggests that COPD aggregates in families.

Risk factors

Tobacco smoking. Tobacco smoking and age account for about 80% to 90% of the risk of developing COPD in the United States. Only homozygous alpha$_1$-protease inhibitor (API) deficiency presents a comparable risk, but this factor accounts for only about 0.1% of patients with COPD in the United States. Data from longitudinal, cross-sectional, and case control studies show that compared with nonsmokers, cigarette smokers have higher COPD mortality. They also have higher prevalence and incidence of productive cough, other respiratory symptoms, and spirometrically shown airways obstruction. A dose-response relationship exists for tobacco smoking; differences between smokers and nonsmokers increase as daily cigarette consumption and number of years smoked increase. Pipe and cigar smokers have higher COPD mortality and morbidity than nonsmokers, although their rates are lower than those of cigarette smokers. For reasons not known, only about 10% to 15% of cigarette smokers develop clinically significant COPD.

Passive, or involuntary, smoking is the exposure of nonsmokers to cigarette smoke indoors. Cigarette smoke in indoor air can produce eye irritation and may incite wheezing in asthmatic persons. An increased prevalence of respiratory symptoms and disease and small but measurable decreases in lung function have been shown in the children of smoking compared with nonsmoking parents. However, the significance of these findings for the future development of COPD is unknown.

Air pollution. It is established that high levels of environmental air pollution are harmful to persons with chronic heart or lung disease. Although the exact role of air pollution in producing COPD is unclear, its role is small compared with that of cigarette smoking.

Occupation. Population-based studies suggest that working in an occupation in which the air is polluted with chemical fumes or a biologically inactive dust leads to increased prevalence of chronic airflow obstruction; increased rates of a decline in forced expiratory volume for 1 second (FEV$_1$), a measure of ventilatory capacity (Chapter 195); and increased mortality from COPD. Interaction between cigarette smoking and exposure to hazardous dust such as silica or cotton dust results in increased rates of COPD. In all these studies, however, smoking effects are much greater than occupational effects.

Miscellaneous. The hypotheses are not proved that the atopic state or nonspecific airways hyperresponsiveness (usually measured as responsiveness to methacholine inhalation) predisposes smokers to the development of airways obstruction. Severe respiratory infection in childhood has been cited as increasing susceptibility to the effects of cigarette smoking.

PATHOLOGY

Chronic bronchitis

Various structural changes, none of which is specific to chronic bronchitis, have been described in the airways of long-time cigarette smokers. The submucosal glands are enlarged and their ducts dilated. Focal areas of squamous metaplasia replace the pseudostratified columnar epithelium. Neutrophils and lymphocytes infiltrate the mucous membranes but are sparse and not a prominent feature. Airways smooth muscle may be hypertrophied. The terminal and respiratory bronchioles show varying degrees of secretory obstruction, goblet cell metaplasia, inflammation with a predominance of macrophages, increased smooth muscle, and distortion from loss of alveolar attachments and fibrosis.

Emphysema

Emphysema is classified according to the portion of the acinus involved by mild disease (see the box on p. 1670). The acinus comprises the respiratory tissues arising from a single terminal bronchiole. Centriacinar emphysema begins as enlargement of the respiratory bronchioles and adjacent air spaces with breakdown of air space walls. Focal emphysema is a form of centriacinar emphysema that occurs in individuals who have had heavy exposure to a biologically inactive dust such as coal dust. The lesions are widespread through the lungs and are infiltrated by pigment-laden macrophages.

Centrilobular emphysema (CLE), a form of centriacinar emphysema, is the most common form of emphysema in smokers. The lesions involve the upper and posterior por-

Respiratory air space enlargement*

I. Simple air space enlargement
   A. Congenital (Down's syndrome)
   B. Acquired (contralateral lung after pneumonectomy; aging lung)
II. Emphysema
   A. Centriacinar emphysema
      1. Focal emphysema (coal workers' pneumoconiosis)
      2. Centrilobular emphysema (main lesion of smokers)
   B. Panacinar emphysema (main lesion in alpha$_1$-protease inhibitor [API] deficiency)
   C. Distal acinar emphysema
III. Air space enlargement with fibrosis (sarcoidosis)

*Examples of each type are given in parentheses.

tions of the lungs more than the lung bases. Panlobular emphysema (PLE), which in diffuse form is the type of emphysema occurring in homozygous API deficiency, involves all the acinus. Focal PLE, which often accompanies CLE in smokers, occurs at the lung bases. Distal acinar emphysema, also known as paraseptal or subpleural emphysema, occurs subpleurally or along fibrous interlobular septa. The remainder of the lung is often spared, so pulmonary function may be well preserved despite the presence of many foci of locally severe disease. This is the type of apical emphysema that causes spontaneous pneumothorax in young people. Air space enlargement with fibrosis, formerly called paracicatricial emphysema, may be an inconsequential lesion adjacent to a scar or it may be severe and clinically important, complicating fibrosing diseases such as tuberculosis, silicosis, or sarcoidosis.

Bullae. Bullae are enlarged air spaces that may reach huge proportions, filling an entire hemithorax. They may be locally severe areas of generalized emphysema, or they may be the focal lesions of distal acinar emphysema. Bullae that are not a part of generalized emphysema may rarely become large enough to severely impair lung function; resectional surgery may result in marked improvement.

Implications of types of emphysema. In addition to the differences in anatomic patterns on which the previous classification of emphysema is based, differences in predilections toward age and sex exist among the types of emphysema. It thus seems likely that differences exist in their etiology and pathogenesis, although little information is available to indicate what these might be. Since the lung parenchyma consists of 300 million air cells circumscribed by a complexly organized vascular tissue, emphysema may represent one of the lungs' stereotyped responses to injury.

Structure-function correlations. Bronchial gland enlargement correlates poorly with airflow obstruction. This is not surprising because the lesion encroaches minimally on the airway lumen. Mild respiratory bronchiolitis, which is the earliest lesion described in smokers, does not cause airflow obstruction. As the lesion increases in severity and is accompanied by terminal bronchiolitis, airflow obstruction supervenes.

Emphysema becomes evident at about the same time as the terminal bronchiolitis and increases steadily in severity as COPD progresses. It is the predominant lesion in most patients with end-stage COPD. Bronchiolitis also increases in severity as COPD runs its course. Its inflammatory component contributes to the reversible elements of airflow obstruction, both by mechanical means and by generating mediators that cause bronchial muscle contraction.

ALPHA$_1$-PROTEASE INHIBITOR DEFICIENCY

Alpha$_1$-protease inhibitor (API), also known as alpha$_1$-trypsin inhibitor, is a serum protein (molecular weight, 52 kD) and is normally found in the lungs. It inhibits several serine proteases, but its main role in the body is inhibition of neutrophil elastase; the deficient state is associated with the premature development of emphysema. API is a glycoprotein composed of 394 amino acids, which is coded for by a single gene on chromosome 14. The serum protease inhibitor phenotype (Pi type) is determined by the independent expression of the two parental alleles. The API gene is highly pleomorphic. About 75 alleles are known, and they have been classified into *normal* (associated with normal serum levels of normally functioning API), *deficient* (associated with serum API levels lower than normal), *null* (associated with undetectable API in the serum), and *dysfunctional* (API present in normal amount but not functioning normally).

The variants of API occur because of point mutations that result in a single amino acid substitution. For example, the Z variant results from the substitution of a lysine for a glutamic acid in the M protein. The substitution changes the charge of the molecule and therefore its electrophoretic mobility. The normal M alleles occur in about 90% of persons of European descent with normal serum API levels; their phenotype is designated PiMM. Normal values of serum API are 150 to 350 mg/dl (commercial standard) or 20 to 48 μM (true laboratory standard).

More than 95% of persons in the severely deficient category are homozygous for the Z allele, designated PiZZ, and have serum API levels of 2.5 to 7 μM (mean, 16% normal). Most of these persons are caucasians of northern European descent because the Z allele is rare in orientals and blacks. Rarely observed phenotypes associated with low levels of serum API include PiSZ and persons with nonexpressing alleles, Pi null. The latter occur in homozygous form, Pi null-null, or in heterozygous form with a deficient allele, PiZ null. Persons with phenotype PiSS have API values ranging from 15 to 33 μM (mean, 52% of normal). The threshold protective level of 11 μM, or 80 mg/dl (35% of normal), is based on the knowledge that PiSZ heterozygotes, with serum API values of 8 to 19 μM (mean, 37% of normal), rarely develop emphysema. PiMZ heterozygotes have serum API levels that are intermediate between levels for normal PiMM and homozygous PiZZ (12 to 35 μM; mean, 57% of normal) and are not at increased risk for emphysema.

Homozygous (PiZZ) API deficiency and lung disease

Homozygous API deficiency is accompanied by the premature development of severe emphysema, with chronic bronchitis occurring in about half of patients. The onset of pulmonary disease is greatly accelerated by smoking; dyspnea begins at a median age of 40 years in smokers compared with a median age of 53 years in nonsmokers. Radiographically, panacinar emphysema, which predominates in PiZ patients, usually begins at the lung bases (Fig. 205-2).

The natural history of API deficiency is incompletely known. In addition to an earlier onset of dyspnea, PiZZ smokers have a lower life expectancy than PiZZ nonsmokers, although the latter have a lower life expectancy than PiMM persons. Severity of lung disease varies greatly; lung function is well preserved in some PiZZ smokers and severely impaired in some PiZZ nonsmokers. Nonindex persons (those discovered in population surveys) tend to have better lung function, whether they smoke or not, than index persons (those discovered because they have lung disease). Nonindex persons may live into their eighth or ninth decade. Airflow obstruction occurs more frequently in men than in women; asthma, recurrent respiratory infections, and familial factors are also risk factors for airflow obstruction.

Diagnosis

The diagnosis of API deficiency is made by measuring serum API level, followed by Pi typing for confirmation. The tests should be ordered in patients with premature onset of COPD and in nonsmokers with COPD. A predominance of basilar emphysema should suggest the genetic defect.

Augmentation therapy

Augmentation therapy with purified human API for patients with severe API deficiency is based on the concept that a deficient protein is being restored to protective levels. It is presumed, but not proved, that augmentation therapy will halt the progression of emphysema. Because emphysema produces a permanent structural change, augmentation therapy cannot improve lung structure or function. The cost of the drug for 1 year of augmentation therapy in a 70 kg patient is about $25,000. Augmentation therapy should be reserved for patients with lung disease whose serum concentration of API is less than 11 μM; it is not indicated for patients with cigarette-smoking-related emphysema who have normal or heterozygous phenotypes. PiZZ persons with normal lung function should be followed but not treated; augmentation therapy should be considered when lung function is abnormal and especially if serial studies show deterioration.

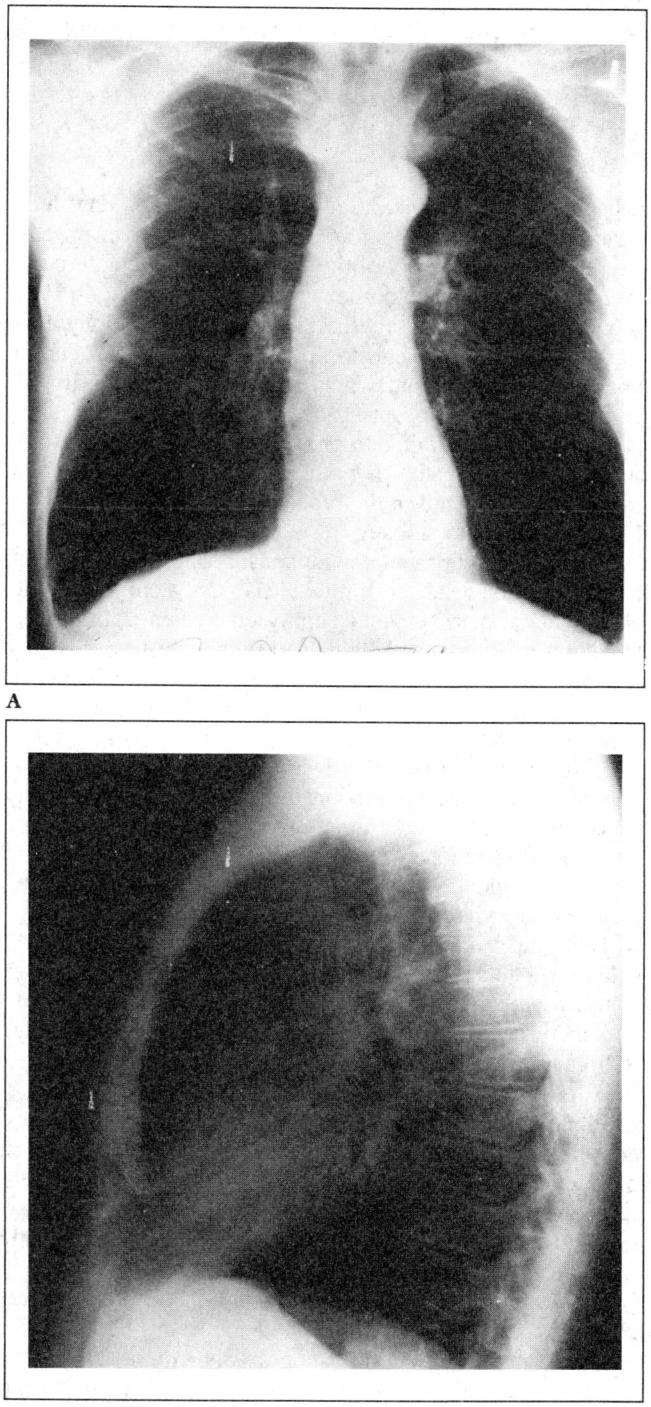

A

B

Fig. 205-2. Chest radiograph of a 66-year-old man with homozygous alpha$_1$-protease inhibitor (API) deficiency. **A,** Frontal view shows a depression and flattening of the diaphragmatic shadow. Areas of hypertransradiancy with poorly defined upper borders occupy the lower lung zones and are patchy in the midlung zones. The cardiac silhouette is narrow. **B,** Lateral view shows marked flattening of the diaphragm and an increase in the retrosternal air space.

For severely impaired persons under age 50, lung transplantation should be considered. The prospect of gene therapy for patients with API deficiency is approaching steadily.

PATHOGENESIS

Emphysema

It has been known since the turn of this century that lung parenchymal elastic fibers are ruptured and frayed in emphysema. The discovery of the association of premature onset of emphysema with homozygous API deficiency in 1963 soon spawned the hypothesis that this form of emphysema was induced by the digestion of lung parenchymal elastic fibers by the individual's own neutrophil elastase. It was postulated that this occurred because the severe API deficiency in the lungs failed to provide a sufficient antielastase shield. Supporting this hypothesis is the observation that free elastase is found in the bronchoalveolar lavage fluid of PiZZ persons who smoke.

Extensive experimental evidence indicates that elastic fiber destruction leads to emphysema. Only enzymes with elastolytic properties induce emphysema when instilled into the lungs of animals; human neutrophil elastase has this property. Emphysema-like changes occur in animals whose elastic fibers do not cross-link normally, either because of a genetic or an induced defect in the cross-linking mechanism. Emphysema has also been induced in experimental animals by repeated induction of pulmonary neutrophilia, especially if at the same time the amount of API is diminished or its functional integrity impaired.

Much work has also been done to relate the elastase-antielastase hypothesis to cigarette smoking. The number of cells that can be lavaged from the lungs is about fivefold higher in smokers than in nonsmokers. The proportion of neutrophils remains at 1% to 3%, but their absolute numbers increase fivefold. In vitro studies have also shown that API can be oxidatively inactivated by oxygen radicals derived either from cigarette smoke or from the neutrophil's myeloperoxidase system. Immuno-ultrastructural studies are purported to show elastase bound to elastin in the lungs of smokers. Thus, although most of it is indirect, compelling evidence supports the concept that elastase-antielastase imbalance is responsible for emphysema in smokers with adequate protective levels of API.

There are also animal models of emphysema in which elastin degradation is not believed to occur. Emphysema has been produced experimentally by hyperoxia and severe starvation; cadmium chloride induces air space enlargement with fibrosis.

Chronic bronchitis

Experimental chronic bronchial injury has been produced with a variety of irritant gases. Sulfur dioxide produces a predominantly central lesion, with submucosal gland and goblet cell metaplasia. Cigarette smoke produces secretory cell metaplasia in both central and peripheral airways. Chronic exposure to low-dose ozone induces injury of the terminal bronchiole and the adjacent respiratory airway.

Serine proteases, which need not be elastolytic but which must be enzymatically active, can induce secretory cell metaplasia in the hamster. Neutrophils are a rich source of serine proteases and are a feature of many bronchial inflammatory processes. The airway goblet cells and serous cells of bronchial glands secrete a 12 kD protein, secretory leukoprotease inhibitor. This protein accounts for more than 80% of the inhibitory capacity of bronchitic sputum and is capable of inhibiting neutrophil elastase. These observations suggest that protease-antiprotease imbalance plays a role in bronchial secretory cell metaplasia and in emphysema.

The development of techniques of studying animal and human airway walls physiologically and in organ culture systems and the development of techniques for culture of dissociated airway cells has begun to unravel the complex ways in which the epithelium responds to injury. Data are emerging on the factors that control desquamation of epithelial cells, the migration and replication of epithelial cells to repair sites of desquamation, water and ion transport through the bronchial wall, and the neurogenic and humoral factors that control vascular and smooth muscle tone.

CLINICAL FEATURES

History

Patients may have a productive cough or an acute chest illness in their fifth decade. Dyspnea on effort of sufficient severity to bring the patient with COPD to the physician usually does not occur until the sixth or seventh decade. A careful history usually reveals that the dyspneic patient has had chronic productive cough and wheezing for many years before the onset of dyspnea. Patients have usually been smoking more than 20 cigarettes per day for more than 35 years before symptoms are sufficiently severe to bring them to the physician.

Sputum production is insidious in its onset. Initially occurring only in the morning, it may later be produced intermittently throughout the day. The daily volume rarely exceeds 60 ml. Sputum is usually mucoid but becomes purulent with an exacerbation.

Acute chest illnesses characterized by increased cough, purulent sputum, wheezing, dyspnea, and occasionally fever may occur from time to time. The history of wheezing and dyspnea may lead to the erroneous diagnosis of asthma. As the disease progresses, the intervals between acute exacerbations tend to become shorter. Late in the course of COPD, an exacerbation may give rise to severe hypoxemia with cyanosis; the latter is accentuated if erythrocytosis is present. Morning headache may be indicative of hypercapnia. Hypercapnia with more severe hypoxemia, sometimes with erythrocytosis, is a feature of many patients with end-stage disease. Weight loss is an important feature in some patients. Cor pulmonale with right-sided heart failure and edema may complicate the course of patients with hypoxemia and hypercapnia.

Since bronchogenic carcinoma occurs with increased frequency in smokers with COPD, an episode of hemoptysis raises the possibility that carcinoma has developed. However, most episodes of hemoptysis complicating chronic bronchitis are caused by mucosal erosion and not by carcinoma. Indeed, hemoptysis complicating chronic bronchitis is currently the most common cause of mucosal erosion in the United States. The need for bronchoscopy and other studies to exclude carcinoma when hemoptysis occurs in a patient with chronic bronchitis is evident.

Physical examination

Early in the course of COPD, physical examination of the chest may not be remarkable except for the auscultation of wheezes. As airways obstruction progresses, hyperinflation of the lungs becomes evident. The chest's anteroposterior diameter is increased because the lungs are near their full inspiratory position. The diaphragm is depressed and limited in its motion. Breath sounds are usually depressed at this stage, and heart sounds often become distant because of the interposition of emphysematous lung between the heart and anterior chest wall. Wheezes are usually heard during only slightly accentuated breathing but may sometimes be audible only during a forced expiration. A few coarse crackles are often heard at the lung bases.

The patient with end-stage COPD often presents a dramatic sight. He stands before a counter or chest of drawers leaning forward, with arms outstretched and weight supported on the palms. The accessory respiratory muscles of the neck and shoulder girdle are in full use. Expiration often occurs through pursed lips. The chest appears overinflated both because of the large total lung capacity of emphysema and because the chest is held near full inspiration. Paradoxic drawing in of the lower interspaces is often clearly evident. Cyanosis may be present.

The signs of pulmonary hypertension and right ventricular hypertrophy are usually not detectable on physical examination in patients with COPD because of the interposition of emphysematous lung between heart and chest wall. An enlarged tender liver indicates heart failure; neck vein distention, especially during expiration, may be observed in the absence of heart failure because of increased intrathoracic pressure. Asterixis may be seen with severe hypercapnia.

LABORATORY FINDINGS

Chest radiography

Since emphysema is defined in anatomic terms, the chest radiograph provides the clearest evidence of its presence. Persistent marked overdistention of the lungs is strongly suggestive of emphysema. Overdistention of the lungs is indicated by a low, flat diaphragm. The lateral view shows an increased retrosternal air space, and the angle formed by the sternum and the diaphragm, instead of being acute, is 90 degrees or greater. The heart shadow tends to be long and narrow. Excessively rapid tapering of the vascular shadows is a sign of emphysema, but it is difficult to be certain about this subjective observation unless it is accompanied by obvious hypertransradiancy of the lungs. Bullae, presenting as radiolucent areas larger than 1 cm in diameter and surrounded by arcuate hairline shadows, are proof of the presence of emphysema. However, bullae reflect only locally severe disease, and their presence does not necessarily indicate widespread emphysema. Computed tomography (CT) clearly shows the hypovascular areas and bullae of emphysema, but because the diagnosis would not ordinarily change management, this test should not be used routinely.

The complication of COPD by right ventricular hypertrophy does not result in cardiomegaly. Comparison with previous chest radiographs may show that the transverse cardiac shadow, although still within normal limits, is wider than before. The heart shadow may be seen to encroach on the retrosternal space as it enlarges anteriorly. The hilar vascular shadows are prominent.

Pulmonary function tests

Pulmonary function measurements are helpful in diagnosis, in assessing the severity of COPD, and in following its progress. Airflow obstruction is an important indicator of impairment of the whole person and of the likelihood of blood gas abnormalities. The FEV_1 is an easily measurable index of airflow limitation that has less variability than other measurements of airways dynamics and that is more accurately predictable from age, sex, and height. Roughly comparable information can be obtained from the peak flow measurement or from the forced expiratory flow-volume curve (Chapter 195). None of these tests can distinguish between chronic bronchitis and emphysema.

The FEV_1 and the FEV_1/forced vital capacity (FVC) ratio fall progressively as the severity of COPD increases. About 30% of COPD patients have an increase of 20% or more in their FEV_1 after treatment in the laboratory with a beta-agonist aerosol; in a few patients the response exceeds 25%. The absence of a bronchodilator response during a single visit to the laboratory should never be used as justification for withholding bronchodilator therapy.

Lung volume measurements show an increase in total lung capacity, functional residual capacity, and residual volume. The vital capacity is decreased. The single-breath carbon monoxide diffusing capacity is decreased in proportion to the severity of emphysema because of the loss of alveolar capillary bed that is part of the destructive process of emphysema. The test is not specific and cannot detect mild emphysema.

Arterial blood gas measurement reveals mild or moderate hypoxemia without hypercapnia in the early stages of COPD. As the disease progresses, hypoxemia becomes more severe and hypercapnia supervenes. Hypercapnia is observed with increasing frequency as the FEV_1 falls below 1 L. Blood gas abnormalities worsen during acute exacerbations and may worsen during exercise and sleep.

Troublesome erythrocytosis is infrequently observed in patients living at sea level who have arterial oxygen tension (PaO_2) levels greater than 55 mm Hg; the frequency of erythrocytosis increases as PaO_2 levels fall below 55 mm Hg. The reasons for failure of the bone marrow to respond to mild or moderate levels of hypoxemia are complex. Matched hypoxemic patients with and without erythrocytosis have no differences in blood erythropoietin levels or in the sensitivity of bone marrow red cell precursors to erythropoietin. Single measures of blood oxygenation are not representative of a patient's mean daily saturation. Intermittent hypoxemia, as during sleep, is a potent stimulus for erythropoietin production. Elevated levels of carboxyhemoglobin contribute to polycythemia in smokers. Given the many factors that influence oxygen delivery to the tissues (hemoglobin concentration, red cell 2,3-diphosphoglycerate concentration, blood carboxyhemoglobin concentration, cardiac output, blood pH and carbon dioxide tension, local tissue blood flow), a variable relation between blood oxygen level and red cell mass in COPD is not surprising.

Sputum examination

In patients with stable chronic bronchitis, sputum is mucoid and the predominant cell is the macrophage. With an exacerbation, sputum usually becomes purulent, and microscopic examination shows an influx of neutrophils. The Gram stain usually shows a mixture of organisms, often gram-positive diplococci, characteristic of *Streptococcus pneumoniae,* and pleomorphic fine gram-negative rods, characteristic of *Haemophilus influenzae*. These are the most frequent pathogens cultured from the sputum. Other oropharyngeal commensal flora such as *Moraxella catarrhalis,* which have been recently shown occasionally to cause exacerbations, can be recovered. However, cultures and even Gram stains are rarely necessary before instituting antimicrobial therapy in outpatients. In hospitalized patients, Gram stains and cultures may reveal infection with a gram-negative rod or rarely a staphylococcus.

DIAGNOSIS

The history and physical examination suggest the possibility of COPD. A chest radiograph excludes other diagnoses (e.g., tuberculosis, lung cancer) that can give rise to the same symptoms and may reveal the findings of emphysema or of a complicating pneumonia. Forced expiratory spirometry and arterial blood gas measurements provide the basic physiologic assessment needed to quantify airways obstruction and the presence and severity of hypoxemia and hypercapnia. A postbronchodilator improvement of the FEV_1 by more than 25% suggests that a trial of corticosteroids may be helpful. Measurements of lung volumes, diffusing capacity, or physiologic responses to exercise usually add little unless the diagnosis is in doubt or surgical risk is being assessed.

TREATMENT

The ambulatory management of patients with COPD is considered here under three headings: specific, symptomatic, and secondary therapy. The management of acute respiratory failure complicating COPD is briefly discussed under that heading; the reader should also refer to a detailed discussion of acute respiratory failure.

Specific therapy

Specific therapy may be considered as dealing with the root causes of COPD. Support during smoking cessation and evaluation and counseling regarding environmental irritants in the workplace or elsewhere fall into this category. Influenza vaccine should be given annually because of the greater risk of serious complications of influenza in these patients. Although some question surrounds its efficacy in COPD, pneumococcal vaccine should be given once every 6 years.

Smoking cessation. Every effort should be made to help the patient with COPD stop smoking, especially if airways obstruction is mild or moderate. Many strategies have been tried to accomplish this aim; hypnotism, behavior modification techniques, group sessions, and nicotine given transdermally or as gum are all in use. No single "best" technique exists. However, it is important to stress the importance of the physician as the initiator of a smoking cessation effort. About 5% of patients stop smoking simply in response to 1 or 2 minutes of such advice. The cessation rate is higher if this advice is supplemented by a self-help manual, such as the one distributed by the American Lung Association, *Freedom from Smoking*. Physicians should also consider referring patients to services in their community that offer smoking cessation programs. Of patients seeking help in smoking cessation programs, only 25% to 39% are not smoking 1 year later.

After smoking cessation, cough and expectoration diminish over a period of a few months; sputum may become more viscid. Understanding what happens to lung function is more complex. Longitudinal studies show that ventilatory function, as measured by the FEV_1 in nonsmokers, declines by 25 to 30 ml/year, along a curvilinear path, beginning at about age 30 (Fig. 205-3). The rate of decline for all smokers is steeper than for nonsmokers. Middle-aged smokers whose FEV_1 is diminished on entry into the study decline at a more rapid rate than the general population of smokers. These persons reach an FEV_1 of 0.8 L, the level at which dyspnea during activities of daily living supervenes, in their sixth decade, whereas most smokers and normal persons do not reach this level even in their tenth decade. After smokers give up the habit, the rate of decline of FEV_1 follows a path that is below but parallel to that of nonsmokers. Thus, although lost lung function is not regained, smoking cessation delays the time of onset of dyspnea on effort, as well as the risk of dying of acute respiratory failure or some other complication of COPD.

Symptomatic therapy

Symptomatic therapy is directed against the reversible elements of airflow obstruction. These result from bronchiolar inflammation, luminal secretions, and smooth muscle spasm.

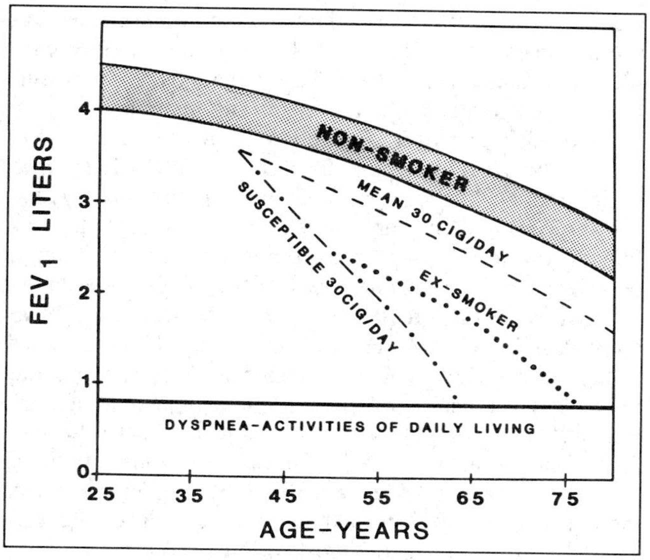

Fig. 205-3. Schema of natural history of COPD. Nonsmokers lose FEV_1 at an accelerating rate with age; the average loss is about 30 ml/year. Smokers of 30 cigarettes/day average a slightly greater rate of decline and have FEV_1 values slightly below average when first studied at age 40. A small proportion of susceptible smokers (10% to 15% of smoking population) lose function much more rapidly (150 ml/year) and have an FEV_1 of 0.8 L at age 65, a level that is so low that they experience dyspnea during activities of daily living. A susceptible smoker who stops smoking at age 50 does not regain any lost function but subsequently loses function at the rate for nonsmokers. Dyspnea on activities of daily living will develop at age 76, 11 years later than if the person had continued to smoke.

Bronchodilator drugs

Sympathomimetics. Although most of the airways obstruction in patients with COPD is fixed and irreversible, there is a high prevalence of partial reversibility with 250 μg of inhaled isoproterenol. The amount of reversibility of the FEV_1 averages 15% of the baseline value, with about one third of patients showing responses of 20% or greater. COPD patients with the greatest bronchodilator responses have the lowest annual decline in FEV_1 and the greatest 5-year survival. The hypothesis that regular bronchodilator therapy may slow deterioration of lung function and provide symptomatic relief is currently under investigation in a large clinical trial, the National Heart, Lung and Blood Institute's Lung Health Study.

The agents of choice are the *beta$_2$-adrenergic agonists,* which are defined as having less cardioaccelerator effect for a given amount of bronchodilation than the less selective beta agonists. The newer agents in this category, such as terbutaline, metaproterenol, and albuterol, are effective both by ingestion and by inhalation and act for up to 6 hours. They relieve smooth muscle spasm and enhance mucociliary clearance.

Administration of the beta$_2$ agonists by inhalation produces a more rapid onset of action and greater bronchodilator effect than oral administration and does so with fewer side effects, such as skeletal muscle tremor. The preferred mode of administration is the metered-dose inhaler (MDI); orally administered beta$_2$ agonists have little place in the treatment of COPD. The MDI should be prescribed on a timed-dose schedule, such as two puffs four or five times daily with the option of using the drugs in additional amounts or additional times on an as-needed basis. Patients should be taught to inhale the aerosol slowly, starting at the resting end-expiratory position, with a brief breath-hold at the end of a full inhalation. When patients cannot perform the MDI maneuver appropriately, the aerosol may be inhaled after delivery into a small chamber or spacer.

Anticholinergics. Anticholinergic agents are time-honored in the treatment of asthma. Their mode of action is not clearly understood; they may act by inhibiting normal, cholinergically mediated bronchomotor tone. Atropine aerosol has bronchodilator properties but is readily absorbed, giving rise to the systemic symptoms of atropinism. The quaternary ammonium compound *ipratropium bromide* is poorly absorbed and is available in an MDI. This agent is effective for 4 to 6 hours, but its peak effect is not reached until 1 to 2 hours. It does not affect mucociliary clearance and has few side effects. In usual doses, ipratropium has had a statistically greater bronchodilating effect in COPD than the beta$_2$ aerosols in many but not all published studies; in absolute terms the differences are not great. In studies in which the agents have been given sequentially in large doses, ipratropium and the beta$_2$ agonist have usually been equipotent.

Beta$_2$ agonists versus ipratropium. Because of their lower cost and more rapid onset of action, it seems reasonable to initiate bronchodilator therapy with a beta$_2$ agonist MDI and to continue such therapy in patients whose airways obstruction is well controlled. Trial of a fixed schedule of inhaled ipratropium seems reasonable for COPD patients who are not doing well with the beta$_2$ agonist, whether because of severe side effects or poor bronchodilator response.

Theophylline. Theophylline has been a mainstay in the management of obstructive airways disease for more than 60 years, but the drug has undergone intensive re-evaluation in the last 2 decades. Its mode of action is poorly understood but appears to be different from that of either the sympathomimetics or the anticholinergics. Theophylline decreases smooth muscle spasm, enhances mucociliary clearance, improves right ventricular function, and decreases pulmonary vascular resistance and arterial pressure. Its role in improving diaphragmatic function and dyspnea on exercise is controversial.

The toxicity of theophylline is weakly related to its blood levels. Sleeplessness and gastrointestinal upset occur often at blood levels less than 20 mg/L and tend to subside with time. More serious toxicity, such as supraventricular and ventricular arrhythmias and seizures, tend to occur at blood levels greater than 20 mg/L. However, individual variation in susceptibility to toxic effects of theophylline is great. Some patients manifest little toxicity at blood levels greater than 30 mg/L; others, especially patients over age 60, may manifest serious toxicity at blood levels that are slightly above 20 mg/L; manifestations of minor toxicity need not precede major toxicity.

Extreme variability exists in hepatic excretion of theophylline by different patients and even by the same patient at different times. Age, cigarette smoking, diet, hepatic dysfunction, severe hypoxemia, and some drugs can influence the rate of theophylline clearance. The only way to be sure that a patient's theophylline blood level is in the therapeutic range is to obtain a blood level after a steady state is achieved, usually 2 to 4 days. Repeat blood levels are infrequently needed in stable, ambulatory patients but are necessary if the patient's clinical state or the treatment regimen has undergone much change.

A linear relation exists between response of the FEV_1 in reversible airways obstruction and the logarithm of the theophylline blood level. Consequently, there is much less responce of the FEV_1 between 15 and 20 mg/L of theophylline than between 10 and 15 mg/L. Given the great variability of theophylline metabolism and the narrow margin between safe and potentially dangerous blood levels, it is appropriate to adjust the theophylline dose to achieve a target blood level of 10 ± 3 mg/L. This provides a reasonable margin between efficacy and toxicity.

A major advance in ambulatory theophylline therapy has been the development of long-acting, slow-release anhydrous theophylline preparations that are well absorbed after oral ingestion and improve patient compliance. A variety of tablet sizes simplifies dose adjustments. Formulations are available that can be given every 12 or 24 hours, although rapid metabolizers may require more frequent dosing. The physician should become familiar with one or two preparations and continue using them unless good reason exists to change. Toxicity can be minimized by combining a low dose of theophylline with a low dose of ipratropium or a $beta_2$ agonist inhaled from an MDI; bronchodilatation after combined therapy is additive rather than synergistic.

Corticosteroids. Most patients with COPD do not respond to corticosteroids when they are in the chronic stable state. However, about 15% of patients show sizable objective responses in ventilatory function after corticosteroid administration. The responders are generally those with improvement of the FEV_1 of 25% or more after a bronchodilator aerosol. A trial of oral corticosteroids should only be initiated after patients have been on an optimum treatment regimen. A 2- to 4-week trial of prednisone in a dose of 0.5 mg/kg body weight (or equivalent) should be instituted. The drug should be continued only if objective evidence of improvement exists. The dose should then be reduced to the lowest level that maintains improvement. The use of aerosolized corticosteroids in patients with COPD remains experimental.

Antibiotics. It is unclear in many exacerbations of COPD whether the bronchial inflammation manifest by the development of purulent sputum is caused by infection or has some other basis, such as exposure for several days to heavily polluted air. Furthermore, it is not usually clear whether the infection is bacterial or viral, and about 25% of exacerbations are believed to be viral. Nevertheless, most clinicians prescribe antibiotics for these exacerbations. Controlled trials in general show that antibiotic-treated exacerbations are briefer and less likely to have serious consequences than placebo-treated exacerbations. Routine cultures are not indicated before instituting treatment.

Frequently employed oral antibiotics to manage a COPD exacerbation include ampicillin (250 to 500 mg four times daily), tetracycline (250 mg four times daily), doxycycline (100 to 200 mg daily), and trimethoprim (160 mg) plus sulfamethoxazole (800 mg) twice daily. Because of the high prevalence of tetracycline-resistant *S. pneumoniae* and a low but increasing frequency of *H. influenzae* resistant to ampicillin (both beta lactamase and non–beta lactamase related), it is logical to use trimethoprim-sulfamethoxazole for most exacerbations. Amoxicillin-clavulanate (Augmentin), ofloxacin (Floxin), and cefuroxime axetil (Ceftin) are also effective against beta lactamase–producing strains of *H. influenzae* and *M. catarrhalis,* but these agents are much more expensive than trimethoprim-sulfamethoxazole and should be reserved for the most seriously ill patients.

Patients should be taught to recognize the change in sputum character from mucoid to purulent and to institute a 10- to 14-day course of antibiotic therapy on their own. Long-term antibiotic prophylaxis should be considered only in patients who have repeated exacerbations on an intermittent regimen.

Thinning and mobilization of secretions. Viscid secretion in peripheral airways is an important mechanism of airways obstruction in COPD. Unfortunately, our ability to effect thinning of secretion or to help patients mobilize their secretions is limited. No drugs, whether administered orally or by inhalation, are effective in thinning secretions. Dehydration causes secretions to become thick, but aggressive hydration does not favorably affect sputum volume or characteristics or ease of expectoration. It is reasonable to advise patients to drink enough fluid to keep the urine pale except for the first morning voiding. Inhaling steam from hot water in the bathroom sink may help patients expectorate secretions. Controlled coughing, consisting of two or three coughs in succession after a deep inhalation, assists in sputum mobilization. Chest wall percussion with cupped hands or an electromechanical percussor, administered in the lateral decubitus, prone, and supine positions, may provide additional assistance in sputum mobilization in the most difficult cases.

Secondary therapy

Secondary therapy is treatment designed to improve the function of the whole person while having little effect on the underlying pulmonary disease. A carefully integrated rehabilitation program, which helps the patient accommodate to physiologic limitations while at the same time providing realistic expectations for improvement, is important in managing patients with severe COPD. The patient's acceptance of responsibility for the treatment regimen is important.

Long-term oxygen therapy. It is now firmly established that long-term oxygen therapy (LTOT) or domiciliary O_2 therapy prolongs life in hypoxemic COPD patients. A 24-hour regimen is better than a nocturnal or 12-hour regimen. In addition to prolonging life, LTOT results in a fall in hematocrit toward normal levels, moderate neuropsychologic improvement, and amelioration of pulmonary hemodynamic abnormalities. LTOT is safe, with no increase in fire hazard. Pulmonary O_2 toxicity is not a problem, and increases in arterial carbon dioxide tension ($PaCO_2$) in patients with hypercapnia are minimal.

Indications. LTOT should be prescribed for patients who have a resting PaO_2 of 55 mm Hg or less while breathing air. For those whose resting PaO_2 is 56 to 59 mm Hg, LTOT is indicated if they demonstrate erythrocytosis (hematocrit, 55% or more) or evidence of cor pulmonale. Stable ambulatory patients should meet these criteria after being on an optimum treatment regimen for at least 30 days. LTOT should be prescribed for hospitalized patients who meet the criteria as soon as they are ready for discharge from the hospital. Their room air PaO_2 should be reassessed after 30 days to determine if they still meet the criteria for LTOT.

Decreases in Pao_2 during brief exercise are probably not harmful. The diffusing capacity for carbon monoxide may be used to predict desaturation with exercise in patients with COPD; desaturation occurs only when the single-breath diffusing capacity is less than 55% of predicted values. It seems reasonable to limit exercise testing to COPD patients with limited exercise tolerance who have a diffusing capacity less than 55% of predicted values, whose room air PaO_2 is 60 mm Hg or higher, and who are highly motivated to work or perform major exercise. O_2 may be prescribed for patients with a PaO_2 greater than 60 mm Hg who desaturate on low-level exercise to a PaO_2 of 55 mm Hg or less.

A sleep study should be considered only for patients with advanced COPD who do not meet the criteria for LTOT but whose clinical assessment suggests the ill effects of hypoxemia. Nocturnal O_2 may be prescribed if a sleep study reveals episodic desaturation to 80% or less for more than 5 minutes, since it would be imprudent to assume that such episodes are harmless. The consequences of nocturnal desaturations include transient periods of pulmonary hypertension and an increase in ventricular ectopy, along with electrocardiographic (ECG) changes of prolonged QT interval, ST-T depression, and bundle branch block.

Modes of oxygen administration. O_2 is administered by nasal cannula at a flow rate sufficient to achieve a PaO_2 greater than 60 mm Hg or saturation more than 90%; this usually requires a flow of 3 L/min or less with the patient at rest. O_2 is supplied by electrically driven O_2 concentrators, as liquid O_2 systems, or in cylinders of compressed gas. Concentrators are the method of choice for patients who spend most of their time at home, since this system is the least expensive of the three. Such patients require small O_2 tanks as backup in the event of an electrical failure and for portable use while walking.

A liquid system is preferable if patients spend much time out of their homes. The portable canisters that are part of liquid systems are easier to carry and have more O_2 capacity than portable cylinders of compressed gas. Large cylinders are the most expensive way of providing O_2 for LTOT and should be used only if no other source is available. All patients must be taught the dangers of smoking during O_2 use.

A variety of devices have been developed that conserve the amount of O_2 used by the patient. These O_2-conserving devices operate either by use of a reservoir system or by permitting O_2 flow only during inspiration. They have been shown to be equivalent to continuous-flow systems. Transtracheal catheter systems have the disadvantage of being invasive but the advantage of being less obtrusive than nasal cannulas. These systems have also been able to correct hypoxemia in patients refractory to high-flow O_2 by nasal cannula.

Exercise programs. Patients who are sedentary because they are dyspneic on exercise or who have undergone a prolonged period of inactivity because they have been hospitalized for respiratory failure develop severe skeletal muscle deconditioning. As a result, they have increased ventilatory and cardiovascular requirements during exercise. These effects can be ameliorated by a program of graded exercise. In seriously deconditioned patients with end-stage COPD, supplemental O_2 therapy is useful in the initial stages of the program. Relief of severe hypoxemia increases exercise tolerance. Training of the respiratory muscles is controversial and seems to have little advantage over exercise training of the whole person. Upper extremity exercises using light weights should be instituted; this approach is based on the observation that unsupported arm exercise results in dyspnea and fatigue at a much lower O_2 uptake than exercise performed by the lower extremities.

These patients should be taught methods of energy conservation during activities of daily living. Difficulties in sexual function should also be explored and advice given on the use of energy-conserving positions for sexual intercourse or noncoital alternatives for sexual gratification.

Noninvasive mechanical ventilation. The use of noninvasive mechanical ventilators in an attempt to rest respiratory muscles is based on the concept that in patients with severe COPD, the respiratory muscles are at the fatigue threshold. Nocturnal resting of the muscles might improve daytime functioning. Although some trials of nocturnal noninvasive ventilation have shown benefit, other long-term trials have not demonstrated improved gas exchange or respiratory muscle function, and many patients did not tolerate the treatment. These methods remain under investigation.

Nutrition. Many patients with advanced COPD experience major but slowly progressive weight loss, and some of them become frankly cachectic. In others the weight loss occurs stepwise, seemingly precipitated by a superimposed acute illness or hospitalization. These patients show no evidence of protein malnutrition; lean body mass is preserved, and serum albumin is normal. The cause of this excessive weight loss is mainly a 15% to 25% increase in resting energy expenditure, perhaps the result of a greatly elevated work of breathing. Increased diet-induced thermogenesis, a higher energy cost of daily activities, and a reduced caloric intake relative to need may be other important factors. One consequence of this excessive weight loss is reduced respiratory muscle strength.

Improved nutrition can restore respiratory and general muscle strength and endurance, but such improvement occurs only after clear-cut weight gain. Unfortunately, this has been consistently accomplished only within a controlled hospital environment, with little success in patients living at home.

Drugs affecting ventilatory control. Drugs that stimulate respiration have never acquired a secure place in the management of COPD in the United States. Acetazolamide, a carbonic anhydrase inhibitor that stimulates ventilation by acidifying plasma and cerebrospinal fluid, does not effectively sustain increased ventilation in hypercapnic COPD patients. Medroxyprogesterone can improve arterial blood gases in patients with modest airways obstruction but is not effective in patients with severe obstruction. Almitrine bismesylate is not available for general use in the United States. The drug increases Pao_2 in about 80% of patients. It is effective during exercise and sleep and acts mainly by improving ventilation-perfusion mismatch. The drug may cause neurotoxicity and weight loss; some investigators have reported pulmonary hypertension as a complication.

Many patients with severe COPD have disabling dyspnea unresponsive to standard therapy. Some of these patients experience a significant reduction in their breathlessness and improve their exercise tolerance after moderate doses of opiates such as dihydrocodeine. These agents seem to reduce respiratory drive and the perception of dyspnea while reducing O_2 consumption during rest and exercise. Arterial blood gases seem to change minimally. Unfortunately, many patients experience intolerable side effects (e.g., nausea, emesis, drowsiness) during long-term use of these drugs, and their ultimate value as a management aid in COPD remains uncertain and experimental.

Pulmonary rehabilitation. Pulmonary rehabilitation may be defined as a program designed to improve the functioning of the whole person once everything possible has been done to improve the function of the lungs. The reader will quickly recognize that many elements of a rehabilitation program for COPD patients have been discussed. However, many important aspects of rehabilitation have not been stressed: the importance of educating the patient and the family about the nature of the illness and how to care for it; the importance of the patient taking as much responsibility for personal care as possible; and finally, the use of specialists in physical therapy, occupational therapy, psychiatry, social services, and vocational counseling.

The benefits of rehabilitation are improved independence and quality of life, decreased hospital days, and improved exercise capacity. Lung function usually is not improved. Every physician who treats end-stage COPD will organize a rehabilitation program for the patient. However, many hospitals and health care organizations have developed formal, multidisciplinary rehabilitation programs with an intensive, focused approach. These programs are especially important for persons who remain ventilator-bound after an episode of acute respiratory failure. Many such patients can attain a few hours per day off the ventilator and can be taught to participate in their own care. Patients can often be sent home on ventilators, receiving care from family members and professional caregivers. Although costs are great for home ventilator care, they are much lower than for such care in the hospital.

STAGING OF THERAPY

The treatment techniques discussed in this chapter need to be applied to ambulatory COPD patients in a graded manner depending on the severity of their airways obstruction, the symptoms they display, their tolerance for the medications, and the reversibility of their airways obstruction. In mild disease a $beta_2$-adrenergic agonist administered by an MDI may be all that is necessary. An alternative is a low dose (5 to 10 mg/kg/day) of a long-acting oral theophylline preparation. For more troublesome complaints, ipratropium by MDI may be tried, or a combination of low-dose theophylline with one of the aerosol medications can be given. As-needed administration of an inhaled $beta_2$ agonist by MDI should always be prescribed. A short trial of oral corticosteroids should be considered in patients with an acute exacerbation of their disease, with rapid tapering of the drugs as the exacerbation subsides. In patients with severe chronic disease a trial of inhaled corticosteroids should be instituted, and if necessary, this can be combined with daily or every-other-day oral prednisone therapy. Oral corticosteroids should be given over long periods only if they have been shown objectively to be effective. Patients should be taught to inspect their sputum and to distinguish between mucoid and purulent secretions. They should begin a course of antibiotics at home as soon as an exacerbation has clearly begun. If cough alone is inadequate to mobilize excessive secretions, chest physical therapy measures should be instituted.

For patients with severe COPD, LTOT should be administered to relieve hypoxemia and the effects of tissue hypoxia, using the guidelines outlined earlier. An exercise program should be instituted, especially for patients who have required a period of hospitalization for an acute medical incident. Lifelong medical supervision and support are an essential part of relieving suffering for these patients.

LUNG TRANSPLANTATION FOR EMPHYSEMA

With the advent of heart-lung or double-lung transplantation, considerable progress has been made over the past 10 years in lung transplantation for obstructive airways disease. Most of the patients who have received transplants had API deficiency. Since 1989, single-lung transplantation has largely replaced double-lung transplantation in these patients. Single-lung transplantation is a much easier procedure to perform than double-lung transplantation. Cardiac bypass is usually not necessary. The surgical, early, and late morbidity and the mortality are lower in single-lung than in double-lung transplantation. Postoperative follow-up is still brief. Also, the FVC and FEV_1 are lower for single-lung than for double-lung transplantation. An excess of ventilation over perfusion occurs in the transplanted lung, but this has little effect on improvement in exercise performance in single-lung compared with double-lung transplantation. Arterial blood gases are similarly improved in the two procedures. Single-lung transplantation is more applicable to an older population than double-lung transplantation. The frequency of transplantable lungs from universal donors is considerably lower than with other solid organs, such as kidneys or livers; thus limited availability of donor lungs is a limiting factor for this expensive treatment.

COMPLICATIONS

Sleep and COPD

A slight decrease in alveolar ventilation is normal during sleep. This is manifest as a 5 to 6 mm Hg increase in $PaCO_2$ and a slightly greater decrease in PaO_2. Patients with COPD have a greater decrease in alveolar ventilation with sleep than normal persons; the increase in $PaCO_2$ and decrease in PaO_2 are also greater than in normal individuals. Since awake PaO_2 is on the shoulder of the oxyhemoglobin dissociation curve in many COPD patients, the decrease in saturation will be much greater in the COPD patient than in the normal person. The decrease in blood O_2 level is greatest during rapid eye movement (REM) sleep and also tends to become greater as the night progresses, perhaps as a result of retention of secretions and worsening ventilation-perfusion relations. Patients with COPD may have hypopnea, but episodes of apnea are distinctly uncommon. The quality of sleep is impaired. Severe nocturnal hypoxemia is associated with increased frequency of cardiac arrhythmias and development of pulmonary hypertension.

Supplemental O_2 therapy alleviates the hypoxemia and its consequences and improves quality of sleep. Relief of hypoxemia by nocturnal O_2 therapy also probably plays a role in the correction of secondary erythrocytosis, the decreased rate of progression of cor pulmonale, and the improved survival that occur with LTOT.

Acute respiratory failure

Acute respiratory failure in patients with COPD may be defined as an exacerbation that is accompanied by a PaO_2 less than 50 mm Hg or a $PaCO_2$ greater than 50 mm Hg. Respiratory depressant drugs, abdominal or thoracic surgery, or complications such as pneumothorax are additional precipitating factors. It is unusual for the $PaCO_2$ to rise above 80 mm Hg unless the patient has received O_2 therapy. The patient's clinical state during an episode of acute respiratory failure is highly variable. Mental state ranges from alert, anxious, agitated and distressed to somnolent, stuporous, or comatose. Cyanosis is usually present unless the patient is receiving O_2 therapy. Diaphoresis and a hyperdynamic circulation typically occur. Breathing is labored, and the accessory muscles are in full use.

The first goal in treatment is to improve hypoxemia and prevent tissue hypoxia. This goal may be quickly reached by administering low, controlled concentrations of O_2 sufficient to raise the PaO_2 to 55 to 60 mm Hg (arterial O_2 saturation, 88% to 90%), which will prevent tissue hypoxia but not completely abolish hypoxic ventilatory drive. The small increase in PaO_2 occurs on the steep part of the oxyhemoglobin dissociation curve, resulting in a large increase in saturation. A Venturi mask that delivers 24% to 28% O_2 or a nasal cannula with an O_2 flow of 1 to 2 L/min may be used. A slight increase in $PaCO_2$ may occur, but since blood bicarbonate levels usually have risen in response to chronic hypercapnia, worsening of acidemia will be slight. Increases in $PaCO_2$ that do not cause decreases in pH below 7.25 are tolerable.

The next step in management is to institute therapy to overcome reversible airways obstruction. Hydration should be started, along with intravenous aminophylline and corticosteroids. Appropriate antibiotic therapy should be given after a Gram stain and culture of sputum have been done. Inhalation therapy with a $beta_2$ agonist should be instituted. Re-evaluation of the patient should be carried out clinically and by blood gas measurement at least every 4 hours. The pH and $PaCO_2$ are the important indices to follow.

A high proportion of patients can be managed by a conservative regimen. Slightly worsening hypoxemia and acidemia are not themselves an indication for instituting mechanical ventilation, as long as they are associated with a stable or improving clinical state. The role of noninvasive methods of mechanical ventilation using intermittent positive pressure by nasal or face mask is under investigation. Deterioration in blood gases associated with clinical deterioration, especially the development of progressive fatigue and difficulty in cooperation, indicates the need for instituting endotracheal intubation and mechanical ventilation.

Once the patient is on a ventilator, it is important not to ventilate so vigorously that the $PaCO_2$ decreases rapidly. Since blood bicarbonate levels are usually high, a steep fall in $PaCO_2$ may result in severe alkalemia with convulsions, coma, and death. Careful attention should be paid to nutrition. Weaning from mechanical ventilation should be carried out as soon as possible, often within a few days. With a good rehabilitation program, many patients can be restored to their former level of function. Patients can be managed with endotracheal tubes for 3 to 4 weeks before a tracheostomy is done.

In managing ambulatory patients who have COPD with severe obstruction, it is important to determine in advance whether, in the event of acute respiratory failure, the patient wishes to be mechanically ventilated and take the risk of becoming tracheotomized and dependent on a ventilator.

Chronic cor pulmonale

Chronic cor pulmonale may be defined as right ventricular hypertrophy caused by pulmonary hypertension. Pulmonary arterial pressures may rise to a mean of 30 to 40 mm Hg at rest and higher on exercise, as opposed to the normal value of 10 to 20 mm Hg. Although loss of capillary bed resulting from emphysema may play some part, the major cause of the pulmonary hypertension in COPD patients is hypoxic vasoconstriction. Acidemia augments hypoxemia and may be important during sleep and exacerbations. Transmission of increased intrathoracic pressure is reflected in pulmonary arterial pressure measurement. Increased viscosity of blood from erythrocytosis is of minor importance, but hypervolemia may play some role. Left ventricular dysfunction is a minor contributor.

Short of right-sided heart catheterization, the diagnosis of pulmonary hypertension and cor pulmonale in COPD is difficult. An R or R′ wave greater than or equal to the S wave in lead V_1, an R wave less than the amplitude of the S wave in lead V_6, and right-axis deviation greater than 110 degrees without right bundle branch block all support the diagnosis of cor pulmonale. Two-dimensional echocardiography, especially with an esophageal transducer, and pulsed Doppler techniques to estimate mean pulmonary arterial pressure are recently developed modalities to assess pulmonary hypertension and right ventricular function. Left ventricular size and performance are generally normal in patients with COPD in the absence of other associated cardiac abnormalities. The right ventricular ejection fraction is frequently abnormal, especially on exercise. The radiographic diagnosis of cor pulmonale is discussed earlier in this chapter.

The treatment of cor pulmonale is the treatment of the underlying lung disease. Correction of hypoxemia by long-term O_2 therapy is essential. Diuretics are useful for the control of edema. Digitalis should be reserved for the management of a supraventricular tachyarrhythmia.

Pneumothorax

Unlike the benign nature of simple spontaneous pneumothorax occurring in a young person with localized bullae, pneumothorax complicating COPD often precipitates severe dyspnea and acute respiratory failure. This condition should be suspected in any patient with sudden worsening of pulmonary status. Physical examination is of limited help because diminished breath sounds, the cardinal sign of a small pneumothorax, also occur with emphysema. The diagnosis is readily made from the chest radiograph. Even a small pneumothorax can cause severe respiratory insufficiency in COPD patients with marginal pulmonary reserve.

Because it is often accompanied by a persistent bronchopleural fistula, pneumothorax complicating COPD is difficult to treat. Most bronchopleural fistulas close after several days of tube thoracostomy, although negative pressures of 30 cm of water or more may be required to expand the lung. If this fails to occur, an open thoracotomy with surgical closure of the fistula, along with bullectomy, pleurodesis, or a parietal pleurectomy, is often necessary. When pulmonary function is severely impaired, thoracotomy may be judged too hazardous to undertake. An attempt to obliterate the pleural space with the instillation of tetracycline is a useful alternative approach. Thoracoscopic intervention should be considered in the difficult case.

Giant bullae

Impairment of function. Large bullae that involve a third or more of one or both hemithoraces may severely disrupt lung function in the involved hemithorax and may even encroach on the opposite lung. Resectional surgery under these circumstances may produce a marked improvement in symptoms and lung function. The functional results of surgery are related to the amount of normal or minimally diseased lung tissue that was compressed by the resected bullae. The results of resection when the released lung tissue is severely emphysematous are disappointing and short-lived. Little improvement occurs in function after excision when bullae occupy less than one third of the hemithorax and lung function is normal or minimally impaired. In general, patients do best when they have large bullae and an FEV_1 of about half the predicted normal value. Serial chest radiographs and CT are most useful in making a decision as to whether compression of viable lung by bullae is responsible for a patient's current functional state or whether the process is part of generalized emphysema.

Infection. Infection with pyogenic organisms or with a fungus such as *Aspergillus* species, causing a mycetoma, may rarely occur within bullae. Treatment with appropriate antibiotics is indicated for pyogenic infection. Mycetomas rarely require therapy unless they are associated with life-threatening hemoptysis. In that event, resectional surgery or bronchial arterial embolization should be considered. Antifungal therapy is not indicated for mycetomas unless clear evidence exists of tissue invasion by the fungus.

COPD and commercial air travel

Because commercial airliners pressurize their flight cabins to an altitude of 5000 to 10,000 feet, COPD patients who fly in the stratosphere are subjected to the added stress of a significantly reduced inspired O_2 partial pressure. At an altitude of 5000 feet, the equivalent inspired fractional concentration of O_2 (FIO_2) is 17.1% and at 10,000 feet 13.9%. This may substantially worsen hypoxemia, since COPD patients have limited ability to increase their resting ventilation. Eucapnic COPD patients with a sea level PaO_2 greater than 68 mm Hg will generally have a flight PaO_2 greater than 50 mm Hg and will not require supplemental O_2. All COPD patients with hypercapnia as well as those with significant anemia (hematocrit < 30) or coexisting cardiac or cerebrovascular disease should use supplemental O_2 during flight.

When making their reservation, patients should notify an airline concerning their diagnosis and the need for in-flight O_2. Patients are not permitted to use their own O_2. The airlines will provide a chemically generated O_2 system at about $50 for each flight segment. Patients should bring their own nasal cannulas because airlines usually provide only face masks.

PROGNOSIS AND COURSE

Not surprisingly, in view of what has already been said about the importance of airways obstruction in causing death and disability, the severity of airways obstruction is related to survival in patients with COPD. Mortality slightly increases at 10 years in persons with moderate airways obstruction but with an FEV_1 greater than 1.0 L. In persons with FEV_1 values less than 0.75 L, the approximate mortality rate at 1 year is 30% and at 10 years 95%. Hypercapnia is an adverse prognostic factor. Recent data suggest that marked reversibility of airways obstruction is a favorable prognostic factor.

Longitudinal studies from several centers have shown that some patients with severe airways obstruction may survive for many years beyond the average, some for as long as 15 years. The reason for this appears to be that death in patients with COPD generally occurs because of some medical complication, such as acute respiratory failure, severe pneumonia, pneumothorax, cardiac arrhythmia, or pulmonary embolism. It is important for these patients to be able to enter the medical care system easily when they are acutely ill. Careful management of COPD patients can be rewarding not only because the physician's involvement in medical care relieves suffering, but also because it prolongs life.

REFERENCES

American Thoracic Society: Standards for the diagnosis and care of patients with chronic obstructive pulmonary disease (COPD) and asthma. Am Rev Respir Dis 136:225, 1987.

Anthonisen NR: Prognosis in chronic obstructive pulmonary disease: results from multicenter clinical trials. Am Rev Respir Dis 133:S95, 1989.

Buist AS et al: Guidelines for the approach to the individual with severe hereditary alpha-1-antitrypsin deficiency: an official statement of the American Thoracic Society. Am Rev Respir Dis 140:1494, 1989.

Clausen JL: The diagnosis of emphysema, chronic bronchitis and asthma. Clin Chest Med 11:405, 1990.

Donahoe M and Rogers RM: Nutritional assessment in chronic obstructive pulmonary disease. Clin Chest Med 11:487, 1990.

Douglas NJ and Flenley DC: Breathing during sleep in patients with obstructive lung disease. Am Rev Respir Dis 141:1055, 1990.

Hodgkin JE: Pulmonary rehabilitation. Clin Chest Med 11:447, 1990.

Hodgkin JE: Prognosis in chronic obstructive pulmonary disease. Clin Chest Med 11:555, 1990.

Hoyos AL et al: Pulmonary transplantation: early and late results. J Thorac Cardiovasc Surg 103:295, 1992.

Lucey EC, Stone PJ, and Snider GL: Consequences of proteolytic injury. In Crystal RG et al, editors: The lung: scientific foundations. New York, 1991, Raven.

Manley MW, Epps RP, and Glynn TJ: The physician's role in promoting smoking cessation among clinic patients. Med Clin North Am 76:477, 1992.

Mathay RA, Niederman MS, and Wiedemann HP: Cardiovascular pulmonary interaction in chronic obstructive pulmonary disease with special reference to the pathogenesis and management of cor pulmonale. Med Clin North Am 74:571, 1990.

O'Donohue WJ: Prescribing home oxygen therapy: what the primary care physician needs to know. Arch Intern Med 152:746, 1992.

Schwartz JL: Methods of smoking cessation. Med Clin North Am 76:451, 1992.

Sherrill DL, Lebowitz M, and Burrows B: Epidemiology of chronic obstructive pulmonary disease. Clin Chest Med 11:375, 1990.

Snider GL: Pulmonary disease in alpha-1-antitrypsin deficiency. Ann Intern Med 111:957, 1989.

Snider GL: Emphysema—the first two centuries—and beyond. Am Rev Respir Dis 146:1334, 1615, 1992.

Snider GL, Faling LJ, and Rennard SI: Chronic bronchitis and emphysema. In Murray JF and Nadel JA, editors: Textbook of respiratory medicine, ed 2. Philadelphia, 1993, Saunders.

Thurlbeck WM: Pathology of chronic airflow obstruction. In Cheriack NS, editor: Chronic obstructive pulmonary disease. Philadelphia, 1991, Saunders.

Transdermal Nicotine Study Group: Transdermal nicotine for smoking cessation: six-month results from two multicenter controlled clinical trials. JAMA 266:3133, 1991.

CHAPTER

206 Interstitial Lung Disease

Jack D. Fulmer

The interstitial lung diseases are diverse disorders grouped together because of common clinical, roentgenographic, and pathologic features. Most patients present with exertional dyspnea, and if the underlying pathologic process is unchecked, destruction of gas exchange units leads to end-stage lung disease.

The nomenclature for these diseases has varied. This chapter uses the term *interstitial* because most of these diseases result in the development of scar tissue in the alveolar interstitium. This term is only partly correct, however, since airways disease, alveolar filling disease, vascular disease, and pleural disease all can coexist with the interstitial disease. The term *infiltrative lung disease* also seems appropriate in some of these diseases, since it implies an abnormal accumulation of cells and noncellular elements in lung tissue. This is particularly applicable in the neoplastic diseases and in some metabolic or inherited interstitial lung diseases.

The objectives of this chapter are to present an overview of the pathologic, pathogenetic, pathophysiologic, and clinical features of these diseases. Then a rational approach to the decision making in the diagnosis and management of these diseases is presented. Finally, specific diseases are briefly discussed. This chapter's overall emphasis, however, is on the interstitial pneumonias.

LUNG PATHOLOGY

An understanding of the pathology of the interstitial lung diseases, particularly the acute injury patterns and the chronic interstitial pneumonias, is critical to diagnosis and management. The pathology of these diseases is remarkably similar and at times difficult for pathologists to classify. In almost all, there is an accumulation of cells within alveolar septae and air spaces, as well as alveolar septal fibrosis with destruction and revision of gas exchange units.

Depending on the etiology, chronicity, and several poorly understood modulating factors, the severity of the alveolitis, degree of fibrosis, and actual tissue destruction vary. In general, early disease is characterized by an active alveolitis with minimum alveolar septal fibrosis and destruction. In contrast, advanced disease is associated with minimum alveolitis but widespread alveolar destruction and fibrosis. If the disease is progressive, end-stage or "honeycomb" lung disease results.

Various pathologic classifications have been used, and when possible, the pathologist makes an etiologic or specific histologic diagnosis. Examples include many of the inorganic dust diseases, the infectious and neoplastic infiltrative diseases, the pulmonary vasculitides, and the pulmonary hemorrhage syndromes. Further, although special techniques may be required, information can be provided on both the natural and the treated history of many interstitial diseases. Some interstitial diseases have a specific histologic pattern, but only through careful clinical and radiographic correlation can a correct diagnosis be made.

The pathologic classification of the interstitial pneumonias has been controversial. One useful classification (see the box on right), which is a modification by Dr. Liebow, is now widely used and can be applied to the idiopathic interstitial pneumonias or the interstitial pneumonias of known etiology. This classification, however, incorrectly includes bronchiolitis obliterans–organizing pneumonia (BOOP). This is primarily an airways disease, not an interstitial disease; BOOP is included because some view it as part of the spectrum of the interstitial diseases, and often an interstitial pattern is evident on the chest roentgenogram. This classification also includes giant cell interstitial pneumonia (GIP), a rare, poorly understood entity. GIP probably is a form of organic dust disease caused by inhalation of heavy metals; this chapter does not discuss this disease further. A description of the interstitial pneumonias is presented in the following sections.

Pathologic classification of interstitial pneumonias

Acute

Acute interstitial pneumonia (AIP)
Bronchiolitis obliterans–organizing pneumonia (BOOP)

Chronic

Usual interstitial pneumonia (UIP)
Desquamative interstitial pneumonia (DIP) (respiratory bronchiolitis)
Chronic interstitial pneumonia–NOS* (CIP)
Lymphoid interstitial pneumonia (LIP)
Giant cell interstitial pneumonia (GIP)

*NOS, Not otherwise specified.

Acute interstitial pneumonia

Acute interstitial pneumonia (AIP) is a rare form of interstitial pneumonia corresponding to the lesion described by Hamman and Rich in 1944. The pathology of AIP is identical to that observed in diffuse alveolar damage (DAD), the pathology of the adult respiratory distress syndrome (ARDS). A single injury seems to occur at one point in time, after which an orderly sequence of events takes place. Initially, there is an exudative phase, which involves capillary congestion, interstitial edema, and alveolar exudation with the formation of hyaline membranes. After approximately 1 week, type II epithelial cells proliferate, and by the second week fibroblasts proliferate, resulting in an organizational phase. Interstitial fibrosis with the formation of end-stage lung disease can occur after 3 to 4 weeks. Thrombi are common in small arteries. The appearance of AIP, depending on the stage when biopsied, usually corresponds to the organizing stage of DAD. Examples of AIP were previously lumped with cases of usual interstitial pneumonia (UIP). However, AIP can be histologically distinguished by the uniformity of the lesions, reflecting an acute injury occurring at a single point in time.

Bronchiolitis obliterans–organizing pneumonia

Previously classified with the chronic interstitial pneumonias, BOOP is primarily a disease in which the fibrosing process involves air spaces and not alveolar interstitium. However, some alveolar septal thickening with an inflammatory cellular infiltrate, as well as type II epithelial hyperplasia, may occur. Ultrastructural studies have demonstrated alveolar epithelial necrosis and collapse, indicating that BOOP is an acute form of lung injury.

The fibrosing process in BOOP is characterized by polypoid plugs of loose connective tissue containing spindle-shaped fibroblasts and a chronic inflammatory cellular infiltrate with a loose, myxoid matrix. These plugs are present in distal bronchioles, alveolar ducts, and peribronchiolar air spaces. These polyps may be covered by a lining of bronchiolar or alveolar epithelial cells. These polypoid lesions may be a minor feature of some other interstitial pneumonia (e.g., UIP), the eosinophilic pneumonias, and Langerhans' cell granulomatosis (eosinophilic granuloma); the presence of these lesions, however, should not mislead the pathologist to make the diagnosis of BOOP. BOOP is usually a steroid-sensitive disease, and many cases of steroid-responsive UIP in the past literature likely represent examples of BOOP.

Usual interstitial pneumonia

UIP is the most common pathologic type of chronic interstitial pneumonia. The characteristic features are microscopic areas of normal lung alternating with areas of active alveolitis and varying degrees of fibrosis. The cellular infiltrate consists of macrophages, lymphocytes, and plasma cells. Although neutrophils are frequently seen on lung lavage cellular analysis, neutrophils are rarely present in tissue. UIP does not represent a specific clinical diagnosis, and the natural history of UIP varies depending on the clinical syndrome. UIP is a common histologic diagnosis in many of the collagen vascular diseases, radiation lung disease, and the late stages of sarcoidosis and some dust diseases. Patients with UIP who have a progressive bibasilar interstitial pattern on chest roentgenogram and no evidence of a systemic illness usually have idiopathic pulmonary fibrosis (IPF).

Desquamative interstitial pneumonia

Desquamative interstitial pneumonia (DIP) is characterized by a homogeneous filling of the alveolar air spaces with macrophages and a few type II epithelial cells. There is minimum alveolar septal infiltration with cells and connective tissue. This lesion was initially thought to represent an early stage of UIP but more likely represents a rare response to some type of parenchymal injury. Most cases are idiopathic, but DIP has been described in drug-induced interstitial disease and in some collagen vascular disorders. Rarely, DIP may progress to end-stage lung disease. Some other interstitial diseases may have an accumulation of macrophages in scattered areas with a "DIP-like reaction," but these differ from DIP by the coexistence of significant interstitial fibrosis and destruction of gas exchange units, a feature not present in DIP.

Although primarily a disease of the airways and more correctly grouped with the inhalation disorders, *respiratory bronchiolitis* may produce an interstitial pattern on the chest roentgenogram. A disease of smokers, respiratory bronchiolitis is characterized by numerous pigmented macrophages in respiratory bronchioles and neighboring alveolar ducts. Alveolar septae may show some fibrous thickening, and some type II epithelial cell hyperplasia may be present. Although most patients do not progress, it has been suggested that DIP may represent a late stage of a progressive form of respiratory bronchiolitis. It has been reported, however, that some patients with respiratory bronchiolitis may show improvement on roentgenograms with cessation of smoking.

Chronic interstitial pneumonia–NOS

A small but significant number of interstitial pneumonias cannot be classified using the previous criteria (NOS, not otherwise specified). Now called chronic interstitial pneumonia (CIP), this lesion was previously classified along with cases of UIP. Histologically, CIP is characterized by a temporally uniform interstitial pattern without the skip areas of normal lung tissue seen in UIP. The interstitial infiltrate consists of chronic inflammatory cells, fibroblasts, and variable degrees of fibrosis. This pattern can be associated with the collagen vascular disorders, drug reactions, organic and inorganic dust diseases, bone marrow transplantation, or acquired immunodeficiency syndrome (AIDS). CIP can also be idiopathic.

Lymphoid interstitial pneumonia

Lymphoid interstitial pneumonia (LIP) was first described as an interstitial disease with a cellular infiltrate consisting of lymphocytes, plasma cells, and an occasional immunoblast. It is now known that LIP usually is a lymphoproliferative disorder, probably a low-grade lymphoma. Some cases of LIP do represent a response to a viral infection; others are associated with an autoimmune disorder. This pattern has also been associated with AIDS, particularly in children. Infrequently, LIP is idiopathic, and progression to end-stage lung disease has been reported.

CLINICOPATHOLOGIC CLASSIFICATION

To approach the interstitial diseases in an orderly manner, some type of clinical or clinicopathologic classification is needed. Ideally, a classification should be based on etiology, but only about one half of these diseases have a defined etiology; the remainder must be classified by careful clinical, laboratory, and pathologic correlation (see the box below). This classification is flawed because several of these diseases have multiple clinicopathologic features. For example, many of the collagen vascular disorders, Wegener's granulomatosis, and several occupational lung diseases can present with diffuse alveolar hemorrhage. In addition,

Clinicopathologic classification of interstitial lung diseases

Known etiologies for interstitial diseases

- Occupational and environmental inhalants
  - Inorganic dusts
  - Organic dusts
  - Gases, fumes, vapors, aerosols
- Drugs
- Poisons
- Infectious agents
- Radiation
- Allergy
- Trauma
- Neoplastic diseases
- Hemodynamic/cardiac diseases
- Metabolic disorders
- Miscellaneous disorders

Interstitial diseases of unknown etiology

- Acute interstitial pneumonia (Hamman-Rich syndrome)
- Idiopathic pulmonary fibrosis
- Collagen vascular diseases
- Sarcoidosis
- Pulmonary vasculitis
- Hemorrhage syndromes
- Langerhans' cell granulomatosis (eosinophilic granuloma)
- Lymphoid infiltrative disorders
- Bronchiolar diseases
- Eosinophilic pneumonias
- Inherited diseases
- Non–collagen vascular immune diseases
- Pulmonary veno-occlusive disease
- Alveolar proteinosis
- Lymphangioleiomyomatosis
- Unclassified interstitial diseases

several alveolar filling diseases can ultimately progress to chronic interstitial fibrosis; these include the eosinophilic pneumonias, pulmonary alveolar proteinosis, and idiopathic pulmonary hemosiderosis.

PATHOGENESIS

Regardless of whether the etiology of the interstitial disease is known or unknown, current concepts are that most follow a common pathogenesis (Fig. 206-1). Initially, some type of stimulus occurs with injury to epithelial or endothelial cells, resulting in edema or cellular death. Proteinases may cause destruction of the basement membrane. As a result of the injury, there is activation of resident lung cells and exudation of serum and cellular debris into alveolar air spaces. Release of cytokines, with serum and cellular breakdown products, recruits inflammatory and immune effector cells into the alveolar interstitium and air spaces (e.g., an alveolitis). Cells of the alveolitis can amplify the injury but are also critical in the reparative process; they recruit and cause proliferation of fibroblasts and type II epithelial cells. The latter ultimately differentiate into type I cells. With a one-time injury, lung repair can be complete, or some residual scarring may occur. In the chronic interstitial pneumonias, there are continuous foci of alveolar injury, inflammation, destruction, and repair.

The injurious agents in these diseases are complex and poorly understood. Even among the interstitial diseases of known etiology, recent advances indicate multiple factors are responsible, including generation of toxic radicals, proteinases, and cationic proteins. Some of these diseases appear to have an immunopathogenesis resulting from immune complex deposition or from tissue-specific or cytotoxic antibodies. Cytokines are important in these diseases; tumor necrosis factor seems important to the initiation of the alveolitis in several types of experimental disease. In some acute and chronic interstitial diseases the alveolar macrophage appears to be central in both the exudative phase and the reparative phase. Previously viewed as only phagocytic cells, macrophages can secrete a variety of polypeptides, complement components, enzymes, lipids, and extracellular matrix proteins. Many of these products appear important in the pathogenesis of the interstitial diseases. Alveolar macrophages harvested from patients with chronic interstitial pneumonias secrete a variety of chemoattractants, including many interleukins and fibronectin, a glycoprotein that can recruit and promote replication of fibroblasts. Additional cytokines include platelet-derived growth factor, a potent mitogenic polypeptide for fibroblasts, and various other growth or competence factors that recruit, activate, and induce proliferation of fibroblasts, type II epithelial cells, and endothelial cells (see Fig. 206-1).

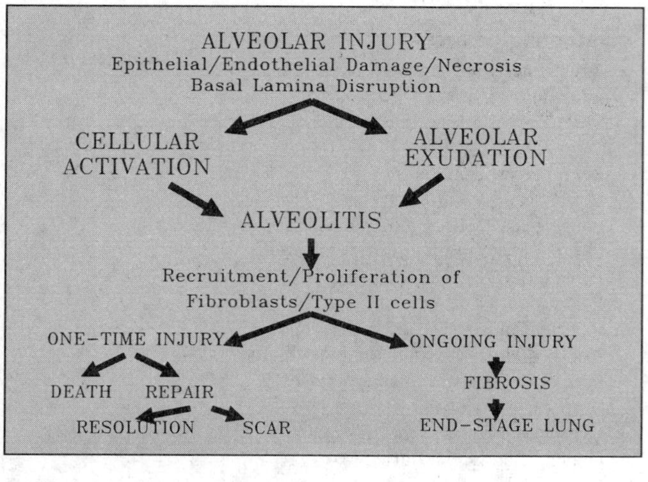

Fig. 206-1. The pathogenesis of interstitial lung disease.

Lung architectural revision and the development of fibrosis have been intensively studied. Whether alveoli can be repaired depends on the intactness of the basement membrane; without it, no scaffolding exists for replacement of denuded cells. Also, proteinases appear important in destroying critical connective tissue macromolecules. Mechanisms of fibrosis are multiple, and the fibroblast is the key cell producing the connective tissue macromolecules. Recruitment of fibroblasts can occur into the alveolar exudate, with subsequent synthesis of collagen and other connective tissue macromolecules. Alternatively, fibroblasts may increase in the alveolar interstitium, with increased connective tissue biosynthesis. Finally, with loss of epithelial cells lining alveoli, alveolar collapse or atelectatic induration and development of fibrosis and volume loss may occur. The result in all these situations is a disorderly deposition of collagen with the formation of epithelial-lined spaces, often called "the honeycomb lung."

PATHOPHYSIOLOGY

The classic physiology of the interstitial diseases is a reduction in lung volumes and compliance, decreased carbon monoxide diffusing capacity (DLCO), and exercise-induced hypoxemia. Airflow obstruction may be present in some patients but is not a common feature.

The earliest physiologic alteration in many patients is a reduction in DLCO and exercise-induced hypoxemia with widening of the alveolar-arterial oxygen gradient. Some patients have a normal roentgenogram and normal lung volumes. Because of thickened alveolar septae, it was initially thought that the major cause of hypoxemia was a diffusion barrier to oxygen. Subsequent research indicated that ventilation-perfusion imbalance was a major cause. Recent re-examination of the etiology of hypoxemia in these diseases, however, suggests that impaired oxygen diffusion may be a significant component of both resting and exercise-induced hypoxemia. As the disease process progresses, loss of gas exchange units from destruction or atelectasis results in increased elastic recoil, causing reduced lung volumes and increased work of breathing.

Vital capacity (VC) and total lung capacity (TLC) are reduced at midcourse in these diseases. Among the alveolar filling diseases and the acute diseases, increased elastic recoil and reduced lung volumes may occur quite early. In the chronic interstitial diseases, residual volume (RV) may not be reduced to the extent of VC, so the RV/TLC ratio is increased. Lung compliance is also reduced midcourse in these diseases, and the volume-pressure relationship is shifted downward and to the right.

Some of the interstitial diseases show morphologic and functional evidence of airways disease. Small airways disease (airways < 2 mm in diameter) may be present in patients with IPF, sarcoidosis, and some collagen vascular diseases. Intraluminal bronchial obstruction caused by granulomatous lesions may be seen in sarcoidosis and in Wegener's granulomatosis. Reversible airflow obstruction may occur in patients with the Churg-Strauss syndrome, in some with eosinophilic pneumonia, and occasionally in those with other interstitial diseases (e.g., sarcoidosis). A few of these diseases may show a major obstructive defect on routine spirometry. These include cystic sarcoidosis, Langerhans' cell granulomatosis, chronic organic dust disease, and lymphangioleiomyomatosis. Exercise-induced hypoxemia is characteristic of early interstitial disease, but resting hypoxemia is typical of advanced disease. In general, most patients with interstitial disease have elevated minute ventilation with hypocapnia. As the disease advances, hypercapnia may result, and large right-to-left intrapulmonary shunts may develop so that oxygenation may be impossible. Pulmonary hypertension with cor pulmonale often occurs in advanced interstitial lung disease.

CLINICAL FEATURES

Most patients present with exertional breathlessness. Depending on the type of interstitial disease, other symptoms may be seen. Some patients may have fever, including some with AIP or BOOP or diseases caused by infectious disorders. Fever may also occur with acute organic dust disease, drug-induced disease, some collagen vascular disorders, some pulmonary vasculitides, and infrequently in IPF. Cough is common at midcourse and in advanced interstitial disease. Wheezes can be auscultated in patients with Churg-Strauss syndrome and eosinophilic pneumonias. Digital clubbing often occurs in the advanced stages.

The physical examination of patients with early interstitial disease may be totally normal. As the disease advances, auscultation may reveal diffuse bronchovesicular breath sounds with bibasilar, coarse crackles. These are often described as "Velcro" crackles by analogy to the sound made by pulling Velcro apart. Interestingly, patients with sarcoidosis can have extensive interstitial disease on the chest roentgenogram but show few physical signs on auscultation. Exertional cyanosis may be present midcourse in these diseases, but resting cyanosis with tachypnea and the use of accessory muscles usually signifies advanced disease. Accentuation of the pulmonic closure sound may initially be present only during exercise, but as the disease advances, pulmonary hypertension and findings of cor pulmonale develop. Right ventricular failure is a late manifestation of these diseases.

IMAGING TECHNIQUES

Some patients with interstitial disease have a normal chest roentgenogram. More often, however, the chest roentgenogram is abnormal and there are minimal symptoms. Four basic roentgenographic patterns have been described: ground glass, nodular, reticulonodular, and reticular. In most of these diseases the infiltrate is predominantly in the lower lobes. A few diseases, such as silicosis and some connective tissue disorders, have predominantly an upper lobe predilection. The roentgenographic pattern in patients with Langerhans' cell granulomatosis typically shows sparing of the costophrenic angles. The ground-glass pattern is characterized by a homogeneous haze of the lung, usually at the bases. This is thought to be produced by confluence of tiny nodular opacities and may represent an early stage of these diseases. A purely nodular pattern is rare but is best described by the pattern of miliary tuberculosis. Nodules can range from a few millimeters up to greater than 10 cm in diameter, as seen in some pulmonary vasculitides. The reticular pattern consists of a network of linear shadows; a series of curvilinear opacities that form rings. This pattern can be further described according to the size of the opacities, using the terms *fine, medium,* and *coarse*. A coarse reticular pattern with intervening air spaces 2 to 10 mm in diameter is typical of honeycomb lung. This pattern corresponds to the presence of thick-walled, epithelial-lined cystic spaces and is mainly seen in advanced IPF, scleroderma, and Langerhans' cell granulomatosis.

The routine chest roentgenogram remains a valuable way to define the lung anatomy, but it is imprecise. In recent years, computer application to lung imaging has enormously improved the precision of diagnostic imaging. High-resolution computed tomography (CT) is currently being investigated as both a diagnostic tool and a staging tool in the interstitial diseases. It is both sensitive and highly specific in demonstrating interstitial and pleural disease. Several diagnostic patterns appear to be emerging, including those associated with lymphangioleiomyomatosis, lymphangitic carcinomatosis, and asbestos-associated pleural disease. Thoracic magnetic resonance imaging (MRI) and nuclear medicine imaging are being investigated but should currently be viewed as research tools.

DIAGNOSIS AND MANAGEMENT

Accurate diagnosis of specific interstitial diseases requires careful clinical, roentgenographic, and laboratory correlation; many require lung biopsy. Advances in imaging and other laboratory tests have greatly improved diagnostic accuracy and in some cases reduced the need for lung biopsy. Most of the interstitial diseases of known etiology can be diagnosed by a very careful history and physical examination along with correlation with imaging techniques. The need for an exhaustive search for an etiologic agent cannot be overemphasized. If a specific etiology can be identified and removed, the disease may regress. High-resolution CT appears to be useful in the diagnosis of some of these diseases. New techniques for detecting antibodies in the collagen vascular disorders have proved to be useful adjunctive measures, and the presence of antineutrophilic cytoplasmic antibody (ANCA) can be helpful in decision making in patients with the pulmonary vasculitides. Additional serum factors that may prove useful in diagnosing and staging various vasculitic syndromes include anti–factor VIII–related antigen, alkaline ribonuclease, and plasma thrombospondin.

Considerable interest continues in the use of *bronchoalveolar lavage* (BAL) cell and fluid analysis in both the diagnosis and the management of interstitial diseases. The procedure has a very low morbidity and has proved to be valuable in the diagnosis of pulmonary infections, particularly in the immunosuppressed patient. BAL cell analysis has been useful in diagnosing some interstitial diseases when ultrastructural studies have been performed or when specific monoclonal antibodies to certain cells have been used. For the average practitioner, however, BAL should be reserved for research purposes and the diagnosis of infectious disorders.

If an accurate diagnosis cannot be established by noninvasive means, *lung biopsy* is indicated. Lung biopsy provides a histologic and at times an etiologic diagnosis and allows for assessment of disease activity and prediction of the natural or treated history of the disease. The latter is of great importance to both patients and families. The initial procedure of choice is fiberoptic bronchoscopy with transbronchial lung biopsy. In patients with suspected IPF or diffuse disease associated with the collagen vascular disorders, some clinicians proceed directly to open lung biopsy because UIP is the most common pathologic pattern and transbronchial biopsy is not reliable in making that diagnosis. Further, almost all pulmonologists would proceed to open lung biopsy in patients with pulmonary hemorrhage or pulmonary vasculitis. This is done to prevent delay in diagnosis and to provide the pathologist with adequate tissue. However, anecdotal reports reveal that these diseases are being diagnosed by transbronchial lung biopsy. If an open lung biopsy is required, areas of end-stage lung should be avoided. Because this is an expensive and invasive procedure, our services use intraoperative frozen sections to ensure that diagnostic tissue has been obtained. It is important for the clinician to provide all clinical and roentgenographic data to the pathologists to maximize the pathologist's diagnostic skills.

The general principles of management of the interstitial diseases are to (1) suppress inflammation to prevent further destruction and fibrosis of lung parenchyma and (2) palliate the complications of the disease. In some of the acute interstitial diseases, avoidance of injurious agents and supportive measures may be sufficient. In other interstitial diseases the use of corticosteroids and/or cytotoxic agents may be required to suppress the inflammatory response. Interstitial diseases associated with circulating antibodies may require plasmapheresis.

In the acute and chronic interstitial pneumonias, once the decision is made to treat the patient, corticosteroids continue to be the mainstay of therapy. The initial treatment of choice is *prednisone,* 1 mg/kg ideal body weight/day (up to 80 mg) given all at one time. Treatment is continued for 6 to 8 weeks at that dosage and then tapered by 5 mg weekly to a maintenance dose of 15 to 20 mg daily. Pulmonary function studies and chest imaging should be obtained serially at intervals of 6 to 8 weeks and are the only objective way to follow patients. Treatment is continued until pulmonary function studies have been stable for 1 year, then the prednisone is slowly tapered off. For patients who progress to prednisone therapy or who cannot tolerate corticosteroids, cytotoxic or immunosuppressive agents have been advocated as alternative therapy. *Cyclophosphamide* at dosages of 1 to 2 mg/kg ideal body weight has been suggested as being useful. Although statistical data supporting the use of cyclophosphamide are lacking, there are anecdotal reports on its usefulness. Azathioprine has also been recommended as an alternative, as have a variety of other agents, such as antimalarials; all are of unproven value.

Preventive and palliative measures are also important in reducing the morbidity and mortality of these diseases. The structural changes constitute a host defense problem, and bacterial pneumonia may be a cause of death. Influenza and pneumococcal vaccines are recommended, and acute bronchitis should be treated. Some patients can have a component of reversible airways obstruction that should be treated with bronchodilators. Supplemental oxygen is recommended for patients who have an arterial oxygen tension of less than 55 mm Hg at rest or exercise, if this therapy has been found to improve oxygenation. Patients with cor pulmonale and right ventricular failure or those with significant hypoxic organ dysfunction (e.g., erythrocytosis) should also be treated. Recurrent pneumothoraces can complicate advanced interstitial disease, and at times, chemical pleurodesis is necessary.

Lung transplantation is now an accepted therapy for selected individuals who are unresponsive to medical therapy. In most patients, single-lung transplantation is used; however, double-lung transplantation has been used in patients with AIP.

KNOWN ETIOLOGIES FOR INTERSTITIAL DISEASES

Occupational and environmental inhalants

Inhalation of a variety of organic and inorganic dusts, vapors, fumes, and aerosols can cause acute or chronic interstitial lung disease. Development of disease depends on the agent's physical properties allowing it to bypass upper airway host defenses and be deposited in gas exchange units. These properties include size, shape, and solubility. In the acute occupational and environmental lung diseases, a short, predictable timetable exists between each exposure and development of lung disease. This predictability, correlated with environmental exposures, may be helpful in diagnosing organic dust disease. In the chronic lung diseases, a lag time of 15 to 20 years often occurs between exposure and development of disease. Chapter 208 discusses the organic dust diseases, and Chapter 211 presents the other occupational and environmental lung diseases.

Drugs

See Chapter 212 for drug-induced lung diseases.

Poisons

The major poison of clinical significance is the herbicide paraquat. Accidental or deliberate ingestion of this agent causes diffuse alveolar damage and adult respiratory distress syndrome (ARDS). The pathogenesis of the injury is unclear but may be caused by the generation of reactive oxygen species. The mortality associated with paraquat-induced lung disease approaches 50%, and treatment is supportive.

Infectious agents

Infections are a common cause of acute interstitial diseases. These are usually self-limited, and patients do not require hospitalization. Diagnosis of viral infections has become important as more effective therapy has become available. In the immunosuppressed host, cytomegalovirus is a common microbe. Acute diffuse interstitial disease is common in AIDS patients. Chapter 242 discusses opportunistic infections in AIDS. Cases of both viral and mycoplasma pneumonias progressing to chronic interstitial disease have been reported.

Radiation

Long recognized as a cause of pneumonitis and fibrosis, most cases of radiation-induced interstitial disease are localized infiltrates from therapeutic radiation for lymphomas or carcinomas. The incidence of radiation-induced lung disease is unknown, but with current refined techniques, clinically significant disease has greatly diminished. Since diffuse lung disease can result from medical or nuclear-related accidents, it is important to recognize the features of this disease. In addition, current data indicate that injury can be amplified by the administration of oxygen or certain cytotoxic drugs. The histology of radiation-induced lung disease does not differ significantly from AIP or, if the disease is chronic, from UIP. Clinical features of pulmonary radiation consist of an acute phase occurring 6 to 12 weeks after exposure, characterized by cough, fever, and breathlessness; remission follows. Chronic interstitial disease develops 6 to 12 months later. Acute radiation-induced pneumonitis can be improved by corticosteroid therapy. However, corticosteroids do not prevent progression to chronic interstitial fibrosis.

Neoplastic diseases

Several neoplasias that invade lymphatics, alveolar air spaces, or pulmonary vasculature can present with a roentgenographic pattern of interstitial disease. Most have a reticular pattern; some have a nodular pattern. Lymphangitic adenocarcinoma generally demonstrates a reticular pattern. A nodular or reticulonodular pattern is more frequently seen in bronchoalveolar carcinomas and lymphomas. Lymphomas are particularly common in treated Hodgkin's disease. Kaposi's sarcoma can present with a diffuse reticular or nodular pattern. Infrequently, mycosis fungoides and some leukemias may demonstrate a diffuse interstitial pattern.

Hemodynamic/cardiac diseases

Chronic pulmonary venous hypertension from mitral stenosis, cor triatriatum, or chronic left ventricular failure can result in a progressive restrictive defect with roentgenographic evidence of interstitial disease. Unless associated with other causes of interstitial disease, primary pulmonary hypertension does not produce detectable pulmonary infiltrates on chest roentgenograms.

Metabolic and miscellaneous disorders

Chronic uremia can result in alveolar inflammation and fibrosis. Typically the roentgenogram shows bilateral perihilar infiltrates. Hypercalcemia can result in deposits of calcium in the alveoli and may rarely be evident on the chest roentgenogram as a ground-glass pattern. Metastatic calcification is seen in some patients undergoing dialysis and can result in a diffuse alveolar calcification. Alveolar amyloidosis is a rare cause for a diffuse reticular pattern; more often, pulmonary amyloidosis is a nodular or airway disease process. Acute allergic reactions and trauma rarely cause diffuse interstitial disease.

INTERSTITIAL DISEASES OF UNKNOWN ETIOLOGY

Acute interstitial pneumonia

AIP occurs infrequently and corresponds to what is usually referred to as the Hamman-Rich syndrome (or disease). The mean age of onset varies, ranging from 13 to more than 70 years of age. In one series, mean age was less than 30 years, and in another, 50 years. No sex predilection has been found. Most patients have a prodromal illness for 1 to 3 weeks. The prodrome consists of a flulike illness that progresses to cough and ultimately to progressive dyspnea. Fever, myalgias, and arthralgias often occur. On initial examination, most patients are tachypneic and cyanotic. The chest roentgenogram shows progressive alveolar filling. Corticosteroids and antibiotics are almost always prescribed, and anecdotal reports are positive concerning their use. The prognosis is variable but generally is considered to be poor, with less than 50% of patients surviving. Many who survive can ultimately have normal or nearly normal pulmonary function.

Bronchiolitis obliterans–organizing pneumonia

Previously confused with UIP or cases of obliterative bronchiolitis, BOOP is a distinct clinical and pathologic entity. Although BOOP is a disease of airways, it is often grouped with interstitial pneumonias (see previous section on pathology), and thus a brief discussion is presented here. BOOP is a specific histologic diagnosis and has been associated with a variety of infections, toxic inhalants, drugs, and other disorders. It is often confused with obliterative bronchiolitis, which is characterized by progressive narrowing and scarring of small airways but without the typical fibrous plugs seen in BOOP. This discussion addresses idiopathic BOOP or BOOP associated with the collagen vascular disorders.

Most patients with BOOP are 40 to 60 years of age and have a flulike illness with fever, sore throat, myalgias, and progressive dyspnea. The duration of symptoms is usually 2 to 10 weeks but in some patients has exceeded 3 months. The chest roentgenogram typically shows bilateral, patchy air space opacities. Lesions are variable on the roentgenogram, however, and can be focal and progressive or nonspecific. The diagnosis often requires open lung biopsy and very careful clinicopathologic correlation. Treatment is with corticosteroids, and the prognosis is usually good, with a high response rate to therapy. Exacerbations of the disease after discontinuation of corticosteroids have been reported; these patients may require indefinite corticosteroid therapy.

Idiopathic pulmonary fibrosis

A common chronic interstitial disease, IPF mainly affects patients in the sixth or seventh decade of life but can occur at any age. No sex predilection exists, and most patients have insidious exertional breathlessness. At times, patients have a constant, nonproductive cough. Although there are reports of a prodromal period, with a flulike illness followed by fever and other constitutional symptoms, many of these reports preceded our current understanding of interstitial pneumonias. Therefore many cases may represent AIP, BOOP, or possibly an undeclared connective tissue disease. Most patients with IPF, however, probably do have fever and constitutional symptoms. Survival can range from 1 to 2 years to longer than 20 years. The mean survival, however, is 4 to 5 years after presentation. IPF represents the prototype of the chronic interstitial pneumonias (see previous section on clinical features for physical findings). Digital clubbing is a late feature of IPF but rarely may antedate the onset of the lung disease.

Initially, the chest roentgenogram may be normal or show a bibasilar reticular or reticulonodular pattern. As IPF advances, infiltrates progressively involve more lung parenchyma, and in the absence of cigarette abuse with coexisting chronic obstructive pulmonary disease (COPD), progressive loss of lung volumes and development of end-stage honeycomb lung occur. Pleural effusions and lymphadenopathy are not features of IPF and, if present, suggest a complication or an alternative diagnosis. The pathology of IPF is UIP. Decision making in IPF is outlined in the previous section on diagnosis and management. Open lung biopsy is generally recommended, but recent use of high-resolution CT holds promise as a useful tool in the diagnosis and staging of IPF. Young patients with minimum fibrosis and active alveolitis appear most responsive to corticosteroid therapy; up to 90% have 5-year survival. By contrast, among patients with severe pulmonary fibrosis with minimum cellularity, less than 25% have a 5-year mean survival.

Sarcoidosis

See Chapter 207.

Collagen vascular disorders

The collagen vascular disorders are a diverse collection of diseases in which the major pathology is inflammation of blood vessels and connective tissue. Thoracic involvement varies and ranges from chest wall disease to parenchymal disease to diaphragmatic disease. Almost every collagen vascular disease can be associated with diffuse interstitial involvement. The pathology in most is that of UIP. The pathogenesis of these diseases is poorly understood but appears to be autoimmune. Although it has been stated that the prognosis in most of these patients is similar, adequate data are not available to support this. Some of the diseases have a course similar to that of IPF and are progressive, whereas others are not progressive and lung disease rarely limits survival. In general, patients with progressive disease are managed as if they have IPF. Initial treatment is with corticosteroids, and if this is not tolerated or the disease is progressive, cyclophosphamide is added.

Rheumatoid arthritis. (See Chapter 304.) Several thoracic manifestations of rheumatoid arthritis exist, with pleuropulmonary manifestations the most common. Approximately 20% of patients have roentgenographic evidence of diffuse interstitial disease. These patients are predominantly males in the sixth decade of life and usually have high titers of rheumatoid factor. The lung disease rarely may antedate the joint disease but usually occurs 5 or more years after the development of rheumatoid arthritis. Prognosis of patients with diffuse interstitial disease varies, but reports indicate that it parallels that of IPF.

Systemic lupus erythematosus. (See Chapter 306.) Presenting with fever, tachypnea, and hypoxemia with diffuse or patchy infiltrates, acute lupus pneumonitis is a well-described entity. In up to 50% of patients, lupus pneumonitis may be the initial presentation of systemic lupus erythematosus (SLE). The incidence of pulmonary infection in SLE far exceeds that in lupus pneumonitis, so it is critical to exclude a treatable microbe. Lung biopsy may be necessary for an accurate diagnosis. Once the diagnosis of acute lupus pneumonitis is made, the disease is generally treated with high-dose intravenous corticosteroids. The addition of cyclophosphamide and/or azathioprine in progressive disease has been reported. Chronic interstitial disease is rare in SLE and is thought to develop from recurrent episodes of acute pneumonitis. The pathology is that of UIP. Death from end-stage chronic interstitial disease appears to be exceedingly rare. When present, it is often responsive to corticosteroids.

Progressive systemic sclerosis. (See Chapter 309.) Interstitial lung disease is common in progressive systemic sclerosis (PSS); it is clinically evident in up to 50% of patients and is seen at autopsy in almost 100%. Generally, a poor correlation exists between the cutaneous manifestations of this disease and the development of interstitial disease. The pathology is that of UIP, and data on treatment are scarce. Currently, the disease is thought to be generally acellular, and corticosteroids are not useful. Some data suggest that penicillamine may be efficacious. Lung and renal disease are the primary conditions that limit survival.

Dermatomyositis-polymyositis. (See Chapter 311.) Diffuse interstitial disease can be seen in up to 5% of patients with dermatomyositis-polymyositis. Among patients who develop progressive interstitial disease, no correlation exists between the pulmonary disease and the severity or duration of the muscle disease. In general, patients with extremely cellular disease respond quite well to steroids and should be managed similar to those with IPF.

Sjögren's syndrome. (See Chapter 305.) Often coexisting with other connective tissue disorders, Sjögren's syndrome can be associated with several types of interstitial diseases, including UIP and LIP. LIP is considered to be a low-grade lymphoma. Little data are available on the natural history of cases with pathology conforming to the UIP pattern, but patients with progressive interstitial disease should be managed similar to those with IPF.

Mixed connective tissue disease. (See Chapter 307.) Presenting with signs and symptoms of several connective tissue disorders, diffuse interstitial disease is frequent in mixed connective tissue disease. There appears to be a female predilection and a trend toward developing many features of SLE. The diagnosis is generally made with clinical correlation and the presence of serum antibodies to extractable nuclear antigens composed of soluble ribonuclear protein and a glycoprotein called SM antigen. Antinative DNA antibodies are rarely present. The clinical course of the interstitial disease in this disorder is variable and, if progressive, should be managed similar to IPF.

Ankylosing spondylitis. (See Chapter 312.) Ankylosing spondylitis is characterized by inflammation and sclerosis of the sacroiliac joints, spine, and costovertebral joints. Patients with ankylosing spondylitis can develop progressive upper lobe fibrocystic disease. The cysts are susceptible to the development of aspergillomas or other mycetomas but may develop invasive aspergillosis. Amphotericin B and more recently fluconazole have been used to treat aspergillomas, but without clear benefit. If invasive disease develops, intravenous amphotericin is indicated. Resection or embolization may be necessary to control massive hemorrhage, a major complication of mycetomas. An identical pattern of upper lobe fibrocystic disease has been described in psoriatic arthritis and seropositive rheumatoid arthritis.

Pulmonary vasculitis

The pulmonary vasculitic syndromes are a diverse group of diseases with overlapping clinical and pathologic features. Most are part of a disseminated vasculitic process, but in a few the lung is the major organ involved. The prototype of these diseases is Wegener's granulomatosis. Only a few of the pulmonary vasculitides present with progressive interstitial disease, but most can ultimately develop significant pulmonary fibrosis. In some vasculitides the lung is the major organ involved; these include Wegener's granulomatosis, the Churg-Strauss syndrome, and necrotizing sarcoid granulomatosis. Previously, lymphomatoid granulomatosis would have been classified with this group; however, it is now known that it is a T cell lymphoma. Pulmonary vasculitis may exist also as part of a diffuse vasculitic process (e.g., Henoch-Schönlein syndrome). Pulmonary vasculitis may be only part of a diffuse spectrum of lung pathology, such as seen with the collagen vascular disorders.

The pathogenesis of the pulmonary vasculitides is not known, but by analogy with other vasculitic syndromes, one cause is believed to be immune complex vascular injury with resulting vasculitis and tissue destruction. Circulating immune complexes have been identified in many of the pulmonary vasculitides, including Wegener's granulomatosis, Behçet's disease, rheumatoid arthritis, and others. In most cases the antigens are unknown, but in several the antigen appears to be molecules derived from microbes. Several factors determine whether or not patients develop immune complex disease. These include the type and size of the immune complex, the immune complex load, and the ability to handle immune complexes. Recent data suggest that when complement deficiencies are present or when defects in complement receptors or immunoglobulin G–Fc (IgG-Fc) receptors exist, the body is unable to handle immune complexes so that disease is more likely to develop. Mechanisms for localization of immune complexes are also poorly understood. Experimental data indicate that agents that alter vascular permeability (e.g., histamine) promote deposition of immune complexes. Once immune complexes are deposited, complement is activated, producing cleavage products that recruit polymorphonuclear leukocytes and cause degranulation of basophils, releasing other soluble mediators, proteolytic enzymes, and toxic radicals. Ultimately, the vessel is infiltrated with polymorphonuclear leukocytes, producing vasculitis and vascular necrosis with tissue damage.

The hallmark of the initial stages of the vasculitides is endothelial cell activation and subsequent endothelial cell damage and sloughing. A prominent feature in some of these diseases is activation of the coagulation cascade with thrombogenesis. Less is known about the chronic granulomatous vasculitides. Evolution from an acute vasculitis is possible, but the development of cell-mediated immunity seems more likely.

Wegener's granulomatosis. (See Chapter 210.)

Churg-Strauss syndrome. (See Chapter 210.)

Pulmonary hemorrhage syndromes

The diffuse alveolar hemorrhage syndromes are characterized by hemoptysis, alveolar filling opacities on chest roentgenograms, dyspnea, hypoxia, and often nephritis with progressive renal failure. Six major disease groups are associated with alveolar hemorrhage:

1. Anti–glomerular basement membrane antibody disease
2. Alveolar hemorrhage associated with vasculitis
3. Alveolar hemorrhage associated with collagen vascular diseases
4. Idiopathic pulmonary hemosiderosis (IPH)
5. Alveolar hemorrhage associated with exogenous agents
6. Alveolar hemorrhage associated with idiopathic, rapidly progressive glomerulonephritis

Principles of diagnosis of these diseases are as follows: (1) document the presence of alveolar hemorrhage, (2) evaluate renal status, (3) search for the presence of serologic abnormalities (anti–glomerular basement membrane [anti-GBM] antibody, antinuclear antibody [ANA], antineutrophil cytoplasm antibody [ANCA], immune complexes), (4) biopsy kidney if vasculitis is not suspected, and (5) biopsy lung if no diagnosis is made. All biopsy material should be studied by light and electron microscopy and by immunofluorescent techniques.

Anti–glomerular basement membrane antibody disease. Previously termed *Goodpasture's syndrome,* anti-GBM antibody disease has only recently been recognized, and the full spectrum of diffuse alveolar hemorrhage and progressive glomerulonephritis is the most common presentation. The disease can affect both sexes and all ages, but it typically occurs in Caucasian males in the third decade of life. Hemoptysis is the most common initial sign, and most patients have cough and dyspnea. Some have subclinical or mild pulmonary hemorrhage and iron deficiency anemia. Most patients have evidence of nephritis initially, and virtually all develop progressive renal failure. Serologic assays for anti-GBM antibody are positive in more than 95% of patients, but in many the diagnosis must be confirmed by immunofluorescent studies of renal tissue. Lung biopsy is usually not necessary.

The etiology of anti-GBM antibody disease is unknown, but interestingly, an association appears to exist between development of this disease and infection with influenza and also with inhalation of hydrocarbons. Renal disease appears to be the limiting factor. The treatment of choice is combined corticosteroids and cytotoxic therapy together with plasmapheresis. The latter is performed daily or three times weekly until the serum levels of anti-GBM antibodies are not detectable. High-dose intravenous corticosteroids for 2 to 3 days are generally recommended for life-threatening alveolar hemorrhage. There are reports of successful renal transplantation in patients with undetectable anti-GBM antibodies.

Alveolar hemorrhage associated with vasculitis. Diffuse alveolar hemorrhage as a presentation of Wegener's granulomatosis occurs infrequently. Reported cases usually involve patients with extensive parenchymal hemorrhage and rapid renal failure. Skin disease, arthritis, and upper airways disease can coexist. The diagnosis is established from lung biopsy and shows a capillaritis; a granulomatous vasculitis may sometimes coexist. Renal biopsy is usually nonspecific. High-dose corticosteroids and cyclophosphamide are recommended for this presentation. The prognosis, however, is poor.

Diffuse alveolar hemorrhage may occur in the *Henoch-Schönlein syndrome*. In reported cases, the extrapulmonary features of this disease were present with palpable purpura, and at times nephritis. Limited studies have shown immunoglobulin A (IgA) granular deposits along the lung's basement membrane. Recommended therapy in life-threatening alveolar hemorrhage is intravenous high-dose corticosteroids. Pulmonary vasculitis with alveolar hemorrhage is also well-described in Behçet's disease. Small vessel vasculitis and necrotizing vasculitis of muscular arteries with aneurysm formation and rupture have been described.

Infrequently presenting as a pure disease, *polyarteritis nodosa* is usually associated with a diffuse immune complex vasculitis. Pulmonary artery involvement is rare but has been reported and can result in alveolar hemorrhage. Alveolar hemorrhage with nephritis has been reported in essential mixed *cryoglobulinemia*.

Alveolar hemorrhage associated with collagen vascular diseases. Diffuse alveolar hemorrhage has been well described in most of the collagen vascular syndromes. The prototype is SLE, and unlike in other alveolar hemorrhage syndromes, hemoptysis is rarely the presenting feature. Most patients with SLE have active disease with fever, arthritis, nephritis, and hypocomplementemia. Infections may complicate the hemorrhage. Alveolar hemorrhage associated with SLE is thought to be caused by immune complexes; however, immune complexes along alveolar septae have only rarely been described. Treatment with high-dose intravenous corticosteroids is usually recommended, but the mortality incidence is high.

Idiopathic pulmonary hemosiderosis. Characterized by recurrent bouts of subclinical or clinical alveolar hemorrhage, IPH has no extrapulmonary manifestations. Mainly a disease of children and young adults, IPH can affect all ages. Patients may present with a single episode of life-threatening alveolar hemorrhage but more often have multiple episodes leading to progressive interstitial fibrosis. Most have an iron deficiency anemia and during bleeds have fever, hyperbilirubinemia, and reticulocytosis. The diagnosis must be established by excluding other causes of alveolar hemorrhage. The pathogenesis of IPH is unknown. The natural history varies, and remissions have been described. Corticosteroids are recommended in high doses during active bleeding and in low maintenance doses until the disease becomes quiescent.

Alveolar hemorrhage associated with exogenous agents and idiopathic, rapidly progressive glomerulonephritis. Inhalation of *trimellitic anhydride* fumes or dust can produce pulmonary hemorrhage. This agent is widely used in the manufacture of plastics, epoxy resins, and paints. Most patients have anemia and pneumonitis, whereas others have recurrent fever, hemoptysis, and hypoxemia. The etiology is unclear but is thought to be immune, with the anhydride functioning as a hapten. Corticosteroid therapy appears useful, but avoidance of the anhydride is recommended. Alveolar hemorrhage has also been described after *lymphangiography,* as a toxic manifestation of *penicillamine* therapy, and with the use of *cocaine*.

Alveolar hemorrhage has been reported in association with idiopathic, rapidly progressive glomerulonephritis. Cases with and without immune complexes have been described. The cause is unknown but may represent part of a spectrum of vasculitis or of the collagen vascular disorders. In general, it is managed similar to lupus nephritis and alveolar hemorrhage.

Langerhans' cell granulomatosis

See Chapter 209.

Lymphoid infiltrative disorders

This infrequently occurring group of diseases was formerly thought to be benign, with some rarely progressing to lymphoma; current data suggest that many are low-grade lymphomas. These include lymphomatoid granulomatosis, a T cell lymphoma; immunoblastic lymphadenopathy; lymphocytic angiitis and granulomatosis; and LIP associated with Sjögren's syndrome, other collagen vascular diseases, or as an idiopathic disorder. Treatment varies according to the disease. Patients with lymphomatoid granulomatosis are generally treated aggressively as having a T cell lymphoma, whereas those with lymphocytic angiitis and granulomatosis are generally treated with chlorambucil. Patients with idiopathic LIP, if progressive, are usually treated with corticosteroids.

Bronchiolar diseases

Several chronic bronchiolar diseases can present with roentgenographic evidence of interstitial disease, usually in the form of a reticular or reticulonodular pattern. BOOP and respiratory bronchiolitis have previously been discussed, but several other bronchiolar diseases can also have similar roentgenographic patterns. A disease described mainly in Japan, *diffuse panbronchiolitis* is characterized by chronic inflammation of respiratory bronchioles. Usually the chest roentgenogram shows hyperinflation, and pulmonary function studies show an obstructive pattern with gas trapping. Some cases, however, show roentgenographic evidence of a bibasilar nodular infiltrate, whereas others show a linear reticular pattern, often with "tram" lines consistent with bronchiectasis/bronchiolectasis. Most patients develop gram-negative bronchial infections, and the prognosis is poor.

Follicular bronchitis/bronchiolitis is a poorly described disease seen primarily in patients with collagen vascular disorders or in immunosuppressed patients. Familial cases also have been reported, and in some patients there appears to be an association with an allergic phenomenon. Most patients have a reticular or reticulonodular infiltrative pattern. Pulmonary function studies may show an obstructive or restrictive pattern or a combined restrictive/obstructive defect. Lung pathology shows reactive lymphoid germinal centers along bronchi and bronchioles, and prominent peribronchial and peribronchiolar fibrosis may be seen. There is no evidence of chronic bronchitis. Therapy is uncertain, with a variable response to corticosteroids.

Lymphangioleiomyomatosis

Lymphangioleiomyomatosis is a rare disease of young females in the third to fourth decade of life and is characterized by proliferation of smooth muscle in a lymphatic distribution without evidence of cancer. The abnormal smooth muscle is seen around the airways, blood vessels, and lymphatic vessels. Lymphatic involvement mainly involves lung, thorax, abdomen, and occasionally lymph nodes. Although mainly a disease of childbearing age with a survival less than 10 years, disease in postmenopausal women has been reported. These latter patients may have a prolonged survival. The clinical features of this disease are progressive dyspnea, hemoptysis, cough, and repeated spontaneous pneumothoraces and chylous effusions. The chest roentgenogram typically shows a diffuse fibrocystic pattern with normal or increased lung volumes. Pulmonary function studies reveal a typical emphysematous presentation. The etiology of lymphangioleiomyomatosis is unknown, but the occurrence of the disease during childbearing years has focused research on sex hormones. Disease remission has been reported after treatment with progesterone, oophorectomy, and synthetic hypothalamic analogs, which produce a medical castration. Successful single-lung transplantation in patients with this disease has been performed. Recurrent pneumothoraces and chylous effusions may require chemical pleurodesis.

Eosinophilic pneumonias

Acute eosinophilic pneumonia can occur in association with a variety of drugs and parasites. Diffuse or patchy infiltrates are related to the migration of parasitic larvae through lungs. The term *Löffler's syndrome* is typically applied to patients with transient pulmonary infiltrates and with peripheral eosinophilia in which no clear etiology is evident. Asthma may be an associated symptom. Chronic eosinophilic pneumonia is a discrete disease characterized by fever, night sweats, exertional breathlessness, and occasional wheezing and peripheral eosinophilia. The chest roentgenogram typically shows peripheral, nonsegmental, fixed infiltrates; however, nodules with cavities and a chronic interstitial infiltrate also have been described. Exquisitely sensitive to corticosteroids, peripheral infiltrates tend to recur in the same location if the disease exacerbates.

Pulmonary alveolar proteinosis

Pulmonary alveolar proteinosis (PAP) is characterized by the deposition of a granular eosinophilic and periodic acid

Schiff–positive material within alveoli. PAP is mainly a disease of the fourth and fifth decades of life. There is a male predominance, and PAP is often associated with dust exposure or respiratory infections. Clinical features are progressive breathlessness, cough, fatigue, and malaise. The chest roentgenogram typically shows bilaterally symmetric, alveolar-filling opacities that spare the costophrenic angles and the apices. Laboratory data are nonspecific, but an elevated lactate dehydrogenase concentration is often present and appears to arise from the lung.

A pathologic reaction resembling PAP has been described in a variety of dust exposures, malignancies, and infections. Acute *silicoproteinosis* is a well-described entity. In animal models a PAP-like reaction can be produced by inhalation of silica, aluminum, and various other dusts. PAP associated with dust exposure is often termed *secondary PAP*. The cause of idiopathic PAP is unknown, but pathogenetic theories speculate that abnormal production or metabolism of surfactin occurs. Some type of derangement seems to exist in either the production or the clearance of the surfactin material produced.

The diagnosis of PAP is established by clinical and pathologic data, often requiring lung biopsy. Treatment is with whole-lung lavage using 40 to 60 L of fluid. Corticosteroids have no value and may increase the incidence of lung infections. Spontaneous remissions have been frequently reported, but progression to advanced fibrotic disease has also been reported.

Other interstitial diseases

Diffuse interstitial disease can occur in a variety of inherited disorders, and a familial form of IPF exists. Von Recklinghausen's disease is associated with progressive interstitial lung infiltrates, with lung biopsy showing UIP. Interstitial disease has been described in Gaucher's disease, Neimann-Pick disease, tuberous sclerosis, and the Hermansky-Pudlak syndrome. Various rare and unusual types of interstitial diseases have been described in relatively common illnesses, including ulcerative colitis, Crohn's disease, primary biliary cirrhosis, chronic active hepatitis, and renal tubular acidosis. The pathology of these diseases has not been well characterized, but in some a vasculitis appears to exist, whereas in others a nonspecific inflammation-fibrotic reaction occurs. Several unclassified interstitial pneumonias exist, and often in the course of patient evaluation, diffuse *nonprogressive* interstitial pneumonia can be identified. These diseases may represent previous infections or cases of respiratory bronchiolitis. Lung biopsy is not indicated unless it is a progressive disorder. Chronic interstitial pneumonia (CIP) is a frequent feature of patients after transplantation and has been increasingly recognized in those with AIDS.

REFERENCES

Burkhardt A: Alveolitis and collapse in the pathogenesis of pulmonary fibrosis. Am Rev Respir Dis 140:513, 1989.

Crouch E: Pathobiology of pulmonary fibrosis. Am J Physiol 259:L159, 1990.

Daniele R et al: Clinical role of bronchoalveolar lavage in adults with pulmonary disease. Am Rev Respir Dis 142:481, 1990.

Fulmer JD and Katzenstein AA: The interstitial lung diseases. In Bone RC, editor: Comprehensive textbook of pulmonary disease, vol 2. St. Louis, 1993, Mosby–Year Book.

Helmers RA and Humminghake GW: Bronchoalveolar lavage in the non-immunocompromised patient. Chest 96:1184, 1989.

Katzenstein AA and Askin F: Surgical pathology of non-neoplastic lung disease. Major Probl Pathol 13:9, 1990.

Katzenstein AA et al: Bronchitis obliterans and usual interstitial pneumonia. Am J Surg Pathol 10:373, 1986.

Kennedy JI and Fulmer JD: Collagen vascular diseases. In Kassiere JP, editor: Current therapy in internal medicine. Philadelphia, 1991, BC Decker.

Kennedy JI and Fulmer JD: Pulmonary vasculitis and interstitial lung disease. In Schwartz MJ and King TE, editors: Interstitial lung disease. Philadelphia, 1993, BC Decker.

Kuhn C III et al: An immunohistochemical study of architectural remodeling and connective tissue synthesis in pulmonary fibrosis. Am Rev Respir Dis 14:1693, 1989.

Leatherman JW: Immune alveolar hemorrhages. Chest 91:891, 1989.

Muller NL and Ostrow DN: High-resolution computed tomography of chronic interstitial lung diseases. Clin Chest Med 12:97, 1991.

Olson J, Colby T, and Elliott C: Hamman-Rich syndrome revisited. Mayo Clin Proc 65:1538, 1990.

Taylor JR et al: Lymphangioleiomyomatosis: clinical course in 32 patients. N Engl J Med 323:1254, 1990.

Wagner PD and Rodrigues-Roisin R: Clinical advances in pulmonary gas exchange. Am Rev Respir Dis 143:883, 1991.

CHAPTER

207 Sarcoidosis

Robert J. Pueringer
Gary W. Hunninghake

DEFINITION

Sarcoidosis is a multisystem disorder of unknown etiology characterized pathologically by the presence of epithelioid granulomas. The diagnosis remains one of exclusion, resting entirely on the demonstration of multiple organ involvement and the absence of other conditions associated with granulomatous disease (see the box at upper right). For these reasons, a careful history coupled with special stains and culture of the biopsied tissue are necessary to exclude granulomatous diseases of known cause.

PATHOLOGY

The epithelial granuloma is the pathologic hallmark of sarcoidosis. The epithelioid granuloma contains two zones: a central compact zone consisting of mature mononuclear phagocytes, epithelioid cells, and giant cells admixed with lymphocytes of the CD4+ type; and a peripheral loose zone consisting of macrophages, monocytes, fibroblasts, and lymphocytes, which, in addition to the CD4+ type, are also

Differential diagnosis of granulomatous lung disease

Infections
Bacteria
- *Brucella*
- *Francisella tularensis*
- *Yersinia enterocolitica*

Mycobacteria
- Tuberculosis
- Atypical tuberculosis

Fungi
- *Histoplasma capsulatum*
- *Blastomyces dermatitidis*
- *Coccidioides immitis*

Spirochetes: *Treponema*

Nonfectious compounds
Organic: hypersensitivity pneumonitis
Inorganic
- Beryllium
- Talc

Drugs
- Methotrexate
- Dilantin

Neoplasms
- Lymphoma
- Germ cell cancer

Idiopathic
Sarcoidosis
Wegener's granulomatosis
Primary biliary cirrhosis
Crohn's disease
Ulcerative colitis

of the CD8+ type. Morphologically, both the mononuclear phagocytes and the lymphocytes appear activated. The granulomas of sarcoidosis are sometimes associated with inclusion bodies, such as Schaumman's bodies and asteroid bodies, and/or small amounts of necrosis, none of which is specific for this disease. For example, Schaumman's bodies are concentrically lamellated structures located in the giant cells of patients with a variety of granulomatous diseases, including hypersensitivity pneumonitis. Likewise, the absence of necrosis is not specific for sarcoidosis, since up to 40% of patients with tuberculosis may have noncaseating granulomas histologically. Once formed, the granulomas can persist, resolve without residua, or undergo fibrotic change.

In the lung, granulomas are primarily localized to areas that parallel lymphatic drainage, including the peribronchial and mediastinal lymph nodes, pleural tissue septa, and along blood vessels. Although compression of the vasculature can occur, frank vasculitis is unusual.

In addition to granulomas, lung specimens from patients with sarcoidosis also contain variable amounts of nongranulomatous pneumonitis or alveolitis. The alveolitis is predominantly composed of macrophages and CD4+ T lymphocytes and appears to precede the development of granulomas. In this regard the degree of histologic cellularity is inversely correlated with the histologic appearance of granulomas.

PATHOGENESIS

Sarcoidosis results from the immunologic persistence of activated monocytes and activated CD4+ lymphocytes at sites of disease. The activated mononuclear cells can affect the host by regulating the initiation, maintenance, and resolution of local granuloma formation and by releasing a variety of mediators that potentially have systemic effects on the host.

The precursor to granuloma formation in sarcoidosis is alveolitis. In the lung this inflammatory process is localized to the interstitium and is reflected in the cells recovered by bronchoalveolar lavage. In normal people, alveolar macrophages make up greater than 85% of the cells, whereas lymphocytes constitute less than 15% of the cells, and both lymphocytes and macrophages are not activated. In contrast, patients with sarcoidosis have greater numbers of both macrophages and lymphocytes in bronchoalveolar lavage, with lymphocytes constituting a much larger percentage of the cells. The lymphocytes recovered are predominantly T helper cells. Furthermore, both sarcoid alveolar macrophages and lymphocytes are activated and possess the ability to initiate and maintain granuloma formation. The activated sarcoid alveolar macrophages have an increased ability to release spontaneously a variety of mediators that attract and activate helper T lymphocytes (interleukin 1 [IL-1], tumor necrosis factor [TNF], interleukin 8 [IL-8]). Likewise, activated sarcoid lymphocytes spontaneously proliferate and also release monocyte chemoattractants, monocyte activators (gamma interferon, granulocyte-monocyte colony-stimulating factor), and interleukin 2 (IL-2). The activated mononuclear cells subsequently organize and differentiate under the control of these mediators into the sarcoid granuloma. The formed granuloma may alter the lung by local destruction and impingement on nearby structures. The resolution of the granuloma can also affect organ function if fibrosis predominates. Activated sarcoid macrophages and lymphocytes may participate in the fibrotic process by releasing mediators that can up-regulate fibroblast proliferation and collagen release.

Activated macrophages and activated lymphocytes can also affect the host by releasing a variety of potent systemically active mediators. The macrophages from patients with sarcoidosis spontaneously release IL-1 and TNF, which can act as pyrogens and stimulate weight loss and acute-phase reactant synthesis. In addition, they can release large quantities of 1,25-dihydroxycholecalciferol. Likewise, activated CD4+ lymphocytes can nonspecifically activate B lymphocytes to differentiate into immunoglobulin-secreting cells in a polyclonal manner. The resultant hypergammaglobulinemia is a common manifestation of sarcoidosis.

In sarcoidosis, granuloma formation is often compartmentalized to specific sites of disease activity. For example, although both macrophages and T helper lymphocytes are increased in number and activated in the lungs of patients with sarcoidosis, these same patients often have a reduction in the circulating number of T helper cells. Furthermore, these patients often exhibit anergy on skin testing despite an exaggerated immune response in the lung. Even within the lung, high-resolution computed tomographic (CT) scanning often reveals disease localized around the central bronchovascular bundles without peripheral parenchymal disease (Fig. 207-1).

ETIOLOGY

Despite advances in our understanding of the immunology of sarcoidosis, the etiology of this disease remains unknown. It is also not known if sarcoidosis is caused by a single agent or by multiple agents that trigger a similar type of granulomatous disease. Various studies examining T cell receptor expression on lymphocytes isolated from the lungs of patients with sarcoidosis support an immunologic reaction to a single agent. These studies have shown that the T lymphocytes from patients with sarcoidosis have a bias toward expression of a specific receptor type on their surface in a subgroup of patients. This suggests that T cell proliferation in sarcoidosis may be directed to a single specific antigen. Potential antigens that have been implicated in stimulating this disease include both exogenous antigens, such as infectious agents (mycobacteria, cell wall deficient cornyebacteria, *Yersinia enterocolitica,* viruses, fungi) and respirable particles (inhaled organic or inorganic antigens), as well as endogenous antigens, such as latent viral or tumor antigens (e.g., germ cell neoplasms). No evidence, however, indicates that any of these agents is the cause of sarcoidosis. Sarcoidosis has also been shown to occur in some families and in some identical twins, suggesting that genetic factors also play a role in expression of this disease.

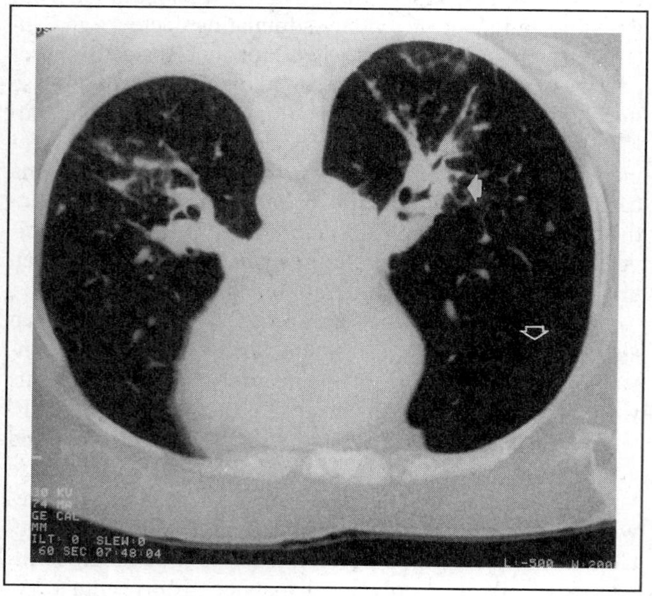

Fig. 207-1. High-resolution computed tomographic (CT) scan of the lung from a patient with sarcoidosis. Disease is localized around the central bronchovascular bundles *(closed arrow),* with sparing of the peripheral parenchyma *(open arrow).*

CLINICAL PRESENTATION

Sarcoidosis is heterogeneous in distribution, presentation, and course. Although worldwide in distribution, sarcoidosis has a predilection for temperate environments. Specifically, sarcoidosis is common in Sweden (prevalence of 64 per 100,000 population). In contrast, sarcoidosis occurs very infrequently in Africa, Southeast Asia, and the Hawaiian Islands. The prevalence in New York has been estimated at 40 per 100,000 population. Likewise, sarcoidosis can occur in any age, race, or sexual group. Classically, however, sarcoidosis appears to be found more frequently in younger people (>70% <40 years of age), blacks, and within the black race, females. These figures, however, represent rough estimates of the true prevalence of sarcoidosis within each group and region, the result of the high prevalence of clinically silent and unrecognized disease. For instance, chest radiographic screening of the population in Denmark detected fourfold more patients with sarcoidosis than did studies that recruited patients who had symptoms. Likewise, 80% of patients with sarcoidosis in a New York study were asymptomatic. Therefore the differences in disease prevalence among countries, age, and race may reflect in part the method used to define and select patients with sarcoidosis.

Sarcoidosis can affect any organ of the body. The disease can present acutely, subacutely, or chronically and can affect a single organ, an organ compartment, or multiple organs (Table 207-1).

The patient's ethnic background has been demonstrated to influence the mode of presentation, organ involvement, and clinical course in sarcoidosis. Women of Swedish, Puerto Rican, and Irish backgrounds often have Löeffler's syndrome, an acute disorder characterized by erythema nodosum, polyarthritis, iritis, and/or fever that has a good prognosis. In contrast, people of West Indian background in London have a later onset of disease and more generalized organ involvement, including the respiratory, ocular, and reticuloendothelial systems, than do Caucasians. Sarcoidosis also has a more chronic presentation with a poorer prognosis in blacks compared with whites in the United States.

Likewise, an individual's genotype may influence disease expression. Human leukocyte antigen B8 (HLA-B8), for example, has been associated with erythema nodosum, arthritis, and early resolution, whereas HLA-B27 is found in a greater percentage of patients with uveitis.

Generalized fatigue, weakness, malaise, weight loss, anorexia, fevers, and sweats are some of the constitutional symptoms that represent the most common presentation of symptomatic sarcoidosis. Generally regarded as benign, sarcoidosis can also involve a number of vital structures, including those in the respiratory, cardiac, endocrine, ophthalmologic, and central nervous systems, with potential life-threatening implications.

Table 207-1. Organ system involvement in sarcoidosis

Organ system	Clinical incidence (% patients)
Thoracic	
Pulmonary	90-95
Hilar nodes	75
Parenchyma	50
Cardiac	5-10
Extrathoracic	
Dermatologic	20-50
Erythema nodosum	15-20
Endocrine	10-50
Hypercalcemia	2-5
Hypercalciuria	20-50
Gastrointestinal	1-2
Genitourinary	1-2
Musculoskeletal	10-20
Nervous system	3-5
Ophthamologic	20-50
Reticuloendothelial	20-30
Liver	20
Lymph nodes	20
Spleen	20
Upper respiratory	5-15
Number of involved organ systems	
Three or more	35
One or two	65

Data from Mayock RL et al: Am J Med 35:67, 1963; and Siltzbach LE et al: Am J Med 57:847, 1974.

The respiratory system is the most frequently involved organ system. Up to 90% of patients with sarcoidosis have pulmonary involvement at some time during the course of their disease. Of these, 60% may develop symptoms of cough, wheezing, or dyspnea. By international convention, chest radiographs are grouped into the following stages: stage 0, normal; stage I, bilateral hilar adenopathy; stage II, bilateral hilar adenopathy with diffuse parenchymal infiltrates; and stage III, diffuse parenchymal infiltrates without bilateral hilar adenopathy. Although useful for communication, the different radiographic stages have not been useful in determining the degree of a patient's symptoms, the progression of the underlying disease, or the histology of the biopsy specimen. The discrepancy between radiographic stage and disease progression partly results from the nonspecific information obtained by the plain chest radiograph. The plain chest radiograph is unable to distinguish fibrosis from alveolitis (see section on prognosis) and also is a two-dimensional representation of a three-dimensional object, the lung. With respect to sarcoidosis, although they may appear as diffuse parenchymal nodules on the plain chest film, with high-resolution CT scanning and autopsy data (see Fig. 207-1) these nodules are localized most frequently to the peribronchovascular bundles, which may be a more accurate representation of disease. The stages demonstrated on chest radiographs do predict resolution of infiltrates in large population studies (Table 207-2).

Table 207-2. Radiographic stage of sarcoidosis and prognosis

Stage	Resolution (%)	Progression (%)
I	54	7
II	31	13
III	4	10

Modified from Siltzbach LE et al: Am J Med 57:847, 1974.

Progressive pulmonary sarcoidosis occurs in up to 20% of patients. The resultant physiologic abnormalities are those seen in most restrictive diseases. Some patients may also have an added obstructive component resulting from endobronchial disease. Often, however, static pulmonary function tests do not correlate with the degree of dyspnea. Exercise testing may be useful in delineating the cause of dyspnea in patients with sarcoidosis. Extrapulmonary factors may cause dyspnea in these patients (e.g., cardiac disease, anemia, myopathy). Finally, although pulmonary function tests do not appear to correlate with the radiographic stage, symptoms, or histology in sarcoidosis (see section on prognosis), they appear to be a sensitive way to follow the course of disease.

The upper airway can also be involved with sarcoidosis, including the nasopharynx, larynx, vocal cords, paranasal sinuses, and nasal bones. Critical narrowing may result in upper airway obstruction, dyspnea, and cough.

Cardiac sarcoidosis, although infrequent, is important because it can be potentially lethal and a major source of symptoms, including dyspnea and cough, without clinical evidence of disease elsewhere. Similar to that of the lung, granulomatous involvement of the heart is patchy. The degree of cardiac compromise depends not only on the extent but also on the location of the disease. Granulomas localized to the conduction system potentially can result in heart block or arrhythmias. Likewise, extensive myocardial involvement may cause a restrictive and dilated cardiomyopathy. The mortality from cardiac sarcoidosis approaches 20% to 30%. Severe pulmonary disease also causes secondary cor pulmonale. Attempts to identify patients with early cardiac involvement, such as by thallium scanning with dipyrimadole infusion, exercise testing with beta blockers, and magnetic resonance imaging (MRI), have resulted in detection of cardiac abnormalities in patients with sarcoidosis at a rate similar to that observed with postmortem examination (25% to 50%). Whether these detected abnormalities contribute to clinical disease remains to be determined.

In addition to direct cardiac involvement, the heart's electrical system also may be altered by hypercalcemia. The mechanism for both the hypercalcemia and the hypercalciuria in sarcoidosis is an increase in 1,25-dihydroxycholecalciferol concentration (see section on pathogenesis), which results in an increase in intestinal calcium absorption. In addition, chronic renal insufficiency from nephrolithiasis and nephrocalcinosis may be the result of a persistent hypercalcemia.

Ocular sarcoidosis, often clinically asymptomatic, can result in blindness. The most common structure involved is the anterior uveal tract. Involvement of any of the ocular structures, however, has been described. Although a careful eye history (altered visual acuity, watering, redness, photophobia) and examination are important, sarcoid eye disease is often asymptomatic and can only be detected by slit-lamp examination. Therefore annual eye examinations by an ophthamologist are recommended.

Likewise, sarcoidosis can involve any portion of the nervous system, including the cranial nerves (most often VII), the peripheral nerves, the skeletal muscle, the basal meninges, and the central nervous system in the form of inflammation or mass lesions. Lesions are more frequently localized at the base of the brain and, if localized to the hypothalamic/pituitary region, may result in diabetes insipidus or galactorrhea/amenorrhea. Seizures are a marker of severe central nervous system disease. Cerebrospinal fluid is typically lymphocytic with an elevated protein concentration, and in 20% of patients, hypoglycorrhachia is present. CT scanning with contrast or MRI with gadolinium is necessary to determine the full extent of disease in most patients.

The reticulendothelial system is frequently involved in sarcoidosis. The liver may be enlarged, but severe hepatic dysfunction with esophagogastric variceal formation is unusual. In addition, these patients may have an unexplained fever or a presentation similar to that seen with primary biliary cirrhosis. The lack of an antimitochondrial antibody has been used to distinguish sarcoidosis from cirrhosis. Finally, splenic enlargement may result in pancytopenia.

Skin manifestations from sarcoidosis can be the result of direct granulomatous involvement of the tissue (lupus pernio, skin plaques, cutaneous nodules) or the result of a vasculitic response. The latter is the mechanism responsible for erythema nodosum in these patients. Lupus pernio is a chronic violaceous lesion of the face that, in contrast to erythema nodosum, has been associated with multiple organ involvement, laryngeal sarcoidosis, and a poor prognosis.

Sarcoidosis can also affect the skeletal, gastrointestinal, and urinary systems. Involvement of the parotid or lacrimal glands in combination with uveitis and fever has been termed *uveoparotid fever* or *Heerfordt's syndrome*.

DIAGNOSIS

The diagnosis of sarcoidosis is made on the basis of the history and radiographic and pathologic findings, with careful exclusion of identifiable causes (see box on p. 1693). Fiberoptic bronchoscopy with transbronchial biopsy is the procedure of choice in patients with suspected pulmonary involvement. The latter can be positive even in the presence of stage I disease. In the patient with asymptomatic bilateral hilar adenopathy, uveitis, and erythema nodosum, the diagnosis presents few uncertainties and may not require tissue confirmation.

Patients with suspected myocardial or central nervous system sarcoidosis present a unique dilemma. These patients have a potentially life-threatening disease that requires specific therapy, and biopsy of symptomatically uninvolved tissue may yield the diagnosis. Gallium-67 (^{67}Ga) scanning may be particularly helpful in selecting the tissue to biopsy. The Kveim test has been used to confirm the diagnosis of sarcoidosis in some patients. However, the 4- to 6-week delay before test interpretation, the 20% false-negative rate, the number of false-positive results, and the lack of a commercially available reagent in the United States make this test impractical for routine use.

COURSE AND PROGNOSIS

The course of sarcoidosis is unpredictable and often organ dependent. Pulmonary sarcoidosis is usually a self-limited condition, with about 50% of patients showing some improvement and 25% remaining unchanged. However, sarcoidosis can progress in 20% of patients and result in pulmonary scarring and fibrosis. Up to 10% of patients may die from their disease. In general, patients with multiple organ involvement, a slower onset of disease, and a more advanced stage on chest radiography (see Table 207-2) do poorly.

In the individual patient, however, conventional clinical, radiographic, and pulmonary function parameters are unreliable in predicting the course of pulmonary sarcoidosis. The failure of chest radiographs and pulmonary function studies to predict the course of sarcoidosis is easily understood in the context of the disease's pathogenesis. The reversible lesion in the lung is the alveolitis, whereas the fibrosis is irreversible. Chest radiographs and pulmonary function tests are nonspecific studies that measure the combined effects of all processes affecting the lungs and do not distinguish alveolitis from fibrosis.

To quantify the degree of alveolitis, investigators have measured markers of alveolar macrophage activation (angiotensin-converting enzyme [ACE] levels, ^{67}Ga scanning) and directly quantified the alveolitis (bronchoalveolar lavage) present in a patient. In general, these studies cannot be recommended for general use to predict the course of disease.

ACE is elevated in up to 80% of patients with sarcoidosis because of the ongoing production of the enzyme by epithelioid cells in the granulomas. ACE levels are not specific for sarcoidosis and are elevated in a variety of other disorders. As such, ACE levels in sarcoidosis may reflect the total granuloma load present in a patient. The latter often differs from disease progression that depends on granuloma location. Progressive sarcoidosis can occur in the absence of elevated ACE levels.

^{67}Ga uptake is a sensitive but nonspecific marker of inflammation. In this respect, most patients with sarcoidosis have a positive scan. Unfortunately, the ^{67}Ga scan may also be positive for reasons unrelated to sarcoidosis (e.g., infection), limiting the study's usefulness.

Finally, in an effort to measure local disease activity directly, bronchoalveolar lavage has been used to assess the degree of lymphocytic alveolitis in these patients. In general, the presence of a lymphocytic alveolitis has reflected disease of shorter duration and does not indicate which patients have functional deterioration. Whether serially performed bronchoalveolar lavages will identify the patient with ongoing pulmonary inflammation and who is more likely to develop progressive disease is unknown.

TREATMENT

Individualizing therapeutic regimens is particularly important in patients with sarcoidosis because the disease has such a heterogeneous presentation and course. Most patients, because of the disease's self-limited nature, do not require therapy but rather simple observation. Occasionally, nonsteroidal anti-inflammatory agents may be symptomatically useful in this group of patients.

Anti-inflammatory therapy is indicated for individuals who have either severe or progressive disease. To determine if progressive disease is present, individuals initially with apparently benign disease should be followed at least at 6-month intervals to observe for evidence of progressive disease. Pulmonary function testing is particularly useful in this regard. Some patients must be treated immediately. These patients usually have critical organ involvement (cardiac disease, central nervous system disease, ocular disease, persistent hypercalcemia or hypercalciuria) or disfiguring skin lesions. Many patients with pulmonary disease need to be treated immediately if progressive pulmonary functional impairment is already evident.

Glucocorticoids are currently the principal anti-inflammatory agents used. Unfortunately, glucocorticoids have several side effects that limit both dosage and duration of therapy. In an attempt to overcome this, glucocorticoid analogs with less toxicity (inhaled steroids) or alternative anti-inflammatory agents (e.g., methotrexate, cyclophosphamide) have been used.

Whom, when, and how long to treat are all unknown. Presently, we observe patients with noncritical organ involvement, including stage I pulmonary sarcoidosis without pulmonary function impairment, at 6-month intervals with serial pulmonary function studies. Patients with critical organ involvement or with evidence of disease progression receive prednisone (1 mg/kg/day) for 4 to 6 weeks, with a rapid tapering (0.25 mg/kg/day) for 3 months more. The prednisone is then tapered to an alternate-day regimen to reduce systemic side effects or to as low a dosage as the patient tolerates. If disease progresses despite prednisone therapy, disease recurs after tapering the prednisone, or severe glucocorticoid-related side effects occur, we institute alternative anti-inflammatory therapy with the agents previously noted.

REFERENCES

Crystal RG et al: Pulmonary sarcoidosis: a disease characterized and perpetuated by activated lung T-lymphocytes. Ann Intern Med 94:73, 1981.

Gilbert SR and Hunninghake GW: Bronchoalveolar lavage in sarcoidosis. In Baughman RP, editor: Bronchoalveolar lavage. Cincinnati, 1992.

Hunninghake GW: Staging of pulmonary sarcoidosis. Chest 89:178S, 1986.

Israel HL et al: Whole-body gallium-67 scans. Am Rev Respir Dis 144:1182, 1991.

Mayock RL et al: Manifestations of sarcoidosis. Am J Med 35:67, 1963.

Moller DR et al: Bias toward use of a specific T-cell receptor B-chain variable region in a subgroup of individuals with sarcoidosis. J Clin Invest 82:1183, 1989.

Muller NL and Miller RR: Computed tomography of chronic diffuse infiltrative disease. Am Rev Respir Dis 142:1440, 1990.

Rosen Y: Sarcoidosis. In Dail DH and Hammar SP, editors: Pulmonary pathology. New York, Springer-Verlag.

Siltzbach LE: Sarcoidosis: clinical features and management. Med Clin North Am 51:483, 1967.

Siltzbach LE et al: Course and prognosis of sarcoidosis around the world. Am J Med 57:847, 1974.

Thomas PD and Hunninghake GW: Current concepts of the pathogenesis of sarcoidosis. Am Rev Respir Dis 135:747, 1987.

Winterbauer RH and Hutchinson JF: The use of pulmonary function tests in the management of sarcoidosis. Chest 78:640, 1980.

CHAPTER

208 Hypersensitivity Pneumonitis

Herbert Y. Reynolds

Repeated inhalation of a variety of small organic particles (as powder or dust or as aerosolized droplets) can cause hypersensitivity pneumonitis, also known as *extrinsic allergic alveolitis*. These dusts can be bacteria or spores from saprophytic fungi that contaminate vegetables, wood bark, water reservoir vaporizers, or dairy and grain products. They can be derived from animal excreta or can be dander. Although the antigen is usually organic, it may be inorganic, such as diphenylmethane di-isocyanate, which acts as a hapten, conjugates to self-proteins, and causes hypersensitivity pneumonitis. Colorful, descriptive names for the diseases underscore the frequent occupational or home environmental nature of exposure (Table 208-1). Two phenomena are implied in the diseases: (1) the affected subject has acquired heightened immunologic reactivity to the inciting agent, and (2) the inflammatory response that occurs is located primarily in the alveolar air exchange portion of the lung and not in the larger conducting airways, which are usually involved in asthmatic diseases. This distinction is important, for extrinsic immunoglobulin E (IgE) antibody–mediated allergic asthma is also a form of hypersensitivity lung disease, which is often associated with airborne organic antigens.

CLINICAL PRESENTATION

Hypersensitivity pneumonitis is a syndrome with a spectrum that varies from acute to chronic, depending on the frequency of antigen exposure. It may vary from mild to

Table 208-1. Hypersensitivity pneumonitis diseases with major antigens and exposure or source

Disease	Major antigens	Exposure or source
Thermophilic bacteria		
Farmer's lung	*Faenia rectivirgula (Micropolyspora faeni)*	Moldy hay
Grain handler's lung	*Thermoactinomyces faeni*	Moldy grain
Mushroom worker's lung	*M. faeni, Thermoactinomyces vulgaris*	Mushroom compost
Bagassosis	*Thermoactinomyces sacchari*	Moldy sugar cane (bagasse)
Humidifier or air conditioner lung	*T. vulgaris, M. faeni* *Aureobasidium pullulans*	Heated water reservoirs
Other bacteria		
Detergent worker's lung	*Bacillus subtilis*	Water
Humidifier lung	*Bacillus cereus*	Water reservoir
True fungi		
Maple bark stripper's lung	*Cryptostroma corticale*	Moldy bark
Malt worker's lung	*Aspergillus clavatus*	Moldy malt, barley
Sequoiosis	*A. pullulans* and *Graphium* species	Moldy redwood dust
Paprika splitter's lung	*Mucor stolonifer*	Moldy paprika pods
Cheese worker's lung	*Penicillium caseii*	Cheese mold
Suberosis	*Penicillium frequentans*	Moldy cork dust
Aspergillosis	*Aspergillus* spores	Water reservoir
Summer-type hypersensitivity	*Trichosporon cutaneum*	House dust, bird droppings
Animal proteins		
Bird breeder's lung	Avian proteins (serum, excreta)	Pigeons, parakeets
Chicken plucker's lung	Chicken feathers (serum)	Chickens
Turkey handler's lung	Turkey feathers (serum)	Turkeys
Duck fever	Duck feathers	Ducks
Rodent handler's disease	Rat urine (serum)	Rats
Pituitary snuff-taker's lung	Porcine and bovine pituitary protein	Pituitary snuff
Ameba		
Humidifier lung	*Acanthamoebea castellani* *Naegleria gruberi*	Water
Bacterial products		
Byssinosis	Lipopolysaccharide	Cotton bract
Bleomycin hypersensitivity (in contrast to fibrosis)	*Streptomyces verticillus* glycopeptides	Bleomycin
Insect products		
Miller's lung (wheat weevil disease)	*Sitophilus granarius*	Contaminated grain
Chemicals		
Chemical worker's lung	Trimellitic anhydride	Plastics
	Toluene di-isocyanate Methylene di-isocyanate	Polyurethane foam or rubber manufacture
Epoxy resin lung	Phthalic anhydride	Heated epoxy resin

Modified from Reynolds HY: Lung, 169:S109, 1991.

severe and even fatal disease depending on the intensity of the immunologic response, the concentration of inhaled antigen, and the duration of exposure. Although many persons can be exposed to these common antigens and many develop specific serum antibodies to them (precipitins are present in 5% of exposed office workers and 30% to 50% of grain handlers, dairy workers, and pigeon or bird handlers), relatively few subjects manifest respiratory disease. Sensitization to an organic dust is often insidious, but repeated exposure can produce lung changes of a lymphocytic alveolitis, but the subject remains asymptomatic. Unique host susceptibility or resistance may influence the individual response, especially in younger patients. Chronic exposure, however, can result in an interstitial, granulomatous, and fibrotic lung disease that is debilitating.

Clinically, three syndromes can occur. First, an acute reaction, occurring 4 to 8 hours after heavy exposure, develops with dyspnea, cough, chills, fever (up to 40° C), and myalgias. In the absence of a repeat exposure, spontaneous recovery occurs in 12 to 24 hours. On physical examination during an acute episode, the patient is dyspneic and has bibasilar crepitant crackles. Leukocytosis, with a left shift in the polymorphonuclear (PMN) differential count, and bibasilar alveolar infiltrates on chest radiographs are common. Pulmonary function tests during an acute attack demonstrate decreases in total lung capacity, vital capacity, and diffusing capacity. Between antigenic exposures, patients are usually asymptomatic, and all clinical tests are normal.

Second, an asymptomatic or subclinical phase of illness may ensue. It is uncertain whether all subjects exposed to an appropriate aerosol antigen manifest the acute symptoms just described or can become sensitized without noticeable respiratory and systemic effects. Since many patients develop serum precipitins to the environmental antigens encountered in dairy and farming operations or after contact with, for example, domesticated birds, a primary host immunologic response may occur without prominent illness. However, when asymptomatic, nonsmoking dairy farmers with serum-precipitating antibodies to *Micropolyspora faeni* antigen were investigated with bronchoalveolar lavage to sample alveolar cells, it was found that they had an increased recovery of lung cells and a higher-than-normal percentage of lymphocytes. Thus these ostensibly sensitized but asymptomatic subjects had subclinical evidence of lymphocytic alveolitis. The long-term effects of this low-grade immunologic response in the lung were apparently well tolerated for up to 2 and 3 years despite continued antigenic exposure. When a group of such farmers were followed with repeat bronchoalveolar lavage analysis, the lymphocytic alveolitis was usually still present. Therefore an unsuspected, asymptomatic phase of illness could be more widespread than clinically evident and represent a reservoir from which some of the chronic-phase patients emerge with much more evidence of lung involvement, with fibrosis and a granulomatous reaction.

Third, if antigen exposure is protracted, a chronic form of disease develops that may no longer feature the acute exacerbation of respiratory symptoms, fever, and so on with re-exposure. Instead, patients can develop breathlessness, dyspnea with exertion, and cough; these symptoms are indistinguishable from those found in many other forms of interstitial pulmonary diseases. Fatigue, poor appetite, and loss of weight can be significant in this stage of disease. Symptoms and evidence of constitutional effects of disease can be evident for months and occasionally for years before the patient comes for evaluation. The chest radiograph is abnormal and has telltale reticulolinear markings attributed to interstitial fibrosis. Pulmonary function tests are characterized by a restrictive ventilatory pattern and a decreased diffusing capacity for carbon monoxide. Such patients with this chronic form of inhalational hypersensitivity disease can be difficult to separate diagnostically from patients with forms of interstitial lung disease of unknown etiology, unless the exposure history is obvious. A serum antibody precipitin screen for hypersensitivity antigens will not establish a diagnosis but, if positive, might direct the clinician to consider a possible environmental exposure.

IMMUNOPATHOLOGIC FINDINGS

Most of the lung pathology studied and bronchoalveolar lavage analyses made of cells and immunoglobulins have been obtained from patients with chronic disease. Often an open lung biopsy is needed to provide an adequate specimen for histologic diagnosis, so these tissue changes are presented first.

Biopsy tissue is obtained from patients with established disease and thus at a time when chronic changes are present in lung tissue. The pathologic findings cited by Reyes and colleagues included 60 biopsies secured from patients with farmer's lung (caused by a variety of thermophilic actinomycetes). All biopsies contained interstitial pneumonitis, described as a patchy infiltrate of the alveolar walls and consisting primarily of lymphocytes and plasma cells and occasionally other inflammatory cells. When the infiltrate was extensive, similar cells were seen within the alveolar spaces. The pathologic pattern was patchy, not uniform, and intervening pulmonary parenchyma did not appear to be involved. In 27 of the 60 biopsies, the degree of interstitial pneumonitis was graded as extensive (3 +), and all biopsies contained some evidence of it. Unresolved pneumonia, featuring a fibrinous exudate and PMN leukocytes, was observed in two thirds of the specimens. Large histiocytes with foamy cytoplasm were observed in more than half the biopsies. Granulomas were usually present; however, none was seen in 18 of 60 biopsies. Other prominent findings in the farmer's lung specimens included interstitial fibrosis (in 65%); bronchiolitis obliterans (in 50 percent); foamy histiocytes (in 65%); granulomas that contained giant cells that in turn contained foreign body material, as determined by polarized light examination (70%); and pleural fibrosis (about 50%). Unfortunately the biopsies were not separated on the basis of clinical stage of disease as to recent versus chronic.

Bronchoalveolar fluid

Although it is generally accepted that hypersensitivity pneumonitis is an immunologic disorder, the exact immunopathogenic mechanisms are unknown. The most characteristic immunologic feature of hypersensitivity pneumonitis is the presence in serum of precipitating antibody against the causative antigen. These precipitins are usually IgG, but IgA and IgM have also been reported. It is important to note that the presence of precipitins is not diagnostic. An occasional patient with hypersensitivity pneumonitis will not have precipitating antibody; however, in these patients, use of concentrated serum or more sensitive assays such as radioimmunoassays may be required to detect antibody. A significant percentage of exposed asymptomatic individuals will have serum precipitins, usually of lower titer than symptomatic patients. Bronchoalveolar lavage fluid has been studied in symptomatic pigeon breeders and those with farmer's lung in subacute or chronic stages of disease without prior or recent exposure to antigen.

Principal changes in blood and lung secretions are given in the box on p. 1700. Peripheral blood values are gener-

Immunologic features of blood and bronchoalveolar lavage fluid in chronic stage of hypersensitivity pneumonitis

Blood

Normal blood cell counts
Normal immunoglobulin levels, usually
Positive serum precipitins (IgG)

Bronchoalveolar lavage fluid

Lung cell recovery increased
High lymphocyte percentages (50% to 70% of bronchoalveolar lavage cells)
- T lymphocytes predominate
- May have increased number of cytotoxic T-suppressor cells (slight reversal of T helper/T suppressor cell ratio)
- T cell division high (10% to 15% in replicating phase)
- Natural killer lymphocytes increased; enhanced cytotoxicity evident; gamma/delta receptors

Large and foamy macrophages, minimum eosinophils, and increased number (up to 1% of all lavage cells) of basophils
Total protein increased
- Elevated IgG and IgM levels
- IgG and IgA antibodies present
- Abnormal surfactant composition

ally normal, in contrast to cellular and protein changes in alveolar lavage fluid. The recovery of respiratory cells is increased, which reflects a substantially higher percentage of T lymphocytes than found in normal persons. Whereas the subtypes of T cells in normals are in a ratio of about 1.5:1.8 for T helper lymphocytes to T suppressor cells (see Chapter 193), a slight excess of T suppressor cells in hypersensitivity pneumonitis can decrease the ratio to less than 1. This decrease has been documented in several studies. In contrast, T helper cells are found in greatly increased numbers in patients with active alveolitis of sarcoidosis such that the ratio may be in the 4 to 8 range. Cytotoxic lymphocytes can be activated in this stage of hypersensitivity disease as well. About 10% of the alveolar macrophages are large and have a peculiar appearance of vacuolated cytoplasm, which have been termed *foamy* macrophages.

Total protein content in lavage fluid is increased but without a disproportionate increase in albumin, which would point to a significant leak of protein across the endothelial-alveolar barrier. Enhanced immunoglobulin content accounts for some of this because IgG and IgM levels are increased; special elevation of IgG_4 was noted in pigeon breeders. Special antibody activity in IgG and IgA classes can be identified. Apparently, surfactant has an unusual composition in hypersensitivity pneumonitis. Specimens show increased levels of phosphatidylinositol compared with phosphatidylcholine, but levels of phosphatidylethanolamine and glycerol are decreased.

DIAGNOSIS

The diagnosis of a typical presentation of acute hypersensitivity pneumonitis can usually be made by history of exposure, subsequent signs and symptoms, chest radiographs, confirmatory serologic studies, and a trial of avoidance. Often the physician may never see someone in an early phase, since an alert person might recognize the precipitating cause and voluntarily remove it from the environment.

The chronic, insidious forms of hypersensitivity pneumonitis are often more difficult to diagnose. The differential diagnosis includes usual interstitial pneumonitis, chronic eosinophilic pneumonia, idiopathic hemosiderosis, sarcoidosis, pulmonary alveolar proteinosis, and interstitial pulmonary disorders caused by infectious agents, mineral dust, chemical fumes, neoplasia, drugs, and collagen vascular disease (Chapter 210). Hypersensitivity pneumonitis involves the lung only; therefore extrapulmonary signs such as hepatosplenomegaly are not compatible with a diagnosis of hypersensitivity pneumonitis. If a specific diagnosis cannot be made by noninvasive tests, a lung biopsy may be required to differentiate hypersensitivity pneumonitis from other forms of interstitial pulmonary disease. Establishing the diagnosis may require considerable detective work, even going into the subject's working or home environment for clues, and may necessitate assessing fellow workers for illness.

Occasionally a challenge with the antigen is indicated for diagnosis. This challenge should be done only if history, physical examination, pulmonary function, chest radiograph, avoidance, and antibody tests have failed to establish a diagnosis. Moreover, challenges should be done only on patients who have recovered lung function and only under the careful supervision of a physician experienced in these procedures. Because patients may become very ill as a result of deliberate challenges, physicians should initiate them with caution and with appropriate plans for observation and therapy in the event that severe immediate or late reaction occurs.

TREATMENT AND PROGNOSIS

Once the offending antigen has been identified, avoidance should be the primary modality of treatment. In a patient with a contaminated ventilation system, for example, cleaning to remove the thermophilic organisms is essential. Since many exposures that cause hypersensitivity pneumonitis are occupational, such measures as improved ventilation, masks, or change in job duties or work site may suffice. Often, however, a change of occupation is necessary to prevent progression to irreversible lung damage. However, some workers can have an unsuspected lymphocytic alveolitis but remain asymptomatic despite continued antigen exposure. Whether to recommend a change in job or avocation for the subject with subclinical, asymptomatic disease can be a difficult decision, since the lung seems to tolerate this smoldering alveolitis for several years at least.

If abnormalities in clinical and pulmonary function occur despite avoidance, corticosteroids in moderate doses (30 to 40 mg of prednisone orally per day) may be required for several weeks or even months to determine whether reversibility of clinical and pulmonary function abnormalities is possible. Cromolyn, antihistamines, and bronchodilators are not helpful. In the patient with an acute episode, corticosteroids significantly ameliorate the severity of an attack. The duration of corticosteroid therapy should be based on patient improvement and objective changes in pulmonary function tests. Avoidance is of paramount importance, and corticosteroids should not be relied on to suppress symptoms caused by repeated exposure.

The prognosis of hypersensitivity pneumonitis depends on two primary factors: the amount of irreversible fibrotic disease at the time of diagnosis and the patient's capability to avoid further antigen exposure. In patients with the acute form of the disease, all clinical abnormalities will reverse and no further attacks will occur if avoidance is practiced. In patients with more chronic forms of the disease, avoidance and corticosteroids produce variable degrees of improvement. Those with permanent, irreversible pulmonary damage from fibrosis or bronchiolitis obliterans unfortunately will have little improvement. This problem underscores the importance of both early detection of clinical disease and identification and avoidance of the causative antigen.

REFERENCES

Campbell JM: Acute symptoms following work with hay. Br Med J 2:1143, 1932.

Cormier Y et al: Abnormal bronchoalveolar lavage in asymptomatic dairy farmers: study of lymphocytes. Am Rev Respir Dis 130:1046, 1984.

Cormier Y, Belanger J, and Laviolette M: Persistent bronchoalveolar lymphocytosis in asymptomatic farmers. Am Rev Respir Dis 133:843, 1986.

Costabel U et al: Ia-like antigens on T-cells and their subpopulations in pulmonary sarcoidosis and in hypersensitivity pneumonitis: analysis of bronchoalveolar and blood lymphocytes. Am Rev Respir Dis 131:337, 1985.

Fournier E et al: Early neutrophil alveolitis after inhalation challenge in hypersensitivity pneumonitis. Chest 88:563, 1985.

Leatherman JW et al: Lung T cells in hypersensitivity pneumonitis. Ann Intern Med 100:390, 1984.

Patterson R et al: IgA and IgG antibody activities of serum and bronchoalveolar fluid from symptomatic pigeon breeders. Am Rev Respir Dis 120:113, 1979.

Reed CE, Sosman A, and Barbee RA: Pigeon breeder's lung. JAMA 193:261, 1965.

Reyes CN, Wenzel FJ, and Lawton BR: The pulmonary pathology of farmer's lung disease. Chest 81:142, 1982.

Reynolds HY: Concepts of pathogenesis and lung reactivity in hypersensitivity pneumonitis. Ann NY Acad Sci 465:287, 1986.

Reynolds H: Hypersensitivity pneumonitis: correlation of cellular and immunologic changes with clinical phases of disease. Lung 169:S109, 1991.

Reynolds HY et al: Analysis of cellular and protein components of bronchoalveolar lavage fluid from patients with idiopathic pulmonary fibrosis and hypersensitivity pneumonitis. J Clin Invest 59:165, 1977.

Semenzato G et al: Lung T cells in hypersensitivity pneumonitis: phenotypic and functional analyses. J Immunol 137:1164, 1986.

Trentin L et al: Mechanisms accounting for lymphocytic alveolitis in hypersensitivity pneumonitis. J Immunol 145:2147, 1990.

CHAPTER

209 Langerhans' Cell Granulomatosis (Histiocytosis X, Eosinophilic Granuloma)

Allan J. Hance
Françoise Basset

DEFINITION AND NOMENCLATURE

Langerhans' cell granulomatosis (LCG) is defined pathologically by the presence of characteristic destructive granulomatous lesions containing Langerhans' cells. Current evidence suggests that LCG results from a granulomatous immune response initiated by Langerhans' cells, although the nature of the antigen(s) involved in this process remains unknown. A wide spectrum of clinical manifestations can be encountered, depending on the number of tissues involved and the specific sites of involvement. Multiple tissue involvement, ranging from diffuse involvement of multiple visceral organs to multifocal involvement of two or more tissues, is more frequently observed in infants and young children. LCG localized to a single tissue (usually bone or lung) is the most common form of LCG observed in older children and adults.

Various names are used for this disease, which may cause confusion. The name *Langerhans' cell granulomatosis* has the virtue of emphasizing the essential role of Langerhans' cells in initiating the process and the granulomatous nature of the lesions. *Histiocytosis X* and *Langerhans' cell histiocytosis* are also frequently used terms. *Letterer-Siwe disease, Hand-Schüller-Christian syndrome,* and *eosinophilic granuloma* are often used, respectively, to describe patients with diffuse visceral and systemic manifestations, multifocal involvement of two or more tissues, or LCG localized to a single organ. In reality, it is often difficult to use this classification because these groupings often overlap.

This discussion is limited to the adult pulmonary form of LCG. Although pulmonary LCG usually is classified among the interstitial lung diseases, the granulomas are centered on small bronchioles, and it may be preferable to consider the process as a bronchiolitis.

EPIDEMIOLOGY

No precise data are available concerning the prevalence of localized pulmonary LCG. Since its description as a discrete nosologic entity in 1951, the disease is being recognized with increasing frequency and probably represents 1% to 5% of all cases of interstitial lung disease. The disease is said to be less common among blacks and Asians. All age groups can be affected, although most patients are 20 to 40 years old. The disease occurs more often in men, which almost certainly reflects the strong association between pulmonary LCG and cigarette smoking. More than 90% of patients are smokers, and patients with LCG tend to smoke more heavily than persons in the general population. Daily cigarette consumption is a more important risk factor than total pack-years, since many patients have smoked for only a limited time.

PATHOGENESIS

Dendritic cells and Langerhans' cells

The initiation of immune responses depends on the participation of "accessory cells," which are required to present antigens to helper T lymphocytes. Two different populations of accessory cells are present in the normal lung: those of monocyte/macrophage lineage (alveolar macrophages) and those of dendritic cell/Langerhans' cell lineage. As with the alveolar macrophages, cells of dendritic cell/Langerhans' cell lineage are derived from bone marrow precursors and probably arrive in the lung through the peripheral circulation. Dendritic cells, present within the alveolar parenchyma and peribronchiolar tissues, have a folded nucleus, multiple long dendritic processes, and contain few phagocytic inclusions. Langerhans' cells, found almost exclusively *within* the bronchiolar epithelium of normal nonsmokers, are morphologically similar to dendritic cells but contain characteristic pentalaminar platelike cytoplasmic organelles called *Birbeck granules,* which can be seen only by electron microscopy. Langerhans' cells also express surface antigens that react with CD1a (T6) monoclonal antibodies. Most pulmonary dendritic cells are CD1a negative but do express CD1c surface antigens. Langerhans' cells are thought to be derived from dendritic cells, and this transformation in lung and other tissues is associated with close contact between the Langerhans' cells and epithelial cells. The differences between the functional capacities of dendritic cells and Langerhans' cells are still under investigation.

Langerhans' cell granulomatosis

The evolution of the pathologic lesions of pulmonary LCG (see following discussion) is highly reminiscent of a granulomatous process and is the most compelling argument that the disease results from an uncontrolled immune response initiated by Langerhans' cells. The virtual absence of Langerhans' cells in late lesions refutes the idea that the disorder is a malignancy or results from the "uncontrolled proliferation" of Langerhans' cells. Langerhans' cells are known to accumulate at sites of pulmonary epithelial hyperplasia and infiltrate some lung carcinomas. Thus bronchiolar epithelial abnormalities may predispose to the development of LCG and could account for heavy cigarette smoking (a common cause of epithelial hyperplasia) being a strong risk factor for this disease.

Langerhans' cells are potent accessory cells and can initiate immune responses against a variety of antigens. The nature of the antigen(s), if any, involved in LCG remains unknown. No associations between LCG and environmental exposures (except cigarette smoking) or infectious agents have been reported. Because of the bronchiolar distribution of the process and the characteristic destruction of bronchiolar epithelium in pathologic lesions, we have suggested that stressed, transformed, or otherwise abnormal epithelial cells may be the target of this immune response, at least in some patients.

PATHOLOGY

Pulmonary involvement by LCG is typically generalized throughout both lungs. However, the process is not diffuse in the sense that the lesions occur almost exclusively adjacent to terminal and respiratory bronchioles and are separated from each other by apparently normal lung tissue. The pathologic appearance of LCG lesions changes considerably as the process evolves. Although the pulmonary lesions in a single biopsy frequently show a spectrum of evolutionary changes, the pathologic appearance of lung tissue is useful in assessing the activity of the process. The center of early lesions is composed primarily of clusters of Langerhans' cells, which are surrounded by variable numbers of lymphocytes, eosinophils, and neutrophils. These foci form adjacent to terminal or respiratory bronchioles and destroy the pre-existing bronchiolar epithelium and wall, from the earliest respiratory bronchiole to the last alveolar duct, in the involved acini.

As the lesions progress, the number of Langerhans' cells usually decreases and other cell types predominate, especially neutrophils, eosinophils, and alveolar macrophages. Fibrotic changes begin to appear at this stage. Most often, scarring results in fibrotic walls, limiting cystic lesions. At other sites, fibrosis develop in the center and results in stellate scars often surrounded by traction emphysema. Scarring predominates in end-stage lesions, and few infiltrating cells are present, although lymphoid aggregates and lipid-laden macrophages may remain; Langerhans' cells are present in very small numbers or may be entirely absent. Although granulomatous lesions of all stages frequently appear cavitary, this does not usually result from necrosis of the center of the granulomatous lesions. Rather, destruction of the wall of bronchioles adjacent to the granulomas typically occurs, such that the distorted lumen of the now unrecognizable bronchiole appears as a cavity. The erosion of such peripheral cavities into the pleural space accounts for the high incidence of pneumothorax seen in patients with pulmonary LCG.

CLINICAL MANIFESTATIONS

Pulmonary LCG may manifest in a variety of ways. The most common presentations include (1) the insidious onset of cough, fatigue, and progressive dyspnea, with or without constitutional symptoms; (2) the presence of systemic symptoms only (e.g., weight loss, malaise, fever); (3) the occurrence of one or several episodes of spontaneous pneumothorax; (4) the discovery of diffuse pulmonary abnormalities on a routine chest roentgenogram; or (5) the identification of lung involvement during evaluation of a patient with extrapulmonary LCG. Only a few adult patients with pulmonary LCG have involvement of other tissues. The most frequent forms of extrapulmonary involvement include isolated bone lesions, skin lesions, and diabetes insipidus resulting from involvement of the hypothalamic/pituitary axis.

In most patients the physical examination of the chest is normal or reveals rales. More rarely, wheezes are present. Clubbing may occur, especially in patients with advanced disease.

Characteristic radiographic findings in the early stages of pulmonary LCG are the presence of bilateral reticular and micronodular infiltrates that are most marked in the upper and middle zones and usually spare the costophrenic angles. In later stages, cystic lesions or small cavitary nodules can be seen. Honeycombing is often observed in advanced cases, frequently associated with the presence of larger bullous changes. Pleural abnormalities are rare, except in patients with a prior history of pneumothorax or thoracotomy. Enlargement of hilar lymph nodes is rarely observed. Recent studies have shown that high-resolution computed tomography (HRCT) is particularly useful in identifying patients with LCG. HCRT permits the detection of characteristic cystic lesions in essentially all patients, even when chest radiographs are interpreted as normal or showing a reticular pattern. Nodular lesions (usually <5 mm diameter) are also identified by HCRT in most patients. ^{67}Ga scans of the thorax are usually normal.

The results of the routine blood tests are often normal, although mild anemia and leukocytosis may be present. Eosinophilia is rare. Increased immunoglobulins and low titers of antinuclear antibodies, rheumatoid factor, and circulating immune complexes have been described in some patients but are of no diagnostic use.

Pulmonary function tests often demonstrate a combined restrictive and obstructive pattern. Total lung capacity and vital capacity are usually reduced or normal; the residual volume/total lung capacity ratio is frequently increased, especially in patients with cystic changes on chest radiographs. The diffusing capacity is reduced in most patients. Evidence of overt airflow limitation is more common in LCG than most other interstitial lung diseases. Hypoxemia occurs frequently and is usually increased with exercise.

Cells recovered by bronchoalveolar lavage from patients with pulmonary LCG typically include clearly increased numbers of eosinophils and neutrophils and a moderate increase in the number of T lymphocytes. Large numbers of alveolar macrophages are also often present but probably reflect that most patients are cigarette smokers; increased numbers of alveolar macrophages need not be present in lavage fluid from nonsmokers with pulmonary LCG. It has been suggested that bronchoalveolar lavage may be used to establish the diagnosis of pulmonary LCG. The identification of large numbers of Langerhans' cells among cells recovered by lavage using CD1a (T6) monoclonal antibodies may be useful in the diagnosis of LCG. Although Langerhans' cells are rarely recovered by lavage from normal individuals, moderate numbers of Langerhans' cells can be recovered from cigarette smokers and patients with other interstitial lung diseases. Furthermore, the percentage of Langerhans' cells recovered by lavage from patients with pulmonary LCG can vary considerably and depends partly on the activity of the process. Thus the test's sensitivity and specificity depend on the threshold used to define a positive result, and this question has not been systematically evaluated. In an appropriate clinical context, however, the presence of more than 5% Langerhans' cells is highly suggestive of LCG. This threshold will be attained in few patients; therefore a negative result does not eliminate the diagnosis.

DIAGNOSIS

The presenting signs and symptoms of pulmonary LCG are usually nonspecific, and it is often difficult to differentiate pulmonary LCG from other, more common forms of interstitial lung disease. Useful differential points in the history include the presence of interstitial lung disease in young patients, especially cigarette smokers; the occurrence of one or more pneumothoraces; or the presence of extrapulmonary involvement. Characteristic findings on chest radiographs or HCRT may raise suspicion of the process. Finally, the presence of combined obstructive and restrictive abnormalities on pulmonary function testing also suggests involvement by pulmonary LCG.

Nevertheless, none of these clinical findings is specific. Histologic examination of lung tissue is required to firmly establish the diagnosis and offers the advantage of providing information concerning the activity of the process. Open lung biopsy is the procedure most often used to obtain lung tissue. It is important that relatively normal lung is biopsied, not tissue with extensive fibrotic changes, which renders pathologic interpretation difficult. Samples of any biopsy should also be processed to permit evaluation by electron microscopy and immunofluorescent techniques, which may be helpful in difficult cases. Transbronchial biopsy is rarely useful, since the lesions of pulmonary LCG are located mainly in the vicinity of terminal or respiratory bronchioles and are not often present in the samples taken through the wall of larger bronchi explored with the fiberoptic bronchoscope.

EVOLUTION

The natural history of pulmonary LCG varies considerably. Approximately 25% to 50% of patients remain asymptomatic or become symptom free with accompanying regression of the radiologic abnormalities. The remaining patients experience a more progressive course, which may be punctuated by periods of remission or relative stability. Although the disease may arrest at any stage, patients with progressive disease are likely to experience persistent respiratory symptoms and have permanent loss of pulmonary function resulting from fibrosis, extensive remodeling of the lung parenchyma, and/or formation of bullous defects. As a general rule, bullous formation with evidence of air trapping and/or airflow obstruction appears to be more common than a purely restrictive defect in patients with significant sequelae. The clinical course is complicated by pneumothorax in 10% to 20% of patients. Unrelenting progression culminating in death from respiratory failure and/or cor pulmonale occurs in few patients.

A variety of factors appears to influence the evolution of pulmonary LCG. Very young or advanced age is often associated with a poor prognosis. The extent of clinical symptoms and radiologic abnormalities at presentation also correlate to some extent with eventual outcome. In particular, repeated episodes of pneumothorax are by themselves a poor prognostic sign, at least partly because they lead to repeated surgical procedures and sometimes to superinfection. The association of pulmonary involvement with evidence of LCG in other tissues, especially cutaneous lesions or diabetes insipidus, can be a particularly ominous sign. However, the association of pulmonary LCG with bone lesions is of less significance, especially when such bone lesions are not widespread.

TREATMENT

Because of the strong association between cigarette smoking and LCG, cessation of tobacco use is imperative, although the effect of discontinuing smoking on the evolution of established LCG has not been studied. In view of the favorable prognosis in most patients, asymptomatic individuals or patients with little functional impairment should be managed conservatively. Similarly, patients whose lung pathology shows only inactive "late" lesions are unlikely to respond to treatment. Systemic corticosteroids (e.g., prednisone 1 mg/kg/day for several months followed by gradually tapering doses) are the usual treatment for patients with progressive symptoms and active pathologic lesions. Although anecdotal reports of favorable responses have been published, corticosteroids have never been proved to improve the course of pulmonary LCG. Recurrent pneumothoraces are adequately treated by pleurodesis.

REFERENCES

Friedman PJ, Liebow AA, and Sokoloff J: Eosinophilic granuloma of lung: clinical aspects of primary pulmonary histiocytosis in the adult. Medicine 60:385, 1981.

Grenier P et al: Chronic diffuse interstitial lung disease: diagnostic value of chest radiography and high resolution CT. Radiology 179:123, 1991.

Hance AJ et al: Pulmonary and extrapulmonary manifestations of Langerhans' cell granulomatosis (histiocytosis X). Semin Respir Med 9:349, 1988.

Valeyre D et al: Langerhans' cell granulomatosis. In Bone RC and Reynolds HY, editors: Pulmonary and critical care medicine, vol 2. St Louis, 1993, Mosby–Year Book.

CHAPTER

210 Primary Granulomatous Pulmonary Vasculitis

Stephen B. Sulavik

Granulomatous vasculitis is the most common *clinically* apparent form of *primary* blood vessel inflammation affecting the lung. Although the inflammatory tissue reaction in these disorders is mainly centered on blood vessels, parenchymal or bronchial involvement, apparently independent of damaged vessels, may also occur in some of these disorders. *Vasculitis* is the initial and dominant inflammatory tissue reaction and may be defined as a *nonmalignant cellular infiltration of the blood vessel walls involving at least the vascular media*. Primary blood vessel involvement, which is mainly associated with vascular endothelial proliferation (scleroderma), vascular wall replacement (amyloidosis), or a sustained increase of pulmonary artery pressure (pulmonary hypertension), is therefore not included.

A *granulomatous* inflammatory tissue response is characterized by the presence of varying *numbers* as well as varied *combinations* of histiocytes (tissue macrophages), lymphocytes, plasma cells, giant cells, eosinophils, or lymphoreticular cells. The specific type of cell (its atypia and/or proliferation) or combination of cells characterizing the *dominant cellular features* of the pathologic lesion identifies the specific disorder in most cases. Unlike other cells that may be involved in the inflammatory process, the histiocyte is virtually always present in abnormal numbers in each of the disorders that make up the granulomatous vasculitides. Furthermore, the granulomatous reaction may take the spatial configuration of a three-dimensional, compact, organized collection of altered mononuclear cells (granuloma) or that of a loosely arranged, amorphous proliferation of these cells (granulomatous reaction). Necrosis (usually fibrinoid) of the vessel wall may or may not result; thus the qualifying terms *necrotizing* or *nonnecrotizing* may be used. A granulomatous vascular inflammatory response therefore may be contrasted to a primary vascular inflammatory response that is predominantly rich in neutrophils, that is, hypersensitivity angiitis (of Zeek) or periarteritis nodosa (PAN), as originally described by Kussmaul and Maier.

It may reasonably be postulated that the immunopathogenesis and etiology of these varied histologic responses differ. Unfortunately at present, the cause of most granulomatous vasculitides is not known, and pathogenetic mechanisms are at best poorly understood, so disease classification on these bases is impossible. Currently, *size* of the blood vessel involved (large, medium, small) is the most widely used parameter in the diagnostic classification of the "systemic" vasculitides, including those involving the lung. Since information pertaining to immunologic and nonimmunologic mechanisms involved in the "trafficking" of specific cells in the lung and their interrelationships in health and disease is rapidly accumulating, this basis for classification does not appear to be appropriate for the *pulmonary* vasculitides; a more rational *cornerstone* therefore is accurate, descriptive tissue histopathology. Although histopathologic interpretation alone at times may be nondiagnostic, when interpreted in conjunction with the chest radiographic appearance and certain distinctive clinical manifestations, rather clear clinical diagnoses generally emerge. Since considerable information is known regarding prognosis and treatment of many of these often life-threatening disorders, clinical suspicion of their presence and accurate histologic diagnosis usually are essential. For these reasons, we have used a combined histologic, chest radiographic, and clinical approach to classify and diagnose these disorders while continuing to retain important historic eponyms (Table 210-1).

In attempting to understand the pulmonary vasculitides, one is confronted with considerable confusion concerning peri(poly)arteritis nodosa and its relationship to the lung. After careful, extensive review (author's) of patients reported to have PAN with "pulmonary" involvement, it is strikingly evident that virtually all would fit the histologic, radiographic, and clinical criteria for either Churg-Strauss syndrome (CSS) or Wegener's granulomatosis (WG), bearing no resemblance to the original histopathologic description of PAN by Kussmaul and Maier. Their classic description included involvement of medium-sized arteries, segmental distribution, and varying stages, from acute *nongranulomatous* inflammation, mainly characterized by neutrophil infiltration, to fibrosis with grossly visible vascular aneurysms and excrescences. These pathologic findings to date have not been described in the low-pressure pulmonary artery system, and they have been observed only rarely in systemic bronchial arteries within the mediastinum. As currently used, the broad term *polyarteritis* is nonspecific and infers only that inflammation involves all layers of a blood vessel wall, which is observed in almost all types of "vasculitides." Unfortunately the word *peri(poly)-arteritis* also tacitly implies the qualifying term *nodosa,* further obscuring the original description of PAN.

EOSINOPHILIC GRANULOMATOUS VASCULITIS

Churg-Strauss syndrome

Clinical and laboratory findings. CSS, also referred to as *allergic granulomatosis* or *allergic vasculitis* (Harkavy syndrome), is a multisystem disorder, the precise mechanism and etiology(ies) of which are unknown. Males and females are affected equally, with a mean age of onset of approximately 35 years. Clinically, CSS is characterized by (1) the presence and/or history of bronchial asthma (rarely, cough-

Table 210-1. Primary granulomatous pulmonary vasculitis (GPV)

Dominant histopathology	Chest radiograph	Unique clinical features
Eosinophilic GPV		
Churg-Strauss syndrome	"Lateral" densities*	Asthma Peripheral blood eosinophilia
Mononuclear-giant cell GPV		
Wegener's granulomatosis		
Complete form (CWG)	Nodule(s),* mass lesion(s)*	Lung; kidney; upper respiratory tract, eye or ear
Limited forms (LWG)	Nodule(s)*, mass lesion(s)*	Variations of complete form
Second-degree *Dirofilaria immitis*	"Solitary" nodule	Limited to lung
Lymphocytic GPV		
"Benign" lymphocytic angiitis and granulomatosis	Nodules, infiltrates	Limited to lung
Behçet's disease, Hughes-Stovin syndrome	Pulmonary artery aneurysms	Eye involvement, phlebitis, orogenital ulcers, systemic phlebitis
Atypical lymphoreticular GPV		
Lymphomatoid granulomatosis	Nodule(s),* mass lesion(s)*	Increased central nervous system and skin involvement
Histiocytic (epithelioid) granuloma GPV		
Necrotizing sarcoid	Nodules, hilar adenopathy	Symmetric nodules
Schistosoma mansoni	Increased size of pulmonary arteries and heart	Pulmonary hypertension
Secondary to talc or starch	Same as above	Same as above
Giant cell GPV		
Takayasu's arteritis	Pulmonary artery narrowing and occlusion	"Aortic branch" syndromes

*Transient-successive radiographic pattern.

equivalent asthma), (2) peripheral blood eosinophilia (PBE), and (3) extrapulmonary signs and/or symptoms resulting from small and medium-sized blood vessel vasculitis, extravascular necrotizing granulomas, or nonvascular tissue infiltration by eosinophils. The erythrocyte sedimentation rate (ESR) and serum immunoglobulin E (IgE) levels are usually elevated, particularly during the "vasculitic" phase of the illness; at this time, anemia, weight loss, temperature elevation, sweats, weakness, and malaise are typically present.

The organ systems most involved clinically in CSS include the respiratory tract (100%), nervous system (65%), skin (60%), gastrointestinal tract (60%), and cardiovascular system (25%). *Respiratory tract* symptoms are dominated by bronchial asthma, with manifestations of other organ involvement usually occurring within the first 2 to 5 years after its onset, although much longer durations have been noted. Since asthma may not clinically be present at the onset of other systemic manifestations, a history of prior asthma assumes diagnostic importance. Sinorhinitis, often accompanied by nasal polyps, typically occurs. Chest pain caused by eosinophilic pleuritis may also occur. Paresthesias, pain, and weakness, mainly resulting from mononeuritis multiplex, are the most common clinical expressions of *nervous system* involvement. Cerebral infarction and hemorrhage, fortunately rare, is one of the more common causes of death. *Skin* manifestations often occur in crops and include purpura (usually palpable), urticaria and angioneurotic edema, and cutaneous or subcutaneous nodules. Biopsy, particularly of the nodular type of lesion (necrotizing CSS granuloma), is often diagnostic. *Gastrointestinal* involvement should be suspected if signs and/or symptoms of ischemia and infarction occur. Angiographic studies of the abdominal arterial system may confirm the diagnosis of vasculitis if aneurysmal dilatation of vessels is found. *Cardiac* manifestations include eosinophilic pericarditis, endomyocardopathy, and coronary vasculitis, with congestive heart failure being the most frequent cause of death. *Renal* failure, quite responsive to corticosteroid therapy, occurs in less than 5% of patients. However, proteinuria and microscopic hematuria, suggesting mild nephritis, typically occur. Arthritis, arthralgia, lymphadenopathy, myositis, and prostatitis may also be observed.

Although tissue biopsy may provide definitive histologic evidence for CSS, in most patients the diagnosis can be made on clinical grounds alone.

Radiographic appearance. Since bronchial asthma is an integral part of CSS, radiographic abnormalities frequently associated with asthma may occur. In addition, in those individuals who develop pericardial, myocardial, or endomyocardial involvement, radiographic changes consistent with such cardiac complications may also be observed.

As the result of massive eosinophil infiltration of the lung parenchyma, distinctive radiographic patterns emerge and serve to differentiate CSS from the other vasculitides. All these patterns have "cloudy shadowing"–like infiltrations that reside almost exclusively in the *lateral* aspects of the posteroanterior (PA) chest radiograph (Fig. 210-1).

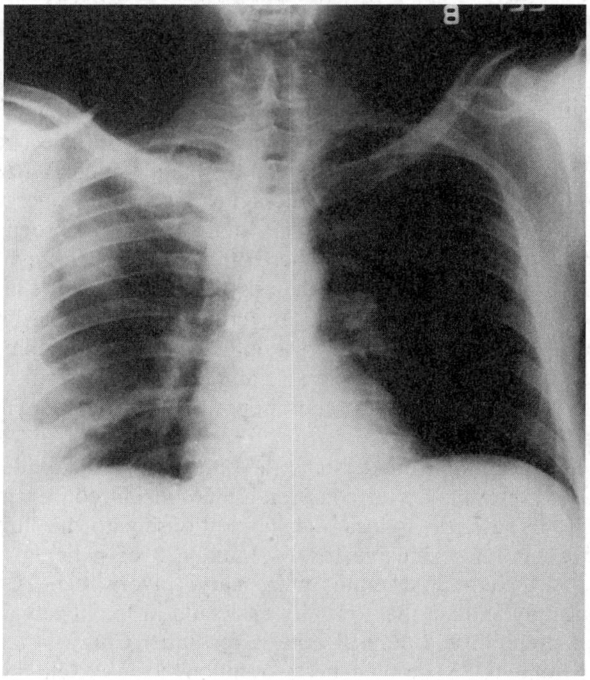

Fig. 210-1. "Cloudy," lateralizing, homogeneous densities occupying the right upper and lower lung fields in a patient with Churg-Strauss syndrome (CSS).

These infiltrations are observed in approximately 40% to 60% of patients at some time during the course of the disease and may assume any of the following patterns:

1. Transient-successive (i.e., on successive radiographs); some densities regress or disappear, whereas others increase in size or new lesions appear
2. Bilateral, symmetric, lateralizing densities extending from the lung apex to base
3. Symmetric variations of pattern 2, involving only the upper, middle, or lower lung fields
4. Unilateral lateralizing densities extending from the apex to the base
5. Most frequent pattern, with multiple lateralizing densities in various lobes and segments. (This pattern may also be observed in an idiopathic *intraluminal* organizing pneumonia referred to as *cryptogenic organizing pneumonia*.)

Although over time all these patterns tend to wax and wane, this aspect may not be appreciated on initial presentation, since they can remain unchanged for considerable periods. Interestingly, these patterns are also characteristic of chronic eosinophilic pneumonia (CEP), and the transient-successive pattern is the hallmark of Löffler's syndrome (LS). Although bronchial asthma and peripheral blood eosinophilia may also be present in CEP and LS, they differ in that no extrapulmonary manifestations exist, and significant vasculitis and necrotizing eosinophilic granulomas are absent. These radiographic features, in addition to peripheral blood and lung eosinophilia, provide a common thread, suggesting a relationship among the clinically benign Löffler's syndrome, the more severe CEP, and the potentially life-threatening CSS. The physician must have a high degree of clinical awareness of the possible presence of CSS in patients with PBE and bronchial asthma alone or in those patients with CEP who develop extrapulmonary manifestations consistent with CSS.

Pathology and immunology. Aneurysmal dilatation of medium-sized arteries may be observed on gross inspection. Other than the usual findings in bronchial asthma, characteristic histopathology includes:

1. *Infiltration* (predominantly by eosinophils) *of blood vessel walls* (venules, arterioles, medium-sized arteries). These lesions are segmental, and different stages, ranging from early eosinophil infiltration with fibrinoid necrosis to more nonspecific scarring, may be observed. The importance of elastic tissue staining to assess the presence and degree of vasculitis in this disease as well as in all the pulmonary vasculitides cannot be overemphasized.
2. *Necrotizing eosinophilic granulomas*. These are composed of an eosinophilic fibrinoid necrotic core surrounded by radially arranged histiocytes and occasional giant cells. The cellular infiltrate surrounding the granuloma consists largely of eosinophils. They are most often found extravascularly but occasionally are seen within walls of the larger blood vessels as well.
3. *Nonvascular tissue infiltration* (predominantly by eosinophils).

It is important to emphasize that these histopathologic lesions are randomly distributed throughout the various organs involved, so biopsy of a single organ rarely demonstrates all three histopathologic changes. The intense tissue eosinophilia readily distinguishes CSS from the other pulmonary vasculitides.

The immunopathology of CSS remains unclear, although some evidence suggests that immune complexes and the eosinophil itself play a role. Recently an antineutrophilic cytoplasmic autoantibody (ANCA) to myeloperoxidase resulting in a *perinuclear* staining pattern (P-ANCA) has been detected in approximately 70% of patients with CSS and other forms of systemic vasculitis. P-ANCA therefore may represent a useful adjunct to the clinical diagnosis and management of CSS.

Treatment. The ultimate mortality from CSS in untreated patients probably exceeds 80% to 90%. The use of corticosteroids and immunosuppressive therapy has reduced this mortality to less than 10% when the disease is diagnosed and treated early. This further emphasizes the importance of accurate, early diagnosis. Most patients respond well to prednisone (60 to 80 mg daily), particularly if heart failure has not supervened. Residual neurologic defects often remain despite therapy. Monitoring of the ESR, eosinophil count, serum IgE, and P-ANCA, if initially detected, provides useful laboratory guidelines for management. Relapses can occur, requiring reinstitution of therapy or an increase in the administered dose. Prolonged therapy of 9 months to 1 year is recommended after an appropriate maintenance dose has been established. For those patients not responding to corticosteroid therapy, cyclophosphamide (2 mg/kg) has proved effective.

MONONUCLEAR-GIANT CELL GRANULOMATOUS VASCULITIS

Wegener's granulomatosis

WG is a multisystem disorder that, as "classically" described, consists of necrotizing vasculitis and aseptic necrosis of (1) the lung and (2) the upper respiratory tract with (3) focal glomerulonephritis of the kidney (complete form [CWG], Wegener triad). Since Wegener's original description, however, patients with identical histopathology, natural history, and response to therapy have been reported with "limited" clinical manifestations (LWG): (1) lung alone or with associated skin involvement; (2) upper respiratory tract, eye or ear (URTE); (3) lung and URTE; (4) lung and kidney; and (5) kidney and URTE. Since focal glomerulonephritis occurs in many other disorders, a diagnosis of CSS based on kidney involvement alone cannot be made. Any of these formes frustes may evolve into another limited form or the classic triad, and since the mortality from these limited forms in untreated patients is exceedingly high, prompt recognition and appropriate therapy are essential.

Clinical and laboratory findings. Males are affected more frequently than females, with a mean age at onset of approximately 40 years. A significant number of patients (20%) are less than age 25, and important clinical differences exist in this younger age group. Typically in CWG, chronic sinusitis or rhinitis, refractory to usual therapy, heralds the onset of the disease. Lung involvement may already be present at this time or follow the upper respiratory tract manifestations. Signs of kidney damage, often culminating in fulminant renal failure, may be present at initial diagnosis but usually occur later in the course of the disease to complete the triad. The ESR and the serum C-reactive protein concentration are usually elevated, and mild anemia and thrombocytosis may be found. Significant peripheral blood eosinophilia is absent.

The following organ systems are the most frequently involved in CWG and LWG. In the *upper respiratory tract,* granulomatous invasion of large bronchi can lead to varying degrees of bronchial, tracheal, or laryngeal stenosis. Chronic ulcerative lesions of the oral mucosa (buccal, palatal, gingival) are particularly frequent in younger patients. Rhinitis (frequently with epistaxis) refractory to usual therapy, with or without ulceration or perforation of the nasal septum, typically occurs. Occasionally a "saddle" nose deformity resulting from cartilage destruction is observed. Chronic sinusitis, also refractory to usual therapy, occurs frequently. Although ulcerations of these areas may be extensive, unlike other granulomatous diseases affecting the midline of the face, WG rarely extends to destroy the overlining skin. Biopsy of bronchial, tracheal, or laryngeal lesions often provides a specific diagnosis. Nasal or sinus biopsy is usually nondiagnostic because of the high prevalence of secondary bacterial infection that occurs in these sites, obscuring the finding of a primary vasculitis.

Other organs of the head, in addition to the pharynx, nose, and sinuses, may also be involved in WG, including the eyes and ears. Since sinorhinitis is so often observed in the general population, recognition of eye and ear involvement may serve to distinguish WG from the other pulmonary vasculitides in which involvement of these organs is exceedingly rare. *Eye* manifestations occur in approximately 40% of patients and, rarely, signal the onset of disease. Proptosis, unilateral or bilateral, caused by orbital granulomatous inflammation (orbital pseudotumor) is the finding most suggestive of WG. Visual loss from corneal scarring, complications of uveitis, or retinal and optic nerve damage can lead to total blindness. *Otologic* manifestations are not only frequent (20% to 40%) but often are the first to appear. Chronic serous or purulent otitis media not responding to therapy is the most common ear manifestation. Mastoiditis, often with destructive bone lesions and associated cranial nerve abnormalities; external otitis; or rarely, ear lobe perforation have also been observed. Such involvement usually results in varying degrees of ear pain and sensorineural deafness.

Symptoms of *lung* involvement include cough, dyspnea, chest pain, or hemoptysis (occasionally massive). In many patients, however, symptoms are absent even in the presence of multiple pulmonary lesions. When present, *renal* abnormalities always appear to follow or occur with lung and/or upper respiratory tract disease. Renal disease may pursue an incredibly fulminant course within even days of onset and is the leading cause of death in patients with this disorder. *Skin* lesions are observed in approximately 40% of patients and include subcutaneous nodules (often resembling erythema nodosa), purpura (usually palpable), and chronic ulcerations. *Nervous system* involvement occurs in less than one fourth of patients. Peripheral nerve (mononeuritis multiplex) and cranial nerves are affected equally. Younger patients appear to have a much higher prevalence of central nervous system manifestations. *Cardiac* involvement, relatively infrequent and occurring in less than 10% of patients, manifests as acute pericarditis or, more rarely, coronary arteritis. Congestive heart failure is rare. Nondeforming *arthritis* and *arthralgia,* usually of large joints, occur in two thirds of patients.

Radiographic appearance. WG, lymphomatoid granulomatosis, "benign" lymphocytic granulomatous vasculitis, and necrotizing sarcoid granulomatosis generally have similar radiographic patterns (i.e., nodule[s] or mass lesion[s]) and therefore cannot radiographically be distinguished one from another. These patterns may mimic primary or metastatic cancer and certain noninfectious and infectious diseases, particularly those associated with a granulomatous reaction. The most common pattern in WG is *bilateral multiple nodules,* defined as oval or round densities 4 cm or less in diameter. They are of varying size and often cavitated. Multiple or single mass lesions, defined as previously but greater in diameter than 4 cm in diameter, are frequently observed and also frequently cavitate (Fig. 210-2). Although radiographic presentation as a solitary pulmonary nodule occurs, a thoracic computed tomographic (CT) scan may reveal more lesions or show that the "solitary" lesion is made up of multiple nodules. Showers of minute nodules may rarely produce a "pneumonic" type of infiltration, either focal or diffuse. When diffuse, which fortunately is rare, the clinical presentation is that of an acute diffuse pulmonary hemorrhage. When this presentation is associated with nephritis, it may mimic Goodpasture's syndrome or "acute lupus lung." The most suggestive radiographic change, however, occurring in about one fourth of patients, is the finding of spontaneous regression of a density in one area while a density in another area is increasing in size or newly develops (i.e., transient-successive) (Fig. 210-3). This peculiar sequence of events also occurs in lymphomatoid granulomatosis. Pleural effusion is observed in approximately 20% of patients.

Pathology and immunology. The most reliable source for tissue diagnosis is the lung. Although radiographically only one lesion may be seen, complete examination at autopsy almost always reveals multiple lesions. The gross appearance suggests pulmonary infarction of a yellow or white-yellow color and should call attention to the possible diagnosis of WG at surgery. These are often pleural based and show multiple or single cavities. Microscopically, numerous plasma cells are found within and around both medium-sized and small veins and arteries; giant cells, mainly of the foreign body type, are characteristically present. Eosinophils are observed only occasionally, as are neutrophils, which are usually seen only within the areas of necrotic debris. The granuloma is characterized by dense aggregates

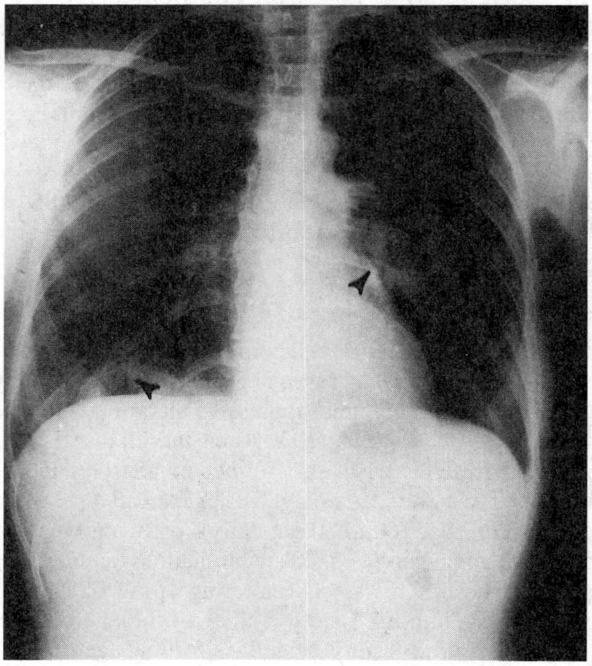

Fig. 210-2. Bilateral, cavitated mass lesions in a patient with Wegener's granulomatosis, complete form (CWG).

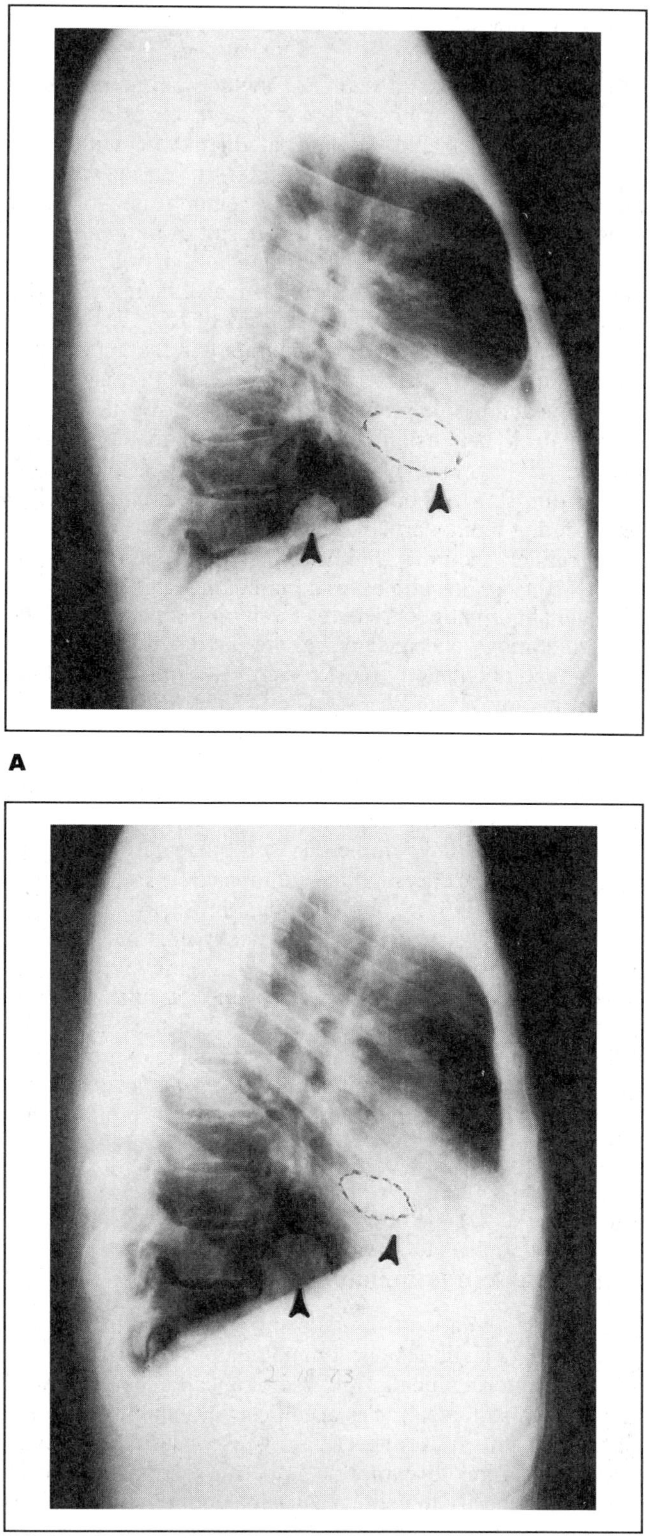

A

B

Fig. 210-3. A, Nodular densities in lower and middle lung lobes in a patient with Wegener's granulomatosis, limited form (LWG). **B,** Six weeks later, lower lobe density has increased in size, whereas the middle lobe density has decreased in size.

of plasma cells as well as giant cells and histiocytes. Scattered epithelioid granulomas (sarcoidlike) occur in approximately 20% to 30% of patients with LWG and lung involvement only. Focal granulomatous glomerulonephritis and necrotizing vasculitis of larger vessels are frequently found in the kidney. Although clinical renal abnormalities are usually absent in the limited form of pulmonary WG, approximately 40% of these patients have the histopathologic changes described.

At present, only conflicting evidence exists concerning the role of immune complex–mediated injury in WG. However, some recent evidence suggests an autoimmune component: Immunoglobulin G (IgG) autoantibodies against extranuclear cytoplasmic components of polymorphonuclear leukocytes (i.e., ANCA). The autoantibodies detected in WG are directed against proteinase-3 of the neutrophil cytoplasmic azurophil granules and produce a diffuse, finely granulated *cytoplasmic* staining pattern (C-ANCA). C-ANCA must be differentiated from ANCA directed against myeloperoxidase and possibly elastase (detected in several systemic vasculitides other than WG, including CSS), which results in P-ANCA (see earlier discussion). C-ANCA has been found to be both sensitive and relatively specific (although not diagnostic) for WG, particularly when the disease is in an "active" phase. C-ANCA therefore appears to be a quite useful clinical *adjunct* to diagnosis, as well as an additional parameter for monitoring the activity of the disease.

Treatment. Before the use of corticosteroids and cyclophosphamide, the 1-year survival of patients with CWG was only 15%. With the administration of these drugs, initial remission occurs in more than 90% of patients, with an ultimate mortality caused by the disease of approximately 20%. Although rare, complete spontaneous remissions may occur. Prednisone (60 to 80 mg daily) and cyclophosphamide (2 mg/kg) are recommended as initial therapy until clinical manifestations have subsided. Prednisone therapy is then reduced to a maintenance dose and then to an alternate-day regimen. Treatment should be continued for approximately 1 year. Relapses (25% to 30%) can occur after a successful course of therapy or when the corticosteroid dose is being reduced. Medical treatment is recommended even when a solitary lung lesion (representing the *only* manifestation of LWG) has been resected, since lung recurrence or renal failure may supervene in untreated patients. Proteinuria may persist for long periods in patients who are otherwise in complete remission. The serum C-reactive protein, ESR, and C-ANCA are useful monitors of disease "activity" in these patients. Trimethoprim-sulfamethoxazole has been used with encouraging results in some patients, raising the question of an infectious etiology. At present, sufficient information does not exist to recommend its routine use.

Dirofilaria immitis granulomatous vasculitis

Pulmonary dirofilariasis is essentially a benign condition that may have histologic features resembling more serious entities. The geographic distribution of *Dirofilaria immitis* (dog heartworm) in the United States is considerable. It not only extends along the seaboard from Maine to Texas but also includes the western coastal states; it penetrates inland to the Mississippi River valley, southern Great Lakes states, and the eastern midwestern states.

Circulating dog microfilaria (infective larval stage) are transported by and injected in the skin of the human by a mosquito vector. The nematode then penetrates the subcutaneous tissue and muscle sheaths. After 3 to 4 months, the infective larvae migrate to and reside in the right ventricle. Since the human environment is an unsuitable host for larvae to develop to adulthood, the larvae die, embolize, and lodge in a branch of the pulmonary artery. Most patients remain asymptomatic; however, some may develop symptoms of pulmonary embolism with infarction (e.g., chest pain, hemoptysis).

Radiographically, the most common finding is a solitary pulmonary nodule. Pathologically, a granulomatous vasculitis develops at the impaction site and may closely resemble the vascular histologic changes of WG or the granulomatous reaction observed in tuberculosis, histoplasmosis, or coccidioidomycosis, all of which may present as an asymptomatic solitary pulmonary nodule. The differentiating feature of dilofilariasis is detection of the larvae on *complete* histologic examination of the excised nodule.

LYMPHOCYTIC GRANULOMATOUS VASCULITIS

"Benign" lymphocytic angiitis and granulomatosis

This disorder shares clinical, radiologic, and therapeutic similarity to LWG (characterized by lung involvement alone). Pathologically, however, lymphocytic angiitis appears to represent a more benign expression of a spectrum observed in angiocentric immunolymphoproliferative lesions (AIL) of T cell type. Necrosis within the lesions is unusual, and although arteries and veins may be heavily infiltrated by lymphocytes, the lumen usually remains patent. Giant cells and atypical lymphoreticular cells are exceedingly rare or absent. Although the prognosis generally appears to be quite good with current therapy, particularly chlorambucil, the process may rarely progress to malignant lymphoma.

Behçet's disease and Hughes-Stovin syndrome

Behçet's disease (BD), although occurring worldwide, has mainly been reported in young men in the Middle East, Eastern Mediterranean basin, and Japan. BD is characterized by relapsing ocular lesions, mainly iridocyclitis with hypopyon, often progressing to blindness, and ulcerations of the mouth and genitalia (Behçet's triad). Many other organ systems, however, including skin, gastrointestinal tract, joints, the blood vessels of the lung, and the systemic veins, may be involved (Chapter 238). Pulmonary involvement is characterized by a necrotizing, predominantly lymphocytic vasculitis of capillaries and all sizes of pulmonary arteries and veins and fortunately is observed in only 5% of patients. Patients who have lung involvement appear to develop fewer eye complications; however, a higher prevalence of relapsing systemic phlebitis is observed in this group of patients.

Clinical manifestations of BD include pulmonary arterial aneurysms; thromboses of pulmonary arteries and veins; obstruction of systemic veins, including those within the mediastinum (e.g., superior and inferior vena cava); and pulmonary infarction. Recurrent hemoptysis or death caused by massive hemoptysis as a result of pulmonary artery aneurysm and bronchial erosion is the frequent outcome, making pulmonary vascular involvement one of the most serious prognostic manifestations of BD. The finding of pulmonary aneurysms by angiography in the appropriate extrapulmonary clinical setting is diagnostic. Perfusion lung scans reveal multiple perfusion defects in most patients, and pulmonary hypertension is noted in approximately 50% of patients at diagnosis. Chest radiographs reveal pleural effusion, unilateral or bilateral infiltrates, or round densities representing pulmonary artery aneurysms. If these densities are parahilar, they may mimic hilar lymphadenopathy. Although BD exhibits clinical and immunologic (T and B lymphocyte abnormalities) features of autoimmune disease, the precise etiology and mechanism are unknown.

Immunomodulation (corticosteroids, immunosuppressives) therapy or surgical excision if the disease is localized to one area of lung are recommended forms of treatment. Anticoagulants have not proved useful and may be harmful in patients with BD as well as in those with Hughes-Stovin syndrome.

Hughes-Stovin syndrome (HSS) is characterized by pulmonary artery aneurysms and pulmonary vessel thromboses associated with systemic venous thrombosis, often involving the large mediastinal and neck veins and cerebral venous sinuses. Since the clinical, angiographic, and histopathologic (vasaculitic) aspects of the vascular manifestations and the clinical course are so similar in BD and HSS, HSS most probably represents an incomplete expression or variant of BD. Systemic phlebitis represents an important clinical finding, differentiating BD and HSS from the other pulmonary vasculitides.

ATYPICAL LYMPHORETICULAR GRANULOMATOUS VASCULITIS

Lymphomatoid granulomatosis

The most enigmatic of the atypical lymphoreticular granulomatous vasculitides is lymphomatoid granulomatosis (LYG), which clinically and radiologically may resemble LWG but histologically has affinities with lymphoma. It appears to manifest as a spectrum of responses from spontaneous remission to evolution into true lymphoma. However, a propensity to cellular invasion and necrosis of veins and arteries in the lung is a striking feature, allowing for inclusion in the pulmonary vasculitides. Clinical features of LYG important in differentiating LYG from WG and typical lymphoma are the frequency of central nervous system involvement and the rarity of lymphadenopathy, upper respiratory tract involvement, and clinical glomerulonephritis.

Clinical and laboratory findings. Males are affected more than females in a ratio of 2 to 3:1, with a mean age of onset of 45 years. All patients with LYG have *lung* involvement, and symptoms of cough, chest pain, and dyspnea are usually the presenting manifestations. The *skin* is often involved in the form of rash or nodules. The nodules are typically tender, are truncal in location, and often resemble erythema nodosa. *Central nervous system* signs and/or symptoms are particularly prevalent (20%) and, with cranial and peripheral neuropathy, make up the neurologic features. *Lymphadenopathy* only is rarely the first manifestation, and glomerulonephritis is rarely observed. Laboratory values are variable and of limited use in diagnosis.

Radiographic appearance. The chest radiograph is abnormal in all patients with LYG. The most frequent finding is that of multiple bilateral nodules. Unilateral nodules, mass lesions, or a single nodule or mass lesion may also be seen, and cavitation may be noted in any of these patterns. These lesions tend to be more vague and irregular than in WG. A thoracic CT scan often reveals the nodular character better than the chest radiograph. The radiodensities in LYG may also wax and wane and thus may be indistinguishable from the radiographic patterns observed in WG. Occasionally a diffuse reticulonodular pattern is seen. Pleural effusion is noted in approximately 20% of patients.

Pathology and immunology. *Vasculonecrosis,* pleomorphic proliferations of atypical cellular elements of the lymphoreticular system (often plasmacytoid) around and within the walls of muscular arteries and/or veins and within the lung parenchyma, characterizes the histology of LYG. Epithelioid granulomas and giant cells are absent. The pathologic process in some patients may arrest or remit, whereas in others it may progress to fulminant lung and/or central nervous system involvement, leading to death, or evolve into a true lymphoma involving lymph nodes. At present the immunopathogenesis of this lymphoproliferative disorder is unknown.

Treatment. Prolonged spontaneous remissions occur in approximately 10% to 15% of patients with LYG. Therapy with corticosteroids and immunosuppressants, although often inducing initial remission, ultimately fails in most patients; the mortality rate even in treated patients is as high as 60%. Further experience with various antilymphoma regimens appears warranted.

HISTIOCYTIC (EPITHELIOID) GRANULOMA GRANULOMATOUS VASCULITIS

Necrotizing sarcoid granulomatosis

Necrotizing sarcoid granulomatosis (NSG) is a comparatively benign disorder, mainly confined to the lung, more frequently seen in women, and with a mean age of onset of approximately 48 years. Approximately one half of all patients are asymptomatic.

Radiographic appearance. Multiple bilateral nodules of varying size represent the most common pattern. Unilateral nodules, a solitary nodule, or solitary or multiple mass lesions may also be observed. Cavitation may occur and occasionally progress to a thin-walled cystic appearance. Two radiographic findings, however, if present, strongly suggest the diagnosis of NSG: (1) exquisite bilateral symmetry of the nodular or mass lesions and (2) bilateral symmetric hilar lymphadenopathy (20% to 30% of patients). Spontaneous waxing and waning of lesions have not been observed in NSG. Examples of sarcoidosis referred to in the literature as "nodular" are most likely examples of NSG.

Pathology and immunology. The walls of arteries and veins of small and medium-sized vessels may undergo replacement by epithelioid granulomas and/or infiltration by histiocytes and giant cells (the latter may closely resemble those changes observed in the giant cell arteritides) or diffuse plasma cell and lymphocyte infiltration with varying degrees of necrosis. Of diagnostic importance is that the background parenchymal lesions are made up of confluent masses of noncaseating epithelioid granulomas. No substantive information exists regarding the immunopathogenesis of NSG. However, since the basic histology, natural history, and response to therapy in NSG are so similar to sarcoidosis, NSG may merely be a clinical variant.

Treatment. Most patients with NSG recover without therapy. Corticosteroids should be reserved for those who have significant systemic and/or pulmonary symptoms.

Schistosoma mansoni granulomatous vasculitis

Worldwide, *Schistosoma mansoni* granulomatous vasculitis occurs more frequently than all the other vasculitides combined (Chapter 282). Signs and/or symptoms of severe pulmonary hypertension with or without cor pulmonale and right-sided heart failure eventually result from widespread impaction of the "embolized" ova form of *S. mansoni*. This occurs in the precapillary arterioles of the lung, where a noncaseating epithelioid granuloma response is generated, resulting in vascular damage and complete vessel occlusion. Finding the egg remnants, usually centrally situated within the granuloma, is diagnostic. Chest radiographs generally demonstrate enlargement of the right ventricle and main pulmonary artery, with relatively clear lung fields. Therefore those patients with pulmonary hypertension not related to intrinsic heart or lung disease who had resided in endemic areas for *S. mansoni* should be suspect. Unfortunately, at the stage of pulmonary hypertension, no specific treatment is available.

Talc and starch granulomatous vasculitis

Signs and symptoms of severe pulmonary hypertension and its complications may also occur in drug abusers who have injected intravenous oral medications containing talc or starch as a filler. Talc crystals or starch granules, initially intraluminal in the precapillary arteriolar system of the lung, are ultimately found in the walls of these vessels, entrapped in epithelioid granulomas of the foreign body type. They may be observed as spindlelike crystals (talc) or maltese crosslike structures (starch) when examined with polarized light. This results in a widespread obliterative arteriolitis resulting in various degrees of pulmonary hypertension. As in *S. mansoni* vasculitis, chest radiographs usually demonstrate right ventricular and main pulmonary artery enlargement, with relatively clear lung fields. No specific effective therapy is available. Interestingly, some patients have only a widespread talc or starch granulomatous response in the lung parenchyma, with relative sparing of the lung vasculature. Chest radiographs in these individuals often reveal a diffuse, infiltrating lung lesion.

GIANT CELL GRANULOMATOUS VASCULITIS

Takayasu's arteritis (pulmonary Takayasu's disease, pulmonary pulseless disease)

Giant cell granulomatous involvement resulting in narrowing and/or occlusion of the pulmonary artery or its branches is mainly observed in young Oriental women and occurs in approximately 50% of patients with Takayasu's arteritis. Varying degrees of pulmonary hypertension is present in most patients with pulmonary vessel involvement. Symptoms of dyspnea and hemoptysis are occasionally observed. The diagnosis of Takayasu's arteritis is initially suggested by the presence of "aortic branch occlusion syndromes." Pulmonary vessel involvement is suggested by loss of lung vasculature on chest radiographs and may be documented by pulmonary angiography.

REFERENCES

Carrington CB and Liebow AA: Limited forms of angiitis and granulomatosis of Wegener's type. Am J Med 41:497, 1967.

Cortes FM and Winters WL: Schistosomiasis cor pulmonale. Am J Med 31:808, 1961.

Hughes JP and Stovin PGI: Segmental pulmonary artery aneurysms with peripheral venous thrombosis. Br J Dis Chest 53:19, 1959.

Kawai C et al: "Pulmonary pulseless disease": pulmonary involvement in so-called Takayasu's disease. Chest 73:651, 1978.

Lanham JG et al: Systemic vasculitis with asthma and eosinophilia: a clinical approach to the Churg-Strauss syndrome. Medicine 63:65, 1984.

Liebow AA: The J. Burns Amberson Lecture: pulmonary angiitis and granulomatosis. Am Rev Respir Dis 108:1, 1973.

Raz I, Okon E, and Chajek-Shaul T: Pulmonary manifestations in Behçet's syndrome. Chest 95:585, 1989.

Risher WH et al: Pulmonary dirofilariasis. J Thorac Cardiovasc Surg 97:303, 1989.

Saldana MJ and Israel HL: Necrotizing sarcoid granulomatosis, benign lymphocytic angiitis, and granulomatosis: do they exist? Semin Respir Med 10:182, 1989.

Wendt VE et al: Angiothrombotic pulmonary hypertension in addicts. JAMA 188:755, 1964.

CHAPTER

211 Occupational Lung Diseases

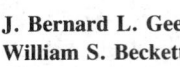

J. Bernard L. Gee
William S. Beckett

Most major categories of respiratory disease may be produced by occupational exposures. Substances in the workplace may produce rhinitis and sinusitis (often mistaken for respiratory infections or "hay fever"); airway disease, including asthma, acute or chronic bronchitis, and chronic airflow limitation; alveolitis leading to diffuse or focal fibrotic or granulomatous interstitial disease; infectious pneumonia, hypersensitivity pneumonitis, or alveolar proteinosis; and primary cancer of the lung or pleura. The one major category of pulmonary diseases not associated with occupational exposures is the primary disease of the pulmonary arteries. In many patients, disease may be chronic and multifactorial in origin. Interactions between exposures often occur. The combined effects of cigarette smoke and inhaled mineral dusts in chronic airflow obstruction and between cigarette smoke and asbestos fibers in bronchogenic carcinoma are perhaps the best understood of these interactions.

Because the normal respiratory system has substantial reserve, considerable injury or loss of function may occur before an individual becomes aware of symptoms and comes to medical attention.

Occupational lung disease results from exposure to a causative agent and host responses, which are a function of the defenses, clearance, and the magnitude of the humoral and cellular immune responses to the agent. Some diseases occur consistently in a graded dose and response manner; others demonstrate marked interindividual variation in severity among patients with apparently equivalent exposures. Because there is no effective therapy for most of these diseases, prevention is also essential. The alert clinician must recognize that for each case diagnosed, many other cases may be about to occur in the same workplace and may be prevented by prompt identification of the cause and the population at risk. Particularly for cancer and the pneumoconioses, a long latency period may elapse between the beginning of exposure and the manifestations of disease. This latency is sometimes measured in decades, and for some diseases the process typically progresses many years after all exposure has ceased.

When approaching the patient with suspected occupational lung disease, detailed information about workplace exposures (substances, air concentrations, particle respirability, duration) may be critical in diagnosis and management and in prevention of further illness. The constituents of industrial materials must now be made available to employees and their physicians in the United States and Canada. This information can be obtained by requesting Material Safety Data Sheets from the employer for the particular employee's work area and the results of any industrial hygiene measurements of exposure levels made in the work area. When the diagnosis of an occupational disease is made, and if others in the workplace are still at risk of becoming ill, it is important to notify (with the patient's prior permission) the employer and appropriate public health agencies (e.g., state health department). The box below is a partial listing of states in which reporting of any occupational disease or certain occupational lung diseases to state officials is now mandatory. If the physician believes that workplace health or safety standards are not being met, the physician may report the workplace to the local office of the federal Occupational Safety and Health Administration (OSHA), while maintaining the patient's confidentiality.

Workers' compensation is a separate health insurance system covering illness and loss of earning power caused by a work-related illness. It depends on the physician accurately identifying the workplace determinants of illness, informing the patient when illness is work related, and sometimes acting as his or her advocate.

AIRWAYS DISEASES

Although occupational exposure may affect the conducting airways anywhere between the nose and alveoli, the airway diseases are grouped into three categories: occupational asthma, chronic bronchitis, and chronic obstructive pulmonary disease.

States in which reporting of any occupational disease or certain occupational lung diseases is mandatory under state law

Alaska
Arkansas
California
Colorado
Connecticut
District of Columbia
Georgia
Iowa
Kansas
Kentucky
Maine
Maryland
Michigan
Missouri
New Hampshire
New Jersey
New Mexico
New York
Oklahoma
South Carolina
Texas
Virginia
West Virginia
Wisconsin

From Freund et al: JAMA 262:3042, 1989.

Occupational asthma

Since dust control measures have reduced new cases of pneumoconiosis, occupational asthma may have become the most common occupational lung disease, the incidence of which may be increasing. It may be considered in two ways. First, in patients without pre-existing asthma, recurrent workplace exposure can produce a new state of sensitization to a substance, thus producing recurrent asthmatic episodes. Second, patients with either clinical asthma or subclinical pre-existing airways hyperresponsiveness may experience exacerbations because of workplace exposure.

Some patients in the first category who continue in their workplace despite symptomatic asthma from sensitization will continue to have symptomatic asthma for years *after* exposure to the sensitizing agent has ceased completely. Because the likelihood of cure may be greater if exposure is ended sooner, some urgency exists for the physician to recognize occupational causes of asthma early and to work in the patient's behalf to end exposure while protecting the patient's livelihood.

More than 100 different workplace agents have been identified as causing occupational asthma, and as new substances are introduced into the workplace, other causative agents will probably be identified. Table 211-1 lists some of the more frequently encountered causative agents by major categories. Most allergens are classic allergic sensitizers, having a molecular weight greater than 1000 daltons and producing a specific immunoglobulin E (IgE) antibody after prolonged or recurrent exposure; on repeat challenge, this antibody binds antigen and leads to release of mediators from inflammatory cells and the reversible bronchoconstriction and mucus hypersecretion of asthma. However, a sizable number of the agents of low molecular weight (less than 1000 daltons) produce a similar clinical picture without an identified IgE, perhaps because the agent acts through a separate mechanism or forms a new antigenic complex with a serum protein. As with nonoccupational asthma, the patient's history alone most frequently leads to the correct diagnosis.

When asthma is caused by a workplace sensitization, the patient will give a history of asymptomatic exposure for months or even years before the gradual onset of symptoms. Once sensitization has occurred, re-exposure may produce an immediate response (within minutes of exposure), a delayed response (several hours after exposure), a dual response combining the immediate and delayed, or a recurrent nocturnal response for several nights after a single exposure. With the delayed response the presenting symptoms may only be a recurrent nocturnal cough and minor wheezing, which, if unrecognized as manifestations of asthma, may progress to recurrent daytime wheezing and eventually to persistent breathlessness. Improvement on weekends or vacations may be the most helpful historic clue to a workplace etiology of asthma but is not invariably present. Correlating airflow obstruction (as measured by a self-administered peak airflow meter) with workplace exposures may be extremely helpful when the history alone is not sufficient. The clinical suspicion of an occupational origin for asthma can usually be confirmed or denied by 1 or 2 weeks

Table 211-1. Listing of selected substances causing occupational asthma

Agents	Industries/occupations
High-molecular-weight compounds	
Laboratory animals	
Rat	Laboratory workers
Mouse	Veterinarians
Rabbit	Animal handlers
Guinea pig	
Birds	
Pigeon	Pigeon breeders
Chicken	Poultry workers
Budgerigar (parakeet)	Bird fanciers
Insects	
Grain mite	Grain workers
Locust	Research laboratory
River fly	Power plants along rivers
Screw worm fly	Flight crews
Cockroach	Laboratory workers
Cricket	Field contact
Bee moth	Fish bait breeders
Moth and butterfly	Entomologists
Plants	
Grain dust	Grain handlers
Wheat/rye flour	Bakers, millers
Buckwheat	Bakers
Coffee bean	Food processors
Castor bean	Oil industry
Tea	Tea workers
Tobacco leaf	Tobacco manufacturing
Hops *(Humulus lupulus)*	Brewery chemists
Biologic enzymes	
Bacillus subtilis	Detergent industry
Trypsin	Pharmaceutical
Pancreatin	Pharmaceutical
Papain	Laboratory Packaging
Pepsin	Pharmaceutical
Flaviastase	Pharmaceutical
Bromelin	Pharmaceutical
Fungal amylase	Manufacturing, bakers
Vegetables	
Gum acacia	Printers
Gum tragacanth	Gum manufacturing
Other	
Crab	Crab processing
Prawn	Prawn processing
Hoya	Oyster farm
Silkworm larva	Sericulture
Low-molecular-weight compounds	
Di-isocyanates	
Toluene di-isocyanate	Polyurethane, plastics, varnish
Diphenylmethane di-isocyanate	Foundries
Hexamethylene di-isocyanate	Automobile spray painting
Anhydrides	
Phthalic anhydride	Epoxy resins, plastics
Trimellitic anhydride	Epoxy resins, plastics
Tetrachlorophthalic anhydride	Epoxy resins, plastics
Wood dust	
Western red cedar *(Thuja plicata)*	Carpentry, construction, cabinetmaking, sawmill
California redwood *(Sequoia sempervirens)*	
Cedar of Lebanon *(Cedra libani)*	
Cocabolla *(Dalbergia retusa)*	
Iroko *(Chlorophora excelsa)*	
Oak *(Quercus robur)*	
Mahogany (*Shoreal* species)	
Abiruana *(Pouteria)*	
African maple *(Triplochiton scleroxylon)*	
Tanganyika aningre	
Central American walnut *(Juglans olanchana)*	
Kejaat *(Pterocarpus angolenisis)*	
African zebra wood *(Microberlinia)*	
Metals	
Platinum	Platinum refinery
Nickel	Metal plating
Chromium	Tanning
Cobalt	Hard metal industry
Vanadium	
Fluxes	
Aminoethyl ethanolamine	Aluminum soldering
Colophony	Electronic
Drugs	
Penicillins	Pharmaceutical
Cephalosporins	Pharmaceutical
Phenylglycine acid chloride	Pharmaceutical
Piperazine hydrochloride	Chemist
Psyllium	Laxative manufacturers
Methyldopa	Pharmaceutical
Spiramycin	Pharmaceutical
Salbutamol intermediate	Pharmaceutical
Amprolium hydrochloride	Poultry feed mixers
Tetracycline	Pharmaceutical
Sulphone chloramides	Manufacturers, brewery
Other chemicals	
Dimethyl ethanolamine	Spray painting
Persulfate salts and henna	Hairdressing
Ethylene diamine	Photography
Azodiacarbonamide	Plastics and rubber
Dioazonium salt	Photocopying and dye
Hexachlorophene (sterilizing agent)	Hospital staff
Formalin	Hospital staff
Urea formaldehyde	Insulation, resin
Freon	Refrigeration
Paraphenylene diamine	Fur dying
Furfuryl alcohol	Foundry mold making

Reprinted with permission of the authors and publisher from Chan-Yeung M and Lam S: Am Rev Respir Dis 133:686-782, 1986.

away from exposure followed by a return to the exposure area. Although the demonstration of IgE antibody specific to the workplace agent by the presence of wheal and flare on intradermal skin tests may be confirmatory, skin testing is not typically required. The demonstration of airway hyperresponsiveness to cholinergic stimulation on methacholine challenge testing may help to distinguish asthma from other forms of airway disease. Inhalation challenge with the substance in question carries the risk of inducing severe bronchospasm or even hypersensitivity pneumonitis and is best performed in specialized centers where exposures can be exactly controlled.

For certain occupational allergens, cigarette smoking appears to be a risk factor that increases the probability of becoming sensitized. A differential diagnosis for occupational asthma may include nonoccupational asthma, industrial bronchitis, and hypersensitivity pneumonitis.

The *reactive airways dysfunction syndrome* (RADS) may be a variant of occupational asthma. This term is used to describe patients who have had a single, usually heavy (e.g., spill, explosion, fire) exposure to inhaled irritants and who have a subsequent chronic symptomatic airways disease characterized by intermittent symptoms and airway hyperresponsiveness. Because the exposure is not repeated, an anamnestic immunologic response cannot be invoked to explain this acquired state of airway hyperreactivity.

Chronic bronchitis (industrial bronchitis)

Daily cough and mucus production 3 or more months of the year for 2 or more years is a functional definition of chronic bronchitis that correlates well with an increase in the thickness of the bronchial mucous gland layer. It may be produced by occupational inhalation as well as cigarette smoking. This may occur without any airways obstruction, is not life-threatening, and can be caused by sufficient exposures to dust in miners, steel foundry workers, cement workers, cotton and other textile workers, welders, and those exposed to a variety of other dusts. In cigarette smokers an interaction often occurs between the effects of smoke and dust. Therapy includes management of acute bacterial superinfections with a short course of a broad-spectrum oral antibiotic and the prevention of further exposure to the offending agent.

Chronic obstructive pulmonary disease

Although chronic obstructive pulmonary disease may occur simultaneously with industrial bronchitis, it may also occur separately. For example, exposure to coal dust alone may be associated with bronchitis, a slight airflow obstruction, or both. The earliest finding on spirometry may be a decreased maximum midexpiratory flow (MMEF). In large epidemiologic studies of certain working groups, small excesses over the normal age-related declines in airflow have been reported in relation to some dust exposures (independently of the effects of cigarette smoking). In the absence of complicated pneumoconiosis, the effect is generally small and clinically unimportant unless other lung disease coexists. An exception is cadmium oxide dust, which some studies have associated with marked emphysema after prolonged exposure.

PARENCHYMAL DISEASE

Acute toxic exposures

In toxic exposures, both the small airways and the alveoli may be affected together as a bronchoalveolar unit. A single overwhelming exposure may cause either acute or chronic airway inflammation, pulmonary edema, and sometimes irreversible pulmonary fibrosis.

The acute disorders result from the inhalation of gases (chemically or thermally active), mists (liquid droplets), or fumes (solid-phase constituents). The depth of penetration, which determines whether alveolar leaks and thus pulmonary edema will occur, depends on the gas solubility in aqueous media or the size of the droplets or fume particulates, with less than 10 μ being critical. Most such materials affect the conjunctival, oronasal, laryngeal, and major bronchial mucosae first, and thus their effects are readily apparent by visual examination of the upper airways. Some other fume materials (e.g., magnesium, cadmium, chromium) usually cause few upper respiratory effects but can have major pulmonary and even systemic effects. Other gases may cause neither external nor intrapulmonary effects but do produce systemic disorders. Examples are organic solvents (which may cause central nervous system manifestations), hydrogen sulfide, carbon monoxide, and oxygen deprivation, which are major hazards for firefighters.

Patients with acute toxic pulmonary edema exhibit the usual manifestations of dyspnea, cough, expectoration, often bloody sputum, profound oxygen desaturation, and patchy radiologic opacification. Cough and sputum from irritation of the upper respiratory tract are more obvious with the more soluble gases (e.g., sulfur dioxide, ammonia) and pulmonary edema with the less soluble ones (e.g., nitrogen dioxide). Many agents produce delayed effects requiring observation up to 24 to 48 hours. Both airway inflammation and obstructive effects are produced by the overtly irritant gases: ammonia, chlorine, nitrogen oxides (from fires, silo filling, shot firing, welding in confined spaces, chemical industries), ozone, formaldehyde, sulfur dioxide, fluoride, sulfuric acid, hydrochloric acid mists, metal fumes (including zinc, copper, magnesium, cadmium, manganese, and occasionally tin and lead), and paraquat. One particular form of hemorrhagic edema results from trimellitic anhydride, a compound used in plastic manufacturing. Finally, isocyanates, particularly those with very high vapor pressure or in association with acute spills or spray aerosols, can cause such airways disease. Isocyanates with lower vapor pressures are less likely to cause airways disease, but they can occasionally cause a hypersensitivity pneumonitis.

Pathologically, acute inflammation and mucosal denudation may be prominent in the larynx and major airways, especially with ammonia. The alveoli may rapidly develop a profound protein leak, fluid transudation, and the mobilization of neutrophils, which themselves contribute to oxidant endothelial and probably alveolar type 1 cell damage and may cause further pulmonary edema.

Management consists in supportive therapy, bronchodilators, and oxygen after immediate removal from the noxious agent. The role of corticosteroids is unclear. Fortunately, many patients recover completely with no demonstrable long-term lung function defects, but long-term effects can occur. These include persistent nonobstructive bronchitis (cough, sputum), more rarely bronchiolitis obliterans (notably with nitrogen dioxide, as in silo filler's disease), and occasionally bronchiectasis.

Metal fume fever is an acute febrile illness caused by inhalation of freshly formed metal fume (metal that has been evaporated by very high temperature and then condensed in air into fine particles). The fever, rigors, and respiratory symptoms that accompany this illness often occur 4 to 6 hours after exposure and usually resolve 12 hours later. Zinc oxide fume is usually the causative agent.

ASBESTOS-RELATED DISEASES

Asbestos was of immense social and economic value, but since its use has recently been somewhat restricted in most industrialized countries (but less so in some developing countries), asbestos-related diseases now largely reflect the sad legacy of its past poorly regulated use. These fibrous silicates exist in two general forms: the serpentine chrysotile and the amphiboles (i.e., crocidolite, amosite, tremolite, anthophyllite). Much experimental and epidemiologic work has examined both these forms of asbestos and the morphologic features associated with both respirability and pathogenicity. Asbestosis, or pulmonary fibrosis, results from all these types of asbestos. However, considerable variation exists in their ability to produce mesothelioma and also in the prevalence of bronchogenic carcinomas in various populations of asbestos workers. The major risks of asbestos-related disorders occur in workers in insulation industries, shipyards, construction, asbestos textiles, mining, the production of friction materials, and sometimes chemical industries. The risk to the general population is exceedingly small, even though in some circumstances judicious, careful asbestos abatement may be appropriate. The disorders associated with asbestos affect the pleura, lung, and peritoneum. Evidence that asbestos causes laryngeal cancer or gastrointestinal cancer is weak or lacking, with the possible exception of stomach cancer with great exposure.

Benign pleural disease

All forms of asbestos cause pleural reactions. The fibrohyaline plaques found on the parietal pleura are most common. These frequently involve the midportion of the thoracic wall, the diaphragm, and occasionally the pericardium. They are lesions that rarely coalesce but typically calcify. Although these radiologic manifestations (Fig. 211-1, *A* and *B*) usually progress, their generally discrete nodular nature by itself does not cause symptomatic restrictive lung function loss. In general, however, patients with plaques have slightly lower lung capacity than similarly exposed individuals without plaques. Plaques are most evident on the lateral aspects of the chest radiograph but, when seen en face, may occasionally need to be distinguished from parenchymal disease, most easily by oblique films or computed tomographic (CT) scanning. Plaques are markers of asbestos exposure but, per se, have little prognostic import. Occasionally they can invade the subjacent lung and cause a nodular mass lesion from lung entrapment known as *rounded atelectasis* (Fig. 211-1, *C*); this may require a differentiation from pleural-based lung tumors. Extensive pleural fibrosis without asbestosis occurs less often than plaques and may rarely lead to a cuirass effect, producing restriction of lung function.

Benign pleural effusions also occur, usually 5 to 15 or more years after exposure. These may be recurrent and rarely may be associated with pleural fibrosis. The fluid is usually an exudate, occasionally bloody. These effusions are generally asymptomatic and resolve spontaneously, but pleuritic pain does occur. The diagnosis is made by the exposure history and the exclusion of other causes of effusions.

Asbestosis

The term *asbestosis* should be reserved for fibrosing alveolitis caused by asbestos deposition in the lung. The clinicophysiologic features are those of other forms of fibrosing alveolitis, even though pathologically the earliest fibrotic lesions occur at the level of the respiratory bronchioles. Although a detailed radiologic classification of stages of asbestosis exists, the radiologic features are also those of other forms of pulmonary fibrosis. In the absence of other causes of such fibrosis, an appropriate exposure history is sufficient for a presumptive diagnosis of asbestosis. However, lung biopsies are occasionally required clinically for differential diagnostic purposes. Asbestosis is characterized by presence of the characteristic iron-staining asbestos bodies seen in association with fibrosis. Asbestosis probably occurs rarely with prolonged exposure to airborne fiber concentrations of less than one fiber per milliliter of air. When severe, progressive fibrosis with secondary pulmonary hypertension and death occur. Among heavily exposed populations, a small subgroup have rapidly progressive fibrosis. Many of those with clinically apparent disease progress slowly over years or decades; those with a low radiologic category of disease frequently remain stable for at least 10 years. Patients with asbestosis who are or have been smokers may have a slightly worse radiographic appearance.

Lung cancer

The incidence of lung cancer in workers at various types of asbestos industries varies widely. It is highest among asbestos textile and insulation workers and only minimally increased over the general population rates in miners, millers, and the friction products trades. Although most studies imply that asbestos causes bronchogenic carcinoma in the absence of smoking, relatively few lung cancers have been reported among nonsmoking workers in epidemiologic studies. The conventional view is that asbestos interacts with such tobacco smoke carcinogens as the polycyclic hydrocarbons. This view is compatible with data from epidemiologic studies. Depending on the population studied, the

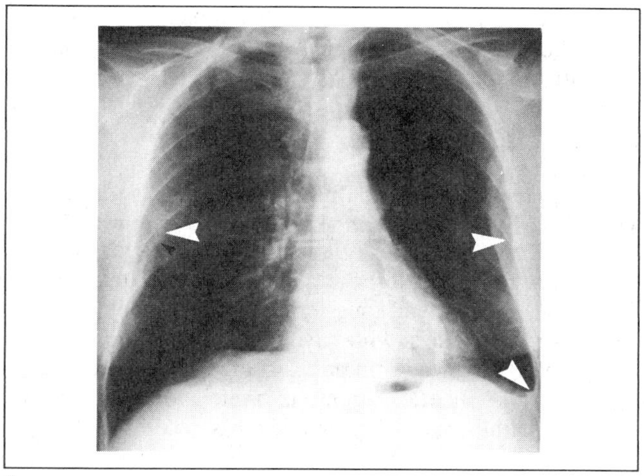

A

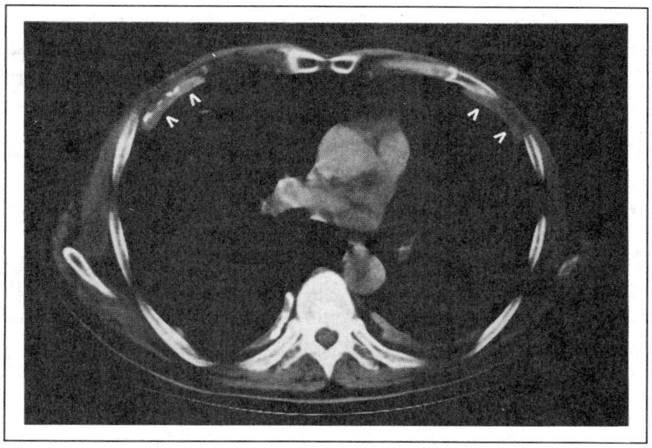

B

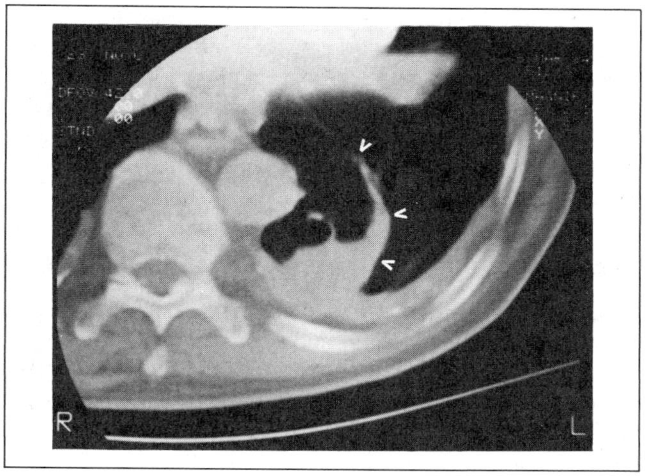

C

Fig. 87-1. Pleural plaques, focal areas of thickened parietal pleura, are the most frequently found pulmonary effects of occupational asbestos exposure. They are usually asymptomatic and are often noted on chest roentgenograms decades after initial exposure to asbestos. They are characteristically seen on the posteroanterior film at the lateral chest margins and on the domes of the diaphragms. This patient was a 75-year-old railroad locomotive mechanic. A. Bilateral plaques are seen (arrowheads), and pleural thickening also blunts the left costophrenic angle. A computed tomogram of his chest in axial section (B) shows partial dense calcification of the right anterior chest wall, and marked pleural thickening posteriorly adjacent to the spine. C. This patient also had rounded atelectasis at the posterior basal segment of the left lower lobe (arrowhead, detail) with folding and entrapment of normal lung within thickened pleura demonstrating the characteristic whorled or "comet tail" appearance in a dense pleural-based mass adjacent to plaques. (Roentgenograms courtesy of Dr. Coralie Shaw.)

amount of asbestos exposure, and the length of follow-up, the lung cancer excess varies from zero to tenfold increases over control smoking populations. Smoking cessation is always appropriate, although tumors present (up to 10 years) before smoking cessation will continue to be manifest. All lung cancer cell types occur in association with asbestos. The attribution of a given lung cancer case to asbestos may be an important legal issue. The presence of associated asbestosis is direct evidence that the fiber burden is sufficient to be a contributing cause of the cancer.

The specific clinical issues in the asbestos-exposed patient with a chest radiograph suggesting cancer are (1) the differential diagnosis of radiologic shadows from plaques and rounded atelectasis and (2) the risks of radiation fibrosis with pre-existing asbestosis, if cancer is diagnosed and radiation therapy is indicated.

Mesothelioma

Mesothelioma is unrelated to cigarette smoking. It takes two forms, the diffuse malignant and benign focal types. The former is a diffusely invasive tumor of either pleura or peritoneum, characterized histologically by combinations of epithelial and mesenchymal cells with fibrous tissue, often with a tubulopapillary pattern. Differentiation from peripheral adenocarcinoma can be difficult. About 80% of cases of malignant mesothelioma are attributable to asbestos exposure, with crocidolite most likely to produce tumors. Long latency between first asbestos exposure and disease is the general rule—from 20 to 30 years. This latency has focused attention on childhood exposure to asbestos in school buildings.

The disease occurs in certain Turkish Cappadocian and Greek villages in epidemic form and has been ascribed to deposits of asbestiform minerals. Family contacts of asbestos workers have also been affected.

Mesothelioma presents with local pain and breathlessness from the tumor mass and/or the associated effusions. Local invasion is the rule; metastases are rarely clinically important. Diagnosis usually requires an open procedure. The prognosis is poor, although some patients have 4- to 6-year survival. Treatment is disappointing; Adriamycin and radiation may be useful palliatives.

SILICOSIS

Crystalline silica (silicon dioxide) exists in many forms with varying toxicity. Exposures occur in mining (gold, coal, flint, bentonite production) and in sandblasting. Thus quarry workers, granite workers, road builders, stone polishers, foundry workers, and those employed in metal casting, ceramics, refractory insulating brick construction, glass making, and slate use are frequently exposed. Silicosis exists in three general forms: acute silicosis, chronic simple silicosis, and progressive massive fibrosis.

Acute silicosis

Acute silicosis is relatively rare, has a fatal course in several months or a few years, and occurs in ceramic workers, silica flour or silica soap workers, and those in poorly regulated tunneling operations. Radiologically a ground-glass appearance is seen, and an irregular nonnodular fibrosis can ensue.

Chronic simple silicosis

Chronic simple silicosis is characterized pathologically by the silicotic nodule, which comprises whorled fibrotic nodules of varying sizes, characteristically occurring in the upper lung zones. These nodules progressively enlarge and become more profuse. In its simple form the diagnosis is based on the history and a chest radiograph, with dense nodulation of varying size. In any patient, nodule size tends to be homogeneous, but the nodulation increases both in size and in profusion with increasing dust exposure, sometimes even after cessation of exposure. Pleural abnormalities are minimal. Radiologically, "eggshell" calcification frequently occurs in the central lymph nodes, in contrast to its rarity in sarcoidosis. Initially, few symptoms of simple silicosis per se are evident, and lung function shows little or no impairment. The lack of symptoms and the good function may contrast sharply with the striking chest radiologic abnormalities. Rarely, and for inapparent reasons, the disorder can have an accelerated course. The best recent studies of Vermont granite workers show minimum or little acceleration of the normal age-related decline in forced expiratory volume in 1 second (FEV_1). Lung cancer rates have not been clearly shown to be increased in patients with silicosis.

Progressive massive fibrosis

Progressive massive fibrosis (PMF, complicated silicosis), although less common than in coal workers' pneumoconiosis, is disabling and life-threatening. It arises on a background of chronic, simple silicosis and is radiographically characterized by the development of bilateral, usually symmetric, progressive mass opacifications greater than 1 cm in diameter in the upper third of the lungs. These may extend and are associated with severe architectural distortion of the unaffected lung with compensatory emphysema. Lung function becomes progressively deranged with restrictive and obstructive components. Arterial desaturation and ultimately right-sided heart failure supervene. The fibrotic material is subject to ischemic necrobiosis with expectoration—*melanoptysis* (black sputum) in silicotic coal workers. The mechanism involved is unknown. The material not only contains collagen but also large amounts of glycosaminoglycans and fibronectin. Therapy, other than general measures, is ineffective.

Tuberculosis

This frequent complication needs evaluation in all patients with silicosis by tuberculin skin tests and sputum cultures. Since silica is cytotoxic for alveolar macrophages, silicotic patients with tuberculosis may be difficult to treat. Many authorities recommend long-term isoniazid prophylaxis for patients with silicosis who have a positive tuberculin reaction, regardless of age. In areas where the incidence of tuberculosis in silicotic patients is high, as in Hong Kong, empiric antituberculosis prophylaxis is recommended, regardless of skin test results. Because of a higher relapse rate among silicotic patients treated with standard regimens, some authorities recommend a prolonged course of antituberculous therapy in active disease from *Mycobacterium tuberculosis*. Necrobiotic cavitation can release entrapped tubercle bacilli, causing serious bronchogenic spread of tuberculosis.

Immune phenomena

More studies on immune reactions in silicotic patients are needed, but several associated disorders are recognized. Scleroderma frequently occurs. Caplan has described the appearance of somewhat larger nodules preceding or coinciding with the development of rheumatoid arthritis (Caplan's syndrome).

Prevention depends on the type of exposure. When heavy, a positive-pressure external air supply respirator is essential. Careful observation of the health-protecting air standards can be successfully achieved in mining, although less effectively in sandblasting.

COAL WORKERS' PNEUMOCONIOSIS

Coal mining has recently become much more mechanized, reducing the overall risks to workers. Nonetheless, those at the coal face (hard-headers) remain at risk.

Pathologically the hallmark of coal workers' pneumoconiosis (CWP) is the coal macule, usually less than 4 mm in diameter. These macules include focal macrophage accumulation, with surrounding reticulin and collagen fibrosis. This leads to bronchiole dilatation and patchy focal emphysema. In those miners exposed to hard-rock coal mining, silicosis also may develop.

Radiographically, CWP appears as fine pinpoint nodulations, which at later stages may become more and more profuse. In this simple form of CWP, symptoms are those of industrial bronchitis, and functional changes are few. In studies of nonsmoking miners, up to 20% increases in residual volume, variable losses of diffusing capacity, little change in the alveolar to arterial oxygen tension gradient or in static compliance, and minor reductions in dynamic compliance were observed. The effect of coal dust exposure on FEV_1 in simple pneumoconiosis, if present, varies from a small acceleration in the age-related FEV_1 loss to an effect (in those most heavily exposed) comparable to that of chronic cigarette smoking; this loss is ascribed to the centrilobular emphysema. Patients with simple CWP have no major changes in exercise capacity, even though breathlessness is a common complaint. Unfortunately, PMF, as in silicosis, is a common problem. This generally occurs in patients with more rapidly progressive CWP. By the time PMF is evident, airway obstruction, increase in residual volume, loss of diffusing capacity, and uneven gas/blood distribution are all evident. Pulmonary hypertension and cor pulmonale supervene when about 50% of the pulmonary vascular bed is lost. No specific therapy exists.

As in patients with silicosis, immunologic abnormalities may occur, notably Caplan's syndrome.

BERYLLIUM DISEASE

Inhalation of the metal beryllium or its salts or compounds may lead to either acute or chronic beryllium disease. Acute beryllium disease is an immediate toxic response, with nasopharyngitis, tracheobronchitis, or pneumonitis. The severity depends on the amount inhaled. Patients may have cough, mucus production, blood-tinged sputum, and dyspnea. Chronic beryllium disease, quite different from the acute form, may occur as a result of lower levels of exposure. It is a systemic, granulomatous disease involving the lung predominantly and has many features of a chronic hypersensitivity lung disease. Pathologically it is an inflammatory disorder with nonnecrotizing epithelioid granulomas involving one or more organs. On physical examination the patient may have no abnormal findings or may have clubbing of the fingers, granulomatous skin lesions, crackles and pleural friction rubs, or an enlarged liver. In cases involving the kidney, hypercalciuria and hypercalcemia may be found. The chest radiograph most frequently shows bilateral, diffuse, small opacities in either a miliary or fibrotic pattern, and pulmonary function testing may show a restrictive ventilatory defect with impairment of gas exchange (as seen in a decreased diffusing capacity or lowered arterial oxygen tension) or in some patients an obstructive defect. It may be extremely difficult to distinguish chronic beryllium disease from sarcoidosis. Patients with berylliosis have not been found to have uveitis and the cystic bone abnormalities sometimes seen in sarcoidosis. Chronic beryllium disease has a worse prognosis than sarcoidosis.

Demonstration of greater than 0.02 μg/g of beryllium in dried lung tissue from open lung biopsy and a marked blast transformation response of the patient's peripheral blood or lavaged lung lymphocytes when cultured in vitro with beryllium salts are usually considered diagnostic of beryllium disease in patients whose exposure history and clinical presentation are consistent.

Specific therapy for patients with acute and chronic beryllium disease consists of high-dose oral corticosteroids. The degree of response to this therapy depends in part on how far the inflammatory and fibrotic lung processes have advanced at the time treatment is started.

HARD METAL DISEASE

"Hard metals," characteristically containing tungsten carbide and cobalt, have great importance in tool grinding, diamond polishing, and the manufacture of jet engines and ferromagnets, as well as in the manufacture of tungsten carbide itself for incorporation in the necessary alloys ("high-speed steels"). Several entities occur in workers with these materials. The most frequent is asthma. Second, persistent, unexplained cough is reported. Finally and most important is a picture clinically and radiologically indistinguishable from other forms of diffuse pulmonary fibrosis without hilar lymph node enlargement. Histologically, this is often characterized by obvious multinucleate giant cells and probably represents the entity first described as giant cell interstitial pneumonia by Liebow (to whom the occupational histories were unavailable). These giant cells can sometimes be detected by examination of bronchoalveolar lavage (BAL) cells. Some improvement results from ending exposure, but progression to severe disability typically occurs. The entity occurs infrequently among tool grinders in general but does occur in those who maintain the sharp grinding bits made of tungsten carbide–cobalt high-speed steels. (Cadmium is sometimes used by such workers as part of a soldering flux and also may cause lung fibrosis patterns but without giant cells.)

OTHER PNEUMOCONIOSES

Many other mineral dusts may also cause pneumoconiosis. Some dusts (barium, antimony, tin, iron oxides), because they avidly absorb the roentgen rays, produce a strikingly abnormal chest radiograph but have little or no measurable effect on pulmonary function. Others (e.g., cement dust) may produce bronchitis and/or airflow obstruction with no radiologic abnormalities. Bauxite and metallic aluminum may produce pulmonary fibrosis. Silicate dusts (talc, kaolin, asbestos, others) are composed of crystalline silica bound to mineral cations. Kaolin appears to be less fibrogenic than either silica or asbestos, but all these may produce pneumoconiosis with sufficient doses.

Siderosis is the pneumoconiosis resulting from inhalation of ferric oxide. By itself it appears to have little effect on lung function. Siderosis may occur in electric arc welders and oxyacetylene cutters, whose inhalation exposures may also include a variety of gases and particulates other than ferrous metals. Metal fume fever (a self-limited febrile illness), chronic bronchitis, and cases of allergic asthma and hypersensitivity pneumonitis have been described in welders as the result of specific exposures encountered in the welding process, the asthma being associated with welding rod materials.

LUNG CANCER (See also Chapter 214.)

Bronchogenic carcinoma attributable to occupational exposures may currently be the most important cause of occupational lung disease mortality in the United States and Canada; an estimated 4% to 5% of the total lung cancer deaths annually in the United States may be occupationally derived. The role for workplace causes of these generally fatal cancers may easily be overlooked if the treating physician limits the exposure history to questions about cigarette smoking.

In heavily exposed working populations, asbestos fibers, coke oven emissions, chloromethyl ether and bischloromethyl ether, mustard gas, the refining of arsenic and nickel ores, and radon daughters (decay products) have all been linked to increased rates of bronchogenic carcinoma. Hexavalent chromium has been associated with nasal and bronchogenic carcinomas. All these cancers are characterized by a long latent period between first exposure to the carcinogen and the eventual clinical appearance of the disease. Thus the tumor may be recognized years or even decades after exposure to the causative agent(s) has ceased. Lung cancers occurring in the present are often the result of past exposures that began before the carcinogenic potential of occupational agents was widely appreciated. The quantitative interactions between cigarette smoke and asbestos are important and have been intensively studied, and it is suspected that other occupational agents also interact with cigarette smoke, producing increased risk for developing lung cancers. Nonetheless, a minority of persons most heavily exposed both to cigarette smoke and occupational carcinogens actually develop lung cancer. Limited data suggest that smoking cessation may reduce the risk of developing lung cancer in populations who have already been heavily exposed to asbestos. Efforts to reduce lung cancer mortality by regular chest radiographs and sputum cytology in middle-aged cigarette-smoking males have not been successful.

In general the lung cancers produced by occupational exposures are indistinguishable histologically from other cancers. An association with occupation is established only by a careful review of the patient's exposure history.

Although identification of the disease-causing potential of these substances should lead to marked reduction in the amount of exposure for individual workers, these substances continue to be used worldwide and sometimes without appropriate regard to their dangers. The potential for preventing deaths from these causes has not yet been realized. The identification of radon daughters as a cause of lung cancer in miners both of uranium and of nonuranium minerals has raised the likelihood that domestic exposure to radon daughters (entering homes through basement walls) may also cause some increase in lung cancer, but the magnitude of this effect is not known.

REFERENCES

Chan-Yeung M and Lam S: Occupational asthma: state of the art. Am Rev Respir Dis 133:686, 1986.

Cugell D and Morgan W: The respiratory effects of cobalt. Arch Intern Med 150:177, 1990.

Cullen M, Cherniack M, and Kaminsky J: Chronic beryllium disease in the United States. Semin Respir Med 7:203, 1986.

Morgan WKC and Seaton A, editors: Occupational lung diseases, ed 2. Philadelphia, 1984, Saunders

Mossman BT and Gee JBL: Asbestos-related diseases (medical progress). N Engl J Med 320:1721, 1989.

Parkes WR: Occupational lung disease, ed 2. London, 1982, Butterworths.

Ziskind M, Jones RN, and Weill H: Silicosis. Am Rev Respir Dis 113:643, 1976.

CHAPTER

212 Adverse Pulmonary Reactions to Drugs and Other Therapeutic Modalities

J. Allen Cooper, Jr.

Administration of various therapeutic modalities has been associated with respiratory alterations (see boxes) ranging from severe parenchymal destruction to reversible chronic cough. Drugs, irradiation, or oxygen therapy can adversely affect the lung. This chapter discusses clinical manifestations of these reactions.

PNEUMONITIS WITH FIBROSIS

Pneumonitis with fibrosis occurs after administration of several drugs and in association with thoracic irradiation. Pa-

Drugs or drug groups that cause pulmonary parenchymal reactions*

- Cytotoxic antibiotics
  - Bleomycin
  - Mitomycin
- Alkylating agents
  - Cyclophosphamide
  - Busulfan
  - Chlorambucil
  - Melphalan
- Nitrosoureas
  - Carmustine (BCNU)
  - Lomustine (CCNU)
  - Methyl-CCNU
  - Chlorozotocin
- Anticonvulsants
  - Diphenylhydantoin
  - Carbamazepine
- Antimicrobials
  - Nitrofurantoin
  - Numerous antibiotics
- Antiarrhythmics
  - Amiodarone
  - Tocainide
  - Lidocaine
- Anti-inflammatory drugs
  - Aspirin
  - Other NSAIDs†
  - Gold salts
  - Penicillamine
- Opiates
  - Heroin
  - Propoxyphene
  - Methadone
- Miscellaneous
  - *Vinca* alkaloids
  - Hydrochlorothiazide
  - Procarbazine
  - Colchicine
  - Oxygen
  - Radiation

*Numerous drugs not listed sporadically cause hypersensitivity pneumonitis.
†Nonsteroidal anti-inflammatory drugs.

Drug groups that induce bronchospasm or cough

Beta-adrenergic antagonists
Aspirin
Other NSAIDs*
Cholinergic agents
Angiotensin-converting enzyme inhibitors

*Nonsteroidal anti-inflammatory drugs.

tients most often have insidious progression of dyspnea and nonproductive cough occurring over weeks or months. Similar symptoms may rarely progress more rapidly. The most common physical finding is bilateral, late inspiratory crackles. Chest radiographs usually demonstrate bibasilar reticular infiltrates; diffuse alveolar infiltrates occur less frequently. Pulmonary function tests show reduced lung volumes consistent with a restrictive ventilatory defect and a decreased diffusing capacity. However, because similar findings can occur from other processes that may affect this patient population, abnormal pulmonary function tests are not sufficient for the definitive diagnosis of pulmonary drug reactions. Pathologically, endothelial damage is an early manifestation of drug-induced pneumonitis. This is followed by type I pneumocyte destruction and type II pneumocyte proliferation with dysplastic changes. Finally, parenchymal inflammation and significant interstitial fibrosis with thickening of the interstitial space occur; the degree of fibrosis probably correlates with irreversibility of the syndrome.

HYPERSENSITIVITY (EOSINOPHILIC) PNEUMONITIS

Patients with drug-induced hypersensitivity pneumonitis have symptoms of cough, fever, and dyspnea developing over several days. Systemic manifestations, including eosinophilia, hepatitis, dermatitis, or nephritis, may also be present. However, some patients may have isolated pulmonary hypersensitivity reactions. Chest radiographs show bilateral alveolar infiltrates that may be peripheral and rarely migratory. Pleural effusions may also be present. Lung tissue shows infiltration of acute inflammatory cells, including eosinophils and neutrophils, into parenchyma with minimum fibrosis. A similar syndrome induced by methotrexate may be associated with pulmonary granulomatous inflammation. The prognosis for patients with drug-induced hypersensitivity pneumonitis is favorable, especially for those with reactions caused by drugs other than methotrexate. Virtually all patients recover with no residual pulmonary abnormalities if the agent is withdrawn and corticosteroids are instituted. Mortality for patients who develop hypersensitivity pneumonitis from methotrexate may approach 10%.

NONCARDIOGENIC PULMONARY EDEMA

Noncardiogenic pulmonary edema can be induced by several drugs and is also a manifestation of pulmonary oxygen toxicity. When associated with drug ingestion, the syndrome usually occurs after overdose. Prognosis is variable but generally better than in patients with other causes of noncardiogenic pulmonary edema, presumably because the offending agent can be removed. Histopathologic specimens from patients with the syndrome show protein and inflammatory cellular exudation into the alveolar space.

COUGH

Recently it has been documented that angiotensin enzyme inhibitors can induce cough in as many as 10% of treated patients. Cough in these patients is generally nonproductive and may be slow in clearing after discontinuation of the drug.

BRONCHOSPASM

Certain drugs also precipitate bronchospasm (see the box at upper left) by varied mechanisms. Nonsteroidal anti-inflammatory drugs (NSAIDs) that inhibit the cyclooxygenase enzyme or arachidonic acid metabolism induce bronchospasm in approximately 15% of adult asthmatic patients. One report indicated an increased incidence of HLA-DQw2 antigen in aspirin-sensitive asthmatic patients. Intolerance to these agents increases with age, may be associated with peripheral eosinophilia, is frequently associated with nasal polyposis and rhinitis, and develops more frequently in females. The associated triad of asthma, nasal polyposis, and aspirin sensitivity was initially described by Samter and Beers. Onset of bronchospasm occurs 30 to 90 minutes after ingestion of the drug. Treatment is similar to that for other forms of bronchospasm. Progressive desensitization with aspirin may be attempted, but this can induce severe bronchospasm if the procedure is done incorrectly.

Cholinergic agents, typically used in the treatment of urologic and ocular disorders, may also occasionally induce bronchospasm in asthmatic patients when these drugs are administered locally to the eye or systemically. Treatment of bronchospasm in these patients consists of drug withdrawal and administration of atropine, parenterally or by inhalation in addition to other bronchodilators.

Beta-adrenergic antagonists may also induce bronchospasm, primarily in patients with pre-existing obstructive airways disease, although apparently normal persons may also rarely be susceptible. The association of timolol with this syndrome is particularly important because patients react to this drug after local ocular treatment, a situation that can be easily overlooked. Symptoms of wheezing and dyspnea occur 1 hour after use of the beta blocker and may be severe. Treatment includes supportive measures, withdrawal of the drug, and administration of bronchodilators. In these patients, anticholinergic bronchodilators such as atropine or ipratropium are the agents of choice, since beta-adrenergic agents may be ineffective because of blocked adrenergic receptors.

RESPIRATORY MUSCLE DYSFUNCTION

Antibiotics, including aminoglycosides, penicillin, polymixin, and occasionally other drugs, can cause acute respiratory failure secondary to respiratory muscle dysfunction. Signs and symptoms include severe dyspnea, orthopnea, hypoxemia, and reduced motion of the diaphragm. The chest radiograph may show an elevated hemidiaphragm and reduced lung volumes. Treatment involves supportive measures, including artificial ventilation. Occasionally, some improvement may occur with calcium or neostigmine therapy.

OTHER SYNDROMES

Pulmonary arterial hypertension can occur after administration of certain agents. Aminorex, an anorectic agent no longer in use, caused a high incidence of such reactions. Granulomatous lung disease with pulmonary hypertension may occur with intravenous injection of talc-containing preparations intended for oral use. The incidence of pulmonary veno-occlusive disease also increases after administration of certain cytotoxic agents. Bronchiolitis obliterans occurs rarely after penicillamine therapy and is manifested primarily by airway obstruction, as documented by pulmonary function testing, although a restrictive component may also be apparent. Finally, a pulmonary-renal syndrome similar to Goodpasture's syndrome has been reported to occur infrequently after penicillamine therapy.

SPECIFIC DRUGS

Bleomycin

The polypeptide antibiotic bleomycin causes pneumonitis with fibrosis in approximately 4% of patients receiving the drug. The incidence of pulmonary reactions to this drug increases with certain well-defined risk factors, including age, oxygen administration, radiotherapy, use of multidrug regimens, and cumulative doses exceeding 450 total units. However, patients developing pulmonary reactions to bleomycin after only one dose have been reported. Although bleomycin most often causes a syndrome of pneumonitis with fibrosis, the drug also rarely induces a hypersensitivity (eosinophilic) pneumonitis.

The diagnosis of bleomycin-induced pulmonary disease usually requires lung biopsy to rule out other causes of lung disease, such as infection or underlying neoplasm. No pathognomonic histologic pattern exists for bleomycin-induced pulmonary damage. Screening for early diagnosis of bleomycin-induced pneumonitis/fibrosis is difficult. Currently, no tests can accurately identify patients at an early stage before onset of irreversible changes. Pulmonary functions tests are either too sensitive or nonspecific, as in the case of carbon dioxide diffusing capacity (DLCO). A percentage of patients who show a decrease in DLCO will never develop clinical bleomycin-induced pneumonitis. In contrast, although relatively more specific, lung volumes are insensitive. Patients with clinical bleomycin-induced pneumonitis generally have reduced total lung capacity, but this occurs late in the process and may indicate irreversibility. Mortality from bleomycin-induced pulmonary disease approaches 50% overall, although the prognosis for patients who develop bleomycin-induced hypersensitivity lung disease is good. Corticosteroids appear to be useful in the treatment of both syndromes of pulmonary toxicity associated with bleomycin.

Methotrexate

This folate antagonist induces pulmonary disease in approximately 7% of patients who receive the drug. Low doses used as part of an anti-inflammatory regimen and higher doses used in the treatment of malignancy have been associated with pulmonary toxicity. Pulmonary reactions have occurred after intravenous (IV) or intrathecal administration of methotrexate. Multidrug regimens, increased frequency of administration, and tapering of corticosteroids or previous adrenelectomy increase the risk of developing pulmonary disease from methotrexate. As noted, the most common clinical syndrome associated with methotrexate is hypersensitivity pneumonitis. However, noncardiogenic pulmonary edema, pneumonitis with fibrosis, and acute pleurisy have also been associated with methotrexate therapy.

Mitomycin

Pulmonary toxicity of the cytotoxic antibiotic mitomycin is manifested by several clinical syndromes. First, the combination of mitomycin with *Vinca* alkaloid treatment can result in acute bronchospasm in the presence or absence of pulmonary infiltrates. The incidence of pulmonary reactions to regimens containing this combination may be as high as 39%. Second, mitomycin can cause a syndrome of microangiopathic hemolytic anemia, pulmonary infiltrates, and uremia that is precipitated by blood transfusions. Finally, mitomycin may induce a pneumonitis with fibrosis that is histopathologically indistinguishable from that caused by other cytotoxic drugs, except for an increased degree of interstitial mononuclear cell infiltrates. The presence of these cells may correlate with the relative responsiveness of patients with this form of mitomycin toxicity to corticosteroid therapy.

Nitrosoureas

Carmustine and other nitrosoureas frequently cause pneumonitis with fibrosis. Symptoms usually progress insidiously, but a few reports have documented a rapid progression. Recently, emphasis has been on the late sequelae of therapy with these agents; reports of pulmonary fibrosis several years after discontinuation of treatment with these agents are relatively frequent. Risk factors for development of nitrosourea-induced pulmonary disease probably include cumulative dose, pre-existing lung disease, younger age, and use of the nitrosourea in multidrug chemotherapy regimens.

Other chemotherapeutic agents

Several alkylating agents have been reported to cause pulmonary injury. In fact, busulfan was the first chemotherapeutic drug to be associated with pulmonary toxicity. Cyclophosphamide causes pneumonitis with fibrosis when used as a single agent and is also an important component of pulmonary-toxic multidrug regimens. Melphalan and chlorambucil rarely cause pulmonary toxicity.

Cytosine arabinoside induces noncardiogenic pulmonary edema in a cumulative dose-dependent manner. Azathioprine and mercaptopurine rarely cause hypersensitivity pneumonitis. Procarbazine has been reported to cause a pulmonary hypersensitivity reaction, with peripheral and pulmonary eosinophilia and skin rash in some patients.

Amiodarone

The antiarrhythmic agent amiodarone causes a syndrome of pneumonitis with fibrosis in 5% to 10% of exposed patients. Elimination half-life of amiodarone from the body may be 30 days. Thus pulmonary toxicity from amiodarone must be recognized promptly and the drug discontinued early in the course of the illness. Risk factors that increase the incidence of pulmonary toxicity to amiodarone are the maintenance dose and previous pulmonary disease. Recent evidence also suggests that the combination of amiodarone and general anesthesia or cardiopulmonary bypass is synergistic for development of acute lung injury. As with bleomycin, pulmonary function tests are relatively poor predictors of early pulmonary disease caused by amiodarone. However, the DLCO is useful in distinguishing between amiodarone pulmonary toxicity and congestive heart failure, a common malady in this patient population. If the DLCO is normal, it is unlikely that pneumonitis resulting from amiodarone is present.

Chest radiographs of patients with amiodarone-induced pulmonary disease typically show both bilateral reticular infiltrates and patchy acinar infiltrates. Infrequent radiographic presentations are focal consolidation, nodular lesions, and isolated pleural effusions. The chest radiograph may be particularly useless in this patient population because of the common occurrence of cardiogenic edema. Positive gallium scans have been reported in several patients with amiodarone-induced pneumonitis, but gallium scans may also be negative.

Histologic findings in patients with amiodarone-induced pulmonary disease are relatively nonspecific, except for the presence of "foamy," phospholipid-laden macrophages. However, the presence of these cells is not pathognomonic for amiodarone-induced lung disease. Moreover, similar abnormal cells may be recovered from patients receiving the drug who have no apparent pulmonary disease. Other pulmonary histopathologic findings associated with amiodarone are pneumocyte atypia, interstitial thickening, and mononuclear cell infiltration.

Mortality in patients who develop amiodarone-induced pneumonitis is high. However, this is caused by the severity of their cardiac disease as much as by the pulmonary reaction to the drug. Many patients who develop amiodarone-induced pneumonitis cannot have the drug discontinued because it is life-saving for them. In these patients a reduction in dosage of amiodarone and institution of corticosteroids may reverse the pulmonary sequelae.

Nitrofurantoin

The urinary antiseptic nitrofurantoin causes two distinct clinical syndromes: (1) a hypersensitivity (eosinophilic) pneumonitis or (2) chronic pneumonitis with fibrosis. The acute syndrome occurs within 1 month of drug initiation and does not predispose to the more chronic syndrome, which occurs after 2 months to 5 years of nitrofurantoin therapy. Both syndromes have been associated with pulmonary tissue eosinophilia and interstitial inflammation, although fibrosis is a more common finding in the chronic form of the disease. Acute pulmonary toxicity from nitrofurantoin carries a lower mortality, and residual pulmonary abnormalities occur infrequently compared with the chronic syndrome.

Gold salts

Chrysotherapy for patients with rheumatoid arthritis may cause hypersensitivity pneumonitis. A more chronic process consistent with pneumonitis/fibrosis or bronchiolitis obliterans has also been described. Approximately 40% of patients with rheumatoid arthritis who develop gold salt–induced pulmonary disease are rheumatoid factor negative. In addition, a recent study has demonstrated a strong association between HLA and complement phenotype and occurrence of pulmonary reactions to gold salts. Lung tissue from patients with gold-induced pulmonary reactions demonstrates interstitial and alveolar infiltration by inflammatory cells, including histiocytes, lymphocytes, and plasma cells. Patients with gold-induced pneumonitis are often responsive to corticosteroid treatment, in addition to discontinuation of the drug.

Sulfasalazine

Sulfasalazine, used in the treatment of inflammatory bowel disorders, has been associated rarely with pulmonary hypersensitivity reactions. The drug also rarely causes chronic pneumonitis with fibrosis, bronchiolitis obliterans, or isolated bronchospasm.

Antiepileptics

Dilantin and carbamazepine have been implicated as causes of pulmonary hypersensitivity reactions. All patients had a similar presentation with cough, myalgia, fever, and peripheral eosinophilia, and most had a maculopapular rash. Some patients developed severe lymphadenopathy and hepatitis. In fact, liver biopsy has been used to diagnose the syndrome.

Opiates

An overdose of heroin, methadone, or propoxyphene causes noncardiogenic pulmonary edema. Pulmonary abnormalities develop acutely over several hours after exposure to the opiate. Signs and symptoms include lethargy, cyanosis, pulmonary crackles, and occasional fever.

Terbutaline and ritrodine

These two tocolytic agents cause noncardiogenic pulmonary edema in less than 1% of patients receiving the drugs for premature labor. Risk factors for developing the syndrome are unclear, although concurrent corticosteroid use, aggressive fluid replacement, and abrupt withdrawal of terbutaline or ritrodine may be important.

Nonsteroidal anti-inflammatory agents

Supratherapeutic serum concentrations of aspirin cause noncardiogenic pulmonary edema. Besides overdose, risk factors include age, a history of smoking, and chronic ingestion of salicylates. Aspirin and other NSAIDs also induce bronchospasm in approximately 0.3% of the normal population as well as 4% to 20% of asthmatic patients (see previous section on bronchospasm). NSAIDs other than aspirin have also been associated with pulmonary hypersensitivity reactions.

Other agents used for benign conditions

Hydrochlorothiazide rarely causes a syndrome of noncardiogenic pulmonary edema. Several patients had previously noted milder symptoms after ingesting the drug, and in all patients, pulmonary symptoms developed within 1 hour of drug ingestion. Penicillamine therapy is associated with pneumonitis/fibrosis, bronchiolitis obliterans, bronchitis, hypersensitivity lung disease, and a pulmonary renal syndrome in less than 1% of the patients at risk, although the role of the underlying disease, usually rheumatoid arthritis, remains to be resolved. Tocainide, an antiarrhythmic agent, has produced three well-documented cases of pneumonitis with fibrosis. Captopril and other angiotensin-converting enzyme inhibitors induce cough in approximately 10% of treated patients. Beta-adrenergic antagonists can induce bronchospasm in asthmatic patients as well as apparently normal individuals.

OXYGEN THERAPY

Delivery of partial pressures of oxygen (O_2) greater than ambient air is associated with lung injury, usually manifested by a syndrome of noncardiogenic pulmonary edema. However, chronic manifestations may occur if the patient survives. It is unclear what O_2 partial pressure is nontoxic to the human lung, although early studies in normal individuals suggest less than 0.50 fraction of O_2 is safe. Concurrent or previous therapy with bleomycin or possibly other cytotoxic agents may lower the tolerance of the lung to O_2 therapy; the lowest possible fraction of O_2 that can be used should be employed at all times. Pathologically the lungs of patients with O_2 toxicity demonstrate an early exudative phase, with loss of normal alveolar lining cells and exudation of protein, and a later proliferative phase, with proliferation of type II pneumocytes and interstitial thickening caused by a fibrotic reaction. To date, no effective therapy exists for pulmonary O_2 toxicity; prevention by use of the lowest possible fraction of O_2 is the best method to avoid the syndrome.

RADIOTHERAPY

Irradiation of the lung causes pulmonary alterations in approximately 10% of patients at risk. Factors that increase the risk of radiation lung injury are dose of radiation and previous or concurrent chemotherapy. The most common clinical manifestation of radiation-induced pulmonary disease is pneumonitis, occurring 1 to 3 months after initiation of radiation therapy. In most patients the pulmonary abnormalities resolve with or without steroid therapy. A few patients progress to chronic irreversible pulmonary alterations. A helpful radiographic manifestation of radiation pneumonitis is the presence of infiltrates only in the location of the irradiation port.

REFERENCES

Cooper JAD Jr, White DA, and Matthay RA: State of the art: drug-induced pulmonary disease. Am Rev Respir Dis 133:321, 488, 1986.

Heffner JE and Sahn SA: Salicylate-induced pulmonary edema: clinical features and prognosis. Ann Intern Med 95:405, 1981.

Jackson RM: Molecular, pharmacologic, and clinical aspects of oxygen-induced lung injury. Clin Chest Med 11:73, 1990.

Kennedy JI Jr: Clinical aspects of amiodarone pulmonary toxicity. Clin Chest Med 11:119, 1990.

Rosenow EC: The spectrum of drug-induced pulmonary disease. Ann Intern Med 77:977, 1972.

Rosiello RA and Merrill WW: Radiation-induced lung injury. Clin Chest Med 11:65, 1990.

Slepian IK, Mathews KP, and McLean JA: Aspirin-sensitive asthma. Chest 87:386, 1985.

CHAPTER

213 Cystic Fibrosis and Bronchiectasis

Robert B. Fick, Jr.

CYSTIC FIBROSIS

Description and genetics

Cystic fibrosis (CF) is a systemic disorder transmitted by an autosomal recessive gene and is still characterized as the most common fatal genetic disease in Caucasians. However, the outlook for patients diagnosed today is greatly improved. CF was originally described as a pathologic entity in 1938, but recently, great advances have been made in understanding the genetics and pathophysiologic mechanisms operant in this common disease. Discovery of elevated concentrations of sodium and chloride (Na^+, Cl^-) in the sweat of patients with CF, reported in 1953, led to the 1959 description of the standard test (pilocarpine iontophoresis) to detect diseased homozygotes. It is now known that virtually every organ in the body is affected (Table 213-1). Although CF is a systemic disorder, lung disease, recurrent pulmonary bacterial infections, and bronchiectasis cause most of the morbidity and account for virtually all the increased mortality from this disease.

Approximately 1:20 in the U.S. Caucasian population is a carrier of the CF gene, and the disease occurs in 1:2000 live births, 1:17,000 black births, and 1:55,000 Oriental births. Carriers of the CF mutation do not manifest symptoms, and a heterozygotus advantage has not been demonstrated. Linkage analysis and the innovations of chromosome "walking" and "jumping" and complementary deoxyribonucleic acid (DNA) hybridization were used to isolate the CF gene, which spans 250,000 base pairs of genomic DNA and contains 27 exons on the long arm of chromosome 7. Sequence analysis predicts a polypeptide of 1480 amino acids. The most characteristic feature of the predicted protein, termed *cystic fibrosis transmembrane conductance regulator* (CFTR), is the presence of two repeat motifs, each of which consists of a domain capable of spanning the membrane six times and another containing the consensus sequence of a nucleotide (adenosine triphosphate, (ATP)-binding domain. The schematic model of the predicted CFTR protein displays much overall structural similarity with mammalian multidrug-resistant P glycoproteins. Seventy percent of the mutations in patients with CF correspond to a specific deletion of three base pairs (ΔF508)), which results in the loss of a phenylalanine from this protein. Since the original 1989 report, more than 200 additional CF mutations have been described. Through major collaborative efforts, the reported CF mutations account for approximately 85% of all CF patients. Continuing analysis of CFTR function will define the basic defect, eventually making possible new, specific therapies.

Table 213-1. Manifestations of cystic fibrosis in adults

Involvement	Frequency (%)
Elevated sweat chloride (>80 mEq/L)	98
Positive family history	70
Chronic sinusitis	100
Nasal polyposis	29-61
Chronic lung disease	90
Recurrent *Pseudomonas* infections	70-90
Bronchiectasis	80
Hemoptysis	
Streaking	40-60
Massive	7-10
Pneumothorax	11-20
Gastrointestinal disease	80
Pancreatic insufficiency (achylia)	80-90
Clinical diabetes	1-5
Cholelithiasis	6-10
Focal biliary cirrhosis	5-15
Intestinal obstruction	20
Azoospermia	95
Heatstroke	1-5

Modified Fick RB: Clin Chest Med 2:91, 1981.

Pathophysiology

The clinical observations that Cl^- and Na^+ concentrations are increased in the sweat of CF patients led investigators to examine the ion transport properties of the sweat duct. They found that in vivo and in vitro sweat ducts in CF patients have a higher transepithelial electrical potential difference than normal ducts. Subsequent studies of transepithelial electrical conductance confirmed the conclusion that the CF sweat duct is Cl^- impermeable. Despite the importance of the sweat duct to our understanding of the basic defect in CF, 75% of all hospitalizations are caused by pulmonary disease, and 95% of CF patients die in respiratory failure. It is somewhat encouraging that much of the pathophysiology described in the CF sweat gland duct also pertains to the secretory apparatus of the CF airway epithelial cell (Fig. 213-1).

As expected, respiratory epithelial cells isolated from CF patients lack protein kinase–dependent Cl^- conductance across their apical membrane. Furthermore, studies in which wild-type and mutant CFTR complement DNAs are expressed in a variety of cell types indicate that the CFTR protein directly mediates this regulatable Cl^- conductance. A prevalent explanation for the molecular basis of CF is that ΔF508 mutation alters nucleotide binding, impairing normal function of the protein and, therefore resulting in failure of secretory CF cells to secrete Cl^-. Transepithelial electrolyte transport controls the quantity and composition of the respiratory tract fluid and therefore is important in effecting normal mucociliary clearance. CF epithelia provide insufficient water to surface liquids to avoid inspissation of periciliary fluids and airway mucus.

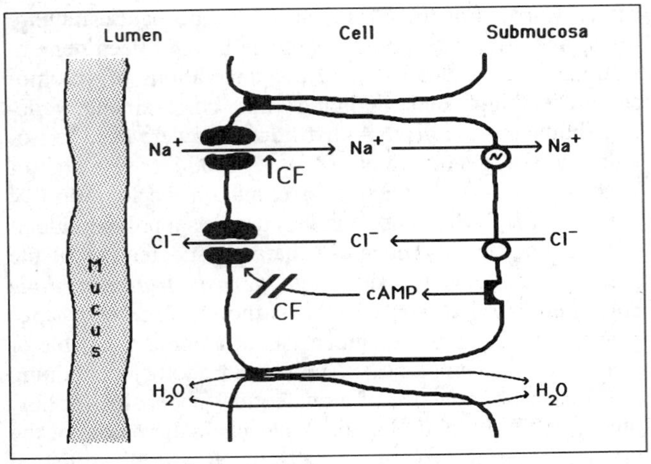

Fig. 213-1. Schematic representation of electrolyte transport by airway epithelium demonstrating the failure in cystic fibrosis *(CF)* cells to secrete Cl^- in response to increased intracellular levels of cyclic 3′,5′ adenosine monophosphate *(cAMP)*. (From Welsh MJ and Fick RB: J Clin Invest 80:1523, 1987.)

Dehydrated airway secretions obstruct the ducts and, in an incompletely understood manner, predispose the adult CF patient to recurrent infections of the upper and lower respiratory tract. After the age of 12 years, these infections are caused by a single pathogen in the overwhelming majority of patients (Fig. 213-2). Although pneumonias in early childhood may be caused by *Staphylococcus aureus, Streptococcus pneumoniae,* or *Haemophilus influenzae,* the mucoid colonial form of *Pseudomonas aeruginosa* is found in the sputum of up to 90% of adult CF patients. Genotyping of CF clinical isolates of *P. aeruginosa* indicates that most patients have a persistent strain in the airway over years.

Pseudomonas adheres to the apical membrane of airway epithelial cells interacting with cellular glycoproteins and respiratory mucins. Damage to the epithelium caused by antecedent viral infection or proteases with loss of fibronectin decrease the adherence of gram-positive organisms, increasing the adherence of gram-negative organisms. The bacterial adhesion responsible for binding may be polar pili, although mucoid pseudomonads are known to adhere more avidly than nonmucoid strains, supporting the notion that alginate, the primary component of the mucoid coat, may serve as an adhesion. This pathogen acquires the iron necessary for growth by secreting a neutral metalloprotease, elastase, which in a nonspecific way frees iron for bacterial use from the serum iron transport proteins. The airway in CF patients is thought to present an iron-restricted milieu to *Pseudomonas,* and these culture conditions are known to induce the release of high levels of elastase and other exoproduct virulence factors such as exotoxin A and exoenzyme S.

Pseudomonas elastase is a potent bacterial protease with broad substrate specificity that is involved in the hydroly-

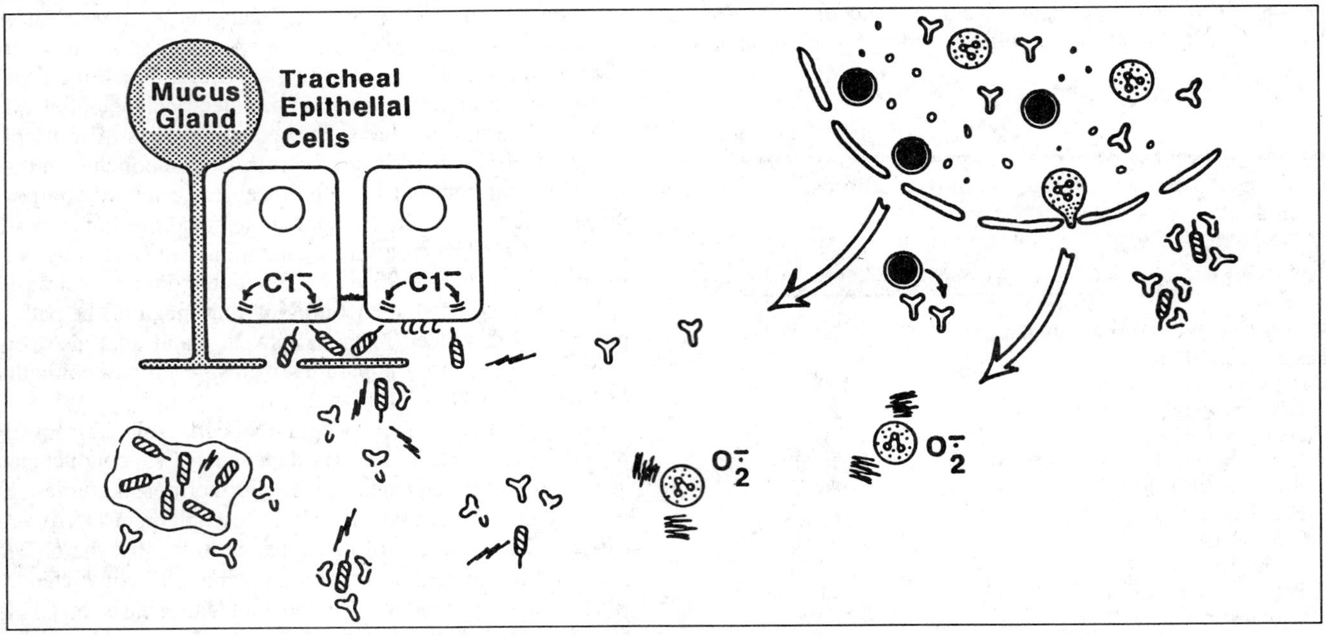

Fig. 213-2. Proposed pathogenetic mechanisms in the establishment and persistence of *Pseudomonas* in airways of patients with CF. *Pseudomonas* adheres to airway epithelial cells through pilus proteins interacting with apical membrane proteins or abnormal mucus. The pathogen survives by cleaving (⫽) immunoglobulin G needed for clearance of *Pseudomonas* in the distal airway and perhaps by forming microcolonies that thwart an immune response. Together with neutrophil elastase (≡) and toxic oxygen products (O_2^-, OH), *Pseudomonas* elastase destroys the airway's connective tissue substrate. The resulting airway ectasia further decreases mucociliary clearance.

sis of immunoglobulin G (IgG) antibodies necessary for pulmonary macrophages to phagocytose and kill *Pseudomonas* optimally. *Pseudomonas* elastase cleaves a low-molecular-weight fragment from $alpha_1$—proteinase inhibitor, thereby partially inactivating the antiprotease screen in the distal airways of patients with CF. Furthermore, *Pseudomonas* releases cell wall constituents that are direct chemotaxins or that stimulate macrophage release of C5a, LTB_4, and interleukin 8 (IL-8). In so doing, *Pseudomonas* moves sheets of neutrophils into the distal airways, augmenting the proteolytic or oxidative damage to the lung in CF patients. Thus, after gaining a foothold on the apical membrane of airway epithelia, pseudomonads grow and produce exoproteins. Through these secretory products, most notably elastase, this pathogen creates defects in host defenses, ensuring its survival, and the same bacterial exoproducts cleave the connective tissue substrate of the airways, contributing to the bronchiectatic lung lesion.

Clinical presentation

Many adults with CF may not appear chronically ill because 44% are at the 50th percentile in height and 32% are at the 50th percentile in weight. The index of suspicion and clinical acumen of the physician seeing these young adults determine the age at which the proper diagnosis is made. Hallmarks of CF (see Table 213-1) include chronic bronchopulmonary infection, chronic sinusitis, pancreatic insufficiency, a high sweat sodium, steatorrhea, and a family history of CF. Not all patients possess all these however, and no consistent abnormalities emerge from routine hematologic and biochemical testing. Involvement of the respiratory tract dominates the clinical picture as the patient grows older and gastrointestinal and pancreatic symptoms become less prominent. Studies attempting to identify correlations between genotype and phenotype are difficult, but ΔF508 is considered a severe mutation usually associated with pancreatic insufficiency when homozygous or associated with another severe allele. Correlation of CF mutations with lung involvement remains controversial.

Pulmonary disease. Hypertrophy of bronchial glands, goblet cell hyperplasia, metaplasia of the bronchiolar epithelium, and mucopurulent plugging of peripheral airways are all part of the early pathologic lesion of CF. Particularly prominent are bronchiolitis, peribronchiolar inflammation, and bronchiectasis. Morphometric work performed on lungs of CF patients, obtained at autopsy indicates that the lung disease and remodeling are irregularly distributed and that the upper lobe segments are disproportionately involved. Careful light and electron microscopic studies have failed to identify a single lesion specific for CF.

The lungs are morphologically normal at birth, and the onset of pulmonary involvement may occur at any time after birth, with varying severity of the respiratory signs and symptoms. CF pulmonary disease may present acutely with staphylococcal pneumonia or insidiously with persistent cough after an upper respiratory infection. Respiratory infection in CF follows a smoldering course punctuated by acute exacerbations (in part caused by viral agents) superimposed on a baseline of chronic productive cough and bacterial colonization most often caused by mucoid *P. aeruginosa*. Curiously, temperature elevations occur infrequently, routine blood counts are generally not helpful, and positive blood cultures are practically unknown. More than 90% of deaths of CF patients occur during one of these pulmonary infections.

Although *P. aeruginosa* is the most common bacterial isolate obtained from the airway of adult patients with CF, new multiresistant organisms have emerged. One nonaeruginosa strain, *P. cepacia,* has been associated with increased morbidity and premature death in some centers. During acute flare-ups of pulmonary symptoms, 5% to 15% of bacterial strains isolated from sputa may be nonaeruginosa *Pseudomonas*. Effective recovery of this *Pseudomonas* species requires use of selective media OF-polymyxin-bacitracin-lactose agar or *P. cepacia* isolation agar.

As the disease progresses, the chest radiograph shows a combination of fibrotic strands, cystic spaces, and radiographic signs of bronchiectasis. The tests of spirometry and lung volumes reveal obstructive physiology with impaired airflows and later a disproportionately greater reduction in forced vital capacity (FVC). Many patients complain of wheezing, and reversible airflow obstruction or increased bronchomotor tone is present in up to 30% of those tested. True emphysema in an anatomic and physiologic sense is unusual in CF because the carbon monoxide diffusing capacity is often preserved. The differential diagnosis to consider when patients have signs as just described is shown in the box below. The younger age of the patient, suppurative nature of the lung disease, the presence of multisystem disease, and marked propensity to recurrent mucoid *Pseudomonas* airway infections usually serve to differentiate CF patients from patients with non-CF chronic obstructive pulmonary disease (COPD).

Differential diagnosis of bronchiectasis

Postpneumonic infection* (tuberculosis; allergic bronchopulmonary aspergillosis; other fungal, postviral, or necrotizing bacterial causes)
Cystic fibrosis
Immotile cilia syndrome (Kartagener's syndrome)
Young's syndrome
Opsonic defects (immunoglobulin deficiencies causing recurrent sinoplumonary infections)
Compensatory (a result of cicatrization of pulmonary parenchyma)
Recurrent gastroesophageal reflux and aspiration
Congenital
 Tracheobronchomegaly
 Williams-Campbell syndrome (short stature, chest deformities, bronchomalacia)
Associated with inflammatory bowel disease
Idiopathic

*Most frequently results in cylindric form (see p. 1730).

Pulmonary complications in CF adults occur often. From 5%, to 10% of adults with CF have clinically evident pneumothoraces; 25% are multiple, and 58% of these pneumothoraces subside spontaneously, not requiring tube drainage. Hypertrophic pulmonary osteoarthropathy (ossifying periostitis) occurs as a complication in older children with severe CF lung disease and causes long bone pain, arthralgias, and occasionally joint effusions. Hemoptysis usually amounts to blood streaking of sputum but may be massive ($>$ 300 ml per episode). The literature shows disagreement as to the prognosis portended by hemoptysis. No one disagrees, however, that pulmonary disease appears in most patients with CF, frequently dominates the clinical picture, is progressive, and determines the fate of most patients.

Gastrointestinal disease. The manifestation of pancreatic exocrine insufficiency, steatorrhea, is much more pronounced in children. Acute pancreatitis is a rare occurrence in adults and may be induced by use of tetracycline antibiotics. Small numbers of patients believed to have a forme fruste of CF because of a positive family history and greatly reduced bicarbonate response to secretin have been reported with high-normal sweat electrolytes (40 to 60 mEq Cl^-/L). Interestingly, these individuals have normal trypsin, chymotrypsin, amylase, and lipase activity in duodenal fluid aspirates. With progression of pancreatic disease, fibrosis distorts the parenchyma, and endocrine pancreatic function becomes impaired as well. An abnormal oral glucose tolerance test is found in up to 42% of adults with CF, but glucosuria occurs much less frequently, and clinical diabetes mellitus is found in less than 5% of older patients. The diabetes tends to be noninsulin dependent (type 2), and ketoacidosis rarely develops.

Fatty liver (steatosis) is the most common hepatic lesion in patients with CF. Focal biliary cirrhosis, characterized by inspissated eosinophilic material in portal bile ductules, ductal proliferation, and chronic inflammation, is characteristic of CF. Hepatic enzymes, usually alkaline phosphatase, are elevated only late in the disease process, and hepatic failure is a rare complication. However, patients with clinical and biochemical liver disease have a high incidence of distal common duct strictures. Microgallbladder, measuring less than 1.5 cm × 0.5 cm, occurs quite often in CF but is more a curiosity and of little clinical importance. More significantly, malabsorption of bile acids interrupts the enterohepatic circulation of bile acids, and thus the secretion of lithogenic bile results. Cholelithiasis is significantly more frequent than in a matched non-CF population, occurring in 6% to 12% of adult CF patients.

Reduced water excretion into the gut leads to thickening of secretions, which in older CF patients results in the syndrome referred to as *meconium ileus equivalent* (distal intestinal obstruction syndrome). These acute attacks of partial small-bowel obstruction cause abdominal pain and bloating, presenting a spectrum of clinical disease from a frequently irritated acute abdomen. Hardened bowel contents may lead to intrussusception.

Abnormalities of reproductive organs. Patients with severe disease have delayed sexual maturation, and full reproductive function may never be achieved. Males show maldevelopment of the seminiferous tubules, plugging and obstruction of the vas deferens and, as a result, are usually infertile. Woman with CF have delayed menarche and thick, sticky cervical mucus, which decrease fertility. However, pregnancy may occur and entails some increased risks to both mother and child. These expectant mothers are best followed in high-risk obstetrics centers with the cooperation of obstetricians, neonatologists, and pulmonologists experienced with CF.

Diagnosis

The diagnosis of CF is often overlooked. A report of a sputum sample obtained from a patient with COPD returning with a growth identified as mucoid *P. aeruginosa* should suggest the diagnosis of CF. Determination of sweat electrolytes by pilocarpine iontophoresis remains the standard test in the diagnosis of CF. The concentration of Na^+ and Cl^- should be determined in a laboratory where the procedure is done often; the tests should be run in duplicate; and at least 100 mg of sweat must be collected for the electrolyte determinations. It has been demonstrated that false-negative and false-positive results are minimized if Na^+ and Cl^- are both measured. In CF patients the Cl^- concentration is usually higher than Na^+, whereas in healthy normal subjects the reverse usually occurs. A sweat chloride concentration greater than 60 mEq/L in a child is considered diagnostic of CF if more than 100 mg of sweat has been collected for analysis. However, it has long been established that sweat chloride concentrations are higher in adults. A large series of healthy normal adults and adults with non-CF COPD yielded sweat chloride values greater than 60 mEq/L in 8% of patients; a small series of 100 normal adults revealed values greater than 80 mEq/L in 4%. Therefore values of 60 to 80 mEq/L may be considered borderline in adults, and support of the diagnosis with a history of recurrent *Pseudomonas* lung infections, pancreatic insufficiency, azoospermia, or a family history of CF is important.

Elevated concentrations of exocrine sweat electrolytes producing false-positive results have been shown in adrenal insufficiency, ectodermal dysplasia, nephrogenic diabetes insipidus, type II glycogen storage disease, dehydration, and hypothyroidism. For these reasons, the diagnosis of CF requires more than a simple elevation of sweat Cl^-, and it is necessary to obtain a compatible clinical history (see Table 213-1) of COPD, pancreatic insufficiency, or a positive family history. An incorrect diagnosis causes much unnecessary stress. Also, approximately 2% of patients with clinical disease compatible with CF and a positive family history will have sweat chloride values of 40 to 60 mEq/L. This situation occurs most often in the CF patient with intact exocrine pancreatic function, as discussed previously.

Routine sweat testing does not differentiate heterozygous carriers of the CF gene from homozygous normal subjects.

Presently, detection of carriers, as with antenatal diagnosis, can only be performed within the framework of family (at risk) studies. The cloning of the CF gene provides a basis for the development of more efficient carrier identification; however, multiple, individually rare mutations rather than a small number of common mutations make carrier testing problematic. Partners of known carriers (obligate heterozygotes) may be tested for all mutations. Individuals with a positive family history may be tested for the mutation known to be in the family. Currently, general population screening is not the standard of care for couples with no documented family history of CF.

Treatment

Replacement of deficient pancreatic enzymes is required in most patients, even if steatorrhea is not a symptom, because pancreatic enzymes will correct the lithogenic bile, tend to prevent gallstones, and lessen chances of meconium ileus equivalent. Patients taking pH-sensitive microspheres (pancrelipase) have significantly less dyspeptic symptoms, decreased stool frequency, better appetite, and greater increments in weight gain than do those treated with powdered pancreatic enzyme preparations. Duodenal postprandial pH in CF patients is too acidic to permit rapid dissolution of current enteric-coated dosage forms of these enzymes, so bicarbonate may be used (5.2 g/m^2 body surface/meal) to enhance the enzymatic activities. Cimetidine (200 to 400 mg) half an hour before meals may be substituted. Fat-soluble vitamins must also be replaced, and during hot weather, some increase in salt intake should be encouraged.

Patients with meconium ileus equivalent are managed conservatively by adjustments to diet and supplemental pancreatic enzymes. More persistent, disruptive symptoms may be treated with *N*-acetylcysteine (5 to 20 ml of 10% solution) three times daily. Meglumine diatrizoate (Gastrografin) by enema may be effective in relieving severe obstruction and simultaneously permits radiographic definition of the obstruction site.

Lung disease. The treatment of acute exacerbations of pseudomonal infections in patients with CF traditionally has consisted of hospitalization and parenteral administration of an aminoglycoside with an antipseudomonal penicillin (carbenicillin, piperacillin). It is important to note that altered gentamicin and tobramycin disposition peculiar to CF precludes application of the standard dosing guidelines widely used in adults without CF. A higher dose administered more frequently is usually required, and peak and trough blood levels must be monitored. Recently, innovations in oral antipseudomonal preparations and outpatient intravenous administration have made home management more effective (Table 213-2) Parenteral antibiotics may be administered at home with significant cost savings, provided adequate nursing and home health care services are available. Additionally, several small clinical trials have demonstrated the safety (low rate of bacterial resistance) and efficacy of aerosolized antibiotics used in chronic, maintenance protocols.

Table 213-2. Antimicrobial protocols in treatment of chronic *Pseudomonas* infections of airways

Route	Agent	Comments
Oral	Ciprofloxacin (500-750 mg q12h)	Not approved for children
Parenteral (home*)	Amikacin (25-50 mg/kg q6-8h)	Peak plasma levels, 15-30 μg/ml
	Gentamicin (6-10 mg/kg q6-8h)	Peak plasma levels, 4-10 μg/ml
Nebulized (outpatient)	Gentamicin (20-80 mg per treatment, bid or tid)	—
Parenteral (hospitalized)	Tobramycin (2.5 mg/kg q8h)	Load, 1.5-2.0 mg/kg; adjust for renal insufficiency
	plus	
	Piperacillin (100-300 mg/kg (maximum 24 g) q4-6h)	Ticarcillin has three times the sodium content

*Accomplished by means of surgically placed Infusaport, PortaCath, or silastic catheter placed at the bedside (Per-Q-Cath).

This route has been used to deliver aminoglycosides, broad-spectrum penicillins, and ceftazidime. This method of administration is controversial but may be used at home and presents another alternative for the treatment of chronic *Pseudomonas* infections of the airways.

Improvement in survival of CF patients largely reflects timely use of newer, more potent antibiotics. Noting the central role *Pseudomonas* plays in the pathogenesis of CF lung disease, many of these new antibiotic protocols are directed at this pathogen. Ciprofloxacin monotherapy (500 to 750 mg two times daily for 14 days) is effective for the acute treatment of CF patients. Ceftazidime is a parenterally administered third-generation cephalosporin that has the best activity against *P. aeruginosa* of all available cephalosporins. Ticarcillin has been combined with clavulanic acid to enhance activity against lactamase-producing bacteria (e.g., *H. influenzae, S. aureus*) frequently found in airways concurrently or antedating *Pseudomonas* infections.

Exercise conditioning programs improve exercise tolerance in normal persons and in adults with non-CF COPD. Similar results have been obtained with adolescents and adults with CF. An exercise program consisting of three 1-hour sessions per week continued for 3 months produces significant increases in exercise tolerance, lowers heart rates at submaximum workloads, and improves respiratory muscle endurance. An added benefit of exercise is that deep breathing facilitates effective clearance of thick respiratory secretions, thereby substituting for more mundane postural drainage. Decreases in oxygen saturations of 5% or greater may occur in those CF patients with forced expiratory volume at 1 second (FEV_1) less than 50% of FVC or with diffusing capacity for carbon monoxide less than 80% of predicted value. These patients should have supervised exercise testing with ear oximetry before undertaking an exercise program.

In an effort to modulate the immune-mediated inflammatory process, a 4-year trial of alternate-day prednisone (2 mg/kg to a maximum of 60 mg/day) has been completed in children with CF who have mild to moderate pulmonary disease. Patients in the prednisone-treated group showed better growth and pulmonary function and reduced morbidity compared with the placebo-treated group. A multicenter trial to evaluate this approach further has recently been completed. Patients were randomized to alternate-day prednisone (2 mg/kg [high dose] or 1 mg/kg [low dose]) or placebo. A high incidence of complications, including an increased frequency of cataracts, growth retardation, and glucose abnormalities, occurred in the high-dose prednisone group after 3 years of study participation. Consequently, the high-dose study treatment was discontinued. It is known that acute daily doses of prednisone (20 to 30 mg/day for 3 weeks) do not significantly increase pulmonary function in those with more advanced disease and may expose these patients to an increased risk of developing a pneumothorax.

Frequently, despite use of antibiotics, exercise, and daily postural drainage, all performed as outpatient procedures, hospitalization is necessary. Nonemergent hospitalization may be warranted because of an insidious downhill clinical course, including cough, dyspnea, anorexia, weight loss, and lack of energy, making daily activities of work or school impossible. Clinical deterioration may be apparent when spirometric values are followed. However, indications for this type of hospitalization and the duration of hospitalization are imprecise.

Massive hemoptysis, a frightening complication of CF lung disease, occurs in up to 8% of adult patients with CF. The bleeding usually arises from the inflamed mucosa overlying the bronchial arterial supply, which is under systemic pressures. Usually, bed rest, antitussives, and treatment of the bacterial infection of the airways with high-dose parenteral antibiotics will be effective treatments. Rarely the profuse bleeding mandates more aggressive treatment; the patient should be provided with an intravenous line and monitored with oximetry during a bronchoscopy procedure intended to localize the site of bleeding. Bronchial angiography, although less successful than bronchoscopy in localizing the site of bleeding, does make arterial embolization possible as an immediate therapeutic option. Embolization can be safely performed only if collaterals to the spinal cord are *not* visualized.

Organ transplantation is an accepted treatment for many causes of organ failure, including CF disease. Many U.S. tertiary care centers have transplantation programs approved for heart-lung transplantation in CF patients. Difficulties still to be overcome include the low number of donor organs and the nature of the chronic infection of the upper and lower respiratory tracts of recipients. Double-lung (without heart) transplantation should help to increase the donor organs available. Twelve-month and 24-month posttransplant survival rates of 58% to 69% have been reported from major transplant centers in North America and England. Additionally, orthotopic liver transplantation is now a therapeutic option in CF patients with biliary cirrhosis.

Prognosis

In developed countries, 20% to 75% of affected individuals reach adult life, the median survival of CF patients is now 28 years, and 25% of patients registered in the 127 U.S. CF centers survive into the third decade. The median life expectancy of children with CF born in 1990 is estimated to be 40 years, double that of 20 years ago. Despite their disability, many CF patients are quite accomplished. In large series of adults with CF, virtually all graduate from high school, many at a time appropriate for their age, and 80% are employed full or part time. Pediatricians continue to treat many CF patients because few internists have had substantial training with CF disease. Adults with CF would benefit greatly from the input of internists experienced with the pharmacokinetics of a wide spectrum of drugs in adults, adult oxygen and nutritional requirements, optimum management of right- and left-sided cardiac failure, and the spectrum of infectious agents causing disease in adults. Mild and atypical cases will go undiagnosed (and untreated) unless internists become aware of the spectrum of the disease and suspect the diagnosis.

BRONCHIECTASIS

Description

Bronchiectasis, abnormal dilatation of bronchial caliber, has been traditionally referred to as *cylindric saccular,* and *varicose*. Although all forms may be seen within a single lobe and present with very similar symptoms, it is important to differentiate cylindric bronchiectasis from the other pathologic subtypes. As discussed later, cylindric bronchiectasis carries a better prognosis. Associated pathologic changes of clinical importance in all forms of bronchiectasis include extensive bronchial and bronchiolar obliterations, which are responsible for the obstruction to flow, and anastomosis of enlarged bronchial arteries with pulmonary arteries, which complicates the episodes of hemoptysis.

Etiologies and clinical presentation

Bronchiectasis is not a single disease entity, and a variety of diseases may cause bronchiectatic lung lesions (see the box on p. 1727). In one third of patients the cause is apparent, usually a severe respiratory infection in childhood (after pertussis, measles, adenovirus). Adenoviruses cause up to 5% of respiratory infections in children, and studies demonstrate that 23% to 27% of those afflicted will develop radiographic bronchiectasis within 10 years. Measles pneumonia produces a profound inflammation of the bronchial wall as well as considerable exudate.

Chronic aspiration in association with pharyngeal or gastrointestinal disorders is also associated with bronchiectatic lung lesions. The intrinsic tone of the lower esophageal sphincter is an important factor contributing to gastroesophageal reflux, and both cigarette and alcohol consumption significantly reduce lower esophageal sphincter pressure. Theophylline also reduces sphincter pressure and simultaneously increases acid secretion. Another gastrointestinal disorder, inflammatory bowel disease, is associated with bronchiectasis, although the mechanism is less clear. This association has not been related to chemotherapeutic agents used in the treatment of ulcerative colitis, and this form of bronchiectasis may be progressive despite colectomy.

Sinusitis is frequently associated with bronchiectasis and should suggest CF, defects in humorally mediated defenses common to the upper and lower respiratory tracts, or the immotile cilia syndrome (Kartagener's syndrome). Patients with common variable hypogammaglobulinemia are particularly prone to chronic infections of the upper and lower respiratory tract leading to bronchiectasis. Deficiencies of IgG subclasses, even though total serum IgG levels may be within normal limits, may predispose individuals to recurrent infections of the airways, leading to bronchiectasis. *Kartagener's syndrome,* described as the triad of bronchiectasis, sinusitis, and situs inversus (Fig. 213-3), is associated with respiratory ciliary abnormalities. The axoneme, which is the central core of the cilium, is altered in the sperm tail as well, resulting in ineffectively beating spermatozoa. Transposition of viscera may be absent in 50% of these patients causing bronchiectasis, sinusitis, and male infertility with recurrent pulmonary infections. This is a presentation that closely resembles CF. It is known that disorganized axonemes and internalized cilia may also be acquired after respiratory infections caused by influenza virus, rhinovirus, myxovirus, or mycoplasma or after inhalation of airway irritants.

Whatever the cause, the principal symptom of bronchiectasis is production of a large amount of purulent sputum. Gross examination of the sputum provides an important clue, since few other disorders (abscess, bronchopleural fistula, bronchoesophageal fistula) produce sputum of this purulence and volume. Daily sputum production of up to 500 ml is not rare, and expectoration is most pronounced in the morning. Clubbing of the digits is found in patients with longstanding bronchiectasis from all causes. Recurrent pneumonias are frequent and caused most often by staphylococci, anaerobic organisms, and *Pseudomonas*. In early bronchiectasis, pulmonary function testing shows an obstructive defect. In severe and extensive involvement, a restrictive ventilatory defect may occur with eventual cor pulmonale. Hemoptysis occurs in nearly half the patients and may be life-threatening.

Diagnosis

Diagnosis of bronchiectasis is occasionally apparent from plain chest radiographs showing cystic spaces ("cluster of grapes"), linear outlines of mucosal edema ("tram tracks," "signet ring"), or dilated bronchi filled with impacted mucus ("finger-glove deformity"). However, the gold standard for the diagnosis of bronchiectasis has been bronchography (see Fig. 213-3), but this method of visualizing the bronchial tree is rapidly being replaced by high-resolution computed tomography (CT) of the chest. CT signs of this lung lesion are (1) air-fluid levels in bronchi; (2) a cluster of cysts; (3) linear, distended peripheral bronchi; and (4) bronchial walls thickened by peribronchial fibrosis (Fig. 213-4). However, CT is most useful for diagnosing saccular bronchiectasis and is less reliable in the identification of varicose and cylindric types.

If pneumonias recur in the same segments, one should investigate the possibility of partial obstruction with localized bronchiectasis caused by anatomic defects in airway

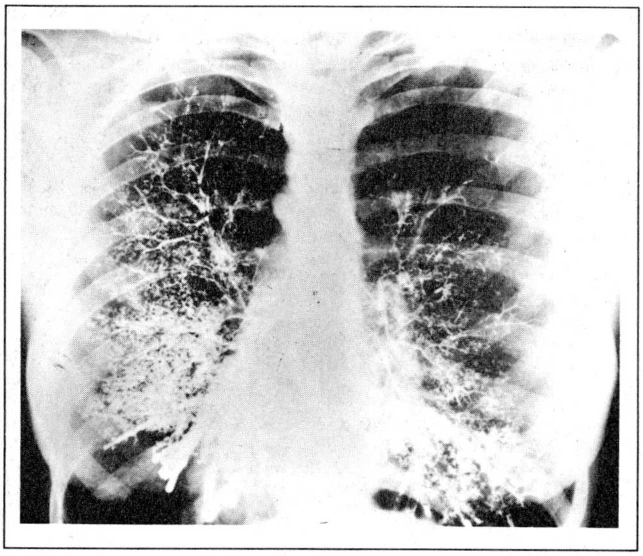

Fig. 213-3. Bronchogram showing extensive bilateral bronchiectasis and dextrocardia in a patient with Kartagener's syndrome.

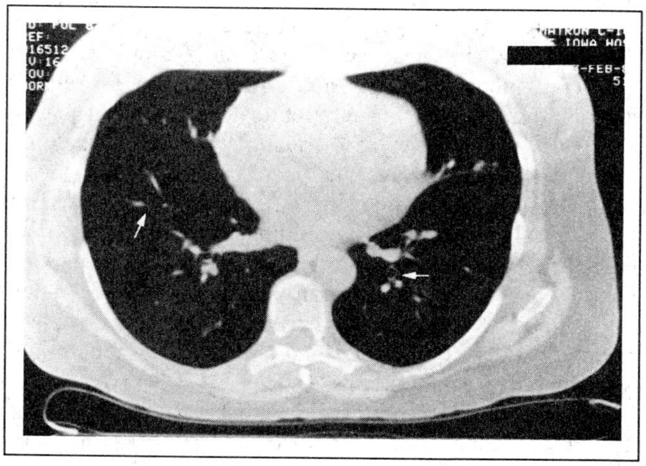

Fig. 213-4. Computed tomographic signs of bronchiectasis shown are a distended linear airway in the periphery with thickened bronchial mucosa *(white arrow, left side),* peribronchial thickening *(white arrow, right side),* and numerous areas of cystic dilatation. Cine CT allows a more thorough evaluation of the lung (3 mm sections), in less time, and with less discomfort to the patient than when conventional CT is employed.

architecture or extrinsic compression. All patients with segmental bronchiectasis should have bronchoscopy to be certain no proximal obstruction exists. In patients with generalized bronchiectasis in combination with sinusitis, CF should be evaluated by determination of sweat chloride; immunoglobulin deficiency diseases should be ruled out with quantitation of serum IgG and IgA levels and, if found to be normal, IgG subclass levels; and immotile cilia syndrome diagnosis may be made by transmission electron microscopic examination of nasal or airway cilia. These specimens must be interpreted by a pathologist experienced with the diagnosis. In Young's syndrome, males tend to be sterile and are recognized by a semen analysis revealing azoospermia in a young male with diffuse bronchiectasis and preserved spermatogenesis. Sweat tests and sperm motility studies are normal in these patients.

Treatment

Using antimicrobial agents and clearing the airway of purulent secretions provide the foundation for effective medical management of most patients with bronchiectasis. Several clinical studies have demonstrated that the bacterial species identified in the culture of an expectorated sputum specimen are representative of the bacteriology obtained from resected lung segments, protected catheter brushes, and percutaneous needle aspirates of these patients' lungs. The selection of antimicrobials should be directed by these culture results and the in vitro sensitivities, although it is well recognized that in vitro sensitivity does not necessarily predict success in clearing the airway of the particular pathogen(s) being treated. All antimicrobial chemotherapeutic agents must be used at high doses because the serum-airway partition coefficient for many classes of antibiotics has reproducibly been shown to be approximately 5:1. That is, the level in airways will be 20% of a simultaneously obtained serum concentration. Therapy should be intermittent, dictated by the quantity and purulence of the sputum produced and the presence of systemic symptoms, rather than continuously administered. Additionally, no reliable data address the issue of duration of therapy, but it is generally 14 days. The value of quantitative sputum cultures in many clinical settings has been argued but may be of value in following both response to therapy and confirming the clinical impression of worsening in patients with bronchiectasis. The greatly distorted airways of these patients continuously harbor bacteria and infrequently yield a sterile sputum culture. In these patients, severity of disease is closely associated with the bacterial burden, as determined by quantitative sputum cultures.

Postural drainage performed with chest percussion and gravity positioning must be performed in the morning on arising, and a daily exercise routine with deep breathing is an effective substitute for the afternoon session of chest percussion. Theophylline has been shown to increase mucociliary clearance in other patients, and hand-held nebulizers may increase the effectiveness of these pulmonary clean-out procedures. The use of expectorants and mucolytics taken orally or by inhalation is regaining popularity, and adequate water intake is important to avoid further inspiration. Bronchoscopy with suctioning and lavage of the airways may rarely be useful for the occasional patient with acute lobar collapse and deterioration in respiratory status.

Surgical treatment is reserved for a few specific indications. Under no circumstances should resectional surgery be undertaken without complete mapping of the bronchial tree. Localized cylindric bronchiectasis may respond to aggressive medical management, and accordingly, surgery in such patients should be delayed 4 to 6 weeks. Surgery is indicated for patients with localized bronchiectasis in whom either hemorrhage or infection causes frequent hospitalizations or great disability.

REFERENCES

Anderson MP et al: Demonstration that CFTR is a chloride channel by alteration of its anion selectivity. Science 253:202, 1991.

Beaudet AL and Buffone GJ: Prenatal diagnosis of cystic fibrosis. J Pediatr 111:630, 1987.

Bolman RM and Wolfe WG: Bronchiectasis and bronchopulmonary sequestration. Surg Clin North Am 60:867, 1980.

Donati MA, Guenette G, and Auerbach H: Prospective controlled study of home and hospital therapy of cystic fibrosis pulmonary disease. J Pediatr 111:28, 1987.

Fernald GW and Boat TF: Cystic fibrosis: overview. Semin Roentgenol 22:87, 1987.

Fick RB and Stillwell PC: Controversies in the management of pulmonary disease due to cystic fibrosis. Chest 95:1319, 1989.

Gilligan PH: Microbiology of airway disease in patients with cystic fibrosis. Clin Microbiol Rev 4:35, 1991.

Hata JS and Fick RB: The *Pseudomonas* lung lesion in cystic fibrosis airways. In Fick RB, editor: Clinics in chest medicine: inflammatory disorders of the airways. Philadelphia, 1988, Saunders.

Higenbottom T et al: Bronchial disease in ulcerative colitis. Thorax 35:581, 1980.

Hunt B and Geddes DM: Newly diagnosed cystic fibrosis in middle and later life. Thorax 40:23, 1985.

Mearns MB: Cystic fibrosis. Arch Dis Child 60:270, 1985.

Penkath AR et al: Cystic fibrosis in adolescents and adults. Thorax 42:526, 1987.

Rommens JM et al: Identification of the cystic fibrosis gene: chromosome walking and jumping. Science 245:1059, 1989.

Rossman CM et al: Immotile cilia syndrome in persons with and without Kartagener's syndrome. Am Rev Respir Dis 121:1011, 1980.

Tablan OC et al: Colonization of the respiratory tract by *Pseudomonas cepacia* in cystic fibrosis: risk factors and outcomes. Chest 91:527, 1987.

Tizzano EF and Buchwald M: Cystic fibrosis: beyond the gene to therapy. J Pediatr 120:337, 1992.

Tsui LC and Buchwald M: Biochemical and molecular genetics of cystic fibrosis. In Harris H and Hirschhorn K, editors: Advances in human genetics. New York, 1991, Plenum.

CHAPTER

214 Neoplasms of the Lung

Michael C. Iannuzzi
Galen B. Toews

At the turn of the twentieth century, lung cancer was a medical curiosity. Today, it is the leading cause of cancer death worldwide. In the United States, lung cancer accounts for more than 140,000 deaths each year, at an annual health care cost of more than $10 billion. Lung cancer has also grown as a major health care problem in women and surpasses breast cancer as the leading cause of female cancer deaths; the ratio of men to women affected is now 2:1, whereas only 1 decade ago it was 5:1.

The diagnosis of lung cancer is generally not difficult. Management focuses on two questions: Is the tumor resectable? and What therapy is suitable to the patient's cardiopulmonary status? Treatment may then be directed at either potential cure or palliation, although cure is largely limited to patients with non–small cell carcinoma resected at an early stage. Despite the progress made in understanding and treating lung cancer, the overall 5-year survival for patients remains about 12%. This dismal fact is particularly disturbing when one recognizes that lung cancer is a preventable disease.

ETIOLOGY AND PATHOGENESIS

The most important etiologic factor in lung cancer is cigarette smoke. Cigarette smoke contains many carcinogens, but the specific components causing lung cancer are not known. Several environmental and occupational exposures also increase the risk of lung cancer (see the box at upper right), and several act synergistically with cigarette smoke. For example, asbestos exposure and radon particle exposure in uranium mining both produce an 8-fold to 10-fold increased risk of developing lung cancer. However, a 50-fold to 60-fold greater risk exists for uranium miners who smoke than for those who do not, and an 80-fold to 90-fold increase exists for smokers previously exposed to asbestos.

Risk factors for lung cancer

A. Cigarette smoke
B. Carcinogens: radon particles—uranium mining
C. Cocarcinogens
   1. Arsenic—smelter, glass, and pesticide workers
   2. Asbestos—insulation workers, textile workers, asbestos users
   3. Coal dust—road workers, coke oven workers, roofers
   4. Chromium—leather, ceramic, and metal workers; tanners
   5. Chlormethyl methyl ether—chemical plant workers
   6. Vinyl chloride—plastic workers
D. Pulmonary fibrosis
   1. Scleroderma
   2. Interstitial pulmonary fibrosis
   3. Pneumoconiosis
   4. Bronchiectasis
   5. Scars secondary to infarcts
   6. Mycobacterial disease
   7. Lung abscess

Genetic predisposition

Differences in genetically controlled processes, such as deoxyribonucleic acid (DNA) repair mechanisms, cellular mitotic control, protease activity, immunocompetence, and metabolic enzymes, are likely reasons why not all individuals who smoke develop lung cancer. The best defined of these genetic factors are the enzymes responsible for the metabolism of carcinogenic substances.

The metabolites of environmental carcinogens rather than the parent compounds appear to initiate malignant transformation. In much the same way that inherited variability exists in drug metabolism, such as fast and slow acetylators of isoniazid (INH), inherited variability also exists in the metabolism or activation of procarcinogenic chemicals to active carcinogens. Among the most important components in carcinogenic metabolism is the family of enzymes, the cytochrome P-450 hydroxylases, and the most extensively studied enzyme in this family is aryl hydrocarbon hydroxylase (AHH). AHH is responsible for the activation of polycyclic aromatic hydrocarbon (PAH) (aromatic hydrocarbons are benzenelike, unsaturated, six-membered carbon rings), a major component of cigarette smoke, to its carcinogenic form. In humans, three degrees of AHH inducibility exist: low, intermediate, and high. Although not all studies agree, several have found that patients with lung carcinoma have a tendency to show intermediate to high inducibility. To clarify the role of carcinogenic metabolism in lung cancer, several groups are examining the DNA sequence of the genes coding for the P-450 gene enzymes. So far more than 40 of the genes encoding these enzymes have been cloned and sequenced.

Besides the P-450 enzymes, certain inherited cancer genes appear to predispose patients to lung cancer. For example, abnormalities in a tumor suppressor gene, the retinoblastoma susceptibility gene, has been found in small cell lung cancer (SCLC). Studies of more than 4000 relatives of patients with retinoblastoma revealed a 15-fold increased risk of lung cancer. Another tumor suppressor gene, P53, as well as other oncogenes, such as *K-ras,* may also be important (Chapter 71).

PATHOLOGY

The histologic classification of primary lung cancer recommended by the World Health Organization is listed in the box on p. 1734. Four histologic types of lung cancer make up 95% of all primary lung neoplasia: squamous cell car-

World Health Organization (WHO) classification of malignant neoplasms

Squamous (epidermoid) carcinoma
Small cell carcinoma
Adenocarcinoma
Large cell carcinoma
Combined cell types
Carcinoid tumors
Bronchial gland tumors
  Cylindromas
  Mucoepidermoid
Papillary tumors

cinoma (30%), adenocarcinoma (25%), small cell (20%), and anaplastic large cell (10% to 15%). It is important to distinguish the cell types because of differences in their natural history and response to treatment. The following is a brief review of the characteristic histologic and pathologic features of the lung cancer cell types.

Squamous cell, or *epidermoid, carcinoma* is the most prevalent lung carcinoma and arises from the central bronchi in about 80% of patients. On light microscopy the neoplastic cells appear flattened to polygonal, tend to stratify, and form intercellular bridges. The presence of keratin "pearls" indicates good to moderate differentiation. Squamous cell lung cancer constitutes more than half the superior sulcus tumors (Pancoast tumors) and is the most common tumor to cavitate. Cavities are generally thick walled and usually without air-fluid levels and portend a poor prognosis. Squamous carcinoma tends to metastasize late. Lymph nodes, adrenal gland, and liver are the favored sites of metastases; bone metastases are lytic and infrequent.

Small cell carcinoma (SCLC) is distinguished by a proliferation of cells with dark, round to oval nuclei that measure more than twice the size of a lymphocyte. These cells have meager cytoplasm in relation to their nuclei, so molding (indentation of one nucleus pressed by another) of adjacent cells occurs, with arrangement of the cells in ribbons, nests, and sheets. The meager cytoplasm is also thought to be responsible for frequently finding "crushing" on biopsy. As with squamous cell carcinoma, SCLC tends to be a central lesion. SCLC is characterized by rapid development, frequent metastases, and low resectability. At presentation, more than 80% of patients have symptoms for less than 3 months. This is in contrast to patients with squamous cell lung carcinoma, in whom symptom duration averages as long as 8 months, and to those with adenocarcinoma, nearly 25% of whom are asymptomatic at presentation. At the time of diagnosis, more than 70% of patients with SCLC have widely metastatic disease.

Adenocarcinoma forms acinar and glandular structures with or without mucin formation. Although squamous and small cell carcinomas are the cell types most closely associated with cigarette smoking, adenocarcinoma has been linked to pulmonary fibrosis and may arise in areas of previous scars in the lung. Unlike squamous cell and small cell carcinoma, most adenocarcinomas occur in the periphery of the lung. The metastatic pattern of adenocarcinoma is not much different from that of small cell carcinoma. Distant metastases occur early and frequently. Bone metastases are frequently blastic.

Bronchiloalveolar carcinoma (BAC) is a variant of adenocarcinoma that constitutes about 5% of all lung carcinomas. BAC is a peripheral, well-differentiated neoplasm that tends to spread locally throughout the air spaces. Because it may be difficult to distinguish BAC from metastatic adenocarcinoma, other supporting criteria that aid diagnosis include the absence of a primary endobronchial carcinoma and the absence of other organ involvement. The cell of origin for this tumor has been controversial. Potential cells of origin are the mucin-secreting bronchial epithelial cells, nonciliated secretory bronchiolar cells, and type 2 alveolar epithelial cells. Other unusual features of this neoplasm include a more common occurrence in women, who account for 30% to 50% of all cases; a chest radiograph that may demonstrate multinodular lesions, which indicate multicentric origin or diffuse fluffy infiltrates; and the least association with tobacco smoke.

Large cell carcinoma is an anaplastic tumor without light microscopic evidence of glandular or squamous differentiation. The cells are large, bizarre, pleomorphic, multinucleated, and round or spindle shaped. Large cell carcinoma generally arises in the lung periphery, is often necrotic and quite large. Large cell carcinoma may invade locally or metastasize widely.

Any combination of the four main cell types may occur. Adenosquamous carcinoma, which is the most common (1% to 2%), tends to occur more peripherally than does squamous cell carcinoma.

MOLECULAR BIOLOGY

The importance of cytogenetic abnormalities and the role of oncogenes in lung cancer are presently being defined. A consistent chromosomal abnormality has been described in SCLC, namely, a deletion in the short arm of chromosome 3. What role the loss of the chromosome 3 segment plays in the malignant process in SCLC is not yet known. One hypothesis is that a gene or gene family in the deleted DNA segment codes for some factor that suppresses a growth-regulating gene or group of genes elsewhere in the genome. This is analogous to mechanisms proposed in the childhood cancers, retinoblastoma and Wilms' tumor. Multiple chromosomal abnormalities have been seen in non-SCLC; however, a specific recurring chromosome defect has not been noted.

Various growth factors secreted by malignant cells in culture have been identified. Some of these growth factors and their receptors are encoded by oncogenes. The endogenous production of growth factors, called *autocrine secretion,* appears to free the cell from external physiologic controls that normally inhibit growth and thus serve as a constant stimulus for cell division. Bombesin, a tetradecapeptide initially isolated from amphibian skin, is one example of an autocrine growth factor for SCLC cells. Monoclonal antibodies to bombesin as well as to other growth factors and their receptors are being studied for potential therapy in lung cancer.

Members of two families of oncogenes, *myc* and *ras*, appear to be important in the development of lung cancer. The *myc* family of oncogenes code for nuclear proteins, and the *ras* gene family code for proteins that bind guanine nucleotides (G proteins) involved in growth-signal transduction. Members of the *myc* family of proto-oncogenes (*c-myc, L-myc,* and *N-myc*) are frequently amplified and overexpressed in SCLC and have been associated with more aggressive and drug-resistant tumors. The *ras* oncogene has been found to be activated in some adenocarcinoma specimens, but the significance of this is yet to be defined. The importance of oncogenes in cancer is discussed further in Chapters 71 and 101.

CLINICAL PRESENTATION

More than 75% of lung cancer patients are affected in their fifth to sixth decade. Lung cancer rarely occurs in persons under 35 years. The initial signs and symptoms (see the box on right) are variable and depend on the location of the tumor, the cell type, rapidity of growth, whether metastasis has occurred, the ectopic production of peptides and hormones, and the presence of underlying pulmonary disease. Systemic symptoms are common and include weight loss and malaise. In a small percentage of patients (5% to 15%), lung cancer is detected before the onset of symptoms, usually by routine chest radiography. The following are the common signs and symptoms of lung cancer:

Cough is the most frequent initial symptom of lung cancer, but since it is a common symptom in many chronic respiratory disorders, it is often overlooked. Cough may be produced by an endobronchial mass acting as a foreign body or by invasion and ulceration of the bronchial mucosa. Patients who have a persistent cough, particularly if they are 40 years or over, should have a chest radiograph. The production of sputum along with cough is of diagnostic value in that it provides material for cytologic examination.

Hemoptysis occurs in about 35% to 45% of patients with bronchogenic carcinoma and may vary from blood-streaked sputum to more significant amounts. Massive hemoptysis in lung cancer patients occurs infrequently. Of all patients with hemoptysis, lung cancer is responsible in about 20%. The absence of roentgenologic abnormalities should not discourage the clinician from ruling out an underlying malignancy, since the cancer may erode the bronchial wall and vessels early, before becoming apparent radiographically.

Chest pain is most frequently described as a dull, intermittent ache, lasting minutes to hours and usually ipsilateral to the tumor. Chest pain may also be severe, constant, penetrating, and pleuritic, indicating metastatic involvement of the pleura. Shoulder and arm pain that is constant may be caused either by a superior sulcus (Pancoast's) tumor or by tumor invading the diaphragm. Other signs of superior sulcus tumors include weakness of the hand and Horner's syndrome. Horner's syndrome, the result of involvement of the sixth cervical segments, consists of a drooping upper eyelid, constricted pupil, and narrowed palpebral fissure.

Clinical presentation and signs and symptoms of lung cancer

Local tumor growth

Cough
Dyspnea
Hemoptysis
Wheezing
Pneumonia
Fever

Local extension

Chest pain
Hoarseness
Dysphagia
Superior vena cava obstruction
Pancoast's syndrome
Horner's syndrome

Metastasis

Bone pain
Headache
Abdominal pain
Pericardial effusion
Lymphadenopathy
Hepatomegaly
Pleural effusion

Paraneoplastic syndromes

Cushing's syndrome
Hypercalcemia
Hypertrophic osteoarthropathy and clubbing
Syndrome of inappropriate antidiuretic hormone (SIADH)
Neuromyopathies
Eaton-Lambert syndrome
Trousseau's syndrome (venous thrombosis)

Hoarseness because of left vocal cord paralysis from carcinoma or nodal metastases involving the left hilum or aortic arch is common. The long, tortuous intrathoracic course of the left recurrent laryngeal nerve makes it more susceptible to tumor involvement than its counterpart on the right.

Wheezing, if unilateral and present in certain body positions, suggests partial bronchial obstruction. A localized wheeze may be heard in the absence of chest roentgenologic abnormalities.

Superior vena cava syndrome is most frequently caused by lung cancer (75% to 80%). The clinical manifestations vary with how quickly obstruction develops. Patients may complain of headache, a feeling of fullness in the head, visual difficulties, dyspnea, cough, dysphagia, or syncope. Physical findings include dilated neck veins, conjunctival edema, plethora and edema of the face and neck, swelling of the arms, and distended veins over the chest. Diagnosis may be confirmed by venogram or contrast-enhanced computed tomography (CT) of the chest. Recent studies have emphasized the relative safety in pursuing a definitive diagnosis rather than initiating emergency empiric treatment. If signs and symptoms are mild and chronic and no evidence exists of increased intracranial pressure, histologic diagnosis may be obtained safely by sputum cytology, fiberoptic bronchoscopy, or mediastinoscopy before treatment.

Pleural involvement with effusion may result in dyspnea (60%) and cough (40%). Lung cancer is the most common cause of malignant pleural effusion, followed by breast cancer and lymphoma. The effusion in lung cancer is most often ipsilateral to the tumor mass, exudative (a ratio of pleural fluid protein to serum > 0.5, lactate dehydrogenase in pleural fluid to serum ratio > 0.6), and frequently hemorrhagic. A low pleural fluid pH (< 7.3) correlates with a greater diagnostic yield on cytology, a worse prognosis, and a poorer response to pleurodesis. Since direct pleural involvement is a contraindication to curative surgery, other mechanisms that may cause pleural effusion in patients with lung cancer should be kept in mind. These other mechanisms include mediastinal lymph node involvement with impaired lymphatic drainage, disruption of the thoracic duct with chylothorax formation, bronchial obstruction with atelectasis or postobstructive pneumonia, and pulmonary embolism.

Cardiac involvement is noted at autopsy in 20% to 25% of patients with SCLC and less frequently with non-SCLC. Patients may complain of dyspnea, which is often mistakenly attributed to coexistent pleural effusion. Other signs of cardiac involvement include atrial arrhythmias, hypotension, pericardial friction rub, pulsus paradoxus, and if cardiac tamponade develops, Kussmaul's sign (increase in jugular venous pressure on inspiration).

THE PARANEOPLASTIC SYNDROMES

Paraneoplastic syndromes are metabolic and neuromuscular disturbances unrelated to the primary tumor, metastasis, or effects of therapy. They are diverse and occur with all the lung cancer cell types, although they are seen most frequently with SCLC. The most common syndromes are the syndrome of inappropriate antidiuretic hormone (ADH) secretion (SIADH), Cushing's syndrome from ectopic adrenocorticotropic hormone (ACTH) production, hypercalcemia, hypertrophic osteoarthropathy, neuromyopathies, and Eaton-Lambert syndrome.

SIADH is caused by neoplasms in more than 50% of patients. SCLC accounts for the vast majority of these neoplasms. SIADH results from the persistent and excessive release of ADH (arginine vasopressin) and is characterized by hyponatremia, volume expansion without edema, renal sodium loss, hypouricemia, and inappropriately high urine osmolarity. SIADH is diagnosed by first excluding hypovolemia and by determining that thyroid and adrenal function are normal. A normal to decreased serum blood urea nitrogen (BUN) and creatinine levels, a urinary sodium concentration that exceeds 30 mEq/L, and a fractional excretion of sodium (FENa) greater than 1% indicate the patient is euvolemic or slightly volume expanded. The inappropriate secretion of ADH in this clinical setting is then recognized by a urine osmolality greater than 120 to 150 mOsm/kg of water in association with a reduced serum osmolality. Treatment of SIADH is aimed at correcting the body water osmolality by first restricting water intake to 600 to 800 ml/day. Alternatively, agents such as lithium or demethylchlortetracycline, which antagonize the renal tubular effect of ADH, may be used.

Cushing's syndrome resulting from ectopic ACTH production may be subtle. Hypokalemic metabolic alkalosis and muscle weakness are usually the predominant manifestations, although glucose intolerance, mild hypertension, hyperpigmentation, and hirsutism may also occur. Physical changes such as moon facies, buffalo hump, and striae occur infrequently, perhaps because of the relatively short survival of these patients. SCLC is the cell type most frequently associated with Cushing's syndrome. Ectopic ACTH levels are very high and not suppressible by high doses of dexamethasone.

Hypercalcemia is a common finding in patients with lung cancer (overall frequency, 12.5%) and varies with the histologic type (25% with squamous, 13% with large cell, and 3% with adenocarcinoma). Hypercalcemia is not associated with SCLC, and if found, another etiology should be sought, such as hyperparathyroidism. The cause of hypercalcemia in solid tumors remains controversial but appears to be primarily mediated by hormonal and/or metabolic mechanisms rather than a direct effect of bone metastasis. In fact, more than half of hypercalcemic patients do not have bone metastases. Furthermore, although bone metastases are frequent in SCLC (66%) and adenocarcinoma (50%), hypercalcemia is infrequent. The clinical features of hypercalcemia include lethargy, psychiatric disturbances, anorexia, nausea, vomiting, abdominal discomfort, constipation, polyuria, thirst, and renal insufficiency.

Hypertrophic osteoarthropathy is characterized by the presence of periosteal new bone formation, arthritis, and clubbing of the digits. Hypertrophic osteoarthropathy (HOA) occurs in up to 30% of patients with lung cancer, although it is rare in those with SCLC. The symptoms are nonspecific and include joint pain, soft tissue swelling, and limitation of motion. HOA may proceed the diagnosis of lung cancer in up to one third of patients, and symptoms are usually relieved by removal of the primary tumor.

Neuromyopathies may occur in association with lung cancer and include encephalopathy, myelopathy, sensory and mixed sensorimotor neuropathies, and polymyositis. Autoimmune, infectious, nutritional, and toxic causes have all been suggested.

Eaton-Lambert syndrome, or myasthenic syndrome, is closely associated with SCLC and may precede the appearance of the tumor by more than a year. Patients generally have easy fatigability and proximal muscle weakness, predominantly in the pelvic girdle and lower extremities. Patients show weakness on first attempts at muscle contraction, but unlike those with myasthenia gravis, repeated efforts increase their muscle strength. Other associated symptoms include dry mouth, muscle discomfort, impotence, and paresthesias. Electromyograms show a pathognomonic increase in amplitude on repetitive stimulation. Successful treatment of the tumor is often associated with relief from the Eaton-Lambert syndrome. Guanidine hydrochloride and plasmapheresis may be beneficial.

NERVOUS SYSTEM METASTASES

Nervous system metastases are a major cause of morbidity and mortality in patients with lung cancer and may be the sole metastatic site. The incidence of brain metastases by histologic type of lung cancer is listed in the box below. For SCLC, the risk increases as survival is prolonged, so brain metastasis occurs in 80% of patients living for more than 2 years after diagnosis. The signs and symptoms are not different from those in patients with other metastatic tumors. Symptoms may have an abrupt onset and include headache, change in mental status, ataxia, focal weakness, and aphasia. Leptomeningeal metastases most frequently occur in SCLC and present with involvement of multiple areas of the neuraxis. Symptoms include headache, cranial nerve palsies, and altered mental status. Lung cancer is also the most common tumor to metastasize to the spine and accounts for up to 30% of these patients. Pain occurs in more than 90% of patients with spinal cord compression, and the onset of pain usually precedes the development of weakness, sensory changes, and autonomic dysfunction by days or weeks. However, once these later symptoms and signs develop, the course is rapid, and the chances for reversing the neurologic changes with treatment greatly diminishes.

DIAGNOSIS AND STAGING

The goal of diagnosis and staging is to answer the following questions: What is the histologic type? Is the tumor resectable? and Is the patient physically able to withstand treatment? This process begins with a thorough history, physical examination, and chest radiograph. The signs and symptoms of lung cancer are discussed earlier. The following is a discussion of the radiographic signs of lung cancer and the techniques used for diagnosis and staging.

The earliest radiographic signs of lung cancer are often overlooked. As many as 90% of peripheral cancers and 75% of central tumors have been reported to be visible in retrospect on prior radiographs. These early signs include enlargement of one hilum, a small homogeneous density with sharp or poorly defined borders, a streaked infiltrate, and signs of volume loss (e.g., atelectasis, displacement of fissure). Other radiographic findings of lung cancer include solitary pulmonary nodule, rounded peripheral mass, cavitary lesion, and pneumonia. A recurrent, persistent, or incompletely resolved infiltrate also suggests malignancy. Lack of air bronchograms in an opacified segment of lung should direct attention to the central bronchi in search of an endobronchial lesion. Volume loss in a consolidated lobe or a large pleural effusion with ipsilateral volume loss suggests bronchial obstruction and should raise suspicion of malignancy.

Incidence of brain metastases in lung cancer

Squamous cell: 15%
Adenocarcinoma: 25%
Large cell: 28%
Small cell: 30%

CT has added to the diagnosis and staging of lung cancer. CT can confirm the presence of a lung mass that was suspected from chest radiograph, define its extent, determine the presence of additional lung lesions, and demonstrate the location of enlarged mediastinal and hilar lymph nodes. The precise indications for CT, however, are debated. To some extent, this debate results from thoracic surgeons' different opinions regarding therapy. For example, in a recent survey, about half of thoracic surgeons believed the presence of tumor in mediastinal nodes (N2 disease) contraindicated resection of the primary tumor.

Sputum cytology, bronchoscopy, and percutaneous needle biopsy are the most common tests used to obtain histologic diagnosis. Sputum cytology is a very useful, noninvasive test that is effective when at least three consecutive specimens are obtained and read by an experienced cytologist. The yield is 30% in the absence of symptoms, 50% when cough is present, and 70% when hemoptysis is present. Respiratory therapists or physiotherapists can frequently help to obtain satisfactory material for sputum examination by using techniques to induce sputum production, such as percussion and inhalation of aerosolized saline solutions. The yield of sputum cytology is also influenced by the histologic type and is most often positive with squamous cell carcinoma and least likely with SCLC. This occurs because squamous cell carcinoma grows as a fungating endobronchial mass, whereas SCLC grows as a submucosal plaque.

Fiberoptic bronchoscopy has proved very useful in the diagnosis of lung cancer. Combining bronchial brushing and biopsy gives a yield of 85% to 95% for bronchoscopically visible lesions. For peripheral masses that are not visible through the bronchoscope, transbronchial biopsy under fluoroscopic guidance is used. The yield with this procedure is a function of tumor size: about 30% for masses less than 2 cm and 65% to 70% for those larger than 2 cm. Thin-needle aspiration via a transtracheal or transbronchial approach has extended the role of bronchoscopy. This method is useful for identifying subcarinal, paratracheal, and parabronchial nodal disease and for aspirating peripheral nodules.

Percutaneous fine-needle aspiration (FNA) may be used to obtain material for cytologic examination, particularly for those lesions not readily accessible by flexible fiberoptic bronchoscopy, such as small peripheral nodules. The incidence of pneumothorax requiring chest tube placement is higher with percutaneous FNA than with bronchoscopic biopsy.

When pleural effusion is detected radiographically, thoracentesis may allow diagnosis. As noted earlier, pleural effusions may arise because of direct pleural invasion by a cancer, metastatic involvement, postobstruction pneumonitis, central lymphatic obstruction, or pulmonary embolism. A positive cytologic diagnosis can be made from pleural fluid in 40% to 75% of patients. If cytologic examination of the pleural effusion is negative, the diagnostic yield of thoracentesis may be increased by repeating it with pleural biopsy. The pleural fluid obtained on repeat thoracentesis often contains freshly denuded cells, which aids cytologic diagnosis. It should be noted that pleural biopsy alone further increases the diagnostic yield by only about 5%.

Routine biopsy of nonpalpable scalene or supraclavicular nodes produces a very low diagnostic yield and is not recommended. However, with palpable supraclavicular nodes, the yield for detection of metastasis is about 90%. The information gained can be valuable for both diagnosis and staging.

A variety of enzyme and hormone tumor products have been investigated as tumor markers. If sensitive and specific tumor markers could be found, they would be useful in screening high-risk populations, diagnosis, staging, prognostication, and monitoring of therapy. At present, tumor markers helpful in the diagnosis of lung cancer do not exist.

Staging guides the physician in assessing prognosis, designing treatment, and comparing treatment protocols between studies and study groups. The approach to staging lung cancer depends on the cell type. In patients with non-SCLC the TNM system (tumor, nodal involvement, metastases), which emphasizes the extent of tumor involvement of surrounding structures, is applied. Stages I and II disease are considered operable and stage III disease, in general, inoperable. However, some patients with stage III disease, because of their young age, cardiopulmonary status, and anatomic location of tumor, may be considered for resection. A reciprocal correlation exists between the anatomic extent of the primary tumor and survivability. In non-SCLC, for $T_1N_0M_0$, patients with all three cell types (squamous, adenocarcinoma, large cell) have a 60% to 80% 5-year survival. For $T_2N_0M_0$, 50% of patients with squamous carcinoma and 40% with adenocarcinoma or large cell survive 5 years. Survival dramatically decreases with nodal involvement and with metastasis: 20% to 40% for stage IIa disease and less than 20% for stage IIIb.

The TNM system is not useful in patients with SCLC, primarily because more than 85% of patients have stage III disease at presentation. For SCLC, a simple two-stage classification is used; patients are classified as having either limited or extensive disease. Limited disease is defined as disease confined to one hemithorax and the mediastinum with or without supraclavicular lymph nodes. The limited-stage group also includes patients with pleural effusions and contralateral hilar and contralateral supraclavicular lymph nodes. The presence of any one or all of these findings does not appear to alter prognosis. Extensive disease is defined as any disease more advanced than limited. Staging and therapy of lung cancer is discussed in detail in Chapter 101.

SCREENING

Once the diagnosis of lung cancer has been made, a staging evaluation eliminates 85% to 90% of patients from curative resection. Because early detection is necessary for cures, several studies have evaluated the role of screening populations at high risk for lung cancer. These studies have examined the role of chest radiographs every 6 months, and chest radiographs combined with sputum cytology have demonstrated that aggressive use of these screening tests can lead to the early detection of limited-stage cancer in a high-risk population. There is no proof, however, that screening decreases overall mortality compared with unscreened groups. Therefore, at this time, insufficient proved benefit exists to recommend intensive mass screening of all high-risk individuals, and screening should be left to those high-risk patients who can be reliably followed by their personal physician.

TREATMENT

Treatment is based on the cell type, stage of disease, and the patient's general condition. The individual roles of chemotherapy, surgery, radiation therapy, and immunotherapy are discussed in Chapter 101. Surgical removal of the tumor is the preferred therapy for patients with non-SCLC. Unfortunately, staging evaluation eliminates 85% to 90% of patients from curative resection. All potentially operable patients should be thoroughly evaluated to determine their ability to undergo lung resection. Despite numerous studies, no firm guidelines are available for criteria that prohibit resectional surgery.

Prior history of cardiac disease doubles the risk of major operative morbidity (20% versus 10%), and pulmonary function may be further compromised by removal of pulmonary tissue. Therefore the preoperative evaluation for any patient in whom surgery is contemplated includes a thorough evaluation of the cardiac and respiratory systems. The box at upper right lists a general approach for determining surgical risk based on clinical assessment, lung spirometry, and arterial blood gas determinations. For patients with marginal lung function, further studies may be necessary. Exercise physiology studies help further define the significance of mildly abnormal arterial blood gases. Ventilation-perfusion scanning may aid in determining the effect of surgical resection on lung function and can be used to help predict the postoperative forced expiratory volume in 1 second (FEV_1).

For patients with unresectable primary lung carcinoma or who are unable to withstand surgery, radiation therapy can achieve complete local control of primary tumor in up to 75% of patients resulting in prolonged survival. Radiation therapy may also be useful as adjuvant therapy together with chemotherapy for SCLC and, along with surgery, for non-SCLC. Radiation therapy is useful for producing symptomatic relief in superior vena cava obstruction and superior sulcus tumors, pain control, neurologic complications such as brain metastases and spinal cord compression, pericardial effusion, and hemoptysis.

Candidates for surgery who have lung cancer

Should probably not undergo resection
Elevated carbon dioxide tension
Dyspnea at rest
Predicted postoperative $FEV_1 < 0.8$ L
Pulmonary hypertension
Cor pulmonale

Should undergo further pulmonary evaluation
Hypoxia
Moderate dyspnea on exertion
Predicted postoperative FEV_1 of 0.8 to 1.2 L
Heart disease

Eligible for resection
Normal arterial blood gases
Good exercise tolerance
$FEV_1 > 50\%$ of predicted value

FEV_1, Forced expiratory volume in 1 second.

Endobronchial obstruction

A common problem during the course of lung cancer is endobronchial obstruction with postobstructive pneumonitis. Radiation therapy is often helpful in relieving obstruction and is generally used for the first occurrence of obstruction. Frequently, endobronchial obstruction is caused by recurrence of neoplasia in an area that had been previously irradiated. Surgical resection is usually contraindicated in these patients because of extent of tumor or poor pulmonary function, and further radiation therapy may not be possible. The development of laser treatment via the bronchoscope has allowed for a new approach to this problem. Endobronchial tumors respond quickly to laser therapy and patients can experience relief of obstruction. The potential complications, however, are serious and include bleeding, perforation, and fistula formation. This procedure is also limited by the rapid recurrence of the tumor. Despite these complications and limitations, it is possible to palliate patients who have failed other therapies and have significant difficulties, particularly dyspnea, because of obstructing tumors.

PREVENTION

The greatest impact on the prevention of lung cancer can be made by helping patients who smoke to quit; after cessation of smoking for 10 to 15 years, the risk for lung cancer decreases to near that of nonsmokers. Tobacco dependence is best conceptualized as a chronic disease that requires that the patient be informed of the medical risks of continued smoking as well as the medical benefits that can be expected from stopping. A treatment plan should be designed according to the individual's needs and may include medication, a self-help manual, behavior modification, and support groups. Several studies have recently shown that nicotine substitution, such as by transdermal nicotine patches, can facilitate tobacco withdrawal by alleviating or even preventing abstinence symptoms.

UNCOMMON "BENIGN" NEOPLASIA

Several uncommon and rare neoplasms may arise in the lung (see the box below). These tumors arise from the epithelium or mesenchyme of lung tissue. Although many appear benign histologically, many are potentially malignant. The radiologic and clinical manifestations depend on the relationship of the neoplasm to the airway. Thus obstructive or nonobstructive findings and symptoms may exist.

Bronchial adenoma

The bronchial adenomas make up about 1% of all primary lung neoplasms. Three histologic types exist: the carcinoid adenoma, mucoepidermoid bronchial tumor, and cylindroma or adenoid cystic carcinoma. Carcinoid adenoma occurs most frequently and constitutes more than 80% of the adenomas. The bronchial adenomas were once classified as benign but are now known to be locally invasive and typically metastasize to regional lymph nodes. Most tumors occur in the mainstem bronchi or in the proximal portion of lobar bronchi, although peripheral bronchial adenomas may occur. Patients have intermittent cough, hemoptysis, and postobstructive pneumonia. The most frequent physical finding is localized dullness with decreased or absent breaths sounds and decreased fremitus caused by bronchial obstruction. A chest radiograph confirms the physical findings, demonstrating volume loss and consolidated lung parenchyma. This is similar to obstructing bronchogenic carcinoma.

Bronchial carcinoid is believed to arise from Kulchitzky's, or K cells of the lung. K cells are also thought to be the cell of origin for SCLC. These cells have amine precursor uptake and decarboxylation (APUD) properties. Bronchial carcinoid infrequently causes the carcinoid syndrome, but when it does, the symptoms are similar to those of intestinal carcinoid. Unlike intestinal carcinoid tumors,

Uncommon "benign" lung neoplasms

Bronchial adenoma
Hamartoma
Papilloma
Fibroma
Lipoma
Hemangioma
Teratoma
Leiomyoma
Chondroma
Endometriosis
Pseudolymphoma

which rarely metastasize to bone and skin and which produce the carcinoid syndrome when liver metastases are present, bronchial carcinoid tumors more often involve the bone and skin and produce the syndrome in the absence of metastases. Substances elaborated by carcinoid tumors may produce sclerosis of cardiac valves downstream from the site of their origin or metastases; right-sided heart valves with abdominal tumors and left-sided heart valves with lung tumors. Symptoms and signs that constitute the clinical carcinoid syndrome include episodic flushing, anxiety, tremulousness, diarrhea, lacrimation, salivation, wheezing, tachycardia, facial edema, and hyperthermia.

Hamartomas

Hamartomas, the most common benign tumors of the lung, result from developmental malformations and are composed of tissues normally found in the lung: cartilage, bronchial epithelia, smooth muscle, fibrous tissue, and fat. Almost all hamartomas lie in the peripheral parenchyma, and less than 10% are found endobronchially. The chest roentgenographic appearance is that of a well-circumscribed solitary nodule, usually less than 4 cm in size. Calcification occurs infrequently (5% to 25% of patients), but a "popcorn" pattern strongly suggests the diagnosis. Hamartomas may enlarge slowly, but more rapid growth can occur, causing a new nodule to appear in adult life. Because of their peripheral location, hamartomas are unlikely to cause symptoms, and hemoptysis is rare.

Papillomas

Papillomas most often present as laryngeal tumors in children but rarely may present in adulthood together with multiple tumors in the tracheobronchial tree. Bronchial papillomas rarely develop in the absence of laryngeal or tracheal lesions. Papillomas contain vascular connective tissue covered by stratified squamous epithelium and occasionally ciliated respiratory epithelia. These tumors characteristically obstruct airways, resulting in peripheral atelectasis and obstructive pneumonia.

PULMONARY METASTASIS

The lung, with its rich vascular and lymphatic networks, is a frequent site of metastasis for a variety of tumors. About 30% of all cases of neoplastic disease metastasize to the lung. The estimated occurrence of pulmonary metastases by primary malignancy is given in the box above. Metastasis may present as a solitary nodular lesion, but in about 75% of patients they are multiple. Certain primary tumors are more likely than others to present as solitary metastasis: sarcomas; colon, kidney, testicular, and breast carcinomas; and melanomas. Endobronchial metastasis is rare compared with parenchymal metastasis and is most frequently caused by breast, kidney, and colon carcinomas and less frequently by melanomas and prostatic, pancreatic, and testicular carcinomas. Lymphangitic pulmonary metastasis is most frequently seen with breast, stomach, thyroid, and pancreatic carcinomas. Metastases to the lung parenchyma infrequently produce respiratory symptoms. Cough and hemoptysis occur very infrequently because metastatic lesions rarely erode the bronchial wall. The most common respiratory symptom is dyspnea, particularly in lymphangitic spread. The treatment of pulmonary metastases includes surgical excision, radiotherapy, chemotherapy, or a combination. Surgical excision results in improved survival when the tumor has a long doubling time (>40 days).

Estimated occurrence of pulmonary metastases by primary malignancy

Choriocarcinoma: 80%
Osteosarcoma: 75%
Kidney carcinoma: 70%
Thyroid carcinoma: 65%
Malignant melanoma: 60%
Breast carcinoma: 55%
Prostatic carcinoma: 45%
Nasopharyngeal carcinoma: 20%
Gastrointestinal carcinoma: 20%
Gynecologic carcinoma: 20%

SUMMARY

Lung cancer is the predominant fatal neoplasm in the United States and is almost totally preventable because it is largely caused by smoking. Other risk factors may act alone or synergistically with tobacco smoke to produce lung cancer and can be identified by eliciting a thorough occupational and past medical history. Although a greater understanding of genetic influences on lung cancer susceptibility may also help to identify those patients particularly at risk to the carcinogenic effect of tobacco smoke, the physician can have a major impact on this disease by helping all patients who smoke to quit.

The presentation and means of diagnosis have been reviewed. Knowledge of the pathologic classification and natural history of the different histologic types of lung cancer is important for deciding which treatment course is best for individual patients. Determining the extent or stage of disease and assessment of the cardiac and respiratory status are necessary to decide on either an aggressive or supportive course. Although a small percentage of patients may be cured of their disease, the vast majority will have intractable, recurrent disease. Certain complications, such as the paraneoplastic syndromes, the superior vena cava syndrome, and endobronchial obstruction with obstructive pneumonia, require specific measures for palliation. Methods for early detection and more effective therapy are desperately needed.

REFERENCES

Aaronchick JM: Lung cancer: epidemiology and risk factors. Semin Roentgenol 25:5, 1990.

Eddy DM: Screening for lung cancer. Ann Intern Med 111:232, 1989.
Geddes DM: The natural history of lung cancer. Br J Dis Chest 73:1, 1979.
Iannuzzi MC and Miller Y: The genetic predisposition to lung cancer. Semin Res Med 7:327, 1986.
Iannuzzi MC and Scoggin CH: Small cell lung cancer: state of art. Am Rev Resp Dis 134:593, 1986.
Lyubsky S and Jacobson MJ: Lung cancer: making the diagnosis. Chest 100:511, 1991.
Mauer LH: Ectopic hormone syndromes in small cell carcinoma of the lung. Clin Oncol 4:67, 1985.
Miller JD, Gorenstein LA, and Patterson GA: Staging: the key to rational management of lung cancer. Ann Thorac Surg 53:170, 1992.
Sachs DPL: Advances in smoking cessation treatment. Curr Pulmonol 12:139, 1991.
Sporn MB and Todaro GJ: Autocrine secretion and malignant transformation of cells. N Engl J Med 303:878, 1980.
Yessner R: Classification of lung cancer histology. N Engl J Med 312:652, 1985.

CHAPTER

215 Solitary Pulmonary Tumor

Thomas Y. Sullivan

DEFINITION AND ETIOLOGY

A *solitary pulmonary nodule* is a small (no more than 5 cm in diameter), rounded, intrapulmonic density with more or less smooth margins. The original term used to describe a solitary nodule, *coin lesion,* has generally been abandoned because the mass is spheric rather than flat. A solitary pulmonary nodule is found in 1 in every 2000 chest radiographs, making this lesion a frequent diagnostic and therapeutic problem. The nodule itself seldom produces symptoms and is often discovered as an incidental finding on a routine chest radiograph. If the patient has respiratory complaints, they are usually attributable to other pulmonary problems such as cigarette smoking, bronchitis, or lower respiratory tract infection.

Many different processes can produce a solitary pulmonary nodule (Table 215-1), and the frequency of each differs among reported series. If the series includes only persons participating in a community chest radiograph screening program, the incidence of lung cancer is very low. If the series includes only patients suspected of having cancer and referred for surgical resection, the incidence of lung cancer is understandably much higher. Benign lesions are usually granulomas associated with tuberculosis, other mycobacteria, or fungi. Fungal granulomas are frequently caused by *Coccidioides immitis* in the southwestern United States and *Histoplasma capsulatum* in the upper Mississippi valley.

The likelihood that a solitary nodule is lung cancer is directly related to the patient's age. Only 1% of solitary nodules are malignant in patients less than 35 years old, but 50% to 60% are malignant in patients age 50 or older. The likelihood that a nodule is lung cancer is also directly related to the amount of previous cigarette smoking. All cell types of lung cancer can present as a solitary nodule, but most malignant nodules are adenocarcinoma or squamous cell carcinoma. Small cell lung cancer rarely presents as a solitary nodule.

Table 215-1. Causes of solitary pulmonary nodules

Cause	Range of reported incidence (%)
Malignant tumors	
Bronchogenic carcinoma	16-52
Bronchial adenoma (certain cell types seem benign and have benign courses)	1-2
Metastatic carcinoma	1-10
Benign tumors	5-12
Hamartoma	1-2
Fibroma	0-1
Granulomas	
Histoplasmosis	5-38
Tuberculosis	10-15
Coccidioidomycosis	2-14
Cryptococcosis	0-1
Miscellaneous	
Bronchogenic cyst	1-3
Arteriovenous malformation	0-1
Bronchopulmonary sequestration	0-1
Sclerosing hemangioma	0-1
Intrapulmonary lymph node	0-1

The average 5-year survival of patients who have resection of a malignant solitary nodule is 30% to 50%. This is clearly better than the 10% survival rate of patients who have surgical resection of more advanced lung cancer. Therefore each solitary nodule represents a potentially resectable and curable lung cancer. In the evaluation it is essential to determine whether the lesion is suspicious for a malignancy and should be removed promptly, or whether it has features that strongly favor a nonmalignant process that can be managed without resection.

DIAGNOSTIC EVALUATION

Separation of benign from probably malignant lesions relies heavily on the chest radiograph. If serial chest radiographs show the development of a nodule during resolution of pneumonia, pulmonary contusion, or pulmonary infarction, the lesion is clearly benign. If vessels are seen entering a nodule, an arteriovenous fistula should be suspected. Other radiographic findings suggesting benignity include small size, increased density, smooth borders, calcification, and absence of growth during a reasonable period of observation.

Reliable radiographic indicators of benign disease are certain calcification patterns noted within the nodule and absence of growth demonstrated by no change on chest radiographs taken 2 or more years apart. The patterns of calcification that indicate benignity include diffuse speckled or "popcorn" pattern (Fig. 215-1), large central nidus (Fig. 215-2), and concentric calcification (Fig. 215-3). A large central nidus or concentric calcification is found in granulomas; popcorn calcification occurs in hamartoma. A small fleck of calcium in the center or periphery of a nodule (Fig. 215-4) is a common finding in a granuloma; therefore this type of calcification suggests a benign disease. However, rarely lung cancer may develop a fleck of calcification or engulf a nearby calcified granuloma. Also, metastatic osteogenic sarcoma may calcify. Because of these unusual examples, a small fleck of calcium within a nodule is not a completely reliable sign of benignity.

Growth rate of a solitary nodule can be estimated from change in size on serial chest radiographs. A small increase in diameter indicates a greater increase in volume. A mass doubling in diameter has increased in volume eightfold, and a mass has doubled in volume when its diameter has increased by about one-fourth. Fig. 215-5 shows how the serial diameter of a nodule can be plotted on semilogarithmic paper against the number of days of observation to determine the doubling time. Doubling time of lung cancer ranges from 15 to 450 days. Thus, if a lesion is malignant, a detectable increase in diameter should be expected within 2 years. Doubling time is the basis of the typically used practice of comparing the size of the lesion on chest radiographs taken 2 or more years apart. Lack of any change in diameter over that time indicates that the lesion has a doubling time greater than 450 days and therefore should be considered benign. Any lesion that increases in diameter during a 2-year period must be considered malignant until proved otherwise.

Benign lesions have their own natural histories and development periods, with doubling times that overlap those of lung cancer. However, lesions with doubling times longer than 450 days are usually granulomas. Lesions with very rapid doubling times (less than 15 days) are almost always inflammatory processes such as pneumonia or vasculitis, if primary or metastatic sarcoma can be excluded.

Several other clinical tests have been employed to help

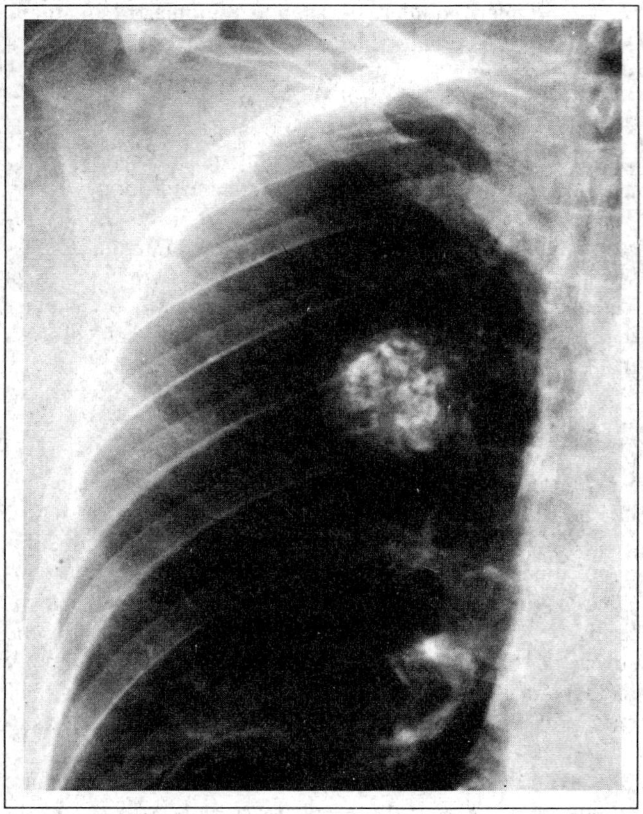

Fig. 215-1. Standard chest radiograph demonstrating a right upper lobe nodule in an asymptomatic patient with diffuse "popcorn" calcification characteristic of a benign hamartoma.

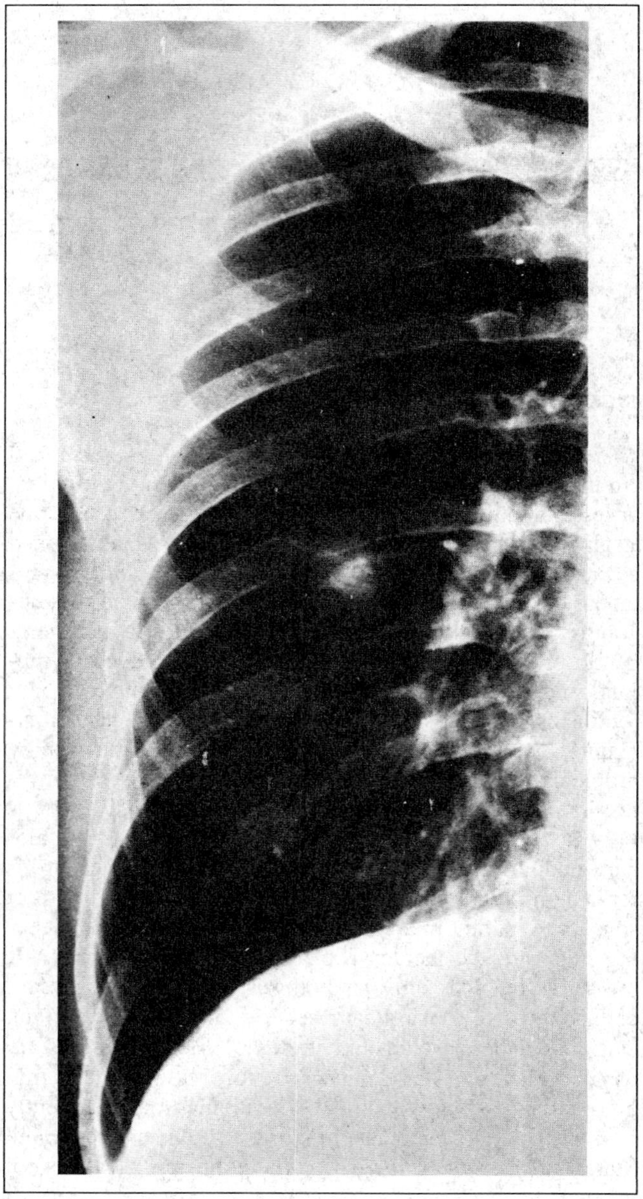

Fig. 215-2. Standard chest radiograph demonstrating a right upper lobe nodule in an asymptomatic patient with a large central nidus of calcium characteristic of a granuloma.

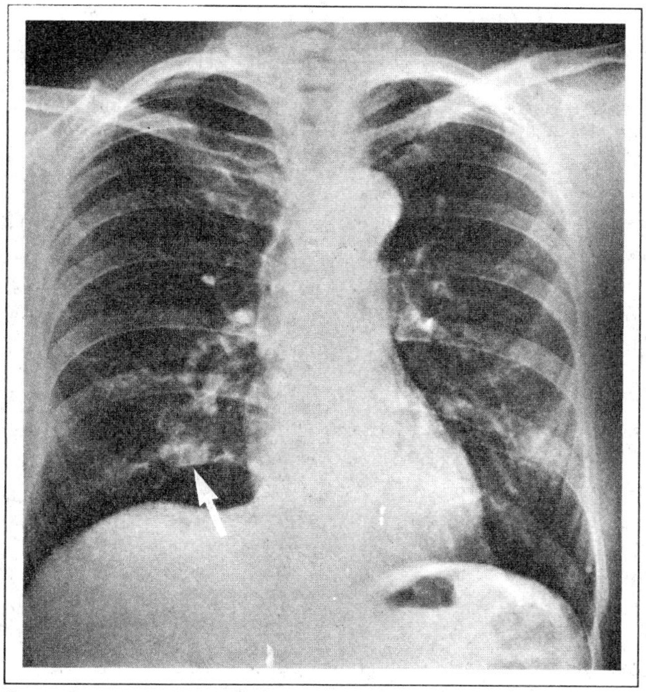

A

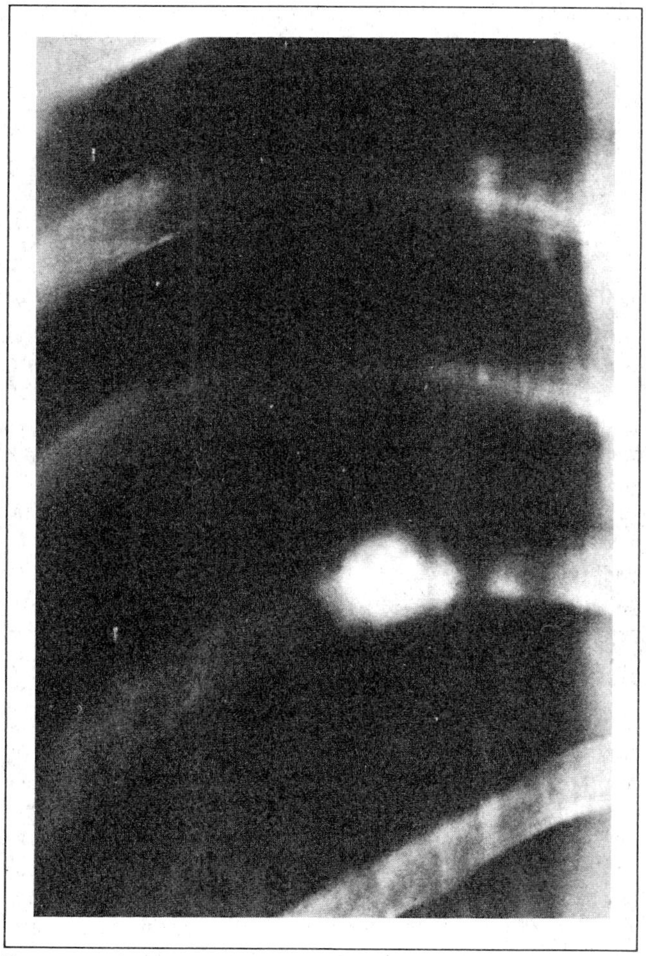

B

Fig. 215-3. A, Standard chest radiograph of a right lower lobe nodule without obvious calcification. **B,** Tomogram of the posterior aspect of the same nodule demonstrating central and concentric calcification characteristic of a granuloma.

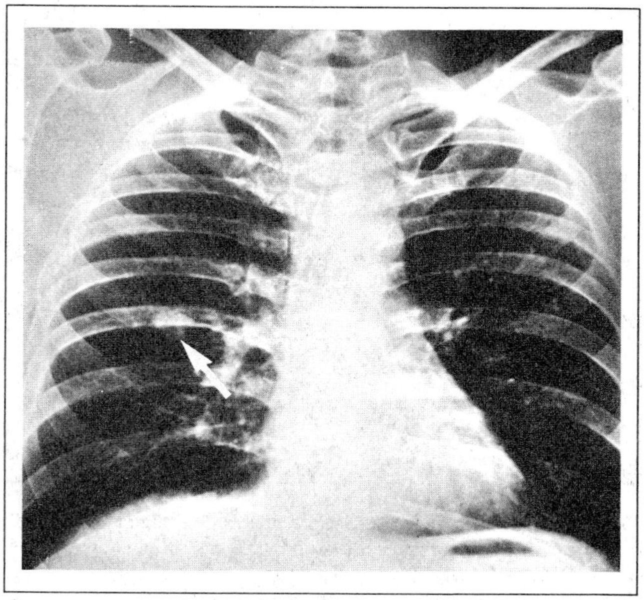

A

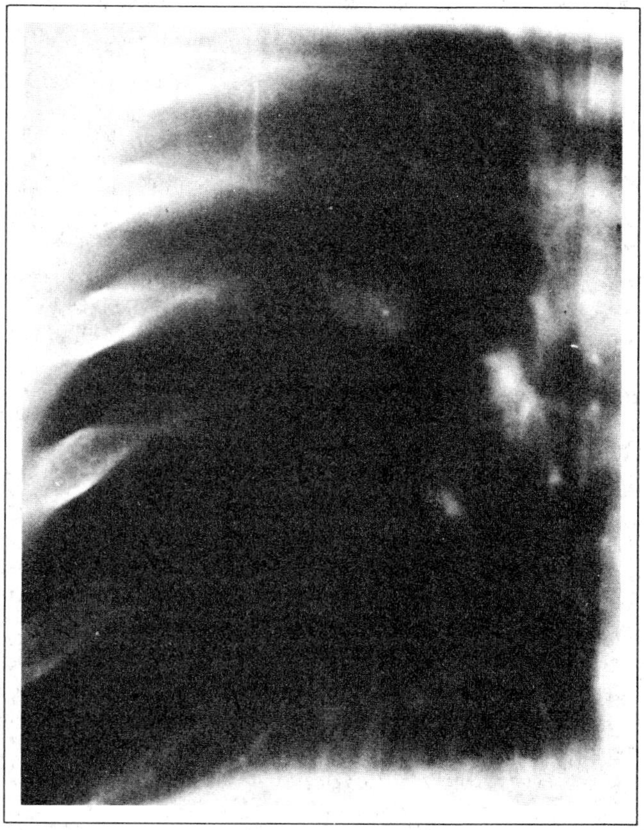

B

Fig. 215-4. A, Standard chest radiograph demonstrating a right mid—lung field nodule *(arrow)* without obvious calcification. **B,** Tomogram of the same nodule showing an eccentric fleck of calcium. This lesion was biopsied by fine-needle aspiration, and a core of cartilage filled the needle on two aspirations. The lesion is a hamartoma.

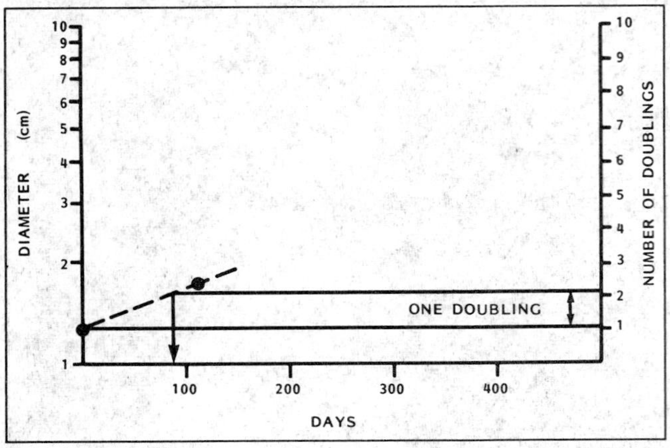

Fig. 215-5. Plot of diameter of a nodule in centimeters and number of doublings on chest radiographs taken 110 days apart. The nodule has increased in diameter from 1.3 to 1.6 cm, indicating that it has a doubling time of approximately 90 days. This lesion should be considered malignant until proved otherwise.

decide whether a solitary nodule is benign or malignant. Skin tests for tuberculous and fungal serologies are often done but may reflect concomitant disease or previous exposures and are not reliable indicators of the etiology of a nodule. Sputum examinations for tuberculosis and fungi may give more specific and reliable information but are seldom positive because small numbers of organisms exist within infectious granulomas. Sputum smears are obtained for cytologic examination but also do not have a high diagnostic yield even in proved cases of malignant solitary nodule. The low yield of sputum cytology probably occurs because the cancer is shedding only small numbers of malignant cells into the airways.

Two additional diagnostic procedures have become useful in the evaluation of a solitary nodule: fiberoptic bronchoscopy with transbronchial brushing, needle biopsy, or forceps biopsy; and transthoracic needle biopsy. Fiberoptic bronchoscopy with transbronchial biopsy has a diagnostic yield of 20% to 40% in patients with malignant nodules. Success decreases with decreasing size of the lesion, more peripheral location, and upper lobe lesions. Risk of hemorrhage or pneumothorax with transbronchial brushing is 5% and increases to 10% to 15% with a forceps biopsy. Transthoracic needle biopsy has an 80% to 95% diagnostic yield in patients with malignant nodules. Risk of pneumothorax is slightly greater than with bronchoscopic biopsy and is much greater if the patient has underlying bullous emphysema. Risk of seeding tumor cells along the needle tract is negligible. To ensure a high diagnostic yield with needle biopsy, it is helpful for a cytopathologist to be present during the aspiration, immediately examine the specimen, and advise the physician doing the aspiration if repeat sampling is indicated.

Characteristics of the borders of the lesion and calcification may be defined with tomograms (see Fig. 215-3) or computed tomography (CT). With CT, density is expressed as relative CT units. Density of the nodule can also be compared with density of a "phantom" nodule with known calcification placed in the scanner. Lesions with calcification density are likely granulomas; less dense lesions can be either benign or malignant. Chest CT or whole-lung tomograms may also show other small nodules that were not apparent on the routine chest radiograph, suggesting metastatic malignancy or a variety of other diseases, including Wegener's granulomatosis, fungal infections, and occasionally sarcoidosis.

In nonmalignant conditions the diagnostic yield of bronchoscopic or needle biopsies varies with the interest and skill of physicians performing the procedures and examining the specimens. The false-negative rate of a cytologic diagnosis of "benign disease" is unclear but of major concern. If acid-fast or fungal organisms are found, one can be secure in a diagnosis of nonmalignant disease; however, a finding of "inflammatory cells" is nonspecific and might be misleading because these types of cells can be found at the edge of a malignancy. Perhaps the major usefulness of biopsy procedures, especially transthoracic needle biopsy because of its higher yield, is in speeding the diagnosis of lung cancer. A rapid diagnosis will decrease the time and cost of hospitalization and prevent delaying necessary surgical resection.

CLINICAL MANAGEMENT

When dealing with a solitary nodule, a logical and sequential management scheme is essential. The first step is examination of previous chest radiographs. It may be possible to show that the lesion has not changed in more than 2 years and therefore can be considered benign. If there are no previous films for comparison, or if a lesion has increased in size within 2 years and does not show any of the patterns of benign calcification, the lesion must be presumed to be cancer. Age and smoking history are important determinants of management. Older patients who smoke should be presumed to have malignant nodules.

The next consideration is that a solitary nodule may represent metastasis from a primary cancer elsewhere in the body. The primary cancer may not be apparent, and the clinician must be suspicious of any symptom or abnormality detected on physical examination. The examination must be thorough and include several tests of stool for occult blood. Laboratory tests should include blood hemoglobin, alkaline phosphatase, and bilirubin, as well as careful microscopic examination of the urine. Abnormal laboratory tests or bleeding into the stool or urine prompt evaluation for an occult malignancy. However, an extensive search for a nonlung cancer that may have metastasized to the lung should be done only when there is a symptom, abnormal physical finding, or other simple clue. Extensive evaluation for occult malignancy in all patients with a solitary nodule is otherwise too often unrewarding and quite expensive.

A solitary nodule occurring in a patient with known nonlung cancer may represent a metastasis but is a second cancer—a primary lung cancer—in slightly more than half the cases. In patients with a solitary nodule and history of previously treated nonlung cancer, it is appropriate to proceed with bronchoscopic or transthoracic needle biopsy without delay. If the cytology from the biopsy shows malignancy, the cell type is compared with the cell type of the previous nonlung cancer to help establish whether the nodule represents metastasis.

If a patient has no evidence of a nonlung cancer, the nodule may represent a primary lung cancer. If so, it may have already metastasized. Symptoms referable to possible metastatic sites require investigation. Brain and bone symptoms and signs should be carefully sought. Supraclavicular fossae should be carefully palpated for enlarged lymph nodes. Liver chemistries and blood calcium are checked. If no symptoms and no abnormal physical findings or blood tests exist, an extensive search for metastasis is generally unrewarding and not recommended. At that point in the evaluation, it is often apparent that the solitary nodule may represent a primary lung cancer without obvious metastasis.

Since the treatment of primary lung cancer is surgical resection, it is imperative to determine the patient's ability to withstand surgery. The patient's general medical health must be evaluated, and many have other medical problems, especially chronic obstructive pulmonary disease. Pulmonary function tests should be measured, and a forced expiratory volume at 1 second (FEV_1) greater than 2000 ml and absence of elevated arterial carbon dioxide tension ($Paco_2$) indicate that the patient can probably tolerate a lobectomy or pneumonectomy. Patients who have lower values of FEV_1 should be evaluated with nuclear lung scan techniques that determine regional lung function. It is important to be certain that lung function is not distributed so that the part with good function may be resected and the poorly functioning part left in the patient. Using these techniques, it is possible to predict postresection pulmonary function, and a predicted postoperative FEV_1 greater than 800 ml is likely adequate to proceed with surgery. If a patient has evidence of significant obstructive lung disease, it is prudent to treat aggressively with bronchodilators and then repeat pulmonary function tests before making a decision about surgery.

If the patient's pulmonary function is adequate to withstand surgical resection of the nodule, it must be decided (1) if the patient should go to surgery promptly, (2) if an attempt should be made to obtain tissue from the lesion to establish a diagnosis, or (3) if the lesion could be watched with serial chest radiographs (i.e., "watchful waiting"). The first approach, prompt resection of the nodule, is often advocated. With larger lesions, greater than 3 cm in diameter, a chest CT scan should be obtained to look for mediastinal lymph nodes that may already harbor metastasis and require biopsy via mediastinoscopy before thoracotomy. A factor always important to consider is the morality and morbidity associated with thoracotomy. Mortality is unusual in young healthy patients but may approach 10% in patients with significant underlying cardiopulmonary disease, and all patients experience significant chest pain and the risk of developing postoperative pneumonia. Selective use of surgery for only malignant lesions is the ideal approach but may or may not be possible. It is often helpful to proceed with either bronchoscopic or needle biopsy. If no specific benign diagnosis is obtained, lung cancer is sufficiently likely that diagnostic/therapeutic surgical resection of the nodule is then appropriate.

Occasionally a patient with a nodule may be at high risk for surgery. Examples might be a patient with a recent myocardial infarction or a patient with multiple medical problems and only marginal pulmonary function to tolerate lung resection. In these extreme cases surgery may be delayed and the nodule followed with repeat chest radiographs. For example, the film could be repeated in 2 weeks. If no change occurs in the size of the nodule, the film is repeated in 4 weeks. The interval between radiographs is progressively increased until a total of 2 years of follow-up has accumulated. If the nodule does not increase in size during that time, it is assumed to be benign. If the nodule increases in size, it likely is malignant, and a decision about surgery must be made. The risk of cancer spreading during such "watchful waiting" is unknown. On one hand, it is likely that most lung cancers have been present for 3 or more years by the time they reach 1 cm in size and can be detected on chest radiograph. It can be argued that during that 3-year period, the cancer had ample opportunity to metastasize, and an additional 2 weeks or months may not alter the prognosis. However, it must be recognized that metastasis occurs at some point in time, after which cure is not possible. Currently, no way exists to predict when metastasis occurs.

FUTURE CONSIDERATIONS

The solitary pulmonary nodule will continue to be a difficult problem for the patient and physician. The smoking habit of the population ensures that concern about lung cancer will be present for many years, and success with treatment for most lung cancers has advanced little over the past 50 years. Since the best results in treatment occur if lung cancer is resected while it is localized as a solitary nodule, there will continue to be keen interest in removing a nodule whenever the clinical picture is not diagnostic of a benign process.

The most promising clinical developments will probably include further standardization and acceptance of CT evaluation of solitary nodules. These may include improvements in CT densitometry techniques, especially nodule simulators or so-called phantom nodules that allow density calibration on each CT scanner. Such developments may allow confident separation of nodules that are very unlikely to be malignant from those that may or may not be malignant. Another development that may prove useful is combining information from the CT with that from bronchoscopic or needle biopsy. A CT-directed biopsy has the advantage of proving that the specimen came directly from the nodule. This might increase the diagnostic yield, especially in nonmalignant nodules, and increase the level of confidence in a cytopathologic diagnosis of "chronic inflammation." Immunologic staining techniques that identify the etiology of previous fungal or other infectious granulomas could also be helpful.

A discouraging aspect in the management of patients with a malignant solitary nodule is that, even after surgical resection, approximately half these patients die of metastatic lung cancer. Obviously, better methods of treatment are necessary, as well as better methods of detection of microscopic metastasis. A method of prevention of most lung cancers has already been discovered—abstinence from cigarette smoking.

REFERENCES

Higgins GA: The solitary pulmonary nodule: ten-year follow-up of Veterans Administration—Armed Forces Cooperative Study. Arch Surg 110:570, 1975.

Lillington GA: Management of solitary pulmonary nodules. DM, May 1991.

O'Keefe ME Jr, Good CA, and McDonald JE: Calcification in solitary nodules in the lung. AJR 77:1023, 1957.

Siegelman SS et al: CT of the solitary pulmonary nodule. AJR 135:1, 1980.

Steele JD and Buell P: Asymptomatic solitary pulmonary nodules: host survival, tumor size, and growth rate. J Thorac Cardiovasc Surg 65:140, 1978.

CHAPTER

216 Pulmonary Hypertension: Primary and Secondary Causes

Lewis J. Rubin
Barbara J. Kircher

The pulmonary circulation is normally a low-resistance, high-flow circuit that has a remarkable capacity for vasoregulation to optimize intrapulmonary gas exchange. Conditions that produce elevations in the pulmonary artery pressure can be classified as either precapillary or postcapillary, based on the primary site of the circulation that is affected (see the box at upper right). Disorders that raise pulmonary venous pressure *(postcapillary)* secondarily raise pulmonary artery pressure. In contrast, *precapillary* pulmonary hypertension is caused by diseases that affect the pulmonary arterial network, either as the primary site of injury or as a consequence of a more widespread process involving the lung parenchyma.

Classification of pulmonary diseases based on site of primary injury

Precapillary

Parenchymal lung diseases
Restrictive chest wall disease
Thromboembolic disease
Primary pulmonary hypertension
Persistent fetal circulation
Congenital heart disease
Pulmonary vasculitis
High-altitude disease
Peripheral pulmonic stenosis
Pulmonary arteriovenous fistula

Postcapillary

Left ventricular failure
Mitral valve disease
Left atrial myxoma or thrombus
Veno-occlusive disease

Pulmonary hypertension is not a disease per se, but rather a hemodynamic abnormality that is common to a variety of diseases. Although the severity of hemodynamic dysfunction may vary among these different conditions, the persistent pressure overload that confronts the right ventricle often leads to right ventricular failure and death. The term *cor pulmonale,* which is often used to describe overt right ventricular failure, is actually better defined as pulmonary hypertension in the absence of valvular, ischemic, or congenital heart disease. Right-sided heart failure is a late manifestation of cor pulmonale and need not be present for the diagnosis of cor pulmonale to be considered.

PRIMARY PULMONARY HYPERTENSION

Primary pulmonary hypertension (PPH) is an uncommon disease characterized by extreme elevations in pulmonary artery pressure in the absence of a demonstrable cause. The diagnosis of PPH requires the confirmation of precapillary pulmonary hypertension by cardiac catheterization and the exclusion of a congenital heart disease, valvular or ischemic heart disease, significant parenchymal lung disease, other conditions that interfere with gas exchange (e.g., sleep apnea), and thromboembolic disease. Although PPH is more frequently found in young or middle-aged women, it can be seen in individuals of either sex and at any age.

PULMONARY HYPERTENSION SECONDARY TO CHRONIC LUNG DISEASE

Pulmonary hypertension can complicate a variety of chronic respiratory diseases, either by reducing the total cross-sectional surface area of the pulmonary circulation as a result of a generalized destructive process or as a result of pulmonary vasoconstriction and subsequent vascular remodeling. The former condition is most frequently seen in diffuse interstitial lung disease, extensive bullous emphysema, and other destructive processes. The latter is characteristic of chronic obstructive lung diseases, sleep-disordered breathing syndromes, or chronic high-altitude exposure. Clearly, overlap between these two mechanisms occurs, particularly as progressive lung destruction leads to greater contribution of hypoxic pulmonary vasoconstriction. This is frequently the sequence of events in patients with cystic fibrosis who survive into adulthood.

It has been known for many years that alveolar hypoxia

produces precapillary pulmonary vasoconstriction, and acidosis or hypercarbia potentiates this phenomenon. Although vasoconstriction to a small region of alveolar hypoxia would optimize ventilation-perfusion ratios by diverting blood to well-ventilated lung units, diffuse alveolar hypoxia produces widespread pulmonary hypertension. Although the mechanism responsible for hypoxic vasoconstriction remains unknown, enhanced calcium entry into the pulmonary vascular smooth muscle cells is an integral feature of the vasoconstrictor response to hypoxia that can be ameliorated with calcium channel blocking agents.

Patients may complain of increasing dyspnea, particularly with exertion, fatigue, and swelling. Physical examination may show cyanosis, jugular venous distention, hepatomegaly, ascites, and edema, particularly in the late stages. A prominent right ventricular impulse may be palpated in the subxiphoid region in individuals with severe obstructive airways disease and hyperinflation.

The presence and severity of pulmonary hypertension in chronic lung disease correlate with the severity of abnormalities in pulmonary function. Pulmonary hypertension is likely to present, at least during exercise, in patients with restrictive lung disease when the vital capacity falls below 50% of predicted values. In patients with obstructive airways disease, pulmonary hypertension is almost invariably present when the forced expiratory volume at 1 second (FEV_1) falls below 1 L. Pulmonary hypertension is also likely to be present when the arterial oxygen tension (Pa_{O_2}) falls below 55 mm Hg; the more severe the hypoxemia, the more severe the pulmonary hypertension.

Several other noninvasive tests may be used to suggest the presence of cor pulmonale. The electrocardiogram (ECG) may show an extreme right-axis deviation $\geq$ 110 to 120 degrees or right ventricular hypertrophy; the chest radiograph may show right-sided heart enlargement and enlarged main pulmonary arteries; and the right ventricular ejection fraction, measured by radionuclide angiocardiography, is depressed. Echocardiography is always indicated to exclude a structural abnormality responsible for pulmonary hypertension, such as a congenital lesion, valvular disorder, or left ventricular dysfunction. It is also valuable as a tool for following the hemodynamic and anatomic consequences of the disease process. The right atrium and right ventricle are usually enlarged, and increased thickness of the right ventricular wall is seen particularly well in subcostal views. Pulmonary artery dilatation can be seen in the short-axis view.

Normally the interventricular septum is displaced toward the right ventricle in late diastole and early systole. With right ventricular pressure overload, the septum flattens or even bows toward the right ventricle (Fig. 216-1). A measurement of the degree of curvature of the septum in the short-axis view is an index of severity of right ventricular pressure elevation.

An estimation of the right ventricular systolic pressure can be obtained by applying the modified Bernoulli equation to the maximum velocity of the tricuspid regurgitation flow. By adding this pressure gradient to the right atrial pressure, obtained from examination of the jugular venous pulse or degree of inspiratory collapse of the inferior vena cava on subcostal views, the right ventricular systolic pressure is determined. The tricuspid regurgitation signal can be augmented by intravenous injection of agitated saline during imaging, a technique that is especially helpful in measuring the pulmonary pressure response to exercise.

A fairly specific but not sensitive sign of pulmonary hypertension is a midsystolic drop or notch in the pulmonary systolic flow velocity curve caused by resistance to right ventricular ejection. The pulmonary artery pressure also correlates with a rapid acceleration time from the onset of pulmonic flow to peak velocity. Since Doppler measurements depend on loading conditions, heart rate, contractil-

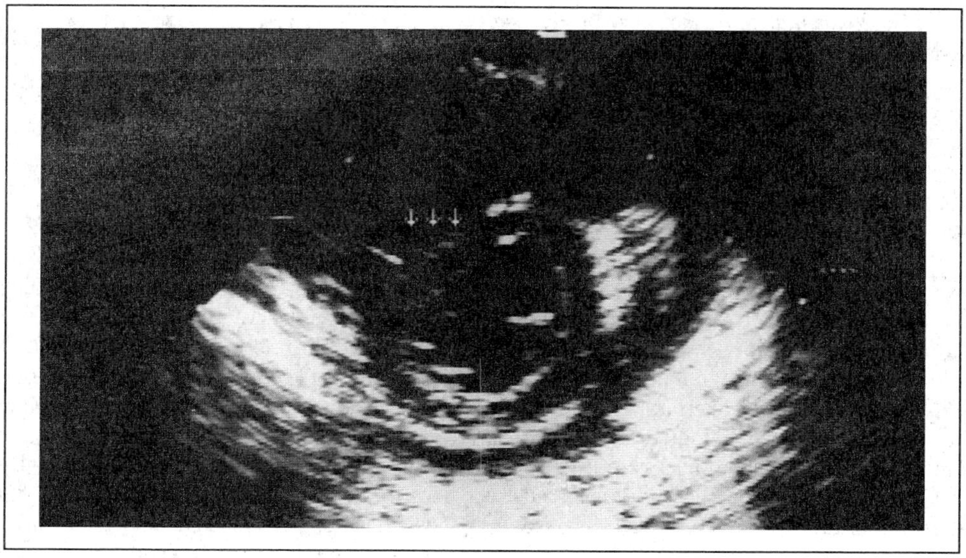

Fig. 216-1. Two-dimensional short-axis echocardiogram demonstrating abnormal septal flattening *(arrows)* at end-diastole in the presence of right ventricular systolic hypertension.

ity, and compliance, they cannot be substituted for invasive hemodynamic measurements of pulmonary artery pressure when following acute or chronic responses to therapy.

Therapy should be aimed at improving gas exchange with bronchodilators, chest physiotherapy, corticosteroids, respiratory stimulants, and mucolytics, as appropriate. Low-flow supplemental oxygen in hypoxemic patients prolongs survival, although its hemodynamic effects are variable. Oxygen should be titrated to achieve a Pao_2 of 60 mm Hg or greater and should be used for a least 18 hours daily to minimize hypoxic vasoconstriction. Vasodilators, particularly the calcium channel blockers, have been shown to reduce pulmonary hypertension in some patients, but their role remains uncertain. Vasodilators can worsen gas exchange by increasing blood flow to poorly ventilated lung units, as well as producing systemic hypotension and salt and water retention.

Diuretics should be used cautiously in patients with cor pulmonale. Although they are useful in controlling excess volume retention, their use can decrease intravascular volume and compromise right ventricular function. Additionally, the hypokalemia and alkalosis induced by excessive diuretic use are poorly tolerated by these patients.

Patients with severe pulmonary hypertension caused by primary pulmonary hypertension, congenital heart disease, or severe obstructive or restrictive lung disease may be candidates for lung transplantation. Patients with pulmonary hypertension and nonreparable, complex congenital heart disease will likely require combined heart-lung transplantation.

MISCELLANEOUS CAUSES

Pulmonary hypertension can be seen in patients with a variety of connective tissue disorders, including scleroderma, systemic lupus erythematosus, and rheumatoid arthritis. Rarely, vasculitis can involve the pulmonary vasculature either solely or in combination with a systemic vasculitis. Parasites, such as *Schistosoma mansoni,* can also produce pulmonary hypertension.

PULMONARY ARTERIOVENOUS FISTULA

Pulmonary arteriovenous (AV) fistula can occur singly, multiply, with hereditary telangiectasia (Osler-Weber-Rendu disease), or as an independent entity. AV fistula should be suspected when cyanosis and hypoxemia occur without evidence of cardiopulmonary disease. The hypoxemia is not corrected by breathing 100% oxygen. Usually no associated pulmonary hypertension or cardiac enlargement occurs unless the patient also has anemia, substantial systemic AV fistulas, or profound hypoxemia.

Particularly when associated with hereditary telangiectasia, AV fistulas may be multiple when discovered, or additional lesions may develop over time. Hemoptysis, pulmonary hemorrhage, and brain abscess may occur as associated complications.

Physical examination may disclose cyanosis and, if the fistula is sufficiently large, a venous hum, which increases with Müller's maneuver and decreases with Valsalva's maneuver. Chest radiography may demonstrate nodular or diffuse vascular lesions with or without connections to the hilum. The lesions generally enhance when visualized by contrast-enhanced computed tomographic (CT) scanning. Diagnosis depends on pulmonary angiography.

Selective embolization of thrombotic material, wire springs designed to induce local thrombosis, or catheter-introduced balloons have been used to close fistulas. Conventional therapy depends on surgical removal either by lobectomy or by wedge resection. In patients with hereditary telangiectasia, surgical therapy should be conservative because of the propensity for development of additional fistulas over time.

REFERENCES

Dawkins KD: Long-term results, hemodynamics, and complications after combined heart and lung transplantation. Circulation 71:919, 1985.

Fuster V et al: Primary pulmonary hypertension: natural history and the importance of thrombosis. Circulation 70:580, 1984.

Hughes JD and Rubin LJ: Primary pulmonary hypertension: an analysis of 28 cases and a review of the literature. Medicine 65:56, 1986.

Matthay RA and Berger HJ: Cardiovascular function in cor pulmonale. Clin Chest Med 4:269, 1983.

Pasque MK et al: Single-lung transplantation for pulmonary hypertension. Circulation 84:2275, 1991.

Rich S and Brundage BH: High-dose calcium blocking therapy for primary pulmonary hypertension: evidence for long-term reduction in pulmonary arterial pressure and regression of right ventricular hypertrophy. Circulation 76:135, 1987.

Schiller NB: Pulmonary artery pressure estimation by two-dimensional and Doppler echocardiography. Cardiol Clin 8:277, 1990.

Terry PB et al: Pulmonary arteriovenous malformations: physiologic observations and results of therapeutic balloon embolizations. N Engl J Med 308:1197, 1983.

CHAPTER

217 Pulmonary Thromboembolism

Charles K. Chan
Richard A. Matthay

Pulmonary thromboembolic disease is a common finding at autopsy. Mortality statistics indicate that pulmonary thromboembolism is the principal cause of death for more than 50,000 patients annually in the United States. Since not all pulmonary thromboembolic events result in death, the true incidence of pulmonary thromboembolism is probably greater than 500,000 per year in the United States. The difficulty in making a firm and correct diagnosis of pulmonary thromboembolism is predominantly because of the lack of specific signs and symptoms. Available data suggest that 25% to 30% of untreated patients die from pulmonary embolism, contrasted with a mortality rate of 5% to 8% in treated patients. Accordingly, prompt diagnosis and appropriate treatment are critical in the management of patients with pulmonary thromboembolism.

This chapter provides an overview of current concepts of the pathogenesis, pathology, and pathophysiology of pulmonary thromboembolism. It also includes a discussion of the clinical manifestations, currently available diagnostic techniques, and appropriate therapy for pulmonary thromboembolism. Finally, prevention of this entity is emphasized.

PATHOGENESIS

Epidemiologic and autopsy data indicate that most pulmonary thromboemboli arise as detached portions of venous thrombi from the deep veins of the lower extremities. Less common sources are the right-sided heart chambers, pelvic veins, and central venous catheters. Several factors have been associated with an increased risk of venous thrombosis: (1) hemostasis, (2) hypercoagulable state, and (3) blood vessel wall abnormalities. Rarely a patient has a hypercoagulable state associated with an inborn error of metabolism, such as antithrombin III deficiency or protein C or S deficiency. More common hematologic conditions associated with thromboembolic disease include polycythemia, thrombocytosis, and sickle cell crisis. Clinical conditions that are generally considered important risk factors for thromboembolic disease are summarized in the box on the right.

Clinical features of pulmonary thromboembolism

Symptoms
Dyspnea
Pleuritic pain
Apprehension
Cough
Hemoptysis
Syncope
Substernal chest pain
Sweats

Signs
Tachypnea
Tachycardia
Reduced breath sounds
Wheezes
Crackles
Pleural rub
Elevated jugular venous pressure
Right ventricular gallop
Right ventricular lift
Loud pulmonic second sound
Pulmonary outflow tract murmur

PATHOLOGY

Autopsy studies reveal that pulmonary thromboemboli are usually multiple, bilateral, and found mainly in the lower lobes. Fewer than 10% of pulmonary thromboemboli cause pulmonary infarction. Infection and left ventricular failure increase the likelihood of pulmonary infarction.

Histologically, a pulmonary infarction appears as an area of coagulative necrosis of alveolar walls with erythrocyte extravasation into alveolar spaces and a mild acute inflammatory response. This type of infarction correlates with an infiltrate on chest radiograph that lasts longer than a week and frequently leaves a linear scar. An incomplete infarction manifests as a transient infiltrate on the chest radiograph and usually clears within a week, leaving no residual scar.

PATHOPHYSIOLOGY

Regardless of the source of the embolic material, the acute pathophysiologic results of sudden pulmonary arterial branch obstruction caused by pulmonary thromboembolism are similar and have been well defined. A total cessation of blood flow to the distal lung zone is the initial effect of embolic obstruction, and this invariably leads to respiratory and hemodynamic consequences.

Respiratory consequences

Embolic obstruction is followed by three primary respiratory events: (1) establishment of an area of lung that is ventilated but not perfused (i.e., alveolar dead space); (2) pneumoconstriction, which is a result of the alveolar hypocapnia after cessation of pulmonary capillary flow; and (3) loss of alveolar surfactant that leads to alveolar collapse and segmental atelectasis in 24 to 48 hours after cessation of pulmonary capillary flow.

In addition to the three primary respiratory abnormalities induced by pulmonary thromboembolism, a secondary consequence is arterial hypoxemia. Arterial hypoxemia is not present in all patients with pulmonary thromboembolism, and accordingly, its absence does not exclude the diagnosis. However, a wide alveolar-arterial oxygen tension difference (PA-ao_2D) and reduced arterial oxygen tension (Pao_2) are common findings, particularly after massive embolism. The principal mechanism responsible for hypoxemia in the early stage of pulmonary thromboembolism is ventilation-perfusion mismatching (i.e., alveolar dead space and pneumoconstriction in the embolized areas of lung). With massive embolic occlusion, arterial hypoxemia may partly result from a reduction of cardiac output and a subsequent drop in mixed-venous Po_2. Later, when emboli begin to resolve, some hypoxemia may persist because of reperfusion of poorly ventilated or nonventilated lung (i.e., intrapulmonary shunt).

Hemodynamic consequences

The principal hemodynamic consequence of pulmonary thromboembolism is a decrease in the functional cross-sectional area of the pulmonary arterial bed causing increased resistance to blood flow through the lungs. A significant increase in pulmonary vascular resistance requires high pulmonary arterial pressures to maintain pulmonary blood flow at the previous level; to maintain the same flow at higher pulmonary artery pressures, the right ventricle must work harder. Thus pulmonary thromboembolism causes an increase in pulmonary arterial resistance, pulmonary arterial pressures, and right ventricular stroke work. Acute right ventricular strain often leads to a decline in cardiac output and a compensatory increase in heart rate.

The severity of these hemodynamic consequences depends on (1) the extent of embolic occlusion of capillary beds, (2) the operation of reflex vasoactive and/or bronchospastic mediators, and (3) the cardiopulmonary status of the patient before the episode of thromboembolism. Because of the large reserve capacity of a normal pulmonary capillary bed, the mean pulmonary artery pressure rarely exceeds 40 mm Hg (normal, ≤ 18 mm Hg) in acute pulmonary embolism. Thus pulmonary artery pressures greater than 40 mm Hg usually indicate the presence of concomitant or pre-existing pulmonary vascular disease or suggest chronic pulmonary thromboembolism.

Infarction

Pulmonary infarction, ischemic necrosis of the parenchyma of the lung, occurs in less than 10% of all patients with pulmonary emboli. The infrequency of infarction is not surprising because the lung has three sources of oxygen: the pulmonary arterial system, the bronchial arterial system, and the airways. Prior studies indicate that the development of a pulmonary infarction is related to the extent of occlusion of the embolized artery and the adequacy of systemic bronchial collateral blood flow in the first few days after the embolic event. Total occlusion of a vessel by an embolus occurs infrequently, and usually some blood flows around the embolus to the distal lung zones. Because this flow is often substantial, the continued perfusion inhibits infarction and moderates the cardiopulmonary events described earlier. Infarction is most common in patients with pre-existing left ventricular failure or pulmonary disease, since bronchial collateral arterial flow and ventilation are most likely to be compromised simultaneously in these individuals. Occasionally and for unclear reasons, infarction does appear in patients without overt cardiopulmonary disease.

Most chest radiographic densities that appear after pulmonary thromboembolism are caused by areas of congestive atelectasis rather than pulmonary infarction. The atelectatic changes usually occur within 72 hours after embolic occlusion, and tissue necrosis does not occur because of the bronchial collateral arterial supply. Histologic studies have revealed restoration of normal parenchyma to such lung zones after several weeks as the embolus resolves.

Resolution of pulmonary thromboembolism

As with venous thrombi, pulmonary thromboemboli resolve rapidly. As in deep vein thrombosis, fibrinolysis and organization control the removal of embolic material from the vascular bed. Whatever the mechanisms involved in the removal of embolic material, vascular patency is generally restored to normal. Studies in dogs have demonstrated substantial resolution within hours and have established that administration of heparin can accelerate the rate of resolution. Radionuclide perfusion lung scans and angiographic studies in humans have confirmed resolution of pulmonary thromboemboli begins within a few days and is well advanced within 2 to 4 weeks. Permanent embolic residuals do occur, although the actual incidence is not known. Fewer than 10% of patients appear to retain perfusion defects on radionuclide perfusion lung scan after 6 weeks. The rate and degree of resolution observed in humans probably is related to age, thrombus composition and volume, and individual difference in fibrinolytic activities. It is noteworthy that even massive emboli are likely to be resolved within days or weeks, particularly in otherwise young and healthy persons without coexisting cardiopulmonary disease. Two groups of patients may develop late pulmonary hypertension: (1) those with major "central" obstruction of main or lobar arteries and (2) those with obstruction of multiple distal vessels that supply a large capillary bed. These embolic events are not always recognized clinically, and incorrect diagnoses ranging from chronic lung disease to primary pulmonary hypertension are made. Early detection of this precapillary form of pulmonary hypertension is often difficult, and the disorder may be recognized only when dyspnea on exertion, effort-related syncope, or overt right ventricular failure develops.

CLINICAL FEATURES (See also Chapter 86.)

To make a diagnosis of pulmonary thromboembolism, a high index of suspicion is necessary, especially in patients with the associated risk factors. Acute onset of unexplained dyspnea is by far the most common and perhaps the most prominent symptom of pulmonary thromboembolism, followed by pleuritic chest pain, apprehension, cough, hemoptysis, syncope, and substernal chest pain.

Characteristic findings on physical examination associated with pulmonary embolism are few. Tachypnea and tachycardia are invariably present, but, as in dyspnea, both may be transient. Other less common physical signs are a reduction in breath sounds and audible wheezing. Atelectasis in the embolic areas may be associated with localized crackles, but in most patients, the lungs are clear to auscultation. If atelectasis or infarction occurs, additional confirmatory findings may include pleural friction rub, presence of a pleural effusion, and fever.

In the event of massive embolism, cardiac findings suggestive of pulmonary outflow tract obstruction may be present. These include a right ventricular diastolic gallop (S_3), a right ventricular "lift," prominent "A" waves in the jugular venous pulse, a scratchy systolic murmur in the pulmonary outflow area, and an accentuated pulmonic second sound. It is prudent to emphasize that none of these physical findings is specific for pulmonary thromboembolic disease because the same clinical syndrome can be present in other cardiopulmonary diseases and other pulmonary embolic disease, such as tumor, septic, and amniotic fluid embolism. Therefore, to establish the diagnosis of pulmonary thromboembolism, clinical features alone cannot be confidently relied on (see the box on p. 1749). It is necessary to obtain additional but crucial paraclinical data.

DIAGNOSIS

Laboratory investigations

Arterial blood gases. Most patients with acute pulmonary embolism have an acute respiratory alkalosis. As stated, PA-ao_2D is typically widened because of an increase in alveolar dead space. Even though 85% of patients with angiographically proved pulmonary thromboembolism have a Pao_2 on room air of less than 80 mm Hg, a Pao_2 within the normal range is not sufficient to exclude this diagnosis. On the other hand, a reduced Pao_2 is by no means specific for this entity.

Electrocardiogram. More than 80% of patients with pulmonary thromboembolic disease have an abnormal electrocardiogram (ECG); however, the abnormalities are usually minor and nonspecific. In patients with massive pulmonary embolism, a classic $S_1Q_3T_3$ pattern, with or without a right bundle branch block pattern, may be present. These changes may be transient and disappear within a few hours.

Chest radiography. Although the chest radiograph is usually abnormal, about 10% of patients with pulmonary thromboembolism have a normal film. A parenchymal infiltrate or pleural reaction and/or effusion may be seen. Parenchymal densities, which vary from patchy infiltrates to platelike atelectasis to round nodular lesions, are present in up to 75% of patients. Comparable vessels in both lungs may be of unequal size, and a "rat tail" appearance of a major pulmonary artery may be indicative of an organizing thrombus within it. Oligemia of a lung zone, particularly in association with increased flow to other lung zones, may also suggest embolic obstruction. A unilateral pleural effusion is found in about 45% of the patients, but bilateral effusions are rare.

Thoracentesis. No specific diagnostic pleural fluid finding has been observed for pulmonary thromboembolism. The effusions can range from transudative to exudative to grossly bloody. The major role of thoracentesis is to exclude an empyema or a malignant effusion.

Other tests. Increased fibrin degradation products are usually found in patients with angiographically proved pulmonary thromboemboli; however, the positive predictive value of this finding is low. Clinical studies evaluating the diagnostic usefulness of circulating cross-linked fibrin degradation products (D-dimers) and plasma thrombin–antithrombin III complexes (TAT) have shown that these two noninvasive diagnostic tests cannot distinguish between patients regarding the likelihood of pulmonary embolism after radionuclide lung scanning. Nonspecific elevations in serum lactic dehydrogenase, glutamic oxaloacetic transaminase, and/or bilirubin have also been described. However, these paraclinical tests have limited diagnostic value in most individuals suspected of having sustained pulmonary thromboemboli.

Diagnostic imaging techniques for pulmonary thromboembolism

Clinical features and routine diagnostic tests may be of little assistance in the diagnosis of pulmonary embolism. However, the combination of a suggestive history in an individual with a known risk factor(s) (see the box on p. 1749), together with consistent changes on arterial blood gases, ECG, and chest radiograph may be persuasive for a probable diagnosis, and therapy may be initiated after this type of evaluation.

However, to establish the diagnosis confidently, more specific diagnostic information is needed. The two pulmonary imaging procedures that provide a reasonably high degree of sensitivity and reliability in the diagnosis of pulmonary thromboembolism are the radionuclide ventilation-perfusion lung scan and pulmonary angiography.

Radionuclide lung scans. Perfusion lung scans are obtained by gamma camera imaging of the distribution of intravenously injected technetium 99m–labeled macroaggregates of albumin. The gamma-emitting radioactive particles are trapped in the pulmonary capillary bed. At least six views from different projections are obtained to help confirm suspicious perfusion defects. Normal perfusion scans show homogeneous distribution of radioactivity throughout both lungs, smooth margins, and configurations that correspond to the normal anatomy of the lungs.

The perfusion lung scan is a sensitive detector of changes in regional blood flow. However, any process that destroys or constricts pulmonary arterial vessels can cause perfusion defects, such as pneumonia, emphysema, or regional hypoventilation. Therefore a good-quality, normal perfusion lung scan virtually excludes the diagnosis of pulmonary thromboembolism, but deviations from normal simply represent an abnormality in blood flow distribution and are not diagnostic for pulmonary thromboembolic obstruction.

An abnormal perfusion lung scan must be interpreted cautiously. The extent of perfusion abnormalities can range from one small subsegmental defect to multiple segmental or even lobar defects, and in these circumstances, a ventilation lung scan is usually performed to determine if ventilation abnormalities exist in the same locations. A ventilation lung scan is usually performed by having patients breathe a radioactive gas such as xenon-133. The radioactive gas is expected to distribute evenly throughout both lungs. Unfortunately, in patients with obstructive airways disease, the xenon-133 is usually trapped in the proximal airways and poorly distributed to the peripheral lung zones, making the interpretation impossible in those patients. A good-quality ventilation lung scan is expected to be normal or mismatched in the regions of perfusion defects because of pulmonary thromboemboli and to be abnormal or matched in the regions of perfusion defects caused by obstructive airways disease.

Data from the Prospective Investigation of Pulmonary

Embolism Diagnosis (PIOPED) study help to define the diagnostic usefulness of radionuclide lung scans. Using lung scanning alone, the positive predictive value for pulmonary embolism at angiography was 88% for high-probability scans, 33% for intermediate-probability scans, 16% for low-probability scans, and a surprisingly high 9% for normal or near-normal scans. Thus the PIOPED data indicate that lung scans cannot replace the conventional "gold standard," pulmonary angiography. However, the PIOPED results also demonstrate that if clinical features and routine diagnostic test results are factored into the interpretation of the lung scans, the diagnostic usefulness of lung scans is enhanced substantially. Specifically, a high level of clinical suspicion coupled with a high-probability lung scan brings the likelihood of pulmonary embolism to 96%. Conversely, a low index of clinical suspicion with a low-probability lung scan yields a 4% likelihood of pulmonary embolism. Except for these extreme settings, patients with intermediate-probability scans and low-probability scans with high levels of clinical suspicion should undergo pulmonary angiography. Also, patients with chronic thromboembolic disease need pulmonary angiography to clarify the development of new embolic episodes.

Pulmonary angiography. Although it is widely accepted that the traditional pulmonary angiogram and, more recently, the intravenous digital subtraction angiogram are the best available methods of visualizing the pulmonary vasculature and thus the diagnostic "touchstones" for pulmonary thromboembolism, angiography is subject to interpretive and technical limitations. Current techniques cannot show obstruction in small subsegmental arterial branches, and thus many small peripheral emboli may be missed. The abrupt cutoff of a major vessel because of an impacted clot is easy to detect. However, by far the more common finding is a filling defect caused by flow of contrast medium around a partially occluded thrombus or an area of segmental hypoperfusion in the lung. Other angiographic signs include "pruning" or "tapering" or absence of small branches, delayed venous emptying, and dilatation of the right ventricle and great vessels. None of these findings is as specific as cutoff and filling defects, particularly in the presence of coexisting cardiopulmonary disease. A well-performed pulmonary angiogram with augmentation techniques, such as subselective injections, magnification radiography, and balloon occlusion angiography, can visualize emboli down to 1 mm in diameter. However, standard angiographic technique without augmentation may completely miss occlusive emboli 2.5 mm in diameter. It is widely accepted that a negative good-quality angiogram confidently excludes pulmonary thromboembolism.

The only investigative procedure for pulmonary embolism that is associated with morbidity or mortality is pulmonary angiography. In high-risk patients (i.e., those with an allergy to contrast material, right ventricular end-diastolic pressure >20 mm Hg, or amiodarone-induced pulmonary toxicity) the use of low-osmolality contrast material may enhance patient safety and comfort. Low-osmolality contrast virtually abolishes the heat sensation and urge to cough, which in turn maximizes the quality of the images. Use of a "pigtail" catheter can also reduce the risk of inadvertent perforation of the right ventricle. In tertiary referral centers, the associated morbidity is only 3% to 4%, and the mortality should not exceed 0.3%. These data attest to the clinical usefulness and safety of this procedure in patients with suspected pulmonary emboli.

Diagnostic tests for peripheral deep venous thrombosis (See also Chapter 22.)

An alternative diagnostic route in patients with suspected pulmonary thromboembolism who have a nondiagnostic ventilation-perfusion lung scan is to search for peripheral deep venous thrombosis. Since the initial treatment for both conditions is identical (i.e., anticoagulation), if the presence of proximal venous thrombosis in the lower extremities is documented by a less invasive technique, therapy can be started without performing a pulmonary angiogram.

The diagnosis of proximal venous thrombosis has traditionally been made by means of contrast venography. However, this procedure is invasive, may cause considerable discomfort, and has been implicated in the generation of venous thrombosis. Critical evaluations of two noninvasive techniques for the detection of proximal venous thrombosis in the legs have been performed. The results of these evaluations suggest that the combination of iodine-125–fibrinogen leg scanning and impedance plethysmography can be used as an alternative to venography, with respectable sensitivity and specificity in patients with clinically suspected venous thrombosis. More recently, high-resolution B-mode ultrasound in combination with color Doppler imaging has been widely applied for the assessment of deep leg veins.

If the noninvasive venous imaging technique reveals proximal venous thrombosis, no need exists to proceed to pulmonary angiography because there is sufficient indication to initiate anticoagulation therapy. On the other hand, if the thrombus is localized below the calf or if no thrombus is revealed, pulmonary thromboembolism cannot be excluded with confidence because more than 20% of patients with pulmonary thromboembolism have no evidence of proximal venous thrombosis at diagnosis. Pulmonary angiography may be necessary in these patients.

DIFFERENTIAL DIAGNOSIS

The differential diagnosis for clinical syndromes suggestive of pulmonary thromboembolism can be subdivided into two parts: infarction and embolism without infarction.

Infarction

The differential diagnosis for pulmonary infarction includes bacterial pneumonia and pleurisy caused by either an infective process (e.g., viral) or an immunologic abnormality (e.g., postmyocardial infarction, Dressler's syndrome).

Embolism without infarction

Pulmonary embolism may result from nonthrombotic material, presenting with the same clinical syndrome as thromboembolism. The differential diagnosis includes septic, tumor, air, fat, bone marrow, and amniotic fluid embolism.

A catastrophic clinical presentation of pulmonary embolism may include circulatory collapse, which usually occurs when a large cross section of the pulmonary vascular tree is obstructed acutely. The differential diagnosis for this condition includes other forms of circulatory collapse, such as acute myocardial infarction, the hyperventilation syndrome, and tension pneumothorax.

Recurrent pulmonary embolism may simulate primary pulmonary hypertension or vasculitis affecting the pulmonary vasculature. Also, patients with acute pulmonary thromboembolism without a clear-cut underlying medical condition or risk factor may have an occult malignancy. Finally, younger patients with acute pulmonary thromboembolism may have an unrecognized specific deficiency of antithrombotic proteins, such as protein S, protein C, or antithrombin III and abnormal forms of fibrinogen.

TREATMENT

Anticoagulation with heparin (See also Chapter 86.)

In addition to heparin or low-molecular-weight heparin, additional supportive measures may be necessary in the acute period. If the patient has arterial hypoxemia, oxygen should be administered. Mild sedation or analgesia may be required to alleviate anxiety or pain, and in the event of circulatory collapse, inotropic agents should be administered; dopamine and isoproterenol are most often used.

Thrombolytic therapy

It has been demonstrated that streptokinase and urokinase, both widely available, are capable of rapidly lysing pulmonary thromboemboli. It is not yet clear, however, whether these agents should be employed in patients with proved pulmonary thromboembolism, even if the pulmonary vascular occlusion is severe enough to cause persistent vascular collapse and profound hypotension. Although long-term studies have shown that stimulation of the plasmin system with enzymes such as streptokinase and urokinase accelerates reversal of physiologic derangements caused by massive embolism, no impact on mortality has been demonstrated. Recent clinical studies on recombinant tissue plasminogen activator (rt-PA) indicate that rt-PA is safer and has more favorable adverse reaction profile than the conventional thrombolytic agents.

Patients in whom thrombolytic therapy may be appropriate are those with massive proximal pulmonary thromboembolism associated with persistent systemic hypotension and those with very little cardiopulmonary reserve. The rationale for thrombolytic therapy is to speed up the lysis of thrombi to restore normal cardiac output and to minimize obliteration of limited pulmonary capillary bed. If streptokinase is used, the dosage is usually 250,000 units (U) given intravenously over 30 minutes, followed by 100,000 U/hr for 24 hours. The dosage for urokinase is 4400 U/kg as a loading dose over 10 minutes, followed by 2200 U/kg/hr for 12 hours. The recommended protocol for rt-PA is 100 mg as a continuous intravenous infusion administered over 2 hours. No dosage adjustment is necessary, and heparin is not given concomitantly. After termination of the thrombolytic agent, heparin can be started when the activated partial thromboplastin time or thrombin time has fallen below twice the control value.

Pulmonary embolectomy

Surgical embolectomy is rarely indicated but may be considered in patients with massive proximal thromboembolic loads. Usually, patients for whom it would be useful die before the surgical team can be mobilized, and those who survive long enough for the procedure to be done usually achieve a stable state before actual emboletomy. Pulmonary embolectomy by a catheter device in selected patients may be a viable alternative at tertiary referral centers, but its widespread use remains to be critically assessed.

Long-term therapy

After the initiation of anticoagulation with heparin, the patient should be changed to maintenance therapy, which should consist of either oral warfarin or adjusted-dose subcutaneous heparin. Traditionally, warfarin is begun on day 3 to 5 after the initiation of heparin therapy. However, recent data indicate that warfarin can be initiated concurrently with heparin, substantially reducing the length of stay in the hospital.

An alternative to oral anticoagulation is to maintain patients on adjusted subcutaneous heparin, usually at about 10,000 U every 12 hours, with the dose tailored to maintain the activated partial thromboplastin time about 1.5 to 2.0 times the control value. This mode of maintenance anticoagulation therapy is perhaps ideal for patients who are pregnant because the heparin molecule does not cross the placenta.

Although no precise data define the necessary duration of anticoagulation, it is prudent to continue this therapy indefinitely in patients who have an ongoing predisposing condition or who have sustained more than one episode of thromboembolism separated by more than a few weeks. On the other hand, it usually seems appropriate to stop anticoagulants after 6 to 8 weeks in patients who are otherwise healthy and have self-limiting predisposing medical problems.

Vena caval interruption

Well-accepted indications for inferior vena caval interruption are (1) an absolute contraindication to anticoagulation, (2) recurrence or major bleeding while receiving effective anticoagulation, and (3) septic pulmonary thromboembolism from an infected pelvic focus. It is unwise to undertake caval interruption without angiographic confirmation of the diagnosis of pulmonary thromboembolism. In addition, it is probably inappropriate to undertake caval interruption unless it has been demonstrated clearly that residual thrombotic material exists in the pelvic or lower venous system.

PREVENTION

The principal strategy in preventing acute pulmonary thromboembolism is to identify high-risk patients and to administer prophylactic measures to prevent deep vein thrombosis. Early ambulation in postpartum and postoperative patients is the best prevention. All patients over age 40 who undergo lower abdominal or gynecologic surgery requiring general anesthesia should be considered for "minidose heparin" therapy (see the box below). The protocol includes an initial dose of 5000 U of heparin subcutaneously to be administered 2 hours before the procedure, followed by a maintenance schedule of 5000 U of heparin administered subcutaneously every 12 hours, and this should be continued until the patient is ambulatory. Evidence has been obtained that this regimen prevents deep vein thrombosis and nonlethal and lethal pulmonary thromboembolism in such patients, and the risk of hemorrhage with this protocol is minimal. This therapy, on the other hand, is neither effective nor safe in patients with hip fracture or replacement, in major trauma patients, or in those facing prostatic surgery. Data on low-molecular-weight heparin administered once daily seem to be at least comparable if not superior to data on conventional minidose or adjusted-dose heparin for the established clinical indications. However, low-molecular-weight heparin remains ineffective in the unworkable clinical settings (see the box).

Current data are not definitive regarding the prevention of nonlethal and lethal pulmonary thromboembolism in other groups of patients known to be at high risk of venous thrombosis. These groups include patients with congestive heart failure, myocardial infarction, varicose veins, and marked obesity, as well as those in the postpartum state and individuals immobilized because of severe illness. Accordingly, the application of heparin prophylaxis should be individualized for such patients. Obese patients with myocardial infarction and congestive heart failure would probably be good candidates, and a postpartum patient with a history of deep vein thrombosis would likely warrant prophylaxis.

The efficacy of other prophylactic drugs such as antiplatelet agents and dextran is unclear. However, preliminary data on intermittent calf compression devices suggest that they may provide a suitable alternative for preventing proximal venous thrombosis in patients at risk for bleeding complications with minidose heparin or in whom minidose heparin is known to be ineffective.

Indications for minidose heparin prophylaxis

Established

Major surgery
- Thoracic
- Abdominal
- Gynecologic

Questionable

Congestive heart failure
Myocardial infarction
Immobilization associated with:
- Marked obesity
- Varicose veins
- Postpartum state
- Malignancy

Unworkable

Total hip replacement
Major trauma
Prostatic surgery

REFERENCES

Carter BL, Jones ME, and Waickman LA: Pathophysiology and treatment of deep-vein thrombosis and pulmonary embolism. Clin Pharm 4:279, 1985.

Chan CK et al: Pulmonary tumor embolism: a critical review of clinical, imaging and hemodynamic features. J Thorac Imaging 2:4, 1987.

Come PC et al: Early reversal of right ventricular dysfunction in patients with acute pulmonary embolism after treatment with intravenous tissue plasminogen activator. J Am Coll Cardiol 10:971, 1987.

European Fraxiparin Study (EFS) Group: Comparison of a low molecular weight heparin and unfractionated heparin for the prevention of deep vein thrombosis in patients undergoing abdominal surgery. Br J Surg 75:1058, 1988.

Fulkerson WJ et al: Diagnosis of pulmonary embolism. Arch Intern Med 146:961, 1986.

Gallus A et al: Safety and efficacy of warfarin started early after submassive venous thrombosis or pulmonary embolism. Lancet 2:1293, 1986.

Gillum RF: Pulmonary embolism and thrombophlebitis in the United States 1970-1985. Am Heart J 114:1262, 1987.

Goldhaber SZ: Recent advances in the diagnosis and lytic therapy of pulmonary embolism. Chest 99:173S, 1991.

Leitha T et al: Pulmonary embolism: efficacy of d-dimer and thrombin-antithrombin III complex determinations as screening tests before lung scanning. Chest 100:1536, 1991.

Lund O et al: Pulmonary embolism: long-term follow-up after treatment with full-dose heparin, streptokinase or embolectomy, Acta Med Scand 221:61, 1987.

Monreal M et al: A prospective double-blind trial of a low molecular weight heparin once daily compared with conventional low-dose heparin three times daily to prevent pulmonary embolism and venous thrombosis in patients with hip fracture. J Trauma 29:873, 1989.

Petti DB, Strom PL, and Melon KL: Duration of warfarin anticoagulant therapy and the probability of recurrent embolism and hemorrhage. Am J Med 81:255, 1986.

PIOPED investigators: Value of the ventilation/perfusion scan in acute pulmonary embolism. JAMA 263:2753, 1990.

Schiff MJ, Feinberg AW, and Naidich JB: Noninvasive venous examinations as a screening test for pulmonary embolism. Arch Intern Med 147:505, 1987.

Steiner RA et al: A prospective randomized trial of low molecular weight heparin-DHE and conventional heparin-DHE (with acenocoumarol) in patients undergoing gynecological surgery. Arch Gynecol Obstet 244:141, 1989.

Timsit JF et al: Pulmonary embolectomy by catheter device in massive pulmonary embolism. Chest 100:655, 1991.

CHAPTER

218 Pleural Diseases

Ian R. G. Dowdeswell

ANATOMY AND PHYSIOLOGY

The pleura is a thin membrane lining the interior surface of the chest wall, the superior surface of the diaphragm, and the lateral aspect of the mediastinum (*parietal* pleura) and enveloping the lungs (*visceral* pleura); the interlobar fissures are also lined by visceral pleura. The visceral and parietal pleurae become continuous at the hila, creating two anatomically distinct potential spaces in each side of the thorax. Each of these pleural spaces contains a small quantity of lubricant fluid, which allows the pleural surfaces to glide smoothly over each other during the movement of respiration. In healthy individuals this fluid is probably less than 10 ml in each pleural space; the fluid contains 1.5 to 2.0 g of protein/dl and about 4500 cells/ml (predominantly mesothelial cells, monocytes, lymphocytes, and a few granulocytes).

The pleura consists histologically of single-cell-thickness mesothelial cells supported by layers of connective tissue, in which networks of lymphatics and capillaries are present. The parietal pleura is supplied by the systemic arterial circulation by way of the intercostal, internal mammary, and phrenic arteries; the visceral pleural capillaries are derived from the pulmonary and bronchial arterial systems. The parietal pleural vessels drain into the intercostal veins, and vessels from the visceral pleura drain into the pulmonary veins. Both parietal and visceral pleurae are liberally supplied with lymphatics, which drain toward the lower mediastinal lymph nodes and hilar nodes, respectively. The parietal pleura derives a rich supply of sensory nerve fibers from intercostal nerves, whereas the visceral pleura is virtually devoid of sensory innervation.

Fluid is formed continuously. Its transport in and out of the pleural space depends on the balance of hydrostatic and oncotic pressures in the capillary networks in the parietal and visceral pleurae. In healthy individuals the oncotic pressures are equal, but the higher hydrostatic pressure in the parietal pleura results in fluid being transferred to the pleural space, where it is reabsorbed by the lower-pressure visceral pleural system. The lymphatics play an important part in removing protein from the pleural space. Even though 600 to 800 ml is formed per day in healthy individuals, the pleural space is kept relatively free of fluid. Excess fluid accumulates if the balance of formation and absorption is upset to favor fluid formation. Excess fluid or pleural effusion is formed in the following situations: (1) when excessive hydrostatic pressure in the visceral pleura exists (e.g., cardiac failure), (2) when reduced osmotic pressure decreases reabsorption of fluid (e.g., nephrotic syndrome), (3) when the lymphatics draining the visceral pleura are obstructed (e.g., central carcinoma), and (4) when the permeability of the visceral or parietal pleura is disrupted (e.g., inflammation, carcinomatous involvement). The first two situations characteristically produce a transudate, but the latter two produce an exudate.

The pleura is normally kept free of gas because the combined partial pressures of oxygen, nitrogen, and carbon dioxide in venous blood lining the pleura are about 54 mm Hg less than atmospheric pressure.

Hydrostatic pleural pressure at functional residual capacity is about 2 mm Hg less than atmospheric pressure. Thus, when air is introduced into the intact pleural space, causing a pneumothorax, it will be reabsorbed steadily by the pleural venous system.

The function of the pleural space is obscure because the parietal pleura can be removed surgically without impairing pulmonary function. However, lining this potential space with stretchable mesothelial cells provides the lungs and other intrathoracic organs with great flexibility to expand, retract, and deform. In addition, the presence of this space allows the development of pleural effusions or pneumothorax in a variety of situations, sometimes with serious or catastrophic results. Large quantities of air or fluid may need to be drained as an emergency, and failure to remove pus or blood from the pleural space may lead to the formation of a fibrothorax with "trapped lung" and subsequent impairment of pulmonary function.

PLEURISY AND PLEURAL EFFUSION

The most common manifestation of pleural disease is pleural effusion, but inflammation of the pleura (pleurisy, or *pleuritis*) can occur in the absence of effusion.

Clinical description

The predominant clinical manifestation of pleural disease is *pleuritic pain,* which is characteristically "sharp" or "cutting" and associated with respiration. Pleuritic pain is often abrupt in onset and is sufficiently severe to induce the patient to seek medical attention. The pain increases on inspiration and decreases on expiration, and respiration may be associated with an expiratory grunt in an attempt to "splint" the chest. Deep breathing, coughing, and sneezing are particularly painful and are often suppressed, but pain may also be exacerbated by body movement. The pain is generally well localized to the adjacent area of disease, but because the lower intercostal nerves supply the abdominal wall as well as the chest, pleuritic pain may be referred to the abdomen. The central portion of the diaphragm has afferent nerve fibers from the phrenic nerve; therefore pain originating in this area may be referred to the shoulder. The combination of low chest pain and ipsilateral shoulder pain is highly suggestive of diaphragmatic pleural disease.

It is important to differentiate pleuritic pain from other causes of chest pain that appear to be related to respiration. Musculoskeletal disorders produce pain exacerbated by breathing, but this type of pain is usually less well localized and less severe than pleuritic pain unless caused by a fractured rib; in the absence of a history of trauma, a rib fracture may result from forceful coughing.

Pain from irritation of inflamed bronchi is dull and more prolonged and is usually associated with coughing rather than with normal respiration. Mediastinal pain tends to be midline and less severe and radiates to the back. Pericardial pain may be associated with respiratory movements but is usually substernal and may be relieved by leaning forward. Myocardial pain may generally be differentiated by its well-known characteristics. When pleuritic pain presents with its classic characteristics, it is generally not difficult to determine its origin, but it may be mistaken for extrathoracic, particularly subdiaphragmatic, pathology.

Other symptoms frequently associated with pleural disease are dyspnea, cough, and fever. *Dyspnea* may be the presenting symptom, since pleuritic pain may have been transient or not present at all in patients with chronic effusions. Dyspnea is often more severe if the effusion has collected rapidly or if a large effusion exists, such as when compression of the lung results in a restrictive ventilatory defect. Dyspnea and cough are often manifestations of "mediastinal shift," when the mediastinal contents are shifted to the unaffected side. *Cough,* when present, produces little or no sputum unless concomitant parenchymal disease is present. *Fever* often accompanies infection but may also be a manifestation of pulmonary infarction or neoplastic or collagen vascular disease.

DIAGNOSTIC TESTS

Physical examination

Examination of the chest should be accompanied by a thorough general examination, including the recording of lymphadenopathy, finger clubbing, skin lesions, signs of cardiac failure, or abdominal features that would help determine the cause of pleural involvement. Examination of the chest may be unrevealing if a small pleural effusion exists, but once the accumulated fluid is more than 500 to 600 ml, there are usually detectable clinical signs: decreased excursion of the chest on the affected side, "dullness" or "flatness" to percussion over the fluid (at the base of the lung when the patient is sitting or upright), diminished breath sounds on the affected side, and decreased vocal fremitus and resonance. Sometimes a creaky *pleural friction rub* is audible during the respiratory cycle, present in both inspiration and expiration; and egobronchophony may be heard over the level of the pleural fluid.

Radiologic manifestations

Conventional radiology is the first approach in evaluating pleural disease but can be aided by ultrasound or computed tomographic (CT) scans in confusing situations. The pleura is generally too thin to be recognized on radiographs unless its layers are doubled or abnormally thickened. The horizontal fissure on the right may be seen in up to 50% of normal posteroanterior (PA) chest films, and the major (oblique) fissures are often visible on lateral views. If pleural disease develops, pleural effusion is the most common radiologic manifestation. On PA films, at least 300 ml of fluid must be present before the costophrenic angle becomes blunted, although a lateral film may reveal a haziness in the posterior costophrenic angle before any abnormality is seen on the PA chest radiograph.

By the time the typical appearance of a small effusion develops in the erect adult, at least 1 L of fluid is present. Radiologically, this appearance includes the loss of the contour of the diaphragm, which is now replaced by a concave opacity located where the upper border of the diaphragm is hazy. In the presence of a large effusion, half the hemithorax or more may be opacified, and the consequent increased pressure may result in displacement of the mediastinum to the contralateral side. A subpulmonic or infrapulmonary effusion is sometimes seen when the hemidiaphragm appears to be elevated; on the left the distance between the diaphragm's upper border and the stomach bubble is increased.

Fluid may be confirmed by a lateral decubitus film with the patient lying on the affected side. In this position, effusions of 100 ml or less may be detected. Atypical appearances of effusions occur when there are pleural adhesions, when the fluid loculates, or when air and fluid are within the pleural cavity (a hydropneumothorax). Occasionally, fluid is present in the interlobar fissures and may form a pseudotumor, which disappears when the fluid is reabsorbed.

Pleural ultrasound

Pleural ultrasound is most often used to elucidate better an abnormality seen on chest radiograph. It is a particularly useful technique for determining the location of fluid in the presence of loculated effusions to help in draining either pus or blood from the pleural space. Also, ultrasound is a sensitive means of detecting fluid in ill patients in whom conventional radiography is limited.

Computed tomography

CT is now widely available and is particularly valuable in evaluating pleural disease in areas not well visualized on conventional radiographs, such as the paraspinous regions, anterior mediastinum, and apical areas. The extent of pleural effusions can be well defined, and mass lesions frequently can be distinguished from fluid to guide needle biopsy or drainage of fluid.

Although conventional radiology remains the main diagnostic procedure in pleural disease, the judicious use of both ultrasound and CT helps in delineating the extent of disease, guiding therapeutic maneuvers, and performing diagnostic procedures such as needle biopsy.

Thoracentesis, pleural biopsy, and thoracoscopy

(See also Chapter 196.)

Thoracentesis should be performed when the cause of the pleural effusion is not apparent, if empyema (accumulation of pus in the pleural space) is suspected, or if the effusion is producing dyspnea. The gross appearance of the fluid is important, particularly in determining if the fluid is uniformly blood stained; a traumatic tap has probably occurred if the fluid clears as more fluid is withdrawn. Empyema or chylous effusions may be recognized at the time of the procedure. The importance of the initial thoracentesis is to differentiate between a *transudate,* which does not require further investigation, and an *exudate,* which indicates inflammation or malignancy. If the cause of an exudate is not determined by initial examination of the fluid, pleural needle biopsy should be undertaken to provide more material for histology and culture. Thoracoscopy, a procedure that provides direct visualization of the visceral and parietal pleura both on the lateral and the diaphragmatic areas, is being increasingly used to evaluate effusions of undetermined etiology and thus increase the diagnostic yield. If these measures are unsuccessful, a limited thoracotomy is sometimes needed to acquire large specimens for analysis.

Despite thorough investigation, 5% to 15% of pleural effusions remain undiagnosed or nonspecific in nature.

SPECIFIC DISEASES

The predominant causes of pleural effusions are congestive heart failure, neoplastic disease, and infections. The box on the right gives a comprehensive list of the causes. Classification into transudate or exudate and specific diagnosis are important to allow appropriate therapy.

Classification of pleural effusions

I. Transudates
- A. Increased hydrostatic pressure
  1. Congestive heart failure
  2. Constrictive pericarditis
  3. Superior vena caval obstruction
- B. Decreased oncotic pressure
  1. Hypoalbuminemia
     a. Nephrotic syndrome
     b. Cirrhosis
  2. Intra-abdominal disease
     a. Cirrhosis with ascites
     b. Peritoneal dialysis

II. Exudates
- A. Infections
  1. Parapneumonic empyema or effusion
  2. Tuberculosis
  3. Fungi
  4. Parasites
  5. Viral
  6. *Mycoplasma*
- B. Neoplasms
  1. Bronchogenic carcinoma
  2. Metastatic carcinoma
  3. Lymphoma and leukemia
  4. Mesothelioma
- C. Pulmonary emboli and infarction
- D. Intra-abdominal disease
  1. Subdiaphragmatic abscess
  2. Pancreatitis
  3. Meigs' syndrome
- E. Connective tissue and hypersensitivity disease
  1. Rheumatoid arthritis
  2. Lupus erythematosus
  3. Dressler's syndrome
  4. Drug reaction
- F. Miscellaneous
  1. Esophageal rupture
  2. Familial Mediterranean fever
  3. Lymphedema
  4. Myxedema
  5. Atelectasis
  6. Uremia
  7. Benign asbestos related
- G. Idiopathic

III. Hemothorax

IV. Lipidic
- A. Chylous
- B. Cholesterol or pseudochylous

Transudates

Congestive heart failure is the leading cause of transudative pleural effusions. Effusions resulting from congestive heart failure are frequently bilateral, but if unilateral, the right side is more frequently affected. If the effusion has been present for some time or if sampled after diuresis, the fluid protein content may be greater than 3 g/dl. However, if the signs of cardiac failure are florid, thoracentesis is not necessary unless another cause is suspected. Effusions secondary to cardiac failure usually decrease with successful treatment of the underlying disease.

Constrictive pericarditis and *superior vena caval obstruction* may be associated with either transudate or exudate.

Transudates caused by a reduced oncotic pressure *(hypoalbuminemia)* are seen in nephrotic syndrome or cirrhosis. Ascites is usually present. Patients with *nephrotic syndrome* usually have bilateral effusions that reaccumulate after thoracentesis unless the underlying cause is treated. The effusion associated with ascites resulting from *cirrhosis* is right sided in two thirds of patients, left sided in one sixth, and bilateral in another sixth. Occasionally, thoracentesis is necessary, but the effusions usually respond to diuretic therapy or when the liver disease improves. The fluid is transported through the diaphragm, so paracentesis may be helpful in relieving the pleural effusion.

Small pleural effusions may develop in patients undergoing peritoneal dialysis. The fluid is similar to the dialysate and is reabsorbed when dialysis is terminated.

Exudates

Infections. Parapneumonic effusions frequently occur with bacterial pneumonias and may also accompany lung abscess or bronchiectasis. These effusions may be sterile or may contain infectious organisms. By definition, an *empyema* is pus in the pleural cavity and frequently contains organisms that may be cultured before therapy is instituted. It is important to examine a parapneumonic effusion early to determine whether it is likely to resolve with appropriate antibiotic therapy or whether tube drainage is required; sterile effusions can usually be managed with thoracentesis alone. A white cell count greater than 15,000/mm^3 or a pH less than 7.3 suggests that tube drainage will decrease the morbidity produced by the effusion. Early antibiotic therapy may obviate the need for pleural drainage. Once empyema has developed, drainage of the pleural space is almost always necessary to effect a bacteriologic cure and preserve pulmonary function; however, fibrinous adhesions in the pleural space may preclude adequate drainage without operative thoracostomy.

The common organisms responsible for empyema reported in recent series are anaerobes (often more than one organism), *Staphylococcus aureus, Pseudomonas* species, and *Escherichia coli*. *Streptococcus pneumoniae* is less often identified as a causative organism since the advent of effective antibiotics, although parapneumonic effusions are seen in 40% to 60% of patients with pneumococcal pneumonia.

Empyema may also be a complication of thoracic surgery, trauma, or ruptured esophagus. Recognition of the underlying condition and drainage of the pleural space are important in the successful management of these patients.

Tuberculosis may produce either a serous exudative effusion or a frank tuberculous empyema. The former is associated with a small inoculation of tubercle bacilli into the pleural space when a subpleural, caseous focus ruptures; usually the pulmonary parenchyma appears normal on chest radiograph. Serous exudative effusion occurs within 3 to 6 months of the primary infection, and most patients are reactive to intermediate-strength tuberculin (purified protein derivative [PPD]), although a negative skin test does not exclude the diagnosis. Clinically the presentation may be acute, with fever and chest pain of a few days' duration, or subacute, with symptoms of up to a month's duration; less frequently the symptoms may have persisted for longer. In the vast majority of patients the effusion is small to moderate in size and unilateral.

Although tuberculous pleurisy is becoming less common in the United States, it is still a frequent finding in the developing world. It is also an important diagnosis to make because, although the natural history of tuberculous pleurisy results in resolution in the early phase, 45% to 65% of patients will proceed to active pulmonary tuberculosis if untreated. The diagnosis is confirmed by culturing sputum, pleural fluid, or pleural biopsy material for mycobacteria. The yield of sputum and pleural fluid cultures is usually about 10% and 25%, respectively. Analysis of the fluid usually shows a very high protein content (more than 5 g/dl) and a lymphocyte predominance in the white cells. Occasionally a polymorphonuclear predominance is seen early in the disease; an eosinophilia of more than 10% is suggestive of another diagnosis. Glucose and lactate dehydrogenase (LDH) levels are not helpful in distinguishing tuberculous from malignant effusions. Needle biopsy of the pleura is particularly helpful and is positive in about 60% of patients; repeat biopsies may increase the yield to as high as 80%.

In contrast, tuberculous empyema occurs in patients with overt pulmonary tuberculosis and is the result of a bronchopleural fistula. The fluid is occasionally green in color and is less viscid than frank pus, or it may appear to be indistinguishable from empyema caused by other organisms. The bacteria are usually seen on direct acid-fast smear; cultures are positive. Tube drainage is necessary and may need to be prolonged. (Specific chemotherapy of tuberculosis is discussed in Chapter 276.)

Fungal diseases are an infrequent cause of small pleural effusions. About 5% of patients with coccidioidomycosis are reported to have pleural effusion. Effusion is not frequently reported in blastomycosis, cryptococcosis, and aspergillosis but may be more common in histoplasmosis than previously recognized.

Pulmonary infections caused by *Actinomyces israelii* and *Nocardia asteroides* are frequently associated with an empyema that may penetrate through the chest wall to present as a subcutaneous swelling or a draining sinus. Both are subacute or chronic diseases; *N. asteroides* is more common in immunosuppressed patients. The diagnosis of *A. israelii* is suggested by the presence of sulfur granules in the pleural fluid or draining sinuses, and confirmation is obtained by culture. Nocardiosis may be associated with hematogenous dissemination and a less favorable outcome. Patients with actinomycosis are best treated with high-dose penicillin but also respond to prolonged tetracyline or lincomycin therapy. Those with nocardiosis are treated with sulfonamides.

Viral diseases and *Mycoplasma* pneumonias may be infrequently accompanied by effusions that are usually small and resolve without specific therapy. Rarely, *Mycoplasma* pneumonia is associated with a larger effusion, and thoracentesis is required to exclude the development of empyema. Coxsackievirus B infection producing pleurodynia may be associated with a small pleural effusion for which no specific therapy is required.

Parasitic infections that may produce pleural exudates include *amebiasis* when the right-sided effusion is the result of either sympathetic effusion or rupture of a liver abscess through the diaphragm to produce an empyema. The diagnosis may be suspected in endemic areas and confirmed by demonstrating a liver abscess in the presence of indirect hemagglutination tests. Treatment is usually satisfactory with antiamebic drugs, but occasionally surgical drainage is required. Hydatid disease of the lungs or liver, caused by *Echinococcus granulosus,* may sometimes be complicated by pleural involvement, as may paragonimiasis, which is caused by the lung fluke *Paragonimus westermani*.

Malignant pleural effusion. Malignant pleural effusion is the most common cause of exudative effusion, particularly in older patients and when the effusion is moderate to massive in extent. The leading cause of malignant effusion is lung cancer, followed by breast carcinoma and then lymphoma; ovarian and other carcinomas, sarcomas, and pleural tumors are less frequent causes. If bilateral effusions are present, the cause is more likely metastatic carcinoma than bronchogenic carcinoma. The mechanisms responsible for malignant effusion are increased permeability caused by pleural metastases involving visceral or parietal pleura and lymphatic obstruction resulting in impaired pleural lymphatic drainage. Atelectasis may also contribute to pleural fluid collection, as may pericardial involvement and postobstructive pneumonia. Most malignant effusions are symptomatic, the most common symptoms being cough, chest pain, and dyspnea; other nonspecific symptoms include anorexia, weight loss, and general malaise.

The diagnosis of malignant pleural involvement may be confirmed by cytologic examination of the fluid or by pleural biopsy. Repeat aspiration and biopsy result in a diagnostic yield of up to 80%. Diagnostic thoracoscopy has increased the yield to more than 90% in some centers. It is important to establish if malignant cells are present in the effusion because this indicates that curative surgery is not feasible. However, if cytology of the fluid and pleural biopsy are negative in the presence of a proximal tumor, a small number may be resectable.

Management of patients with malignant effusion caused by lung cancer depends on the identification of the primary tumor; if the primary is likely to be responsive to chemotherapy, this treatment may provide cure or long-term palliation. If the primary tumor is not chemosensitive and the effusion is causing symptoms, drainage of the pleural space may be helpful. Determining the rate of reaccumulation of fluid helps determine whether pleurodesis should be attempted. Removal of the pleura surgically is seldom indicated but is usually successful in patients who are found to have malignant pleural involvement at thoracotomy. If the lung re-expands well with thoracentesis, chemical pleurodesis is worth attempting in selected patients. Various chemical irritants have been tried, including tetracycline, bleomycin, and doxycycline, with similar results. More recently, insufflation of talc at thoracoscopy has been reported to be very effective in producing pleurodesis in patients whose effusions can be drained with good expansion of the underlying lung. Occasionally, radiation therapy to the mediastinum is useful when lymphatic obstruction plays a significant role in the pathogenesis of the effusion.

The management of patients with metastatic carcinomas and lymphomas producing pleural effusion depends on the treatment of the primary tumor. Chemical pleurodesis or radiation therapy may be useful in controlling symptoms. Small effusions that do not produce significant symptoms do not need specific therapy.

Pulmonary infarction. Pulmonary infarction, which occurs in 30% to 50% of patients with pulmonary embolism, is often accompanied by a pleural effusion. Pleuritic chest pain, usually of abrupt onset and associated with dyspnea, is present in about 80%. Radiologically the effusion may be associated with a parenchymal infiltrate, and bilateral effusions may be seen. The fluid usually has the characteristics of an exudate and is blood stained in 50% of patients. (Further details of diagnosis and management are discussed in Chapter 217.)

Intra-abdominal diseases. Diseases of the gastrointestinal tract sometimes produce exudative pleural effusion. *Pancreatic disease* is frequently complicated by effusion; acute pancreatitis is associated with pleural effusion in nearly 20% of patients. The effusion is most often on the left but may be right sided or bilateral. The mechanism may be (1) transdiaphragmatic transfer of fluid arising from the pancreatic inflammation or (2) a sinus tract formation between the pancreatic bed and the pleura. The fluid, which is often serosanguineous, frequently has amylase levels that are elevated for longer than the serum amylase levels and may be very high. Persistence of the effusion after the pancreatitis has resolved suggests the possibility of pancreatic abscess or pseudocyst. In these patients the effusion may be resolved only by a surgical approach to the pancreatic disease; if a sinus tract is found, it should be ligated or excised.

Subphrenic abscess is a complication of gastrointestinal surgery, splenectomy, and exploratory laparotomy for trauma. Approximately 50% of subphrenic abscesses are associated with a pleural effusion, which usually has a high white cell count and is sterile. CT scan or ultrasound may be helpful in demonstrating the subphrenic fluid collection. If a right-sided effusion is present, the possibility of intrahepatic abscess, either pyogenic or amebic, should be considered.

Meigs' syndrome is the association of a pelvic neoplasm with ascites and pleural effusion. It was originally described with benign fibromas of the ovary but has been associated with other benign pelvic tumors. The exudative effusion is characteristically right sided but may be bilateral. The ascites is not always detected clinically unless the pelvic tumor is large. The syndrome resolves after removal of the tumor.

Connective tissue disease. Connective tissue diseases may be associated with pleural effusion during the course of the disease. About 5% of patients with *rheumatoid arthritis* develop pleural effusions; this finding is more common in males and in older patients with a long history of arthritis and subcutaneous nodules. The effusion characteristically produces symptoms of pleuritic pain and usually is small to moderate in size and unilateral. One third of patients have associated intrapulmonary manifestations of rheumatoid arthritis. The fluid generally is yellow and may be turbid; lymphocytes predominate. Characteristically the fluid glucose level is very low (usually <20 mg/dl), the pH is low (< 7.20), and LDH and rheumatoid factor titers are high. Another interesting feature is the fluid tends to contain cholesterol crystals or high levels of cholesterol. Closed pleural biopsy is of limited value in diagnosing rheumatoid disease because of the infrequency of finding rheumatoid nodules but may be useful in excluding other etiologies for effusion. Rheumatoid effusions tend to resolve slowly and respond poorly to therapy; occasionally, decortication is required.

Both *systemic lupus erythematosus* (SLE) and *drug-induced LE* may affect the pleura, producing an effusion in 16% to 40% of patients, although almost 60% report episodes of pleuritic chest pain during the course of their disease. The effusions tend to be small, evanescent, and recurrent; they are frequently bilateral. The fluid is a yellow exudate in which either polymorphs or lymphocytes may predominate; complement levels are usually low. Unlike rheumatoid pleuritis, glucose level and pH tend to be near serum levels, and antinuclear antibody (ANA) may be demonstrated. Also, in contrast to those with rheumatoid effusion, patients with pleural disease of SLE respond to corticosteroid therapy.

Drug hypersensitivity reactions account for only a small percentage of all pleural effusions, but it is an important cause to consider in the differential diagnosis of an exudate because there is usually rapid resolution after withdrawal of the drug. In addition to drugs that induce a lupus syndrome (i.e., hydralazine, procainamide, phenytoin, isoniazid), nitrofurantoin, methysergide, procarbazine, and methotrexate have been reported to produce pleural reactions.

Dressler's syndrome is characterized by pericarditis, pleuritis, and pneumonitis occurring after pericardial injury caused by trauma, surgery, or myocardial infarction. Pleural effusion may develop; the fluid is yellow or sanguineous. The diagnosis is suggested in the appropriate clinical setting and is confirmed by excluding pulmonary infarction or pneumonia. The patient's symptoms usually respond to nonsteroidal anti-inflammatory drugs.

Miscellaneous disorders. *Asbestos* exposure has been associated with benign exudative pleural effusions that are sometimes persistent or recurrent and may lead to pleural fibrosis; occasionally, these effusions are followed by the development of mesothelioma. The diagnosis is one of exclusion.

Esophageal rupture, although infrequent, should always be considered in the differential diagnosis of pleural effusion because the mortality is very high if the condition is not treated rapidly. The diagnosis should be suggested if the fluid examination reveals a high amylase (salivary) level, a low pH, squamous epithelial cells, and occasionally, food particles.

Other, less common causes of pleural effusion are listed in the box on p. 1757. Even after intensive diagnostic efforts, the etiology in some patients remains obscure, and it may be necessary to follow the clinical course of these patients. If the only positive finding has been a positive tuberculin skin test in the absence of other confirmatory evidence for tuberculosis, it is appropriate to give a course of antituberculous therapy followed by serial radiographs.

Hemothorax

Hemothorax occurs when a significant amount of blood is present in the pleural space, as opposed to a serosanguineous effusion. The hematocrit is usually more than 50% of the blood level. The most common cause of hemothorax is trauma, either penetrating or nonpenetrating, and is often associated with a pneumothorax. Occasionally, spontaneous pneumothorax is complicated by a small hemothorax. Iatrogenic hemothorax is being reported more frequently with placement of central venous catheters; thoracentesis or pleural biopsy is occasionally complicated by hemothorax. Nontraumatic hemothorax occurs infrequently but is seen in metastatic pleural disease and as a complication of anticoagulant therapy. Rupture of an aortic aneurysm rarely presents as hemothorax. Treatment is directed to the underlying condition and to evacuating the blood from the pleural space, usually by intercostal tube drainage, so that blood loss can be monitored and development of a secondary blood infection or subsequent fibrothorax can be prevented. Occasionally, bleeding persists and a thoracotomy is necessary.

Lipid effusions

When high levels of lipid accumulate in the pleural space, the fluid appears milky or turbid. Lipid effusions occur in two situations: (1) a *chylothorax* forms when the thoracic duct is disrupted and chyle enters the pleural space; and (2) in longstanding effusions, large amounts of cholesterol or lecithin-globulin complexes accumulate to produce a chyliform effusion, and the patient is said to have a *pseudochylothorax*. It is important to distinguish between these two conditions because the etiology and management are completely different.

The most common cause of chylothorax is tumor, predominantly lymphoma. The second most frequent cause is trauma, generally in a postoperative situation after cardiovascular surgery. In about 15% of patients, the cause is said to be idiopathic, including congenital. Chyle is bacteriostatic, so infection occurs infrequently. Symptoms of chylothorax are related to the presence of space-occupying fluid, and patients develop dyspnea. The fluid is milky white and odorless, and the constituents can be confirmed by staining with Sudan III and analyzing the triglyceride content, which is usually greater than 150 mg/dl. The demonstration of chylomicrons in the fluid establishes the diagnosis. The pleural surfaces are normal. Treatment is directed to the cause because the fluid tends to recur after aspiration. Repeated aspiration is not advisable because the patient may become nutritionally depleted. Treatment of patients with progressive chylous effusions includes dietary modification and thoracic duct ligation if conservative measures fail.

The pathogenesis of pseudochylothorax is not known, but most patients with chyliform effusion have longstanding effusion with thickened, occasionally calcified pleura. The fluid is negative when stained with Sudan III dye and has a high-cholesterol content, sometimes greater than 1000 mg/dl. These effusions may result from rheumatoid arthritis or tuberculosis but are often idiopathic. Treatment is directed toward the underlying condition; occasionally, decortication is indicated.

Pneumothorax

Pneumothorax is defined as the presence of air in the pleural space, occurring either spontaneously or as a result of trauma. A classification of pneumothorax is shown in the box at upper right.

Pathogenesis. *Spontaneous* pneumothorax, which occurs without antecedent trauma, may be classified as primary

Classification of pneumothorax

Spontaneous pneumothorax
- Primary (no previous lung disease)
- Secondary
  - Pre-existing lung disease
  - Catamenial

Traumatic pneumothorax
- Chest trauma
  - Penetrating
  - Nonpenetrating
- Iatrogenic

pneumothorax or secondary pneumothorax; the latter occurs with associated underlying lung disease. *Primary* spontaneous pneumothorax results from rupture of subpleural blebs, which are usually located at the apices. The cause of these blebs and why they rupture are unclear, but patients with this disorder have been reported to be taller and thinner than age-matched control subjects. It is reported that primary spontaneous pneumothorax is more common in smokers. *Secondary* spontaneous pneumothorax occurs most often in patients with chronic obstructive lung disease, including asthma, and less frequently in patients with granulomatous disease such as tuberculosis or sarcoidosis. Bronchogenic carcinoma, suppurative lung disease, and pulmonary fibrosis may also be associated with pneumothorax. Rarely, pneumothorax is associated with menstruation (*catamenial* pneumothorax).

Traumatic pneumothorax may be iatrogenic in origin or result from penetrating or nonpenetrating injuries. Iatrogenic pneumothorax is becoming increasingly common with the widespread use of invasive procedures such as transbronchial biopsy, percutaneous fine-needle aspiration of the lung, mechanical ventilation with positive end-expiratory pressure, and subclavian vein catheterization. Nonpenetrating trauma causing pneumothorax may be associated with fractured ribs and thus laceration of the lung. Sudden compression of the chest is thought to cause raised intra-alveolar pressure and rupture. Occasionally the trachea or major bronchi are ruptured, and it is important to recognize this complication because surgical repair is often necessary. This complication is usually associated with severe trauma involving fracture of one or more of the first three ribs.

Clinical manifestations. The symptoms and physical findings depend largely on the volume of gas in the pleural space and the extent of any underlying lung disease. The onset of dyspnea and pleuritic chest pain is usually sudden, with chest pain usually localized to the affected side. Primary spontaneous pneumothorax occurs most often in thin, asthenic men 30 to 40 years of age and, interestingly, occurs infrequently during vigorous exercise. Many of these patients do not seek medical attention immediately. Dyspnea is more prominent if the pneumothorax is large, and the clinical signs of decreased excursion of the affected hemithorax, with diminished breath sounds in the presence of normal or hyperresonant percussion, are characteristic. Arterial hypoxemia may be present early, but a subsequent decrease of both perfusion and ventilation to the affected lung may result in almost-normal arterial blood gases in subjects with otherwise healthy lungs.

Patients with secondary spontaneous pneumothorax, however, more frequently seek assistance early because symptoms are more severe. The severity of the symptoms appears out of proportion to the size of the pneumothorax, particularly in those with obstructive pulmonary disease, and the clinical signs are more difficult to elicit. In patients being supported by positive-pressure ventilation, the development of a pneumothorax is frequently associated with positive end-expiratory pressure and is manifested by the development of high peak inspiratory pressure with decreased lung compliance. Chest radiographs are essential to confirm the diagnosis and to quantitate the volume of the pneumothorax.

Treatment. For patients with primary spontaneous pneumothorax, treatment depends on the severity of symptoms and the size of the pneumothorax. Air leaks usually seal spontaneously, and the air is gradually reabsorbed. However, recurrence develops in about 50% of patients after the first pneumothorax; after the second the recurrence rates increase. If the pneumothorax is more than 40%, tube thoracostomy is required to allow the lung to re-expand and to seal the air leak. In recurrent pneumothorax or if an air leak persists, thoracotomy, with oversewing of the blebs and pleural scarification, is effective in preventing further episodes. The role of chemical pleurodesis remains controversial, but this approach should be considered in managing patients with secondary pneumothorax who are poor surgical candidates. More recently the use of the thoracoscope for chemical pleurodesis or pleural scarification provides the opportunity to avoid a thoracotomy; subpleural blebs may also be resected or oversewn using this technique. Iatrogenic pneumothorax can be managed conservatively unless the pneumothorax is large or unless the patient is on a positive-pressure ventilator, in which case tube thoracostomy is mandatory. Also, it may be necessary to reduce positive end-expiratory pressure to allow the air leak to seal.

Complications

Tension pneumothorax. A tension pneumothorax is present when air in the pleural space exceeds atmospheric pressure during expiration and often during inspiration. This abnormality produces major collapse of the lung and displacement of the mediastinum to the unaffected side, progressing to shock, which is probably on the basis of hypoxemia rather than decreased venous return. The progression of tension pneumothorax is thought to be caused by a one-way valve effect resulting in air entering the pleural space during inspiration and being trapped during expiration. Although tension pneumothorax occasionally develops after spontaneous pneumothorax, it occurs more often after traumatic pneumothorax or when a patient is on a positive-pressure ventilator. The clinical manifestations include tachypnea, central cyanosis, and a larger hemithorax on the affected side, with a shift of the trachea to the contralateral side. Tension pneumothorax is a medical emergency and requires prompt decompression with a needle, catheter, or tube thoracostomy.

Pulmonary edema. Pulmonary edema can occur after rapid re-expansion of a lung following drainage of either a pneumothorax or a pleural effusion. The mechanism remains obscure, but controlled removal of air or fluid from the pleural space is likely to reduce the incidence of pulmonary edema.

Pyopneumothorax is seen as a complication of suppurative lung disease, tuberculosis, or ruptured esophagus. Large-tube thoracostomy drainage is required to prevent the development of fibrothorax. *Hemopneumothorax* may occur after trauma to the chest, and chest tube drainage is required, as for hemothorax.

Malignant mesothelioma

Malignant mesothelioma is a rare tumor being recognized more frequently because of its association with asbestos exposure and the widespread use of asbestos until 1970. It occurs most frequently in asbestos workers, particularly in the manufacturing industries (Chapter 211). The interval between first exposure and presentation with the tumor is usually 25 to 45 years, but periods varying from 10 to 60 years have been reported. Pathologically, marked variation within a single tumor is characteristic, and differentiation from the much more common adenocarcinoma may be difficult, particularly early in the disease. Histologically, these tumors have been classified as epithelial, mesenchymal (sarcomatoid), or mixed. Initially, discrete plaques and nodules of firm, grayish tumor occur in the pleura; these progress to produce adherent parietal and visceral pleura, which encases and constricts the lung. Invasion of the chest wall or pericardium may occur. Lymphatic or hematogeneous spread is a late feature, but at autopsy, peritoneal involvement is not unusual. The diagnosis may only be confirmed by extensive sampling or at open biopsy. Special stains and electron microscopy may be necessary to differentiate the tumor from adenocarcinoma.

Clinical presentation usually occurs in patients over age 40 years, with insidious onset of dyspnea, chest pain, or both. Weight loss and a dry, hacking cough develop with progression of the disease. Clinically and radiologically, a pleural effusion usually is found. After drainage, irregular pleural thickening may be seen in association with loss of volume of the underlying lung. This may be better visualized on a chest CT scan, when any pericardial or mediastinal involvement can also be appreciated. The pleural fluid is yellow or serosanguineous and contains a mixture of normal mesothelial cells with other cells of varying differentiation. It is seldom possible to confirm the diagnosis on cytologic examination alone. The outlook is generally poor because these tumors are relatively unresponsive to chemotherapy or irradiation. Occasionally, excision of the pleura is successful in prolonging survival, and this modality should be considered if an open biopsy is undertaken. Although these tumors may metastasize, death usually results from intrathoracic complications.

Benign mesotheliomas remain localized and produce large, well-circumscribed globular masses, and only 10% are associated with pleural effusions. About 50% of these tumors are asymptomatic, but 20% are associated with hypertrophic osteoarthropathy. Diagnosis is made at thoracotomy, when the treatment is surgical excision; the lung parenchyma sometimes must be resected as well. Recurrence has been reported.

Pleural calcification

Unilateral pleural calcification may develop after hemothorax, empyema, and tuberculous effusions. Calcified plaques, often on the diaphragmatic surface, may be seen in subjects exposed to asbestos and talc or in association with asbestosis.

REFERENCES

American College of Physicians, Health and Public Policy Committee: Diagnostic thoracentesis and pleural biopsy in pleural effusions. Ann Intern Med 102:799, 1985.

Boutin C et al: The role of thoracoscopy in the evaluation and management of pleural effusions. Lung 168(suppl):1113, 1990.

Chretien J et al, editors: The pleura in health and disease. New York, 1985, Marcel Dekker.

Light RW: Pleural diseases, ed 2. Philadelphia, 1990, Lea & Febiger.

Sahn SA: The pleura—state of the art. Am Rev Respir Dis 138:184, 1988.

CHAPTER

219 Diseases of the Mediastinum

Ian R. G. Dowdeswell

ANATOMY AND PHYSIOLOGY

The mediastinum comprises the part of the thorax that lies between the lungs. Its contents can become involved in various diseases. The mediastinum is bounded superiorly by the thoracic inlet, anteriorly by the sternum, laterally by the parietal pleura, inferiorly by the diaphragm, and posteriorly by the spine and ribs. Within the mediastinum lie the heart and central vessels, the major airways, the esophagus, phrenic nerves, vagus nerves, sympathetic trunks, lymph nodes, and the main channel of the lymphatic system. All these structures can be affected primarily or secondarily by diseases involving the mediastinum.

Classically the mediastinum is divided into three compartments. The anterior, or anterosuperior, mediastinum extends from the thoracic inlet superiorly, along the anterior spinal ligament of the first four vertebrae posteriorly, forward to the anterior aspect of the pericardium and small portion of the anterior diaphragm inferiorly, and is bounded by the sternum anteriorly. The middle mediastinum extends from the level of the fourth thoracic vertebra superiorly and is bounded by the posterior pericardium, diaphragm, and anterior pericardium. The posterior mediastinum lies behind the middle mediastinum, extending up to the anterior mediastinum, and is bounded by the posterior chest wall. The contents of each compartment are listed in the box below.

The mediastinum is not a rigid compartment and may be displaced from its central position if the pressures in the pleural spaces are disrupted, such as by tension pneumothorax, pleural effusion, or pneumonectomy. Abrupt displacement of the mediastinum can impair cardiorespiratory function, but insidious growth of a mediastinal mass can also compress vital structures, producing symptoms indicative of cardiorespiratory impairment. The elasticity and compliance of the mediastinum decrease with age or disease (e.g., neoplasm, chronic inflammation).

CLINICAL MANIFESTATIONS

Symptoms of central chest pain, cough, hoarseness, stridor, or dyspnea may indicate mediastinal abnormality. In adults, almost 50% of mediastinal masses are asymptomatic; inflammatory disease is more likely to be symptomatic. In children, however, mediastinal lesions are more likely to cause symptoms and findings. About 50% of symptomatic mediastinal masses prove to be malignant, whereas about 90% of asymptomatic masses are benign.

Contents of the mediastinum

Anterior or anteroposterior

Thymus gland
Aortic arch and major branches
Innominate veins
Lymphatic and areolar tissue
Thyroid gland (occasionally)
Upper trachea and upper esophagus

Middle

Heart
Pericardium
Trachea
Hilum of each lung
Tracheobronchial lymph nodes
Phrenic nerves

Posterior

Esophagus
Vagus nerves
Sympathetic nerve chains
Thoracic duct
Descending aorta
Azygos and hemiazygos venous systems
Paravertebral lymph nodes

The most frequent symptoms are chest pain, cough, dyspnea, recurrent respiratory infection, and dysphagia, all usually resulting from compression by a mediastinal lesion or invasion of adjacent structures. Less frequent local symptoms include superior vena caval obstruction, vocal cord paralysis, Horner's syndrome, and spinal cord compression. A few patients have tumors or cysts that impinge on the heart or great vessels and produce symptoms simulating cardiac disease (e.g., pericardial involvement, pericardial tamponade). The presence of cough, hemoptysis, or stridor with a mediastinal mass suggests malignancy; hemoptysis is particularly suggestive of a bronchogenic carcinoma. Inspiratory stridor may occur with narrowing of the extrathoracic trachea or bilateral vocal cord paralysis and is an ominous finding. Usually, tumors grow to a large size before pain develops, but retrosternal pain suggests malignancy or inflammatory disease. Dyspnea may be caused by compression of the major airways, involvement of the phrenic nerve paralyzing diaphragmatic function, or a concomitant pleural effusion. The box below lists manifestations of local compression or invasion.

Some patients have systemic symptoms. These symptoms may result from endocrine secretion by the tumor, such as manifestations of hyperthyroidism caused by intrathoracic thyroid adenoma, hypercalcemia secondary to parathyroid adenoma, and systemic hypertension in association with neurogenic tumor. Myasthenia gravis occurs with thymoma, and fever occurs with Hodgkin's disease (Table 219-1).

Superior vena caval obstruction

Obstruction of the superior vena cava produces a characteristic syndrome that often appears abruptly with headache, swelling, and venous engorgement of the face, chest, and arms. Patients with superior vena caval obstruction have distended, nonpulsatile jugular veins and often prominent upper thoracic collateral venous circulation. Obstruction below the junction of the azygos vein usually produces greater obstructive symptoms and results in more extensive collat-

Manifestations of compression and invasion by mediastinal masses

Cough
Hemoptysis
Stridor
Dyspnea, especially with phrenic nerve palsy
Hoarseness (vocal cord paralysis)
Superior vena caval obstruction
Pain (usually retrosternal)
Dysphagia
Pleural effusion, including chylothorax
Spinal cord compression
Pericarditis and pericardial tamponade
Horner's syndrome

Table 219-1. Systemic syndromes associated with mediastinal tumors

Tumor	Syndrome
Thymoma	Myasthenia gravis, red cell aplasia, hypogammaglobulinemia, Cushing's syndrome
Germ cell tumor	Gynecomastia
Substernal goiter	Thyrotoxicosis
Lymphoma (e.g., Hodgkin's disease)	Fever of undetermined origin, hypercalcemia
Neurofibroma, neurilemmoma	Osteoarthropathy
Pheochromocytoma	Hypertension
Ganglioneuroma	Hypertension, diarrhea
Parathyroid adenoma	Hypercalcemia

eral routes through the abdominal wall to enter the drainage system of the inferior vena cava. Obstruction above the azygos veins results only in the development of collateral drainage into the azygos system and thus the right atrium. Conjunctival edema and even chemosis can occur when obstruction has been rapid in onset.

Caval obstruction is usually readily apparent clinically, but identification of the cause of the obstruction may be more difficult. In patients with a history of cigarette smoking, especially middle-aged males, the diagnosis is almost always bronchogenic carcinoma. Attempts to confirm the diagnosis histologically must be undertaken with care because of the risks of bleeding from the engorged and extensive venous bed. Sputum cytology may be helpful. If cytology is negative, bronchoscopy may be undertaken with reasonable safety. Evidence of disease elsewhere, such as in lymph nodes, should be sought because scalene lymph node biopsy or mediastinoscopy may be accompanied by bleeding. However, fine-needle aspiration of supraclavicular nodes or of a mediastinal mass has been shown to be safe in these patients. Venography is seldom indicated unless the signs are equivocal, since it may be complicated by chemical phlebitis resulting from sluggish flow in the obstructed venous system.

In younger patients, in patients with bilateral hilar masses, or in those with findings compatible with lymphoma elsewhere, it is particularly important to establish a histologic diagnosis because therapy depends on a specific diagnosis. In such patients, more material for histology is necessary than can be obtained by fine-needle aspiration, and tissue from extrathoracic sites should be sought. In young patients without an identifiable mass, fibrosing mediastinitis is possible. This condition may be associated with pulmonary artery or venous involvement, which may be demonstrated by angiography or perfusion lung scans. Fibrosing mediastinitis has been attributed to histoplasmosis, and therefore serologic evidence should be sought.

Once the diagnosis of caval obstruction has been established, treatment is determined by the nature of the primary disease. Adjunctive therapy includes elevation of the head of the bed, diuretic therapy, and corticosteroids. Emergency treatment with chemotherapy or radiotherapy is often advocated for this condition, but sufficient satisfactorily controlled trials to substantiate benefit are lacking. As with other thoracic malignancies, therapy should be dictated by cell type and stage rather than site, although caval obstruction does indicate inoperability. Whatever form of therapy is used, relief of obstructive symptoms is usually satisfactory because collateral vessels develop, even in the absence of resolution of the caval obstruction.

Surgical relief of caval obstruction in patients with nonmalignant disease is tempting and has been tried with occasional success. In general, however, surgical procedures offer little therapeutic help. It is best to allow collateral routes provide relief of symptoms. Sometimes surgical exploration is indicated to confirm the diagnosis of fibrosing mediastinitis or to exclude other etiologies.

Hoarseness

Hoarseness associated with a mediastinal mass usually results from paralysis of the left recurrent laryngeal nerve. This paralysis is most often associated with malignancy but is occasionally caused by an aortic aneurysm and, rarely, by an enlarged pulmonary artery from pulmonary hypertension.

Horner's syndrome

Tumors of the anterior mediastinum may produce Horner's syndrome: unilateral pseudoptosis, enophthalmos, constricted pupil, and warmth and dryness of the face on the affected side. In the mediastinum, Horner's syndrome results from involvement of the inferior cervical or superior thoracic sympathetic ganglia. The most common cause of Horner's syndrome is bronchogenic carcinoma.

DIAGNOSTIC TESTS

Diagnostic studies are aimed at localizing the lesion, determining its site of origin, and obtaining a tissue diagnosis. With the expanding number of diagnostic modalities, the investigation of mediastinal lesions should follow a logical sequence from simpler, inexpensive techniques to more complex, more expensive, and sometimes less comfortable techniques.

Since localization is of major importance, radiographic techniques play a crucial role in the evaluation of mediastinal lesions. A good chest film, particularly the lateral view, is the initial diagnostic test, providing information on the size and anatomic location of the mass; calcification may also be identified. Although oblique views and fluoroscopy can be helpful in equivocal chest radiographs, computed tomography (CT) is most valuable because masses of different density can be identified, and fatty tissue and cysts can be delineated. With the use of contrast materials, vascular lesions can be distinguished from nonvascular structures. CT is widely used to assess mediastinal lymphadenopathy and is particularly valuable in the posterior mediastinum. A barium contrast study of the esophagus may distinguish intrinsic pathology from extrinsic compression or may demonstrate a fistula. Magnetic resonance imaging (MRI) may be used to complement a CT scan, but its routine use remains limited in providing more information than CT. Additional tests include angiography for suspected vascular lesions and radiolabeled iodine scans for thyroid tumors.

Nonvascular mediastinal masses usually require a histologic diagnosis; several techniques are available for obtaining tissue. In the appropriate setting, not only may bronchoscopy and esophagoscopy reveal compression, but a biopsy may also be obtained if invasion of these structures has occurred. Transthoracic fine-needle aspiration for cytology is a useful technique because it is accompanied by relatively minor morbidity, and it may obviate the need for more invasive procedures. However, the small amount of material obtained is less useful for diagnosing lymphoma or benign lesions.

Mediastinoscopy is performed through an incision just above the sternal notch and is a valuable procedure for obtaining adequate amounts of tissue for specific diagnosis. Only lesions in the upper anterior mediastinum can be explored by this technique, and it is less useful on the left side because the great vessels interfere with the procedure. Lesions beyond the reach of the mediastinoscope can be approached by anterior mediastinotomy. This approach does not preclude a thoracotomy for resection of a cyst or tumor, if indicated, or if the diagnosis is still not established. A period of observation for a patient with an undiagnosed mediastinal lesion is seldom indicated, and chemotherapy or irradiation should not be prescribed without a tissue diagnosis.

SPECIFIC DISEASES

Tumors

The location of mediastinal tumors is important in diagnosis because of the predilection of certain mediastinal lesions to arise in specific compartments of the mediastinum. The box at upper right summarizes the common tumors found in the three divisions of the mediastinum.

Anterior mediastinal tumors. *Thymoma* is the most common tumor originating in the anterior mediastinum. Benign and malignant thymomas are distinguished by their invasive features rather than by their microscopic appearance. About 30% of thymic tumors are malignant and tend to invade locally rather than by hematogeneous spread. Approximately 70% of thymomas are associated with systemic symptoms, of which the most common is myasthenia gravis, associated with up to 50% of thymomas; conversely, 10% to 15% of patients with myasthenia have a thymoma. The treatment of choice for a thymoma is surgical removal. A patient with myasthenia has a significant chance of improvement. Malignant thymomas may respond to radiation therapy, occasionally used in conjunction with surgery.

Germ cell tumors of the mediastinum occur primarily in adolescents or young adults and may be classified into benign teratomas, malignant teratomas (e.g., embryonal carcinomas, teratocarcinomas, choriocarcinomas), and seminomas. About 20% of these tumors are malignant and occur more frequently in males. The cystic teratomas, or *dermoids,* are usually benign, whereas almost one third of solid tumors are malignant. Benign teratomas may be identified because calcification, hair, or teeth are found within the cyst. Occasionally the cysts rupture into a bronchus or the pericardium, causing severe symptoms. Ninety percent of patients with malignant teratomas have elevated levels of beta human chorionic gonadotropin or alphafetoprotein; these tumor markers should be measured in young male patients with masses in the anterior mediastinum. Benign teratomas are usually easily resected, but complete removal of malignant teratomas may be impossible. Treatment for malignant teratomas is primarily with chemotherapeutic agents. Seminoma is the most common form of malignant germ cell tumor to affect the mediastinum primarily and the anterior compartment exclusively. Treatment of patients with seminoma should include surgical extirpation and radiation therapy; chemotherapy is usually reserved for those patients with advanced disease or recurrence.

Substernal goiters are an important cause of anterior mediastinal masses. The routine chest film is occasionally diagnostic, with evidence of displacement and/or compression of the trachea, a smooth outline, and some calcification within the mass. Radioisotope scanning is often helpful, but some substernal goiters are nonfunctional. CT is often most helpful, demonstrating continuity of the mass

Classification of mediastinal masses

Anterior or anterosuperior

Thymoma
Germ cell tumor
Lymphoma
Substernal goiter
Enlarged fat pad or lipoma
Aneurysm of ascending aorta
Parathyroid adenoma

Middle

Bronchogenic carcinoma
Bronchogenic cyst
Lymphoma
Metastatic tumor
Systemic granuloma (sarcoid, histoplasmosis, tuberculosis)
Pericardial cyst

Posterior

Neurogenic tumor
Bronchogenic cyst
Enteric cyst
Aneurysm of descending aorta
Diaphragmatic hernia
Paravertebral abscess
Meningocele
Achalasia

with the cervical thyroid and confirming calcification. Calcification does not exclude malignancy, which is present in about 2% of patients with substernal goiters; hyperthyroidism also occurs infrequently. Surgical excision is the treatment of choice unless surgical risks are unacceptable.

Aneurysms of the ascending aorta, now usually arteriosclerotic in origin, usually present as anterior mediastinal masses; occasionally, aneurysms of the subclavian or innominate arteries also appear in this compartment. They are characterized by a smooth border, and continuity with other vascular structures may be recognized on the plain chest film. Angiography is often required to define the full extent of the aneurysm and assess the feasibility of surgery.

Patients with spontaneous or iatrogenic Cushing's syndrome often have radiographic evidence of fullness of the anterior mediastinum, best visualized on the lateral chest film. This fullness is usually caused by an enlarged mediastinal fat pad, and no therapy is indicated. CT is particularly useful in identifying fatty tissue in these patients or when a lipoma is present.

Lymphomas may present as anterior mediastinal masses because of forward growth of the mediastinal node group. Diagnosis must be confirmed histologically. Fibromas, hemangiomas, and lymphangiomas are rare, usually benign masses that require surgical excision to confirm the diagnosis.

Middle mediastinal tumors. *Lymph node enlargement* is a common cause of a mass in the middle mediastinum and is seen in many conditions. Many patients with mediastinal lymph node involvement have malignancies, either lymphoma or metastatic carcinoma. Small cell carcinoma of the lung may also present as a middle mediastinal mass, with a central bronchial tumor and mediastinal lymph node involvement. Benign disorders involving mediastinal nodes include sarcoidosis, histoplasmosis, coccidioidomycosis, and primary tuberculosis. These conditions should always be considered when investigating patients with mediastinal disease; evidence for disease elsewhere should be sought and appropriate serologic studies undertaken. When the diagnosis cannot be made by noninvasive means, mediastinoscopy is often successful in obtaining adequate tissue for histology.

Congenital cysts. Cysts, including those of pericardial, bronchogenic, enteric, thymic, and thoracic duct origin, account for about 20% of mediastinal masses. Most are discovered incidentally on routine chest radiographs in asymptomatic individuals and are confirmed to be cystic on a CT scan.

Pericardial cysts are the most common congenital cysts of the mediastinum. They seldom produce symptoms even though they occasionally contain several liters of fluid. They are usually solitary and characteristically are seen in the right cardiophrenic angle. Pericardial cysts may appear teardrop shaped on lateral projection; their contour may alter with respiration or positional change. The clear fluid they contain accounts for the term *springwater cysts.* CT and ultrasonography assist in the diagnosis. Surgical excision is usually undertaken.

Bronchogenic cysts occur in the lung or mediastinum. In the adult they are usually asymptomatic, whereas in children they may cause tracheobronchial compression with cough, stridor, wheezing, dyspnea, and occasionally atelectasis. Cysts sometimes become secondarily infected and produce a mediastinal abscess. Surgical removal of the cyst is indicated to exclude malignancy and to relieve compression of adjacent structures.

Enteric cysts are located adjacent to the esophagus in the posterior mediastinum. They are lined with esophageal, gastric, intestinal, or respiratory epithelium but rarely communicate with the esophageal lumen. Enteric cysts lined with gastric epithelium may develop peptic ulceration and bleed or perforate. More than 50% of enteric cysts are found in infants and produce symptoms by compressing adjacent structures. They have a solid appearance with a smooth contour radiographically. Barium swallow may be helpful because a localized defect in the lumen is common. Surgical extirpation is indicated in symptomatic patients and to establish a diagnosis.

Thymic cysts and those of thoracic duct origin are rare; they occur in the anterior and posterior mediastinal compartments, respectively. The diagnosis is established at surgery.

Posterior mediastinal tumors. *Neurogenic tumors* are the most common posterior mediastinal tumors, accounting for about one fifth of all mediastinal tumors. Less frequently seen are enteric cysts, esophageal tumors, achalasia, and lesions of the thoracic spine. Neurogenic tumors include all benign and malignant neoplasms arising from the intercostal nerves, sympathetic ganglia, and chemoreceptor cells. These tumors can occur at any age; however, in adults, most are asymptomatic and benign, whereas in children, 50% are symptomatic and malignant. Symptoms are occasionally caused by hormonal activity of the tumor (e.g., pheochromocytoma). The neural tumors are differentiated by the cells of their origin, (e.g., neurilemmoma, neurofibroma, ganglioneuroma, neuroblastoma [predominantly in children], pheochromocytoma). Radiographically, neurogenic tumors are smooth, rounded, homogeneous, and well circumscribed and are seen in the paravertebral sulcus; occasionally, calcification is seen. Erosion of the vertebral bodies or ribs can occur, and enlargement of the spinal neural foramen is a useful diagnostic sign. About one third of these neural tumors become malignant; therefore all should be excised.

Pneumomediastinum

Pneumomediastinum, or mediastinal emphysema, is the presence of gas in the interstices of the mediastinum. It can occur spontaneously, from trauma, or from dissection of air from the neck or retroperitoneal space. Infections with gas-forming organisms are very rare and are usually related to trauma.

Spontaneous pneumomediastinum. In the absence of an obvious cause, pneumomediastinum is said to be spontaneous. Air is thought to leak from alveoli under high pressures into the interstitium of the lung and then into the perivascular sheaths, the hilar regions, and subsequently the mediastinum. The condition may be precipitated by a sudden rise in intrathoracic pressure during vigorous coughing or after a Valsalva maneuver.

Spontaneous pneumomediastinum is relatively common in the newborn and is associated with mucous or meconium plugging, respiratory infections, and use of positive-pressure ventilators. In adults, this condition can occur in young, otherwise healthy individuals, or it may be associated with asthma, pneumonia, bronchitis, emphysema, or pulmonary fibrosis. Pneumomediastinum can also occur during obstetric labor or as a result of rapid decompression while diving, and it may be a complication of positive-pressure ventilator therapy.

The air may spread from the mediastinum to the subcutaneous tissues of the neck or axilla, producing subcutaneous emphysema; and it may leak into the pleural space, producing pneumothorax.

Patients with spontaneous pneumomediastinum may be asymptomatic or have retrosternal chest pain and dyspnea; occasionally, sore throat is present because of dissection of air to the retropharyngeal space. Physical examination may demonstrate distant heart sounds and a crunching sound synchronous with the heart (Hamman's sign). Both these signs may accompany pneumothorax without evident mediastinal emphysema. Evidence for subcutaneous emphysema in the neck and axilla should be sought.

The diagnosis is usually made by radiography. A thin line of air is seen along the border of the mediastinum; sometimes this line of air is more clearly seen on the lateral chest film. Occasionally, large amounts of air produce mediastinal widening. The presence of a concomitant pneumothorax should be sought.

Most patients with spontaneous pneumomediastinum do not require specific therapy; occasionally, however, severe symptoms develop, with signs of cardiac decompensation and tamponade. Decompression is then indicated and may be accomplished by either needle aspiration or mediastinotomy.

Traumatic pneumomediastinum. The most common cause of traumatic pneumomediastinum is rupture of the esophagus, which can occur during an episode of severe vomiting or, less frequently, after esophageal instrumentation. Traumatic pneumomediastinum can also occur after penetrating wounds of the chest or after fracture of the trachea or main bronchus after blunt trauma to the chest.

Rupture of the esophagus is usually associated with severe, boring chest pain and may be complicated by acute mediastinitis. Traumatic pneumomediastinum requires thoracotomy, with repair of the esophagus or tracheobronchial tree. Esophageal rupture is associated with high morbidity and mortality, which may be reduced if surgery is undertaken promptly.

Mediastinitis

Acute mediastinitis. Acute infections of the mediastinum are usually the result of introduction of organisms into the mediastinum after perforation of the esophagus during vomiting or instrumentation. The diagnosis should be suspected when substernal pain, fever, and radiographic evidence of mediastinal air develop after a bout of vomiting or instrumentation. This setting represents an emergency requiring antibiotic therapy directed at gram-positive, gram-negative, and anaerobic organisms as well as early surgical drainage and repair. Occasionally, mediastinal lymph nodes perforate, with drainage into the mediastinum and consequent acute suppurative mediastinitis. This situation is rare, however, and most often discovered only at autopsy. Perforation of mediastinal lymph nodes should be suspected if a patient with mediastinal lymphadenopathy develops substernal chest pain, fever, and hypotension. Therapy should include antibiotics to cover both gram-positive and gram-negative organisms and surgical exploration. An important consideration in the differential diagnosis is bleeding from or further dissection of an aneurysm.

Chronic mediastinitis. Chronic mediastinitis is a condition usually of unknown cause that produces fibrosis in the mediastinum, with compression and restriction of vascular structures entering and leaving the mediastinum. Occasionally, bronchial obstruction occurs. It was previously thought that tuberculosis was the chief cause of chronic fibrosing mediastinitis, but other granulomatous diseases, particularly histoplasmosis, may also cause this syndrome. Precise etiologic diagnosis is seldom possible because the initial infection may precede the chronic condition by months or years. Symptoms are nonspecific and include chest pain. Superior vena caval obstruction may develop, and bronchial obstruction with distal infection and cough may be troublesome. Pulmonary hypertension from constriction of the pulmonary arteries can occur, and regional venous hypertension from focal venous obstruction is sometimes a feature.

Full evaluation of the patient includes bronchoscopy and ventilation-perfusion lung scans, in addition to skin testing for tuberculosis and complement-fixation tests for histoplasmosis. Treatment is very limited once vascular obstruction has developed, although surgical decompression has been attempted. Often, however, fibrosis is too advanced to be amenable to surgical repair.

Mediastinal fibrosis is sometimes a complication of methysergide therapy.

REFERENCES

Adkins RB, Maples MD, and Hainsworth JD: Primary malignant mediastinal tumors. Ann Thorac Surg 38:648, 1984.

Brown K et al: Current use of imaging in the evaluation of mediastinal masses. Chest 98:466, 1990.

Cohen AJ et al: Primary cysts and tumors of the mediastinum. Ann Thorac Surg 51:378, 1991.

Davis RD Jr, Odham HN Jr, and Sabiston DC Jr: Primary cysts and neoplasms of the mediastinum: recent changes in clinical presentation, methods of diagnosis, management and results. Ann Thorac Surg 44:229, 1987.

Lloyd JE et al: Mediastinal fibrosis complicating histoplasmosis. Medicine (Baltimore) 67:295, 1988.

Newell JD: Evaluation of pulmonary and mediastinal masses. Med Clin North Am 68:1463, 1984.

CHAPTER

220 Pulmonary Transplantation

James H. Dauber
Irvin L. Paradis
Penny Williams

HISTORICAL CONSIDERATIONS

The first successful canine pulmonary transplant was performed in 1905. Refinement of surgical techniques and a better understanding of transplantation immunology permitted the first human lung transplant in 1963. In the next 15 years a total of 38 lung transplants were reported, but none of the recipients was discharged from the hospital, and survival did not exceed 6 months. The principal causes of death were infection and breakdown of the airway anastomoses. Such frustrating results lead to a virtual abandonment of the technique by 1978. Much of the blame for this dismal record fell on corticosteroids, which were used in high doses for immunosuppression. The group at Stanford ushered in the modern era of lung transplantation in 1981 when they achieved long-term survival in recipients of heart-lung allografts in whom the principal immunosuppressant was cyclosporine A (CsA). Nearly a decade would pass, however, before 1-year survival rates approached those of other major organs. By 1992 this goal was achieved, which has firmly established pulmonary transplantation as the pre-eminent therapy for end-stage lung disease.

DEFINITION

The term *pulmonary transplantation* is used to cover three major procedures: single-lung, double-lung, and heart-lung allografting. The indications and operative techniques for each are still evolving. Much of the impetus to pursue single-lung transplantation emanated from the ever-increasing shortage of donors. This forced a reconsideration of earlier dictums about the use of such a scarce resource. Whereas heart-lung allografting was the principal form of pulmonary transplantation in the early to mid 1980s, it is a much less frequently performed procedure in the 1990s. If not for cystic fibrosis, in which a double-lung allograft is essential, most pulmonary transplantation today would involve just one lung.

INDICATIONS

Indications for various forms of pulmonary transplantation are undergoing refinement. Some differences of opinion among principal transplant centers still remain, but the following information represents the current consensus. Table 220-1 matches diseases to forms of pulmonary transplantation.

Table 220-1. Matching diseases to forms of pulmonary transplantation

Procedure	Established indications	Under evaluation
Single lung	Pulmonary fibrosis Idiopathic Collagen vascular diseases Pneumoconioses Sarcoidosis Histiocytoses Emphysema Lymphangiomyomatosis	Pulmonary hypertension Primary with good left ventricular function Secondary with correctable cardiac defect
Double lung	Septic lung disease Cystic fibrosis Bronchiectasis	Pulmonary hypertension with systemic pressures Emphysema from alpha, antitrypsin deficiency
Heart-lung	Eisenmenger's syndrome with uncorrectable cardiac defect End-stage lung or pulmonary vascular disease with irreversible cardiomyopathy	

Single-lung allograft

Single-lung allografting is suitable for most types of advanced parenchymal lung disease that are not complicated by chronic infection or irreversible cardiac dysfunction. Restrictive disease from a wide array of causes and obstructive disease from emphysema or lymphangiomyomatosis fall into this category. Primary pulmonary hypertension (PPH) and many types of secondary pulmonary hypertension are also amenable. The foremost consideration in the latter group is adequacy of cardiac reserve and ability to correct the associated cardiac anomaly. If these conditions are met, short-term results for recipients with vascular disease parallel those for uncomplicated end-stage parenchymal lung disease.

Double-lung allograft

Today, double-lung allografting is reserved mainly for end-stage septic lung disease. The main population undergoing this procedure is patients with cystic fibrosis. Bronchiectasis that is not a result of cystic fibrosis also requires double-lung allografting. Whether transplantation will be successful in patients with bronchiectasis caused by an immunologic deficiency requires further clinical testing. Some programs use a double-lung allograft in patients with pulmonary vascular disease whose pulmonary artery pressures reach systemic levels, since concern exists that a single lung will be injured by exposure to high pressures and flow rates in the early postoperative period. Whether single-lung allografting will be adequate in such patients remains to be established, but preliminary results are encouraging.

Heart-lung allograft

This type of allografting is performed less frequently today because an insatiable demand for hearts rarely permits availability of an intact heart-lung block. Nonetheless, this approach is indispensable for patients with intractable heart and lung disease. The cardinal indication is Eisenmenger's syndrome with an uncorrectable cardiac defect. Other lung diseases complicated by inadequate left ventricular function require this approach as well. To date there are no reports that a heart and *single* lung have been grafted instead of a heart and two lungs. Such a procedure would permit more efficient use of organs but is technically very challenging.

SELECTION OF DONOR AND RECIPIENT

Donor

Relatively few requirements exist for suitable donors, but they are sufficiently stringent that the number of donors does not exceed 600/year in the United States. Lung function must be satisfactory (see the box below) and the donor free of neoplastic disease and infection with human immunodeficiency virus (HIV) and hepatitis B virus. Preferably the patient should have no history of heavy smoking or severe asthma. The age cutoff for most donors is 40 years, but "chronologic" age may be less important than "physiologic" age.

Recipient

Although many more requirements seem to exist for a suitable recipient than for the ideal donor (see the box at upper right), the number of potential recipients far exceeds the number of donors. Consequently, criteria for selection of recipients have been more stringent in recent years to improve outcome. The criteria listed here are widely employed, but the degree to which they are adhered varies from center to center. A previous thoracotomy or pleurodesis is an absolute contraindication for heart-lung transplantation because of the risk of severe perioperative hemorrhage from anticoagulation. Cardiopulmonary bypass is not required for single-lung transplantation and can be avoided in double-lung transplantation when it is performed as "sequential" single-lung transplants. Diabetes mellitus per se is not an absolute contraindication to pulmonary transplantation. Secondary end-organ damage, however, may disqualify the candidate.

Potential candidates must be evaluated systematically and criteria applied consistently to ensure proper selection. Given the disability imposed by the underlying diseases, this process is completed most expeditiously and comfortably by admitting patients to the hospital. Once selected, candidates must be monitored closely for developments that might complicate transplantation or disqualify them altogether. In addition, rehabilitation during the waiting period should be practiced whenever feasible and safe. The entire selection process is best handled by a qualified team of health care providers with relevant expertise.

Criteria for recipient selection

1. Age
   a. Less than 60 for single-lung or double-lung allograft*
   b. Less than 50 for heart-lung allograft*
2. Adequate function of left ventricle for lung allograft
3. From 80% to 120% of ideal body weight
4. Never smoker or exsmoker (stopped smoking at least 3 months before listing)
5. No substance abuse
6. On less than 10 mg/day of prednisone
7. No severe osteoporosis
8. No evidence of active tuberculosis or hepatitis B and human immunodeficiency virus (HIV) infection
9. No hepatic or renal insufficiency
10. No evidence of active neoplastic disease (long-term remission from previous neoplastic disease acceptable)
11. No severe psychiatric disease
12. Adequate support group at home
13. Available within 4 hours of being called

*See text for recommendations regarding acceptability of previous thoracotomy for each type of allograft.

Indicators of adequate function in donor lung

1. Normal chest radiograph
2. Arterial oxygen tension (PaO_2) greater than 300 mm Hg with fractional inspired oxygen (FIO_2) of 100%
3. No significant chest wall contusion
4. No evidence of recent aspiration by bronchoscopy
   a. Blood
   b. Cerebrospinal fluid
   c. Food
   d. Foreign bodies

SURGICAL CONSIDERATIONS

The purpose of this section is to indicate how the surgical approach influences the medical management of recipients. Actual techniques will not be described, but selected complications will.

Heart-lung transplantation

This approach requires cardiopulmonary bypass and subjects the recipient to risks of hemorrhage (see earlier) and air embolism. Phrenic and vagal nerve injury occasionally lead to diaphragmatic paralysis and gastric atony. These complications cause difficulty in weaning and erratic absorption of oral drugs in the early postoperative period.

Single-lung transplantation

Although this approach rarely requires cardiopulmonary bypass, it demands a wide thoracotomy. This incision causes considerable pain, which interferes with pulmonary toilet and early mobilization of the recipient. In addition to parenteral narcotics, local nerve block is often required. Vigorous pulmonary toilet is essential for prevention of atelectasis and infection of the graft. Extensive injury to the graft results in severe respiratory insufficiency and the need for differential mechanical ventilation to prevent overinflation of the highly compliant native lung.

Double-lung transplantation

Preferably, this is performed as sequential single-lung transplants to avoid cardiopulmonary bypass. This can be achieved if one native lung and the first allograft sufficiently oxygenate the recipient's blood during surgery but entails continuous bilateral thoracotomies (referred to as a *"clamshell"* procedure). Incisional pain is substantial, and without proper fixation, the sternum may be unstable. These complications interfere with pulmonary toilet. Injury to the phrenic and vagal nerves is less frequent than with heart-lung transplantation.

IMMUNOSUPPRESSION

Induction

Most regimens employ intravenous (IV) CsA in sufficient doses to achieve whole-blood levels of 500 to 1000 ng/ml by radioimmunoassay. Many regimens also use parenteral azathioprine, 1 to 2 mg/kg/day. The amount of methylprednisolone given in the perioperative period is more variable. A dose of 125 mg IV every 8 hours for two to three doses is often used, but most centers still avoid corticosteroids in the early postoperative period unless the recipient was receiving maintenance doses preoperatively. Several programs contend, however, that routine use of low doses of corticosteroids in the early postoperative period are not detrimental. Even more variable is the use of antilymphocyte globulins. A variety of antisera have been employed that appear to be effective. Because they may cause lung injury, serum sickness, and enhanced susceptibility to infection, however, their use is generally confined to recipients in whom adequate levels of CsA cannot be achieved. Controlled trials that compare the efficacy and toxicity of various induction regimens remain to be done.

Maintenance

Here the field is more uniform, with most centers using a combination of oral CsA, azathioprine, and prednisone. CsA is administered every 12 hours to achieve a trough level of 500 to 750 ng/ml in whole blood. A single daily dose of azathioprine is given that maintains the total white blood cell count greater than $5000/mm^3$. The dose of prednisone varies from 5 to 15 mg/day. Lower doses are preferable for recipients with osteoporosis and diabetes mellitus.

OUTCOME

Survival

Recipient survival is essentially equivalent to graft survival, since if the allograft fails, the outcome is usually death given the scarcity of donor lungs for retransplantation. Before 1990 limited information was available on long-term survival, and most results were based on heart-lung recipients. One-year survival compiled by the United Network for Organ Sharing (UNOS) was in the range of 55% to 60%. Because activity with single-lung and double-lung transplantation has increased substantially since 1990, more accurate survival rates are becoming available for these procedures. Results from experienced centers performing more than 20 procedures per year suggest that 1-year actuarial survival now exceeds 70% for all three forms of pulmonary transplantation and may approach 85% to 90% for selected patients undergoing single-lung or double-lung transplantation. Long-term survival rates are less reliable given the relatively small numbers of recipients who have survived more than 3 years. Present trends, however, point to ongoing loss of life from infection and rejection in the late postoperative period, leading to a 5-year survival in the range of 50%.

INTRODUCTION TO COMPLICATIONS

The ensuing sections focus on the most common problems likely to be encountered by internists and medical subspecialists. The three principal complications are preservation injury, infection, and rejection. The lung allograft appears to have a greater susceptibility to infection than do other solid-organ allografts, probably partly the result of direct exposure to the environment. The three major complications may occur contemporaneously in the early postoperative period, and later, infection and rejection are often intertwined. Distinguishing between them is essential for proper therapy.

PRESERVATION INJURY

Sometimes referred to as the *reimplantation response,* this complication occurs very early in the postoperative course. Characteristically diffuse interstitial and alveolar radiographic infiltrates develop in the first 12 to 72 hours, particularly after cessation of positive-pressure ventilation, and are often associated with a decline in lung function. The pathogenesis remains incompletely defined but is believed to involve several mechanisms. The inciting event probably is an ischemia-reperfusion injury, but this process may be aggravated by disruption of pulmonary lymphatics and pulmonary venous hypertension from volume overload and stenosis of pulmonary venous anastomoses. Histologic abnormalities are typical of diffuse alveolar damage. Hyaline membrane formation, intra-alveolar edema, and hyperplasia of type II pneumocytes eventually give way to organization, which is followed by resolution if infection does not supervene. The differential diagnosis includes acute rejection and infection. Bronchoalveolar lavage is useful to evaluate for infection, but a lung biopsy is required to exclude acute rejection. This syndrome is usually a self-limited process from which the recipient will recover. However, careful monitoring for infection and rejection, institution of broad-spectrum antibacterial prophylaxis, and early specific therapy are essential. Avoidance of infection is aided by reducing the level of immunosuppression, but this necessitates vigilance for rejection. Fortunately the allograft afflicted with mild to moderate injury does not seem more prone to acute rejection than an uninjured allograft. Overwhelming injury of this type, however, may lead to multisystem organ failure and death if new lungs are not implanted.

BACTERIAL PNEUMONIA

Time course

Bacterial pneumonia is the most common infection in the early postoperative period. Before intensive prophylaxis and pulmonary toilet, nearly half of all recipients surviving more than 48 hours contracted pneumonia in the first 2 weeks, but after institution of these measures the rate declined to about 10%. Most cases now are associated with severe preservation injury and pre-existing septic lung disease. Bacteria are also the most common cause of pneumonia after the sixth postoperative month. In such patients, chronic rejection appears to be an important associated condition.

Agents

Most bacterial pneumonias are caused by gram-negative rods. In the early postoperative period, various species have been implicated. In the late postoperative period, *Pseudomonas* predominates. In recipients with cystic fibrosis the allograft may become infected with organisms that colonize the airway of these individuals. This is particularly threatening if the organism is resistant to antibiotics. In fact, colonization with resistant bacteria is a relative contraindication to transplantation. A smaller but still substantial proportion of pneumonias are caused by *Staphylococcus aureus*. This pathogen must still be respected because it produces a highly destructive pneumonia.

Diagnosis

Culturing the trachea of the donor lung at harvest may provide useful information about subsequent complications. Isolation of mouth flora indicates an aspiration event before harvest and is often associated with significant preservation injury. Isolation of *S. aureus,* on the other hand, is a harbinger of infection with this agent in the allograft. Isolation of *Candida* species deserves attention as well (see later discussion).

Sputum and blood should be obtained for culture whenever a pneumonia is suspected and daily for surveillance in the first 72 hours. The sputum must also be examined for bacteria by conventional stains and the direct fluorescent antibody technique for *Legionella* species. Not infrequently, this information is sufficient for an accurate bacteriologic diagnosis. When the pneumonia occurs in patients with preservation injury or diffuse radiographic infiltrates from other causes, more invasive techniques for obtaining secretions from the lower airways are often required. If properly standardized, bronchoalveolar lavage can yield valuable information about not only bacterial but also viral and protozoal pathogens. Quantitative bacterial cultures of specimens obtained by protected brush catheter may also be used.

Treatment

Some form of prophylaxis should be employed in all recipients in the early postoperative period. Initially a combination of ceftazidime and clindamycin is sufficient (Table 220-2). This regimen should be employed until results of cultures from the donor trachea become available. Antibacterial coverage needs be continued after this time if severe ischemic injury to the allograft, positive donor trachea culture, or clinically significant infection occurs. In the latter two instances the regimen should be tailored to the sensitivities of bacterial isolates. If *S. aureus* is isolated from the donor trachea or from a surveillance sputum culture in the first 48 hours, vancomycin should be given for 7 days. When the recipient was transplanted for septic lung disease associated with *Pseudomonas* species, prophylaxis with three antipseudomonal drugs for 1 to 2 weeks is indicated (Table 220-2). Obtaining cultures from the *recipient's* native lungs at the time of transplantation will often provide information about potential pathogens in the postoperative period and should be done routinely for septic lung disease. Prophylaxis in the patient with multiply resistant organisms is more controversial, but it is not unreasonable to employ standard prophylaxis to prevent infection with sensitive organisms.

Specific antibiotic coverage is the backbone of treatment for bacterial pneumonia that supervenes in the early postoperative period. For infections with *Pseudomonas* species, two drugs are indicated, one being an aminoglycoside. Drug therapy should not be relied on solely. The contribution of airway injury and denervation to initiation and resolution of infection cannot be underestimated. Pulmonary toilet in this period is essential. Postural drainage and chest percussion should be employed routinely. Repeated therapeutic fiberoptic bronchoscopy appears to be helpful in recipients with poor cough and large volumes of sputum. When bacterial pneumonia is extensive or occurs with moderate to severe preservation lung injury, reduction of immunosuppression should be strongly considered.

Bacterial pneumonia in the late postoperative period almost always occurs in concert with chronic rejection. Colonization of the airways with bacteria supervenes in such recipients. Most often the organisms are gram-negative rods with *Pseudomonas* species dominating, but *S. aureus* may also be isolated. The colonizing organism is usually the pathogen in these patients. Treatment is similar to that for infection in the early postoperative period. After resolution of infection, however, it is often useful to keep the recipient with repeated infections on a regimen of rotating antibiotics, some of which may be given by inhalation. Chronic postural drainage may also

Table 220-2. Prophylaxis for infection

Organism	Peak prevalence in postoperative period	Starting point	Antimicrobial agents	Dosage	Duration
Bacteria	Days 1-14	Postoperative day (POD) 1	Ceftazidime Clindamycin	1 g IV q8h 600 mg IV q8h	3-14 days (see text)
Herpes simplex virus	Days 1-7	POD 1	Acyclovir*	600 mg PO tid	3 months unless ganciclovir given for cytomegalovirus
Candida species	Days 7-30	As soon as organisms identified in donor trachea or isolated from lower airway of allograft	Amphotericin B* + 5-Flucytosine*† or Fluconazole	25 mg IV daily 1 g PO bid 400 mg IV/PO qd	21 days With amphotericin 4-6 weeks
Toxoplasma	Days 7-30	When mismatch identified (positive donor to negative recipient)	Sulfadiazine* Pyrimethamine Folinic acid Pyrimethamine Folinic acid	1 g PO qid 25 mg PO qd 10 mg PO qd 25 mg PO weekly 10 mg PO weekly	Initial 14 days For following 6 months
Cytomegalovirus (CMV)	Days 30-40	POD 7 POD 21	Ganciclovir*†	5 mg/kg IV bid 5 mg/kg IV daily	14 days 6 weeks for CMV-positive recipients; 3 months for CMV-negative recipients of CMV-positive organs
Pneumocystis carinii	Month 3	POD 30	Trimethoprim/ sulfamethoxazole (160 mg/800 mg) Dapsone	1 tablet qod or bid for 7 day/mo or bid for 2 wk/3 mo 100 mg PO weekly	Indefinite Indefinite
Mycobacterium tuberculosis	?	Before transplant or immediately after surgery	INH	300 mg PO qd	1 year

*Dosage adjustment required for renal insufficiency.
†Dosage adjustment required for leukopenia.

be helpful. The issue regarding immunosuppression in these individuals is more complex. Transient reductions may be possible, but intermittent augmentation is often necessary to control underlying rejection.

Outcome

Bacterial pneumonia continues to be one of the leading causes of death in the early postoperative period. Aggressive prophylaxis and improved diagnosis and treatment have greatly reduced its toll, but despite these improvements, the mortality rate from infection at this time remains about 25%. It is also a leading cause of death in the late postoperative period. Recipients with far advanced chronic rejection are those mainly affected. Because the number of long-term survivors who develop chronic rejection is increasing, this complication will have an even greater impact in the future.

CYTOMEGALOVIRUS INFECTION

Prevelance

Infection with cytomegalovirus (CMV) may be detected as early as 3 weeks after transplantation. In recipients who do not receive prophylaxis, the onset is most often around the 40th postoperative day. Prophylaxis with ganciclovir delays the onset of infection, with the degree of delay depending on the duration and effectiveness of prophylaxis. Primary CMV infection occurs in recipients who were seronegative at transplantation and receive an organ or blood products from seropostive donors. Infections in recipients who were seropositive before transplantation usually represent reactivation of latent virus and are called *secondary* infections, but such recipients may also be infected with a new strain of virus. The prevalence of infection therefore depends on the serologic status of both recipient and donor pools and the extent to which primary infection is prevented by using allografts and blood products from CMV-negative donors in CMV-negative recipients. In the past the bulk of primary infections arose through the use of CMV-positive blood products in seronegative recipients. Restricting exposure of seronegative recipients to CMV-positive blood products greatly reduces the overall rate of primary infections. Since no effort is presently made to match the CMV status of the donor organ and recipient, primary infection will continue to arise through this mechanism. In the absence of prophylaxis, about 80% of seropositive recipients become infected. Thus, without effective prophylaxis, a substantial proportion of lung recipients will develop infection with this agent.

Clinical manifestations

Before prophylaxis, about 25% of patients with CMV infections were totally asymptomatic, with the virus isolated from the buffy coat, urine, or bronchoalveolar lavage (BAL) fluid. Most of these patients had secondary infections. About two thirds of symptomatic infections are caused by involvement principally in the lung allograft. The rate of CMV pneumonia in the allograft greatly surpasses that in other solid-organ recipients, and most patients have primary infections. The remainder of infections are associated with a viral syndrome, esophagitis, or disseminated disease involving more than one organ. Overall the severity of symptoms and organ dysfunction tends to be greater in primary infection than in secondary infection.

Diagnosis

Diagnosis is confirmed by isolating CMV from blood, urine, or BAL fluid or by finding specific inclusion bodies in cytologic or histologic preparations from affected organs. With the lung allograft, fiberoptic bronchoscopy with transbronchial lung biopsy is probably the approach with the highest diagnostic yield. It should be used when infection is suspected on clinical grounds. Sometimes a surveillance procedure will reveal CMV pneumonitis in an asymptomatic recipient who is at risk for infection. This result and the striking predilection of the lung allograft to infection are strong rationales for the use of surveillance bronchoscopy in this population. In complex situations when several processes may coexist in the allograft, an open lung biopsy may be required to confirm the presence of CMV.

Treatment

Acyclovir in high doses may provide protection against symptomatic CMV infection but is not useful in the treatment of established disease. Reducing the level of immunosuppression improves host defenses but usually is not sufficient for recovery and increases the risk of acute rejection. Ganciclovir is highly effective as both a prophylactic and a therapeutic agent. Although uncertainty exists about the optimum prophylactic regimen with this agent, it is universally agreed that it delays the onset of infection, and encouraging signs suggest that it may even prevent infection. Doses and duration of prophylaxis are outlined in Table 220-2. It should be noted that "breakthrough" infection with ganciclovir prophylaxis occasionally develops.

Symptomatic infection is treated with the same regimen of ganciclovir as outlined in Table 220-2 except for the addition of immune globulin, 0.5 g/kg IV every other day for 10 doses. Duration of therapy usually is 3 weeks. Marked reduction in the level of immunosuppression is usually not called for unless the infection is severe. Because subclinical infection may linger in the allograft for weeks, follow-up bronchoscopy is usually indicated. Persistence of active infection (inclusion bodies on cytology or histology) or viral shedding requires additional therapy because the infection can become more severe without it. Foscarnet may be employed in particularly stubborn cases or when resistance to ganciclovir is strongly suspected. CMV-specific immuneglobulin may play a role in treatment or prophylaxis of CMV in the future, but remains to be studied.

Outcome

Before the availability of ganciclovir, prevention and treatment of CMV were relatively ineffective. The mortality rate from pneumonia in primary infection exceeded 50%. Prophylaxis with ganciclovir has dramatically reduced the prevalence of infection, and specific therapy with this drug for established pneumonia is highly effective in inducing a remission. Consequently the overall mortality rate has declined from 22% before the availability of ganciclovir to less than 5%. Nonetheless, infection with CMV and CMV pneumonia in particular continue to be an important cause of morbidity. Also, disturbing evidence suggests that infection of the allograft is frequently associated with chronic rejection and an accelerated decline in allograft function. For this reason, efforts to eradicate completely CMV infection in lung allograft recipients are indicated.

PNEUMOCYSTIS CARINII PNEUMONIA

Before aggressive prophylaxis with trimethoprim (TMP) and sulfamethoxazole (SMX) (co-trimezole) the frequency of *P. carinii* infection in the allograft was 85% at the University of Pittsburgh. Most of these infections were subclinical, but several proved fatal. Infection is first encountered around the third to fourth postoperative month and recurs after successful treatment if prophylaxis is not instituted. With effective prophylaxis, this infection is a rarity and tends to be encountered late in the postoperative course. Most recipients who contract it today have not been following the prescribed regimen of prophylaxis. If properly prepared, specimens from BAL fluid reliably detect both clinical and subclinical infection. Transbronchial or open lung biopsy is rarely necessary. Subclinical infection responds to oral co-trimezole, one double-strength (DS) tablet of 160 mg TMP and 800 mg of SMX twice a day. Clinically significant infection demands IV therapy with sulfa drugs or pentamidine. A variety of prophylactic regimens have proved successful (see Table 220-2). Experience with inhaled pentamidine as prophylaxis in lung allograft recipients is too limited to draw conclusions about safety and efficacy.

OTHER INFECTIONS

Herpes simplex

For the most part, herpes simplex infection is clinically insignificant. Herpetic lesions of mild severity typically develop on the lips and buccal mucosa during the first postoperative week and should be treated with acyclovir. In the occasional recipient with no previous exposure, a primary infection can develop and produces a devastating pneumonia in the allograft in the absence of prompt therapy. For this reason the recipient's serologic status for this virus should be routinely established before transplantation and the donor trachea cultured for virus. If at risk for organ-transmitted HSV, recipients who will not receive ganciclovir for CMV prophylaxis should be given acyclovir for the first 3 months beginning on the second postoperative day.

Epstein-Barr virus and posttransplant lymphoproliferative disease

The principal rationale for discussing Epstein-Barr virus (EBV) is the very strong association between primary, and to a lesser extent secondary, infection and posttransplant lymphoproliferative disease (PTLD). The frequency of primary infection depends primarily on the proportion of recipients who are seronegative at the time of transplantation. Most seronegative recipients will seroconvert in the early postoperative period. Primary infection manifests as a self-limited mononucleosis syndrome of variable severity in the second to fourth month. Unfortunately, as many as 75% of recipients with primary infection will subsequently develop PTLD, which in up to two thirds of patients presents in the allograft. The second most common site is the bowel, followed by the liver, then abdominal and peripheral lymph node groups. A biopsy is needed to confirm the diagnosis. It reveals B cell proliferation, which is polyclonal or monoclonal in origin. EBV is usually detected in cells that are pleomorphic and focally necrotic. Distinction between a benign proliferative process and PTLD in these patients is often difficult.

PTLD usually involutes quickly after the level of immunosuppression is drastically reduced. After involution, immunosuppression may be increased, but not to previous levels. Unfortunately, this manipulation is sometimes associated with development of acute and chronic rejection, which demands augmentation of immunosuppression. In such patients the lymphoma may recur. If PTLD fails to be controlled by manipulation of immunosuppression or if there is relapse, radiation therapy and chemotherapy may be undertaken, but the results are frequently disappointing. Given the magnitude of the problem with PTLD, efforts to avoid and treat primary infection with EBV are clearly warranted, but to date no highly effective measures have been reported.

PTLD may also develop much later in the postoperative course. In these patients, association with clinical EBV infection usually is less obvious and reduction of immunosuppression less effective in producing a remission. In such patients, radiation and chemotherapy may be employed but fail to induce a long-term remission in most.

Candida species

The presence of *Candida* organisms in the airway at the time the donor lung is harvested is a predictor for infection in the early postoperative period. Other conditions permissive to infection include ischemic injury to the airway mucosa and lung, use of broad-spectrum antibiotics, generalized debility of the recipient, need for chronic central venous lines, and the development of oral thrush. Most infections are relatively superficial and clinically insignificant. However, these organisms may infect the aortic anastomoses of the heart-lung allograft, creating a mycotic pseudoaneurysm that is usually fatal. In addition, they may cause a mediastinal abscess around a dehisced bronchial anastomosis. This type of infection usually responds to therapy if not widely disseminated. Multiple parenchymal abscesses are rare and develop in the lung allograft only with disseminated infection. Amphotericin B may be given prophylactically in a dose of 25 mg IV daily for up to 3 weeks when organisms are isolated from the donor trachea at harvest or when organisms are isolated from several sites in the absence of signs of disseminated infection. Fluconazole appears to be effective as well, with less risk of renal insufficiency (see Table 220-2). Deep-seated but isolated infection and disseminated infection demand the usual therapeutic doses of amphotericin B (1 to 2 g IV) together with 5-flucytosine. The latter can be given only by the oral route, and lower-than-usual doses usually achieve adequate serum levels. Prophylaxis for thrush and esophagitis with anticandidal troches or mouthwashes is advisable during the initial hospital stay, particularly in recipients who were treated with broad-spectrum antibiotics before transplantation. Prospective bronchoscopic examination within the first 10 days is advisable because it may detect unsuspected infection of the airways.

Aspergillus species

Infection with *Aspergillus* organisms is rare in the early postoperative period but begins to pose dilemmas for the clinician after the third postoperative month. Organisms may be detected in the lavage fluid obtained from asymptomatic recipients during surveillance bronchoscopy. Some of these recipients will develop clinical infection in the allograft later, but the ability to predict this event is inadequate at present. Recovery of *Aspergillus* in lavage fluid from recipients with pulmonary infiltrates is much more ominous, but confirming that the infiltrates are caused by infection with this agent may prove difficult. Transbronchial lung biopsy usually does not document invasive disease, and this diagnosis may not even be evident on open lung biopsy. Invasive pulmonary aspergillosis is not always a fulminant process but, when suspected, demands treatment with amphotericin B until confirmed or excluded. Unfortunately, amphotericin B usually does not eradicate well-established disease, and the outcome in such patients is death. Optimum therapy for recipients with colonization of the allograft airways remains to be defined. Treatment with amphotericin B and the oral agent itraconazole has been successful in preventing dissemination of organisms but probably does not totally eliminate them. One source of organisms that may be overlooked initially is the native lung in a recipient of a single-lung allograft. If the native lung contains cystic spaces or cavities, *Aspergillus* may colonize these poorly defended regions first and then disseminate endobronchially into the allograft. One possible future approach to *Aspergillus* colonization in the transplant patient may be to use nebulized Amphotericin B (5 to 10 mg tid).

Other infections

Because the lung allograft is susceptible to a wide range of pathogens and opportunistic agents, less common agents occasionally cause clinically significant infection. In the program at the University of Pittsburgh the allograft has been invaded by *Cryptococcus neoformans, Rhizopus* species, and *Pseudoallescheria boydii*. If such agents are isolated from the allograft, they should never be considered contaminants. Infections with the former two organisms respond to early and aggressive treatment with amphotericin B, whereas the latter requires miconazole or itraconazole. Prolonged or even continuous therapy may be needed to control such infections. Toxoplasmosis infrequently causes illness in lung recipients, but growing concern exists that an organ from a positive donor may transmit this disease to a seronegative recipient. For this reason the serologic status of the donor and recipient should be established and prophylaxis provided when such a mismatch occurs (see Table 220-2). Pulmonary tuberculosis has not been a significant problem to date; careful screening of potential recipients and appropriate prophylaxis in the preoperative period appear to be the reasons.

Allograft rejection

The lung allograft is a highly immunogenic organ that will reject rapidly in the absence of an identical match. Because living related donor programs for pulmonary transplantation in adults will likely never become a source of organs, and because the supply of adult organs is too limited to attempt close matching for HLA loci, immunosuppression to prevent rejection of mismatched organs will be essential in the future. Even in the face of what is considered relatively intense immunosuppression, the rate of rejection in the early postoperative period exceeds 75%. The pathogenesis of rejection involves the infiltration of the graft by lymphocytes that recognize antigens of the donor. The principal donor antigens in the lung allograft that appear to initiate acute rejection are the HLA DR subsets of class II major histocompatibility complex (MHC). Antigens of the class I MHC subsets and other yet to be defined antigens probably play a role as well, particularly in chronic rejection.

The histologic and clinical manifestations of rejection appear to take two forms. In the early posttransplant period the endothelium and surrounding vessels seem to be the main target. As the intensity of this response escalates, it spills into the interstitium, and pulmonary compliance increases while gas exchange deteriorates. These physiologic changes are associated with diffuse radiographic infiltrates and symptoms. The response to augmentation of immunosuppression is typically brisk and substantial. Relapse may occur, but additional therapy almost always brings this form of rejection under control and restores allograft function. As early as 3 months after transplant but typically much later, a different form of rejection supervenes in up to half of long-term survivors. In this instance the target of injury is principally the airways, particularly the bronchioles. Histologically the principal finding is bronchiolitis obliterans. Physiologically the most prominent abnormality is obstruction to airflow, but a restrictive impairment also develops. The chest radiograph reveals no new abnormalities until late in the course. Response to augmented immunosuppression is variable, with only a minority of treated recipients regaining most lost lung function. Relapse is almost the rule, and response to additional therapy is often unsatisfying. Progressive loss of graft function occurs in about 25% of affected recipients, who will eventually die from respiratory failure and infection unless they receive a second transplant. This syndrome has been termed *posttransplant bronchiolitis obliterans* and is considered synonymous with chronic rejection. These two forms of allograft rejection are discussed in more detail later.

Acute rejection

Time course and frequency. Acute rejection is encountered as early as the third postoperative day but most often presents in the second to third week. It can also be seen later if the level of immunosuppression dramatically decreases. The prevalence depends on several factors. The most important appears to be the intensity of the induction and maintenance phases of immunosuppression. The degree of mismatch at HLA loci, the method for detecting rejection, and the philosophy about treatment also influence frequency of reported acute rejection. Despite minor differences in frequency from center to center, acute rejection is a common event, occurring in nearly all recipients to at least a minor degree sometime in the early postoperative course.

Clinical manifestations and diagnosis. Recipients with acute rejection may be asymptomatic, but most experience symptoms such as cough, dyspnea, chest tightness, fever, fatigue, and malaise. Fulminant acute rejection rarely even mimics bacterial sepsis. The most sensitive laboratory abnormality is a decline in the arterial oxygen tension. Leukocytosis with a left shift typically occurs, as do new interstitial radiographic infiltrates and pleural effusions. If formal pulmonary function tests can be performed, the principal finding is a decline in lung volumes with preservation of the forced expiratory volume at 1 second/forced vital capacity (FEV_1/FVC) ratio. None of these routine evaluations posseses sufficient specificity, however, to permit a clear-cut diagnosis. For this reason a lung biopsy is required. The transbronchial route is usually sufficient if the specimens are adequate in quantity and quality. From 8 to 10 generous pieces should be obtained from upper and lower lobes. The availability of a pathologist experienced in reading transbronchial lung biopsy specimens favorably influences the yield of this approach. If the recipient is too ill to undergo a transbronchial biopsy or other extenuating circumstances exist, an open lung biopsy may be required. Results from BAL fluid are helpful in establishing the presence of infection, but presently no markers exist in lavage fluid that are diagnostic for this complication.

The histologic changes encountered in the rejecting lung allograft have recently been classified and graded in severity. This scheme, which is being widely adopted (see the box below), is useful for following a single recipient longitudinally and for facilitating comparisons of recipients within a single center and between different centers. A depiction of histologic abnormalities in moderate acute cellular rejection is shown in Fig. 220-1. Mononuclear inflammatory cell infiltrates are found mainly around and in the wall of the blood vessel but also occur in large and small airways. However, organization and fibrosis in the latter sites are rare. Generally a good correlation exists between the histologic score of rejection and the clinical manifestations it causes.

Treatment. Clinically evident acute rejection associated with grade III or IV changes on biopsy requires acute augmentation of immunosuppression. Most centers employ pulsed doses of corticosteroids. Recipients typically receive 1 g of methylprednisolone IV daily for 3 days, although half to three quarters of that dose is effective in smaller or younger recipients. Symptoms often improve hours after the first dose. Radiographic and laboratory abnormalities revert more slowly but usually resolve soon after completion of therapy. A repeat biopsy 10 to 14 days after completion of therapy is indicated. The interval should be shorter if the response has not been satisfying. A good response is usually associated with almost complete clearing of the inflammatory cell infiltrates. A less favorable clinical response associated with persistent histologic infiltrates of grade II or higher on biopsy requires a second course of corticosteroids. In most patients, two courses of pulsed doses of corticosteroids are sufficient to bring acute rejection under control. If not, additional treatment with antilymphocyte globulins should be undertaken and nearly always is successful.

Treatment of subclinical acute rejection associated with grade II or lower changes is somewhat controversial. Many centers elect to withhold therapy, continue to observe, and repeat the biopsy later if this is the first episode of rejection. On the other hand, if the recipient had recently received pulsed doses of corticosteroids for a more serious histologic grade of rejection and Grade II infiltrates persist, original treatment would likely be considered inadequate. Accordingly, additional therapy would be given.

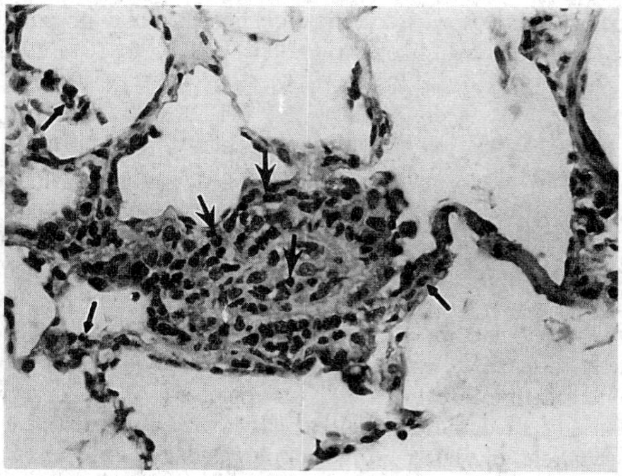

Fig. 220-1. Histologic grade III acute rejection. A small vein is infiltrated by inflammatory cells, which extend into the alveolar interstitium. Most of the infiltrating cells are lymphocytes *(broad arrows),* which have a pleomorphic appearance characteristic of cellular activation. Occasional polymorphonuclear leukocytes are also seen *(thin arrows).*

Histologic grades of acute rejection*

Grade I: minimum acute rejection
Infrequent lymphocytic infiltrates surrounding blood vessels, but principally venules. Lymphocytes have variable appearance, with some undergoing transformation.
Grade II: mild acute rejection
Frequent perivascular infiltrates of activated lymphocytes, macrophages, and eosinophils invade vessel walls and alter appearance of endothelial cells ("endothelialitis").
Grade III: moderate acute rejection
Perivascular infiltrates extend into alveolar septi and air spaces adjacent to bronchioles and vessels. Eosinophils are more prominent, and neutrophils may be seen.
Grade IV: severe acute rejection
Diffuse infiltration of interstitium and air spaces with alveolar pneumocyte injury, alveolar hemorrhage, and hyaline membrane formation (acute alveolar damage). A necrotizing vasculitis may cause infarction.

*All grades may be associated with inflammation and injury of cartilaginous bronchi and bronchioles.

Outcome. This complication contributes to morbidity in the early postoperative period but rarely is fatal. Care must be exercised, however, not to immunosuppress the recipient too greatly during this time in order to avoid opportunistic infection and the emergence of PTLD in susceptible hosts. If serious infection is not encountered and only one or two courses of treatment bring the episode under control, the outcome is uniformly good. Recipients with persistent acute rejection that requires multiple courses of treatment or is complicated by infection seem to be at greater risk for developing chronic rejection in the ensuing months to years, as discussed next.

Chronic rejection

Time course and prevelance. Chronic rejection syndrome is sometimes encountered as soon as 3 months after transplantation but more often occurs after the sixth to twelfth month. The time of onset is highly variable, however, since some recipients with excellent graft function will be affected in the fourth to sixth year. The overall prevalence depends partly on the number of long-term survivors and the duration of follow-up. Because these numbers are steadily increasing worldwide, a better approximation of prevalence should emerge. Presently, however, 25% to 50% of long-term survivors will develop this complication.

Clinical findings and diagnosis. The onset of symptoms is usually insidious. The afflicted recipient may first notice only a decline in flow rates that may be easily monitored with hand-held spirometers in the home. The earliest symptoms are cough and dyspnea. The cough initially is productive of mucoid sputum, but as the disorder progresses, the sputum may become purulent. Dyspnea is usually encountered only with exertion unless the level of obstruction becomes severe. Physical examination in early disease is normal. In more advanced disease, rhonchi and expiratory wheezes may be heard. The chest radiograph remains unchanged from baseline until late in the course, when both nodular and reticular interstitial markings appear. Segmental infiltrates usually indicate superimposed bacterial or fungal infection. Pulmonary function testing reveals a combined obstructive and restrictive impairment with a variable decline in diffusing capacity and increase in the alveolar-arterial oxygen gradient. Most often the decline in FEV_1 exceeds that of the FVC, resulting in reduced FEV_1/FVC ratio. Despite relatively large declines in the FVC, lung volumes on chest radiograph typically are well preserved, suggesting air trapping.

Although these findings indicate chronic rejection, they lack diagnostic specificity. Infection with bacteria and CMV may produce similar abnormalities and obviously require different therapy. Consequently the diagnosis must be confirmed with a lung biopsy. The transbronchial route is usually adequate, but since the histologic abnormalities have a patchy distribution, at times this approach will not yield the expected diagnosis. In such patients it may be necessary to perform a thoracoscopic or open lung biopsy. The constellation of findings required by most pathologists to make a diagnosis includes lymphocytic bronchiolitis, denudation of bronchiolar epithelium, plugs of granulation tissue in the lumen of the brochioles, and collections of foamy macrophages in the alveoli of affected lobules (Fig. 220-2, *A*). The presence of perivascular lymphocytic infiltrates of the type seen in acute rejection is variable. However, lymphocytic infiltrates around arteries may be prominent, along with sclerosis of veins. In addition, there may be lymphocytic infiltrates in larger airways and evidence of injury to cartilage. The number of neutrophils in the inflammatory infiltrates is typically small. Prominence of these cells suggests infection. Special stains for bacteria and fungi should be performed routinely to detect microorganisms in the infiltrates. BAL is very useful in clarifying infection. Even in the absence of infection, the proportion of neutrophils in BAL fluid is usually much greater than expected, but the presence of bacteria in these cells (Gram stain) and isolation of pathogens by culture of BAL fluid indicate superimposed infection, which may occur simultaneously with chronic rejection or alone.

Pathogenesis. Chronic rejection of the lung allograft belongs in the syndrome of bronchiolitis obliterans, which can result from several other causes. Whether the form encountered in the lung allograft, which is often called posttransplant bronchiolitis obliterans (PTBO), has a unique immunologic pathogenesis is still somewhat controversial. Recipients of a lung allograft are susceptible to recurrent infection and repeated aspiration, both of which are known causes of bronchiolitis obliterans. In addition, the bronchial

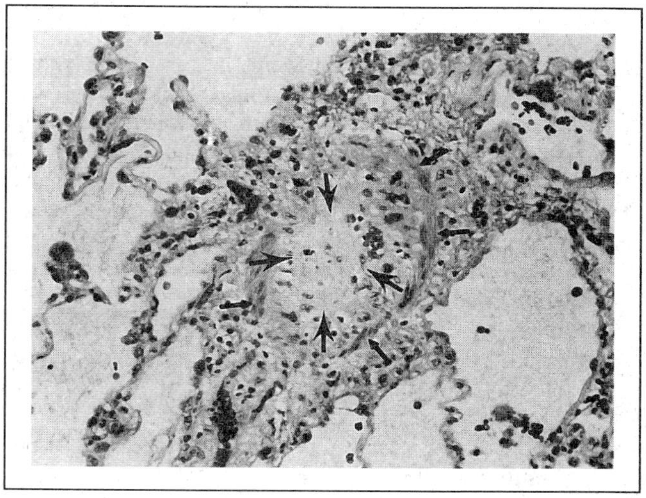

A

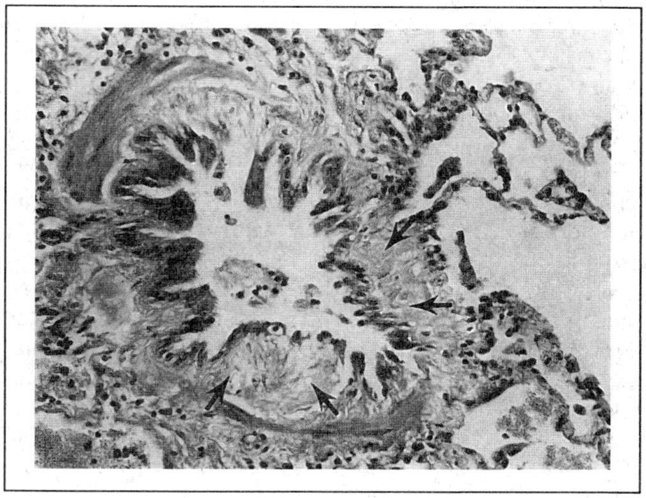

B

Fig. 220-2. **A,** Posttransplant bronchiolitis obliterans. The lumen of this small bronchiole, which is surrounded by a mononuclear inflammatory infiltrate, is totally occluded by granulation tissue *(broad arrows)*. The epithelium is virtually absent in this section. The smooth muscle cells *(thin arrows)* indicate that this destructive process involves a small airway. **B,** Inactive bronchiolitis obliterans. The lumen of this airway no longer contains granulation tissue, and the epithelium is basically intact. Nonetheless, eccentric collections of mature fibrous tissue *(broad arrows)* narrow the lumen. This histologic abnormality is usually associated with an obstructive impairment of lung function circulation is disrupted during harvest but is not re-established during engraftment. Loss of this blood supply likely plays a role, but because not all recipients contract PTBO and yet their bronchial circulation is nearly always compromised, this clearly is not the principal cause. Despite the potential importance of nonimmunologic factors, a growing consensus exists that PTBO represents chronic rejection for the following reasons:

1. A syndrome characterized by chronic inflammation and dysfunction of the allograft occurs with other transplanted organs (e.g., kidney, liver) where epithelium is prominent and eventually becomes damaged.
2. Bone marrow transplant recipients with graft versus host disease develop bronchiolitis obliterans.
3. Lymphocytes, which recognize donor-derived antigens and exhibit proliferation and cytotoxicity in vitro, can often be detected in BAL fluid and grown from transbronchial lung biopsy specimens of recipients with PTBO.
4. Recipients with recurrent acute rejection that is difficult to control seem to be more prone to developing PTBO.
5. Finally, augmentation of immunosuppression frequently stems the decline of lung function seen during PTBO and, in about 50% to 75% of affected recipients, seems to restore at least some of the function that was lost.

Taken together, these findings strongly support a role for alloreactivity in the pathogenesis of this disorder. Nonetheless, recent findings that identify airway ischemic injury in the early postoperative period, pneumonitis with CMV, and bacterial pneumonia in the late postoperative period as "risk factors" for occurrence of chronic rejection raise the possibility that modifying influences are present in this process.

Treatment and outcome. General agreement exist that chronic rejection associated with a significant decline in lung function demands treatment with augmented immunosuppression. Untreated chronic rejection of this severity almost always results in a progressive deterioration in graft function and death. Corticosteroids, either orally (100 mg prednisone initially then tapered by 10 mg/day until maintenance dose is reached) or intravenously (1 g methylprednisolone IV daily for 3 days), and parenteral antilymphocyte globulin (rabbit antithymocyte globulin, Minnesota antilymphocyte globulin, or OKT-3) are the most widely employed. Often, several separate courses of both corticosteroids and antilymphocyte globulin must be given before lung function stabilizes or improves (Fig. 220-3, *A*). This goal can be achieved in up to 75% of affected recipients. The remainder tend to suffer continued decline in graft function and succumb to respiratory failure or infection (Fig. 220-3, *B*). unless they receive a new allograft.

The rate of improvement in graft function differs for the two major treatments. A response to corticosteroids usually becomes apparent within 2 weeks, whereas there is a lag of up to 6 weeks with polyclonal antilymphocyte globulins. On follow-up biopsy, inflammation and fibrosis may be completely resolved, but this is not the rule. More often, inflammation resolves but fibrosis persists, causing concentric or eccentric narrowing of the lumina of small airways (Fig. 220-2, *B*). In the later case, flow rates, although higher than their lowest values, usually do not return to premorbid levels. If the follow-up biopsy reveals residual inflammation, another course of augmented immunosuppression should be given, maintenance immunosuppression should be maximized, and the biopsy repeated in 4 to 6 weeks. In most patients, two or three treatments of augmented immunosuppression and maximization of maintenance therapy will arrest inflammation and fibrosis. The duration of this remission is variable, however, and most recipients relapse and require additional therapy. For the few recipients in whom this approach fails to stem bronchiolar inflammation and fibrosis, other forms of therapy have been tried. These include inhalation of cyclosporine A, total nodal irradiation, and colchicine and other cytotoxic drugs. Clearly, such approaches are experimental and must be performed under a protocol. Retransplantation is the ultimate treatment for end-stage disease in properly selected recipients. Because the number of potential and actual recipients of this type is presently very small, the feasibility and overall efficacy of this approach with its many medical and ethical implications remain to be defined.

Augmentation of immunosuppression in recipients with chronic rejection is not without risk. The airways of most of these individuals, particularly those with cystic fibrosis, become colonized with bacteria (*Pseudomonas* species, *S. aureus*). Efforts to limit the burden of bacteria in these recipients are indicated because these organisms lead to recurrent bacterial pneumonia. Such measures may include repeated surgical drainage of the paranasal sinuses, especially in recipients with cystic fibrosis. A staphylococcal pneumonia in these patients is nearly always life-threatening and often irreversibly injures the allograft. Reactivation of CMV typically is clinically insignificant, but it may accelerate or promote the rejection process. Recipients with PTLD that has previously gone into remission may experience a relapse with devastating consequences. Finally, invasive fungal infection occasionally ensues. The high risk of superinfection in recipients with far advanced chronic rejection is often a deterrent to additional immunosuppressive therapy. It also raises a question about the need to treat early asymptomatic chronic rejection as aggressively as more established disease. However, whether the option of withholding treatment in recipients with asymptomatic chronic rejection is viable remains to be proved.

FUTURE TRENDS

The achievement of acceptable 1-year survival rates for pulmonary transplantation has ensured a future, at least in the near term, for this practice. The extent to which pulmonary transplantation eventually is adopted depends principally on the supply of organs. Because demand is growing more rapidly than is supply, many suitable candidates in the near term will die before they can be transplanted. Thus efforts to improve the rate of donation must be increased

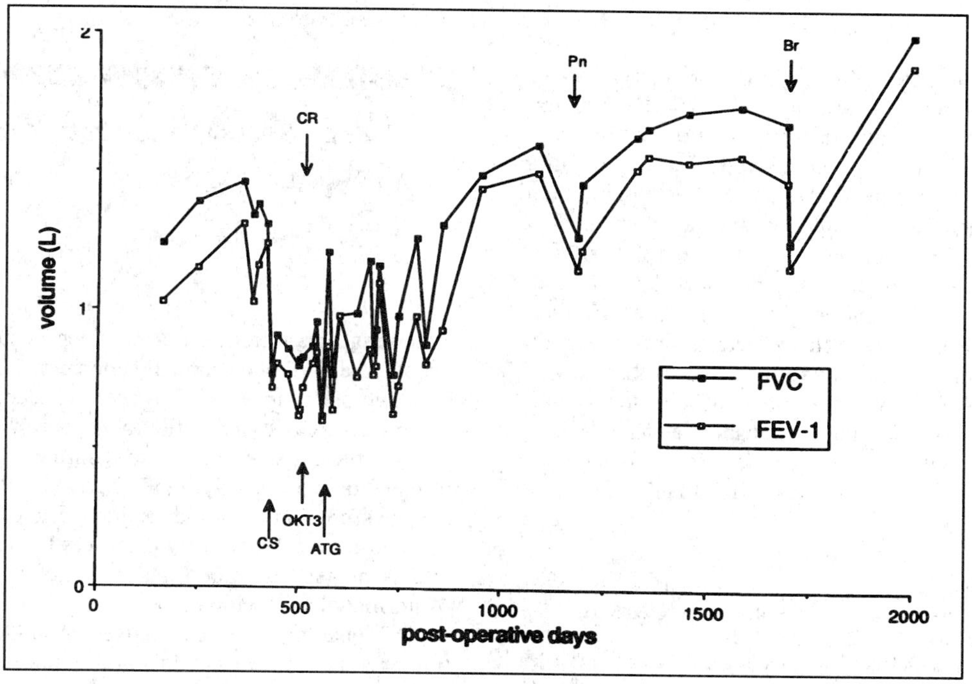

A

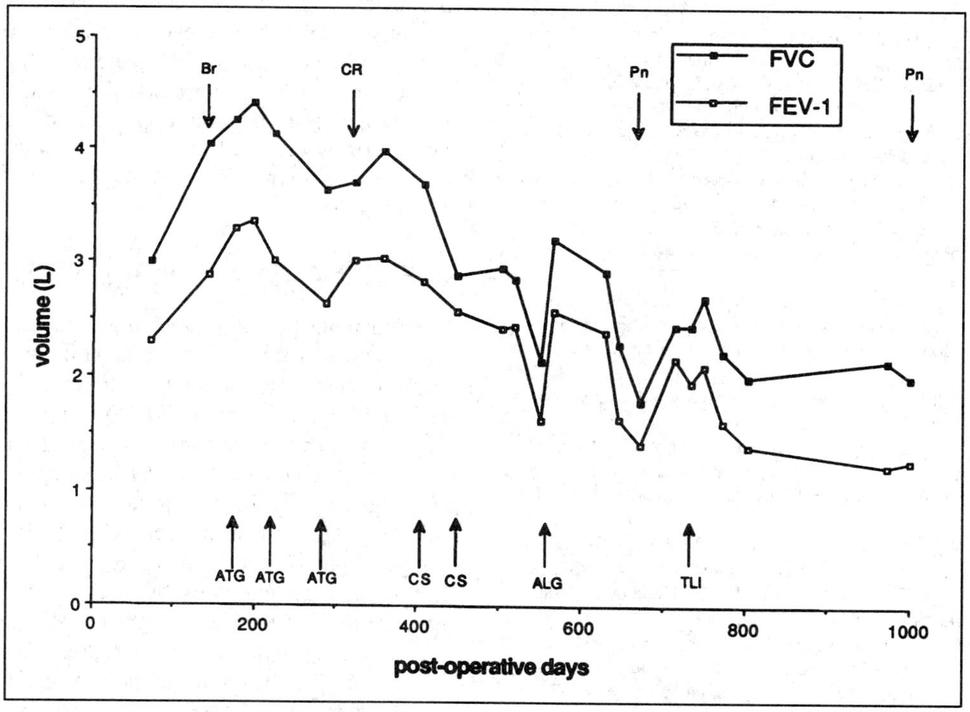

B

Fig. 220-3. **A,** Improvement in lung function after treatment of chronic rejection *(CR)* in a 10-year-old recipient of a heart-lung allograft. A marked decline in lung function occurred around the 400th postoperative day because of emergence of CR. After treatment with corticosteroids *(CS),* OKT-3, and antithymocyte globulin *(ATG),* lung function gradually improved in concert with resolution of obliterative bronchiolitis. Later episodes of infectious pneumonia *(Pn)* and bronchitis *(Br)* were also associated with a decline in lung function, which was quickly restored after treatment with appropriate antimicrobial therapy. **B,** Progressive decline in lung function despite multiple treatments for CR in a recipient of a double-lung allograft. Although CR was not diagnosed unequivocally until nearly the first postoperative year, it probably had begun several months earlier and was clinically suspected at that time. Multiple modes of augmented immunosuppression, including Minnesota antilymphocyte globulin *(ALG)* and total lymph node irradiation *(TLI)* achieved transient responses, but overall lung function declined inexorably. This recipient also had infectious pneumonias after the onset of CR, the last of which was fatal.

dramatically. Failure to improve the donor supply will severely limit the number of patients who would benefit from this procedure. A more efficient exploitation of the existing donor supply must also be achieved. The implantation of a single lung must be performed whenever possible, and the major complications of infection and rejection must be better controlled. Whether retransplantation for graft failure from any cause is effective and reasonable must be established. Despite the daunting challenges posed by these objectives, their achievement in the near future is realistic. In addition, prevention and control of diseases that now require transplantation may prove more difficult than anticipated. For this reason, pulmonary transplantation will likely continue to be the pre-eminent treatment for end-stage pulmonary and cardiopulmonary disease for many years.

REFERENCES

Armitage JM et al: Posttransplant lymphoproliferative disease in thoracic organ transplant patients: ten years of cyclosporine-based immunosuppression. J Heart Lung Transplant 10:877, 1991.

Burke CM et al: Post-transplant obliterative bronchiolitis and other late lung sequelae in human heart-lung transplantation. Chest 86:824, 1984.

Dauber JH, Paradis IL, and Dummer JS: Infectious complications in pulmonary allograft recipients. Clin Chest Med 11:291, 1990.

Duncan SR et al: Ganciclovir prophylaxis for cytomegalovirus infections in pulmonary allograft recipients. Am Rev Respir Dis (in press).

Duncan SR et al: Sequelae of cytomegalovirus pulmonary infections in lung allograft recipients. Am Rev Respir Dis 146:1419, 1992.

Fremes SE et al: Single lung transplantation and closure of patent ductus arteriosis for Eisenmenger's syndrome. 100:1, 1990.

Griffith BP et al: Immunologically mediated disease of the airways after pulmonary transplantation. Ann Surg 208:371, 1988.

Gryzan S et al: Unexpectedly high incidence of *Pneumocystis carinii* infection after lung-heart transplantation. Am Rev Respir Dis 137:1268, 1988.

Higenbottam T et al: Transbronchial lung biopsy for the diagnosis of rejection in heart-lung transplant patients. Transplant 46:532, 1988.

Hutter JA et al: Heart-lung transplantation: better use of resources. Am J Med 85:4, 1988.

Levin SM et al: Single lung transplantation for primary pulmonary hypertension. Chest 98:1107, 1990.

Rabinowich H et al: Alloreactivity of lung biopsy and bronchoalveolar lavage–derived lymphocytes from pulmonary transplant patients: correlation with acute rejection and bronchiolitis obliterans. Clin Transplant 4:376, 1990.

Reitz BA et al: Heart-lung transplantation: successful therapy for patients with pulmonary vascular disease. N Engl J Med 306:557, 1982.

Trulock EP et al: The Washington University–Barnes Hospital experience with lung transplantation. *JAMA* 266:1943, 1991.

Veith FJ: Lung transplantation. Surg Clin North Am 58:357, 1978.

Yousem SA, Burke CM, and Billingham M: Pathologic pulmonary alterations in long term human heart-lung transplantation. Hum Pathol 16:911, 1985.

Yousem SA et al: Efficacy of transbronchial lung biopsy in the diagnosis of bronchiolitis obliterans in heart-lung transplant recipients. Transplantation 47:893, 1989.

Yousem SA et al: A working formulation for the standardization of nomenclature in the diagnosis of heart and lung rejection: lung rejection study group. J Heart Lung Transplant 9:593, 1990.

CHAPTER

221 Sleep-Related Respiratory Disorders

Laurel Wiegand

Breathing abnormalities during sleep occur often and contribute to a variety of clinical syndromes. These include obstructive sleep apnea (OSA), central sleep apnea, and the central alveolar hypoventilation syndromes. Irregular respiration during sleep may also complicate the management of patients with underlying restrictive or obstructive pulmonary dysfunction or cardiac failure. The clinical importance of sleep-related respiratory disorders relates to the systemic effects of periodic blood gas derangements and disruption of normal sleep architecture.

This chapter primarily focuses on OSA, a disorder with tremendous medical, social, and economic consequences. The incidence of OSA is unknown, but it is estimated to affect 1% to 4% of adult men over age 40 years. Although described in the lay literature for centuries, OSA has only recently received widespread clinical recognition, since most patients with sleep apnea breathe normally while awake and must be examined during sleep for the breathing instability to become apparent. In addition, the importance of a good sleep history as a fundamental part of the comprehensive medical evaluation has traditionally been overlooked.

INFLUENCES OF SLEEP ON RESPIRATION

Various neurophysiologic changes occur during sleep. Normal sleep has a cyclic pattern with two major alternating components: non–rapid eye movement (non-REM) sleep and rapid eye movement (REM) sleep. These states are defined by characteristic electrophysiologic patterns. Sleep normally begins with a non-REM sleep period with progression through several non-REM sleep stages over about 90 minutes. The transition from *light* (stage 1) through *deep* (stages 3 and 4) non-REM sleep involves progressive slowing of the electrical activity recorded over the brain cortex by surface electroencephalography (EEG) and corresponding decreases in skeletal muscle tone (recorded by electromyography, EMG) and autonomic responses. The deepest stages of non-REM sleep are also referred to as *slow-wave sleep,* based on a slow, highly synchronized EEG pattern. REM sleep follows the non-REM sleep period and completes each cycle. Non-REM and REM phases alternate several times over the course of a normal sleep period. REM sleep is also known as *dream, paradoxical,* or *desynchronized sleep*. REMs and a marked decline in chin EMG activity help to identify REM sleep on electrophysiologic recordings. The eye movements are identified by electrooculogram (EOG) recordings and occur in phasic bursts in association with irregular respiration. The REM sleep EEG resembles that recorded during wakefulness and stage 1 non-REM sleep. Except for certain critical muscles such as the diaphragm, generalized skeletal muscle atonia occurs in REM sleep. Thus the "paradoxical" nature of the state: a highly active brain cortex in conjunction with inactive somatic musculature.

Important changes in respiration occur during sleep. With sleep onset, ventilation declines and arterial carbon dioxide increases. These changes result from true alveolar hypoventilation relative to the awake state because metabolic rate and carbon dioxide production decrease during sleep. Although ventilatory drive tends to decrease during sleep, the fall in alveolar ventilation may be more importantly related to a sleep-associated change in ventilatory mechanics. For instance, at sleep onset, partial pharyngeal collapse causes an increase in inspiratory resistance. This change most likely results from sleep-related changes in upper airway muscle activity. Ventilation during sleep depends on autonomic carotid and medullary chemoreceptor control systems because of the loss of behavioral input or the so-called wakefulness stimulus to breathe. Since cortical influences are diminished, the ventilatory response to perturbing influences such as increased upper airway resistance may be slower during sleep than during wakefulness.

Unlike other species, humans have a long pharyngeal segment that is unsupported by rigid structures. Although many factors have been postulated to affect pharyngeal patency, upper airway dilator muscles surrounding the pharynx have received the most attention. These muscles include the geniohyoid, genioglossus, and tensor veli palatini, which control the hyoid, tongue, and palate regions. Coordinated activation of these upper airway muscles stiffens or dilates the collapsible pharynx as intraluminal pressure decreases during inspiration. Inspiratory upper airway muscle activation slightly precedes that of the diaphragm and peaks earlier, presumably to prepare the extrathoracic upper airway for the impending collapsing force. The activities of most upper airway dilator muscles are diminished during sleep, rendering the upper airway more collapsible. A sleep-associated perturbation of the balance between upper airway and thoracic muscle forces could account for the observed increase in upper airway resistance. The relative importance of sleep-related changes in the activity of specific upper airway muscle groups remains poorly understood and may vary with individual upper airway anatomy.

BREATHING IRREGULARITIES DURING SLEEP

Apnea is defined as complete cessation of airflow for 10 or more seconds. Apneas may be obstructive, mixed, or central. During obstructive apneas, airflow is impeded by a completely collapsed upper airway despite continued effort to breathe. During central apneas, no effort is made to breathe, the diaphragm is inactive, and ventilation ceases. Mixed apneas begin with a central respiratory pause, followed by inspiratory effort against an obstructed airway.

The term *hypopnea* is applied when airflow decreases enough to lower oxygen saturation, although airflow does not completely cease. Hypopneas may also be obstructive, mixed, or central. During obstructive hypopneas the upper airway partially collapses. The patient does not fully compensate for the added breathing resistance, and hypoventilation results in oxyhemoglobin desaturation. Sustained periods of hypoventilation may also occur during sleep, particularly in patients with underlying cardiopulmonary or neurologic disease.

Apneas and hypopneas are referred to as *sleep-disordered breathing events*. They cause asphyxia and provoke arousal from sleep. The degree of asphyxia produced depends on the baseline arterial oxygen saturation, underlying cardiopulmonary function, and the duration of compromised breathing. Most apneas and hypopneas are terminated by arousal, which serves a protective function. Duration of the apnea or hypopnea depends on the patient's *arousal threshold,* which can be influenced by many factors. Although apneas, hypopneas, and sustained periods of hypoventilation may occur in any sleep stage, they tend to be most frequent and severe during REM sleep, when ventilation is inherently most irregular. Breathing irregularities are also common after the transition from wakefulness to light non-REM sleep because of the transitional state-related changes in ventilation already described.

CLINICAL DISORDERS ASSOCIATED WITH SLEEP-DISORDERED BREATHING

Many patients with underlying pulmonary dysfunction (chronic obstructive pulmonary disease, chest wall deformities, diseases associated with respiratory muscle paresis) develop clinically important oxygen desaturation during the night. This likely results from a combination of sleep-induced hypoventilation, reduced lung volumes, and ventilation-perfusion mismatching. These patients may benefit from a sleep laboratory study to determine the severity of sleep-disordered breathing and the effect of therapeutic intervention. The therapeutic approach to such disorders involves optimizing pulmonary function and the cautious use of ventilatory assist devices or oxygen.

Central sleep apnea (CSA) is an infrequent clinical disorder. Central apneas caused by the cessation of respiratory drive result from a defect or an instability in the ventilatory control apparatus. Congestive heart failure is probably the most common cause of CSA. CSA may also occasionally be seen in patients with neurologic disorders involving brainstem respiratory control centers. Although these patients typically exhibit chronic alveolar hypoventilation while awake, sleep provides a further destabilizing influence on respiration. This is caused by the loss of the stimulatory effect of wakefulness on breathing and by fluctuations in ventilatory stimuli that accompany transitions from wakefulness to sleep. The clinical sequelae of CSA relate to the severity of the respiratory control abnormality and are similar to those described for OSA (Table 221-1). Therapeutic options include supplemental oxygen, acetazolamide, nocturnal mechanical ventilation, and nasal continuous positive airway pressure (CPAP) therapy. Nasal CPAP is primarily used for the treatment of OSA. The mechanism by which it abolishes central apneas is not clear.

Table 221-1. Clinical sequelae in obstructive sleep apnea

Sleep disturbance	Clinical sequelae
Sleep fragmentation by frequent arousals and loss of "deep" non-REM sleep	Repeated arousals Restless sleep Nonrestorative sleep Daytime sleepiness Cognitive impairment Personality changes Morning headaches
Recurrent hypoxemia	Cardiac arrhythmias Pulmonary hypertension Right-sided heart failure Systemic hypertension Polycythemia Chronic respiratory failure Sudden death

OSA is the sleep-disordered breathing syndrome encountered most frequently. Patients with the OSA syndrome have alveolar hypoventilation during sleep in the form of repetitive obstructive or mixed apneas and hypopneas.

PATHOPHYSIOLOGY OF OBSTRUCTIVE SLEEP APNEA

The fundamental problem in OSA is excessive sleep-induced upper airway collapsibility. In most patients, upper airway obstruction during sleep occurs in the pharynx somewhere between the posterior edge of the hard palate and the epiglottis. The specific site of collapse varies among patients, with obstruction most often occurring behind either the soft palate or the tongue base. Why patients with OSA have complete occlusion of the upper airway whereas nonapneic subjects simply have an increase in upper airway resistance during sleep remains unknown. A central question is whether the problem is primarily caused by upper airway structural abnormalities or by abnormal sleep influences on factors controlling upper airway patency.

The most popular hypothesis is that obstructive apneas and hypopneas result from the normal sleep-induced attenuation in upper airway dilator muscle activity in individuals with a structurally small or excessively collapsible upper airway. A minority of OSA patients have upper airway structural abnormalities on physical examination. Nasal obstruction, tonsillar and adenoid hypertrophy, enlarged soft palatal structures, micrognathia, and macroglossia have all been associated with obstructive apneas and hypopneas. Surgical correction of these problems can eliminate or improve the sleep-disordered breathing. These anatomic abnormalities result in airway narrowing, requiring greater inspiratory pressure generation to achieve adequate airflow. Collapse occurs when the intrapharyngeal pressure decrease exceeds the dilating forces of the upper airway muscles. However, visual inspection does not reveal specific upper airway abnormalities in most OSA patients. Small pharyngeal lumina have been demonstrated in OSA patients by computed tomography, acoustic reflection, and cephalometric imaging techniques, although few well-controlled studies are available. Obstructive breathing events may also be related to excessive airway compliance or "floppiness" caused by altered soft tissue characteristics from adipose deposition or other factors. An alternative hypothesis is that OSA patients have a defect in ventilatory control that, coupled with the normal changes in upper airway mechanics, promotes airway instability during sleep.

The OSA syndrome involves the sequence of cyclic events illustrated in Fig. 221-1. With the initial onset of sleep, the pharyngeal airway collapses and airflow decreases despite continuing ventilatory effort. Hypoventilation results in progressive asphyxia, which increasingly stimulates ventilatory efforts against the occluded airway, typically until arousal occurs. With arousal, the upper airway opens and airflow is restored. Arousal coincides with a surge in upper airway muscle activity, which may help to restore airway patency. Hyperventilation in response to the accumulated chemical ventilatory stimuli (hypercapnia, hypoxia) initially follows upper airway deocclusion. The subsequent hyperventilation-induced hypocapnia and return to the sleeping state are followed by a decrease in pharyngeal dilator muscle activity and recurrent pharyngeal collapse, which begins the cycle again. This series of events may be repeated hundreds of times each night.

CONSEQUENCES OF SLEEP-DISORDERED BREATHING

We all have occasional apneas and hypopneas during sleep. However, when they become frequent and prolonged, clinical consequences develop that establish the diagnosis of the

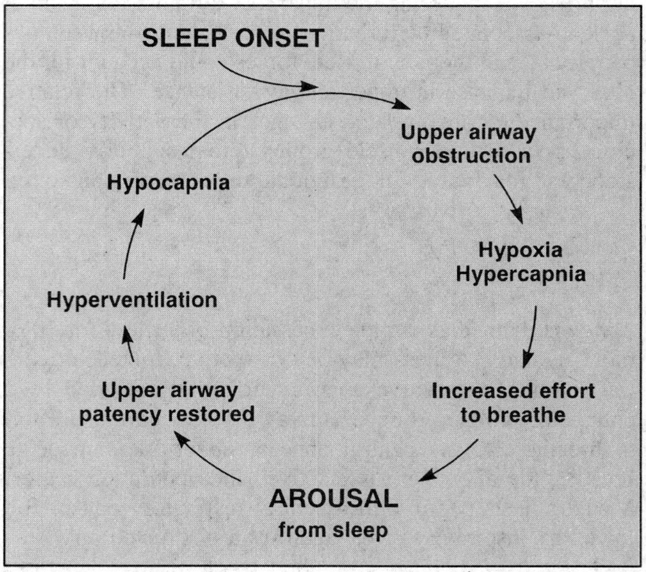

Fig. 221-1. Diagram of the cycle of events that occurs in a patient with obstructive apnea during sleep.

OSA syndrome. The term *syndrome* is reserved for patients with clinical sequelae of the disordered breathing.

Patients with the OSA syndrome have many associated neuropsychologic and cardiovascular problems, related both to long-term exposure to asphyxic stimuli during sleep and to disruption of normal sleep architecture (see Table 221-1). Such sequelae include excessive daytime sleepiness, impaired cognition and performance, pulmonary hypertension, and right ventricular failure. The specific factors responsible for the development of these sequelae are not well established. In addition, the severity of symptoms is often poorly correlated with the degree of nocturnal breathing disturbance.

Excessive daytime sleepiness and related neuropsychologic sequelae are probably caused by disruption of normal sleep patterns. Apneas and hypopneas are frequently terminated by arousals of short duration (< 15 seconds), but patients are typically unaware of their occurrence. These apnea-related arousals fragment normal sleep architecture and prevent OSA patients from achieving normal quantities of the deeper stages of non-REM sleep. This leads to progressive sleep deprivation. In severe cases, patients never achieve sustained or deep sleep and experience the symptoms of profound chronic sleep deprivation, which include depression, personality changes, cognitive impairment, decreased vigilance, and irresistible sleepiness. These sequelae affect the individual's quality of life, family relations, job performance and safety, and public safety. For example, concern exists that OSA patients have a higher rate of motor vehicle and industrial accidents.

Hemodynamic and cardiac abnormalities are related to repeated episodes of asphyxia and to fluctuations in intrathoracic pressure and autonomic activity during obstructed breaths. Complex neurohumoral changes occur that may eventually contribute to sustained pulmonary and systemic hypertension and ventricular dysfunction. It remains controversial whether a causal relationship exists between OSA and systemic hypertension. Debate also surrounds whether OSA patients are at increased risk for malignant cardiac arrhythmias and sudden death. Cardiac arrhythmias, including sinus and atrial arrhythmias, atrioventricular blocks, and ventricular arrhythmias, have been reported and occur predominantly during apneic spells. One recent study showed a higher mortality in OSA patients with more severe sleep-disordered breathing. Effective treatment appeared to have a positive influence on cumulative survival rates.

CLINICAL ASPECTS OF OBSTRUCTIVE SLEEP APNEA

Risk factors for OSA include structural upper airway abnormalities, male gender, and obesity. Approximately 4 to 10 times as many men as women have OSA. The male predominance of OSA suggests that important gender differences may exist in upper airway anatomy or in sleep influences on upper airway stability. Of interest, several studies have reported that most women with OSA are postmenopausal, suggesting that a hormonal influence may be important. Premenopausal women with OSA are often morbidly obese and amenorrheic.

OSA affects people of all ages but is most common from ages 40 to 70 years. In addition, a higher incidence of OSA occurs in patients with various congenital disorders (Prader-Willi and Downs syndromes), acromegaly, hypothyroidism, and neuromyopathic diseases affecting upper airway muscle function. However, these patient groups account for a minority of OSA patients.

Patients may notice several symptoms during wakefulness. Excessive daytime sleepiness is the most common complaint. Initially, daytime sleepiness may be mild and develop under benign conditions such as while watching TV. As the disorder progresses, daytime sleepiness becomes increasingly irresistible, debilitating, and potentially dangerous. For example, unwanted sleep may interrupt specific high-risk tasks such as driving a motor vehicle. By-products of excessive daytime sleepiness, such as inability to concentrate, memory and judgment impairment, irritability, depression, and personality changes, also become more common as the disorder progresses. Decreased libido and impotence are common complaints, although the etiology is undetermined. Early-morning headache is occasionally reported and may be related to the nocturnal episodes of hypercapnia and associated changes in cerebral blood flow.

Patients do not always report sleep-related complaints or realize that their sleep is disrupted by frequent, brief arousals. However, patients may complain of restless sleep or episodic choking spells. The sleeping partner is often a better historian and invariably reports loud or intolerable snoring, although not all snorers have sleep apnea. The sleeping partner may also describe periodic apneas terminated by snorting, gasping, or abnormal motor activity.

On physical examination, patients are often but not invariably obese. The neck may be short and well endowed with redundant soft tissue. The upper airway should be examined for structural abnormalities such as nasal polyps, a deviated nasal septum, chronic rhinitis, hypertrophied tonsils, macroglossia, micrognathia, or pharyngeal tumor or mass. Patients may exhibit systemic hypertension. As the disorder progresses, signs of pulmonary hypertension, right-sided heart failure, left ventricular dysfunction, polycythemia, and chronic alveolar hypoventilation may appear. Neurologic examination may reveal signs of excessive sleepiness and its by-products (e.g., impaired cognition).

Standard laboratory tests are of limited value in the diagnosis of OSA. Only 5% to 10% of OSA patients have chronic alveolar hypoventilation with elevated arterial carbon dioxide tension during wakefulness. These patients have the so-called pickwickian or obesity-hypoventilation syndrome. They tend to have severe OSA, morbid obesity, sustained pulmonary hypertension, and right-sided heart failure. A few patients are polycythemic. Although the pathophysiology of the obesity hypoventilation syndrome remains poorly understood, awake hypoventilation often resolves after effective treatment of the obstructive breathing events during sleep.

DIAGNOSIS OF OBSTRUCTIVE SLEEP APNEA

When a reasonable clinical suspicion exists that OSA is present, evaluation of sleep structure and respiratory function with *polysomnography* is indicated. Indications for nocturnal polysomnography for persons with suspected OSA include (1) unexplained excessive daytime sleepiness, (2) unexplained pulmonary hypertension or polycythemia, and (3) unexplained alveolar hypoventilation with chronic hypercapnia. Polysomnography involves recording electrophysiologic variables, such as electrical activity in the brain (EEG), eye movements (EOG), and chin muscle tone (EMG). This information allows sleep quantity and quality to be characterized. The electrocardiogram (ECG) is also usually recorded. Standard measurements of respiration include recordings of thoracic displacement, nasal and oral airflow, and arterial oxyhemoglobin saturation. The number of apneas and hypopneas, their type and duration, and their sequelae (e.g., amount of hypoxia, associated sleep fragmentation) can then be quantified. Periods of sustained hypoventilation may also be identified. By defining the type and severity of sleep-disordered breathing and associated sleep fragmentation, polysomnographic data help the clinician to develop a therapeutic strategy.

Standardized overnight polysomnography performed in a sleep laboratory by a trained technician is currently recommended as the diagnostic "gold standard." However, this test is labor intensive and expensive. Accordingly, clinicians are interested in developing simplified techniques for screening purposes. Proposed approaches have included analysis of self-reported symptoms and home monitoring with oximetry or an abbreviated polysomnographic montage. However, further study of the sensitivity, specificity, and cost-effectiveness of such approaches is required before firm recommendations can be made regarding their use.

THERAPEUTIC OPTIONS FOR OBSTRUCTIVE SLEEP APNEA

No large-scale prospective studies have been conducted to allow characterization of the natural history of OSA or of the clinical consequences for the untreated individual. Levels of sleep-disordered breathing formerly considered pathologic (more than five apneas per hour of sleep) have been reported in healthy, largely asymptomatic persons, particularly over 40 years of age. Because the natural history of OSA is poorly understood, no absolute indices of apnea frequency, severity of oxyhemoglobin desaturation, or sleep fragmentation currently mandate treatment. Most clinicians would agree that symptomatic patients with greater than 30 apneas and hypopneas per hour of sleep or severe oxyhemoglobin desaturation should be treated; however, symptomatic patients with fewer sleep-disordered breathing events may also benefit from treatment. The decision to treat is based on an overall assessment of the severity of hypersomnia and related neuropsychologic symptoms, cardiac sequelae, and the severity of sleep-disordered breathing documented on polysomnography.

The first step in OSA therapy involves a search for reversible factors that exacerbate sleep-disordered breathing. For example, ethanol and sedative-hypnotic use should be eliminated because these agents have been shown to worsen sleep-disordered breathing in most patients. Weight loss should be encouraged in obese patients and may correct or reduce the quantity of sleep-disordered breathing, particularly if the obesity is moderate. However, dietary weight reduction is often difficult to achieve and even more difficult to sustain. Surgical procedures such as gastric stapling have been successful in morbidly obese patients. Some patients benefit from adjustment of sleeping position because upper airway collapse is less likely in the lateral than in the supine position. Reversible causes of nasal congestion (e.g., chronic rhinitis) should be treated. High nasal resistance exacerbates pharyngeal collapse by requiring larger subatmospheric swings in intraluminal airway pressure to maintain airflow. In addition, two endocrine conditions, hypothyroidism and acromegaly, should be considered. Cautious thyroid replacement may lead to marked improvement in hypothyroid patients with sleep apnea. Since the clinical effect of modifying these risk factors is often unpredictable, follow-up polysomnography should be considered to assess the response to intervention.

Supplemental *oxygen* has been used with mixed results in selected OSA patients. Some patients have less sleep-disordered breathing and improved oxygen saturation when receiving supplemental oxygen. However, oxygen must be used with caution because it may aggravate apneas in a minority of patients. It should not be considered definitive therapy for OSA and does not address the fundamental problem of upper airway collapse. The response to supplemental oxygen should be tested during sleep in a monitored setting before it is prescribed for home use.

Pharmacologic therapy for OSA has generally been disappointing. The greatest experience has been with *protriptyline,* a tricyclic antidepressant. Protriptyline reduces the amount of REM sleep and may also stimulate upper airway muscle activity. The drug may be effective in mild OSA but has substantial side effects. Ventilatory stimulants (e.g., medroxyprogesterone) are occasionally used to improve gas exchange in the minority of OSA patients with the obesity-hypoventilation syndrome. However, chronic alveolar hypoventilation usually resolves with definitive therapy of the sleep-induced upper airway collapse, and long-term use of ventilatory stimulants is rarely necessary.

Several small studies have reported success with various *dental appliances* for the treatment of OSA. Most are designed to stabilize mandibular position and reduce tongue prolapse into the pharynx during sleep. Although this approach may be useful for selected patients with mild OSA, polysomnography is recommended to assess the response in individual patients. More experience with dental devices is needed before they can be widely recommended.

Other therapeutic modalities include tracheostomy and various surgical procedures designed to alter upper airway structure. *Tracheostomy* was once standard and highly effective therapy for OSA because the pharynx is completely bypassed. However, with the advent of better-tolerated options, tracheostomy is now reserved for morbidly ill patients. *Uvulopalatopharyngoplasty* (UPPP) is designed to augment upper airway patency by removing the uvula, part of the soft palate, and redundant pharyngeal tissue. Enthusiasm for UPPP surgery has waned as numerous studies have demonstrated that the success rate is highly variable in OSA patients. In addition, practical means of preoperatively predicting who will benefit from surgery are lacking. *Surgical correction* of specific upper airway abnormalities, such as a deviated nasal septum, tonsillar and adenoid hypertrophy, or maxillary and mandibular hypoplasia, has been shown to produce demonstrable improvement in sleep-disordered breathing in carefully selected OSA patients.

Introduced by Sullivan and colleagues in 1981, *nasal continuous positive airway pressure* has become the most popular therapy for patients with OSA and is in widespread use. Nasal CPAP is produced by a high flow blower that delivers a continuous stream of room air into a sealed nasal mask that the patient wears during sleep. The positive pressure created in the circuit pneumatically splints the pharyngeal airway open. Nasal CPAP abolishes apneas and hypopneas, oxygen desaturation, and apnea-related sleep fragmentation in most patients. Patients should be studied in the sleep laboratory to determine the optimum CPAP level, which varies with individual upper airway compliance. CPAP pressures in the range of 5 to 15 cm H_2O are typically required. After the initiation of effective nasal CPAP therapy, patients immediately experience a marked rebound in the deep stages of non-REM sleep and REM sleep. The sleep pattern gradually normalizes over the first few weeks of therapy, in association with dramatic symptomatic improvement, particularly in terms of daytime function. Side effects are minimal. Long-term compliance is the major concern with nasal CPAP therapy, since sustained use of the apparatus requires considerable patient commitment.

REFERENCES

American Sleep Disorders Association: The international classification of sleep disorders: diagnostic and coding manual. Lawrence, Kan, 1990, Allen Press.

American Thoracic Society Consensus Conference: Indications and standards for cardiopulmonary sleep studies. Am Rev Respir Dis 139:559, 1989.

Guilleminault C, Van den Hoad J, and Mitler M: Clinical overview of the sleep apnea syndrome. In Guilleminault C and Dement WC, editors: Sleep apnea syndromes. New York, 1978, Alan R Liss.

Lydic R, Wiegand L, and Wiegand D: Sleep-dependent changes in upper airway muscle function. In Lydic R and Biebuyck JF, editors: Clinical physiology of sleep. Bethesda, Md, 1988, American Physiologic Society.

Robinson RW and Zwillich CW: The effects of drugs on breathing during sleep. In Kryger MH, Roth T, and Dement WC, editors: Principles and practice of sleep medicine. Philadelphia, 1989, Saunders.

Sullivan CE et al: Reversal of obstructive sleep apnoea by continuous positive airway pressure applied through the nares, Lancet 1:862, 1981.

Thawley SW: Surgical therapy of obstructive sleep apnea. Med Clin North Am 69:1337, 1985.

White DP: Central sleep apnea. Med Clin North Am 69:1205, 1985.

PART SEVEN

Infectious Diseases

I BASIC PRINCIPLES

CHAPTER

222 Basic Principles of Infectious Diseases

Peter Densen
Merle A. Sande

Microorganisms surround us; they abound in our environment, on our skin, and on our mucosal membranes. Their acquisition from natural reservoirs in the environment, animals, or other humans requires an effective mode of transmission from and return to the reservoir. Transmission may occur by direct contact or through a common vehicle, or the microorganism may be airborne and vectorborne. For transmission to be successful, organisms must either adhere to body surfaces or gain access to subepithelial tissues directly. Acquisition may manifest itself as colonization (asymptomatic, little or no immune response), subclinical infection (asymptomatic, accompanied by an immune response), or active disease (symptomatic with or without an immune response). Delineation of the mode of transmission provides an opportunity for control of infection through the institution of primary preventive measures, such as hand washing or mosquito control. Identification of the biochemical determinants that account for adherence, invasiveness, and virulence coupled with an understanding of the host immune response to these pathogenic features provides the basis for primary prevention of infection through vaccination. The emergence of active clinical infectious disease heralds the need for therapeutic intervention (e.g., incision and drainage or specific antimicrobial therapy).

Microbial agents possess the capacity for genetic change in response to environmental and evolutionary pressures. This feature in conjunction with a short multiplication time permits the relatively rapid expression of new genetic information. The interaction of this genetic process with environmental, behavioral and technologic changes within society provides a dynamic situation in which new agents emerge to cause new diseases (e.g., acquired immunodeficiency syndrome [AIDS]), old agents acquire resistance to standard therapy (e.g., plasmid-mediated antimicrobial resistance), and old agents can be transmitted in new ways to cause typical disease in an atypical setting (e.g., corneal transplant-associated rabies).

In the face of such varied and constant exposure, it is amazing that active disease is as uncommon as it is. Most microorganisms, however, are relatively avirulent, and these "nonpathogens" are restricted to their interface with the human host by an array of both nonspecific and specific host defense mechanisms (Table 222-1). Relatively few microorganisms are pathogenic for the normal host. These organisms possess unique surface structures or secrete products that enhance their virulence. For a given organism, the risk of infection can be expressed by the following relationship:

$$\text{Risk of infection} \propto \frac{\text{Dose (\# of organisms)} \times \text{Virulence}}{\text{Host resistance}}$$

or

$$\text{Infectious diseases} \propto \frac{\text{Epidemiology} \times \text{Microbiology}}{\text{Anatomy} \times \text{Immunology}}$$

In some situations, a single factor dwarfs the importance of the other variables in these equations. For example, a nationwide outbreak of sepsis caused by *Enterobacter cloacae* and *Enterobacter agglomerans* was associated with commercially available intravenous fluid that had become contaminated during preparation. In this situation, ready access to the bloodstream by large numbers of relatively avirulent bacteria was a critical factor in the outbreak and overrode otherwise intact host defenses. More commonly, however, the balance between microbial factors and host resistance is shifted by disturbances in several variables simultaneously rather than by selective alteration of a single factor.

These principles also apply to patients with inherited or acquired immunodeficiency. These patients become infected at the same sites and with many of the same organisms as do normal individuals. Features that often characterize infection in these patients are increased frequency and severity, rapidity of onset, and slow resolution despite appropriate therapy. Relatively nonpathogenic organisms commonly cause infection in these patients and in individuals in whom local anatomic barriers to infection are breached by catheters, cytotoxic chemotherapy, or obstruction of a hollow viscus. The defect in host defenses permits these common "nonpathogens" to make their presence known.

Most organisms can be classified as either extracellular or intracellular pathogens. The former, typified by pyogenic cocci such as the pneumococcus, cause infection only while located extracellularly and are readily killed upon ingestion by phagocytic cells. Intracellular pathogens like *Mycobacterium tuberculosis* possess virulence factors that inhibit the killing mechanisms of phagocytic cells. In their intracellular location they enjoy protection from humoral defense mechanisms as well as from many antibiotics. Such organisms generally cause chronic infection. Some organisms (e.g., *Staphylococcus aureus* and *Salmonella typhi*) are well adapted for an existence in either milieu.

An additional relationship exists between the site of infection, the microorganism, and the type of host defense primarily responsible for control of the infection (Table 222-1). Most infections arise at the interface between the host and the environment. Thus knowledge of the organisms that colonize the skin and the various mucosal surfaces is valuable in predicting the range of likely causative organisms when infection arises from these sites. Con-

Table 222-1. Patterns of infection in patients with impaired host defense mechanisms

Host defense mechanism impaired	Cause of impairment	Site of infection	Common infecting agents
I. Anatomic and physiologic barriers to infection		Recurrent at site of abnormality	
A. Skin	Dermatitis Burns IV catheters	Skin → blood	Staphylococci, streptococci, GNR*
B. Skull	Skull fracture Cerebral spinal fluid leak	Meninges	Depends on site of leak: predominantly pneumococci but occasionally staphylococci or GNR if a dermal sinus is present
C. Mucociliary elevator	Alcohol Smoking Endotracheal tube Obstruction Immotile cilia (Kartagener's syndrome)	Bronchi, lungs	Colonizing flora
D. Gastric acid	Surgery, pernicious anemia, antacids	Intestine	*Salmonella* *Mycobacterium tuberculosis* Cholera
E. Intestinal motility or mucosal barrier	Blind loop syndrome, obstruction, tumor	Intestine → blood	Colonizing flora (*Streptococcus bovis,* clostridia, usually in the presence of a colonic neoplasm)
F. Urinary tract	Obstruction Catheterization Stones	Upper or lower urinary tract → blood	*Escherichia coli* "Urea splitters": *Proteus, Providencia*
G. Lymphatics	Obstruction	Lymphangitis	Group A streptococci
II. Immunologic barriers to infection			
A. Antibody IgG		Blood, meninges, bronchopulmonary tree, sinuses, ears, intestine	Encapsulated bacteria† Enteroviruses *Giardia lamblia* *Pneumocystis carinii*
IgM	Acquired or inherited	Blood	Meningococci, GNR
IgA		Bronchopulmonary tree, sinuses	Colonizing flora
B. Complement	Acquired or inherited	Blood, meninges, bronchopulmonary tree, sinuses, ears	Encapsulated bacteria Disseminated gonococcal infection
C. Cell-mediated immunity	Acquired or inherited	Lungs, meninges, gastrointestinal tract	Bacteria *Listeria* *M. tuberculosis* Atypical mycobacteria Viruses Herpes simplex Cytomegalovirus Varicella zoster (shingles) Fungi *Candida* *Cryptococcus* Protozoa *P. carinii* *Toxoplasma gondii* *Cryptosporidium*
D. Phagocytic function			
1. Neutrophils			
Deficient numbers ($<500/mm^3$)	Neoplasia Cytotoxic chemotherapy Autoimmune neutropenia	Skin, soft tissue, lung, blood	Staphylococci, GNR, *Candida, Aspergillus*
Defective function	Chronic granulomatous disease	Skin, soft tissue, lung, blood, bone, liver	Staphylococci, GNR, *Nocardia, Candida Aspergillus*
	Job's (hyperimmunoglobulinemia E) syndrome	Skin, soft tissue	Staphylococci
	Chediak-Higashi syndrome	Skin, soft tissue	Staphylococci
	Myeloperoxidase deficiency	Lung	*Candida*
2. Reticuloendothelial function	Asplenia Hemoglobinopathies	Blood	Encapsulated bacteria†
	Cirrhosis	Blood	GNR

*GNR, gram-negative rods.

†*Streptococcus pneumoniae, Haemophilus influenzae, Neisseria meningitidis.*

versely, identification of the infecting organism provides an important clue to the site of infection. Knowledge of these relationships is particularly useful when bacteremia is suspected as a complication of local infection or when it has been identified in the absence of an apparent site of infection.

The propensity of certain bacteria to cause infection affecting predominantly one organ system is known as tissue tropism. Examples of this phenomenon are the striking tendency of the meningococcus to cause meningitis, of viridans streptococci to cause subacute bacterial endocarditis, and of herpes simplex type I to cause encephalitis while a close relative herpes simplex type II, causes primarily genital tract infection. Factors that contribute to tissue tropism include (1) specific biochemical moieties on the surface of organism that are recognized by complementary structures on the surface of cells in the target organ; (2) the relative absence in the target organ of host defenses relevant for the organism in question; (3) the presence in the target organ of a specific nutrient critical for the growth of the organism; and (4) the local chemical environment as reflected by pH, tonicity, and redox potential. Sites in the human host that are partially immunocompromised include the relatively avascular heart valves; the cerebrospinal fluid, which contains few phagocytic cells and low levels of antibody and complement; bone; and the renal medulla. Treatment of infection in these sites generally necessitates administration of high dose, parenteral, bactericidal antibiotics for a prolonged time.

The host is not indiscriminately assailed by a multitude of organisms when anatomic abnormalities or genetic accidents create a specific rent in the host's armamentarium. Rather, infection usually is caused by a group of organisms with similar characteristics (Table 222-1). Anatomic abnormalities frequently manifest as recurrent infection at the exact same site. Defects in humoral immunity or in the complement cascade are associated with recurrent infection caused by encapsulated bacteria while infections caused by *S. aureus* or gram-negative bacilli are common in patients with defective neutrophil function. Patients with defective cell-mediated immunity (e.g., as occurs in AIDS) become infected with intracellular pathogens such as the herpes type viruses, toxoplasmosis, or *Pneumocystis carinii*. When host defense is simultaneously impaired in different arms of the immune system, the pattern of infection reflects the sum of the defects. Thus patients with impaired humoral and cellular immunity (e.g., severe combined immunodeficiency) experience recurrent infections caused by pyogenic cocci and intracellular pathogens. Combined patterns of infection are also observed when therapy of the underlying disorder has a toxic effect on other arms of the immune system, as may occur during treatment of hematologic malignancies. Patterns of infection also blur when concomitant broad-spectrum antibiotic therapy leads to the elimination of the critically important, protective, nonpathogenic organisms, thereby providing for overgrowth of mucosal surfaces with resistant organisms. Nevertheless, the pattern of infections is an extremely valuable clue pointing to the site of immunologic or anatomic impairment and is important in directing the initial evaluation of patients efficiently and cost effectively.

Redundancy and multiplicity are important characteristics of the immune system. Hence, a single organism can be eliminated effectively by diverse but often overlapping mechanisms (Table 222-1). The contribution of an individual mechanism to the defense against a given organism is determined by the specific location and the organism. For example, complement-dependent bactericidal activity is most important in protecting the bloodstream, whereas neutrophil phagocytic activity is more important in the soft tissues.

Infectious injury is produced in the host through a wide variety of mechanisms. Injury may occur systemically as well as locally and may be immediate or delayed. Local damage may be produced by cell-bound or secreted toxins that are cytotoxic or interfere with the normal function of a particular organ system in the absence of obvious anatomic disruption. The normal inflammatory response plays an important role in containing infection. The development of an exuberant response, however, contributes to tissue destruction through the unchecked action of cytokines, inflammatory proteases, and toxic metabolites released from phagocytic cells in response to microbial invasion. Damage is particularly likely to occur when infection occurs in a closed space (e.g., in a joint or in the brain) or when large numbers of different organisms are present (e.g., in the development of an anaerobic lung abscess). Resolution of the inflammatory response results in fibrosis or scarring and occasionally calcification. These healing processes may be responsible for delayed injury to the host (e.g., sterility in women recovering from pelvic inflammatory disease), the development of a new heart murmur during the healing phase of endocarditis, or the onset of seizures in patients with calcified intracerebral pork tape worm larvae (cerebral cysticercosis).

The expression of microbial antigens on the surface of epithelial and endothelial cells during intracellular replication of the pathogen can elicit the immune destruction of these cells. Other immunologic mechanisms of tissue injury include immune complex formation (endocarditis) and autoimmune hemolytic anemia, thrombocytopenia, or neutropenia that may occur during the polyclonal antibody response induced by infection of B lymphocytes with Epstein Barr virus during infectious mononucleosis. Finally, systemic injury may be initiated by ischemia and disseminated intravascular coagulopathy during septic shock.

It is clear from the foregoing discussion that the outcome of the encounter between the host and the microbe lies in dynamic balance. Infection with one organism (e.g., influenza virus) can alter this balance and set the stage for another infection (e.g., postviral bacterial pneumonia) caused by bacteria previously residing in symbiotic bliss in the host's oropharynx. It is also apparent that microorganisms owe their pathogenicity to virulence factors that enable the organism to colonize the host and elude host defense mechanisms. The value of specific immunity to the host is to negate the effect of microbial virulence factors by establishing an immune reaction on the organism itself or to its toxic products.

The remainder of this section deals with the interaction between the human host and infectious agents. The chapters are grouped into four subsections: The subsections Laboratory Tests provide a description of the specific host defenses, address the issue of the antibiotics used to aid these defenses, and describe methods used for identifying pathogens. The subsection Clinical Syndromes describes common clinical syndromes that result when infection occurs, the syndromes being enumerated and detailed according to how they are presented to the physician by the patient. In the subsection Organisms Infective to Humans, each agent that produces disease in humans—from the viruses to the helminths—is described in detail: its ecology, the host defenses it must overcome, how it produces infection, the specific disease it causes, and how the disease is diagnosed and most appropriately treated and prevented. The format of this section should enable the clinician to quickly obtain necessary information derived either from the clinical setting (the patient) or from the microorganism (a positive culture). Cross-referencing has been used liberally to aid in the appropriate work-up or therapy.

REFERENCE

Lorber B: Changing patterns of infectious diseases, Am J Med 84:569, 1988.

CHAPTER

223 Host Defense Against Infection: The Roles of Antibody, Complement, and Phagocytic Cells

Peter Densen
David L. Weinbaum
Gerald L. Mandell

HUMORAL IMMUNITY

Humoral immunity reflects protection from infection mediated by specific antibody. Protection depends on the highly specific capacity of a given antibody to recognize a given antigen and to trigger other aspects of host defense.

Properties and distribution of antibody

There are five classes of immunoglobulins: IgG, IgA, IgM, IgD, and IgE. Although IgE may play a role in limiting disease caused by some helminths, its function and that of IgD in host defense against infection has not been clearly delineated and will not be considered further here. IgG, which accounts for about 76% of the total plasma immunoglobulin, is distributed equally between the plasma and soft tissues and is the only immunoglobulin transported across the placenta to the fetus. There are four subclasses of IgG, numbered according to their decreasing concentration in plasma. Only IgG1 and IgG3 are efficient activators of complement and bind to neutrophils. The capacity of infants to synthesize different classes and subclasses of immunoglobulins matures at different rates. IgG2 and IgG4 synthesis matures more slowly than IgG1 and IgG3 and low levels of the former two are present for the first 18 to 24 months of life. Among the subclasses, IgG2 is particularly important in the response to polysaccharide antigens. These physiologic and functional attributes of IgG2 probably contribute to the high incidence of infection caused by encapsulated bacteria in young children and to the poor immunologic response of children under the age of 2 years to polysaccharide vaccines.

IgA, which accounts for 15% of the total plasma immunoglobulin, is distributed approximately equally between plasma and mucosal surfaces. Two subclasses are recognized: IgA1 predominates over IgA2 in serum (6:1), whereas the concentrations of the two subclasses are more nearly equal (2:1) on mucosal membranes. IgA is not transported transplacentally and although it may activate complement, its primary role is to prevent colonization of mucosal surfaces by microbial pathogens.

IgM accounts for just 8% of the total plasma immunoglobulin and is confined principally (75%) to plasma. Much of the "natural" antibody present in serum against gram-negative organisms is found in the IgM class and presumably arises in response to unrecognized exposure to lipopolysaccharide antigens derived from gut flora. IgM is not transported transplacentally and IgM receptors are not present on phagocytic cells. Nevertheless, because of its pentameric structure, it is an efficient activator of complement.

The highly specific nature of the recognition of antigen by antibody imposes a requirement for antibody synthesis during the initial presentation of antigen. Consequently, a delay occurs before the beneficial effects of specific antibody are felt. The primary immune response is characterized by the synthesis of IgM followed by IgG. Subsequent exposure to the same antigen results in an anamnestic response with the rapid production of antibody, mainly IgG. This pattern is useful clinically in the serologic diagnosis of acute (elevated titer of specific IgM followed by an elevated titer of specific IgG) versus recurrent or chronic infection (elevated titer of specific IgG only). In addition, because IgM does not cross the placenta and because the capacity to synthesize IgM in response to a specific stimulus is acquired in utero, the presence in cord serum of IgM specific for a particular infectious agent, for example, *Toxoplasma gondii,* is indicative of in utero acquisition of infection.

Antibody function in infectious diseases

Antibodies are bifunctional molecules, one end of which (Fab) recognizes and binds to antigen. The other end (Fc) triggers the biologic response of the host. Antibodies with differing antigenic specificities are produced by the host in response to the many antigens presented by an individual infectious agent. Thus more than one type of functional antibody may be produced during a single infection; conversely, a single antibody can mediate different functions, for example opsonic and bactericidal. The triggering function of an antibody is determined in part by the chemical nature of the antigen, protein, or polysaccharide; by the state of the antigen, soluble, or particulate; by the properties of the antibody, class, or subclass and complement or noncomplement fixing; and by its distribution.

IgA inhibits microbial attachment to the surface of mucosal cells by reacting with specific adhesion molecules on the microbial surface. *Neisseria gonorrhoeae, Neisseria meningitidis, Haemophilus influenzae,* and *Streptococcus sanguis* secrete a protease that specifically cleaves IgA1 into its component Fab and Fc fragments and probably contributes to the predilection of these organisms to cause mucosal infection or dental caries. Neutralizing antibodies are predominantly IgG molecules that neutralize microbial toxins, for example tetanus or diphtheria toxins. They bind to the toxin and prevent its attachment or entry into the target cells of the host. Bactericidal antibodies (IgM and IgG) promote complement-dependent killing of susceptible gram-negative bacteria. Bactericidal activity requires recognition of specific (lytic) epitopes on the bacterial surface. For example, IgM specific for gonococcal lipopolysaccharide promotes killing of that organism, whereas IgM specific for outer membrane proteins does not. Opsonic antibodies promote ingestion of microorganisms by interacting with specific receptors on phagocytic cells. The interaction of antibody with its specific receptor also activates the microbicidal mechanisms of these cells. Only IgG1 and IgG3 function in this capacity by themselves. However, there are also neutrophil receptors for C3b and C3bi, opsonic molecules generated during complement activation. Thus both IgM and IgG also function as opsonins by virtue of their ability to activate complement. Opsonization requirements vary from organism to organism but in general, phagocytic uptake is most efficient when the organism is coated with both IgG and C3.

Immunoglobulin deficiencies

Acquired immunoglobulin deficiencies result from decreased production, increased catabolism, or both. Decreased synthesis of immunoglobulin is most commonly observed in the setting of hematologic or lymphatic malignancy. Rarely, these deficiencies may arise as a postinfectious complication of certain viral infections (e.g., Epstein-Barr virus) in which the virus infects B cells and appears to initiate an uncontrolled suppressor T cell response. Increased catabolism of antibody is a well-described consequence of excessive protein loss (e.g., the nephrotic syndrome, third-degree burns, or protein-losing enteropathies).

Inherited immunoglobulin deficiencies are relatively common, occurring in about 1 in 600 in the general population. Alone or in conjunction with an associated defect in cell-mediated immunity these disorders constitute the majority (50% and 70%, respectively) of the primary immunodeficiency syndromes. The severity of these disorders is a function of whether all, several, or only one of the antibody classes or subclasses is affected and whether they are associated with defects in cell-mediated immunity. Patients with a global deficiency of IgG, IgA, and IgM experience recurrent pyogenic infections involving the sinopulmonary tract, ears, meninges, and bloodstream. These infections are caused predominantly by encapsulated organisms. Chronic or recurrent diarrhea occurs in many individuals with common variable hypogammaglobulinemia. An infectious etiology, primarily *Giardia lamblia,* is responsible for about 60% of these cases, whereas noninfectious causes, for example gluten enteropathy, account for the remainder. Occasionally, plasma immunoglobulins will be normal in patients with this clinical history. In this situation, a selective deficiency of one of the IgG subclasses, in particular IgG2, should be sought. These patients may have a total plasma IgG within the normal range, as IgG1 accounts for an average of 70%, whereas IgG2 accounts for about 25%, of the total IgG.

Most patients with IgA deficiency are healthy, but some have atopic disease, gastrointestinal disorders, autoimmune disease, malignancy, or recurrent infection. When recurrent infection does occur, it usually involves the sinopulmonary tract, but an association with a specific group of organisms is reported infrequently. A high proportion of individuals with IgA deficiency and recurrent infection also has a selective deficiency of IgG2 or IgG4 or both.

Patients with a deficiency of IgM are at risk for bacteremia caused by gram-negative bacteria, in particular the meningococcus. This observation attests to the primary importance of IgM in host defense of the vascular space.

Therapy

Stable nonaggregating preparations of IgG that maintain their functional activity have recently been developed for intravenous infusion. Their use has been effective in decreasing the incidence of infection in patients with IgG deficiency. The increasing availability of preparations obtained from individuals with high titers of IgG against likely infectious agents, the ease of administration, and the low frequency of side effects have made these preparations the therapy of choice for deficient individuals. The optimal dosage has not been rigorously established, but 400 mg/kg given IV once a month has resulted in adequate levels and calculated half-lives in the 25- to 40-day range for all four IgG subclasses. Infusions of fresh-frozen plasma or IgG should not be given to patients with a selective deficiency of IgA because there is an increased risk of anaphylactic reactions due to the synthesis of antibodies to IgA.

The complications of chronic infection, pulmonary fibrosis, and bronchiectasis may progress despite immunoglobulin replacement therapy. Appropriate antibiotics should be used during periods of infection. Chronic antibiotic administration is not successful in preventing infection and may predispose to infection with resistant organisms. Close attention to good pulmonary drainage is important during periods of active infection as well as infection-free intervals.

HUMORAL IMMUNITY AND THE SPLEEN

Anatomically, the spleen is unique because it constitutes a quarter of the fixed lymphoid tissue and sits, not in the lymphatic drainage, but in the systemic circulation. As a consequence of its content of macrophages, dendritic cells, and lymphocytes, the spleen plays a major role in filtration of the arterial circulation and is critical for the generation of a primary immune response to blood-borne antigens, especially when the antigen is a polysaccharide.

Absent splenic function occurs in cases of inherited or postsurgical asplenia. Decreased function has also been reported after infarction or irradiation, in systemic lupus erythematosus, inflammatory bowel disease, adult celiac disease, dermatitis herpetiformis, and in the hemoglobinopathies. The spleens of patients with sickle cell disease are nonfunctional by an average age of 13 months. The hyposplenic state can be readily established by examination of the peripheral blood smear for Howell-Jolly bodies.

Patients with splenic dysfunction are at increased risk of overwhelming sepsis caused by encapsulated bacteria. The overall risk of infection is increased 250-fold and is influenced by the underlying disease, ranging from 58 to 1000 times that in the general population for patients splenectomized for trauma or thalassemia, respectively. The risk is greatest if splenectomy is performed during the first 3 years of life. The median time from splenectomy to infection is 5 years, but cases of overwhelming infection have been reported as many as 40 years after surgery. The pneumococcus is the most common pathogen and together with *H. influenzae* and the meningococcus accounts for 70% to 90% of the cases. The bulk of the remaining cases are accounted for by *Staphylococcus aureus* and *Escherichia coli*.

As many as 70% of patients with postsplenectomy sepsis have no apparent primary site of infection. Gram stain of the buffy coat from peripheral blood will demonstrate organisms in one third of patients. A positive smear indicates at least 10,000 organisms per milliliter of blood, approximately 100 times that in the blood of the patients with intact spleens and bacteremia. Consequently, infection is fulminant and disseminated intravascular coagulopathy occurs in 60% to 70% of patients. The overall mortality rate is about 50%, but ranges from 40% to 90% depending on the underlying disease.

Experiments in animals have shown that in the absence of specific anticapsular antibody, the spleen is essential for the removal of encapsulated pneumococci from the circulation and that this dependence increases with the degree of encapsulation. The effect of specific anticapsular antibody is to shift the major responsibility for bacterial clearance from the spleen to the liver.

These findings have led to the use of prophylactic antibiotics in children splenectomized before they are capable of responding to polysaccharide vaccines. In older children and adults, emphasis has been placed on vaccination with the multivalent pneumococcal and the tetravalent meningococcal vaccines. The response of splenectomized individuals to polysaccharide vaccines is affected by the underlying disease and, in general, is not as good and does not persist as long as in normal individuals. Consequently, it may be advisable to periodically evaluate specific antibody titers and to consider repeating vaccination as necessary. Due to the possibility of intense local reactions, pneumococcal vaccination should not be repeated routinely.

THE COMPLEMENT SYSTEM IN INFECTIOUS DISEASES

The complement cascade functions chiefly as an amplification system. A recurrent theme is the cleavage of one component into two fragments, the smaller of which floats free while the larger is bound to the cell surface. The smaller fragments are potent mediators of the inflammatory response. These anaphylatoxins promote vascular dilatation and enhance permeability (C3a, C5a) or act as a chemoattractant stimulus (C5a) for neutrophils, monocytes, and eosinophils. The larger cleavage products promote the continued sequential activation of the complement cascade, enhance phagocytosis (C3b, C3bi), and through the insertion of the membrane attack complex (C5b to C9) promote killing of susceptible organisms. Other actions include modulation of the immune response, promotion of neutrophil release from the bone marrow, and inhibition of precipitation and promotion of solubilization of immune complexes.

Complement activation proceeds by either the classical or alternative pathway. These pathways converge at the level of C3 and share a final activation sequence from C5 to C9. Due to positive feedback at the level of C3, activation of the classical pathway facilitates alternative pathway activation. A major feature of the classical pathway is its activation by antibody. As a consequence, activation occurs rapidly and efficiently, even at low concentrations of both antibody and complement. Antibody directs complement deposition to nearby structures and may itself serve as a site for complement binding. Proximity between antibody and complement on the microbial surface enhances the effector functions of these molecules.

Activation of the alternative pathway can occur in the absence of antibody. Hence the beneficial effects of complement as an amplification system can be expressed early in the course of microbial invasion before the synthesis of specific antibody. Although not required, antibody does facilitate alternative pathway activation. Activation is slow, taking two to three times as long as the classical pathway to achieve maximal activity and requiring a higher concentration of components for initiation.

Unlike the classical pathway, activation of the alternative pathway occurs continuously in the fluid phase, but its products are dissipated in a highly regulated manner by factors H and I, which interfere with the formation and function of C3bBb, the C3 convertase that is the critical product of alternative pathway activation. Properdin, another component, is a positive regulator of the alternative pathway and stabilizes C3bBb. Introduction of an appropriate cell surface shifts the balance from fluid phase control to complement activation and deposition. Thus the biochemical composition of the microbial surface is another determinant of activation. For example, the presence of sialic acid or sulfated acid mucopolysaccharides (heparin sulfate) on some cells enhances the binding of factor H to C3b, thereby promoting both the dissociation of Bb from C3bBb and the inactivation of C3b by factor I. Sialic acid is a prominent chemical constituent of the capsular polysaccharides of type III group B streptococci, *K1 E. coli,* and group B and C meningococci, whereas the capsule of K5 *E. coli* is composed of disulfoheparin. Thus the capsules of these organisms are nonactivators of the alternative pathway. It is noteworthy that these organisms are prominent causes of neonatal and infant sepsis. In these young individuals the absence of specific antibody to activate the classical pathway coupled with capsular polysaccharide-mediated inhibition of complement consumption via the alternative pathway may provide the ideal setting for infection with these organisms.

Recently, a number of host cell membrane proteins have been identified that interact with specific activated complement components. These proteins fall into two general categories. The first group are complement receptors, which exhibit limited cellular distribution and subserve cell-specific functions. For example, CR-3 receptors are found primarily on phagocytic cells. Their genetic absence is associated with severe infections and death shortly after birth as a consequence of impaired neutrophil function. CR-2 receptors are present primarily on B lymphocytes. Ligand interaction with this receptor augments antibody production. Epstein-Barr virus uses the CR-2 receptor to enter B lymphocytes, thereby stimulating the polyclonal antibody response that characterizes the early phase of infectious mononucleosis. The second group of molecules are membrane proteins that inhibit complement activation. These proteins are widely distributed and prevent complement-mediated damage to host cells. They exert their influence by inhibiting either the cell-bound C3 convertases or assembly of the membrane attack complex. The deficiency of two of these membrane proteins, decay-accelerating factor and CD59, is the functional basis for the syndrome of paroxysmal nocturnal hemoglobinuria. Some microbial organisms (e.g., *Candida albicans* and herpes simplex type 1) express C3 binding proteins on their surface, which both protect the organism from complement activation and alter the ability of bound C3 to promote phagocytosis of the organism.

Complement deficiency states

Complement deficiencies may be acquired or inherited. Acutely acquired deficiencies most commonly reflect consumption of complement components as occurs during overwhelming infection, severe burns, or hemodialysis. Total hemolytic complement is low and there is a global reduction of most of the individual components, which returns to normal after the acute event has subsided. Acquired chronic depression of complement activity is usually due to circulating immune complexes or, in rare situations, to antibody reacting with one of the components. These patients exhibit the same patterns of infection seen in individuals with inherited deficiencies of complement.

Homozygous complement deficiencies are found in approximately 1 in 10,000 persons, but the frequency is higher among patients with collagen vascular disease or certain infections. The pattern of infection varies with the deficiency and the nature of the accompanying defect in host defense effector mechanisms. For example, only 20% of patients with a classical pathway defect (C1, C2 or C4) experience infection, probably because their alternative pathway is intact. Infection occurs early in life and is usually caused by encapsulated bacteria. On the other hand, immunologic diseases appear to be more common than infection, affecting 85% of these individuals.

Inherited defects of the alternative pathway are rare. The distinguishing feature of properdin deficiency is its X-linked mode of inheritance, which is reflected in a family history of fulminant meningococcal infection occurring predominantly in teenage boys in skipped generations.

C3 deficient individuals experience both recurrent infection and immunologic disease. Opsonic, chemotactic, and serum bactericidal activity are defective in these patients. Infection typically occurs early in life, is recurrent, and is caused primarily by encapsulated bacteria. Patients with factor I or H deficiency are unable to inhibit the formation and activity of the alternative pathway C3 convertase, C3bBb. Hence their serum contains low levels of C3, and they exhibit a pattern of infection similar to that in patients with primary C3 deficiency.

Serum from patients with a deficiency of one of the terminal complement components (C5 to C9) lacks bactericidal activity but is capable of opsonizing organisms normally. Approximately half of these individuals never experience infection and a minority develop immunologic disorders. The other half experience systemic meningococcal or gonococcal disease; of these, half suffer recurrent bouts of neisserial infection. Compared with the general population, meningococcal disease in these individuals is distinguished by (1) a 5- to 10,000-fold greater risk of infection, (2) a higher male/female ratio (3:1 vs 1:1), (3) a higher median age of first infection (17 vs 3 years), (4) a tenfold greater relapse rate, (5) a higher recurrence rate (45% vs <1%), (6) a higher rate of infection caused by group Y meningococci (44% vs 10%), and (7) a paradoxically lower case fatality rate (2.9% vs 19%). (Chapter 287).

Serum bactericidal activity plays a major role in protection against blood-borne infections. Both antibody and complement are critical for the expression of this activity and in their presence invasion of bloodstream is restricted to organisms that are naturally resistant to it. The physiologic nadir of antibody that occurs during the first year of life is reflected by absent serum bactericidal activity and the highest age-specific incidence of bacteremia and meningitis due to *H. influenzae* and *N. meningitidis*. These bacteria are readily killed by most adult sera. At the other end of the spectrum are patients with absent serum bactericidal activity due to a deficiency of one of the terminal complement components and who experience an inordinate number of neisserial infections.

The frequency with which patients with hypogammaglobulinemia, hyposplenia or complement deficiency experience infection caused by encapsulated bacteria, in particular *Streptococcus pneumoniae, H. influenzae,* and *N. meningitidis,* underscores the interplay between these host defense systems. In animal models of infection, elimination of these organisms from the bloodstream occurs in three phases: an early phase (0 to 1 hour) during which the bulk of the organisms are removed in an antibody-modulated manner by phagocytic cells within the spleen, liver, and lung; an intermediate phase during which further sterilization of the blood occurs as a consequence of complement-dependent killing of susceptible organisms; and a late phase, which is critically dependent on the contribution of the complement system to opsonization. In the absence of anticapsular antibody, complement fixation is less effective in promoting phagocytosis because C3b is deposited beneath the antiphagocytic polysaccharide capsule. Specific antibody promotes C3b fixation to the capsule itself. In this location, the cooperative opsonic function of C3b and antibody promotes ingestion and killing of these organisms. Patients with defective neutrophil function do not experience a higher frequency of these infections probably because of the large number of phagocytic cells and variety of mechanisms by which these cells can kill ingested organisms.

Diagnosis and treatment of complement deficiency states

From the standpoint of infectious diseases, complement assays are used most commonly to evaluate the possibility of complement deficiency as an explanation for recurrent infection. In this setting, the most important screening test is the assay for total hemolytic complement (CH50). This assay measures the functional integrity of all nine proteins in the classical pathway. It is important to realize that a normal result in the more commonly available antigenic assays for C3 or C4 does not exclude a defect elsewhere in the cascade.

Patients with complement deficiency states should receive the pneumococcal and meningococcal polysaccharide vaccines as well as the *H. influenzae* conjugate vaccine. Use of the classical pathway in patients with a defect in the alternative pathway is improved by vaccination. Conversely, the ability of specific antibody to facilitate alternative pathway activity independent of complement activation by the Fc portion of the immunoglobulin molecule provides a rationale for vaccinating patients with a defect in the classical pathway. Patients missing one of the terminal components benefit from vaccination as a consequence of improved opsonization and a shifting of the burden of host defense from complement-dependent bactericidal activity to phagocytosis. Fresh-frozen plasma can be used to restore complement component levels to normal but because of the short half-life of the components and development of antibody to the missing component, this approach should be reserved for life-threatening infections. Prophylactic antibiotics are necessary only rarely.

PHAGOCYTIC CELLS

Neutrophils, eosinophils, basophils, monocytes, and macrophages are all capable of ingesting invading pathogens and are classified as phagocytes. Neutrophils, eosinophils, and basophils are granulocytic phagocytes; monocytes and macrophages constitute the mononuclear phagocytic system. The cellular immune system (monocytes and macrophages) is discussed in detail in Chapter 286.

Neutrophils

Neutrophils are the most common phagocyte in the blood, constituting approximately 60% of the leukocytes on a blood smear. Development in the bone marrow consists of (1) a mitotic phase, in which myeloblasts divide and mature through promyelocytes and myelocytes, and (2) a nonmitotic phase of maturation, in which metamyelocytes mature to band cells and then to segmented neutrophils. The majority of mature neutrophils in the body are found in the nonmitotic compartment (i.e., the bone marrow reserve). It takes 9 to 11 days for the progeny of a myeloblast to leave the marrow, and in the adult up to 10^{11} mature neutrophils per cubic millimeter enter the circulation per day. Once in the blood, neutrophils separate into two equal classes, actively circulating neutrophils and marginated neutrophils that adhere to blood vessel walls. The intravascular neutrophil half-life is 6 to 8 hours, after which neutrophils pass out of the bloodstream and migrate to mucosal surfaces or localize in areas of inflammation. Senescent neutrophils are themselves phagocytized by fixed tissue macrophages. Extravascular survival varies from hours to 4 days. Granulocyte-monocyte colony-stimulating factor (GM-CSF) increases total neutrophil production by acting at the pluripotent stem cell. Recombinant human granulocyte colony-stimulating factor (G-CSF) is also available and shortens periods of chemotherapy-induced neutropenia.

The mature neutrophil possesses two types of morphologically distinct cytoplasmic granules. The primary granule is a true lysosome, as it contains acid hydrolases in addition to myeloperoxidase, elastase, cationic proteins, lysozyme, and defensins. This granule appears to serve a microbicidal function. The specific granules outnumber the primary granules by 3:1 and contain lysozyme, lactoferrin, collagenase, and vitamin B_{12}-binding proteins. Specific granules discharge their contents into the extracellular fluid and may therefore function in part in the secretory regulation of the inflammatory response. The neutrophil membrane has surface receptors capable of binding the iC3b (CR3 receptor) and C5a components of complement, as well as the Fc end of immunoglobulin G.

The neutrophil's response in host defense against invading microbes may be divided into mobilization, adherence, locomotion, chemotaxis, phagocytosis, and intracellular killing. Although each of these events will be considered separately, they form a continuous process that may exist in all stages at once. Microbial invasion is followed by mobilization of both mature and band forms from the bone marrow, resulting in the leftward shift noted with many acute bacterial infections. These neutrophils become sticky and adhere to the vascular endothelium (margination). The cell then enters the tissues by locomoting between the endothelial cells (diapedesis). Once it is in the tissues, the neutrophil moves, by chemotaxis (directed migration), in the direction of increasing concentrations of attractants (chemotactic factors). A large number of substances act as chemotactic factors for the neutrophil. The most important include (1) bacterial products, (2) complement components C3a and C5a obtained through either classical or alternative complement pathway activation, and (3) cellular products such as leukotrienes and cytokines derived from other neutrophils, lymphocytes, and macrophages. These factors include arachidonic acid metabolites, interleukin 1 (IL-1) (endogenous pyrogen), and tumor necrosis factor (cachectin). At the site of inflammation, the concentration of chemotactic factors is so strong that neutrophil chemotaxis is actually stopped and the cell becomes hyperadhesive.

Contact with the microorganisms initiates phagocytosis. Many virulent organisms resist ingestion by neutrophils. These organisms can be engulfed only by being trapped against a surface (surface phagocytosis) or by being opsonized. Once the microbe is bound to the neutrophil surface, the neutrophil membrane flows around it and encloses it in a vacuole called the *phagosome*.

Microbial attachment to the neutrophil initiates two events involved in intracellular killing, the "oxidative post-phagocytic burst" and degranulation. The *oxidative burst* refers to a large increment in oxygen consumption and related metabolic changes by phagocytizing neutrophils. Most of this oxygen is converted to superoxide anion (O_2^-) and then hydrogen peroxide (H_2O_2). These oxygen metabolites are released into the phagosome, where they exert a microbicidal effect.

Degranulation, the other event in intracellular killing, begins before the phagosome is completely closed. The specific granules fuse with the developing phagosome and fire their contents. Because this fusion occurs before closure of the phagosome, specific granule contents are released into the extracellular fluid. The specific granule contains factors that generate chemoattractants for polymorphonuclear neutrophils (PMNs) and monocytes, have antimicrobial activity, and cause platelet activation. The primary granules fuse with the completed phagosome, and thus the contents of these granules usually stay in the phagosome. Inside the phagosome, granule contents and oxygen metabolites interact to kill microbes. Oxygen-dependent microbial substances include the active metabolites of oxygen (H_2O_2, O_2^-, the hydroxyl radical [OH^-], and singlet oxygen [O.]) and myeloperoxidase from the primary granule. Hydrogen peroxide, a halide (iodide, bromide, or chloride), and myeloperoxidase act synergistically, increasing the microbicidal capabilities of H_2O_2 50-fold. Oxygen-independent microbicidal systems include the products of primary and specific granule fusion with the phagosome, namely, acidity, lactoferrin, lysozyme, cationic proteins, and defensins.

The multiple killing mechanisms of neutrophils are important, because microbes vary in their susceptibility to the different systems. Numerous defects of neutrophil function have now been identified (see accompanying box), and most lead to increased susceptibility to infection.

Mobilization. Problems in mobilizing sufficient numbers of neutrophils from the bone marrow to inflammatory sites usually result from insufficient bone marrow reserves. Neutropenia is the most common granulocyte abnormality seen in clinical practice. Cytotoxic drug-induced neutropenia accounts for the majority of cases, and infection remains the most important complication of the chemotherapy of malignant disease. The risk of infection increases with decreasing neutrophil counts, rising dramatically at peripheral blood neutrophil counts of less than 0.5×10^9 per liter (Chapter 229). Gram-negative rods, staphylococci, and fungal species account for the majority of infections in neutropenic patients. The lung, gut, skin, and urinary tract are

Functional defects of neutrophils

Mobilization
- Acquired neutropenia: drug-induced (i.e., by cytotoxic agents), autoimmune, leukemias
- Congenital neutropenia: cyclic neutropenia, familial neutropenia, infantile genetic agranulocytosis

Adherence
- Acquired: drug-induced (e.g., by corticosteroids), diabetes mellitus, leukemia
- Congenital: CR3 deficiency

Locomotion
- Actin dysfunction
- Bacteria-induced dysfunction
- CR3 deficiency

Chemotaxis
- Humoral defects: complement deficiency (C3 and C5), cell-derived agent deficiencies (e.g., lymphokines)
- Inhibitors: Hodgkin's disease, sarcoidosis, lepromatous leprosy
- Cellular defects: cells from neonates, Chédiak-Higashi syndrome, hyperimmunoglobulin E syndrome, thermal injury, hypophosphatemia

Phagocytosis (ingestion)
- Opsonic defects: complement C3 deficiency, hypogammaglobulinemia, asplenia
- Cellular defects: diabetes mellitus, systemic lupus erythematosus, hypophosphatemia

Intracellular killing
- Oxidative burst abnormalities: chronic granulomatous disease, glucose 6-phosphate dehydrogenase deficiency, glutathione peroxidase deficiency
- Granule abnormalities; Chédiak-Higashi syndrome, myeloperoxidase deficiency

common sites of local and disseminated infection, although bacteremia in which there is no demonstrable portal of entry is also common. Fever is usually present, but local signs of inflammation may be minimal because of the paucity of neutrophils.

Defects of adherence and locomotion. Abnormalities in adherence not only affect the neutrophil's ability to marginate and leave the bloodstream but also inhibit migration to infected tissue. Drug-induced defects are the most common and are often reversible when the drug is discontinued. Corticosteroids and ethanol are prime offenders and may help explain the increased incidence of infection with the use of these agents. Rare congenital defects have been described in which the cells have abnormal surface glycoproteins. CR3 deficiency is an example.

Defects of locomotion. Once adherent, the cell must be capable of moving out of the intravascular space. Defects of locomotion, such as the actin dysfunction syndrome, are separated from chemotactic defects by the inability of the neutrophil to move randomly as well as directionally (chemotaxis).

Chemotactic defects. Inability of neutrophils to respond to chemotactic stimuli may be due to abnormal cells, absent or abnormal humoral factors, or humoral inhibitors of chemotaxis. Humoral defects include both congenital and acquired deficiency of the C3 and C5 complement components, as well as defective chemotactic lymphokines. Humoral inhibitors may be found in Hodgkin's disease, sarcoidosis, lepromatous leprosy, cirrhosis, uremia, and glomerulonephritis. Intrinsic cellular defects have been described in diabetes mellitus, the Chédiak-Higashi syndrome, thermal injury, neutrophil cytoskeletal defects, hypophosphatemia, and cells from neonates. Job's syndrome patients have defective neutrophil and monocyte chemotaxis and are characterized by markedly elevated levels of IgE, eczema, and recurrent "cold" staphylococcal skin infections (lacking signs of inflammation).

Although defective chemotaxis results in a delay in the establishment of an inflammatory focus, in most of these syndromes adequate numbers of neutrophils eventually reach the site of infection. Bacteremia, pneumonia, and deep visceral infections are uncommon. Abscesses of skin and soft tissue with regional adenopathy are the usual manifestations. Some patients suffer from otitis media and periodontal disease. *S. aureus* is the most common offending organism. Therapy consists of prolonged treatment with appropriate antimicrobials and surgical drainage of abscesses.

Defects of phagocytosis. Decreased phagocytosis is most often related to opsonin defects, such as complement or immunoglobulin deficiencies. Rarely, a cellular defect is found. Anatomic or functional asplenia (i.e., sickle cell disease) may cause a deficiency of opsonic factors. Patients with these disorders have recurrent serious and, at times, life-threatening infections from encapsulated bacteria, primarily the pneumococcus and *H. influenzae*. Patients in this group should receive the pneumococcal and perhaps the *H. influenzae* vaccines, although the efficacy for these patients is unproved (Chapter 260).

Defects of intracellular killing. Defects of intracellular killing involve abnormalities of either the oxidative burst or granule function. Chronic granulomatous disease (CGD) of childhood is a syndrome characterized by abnormal neutrophil oxidative metabolism. Affected persons suffer repeated severe infections involving the skin, lymph nodes, lungs, bones, liver, and spleen. Physical findings include an eczematoid dermatitis, lymphadenopathy, and hepatosplenomegaly. Laboratory abnormalities include leukocytosis, anemia, and hyperglobulinemia. Chest x-ray films often reveal pulmonary scarring from recurrent pneumonia. Noncaseating granulomas are a prominent histopathologic feature. *S. aureus* is the most common organism causing these lesions, followed by gram-negative rods (especially *Serratia marcescens*), *Nocardia,* and *Aspergillus* species. The usual course of the disease is one of recurrent infection leading to death in childhood, although some patients have milder forms of the disease. Chronic granulomatous disease occurs with a frequency of 1 in 1 million individuals. Classic CGD is an X-linked recessive disease with identifiable female carriers and accounts for two thirds of the cases. Autosomal recessive cases account for most of the remaining third.

The granulocytes and monocytes in this disease fail to exhibit a burst in oxygen uptake during phagocytosis, resulting in phagosomes that lack the microbicidal activity of superoxide anion and hydrogen peroxide. Neutrophils from X-linked CGD lack cytochrome b 558. This defect results in a failure of membrane-associated pyridine nucleotide oxidase to generate active oxygen metabolites during and after phagocytosis. Infection by catalase-negative organisms (pneumococci and streptococci) is rare in all cases of CGD, as these microbes generate H_2O_2, replacing the defective neutrophil H_2O_2-generating system. This microbial H_2O_2 can react with normally released myeloperoxidase and halide ions in the phagosome, resulting in microbial death. Catalase-positive microorganisms break down their endogenous H_2O_2, preventing the neutrophil from using it.

The diagnosis of CGD is made by demonstrating an abnormal oxidative burst during phagocytosis. A slide test that measures nitroblue tetrazolium reduction by neutrophils from a drop of patient blood is a sensitive screening test. Neutrophils from CGD patients cannot reduce the dye because they do not generate superoxide. The management of the disease is aimed at its infectious complications and includes antimicrobials and surgical drainage of lesions when indicated. Trimethoprim-sulfamethoxazole has been an effective prophylactic agent. The use of rifampin, which penetrates inside neutrophils and aids in intracellular killing, in conjunction with other antistaphylococcal antibiotics, has been advocated for severe staphylococcal infections. Gamma interferon improves phagocyte oxidative metabolism in some patients with CGD and has been shown to reduce infectious complications.

The granule abnormalities include myeloperoxidase deficiency and the Chédiak-Higashi syndrome. Myeloperoxidase deficiency may be the most common neutrophil functional defect occurring as either total (approximately 1 in 4000 persons) or partial (1 in 2000 persons) absence of myeloperoxidase in neutrophils and monocytes. The majority of patients with myeloperoxidase deficiency are free of infectious complications, although there is an association with systemic candidiasis and diabetes. In most patients, the disease is inherited in an autosomal recessive pattern.

The Chédiak-Higashi syndrome is a rare autosomal recessive disease characterized by the presence of abnormal giant granules in all granule-containing cells. The clinical features include partial oculocutaneous albinism; rotatory nystagmus; peripheral neuropathy; recurrent skin, soft tissue, and respiratory tract infections; and an accelerated lymphoma-like phase characterized by widespread tissue infiltration by lymphoid cells. The diagnosis is made by the demonstration of giant granules in the neutrophils on the blood smear. Chemotaxis and intracellular killing are diminished, even though phagocytosis and the oxidative burst occur normally. Impaired killing is due to defective degranulation into the phagosome.

Neutrophil mediation of tissue injury. The same microbicidal events used by PMNs to kill invading microbial pathogens can also act on host tissue to cause injury. The accompanying box lists some noninfectious diseases in which neutrophils play a role. In the inflammatory arthritides, PMNs are attracted by nonmicrobial chemoattractants (complement components, leukotrienes, and cytokines). Escape from the neutrophil of both oxidative and nonoxidative factors causes destruction of adjacent tissue. This injury then attracts more PMNs. Similar events occur in autoimmune vasculitis. A role for the PMN has been proposed in potentiating tissue injury in inflammatory bowel disease and myocardial infarction as well.

The PMN appears to play a central role in pathogenesis of the adult respiratory distress syndrome (ARDS). Pulmonary vessels and parenchyma usually show large numbers of PMNs, suggesting that they are the major mediator of lung damage in this condition. ARDS can occur in the presence of severe neutropenia, however, and a unifying hypothesis suggests that a variety of stimuli (infection, trauma, toxic chemicals) triggers release of cytokines (IL-1, tumor necrosis factor, etc), which activate PMNs and endothelial cells and causes ARDS.

Noninfectious diseases in which polymorphonuclear neutrophils play a role in tissue damage

Gout
Rheumatoid arthritis
Immune vasculitis
Neutrophil dermatoses
Glomerulonephritis
Inflammatory bowel disease
Myocardial infarction
ARDS
Asthma
Emphysema
Malignant neoplasms at area of chronic inflammation

Modified from Malech HL and Gallin JI. Neutrophils in human diseases, N Engl J Med 317:687-693, 1987.

Evaluation of neutrophil function. Most patients referred for evaluation because of "frequent infections" do not have identifiable defects of neutrophil function. However, a careful history, including a detailed family history, and physical examination will often identify patients who are most likely to have a significant defect. Clues include a positive family history, deep visceral infections requiring hospitalization, and multiple scars representing previous skin infections and drained abscesses. Determination of total white blood cell count with differential counts, total hemolytic complement, and immunoglobulin levels, and a nitroblue tetrazolium test will screen several of the more common previously mentioned defects. If suspicion is high and expertise is available, the more sophisticated studies to evaluate adherence, chemotaxis, phagocytosis, oxidative activity, and microbicidal activity can be performed.

Eosinophils

Eosinophils develop from a common granulocyte-monocyte stem cell in the bone marrow and function as tissue-based granulocytes. Their characteristic red-staining granules contain a myeloperoxidase distinct from that of the neutrophil and a crystalloid core. Their half-life in circulating blood is 3 to 8 hours, after which they migrate to tissues. Eosinophils are less efficient at phagocytosis than are neutrophils. They are selectively attracted by an eosinophil chemotactic factor of anaphylaxis, histamine, and certain lymphokines. Eosinophils appear to be the most effective killer cells for helminths. Eosinophils are also involved in allergic responses.

The causes of eosinophilia ($>500/mm^3$ of blood) include drug reactions, helminthic infections, allergic disorders, collagen vascular diseases, malignancy, and idiopathic hypereosinophilic syndrome. Low-grade eosinophilia is often seen in Addison's disease. Charcot-Leyden crystals, a product of eosinophil degeneration, are seen in areas of eosinophil accumulation, such as respiratory secretions from patients with asthma.

Basophils

Basophils are also tissue-based granulocytes and are the least common blood granulocyte. They are related to mast cells and have IgE bound to their surface. Their granules are rich in histamine. Although basophils are capable of phagocytosis, they do not play a primary role in infection control but are involved in IgE-mediated allergic reactions.

Mononuclear phagocytes

The mononuclear phagocyte system is composed of peripheral blood monocytes and their tissue counterparts, macrophages (see chapter 227 for a more detailed discussion). Like the neutrophil, monocytes and macrophages are capable of adherence, chemotaxis, phagocytosis, and intracellular killing. They function at a slower rate, as evidenced by their later arrival at infected areas and by their slower chemotaxis and phagocytosis in vitro.

The mononuclear phagocytes have three major functions: (1) they clear the body of damaged cells and cellular debris; (2) they are the first line of defense against intracellular pathogens that are not destroyed by neutrophils, such as *Mycobacterium tuberculosis* and *Histoplasma capsulatum;* and (3) they interact with lymphocytes to produce antibody (Chapter 222) and to form the cell-mediated immune system (Chapter 286). The final stage of development of the mononuclear phagocyte is the giant cell. This cell characterizes inflammatory responses to organisms that require intact mononuclear phagocytes and cell-mediated immunity (see the accompanying box). Both monocytes and macrophages appear before giant cells, and it is felt that these cells fuse to form the multinucleated cells.

Cell-mediated immunity. In 1891, Koch showed that inoculation of tubercle bacilli into guinea pigs led to rapidly disseminated and often fatal infection, yet when the survivors were rechallenged with the same bacilli, dissemination did not occur. In the 1940s this mechanism of resistance was further defined by showing that immunity to the tubercle bacillus could be transferred by lymphoid cells but not by serum (antibody) from immunized animals. This mechanism of host defense is now called the *cell-mediated immune system* (Chapter 227). By complex interactions between T cells and mononuclear phagocytes, this system kills organisms resistant to the usual humoral and phagocytic (neutrophil) microbicidal mechanisms. Some of the infections against which the cell-mediated immune system is important and defects are listed in the box.

Infections found in patients with impaired cell-mediated immunity

Tuberculosis and atypical mycobacteria
Leprosy
Listeriosis
Herpes simplex and herpes zoster infections
Cytomegalovirus infections
Vaccinia infections
Aspergillosis
Cryptococcosis
Histoplasmosis
Coccidioidomycosis
Toxoplasmosis
Pneumocystigis infections
Salmonellosis
Cryptosporidisis

Lymphocyte defects

Primary disorders of T cells. Thymic hypoplasia (DiGeorge's syndrome) is the prototype of disordered cell-mediated immunity. Patients with this disease are born lacking the thymus and parathyroid glands. The resultant defective cell-mediated immunity is associated with specific life-threatening infections (see the box at lower left). The Wiskott-Aldrich syndrome is an X-linked disorder characterized by eczema, thrombocytopenia, and recurrent infections. There is progressive T-cell dysfunction with actual T-cell lymphopenia. Affected males rarely survive past the first decade. In other syndromes, such as chronic mucocutaneous candidiasis, ataxia-telangiectasia, and purine nucleoside phosphorylase deficiency, T-cell dysfunction with altered cell-mediated immunity is present.

Defects in the cell-mediated immune system

- Monocytes
  - Chemotactic defects
    - Complement deficiencies (newborns)
    - Chédiak-Higashi syndrome
    - Chronic mucocutaneous candidiasis (thermal injury)
    - Malignancy
    - Viral infections
- Microbicidal defects
  - AIDS
  - Chronic granulomatous disease
  - Chédiak-Higashi syndrome
  - Malignancies
  - Myeloperoxidase deficiencies
  - Viral infections
- Lymphocytes
  - Primary
    - Thymic hypoplasia (DiGeorge's syndrome)
    - Wiskott-Aldrich syndrome
    - Chronic mucocutaneous candidiasis
    - Purine nucleoside phosphorylase deficiency
    - Severe combined immunodeficiency
    - Common variable immunodeficiency
- Secondary
  - Infections
    - Viral: measles, mumps, chicken pox, influenza, mononucleosis, HIV (AIDS)
    - Bacterial: tuberculosis, leprosy, syphilis, typhoid fever
    - Fungal: coccidioidomycosis, histoplasmosis, blastomycosis
    - Parasitic: schiostosomiasis, toxoplasmosis
- Malignancies
  - Hodgkin's disease
  - Melanoma
  - Others
- Drugs: cyclophosphamide, azathioprine, corticosteroids, antilymphocyte serum

Primary disorders of both B and T cells. Severe combined immunodeficiency is an X-linked or autosomal recessive disorder. Because affected persons lack both T and B cells, both humoral and cell-mediated immune mechanisms are impaired. The disease is rapidly fatal, with few patients surviving beyond 2 years of age. Common variable immunodeficiency is an acquired disease of unknown cause that affects B cells and sometimes T cells. Antibody production, and sometimes T-cell function, is abnormal. A malabsorptive syndrome, often caused by *G. lamblia* infection of the small intestine, may be seen (Chapter 280).

Secondary defects of T-cell function. T-cell function in secondary cell defects is suppressed by other conditions (see the box on p. 1799). The most common cause of secondary T-cell defects is infection. Suppression of both delayed hypersensitivity skin test reactions and in vitro lymphocyte transformation has been associated with many viral, bacterial, and fungal infections. Cure of the underlying infection results in a return of normal cell-mediated immunity.

AIDS is described as a condition in which helper T cells are selectively infected and destroyed by a retrovirus (the human immunodeficiency virus [HIV]) resulting in profound depression of the cell-mediated immune system (Chapters 242 and 252).

Various malignancies can also depress T-cell function and cell-mediated immunity. Hodgkin's disease is the best studied of these. The delayed hypersensitivity skin test reaction and lymphocyte transformation are often abnormal. The mechanism behind these defects is not known. Immunosuppressive drugs, including azathioprine, cyclophosphamide, corticosteroids, and antilymphocyte serum, make up the third group of causes. T-cell function and cell-mediated immunity usually return to normal when the drugs are stopped.

REFERENCES

Brown EJ, Joiner KA, and Frank MM: The role of complement in host resistance to bacteria, Springer Semin Immunopathol 6:349-360, 1983.

Buckley RH: Immunodeficiency diseases, JAMA 258:2841-2850, 1987.

Crawford J et al: Reduction by granulocyte colony-stimulating factor of fever and neutropenia induced by chemotherapy in patients with small-cell lung cancer, N Engl J Med 325:164-170, 1991.

Densen P et al: Familial properdin deficiency and fatal meningococcemia, N Engl J Med 316:922-926, 1987.

Densen P and Mandell GL: Phagocyte strategy vs. microbial tactics, Rev Infect Dis 2:817-838, 1980.

Densen P and Mandell GL: Granulocytic phagocytes. In Mandell GL, Douglas RG Jr, and Bennett JE, editors: Principles and practice of infectious diseases, ed 3, New York, 1990, Churchill Livingstone.

Fearon DT: Complement, J Allergy Clin Immunol 71:520-529, 1983.

Figueroa JE and Densen P. Infectious diseases associated with complement deficiencies, Clin Microbiol Rev 4:359-395, 1991.

International Chronic Granulomatous Disease Cooperative Study Group: A controlled trial of interferon gamma to prevent infection in chronic granulomatous disease, N Engl J Med 324:510-516, 1991.

Johnston RB Jr: Current concepts: recurrent bacterial infections in children, N Engl J Med 310:1237-1242, 1984.

Johnston RB Jr: Monocytes and macrophages, N Engl J Med 318:747-752, 1988.

McCleod R, Wing EJ, and Remington JS: Lymphocytes and macrophages in cell-mediated immunity. In Mandell GL, Douglas RG Jr, and Bennett JE, editors: Principles and practice of infectious diseases, ed 3, New York, 1990, Churchill Livingstone.

Sawyer DW, Donowitz GR, and Mandell GL: Polymorphonuclear neutrophils: an effective antimicrobial force, Rev Infect Dis 2(7):S1532-S1544, 1989.

Schifferli JA, Ng YC, and Peters DK: The role of complement and its receptors in the elimination of immune complexes, N Engl J Med 315:488-495, 1986.

Schur PH et al: Selective gamma globulin deficiencies in patients with recurrent pyogenic infections, N Engl J Med 283:631-634, 1970.

Singer DG: Postsplenectomy sepsis, Perspect Pediatr Pathol 1:285-311, 1973.

Stiehm ER, Chin TW, Haas A, Peerless AG: Infectious complications of the primary immunodeficiencies, Clin Immunol Immunopathol 40:69-86, 1986.

Wara DW: Host defense against *Streptococcus pneumoniae:* the role of the spleen, Rev Infect Dis 3:299-309, 1983.

Wedgwood RJ: Intravenous immunoglobulin, Clin Immunol Immunopathol 40:147-150, 1986.

Weller PF: The immunobiology of eosinophils, N Engl J Med 324:1110-1118, 1991.

Yang KD and Hill HR: Neutrophil function disorders: pathophysiology, prevention, and therapy, J Pediatr 119:343-354, 1991.

CHAPTER

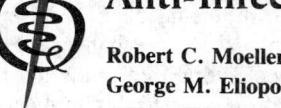

224 Principles of Anti-Infective Therapy

Robert C. Moellering, Jr.
George M. Eliopoulos

The introduction of sulfonamides into clinical use in the mid-1930s marked the beginning of the modern era of antimicrobial therapy. Few other advances in medicine have had such a striking impact on the morbidity and mortality of human disease. In the subsequent five decades, an impressive armamentarium of antimicrobial agents has become available; however, antibiotics have not been a panacea for clinical infections. The development of resistance to antimicrobial agents among pathogenic bacteria and the toxicity related to their use have remained significant problems, providing impetus for the development of new therapeutic agents. As a result, the annual cost of antibiotic use in this country has grown enormously, and they are now administered to more than a third of all hospitalized patients. The increased costs of antibiotics contribute significantly to the costs of caring for hospitalized patients. For these reasons, the appropriate use of antimicrobial agents has been the subject of intense interest in recent years.

MECHANISMS OF ANTIMICROBIAL ACTION

An effective antimicrobial agent should be selectively toxic for the microbial pathogen, with little toxicity for the human host. Several structures or metabolic pathways within a bacterium are susceptible to such selective attack, either because they lack a counterpart in mammalian cells or because their sensitivity to antibiotic action greatly exceeds that of the mammalian cell. Categorization of antimicrobials by major site of action (Fig. 224-1) allows a useful overview of the ever-expanding number of available agents.

Cell wall synthesis

Bacteria are hyperosmolar with respect to mammalian tissue and interstitial fluid; thus they require a rigid cell wall to maintain their integrity when they colonize or infect humans. With no counterpart in the mammalian cell, this unique structure provides an ideal target for antibiotic action; inhibition of cell wall synthesis usually is bactericidal (i.e., results in bacterial cell death rather than simple inhibition of growth). The backbone of the cell wall, a polymer called *peptidoglycan,* is synthesized in three major steps, each inhibited by specific antimicrobial agents.

In the first step, uridine diphosphate (UDP)-*N*-acetylmuramyl-pentapeptide is assembled in the bacterial cytoplasm. Cycloserine, a structural analog of alanine, inhibits the assembly of the pentapeptide chain. Next, UDP-*N*-acetylmuramyl-pentapeptide and *N*-acetylglucosamine are polymerized into linear peptidoglycan strands, which are then transferred across the plasma membrane and linked to the growing point of the bacterial cell wall. Three antibiotics, namely, vancomycin, bacitracin, and ristocetin, inhibit this phase of cell wall synthesis. Finally, outside the cell, the peptidoglycan strands are cross-linked via their pentapeptide side chains to create a three-dimensional polymer. Penicillins, cephalosporins, and other beta-lactam antibiotics inhibit this final polymerization step, called the *transpeptidation reaction*.

Penicillin binds to several distinct proteins in the bacterial cytoplasmic membrane. Each of these "penicillin-binding proteins" is believed to represent a distinct penicillin-sensitive enzyme involved in the final stage of peptidoglycan synthesis. One or more of these proteins would function as a transpeptidase that catalyzes the final cross-linking step, and others serve as carboxypeptidases on transglycosylases, but the function(s) of most penicillin-binding proteins in cell wall synthesis and remodeling is currently unknown.

The bactericidal effect of penicillin is an indirect process rather than a direct consequence of inhibition of wall synthesis. Penicillin-induced inhibition of peptidoglycan synthesis is followed by activation of an autolytic enzyme system within the bacterium. Presumably, this system normally functions to break down the cell wall at points of growth or cell division; when triggered by penicillin, however, the autolytic system functions more extensively and is responsible for cell death and lysis. Mutants of bacteria defective in the autolytic system may demonstrate the phenomenon of tolerance; that is, their growth is inhibited by penicillin, but the cells are not killed.

Cell membrane

The bacterial cytoplasmic membrane is an important regulator of the internal environment of the cell. The polymyxins are cationic detergents with specificity for polyphosphate-binding sites in bacterial membranes. Because disruption of the membrane is a lethal event, these antibi-

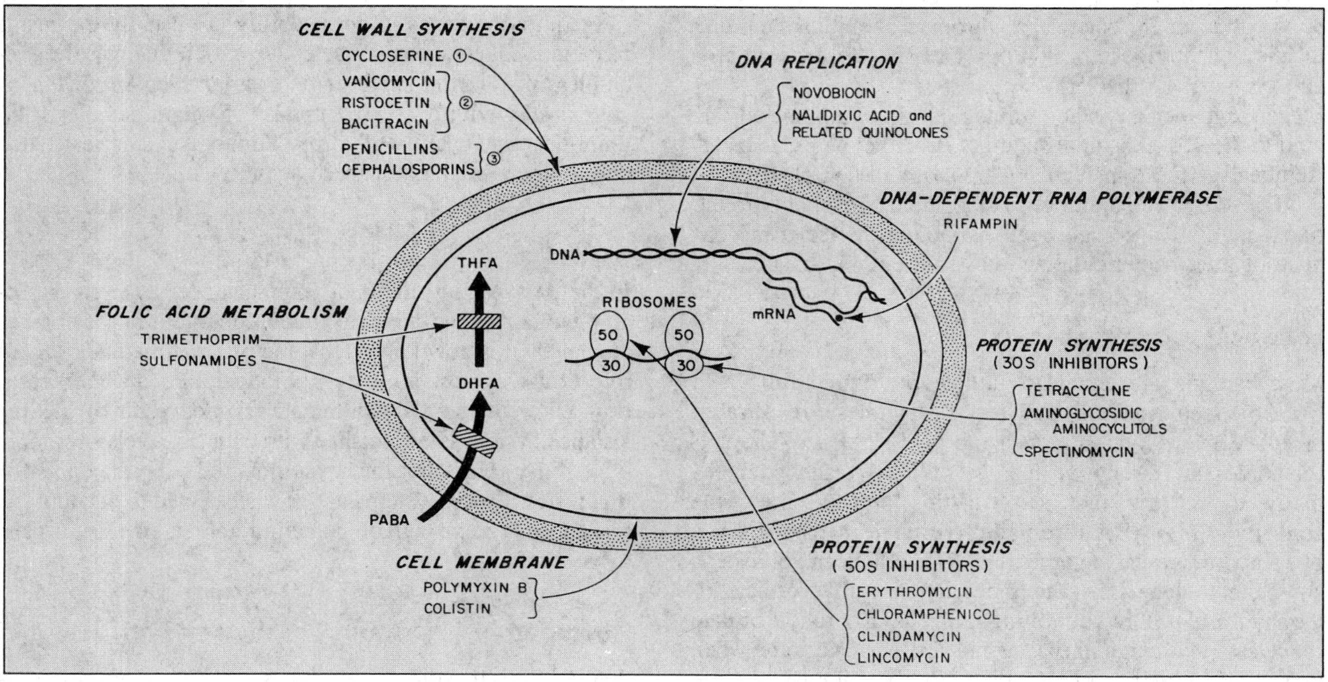

Fig. 224-1. Mechanisms of action of the antibacterial agents. PABA, para-aminobenzoic acid; DHFA, dihydrofolic acid; THFA, tetrahydrofolic acid.

otics are bactericidal. Unfortunately, however, mammalian cell membranes also bind the polymyxins, and, as a result, these antibiotics are toxic.

DNA synthesis and replication

Novobiocin, nalidixic acid, and the newer fluoroquinolone antimicrobials inhibit the replication of bacterial deoxyribonucleic acid (DNA), probably through interaction with the enzyme DNA gyrase. Despite intensive investigation, the precise mechanism of action of these drugs is not completely understood. At low concentrations, these antimicrobials are bactericidal, but at very high concentrations, ribonucleic acid (RNA) and protein synthesis are also inhibited, and they become bacteriostatic.

DNA-dependent RNA polymerase

Rifampin selectively inhibits the enzyme DNA-dependent RNA polymerase, which catalyzes the transcription of genetic information onto messenger RNA (mRNA). Against most bacterial species, this effect is bactericidal.

Protein synthesis

A number of antibiotics inhibit bacterial protein synthesis by binding to ribosomes and blocking translation of messenger RNA. The bacterial ribosome is smaller than its mammalian counterpart and consists of two subunits, designated *50s* and *30s*. Four antibiotics bind to the 50s subunit: erythromycin, clindamycin, lincomycin, and chloramphenicol. It appears that all four may share a similar binding site. Clindamycin, lincomycin, and chloramphenicol block the transfer of new amino acids onto the growing polypeptide chain, whereas erythromycin inhibits the translocation of the ribosomes on mRNA. These effects on protein synthesis are bacteriostatic.

Tetracycline and the aminoglycosidic aminocyclitols bind to the 30s ribosomal subunit. Tetracycline prevents attachment of the transfer RNA-amino acid complex and is bacteriostatic. The aminoglycosides bind irreversibly to the ribosome and cause cell death, although the exact mechanism of their bactericidal action is not entirely clear.

Folic acid metabolism

Most bacteria are unable to utilize preformed folic acid from their environment and rely on synthesis of tetrahydrofolate from para-aminobenzoic acid (PABA). The sulfonamides are structural analogs of PABA and competitively inhibit the first step in this process, i.e., the conversion of PABA to dihydrofolic acid in the presence of dihydropteroate synthetase. Trimethoprim blocks a subsequent step (i.e., the reduction of dihydrofolate to tetrahydrofolate) by inhibiting the enzyme dihydrofolate reductase. Although these agents are bacteriostatic when given individually, in combination they are frequently synergistic and bactericidal.

Miscellaneous mechanisms

Methenamine is a condensation product of formaldehyde and ammonia. It dissociates to release free ammonia and formaldehyde only at a pH of 5.5 or less. This characteristic restricts its antibacterial effect to the urinary tract and then only in an acid urine. Nitrofurantoin, another urinary antiseptic, acts by a mechanism as yet unknown.

MECHANISMS OF ANTIMICROBIAL RESISTANCE

Bacterial resistance to an antibiotic may be either an intrinsic property of a species or an acquired characteristic of an individual organism. Acquired resistance may result either from a chromosomal mutation or from the acquisition of exogenous DNA on a resistance plasmid, an extrachromosomal piece of DNA that codes for antibiotic-resistance genes, or on a transposon, a segment of DNA capable of insertion into either the bacterial chromosome, resident plasmids, or both. Most acquired resistance in clinical isolates is plasmid-mediated. Mechanisms of antimicrobial resistance may be broadly viewed in three major classes.

Decreased permeability

Decreased permeability to an antibiotic is the most common form of intrinsic resistance. Examples include the resistance of gram-negative bacilli by virtue of the relatively impermeable outer cell envelope to penicillin G, erythromycin, clindamycin, and vancomycin; the resistance of streptococci to the aminoglycosidic aminocyclitols; and the resistance of all gram-positive organisms to the polymyxins.

Acquired changes in permeability are usually the result of mutational events under selective antibiotic pressure. Examples include the small-colony variants of *Staphylococcus aureus,* with decreased uptake of gentamicin, and the gram-negative bacilli with broad aminoglycoside resistance due to altered uptake of these agents.

Active efflux

In the past, tetracycline resistance has been cited as an example of a plasmid-mediated alteration of antibiotic uptake. However, it is now known that the plasmid mediates an active efflux system for the antibiotic rather than affecting drug entry per se. Thus although the net result of this resistance system is diminished intracellular levels of antibiotic, active removal rather than impaired entry accounts for this result. Efflux systems are now suspected to account for resistance to fluoroquinolone antimicrobials in some organisms.

Alteration or inactivation of the antibiotic

Alteration or inactivation of the antibiotic is the most common mechanism of acquired antimicrobial resistance and is frequently plasmid-mediated. Several examples are found in both gram-positive and gram-negative organisms.

Beta-lactamases. Acquired resistance to the beta-lactam antibiotics (the penicillins and cephalosporins) is largely determined by the production of enzymes (beta-lactamases) that hydrolyze the beta-lactam ring and inactivate the corresponding antibiotic. The genetic information for these enzymes may be carried either on the chromosome or on a plasmid, and their production may be either constitutive (produced at a constant rate) or inducible in the presence of an appropriate substrate.

The resistance of *S. aureus* to penicillin G was recognized in the 1940s, shortly after the introduction of penicillin into clinical use. Resistant strains were characterized by a plasmid-mediated, inducible penicillinase that cleaved the beta-lactam ring of penicillin G. Fortunately, this staphylococcal beta-lactamase proved to have a narrow range of substrate specificity, and compounds such as the "penicillinase-resistant" penicillins (e.g., methicillin, nafcillin, oxacillin) and the cephalosporins were resistant to inactivation; these compounds rapidly became the preferred agents for therapy of infections due to penicillinase-producing staphylococci. Although four physicochemically distinct beta-lactamases have been described in staphylococci, all appear to have similar substrate ranges and clinical significance.

The situation in gram-negative bacilli, however, is much more complicated, and many different types of beta-lactamases have been described. Unlike the gram-positive penicillinase, which has a narrow spectrum, these enzymes frequently have a broad-substrate range and may be active against most of the available beta-lactam antibiotics. The development of beta-lactamase-resistant semisynthetic derivatives effective against gram-negative bacilli that produce these enzymes has been much more difficult than for *S. aureus*. The introduction of a new derivative has often been followed by prompt recognition of a beta-lactamase capable of inactivating it.

Another important feature of the gram-negative beta-lactamases is their broad dissemination and relative ease of transfer, both within and between species. The widespread emergence of high-level penicillin and ampicillin resistance in *Haemophilus influenzae* and *Neisseria gonorrhoeae* is the result of acquisition by these organisms of a beta-lactamase common in enteric gram-negative bacilli. Although rare, this enzyme has also been detected in penicillin-resistant clinical isolates of *Neisseria meningitidis*.

Chloramphenicol acetyltransferase. Plasmid-mediated resistance to chloramphenicol is common in staphylococci, streptococci, and gram-negative bacilli. The mechanism of resistance involves inactivation of the antibiotic by plasmid-mediated acetylation.

Aminoglycoside-modifying enzymes. The aminoglycosides are important antibiotics in the treatment of gram-negative bacillary infections. Increasing resistance to the aminoglycosides, however, has paralleled their increasing use in clinical medicine. Resistance of clinical isolates to the aminoglycosides is largely determined by plasmid-mediated production of aminoglycoside-modifying enzymes. Three types of modification have been described:

1. Phosphorylation of hydroxyl (-OH) groups, with adenosine triphosphate as the phosphate donor
2. Adenylylation of hydroxyl groups, with adenosine triphosphate as the nucleotide donor
3. Acetylation of amino groups (-NH_2), with acetyl coenzyme A as the acetyl donor

Because the aminoglycosides contain many hydroxyl and amino groups potentially available for modification, a number of different aminoglycoside-modifying enzymes have been described. Bacterial strains are generally resistant to aminoglycosides against which their modifying enzymes are active. Semisynthetic aminoglycosides, such as netilmicin and amikacin, have been specifically tailored to resist modification by the more common enzymes and enhance their spectrum against many plasmid-containing strains.

Alteration in the target site

Resistance to an antimicrobial may also result from a change in the target site at which it acts. This resistance may take one of three forms.

Increased concentration of a competing substance. Sulfonamide inhibition of dihydropteroate synthetase may be overcome by increased concentrations of PABA, the natural substrate of the enzyme. A direct increase in PABA production is the mechanism of sulfonamide resistance in *S. aureus* and *N. gonorrhoeae*.

Synthesis of a resistant target. Bacteria may acquire a target resistant to antimicrobial action either by a mutation in the structural gene for that target or by plasmid-mediated modification of the target site. Rifampin resistance, for example, is mediated by a chromosomal mutation in the structural gene for the RNA polymerase such that it no longer effectively binds rifampin. There are similar mechanisms for nalidixic acid resistance, penicillin and sulfonamide resistance in pneumococci, and streptomycin resistance in enterococci.

Plasmid-mediated modification of a target site is exemplified by erythromycin and clindamycin resistance in *S. aureus*. In this situation, the plasmid codes for an enzyme that methylates adenine residues in the ribosomal RNA of the 50s ribosomal subunit. This alteration of the 50s subunit blocks binding by erythromycin and clindamycin and confers resistance to these antibiotics.

Resistance to vancomycin in enterococci (which may be encoded by genes on pasmids or on the chromosome) is due to the production of a ligase with altered specificity that causes synthesis of cell wall precursors that do not have the D-ala-D-ala sequence to which vancomycin normally binds.

Synthesis of an alternative target. Plasmid-mediated sulfonamide resistance in *Escherichia coli* results from the production of a second dihydropteroate synthetase enzyme, encoded by the plasmid and insensitive to sulfonamide inhibition. A similar mechanism of plasmid-mediated trimethoprim resistance is also well established.

CHOICE OF AN APPROPRIATE ANTIMICROBIAL AGENT

Armed with the basic information outlined here, the clinician can proceed to choose an appropriate antimicrobial agent for a given clinical setting. Three factors enter into the choice: (1) the identification of the infecting organism, or a clinical estimate of the probability that a given organism is present; (2) knowledge of the antimicrobial susceptibilities of the organism(s); and (3) consideration of host factors that may affect the efficacy or toxicity of particular antimicrobial agents.

Identification of the organism

In cases of suspected bacterial infection, cultures of appropriate sites should always be obtained before antibiotic therapy is begun. The results of these studies, however, are ordinarily not available for 24 to 48 hours. In situations in which immediate antimicrobial therapy is warranted, more rapid identification of the infecting organism is needed. A Gram-stained smear of clinically infected material may provide useful preliminary information. Even if the Gram-stained appearance is not diagnostic of a particular organism, it may limit the possibilities and guide initial choice of an antibiotic regimen. In fluids that are normally sterile, detection of bacterial antigens may be useful.

In certain situations, no material will be available for either Gram stain examination or attempts at bacterial antigen detection. In these cases, the physician must use clinical experience in arriving at an estimate of the possible infecting organisms. For example, in a young child presenting with acute otitis media, the likely pathogens would be a virus, *H. influenzae,* the pneumococcus, or a group A streptococcus. Knowing these probabilities, the physician could choose appropriate initial antimicrobial therapy directed at this spectrum. Information presented in the later chapters on clinical infectious disease syndromes will be of help in selecting appropriate initial antimicrobial therapy in patients in whom rapid presumptive identification of the pathogen cannot be made.

Antimicrobial susceptibility testing

Once an infecting organism has been either presumptively or definitely identified, knowledge of its antimicrobial susceptibilities will be helpful. There is significant local variation in the pattern of antibiotic susceptibilities of most bacterial pathogens, and the physician should be aware of the latest information available in his or her particular area. Table 224-1 presents a listing of the drugs of choice and alternatives for infections caused by a variety of pathogens.

For certain organisms, susceptibility to particular antibiotics can be reliably predicted, and no specific testing is necessary. For example, the group A streptococcus is uniformly sensitive to penicillins and cephalosporins, whereas meningococci are susceptible to penicillin, ampicillin, and chloramphenicol. If erythromycin is used to treat a streptococcal infection, however, susceptibility to this drug should be determined, because resistance is known to occur. In addition, some species that previously did not require susceptibility testing are now routinely checked because of the recent emergence of antibiotic resistance. The pneumococcus, for example, is checked for penicillin susceptibility when isolated from spinal fluid or blood, based on the worldwide appearance of strains that are resistant or relatively resistant to penicillin. (Chapter 260) Similarly, *H. influenzae* is now routinely screened for ampicillin resistance because of the acquisition of a beta-lactamase, which has led to ampicillin resistance in as many as 40% of strains isolated in certain parts of the United States (Chapter 265).

The organisms most frequently tested for antibiotic susceptibilities are the gram-negative bacilli and *S. aureus*. These organisms have a variety of antimicrobial resistance mechanisms, and susceptibility cannot be reliably predicted without specific testing. In addition, therapeutic choices may be limited or may require the use of toxic agents. Susceptibility testing is mandatory to optimize these decisions.

A common method of susceptibility testing in the clinical laboratory is the disk-diffusion, or Bauer-Kirby, method. In this procedure, a suspension of the bacterium to be tested is adjusted to a standard density and inoculated on the surface of a Mueller-Hinton agar plate. Filter paper disks impregnated with standard amounts of antibiotics are placed on the surface of the plate, which is then incubated overnight at 35° C. The diameter of the zone of inhibition around each antibiotic disk is measured and compared with a reference value. Organisms are scored as susceptible, intermediate, or resistant, based on the zone sizes of a large number of control organisms with known quantitative susceptibilities. A susceptible organism is one that is inhibited by a concentration of antibiotic achievable in serum (for most drugs) or urine (for drugs such as sulfonamides, nitrofurantoin, and nalidixic acid the use of which is largely restricted to treatment of urinary tract infections). The disk-diffusion method is well suited for screening large numbers of organisms but provides only semiquantitative information and is not applicable to slowly growing or fastidious organisms.

Quantitative antibiotic susceptibilities may be determined by either the agar or broth dilution technique. The latter is now widely available for use in clinical laboratories with the advent of commercially prepared microdilution panels. Serial dilutions of antibiotic are made in either agar or broth medium, and a standard inoculum of bacteria is added. The lowest concentration of antibiotic preventing any visible growth after overnight incubation is termed the *minimum inhibitory concentration*. With the broth dilution method, the inhibited tubes can then be subcultured for the determination of the minimum bactericidal concentration (i.e., the lowest concentration of antibiotic that sterilizes

Table 224-1. Antimicrobial drugs of choice*

Infecting organism	Antimicrobial of choice	Alternative drugs
Gram-positive cocci		
S. aureus or *epidermidis*		
Non-penicillinase-producing	Penicillin G or V	Cephalosporin,† vancomycin, clindamycin, erythromycin
Penicillinase-producing	Penicillinase-resistant penicillin‡	Cephalosporin,† vancomycin, clindamycin, erythromycin, imipenem
Methicillin-resistant	Vancomycin (± gentamicin and/or rifampin)	Trimethoprim-sulfamethoxazole, monocycline
Beta streptococci (groups A, B, C, G)	Penicillin G or V	Erythromycin, cephalosporin,† vancomycin
Streptococcus, viridans group	Penicillin G	Cephalosporin,† vancomycin, erythromycin
Streptococcus bovis	Penicillin G	Cephalosporin,† vancomycin, erythromycin
Enterococci		
Uncomplicated urinary tract infection	Ampicillin or amoxicillin	Nitrofurantoin, quinolone§
Endocarditis or other serious infection	Penicillin G (or ampicillin) plus gentamicin or streptomycin	Vancomycin plus gentamicin or streptomycin
Pneumococcus	Penicillin G or V	Erythromycin, cephalosporin,† chloramphenicol, vancomycin
Gram-negative cocci		
N. gonorrhoeae	Ceftriaxone	Ampicillin, amoxicillin, penicillin G, spectinomycin, cefoxitin, cefuroxime, cefotaxime, ceftizoxime, quinolone,§ erythromycin
N. meningitidis	Penicillin G	Chloramphenicol, cefuroxime, ceftriaxone, ceftizoxime, cefotaxime, sulfonamide, trimethoprim-sulfamethoxazole
Gram-positive bacilli		
Bacillus anthracis (anthrax)	Penicillin G	Erythromycin, tetracyline
Corynebacterium diphtheriae	Erythromycin	Penicillin G
Listeria monocytogenes	Ampicillin or penicillin G (± gentamicin)	Trimethoprim-sulfamethoxazole, chloramphenicol, tetracycline, erythromycin
Gram-negative bacilli		
Acinetobacter sp.	Imipenem	Aminoglycoside,‖ broad spectrum penicillin, trimethoprim-sulfamethoxazole, doxycycline
Bordetella pertussis (whooping cough)	Erythromycin	Trimethoprim-sulfamethoxazole, ampicillin
Brucella sp. (brucellosis)	Tetracycline (± streptomycin)	Chloramphenicol (± streptomycin)
Campylobacter jejuni	Erythromycin	Tetracycline, gentamicin, quinolone§
Enterobacter sp.	Aminoglycoside,‖ imipenem broad spectrum penicillin,** trimethoprim-sulfamethoxazole	Quinolone§, cefotaxime, ceftizoxime, ceftriaxone, chloramphenicol, tetracycline
E. coli		
Uncomplicated urinary tract infection	Trimethoprim-sulfamethoxazole or amoxicillin clavulanate	Cephalosporin,† tetracycline, ampicillin, amoxicillin, trimethoprim, quinolone§
Systemic infection	Aminoglycoside‖ or cephalosporin†	Ampicillin,† broad-spectrum penicillin,** trimethoprim-sulfamethoxazole, chloramphenicol, ampicillin-sulbactam, ticarcillin-clavulanate
Francisella tularensis (tularemia)	Streptomycin	Tetracycline, chloramphenicol
H. influenzae		
Meningitis, epiglottitis, bacteremia	Ceftriaxone, cefotaxime, or ceftizoxime	Trimethoprim-sulfamethoxazole, ampicillin plus chloramphenicol initially (Chapter 265)
Other infections	Ampicillin or amoxicillin, ampicillin-sulbactam, amoxicillin-clavulanate	Trimethoprim-sulfamethoxazole, cefamandole, cefixime, cefprozil, cefuroxime, cefonicid, cefaclor, ceftriaxone, cefotaxime, ceftizoxime, sulfonamide, tetracycline, quinolone†
Klebsiella pneumoniae	Aminoglycoside‖ (for serious infections, cefotaxime, ceftizoxime, ceftazidime, or ceftriaxone)	Cephalosporin† (for serious infections, cefotaxime, ceftizoxime, ceftazidime, or ceftriaxone), ampicillin-sulbactam, trimethoprim-sulfamethoxazole, quinolone†, extended spectrum penicillin, chloramphenicol, tetracycline, ticarcillin-clavulanate
Legionella pneumophila	Erythromycin	Add rifampin, quinolone
Pasteurella multocida	Penicillin G	Tetracycline, cephalosporin,† amoxicillin-clavulanate
Proteus mirabilis	Ampicillin	Cephalosporin,† aminoglycoside,‖ broad spectrum penicillin,** trimethoprim-sulfamethoxazole, chloramphenicol, quinolone†
Proteus, indole-positive	Aminoglycoside‖	Cefotaxime, ceftizoxime, ceftriaxone, ceftazidime, ticarcillin-clavulanate, broad spectrum penicillin,** trimethoprim-sulfamethoxazole, chloramphenicol, tetracycline, quinolone,§ imipenem

Continued.

Table 224-1. Antimicrobial drugs of choice*—cont'd

Infecting organism	Antimicrobial of choice	Alternative drugs
Pseudomonas aeruginosa		
Urinary infection	Broad spectrum penicillin,** quinolone†	Aminoglycoside,‖ ceftazidime, imipenem
Other infection	Aminoglycoside‖ ± broad spectrum penicillin**	Ceftazidime ± aminoglycoside, imipenem ± aminoglycoside, ciproflaxacin
Salmonella sp.	Quinolone† or ceftriaxone or cefotaxime	Ampicillin, amoxicillin, chloramphenicol, trimethoprim-sulfamethoxazole
Serratia marcescens	Aminoglycoside‖ or cefotaxime, ceftazidime, ceftizoxime	Trimethoprim-sulfamethoxazole, broad spectrum penicillin,** chloramphenicol, quinolone,† imipenem
Shigella sp.	Quinolone§	Trimethoprim-sulfamethoxazole, ampicillin, chloramphenicol, tetracycline
Yersinia pestis (plague)	Streptomycin	Tetracycline, chloramphenicol
Anaerobes		
Anaerobic streptococci	Penicillin G	Clindamycin, chloramphenicol, cephalosporin,† erythromycin
Bacteroides sp.		
Oropharyngeal strains	Penicillin G	Clindamycin, cefoxitin, chloramphenicol, metronidazole, cefotetan, cefmetazole, imipenem, ampicillin-sulbactam, ticarcillin-clavulanate
Gastrointestinal strains	Clindamycin or metronidazole	Cefoxitin, chloramphenicol, cefotetan, cefmetazole, imipenem, ampicillin-sulbactam, ticarcillin-clavulanate
Clostridium sp.	Penicillin G	Chloramphenicol, clindamycin, metronidazole

*Not all drugs listed are approved for that indication by the US Food and Drug Administration.
†A first-generation cephalosporin (cephalothin, cephapirin, cefazolin, cephradine, cephalexin, cefadroxil, cefaclor) is preferred. Enteric gram-negative bacilli resistant to these agents may be susceptible to second or third generation cephalosporins.
‡Methicillin, nafcillin, oxacillin, cloxacillin, dicloxacillin.
‖Gentamicin, tobramycin, netilmicin, amikacin.
**Carbenicillin, ticarcillin, mezlocillin, piperacillin, azlocillin.
§Ciprofloxacin, Lomefloxacin, Ofloxacin or (for urinary tract infections only) norfloxacin, enoxacin.

the original inoculum). Determination of quantitative susceptibilities may be important in infections that are difficult to eradicate, such as endocarditis (Chapter 15) and osteomyelitis (Chapter 237).

Host factors

Despite precise identification of an infecting organism and determination of its antimicrobial susceptibility, several factors related to the host are of paramount importance in choosing an antimicrobial.

History of allergy or previous reaction. Patients with a past history of a major adverse reaction to an antibiotic should not ordinarily receive that agent again. Allergy to one member of an antibiotic class, such as the penicillin family, ordinarily implies allergy to all members of that group. Patients with a history of penicillin allergy may be given cephalosporins cautiously if the past allergy was not immediate or life-threatening. Cross allergenicity has been reported between these two groups of compounds.

Age. Even in patients without clinical evidence of renal disease, there is a progressive decrease in glomerular filtration (measured as creatinine clearance) with age. Because muscle mass also diminishes with age, the serum creatinine level often remains normal in this circumstance. Antimicrobials with a predominantly renal mechanism of excretion (see Impaired Renal Function) should be administered to elderly patients in diminished dosage. In addition, the incidence of adverse effects associated with many antimicrobials increases with age. An example is isoniazid hepatitis, which is very unusual under the age of 20 years but may occur in more than 2% of patients over the age of 50 years.

Genetic and metabolic disorders. Deficiency of the enzyme glucose 6-phosphate dehydrogenase may be associated with hemolytic episodes in response to oxidant stress. Antibiotics that may cause hemolysis in patients with this deficiency include the sulfonamides, nitrofurantoin, nalidixic acid, and chloramphenicol.

The rate of liver metabolism of certain drugs, such as isoniazid, is genetically determined. Persons who are "slow acetylators" of isoniazid have higher and more prolonged blood levels of the parent compound than others and an associated higher risk of isoniazid peripheral neuropathy. Persons who are "rapid acetylators," on the other hand, generate greater amounts of a toxic metabolite and may be more prone to the development of isoniazid hepatitis.

Patients with diabetes mellitus, especially those with associated vascular disease, absorb intramuscular medications very poorly; if parenteral administration of a drug is required, the intravenous route is preferred in the diabetic patient. In addition, certain antibiotics, such as the sulfonamides and chloramphenicol, may potentiate the effect of oral hypoglycemic agents and should be used with caution in diabetic patients maintained on these drugs.

Pregnancy and lactation. Virtually all antibiotics cross the placenta and, as with other medications, should be avoided during pregnancy unless absolutely indicated. Moreover, certain antibiotics are associated with specific risks in this setting, and an alternative should be used if antimicrobial therapy is necessary. Trimethoprim and rifampin are teratogenic in rodents, and metronidazole is mutagenic in vitro; these agents should be avoided during gestation. The tetracyclines, including both minocycline and doxycycline, bind to growing bone and teeth. This effect may result in dysplastic changes of bone or enamel and discoloration of the teeth. In addition, pregnant women have an increased risk of tetracycline-induced hepatotoxicity. Because many alternatives are available, these agents should be avoided throughout pregnancy. The sulfonamides are probably safe in early pregnancy but should be discontinued before delivery. In fetal serum, they compete with unconjugated bilirubin for albumin-binding sites and may increase the risk of kernicterus in the neonate. The aminoglycosides carry the theoretic risk of toxicity to the developing fetal ear. This risk has been documented only with streptomycin, however, and the ototoxicity was mild. Thus if these agents are required for the treatment of severe infections, they probably are reasonably safe in the latter half of pregnancy.

When therapy with an antibiotic is required in the pregnant woman, certain agents are preferred for use. These agents include the penicillins, the cephalosporins, and erythromycin. Data on other agents, such as clindamycin, chloramphenicol, vancomycin, and nitrofurantoin, are insufficient for an assessment of their safety during pregnancy.

The nursing mother also warrants special consideration in the selection of an antimicrobial agent. Many antibiotics appear in breast milk if administered to lactating women and may be associated with adverse effects in the infant; for example, because of the risk of kernicterus, sulfonamides should be avoided shortly after delivery if the mother is breast-feeding. Nitrofurantoin, nalidixic acid, and the sulfonamides may cause hemolysis in the infant with glucose 6-phosphate dehydrogenase deficiency. Chloramphenicol may reach relatively high levels in breast milk, which could result in the "gray syndrome" in a nursing infant. Perhaps the best approach is to discontinue breast-feeding temporarily during antibiotic administration while maintaining milk flow via a breast pump. When the antibiotic course is complete, breast-feeding may then be resumed.

Impaired renal function. The clinical use of drugs that are excreted primarily by the kidney may be affected in at least three ways by impairment of renal function. First, the dosage schedule for several of these antimicrobials will require a change. Table 224-2 presents dosage recommendations for the major antibiotics and suggested modifications in patients with various degrees of renal impairment. Second, the risk of toxicity associated with a drug may increase in patients with delayed excretion. Examples include impaired platelet function due to carbenicillin, tetracycline hepatotoxicity, and peripheral neuropathy caused by nitrofurantoin. Third, the efficacy of an agent in treating urinary tract infections may diminish as glomerular filtration of the drug falls. This is particularly important for the "urinary antiseptics" nitrofurantoin, nalidixic acid, and methenamine. Because of these considerations, an antimicrobial with a nonrenal route of excretion may be preferable for systemic infections in the patient with severe renal impairment.

Impaired hepatic function. Similarly, drugs that are predominantly metabolized in the liver should be used with caution in the patient with hepatic insufficiency. Included in this group are erythromycin, chloramphenicol, and clindamycin. In addition, the tetracyclines may exacerbate preexisting liver disease, and their use in this setting requires careful monitoring.

Site of infection. To be effective, an antimicrobial agent must reach the site of an infection in a concentration adequate to inhibit the bacterial pathogen. For mild infections, this goal can often be achieved with oral therapy. For more serious infections, however, the parenteral route is usually preferable. For infections in the pleural, pericardial, peritoneal, and synovial spaces, antibiotic penetration is relatively good, and parenteral administration of an effective drug is usually adequate for cure; direct, local instillation of the antibiotic is not necessary. For other sites of infection, however, antibiotic penetration is more marginal, and cure may require either the use of high-dose, prolonged parenteral therapy or the direct, local instillation of the drug. Examples of these sites include the vegetations of bacterial endocarditis, areas of devitalized tissue, bone, the vitreous humor of the eye, and the cerebrospinal fluid (CSF). Knowledge of the achievable CSF concentrations of antimicrobials is an important factor in designing appropriate therapy for infections of the central nervous system (Chapters 233 and 234).

Concentration of antimicrobial agents in the bile may be an important factor in treating infections of the hepatobiliary system (Chapter 232). In Table 224-3, antibiotics are classified into two groups, based on whether biliary levels exceed those of serum in the unobstructed biliary tree. None of the antibiotics reliably achieves adequate biliary levels in the presence of obstruction, which usually requires surgical drainage.

Almost all antimicrobial agents are concentrated in the urine (Chapter 240). The pH of the urine, however, may significantly affect the activity of particular drugs; methenamine, nitrofurantoin, and chlortetracycline are all more efficacious at an acid pH. In contrast, erythromycin, clindamycin, and the aminoglycosides are more active at an alkaline pH. In difficult therapeutic situations, adjustment of the urine pH may increase the effectiveness of therapy. Unfortunately, antibiotic penetration of the prostate gland is

Table 224-2. Dosage of antimicrobial agents

Drug	Normal unit dose (route)	Normal dose interval (h)	Adjusted maximum dose in renal failure: GFR >50 ml/min	GFR 10-50 ml/min	GFR <10 ml/min	Removal by dialysis
Aminoglycosides						
Gentamicin, tobramycin*	1.0-1.7 mg/kg (IM,IV)	8	1.0-1.7 mg/kg q(8 × creatinine)h or (1.0-1.7 mg/kg ÷ creatinine) q8h†			Yes(H,P)†
Netilmicin*	1.3-2.2 mg/kg (IM,IV)	8	1.3-2.2 mg/kg q(8 × creatinine)h or (1.3-2.2 mg/kg ÷ creatinine) q8h†			Yes(H,P)§
Kanamycin, amikacin*	5 mg/kg (IM,IV)	8	5 mg/kg q(8 × creatinine)h or (5 mg/kg ÷ creatinine) q8h†			Yes(H,P)‖
Azithromycin	250-500 mg (PO)	24	Unknown	Unknown	Unknown	Unknown
Carbapenems						
Imipenem	0.5-1(IV)	6	0.5 q6h**	0.5 q8-12h	0.25-0.5 q12h††	Yes(H)
Cephalosporins						
Cefaclor	0.25-0.5 g (PO)	8	NC	NC	NC	Yes(H)
Cefadroxil	0.5-1.0 g (PO)	12	NC	0.5 g q12-24h	0.5 g q36h	Yes(H)
Cefamandole	1-2 g (IM,IV)	4	1-2 g q6h	1-2 g q6-8h	0.5-1.0 g q8-12h	Yes(H), No(P)
Cefazolin	0.5-1.5 g (IM,IV)	8	0.5-1.0 g q8h	0.5-1.0 g q12h	0.5-1.0 g q24-48h	Yes(H), No(P)
Cefixime	400 mg (PO)	24	NC§§	300 mg q24h‖‖	200 mg q24h***	No(H,P)
Cefmetazole	2 g (IV)	6-12	1-2 g q12h	1-2 g q16-24h	1-2 g q48h	Yes(H)
Cefonicid	1-2 g (IM,IV)	24	NC	1 g q24-48h	0.25-1.0 g q72-120h	No(H)
Cefoperazone	1-3 g (IM,IV)	8	NC	NC	NC	Yes(H)
Ceforanide	0.5-1.0 g (IM,IV)	12	NC	1 g q24-48h	1 g q48-72h	Yes(H)
Cefotaxime	1-2 g (IM,IV)	6	NC	1-2 g q6-12h	1-2 g q12-24h	Yes(H), No(P)
Cefotetan	2 g (IV,IM)	12	NC	1-2 g q12-24h	1-2 g q48h	Yes (H)
Cefoxitin	1-2 g (IM,IV)	4	1-2 g q6h	1-2 g q8-24h	0.5-1.0 g q12-48h	Yes(H), No(P)
Cefprozil	250-500 mg (PO)	12-24	NC	125-250 mg q12-24h‡‡	125-250 mg q12-24h	Yes(H)
Ceftazidime	0.5-2.0 g (IM,IV)	8	0.5-2.0 g q8h	0.5-2.0 g q12-24h	0.5-2.0 g q36-48h	Yes(H,P)
Ceftizoxime	1-2 g (IM,IV)	6	1-2 g q8h	1 g q12h	0.5 g q12-24h	Yes(H), No(P)
Ceftriaxone	1-2 g (IM,IV)	12-24	NC	NC	NC	No(H)
Cefuroxime	0.75-1.5 g (IM,IV)	6	NC	0.75-1.5 g q8-12h	0.75 g q24h	Yes(H,P)
Cephalexin	0.25-0.5 g (PO)	6	NC	NC	NC	Yes(H,P)
Cephalothin	1-2 g (IV)	4	1-2 g q6h	1-2 g q6h	1 g q8-12h	Yes(H,P)
Cephapirin	1-2 g (IV)	4	1-2 g q6h	1-2 g q6h	1 g q8-12h	Yes(H,P)
Cephradine	1-2 g (IV)	4	1-2 g q6h	1 g q6h	1 g q12h	Yes(H,P)
	0.25-0.5 g (PO)	6	NC	NC	NC	
Chloramphenicol	0.25-1.0 g (PO,IV)	6	NC	NC	NC	Yes(H), No(P)
Clarithromycin	250-500 mg (PO)	12	Unknown	Unknown	Unknown	Unknown
Clindamycin	0.6 g (IM,IV)	6-8	NC	NC	NC	No(H,P)
	0.15-0.3 g (PO)	6	NC	NC	NC	
Erythromycin	0.5-1.0 g (IV)	6	NC	NC	NC	No(H,P)
	0.25-0.5 g (PO)	6	NC	NC	NC	
Metronidazole	15 mg/kg load (IV), then 7.5 mg/kg (IV)	6	NC	NC	NC	Yes(H), No(P)
Monobactams						
Aztreonam	1-2 g (IV)	8	NC	1 g q8h	0.5 g q6-12h	Yes(H,P)
Nitrofurantoin	50-100 mg (PO)	6	NC	Avoid	Avoid	Yes(H)
Penicillins						
Amoxicillin	0.25-0.5 g (PO)	8	NC	0.25-0.5 g q12h	0.25 g q12h	Yes(H), No(P)

Ampicillin	0.5-2.0 g (IM,IV)	4	NC	0.5-2.0 g q8h	0.5-2.0 g q12h	Yes(H), No(P)
	0.25-0.5 g (PO)	6	NC	0.25-0.5 g q8h	0.25-0.5 g q12h	
Azlocillin	2-3 g (IM,IV)	4	NC	3 g q6h	3 g q12h	Yes(H), No(P)
Carbenicillin	2-5 g (IM,IV)	4	NC	2-5 g q6h	2 g q8-12h	Yes(H,P)
Indanyl-carbenicillin	0.5-1.0 g (PO)	6	NC	NC	Avoid	
Cloxacillin	0.5-1.0 g (PO)	6	NC	NC	NC	No(H,P)
Dicloxacillin	0.25-0.5 g (PO)	6	NC	NC	NC	No(H,P)
Methicillin	1-2 g (IM,IV)	4	NC	NC	1-2 g q8-12h	No(H,P)
Mezlocillin	2-3 g (IM,IV)	4	NC	3 g q6-8h	2 g q6-8h	Yes(H), No(P)
Nafcillin	1-2 g (IM,IV)	4	NC	NC	NC	No(H,P)
Oxacillin	1-2 g (IM,IV)	4	NC	NC	NC	No(H,P)
	0.5-1.0 g (PO)	6	NC	NC	NC	
Penicillin G	0.4-4.0 million units (IM,IV)	4	NC	NC	2 million units q4h	Yes(H), No(P)
Penicillin V	0.25-0.5 g (PO)	6	NC	NC	NC	Yes(H), No(P)
Piperacillin	2-3 g (IM,IV)	4	NC	3 g q6h	3 g q8h	Yes(H)
Ticarcillin	2-3 g (IM,IV)	4	NC	2-3 g q6h	2 g q12h	Yes(H,P)
Polymyxins						
Polymyxin B	1.5-2.5 mg/kg/day (IV)	Continuous infusion	Avoid	Avoid	Avoid	No(H), Yes(P)
Colistin	0.8-1.7 mg/kg (IM)	8	Avoid	Avoid	Avoid	No(H), Yes(P)
Quinolones						
Nalidixic acid	0.5-1.0 g (PO)	6	NC	NC	Avoid	Unknown
Ciprofloxacin	250-750 mg (PO)	12	NC	250-500 mg q12h†††	250-500 mg q18h‡‡‡	
	200-400 mg (IV)	12	NC	200-400 mg q18-24h‡‡‡	200-400 mg q18-24h‡‡‡	No(<14%) (H,P)
Lomefloxacin	400 mg (PO)	24	NC	200 q24h	Unknown	No(<14%) (H,P)
Norfloxacin	400 mg (PO)	12	NC	400 q24h	400 q24h	No(<14%) (H,P)
Ofloxacin	200-400 mg (PO,IV)	12	NC	200-400 mg q24h	100-200 mg q24h	No(<14%) (H,P)
Sulfisoxazole	1 g (PO)	6	NC	1 g q8-12h	1 g q12-24h	Yes(H,P)
Tetracyclines						
Tetracycline	0.25-0.5 g (PO,IV)	6	0.25-0.5 g q8-12h	Avoid	Avoid	No(H,P)
Doxycycline	100 mg (PO,IV)	12-24	NC	NC	NC	No(H,P)
Trimethoprim-sulfamethoxazole	2-3 mg TMP/kg (IV)	6	NC	2-3 mg TMP/kg q12h	Avoid	Yes(H), No(P)
	160/800 mg (PO)	12	NC	160/800 mg q24h	Avoid	
Trimethoprim	100 mg (PO)	12	NC	100 mg q24h	Avoid	Yes(H), No(P)
Vancomycin*	1 g (IV)	12	1 g q24-72h	1 g q72-240h	1 g q240h	No(H,P)

GFR, glomerular filtration rate; H, hemodialysis; P, peritoneal dialysis; NC, no change; TMP, trimethoprim.

*Serum level monitoring is recommended for therapy of the patient with renal impairment.

†When using the latter formula, a normal unit dose is necessary initially.

‡Following an initial loading dose, therapeutic levels can be maintained by administering a dose of 1 mg/kg after each hemodialysis or by adding 5 μg/ml to the peritoneal dialysis fluid.

§Following an initial loading dose, therapeutic levels can be maintained by administering a dose of 1.5 mg/kg after each hemodialysis or by adding 7.5 μg/ml to the peritoneal dialysis fluid.

‖Following an initial loading dose, therapeutic levels can be maintained by administering a dose of 3.5 mg/kg after each hemodialysis or by adding 20 μg/ml to the peritoneal dialysis fluid.

**Dose adjustment generally required for C_{cr} <70 ml/min/1.73m^2.

††This range applies to C_{cr} 6-20 ml/min/1.73m^2; the upper range may be associated with increased risk of seizures. The drug should not be used when C_{cr} <5ml/min/1.73m^2 unless the patient is on hemodialysis.

‡‡50% standard dose recommended for GFR ≤30 ml/min.

§§If C_{cr}≥60ml/min.

‖‖If C_{cr} 21-60 ml/min.

***If C_{cr} <20 ml/min.

†††If C_{cr} 30-50 ml/min.

‡‡‡If C_{cr} 5-29 ml/min.

Table 224-3. Biliary concentration of antimicrobials*

Concentration	Antimicrobial
Exceeds serum levels	Penicillins (particularly nafcillin, ampicillin, azlocillin, mezlocillin, piperacillin), cephalosporins (particularly cefazolin, cefamandole, cefoxitin, cefoperazone, cefotaxime, moxalactam), tetracyclines (particularly doxycycline, minocycline), clindamycin, eythromycin, azithromycin, clarithromycin, metronidazole
Less than serum levels	Chloramphenicol, aminoglycosides, vancomycin, polymyxins, sulfonamides

*Assumes no obstruction is present.

not related to high urinary levels of drug. Erythromycin, trimethoprim, and various fluoroquinolones have produced satisfactory tissue levels at this site.

Host defense mechanisms. In the presence of normal host defense mechanisms, there appears to be no difference in outcome whether patients are treated with a bactericidal or a bacteriostatic antibiotic. If host defenses are impaired, however, bacterial killing may be largely dependent on antibiotic action, and simple bacteriostasis alone may be insufficient for cure. Such impairment of host defense may be either local, as in the vegetations of bacterial endocarditis or the open spaces of the CSF in meningitis, or global, as in the patient with neutropenia. In these situations, the patient is best treated with bactericidal antibiotics.

SPECIFIC ANTIMICROBIAL AGENTS

Antimicrobial agents differ in their spectrum of activity, pharmacokinetic properties, and potential adverse effects. These considerations are important in selecting appropriate therapy.

Penicillins

Benzylpenicillin (penicillin G) was introduced into clinical use in the early 1940s. Since then, a number of derivatives of the basic penicillin nucleus have been developed in an attempt either to improve pharmacokinetic properties or to alter the spectrum of activity of the compounds. All these agents, however, share common toxic effects and cross allergenicity.

Spectrum of activity. Penicillin G is highly active against most gram-positive cocci, with the exceptions of penicillinase-producing *S. aureus,* the enterococci, and penicillin-resistant pneumococci. It is also effective against the following organisms: gram-positive bacilli, including *Corynebacterium diphtheriae,* variable numbers of other diphtheroids, *Listeria monocytogenes, Bacillus anthracis,* and *Erysipelothrix rhusiopathiae;* some gram-negative organisms, including many beta-lactamase-negative gonococci, meningococci, *Pasteurella multocida,* and *Streptobacillus moniliformis;* the spirochetes, including *Treponema pallidum,* leptospiras, and *Spirillum minus;* and most anaerobes except *Bacteroides* species. Penicillin V (phenoxymethylpenicillin) has a similar spectrum, except it has less activity against *Neisseria* and should not be used for the treatment of gonorrhea.

One of the important deficiencies in the spectrum of penicillin G is its ineffectiveness against penicillinase-producing *S. aureus*. Several derivatives of the penicillin nucleus have been developed to resist inactivation by the staphylococcal beta-lactamase; these include methicillin, nafcillin, oxacillin, cloxacillin, and dicloxacillin (Fig. 224-2). These agents are active against staphylococci, but methicillin-resistant strains, which are cross resistant to the other penicillins and cephalosporins, have been recognized with increasing frequency in recent years. The mechanism of this resistance relates to an alteration in the penicillin-binding protein targets rather than to the production of penicillinase. The other organisms inhibited by penicillin G are generally less susceptible to the penicillinase-resistant derivatives. The high blood levels achievable with these derivatives, however, are usually sufficient to inhibit most strains. *Enterococci, Listeria,* and *Neisseria* are exceptions; these organisms are not adequately treated with the antistaphylococcal penicillins.

Modifications have also been made in the penicillin nucleus to expand the spectrum of gram-negative coverage (Fig. 224-3); none of these broader spectrum penicillins, however, is effective against penicillinase-producing *S. aureus*. Ampicillin and amoxicillin (as well as the closely

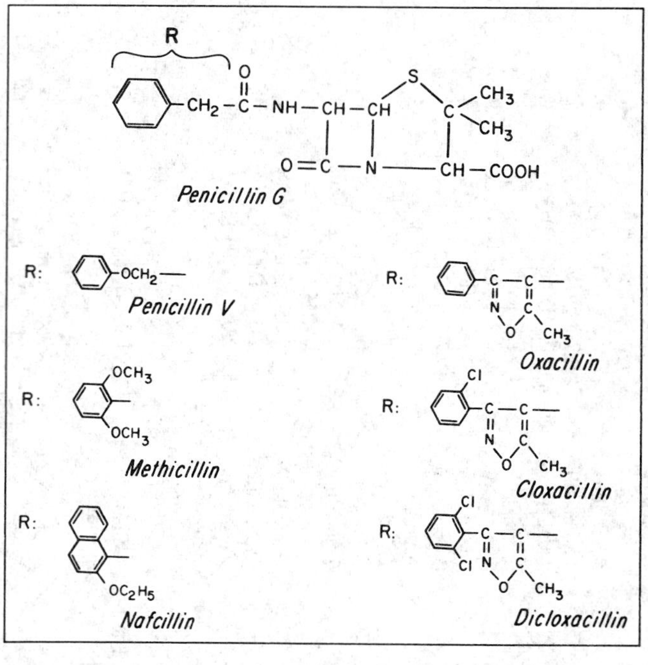

Fig. 224-2. Structural formulas of penicillin and the penicillinase-resistant penicillins.

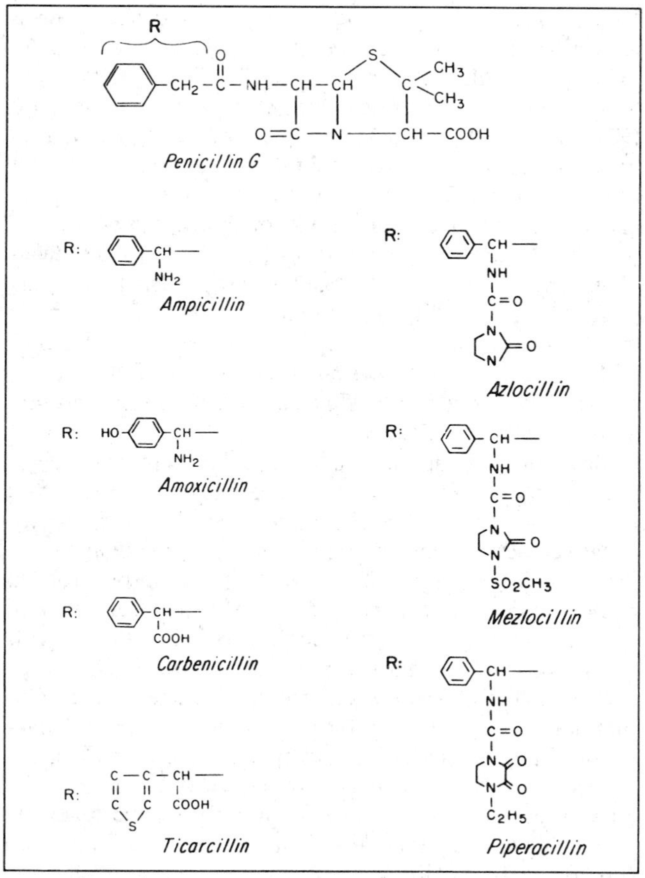

Fig. 224-3. Structural formulas of the broader spectrum penicillins.

related drugs bacampicillin and cyclacillin) provide excellent coverage for the same organisms as penicillin G. In addition, a majority of strains of *H. influenzae, E. coli, Proteus mirabilis, Salmonella,* and *Shigella* are susceptible. The widespread acquisition of a beta-lactamase in *H. influenzae* makes susceptibility testing for ampicillin mandatory. There is no significant difference between the spectrum of ampicillin and that of amoxicillin, except that the latter is less effective clinically for shigellosis.

Carbenicillin, ticarcillin, azlocillin, mezlocillin, and piperacillin are five other penicillins with enhanced spectra. Although often less active than ampicillin on a weight basis, they are effective against the same organisms. In addition, they are relatively resistant to certain gram-negative beta-lactamases and inhibit most strains of indole-positive *Proteus* species, *Enterobacter* species, and *Pseudomonas aeruginosa*. The minimum inhibitory concentrations of carbenicillin for *P. aeruginosa* are usually high (e.g., 75 to 100 μg/ml), but serum levels above this range are easily achieved with high doses. Ticarcillin is twice as active by weight as carbenicillin against *P. aeruginosa* and may therefore be used in a lower dose; for other organisms, the spectrum of activity of ticarcillin and carbenicillin is similar. Mezlocillin and piperacillin are more active against Enterobacteriaceae than the other two agents, particularly against strains of *Klebsiella pneumoniae*. Against strains of *P. aeruginosa,* the activity of mezlocillin parallels that of ticarcillin, whereas azlocillin and piperacillin are more active. In the treatment of serious gram-negative infections beyond the urinary tract, these drugs are often combined with an aminoglycoside both to extend the antibacterial spectrum and to minimize the risk of the development of resistance.

Ampicillin has been combined with the beta-lactamase inhibitor sulbactam, whereas both ticarcilin and amoxicillin are marketed with the beta-lactamase inhibitor potassium clavulanate, in order to extend the spectrum of each penicillin against some beta-lactamase-producing organisms. Such combinations typically demonstrate activity against *E. coli* and *K. pneumoniae*. Unfortunately, these inhibitors are inactive against the chromosomal beta-lactamases of several gram-negative bacilli, which are troublesome nosocomial pathogens, such as *Enterobacter* species and *P. aeruginosa*.

Pharmacokinetics. Penicillin G is unstable in gastric acid and therefore unreliably absorbed by the oral route. Penicillin V is more acid-stable and is preferred to penicillin G if oral therapy is appropriate. Methicillin and nafcillin are also poorly absorbed by mouth, but oxacillin and especially cloxacillin and dicloxacillin are fairly well absorbed. One of the latter two agents is generally preferred for oral therapy of staphylococcal infections. Oral ampicillin and amoxicillin are well absorbed, but the latter is more completely absorbed, with consequent higher and more prolonged blood levels. Amoxicillin may be given every 8 hours by mouth, compared with every 6 hours for ampicillin. Amoxicillin is also available in combination with potassium clavulanate for administration by mouth. Carbenicillin, ticarcillin, azlocillin, mezlocillin, and piperacillin are not absorbed orally, but the indanyl ester of carbenicillin is well absorbed and achieves adequate urine levels for the therapy of urinary tract infections due to susceptible organisms. It does not provide serum levels high enough for the treatment of systemic infections.

The penicillins are well absorbed intramuscularly, but intravenous infusion is generally preferred if large doses are required. Two repository forms of penicillin G are available for intramuscular use. Procaine penicillin G achieves therapeutic serum and tissue levels for up to 12 hours after intramuscular injection, and benzathine penicillin G achieves detectable serum levels for up to 30 days. The latter levels are low, however, and are useful only for exquisitely sensitive organisms.

All the penicillins except nafcillin are primarily cleared by the kidney. In general, active tubular secretion is more important than glomerular filtration. Most of these agents require dosage adjustment in the presence of severe renal disease (see Table 224-2). Nafcillin, on the other hand, is primarily metabolized by the liver and does not require a dosage change in renal failure. Similarly, oxacillin can be given in full doses in renal failure, as in this setting it can be excreted by the liver.

Adverse effects. The most common important adverse reactions to the penicillins involve systemic drug allergy; these reactions include anaphylaxis, various forms of skin rash, drug fever, and serum sickness. In addition, organ- and tissue-specific hypersensitivity may occur. Coombs-positive hemolytic anemia, immune thrombocytopenia, neutropenia, pulmonary infiltrates with eosinophilia, and drug-induced lupus may occasionally occur with any of the agents. Methicillin is the penicillin that has most commonly caused acute allergic interstitial nephritis, and oxacillin has been associated with hypersensitivity hepatitis. Ampicillin is a frequent cause of pseudomembranous colitis secondary to colonic overgrowth of toxigenic *Clostridium difficile* (Chapter 262). Any of these drugs can cause milder forms of diarrhea or other gastrointestinal upset. Carbenicillin and ticarcillin in high doses may cause volume overload (sodium content 5 mEq/g antibiotic), hypokalemic alkalosis (by acting as a nonresorbable anion in the distal renal tubule), and interference with platelet function, with clinical bleeding. High CSF levels of any penicillin may cause neurotoxicity, with coma, myoclonus, and seizures.

Cephalosporins

The first cephalosporin commercially available, cephalothin, was released in this country in 1964. Since then, many additional cephalosporins and related antibiotics have been approved for clinical use. All except cefoxitin, cefotetan, cefmetazole, and moxalactam are semisynthetic derivatives of the same basic nucleus, 7-amino cephalosporanic acid.

Spectrum of activity. Seven available cephalosporins (cephalothin, cephapirin, cefazolin, cephradine, cephalexin, cefadroxil, cefaclor) have very similar spectra of activity and have been termed *first-generation cephalosporins* (Fig. 224-4). In vitro susceptibility to these agents is routinely tested with a class antibiotic disk containing either cephalothin or cefazolin. Most gram-positive cocci are susceptible to these drugs, including penicillinase-producing *S. aureus*. However, enterococci, methicillin-resistant staphylococci, and *L. monocytogenes,* are resistant. Among gram-negative bacilli, most strains of *E. coli, P. mirabilis,* and *K. pneumoniae* are susceptible, as are most anaerobes, with the exception of *Bacteroides* species. Cefaclor has greater activity against *H. influenzae* than do the other oral derivatives in this class.

Seven cephalosporins (cefamandole, cefonicid, ceforanide, cefmetazole, cefuroxime, cefoxitin, and cefotetan) have expanded spectra of activity against certain gram-negative bacteria and are termed *second-generation cephalosporins* (Fig. 224-5). These agents, particularly cefotetan and cefoxitin, are less active than first-generation cephalosporins against gram-positive organisms. All of these agents are active against *Klebsiella* species, *P. mirabilis,* and *E. coli*. Four (cefamandole, cefonicid, ceforanide, and cefuroxime) of them also inhibit most strains of *Enterobacter* species, indole-positive *Proteus* species, and *H. influenzae*. Cefuroxime is more active against *H. influenzae* than the other three agents and has been approved for the treatment of meningitis due to selected pathogens. The other two compounds (cefoxitin and cefotetan) are cephamycins and inhibit most strains of indole-positive *Proteus* species,

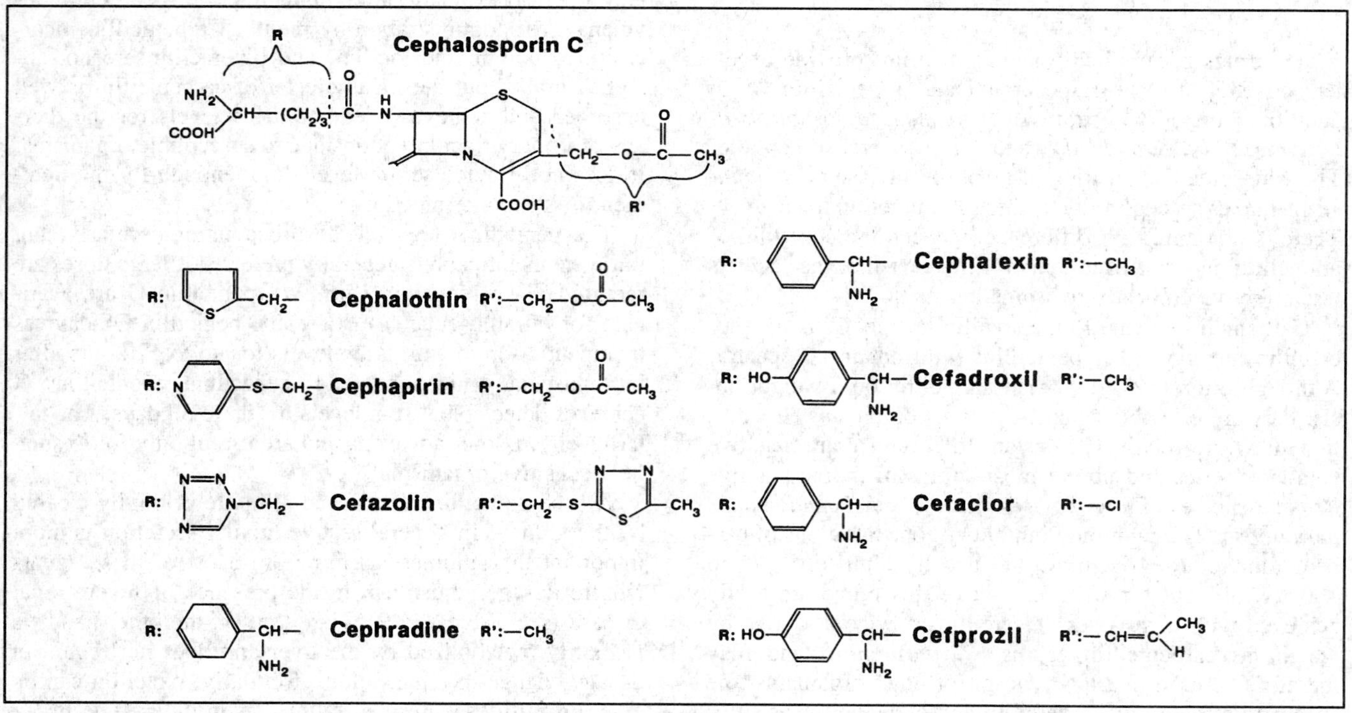

Fig. 224-4. Structural formulas of the first-generation cephalosporins.

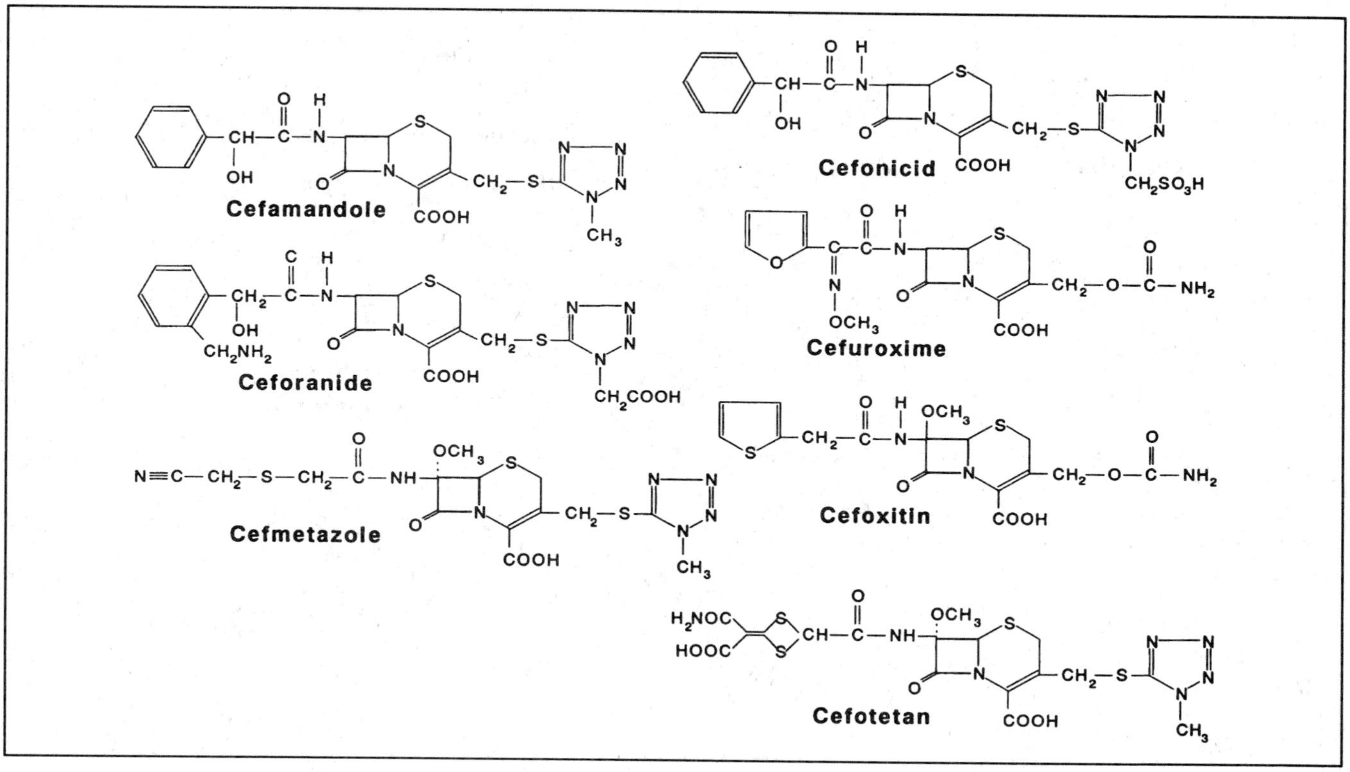

Fig. 224-5. Structural formulas of the second-generation cephalosporins.

Bacteroides species, and *N. gonorrhoeae* (including penicillinase producers). Cefotetan inhibits a spectrum of organisms similar to that of cefoxitin; some species of *Bacteroides* are more resistant to cefotetan, whereas some *Enterobacter* species are more susceptible. Cefmetazole, like cefoxitin and cefotetan, demonstrates notable activity against *Bacteroides fragilis* and other anaerobic bacteria and is also active against various streptococci and facultative gram-negative organisms. Cefotaxime, ceftizoxime, moxalactam, ceftriaxone, cefoperazone, and ceftazidime are termed *third-generation cephalosporins* (Fig. 224-6). These compounds are much more potent against gram-negative bacteria than were earlier cephalosporins and are more resistant to degradation by beta-lactamases. Cefotaxime, ceftizoxime, moxalactam, and ceftriaxone are highly active against most strains of Enterobacteriaceae, as well as *H. influenzae,* and *N. gonorrhoeae*. They have poor activity however, against *Acinetobacter* species and *P. aeruginosa,* and are generally less active than cefoxitin or cefotetan against *Bacteroides* species. Ceftazidime is the most potent of these drugs against *P. aeruginosa*. Cefoperazone is less stable to beta-lactamase hydrolysis than the other third-generation agents and is less active against Enterobacteriaceae. However, it is more active against *P. aeruginosa* than the other cephalosporins. Ceftazidime is highly active against Enterobacteriaceae, *N. gonorrhoeae,* and *H. influenzae*. It is the most active of the available cephalosporins against *P. aeruginosa*. The third-generation cephalosporins are less active than first-generation agents against many gram-positive organisms. Nevertheless, cefotaxime, ceftizoxime, and ceftriaxone are highly active against most streptococci, including pneumococci. Cefixime, an oral agent classified as a third-generation drug based on activity against some gram-negative bacteria, is inactive against staphylococci.

Pharmacokinetics. Several of the available cephalosporins are absorbed by the oral route. Cephalexin, cephradine, and cefaclor are well absorbed and are similar pharmacokinetically. Cefadroxil has a longer serum half-life than these agents and may be given every 12 hours rather than every 6 hours. In other respects, it is similar to cephalexin.

Cefuroxime axetil is an ester prodrug of cefuroxime available for oral administration. Upon absorption, the compound is hydrolyzed to the parent drug cefuroxime. The drug is usually administered twice daily. Cefprozil is well absorbed after oral administration and is eliminated primarily by renal mechanisms with a half-life of approximately 1.2 hours. It can be administered once or twice daily, depending on clinical circumstances. Cefixime is partially (40% to 50%) absorbed after oral administration. Absorption of the oral suspension is superior to that from tablets. A long serum half-life permits once or twice a day dosing, and dose adjustment is required for patients with renal dysfunction.

The remaining cephalosporins are approved for parenteral use (cephradine is available for both oral and parenteral administration). Three of the agents—cephalothin,

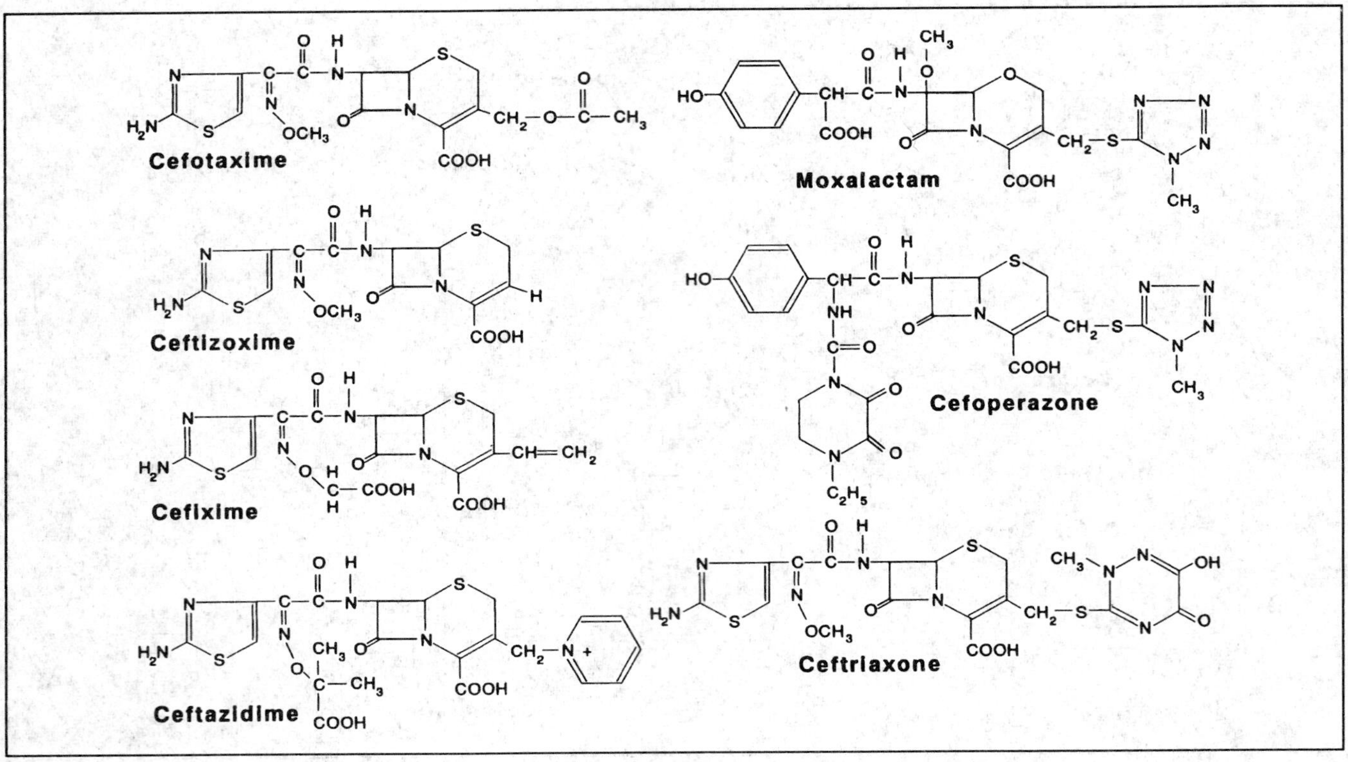

Fig. 224-6. Structural formulas of the third-generation cephalosporins.

cephapirin, and cephradine—are painful when administered intramuscularly and are usually given only by vein. These agents have similar pharmacokinetics and may be considered interchangeable. Data are not available regarding intramuscular administration of cefmetazole. The remaining parenteral cephalosporins may be given either intramuscularly or intravenously. Several of the agents have a significantly longer half-life than that of cephalothin and may be administered at less frequent dosing intervals (Table 224-2). Ceftriaxone has a uniquely long half-life (6 to 8 hours) and can be administered intramuscularly or intravenously once or twice a day. The third-generation cephalosporins achieve excellent levels in CSF in the presence of meningeal irritation and (with the exception of cefoperazone, which is not approved for use in meningitis) have become the agents of choice for meningitis caused by the Enterobacteriaceae. Ceftriaxone, cefotaxime, and cefuroxime have also been used successfully in childhood meningitis.

Most of the cephalosporins are primarily excreted by the kidney, both by active tubular secretion and by glomerular filtration. Doses are modified in the presence of renal failure, as suggested in Table 224-2.

Adverse effects. As with the penicillins, the most common major reactions to the cephalosporins involve systemic drug allergy. In addition, neutropenia and immune thrombocytopenia are occasionally seen. Cephalosporins rarely cause renal injury by themselves but appear to potentiate the nephrotoxicity of concurrently administered aminoglycosides.

Moxalactam, which is now infrequently used, was associated with a bleeding diathesis. This is believed to be related in part to the presence of a labile methylthiotetrazole side-chain. This moiety, which has also been associated with a disulfiram-like reaction after ingestion of alcoholic beverages, is also present on cefoperazone, cefamandole, cefmetazole, and cefotetan. Bleeding diatheses have not been common with these other agents in standard clinical use.

Other beta-lactams

Two other beta-lactam antibiotics, which are neither penicillins nor cephalosporins, are also available for clinical use. Imipenem, the first carbapenem antibiotic approved for human use, is formulated in combination with the dehydropeptidase I enzyme inhibitor, cilastatin, which prevents renal metabolism of the drug. Aztreonam is the first available monobactam antibiotic. In contrast to penicillins, cephalosporins and carbapenems, the nucleus of this agent contains only the single (beta-lactam) ring (Fig. 224-7).

Spectrum of activity. Imipenem is active against a wide variety of gram-positive and gram-negative, aerobic and anaerobic pathogens. Notable exceptions include methicillin-resistant strains of *S. aureus*, some enterococci (especially *E. faecium*), and *Xanthomonas maltophilia*. The

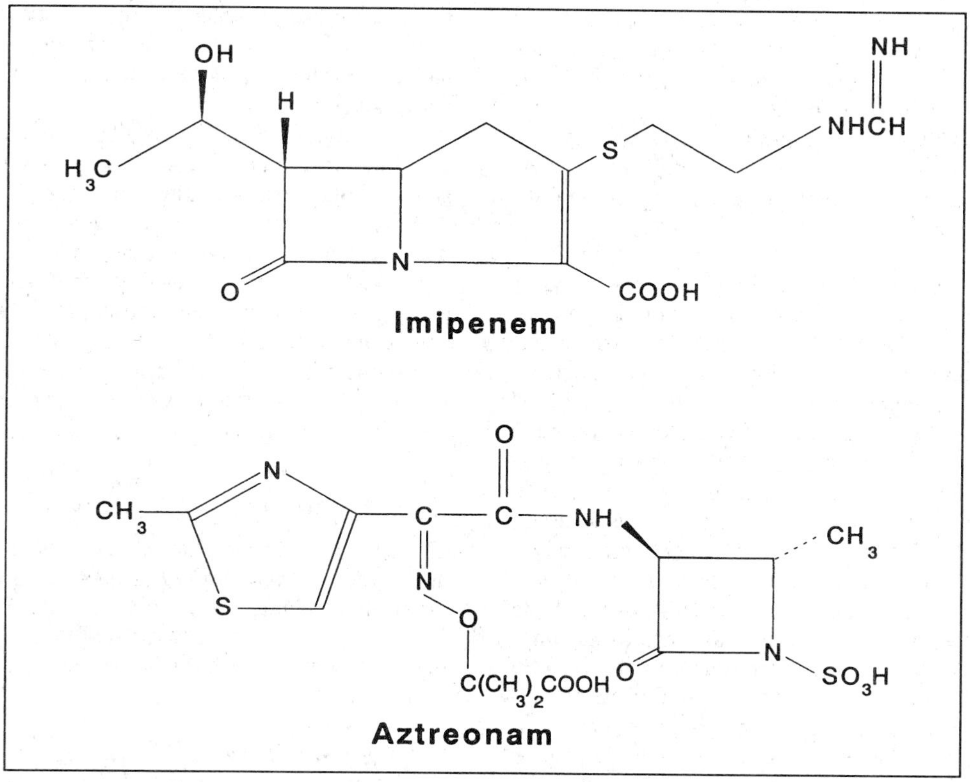

Fig. 224-7. Structural formulas of imipenem and aztreonam.

latter produces a beta-lactamase, which inactivates the drug. Although most strains of *P. aeruginosa* are susceptible to imipenem, resistance to the drug has emerged during therapy. The antimicrobial spectrum of aztreonam is limited to aerobic and facultative gram-negative bacteria. The drug is relatively resistant to hydrolysis by many common beta-lactamases, but enzymes capable of inactivating the drug do exist.

Pharmacokinetics. Imipenem is usually administered intravenously, which is appropriate for its use in severely ill patients. A formulation for intramuscular injection however, is available. The drug is eliminated primarily by the kidneys; doses are usually administered every 6 hours in adults with normal renal function. Adjustments in dosage are needed when renal function is decreased. Aztreonam can be given either intravenously or intramuscularly. Elimination is via the kidneys, with contributions of both glomerular filtration and tubular secretion. In healthy volunteers, the serum elimination half-life is approximately 1.5 to 2 hours. Dose adjustment is necessary in patients with impaired renal function.

Adverse effects. Adverse reactions to imipenem are similar to those seen with other beta-lactam antibiotics. Nausea is a significant symptom in some patients. Adherence to dosing guidelines is recommended to minimize the risk of seizures or other adverse central nervous system effects, particularly when imipenem is used in patients with renal dysfunction. Although some penicillin-allergic patients will prove to be allergic to aztreonam as well, it appears that the new drug can be given safely in most patients allergic to penicillin. In our experience this feature has been a major factor in decisions to choose aztreonam from among alternative agents in selected beta-lactam allergic patients.

Aminoglycosidic aminocyclitols

Eight currently available antibiotics contain an aminocyclitol ring. They all share certain pharmacologic and antimicrobial properties. Seven of these antibiotics are aminoglycosidic aminocyclitols (usually referred to as *aminoglycosides*); that is, they have amino-containing sugars linked to an amino-cyclitol ring by glycosidic bonds. The eighth, spectinomycin, is a nonaminoglycoside aminocyclitol. Although its mechanism of action and antimicrobial spectrum are roughly similar to those of the aminoglycosides, the rapid development of resistance in vivo limits its current application to the therapy of gonorrhea.

Streptomycin was the first aminoglycoside available for clinical use. The rapid development of resistance and the occurrence of irreversible ototoxicity account for its less frequent use today. However, it is still recommended for the therapy of brucellosis, tularemia, plague, tuberculosis, and, in combination with penicillin, for streptococcal and enterococcal endocarditis. The second aminoglycoside, neomycin, was used parenterally in the early 1950s. Its use by this route, however, was rapidly abandoned because of the frequent occurrence of severe ototoxicity and nephrotoxicity. It is currently approved only for oral or topical administration. Neomycin should not be used to irrigate serosal cavities, such as the peritoneum, as significant systemic absorption may result in severe toxicity. The remaining five aminoglycosides—kanamycin, gentamicin, tobramycin, netilmicin, and amikacin—are currently the commonly used parenteral agents.

Spectrum of activity. The aminoglycosides require oxygen-dependent, active uptake by the bacterial cell. Accordingly, anaerobes and facultative organisms grown under anaerobic conditions are resistant. Streptococci, enterococci and *L. monocytogenes* are resistant, although a combination of a penicillin and an aminoglycoside may produce synergism against these organisms. Staphylococci are usually sensitive initially, but the emergence of resistant small-colony variants makes the therapy of staphylococcal infection with the aminoglycosides as single agents ineffective. The main group of organisms effectively inhibited are the aerobic and facultative gram-negative bacilli. Among the Enterobacteriaceae, the incidence of resistance to kanamycin is higher than that to the other four commonly used agents. In addition, *P. aeruginosa* is virtually always resistant to kanamycin. Gentamicin and tobramycin are similar in efficacy, and organisms resistant to one are usually cross-resistant to the other. Exceptions are *P. aeruginosa,* for which tobramycin is more active, and *S. marcescens,* for which gentamicin is more active. Netilmicin and amikacin are semisynthetic aminoglycosides designed to resist inactivation by many plasmid-mediated aminoglycoside-modifying enzymes. Amikacin has the broadest spectrum of activity of the currently available compounds.

Pharmacokinetics. None of the aminoglycosides is absorbed in clinically useful amounts by the oral route. Intramuscular and intravenous administration produce similar blood levels. Intravenous infusion should be slow, given over 30 minutes. The four commonly used parenteral agents have nearly identical pharmacokinetics. Kanamycin and amikacin, however, are less active on a weight basis than are gentamicin, netilmicin, and tobramycin and consequently are given in higher doses. Therapeutic serum concentrations of kanamycin and amikacin are 20 to 25 μg/ml after a dose and less than 7 μg/ml before the next dose. For gentamicin, netilmicin, and tobramycin, therapeutic postdose levels are 4 to 8 μg/ml (6 to 10 μg/ml for netilmicin), and predose levels are less than 2 μg/ml.

The aminoglycosides are excreted solely by glomerular filtration. Careful dosage adjustment is mandatory in the presence of renal impairment (see Table 224-2). Serum levels should be monitored to ensure appropriate therapy in this circumstance.

Adverse effects. All the aminoglycosides are ototoxic. Streptomycin, gentamicin, and tobramycin affect predominantly the vestibular system, whereas kanamycin, neomycin, netilmicin, and amikacin affect mainly auditory function. The risk of ototoxicity increases with age, longer duration of therapy, higher total dose, renal impairment, high serum levels of the drug, previous aminoglycoside therapy, and concurrent use of loop diuretics. Ototoxicity may be irreversible.

The aminoglycosides are also direct renal tubular toxins, most commonly producing a picture of nonoliguric acute tubular necrosis. The same factors that enhance ototoxicity also appear to worsen nephrotoxicity. Concurrent use of cephalosporins may increase the risk of renal injury.

When given rapidly in very high doses, the aminoglycosides may produce neuromuscular blockade. This blockade is much more likely to occur with concomitant use of neuromuscular blocking agents for anesthesia or with preexisting impairment of neuromuscular transmission, as with myasthenia gravis.

Tetracyclines and chloramphenicol

The tetracyclines and chloramphenicol are often referred to as *broad-spectrum antibiotics* because of the wide range of organisms that may be sensitive to them. Resistance to these agents is common, however, and they may produce a number of adverse effects. Alternative agents are often preferred.

Spectrum of activity. All the tetracycline analogs have similar spectra of activity, although the newer derivatives, minocycline and doxycycline, may be more active. Many gram-positive organisms are susceptible, but *S. aureus* and group A streptococci are often resistant, as are most enterococci. Significant numbers of pneumococci and gonococci are now resistant to tetracyclines. *H. influenzae* and meningococci are usually susceptible, as are a number of less common gram-negative organisms, such as *P. multocida, Vibrio cholerae, Yersinia pestis, Francisella tularensis, Brucella species, Pseudomonas pseudomallei, Haemophilus ducreyi,* and *Calymmatobacterium granulomatis.* Enteric gram-negative bacilli may be sensitive, especially to levels achieved in urine, but *P. aeruginosa, P. mirabilis,* and *S. marcescens* are nearly always resistant. On occasion, some strains of *P. aeruginosa* may respond to the concentrations of tetracycline that are achievable in the urine. Anaerobes may be susceptible, but other agents are usually preferred for the treatment of *B. fragilis* infections. Rickettsiae, chlamydiae, mycoplasmas, and spirochetes are generally inhibited by the tetracyclines.

Chloramphenicol is similarly active against a variety of organisms, including rickettsiae, chlamydiae, mycoplasmas, spirochetes, and most gram-positive and gram-negative bacteria, including anaerobes. Less toxic agents are usually preferred, however, and chloramphenicol is useful mainly for brain abscess, beta-lactamase-producing *H. influenzae* infections, meningococcal or pneumococcal meningitis in a penicillin-allergic patient, invasive salmonellosis, and infections involving *B. fragilis*. *P. aeruginosa* is uniformly resistant.

Pharmacokinetics. Based on differences in pharmacokinetics, the tetracyclines can be divided into three groups:

(1) the short-acting agents, chlortetracycline, oxytetracycline, and tetracycline, which are given every 6 hours; (2) the intermediate group, methacycline and demeclocycline, which are given every 12 hours; and (3) the long-acting compounds, minocycline and doxycycline, which are administered at 12- to 24-hour intervals. All the compounds are well absorbed by mouth, although food, antacids, and iron therapy may interfere. Intramuscular injection is too painful, but the short- and long-acting agents can be given intravenously, in doses equivalent to those by mouth. The tetracyclines are excreted in the bile but reabsorbed from the intestine and eventually eliminated by the kidney. All the agents except doxycycline accumulate in the serum in the presence of renal failure and thus should be avoided in this setting.

Chloramphenicol is equally effective orally or intravenously. It is not approved for intramuscular administration. The drug is mainly metabolized in the liver, and dosage reduction may be necessary in hepatic insufficiency.

Adverse effects. The tetracyclines may be associated with systemic drug allergy, photosensitization, aggravation of uremia, and dose-related hepatotoxicity, especially during pregnancy or in the presence of renal failure. Demeclocycline may cause nephrogenic diabetes insipidus. The potential for dysplasia and staining of teeth makes them unsuitable for use in children and pregnant women.

Chloramphenicol produces two forms of bone marrow toxicity. One common form, reversible bone marrow suppression, is related to the dose and duration of therapy. The more serious toxicity, aplastic anemia, is rare (1 in 20,000 to 1 in 40,000) but usually fatal.

Erythromycin and clindamycin

Although chemically unrelated, erythromycin and clindamycin have similar mechanisms of action and resistance, spectra of activity, and pharmacokinetics.

Spectrum of activity. Erythromycin is active against most gram-positive cocci, but some strains are resistant, including 50% to 90% of enterococci. It is not recommended for the treatment of severe staphylococcal infections because of the potential development of resistance during therapy. In some parts of the world, significant resistance to erythromycin has emerged among *S. pyogenes* as well. Erythromycin is also effective against the following organisms: many gram-positive bacilli, including *C. diphtheriae,* other diphtheroids, *L. monocytogenes, E. rhusiopathiae,* and *B. anthracis;* some gram-negative organisms, such as gonococci, meningococci, *Bordetella pertussis, Campylobacter jejuni,* and *Legionella pneumophila;* many anaerobes; treponemes; *Mycoplasma pneumoniae;* and some strains of *Chlamydia* and *Rickettsia*. Enterobacteriaceae are resistant except as the pH approaches 8.5.

Clindamycin is a chemical derivative of the older antibiotic lincomycin, which it has now largely replaced because of better oral absorption and increased potency. It has activity against gram-positive cocci similar to that of erythromycin; enterococci, however, are nearly always resistant. In addition, erythromycin-resistant staphylococcal infections should not be treated with clindamycin, even if the organisms are initially sensitive, because of the likely emergence of resistance during therapy. Clindamycin is more active than erythromycin against anaerobes and is an excellent drug for *B. fragilis* infections (Chapter 270). Some strains of peptococci and *Clostridium* may be resistant, as are virtually all aerobic gram-negative bacilli. Clindamycin is not active against gonococci.

Pharmacokinetics. Both erythromycin and clindamycin are adequately absorbed by mouth and are primarily metabolized by the liver. Clindamycin may also be given intramuscularly or intravenously, but parenteral erythromycin is only given intravenously because of pain on intramuscular injection. Neither drug is given in altered dose in renal failure, but both may require adjustment of the dose with severe liver disease. Clindamycin achieves particularly high concentrations in bone and has been suggested as a useful alternative to the penicillins and cephalosporins in the treatment of osteomyelitis (Chapter 237).

Adverse effects. Erythromycin is an exceptionally safe antibiotic. Apart from phlebitis with intravenous use, the only major adverse effect is a hypersensitivity cholestatic hepatitis, seen exclusively with erythromycin estolate. Drug fever and rash are rare complications of erythromycin use.

The major complication of clindamycin therapy is pseudomembranous colitis, a severe and sometimes fatal inflammatory colitis caused by *C. difficile* that may occur in 2% to 10% of patients taking the drug (Chapter 262). Rarely, clindamycin is associated with drug fever, rash, or leukopenia.

New macrolides

The macrolide antibiotics are naturally occurring agents that have a large 14-, 15-, or 16-member lactone ring. Erythromycin is the best known macrolide and has a 14-member ring (Fig. 224-8). One of the major drawbacks of erythromycin is its lack of stability under acid conditions. The breakdown products on exposure to gastric acid are not only inactive, but also are responsible in large part for the gastrointestinal side effects seen in many patients who receive this drug. Chemical modification to prevent acid breakdown has resulted in the synthesis of a variety of new macrolides, including roxithromycin, dirithromycin, clarithromycin, and flurithromycin, which are more resistant to acid hydrolysis, better absorbed when given by the oral route, and produce fewer gastrointestinal side effects than erythromycin. A number of these agents are undergoing clinical trials, and one of them, clarithyromycin, has recently been released for clinical use in the United States. In addition, the 15-member azalide, azithromycin, has also recently been approved for use in the United States. This 15-member macrolide has a nitrogen atom in the ring structure, and as a result, it possesses some unique characteristics.

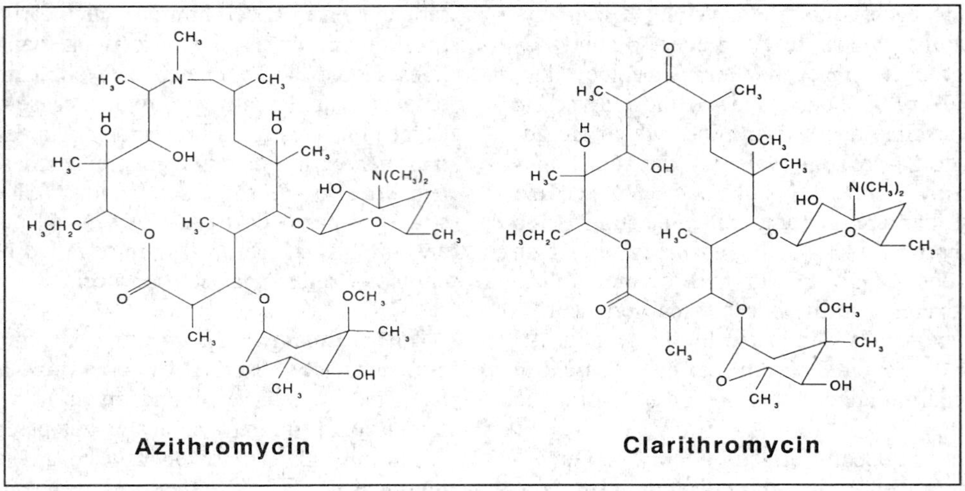

Fig. 224-8. Structural formulas of azithromycin and clarithromycin.

Spectrum of activity. The new 14-member macrolides, including clarithromycin, are generally similar to erythromycin in spectrum of activity, and, as a result, the reader can refer to the section on erythromycin for more specifics. Because the 14-hyroxy metabolite of clarithromycin exhibits enhanced activity against *H. influenzae,* this drug appears more potent in vivo than erythromycin against *Haemophilus* species. In general, the spectrum of azithromycin against gram-positive organisms is similar to that of erythromycin as well, although on a weight basis, it is slightly less active. It is approximately four times more active against *H. influenzae* than erythromycin and shows activity against a variety of Enterobacteriaceae and other gram-negative organisms. It is also quite active against *Chlamydia trachomatis* and other *Chlamydia* species (as is true for most of the macrolides). Both azithromycin and clarithromycin possess in vitro activity against *Mycobacterium,* including *Mycobacterium avium-intracellulare* complex.

Pharmacokinetics. Both azithromycin and clarithromycin are well absorbed from the gastrointestinal tract, and clarithromycin, on a weight basis, produces higher serum levels than erythromycin. Both of these new agents are rapidly taken up by a variety of tissues and are concentrated in macrophages and other professional phagocytes. Indeed, the tissue uptake of azithromycin is so rapid and complete that it produces considerably lower serum levels than erythromycin when given in similar doses. Because of its high concentration in tissues and slow release therefrom, azithromycin may produce therapeutic concentrations in tissues for a number of days after therapy. Like all macrolides, these new agents are primarily excreted via the liver.

Adverse effects. Although azithromycin and clarithromycin produce fewer and less severe gastrointestinal side effects than erythromycin, they are not devoid of this adverse effect. Diarrhea, nausea, and abdominal pain are the most commonly reported adverse effects.

Polymyxins

The polymyxins are cyclic polypeptide antibiotics; all derivatives except polymyxin B and E (colistin) are too toxic for human use.

Spectrum of activity. Polymyxin B and colistin have identical spectra of activity. Gram-negative bacilli, particularly *P. aeruginosa,* are usually susceptible. *Proteus* species, *Providencia stuartii (Proteus inconstans),* and *S. marcescens* are nearly always resistant, as are gram-positive and anaerobic organisms. The availability of the aminoglycosides, newer beta-lactams, and fluoroquinolones for *P. aeruginosa* infections has relegated these toxic agents to infrequent use.

Pharmacokinetics. Neither agent is absorbed by mouth. Polymyxin B is usually given as a continuous intravenous infusion in a dose of 1.5 to 2.5 mg/kg/day. Colistin is given intramuscularly two or three times a day, in a total daily dose of 2.5 to 5.0 mg/kg. These drugs have poor tissue penetration and may not be effective in systemic infections; their main use now is for resistant urinary tract infections. In addition, polymyxin B can be given intrathecally, in a daily dose of 5 to 10 mg for adults for the treatment of gram-negative meningitis. Both drugs are excreted by glomerular filtration and require major dosage change with renal insufficiency (see Table 224-2).

Adverse effects. Nephrotoxicity, in the form of acute tubular necrosis, occurs in 20% of patients treated with these drugs. In addition, neurotoxicity is common, ranging from circumoral paresthesias to neuromuscular blockade, apnea, and seizures.

Vancomycin

Vancomycin was introduced in the mid-1950s for therapy of infections due to penicillinase-producing *S. aureus*. With the development of the penicillinase-resistant penicillins, however, it was relegated to a secondary role because of its apparent toxicity. The emergence of methicillin-resistant staphylococci, which remain susceptible to vancomycin, and the availability of a purer compound with less toxicity have led to a resurgence of interest in this agent.

Spectrum of activity. Most gram-positive organisms are susceptible, including penicillinase-producing *S. aureus,* methicillin-resistant *S. aureus,* enterococci, *S. epidermidis,* and penicillin-resistant pneumococci. Gram-negative bacilli and *Bacteroides* are resistant. Strains of enterococci that are resistant to high concentrations of vancomycin have been reported. Resistance is often plasmid-mediated and transferable and appears to result from target-site modification. There is increasing awareness of rare pathogens that are intrinsically resistant to vancomycin, including *Leuconostoc, Pediococcus,* and *Lactobacillus* species.

Pharmacokinetics. Vancomycin is usually not absorbed by mouth, and it is given by this route only for bowel sterilization or treatment of pseudomembranous colitis. In rare patients with intense colitis, some systemic absorption can occur from the enteral route. Intramuscular injection is painful; therefore, vancomycin is given intravenously at 6- to 12-hour intervals. Therapeutic serum levels are 20 to 30 μg/ml after a dose and 5 to 10 μg/ml before a dose. Elimination is by glomerular filtration, and the dosage is changed with impaired renal function (see Table 224-2).

Adverse effects. With current preparations of this drug, toxicity seems less common than it was in the 1950s and 1960s. The major adverse effect is ototoxicity, which is dose-related but very rare if serum levels are kept below 50 μg/ml. Phlebitis may result from rapid intravenous administration, and rapid intravenous infusion may produce a syndrome of hypotension and diffuse erythematous rash. Nephrotoxicity may occur but seems relatively uncommon. In an occasional patient, fever, rash, or leukopenia may develop.

Sulfonamides and trimethoprim

Spectrum of activity. The sulfonamides have a broad spectrum of activity, including most gram-positive cocci (except enterococci), many gram-negative bacilli (except *P. aeruginosa* and *S. marcescens*), most *H. influenzae,* gonococci and meningococci, and *Chlamydia* and *Nocardia.* Although sulfonamides are active in vitro against the group A streptococcus, they do not eradicate this organism from the throat or prevent the nonsuppurative sequelae. Trimethoprim has a spectrum similar to that of the sulfonamides, and the combination is frequently synergistic, especially against the Enterobacteriaceae. The combination is also frequently used in the prophylaxis and therapy of *Pneumocystis carinii* pneumonia.

Pharmacokinetics. The sulfonamides are well absorbed by mouth and are distributed to most body tissues in high concentrations. Sulfadiazine has the lowest protein binding of this class and achieves the highest levels in spinal fluid. It is less soluble than the newer agents, however, and may produce crystalluria. Sulfisoxazole, sulfamethoxazole, sulfamethizole, and sulfacytine are more soluble derivatives used for treatment of urinary infections. Sulfisoxazole is available for intravenous administration. The sulfonamides are metabolized by the liver, as well as filtered and secreted by the kidney; doses are changed in the presence of renal impairment (see Table 224-2). Trimethoprim is also well absorbed by mouth and is available alone for oral use and in fixed combination with sulfamethoxazole for oral or intravenous administration.

Adverse effects. The sulfonamides are associated with fairly frequent systemic drug allergy, including anaphylaxis, severe skin rash, vasculitis, and drug fever. In addition, they may occasionally cause aplastic anemia, agranulocytosis, immune hemolytic anemia, neutropenia or thrombocytopenia, pulmonary infiltrates with eosinophilia, and granulomatous hepatitis, sometimes with progression to chronic active hepatitis. Sulfadiazine may cause crystalluria and acute renal failure, but this is rare with the more soluble agents. Trimethoprim occasionally causes megaloblastic anemia.

Metronidazole

Spectrum of activity. Metronidazole is highly active against the gram-negative anaerobic organisms (including *B. fragilis*), *Clostridium* species, and most strains of anaerobic gram-positive cocci. The anaerobic nonsporulating gram-positive bacilli and microaerophilic streptococci are often resistant, as are aerobic bacteria with the exception of *C. jejuni* and *Gardnerella vaginalis.* Metronidazole may be ineffective as a single agent for mixed aerobic-anaerobic infections.

Pharmacokinetics. Oral metronidazole is well absorbed, giving serum levels similar to those after intravenous administration. The drug diffuses well into tissues and body fluids, including the CSF and bile. The liver is the main site of metabolism, and no change in dose is necessary in the presence of renal failure. The presence of severe hepatic disease, however, may require a dosage reduction.

Adverse effects. Frequent, minor side effects of metronidazole administration include nausea, dry mouth, an unpleasant metallic taste, and a disulfiram-like interaction with alcohol. A peripheral neuropathy may complicate high-dose therapy, but is generally reversible if the drug is stopped promptly. Transient neutropenia has been observed with longer durations of therapy. Metronidazole is mutagenic in vitro and carcinogenic in rodents; the relevance of these observations to human use of the drug is unknown.

Quinolone antibiotics

Nalidixic acid was synthesized in 1962 and is the prototypic drug of a class of antimicrobial agents referred to as the quinolones. The original representatives of this class lacked activity against gram-positive bacteria, anaerobes, *Pseudomonas aeruginosa,* and *Serratia* species. Several important chemical modifications, including the addition of a fluorine atom at position 6 in the quinolone ring, and key substitutions at positions 1 and 7, have resulted in a variety of new compounds with enhanced spectra of activity and decreased toxicity, and against which bacteria are less likely to develop mutational resistance (Fig. 224-9). At the present time, norfloxacin, ciprofloxacin, ofloxacin, enoxacin, and lomefloxacin have been approved for use in the United States. Other new quinolones, such as pefloxacin and tosufloxacin are available in other countries, and a variety of additional compounds are currently undergoing clinical trials in the United States and elsewhere.

Spectrum of activity. In general, the new fluoroquinolones all possess outstanding activity against Enterobacteriaceae and most other gram-negative bacilli, including *P. aeruginosa* and *Legionella* species. Of the currently available compounds, ciprofloxacin is most active against *P. aeruginosa*. They are also active against gram-positive organisms, but their activity against these bacteria, particularly that against streptococci, including *S. pneumoniae,* is not as impressive as their activity against gram-negative bacilli. Of the currently available compounds, ofloxacin appears to have the greatest activity against the pneumococcus. Gram-negative diplococci, such as gonococci and meningococci, are generally susceptible to the new fluoroquinolones, as are *Chlamydia, Mycoplasma,* and *Rickettsia.* Although these antimicrobial agents possess excellent activity against methicillin-susceptible staphylococci, in many areas, the majority of methicillin-resistant staphylococci are now resistant to the new fluoroquinolones. The activity of these compounds against anaerobes is limited. Likewise, none has outstanding activity against enterococci.

Pharmacokinetics. As a rule, the new fluoroquinolones are all well absorbed when given orally. Indeed, the oral bioavailability exceeds 50% for all of these compounds, and, in some cases (such as ofloxacin), it exceeds 95%. Although serum concentrations of most of these drugs are only modest, they penetrate well into a variety of tissues, including the prostate. Protein binding is low for all of the quinolones, and with the exception of enoxacin, none is more than 25% bound to serum proteins. Elimination of the ofloxacin is almost entirely by the renal route while both renal and nonrenal mechanisms are important for norfloxacin, ciprofloxacin, enoxacin, and lomefloxacin. All of the new fluoroquinolones are available for oral administration, and intravenous preparations of ciprofloxacin and ofloxacin are also available.

Adverse effects. In general, the fluoroquinolones are relatively free of serious adverse effects. The lone exception so far has been temafloxacin, which was taken off the market because its use was occasionally associated with thrombocytopenia, hemolytic anemia, and renal failure. In many clinical trials, the overall prevalence and severity of adverse effects to the quinolones has been lower than those to the comparative agents, including penicillins and sulfonamides. The majority of side effects are gastrointestinal (nausea, abdominal discomfort, vomiting, and diarrhea) followed by central nervous system symptoms (headache, dizziness, nervousness, and insomnia). Photosensitivity is occasionally seen in patients receiving fluoroquinolones. Although they cause cartilage erosions in the weight-bearing joints of certain experimental animals, these findings have not been documented in humans. These agents are *not* recommended for use in children or pregnant women.

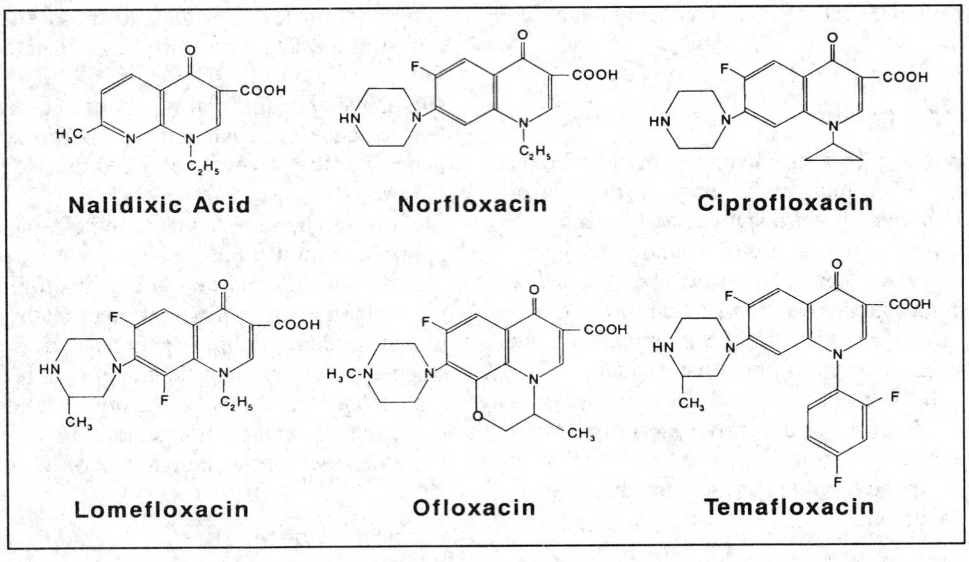

Fig. 224-9. Structural formulas of nalidixic acid and the newer fluoroquinolone antimicrobial agents.

Urinary antiseptics

Nitrofurantoin. Nitrofurantoin inhibits many enterococci and Enterobacteriaceae at concentrations achievable in the urinary tract. The majority of *Proteus* species, however, and all *P. aeruginosa* strains are resistant. Achievable blood levels are low and are not effective for systemic therapy. Therefore the use of nitrofurantoin is limited to acute infections of the urinary tract and prophylaxis of recurrent infections. Toxic reactions include an acute pneumonic syndrome with eosinophilia as well as chronic pulmonary fibrosis. In addition, nitrofurantoin may cause a hypersensitivity hepatitis and a peripheral neuropathy that is more common in patients with renal impairment. Gastrointestinal distress with nitrofurantoin is reduced when the macrocrystalline preparation (Macrodantin) is used.

Methenamine. Methenamine is active against most gram-positive and gram-negative organisms but only at a urine pH of 5.5 or less. Urea splitters, such as *Proteus* species, raise urine pH and may be resistant because they make it impossible to acidify the urine. Methenamine is effective only as a urinary suppressant and is not used for the therapy of acute infection. It is contraindicated in the setting of hepatic insufficiency because of the free ammonia generated as the compound dissociates.

ANTIMICROBIAL COMBINATIONS

A combination of antimicrobial agents may interact in four possible ways against a microorganism. The interactive effect may be (1) neutral (or indifferent) (i.e., no different than the most effective agent alone), (2) antagonistic (i.e., less than the most effective agent individually), (3) additive (i.e., equal to the sum of the actions of the individual drugs), or (4) synergistic (i.e., more than the sum of actions).

The use of synergistic antimicrobial combinations has been advocated for the treatment of endocarditis (Chapter 15) caused by drug-resistant organisms, such as the enterococcus or *P. aeruginosa,* and for the therapy of infections in settings in which bacterial killing by the host may be defective, as in the neutropenic patient (Chapter 229). Combinations of agents may produce synergy in several ways. They may inhibit serial or sequential steps in a biochemical pathway, as with trimethoprim-sulfamethoxazole. One of the drugs may block bacterial inactivation of the other, as exemplified by the combination of a beta-lactamase inhibitor, such as clavulanic acid, with a beta-lactam antibiotic. The best studied mechanism involves enhancement of aminoglycoside uptake by a cell wall inhibitory agent, such as penicillin. This is the mechanism that underlies penicillin-aminoglycoside therapy of serious enterococcal infections and that probably accounts for beta-lactam aminoglycoside synergism against *P. aeruginosa,* and other gram-negative bacteria.

The use of more than one antibiotic in therapy, however, increases the risk of an adverse drug reaction and enhances the selective pressure for the emergence of resistant organisms. In addition, the possibility of antagonism between the agents, as previously mentioned, must be considered. The best studied example of antibiotic antagonism involves the combination of a bacteriostatic agent, particularly tetracycline or chloramphenicol, with a beta-lactam, such as penicillin. In vitro, the simultaneous use of these agents results in clear-cut antagonism against a variety of species. In a clinical study of patients with pneumococcal meningitis, a group receiving both penicillin and chlortetracycline had nearly four times the mortality of a group treated with penicillin alone. In animal studies, this effect is evident only if the static agent is given first. It is assumed that inhibition of bacterial growth by tetracycline or chloramphenicol may interfere with the mechanism of bacterial killing by the beta-lactam.

Other examples of potential antimicrobial antagonism include (1) the simultaneous use of more than one 50s ribosomal subunit inhibitor, which may produce competition for binding to the same site of action; and (2) the combination of the bacteriostatic agents tetracycline or chloramphenicol with the bactericidal aminoglycosides. In the second example, the bacteriostatic agent may interfere with active aminoglycoside transport into the cell and inhibit bacterial killing. The phenomenon of antimicrobial antagonism is probably of clinical significance only in situations of impaired host defense, in which bacterial killing is most dependent on antibiotic action. Examples include local impairment of host defense (e.g., endocarditis and meningitis, and systemic impairment, as with neutropenia).

Whenever possible, a single antimicrobial agent is preferred for therapy of infectious diseases. Use of combination therapy has been advocated only in the following specialized situations: (1) prevention of emergence of resistant organisms, when this is common with a single agent; (2) polymicrobial infections; (3) initial therapy of sepsis of unknown cause, pending identification of the pathogen; and (4) infections in which synergistic killing has been shown to be of benefit.

EVALUATION OF RESPONSE TO ANTIMICROBIAL THERAPY

As with any medical intervention, careful follow-up of a patient receiving an antimicrobial is essential for assessing clinical response and the possibility of drug toxicity. In the patient who is not responding appropriately to the therapy, the following possibilities should be considered:

1. The presence of a nonbacterial infection (e.g., viral, fungal, tuberculous, parasitic) or the presence of a noninfectious process that might mimic an infection (e.g., vasculitis, lymphoma)
2. Inadequate dose of the antimicrobial chosen
3. Incorrect drug for the site of infection (e.g., cephalothin for meningitis, oral carbenicillin for systemic *P. aeruginosa* infection)
4. Development of antibiotic resistance
5. Failure to drain purulent collections, relieve obstruction, or remove a foreign body
6. Superinfection with a new pathogen

7. Adverse reaction to the antimicrobial agent (e.g., drug fever, vasculitis)
8. Impairment of host defense that may delay or interfere with the response to antibiotics

The choice of appropriate antimicrobial therapy is best made with a detailed knowledge of the anatomic and pathophysiologic correlates of the specific infectious disease processes. This material is reviewed in subsequent chapters on specific infectious diseases.

REFERENCES

Abramowicz, M, editor: Handbook of antimicrobial therapy. New Rochelle, NY, Medical Letter, 1992.

Bennett, WM et al: Drug prescribing in renal failure: dosing guidelines for adults, Am J Kidney Dis 3:155, 1983.

Calderwood SB and Moellering RC Jr: Common adverse effects of antibacterial agents on major organ systems, Surg Clin North Am 60:65, 1980.

Donowitz GR and Mandell GL: Beta-lactam antibiotics, N Engl J Med 318:419-426, 490-500, 1988.

Fass, RJ et al: Platelet-mediated bleeding caused by broad-spectrum penicillins, J Infect Dis 155:1242-1248, 1987.

Geddes AM and Stille W: Imipenem: the first thienamycin antibiotic, Rev Infect Dis 7:(Suppl 3), 1985.

Goldman P: Metronidazole, N Engl J Med 303:1212, 1980.

Hooper DC and Wolfson JS: Fluoroquine antimicrobial agents, N Engl J Med 324:384, 1991.

Hooper DC and Wolfson JS: The fluoroquinolones: pharmacology, clinical uses, and toxicities in humans, Antimicrob Agents Chemother 28:716, 1985.

Kirst H and Sides GD: New directions for macrolide antibiotics, Antimicrob Agents Chemother 33:1413, 1989.

Kitzis MD et al: Dissemination of the novel plasmid-mediated β-lactamase CTX-1, which confers resistance to broad-spectrum cephalosporins, and its inhibition by β-lactamase inhibitors, Antimicrob Agents Chemother 32:9-14, 1988.

Mandell GL and Sande MA: Antimicrobial agents. Drugs used in the chemotherapy of tuberculosis and leprosy. In Gilman AG et al, editors: The pharmacological basis of therapeutics, ed 8, New York, 1990, Macmillan.

Mandell GL and Sande MA: Antimicrobial agents. Penicillins, cephalosporins, and other beta-lactam antibiotics. In Gilman AG et al, editors: The pharmacological basis of therapeutics, ed 8, New York, 1990, Macmillan.

Mandell GL and Sande MA: Antimicrobial agents. Sulfonamides, trimethoprim-sulfamethoxazole, and agents for urinary tract infections. In Gilman AG et al, editors: The pharmacological basis of therapeutics, ed 8, New York, 1990, Macmillan.

Moellering RC Jr, editor: Tissue-directed antibiotic therapy, Am J Med (Suppl 3A): 1S-45S, 1991.

Moellering RC Jr, Elipoulos GM, and Sentochnik DE: The carbapenems: new broad-spectrum beta-lactam antibiotic, J Antimicrob Chemother (Suppl A):1-8, 1989.

Moellering RC Jr, Krogstad DJ, and Greenblatt DJ: Vancomycin therapy in patients with impaired renal function: a nomogram for dosage, Ann Intern Med 94:343, 1981.

Neu HC, editor: Aztreonam: a monocyclic beta-lactam antibiotic, Am J Med 78(2A):1-80, 1985.

Ristuccia AM and Cunha BA: The aminoglycosides, Med Clin North Am 66:303, 1982.

Sande MA and Mandell GL: Antimicrobial agents. The aminoglycosides. In Gilman AG et al, editors: The pharmacological basis of therapeutics, ed 7, New York, 1985, Macmillan.

Sande, MA, and Mandell, GL: Antimicrobial agents. In Gilman AG et al, editors: The pharmacological basis of therapeutics, ed 8, New York, 1990, Macmillan.

Sanford JP, editor: Guide to antimicrobial therapy 1992, Dallas, 1992, Antimicrobial Therapy, Inc.

Smith LG and Sensakovic J: Trimethoprim-sulfamethoxazole, Med Clin North Am 66:143, 1982.

Tartaglione TA and Polk RE: Review of the second-generation cephalosporins: cefonicid, ceforanide, and cefuroxime, Drug Intell Clin Pharm 19:188-198, 1985.

Ward A and Richards DM: Cefotetan. A review of its antibacterial activity, pharmacokinetic properties, and therapeutic use, Drugs 30:382-426, 1985.

Weber DJ, Tolkoff-Rubin NE, and Rubin RH: Amoxicillin and potassium clavulanate: an antibiotic combination, Pharmacotherapy 4:122-133, 1984.

Wolfson JS and Hooper DC: The fluoroquinolones: structures, mechanisms of action and resistance, and spectra of activity in vitro, Antimicrob Agents Chemother 28:581, 1985.

Yost RL and Ramphal R: Ceftazidime review, Drug Intell Clin Pharm 19:509-513, 1985.

CHAPTER

225 Hospital Infection Control

R. Michael Massanari
Richard P. Wenzel

Modern health care has been acclaimed for accomplishments in preserving life and sustaining dysfunctional organ systems; however, these advances are not achieved without a price. Intervention in the natural history of disease, whether with highly technical surgical procedures or with sophisticated, toxic chemicals, is often accompanied by adverse events with serious sequelae for the patient. In general, the risk of adverse events and the impact of adverse outcomes are poorly understood. Nosocomial infections are an exception to this generalization, for this subset of adverse outcomes of medical care has been the subject of intense investigation for several decades.

Nosocomial infections are infections that occur in the course of health care delivery. Because these infections usually occur during hospitalization, they have been designated hospital-acquired infections. This term is used rather than iatrogenic infections, which inappropriately implicates the physician in the causation of infection. Estimates of the frequency of nosocomial infections suggest that 5% of patients admitted to acute care institutions in the United States will acquire an infection. Approximately 2 million patients will acquire a nosocomial infection per annum. The impact of hospital-acquired infections on the patient and on society is significant. Annually, 20,000 to 40,000 patients die as a direct result of nosocomial infections. For those who recover, 4 days will be added to the hospital stay, with an overall cost to society of $2 billion.

Nosocomial infections are not an inevitable consequence of health care. With proper attention to prevention and proactive medical care, up to 33% of nosocomial infections can be prevented. Before considering prevention, the complexity of the problem and the factors that contribute to the risk of nosocomial infections must be understood. A conceptual model of disease may be helpful in analyzing hospital-acquired infections. The "triangular" model of disease (Fig. 225-1) comprises three components: the host or infected patient, the agent or nosocomial pathogen, and the environment or context in which the disease occurs. To understand causation of nosocomial infections, one must recognize the interplay of these components.

THE HOST

Hospitalized patients are a unique subset of the population in terms of risk for infection. Conditions that predispose the host to infection can be categorized into those that are intrinsic to the patient and those that are imposed by the health care system.

Intrinsic conditions

Age is generally considered an important determinant of risk for nosocomial infections. Neonates, particularly low-birth-weight infants, are at considerable increased risk for infection. Immature mechanisms of host defense are important determinants of host susceptibility. Whether age is an independent risk factor for patients in the eighth and ninth decades is still a matter of debate.

The nutritional status of the patient has also been considered an important risk factor for infection. Undernutrition results in significant alterations in immunologic responses, and cellular immunity is particularly impaired among patients with severe malnutrition; however, the importance of malnutrition as an independent risk factor for hospitalized patients has not been well documented. Overnutrition or obesity also contributes to infection, particularly to postoperative wound infections.

The most significant risk factors for infection in hospitalized patients are the underlying diseases. In patients with severe burns, the skin is denuded, depriving the host of a vital mechanical barrier that prevents invasion by environmental microorganisms. Nosocomial infections constitute a major threat to survival for burn patients. Patients with leukemia and aplastic anemia are at risk for nosocomial infections because the underlying disease interferes with the production of phagocytic cells, which are essential in the defense against infection. Finally, patients with the acquired immunodeficiency syndrome (AIDS) are at increased risk for nosocomial infection by virtue of impairment of cellular immune responses. Thus any disease that interferes or impairs normal mechanical or physiologic host defense mechanisms will increase susceptibility to nosocomial infections.

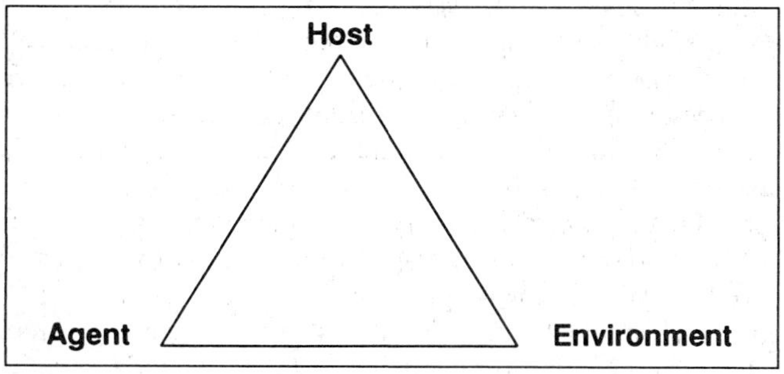

Fig. 225-1. Triangular model of disease showing that the interplay of host, agent, and environment is important in understanding the causation of disease and its control.

Conditions imposed by the health care system

Every diagnostic and treatment modality used by the physician, however simple and seemingly harmless, is accompanied by a risk of adverse reaction(s). Pertinent to nosocomial infections, medications used to treat malignant diseases or to modulate immunologic responses alter the capacity of the patient to control infection. Some medications augment the risk of infection as a direct consequence of the pharmacologic effects. Antacids and beta-2 blockers, routinely administered to patients in intensive care units to reduce the risk of gastrointestinal bleeding, may increase the risk of gram-negative lower respiratory infections by interfering with the secretion of gastric acid.

An assortment of paraphernalia, usually plastic or metal cannulae and tubes, is introduced through normal protective barriers such as skin and mucous membranes or into a hollow viscus. These foreign bodies interfere with normal physical barriers and protective mechanisms. Intravenous cannulae, urinary catheters, pressure monitoring devices, dialysis catheters, and intubation tubes predispose to severe and sometimes fatal nosocomial infections.

Finally, it is routine during surgical interventions to enter the sterile internal milieu of the host. Despite the most sophisticated techniques to maintain a sterile environment, inoculation of even small numbers of organisms into the operative site may be sufficient to establish a nidus of infection.

AGENTS

The biologic agents capable of producing nosocomial infections are myriad. Viruses, bacteria, fungi, protozoa, and arachnids have all been implicated. Nosocomial bacterial and fungal infections are most significant in terms of frequency, morbidity, and mortality. Although many species of bacteria and fungi have been associated with nosocomial infections, a few common pathogens account for most of the infections. The Centers for Disease Control maintains the only national database on nosocomial infections in the United States. More than 100 hospitals voluntarily report summary information on nosocomial infections to the National Nosocomial Infection Surveillance (NNIS) System. The distribution of nosocomial pathogens isolated from the bloodstream and reported by NNIS between 1986 and 1989 are summarized in Fig. 225-2. The four most frequent pathogens isolated from blood cultures account for more than 50% of bacteremias: coagulase-negative staphylococci, *Staphylococcus aureus*, enterococci, and *Escherichia coli*. The relative frequency with which specific strains of pathogens have been associated with nosocomial infections

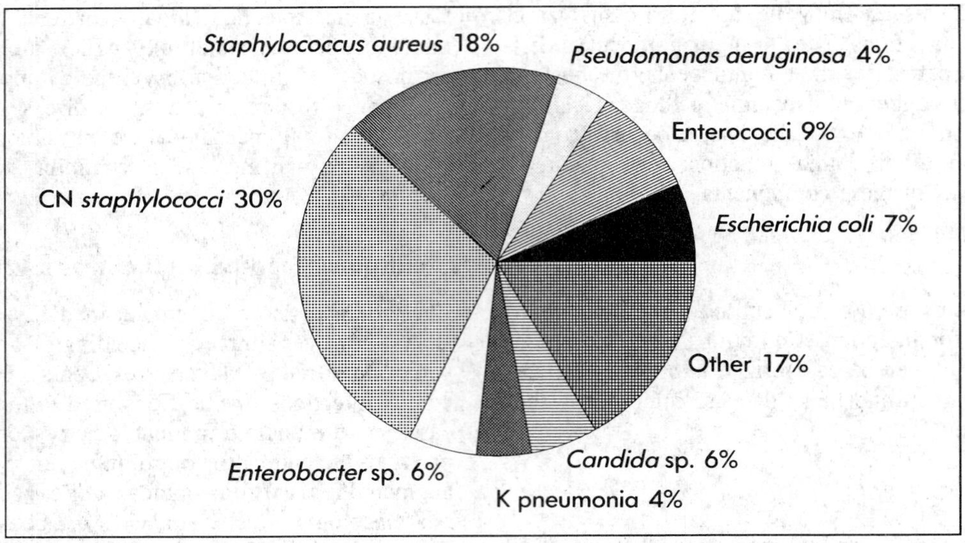

Fig. 225-2. Distribution by species of more than 10,000 bloodstream isolates from the National Nosocomial Infection Surveillance System, 1986-1989.

has changed over time. Group A beta-hemolytic streptococci, presently a rare cause of nosocomial infections, were a frequent source of serious infections in the early twentieth century. From the 1940s through the 1960s, *S. aureus* was the predominant pathogen. During the next two decades, gram-negative bacilli such as *E. coli, Enterobacter* species, *Klebsiella* species, and *Pseudomonas* species emerged as predominant pathogens. During the past decade, coagulase-negative staphylococci and *Candida* species, commensal flora and once regarded as contaminants, have emerged as increasingly important pathogens.

The changing ecology of nosocomial pathogens during the latter half of the twentieth century reflects changing technologies and the ability to care for and preserve patients with severe chronic diseases. Use of antibiotics, in particular, has changed the distribution of nosocomial pathogens. Commensurate with changes in species of nosocomial pathogens has been the emergence of expanding patterns of multiple antimicrobial resistance. Paradoxically, the emerging pathogens are less virulent as measured by their capacity to produce disease in healthy hosts. Nevertheless, several factors render these organisms virulent in the hospital environment.

Adherence

The first step in the infectious process is adherence of the microbe to host tissue. Intrinsic properties of the agent that facilitate adherence enhance the capacity of an organism to produce disease. *E. coli, Proteus mirabilis,* and other gram-negative bacteria contain fimbriae (pili), which are tiny projections on the surface of the bacterium. Specific chemicals located on the tips of pili enable organisms to attach to selected sites in tissues of the host (e.g., *E. coli* to urinary tract endothelium). Similarly, the cell walls of *S. aureus* contain teichoic acids that adhere to host epithelial cells (Chapter 257). *Staphylococcus epidermidis* produces a layer of "slime," a biofilm consisting of glycocalyx that surrounds the organism (Chapter 258). A potentially important property of the biofilm is attachment to foreign material such as intravascular cannulae, prosthetic valves, and prosthetic joints. This intrinsic property of *Staphylococcus epidermidis* may explain, in part, why this organism has emerged as one of the most frequent nosocomial pathogens.

Toxin production

Microbes produce toxic substances that may be important in the pathogenesis of nosocomial infections. *S. aureus* produces several exotoxins such as leukocidin, which is cytotoxic for neutrophils. *S. aureus* also produces enterotoxin F, a toxin responsible for toxic shock syndrome, and exfoliatin, a toxin responsible for the "scalded skin syndrome." Exotoxin A is an enzyme released by *Pseudomonas aeruginosa* that produces diphtheria toxin-like effects on cells. The toxin is lethal for mammalian cells and may be important in the pathogenesis of disease in humans. A virulence factor common to all gram-negative bacteria is endotoxin (Chapter 239). The active component of endotoxin is lipid A, a structural component of gram-negative bacterial cell walls. Endotoxin plays a pivotal role in gram-negative septicemia and shock by triggering the release of endogenous mediators of inflammation, such as tumor necrosis factor and leukotrienes, and by activating several host protein "cascades" including complement, coagulation, kallikrein-kinin, and other pathways. Despite the role of toxic substances in the pathogenesis of nosocomial infections, it should be apparent that these "virulence" factors are not imperative for inducing disease. Bacteria such as enterococcus and coagulase-negative staphylococci produce little in the way of toxic substances. Despite this apparent impotence, these organisms are among the most frequent pathogens responsible for nosocomial infections and may be associated with significant morbidity and mortality.

Antimicrobial resistance

To ensure survival in "hostile" environments, bacteria have acquired several mechanisms for combating the toxic effects of antimicrobial agents. In an environment where antibiotics are used frequently, this intrinsic property is important to ensure survival of nosocomial pathogens. Antibiotic resistance coupled with the capacity to rapidly transmit this genetic information to other bacteria by conjugation and transduction accounts for the emergence of endemic strains of multiply resistant bacteria in the hospital environment.

Environmental adaptability

Several of these pathogens are able to adapt to a variety of environmental temperatures. *Legionella pneumophila* will survive in water in which the temperature varies between 5° C (41° F) and 45° C (113° F). The capacity to withstand changes in ambient temperatures enhances the opportunity for transmission from one environmental niche to another. Both *Pseudomonas* and *Legionella* species are capable of surviving in water reservoirs with minimal energy requirements. Thus organisms are able to establish a niche in a variety of sites within a hospital.

ENVIRONMENT

The third component of the model that determines susceptibility to nosocomial infections is the biologic and physical environment in which the patient receives care.

Biologic environment

A reservoir is that site in the environment where microbes reside. The reservoir provides a source of nutrients and a niche conducive to survival and replication of the organism. Microbes are found in humans, animals, plants, and inert material in the environment. Reservoirs may be categorized with reference to the patient as exogenous or endogenous.

Exogenous reservoirs include air, water, food, equipment, medications, and animate sources (i.e., the health care worker). Epidemics associated with *Aspergillus* in air, *L. pneumophila* in water, and *Salmonella* in food have been reported in hospitals. Past experience and attention to hospital design have eliminated many exogenous reservoirs; however, sometimes elusive reservoirs continue to create problems for the immunocompromised patient. Once identified, these reservoirs can usually be controlled, but often at considerable cost to the hospital. Medical equipment, particularly that which uses water reservoirs or nebulizers, provides potential reservoirs for aquaphilic nosocomial pathogens. Medical personnel constitute a critically important reservoir and contribute to infections by carrying and shedding organisms or by serving as vectors who carry organisms from reservoirs to the uninfected patient. For example, 15% to 20% of the population carry *S. aureus* in the nasal antrum. A subgroup of carriers are prone to shed organisms into the environment, thereby creating a risk for patients. Health care workers also transmit disease during acute infections with communicable agents (e.g., influenza, rotavirus, and respiratory syncytial virus).

The most important reservoir for nosocomial pathogens is endogenous flora found in or on the patient. Humans are colonized with a myriad of gram-positive and gram-negative bacteria. This symbiotic relationship between host and commensal is easily disturbed during hospitalization. The severity of the underlying disease and frequent use of antibiotics alter the normal flora that reside on the skin and in the upper airway and bowel. When antibiotic-susceptible flora are eradicated during the course of antibiotic therapy, patients become colonized with large numbers of intrinsically resistant flora such as enterococci, *S. epidermidis, Candida* species, or with resistant Enterobacteriaceae and *Pseudomonas*. In the compromised host, these "new" flora invade and establish a nidus of infection. Unlike exogenous reservoirs that can be disinfected or eradicated, little can be done to eradicate nosocomial pathogens from endogenous reservoirs.

Transmission of microorganisms from exogenous reservoirs to the patient occurs via several mechanisms. Some organisms (e.g., *Mycobacterium tuberculosis*) remain viable when suspended in air and are spread by aerosols. Aerosolized particles may be as small as 1 to 5 μm in diameter so that on inhalation, the organism is carried to and deposited in the alveoli of the lung. Organisms are also spread by direct contact between persons. The most frequent person-to-person contact in hospitals is between health care worker and patient. Without vigorous hand washing, staphylococci and a variety of gram-negative bacilli may easily be carried as superficial flora on the hands and spread from one patient to another.

Physical environment

Once the importance of reservoirs and modes of transmission in nosocomial infections is recognized, the role of the structural environment should be apparent. Improper ventilation may disseminate airborne organisms from patient to patient or patient to employee. Potable water, which harbors *Legionella*, can aerosolize bacteria from shower heads and water spigots. Finally, inadequate space allocation or inadequate attention to traffic patterns in the hospital may contribute to spread of organisms from reservoir to patient.

Medical equipment, particularly that which comes into intimate contact with the patient such as respirators, dialyzers, and endoscopes, may predispose to infections when improperly cleaned and disinfected. This situation is a particular problem when a new technology is introduced. Sophisticated new technologies often limit alternatives for disinfection and simultaneously introduce unsuspected reservoirs and new modes of transmission.

INFECTION SITES

Nosocomial infections may occur at any conceivable anatomic site. Most (80%) occur in one of four sites: urinary tract, surgical wound, lower respiratory tract, or bloodstream. Lower respiratory infections are discussed elsewhere in the text (Chapter 231).

Urinary tract infections

The urinary tract is the most frequent site of infection, accounting for 40% of nosocomial infections. Most infections are associated with some form of instrumentation of the urinary tract. Four factors have been identified as independent risk factors for infection with indwelling urinary catheters: duration of catheterization, breaches in proper care of catheters, absence of systemic antibiotics, and female gender. Nosocomial urinary tract infections are associated with increased risk of septicemia and mortality. Because of the morbidity and mortality associated with urinary tract infections, the physician must be sure that the benefits of catheterization outweigh the risks of the intervention (Chapter 240).

Postoperative wound infections

Wound infections after surgical procedures have a significant impact on morbidity by prolonging hospitalization and convalescence. Contamination of the wound by the inciting pathogen may occur from endogenous or exogenous reservoirs. Endogenous reservoirs include the skin and flora of the bowel or airways when mucous membranes are transected during surgical procedures. Exogenous sources include operating room personnel and surgical equipment. Contamination often occurs during a breakdown in surgical technique.

Several factors or conditions have been associated with increased risk of wound infections. Some of these conditions are summarized in the accompanying box. The most consistent predictors of risk of postoperative wound infections include (1) severity of illness of the patient as reflected in the American Society of Anesthesiologists' preoperative assessment score, (2) duration of the operative procedure (a reflection of the complexity of the operative procedure and skill of the surgeon), and (3) level of contamination as classified by a contaminated or dirty wound (e.g., perforated bowel, compound fracture).

Several of the factors that predispose to wound infections can be controlled or managed. Results from the Study for Efficacy of Nosocomial Infection Control (SENIC) conducted by the Centers for Disease Control suggested that at least 33% of wound infections are preventable by careful attention to techniques. Furthermore, prophylactic antibiotics reduce the incidence of wound infections. Optimal chemoprophylaxis requires that the antibiotic inhibit the growth of potential nosocomial pathogens, that it penetrate the site of infection, and that administra tion precede the operative procedure. Prophylactic antibiotics should be initiated within 2 hours before the incision is made and continued for no longer than 24 hours after the procedure is completed.

Conditions that increase the risk of postoperative wound infections

Preoperative
- Age
- Underlying disease, e.g., obesity, remote infection
- Duration of preoperative hospital stay
- No preoperative shower
- Shaving the operative site

Intraoperative
- Duration of the procedure
- Use of electrocautery
- Use of surgical drains
- Technical care of the wound

From Mayhall CG: Surgical infections including burns. In Wenzel RP, editor: *Prevention and control of nosocomial infections,* ed 2, Baltimore, 1993, Williams & Wilkins.

Bacteremia

Hospital-acquired bloodstream infections occur less frequently than infections at other sites, accounting for approximately 10% of nosocomial infections. These infections are more serious, however, resulting in 7 to 14 additional days of hospitalization and an attributable mortality rate of 25%. Bacteremias may occur without an apparent source (primary) or secondary to infection at a distal site. The distinction between primary and secondary bacteremia is important for epidemiologic as well as clinical reasons. Secondary bloodstream infections occur as a complication of 1% to 5% of urinary tract infections, 3% of postoperative wound and pulmonary infections, and 5% of cutaneous infections. The usual pathogens are *E. coli, S. aureus, Klebsiella pneumoniae,* and *P. aeruginosa.* Identification of the source allows one to treat both the underlying condition and the complicating bacteremia. For example, bacteremia developing in patients with a urinary tract infection should always suggest the possibility of obstruction, which may require surgery as well as antibiotics.

Primary bacteremias are often associated with intravascular cannulas. In large referal hospitals, 80% of patients receive intravenous infusions. When primary bacteremias occur, cannulas should lead the list of suspected sources of infection. Increasing reliance on technologies such as hyperalimentation, and arterial monitors, Swan-Ganz and tunneled catheters has added to the risk of nosocomial bacteremia. Prevention of this hazardous infectious complication requires discretion in deciding when patients will benefit from the technology and careful attention to asepsis when inserting and maintaining intravascular cannulas.

PREVENTION

As knowledge regarding risk factors and causation in nosocomial infections increased, a discipline emerged that is dedicated to the study and prevention of these untoward events. Infection control programs have become the standard of care in acute care hospitals. The components of these programs are summarized here.

Infection control committee

The committee provides the authority for control programs. It is usually appointed by the hospital administration and includes representatives from the physician staff, nursing, administration, engineering-maintenance, central sterilizing, pharmacy, and other departments deemed appropriate by the administrator. The charge to the committee is to formulate and execute policies related to the control of hospital-acquired infections.

Infection control staff

The committee retains a staff who is responsible for implementing committee policies. In most smaller hospitals, the staff includes the committee chairperson, usually a physician with interest in infectious diseases, who serves as "hospital epidemiologist." In larger institutions, hospital epidemiologists are specially trained for this task and commit a significant portion of professional time to this effort. In most hospitals, the principal staff person is the infection control practitioner, usually a nurse or microbiologist who has received specific training for this task and who commits most of his or her professional time to this effort. For larger hospitals, it has been recommended that optimal staffing should include one practitioner for every 250 beds. The tasks of the infection control staff are described in the next sections.

Surveillance

Surveillance is a method for identifying, counting, and monitoring nosocomial infections. It is used to establish endemic rates of nosocomial infections and to identify epidemics. The success of surveillance programs depends on establishing explicit definitions for infections and adhering to the definitions over time. Surveillance data are most useful when converted to rates, for example, the number of events per patients at risk (number of infections per 100 admissions) or number of events per time at risk (number of events per 1000 patient-days). The data are usually reported monthly (when), by service or by physician (who), by patient care area (where), by pathogen (what), and by procedure (how). The information is used by the infection control committee to analyze problems, establish program priorities, and design interventions. The information may also be disseminated to health care providers in the institution to increase awareness regarding methods for preventing nosocomial infections.

Control programs

A second important component of the infection control program is the implementation of effective interventions to control the spread of infection in hospitals. In most circumstances, this effort entails implementation of guidelines set forth by the Centers for Disease Control or the American Hospital Association. These guidelines for the control of nosocomial infections are usually based on scientific studies that have passed the scrutiny of experts in the field. Some controls emerge from local efforts to control institution-specific problems. These measures can be equally important as long as they have been demonstrated to be effective. Controls are generally designed to disinfect, to contain known reservoirs, or to interfere with known modes of transmission. Methods for containing hospital biohazards may be categorized into engineering or administrative controls.

Engineering controls. Engineering controls are incorporated into the design and structure of the hospital. They include everything from the proper design of ventilation systems to the simple placement of hand-washing sinks in convenient, "unavoidable" locations. Protection of the environment in high-risk areas, such as operating suites, includes the proper exchange of fresh air (20 L/hr) through high-efficiency filters to remove potential airborne pathogens. For hospitals in which outbreaks of legionellosis have been documented, special engineering controls may be required to eradicate and control *Legionella* in the potable water system. Currently available options include hyperchlorination, raising the hot water temperature, and ultraviolet light. Infection control staff must be cognizant of these important aspects of control programs and review all new construction plans to ensure that these measures have been addressed.

Administrative controls. Administrative controls must be implemented at the volition of the health care worker. Because the success and efficacy of administrative controls depend on the knowledge and initiative of health care workers, education and reinforcement are important elements in a successful prevention program. Examples of administrative controls include the following:

Guidelines for procedures. The insertion of an intravenous line (e.g., intravenous cannula) is accompanied by a measurable risk of infection. The risk of infection may be reduced by adhering to certain guidelines regarding insertion, maintenance, and removal. Guidelines for proper insertion of an intravenous line are summarized in the box on p. 1828. Similarly, infection control programs must ensure adherence to proper guidelines for all procedures that impose a risk of infection for patients.

Isolation and universal precautions. Isolation/segregation precautions are procedures that have been traditionally used in hospitals to contain transmissible pathogens and protect employees and other patients. These administrative controls are implemented after establishing a presumptive diagnosis of a transmissible disease.

The AIDS epidemic has heightened concern for the risk of transmission of disease from patients to health care workers and from health care workers to patients. Blood-borne nosocomial pathogens such as hepatitis B, human immunodeficiency virus, and the agent of Creutzfeldt-Jakob disease pose a particular risk to health care workers because

Guidelines for intravenous line use

1. Use only when indicated
2. Choose a low-risk site (upper extremity)
3. Use good technique
   a. Wash hands
   b. Use aseptic prep
   c. Date and label the site
4. Maintain appropriately
   a. Discontinue emergency sites within 24 hours
   b. Observe daily
   c. Change q48h
5. Discontinue as early as possible
6. With unexplained sepsis, suspect the intravenous site

Universal precautions to reduce risk of infection

1. All health care workers should use barrier precautions* when contact with infectious body fluids is anticipated.
2. Wash hands if contaminated and immediately after removing gloves.
3. Avoid sharp injuries.
4. Use mouthpieces, resuscitation bags, or other ventilation devices for emergency resuscitation.
5. Health care workers who have exudative lesions or weeping dermatitis should refrain from direct patient care.
6. Pregnant health care workers should be especially familiar with and strictly adhere to precautions to minimize risk of exposure to blood-borne agents.

*Gloves (routine); goggles, masks, and gowns (when indicated). From Centers for Disease Control: Recommendations for prevention of HIV transmission in health-care settings, MMWR 36(Suppl 2S):2, 1987.

of their exposure to body fluids and secretions. These exposures often occur when health care workers encounter patients with undiagnosed, asymptomatic disease. To reduce the risk of infection, it has been recommended that health care workers avoid direct contact with body fluids by exercising universal precautions with all patients. These precautions, summarized in the accompanying box, include the routine use of gloves when exposure to potentially infectious fluids is anticipated and use of goggles and masks when there is risk of droplet contact with mucous membranes. Special attention must be given to reducing accidental needle sticks (e.g., no recapping of used needles and using puncture-resistant containers for disposal of used needles). It is assumed that when universal precautions are used as part of routine patient care practices, an added level of protection against transmission of blood-borne pathogens is afforded both health care workers and patients.

Hand washing. Hand washing is a simple hygienic measure that interrupts the transmission of nosocomial pathogens from a patient reservoir to an otherwise uninfected, uncolonized patient. Despite repeated reports that confirm Semmelweis' original observation on the efficacy of hand washing in 1840, clusters of preventable nosocomial infections continue to occur because of careless inattention to hand washing by health care personnel.

Employee health. Two important objectives of an employee health program include protection of patients from transmissible diseases carried by health care workers and protection of the employee against communicable diseases in patients. These objectives may be accomplished by screening employees for disease (e.g., tuberculosis) at the time of job entry and periodically during the term of employment. The latter is especially important in the current era of multiple antibiotic-resistant strains of tuberculosis (Chapter 276). Employee health programs also screen employees to ensure that they are protected by vaccination against a variety of communicable diseases. When previous exposure or vaccination cannot be documented, many institutions will provide vaccination against hepatitis B and rubella for employees. The employee health program should also include counseling, volunteer testing, and follow-up for health care workers parenterally exposed to human immunodeficiency virus or other blood-borne pathogens. Finally, the programs should have provisions for evaluation of acute illnesses to ensure that employees with acute transmissible infections are excused from work.

Efficacy of infection control programs. It has been estimated that the cost of an effective infection control program in a 250-bed hospital is approximately $78,000 (1989 dollars). Because infection control programs do not generate revenue, one may query whether prevention programs can be justified. In a large national study (SENIC) conducted by the Centers for Disease Control in the mid-1970s, it was observed that hospitals incorporating all elements of an infection control program had a 33% reduction in the rates of nosocomial infections. Based on estimates of cost for increased lengths of stay following nosocomial infections, the program should "break even" when the infection rate is reduced by as little as 10%. Thus effective infection control programs are not only effective in reducing rates of nosocomial infection but also are cost-effective. This observation is all the more pertinent under prospective reimbursement where costs of additional hospitalization due to nosocomial infections must be absorbed by the institution.

REFERENCES

Bennett JV and Brachman, PS, editors: Hospital infections, ed 3, Boston, 1992, Little, Brown.

Centers for Disease Control: Recommendations for prevention of HIV transmission in health-care settings, MMWR 40:1-9, 1991.

Classen DC et al: The timing of prophylactic administration of antibiotics and the risk of surgical wound infection, N Engl J Med 326:281-286, 1992.

Cruse PJE and Foord R: The epidemiology of wound infection. A 10-year prospective study of 62,939 wounds, Surg Clin North Am 60:27-40, 1980.

Doebbeling BN, Stanley GL, Sheetz CT et al: Comparative efficacy of alternative handwashing agents in reducing nosocomial infections in intensive care units, N Engl J Med 327:88-93, 1992.

Driks MR, et al: Nosocomial pneumonia in intubated patients given sucralfate as compared with antacids or histamine type 2 blockers: the role of gastric colonization, N Engl J Med 317:1376-1382, 1987.

Haley RW et al: The nationwide nosocomial infection rate: a new need for vital statistics, Am J Epidemiol 121:159-167, 1985.

Haley RW et al: The efficacy of infection surveillance and control programs in preventing nosocomial infections in U.S. hospitals, Am J Epidemiol 121:182-205, 1985.

Helms CM et al: Legionnaires' disease associated with a hospital water system: a 5-year progress report on continuous hyperchlorination, JAMA 259(16):2423-2427, 1988.

Ishak MA et al: Association of slime with pathogenicity of coagulase-negative staphylococci causing nosocomial septicemia, J Clin Microbiol 22:1025-1029, 1985.

Kunin CM: Detection prevention and management of urinary tract infections, ed 4, Philadelphia, 1987, Lea & Febiger.

Maki DG: Nosocomial bacteremia: an epidemiologic overview, Am J Med 70:719-732, 1981.

Martone WJ and Garner JS, editors: Proceedings of the Third Decennial International Conference on Nosocomial Infections, Am J Med 91 (3B):1-333, 1991.

Massanari RM et al: Reliability of reporting nosocomial infection in the discharge abstract and implications for receipt of revenues under prospective reimbursement, Am J Public Health 77:1-3, 1986.

Miller PJ and Wenzel RP: Etiologic organisms as independent predictors of death and morbidity associated with bloodstream infections (BSI), J Infect Dis 156:471-477, 1987.

Selden R, Lee S, and Wang WL: Nosocomial *Klebsiella* infections: intestinal colonization as a reservoir, Ann Intern Med 74:657-664, 1971.

Sheth NK, Franson TR, and Sohnle PC: Influence of bacterial adherence to intravascular catheters on in vitro antibiotic susceptibility, Lancet 2:1266-1268, 1985.

Stamm WE: Catheter-associated urinary tract infections: epidemiology, pathogenesis, and prevention, Am J Med (Suppl 3B)91:65S-71S, 1991.

Wadowsky RM et al: Effect of temperature, pH, and oxygen level on multiplication of naturally occurring *Legionella pneumophila* in potable water, Appl Environ Microbiol 49:1197-1205, 1985.

Wenzel RP, editor: Prevention and control of nosocomial infections, ed 2, Baltimore, 1993, Williams & Wilkins.

Wenzel RP, editor: Assessing quality health care. Perspective for clinicians, Baltimore, 1992, Williams & Wilkins.

II Laboratory Tests

CHAPTER

226 Use of Laboratory Tests in Infectious Diseases

Thomas A. Drake

Identification of an etiologic agent is essential for the diagnosis of and choice of therapy for most infectious diseases. Laboratory techniques to identify etiologic agents can be grouped into three categories: isolation of the organism in culture, demonstration of the organism or its specific components at sites of infection, and measurement of specific immune response.

Isolation of pathogenic organisms in culture, except when culture is not feasible, has long been the mainstay of diagnostic methods, with other techniques providing supportive information. A major drawback with culture and serologic techniques, however, is the length of time normally required to establish a diagnosis. The need for more immediately available information, coupled with recent technologic developments, has dramatically increased interest in direct detection techniques, techniques encompassing a variety of tests ranging from simple morphologic stains on direct specimens to the newly developed tests of antigen detection by monoclonal antibodies and pathogen-specific DNA detection by hybridization. Although relatively few of these procedures have replaced culture as the standard diagnostic technique, they will be used more and more as methodologies are improved to provide timely results.

TEST INTERPRETATION

The usefulness of any laboratory technique varies with the nature of the infection and must be evaluated clinically in terms of predictive value, timeliness, and cost. The *predictive value* of a test is the frequency with which a disease is accurately predicted to be present or absent by a particular positive or negative test result, respectively. (A positive predictive value of 60% means that of 100 patients with positive tests, 60 will actually have the disease and 40 will not.) To assess predictive value, test sensitivity (frequency of positive test result among patients with the disease), test specificity (frequency of negative test results among persons without the disease), and disease prevalence (probability of the presence of disease in the population being evaluated) must be known or reasonably approximated. The details of predictive value theory are available elsewhere and will not be presented here (see References). The concepts involved, however, are directly applicable to testing in clinical microbiology.

For tests in which the ranges of values obtained from reference and patient populations overlap, test sensitivity and specificity are determined by the cutoff value chosen to separate positive and negative results; a gain in one will result in a loss in the other. One can illustrate this relationship by reference to coliform urinary infections (the presence of coliform bacteria in urine obtained by suprapubic aspiration or catheterization) in symptomatic women. The traditional diagnostic criterion of $\geq 10^5$ bacteria per milliliter of midstream urine yields 99% specificity but only 51% sensitivity (Chapter 240) for this group of patients (in which the prevalence of infection is 50%). In this setting, predictive values of positive and negative results are 98% and 67% respectively. If the criterion for a positive test in this group is revised to $\geq 10^2$ bacteria per milliliter, specificity is 85%, sensitivity is 95%, and predictive values of positive and negative results are 86% and 94%, respectively. Thus use of the lower cutoff produces more clinically acceptable predictive values of positive and negative results. Other tests for which established cutoff values are of comparable import include purified protein derivative (PPD) skin testing (diameter of induration), some enzyme and radioimmunoassays (degree of enzymatic activity or radioactivity measured), and many titrated serologic tests.

A second important aspect of laboratory testing, which is often not appreciated intuitively, is the significant influence that the probability of disease has on a test's predictive value. To continue the preceding example, although the cutoff of $\geq 10^2$ bacteria per milliliter was clinically useful in a high-prevalence (50%) population, application of this criterion in a low-prevalence setting (e.g., 6% in certain asymptomatic patients) would result in an unacceptably low predictive value of a positive result (29%). The predictive value of a negative result, however, would be high (>99%). In low-prevalence settings test specificity becomes a critical determinant of positive predictive value. With 1% prevalence, the latter drops from 91% to 50% to 17% when test specificity changes from 99.9% to 99%, to 95% respectively. Because many tests do not have 99.9% sensitivity or are used in even lower disease prevalence populations, positive results may need to be confirmed by independent means as is accepted practice for the serologic diagnosis of syphilis and human immunodeficiency virus (HIV) infection. In general, in low-prevalence settings positive results should be questioned, whereas in high-prevalence settings negative findings should prompt further investigation.

Do's and don'ts of specimen collection and handling

1. Collect specimen from site of infection.
2. Use appropriate collection technique to avoid contamination by indigenous flora.
3. Do not use swabs for anaerobic cultures.
4. Avoid contaminating specimen for culture when Gram stain or other stain is prepared at the time of collection.
5. Use proper technique when culture medium is directly inoculated.
6. Label specimen and provide a specific description of the source and the testing desired.
7. Use appropriate transport medium to preserve organism viability.
8. Avoid delays in specimen transport.
9. Never freeze specimen or expose to heat; refrigerate only stool and urine; incubate only blood and CSF.

CULTURE OF PATHOGENIC MICROORGANISMS IN CLINICAL MEDICINE

Bacteria

Specimen collection and handling. Avoidance of contamination, adequacy of sampling, and preservation of viability are critical factors in proper specimen collection and handling. Effort must always be made to obtain appropriate specimens before the institution of antibiotic therapy. Details regarding specimen collection from specific body sites are presented in other chapters; general guidelines are presented in the accompanying box. Submission of inappropriate, contaminated, or mishandled specimens creates potentially confusing and dangerous clinical situations. The patient is placed at risk if effective therapy is withheld or if unnecessary therapy administered, and the cost of care is increased.

The human body harbors abundant flora of commensal bacteria on the skin and mucous membranes and in the intestinal tract (Table 226-1). Skin should be disinfected with tincture of iodine, iodophor, chlorhexidine, or alcohol before being traversed to obtain specimens. Alcohol is the least rapidly acting, requiring 1 to 2 minutes of contact to afford maximum antibacterial effect. The practice of replacing needles on syringes before inoculating blood culture bottles should be abandoned, as it does not reduce contamination and increases the risk of needle stick injury. When sites of infection are in continuity with the skin (e.g., via sinus tracts or open wounds), superficial or sinus tract material should be considered contaminated, and acceptable samples are those taken only at deep sites.

Specimens may be collected directly into sterile containers (cerebrospinal fluid [CSF], urine, stool, tissue) via syringe (blood, body fluid, and tissue aspirates) or with a swab (mucous membranes). Cotton swabs are adequate for most purposes but Dacron- or calcium alginate-tipped swabs should be used when *Neisseria gonorrhoeae, Bordetella pertussis,* or *Corynebacterium diphtheriae* are sought. The volume of a specimen submitted is important in situations where pathogenic bacteria may be present in low numbers. Maximum recovery of organisms from blood is obtained by culturing a total of 30 ml of blood in two or three draws. At least 5 ml of CSF should be obtained for routine bacterial culture and 10 ml for mycobacterial culture. In addition, bulk stool samples more frequently yield pathogens than do rectal swabs.

Procedures for specimen transport must ensure viability of pathogens, as well as limitation of contaminant growth. The best means to accomplish these goals are through use of appropriate transport systems and prompt delivery to the laboratory. Transport media such as Stuart and Amies media are formulated to maintain organism viability but restrict rapid growth and should be used for swabs and tissue samples. Urine and stool should be transported in sealed sterile containers and refrigerated if not processed within 1 hour of collection. In contrast, blood and CSF should be incubated at 37° C if processing is delayed. All other specimens, including sputum, should be kept at room temperature. Certain pathogens such as *Neisseria* and *Haemophilus* species are killed when exposed to the cold, whereas others such as group A streptococci are quite hardy.

Blood specimens are inoculated immediately into culture bottles to optimize organism recovery. Adequate dilution (1:5 to 1:10) in medium is important to minimize natural antibacterial properties of blood. This is also facilitated by having sodium polyethylene sulfonate (SPS) as a component of blood culture medium, which serves additionally as an anticoagulant. *Neisseria* species and *Peptostreptococcus anaerobius* are inhibited by SPS, however, and SPS-free media should be used when these organisms are suspected.

Sucrose-supplemented media designed for recovery of cell wall-deficient organisms have not proved useful for routine use. Media containing resins to absorb and inactivate antibiotics are of limited benefit; these methods appear to be most advantageous when used with small-volume systems like the BACTEC (Becton-Dickinson Diagnostic Instrument Systems, Towson, Md). One novel blood culture system, the lysis centrifugation method (Isolator, DuPont Co., Wilmington, Del) avoids the use of liquid culture media. Blood is drawn directly into an evacuated tube containing a blood cell lysing solution. Tubes are centrifuged to sediment bacteria, and the bottom layer plated directly to agar media.

The recognized spectrum of disease associated with anaerobic bacteria has broadened as improved techniques for recovery, isolation, and identification have been developed. Although some anaerobes can survive extended exposure to oxygen, others are oxygen-sensitive; thus specimens that may harbor such anaerobes should not be exposed to air. Fluids should be collected in a syringe, the air immediately expressed, and the end plugged with a rubber stopper or the contents injected into an anaerobic transport tube. Swabs should not be used because air remains trapped among the fibers. Tissue specimens should be placed in anaerobic transport containers. A variety of these systems is currently commercially available; the simplest of them is the carbon dioxide-filled, stoppered tube. When the tube is held upright during opening and insertion of the specimen, the carbon dioxide will not flow out of the bottle, and the atmosphere will remain anaerobic if the container is recapped quickly. Preservation of *N. gonorrhoeae* requires carbon dioxide added to the incubation atmosphere, as is provided by the traditional candle jars or various commercially available systems.

Isolation and identification. Inoculation of agar plates, properly streaked, allows isolation of separate colonies. This separation is essential for identification of bacteria and may also provide a crude estimate of relative numbers of bacteria. The concentration of organisms in a liquid sample (such as urine) can be determined by plating a defined amount of dilution of the sample uniformly over the surface of an agar plate. Inoculation of broth medium precludes quantitation but permits culture of a larger sample volume and may be more conducive to growth. Specimens from normally sterile body sites should be inoculated to a medium that will support the growth of suspected pathogens. Usually, this medium includes blood and chocolate (laked blood) agar plates and a nutrient broth. When specimens are obtained from areas of the body normally harboring bacteria, selective culture media and environments are often necessary. In selective media, the nutrient, chemical, and inhibiting composition are varied to allow growth of only certain organisms. These media are necessary for isolation of certain enteric pathogens and are commonly used to improve recovery of group A streptococci from throat cultures.

The time needed to grow, isolate, and identify different organisms varies considerably. The more common aerobic pathogens grow rapidly, and preliminary reports can be expected from the laboratory within 24 hours. Anaerobes generally grow more slowly, and plates are not usually examined for 48 hours. Most pathogenic mycobacteria require at least several weeks of incubation before identification is possible. Several species of pathogenic bacteria (e.g., *Treponema pallidum, Borrelia* species, and *Mycobacterium leprae*) cannot be isolated on artificial media. Assessments of mixed organism growth as "normal (e.g., fecal, oral) flora" in specimens from contaminated sites are made simply by inspection of culture plates, without specific organism identification.

Blood cultures are incubated in the collection bottle and monitored regularly, with Gram stain and subcultures performed if there is evidence of bacterial growth. The BACTEC system (Becton-Dickinson Diagnostic Instrument Systems, Towson, Md) and the BacT/Alert system (Organaon Technika Corp., Durham, NC) have automated monitoring based on CO_2 production by growing organisms, which reduces the time needed for a culture to be recognized as positive. The Septi-chek system (Roche Diagnostics Systems, Nutley, NJ) consists of a device with an enclosed agar paddle that is attached to the top of the blood culture bottles after inoculation. When the bottles are inverted, the paddle is flooded; hence one is effectively performing a subculture without entering the system. This technique reduces the time needed to make bacterial colonies available for identification and susceptibility testing. Blood cultures are held for at least 7 days before being reported as negative and discarded. The laboratory should be notified if a longer incubation is indicated, as for suspected brucellosis.

Laboratory personnel should always be notified if plague *(Yersinia pestis)* or tularemia *(Francisella tularensis)* is suspected. These agents are highly infectious in culture, and isolation should be attempted only in laboratories using adequate safety precautions. Usual laboratory precautions are also insufficient for safe handling of specimens that contain *Coccidioides immitis* or hemorrhagic fever viruses (see accompanying box).

Management of specimens from specific body sites. Principal discussions of these aspects are found in the following chapters presenting the major clinical syndromes associated with each: blood, Chapter 274 and 280; CSF, Chapter 233; upper respiratory tract specimens, Chapter 230; lower respiratory tract specimens, Chapter 231; gastrointestinal tract specimens, Chapter 236; urine, Chapter 240; gen-

Organisms hazardous to laboratory personnel if handled without special precautions

Francisella tularensis (tularemia)
Yersinia pestis (plague)
Coccidioides immitis (coccidioidomycosis)
Hemorrhagic fever viruses (Lassa fever and others)

Table 226-1. Normal human microbial flora*

Organism	Gram stain/ morphology†	Skin	Nose/ nasopharynx	Mouth/ oropharynx	Conjunctiva	Colon	Vagina	External genitalia	Anterior urethra
Aerobic and facultative anaerobic bacteria									
Staphylococcus									
Coagulase-negative	+/c	++	++	++	++	±	++	++	+
S. aureus	+/c	+	+	+	+	±	±	+	+
Streptococcus									
Beta-hemolytic	+/c	±	±	±		+		+	
S. pneumoniae	+/c		±	+					
Enterococci	+/c			+		+	+	+	+
Viridans	+/c	±		++	±	+	++	+	+
Corynebacterium	+/cb	++	+	++	+	+	++	+	+
Branhamella	−/c		+	+					
Neisseria	−/c		+	+	±		±		+
Haemophilus	−/cb		++	+	±				
Gardnerella	−/cb						+		
Enterobacteriaceae	−/b	±	±	+	±	++	+	+	±
Acinetobacter	−/b	±		±		+	+		
Moraxella	−/b	±	±		±		±		
Pseudomonas	−/b	±				±			
Treponema	/s		+	++		+			
Mycobacterium	af/b	±	+	±		±			
Mycoplasma, Ureaplasma				+			+		+

Anaerobic bacteria									
Peptococcus, Peptostreptococcus	+/c	+	+	++		++	++	+	±
Actinomyces	+/b		+	+		±	+		
Bifidobacterium	+/b			+		++	+		
Clostridium	+/b	±		±		++	±		±
Eubacterium	+/b					+	+		
Lactobacillus	+/b	±		+		+	++		±
Bacteroides	−/b		+	++		++	+	+	+
Fusobacterium	−/b		+	++		++	±	+	+
Propionibacterium	−/b	++	+	±		±	±		±
Veillonella	−/b			++			±		
Fungi									
Candida		±	+	++	+	+	+		
Torulopsis		±		+		±	±		
Rhodotorula		±		+	+				
Cryptococcus		±		±					
Aspergillus		±		+	+				
Penicillium		+		+	+				
Pityrosporon		+							

*Relative presence at each body site is indicated: ++, prominent; +, common; ±, irregular.
†Gram stain/morphology: +, gram-positive; −, gram-negative; af, acid-fast; c, coccus; cb, coccobacillus; b, bacillus; s, spirochete.

ital tract specimens, Chapter 238; and skin and soft tissue specimens, Chapter 235.

Clinicians should familiarize themselves with specimen handling and culture protocols in the clinical microbiology laboratory they use to ensure that they will obtain the clinical information needed without excessive testing (and its attendant cost). For example, throat cultures may routinely include only a search for group A streptococci or, conversely, might entail identification and susceptibility testing of all possible pathogens. Another example is urine cultures, where a screening procedure may or may not be used and policies for detection and susceptibility testing of fewer than 10^4 or 10^5 organisms per milliliter can vary.

Viruses

It is possible to culture viruses through the use of tissue culture systems. Viruses causing human disease that can be routinely cultured are listed in Table 226-2, and those primarily detected by nonculture techniques are listed in Table 226-3. Viral diagnostic services are now available in many hospital and commercial laboratories. A discussion with laboratory personnel is always the best way to ensure proper and expeditious treatment of specimens.

Table 226-2. Appropriate agents and specimens for diagnostic viral culture

Agent	Specimens
Enteroviruses	Feces, throat swab; CSF if indicated
Influenza viruses	Throat swab
Parainfluenza virus	Throat swab
Respiratory syncytial virus	Nasopharyngeal wash (preferable to throat swab)
Mumps virus	Throat swab, urine; CSF if indicated
Measles virus (rubeola)	Throat swab
Rubella virus	Throat swab, urine
Herpes simplex virus	Skin or mucosal lesion (swab from base); involved tissue (e.g., brain)
Varicella-zoster virus	Vesicle fluid or swab
Cytomegalovirus	Throat, urine, blood leukocytes
Adenovirus	Throat swab, feces

Table 226-3. Human viruses detected primarily by nonculture techniques

Direct detection	Serologic diagnosis
Hepatitis B	Hepatitis A, B, C
Human immunodeficiency virus	Human immunodeficiency virus
Papilloma virus	Epstein-Barr virus
Polyoma virus	Arboviruses
Rotavirus	Human T lymphotrophic virus I, II
Norwalk virus	
Rabies virus	

Specimen collection and handling. Maximum recovery of virus depends on obtaining samples as early as possible in the course of the patient's illness and minimizing the time from specimen procurement to laboratory processing. In contrast to most bacterial infections, sampling of sites other than the focus of infection may yield the causative virus (Table 226-2).

Swabs are convenient for obtaining specimens from the throat, nasopharynx, rectum, external urogenital tract, conjuctiva, and skin lesions. Because viruses multiply intracellularly, recovery depends on obtaining a sufficient number of infected cells when sampling. Swabs should be placed in appropriate transport media, preferably a specific viral transport medium (usually buffered saline with added protein and antibiotics). If samples are to be processed within 4 hours, a routine transport medium (e.g., Stuart or Amies medium or the Culturette system [Marion Scientific Corp., Rockford, Ill]) is acceptable. CSF, urine, feces, and tissues can be placed directly in sterile containers, as for bacterial culture. Vesicular skin lesions can be aspirated and the fluid injected into a small volume of liquid viral transport medium (and the syringe flushed with same) before the base of the lesion is swabbed. Blood for viral culture should be collected in heparinized tubes to allow recovery of leukocyte fractions.

Delays in transport before processing should be minimized; in some instances it may be desirable to inoculate tissue culture tubes at the bedside. Respiratory syncytial virus, varicella-zoster virus, and cytomegalovirus are particularly labile. Otherwise, specimens should be kept at 4° C until processed; blood should be held at room temperature. Freezing is detrimental to most viruses and should be avoided unless samples must be held for more than several days.

Isolation and identification. Viruses are cultured in living mammalian cells. Because no single type of cultured cells will support the growth of all viruses, specimens are inoculated to two or more types of cells (usually including primary monkey kidney cells and human fetal diploid fibroblast cells). Culture medium is biochemically complex to maintain cell viability and contains antibiotics to prevent growth of bacteria or fungi. Highly contaminated specimens such as stool are pretreated with antibiotics, and a filtrate of centrifuged supernatant is used to inoculate cell cultures.

Characteristics used to identify specific viruses include the cell lines that support replication, the morphology of the cytopathic effect, and the results of a variety of tests, (e.g., hemadsorption to infected cells, hemagglutination inhibition, and direct immunofluorescence). Providing a brief statement of the clinical situation will assist laboratory personnel in choosing appropriate cell lines for inoculation and tests to perform to identify likely pathogens. The time required to isolate and identify viruses varies considerably, depending on the type of virus and the infecting inoculum (Table 226-4). In many instances, these times may be shortened to 24 hours for herpes simplex virus and 72 hours for cytomegalovirus if direct immunofluorescence with specific

Table 226-4. Time to detection for viruses in tissue culture

Agent	Usual time (days)	Range (days)
Enteroviruses	2-5	1-14
Influenza viruses	5-7	3-14
Parainfluenza virus	5-10	3-14
Respiratory syncytial virus	5-7	2-10
Mumps virus	5-10	3-14
Measles virus (rubeola)	5-10	3-14
Rubella virus	10-14	10-21
Herpes simplex virus	1-4 (1)*	1-10
Varicella-zoster virus	7-10	5-21
Cytomegalovirus†	5-28(3)*	3-42
Adenovirus	5-10	3-28

*Using direct immunofluorescence on inoculated cell monolayers.
†Time varies considerably depending on patient population.

antibody rather than cytopathic effect is used to detect viral replication in inoculated cell cultures.

Fungi

Nearly all pathogenic fungi are readily cultured when appropriate media are used. Methods of procurement and transport of most specimens are similar to those for bacteria. Skin lesions should be sampled by obtaining scrapings, preferably from the margins of the lesion. As with mycobacteria, recovery of fungal material is greater with larger volumes of fluids (CSF, urine, effusions) than are normally obtained for culture of the usual bacteria. If fungemia is suspected, blood should be inoculated in special culture bottles containing a biphasic medium (broth plus agar slant) or collected using the Isolator system (DuPont Company, Wilmington, Del), which may provide optimum recovery. Specimens should never be frozen. The time required for growth and identification varies considerably among species, ranging from only several days (or less) for some, such as *Candida* species, to several weeks for others, such as *Histoplasma capsulatum*. Characteristics used for identification include growth rate, colony and microscopic morphology, and, for yeasts, biochemical reactions, such as carbohydrate assimilation and fermentation.

Penicillium is a frequently encountered contaminant. Although *Candida* and *Aspergillus* species are potentially pathogenic, isolation of these fungi from normally nonsterile sites commonly represents only colonization and should prompt further attempts to document true infection.

Chlamydiae, Rickettsiae, Mycoplasmas

Laboratories providing viral diagnostic services will usually also isolate *Chlamydia trachomatis,* as these grow intracellularly and are cultured in cell monolayers. However, direct antigen or nucleic acid detection methods are more commonly used, and *C. psittaci* and *C. pneumoniae* are best diagnosed by serologic means (Chapter 254). Rickettsiae are also obligate intracellular parasites that can be cultured only in animals, embryonated eggs, or tissue culture. Diagnosis rests on serologic testing or direct detection in infected tissue (Chapter 256). *Mycoplasma* species can be isolated on artificial agar-based media, but the availability of services for their culture remains limited (Chapter 255). Swabs may be used to collect specimens and are best transported in a protein-containing medium formulated specifically for *Mycoplasma* species.

DIRECT DETECTION TECHNIQUES

These techniques, of widely varying complexity and cost, are capable of rapid, direct detection of microorganisms in body samples and in some instances supplant culture as the diagnostic method of choice. They often complement culture techniques, however, particularly in cases in which culture is the more sensitive technique or when isolation of the organism is necessary for further characterization (e.g., antibiotic susceptibility testing). These techniques are also used to more rapidly identify organisms isolated in culture.

Microscopy

Wet mounts. The wet mount is the simplest of microscopic methods and allows for observation of the motility and morphology of the living organism (Plate V-1). A drop of fresh specimen is placed on a slide, and a cover glass is added (with margins petrolatum-sealed to prevent desiccation, if desired). Samples may be examined with bright-field (this is the usual way; lowering the condenser provides the necessary contrast) or phase-contrast microscopy. Stool and vaginal pool specimens are commonly examined by this method. Use of the dark-field condenser provides a clearer outline of organisms—although internal detail is lacking—and is most commonly used in examining exudates for *T. pallidum* to diagnose syphilis (Plate V-2). Contrast can also be provided by the addition of India ink (traditionally used for demonstration of *Cryptococcus neoformans* in CSF [Fig. 279-1]) or methylene blue (see box, p. 1836). Potassium hydroxide solution dissolves host cells and keratinous debris and facilitates visualization of fungi in skin scrapings and vaginal secretions (see box, p. 1836). Iodine solution, although it renders trophozoites immotile, is also useful, especially for identification of ova and parasites in stool samples. For Neufeld's reaction, or quellung reaction, a highly sensitive and specific test for identifying pneumococci in clinical specimens, the specimen is prepared as a wet mount to which antibody to the capsular polysaccharide is added, making the capsule refractile and thereby visible (Plate V-3).

Stains for smears and imprints. A variety of stains are available for use on air-dried or alcohol-fixed smears or touch preparations (see box, p. 1836). Gram stain, the most widely used, should be performed on specimens submitted for bacterial or fungal culture (Plates V-4 through V-9). Organisms are grouped as gram-positive or gram-negative based on their ability to retain crystal violet dye after ex-

Wet-mount microscopic procedures

India ink preparation

1. Place a drop of specimen on a clean glass slide.
2. Cover with coverslip, preferably a larger size.
3. Place a small drop of India ink on the slide, touching the coverslip; it will be drawn under the coverslip and provide a gradient suspension of the ink particles.
4. Examine using bright-field microscopy; scan the slide to find the point at which suspension is optimal for observing capsules or organisms.

Potassium hydroxide preparation

1. Place a small portion of specimen on a clean glass slide.
2. Add a drop of 10% potassium hydroxide solution; if necessary, mix with specimen using an applicator stick.
3. Cover with a coverslip, then heat gently by passing through a flame (do not heat excessively; several minutes or more of setting may be necessary to dissolve material composed of keratin).
4. Examine using bright-field microscopy; adjust substage condenser to optimize contrast.

Methylene blue stain for fecal leukocytes

1. Place a small portion of liquid stool on a clean glass slide.
2. Add a drop of methylene blue stain and mix with the specimen; place coverslip.
3. Let stand several minutes, then examine with bright-field microscopy.

Staining procedures for smears and imprints

Gram stain procedure

1. Air dry the smear, and fix by heating.
2. Flood with crystal violet solution, let stand 1 minute, and then rinse briefly with tap water.
3. Flood with iodine solution, let stand 1 minute, and then wash with tap water as before.
4. Flush the slide with decolorizer solution until the stain no longer elutes from the thinner areas of the smear, and then rinse with tap water.
5. Apply safranine counterstain, let stand 10 seconds, and then flush with tap water and blot dry.

Kinyoun acid-fast stain procedure

1. Air dry the smear, and fix well by heating.
2. Flood with Kinyoun carbol-fuchsin, let stand 2 minutes (no heating), and then wash briefly with tap water.
3. Flush with acid alcohol decolorizer for 1 minute, and then wash with tap water.
4. Apply methylene blue counterstain for 20 to 30 seconds, flush with tap water, and blot dry.

Wright's stain

1. Make a thin peripheral blood smear on a clean glass slide and allow to air dry.
2. Flood horizontally placed slide with undiluted stain solution and let sit for 5 minutes.
3. Without removing stain, add an equal volume of buffer and mix by blowing gently on the liquid surface; let sit 10 to 20 minutes.
4. Wash off stain thoroughly with water and air dry.

Tzanck preparation

1. Obtain cells from the base of a lesion or mucosal surface by gentle scraping or with a swab moistened in saline.
2. Apply to a limited area of a clean glass slide (do not smear); if using a swab, roll it across the surface.
3. Allow specimen to air dry (fix in methyl alcohol for 1 minute or more if using Giemsa stain).
4. Stain as described for Wright's stain.

posure to an acetone-alcohol solution. Reactivity is dependent on cell wall characteristics. Bacteria stain positively or negatively (with a few exceptions such as *Legionella* in clinical specimens and mycobacteria, which will not stain at all). Fungi are uniformly gram-positive. Carbol-fuchsin stain (1% solution) can be substituted for safranine as a counterstain to provide more intense staining of gram-negative organisms that may otherwise be difficult to see. Although the stain is easy to accomplish and its interpretation is often straightforward, it must be examined critically. Whether or not the material is representative of the site of infection (e.g., sputum versus saliva) and whether or not the staining was properly performed should be determined. Overdecolorization is often feared but is easily evaluated by examining the degree of staining of neutrophils or other cells (nuclei should stain purple, cytoplasm pink). Morphology is as important as the staining because both aging and exposure to antibiotics may alter an organism's reactivity to stain; antibiotics may also distort the organism's usual morphology. Gram stain aids in determining whether an infection is present and, if so, what organisms are present. The findings should also be used to interpret the culture results: Anaerobes, other fastidious organisms, or organisms exposed to antibiotics may be seen with Gram's stain but fail to grow in culture.

Mycobacteria stain with the Ziehl-Neelsen and Kinyoun methods (please refer to the box above), as well as with auramine-rhodamine fluorescent stain. The latter stain requires the use of a fluorescence microscope, but is more sensitive than the former methods and permits rapid screening of slides. *Nocardia* species and some nontuberculous mycobacteria may be less acid-fast, requiring a modified staining procedure. Acridine orange is a fluorescent stain that stains all bacteria. Methenamine silver and toluidine blue stain fungi and *Pneumocystis carinii* cysts (Plate V-10). Giemsa stain (Plates V-11 and V-12) provides excellent cellular detail and demonstrates fungi, many parasites including *Toxoplasma* species and *P. carinii* trophozoites, and viral inclusions (Tzanck cell test) (Plate V-13). Wright's stain (see the box above) can also be used for Tzanck preparations and is generally more available to the clinician. Iron hematoxylin and trichrome stains are useful in screening for intestinal parasites. Wright's and Giemsa stains demonstrate parasites in blood (Plates V-14 through V-17), with the exception of leptospiras. Antibody staining for direct fluorescence microscopy (discussed next) is applicable to smears, imprints, and many histologic sections.

Immunologic tests

Direct immunofluorescence and related methods. These methods identify microorganisms or viral-infected cells on slide preparations of specimens and thus are similar to routinely stained smears, except that selectivity and visualization of staining are achieved by using labeled, specific antibody. Slides are prepared by rolling a swab over a limited area of the surface or applying a drop of sediment from centrifuged fluid specimens; they are then air-dried and fixed. Specific antibody labeled with fluorescent compound is layered over the slide, which is then incubated and washed. Specifically bound antibody remains attached, and the organisms or cells carrying the antigen appear brightly stained against a dark background when viewed through a fluorescence microscope. The alternative use of enzyme-conjugated antibody eliminates the need for a fluorescence microscope but requires the additional step of incubating with enzyme substrate, which is deposited as a colored precipitate. The technique is also applicable to frozen or paraffin-embedded histologic sections of tissue.

Direct immunofluorescence and immunoenzyme techniques are used to detect *C. trachomatis* in genital and conjunctival specimens, *Legionella* species, *B. pertussis, P. carinii,* and various viruses (respiratory syncytial, influenza, parainfluenza, cytomegalovirus, and adenovirus) in respiratory samples, *Cryptosporidium* in stool, and herpes simplex virus in skin and mucous membrane samples and tissue biopsies.

Agglutination tests. Antigen-antibody interactions in agglutination tests are observed as visible clumping of microscopic particles in suspension. A particulate-phase suspension is mixed with a soluble-phase solution in test tubes or on flat surfaces, and visible clumping is assessed in minutes to hours. Direct agglutination tests are those in which a particulate antigen (e.g., bacteria in suspension) reacts directly with specific antibody in solutions. Indirect (or passive) agglutination tests have antibody in the particulate phase (e.g., coating latex beads) reacting with antigen in solution or suspension. Semiquantitative results can be obtained by titrating samples. In both the direct and indirect tests, interacting antigen and antibody bridge adjacent particles, causing visible agglutination.

These methods are rapid and sensitive and have been applied to direct detection of microorganisms and their soluble antigens in various clinical specimens, having replaced counterimmunoelectrophoresis (CIE) methods. Applications include detection of group A streptococci in throat swabs, capsular polysaccharide antigens of *Streptococcus pneumoniae, Haemophilus influenzae, Neisseria meningitidis,* group B streptococci, and *Cryptococcus neoformans* in CSF, serum, and urine, and *Clostridium difficile* toxin in stool. False-positive reactions may occur (often due to rheumatoid factor in serum samples) but should be detected in most cases by the use of proper controls.

Radioimmunoassays and enzyme immunoassays. Radioimmunoassay (RIA) and enzyme immunoassay (EIA) procedures are extremely sensitive techniques, analogous in principle and differing only in the "label" that is measured. Fluorescent compounds are less commonly used alternative labels. Enzyme immunoassays can be as sensitive as RIAs and are often preferred. Enzymes and substrates are chosen to yield a colored product, thus permitting quantitation using spectrophotometry or qualitative results by visual inspection. The numerous exact RIA and EIA methodologies are variants of two basic methods, competitive binding and immunosorbent assays.

The enzyme-linked immunosorbent assay (ELISA) is the most widely used immunosorbent, or "sandwich," technique (Fig. 226-1). Specific antibody is bound to a solid substrate of the reaction system, which may be the wall of

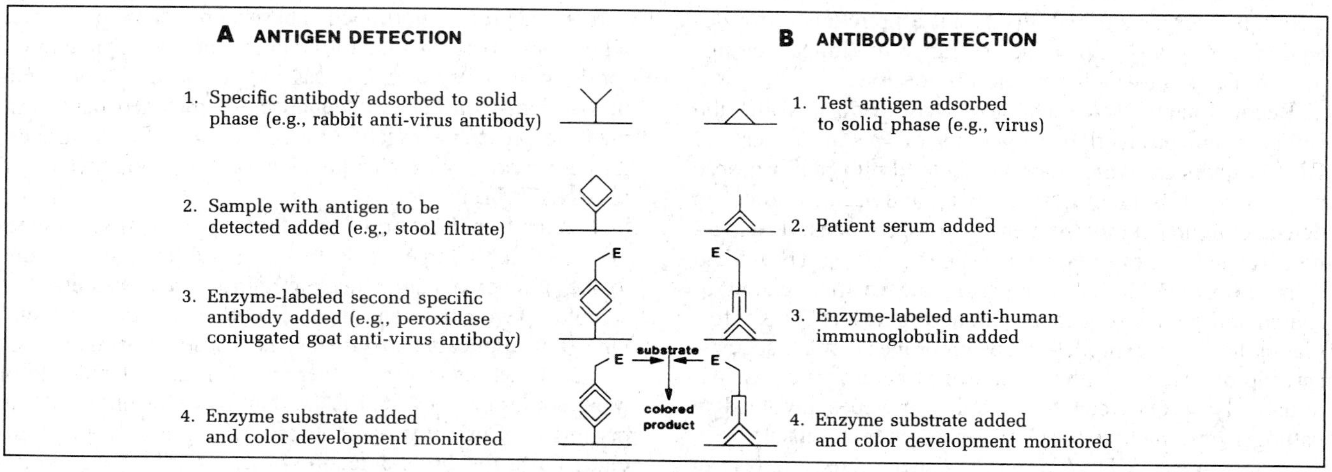

Fig. 226-1. Technique of solid phase ELISA for antigen (**A**) or antibody (**B**). Washes are performed after steps 2 and 3 to remove unbound reactants.

the chamber itself (tubes or microtiter plate wells) or a removable component (e.g., beads, a stick, or a disk). The test sample is incubated in the chamber; the antigen, if present, binds to the fixed antibody. Radio- or enzyme-labeled antibody directed against the antigen is then added, and unbound antibody is removed by washing. The amount of specifically bound labeled antibody is proportional to the amount of antigen present in the test sample. Quantitation is made by comparison with a standard curve that is prepared by assaying known quantities of antigen.

In competitive binding assays, antigen in test samples competes with an added known amount of purified labeled antigen for binding to specific antibody. After separation of antigen-antibody complexes from free antigen, the amount of antibody-bound, labeled antigen (which is inversely proportional to the concentration of antigen in the test sample) is measured.

Although these techniques have enjoyed widespread application in the research setting, their use in the routine clinical microbiology laboratory for direct detection of antigen is just now increasing. RIAs and EIAs are established methods for detecting hepatitis B surface and core antigens in serum and of rotavirus in stool. Other commercially produced assays that have become available will detect chlamydia, gonococci, and herpes simplex virus in genital specimens, group A streptococci in throat specimens, respiratory syncytial virus in nasal secretions, *Legionella pneumophila* antigen in urine, enteric adenoviruses in stool, and HIV antigens in serum.

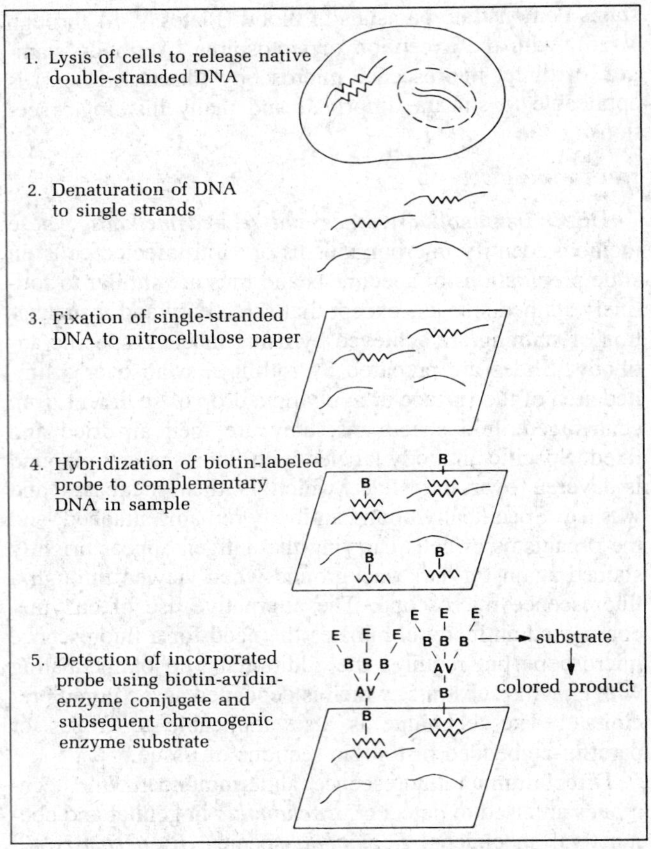

Fig. 226-2. Steps in nonradioactive probe detection of pathogen-specific DNA. Washes are performed at steps 4 and 5 to remove unbound reactants. Steps 1 and 2 can be performed concurrently on samples initially spotted to nitrocellulose paper.

Nucleic acid hybridization

The application of molecular biologic techniques for detection of microorganisms holds great promise and is beginning to takes its place as a routine technique in the clinical microbiology laboratory. Although the majority of current applications available commercially simply provide an alternative to existing technologies (e.g., detection of *N. gonorroheae* genital infection), novel applications will ultimately facilitate rapid detection of organisms where that is currently not possible. As with immunologic detection techniques, organism viability is not a prerequisite for detection, potentially expanding the range of clinical settings or time frame in which detection is feasible.

Recombinant DNA technology has made possible the isolation and production in quantity of specific genes and DNA sequences, which can be labeled (with radioisotopes or a variety of nonradioactive labels) and used as probes to detect complementary sequences in specimens. Phylogenetic relatedness of organisms has been extensively studied using ribosomal RNA, comparing the relative extent of shared and unique sequences among organisms. This information has been exploited to design probes that are species-specific or reactive with a group of related organisms. Alternatively, probes can be specific for genes involved in pathogenesis, such as those encoding enterotoxins.

Complementary DNA or RNA sequences in samples can be detected by hybridization with labeled DNA probes (Fig. 226-2). Under certain conditions, native double-stranded DNA in samples can be released from cells and separated into single strands. On reversal, complementary DNA strands (native DNA or exogenously added probe) will anneal (hybridize) by reforming hydrogen bonds between matched base pairs. Complexed DNA can be separated from remaining single-stranded DNA and the amount of incorporated probe determined. These steps can be performed with DNA fixed to a solid support (such as a membrane for dot blot or Southern blot assays) or with all components in solution. Consecutive sequences of matched base pairs must be present for stable reassociation of DNA strands, thus accounting for the exquisite specificity of assays based on DNA hybridization.

Practical application of this technique for direct detection has been hampered by test sensitivity limitations due to the number of target nucleic acid sequences present in samples. Two approaches have circumvented this problem. One (not applicable to viruses) is to use ribosomal RNA sequences as the target, as there are generally 1000-fold or more copies of ribosomal RNA than chromosomal DNA in organisms. Currently available tests using this technique include those for direct detection of *Legionella, N. gonorroheae*, and *C. trachomatis*.

Gene amplification is the other approach that is somewhat more complicated but more broadly applicable. Both the polymerase chain reaction (PCR) and self-sustained sequence replication (3SR) techniques can achieve greater than 100,000-fold amplification of target DNA or RNA in a matter of hours. Short synthetic DNA sequences (primers) are used, which are complementary to the sequences present on either end of a target sequence in the organism. Sequential and repetitive activity of nucleic acid replicating enzymes, replicate exponentially the intervening sequence between the primers. A large amount of specific target derived from as little as a single copy of a sequence is then available for detection. Gene amplification is a commonly used research technique, and numerous studies demonstrate its feasibility and value for infectious disease diagnosis. Theoretically, any pathogen in any sample could be detected in less than a day. Use of the technique, however, will be limited to research centers until simplified assay formats are developed that can be easily performed in the routine laboratory setting.

SEROLOGY

The primary humoral immune response to an antigenic stimulus is an initial production within 1 to 2 weeks of IgM antibodies, followed by a more prolonged production of IgG and a gradual fall in specific IgM levels. The secondary response occurs several days after reexposure to an antigen and consists predominantly of IgG production. The nature of the primary and secondary responses has important implications for the use of serologic testing as a diagnostic tool. Given the time necessary to mount a response to a primary infection, antibody may not be demonstrable until several weeks after the onset of the illness, often too late to be of practical diagnostic use. For certain agents with a significant latent period, such as hepatitis A, the appearance of antibody precedes or coincides with the clinical syndrome (Chapter 57). Persistence of IgG antibody may preclude the association between detectable antibody and the current illness in patients in whom previous infection has occurred with the same or an antigenically related organism. In these instances detection of IgM-specific antibody may distinguish between recent and remote infections, as is possible for hepatitis A and toxoplasmosis. Otherwise, one relies on demonstration of a fourfold increase in titer between acute and convalescent sera (2 to 3 weeks or more apart) or a standing titer that is significantly higher than that found in the general population. Specific titers obtained for the same sample may vary among laboratories or even in one laboratory if assayed at different times. Therefore when serial titered serologic tests are used to document or follow an infection, samples should be tested in parallel in the same laboratory.

All microorganisms are antigenically complex, and the onset, nature, and duration of the antibody response can vary for each antigenic component. In some cases advantage can be taken of this spectrum of response by varying either the antigen or the method used (e.g., precipitin versus complement-fixation procedures), as in serologic tests for rubella.

Precipitin reactions

Precipitin reactions are based on direct visualization of a precipitated antigen-antibody complex. The reaction can occur in either liquid medium (tube precipitin tests) or, more commonly, in gel medium (radial and Ochterlony immunodiffusion tests). Except for radial immunodiffusion, reactions are qualitative, and serial dilutions of the test sample must be run to obtain a semiquantitative result ("antibody titer"). Precipitin and immunodiffusion assays are commonly used in the serologic diagnosis of systemic mycoses and various parasitic infections.

Agglutination reactions

The principle and performance of these assays are similar to those for direct detection of antigens. When designed for detection of specific antibody, however, the solid phase carries the appropriate antigen, which may be intact organisms (e.g., formalinized bacteria) or soluble antigen bound to carrier particles such as erythrocytes or latex beads. Common uses of these techniques are the nontreponemal tests for syphilis (Chapter 273) and the detection of heterophilic antibodies in infectious mononucleosis (Chapter 251). A related technique, hemagglutination inhibition, is used to detect antibodies to rubella (Chapter 246).

Neutralization tests

Neutralization tests are used to detect protective antibody to viruses, including rubella, polio, and rabies. Dilutions of serum are incubated with given amounts of virus, and ability to block infection in cell culture is determined. Neutralization of hemolytic or enzymatic activity is also the basis for detecting antistreptolysin O, antideoxyribonuclease B, and antihyaluronidase antibodies in group A streptococcal infection (Chapter 259).

Complement-fixation assays

Although technically complicated, complement-fixation assays are used extensively in serologic testing, particularly in reference laboratories. The assays are performed in two phases. The first phase is based on the ability of certain immunoglobulins to bind, or fix, complement when they form antigen-antibody complexes; the second is based on the ability of unbound complement to lyse red blood cells. Results are reported as the maximum dilution of serum causing a given degree of complement inhibition. Assays require several days to complete and are not usually performed in routine clinical microbiology laboratories.

The technique has been widely applied but for many pathogens has been supplanted by other, more rapid and easily performed assays. However, complement-fixation assays are still commonly used for detecting antibody to *C. immitis, Histoplasma capsulatum* (Chapter 278), and various viruses.

Indirect immunofluorescence assays

Indirect immunofluorescence assays are designed to detect specific antibody and are similar in performance to the direct immunofluorescence assays described for detection of antigen. For indirect assays the antigen in question, usually intact organisms or virus-infected cells, is fixed to microscope slides. Dilutions of test serum are incubated over the surface, and unbound antibody is removed by washing. Bound antibody is detected by a second incubation with a fluorescence or enzyme-labeled antihuman immunoglobulin. The latter may be selected or prepared to detect bound IgG or IgM, or both. Results are reported as the maximum dilution of serum producing a given degree of specific fluorescence. These assays are sensitive and relatively simple to perform and are used for detection of antibody to *Legionella* species, *T. pallidum,* chlamydiae, rickettsiae, Epstein-Barr virus, HIV, toxoplasma, and *Entamoeba histolytica*.

Radioimmunoassays and enzyme immunoassays

RIAs and EIAs for antibody detection are usually immunosorbent type assays. Their design and execution is similar to that described for direct detection of antigen, but the sequence of steps is altered, being analogous to those of indirect immunofluorescence assays (Fig. 226-1). First, antigen is bound to a solid phase of the system. A dilution of test serum is then incubated with the solid phase; a second incubation using labeled antihuman immunoglobulin follows, with washes after each. Labeled staphylococcal protein A, which binds to the Fc portion of IgG, may also be used to detect bound antibody.

Results are reported as positive or negative by comparing the amount of label activity from a given test serum dilution with the range of activities found in negative control sera at the same dilution. The sensitivity and specificity of these assays depend on the cutoff level chosen to separate positive from negative samples. In some cases this necessitates establishing an indeterminate range if the separation is not clear-cut. Quantitative results, if reported, may be expressed as absolute activity units (counts per minute for RIAs, or optical density or absorbance for EIAs) or as a ratio of sample activity to that of a strongly positive reference serum.

These techniques have broad application, but in the clinical serology laboratory they have generally not replaced assays that were well established before EIA development. RIA and EIA are the primary methods for detecting antibody to hepatitis A, B, and C and the HIV (Chapter 242) and are alternative techniques for detecting many other agents, including toxoplasma, rubella, cytomegalovirus, herpes simplex virus, and the Lyme disease spirochete (Chapter 275).

Western blot assay

This technique, common in research laboratories, has become a diagnostic test for confirmation of HIV antibody in serum. In the procedure, proteins in a mixture extracted from cultured virus are separated electrophoretically according to molecular weight then replica transferred ("blotted") to nitrocellulose paper. After incubation with the patient's serum, bound antibody is detected, which allows determination of the specific proteins that antibodies are directed against. Because some are more specifically associated with infection than others, test specificity is better than that of EIAs, which use whole virus homogenates as the substrate antigen. Simpler procedures, such as EIAs, using purified proteins or protein fragments are likely to supplant this test for diagnostic purposes in the future.

SKIN TESTING

In contrast to the many in vitro methods available to measure the antibody response to infection, the in vivo delayed hypersensitivity skin test is still the only routinely used method for evaluating the cellular immune response to infection. The test is performed by placing 0.1 ml of antigen solution intradermally using a 25- or 27-gauge needle. The site of inoculation is marked and is examined 24, 48, and sometimes 96 hours later, and the diameter of the area of induration is measured. Erythema often occurs but is generally not of significance in interpreting the test, except in the case of mumps antigen (Chapter 246). Other methods, such as multiple puncture devices, are less well standardized, and the results are therefore less reliable. By convention, induration of 5 mm or more in diameter is considered a positive reaction, although 10 mm is the accepted cutoff for tuberculin testing (Chapter 276). It should be realized that in a truly positive population (i.e., those infected with or exposed to the organism), the measured values form a continuum, including those of persons with no response. Interpretation in any given case should be flexible, depending on the question being asked, because sensitivity varies inversely with specificity, depending on the cutoff set.

The optimum concentration of each antigen for testing has been standardized, and for some antigens, such as tuberculin, lower and higher concentrations are available. In patients in whom a severe reaction may be anticipated, the lower dose may be used initially; if the reaction is negative, the test is repeated with a standard dose. When no reaction occurs with the standard concentration, a negative response to a higher (×10) dose is more definitive evidence of anergy or lack of primary exposure. However, interpretation of a measurable response to the higher concentration must be made with caution. Negative responses in the presence of current or past infection may be secondary to local skin abnormalities, anergy, or technical faults in test administration. Antigen should not be injected into areas of skin with dermatologic lesions, such as atopic dermatitis.

Anergy is associated with numerous conditions, including congenital and acquired immune deficiencies and a variety of infections, especially extensive tuberculous and fungal infections. If anergy is suspected, a battery of skin tests is used to determine its presence or absence. The battery includes at least three antigens to which most persons have been exposed and to which they will react. Those currently available for use include *Candida, Trichophyton,* streptokinase-streptodornase, mixed respiratory vaccine, and staph-phage lysate. Mumps antigen has been used extensively because of the high frequency of reactivity to it in the population.

Administration of skin tests generally does not immunize the patient, although serologic responses may occur after histoplasmin, *Brucella,* mumps, and lymphogranuloma venereum testing; these antigens should be avoided in situations in which serologic testing has greater diagnostic value. The Frei test for lymphogranuloma venereum is now obsolete.

REFERENCES

Balows, A. et al, editors. Manual of clinical microbiology, ed 5, Washington, DC, 1991, American Society for Microbiology.

Cumulative techniques and procedures in clinical microbiology, Washington, DC: American Society for Microbiology.

Drew WL: Controversies in viral diagnosis, Rev Infect Dis 8:814, 1986.

Hilborne LH and Grody WW: Diagnostic applications of recombinant nucleic acid technology: basic techniques, Lab Med 22:849, 1991.

Hilborne LH and Grody WW: Diagnostic applications of recombinant nucleic acid technology: infectious diseases, Lab Med 23:89, 1992.

Needham CA: Rapid detection methods in microbiology: are they right for your office? Med Clin North Am 71:591, 1987.

Rose NR, et al, editors: Manual of clinical laboratory immunology, ed 4, Washington, DC, 1992, American Society for Microbiology.

Sox HC, Jr: Probability theory in the use of diagnostic tests, Ann Intern Med 104:60, 1986.

III CLINICAL SYNDROMES

CHAPTER

227 Fever of Unknown Origin

Martin G. Täuber

Body temperature is one of the most frequently monitored physical signs in modern day medicine. The normal upper limit of orally measured temperature is generally considered to be 98.6° F (37.0° C). Normal temperature varies among healthy individuals, however, so that many persons, particularly younger adults and women in the second half of their menstrual cycle, may have temperature readings up to 1.5° F (0.8° C) higher. Physical exercise and heavy meals also increase body temperature. In addition, body temperature physiologically shows diurnal changes of up to 1.8° F (1° C). The lowest temperatures are in the early morning hours, and the highest are in the late afternoon. Axillary temperature is usually about 1° F (0.6° C) lower, and rectal temperature is approximately the same amount higher than oral temperature.

FEVER

Fever is defined as an elevation of body temperature above normal limits induced by regulatory processes of the nervous system that originate in the hypothalamus. The rise of body temperature to a higher level is achieved by a combination of increased internal heat production and reduced external heat loss. Shivering in skeletal muscles is the major source of increased heat production; peripheral vasoconstriction results in conservation of body heat.

The key pathophysiologic factor in the patient with fever is the adjustment of the hypothalamic temperature set point to a higher than normal level by a disease process usually distant to the hypothalamus. The release of prostaglandins, primarily of the E class, from endothelial cells of the cerebral microvasculature in the vicinity of the thermoregulatory area appears to be instrumental in increasing the temperature set point. This release can be stimulated by two classes of substances circulating in the bloodstream of febrile patients: endogenous and exogenous pyrogens. Several members of the family of cytokines function as endogenous pyrogens, including interleukin-1 and -6, cachectin/tumor necrosis factor, and interferons. Prototype exogenous pyrogens are the lipopolysaccharides (endotoxin) that are released from gram-negative bacteria during infection, but gram-positive organisms also release potent pyrogens.

In the great majority of illnesses associated with fever, the underlying disease process stimulates the release of pyrogenic cytokines which then act on the hypothalamus. The primary sources of cytokines are phagocytic monocytes/macrophages, although other leukocytes and other types of cells have also been shown to release endogenous pyrogens. Furthermore, some evidence suggests that pyrogenic cytokines may be released locally in the hypothalamus under the influence of other pyrogens. A large variety of disease processes, such as infections, tumors, and immunologic reactions, can precipitate the secretion of pyrogenic cytokines from macrophages and other sources. Exogenous pyrogens act both directly on the thermoregulatory center and stimulate the release of cytokines from macrophages. Consequently, it is evident that the pathogenesis of fever follows the same final pathway in many different, pathologically unrelated diseases. This makes fever a highly nonspecific sign, a fact that should be kept in mind when considering fever of unknown origin.

Pathologic states other than fever may also result in an elevation of body temperature. In hyperthermia, for instance, impairment of peripheral heat-dissipating mechanisms or unusual internal heat production results in a body temperature above that set by the central regulation. Hyperthermia due to disturbed heat dissipation is found in heat stroke or in states of prolonged peripheral vasoconstriction caused by pheochromocytoma, Addison's disease, or anticholinergic drugs. Malignant hyperthermia, a rare disorder characterized by excessive muscular heat production induced by some anesthetics, is a typical example of hyperthermia due to excessive heat production. Primary or metastatic tumors, trauma, and inflammatory processes that directly involve the thermoregulatory center in the hypothalamus may also alter body temperature. In these patients hypothermia is usually observed, whereas hyperthermia is extremely rare.

FEVER OF UNKNOWN ORIGIN

The wide variety of diseases that can cause fever makes the medical evaluation of a febrile patient a constant challenge. A thorough medical history and a physical examination, supplemented by routine laboratory tests, enable identification of the cause of fever in most patients. In a few febrile patients, however, the underlying disease eludes diagnosis even after a prolonged period of illness and despite careful medical evaluation. These patients are then given the tentative diagnosis of having a fever of unknown origin (FUO).

Diagnostic criteria for FUO have been strictly defined for study purposes. Although details of these definitions may need adjustments to account for changing practices in medicine, the three principles defining the concept of FUO have retained their validity. Febrile patients should be given this diagnosis only if the illness has persisted long enough to make the presence of a common, self-limiting viral disease unlikely (usually at least 3 weeks); the patient must have been carefully examined, which includes routine laboratory tests and chest radiographs, in order for all readily detected causes of fever to have been ruled out. Finally, the fever has to be significant on several occasions (usually above 101° F [38.3° C]). This final point is particularly important, as many patients may have slightly elevated body temperatures for many months or years without evidence of serious underlying diseases. In some cases, exaggerated diurnal temperature variations are interpreted as fever ("habitual hyperthermia"). Patients with the *chronic fatigue syndrome,* a syndrome of undetermined etiology, also often complain of low-grade fever, although the predominant symptom is disabling fatigue. It is important in these instances to avoid the extensive and invasive evaluations that have to be considered in patients with FUO.

The large majority of FUOs are caused by infections, neoplasias, and collagen vascular diseases. A fourth group includes diseases categorized as granulomatous disorders. Numerous miscellaneous diseases are responsible for the rest of the patients in whom a cause for FUO can be identified (Table 227-1).

The spectrum of diseases found in several series examining FUO shows some variation according to the population studied and the study period (Table 227-1). In children, infections tend to be the most frequent cause of FUO, whereas neoplasms and connective tissue disorders are more frequent in the elderly. In patients with FUO lasting more than 1 year, infections and neoplasias decrease in frequency, whereas granulomatous diseases are the single most important category. Diagnostic advances may continuously change the spectrum of causes of FUO. For example, serologic tests have reduced the importance of systemic lupus erythematosus as a cause of FUO, and modern imaging techniques facilitate early detection of abscesses and solid tumors.

In all studies, a substantial number of patients evaluated for FUO remained without a definite diagnosis (Table 227-1). A follow-up of these patients usually shows a benign long-term course, especially in those patients whose fever is not accompanied by a substantial weight loss or by other signs of a serious underlying disease. This pattern suggests that intensive diagnostic evaluation of patients with FUO results in identification of most serious diseases that initially manifested themselves with a FUO.

Causes

Factitious fever. The possibility of factitious fever should be considered in every patient with prolonged fever before engaging in extensive and invasive procedures. Factitious fever is responsible for up to 10% of the cases of FUO and is most commonly encountered among young adults within the health professions. Frequently, there is evidence of psychiatric problems or a history of multiple hospitalizations in different institutions. Rapid changes of body temperature without associated shivering or sweating, large differences between rectal and oral temperature, and discrepancies between fever and pulse rate or general appearance are typically seen in patients who manipulate or exchange their thermometers, the most common cause of factitious fever. Alternatively, fever may be caused by injection of nonsterile material, such as feces or milk, resulting in atypically localized abscesses or polymicrobial infections.

Infections

Bacterial diseases

Abscesses. Abscesses are most frequently located intraabdominally and must be considered in patients with FUO even in the absence of localizing symptoms (Chapter 232). Previous abdominal operations, trauma, or a history of diverticulosis, peritonitis, endoscopy, or gynecologic procedures all increase the likelihood of an occult intraabdominal abscess. The most common abscess locations are the subphrenic space, the liver, the right lower quadrant, the retroperitoneal space, and in women, the pelvis.

Tuberculosis. Tuberculosis continues to be an important cause of FUO (Chapter 276). Several factors may prevent its prompt diagnosis. Dissemination, which typically occurs in patients with reduced immunocompetence, may initially be present with constitutional symptoms lacking localized signs, and with normal chest radiographs. Patients with disseminated tuberculosis or with early tuberculosis may have negative purified protein derivative (PPD) tests, and cultures take 4 to 6 weeks to become positive. Tuberculous infections of the kidney, female genitalia, or mesenteric lymph nodes tend to manifest themselves as FUO because of a lack of characteristic, localized manifestations. Disseminated, visceral infections with atypical mycobacteria have also been implicated as a cause of FUO. Most of these patients have some underlying hematologic malignancy or are infected with the human immunodeficiency virus (HIV) (see below).

Hepatobiliary infections. Cholangitis sometimes occurs without local signs and with only mildly elevated or nor-

Table 227-1. Causes of fever of unknown origin

Disease category	Petersdorf and Beeson (100 patients, 1952-1957)	Howard et al (100 patients, 1969-1976)	Larson et al (105 patients, 1970-1980)	Knockaert et al (199 patients, 1980-1989)
Infections	**36 (36%)**	**37 (37%)**	**32 (30.5%)**	**45 (22.6%)**
Tuberculosis	11	3	5	10
Abdominal abscess	4	9	8	4
Hepatobiliary	7	7	4	1
Endocarditis	5	9	0	3
Urinary tract	3	4	3	1
Cytomegalovirus	0	0	4	8
Others	6	5	8	18
Malignancies	**19 (19%)**	**31 (31%)**	**33 (31.4%)**	**14 (7.0%)**
Lymphoma	6	20	11	2
Leukemia	2	3	5	4
Solid tumors	9	8	6	7
Others	2	0	11	1
Collagen-vascular and autoimmune disorders	**13 (13%)**	**13 (13%)**	**8 (7.6%)**	**21 (10.6%)**
Juvenile rheumatoid arthritis	2	1	4	6
Systemic vasculitis	0	5	1	6
Lupus erythematosus	5	3	0	1
Rheumatic fever	6	0	1	0
Others	0	4	2	8
Granulomatous disorders	**6 (6%)**	**7 (7%)**	**9 (8.6%)**	**28 (14.1%)**
Granulomatous hepatitis	2	0	4	3
Crohn's disease	0	4	2	4
Sarcoidosis	2	0	2	4
Giant cell arteritis	2	3	1	17
Miscellaneous	**19 (19%)**	**7 (7%)**	**10 (9.5%)**	**43 (21.6%)**
Factitious fever	3	0	3	7
Periodic fever	5	0	0	2
Pulmonary emboli	3	0	1	5
Drug fever	0	2	0	6
Others	8	5	6	23
Undiagnosed	**7 (7%)**	**5 (5%)**	**13 (12.4%)**	**48 (24.1%)**

Data from Petersdorf RG and Beeson PG: Fever of unexplained origin: report of 10 cases, Medicine (Baltimore) 40:1, 1961.
Howard P et al: Fever of unknown origin: a prospective study of 100 patients, Tex Med 73:56, 1977.
Larson EB, Featherstone HJ, and Petersdorf RB: Fever of undetermined origin: diagnosis and follow-up of 105 cases, 1970-1980, Medicine (Baltimore) 61:269, 1982.
Knockaert DC et al: Fever of unknown origin in the 1980s: an update of the diagnostic spectrum, Arch Intern Med 152:51, 1992.

mal liver function tests (Chapter 65). Similarly, acute cholecystitis or gallbladder empyema (Chapter 65) has been responsible for cases of FUO because of the lack of right upper quadrant pain or jaundice, especially in elderly patients. A rare cause of FUO is bacterial hepatitis, caused by alpha-hemolytic streptococci, *Propionibacterium acnes,* or *Actinomyces israelii.* The only abnormal finding in these patients may be an elevated alkaline phosphatase.

Urinary tract infections. These infections are rare causes of FUO because urine analysis is an easily performed routine test that detects most cases of urinary tract infections. In young children, however, the collection of clean-catch urine specimens may be difficult. Furthermore, perinephritic abscesses sometimes fail to communicate with the urinary system and can thus yield a normal urine analysis (Chapter 240). Anatomic abnormalities of the urinary tract in a patient with FUO should raise the possibility of an occult urinary tract infection.

Endocarditis. Endocarditis (Chapter 15) has become a rare cause of FUO. Failure to diagnose endocarditis may be due to the absence of a murmur, or the failure of blood cultures to yield the organism. Culture-negative endocarditis is reported in 5% to 10% of endocarditis cases in the literature. Prior antibiotic therapy is the most frequent reason for negative blood cultures. Manifestations of endocarditis (such as cerebrovascular stroke, nephritis, or musculoskeletal symptoms) involving organs other than the heart may detract from the correct diagnosis in febrile patients with sterile blood cultures.

Osteomyelitis. Osteomyelitis almost always causes localized pain or discomfort at least intermittently (Chapter 237). The most frequent reason that this diagnosis is missed is the failure to consider osteomyelitis in a febrile patient with musculoskeletal symptoms. A typical example is the elderly patient with back pain, in whom degenerative changes are thought to be responsible. Low-grade fever or a history of urinary tract infection should raise the possibility of vertebral osteomyelitis in these patients. Radiographs fail to show changes suggestive of osteomyelitis sometimes for weeks after the development of symptoms. Radionucleotide studies (technetium 99m bone scanning) are more sensitive than conventional radiology but lack specificity.

Other bacterial diseases. Some systemic bacterial illnesses may occasionally manifest themselves as FUO. Among these, brucellosis, which is still prevalent in Latin America and the Mediterranean, is the most important (Chapter 269). It should be considered in patients with persisting fever and a history of contact with cattle, swine, goats, and sheep, or consumption of raw milk products. Systemic infections due to *Salmonella* (Chapter 268), *Neisseria meningitidis* (Chapter 263), or *N. gonorrhoeae* (Chapter 264) have been described as causes of FUO. Cutaneous changes may be the only sign other than fever in neisserial infections. Cultures and serologic tests are necessary to establish the diagnosis of these infections. Finally, spirochetes also occasionally cause FUO. The most important among these is *Borrelia recurrentis,* which is transmitted by ticks and is responsible for causing sporadic cases of relapsing fever (Chapter 275). Febrile episodes lasting 3 days with intervals of approximately 7 days occur in these patients. Ratbite fever, caused by *Spirillum minor,* has also been described as a cause of FUO (Chapter 30). *Borrelia burgdorferi* (responsible for Lyme disease) (Chapter 275) and *Treponema pallidum* (causing syphilis) (Chapter 273) are other spirochetes that rarely can cause FUO.

Viral diseases

Herpes viruses. Two members of the herpesvirus family, the cytomegalovirus and the Epstein-Barr virus, can cause prolonged febrile illnesses with constitutional symptoms and no prominent organ manifestations, particularly in the elderly (Chapter 251). Infections by each of these viruses typically cause enlarged lymph nodes, but these may be missed on physical examination when they are small. Lymphocytosis with atypical lymphocytes should direct attention to the correct diagnosis, which can be confirmed by appropriate serologic tests. These tests may initially be negative and should be repeated in suspected cases 2 to 3 weeks after the onset of illness.

Human immunodeficiency virus. Prolonged febrile episodes are frequent in patients with advanced HIV infection (Chapter 242). In these patients, fever may be caused by a large variety of opportunistic infections, by lymphomas, or by the HIV itself. Typical and atypical mycobacteria and cytomegalovirus are opportunistic infections that frequently cause prominent constitutional symptoms, including fever, with few localizing or specific signs. Rarely, other opportunistic infections, such as salmonellosis, histoplasmosis, or toxoplasmosis, can also elude rapid diagnosis in febrile AIDS patients and thus present as FUO. Lymphomas involve extranodal sites, including the brain, in over 80% of AIDS patients and can at times be difficult to diagnose promptly. Extensive diagnostic work-up, including imaging studies, are necessary to exclude these opportunistic diseases in HIV-infected patients with prolonged fever, before the fever can be attributed to the HIV infection itself (Centers for Disease Control stage IVA).

Other infectious causes

Fungi. Immunosuppression, the use of broad-spectrum antibiotics, and intravascular devices all predispose to disseminated infections with opportunistic fungi, such as *Candida albicans* (Chapter 278). Systemic infection can remain undiscovered in these patients because blood cultures are negative in approximately 50% of cases. *Malassezia furfur* has caused FUO and line infections in patients on total parenteral nutrition receiving intravenous lipid preparations. Fever can sometimes be the most prominent symptom in patients who have reticuloendothelial involvement by histoplasmosis without clinical manifestations in other organs (Chapter 278).

Parasites. Toxoplasmosis should be considered in febrile patients with lymph node enlargement, but because the lymph nodes may be small, diagnosis is sometimes difficult (Chapter 280). Rising antibody titers and IgM antibodies confirm the diagnosis. Malaria can be missed as a cause of fever if the physician is unaware of a history of recent travel to an endemic area and if the fever pattern is nonsynchronized. Other parasites (Chapter 280) that can rarely cause FUO include *Trypanosoma, Leishmania,* and *Ameba.*

Chlamydia. *Chlamydia psittaci,* the cause of psittacosis, should be considered in a patient with FUO who has a history of contact with birds (Chapter 254). Lymphogranuloma venereum may on rare occasions also manifest itself as FUO. Serology is essential for the diagnosis of these chlamydial infections.

Rickettsia. Chronic infections with *Coxiella burnetii,* chronic Q fever, or Q fever endocarditis have been identified in patients with FUO (Chapter 256). Signs of hepatic involvement are frequent. The infection is transmitted from cattle and sheep, and serologic tests should be performed in suspected cases.

Neoplastic diseases

Lymphomas. Both Hodgkin's disease (Chapter 94) and non-Hodgkin lymphomas (Chapter 94) frequently cause fever, night sweats, and weight loss. The correct diagnosis can be delayed if the tumor is difficult to detect, as is the case when the disease is confined to the retroperitoneal lymph nodes. Anemia may be the most prominent laboratory abnormality in patients with lymphomas.

Malignant histiocytosis. This rare, rapidly progressive malignant disease that manifests itself with high fevers; weight loss; and enlargement of lymph nodes, liver, and spleen is occasionally found in patients with FUO (Chapter 92).

Leukemias. Acute leukemias are another important neoplastic cause of FUO. In aleukemic or preleukemic states, the peripheral blood smear and bone marrow aspirate may not reveal the correct diagnosis, and a bone marrow biopsy is necessary (Chapter 93).

Solid tumors. Among the solid tumors, hypernephromas are most commonly associated with FUO, with fever as the only presenting symptom in 10% of the cases (Chapter 364). Hematuria may be absent in about 40% of cases, whereas anemia and a highly elevated sedimentation rate are frequent. Other solid tumors that may cause fever as the presenting symptom include primary liver carcinomas; adenocarcinomas of the breast, colon, or pancreas with metastases to the liver; and sarcomas of the retroperitoneum. If bronchogenic carcinomas cause fever, it is usually because of bronchial obstruction with subsequent pneumonia. Benign leiomyomas can sometimes cause fever and may be difficult to detect when they originate in the gastrointestinal tract.

Myxomas are rare tumors of the heart that are well recognized as a cause of FUO (Chapter 24). They frequently cause fever along with a high sedimentation rate and anemia, whereas a cardiac murmur may be absent or intermittent. Myxomas are easily detected by echocardiography.

Collagen vascular and autoimmune diseases. A variety of different diseases of uncertain etiology are summarized as collagen vascular and autoimmune diseases. These diseases can present as FUO if fever precedes other, more specific manifestations, such as arthritis, pneumonitis, or renal involvement. Systemic lupus erythematosus (Chapter 306) was a relatively common cause of FUO 20 years ago. Today, it is readily diagnosed in most cases by demonstration of antinuclear antibodies. In this group, systemic-onset juvenile rheumatoid arthritis is a cause of fever difficult to diagnose (Chapter 304). High-spiking fevers, nonpruritic rashes, arthralgias and myalgias, pharyngitis, and lymphadenopathy are typically present. Laboratory abnormalities include pronounced leukocytosis, elevated sedimentation rate, anemia, and abnormal liver function tests. All these findings prompt the search for an infectious cause and thus delay the correct diagnosis.

Other collagen vascular diseases that need to be considered because of their potential for nonspecific presentations are periarteritis nodosa, rheumatoid arthritis, and mixed connective tissue disease. Rheumatic fever can be difficult to diagnose because it has become rare in the developed world, despite an apparent recent increase in some areas in the United States, and because some of the classic criteria may be absent (Chapter 316).

Granulomatous diseases

Giant-cell arteritis. This disease occurs in elderly persons, usually over 60 years of age (Chapter 307). The diagnosis may be obscured when typical symptoms such as headache, tender temporal arteries, and polymyalgia rheumatica are absent. Anemia, a high sedimentation rate, and elevation of alpha-2 serum proteins are typical laboratory findings. The diagnosis can usually be confirmed by biopsy of an involved artery, but therapy with corticosteroids should be instituted in all suspected cases.

Regional enteritis. Crohn's disease is the most common gastrointestinal cause of FUO. Diarrhea and other abdominal complaints may be absent in a few patients, particularly in young adults (Chapter 43). The diagnosis is made in these patients by endoscopy and biopsy.

Sarcoidosis. Very rarely, sarcoidosis manifests itself with fever and malaise in the absence of evidence of lymph node and pulmonary involvement (Chapter 207). Erythema nodosum is sometimes present. The diagnosis should be suspected if noncaseous granulomas are found in the liver.

Granulomatous hepatitis. In some patients with hepatic granulomas, none of the diseases usually associated with this nonspecific reaction, such as tuberculosis, syphilis, brucellosis, sarcoidosis, Crohn's disease, or Hodgkin's disease, can be found. These patients often have fever that may be accompanied by slight hepatomegaly, asthenia, and sometimes arthralgias and myalgias for many months or years (Chapter 60). Elevated alkaline phosphatase is the most consistent laboratory abnormality. The long-term prognosis is excellent, with about half of the patients recovering spontaneously. The other half responds to corticosteroid treatment ranging from a few weeks to several years.

Idiopathic granulomatosis. Noncaseating granulomas involving multiple organs are associated with fever and other nonspecific signs and symptoms in patients with this recently described disease. The etiology is unclear and the disease runs a prolonged course with a fairly good prognosis. Many patients have been treated with corticosteroids or other immunosuppressive agents.

Miscellaneous causes

Inherited diseases. Familial Mediterranean fever is most often, but not exclusively, found in patients of Mediterranean descent (Chapter 313). Recurrent febrile episodes at varying intervals are associated with pleural, abdominal, or joint pain due to polyserositis. The diagnosis can be made only after exclusion of other causes of fever and polyserositis. Other inherited diseases that cause febrile episodes and have been reported as causing FUO include Fabry's disease and hypertriglyceridemia.

Drug fever. Although a wide variety of drugs can cause drug fever, those more frequently involved include alphamethyldopa, quinidine, diphenylhydantoin, beta-lactam antibiotics, procainamide, and isoniazid. A history of allergy, skin rashes, or eosinophilia is often absent in cases of drug fever; and neither the fever pattern nor the duration of previous therapy is a helpful parameter in establishing the diagnosis. Whenever drug fever is suspected, the incriminated drug should be discontinued. This cessation leads to defeverescence within 2 days in the vast majority of cases if the drug was in fact responsible for the fever.

Others. Peripheral pulmonary emboli as well as occult thrombophlebitis can cause FUO. These diagnoses should be considered in patients with predisposing conditions, particularly previous surgery, traumas, or prolonged bed rest. Another possible cause of fever in a patient after surgery or trauma is an undiscovered hematoma, usually located intra-abdominally.

A self-limiting necrotizing lymphadenitis (Kikuchi's disease) has recently been described as cause of FUO. It causes prolonged fever, constitutional symptoms, laboratory evidence of chronic inflammation, and sometimes liver function abnormalities. The etiology of the disease is not known.

Fever can occur in patients with Laennec's cirrhosis (Chapter 59). If there is lack of evidence for a hepatic disease, it may be classified as FUO. Whipple's disease should be considered in a patient with abdominal complaints and central nervous system symptoms (Chapter 42). Other diseases that on rare occasions may cause FUO include idiopathic pericarditis, thyreoiditis, renal angiomyolipoma, and complex partial status epilepticus.

Diagnostic approach to adults

The numerous possible causes of FUO in an individual patient combined with the availability of a broad armament of diagnostic tests make the rational evaluation of a patient with FUO a demanding task. Experiences of many investigators document the best strategy for the initial approach to such patients as being a careful clinical examination combined with a limited set of diagnostic "routine" tests (see the accompanying box). Based on a detailed knowledge of the possible causes of FUO, these basic evaluations usually provide the clinician with clues to the nature of the underlying disease. The subsequent evaluations should then attempt to confirm or refute the diagnostic possibilities raised by the initial evaluation. Nonselective application of numerous tests within a short time is likely to result in high costs, a heavy burden to the patient, and findings that may be difficult to interpret.

History. The history of a patient with FUO is best structured to cover three areas.

1. Inquiries regarding symptoms from all major organ systems should be made, including a detailed history of general complaints such as fever, weight loss, night sweats, headaches, and rashes. All complaints should be recorded, even if they have disappeared before the examination.
2. Previous illnesses are important including surgery, dental history, and psychiatric illnesses.
3. A detailed evaluation should include the family history; immunization status; the work place situation; travel; nutrition, including consumption of dairy products; drugs; a sexual history; recreational habits; and animal contacts, including possible exposure to ticks and other vectors.

Physical examination. The unambiguous documentation of fever and the exclusion of factitious fever are obvious early steps in the physical examination of a patient with FUO. Over 25% of the patients evaluated for FUO at the National Institutes of Health were ultimately found to have no fever, whereas another 9% had factitious fever. Fever should be measured more than once in the presence of a nurse to exclude manipulation of thermometers. Electronic thermometers facilitate the rapid and unequivocal documentation of fever.

The pattern of fever (continuous, remittent, or intermittent) is usually of little help in the evaluation of a patient with FUO, as, in general, there is a weak correlation between fever patterns and specific diseases. Exceptions are tertian and quartan malaria (Chapter 280), but these should not present as FUO because of their suggestive fever pattern. Other diseases, such as brucellosis, borreliosis, or Hodgkin's disease, tend to cause recurrent episodes of fever; but the fact that these diseases are typical causes of FUO underscores the limited diagnostic value of fever patterns.

Stage-specific diagnostic approach to FUO

Stage 1: Screening (in all adult patients with FUO)
- History: Specific symptoms; review of systems; immunization; travel; animal exposure; medications and drugs; sex; work; recreation
- Physical examination: Fever documentation, general examination with special attention to skin, lymphnodes, fundi, heart and lungs, abdomen, joints
- Hematology: Complete blood count and differential, ESR
- Chemistry: Liver function tests, protein electrophoresis
- Urine analysis: Cells; chemistry
- Cultures: Blood (aerob and anaerob, mycobacteria, fungi, viruses); urine; CSF and other body fluids, if obtained
- Serologies: Brucellosis, syphilis, Lyme, HIV, CMV, EBV, amebiasis, toxoplasmosis, chlamydia; ANA, rheumatoid factors, antistreptolysin-O
- Imaging: Regular chest radiogram; abdominal ultrasound
- Others: Skin tests (PPD and control); ECG; bone marrow aspirate (?)

Stage 2: Noninvasive approach to suspected diagnoses
- CT scan: Abdomen (intraabdominal tumors or abscesses; liver abscesses); chest (lung tumors); head (lymphoma, toxoplasmosis, abscess)
- Radiograms: Intravenous pyelogram (urinary tract abnormalities); bone films (osteomyelitis); retrograde cholangiography (cholangitis)
- Endoscopies: GI-tract (Crohn's disease); bronchial tree (bronchus tumors)
- Radionucleotide studies: Bone (osteomyelitis); thyroid gland (thyreoiditis); pulmonary perfusion/ventilation (emboli)
- Echocardiogram: (Cardiac tumors, endocarditis)

Stage 3: Invasive approach to suspected diagnosis
- Biopsies: Lymph nodes, tumors, skin lesions, liver, bone marrow
- Laparascopy (if evidence for intra-abdominal process obtained during stage 1 or 2)

Stage 4: Failure to establish a diagnosis
- Reevaluate patient at regular intervals (if clinical status not rapidly deteriorating)
- Empiric therapy: Nonsteroidal anti-inflammatory drugs; corticosteroids; antituberculous drugs; antibiotics

ESR, erythrocyte sedimentation rate, CMV, cytomegalovirus, EBV, Epstein-Barr virus.

A regular physical examination should be repeated daily while the patient is hospitalized for the evaluation of FUO. Special attention should be directed to rashes, new or changing cardiac murmurs, signs of arthritis, abdominal tenderness or resistances, lymph node enlargement, and funduscopic changes. The latter may be the only localized physical finding in patients with disseminated mycobacterial or fungal infections.

Basic laboratory tests and procedures. Despite the rationale for a carefully selected approach to the patient with FUO, it is reasonable to routinely perform a set of basic laboratory tests and procedures (refer to the box at left). These tests and procedures are discussed below.

Blood count and microscopic examination. Anemia is an important sign and suggests a serious underlying disease in a patient with FUO. Leukemias can be missed in aleukemic cases. Lymphocytosis with atypical cells should raise the suspicion of a herpesvirus infection. A leukocytosis with a "left shift" (increase in band forms) suggests an occult bacterial infection. Malaria and spirochetal diseases can be diagnosed by direct examination of the peripheral blood smear, but repeated examinations are often necessary.

Urine analyses. It is important to exclude urinary tract infections and malignant tumors of the urinary tract. Not all urinary tract infections or tumors are consistently associated with pathologic findings in the urine, however, and a single normal urine analysis is insufficient to exclude a urinary tract infection.

Serum chemistry. At least one liver function test is usually abnormal in patients with FUO, in whom the underlying disease originates in the liver or causes nonspecific alterations of the liver, such as granulomatous hepatitis. Most other chemistry tests rarely contribute to the diagnosis in patients with FUO, although they are frequently ordered. Protein electrophoresis is almost routinely performed and can sometimes suggest a specific diagnosis, such as giant-cell arteritis.

Cultures. Blood cultures for aerobic and anaerobic pathogens are essential in the evaluation of all patients with FUO (Chapter 226). However, more than a total of approximately six blood cultures are not required. Urine should also be cultured routinely; cultures of sputum and stool (Chapter 226) may be helpful in the presence of signs or symptoms suggestive of pulmonary or gastrointestinal disease. All normally sterile tissues and liquids that are sampled during the further work-up of patients with FUO need to be cultured for bacteria, mycobacteria, and fungi. These tissues and liquids include CSF, pleural or peritoneal fluid, liver, bone marrow, and lymph nodes (Chapter 226).

Serologies. Serologies are most helpful if paired samples show a significant, usually fourfold increase of antibodies specific to an infectious microorganism (Chapter 226). Causes of FUO that can be diagnosed by serology include brucellosis, lues, cytomegalovirus, infectious mononucleosis, HIV infection, amebiasis, toxoplasmosis, and chlamydial diseases. In the majority of patients with FUO, however, serologic tests are of limited diagnostic value.

Antibodies directed against host-specific tissue components, rheumatologic tests, and the detection of circulating immune complexes are frequently performed tests in patients with FUO. These tests are helpful in diagnosing a few diseases such as systemic lupus erythematosus or thyroiditis, but their diagnostic accuracy is limited in other autoimmune and collagen vascular diseases.

Imaging. Chest radiographs are routinely performed in all patients with FUO. Routine abdominal ultrasound examinations may also be justified, even in the absence of signs of an intra-abdominal process. However, in a patient with signs or symptoms suggestive of an intra-abdominal process, a negative ultrasound examination should not give rise to the exclusion of such a process.

Additional noninvasive procedures. The use of additional noninvasive procedures in patients with FUO should be guided by clinical or laboratory findings. The relative diagnostic value of these noninvasive procedures in the evaluation of a patient with FUO has been studied only to a limited degree. In general, adding a second or even third test to the evaluation of the same organ or body region increases the likelihood of detecting a disease process. The possibility that at least one of the tests will be false-positive, however, also increases. Thus the choice of these procedures should be carefully considered.

Computed tomography scans. If ultrasound studies fail to reveal the diagnosis, computed tomography (CT) scans of the abdomen are indicated in all patients with symptoms suggestive of an intra-abdominal process, in patients with suspected retroperitoneal tumors or infections, or in those with abnormal liver function tests. Intravenous pyelography may be more sensitive than the CT scan in detecting processes involving the descending urinary tract, but for most other processes of the retroperitoneal space, the CT scan is the preferred method today. The little data comparing CT scanning and magnetic resonance imaging (MRI) currently provide no evidence for the superiority of MRI in patients with FUO. There is no reason to routinely perform both examinations in these patients.

Endoscopy. Endoscopic examination of the upper and lower gastrointestinal tract, including retrograde cholangiography where indicated, must be performed when searching for Crohn's disease, Whipple's disease, biliary tract diseases, and gastrointestinal tumors. Sometimes, it may be necessary to complement these endoscopic studies with barium enemas or upper gastrointestinal series.

Radionucleotide studies. Ventilation and perfusion radionucleotide studies are necessary to document pulmonary emboli. If suspicion of pulmonary emboli persists despite negative scanning studies, pulmonary angiography is indicated. If osteomyelitis is suspected in a patient without compatible changes in conventional radiography, technetium bone scan may be a more sensitive method for documenting skeletal involvement. Radionucleotide studies using gallium citrate or indium-111-labeled granulocytes are recommended by some authors for the diagnosis of occult abscesses. Although these techniques have been successful in some studies, other authors have found a high number of false-positive and false-negative results with both of these techniques.

Echocardiography. This technique is highly sensitive in diagnosing cardiac tumors, such as myxomas. In addition, the diagnosis of endocarditis is frequently possible by echocardiography, particularly when transesophageal echocardiography is available (Chapter 15).

Invasive procedures and biopsies. In many instances of FUO, the final diagnosis is based on direct examination of involved tissue. Therefore any indication of organ involvement should raise the question of a biopsy. Biopsies are readily performed in enlarged, accessible lymph nodes, other peripheral tissues, and the bone marrow. For the latter, there may be some justification for routine examination in all patients with FUO, independent of signs of bone marrow involvement. The decision to biopsy is more difficult if it necessitates an exploratory surgical procedure, such as laparatomy. Experiences with modern imaging techniques suggest that laparatomy should be performed only in those patients in whom noninvasive testing has revealed an indication of an intra-abdominal process. If all noninvasive examinations are negative, it is unlikely that the laparatomy will reveal a diagnosis. The same holds true for liver biopsy. Liver biopsy rarely results in important information in patients without abnormal liver findings, although it is a valuable tool in patients with abnormal liver function tests or morphologic alterations of the liver.

Empiric treatment

If all efforts to establish a cause of FUO fail, empiric treatment may be considered. The decision to treat should depend on the general condition of the patient, on symptoms associated with fever, and on clinical considerations about the underlying illness. In general, empiric therapy with antibiotics or antituberculous drugs rarely produces favorable results. Most often, corticosteroids are used as initial empiric therapy. As an alternative, nonsteroidal anti-inflammatory drugs may be used. It appears, however, that in the patient lacking symptoms making an empiric therapy mandatory, repeated clinical evaluation is more prudent than empiric therapy.

REFERENCES

Aduan RP et al: Factitious fever and self-induced infection: a report of 32 cases and review of the literature, Ann Intern Med 90:230, 1979.

Calamia KT and Hunder GG: Giant cell arteritis (temporal arteritis) presenting as fever of undetermined origin, Arthritis Rheum 24:1414, 1981.

Davis SG and Gravie NW: The role of indium-labelled leukocyte imaging in pyrexia of unknown origin, Br J Radiol 63:850, 1990.

Dinarello CA, Cannon JG, and Wolff SM: New concepts on the pathogenesis of fever, Rev Infect Dis 10:168, 1988.

Dinarello CA and Wolff SM: Fever of unknown origin. In Mandell GL, Douglas RG Jr, and Bennett JE, editors: Principles and practice of infectious diseases, ed 3, New York, 1990, Churchill Livingstone.

Durack DT, and Street AC: Fever of unknown origin-reexamined and redefined. In Remington JS, and Swartz MN, editors: Curr Clin Top Infect Dis 11:35, 1991.

Howard P et al: Fever of unknown origin: a prospective study of 100 patients, Tex Med 73:56, 1977.

Knockaert DC et al: Fever of unknown origin in the 1980s. An update of the diagnostic spectrum, Arch Intern Med 152:51, 1992.

Larson EB, Featherstone HJ, and Petersdorf RG: Fever of undetermined origin: diagnosis and follow-up of 105 cases, 1970-1980, Medicine (Baltimore) 61:269, 1982.

Mackowiak PA and LeMaistre CF: Drug fever: a critical appraisal of conventional concepts, Ann Intern Med 106:728, 1987.

McNeil BJ et al: A prospective study of computed tomography, ultrasound, and gallium imaging in patients with fever, Radiology 139:647, 1981.

Petersdorf RG and Beeson PB: Fever of unexplained origin: report of 100 cases, Medicine (Baltimore) 40:1, 1961.

Telenti A and Hermans PE: Idiopathic granulomatosis manifesting as fever of unknown origin, Mayo Clin Proc 64:44, 1989.

Welsby PD: Pyrexia of unknown origin sixty years on, Postgrad Med J 61:887, 1985.

Zoutman DE, Ralph ED, and Frei JV: Granulomatous hepatitis and fever of unknown origin. An 11 year experience of 23 cases with three years' follow-up, J Clin Gastroenterol 13:69, 1991.

CHAPTER

228 Fever and Rash

Randy Taplitz
Merle A. Sande

The clinical syndrome of fever and rash presents a challenging and often urgent diagnostic problem. Because a wide variety of disease processes can present in this manner, the clinician must have both a complete grasp of the differential diagnosis and the ability to recognize specific disease entities, especially those that are potentially life-threatening. A careful history, close observation of the rash itself, recognition of relevant clinical findings, and judicious use of laboratory tests are necessary components of a successful evaluation. Therapy may be specific, as in the case of recognized bacterial infection, supportive, as in most viral infections, or presumptive, as in the toxic patient with petechial skin lesions.

PATHOGENESIS

Exanthems may be caused by the direct effects of a pathogen or by the immunologic response of the body toward an antigen. Bloodstream spread of an infecting organism can lead to multiplication in the skin itself or to invasion of the cutaneous vessels. The vesicular rash of the herpesviruses is an example of direct cutaneous invasion with a cellular response characterized by multinucleated giant cells and inclusion bodies. In Rocky Mountain spotted fever (RMSF), the rickettsiae invade the vasculature of the integument via endothelial cells as well as other organs (Plate V-18) and can be demonstrated in vessel walls by immunofluorescence. The recognition of direct invasion of the skin or cutaneous vessels is important because a direct aspirate or biopsy may lead to an immediate definitive diagnosis (Chapter 256) (Plate V-19). Bacterial toxin production is another mechanism of cutaneous injury, as seen in staphylococcal scalded skin syndrome and toxic shock syndrome (TSS).

Infectious organisms or other antigens may invoke an immune response that leads to the development of a rash. This rash can represent an antigen-antibody reaction, delayed hypersensitivity, or, less commonly, an immediate hypersensitivity reaction. The erythematous rashes of drug reactions, measles, mononucleosis, hepatitis B infection, leptospirosis, typhoid fever, and rheumatic fever are examples of exanthems mediated largely by antigen-antibody reactions. The rash of a drug reaction may also be initiated by a nonimmunologic mechanism. Delayed hypersensitivity has been shown to be essential to vesicle formation in vaccinia infection and may be important in other vesicular eruptions. Urticarial rashes, such as those seen with serum sickness or drug ingestion, are probably mediated by an "allergic" reaction, although this mechanism is not common in exanthems caused by infectious agents. Systemic lupus erythematosus (SLE), dermatomyositis, and the skin lesions of inflammatory bowel disease are examples of proved or suspected autoimmune phenomena, such as Behçet's disease, Sjögren's and Reiter's syndromes, and juvenile rheumatoid arthritis.

DIFFERENTIAL DIAGNOSIS

The differential diagnosis of fever and a rash includes a wide variety of disease processes, some of which are potentially life-threatening (Tables 228-1 and 228-2). The approach to the patient must include an initial evaluation of clinical severity. As a corollary the clinician must judge whether the patient needs emergent empiric antibiotics.

The history should focus on travel history, exposure to other ill individuals, rural habitats, pets, toxins, and so forth; an STD history, including HIV risk factors; recent drug ingestions; and, a history of drug allergies. In addition to the history, evaluation must include an appreciation of the clinical setting, a detailed evaluation of the rash, an assessment of associated physical findings, and a judicious use of diagnostic tests.

Knowledge of the season, geographic setting, exposure, clinical setting, and associated symptoms is critical for diagnosis. RMSF is almost exclusively a disease of late spring to early fall, coinciding with increased exposure to the tick vector. Outbreaks of exanthems caused by enteroviruses (Chapter 244) also occur in the warmer months, whereas meningococcal and streptococcal diseases usually occur in late winter and early spring. Lyme disease occurs most commonly in the summer months, but also in the spring, coinciding with exposure to the infected tick nymph in distinct areas of the United States where the tick vector is found (Northeast, Midwest [Minnesota/Wisconsin], and West [California/Oregon]). The geographic setting is also important for RMSF, which is heavily concentrated in the middle Atlantic states. A history of travel to endemic areas will usually be found in cases of coccidioidomycosis (southwestern United States), and in viral hemorrhagic fever and scrub typhus (Southeast Asia).

To elicit an exposure history one must inquire about contact with other ill persons, animals, insects, contaminated food or water, drugs or vaccines, sexual partners, and living and working conditions. Most viral, streptococcal, gonococcal, meningococcal, and chlamydial infections are transmitted from person to person. Contact with livestock or contaminated water should raise the possibility of leptospirosis, whereas exposure to rodents might suggest rat-bite fever. A history of tick exposure is obtainable in 60% to 75% of patients with RMSF and in approximately 30% of patients with Lyme disease. *Erysipelothrix* is seen primarily in patients having contact with fish, swine, or cattle. Ingestion of undercooked pork or bear meat may result in trichinosis. Previous vaccination with killed measles vaccine may result in altered immunity and the development of atypical measles after exposure to live virus. Intravenous drug abuse and rash suggest hepatitis B infection or infective endocarditis. Sporotrichosis is usually seen in farmers, gardeners, or florists who have extensive contact with soil or vegetation. Toxic shock syndrome is frequently associated with tampon use during menstruation.

The hospitalized patient in whom fever and rash develop presents a special situation. Neutropenic or immunosuppressed patients are at particular risk of bacteremia, disseminated herpesvirus infection, or fungal infection. Fever and rash developing during broad-spectrum antibiotic therapy or parenteral hyperalimentation should suggest the possibility of systemic candidiasis. Indwelling intravascular catheters, pacemakers, prosthetic heart valves, and dialysis shunts create a significant potential of bacteremia or endocarditis.

Almost any drug may produce fever and cutaneous eruption. The diagnosis of drug eruption, however, is usually one of exclusion. A careful medication history (including nonprescription drugs) should be taken. Hospitalized patients receiving multiple medications are a particularly susceptible group. Drug reactions produce myriad cutaneous manifestations that may be maculopapular (morbilliform), urticarial, vesiculobullous, petechial, purpuric, nodular, acneiform, or desquamating. The same drug may cause different findings in different patients. Frequently implicated medications include penicillins, phenytoin, sulfonamides, sulfones, and barbiturates.

Associated symptoms may provide important clues in considering many of the disease processes included in the differential diagnosis of fever and rash. Usually, RMSF begins after a 3- to 12-day incubation period with fever, headache, and myalgias, with the rash appearing on or about the fourth febrile day (range 2 to 6 days). Disseminated gonococcal infection is more common in females than in males, and the onset is often related to menstruation. Low-grade fever, migratory polyarthralgia, and tenosynovitis often accompany the rash (Chapter 264). Prominent articular symptoms accompanying a rash should also suggest a primary immunologic process, such as collagen vascular disease, serum sickness, or inflammatory bowel disease. Me-

Table 228-1. Identification of life-threatening diseases associated with fever and rash

Disease	History	Characteristics of rash	Distribution of rash	Associated clinical findings	Diagnostic aids
Rocky Mountain spotted fever	Tick exposure (75%) May-September occurrence in temperate-zone states Heaviest endemic area middle Atlantic states and Southeast	Initial maculopapular petechiae appearing on 2nd to 6th febrile day and usually painless (Plates V-18 and V-19)	Begins on wrists, ankles, forearms, spreading within 6-8 hours to palms, soles, trunk	Prodrome of fever, headache, myalgias Hyponatremia, normal to slightly increased WBC, thrombocytopenia, hypoalbuminemia	Biopsy of involved skin with immunofluorescence and other serologic tests Serology: Complement-fixation more sensitive and more specific than Weil-Felix agglutination
Meningococcemia*	Tends to occur in late winter, early spring Outbreaks in military recruits, crowded living conditions	*Acute:* May be maculopapular initially. Small petechiae with irregular borders ("smudging"), at times with vesicular or grayish ulcer. May coalesce. Painful (Plates V-20 and V-21)	*Acute:* Extremities and, trunk in random fashion	*Acute:* Meningitis, disseminated intravascular coagulation, shock, acidosis	*Acute:* Aspiration of center of skin lesions for Gram stain, culture (up to 60% positive). Blood cultures. Cerebrospinal fluid culture and Gram stain
		Chronic: Maculopapules, petechial vesicles, or pustules; tender nodules	*Chronic:* Extremities, particularly over joints	*Chronic:* Rash appears with recurrent cycles of fever over 2-3 months	*Chronic:* Blood culture usually positive during febrile episode. Biopsy findings resemble leukocytoclastic angiitis
Disseminated gonococcal infection	Incidence higher in women than in men Young, sexually active Onset often related to menstruation	Pustules on erythematous base most characteristic. Also, macules, papules, pustules, and bullae less commonly (Plate V-22)	Over extremities, with relative sparing of face and trunk. Usually few (5-40) lesions	Migratory polyarthralgia, tenosynovitis, septic arthritis	Gram stain of lesion Blood, joint fluid culture (50%) prove diagnosis Cervical, rectal, throat cultures support diagnosis
Staphylococcal septicemia	Nosocomial: indwelling catheters, pacemakers, dialysis shunts, wound infections Drug abuse	Pustules, purulent purpura, subcutaneous nodules, infarcts	Widespread, with infracts having predilection for distal extremities	Endocarditis, with valvular incompetence, meningitis, multiple-organ involvement	Aspiration of lesions for Gram stain culture Blood, cerebrospinal fluid (where indicated) cultures Teichoic acid antibody suggestive of deep-seated infection
Pseudomonas septicemia	Hospitalized patients, especially with neutropenia or burns	*Vesicles:* Isolated or in small clusters rapidly becoming hemorrhagic	Random	Generally extremely toxic, with fever; septic picture	Aspiration of lesion for Gram stain, culture
		Ecthyma gangrenosum: Round, indurated,	Axillary or anogenital area, thigh		Cultures of blood, urine, sputum, etc.

		ulcerated painless lesion with central gray eschar (Plate V-23) *Maculopapular lesion:* Small erythematous lesion resembling "rose spots" Gangrenous cellulitis	Trunk Localized		
Candida septicemia	Broad-spectrum antibiotics, leukemia, immunosuppression, hyperalimentation, cardiac surgery	Multiple discrete pink maculopapular lesions 2-5 mm in diameter	Trunk and extremities	Toxic state; associated ophthalmitis, esophagitis, cystitis	Punch biopsy of lesion with stains for fungus Buffy coat of blood Blood cultures (definitive diagnosis) Examination and culture of stool, urine, sputum (supportive of diagnosis with multiple-site involvement) Barium or endoscopic examination of esophagus
Infective endocarditis	Indwelling catheters, pacemakers, dialysis shunts, valvular heart disease, prosthetic valves, intravenous drug abuse, preceding dental or surgical manipulations	*Petechiae:* often in small groups *Osler's nodes:* pea-sized, tender, erythematous nodules *Janeway's lesions:* small erythematous or hemorrhagic macules	Conjunctivae, palate, upper chest, distal extremities Pads of fingers and toes Palms and soles	Heart murmur, valvular incompetence, metastatic abscesses, infracts, Roth's spots, splenomegaly, hematuria, glomerulonephritis, etc.	Serology not yet reliable Blood cultures (3-5 sets) Echocardiogram Circulating immune complexes
Toxic shock syndrome	Young female predominance 1-4 days prodrome of fever, myalgias, arthralgias, and diarrhea Onset during or soon after menses (has also been reported in men and unassociated with menses in women)	*Erythroderma:* Seen at presentation. Diffuse, blanching, macular (deep-red "sunburned" appearance). Resolves within 3 days, followed 5-12 days later by desquamation, most commonly of hands and feet (Plate V-24) *Mucosal hyperemia:* pharynx, conjunctivae, vagina	Diffuse, hands and feet predominantly	Fever, severe hypotension, multisystem involvement (gastrointestinal, muscular, renal, hepatic, hematologic, central nervous system)	Clinical criteria (see text) Negative serology for RMSF, leptospirosis, measles Identification of toxin-producing strain of *S. aureus*
Lyme disease	From endemic areas—Northeast, Midwest (Minnesota/Wisconsin), and West (California/Oregon) Usually begins in summer	*Erythema chronicum migrans:* Expanding annular erythema (median diameter 15 cm) from central macule or papule. Secondary annular lesions seen	Commonly thigh, groin, axilla. Any site can be involved	Fever, chills, malaise, myalgias, lymphadenopathy Late (weeks to months) central nervous system, cardiac, and joint involvement	Primarily history and clinical criteria Organism can be cultured (difficult, special media) Serology

*Acute syndrome may occasionally be caused by *Haemophilus influenzae* and *Streptococcus pneumoniae*, especially in splenectomized patients.

Table 228-2. Differential diagnosis of fever and rash based on appearance of rash

Macules or macules and papules	*Bacterial:* Scarlet fever, erysipelas, meningococcemia, *Pseudomonas* septicemia, secondary syphilis, infective endocarditis (Osler's nodes), leptospirosis, toxic shock syndrome, Lyme disease, chlamydia *Viral:* Rubeola, rubella, enteroviruses, erythema infectiosum, mononucleosis, cytomegalovirus, hepatitis B, roseola, adenovirus, atypical measles, HIV, coxsackie *Rickettsial:* Rocky Mountain spotted fever (early), murine and scrub typhus *Fungal:* Disseminated candidiasis, coccidioidomycosis, sporotrichosis, cryptococcosis, histoplasmosis, blastomycosis *Other:* Drug reactions, mycoplasmal pneumonia, toxoplasmosis, trichinosis, erythema multiforme, erythema marginatum, erythema nodosum, systemic lupus erythematosus, dermatomyositis, serum sickness, sarcoidosis, Behçet's syndrome, Reiter's syndrome, inflammatory bowel disease, familial Mediterranean fever
Vesicles	*Bacterial:* Staphylococcal scalded skin syndrome, bullous impetigo, *Pseudomonas* septicemia *Viral:* Herpes simplex, varicella-zoster, hand-foot-and-mouth disease, eczema herpeticum, disseminated vaccinia *Rickettsial:* Rickettsialpox *Other:* Drugs, mycoplasmal pneumonia, Stevens-Johnson syndrome, inflammatory bowel disease, porphyria, pemphigus, pemphigoid
Petechiae, purpura, or purpuric macules, papules or pustules	*Bacterial:* Meningococcemia, sepsis with disseminated intravascular coagulation, gonococcemia, *Pseudomonas* sepsis, staphylococcal sepsis, infectious endocarditis, listerosis *Viral:* Atypical measles, viral hemorrhagic fevers, enterovirus (occasional) *Rickettsial:* Rocky Mountain spotted fever, epidemic typhus *Other:* Drug, trichinosis, Henoch-Schönlein purpura, thrombotic thrombocytopenic purpura

ningococcemia may present as a mild febrile illness, with headache, weakness, and general malaise but can very rapidly accelerate to fulminant sepsis. Staphylococcal bacteremia may be associated with symptoms of cardiac, central nervous system, or pulmonary involvement.

Toxic shock syndrome is characterized by fever, severe hypotension (systolic blood pressure less than 90 mm Hg), diffuse myalgias/arthralgias, and a characteristic deep-red diffuse macular erythroderma (Chapter 257). The rash fades over 3 to 4 days, followed 5 to 12 days later by desquamation, usually of the hands and feet (Plate V-24). Other skin manifestations of TSS include papulopustular lesions, petechiae, and bullae. Multisystem involvement is seen, with central nervous system, renal, hepatic, gastrointestinal, hematologic, and musculoskeletal abnormalities. Although TSS was initially described in young women in association with menstruation and tampon use, it is now recognized that up to 13% of cases of TSS are unrelated to menses and may be associated with a variety of staphylococcal infections such as abscesses, postoperative and postpartum infections, cutaneous infections, and those associated with burns. The syndrome is caused by strains of *Staphylococcus aureus* producing a toxin called toxic shock syndrome toxin-1. Initially reported mortality rates of 10% to 15% have declined to less than 5%, presumably due to increased recognition and appropriate therapy. Toxic shocklike syndrome associated with concurrent group A streptococcal infection is also characterized by hypotension or shock, fever, multiorgan system involvement, and erythroderma. This syndrome appears to be associated with a more invasive group A streptococcal disease; exotoxin A may be a causal factor in the pathogenesis of this syndrome (Chapter 259).

Lyme disease is an infection with a characteristic cutaneous presentation and frequently an accompanying systemic illness (Chapter 275). Erythema chronicum migrans, the classic eruption of Lyme disease, is observed in 50% to 75% of patients. It begins as a small red papule followed by a gradually expanding ringlike erythema, often with central clearing. The axilla, thigh, and groin are most commonly involved; but any site may be affected. Within several days half of the patients will develop distant secondary annular lesions similar to, though smaller than, the primary erythema. The presenting skin involvement may be accompanied by fevers, chills, myalgias, arthralgias, myocarditis, hepatitis, conjunctivitis, meningitis, meningoencephalitis, or other organ involvement. Although most of these symptoms are transient, some may last for months or recur. "Late" (weeks to months) systemic manifestations include central nervous system disease (meningoencephalitis, cranial and peripheral nerve palsies) and cardiac involvement (atrioventricular block, diffuse myocarditis, and, rarely, pericarditis); arthritis, usually involving the knee, may occur even later (months to 2 years); and, cutaneous involvement (acrodermatitis chronic atrophicans). The syndrome is caused by the spirochete *Borrelia burgdorferi,* which is transmitted in the United States by the tick vector *Ixodes dammini* or *Ixodes pacificus*. Diagnosis of Lyme disease relies primarily on a clinical constellation of findings in the appropriate epidemiologic setting, and secondarily on serology. The treatment of choice is doxycycline for early or mild disease and penicillin or ceftriaxone for late or severe disease.

DIFFERENTIAL DIAGNOSTIC VALUE OF THE RASH

The skin responds to infection or immunologic challenge in limited ways. Exanthems can be generally divided into three groups: (1) macular and maculopapular lesions, (2) vesicular or bullous lesions, and (3) pustular, petechial, or purpuric lesions (Table 228-2). It should be realized, however, that although these divisions are helpful in the initial appraisal of the patient, they do not represent absolute distinctions. Not only do many processes present with a similar rash, but also one agent may produce more than one type of rash. Exanthems may also change with time; for example, RMSF progresses from an erythematous maculopapular eruption to a petechial rash.

A macular or maculopapular rash is the most common exanthem elicited by nonherpetic viruses, but such a rash does not always signify a benign process. Examples of more serious infections that may present with a maculopapular rash include RMSF, meningococcemia, gonococcemia, *Pseudomonas* septicemia, typhoid fever, and disseminated candidiasis. Lyme disease presents with the classic erythema chronicum migrans. Drugs typically produce maculopapular exanthems that are frequently cherry red in color. The "slapped-face" rash of erythema infectiosum, the "iris" lesion of erythema multiforme, and the rapidly spreading macule around a pale center of erythema marginatum are examples of maculopapular lesions distinctive enough to suggest a specific diagnosis. Desquamation is common with scarlet fever, Kawasaki disease, TSS, and severe erythroderma caused by drug reactions.

Vesicular lesions are caused by a number of viruses including herpes simplex, varicella-zoster, vaccinia, and some enteroviruses. Similar lesions may also be seen with mycoplasmal infections, usually associated with ulcerative stomatitis. The staphylococcal scalded skin syndrome is characterized by large bullae that rupture, leaving areas of bright-red, denuded skin resembling a burn. *Pseudomonas* septicemia may be associated with single or clustered vesicles that rapidly become hemorrhagic or with the centrally necrotic lesions of ecthyma gangrenosum. Vesicular lesions of the Stevens-Johnson syndrome prominently involve the oral mucosa as well as the skin. Ulcerative colitis or regional enteritis may be associated with vesicular lesions that progress to chronic ulceration and may also have prominent mucosal involvement in the form of aphthous stomatitis.

Petechial, purpuric, or pustular skin lesions frequently indicate life-threatening disease. The identification of such a rash should immediately direct the clinician's attention to treatable bacterial or rickettsial infections, such as meningococcemia (Plate V-20), gonococcemia (Plate V-22), RMSF (Plate V-18), infectious endocarditis, and disseminated intravascular coagulation associated with septicemia. The petechial rash of atypical measles, which may also have vesicular and urticarial components, may mimic RMSF. Rarely, enterovirus infections produce petechial lesions. Other causes include various collagen vascular diseases, Henoch-Schönlein purpura, and thrombotic thrombocytopenic purpura.

The distribution of an exanthem is also of diagnostic significance. A nonvesicular rash involving the palms and soles should suggest RMSF, meningococcemia, infective endocarditis, mycoplasmal infection, scarlet fever, or bacteremia. The copper-colored, scaly macules and papules of secondary syphilis, as well as drug exanthems, atypical measles, and Kawasaki disease, may also affect these sites. Kawasaki disease, or mucocutaneous lymph node syndrome, has recently been described in adults. Skin involvement is characterized by an indurative, erythematous, desquamative rash of the palms and soles and a polymorphous, nonvesicular rash. Maculopapular rashes due to viruses usually spare the palms and soles, whereas these sites may be involved in vesicular exanthems caused by the herpesviruses and certain coxsackievirus strains (e.g., hand-foot-and-mouth disease). Exanthems that have a predilection for the extremities include gonococcemia, Henoch-Schönlein purpura, dermatomyositis, ecthyma gangrenosum (Plate V-23), and sporotrichosis (Plate V-25). The rash of scarlet fever begins on the face and neck and spreads to the trunk and extremities within 36 hours to localize in body folds and antecubital areas, and on the palms and soles. Rubeola usually begins behind the ears, spreads first to the forehead, then involves the entire body within 1 day, without confluence. The "rose spots" of typhoid fever and the maculopapular lesion associated with *Pseudomonas* septicemia are generally confined to the trunk.

Patients with HIV infection frequently present with a fever and a rash. An exanthem associated with a "viral syndrome" (fever, headache, aseptic meningitis, pharyngitis, myalgias) may be associated with acute HIV seroconversion (Chapter 242). Common dermatologic disorders in HIV-infected individuals include seborrheic dermatitis, eosinophilic folliculitis, papular dermatitis, and psoriasis. Common bacterial infections such as pyoderma furunculosis and folliculitis may complicate HIV disease. Cutaneous manifestations of systemic infections may occur, and cutaneous infections may occur in severe forms. Varicella zoster and herpes simplex lesions are common, and sometimes severe, in HIV-infected patients. Cryptococcal, histoplasmal, candidal, and coccidioidal fungal infections may involve the skin; mycobacterial infections may rarely involve the skin. Neoplasms that affect the skin include Kaposi's sarcoma and, occasionally, malignant lymphomas. Bacillary angiomatosis, a recently described disease in HIV-infected patients, is caused by a rickettsia, *Rochalimaea henselae* or *Rochalimaea quintana*. The clinical syndrome can be varied and may include skin lesions (usually friable red papules or nodules) with or without systemic involvement such as fever, malaise, hepatosplenomegaly, lymphadenopathy, and lytic bone lesions. Infection caused by *R. quintana* or *R. henselae* can also cause fever, bacteremia, and hepatosplenomegaly with blood-filled cysts (peliosis hepatis and peliosis splenis) in the absence of cutaneous findings. The diagnosis can be made by Warthin-Starry stain of affected tissue. Recently, detection by the polymerase chain reaction and culture has become available in some research laboratories. Treatment is with erythromycin or tetracycline.

Drug reactions are common in HIV-infected patients and may commonly present as fever with a rash. Trimethoprim-sulfamethoxazole is a common offender; some studies have reported that greater than 50% of patients taking this drug developed a rash and up to 30% of patients need to change therapy because of severe skin toxicity. Rash with or without fever has also been reported to accompany treatment with dapsone, pentamadine, clindamycin, fluconazole, foscarnet, sulfadiazine, DDI, and AZT.

ASSOCIATED PHYSICAL FINDINGS

Associated physical findings may be of diagnostic value. Many processes that involve the skin also involve the mucous membranes. Thus a careful search for exanthems should be undertaken. Koplick's spots, which are diagnostic of rubeola, are bluish-gray specks on a red base, resembling a "grain of sand" on the buccal mucosa opposite the second molar. A "strawberry tongue" suggests Kawasaki disease, TSS, or scarlet fever; and in the latter may be associated with purpuric macules on the soft palate. Palatal petechiae are seen in up to 50% of patients with infectious mononucleosis, usually at the junction of the hard and soft palate; they are also seen in patients with infective endocarditis. Vesicular or ulcerative mucosal lesions may be seen in hand-foot-and-mouth disease, Behçet's syndrome, Reiter's syndrome, inflammatory bowel disease, and the Stevens-Johnson syndrome.

Meningitis or neurologic changes may be seen with meningococcemia, RMSF, staphylococcal bacteremia, leptospirosis, Kawasaki disease, TSS, the "aseptic meningitis" caused by enterovirus infection, and as a late finding in Lyme disease. Generalized adenopathy may be prominent in mononucleosis, toxoplasmosis, syphilis, sarcoidosis, SLE, and drug hypersensitivity. Cervical adenopathy is common in scarlet fever with streptococcal pharyngitis, rubella, and mucocutaneous lymph node syndrome. Hilar adenopathy may be prominent in sarcoidosis and atypical measles. Prominent joint involvement is suggestive of disseminated gonococcal infection or immunologic disorders (e.g., collagen vascular diseases, drug reactions, the prodrome of hepatitis B, or inflammatory bowel disease). The rash of the inflammatory bowel disease generally accompanies exacerbations of gastrointestinal symptoms. Rash, fever, and pneumonia should suggest mycoplasmal infection, atypical measles, RMSF, mononucleosis, coccidioidomycosis, or septicemia associated with staphylococcal or *Pseudomonas* pneumonia. Multisystem involvement is frequently seen in SLE and TSS.

LABORATORY DIAGNOSIS

Diagnostic attempts should be directed initially toward procedures that may give immediate results (Table 228-3). Pustular, petechial, and purpuric lesions should be aspirated or scraped, and any obtainable fluid cultured and examined microscopically. Gram-negative, biscuit-shaped cocci can be found in the skin lesions of up to 60% of patients with meningococcemia. Vesicular lesions should be unroofed with a scalpel blade and the contents examined with Wright or Giemsa stain for multinucleated giant cells or inclusion bodies characteristic of herpesvirus infection. In the immunocompromised patient, aspiration of maculopapular lesions may reveal gram-negative *Pseudomonas aeruginosa* bacilli, and strong consideration should also be given to performing a punch biopsy with fungal staining for *Candida*. Biopsy may also be helpful in identifying vasculitis or granulomatous disease. Immunofluorescence of skin biopsy specimens in RMSF may be positive as early as the fourth day of illness and should be considered an early diagnostic aid. Immunofluorescence is also valuable in the diagnosis of SLE, pemphigus vulgaris, and pemphigoid.

Table 228-3. Diagnostic tests useful in fever and rash

Test	Application
Aspirate of lesion for Gram stain and culture	Most helpful in pustular or petechial lesions. Positive in up to 60% of meningococcemias
Wright or Giemsa stain of vesicular fluid	Up to 70% of herpesvirus infections will show multinucleated giant cells or cytoplasmic inclusion bodies
Biopsy	Fungal infections, vasculitis, granulomatous disease Immunofluorescence: RMSF, SLE
Cultures of distant sites	
Blood	All cases of possible bacteremia, fungemia
Throat, rectal swab	Viral infections
Throat, rectum, urethra, cervix, joint	Disseminated gonococcal infection
Serologic testing	Streptococcal and rickettsial infections, syphilis, typhoid fever, leptospirosis, Lyme disease (*B. burgdorferi* spirochete), *Mycoplasma,* coccidioidomycosis, hepatitis B, Epstein-Barr virus, cytomegalovirus, measles, atypical measles, SLE, trichinosis, enterovirus and adenovirus infections

Examination and culture of cerebrospinal fluid, joint fluid, or urethral or cervical discharge may yield a bacteriologic diagnosis, especially in meningococcal or gonococcal infection. Blood cultures should be performed in all cases in which bacteremia is considered. Throat, rectal, and cerebrospinal fluid cultures for viruses are becoming increasingly useful and available. Throat, rectal, urethral, and cervical cultures should be performed in patients suspected of having disseminated gonococcal infection. Serologic tests may be useful in selected cases. A list of diseases in which they may be helpful is given in Table 228-3.

REFERENCES

Barbour AG: Laboratory aspects of Lyme borreliosis, Clin Microbiol Rev 1(4):399-414, 1988.

Berger T and Perkocha LA: Bacillary angiomatosis, AIDS Clin Rev 81-95, 1991.

Bohach GA et al: Staphylococcal and streptococcal pyrogenic toxins involved in toxic shock syndrome and related illnesses, Crit Rev Microbiol 17(4):251, 1990.

Buchstein SR and Gardner P: Lyme disease, Infect Dis Clin North Am 5(1):103, 1991.

Cone LA et al: Clinical and bacteriologic observations of a toxic shock-like syndrome due to *Streptococcus pyogenes,* N Engl J Med 317(3):146, 1987.

Gordin F et al: Adverse reactions to trimethoprim-sulfamethoxazole in pa-

tients with the acquired immunodeficiency syndrome, Ann Intern Med 100:495, 1984.
Heymann WR: Noninfectious causes of fever and a rash, Int J Dermatol 28(3):145, 1989.
Kingston ME and Mackey D: Skin clues in the diagnosis of life-threatening infections, Rev Infect Dis 8(1):1, 1986.
LeBoit P: Dermatopathologic findings in patients infected with HIV, Dermatol Clin 10(1):59, 1992.
Lee BL and Safrin S: Drug interactions and toxicities in patients with AIDS. In Sande MA and Volberding PA editors: The medical management of AIDS, ed 3, Philadelphia, 1992, WB Saunders.
MacKowiak PA and LeMaistre CF: Drug fever: a critical appraisal of conventional concepts, Ann Intern Med 106:728, 1987.
Mastin DB et al: Atypical measles in adolescents and young adults, Ann Intern Med 90:877, 1979.
McCalmont C and Zanolli M: Rickettsial diseases, Dermatol Clin 7(3):591, 1989.
Medina I et al: Oral therapy for *Pneumocystis carinii* pneumonia in the acquired immunodeficiency syndrome, N Engl J Med 323(12):776, 1990.
Milgrom H et al: Kawasaki disease in a healthy young adult, Ann Intern Med 92:467, 1980.
Millikan LE: Drug eruptions (dermatitis medicamentosa). In Moschella SL, and Hurley HJ, editors Dermatology, vol I, Philadelphia, 1985, WB Saunders.
Spencer LV and Callen JP: Cutaneous manifestations of bacterial infections, Dermatol Clin 7(3):579, 1989.
Todd JK: Toxic shock syndrome, Clin Microbiol Rev 1(4):432-446, 1988.
Toews WH and Bass JW: Skin manifestations of meningococcal infection, Am J Dis Child 127:173, 1974.
Wilfert CM: Epidemiology of Rocky Mountain spotted fever as determined by active surveillance, J Infect Dis 150(4):469, 1984.

CHAPTER 229 Fever in the Compromised Host

Lowell S. Young

Many patients who are immunologically compromised are at risk of developing serious infection. The initial clinical manifestation of this infectious process is usually fever. For the purposes of definition, fever represents an elevation in core body temperature in excess of 38° C or 100.2° F. Such definitions are arbitrary, however, and some individuals may have a normal body temperature within 1 degree above or below 37° C. Fever is the hallmark of infection but is not diagnostic of it. Indeed, the opposite of fever—hypothermia—can occasionally be an important clinical finding that suggests infection in markedly debilitated patients. Perhaps most important, a change in body temperature in a compromised patient—particularly if measured at a rectal source, which approximates core body temperature—should alert the clinician to the possibility of an incipient infectious process, should prompt an immediate and comprehensive clinical evaluation, and should lead to the consideration of empiric antimicrobial therapy.

More difficult to define than an actual elevation in body temperature is the term *compromised,* or *immunocompromised*. The term implies an impaired ability to resist infection. Susceptibility to infection can result from purely mechanical factors such as major trauma or damage to the integument. However, the term compromised usually refers to patients who have some impaired ability to resist infection that results from an immunologic defect. The prime examples of compromised hosts are individuals with hematologic malignancies (e.g., acute leukemia), recipients of organ transplants, and patients treated with corticosteroids or ionizing radiation. Some individuals are born with congenital immunodeficiencies and obviously qualify for the classification.

The nature of the immunologic defects predisposing to infection has been covered in other chapters but may be categorized under the following concepts. First, the number of the phagocytic cells belonging to the neutrophil or polymorphonuclear leukocyte series may be reduced or their function impaired. These cells respond to acute infection, and severe impairment in the function of such cells either qualitatively (as in chronic granulomatous disease of childhood) or quantitatively (as in the case of acute leukemia in which blast cells exceed the production of normal functioning neutrophils in the bone marrow) results in markedly increased susceptibility to bacterial infection. Second, a relatively slower acting population of phagocytic cells includes circulating monocytes and tissue macrophages, and the fixed mononuclear phagocytes of the reticuloendothelial system may be functionally impaired. These cells collaborate with T-helper cells in defense against intracellular pathogens, particularly slow-growing bacteria such as *Mycobacterium tuberculosis*. This component of immunity, often referred to as cell-mediated immunity, seems critical in the defense against a variety of viral, parasitic, and fungal pathogens. Third, there may be quantitative defects in humoral factors that are important in host defense. These include circulating antibodies of the IgA, IgG, and IgM class as well as an enzymatic system such as the complement cascade, which results in direct lysis of some bacteria and viruses. Clearly, however, this segregation of the components of host defense is artificial. To optimize host defense, antibodies bind to bacteria or other microbes (a process known as *opsonization*) and prepare them for ingestion by phagocytic cells. The great majority of patients who are immunologically compromised have defects of one or more of these components in host defense. Not to be overlooked, however, is the fact that therapeutic intervention with cytotoxic anticancer drugs or the use of immunosuppressing medications such as corticosteroids can have profound effects on both humoral antibody production and can reduce the number or impair function of phagocytic cells and lymphocytes. Quite often combinations of defects are present. Therapy with cytotoxic or immunosuppressive medications superimposed on a preexisting immunologic defect results in markedly enhanced infection risk.

PATHOGENESIS OF FEVER

The mechanisms of inflammation leading to fever are much better understood now than when earlier investigators identified a crude substance elaborated by phagocytic cells that, different from endotoxin, triggered fever in experimental animals. Initially termed *endogenous pyrogen,* it was hypothesized that phagocytosis led to the elaboration of a humoral factor that then acted centrally on brain centers that regulate body temperature. Elaboration of endogenous pyrogen would then be the signal to hypothalamic temperature control centers for the triggering of muscular activity (e.g., shivering) that results in elevation of core temperatures. It is now recognized that *endogenous pyrogen* is a term that describes the effects of several cytokines elaborated by mononuclear phagocytes. The best known is interleukin-1 (IL-1), a chemically sequenced protein that will trigger fever in experimental animals and in humans. Endotoxin administration as well as other stimuli causes release of IL-1. Other pyrogenic substances, however, are elaborated by mononuclear phagocytes after exposure to infectious stimuli such as bacteria, viruses, and parasites. These inflammatory mediators include tumor necrosis factor (also known as cachetin) and the interferons. It seems probable that antigen-antibody complexes, as may occur in collagen vascular diseases, can trigger the elaboration of endogenous pyrogens such as IL-1. Furthermore, various neoplastic processes seem also to result in the release of pyrogens from the reticuloendothelial system. Thus a variety of mechanisms, from the progression of underlying disease to a hypersensitivity reaction, can provoke fever in both normal and compromised patients.

CLINICAL APPROACH TO THE PATIENT

The clinician must be alert to the fact that the development of fever in a patient with impaired immunity may be due to multiple causes, and that multiple infectious processes may be present simultaneously. The cardinal principle with regard to clinical management is that infection should clearly be suspected as the most likely cause of fever, and, depending on the immune status of the host, measures to diagnose and treat infection should be rapidly initiated.

The onset of fever should prompt a meticulous yet expeditious bedside evaluation of the patient that should be completed in a matter of minutes. Particular areas of concern during the physical examination should be the head and neck for evidence of central nervous system infection, the oropharynx for evidence of bacterial pharyngitis, the lungs for evidence of any infectious process therein, the abdomen, the urinary tract, the perirectal area, and the integument. If a patient has a foreign body in place, such as an intravenous or intra-arterial catheter, it should be carefully examined and cultures drawn through the catheter channel(s). Immunosuppressed patients are likely to have a limited or impaired inflammatory response. A frank purulent reaction (abscess or sputum production) is rare in severely neutropenic patients. Laboratory studies should focus on studies that give prompt results (e.g., Gram stains of body fluids and aspirates). Some processes involving the lung or brain are notoriously difficult to diagnose without a biopsy, and empiric therapy may have to be initiated before invasive diagnostic measures. Cultures for suspected aerobic and anaerobic organisms and for fungi should be taken immediately. Blood cultures should be obtained before the initiation of any antimicrobial therapy and before appropriate serologic tests are obtained. One cannot criticize the latter measures, but serologic results will not be forthcoming for days, so such studies are largely for confirmatory purposes. If the patient has any central nervous system finding, a chest x-ray film of the lung, routine urinalysis, and lumbar puncture should be obtained as quickly as possible, depending on the underlying clinical urgency. In a hypotensive patient, treatment should be initiated within a matter of minutes.

Epidemiology

The source of infectious fever may be categorized as either endogenous or exogenous. Normal hosts are colonized by myriad microorganisms that generally are harmless. Given the presence of impaired immunity, staphylococci colonizing the skin (coagulase negative) or nares *(Staphylococcus aureus)* can invade and cause life-threatening diseases. This process may be abetted by foreign bodies such as vascular or urinary catheters. Perhaps more than the majority of documented infections in compromised individuals are endogenous, with the natural reservoir being the skin or gastrointestinal tract. Gram-negative bacilli, the most common cause of life-threatening bloodstream invasion, are usually regarded as endogenous pathogens, and the same concept applies to *Candida* species. The great majority of normal individuals, however, are not carriers of *Pseudomonas aeruginosa* or *Klebsiella* species. Careful studies have shown that compromised individuals acquire these organisms from food or environment and are often colonized in the gut before systemic invasion. In a hospital setting, the potential for transmission of infection from person to person or from an environmental source to a high-risk patient is increased when the host is immunocompromised. Additional examples of exogenous infections are *Aspergillus* pneumonia or transfusion-associated infection. The setting of a critical care unit unfortunately presents many opportunities for transmission of infection from patient to patient or from the inanimate environment to patient.

DIFFERENTIAL DIAGNOSIS OF INFECTIOUS DISEASE SYNDROMES IN THE COMPROMISED HOST

Table 229-1 attempts to summarize some of the major clinical syndromes and the causative agents that the clinician should seek to identify in febrile, immunocompromised patients. They can be conveniently categorized in terms of anatomic localization of symptoms: central nervous system, respiratory, gastrointestinal, and skin and soft tissues. Some febrile patients, however, may not demonstrate any localizing signs of infections, and these patients may be among those who are most seriously ill.

Table 229-1. Etiology of infectious disease syndromes in the compromised host

	Pathogens to consider			
Pattern of involvement	**Bacteria**	**Fungi**	**Viruses**	**Parasites**
Disseminated disease with skin lesions (vasculitis or abscesses, or both)	*Staphylococcus aureus* *Pseudomonas aeruginosa* *Aeromonas hydrophila* Other gram negative bacteria *Nocardia* *Noncholera vibrios* *Mycobacteria*	*Candida* sp. *Aspergillus* Phycomycetes *Trichosporon* sp.	Herpes simplex Varicella-zoster	
Diffuse interstitial pneumonia*	Any gram-negative or gram-positive, including *Nocardia* and mycobacteria	*Aspergillus* *Candida* *Mucor* sp. *Cryptococcus*	Herpes simplex Varicella-zoster Cytomegalovirus Measles	*Pneumocystis carinii* *Toxoplasma gondii* *Strongyloides stercoralis* *T. gondii*
Central nervous system infection, meningoencephalitis, possibly brain abscess	*Listeria monocytogenes* *Nocardia* *S. aureus* *P. aeruginosa* *Mycobacterium tuberculosis*	*Cryptococcus neoformans* *Aspergillus fumigatus* *Phycomycetes* *Candida* sp.	Varicella-zoster	*T. gondii*
Oroesophageal syndromes	Anaerobes Aerobes: streptococci and gram-negative rods, particularly *P. aeruginosa*	*Candida* *Aspergillus*	Herpes simplex Cytomegalovirus	
Diarrhea	*Clostridium difficile* *Campylobacter* *Salmonella* *Shigella*		Adenovirus Coxsackievirus Rotavirus	*Giardia lamblia* *Cryptosporidium* *Microsporidia* *Isospora belli*

*Consider also underlying disease, radiation, and drug reactions.

Central nervous system infection

In the immunocompromised host both gram-positive and gram-negative bacillary pathogens cause brain abscess or meningitis, but one organism should always be considered: *Listeria monocytogenes*. In many series this organism is the most common cause of bacterial meningitis. However, encapsulated bacteria such as pneumococci and staphylococci (usually from a bacteremic source) may cause metastatic central nervous system disease. Patients with compromised cell-mediated immunity (Hodgkin's disease or acquired immunodeficiency syndrome [AIDS]) are at particular risk for developing cryptococcal or even *Listeria* meningitis. The cryptococci are probably the most important fungal pathogens, but occasionally *Candida* and *Aspergillus* can cause central nervous system disease. The herpes viruses including cytomegalovirus, Epstein-Barr, and herpes simplex may cause central nervous system disease although the exact proportion of attributable causes is a matter of controversy. The human immunodeficiency virus (HIV-I) can cause central nervous system reactive pleocytosis. Reactivated or quiescent central nervous system syphilis should also be considered in patients with severe immunologic impairment. Parasites rarely cause central nervous system disease in immunocompromised patients.

Respiratory

The lungs offer a particular challenge for the evaluation of fever in the compromised patient. Often, it is clear that the patients have respiratory symptoms manifested by cough, hypoxia, and shortness of breath. Despite the ready detection of pulmonary abnormalities, diagnosis is difficult because of problems in accurately obtaining pulmonary secretions or in obtaining an adequate sampling of lung parenchyma. Community-acquired pathogens such as pneumococcus and *Haemophilus influenzae* can cause lobar and sometimes even diffuse pneumonia. Gram-negative bacilli are often associated with opportunistic pneumonia in intubated patients; these lung infections are associated with extraordinarily high mortality rates. Depending on epidemiologic circumstances, *Legionella* species may cause life-threatening infections in patients who are debilitated, receiving organ transplants, or receiving immunosuppressive therapy associated with transplantation or cancer treatment. The primary parasitic cause of diffuse pneumonia in immunocompromised patients has clearly been *Pneumocystis carinii*. However, *Toxoplasma* and *Strongyloides* can cause pulmonary infiltrates.

The most common opportunistic fungi causing lung infection include the *Aspergillus* species and cryptococci. Even *Candida*, however, may involve the lung on a fungemic basis. One should not overlook the possibility of mycobacterial disease, particularly in patients with impaired cell-mediated immunity. The pulmonary involvement is usually primary for tuberculosis but can be secondary for the atypical mycobacteria (e.g., *Mycobacterium avium* complex).

Viral infections are often difficult to diagnose in immunocompromised patients. Respiratory pathogens such as adenovirus, measles, and respiratory syncytial virus have long been known to complicate immunosuppression. However, the predominant pathogen in patients after organ transplantation is cytomegalovirus (CMV). This agent can cause a diffuse interstitial pneumonitis that is indistinguishable from *Pneumocystis* infection; indeed, CMV may coexist with pneumocystosis. Other viral causes of lung disease in compromised patients include varicella-zoster virus. Interestingly, mycoplasma and chlamydia—despite their major role as a cause of pneumonia in young adults—are not common pathogens in immunosuppressed patients.

Gastrointestinal tract

The multiple causes of diarrhea in immunosuppressed patients are listed in Table 229-1. Conventional enteric pathogens such as *Salmonella, Shigella,* and *Campylobacter* should be considered;, but it should be borne in mind that diarrhea can stem from the toxins of *Clostridium difficile,* whose overgrowth is a result of selection by antimicrobial therapy, *Isospora belli* and *Cryptosporidium* are two acid-fast-staining parasites associated with impaired cell-mediated immunity, especially AIDS. Their role as a cause of diarrhea has been appreciated in other immunosuppressed patients. Pain on swallowing has commonly been linked to *Candida* mucosal overgrowth (thrush and esophagitis). Herpes simplex and CMV, however, may cause identical symptomatology as well as a similar radiologic appearance on esophagram. Occasionally, severe cellulitis of the posterior pharynx can be caused by streptococci and even *P. aeruginosa* in the markedly neutropenic host.

Cutaneous syndromes

Occasionally the sudden onset of bacteremia, such as due to streptococci or staphylococci, may be manifested by cutaneous involvement. Ascending cellulitis of an extremity due to streptococci can occur in immunosuppressed as well as normal patients. Metastatic abscesses are common with *S. aureus* bacteremia. In systemic gram-negative infections, necrotizing vasculitis such as the ecthyma gangrenosum of *P. aeruginosa* infection is considered to be virtually diagnostic of this particular pathogenic disease (Plate V-23). Fungal pathogens such as *Aspergillus* or *Candida,* however, have been associated with metastatic lesions, and their appearance may be indistinguishable from gram-negative vasculitis. The obvious approach in this situation is not to rely on morphologic interpretation of the findings but to carry out aspirations and biopsies of suspicious lesions. The information gained therefrom may be more valuable than a blood culture, and the results may be back far sooner than the results of blood cultures.

EMPIRIC ANTIMICROBIAL THERAPY

One of the major important decisions that the clinician must make at the bedside is whether to initiate empiric therapy for the patient who has fever. In some patients, it is not possible to discern, on clinical grounds alone, the difference between infectious fever and fever secondary to a neoplasm, drug reaction, or hypersensitivity reaction (including reactions to blood products). Whereas the recent administration of blood products might lead the clinician to temporize in the administration of empiric antimicrobial therapy, the basic tenet that underlies all major initial therapeutic choices should be the clinical status of the host. If the patient's immunologic status is severely impaired, as manifested by a circulating normal neutrophil count of less than 500 per μl, and the patient's overall clinical condition appears to be deteriorating, then it is prudent to obtain diagnostic studies mentioned previously and begin broad-spectrum antimicrobial treatment. If a reasonable likelihood exists that the fever is due to a hypersensitivity reaction or underlying disease, then diagnostic measures including cultures should be obtained and the patient very carefully observed over the ensuing hours. For the patient who is markedly neutropenic (white count less than 100 μl) or severely neutropenic (white count less than 500 μl), a broad-spectrum regimen is preferred as initial therapy unless specific clues identify a likely causative microorganism. Examples of the latter might be transtracheal aspirates, urine Gram stains, or the aspiration of infected material from an abscess.

Choice of empiric therapy

Despite many advances in laboratory diagnosis, there is no clear-cut way to distinguish between gram-negative sepsis and gram-positive infection. Therefore, an initial choice of antimicrobial agents should provide broad-spectrum coverage (Fig. 229-1) (Chapter 224). Traditional choices have included an aminoglycoside such as gentamicin, tobramycin, or amikacin for gram-negative activity paired with another broad spectrum agent of another class that covers *P. aeruginosa*. That broad-spectrum agent may be a beta-lactam compound such as carbenicillin, ticarcillin, azlocillin, or mezlocillin, or one of the cephalosporins with reliable anti-pseudomonal activity (cefoperazone or ceftazidime). Alternative choices would include imipenem, aztreonam, or one of the intravenous quinolones. The gram-positive activity of the aforementioned compounds is variable, and some clinicians would consider the additional use of vancomycin as initial therapy if the likelihood of gram-positive infection is significant.

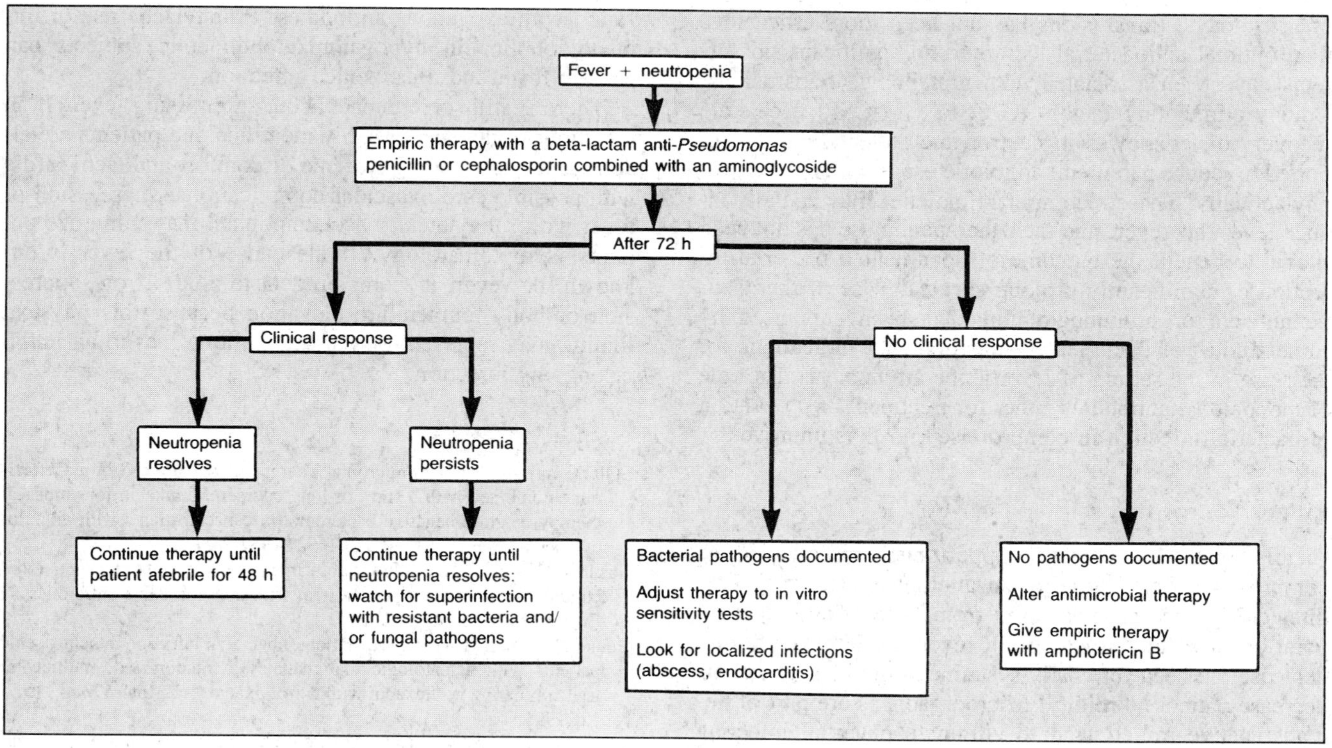

Fig. 229-1. Empiric approach in febrile neutropenic patients.

Many therapeutic trials have been carried out to evaluate the efficacy of one, two, or three antimicrobial agents as empiric therapy. No convincing evidence suggests that three or more antimicrobial compounds are more effective than double-agent therapy. Several studies performed over the last decade suggest that dual-agent combination therapy may provide synergistic antibacterial activity and minimize the emergence of resistance. Some recent reports, however, suggest that monotherapy with an agent such as ceftazidime or imipenem may be adequate to sustain a neutropenic immunocompromised patient for the first 48 hours until the results of cultures may identify the target of specific antimicrobial therapy. Such a decision should be based on the predictability that most disease-causing bacteria in an institution will be susceptible in vitro. For relatively susceptible organisms such as *Escherichia coli* or *Klebsiella* species, a potent beta-lactam compound may be sufficient as monotherapy. For *P. aeruginosa* infections, the weight of evidence favors the continued use of combinations. For *S. aureus* bacteremia, the evidence points toward the continuing efficacy of monotherapy providing that the organism is susceptible in vitro. For deep-seated staphylococcal infections, however, the combination of a beta-lactam penicillinase—stable agent plus rifampin or an aminoglycoside—may lead to more rapid clinical improvement.

The identification of a specific infecting agent may permit more targeted treatment. A therapeutic dilemma, however, relates to patients who manifest persistent neutropenia and yet no organism is identified as the cause of pyrexia (see Fig. 229-1). Indeed, between 50% and 80% of febrile neutropenic patients may have no identified cause of fever yet respond to broad-spectrum therapy. It has been suggested that such patients have incipient nonbacteremic infection (e.g., from a gastrointestinal source), and that early treatment arrests further spread of infection. Some clinicians prefer to continue antibiotics until the neutrophil count rises above 500 μl. Usually, however, antibiotics may be discontinued after 3 to 5 afebrile days and patients are very carefully followed. If this regimen is followed, patients must be monitored to avoid the development of a catastrophic "rebound" septicemia. A greater challenge, however, is what to do for the persistently febrile patient who has undocumented infection. Some controlled studies suggest that in the face of persistent immunosuppression and fever, the most prudent choice after the initiation of antibacterial treatment is to initiate empiric antifungal therapy with amphotericin B (see Fig. 229-1). Unfortunately, the agents that are active against the opportunistic fungi (such as amphotericin B with or without flucytosine) are toxic, and the decision to initiate empiric antifungal therapy should not be made lightly. On the other hand, controlled clinical studies suggest the benefits of such empiric treatment with amphotericin alone in the febrile neutropenic patient who has not responded to 5 to 7 days of empiric antibacterial therapy and in whom no apparent cause of the fever is identified. The role of the new azoles, fluconazole or itraconazole, for empiric therapy in place of amphotericin B, requires further evaluation.

Augmentation of host defenses in compromised patients is a highly desirable goal. In practice, however, routine use of granulocyte transfusions has not been more efficacious than optimal antibacterial therapy, and significant side effects have been associated with granulocyte transfusions. Colony stimulating factors (G-CSF, GM-CSF) accelerate recovery of leukocytes in neutropenic patients and are reported to reduce parenteral antibiotic usage when given prophylactically. These recombinant moieties may actually induce fever, however, and their therapeutic use has not been shown to benefit the outcome of documented bacterial infection or significantly prolong survival. Use of therapeutic antisera or immunoglobulins has been supported by some studies of documented infection, but indications for their use in the setting of fever alone are unclear. The role of monoclonal antibodies either for treatment or prevention of bacterial infection in compromised hosts is unproven.

Prevention of fever and infection

Clearly, measures of treating opportunistic infection in the compromised host represent an attempt to deal with life-threatening emergencies, but from a cost-effectiveness point of view, the prevention of fever and infection would decrease the need for costly systemic antibiotics as well as decrease patient morbidity. Microorganisms are part of humans' native milieu, and to eliminate potential infecting pathogens entirely would be unrealistic and unfeasible. On the other hand, a number of epidemiologic studies have determined that the gastrointestinal tract is often the site of colonization by potential disease-causing microorganisms, particularly *P. aeruginosa, Klebsiella* species, *Proteus, Serratia,* and gram-negative organisms that are not normally found in the stool of healthy individuals. Measures to decrease gastrointestinal carriage via the monitoring of food products given to patients, restriction of diets to cooked food products, and use of prophylactic antibiotics have gained favor. Some prophylactic antibiotic approaches have significant side effects. The advent of the quinolones may provide both local and systemic prophylaxis against the majority of gram-negative and many of the important gram-positive opportunistic bacterial pathogens. More extensive use of prophylactic agents to "decontaminate" the gastrointestinal tract with nonabsorbable antibiotics has not met with uniform success. Anticandidal prophylaxis may be accomplished with agents such as clotrimazole (topically) or fluconazole (systemically). Acyclovir provides prophylaxis against viral opportunistic infections caused by herpesviruses. Agents such as trimethoprim-sulfamethoxazole will prevent *P. carinii* pneumonia in patients with leukemia or impaired cell-mediated immunity. Attempts to minimize the environmental acquisition of potential pathogens have met with limited success. Nonetheless, meticulous infection measures (hand washing, reverse isolation, avoidance of unnecessary procedures) appear to have some effect in reducing the opportunistic infection.

Immunoprophylaxis has clear-cut appeal, and use of killed or recombinant vaccines such as those directed against pneumococci or hepatitis B is justified. However, humoral antibody responses in immunosuppressed patients are often poor. An alternative approach is passive immunization with exogenous antibodies. Prophylactic use of immunoglobulins in hypogammaglobulinemic subjects can prevent fever and documented infection.

There is still some debate about suppressing fever. If an infectious organism is readily identified and patients are elderly and experiencing extreme discomfort and tachycardia with possible cardiovascular complications, suppression of fever with salicylates or acetaminophen may minimize patients' symptomatology. If the cause of the fever is unknown, however, it seems prudent to hold off on suppression of body temperature elevation because this physical finding may represent one of the earliest clues to an initial or ongoing infection.

REFERENCES

EORTC International Antimicrobial Therapy Cooperative Group: Ceftazidime combined with a short or long course of amikacin for empirical therapy of gram-negative bacteremia in cancer patients with granulocytopenia, N Engl J Med 317:1692, 1987.

Gastinne H et al: A controlled trial in intensive care units of selective decontamination of the digestive tract with nonabsorbable antibiotics, N Engl J Med 326:594-599, 1992.

Ginema Infection Program: Prevention of bacterial infection in neutropenic patients with hematologic malignancies: a randomized, multicenter trial comparing norfloxacin with ciprofloxacin, Ann Intern Med 115:7-12, 1991.

Infectious Diseases Society of America: Guidelines for the use of antimicrobial agents in neutropenic patients with unexplained fever, J Infect Dis 161:381-396, 1990.

Lieschke GJ and Burgess AW: Drug therapy: granulocyte colony-stimulating factor and granulocyte-macrophage colony-stimulating factor, N Engl J Med 327:28-35, 99-106, 1992.

Mackowiak PA, editor: Fever: basic mechanisms and management, New York, 1991, Raven Press.

Pizzo PA et al: Empiric antibiotic and antifungal therapy for cancer patients with prolonged fever or granulocytopenia, Am J Med 72:101-111, 1982.

Rubin RH and Young LS: Clinical approach to infection in the compromised host, ed 2, New York, 1992, Plenum.

CHAPTER

230 Upper Respiratory Infections (Colds, Pharyngitis, Sinusitis)

Birgit Winther
Jack M. Gwaltney, Jr.

Acute respiratory infections are a major cause of morbidity in all age groups. They are caused by a large variety of viruses and bacteria that, either alone or in combination, produce illness. The mechanisms by which viruses and bacteria interact to cause respiratory disease are poorly understood. The major pathogenic respiratory viruses include the rhinovirus, myxovirus, paramyxovirus, adenovirus, and coronavirus groups. Most viral infections follow a short, self-limited course.

Bacterial colonization is generally limited to the nostrils, nasopharynx, mouth, and throat, whereas clinical infection may occur both in colonized areas and in normally sterile areas, such as the middle ear and paranasal sinuses. *Streptococcus pneumoniae, Haemophilus influenzae,* and group A beta-hemolytic streptococci are the most common bacterial pathogens in upper respiratory infection. Other important, though less common, bacterial pathogens include *moraxella catarrhalis, Staphylococcus aureus,* other streptococcal species, and anaerobic species, including *Fusobacterium* and *Bacteroides*.

THE COMMON COLD

Despite its mild and self-limited nature, the common cold is the leading cause of acute morbidity in the United States. As such, it is the most frequent reason for nonelective physician visits, as well as for industrial and school absenteeism. The most important common cold viruses are the rhinoviruses (Chapter 244) and coronaviruses (Chapter 246), although other respiratory viruses may also cause the syndrome (Table 230-1). The cause of approximately one third of colds in adults remains unknown—presumably they are caused by undiscovered viruses.

One reason colds occur frequently is because of the large number of pathogenic viruses. There are currently 100 antigenically different types of rhinovirus producing specific immunity. In some studies, over three fourths of persons with coronavirus colds had neutralizing antibody, indicating a previous infection.

Epidemiology

Observation of families in the home has provided important information on the frequency and epidemiology of colds. Overall, children average 6 to 8 colds per year; however, young children in nursery school can have up to 10 to 12 colds per year. Adults average only 2 to 3 per year. Males have a slightly higher incidence of colds through adolescence. Most frequently, school children introduce respiratory viruses into the home. After a cold is introduced, the spread among family members depends on both the age of the index case and the age and immune status of the exposed person. Adults without children in the home have fewer colds than do persons with this exposure.

Table 230-1. Viruses associated with the common cold

Virus group	Percentage of cases
Rhinovirus	30-35
Coronavirus	≥10
Parainfluenza virus, Respiratory syncytial virus, Influenza virus, Adenovirus	10-15
Other known viruses	5
Presumed undiscovered viruses	30-35

Different respiratory viruses tend to predominate during specific times of the year (Table 230-2). Rhinovirus colds are most common in the early fall and late spring; parainfluenza virus infections peak in late fall; and coronavirus colds are most often seen in midwinter. Other viruses, such as influenza and respiratory syncytial virus, usually produce a distinct annual outbreak, which usually occurs during the winter or early spring.

The mechanism(s) for the spread of respiratory viruses has not been well established. Transmission may occur by large or small aerosol spread or by direct contact with infectious secretions on skin and environmental surfaces. Rhinovirus is produced primarily in the nose and nasopharynx and is shed in highest concentration in nasal secretions (Chapter 244). Peak viral titers in nasal mucus usually occur on the third day of experimental infection and coincide with the period of maximum symptoms. Many persons with natural or experimental rhinovirus colds have recoverable virus on the hands. From there, virus can be transmitted experimentally to the hands of other susceptible persons, in whom colds can be initiated by self-inoculation of the nasal or conjunctival mucosa. These findings suggest that direct contact may be an important mode of rhinovirus transmission. Other respiratory viruses, such as rubeola and coxsackievirus A21, are believed to spread by droplet nuclei as true airborne infections. Influenza and adenovirus are also thought to be transmitted by the airborne route in some cases. More experimental studies will be required to establish with certainty the natural mechanism of transmission of each of the common respiratory viruses.

Pathogenesis

The pathogenesis of rhinovirus colds has become better understood in recent years but much remains to be learned. Indeed, little research has focused on the pathogenesis of other cold viruses. Viral deposition into the nose is the first step in rhinovirus pathogenesis. Virus may reach the nose directly or by way of the eye and lacrimal duct. A very small amount of virus is sufficient to initiate infection. After deposition into the nose, virus is carried posteriorly by the mucociliary escalator to the adenoid where it is thought to initially infect M cells, specialized epithelial cells lining the adenoid crypts. These cells are richly supplied with the ICAM-1 rhinovirus receptor. Viral cytopathic effect on the nasal epithelium is minimal in rhinovirus infection but is believed important as the stimulus for triggering various inflammatory events in the airway. These inflammatory reactions, which are associated with both soluble mediators and neurogenic reflexes, result in vasodilation, vascular transudation, mucous gland secretion, pain, cough, and sneezing. Symptoms begin approximately 16 hours after viral inoculation. Over the second and third day of infection, the virus appears to spread anteriorly from the nasopharynx to ciliated epithelial cells in the nasal passages. The amount of viral excretion from the nose is reduced after several

Table 230-2. Seasonal incidence of colds due to different respiratory viruses

Month	Rhinovirus	Coronavirus	Respiratory syncytial virus	Parainfluenza virus	Adenovirus	Influenza virus
September	++++			+	++	
October	++			++	+	
November	+	++	+	++	+	+
December	+	+++	++	+	++	+++
January	+	+++	+++	+	++	+++
February	+	+++	+++	+	++	+++
March	++	+	++	+	++	+++
April	+++			+	+	++
May	++			+	+	
June	++				++	
July	++				++	
August	+++				++	

Relative frequency: ++++, most common; +, least common.

days, but viral shedding persists on average for 3 weeks and then ceases. Inflammatory mechanisms activated in rhinovirus colds include alpha-adrenergic and parasympathetic nervous pathways, and interleukin-1, prostaglandin, and kinin systems.

Clinical features

The incubation period of rhinovirus colds is generally 16 to 20 hours. The most prominent symptoms include nasal discharge, nasal congestion, sore throat, sneezing, and cough. Malaise and myalgias may be present, but constitutional symptoms are not prominent in rhinovirus and coronavirus infections. A temperature elevation of more than a degree is distinctly uncommon in adults; infants and young children may have more marked febrile responses. The nasal and pharyngeal symptoms reach their peak on the second and third day of illness and rapidly decline thereafter. Cough and laryngeal symptoms, when present, subside more slowly. One fourth of rhinovirus colds last longer than 1 week.

The clinical manifestations of the common cold are so typical that the diagnosis is usually made by the patient. The only conditions that frequently mimic these symptoms are allergic and vasomotor rhinitis, which may be recognized by their recurrent or chronic clinical history. Findings on physical examination may be minimal, despite the patient's subjective discomfort, but the patient may look congested with oral respiration and have the characteristic nasal voice (rhinolalia clausa). Anterior rhinoscopy may show secretions in the nasal cavity, but the mucous membrane appears normal. Mild pharyngeal and tonsillar injection without exudate are considered typical but may not be prominent. Pulmonary abnormalities are limited to rhonchi without rales or other evidence of pulmonary alveolar consolidation. No clinical features have been found that distinguish between infections caused by different rhinovirus types or between rhinovirus colds and those due to other viruses. Diagnosis of the specific viral causative agent is usually not possible on the basis of clinical findings. In certain epidemiologic settings, some acute respiratory infections, such as influenza and pharyngoconjunctival fever, can be recognized without viral culture or serologic tests. Knowledge of the characteristic seasonal patterns for the different viruses may aid in the identification of a particular infection (see Table 230-2).

Diagnosis

The main challenge to the physician is to distinguish the uncomplicated cold from the 10% of cases of streptococcal pharyngitis and the estimated 5% to 10% of cases of secondary acute bacterial sinusitis or otitis media. Streptococcal antigen detection tests and throat cultures are useful for diagnosing streptococcal pharyngitis, but recognizing bacterial infection of the sinus and ear is difficult because of the lack of simple, noninvasive diagnostic tests for these complications.

The pharynx, nasal cavity, ears, and sinuses should be thoroughly examined. Pharyngeal or tonsillar exudate should raise suspicion of streptococcal or adenovirus infection, mononucleosis, Vincent's angina, or diphtheria. A vesicular eruption on the soft palate is characteristic of herpes simplex and coxsackievirus A infection. Transillumination of the maxillary and frontal sinuses is a valuable procedure in the diagnosis of acute sinusitis, but limited CT scan of the sinuses or sinus radiography should be performed when suspicion of acute sinusitis is high (see Acute Sinusitis). It has been recognized that sinus x-ray examination is not adequate for detecting ethmoid sinusitis. Examination of the ears is directed at pathologic features of the tympanic membrane during acute otitis media. Pneumatic otoscopy is helpful in differentiating chronic middle ear effusion (secretory otitis media) from acute otitis.

Most respiratory viruses can be grown in cell culture, but this is currently not possible in most labs. Rapid techniques of viral identification using nucleic acid probes, fluorescent-antibody, and other immunodiagnostic procedures on respiratory secretions are being developed and will be useful if antiviral chemotherapy becomes available. The serologic diagnosis of influenza, parainfluenza, respiratory syncytial virus, and adenovirus infection may be made retrospectively with paired sera obtained in the acute phase of illness and approximately 3 weeks later. A fourfold or greater rise in antibody titer is indicative of infection. Serologic diagnosis of rhinovirus infection is not practical because of the numerous antigenic types.

Treatment

Treatment of patients with an uncomplicated common cold is symptomatic. Rest during the initial day or so of illness is advisable, not only for the comfort of the patient, but also to reduce the exposure of others during the period of maximum virus shedding. Regular hand washing and care to avoid contamination of the environment with nasal secretions may help to prevent spread. Aspirin and acetaminophen are standard treatments for the systemic symptoms of colds. Recently, naproxen has been shown to have a beneficial effect on malaise, myalgia, headache, and cough in rhinovirus colds. Saline gargles or topical anesthetics help alleviate sore throat. Nasal decongestants such as 0.5% phenylephrine or 1% ephedrine provide symptomatic relief of nasal obstruction and provide drainage of nasal secretions. Topical decongestants may be used every 4 hours on a regular basis for not more than 3 to 4 days because of the risk of rebound effect. Topical ipratropium, an active parasympatholytic agent, has recently been shown to reduce the watery nasal secretions during the first days of the cold.

Nonsedating antihistamines have been shown to provide some minimum benefit in the symptomatic management of sneezing and rhinorrhea. Antibiotics have no place in the treatment of uncomplicated colds. Evaluation of published studies suggests that vitamin C is not effective in either prophylaxis or treatment of colds.

The topical intranasal administration of interferon-α2b made by the recombinant technique is effective when given prophylactically in experimental rhinovirus colds. In addition, contact prophylaxis with interferon-α2b prevented natural rhinovirus colds in the family setting. Work is in progress on experimental treatments for rhinovirus colds that combine antivirals with drugs that block inflammatory reactions, thus simultaneously reducing viral replication and blocking its associated airway inflammation.

Attempts to develop vaccines have been thwarted by the great number of causative viruses.

ACUTE PHARYNGITIS

A variety of respiratory viruses and a number of bacteria cause acute pharyngitis. The majority of cases are of viral origin and are self-limited in their clinical course. Accurate diagnosis of these infections is important for two reasons: first, to recognize infections that are amenable to treatment, specifically group A beta-hemolytic streptococcal infection and its major postinfectious complication; and second, to detect the causes of pharyngitis that may be associated with serious systemic illness, such as infectious mononucleosis and diphtheria.

Etiology

The results of epidemiologic investigations are influenced by the season, the age of the population, the severity of the illness, and the diagnostic methods employed. In most studies common cold viruses cause about 25% of all cases of pharyngitis while other recognized respiratory viruses account for an additional 10% to 15% (Table 230-3). Pharyngitis due to rhinovirus and coronavirus infections is generally mild, whereas pharyngitis produced by adenoviruses and herpes simplex virus may be severe.

Streptococcus pyogenes (group A beta-hemolytic streptococci) is the leading bacterial pathogen, accounting for 15% to 30% of all cases of acute pharyngitis (Chapter 259). The importance of non-group A beta-hemolytic streptococci as a cause of pharyngitis remains uncertain. Infection with these strains does not carry the risk of acute rheumatic fever or poststreptococcal glomerulonephritis. Other causes of bacterial pharyngitis include mixed anaerobic infection (Vincent's angina), *Corynebacterium diphtheriae, Mycoplasma pneumoniae,* and *Neisseria gonorrhoeae*. The role of *Chlamydia pneumoniae* as a cause of pharyngitis is not defined but has been suggested in some studies.

Clinical features of the various types

The common cold frequently produces mild or moderate pharyngeal discomfort. Additional respiratory symptoms, especially nasal complaints and coughs, usually accompany the sore throat. Posterior pharyngeal erythema and edema, if present, are mild. Pharyngeal and tonsillar exudate and painful regional adenopathy are not present. Temperature elevation is not usually seen in adults and adolescents.

Influenza virus infection may produce moderate to severe pharyngeal discomfort in addition to systemic complaints of myalgia, headache, and cough (Chapter 245). Fever is common in adults as well as children and may reach 101.3° F (38.5° C) or higher. Pharyngeal exudate and painful adenopathy are not present. Defervescence occurs in 3 to 4 days, but fever may last for over a week.

Adenovirus generally produces more severe pharyngeal and systemic symptoms than do the common cold viruses (Chapter 253). In addition to the prominent sore throat, accompanied by malaise, myalgia, headache, dizziness, and chills, conjunctivitis occurs in up to half of the patients. Such cases of so-called pharyngoconjunctival fever may occur as summertime waterborne epidemics, as well as during the respiratory disease season. Tonsillar or pharyngeal exudate may be present. The duration of fever and symptoms averages 5 to 7 days.

Mild cases of herpes simplex pharyngitis cannot be distinguished from other viral causes of pharyngitis (Chapter 251). Severe disease is marked by a prominent ulcerative and exudative pharyngitis. Coxsackievirus pharyngitis, also known as herpangina, may be recognized by a relatively sparse vesicular eruption on the soft palate, uvula, and anterior tonsillar pillars, primarily in children with prominent fever and dysphagia (Chapter 244).

Table 230-3. Microbial causes of acute pharyngitis

Type of microorganism	Syndrome or disease	Estimated incidence (%)
Viral		
Rhinovirus	Common cold	20
Coronavirus	Common cold	5
Adenovirus	Pharyngoconjunctival fever	5
Herpes simplex virus	Gingivitis, stomatitis, pharyngitis	4
Parainfluenza virus	Common cold, croup	2
Influenza virus	Influenza	2
Coxsackievirus A	Herpangina	<1
Epstein-Barr virus	Infectious mononucleosis	<1
Cytomegalovirus	Infectious mononucleosis	<1
Human immunodeficiency virus	Primary HIV infection	<1
Bacterial		
Streptococcus pyogenes	Pharyngitis, tonsillitis	15-30
Mixed anaerobic infection	Gingivitis, stomatitis (Vincent's angina), peritonsillitis, peritonsillar abscess (quinsy)	<1
Neisseria gonorrhoeae	Pharyngitis	<1
Corynebacterium diphtheriae	Diphtheria	<1
Mycoplasmal		
Mycoplasma pneumoniae	Pneumonia, bronchitis, pharyngitis	<1
Unknown		40

Infectious mononucleosis due to Epstein-Barr virus is associated with an exudative pharyngitis or tonsillitis in half the patients, in addition to the characteristic systemic symptoms and signs of persistent anorexia, malaise, fatigue, generalized adenopathy, and splenomegaly (Chapter 251). The mononucleosis syndrome is also associated with cytomegalovirus infection, but exudative pharyngitis is typically absent.

Acute streptococcal pharyngitis varies greatly in severity. It may be mild and indistinguishable from the pharyngitis associated with the common cold. In contrast, the severe disease is characterized by marked pharyngeal pain, dysphagia, and fever, with the physical findings of exudative posterior pharyngitis and tonsillitis with tender cervical lymphadenitis. Strains of *S. pyogenes* that produce erythrogenic toxin also cause the characteristic rash of scarlet fever.

Another bacterial pharyngitis that may have distinguishing clinical features is Vincent's angina, caused by mixed anaerobes and spirochetes. It produces necrotic tonsillar ulceration with a gray membrane and foul breath. Peritonsillar abscess (quinsy) is also a mixed anaerobic infection that occurs most commonly in young adults. Pharyngeal discomfort is severe, with associated dysphagia. The characteristic physical findings include peritonsillar swelling with medial displacement of the tonsil on the involved side. Bilateral involvement may occur.

In unimmunized persons, diphtheritic pharyngitis continues to occur (Chapter 261). The onset of symptoms tends to be insidious, and pharyngeal discomfort is mild. The characteristic tonsillar membrane is gray and firmly adherent to the mucosa.

Diagnosis

Diagnosis of streptococcal pharyngitis by the clinical features of the illness, even with the aid of explicit scales and prediction rules, is often difficult. The diagnosis can be made in cases with pharyngeal exudate, fever, and tender adenopathy, although a similar presentation may occur with adenoviral and herpetic pharyngitis. In cases without exudate, it is difficult to distinguish streptococcal pharyngitis from that due to common cold viruses and influenza. Therefore, laboratory confirmation of the diagnosis is often necessary. Rapid diagnosis by streptococcal antigen detection with latex agglutination is highly specific but only moderately sensitive compared to throat culture. Specimens with only sparse growth on culture are likely to have a false-negative latex test. A substantial proportion of patients with falsely-negative latex tests develop serologic responses to group A streptococci, indicating an invasive infection. For this reason, throat culture should be performed on patients with pharyngitis who have negative streptococcal antigen tests.

A crystal violet-stained smear of pharyngeal exudate will demonstrate the presence of numerous *Fusobacterium* organisms and spirochetes in Vincent's angina. Throat culture on Loeffler medium should be obtained in all suspected cases of diphtheria. Cultures and serologic tests for influenza viruses, adenovirus, herpes simplex virus, cytomegalovirus, and *M. pneumoniae* are available in some large laboratories.

Treatment

Although streptococcal pharyngitis is ordinarily self-limited, antibiotic therapy has been shown to shorten the duration of clinical illnesses. Antimicrobial therapy will prevent suppurative complications and will reduce the risk of the subsequent development of acute rheumatic fever. Because initiation of antimicrobial therapy within a week of the onset of streptococcal pharyngitis will prevent the subsequent development of acute rheumatic fever, therapy may be withheld until the result of the throat culture is known. For patients not allergic to penicillin, oral therapy should include penicillin V, 250,000 units every 6 to 8 hours in adults and 50,000 units/kg/24 hours in four divided doses in children for 10 days. A single dose of long-acting benzathine penicillin (1.2 million units intramuscularly in adults) is also effective. Penicillin-allergic patients should be treated with a 10-day course of erythromycin.

Oral penicillin in the preceding doses is also the treatment of choice for peritonsillitis and Vincent's angina. Peritonsillar abscess also generally requires surgical drainage. The treatment of viral pharyngitis remains symptomatic, but amantadine is beneficial when given early in the course of illness in patients with presumed influenzal pharyngitis occurring during known influenza A epidemics. Chronic oropharyngeal herpetic infection in an immunosuppressed patient should be treated with acyclovir, but acyclovir is not recommended in otherwise healthy persons with acute herpetic pharyngitis.

The standard supportive measures of bed rest, saline gargles, minor analgesics, and adequate hydration are sufficient in most cases of viral as well as streptococcal pharyngitis.

Active immunization is available for types A and B influenza and diphtheria. Attenuated adenovirus vaccines have been successful in certain high-risk populations, such as military recruits, but are not available for general use.

ACUTE LARYNGITIS, CROUP, AND EPIGLOTTITIS

Acute laryngitis usually occurs as part of more generalized upper respiratory illnesses. Hoarseness may be a major complaint during infection with any of the respiratory viruses. It is not known whether secondary bacterial infection plays a role in cases of acute laryngitis. *M. catarrhalis* has been isolated from the nasopharynx of a majority of a group of adults with acute laryngitis. The significance of this finding remains to be determined. The diagnosis of acute laryngitis is usually evident from the clinical history and is confirmed when mirror examination of the larynx reveals hyperemia and edema. There is no evidence that antimicrobial agents are of value in the treatment of acute laryngitis. Supportive care includes humidification of inhaled air and resting the voice.

Croup is a clinical syndrome in children, characterized by inspiratory stridor and a barking cough. Viral laryngotracheobronchitis is most commonly responsible, with parainfluenza viruses the most frequently identified pathogens. The diagnosis depends on recognition of the clinical syndrome and exclusion of acute bacterial epiglottitis or the presence of a laryngeal foreign body.

Acute epiglottitis caused by group B *H. influenzae* is primarily a disease of childhood and may be mistaken for croup or laryngitis. Clinical differentiation is not always possible, although in this condition the patient appears toxic, and the clinical course is more rapidly progressive (Chapter 265). Visualization of the inflamed epiglottis with either a tongue blade or a laryngoscope must be undertaken with extreme care to avoid precipitating acute airway obstruction. Blood cultures are frequently positive for *H. influenzae*. Hospitalization, nasotracheal intubation, and intravenous chloramphenicol (50 to 75 mg/kg/day in four divided doses) has been the standard treatment. Intravenous cefuroxime (100-200 mg/kg/day in three divided doses) or a third-generation cephalosporin such as cefotaxime (100-150 mg/kg/day in four doses) are also acceptable treatments for acute epiglottitis.

ACUTE SINUSITIS

The majority of cases of acute sinusitis occur as a complication of viral upper respiratory tract infection. A smaller proportion of cases are associated with dental infection, allergic rhinitis, or nasal anatomic abnormalities. An important new concept in understanding the pathogenesis of sinusitis is the recognition of the importance of the osteomeatal area of the nasal cavity. Obstruction of this narrow passageway, into which drains the frontal, maxillary, and ethmoid sinuses, is recognized as a major risk factor for inflammatory sinus disease. The sinuses normally remain sterile as a result of continuous mucociliary clearance of particulate matter entering the sinus cavity. Colds, influenza, and other acute respiratory infections cause inflammation in the nasal passages, which may lead to narrowing or obstruction of the osteomeatal area. In addition, respiratory viruses have been recovered from sinus aspirates of patients with acute sinusitis and may infect the ciliated epithelial cells lining the sinus cavities. Both of these processes could disrupt the normal cleansing mechanism and increases the susceptibility of the sinus to secondary bacterial invasion. The resulting exudative effusion usually contains more than 5000 polymorphonuclear leukocytes per cubic millimeter, with bacterial titers usually exceeding 10^5 CFU per milliliter. The maxillary sinus may also be infected by direct extension of dental root abscesses of the upper molars or bicuspids.

Etiology

The infectious agents responsible for acute maxillary sinusitis in adults have been identified by direct sinus puncture and culture of the aspirated fluid (Table 230-4). This ap-

Table 230-4. Causative organisms in acute maxillary sinusitis and acute otitis media

Organism	Acute maxillary sinusitis (%)	Acute otitis media (%)
Streptococcus pneumoniae	30	50-60
Haemophilus influenzae	25	20
Anaerobic bacteria	6	
Staphylococcus aureus	4	2
Streptococcus pyogenes	2	5-10
Moraxella catarrhalis	2	5-10
Gram-negative bacteria	9	10

proach avoids contamination of the culture specimen by nasopharyngeal flora. *S. pneumoniae* and unencapsulated strains of *H. influenzae* account for approximately half the cases, with smaller numbers of cases being due to *S. aureus, S. pyogenes, M. catarrhalis,* and gram-negative bacteria. Mixed anaerobic infection is usually associated with contiguous dental disease. Respiratory viruses, including rhinovirus, influenza virus, and parainfluenza virus, have been recovered alone or in combination with bacteria in about 20% of patients. A small proportion of sinus disease results from fungal infections, particularly aspergillosis, phaeohyphomycosis, zygomycosis (mucormycosis), pseudallescheriasis, and hyalohyphomycosis (penicillosis). Presumably, the causes of infections of the frontal, ethmoidal, and sphenoidal sinuses are similar to those of the maxillary antra.

Diagnosis

The clinical features of acute sinusitis may be difficult to distinguish from those of a prolonged cold. Uncomplicated colds on average last about a week, thus illnesses lasting longer probably have sinus involvement. Facial discomfort, purulent nasal discharge or postnasal discharge, and tonal changes in the voice are common features of sinusitis, and these symptoms may be accompanied by moderate headache. The findings on physical examination are variable. Temperature elevation occurs in less than half of adults with acute maxillary sinusitis documented by sinus aspiration. Erythema, swelling, and tenderness may be found over the involved sinus but are not present in most patients, and their absence does not exclude the diagnosis. Periorbital edema and increased lacrimation are characteristic findings in ethmoid sinusitis.

Transillumination of the maxillary and frontal sinuses is useful in a patient with previously normal sinuses. The procedure should be undertaken in a completely darkened room using a sinus transilluminator. For examination of the maxillary sinuses, the tip of the instrument is placed on the infraorbital ridge and is directed downward toward the hard palate. The finding of complete opacity is strong evidence for the presence of active infection. The presence of "dullness" (diminished but not complete absence of light transmission) is also suggestive of infection. The finding of normal transillumination is good evidence that no infection is present. Transillumination is less helpful in patients with chronic sinusitis, in whom reduced light transmission may be a persistent finding. Normal variations in bone thickness may cause different intensity of transillumination among different individuals.

X-ray examination of the sinuses has traditionally been the gold standard for diagnosis. The finding of complete opacification, an air-fluid level, or mucosal thickening is strong evidence for the presence of active infection (Fig. 230-1). It is now recognized that although standard radiographs are satisfactory for detecting disease of the frontal, antral, and sphenoid sinuses, they are insensitive for diagnosing ethmoid sinusitis. For this reason, limited computed tomography (CT) examination of the sinuses is now being offered by some radiology departments at costs comparable to those of a standard sinus x-ray series. CT examination also allows evaluation of the osteomeatal complex for evidence of narrowing and anatomic obstruction. In patients with chronic sinusitis, the presence of persistent radiographic abnormalities limits the usefulness of imaging techniques in the diagnosis of active infection.

Culture of nasal secretions or sinus washings obtained through the natural ostium are not of diagnostic usefulness because of contamination with the resident nasopharyngeal flora. Specimens for culture that are collected from the mouth of the sinus ostium under direct vision by endoscopy have not been compared to those obtained by sinus puncture and cannot be considered as free from extraneous mi-

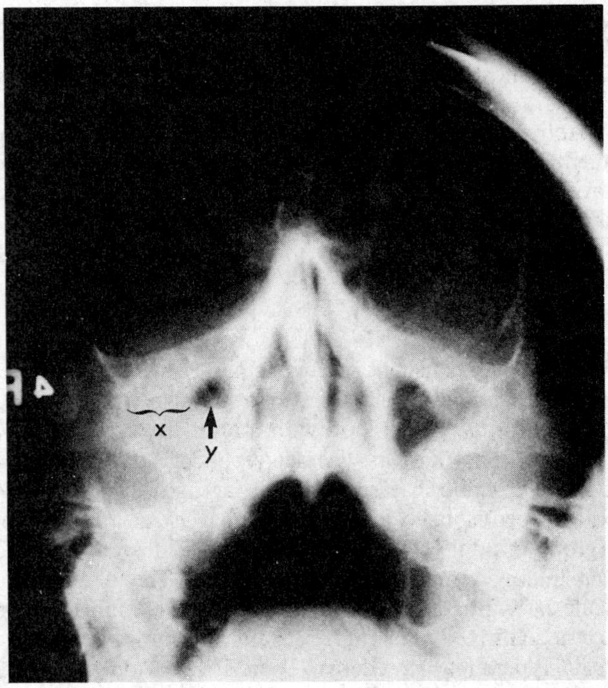

Fig. 230-1. Waters' projection x-ray of a patient with acute maxillary sinusitis. The right maxillary sinus shows evidence of significant mucosal thickening *(x)* and an air-fluid level *(y)*.

crobial contamination. Direct sinus puncture is the accepted way to collect specimens for culture but is not practical in the usual case of sinusitis. Sinus puncture is generally reserved for patients with unusually severe infection, those not responding to therapy, or those in whom intracranial spread of infection is suspected. Because routine bacteriologic diagnosis is not possible, it is necessary to base antimicrobial treatment on the known causes of sinusitis (Table 230-4).

Treatment

Treatment of acute community-acquired sinusitis is a course of antimicrobial therapy that covers the major known causes of infection. The ampicillins recommended previously are no longer considered adequate because of the increasing importance of β-lactamase-producing strains of *H. influenzae* and *M. catarrhalis*. Several antimicrobials have been shown effective by pre- and post-treatment sinus puncture studies for treating the usual bacterial causes of acute sinusitis, including the beta-lactamase-producing strains (Table 230-5). In selecting among these agents, cost and the potential for side effects are the major considerations, as all appear equally effective, with bacteriologic cure rates of over 90%. A 10-day course of treatment is recommended in the usual case. Supportive therapy generally includes nasal decongestants and analgesics if required.

Management of therapeutic failures can be difficult. If the response to the initial course of treatment is not satisfactory, a sinus puncture is recommended to provide a specimen for bacterial culture and antimicrobial sensitivities and to obtain the therapeutic benefits of sinus lavage. An additional and more prolonged course of antimicrobial treatment, based on culture results if available, is then recommended. Topical steroids are also used in the hope of reducing swelling and promoting sinus drainage, although their effectiveness is unproven. If the condition still does not clear, allergy and immunology evaluations may be helpful. Most important, CT imaging of the osteomeatal complex and sinuses should be performed to determine if there are anatomic abnormalities that require surgical correction.

Repetitive bacterial infections, particularly when untreated or inadequately treated, may produce irreversible changes in the sinus mucosa. In chronic sinus disease squamous cells may replace the normal ciliated epithelium, and sinus sterility cannot be maintained by the normal clearance mechanisms. Although the sinus becomes colonized with bacteria, antimicrobial therapy is usually not helpful for controlling the symptoms of chronic sinus disease. Exacerbations of acute infection can occur, however, and should be treated in the same way as an acute infection in persons with normal sinuses. Surgical correction of obstructive lesions is most important in the treatment of chronic sinus disease.

Table 230-5. Antimicrobials for treating acute community-acquired sinusitis

Antimicrobial	Adult dose
Trimethoprim-sulfmethoxazole double strength	1 bid
Cefuroxime axetil	250 mg bid
Amoxicillin/clavulanate	500/125 mg tid
Loracarbef	400 mg bid

OTITIS MEDIA

Acute otitis media is an inflammation of the middle ear mucosa and may be classified as suppurative or nonsuppurative based on the characteristics of the fluid present in the middle ear. The most important predisposing factor in the development of this disease is an acute infection, usually viral, involving the eustachian tube in the posterior nasopharynx. Eustachian tube dysfunction and abnormal middle ear pressures have recently been observed in young adults with experimental rhinovirus infection. If local host defense mechanisms are inadequate, microbial proliferation results in infection.

Etiology

Several viruses have been isolated from middle ear fluid, either alone or in combination with bacteria. These include rhinovirus, adenovirus, respiratory syncytial virus, parainfluenza virus, and coxsackievirus. Bacterial pathogens identified by diagnostic tympanocentesis include many common inhabitants of the nasopharynx. *S. pneumoniae* is the most important, accounting for over half of the cases. Next in importance are *H. influenzae, M. catarrhalis,* and *S. pyogenes* (see Table 230-4). Nose and throat cultures obtained at the time of tympanocentesis have yielded a variety of potential pathogens, but are not useful in determining the bacterial cause of acute otitis media. In infants less than 6 weeks of age, a considerable fraction of cases are due to coliform organisms and *S. aureus,* in addition to the more common pathogens, such as *S. pneumoniae* and *H. influenzae*.

Clinical features and diagnosis

Acute otitis media is often preceded by an upper respiratory illness. In the typical history, an earache develops in a patient with a cold that has been improving. Fever is often present and the hearing slightly impaired. The diagnosis of acute otitis media is based on an otoscopic examination of the tympanic membrane that typically in the early phase shows a bright-red bulging of the posterior-superior part of the drum. Later the redness extends to most of the tympanic membrane, and the landmarks disappear. Within hours to days a spontaneous perforation may occur with normalization of the temperature and relief of pain. The characteristics of the fluid in the middle ear vary from clear to mucopurulent, and it may be blood tinged at the time of perforation. Closure of the perforation and normalization of the hearing usually occur within 1 to 2 weeks. Small children under 1 year of age may have a more prolonged illness. Tympanocentesis is required for an etiologic diagnosis but is not routinely performed in clinical practice. Its use is generally limited to neonates, other children, or adults with complications that require identification of the pathogen to guide antimicrobial therapy.

Treatment

Antimicrobial therapy in the uncomplicated case of acute otitis media should be directed against *S. pneumoniae, H. influenzae,* and *M. catarrhalis*. Augmentin, cefuroxime axetil, and trimethoprim-sulfamethoxazole provide such coverage or other agents may be chosen on the basis of examination of the middle ear fluid. Myringotomy may be beneficial in patients with severe earache caused by a bulging tympanic membrane. The usefulness of symptomatic therapy, including oral antihistamines and decongestants, is controversial.

Complications following acute otitis media are rare but include acute mastoiditis, labyrinthitis, and meningitis. Chronic middle ear effusion (secretory otitis media) may persist for several months and may be caused by eustachian tube dysfunction probably due to persistent adenoiditis. Chronic effusions may produce a degree of conductive hearing loss that requires treatment by the placement of pneumatic equalization tubes. However, surgery should be withheld for 3 or more months to permit the highest rate of spontaneous resolution.

Prophylactic antibiotics have been shown to be of value in the prevention of recurrent infections in selected patients. Steroid treatment in addition to antibiotics has not been beneficial.

In children with recurrent acute otitis media and chronic middle ear effusion (secretory otitis media), locally produced secretory immunoglobulin A (IgA) antibody is usually present in the nasopharynx. However, patients who have repeated bacterial infections of the middle ears and/or sinuses should be evaluated for immunoglobulin deficiency.

REFERENCES

de Arruda E et al: Localization of rhinovirus replication in vitro with in situ hybridization, J Med Virol 34:38, 1991.

Gwaltney JM Jr et al: The microbial etiology and antimicrobial therapy of adults with acute community acquired sinusitis: a 15-year experience at the University of Virginia and review of other selected studies, J Allergy Clin Immunol 90:457, 1992.

Gwaltney JM Jr: Viral vaccines in the control of otitis media. Workshop on Vaccines for Otitis Media, Children's Hospital of Pittsburgh, Pediatr Infect Dis J 8:578, 1989.

Hayden FG et al: Prevention of natural colds by contact prophylaxis with intranasal alpha$_2$-interferon, N Engl J Med 312:71, 1986.

McBride TP et al: Alterations of eustachian tube, middle ear and nose in rhinovirus infection, Arch Otolaryngol Head Neck Surg 115:1054, 1989.

Naclerio RM et al: Kinins are generated during experimental rhinovirus colds, J Infect Dis 157:133, 1988.

Sperber SJ et al: Effects of naproxen in experimental rhinovirus colds, Ann Intern Med (in press).

Turner BW et al: Physiologic abnormalities in the paranasal sinuses during experimental rhinovirus colds, J Allergy Clin Immunol 90:474, 1992.

Winther B et al: Sites of rhinovirus recovery after point inoculation of the upper airway, JAMA 256:1763, 1986.

Winther B et al: Distribution of the human rhinovirus receptor, ICAM-1, on epithelia of the upper airways, (unpublished).

CHAPTER

231 Pneumonia

Harold C. Neu

Pneumonia is an inflammatory process of the pulmonary parenchyma that can be produced by many different microorganisms. These microorganisms can be either highly virulent bacteria or organisms of extremely low pathogenicity, which normally colonize the oral pharynx of healthy individuals. Pneumonia is a major cause of morbidity and mortality, particularly in hospitalized patients. Approximately 1% of patients admitted to a university hospital develop nosocomial pneumonia, and overall 35% of patients who develop nosocomial pneumonia die. The diagnosis of pneumonia remains difficult despite great progress in clinical medicine. Antimicrobial therapy must be initiated before a definitive microbiologic diagnosis is established; and it requires collection of specimens and interpretation of numerous clinical, laboratory, and radiologic clues to make an acute diagnosis so that the proper antimicrobial agent may be used.

PATHOGENESIS

Pneumonia results from a failure of a series of host defense mechanisms that keep the respiratory tract free of infection (see the accompanying box). Pathogens must reach the distal airway and multiply to produce pneumonia. Organisms can reach the lung by three methods: aspiration, aerosolization, or hematogenous spread. The most important mechanisms are by aspiration of fluids transversing the oral pharynx or via inhalation of droplet nuclei. Although there

Pathophysiology of pneumonia

Colonization of oropharynx
- Increased with illness, underlying respiratory disease, broad-spectrum antibiotic therapy

Microaspiration
- Increased in alcoholism, central nervous depressant drugs, nasogastric tubes, cerebrovascular disease

Pneumonia
- Massive inoculum, decreased host defenses, virulent organisms

is frequent aspiration of oral pharyngeal material, the incidence of pneumonia is low due to host defenses and the low pathogenicity of the organisms that are aspirated. Bacteria are present in air at a level of 15 to 30 organisms per cubic meter of air. The likelihood of large numbers of bacteria reaching the distal airways is small. Normally, aerodynamic filtration of air through the vibrissae in the nose and through the nasopharynx will remove most particles >10 μm in diameter as well as many toxic soluble gases. Particles that are between 3 and 10 μm in diameter will strike the trachea above the carina and be trapped in mucus. Particles smaller than 0.5 μm are not retained in the lung, but are removed in expired gas. Thus the particles that reach the distal part of the lungs are between 0.5 and 3 μm in diameter, the size of many bacteria and other microorganisms.

Normally, mechanical mechanisms exclude particulate matter from reaching the large airways by the anatomic barrier of the epiglottis and the reflex closure of the glottis. Furthermore, branching of the pulmonary tree causes large particles to impact the mucosal surface, which is covered with mucus that entraps material. The cough response causes aspirated material to be cleared from the tracheal bronchial tree. Bacteria or other particles trapped in mucus are removed via ciliary action by what has been referred to as a mucociliary escalator activity. Unfortunately, alveoli do not contain ciliated epithelia or mucus-secreting goblet or mucus gland cells. Therefore other mechanisms are required to remove bacteria that have reached these areas.

Bacteria that contain lipoprotein and glycoprotein projections on their surface are trapped in the mucus. Fibronectin also aids in the phagocytosis of bacteria by alveolar macrophages. In addition, immunoglobulins may be present in the lung, either as the result of immunization or exposure to pathogens by other mechanisms, and the complement system may be activated. In general, alveolar macrophages ingest bacterial particles much less readily than inert particles. Being long-lived cells, they can respond to multiple exposures of microorganisms and can process antigens to activate lymphocytes within the lung. This process produces secretory substances such as cytokines that activate macrophages and produce chemotactic substances such as leukotriene B4, which together with C5a, attract polymorphonuclear cells from pulmonary capillaries. In this way alveolar spaces are consolidated. As white cells die, proteolytic enzymes are released, which damages the lung tissue. Inhibitor proteins have been identified within the lung that to some extent can prevent lung destruction. With early initiation of therapy (or with infection due to certain organisms), the ultimate damage to the lung may be minimal, and the lung will resume its normal gas exchange mechanisms.

Although not all pneumonia occurs as a result of a defective host defense, most pneumonias are the result of some damage to one of the normal pulmonary host defense mechanisms, Table 231-1. In certain situations, a particular host defense results in a specific type of pneumonia.

The normal microbial flora of the upper respiratory tract consists of a variety of streptococcal species, which are facultative, that is, able to grow in aerobic or anaerobic conditions, and organisms such as *Streptococcus pneumoniae, Haemophilus influenzae* (nontypeable strains), *Moraxella catarrhalis,* various *Neisseria* species, and occasionally staphylococci. Large numbers of anaerobic organisms such as oral *Bacteroides* species, *Fusobacteria* species, and some spirochetes are present in the areas around teeth.

Normally, viruses and fungi are not part of the normal flora of the oral pharynx. In normal individuals, the oral pharyngeal flora remains remarkably constant. New species rarely colonize the pharynx due to the normal physiochemical milieu of the oropharynx and the elaboration of inhib-

Table 231-1. Factors altering pulmonary host defenses

Alteration	Factor
Upper airway	
Bypass nasal filtration and humidification	Tracheostomy
Deficient secretory IgA	Congenital or acquired deficiency
Alteration of normal flora	Debility, antibiotics, periodontal disease, institutionalization
Depressed glottis	Coma, seizure, corticobulbar disease, anesthesia, alcoholism
Lower airway	
Inadequate cough	Central nervous system depression, respiratory muscle weakness, postoperative pain
Impaired mucociliary transport	Cigarette smoking, pollutants, anesthetics, alcohol, hypoxia, endobronchial lesion, viral or mycoplasmal infection, chronic bronchitis, bronchiectasis
Abnormal cilia	Kartagener's syndrome, immotile cilia syndrome
Abnormal mucus	Cystic fibrosis
Impaired reflex bronchoconstriction	Bronchiectasis
Alveolus	
Impaired macrophage	Cigarette smoking, pollutants, hypoxia, acidosis, alveolar proteinosis, uremia
Deficient or abnormal immunoglobulins (IgG, IgM)	Myeloma, lymphoproliferative disease, nephrosis, congenital deficiencies, nephrotic syndrome, HIV
Impaired cell-mediated immunity	Hodgkin's disease, malnutrition, steroids, congenital and acquired deficiencies
Inadequate neutrophil function	Neutropenic states, corticosteroids, chronic granulomatous disease
Deficient complement	Deficiencies (rare)
Deficient surfactant	Hyperoxia, adult respiratory distress syndrome

itory substances by the resident bacterial flora. Colonization of mucosal surfaces is mediated by bacterial adherence to local epithelial cells and numerous pathologic factors can alter these bacterial-cell surface binding sites, leading to adherence by nonresident bacteria to the epithelial cells.

Cigarette smoking and chronic bronchitis are known to increase colonization of the oral pharynx with *S. pneumoniae* and nontypeable strains of *H. influenzae*.

Hospital-acquired pneumonia is similar to many community-acquired pneumonias and results from aspiration. Blood-borne infection is distinctly uncommon, and aerosol pneumonia is seen only occasionally with *Legionella* in immunocompromised patients. This alteration in bacterial adherence and pharyngeal colonization also explains, in part, the unique microbiology of nosocomial pneumonia.

Aerobic gram-negative organisms such as *Klebsiella pneumoniae, Pseudomonas aeruginosa, Acinetobacter* species, *Enterobacter,* and other members of the Enterobacteriaceae are known to colonize hospitalized patients. Less than 15% of normal healthy ambulatory individuals have any of the aforementioned species in their oropharynx, whereas over 40% of patients in intensive care units (ICUs) are colonized with gram-negative bacteria within 3 to 5 days of admission. Although the reason for colonization with these organisms has not been fully elucidated, increased levels of salivary protease and depletion of cell surface fibernectin seem to be the pathogenic mechanism.

It has also been shown that nutritional impairment will increase the adherence of some gram-negative organisms, particularly *P. aeruginosa* to tracheal epithelial cells. Upper airway squamous epithelial cells of ill individuals absorb many more gram-negative organisms than do the epithelial cells of normal individuals. Thus when aspiration occurs in hospitalized patients, a much larger number of organisms reach the alveoli. Many of these organisms are serum resistant and are not opsonized by the nonspecific antibody present in the lung, because there is depletion of glycoproteins and fibernectin.

Individuals who have underlying structural defects of the pulmonary system, such as may occur from previous chronic lung disease particularly in chronic smokers or in those who have undergone surgery of the upper abdomen or chest, are extremely likely to develop pneumonia. Obtundation as a result of medications for sleep will depress glottic closure and result in aspiration similar to that which occurs in individuals with a seizure disorder or alcoholism. Tracheal intubation of patients prevents normal ciliary function and results in difficulty in clearing aspirated microorganisms. Although the theory is somewhat controversial, it has been postulated that the use of H_2 blockers and antacids elevates gastric pH causing increased growth of bacteria in gastric secretions. These organisms then are aspirated and result in pneumonia.

EPIDEMIOLOGY

Pneumonias may be either community-acquired (ambulatory, nonhospitalized individuals) or hospital-acquired. Such a classification is useful, but has several defects. With an increasingly aged population, many individuals living in chronic care facilities are exposed to antimicrobial agents to treat urinary tract infections or other minor problems that occur in this setting. These individuals have more in common with hospitalized patients. Thus this distinction between community and hospital must take into consideration whether individuals live by themselves or in a setting with others.

A relatively small number of organisms cause community-acquired pneumonia (Table 231-2). *S. pneumoniae* is responsible for most community-acquired pneumonias that require hospitalization. Other organisms that are important causes of community-acquired pneumonia include *Legionella pneumophila* and in certain age populations *Mycoplasma pneumoniae*. Recently, it has been suggested that the organism *Chlamydia pneumoniae* (formerly called TWAR) may account for a number of cases of community-acquired pneumonia.

Hospital-acquired pneumonia is caused by a combination of aerobic gram-negative bacteria and anaerobic species in 60% of patients, by aerobic species alone in 20% of patients, and by anaerobic species alone in 20% (Table 231-3). The precise aerobic organism depends to a major extent on the microbial flora of the hospital or ICU in which the pneumonia develops or of the flora of other patients or hospital personnel involved in the care of the patient. Nosocomial outbreaks due to species such as *Acinetobacter, P. aeruginosa, Xanthomonas maltophilia,* or *Pseudomonas cepacia* frequently follow the use of broad-spectrum antibiotics for the treatment of other infections.

FACTORS THAT AID IN THE DIAGNOSIS OF PNEUMONIA

Pneumonia usually presents with prominent symptoms of a fever, cough, sputum production, and pleuritic chest pain or chills. Occasionally, the initial symptoms of the patient may suggest illness in the abdomen or symptoms such as those of heart failure. At other times disease in another part

Table 231-2. Causes of community-acquired pneumonia

Organism	Frequency (%)
S. pneumoniae	50-80
Aerobic gram-negative bacilli	3-11
K. pneumoniae	2-6
S. aureus	1-10
Mixed anaerobes	2-12
M. pneumoniae	3-44 (increased in young adults)
H. influenzae	2.5-15
Viral (influenza A and B, parainfluenza, adenovirus)	1-16 (dependent on epidemics)
S. pyogenes	0-1
L. pneumophila	5-20
P. carinii	Rare except in AIDS patients

Table 231-3. Nosocomial pneumonias: frequency of various pathogens

Organism	Frequency (%)
Gram-negative	
Klebsiella sp.	5-13
P. aeruginosa	10-22
E. coli	4-7
Enterobacter	5
Proteus and *Providencia*	5
Serratia	5
Acinetobacter	5
Bacteroides	10-50
Gram-positive	
S. aureus	5-10
S. pneumoniae	10
Enterococci	1
Anaerobic cocci	10-50
Fusobacterium	10-20

of the body may overshadow the pneumonia such as might occur with peritonitis, meningitis, or septic arthritis.

A complete and accurate account of symptoms, especially with regard to the duration of symptoms and tempo of development of disease, may be particularly useful in making a diagnosis. Underlying medical problems, previous pulmonary disease, antibiotic use, occupational or animal exposure, and travel may focus attention on a particular form of pneumonia. Illnesses that predispose to aspiration such as neurologic defects, seizures, drug overdose, alcoholism, recent dental procedures, and anesthesia suggest an aspiration pneumonia caused by oral anaerobic bacteria. Infrequent causes of community pneumonia are suggested on the basis of an exposure or travel history (Table 231-4). Furthermore, a number of noninfectious diseases of the chest or abdomen have all of the symptoms of pneumonia (see accompanying box). The age of the patient may suggest a particular form of pneumonia. For example, *M. pneumoniae* is seen much more frequently in adolescents and young adults than in older patients. The particular season of the year may influence the cause of the pneumonia. For example, during winter months and particularly after outbreaks of influenza, pneumonia is due to *S. pneumoniae, S. aureus, H. influenzae,* and less frequently *Staphylococcus pyogenes*. Legionella disease often occurs during summer months, but can occur throughout the year. As already noted, hospital or nursing home residents are predisposed to gram-negative bacillary gram-negative pneumonia. Intravenous drug abuse and soft tissue infections associated with *S. aureus* should suggest that form of pneumonia. Although *Pneumocystis carinii* pneumonia is frequently a presentation of patients with AIDS, these individuals are also particularly prone to develop pneumococcal pneumonia with bacteremia (see Chapter 242).

Table 231-4. Key epidemiologic factors associated with the history in unusual pneumonias

Pneumonia	Epidemiologic factor
Tularemia	Hunters, butchers, or any exposure to small animals (e.g., muskrats, rabbits)
Plague	Exposure to small animals (rats or ground squirrels in endemic areas, such as western United States)
Neisseria meningitidis	Military recruits (similar population for *M. pneumoniae* and adenovirus)
Anthrax	Wool sorters, butchers, tanners, or exposure to infected hides or skins
Melioidosis	Residence in or travel to Southeast Asia or the Far East
Tuberculosis	Family contact, alcoholics, blacks, miners
Atypical mycobacteriosis	Sand blasters, arc welders, AIDS patients
Cryptococcosis	Exposure to pigeon droppings or infected roosts, AIDS patients
Histoplasmosis	Residence in river valleys, especially in southeastern United States, or exposure to chicken coops or bat droppings
Coccidioidomycosis	Residence in or travel to southwestern United States, expecially San Joaquin Valley
Sporotrichosis	Gardeners, florists, miners
Psittacosis	Exposure to birds (e.g., parakeets, turkeys, parrots)
Q fever	Infected dusts from hides or milk
Parasites	Tropical residence or travel
Pneumocystis carinii	AIDS patients

Noninfectious causes of pneumonia syndromes

- Pulmonary infarction, hemoglobinopathy (chest syndrome)
- Congestive heart failure
- Neoplasia (primary, metastatic, lymphoma)
- Lymphomatoid granulomatosis
- Collagen vascular disorder (lupus, rheumatoid arthritis, vasculitis)
- Hypersensitivity (allergic alveolitis, PIE syndromes)
- Granulomatous disease (sarcoid, Wegener's)
- Drug reaction (phenytoin sodium, heroin, cytotoxic drugs)
- Toxic inhalation
- Radiation

PIE, pulmonary infiltrates with eosinophilia.

CLINICAL PRESENTATION

Many patients with pneumonia will have had mild upper respiratory symptoms and malaise for several days before the onset of the pneumonia. Bacterial pneumonia caused by organisms such as *S. pneumoniae* usually have an abrupt onset with chills and, in many cases, often a single dramatic rigor. There is sustained fever and cough becomes productive of mucopurulent sputum. There may be pleuritic chest pain in pneumococcal pneumonia, although this manifestation is also seen in staphylococcal pneumonia. Multiple chills tend to occur with staphylococcal disease or pneumonia due to group A streptococci. With *M. pneumoniae* infection, there often is a much more gradual onset with a longer prodromal respiratory phase and very prominent headache, malaise, and nonproductive cough, which gradually gives way to a productive cough. The chest pain associated with viral or *Mycoplasma* pneumonia often is more of a chest tightness or a substernal discomfort that follows an episode of coughing. In the case of Legionnaire's pneumonia, severe malaise, myalgias, headache, and diarrhea may precede the pulmonary symptoms. The individual may be markedly dehydrated or is neutropenic, and there may be no purulence to the sputum. Hemoptysis is frequently present in patients with *K. pneumoniae* or pneumonia due to *S. aureus* but can occur in pneumonia due to other organisms as well. Characteristically, the sputum of patients with pneumonia is reported to be blood-streaked to rusty. Putrid and foul smelling sputum would be more characteristic of anaerobic bacteria, either alone or in combination with aerobic strains. However, some anaerobic organisms, particularly microaerophilic organisms, do not produce a pneumonia that causes a purulent sputum.

The clinical manifestations of pneumonia in the hospitalized patient may be quite different. The classic signs and symptoms of fever, cough, sputum production, tachypnea, and altered breath sounds (rales) may not develop. Elderly or severely ill patients may be unable to produce sputum and often have no fever. Many hospitalized patients who develop nosocomial pneumonia have no specific signs that localize the infection to the chest when they develop a fever.

PHYSICAL FINDINGS

Most patients with pneumonia have significant tachypnea, and some will have splinting of the chest in an effort to decrease pain caused by pleuritic friction. There may be a pulse-temperature deficit; the pulse should increase by 10 beats per degree Celsius except in viral, *Mycoplasma,* early Legionnaire's and psittacosis pneumonia. Hypothermia may occur in pneumonia, especially in the elderly patient. Percussion and auscultation of the chest frequently reveal signs of consolidation in individuals with pneumococcal pneumonia. Egophony, dullness to percussion, and increased vocal and tactile fremitus may be noted. If there is a pleural effusion, there will be suppression of breath sounds and dullness to percussion over the area of the effusion. Pulmonary consolidation may be absent in pneumonia due to *S. aureus* and is infrequent at the onset of pneumonia due to *L. pneumophila*. Patients with *Mycoplasma* pneumonia may not have any significant oscillatory signs. Examination of the teeth and gingiva combined with a history of alcohol use may suggest that aspiration has occurred. Examination of the heart with the presence of murmurs and cutaneous signs indicating present or former drug use would suggest staphylococci (see Chapter 222). There may be abdominal distention due to ileus in severe pneumonia involving the lower lobes. An altered mental status suggests complications such as meningitis or hypoxemia.

DIAGNOSTIC STUDIES

Examination of sputum material and a chest radiograph are essential to determine the presence of pneumonia and may aid in suggesting an etiologic agent. It is critical to attempt to obtain a good sputum sample. Freshly expectorated sputum should be carefully Gram stained, and the morphology of the microorganisms associated with the polymorphonuclear cells determined (see Chapter 226). The presence of more than five squamous cells per high power field indicates that the specimen is inadequate and represents primarily oral pharyngeal contamination. Adequate sputum specimens representing lower respiratory tract infection will contain polymorphonuclear cells, provided the patient is not neutropenic, and occasionally alveolar macrophages, but rarely squamous epithelial cells. If the patient is not producing sputum, attempts should be made to induce sputum through the use of ultrasonic nebulization of saline. This approach stimulates the patient to cough and should produce adequate material.

If more than 10 gram-positive diplococci are found in a microscopic high power field (× 1,000), the specificity of the diagnosis of pneumococcal pneumonia is approximately 85%, with a sensitivity of 60% (Plate V-26). Use of pneumococcal antiserum can improve the Gram stain correlation to approximately 90% if refractile halos are seen around organisms, a Quellung reaction (Plate V-3). *H. influenzae* are small gram-negative coccal bacillary forms that stain variably and sometimes are difficult to recognize in the red background of the Gram stain (Plate V-5). Staphylococci will be identified as clusters of gram-positive organisms (Plate V-4), and *M. catarrhalis* will be seen as small gram-negative rods. The presence of large gram-negative rods would suggest organisms such as *K. pneumoniae,* other members of the Enterobacteriaceae, or *P. aeruginosa* (Plate V-6). Specific fluorescent stains are available to identify *L. pneumophila*. Expectorated sputum from patients with aspiration anaerobic pneumonia will show a mixture of gram-positive cocci and gram-negative, bizarre-shaped bacilli (Plate V-7).

Examination of sputum for the presence of gram-negative bacteria may not be helpful in many hospital-acquired pneumonias, as it will not be possible to distinguish between colonization and pneumonia. The presence of elastin fibers demonstrated by hydroxide preparation of tracheal aspirates in intubated patients has correlated with the presence of nosocomial pneumonia.

Several other techniques are available to obtain sputum samples. Transtracheal aspiration, that is, aspiration through a puncture of the cricothyroid membrane, will in most situations bypass oral pharyngeal contamination. It may be of less value in individuals who have received antibiotics, patients with chronic bronchitis, or patients with bronchogenic carcinoma. Transtracheal aspiration is infrequently performed today and should be considered only if it can be performed by an experienced operator and if the patient is highly cooperative and has no underlying thrombocytopenia or other coagulation disorder. Potential complications of transtracheal aspiration include hemoptysis, soft tissue infection, subcutaneous and mediastinal emphysema, bradyarrhythmias, aspiration, bleeding, asphyxiation, and severe hypoxemia.

Nasal tracheal aspiration frequently results in contamination of the specimen with saliva (oral flora) as the catheter passes through the nasal pharynx. The use of fiberoptic bronchoscopy with bronchoalveolar lavage and use of a protected brush catheter has resulted in excellent specimens and provides a very small risk to the patient. The cost of such a procedure, however, is significant and should only be considered in patients in whom a diagnosis cannot be made by other means. Bronchoscopy may be particularly useful to exclude endobronchial obstruction in patients with unresponsive or recurrent pneumonia that is due to aspiration.

Transthoracic lung aspiration can be performed under radiologic guidance through CT for discrete lung infiltrates. It should be considered in patients who have failed to respond to therapy or in whom unusual organisms are suggested. Transthoracic lung aspiration may produce a pneumothorax, especially if the lung is not consolidated.

Pleural effusions are common in bacterial pneumonia. Sterile, purulent, exudative collections complicate anywhere from 10% to 50% of cases of pneumococcal pneumonia. Small effusions are encountered in 20% to 25% of pneumonias due to *M. pneumoniae* and in up to 90% of pneumonias due to *S. pyogenes*. Pleural effusions are found in 15% to 40% of patients with pneumonia due to *L. pneumophila*. Any pleural effusion should be aspirated and the fluid Gram stained, cultured, and examined for cell count, glucose, protein, lactate dehydrogenase, and pH. Effusions with a pH <7.2 should be completely drained via a chest tube to avoid entrapment of the lung and other inflammatory complications (see Chapter 218).

Blood cultures should be obtained in patients with acute bacterial pneumonia. Approximately 25% of patients with pneumococcal pneumonia will have a positive blood culture, and 80% of the patients with AIDS and who have pneumococcal pneumonia have positive blood cultures. It is rare for pneumonia due to anaerobic organisms or to *Haemophilus* or *Moraxella* to yield positive blood cultures. Blood cultures also are infrequently positive in hospital-acquired pneumonia (<20%); nonetheless it is appropriate to obtain a blood culture.

Other tests that may aid in the diagnosis of pneumonia are the use of latex agglutination or counter immunoelectrophoresis tests to detect specific microbial antigens in blood, urine, sputum, pleural fluid, or other body fluids. These tests can detect pneumococcal antigens. Cold agglutinin tests may be useful in patients with *M. pneumoniae* infection. Specific DNA probes are available to detect *Mycoplasma* and *Legionella* from sputum samples. However, these tests are fairly expensive and the yield has been variable. Serologic studies to diagnose pneumonia usually are not helpful except retrospectively, as it will take several weeks for most tests to become positive.

RADIOGRAPHIC STUDIES

Posteroanterior and lateral chest radiographs should be obtained. It is important to realize that the extent of the pneumonia or the type of configuration seen on an x-ray film may not provide a specific diagnosis. However, lobar consolidation cavitation, large pleural effusions, and bronchopulmonary involvement may suggest a particular bacteria or other etiology. Pneumonia due to pneumococci most often produces lower lobe consolidation. Cavitation is rare unless the pneumonia is due to type 3 pneumococcus.

A number of different radiographic patterns, including patchy bronchopneumonia or even interstitial infiltrates, particularly in patients with underlying chronic pulmonary disease or congestive failure, are caused by pneumococcal pneumonia. Cavitation in the lung is seen most often with anaerobic pneumonia or with aerobic gram-negative bacilli. However, organisms such as *S. aureus, Nocardia asteroides,* and *Mycobacterium tuberculosis* also cause cavitary disease. Staphylococcal pneumonia may be multilobar and patchy or may produce pneumoatoceles, empyema, or cavitation. Anaerobic pneumonia occurs in the dependent portions of the lung, such as the basilar or superior segments of the lower lobes or the posterior sections of the upper lobes. Pneumonia caused by *H. influenzae* often is multilobar without cavitation. *S. pyogenes* produces a lower lobe pneumonia with early formation of large effusions. *M. pneumoniae* often produces a lower lobe or perihilar infiltrate of a patchy nature, although lobar consolidation has been noted. The x-ray findings in *Mycoplasma* pneumonia frequently are much more impressive than are the physical findings on auscultation of the chest. *Mycoplasma, P. carinii,* and viruses such as adenovirus often cause inflammation of alveoli which leads to a reticular radiographic appearance. The association of hilar adenopathy with pneumonia may suggest tuberculosis, fungal infection, or associated malignancy. It is important to realize that pulmonary emboli with infarction, neoplasms, and congestive heart failure can produce a radiographic appearance, suggestive of pneumonia (see box below).

Conditions that mimic hospital-acquired pneumonia

- Congestive heart failure
- Pulmonary infarction
- Atelectasis without infection
- Pulmonary contusion and hematoma
- Sympathetic effusion from intra-abdominal infection, surgery, pancreatitis, etc.

OTHER LABORATORY TESTS

The white blood cell count is elevated in the majority of patients with community-acquired bacterial pneumonias and exceeds 10,000/mm^3. In approximately 25% of *Mycoplasma* pneumonias, there will be a leukocytosis. Elderly individuals with community-acquired pneumonia, particularly when acquired in the hospital, may not develop leukocytosis similar to their failure to develop a fever. There may be hyperbilirubinemia, particularly in patients with severe pneumococcal pneumonia and moderate elevations of serum transaminase values. Hematuria, elevated serum creatinine phosphokinase, hyponatremia, and hypophosphatemia occur fairly frequently in patients with pneumonia due to *Legionella* species.

TREATMENT

The first aspect of treatment of pneumonia is the decision whether the patient requires hospitalization and parenteral therapy, or whether it is possible to treat the pneumonia on an outpatient basis (see accompanying box). Whenever respiratory insufficiency compromise is suspected, blood gas determinations should be made. Physical findings will often not adequately predict the degree of hypoxemia or hypercapnia. The severity of the hypoxemia may be disproportionate to the size of the infiltrate. Pneumonia will produce a mild hypoxemia associated with respiratory alkalosis due to ventilation-perfusion mismatching.

In many situations, particularly in hospital-acquired pneumonia, therapy is initiated before a definitive diagnosis is made. Antibiotic therapy should be based on the history, physical findings, chest radiographic appearance, and examination of the sputum. It is not cost-effective or helpful to obtain daily sputum samples in hospitalized patients who have an endotracheal tube or who have a tracheostomy in anticipation of developing infection. Knowledge of organisms that have caused pneumonia in other patients in an ICU or what bacteria have been isolated in wounds or urinary tract infections in patients in a multibedded room may be helpful in selecting the most appropriate antimicrobial agent(s).

Indications for hospitalization for pneumonia

Old age
Shock, dehydration
Vomiting, requirement for parenteral therapy
Multilobar disease
Low white blood cell count
PO_2<55 mm Hg
Respiratory acidosis
Significant concomitant disease
Uncertain etiology
Suspected extrapulmonary complications (empyema, pericarditis, endocarditis, meningitis, peritonitis, arthritis)

ANTIMICROBIAL THERAPY

The choice of antimicrobial therapeutic treatment of pneumonia depends on a number of different factors: the patient's age, immune status, underlying medical conditions, and allergies, as well as the seriousness of the infection and the etiologic agent suspected. Initial antimicrobial therapy should be specific, realizing that in many situations it will be necessary to use antimicrobial agents that would inhibit a number of different microorganisms. Therapy for a short time with antimicrobial drugs that inhibit many different bacteria will not result in the selection of resistant organisms. Antimicrobial therapy can be adjusted to specific narrow-spectrum agents once the results of cultures and antimicrobial susceptibility tests are available (Table 231-5).

Pneumonia thought to be due to *S. pneumoniae* that does not require hospitalization can be treated with penicillin orally, or in the penicillin-allergic patient, an oral cephalosporin or erythromycin. More critically ill patients who require hospitalization, in view of the increasing relative resistance of *S. pneumoniae* to penicillin, should be treated with a second- or third-generation cephalosporin such as cefuroxime 750 mg intravenously every 8 hours, cefotaxime 1 g intravenously every 8 hours, or ceftriaxone 2 g once a day. This approach provides therapy not only for *S. pneumoniae* but for *Haemophilus* species and *S. aureus* as well. Such a program does not provide antimicrobial activity against Legionella or *M. pneumoniae*. When these organisms are suspected, use of a macrolide, erythromycin, would be appropriate. The newer macrolides, clarithromycin and azithromycin, have increased activity against *Haemophilus* species and as a result could be used in therapy of outpatient pneumonia caused by *S. pneumoniae, L. pneumophila, M. pneumoniae,* or *C. pneumoniae*. Adults in whom one suspects that the pneumonia could be due to *K. pneumoniae,* on the basis of seeing large gram-negative bacilli in the sputum, would appropriately be treated with a third-generation cephalosporin.

Aspiration pneumonia due to mouth anaerobic species occurring in the community will respond to penicillin, although many studies have suggested that use of an agent such as clindamycin may be more appropriate due to the presence of beta-lactamases in the oral *Bacteroides* species. A penicillin beta-lactamase inhibitor combination, such as ampicillin/sulbactam, or oral therapy with amoxicillin-clavulanate would also be appropriate for aspiration pneumonitis due to anaerobic mouth flora and in addition would provide activity against *Klebsiella* organisms.

In the treatment of hospital-acquired pneumonia, it is useful to make an initial appraisal whether the patient could have a *P. aeruginosa* pneumonia or whether *S. aureus* is present (Table 231-6). A Gram stain is helpful with regard to staphylococci, but will not differentiate *Pseudomonas* from the members of the Enterobacteriaceae. The antibiotics traditionally used in treatment of pneumonia in the hospital were an aminoglycoside combined with a penicillin or cephalosporin. The pH of the infected lung is acidic in the range of approximately 6.4, and bronchi are filled with

Table 231-5. Treatment of community-acquired pneumonia

Cause	Primary antibiotic	Alternative antibiotic
S. pneumoniae	Hospitalized cefuroxime 750 mg q12h penicillin V, 500 mg qid po until afebrile for 4 d	Erythromycin, 500 mg po or IV q6h, or cefotaxime or ceftriaxone
Aerobic gram-negative bacilli		
H. influenzae	Cefuroxime or a third-generation cephalosporin for 10-14 days (switch to ampicillin if sensitive)	Trimethoprim-sulfamethoxazole (see below) Fluoroquinolone
S. aureus	Nafcillin or oxacillin, 2 g IV q1 to 6h for 14 days	Vancomycin, 1 g IV q12h
S. pyogenes	Aqueous procaine penicillin G, 600,000 U IM q12h until afebrile for 3 days then penicillin V, 500 mg po qid for 2-3 wk	Erythromycin 500 mg po or IV q6h, or a cephalosporin
Necrotizing pneumonia or lung abscess	Clindamycin, 600 mg IV q8h until afebrile, then 300 mg po q8h; penicillin G, 10-20 million U/d IV until response, then penicillin V, 500-750 mg qid for 6-12 wk	Cefoxitin, 2 g IV q6h
M. pneumoniae	Erythromycin, 250-500 mg po q6h for 10-14 days, clarithromycin, 500 mg po q12h, or azithromycin, 250 mg po qd for 10 d	Tetracycline, 250-500 mg po q6h
L. pneumophila	Erythromycin, 1 g IV q6h until afebrile for 48 h, then 500 mg po q6h for total 3 wk or Rifampin 600 mg po qd for severely ill	Ciprofloxacin, 750 mg po q12h or Ofloxacin, 400 mg po q12h
P. carinii	Trimethoprim-sulfamethoxazole, 20 mg trimethoprim/100 mg sulfamethoxazole/kg/d IV in four divided doses daily, or pentamidine 4 mg/kg/day IV	Trimethoprim plus dapsone

Table 231-6. Therapeutic choices for gram-negative bacillary pneumonias

Organism	Drugs of choice	Combination therapy	Alternative therapies
Acinetobacter anitratus	Imipenem	Tobramycin	Timentin, ampicillin/sulbactam
Citrobacter sp.	Aminothiazolyl cephalosporin		Aztreonam, imipenem
Enterobacter sp.	Imipenem	Gentamicin or amikacin	TMP-SMX
E. coli	Aminothiazolyl cephalosporin		Aztreonam, imipenem
H. influenzae	Aminothiazolyl cephalosporin		Aztreonam
K. pneumoniae or *K. oxytoca*	Aminothiazolyl cephalosporin		Aztreonam, imipenem
Providencia sp.	Aminothiazolyl cephalosporin		Aztreonam
Proteus mirabilis	Aztreonam		Aminothiazolyl cephalosporin
P. aeruginosa	Antipseudomonas penicillin, aztreonam, ceftazidime, or imipenem	Tobramycin or amikacin	Ciprofloxacin
P. cepacia	Ceftazidime or TMP-SMX		
X. maltophilia	TMP-SMX		Timentin
Serratia marcescens	Ceftazidime or aztreonam	Gentamicin or amikacin	TMP-SMX imipenem

Aminothiazolyl cephalosporin, cefotaxime, ceftizoxime, ceftazidime, or cefoperazone; TMP-SMX, trimethoprim-sulfamethoxazole; Antipseudomonas penicillins, azlocillin, piperacillin, ticarcillin.

white cells and cellular debris. These factors markedly reduce the activity of aminoglycosides.

Extended spectrum penicillins, cephalosporins, aztreonam, or imipenem, should be the choice for initial therapy of hospital-acquired pneumonia. If an agent such as aztreonam is used, it is necessary to add clindamycin as aztreonam does not inhibit gram-positive or anaerobic species. It is not established whether an aminoglycoside should routinely be combined with an antipseudomonas cephalosporin or with an antipseudomonas penicillin when treating *Pseudomonas* infection of the lung. Such a program has been advocated to reduce more rapidly the number of infecting organisms, thereby decreasing lung destruction and preventing the emergence of resistance to the beta-lactamase agent.

In general, two agents would be used in treating bacteremic gram-negative pneumonia acquired in the hospital, as the mortality rate in this illness exceeds 50%. *S. aureus* pneumonia should be treated with antistaphylococcal penicillin such as oxacillin and nafcillin or with a first-generation cephalosporin if the patient is allergic to penicillin. Methicillin-resistant *S. aureus* would be treated with vancomycin or teicoplanin.

Most community-acquired pneumonia will be adequately

treated with 7 days of therapy. In contrast, nosocomial pneumonia usually requires 2 to 3 weeks of therapy and *S. aureus* pneumonia should always be treated for at least 3 weeks. It has been suggested that pneumonia due to *M. pneumoniae* or *C. pneumoniae* be treated for a minimum of 2 weeks and preferably for 3 weeks.

In a number of situations in which pneumonia is due to gram-negative organisms, it is now possible to initiate oral therapy at an earlier period using one of the fluoroquinolones such as ciprofloxacin or ofloxacin. After 5 to 7 days of parenteral therapy, many patients could be treated with one of these agents twice a day.

Aerosolization of antimicrobial agents has been tried as a means to deliver more antibiotic in patients with hospital-acquired pneumonia. In general approach this has not proved successful, but with new aerosol equipment may be feasible for the aminoglycosides.

SUPPORTIVE TREATMENT

It is extremely important to provide supplemental oxygen to hospitalized patients to provide a Pao_2 of more than 60 mm Hg and to correct any acid-base disorder or electrolyte disorders, as well as hypovolemia. Chest physiotherapy and postular drainage may be useful in mobilizing secretions but probably are unimportant in uncomplicated cases of pneumonia. Chest radiographs should be used to follow the progression of pneumonia and detect worsening or improvement in the patient with hospital-acquired pneumonia, but are frequently not necessary in uncomplicated community-acquired pneumonia, as it may take up to 3 to 4 weeks to achieve full resolution of a pulmonary infiltrate. Failure of the patient to become afebrile and show a decrease in a white cell count and improvement of blood gases should prompt repeat radiography to eliminate possible obstruction by secretions or the presence of a large pleural effusion, which needs to be drained. In many patients it may be necessary to provide tracheal intubation to achieve adequate ventilation and to provide removal of inspissated secretions.

COMPLICATIONS

Unfortunately, significant mortality is associated with pneumococcal pneumonia, particularly in the elderly with underlying bacteremia and multilobar disease. Mortality rates associated with pneumococcal disease have not changed over the past 30 years in spite of major advances in antimicrobial therapy and significant advances in intensive care support. The mortality rate in aerobic gram-negative bacteremia pneumonia is as high as 50%, primarily due to the underlying disease of the patient. The exact mortality in pneumonia due to *Legionella* species is unknown, but it probably approaches 15%. Pneumonia may result in meningitis, pericarditis, or septic arthritis, depending on the organism involved. Although pneumococcal pneumonia shows a rapid response in otherwise fairly healthy individuals, the response may be delayed, and in the elderly fever may remain for as long as a week. This delay is important to remember, as there may be a tendency to change therapy inappropriately. The indiscriminant addition of broad-spectrum antibiotics to treat pneumonia should be avoided.

PREVENTION

A 23-capsular-type polyvalent pneumococcal vaccine is currently available. Recommendations for its use include adults with chronic respiratory illness, cardiopulmonary disease, and illnesses specifically associated with an increased risk of pneumococcal disease such as splenic dysfunction and anatomic asplenia. Unvaccinated patients admitted to a hospital with pneumonia should receive vaccination before they are discharged. Patients who have received the 14-valent vaccine should not be revaccinated with the 23-valent vaccine. In addition, individuals at risk to develop pneumonia should receive an influenza vaccine annually in the fall to prevent influenza, which is a precursor of pneumonia in many patients.

Prevention of hospital-acquired pneumonia remains a difficult problem. Avoidance of excessive use of H_2-blocking agents in patients who are intubated to avoid colonization of the gastric tract with gram-negative organisms has been suggested. Antimicrobial prophylaxis of patients with oral and/or parenteral antibiotics in an ICU has been shown to be effective only in patients who have undergone recent traumatic injury. Patients who smoke should be strongly encouraged to stop smoking before entering the hospital for elective surgical procedures. Patients with viral respiratory infections should not undergo elective surgery for at least 3 weeks after the viral respiratory infection, as it takes this long for small bronchial function and ciliary clearance to return to normal.

The following recommendations are made to reduce hospital pneumonia:

1. Mainstream humidifiers are safer than nebulizers, as the latter create small droplets capable of carrying organisms to the alveoli.
2. Management of the tracheal cuff, with particular attention to balloon pressure, to prevent deflation may minimize the risk of aspiration and subsequent pneumonia.
3. All medications and diluents for respiratory therapy should be in small-volume, sterile-unit dose.
4. Respiratory equipment should be sterilized before use, and tubing should be changed every 24 hours during the initial phase of the illness and every 48 hours when secretions have diminished.
5. Tracheostomy should be an elective procedure under aseptic conditions. Careful attention to postoperative wound care is critical, and inner cannular tubes should be changed frequently if secretions are profuse.
6. Patients on respirators should be properly suctioned to maintain a clear airway. Gloves must always be worn to prevent cross-contamination of patients. Additional measures to minimize the collection of secretions are adequate humidification, rotation of the patient from side to side, and physical therapy.
7. Proper hand washing to minimize cross infection is

essential. Nurse/patient ratios of 1 : 1 are optimal in ICUs.

8. Use of filters on inspired or expired air is not necessary, as there is no evidence that inspired oxygen leads to infection. Transmission from the ventilator surface is not a problem, but the surfaces of ventilators used on patients infected with *S. aureus* and multiply-resistant, gram-negative bacteria should be cleaned before use on another patient.

REFERENCES

Broughton WA et al: Bronchscopic protected specimen brush and bronchoalveolar lavage in the diagnosis of bacterial pneumonia, Infect Dis Clin North Am 5:437-452, 1991.

Bryan CS et al: Bacteremic nosocomial pneumonia, Am Rev Respir Dis 129:668, 1984.

Cohn DL: Bacterial pneumonia in the HIV-infected patient, Infect Dis Clin North Am 5:485-507, 1991.

Craven DE et al: Risk factors for pneumonia and fatality in patients receiving continuous mechanical ventilation, Am Rev Respir Dis 133:792, 1986.

Craven DE et al: Nosocomial pneumonia in the intubated patient, Semin Respir Infect 2:20, 1987.

Fang GD et al: New and emerging etiologies for community-acquired pneumonia with implications for therapy, Medicine 69:307-314, 1990.

Fine MJ et al: Prognosis of patients hospitalized with community-acquired pneumonia, Am J Med 88:1N-6N, 1990.

Fine MJ, Smith DN, and Singer DE: Hospitalization decision in patients with community-acquired pneumonia: a prospective cohort study, Am J Med 89:713-721, 1990.

Gross PA et al: Deaths from nosocomial infections: experience in a university hospital and a community hospital, Am J Med 68:219, 1980.

Johanson WG Jr et al: Bacteriologic diagnosis of nosocomial pneumonia following prolonged mechanical ventilation, Am Rev Respir Dis 137:259, 1988.

Johanson WG et al: Prevention of nosocomial pneumonia using topical and parenteral microbial agents, Am Rev Respir Dis 137:265, 1988.

Levison ME et al: Clindamycin compared with penicillin for treatment of anaerobic lung abscess, Ann Intern Med 98:466, 1983.

Macfarlane JT et al: Hospital study of adult community-acquired pneumonia, Lancet 2:255, 1982.

MacFarlane JT et al: Prospective study of aetiology and outcome of adult lower-respiratory tract infections in the community, Lancet 341:511, 1993.

Mansel JK et al: *Mycoplasma pneumoniae* pneumonia, Chest 95:639, 1989.

Martin LF et al: Post-operative pneumonia: determinants of mortality, Arch Surg 119:379, 1984.

Piefenthal HC and Tashijian J: The role of plain films, CT, tomography, ultrasound, and percutaneous needle aspiration in the diagnosis of inflammatory lung disease, Semin Respir Dis 3:83, 1988.

Salata RA et al: Diagnosis of nosocomial pneumonia in intubated, intensive care patients, Am Rev Respir Dis 135:426, 1987.

Verghese A and Berk SL: Bacterial pneumonia in the elderly, Medicine (Baltimore) 62:271, 1983.

Verghese A and Berk SL: *Moraxella* (Branhamella) *catarrhalis*, Infect Dis Clin North Am 5:523-538, 1991.

Williams WW et al: Immunization policies and vaccine coverage among adults, Ann Intern Med 108:616, 1988.

CHAPTER

232 Intra-Abdominal Infections

Matthew E. Levison

Intra-abdominal infection due to bacteria and fungi may take several forms. Infection may be in the retroperitoneal space or within the peritoneal cavity. Intraperitoneal infection may be diffuse or localized in one or more abscesses. Intraperitoneal abscesses may form in dependent recesses, such as the pelvic space or pouch of Morison, in the various perihepatic spaces, within the lesser sac, and along the major routes of communication between intraperitoneal recesses, such as the right paracolic gutter. Abscesses also often form about diseased viscera—pericholecystic, periappendiceal, pericolic, and tubo-ovarian—and between adjacent loops of bowel (i.e., interloop abscesses). In addition, infection may be contained within the intra-abdominal viscera, such as in hepatic, pancreatic, splenic, or renal abscesses.

Intraperitoneal infection has been divided into two categories: primary, in which an intra-abdominal source is not clinically evident, and secondary, in which an intra-abdominal source is evident. Secondary intraperitoneal infection is far more common than the primary variety.

PRIMARY INTRAPERITONEAL INFECTION

Pathogenesis

Primary peritonitis usually is seen in children with nephrosis or adults with cirrhosis. The presence of ascites appears to be the common feature among the various underlying conditions associated with primary peritonitis. The route of infection in primary peritonitis is presumed to be hematogenous, lymphogenous, or transmural migration through an intact gut wall from the intestinal lumen or the lumen of the fallopian tubes from the vagina. The hematogenous route is most likely in patients with cirrhosis, as the reticuloendothelial system of the liver is known to be normally a major site for removal and destruction of bacteria from blood. The transmural migration of bacteria is the probable route of infection in the majority of patients with anaerobic primary peritonitis.

A single species of bacteria is usually isolated. The organisms that most commonly cause primary peritonitis in children are *Streptococcus pneumoniae* and group A streptococci, followed in frequency by gram-negative enteric bacilli. In cirrhotic patients, enteric organisms, especially *Escherichia coli,* account for up to 69% of the pathogens, followed by streptococci (e.g., *S. pneumoniae* and group A streptococci) and anaerobes.

Other causes of primary peritonitis include *Neisseria gonorrhoeae, Chlamydia trachomatis,* and *Mycobacterium tuberculosis*. Gonococcal or chlamydial perihepatitis (Fitz-Hugh-Curtis syndrome) may develop in women, presumably from asymptomatic infection of the fallopian tubes that spreads from the pelvic space along the right paracolic gutter to the perihepatic space. Tuberculous peritonitis may result from the direct entry into the peritoneal cavity of tubercle bacilli from the lymph nodes, intestines, or genital tract or via hematogenous dissemination from remote foci.

Clinical manifestations

Primary peritonitis occurs at all ages. In the preantibiotic era, it accounted for about 10% of all pediatric abdominal emergencies but now is responsible for less than 1% to 2%. Primary peritonitis in children usually accompanies postnecrotic cirrhosis or the nephrotic syndrome. It may precede other manifestations of nephrosis, and repeated episodes may occur. Primary peritonitis may present as an acute febrile illness that is often confused with appendicitis. In adults, primary peritonitis occurs in about 10% of those presenting with cirrhosis and ascites. The onset may be insidious, and findings of peritoneal irritation may be absent in an abdomen distended with ascites. Indeed, ascitic fluid with a positive culture, but few leukocytes, has been noted in patients without clinical findings of peritonitis (so-called bacterascites) and may represent early infection of the peritoneum, before a host response. Primary peritonitis in cirrhotic patients is generally associated with other features of end-stage liver disease (hepatorenal syndrome, progressive encephalopathy, variceal bleeding).

Gonococcal or chlamydial perihepatitis most often occurs in women and simulates acute cholecystitis. It presents with the sudden onset of pain in the right upper quadrant of the abdomen; at times, the pain is referred to the right shoulder. There may be low-grade fever, right upper quadrant tenderness, guarding, and a friction rub over the liver. In patients with primary gonococcal or chlamydial peritonitis, the source would not be clinically evident, but in other patients the peritonitis may be secondary to clinically apparent uterine cervicitis and/or salpingitis.

Primary tuberculous peritonitis usually is gradual in onset, with fever, weight loss, malaise, night sweats, and abdominal distention. The abdomen may not be rigid and is often characterized as being "doughy" on palpation.

SECONDARY INTRAPERITONEAL INFECTION

Pathogenesis

Secondary intraperitoneal infection may occur as a result of any one of a variety of primary intra-abdominal processes (see the accompanying box). Most have in common contamination of the peritoneal cavity with organisms that normally reside on the mucosal surfaces of the gastrointestinal tract or vagina. The resultant infection is usually polymicrobial, and the composition reflects the predominantly anaerobic mucosal microflora at these sites.

The surface microflora of the digestive tract varies quantitatively and qualitatively from region to region along its length and is different again from that of the vagina. For example, the gingival crevice in the oral cavity has an enormous microflora, with over 100 different species in total numbers of 10^{11} to 10^{12} organisms per gram. (By way of comparison, a colony of solid-packed bacteria on the surface of an agar plate has a density of 10^{12} organisms per gram.) Obligate anaerobes outnumber the aerobes in the gingival crevice.

Primary intra-abdominal processes leading to peritonitis

- Perforation of peptic ulcer
- Traumatic perforation of uterus, urinary bladder, stomach, bowel
- Spontaneous bowel perforation (typhoid, tuberculosis, amebic or *Strongyloides* ulcers)
- Appendicitis, diverticulitis
- Intestinal neoplasms
- Gangrene of bowel (strangulation, obstruction, vascular insufficiency)
- Suppurative cholecystitis
- Bile peritonitis
- Pancreatitis
- Operative contamination or disruption of surgical anastomosis
- Female genital abnormalities (septic abortion, puerperal sepsis, postoperative uterine infection, endometritis from IUD, nongonococcal salpingitis, etc.)
- Suppurative prostatitis
- Rupture of any intraperitoneal abscesses
- Chronic ambulatory peritoneal dialysis
- Peritoneovenous and ventriculoperitoneal shunts

The stomach, due to its acidity, normally has a sparse flora (less than 10^3 organisms/ml), which consists of the more acid-tolerant species of mouth organisms such as lactobacilli and yeast. In the presence of achlorhydria or gastric obstruction, however, an abundant flora may be in the stomach that is derived from the oral cavity or from contaminated food or water.

Similarly, few organisms normally inhabit the upper small bowel, but in the presence of slowing of small bowel motility (as occurs in scleroderma), small bowel obstruction (as may occur in Crohn's disease), blind loops, diverticula, and gastric achlorhydria or gastric obstruction, an abundant flora may be present in the small bowel. Patients with cirrhosis, intestinal pseudo-obstruction, gastrocolic or jejunocolic fistula, immunoglobulin deficiencies, or malnutrition and some elderly patients with malabsorption also may have more than normal numbers of bacteria in the small bowel.

Members of the large bowel flora may be found in the terminal ileum in counts of 10^6 to 10^7 per milliliter, but only in the relatively stagnant large bowel is an enormous, predominantly anaerobic microflora normally present. The colonic microflora is similar in density (10^{11} to 10^{12} per gram) and complexity (over 200 different species) to that of the gingival crevice; however, the species differ at the two sites. For example, the oral microflora contains bile-sensitive *Bacteroides* species (the *Bacteroides melanino-*

genicus group: *B. melaninogenicus, B. intermedius, B. asaccharolyticus*), whereas the colonic microflora contains bile-resistant *Bacteroides* species (the *Bacteroides fragilis* group: *B. fragilis, B. thetaiotaomicron, B. vulgatus, B. distasonis,* and *B. ovatus*). *Clostridium perfringens,* another important pathogen, is not normally isolated from the mouth, stomach, or small bowel, but is usually found in the fecal flora. The predominant aerobes in colonic flora include *E. coli* and enterococci, which are usually not found in the oral microflora. The large bowel flora is relatively stable but may be altered by antibiotic therapy.

The vaginal microflora is much less dense (10^7 to 10^8 organisms/ml) and less complex than the oral or colonic flora. It consists predominantly of anaerobic lactobacilli and to a lesser extent of non-*fragilis* species of *Bacteroides*. As with the gingival crevice flora, the vaginal flora is normally characterized by the absence of *B. fragilis, E. coli,* and enterococci in large numbers. However, the vaginal microflora may resemble that of the colon in certain circumstances, such as soon after gynecologic surgery.

Not all members of the microflora are found in an established intra-abdominal infection. The extremely oxygen-sensitive components of the anaerobic flora do not seem to be as pathogenic as the relatively aerotolerant anaerobes (e.g., *B. fragilis* and *B. melaninogenicus*), which are encapsulated by a surface polysaccharide, their presumed virulence factor. These two *Bacteroides* species, together with *Fusobacterium nucleatum,* various anaerobic gram-positive cocci (including *Streptococcus milleri*), and *C. perfringens,* account for over 80% of anaerobic isolates. As part of the polymicrobial flora characteristic of established infection, the facultative anaerobic copathogens include *E. coli* and enterococci, especially when the intra-abdominal infection is of colonic origin. Together with highly antibiotic-resistant strains of enteric gram-negative bacilli, *Pseudomonas aeruginosa* is more frequently isolated from patients who develop their intra-abdominal infection while in the hospital, after having received broad-spectrum parenteral antimicrobials. However, recent studies have noted *P. aeruginosa* to compose a more significant portion of the aerobic isolates in community-acquired intra-abdominal infection than had been noted previously. Anaerobic gram-positive cocci, *B. melaninogenicus, B. disiens,* and *B. bivius,* are found more frequently than *B. fragilis, E. coli,* and enterococci in intra-abdominal infections of gynecologic origin, as would be predicted from the composition of normal vaginal flora. These anaerobes may be found with or without *N. gonorrhoeae*. However, *B. fragilis* may be a more common pathogen when a tubo-ovarian abscess is present.

Peritonitis that occurs in patients receiving chronic ambulatory peritoneal dialysis is usually due to contamination of the catheter with skin microflora, since gram-positive organisms (most commonly *Staphylococcus epidermidis,* followed by *Staphylococcus aureus, Streptococcus* species, and diphtheroids) constitute 60% to 80% of isolates. Gram-negative organisms account for 15% to 30% of isolates, in which case, enteric bacteria presumably gained access to the peritoneal cavity by transmural migration through an intact intestinal wall after the introduction of dialysis solutions into the peritoneum.

Candida peritonitis has also been observed as a complication of peritoneal dialysis, gastrointestinal surgery, or perforation of a viscus, and its occurrence in the latter two instances is related to numerous factors that increase the rate of *Candida* colonization in the gastrointestinal tract. These include immunosuppression, prolonged hospitalization, and antimicrobial and/or antacid therapy.

Endogenous infections depend primarily on defects of local host defense mechanisms that otherwise limit the invasive activities of indigenous bacteria. Disruption of the mucosal surface would allow escape of indigenous bacteria. Once in tissues beneath the epithelium, pathogenic anaerobes require low oxidation-reduction potential, low oxygen concentration, and abundant nutrients to support optimum growth. These requirements are usually met by tissue devitalized by ischemia, trauma, neoplastic growth, or previous infection with facultative organisms. In this environment, anaerobic organisms can attain growth rates similar to those seen with aerobic enteric bacilli. The rapidly expanding bacterial and inflammatory cell mass, frequently accompanied by gas production, can then interrupt blood supply to the surrounding tissue and cause further tissue necrosis. The organisms themselves possess several virulence factors, such as polysaccharide capsules, endotoxin, and the production of proteolytic enzymes and heparinase, which promote additional tissue necrosis, local spread, and hematogenous dissemination.

Each component of the pathogenic mixture of organisms may contribute in different ways to produce the clinical picture. For example, after implantation of fecal contents in rats, *E. coli* is responsible for bacteremia and early mortality, whereas *B. fragilis* is responsible for late abscess formation.

Infectious material can be spread over much of the peritoneal cavity within a short time by gravity, movement of the diaphragm, and peristaltic movement of the gastrointestinal tract. The extent and rate of intraperitoneal spread of contamination depend on the volume and nature of the exudate, the course of the primary disease process, and the effectiveness of the localizing processes. If peritoneal defenses, aided by appropriate supportive measures, control the inflammatory process, the disease may end by resolution; abscesses may develop only about diseased organs, such as the appendix or gallbladder; or an abscess may be confined in the peritoneal space, usually in the pelvis, perihepatic spaces, or right paracolic gutter. When the peritoneal and systemic defense mechanisms cannot localize the inflammation, diffuse peritonitis results.

Clinical manifestations

Peritonitis. Primary and secondary peritonitis may present clinically in an identical way, but on occasion the clinical presentation is masked either by the underlying disease in patients with primary peritonitis (e.g., hepatic encephalopathy in patients with ascites and end-stage cirrhosis) or by the primary disease process in patients with secondary peritonitis. Moderately severe abdominal pain is almost always the predominant symptom. The pain is aggravated by any motion, including respiration. The progression of abdominal pain is a function of the rate of dissemination of the material producing the pain stimulus. Rupture of a peptic ulcer, with massive spillage of gastric contents, produces catastrophic epigastric pain, which, within minutes, may spread to involve the entire abdomen. The spread of pain from a lesion such as a ruptured appendix is much more gradual. Decreased intensity and extent of pain with time usually suggests localization of the inflammatory process.

Anorexia, nausea, and vomiting commonly accompany abdominal pain. Patients may also complain of feverishness, sometimes with a chill, thirst, scanty urination, inability to pass feces or flatus, and abdominal distention.

Body temperatures may reach 106° F (41° C). Subnormal temperature in the range of 95° F (35° C) is often seen in the early stages of chemical peritonitis (e.g., bile peritonitis) and late in the course of continuing intra-abdominal sepsis or septic shock and is a grave sign.

Initially in peritonitis, there is hypermotility, which is followed by paralysis of the bowel and accumulation of fluid and electrolytes in the lumen of the adynamic bowel. Marked abdominal tenderness to palpation is present and is usually maximum over the organ in which the process originated. Rebound tenderness, both direct and referred, signifies parietal peritoneal irritation. This finding is sometimes more accurate than direct palpation in locating the point of maximum tenderness, as well as in delineating the extent of peritoneal irritation.

Muscular rigidity of the abdominal wall is produced both by voluntary guarding and by reflex muscle spasm. Hyperresonance due to gaseous intestinal distention can usually be demonstrated by percussion. Pneumoperitoneum from a ruptured hollow viscus may produce decreased liver dullness to percussion. Rectal and vaginal examination may reveal tenderness and the presence of a pelvic abscess and may indicate a primary focus in the female pelvic organs.

Abdominal muscle spasm may be deceptively absent in some patients. Those with lax abdominal musculature (e.g., patients in the postpartum period, with ascites due to cirrhosis, or with marked cachexia) may not have abdominal rigidity. Similarly, patients in shock or receiving glucocorticosteroid therapy, or in whom loculated intra-abdominal abscesses are not in contact with the anterior abdominal wall (e.g., subphrenic, lesser sac, and pelvic abscesses) may not exhibit marked abdominal wall spasm. Absent bowel sounds may be the only manifestation of peritonitis; a high index of suspicion is necessary to make a diagnosis in such patients.

Shifts of isotonic, protein-rich fluid into the peritoneal cavity as a consequence of inflammation, combined with fluid shifts into the bowel lumen, can produce a profound fall in circulating blood volume and elevation of the hematocrit. Fluid and electrolyte losses are further exaggerated by coexisting fever, vomiting, occasional diarrhea, and loss of gastrointestinal fluid via intestinal intubation. As the process continues, the decreased venous return to the right heart results in a drop in cardiac output, causing hypotension. In addition, endotoxic or bacteremic shock may develop (Chapter 239).

The intraperitoneal inflammation results in a relatively high and fixed diaphragm and considerable pain on respiration, leading to basilar atelectasis with intrapulmonary shunting of blood. In some patients, pulmonary edema develops due either to increased pulmonary capillary leakage as a consequence of hypoalbuminemia or to the direct effects of bacterial toxins (adult respiratory distress syndrome). In these patients, progressive hypoxemia develops with decreasing pulmonary compliance and requires volume-cycled ventilatory assistance with increasingly higher concentrations of inspired oxygen.

INTRAPERITONEAL ABSCESS

The clinical picture associated with the formation and progression of an intraperitoneal abscess may be acute but is often gradual: The patient who seemed to be recovering from peritonitis or an abdominal operation stops improving; fever returns, and localizing symptoms may develop. Local symptoms and signs vary widely with the location and source of the abscess. Subphrenic abscesses are usually accompanied by pleural or pulmonary involvement, whereas subhepatic abscesses have more dominant signs in the upper abdominal or subcostal area and fewer pulmonary changes.

RETROPERITONEAL ABSCESSES

Abscesses in the retroperitoneal spaces have been associated with prolonged morbidity and high mortality because of their insidious course and frequently vague clinical manifestations, which have resulted in delayed diagnosis and delayed or inadequate treatment. These infections arise most commonly from disease in organs that lie within or adjacent to one of the spaces in the retroperitoneum. Less commonly, retroperitoneal abscesses result from hematogenous dissemination of infection at a distant site.

The retroperitoneum extends from the diaphragm to the brim of the true pelvis. The lateral borders of the quadratus lumborum muscles correspond to its lateral margins. It is divided into anterior and posterior spaces by the anterior layer of the renal fascia. The anterior space contains the pancreas and retroperitoneal portions of the duodenum and colon. Abscesses in the anterior retroperitoneal space may originate, for example, from perforation of the duodenum as a result of peptic ulceration or trauma, from trauma or inflammation of the pancreas, from appendicitis, or from colonic perforation due to diverticulitis, inflammatory bowel disease, or carcinoma. The posterior retroperitoneal space contains on each side a kidney and ureter surrounded by renal fascia, and in the midline the abdominal aorta, inferior vena cava, lymphatics, and lymph nodes surrounded by renal fascia.

Infections of the abdominal aorta or suppurative lymphadenitis may be the cause of abscess in the medial portion of the posterior retroperitoneum. Pyelonephritis is the usual cause of abscesses in the perinephric space (Chapter 240).

Most retroperitoneal space infections lateralize to one side or the other, but extension across the midline can cause bilateral abscesses. Lack of an anatomic barrier inferiorly favors spread of infection downward into the pelvis.

Posterior to the retroperitoneum are the retrofascial spaces, which are occupied by the quadratus lumborum and psoas muscles. Abscesses in the retrofascial spaces arise from infection in the disk spaces or vertebral bodies or from infection in the retroperitoneum. Osteomyelitis of the lumbar spine can be associated with contiguous infection of the abdominal aorta.

The clinical course of retroperitoneal and retrofascial infection is frequently chronic. In over 50% of patients symptoms are present for more than 3 weeks before diagnosis and consist of fever, sweats, generalized malaise, cachexia, and back, flank, or hip pain, which may radiate into the legs. A tender mass may be palpable in the flank or back. Scoliosis and abdominal disturbance are less common. The thigh may be held in a flexed position and pain elicited by extension and internal rotation of the thigh, which indicates involvement of the psoas space (psoas sign). Retrofascial infection points into the groin, either above Poupart's ligament or in the inguinal region of the thigh. Infection may also extend into the pleural space, mediastinum, or peritoneal cavity. Periureteral inflammation may result in sterile pyuria.

Polymicrobial infection involving obligate and facultative anaerobes would be expected in abscesses arising from disease in the duodenum or colon, whereas single species, either *E. coli* or *S. aureus,* would be expected in abscesses secondary to either ascending or hematogenous pyelonephritis, respectively, or to vertebral osteomyelitis.

VISCERAL ABSCESSES

Liver abscess

For a discussion of liver abscess, see Chapter 62.

Splenic abscess

Pathogenesis. Splenic abscesses are uncommon lesions and are usually multiple. The multiple small abscesses usually develop as a complication of hematogenous dissemination. Splenic abscesses that develop during the course of bacterial endocarditis are usually due to *S. aureus* or streptococci. Enterobacteriaceae (e.g., *Salmonella*) and anaerobic microorganisms have also been recovered. Some are related to infection in contiguous organs and others result from infected traumatic hematomas or infarcts of the spleen (e.g., in patients with sickle cell hemoglobinopathies). Positive blood cultures have been reported in 70% of patients with multiple splenic abscesses but in only 14% with solitary abscesses. Fungal splenic abscesses, often occurring as part of the syndrome of hepatosplenic candidiasis, have been noted recently in patients predisposed to candidial infections (e.g., patients on high-dose corticosteroids or cancer chemotherapy).

Clinical manifestations. Left upper quadrant abdominal pain and fever are the usual manifestations of splenic abscesses. Irritation of the adjacent diaphragm may result in pain referred to the left shoulder. Splenic enlargement and tenderness are usually present, with high, spiking temperatures, and occasionally a splenic rub is heard. Clinical findings may be absent in some patients with multiple small splenic abscesses.

Pancreatic abscess

For a discussion of pancreatic abscess, see Chapter 67.

Pathogenesis. Pancreatic abscesses develop in about 1% to 9% of patients following acute pancreatitis, which may be either biliary, alcoholic, postsurgical, or posttraumatic in origin. A pancreatic abscess occasionally follows penetration by a peptic ulcer or as a complication of endoscopic retrograde cholangiopancreatography.

About one third to one half of pancreatic abscesses have been reported to be polymicrobial, involving mainly facultative microorganisms, such as *E. coli* and other Enterobacteriaceae, enterococci, viridans streptococci, and occasionally *S. aureus*. Modern anaerobic bacteriologic techniques have also documented the presence of anaerobes. The mixed enteric bacterial origin of many pancreatic abscesses suggests that bacteria may reach the pancreas by reflux of contaminated bile. The hematogenous route probably accounts for infections due to *S. aureus*.

Clinical manifestations. The clinical presentation of pancreatic abscesses varies. The patient may fail to respond to therapy for pancreatitis, or 1 to 3 weeks after the onset of pancreatitis, the patient's condition may deteriorate after an initial response. Nausea, vomiting, and abdominal pain that frequently radiates to the back are present in more than 80% to 90% of patients. A body temperature of more than 101° F (38.3° C) and abdominal tenderness are usually present. Less frequently, jaundice, abdominal distention, or an abdominal mass or signs of generalized peritonitis may be present. The serum amylase level is elevated in 20% to 70% of patients and may remain elevated.

ACUTE CHOLECYSTITIS AND CHOLANGITIS

For a discussion of cholecystitis and cholangitis, see Chapter 65.

DIAGNOSIS OF INTRA-ABDOMINAL INFECTION

The diagnosis of primary peritonitis is one of exclusion of a primary intra-abdominal source of infection (Chapter 44) and can be made with certainty only after a thorough laparotomy. Under certain circumstances, however, laparotomy may be avoided on the basis of an appropriate clinical setting, such as cirrhosis or nephrosis, and findings in peritoneal fluid obtained by paracentesis (e.g., if gram-positive organisms are found, a diagnosis of primary peritonitis can usually be made and exploratory laparotomy deferred). In children, if gram-negative organisms, a mixed flora, or no organisms are obtained, full exploratory laparotomy is indicated to rule out possible intra-abdominal sources of peritoneal contamination. In patients with end-stage cirrhosis, exploratory laparotomy may be very life-threatening, and the likelihood of finding a primary intra-abdominal focus may be small. It is best to defer operation in these patients while awaiting a response to antimicrobial therapy. Patients with primary peritonitis usually respond to appropriate antimicrobial therapy within 48 hours. Paracentesis for smear and culture is indicated in all cirrhotic patients with ascites and in children with marked proteinuria and abdominal pain, whether or not the diagnosis of nephrotic syndrome has been previously established.

Paracentesis is not without hazard, especially in patients with hemorrhagic tendencies or bowel distention. Rarely, major complications can occur, including perforation of the bowel followed by generalized peritonitis, abdominal wall abscess, and serious hemorrhage. If no fluid can be aspirated, peritoneal lavage with Ringer's lactate solution can provide fluid for examination. Taps should not be attempted in the region of abdominal scars, where bowel may be adherent to the underside of the scar. The aspirate should be examined for blood, pus, bile, digested fat, and amylase; the sediment should be Gram-stained, and the fluid should be cultured aerobically and anaerobically (Chapter 226).

In patients with primary peritonitis, the leukocyte count in peritoneal fluid usually is greater than $300/mm^3$, with granulocytes predominating unless *M. tuberculosis* is the pathogen. Gram stain of the sediment is frequently diagnostic but may be negative in up to 60% or more of patients with cirrhosis and ascites.

The diagnosis of tuberculous peritonitis often requires operation or laparoscopy and is confirmed by histologic study of the peritoneal biopsy and bacteriologic examination of the peritoneal biopsy specimen and fluid. Multiple nodules scattered over the peritoneal surface and omentum are observed. Adhesions and a variable amount of peritoneal fluid are usually present. Ascitic fluid may have an elevated protein concentration (> 3 g/dl) and a lymphocytic pleocytosis, but neither may be present. *Coccidioides immitis* can cause a similar granulomatous peritonitis with a variable clinical presentation. The diagnosis of *C. immitis* peritonitis can be made from a wet mount of ascitic fluid, on finding *C. immitis* by culture, and histologic examination.

A peripheral leukocytosis of 17,000 to $25{,}000/mm^3$ is usual in acute intra-abdominal infections, the differential count showing polymorphonuclear predominance and a moderate to marked shift to the left. Although there may be fewer than 5000 white $cells/mm^3$ in the circulating blood, the differential smear usually shows an extreme shift to immature polymorphonuclear forms. Hematuria and pyuria without bacteriuria may reflect intra-abdominal inflammatory disease (e.g., appendicitis, adjacent to the urinary tract). Elevated serum amylase may be seen in peritonitis due to almost any cause, but very high levels are seen only in acute pancreatitis. Hyponatremia may be seen in patients given water to replace isotonic fluid losses, but it is also characteristic of porphyria. Acidosis is present in severe and late peritonitis.

Supine, upright, and lateral decubitus radiographs of the abdomen may reveal distention of both small intestine and colon, with adynamic loops of bowel or features of mechanical intestinal obstruction, volvulus, intussusception, or vascular occlusion. Inflammatory exudate and edema of the intestinal wall produce a widening of the space between adjacent loops. Peritoneal fat lines and psoas shadows may be obliterated. Free air may be visible if a viscus is ruptured. Chest radiographs should always be taken to rule out a pulmonary or thoracic problem as the cause of the abdominal distress and best determine the presence of air beneath the diaphragm.

Gas with a fluid level, or mottling due to gas, may also be visible in intraperitoneal or visceral abscesses. Calcification in the gallbladder or other organs may also be observed on x-ray film.

The search for intraperitoneal or visceral abscesses may be aided by routine and contrast radiography, radionuclide scanning, ultrasonography, angiography, and computed tomography (CT). Some radiographic findings of a right subphrenic or liver abscess include right-sided pleural effusion, basilar atelectasis, elevation of the diaphragm, and loss of diaphragmatic movement on fluoroscopy. Left subphrenic, splenic, or pancreatic abscess may be accompanied by left-sided pleuropulmonary findings. Radiography may also reveal displacement of viscera by an abscess; for example, the stomach may be outlined with barium or air to reveal displacement due to a left perihepatic, lesser sac, or pancreatic abscess. Intravenous cholangiography has been replaced by sensitive and specific hepatobiliary scanning with one of the ^{99m}Tc-labeled acetanilid iminodiacetic acid (IDA) derivatives for the diagnosis of acute cholecystitis, even in the presence of moderately severe liver dysfunction. In acute cholecystitis, the common duct and small bowel are visualized, but because the cystic duct is occluded, the gallbladder is not visualized. Obstruction of the common bile duct also can be diagnosed by hepatobiliary scanning. In this case, no component of the biliary system or small bowel is visualized, despite adequate hepatic uptake. In obstructive cholangitis, however, ultrasonography is preferred due to decreased dependability of IDA scintigraphy in the presence of severe jaundice. Percutaneous transhepatic cholangiography and endoscopic retrograde cholangiography are extremely valuable in evaluating bile duct obstruction. However, it is seldom feasible to use these techniques in the acutely ill patient with cholangitis.

Technetium 99m sulfur colloid liver-spleen scan visualizes the entire organ and delineates abnormal areas as "cold spots" due to decreased uptake of the isotope. Combined ^{99m}Tc scanning of the lungs and liver is especially useful for evaluating the right subphrenic space. Normally, the image of the lung and liver blend uniformly in all views. With subphrenic collections, there is a clear separation of the liver from the right lung base. Separation of the lung and liver image also may occur in patients with a right pleural effusion or pulmonary perfusion defect or in patients with ascites, but they do not cause the defects in the contour of the liver that occur with a subphrenic abscess.

Gallium-67 (Ga 67) and Indium-111 (In 111)-tagged leukocytes are two other radionuclide scans that are at times helpful in detecting intra-abdominal abscesses. Unlike ^{99m}Tc, Ga 67 and In 111 accumulate in areas of inflammation and appear as areas of increased radioactivity or "hot spots." Gallium is excreted into the intestinal tract and Ga 67 and In 111 can accumulate in any inflammatory process. For these reasons, false-positive scans may result from misinterpretation of radioactivity within the lumen of the bowel, within the wall of an inflamed bowel, or within a noninfected operative site in the process of healing.

Ultrasound is helpful in determining the size, shape, consistency, and anatomic relationships of an intra-abdominal abscess or collection of peritoneal fluid. Ultrasound can be used to determine gallbladder size and the presence of stones and bile duct dilatation; however, common duct obstruction can be present without bile duct dilatation. CT has proved to be especially well suited for the diagnosis of intra-abdominal abscess. Definition is unimpeded by intraluminal gas and postoperative changes, except in the presence of metallic surgical clips or residual barium, which may disrupt the image. Observed findings consistent with abscess include a low-density tissue mass and a definable capsule. CT can detect extraluminal gas, a finding highly suggestive of abscess. Contrast material is commonly administered orally, rectally, and intravenously when an attempt is being made to diagnose intra-abdominal abscess. The intraluminal contrast helps to distinguish loops of bowel from abscess cavities, and the parenteral contrast may enhance a surrounding capsule, thus allowing for easier identification.

Magnetic resonance imaging (MRI), the newest imaging modality, requires no administration of contrast material and eliminates exposure to radiation but is costly, and its usefulness in relation to CT and ultrasound remains to be demonstrated.

Under favorable circumstances, percutaneously placed catheters, guided by CT and ultrasonography, can be used to drain intra-abdominal abscesses and thus confirm the presence and position of the abscess with certainty. Gram stain and culture of the purulent material obtained allow specific antibiotic therapy to be initiated earlier in the course of illness.

With these new methods of determining the location and extent of intra-abdominal infection, subsequent operative treatment can be more direct. In some cases percutaneous catheter drainage and antibiotic therapy may avert the need for surgery. Overreliance on any single technique is dangerous, and the diagnosis should be confirmed by other methods and by clinical findings.

TREATMENT OF INTRA-ABDOMINAL INFECTION

Antimicrobial therapy should be initiated immediately after appropriate specimens (e.g., blood and peritoneal fluid) are obtained for Gram stain and culture. Initial antimicrobial therapy is therefore empiric, based on the predicted sensitivities of the most likely pathogens. In vitro sensitivity reports will allow subsequent adjustment of the initial regimen to more specific therapy.

Primary bacterial peritonitis due to either *S. pneumoniae* or group A streptococci is best treated with penicillin G. Suspected *S. aureus* peritonitis should be treated with a penicillinase-resistant penicillin or a first-generation cephalosporin (e.g., cefazolin), unless a methicillin-resistant strain is identified, when vancomycin is appropriate. Suspected Enterobacteriaceae or *P. aeruginosa* infection should be treated initially with an appropriate beta-lactam antibiotic, such as ampicillin, ticarcillin, a ureidopenicillin, aztreonam, imipenem, or a cephalosporin with or without gentamicin or tobramycin.

If the infection is community-acquired, Enteroacteriaceae, such as *E. coli, Proteus mirabilis,* or *K. pneumoniae,* are likely to be involved, and if hospital-acquired, more antibiotic-resistant Enterobacteriaceae, such as *Enterobacter* or *Serratia,* or *P. aeruginosa* may be involved. The antimicrobial activity that can be expected from agents used in empiric regimens against commonly encountered facultative gram-negative bacillary pathogens is shown in Table 232-1. Up to 30% to 40% of both community and nosocomial *E. coli* are resistant to ampicillin, on the basis of beta-lactamase production, and even over 10% may be resistant to first-generation cephalosporins. *P. mirabilis* is likely to be sensitive to ampicillin, first-, second-, and third-generation cephalosporins, imipenem, and aztreonam. *K. pneumoniae* is sensitive to all of the forementioned, except ampicillin, to which it is resistant on the basis of beta-lactamase production.

Beta-lactamases produced by *E. coli* and *K. pneumoniae* are inhibited, as are the beta-lactamases produced by *B. fragilis* and *S. aureus,* by clavulanic acid and sulbactam. When these beta-lactamase inhibitors are combined in formulations with ticarcillin (Timentin), amoxicillin (Augmentin), and ampicillin (Unasyn), the antibiotics become active against these beta-lactamase-producing organisms. These inhibitors, however, do not inhibit the inducible, chromosome-encoded beta-lactamases produced by commonly encountered nosocomial pathogens, such as *Enterobacter cloacae, Serratia marcescens, Citrobacter freundii, Morganella morganii,* and *P. aeruginosa.* Addition of clavulanic acid therefore does not improve the activity of ticarcillin against these beta-lactamase producers. These organisms are resistant to ampicillin or amoxicillin, first-generation cephalosporins, and frequently second-generation cephalosporins on the basis of mechanisms other than beta-lactamase, so that addition of beta-lactamase inhibitors, does not improve the activity of ampicillin or amoxicillin against these organisms.

These nosocomial pathogens have an additional mechanism for resistance to beta-lactam antibiotics: They have a sufficiently high rate of mutational loss of the genetic expression for production of these lactamases so that about 1 in 10^7 CFU are "stable derepressed" mutants, which constitutively produce large amounts of beta-lactamase. In in-

Table 232-1. Susceptibility of clinically important pathogens to antimicrobial agents used in empiric regimens

	Ampicillin	Cefazolin	Cefamandole	Cefoxitin	Third-generation cephalosporin	Ceftazidime
E. coli	R	R	S	S	S	S
P. mirabillis	S	S	S	S	S	S
Klebsiella	R	S	S	S	S	S
Enterobacter	R	R	S	R	R*	R*
Serratia	R	R	R	R	R*	R*
P. aeruginosa	R	R	R	R	R*	R*
B. fragilis	R	R	R	R	R	R

R, Clinically significant resistance (> 10% of isolates); S, sensitivity.
*Inducible, chromosome-encoded beta-lactamases producers.

fected tissue that usually contain $10^{8\text{-}10}$ CFU/g, there are large numbers of these stable-derepressed mutants even before initiation of antimicrobial therapy. These mutants cause persistent infection during therapy with third-generation cephalosporins, including ceftazidime, and are highly resistant to all beta-lactam antibiotics, except imipenem. There is no cross-resistance among these strains to quinolones, aminoglycosides, or trimethoprim/sulfamethoxazole. If anaerobic bacteria are suspected, antibiotics active against *B. fragilis* (see later discussion) should also be used initially.

The role of antimicrobial therapy in the outcome of localized infection due to anaerobes or a mixture of anaerobes and facultative micro-organisms is extremely difficult to assess, as there is usually a dramatic response to surgical drainage and debridement alone. Antimicrobial therapy significantly reduces mortality among patients with bacteremic infections due to Bacteroidaceae or Enterobacteriaceae. Antimicrobial drugs will also control early metastatic foci of infection, reduce suppurative complications if given early, and prevent local spread of existing infection. Once an abscess has formed, antimicrobial drugs alone, without drainage, will not eliminate the infection, but they may mask some of the clinical manifestations of abscess formation.

Because anaerobic infections are commonly polymicrobial, a broad spectrum of antimicrobial activity is required. Drugs active against anaerobic bacteria may be inactive against the accompanying aerobic or facultative pathogens in mixed infections, and vice versa. For this reason, combinations of two or three drugs are used. However, some drugs, such as imipenem, ticarcillin plus clavulanic acid, or ampicillin plus sulbactam, are active against both aerobes and *B. fragilis* and can be used alone. Drugs are selected for their activity against most of the more virulent pathogens in the infective mixture, for example, the Enterobacteriaceae and *B. fragilis,* which frequently cause bacteremia and abscesses in these patients. However, the antibiotics need not be active against every pathogen isolated. It is apparent that if most of the organisms are eliminated, their synergistic effect is removed, and the patient's defenses may be able to eradicate the remaining organisms. Although enterococci were not considered significant pathogens in polymicrobial infection in the past, this organism may be the sole intra-abdominal pathogen, at times associated with enterococcal bacteremia, especially in patients with polymicrobial intra-abdominal infection who were treated with an antimicrobial agent that lacked activity against the enterococcus.

If present, enterococci may be treated with ampicillin, penicillin G, imipenem, or a ureidopenicillin. Enterococci are less susceptible to other beta-lactam antibiotics, such as carbenicillin or ticarcillin and are least susceptible to the antistaphylococcal penicillins and cephalosporins. Recently, enterococci have been identified with increasing frequency in monomicrobial and polymicrobial infections and nosocomial outbreaks. These organisms frequently are (1) highly resistant to ampicillin, either secondary to beta-lactamase production in *E. faecalis* or to loss of affinity of penicillin-binding bacterial cell membrane protein in *E. faecium;* (2) resistant to glycopeptides (i.e., vancomycin or teicoplanin) due to plasmid-encoded synthesis of a membrane protein in both *E. faecalis* and *E. faecium;* or (3) resistant to aminoglycosides due to the presence of plasmid-encoded aminoglycoside inactivating enzymes.

Some strains of enterococci are resistant to all penicillins, glycopeptides, and aminoglycosides. Emergence of clinically significant infection due to strains that are resistant to traditional antibiotic therapy requires routine antimicrobial susceptibility testing of enterococci, which may have been abandoned in the recent past. Either combinations of beta-lactamase inhibitors with a beta-lactam antibiotic, such as sulbactam/ampicillin (Unasyn), clavulanic acid/amoxicillin (Augmentin) or clavulanic acid/ticarcillin (Timentin), or glycopeptides are effective for treatment of infection due to beta-lactamase-producing *E. faecalis*. Glycopeptides are effective for treatment of infections due to *E. faecium* that is highly resistant to ampicillin. Treatment of infections due to multiresistant strains should be based on results of susceptibility tests; potential antimicrobial agents include fluoronated quinolones, rifampin, chloramphenicol, erythromycin, or doxycycline.

Nearly 100 percent of strains of *B. fragilis* are sensitive to imipenem (0.5 to 1.0 g IV q6h), chloramphenicol (50 to 100 mg/kg/day), ticarcillin plus clavulanic acid (3 g ticarcillin IV q4-6h), ampicillin plus sulbactam (2 g ampicillin

Aztreonam	Amoxicillin/clavulanate Ampicillin/sulbactam	Broad-spectrum penicillins	Ticarcillin/clavulanate	Imipenem	Aminoglycoside quinolones
S	S	S	S	S	S
S	S	S	S	S	S
S	S	R	S	S	S
R*	R	R*	R*	S	S
R*	R	R*	R*	S	S
R*	R	R*	R*	S	S
R	S	R	S	S	R

IV q6h), or metronidazole (loading dose of 15 mg/kg IV and then 7.5 mg/kg q6h IV or po). However, chloramphenicol may be active against these organisms only at concentrations that are close to serum levels (i.e., 20 to 25 μg/ml), above which predictable bone marrow suppression occurs if therapy is longer than 1 week. Clindamycin (300 to 600 mg IV q6-8h) and cefoxitin (1 to 2 g q4h) are active against anaerobic gram-negative bacilli, although resistance has been reported at some medical centers.

Only about 85% of *B. fragilis* strains are sensitive to cefoxitin; 90 percent are sensitive to carbenicillin or ticarcillin (400 to 500 mg/kg/day), or ureidopenicillins, but this species is usually resistant to other beta-lactam antibiotics. At present, in most clinical microbiology laboratories, no standardized in vitro method is available to determine the antibiotic sensitivity of anaerobes. Thus in seriously ill patients with *B. fragilis* infection, the use of imipenem, ticarcillin-clavulanic acid, ampicillin-sulbactam, or metronidazole, which has almost 100% predictable activity against *B. fragilis,* is advised.

The other anaerobic pathogens in polymicrobial infections are usually sensitive to beta-lactam antibiotics, clindamycin, or chloramphenicol. However, anaerobic and microaerophilic gram-positive cocci may not be sensitive to metronidazole. If this agent is used for its *B. fragilis* activity, an additional antibiotic (e.g., ampicillin) should be given for the treatment of these gram-positive cocci. The facultative or aerobic components (e.g., *E. coli* or *P. mirabilis*) may not be sensitive to some of the antibiotics active against *B. fragilis,* and initial therapy should include an aminoglycoside (e.g., 1.7 mg gentamicin or tobramycin/kg q8h IV or IM in patients with normal renal function). A beta-lactam antibiotic (ampicillin or cephalosporin) should be substituted for the potentially nephrotoxic and ototoxic aminoglycoside if sensitivity testing indicates appropriate activity.

The newer cephalosporins (e.g., cefotaxime, ceftizoxime, ceftazidime, and ceftriaxone) and other, similar beta-lactam antibiotics (e.g., imipenem) have demonstrated significantly better activity against the Enterobacteriaceae than the older cephalosporins, but, except for imipenem, they have poor activity against *B. fragilis*. Thus the newer cephalosporins can be used to replace aminoglycosides in empiric regimens, combined with either metronidazole or clindamycin, and avoid the risk of aminoglycoside toxicity. Imipenem or ticarcillin-clavulanic acid can be used as a single empiric agent because of broad-spectrum antimicrobial activity. The duration of therapy is usually prolonged to prevent relapse, as host defenses may not eradicate the pathogens from sequestered areas of extensive tissue necrosis and abscess formation. Not all these areas are accessible to adequate surgical drainage.

Operation for peritonitis is performed to stop continuing contamination, to remove foreign material from the peritoneal cavity, and to provide drainage of purulent collections. Operation is generally not indicated in the following situations:

1. Primary peritonitis
2. Moribund patients whose condition continues to deteriorate despite vigorous supportive therapy
3. Patients in whom the disease process subsides and localizes while they are being prepared for surgery
4. Patients with peritonitis secondary to pelvic inflammatory disease (which usually responds to nonsurgical therapy)

In localized pyogenic infection, such as intraperitoneal or visceral abscess, surgical drainage is usually required. Immediate operation is indicated for the suppurative complications of acute cholecystitis and for severe forms of cholangitis.

Percutaneous catheter drainage guided by ultrasonography or CT has been used successfully as an alternative to surgery and appears most effective with unilocular abscess cavities when a safe route of approach is present. Surgery may be required for more complete drainage of multiloculated or highly viscous abscesses, for abscesses not in contact with the abdominal wall (e.g., interloop or mesenteric abscesses), or for correction of instigating factors (e.g., biliary tract obstruction or perforated bowel). Complications or percutaneous catheter drainage may occur in up to 15% of patients and include septicemia, hemorrhage, peritoneal spillage, and fistula formation. However, the morbidity and mortality associated with percutaneous drainage may be less than that associated with surgery.

Drainage of the general peritoneal cavity is physically impossible, as exudate and adhesions rapidly isolate and occlude the drains and may increase the risk of secondary infections. However, drains are often placed in a dependent point to which fluid can be expected to gravitate or in an area of devitalized tissue that cannot be removed.

REFERENCES

Dellinger EP et al: Surgical infections stratification system for intra-abdominal infection, Arch Surg 120:21, 1985.

Dunn DL and Simmons RL: The role of anaerobic bacteria in intraabdominal infections, Rev Infect Dis 6(suppl 1):S139, 1984.

Finegold SM and Lance WL, editors: Anaerobic infections in humans. San Diego, 1989, Academic.

Finegold SM and Wexler JM: Therapeutic implications of bacteriologic findings in mixed aerobic-anaerobic infections, Antimicrob Agents Chemother 32:611, 1988.

Gerzof SG, Robbins AH, and Johnson WC: Percutaneous catheter drainage of abdominal abscesses, N Engl J Med 305:653, 1981.

Joiner KA and Gorbach SL: Acute septic complications in gastrointestinal emergencies, Clin Gastroenterol 10:93, 106, 1981.

Mandel SR et al: Drainage of hepatic, intra-abdominal, and mediastinal abscesses guided by computerized axial tomography. Successful alternative to open drainage, Am J Surg 145:120, 1983.

Nichols RL: Intra-abdominal infections: an overview, Rev Infect Dis 7(suppl 4):S709, 1985.

Root RK, Trunkey DD, and Sande MA, editors: Contemporary issues in infectious diseases, vol 6, Focus on infection: new surgical and medical approaches, New York, 1986, Churchill Livingstone.

Sanford JP: Guide to antimicrobial therapy. Dallas, 1993, Antimicrobial Therapy.

Wilcox CM and Dismukes WE: Spontaneous bacterial peritonitis: a review of pathogenesis, diagnosis and treatment, Medicine (Baltimore) 66:447, 1987.

Wilson SE, Finegold SM, and Williams RA, editors: Intraabdominal infection, New York, 1982, McGraw-Hill.

CHAPTER

233 Acute Meningitis

Allan R. Tunkel
W. Michael Scheld

Acute inflammation of the central nervous system (CNS) may be caused by a wide variety of etiologic agents. Because of their overall frequency, this chapter focuses on meningitis due to the most important pathogens: bacteria, viruses, and fungi.

EPIDEMIOLOGY AND ETIOLOGY

Bacterial meningitis

Although the exact incidence of bacterial meningitis in the United States is not known, in a surveillance study of 27 states in the United States from 1978 through 1981, the overall attack annual rate was 3.0 cases per 100,000 population. Attack rates have been reported to vary by age, sex, and geographic area with the highest rates in the Pacific region (Washington and Oregon) and lowest rates in the mid-Atlantic region (Arkansas and Louisiana). The disease is more common worldwide, especially in certain regions, such as the sub-Saharan "meningitis belt" of Africa. In addition, a recent review of all cases (~ 4100) of bacterial meningitis admitted to an isolation-fever hospital in Salvador, Brazil, between 1973 and 1982 revealed an average annual incidence of 45.8 cases per 100,000 population, illustrating the global importance of the meningitis problem.

Over 80% of all cases of bacterial meningitis are due to one of three major organisms: *Haemophilus influenzae, Neisseria meningitidis,* and *Streptococcus pneumoniae*. All are more common in the winter months except *H. influenzae,* which demonstrates a biphasic pattern in the northern states with peak incidences in spring and fall, although in southern states the peak incidence is also in the winter months. The attack rate is higher in members of the lower socioeconomic groups. The frequency of bacterial meningitis is age-related (Table 233-1). Nearly 75% of cases occur in children under 6 years of age, and males are affected more commonly than females in all age groups (1.5 to 2:1). In infants 2 months old or younger, the most common etiologic agents are *Escherichia coli,* other gram-negative bacilli, and group B streptococci *(S. agalactiae)*. Between the ages of 2 months and 6 years, *H. influenzae* is the predominant pathogen. Beyond age 6, meningococci and pneumococci cause the majority of cases, with a second peak after age 50 years for pneumococci and gram-negative bacilli.

H. influenzae (Chapter 265) is the most common cause of meningitis in the United States (40% to 50% of cases), and capsular type b strains account for over 90% of serious *H. influenzae* infections. Over 50% of patients with *H. influenzae* meningitis have concurrent pharyngitis or otitis media on presentation. Disease due to this organism after age 6 is rare and suggests an underlying host defect; for example, chronic parameningeal foci of infection (sinus or mastoids), sickle cell disease, splenectomy, diabetes mellitus, hypogammaglobulinemia, CNS trauma with a cerebrospinal fluid (CSF) leak, or alcoholism. This disease appears to be increasing in frequency in both children and adults. Recently, it has been recognized that unencapsulated *H. influenzae* strains may also cause meningitis.

Meningococcal meningitis (Chapter 263) is primarily an illness of children and young adults; less than 10% of cases

Table 233-1. Causes of bacterial meningitis: age-related incidence (%)

Organism	Under 2 months of age	2 months to 6 years of age	Over 6 years of age
H. influenzae	0-2	40-60	5
N. meningitidis	0-1	20-30	25-40
S. pneumoniae	1-4	10-20	40-50
E. coli (and other gram-negative bacilli)	30-50	1-4	5-10
S. agalactiae	30-40	2-5	1-3
Staphylococci	2-5	1-2	5-10
Listeria monocytogenes	2-8	1-2	5
Others (including unidentified organisms)	5-10	5-10	5-10

occur after age 45. It differs from other types of bacterial meningitis in that it may occur in epidemics (usually due to serogroups A and C), now primarily outside of the United States. Deficiency of the terminal complement components (C5, C6, C7, C8, and perhaps C9) predisposes to disseminated *Neisseria* infections, including gonococcemia and meningococcemia. The distribution of meningococcal serogroups in a surveillance study of 27 states from 1978 through 1981 was as follows: A, 4.7% (especially in the skid row populations of Seattle and Anchorage); B, 51.1%; C, 22.3%; Y, 5.8% (higher incidence in military personnel with a predilection for pneumonia); others (especially W135), 6.4%; unclassifiable, 9.7%.

Pneumococcal meningitis is the most common form in adults and is frequently associated with other suppurative foci: pneumonia (25%), otitis media or mastoiditis (30%), sinusitis (10% to 15%), and endocarditis (<5%) (Chapter 15). Previous head trauma (with or without a CSF leak) is found in approximately 10% of patients with pneumococcal meningitis, and the pneumococcus causes the overwhelming majority of recurrent meningitis cases. Other conditions (sickle cell disease, splenectomy, hypogammaglobulinemia, multiple myeloma, alcoholism) also predispose to systemic pneumococcal infection, including meningitis. Among the 84 known serotypes of pneumococci, 18 cause the majority (82%) of bacteremic pneumococcal pneumonia, and there is a close correlation between bacteremic serotypes and those responsible for meningitis.

Gram-negative bacillary meningitis is encountered only in specific clinical settings: in neonates, in head trauma, after neurosurgical procedures, during gram-negative septicemia, in underlying defects in host defenses, and in association with strongyloidiasis (Chapter 282). The most common etiologic agents, in approximate order of frequency are *Klebsiella* species, *E. coli,* and *Pseudomonas aeruginosa,* although a wide variety of other organisms may be responsible. Nosocomial meningitis is increasing in frequency, as is the proportion due to aerobic gram-negative bacilli.

Group B streptococcal disease (Chapter 260) in neonates has been divided into two types: early-onset septicemia, associated with premature rupture of the membranes and low-birth-weight infants, and late-onset (>7 days after birth) meningitis. In early-onset disease, the organism is acquired from the maternal genital tract. Intrapartum chemoprophylaxis with penicillin or ampicillin directed at parturient women with high-risk factors (colonized with group B streptococci, prolonged rupture of amniotic membranes >18 hours, fever, and low-birth-weight infant [<2.5 kg]) could effectively reduce the incidence of early-onset disease. The source of the organism (nearly always serotype III) in late-onset disease remains unknown, as 40% of affected infants are born to culture-negative mothers. Nosocomial transmission from other colonized infants or nursery personnel is possible. This organism is the most common cause of serious neonatal infection in many large centers. Although the incidence of group B streptococcal infection varies in different geographic areas, the overall incidence has remained the same (≅ 1 to 3 cases per 1000 live births) in recent years. An estimated 12,000 cases occurred in the United States in 1979.

The other bacterial etiologic agents of meningitis are relatively uncommon. *Listeria monocytogenes* causes disease in neonates and immunosuppressed adults (especially renal transplant recipients) but should also be considered in the elderly, alcoholic, or cancer patient (Chapter 261). Thirty percent of all cases occur in presumably normal persons. Outbreaks have been associated with the consumption of contaminated food, especially dairy products. More than 300 patients with listeriosis have been reported in two separate outbreaks in California and Switzerland in the late 1980s from contaminated cheese. An encephalitis, especially involving multiple cranial nerves, is relatively common with *Listeria* meningitis. *Staphylococcus aureus* may initiate meningitis after open head trauma, a neurosurgical procedure, or in association with endocarditis. *Staphylococcus epidermidis* is the most common cause of an infected CSF shunt, followed in frequency by *S. aureus,* gram-negative bacilli, and diphtheroids.

Viral meningitis

The exact incidence of viral meningitis is unknown. It peaks in incidence in late summer and early autumn (for the enteroviruses), and nearly all patients are under 40 years of age. A wide variety of etiologic agents is responsible, but the enteroviruses (Chapter 244) are most commonly implicated in the United States. Frequently encountered enteroviral isolates are ECHO virus 9,4,6,11,18,33 and coxsackievirus A9 or B4. Mumps is particularly common in Scandinavian series, but the incidence in the United States has declined dramatically since the introduction of mumps vaccine in 1967. A wide variety of other viruses may be responsible: herpes simplex types 1 and 2, poliovirus, adenoviruses, measles virus, cytomegalovirus, herpes zoster virus, lymphocytic choriomeningitis virus (LCM), hepatitis viruses, Epstein-Barr virus, and various arboviruses. The arboviruses produce an encephalitic clinical picture (Chapter 249). In addition, the human immunodeficiency virus type 1 (HIV-1) may cause aseptic meningitis, more commonly in the otherwise asymptomatic seropositive patient. Some specific clues may aid in determining the causative organism: parotitis, pancreatitis, orchitis, or oophoritis with mumps; contact with mice or hamsters (winter peak) with LCM (Chapter 248); a coexisting typical skin rash with varicella-zoster and measles; and genital lesions with herpes simplex type 2. Despite vigorous virologic culturing techniques, the cause of aseptic meningitis remains unknown in up to 70% of cases.

Fungal meningitis

Numerous fungal species may infect the nervous system and produce meningitis, encephalitis, or brain abscess (Chapter 277). Some are encountered nearly exclusively in immunocompromised hosts or diabetic patients (e.g., *Aspergillus* species, *Mucor* species) (Chapter 277). Two species cause most fungal meningitis in the United States. Meningitis due to *Cryptococcus neoformans* (Chapter 279) is encountered in patients with lymphoma, the acquired immunodeficiency syndrome (AIDS), sarcoidosis, organ transplantation, collagen vascular diseases, diabetes mellitus, chronic hepatic failure, chronic renal failure, and patients receiving corticosteroid therapy; up to 50% of patients have no underlying disease. Currently, patients with AIDS are in the highest risk group; clinical studies suggest that 6% to 13% of AIDS patients develop cryptococcal meningitis. *Candida albicans* meningitis is rare but may develop in debilitated patients receiving hyperalimentation or broad-spectrum antibiotics, including recent therapy for bacterial meningitis, and is also associated with prematurity, malignancy, chronic granulomatous disease, diabetes mellitus, thermal injuries, and insertion of central venous catheters. Disseminated coccidioidomycosis, histoplasmosis, or blastomycosis may involve the nervous system and present as a subacute or chronic meningitis (Chapter 277).

PATHOGENESIS AND PATHOPHYSIOLOGY

Several factors affect the pathogenesis of bacterial meningitis: (1) host defense mechanisms; (2) microbial virulence factors; (3) microbial route of invasion of the CNS; and (4) pathophysiologic alterations as a result of CNS infection.

Mucosal colonization and systemic invasion

Multiple defects in host defense (splenectomy, hypogammaglobulinemia, complement-deficiency states, defects in cell-mediated responses) may predispose the patient to the development of bacterial meningitis. The most important predisposing factors, however, are recent colonization of the nasopharynx by an appropriate pathogen and the absence of specific antibody. Many of the major meningeal pathogens possess surface characteristics that enhance mucosal colonization. The fimbriae of *N. meningitidis* mediate adhesion of the organism to nasopharyngeal epithelial cells. After attachment via a specific cell-surface receptor, meningococci are then transported across nonciliated nasopharyngeal columnar epithelial cells within a phagocytic vacuole. This series of events appears to be essential for development of invasive meningococcal disease. Fimbriae have also been implicated in the adhesion of *H. influenzae* to upper respiratory tract epithelial cells, although fimbriae have not been found on CSF or blood isolates of *H. influenzae* type b in patients with invasive disease.

Bacterial meningitis is more likely to occur if the nasopharynx has been recently colonized by *H. influenzae,* pneumococci, or meningococci when circulating bactericidal or opsonizing antibody against the appropriate serotype is absent. The common occurrence of *E. coli* sepsis and meningitis in the premature infant may be related to delayed passage of opsonizing IgG2 antibody to K1, which crosses the placenta only in the late stages of gestation.

Bacteremia

Once bacteria gain access to the bloodstream, they must overcome additional host defense mechanisms for survival. An important virulence factor in this regard is bacterial capsule, which through its ability to resist classical complement pathway bactericidal activity and inhibit neutrophil phagocytosis, facilitates development of a high-grade bacteremia. The host possesses several defense mechanisms to counteract the antiphagocytic activity of bacterial capsule. One is the alternative complement pathway, which is activated by the capsular polysaccharides of pneumococci, resulting in cleavage of C3 with attachment of C3b to the bacterial surface, thereby facilitating opsonization, phagocytosis, and intravascular clearance of the organism.

Meningeal invasion

There are three potential bacterial routes of entry into the CSF: hematogenous, via a contiguous structure, and direct implantation. The hematogenous route is the most common; the primary foci of infection may be the nasopharynx, skin, lung, heart, gastrointestinal or genitourinary tract, umbilical stump, or elsewhere. Bacteria may enter the CSF through the dural sinuses or the choroid plexus—the precise mode of penetration is unknown. There is evidence that preexisting sterile inflammation (as in the cribriform plate area after nasopharyngeal colonization) may selectively localize organisms in these areas if bacteremia occurs.

Recent studies have shown that cells in the choroid plexus and/or cerebral capillaries possess receptors capable of mediating adherence of some meningeal pathogens, with subsequent transport into the subarachnoid space. For example, *E. coli* strains expressing S fimbriae bind to the luminal surface of the vascular endothelium and to the epithelium lining the choroid plexus and brain ventricles. When bacteria reach the CSF from contiguous structures (sinusitis, otitis media, mastoiditis, dental infection, petrositis, facial or scalp infections), three routes are possible: septic thrombosis of emissary veins with intracranial spread; association with secondary osteomyelitis; or via paraspinal lymphatics (not applicable to intracranial infection when lymphatics are absent). Bacteria may also be directly implanted within the CSF by a skull fracture (recent or remote, with CSF leak), lumbar puncture, neurosurgical procedure, or skin communication (meningomyelocele, dermal sinus, decubitus ulcer).

Alterations of the blood-brain barrier

A major host defense against the development of meningitis is the integrity of the blood-brain barrier. The barrier separates the brain from the intravascular compartment and functions as a regulatory interface. An experimental rat model has been used to investigate the blood-brain barrier alterations that occur during bacterial meningitis. After the intracisternal inoculation of meningeal pathogens, there was a uniform host response at the level of the cerebral capillary endothelial cell characterized morphologically by an early and sustained increase in pinocytotic vesicle formation and a progressive increase in separation of intercellular tight junctions. These morphologic changes correlated functionally with increased penetration of albumin across the blood-brain barrier. Increased permeability occurred in the near absence of CSF leukocytes, although the presence of leukocytes augmented changes in permeability late in the disease course. The major bacterial virulence factor responsible for this increased permeability after challenge with gram-negative organisms is lipopolysaccharide (LPS), likely through LPS-induced release of various inflammatory cytokines (e.g., interleukin-1, tumor necrosis factor) within the CNS.

Bacterial survival within the subarachnoid space

Once bacteria enter the subarachnoid space, host defense mechanisms are inadequate to control the infection. Concentrations of antibody and complement are extremely low in normal CSF and in infected CSF early in the disease course; functional opsonic and bactericidal activity are essentially absent in CSF. These properties are necessary for adequate phagocytosis and killing of encapsulated organisms, including the most common etiologic agents of bacterial meningitis. It has been suggested that during bacterial meningitis, leukocyte proteases degrade complement components crossing the blood-brain barrier, further resulting in inefficient phagocytic activity at the site of infection.

Bacterial meningitis produces an inflammatory exudate within the subarachnoid space that may exert both beneficial and detrimental effects. A high bacterial concentration with a low leukocyte concentration in purulent CSF is associated with a poor prognosis in meningitis. However, a study of experimental pneumococcal meningitis in leukopenic animals found no differences in bacterial growth rates in normal as compared to leukopenic animals, suggesting that bacterial eradication from the CSF during the early phase of bacterial meningitis is not leukocyte dependent.

The pathway of neutrophil traversal into the CSF is unknown. Adherence of neutrophils to vascular endothelium may be a necessary prerequisite. Pretreatment of endothelial cells with various inflammatory cytokines has induced formation of specific adhesion molecules such as endothelial leukocyte adhesion molecule 1, although these adhesion molecules have not yet been demonstrated conclusively in cerebral endothelium. Recent studies in an experimental rabbit model have suggested that the intravenous inoculation of a monoclonal antibody (IB4) against the CD18 family of integrin receptors on leukocytes blocks accumulation of leukocytes in CSF despite intracisternal challenge with meningeal pathogens or their potential virulence factors. Although the site of leukocyte traversal into CSF is unknown, most evidence supports entry through postcapillary venules. Purulent CSF is chemotactic for leukocytes in vitro. One putative substance has been identified as C5a, and the intracisternal inoculation of C5a into rabbits causes a rapid, early influx of leukocytes into CSF.

Induction of subarachnoid space inflammation

The induction of a subarachnoid space inflammatory response is a critical event leading to many of the pathophysiologic consequences of bacterial meningitis. Although bacterial capsule is crucial for intravascular and subarachnoid space survival of meningeal pathogens, capsular polysaccharides are remarkably noninflammatory. Recent studies have investigated the surface-exposed virulence factors of meningeal pathogens responsible for induction of this inflammatory response. For *S. pneumoniae* it is predominantly the cell wall, and for *H. influenzae* type b it is LPS. Release of these virulence factors after bacteriolytic therapy may further augment the subarachnoid space inflammatory response. In addition, these virulence factors elicit inflammation through the CSF release of inflammatory cytokines such as interleukin-1 and tumor necrosis factor. In fact, increased CSF concentrations of tumor necrosis factor may be specific for bacterial meningitis, as tumor necrosis factor concentrations, measured in mice and humans with either bacterial or viral meningitis, were elevated in CSF only during bacterial meningitis. Other inflammatory cytokines, such as interleukin-6, have also been detected in the CSF of patients with bacterial meningitis, although additional studies are needed to precisely define its contribution to disease. Elevated CSF concentrations of platelet-activating factor have been observed in children with *H. influenzae* meningitis, correlating with bacterial density, and CSF LPS and tumor necrosis factor (TNF) concentrations; these elevated concentrations of TNF and platelet-activating factor were associated with severity of disease.

Increased intracranial pressure

A major pathophysiologic consequence of bacterial meningitis is the development of increased intracranial pressure, primarily due to the development of cerebral edema; the edema may be vasogenic, cytotoxic, and/or interstitial in origin. Vasogenic cerebral edema is primarily a consequence of increased blood-brain barrier permeability (see earlier discussion). Cytotoxic cerebral edema results from swelling of the cellular elements of the brain, most likely due to release of toxic factors from neutrophils and/or bacteria. Interstitial edema occurs secondary to obstruction of normal CSF pathways as in hydrocephalus. CSF outflow resistance (defined as factors that inhibit the flow of CSF from the subarachnoid space to the major dural sinuses) has been shown to be markedly elevated in experimental animal models of bacterial meningitis, suggesting that attenuation of the normal CSF absorptive mechanisms during meningitis may decrease the ability of the brain to compensate in situations of increased intracranial pressure. These concepts have been solidified in greater detail by measuring brain water content (indicative of cerebral edema if elevated), CSF lactate, and CSF pressure in animals with pneumococcal meningitis. All three parameters were elevated in infected animals, and early, specific antibiotic therapy normalized CSF pressure and brain edema.

Alterations in cerebral blood flow

Cerebral blood flow may also be altered in patients with bacterial meningitis. Intracranial vessels passing through the inflammatory exudate are often involved with secondary parenchymal changes (e.g., infarction, hemorrhage, abscess). In an infant rhesus monkey model of *H. influenzae* meningitis, certain areas of the cerebral cortex (postcentral, temporal, and occipital) were hypoperfused relative to the hypothalamus and midbrain, whereas the brainstem may be hyperperfused, suggesting that one of the initial physiologic changes in *H. influenzae* meningitis is cerebral cortical hypoperfusion with resultant cerebral anoxia. Recent studies in an experimental model of pneumococcal meningitis have demonstrated disturbances in cerebral autoregulation, in which even minor fluctuations of mean arterial blood pressure are likely to have adverse consequences for patients with meningitis, with risk of brain injury from either transient hypotension or hypertension. Blood flow alterations may lead to regional hypoxia, increased brain lactate concentration secondary to utilization of glucose by anaerobic glycolysis, and CSF acidosis, which may be precursors to encephalopathy.

The transport capacity of the barrier is also disturbed, and this, in concert with an increased utilization by intracranial tissues, is the major cause of the depressed CSF glucose content (hypoglycorrhachia) seen in bacterial meningitis. Glucose utilization by microorganisms or leukocytes within the CSF appears to play only a minor role in this process.

CLINICAL MANIFESTATIONS

The classic findings in adults with meningitis (Table 233-2) include fever, headache, nuchal rigidity, and signs of cerebral dysfunction. Shaking chills, profuse sweats, weakness, anorexia, nausea, vomiting, myalgias of the lower extremities or back (especially with meningococcal disease), and photophobia are common. Patients able to speak usually describe the headache as generalized and extremely severe. Neck stiffness may be subtle or marked and accompanied by Brudzinski's and Kernig's signs. Cerebral dysfunction is manifested as confusion, delirium, or a declining level of consciousness, from lethargy to coma. Cranial nerve palsies (principally involving cranial nerves III, IV, VI, and VII) occur in approximately 10% of patients, whereas seizures (due to the underlying disease, fever in infants, or penicillin neurotoxicity) are somewhat more frequent. Focal cerebral signs are unusual (10% to 20%) and include hemiparesis, visual field defects, and dysphasia. These may be transitory (e.g., Todd's paralysis) or may appear late in the disease course as a result of the development of intracranial venous thrombophlebitis, subdural empyema, brain abscess, hemorrhage, or infarction. Signs of increased intracranial pressure (coma, hypertension, bradycardia, third nerve palsy) appear late in the disease course and are ominous prognostic signs. Papilledema is rare and should suggest an alternate diagnosis (e.g. intracranial mass lesion).

Table 233-2. Symptoms and signs in bacterial meningitis

Findings	Relative frequency (%)
Headache	≥90
Fever	≥90
Meningismus	≥85
Brudzinski's sign	≥50
Kernig's sign	≥50
Altered sensorium	>80
Vomiting	~35
Seizures	~30
Petechiae	~50
Focal findings	10-20
Cranial nerves	~10
Hemiparesis	<5
Papilledema	<1
Myalgia	30-60
Other suppurative foci (pneumonia, otitis, sinusitis, etc.)	0-30

A rash develops in approximately 50% of meningococcal infections. An erythematous maculopapular eruption, chiefly centrifugal in location (e.g., volar aspect of the forearms, wrists, ankles, occasionally the palms and soles), is present early and is easily confused with numerous other entities, including enteroviral aseptic meningitis syndromes. A petechial, purpuric, or ecchymotic rash is suggestive of meningococcal infection but may be seen in other types of meningitis due to ECHO virus type 9, *Acinetobacter* species, *S. aureus,* and, rarely, *H. influenzae* or *S. pneumoniae*. An indistinguishable skin rash may be present in Rocky Mountain spotted fever, *S. aureus* endocarditis, and rapidly overwhelming *S. pneumoniae* or *H. influenzae* bacteremia in patients who have undergone splenectomy. In patients who have suffered basilar skull fractures in which a dural fistula is produced between the subarachnoid space and the nasal cavity, paranasal sinuses, or middle ear, meningitis is usually caused by *S. pneumoniae*. These patients commonly present with rhinorrhea or otorrhea due to a CSF leak, and a persistent defect is a common explanation for recurrent bacterial meningitis.

The classic findings may be less apparent in several clinical settings. Neonates usually do not demonstrate nuchal rigidity and may have normal temperatures. The only clues may be listlessness, high-pitched crying, fretfulness, refusal to feed, irritability, and other nonspecific abnormalities. Full or tense fontanelles are a late sign of disease and are often absent. Similarly, elderly patients with various underlying conditions (e.g., diabetes mellitus, cardiopulmonary disease) may become lethargic or obtunded, and thus other clues to the meningitis, including fever, may not be revealed. Signs of meningeal irritation are variable, and the onset may be insidious. The postneurosurgical patient or the patient who has undergone head trauma also presents a unique clinical situation, as these patients already have many of the symptoms and signs from their underlying disease process that are similar to those seen in patients with meningitis. When doubt arises, lumbar puncture is indicated. Meningitis is more common in the febrile alcoholic patient, and an altered mental state should not be ascribed to delirium tremens or other causes unless meningitis has been excluded by CSF examination.

Nearly all the preceding findings may be present with viral meningitis (Chapter 244), although the illness is usually milder, with less derangement of higher integrative functions, and less cranial nerve palsies, focal neurologic deficits, and seizures. Extracranial manifestations, such as herpangina, exanthems, parotitis, or pleurodynia, may suggest a viral cause.

The mode of onset has important diagnostic and prognostic implications. Approximately 20% of all patients present with acute disease of less than 24 hours and rapidly progressive signs. In almost all these patients, the disease is due to pyogenic bacteria and requires rapid therapeutic intervention (see Treatment). Despite such intervention, however, mortality remains high (≥50%). In the subacute form, signs and symptoms have been present for 1 to 7 or more days, the differential diagnosis is extensive, and mortality, even when a bacterial cause is established, is lower (≤25%). The disease in these patients is commonly preceded by an upper respiratory infection (e.g., pharyngitis), which may have resolved by the time meningitis becomes evident. The symptoms and signs of another infectious focus (e.g., otitis, sinusitis, mastoiditis, pneumonia, endocarditis) may be evident on admission.

A variety of epidemiologic and clinical features may be useful in predicting the etiologic agent in meningitis (Table 233-3).

LABORATORY INVESTIGATION

Blood studies

Certain serum chemistries and blood tests are helpful in the diagnosis and management of meningitis. Hyponatremia is common and may indicate the presence of the syndrome of inappropriate antidiuretic hormone secretion. Severe renal failure necessitates an alteration in dosage of many antibiotics. A leukocytosis with a shift to the left suggests a bacterial origin, but there is a large overlap. In patients with petechiae, purpura, hypotension, or shock, clotting variables may reflect disseminated intravascular coagulation. Blood cultures should be obtained in all patients; they are positive in 40% to 80% of cases of bacterial meningitis and are occasionally positive when CSF cultures are negative. If a petechial rash is present, aspiration of the lesion may demonstrate the pathogen when examined by Gram stain. Wright's stain of the buffy coat (or even a peripheral blood smear) may reveal intraphagocytic meningococci (or pneumococci) in fulminant cases, even when the CSF stains are negative.

X-ray studies

If pyogenic meningitis is suspected or established, radiographic studies of the sinuses, mastoids, and chest should be obtained to exclude suppurative foci in these locations. When papilledema or focal neurologic signs are present, a computed tomographic (CT) scan is necessary in the initial evaluation to exclude a space-occupying intracranial lesion (e.g., brain abscess, subdural empyema) before attempting lumbar puncture. CT or magnetic resonance imaging (MRI) may also be useful in patients with prolonged fever several days after initiation of antimicrobial therapy, or in those with prolonged obtundation or coma, new or recurrent seizure activity, signs of increased intracranial pressure, or focal neurologic deficits. MRI is better than CT for evaluation of subdural effusions, cortical infarctions, and cerebritis, although it is more difficult to obtain an MRI scan in a critically ill patient, limiting its usefulness in many patients with bacterial meningitis.

CSF examination

The diagnosis of meningitis rests on careful examination of the CSF. The opening pressure is elevated (e.g., 200 to 300 mm H_2O) in virtually all cases of meningitis. Values over 600 mm H_2O suggest extensive cerebral edema, intracranial suppurative foci, or communicating hydrocephalus due to the exudate in the subarachnoid space.

In acute, untreated, bacterial meningitis, the CSF white cell count usually ranges from 100 to 10,000/mm^3, with a median of approximately 2000 and polymorphonuclear leukocyte predominance. About 10% of patients will present with over 50% lymphocytes in the CSF. Very high white cell counts (≥50,000/mm^3) are unusual and suggest intraventricular rupture of a brain abscess. Occasionally, the white cell count may be very low (0 to 20/mm^3) while the CSF is turbid because of a high bacterial concentration; the prognosis is poor in such cases. Therefore, a Gram stain and culture should be performed on the CSF from all patients with suspected meningitis even if the cell count is zero. A lymphocytic predominance is found in the majority of cases with the aseptic meningitis syndrome (Table 233-4), and this may be helpful in differential diagnosis. The CSF protein concentration is elevated in virtually all types of meningitis (Table 233-4) and often exceeds 100 mg/dl. Huge elevations (>1000 mg/dl) suggest subarachnoid block or inadvertent insertion of the spinal needle into an epidural or subdural abscess instead of the subarachnoid space. Similar elevations are also commonly seen in gram-negative bacillary ventriculitis in infants. A CSF glucose value of 40 mg/dl or less, or a CSF blood sugar ratio of less than 0.5, is found in approximately 60% of bacterial meningitis patients and suggests this diagnosis. However, a wide variety of other conditions can produce hypoglycorrhachia of this magnitude (Table 233-4) and must be considered: fungal or tuberculous meningitis and rare cases of viral meningitis, sarcoidosis, meningeal carcinomatosis, hypoglycemia, and subarachnoid hemorrhage. A recent analysis found that a CSF glucose <34 mg/dl, a CSF blood glucose ratio < 0.23, a CSF protein > 220 mg/dl, more than 2000 CSF leukocytes/mm^3, or more than 1180 CSF neutrophils/mm^3 were individual predictors of bacterial, as opposed to viral, meningitis with 99% certainty or better.

Bacterial concentration is usually very high (generally, $\geq 10^5$ CFU/ml and often $\geq 10^7$ CFU/ml) and correlates directly with the antigen titer in the CSF. Higher values are associated with a more prolonged and severe illness and perhaps a worse prognosis. Gram stain permits identification of the causative agent in about 80% of patients with untreated bacterial meningitis (Plates V-8 and V-9). The probability of detecting the organism through staining techniques correlates with bacterial concentrations in CSF; CSF bacterial concentrations $\leq 10^3$ CFU/ml are associated

Table 233-3. Epidemiologic and clinical clues to the etiologic agent in acute meningitis

Feature	Microorganism(s) suspected
Age	See Table 233-1
Seasonal incidence	
Winter, spring	Meningococci, pneumococci, mumps, LCM
Late summer, fall	Enteroviruses, arboviruses, leptospires
Sibling with meningitis	Meningococci, *H. influenzae*
Military recruit	Meningococci, *Mycoplasma,* adenovirus
Epidemic	Meningococci, enteroviruses, arboviruses
Swimming, freshwater lake	Amebas (*Naegleria* sp.)
Contact with water, rats, domestic animals	Leptospires
Contact with mice, hamsters	LCM virus
Contact with tuberculosis	*Mycobacterium tuberculosis*
Contact with pigeon excreta	*C. neoformans*
Recurrent meningitis	Pneumococci
During, after treatment of bacterial meningitis	*Candida* sp.
Geographic area	*Coccidioides immitis*
Homosexuality, intravenous drug abuse	HIV
Associated condition	
Alcoholism	Pneumococci, *Listeria, H. influenzae*
Diabetes mellitus	Pneumococci, Enterobacteriaceae, *S. aureus, Cryptococcus,* rhinocerebral mucormycosis (with acidosis)
Cancer	Enterobacteriaceae, pneumococci, *Listeria, Cryptococcus, S. aureus,* carcinomatous abscess (*Aspergillus* + *Nocardia*)
Steroids, immunosuppressives	*Listeria, Cryptococcus, M. tuberculosis*
AIDS	*Cryptococcus,* toxoplasmosis, PMLE, and others
Sickle cell anemia	Pneumococci
Splenectomy	Pneumococci, *H. influenzae*
Hypogammaglobulinemia	Pneumococci, *H. influenzae*
Skull fracture (closed)	Pneumococci, *H. influenzae,* Enterobacteriaceae
Skull fracture (open) or craniotomy	Enterobacteriaceae, *S. aureus,* pneumococci, clostridia (rare)
CSF otorrhea or rhinorrhea	Pneumococci, *H. influenzae,* Enterobacteriaceae, *S. aureus*
CSF shunt	*S. epidermidis, S. aureus,* Enterobacteriaceae, diphtheroids
Strongyloidiasis	Enterobacteriaceae
Associated infections and physical findings	
Pharyngitis	Viruses, *H. influenzae,* meningococci, pneumococci
Otitis media	*H. influenzae,* pneumococci, mixed anaerobes
Malignant otitis externa	*P. aeruginosa*
Sinusitis	Pneumococci, *H. influenzae,* anaerobes
Pneumonia	Pneumococci, meningococci
Endocarditis	Pneumococci, *S. aureus*
Cellulitis	Streptococci, *S. aureus*
Arthritis	Meningococci, pneumococci, *S. aureus, H. influenzae* (rare)
Brain abscess, subdural empyema	Anaerobes, *S. aureus,* Enterobacteriaceae
Petechiae, purpura	Meningococci, ECHO virus 9, Rocky Mountain spotted fever, *S. aureus* endocarditis, pneumococci or *H. influenzae* (splenectomy)
"Typical" skin rash	Measles, varicella
Herpes progenitalis	Herpesvirus type 2
Conjunctival suffusion	Leptospires
Parotitis	Mumps
Choroid tubercles	*M. tuberculosis*

PMLE, progressive multifocal leukoencephalopathy.

with poor microscopic results (organisms seen 25% of the time), whereas microscopy is positive in 97% of cases when CSF bacterial concentrations are $\geq 10^5$ CFU/ml. The recent administration of antibiotics reduces this frequency to approximately 60% and may result in diagnostic confusion. If sufficient numbers of organisms are present, a positive Quellung reaction with specific antisera establishes a pneumococcal etiology. Cultures are positive in 70% to 85% of cases of bacterial meningitis but are often negative in tuberculous or fungal meningitis (Table 233-4).

Many CSF enzymes (e.g., lactate dehydrogenase, glutamic-oxaloacetic transaminase, creatine kinase) are increased in bacterial meningitis, but the precise tissue(s) of origin remains unknown. Because these elevations may also accompany other conditions, none of these enzymatic assays is used in routine diagnosis. Lysozyme is present in

Table 233-4. Typical CSF findings in acute meningitis

Test	Bacterial meningitis	Aseptic meningitis syndrome
Cell count	<100->10,000, usually 1000-5000	<10->1000, usually 100-500
Percentage of granulocytes	≥80	≤50*
Protein	100-500, occasionally >1000	100-500
Glucose	≤40	Normal†
Gram stain	Positive 75%-80%	Negative‡
Culture	Positive 70%-85%	Negative§
Acid-fast stain	Negative	Positive in tuberculosis (15%->60%)
India ink	Negative	Positive in cryptococcal disease (50%-75%)
Cytology	Negative	Positive in cryptococcal or neoplastic (≥70%) disease
Wet mount	Usually negative	Positive in amebic meningitis
Counterimmunoelectrophoresis	Positive‖	Negative
Lactate	Positive (≥35 mg/dl)	Negative
Limulus lysate	Positive**	Negative
Cryptococcal antigen	Negative	Positive in cryptococcal (≥95%) disease
Enzymes (e.g., lactate dehydrogenase)	Often elevated	Often elevated
Cyclic adenosine monophosphate	Decreased	Unknown
Adenosine deaminase	Negative	Positive in tuberculosis (≥80%)
C-reactive protein	Positive	Negative

*May be ≥50% in early tuberculous, fungal, amebic, spirochetal, or viral meningitis.
†Commonly, CSF glucose is low in meningitis due to *M. tuberculosis, C. neoformans,* and other fungi; neoplasia; chemicals; sarcoidosis (~10%); syphilis (50%-55%); and subarachnoid hemorrhage. It is under 40 mg/dl in less than 5% of viral cases (especially mumps and LCM).
‡May be positive in fungal meningitis (e.g., 40% with *Candida* sp.).
§Positive in tuberculous (≥80%) and cryptococcal (50%) meningitis, and, rarely, in viral syndromes.
‖Positive response rates on CIE, staphylococcal coagglutination, and latex agglutination vary with infecting organisms (see text).
**The *Limulus* lysate test is positive only in gram-negative meningitis (≥90%).

increased concentrations in the CSF in a wide variety of CNS infections and is not diagnostically useful. The CSF lactic acid concentration is increased in bacterial meningitis, whereas it is usually normal in "aseptic" meningitis due to viruses. This test may be helpful (measured by gas-liquid chromatography or various simpler chemical methods) in differentiating partially treated bacterial meningitis (or others with a negative Gram stain) from a viral syndrome. In hospitals where the facilities for enzymatic determination of lactate are not available, the same information may be provided by measurement of the anion gap in CSF: $[Na^+] + [K^+] - [Cl^-] - [HCO^-{}_3]$. This value is usually above 6 mEq/L in bacterial, but not viral, meningitis.

Several specific diagnostic tests have been developed. The lysate of the amebocytes of the horseshoe crab *(Limulus)* gels on exposure to small quantities of bacterial endotoxin (≤10 ng/ml). A positive *Limulus* lysate test indicates that a gram-negative organism is the cause of the meningitis (e.g., meningococci, *H. influenzae,* gram-negative bacilli), but speciation is not possible.

Counterimmunoelectrophoresis (CIE) is available for the detection of specific antigens in the CSF due to meningococci (serogroups A or C), *H. influenzae* type b, pneumococci (omniserum representing 83 serotypes), type III group B streptococci, and *E. coli* K1. These tests are variably sensitive (positive in 62% to 95%) but highly specific. Cross reactions may occur. The tests may be useful in the rapid diagnosis (results generally available in 1 hour) of suspected bacterial meningitis when Gram stains are negative.

Recently, several new tests using staphylococcal coagglutination or latex agglutination have been described for detection of bacterial capsular polysaccharide antigen in the CSF of patients with meningitis due to one of the three major pathogens. These newer tests are both more rapid and more sensitive (they detect ≅1 ng/ml) than CIE and are commercially available (e.g., Directigen, Bactigen, Wellcogen). They are less expensive than CIE, require less technical sophistication for performance in the laboratory, and can be applied in outpatient (and even field) settings. These procedures should be performed on compatible CSF specimens with a negative Gram stain.

Because culture and India ink preparations are positive in only ≃50% of cases of cryptococcal meningitis, detection of cryptococcal polysaccharide antigen in CSF, serum, or urine is very helpful in the diagnosis of this infection (Chapter 226).

DIFFERENTIAL DIAGNOSIS

As noted, multiple infectious and noninfectious processes may be responsible for the acute meningitis syndrome. Bacterial meningitis must be recognized rapidly and separated from the aseptic meningitis syndrome by the epidemiologic, clinical, and laboratory clues that have been enumerated. This differentiation will often depend on a thorough examination of the CSF (see Table 233-4). Because many other causes of the aseptic meningitis syndrome also require aggressive therapy, up to 50% of patients with a presumptive diagnosis of bacterial meningitis will have received antibiotics before the initial lumbar puncture. Although this practice may obscure Gram stain or culture results (usually, 60% or more positive), usually a granulocytic pleocytosis, high protein, and hypoglycorrhachia persist in the CSF and suggest this diagnosis. Other procedures (e.g., CIE, staphylococcal coagglutination, and latex agglutination; *Limulus* lysate test; lactate) may be very helpful in differentiating this entity from viral, tuberculous, or fungal meningitis.

Tuberculous meningitis (Chapter 276) usually presents in a subacute or chronic aseptic form, but an acute presentation with a granulocytic predominance in the CSF may occur in immunosuppressed hosts or during the course of miliary tuberculosis. Cranial nerve palsies (presumably due to the predominantly basilar exudate) are common. The CSF protein may be high, and hypoglycorrhachia is usual. Smears of the CSF for acid-fast bacilli are usually negative (≥75%), and cultures, although eventually positive in more than 80% of cases, are not helpful in the acute situation. Other procedures may be necessary to secure this diagnosis (e.g., a tuberculin skin test, a chest x-ray, or bone marrow or liver biopsies). The occurrence of meningitis with hyponatremia and a negative CSF Gram stain is suggestive of tuberculous meningitis. Several rapid diagnostic tests are under development, the most promising of which is the presence of tuberculostearic acid in CSF. High CSF concentrations of adenosine deaminase may support this diagnosis.

Meningitis due to fungi is also usually chronic and progressive, but acute presentations do occur. Epidemiologic features, such as treatment for bacterial meningitis, hyperalimentation *(Candida),* geographic locale *(Coccidioides;* rarely, *Histoplasma*), lymphoma, or immunosuppression (cryptococci), may suggest the diagnosis. In the acute presentation, the CSF findings may be indistinguishable from those of bacterial or tuberculous meningitis, but a lymphocytic pleocytosis or an aseptic picture is usually evident. Cryptococci may be seen on India ink or cytologic preparations; they are cultured in the majority of cases. The yield is enhanced if large volumes of CSF (e.g., >10 ml) are cultured. Cultures of blood, urine, sputum, or stool may also be positive. Cryptococcal polysaccharide antigen can be detected in the CSF by latex fixation in approximately 95% of cases; the yield may increase if latex fixation is also performed on serum and urine. Yeast cells are present on CSF smear in 40% of cases of *Candida* meningitis, and most cases are confirmed rapidly by culture. Coccidioidal meningitis is rarely acute, and the CSF usually demonstrates a lymphocytic predominance. The skin test is usually negative, but the presence of complement-fixing antibody to the causative organism in the CSF is confirmatory in approximately 95% of cases.

Parameningeal foci of infection, such as epidural abscess, subdural empyema, or brain abscess, are often suggested by the clinical setting (Chapter 234), but they may also produce the CSF findings typical of aseptic meningitis. Other procedures (e.g., CT or MRI, myelograms) are necessary for diagnosis. A combined surgical and medical (antibiotic) approach is usually required.

CNS syphilis (Chapter 273) may be manifested in many different ways; an acute meningitis may be the first clue to this disease in 25% of patients. The CSF reflects the typical abnormalities of the aseptic meningitis syndrome, although hypoglycorrhachia is present in 55% of patients. The presentation is usually subacute, and cranial nerve palsies or seizures are common. Serologic tests for syphilis must be performed on the serum and CSF in all cases of the aseptic meningitis syndrome. A transient deterioration in neurologic function on initiation of penicillin therapy (Jarisch-Herxheimer reaction) also suggests this diagnosis. Lyme disease, due to *Borrelia burgdorferi,* may produce meningitis during its second stage (weeks to months after the initial infection) in which patients have symptoms of headache, stiff neck, nausea, vomiting, malaise, and fever of several weeks duration that may alternate with periods of milder symptoms. Serum tests for antibodies to *B. burgdorferi* are usually positive in the majority of cases during this stage (Chapter 275).

Free-living amebas *(Naegleria)* may produce a fulminant, acute purulent meningitis with a high fatality rate (Chapter 280). The diagnosis is suggested by a history of swimming in warm freshwater lakes or swimming pools and is confirmed by noting freely motile amebas on fresh preparations of unrefrigerated, unspun CSF. Despite therapy with amphotericin B or miconazole, mortality remains high.

Herpes simplex type 1 infection of the CNS usually produces progressive, often fatal encephalitis, whereas herpes simplex type 2 infection may present as a progressive meningoencephalitis in neonates or immunosuppressed patients or as a benign aseptic meningitis in normal adults (Chapter 251). The diagnosis of type 1 infections usually requires a brain biopsy, although CT, MRI, or electroencephalogram findings localizable to the temporal lobe are suggestive. Adenine arabinoside and acyclovir have reduced mortality in these infections.

Neurologic disease associated with HIV may take the form of encephalitis, meningitis, ataxia, or myelopathy. Aseptic meningitis usually occurs in the asymptomatic seropositive patient, although it may manifest before seroconversion or in patients with full-blown AIDS. The CSF typically shows a mononuclear pleocytosis with normal glucose and slightly elevated protein. Direct HIV infection of the meninges is the presumed cause of the meningitis, as the virus is readily isolated from the CSF.

The neurologic complications of bacterial endocarditis (Chapter 15) are myriad and may overshadow other stigmata of the disease. An acute meningitis syndrome with a purulent CSF (often negative on culture) may represent the "cerebritis" that is particularly common in acute staphylococcal endocarditis. Careful attention to other peripheral manifestations of this disease, heart murmurs, or splenomegaly will usually suggest this disorder.

Multiple causes of the aseptic meningitis syndrome do not require antimicrobial or surgical therapy; the most important of these are viral (Chapter 244) and leptospiral (Chapter 274) meningitis. The epidemiologic clues to these infections are outlined in Table 233-3; the CSF findings are usually typical of the aseptic meningitis syndrome (see Table 233-4), with a lymphocytic CSF pleocytosis, mildly elevated protein, and normal glucose. Occasionally, the CSF white cell count is high (e.g., $\geq 1000/mm^3$ with LCM virus), and glucose is depressed in ≤5% of cases (mumps, LCM, occasionally ECHO viruses). Viral isolation should be attempted by throat, stool, and CSF cultures, although the CSF culture is rarely positive. If an agent is isolated, diagnosis is confirmed by a fourfold difference in antibody between acute and convalescent sera. Although leptospires can occasionally be cultured on special media or seen by dark-field examination (e.g., of urine), the diagnosis usually rests on specific serologic procedures.

A wide variety of other, presumably noninfectious processes may produce the aseptic meningitis syndrome, including neoplasia, cerebritis in systemic lupus erythematosus, granulomatous angiitis, sarcoidosis, lymphomatoid granulomatosis, cyst-related meningitis, chemically induced meningitis (e.g., radiographic dyes or anesthetics), and various poorly understood chronic or recurrent syndromes (Mollaret, Behçet, Vogt-Koyanagi-Harada). These are rarely confused with acute bacterial meningitis.

TREATMENT

The successful management of the acute meningitis syndrome is based on the following principles: (1) recognition that meningitis is present (through an appreciation of the clinical setting, physical findings, and presumed etiologic agents) (see Table 233-4); (2) rapid identification of the pathogen (through rapid techniques of CSF examination, for example, Gram stain, CIE and agglutination tests, *Limulus* lysate test, lactate); (3) rapid initiation of therapy; and (4) observation and treatment of complications (e.g., shock, disseminated intravascular coagulation) and sequelae.

Initial approach

Once meningitis is recognized, the initial approach is designed to optimize early therapy. If the mode of onset is acute, pyogenic meningitis is likely, and the prognosis is less favorable than if the onset had been more prolonged. The first consideration is the rapid (within 30 minutes of encountering the patient) initiation of therapy. The same procedure should be followed if the patient is comatose.

If focal neurologic signs are absent, the next step is rapid evaluation of the CSF through a lumbar puncture and appropriate diagnostic tests. If focal neurologic signs are present, a CT scan should be obtained immediately to exclude a brain abscess or other intracranial mass lesion, as lumbar puncture is relatively contraindicated in this setting. If there is any delay in obtaining a CT scan, empiric antibiotics should be started immediately, with the choice based on age and the underlying disease status of the patient (see later discussion).

The diagnosis of bacterial meningitis will rest on the initial battery of tests (e.g., CSF Gram stain, lactate, CIE or agglutination tests, *Limulus* lysate, examination of peripheral blood or skin lesions for organisms, purulent CSF without a positive Gram stain) and clinical judgment. Antimicrobial therapy should be started on the basis of the most likely etiologic agent. If pyogenic meningitis is unlikely and the diagnosis is consistent with the aseptic meningitis syndrome (e.g., CSF pleocytosis with a lymphocytic predominance, normal glucose), treatable causes must be ruled out (e.g., partially treated bacterial meningitis, parameningeal foci, fungal or tuberculous meningitis, herpes simplex encephalitis, as previously outlined). If one of these treatable conditions is likely, specific therapy (antibiotics with or without surgery) should be started; if they are not, careful observation, often with a follow-up lumbar puncture in 6 to 8 hours, is a reasonable approach.

Finally, complications may be present and adjunctive measures may be required. If the patient is comatose and/or signs of increased intracranial pressure are present, the intracranial pressure should be monitored and kept in the normal range (see Adjunctive Therapy). If shock, disseminated intravascular coagulation, or suppurative complications are present, the patient should be placed in an intensive care environment, monitored, and aggressively treated.

Antimicrobial therapy

Because host defenses are relatively inadequate at the site of infection in bacterial meningitis, only parenteral bactericidal antibiotics should be used. The choice of a particular agent is influenced by its ability to penetrate the blood-brain barrier (Chapter 224). In addition, bacterial meningitis is the only infection in which definite in vivo antibiotic antagonism has been demonstrated. Thus potentially antagonistic combinations of a bactericidal and a bacteriostatic agent, such as chloramphenicol-gentamicin for gram-negative bacilli, or penicillin-tetracycline for pneumococci, should be avoided in the treatment of this disease. The current antimicrobial agents of choice (with alternative agents) for the treatment of meningitis are listed in Table 233-5, with recommended dosages for adults in Table 233-6. In the patient with presumed bacterial meningitis and a negative CSF Gram stain, treatment is directed at the most likely etiologic agent, depending on age, as shown in Table 233-7.

Penicillin (20 to 24 million units/day IV) and ampicillin (12 g/day IV) are equally effective against both pneumococci and meningococci. In the penicillin-allergic patient, or when relatively penicillin-resistant strains of pneumococci (minimal inhibitory concentration [MIC] = 0.1 to 1.0 μg/ml) are isolated or suspected, cefotaxime or ceftriaxone should be used. Absolute resistance of pneumococci to penicillin (MIC of 2 μg/ml or greater) has been documented in South Africa and in some areas in the United States where vancomycin is the treatment of choice in pneumococcal meningitis. However, a recent report documented therapeutic failure of vancomycin in 4 of 11 patients with CSF-culture-proven pneumococcal meningitis, indicating the need for careful monitoring of patients receiving vancomycin therapy for pneumococcal meningitis. Meningococci have been found in Spain that are relatively resistant to penicillin due to decreased affinity of penicillin to penicillin-binding protein 3. The clinical significance of these isolates is unclear because patients have recovered uneventfully with standard penicillin therapy. In addition, beta-lactamase-producing isolates have been reported in Africa. Although they have not yet been reported in the United States, it would seem prudent to analyze the MICs for all meningococcal isolates.

Therapy of meningitis due to *H. influenzae* type b has

Table 233-5. Antibiotics of choice for bacterial meningitis

Organism	Antibiotic(s) of choice	Alternatives
N. meningitidis	Penicillin G	Ampicillin, chloramphenicol, cefuroxime, third-generation cephalosporin
S. pneumoniae	Penicillin G	Same as above, vancomycin
H. influenzae (beta-lactamase—negative)	Ampicillin	Chloramphenicol, cefuroxime, third-generation cephalosporin
H. influenzae (beta-lactamase—positive)	Cefotaxime or ceftriaxone	Chloramphenicol, cefuroxime
Enterobacteriaceae	Third-generation cephalosporin	Aminoglycosides, extended-spectrum penicillins, aztreonam, quinolones
P. aeruginosa	Ceftazidime (? plus an aminoglycoside*)	Extended-spectrum penicillin plus an aminoglycoside, aztreonam, quinolones
S. agalactiae	Penicillin G or ampicillin (? plus an aminoglycoside*)	Third-generation cephalosporin, chloramphenicol
L. monocytogenes	Ampicillin (? plus an aminoglycoside*)	Trimethoprim-sulfamethoxazole, chloramphenicol
S. aureus (methicillin-sensitive)	Nafcillin or oxacillin	Vancomycin (? plus rifampin)
S. aureus (methicillin-resistant)	Vancomycin	Trimethoprim-sulfamethoxazole, quinolones (?)
S. epidermidis	Vancomycin (? plus rifampin)	Penicillin G
M. tuberculosis	Isoniazid plus rifampin (? plus ethambutol or pyrazinamide)	
Candida sp.	Amphotericin B	Fluconazole
C. neoformans	Amphotericin B (? plus 5-fluorocytosine)	Fluconazole
C. immitis	Amphotericin B†	Fluconazole

*Value of aminoglycoside addition unproved.
†Intraventricular administration is usually required in addition to systemic route.

been markedly altered due to the emergence of beta-lactamase-producing strains, accounting for approximately 24% and 32% of CSF isolates overall in the United States in 1981 and 1986, respectively. Resistance to chloramphenicol has also been described, although it occurs more commonly in Spain (>50% of isolates) than the United States (<1% of isolates). Currently third-generation cephalosporins (cefotaxime or ceftriaxone) are recommended as therapy when beta-lactamase-producing strains of *H. influenzae* type b are suspected or isolated. Despite initial studies suggesting its efficacy, cefuroxime should not be used for the treatment of bacterial meningitis based on findings in a recent prospective, randomized study in which ceftriaxone was found superior to cefuroxime in rapidity of CSF ster-

Table 233-6. Dosages of antimicrobials in meningitis (adults with normal renal function)

Drug	Daily dose	Dosing interval
Penicillin G	20-24 million U	Continuous infusion or 4 million U q4h
Ampicillin	12-16 g	2 g q4h
Chloramphenicol	4-6 g*	1.0-1.5 g q6h
Nafcillin, oxacillin	12 g	2 g q4h
Cefotaxime	12 g	2 g q4h
Ceftriaxone	4 g	2 g q12h
Ceftazidime	6 g	2 g q8h
Vancomycin	2-3 g	1 g q8-12h
Gentamicin, tobramycin	3-5 mg/kg	1.7 mg/kg q8h
Amikacin	7.5 mg/kg	2.5 mg/kg q8h
Isoniazid	300 mg	Daily (p.o.)
Rifampin	600 mg	Daily (p.o.)
Amphotericin B	0.3-0.7 mg/kg	Daily
5-Fluorocytosine	100-150 mg/kg	q6h
Fluconazole	200-400 mg	Daily

*Higher dose recommended if used for pneumococcal meningitis.

Table 233-7. Empiric therapy of purulent meningitis

Age	Standard therapies	Alternative therapies
0-3 wk	Ampicillin plus cefotaxime	Ampicillin plus an aminoglycoside
4-12 wk	Cefotaxime or ceftriaxone plus ampicillin	
3 mo-18 yr	Cefotaxime or ceftriaxone	Cefuroxime, ampicillin, chloramphenicol, ampicillin plus chloramphenicol
18 yr-50 yr	Cefotaxime or ceftriaxone	Chloramphenicol
>50 yr	Third-generation cephalosporin plus ampicillin	Ampicillin plus an aminoglycoside, trimethoprim-sulfamethoxazole

ilization in children with bacterial meningitis. In addition, ceftriaxone was associated with a reduction of hearing impairment when compared with cefuroxime.

Ampicillin is generally recommended for the therapy of meningitis due to group B streptococci or *L. monocytogenes*. However, the combination of ampicillin and gentamicin is synergistic in vitro and in vivo, and such treatment appears reasonable for these infections. Alternatively, trimethoprim-sulfamethoxazole can be used for the treatment of *L. monocytogenes* meningitis.

In patients with a CSF shunt, meningitis is most commonly caused by coagulase-negative staphylococci. Initial therapy should consist of vancomycin with close monitoring of CSF levels during treatment. If the patient fails to improve, the addition of rifampin may be warranted. Removal of the shunt is important adjunctive therapy. *S. aureus* meningitis should be treated with nafcillin or oxacillin, with vancomycin reserved for patients allergic to penicillin or when methicillin-resistant organisms are isolated or suspected.

The therapy of gram-negative bacillary meningitis remains problematic. Most strains are resistant to ampicillin, and chloramphenicol is bacteriostatic. Until recently, the aminoglycosides were considered the drugs of choice. However, these agents penetrate poorly into the CSF during parenteral therapy alone, and intrathecal administration (via lumbar puncture) fails to produce reliable antibiotic concentrations at a site where infection (ventriculitis) is usually present.

The introduction of the third-generation cephalosporins has changed the approach to therapy of gram-negative bacillary meningitis in many patients. These agents have excellent in vitro activity against the major gram-negative meningeal pathogens and enter purulent CSF in bactericidal concentrations. Therapy with cefotaxime for gram-negative bacillary meningitis (due to susceptible strains) in adults results in cure rates of 74% to 94% in contrast to the mortality rates of 40% to 90% or more achieved with older regimens (e.g., aminoglycosides and/or chloramphenicol). These agents must be considered the drugs of choice for this disease. One particular agent, ceftazidime, has been shown to be efficacious for the treatment of *P. aeruginosa* meningitis, resulting in cure in 19 of 24 patients in one study when administered either alone or in combination with an aminoglycoside. Intrathecal or intraventricular aminoglycoside therapy should be considered only if there is no response to systemic therapy. This mode of administration is rarely needed at present. The fluoroquinolones (e.g., ciprofloxacin or pefloxacin) have been used successfully in some patients with gram-negative bacillary meningitis, but at present should only be used in adult patients with gram-negative bacterial meningitis who are failing conventional therapy or when the causative organism is resistant to standard drugs. Due to the poor activity of third-generation cephalosporins against some major meningeal pathogens (all agents of this class against *L. monocytogenes*), none of these agents should be used alone for purulent meningitis of unclear etiology.

Treatment for acute bacterial meningitis is usually continued for 10 to 14 days for the more common forms of meningitis and often longer (e.g., 3 weeks) for gram-negative bacillary meningitis. Several studies have demonstrated the efficacy and safety of short-course therapy (7 days) in infants and children with *H. influenzae* meningitis, but despite successes, the duration of therapy should be individualized.

Tuberculous meningitis is best treated with two tuberculocidal agents: isoniazid (300 to 600 mg po daily) and rifampin (600 mg po daily) (Chapter 276). Both attain excellent CSF concentrations. More recently, regimens have taken advantage of the newly appreciated merits of pyrazinamide and its intracellular microbicidal activity. For tuberculous meningitis in nonimmunocompromised patients, a 6-month treatment regimen is recommended consisting of isoniazid, rifampin, and pyrazinamide for the first 2 months, followed by 4 months of isoniazid and rifampin. Some authors, however, recommend 9 months of treatment for CNS tuberculosis. In addition, HIV-1 infected patients may require longer courses of treatment. Ethambutol should be added in cases of suspected drug resistance.

Steroids appear to exert a beneficial effect in this disease and should be administered in selected cases with extreme neurologic compromise, elevated intracranial pressure, impending herniation, or impending or established spinal block. Some authors also recommend corticosteroids in patients with CT evidence of either hydrocephalus or basilar meningitis. Prednisone, 1 mg/kg/day, tapered over 1 month, is often recommended, although varying doses of dexamethasone or hydrocortisone have also been used.

Amphotericin B is the mainstay of therapy for fungal meningitis (Chapter 278). Intravenous therapy alone (0.5 to 0.7 mg/kg/day IV) is indicated for *Candida* meningitis (Chapter 278). The addition of 5-fluorocytosine allows a reduction in dosage of amphotericin B to 0.3 mg/kg/day for the treatment of cryptococcal meningitis. This combination of fluorocytosine and amphotericin B for 6 weeks is as efficacious (with more rapid sterilization of the CSF) as 0.4 mg/kg/day of amphotericin B alone for 10 weeks. Fluorocytosine alone cannot be recommended because of the development of resistance and a low cure rate. Leukopenia, thrombocytopenia, and diarrhea may occur with peak fluorocytosine serum levels of 100 μg/ml or more. It is advisable to monitor complete blood counts biweekly and reduce the fluorocytosine dose if azotemia occurs. In a recent study a shorter course of combined amphotericin B and fluorocytosine therapy for 4 weeks was recommended for patients with the following characteristics: no underlying disease or immunosuppressive therapy; meningitis that is recognized early and not complicated by neurologic abnormalities; a CSF white cell count before treatment of greater than or equal to 20/mm^3; a pretreatment serum cryptococcal antigen titer less than 1:32; a negative CSF India ink preparation after 4 weeks of therapy; and serum and CSF cryptococcal antigen titers less than 1:8 at 4 weeks (Chapter 280).

Fluconazole, a new triazole antifungal agent, has been evaluated in the treatment of cryptococcal meningitis in patients with AIDS. In one trial the failure rate with fluconazole (8 of 14 patients) was much greater than in patients receiving combination therapy with amphotericin B plus 5-fluorocytosine (0 of 6 patients). A subsequent study by the Mycoses Study Group found no significant differences in the number of patients who were cured, improved, or died whether they received treatment with amphotericin B (at least 0.3 mg/kg/day) or fluconazole (200 mg/day). However, there was a trend toward early mortality in patients who were initially randomized to therapy with fluconazole. Based on these findings, we recommend that AIDS patients with cryptococcal meningitis receive initial therapy with amphotericin B (0.5-0.7 mg/kg/day) with or without 5-fluorocytosine for a period of about 2 weeks. This regimen is then followed by fluconazole (400 mg/day) to complete a 10-week course (Chapter 242). Due to the high rate of relapse in AIDS patients with cryptococcal meningitis, maintenance antifungal therapy should then be instituted; the maintenance therapy of choice is fluconazole, 200 mg/day.

Intraventricular administration of amphotericin B is usually necessary for meningitis due to *Coccidioides immitis* but is rarely required for cryptococcal disease. The benefit of adding agents other than 5-fluorocytosine (e.g., rifampin, tetracyclines) to amphotericin B remains unproved, despite in vitro susceptibility studies with strains of *Histoplasma* or *Aspergillus*. In patients who fail to respond to amphotericin B, the newer antifungal agents (e.g., fluconazole) in maximum tolerated doses may be considered (Chapters 277 and 278).

Adjunctive therapy

The value of corticosteroid therapy in bacterial meningitis has recently been examined in three controlled clinical trials. In one double-blind, placebo-controlled trial, infants and children with predominantly *H. influenzae* type b meningitis were randomized to receive antibiotics (cefuroxime or ceftriaxone) with either dexamethasone or placebo. The patients who received antibiotics plus dexamethasone became afebrile sooner, had more rapid normalization of CSF parameters, and were significantly less likely to acquire moderate to severe sensorineural hearing loss. The benefits in terms of morbidity, however, were statistically significant only in the patients receiving antibiotic therapy with cefuroxime, not in those receiving ceftriaxone.

In a second study from Egypt performed in children and adults with bacterial meningitis, there was a significant reduction in mortality rate and overall neurologic sequelae in patients with pneumococcal meningitis who received adjunctive dexamethasone concomitant with antibiotics (ampicillin plus chloramphenicol). However, no significant differences were observed in time to afebrility or improvement in CSF parameters. The antibiotics were given intramuscularly, and an extraordinarily high percentage of patients presented in a comatose state.

In a third recently published trial from Costa Rica, infants and children with bacterial meningitis were treated with cefotaxime with or without adjunctive dexamethasone administered 15 to 20 minutes before the first antibiotic dose. At 24 hours the clinical condition and mean prognostic scores were significantly better among the patients who received adjunctive dexamethasone therapy. When the patients were followed up for a mean of 15 months, those who received adjunctive dexamethasone had a significantly decreased incidence of one or more neurologic sequelae, although there was only a trend in reduction of audiologic impairment.

Based on these data, the use of adjunctive dexamethasone therapy (0.15 mg/kg every 6 hours for 4 days) is recommended for infants and children with *H. influenzae* type b meningitis. Routine dexamethasone therapy cannot be recommended in adults, pending results of ongoing studies. If dexamethasone is to be used, however, administration before or concomitant with antibiotics is optimal to attenuate the inflammatory response in the subarachnoid space.

When cerebral edema and raised intracranial pressure appear likely (e.g., by CT scan or neurologic examination) and the patients are comatose or have markedly abnormal neurologic examinations, making the detection of further deterioration difficult, a pressure-monitoring device should be placed intracranially. The patient should be monitored regularly in an intensive care environment and measures instituted to maintain the intracranial pressure in the normal range. These measures may include forced hyperventilation with respiratory muscle paralysis, hypothermia, osmotic agents such as mannitol or glycerol, and dexamethasone.

If shock complicates acute bacterial meningitis, vigorous supportive measures are necessary. The use of pressor agents, heparin for disseminated intravascular coagulation, and corticosteroids is discussed in Chapter 85. The septic arthritis that develops occasionally usually responds to systemic antibiotics and repeated needle aspiration, but open surgical drainage is indicated in a minority of patients. Seizures can be managed acutely with anticonvulsant therapy, and the presence of focal seizures should raise the question of brain abscess or subdural empyema.

PROGNOSIS

With appropriate therapy, mortality for the various forms of meningitis in the United States is as follows: *H. influenzae,* 3% to 6%; *N. meningitidis,* 5% to 10%; *S. pneumoniae,* 20% to 35%; *E. coli,* 30%; *L. monocytogenes,* 15% to 40%; group B streptococci, 10% to 30%; viruses, less than 1%; and fungi, 10% to 50% or more, depending on the organism. The rates are higher in neonates and in adults over 50 years of age. Coma and selected CSF abnormalities (high bacterial concentrations, low leukocyte counts, glucose $\leq$13 mg/dl, lactate $>$10 mEq/L) all adversely influence the prognosis. Sequelae such as mental retardation, deafness and other cranial nerve abnormalities, and seizures are present in up to half the survivors of neonatal or childhood meningitis. The development of hydrocephalus may necessitate CSF shunt insertion.

REFERENCES

Barnes PF et al: Tuberculosis in patients with human immunodeficiency virus infection, N Engl J Med 324:1644-1650, 1991.

Berenguer J et al: Tuberculous meningitis in patients infected with the human immunodeficiency virus, N Engl J Med 326:668-672, 1992.

Bozzette SA et al: A placebo-controlled trial of maintenance therapy with fluconazole after treatment of cryptococcal meningitis in the acquired immunodeficiency syndrome, N Engl J Med 324:580-584, 1991.

Bryan JP et al: Etiology and mortality of bacterial meningitis in Northeastern Brazil, Rev Infect Dis 12:128-135, 1990.

Dismukes WE et al: Treatment of cryptococcal meningitis with combination amphotericin B and flucytosine for four as compared with six weeks. N Engl J Med 317:334-341, 1987.

Geisler PJ et al: Community-acquired purulent meningitis: a review of 1,316 cases during the antibiotic era, 1959-1976, Rev Infect Dis 2:725-745, 1980.

Girgis NI et al: Dexamethasone treatment of bacterial meningitis in children and adults, Pediatr Infect Dis J 8:848-851, 1989.

Hollander, H and Stringari, S. Human immunodeficiency virus–associated meningitis. Clinical course and correlations. Am J Med 83:813-816, 1987.

Larsen RA et al: Fluconazole compared with amphotericin B plus flucytosine for cryptococcal meningitis in AIDS. A randomized trial, Ann Intern Med 113:183-187, 1990.

Lebel MH et al: Dexamethasone therapy for bacterial meningitis: results of two double-blind, placebo-controlled trials, N Engl J Med 319:964-971, 1988.

Odio CM et al: The beneficial effects of early dexamethasone administration in infants and children with bacterial meningitis, N Engl J Med 324:1525-1531, 1991.

Powderly WG et al: A controlled trial of fluconazole or amphotericin B to prevent relapse of cryptococcal meningitis in patients with the acquired immunodeficiency syndrome, N Engl J Med 326:793-798, 1992.

Radetsky M: Duration of treatment in bacterial meningitis: a historical inquiry, Pediatr Infect Dis J 9:2-9, 1990.

Saag MS et al: Comparison of amphotericin B with fluconazole in the treatment of acute AIDS-associated cryptococcal meningitis, N Engl J Med 326:83-89, 1992.

Sande MA et al: Pathophysiology of bacterial meningitis: summary of a workshop, Pediatr Infect Dis J 8:929-933, 1989.

Schaad UB et al: A comparison of ceftriaxone and cefuroxime for the treatment of bacterial meningitis in children, N Engl J Med 322:141-147, 1990.

Scheld WM and Wispelwey B, editors: Meningitis, Infect Dis Clin North Am 4:555-854, 1990.

Schlech WF et al: Bacterial meningitis in the United States, 1978 through 1981. The national bacterial meningitis surveillance study, JAMA 253:1749-1754, 1985.

Schlesinger LS et al: *Staphylococcus aureus* meningitis: a broad-based epidemiologic study, Medicine (Baltimore) 66:148-156, 1987.

Spanos A et al: Differential diagnosis of acute meningitis. An analysis of the predictive value of initial observation, JAMA 262:2700-2707, 1989.

Tunkel AR and Scheld WM: Therapy of bacterial meningitis: principles and practice, Infect Control Hosp Epidemiol 10:565-569, 1989.

Tunkel AR and Scheld WM: Acute therapy of bacterial meningitis, J Intensive Care Med 6:229-237, 1991.

Tunkel AR et al: Bacterial meningitis: recent advances in pathophysiology and treatment, Ann Intern Med 112:610-623, 1990.

Viladrich PF et al: Characteristics and antibiotic therapy of adult meningitis due to penicillin-resistant pneumococci, Am J Med 84:839-846, 1988.

Viladrich PF et al: Evaluation of vancomycin for therapy of adult pneumococcal meningitis, Antimicrob Agents Chemother 35:2467-2472, 1991.

Wenger JD et al: Bacterial meningitis in the United States, 1986: report of a multistate surveillance study, J Infect Dis 162:1316-1323, 1990.

CHAPTER

234 Brain Abscess and Perimeningeal Infections

Adam P. Brown
Colin Derdeyn
Ralph G. Dacey, Jr.

Localized intracranial and intraspinal infections present formidable difficulties in diagnosis and treatment. Despite recent improvements in the antimicrobial chemotherapy and neuroradiology of central nervous system (CNS) infections, mortality from brain abscess and perimeningeal infections remains high. Optimum management of the patient with these conditions therefore demands close cooperation between the primary physician and neurosurgeon.

BRAIN ABSCESS

Pathophysiology and etiology

In 80% of patients, brain abscess is associated with known extracerebral sources of infection. The most common primary sites of infection are found either in close proximity to the CNS (e.g., in the paranasal sinuses) or in distant locations, usually within the chest (Table 234-1). In addition to gram-positive cocci and Enterobacteriaceae, microaerophilic and anaerobic organisms form brain abscesses up to 40% of the time and anaerobic cultures should therefore be obtained in all patients. The causative organism can often be predicted from the site of the abscess—an important fact when choosing initial antibiotic therapy.

Bacteria may gain access to the brain from contiguous sites of infection by direct spread or presumably via infected thrombi in the emissary veins that penetrate the cranial vault. Otitis media and complicating mastoiditis may cause abscesses in the adjacent temporal lobe or cerebellar hemisphere. Common bacterial isolates from otogenic abscesses are aerobic and anaerobic streptococci, *Bacteroides fragilis*, and Enterobacteriaceae, often in mixed culture. Frontal lobe abscess is usually associated with frontal, ethmoidal, or sphenoidal sinusitis. The most common bacterial isolates in frontal lobe abscesses are aerobic and anaerobic streptococci (especially the *Streptococcus milleri* group), although Enterobacteriaceae, *Bacteroides* species, and other organisms are also reported. In brain abscess resulting from penetrating craniocerebral trauma or neurosurgical wound infection, *Staphylococcus aureus* is usually the causative agent, although Enterobacteriaceae and *Clostridium* species are also found.

Brain abscess in association with a distant primary source of infections is the result of hematogenous dissemination of the infecting organism. Such abscesses are often multiple. These metastatic abscesses may occur at any location within the brain, although there appears to be a predisposition for sites in the distribution of the middle cerebral artery. Most metastatic brain abscesses occur as a re-

Table 234-1. Brain abscess: predisposing conditions, locations, and microbiology

Predisposing condition*	Site of abscess	Usual isolate(s) from abscess
Contiguous site of primary infection		
Otitis media and mastoiditis	Temporal lobe or cerebellar hemisphere	Streptococci (anaerobic or aerobic) *Bacteroides fragilis,* Enterobacteriaceae
Frontoethmoidal sinusitis	Frontal lobe	Predominantly streptococci: *Bacteroides,* Enterobacteriaceae, *Staphylococcus aureus,* and *Haemophilus* species
Sphenoidal sinusitis	Frontal or temporal lobe	Same as in frontoethmoidal sinusitis
Dental sepsis	Frontal lobe most common	Mixed *Fusobacterium, Bacteroides,* and *Streptococcus* species
Penetrating cranial trauma or postsurgical infection	Related to wound	*S. aureus;* streptococci, Enterobacteriaceae, *Clostridium* species
Distant site of primary infection		
Congenital heart disease	Multiple abscess cavities; middle cerebral artery distribution common but may occur at any site	Streptococci (*viridans,* anaerobic, and microaerophilic), *Haemophilus* species
Lung abscess, empyema, bronchiectasis	Same as in congenital heart disease	*Fusobacterium, Actinomyces, Bacteroides,* streptococci, *Nocardia asteroides*
Bacterial endocarditis	Same as in congenital heart disease	*S. aureus,* streptococci
Compromised hosts (immunosuppressive therapy or malignancy)	Same as in congenital heart disease	*Toxoplasma,* fungi, Enterobacteriaceae
Acquired immunodeficiency syndrome	Any location	*Toxoplasma;* less likely are *Cryptococcus,* TB, cytomegalovirus encephalitis (consider PML,† and primary lymphoma)

*Predisposing conditions identified in approximately 80% of cases.
†PML, progressive multifocal leukoencephalopathy.

sult of suppurative pulmonary disease, such as lung abscess, empyema, or bronchiectasis. Isolates from this group of patients include *Fusobacterium, Actinomyces, Nocardia asteroides, Bacteroides,* and *Streptococcus* species. Brain abscess occurs in patients with congenital heart disease with right-to-left shunting. Streptococci (aerobic, microaerophilic, and anaerobic) are isolated from most brain abscesses in patients with congenital heart disease. Brain abscess is rare in bacterial endocarditis.

The compromised host is also at increased risk for the development of brain abscess, as a result of either immunosuppressive therapy or underlying malignancy. Fungi and parasites are important diagnostic considerations in this group of patients.

Patients with acquired immunodeficiency syndrome (AIDS) have CNS involvement in about 40% of cases, whereas 10% of AIDS patients will present initially with neurologic symptoms. Many of these patients have focal mass lesions identified by computed tomography (CT) or magnetic resonance imaging (MRI) caused by *Toxoplasma gondii,* primary CNS lymphoma, progressive multifocal leukoencephalopathy (PML), or fungal sources (Chapter 280). Biopsy of these disparate lesions may be indicated, as appropriate therapy varies drastically depending on histologic and culture data. Recently, however, an empiric trial of antitoxoplasmal chemotherapy followed by serial CT scanning (every 2 to 3 weeks) has been recommended as an initial step in managing these patients (Chapter 242).

Patients who have lived in or traveled to Mexico or Central or South America, and who have enhancing lesions on CT/MRI, must be considered at risk for cysticercosis (Chapter 282).

Clinical manifestations and differential diagnosis

The correct diagnosis of brain abscess is often delayed because patients with this disease may manifest little neurologic deficit and few signs of an infectious process. Therefore, any neurologic illness in a patient with one of the predisposing conditions (Table 234-1) should suggest the diagnosis of brain abscess at an early point in the course of the disease. The classic triad of fever, headache, and focal neurologic deficit is present in less than 50% of patients. The single most common symptom is headache, which is seen in approximately 70% of patients. Fever occurs in 50% to 60% of adults, but is more common in children. The focal nature of brain involvement by the abscess is demonstrated in approximately 80% of patients by either a localizable neurologic deficit or seizures. Other indicators of increased intracranial pressure, such as nausea, vomiting, and lethargy, are less common but important, as they may point to incipient decompensation and require urgent surgical management. Papilledema and cranial nerve deficits are seen in a minority of patients. Brain abscess may sometimes mimic bacterial meningitis in its presentation, with signs of meningeal inflammation that may indicate close proximity of the abscess to the ventricles or subarachnoid space. A slight male predominance exists.

Brain abscess must be differentiated from other intracranial infections, such as meningitis, subdural empyema, mycotic aneurysm, and epidural abscess. CT and/or MRI are essential for accomplishing this differentiation. Other conditions to be distinguished from brain abscess include primary or metastatic cerebral tumors, cerebral infarction, viral encephalitis (predominantly herpes simplex), and chronic subdural hematoma.

Laboratory diagnosis and radiologic evaluation

Lumbar puncture should not be performed in patients with known or suspected intracranial abscess for two reasons. First, the analysis of the cerebrospinal fluid (CSF) is nondiagnostic. Findings include elevated CSF protein, variable pleocytosis, and a normal glucose. Second, lumbar puncture may precipitate brain herniation if a mass lesion is present. Consequently, the diagnosis of intracranial abscess rests with the patient's history and the imaging studies, either CT or MRI. In a patient with an apparent intracranial infection and a focal neurologic deficit, or history of a predisposing condition (Table 234-1), a CT or MRI scan should be obtained to exclude an abscess before lumbar puncture.

CT is more quickly obtained and more safely performed than MRI in the acutely ill patient. Its sensitivity is comparable to MRI; however, CT may miss early inflammatory changes. This fact is rarely clinically significant because few patients present in the early cerebritis stage of abscess formation. Noncontrasted images usually show white matter edema and mass effect. Depending on the location, hydrocephalus may also be present. With the infusion of intravenous contrast, ring enhancement is observed in the mature abscess (Fig. 234-1). This pattern of edema and enhancement, however, is similar to that observed in some tumors. Therefore the diagnosis must often be made by aspiration or biopsy.

CT is particularly helpful in defining paranasal sinus disease. The standard transaxial examination may detect the underlying frontal, ethmoid, sphenoid, or mastoid sinus infection responsible for the intracranial abscess. Coronal images of the sinuses provide an even more detailed examination for underlying sinus disease. This examination is more expensive but more sensitive than plain films.

MRI provides greater definition of the intracranial anatomy and better sensitivity for edema and early inflammatory changes, such as those seen in cerebritis. In addition, it is not limited by bone artifact in the posterior fossa. The pattern and timing of enhancement with gadopentate dimeglumine (gadolinium-DPTA) is similar to iodinated contrast in CT; therefore, a mature abscess will ring en-

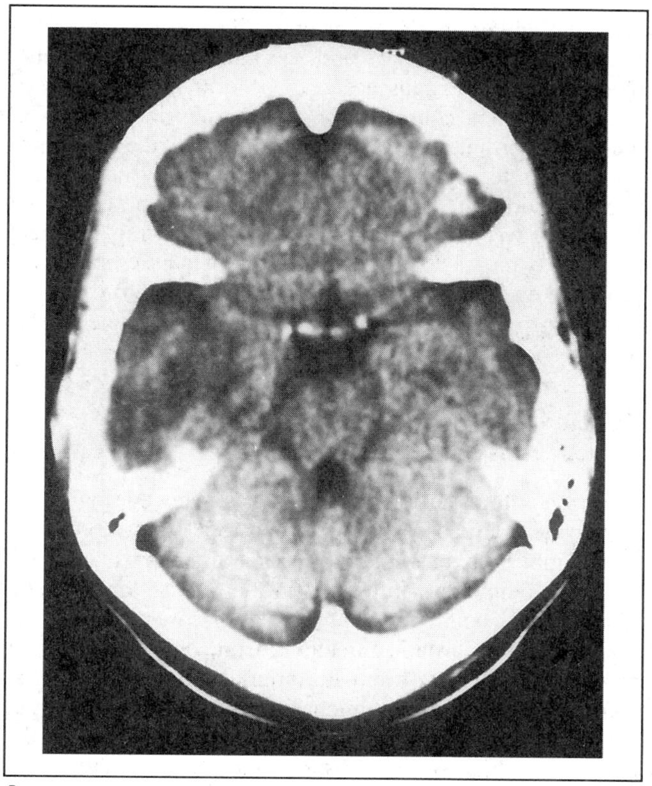

A

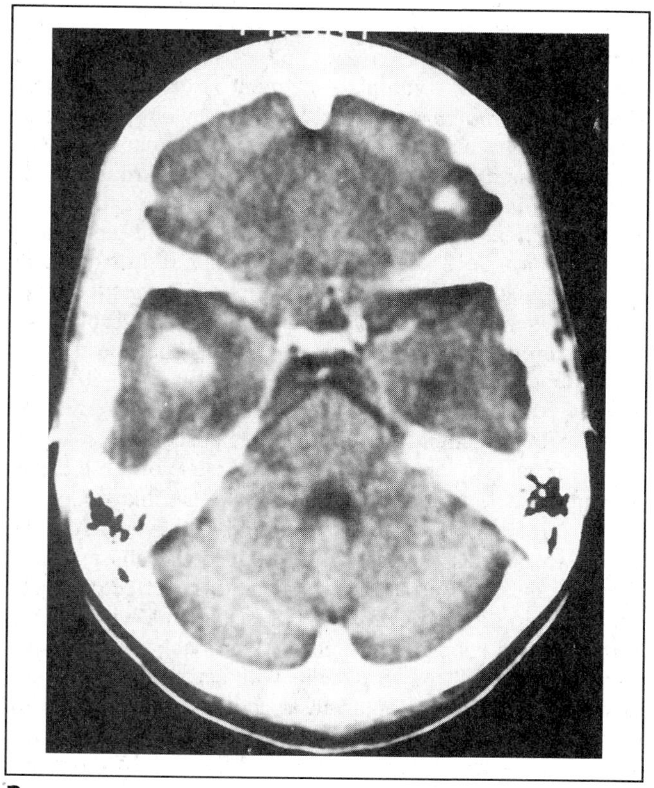

B

Fig. 234-1. This 38-year-old alcoholic presented with a chronic cough and headache. Systemic evaluation revealed a right lung abscess. **A,** Noncontrast CT scan demonstrates an area of low attenuation in the right temporal lobe with mass effect on the temporal tip of the lateral ventricle. **B,** Postcontrast CT demonstrates a ring-enhancing lesion with a thick rim, consistent with an intracranial abscess.

hance (Fig. 234-2). This appearance, however, is not specific and a neoplasm must still be ruled out.

Both MRI and CT may be used for stereotactic biopsies or aspirations of suspicious lesions. In addition, repeat scanning is useful for postoperative follow-up and mandatory for those patients managed by antimicrobial chemotherapy alone.

Treatment

Most patients with brain abscess require a combination of surgical and antibiotic therapy. Despite adequate treatment, mortality in brain abscess may be as high as 25% to 30%, with permanent neurologic sequelae occurring in 30% to 55%. However, with current access to noninvasive neuroimaging, which allows early and accurate localization of the lesion, mortality and morbidity may become significantly lower.

The initial choice of antibiotic therapy should be based on the location of the abscess and the underlying primary infection (if one can be identified), because these features can be used to predict the probable bacteriologic isolate. Specific therapy should then be prescribed when abscess cavity culture data become available. Before surgical drainage, therapy should be initiated with penicillin G, 20 to 24 million units per day and metronidazole, 500 mg IV every 6 hours. Metronidazole may be preferable to chloramphenicol in this setting because it achieves a higher concentration into the abscess cavity, and is bactericidal versus *Bacteroides*. This combined treatment is effective against streptococcal, *Bacteroides,* and *Fusobacterium* species, and many Enterobacteriaceae, although recent increases in these organisms, and in *Pseudomonas aeruginosa* (chronic ear infections), may suggest adding stronger gram-negative coverage, such as an aminoglycoside or a third-generation cephalosporin such as ceftazidime. Methicillin or nafcillin (8 to 12 g/day IV) should be substituted for penicillin G when *S. aureus* is the likely causative organism (Table 234-1). Vancomycin (1 g IV every 12 hours) may be used if the patient is penicillin allergic. Dexamethasone, 20 to 30 mg/day, or methylprednisolone, 100 to 150 mg/day, appears to be beneficial in reducing periabscess edema and hence intracranial pressure, although the use of these drugs in brain abscess is controversial because they may slow the macrophage and glial response. Steroids, however, do not appear to decrease antibiotic delivery to the abscess. Pyrimethamine and sulfadiazine appear to be effective therapy for toxoplasmosis of the CNS in patients with AIDS, but prolonged suppressive therapy is probably necessary to prevent relapse. In AIDS patients with acute intracranial lesion(s) suggesting toxoplasmosis, empiric coverage with the previous agents should be initiated. A clinical and radiologic response should be noted by 10 and 14 days, respectively; otherwise a biopsy should be performed to rule out other diagnoses. A biopsy should be performed initially in AIDS patients if the CT/MRI scan is atypical for toxoplasmosis. Antiepileptic therapy is usually instituted in patients with brain abscess(es).

There are two accepted methods for the surgical treatment of brain abscess—complete excision and stereotactic needle aspiration. Complete excision of the well-encapsulated abscess in an accessible location may be superior to stereotactic aspiration, but results with either excision or aspiration appear equivalent. Surgical excision is preferred for posterior fossa lesions, as well as for brain abscesses caused by fungi because available antifungal therapy is unsatisfactory. The use of CT/MRI in following patients with brain abscess and in facilitating stereotactic biopsy in selected patients may potentially lower mortality rates in this disease. Several recent series document a diagnostic yield of 94% to 96% with a low transient morbidity (4% to 6%) associated with stereotactic biopsy. Repeat aspiration is occasionally necessary. Surgical drainage should be accomplished immediately in patients who demonstrate a progressive neurologic deficit or a decreasing level of consciousness.

Recent reports suggest that selected patients with brain abscess may be managed with antibiotic therapy alone. Patients with early abscess or cerebritis, patients with small abscesses (i.e., diameter less than 2 cm), and alert patients without neurologic deficits may be candidates for nonsurgical therapy; but they should be followed closely for clinical or radiologic deterioration, which would indicate the need for surgical drainage. Nevertheless, this nonsurgical approach to treating brain abscesses poses several potential problems. Because the causative agent is not identified, the choice of antibiotic may be incorrect. Moreover, the proper treatment of brain tumors and vascular lesions mistakenly diagnosed as brain abscess may be critically delayed. If such a treatment course is chosen, the physician must exercise extraordinary care in monitoring the patient's neurologic status to detect subtle changes that may herald sudden deterioration. Antibiotic therapy should be continued for 4 to 6 weeks parenterally, followed by oral treatment for 2 to 6 months, although this regimen is empiric and probably excessive for some organisms. Therefore the decision to treat the patient by medical means alone should be made jointly with the neurosurgeon.

INTRACRANIAL SUBDURAL EMPYEMA

Pathogenesis and etiology

Infection within the subdural space has many etiologic similarities to brain abscess. Most cases (35% to 60%) of subdural empyema are related to paranasal sinusitis, most often frontoethmoidal. Infections in the middle ear and temporal bone account for around 15% of cases, and the remainder are metastatic infections from distant sources or related to surgery or traumatic injuries. Most of the metastatic cases arise from purulent bronchopulmonary disease.

The most common site for subdural empyema is in the anterior cranial fossa, as a result of paranasal sinusitis. Otogenic subdural empyema occurs over the temporal and occipital lobes or in the posterior fossa. Frontal subdural empyema may be bilateral and/or situated between the two hemispheres. Infection in the subdural space is often associated with septic venous thrombosis and subsequent hemorrhagic cortical infarction. This pathologic finding may be

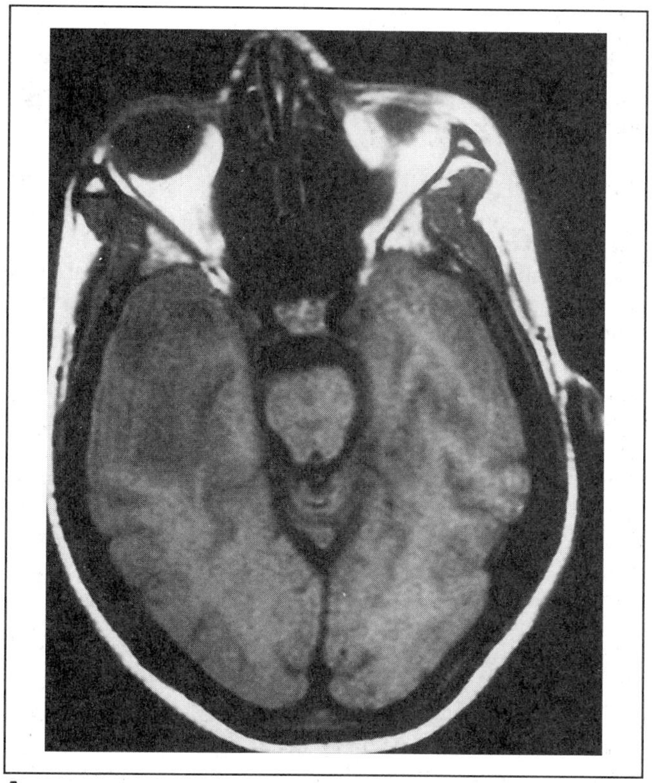

A

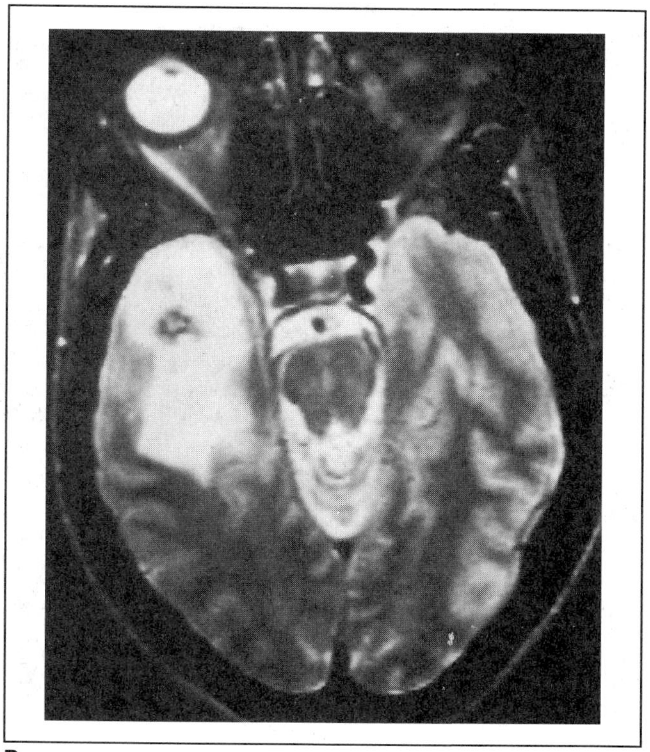

B

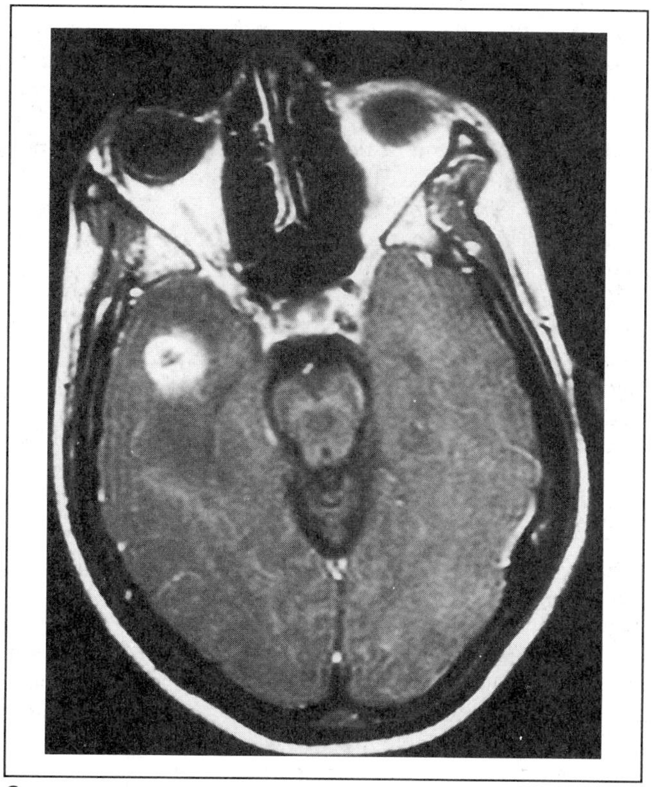

C

Fig. 234-2. Same patient as in Fig. 234-1. **A,** T_1-weighted image shows swelling of the right temporal lobe. **B,** T_2-weighted image shows extensive high signal intensity consistent with edema. The low intensity center may be cellular debris within the abscess cavity. **C,** After intravenous gadolinium the image demonstrates a ring-enhancing abscess centered in the temporal lobe. Given the patient's history and the chronic antibiotic regimen required for the lung abscess, this lesion was treated medically. No recurrence was seen on MRI at 6 months.

responsible for the high incidence of focal seizures in this condition.

Aerobic, microaerophilic, and anaerobic streptococci, Enterobacteriaceae, and *B. fragilis* are the most common bacterial isolates. Subdural empyema in infants is almost always associated with meningitis caused by *Haemophilus influenzae* or gram-negative bacteria.

Clinical manifestations

Most patients with subdural empyema are males with paranasal sinusitis (the male/female ratio is 3:1). There is a peak incidence in the second and third decades. The presence of localized severe headache (75%) and fever (85%), later becoming associated with lethargy and focal seizures (50%), should suggest the diagnosis of subdural empyema. Papilledema is noted in fewer than half the patients, but other indicators of increased intracranial pressure (e.g., lethargy, nausea, and vomiting) are common.

Laboratory diagnosis and radiologic evaluation

CSF findings in subdural empyema are nonspecific, as is the case with brain abscess. Lumbar puncture therefore is often not useful and may be dangerous, as intracranial pressure may be elevated and herniation may follow lumbar puncture.

MRI is superior to CT in detecting extracerebral infections such as subdural or epidural empyemas. Small amounts of extracerebral fluid or pus may be difficult to detect with CT but are visible with MRI because of the lack of bone artifact, the better separation of CSF and brain, and the capability of multiplanar imaging. The signal characteristics of the fluid collection can also be used to differentiate a benign effusion from a more complex purulent collection.

The CT scan typically demonstrates an extracerebral fluid collection with surrounding low attenuation and enhancement. MRI detects even more subtle amounts of parenchymal edema as high signal on T_2-weighted images. The T_1-weighted images delineate the extracerebral collection. Gadolinium enhancement is similar to that seen on CT (Fig. 234-3).

Treatment

The clinical suspicion or radiologic diagnosis of subdural empyema requires the immediate use of antibiotic therapy. Either penicillin G, nafcillin, or vancomycin, and metronidazole and a third-generation cephalosporin should be initiated after appropriate cultures are made. Beta-lactamase-resistant antibiotics should be used in traumatic or postsurgical cases in which *S. aureus* is likely. Steroids may be useful in patients with increased intracranial pressure. Antiepileptic therapy is usually instituted.

Burr holes and irrigation will accomplish adequate drainage in some patients, but craniotomy is usually necessary for thorough evacuation of pus. Fluid for aerobic and anaerobic cultures must be obtained intraoperatively. Parenteral antibiotic therapy is continued for 4 to 6 weeks after surgical drainage.

Despite medical and surgical therapy, mortality in subdural empyema is 15% to 30% primarily because the diagnosis is often delayed.

INTRACRANIAL EPIDURAL ABSCESS

Intracranial epidural abscess has an incidence of 10%, with the remainder of these epidural infections occurring in the spine. This abscess shares with subdural empyema the common causes of sinusitis, mastoiditis, and postoperative wound infection. Subdural empyema and osteomyelitis commonly coexist with epidural abscesses. Epidural abscess should be suspected in patients with sinusitis or otitis who present with cellulitis of the face or scalp. Treatment should consist of appropriate antibiotic therapy and drainage of pus by burr holes or craniectomy. If a communication between the epidural space and a sinus cavity exists, proper closure should be accomplished to prevent recurrent infection.

SPINAL EPIDURAL ABSCESS

Etiology and pathogenesis

Intraspinal bacterial infections occur most often within the posterior epidural space. Bacteria may gain access to the epidural space by hematogenous spread from distant infections, usually in the skin or pelvic structures. Alternatively, vertebral osteomyelitis may progress to involve the epidural space directly, or penetrating injuries may implant bacteria in the epidural space.

S. aureus is the most common causative organism, being isolated in 60% to 90% of cases. *Escherichia coli, P. aeruginosa, Streptococcus pneumoniae,* and *Klebsiella* and *Proteus* species have been reported. Tuberculosis of the spine may involve the epidural space.

The thoracic spine is the site of the abscess in 50% to 80% of patients, followed in frequency by the cervical and lumbar spine. Spinal epidural abscess may extend over many spinal levels. The epidural mass may consist of pus and granulation tissue in acute cases or of fibrous granulation tissue in chronic cases.

Clinical manifestations

The triad of fever, back pain, and neurologic symptoms of spinal cord dysfunction should immediately suggest the diagnosis of spinal epidural abscess. Patients will often note localized back pain that subsequently becomes associated with a radicular component. Weakness, dysesthesia, and urinary or fecal incontinence or retention may subsequently be followed by complete paralysis. Physical examination will almost always demonstrate spinal percussion tenderness (unless the infection is predominantly subdural) and signs of root or cord compression.

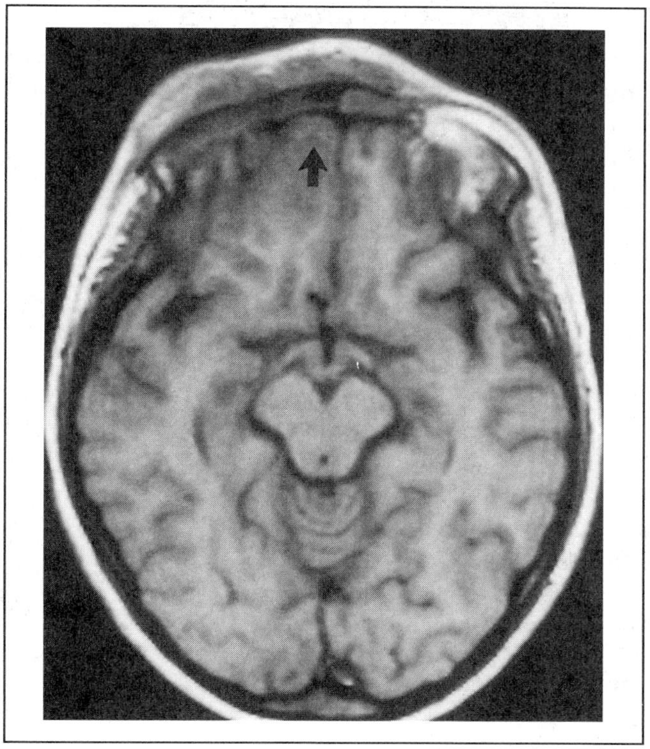

A

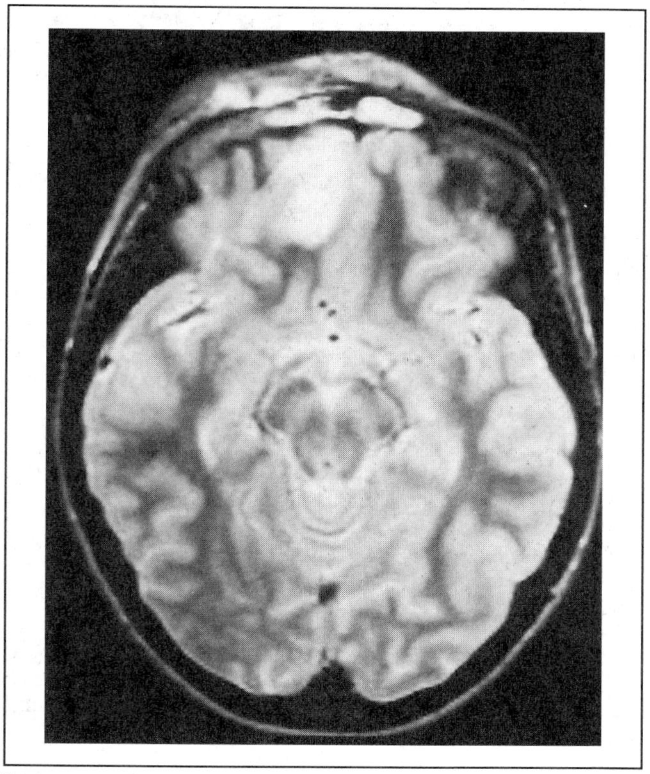

B

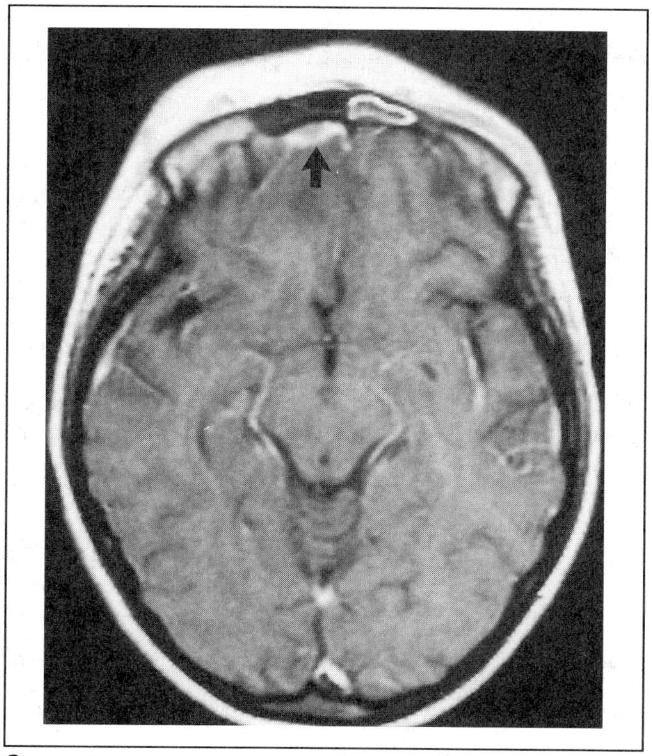

C

Fig. 234-3. A 19-year-old man with a several week history of sinusitis experienced a generalized seizure. **A,** T_1-, **B,** T_2-, and **C,** T_1-weighted postgadolinium images demonstrate a subtle, enhancing subdural empyema anterior to the right frontal lobe (*arrow* in **A** and **C**). This fluid collection was missed on CT. Marked edema of the adjacent frontal lobe is especially prominent in the T_2 image, **B.** Fluid is also present in the right frontal sinus. The left sinus enhances, consistent with chronic sinusitis. The thickened overlying scalp represents cellulitis.

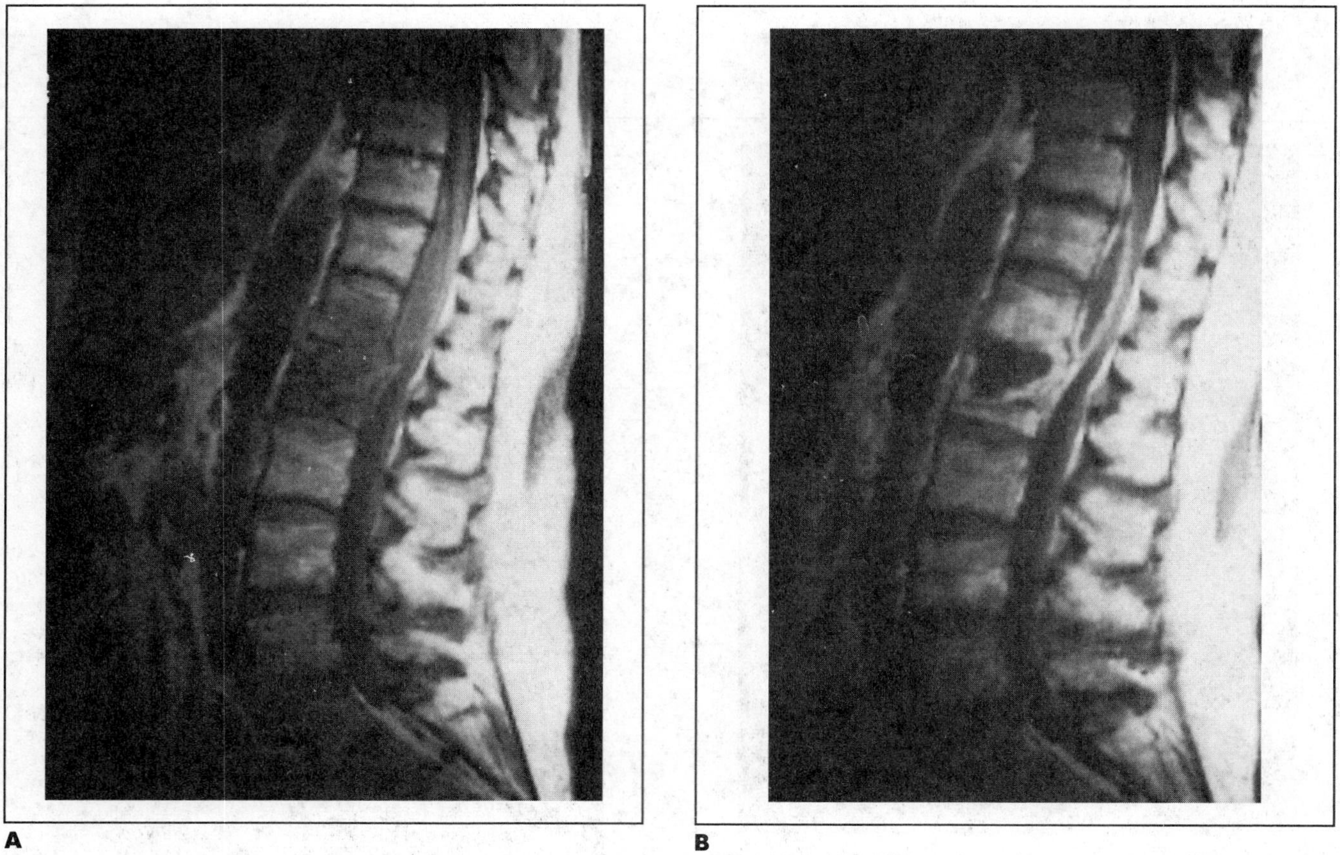

Fig. 234-4. A 65-year-old woman presented with low back pain and fever. **A,** Sagittal T_1-weighted and **B,** T_1-postgadolinium scans reveal a large anterior, peripherally enhancing epidural abscess in the region of the conus medullaris. Disk-centered osteomyelitis is also present at L1-L2. Intraoperative cultures grew *S. aureus*.

Laboratory diagnosis and radiologic evaluation

MRI has replaced CT myelography as the radiologic procedure of choice for the detection of epidural abscess. Although both techniques are equally sensitive, MRI is superior to CT myelography in specificity. MRI better defines the rostral and caudal extent of the abscess, as well as the degree of cord compression (Fig. 234-4). In addition, MRI is equal to combined bone and gallium scans in sensitivity (96%) and specificity (92%) for underlying vertebral osteomyelitis. MRI offers the additional advantage of not requiring a lumbar puncture. Plain films continue to serve as the screening examination for suspected disk space infection or a paravertebral soft tissue mass.

Treatment

As with other perimeningeal infections, treatment should be instituted as soon as the diagnosis is made and should consist of a combination of antibiotic therapy and surgical drainage. Antistaphylococcal therapy (methicillin, nafcillin, or vancomycin) should initially be combined with aminoglycosides or third-generation cephalosporins until intraoperative culture data are available. Steroids probably should be given perioperatively to patients with spinal epidural abscess to reduce edema.

Surgical drainage should be performed as an emergency procedure consisting of laminectomy and irrigation of the epidural space. The subdural space should not be violated. Despite combined therapy, mortality rates remain as high as 10% to 20%, and morbidity can be catastrophic (e.g., paraplegia). Early diagnosis and rapid treatment offer the best chance for reducing mortality and morbidity.

REFERENCES

Baker AS et al: Spinal epidural abscess, N Engl J Med 293:463, 1975.

Brant-Zawadzki M et al: Magnetic resonance imaging and characterization of normal and abnormal intracranial cerebrospinal fluid spaces: initial observations, Neuroradiology 27:3, 1985.

Brant-Zawadzki M et al: NMR imaging of experimental brain abscess: comparison with CT, Am J Neuroradiol 4:250, 1983.

Chun CH et al: Brain abscess. A study of 45 consecutive cases, Medicine (Baltimore) 65:415, 1986.

Ciricillo SF and Rosenblum ML: Imaging of solitary lesions in AIDS (letter), J Neurosurg 74:1029, 1991.

Ciricillo SF and Rosenblum ML: Use of CT and MR imaging to distinguish intracranial lesions and to define the need for biopsy in AIDS patients, J Neurosurg 73:720, 1990.

Cowie R and Williams B: Late seizures and morbidity after subdural empyema, J Neurosurg 58:569, 1983.

Dacey RG Jr: Central nervous system infections (brain abscesses and shunt infection). In Root RK, Trunkey DD, and Sande MA, editors: Contemporary issues in infectious diseases, vol. 6, Focus on infection: new surgical and medical approaches, New York, 1986, Churchill Livingstone.

DeLouvois JD et al: Bacteriology of abscesses of the central nervous system: a multicentre prospective study, Br Med J 2:981, 1977.

Harrison MJ: The clinical presentation of intracranial abscesses, Q J Med 51:4611, 1982.

Hlavin ML et al: Spinal epidural abscess: a ten year perspective, Neurosurgery 27:177, 1990.

Itakurg T et al: Stereotactic operation for brain abscess, Surg Neurol 28:114, 1987.

Kagawa M et al: Brain abscess in congenital cyanotic heart disease, J Neurosurg 58:913, 1983.

Kaufman DM, Miller MH, and Steigbigel MH: Subdural empyema: analysis of 17 cases and review of the literature, Medicine (Baltimore) 54:485, 1975.

Levy RM et al: Neuroepidemiology of acquired immunodeficiency syndrome, J Acquir Immune Defic Syndr 1:31, 1988.

Levy RM, Pons VG, and Rosenblum ML: Central nervous system mass lesions in the acquired immunodeficiency syndrome (AIDS), J Neurosurg 61:9, 1984.

Luft BJ and Remington JS: Toxoplasmic encephalitis, J Infect Dis 157:106, 1988.

Lunsford LD: Stereotactic drainage of brain abscesses, Neurol Res 9:270, 1987.

McAlister WH, Lusk R, and Muntz HR: Comparison of plain radiographs and coronal CT scans in infants and children with recurrent sinusitis, Am J Roentgenol 153:1259, 1989.

Modic MT, Feiglin DH, and Piraino DW: Vertebral osteomyelitis: assessment using MR, Radiology 157:157, 1985.

Rodesch G et al: Nervous system manifestations and neuroradiologic findings in acquired immunodeficiency syndrome (AIDS), Neuroradiology 31:33, 1989.

Rosenblum ML, Mampalam TJ, and Pons VG: Controversies in the management of brain abscesses, Clin Neurosurg 33:603, 1986.

Rosenblum ML et al: Nonoperative treatment of brain abscesses in selected high risk patients, J Neurosurg 52:217, 1980.

Salzman C and Tuazon CU: Value of the ring-enhancing sign in differentiating intracerebral hematomas and brain abscesses, Arch Intern Med 147:951, 1987.

Schroth G et al: Advantage of magnetic resonance imaging in the diagnosis of cerebral infections, Neuroradiology 29:120, 1987.

Smith AS and Blaser SI: Infectious and inflammatory processes of the spine, Radiol Clin North Am 29:809, 1991.

Sze G and Zimmerman RD: The magnetic resonance imaging of infections and inflammatory diseases, Radiol Clin North Am 26:839, 1988.

Wingarten K et al: Subdural and epidural empyemas: MR imaging, Am J Neuroradiol 10:81. 1989.

Wispelwey B and Scheld WM: Brain abscess, Clin Neuropharmacol 10:483, 1987.

Yildizhan A, Pasoglu A, and Kandemir B: Effect of dexamethasone on various stages of experimental brain abscess, Acta Neurochir 96:141-148, 1989.

CHAPTER

235 Skin and Subcutaneous Infections

Richard E. Bryant

PRIMARY INFECTIONS OF SKIN

Impetigo

Impetigo is a superficial pyoderma that is usually caused by *Staphylococcus aureus,* mixtures of *S. aureus* and group A streptococci, or less often by group A streptococci alone. Impetigo is rarely caused by group C or G streptococci. In neonates it may be caused by group B streptococci. Impetigo is highly contagious in families or institutions where crowding, poor hygiene, and recurrent abrasions enhance the likelihood of infection, especially in preschool children.

Bacteria colonize the skin several weeks before initiation of disease after minor trauma (Chapter 259). Lesions start as small vesicles beneath the stratum corneum and quickly become pustules and rupture to produce the characteristic honey-colored "stuck-on" crusts. Lesions on exposed surfaces often coalesce to form large crusts. Autoinoculation frequently produces separate lesions. Lymphadenopathy occurs often, but constitutional symptoms are mild or absent.

Diagnosis is usually suspected by clinical appearance and confirmed by Gram stain and by culture. Serologic confirmation of group A streptococcal skin infection is obtained by a rising titer of antibody to antideoxyribonuclease B or antihyaluronidase. Antistreptolysin O titers do not rise predictably after impetigo. The differential diagnosis of impetigo includes secondary infection of primary skin lesions, such as insect bites, eczema, or dermatophytosis. Early lesions of varicella or herpes simplex are usually larger and persist longer than do vesicles associated with impetigo. Viral diagnosis can be confirmed by Tzanck test, fluorescent antibody test, or viral culture. Cost-effective treatment options include oral erythromycin, topical mupirocin, or oral cephalosporins given twice daily.

Bullous impetigo

Bullous impetigo is caused by *S. aureus* strains that produce an exfoliative exotoxin. The staphylococci are in phage group II, usually type 71. Nasal colonization is usually the reservoir from which bacteria spread to the skin, where invasion occurs after minor trauma. Bullous impetigo occurs primarily in neonates and young children and is less common than nonbullous impetigo.

Lesions begin as small vesicles and progress to large, flaccid blisters containing clear yellow fluid. Bullae rupture to form a thin, light-brown crust. Lymphadenopathy is rare, and systemic symptoms are usually mild. Diagnosis is made from a Gram stain showing clusters of gram-positive cocci and cultures growing *S. aureus.* Staphylococcal impetigo is easily differentiated from primary bullous diseases such as pemphigus because in patients with impetigo, cultures and smears are positive and Nikolsky's sign is negative. A penicillinase-resistant penicillin given orally is the treatment of choice. Erythromycin or mupirocin may be used for penicillin-allergic patients.

Ecthyma

Ecthyma is an ulcerative crusting infection caused by group A streptococci that occurs on exposed skin areas, especially the legs of children after abrasions, cuts, or insect bites. It may affect all sites and age groups but in adults usually is associated with poor hygiene.

Lesions begin as vesicles that become pustular and rupture to form dried, grayish, "punched-out," crusted lesions on a red, indurated base. Lesions extend below the epidermis and therefore heal more slowly than do those of impetigo and often leave scars. Patients with acquired immunodeficiency syndrome (AIDS) may have severe infection and bacteremia. Penicillin is the treatment of choice.

Erysipelas

Erysipelas is a distinctive superficial cellulitis of the skin usually caused by group A streptococci, (rarely by group B, C, G, or D streptococci), by *S. aureus,* or by *Haemophilus influenzae*. Infection may occur at any age but is more common in infants, young children, and the elderly. Infants may develop abdominal erysipelas from umbilical infection, whereas in children and adults the face and lower extremities are more often involved. Infection may occur at sites of minor trauma or surgery. Pelvic erysipelas may occur after surgery or radiotherapy. Erysipelas of the vulva may be caused by group B streptococci. Erysipelas often represents a complication of lymphatic obstruction that may be congenital (Milroy's disease) or iatrogenic (e.g., saphenous vein donor graft sites, cancer surgery, irradiation).

Illness usually begins as a localized, tender, red lesion that rapidly becomes bright-red, hot, painful, and indurated and develops a raised, advancing border reflecting the dermal involvement (Color Plate V-27). Malaise, headaches, and fever are common, and chills may occur. Lymphatic obstruction during infection produces the peau d'orange appearance of the skin. Lymphatic obstruction may persist after therapy and predispose to recurrent erysipelas at the same site.

Erysipelas is diagnosed by its distinctive clinical appearance, blood and throat cultures, or serologic confirmation of a group A streptococcal infection.

Early stages of herpes zoster may mimic erysipelas but are distinguished by pain and hyperesthesia, which precede development of vesicular lesions. Angioedema and severe contact dermatitis may mimic erysipelas.

Early in its course, erysipelas can usually be managed with oral antibiotics. Penicillin is the drug of choice and erythromycin, newer macrolide analogs, or cephalosporins are alternatives. Patients with extensive disease and systemic symptoms should be hospitalized and receive parenteral antibiotics. Bacteremia occurs in 20% of patients. Superficial desquamation may be seen at the site of infection.

Cellulitis

Cellulitis is an acute infection of the skin with prominent involvement of subcutaneous tissue. *S. aureus* and group A streptococci are the most common infecting organisms. In young children, *H. influenzae* causes a distinctive violaceous cellulitis of the face, neck, or upper body (Color Plate V-28). The etiology of cellulitis is suggested by circumstances, bacterial features, and host-specific features of clinical presentation. Intravenous drug addicts have a high frequency of infection caused by *S. aureus* and *Streptococcus pyogenes* and more rarely by gram-negative bacilli or anaerobes. Diabetic patients have recurrent cellulitis and polymicrobial anaerobic infection of their insensate, traumatized feet. Deep-seated polymicrobial infections of the oropharynx or perirectal areas may present as cellulitis. Leukemic patients with neutropenia may have cellulitis caused by gram-negative bacilli, anaerobes, or fungi. Cellulitis after surgery is usually staphylococcal or streptococcal but may be polymicrobial and anaerobic if associated with gastrointestinal procedures or fecal soilage. Cellulitis after animal bites is usually caused by streptococci, staphylococci, or *Pasteurella multocida* and less often by anaerobic or polymicrobial infections. Human bites are often polymicrobial and have a higher frequency of anaerobic pathogens. Cellulitis after trauma in aqueous environments may be caused by *Erysipelothrix rhusiopathiae, Aeromonas hydrophila,* or *Vibrio* species. Cellulitis may be a presenting sign of bacteremia caused by *Vibrio vulnificus* in the chronic alcoholic or immunocompromised patient after ingestion of raw seafood.

Cellulitis usually originates at sites of previous injury of the skin or more rarely by hematogenous spread *(H. influenzae)*. Initial local tenderness and erythema are followed by rapid intensification of heat, swelling, and pain. Involved skin is red and hot but, unlike erysipelas, has indistinct borders because of the depth of infection. Central areas may become necrotic or blister. Regional lymphadenopathy, chills, and fever often occur, and lymphangitis may be present.

Information gained by microscopic examination of smears and Gram stains can direct initial antibiotic therapy and should be modified by results of cultures and sensitivity studies. Representative material is usually obtained from the more central, purulent areas of infection rather than from the advancing borders of cellulitis. Skin biopsies are especially helpful for diagnosing fungal infection in immunocompromised patients.

The type and route of antibiotic administration are determined by the infecting organism and the extent and severity of infection. More extensive disease may require surgical debridement. Patients with cellulitis complicating dermatophytosis should have treatment for their underlying fungal infection.

Patients with recurrent cellulitis associated with lymphatic obstruction often benefit from prolonged therapy with oral penicillin.

Lymphangitis

Lymphangitis is an infection of the lymphatic vessels, usually involving an extremity. Group A streptococci and *S. aureus* are the most common causative organisms. The site of entry is often less conspicuous than the red, tender streaking of the skin overlying the inflamed lymphatic channels. Proximal lymph nodes are enlarged and usually tender. Fever and leukocytosis typically occur. Diagnosis is made by clinical appearance and confirmed by Gram stains of the primary lesion or by blood cultures. Antibiotic therapy is directed toward suspected bacterial pathogens. Since lymphangitic streaking can also occur with herpetic infection, it is important to exclude that entity by careful history and follow-up examination.

Folliculitis

Folliculitis is an infection of hair follicles usually caused by *S. aureus,* but it may be caused by streptococci, Enterobacteriaceae, Pseudomonadaceae, fungi, and viruses or may be sterile. Involvement of the follicle may be superficial or deep and may follow mechanical occlusion of follicles after superficial irritation. Sycosis barbae is deeper folliculitis of the bearded area caused by *S. aureus. Pseudomonas aeruginosa* is a common cause of folliculitis on the buttocks, hips, or axillae that may be acquired from "hot tubs" or from heavily contaminated water (Color Plate V-29). This lesion may be preceded by pruritic and papular lesions. Folliculitis adjacent to intertriginous yeast infection may be caused by *Candida*. Patients with bone marrow transplants can have lesions mimicking folliculitis caused by *Pityrosporum* organisms. Severely immunocompromised patients may have folliculitis caused by *Malassezia furfur*.

Superficial folliculitis usually responds to local measures such as cleansing and topical antibiotics, but oral antibiotics may be required for management of deep or recurrent folliculitis. Some patients may require ciprofloxacin therapy for *Pseudomonas* folliculitis.

Patients with AIDS may have a widespread acneiform eruption, recurrence of adolescent acne, necrotizing folliculitis, or eosinophilic pustular folliculitis.

Noninfectious folliculitis may be seen with pustular psoriasis, acne, occupational acne, corticosteroid or lithium therapy, acne rosacea, and a variety of disorders of uncertain etiology.

Furuncles and carbuncles

These lesions are abscesses (boils) of deeper skin structures caused by *S. aureus*. Lesions usually begin as folliculitis and are found in hairy areas of the face, neck, buttocks, extremities, or axillae that are sites of heavy perspiration and frequent irritation. Furuncles begin as painful, red nodules that expand and liquefy centrally in the characteristic stages of development of a "boil." Deeper lesions with multiple interconnecting subcutaneous furuncles are termed *carbuncles*. These lesions usually drain to overlying skin at several sites. Carbuncles are most common on the back of the neck, the back, and the thighs.

Furuncles appear to be more common in obese and diabetic patients and are recognized as complications of corticosteroid therapy or underlying immunologic disease, immunoglobulin deficiency, or neutrophil dysfunction. Linkage between iron deficiency and recurrent furunculosis remains unproved. Leukocytosis, fever, and constitutional symptoms usually reflect more extensive cellulitis and tissue involvement.

Recurrent furunculosis may be caused by the predisposing conditions already cited but more often reflects persistent colonization and/or reinfection of a normal host. Nasal colonization is usually the site of primary carriage. Less often, patients may be colonized in perineal or other skin sites as well. Recurrent furunculosis may be perpetuated in some patients by recolonization through cross-contamination from family members.

Topical application of moist heat that promotes localization and drainage is often adequate treatment for simple furuncles. Antistaphylococcal antibiotics are recommended for extensive involvement or lesions located on the midface or for patients thought to have bacteremia or those at risk of colonizing previously damaged heart valves or prosthetic devices.

Patients with boils and compromised host defenses from diabetes mellitus, rheumatoid arthritis, organ transplantation, or leukemia should receive antistaphylococcal antibiotics. Patients requiring parenteral therapy for infection with methicillin-resistant staphylococci (MRSA) should receive vancomycin. Surgical drainage is an integral part of managing large furuncles or carbuncles. Furunculosis is usually a self-limited process. Patients with recurrent furunculosis are best treated with regimens containing rifampin to eradicate staphylococcal carriage (Chapter 257). Topical application of antibiotics to the nose or use of various staphylococcal vaccines are not of proven value. However, topical mupirocin is an effective means of eradicating staphylococcal colonization of the nose and is active against MRSA. Prolonged therapy with oral clindamycin or ciprofloxacin eradicates carriage in some patients.

Staphylococcal scalded skin syndrome

In this syndrome, extensive bullae formation and exfoliation of the skin (Chapter 257) are caused by phage group II *S. aureus* organisms that produce an exfoliative exotoxin. Toxin-producing staphylococci may primarily involve the conjunctivae, pharynx, umbilicus, abscesses, or the bloodstream, but in contrast to bullous impetigo, the lesions of the scalded skin syndrome are sterile. Lesions are characterized histologically by a cleavage plane high in the epidermis. This feature aids in differentiating this disease from toxic epidermal necrolysis, which involves subepidermal layers that can be distinguished histologically (Color Plate V-30).

Staphylococcal scalded skin syndrome is seen almost exclusively in young children and has caused epidemics in neonatal nurseries. The disease appears rapidly but may follow a recognized staphylococcal infection by several days. Pain, fever, and a generalized erythema and edema of the skin are followed by development of large, flaccid bullae that are easily ruptured and demonstrate a positive Nikolsky's sign. Skin sloughs off with light lateral pressure (Chapter 258). Extensive denudation of skin may cause problems with fluid and electrolyte balance. There is little difficulty differentiating this disease from toxic epidermal necrolysis. The latter is usually caused by drug allergy, may involve mucous membranes, occurs most often in adults, and involves the subepidermis.

Treatment of the staphylococcal scalded skin syndrome includes penicillinase-resistant penicillins (nafcillin) and supportive therapy. Corticosteroids are not recommended.

Scarlet fever

Scarlet fever is a classic exanthematous disease of childhood associated with acute group A streptococcal pharyngitis. The erythrogenic toxin responsible for the rash is coded for by a bacteriophage infecting the streptococcus. Immunity to the toxin precludes recurrence of this syndrome (Chapter 259).

Symptoms of pharyngitis usually develop 1 to 2 days before appearance of the rash. Headache, fever, malaise, and submandibular adenopathy are often present. The pharynx is erythematous, with enlarged tonsils and a purulent exudate. The tongue has prominent papillae that protrude through a whitish coating. Over several days, this coating clears, leaving a bright-red tongue with accentuated papillae, giving rise to the term *strawberry tongue*. The exanthem begins on the upper chest, with subsequent spread to the neck and extremities. It is a confluent erythema composed of small puncta that impart a rough feel to the skin. The rash is accentuated in the flexural creases, where it may assume a linear petechial appearance (Pastia's lines). The exanthem persists for 5 to 10 days and desquamates on clearing. Desquamation begins on the face, where it produces a fine scale, and subsequently progresses to the trunk and limbs. Desquamation is often most marked on the hands and the feet, where large areas of skin may slough. Scarlet fever is often accompanied by an elevated white blood cell count. Throat cultures grow group A streptococci, and serologic evidence of infection is provided by rising titers to antistreptolysin O. Penicillin is the drug of choice.

Staphylococcal scarlet fever may mimic many of the features of streptococcal scarlet fever. The syndrome is presumed to represent an incomplete form of the staphylococcal scalded skin syndrome caused by exfoliative exotoxin. The rash can be identical, but staphylococcal scarlet fever does not produce an exanthem and is not associated with pharyngitis but may arise from a surgical wound infection. The treatment of choice is a penicillinase-resistant penicillin.

Streptococcal toxic shock

Streptococcal toxic shock is a term applied to fulminant streptococcal infection associated with progressive multiorgan failure and a mortality of 30% to 60% (Chapter 259). One study found positive tissue cultures in 95% and bacteremia in 65% of patients. None of the patients had a classic rash of scarlet fever. Patients had a brief, nonspecific prodrome that was quickly followed by hypotension, renal failure, adult respiratory distress syndrome, mental status changes, and disseminated intravascular coagulation.

The primary site of infection may be inapparent or may be marked by slight local tenderness. Streptococcal toxic shock syndrome has occurred with pharyngitis, cellulitis, otitis, osteomyelitis, necrotizing fasciitis, myositis, postpartum myometritis, endocarditis, and peritonitis. Women may have this syndrome as a complication of pregnancy, gynecologic surgery, or pelvic inflammatory disease. Patients with fulminant pneumonia may have rapidly progressive pleural effusions and empyema.

Toxic shock syndrome

The multisystem toxic shock syndrome is caused by a pyrogenic exotoxin producing staphylococci and occurs in conjunction with menstrual and nonmenstrual illness (Chapter 257). Criteria for diagnosis include a temperature of 102° F or greater, a diffuse erythroderma, hypotension, involvement of three or more organ systems, and desquamation of the skin on the palms and/or soles late in the course of illness (Chapters 257 and 228). The rash is scarlatiniform, may be evanescent, and may resemble a sunburn. There is often prominent mucous membrane involvement, with conjunctivitis, pharyngitis, and vaginal hyperemia or erythema. Changes in cognitive function may be severe. Leukocytosis, thrombocytopenia, and microscopic hematuria are often present. Elevation of creatinine and liver function test abnormalities are common. Myoglobinuria and increased serum creatine kinase levels occur in patients with muscle injury. By definition, patients with bacteremia are excluded from this syndrome complex, but identical symptoms may occur in patients with deep-seated staphylococcal infection or postoperative staphylococcal infection. Infected wounds causing toxic shock are uniquely devoid of signs of inflammation and must be explored to confirm the diagnosis by culture and Gram stain.

Toxic shock syndrome usually occurs within 2 days but may occur more than a week after surgery. Virtually all wounds, lesions, or bites are at risk of this complication. Toxic shock associated with nasal packing for epistaxis appears analogous to tampon-related disease but has occurred in the absence of absorbent materials. Approximately 50% to 70% of toxic shock cases occur in association with menstruation and tampon use. Most patients are young white women. Black and Hispanic women rarely develop toxic shock syndrome unless it complicates surgery or deep-seated infection. The syndrome may occur in conjunction with influenza, sinusitis, pharyngitis, tracheitis, infected burns, or abscesses.

Appropriate management includes removal of tampons and vaginal irrigation or drainage of infected sites in patients with associated deep-seated infection. Patients should receive aggressive fluid volume replacement and monitoring and general measures to treat shock and maintain ventilatory function. Corticosteroids are probably helpful early in the course of shock. Antistaphylococcal therapy is helpful in eradicating toxin-producing organisms and reduces the likelihood of recurrent disease.

Erythrasma

Erythrasma is a chronic superficial infection of the skin caused by *Corynebacterium minutissimum*. It generally affects the intertriginous zones, such as the groin, axillae, toe clefts, and inframammary folds, but occasionally may be widespread. The clinical lesion appears as a well-demarcated brownish-red patch with a fine scale. Patients are usually asymptomatic or mildly pruritic. Erythrasma is a common condition that occurs more often in men and is seen more frequently in a humid climate.

Tinea cruris may resemble erythrasma, although tinea may appear more inflammatory. The distinction between the two is made by a positive potassium hydroxide examination in tinea and by Wood's light examination, which shows a characteristic coral-red fluorescence, in erythrasma. Erythromycin, 1 g/day for 1 week, produces excellent therapeutic results.

Trichomycosis axillaris

Trichomycosis axillaris is a superficial infection of the axillary and pubic hairs caused by diphtheroids. Although the etiologic agent has been said to be *Corynebacterium tenuis,* multiple types of organisms appear to be responsible, sometimes in the same patient. This asymptomatic condition presents with the formation of yellow, red, or black nodules on the hair shaft. The sweat may be similarly colored. Treatment consists in shaving the affected area and applying a topical erythromycin ointment.

NECROTIZING SOFT TISSUE INFECTIONS

Many infections may lead to necrosis of skin and soft tissues. These diseases should be classified primarily on the basis of their anatomic involvement and secondarily on their microbial etiology. Thus they may be divided into superficial cellulitis, fascial level infection, or myonecrosis and are best characterized at surgery. Deep infections may dissect along fascial planes and involve muscles and fat to a greater extent than is suspected clinically. Prompt and aggressive surgical intervention, deep biopsy, and adequate debridement are the key to reduced mortality. Broad-spectrum antibiotics are selected empirically and changed on the basis of smears and culture results. These infections have been linked with group A streptococcal infection but may occur with staphylococci, gram-negative bacilli, *Vibrio vulnificus,* mucormycosis, or *Aspergillus*. Polymicrobial infection with anaerobic and aerobic organisms is probably the most common cause of these diseases.

Necrotizing fasciitis

Necrotizing fasciitis is a life-threatening infection of subcutaneous tissue and fascial planes. It may occur in normal persons after minor trauma or may occur in surgical wounds. Such infections occur more frequently in elderly debilitated diabetic patients, indigent alcoholic or homeless patients, or drug abusers. Tissue necrosis follows hemorrhage and dissection of infection along fascial planes, with secondary vascular thrombosis and gangrene. Lesions begin as tender, red, swollen areas that may spread over 24 to 48 hours to become indurated and cyanotic with blisters containing reddish black fluid. Lesions are tender but may become anesthetic in gangrenous areas. Black eschar formation may resemble a deep burn (Color Plate V-31). Surrounding skin is often undermined and can be easily separated from deep fascia by manipulation with a probe. Patients manifest chills, fever, and prostration. Despite apparently adequate antibiotic therapy, persistent fever and clinical deterioration typically occur because tissue-space fluid collections are overlooked.

Cultures of blood and involved tissue are usually positive, and diagnosis can be confirmed by Gram stain, biopsy of involved skin, or computed tomography–guided or ultrasound-guided aspiration of tissue fluid collections. Leukocytosis is marked, and anemia requiring transfusion may be present.

Necrotizing fasciitis must be distinguished from other acute cutaneous infections. The necrotic areas of skin separate it from simple erysipelas or cellulitis. Clostridial cellulitis and nonclostridial crepitant cellulitis usually have more crepitus and few cutaneous changes. Gas gangrene characteristically affects underlying muscle, whereas necrotizing fasciitis does not. Radiographic evidence of gas suggests a diagnosis other than necrotizing fasciitis. Since both gangrene and necrotizing fasciitis require surgery, the differential diagnosis is often best made at surgery. Needle aspiration of fluid after demonstration of fluid collections by imaging techniques may be especially useful in streptococcal gangrene but is not adequate for management of other forms of fasciitis. Surgery should be done promptly.

One must remember that aggressive surgical debridement is the key to effective therapy of necrotizing fasciitis and that appropriate parenteral antibiotic therapy plays a vital but ancillary role. Although diabetes and atherosclerosis may adversely affect survival, the worst prognostic factors include delayed recognition or incomplete surgical debridement.

Clostridial cellulitis

Clostridial cellulitis (Chapter 262) is a superficial infection that does not extend to involve muscles. It is characterized by a longer incubation period, but less pain, edema, and systemic toxicity than gas gangrene. A thin discharge is present, and crepitus and gas formation are often prominent.

A Gram stain and culture of the exudate establish the clostridial nature of the process. Radiographs show the presence of gas without involvement of muscle. Diagnosis is confirmed at surgery. Therapy consists of simple wound debridement and administration of penicillin, cefoxitin, or a beta-lactamase inhibitor combination.

Nonclostridial crepitant cellulitis

Nonclostridial crepitant cellulitis, a gas-forming infection, probably occurs more often than gas gangrene. It frequently mimics clostridial cellulitis. The infection is usually polymicrobial and may contain coliforms, streptococci, and bacteroides. Diabetic patients are predisposed to this syndrome and often have a more aggressive course than do nondiabetic patients. There may be abundant gas dissecting along tissue planes, but there is characteristically little systemic toxicity and no muscle involvement (Chapter 270).

Local surgical debridement and drainage are indicated. Antibiotics are eventually dictated by culture results, but broad-spectrum coverage should be instituted initially because of the variable causes of the infection.

Gas gangrene

Gas gangrene is a fulminant, life-threatening infection of subcutaneous tissue and muscle caused by *Clostridium* (usually *C. perfringens*) (Chapter 262). It follows trauma complicated by wound contamination and may be associated with cholecystectomy or other surgical procedures, compound fractures, or vascular insufficiency. Contamination may originate from soil containing spores of *C. perfringens* or may arise from normal skin flora that contains this organism in large numbers. Invasiveness of this pathogen is enhanced by its production of more than a dozen exotoxins, of which the alpha toxin is the most important. Infectivity is increased a millionfold when organisms lodge in injured muscle tissue with a compromised vascular supply. Thus both contamination and a properly anaerobic environment are necessary for development of overt disease.

Onset of infection may occur within a few hours to a few days after the inciting event. Pain may increase dramatically after an initial improvement and appear disproportionate to early changes in the wound appearance. Marked edema soon follows, muscle may herniate through wounds, and surrounding skin may form dark blisters and undergo necrosis. Crepitus is rarely prominent early, and gas may be obscured by extensive edema. The wound has a foul-smelling, thin discharge. Gram stain of this material shows many large, gram-positive bacilli but very few neutrophils. Delirium, tachycardia, and shock may follow rapidly, but fever may be mild. In overwhelming infection, this process may evolve and result in death in several hours.

The diagnosis of gas gangrene is made on clinical grounds, is substantiated by Gram stain smears and by radiographs showing gas spreading linearly along muscle and fascial planes, and is proved at surgery by demonstration of gas in tissues and myonecrosis. Bacteremia is rare.

Prompt and aggressive surgical debridement, with removal of all involved tissue, is required for successful therapy. Although high-dose penicillin is the drug of choice for gas gangrene, empiric therapy is usually broadened to cover polymicrobial infection, including gram-negative bacilli and anaerobes. Clindamycin has been suggested to reduce toxin elaboration by clostridia and may enhance efficacy of alternative regimens, including cefoxitin, imipenem, or beta-lactamase inhibitor combinations. Hyperbaric oxygen therapy, when available, may be valuable as an additional mode of therapy.

Synergistic nonclostridial anaerobic myonecrosis

This disease may involve subcutaneous tissue, fascia, and muscle. It is caused by combinations of aerobic gram-negative bacilli (e.g., *Escherichia coli, Klebsiella, Enterobacter, Proteus*) and anaerobes (*Bacteroides* and/or anaerobic streptococci).

Synergistic necrotizing cellulitis occurs most frequently in the perineal region or lower extremities of patients with diabetes and/or renal disease and vascular disease. A variant, Fournier's gangrene, which can be caused by staphylococci and streptococci in addition to the organisms just cited, involves prominent necrotizing fasciitis of male genitalia. The distinction is artificial because Fournier's gangrene may be predominantly cellulitis or may extend to involve muscles of the abdominal walls and extremities.

The infection may begin as vesicles that form tender skin ulcers that drain thick, foul-smelling, "dishwater" pus. Necrotic skin is quite tender and is surrounded by florid erythema and edema. Crepitus may be present. Patients appear toxic, and many are bacteremic.

Radical surgical debridement is the cornerstone of successful therapy. Amputation may be necessary, but tissue recovery is often better than expected. Broad-spectrum antimicrobial therapy is started empirically and is modified by the results of smears and cultures. Mortality is high even with adequate management.

Progressive bacterial synergistic gangrene

Progressive bacterial synergistic gangrene was first described by Meleney, who was thought to have produced similar lesions in animals by combined infection with staphylococci and streptococci but not by either alone. The synergistic infection induced in animals was a more fulminant infection than the disease described by Meleney and led some observers to suggest that Meleney's synergistic gangrene was actually cutaneous amebiasis. The disease is a rare complication of surgical or traumatic wounds caused by microaerophilic or anaerobic streptococci along with *S. aureus* or, rarely, a gram-negative bacillus.

The lesion begins as a painful ulcer that classically enlarges to contain three discrete parts. The central necrotic

Table 235-1. Distinctive skin signs and risk factors associated with specific infections

Disease (infectious agent)	Risk factors	Skin signs and presentation
Ecthyma gangrenosum *(Pseudomonas aeruginosa)* (Chapter 229)	Immunocompromised patients, especially those with neutropenia and leukemia or lymphoma; prognosis significantly better if not bacteremic	Single or multiple lesions evolving from vesicles to round indurated necrotic ulcers or eschars, often involving skin folds (Color Plate V-23)
Toxic shock syndrome (TSS) *(Staphylococcus aureus)* (Chapter 259)	Menstruating women (usually young Caucasians); may occur postpartum	Sunburnlike rash, conjunctivitis, "strawberry tongue," pharyngitis with fever, hypotension, and prostration; desquamation of palms and soles several days to 1 to 2 weeks later (Color Plate V-24)
	TSS related to wound, medical procedure, or injury (any sex or race)	Wound usually only slightly red, indurated, and not purulent
Vibrio vulnificus–related *Vibrio* species cellulitis (Chapter 267)	Immunocompromised patients: alcoholism, cirrhosis, diabetes, leukemia, renal failure, or steroid recipient having contact with sea water, brackish water, or shellfish	May begin as pustules, cellulitis, or lymphangitis, progressing to large hemorrhagic bullous lesions that ulcerate
Anthrax *(Bacillus anthracis)* (Chapter 261)	Contact with infected animals or animal products (wool, hides, ivory, hair) imported from countries with endemic disease (e.g., Africa, India, Pakistan, Haiti)	Malignant pustule usually on exposed skin of face, neck, hands, or arms; bullae develop in 1 to 5 days with edema and erythema; signs of sepsis possibly severe
Plague *(Yersinia pestis)* (Chapter 269)	Fleaborne disease from infected animals (rabbits, bobcats, prairie dogs) in Southwest United States to sightseers, hunters, or vacationers or to pets, from which owners are secondarily infected	Rarely prominent flea bite with papule or vesicopustule; may have associated tender lymphadenopathy (buboes) and serious systemic illness
Tularemia *(Francisella tularensis)* (Chapter 269)	Avocational, vocational, or domestic exposure to ticks or infected animals	Ulcerative lesion with raised margins at site of injury; may have marked regional adenopathy and systemic illness; may have oculoglandular syndrome
Cutaneous diphtheria *(Corynebacterium diphtheriae)* (Chapter 261)	Poor hygiene; more common in "skid row" population of South and Northwest United States	Lesions may be primarily or secondarily infected; often a persistent punched-out ulcer with a pustule or gray shaggy membrane
Lyme disease *(Borrelia burgdorferi)* (Chapter 275)	Tick bite that usually goes undetected in endemic area	Quite variable: characteristic lesion of erythema chronicum migrans begins as red macule or papule, developing bright-red outer margins with central clearing
Hot tub folliculitis	Recent use of hot tubs, whirlpools, or spa pools (usually within 1 to 4 days); diagnosed by culture of lesion	Folliculitis with papules, vesicles, or pustules over exposed areas; spares face and neck; may have fever, adenopathy, and mastitis; usually self-limited (Color Plate V-29)
Elephantiasis nostras	Chronic cellulitis and edema of extremity caused by lymphangitis and lymphadenitis	Progressively worsening lymphedema with recurrent infection; thickening and hardening of skin with nodulation, ulceration, and hypertrophy of skin to form pachydermatosus appearance (Color Plate V-32)
Clostridium septicum sepsis	Gas gangrene caused by hematogenous spread, usually from underlying malignancy that may be inapparent	"Spontaneous" gas gangrene with rapid development of edema, blisters, bulla formation, and subcutaneous air
Erysipeloid *(Erysipelothrix rhusiopathiae)*	Usually secondary infection of cut or abrasion by contact with fish, crustaceans, or meat products	Violaceous, warm, and tender lesion with raised margins; lesion may clear centrally with brownish discoloration; few constitutional symptoms
Epithelioid (bacillary) angiomatosis	Disseminated cutaneous and multiorgan bacillary infection of patients with AIDS	Vascular lesion with 2 to 6 mm papules resembling Kaposi's sarcoma or pyogenic granuloma; silver-staining bacilli seen in areas of necrosis
Sporotrichosis *(Sporothrix schenckii)* (Chapter 277)	Secondary infection of abrasion or cut of skin from thorns, splinters, sphagnum moss, or mine timbers colonized with fungus	Papules, pustules, or nodules that become indurated and ulcerate, producing multiple lesions by lymphangitic spread (Color Plate V-25)
Mycobacterium marinum (Chapter 276)	Exposure to fish, aquariums, or swimming pools	Violaceous papule, ulcer, or scaling lesion at site of injury; lesions may resemble sporotrichosis (Color Plate V-33)

Table 235-2. Antimicrobial therapy of dermal infection

Infection	Usual organisms	Antibiotic treatment
Impetigo		
Nonbullous	*Staphylococcus aureus* more than *Streptococcus pyogenes*	Oral macrolide, mupirocin, antistaphylococcal beta lactam (ASB)
Bullous	*S. aureus*	As above
Ecthyma	*S. pyogenes*	Oral Pen-G or Pen-V (parenteral Pen for sepsis)
Erysipelas	*S. pyogenes*	Oral Pen (parenteral for sepsis)
	S. aureus	Antistaphylococcal beta lactam (parenteral for sepsis or associated vascular insufficiency)
Cellulitis		
Usual	*S. aureus, S. pyogenes*	ASB (parenteral for sepsis, associated vascular insufficiency, or compromised host, followed by specific oral therapy)
Water injury	*Vibrio vulnificus*	Tetracycline + Imi, Cipro, or chloramphenicol
	Aeromonas hydrophila	Cipro, SMX/TMP, Imi, or ESC
	Erysipelothrix rhusiopathiae	Pen-G, Amp, Erythro, oral cephalosporin
Diabetic foot		
Early	Aerobic gram-positive cocci	Pen-G, Pen-V, Clind
Late	Anaerobes, aerobic gram-negative bacilli, streptococci	Ticar/Clav, Imi, Amp/Sul ± Aztreo (parenteral for severe disease and sepsis)
		Oral Amox/Clav, Clind + Cipro, Metro + Cipro or ASB
Bite wound	*S. pyogenes, S. aureus, Pasteurella multocida, Eikenella corrodens, Capnocytophaga canimorsus*	Amox/Clav, Amp/Sul, ESC, tetracycline
Necrotizing dermatitis	—	*Agressive surgery for diagnosis and therapy*
Necrotizing fasciitis	*S. pyogenes*	Parenteral Pen-G
	Polymicrobial anaerobic and aerobic gram-negative bacilli	Imi, Ticar/Clav, Amp/Sul + Aztreo, or Amp + Clind + Gent
Clostridial	Clostridial cellulitis	Pen-G, Cefox, Ticar/Clav, Amp/Sul
	Gas gangrene	Imi + Clind, Pen-G + Clind
Synergistic nonclostridial anaerobic myonecrosis	Anaerobes, aerobic gram-negative bacilli and streptococci	Imi, Ticar/Clav, Amp/Sul + Aztreo, Amp + Clind + Gent
Meleney's ulcer	Combined infection: *S. aureus,* microaerophilic streptococci (± *Entamoeba histolytica)*	ASB (Metro if *E. histolytica* present)

Drug grouping	Commentary and abbreviations
Beta lactams	Penicillins, cephalosporins, carbopenems, or monobactam
Macrolides	Erythromycin (Erythro): cheapest to use, less well tolerated
	Clarithromycin, azithromycin: active versus *Haemophilus influenzae,* broader spectrum but not active versus Erythro-resistant *S. aureus* or *S. pyogenes*
	Clindamycin (Clind): good anaerobic spectrum, poor versus *H. influenzae*
Antistaphylococcal beta lactams (ASB)	
Oral penicillins	Dicloxacillin, amoxicillin/clavulanate (Amox/Clav)
Oral cephalosporins	Cephradine, cefadroxil, cefuroxime, axetil, cefaclor
Parenteral penicillins	Nafcillin, ampicillin/sulbactam (Amp/Sul), ticarcillin/clavulanate (Ticar/Clav), imipenem (Imi)
Parenteral cephalosporins	Cephalothin, cephapirin, cefazolin, cefuroxime
Penicillin	Penicillin G (Pen-G): oral or parenteral
	Penicillin V (Pen-V): oral
Expanded-spectrum cephalosporins (ESC)	Cefmenoxime, cefotaxime, ceftizoxime, ceftriaxone, ceftazidime
	Sulfamethoxazole/trimethoprim (SMX/TMP), ciprofloxacin (Cipro), cefoxitin (Cefox), aztreonam (Aztreo), gentamicin (Gent), metronidazole (Metro)

ulcer and gangrenous skin is surrounded by a zone of intense purplish discoloration; cellulitis and erythema form the outside of the three-part lesion. Untreated lesions expand to involve contiguous areas, with subsequent systemic complications. Cultures show that the outer edge of the infection contains streptococci, whereas central ulcerated lesions contain staphylococci. Lesions should be carefully examined for amebae, and amebic serologic studies should be done.

Radical surgical debridement and intensive antibiotic therapy are needed for optimum management of patients with affected wounds.

• • •

Table 235-1 lists the skin signs and risk factors for specific infections. Table 235-2 lists antimicrobial therapy for various dermal infections.

REFERENCES

Ahrenholz DH: Necrotizing soft tissue infections. Surg Clin North Am 68:199, 1988.

Allen TA et al: Toxic shock syndrome associated with use of latex nasal packing. Arch Intern Med 150:2587, 1990.

Bufill JA et al: *Pityrosporum* folliculitis after bone marrow transplantation. Ann Intern Med 108:560-563, 1988.

Caplan ES and Kluge RM: Gas gangrene: review of 34 cases. Arch Intern Med 136:778, 1976.

Chartier C and Grosshans E: Erysipelas. Int J Dermatol 29:458, 1990.

Davson J, Jones DM, and Turner L: Diagnosis of Meleney's synergistic gangrene. Br J Surg 75:267, 1988.

Demidovich CW et al: Impetigo: current etiology and comparison of penicillin, erythromycin, and cephalexin therapies. Am J Dis Child 144:1313, 1990.

Farmlett EJ et al: Computed tomography in the assessment of myonecrosis. J Am Assoc Radiol 38:278, 1987.

Feingold DS: Gangrenous and crepitant cellulitis. J Am Acad Dermatol 6:289, 1982.

Harawi SJ et al: Cutaneous diseases associated with HIV infection. Pathol Annu 26:265, 1991.

Herman LE et al: Folliculitis: a clinicopathologic review. Pathol Annu 26:201, 1991.

Hewitt WD and Farrar WE: Care report: bacteremia and ecthyma caused by *Streptococcus pyogenes* in a patient with acquired immunodeficiency syndrome. Am J Med Sci 295:52, 1988.

Kingston D and Seal DV: Current hypotheses on synergistic microbial gangrene. Br J Surg 77:260, 1987.

Neefe LI et al: Staphylococcal scalded-skin syndrome in adults: case report and review of the literature. Am J Med Sci 277:99, 1979.

Riseman JA et al: Hyperbaric oxygen therapy for necrotizing fasciitis reduces mortality and the need for debridements. Surgery 108:847, 1990.

Sanders LJ, Slomsky JM, and Berger-Caplan C: Elephantiasis nostras: an eight-year observation of progressive nonfilarial elephantiasis of the lower extremity. Cutis 42:406, 1988.

Sarkany I, Taplin D, and Blank H: The etiology and treatment of erythrasma. J Invest Dermatol 37:283, 1961.

Stamenkovic I and Lew PD: Early recognition of potentially fatal necrotizing fasciitis: the use of frozen-section biopsy. N Engl J Med 310:1689, 1984.

Stevens DL et al: Severe group A streptococcal infections associated with a toxic shock-like syndrome and scarlet fever toxin A. N Engl J Med 321:1, 1989.

Stevens DL et al: Spontaneous, nontraumatic gangrene due to *Clostridium septicum*. Rev Infect Dis 12:286, 1990.

Sudarsky LA et al: Improved results form a standardized approach in treating patients with necrotizing fasciitis. Ann Surg 206:661, 1987.

CHAPTER

236 Gastrointestinal Infections

Herbert L. DuPont

Although diarrheal illness is a major cause of absenteeism from work and school in industrialized regions, it is of greater importance in developing nations, where it is often the major cause of infant mortality and serious morbidity in travelers from areas of lower disease endemicity. Laboratory procedures available during the past decade have provided convincing evidence that most of the acute diarrhea occurring throughout the world is of infectious origin. Thus with these laboratory techniques, the disease is now subject to study with the aim of defining etiology, describing specific epidemiologic modes of spread and patterns of susceptibility, and developing effective means of treating, controlling, and even preventing the disease. This chapter focuses on the responsible etiologic agents in gastrointestinal infection; discusses their mechanisms of disease production; and offers a perspective on diagnosis, therapy, and prevention. Acute diarrhea is the primary focus. The other important clinical presentation of intestinal infection, enteric (typhoid-like) fever, also is discussed briefly.

PATHOPHYSIOLOGY (also see Chapter 41)

Most forms of enteric infection lead to the occurrence of diarrhea with variable associated symptoms. Diarrhea is generally defined as the passing of a greater number of stools of decreased form than is customary. A more rigid definition is not practical. Three factors acting together or separately lead to the passage of unformed stools: intestinal secretion, malabsorption of dietary constituents (often disaccharides), and altered intestinal motility. In acute infectious diarrhea, available evidence would suggest that the first two mechanisms are important, and the third, which is largely unstudied in acute diarrhea states, is of particular importance in chronic diarrhea of noninfectious origin (i.e., irritable bowel syndrome and idiopathic ulcerative colitis). The ways infectious microorganisms produce increased luminal fluid are reviewed briefly when the specific etiologic agents are described.

ETIOLOGIC AGENTS AND THEIR VIRULENCE PROPERTIES

The various microbial agents capable of producing active infection of the intestinal tract make up a formidable list, which will not be reviewed in its entirety in this chapter. Rather, the focus will be on the more important agents that are recognized to produce a measurable amount of illness or on newly described organisms that might soon be shown to play important roles in disease occurrence.

Bacterial agents

Bacterial enteropathogens probably account for between 50% and 80% of acute diarrhea, depending on the setting. The bacterial agents appear to be particularly important in tropical areas and are responsible for most of the morbidity among persons traveling from low- to high-risk areas ("traveler's diarrhea"). Table 236-1 lists the more important bacterial causes of acute diarrhea. Additional bacterial enteropathogens are discussed later in the chapter.

Vibrio cholerae. Cholera characteristically is a severe, dehydrating illness caused by *V. cholerae* O1 and occurs in certain endemic areas of Asia, Africa, the Middle East, and Latin America. Within the past 15 years, cholera has been endemic along the US Gulf Coast (Chapter 267). The *V. cholerae* found in the United States has been hemolytic, biotype El Tor, serotype Inaba. An important widespread epidemic of cholera is currently occurring in South and Central America. Cases have been imported into the United States primarily through foods obtained in outbreak area. Diarrhea caused by non-O1 strains of *V. cholerae* may be severe, and in many cases these strains produce septicemia, particularly in those who are compromised. The source of non-O1 infection in this country has generally been uncooked oysters, although infection has also been acquired by world travelers. To isolate *V. cholerae* the laboratory must use a Vibrio-selective medium (e.g., thiosulfate citrate bile salts sucrose [TCBS]).

E. coli. Discussing *E. coli* as a cause of diarrhea is a complex task and is getting more so daily. A growing body of evidence suggests that the rubric *E. coli* encompasses a variety of unrelated agents showing biochemical similarities but strikingly different virulence properties, epidemiology, and clinical features. The organisms collectively might be referred to as diarrheagenic *E. coli*.

E. coli was first described as a cause of diarrhea in the 1940s and 1950s, when a limited number of serotype-identified organisms were shown to produce diarrhea outbreaks in hospital newborn nurseries. Serologic schemes were developed in the 1950s to type the *E. coli* by the somatic and flagellar antigens, and the serotypes epidemiologically implicated in nursery outbreaks were collectively called enteropathogenic *E. coli* (EPEC). Although it is currently thought that these strains are important causes of infantile diarrhea, their rate of occurrence and general epidemiology need additional study. A factor limiting such study has been the lack of reliable reagents for serotype identification. Recently, EPEC strains have been shown to commonly adhere to HEp-2 tissue culture cells; this property may serve as screening procedure (Fig. 236-1). The property of adherence has also been shown for EPEC in infants with diarrhea, where the organism has been shown to adhere to the epithelial surface and produce damage to microvilli, terminal web, and glycocalix without invasion. *E. coli* strains showing various patterns of attachment to tissue culture cells (local, diffuse, or aggregative types) not belonging to EPEC serotypes have been associated with diarrhea. The biologic significance of these strains and their relationships are currently being studied.

In the early 1970s, strains of *E. coli* were identified as causes of diarrhea in persons from the United Kingdom or the United States during military stationing in the Middle East and Southeast Asia. These strains, shown to variably produce heat-labile choleralike toxin (LT) or heat-stable enterotoxins (ST), have been called enterotoxigenic *E. coli* (ETEC). Both LTs and STs produce transudation of fluid and electrolytes and thus lead to dilatation of the bowel (Fig. 236-2). Strains of ETEC are now known to be a major cause if not the most important cause of diarrhea among infants living in tropical areas and are also responsible for just under half the cases of traveler's diarrhea. The ETEC organisms possess colonization fimbriae, which render them adherent to the upper gut of the infected host. Host specificity of the various colonization fimbriae or pili may

Table 236-1. Important bacterial enteropathogens, their virulence properties and world occurrence

Etiologic agent	Virulence properties	Occurrence
Vibrio cholerae	Heat-labile enterotoxin	Endemic areas primarily in Asia, Africa, and Latin America
Enteropathogenic and enteroadherent *E. coli*	HEp-2 cell adherence	Infantile diarrhea, worldwide
Enterotoxigenic *E. coli*	Colonization factor antigen, heat-stable and heat-labile enterotoxins	Developing regions, tropical countries, infants, and travelers
Invasive *E. coli*	*Shigella*-like invasiveness	Rare epidemics, endemic in South America and Eastern Europe
Hemorrhagic colitis *E. coli*	Shigalike toxin	Beef source in industrialized areas
Shigella	Shigalike toxin, invasiveness	Worldwide
Salmonella	Cholera-like toxin production, invasiveness	Worldwide
Campylobacter jejuni	Cholera-like toxin production, invasiveness	Worldwide
Aeromonas species	Hemolysin, cytotoxin, enterotoxin	Worldwide, especially Thailand, Australia, and Canada
Yersinia enterocolitica	Heat-stable enterotoxins, invasiveness	Worldwide, primarily Scandinavia, Canada, and South Africa

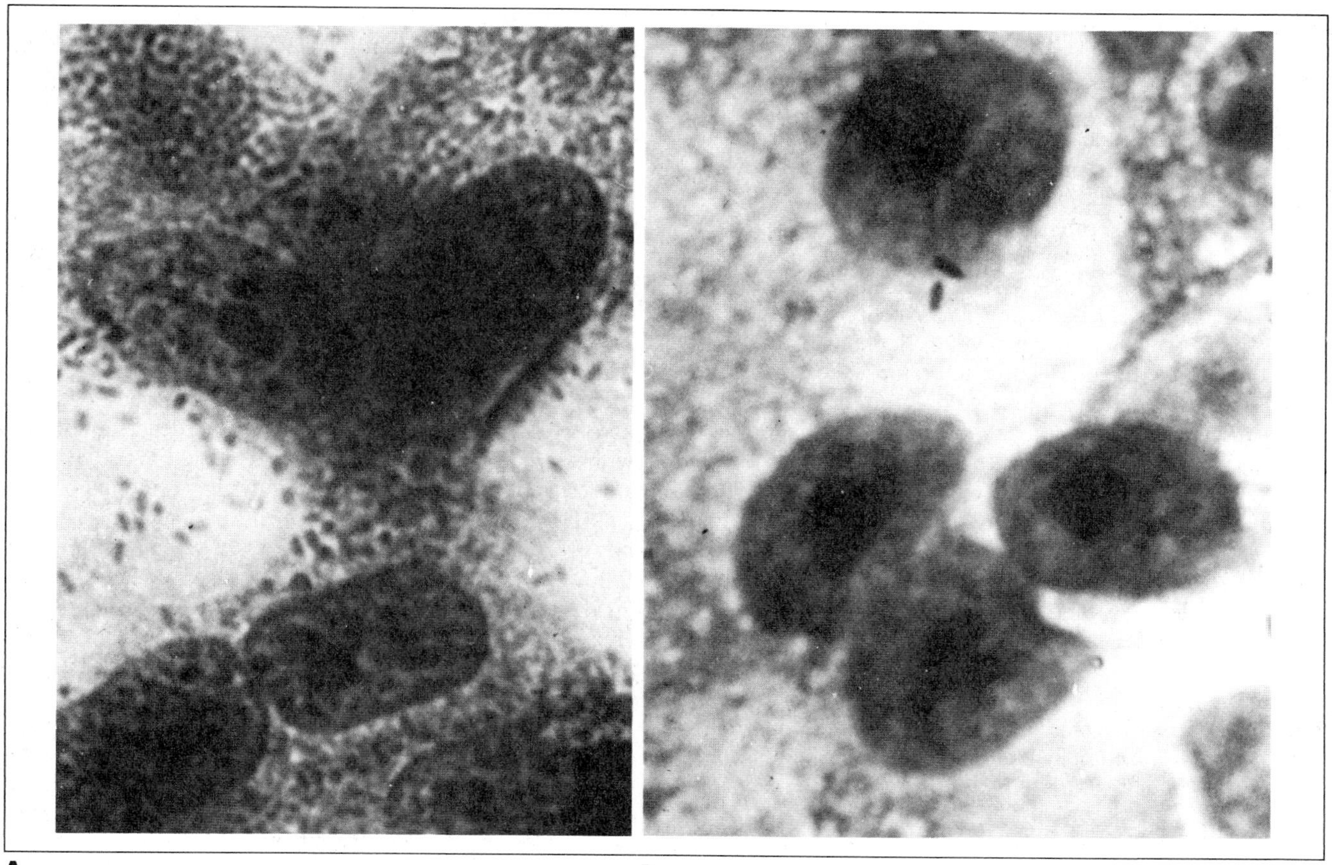

A **B**

Fig. 236-1. HEp-2 cell adherence assay. **A,** An enteropathogenic. *E. coli* (serogroup O119) is shown to be adherent to the tissue culture cells while a nonpathogenic strain of *E. coli* remains nonadherent. **B,** (Wright-Giemsa, × 1000)

prevent transmission of ETEC between animals and humans.

When ETEC were first studied, a large outbreak of diarrhea occurred in the United States due to *E. coli,* which possessed the property of *Shigella*-like invasiveness. The organism had contaminated Camembert and Brie cheese imported from France. The clinical disease resembled shigellosis; persons affected commonly complained of fever, severe abdominal pain, and bloody diarrhea. These invasive *E. coli* have not been shown to be important causes of endemic diarrhea, although they seem to be regularly found in urban Brazil and some areas in Eastern Europe. The property of invasiveness of these strains of *E. coli,* like strains of *Shigella,* is associated with a mixture of soluble bacterial proteins encoded by a 140-megadalton plasmid. In some strains, a portion of the chromosome also controls the property of invasiveness.

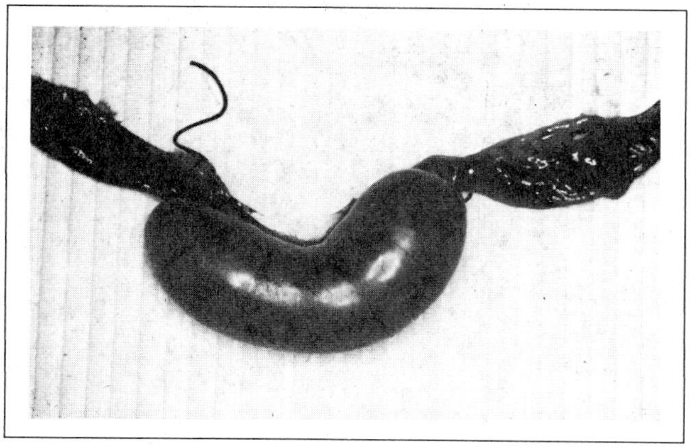

Fig. 236-2. Rabbit ileal intestinal loop test for *E. coli* enterotoxin. Dilatation has occurred 18 hours after injection of a filtrate containing heat-labile enterotoxin. (From DuPont HL: Med Clin North Am 62:945, 1978.)

The most recent addition to the growing list of diarrheagenic *E. coli* has been associated with diarrhea outbreaks traced to contaminated beef. The illness is distinctive: Patients are afebrile or have low-grade fever yet commonly pass grossly bloody stools. An intense colitis is characteristically found by endoscopy. The clinical syndrome (bloody diarrhea without fever) has been called hemorrhagic colitis. The implicated etiologic agents, an O157:H7 and less commonly an O26:H11 *E. coli,* have been shown to produce a cytotoxin immunologically related to if not the same as that produced by the Shiga bacillus (*Shigella dysenteriae* type 1). This organism, including others that produce Shigalike toxin, may produce the hemolytic uremic syndrome during the course of infection.

Shigella. For *Shigella* strains, with worldwide distribution, the human is the only important reservoir (Chapter 268). The most important virulence property of this organism is invasiveness, although a Shigalike toxin is also produced and may play a role in the early, watery, small-bowel phase of the illness. Later in the disease the colon is the target organ, and here extensive mucosal invasion occurs, leading to the passage of many small-volume stools containing blood and polymorphonuclear leukocytes and patient complaints of abdominal pain, cramps, fecal urgency, and tenesmus. Because of the low dose of *Shigella* required to transmit the illness, secondary spread from an index case characteristically occurs.

Salmonella. *Salmonella* also occurs throughout the world in both the human and an important animal reservoir (Chapter 268). The strains are invasive to the intestinal mucosa but are less destructive locally than *Shigella*. In *Salmonella* gastroenteritis, an intestinal polymorphonuclear leukocyte reaction occurs after invasion by the organisms, and the organisms are contained locally. In typhoid or enteric fever, the organisms stimulate an intestinal mononuclear leukocyte reaction, which may facilitate the dissemination of the infecting strain into the regional and then systemic circulation.

Campylobacter jejuni. This microaerophilic *Vibrio* organism is a major cause of diarrhea in all regions of the world (Chapter 266). The reservoir most closely resembles that of *Salmonella;* animals, particularly poultry, and unpasteurized milk, are important vehicles of transmission. The organism is invasive to intestinal mucosa, which explains the occurrence of bloody stools and an inflammatory intestinal exudate. The importance of the cholera-like toxin produced by *C. jejuni* strains is not known.

Aeromonas and Plesiomonas shigelloides. *Aeromonas* species (especially *A. hydrophila* and *A. sobria*) have been associated with diarrhea in all regions. A high frequency of occurrence has been seen only for certain areas, however, including Thailand, western Australia, and Canada. The organisms produce a number of impressive virulence properties as demonstrated in the research laboratory: hemolysins, a cytotoxin in adrenal cells, and an enterotoxin in the suckling mouse model; and invasiveness in rabbit ileal loops has been shown for one strain. Yet *Aeromonas* is often found in stools of asymptomatic persons living in endemic areas, and several strains possessing the virulence characteristics in laboratory studies failed to produce illness when ingested by adult volunteers in high doses. *P. shigelloides* is an occasional cause of diarrhea.

Yersinia enterocolitica. *Y. enterocolitica* clearly shows geographic preferences (Chapter 269). It likes colder regions of the world, such as Canada and Scandinavia, although it is characteristically a summer pathogen in these areas. The organism produces heat-stable enterotoxins differing in methanol solubility, and it can be invasive to intestinal mucosa.

Viral agents

Viruses play important roles in producing diarrheal diseases. Two unrelated viruses, rotavirus and Norwalk agent, are particularly noteworthy. Enteric adenoviruses, astroviruses, and caliciviruses cause diarrhea, but their frequency and epidemiology are largely unstudied.

Rotavirus. No agent can rival rotaviruses as important causes of gastroenteritis in industrialized areas (Chapter 250). Rotaviruses probably produce more deaths associated with diarrhea than any other single agent. Those affected are less than 3 years of age, and vomiting is the major clinical feature. Because of the frequent involvement of small-bowel brush border, disaccharidase deficiency commonly follows rotavirus infection. Rotaviruses are detected in diarrheal stools as a 70-nm particle by electron microscopy (Fig. 236-3). Serologic procedures such as the enzyme-linked immunosorbent assay are available and are quite sensitive means of diagnosing the etiologic agents.

Norwalk-like agents. The Norwalk agent and related viruses, 26- to 27-nm particles seen by immune electron microscopy, probably explain a majority of the water-borne outbreaks of gastroenteritis in the world (Chapter 250). All age groups appear to be susceptible. Patients characteristically report previous ingestion of seafood or travel to a tropical region in the United States, whereas in developing tropical countries Norwalk virus infects a majority of persons by the time they reach 3 years of age (like rotavirus). Vomiting is common, as is secondary disaccharidase deficiency. Two US laboratories have cloned the Norwalk virus, which

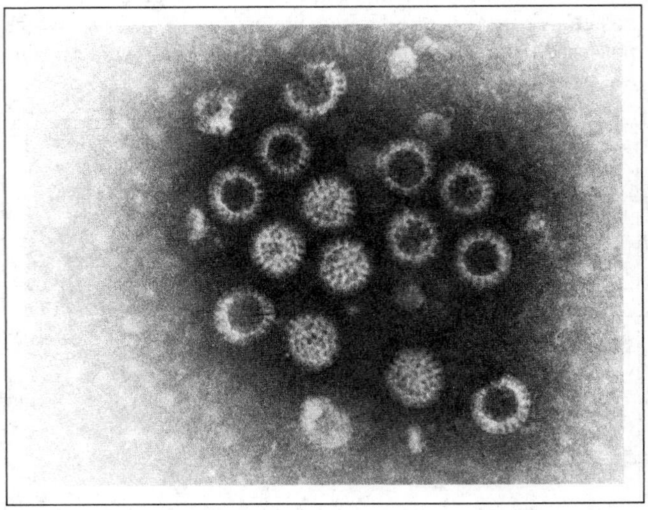

Fig. 236-3. Representative electron micrograph of rotavirus in diarrheal stool from a 10-month-old infant from rural Central America. (Phosphotungstic acid hematoxylin, ×259,000.) (From DuPont HL, Portnoy BL, and Conklin RH: Annu Rev Med 28:167, 1977.)

will be important in producing the reagents needed for organism detection.

Parasitic agents

Although numerous parasites are capable of producing diarrhea, and their ubiquity, particularly in the developing regions of the world, makes them all potentially important, only three agents will be considered briefly here, as their importance is established as enteric pathogens: *Giardia lamblia, Entamoeba histolytica,* and *Cryptosporidium*. It appears likely that occasionally patients will have symptomatic infection due to *Blastocystis hominis, Trichomonas hominis,* or *Dientamoeba fragilis*.

Giardia lamblia (Fig. 236-4). In the developing world this protozoan is so commonly encountered that it is impossible to implicate it as a common cause of acute diarrhea (Chapter 280). It does cause acute diarrhea in industrial areas, particularly in persons exposed to water in mountainous areas or in infants attending day care centers. The reservoir includes infected persons, although animals may play an important role as sources of infection in certain areas. The relationship between animal and human strains of *G. lamblia* needs additional study.

Entamoeba histolytica (Fig. 236-5). *E. histolytica* is a cause of morbidity primarily in less developed areas. All age groups are affected in these regions, and chronic or recurrent symptoms occur. The potential for development of liver abscess is a fact about which all students of medicine need to be aware (Chapter 280).

Cryptosporidium (Fig. 236-6). This Coccidia organism is a cause of acute diarrhea in rural populations of developing nations living in proximity to a variety of animals. It is an important cause of severe, cholera-like diarrhea in patients with acquired immunodeficiency syndrome (AIDS) (Chapter 243) (Plates V-34 and V-35) and in infants attending day care centers. The important reservoir of *Cryptosporidium* is probably drinking water.

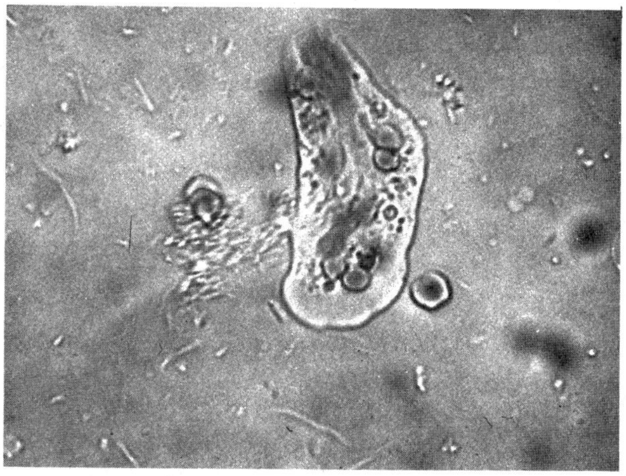

Fig. 236-5. Live *Entamoeba histolytica* trophozoite with ingested red blood cells. Unidirectional movement along with cytoplasmic streaming was noted. This photomicrograph was taken directly from stool specimen from a patient with diarrhea. Prepared by Bernard J. Marino of the Houston City Health Department; saline preparation, × 1000. (From DuPont HL and Pickering LK: Infections of the gastrointestinal tract, New York, 1980, Plenum.)

FREQUENCY OF OCCURRENCE OF ETIOLOGIC AGENTS

Endemic diarrhea

The relative importance of the various enteropathogens in endemic settings differs according to patient age, time of year, and geographic location. Table 236-2 summarizes the results of a number of studies that attempted to characterize the occurrence of the different pathogens as causes of endemically acquired diarrhea. Three groups or settings are

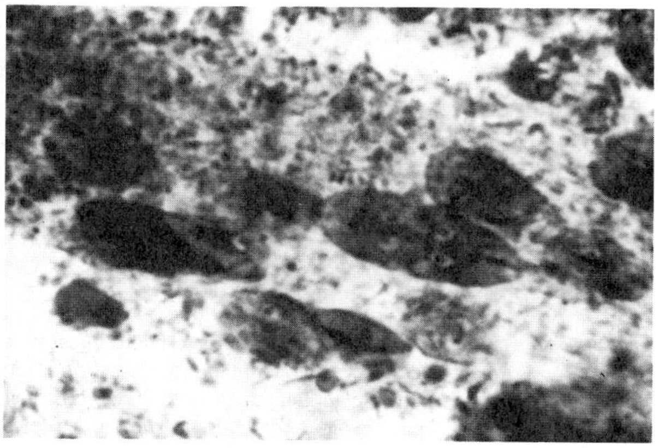

Fig. 236-4. *Giardia lamblia* trophozoites from an asymptomatic infant attending a Houston day care center. The trophozoites are entangled in debris. (Trichrome, ×1000.)

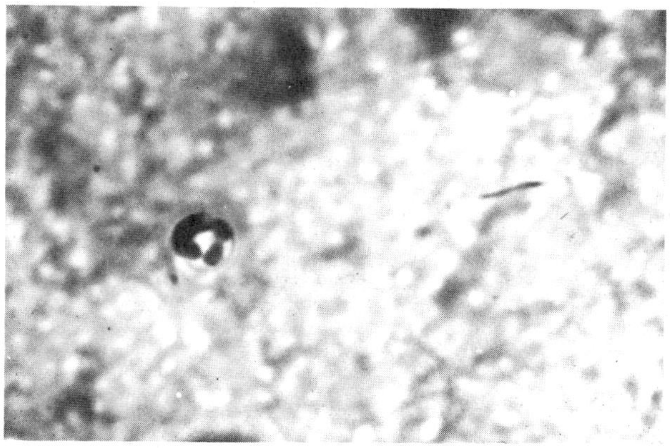

Fig. 236-6. *Cryptosporidium* oocyst in diarrheal stool obtained from a patient with AIDS. Permanent modified Kinyoun acid-fast stain.

Table 236-2. Relative importance of enteropathogens in endemically acquired diarrhea

Agent Δ	Industrialized regions: children (%)	Developing areas*: children (%)	Traveler's diarrhea† (%)
Rotavirus	20-30	15-30	<10
Enterotoxigenic *E. coli*	4	20-30	40
Enteropathogenic *E. coli*	4	4	<1
Shigella	3-15	3-12	15
Salmonella	4	4	7
Campylobacter jejuni	3-12	3-12	3
Giardia lamblia	4	4	<3
Unknown	40	<40	20

*Non-cholera endemic areas.
†US adults traveling to Mexico.

identified in the table: diarrhea in children in industrialized regions such as the United States; diarrhea occurring in children in developing areas where cholera is not endemic; and finally, diarrhea that occurs among US adults traveling to Mexico (traveler's diarrhea). Rotavirus is an important cause of diarrhea in infants and children under 3 years of age in all areas. It shows an impressive wintertime predisposition in temperate areas; this seasonal peak is blunted in more tropical regions. The less developed the region, the more important ETEC becomes, again primarily in infants and children. These strains usually are the most important causes of diarrhea in infants and children in the less developed areas, which explains their presence and importance as causes of traveler's diarrhea. Immunity occurs secondary to rotavirus and ETEC infections. Travelers from the United States are susceptible to ETEC because of the rarity of these strains in the United States; they are less susceptible to rotavirus, which is endemic to both areas. *Shigella* and *Campylobacter* are important in all settings and often show an inverse pattern of occurrence.

Food-borne diarrhea

Food is an excellent culture medium for enteric pathogens and represents an extremely important vehicle of disease transmission, particularly in tropical areas. Development of clinical symptoms when a contaminated food is ingested by a healthy person depends on one of two factors: (1) the number of organisms in the food and (2) the presence of a highly virulent organism in the vehicle. Nearly any bacterial species is capable of producing at least mild diarrhea and other intestinal complaints if swallowed in sufficient numbers. A far smaller inoculum is necessary to produce symptoms if the agent is a high-grade (virulent) pathogen, such as *Shigella, Salmonella,* or *Campylobacter*. Table 236-3 summarizes the clinical features of the most common forms of food-borne diarrhea, which are useful in separating the various etiologic agents. Determining the presence of associated cases, constructing the incubation period, and assessing the degree of vomiting and fever can suggest the etiologic diagnosis of food-borne illness before laboratory confirmation is received. In the United States the most common forms of food-borne diarrhea outbreaks unassociated with fever in the affected are *Staphylococcus aureus* (a true food poisoning) and *Clostridium perfringens;* the incubation period usually allows differentiation. *Bacillus cereus* produces two forms of food-borne illness, which resemble either *S. aureus* food poisoning or *C. perfringens* disease. Isolation of the organism is necessary to determine the presence of *B. cereus*. Finding fever in a percentage of cases suggests strongly that an invasive agent is responsible (i.e., *Salmonella, Shigella,* or *Campylobacter*). *Vibrio parahaemolyticus* is a possible agent in diarrhea outbreaks (which may be extensive) secondary to ingestion of contaminated seafood. Laboratory identification of one of the invasive pathogens from stool and/or less commonly from food is required to make a definitive diagnosis.

Gay bowel syndrome

Certain male homosexual patients experience diarrhea with a high frequency. Diarrhea in male homosexual persons should be approached in a special way. Because of sexual practices of many of these patients, they more frequently

Table 236-3. Major forms of food-borne diarrhea

Agent	Incubation period (H)	Fever	Vomiting	Diagnosis
S. aureus	1-5	Absent	Profuse	Characteristic epidemiologic and clinical picture
B. cereus	2-5	Absent	Profuse	Isolation of organism from food and/or stool
	8-22	Absent	Yes	Isolation of organism from food and/or stool
C. perfringens	8-22	Absent or low-grade	Minimal	Characteristic epidemiologic and clinical picture
Salmonella	8-24	Common	Common	Isolation of organism from food and/or stool
Shigella	7-120	Common	Occasional	Isolation of organism from food and/or stool
V. parahaemolyticus	12-24	Occasional	Occasional	Isolation of organism from seafood and/or stool

experience fecal-oral contamination and therefore show accelerated transmission of all the agents spread by this route (*Shigella, Salmonella, Campylobacter, G. lamblia, E. histolytica,* etc.). Also, they may experience unique enteric infections. Perhaps through direct rectal inoculation, proctitis occurs, which may be due to *Neisseria gonorrhoeae, Chlamydia trachomatis,* herpes simplex, or *Treponema pallidum*. Finally, male homosexual patients with AIDS may present with diarrhea due to intestinal infection secondary to *Cryptosporidium, Isospora,* Microsporidia, *Salmonella,* herpes viruses (herpes simplex and cytomegalovirus), and *Mycobacterium* of the *avian-intracellulare* complex.

Persistent diarrhea

Most patients with enteric infection experience diarrhea for no more than a week. When diarrhea lasts 2 weeks, certain agents or processes should be considered (see accompanying box). Although *G. lamblia* is the cause of diarrhea in no more than 4% of unselected cases of acute illness, this protozoan can be found in one third or more cases of persistent illness, as defined here. The agents that infect the small bowel (rotavirus, Norwalk agent, and *G. lamblia*) may lead to a disruption of disaccharidase production by cells of the intestinal brush border. Failure to split disaccharides, most particularly milk lactose, may lead to an osmotic and fermentative diarrhea. Alteration of diet with restriction of milk consumption may be all that is necessary to control symptoms. In selected cases of acute diarrhea, small-bowel motility patterns are disturbed, leading to stasis in the upper gut and overgrowth of colonic bacteria. Bacterial species in high numbers in the small bowel interfere with absorption of dietary constituents at least partially through deconjugation of bile salts. Small bowel intubation will reveal heavy growth ($>10^5$ colonies/cc) of normally nonpathogenic bacteria in these cases. A favorable response of the subacute illness to empiric anti-*Giardia* therapy with metronidazole may represent treatment of giardiasis or may be secondary to an anaerobic bacterial overgrowth syndrome responding to antimicrobial properties of the drug rather than actual giardiasis. Finally, the conventional bacterial enteropathogens (*Shigella, Salmonella, Campylobacter, Yersinia,* and EPEC) may occasionally produce more protracted diarrhea, as has been seen most clearly for EPEC and other adherent *E. coli* in young infants. Stool culture should reveal one of these agents.

Causes of diarrhea lasting more than 1 to 2 weeks (persistent illness)

Giardia lamblia enteritis
Disaccharidase deficiency
Bacterial overgrowth syndrome
Bacterial enterocolitis (due to a *Shigella, Salmonella, Campylobacter, Yersinia,* or EPEC)
Less defined agents (Cyanobacteria-like organisms, Brainerd agent)
Host deficiencies (immunodeficiency, micronutrient deficiency)

ETIOLOGIC DIAGNOSIS OF ENTERIC INFECTION

Clinical aspects

Certain enteric pathogens tend to produce characteristic clinical symptoms. In general, invasive bacterial enteropathogens (*Shigella, Salmonella, Campylobacter*) produce more intense diarrhea when compared with the viral or parasitic agents and infections. *Shigella* and *Campylobacter* strains characteristically lead to the passage of bloody stools (occurring in about 30% to 50% of cases). Bloody stools are passed in about 8% of patients with salmonellosis. Other less common causes of dysentery (bloody stools) are *E. histolytica, V. parahaemolyticus, A. hydrophila,* and *Y. enterocolitaca*. Viral agents (rotaviruses and Norwalk-like agents) produce vomiting in most cases. In classic giardiasis, the patient describes intermittent diarrhea associated with abdominal pain and cramping, bloating, and flatulence. Despite these clinical characteristics of enteric infection when in the classic presentation, it is extremely difficult to diagnose clinically the etiology of most cases of diarrhea. For this reason laboratory diagnosis is necessary.

In most patients with persistent diarrhea, an etiologic agent cannot be identified. With further research, new agents will be identified. Cyanobacteria-like organisms or so-called blue-green algae have been identified in patients with persistent or chronic diarrhea, particularly in patients who are immunosuppressed. An interesting syndrome known as "Brainerd diarrhea," first described during an outbreak in Brainerd, Minnesota, is associated with consumption of unpasteurized milk or untreated surface water. The illness characteristically lasts longer than 1 year and is unresponsive to antimicrobial agents. The cause of the syndrome remains undefined. Finally, in developing regions where malnutrition is common, deficiency in micronutrients such as zinc, vitamin A, or folic acid may lead to protracted diarrhea.

Typhoid or enteric fever is seen in patients with systemic *Salmonella* infection (Chapter 268). In Latin America, Asia, and Africa, it usually corresponds to bacteremic infection by *Salmonella typhi,* or less commonly *Salmonella paratyphi*. In the United States, bacteremia and typhoidlike disease are more frequently caused by nontyphoid strains of *Salmonella*. Symptoms and signs include fever, which may be impressive, headache, and abdominal symptoms. The abdominal findings are variable and may consist of constipation, diarrhea, pain and cramps, distention, and ileus. On physical examination patients may have small, delicate erythematous macules that blanch on pressure, clustered in small numbers usually around the abdomen (rose spots). In addition, steady deep palpation of the abdomen often reveals segmental ileus, felt as air and fluid being displaced by the pressure. Patients typically have a leukopenia and a pulse-temperature deficit. Other infections resembling typhoid fever are rickettsial infection, brucellosis, tularemia, yersiniosis, babesiosis, leptospirosis, and *Campylobacter fetus* infection.

Use of the laboratory

For most cases of mild to moderately severe diarrheal disease (≤5 unformed stools without fever and/or without bothersome cramps, pain, nausea, and vomiting), an etiologic assessment is unnecessary and treatment can be given empirically. For more severe diarrhea (≥6 unformed stools or the other clinical findings are of concern or are disabling to the patient), the laboratory can offer invaluable help in determining how best to manage the patient. Table 236-4 summarizes the tests described below (Chapter 226).

Fecal leukocyte test. In patients to be further evaluated, the fecal leukocyte test can give rapid useful information. By mixing stool (if present, mucus is preferred) with dilute methylene blue and looking at the wet-mount preparation under a coverslip, or after heat-fixing the specimen, adding the same stain, and allowing it to dry, one can determine microscopically the presence of leukocytes and a rough quantitation of their number. The finding of numerous leukocytes (Fig. 236-7) indicates diffuse colonic inflammation rather than a specific etiology. Thus the test is useful in defining the pathology of the infection. Not all patients with invasive bacterial diarrhea will have numerous leukocytes on fecal smears. Early in a *Shigella* infection the small bowel is the site of infection, and late in the disease the inflammatory character of the colitis is reduced. In both situations stools are positive for *Shigella,* but the stool examination for leukocytes may be negative. The infectious process also may be focal (e.g., in selected cases of antibiotic-associated colitis), and leukocytes will be sparse due to dilution by the luminal contents. Understanding these limitations of the test, one can consider the agents that are likely to produce diffuse colonic inflammation and therefore characteristically produce a fecal leukocyte exudate. The three most common causes of leukocyte-positive stools are *Shigella, Salmonella,* and *Campylobacter*. Other recognized causes of numerous stool leukocytes are *Clostridium difficile* (antibiotic-associated colitis), *Y. enterocolitica, A. hydrophila, V. parahaemolyticus,* and invasive or hemorrhagic colitis *E. coli*. Patients with idiopathic ulcerative colitis and certain patients with other forms of allergic colitis will also be found to have fecal leukocytes. Finding stools with many leukocytes in the presence of moderate to severe diarrheal illness generally is an indication for either performing a stool culture or treating the patient empirically with an antimicrobial agent.

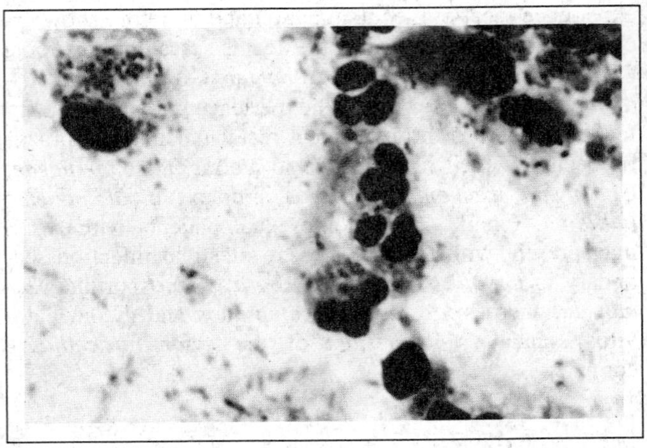

Fig. 236-7. Fecal leukocytes in a patient with diffuse colitis of unknown etiology. (Methylene blue permanent, ×1000.)

Stool culture. It should be realized that the routine laboratory should be able to recover *Shigella, Salmonella,* and *Campylobacter* from culture of stool. The indications for performing a stool culture include moderate to severe illness (particularly those with fever or requiring hospitalization) and cases positive for fecal leukocytes. In selected cases, the laboratory can be instructed to culture stool for *V. cholerae, V. parahaemolyticus* (on TCBS agar), *Y. enterocolitica,* or *C. difficile*.

Blood culture. In patients with clinical typhoid or enteric fever or in any ill, hospitalized patient who has intestinal symptoms, blood cultures should be performed. The diagnosis of typhoid fever is generally made in the proper clin-

Table 236-4. Use of the laboratory in determining etiology of sporadic cases of diarrhea

Laboratory test	Indications	Probable diagnosis if test is positive
Fecal leukocytes	All moderately to severely ill cases	Diffuse colonic inflammation (see text)
Stool culture	Moderately to severely ill cases; those with fever or positive fecal leukocytes; male homosexuals	*Shigella; Campylobacter; Salmonella*
Blood culture	Enteric fever and all clinically septic patients	*Salmonella* bacteremia; less likely, sepsis associated with *Campylobacter* or *Yersinia*
Parasite examination (stool or small-bowel fluid)	Diarrhea of >1 week's duration; travel to special areas (see text); day care center–associated case; male homosexuals	*G. lamblia; E. histolytica; Cryptosporidium*
Rotavirus antigen	Hospitalized infants <3 years of age	Rotavirus

ical setting by a positive blood culture for the causative agent. If the patient has received antimicrobial therapy preceding the evaluation, culturing bone marrow aspirate material will give a higher yield. Other systemic enteric infections are diagnosed etiologically by blood culture. Nontyphoid salmonellae, *C. fetus*, and *Y. enterocolitica* are included in this category.

***Parasite examination* (Figs. 236-4 to 236-6).** Indications for parasite examination include (1) all patients with diarrhea lasting more than a week, (2) illness originating during travel to the Rocky Mountains, Russia, or developing regions of the world, (3) diarrhea in a person exposed to day care centers, or (4) a male homosexual patient. Evidence suggests that in *G. lamblia* infection, stools are negative for the protozoan in half the cases. When *Giardia* infection is strongly suspected and stools are negative, it is advisable to collect small bowel fluid or mucus, perform a small bowel biopsy to look for the agent, or treat the patient empirically without establishing a diagnosis. The nylon string test (Entero-Test) can be tried to sample small bowel mucus but will be helpful in a limited number of patients.

Special tests. Commercial kits for rotavirus detection (e.g., Rotazyme) are readily available. Because there is no specific treatment for viral gastroenteritis, the test has limited applicability. The major indication for the serologic study for rotavirus is hospitalization of an infant under 3 years of age with gastroenteritis. Here the test is used in a negative way. A positive rotavirus antigen test result in such a patient should lead to fluid, but not antimicrobial therapy. The best laboratory test for diagnosing antibiotic-associated colitis is to assay for *C. difficile* toxin by tissue culture or serologic procedure (Chapter 226 and Chapter 262). This is a reliable indicator of antibiotic-associated colitis in the older child and adult. Young infants and children may have toxin in stool without evidence of a pathologic process. In the patient with typhoid or enteric fever, serologic studies are of limited value in making a diagnosis. Serologic diagnosis of typhoid fever (Widal's reaction) is useful in parts of the world where the illness is endemic, because of the relative importance of *S. typhi*. In areas where typhoid fever is unusual (e.g., the United States), serologic changes suggesting typhoid fever are more likely to be due to exposure to other cross-reacting gram-negative rods than to the typhoid bacillus.

TREATMENT OF DIARRHEA

For all patients with diarrhea, fluid and electrolyte replacement is advisable. Although this treatment is not usually critical to well-nourished adults with mild to moderate diarrhea, it can be lifesaving to the very young or the elderly patient with dehydrating illness. All patients with active diarrhea should be encouraged to drink Gatorade, Pedialyte, Lytren, or soft drinks augmented with saltine crackers. In dehydrating illness, oral rehydration salts or intravenous fluids should be given. Packets of salts containing NaCl 3.5 g, $NaHCO_3$ 2.5 g, NaHCO 2.5 g, KCl 2.5 g, and glucose 20 g are available to add to 1 liter of fluid, giving the following chemical composition: Na^+ 90 mmol, Cl^- 80 mmol, K^+ 20 mmol, HCO_3^- 30 mmol, and glucose 111 mmol. Diet alteration during the height of acute illness includes taking fluids only (bottled water, soft drinks, soups, etc.) and avoiding milk (except for breast-feeding). As stool rate decreases and appetite improves, bread, toast, rice, and baked fish or chicken can gradually be added to the diet. In most cases full diet can be resumed within 2 or 3 days, when stools are no longer liquid in composition.

Empiric therapy

In mild to moderate diarrhea or when illness develops in a person away from home, it is often not practical to use the laboratory to help establish an etiologic diagnosis. In this instance, therapy can be given empirically based on clinical features of illness (Table 236-5). Although mild symptoms need not be treated with anything other than fluids, moderate illness may be optimally managed with a drug to nonspecifically improve the illness, such as bismuth subsalicylate (Pepto-Bismol) or loperamide (Imodium). Bismuth subsalicylate will reduce the diarrhea by 50% and is most effective in treating a secretory type of illness. The dose is 30 ml every 30 minutes for eight doses (one 8-ounce bottle over 3½ hours). This therapy can be repeated on the second day. Loperamide even more impressively reduces symptoms and is given in a dose of two capsules (4 mg) initially followed by one capsule after each unformed stool not to exceed eight capsules in 24 hours; prescription dosing—16 mg/day maximum dose or 4 mg initially followed by 2 mg (liquid or caplet) after each unformed stool not to exceed 8 mg (over-the-counter dosage not requiring a prescription). Patients with fever or dysentery (bloody stools), or those worsening on therapy, should not receive loperamide-like drugs.

Antimicrobial agents are given to patients with severe diarrhea or those with fever and perhaps to those found to have fecal leukocytes on microscopic examination. For adults with traveler's diarrhea acquired in the interior of Mexico during rainy summer months or for any person meeting these criteria for therapy in an area of high *Shigella* endemicity, trimethoprim-sulfamethoxazole (TMP-SMX) is the optimal empiric therapy. The dose is one double-strength tablet (160 mg TMP/800 mg SMX) twice daily for 3 days. If the severe illness occurs in an area where *Campylobacter* is more common than *Shigella* but where laboratory testing is not available, erythromycin (500 mg four times a day for 3 to 5 days) can be given by mouth. Drugs effective for both forms of diarrhea (*Shigella* and *Campylobacter*) are norfloxacin 400 mg twice a day by mouth or ciprofloxacin 500 mg twice a day by mouth or ofloxacin 300 mg twice a day by mouth for 3 days for adults. For traveler's diarrhea occurring outside of the Mexican interior (noncoastal areas) or anywhere during the winter, one of the three quinolones should be used (norfloxacin, ciprofloxacin, or ofloxacin).

Table 236-5. Therapy of acute diarrhea according to clinical and laboratory findings (see text for details)

Laboratory results	Clinical aspects	Therapy
None performed	Mild diarrhea (≤3 unformed stools/day, little associated symptomatology)	Fluids only
	Moderate diarrhea (≥4 unformed stools/day and/or associated symptomatology)	Loperamide or bismuth subsalicylate (Pepto-Bismol)
	Severe diarrhea (≥6 unformed stools/day and/or temperature ≥101° F and/or severe symptomatology and/or numerous fecal leukocytes)	Antimicrobial therapy
Culture positive for *Campylobacter*	Any situation	Erythromycin or quinolones
Culture positive for *Shigella*	Any situation	TMP-SMX or quinolone
Culture positive for *Salmonella*	Asymptomatic or mild to moderate gastroenteritis	Fluids only
	Severe gastroenteritis, septic or hospitalized patient	Quinolone, TMP-SMX, ampicillin, or chloramphenicol

Specific therapy

Ideally, the laboratory can be used to make a presumptive or definitive diagnosis. Culture-positive cases of campylobacteriosis are best treated with erythromycin. When stool cultures are positive for *Shigella,* TMP-SMX is given unless TMP-resistant *Shigellae* are common in the area. For patients with *Salmonella* gastroenteritis, no antimicrobial therapy is given for mild to moderate or asymptomatic cases. If, on the other hand, the patient is clinically septic, has a severe bout of illness due to *Salmonella,* or is ill enough to justify admission to the hospital, antimicrobial agents should be given to treat bacteremic illness. For typhoid (enteric) fever, TMP-SMX (160 mg TMP/800 SMX twice daily), ampicillin (1.5 g IV every 4 hours), or chloramphenicol (1 g every 8 hours by mouth or intravenously) is given for 2 weeks. Relapses occur in typhoid fever and should be treated with a second short course of therapy. For nontyphoid bacteremic salmonellosis, TMP-SMX or chloramphenicol is preferred because ampicillin-resistance among these strains is common. Many persons feel that 10 days of fluoroquinolone represents optimal therapy for bacteremia *Salmonella* (typhoid or nontyphoid).

PROPHYLAXIS FOR TRAVELER'S DIARRHEA

Diarrhea occurs in approximately 40% of persons traveling from low-risk (United States, Canada, northwestern Europe) to high-risk areas (Latin America, Asia, and Africa) (Chapter 242). The problem can be reduced by exercising care about where and what one eats. Heat kills microbes, and steaming hot foods should be sought. Other usually safe items include bread and other dry goods, citrus fruit, and bottled (particularly carbonated) liquids.

For certain travelers, drug prophylaxis (antimicrobial drugs or bismuth subsalicylate) can be given. Because of side effects of the conventional antimicrobials (intestinal reactions, skin rashes, acquisition of resistance by intestinal flora, etc.), we currently advise that they be used only for a minority of persons making critical trips and for persons at risk of developing a more serious illness or suffering greater consequence if they acquire an illness. Persons with achlorhydria, or those who have had gastric resection or regularly take maximum doses of H_2 blockers (cimetidine-like agents) or omeprazole might be considered in the latter category. A traveler should use this form of prophylaxis only after receiving approval from a physician and after the risks and benefits are clearly understood. Three agents are currently recognized as useful in preventing the illness: TMP-SMX, a quinolone, and bismuth subsalicylate. The antimicrobial agents are 80% to 90% effective and are given in the dose of one double-strength tablet of TMP-SMX (160 mg TMP/800 mg SMX) during summertime travel to the interior of Mexico and other areas where TMP-resistance among bacterial enteropathogens is unusual, norfloxacin 400 mg, ciprofloxacin 500 mg, or ofloxacin 300 mg once daily beginning the day of travel and continuing for 1 to 2 days after returning home. Studies to determine the optimum dose of the tablet form of bismuth subsalicylate (Pepto-Bismol) for use in treatment and prophylaxis indicate that bismuth subsalicylate is between 60% and 65% effective in preventing the illness and should be administered in a dosage of two tablets just before meals and at bedtime four times a day. Prophylactic agents are most practical for short-term use (less than a week) and probably should be restricted to trips of 3 weeks or less. For many international travelers, cautious food selection and early treatment of illness (fluids, nonspecific drugs, or antimicrobials, depending on severity of symptoms) are the optimum ways to prevent or treat diarrhea.

REFERENCES

Blacklow NR and Greenberg HB: Viral gastroenteritis, N Engl J Med 325:252-263, 1991.

Blaser MJ and Reller LB: *Campylobacter* enteritis, N Engl J Med 305:1444, 1981.

DuPont HL et al: Pathogenesis of *Escherichia coli* diarrhea, N Engl J Med 285:1, 1971.
DuPont HL and Pickering LK: Infections of the gastrointestinal tract. Microbiology, pathophysiology, and clinical features, New York, 1980, Plenum.
DuPont HL et al: Emporiatric enteritis: lessons learned from US students in Mexico, Trans Am Clin Climatol Assoc 97:32, 1985.
Guerrant RL and Bobak DA: Bacterial and protozoal gastroenteritis, N Engl J Med 325:327-339, 1991.
Harris JC, DuPont HL, Hornick RB: Fecal leukocytes in diarrheal illness, Ann Intern Med 76:697, 1972.
Hornick RB et al: Typhoid fever: pathogenesis and immunologic control, N Engl J Med 283:686, 739, 1970.
Koopman JS et al: Patterns and etiology of diarrhea in three clinical settings, Am J Epidemiol 119:114, 1984.
Navin TR and Juranek DD: Cryptosporidiosis: clinical, epidemiologic, and parasitologic review, Rev Infect Dis 6:313, 1984.
Paisley JW et al: Dark-field microscopy of human feces for presumptive diagnosis of *Campylobacter fetus* subspecies jejuni enteritis, J Clin Microbiol 15:61, 1982.
Pickering LK et al: Prospective study of enteropathogens in children with diarrhea in Houston and Mexico, J Pediatr 93:383, 1978.
Quinn TC et al: The polymicrobial origin of intestinal infections in homosexual men, N Engl J Med 309:576, 1983.

CHAPTER

237 Osteomyelitis

Jon T. Mader

Based on etiologic and clinical considerations, bone infections have traditionally been classified as either hematogenous osteomyelitis or osteomyelitis secondary to a contiguous focus of infection. Contiguous focus osteomyelitis has been further subdivided into osteomyelitis in patients who have relatively normal vascularity and osteomyelitis in patients with generalized vascular insufficiency.

Osteomyelitis may be acute or chronic. The acute disease is characterized by a suppurative infection accompanied by edema, vascular congestion, and small-vessel thrombosis. The vascular supply to the bone is compromised as the infection extends into the surrounding soft tissue. Large areas of dead bone (sequestra) may be formed when both the medullary and periosteal blood supplies are compromised. Viable colonies of bacteria may be harbored within the necrotic and ischemic tissues even after an intense host response, surgery, and therapeutic antibiotics. Once the antibiotics are discontinued or the host response declines, the organisms may again proliferate and lead to a recurrence of the infection. The hallmarks of chronic osteomyelitis are a nidus of infected dead bone or scar tissue, an ischemic soft tissue envelope, and a refractory clinical course.

HEMATOGENOUS OSTEOMYELITIS

Long bone hematogenous osteomyelitis occurs mainly in infants and children. The metaphysis of the long bones (tibia, femur) are most frequently involved. The anatomy in the metaphyseal region seems to explain this clinical localization. Nonanastomosing capillary ends of the nutrient artery make sharp loops under the growth plate and enter a system of large venous sinusoids where the blood flow becomes slow and turbulent. The metaphyseal capillaries lack phagocytic lining cells, and the sinusoidal veins contain functionally inactive phagocytic cells. These capillary loops are essentially end-artery branches of the nutrient artery. Any end-capillary obstruction could lead to an area of avascular necrosis. Minor trauma probably predisposes the infant or child to infection by producing a small hematoma, vascular obstruction, and a subsequent bone necrosis that is susceptible to inoculation from a transient bacteremia. The acute infection initially produces a local cellulitis, which results in a breakdown of leukocytes, increased bone pressure, decreased pH, and decreased oxygen tension. The cumulative effects of these physiologic factors further compromise the medullary circulation and enhance the spread of infection.

The infection may proceed laterally through the haversian and Volkmann's canal systems, perforate the bony cortex, and separate the periosteum from the surface of the bone. When this process is coupled with the presence of medullary extension, both the periosteal and endosteal circulations are lost, and large segments of dead cortical and cancellous bone are formed. In the infant, the medullary infection may spread to the epiphysis and joint surfaces through capillaries that cross the growth plate. In the child over 1 year of age, the growth plate is avascular, and the infection is confined to the metaphysis and diaphysis. The joint is usually spared unless the metaphysis is intracapsular. Thus cortical perforation at the proximal radius, humerus, or femur infects the elbow, shoulder, or hip joint, respectively, regardless of the age of the patient.

A single pathogenic organism is almost always recovered from the bone in hematogenous osteomyelitis. Polymicrobic hematogenous osteomyelitis is rare. In the infant, *Staphylococcus aureus, Streptococcus agalactiae,* and *Escherichia coli* are the most frequently recovered bone isolates; in children over 1 year of age, *S. aureus, Streptococcus pyogenes,* and *Haemophilus influenzae* are the most common organisms isolated. After age 4, however, the incidence of *H. influenzae* osteomyelitis decreases.

Infants and children have clinically different presentations of osteomyelitis. Neonatal osteomyelitis is characterized by a paucity of systemic and local findings. Local findings that may be present include edema and decreased motion of a limb. A joint effusion or septic joint adjacent to the bone infection is present in 60% to 70% of cases. Classically, children with hematogenous osteomyelitis present with abrupt fever, irritability, lethargy, and local signs of inflammation 3 weeks or less in duration. However, 50% of children now present with vague complaints including pain in the involved limb of 1 to 3 months in duration and minimal if any temperature elevation.

Because infants and children with hematogenous osteomyelitis usually have normal soft tissue enveloping the infected bone and are capable of a very efficient metabolic response to infection, they have the potential to resorb large sequestra and generate a significant periosteal response to the infection. This latter feature leads to substantial formation of bone at the margin of the infection called involucrum. The involucrum affords skeletal continuity and a maintenance of function during the healing phase. If antimicrobial therapy directed at the responsible pathogen is begun before extensive bone necrosis, the patient has an excellent probability for arrest of the infection.

Hematogenous osteomyelitis is also found in the adult population. The infection usually begins in the diaphysis but may spread to involve the entire medullary canal. Extension into the joint may occur because the growth plate has matured and once again shares vessels with the metaphysis. Cortical penetration usually leads to a soft tissue abscess as the periosteum is firmly adherent to the bone. In time, sinus tracts will form, connecting the sequestered nidus of infection to the skin by way of the soft tissue extension(s). In the adult, *S. aureus, Staphylococcus epidermidis,* and aerobic gram-negative organisms account for the majority of the bone or blood isolates.

The adult usually presents with vague complaints consisting of nonspecific pain and few constitutional symptoms, 1 to 3 months in duration. However, acute clinical presentations with fever, chills, swelling, and erythema over the involved bone(s) are sometimes seen. The clinical signs resulting from soft tissue extension often dominate the findings at presentation and can lead to inappropriate diagnostic and therapeutic measures unless the possibility of an osseous etiology is considered.

VERTEBRAL OSTEOMYELITIS

Vertebral osteomyelitis in the adult patient population is usually hematogenous in origin but may be secondary to trauma. A preceding history of urinary tract infection or intravenous drug abuse often is present. An early involvement of the anterior-inferior edge of the vertebral body suggests spread from the bony entrance of the anterior spinal artery; however, retrograde infection via Batson's plexus of veins is also postulated. The lumbar vertebral bodies are most often involved, followed in frequency by the thoracic and cervical vertebrae. Spread to adjacent vertebral bodies may occur rapidly through the rich venous networks in the spine. Posterior extension may lead to epidural and subdural abscesses or even meningitis. Extension anteriorly or laterally may lead to paravertebral, retropharyngeal, mediastinal, subphrenic, retroperitoneal, or psoas abscesses.

Clinically, the patient usually presents with vague symptoms and signs consisting of dull constant back pain and spasm of the paravertebral muscles. More specific complaints may localize to a soft tissue abscess. The presence of point tenderness over the involved vertebral body is a characteristic finding. Fever may be low grade or absent.

The infection is usually monomicrobic when hematogenous in origin. The most common organism isolated is *S. aureus*. However, aerobic gram-negative rods are found in 30% of the cases. *Pseudomonas aeruginosa* and *Serratia marcescens* have a high incidence of isolation among intravenous drug abusers.

CONTIGUOUS FOCUS OSTEOMYELITIS WITH NO GENERALIZED VASCULAR INSUFFICIENCY

In contiguous focus osteomyelitis, the organism may be directly inoculated into the bone at the time of trauma or may extend from adjacent soft tissue infections. Common predisposing conditions include open fractures, surgical reduction and internal fixation of fractures, and chronic soft tissue infections. In contrast to hematogenous osteomyelitis, multiple bacterial organisms are usually isolated from the infected bone. The bacteriology is diverse, but *S. aureus* remains the most commonly isolated pathogen. In addition, aerobic gram-negative bacilli and anaerobic organisms are frequently isolated. Bone necrosis, soft tissue damage, and loss of bone stability occur regularly, which makes this form of osteomyelitis difficult to manage.

CONTIGUOUS FOCUS OSTEOMYELITIS WITH GENERALIZED VASCULAR INSUFFICIENCY

The small bones of the feet are commonly involved in this category of osteomyelitis. Inadequate tissue perfusion predisposes the patient to the infection by blunting the local inflammatory response. The infection commonly develops after minor trauma to the feet, infected nail beds, cellulitis, or trophic skin ulceration. Multiple bacteria are usually isolated from the infected bone. The most common organisms are *S. aureus, S. epidermidis, Enterococcus,* gram-negative rods, and anaerobes. Although cure is desirable, a more attainable goal of therapy is to suppress the infection and maintain the functional integrity of the involved limb. Even after successful treatment, recurrent or new bone infection occurs in the majority of patients. In time, resection of the infected bone is almost always necessary.

CHRONIC OSTEOMYELITIS

Both hematogenous and contiguous focus osteomyelitis can progress to a chronic bone infection. No exact criteria separate acute from chronic osteomyelitis. Clinically, newly recognized bone infections are considered acute, whereas a relapse of a treated infection represents a chronic process; however, this simplistic classification is clearly inadequate. As mentioned, the hallmark of chronic osteomyelitis is the simultaneous presence of organisms, necrotic bone, and a compromised soft tissue envelope. The infection will not regress until the nidus for the persistent contamination is removed. Persistent drainage and/or sinus tract(s) are common. Antibiotic therapy alone is usually unsuccessful in the treatment of chronic osteomyelitis.

Multiple species of bacteria are usually isolated from biopsies of infected granulations from deep within the wound, except in chronic hematogenous, where a single organism is often recovered from patients even after years of intermittent drainage. The prospects of arresting the infection are reduced when the integrity of the soft tissue surrounding the infection is poor or the bone itself is unstable secondary to an infected nonunion or an adjacent septic joint.

DIAGNOSIS OF BACTERIAL OSTEOMYELITIS

The bacteriologic diagnosis of long-bone bacterial osteomyelitis rests on the isolation of the causative bacteria from bone or blood. In hematogenous osteomyelitis, positive blood cultures can often obviate the need for a bone biopsy when there is associated radiographic or radionuclide scan evidence of osteomyelitis. Chronic osteomyelitis is rarely associated with a bacteremia unless there is an acute extension of the infection into the soft tissues. Sinus tract cultures are not reliable for predicting which organisms will be isolated from the infected bone. Antibiotic treatment of osteomyelitis should be based on deep-bone biopsy cultures and specific antimicrobial susceptibilities.

Radiographic changes in acute hematogenous osteomyelitis are often difficult to interpret and lag at least 2 weeks behind the evolution of infection. The earliest radiographic changes are soft tissue swelling, periosteal thickening and/or elevation, and focal osteopenia. These findings are subtle and may be missed. The more diagnostic lytic changes are delayed and often associated with an indolent infection of several months' duration. Later, when the patient is receiving appropriate antimicrobial therapy, radiographic improvement may lag behind clinical recovery. In contiguous focus and chronic osteomyelitis, the radiographic changes are even more subtle, often found in association with other nonspecific radiographic findings, and require a careful clinical correlation to achieve diagnostic significance.

An earlier diagnosis of osteomyelitis may be achieved with radionuclide imaging. However, the actual mechanism of labeling bone with radiopharmaceuticals is still unclear. The technetium polyphosphate ^{99m}Tc scan demonstrates increased isotope accumulation in areas of increased blood flow and reactive new bone formation. It is usually positive in biopsy-confirmed cases of hematogenous osteomyelitis as early as 48 hours after the initiation of the bone infection. Negative ^{99m}Tc scans reported in documented osteomyelitis may relate to impaired blood supply in the infected area.

A second class of radiopharmaceuticals used for the evaluation of osteomyelitis includes gallium citrate and indium chloride. Gallium/indium attach to transferrin, which leaks from the bloodstream into areas of inflammation. Gallium/indium scans also show increased isotope uptake in areas concentrating polymorphonuclear leukocytes, macrophages, and malignant tumors. Because these scans do not show bone detail well, it is often difficult to distinguish between bone and soft tissue inflammation; a comparison with a ^{99m}Tc scan helps resolve this problem. In contrast to gallium citrate, indium chloride is more heavily concentrated by hematopoietic tissue. When first evaluating a suspected case of osteomyelitis, x-ray studies, technetium bone scans, and gallium or indium scans are selectively ordered to assist in the diagnosis, assess the extent of involvement, and guide the site selection for the bone biopsy.

Indium-labeled leukocyte scans are less useful in the evaluation of osteomyelitis. Indium leukocyte scans are positive in about 40% of patients with acute osteomyelitis and 60% of patients with septic arthritis. Patients who had chronic osteomyelitis, bony metastases, and degenerative arthritis often have negative scans.

Computed tomography (CT) may have a role to play in the diagnosis of osteomyelitis. Increased marrow density occurs early in the infection, and intramedullary gas has been reported in patients with hematogenous osteomyelitis. The CT scan is also useful to help identify areas of necrotic bone and to assess the involvement of the surrounding soft tissues. In a recalcitrant infection, the CT scan may identify the surgical approach and augment a thorough debridement. One disadvantage of this study is the scatter phenomenon that occurs when metal is present in or near the area of bone infection. The scatter results in a significant loss of image resolution.

Magnetic resonance imaging (MRI) is a useful modality for differentiating between bone and soft tissue infection. Initial MRI screening usually consists of a T_1-weighted and a T_2-weighted spin-echo pulse sequence. In a T_1-weighted study tissue edema is dark and fat is bright. In a T_2-weighted study the reverse is true. The typical appearance of osteomyelitis is a localized area of abnormal marrow with decreased signal intensity on T_1-weighted images and increased signal intensity on T_2-weighted images. On occasion there may be decreased signal intensity on T_2-weighted images. Post-traumatic and surgical scarring of the bone marrow show a region of decreased signal intensity on T_1-weighted images with no change on the T_2-weighted image. Sinus tracts are seen as areas of high signal intensity on the T_2-weighted image extending from the marrow and bone through the soft tissues and skin. Differentiation of infection from neoplasm on the basis of the MRI may be difficult; therefore, clinical and radiographic correlation is mandatory. Metallic implants in the region of interest may produce focal artifacts decreasing the utility of the image.

Sedimentation rates and leukocyte counts are frequently elevated before therapy in the acute disease. The white blood cell count rarely exceeds 15,000/mm^3. The leukocyte count is usually normal in patients with chronic osteomyelitis. The sedimentation rates and leukocyte counts may fall with appropriate therapy; however, both values may elevate contemporaneously around each debridement surgery. A sedimentation rate that returns to normal during the course of therapy is a favorable prognostic sign. This laboratory determination, however, is not reliable in the compromised host, as these patients are constantly challenged by minor illnesses and peripheral lesions that may elevate this index.

The diagnosis of vertebral osteomyelitis relies on the isolation of a causative organism from the infected vertebral body, disk space, paravertebral abscess, or blood. A closed biopsy for culture and histology may be performed under fluoroscopy or CT guidance. An open biopsy is indicated when a closed biopsy carries a high risk of possible complications. Tissue must be sent both for cultures and histologic confirmation as the differential diagnosis includes metastatic or primary tumors, mycoses, and tuberculosis. The earliest radiographic change is a subtle rarefaction of the vertebral end plate. Narrowing of the adjacent joint and involvement of the vertebral body occur later in the course of the disease.

The technetium scan is useful in vertebral infection and is usually positive in biopsy-confirmed cases of axial osteomyelitis. The gallium/indium scans are difficult to interpret because of the high concentrations of hematopoietic tissue in the vertebral bodies. CT and MRI are used to assess the extent of vertebral, paravertebral, and soft tissue involvement.

THERAPY

Acute hematogenous osteomyelitis

Acute long bone hematogenous osteomyelitis is primarily a medical disease in children. In the adult, debridement surgery and/or incision and drainage of soft tissue abscesses are often required. Identification of the causative pathogen is essential. The infection is usually susceptible to specific antimicrobial therapy (Chapter 224). Mismanagement with inappropriate antibiotic(s) encourages disease extension, sequestra formation, and the development of a refractory infection. Surgical intervention is indicated if the patient has not responded to specific antimicrobial therapy within 48 hours, has evidence of a persistent soft tissue abscess, or joint sepsis is diagnosed or suspected. The first step is to obtain appropriate culture material. A bone biopsy is necessary unless the patient has positive blood cultures along with x-ray studies or bone scan findings consistent with osteomyelitis. After cultures are obtained, a parenteral antimicrobial regimen is initiated to cover the clinically suspected pathogens. Once the organism is obtained, the antibacterial activity of different antibiotic classes can be determined by appropriate sensitivity methods. The disk diffusion method is often a sufficient guideline for antibiotic therapy. However, quantitative antibiotic sensitivity testing by the macrodilution or microdilution techniques on all aerobic bone isolates is a prerequisite to determine the minimum concentration of the antibiotic to inhibit (minimum inhibitory concentration [MIC]) and kill (minimum bactericidal concentration [MBC]) the pathogenic organism(s). It is best to choose an antibiotic or antibiotic combination that has a low MIC/MBC ratio relative to its expected serum concentration. The antibiotic regimen may be continued or changed on the basis of sensitivity results. The patient is treated for 4 to 6 weeks with appropriate parenteral antimicrobial therapy dated from the initiation of therapy or after the last major debridement surgery. The goal of the therapy is to prevent a refractory infection. If the initial medical management fails and the patient is clinically compromised by a recurrent infection, medullary and/or soft tissue debridement will be necessary in conjunction with another course of antibiotics.

Occasionally, oral antibiotic therapy can be used for treatment of childhood osteomyelitis. However, it is recommended that the patient first receive 2 weeks of parenteral antibiotic therapy before changing to an oral regimen. In addition, the patient must be compliant and agree to close outpatient follow-up. Absorption and activity of the orally administered antibiotic should be monitored by the measurement of the serum bactericidal activity against the causative pathogen. A peak bactericidal dilution of at least 1:8 or greater should be present and maintained. Oral therapy is possible in pediatric hematogenous osteomyelitis because of an increased bone blood flow and the aggressive mesenchymal and immunologic responses found in this age group. Pediatric patients cannot be given oral antimicrobial therapy with the quinolone class of antibiotics.

Vertebral osteomyelitis

The therapy of vertebral osteomyelitis requires parenteral antibiotics and may include early surgery and stabilization. The choice of an antibiotic is guided by the biopsy or debridement culture results. The antibiotic is given for 4 to 6 weeks and is usually dated from the initiation of therapy or from the last major debridement surgery. The indications for surgery are the same as for all other hematogenous infections of bone: failure of medical management, soft tissue abscess formation, and an impending instability. The neurologic status of the patient must be closely monitored at frequent intervals. Fusion of adjacent infected vertebral bodies is a major goal of therapy. The decision to advise an orthosis as opposed to internal fixation or bed rest is best individualized. The failure rate with bed rest alone is not statistically different from that of patients stabilized with a cast, corset, or brace.

The therapy of vertebral osteomyelitis has improved over the years. The current mortality rate is approximately 5%. Nearly 90% of patients treated for vertebral osteomyelitis recover uneventfully. About 6% have permanent neurologic defects.

Osteomyelitis secondary to contiguous focus infection or chronic osteomyelitis

These types of osteomyelitis share the common denominators of infected necrotic bone and poorly perfused soft tissue enveloping the bone. Adequate drainage, thorough debridement, obliteration of dead space, wound protection, and specific antimicrobial coverage are the mainstays of therapy. After the diagnostic evaluation, a bone biopsy is performed. Aerobic and anaerobic cultures are taken from these bone samples. The patient receives antibiotics only after the results of the cultures and their sensitivities are known. If immediate debridement surgery is required, however, the patient may receive antibiotics to cover the clinically suspected pathogens before the bacteriologic data are reported. These antibiotics may be modified, if necessary, when results of the debridement cultures and sensitivities are determined.

When possible, debridement surgery is performed after specific antibiotic therapy has begun. Antimicrobial therapy initiated before surgery decreases the risk of bacteremia at surgery, helps marginate the wound, and produces more supple soft tissues at the time of surgery. Surgical exposure is direct and atraumatic and is designed to avoid unnecessary devitalization of bone and soft tissue. If necessary, the wound is debrided every 48 to 72 hours until all nonviable tissue and superfluous hardware have been removed. The cortical and cancellous bone remaining in the wound after debridement surgery must bleed uniformly to ensure antibiotic perfusion and avoid continued sequestration.

Appropriate management of the dead space created by debridement surgery is mandatory to arrest the disease and maintain the integrity of the skeletal part involved. The goal of dead space management is to replace dead bone and scar with durable vascularized tissue. For this reason, secondary infection healing is discouraged because the scar tissue that fills the defect may later become avascular. Suction irrigation systems are now rarely used because of the high incidence of associated nosocomial infections and the unreliability of these setups. Complete wound closure should be attained whenever possible. Local tissue flaps or free flaps may be used to fill dead space. Cancellous bone grafts may be placed beneath local or transferred tissues when structural augmentation is necessary. Careful preoperative planning is crucial to make efficient use of the patient's limited cancellous bone reserves. Open cancellous grafts without soft tissue coverage are useful when a free tissue transfer is not a treatment option and local tissue flaps are inadequate. Finally, if motion is present at the site of infection, measures must be taken to achieve permanent stability of the skeletal unit. Antibiotic-impregnated acrylic beads are occasionally used to sterilize and temporarily maintain a dead space. The beads are usually removed within 2 to 4 weeks and replaced with a cancellous bone graft. The evolution of local antibiotic therapy is rapidly taking place.

Most recently, bone reconstruction of segmental defects and difficult infected nonunions has been accomplished using the Ilizarov external fixation method. This method uses distraction or compression histogeneses, a process of bone regeneration to fill bone defects or to compress nonunions and correct malunions. In one clinical series, 92% were of patients with chronic osteomyelitis with segmental defects, ranging from simple nonunions to 8-cm gaps, that were successfully reconstructed. The technique is labor intensive and required a long period of treatment (average of 8.5 months in the device).

Antibiotics are used to treat live infected bone and to protect bone undergoing revascularization, as it takes bone 3 to 4 weeks to revascularize after debridement surgery. The patient is treated with 4 to 6 weeks of parenteral antimicrobial therapy usually dated from the last major debridement surgery; however, the length of antibiotic administration for osteomyelitis remains controversial. Outpatient intravenous therapy is now possible and feasible. The long-term intravenous access catheters make outpatient intravenous treatment possible and decrease hospitalization time. A responsible patient or visiting nurse can be taught to administer the antibiotic at home using the implanted catheter. Outpatient intramuscular antibiotic administration is also feasible. Oral therapy using the quinolone class of antibiotics is currently being evaluated in adult patients with osteomyelitis. Effective oral therapy would make the treatment of adult osteomyelitis less cumbersome and expensive for the patient.

Osteomyelitis secondary to contiguous focus infection with vascular disease

Osteomyelitis associated with vascular insufficiency is difficult to treat due to the relative inability of the host to participate in the eradication of the infection process. As these infections are insidious, they are often beyond simple salvage by the time the patient seeks medical therapy.

The determination of the vascular status of the tissue at the infection site is crucial in the evaluation of these patients. Several methods are used to determine the vascular status. The measurement of cutaneous oxygen tensions and pulse pressures, however, are most commonly used. Cutaneous oxygen tensions are obtained by a modified Clark electrode, which is applied to the skin surface. Cutaneous oxygen tensions provide guidelines for determining the location of adequate tissue perfusion. The values also aid in the assessment of whether local debridement surgery can be performed and in selecting surgical margins where wound healing can be expected to occur. Hyperbaric oxygen therapy may allow healing in areas where marginal tensions are present.

The patient may be managed by suppressive antibiotic therapy, local debridement surgery, or ablative surgery. Judgment regarding which type of treatment to offer the patient depends on tissue oxygen perfusion at the infection site, extent of the osteomyelitis, and the preference of the patient.

The patient may be given long-term suppressive therapy when a definitive surgical procedure would lead to unacceptable patient morbidity or disability, or when the patient refuses local debridement or ablative surgery. Even with suppressive antibiotic therapy, in time, most of these patients will require ablative surgery.

Local debridement surgery and a 4-week course of antibiotics may be used in the patient who has localized osteomyelitis and good tissue oxygen perfusion. If these criteria are not present, the wound will fail to heal and ultimately an ablative procedure will be necessary.

The patient with extensive osteomyelitis and poor tissue oxygen perfusion usually requires some type of ablative surgery. Digital and ray resections, transmetatarsal amputations, midfoot disarticulations, and Syme's amputations allow the patient to ambulate without a prosthesis. The amputation level is determined by the vascular status of the tissues proximal to the site of infection and the requirements of a thorough debridement. The patient is given 4 weeks of antibiotics when infected bone is surgically transected. Antibiotics are given for 2 weeks when the infected bone is completely removed, but some residual soft tissue infection remains. When the amputation if performed proximal to the bone and soft tissue infection, the patient is given standard prophylaxis.

STAGING OF OSTEOMYELITIS

Four major factors influence the treatment and prognosis of osteomyelitis: (1) the degree of necrosis, (2) the condition of the host, (3) the site and extent of involvement, and (4) the disabling effects of the disease itself. These factors must be considered when assessing treatment results and efficacy of treatment alternatives.

The current classification of hematogenous and contiguous focus osteomyelitis with or without generalized vascular insufficiency is vague and does not adequately define the anatomic nature of the disease, take into account the quality of the host, determine treatment, or identify prognostic factors. Cierny and Mader have developed an alternate classification, which includes these factors (see accompanying box). In this approach the infection and host are staged using four anatomic types and three physiologic classes. The paradigm is determined by the status of the disease process regardless of its etiology or regionality. The anatomic types of osteomyelitis are medullary, superficial, localized, and diffuse. Medullary osteomyelitis denotes infection confined to the intramedullary surfaces of the bone. Hematogenous osteomyelitis and infected intramedullary rods are examples of this anatomic type. Superficial osteomyelitis, a true contiguous focus infection of bone, occurs when an exposed infected necrotic surface of bone lies at the base of a soft tissue wound. Localized osteomyelitis is usually characterized by a full-thickness, cortical sequestration, which can be removed surgically without compromising bony stability, whereas diffuse osteomyelitis is a through-and-through process that usually requires an intercalary resection of the bone for cure. Diffuse osteomyelitis includes those infections with a loss of bony stability either before or after debridement surgery.

The patient is classified as an A, B, or C host. An A host represents a patient with normal physiologic, metabolic, and immunologic capabilities. The B host (Table 237-1) is either systemically compromised, locally compromised, or both. When the morbidity of treatment is worse than that imposed by the disease itself, the patient is given the C host classification. The terms *acute* and *chronic osteomyelitis* are not used in this staging system, as areas of macronecrosis must be removed regardless of the acuity or chronicity of the infection. The stages are dynamic and interact according to the pathophysiology of the disease; they may be altered by successful therapy, host alteration, or treatment. This staging system provides a framework for describing and developing experimental models of osteomyelitis, planning medical and surgical treatments, and comparing the results of therapy among institutions.

Cierny and Mader classification of osteomyelitis

Anatomic type

Stage 1-	Medullary osteomyelitis
Stage 2-	Superficial osteomyelitis
Stage 3-	Localized osteomyelitis
Stage 4-	Diffuse osteomyelitis

Physiologic class

A Host-	Normal host
B Host-	Systemic compromise (Bs) Local compromise (B1)
C Host-	Treatment worse than the disease

Systemic or local factors that affect immune surveillance, metabolism, and local vascularity

Systemic (Bs)	Local (B1)
Malnutrition	Chronic lymphedema
Renal, liver failure	Venous stasis
Diabetes mellitus	Major vessel compromise
Chronic hypoxia	Arteritis
Immune disease	Extensive scarring
Malignancy	Radiation fibrosis
Extremes of age	Small vessel disease
Immunosuppression or immune deficiency	Complete loss of local sensation
Tobacco abuse	

SKELETAL TUBERCULOSIS

Skeletal tuberculosis is the result of hematogenous spread of *Mycobacterium tuberculosis* early in the course of a primary infection (Chapter 276). In rare instances, skeletal tuberculosis may result from the contiguous spread of infection from a caseating lymph node or from direct inoculation. A primary or recurrent bone infection initially elicits an acute inflammatory reaction that gradually matures to an indolent, granulomatous process. Bony sequestration is not uncommon. Cartilage and bone are destroyed slowly by granulation tissue. Thus articular cartilages are retained and recognizable both clinically and radiographically late in the disease process. The symptoms are usually related to biomechanical alterations in articular function, fractures, or the sequela of extraosseous extension of the infection.

Any bone may be involved in skeletal tuberculosis; however, the infection is usually monostotic. In children and adolescents the metaphyses of the long bones are the most frequently infected sites as in any pyogenic infection. In the adult, axial skeleton involvement is most common, followed in frequency by the proximal femur, knee, and small bones of the hands and feet. A vertebral infection usually begins in the anterior portion of a vertebral body adjacent to an intervertebral disk in a thoracic vertebral body. The lumbar and cervical vertebrae are less commonly involved. Adjacent vertebral bodies may become infected and a soft tissue abscess may develop. Fifty percent of the patients with skeletal tuberculosis have evidence of extraosseous infection.

Tissue for culture and histology is almost always required for the diagnosis of skeletal tuberculosis. Cultures for tuberculosis are positive in approximately 80% of the cases, but 6 weeks may be required for growth and identification of the organism. Histology showing granulomatous tissue compatible with tuberculosis and a positive tuberculin skin test is sufficient evidence to begin tuberculosis therapy. However, a negative skin test does not rule out skeletal tuberculosis. Therapy involves prolonged chemotherapy and in some cases surgical debridement surgery and/or stabilization.

FUNGAL OSTEOMYELITIS

Bone infections may be caused by a variety of fungal organisms, including coccidioidomycosis, blastomycosis, cryptococcus, histoplasmosis, and sporotrichosis (Chapters 277 and 279). The most common presentation is a cold abscess overlying an osteolytic lesion. Joint extension occurs most frequently in coccidioidomycosis and blastomycosis. Therapy for fungal osteomyelitis involves surgical debridement and antifungal chemotherapy.

REFERENCES

Cierny G and Mader JT: Adult chronic osteomyelitis, Orthopedics 7:1557, 1984.

Cierny G, Mader JT, and Penninck JJ. A clinical staging system of adult osteomyelitis. Contemp Orthopedics 10:17, 1985.

Calhoun JH, Anger DM, and Mader JT: The Ilizarov technique in the treatment of osteomyelitis, Tex Med 87:56, 1991.

Calhoun JH and Mader JT: Osteomyelitis of the diabetic foot. In Fryberg RG, editor: The high risk foot in diabetes mellitus, New York, 1991, Churchill Livingstone.

Davidson PT and Horowitz I: Skeletal tuberculosis. A review with patient presentations and discussion, Am J Med 48:77, 1970.

Sapico FL and Montgomerie JZ: Pyogenic vertebral osteomyelitis: report of nine cases and review of the literature, Rev Infect Dis 1:754, 1979.

Waldvogel FA, Medoff G, and Swartz MM: Osteomyelitis: a review of clinical features, therapeutic considerations, and unusual aspects, N Engl J Med 282:198, 260, 316, 1970.

CHAPTER

238 Sexually Transmitted Diseases (Urethritis, Vaginitis, Cervicitis, Proctitis, Genital Lesions)

Michael F. Rein

EPIDEMIOLOGY

A variety of microorganisms can be transmitted during sexual contact (see accompanying box). They differ markedly in their taxonomy, virulence factors, growth requirements, and response to therapy. They are grouped together because sexual transmission plays an important role in their overall epidemiology. None of the sexually transmitted diseases (STD) is acquired solely via coitus. In some cases (e.g., shigellosis and candidiasis), sexual transmission plays a relatively minor role, although for other conditions, such as infection with *Chlamydia trachomatis,* sexual transmission is the major route of acquisition in the United States.

Recognizing a disease as sexually transmitted has several practical consequences for the clinician. It allows one to identify a population at very high risk for the same infection, specifically the sexual partners of the infected patient. Rough estimates of the prevalence of infection among sexual partners of patients with sexually transmitted diseases are listed in Table 238-1. The figures are averages and do not reflect the risk of acquiring a STD from a single exposure to an infected sexual partner. Some sexual partners will have been exposed but once, and these people are at considerably lower risk of infection than are those who have had frequent contact with the infected patient. In most cases, the rates of infection among sexual partners are so high that, when identified as such, they are immediately treated for the infection even before the diagnosis has been confirmed. The rationale for such "epidemiologic treatment" is that complications may develop in these patients,

Table 238-1. Prevalence of infection among sexual partners of heterosexual patients with sexually transmitted diseases

Type of infection in index patient	Percentage of consorts infected	
	Male	Female
Gonorrhea	60 (40-90)	60 (37-92)
Syphilis	30-50	30-50
Chlamydia trachomatis	30	60-75
Trichomoniasis	30-70	90
Herpes genitalis	75	75
Venereal warts	60	60
Donovanosis	0.4-60.0	0.4-60.0

Sexually transmitted microbial pathogens

Viruses
- Herpes simplex
- Cytomegalovirus
- Molluscum contagiosum (poxvirus)
- Wart virus (papillomavirus)
- Epstein-Barr
- Hepatitis A, B, C*
- Human immunodeficiency virus (HIV)

Mycoplasmas
- *Mycoplasma hominis*
- *Ureaplasma urealyticum**
- *Mycoplasma genitalium*

Bacteria
- *Neisseria gonorrhoeae**
- *Neisseria meningitidis*
- *Treponema pallidum**
- *Haemophilus ducreyi**
- Shigellae
- Group B streptococci?
- *Gardnerella vaginalis*
- Salmonellae?
- *Listeria monocytogenes?*
- *Calymmatobacterium granulomatis**
- *Campylobacter fetus*

Chlamydiae
- *Chlamydia trachomatis**

Fungi
- *Candida* species

Endoparasites
- *Entamoeba histolytica**
- *Trichomonas vaginalis**
- *Giardia lamblia**

Ectoparasites
- *Phthirus pubis**
- *Sarcoptes scabiei**

*Epidemiologic treatment is appropriate

or they may further transmit the infection while awaiting the results of confirmatory laboratory tests. In this setting, the risks of antibiotic administration are outweighed by the risks of waiting to confirm the diagnosis. Epidemiologic treatment is a cornerstone of control of many STDs (see box).

Failure to treat sexual partners simultaneously for many of these infections may permit them to reinfect each other sequentially, resulting in so-called ping-pong infection. Apparent relapse or treatment failure often results from one sexual partner's remaining untreated. Sympathetic, nonjudgmental questioning about sexual partners and practices may yield information about an untreated sexual partner that is essential to eradicating the disease in a patient.

The STDs are largely diseases of life-style, and their incidence is higher among patients with multiple sexual partners. As a consequence, the coexistence of many STDs is prevalent in groups with high levels of sexual activity. Patients whose patterns of sexual behavior predispose them to one STD predispose them to others. Thus multiple venereal infections are common. Faced with the diagnosis of a single sexually transmitted infection in a patient, the clinician should carefully rule out others. Patients with any sexually transmitted disease should be considered at increased risk for infection with human immunodeficiency virus (HIV) and should be offered antibody testing (Chapters 242 and 252).

Infections dependent on sexual contact for their transmission occupy their epidemiologic niche for a number of reasons. In general, the organisms do not survive well in the environment, and transmission by fomites is rare. Additionally, the organisms tend to have somewhat restricted anatomic range. Cornified squamous epithelium is, for example, resistant to primary infection with *Neisseria gonorrhoeae* or *C. trachomatis,* organisms that can infect the epithelium of the urethra, endocervix, pharynx, rectum, and conjunctiva. *Trichomonas vaginalis* can infect only the urogenital tract. Organisms must be inoculated into these sites to produce disease. The lesions or discharges that characterize most STDs and that contain the highest concentration of organisms tend to occur on the genitalia. Transmission of these infections therefore requires intimate contact of susceptible epithelia with anatomic sites containing relatively larger numbers of fresh organisms.

Sexually transmitted diseases generally enter into the differential diagnosis of signs and symptoms affecting the genitalia. The primary lesions of STDs may, however, also affect the mouth, eye, and rectum, and disseminated infection may involve distant sites.

DIAGNOSIS

History

The patient should be asked about the onset and progression of symptoms, with specific emphasis on skin lesions, discharges, and discomfort. Association of symptoms with the menstrual period and sexual activity should be investigated, and specific details of the methods of contraception and recent antibiotic use should be obtained. It is helpful to ask whether the patient has a specific reason to suspect an STD. An estimate of the incubation period may be obtained by determining the patient's last sexual contact or last contact with a new partner. It is important not to assume that patients are heterosexual. The history should be taken referring to sexual partners in gender-neutral terms until the sexual preference of the patient has been established. Sympathetic questioning with regard to the sex of partners and the orifices used for sexual contact is essential to the management of patients with STD.

Physical examination

Male genitalia are best examined with the patient standing in front of the seated examiner. The entire genital area should be evaluated, noting inguinal adenopathy and skin lesions involving the pubis, thighs, and buttocks. The penis should be examined for skin lesions, and one should note the presence of perimeatal erythema, which can suggest urethritis, and the quantity and character of urethral discharge. The patient's underwear may reveal staining and give an indication of the amount of discharge, particularly in a patient who has urinated shortly before examination; recent micturition can eliminate much inflammatory discharge. If no urethral discharge is spontaneously present, the urethra should be gently stripped. This is best accomplished by grasping the penis firmly between the thumb and forefinger with the thumb pressing on the ventral surface. The examiner's hand is then moved distally, compressing the urethra. This maneuver will express small amounts of discharge. The urethral meatus can be gently spread, and the degree of erythema of the urethra can be estimated. If no urethral discharge is expressed, a calcium-alginate urethral (or nasopharyngeal) swab should be inserted at least 2 cm into the urethra. The use of cotton-tipped swabs is contraindicated because their large size makes insertion extremely uncomfortable, and the cotton fibers may inhibit the growth of certain fastidious organisms. Scrotal contents should be palpated for masses or tenderness. In men practicing receptive anal intercourse, the anus and perianal skin should be carefully examined. Anoscopy is a helpful addition to the diagnostic work-up in selected patients.

The female genitalia are best examined with the patient in the lithotomy position. Lesions around the labia are sought, and labial edema, erythema, or excoriation is noted. The labia minora are spread and the urethral orifice examined. Periurethral erythema suggests urethritis. Urethral discharge can be expressed by gently stripping the urethra with the forefinger inserted into the vagina. The examiner should attempt to palpate Bartholin's glands in the labia minora; they should be neither palpable nor tender. Any discharge expressible from the orifices of these glands should be carefully examined.

A vaginal speculum is then inserted using warm water as the only lubricant, as jelly contains antibacterial substances that can interfere with the recovery of fastidious pathogens. The cervix should be visualized and cervicitis or cervical discharge noted. The vaginal walls are also examined for erythema, punctate hemorrhages, or tiny ulcerations. The character (e.g., color, adherence, frothiness) and amount of vaginal discharge should be noted. Endocervical specimens are obtained by inserting a swab into the endocervix. Vaginal specimens are obtained by sweeping a swab through the anterior and posterior vaginal fornices. After obtaining all suitable specimens for cultures and microscopic examination, the speculum is removed, and discharge collected in the blade is examined as described in the next section. A bimanual examination is conducted. Specific attention should be directed to tenderness in the adnexae or discomfort on cervical traction. The vaginally contaminated finger should not be inserted into the rectum; the examiner should change gloves between the vaginal and rectal examinations. Rectal mucosa is susceptible to infection with a variety of sexually transmitted pathogens, and it is possible that these organisms could be transmitted from the vagina to the rectum on the examiner's glove. Inguinal adenopathy and lesions of the pubic area, thighs, and buttocks should be sought in patients of either sex.

Laboratory examinations

Urethral discharge should be applied to a microscope slide by rolling the swab across the slide. This material should be Gram stained and examined with the oil immersion objective. Squamous epithelial cells from the distal portion of the urethra will be seen, and cuboidal epithelial cells will be observed if the specimen has been obtained by inserting a swab into the urethra. The distal portion of the urethra is colonized by skin flora (i.e., a variety of gram-positive and gram-negative organisms), but they have no specific diagnostic significance. The presence of polymorphonuclear neutrophils (PMNs) is abnormal. Although a strong association between the presence of five PMNs per oil immersion field and acute urethritis has been suggested, many patients with urethritis may display fewer PMNs, particularly if they have urinated shortly before the examination. The slide should be carefully scanned for gram-negative cell-associated diplococci, which will confirm a diagnosis of gonorrhea in 95% of infected, symptomatic men (Chapter 264).

Endocervical discharge collected on a cotton swab should be examined against a white background. A yellow or green tinge suggests mucopurulent cervicitis. The swab is then rolled over an area of 2 cm^2 on a microscope slide and Gram stained. PMNs are normally found in the endocervical mucus, but they should arouse suspicion of mucopurulent cervicitis if present in sheets. Vaginal flora always contaminates the endocervical specimen, and rigid criteria must be applied to the diagnosis of gonorrhea on the basis of an endocervical smear. The smear will be positive in only 50% of infected women.

The pH of vaginal discharge should be assessed by inserting a piece of indicator paper in the discharge that has pooled in the speculum. We have found nitrazine paper useful because it has a pH range of 4.5 to 7.0. The normal vaginal pH is 4.5, and this pH is preserved in vulvovaginal candidiasis. On the other hand, an elevated vaginal pH is associated with trichomoniasis or bacterial vaginosis. The apparent pH can be artifactually elevated by contamination with cervical discharge or semen.

After testing the pH, one should add one or two drops of 10% potassium hydroxide (KOH) to the discharge. The preparation is then examined for the presence of a pungent, fishy, aminelike odor. This odor constitutes a positive whiff test and suggests trichomoniasis or bacterial vaginosis. The whiff test is negative in candidiasis.

Vaginal discharge should be examined as a wet mount, which may be prepared by agitating the swab carrying vaginal discharge in a test tube containing a small amount of normal saline. A drop of this material is then transferred to the microscope slide, a coverglass is applied, and the preparation is examined at 100× and 400×, with the substage condenser racked down to increase contrast; vaginal squamous epithelial cells are transparent, and their edges are sharp and easily discerned. The presence of large numbers of coccobacilli adhering to the surface of these cells (clue cells) and obscuring their edges suggests bacterial vaginosis. The presence of approximately one polymorphonuclear leukocyte per epithelial cell is normal; increased numbers are distinctly unusual in bacterial vaginosis but are seen with some other forms of vaginitis and with cervicitis. The appearance of an excessive number of PMNs in a specimen containing clue cells should suggest a second process.

The normal flora consists of large rods. In bacterial vaginosis the flora consists primarily of sheets and clumps of coccobacilli. Motile trichomonads are approximately the size of a PMN, are most easily recognized by their characteristic twitching motility, and are seen in about 70% of infected women. Spermatozoa may be seen up to 10 days after the last sexual contact; motile spermatozoa suggest coitus within 24 hours. *Candida* organisms are recognized as budding, ovoid yeasts or as elongated pseudohyphae.

A KOH preparation is prepared by combining a drop of the wet-mount suspension with a drop of 10% KOH, applying a coverslip, and gently warming before microscopic examination. All cellular elements except bacteria and fungi are destroyed. The KOH preparation is more sensitive and more specific than the wet mount for the diagnosis of candidiasis but obviously cannot be used to diagnose other genital infections. Vaginal discharge can be examined with Gram stain, and bacterial vaginosis can be diagnosed therefrom, but *Candida* and trichomonads are best recognized on the wet-mount preparation.

A Gram stain from the rectal mucosa will reveal large numbers of bacteria; gonococci can be identified in about 50% of rectal infections. The sensitivity can be increased by taking the specimen through an anoscope, recovering flecks of mucus or mucopus for microscopic examination.

Material from lesions can be examined with the Tzanck preparation for multinucleated giant cells, which is diagnostic of herpesvirus infection (Chapter 251) or by dark-field microscopy for the spirochete of syphilis (Chapter 273).

Cultures for *N. gonorrhoeae* should be taken from the urethra of men, from the endocervix and possibly from the rectum in women, and from any mucosal surface used for sexual contact. Thus the throat and rectum should be cultured in homosexual men who have participated in receptive oral or anal intercourse. Vaginal discharge can be cultured for *Candida, Trichomonas,* and *Gardnerella vaginalis* (previously called *Haemophilus vaginalis;* an agent of bacterial vaginosis) on appropriate media. In special circumstances, cultures can be taken for herpes simplex or for *C. trachomatis,* although these organisms can be recovered only with tissue culture techniques.

C. trachomatis can be recovered from the urethra, endocervix, or other sites by tissue culture (Chapter 254). Direct fluorescence microscopy with monoclonal antibodies, ELISA, and DNA probes have been used to identify *C. trachomatis* in genital smears with high accuracy, rapid turnaround time, and low cost compared to culture (Chapter 254).

SPECIFIC CLINICAL SYNDROMES

Sexually transmitted diseases often enter into the differential diagnosis of specific syndromes associated with genital infections.

Urethritis

Patients with urethritis generally present with some combination of urethral discharge and dysuria (Table 238-2).

Gonococcal and nongonococcal urethritis. Gonorrhea accounts for approximately half of the urethritis seen in STD clinics but for as little as 10% of the acute urethritis seen in private practice and student health settings. Acute urethritis of any other etiology is referred to as nongonococcal urethritis (NGU). The clinical spectrum of gonorrhea differs from that of NGU (Table 238-2); unfortunately, there is sufficient clinical overlap that accurate differential diagnosis must be based on microscopic examination of the urethral specimen.

Shorter incubation periods tends to be associated with gonorrhea; longer incubation periods are more suggestive of NGU. The onset of symptoms in gonorrhea is often abrupt, whereas the symptoms of NGU are generally subacute. They may increase gradually over several days or may fluctuate, sometimes almost completely disappearing, only to reappear 2 to 3 days later. These stuttering symptoms often greatly prolong the time until patients seek medical care. Most men with gonorrhea seek attention within 2 to 3 days of the development of symptoms, whereas delays of more than a week are common with NGU. The symptoms of gonorrhea tend to be more severe than those of NGU, with almost three-fourths of the patients complaining of discharge and dysuria. Patients with NGU tend to complain of discharge or dysuria rather than both. Most commonly, patients present with dysuria and do not note the discharge, which is revealed on examination.

The discharge of acute gonococcal urethritis is usually purulent; a purulent discharge visible at the meatus on initial examination strongly suggests gonorrhea. The discharge of NGU may be equally purulent but is more likely to be mucoid or mucopurulent, that is, clear with purulent flecks. The discharge of NGU is usually not obvious until it is expressed from the urethra.

Even if untreated, the symptoms of urethritis will grad-

Table 238-2. Clinical features of acute gonococcal and nongonococcal urethritis

Clinical feature	Gonococcal	Nongonococcal
Incubation period	Shorter:	Longer:
	≤4 d 70%	≤4 d 40%
	≤2 wk 90%	2-3 wk ~30%
Onset of symptoms	Abrupt	Gradual, fluctuating
Discharge and dysuria	70%	40%
Discharge	Purulent	Mucoid or mucopurulent

ually subside over months. Untreated gonorrhea may progress to *gleet,* a chronic inflammatory condition characterized by very little dysuria and a mucoid discharge reminiscent of NGU.

The definitive diagnosis is made on the basis of a Gram stain of the urethral discharge. Gram-negative, cell-associated diplococci are seen in 95% of patients whose discharge will subsequently grow gonococci. Since the sensitivity of the culture is less than 100%, discrepancies between the Gram stain and the culture may indicate a failing of the culture rather than of the Gram stain. A patient with acute urethritis and a Gram stain suggestive of gonorrhea should be treated for that disease, whereas a patient with a Gram stain revealing PMNs but no gram-negative, cell-associated diplococci should be treated for NGU. An important shortcoming of the urethral Gram stain is its inability to detect coincident NGU in the presence of gonorrhea. Miscellaneous bacteria often observed on Gram stain represent the normal flora of the anterior urethra and are of no diagnostic significance.

Nongonococcal urethritis actually includes several different infections. *Chlamydia trachomatis* (Chapter 194) causes somewhat less than half of cases of NGU, and *Ureaplasma urealyticum* is responsible for some fraction of the remainder. From the practical standpoint, these two organisms account for more than 80% of cases of NGU and can be effectively treated with regimens consisting of tetracycline or macrolide antibiotics. Thus when a Gram stain of urethral discharge does not display gram-negative, cell-associated diplococci, the disease is probably caused by a tetracycline-sensitive infection. *Trichomonas vaginalis* is usually carried asymptomatically by men but may be responsible for 5% of cases of NGU. Syphilis, lymphogranuloma venereum, and occasionally herpes genitalis can cause urethral discharge. Urinary tract infection (UTI) in the presence of urethral stricture has also been associated with urethral discharge. All these conditions are rare.

Postgonococcal urethritis. *C. trachomatis* is not eradicated by the single doses of antimicrobials usually used to treat gonococcal urethritis. Because these agents are extremely prevalent in sexually active populations, men may acquire gonococci and chlamydiae from the same sexual exposure. Such patients initially respond to appropriate single-dose therapy, but a re-exacerbation of symptoms occurs in the absence of re-exposure. Treatment with a tetracycline eradicates the chlamydiae and cures the patient. Patients suffering a recurrence of urethral symptoms after treatment for gonorrhea, however, may be reinfected or may be true treatment failures. Thus a workup with a urethral Gram stain and culture is necessary in a patient presenting with a recrudescence of symptoms.

Asymptomatic urethral infections. The gonococcus and the agents of NGU can be carried asymptomatically. In about 3% of men acquiring gonococcal infection of the urethra, symptoms never develop. Because these men do not seek treatment, their number tends to grow. They are usually identified because of the development of the complications of gonorrhea or because the diagnosis is made in a sexual partner. Women whose gonorrhea is diagnosed because complications have developed or because a routine screening culture was positive are likely to have acquired the infection from an asymptomatic male. Up to 40% of the asymptomatic male sexual partners of such women are infected, and all the sexual partners of a patient with gonorrhea should receive medical attention. It has been shown that 5% of asymptomatic men in venereal disease clinics carry *C. trachomatis*. The asymptomatic male sexual partners of women known to have chlamydial infection should receive epidemiologic treatment. Asymptomatic carriers of *N. gonorrhoeae* or *C. trachomatis* may have small numbers of PMNs on Gram-stained smears of material recovered from urethral swabs. Trichomonal infestation of the urethra is usually asymptomatic.

Urethritis in women and the urethral syndrome. Dysuria in women may be a symptom of classic upper or lower urinary tract infection (UTI). Among sexually active women, however, it is a relatively nonspecific complaint and is actually more likely to result from vulvovaginitis than from UTI. Fifty percent of women with symptomatic UTI actually have levels of bacteriuria far lower than the traditional $10^5/mm^3$. Women with dysuria who do not have vaginitis or routine UTI have been said to have the urethral syndrome. Some of these women also have pyuria as defined by placing some uncentrifuged midstream urine in a hemacytometer and finding more than eight white blood cells per cubic millimeter. It is now clear that many of these symptomatic women with pyuria actually have sexually transmitted urethritis caused by *N. gonorrhoeae* or *C. trachomatis*. Women are generally unaware of urethral discharge, although it can sometimes be identified on physical examination. These same organisms are likely to cause coincident cervical infection, and detection of mucopurulent cervicitis on physical examination lends support to the diagnosis. Unless the sexually transmitted nature of these infections is recognized, asymptomatic male sexual partners of these women will not be treated, and frequent, frustrating recurrence of symptoms from reinfection will result. As chlamydial and gonococcal infection may well respond, at least initially, to regimens prescribed for UTI (e.g., quinolones, SMX/TMP, amoxycillin), the clinician should consider sexually transmitted disease in the patient with recurrent "culture negative" UTI. Even if the initial infection were, in fact, cured by the urinary tract regimen, recurrence could result from reinfection by an untreated sexual partner (Chapter 240).

Treatment of acute urethritis. Nongonococcal urethritis, which is most likely due to a tetracycline- or erythromycin-sensitive organism, should be treated orally with doxycycline, 100 mg twice a day or erythromycin, 500 mg four a day, either for 7 days. Urethritis or cervicitis that is known to be chlamydial can also be treated with a single, 1 g, oral dose of azithromycin (the only single-dose regimen effective in this setting), or with ofloxacin, 300 mg orally, twice a day for 7 days. These regimens are currently far more expensive than the first two. The treatment of gonorrhea is discussed in Chapter 264. The tetracycline regimens once highly effective in gonorrhea are now associated with high failure rates in certain areas. Treatment for urethritis of unknown etiology should include a single dose effective for gonorrhea and a regimen active against the agents of NGU.

The patterns of recurrent NGU can be helpful in deciding on future therapy. Some patients have a prompt resolution of symptoms but note recurrence after sexual exposure. Such cases probably represent reinfection, and the patient can be retreated with the initial regimen. It is of course important to ensure that all sexual partners receive appropriate treatment. Other patients note an initial symptomatic response, but their symptoms return after discontinuation of therapy, even though they have not been re-exposed. Such patients are often successfully treated with longer courses of doxycycline (e.g., 100 mg twice a day for 4 weeks). Alternatively, one can use erythromycin in doses of 500 mg, four times daily for the same interval. A few patients note no response of symptoms to doxycycline. These patients are likely to be infected with a tetracycline-resistant organism, principally *T. vaginalis* or tetracycline-resistant *U. urealyticum*. Trichomoniasis is diagnosed with great difficulty in men, usually depending on the culture results rather than on direct microscopic examination. Trichomoniasis responds to metronidazole, 2 g as a single, oral dose and ureaplasmal infection to erythromycin, 500 mg orally four times a day for 7 days. Persistent relapses or treatment failures should prompt referral to a urologist.

Because up to 40% of men with acute gonococcal urethritis are also infected with *C. trachomatis,* gonorrhea might best be treated with a single dose of an appropriate drug (see Chapter 264) followed by a regimen of doxycycline, erythromycin, or azithromycin effective against chlamydia. Ofloxacin in a regimen of 300 mg orally, twice a day for 7 days will cure both chlamydial and gonococcal infection, but the cost is higher than those two drug regimens using doxycycline or erythromycin.

Other urethritides. Nongonococcal urethritis can accompany Stevens-Johnson syndrome and is a part of Reiter's syndrome. In both cases, the diagnosis is made on the basis of extragenital manifestations (Chapter 312). Many cases of Reiter's syndrome seem to follow urethral infection with *C. trachomatis* and probably represent a disordered immune response to the pathogen. Because of this association, patients with Reiter's syndrome should initially receive a course of doxycycline.

Cervicitis

Under the influence of estrogens, the vaginal epithelium cornifies and becomes resistant to several important sexually transmitted pathogens. Thus a number of venereal diseases involve the cervix while sparing the vagina. Acute cervicitis usually is manifested by an increased cervical discharge, mucoid or purulent, and inflammation around the cervical os.

Increased cervical discharge is seen in pregnancy, during the use of oral contraceptives, and in some patients wearing an intrauterine contraceptive device. The discharge is generally mucoid rather than purulent and does not contain abnormally large numbers of PMNs. Cervical erythema can result from the outgrowth of columnar epithelium onto the cervix. Such "erosion" is usually symmetric around the os.

Purulent or mucopurulent cervical discharge usually accompanies cervicitis of gonococcal or chlamydial origin. A Gram stain of the discharge reveals large numbers of PMNs and will reveal gram-negative, cell-associated diplococci in about 50% of women with gonorrhea; a negative Gram stain does not rule out gonococcal infection. The smear may be misleading because of the presence of other gram-negative diplococci in normal vaginal secretions.

Gonococci or chlamydiae are isolated from 60% to 90% of the sexual partners of men with gonococcal or chlamydial urethritis. Chlamydiae have been isolated from 50% to 90% of sexually active patients with a specific form of cervicitis characterized by erosion, congestion, edema, and hypertrophy about the cervical os. The lesion is generally intensely red, asymmetric about the os, and often friable, bleeding when it is abraded during the examination. A purulent cervical discharge usually accompanies this type of cervicitis. Women presenting with the syndrome of hypertrophic cervicitis (and their sexual partners) should be given a course of doxycycline. After adequate treatment, the hypertrophic cervicitis usually resolves to a simple cervicitis. About 50% of women with gonorrhea also have chlamydial infection, and women with gonococcal cervicitis should be treated with a double regimen as described for gonococcal urethritis.

Herpes simplex virus is recovered from the cervix of 80% of women with primary herpes genitalis and can cause an acute cervicitis that may not be associated with lesions of the external genitalia. The cervix may show discrete, grouped, or coalescent ulcerations; and there may be frank cervical necrosis. This type of cervicitis is often accompanied by a mucoid discharge.

Vulvovaginitis

Vulvovaginitis is a common clinical syndrome and is the most frequent cause of genital symptoms in women. Treatment should be based on a specific etiologic diagnosis, which can usually be made at the time of initial evaluation. Nonspecific local treatments, such as sulfanilamide or triple sulfa preparations are considerably less effective than specific therapies and have no role. Although the infectious vaginitides have different manifestations (Table 238-3), there is so much clinical overlap that initial evaluation must include bedside laboratory evaluation.

Candidiasis. *Candida albicans* causes most of the symptomatic vulvovaginitis in the United States (Chapter 277). The problem of diagnosing this infection is compounded by the fact that *Candida* can be isolated from approximately 50% of the vaginas of healthy, asymptomatic women. Thus its presence in an inflamed vagina does not prove that the organism is responsible for the disease. Broad-spectrum an-

Table 238-3. Vulvovaginitis

Clinical and laboratory finding	Trichomoniasis	Candidiasis	Bacterial vaginosis
Symptoms			
Pruritus	+++	+++	+
Discharge	+++	+	++
Odor	+	+	+++
Menses	Increased after	Increased before	Not related
Discharge	Thin, purulent	Thick, adherent	Thin, adherent
Froth	++		+
Color	White, yellow, green	White	Grayish white
pH	Elevated	4.5	Elevated
Whiff test	++		++++
Microscopy			
Flora	Rods or coccobacilli	Rods, yeasts, pseudohyphae	Coccobacilli
PMNs	+++	May be present	
Epithelial cells	Normal	Normal	Clue cells

tibiotics predispose to the development of vulvovaginal candidiasis by reducing the normal bacterial content of the vagina and allowing the yeasts to overgrow. The balance between bacteria and yeasts in the vagina is obviously under some hormonal influence. *Candida* organisms are carried more frequently by women on oral contraceptives, and these women have a higher incidence of candidal vulvovaginitis. The disease is also more common in diabetic patients and during pregnancy, and many women describe a recrudescence or exacerbation of symptoms in the immediate premenstrual period.

Patients with candidal vulvovaginitis generally complain of perivaginal pruritus and relatively little discharge. Dysuria is occasionally described. On examination, the labia minora may be pallid or erythematous. The vulva is often intensely red, and excoriation attests to the marked pruritus. Satellite lesions, tiny papulopustules located beyond the main erythematous border may be observed. The discharge is characteristically thick and adherent to the vaginal walls. On speculum examination, it often manifests curds resembling cottage cheese. Rarely, a thin discharge may be seen. Vaginal pH is normal, and the whiff test is negative. Wet mount and KOH examinations often but by no means always reveal budding yeasts and variable, often normal numbers of PMNs. The diagnosis of candidal vulvovaginitis is best based on a combination of clinical and microscopic findings, since up to 50% of infected, symptomatic women have negative microscopic examinations for yeasts. Culture may be useful in these cases.

The infection is usually treated by the local application of an antifungal drug. Commercial preparations of imidazole antifungals (miconazole, clotrimazole, butoconazole, terconazole) are the most effective agents. Seven-day, three-day, and single-dose regimens have been shown to be reasonably effective. Polyene drugs (nystatin) are also in common use. Treatment with a single oral dose of fluconazole, 200 mg, is also highly effective and may be useful in certain circumstances, such as when the patient suffers from concurrent herpetic infection, and topical preparations should be avoided. Recurrence is a major problem and should cause a search for risk factors that can be eliminated. Unnecessary use of antibiotics should be avoided, and switching to a lower dosage oral contraceptive may be useful. Sequential contraceptives may predispose the patient to recurrences less than do combination regimens. There is no good evidence that simultaneous treatment of a rectal focus with oral nystatin reduces the frequency of relapse.

Sexual transmission seems to contribute relatively little to the overall epidemiology of vulvovaginal candidiasis. In up to 10% of the sexual partners of infected women, however, a candidal balanitis may develop that is characterized by an intense erythema and pruritus of the glans. This condition appears to be sexually transmitted and responds to topical anticandidal medication.

Trichomoniasis. Estimates based on the amount of metronidazole sold in this country suggest that 3 million Americans are infected with *T. vaginalis* each year. This infection is almost always sexually transmitted, although trichomonads can survive for several hours on wet surfaces, and nonvenereal transmission probably occurs in certain rare instances. Affected women usually complain of pruritus and discharge, which may begin or be exacerbated during or immediately after the menstrual period. Dysuria is relatively common, and trichomonal involvement of the urinary tract is one of the causes of dysuria associated with negative cultures for routine pathogens.

On examination, the labia are often erythematous, and there may be a discharge present on the perineum. Through the speculum, the vaginal walls are seen to be erythematous, sometimes manifesting punctate hemorrhages, which give a granular appearance to the mucosa. The discharge is loose and collects in the posterior fornix. It is frothy in about 40% of cases. The diagnosis is best made by wet-mount examination of the discharge, which contains numerous PMNs and will reveal motile trichomonads in about

70% of cases. Of women coming to venereal disease clinics, 25% of those in whom trichomonads are isolated from the vagina will be asymptomatic. These women should be treated, however, because symptoms will develop in about half of them within the next 6 months, and they constitute an important reservoir of infection.

Treatment of trichomoniasis is with metronidazole, which can be administered as a single 2-g dose or in doses of 250 mg orally three times daily or 500 mg twice daily for 7 days. Metronidazole, like disulfiram, causes nausea, vomiting, and flushing if consumed with alcohol, and patients should be suitably cautioned. The drug is contraindicated in early pregnancy, and treatment of trichomoniasis in this setting is less than ideal. Clotrimazole, 100 mg intravaginally each night, may relieve symptoms and occasionally produces a cure. Just before delivery, infected women should be definitively treated with metronidazole to prevent possible spread of infection to the infant during the birth process. Trichomonads resistant to metronidazole are being recognized with increasing frequency. Infections with these organisms are very difficult to cure but are sometimes eradicated by a 2-week course of metronidazole, 2 g orally per day, along with 500 mg (broken tablet) intravaginally each night.

Trichomonads can be isolated from 30% to 70% of the male sexual partners of infected women. Most of these men are asymptomatic, but they should be treated as a public health measure and because the long-term effects of chronic trichomonal carriage are unknown.

Bacterial vaginosis. Affected women are sexually active and complain of a vaginal discharge that may be relatively scanty and, unlike that of trichomoniasis, is usually nonirritating. More so than with the other vaginitides, affected women complain of a vaginal odor that they often describe as "fishy." Symptoms bear little relation to the stage of the menstrual cycle, and there is very little vulvar inflammation. The discharge is loose but often adheres to the vaginal walls. There may be enough to pool in the posterior fornix, and it is often seen to contain small bubbles. If present in smaller amounts, it appears as increased moistness of the vaginal walls, often yielding a light reflex during examination. The vaginal pH is elevated, usually to 5.0 or higher, and the whiff test is positive. Microscopic examination of the discharge reveals clue cells, vaginal epithelial cells studded with tiny coccobacilli. These organisms often obscure the nucleus or the edges of the cells. Among the epithelial cells there are relatively few PMNs; the presence of large numbers of PMNs suggests a coincidental inflammatory process. The bacterial flora consists of sheets or clumps of weakly gram-negative coccobacilli.

The coccobacilli that are present in large numbers are *Gardnerella vaginalis* and are one component of a synergistic infection with vaginal anaerobes that produce the

Table 238-4. Differential diagnosis of genital lesions

Morphology	Number	Distribution	Surface	Base
Ulcers	?Single (55%) or multiple	Penis, labia, cervix	Clean	Indolent
	Single	Penis	Purulent	Inflamed
	Single	Penis, labia	Beefy red, granulation tissue	Friable
	Single	Penis, labia	Eroded papule	Benign
	Multiple	Penis, vulva, thigh, cervix, grouped	Clean	Clean, all same size
	Multiple (30%) or single (70%)	Penis, vulva, thigh	Necrotic	Variable size, ragged
Papules	Single	Penis, labia	Clean or small erosion	Benign
	Multiple	One or more rows behind corona	Clean	Benign
	Multiple	Penis, labia, vagina, often grouped	Verrucous	Benign
	Multiple	Penis, labia, pubic hair, thighs, buttocks	Umbilicated, with tiny plug	Benign
	Multiple	Disseminated, palms, soles	Coppery	Benign
	Multiple	Penis, labia, thighs, buttocks, wrists, and ankles	Crusted	
Vesicles	Multiple	Penis, labia, thighs, cervix, grouped	Umbilicated	Erythema
Crusts	Multiple	Grouped		Erythema
	Multiple	Disseminated		Erythema may be present
Erythema	Patches	Glans, shaft of penis, labia, vulva	Intense erythema	

amines responsible for the characteristic odor. Carriage of *G. vaginalis* alone does not produce clinical disease. The role of curved anaerobic rods such as *Mobiluncus curtisii* is a matter of current controversy and investigation.

Treatment of bacterial vaginosis consists of metronidazole, presumably active against vaginal anaerobes, in doses of 500 mg orally twice a day for 7 days. Recent work suggests that a single 2-g dose may be as effective. Pregnant women may be treated with clindamycin, 300 mg orally, twice a day for 7 days. Topical clindamycin and topical metronidazole are now available and are acceptably effective. Somewhat surprisingly, initial management of infected women need not involve treatment of male sexual partners. Some women with recurrent disease, however, can be cured only by simultaneous treatment of sexual partners.

Other specific infections. True vaginal infections with other specific agents, such as *Mycobacterium tuberculosis*, salmonellae, Enterobacteriaceae, staphylococci, and schistosomes are rare and usually occur in patients with underlying diseases who are systemically ill. Actinomycetes have been isolated from women wearing intrauterine devices and should be treated by removing the device. Pinworms are an occasional cause of perivaginal itching, especially in children, and this diagnosis may be suggested by perianal pruritus that becomes worse at night.

Pre-existing lesions due to other diseases may become secondarily infected with a mixed anaerobic flora. Such "fusospirochetal" infections are sometimes rapidly progressive and necrotizing.

Skin and mucous membrane lesions

The skin of the genital area is involved in many generalized dermatoses, but STDs are a frequent cause of genital lesions among adults. One can occasionally estimate the incubation period of STDs by obtaining a history of a single recent sexual contact or a recent contact with a new sexual partner. When available, an estimate of the incubation period can be helpful in the differential diagnosis of genital lesions (Table 238-4).

Recently, there has been an increase in the incidence of chancroid in the United States, but chancroid and lymphogranuloma venereum are still considerably more common in the Far East and Africa than in the United States. Donovanosis is endemic in India, New Guinea, the West Indies, and some parts of Africa and South America. It is now extremely rare in the United States. In these days of rapid intercontinental travel, recent sexual exposure in an endemic area can increase the probability of these otherwise rare diseases.

Medications occasionally produce a fixed drug eruption involving the genitalia, and broad-spectrum antibiotics may predispose to the development of candidiasis and may alter or completely eliminate the lesions of syphilis.

Although the typical syphilitic chancre (Plate V-36) is described as nontender, up to 30% of patients with primary

Edge	Pain	Adenopathy	Incubation period	Suggested diagnosis
Indurated	Mild (30%)	Moderate	<21 d (up to 90 d)	Syphilis
Ragged	Mild to severe	Mild or absent	<24 h	Human bite, other trauma
Serpiginous		Inguinal granulomas	1-12 wk	Donovanosis
Benign	Lesion often goes entirely unnoticed	Moderate, but usually appears after lesion resolves	2 wk	Lymphogranuloma venereum
Erythema	Severe: prodome of paresthesia	Moderate, tender	3-7 d, recurrent	Herpes genitalis
Undermined erythema	Moderate	Moderate, tender	2-5 d	Chancroid
Benign			2 wk	Early lymphogranuloma venereum
Benign				Pearly penile papules
Benign			3-30 wk	Venereal warts
Benign			2-26 wk	Molluscum contagiosum
Benign	Occasional, mild	Prominent	6-12 wk	Secondary syphilis
Linear tracks may be seen	Intense pruritus	Rare superinfected excoriation	4 wk	Scabies
	Mild	Moderate, tender	2-5 d	Herpes genitalis
	Mild	Mild	2-5 d	Healing herpes genitalis
	Pruritus	Mild or absent	4 wk	Scabies
Satellite lesions	Pruritus		Undefined	Candidiasis

syphilis describe either pain or tenderness of the lesions. Significant pain usually accompanies the lesions of chancroid, herpes genitalis, and tularemia.

Because lesions often change over time, a history of the initial manifestation may be crucial to making the diagnosis. Genital ulcerations that began as vesicles point to a diagnosis of herpes genitalis.

Morphologic characteristics of genital lesions. In many cases, the appearance of genital lesions will be sufficiently distinctive to permit accurate differential diagnosis without resorting to laboratory tests (see Table 238-4). Herpes genitalis and chancroid both produce painful genital ulcerations. Grouped clusters of vesicles or small ulcerations are characteristic of herpes genitalis. These lesions tend to be of approximately the same size and appear relatively clean; the ulcers of chancroid tend to vary in size and look ragged and necrotic. Herpes characteristically begins as umbilicated vesicles, although by the time the patient comes to the physician, all of these may have ruptured to form shallow ulcers. Recurrence is characteristic of herpes genitalis but not of chancroid. Patients with the former sometimes note a prodrome of local paresthesias preceding the eruption of vesicles by about 12 hours. Vesicles are not a manifestation of chancroid, and a history of vesicles can simplify the differential diagnosis. If the differential diagnosis is in doubt, material from the edge of an ulcer can be Gram stained and examined for the characteristic pallisading gram-negative coccobacilli suggestive of *Haemophilus ducreyi*. Material from an ulcer can be stained with Giemsa or Wright stain and examined for the presence of the multinucleated giant cells diagnostic of herpetic infection. Unfortunately, both these techniques have very low sensitivity, and the physician is generally obliged to arrive at a diagnosis on clinical grounds or to await the results of culture for the organisms, which usually involves considerable delay.

Pruritic patches in the groin may represent candidiasis or dermatophytosis. Candidiasis is usually intensely red rather than the brown to violet discoloration that accompanies *Tinea* infection. Dermatophytes usually spare the scrotum, whereas *Candida* involves it. Satellite lesions, tiny papulopustules beyond the main area of erythema, strongly suggest candidiasis. A potassium hydroxide preparation of skin scrapings will establish the diagnosis.

Healing herpes genitalis and scabies both result in crusted lesions in the genital area. Intense itching, often worse at night or immediately after bathing, is characteristic of scabies. Herpetic lesions are usually restricted to the genitalia, whereas itching around the ankles or wrists or in the interdigital webs strongly suggests a diagnosis of scabies.

The lesions of STDs may be found in the perianal region in patients practicing receptive anal intercourse and in the perioral or oral area in patients engaging in orogenital contact.

Other conditions should be considered in the differential diagnosis of genital lesions, including Behçet's syndrome, in which recurrent genital ulcerations are associated with recurrent lesions in the mouth and systemic symptoms. Malignancy is part of the differential diagnosis of subacute or chronic lesions, particularly in older patients. In endemic areas, tick-borne tularemia can produce a painful genital ulcer that is usually associated with regional adenopathy and systemic toxicity.

Inguinal adenopathy

Inguinal adenopathy accompanies a variety of genital lesions in STDs (see Table 238-4). Tender adenopathy is more common with gonococcal than with nongonococcal urethritis, but is not a common finding with either disease. Adenopathy, usually bilateral, is seen in about 80% of patients with primary herpes genitalis and usually begins during the second week of illness. Tender adenopathy usually accompanies lesions of chancroid as well. Occasionally, patients with infectious mononucleosis will present with isolated inguinal adenopathy, although generalized lymphadenopathy is more common. Relatively painless inguinal adenopathy accompanies primary syphilis, and the involved nodes are discrete, firm, and freely movable. Suppuration is rare.

The inguinal adenopathy of lymphogranuloma venereum usually appears some weeks after resolution of the primary lesion. Indeed, the primary lesion is so subtle that it is described by only about 30% of infected men and by virtually no infected women. The adenopathy of lymphogranuloma venereum may be extensive and may involve nodes above and below the inguinal (Poupart's) ligament. This adenopathy gives the appearance of a single mass of nodes bisected by a groove, a sign highly suggestive of lymphogranuloma venereum. The nodes in lymphogranuloma venereum may eventually suppurate and drain, and they are sometimes described as giving a bluish discoloration to the overlying skin. The complement-fixation test for lymphogranuloma venereum is sensitive by the time nodes have appeared, and a negative test goes far to ruling out the disease. The test is positive, however, in patients who have had other chlamydial exposure, and because NGU is relatively common in sexually active populations, a positive test is not by itself diagnostic of lymphogranuloma venereum. Serologic tests may be of assistance in diagnosing plague and tularemia. The diagnosis of syphilitic adenopathy is often confirmed serologically.

Patients with inguinal adenopathy should be carefully examined for associated findings suggesting STD, as well as for evidence of infection of the lower extremities. The diagnosis may be assisted by needle aspiration of nodes. Material recovered should be examined by darkfield microscopy for *Treponema pallidum* and by Gram stain and cultured for bacteria and chlamydiae (Plate V-2).

In endemic areas, plague and tularemia must be considered in the differential diagnosis of acute inguinal adenopathy in a young person. Affected patients are usually systemically ill, and their diseases represent medical emergencies. In appropriate areas, the diagnosis should be pursued vigorously. In young children, staphylococci and streptococci, spreading from infections of the lower extremities, are the most common cause of inguinal adenopathy.

Miscellaneous syndromes

Acute epididymitis has been associated with gonococcal and chlamydial infection. Patients with chlamydial epididymitis usually have an accompanying nongonococcal urethritis (Chapter 240). Older men with epididymitis may be infected with gram-negative rods. These men usually do not have a urethral discharge but may notice scrotal swelling and erythema. Various viruses can also cause acute orchiepididymitis.

Bartholinitis has been associated with gonorrhea as well as with various aerobic and anaerobic bacteria. Material expressed from Bartholin's glands should be cultured on a medium selective for gonococci as well as on routine media. Gram stain of expressed discharge may be extremely helpful in determining the cause.

Acute proctitis can be caused by *N. gonorrhoeae* and is usually manifested as a mild change in bowel habits and the appearance of mucus or pus in the stool. Most rectal gonococcal carriers are completely asymptomatic, and gonococci can be isolated from the rectums of 40% of women with gonorrhea. At the other end of the spectrum is a rare colitis syndrome with bloody diarrhea. *C. trachomatis* has also been isolated from the rectums of asymptomatic men and men with acute colitis. Lymphogranuloma venereum may involve the rectum years after genital symptoms have subsided, with the development of rectal strictures that sometimes require operation. Herpetic proctitis has been described in homosexual men. Amebic proctocolitis is associated with homosexual practices and should enter into the differential diagnosis of homosexual men presenting with large bowel symptoms. *Shigella* dysentery has also been acquired by homosexual practices. Recently, infection with *Campylobacter* and so-called *Campylobacter*-like organisms have been associated with diarrheal disease in homosexual men (Chapter 266). Giardiasis is a common cause of small bowel symptoms in this same population. All these infections are components of what has been termed the *gay bowel syndrome*.

REFERENCES

Bowie WR et al: Etiology of non-gonococcal urethritis: evidence for *Chlamydia trachomatis* and *Ureaplasma urealyticum*, J Clin Invest 59:735, 1977.

Brown ST et al: Molluscum contagiosum, Sex Transm Dis 8:227, 1981.

Brunham RC et al: Mucopurulent cervicitis—the ignored counterpart in women of urethritis in men, N Engl J Med 311:1, 1984.

Centers for Disease Control: Sexually transmitted diseases treatment guidelines 1989, MMWR—Morb Mortal Wkly Rep 38(Suppl 8):S1, 1989.

Corey L et al: Genital herpes simplex infection: clinical manifestations, course, and complications, Ann Intern Med 98:958, 1983.

Holmes KK et al, editors: Sexually transmitted diseases, ed 2, New York, 1990, McGraw Hill.

Jacobs NF et al: Gonococcal and nongonococcal urethritis in men: clinical and laboratory differentiation, Ann Intern Med 82:7, 1975.

Lugo-Miro VI: Comparison of different metronidazole therapeutic regimens for bacterial vaginosis, JAMA 268:92, 1992.

Oriel JD: Natural history of genital warts, Br J Vener Dis 147:1, 1971.

Rein MF et al: Section on infections of the reproductive organs and sexually transmitted diseases. In Mandell GL et al, editors: Principles and practice of infectious diseases, ed 3, New York, 1990, Churchill Livingstone.

Sobel JD: Epidemiology and pathogenesis of recurrent vulvovaginal candidiasis, Am J Obstet Gynecol 152:924, 1985.

Spiegel CA et al: Anaerobic bacteria in nonspecific vaginitis, N Engl J Med 303:601, 1980.

Stamm WE et al: *Chlamydia trachomatis* urethral infections in men: prevalence, risk factors, and clinical manifestations, Ann Intern Med 47:100, 1984.

zur Hausen H: Genital papillomavirus infections, Prog Med Virol 32:15, 1985.

CHAPTER

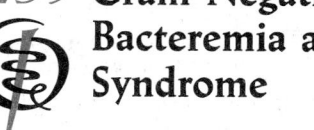

239 Gram-Negative Bacteremia and the Sepsis Syndrome

Lisa J. Istorico-Sanders
C. Glenn Cobbs

This chapter discusses gram-negative bacteremia, sepsis, and septic shock. When infectious disorders caused by gram-negative bacilli result in bloodstream invasion, so-called gram-negative bacteremia occurs. Fever and toxicity due to microbial disease is sometimes referred to as sepsis. Septic shock implies hypotension and decreased tissue perfusion due to microbial disease. The sepsis syndrome is now the thirteenth leading cause of death in the United States, accounting for $5 to $10 billion in annual health care expenditures. Fig. 239-1 illustrates the relationship among these three disorder.

Enterobacteriaceae (including *Escherichia coli, Klebsiella, Proteus,* and others) and *Pseudomonas* are the microorganisms most commonly responsible for gram-negative bacteremia. When gram-negative bacteremia occurs, it appears that endotoxin, a component of gram-negative bacterial cell walls, triggers a cascade of host inflammatory responses and is responsible for the major detrimental effects. Gram-positive bacteria, fungi, and even viruses can produce a disorder that is clinically indistinguishable from gram-negative sepsis. Nevertheless, it is useful to consider gram-negative bacteremia as a distinct entity because of its characteristic epidemiology, pathogenesis, pathophysiology, and treatment.

EPIDEMIOLOGY

The true incidence of gram-negative bacteremia and the sepsis syndrome can only be estimated, as neither are presently reportable illnesses. The best estimates of incidence come from certain medical centers that have tracked bloodstream infections over a number of years and from data collected nationwide from sentinel hospitals by the Centers for

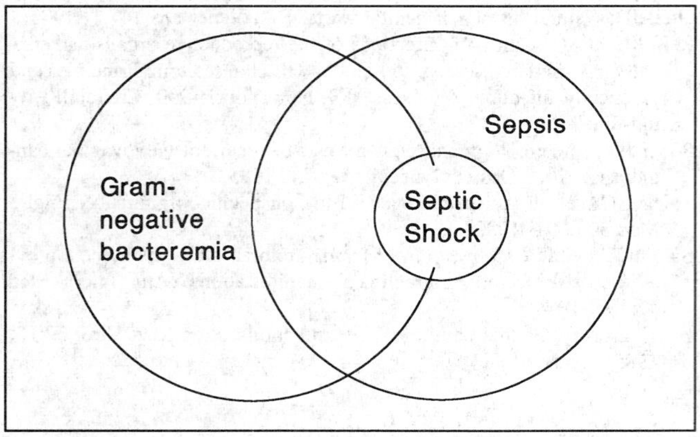

Fig. 239-1. Relationship between gram-negative bacteremia, sepsis, and septic shock.

Disease Control (CDC). Both sources indicate the incidence of gram-negative bacteremia has increased. At Boston City Hospital, the incidence of gram-negative bacteremia between 1935 and 1972 rose from less than 1 to 10 cases/1000 medical/surgical admissions. During a 20-year study at St. Thomas' Hospital in London, the annual incidence of all bacteremias increased from 3.8 episodes/1000 admissions in 1970 to 8.7/1000 in 1987, with gram-negative bacteria accounting for more than 40%. The CDC has estimated that annual cases of septicemia in the United States more than doubled from 1979 to 1987, increasing from 164,000 cases to 425,000. The proportion of these cases attributable to gram-negative bacteria was not stated, but current estimates indicate that about 200,000 cases of gram-negative bacteremia occur yearly in the United States.

Numerous factors may account for this increase. Invasive devices such as central venous catheters are being used more frequently in both inpatient and outpatient settings. Large numbers of patients are now being treated with immunosuppressive and cytotoxic therapies. The proportion of elderly patients and patients with serious underlying diseases in our society is steadily increasing.

Bacteremia may be classified as either community-acquired or hospital-acquired (nosocomial). The incidence of community-acquired gram-negative bacteremia has increased slightly in the past few years. Most cases still occur as a complication of urinary tract infection in otherwise healthy individuals. In contrast, hospital-acquired gram-negative bacteremia has increased steadily over the past 25 years (Chapter 231). More episodes of polymicrobial bacteremia and multiple bacteremic episodes in the same patient have also been noted. Although gram-negative bacteria still account for a significant proportion of nosocomial infections, coagulase-negative staphylococci, enterococci, and yeast have emerged as important bloodstream pathogens as well.

The incidence of gram-negative bacteremia varies in different hospital settings. Tertiary care institutions generally have twofold to fourfold higher rates of bacteremia than do smaller community hospitals. Moreover, the percentage of bacteremia episodes that are nosocomially acquired is much higher for tertiary care centers (up to 75% versus 40% to 50% for community hospitals). These differences presumably reflect the relative severity of patient illness as well as the average length of stay at the two types of institutions.

The present in-hospital mortality rate for patients with gram-negative bacteremia is approximately 30%. The most important factor predicting mortality is the presence of severe underlying disease. In their study of outcome in patients with gram-negative bacteremia, McCabe and Jackson classified patients into risk categories: rapidly fatal disease (e.g., terminal malignancy), ultimately fatal disease (death anticipated within 4 years), and nonfatal disease. The mortality rate in these three groups was 91%, 66%, and 11%, respectively. Additional predictors of poor prognosis identified in more recent studies include the presence of shock, organ system failure, nosocomial infection source, granulocytopenia, hypothermia, and inappropriate antimicrobial therapy.

MICROBIOLOGY

The genitourinary tract is the site of origin of disease that leads to gram-negative bacteremia in approximately 35% of patients. In otherwise healthy individuals, urinary tract infections are most often caused by *E. coli*. In contrast, individuals with urinary tract obstruction or those who develop infection after instrumentation frequently become infected with bacteria such as *Enterobacter, Klebsiella, Proteus, Serratia,* and *Acinetobacter*. Prior antimicrobial therapy, especially in the presence of foreign bodies in the urinary tract, predisposes to uropathogens with multiple antimicrobial resistance patterns (Chapter 361). The presence of the sepsis syndrome associated with a urinary tract infection should raise suspicion for urinary tract obstruction.

Pulmonary infections are responsible for 10% to 15% of episodes of gram-negative bacteremia. *E. coli, Klebsiella,* and resistant microorganisms such as *Pseudomonas, Serratia,* and *Acinetobacter* are frequently encountered. The upper respiratory tract may be colonized by gram-negative bacteria in patients with chronic illnesses, recent hospitalizations, or recent antibiotic therapy and the majority of nosocomial gram-negative bacillary pneumonias result from aspiration of infecting strains. When gram-negative bacillary pneumonia occurs, bacteremia complicates the disease in approximately 15% of patients. It occurs most often when there is associated lung abscess and/or endobronchial obstruction (Chapter 361).

An intra-abdominal source (including perforated appendix, perforated diverticulum, ischemic bowel, peritonitis, liver abscess, and biliary tract disease) is found in approximately 15% of patients with gram-negative bacteremia. In such cases, the microorganism isolated from the blood presumably reflects the pre-existing bowel flora. Anaerobic species, especially *Bacteroides,* may also cause bacteremia in this setting, and polymicrobial bacteremia is also encountered with serious intra-abdominal disease (Chapters 236 and 270).

Patients with burns are at particular risk for microbial invasion of skin, both because of the loss of this natural barrier to infection and because of perturbations of their immune defenses as a consequence of the injury. Care in burn centers is directed at prevention of skin colonization by using topical creams with broad activity against many species of bacteria, rigorous debridement of necrotic tissue, and use of parenteral antibiotics. The microorganisms that colonize a particular unit are usually isolated when infection occurs.

Gram-negative bacilli are also important etiologic agents of nosocomial intravascular catheter infections, accounting for approximately one half of bacteremic episodes arising as a result of these infections. The genera encountered reflect the particular hospital's ecology and include *Klebsiella, Enterobacter, Acinetobacter, Pseudomonas,* and *E. coli*.

Patients with profound granulocytopenia are susceptible to bacteremia as a result of invasion of mucosal surfaces by resident flora. The oropharynx and gut appear to serve as sites of bacterial invasion in the granulocytopenic patient with occult gram-negative bacteremia (Chapter 229).

Despite thorough evaluation, a primary source cannot be determined in up to 30% of patients with gram-negative bacteremia.

PATHOGENESIS

Host/parasite interactions

The pathogenesis of bacterial infection is a dynamic process in which colonizing microorganisms interact with host defenses. The virulence of the particular bacterial species and the status of the host's immune system are the variables that determine the likelihood of subsequent disease. The general principles of host defense against infection are discussed in detail in Chapter 222; specific factors related to gram-negative infection are discussed here.

Host defense factors

Anatomic barriers are an important first line of defense against bacterial infection. Disruption of the skin barrier due to trauma, burns, or intravascular catheterization may allow entry of gram-negative bacteria as does urinary tract catheterization.

Both the humoral and cell-mediated arms of the immune system play a role in preventing gram-negative infection. Burn patients have numerous defects in their immune defenses, which further predispose them to infection. These patients have low levels of immunoglobulins, increased suppressor T-cell activity, decreased helper T-cell activity, and perhaps, most important, defects in neutrophil function.

Polymorphonuclear leukocytes are the host's primary defense against pyogenic bacteria that have penetrated external mechanical barriers. Patients with profound granulocytopenia are especially susceptible to invasive bacterial infection.

Occasionally, therapy directed at preventing other nosocomial complications may predispose to infection. Gastric alkalization used to prevent stress ulceration in ill patients may allow bacterial overgrowth in the upper gastrointestinal tract leading to an increased risk of nosocomial pneumonia should aspiration occur.

Microbial virulence factors

For a potential pathogen to cause bacteremia, it must (1) attach to host epithelial surfaces, (2) evade local defenses, (3) multiply, and (4) disseminate from the site of primary infection (Table 239-1).

Attachment of invading microorganisms frequently involves specific interactions between receptors on the bacterial surface and carbohydrate moieties or other ligands on the host cell membrane. Fimbriae are cellular appendages that bacteria use to attach to epithelial or environmental surfaces. P fimbriae of *E. coli* allow attachment to susceptible uroepithelial cells and *Vibrio cholerae* likely attach to intestinal epithelial cells via fimbriae before delivery of toxin.

Bacterial proliferation and invasion at local sites are facilitated by the production of a variety of extracellular bacterial enzymes and toxins. Many species of gram-negative bacilli produce hemolysins, proteases, and elastases, which break down tissue barriers, degrade immunoglobulins, and damage phagocytic cell membranes. Fibronectin normally coats mucosal cells in the oropharynx and covers cell surface receptors for gram-negative bacilli, thereby blocking their adherence. In ill patients, fibronectin may be digested by elastase released by inflammatory cells and gram-negative colonization may occur. A pseudomonal toxin, exotoxin A, inhibits host cell protein synthesis by inactivating elongation factor 2, a necessary co-factor for ribosome function.

Some gram-negative bacteria possess extracellular capsules composed of long-chain acidic polysaccharides. In the

Table 239-1. Virulence factors of gram-negative bacteria

Virulence factor	Activity	Example
Fimbriae	Promote adherence	P fimbriae of *E. coli*
Enzymes, exotoxins	Degrade immunoglobulins, damage phagocytes	Pseudomonas exotoxin A, Shiga toxin
Capsules	Inhibit opsonization and phagocytosis	*Haemophilus influenzae*, type B *Klebsiella* species K1 capsule of *E. coli*
O-polysaccharides	Impair antibody-mediated complement killing	Present in virulent gram-negative bacilli
Endotoxin-Lipid A	Triggers sepsis cascade	Most gram-negative bacilli

absence of specific antibody, these capsules act as virulence factors by protecting the microorganism from the opsonic effects of alternative complement pathway components. Moreover, capsular polysaccharide is often poorly immunogenic, leading to an inadequate host antibody response. For example, *E. coli* K5 capsule is structurally quite similar to an intermediate molecule in the biosynthesis of heparin and the capsule apparently is perceived as a "self" antigen by the host immune system.

Cell wall components of gram-negative bacilli clearly contribute to their virulence. Endotoxin (LPS) is a lipopolysaccharide component of gram-negative bacterial outer membranes. It is composed of three segments (Fig. 239-2), an outermost series of oligosaccharides that are antigenically diverse and determine the O serotype of the bacteria, a connecting series of core oligosaccharides, which are relatively conserved among gram-negative bacteria, and an innermost lipid segement, lipid A. Lipid A is the toxic portion of the molecule and directly or indirectly appears to trigger many of the systemic effects associated with gram-negative bacteremia (see later discussion). The O-polysaccharide side chains also contribute to the microorganism's virulence. Strains that lack these polysaccharide antigens have a characteristic rough colony appearance and may be more susceptible to the lytic action of complement and other products that attack the bacterial cell wall.

PATHOPHYSIOLOGY

The complex pathophysiologic events that lead from localized gram-negative bacterial disease to the sepsis syndrome remain incompletely understood. LPS has received the most attention as a virulence factor. When injected into experimental animals, purified LPS can produce many of the signs of septic shock including fever, chills, hypotension, coagulopathy, and death. Recent studies have shown that LPS in the circulation binds via its lipid A moiety with high affinity to a host protein, LPS-binding protein (LBP). The LPS-LBP complex then attaches to monocytes and macrophages via a specific cell surface receptor, CD14, inducing release of tumor necrosis factor (TNF-α) from these mononuclear cells (Table 239-2).

Evidence implicating TNF-α in the pathogenesis of the sepsis syndrome includes increases in TNF-α levels in animals and human volunteers given endotoxin, the duplication of signs and symptoms of sepsis by TNF-α infusion, and the finding of elevated TNF-α levels in patients with the sepsis syndrome. TNF-α stimulates macrophages to release interleukin 1 (IL-1), and there appear to be at least two important results of the interaction of TNF-α and host endothelial cells, induction of procoagulant activity, which may trigger the coagulation cascade (see discussion later), and increased expression of adhesion molecules promoting white blood cell adherence. In some instances, TNF-α may not be uniquely responsible for the sepsis syndrome, as TNF-α levels may be elevated in patients with a variety of conditions unrelated to sepsis, including rheumatoid arthritis, leprosy, and AIDS. TNF-α is not detectable in some patients with the sepsis syndrome.

IL-1 shares many biologic activities with TNF-α, including pyrogenic effects, and induction of procoagulant activity and adhesions on endothelial cells. IL-1 also results in release of platelet-activating factor (PAF) and an inhibitor of tissue plasminogen activator. This latter effect results in increased platelet aggregation and coagulation. In addition, IL-1 plays a role in the host immune response by initiating activation of T lymphocytes, aiding in B-cell replication and antibody production, and activating polymorphonuclear leukocytes.

A variety of important inflammatory mediators and reg-

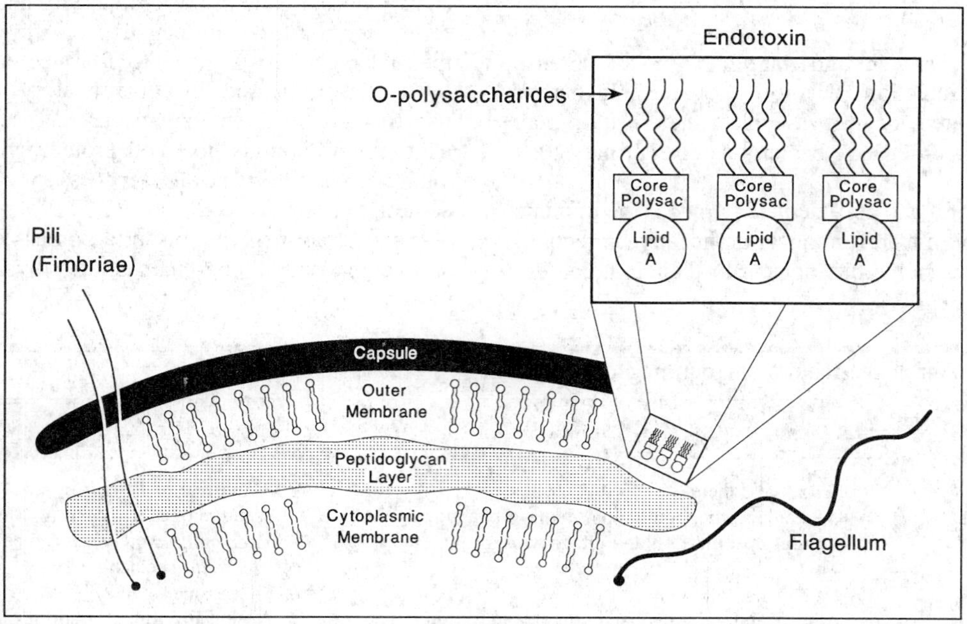

Fig. 239-2. Cell wall structure of a typical gram-negative microorganism.

Table 239-2. Mediators of the biologic effects of endotoxin

Mediator	Effects
Tumor necrosis factor (TNF)	Stimulates release of cytokines; pyrogenic; promotes cellular adhesion; induces procoagulant activity
Interleukin-1 (IL-1)	Endogenous pyrogen; regulates lymphocyte proliferation; activates other inflammatory mediators
Platelet-activating factor (PAF)	Stimulates release of TNFα, leukotrienes, thromboxane A_2; causes platelet aggregation; increases microvascular permeability
Arachidonic acid metabolites:	
Prostaglandins	Pyrogenic; cause vasodilatation; increase vascular permeability
Leukotrienes	Promote neutrophil chemotaxis; increase vascular permeability
Thromboxane A_2	Causes platelet aggregation; promotes release of endothelium-derived relaxing factor (EDRF); causes vasoconstriction
Hageman factor (XII)	Initiates coagulation cascade; stimulates bradykinin production
Complement	Causes vasodilatation; increases vascular permeability; promotes leukocyte chemotaxis
Endothelial factors:	
EDRF	Causes vasodilatation; inhibits platelet aggregation
Endothelin-1	Causes intense vasoconstriction
Myocardial depressant substance	Causes reversible ventricular dilatation; decreases myocardial contractility

ulatory hormones (PAF, arachidonic acid metabolites [prostaglandins, leukotrienes], and related molecules) are derived from the phospholipid component of cell membranes. Endotoxin, directly or indirectly through the effects of TNF-α and IL-1, leads to generation of a number of these molecules.

PAF is released from cell membranes of many cell types including monocytes, macrophages, platelets, neutrophils, and endothelial cells in response to endotoxin. PAF causes platelet aggregation and thrombosis as well as a marked increase in microvascular permeability. It also has a negative ionotropic effect on the heart and causes hypotension. Finally, it leads to increased production of arachidonic acid metabolites in a similar manner to TNF-α and IL-1.

Arachidonic acid, generated from cell membrane phospholipids, may be metabolized to produce prostaglandins via the cyclo-oxygenase pathway or leukotrienes via the lipoxygenase pathway and prostaglandins and leukotrienes appear to mediate many of the systemic effects of TNF-α and IL-1. Specific inhibitors of cyclo-oxygenase will blunt the effects of experimentally administered endotoxin in humans and lipoxygenase inhibitors have similar effects in animals. Prostaglandin I_2 is a potent vasodilator that at least contributes to the hypotension seen during gram-negative sepsis. Prostaglandin E_2 is mainly responsible for the fever seen in gram-negative sepsis through its effects on the hypothalamus. Leukotriene B_4 is a powerful chemotactic and activating factor for polymorphonuclear leukocytes, and other leukotrienes such as C_4 affect vascular tone and permeability.

Myocardial depressant substance, a poorly characterized moiety found in the serum of experimental animals after administration of endotoxin, works in concert with TNF-α, PAF, and other cytokines to suppress myocardial function. Hemodynamic stability is further compromised by the endothelial factors endothelin-1, an intense vasoconstrictor, and endothelium-derived relaxing factor (recently identified as nitric oxide), a vasodilator.

Additional humoral mediators of the sepsis syndrome include components of the coagulation and complement cascades. Endotoxin directly activates Hageman factor (factor XII of the coagulation cascade), which triggers the intrinsic coagulation pathway through activation of factor XI and the extrinsic pathway by stimulating release of tissue factor from endothelial cells and macrophages. Hageman factor also converts plasminogen to plasmin, activating the fibrinolytic system. This characteristic may be responsible for the disseminated intravascular coagulation seen in some patients with sepsis. Finally, Hageman factor stimulates the conversion of prekallikrein to kallikrein, which converts kininogen to circulating bradykinin. Kinins then play a role in the hypotension and increased vascular permeability encountered during bacteremia.

Complement components are another important group of humoral mediators activated during the sepsis syndrome. Complement may be activated during bacteremia by the classic pathway (interaction of microbial antigens and specific antibodies) or the alternative pathway (nonspecific activation by bacterial cell wall components). Complement may also be activated through interaction with the coagulation or fibrinolytic pathways. C3a and C5a function as anaphylatoxins causing vasodilatation, increased vascular permeability, and histamine release from mast cells. C5a is a potent chemotactant for neutrophils and may lead to local aggregation of these effector cells with subsequent tissue damage from released granular products. C5a has been further implicated as a stimulus for producing prostaglandins and other bioactive arachidonic acid products.

The net result of the complex interactions described here are fever, hypotension, myocardial depression, disseminated intravascular coagulation (DIC), and altered organ system function, the clinical manifestations of the sepsis syndrome. Fig. 239-3 is an attempt to illustrate the proposed interaction of (LPS) and cellular and humoral factors.

CLINICAL MANIFESTATIONS

Fever, often accompanied by shaking chills, is the most common clinical manifestation of bacteremia (Table 239-3). In a series of 612 patients with gram-negative bacteremia reported by Kreger et al, fever (temperature >99.6° F) was seen in 82% of patients. Thirty patients did not mount

Table 239-3. Clinical and laboratory manifestations of gram-negative bacteremia

Finding	Comment
Physical examination	
Fever	Hypothermia also occurs
Tachypnea	Occurs early via direct stimulation of central respiratory center by endotoxin
Altered mental status	Multifactorial
Hypotension	Related to decreased systemic vascular resistance, decreased myocardial contractility
Cyanosis	Low cardiac output syndrome
Petechiae, purpura	Manifestation of DIC
Muscle tenderness	Associated with bacteremic localization in muscle
Laboratory studies	
Leukopenia	May occur transiently early or later with overwhelming infection
Leukocytosis	Common
Thrombocytopenia	Present to some degree in 50% of patients
Hypoglycemia	Depletion of glycogen stores
Abnormal renal or liver function	Secondary to poor perfusion
Respiratory alkalosis	Direct stimulation of central respiratory center
Hypoxemia	Multifactorial; right-to-left shunt, noncardiogenic pulmonary edema
Metabolic acidosis	Due to lactate accumulation

a febrile response within the first 24 hours after the onset of bacteremia. These patients had a higher incidence of shock and death than those with fever. Hypothermia (temperature <97.6° F) was seen in 83 bacteremic patients (13%). These patients had outcomes similar to those patients who presented with fever. Although the majority of bacteremic patients have fever, a significant percentage of patients who present with hypothermia are also found to be bacteremic. Of 85 consecutive patients with hypothermia admitted to San Francisco General Hospital, 33 were bacteremic, 19 with gram-negative microorganisms. In patients with unexplained hypothermia, blood cultures should be obtained and consideration given to beginning empiric antibiotics. Age, renal insufficiency, corticosteroid or antipyretic administration, and malignancy all increase the likelihood that a bacteremic patient will not mount a febrile response.

Respiratory manifestations frequently accompany gram-negative bacteremia, and acute onset of tachypnea with respiratory alkalosis is among the earliest and most consistent finding. The adult respiratory distress syndrome (ARDS) occurs in as many as 20% of patients with gram-negative sepsis, and the mortality rate approaches 90% in this subgroup.

Mental status changes may occur in patients with gram-negative bacteremia. Changes may range from mild anxiety or restlessness to profound confusional states. Change in mentation is a particularly important diagnostic clue in elderly patients who may exhibit few other early signs of disease.

Shock develops in up to 40% of patients with gram-negative bacteremia, and its presence is a predictor of in-

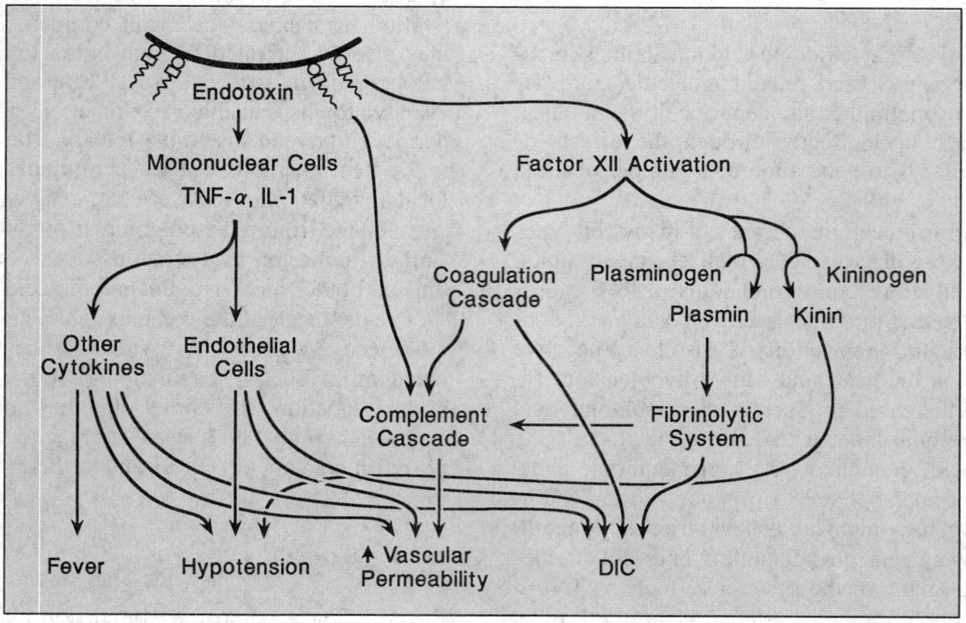

Fig. 239-3. Diagram of the interaction of host inflammatory mediators during gram-negative sepsis. TNF-α, tumor necrosis factor; IL-1, interleukin 1; DIC, disseminated intravascular coagulation.

creased mortality. The characteristic hemodynamic findings early in septic shock are an increased cardiac index and decreased systemic vascular resistance. Studies have also shown a decreased left ventricular ejection fraction and acute left ventricular dilatation, perhaps due to circulating myocardial depressant factor. These abnormalities usually revert to normal by 7 to 10 days. Of course, prolonged hypotension may lead to development of end-organ failure, including acute myocardial infarction, acute renal tubular damage, and respiratory failure.

A number of dermatologic manifestations have been described in patients with gram-negative bacteremia. Skin may be the primary site of disease leading to bacteremia (especially in the presence of percutaneous intravascular devices), or skin manifestations may develop secondary to hematogenous seeding. Metastatic skin lesions are especially prominent with infections caused by certain *Vibrio* species. Ecthyma gangrenosum is characterized by erythematous, maculopapular lesions with central necrosis. On histologic examination, large numbers of microorganisms are seen, some within blood vessel walls, and few inflammatory cells are present. Ecthyma gangrenosum was once thought to be diagnostic of pseudomonal bacteremia, but similar lesions have been caused by *Aeromonas* or other gram-negative species. Dermatologic lesions associated with sepsis not due to direct bacterial invasion of the skin include petechiae, purpura, and peripheral gangrene from DIC, immune injury, or vasoconstriction, respectively.

LABORATORY FINDINGS

Results of routine laboratory studies are seldom pathognomonic of bacteremia, but certain findings may suggest primary or secondary sites of focal infection (e.g., pyuria with urinary tract infection). In addition, a number of nonspecific laboratory abnormalities have been reported in association with gram-negative sepsis (see Table 239-3).

Polymorphonuclear leukocytosis with an increase in immature forms typically develops soon after the onset of pyogenic bacterial infection. Leukopenia may occasionally develop in patients with overwhelming infections due to rapid destruction or aggregation of granulocytes or possibly suppression of bone marrow function by bacterial toxins or host inflammatory mediators. Leukopenia is more commonly seen in infants, the elderly, alcoholics, and others with decreased bone marrow reserve. Morphologic changes in polymorphonuclear cells may occur with sepsis, including the nonspecific findings of toxic granulations and Döhle's bodies and the more specific finding of vacuolization.

Abnormalities of coagulation are common during bacteremia. In one series, 126 of 222 bacteremic patients had laboratory evidence of thrombocytopenia. DIC with increased fibrin split products and depressed levels of clotting factors was noted in 25 (11%) patients in the same report. Clinically, however, significant bleeding was uncommon (3%). If very sensitive tests for detection of thrombin and plasmin activation are used, evidence of DIC can be found in almost all patients with bacteremia and less than 50,000 platelets/μL.

A number of metabolic derangements have been described during gram-negative bacteremia. Insulin resistance may be an early clinical sign of bacteremia in diabetic patients, but hypoglycemia has also been reported. Serum amino acid levels rise as a result of muscle proteolysis, and serum triglycerides are characteristically elevated due to increased fat breakdown and alterations in use. Increases in blood urea nitrogen and creatinine coincide with renal hypoperfusion and acute tubular damage. Immunologically mediated renal injury with abnormalities of urinary sediment may also occur. A recent series reported depressed serum levels of ionized calcium in 12 of 40 patients with gram-negative bacteremia versus none of 20 patients with gram-positive bacteremia.

Elevation of serum bilirubin disproportionate to other liver function tests has been described during bacteremia, even among patients with nonabdominal primary sites. Hemolysis and increased tissue breakdown as well as toxic or metabolically mediated hepatocellular dysfunction may be responsible. Serum transaminase levels may also be elevated from long-standing hypotension and ischemic hepatic injury.

Varying degrees of hypoxemia may develop during sepsis as a result of pneumonia, ARDS, or other causes of intrapulmonary arteriovenous shunting. At the same time, the arterial/venous oxygen difference is often decreased. This apparent inefficiency in blood oxygen extraction by the tissues may be caused by derangement of microvascular blood flow regulation and/or a poorly characterized primary defect in cellular oxidative metabolism. Unless cardiac output is maintained or increased, tissue oxygen delivery may become impaired at a time when fever and stress of infection greatly raise cellular energy requirements. Lactic acidosis is often a manifestation of bacteremic shock reflecting both an increase in anaerobic glycolysis and impairment of hepatic lactate clearance.

DIAGNOSIS

The diagnosis of bacteremia ultimately rests on the isolation of the causative microorganism from blood cultures. At least two aerobic and anaerobic blood cultures should be obtained before antibiotic administration. In gram-negative sepsis, the majority of such specimens will be positive, but bacteremia may occasionally be intermittent and is usually low grade (<10 organisms/ml blood). Hypertonic blood culture media of culture systems using antibiotic removal devices may increase the yield of positive cultures in those patients already receiving antimicrobial therapy. It is important to note that the entire spectrum of septic shock may develop in the absence of demonstrable bloodstream invasion if sufficient quantities of bacterial cell wall fragments or toxins are absorbed.

Because blood culture results may not be available for 24 to 48 hours, empiric diagnosis and therapy must often be based on a clinical judgment. Physicians must be alert for early clinical manifestations of the sepsis syndrome, including fever, changes in mentation, and hyperventilation. A number of large studies of patients with suspected gram-negative sepsis, including two recent ones, have shown that only about 30% to 40% of patients suspected clinically will have gram-negative organisms isolated from their blood. Because of the imprecise nature of a clinical diagnosis of gram-negative sepsis and delay in obtaining blood culture data, other methods for confirming a diagnosis have been studied. Several assays have been developed to detect circulating endotoxin, the most sensitive and widely studied of which is the limulus gelatin reaction. This test is currently used only as a research tool, but in the future more rapid and precise endotoxin assays may be available to confirm the diagnosis.

The evaluation of any patient with suspected bacteremia should include a diligent search for evidence of a primary focus of infection. Examination should include the skin surface, including the perirectal area. In addition to blood cultures, a chemistry profile, urinalysis, and complete blood count with differential should also be obtained. Arterial blood gas determination may reveal respiratory alkalosis, evidence of hypoxia, or metabolic acidosis. Radiographic evaluation should include chest x-ray film and possibly abdominal films. For patients with a suspected abdominal (including renal) source, sonography, or computed tomography (CT) may also be indicated.

Hemodynamic monitoring with a pulmonary artery catheter may be diagnostically and therapeutically useful in selected patients presenting with hypotension. The characteristic findings of sepsis, viz increased cardiac output with very low systemic vascular resistance are seen in only a small number of other conditions (e.g., hypotension caused by drugs such as nitroprusside, narcotics, and psychotropic drugs). These findings may also occur in patients with anaphylaxis, Addisonian crisis (see later discussion), or shock resulting from neurogenic injury.

Differential diagnosis

Infections with gram-positive bacteria, viruses, fungi, protozoa, and metazoa can mimic gram-negative sepsis. Toxic shock syndrome due to either staphylococcal vaginal colonization, staphylococcal cellulitis, staphylococcal pneumonia (Thucidides syndrome), or to group A streptococcal disease may produce the signs and symptoms of sepsis (Chapters 257 and 259). A characteristic "sunburn" rash, mucosal erythema, and multiorgan failure should suggest this diagnosis. Pneumococcal bacteremia in the asplenic host, overwhelming staphylococcal disease without rash, and meningococcal bacteremia syndrome without meningitis may closely resemble gram-negative bacteremia and shock. Rickettsial disease, particularly Rocky Mountain spotted fever and epidemic typhus, may mimic gram-negative bacteremia early on. History of tick bite, headache, and rash developing several days after fever support Rocky Mountain spotted fever. Other infectious diagnoses to be considered include disseminated fungal infection (e.g., *Candida* or related species in leukopenic patients or *Histoplasma capsulatum* in HIV-infected patients), disseminated tuberculosis, falciparum malaria, and disseminated viral infection (e.g., cytomegalovirus in transplant recipients).

Several important noninfectious conditions must be differentiated from gram-negative bacteremia. Myocardial infarction may present with hypotension and occasionally fever. In this setting cardiac output is initially low, with elevated systemic vascular resistance.

Pulmonary embolus may be especially difficult to differentiate from bacteremia; fever, hypoxia, tachypnea, and hypotension may all be present. Usually, fever is low grade, and pulmonary and systemic vascular resistance are both increased. Leukocytosis with left shift is usually absent.

Several endocrine disorders, including adrenal insufficiency and thyroid storm, may mimic the findings of bacteremia. Acute adrenal insufficiency, in particular, may present with hypotension, mental status changes, and fever.

Some collagen vascular diseases may be confused with the sepsis syndrome. Vasculitis may present with fever, skin lesions, and end-organ damage. Hypotension and decreased vascular resistance, however, are not typical features of systemic vasculitis.

Chronic salicylate intoxication can result in a "pseudosepsis" syndrome characterized by fever, leukocytosis, hypotension, increased cardiac output, decreased systemic vascular resistance, and multiple system organ failure. This syndrome should be considered in older adults who are taking aspirin regularly for chronic pain or inflammatory conditions and in whom a source of infection cannot be identified.

THERAPY

The treatment of gram-negative bacteremia has traditionally involved three basic principles: (1) identification and management of the primary focus of infection, (2) ongoing assessment of physiologic parameters with intervention to support vital organ perfusion, and (3) specific antimicrobial therapy (see the accompanying box). Recently, attention has focused on a fourth method, modulation of the host inflammatory response through use of genetically engineered molecules.

General measures

The physician should always attempt to identify primary sites of infection, as the resolution of bacteremia may depend on successful management of such a focus. Rapid identification of the microorganism responsible for bacteremia may also be possible based on Gram stain of clinical specimens (sputum, urine, cerebrospinal fluid, synovial fluid, etc.). Specific therapeutic goals should include drainage of abscesses, relief of obstruction (e.g., an obstructed ureter in pyelonephritis), excision of dead tissue (e.g., infarcted bowel), and removal of infected prosthetic devices.

All patients with suspected gram-negative bacteremia should be hospitalized. Although some patients with gram-negative bacteremia have relatively mild symptoms, many

Management of gram-negative bacteremia

Seek to identify a primary site of gram-negative disease
- Gram stain and culture inflammatory material, sputum, urine, etc.

Monitor physiologic parameters
- Vital signs, mental status, urine output, arterial blood gases, electrolytes, creatinine, coagulation studies

Maintain tissue perfusion if hypotensive
- Expand intravascular volume
- Sympathomimetic amines if volume expansion fails
  - Dopamine—begin at 2-5 μg/kg/min
  - Norepinephrine—0.05 μg/kg/min if dopamine ineffective
    - Causes intense vasoconstriction
- Consider physiologic monitoring with Swan-Ganz catheter

Administer antibiotics
- See text and Table 239-4

Consider modulation of host inflammatory response
- See text and Table 239-5

Support if organ system failure develops
- Mechanical ventilation, hemodialysis, etc.

require aggressive supportive care in an intensive care unit setting. Vital signs, including temperature, pulse, blood pressure, and respiratory rate, should be monitored continuously or determined at frequent intervals. Intravenous and oral fluid intake and urinary, stool, and gastric outputs should also be recorded. Invasive monitoring of pulmonary artery pressure may be required for optimal management of patients with severe hypotension or ARDS.

For the patient with septic shock, aggressive repletion of circulatory volume may be lifesaving. Vascular pooling and increased vascular permeability during sepsis lead to decreased effective blood volume. An isotonic fluid challenge should be administered promptly. Normal saline is appropriate, although some authorities believe that colloid solutions such as albumin or hetastarch are more effective volume expanders. Packed red blood cells provide effective volume replacement for patients with significant anemia.

Due to pulmonary artery constriction during sepsis, simple central venous pressure determinations cannot be relied on to accurately reflect volume status. Monitoring pulmonary capillary wedge pressure (PCWP) with a Swan-Ganz catheter may be useful in guiding the volume expansion of severely hypotensive patients, patients with underlying cardiac dysfunction, and ventilatory-dependent patients requiring positive end-expiratory pressure. Cardiac output is usually optimal at a PCWP of approximately 12 cm H_2O. Critics of "routine" use of a pulmonary artery catheter point out that adequate controlled trials have not been performed to demonstrate that patient survival is improved by the use of these devices. Furthermore, complications due to pulmonary artery catheterization include bleeding, pneumothorax, catheter-related infection, and dysrhythmias. Clearly, the pulmonary artery catheter is a potentially valuable tool, but should be used judiciously and only by a physician adequately trained in its proper use. Retrospective studies have shown that patients managed in intensive care units by trained critical care physicians have improved survival rates over those who are not managed in this way.

Vasopressors may be beneficial for patients who remain hypotensive despite fluid replacement. Dopamine, at a starting dose of 2 to 5 μg/kg/min, is the agent preferred by most authorities; the final dose must be titrated for each patient. Occasional patients may require the use of more potent agents, such as norepinephrine, but excessive vasoconstriction may further impair tissue perfusion and lead to gangrene.

Renal function may be severely impaired during sepsis due to poor renal perfusion pressure. Dopamine augments renal blood flow when used in a dose up to about 10 μg/kg/min, but higher doses lead to renal vasoconstriction. Patients who remain oliguric after fluid challenge and correction of hypotension should be monitored closely for signs of acute renal failure. Hemodialysis may be required to correct fluid and electrolyte imbalances in some patients.

Many patients with pneumonia or ARDS require intubation and mechanical ventilatory support. Maintenance of adequate blood oxygenation is critical, as tissue oxygen delivery in sepsis is highly dependent on oxygen delivery. Positive end-expiratory pressure may be necessary for patients with severe ARDS, but must be used with caution in patients with depressed cardiac outputs.

Lactic acidosis often complicates tissue hypoperfusion during sepsis. Although the administration of bicarbonate solutions should be considered for patients with arterial pH of less than 7.0, management is primarily directed toward restoring tissue oxygen delivery. Bicarbonate infusion may correct acidemia, but a controlled trial has shown that it does not improve hemodynamics.

Antimicrobial therapy

In patients with suspected gram-negative bacteremia, antimicrobial therapy is almost always begun before the precise bacterial pathogen and its antimicrobial susceptibilities are known. Initial therapy in this clinical situation usually involves the use of two or more antimicrobial agents. Combination antimicrobial therapy is used to provide coverage against a broad spectrum of pathogens, to help prevent the emergence of resistant strains during therapy, and to provide possible synergistic bactericidal activity against specific microorganisms. An example of this synergism is that produced by the combination of an aminoglycoside and an antipseudomonal penicillin for treatment of *Pseudomonas aeruginosa* infection.

Table 239-4 indicates examples of initial antimicrobial therapy in patients with suspected gram-negative bacteremia associated with disease at various sites. In most situations, an aminoglycoside is recommended in combination with a beta-lactam agent with activity against gram-negative bacilli (penicillin, cephalosporin, carbapenem, or monobactam) (Chapter 224). Among patients at high risk for nephrotoxicity or ototoxicity, a broad-spectrum beta-lactam,

Table 239-4. Suggested initial drug therapy based on suspected site of origin of gram-negative bacteremia*

Site	Antibiotics	Comment
Urinary tract	—Ampicillin† plus aminoglycoside‡	Combination also covers enterococcus
Respiratory tract:		
Community-acquired	—Erythromycin† and third-generation cephalosporin§ OR first- or second-generation cephalosporin‖ plus aminoglycoside	Gram-negative bacteria cause 10%-20% community pneumonias requiring hospitalization. *Haemophilus influenzae, Klebsiella pneumoniae,* and others implicated. Consider *Legionella* if elderly or immunosuppressed.
Hospital-acquired	—Anti-pseudomonal beta-lactam** plus aminoglycoside	Must treat for more resistant organisms including *P. aeruginosa*
Intra-abdominal and biliary tract	—Ticarcillin-clavulanate† plus aminoglycoside OR —Imipenem plus aminoglycoside	Use regimen active against enteric gram-negative bacteria and anaerobes
Burns	—Anti-pseudomonal beta-lactam plus aminoglycoside	Choose agent with greatest anti-peudomonal activity at particular hospital
Catheter infection	—Vancomycin† plus ceftazidime OR —Vancomycin plus aminoglycoside	Include vancomycin for methicillin-resistant staphylococci
Granulocytopenia	—Anti-pseudomonal beta-lactam plus aminoglycoside	Add vancomycin for *Staphylococcus* species if intravascular catheter present

*If source unknown, consider imipenem or ticarcillin-clavulanate plus aminoglycoside. Add vancomycin if gram-positive infection is a consideration.
†Others: Ampicillin 1-2 g every 4-6 hr; erythromycin 0.5-1 g every 6 hr; ticarcillin-clavulanate 3.1 g every 4-8 hr; vancomycin 1 g every 12 hr.
‡Gentamicin, tobramycin 3-5 mg/kg/day divided every 8 hr; amikacin 15 mg/kg/day divided every 8 hr. Must adjust for renal dysfunction.
§Cefotaxime 1-2 g every 6-8 hr; ceftriaxone 1-2 g every 24 hr; ceftazidime 1-2 g every 8 hr.
‖Cefazolin 1 g every 8 hr; cephalothin 1-2 g every 4-6 hr; cefuroxime 1 g every 8 hr.
**Pipracillin, mezlocillin, ticarcillin 3 g every 4 hr; ceftazidime 1-2 g every 8 hr; imipenem 500 mg every 6 hr.

such as a third-generation cephalosporin or imipenem, may be used alone initially. For the penicillin-allergic patient, aztreonam, which appears to have a low incidence of cross-reactivity with other beta-lactam drugs, or a parenteral quinolone may be used with or without an aminoglycoside.

An educated guess as to the etiology of suspected gram-negative bacterial disease may be possible on the basis of clinical setting, ancillary culture data such as a urinary tract pathogen, skin or other surveillance cultures, or examination of inflammatory material. After isolation and identification of the etiologic microorganism and determination of its sensitivities, the physician should re-evaluate antimicrobial therapy to select the safest and most effective therapeutic regimen.

Bacteremia may persist or recur in up to 10% of patients despite appropriate therapy and may be a clue to the presence of an occult abscess or intravascular site of infection. In addition, persistent bacteremia may indicate inadequate serum antimicrobial concentrations and prompt the assessment of serum bactericidal activity.

Therapies directed toward modulation of host immune response

Despite the availability of broad-spectrum antimicrobial agents, the mortality rate associated with gram-negative bacteremia has remained at about 30% for the past three decades. Further advances in the treatment of gram-negative bacteremia will likely depend on interrupting the underlying pathophysiologic mechanisms responsible for tissue damage. Strategies currently undergoing investigation include neutralization of the endotoxin portion of gram-negative cell membrane by specific antibodies or chemical binding agents and blocking activation or function of host inflammatory mediators through similar means (Table 239-5).

Corticosteroids have been studied extensively in gram-negative sepsis because of their ability to attenuate the inflammatory response. In animal studies pretreatment with corticosteroids prevented lethal effects of injected endotoxin. Among more than 600 bacteremic patients evaluated in several large human trials, however, mortality rates for patients receiving corticosteroids and those receiving placebo were similar.

Opiate receptor blockers such as naloxone have also received considerable attention. As with corticosteroids, animal models suggest improved survival when naloxone is administered early in the course of septic shock. However, at least one small prospective human trial failed to show any significant difference in outcome among patients receiving naloxone versus those receiving placebo.

Inhibitors of cylco-oxygenase and lipoxygenase may prove to be clinically useful in the treatment of the sepsis syndrome because prostaglandins and leukotrienes appear to mediate many of the metabolic effects of TNF-α. In a recent human trial, ibuprofen was shown to blunt many of

Table 239-5. Agents under investigation that may modify host response to gram-negative infection

Agent	Comment
Corticosteroids	No benefit in two large, randomized trials of gram-negative sepsis.
Naloxone	Conflicting data in animal and human studies.
Ibuprofen	Blocks cyclo-oxygenase. Some efficacy in animals, humans.
Pentoxifylline	Attenuates neutrophil function, blocks TNF-α production, improved survival in animals.
J5 Antiserum	Pooled serum from volunteers immunized with J5 mutant *E. coli*. Technical problems with production; potential to transmit infection.
HA-1A	Chimeric human-mouse monoclonal IgM antibody to lipid A.
E5	Murine monoclonal IgM antibody to lipid A.
Lipid A precusors	In vitro data, animal studies show efficacy in blocking endotoxin.
Monoclonal antibody to TNF-α	Decreases mortality in sepsis model in rats.
IL-1 receptor antagonists	Decrease mortality in animals and humans with sepsis. May be effective in both gram-positive and gram-negative infections.
PAF receptor antagonists	Block vasoconstriction in animals.

the physiologic effects of injected endotoxin. Selective leukotriene inhibitors have also attenuated the effects of injected endotoxin in animals.

Initial studies in humans utilizing antibodies to endotoxin involved the administration of human polyclonal antisera raised against the core polysaccharide and lipid regions of endotoxin. This antiserum was produced in human volunteers who were immunized with mutant rough bacterial strains (such as *E. coli* J5) that lack the antigenically diverse external O-polysaccharides. In a human study of more than 200 bacteremic patients, mortality was significantly reduced among patients receiving adjunctive treatment with antisera directed against *E. coli* J5 as compared with controls. Problems with production of antisera and the potential for transmission of infection prevented the widespread use of this product. Recently developed hybridoma technology has made possible the production of specific monoclonal antibodies directed against lipid A, which have overcome the feasibility problems of human antisera.

Two monoclonal antibodies, HA-1A (Centocor Corp.) and E5 (Xoma Corp.), have undergone phase III testing and are awaiting FDA approval. More will likely follow. HA-1A and E5 have been shown to bind mainly to antigens located in the deep core and lipid A regions of endotoxin. Each has also been shown to be effective in animal models of gram-negative sepsis. In two large randomized, controlled trials involving patients with suspected gram-negative sepsis, benefit has not been shown with either HA-1A or E5 when outcome in all patients was pooled; however, certain subgroups in each study have benefited from these drugs. In the HA-1A study, those patients with gram-negative bacteremia (37% of those enrolled) had improved survival with drug, whether or not they were in shock at the time of enrollment. The most recently conducted HA-1A trial (results were published in early 1993) actually showed a trend toward decreased survival in the treated group. In contrast, E5 is associated with decreased mortality only in those patients with gram-negative bacteremia or focal infection who were not in shock at study entry. Side effects with both agents have been minimal. The major drawbacks to use of all monoclonal antibodies against endotoxin include the anticipated cost ($3000 to $4000) and an inability to identify prospectively those patients who will benefit.

Another approach to blocking the toxic effect of endotoxin is the administration of nontoxic lipid A precursor molecules, which appear to enhance survival of experimental animals with gram-negative bacteremia. Such precursors probably do not compete for receptors with lipid A, but rather block lipid A-induced cytokine release. Other factors such as nonspecific activation of the immune system may also be involved.

Monoclonal antibodies to recombinant TNF-α have been shown to decrease mortality in endotoxin-challenged rats. When infused into humans with severe septic shock, mean arterial blood pressure improved without significant side effects. A controlled trial with this agent is underway. Other monoclonal antibodies under study include antibodies to IL-1, C5a, and adhesion molecules.

A recombinant IL-1 receptor antagonist has been developed that in animal studies decreases mortality associated with endotoxin infusion. A preliminary study in humans has shown decreased mortality in small numbers of patients with both gram-negative and gram-positive bacteremia. However, a recently ongoing larger study was discontinued when the drug failed to demonstrate any benefit. Other similar molecules under study include receptor antagonists to PAF, bradykinin, TNF-α, and thromboxane A_2.

It is currently unclear which, if any, of these biologic products will be available and indicated for use in the near future. Products that bind to the lipid A moiety of endotoxin would not be expected to work after endotoxin has started the release or elaboration of secondary mediators. Theoretically, monoclonal antibodies may even accelerate the uptake of an endotoxin-antibody complex through greater release of cytokines by monocytes and neutrophils. The problem of cost-benefit ratio associated with some of these products has already stimulated spirited debate. By the time of approval, it is hoped that guidelines will be available to assist the physician in choosing among products.

PREVENTION

Because gram-negative bacteremia is a potentially lethal disorder, even with appropriate therapy, prevention is crucial. Simple procedures, such as strict adherence to approved hand-washing techniques and meticulous care of intravascular catheters, are important in decreasing the incidence of nosocomial infection. Moreover, both intravascular and urinary tract (Foley) catheters should be used only when needed and removed as soon as possible. Surgical correction of anatomic defects may be useful in preventing bacteremia in selected patients with recurrent urinary tract infections.

Colonizing oropharyngeal and gastrointestinal bacteria are often implicated in gram-negative infections; hence, strategies to reduce colonization have been attempted. Aerosolized polymyxin B sulfate and endotracheal gentamicin have been shown to decrease colonization; however, resistant organisms may emerge. Other studies have assessed selective decontamination of the digestive tract with topical nonabsorbable antibiotics. Results of these studies are conflicting but a recent study of 445 intubated patients in Europe demonstrated no difference in the incidence of pneumonia or in mortality rates. Finally, prophylactic oral antibiotics are occasionally used to prevent gram-negative infections. Trimethoprim-sulfamethoxazole has been shown to prevent urinary tract infections in renal transplant patients and in patients with recurrent urinary tract infections. This agent and, more recently, quinolones have been used to prevent infections in neutropenic cancer patients.

REFERENCES

Banerjee SN et al: Secular trends in nosocomial primary bloodstream infections in the United States, 1980-1989, Am J Med 91:S86, 1991.

Bone RC et al: A controlled clinical trial of high-dose methylprednisolone in the treatment of severe sepsis and septic shock, N Engl J Med 317:653, 1987.

Bone RC: The pathogenesis of sepsis, Ann Intern Med 115:457, 1991.

Centers for Disease Control: Increase in national hospital discharge survey rates for septicemia—United States, 1979-1987, MMWR 39:31, 1990.

Eykyn SJ, Gransden WR, and Phillips I: The causative organisms of septicaemia and their epidemiology, J Antimicrob Chemother 25:S41, 1990.

Glauser MP et al: Septic shock: pathogenesis, Lancet 338:732, 1991.

Greenman RL et al: A controlled clinical trial of E5 murine monoclonal IgM antibody to endotoxin in the treatment of gram-negative sepsis, JAMA 266:1097, 1991.

Harris RL et al: Manifestations of sepsis, Arch Intern Med 147:1895, 1987.

Kreger BE, Craven DE, and McCabe WR: Gram-negative bacteremia. IV. Re-evaluation of clinical features and treatment in 612 patients, Am J Med 68:344, 1980.

McCabe WR and Jackson GG: Gram-negative bacteremia, Arch Intern Med 110:83, 1962.

McGowan JE: Changing etiology of nosocomial bacteremia and fungemia and other hospital-acquired infections, Rev Infect Dis 7:S357, 1985.

Michie HR et al: Detection of circulating tumor necrosis factor after endotoxin administration, N Engl J Med 318:1481, 1988.

Morris DL et al: Hemodynamic characteristics of patients with hypothermia due to occult infection and other causes, Ann Intern Med 102:153, 1985.

Morrison DC and Ryan JL: Endotoxins and disease mechanisms, Ann Rev Med 38:417, 1987.

Rackow EC and Astiz ME: Pathophysiology and treatment of septic shock, JAMA 266:548, 1991.

Scheckler WE, Scheibel W, and Kresge D: Temporal trends in septicemia in a community hospital, Am J Med 91:S90, 1991.

Schumann RR et al: Structure and function of lipopolysaccharide binding protein, Science. 249:1429, 1990.

Veterans Administration Systemic Sepsis Cooperative Study Group: Effect of high-dose glucocorticoid therapy on mortality in patients with clinical signs of systemic sepsis, N Engl J Med 317:659, 1987.

Wenzel RP et al: Antiendotoxin monoclonal antibodies for gram-negative sepsis: guidelines from the IDSA, Clin Infect Dis 14:973, 1992.

Zeigler EJ et al: Treatment of gram-negative bacteremia and septic shock with HA-1A human monoclonal antibody against endotoxin, N Engl J Med 324:429, 1991.

Zeigler EJ et al: Treatment of gram-negative bacteremia and shock with human antiserum to a mutant *Escherichia coli,* N Engl J Med 307:1225, 1982.

CHAPTER

240 Urinary Tract Infections

Donald Kaye
Allan R. Tunkel
George R. Fournier, Jr.

Infection of the urinary tract indicates the presence of microorganisms (almost always bacteria) within the urinary system. The definitive diagnosis depends on the isolation of these organisms from the urine. Under normal circumstances urine within the bladder is sterile. On voiding, however, it becomes contaminated by the bacterial flora that normally colonize the mucosal surface of the anterior urethra. Other sources of contamination are the vagina and surrounding skin. Therefore in culturing voided urine, it is necessary to make a decision about what numbers of bacteria in the urine indicate probable infection of the urinary tract and which are likely to be due to contamination from the urethra. Although specimens collected by urethral catheterization or suprapubic aspiration more accurately reflect the microbiologic status of the urine, such procedures are invasive and uncomfortable; thus it is usually necessary to rely on cultures of voided urine for diagnosis of urinary tract infection. In the majority of patients with urinary tract infection, voided urine contains at least 10^5 organisms/ml of urine. In contrast, urine from healthy subjects usually contains less than 10^4 organisms/ml of urine. Significant bacteriuria therefore means 10^5 or more organisms/ml of urine. Its presence defines a high probability of the existence of a urinary tract infection. Other studies suggest that a threshold of 10^2 coliform bacteria/ml of urine may be a more sensitive indicator of infection in acutely symptomatic women while yielding only slightly more false-positives than a value of 10^5 organisms/ml. Thresholds of 10^3 and 10^2 organisms/ml have been suggested as significant bacteriuria in symptomatic men and catheterized patients, respectively.

Urinary tract infection includes the clinical entities of *cystitis,* reflecting symptoms related to the bladder and urethra (lower tract), and *pyelonephritis,* reflecting symptoms related to the kidneys (upper tract). Cystitis is associated with the presence of dysuria (Chapter 344), frequency, urgency, and occasionally suprapubic tenderness. Acute pyelonephritis describes the clinical syndrome characterized by flank pain, fever, and flank tenderness and is often associated with dysuria, frequency, and urgency.

It is important to recognize, however, that the correlation between symptoms and the presence of infection can be very poor. Urinary tract infections (upper or lower tract) may be asymptomatic (asymptomatic bacteriuria), and patients with upper tract infection may have only lower tract symptoms. Lower urinary tract symptoms may occur in patients (usually females) with less than 10^5 bacteria/ml of urine. The term *urethral syndrome* has been used to describe this entity. Of patients with urethral syndrome (after excluding vaginitis and herpes as causes of the frequency, urgency, and/or dysuria), some—about one third of sexually active women—are found to have bacteria in bladder urine and therefore have urinary tract infection (presumably lower tract infection); the remaining patients with the urethral syndrome have *Chlamydia trachomatis* (Chapter 254) or less commonly *Neisseria gonorrhoeae* urethritis or symptoms of unknown etiology. *Ureaplasma urealyticum* and noninfectious etiologies of urethritis (trauma, psychological, allergic, and chemical) have been postulated as possible causes. Bacterial urinary tract infection and *C. trachomatis* or *N. gonorrhoeae* urethritis are associated with pyuria (greater than or equal to eight leukocytes/mm^3 uncentrifuged urine), whereas the other causes of the urethral syndrome are not associated with pyuria. Upper tract symptoms may also occur in the absence of infection and may be associated with renal infarction or renal calculi.

A urinary tract infection may occur as a single event or as part of a pattern of recurrent infections. Recurrences may be either relapses or reinfections. The term *relapse* means that the same infecting organism is causing recurrent infection in spite of appropriate therapy and implies that the organism is being harbored somewhere within the urinary tract. Relapses occur within 1 to 2 weeks after stopping antimicrobial therapy and are often associated with renal infection, underlying structural abnormalities of the urinary tract (e.g., stones), or the presence of chronic bacterial prostatitis. In *reinfection,* different organisms cause the recurrence each time; therefore reinfection is a new infection. Occasionally, a reinfection with the same microorganism, which may have persisted in the vagina or feces, may occur within 2 weeks and may be mistaken for a relapse.

The terms *chronic urinary tract infection* and *chronic pyelonephritis* are confusing, meaning different things to different authors. Chronic urinary tract infection literally means a continuing infection, and this definition fits the patient with persistent urinary tract infection who relapses. However, multiple reinfections should not be categorized as "chronic." Chronic pyelonephritis has come to refer to a morphologic appearance of the kidney that may be caused by bacterial infection but is also seen in other disease entities, such as chronic urinary tract obstruction, analgesic nephropathy, and uric acid nephropathy. The situation would be clearer if these morphologic findings, which are really nonspecific, were termed *chronic interstitial nephritis,* with the term *chronic pyelonephritis* reserved for cases with a proven bacteriologic cause.

PATHOGENESIS

Bacteria can presumably gain access to the urinary tract and cause infection through three pathways: through the bloodstream to the kidneys; by lymphatic channels to the kidneys from a possible source in the bowel or pelvis, or by ascending from the urethra into the bladder and then up to the kidneys through the ureters. There is variable clinical and experimental evidence to support each of these pathways. The kidney is frequently a site of abscesses in patients with staphylococcal bacteremia or endocarditis. Experimental pyelonephritis can be induced by intravenous inoculation of large numbers of *Candida, Staphylococcus aureus,* or enterococci. It is difficult, however, to produce pyelonephritis in animals by the intravenous injection of gram-negative bacilli (the organisms that usually cause infection in humans) unless the kidney is manipulated in some way to produce either extrarenal or intrarenal obstruction (e.g., by ureteral ligation or renal cautery). Extrapolating this evidence to humans, together with clinical observations, suggests that pyelonephritis caused by gram-negative organisms rarely occurs by the hematogenous route.

The role of lymphatic spread of bacteria in the pathogenesis of pyelonephritis is based on indirect (and tenuous) evidence consisting of the demonstration in animals of lymphatic connections between the upper and lower urinary tracts and the possible existence of lymphatic channels between the colon and right kidney.

Most clinical and experimental evidence clearly supports the ascending pathway in the vast majority of urinary tract infections. Organisms that cause urinary tract infection in women usually colonize the vaginal introitus and periurethral area from a fecal reservoir before urinary tract infection occurs. The female urethra, by virtue of its anatomic location in proximity to the warm, moist vulvar and perirectal areas, is very prone to contamination; and its short length provides easy access to the bladder. Men appear to be relatively immune to ascending infection because of the male urethra's obviously different anatomic location and also perhaps because of prostatic secretions that exhibit antibacterial activity. These facts may help explain the much higher incidence of urinary tract infections in females as compared with males. Further clinical evidence for the importance of the ascending route is provided by the fact that urethral catheters with open drainage systems result in urinary tract infections in essentially all patients within 96 hours. Presumably, bacteria enter the bladder by moving up through the lumen of the catheter from the collecting bag or along the exudative material between the urethral mucosa and catheter.

Colonization of the periurethral areas and subsequent urinary tract infection depend on an interplay between the infecting organism and the host defense mechanisms. Inoculum size certainly is important, having a positive correlation with the risk of infection. Certain virulence factors have been identified in bacteria. The presence of fimbriae has been demonstrated to be important for attachment of *Proteus mirabilis* and *Escherichia coli* to urinary tract epithelium. These hairlike structures project outward from the organism and contain highly specific polysaccharides that attach to specialized receptors on the uroepithelium. The adhesins most commonly and specifically expressed by pyelonephritic strains of *E. coli* are P and S fimbriae, whereas type 1 fimbriae appear to play a more important role in colonization of the vagina, perineum, and bladder. Changes in just one simple sugar render the organism unable to attach and avirulent in producing urinary tract infections. Bacterial lipopolysaccharide likely plays an important role in inducing the local inflammatory response and in producing constitutional symptoms and signs during both cystitis and pyelonephritis. *E. coli* organisms possessing high quantities of certain K antigens (K1, K2, K5, and K13 or K51) appear to be more virulent pathogens than other *E. coli* strains, as they are more likely to infect the kidney. Resistance to serum bactericidal activity, presence of aerobactin, and hemolysin production are other potentially important virulence factors. Bacterial production of urease has also been shown to increase the risk of pyelonephritis in experimental animals. Urease production, together with the presence of bacterial motility and fimbriae, may favor the production of upper tract infection by organisms such as *Proteus*.

The host in turn possesses mechanisms that defend against bacterial invasion. The urine is a good but variable culture medium. Anaerobic bacteria and other fastidious organisms that make up most of the normal urethral flora do not generally multiply well in urine. Extremes in urine osmolality, a low pH, and a high urea concentration inhibit growth of many bacteria. The bladder mucosa appears to have its own intrinsic antibacterial defense mechanisms. Uromucoid or urinary slime (Tamm-Horsfall protein) rich in mannose residues avidly binds *E. coli* and may prevent attachment of *E. coli* to uroepithelial cells; the increased risk of urinary infection in the elderly has been attributed, in part, to the lower urinary excretion rates of Tamm-Horsfall protein found in the elderly. Natural antiadherence mechanisms have also been identified in the bladders of several animal species (dogs, rabbits, rats, and mice). These mechanisms can be reversed after brief treatment of the bladder with dilute hydrochloric acid, supporting the concept of a superficial acid-sensitive natural antiadherence mechanism. Further information is needed, however, to precisely define the importance of antiadherence mechanisms as defense mechanisms against urinary tract infections. In addition, the flushing mechanism of the bladder is an important defense mechanism. Urine flow first dilutes the bacterial inoculum, and then voiding flushes it from the bladder. Any interference with normal voiding, such as obstruction, the presence of a foreign body, or incomplete bladder emptying, can compromise these bladder defense mechanisms and lead to bacterial retention and multiplication.

The different regions of the kidney have different susceptibilities to infection. Animal studies have shown that the medulla is generally much more susceptible to bacterial infection than the cortex. This same susceptibility correlates with human kidney disease in which the earliest lesions occur in the renal pelvis, with an area of inflammation and exudate extending from the pelvis and medulla to the cortex in a triangular wedge. This particular vulnerability of the medulla has been attributed to the high concentration of ammonia, which may inactivate complement, and to high osmolality, low pH, and low blood flow, which inhibit leukocyte mobilization to the area.

PATHOLOGY

Morphologically, the acutely infected kidney may be enlarged, with small abscesses scattered throughout the parenchyma. Abscesses that occur beneath the capsule give the surface a studded, nodular appearance. They may coalesce, producing a renal carbuncle that can perforate through the capsule and result in a perinephric abscess. The pelvis appears hemorrhagic and ulcerated. An intense neutrophilic infiltrate surrounds the tubules and eventually produces areas of necrosis. White cell casts may be found within the tubules and become hallmarks for the laboratory diagnoses of acute pyelonephritis when they are detected in the voided urine. Generally, the glomeruli and blood vessels are spared in the acute inflammatory process.

The circulation to the most distal part of the medulla and papilla is easily compromised. In certain populations—specifically patients with diabetes mellitus, sickle cell disease, or chronic obstruction or analgesic abusers—vascular disease is present and can lead to ischemia and infarction of the papilla. In these patients, papillary necrosis can become a serious complication of acute pyelonephritis (and can also occur in the absence of infection). The papilla may slough, with the remnant being voided in the urine. The papilla can also obstruct, producing renal colic, oliguria, and suppurative hydronephrosis. Death may follow from rapidly progressive renal insufficiency or bacteremia.

Chronic pyelonephritis is characterized morphologically by caliceal dilatation and cortical scarring. Involvement of the kidney is focal and unequal, and kidney size may be variable, ranging from large (early) to small shrunken kidneys (late). Microscopically, lymphocytes, plasma cells, and macrophages are present in the interstitium. The tubules are atrophied and dilated and may be filled with casts, giving the appearance of thyroid tissue. The glomeruli and blood vessels are spared until late in the disease course, when the glomeruli exhibit sclerosis, and fibrotic thickening of the intima of the small arteries develops. As mentioned previously, these morphologic changes are nonspecific and have multiple causes. In a strict sense, the term *chronic pyelonephritis* should be applied only to patients in whom past or present infection can be documented.

Most patients in whom urinary tract infections develop have anatomically and functionally normal urinary tracts, but many predisposing factors increase the risk that infection will develop. Obstruction to urine flow with impairment of normal bladder function and stasis within the urinary system is the most important factor. It markedly increases the risk of urinary tract infection from the hematogenous as well as the ascending route. Obstruction can be caused by any number of factors. Extrarenal obstruction may be the result of (1) congenital anomalies of the ureters or urethra (valves, bands); (2) calculi (which also harbor bacteria, making eradication of infection extremely difficult); (3) extrinsic ureteral compression; and (4) an enlarged prostate gland. Obstruction may also be intrarenal in conditions such as nephrocalcinosis, uric acid nephropathy, polycystic kidney disease, and scars. Males of any age appear to be much more prone to obstructive lesions of the urinary tract than are women.

The importance of vesicoureteral reflux in the pathogenesis of urinary tract infection and the development of subsequent renal damage has become apparent in recent years. Reflux of contaminated urine from the bladder provides a direct route to the pelvicaliceal system and obviously predisposes to ascent of infection. Reflux also tends to perpetuate infection by maintaining a residual pool of infected urine in the bladder after voiding. Reflux, most common in young children, can be due to a congenital abnormality or to bladder overdistention, such as occurs in bladder outlet obstruction. In children and young adult women, it can be caused by bladder infection alone, the inflammation and edema inhibiting the competency of a marginally competent vesicoureteral junction. Reflux in the presence of infection in a child is associated with development of renal scarring and lack of growth of the kidney. Infants and preschool-aged children are at the highest risk for developing renal damage. These children may have severe degrees of reflux, which may eventually cause enough scarring to lead to end-stage renal disease. The progression of scars or the development of new ones becomes less common after the age of 5 years and is rare after full growth of the kidney. There is thus a population of patients (infant or preschool-aged) in whom bacteriuria and reflux can produce significant renal damage. On the other hand, it is clear that sterile reflux per se can result in renal scarring. Reflux tends to decrease with the treatment of bacteriuria, and mild to moderate degrees disappear over time, even with persistent infection, probably because of the maturation of the vesicoureteral junction. Progressive renal disease rarely develops in adults in association with urinary tract infections, except in the presence of obstruction or other significant renal disease that in itself can cause renal damage.

BACTERIOLOGY

Enterobacteriaceae are the most common pathogens involved in urinary tract infection. *E. coli* is responsible for the vast majority (85%) of the cases of acute urinary tract infection. Patients with recurrent infections, those with structural abnormalities of the urinary tract, those who have had urethral instrumentation, and those whose infections were acquired in the hospital have an increased frequency of infection caused by *Proteus, Klebsiella-Enterobacter* species, *Pseudomonas,* enterococci, and staphylococci. *E. coli* accounts for about 50% of urinary tract infections in hospitalized patients. Generally, gram-positive organisms are much less important as causes of urinary tract infection than are gram-negative bacilli. When *S. aureus* causes infection, the illness may be acute, and renal infection may be secondary to bacteremia. Coagulase-negative staphylococci (usually *S. saprophyticus*) currently account for up to 10% to 15% urinary tract infections, mainly in young, sexually active females. Anaerobic organisms rarely cause urinary tract infection.

EPIDEMIOLOGY

As previously stated, urinary tract infection is much more common in females than in males. It is interesting to note, however, that infant males have a higher prevalence of infection than do infant females. In one study, the prevalence of bacteriuria was 2.7% in male infants, with no bacteriuria or pyuria found in females. This higher frequency is presumably secondary to the higher incidence of anomalies of the urinary tract in male infants. In addition, studies have suggested that uncircumcised male infants are more likely than circumcised infants to have urinary tract infections during the first year of life. After infancy, the prevalence of urinary tract infection in males drops to less than 0.1% until the ages when prostatic disease occurs. In these later years, the prevalence of urinary tract infection in men increases to 4% to 10%.

Urinary tract infection in males is frequently associated with urologic abnormalities. However, a small number of men between 20 and 50 years suffer acute, uncomplicated urinary tract infections. The exact reason for such infections is unclear, but possible explanations are homosexual intercourse and intercourse with a female partner who has a urinary tract infection.

In males with infection, it is usually important to evaluate for structural abnormalities of the urinary tract. Ultrasonography should be performed to rule out nephrolithiasis and obstructive uropathy. Further evaluation, including intravenous pyelography with postvoiding views of the bladder, cystoscopy, and radionuclide evaluation utilizing DPTA technetium may also be necessary. When infection is eradicated in a man, he tends not to become infected again unless there is catheterization or instrumentation of the urethra.

At least 10% to 20% of the female population have a symptomatic urinary tract infection sometime during their lives, and up to one third of elderly women have asymptomatic urinary tract infections when populations are screened. During the preschool years, the period prevalence (i.e., percentage with infection sometime during the preschool years) of significant bacteriuria has been reported to be 4.5% for girls and 0.5% for boys. Infection during this period is often symptomatic, and it is believed that much of the renal damage that occurs from infection in both males and females occurs at this time.

Bacteriuria is common in females of school age, is often asymptomatic, and frequently recurs. The prevalence of bacteriuria is about 1%, and about 5% of schoolgirls have significant bacteriuria at least once before leaving high school. Each year on resurvey, about 25% of those reported as infected in the previous year's survey are cured either spontaneously or with antibiotics but are replaced by an equal number in whom bacteriuria has developed. The same girls tend to have multiple reinfections. Thus the prevalence remains the same from year to year. Within 3 months after marriage, over 50% of the women who had childhood bacteriuria have bacteriuria again. From these data it appears that in women, bacteriuria in childhood defines a population at increased risk for the development of bacteriuria in later life.

Once adulthood is reached, the prevalence of bacteriuria increases in the female population, the increase being positively correlated with increasing age and parity. Sexual activity is associated with an increased risk of urinary tract infection and probably plays a permissive role in facilitating inoculation of bladder urine with urethral flora. Recently, it has been demonstrated that use of the diaphragm with spermicidal jelly or use of spermicidal foam with a condom markedly alters normal vaginal flora and strongly predisposes users to developing vaginal colonization and *E. coli* bacteriuria.

The prevalence of bacteriuria in young nonpregnant women is about 1% to 3%, rising to 33% in elderly women. On yearly resurveys of populations, bacteriuria has cleared in about 25% of bacteriuric women, and they are replaced by an equal number who have become infected. The same women tend to become infected repeatedly. Therefore, it is apparent that "cure" of urinary tract infection in a female applies only to the episode being treated. It is likely that it will be followed by future infections.

The prevalence of asymptomatic bacteriuria during pregnancy ranges from 4% to 7%, with much of the bacteriuria already present during the first trimester. Symptomatic pyelonephritis develops during pregnancy in about 20% to 40% of bacteriuric patients. Most cases of acute pyelonephritis can be prevented by treating and eliminating asymptomatic bacteriuria in the early stages of pregnancy. This fact is very significant, not only because of the decrease in maternal morbidity but also because of the apparent association between acute pyelonephritis of pregnancy and an increased frequency of premature delivery and infant morbidity and mortality. Asymptomatic bacteriuria per se may also increase the frequency of prematurity and fetal wastage. Therefore it seems justified to screen for urinary tract infection in pregnancy and to treat bacteriuria in pregnant women.

CLINICAL SYMPTOMS AND DIAGNOSIS

The manifestations of urinary tract infections in adults are usually easy to recognize. The lower tract symptoms result from inflammation and irritation of the urethral and bladder mucosa, causing frequent and painful urination of small amounts of turbid urine. Patients sometimes complain of suprapubic heaviness or pain. Occasionally, the urine is blood tinged or grossly bloody, reflecting damage to superficial blood vessels in the bladder mucosa. Fever tends to be absent, with infection limited to the lower tract. The classic clinical manifestations of upper tract involvement include fever, sometimes accompanied by chills, flank pain, flank tenderness, and often by lower tract symptoms of frequency, urgency, and dysuria. The lower tract symptoms may antedate the appearance of fever and upper tract symptoms by 1 or 2 days. Pain from the kidney can occasionally be localized near the epigastrium and can radiate to one of the lower quadrants.

As previously mentioned, there can be a poor correlation between symptoms and the presence of infection. About 40% of sexually active females presenting with lower tract symptoms have the urethral syndrome with sterile urine or insignificant bacteriuria. Only about one third of these patients have urinary tract infection; the rest have urethritis caused by *Chlamydia* (Chapter 254) or other infectious or noninfectious etiologies. There is also a poor correlation between symptoms and signs and the site of infection. About one third of patients with no symptoms or with only symptoms of cystitis have renal bacteriuria.

The definitive diagnosis of a urinary tract infection depends on the isolation of bacteria from the urine in significant numbers. Microscopic examination of the urine can be helpful. The presence of at least one bacterium per high power field in a properly collected midstream clean-catch, Gram-stained, uncentrifuged urine correlates with 10^5 or more bacteria/ml of urine (i.e., significant bacteriuria). The absence of bacteria in several fields of a stained sedimented specimen indicates the probability of less than 10^4 bacteria/ml and is evidence against significant bacteriuria.

The major reason for obtaining a urine culture before therapy in a woman with apparent lower urinary tract infection is to detect those with the urethral syndrome (who will have $<10^5$ bacteria/ml urine). In this group are patients with chlamydial urethritis, which often has more serious implications than urinary tract infection (Chapter 254). Therefore if significant bacteriuria is present by microscopic examination, it is reasonable in the nonpregnant adult female with lower tract symptoms to take a culture only if symptoms do not respond to therapy or recur after therapy is discontinued. Isolates can then be submitted for antimicrobial susceptibility testing.

The presence or absence of pyuria, as defined by at least 5 to 10 leukocytes per high power field in sedimented urine, correlates poorly with bacteriuria. About 20% of urine samples with pyuria have less than 10^5 bacteria/ml. Conversely, about 30% of the specimens with at least 10^5 bacteria/ml do not have increased numbers of white cells. However, the vast majority of patients with symptomatic infection have pyuria. According to a stricter definition of pyuria (at least 10 leukocytes/mm^3 of midstream urine), the vast majority of patients with either symptomatic or asymptomatic bacteriuria will have pyuria; however, pyuria without infection remains common.

The measurement of pyuria has been simplified by the use of a rapid assay to determine the presence in the urine of leukocyte esterase, an enzyme found in primary neutrophil granules. The assay is a reasonable method to quickly determine the presence of significant pyuria, and it is used most appropriately as a screening test to determine the need for urine cultures in symptomatic patients for whom routine microscopy is either unavailable or impractical.

White cell casts in the presence of urinary tract infection are strong evidence for pyelonephritis. Although mild proteinuria is common in urinary tract infections, excretion of 3 g or more of protein in 24 hours suggests the presence of glomerular disease and should not be attributed to infection alone. Occasionally, microscopic or gross hematuria is seen in the urine of patients with infection, reflecting hemorrhagic cystitis. Red cells, however, may indicate other disorders, such as the presence of calculi, vasculitis, glomerulonephritis, or renal tuberculosis.

Interpretation of a culture depends on both the clinical setting and the manner in which the specimen was obtained. The standard urine culture in most laboratories is performed on midstream, clean-catch specimens collected in sterile containers. In women, the external genitalia are washed two to three times with a cleaning agent to reduce urethral contamination. This cleaning procedure is of questionable value in men, although it is widely practiced. After collection, specimens should be processed expeditiously. A urine specimen that is allowed to sit at room temperature for several hours may yield falsely elevated bacterial colony counts. Counts of bacteria are relatively stable for up to 24 hours when urine is stored at 4° C.

In general, there are two separate but overlapping populations. One has bacterial counts between 0 and 10^4 bacteria/ml of urine, which usually represents contamination. The second, which represents true bacteriuria, has counts of more than 10^5 bacteria/ml. The two populations overlap mainly between 10^4 and 10^5 bacteria/ml. If there are more than 10^5 bacteria/ml in a clean-catch urine specimen from an asymptomatic female, there is an 80% probability that this represents true bacteriuria. If two different specimens demonstrate at least 10^5 of the same bacterium per milliliter, the probability increases to 95%. Thus two clean-catch specimens should be obtained in an asymptomatic female to confirm the diagnosis. In a symptomatic patient, one titer of 10^5/ml or more is sufficient to establish the diagnosis. When the number of bacteria per milliliter is between 10^4 and 10^5 in an asymptomatic female, a confirmatory second specimen (preferably a first-voided morning specimen) will contain 10^5 bacteria/ml in only 5% of instances. Thus 95% of the time, titers between 10^4 and 10^5 bacteria/ml represent contamination. However, in males, in whom contamination is less likely, a titer of 10^4 organisms/ml is more suggestive of infection. These criteria apply only to the Enterobacteriaceae. Gram-positive organisms, fungi, and bacteria with fastidious growth requirements may not reach titers of 10^5/ml in patients with infection and may be in the range of 10^4 to 10^5/ml. Isolation of Enterobacteriaceae in low-titer counts (e.g., 10 to 10^4/ml) in patients with frequency, urgency, and dysuria (i.e., the urethral syndrome) usually indicates lower tract infection caused by these organisms.

Localization of infection

Several methods have been used to localize the site of infection in the urinary system. One method involves inserting an indwelling catheter and sterilizing the bladder by washing it with antibiotic solutions. Serial quantitative urine cultures are then taken at frequent intervals through the catheter. Because all bacteria previously in the bladder have theoretically been killed, organisms found in the early serial specimens will have collected in the bladder from the ureters, thus localizing infection to the upper tract. Another method involves direct catheterization of the ureters for quantitative cultures. These two methods, though reliable, are invasive techniques and not routinely recommended.

A noninvasive technique has been developed based on the fact that bacteria in urine of renal origin are coated with antibody. Fluorescein-conjugated antihuman globulin is added to the bacteriuric urine, and the urine is examined under a fluorescence microscope. Fluorescence indicates antibody-coated bacteria and usually correlates with upper tract infection. The predictive value of associating a positive test for fluorescence with upper tract infection is 88% as established by several studies. The predictive value of associating a negative test with bladder infection is 76%. The relatively high false-positive and false-negative rates render this test useful mainly for clinical studies and not for management of individual patients. False-positive results may be observed in children, in men with a prostatic focus of infection, in women whose urine becomes contaminated with vaginal contents, in men and women with proteinuria, and with hemorrhagic cystitis, bladder tumors, bladder stones, indwelling catheters, and organisms that fluoresce even if not coated (e.g., yeasts and pseudomonads). False-negative results may be observed in children, in early acute pyelonephritis, and with inability of antibody to combine with certain bacteria (e.g., mucoid-coated pseudomonads).

MANAGEMENT

All antimicrobial agents have side effects, and the associated possible morbidity must be weighed against the anticipated benefit to the patient. Infections in nonpregnant adult (especially elderly) women are characterized by their frequency and propensity to reinfect and/or relapse. The prognosis in this population is good in that progressive renal impairment and damage are rare after recurrent infections except when there is obstruction or other underlying abnormality that by itself can cause damage. Although several studies have demonstrated increased mortality (not resulting from renal failure) in patients with asymptomatic bacteriuria, a cause-effect relationship has not been demonstrated. Furthermore, other studies have not confirmed increased mortality. The increased mortality, if real, may be related to the increased frequency of bacteriuria in patients more prone to both bacteriuria and to death, such as those with dementia or those who are bedridden. No study has demonstrated decreased mortality resulting from treatment of patients with asymptomatic bacteriuria. With present information, considering that the cost and toxicity of antimicrobial therapy may be more significant than the infection itself, therapy may not be warranted in the nonpregnant woman who presents with asymptomatic bacteriuria. It is necessary, however, to treat symptomatic patients to relieve their symptoms even though infection may recur.

In contrast to the benign course in nonpregnant women, bacteriuria in preschool-aged children of either sex (and to a lesser degree in older children) can result in significant morbidity, with impaired kidney growth, scar formation, and even renal insufficiency. Similarly, in pregnant women, bacteriuria has significant consequences for the health of the newborn. Therapy in children and pregnant women is beneficial and should be aggressively undertaken.

Bacteriuria in males is uncommon except in the elderly, as previously described, and its presence implies a structural abnormality of the urinary system (e.g., obstruction). These patients therefore must have a diagnostic workup for structural abnormalities. Children and males of any age experiencing their first episode of urinary tract infection, and women who have a relapse after appropriate therapy, are at risk of urologic abnormalities and should have an intravenous pyelogram and a postevacuation view of the bladder to evaluate for residual urine. Ultrasonography studies and/or radionuclide evaluation utilizing DTPA technetium may also be sufficient. These studies are unnecessary in women with their first episode of urinary tract infection, but after three or four reinfections, evaluation may be indicated.

Management of urinary tract infection (Fig. 240-1) includes nonspecific and specific antimicrobial therapy. Forcing fluids has been advocated as a part of therapy. Theoretically, hydration results in a rapid reduction of bacterial counts and flushes bacteria from the bladder. It also decreases renal medullary hypertonicity, thus enhancing leu-

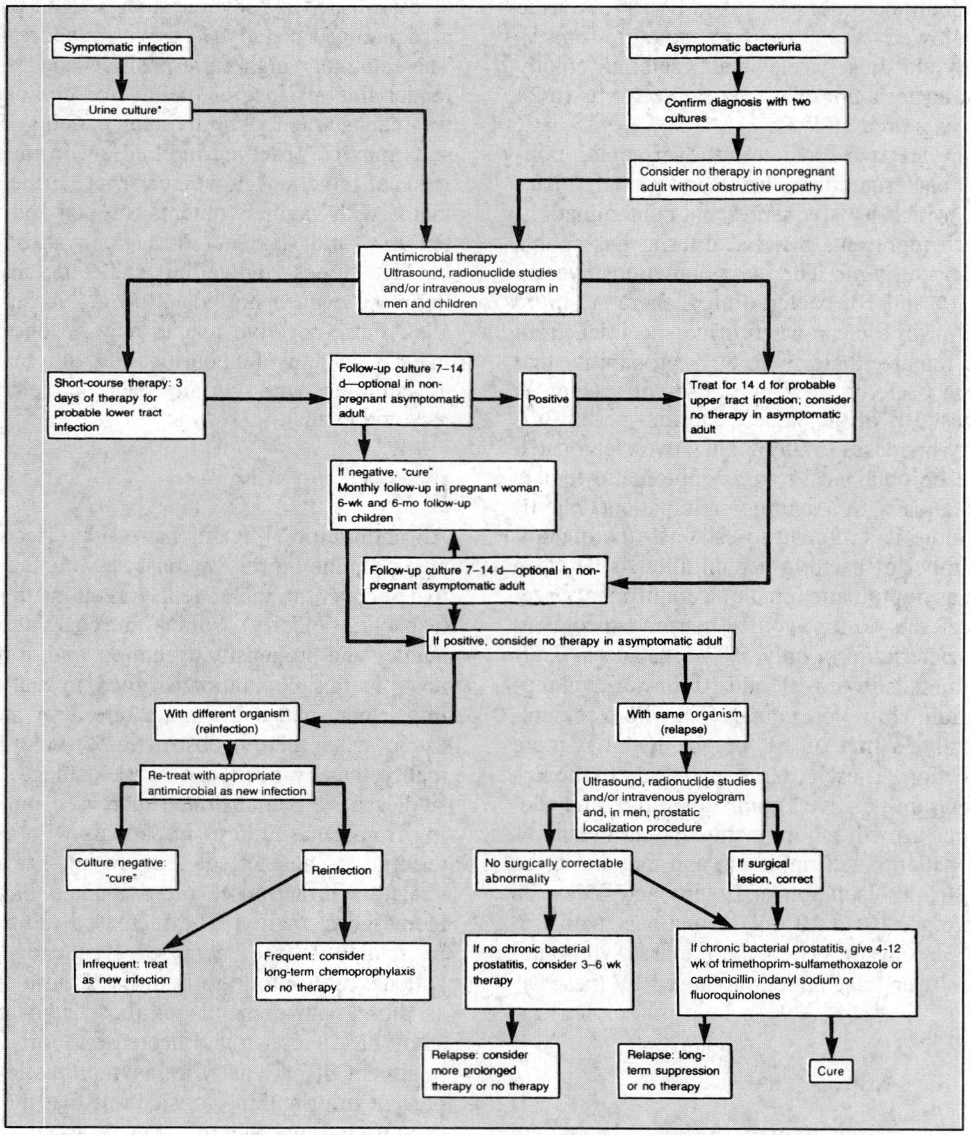

Fig. 240-1. Management of urinary tract infections.* Not mandatory in women with only lower tract symptoms.

kocyte migration to the area. It may, however, hinder therapy by producing increased urine output, thereby lowering urinary concentrations of antimicrobial agents. Because there is no evidence that hydration improves the results of appropriate antimicrobial therapy, its routine use is not recommended.

Changing the urinary pH has also been recommended as an adjunct to therapy. Lowering urinary pH enhances the antibacterial activity of urine by increasing the concentration of undissociated molecules of organic acids normally found in urine. The undissociated molecules probably penetrate better into the bacterial cell than do those in the ionized form present at a high pH. Urinary pH also affects the activity of many chemotherapeutic agents. The activity of methenamine mandelate, methenamine hippurate, and nitrofurantoin is increased at low urinary pH, whereas the aminoglycoside antibiotics are more effective at an alkaline pH. However, pH change is not necessary or even desirable except when methenamine mandelate or methenamine hippurate is used. For these agents to be effective, the urinary pH must be maintained at 5.5 or less. Acidification can be achieved by the use of ascorbic acid or methionine; by a modification of diet; and by restricting milk, sodium bicarbonate, and fruit juices except for cranberry juice; cranberry juice increases the urinary concentration of hippuric acid, which has antibacterial activity at low urine pH. Urinary acidification can be difficult to achieve and can cause precipitation of urate stones. Urinary analgesics, for example phenazopyridine hydrochloride (Pyridium), have little place in the routine management of symptomatic infections. The dysuria usually responds rapidly to antibacterial therapy.

Selection of an appropriate antibiotic has become complex because of the increasing number of compounds available. Ideally, the agent chosen should not affect anaerobic bacteria (to avoid *Candida* vaginitis and *C. difficile* colitis) and should have low toxicity. There is no evidence to support any superiority of bactericidal over bacteriostatic drugs. It is also important to note that the correlation between the response of bacteriuria and inhibitory blood levels of antimicrobial agents is poor. In contrast, inhibitory urine levels are essential. Many oral antimicrobial agents in the dosages commonly used for urinary tract infection do not achieve serum levels above the minimum inhibitory concentration for most urinary pathogens. Yet these agents are effective because concentration in the urine results in high urinary levels. Achieving blood levels therefore does not seem to be important in treating most urinary tract infections, although adequate blood levels are necessary in bacteremia. In patients with renal insufficiency, dosage modifications are necessary for agents that are excreted primarily by the kidneys and cannot be cleared by any other mechanism. In renal failure, there is also an inability of the kidney to concentrate antibiotics in the urine, making it difficult to eradicate bacteriuria. This fact may be a particularly important factor when using aminoglycosides, but with the penicillins and cephalosporins, adequate urine concentrations are generally attained in spite of impaired renal function.

Symptomatic urinary tract infection

Most patients with symptomatic urinary tract infection are women of childbearing age. The onset of symptoms is frequently related to sexual intercourse. No one chemotherapeutic agent is unequivocally the drug of choice in these patients. Some useful agents are ampicillin, amoxicillin, cephalexin, tetracycline, trimethoprim-sulfamethoxazole, trimethoprim alone, norfloxacin, ciprofloxacin, ofloxacin, and nitrofurantoin. Effective therapy will result in a marked decrease in bacterial titers within 48 hours after the onset of treatment. Many of the organisms commonly causing community-acquired urinary tract infections are now resistant to amoxicillin. Amoxicillin-clavulanic acid, trimethoprim-sulfamethoxazole, and the newer fluoroquinolones are active against the great majority of these organisms. Trimethoprim-sulfamethoxazole and the fluoroquinolones have the added advantage of having poor activity against the anaerobic flora of the vagina and gut.

A symptomatic response can be an unreliable index of efficacy, as symptoms can abate spontaneously without chemotherapy, although bacteriuria persists. In patients with pyelonephritis severe enough for hospitalization and when gram-negative bacillary bacteremia is suspected by the presence of high fever, shaking chills, and/or hypotension, antibiotic therapy should be parenteral and must have activity against all potential pathogens (Chapter 239).

Evidence has accumulated that upper urinary tract infection requires more prolonged therapy than lower tract infection. A number of workers have demonstrated that with infections limited to the lower urinary tract, single doses of antibacterial therapy have been sufficient to eradicate bacteriuria in women. To date, a number of agents (i.e., various sulfonamides, kanamycin, amoxicillin, trimethoprim-sulfamethoxazole, and trimethoprim alone) have been shown to be effective in single-dose regimens. It is likely that short courses of any antimicrobial agent active against the infecting organism will be effective in lower urinary tract infection. In patients with lower tract infection, 1 to 3 days of therapy or, in fact, only one dose (e.g., 3 g of amoxicillin or four tablets of regular strength trimethoprim-sulfamethoxazole) is usually sufficient for cure. It seems reasonable therefore to treat patients who have only lower tract symptoms (i.e., no fever, flank pain, or flank tenderness) with such short-term therapy. In contrast to lower tract infection, patients with upper tract infection require at least 2 weeks of treatment. We use 3 days of therapy rather than single doses as short-course therapy. Three days may cure some unsuspected upper tract infection and is more likely to eliminate the organism from the gut and vagina, decreasing the risk of reinfection.

Urine cultures should be obtained in all children, all men, and women with upper tract symptoms or fever before initiating therapy. Cultures are not mandatory in women with lower tract symptoms.

A follow-up urine culture may be obtained 1 to 2 weeks after the discontinuance of therapy to detect relapses. A patient who relapses after short-course therapy may have upper tract infection, and a 2-week course is indicated. In children and pregnant women, follow-up cultures should be obtained again at 6 weeks and 6 months (children) or monthly (pregnant women) to detect reinfections. In the nonpregnant adult who remains asymptomatic after therapy, a follow-up culture is probably not cost-effective.

Asymptomatic bacteriuria

Most patients with asymptomatic bacteriuria are women, usually in the older age group, with reinfection (and occasionally relapse) occurring very commonly after therapy. As previously discussed, potentially toxic and expensive therapy in this type of patient must be weighed against the apparently benign nature of the infection. In general, asymptomatic bacteriuria in the elderly should not be treated, particularly in view of the high rate of reinfection or relapse, and the high rate of adverse drug reactions in this population. If there are pressing reasons to treat asymptomatic bacteriuria, short-course therapy with a nontoxic antibiotic (e.g., a penicillin or cephalosporin) should be the first approach.

Asymptomatic infection in children, pregnant women, and adults with evidence of obstruction should not be ignored because of the associated morbidity. These patients should be managed as described for symptomatic infection, with initial therapy directed at lower tract infection (i.e., short-course therapy).

Relapsing urinary tract infection

If there is a relapse after appropriate antimicrobial therapy, renal infection (the usual cause of relapse in women), a structural abnormality of the urinary tract such as stone or obstruction, or chronic bacterial prostatitis must be considered. The ultimate success of therapy in the presence of a significant abnormality depends on its correction. Many recurrent infections in men are relapses, presumably because of a persistent focus in the prostate (i.e., chronic bacterial prostatitis). These patients usually have no prostatic signs or symptoms but have recurrent urinary tract infections, always with the same organism. Recurrences of urinary tract infection may be frequent or as infrequent as every several months.

In all patients who have a relapse, an investigation for structural abnormalities should be considered with radiographic evaluation and, in males, an attempt to diagnose chronic bacterial prostatitis should be made using a quantitative bacterial localization technique (see Chronic Bacterial Prostatis later in the chapter).

Women without structural abnormalities who have a relapse (presumably from a renal focus) have a higher cure rate with long courses of therapy. In a woman who has a relapse after a 14-day course and who has no structural abnormalities, a more prolonged course (e.g., 3 to 6 weeks) should be considered. Even longer-term therapy (e.g., 6 weeks to 6 months) may be given but only in selected patients, such as adults with continuous symptoms or those who are at high risk for the development of renal damage, such as children. Asymptomatic adults without obstruction probably should not receive these longer courses. If bacteriuria persists or relapses during chemotherapy, indicating the development of resistance, the antimicrobial agent should be changed. All patients should be followed with urine cultures every 1 to 2 months while on therapy. The chemotherapeutic agents that can be used for long-term therapy include ampicillin, amoxicillin, sulfisoxazole, cephalexin, trimethoprim-sulfamethoxazole, trimethoprim alone, nitrofurantoin, carbenicillin indanyl sodium, norfloxacin, ciprofloxacin, and ofloxacin.

Trimethoprim-sulfamethoxazole is effective therapy for chronic bacterial prostatitis because of its superior penetration into the noninflamed prostate. Oral carbenicillin indanyl sodium may also be useful. Nevertheless, only about a third of patients with chronic bacterial prostatitis can be cured with these agents, even with 12-week courses. The newer fluoroquinolones are also concentrated in the noninflamed prostate and are useful in chronic bacterial prostatitis. Patients with chronic bacterial prostatitis or relapsing urinary tract infection who are not cured can be managed by treating each flare-up of urinary tract infection or by daily low-dose suppressive therapy with an agent that is active against the infecting organism.

Reinfection of urinary tract

Patients with reinfections can be divided into two groups: those who have relatively infrequent reinfections, perhaps every 2 to 3 years or up to several times each year, and those in whom frequent reinfections develop. Of recurrent urinary tract infections in women, 80% are reinfections. Reinfections are uncommon in men. Patients with infrequent reinfections can be treated with a short course of therapy for each recurrence as a new episode of infection.

Many patients with frequent reinfections are middle-aged or elderly women with infection limited to the lower urinary tract. Most asymptomatic reinfections in this group need not be treated. If, however, the episodes are very frequent and symptomatic, or if there is the likelihood of renal damage (i.e., the presence of uncorrectable obstruction), these patients should be treated on a long-term basis. Long-term therapy should also be instituted in children because of the risk of the development of renal parenchymal damage. This approach is actually prophylactic and is aimed at decreasing the number of reinfections. Trimethoprim-sulfamethoxazole and nitrofurantoin are particularly useful agents for long-term prophylaxis, because, with prolonged use, they are unlikely to allow the emergence of antimicrobial-resistant bacteria in the periurethral area. Trimethoprim-sulfamethoxazole also has the ability to penetrate into vaginal secretions, helping prevent colonization of the periurethral area with bacteria from a fecal source. As little as 40 mg of trimethoprim and 200 mg of sulfamethoxazole (half of a regular-strength tablet) three times a week at bedtime is effective in preventing recurrent infection. Patients receiving long-term prophylaxis should be followed with urine cultures every 1 to 2 months. Therapy is continued with the same agent as long as the patient remains abacteriuric. If bacteriuria persists or recurs, the therapy should be altered, using the response of the bacteriuria as the criterion of efficacy.

Most authorities advocate a 6-month trial of prophylaxis, after which the regimen is discontinued and the patient observed for further infection. Others have advocated a longer period of prophylaxis of 2 years or more in women who continue to have symptomatic infections. Use of trimethoprim, trimethoprim-sulfamethoxazole, or nitrofurantoin for as long as 5 years has been reported to be effective and well tolerated. Some women, however, do not want to take antimicrobial agents over an extended period of time. If such women are reliable and have clearly documented recurrent infections, they may be candidates for self-administration of a single-dose or 3-day antimicrobial regimen at the onset of symptoms of urinary tract infection.

In some women, symptomatic reinfections are associated with sexual activity. These episodes may be prevented by voiding within 15 minutes after intercourse and/or by the administration of a single dose of an antimicrobial agent immediately before or after coitus.

PREVENTION

Catheterization of the urinary bladder should be avoided if possible (Chapter 225). The risk of infection after a single catheterization in an ambulatory patient is about 1% but is higher in elderly or debilitated patients, patients with urologic abnormalities, and pregnant women. Patients with indwelling catheters have a much greater risk of infection. Infection will develop within 4 days in essentially all patients with an open drainage system. The use of a triple-lumen catheter with a continuous rinse of neomycin plus polymyxin B or use of a closed sterile drainage system will delay the development of bacteriuria for up to 10 days in most patients. One of these systems should be used when an indwelling catheter cannot be avoided. Other alternatives include intermittent catheterization by insertion of a sterile or clean catheter every 3 to 6 hours for periodic bladder emptying, and suprapubic catheterization, which yields lower rates of bacteriuria because of the lower density of bacteria on the anterior abdominal skin than the urethra. Catheters coated or impregnated with silver ions, which are bactericidal, have shown reduced incidence of catheter-associated urinary tract infections in some studies but not others.

Although it is possible to eradicate urinary tract infection with antimicrobial therapy in the presence of a sterile drainage system, reinfection is the rule. The patient in whom symptoms of infection develop in the presence of an indwelling catheter must be treated. In the absence of symptoms, however, it is better to avoid treatment until removal of the catheter, at which time eradication of infection becomes easier.

PROSTATITIS

The term *prostatitis* means prostatic inflammation and should be interpreted as a generic term having four major subcategories: acute bacterial prostatitis, chronic bacterial prostatitis, nonbacterial prostatitis, and prostatodynia. Acute bacterial prostatitis is an acute, usually gram-negative, bacterial infection of the prostate gland that coexists in the majority of cases with acute bacterial cystitis. Chronic bacterial prostatitis is a subclinical or indolent chronic infection of the prostatic acini by bacteria that can be localized to the prostatic secretions. Nonbacterial prostatitis is a chronic inflammatory condition of the prostatic acini for which there is no identifiable etiologic organism; associated symptoms can be indolent or totally subclinical. Prostatodynia refers to a clinical condition in which irritative voiding symptoms and pelvic pain suggest an acute inflammatory process but with minimum or no evidence of inflammatory cells in the prostatic secretions. In all forms of prostatitis except prostatodynia there are usually more than 10 white blood cells per high power field on examination of the expressed prostatic secretions.

Acute and chronic bacterial prostatitis constitute the two conditions of greatest general medical interest. Both conditions can result from ascent of bacteria in the urethra, reflux of infected urine into the posterior urethral prostatic ducts, lymphatogenous spread of bacteria from the rectum, or hematogenous spread. The first two routes of infection are thought to be the most common. In acute bacterial prostatitis, marked inflammation is present in part or all of the gland, with diffuse stromal hyperemia and edema, polymorphonuclear leukocyte infiltration within and around the acini, varying degrees of lymphocyte and macrophage invasion, intraductal glandular cell desquamation, and microabscess formation. Large abscesses are a late complication.

In chronic bacterial prostatitis, the inflammatory reaction is less pronounced, more focal, and characterized by lymphocyte, plasma cell, and macrophage infiltration within and around the acini and stroma. Because such changes have also been observed to lesser and greater degrees in 98% of prostatectomy specimens from patients with prostatic hypertrophy, the diagnosis of this form of prostatitis rests on the demonstration of bacteria in the prostatic secretions and not merely on the presence of inflammatory changes in the tissue.

The bacteriology of both forms is similar, with *E. coli*, *Pseudomonas* species, and enterococci being the most common pathogens. Cases resulting from nosocomial infections following instrumentation may be due to highly resistant gram-negative organisms.

Acute bacterial prostatitis

Clinical manifestations. In acute bacterial prostatitis the symptoms are usually of short duration before presentation and typically consist of perineal pain, dysuria, frequency, urgency, and nocturia, all of which may at times be complicated by urinary retention. The perineal pain may radiate to the sacral region of the back, down the penis and suprapubic area, or to the rectal area. Less severe obstructive symptoms (e.g., urinary hesitancy and a decreased force and caliber of the stream) may occur. Gross or microscopic hematuria may be present, as may a purulent urethral discharge. Fever with or without chills and malaise are almost always present. In the more severe form of infection, the patient appears ill and may be frankly septic, with positive blood cultures. The prostate is typically painful to palpation, but in subacute cases the pain may be minimal. Complications of acute bacterial prostatitis include formation of abscesses (which may rupture into the urethra, perineum, or rectum), pyelonephritis, acute epididymitis and orchitis, and septic shock. Although uncommon, progression to chronic bacterial prostatitis can occur if the acute phase is not adequately treated.

Diagnosis. Vigorous prostatic massage may produce serious complications, such as spread of infection to the epididymis or kidney, or bacteremia. However, a careful rectal examination of the prostate to ascertain degree of tenderness, determine consistency of the gland, and rule out the presence of a perirectal abscess, tumor, or foreign body is indicated. It is not necessary to express prostatic secretions to make the diagnosis of acute bacterial prostatitis because the urine is almost always infected and culture of a voided specimen will identify the offending organism. Likewise, instrumentation of the urethra should be avoided in cases complicated by urinary retention. In such situations urologic consultation should be obtained for suprapubic urinary diversion.

Chronic bacterial prostatitis

Clinical manifestations. Chronic bacterial prostatitis is usually asymptomatic when the infection is confined to the prostate proper, but should be suspected when chronic relapsing cystitis secondary to infections with bacteria of the same serotype is documented. Eradication of the bladder bacteria leads to disappearance of symptoms, despite the fact that bacteria can still be cultured from the prostatic secretions.

Diagnosis. The diagnosis is established by performing the bacterial localization studies described by Meares and Stamey, which demonstrate a higher bacterial count in the expressed prostatic secretions, or preferably an ejaculate, as compared to that in the urine (quantitative methods that will detect small numbers of bacteria must be used). In brief, the localization test, performed after eradicating bladder bacteria with an antibiotic that does not diffuse into the prostatic secretions (e.g., nitrofurantoin, ampicillin, or cephalexin), consists of three sets of cultures: (1) an initial 10-ml aliquot and an additional 10-ml aliquot of urine (voided bladder urines, or VB_1 and VB_2, respectively) are cultured separately; (2) the expressed prostatic fluid following prostatic massage is cultured; (3) a 10-ml aliquot of urine is subsequently collected and cultured (VB_3). The infection is localized to the prostatic secretions if the bacterial count in the secretions is tenfold greater than the count in the VB_2 urine culture. If the bacterial count in VB_2 exceeds 10^3 bacteria/ml, the infection cannot be localized and the localization procedure must be repeated after additional antimicrobial administration. Because chronic inflammation and fibrosis are present in the gland, the prostate may be firm and irregular and thus suggestive of cancer; the demonstration of infected prostatic secretions does not rule out this possibility. If the consistency of the gland does not return to normal after adequate antibiotic therapy or if a nodule persists, a transrectal ultrasound examination with guided biopsies is indicated to rule out cancer.

Chronic granulomatous prostatitis is a rare inflammatory condition (0.8% of all benign inflammatory diseases) frequently associated with a recent urinary tract infection. This condition is notable in that it mimics prostate cancer on digital rectal examination and is rarely due to specific granulomatous disease. Irritative voiding symptoms are the most common symptoms and in most patients tend to resolve within a few months.

Therapy of acute and chronic bacterial prostatitis. As a general rule, treatment should be guided by the results of bacterial cultures and the overall clinical situation. Therapy of serious acute bacterial prostatitis may require parenteral antibiotics until the acute phase of the infection has been overcome, followed by a 1-month course of oral antibiotic therapy. Therapy of less serious bouts of acute prostatitis consists of a 3- to 4-week course of oral antibiotics. Because penetration by most antibiotics is good in the acute phase of infection, any antibiotic demonstrated to be effective on sensitivity studies can be used.

Therapy of chronic bacterial prostatitis is less clear-cut, because this form of prostatitis is notoriously refractory to treatment. Most urologists would treat for a minimum of 4 weeks with trimethoprim-sulfamethoxazole or indanyl carbenicillin sodium and then repeat cultures. Because of their wide spectrum of activity and ability to concentrate in the prostate (up to 14 times serum concentration), the newer fluoroquinolones (ciprofloxacin, norfloxacin, and ofloxacin) constitute a very effective alternative therapy for cases refractory to other antimicrobial agents. Treatment dosages are 500 mg twice a day for ciprofloxacin and 400 mg twice a day for norfloxacin for periods of 2 to 6 weeks. Infections due to *Pseudomonas aeruginosa* and enterococci can be refractory to fluoroquinolone therapy.

Longer periods of therapy are justified if initial therapy fails. If the infection persists after 12 weeks despite appropriate antibiotic therapy, switching to another of the aforementioned drugs is reasonable. Unfortunately, some patients with this form of prostatitis are not cured with chemotherapy alone and at the same time do not have clear indications for surgery, such as secondarily infected prostatic calculi or significant benign prostatic hypertrophy. In these patients consideration should be given to treating symptomatic infection when it occurs or to instituting a regimen of chronic suppressive therapy (e.g., low daily doses of trimethoprim-sulfamethoxazole or nitrofurantoin) to avoid episodes of cystitis (which is the major source of symptoms).

Chronic nonbacterial prostatitis and prostatodynia

In general the symptoms of chronic nonbacterial prostatitis and prostatodynia are the same and include chronic irritative symptoms along with varying degrees of perineal pain and discomfort in the absence of any conventionally demonstrable infection. Chronic nonbacterial prostatitis is often associated with symptoms that can be indolent or totally subclinical, although in symptomatic cases irritative voiding symptoms are present. Symptoms associated with prostatodynia tend to be more severe (irritative voiding symptoms, pelvic pain) and in unusual cases incapacitating. In both conditions various urodynamic derangements of voiding are observed, leading to hyperirritability of the bladder and incoordination of the urethral sphincteric mechanism. Symptoms associated with nonbacterial prostatitis probably result from the chronic inflammatory process within glandular acini; the observed urodynamic abnormalities associated with prostatodynia may result from a primary neurologic (sensory or motor) disorder. The major difference between these two forms of prostatitis is that the white blood cell count in prostatic secretions is by convention higher in chronic nonbacterial prostatitis (more than 10 white blood cells per high power field) than in prostatodynia. Thus the distinction between the two entities can be rather vague and arbitrary. Because symptoms of transitional carcinoma of the prostatic urethra can mimic symptoms of chronic prostatic irritation (i.e., frequency, urgency, and nocturia), a urologic consultation should be obtained and urinary cytologies performed. From a practical standpoint, as long as serious disorders (such as adenocarcinoma of the prostate or transitional cell carcinoma of the prostate, bladder, or urethra) and surgically correctable anatomic abnormalities (such as urethral strictures) are ruled out, then in the vast majority of cases the long-term morbidity to the patient is minimal. Tuberculosis of the prostate can masquerade as nonbacterial prostatitis, but in this condition it would be expected that other upper tract stigmata indicating a more generalized genitourinary tubercular infection would also be present. Antibiotic therapy is of no value in the management of these forms of prostatitis.

REFERENCES

Andriole VT: Use of quinolones in treatment of prostatitis and lower urinary tract infections, Eur J Clin Microbiol Infect Dis 10:342-350, 1991.

Boscia JA, Abrutyn E, and Kaye D: Asymptomatic bacteriuria in elderly persons: treat or do not treat? Ann Intern Med 106(5):764-766, 1987.

Childs SJ: Ciprofloxacin in treatment of chronic bacterial prostatitis, Urology 35:15-18, 1990.

Hooton TM et al: *Escherichia coli* bacteriuria and contraceptive method, JAMA 265:64-69, 1991.

Johnson JR et al: Prevention of catheter-associated urinary tract infection with a silver oxide-coated urinary catheter: clinical and microbiologic correlates, J Infect Dis 162:1145-1150, 1990.

Johnson JR and Stamm WE: Urinary tract infections in women: diagnosis and treatment, Ann Intern Med 111:906-917, 1989.

Kaye D, editor: Urinary tract infections, Med Clin North Am 75:241-520, 1991.

Komaroff AL: Urinalysis and urine culture in women with dysuria, Ann Intern Med 104:212-218, 1986.

Lipsky BA: Urinary tract infections in men. Epidemiology, pathophysiology, diagnosis, and treatment, Ann Intern Med 110:138-150, 1989.

Meares EM: Prostatitis, Med Clin North Am 75(2):405-424, 1991.

Meares EM and Stamey TA: Bacteriologic localization patterns in bacterial prostatitis and urethritis, Invest Urol 5:491, 1968.

Sobel JD and Kaye D: Urinary tract infections. In Mandell GL, Douglas RG Jr, and Bennett JE, editors: Principles and practice of infectious diseases, ed 3, New York: 1990, Churchill Livingstone.

Spach DH, Stapleton AE, and Stamm WE: Lack of circumcision increases the risk of urinary tract infection in young men, JAMA 267:679-681, 1992.

Stamm WE: Catheter-associated urinary tract infections: epidemiology, pathogenesis, and prevention, Am J Med 91(3B):65S-71S, 1991.

Stamm WE, et al: Natural history of recurrent urinary tract infections in women, Rev Infect Dis 13:77-84, 1991.

Stapleton A et al: Postcoital antimicrobial prophylaxis for recurrent urinary tract infection. A randomized, double-blind, placebo-controlled trial, JAMA 264:703-706, 1990.

Stillwell TJ, Engen DE, and Farrow GM: The clinical spectrum of granulomatous prostatitis: a report of 200 cases, J Urol 138:320-323, 1987.

CHAPTER

241 Fever and Infections in Travelers

Henry F. Chambers III

Infections usually come to the attention of a physician for one of four reasons: diarrhea, fever, eosinophilia, or rash or other cutaneous disorder.

DIARRHEA

By far the most common problem, diarrhea affects 50% or more of travelers to developing countries. Incubation periods generally are short, so most diarrheal illnesses begin during or soon after the trip (Table 241-1). Characteristically, acute diarrhea will be one of two types: (1) bloody diarrhea, or dysentery, with fecal blood and white cells present or (2) watery diarrhea, with blood and white cells absent (Table 241-2) (Chapter 236). Bloody diarrhea is usually caused by invasive organisms, predominantly amebas, *Salmonella,* or *Shigella,* that infect the terminal small bowel or colon. Watery diarrhea is usually of unknown cause or due to viruses or toxigenic *Escherichia coli.* Although *Entamoeba histolytica* can cause dysentery, more often symptoms are milder and the diarrhea is watery. Chronic diarrhea or diarrhea commencing a week or more

Table 241-1. Causes of infectious diarrhea in travelers according to clinical presentation

Watery diarrhea	Dysentery
Entamoeba histolytica	*Campylobacter jejuni*
Giardia lamblia	*E. histolytica*
Non-cholera vibrios	Invasive *E. coli*
Norwalk agent	*Salmonella* sp.
Rotavirus	*Shigella* sp.
Salmonella sp.	*Yersinia enterocolitica*
Toxigenic *E. coli*	
Vibrio cholerae	
Vibrio parahaemolyticus	

Table 241-2. Infectious disease in travelers categorized according to approximate time after exposure when patients are likely to present with evidence of disease

3 days or less	3 to 28 days	1 to 6 months	6 to 18 months	Several years
Cholera	Amebiasis	Amebiasis	Amebiasis	Amebiasis
Diarrhea from *Campylobacter, E. coli,* or *Vibrio* sp.	Bartonellosis	Ascariasis	Ascariasis	Chagas' disease, chronic phase
Plague	Brucellosis	Bartonellosis	Clonorchiasis	Clonorchiasis
Salmonellosis	Chagas' disease, acute phase	Brucellosis	Cutaneous leishmaniasis	Hookworm infection
Shigellosis	Dengue fever	Chagas' disease, acute phase	Fascioliasis	Mucocutaneous leishmaniasis
Viral gastroenteritis	Diarrhea from *Campylobacter*	Clonorchiasis	Fasciolopsiasis	Paragonimiasis
	Giardiasis	Cutaneous leishmaniasis	Loiasis	Schistosomiasis, chronic
	Hemorrhagic fevers	Fascioliasis	Malaria	Strongyloidiasis
	Hepatitis A	Fasciolopsiasis	Onchocerciasis	Tapeworm infection
	Leptospirosis	Hepatitis A	Paragonimiasis	Tropical sprue
	Malaria	Hepatitis B	Sleeping sickness	
	Meningococcal disease	Hookworm disease	Strongyloidiasis	
	Paragonimiasis	Kala-azar	Tropical sprue	
	Plague	Malaria		
	Polio	Paragonimiasis		
	Relapsing fever	Relapsing fever		
	Sleeping sickness	Schistosomiasis, acute		
	Tularemia	Sleeping sickness		
	Typhoid fever	Strongyloidiasis		
	Typhus	Tropical sprue		

after the return home is likely due to either *E. histolytica* or *Giardia lamblia*.

Since 1991, a cholera epidemic has been spreading throughout South and Central America. Most cases have occurred in Peru, but some have been imported into the United States. Physicians should be alert to the possibility of cholera in patients who acutely develop profuse, watery diarrhea without fever after travel to Latin American countries.

Helminthic parasites rarely cause diarrhea, although *Strongyloides stercoralis* can, because of its unique ability to multiply in the host. With few exceptions, other helminths do not multiply in the host; consequently, the parasitic load is light unless the exposure has been repeated or especially intense. Intestinal helminths (e.g., *Ascaris,* hookworms) or schistosomes can cause diarrhea if large numbers of worms are present (Chapter 282).

Occasionally, diarrhea is chronic or recurrent or there is malabsorption. If no cause is found after several examinations for fecal pathogens, the logical next step is upper gastrointestinal endoscopy with biopsy or an empiric trial of quinacrine or metronidazole to differentiate infection by *G. lamblia* from tropical sprue and other noninfectious causes of diarrhea.

FEVER

Malaria, viral hepatitis, typhoid or other enteric fever, and amebic liver abscess are responsible for most of the fevers for which a cause is found (Table 241-3). Except for malaria, the risk of these diseases is determined not by geographic location but rather by the adequacy of public health measures. Where these measures are inadequate, as is the case in many developing countries, contaminated food and drink are the source for most infections.

Table 241-3. Infectious causes of fever in travelers

Common	Unusual
Amebic liver abscess	Bartonellosis
Hepatitis A	Brucellosis
Hepatitis B	Chagas' disease, acute
Malaria	Dengue fever
Typhoid fever	Kala-azar
	Leptospirosis
	Measles
	Meningococcal disease
	Plague
	Polio
	Relapsing fever
	Schistosomiasis, acute
	Sleeping sickness
	Tularemia
	Typhus
	Viral hemorrhagic fevers
	Yellow fever

Exotic infections typically are acquired by means other than contaminated food or drink (e.g., insect vectors, repeated exposures). Consequently, these infections are more likely to occur in persons who have resided for months or years in a developing country, in those who have traveled to rural villages, rivers, savannas, jungles, and forests, and in those exposed to wild animals.

Common causes of fever

Malaria should be suspected in anyone who develops fever after travel to an endemic area (Chapter 280). Despite prophylaxis, malaria can still occur. A weekly dose of medication may easily be missed or forgotten, or the patient may not have completed the prescribed 6 weeks of treatment after return from the endemic area. Chloroquine, the recommended drug for malaria prophylaxis, is not effective against chloroquine-resistant *Plasmodium falciparum* malaria. Mefloquine (one 250 mg tablet one time per week starting 1 week before and continuing through 4 weeks after travel) is recommended for prophylaxis during travel to areas where chloroquine-resistant falciparum malaria occurs. Although rare, mefloquine-resistant strains have been reported in Southeast Asia. Finally, chloroquine is ineffective against the exoerythrocytic stages of *Plasmodium ovale* and *Plasmodium vivax,* and unless primaquine is taken, malaria may relapse for up to 3 years after exposure. Diagnosis is made from thick and thin smears of peripheral blood. Because the degree of parasitemia may be low when the patient is first seen, examination of several smears of peripheral blood taken every 6 to 12 hours on two successive days may be necessary to make the diagnosis. Diagnosis of falciparum malaria is extremely important because it can be rapidly fatal. Falciparum malaria usually occurs within 2 months of traveling to an endemic area.

The next diagnosis to consider is enteric fever due to *Salmonella typhi* or, occasionally, other Salmonella species. Fever usually occurs 1 to 3 weeks after exposure, and other findings may be few or absent (Chapter 268). Serologic tests are unreliable for diagnosis, which requires isolation of the organism in blood cultures.

Like enteric fever, hepatitis A, hepatitis B, and non-A, non-B hepatitis are endemic in developing countries where public health measures are inadequate or nonexistent. The risk of hepatitis A is greatest for those traveling off ordinary tourist routes or for 3 months or more. Hepatitis B is unlikely to be acquired abroad unless risk factors are present, such as travel to regions where carrier rates exceed 5%, plus either direct contact with blood or secretions of carriers or infected persons or sexual contact (Chapter 57). The risk of non-A, non-B hepatitis to the traveler is not well characterized.

Amebic liver abscess is the least common of the usual causes of fever. Amebic liver abscess should be considered if a patient has fever, right upper quadrant pain, and a history of travel (recent or remote) to a developing country, which for United States residents is usually Mexico. Diarrhea accompanies the abscess in only a third of cases, and amebas are usually not found in the stool. Serologic tests are almost always positive except very early in the disease (Chapter 280).

Unusual causes of fever

Bacterial infections. Meningococcal disease is endemic throughout the world. The disease is rare in travelers, but the risk can be significant during epidemics, which regularly occur in developing countries (e.g., Brazil and sub-Saharan Africa). The risk is greatest for persons in close contact with large numbers of people and for those in health care settings.

Plague, tularemia, leptospirosis, relapsing fever, and brucellosis generally pose no threat to the traveler. Persons who have traveled to rural areas and who have been exposed to rodents, lice, fleas, ticks, or wild animals are at increased risk for plague, tularemia, leptospirosis, and relapsing fever. Brucellosis occurs in tropical South America, southern Europe (Spain and Portugal), and eastern Asia, and is a consideration in individuals who have consumed local (unpasteurized) milk or milk products (e.g., cheese) and who have fever, chills, and no localizing signs or symptoms.

Rickettsial infections. Infections caused by these organisms should be suspected in persons who have fever accompanied by a macular or petechial rash, which is usually central in distribution. An eschar may be present in tick-borne typhus or scrub typhus but is absent in epidemic or murine typhus. A positive Weil-Felix test result is suggestive of these infections.

Except for epidemic (louse-borne) or murine typhus and Q fever, which are worldwide in distribution, rickettsial diseases are transmitted by either ticks or mites and are restricted to certain geographic areas (Chapter 256). A history of travel to these areas and conditions of possible exposure to ticks or mites raise suspicion of the diagnosis.

Viral infections. Polio and measles are endemic throughout developing nations, and the unimmunized traveler is at relatively high risk for either infection. Measles is a particular concern because a substantial number of individuals, including some who have been vaccinated, may be susceptible.

Dengue fever occurs throughout tropical regions of the world. Clinical manifestations are fever, chills, headache, retro-orbital pain, myalgias, and arthralgias followed by a diffuse rash. A hemorrhagic form occurs and is a more severe illness characterized by thrombocytopenia, hemoconcentration, and hemorrhagic phenomena (Chapter 249).

Hemorrhagic fever in travelers to central or western Africa may be due to Lassa, Marburg, or Ebola virus. These diseases are rare but rapidly fatal. Recognition is important so that patients can be isolated to prevent secondary spread of the infection. Hemorrhagic fevers due to other viruses occur throughout Asia, Africa, and South America (Chapter 248).

Yellow fever is endemic in Africa and South America, but no cases have been imported into the United States in over 50 years. This success is almost certainly due to effective immunization policies.

Travelers from areas where seroprevalence of human immunodeficiency virus (HIV) is high, such as some central and east African countries, may be at risk for this infection. Persons from these areas who have had heterosexual contacts, especially with prostitutes, or who have received blood transfusions are at increased risk of HIV infection and its associated infections (Chapter 242).

Protozoal infections. African sleeping sickness, caused by either *Trypanosoma gambiense* or *Trypanosoma rhodesiense,* is transmitted by the tsetse fly. Its distribution is confined to tropical Africa between 15 degrees north and 20 degrees south latitude. Wild animals are an important reservoir of the organism, and most infections have occurred after visits to game parks. Diagnosis is made by observation of the trypanosomes in peripheral blood smear or cerebrospinal fluid (Chapter 280).

Chagas' disease, or American trypanosomiasis, is caused by *Trypanosoma cruzi*. Infection in travelers is rare but is more likely after travel for extended periods to rural areas of Central and South America, where reduviid bugs, vectors of the parasite, are numerous. In the acute phase, fever, lymphadenopathy, hepatosplenomegaly, and occasionally myocarditis and/or meningoencephalitis occur. Only early in the disease can *T. cruzi* be found on direct examination of thick smears of blood.

Visceral leishmaniasis, or kala-azar, is caused by *Leishmania donovani* and transmitted by *Phlebotomus* flies. Over weeks to months, the patient develops fever and a wasting illness accompanied by a large liver and spleen, which can be massive. Diagnosis is made by detection of the organism in macrophages from bone marrow, liver, or spleen tissue.

Acute toxoplasmosis resembles mononucleosis with fever, diffuse lymphadenopathy, and atypical lymphocytosis. It may be acquired by eating raw or poorly cooked meat.

EOSINOPHILIA

Eosinophilia of an infectious cause is due to worms: intestinal roundworms, filariae, tissue roundworms, flukes, and tapeworms. In general, bacterial and protozoal infections do not cause eosinophilia. Parasites that cause eosinophilia usually do not cause fever.

Intestinal parasites

Eosinophilia, usually in the range of 10% to 20% of the total white cell count, may be the only indication of a helminthic infection. Other symptoms typically are absent because most helminths cannot multiply in the host and, unless exposure has been repeated or intense, only a few parasites are present. Examination of stool for ova and parasites usually will establish the cause.

Unlike most other parasites, *Strongyloides stercoralis* can multiply in the host and reinfect. Therefore large numbers of adult worms may be present and infection can last 20 years or more. Eosinophilia is moderate but can range as high as 25% or 50%. Most patients are asymptomatic; but a few may experience bouts of abdominal pain, diarrhea, pneumonia, and urticarial skin rashes. A hyperinfection syndrome characterized by pulmonary infiltrates and septicemia occurs in individuals who are immune compromised, often as a result of steroid therapy. Diagnosis requires examination of fresh stool, either directly or concentrated, for larval forms. If feces are negative in suspected cases, duodenal aspirates should be examined because the yield is higher (Chapter 282).

Filariae

Filarial infections are an important cause of significant and persistent eosinophilia, at times as high as 80%.

Filariasis caused by *Wuchereria bancrofti* and *Brugia malayi* occurs worldwide in tropical and subtropical countries. Because of an exuberant immune response in the naive host, microfilariae commonly are not found in the blood. The syndrome of tropical pulmonary eosinophilia, characterized by hypereosinophilia, pulmonary infiltrates on chest radiograph, and paroxysms of cough and wheezing, is probably also caused by either *W. bancrofti* or *B. malayi*. No microfilariae are detected in this disorder, presumably because they are trapped in lymph nodes or the lung, giving rise to allergic pulmonary symptoms.

Loa loa, Onchocerca volvulus, and *Dipetalonema perstans* are tissue filarial species endemic to western and central equatorial Africa and parts of Central and South America (*Onchocerca* species only). *Loa loa* causes transient localized subcutaneous swellings, and the worm can be seen in conjunctivae during migration. *Onchocerca volvulus* causes river blindness. Adult worms reside in subcutaneous nodules in the host, and microfilariae migrate in subcutaneous tissues. *Dipetalonema perstans* causes little tissue reaction and is a relatively common cause of asymptomatic eosinophilia.

Because microfilariae may not be readily demonstrable in blood (even after microfilter concentration techniques) or in skin snips (for *Onchocerca* microfilariae), a clinical trial of diethylcarbamazine, 3 mg/kg orally three times daily for 3 weeks, may be indicated for suspected filariasis in a patient with the appropriate travel history and otherwise unexplained eosinophilia.

Flukes

Intestinal (*Fasciolopsis buski* and others), lung *(Paragonimus westermani),* and liver *(Fasciola hepatica* and *Clonorchis sinensis)* flukes can all cause eosinophilia but rarely cause infection in the traveler. All are transmitted by eating either raw or poorly cooked fish *(Clonorchis),* crab *(Paragonimus),* or aquatic plants *(Fasciolopsis),* particularly watercress in the case of *Fasciola hepatica*. *F. hepatica* is found throughout the world wherever sheep and cattle are raised, but the other flukes are restricted mostly to China and Southeast Asia.

Schistosomiasis is acquired by travelers who drink, swim, wade, or wash in fresh water from an endemic region (Chapter 282). Heavy infections are characterized by fever, marked eosinophilia, cough and pulmonary infiltrates, acute hepatitis, and abdominal discomfort (Katayama fever) as larvae migrate through the lungs to the portal veins. Eosinophilia plus either hematuria *(Schistosoma haematobium)* or abdominal pain and diarrhea *(Schistosoma mansoni* and *Schistosoma japonicum)* commence as adult worms begin to lay eggs. Schistosomiasis in the traveler is almost always due to *S. mansoni*. Serologic tests are useful to screen for all types of schistosomiasis, but swimmer's itch (see later discussion) may cause false-positive results, so treatment should not be given unless eggs are found.

Tapeworms

Tapeworms may cause mild eosinophilia. All are transmitted to the host by eating raw or poorly cooked beef *(Taenia solium),* pork *(Taenia saginata),* or fish *(Diphyllobothrium)*. Infection usually goes unnoticed until one or several proglottids are regurgitated or passed in stool (Chapter 282).

CUTANEOUS DISORDERS

Primary diseases of the skin include cutaneous leishmaniasis, onchocerciasis, loiasis, cutaneous larva migrans (caused by the dog or cat hookworm), swimmer's itch (caused by invasion of human skin by schistosomal species of birds or mammals), and myiasis (infestation of skin by larvae of dipterous flies). These diseases tend to occur in persons (e.g., anthropologists, archaeologists, missionaries, geologists, construction workers) who reside for extended periods of time in areas where insect vectors or contaminated soil are present.

Urticarial rashes may be part of an allergic reaction to nonprotozoal parasitic infections (e.g., schistosomiasis, hookworm, and *Strongyloides*) and to circulating immune complexes in hepatitis B infection. A petechial rash is characteristic of meningococcal disease but may also occur in relapsing fever, rickettsial infections, and viral hemorrhagic fevers. Maculopapular rashes occur in measles, typhoid fever, dengue fever, relapsing fever, and typhus. Rash accompanied by hemorrhagic phenomena suggests meningococcal disease or one of the hemorrhagic fevers.

CLINICAL EVALUATION OF THE TRAVELER FOR SUSPECTED INFECTION

Most important in the evaluation of a traveler or any other patient who presents with what may be an infectious disease is a meticulous history that includes a list of all countries traveled (including layovers, even if the patient only remained at the airport); whether travel was restricted to cities or included rural areas, villages, or famine or war zones; activities during the trip; and conditions of travel. The patient should be asked about exposure to raw fruits and vegetables, particularly any local "delicacies"; to unpasteurized milk or milk products; to raw pork, beef, or fish; to potentially contaminated water sources (including swimming in any freshwater lakes, streams, and rivers); and to biting ticks, flies, mosquitoes, or other vectors. Exposure to epidemics, persons with similar symptoms, vaccination history, and whether or not immunoglobulin and chemoprophylaxis for malaria or other infections were taken should be ascertained. Duration of stay in each country and first occurrence of symptoms can help to narrow the diagnostic possibilities.

In addition to a thorough physical examination, a complete blood count with differential should be obtained in all patients. If eosinophilia is present, stool samples should be examined for ova and parasites. If ova and parasites are not found, then blood smears (and occasionally skin biopsies) should be examined for filariae.

For patients with acute diarrhea, a useful first step is examination of methylene blue-stained fecal smears. The finding of white or red cells in the stool makes infection by an organism that causes dysentery likely (see Table 241-2). Once bacterial cultures and examinations of stool specimens for ova and parasites have been performed, empiric therapy with one double-strength tablet of trimethoprim-sulfamethoxazole twice a day or ciprofloxacin 500 mg twice a day can be initiated.

If the diarrhea is watery, a bacterial cause is less likely than if dysentery is present. Therapy should be withheld until a pathogen is identified. Stool examination for ova and parasites is more likely to reveal the cause in these cases. Infection by *Vibrio* species (including cholera) is a possibility if there is a history of exposure to brackish or sea water, ingestion of shellfish, or travel to an epidemic area. Special media (e.g., thiosulfate citrate bile salt sucrose) is required for their isolation.

Differentiation of benign, self-limited, and presumably viral fevers (which account for most cases of fever in travelers) from those due to serious illness can be difficult, at least initially. A detailed travel history and search for associated signs and symptoms are invaluable in determination of whether a fever is likely to be benign, due to one of the other common causes (malaria, hepatitis, typhoid fever, or amebic disease), or caused by an exotic infection.

Malaria, if the patient has traveled to an endemic area, and typhoid fever should be excluded early in the evaluation by examination of thick and thin blood smears and by blood culture, respectively. If hepatitis is a possibility, then liver function tests followed by specific serologic testing for hepatitis A and B should be obtained. Amebic liver abscess should be suspected if the patient complains of liver pain or tenderness. Serologic testing and an imaging study of the liver, such as computed tomography, sonography, or a nuclear scan, to identify an abscess is recommended for these patients. Stool examination for ova and parasites is not useful for diagnosis or exclusion of amebic liver abscess. If helminths are detected in the stool, these should not be assumed as the cause of fever.

If features from the travel history suggest other possibilities or if none of the usual causes is found and the fever persists, then a more extensive workup should be undertaken (e.g., blood smears for filariae or trypanosomes, serology for schistosomiasis, brucellosis, or rickettsia).

Ulcerative and/or papular skin lesions, particularly if satellite lesions are present, should be biopsied for histopathologic examination and, if available, for culture for *Leishmania*. Stains and culture to exclude fungal infection are also recommended. Nodular lesions not due to myiasis should be excised and examined if onchocerciasis is a possibility. Biopsy of urticarial or macular lesions is not likely to be helpful because these are usually manifestations of systemic illnesses.

PREVENTION OF DISEASE IN TRAVELERS

Most of the diseases likely to affect the traveler are food and water borne. Simply by avoiding hazardous food and contaminated water, the traveler can prevent most illnesses. Raw fruits and vegetables, salads, uncooked or poorly cooked beef, pork, fish, seafood, and unpasteurized milk and local dairy products should be considered unsafe in developing countries. Water should be drunk only if boiled, as for tea and coffee. Soft drinks are safe, but the ice cubes are not. Swimming in fresh water (unchlorinated) is ill-advised in areas where schistosomiasis is endemic.

By minimizing exposure to arthropod vectors, travelers can protect themselves against disease transmitted by these pests. Adequate clothing, liberal use of insect repellent, frequent checks for the presence of ticks, and the use of mosquito netting at night are simple and effective methods to reduce risk.

Despite the most conscientious measures, traveler's diarrhea is still likely to occur. Prophylactic regimens of tetracyclines or trimethoprim-sulfamethoxazole have been effective, but side effects make their use impractical. Because many episodes of diarrhea are self-limited and not all patients are affected, perhaps the best strategy is to provide the patient with a supply of trimethoprim-sulfamethoxazole (160 mg trimethoprim/800 mg sulfamethoxazole per dose), or ciprofloxacin 500 mg to be taken twice daily for 3 to 5 days, should significant diarrhea occur during the trip.

Prophylaxis of malaria

Malaria prophylaxis is recommended for all travelers to regions where malaria is endemic. The regimen will vary depending on length of stay and on whether or not the itinerary includes countries where chloroquine-resistant falciparum malaria is present (Chapter 280). Up-to-date information about the occurrence of resistant malaria is also available from the Centers for Disease Control in Atlanta, Georgia, on request (telephone 404-488-4046).

Recommended immunizations

Because the prevalence of polio, measles, mumps, rubella, diphtheria, and tetanus has been greatly reduced in the United States by immunization programs, unimmunized susceptible individuals are at low risk for these diseases.

Table 241-4. Recommended vaccinations for international travel

Vaccine	Indications	Dose
Measles/mumps/rubella	Susceptible persons born after 1957* Contraindicated in pregnancy	One dose of combined vaccine‡
Polio		
Inactivated polio vaccine (IPV)†		
Primary series	For unimmunized adults and immunocompromised individuals. Safe in pregnancy	Three doses, 1-2 months apart
Booster series		One dose before departure
Oral polio vaccine (OPV)†		
Primary series	Not recommended in adults‡	
Booster series	For immunocompetent, immunized adults at increased risk. Safe in pregnancy	One dose before departure
Tetanus/diphtheria		
Primary series	All unimmunized adults	One dose of combined vaccine at 0, 2, and 6-12 months
Booster series		One dose every 10 years
Typhoid		
Primary series	Travelers to developing countries, particularly rural areas where food and water sanitation are poor	Oral vaccine: one capsule every other day for four doses Parenteral vaccine: 0.5 ml subcutaneously at 0 and ≥ 4 weeks§
Booster series		Oral vaccine: repeat primary series every 5 years Parenteral vaccine: 0.5 ml every 3 years

*Persons born before 1957 can be considered immune to measles and mumps; others are susceptible unless immunized or the presence of specific antibody is demonstrated. Rubella vaccine is recommended for all unvaccinated individuals without serologic evidence of previous immunity.

†The risk of adverse effects from OPV is slightly increased in adults compared with IPV. If protection is needed for these individuals within 4 weeks, however, a single dose of OPV is recommended. If protection is needed within 4 to 8 weeks, two doses of IPV 4 weeks apart are recommended; remaining dose can be administered at recommended intervals at a later time.

‡The current recommendation for measles vaccination is that two doses of vaccine be given at least 1 month apart to all persons born after 1957. Many individuals have never received the second dose and unless this can be documented, administration of measles vaccine is recommended.

§If less than 4 weeks are available before departure, 0.5 ml can be administered weekly for three doses but is slightly less effective than the standard regimen. Alternatively, the oral vaccine can be used.

In countries where immunization programs do not exist, however, these diseases are endemic and the risk to the unimmunized traveler is correspondingly increased. Therefore the occasion of travel is a good opportunity to review a patient's immunization record and to administer the recommended primary or booster vaccines (Table 241-4).

Vaccination against typhoid fever is not required but may be advised for travelers to most developing countries of Africa, Asia, and South and Central America, where typhoid is endemic. Vaccination of travelers to epidemic areas and to villages and rural areas is recommended. An oral, live-attenuated typhoid Ty21a vaccine is available. Although it is no more effective than the parenteral, heat-killed vaccine preparation, it is more easily administered and better tolerated (see Table 241-4). Vaccine confers protection in 70% to 90% of recipients at best, therefore, even vaccinated persons should be advised to avoid contaminated food and water sources.

Required immunizations

Smallpox vaccine is no longer required for international travel and should not be given. An International Certificate of Vaccination against cholera is required for entry into some countries, and vaccination is recommended for persons traveling to these areas (Table 241-5). One dose satisfies the requirement. The complete primary series is not recommended, except for individuals who will travel to regions where cholera is highly endemic or epidemic or who have a medical condition (e.g., achlorhydria, gastric resection, antacid therapy) that predisposes to cholera. Cholera vaccine is not always effective, so vaccinated individuals should continue to avoid potentially contaminated food and water.

An International Certificate of Vaccination against yellow fever is required for entry into some countries. Yellow fever vaccine is recommended for persons traveling to countries that require a Certificate of Vaccination for entry and for persons traveling to areas where yellow fever is endemic. Yellow fever is endemic in South America and Africa between 15 degrees north and 15 degrees south latitude. A valid Certificate of Vaccination can be obtained only after vaccination at a designated yellow fever vaccination center. Information about which countries require vaccination and the location of vaccination centers can be obtained from the local health department.

Table 241-5. Required vaccination for international travel

Vaccine	Indication	Adult dose
Cholera		
Single dose	To fulfill requirement for entry into a country	0.5 ml
Primary series	For persons at increased risk for cholera in countries where cholera is endemic or epidemic	0.5 ml, two doses 1-4 weeks or more apart
Booster		0.5 ml every 6 months
Yellow fever		
Primary series	To fulfill requirement for entry into a country; for travel to endemic area	0.5 ml once
Booster		0.5 ml every 10 years

Table 241-6. Immunizations against hepatitis

Immunization	Indications	Dose*
Immune serum globulin	Protection against hepatitis A; repeat higher dose every 4-6 months for prolonged travel	For travel ≤3 months: 2.0 ml For travel ≥ 3 months: 5.0 ml
Hepatitis B vaccine	For persons exposed to blood, secretions, or intimate sexual contact in countries where 5% to 10% of the population are carriers of hepatitis B; for health care workers traveling to developing countries	1.0 ml at 0, 1, and 6 months

*For adults weighing < 45 kg, give half the dose.

Other immunizations

The risk of hepatitis A varies considerably depending on the living conditions and length of stay. Immune serum globulin is recommended for those who plan to visit developing countries for 3 months or longer or who plan excursions outside of tourist areas in these countries (Table 241-6).

Hepatitis B is common throughout sub-Saharan Africa, China, Southeast Asia, the South Pacific, and the Caribbean. The risk to travelers is small, however, in the absence of other risk factors (sexual contact, exposure to blood or secretions of carriers). Vaccination is recommended for persons who may have one or more risk factors or who plan extended travel to countries where the carrier rate exceeds 5% to 10%.

Vaccinations against meningococcal disease, rabies, typhus, and plague, though available, are rarely indicated. Certain individuals (health care workers, laboratory personnel, persons exposed to wild game, wild rodents, or their fleas) may be at increased risk depending on their particular situation, and vaccination may be advisable in some instances. Recommendations and information concerning these vaccines are available from the Centers for Disease Control in Atlanta, Georgia.

REFERENCES

Brown HW and Neva FA: Basic clinical parasitology, ed 5, Norwalk, Conn, 1983, Appleton-Century-Crofts.

Gove S and Slutkin G: Infectious diseases of travelers and immigrants, Emerg Med Clin North Am 2:587, 1984.
Hill DR and Pearson RD: Health advice for international travel, Ann Intern Med 108:839, 1988.
Katzenstein D, Rickerson V, and Braude A: New concepts of amebic liver abscess derived from hepatic imaging, serodiagnosis, and hepatic enzymes in 67 consecutive cases in San Diego, Medicine (Baltimore) 61:237, 1982.
Lange WR: Viral hepatitis and international travel, Am Fam Physician 36:179, 1987.
National Institutes of Health Consensus Development Conference: Travelers' diarrhea, Rev Infec Dis 8(Suppl 2):S104, 1986.
Steffen R: Health problems after travel to developing countries, J Infect Dis 156:84, 1987.
Tauxe RV and Blake PA: Epidemic cholera in Latin America, JAMA 267:1388-1390, 1992.

CHAPTER

242 Acquired Immunodeficiency Syndrome

Julie Louise Gerberding
Merle A. Sande

In 1981 a group of homosexual men with an unusual presentation of Kaposi's sarcoma and *Pneumocystis carinii* pneumonia were identified in the United States. This cluster of cases proved to be the beginning of what has become an enormous pandemic. The term AIDS (acquired immunodeficiency syndrome) was defined by the Centers for Disease Control (CDC) to describe patients who lacked other causes for impaired immunity and who developed unusual malignancies such as Kaposi's sarcoma or opportunistic infections. It is now obvious that human immunodeficiency virus (HIV) is responsible for AIDS as well as a myriad of earlier and less severe manifestations of progressive immunodeficiency. This chapter describes the spectrum of disease associated with HIV infection.

ETIOLOGY AND PATHOPHYSIOLOGY

HIV (type 1) infection and the human diseases it causes appears to be new, although some studies have demonstrated antibodies to this retrovirus in sera obtained in Africa as early as the mid-1950s. HIV is found in many body fluids including blood, semen, saliva, vaginal secretions, and breast milk and is transmissible by direct inoculation of any of these fluids. It is trophic for T-cell lymphocytes and other cells that possess CD4 surface receptors, including macrophages, promyelocytes, intestinal immunocytes, astrocytes, oligodendrocytes, epidermal Langerhans cells, and certain fibroblasts (Chapter 252). The manifestations of HIV infection are a consequence of the immune defects that result from dysregulation and destruction of T-helper cells (CD4 lymphocytes) and other target cells. Infection is associated with a release of lymphokines, nonspecific stimulation of B-cells, and an initial increase in the number of suppressor and T-killer cells (CD8 lymphocytes) that is followed by a progressive decline in the number of circulating CD4 lymphocytes over several years (mean 10.5 years from infection to CD4 count less than 200/mm^3). Although infection leads to abnormal B-cell function, the predominant clinical manifestations reflect severe deficiencies in the cellular immune system. To date, attempts to reconstitute the immune defects have been largely unsuccessful. Once the reduction in CD4 lymphocytes has occurred it appears to be essentially irreversible.

EPIDEMIOLOGY

HIV infection is a global disease and the pandemic is expected to spread to more than 40 million persons by the end of this century. Infection is transmitted by three main mechanisms: (1) sexually, through unprotected heterosexual or homosexual contact with an infected partner; (2) parenterally, by direct inoculation of infected blood (transfusion of blood products, sharing contaminated injection drug equipment, occupational injury among health care workers); and (3) perinatally, from infected mothers to their offspring. Early in the epidemic, infection appeared to be confined to individuals populating "high risk groups." It is now clear, however, that activities leading to infection do not necessarily correlate with these risk groups and it is more appropriate to assess HIV risk in terms of high risk behaviors.

The importance of these risk behaviors in perpetuating the epidemic varies throughout the world. Three main epidemiologic patterns have been described by the World Health Organization. The first pattern predominates in developed countries including the United States and is primarily related to sexual transmission among homosexual men and contact with contaminated blood among injection drug users. The second pattern is evident in Africa, Latin America, and the Caribbean where heterosexual and perinatal transmission predominate. In these areas, HIV has penetrated into the general population to such an extent that more than 20% of the adult population in some locales is seropositive, and the number of cases among women equals or exceeds that among men. The third pattern of transmission is seen in Asia, India, Eastern Europe, and the Pacific rim, where the epidemic became apparent in the late 1980s and is now spreading rapidly among sexually active heterosexual and homosexual adults as well as injection drug users. A distinct but genetically related virus, HIV type 2 (HIV 2), is found in western Africa and has not yet spread extensively outside of this region. Although the clinical presentation and natural history of infection with HIV 2 are not as clearly defined as for HIV 1, there appear to be few if any differences in the outcome of infection with these retroviruses. To date, the only cases of HIV 2 infection in the United States have occurred in persons previously residing in HIV 2 endemic areas and no secondary cases have been detected. Nevertheless, the blood supply is now screened with tests that will detect infection with both agents.

It is difficult to determine factors that influence transmissibility, but some helpful information has accumulated. Among homosexual men, rectal receptive intercourse without condom protection, traumatic intercourse, and multiple sexual partners are factors highly correlated with transmission. Among intravenous drug users, exposure to contaminated blood via shared needles, contaminated drug paraphernalia, and possibly even contaminated drug increases transmission risk. Sexual transmission is also important in this population, especially when prostitution is practiced to finance drug use. With the advent of donor screening protocols recommended by the blood bank community, the current risk of acquiring HIV from blood transfusion in the United States is estimated to be less than 1/50,000 units transfused, a rate that reflects the low but "nonzero" frequency of blood collection from recently infected donors who have not yet seroconverted. Infected blood products such as clotting factor preparations were an important source of infection among hemophiliacs and other blood product recipients early in the epidemic, but these products are now prepared from rigorously screened donors and are treated with a process proven to reliably inactivate HIV and other blood-borne pathogens. Unfortunately, transfusions continue to transmit HIV at an alarming rate in the developing world where donor screening is not always available.

Children acquire HIV perinatally or from infected blood products. The exact mode(s) of perinatal transmission have not been clearly delineated, but infection in the first trimester of pregnancy has been documented. Overall, a significant proportion, about 60% to 80%, of children born to infected mothers are not infected, but once one child has been infected the risk to the next child increases dramatically. Breastfeeding is also a proven route of HIV transmission. Current recommendations in the United States argue against breastfeeding when maternal infection is documented, but this approach has not been advocated in developing countries where it is believed that the benefits of breastfeeding may outweigh the risks of HIV transmission.

Heterosexual partners of individuals in all risk categories have acquired HIV, but transmission appears to be more efficient from man to woman. About 40% of steady male sexual partners of infected women have HIV infection, whereas about 60% of female partners of infected men acquire the disease. The efficiency of sexual transmission is believed to increase in the presence of concomitant genital lesions such as chancroid, syphilitic chancres, and perhaps herpes virus infections that disrupt the integrity of the mucosal barrier. In Africa, lack of circumcision is likely to be an independent risk for infection, but this is not established with certainty in the United States.

There is no evidence to suggest that HIV is spread by casual contact, by the airborne route, by insects, by direct exposure to tears or saliva, or by environmental contamination. Nonsexual household contacts of infected individuals do not acquire antibodies to the virus or exhibit disease manifestations, even with close contact among infected children or adults.

Occupational transmission to health care workers is now well documented and poses a challenge to those responsible for providing care to the increasing number of infected patients. Prospective studies of providers who sustained exposure to HIV through needlesticks or similar percutaneous injuries demonstrate that the magnitude of risk is 0.2% to 0.3%. Although these data are useful in defining the average risk among populations of exposed workers, care must be taken to avoid ascribing this average risk to individual exposures. Factors that may increase transmission risk include exposure to large volumes of blood (injections, large-bore hollow needles, deep penetration) or exposure to blood containing high titers of HIV (e.g., source patients with advanced stages of HIV infection). Risk may be lower when the exposure involves minimum amounts of blood (superficial injuries, suture needlesticks, needles passing through gloves before contacting the skin) or when the source patient has early stages of HIV infection and is not highly viremic. The risk from contamination of mucous membranes or nonintact skin is too low to be reliably quantified in the studies that have been performed to date, but most authorities agree that these exposures are less risky than percutaneous exposures unless prolonged contact with relatively large volumes of blood occurs via a break in the integument or some other portal of entry.

CLINICAL STAGES OF HIV INFECTION

The availability of serologic testing for antibody to HIV has expanded our understanding of the wide variability in clinical presentations. Several distinct stages of infection have been identified, but significant overlap occurs and the rate of progression from one phase to another is not uniform. The degree of immunosuppression as measured by the loss of CD4 lymphocytes and cutaneous anergy is the major determinant of disease and correlates well with the severity of illness and long-term prognosis.

Asymptomatic infection (stage 1)

Many individuals are infected with HIV but have not yet developed symptoms. Although the proportion of these individuals who will ultimately progress to AIDS is not known, the vast majority will eventually develop signs of infection. Even though both cell-associated and cell-free virus titers are lower during the early stages of infection than after AIDS develops, most if not all asymptomatic individuals remain infectious and can transmit HIV to susceptible persons.

Acute viral syndrome (stage 2)

A majority of patients infected with HIV develop an acute mononucleosis-like illness characterized by fever, headache, lymphadenopathy, pharyngitis, macular rash, and malaise within several weeks of exposure. Aseptic meningitis, hepatosplenomegaly, extreme fatigue, weakness, arthralgias, and myalgias are also frequently associated with this syndrome. Symptoms usually resolve within 2 to 4 weeks, but occasionally rapid progression with early development of an AIDS-defining condition has been described. The acute illness is temporally associated with seroconversion and viremia. Immune complex disease may also play a role in pathogenesis. Some authorities have speculated that this illness could also be caused by lymphokines released during nonspecific activation of multiple clones of lymphocytes by HIV antigens that behave as superantigens. Regardless of the mechanism, HIV infection should be suspected in any person at risk who presents with an unexplained febrile viral-like illness. Initially, HIV screening tests may not demonstrate antibody. However, tests for HIV p24 antigen are usually positive early in the course of this illness and should be performed when the index of suspicion is high. Currently no data suggest that treatment with antiretroviral agents will abort infection or affect the long-term outcome when instituted during the acute illness.

Persistent generalized lymphadenopathy (stage 3)

Lymphadenopathy, defined in this setting as enlargement of the lymph nodes in at least two extrainguinal sites for a minimum of 3 months in the absence of any illness or drug known to cause lymphadenopathy, is usually present and may be caused by an immunologic response to infection with HIV. In and of itself, persistent lymphadenopathy does not influence prognosis. A progressive decrease in the size of the involved nodes correlates with the onset of AIDS and portends a bad prognosis.

Symptomatic infection (stage 4)

Nonspecific complaints of fever, weight loss, diarrhea, and malaise; lymphadenopathy; and oral thrush are frequently noted in patients who have been infected with HIV for more than 5 years. In the past, these symptoms and signs defined a condition known as AIDS-related complex (ARC). Use of this clinical designation has largely been abandoned, as there is no clear distinction between symptomatic HIV infection, ARC, and AIDS; and CD4 counts have emerged as a somewhat more objective determinant of clinical stage.

A distinct subgroup of patients develop immune thrombocytopenic purpura (ITP), which is clinically similar to ITP in other patients. Although platelet counts less than 50,000 are common, bleeding is rare unless other drugs adversely affecting platelet function are administered. Optimal treatment for AIDS-related ITP remains controversial. Platelet counts improve after antiretroviral therapy with zidovudine is instituted in some patients; others seem to benefit from corticosteroids. Splenectomy is rarely necessary.

Diseases suggestive of modest immune deficiency, such as dermatomal varicella zoster infection, chronic herpes simplex lesions, cutaneous fungal infections, and oral leukoplakia portend progression to AIDS-defining infections. Recurrent infection with encapsulated bacteria and nontyphoid *Salmonella* species also occurs in these patients. The risk of reactivating tuberculosis is increased (Chapter 276) Tuberculosis may present as upper lobe pulmonary disease similar to infection in nonimmunosuppressed adults, but nonupper lobe pulmonary involvement and extrapulmonary disease occur in those with lower CD4 counts.

The diagnosis of AIDS is readily established when the patient presents with obvious manifestations such as Kaposi's sarcoma or *P. carinii* pneumonia. In many patients, however, the initial symptoms and signs are subtle and necessitate careful evaluation to establish a definitive diagnosis. The CDC surveillance definition of the syndrome was initially based solely on clinical manifestations, was later expanded to incorporate HIV antibody positivity as a requirement in certain instances, and now includes CD4 lymphocyte counts as criteria for diagnosis.

Onset of AIDS may be gradual or abrupt. In most patients a history of prodromal symptoms is elicited for variable periods of time before diagnosis. Some patients present with isolated Kaposi's sarcoma lesions and no evidence of prodrome or opportunistic infection and overall have a better short-term prognosis than those who present with opportunistic infections or neurologic disease.

A rational approach to evaluating individuals with suspected HIV disease has several objectives: (1) to diagnose HIV infection early at a point where medical intervention is effective; (2) to establish the presence and severity of immune deficiency, (3) to exclude other etiologies of the clinical findings, (4) to identify preventable and/or treatable components of the illness, and (5) to diagnose life-threatening complications expediently. No single protocol can be provided to accomplish these objectives in all patients, but the following general approach can be individualized.

DIAGNOSING HIV INFECTION

In the AIDS era, it is essential to incorporate a careful history to elicit information about risk behaviors for acquiring HIV infection into the routine medical history for all adult patients. Sufficient information should be sought to accurately assess risk from sexual practices, recreational drug use, and blood product transfusions. All patients for whom HIV infection cannot be excluded with reasonable certainty on the basis of history should be offered HIV counseling and testing, or at the very least, they should be referred to appropriate community resources for such testing. History alone is actually an unreliable method for excluding HIV infection; many patients are reluctant to disclose risk behaviors, and many (especially women) may not realize that their sexual partners are at risk for infection.

Pretest counseling should assess individual risk, provide risk reduction education, and explain the importance of testing and the meaning of a positive and negative test. Third-party risks should also be addressed. The procedures for recording test results and protecting the patient's confidentiality are important components of this process as well.

Licensed tests for HIV use three general techniques for detection of the antibody: ELISA (enzyme-linked immunoabsorbant assay), IFA (immunofluorescent assay), and Western Blot. The commercially available ELISA tests are extremely sensitive but relatively nonspecific, whereas the

IFA and Western Blot are more specific but are more labor intensive and expensive to perform. The ELISA tests are useful screening tests; the Western Blot or IFA is then used as a confirmatory test for repeatedly reactive ELISA-positive serum. Using this protocol, HIV testing is one of the most accurate laboratory procedures currently available. Rapid tests for HIV antibody are not yet in widespread use, but may prove useful in settings where delays in obtaining test results are problematic.

Although a negative antibody test does not exclude the diagnosis of HIV, it makes it extremely unlikely unless the individual has been exposed in the previous 6 months. If such is the case, a repeat test should be offered 3 to 6 months later. Although documented cases of delayed seroconversion (after 1 year) have appeared, this phenomenon is rare, and the vast majority of patients will have antibody within 6 months of initial infection. Antibody to HIV may disappear in the preterminal phases of the disease in some patients. Obviously, antibody to HIV is not protective, and its presence is highly correlated with persistent viremia.

There is little utility in performing p24 antigen tests for detecting HIV infection. The initial antigen test procedures are not highly sensitive and false-negative results are a serious problem. The sensitivity of antigen detection, however, may improve with methods that dissociate antigen-antibody complexes and a role for antigen detection may be established. Special tests, including gene amplification studies to detect HIV in peripheral lymphocytes or serum, and virus cultures are rarely required and should be reserved for situations where the index of suspicion is high and antibody tests are negative. These procedures may also facilitate diagnosis of perinatal HIV infection, which is otherwise complicated by the presence of maternal antibody in the infant.

Care should be taken to present HIV test results in person to the patient. Post-test counseling should include an assessment of mental status (especially if a positive test result was obtained), an explanation of the meaning of the result, a review of third-party risks and confidentiality procedures, appropriate referral for psychologic support and drug rehabilitation if needed, and a follow-up appointment. If a positive result is returned from a patient at low risk, testing should be repeated.

INITIAL EVALUATION AND MANAGEMENT OF THE INFECTED PATIENT

A comprehensive medical evaluation should be performed for all newly diagnosed patients with HIV infection. The history should include assessment of general health status; immunizations, drug and medication history; sexual history (including obstetric and gynecologic information in women); and assessment of travel, geographic, and occupational exposures that increase the risks of specific opportunistic infections. The physical examination should document initial height and weight and include a careful funduscopic, oral, lymphatic, cutaneous, and genital examination (including pelvic with Pap smear).

Laboratory studies are helpful in establishing the presence of immune dysfunction and overall health status. The CD4 lymphocyte count provides essential prognostic information and is necessary to guide medical interventions. However, significant diurnal variation in CD4 count is well documented, and results can vary significantly among laboratories. Many clinicians recommend repeating CD4 counts when they are used as the sole criterion for clinical decisions. In some cases, measuring the CD4 cell count as a percentage of total lymphocyte count is a more useful index of immunosuppression. Quantitative measurement of serum HIV titer is investigational, but in some research studies such measurement has provided useful evidence of drug efficacy and clinical response. Nonspecific markers of disease progression include elevated erythrocyte sedimentation rate and beta-2-microglobulin, but these tests have largely been rendered obsolete by more specific CD4 count testing.

Hematologic abnormalities are common in HIV infection and may be multifactorial. A decreased white cell count ($<3000/mm^3$) is often seen, usually with concomitant absolute lymphopenia ($<1500/mm^3$). Lymphopenia correlates somewhat with the immune suppression but is by no means diagnostic. Pancytopenia or decreases in individual cell lines can be ascribed to nutritional deficiency or the presence of fever and chronic disease in some patients. Thrombocytopenia may be induced by antiplatelet antibodies as in ITP (see earlier discussion). In addition, many of the chemotherapeutic and other therapeutic agents administered to patients are toxic to the bone marrow. The bone marrow should be examined if the etiology is in doubt since disseminated fungal, *Mycobacterium tuberculosis* and *Mycobacterium avium-intracellulare* infection and lymphoma can be associated with pancytopenias and are often detected in the bone marrow.

Minor abnormalities in liver function tests are not uncommon. Hepatitis B and hepatitis C virus infection should be identified, as these concomitant infections may have a more severe course in patients with HIV. Serum lactate dehydrogenase enzyme may also be increased, and many clinicians obtain this test at the time of initial evaluation so that the baseline value can be compared to that obtained when pneumocystic pneumonia is later suspected. A polyclonal gammopathy is typically present. A serologic test for syphilis, antitoxoplasma IgG titer, and a chest radiograph are also advisable.

Most but not all AIDS patients are anergic when a battery of a least four intradermal skin tests for delayed hypersensitivity are applied. A smaller proportion of those with earlier stages of infection are anergic and purified protein derivative (PPD) testing should be routine for all patients. Those with a PPD response greater than 5 mm and those exposed to active cases of tuberculosis are at high risk for active disease and should be given isoniazid prophylaxis, regardless of age.

Initial health care maintenance is directed toward improving overall health status. Nutrition, smoking cessation, drug rehabilitation, safer sex, and psychosocial issues should be explored. Reproductive counseling is extremely important and all too often overlooked. Pneumococcal vaccine, influenza vaccine (annually), hepatitis B vaccine (especially if the patient is sexually active or sharing needles), and hemophilus B vaccine are recommended. Although the response to these vaccines declines as immunodeficiency develops, a proportion of patients will achieve protective titers and immunization is strongly encouraged. There is no evidence that immunization accelerates disease progression.

Antiretroviral therapy

If the CD4 count is above 500 and the patient is relatively asymptomatic, no specific antiretroviral or prophylactic therapy for opportunistic infection is currently indicated, but recommendations could change as research data become available. If the CD4 count is less than 500, treatment with zidovudine (ZDV) is recommended (500 to 600 mg/day). Most patients on this regimen will develop macrocytosis and mild decreases in hemoglobin, but careful monitoring is warranted to detect clinically significant anemia or other toxicities (cytopenias, severe gastrointestinal complaints, headache, sleep disturbance) that will develop in a minority of patients. Periodic transfusions or treatment with erythropoitin-A can improve tolerance to ZDV in some cases, but the availability of new antiretroviral drugs provides a more attractive alternative.

Dideoxyionosine (DDI) has been shown to decrease the rate of disease progression in patients previously exposed to ZDV and appears to be similar to ZDV in some efficacy studies.

Although dideoxycytosine (DDC) is not as effective as ZDV when used alone, in combination with ZDV clinical benefit is evident. These drugs rarely cause cytopenias, but are associated with neurologic toxicity and, rarely, severe pancreatitis. The best antiretroviral regimen for ameliorating disease progression has not yet been established, and clinicians should consult the medical literature as data from the myriad of ongoing studies becomes available. Evidence mounts to implicate emergence of drug-resistant virus isolates as an explanation for the eventual decline in efficacy of single drug regimens.

Combination therapy, either sequential or simultaneous, may prove to be more effective than single drug therapy, perhaps by preventing the emergence of drug resistance. Use of simultaneous combination therapy using drug doses lower than that required for single drug therapy is an attractive approach (especially if central nervous system [CNS] drug levels sufficient to ameliorate CNS disease are achieved) because less toxicity is expected. Indications for combination therapy or for changing from one to another agent are yet to be defined. At present, most clinicians begin patients on ZDV and then change to DDI or add DDC when CD4 counts decline, when ZDV toxicity occurs, or when the clinical course deteriorates.

Prophylaxis for opportunistic infections

When the CD4 count is less than 200, patients are at high risk for the development of pneumocystic pneumonia. Prophylaxis with trimethoprim sulfamethoxazole (1 DS tablet everyday or three times a week) is advised. Dapsone (50 to 100 mg everyday) may also be effective, but monitoring for methemoglobinemia is required and G-6PD deficiency contraindicates treatment. Several other regimens have also been tested and appear promising (Chapter 281). These oral regimens are now believed to be superior in efficacy to aerosolized pentamidine, which has been relegated to second line drug status. The decline in incidence of pneumocystic pneumonia as the index diagnosis for AIDS attests to the benefit of routine primary prophylaxis.

The value of prophylaxis of other common opportunistic infections is under investigation. The incidence of toxoplasmosis in the United States is probably too low to justify routine primary prophylaxis at this time, especially because current tests do not allow easy identification of a higher risk subpopulation. Moreover, pneumocystis prophylaxis with trimethoprim sulfamethoxazol appears to simultaneously decrease the incidence of toxoplasmosis. In areas such as France where toxoplasmosis is highly endemic and reactivation and/or primary infection rates are high, prophylaxis for toxoplasmosis may be warranted. Prophylaxis for cryptococcal meningitis is not yet recommended, but periodic screening for serum cryptococcal antigen among patients with CD4 counts less than 200 may be useful in detecting early disease. Prophylaxis for atypical mycobacterial infection is being studied in patients at high risk for this infection (those with CD4 counts less than 100), but specific recommendations are not yet developed.

CLINICAL SYNDROMES ASSOCIATED WITH HIV

Improvement in the quality of life and survival of HIV-infected patients through appropriate antiretroviral therapy, prophylaxis for common infectious complications, and prompt treatment of complicating illnesses is a realistic goal. Recognition of the wide variability in presentation and the more common manifestations of involvement of the various organ systems is necessary to rationally approach diagnosis and management.

Fever

Fever is not uncommon in HIV-infected patients with CD4 counts less than 500 and night sweats are frequently associated. When fever accompanies an accelerated catabolic state with weight loss and anorexia, the presence of opportunistic infection or malignancy signifying the onset of AIDS should be suspected.

In sexually active adults, sexually transmitted diseases and anorectal infections often go unrecognized as sources of fever. Serologic tests for syphilis and proctologic examination with cultures for *Neisseria gonorrhoeae, Chlamydia trachomatis,* and *herpes simplex* virus should be performed. Blood cultures should be obtained and processed for isolation of bacteria, mycobacteria, and fungi. In the absence of other symptoms infection with disseminated *M. tuberculosis* (Chapter 276), *M. avium-intracellulare, Histoplasma capsulatum, Coccidioides immitis* (Chapter 277), and *Cryptococcus neoformans* (Chapter 279) should be excluded. Nontyphoid salmonella bacteremia can also present with fever alone and is often recurrent despite appropriate treatment.

Cytomegalovirus (CMV) infection is a cause of fever and CMV may be cultured from the blood and urine (Chapter 251). Because this organism is prevalent in HIV-infected persons, a causal relationship to fever can be implied only when no other pathogen is detected.

Hypotension suggests hypoadrenalism, especially if electrolyte disturbances are noted. Adrenal insufficiency is very common in AIDS patients and has been attributed to HIV-induced abnormalities in steroid synthesis, adrenalitis from CMV infection, and ketoconazole therapy.

Lymphadenopathy

In patients with HIV lymph node biopsy typically reveals reactive hyperplasia (Color Plate V-37), and biopsy of nodes in patients with persistent generalized lymphadenopathy is not routinely required. Biopsy should be performed to exclude disseminated tuberculosis, *M. avium-intracellulare* infection (Color Plate V-38), histoplasmosis, toxoplasmosis, bacillary angiomatosis (Chapter 269), lymphoma, and Kaposi's sarcoma, when asymmetric, regional, or painful lymphadenopathy occurs. Increasing numbers of patients with aggressive B-cell lymphomas have been recognized in the past several years (as many as 30% of patients on retroviral therapy followed for more than 3 years in one study).

Enlargement of the hilar or mediastinal nodes is unusual and should suggest a diffuse lymphoma, mycobacterial infection, or pulmonary Kaposi's sarcoma. If no other tissue is available for examination, these nodes should also be biopsied.

Although hepatosplenomegaly in combination with lymphadenopathy and fever may be a manifestation of HIV, it may also be a sign of disseminated fungal or mycobacterial infection or lymphoma. Liver biopsy should be considered if blood cultures are negative, peripheral lymph nodes are not enlarged, and no contraindications are present.

Dysphagia

Complaints of dysphagia or odynophagia usually signify mucosal infection with *Candida albicans* (Chapter 278) or *herpes simplex* virus. Infection may extend from the oral mucosa into the esophagus or upper respiratory tract and often results in anorexia and weight loss from decreased caloric intake. Candida infection may be presumptively diagnosed by scraping the typical patchy white mucosal lesions and identifying hyphae after wet-mount in 10% potassium hydroxide. Virus cultures should be performed if wet-mount preparations are negative. Cytomegalovirus may be cultured in both symptomatic and asymptomatic patients, and should be considered pathogenic only when other causes have been excluded and histologic findings are consistent.

Oral candidiasis can be treated topically with nystatin in oral suspension or clotrimazole troches. With more extensive mucosal involvement systemic therapy with ketoconazol or fluconazole should be considered. Acyclovir should be administered intravenously to patients with documented herpes simplex esophagitis (Chapter 251).

Diarrhea

Diarrhea is a frequent complaint. Symptoms range from frequent loose stools to fulminate diarrhea producing profound weight loss and malabsorption. A thorough evaluation is warranted as virtually any gastrointestinal pathogen may be found (see the accompanying box) (Chapter 236). Stool for bacterial cultures, testing for ova and parasites including microsporidia and cryptosporidia (Chapters 41, 48, and 280), and proctosigmoidoscopy should be included in the initial diagnostic work-up.

Common bacterial pathogens cultured include *Campylobacter* species (Chapter 266), *Salmonella* species, *Shigella* species (Chapter 268), and *Yersinia* species. If any of these organisms is isolated, specific antibiotic treatment is indicated.

Although parasites are frequently identified in stool specimens from asymptomatic homosexual men, they may produce diarrhea and treatment is indicated. In addition to *Giardia lamblia* and *Entamoeba histolytica* (Chapter 280), unusual parasites such as *Isospora belli, Blastocystis hominis,* micropsoridium, and *Cryptosporidium* may produce symptoms. Cryptosporidia are readily demonstrated by direct examination of the stool with a modified Kinyoun stain (Color Plate V-34). Therapy with trimethoprim-sulfamethoxazole is usually effective in eradicating *Isospora* organisms. To date, treatment for cryptosporidiosis

Gastrointestinal infections commonly associated with AIDS and the pathogens frequently causing these infections

Proctitis

Herpes simplex virus
Neisseria gonorrhoeae
Treponema pallidum
Chlamydia trachomatis

Colitis

Salmonella species
Campylobacter species
Shigella species
Entamoeba histolytica
Cytomegalovirus

Enteritis

Cryptosporidium
Isospora belli
Giardia lamblia
Strongyloides stercoralis
Mycobacterium avium-intracellulare
Cytomegalovirus

has been disappointing, and diarrhea in these patients may persist or wax and wane indefinitely. Reports of limited success with paramomycin, spiramycin (a macrolide antibiotic not available in the United States), or a combination of clindamycin and quinine have surfaced but have not been confirmed.

When stool examination and culture fail to reveal a pathogen, more invasive diagnostic tests are indicated. Sigmoidoscopy and colonoscopy with mucosal biopsy are necessary to thoroughly evaluate the lower intestinal tract. Duodenal aspirate may be necessary to definitively diagnose *G. lamblia* and *I. belli* infection. Small bowel biopsy may reveal evidence of parasitic infection, Kaposi's sarcoma, *M. avium-intracellulare* infection, Whipple's disease, or intestinal lymphoma. Cytomegalovirus has been implicated as a cause of diarrhea when mucosal biopsy reveals histologic evidence of intracellular inclusions in areas of active inflammation and no other cause is found (Color Plate V-39).

A history of recent antibiotic use should stimulate a search for *Clostridium difficile* toxin, and evidence of pseudomembrane formation and mucosal inflammation are usually seen on lower endoscopy (Chapter 262).

An etiology for the diarrhea in AIDS patients will often not be found despite extensive evaluation. Symptomatic treatment with antimotility drugs may afford some relief to some patients, but the diarrhea may persist relentlessly, resulting in profound weight loss and debilitation.

Perirectal pain

Anorectal pain with purulent discharge usually signifies localized infection. Anoscopic examination with cultures for herpes simplex virus and *N. gonorrhoeae* may be diagnostic. The presence of mucosal ulcerations suggests herpes simplex virus, *Treponema pallidum,* or *C. trachomatis* infection. Perirectal abscesses are occasionally seen, particularly in the homosexual population (Chapter 22). Rectal malignancies such as squamous cell carcinoma and cloacagenic carcinoma are increasingly found in individuals with AIDS, and these patients may present with proctologic symptoms. Kaposi's sarcoma lesions can also be etiologic.

Acute abdominal pain

Patients with AIDS occasionally develop symptoms of intra-abdominal catastrophe or peritonitis. Bowel perforation secondary to gastrointestinal lymphoma accounts for the findings in the majority of these cases, and prognosis is poor. Symptoms of peritoneal irritation as an isolated finding may also occur. Gastrointestinal tuberculosis, CMV infection, and disseminated fungal infections have been reported in this setting.

Cutaneous lesions

The lesions of Kaposi's sarcoma are often the first sign of AIDS to appear, particularly in homosexual men. These nontender, raised, violescent tumors may occur on any part of the body (Color Plate V-40), and a scrupulous search for lesions should be undertaken during the initial evaluation of any patient suspected of having AIDS. Kaposi's sarcoma may initially present in the oral cavity, on the soles of the feet, and in the rectal mucosa and other inconspicuous sites, as well as in the gastrointestinal tract (Color Plate V-41). Biopsy of any suspicious lesion will be diagnostic if Kaposi's sarcoma is present.

Bacillary angiomatosis should be considered in patients with raised tender nonblanching angiomatous lesions on the skin (Color Plate V-42). These patients usually have fever and may also present with hepatomegaly (peliosis hepatitis). The infection results from infection with *Rochalimaea henslei* or *R. quintana,* which induces proliferation of vascular endothelial cells. These bacteria can now be cultured from the skin or blood in some laboratories. The Warthin-Starry silver stain will also reveal the bacilli in biopsied tissue. Treatment with erythromycin is often effective (Chapters 48 and 269).

Herpesvirus infection can be diagnosed by viral culture of the typical cutaneous vesicles and mucosal ulcerations. Herpes simplex (types I and II) produces localized or disseminated lesions, which are not always distinguishable from varicella zoster infection without culture. Therapy with acyclovir may be useful in severe local infections or disseminated disease (Chapter 251).

Cutaneous bacterial infections including impetigo, folliculitis, and ecthyma caused by *S. aureus* occur in many patients. These conditions usually respond to oral systemic therapy, but tend to recur. Psoriasis, maculopapular rashes, and basal cell carcinomas also appear with increased incidence in HIV-infected patients. *C. neoformans* and, rarely, other fungi can produce chronic cutaneous infections of the skin, nailbeds, and genitalia. Fungal cultures should be obtained any time such an infection does not respond promptly to antibacterial therapy.

Dyspnea

The onset of shortness of breath with exertion in a patient with risk factors for acquiring AIDS usually signifies the onset of *P. carinii* pneumonia (Chapter 281). A dry hacking cough, fever, and tachypnea are also common presenting complaints; but any symptom suggestive of respiratory involvement should initiate a diagnostic evaluation aimed at identifying this opportunistic pathogen. Symptomatic patients should be evaluated with a chest radiograph and arterial blood gas determination. Pulmonary function tests and gallium scanning are no longer routine, but may be indicated in symptomatic patients with normal chest radiographs.

The chest radiograph usually reveals bilateral diffuse interstitial infiltrates, but infiltrates may also be alveolar or well localized. Occasionally, the chest radiograph is entirely normal. Pleural effusion is atypical for pneumocystis infection and suggests pleural involvement with Kaposi's sarcoma or other opportunistic pathogens. Pleuritic chest pain suggests pneumothorax, a complication of recurrent pneumocystic pneumonia, which may also be more common in patients who received aerosolized pentamidine prophylaxis. Arterial blood gas analysis usually demonstrates a mild respiratory alkalosis and hypoxemia (Po_2 50 to 60 mm Hg). A restrictive pattern with abnormal diffusing capacity to carbon monoxide is almost always demonstrated on pulmonary function tests. An increased uptake of gallium in the lungs is found on scanning in more than 90% of patients with pneumocystis pneumonia.

The organism can be identified on direct examination of induced sputum (induced with saline nebulization) with Giemsa staining (Chapter 226) (Color Plate V-10) in over half of the patients. Bronchoscopy performed with transbronchial lavage followed by immediate examination of specimens with Giemsa, silver methionine, and fluorescent antipneumocystis antibody tests will reveal the diagnosis in more than 80% of patients. Bronchoscopic biopsy may increase the yield of this approach but is not usually required. Open lung biopsy is rarely indicated.

P. carinii pneumonia still contributes to the morbidity and mortality of HIV infection despite effective prophylactic therapy. Treatment with trimethoprim-sulfamethoxazole or pentamidine is effective in the majority of patients, but the infection is fatal in up to 30% of initial episodes. Relapse occurs in at least 20% and mortality increases with recurrent infection.

In addition to *P. carinii,* a multitude of other organisms may invade the respiratory tract in AIDS patients. *M. tuberculosis, M. avium-intracellulare, H. capsulatum, C. immitis, C. neoformans,* and CMV are not uncommonly detected; infection with *Legionella* species has also been reported. These organisms can usually be identified by careful culturing of specimens obtained at bronchoscopy and by histologic examination with special stains (acid-fast, PAS, Geimsa, and silver methionine). Procedures for processing specimens should be carefully coordinated with the microbiology and pathology services to facilitate diagnosis. Infection with *Streptococcus pneumoniae* or other common respiratory bacterial pathogens should be considered when the chest radiograph reveals lobar consolidation, as this radiographic pattern is not common in pnuemocystis or fungal pneumonias.

Not all pulmonary disease in AIDS patients is directly related to the immune deficiency. Pulmonary embolism should be considered, particularly after prolonged bed rest. Diagnosis usually requires arteriography because many patients have other pulmonary abnormalities making ventilation-perfusion scanning nondiagnostic.

Headache

The symptoms and signs of CNS involvement in AIDS patients are often subtle, and opportunistic infections of the CNS therefore may go unrecognized unless careful history and neurologic examinations are performed. Chronic or progressive headache is the most prevalent symptom suggesting CNS involvement.

Toxoplasma gondii has emerged as the most frequent cause of encephalitis in AIDS patients (Chapter 280). Headache and focal neurologic signs and seizures are typical, although patients may have no localizing findings. A wide array of serologic studies to facilitate diagnosis of toxoplasmosis have been developed. The absence of antitoxoplasma antibody as assayed by the Sabin-Feldman dye test or other equally sensitive test for IgG makes the diagnosis less likely but does not exclude it entirely because histopathologic evidence of toxoplasmosis has been reported in up to 15% of individuals with negative serology.

Computed tomography (CT) usually demonstrate single or multiple ring-enhancing lesions, but other findings such as focal edema and large lesions with mass effect have also been described (Fig. 242-1). Delayed scanning after double-dose contrast infusion improves the yield of the procedure. CT scans may be completely normal in some patients with documented toxoplasmosis at autopsy. Magnetic resonance imaging (MRI) is more sensitive than CT and may reveal lesions not evidenced on conventional scans (Fig. 242-2).

In patients with HIV infection and less than 200 CD4 cells/mm^3, a trial of treatment for toxoplasmosis with pyramethamine and sulfadiazine may be justifiable without obtaining a tissue diagnosis, providing the clinical and radiographic findings are consistent with the diagnosis. However, brain biopsy is recommended by most investigators if the diagnosis of AIDS is not established, if the CT scan or MRI scan is atypical, or if the patient deteriorates on therapy. If brain biopsy does not reveal other etiologies to explain the clinical findings, therapy with pyramethamine

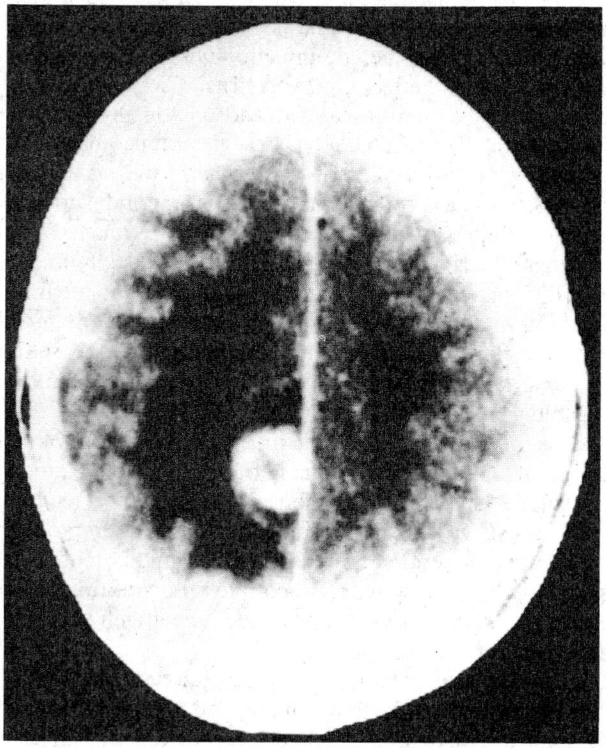

Fig. 242-1. Computer tomography brain scan of patient with biopsy-proved *Toxoplasma* infection.

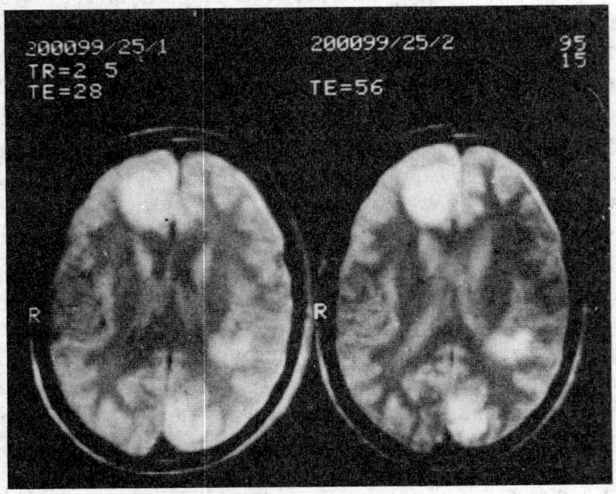

Fig. 242-2. Magnetic resonance imaging of patient with multiple *Toxoplasma* lesions in the central nervous system.

and sulfadiazine should be continued because toxoplasmosis has been diagnosed at autopsy in a number of patients with negative brain biopsies. In patients who present with a high probability of toxoplasmosis based on clinical findings and in whom scans reveals large lesions with mass effect, dexamethasone for 5 to 7 days is useful. If deterioration is noted after dexamethasone is discontinued biopsy is recommended.

Other pathophysiologic processes that have been identified in patients with headache or other CNS symptoms and abnormal CT scans include infection with *M. tuberculosis, H. capsulatum,* herpes simplex virus, CMV, HIV itself, and progressive multifocal leukencephalopathy (see later discussion). The most likely cause is primary CNS lymphoma, which may present with exactly the same symptoms as toxoplasmic encephalitis. It is important to establish this diagnosis, as most patients will respond to radiation therapy. Headache is also the most frequent complaint of AIDS patients with meningitis. Evidence of meningeal irritation may be subtle or absent. Because it is often difficult to exclude elevated intracranial pressure in this setting, CT scan should be performed before lumbar puncture, if feasible.

C. neoformans is by far the most common cause of meningitis in AIDS patients (Chapter 279). India ink preparation of the spinal fluid demonstrates the typical encapsulated fungus in about 75% of cases, but the cryptococcal antigen test of serum and cerebrospinal fluid is more sensitive (>95%). The spinal fluid culture will confirm the presence of *C. neoformans*. Rarely, the CSF antigen test is negative but cultures are positive.

Once the diagnosis is established, therapy with amphotericin or fluconazole is recommended. Most patients will respond to conventional therapy, the organism will disappear from the cerebrospinal fluid, and antigen titers will decrease. Definitive cure, however, is almost never achieved, and relapse will occur within 4 to 6 months. Maintenance therapy with fluconazole will decrease relapse rates. Sequential analysis of serum titers of cryptococcal antigen should be performed periodically during maintenance therapy, as rising titers correlate with relapse.

Other opportunistic fungi, *M. tuberculosis,* lymphoma, and, rarely, *Listeria monocytogenes* also produce meningitis in AIDS patients. HIV can be cultured from the spinal fluid but pleiocytosis is unusual and isolated elevation of protein is the only clue to diagnosis. Bacterial meningitis caused by *Pneumococcus, Haemophilus, Listeria,* or *Meningococcus* organisms also occurs and present in typical fashion.

Seizures

CNS involvement in AIDS patients may first be manifested by seizures. By far the most common cause of seizures is toxoplasma encephalitis, although CNS lymphoma and herpesvirus infection may also produce seizures. CT should be performed before lumbar puncture to avoid precipitating herniation. Therapy is aimed at treating the underlying disorder and preventing seizure activity with anticonvulsants.

Dementia

More than half of all AIDS patients will have evidence of neurologic abnormalities on initial presentation when careful mental status and neurologic examination is performed. Mild to moderate dementia is not uncommon, but the true incidence may have been overestimated in early reports. Psychiatric disturbances secondary to the stress inherent in coping with this debilitating and ultimately fatal disease or unmasking of underlying psychiatric problems certainly contribute to the high incidence of neurologic abnormalities in these patients, but opportunistic infection must be excluded.

Histopathologic studies of brain tissues from biopsy specimens or autopsy have provided convincing evidence to support a role for viral infection in many of these patients. HIV has been identified in some patients with progressive encephalopathy or coma and may also produce sensory neuropathy and vacuolating myelopathy. Likewise, CMV inclusions have been associated with a more acute syndrome characterized by psychosis and rapid death. Papova viruses, particularly SV-40 and JC viruses, have been implicated in progressive multifocal leukencephalopathy in several patients (Chapter 121).

Blindness

Visual disturbances, a serious complication of HIV infection, are usually the result of CMV infection (Chapter 251). CMV produces a progressive retinochoroiditis, which may rapidly progress to visual field defects and ultimately blindness (Color Plate V-43). Ophthalmologic examination reveals white plaques and focal hemorrhages. Early lesions are commonly asymptomatic. The use of 9-(1,3-dihydroxy-2-propoxymethyl) guanine (ganciclovir) is helpful in some patients, but treatment may be limited by drug toxicity. Foscarnet is an alternative agent that is at least as effective as ganciclovir but has a high frequency of side effects in patients with renal impairment. *Candida* species and *T. gondii* also produce patchy retinal exudates which may interfere with vision. Treatment is indicated but requires close ophthalmologic follow-up.

Miscellaneous conditions

Pericardial effusions have been seen in AIDS patients and are most often secondary to Kaposi's sarcoma invading the pericardial surfaces. Hemodynamic compromise is uncommon, and the diagnosis is often apparent only after postmortem examination. Murantic endocarditis without clinical manifestations has also been described as an incidental finding at autopsy.

Primary renal disease is not common in AIDS patients, although nephrosclerosis progressing to renal failure and immune complex glomerulonephritis have been reported by some centers. Impaired kidney function secondary to nephrotoxic drugs often complicates therapy.

A peculiar oral lesion termed hairy cell leukoplakia has been identified in patients with HIV. This condition produces whitish plaques on the lateral borders of the tongue, which may be confused with thrush (Color Plate V-44). Epstein-Barr and papilloma viruses are both present within the lesion. The condition temporarily responds to high doses of acyclovir, but relapse is expected and treatment is not indicated unless symptoms are present.

Infection of the paranasal sinuses may produce symptoms of acute sinusitis in AIDS patients. Although common bacterial pathogens are often isolated, antral aspirates from these patients have demonstrated a high incidence of *Candida* species and *Pseudallescheria boydii* (a normally saprophytic fungus, which has only rarely been associated with sinusitis in immunocompromised hosts). Otolaryngologic consultation should be obtained therefore if symptoms do not respond to antibacterial therapy.

PROGNOSIS AND TREATMENT GOALS

The course of AIDS is dictated by the severity of the immune deficiency and the resulting clinical manifestations. Patients who present with Kaposi's sarcoma tend to have a longer median survival period than do those presenting with opportunistic infections. Although individual infections can be treated with varying degrees of success, the course is usually relentless in its progression. Typically, the patient eventually becomes infected with multiple pathogens including *P. carinii, M. avium-intracellulare, T. gondii,* and aggressive CMV. Death is most often the result of progressive wasting, respiratory insufficiency, or CNS involvement.

Medical care should focus on providing comfort and education. Although antiviral drugs have improved the prognosis, there is currently little reason to be optimistic that these agents will ever be curative. Treatment of the infections and malignancies associated with the disease is largely palliative and should be instituted only after careful consideration of the potential complications of therapy. A thorough discussion of these facts with the patient will facilitate realistic treatment expectations. The use of life-support measures, including cardiopulmonary resuscitation and artificial ventilation, should also be addressed as early as possible. The survival rates for AIDS patients with respiratory failure has actually improved in the last few years, and intensive care is certainly not contraindicated; but the expected benefit from aggressive measures must be balanced against the overall quality of life in the face of a progressive disease.

An organized team approach with involvement of counselors, nurses, and physicians can offer valuable contributions to the medical and psychosocial care of the patient with AIDS. Home health aids and hospice care can maximize the number of days that patients remain outside of the hospital and in their own environment. Involvement of family members and loved ones can also contribute dramatically to the patient's ability to cope with the disease.

PREVENTION

Vaccine against the AIDS retrovirus is not yet available, and prevention of infection depends preventing transmission of the virus. Family members and household contacts should be reassured that the disease is not transmitted by casual contact and instructed in the use of good hygienic practices. Patients and their sexual partners should be counseled about the potential for sexual transmission of the virus. Women with HIV infection should be advised of the possibility of transplacental transmission.

REFERENCES

Kahn JO et al: A controlled trial comparing continued zidovudine with didanosine in human immunodeficiency virus infection, N Engl J Med 327:581-587, 1992.

Porter SB and Sande MA: Toxoplasmosis of the central nervous system in the acquired immunodeficiency syndrome, N Engl J Med 327:1643-1648, 1992.

Sande MA, section editor: HIV infection and AIDS, Curr Opin Infect Dis 5:187-188, 1992.

Sande MA and Volberding PA, editors: The medical management of AIDS, ed 3, Philadelphia, 1992, WB Saunders.

Sanford JP et al, editors: The Sanford guide to HIV/AIDS therapy 1992, Dallas, 1992, Antimicrobial Therapy.

Volberding PA et al: Zidovudine in asymptomatic human immunodeficiency virus infection: a controlled trial in persons with fewer than 500 CD4-positive cells per cubic millimeter, N Engl J Med 322:941-949, 1990.

CHAPTER

243 Fever in the Hospitalized Patient

John E. McGowan, Jr.
Rafael Jurado

Many patients have fever while hospitalized; a study in a county hospital in Atlanta, Georgia, found that 29% of hospitalized patients had oral temperatures ≥38° C during the course of their hospital stay, with the highest frequencies of occurrence in patients on medicine and surgical services. Although many published studies focus on the problem of prolonged fever or fever of unknown origin (Chapter 227), management of fever of short duration represents the problem for the majority of patients who experience hospital-acquired (nosocomial) fever. The likely sources of such fevers differ from those of fevers acquired before hospitalization and those of extended duration.

On occasion the source of fever is readily apparent, such as in surgical wound infection with copious exudate. More often, the source of the fever is at first obscure. Careful history and physical examination of the febrile patient must be combined with consideration of the procedures and instrumentations that the patient has experienced and the medications initiated during the hospitalization to make an effective plan for diagnosis. In many cases the fever is alleviated by removing one or more of these elements from the patient's care (e.g., an intravenous catheter or a drug) rather than by adding new therapies.

ETIOLOGY OF HOSPITAL-ACQUIRED FEVER

Likely sources of fever vary for patients on different hospital services. This chapter focuses on the causes most often associated with patients admitted to an internal medical service. Both infectious and noninfectious processes have been associated with nosocomial fever in these patients. The relative proportion of each can vary dramatically from center to center (Table 243-1). Such distribution depends largely on the patient population served, the types of services offered at the facility, and the availability and use of diagnostic procedures to determine cause. Relevant diagnostic possibilities are discussed in the following sections.

Table 243-1. Sources of hospital-acquired* fever episodes in medical service patients

	Grady Memorial Hospital, Atlanta	VA Hospital, Minneapolis
Total fever episodes	184	123
Proportion caused by		
Infection	50%	66%
Inflammatory diseases	4%	12%
Malignancy	16%	10%
Vascular diseases	10%	6%
Procedure complications	6%	2%
Drug reactions	3%	3%
Miscellaneous and unknown sources	11%	1%

Grady Memorial Hospital data from McGowan et al: Am J Med 82:580, 1987; VA Hospital data from Filice et al: Arch Intern Med 149:319, 1989.
*Episodes with onset after first 24 hours of hospitalization.

Infections commonly leading to nosocomial fever

1. *Sepsis associated with intravascular therapy:* Infection at the cannula, in the subcutaneous tunnel, or in the fluid delivery system is frequently a source of febrile episodes in patients who have received intravascular therapy for 48 hours or more. Fever caused by septic thrombophlebitis is particularly difficult to identify, as development of the typical signs of abscess formation in the underlying vein may require an extended period. Incision and drainage of the loculated exudate inside the vessel often are required for management.
2. *Catheter-associated bacteriuria:* Colonization of the bladder with micro-organisms is the most frequent nosocomial infection today and is closely associated with catheterization of the bladder, whether indwelling or periodic. Many patients with newly acquired bacteriuria remain asymptomatic but in some infection manifested by fever develops (Chapter 240).
3. *Lower respiratory infection:* Lower respiratory infection is the third most frequent site of nosocomial infection today. It is especially likely in patients who have been on ventilator therapy (Chapter 231). Especially susceptible are postoperative patients who received general anesthesia, patients with respiratory insufficiency, and elderly patients (all of whom are likely candidates for aspiration). Fever usually accompanies these pneumonias or other pulmonary infections.
4. *Surgical wound infection:* Infection of surgical wounds afflicts those who have undergone operative procedures; overall it occurs in about 1 of 200 hospitalized patients. Fever associated with superficial wound infections (stitch abscess, etc.) often has few associated systemic signs such as fever, but abscess or infection deeper in the wound is often accompanied by fever.
5. *Cardiac bypass:* Cardiac bypass procedures subject patients to postperfusion syndrome, caused by cytomegalovirus or Epstein-Barr (EB) virus (Chapter 251).
6. *Upper respiratory infection:* Upper respiratory infection may be manifested as a general malaise with fever, especially before localizing signs or symptoms appear. For example, sinusitis can be relatively hard to identify as a fever source. Paranasal sinusitis is especially prominent in patients hospi-

talized in an intensive care unit and is associated with obstruction created by the devices inserted through the patient's nose, such as gastric tube or nasotracheal tube. Viral infections transmitted within the institution can appear after several days of hospitalization; these can be as serious as influenza or as trivial as a common cold (Chapter 230).

7. *Pacemaker and prosthesis infections:* Infection caused by pacemakers and other prosthetic devices may be manifest only by onset of fever. Data pointing to the source may not be obtained until the infection has continued for an extended period.
8. *Skin or soft tissue infection:* Skin or soft tissue infection, especially at points where pressure is applied during hospital stay, is likely to worsen during a hospital stay. Sometimes these sites produce fever as their presenting manifestation (Chapter 235).
9. *Incubating infections:* Infections that are incubating at the time of admission may be responsible for fever during hospital stay, especially when the incubation period is prolonged. For example, development of illness associated with varicella or hepatitis infection acquired in the community may occur only after a patient has been admitted. In addition, fevers associated with some infections tend to be intermittent or low-grade and may be absent or unremarkable at the time of hospital admission. Increased activity of these processes may lead to the conclusion that the fever and the process have begun after hospitalization.
10. *Bacteremia:* Bacteremia without an apparent underlying source may have fever as its only indicator. Peduzzi and colleagues have documented that detecting such cases is difficult, and the only defense against overlooking such a potentially severe source is routinely obtaining blood cultures of patients whose fever with hospital onset is not readily explained. Endocarditis, especially on the tricuspid valve, may account for this clinical manifestation but remain unapparent until specific search is made for this possibility (Chapter 15).

Likely noninfectious causes

Reactions to therapeutic agents (medications, contrast dyes, etc.) frequently are manifested by development of fever. Approximately 15% of hospitalized patients experience some drug-related side-effect. Usually this cause is recognized because other signs of drug toxicity, such as rash or eosinophilia, are present concurrently. Of special interest are those begun recently and those for which fever is a frequent adverse effect (e.g., beta lactams, isoniazid, phenytoin). Some drugs are more likely than others to produce inflammation at the site of administration when given parenterally. For example, erythromycin compounds for parenteral administration, which have inherently low pH, often cause phlebitis at the intravascular cannula site, and this occurrence should be sought if a patient has fever after parenteral erythromycin therapy is begun. Therapeutic immunoglobulins or immunologic products such as interferon also may lead to fever. Many affected patients have no history of prior drug reactions, and some will manifest no other symptoms or signs that suggest the diagnosis of drug-induced fever.

Surgical procedures commonly are followed by fever. In a study of 81 surgical patients who had unexplained fever after operation, Garibaldi and colleagues found that fevers that developed more than 48 hours after the procedure usually were due to infection. Of those fevers occurring in the first 48 hours, most resolved without specific antimicrobial or other therapy. Cases in this group not associated with atelectasis were attributed to intraoperative tissue trauma and concomitant release of pyrogens into the circulation. Postcardiotomy syndrome is a special case of postoperative fever that should be considered in patients who have undergone this type of procedure. Pleural or pericardial rub may help indicate the source.

Intravascular-catheter-induced inflammation without concurrent infection can serve as a source of fever in patients who have received intravascular therapy. Only about half of patients with positive intravenous catheter tip culture findings have phlebitis at the site of catheter insertion at the time the catheter is removed.

Transfusion of blood products is associated with febrile reactions in a small number of cases. On occasion, fever is the only manifestation of reaction. Such reactions usually are of small clinical import, as they usually are benign and self-limited. Because such reactions occur more frequently in patients who have received several transfusions, they probably are associated with reactions to protein.

Thrombophlebitis is a potential threat to any hospitalized patient, as enforced bedrest and inactivity increase the risk of venous stasis. Local inflammation of veins in legs or pelvis is a particular concern in patients who have diseases that increase pressure on vessels, have undergone extensive abdominal or pelvic surgery, or have experienced other procedures that make phlebitis more likely (Chapters 22 and 86). Infection may be present, but inflammation in the absence of infection is common. Abdominal or pelvic tenderness may provide the clue to this process.

Pulmonary embolus can be associated with fever in the absence of readily apparent signs of phlebitis, endocarditis, or other predisposing factors. As the pulmonary signs and symptoms associated with embolus and the accompanying infarction of lung tissue are often mild or absent, only a high index of suspicion will lead to the testing that documents this reason for hospital onset of fever in some cases. The fever often lasts 2 to 3 days after the acute event, but recurrent emboli can prolong the period.

Instrumentation other than that described previously can lead to fever in hospitalized patients. Inflammation may develop at the site of hemodialysis catheters, in the presence or absence of active infection. Angiography, colonoscopy, duodenoscopy, fiberoptic bronchoscopy, endoscopic retrograde cholangiopancreatography, and so on, all have been associated with fever episodes after their performance.

Therapeutic devices and procedures can cause fever in

the hospital setting. For example, fever can be associated with nasotracheal intubation even if no infection develops in the area of physical trauma to the upper airways. This is especially likely when the devices are used improperly. For example, incorrect setting of a water mattress used for care of a patient with decubitus ulcers has been reported by Gonzalez et al as a cause of nosocomial fever. Fever arising later in the hospital course also can arise from sterile abscesses or other inflammation associated with repeated intramuscular injections.

Noninfectious illnesses can have their onset during hospitalization, and fever may result. Similarly, diseases producing fever only intermittently may demonstrate this manifestation only after the patient has been hospitalized for an extended period. Immune-mediated diseases such as arthritis and neurologic events such as subarachnoid or subdural hemorrhage, intracerebral bleeding, or seizure must be considered. Hepatitis, cholangitis, appendicitis, pancreatitis, myocardial infarction, vascular ischemia of an extremity, perforation of a gastrointestinal ulcer, acute gout or pseudogout, and similar events unrelated to hospital care also can produce episodic fever that sometimes appears during the hospital stay. The relationship between malignancy and fever is considered in Chapter 227; nonhematologic malignancies were associated with fever as often as leukemia and lymphoma in the investigation of Filice et al. Fever associated with ethanol withdrawal may be delayed for a day or two after admission, depending on circumstances leading to the patient's hospitalization and details of recent alcohol consumption.

Factitious (self-induced) fever may be produced at any time, and on occasion appears to be nosocomial in onset. Contamination of intravascular delivery lines with mouth or other endogenous flora, alteration of thermometry, self-injection of skin and joint spaces, and use of nonprescribed drugs all may be sources of fever in hospitalized patients.

Hospital-acquired fever in selected populations of patients

Fever has been investigated in selected groups of hospitalized patients, including those who have malignancy and who fulfill the strict criteria for fever of unknown origin (Chapter 227). Causes also have been investigated for newborns in the first 4 days of life, patients seen by an infectious disease consultation service, drug addicts, patients with burns, those with spinal cord injury, and those with endocarditis. Fever after surgical and other procedures also has been studied. In each of these special groups the most likely sources vary greatly from those recorded for hospital populations in general, and presence of any of these factors or settings must be taken into account in making the determination of likely sources.

DIAGNOSTIC APPROACH

When a patient becomes febrile in the hospital, the following steps should be included in the evaluation:

1. Quickly evaluate the patient for a localizing sign or symptom that indicates the fever source. Signs and symptoms such as a new cough productive of purulent sputum or a hot, swollen joint obviate extensive investigations of other possible causes. Bornstein stresses that the nature of the patient's underlying illness often provides clues. For example, concomitant esophageal stricture or altered mental status may make the possibility of mixed aerobic/anaerobic aspiration pneumonia more likely.
2. The next most important step is detailed review of the patient's clinical course since hospitalization, with particular attention to procedures, instrumentation, medications, and other interventions that have been part of clinical care. Because many sources of nosocomial fever are linked to procedures or instruments, this can be an efficient way to determine the source.
3. If the patient is receiving intravascular therapy, inspect the site of cannula insertion for phlebitis. Determine whether the cannula has been in place longer than the recommended period (Chapter 225). If so, or if no other steps define the likely fever sources, remove the entire intravascular therapy system and, if such therapy is still required, insert a new system at a different location. Send the cannula tip for semiquantitative bacterial culture evaluation. Examine the site of cannulation carefully for signs of venous thrombophlebitis that might require incision and drainage or ligation of the infected vein. Milk the vein backward to the point of catheter insertion to see whether pus can be expressed. If it can, septic thrombophlebitis is possible. Fluid-associated sepsis is more rare, so culture of the fluid being administered is less frequently requested or found to be the source. Examine the fluid container for cracks, cloudy fluid, blood, or other signs of contamination, and send the fluid for culture evaluation if any of these findings is present.
4. If the patient currently has an indwelling urinary catheter or was subjected to bladder catheterization earlier in the hospitalization, examine a urine specimen for presence of white blood cells, bacteria, and yeast. If any of these is present, obtain a culture specimen of the urine for evaluation for bacteria and yeast. Evaluate the urine sediment for presence of casts or other evidence of inflammatory diseases of the urinary tract. Presence of periurethral abscess or epididymitis can be detected by careful examination.
5. Patients currently or previously on ventilator therapy should be evaluated for the presence of pneumonia by physical and radiologic examination. Respiratory secretions obtained through the endotracheal tube (or any sputum being produced, if the patient is not intubated) should be examined and, if findings warrant, cultures evaluated for bacteria and yeast. Consider the possibility of pulmonary embolus in any patient with hospital-acquired fever, as only high suspicion allows diagnosis of this poten-

tially lethal process to be made in patients when other manifestations are relatively weak or absent.

6. Operative or traumatic wounds should be inspected for signs of inflammation, and any drainage present should have culture evaluation for bacteria and fungi. Signs and symptoms suggestive of deep abscess in the trauma or operative region should be sought, and imaging or other tests undertaken if this possibility remains likely (Chapter 232). In particular, perirectal or prostatic abscess can be overlooked if meticulous attention is not given to physical examination. Fever early (within the first 48 hours) after surgical procedures may be due to atelectasis or release of pyrogens after intraoperative tissue trauma, but these should be considered only after other potentially severe possibilities have been eliminated. Sensitization resulting from exposure to halothane or other anesthetic agents that produce severe pyrexia may be recognized as such, but less dramatic increases still may be produced by general anesthetic agents and should be considered.
7. Special aspects of the patient's care should be evaluated if the surgery has been performed. For example, use of certain anesthetic agents can produce sensitization manifested in part by fever (e.g., halothane reaction). Likewise, thyroid storm can be precipitated by surgery on this gland. Malignant hyperthermia is a dramatic event manifested by acute hyperpyrexia and muscle rigidity after exposure to certain anesthetics.
8. The patient's list of medications should be surveyed for drugs known to be associated with fever production. All nonessential medications should be discontinued, especially those that have recently been prescribed. Parenteral drugs likely to produce inflammation at the site of administration (e.g., erythromycin) should be discontinued or replaced, if possible. Because fever will not necessarily remit within 24 to 48 hours of the time that the drug is discontinued, patience in observing the patient's response may be needed.
9. Review the patient's record and laboratory testing summaries to determine whether blood or blood product transfusion has taken place. Febrile reac-

Work flow approach to history and physical examination in diagnosis of hospital-acquired fever

History

—What procedures, instrumentations, or other interventions have been performed since this patient was hospitalized? Has anesthesia been administered?

—What new medications, immunoglobulins, or transfusion products has the patient received since hospitalization?

—Has the patient been treated with antipyretics or other drugs that affect fever?

—Have contrast dyes or other diagnostic products been administered as part of imaging or other diagnostic procedures?

—What underlying diseases has the patient that may be manifested by intermittent fever, which may have created the false appearance of fever as nosocomial?

—Has the patient manifested new symptoms that may signal acquisition of a likely nosocomial pathogen (e.g., nosocomial diarrhea as a manifestation of *Clostridium difficile* infection, sputum production as a manifestation of nosocomial pneumonia)?

Physical examination

Head

—Nasogastric or gastric tube in place? Evaluate for sinusitis.

Chest

—On ventilator now or recently? Operative procedure with general anesthesia since admission?

—New onset or change in character of sputum production or of respiratory function? Careful chest examination for infection or inflammation, follow-up diagnostic studies (radiograph, scanning, etc.) as warranted.

—Murmur or other sign of cardiac dysfunction? If operative or invasive diagnostic procedure performed, evaluate possibility of endocarditis, especially if prophylaxis for the procedure was suboptimum. Blood culture evaluation should be made if there is any suspicion that the fever represents bloodstream invasion.

—Are the patient's prior course and care consistent with a focus for pulmonary emboli?

Gastrointestinal

—Onset of diarrhea in the hospital? Evaluate for *Clostridium difficile* infection, especially if the patient has recently been treated with antimicrobial agents. Perhaps more likely, which new medication could be causing local irritation of the gut?

Genital

—Urinary catheter in place now or recently? Obtain urine specimen for microscopic examination (pyuria, hematuria, bacteriuria); if appropriate, follow with Gram's stain and culture.

Operative site or site of trauma

—Signs of superficial or deep infection? Possibility of loculated areas requiring imaging techniques for evaluation?

Extremities

—Are signs of thrombophlebitis or manifestations of extremity ischemia present?

Skin

—Skin rashes are probably the most common and easily noted manifestations of febrile drug reaction, transfusion reaction, and viral or other infections

—Intravascular therapy administered now or recently? Examine closely for phlebitis or exudate at the site of cannulation. Attempt to milk fluid back from vein, and palpate for possible septic thrombophlebitis. Examine fluid container for cracks or cloudy fluid.

—Signs of decubitus or other ulcer, especially one that has broken down since hospital stay began?

tions associated with this procedure usually occur during or just after transfusion, but fever with onset months afterward may be associated with infection produced by hepatitis viruses, especially hepatitis C virus, acquired at the time of transfusion.

10. Of hospital-acquired fevers 10% to 20% may remain undiagnosed. Some resolve spontaneously. With long-term follow-up evaluation, causes of others eventually become clear as new symptoms or findings appear. Collagen diseases, factitious fever, lymphoma, chronic granulomatous disease of the liver, and chronic viral infections such as those produced by Epstein-Barr virus (EBV) or cytomegalovirus (CMV) often become more obvious as time progresses.

These 10 general approaches to evaluation of nosocomial fever are related to aspects of the history and physical examination listed in the box on p. 1983.

THERAPY AND PREVENTION

Therapy and preventive measures depend on the findings of the diagnostic evaluation. Use of antipyretics often is discouraged until the source of the fever has become clear, although Styrt and Sugarman note that in some patients the comfort produced by antipyretics outweighs the relative benefit of observing fever pattern, and in some patients the drugs are needed to reduce the risk of adverse effects associated with underlying cardiac disease.

Because hospital-acquired fever frequently has noninfectious causes, routine use of antimicrobial agents when fever begins is not recommended. Of course, if a patient has hypotension or other manifestations of suspected bacterial infection, empiric antimicrobial therapy may be wise. Organisms causing nosocomial infections frequently are resistant to many commonly used antimicrobial agents, so the choice of empiric therapy depends on patterns of resistance in the specific institution. The most important step in many cases is removal of the predisposing catheters and other devices that have been listed.

REFERENCES

Bor DH et al: Fever in hospitalized medical patients: characteristics and significance. J Gen Intern Med 3:119, 1988.

Bornstein DL: Fevers of nosocomial origin. J Med 11:275, 1980.

Filice GA et al: Nosocomial febrile illness in patients on an internal medicine service. Arch Intern Med 149:319, 1989.

Garibaldi RA et al: Evidence for the non-infectious etiology of early postoperative fever. Infect Control 6:273, 1985.

Gonzalez EB, Suarez L, and Magee S: Nosocomial (water bed) fever. Arch Intern Med 150:687, 1990.

Knodel AR and Beekman JF: Unexplained fevers in patients with nasotracheal intubation. JAMA 248:868, 1982.

McGowan JE Jr et al: Fever in hospitalized patients, with special reference to the Medical Service. Am J Med 82:580, 1987.

Peduzzi P et al: Predictors of bacteremia and gram-negative bacteremia in patients with sepsis. Arch Intern Med 152:529, 1992.

Styrt B and Sugarman B: Antipyresis and fever. Arch Intern Med 150:1589, 1990.

Young EJ, Fainstein V, and Musher DM: Drug-induced fever: cases seen in the evaluation of unexplained fever in a general hospital population. Rev Infect Dis 4:69, 1982.

ORGANISMS INFECTIVE TO HUMANS IV

VIRAL DISEASES

CHAPTER

244 Picornavirus Infections (Enterovirus and Rhinovirus)

R. Gordon Douglas, Jr.

The picornavirus family consists of a large number of serologically distinct viruses that are similar in structure and physical and chemical properties. They are responsible for many asymptomatic infections, as well as for a spectrum of illnesses ranging from common colds to pneumonia, myopericarditis, aseptic meningitis, paralytic poliomyelitis, and hepatitis.

CLASSIFICATION

Picornaviruses are very small, nonenveloped ribonucleic acid (RNA) viruses. Three genera infect humans: enterovirus, rhinovirus, and hepatitis A virus. The enterovirus genus consists of 67 immunotypes, including three poliovirus types, 23 coxsackievirus types A and 6 types B, 30 echoviruses, and 5 enteroviruses. More than 100 immunotypes of rhinovirus have been described (Table 244-1). Hepatitis A virus was originally classified as enterovirus type 72 but now is thought to represent a new genus (Chapter 57).

Originally, the enteroviruses were subdivided into three groups, namely, polioviruses, coxsackieviruses, and echo-

Table 244-1. Human picornaviruses

Genera and species	Number of immunotypes
Enteroviruses	
Poliovirus	3
Coxsackievirus A	23
Coxsackievirus B	6
ECHO virus	30
Enterovirus	5
Rhinovirus	>100
Hepatitis A virus	1

viruses, on the basis of antigenic relationships and differences in host range. In recent years, as new enteroviruses have been isolated, it has become clear that basing their classification on host range is not the best approach. Thus newly discovered enteroviruses have been given the designation of enterovirus types 68 to 72, whereas the enterovirus immunotypes previously classified as poliovirus, coxsackievirus group A, coxsackievirus group B, and echoviruses have retained the previous classification.

CHARACTERISTICS

Picornaviruses are small icosahedral, nonenveloped, ether-resistant viruses. The capsid, which is 20 to 30 nm in diameter, is composed of 60 subunits (capsomers) that are synthesized from four structural polypeptides (VP1 through VP4); VP1 is the dominant antigen. The capsid encloses a linear, single-stranded RNA genome with a molecular weight of 2.6×10^6. The RNA functions as a monocistronic messenger, yielding a polyprotein of molecular weight 2.5×10^5 that subsequently undergoes specific cleavages to form the structural polypeptides of the capsomers. In addition, a virus-coded RNA polymerase and other polypeptides required for viral replication are produced.

EPIDEMIOLOGY

Enteroviruses

The epidemiologies of most enteroviruses are similar. Enteroviruses are distributed worldwide, but their epidemiologic behavior is affected by climate, season, age, and socioeconomic and other factors. In temperate climates, enteroviruses are strikingly more prevalent in the summer and autumn months, predominantly August through October, but often beginning earlier and extending well into winter months. This seasonal periodicity has never been satisfactorily explained, but it is not observed in the tropics, where enteroviruses are endemic year-round. Age is another important epidemiologic factor. Outbreaks of enteroviral infections are highest in children less than 1 year of age, and children invariably have higher attack rates than adults. Antibody incidence is at least three to six times higher in the lower socioeconomic classes, and multiple infections are common in such situations, where such conditions as poor hygiene and overcrowding may be present.

In urban areas of the United States, several immunotypes of enteroviruses usually dominate each season, but the types may vary from city to city or region to region and, further, from year to year. Occasional epidemics with a single immunotype (e.g., echovirus type 9) have occurred nationwide or even worldwide. The most frequent nonpolio isolates reported to the World Health Organization and the Centers for Disease Control in recent years include echovirus types 11, 9, 4, 6, 3, and 7; coxsackievirus types B5, B2, B4, and B3; and coxsackievirus type A9. These types accounted for two thirds of all isolates.

Enteroviruses are spread predominantly via the fecal-oral route, principally from person to person directly, although enteroviruses have been isolated from flies, cockroaches, food naturally exposed to flies, dog feces, and a number of other vehicles. Direct person-to-person, fecal-oral transmission is consistent with the higher antibody incidence in children and in the lower socioeconomic groups. Enterovirus infections often cluster in families, and the home may be the setting where most transmission takes place. The period of maximum contagiousness corresponds to the period of maximum virus excretion. Once virus has been introduced into a household, secondary attack rates are close to 100% for wild polioviruses, about 75% for coxsackieviruses, and 50% for echoviruses. Presumably, the lower rate for echoviruses is due to their being shed for shorter periods and in lower quantities than polioviruses or coxsackieviruses. There are exceptions (e.g., coxsackievirus A21 behaves like a respiratory virus). Respiratory spread of other enteroviruses may occasionally be important. Enterovirus type 70, the agent of acute hemorrhagic conjunctivitis, appears to be spread by fomites, fingers, and ophthalmologic instruments contaminated with virus.

The last case of endemic poliomyelitis in the United States occurred in 1979. All of the 5 to 10 cases that occur annually are associated with the use of live oral polio vaccine. Approximately 40% occur in vaccine recipients and 60% in controls of recipients.

Rhinoviruses

The epidemiology of rhinovirus infections differs considerably from that of enteroviruses. The seasonal pattern is not so abrupt. Rhinovirus infections tend to occur year-round, with fall and spring peaks of infection. In the United States, an early fall peak occurs shortly after the opening of school and a second peak occurs in the early spring. However, continuing rhinovirus infections are observed each month of the year.

Like enteroviruses, rhinoviruses are worldwide in distribution. In a given geographic area, one or several immunotypes may be prevalent at any time, only to be replaced during the next peak by one or several other immunotypes. Studies of the incidence of antibody show rapid acquisition of antibody during childhood and adolescence, with a peak incidence in young adults. There is little evidence that any of the more than 100 immunotypes predominates. Rhinovirus infections are among the most common human virus infections. Studies indicate infection rates of at least 1.2 per person per year in children under the age of 1 year and 0.7 in young adults.

Recent studies have elucidated the mechanisms of transmission. Most rhinovirus infections appear to be transmitted in the home after introduction of infection by a child of school age. The incubation period is 2 to 6 days, and secondary attack rates in family members range from 25% to 70%. Infection is initiated via the respiratory tract. Virus spreads from person to person by transfer of contaminated secretions from an infected donor to a susceptible recipient. Such transfer may occur from hand to hand or from hand to fomite to hand, followed by autoinoculation of nasal or conjunctival mucosa by the susceptible subject. Infection also may be transmitted by large or small particle aerosols.

PATHOGENESIS

Most enteroviruses initially produce infection of the mucosal and lymphoid tissue of the pharynx and gut. In some instances, viremia occurs, with subsequent involvement of other target organs, such as the heart, brain, meninges, and skin. In contrast, rhinoviruses exclusively infect the upper respiratory tract; they have not been demonstrated to disseminate to distant sites in the body.

Rhinovirus

The pathogeneses of enterovirus and rhinovirus infections are contrasted in Table 244-2. There is no apparent effect of exposure to cold on the frequency and severity of common colds resulting from rhinovirus infection in humans. The pathologic findings of rhinovirus infection include hyperemia and edema of the mucous membranes, with exudation of serous and mucinous fluid and engorgement of the turbinates. On histologic examination, subepithelial edema with sparse cellular infiltrates is seen. Virus is recovered from the nose, throat, and saliva, but the nose appears to be the predominant site of replication. The severity of the illness parallels the quantity of virus shed in the nasopharyngeal secretions. Direct viral damage to the epithelium is slight, and symptoms most likely result from the release of chemical mediators such as bradykinin and lysylbradykinin.

Poliovirus

Among enteroviruses, the pathogenesis of poliovirus infection has been most clearly worked out, and the pathogenesis of most other enteroviruses probably resembles that of poliovirus. The initial infection with poliovirus involves the mucosal and lymphoid tissue of the pharynx and gut. Virus shortly thereafter disseminates to regional lymph nodes, and replication in these sites leads to viremia, which may correspond clinically to mild illness. Viremia may or may not result in infection of the central nervous system and other susceptible sites. In only 1% to 2% of the cases does the virus penetrate the central nervous system. Although it is most likely that the central nervous system is invaded across the blood-brain barrier, the possibility of transmission of virus along nerve fibers has never been completely excluded. The prominent lesion of poliomyelitis results from infection of neurons, particularly the anterior horn cells. Inflammation is secondary and consists of perivascular cuffing and diffuse infiltration of mononuclear cells. In other enterovirus infections, the target organ of the viremia may be the meninges, skeletal muscle, testicle, skin, heart, or other sites.

It is clear that there are differences in virulence among strains of poliovirus, which may in part explain differences in paralysis attack rates. In addition, a number of host factors have been associated with an increased risk of paralysis. Boys are more commonly paralyzed than girls. Fatigue and strenuous exercise during the first 3 days of the major illness substantially increase the incidence and severity of paralysis. Conversely, strict bed rest during this period has a sparing effect on paralysis. Intramuscular injection, trauma, or surgery within 2 weeks of the onset of illness tends to localize paralysis to the involved limb. Tonsillectomy, even in the remote past, increases the incidence of bulbar poliomyelitis. The incidence, but not the severity, of poliomyelitis is increased in pregnancy. Finally, genetic factors appear to increase the incidence of paralysis; histocompatibility antigens human leukocyte antigen 3 (HLA3) and HLA7 are associated with an increased risk of paralysis.

In the last decade, 14% of cases of paralytic poliomyelitis in the United States have occurred in children with hereditary immunodeficiencies either as vaccine recipients or their contacts. Most cases have occurred with type 2 or type 3 oral poliovirus vaccine. Both isolated B cell immunodeficiency and severe combined immunodeficiency syndrome have been implicated.

Table 244-2. Comparative pathogenesis of enterovirus (poliovirus) and rhinovirus infections

Pathogenesis	Poliovirus	Rhinovirus
Method of transmission	Fecal-oral	Respiratory
Site of viral deposition	Gastrointestinal mucosa	Upper respiratory mucosa
Virus isolation	Throat and feces	Nose and throat
Viremic	Yes	No
Central nervous system involvement	Yes	No

Other enteroviruses

The pathogenesis of coxsackievirus and echovirus infections may be similar to either the poliovirus or the rhinovirus model, depending on the strain and other factors. In the case of viruses that produce primarily upper respiratory infections, the pathogenesis is presumed to be similar to that described for rhinovirus infection. In the case of enterovirus infections that result in aseptic meningitis with or without exanthema, the pathogenesis may be similar to that for poliovirus, except that the target tissue in the final phase is the meninges and skin instead of the spinal cord gray matter.

Host risk factors, such as those identified with poliovirus infections, have not been observed in other human enterovirus infections. However, in experimental coxsackievirus myopericarditis in mice, adrenal corticoids, exercise, exposure to cold, alcohol, male sex, genetic factors, and chronic undernutrition have been associated with increased virulence of infection. It is not known whether or not these factors play a role in coxsackievirus infection in humans.

In both poliovirus and rhinovirus infection, the mechanism of cellular injury is believed to be the cytolysis that results from virus replication. Immunologic mechanisms may also be involved in some enterovirus infections. Patients with isolated agammaglobulinemia have persistent enterovirus infections. In patients with myopericarditis, coxsackievirus can be detected in the myocardium or pericardium, and cytolysis may result directly from viral replication early in the illness. Later in the illness, an immunologic basis for continuing lesions is suggested by the absence of infectious virus and the presence of immunoglobulins and complement on immunofluorescent staining in the heart of patients with myopericarditis. An immunologic pathogenesis is consistent with the findings in experimental coxsackievirus myocarditis in mice: an early "infectious phase" and a later "immunologic phase."

DISEASES IN HUMANS

All the picornaviruses produce subclinical infection in humans (Table 244-3). In the case of the enteroviruses, the majority of infections are asymptomatic, whereas for rhinoviruses the proportion of asymptomatic infections is probably around 30% to 40%. Picornaviruses contribute to a broad clinical spectrum of illnesses.

Common colds and other respiratory illnesses

The predominant illness resulting from rhinovirus infection is a typical common cold, which is indistinguishable from that produced by other respiratory viruses (Chapter 230). Rhinoviruses are the single most important cause of common colds in older children and adults. Although all picornaviruses presumably contribute to the total causes of common colds, the relative proportion of colds attributable to enteroviruses is small.

Acute febrile undifferentiated illness

Undifferentiated febrile illnesses caused by most enterovirus immunotypes may be accompanied by upper respiratory symptoms, such as sore throat and occasionally cough and coryza. These illnesses are clinically indistinguishable from the "flu-like" syndromes caused by rhinoviruses, parainfluenza viruses, adenoviruses, and influenza viruses, except for their common occurrence in the summer months, when influenza, for example, is almost entirely absent in the northern hemisphere. These illnesses may be unaccompa-

Table 244-3. Diseases associated with picornaviruses*

Syndrome	Polioviruses	Coxsackieviruses Group A	Coxsackieviruses Group B	Echoviruses	Enteroviruses	Rhinoviruses
Asymptomatic infection	1-3	All types	All types	All types	All types	All types
Common cold	1-3	All types	All types	All types	All types	All types
Acute febrile, undifferentiated illness	1-3	All types	All types	All types	All types	
Paralysis	1-3	4,6,7,9,11,14,21	1-6	1-4,6,7,9,11,14, 16,18,19,30	70,71	
Aseptic meningitis	1-3	1-11,14,16-18,22,24	1-6	All except 24,26, 29,32	70,71	
Encephalitis		2,5-7,9	1-5	2-4,6,7,9,11,14, 17-19,25	70,71	
Herpangina		2-6,8,10,22				
Hand-foot-mouth syndrome		5,7,9,10,16			71	
Lymphonodular pharyngitis		10				
Exanthem		2,4,5,9,16	1,3-5	1-9,11,14,18,19,25, 30,32,33	71	
Pleurodynia			1-5			
Myopericarditis			1-5			
Generalized disease of the newborn			1-5			
Orchitis			1-5			
Neonatal diarrhea				11,14,18		
Chronic meningoencephalitis in agammaglobulinemics				2,3,5,9,11,19,24, 25,30,33		
Acute hemorrhagic conjunctivitis		24			70	

*Numbers indicate the immunotype associated with indicated syndrome. Hepatitis produced by hepatitis A virus (enterovirus 72) is excluded from this table.

nied by any respiratory signs or symptoms. Their occurrence in the summer months is suggestive of enterovirus infection, especially when other evidence of enterovirus infection (i.e., aseptic meningitis, exanthem) is in the community.

Enteroviruses occasionally also produce the syndromes attributable to other respiratory viruses, such as pharyngitis, laryngitis, tracheobronchitis, and pneumonia. During outbreaks of other types of enteroviral disease (e.g., aseptic meningitis, pleurodynia), cases of viral respiratory illness such as viral pneumonia are encountered.

Paralytic poliomyelitis

Clinical findings. The incubation period of paralytic poliomyelitis is 9 to 12 days. The manifestations are extremely variable, ranging from inapparent infection to severe paralysis and death. Approximately 95% of poliovirus infections are subclinical. In 4% to 8% of infections, an illness known as abortive poliomyelitis, in which there is fever, headache, sore throat, listlessness, anorexia, vomiting, and pain in the muscles or abdomen, occurs. The physical findings are normal, and the illness lasts only a few hours to days. Nonparalytic poliomyelitis occurs in 1% to 2% of all infections and differs from abortive poliomyelitis in that aseptic meningitis is present. In addition to stiffness of the neck and back, the patient generally has more headache and higher fever and appears more toxic than in abortive poliomyelitis. Frank paralysis occurs in roughly 0.1% of all poliovirus infections in children. There is a biphasic course in a third of affected children, beginning with a "minor" illness, resembling abortive poliomyelitis, which coincides with viremia and lasts 1 to 3 days. The patient then appears to be recovering and remains symptom-free for 2 to 5 days before the abrupt onset of meningitic symptoms and signs of "major" illness: headache, fever, malaise, vomiting, and neck stiffness. The temperature is generally 98.6 to 102.2° F (37 to 39° C) and is often accompanied by chilliness and, rarely, by rigors. In older children and in most adults, the illness consists of a single phase, with a more prolonged prodrome and a more gradual onset of paralysis.

The occurrence of spontaneous muscle pain is the most important characteristic of the major illness. Most commonly involved are muscles of the neck and lumbar region, but muscles of the flank, abdomen, or limbs also may be involved. The pain is relieved by motion, and the patient may pace nervously to work it off.

The meningitic phase of the major illness, accompanied by muscle pain, is generally present for 1 to 2 days before the characteristic asymmetric paralysis ensues. The proximal muscles of the extremities tend to be more involved than the distal muscles. The legs are more commonly involved than the arms, and large muscle groups of the hand are at greater risk than small ones. Any combination of limbs may be paralyzed; the most common pattern is involvement of one leg, followed by involvement of one arm or both legs and both arms. Both the extent and rapidity of paralysis are highly variable. Most commonly, paralysis progresses over 2 to 3 days and almost invariably halts when the patient becomes afebrile. Sensory loss does not occur in poliomyelitis, and its presence should strongly suggest other diagnoses, such as Guillain-Barré syndrome.

In bulbar poliomyelitis, there is paralysis of muscle groups innervated by cranial nerves, especially the muscles of the soft palate, pharynx, and larynx. Other cranial nerve nuclei are frequently involved but rarely pose a threat to life. The frequency of the bulbar form of the disease varies between 5% and 35%.

Encephalitis, manifested primarily by confusion, disturbances of consciousness, and seizures, is an uncommon form of poliomyelitis occurring principally in infants.

Coxsackievirus A7 and enterovirus 71 are neuropathogenic in monkeys and have been recognized as the cause of small outbreaks of poliomyelitis. Other enterovirus immunotypes, as indicated in Table 244-3, have also been associated with sporadic cases of paralytic disease that is usually milder than poliomyelitis. Frank paralysis, which is less common than muscle weakness, is usually not permanent. Poliomyelitis caused by administration of oral poliomyelitis vaccines to children with hereditary immunodeficiencies occurs after an incubation period of 7 to 21 days. In contacts, usually young adults, the incubation period is 20 to 29 days. In immunocompromised children, the illness is protracted, and paralysis may progress over several weeks. Mortality is high (40%) and prolonged fecal excretion of virus is characteristic.

Complications. The complications of poliomyelitis include respiratory failure caused by paralysis of the respiratory muscles, and airway obstruction from involvement of cranial nuclei or lesions in the respiratory center. Other complications include aspiration pneumonia, pulmonary edema, pulmonary embolism, viral myocarditis, gastrointestinal hemorrhage, paralytic ileus and gastric dilatation, and development of urinary calculi.

Differential diagnosis. Poliomyelitis usually presents a clear-cut clinical picture that differs from that of Guillain-Barré syndrome. In Guillain-Barré syndrome, paralysis is symmetric and is accompanied by sensory loss; facial diplegia is common, and paralysis may progress over a period of up to 2 weeks. Hysteria, diphtheria, botulism, tick paralysis, pseudoparalysis, and encephalitis may mimic poliomyelitis in some instances.

Laboratory findings. The peripheral white cell count may be normal or elevated. Cerebrospinal fluid findings are similar to those of aseptic meningitis, with pleocytosis and a minimally elevated protein concentration. The cell count usually returns to normal within 2 to 3 weeks, but minor protein abnormalities may last longer. Polioviruses can be isolated from throat secretions in the first week of the illness and may often be isolated from feces for several weeks (Chapter 226). They are rarely isolated from cerebrospinal fluid.

Prognosis. The overall mortality of paralytic poliomyelitis in epidemics in the past was 5% to 10%. In bulbar poliomyelitis, mortality is high and most patients with poliovirus encephalitis die. Some degree of permanent damage is observed in about a third of poliomyelitis victims. Full return of function is less likely in severely paralyzed muscles than in mildly paralyzed ones. Patients requiring mechanical ventilation because of spinal respiratory paralysis rarely recover without some sequelae. Although bulbar poliomyelitis causes the greatest threat to life in the first week of illness, it is rarely responsible for permanent damage in surviving patients. Some estimate of the eventual outcome can be made at 1 month. No additional return of function can be expected beyond 9 months. New onset of weakness in the previously affected muscle groups has been reported years later and is apparently due to gradual deterioration of motor neurons and not infections or immunologic mechanisms.

Treatment. There is no specific antiviral treatment, and therapy is therefore supportive and symptomatic and includes hospitalization, bed rest, a bed board and footboard, moist heat packs, and management of problems threatening the respiratory tract, including the use of mechanical ventilators.

Aseptic meningitis

Clinical findings. Acute aseptic meningitis (acute viral meningitis) is a syndrome characterized by signs and symptoms of meningeal irritation with mononuclear pleocytosis of the cerebrospinal fluid (Chapter 233). The attack rates for aseptic meningitis are highest in children less than 1 year of age. The disease is also seen in older children and young adults, but enteroviral aseptic meningitis after the age of 40 is rare.

The onset may be gradual or abrupt. Typically, the patient feels chilly and has fever and headache for only a few hours before frank signs of meningitis are present. Nausea and vomiting are common, especially in children. Some patients also complain of sore throat. The illness may be biphasic, as in poliomyelitis, and fever and myalgia are present for a few days, followed by defervescence and absence of symptoms for 2 to 10 days before the sudden reappearance of fever, headache, and stiff neck. Signs of meningeal irritation may be absent in neonates, and even in older children and adults these signs are usually mild. Stiffness of the neck and back, sometimes with muscle spasms, is the only neurologic sign in most cases. Kernig's and Brudzinski's signs are present in about a third of patients.

Laboratory findings. The peripheral white blood cell count is usually normal. The cerebrospinal fluid is clear but may be under mildly increased pressure. The total white cell count is usually 30 to 300 per cubic millimeter but may on occasion exceed 1000. Cell counts less than 10 or even normal are not rare, especially in neonates. Typically, the white cells are predominantly lymphocytes, but in the first 24 hours of illness, polymorphonuclear leukocytes may outnumber lymphocytes. The cerebrospinal fluid glucose and protein concentrations are usually normal.

Echoviruses and coxsackieviruses can be isolated from the cerebrospinal fluid in the first few days after the onset of meningitis but rarely after the first week. More frequently, and for longer periods, such viruses may often be isolated from throat or anal swab specimens. Because of the multiplicity of immunotypes, serologic diagnosis is not practical in most hospital viral diagnostic laboratories.

Treatment. Treatment of the patient with aseptic meningitis is symptomatic. Fever and signs of meningeal irritation subside in a few days to 1 week. Cerebrospinal fluid pleocytosis may persist for some time after the fever and signs of meningeal irritation are resolved.

Encephalitis

In some patients with enteroviral infection, in addition to meningitis, confusion and changes in the highest integrative functions that are indicative of encephalitis develop. In neonates, disseminated disease, including encephalitis with lethargy, convulsions, bulging fontanelles, and cerebrospinal fluid pleocytosis, may develop.

Herpangina

Herpangina is a specific infectious disease characterized by a vesicular enanthem of the fauces of the soft palate, accompanied by fever, sore throat, and pain on swallowing. It is caused predominantly by group A coxsackieviruses but has also infrequently been associated with other enterovirus infections. It primarily affects children between the ages of 3 and 10 years but is occasionally seen in older children and adults. The illness begins suddenly with a fever of 99.8° F (37.7° C) to 104.9° F (40.5° C). Vomiting, myalgia, and headache are common at onset but generally do not persist. Sore throat and pain on swallowing are the most prominent symptoms and precede the appearance of the enanthem by several hours to a day. Inspection of the throat reveals erythema, a mild exudate on the tonsils, and the characteristic enanthem, which must be carefully sought to avoid missing it. The lesions, usually 2 to 6 in number (rarely, 12) are painful. They are located on the soft palate, on the free-hanging margin between the tonsils and the uvula; less commonly, they are on the surface of the tonsils or the posterior pharyngeal wall. They begin as punctate macules that evolve over a 24 hour period to 2 to 4 mm papules that vesiculate centrally and eventually ulcerate. The usual clinical laboratory diagnostic tests are not helpful. Management is symptomatic.

Lymphonodular pharyngitis

Lymphonodular pharyngitis is a variant of herpangina. It consists of tiny nodules of packed lymphocytes, which eventually recede without undergoing vesiculation or ulceration.

Hand-foot-mouth syndrome

Hand-foot-mouth syndrome is a distinctive vesicular eruption that most commonly is caused by coxsackievirus A16, also by enterovirus 71, and less commonly by other enteroviruses. The illness is mild and lasts for 1 week or less. It occurs predominantly in children and consists of sore throat or mouth, refusal to eat, fever of 100.4 to 102.2° F (38 to 39° C), which lasts for 1 to 2 days, and vesicles in the oral cavity, chiefly on the buccal mucosa and tongue. Several lesions may coalesce to form bullae that frequently ulcerate by the time they are seen by a physician. Lesions of the skin are less constant, occurring in 75% of patients. They are most commonly seen on the hands and feet, where either the extensor surfaces or the palms or soles may be involved. Less commonly, lesions occur more proximally in the extremities or buttocks and, rarely, on the genitalia.

The cutaneous lesions of hand-foot-mouth disease are tender and consist of mixed papules and clear vesicles with a surrounding zone of erythema. They are located subepidermally and are accompanied by mixed lymphocytic and polymorphonuclear inflammation and extensive acantholysis of the overlying epidermis. The lesions may resemble those caused by herpes simplex or varicella-zoster viruses, but they can be usually distinguished clinically by the number and distribution of lesions.

Exanthems

One of the most interesting features of enteroviral infections is the occurrence of exanthems. Once recognized, they are important as indicators of the prevalence of enterovirus infections in the community. On the other hand, they may be confused with other infective exanthems of greater medical significance (Chapter 228). Fine maculopapular rashes resembling rubella but occurring during summer epidemics have been reported with echovirus type 9, although a number of other enteroviruses may produce this syndrome. The rash characteristically occurs simultaneously with fever and begins on the face, then spreads to the neck, chest, and extremities. It consists of innumerable faint, pink macules that do not itch or desquamate. The rash is transient, but it may last 5 days or more on the face. Lesions may coalesce, giving the cheeks a violaceous hue. Helpful features in distinguishing enteroviral rash from rubella are the summertime occurrence and absence of lymphadenopathy in the posterior cervical and postauricular regions. Rash associated with echovirus type 9 and coxsackievirus A9 may have a petechial component. Petechial enteroviral exanthem associated with signs of meningeal irritation can be confused with meningococcemia.

A number of enterovirus infections may produce roseoliform exanthems. As in roseola, the rash does not appear until defervescence. The prototype is the Boston exanthem, first of the known enterovirus exanthems to be recognized and now known to be caused by echovirus type 16. Multiple cases often occur sequentially in families, and the mean age of those affected is 3 years. Before the rash, the temperature is 100.4 to 102.2° F (38 to 39° C), and there may be pharyngitis without cough or coryza.

Epidemic pleurodynia (Bornholm disease)

Epidemic pleurodynia is an acute infectious disease characterized by fever and sharp spasmodic pain of the chest or abdomen. It is a disease of muscle, not of the pleura or peritoneum. Group B coxsackieviruses are the most important cause of epidemic pleurodynia. The illness occurs mainly in children 5 to 15 years of age and their parents.

There is no prodrome. The illness begins with the abrupt onset of spasmodic pain, typically over the lower rib cage or upper abdomen. Fever of 100.4 to 103.1° F (38 to 39.5° C) reaches its peak within 1 hour after the onset of each paroxysm and subsides as the pain recedes. In some outbreaks, sore throat and headache have been prominent, but cough and nasopharyngeal symptoms are usually notably absent. The intensity of the discomfort varies from a mild ache to severe pain. It is most often described as stabbing or constricting pain, occurring along the costal margin or occasionally the subxyphoid region. Half of the patients, especially adults, have pain primarily in the thorax. In the other half, pain primarily occurs in the upper abdomen. Periumbilical pain or pain in the lower abdominal quadrants is more common in children. In an individual patient, only one site or at most two are usually involved.

The spasmodic and paroxysmal character of the pain is characteristic of this disease. Each paroxysm typically lasts 2 to 10 hours. The first paroxysm is the most severe; subsequent paroxysms are shorter and are accompanied by less fever. During a paroxysm, if the pain is mild and the patient is ambulatory, he or she stoops forward or leans to the side, splinting the chest. With more severe pain, the patient lies in bed, resists being turned, and appears acutely ill and apprehensive. Chest pain limits deep inspiration; consequently, respirations are rapid and shallow. In most patients, tenderness mimicking the spontaneously occurring pain is elicited by pressing on the affected muscles, and palpable, often visible muscle swelling may be observed. Auscultation of the chest reveals nothing abnormal. Pleural friction rubs are rare. As the pain subsides and the temperature drops to normal, profuse sweating may occur. Although dull aching of muscles often persists, the patient may look and feel entirely healthy between paroxysms. About a fourth of patients experience multiple recurrences, often after they have been free of pain for a day or more and have felt well enough to return to work or school. Most patients are ill for 6 days or less. In keeping with the multiple disease manifestations of enteroviruses, during any given outbreak of pleurodynia caused by a particular enterovirus, a number of patients may appear with aseptic meningitis, pericarditis, and mildly symptomatic disease caused by the same immunotype.

Pleurodynia may be confused with many other illnesses because of the variable location of the disease. The usual clinical laboratory findings are normal. Therefore during the enterovirus season, pleurodynia should be considered in adults or children who have acute onset of fever and pain in the chest or abdomen.

Myopericarditis

Coxsackieviruses rarely attack the myocardium without attacking the pericardium; however, signs of either myocarditis or pericarditis may be dominant. In infants, myocarditis tends to be predominant and the disease fulminant. In contrast, the disease is usually much milder in adults and consists clinically of signs and symptoms of pericarditis or a mixed picture of myocarditis and pericarditis. Most cases are due to group B coxsackievirus types 1 to 5, although other enteroviruses may produce this syndrome.

In the newborn, the illness typically begins abruptly at about 1 week of age with listlessness, anorexia, and fever. These symptoms persist for about 2 days before clinical evidence of heart disease becomes apparent. In a third of patients, the illness is biphasic, with a hiatus of 1 to 7 days of apparent well-being between the initial febrile illness and the appearance of frank myocarditis. With the onset of heart failure, respiratory distress, marked tachycardia, cardiomegaly, a systolic murmur, and electrocardiographic evidence of myocardial injury are seen. Clinical or electrocardiographic evidence of pericarditis is usually absent. In severely affected infants, cyanosis and circulatory collapse develop rapidly. In fatal cases, disseminated viral infection involving the central nervous system, liver, pancreas, and adrenal glands is often seen.

In older children and adults, the disease occurs at least twice as frequently in men as in women. An upper respiratory tract illness usually precedes the onset of cardiac manifestations by about 2 weeks. Symptoms include dyspnea, chest pain, fever, and malaise. Pain in the precordial area is usually dull, but it may resemble angina pectoris or be sharp, pleuritic, aggravated by lying down, and relieved by sitting up and leaning forward. There is a pericardial friction rub in 35% to 85% of patients. Enlargement of the cardiac silhouette on chest radiographs may be due either to effusion or to dilatation. Signs of frank congestive heart failure are observed in 20%. Electrocardiographic abnormalities are invariably present. These consist of S-T segment elevation or nonspecific S-T and T wave abnormalities. More severe myocardial disease may lead to the development of Q waves, arrhythmias, and heart block. Serum levels of myocardial enzymes and white blood cell counts are frequently elevated.

Neonatal coxsackievirus myocarditis has a mortality rate of about 50%, and death usually occurs within 1 week of onset. Most older children and adults recover uneventfully. However, there may be one or more recurrences of myopericarditis several weeks to more than 1 year after the initial illness in 20%. Persistent electrocardiographic abnormalities, cardiomegaly, and chronic congestive heart failure indicate that permanent myocardial injury sometimes occurs. Chronic constrictive pericarditis has occurred after coxsackievirus myopericarditis after intervals of 5 weeks to 1 year.

Virus has been isolated rarely from myocardium or pericardial fluid in adults and only occasionally from other sites. The diagnosis can be established only by demonstrating a fourfold rise in antibody titer. The presumptive diagnosis is based on high titers of antibody titers in convalescent sera specimens.

Specific antiviral agents are not available, and therapy must be symptomatic. Corticosteroids are of no proven benefit.

Chronic meningoencephalitis in agammaglobulinemias

Echoviruses have been responsible for persistent, sometimes fatal infection of the central nervous system in patients with agammaglobulinemia. The illness is commonly associated with a syndrome resembling dermatomyositis.

Acute hemorrhagic conjunctivitis

Acute hemorrhagic conjunctivitis is a newly recognized ocular infection caused by enterovirus type 70 and coxsackievirus A24. Unlike most enteroviral infections, it is probably transmitted primarily from fingers or fomites directly to the eye.

Acute hemorrhagic conjunctivitis emerged as a newly recognized disease in 1969, simultaneously in Ghana and Indonesia. Since then, its spread has been explosive and pandemic. It has reached all parts of the world including North America, but the western hemisphere has not experienced the same widespread epidemics as have Asia and Africa. The disease apparently spreads more rapidly in crowded and unsanitary conditions.

Acute hemorrhagic conjunctivitis begins abruptly, and the illness reaches its peak on the first day. Symptoms appear first in one eye and then a few hours later in the other. The major symptoms are a burning sensation, ocular pain, photophobia, swelling of the eyelids, and a watery discharge. Constitutional symptoms, such as fever, malaise, and headache, are observed in a fifth of patients. The most distinctive sign is subconjunctival hemorrhage, which is present in 70% to 90% of patients with enterovirus type 70 infection, but it is seen much less frequently in disease caused by coxsackievirus A24. The hemorrhages may be pinpoint or may occupy the entire bulbar conjunctiva and are precipitated by everting the upper lid or rubbing the eye. Small follicles appear on the tarsal conjunctiva after 3 to 5 days in 90% of the patients. Corneal erosions or a fine punctate epithelial keratitis is also present in most patients. The ocular discharge is serous or seromucous. The preauricular lymph nodes are often enlarged and tender. Recovery usually begins by the second or third day and is complete by 10 days.

Fortunately, serious complications are very rare. Some cases of motor paralysis (poliomyelitis) have occurred in association with the disease. Treatment is symptomatic. Antimicrobial agents are not indicated, and antiviral agents are not available. Attention to aseptic technique should decrease the transmission.

Hepatitis

Hepatitis A is caused by hepatitis A virus, a picornavirus belonging to a separate genus (Chapter 57).

Other illnesses

Enteroviral infections have been associated with a number of other illnesses. In most instances, the evidence that such associations are causal is lacking. For example, many reports indicate recovery of enteroviruses from stool specimens of patients with nonbacterial gastroenteritis. In most controlled studies, however, the rate of isolation of enteroviruses from control subjects is about the same as that from ill subjects. There is stronger evidence that echovirus types 11, 14, and 18 are associated with epidemic diarrhea of the newborn. Overall, it appears that the role of enteroviruses in diarrheal diseases is minor.

Hepatitis has occurred in disseminated enteroviral infections, generally those produced by group B coxsackieviruses, but there is no known relationship between enteroviral infections (other than hepatitis A virus) and hepatitis occurring in the absence of other manifestations. Pancreatitis and orchitis have occurred in patients with group B coxsackievirus infections. A role for coxsackievirus B4 in the pathogenesis of juvenile diabetes mellitus has been suggested.

PREVENTION

Vaccines

No vaccines exist for rhinovirus, coxsackievirus, echovirus, or the more recently discovered enterovirus infections. However, one of the most dramatic demonstrations of vaccine efficacy has been the eradication of paralytic poliomyelitis in much of the world by use of oral and inactivated poliovirus vaccines. Both vaccines have excellent records of safety and efficacy.

Oral poliovirus vaccine elicits both circulatory and secretory antibodies and induces immunity that may be lifelong. One advantage of this vaccine is that nonvaccinated persons may become immunized by contact with vaccinated persons, and the circulation of wild viruses is prevented by alimentary immunity.

At present in the United States, three doses of trivalent oral polio vaccine are given. The first is given at 2 months of age, the second at 4 months of age, and the third at 12 to 18 months of age. In addition, a booster dose is advised for children entering school. This vaccine is safe in pregnancy. Its main disadvantage is its potential, albeit rare, for paralytic disease among recipients and their contacts. Immunodeficient children are particularly susceptible to this complication.

Wild poliovirus infection has been eliminated from the United States and is targeted for elimination in Latin America in the next few years by the use of vaccines. Global eradication is projected by the year 2000 by the World Health Organization.

Recently a more potent inactivated poliovirus vaccine was licensed. It confers humoral but not secretory immunity, provided three initial doses and subsequent boosters are given. Its advantages are that it cannot undergo mutation or reversion to virulence, and it is safe to administer to immunodeficient or immunosuppressed persons. It is the preferred vaccine for previously unvaccinated adults as well as immunodeficient persons.

Inactivated hepatitis A vaccines that confer protection after one or two doses are in clinical trials and are expected to be approved for use in the United States in the near future.

Alpha$_2$-interferon administered intranasally has shown significant protection against rhinovirus infection and illness. However, long-term prophylaxis results in epistaxis and nasal erosions, thus limiting its potential usefulness.

REFERENCES

Centers for Disease Control: Poliomyelitis prevention: enhanced-potency inactivated poliomyelitis vaccine—supplementary statement. MMWR 36:795, 1987.

Dalakas MC et al: A long-term follow-up study of patients with post-poliomyelitis neuromuscular symptoms. N Engl J Med 314:959, 1986.

Doyle WJ et al: A double-blind placebo-controlled clinical trial of the effect of chlorpheniramine on the response of the nasal airway, middle ear and eustachian tube to provocative rhinovirus challenge. Pediatr Infect Dis 7:222, 1988.

Hendley JO and Gwaltney JM Jr: Mechanisms of transmission of rhinovirus infections. Epidemiol Rev 10:242, 1988.

Hinman AR et al: Live or inactivated poliovirus vaccine: an analysis of the benefits and risks. Am J Public Health 78:291, 1988.

McBean AM et al: The serologic response to oral polio vaccine and enhanced potency inactivated polio vaccines. Am J Epidemiol 128:615, 1988.

McKinney RE Jr, Katz SL, and Wilfert CM: Chronic enteroviral meningoencephalitis in agammaglobulinemic patients. Rev Infect Dis 9:334, 1987.

Naclerio RM et al: Kinins are generated during experimental rhinovirus colds. J Infect Dis 157:133, 1988.

Nkowane BM et al: Vaccine-associated paralytic poliomyelitis: United States: 1973 through 1984. JAMA 257:1335, 1987.

O'Neil KM et al: Chronic group A coxsackievirus infection in agammaglobulinemia: demonstration of genomic variation of serotypically identical isolates persistently excreted by the same patient. J Infect Dis 157:183, 1988.

Rose NR et al: Post-infectious autoimmunity: two distinct phases of coxsackievirus B3–induced myocarditis. Ann NY Acad Sci 475:146, 1986.

Sperber SJ and Hayden FG: Minireview: chemotherapy of rhinovirus colds. Antimicrob Agents Chemother 32(4):409, 1988.

Strikas RA, Anderson LJ, and Parker RA: Temporal and geographic patterns of isolates of nonpolio enteroviruses in the United States. J Infect Dis 153:346, 1986.

Wright PF: Strategies for the global eradication of poliomyelitis by the year 2000. N Engl J Med 325:1774, 1991.

CHAPTER

245 Orthomyxovirus Infections (Influenza)

Robert B. Couch

The orthomyxoviridae contain only one genus, influenza, and three types (species), A, B, and C. Types A and B cause a variety of acute respiratory disease syndromes in humans, the most notable being influenza, an acute respiratory disease with fever and prominent systemic symptoms. Both types A and B viruses cause recurring epidemics of varying severity in human populations. In temperate climates these epidemics typically occur during the cold weather months and involve persons in all age groups. Complicating pneumonia occurs with significant frequency in persons with underlying chronic disease and may lead to death. Vaccines are effective for the prevention of types A and B influenza, and the drug amantadine is effective for both prevention and treatment of type A disease.

Type C virus appears to be endemic and primarily to cause minor respiratory illness in young children.

CHARACTERISTICS

Influenza virus particles are spherical, with a diameter of 80 to 120 nm; however, filamentous particles of varying lengths may also be seen. An electron micrograph and diagrammatic representation of an influenza virus particle (Fig. 245-1) show a helical viral nucleocapsid that is composed of nucleoprotein and ribonucleic acid (RNA). The RNA genome is single stranded and divided into separate segments. There are eight segments for types A and B and seven for type C. Structural stability is provided by matrix protein, and the viral core is surrounded by an outer lipid bilayer into which the surface subunits are inserted. Two different surface subunits, hemagglutinin and neuraminidase glycoproteins, are present on types A and B particles, whereas a single glycoprotein, a hemagglutinin-esterase glycoprotein, is present on type C particles.

Attachment of the virus to susceptible cells is mediated by the hemagglutinin subunit. The red blood cell receptor is a neuraminic acid–containing glycoprotein; it is presumed that a similar receptor is involved in initiation of infection of eukaryotic cells, although a receptor with different specificity may be involved. Penetration is by pinocytosis, and uncoating results from fusion with the endosomal membrane. RNA polymerase activity increases over the first 2 hours. New viral RNA is replicated through a complementary RNA messenger, and this takes place in the cell nucleus. Newly synthesized host cell messenger RNA (mRNA) provides a source of cap for viral mRNA. Viral proteins are synthesized in the cytoplasm. Nucleocapsid assembly takes place in the cell nucleus and virion assembly takes place at the cell surface. Virion surface subunits orient on the cell plasma membrane, and virus is released by budding through the membrane. During the latter process the lipid bilayer is acquired.

Newly synthesized virus contains neuraminic acid residues that promote aggregation at the cell surface. Neuraminidase activity disrupts or prevents occurrence of these aggregates, a phenomenon that results in an increase in free infectious particles. From initiation to completion, replica-

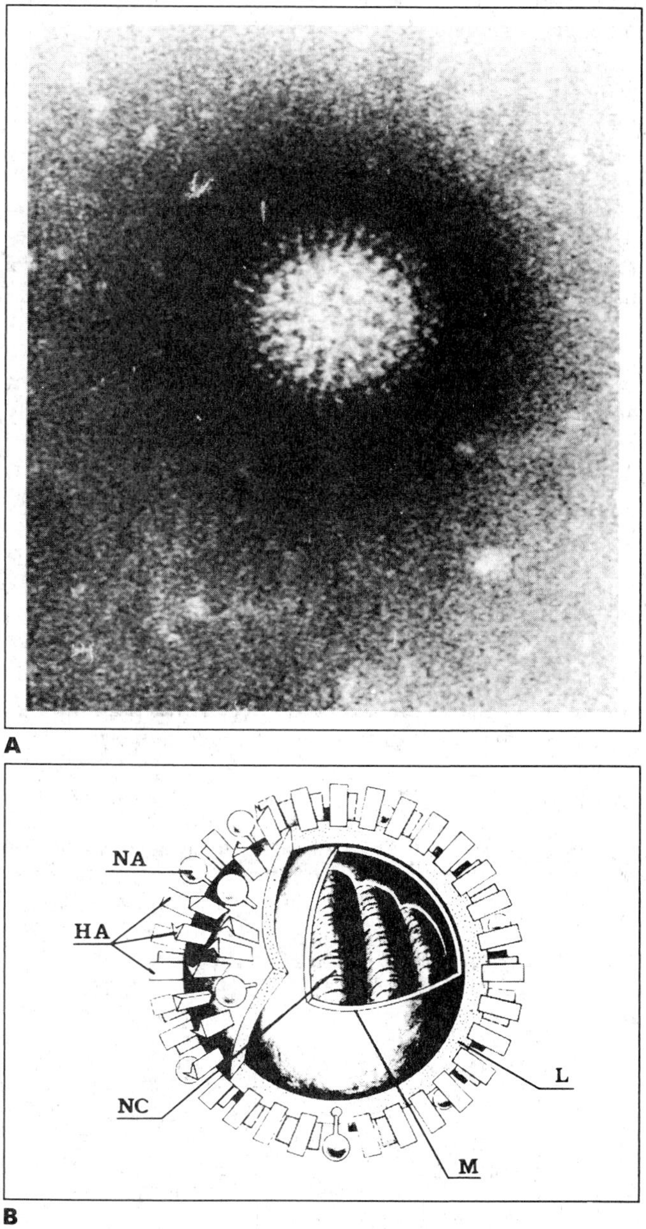

Fig. 245-1. Electron micrograph and diagrammatic representation of influenza virus. **A,** Electron micrograph; **B,** diagrammatic representation. HA and NA, hemagglutinin and neuraminidase subunits, respectively; NC, nucleocapsid that consists of nucleoprotein and viral RNA; M, matrix protein; L, lipid bilayer. (Electron micrograph from Gerin JL. Diagram from Stuart-Harris CH and Schild GC: Influenza: The viruses and the diseases. Littleton, MA, 1976, Publishing Sciences Group.)

tion takes about 6 hours. Infected cells produce new virus over a period of several hours, then cell death ensues.

CLASSIFICATION

The human influenza viruses are classified as shown in Table 245-1. All three types are similar in biochemical and biophysical properties. However, distinctive differences in antigenic determinants of major structural subunits provide a basis for a classification that reflects biologic and epidemiologic behavior.

Types A, B, and C viruses contain different but antigenically stable nucleoprotein antigens. Type A viruses may exhibit major and minor antigenic variation of their surface hemagglutinin and neuraminidase subunits. When new type A viruses that lack serologic cross reactivity with one of the surface subunits of earlier viruses (major change) appear, a subtype designation is assigned. This phenomenon has been called antigenic shift, and each occurrence has led to widespread epidemic or pandemic influenza. Three distinct human subtypes have been described.

Separate and distinct subtypes of type A virus have also been described for equine and avian species. Because of antigenic relatedness, type A viruses of swine (formerly $H_{SW}1N1$) have now been designated as H1N1 viruses. Types B and C viruses have not exhibited antigenic shift, and no indigenous occurrence in animals has been described.

The prevalent concept to explain antigenic shift among type A viruses is that new surface antigens are acquired from an animal virus by recombination, and this is followed by subsequent spread among humans. The existence of a segmented genome would facilitate a reassortment of genes (recombination) in a mixed infection.

Both types A and B viruses exhibit minor antigenic change of the hemagglutinin and neuraminidase subunits; in these instances, serologic cross reactivity between subunits is demonstrable. This type of change has been called antigenic drift and is presumed to result from mutability of the virus genome and selective pressure of population immunity. Such changes may lead to epidemic influenza. A prototype strain representative of each of these variants is designated by geographic origin, strain number, and year of isolation (see Table 245-1).

Antigenic differences among type C viruses have thus far been minimal.

Table 245-1. Classification of human influenza viruses

Type	Subtype	Years of prevalence	Representative variants*
A	H1N1†	1918-1957‡	Puerto Rico/8/34 A/FM/1/47
	H2N2	1957-1967	A/Japan/305/57
	H3N2	1968-	A/Hong Kong/1/68 A/Victoria/3/75 A/Beijing/32/92
	H1N1	1977-	A/USSR/92/77 A/Taiwan/1/86 A/Texas/36/91
B	None determined	1940-§	B/Hong Kong/5/72 B/Panama/45/90
C	None determined	1949-‖	C/JHB/2/66

*Variants are monitored by using a reference strain described by type, geographic origin/strain number/year of isolation.

†Earlier classifications of this subtype included the separate designations $H_{SW}1N1$, H0N1, and H1N1. All are now designated as the H1N1 subtype.

‡An influenza virus was first isolated from swine in 1931 and from humans in 1933; retrospective serologic studies indicated that a virus resembling swine/31 became prevalent in humans in 1918.

§First isolated from humans in 1940.

‖First isolated from humans in 1949.

EPIDEMIOLOGY

Epidemic history

Influenza viruses were probably a cause of disease in ancient times; retrospective tracing has dated the occurrence of influenza epidemics at least to 1173. Thereafter there is a nearly continuous record of epidemics, which are periodically interspersed with extensive pandemics (worldwide epidemics). During the past century, serologic tests of sera from elderly persons have permitted a more certain assessment of epidemic disease. In 1889 a pandemic occurred with a type A virus containing an H3-like hemagglutinin and an equine 2 (now N8)–like neuraminidase. Little is known of influenza in the intervening years preceding the devastating pandemic of 1918, which was caused by an H1N1 (formerly called swine) virus. In that pandemic, about 20 million persons in the world and about 500,000 in the United States died as a consequence of influenza.

The modern history of influenza began with isolation of influenza virus from humans in 1933. Since that time two shifts causing pandemics have occurred, one in 1957, caused by H2N2 (Asian) virus, and a less extensive one in 1968, caused by H3N2 virus. In the intervening years antigenic drift and epidemics of varying severity have occurred.

Patterns of epidemics

The pattern exhibited by a typical type A epidemic in an urban community is shown in Fig. 245-2. In the initial phases of an epidemic, infection and illness appear predominantly in schoolchildren, and this is reflected by a sharp rise in school absenteeism, physician visits, and pediatric hospital admissions. These children carry the virus into the home, where preschool children and adults acquire the infection. Infection and illness among adults are then reflected in industrial absenteeism, adult hospital admissions, and mortality associated with influenza or pneumonia.

The duration of an epidemic is generally 3 to 6 weeks, although virus is present in the community for a variable number of weeks before and after the epidemic period. During the epidemic period the duration of an outbreak in subsegments of the population may be brief (e.g., the com-

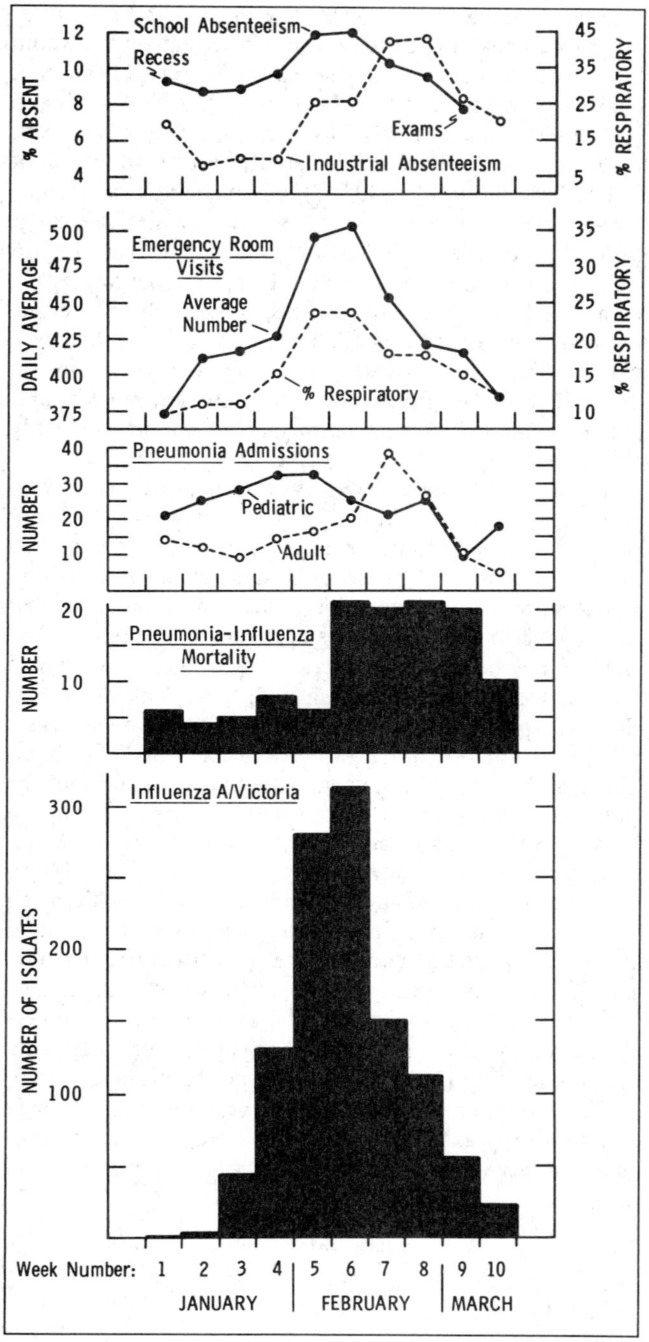

Fig. 245-2. Correlation of the nonvirologic indices of epidemic influenza with the number of isolates of influenza A/Victoria virus according to week, Houston, 1976. (From Glezen WP and Couch RB: N Engl J Med 298:587, 1978.)

plete course of epidemic influenza may occur in an institutionalized population in a period of 2 weeks).

Influenza type B presents a similar pattern of epidemic occurrence, except that excess mortality may not be apparent. Influenza type C has not been shown to produce epidemic disease.

Epidemics in temperate climates typically occur in winter, although fall and spring epidemics may also be seen. Both types A and B (and probably C) viruses cause infections and illness every winter; however, an epidemic does not occur unless the constellation of factors required for epidemic spread occurs. The relative significance of crowding, environmental conditions, and so forth, for development of an epidemic is uncertain, but the most significant factor is population susceptibility, an occurrence primarily attributable to antigenic variation.

Antigenic shift occurs at a point location, and the new virus then spreads throughout the world along transportation routes; the source and spread of antigenic drift viruses are less certain. Community "seeding" with a new virus may occur during the "off season," and as much as 2 years may precede the occurrence of epidemic disease. Such a pattern of infection would imply a summer survival mechanism or repeated community introductions of new viruses; evidence favors the latter.

Attack rates of illness during epidemics vary between 10% and 50%. The highest attack rates during types A and B epidemics are in the 5 to 19 year age group; however, high frequencies occur in preschool children and adults of all ages. Attack rates are usually lower for type B in preschool children and adults.

Mortality attributable to influenza has proved to be a reliable index of epidemic influenza, but it tends to minimize the magnitude of a type B epidemic because there may be no excess mortality. The severity and frequency of influenza epidemics are variable. Only in a general way can the magnitude be related to the occurrence of antigenic shift. Thus the consequences of antigenic drift must be considered of equal significance.

PATHOPHYSIOLOGY

Epidemic influenza is transmitted primarily by the airborne route, but the occurrence of cases in almost all circumstances of human interaction suggests that it may also be transmitted by contact. The initial deposition site of inhaled aerosol particles is the tracheobronchial mucosa. The covering mucous blanket includes mucoproteins that contain the neuraminic acid receptor. Binding undoubtedly occurs, but the action of viral neuraminidase could induce release and liquefaction of mucus, thereby further promoting access of virus to the mucosal surface. The primary site of infection is the superficial columnar epithelium. Completion of the viral replicative cycle in these cells results in cellular death and desquamation. Edema and mononuclear cell infiltration of involved areas result, and these changes are accompanied by a prominent cough. A similar sequence occurs in the nasopharynx, where virus may also be deposited. Changes at these sites lead to nasal and pharyngeal symptoms.

The incubation period varies between 1 and 5 days. During this interval the extent of involvement of the cellular mucosa increases, and this change is reflected in an increase in the quantity of virus detected in secretions. There is a direct relationship between the quantity of virus detected and the severity of the illness in uncomplicated cases. After a 2 to 3 day period, a fall in the quantity of virus in secretions occurs; this fall is accompanied by an improvement in symptoms, but virus shedding and symptoms may last for 5 to 8 days. Although severe myalgias are a feature of acute influenza, viremia has rarely been detected.

Recovery from acute influenza generally ensues before antibody is detectable in either serum or secretions. A role for interferon in recovery is suggested by its appearance in secretions just as the progressive reduction in the quantity of virus ensues. Cell-mediated cytotoxicity for virus-infected cells has been demonstrated; T cells, natural killer cells, and cells mediating antibody-dependent cellular cytotoxicity may contribute to clearance of the localized infection. When antibody appears in secretions, virus is no longer detectable, suggesting a role for local antibody in the final clearance of virus.

On occasion, particularly in persons with underlying heart or lung disease, viral involvement of alveolar tissues of the lung may occur and produce an interstitial pneumonia. Virus titers in secretions from these patients may be very high ($10^{7-9}TCID_{50}$/ml) and the duration of viral shedding prolonged. Sometimes, marked accumulation of lung edema, with hemorrhage, hyaline membrane formation, extensive mononuclear infiltration, and pulmonary fibrosis, may be seen.

Pneumonia in association with influenza is most commonly caused by bacteria. In these cases, viral infection has presumably impaired the normal lung defense mechanisms so that invasion by pneumococci, staphylococci, and gram-negative bacteria is promoted (Chapter 231). Such cases exhibit the histologic features of bacterial pneumonia, although, if the pneumonia occurs early in the course of influenza, the histologic features of both viral and bacterial pneumonia may be exhibited.

Antibody is the primary defense mechanism against acquisition of infection. Locally synthesized immunoglobulin A (IgA) antibody is the primary mediator of protection for the upper respiratory passages, whereas serum-derived IgG antibody mediates protection of the lower respiratory passages. The latter measure is used to assess immunity, because a direct correlation exists between serum antibody titer and resistance to infection. In general, a hemagglutination-inhibition titer of 1:32 against the epidemic virus is associated with substantial resistance. Antibody directed toward the hemagglutinin is required to prevent infection, whereas antibody directed toward either the hemagglutinin or the neuraminidase reduces the level of infection, the likelihood of occurrence of illness, and the severity of any illness.

The risk of febrile illness in persons lacking either hemagglutinin or neuraminidase antibody is about 80%, whereas in most circumstances some antibody is present, and the febrile illness risk is about 50%.

DISEASES IN HUMANS

Uncomplicated influenza

The influenzal syndrome is a febrile illness of sudden onset, with tracheitis and marked myalgias. The case of a typical patient treated with amantadine appears in Fig. 245-3. After an incubation period of 1 to 5 days, patients in whom this syndrome develops have a sudden onset of headache, chilly sensations, fever, malaise, myalgias, anorexia, and sore throat. Shaking chills may occur, but they rarely recur after the onset of fever. Fever rapidly ascends to a level of 101 to 104° F (38.3 to 40.0° C), and respiratory symptoms ensue. A nonproductive cough is characteristic; sneezing, rhinorrhea, and nasal obstruction are common. The nonproductive cough frequently occurs in paroxysms and is accompanied by substernal soreness; these findings indicate the presence of tracheitis. Patients may also report photophobia, hoarseness, nausea, vomiting, diarrhea, and abdominal pain. Gastrointestinal symptoms are more prominent in children than in adults and are noted more frequently with type B than with type A infection.

Physical examination reveals an acutely ill patient who is usually coughing. Lid slits may be narrowed, as a result of eye pain, and minimum to moderate nasal obstruction or discharge may be present. Despite complaints of sore throat, minimum inflammation is seen on examination, but tender anterior cervical nodes are commonly present. The trachea may be tender on lateral motion, and cough that is precipitated by deep breathing with the mouth open confirms the presence of tracheitis. Examination of the chest reveals nothing abnormal or an occasional dry rale. Muscles may be tender on palpation, but the remainder of the physical findings are unremarkable.

Most adults ill with influenza virus infection do not exhibit the exact syndrome that has been described. Moreover, the influenzal syndrome is uncommon in children and is not seen in infants. Predominant symptoms in a particular patient may be sneezing, nasal obstruction, and discharge (common cold); nasal obstruction, discharge, and sore throat (upper respiratory illness); sore throat with erythema (pharyngitis); hoarseness (laryngitis); or cough (tracheobronchitis). Fever may or may not be present.

The duration of prominent respiratory and systemic symptoms is 1 to 5 days. Thereafter a progressive improvement ensues, although the nasal symptoms, malaise, and

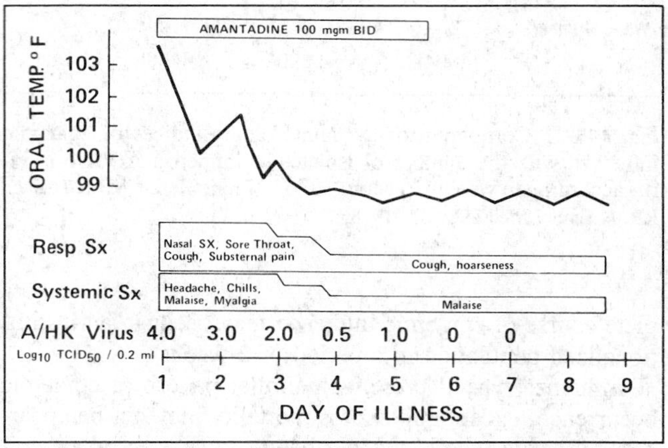

Fig. 245-3. Case of uncomplicated acute influenza in a healthy 24-year-old man. (Courtesy of Dr. V. Knight.)

cough may continue for several days. The total duration of overt illness rarely exceeds 10 days, although many patients complain of lassitude for an additional 1 to 2 weeks.

The clinical presentations of influenza are summarized in the box below.

COMPLICATIONS

Pulmonary complications

Although lung involvement is generally considered a complication of influenza in many patients, it merely represents more extensive disease or influenza in a patient with preexisting chest disease. Some patients with influenza exhibit moist or dry rales over a localized area of the lung on physical examination, and some exhibit diffuse inspiratory and expiratory wheezes. The moist or dry rales are usually over a lower lobe and represent a segmental pneumonia that may or may not be apparent on the chest radiograph; the wheezes represent bronchiolitis. Such patients initially appear very ill, but, apart from a tendency to remain febrile and acutely ill for a longer period than usual, the course of their illness is similar to that of patients without chest findings. Fewer than 5% of healthy adults exhibit one of these disease patterns, but they are common in infants and small children.

As a consequence of influenza infection, exacerbations of acute respiratory insufficiency may occur in patients with chronic obstructive pulmonary disease. Such patients may have increased coughing and sputum production and new chest findings, or they may simply exhibit fever and respiratory insufficiency. Some permanent deterioration in lung function may result from the infection.

Extensive influenzal pneumonia was a prominent disease during the pandemics of 1918 and 1957. The disease is most likely to occur in persons with underlying heart or lung disease, but about half of the cases in recent years have occurred in persons thought to be otherwise healthy. A case in an otherwise healthy person is shown in Fig. 245-4. The disease at onset is similar to other cases of influenza, but instead of improving by the third to fifth day of illness, patients continue to be febrile, and progressive air hunger and cyanosis develop. Chest examination initially reveals bilateral moist rales and wheezes without signs of consolidation; chest radiographs reveal bilateral interstitial disease, sometimes accompanied by areas of local consolidation. Sputum is often scanty but may be copious, frothy, and pink tinged if the patient has underlying heart disease. Bacteriologic tests reveal normal flora, and such patients do not respond to antibiotics. Blood gas studies reveal marked hypoxia, and ventilatory assistance may be required. Mortality rate is very high.

Mixed viral and bacterial pneumonia may also occur. The clinical appearance is of typical influenza at onset, but after 2 to 5 days, a cough productive of purulent or bloody sputum and chest pain that is sometimes pleuritic develop. These findings usually indicate the onset of a superimposed bacterial pneumonia. Chest examination reveals an area of consolidation, and examination of sputum reveals predominance of a lung pathogen. The most likely cause of the bacterial pneumonia is the pneumococcus, but staphylococci and *Haemophilus influenzae* also are commonly found. If the patient was receiving antibiotics or was hospitalized before the onset of bacterial superinfection, a gram-negative organism may be responsible. Mortality is variable, depending on the presence of an underlying disease and the bacterium responsible for the pneumonia.

The most common pattern of pneumonia with influenza is postinfluenzal bacterial pneumonia. This disease occurs most commonly in persons with an underlying chronic disease, particularly cardiovascular or lung disease. Patients have influenza, and remission of fever and symptoms ensues. Then during or just after recovery they experience the reappearance of fever and the onset of chest pain, which

Clinical presentations of influenza

- Uncomplicated influenza
  - Common cold
  - Upper respiratory illness
  - Pharyngitis
  - Laryngitis
  - Tracheobronchitis
  - Influenzal syndrome
- Complications of influenza
  - Pneumonia
    - Segmental influenzal
    - Extensive influenzal
    - Mixed viral bacterial
    - Postinfluenzal bacterial
    - Exacerbation of acute respiratory insufficiency
  - Neurologic
    - Encephalitis, encephalopathy
    - Reye's syndrome
    - Guillain-Barré syndrome
    - Transverse myelitis
  - Other
    - Sinusitis, otitis

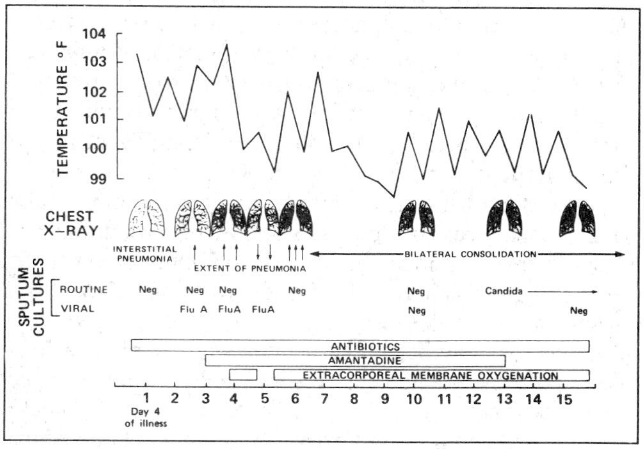

Fig. 245-4. Case of fulminant influenzal pneumonia leading to death in an otherwise healthy 48-year-old man. Day 1 of hospitalization was day 4 of the illness. (Modified from Lefrak EA et al: Chest 66:385, 1974.)

may be pleuritic, and a cough productive of purulent or bloody sputum. The physical examination, chest radiograph, sputum studies, and leukocyte counts reveal findings typical of a bacterial pneumonia (Chapter 231). These patients respond to appropriate antibiotics, and mortality rate is low.

Neurologic complications

The occurrence of encephalitis and encephalopathy in association with acute influenza, particularly in children, is well documented, although rare. Virus is not isolated from the cerebrospinal fluid, and the pathogenesis is uncertain.

Reye's syndrome (Chapter 60) may be seen after both type A and type B influenza. It is most prominent after influenza in older children but occurs in young adults as well.

Guillain-Barré syndrome and transverse myelitis have also been reported after influenza, but the absence of a relationship between epidemic influenza and the incidence of Guillain-Barré syndrome suggests that influenza infection is rarely associated with this disease.

Other complications

Sinusitis and otitis media may occur as a consequence of upper respiratory illness (Chapter 230). Although otitis is reported to be caused by influenza virus directly, in most cases the ear and sinus symptoms are probably caused by pressure changes secondary to obstruction of the eustachian tube or sinus foramina. Frank secondary bacterial sinusitis and otitis media may, however, occur.

Myositis may be seen in children, particularly with influenza type B infection.

Myocarditis, pericarditis, disseminated intravascular coagulation, and myositis with myoglobinuria have accompanied acute influenza but are rare.

DIAGNOSTIC TESTS

A presumptive diagnosis of influenza may be made if a patient has an acute respiratory disease with fever and without pneumonia during a community epidemic of influenza. Supporting information is provided by a throat culture finding negative for group A streptococci in patients with prominent pharyngitis and by the absence of significant peripheral blood leukocytosis and neutrophilia.

A definite diagnosis of influenza requires demonstration of influenza virus in a patient's respiratory secretions or a rise in titer of specific antibody. The optimum specimen for virus detection is a combined nasal wash and throat swab specimen, but a nose and throat swab specimen will do. Methods for rapid detection of virus are being increasingly used and some methods are commercially available. Specificity for types A and B viruses is high; sensitivity is also high for acutely ill hospitalized children but data for outpatients and adults are limited.

For virus isolation a protein stabilizer must be added to nasal wash specimens with saline, but a swab specimen may be directly inserted into a protein-containing medium. Storage at 4° C for up to 5 days does not alter isolation rates from febrile patients, but testing should be done as early as possible (Chapter 226).

Both tissue cultures and embryonated chicken eggs are suitable for isolation, with the optimum system varying for the different influenza viruses. Virus is detected after a 3 day period of incubation in 85% to 90% of cases, although 7 to 10 days may be required. Methods for rapid detection of virus in respiratory epithelial cells or respiratory fluids can provide a specific diagnosis on the day of collection.

A rise in titer of antibody between acute and convalescent sera may be detected with several serologic procedures. The most readily available test is complement fixation; because this test generally uses nucleoprotein antigen, recall antibody rises may appear early. Hemagglutination inhibition, neutralizing antibody, and enzyme-linked immunosorbent tests are generally more sensitive but less available. Neuraminidase antibody may be determined by enzyme inhibition tests, and antibody to both hemagglutinin and neuraminidase may be detected in immunodiffusion tests.

TREATMENT

Nonspecific treatment designed to ameliorate distressing symptoms should be individualized. Bed rest, adequate fluid intake, and judicious use of acetaminophen in 0.6 g doses at 3 to 6 hour intervals are indicated for high fever, headache, and myalgias. Acetylsalicyclic acid is not recommended because of its association with Reye's syndrome after influenza. Significant nasal obstruction may be alleviated with 0.25% phenylephrine three to four times daily or 0.1% xylometazoline twice daily by nasal spray or drops. Significant cough may be relieved by guaifenesin syrup with dextromethorphan in doses of 5 to 10 ml every 3 to 4 hours.

Specific treatment is available for type A influenza. Amantadine hydrochloride in doses of 100 mg twice daily hastens the disappearance of fever and symptoms, but, to be effective in uncomplicated influenza, it must be started within the first 48 hours of illness. When type A influenza is known to be the cause of disease in a community, amantadine is recommended for all persons with a chronic underlying disease who have acute influenza and for healthy persons with clinically severe influenza. Central nervous system side-effects, such as drowsiness, dizziness, nervousness, and insomnia occur in 5% to 7% of healthy persons. Such symptoms are not generally apparent in acutely ill persons. Because of renal excretion of the drug, caution must be used in persons with compromised renal function, and reductions in dosage are indicated. Schedules for dosages based on level of renal function are available. Because of the general reduction in renal function among elderly persons, therapy with only 100 mg per day is recommended for persons 65 years and older. Caution must be exercised in medicating persons with central nervous system disease and in those receiving drugs with central nervous system activity.

Persons presumed to have primary influenzal pneumonia or mixed influenza and bacterial pneumonia should also receive amantadine, in the doses indicated, although the benefit is uncertain. Patients with mixed viral-bacterial pneumonia and bacterial pneumonia after influenza should receive appropriate antibiotics (Chapter 224).

Rimantadine, an analog of amantadine, has a similar mechanism of action and spectrum of activity to those of amantadine but is not yet approved for use. Because of slower absorption, it may require a loading dose for comparable activity but is otherwise recommended at dosages similar to those for amantadine.

Because of emergence of viral isolates resistant to amantadine and rimantadine among treated patients, some concern has been expressed about use of these drugs for treatment. However, all practical and theoretical concerns for this circumstance have been discounted except for the circumstance of treatment of an otherwise healthy person where there is an unhealthy or elderly person in the same household who might acquire influenza from that person and need treatment. A single question by the prescribing physician can prevent this use of drug. Alternatively, it has been suggested that a shorter duration of treatment than the usual 5 days may reduce emergence of resistant virus without loss of clinical benefit.

Ribavirin, a nucleoside analog, is approved for small-particle aerosol treatment of severe respiratory syncytial virus infections in infants. It has also been shown to be effective for treatment of uncomplicated type A and B influenza in healthy adults, and results of treatment of severe disease are encouraging. It is not yet approved for treatment of acute influenza.

PREVENTION

Vaccines

Inactivated influenza virus vaccines are prepared as follows: Virus is grown in embryonated chicken eggs, inactivated by formalin, and partially purified to remove adventitial egg material. The resulting virus is either left intact (whole virus vaccine) or disrupted and sometimes further purified (split product and subunit vaccines). The formulation is determined by immunization advisory committees of the World Health Organization and the Centers for Disease Control in Atlanta. Currently circulating types A and B viruses are included annually, with selection of particular variants based on antigenic novelty and recent epidemiologic experience. Because of the persistence of H3N2 viruses since the appearance of H1N1 virus in 1977, recent vaccines have contained H3N2, H1N1, and B variants. The dosage is standardized for hemagglutinin content.

Protection against influenza among persons given influenza virus vaccine generally varies between 50% and 90%. The degree of protection has varied with the potency of the vaccine, the extent of influenza activity, and the degree of antigenic relationship of the vaccine virus to the challenge virus. For most years, the vaccine may be assumed to convey about 70% protection against illness caused by influenza virus infection.

Annual vaccination is recommended for persons with a chronic underlying disease that increases the likelihood that they will have pneumonia and die of influenza. These diseases include cardiovascular and pulmonary disease, renal disease, metabolic disease, severe anemia, and diseases with compromised immune function. In the United States a priority list has recently been established (see the box below).

Vaccine is given by intramuscular injection, and any of the different types may be used in adults, but split product only is recommended for those 6 months to 12 years of age. Persons with previous exposure to the vaccine components need be given only one dose, whereas those without previous exposure to one of the components should be given two doses of that component 1 month apart. Two doses of the 1992 formulation are recommended for persons less than 9 years of age who are receiving influenza vaccine for the first time.

Current vaccines have minimum side-effects. Persons with allergy to eggs or egg products should not be given vaccine. In the past some pain, redness, or swelling at the vaccination site was reported by about 10% of adults in the 48 hours after vaccination, and systemic symptoms in about 2%. Such reactions were usually mild, but moderately severe local and systemic reactions occurred. More recent reports of U.S. vaccines indicate still fewer reactions; among elderly populations there is little to no detectable reactogenicity. During the 1976 national immunization program for swine influenza in the United States, an increase in the incidence of the Guillain-Barré syndrome was noted in the 8 week period after vaccination. The risk that the syndrome would develop was about 1 in 100,000 vaccinations and increased with increasing age. However, 3 subsequent years of vaccine monitoring did not reveal a similar increased risk and no increased risk was noted in the military vaccine program. Thus the basis of the association of Guillain-Barré syndrome with swine influenza immunization is uncertain,

Influenza virus vaccine

Recommended for
- Patients with compromised heart or lung function
- Residents of nursing homes
- Persons with extensive "high-risk" contacts, including household members
- Those over age 65
- Chronic metabolic disease, kidney disease, anemia, and immunosuppression requiring regular care
- Children and teenagers on long-term aspirin therapy

May be used for
- Persons rendering essential community services
- Any person wishing to prevent influenza

but it does not appear to be a complication attributable to all influenza vaccines.

Chemoprophylaxis

Amantadine, if given before exposure, prevents about 50% of type A influenza virus infections and about 70% of illnesses. It is not effective for type B influenza. It is recommended for the same persons for whom vaccine is recommended if they are unvaccinated or were vaccinated with a variant unrelated to the epidemic virus. The drug should be given in a dosage of 100 mg twice daily, starting administration at the beginning of a type A epidemic and continuing until the epidemic ceases, generally for 4 to 6 weeks. Data suggest that 100 mg daily may produce blood levels among elderly persons comparable with those seen among healthy young adults receiving 200 mg daily. Persons 65 years and older should be given 100 mg daily; side-effects should be less of a problem among elderly persons at this lower dosage, yet effectiveness should remain high.

An alternative use for amantadine is to provide prophylaxis against epidemic type A disease during the early phase of an epidemic while an antibody response to vaccine given at the beginning of the epidemic develops. For this purpose, a 14 day course is recommended.

Amantadine may also be used for influenza A outbreak control in nursing homes. When used in this way, it should be administered to all residents regardless of whether they have received vaccine for the duration of the community epidemic. Dosage is 200 mg daily for young persons and 100 mg daily for elderly persons; reductions in these dosages may be needed, depending on renal function.

Nausea, headache, and central nervous system side-effects (see Treatment), which may occur with amantadine therapy, are usually mild and begin within the first 48 hours of drug use. They may disappear with continued drug usage and cease on withdrawal of the drug. Severe central nervous system side-effects, including seizures and hallucinations, may occur with high blood levels in patients with reduced renal function.

REFERENCES

Barker WH and Mullooly JP: Pneumonia and influenza deaths during epidemics: implications for prevention. Arch Intern Med 142:85, 1982.

Beare AS: Basic and applied influenza research. Boca Raton, FL: CRC Press, 1982.

Couch RB and Kasel JA: Immunity to influenza in man. Annu Rev Microbiol 37:529, 1983.

Couch RB et al: Influenza: its control in persons and populations. J Infect Dis 153:431, 1986.

Glezen WP: Serious morbidity and mortality associated with influenza epidemics. Epidemiol Rev 4:25, 1982.

Glezen WP and Couch RB: Interpandemic influenza in the Houston area, 1974-76. N Engl J Med 298:587, 1978.

Hayden FC and Couch RB: Clinical and epidemiological importance of influenza A viruses resistant to amantadine and rimantadine. Rev Med Virol 2:89, 1992.

Nichol KL et al: Achieving the national health objective for influenza immunization: success of an institution-wide vaccination program. Am J Med 89:156, 1990.

Shaw MW, Arden NH, and Maassab HF: New aspects of influenza viruses. Clin Microbiol Rev 5:74, 1992.

Stuart-Harris CH, Schild GC, and Oxford JS: Influenza: the viruses and the diseases, ed 2. Baltimore, 1985, Arnold.

CHAPTER

246 Paramyxovirus (Measles, Parainfluenza, Mumps, and Respiratory Syncytial Virus), Rubella Virus, and Coronavirus Infections

Frederick G. Hayden
Gregory F. Hayden

PARAMYXOVIRUS INFECTIONS

Classification

The paramyxoviridae family is a group of medium-sized (150 to 300 nm) pleomorphic ribonucleic acid (RNA) viruses that include several important human (Table 246-1) and veterinary pathogens. Their common characteristics include a helical nucleocapsid that contains a linear, single-stranded RNA; a lipid-containing envelope; cytoplasmic replication; and, unlike influenza viruses, antigenic stability without recognized genetic recombination. One glycoprotein (HN) on the surface of paramyxoviruses has hemagglutinin and sometimes neuraminidase activity and is responsible for adsorption of virus to host cell receptors. Another protein (F), which has hemolyzing and membrane-fusing activity, is responsible for viral penetration into cells and the formation of multinucleated giant cells, a major cytopathic effect of paramyxoviruses.

The family is subdivided into three genera: (1) The paramyxovirus genus includes parainfluenza viruses types 1 to 4, mumps virus, and Newcastle disease virus, which causes respiratory tract disease in chickens and may accidentally infect humans. These viruses have both hemagglutinin and neuraminidase activities. (2) Measles virus has a hemagglutinin but no neuraminidase and is grouped in the morbillivirus genus. (3) Respiratory syncytial virus has neither hemagglutinin nor neuraminidase and is classified in the pneumovirus genus. There is no antigen common to all paramyxoviruses, but considerable cross reactivity in complement fixation or neutralization tests is present in members of the paramyxovirus genus. Recently an unusual form of severe hepatitis characterized histologically by giant multinucleated syncytial hepatocytes has been linked to a paramyxoviral infection of undefined type.

Table 246-1. Human paramyxoviridae

Virus	Types	Clinical syndromes	Virus detection: Specimen	Virus detection: Method	Serologic tests	Vaccine
Parainfluenza	1-4	Colds Pharyngitis Croup Bronchitis Bronchiolitis Pneumonia	Nasal aspirate/wash, throat/NP swabs, sputum	VI, IF, EIA	NT, CF, HAI, ELISA	No
Mumps	1	Parotitis Orchitis Oophoritis Pancreatis Aseptic meningitis Encephalitis Arthritis	Saliva, urine, CSF	VI	CF, NT, HAI, IF, ELISA	Live virus
Measles	1	Typical measles Modified measles Atypical measles Pneumonia Encephalitis	Throat/NP swabs, urine, blood	VI, IF	CF, HAI, NT, ELISA	Live virus
Respiratory syncytial	1 (2 subgroups)	Colds Bronchitis Bronchiolitis Pneumonia	Nasal aspirate/wash, sputum, NP/throat swabs	VI, IF, EIA	CF, NT, ELISA	No

PARAINFLUENZA VIRUSES

Characteristics

The human parainfluenza viruses are separated into types 1 to 4 and type 4 into subtypes A and B on the basis of antigenicity. These serotypes differ in their epidemiologic characteristics and patterns of clinical illness.

Parainfluenza viruses 1 to 3 can often be isolated within 3 days and usually within 10 days after inoculation from specimens taken from infants and children. Isolation of type 4 virus or virus from specimens during reinfections, as in adults, may require 2 to 3 weeks. Viral presence is usually detected by hemadsorption of guinea pig erythrocytes and confirmed by immunoassays.

Epidemiology

Parainfluenza viruses have a worldwide distribution and infect most persons initially during childhood. They are the most commonly identified cause of acute laryngotracheobronchitis (croup) in children and are second only to respiratory syncytial virus as a cause of lower respiratory tract disease causing hospitalization of infants. Parainfluenza virus infection is documented in 31% to 42% of croup, 7% to 17% of pneumonia, and 7% to 18% of bronchiolitis cases in children. The incidence of croup and other lower respiratory tract disease produced by parainfluenza virus type 1 or 2 infection is highest between 4 months and 4 to 6 years. Parainfluenza virus type 3 can cause bronchiolitis or pneumonia in very young infants despite the presence of maternal antibody. Reinfections with parainfluenza viruses are common, are rarely severe, and account for nearly all the parainfluenza viral illness of adults. In children, reinfections with the same serotype have occurred within months.

Parainfluenza types 1 and 2 typically cause epidemics lasting up to several months during alternate years in the fall. Overlapping outbreaks involving both types 1 and 2 may occur. Parainfluenza type 3 causes sporadic infection throughout the year but also epidemics in spring and summer months. Transmission of parainfluenza viruses occurs within families, and outbreaks with high attack rates have occurred in closed populations, such as nurseries, day care centers, and hospitals.

The virus is transmitted from person to person in infected respiratory secretions by direct contact or by large droplets. The incubation period ranges from 2 to 8 days. The duration of viral shedding is 3 to 10 days, although persistent shedding of parainfluenza types 1 and 3 for months has been reported.

Pathogenesis

Although dissemination of infection has been reported rarely, the principal features of parainfluenza virus infection are replication and cytolytic change in the respiratory tract mucosa. The virus can be localized to ciliated columnar epithelial cells. Viral shedding tends to reflect the severity of illness. Severe giant cell pneumonia has developed in patients who have deficits in cell-mediated immune function.

Levels of serum neutralizing antibody correlate partially with protection against infection and illness, but immunity is more closely associated with neutralizing antibody levels in the respiratory tract secretions. The nasopharyngeal secretion concentrations of parainfluenza virus–specific IgE and of histamine are higher in patients with croup or wheezing than in those with upper respiratory illness alone.

Clinical features

Initial infections with parainfluenza virus types 1 to 3 commonly cause febrile rhinitis, pharyngitis, laryngitis, and/or bronchitis. Up to 30% of children with primary infections have evidence of lower respiratory disease. Fatal laryngeal obstruction has occurred. The principal severe form of illness in type 1 and 2 infection is croup, manifested by inspiratory stridor, barking cough, and hoarseness caused by subglottic edema. Bacterial suprainfections are rare in croup but may complicate other respiratory tract infections produced by parainfluenza viruses. Type 3 infection causes croup, bronchiolitis, or pneumonia. Type 4 infections are mild and are infrequently recognized.

Reinfection with parainfluenza virus is frequently asymptomatic, but it may be associated with lower respiratory disease in children. Symptomatic infections in adults are manifested as common colds, usually without fever, pharyngitis, tracheobronchitis, influenza-like illness, exacerbations of chronic bronchitis and rarely pneumonia. Parainfluenza virus has been associated with parotitis and has been isolated from patients with Guillain-Barré syndrome, aseptic meningitis, and acute renal transplant rejection.

Diagnosis

Throat and nasopharyngeal swabs or nasal washings contain the virus at the onset of symptoms. The duration of viral shedding averages 8 days, but it decreases significantly in reinfections. Immunofluorescence of respiratory tract cells has been used successfully for rapid diagnosis of parainfluenza virus infection.

Antibodies to parainfluenza viruses can be measured by a variety of serologic techniques (Table 246-1). A fourfold or greater titer rise constitutes evidence of infection, but a serotype-specific diagnosis cannot be reliably made because of the common occurrence of heterotypic antibody responses. Complement fixation or hemagglutination inhibition antibodies increase in only one half of adults infected with type 1 or type 3 virus. A combination of virus isolation and serologic testing provides the most sensitive means of deleting infection.

Treatment

Supportive care and close monitoring are indicated in patients with severe lower respiratory involvement. Management of croup typically consists of mist therapy and supplemental oxygen as indicated. Racemic epinephrine nebulization is commonly used in hospitalized patients under close observation. Short-term, high-dose systemic corticosteroids appear beneficial and may reduce the need for intubation. Aerosolized ribavirin has been used in immunodeficient children with severe parainfluenza virus infection.

MUMPS VIRUS

Characteristics

Only one serotype of mumps virus is known to exist, although antigenic differences between strains have been detected by monoclonal antibodies. The soluble (S) antigen derived from the nucleocapsid and the viral (V) antigen associated with the envelope elicit complement-fixing antibodies detectable early and late after infection, respectively. Mumps virus can be propagated in embryonated eggs and a variety of cell cultures, including monkey kidney, human embryonic kidney, or HeLa cells, and can be detected by cytopathic effects and hemadsorption of guinea pig red blood cells.

Epidemiology

Mumps virus is endemic worldwide and humans are the only known natural host. Before wide-scale immunization, mumps was primarily a disease of childhood with 90% of the cases occurring in those less than 14 years. Since the introduction of the live attenuated vaccine, the annual reported incidence of mumps has decreased over 95% in the United States. However, a relative resurgence of mumps related to failure to vaccinate and vaccine failure has been recognized since 1986. Nearly 40% of cases have been reported in those 15 years and older. Serum neutralizing antibody testing indicates that 10% to 20% of adults are susceptible. Outbreaks, some involving highly immunized populations, have occurred among groups of high school and college students, in work settings including hospitals, and in other closed populations such as those in military barracks or prisons. The disease occurs throughout the year, with a peak incidence in late winter to early spring in temperate climates.

Mumps virus is transmitted in infected saliva or respiratory secretions by direct contact or droplets that enter the upper respiratory tract. More intimate contact is needed than for transmission of measles or varicella. The infection rates in outbreaks involving susceptible, closed populations have been as high as 80%. The period of peak communicability extends from several days before to several days after the onset of parotitis, but virus has been isolated as long as 7 days before and 9 days after the appearance of parotitis. Virus can be present in saliva in cases of inapparent infection or in those without parotitis, and these persons may be contagious. The incubation period averages 14 to 18 days, with a range of 7 to 25 days. Natural mumps infection is thought to confer lifelong immunity. The frequency and manifestations of reinfection are uncertain.

Pathophysiology

After primary infection, the virus is thought to proliferate in the upper respiratory tract epithelium and regional lymph nodes during the incubation period. Viremic dissemination then leads to secondary localization in glandular and neural tissue and to subsequent clinical disease. Infection has been produced experimentally by direct instillation of the virus into the parotid (Stensen's) duct.

The infected salivary glands show a diffuse interstitial edema, with a serofibrinous exudate containing mononuclear cells. The ductal epithelium shows degenerative changes, but the glandular cells are relatively spared. Involved pancreas or testes show similar changes with more hemorrhage and polymorphonuclear cell infiltration. Local areas of infarction may develop because of vascular compromise, and atrophy of the germinal epithelium with hyalinization and fibrosis can ensue.

In mumps encephalitis the brain may show widespread neurolysis typical of a primary viral encephalitis or changes consistent with a postinfectious encephalitis (i.e., perivenous demyelination, perivascular mononuclear cuffing, and an increase in microglial cells, with relative sparing of neurons). Virus-specific cytotoxic T lymphocytes have been demonstrated in peripheral blood and cerebrospinal fluid of children recovering from mumps meningitis. Unlike in other paramyxovirus infections, severe illness is not recognized in immunosuppressed patients.

Clinical features

Mumps virus causes an acute, generalized infection in susceptible hosts, with characteristic involvement of the salivary glands and other organ systems. Approximately a third of infections are asymptomatic. The prodromal symptoms are nonspecific and include fever, anorexia, malaise, and headache. The higher frequency of complications in postpubertal persons is important with respect to the recent increase in mumps cases in older age groups.

Sialitis. Most patients with clinical mumps have parotitis. Other salivary glands can be affected in 10% of cases, but they are rarely affected alone. Parotid involvement usually begins with complaints of earache or jaw tenderness on mastication. Pain worsens over a 2 to 3 day period, as the gland reaches maximum size, and is exacerbated by sour stimuli, such as citrus fruit.

Parotid involvement is bilateral in three fourths of patients. Swelling in one gland usually precedes that in the other by 1 to 5 days. It occurs at the angle of the jaw, with eventual obliteration of the angle. The lower portion of the ear is lifted up and out, increasing the angle between the earlobe and the side of the neck. Neck asymmetry is particularly obvious when viewed from behind, and a bull-neck appearance may be seen. The gland feels doughy and edematous, with indistinct borders. The orifices of Stensen's ducts may be red and swollen, with petechial hemorrhages. Pus cannot be expelled from the affected ducts; this characteristic helps to distinguish this disease from bacterial sialitis. In the presence of submandibular gland involvement, the distinction between mumps and cervical adenitis may be difficult. Although uncommon, sublingual gland involvement is usually bilateral and causes submental swelling, which also can involve the floor of the mouth and the tongue. Presternal edema has been described, possibly secondary to obstruction of cervical lymphatic drainage. During the first 3 days of illness, the temperature may range from normal to 104° F (40° C). Defervescence and resolution of parotid tenderness and swelling occur within 1 week. Late complications of parotitis (sialectasia and recurrent sialadenitis) are rare.

Orchitis-epididymitis and oophoritis. Mumps orchitis is rare before adolescence but occurs in 20% to 30% of postpubertal males and is bilateral in a fourth of the patients. Epididymitis precedes or accompanies orchitis in 85% of cases. Orchitis usually occurs 1 to 2 weeks after the onset of parotitis, but it may precede or occur without parotitis. Symptoms begin abruptly, with fever, nausea, vomiting, and headache, followed by testicular swelling and tenderness. The testicle may enlarge to three or four times normal size. Pain and swelling diminish in conjunction with defervescence, usually by 7 to 10 days. Some degree of atrophy develops in approximately 50% of affected testicles. Although abnormalities in sperm count follow mumps orchitis, sterility is a rare sequela, and impotence is not a recognized complication. An increased risk of testicular neoplasia after mumps orchitis has been debated.

Oophoritis is reported to occur in 5% of postpubertal females. Involvement of the right ovary can mimic appendicitis. Infertility or premature menopause after mumps oophoritis has been reported rarely.

Central nervous system. Asymptomatic cerebrospinal fluid (CSF) pleocytosis can be found in up to a half of patients with mumps. Clinical meningitis accompanies mumps parotitis in up to 15% of patients, more frequently in males than in females. Meningeal symptoms develop between 1 week before and 2 weeks after parotitis, but up to half of the cases occur in the absence of parotitis.

The clinical manifestations are typical of viral meningitis (Chapter 233). Lymphocytic pleocytosis, with less than 500 cells per cubic millimeter, is usual, but CSF white counts may increase to over 2000 per cubic millimeter. Up to a fourth of patients have an initial polymorphonuclear predominance. Glucose level is usually normal, but hypoglycorrhachia occurs in 6% to 30% of patients. Protein concentration is normal to slightly elevated. Clinical and laboratory abnormalities usually return to normal in 7 to 10 days. Sequelae of mumps meningitis are rare.

Encephalitis is estimated to occur in 1 in 400 to 6000 cases. Manifestations usually develop 7 to 10 days after parotitis and include high fever, alterations in the sensorium, seizures, focal neurologic signs, ataxia, movement disorders, and rarely cortical blindness. Although recovery is usually complete, death occurs in approximately 1% and is more likely in adults, and sequelae of psychomotor retardation, seizures, and aqueductal stenosis with hydrocephalus have been reported. Other neurologic syndromes associated with mumps include cerebellar ataxia, facial palsy, polyradiculitis, transverse myelitis, and cranial neuropathies.

Other complications. Acute pancreatitis, manifested by nausea, vomiting, deep epigastric pain, fever, and chills, occurs in approximately 5% of patients. Recovery usually occurs over 5 to 7 days but in severe cases may take several weeks (Chapter 67).

Electrocardiographic abnormalities, including altered

atrioventricular conduction, depressed S-T segment, and inverted T waves, occur in 4% to 15% of adults with mumps, but symptomatic myocarditis is rare. Sudden infant death and fatalities caused by heart failure have occurred.

Arthritis following mumps occurs in less than 1% of patients. Adult males are most commonly affected, and in about three fourths of the cases arthritis follows parotitis by 1 to 3 weeks. It can occur before or in the absence of parotitis. Although it is usually a nondeforming, migratory polyarthritis involving large joints, arthralgia and monoarticular arthritis have also been described. Arthritis is commonly accompanied by fever, leukocytosis, and elevated erythrocyte sedimentation rate, as well as by other, visceral complications (orchitis, pancreatitis). Resolution usually occurs within 1 month.

Transient high-frequency hearing loss occurs in less than 5% of patients. Complete, permanent hearing loss occurs in approximately 1 in 20,000 patients with mumps and is occasionally associated with vestibular dysfunction. The hearing loss is unilateral in three fourths of patients. Onset is usually sudden, with vertigo, tinnitus, nausea, and vomiting, followed by permanent deafness. The cause is likely either acoustic neuritis or an endolymphatic labyrinthitis.

Mumps in pregnant women is generally no more severe than in nonpregnant females. Transplacental infection can occur, but no increase in the incidence of congenital malformation following maternal infection is proven. An increase in fetal mortality rate and possibly an increased frequency of low birth weight may follow maternal mumps infection during the first trimester.

Mumps virus has been implicated as a cause of juvenile-onset diabetes mellitus. Many reports document the onset of diabetes from 10 days to 5 weeks after clinical mumps. A similar 7-year periodicity of mumps and diabetes with a period of 3 to 4 years between peaks has been found in epidemiologic studies. Other reported complications of mumps virus infection include ocular disease (conjunctivitis, iritis, retinitis, uveitis, optic neuritis), hemolysis, thrombocytopenia, thyroiditis, prostatitis, nephritis, splenic rupture, and neonatal pneumonia.

Diagnosis

The peripheral white blood cell count is variable, but relative lymphocytosis is common. In the presence of orchitis or meningitis, the white count may exceed 20,000 per cubic millimeter with a polymorphonuclear predominance. The level of serum amylase, principally the salivary isoenzyme, is elevated in 90% of patients with parotitis. A normal serum lipase level may be helpful in differentiating the high amylase level from that seen in pancreatitis. The levels of salivary and pancreatic amylase isoenzymes may not correlate well with the clinical diagnosis of mumps pancreatitis. Transient hematuria and decreased urine concentrating ability and creatinine clearance are common during the course of mumps.

Saliva, urine, and, in the cases of central nervous system disease, CSF all contain virus. Virus is usually present in saliva for 4 to 5 days after the onset of parotitis. It is usually present in urine during the first 5 days and occasionally up to 2 weeks. Cerebrospinal fluid culture results may be positive during the first 6 days of illness.

Serologic tests are useful in diagnosis and determination of immune status. S antigen complement-fixation antibody titer levels rise in the first week of illness and disappear over several months. V antigen complement-fixation antibody titer levels rise 1 to 2 weeks later and persist at low levels for years. A fourfold rise in convalescent titer level is diagnostic. An acute phase serum that contains an elevated anti-S titer level and a low anti-V titer level is presumptive evidence of acute mumps infection. Detection of mumps-specific IgM by ELISA or immunofluorescence assay is a sensitive and specific means of establishing the diagnosis with a single serum specimen. Measurement of virus-specific IgG by ELISA has been found to be more sensitive than conventional assays for assessment of immune status. Skin testing is not reliable for the diagnosis or assessment of immune status and may provoke an antibody rise that can obscure the serologic diagnosis.

Treatment

Specific therapy is not available for mumps virus infection, and treatment remains symptomatic. Treatment of mumps orchitis has included scrotal elevation or support, ice packs, and anti-inflammatory agents. Glucocorticoids, diethylstilbestrol, anesthetic block of the spermatic cord, and incision of the tunica albuginea have not been proved beneficial.

Prevention

A live attenuated mumps vaccine prepared in chick embryo cell culture has been available in the United States since 1968 and is 75% to 95% effective in the prevention of mumps. Immunization can be given any time after 1 year of age and is usually given at 15 months in combination with measles and rubella vaccination. Mumps vaccine should be given to all susceptible persons, unless contraindicated by documented anaphylactic reaction to egg proteins or to neomycin, immunodeficiency states, or pregnancy. In particular, susceptible adults should be immunized because of the increased risk of mumps-associated complications. Previous infection or immunization does not increase the risk of vaccine reactions. Immunization may be ineffective if given within 3 months of blood transfusions or treatment with immunoglobulin for any reason.

Complications following vaccination are rare. Parotitis, rash, pruritus, febrile seizures, unilateral deafness, and meningoencephalitis with virus recovery from CSF have been reported in the 30 days following vaccination.

Postexposure administration of mumps immune globulin is of doubtful value in preventing mumps, although its use has been reported to decrease the risk of orchitis in men with mumps. The globulin is not licensed or available in the United States. Immune serum globulin is not recommended for postexposure prophylaxis. Postexposure administration of mumps vaccine may not be protective, but there is no contraindication to its administration.

Patients with mumps should be considered to be infectious until parotid swelling has subsided.

MEASLES VIRUS

Characteristics

Wild measles virus is pathogenic only for humans and certain old world primates. Only one strain of wild measles virus is recognized. Virus isolation from clinical specimens can be performed in several types of cell culture (human embryonic kidney, primary monkey kidney). The characteristic cytopathic effects of multinucleated giant-cell formation usually develop in 5 to 10 days. Spin amplification in A549 cells followed by immunofluorescence assay can reduce the detection time to 1 to 2 days.

Epidemiology

In the prevaccine era, measles caused epidemics of 3 to 4 months' duration every 2 to 5 years, especially in populous areas. In the United States 90% of reported cases occurred in those less than 10 years old. Vaccine use has been associated with over 95% decrease in the incidence of measles and a marked change in the age distribution of cases. The recent upsurge in measles incidence in the United States has been related to outbreaks in unimmunized preschool children, but persons aged 15 years and older, particularly high school college students with prior immunization, have accounted for 30% or more of cases. Maternal antibody usually protects infants for at least 6 months. Infection confers lifelong protection against repeated measles, although asymptomatic reinfections can occur and may contribute to the persistence of antibody.

Measles is highly communicable and can spread despite high levels of herd immunity. Measles transmission occurs primarily in schools or households, although up to 4% of measles cases are nosocomially acquired. While immunization rates above 80% have been associated with protection against outbreaks in urban populations, rates over 95% have not prevented outbreaks in closed populations, such as schools. Airborne transmission without face-to-face contact has been implicated in outbreaks linked to physicians' waiting rooms and other medical settings.

Measles virus is transmitted to the respiratory tract or conjunctiva by airborne droplets or by direct contact with infectious secretions. The virus remains infectious in small-particle aerosols for several hours. Patients are most infectious during the late prodrome, when sneezing and coughing contribute to dissemination of infected respiratory secretions, but virus may be shed for several days after the onset of rash. Although virus is present in blood and urine, transmission by these sources is believed to be uncommon. The incubation period is usually 10 to 14 days but may last up to 3 weeks in adults.

Pathogenesis

Measles virus initially infects the respiratory epithelium. Viremia then leads to infection of reticuloendothelial cells. A secondary viremia corresponding to the prodromal stage of illness results in virus dissemination to the skin, respiratory tract, and other sites. Giant cells may be present in the tonsils, appendix, other lymphoid organs, and multiple sites in the respiratory tract. Leukopenia, particularly lymphocytopenia, may be secondary to direct infection and destruction of leukocytes.

Skin and mucous membrane lesions contain multinucleated giant cells and other markers of viral replication. The onset of the exanthem corresponds temporally to the appearance of specific immune responses. Cellular immunity plays a major role in viral clearance. Measles infection is associated with both immune activation and suppression, in part manifested by suppression of delayed hypersensitivity reactions and depressed natural killer cell activity for at least 3 weeks after rash onset. Skin rash develops in agammaglobulinemic patients with measles, whereas in patients with deficient cell-mediated immunity, progressive giant-cell pneumonia without rash may occur.

The histopathologic changes in involved organs include lymphoid hyperplasia, mononuclear cell exudates, and multinucleated giant cells with eosinophilic intranuclear and intracytoplasmic inclusions. Severe lower respiratory tract involvement is marked by destruction of ciliated respiratory epithelium, interstitial pneumonia, epithelial cell hyperplasia, and giant-cell formation.

Clinical features

Typical measles. The prodrome of measles lasts 2 to 4 days (range up to 8 days) and is characterized by fever up to 105° F (40.5° C), malaise, anorexia, cough, coryza, and conjunctivitis with photophobia and excess lacrimation. Koplik's spots, red-based lesions with central bluish gray specks, appear on the buccal or labial mucosa, typically opposite the second molars, toward the end of the prodromal period and last for several days. The enanthem may involve the soft or hard palate or may become hemorrhagic in more extensive cases. The skin eruption begins about the face and neck behind the ears as discrete erythematous macules, which proceed downward to cover the trunk and extremities, including the palms and soles. Lesions enlarge, become maculopapular, and often coalesce on the face, shoulders, and upper trunk. In adults, gastrointestinal (abdominal pain, vomiting, diarrhea) and musculoskeletal complaints are common. The eruption clears after 5 to 6 days in its order of appearance, often with brownish discoloration and fine desquamation. Defervescence and symptomatic improvement usually occur several days after the appearance of the rash, but cough may persist.

Modified measles. The administration of immune serum globulin after measles exposure may alter the course by prolonging the incubation period, shortening the prodrome, and ameliorating the clinical manifestations, including conjunctivitis, Koplik's spots, and rash.

Atypical measles. In adults who received the inactivated measles vaccine between 1963 and 1968, an unusual, often severe constellation of clinical manifestations may develop 1 to 2 weeks after exposure to wild virus. This syndrome has also occurred after sequential killed live virus immunizations or, rarely, after live vaccine alone. The illness begins abruptly with fever, headache, myalgia, vomiting, abdominal pain, and nonproductive cough. Dyspnea, coryza, sore throat, and pleuritic pain are common. After 3 to 4 days, an erythematous maculopapular rash (Plate V-45) begins on the distal extremities and spreads proximally for 3 to 5 days. Vesicles singly or in crops, petechiae (Plate V-46), purpura, and/or urticarial lesions can develop, along with peripheral edema. Because of the polymorphous nature of the eruption, atypical measles may be mistaken for varicella, scarlet fever, meningococcemia, or Rocky Mountain spotted fever. The face is often spared, Koplik's spots are absent, but conjunctivitis and glossitis with strawberry tongue (Plate V-47) may occur. Pneumonia occurs in most cases, and chest radiograph changes include patchy, diffuse, or dense lobar infiltrates; pleural effusion; and hilar adenopathy. Leukocyte counts are low to normal, but left shift, eosinophilia, increased transaminase levels, coagulopathy and elevated erythrocyte sedimentation rate are common. The fever and other symptoms resolve in 1 to 3 weeks. The course is self-limited, although acute respiratory failure has been described. Residual nodular pulmonary infiltrates may persist for years.

Serologic studies show low or absent initial measles antibody titers, with high titers in convalescent samples. Measles virus has been isolated rarely from these patients. This syndrome is probably the result of an altered immune response to wild measles virus exposure in a previously sensitized host. Skin biopsy specimens demonstrate small vessel vasculitis with a mixed cellular infiltrate. Failure to develop antibody to the measles hemolysin (F protein) after administration of killed vaccine has occurred. Recurrences have not been documented.

Complications

Immunologic status, nutrition, age, race, and availability of medical services influence the outcome of infection. The mortality rate of measles in developed areas with good medical services is usually 0.03% to 0.1% but is 10- to 100-fold higher in the developing world. Morbidity rate is highest in the very young, adults, one third of whom are hospitalized, and those with underlying immunodeficiency or malnutrition. Most deaths follow respiratory tract and/or neurologic complications. Fatalities occur in about one half of those with underlying malignancy or HIV infection, in whom rash is not apparent in up to 40% on presentation.

Respiratory tract. Lower respiratory tract complications develop in 4% to 50% of patients. Direct viral infection of the respiratory tract is manifested as bronchitis, pneumonia, and, in children, croup or bronchiolitis. In young adults, a multilobar reticulonodular infiltrate is the most common radiographic finding, and pleural effusion or lobar consolidation is uncommon. In immunocompromised hosts and, rarely, in normal persons, measles can cause fatal giant cell pneumonia with or without rash. Secondary bacterial pneumonia is commonly associated with measles pneumonia, and acute sinusitis and serous or suppurative otitis media often follow measles.

Central nervous system. Electroencephalograph abnormalities with slowing occur transiently in over half of patients with uncomplicated measles. Lymphocyte pleocytosis occurs in about one third of ordinary measles cases. Acute encephalitis, manifested by fever, headache, seizures, altered sensorium, and sometimes focal signs, occurs in 1 in 1000 to 2000 patients. Onset is usually 4 to 7 days after the appearance of the exanthem, but it may precede the rash by 10 days. Cerebrospinal fluid findings include mild elevations in protein level and lymphocytic pleocytosis. Although virus has been demonstrated rarely in the brain of patients who died, in most cases the pathologic changes of demyelination, gliosis, and mononuclear cell infiltrate suggest an immune-mediated, postinfectious encephalomyelitis. Cell-mediated immune responses to myelin basic protein are present in about one half of patients. Death occurs in about 10% of affected persons. The sequelae include behavioral and intellectual changes, seizures, and motor deficits. A fatal inclusion-body encephalitis related to persistent measles virus infection may develop 1 to 6 months after initial exposure in immunocompromised hosts. The CSF may be normal and serologic studies nondiagnostic. Subacute sclerosing panencephalitis is a rare, late complication of measles infection.

Other clinical presentations. Viral mesenteric adenitis or appendicitis can cause abdominal pain and signs of peritonitis. Such an occurrence during the prodromal stage may present a particularly confusing differential diagnostic problem. Mild viral keratitis occurs commonly and may progress to corneal ulceration in a small portion of cases. Blindness has been reported in 1% of those with ocular involvement. Icteric hepatitis occurs in up to 5% of adult cases and two- to threefold elevations of serum AST, LDH, and/or CPK values are common in adults with measles. Transient electrocardiographic changes occur in about 20% of patients, but clinical signs of cardiac disease are rare. Although not a recognized cause of congenital anomalies, measles infection during pregnancy has been associated with spontaneous abortion, premature delivery, and perinatal mortality. Tuberculin reactivity may be depressed for up to 4 weeks after infection. Measles may activate tuberculosis.

Laboratory diagnosis

Leukopenia is common during the prodrome and early eruptive stage of measles, and if it is pronounced (< 2000 cells/mm^3), is associated with a poor prognosis. The development of leukocytosis suggests bacterial superinfection or other complications. Measles virus may be isolated from the blood, urine, and throat or conjunctival secretions during the prodrome and up to several days after the exanthem appears. Virus isolation should be attempted in unusual circumstances, such as in encephalitis after measles vaccine and in encephalitis or pneumonia without rash in immunocompromised patients. Cytologic studies of respiratory and conjunctival secretions or urinary sediment may reveal multinucleated giant cells with characteristic intranuclear inclusions. Immunofluorescence staining of cells from these sites may demonstrate measles virus antigens.

Serologic studies of paired specimens constitute the most practical method of laboratory diagnosis of acute and atypical measles. Antibody appears rapidly, so that specimens collected within several days in the first week of rash may demonstrate seroconversion. Because of its technical simplicity and greater sensitivity than the complement-fixation test, the hemagglutination-inhibition method is commonly used for antibody measurement. Other assays (see Table 246-1) are reliable for serodiagnosis and determination of immune status. Detection of measles-specific immunoglobulin M (IgM) by enzyme-linked immunosorbent assay (ELISA) is a sensitive indicator of recent infection and can yield positive findings within 1 week of rash onset. For the diagnosis of subacute sclerosing panencephalitis, CSF antibody measurements should also be obtained.

Prevention

The live attenuated measles virus vaccine currently used in the United States is prepared in chick embryo cell culture. This vaccine provides durable immunity in at least 95% of recipients vaccinated at 15 months or older. Antibody titers elicited by immunization tend to decrease with time, and secondary vaccine failures occur. All school-aged children, including college and high school students, and health care workers should have documented immunity to measles (birth before 1957, physician-diagnosed measles, prior immunization with two doses of vaccine, or seropositivity). Combined measles-mumps-rubella (MMR) vaccine is preferred because mumps can also occur in highly vaccinated populations. A two dose schedule is now advocated for all children, with the first dose at age 15 months and the second at entrance to school. Immunization is indicated for asymptomatic human immunodeficiency virus– (HIV)-infected children and should be considered in symptomatic ones. Administration of monovalent measles vaccine at 6 to 12 months of age, followed by revaccination with MMR at 15 months, is indicated for children, including HIV-infected ones, at high risk of measles exposure. In such children the second vaccination may not elicit protective antibody levels, and a third dose on school entry is recommended. Persons whose initial vaccine may have been ineffective are also candidates for revaccination. This includes those who received inactivated measles vaccine (available 1963 to 1968), a close sequence of inactivated and live virus vaccines (3 months between injections), concurrent administration of immune serum globulin, vaccine before 12 months of age when maternal antibody may suppress an active response, and in general those whose immunization status cannot be documented. Most persons born before 1957 are likely to have been naturally infected.

The most common side-effects associated with measles vaccination are fever, rash, or both, occurring in 5% to 15% of recipients between 5 and 12 days after inoculation. Febrile convulsions, and, rarely, meningoencephalitis have also been described. Contraindications to live measles vaccine include pregnancy; primary or acquired immunodeficiency states; recent immunoglobulin therapy; anaphylactic reaction to egg ingestion or neomycin; and intercurrent febrile illness, which may increase the rate of primary vaccine failure. Revaccination of those who previously received inactivated vaccine is sometimes accompanied by fever, rash, and localized induration, erythema, and vesiculation at the injection site.

Postexposure prophylaxis of measles with passive immunization is indicated for susceptible persons who are at increased risk of complications, including pregnant women and immunocompromised patients. Immunoglobulin may prevent or modify measles if given within 6 days of exposure. The recommended dose of immunoglobulin is 0.25 ml/kg (0.5 ml/kg for immunocompromised individuals) to maximum of 15 ml. Exposed symptomatic HIV-infected patients should receive immunoglobulin regardless of vaccine status. In normal hosts, postexposure administration of vaccine usually prevents disease if administered within 3 days after exposure to natural measles. Hospitalized patients require respiratory isolation.

Treatment

Vitamin A administration may reduce morbidity and mortality in severe measles in children. Parenteral and/or aerosolized ribavirin and immunoglobulin have been used in immunocompromised patients with measles pneumonia.

RESPIRATORY SYNCYTIAL VIRUS

Characteristics

Two major subgroups (A and B) are distinguished principally by antigenic differences in the G surface glycoprotein, which mediates attachment to host cells. The importance of strain variation in clinical or immunologic responses is unresolved, but infections by subgroup A strains may be more severe. Natural infection occurs only in humans and chimpanzees. Respiratory syncytial virus (RSV) grows well in several human heteroploid cell lines (HEp 2, HeLa), in which it causes characteristic syncytia formation. On primary isolation, RSV can be detected after an average of 3 to 5 days.

Epidemiology

Respiratory syncytial virus has worldwide distribution. In temperate climates, it causes annual outbreaks up to 6 months in the late fall, winter, and spring months. Most children have specific serum antibody by 4 years of age, but reinfections in children and adults are common. Strains of both subgroups of RSV appear to cocirculate during epidemic periods but in varying proportions.

Respiratory syncytial virus is the major cause of lower respiratory tract illness in infants and young children. It accounts for 60% to 90% of bronchiolitis and up to 40% of pneumonia cases in this age group. Most severe infections occur in infants less than 6 months old, although high levels of maternal RSV antibody may be associated with protection against lower respiratory tract disease. Other risk factors for lower respiratory tract disease include male gender, lack of breast feeding, crowding, lower socioeconomic status, day care attendance, and parental smoking. RSV activity correlates with winter peaks in respiratory deaths of infants less than 1 year of age. Secondary infection in family contacts of an index case are common. RSV is a major nosocomial pathogen, and high attack rates occur in patients and staff during outbreaks in hospitals, day care centers, and geriatric units. Nosocomial outbreaks of RSV infection have involved up to one half of hospital staff and patients. The average incubation period is 5 days, with a range of 2 to 8 days. RSV transmission requires close contact, with spread either by large-particle aerosols or by contamination of hands with infectious secretions and inoculation into the eye or nose.

Pathogenesis

Respiratory syncytial virus primarily infects the respiratory tract, and cell-to-cell spread of the virus may lead to involvement of the entire length of the respiratory mucosa. Lymphocytic peribronchiolar inflammation and later necrosis and proliferation of the bronchiolar epithelium contribute to small airway obstruction in RSV bronchiolitis. Air trapping with hyperinflation or atelectatic collapse results. Eosinophilic cytoplasmic inclusions in epithelial cells and multinucleated giant cells, severe fibrosis, and hyaline membrane formation may occur in fatal RSV pneumonia. The possibility that immunologic mechanisms may contribute to disease pathogenesis in infants is unresolved. Increased nasopharyngeal secretion titer levels of RSV-specific IgE and histamine correlate with the occurrence of wheezing and the degree of hypoxia in infected infants.

Naturally acquired immunity to RSV is incomplete and of short duration, but the severity of the illness decreases with reinfections. Local antibody concentration correlates better with protection from illness than does serum antibody level. The role of cell-mediated immunity in recovery from infection is unresolved, but severe infections may occur in immunocompromised children and adults.

Clinical features

The majority of infections in both children and adults are symptomatic. In infants and young children, upper respiratory illness accompanied by fever and otitis media is common. Lower respiratory tract involvement is manifested as pneumonia, bronchiolitis, tracheobronchitis, or, less often, croup. Bronchiolitis in infancy has been associated with an increased risk of subsequent recurrent wheezing, and lower respiratory RSV disease early in life may be followed by chronic alterations in pulmonary function. Infants with congenital heart disease or prematurity-associated lung disease and immunocompromised hosts of any age are at risk for severe infection. RSV infection has been associated with apneic spells, particularly in premature infants, and with sudden infant death syndrome.

The most common syndrome observed in adults is upper respiratory illness with coryza and cough, often accompanied by low-grade fever. The illness tends to be more severe and prolonged than rhinovirus colds. Bronchitis, influenza-like symptoms, pneumonia, sinusitis and otitis, and exacerbations of asthma and chronic bronchitis have also been associated with RSV infection in adults. Bronchial hyperreactivity measured by pulmonary function testing may last for several months after infection in previously healthy adults. Bronchopneumonia or secondary bacterial pneumonia complicates a high proportion of infections in the elderly. Rarely, RSV infections may be associated with diffuse, life-threatening pneumonia or with cardiac or central nervous system disease in previously healthy adults. Immunocompromised hosts, particularly bone marrow transplant recipients in the early transplant period, have an increased risk of severe RSV infection with high mortality rate.

Diagnosis

Nasal secretions obtained by nasopharyngeal aspiration or washing, as well as sputum or lower respiratory samples, are appropriate specimens for virus isolation. Because the virus is heat-labile, freezing and delays in processing of clinical specimens should be prevented. Various techniques for detection of viral antigens in clinical specimens are commercially available. Immunofluorescence staining of exfoliated respiratory cells is a sensitive method of rapid (less than 2 hours) diagnosis. Detection of RSV antigens by enzyme immunoassays is also sensitive and specific. Antibodies in paired sera can be measured by various methods (Table 246-1), although infections may occur without significant titer level rises in infants and during reinfections in adults.

Treatment

Management of lower respiratory disease includes correction of hypoxemia and close monitoring of respiratory status. Bronchodilators have not been found to be beneficial. Aerosol delivery of the synthetic nucleoside ribavirin is effective in reducing viral shedding, illness severity, and blood gas abnormalities in previously healthy and high-risk infants hospitalized with RSV bronchiolitis or pneumonia. Aerosol ribavirin has been shown to reduce hospitalization duration in intubated infants and has been used in severe infections in immunocompromised patients with variable success. Aerosolized ribavirin is generally well tolerated, but its administration requires prolonged periods of exposure. Intravenous immunoglobulin therapy has antiviral effects in animal models and is being assessed for prophylaxis and treatment of severe RSV infections in infants.

Prevention

No vaccine against RSV is currently available. Thorough hand washing and regular use of eye-nose goggles may be effective in preventing nosocomial RSV spread. Use of gowns and gloves, decontamination of surfaces and fomites, cohorting of infected cases, and perhaps protective isolation of high-risk contacts are additional control measures.

RUBELLA VIRUS

Classification

Rubella is a spherical, enveloped, RNA-containing virus. Although its clinical and epidemiologic behavior is more similar to that of the paramyxoviruses, rubella is grouped morphologically in the togavirus family, along with the arthropod-borne alphaviruses and flaviviruses. Only one serologic type is recognized.

Epidemiology

During the prevaccine era in the United States, epidemics of rubella occurred every 6 to 9 years, and most reported cases occurred in children under 10 years of age. A major epidemic in 1964 resulted in the birth of approximately 20,000 infants with congenital rubella defects, and, on the basis of the periodicity of reported rubella, another significant epidemic was forecast for the early 1970s. When live attenuated rubella virus vaccine became available in 1969, mass vaccination of children 1 year of age and older was recommended to reduce transmission of rubella from children to susceptible pregnant women. This approach has dramatically altered the epidemiology of rubella in this country. The predicted epidemic did not occur, and the incidence of rubella has dropped to all-time low levels, with fewer than 175 cases reported during 1992. This represents a decline of over 99% compared to the prevaccine era. The seasonal pattern of rubella, with the peak incidence in the late winter and early spring, has been less prominent in recent years.

Unfortunately, disease activity during the 1970s remained relatively constant among adolescents and young adults, and outbreaks of rubella were described among high school and college students, military trainees, prison inmates, hospital employees, and even discotheque clientele. Several outbreaks occurred among populations with rates of immunity greater than 90%; moderate levels of herd immunity have not reliably prevented transmission. Increased emphasis was therefore placed on the identification and vaccination of susceptible adolescents and adults, especially women, and levels of reported rubella in these older age groups dropped markedly in the 1980s.

Pathogenesis

Transmission of rubella is primarily via respiratory droplets or direct contact with an infected patient. The period of communicability is from approximately 7 days before to 5 days after rash onset. Patients differ markedly in their ability to spread infection, perhaps related to the presence of respiratory symptoms, such as sneezing and coughing, that facilitate dissemination. Persons with subclinical rubella can nevertheless transmit infection. Infants with congenital rubella often shed large amounts of virus for prolonged periods (in some cases, over 1 year) and can therefore pose an important infection hazard to nonimmune caretakers in the home or hospital setting.

After infection of the upper respiratory tract, the virus multiplies locally, and eventually viremia results. The incubation period averages 18 days (range 14 to 21 days). The rash is believed to be immunologically mediated. Rubella virus can be isolated from rash lesions and also from adjacent areas of normal skin. Virus has also been isolated from joint effusions in persons with rubella arthritis.

Naturally acquired immunity against rubella is usually permanent, but reinfections, mostly subclinical, have been reported. Such reinfections are more common in persons with vaccine-induced immunity, especially those with low antibody titer levels. Viremia is probably extremely rare in such persons, and gestational reinfection appears to pose minimum risk to the fetus.

Clinical features

Rubella is commonly inapparent. When clinical illness occurs, it is generally benign and is manifested by rash and lymphadenopathy, with mild constitutional symptoms. Discrete, pink maculopapules appear first on the face and then spread to the chest, abdomen, and extremities. The lesions may coalesce, especially on the face, and may desquamate during convalescence. An enanthem of punctate or larger red macules (Forchheimer spots) may appear on the soft palate before or coincident with the rash onset. The usual duration of rash is 2 to 5 days. Rash may be totally absent. The postauricular, posterior cervical, and suboccipital lymph nodes are often tender and swollen; the discomfort is usually short-lived, but palpable nodal enlargement may persist for weeks. Splenomegaly may be observed. In children, rash is usually the first sign of the illness, but many adults experience a prodrome consisting of low-grade fever, malaise, anorexia, headache, sore throat, and, in severe cases, cough, coryza, and conjunctivitis, as seen in rubeola. Arthralgia and arthritis are infrequent in children, but are more common among adult women. Joint symptoms usually appear 2 to 3 days after the onset of rash and persist only a few days. Thrombocytopenic purpura and encephalitis are infrequent complications. Testalgia has been reported in recent outbreaks and may indicate orchitis.

Congenital infection. In marked contrast to the usually mild nature of postnatal rubella, gestational rubella can be potentially devastating to the developing fetus and may produce the congenital rubella syndrome. Defects of virtually every organ system have been described, but the most notable involvement is of the eyes (e.g., cataract, glaucoma), heart (especially patent ductus arteriosus and pulmonary stenosis), and central nervous system (e.g., sensorineural deafness, psychomotor retardation). A fulminant neonatal presentation, with hepatosplenomegaly, jaundice, thrombocytopenic purpura, and radiolucent bone lesions, may also occur. More subtle changes, such as learning disabilities and behavioral disturbances, may not be recognized until years after birth. Endocrinopathies, especially diabetes mellitus, and a late-onset, progressive encephalitis may be other late manifestations. The clinical expression of congenital rubella is intimately related to the gestational timing of infection. The risk of major anomalies is greatest for infection during the first trimester.

Diagnosis

Because of the nonspecific nature of the signs and symptoms, clinical diagnosis of postnatal rubella is often difficult or impossible in a nonepidemic setting. The virus can often be detected in throat, blood, or urine specimens, but viral isolation is expensive and time-consuming.

Diagnosis is usually best accomplished by serologic demonstration of a significant rise in antibody level in acute and convalescent sera. Several serologic methods are available. The hemagglutination inhibition (HI) technique is reliable and was the standard, benchmark method for many years. With this assay, a fourfold rise in titer level indicates recent infection. Many newer serologic techniques for rubella offer certain technical advantages and have become widespread in recent years. These methods include enzyme immunoassay, latex agglutination, immunofluorescence assay, passive hemagglutination, hemolysis in gel, and virus neutralization. Using these newer methods, the criteria for a significant rise in antibody level vary by type of assay and by laboratory. When the first serum specimen is not obtained until several days to weeks have elapsed after the onset of the rash, two other strategies are sometimes useful. Complement-fixing antibodies usually appear 7 to 10 days after hemagglutination inhibition antibodies, so complement-fixation testing in such cases may still allow demonstration of a significant titer rise. Alternatively, the presence of rubella-specific IgM antibodies in a single specimen obtained during the subacute stage strongly suggests recent primary infection.

The diagnosis of congenital rubella infection may be strongly suggested in some instances by the history and physical examination. In other instances, however, the clinical presentation does not allow easy differentiation of rubella from other types of congenital infection, including toxoplasmosis, cytomegalovirus, herpes simplex, and syphilis.

The diagnosis of congenital rubella infection in an infant can be confirmed by the presence of rubella-specific IgM antibodies or by a significant titer level of rubella antibody between 6 and 11 months of age (by which time levels of passively acquired maternal antibody should be negligible). Viral isolation is also diagnostic and can be helpful even after the immediate neonatal period, because viral persistence and shedding may be prolonged for 6 months or longer after birth.

Prevention and treatment

There is no specific therapy for rubella, but symptomatic treatment may be helpful for patients with significant fever, malaise, or arthritis.

Since the time of its licensure in 1969, over 180 million doses of live attenuated rubella virus vaccine have been distributed in the United States. The vaccine strain currently available in this country (RA 27/3) is grown in a human diploid cell line and, though more immunogenic than the previously used strains, has no increase in side-effects. Rubella vaccine is available as a monovalent antigen or in combination with live measles and/or mumps vaccines.

Vaccine reactions are uncommon in children but may include fever, rash, lymphadenopathy, arthralgia, arthritis, and peripheral neuritis. Joint symptoms are more common in adult women than in children and begin 1 to 10 weeks after immunization. These symptoms are usually short-lived and do not result in permanent disability or deformity. Recurrent joint symptoms and frank arthritis are very unusual but have been reported. All joint reactions are less frequent and less severe with rubella vaccine than with rubella illness.

The durability of vaccine-induced immunity is of crucial importance, because it was hoped that vaccination during childhood might protect a woman through her childbearing years. In the largest ongoing study, 92% of vaccinees with seroconversion have had persistent serologic immunity after 16 years, and the few whose titer levels had dropped to undetectable levels have shown booster-type immune responses when revaccinated. Other, smaller studies, however, have demonstrated loss of serologic immunity in a disturbingly large percentage of vaccinees. Continued follow-up observation will be necessary to determine the durability of clinical immunity and the possible need for booster vaccinations.

Rubella vaccine can cross the placenta and infect the fetus of a susceptible vaccinee. Its teratogenic potential has been suggested by the observation of a probable early cataract in an aborted, infected fetus of a susceptible vaccinee. However, more than 320 susceptible women have been vaccinated inadvertently within either 3 months before or 3 months after their presumed dates of conception and have carried their pregnancies to term. None of the infants had defects compatible with congenital rubella syndrome. Thus the risk, if any, of major malformation appears to be less than 2%. A few of these infants have shown serologic evidence of subclinical rubella infection. Although the risk of major defects appears low, vaccination remains contraindicated during pregnancy. Females of childbearing age should be vaccinated only if they are not pregnant and they agree to take responsible precautions to prevent pregnancy for 3 months after vaccination. Vaccine may be given to children whose mothers are pregnant, because the vaccine virus is nontransmissible.

Rubella vaccination is currently recommended for all children, many adolescents, and some adults, particularly women, unless it is otherwise contraindicated. Careful attention to routine vaccination of infants, along with enthusiastic enforcement of state laws requiring immunization of schoolchildren, should ensure continuously high levels of immunity among young children. Many persons who receive the currently recommended second dose of measles vaccine are given the combined measles-mumps-rubella vaccine. Ideally this second dose of rubella vaccine will serve to increase the overall level of rubella immunity. The effective identification and vaccination of susceptible adolescent and adult women are also essential for optimum rubella control. Situations that lend themselves well to serologic screening for rubella susceptibility include the premarital examination, entrance into educational or training institutions (such as colleges or military bases), and visits to family-planning clinics and employee health services. Serologic documentation of susceptibility in potential vaccinees of childbearing age is sometimes desirable but should not be considered mandatory, especially in outbreaks. No known ill effects result from vaccination of persons with pre-existing immunity. Screening at prenatal visits allows vaccination of susceptible persons immediately after delivery. Breast-feeding and previous administration of $Rh_0(D)$ immune globulin or blood products are not contraindications to postpartum vaccination. In this latter instance, however, serologic testing is recommended 6 to 8 weeks later to ascertain whether seroconversion has occurred.

The traditional concern with nosocomial rubella has been that a pregnant hospital employee would contract rubella from an infected patient. Female hospital employees of childbearing age who are in contact with patients should be required to prove rubella immunity for their own protection. In several recent outbreaks, hospital employees with rubella have exposed large numbers of susceptible pregnant patients. It is therefore advisable for all hospital employees, male or female, who are in contact with pregnant patients to undergo similar screening for patient protection.

In screening for rubella susceptibility using the time-honored hemagglutination-inhibition technique, the presence of any level of rubella antibody has generally been considered to indicate previous infection (or immunization) and presumed immunity; the absence of such antibody indicates probable susceptibility. Clinical experience with the newer serologic methods is less extensive, but any antibody level above the standard positive cut-off value for that particular assay is likewise generally considered presumptive evidence of immunity. The clinical significance of low antibody levels remains under careful study, however, especially for levels detectable only by newer assays that are extremely sensitive. Limited data suggest that infection with viremia has occurred, although very rarely, among persons with such low antibody levels; very rare occurrences of congenital rubella infection after reinfection have likewise been reported. An undocumented history of rubella illness is unreliable and should not be accepted as evidence of immunity.

There is no evidence that rubella vaccine is either helpful or harmful in the management of patients recently exposed to rubella, but it is often given to provide future protection if the recognized exposure has not resulted in incubating infection. Immune serum globulin given after exposure may suppress or modify symptoms but does not reliably prevent infection or viremia. Limited experience with high-titer-level human rubella immunoglobulin has been favorable, but this material is not generally available. Prophylactic use of immune serum globulin after exposures during early pregnancy is not of proven benefit and should be considered only among women who would not contemplate therapeutic abortion under any circumstances. Serologic testing done promptly after such exposures often establishes pre-existing immunity and reassures the involved persons.

CORONAVIRUS INFECTIONS

Classification and characteristics

Coronaviruses are medium-sized, pleomorphic, lipid-enveloped viruses that contain a single-stranded RNA genome. The term coronavirus refers to the widely spaced, club-shaped spikes that radiate from the virus surface in electron microscopic preparations and impart a crown-like appearance. The surface projections, or peplomers, contain glycoproteins that have cell receptor binding, membrane fusing, and in some strains, hemagglutinating activities. They replicate in the cytoplasm of infected cells and cause a cytocidal effect. At least five human serotypes have been described, of which strains 229E and OC43 are the best characterized. Most isolates from the respiratory tract are antigenically similar to one of these two strains. Human enteric coronaviruses have been recovered from cases of acute gastrointestinal infection, and coronavirus-like particles (CVLPs) detected by electron microscopy in the stool of both symptomatic and asymptomatic persons. In addition, the coronavirus genus contains at least 10 animal coronaviruses, including important veterinary pathogens. Disease syndromes in different species include bronchitis, pneumonitis, gastroenteritis, hepatitis, encephalomyelitis, demyelinating disease, and genitourinary infection.

Epidemiology

Coronaviruses are the second most frequently recognized cause of the common cold and account for approximately 15% of all colds. Coronaviruses have been found throughout the world. In temperate climates, infection occurs principally in the winter and spring months, although outbreaks have been described during summer. The proportion of colds caused by coronaviruses is as high as 35% during periods of peak activity. Strain 229E causes outbreaks at 2 to 4 year intervals. The prevalence of antibody rises rapidly during the first 5 years of life, and most adults have antibody to OC43 and 229E. Reinfection with the same serotype appears to be common, and the level of circulating antibody correlates to a limited extent with protection from infection.

Coronaviruses are transmitted by the respiratory route, whereas enteric coronaviruses are presumably spread by the fecal-oral route. The seasonal (fall-winter) and age (2 years old) patterns of diarrhea associated with fecal shedding of CVLPs are similar to those with rotaviruses. There are no recognized animal reservoirs or vectors of human coronaviruses.

Clinical features

The full spectrum of human coronavirus infections has not been determined. One third to one half of respiratory coronavirus infections are asymptomatic. The usual manifestations of infection are typical common colds (Chapter 230). In experimentally induced infections, the incubation period (2 to 5 days) is longer than in rhinovirus colds. The average duration of illness (6 to 7 days) is several days shorter. Low-grade fever occurs in about one fifth of infected persons. In addition to nasal symptoms, cough and sore throat occur frequently. Virus multiplication is probably limited to the respiratory tract. Virus excretion is detectable at the time symptoms begin and lasts for 1 to 4 days. Coronavirus infections have been associated with exacerbations of asthma and chronic bronchitis, recurrent wheezy bronchitis in children, and, uncommonly, lower respiratory tract disease or pneumonia in selected groups, including infants, young children, and military recruits.

The etiologic role of enteric coronaviruses in diarrheal disease is unresolved. Coronaviruses have been implicated as causes of acute gastroenteritis in young children and rarely of outbreaks of necrotizing enterocolitis in neonates. In addition to diarrhea, fever, and vomiting, more severely affected infants may show abdominal distention, blood in the stool, and radiologic evidence of pneumatosis intestinalis. CVLPs have been detected in adults with diarrhea, including some acquired immunodeficiency syndrome (AIDS) patients, but also in a high proportion of asymptomatic persons. CVLP excretion may be prolonged and has been associated with poor hygienic conditions.

Diagnosis

Laboratory diagnosis of coronavirus infections is technically difficult. Human coronaviruses have fastidious growth requirements and usually require human organ culture for primary isolation, where detection depends on electron microscopy, immunologic techniques, or production of disease in volunteers. Immunoassays and nucleic acid hybridization assays have been described for detection of coronavirus in nasopharyngeal secretions. Serologic diagnosis of 229E and OC43 infections is possible but not generally available.

Treatment and prevention

Intranasal interferon protects against experimental coronavirus infection, but no specific antiviral therapy or vaccine is currently available. Treatment is symptomatic.

REFERENCES

Baum SC and Litman N: Mumps virus. In Mandell GL, Douglas RG Jr, and Bennett JE, editors: Principles and practice of infectious diseases, ed 3. New York, 1990, Churchill Livingstone.

Best JM: Rubella vaccines: past, present and future. Epidemiol Infect 107:17, 1991.

Centers for Disease Control: Rubella prevention: recommendations of the Immunization Practices Advisory Committee (ACIP). MMWR 39:1, 1990.

Centers for Disease Control: Measles prevention: recommendations of the Immunization Practices Advisory Committee. MMWR 38:1, 1989.

Centers for Disease Control: Mumps prevention: recommendations of the Immunization Practices Advisory Committee (ACIP). MMWR 38:388, 1989.

Cradock-Watson JE: Laboratory diagnosis of rubella: past, present and future. Epidemiol Infect 107:1, 1991.

Gershon AA: Measles virus (rubeola). In Mandell GL, Douglas RG Jr, and Bennett JE, editors: Principles and practice of infectious diseases, ed 3. New York, 1990, Churchill Livingstone.

Giladdi M et al: Measles in adults: a prospective study of 291 consecutive cases. Br Med J 295:1314, 1987.

Hall CB: Respiratory syncytial virus. In Mandell GL, Douglas RG Jr, and Bennett JE, editors: Principles and practice of infectious diseases, ed 3. New York, 1990, Churchill Livingstone.

Hendley JO: Parainfluenza viruses. In Mandell GL, Douglas RG Jr, and Bennett JE, editors: Principles and practice of infectious diseases, ed 3. New York, 1990, Churchill Livingstone.

Hersh BS et al: Mumps outbreak in a highly vaccinated population. J Pediatr 199:187, 1991.

Hertz MI et al: Respiratory syncytial virus–induced acute lung injury in adult patients with bone marrow transplants: a clinical approach and review of the literature. Medicine 68:269, 1989.

Johnson RT et al: Measles encephalomyelitis—clinical and immunologic studies. N Engl J Med 310:137, 1984.

Kaplan LJ et al: Severe measles in immunocompromised patients. JAMA 267:1237, 1992.

Kelley PW et al: The susceptibility of young adult Americans to vaccine-preventable infections. JAMA 266:2724, 1991.

McIntosh K: Coronavirus. In Mandell GL, Douglas RG Jr, and Bennett JE, editors: Principles and practice of infectious diseases, ed 3. New York, 1990, Churchill Livingstone.

Phillips MJ et al: Syncytial giant-cell hepatitis: sporadic hepatitis with distinctive pathological features, a severe clinical course, and paramyxoviral features. N Engl J Med 324:455, 1991.

Smith DW et al: A controlled trial of aerosolized ribavirin in infants receiving mechanical ventilation for severe respiratory syncytial virus infection. N Engl J Med 325:24, 1991.

Weber DJ, Rutala WA, and Orenstein WA: Prevention of mumps, measles, and rubella among hospital personnel. J Pediatr 119:322, 1991.

Werdt CH et al: Parainfluenza virus respiratory infection after bone marrow transplantation. N Engl J Med 326:921, 1992.

CHAPTER

247 Rabies

Steven L. Chuck

CHARACTERISTICS

The rabies virus is one of four rhabdoviruses known to infect humans. The other three viruses, Mokola virus, Duvenhage virus, and vesicular stomatitis virus, are much less common human pathogens. These four viruses, along with the many other rhabdoviruses, have a characteristic bullet shape that imparts the name of the group.

The rabies virus contains a single nonsegmented negative strand of genomic RNA with five nonoverlapping genes, each of which encodes a single, distinct protein. The order of the genes is similar to that of other rhabdoviruses: from the 3′ end, nucleoprotein, phosphoprotein, matrix protein, glycoprotein, and transcriptase. The nucleoprotein, phosphoprotein, and transcriptase, together with the genomic RNA, form the helical core of nucleocapsid. Antibody directed against the nucleocapsid is useful for detecting intracytoplasmic inclusions of rabies virus (Negri bodies). In addition, vaccination with epitopes from the nucleoprotein protect against experimental infection. An envelope of lipid bilayer covers this core. The matrix protein may be anchored on the inner aspect of the lipid membrane, and the glycoprotein coats the outer surface of the virus. This glycoprotein plays a large role in the virulence of the virus. Point mutations leading to a single amino acid substitution at one critical location in the glycoprotein can render the virus nonlethal in a mouse model, and neutralizing antibodies directed against the glycoprotein spikes confer immunity.

The virus is susceptible to inactivation by drying, heating, or exposure to sunlight, ultraviolet light, ethanol, formalin, and quaternary ammonium compounds. Importantly, the virus can also be inactivated by 20% soap solutions.

EPIDEMIOLOGY

Rabies virus exists in an enzootic cycle of warm-blooded animals transferred by bite from one animal to another. Worldwide, domestic dogs and cats account for the majority of cases. In areas where vaccination programs have been successfully implemented, the principal reservoir of rabies is in wild animals. In the United States the infected animals reported most commonly are skunks, raccoons, bats, foxes, and dogs. Although skunks are the most common carrier of rabies, bats are more widely distributed, being found in 48 states. Along the Mexican–United States border, stray dogs are a major carrier of rabies virus. Among domestic animals in the United States, cattle, cats, and dogs are most commonly infected. In Europe, foxes are the principal vector. Vampire bats, mongooses, jackals, and wolves are prominent sources of rabies elsewhere in the world. Rabies has rarely been reported in rodents, and no cases of human rabies have resulted from a rodent bite. Control of rabies in wild or domestic animal populations can be achieved with vaccination.

Human rabies usually results from the bite of an infected animal. Contamination of an open wound or inhalation of the virus, however, can lead to rabies; cases have been reported in spelunkers investigating bat-infested caves and laboratory workers preparing homogenates of infected brain. Furthermore, cases of rabies have been reported in which no exposure to animals could be recalled. Human-to-human transmission has been documented only in recipients of corneal transplants from donors who died of undiagnosed rabies.

PATHOPHYSIOLOGY

The saliva of diseased animals contains infective rabies virus for several days before outward manifestations of illness, so bites from seemingly normal animals may lead to rabies. Most animals die of rabies, although some do recover and then no longer secrete the virus in their saliva. Some bats have been found with virus in their fat and apparently secrete the virus in their saliva during periods of stress.

After a bite by a rabid animal, the virus may replicate in nearby striated muscle cells or directly enter exposed nerve endings. After a period of replication and amplification in muscle cells, the virus enters unmyelinated peripheral nerves unless it is inactivated by antibody-mediated host defenses. Rabies virus moves through peripheral nerves passively via axoplasmic flow toward the central nervous system. Once it reaches the first cell body, such as in the dorsal root ganglia, the virus replicates, infects adjacent cells, and continues to move proximally. In the brain, the virus involves the neurons of the limbic system early on but replicates and spreads rapidly, causing widespread neural dysfunction. Rabies virus then disseminates centrifugally from the central nervous system through nerves to many tissues. Subsequently, the virus may be demonstrated in saliva, urine, cerebrospinal fluid, corneal cells, and skin.

Infected brains typically are edematous and infiltrated in either a focal or diffuse manner with lymphocytes, particularly around small blood vessels. Diffuse degenerative changes are seen in the neurons of the brain and spinal cord. Pathognomonic Negri bodies are seen in three fourths of cases. These eosinophilic, oval cytoplasmic inclusions may be stained with fluorescent antibodies for nucleocapsid material (Plate V-48). Negri bodies are most often seen in the ganglion cells of Ammon's horn in the hippocampus but may also be seen in neurons of the cerebellum, cortex, and spinal cord.

CLINICAL MANIFESTATIONS

After an incubation period, human rabies occurs in three stages: a prodrome, acute neurologic phase, and coma followed by death. Incubation usually occurs over 20 to 60 days, but periods of 10 days to longer than 1 year have been reported. The incubation period tends to be shorter in children, when the bite is on the head or neck, and after a severe, deep bite. Symptoms are related only to the wound during the incubation period.

The nonspecific prodromal symptoms consist of apathy, malaise, anorexia, fatigue, fever, chills, and headache. Anxiety, irritability, and depression may occur. At the wound, hyperesthesia, pruritus, or pain radiating proximally may all occur. Other less common symptoms include cough, sore throat, abdominal pain, nausea, vomiting, diarrhea, and dysuria; an upper respiratory tract infection or gastroenteritis may be diagnosed initially. The prodrome may last from 1 to 10 days.

In 80% of patients, the disease progresses to "furious" rabies, so named because of the neurologic hyperactivity. Agitation, excitement, and marked motor activity are soon followed by dysphagia and hydrophobia. Pathognomonic of rabies, hydrophobia results from fear of pain and choking produced by laryngeal and pharyngeal muscle spasms. Drooling may result from increased salivation and avoidance of swallowing. Hypersensitivity of the skin may lead to avoidance of stimulation even by air (aerophobia). Cortical hyperactivity is manifested in bursts of aggressiveness marked by thrashing, biting, hallucinations, and disorientation lasting 1 to 5 minutes separated by periods of full orientation and calmness. Seizures may also occur. Autonomic hyperactivity is common and may consist of supraventricular arrhythmias, deregulation of blood pressure, and tachypnea. If death does not occur abruptly as a result of cardiopulmonary arrest, a paralytic phase may occur. Typically 2 to 7 days after the onset of symptoms, death supervenes.

In 20% of patients, however, hyperactivity is not prominent, and the prodrome is followed instead by predominantly "paralytic" or "dumb" rabies. This form is most common in patients bitten by vampire bats or given postexposure vaccination. Paresis or paralysis accompanied by pain may develop either predominantly in the bitten extremity, diffusely, or in an ascending fashion similar to the Guillain-Barré syndrome. Hydrophobia occurs late if at all. The mental status declines leading to disorientation, obtundation, and then coma. Death occurs an average of 12 days after the onset of symptoms.

Once symptoms have begun, survival is unusual. Three cases of nonfatal rabies developing after pre-exposure or postexposure prophylaxis have been reported. Two persons developed rabies after postexposure prophylaxis had been given, and in both persons, recovery was reportedly complete. A third person who had been immunized prior to exposure recovered with some permanent loss of speech and motor function.

COMPLICATIONS

Neurologic, cardiac, and pulmonary complications are most common. Cerebral edema, increased intracranial pressure, seizures, inappropriate secretion of antidiuretic hormone or diabetes insipidus, and autonomic dysfunction resulting in alterations in blood pressure, heart rate and rhythm, or temperature regulation are the most frequent neurologic complications. Cardiac arrhythmias include atrial premature contractions, sinus bradycardia, and sinus arrest. Hypotension may develop from myocarditis, bradyarrhythmias, autonomic dysfunction, fluid depletion, or congestive heart failure. Hyperventilation with respiratory alkalosis is common. Hypoxia, hypoventilation, and abnormalities in the pattern of breathing may culminate in respiratory arrest. Aspiration, superinfection, or pulmonary edema from congestive heart failure or the adult respiratory distress syndrome may develop.

DIFFERENTIAL DIAGNOSIS

Antemortem diagnosis can be difficult if a clear history of exposure is absent and symptoms are atypical. The differential diagnosis encompasses all forms of encephalitis (Chapter 249), including infections from arboviruses, enteroviruses, and herpesviruses. Delirium tremens and toxic ingestions should also be considered.

Unfortunately, no tests are available to diagnose infection with rabies virus before the onset of disease. The diagnosis may be confirmed antemortem by isolation of the virus, antibody testing, and immunofluorescent staining of viral antigens in tissues. During the first 2 weeks of illness, the virus may be found in saliva, cerebrospinal fluid, or urine. Isolation of the virus, however, is not a very sensitive test and requires an incubation period in the laboratory of up to 3 weeks. Rabies antibody can be detected in serum 6 to 13 days after the onset of illness in both vaccinated and unvaccinated patients. Such neutralizing antibodies are first found around day 10 in unvaccinated patients and then sharply increase to levels significantly higher than those seen in vaccinated patients. Vaccinated patients develop measurable titers of antibody in their serum about 8 days after vaccination. The presence of rabies antibody in the cerebrospinal fluid is diagnostic. These antibodies appear a few days after the rise in serum antibodies. Unfortunately, many patients die before developing appreciable titers of neutralizing antibody. Finally, viral antigens may be detected by immunofluorescent staining of full-thickness punch biopsies of the skin overlying the back of the neck above the hairline. This tissue is optimum because it is close to the central nervous system, it is readily accessible, and hair follicles are densely innervated; corneal impressions are no longer recommended. Immunofluorescent staining of neck skin, however, rarely yields positive findings before the development of measurable serum antibodies.

TREATMENT

Because specific therapy does not improve outcome once clinical signs are noted, treatment of human rabies, except for postexposure prophylaxis, consists of supportive care. A variety of antiviral agents have been tried, including human leukocyte interferon, but none has been beneficial when given after the onset of illness. Because the virus may be present in the saliva, urine, and cerebrospinal fluid of an infected patient, these fluids should be handled and disposed properly. Although virus has not been isolated from blood of infected humans, precautions are warranted. Exposed personnel should be given the standard postexposure prophylaxis.

PROPHYLAXIS

Prevention of rabies involves vaccination of domestic animals and administration of immunoprophylaxis to exposed persons. Since the institution of legal requirements for vaccination of dogs, the incidence of human rabies has dropped markedly in the United States. Domestic cats, however, are less often required to be vaccinated and remain a potential transmitter of rabies.

Vaccination of humans dates back to 1881, when Louis Pasteur developed the first successful vaccine for a human infection from dried spinal cords of rabid animals. Modified phenol-inactivated nerve tissue vaccines are still used in some countries in Africa and Asia because of their low cost and ease of preparation. Other vaccines, such as those derived from suckling mouse brain (SMB) and duck embryos (DEV), were developed because of the high rate of neurologic side-effects associated with nerve tissue vaccines. Because of the neurologic side-effects of SMB and low potency of DEV, however, these vaccines are no longer distributed, and human diploid cell vaccine (HDCV), composed of inactivated whole virions, currently is the main vaccine used in the United States. A new cell culture–derived, adsorbed vaccine (rabies vaccine, adsorbed or RVA) was approved in 1988, but is not widely available.

Immunoprophylaxis against rabies in humans may occur before or after exposure to the virus. The effectiveness of these regimens has been well demonstrated in animals and humans. Successful pre-exposure vaccination protects the host against subsequent infection with rabies virus. Postexposure protection consists of both early passive immunity conferred via injection of immunoglobulins and long-lasting immunity induced simultaneously with HDCV. Without postexposure prophylaxis, the risk of developing human rabies after an animal bite has been estimated at 15% to 40%; after the administration of serum and HDCV, the incidence is much less than 1%.

Pre-exposure prophylaxis

Pre-exposure prophylaxis with HDCV is indicated for persons at high risk of subsequent exposure to rabies, such as veterinarians, animal handlers or trainers, some laboratory workers, spelunkers, travelers, or any other persons likely to contact rabid animals. Three 1 ml injections of HDCV given intramuscularly into the deltoid on days 0, 7, and 21 or 28 have led to adequate antibody responses in all persons vaccinated.

Pre-exposure prophylaxis has also been administered intradermally in the lateral upper arm also with three 0.1 ml doses on days 0, 7, and 21 or 28. The intradermal route should not be used if the patient is concomitantly receiving chloroquine phosphate for malaria prophylaxis or if all three intradermal doses of vaccine cannot be given 30 days before travel to an area with endemic rabies.

Serologic testing for adequate antibody after pre-exposure prophylaxis is not recommended for routine cases, but antibody titers can be checked if the patient is immunosuppressed or an atypical regimen is used. Additionally, persons with ongoing exposure to rabies should have measurements of antibody every 2 years. If the titer is inadequate, they should receive a booster dose of either 1 ml intramuscularly or 0.1 ml intradermally. Booster injections should be given only when clearly indicated because they have been associated with serum sickness reactions in approximately 6% of patients.

Postexposure prophylaxis

Postexposure prophylaxis (Fig. 247-1) includes thorough cleaning of the wound, passive immunization with human rabies immunoglobulin (HRIG), and active immunization with HDCV. Persons with a known immune response to pre-exposure prophylaxis should receive HDCV on day 0 and again on day 3 in addition to meticulous wound care. All other persons, including those with an unknown antibody response to pre-exposure prophylaxis, should receive the full postexposure regimen.

Initiation of postexposure prophylaxis should begin after consideration of the type of exposure (bite or nonbite), the species of the animal involved, the vaccination status of the animal, the local epidemiology of rabies, the appearance of the animal, and whether the attack was provoked. Postexposure prophylaxis is recommended after any bite by a known or suspected rabid dog, cat, skunk, bat, raccoon, fox, or other carnivore unless the animal is shown to be nonrabid by fluorescent-antibody staining of the brain. Healthy dogs or cats should be confined if possible for 10 days; rabies prophylaxis should be given only if the animal develops rabies in that time. If the dog or cat has escaped, local public health officials can be consulted regarding the occurrence of rabies in the area. Bites by rodents and rabbits virtually never require postexposure prophylaxis. Recommendations for other types of exposure, such as to aerosolized laboratory specimens or livestock, may require the consultation of local public health officials.

Thorough cleansing of the wound is an essential part of postexposure prophylaxis. Too often, this aspect is overlooked in the haste to vaccinate the patient. The wound should be washed with liberal amounts of soap and water, devitalized tissue debrided, and tetanus vaccine and antibiotics given if indicated. Soap can inactivate the virus, and aggressive cleansing of wounds has been shown to reduce the incidence of rabies markedly in inoculated experimental animals.

Passive immunity should be given as soon after exposure as possible, preferably with HRIG although equine antirabies serum is the only form available in some areas. HRIG is available in preparations containing 150 IU per milliliter and is given once in a dose of 20 IU per kilogram. Half of the rabies immunoglobulin should be infiltrated into the area around a nonmucosal wound, and the second half injected intramuscularly. The entire dose is administered intramuscularly if a mucous membrane is the site exposed. The recommended dose of HRIG should not be exceeded because HRIG may partially suppress the induction of active antibodies. HRIG provides rapid but temporary immunity; the half-life of the antibodies is approximately 21 days.

Immunization with HDCV should also be initiated as soon as possible after exposure and is completed with four subsequent doses on days 3, 7, 14, and 28 after the first dose. The vaccine should not be given at the same site as HRIG or antirabies serum. In adults, HDCV should be injected into the deltoid; in children, the anterolateral thigh may also be used. Lower titers of antibody and even failure of protection have been associated with gluteal injections. The intradermal route should not be used for postexposure prophylaxis. Active immunity induced by HDCV occurs 7 to 10 days after vaccination. Antibody testing after vaccination is not recommended except in immunosuppressed patients.

Postexposure prophylaxis is recommended regardless of the time between exposure and treatment. Both HRIG and HDCV must be given for optimum protection. HDCV is

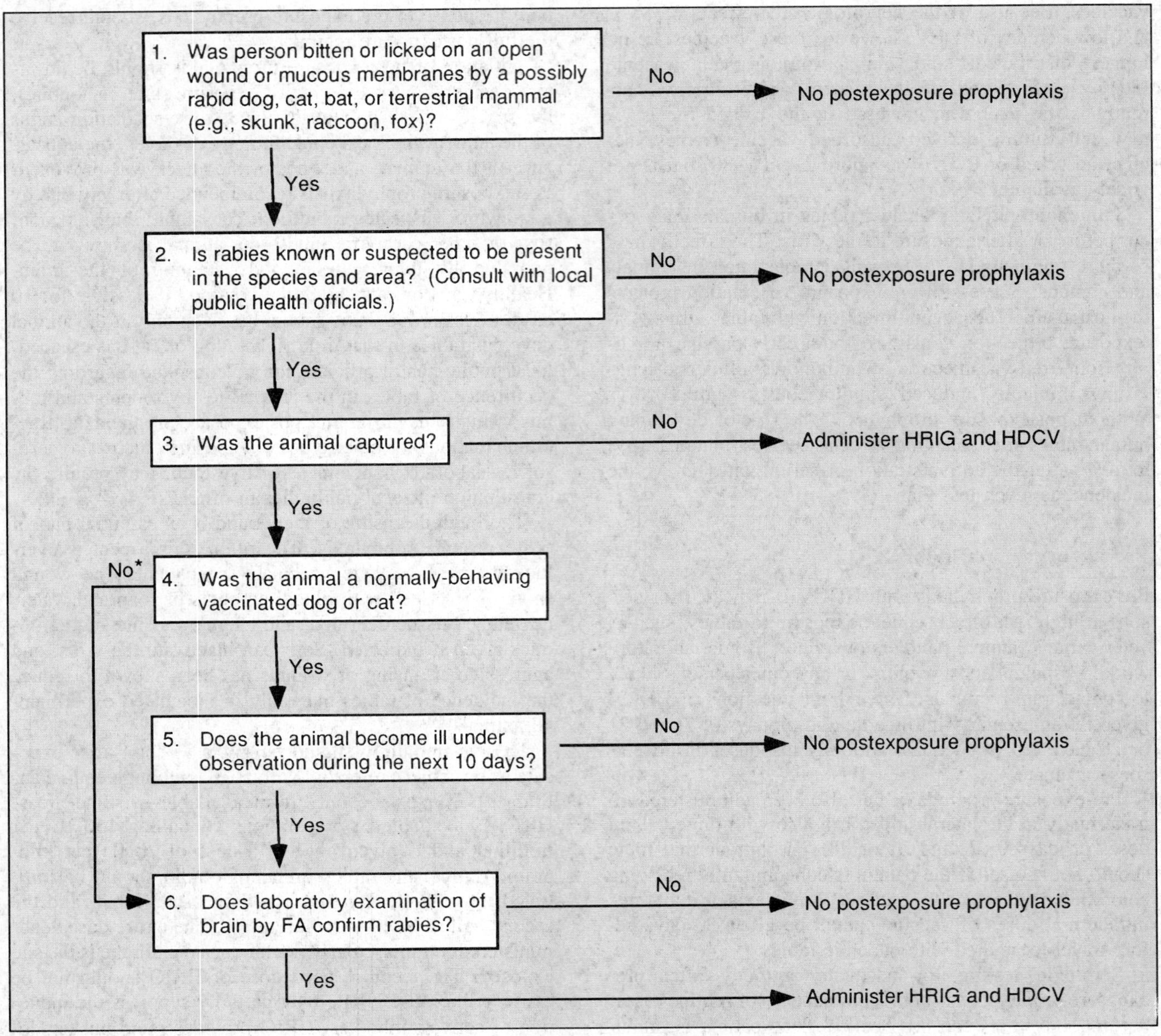

Fig. 247-1. Algorithm for postexposure prophylaxis of rabies. *If the captured animal is not a normally behaving vaccinated dog or cat, postexposure prophylaxis may be initiated pending quarantine or examination of the brain.

prepared from inactivated virus and is not contraindicated in exposed pregnant patients.

Both systemic and local complications have been reported in association with HDCV. Up to one half of patients experience local swelling, erythema, induration, or pain at the site of injection. Approximately 20% have mild systemic reactions including nausea, myalgias, malaise, fever, headache, adenopathy, or nonspecific abdominal pain. Two cases of Guillain-Barré syndrome have occurred, and both recovered without sequelae within 2 weeks. Anaphylaxis is rare; fatal anaphylaxis has not been reported. Booster injections of HDCV have been often associated with serum sickness.

REFERENCES

Immunization Practices Advisory Committee (ACIP): Rabies prevention—United States, 1984: recommendation of the Immunization Practices Advisory Committee. MMWR 33:393, 1984.

Immunization Practices Advisory Committee (ACIP): Rabies prevention: a supplementary statement on the preexposure use of human diploid cell rabies vaccine by the intradermal route. MMWR 35:767, 1986.

Anderson LJ et al: Human rabies in the United States 1960-1979: epidemiology, diagnosis, and prevention. Ann Intern Med 100:728, 1984.

Baer GM and Fishbein DB: Rabies post-exposure prophylaxis. N Engl J Med 316:1270, 1987 (editorial).

Bernard KW and Fishbein DB: Rabies virus. In Mandell GL, Douglas RG Jr, and Bennett JE, editors: Principles and practice of infectious diseases, ed 3. New York, 1990, Wiley.

Bernard KW and Fishbein DB: Pre-exposure rabies prophylaxis for travellers: are the benefits worth the cost? Vaccine 9:833, 1991.
Brochier B et al: Large-scale eradication of rabies using recombinant vaccinia-rabies vaccine. Nature 354:520, 1991.
Centers for Disease Control: Rabies vaccine, adsorbed: a new rabies vaccine for use in humans. MMWR 37:217, 1988.
Fishbein DB: Rabies. Infect Dis Clin North Am 5:53, 1991.
Fishbein DB and Baer GM: Animal rabies: implications for diagnosis and human treatment. Ann Intern Med 109:935, 1988.
Fishbein DB et al: Administration of human diploid-cell rabies vaccine in the gluteal area. N Engl J Med 318:124, 1988 (letter).
Fu ZF et al: Rabies virus nucleoprotein expressed in and purified from insect cells is efficacious as a vaccine. Proc Natl Acad Sci USA 88:2001, 1991.
Helmick CG, Tauxe RV, and Vernon AA: Is there a risk to contacts of patients with rabies? Rev Infect Dis 9(3):511, 1987.
National Association of State Public Health Veterinarians, Inc: Compendium of animal rabies control, 1991. J Am Vet Med Assoc 198:37, 1991.
Pappaioanou M et al: Antibody response to preexposure human diploid-cell rabies vaccine given concurrently with chloroquine. N Engl J Med 314:280, 1986.
Smith JS et al: Unexplained rabies in three immigrants in the United States: a virologic investigation. N Engl J Med 324:205, 1991.

CHAPTER

248 Arenavirus Infections (Lymphocytic Choriomeningitis, Lassa Fever, Hemorrhagic Fevers), Colorado Tick Fever, and Parvovirus Infection

Charles J. Schleupner

ARENAVIRUSES

The arenaviruses are a group of single-stranded ribonucleic acid (RNA) viruses that are similar morphologically and, to a lesser extent, antigenically, indicated by complement-fixation and immunofluorescence assays. The electron-dense granules within the virion account for the name arenavirus (from the Latin *arenaceus,* meaning "sandy"). The group includes lymphocytic choriomeningitis (LCM) virus, Lassa fever virus, a group of four Lassa-like viruses from Central and South Africa, and the Tacaribe group of nine viruses. Only LCM virus, Lassa virus, and two members of the Tacaribe group, Junin and Machupo viruses, are pathogenic for humans under natural circumstances. Junin virus infection results in Argentinian hemorrhagic fever, and infection with Machupo virus produces Bolivian hemorrhagic fever. Lymphocytic choriomeningitis virus, first isolated in 1933, is the prototype of the arenavirus group.

Epidemiology

Rodents are the natural reservoirs for most of the arenaviruses, in which there is an enzootic viral cycle of replication. Human infection represents accidental transmission through rodent bites or through contact with or aerosol exposure to their excreta. Exceptions to these routes of exposure may include Lassa fever and, rarely, Argentinian or Bolivian hemorrhagic fever, for which human-to-human transmission is also believed to occur via similar mechanisms.

Lymphocytic choriomeningitis

Lymphocytic choriomeningitis virus infection occurs worldwide. Latent inapparent infection of wild and laboratory mice is the primary natural reservoir for sporadic LCM. Estimates of the virus carrier rate in mice have ranged from 4% in New York City to 27% in Washington, D.C. Isolated cases have also been related to infected dogs and guinea pigs. Syrian golden hamsters, found both in the laboratory setting and as household pets, have been epidemic sources. Lymphocytic choriomeningitis has been noted to occur less frequently in the summer months than in the other seasons of the year. This may be related to entry of field mice into homes during the colder months.

Although both acute illness, followed by recovery or death, and chronic infection are observed in rodents, persistent infection with LCM virus is not seen in humans. Furthermore, few acute cases have been studied in sufficient detail to define the pathogenesis of LCM. Because an influenza-like illness predominates at least early in the course of disease in most patients, the route of acquisition of LCM virus is assumed to be most often pulmonary, with subsequent viral replication in the respiratory epithelium. A secondary viremia is then presumed to lead to multisystem involvement, including the central nervous system, when meningitis develops. Intact cell-mediated immunity is believed to be most important for host defense and recovery, as defined in the murine model of this infection. The correlations of interferon levels with the severity of illness and the cytotoxic lymphocyte response with recovery in the mouse have not yet been established in humans.

Subclinical disease appears to be common. When symptomatic, LCM presents initially as an influenza-like illness of varying severity, with an incubation period of 5 to 12 days. The initial phase of the illness lasts 3 to 7 days. In the 25% to 50% of patients with a biphasic illness, a period of remission for 3 to 5 days then ensues and is followed by a less severe recrudescence of illness lasting another 3 to 5 days, during which clinically evident meningitis or meningoencephalitis develops in 5% to 15% of patients.

The initial influenza-like illness and the second phase of illness are typified by the signs and symptoms presented in Table 248-1. In the initial phase, myalgias are usually severe; headache, often retrobulbar, is associated with pain on eye motion. Less common complaints include testicular and parotid pain, dysesthesias, chest pain, and nonproduc-

Table 248-1. Frequency of signs and symptoms during lymphocytic choriomeningitis virus infection

Characteristics	Frequency (%)
Fever with rigors	90-100
Malaise	100
Myalgias	80-93
Headache	85
Anorexia, nausea	50-80
Photophobia	25-80
Sore throat	25-70
Arthralgias	60
Vomiting	35-40
Scalp hair loss	≤47

tive cough. Physical findings are limited to a relative bradycardia, apathy (90%), and pharyngeal injection without exudate (65%).

The second phase of the illness, though generally milder, is typified by more severe headache; other findings include varied types of skin eruptions (10% to 20%), arthritis (10% to 20%), orchitis, parotitis, alopecia, and meningeal or encephalitic signs (5% to 15%), including confusion and nuchal stiffness. Convalescence lasts 2 to 4 weeks and is characterized by easy fatigability, excessive need for sleep, and myasthenia. Recovery is usually complete, and death is rare. Encephalitis may leave neurologic residua in 25% of cases. During pregnancy, LCM may lead to spontaneous abortion or congenital infection with anomalies.

Laboratory abnormalities include leukopenia (<4000 white blood cells/mm^3 in 90% of cases), thrombocytopenia (<150,000 platelets/mm^3 in most cases), and modest elevations of serum levels of enzymes (aspartate aminotransferase [AST] and lactic dehydrogenase). Abnormalities of spinal fluid include a pleocytosis (100 to 1500/mm^3, predominantly mononuclear), an elevated protein level (50 to 300 mg/dl), and hypoglycorrhachia (25% to 50% of cases).

The diagnosis of LCM is suggested in a patient who has leukopenia and thrombocytopenia with a nonspecific, biphasic, febrile illness associated with severe myalgias. Meningeal symptoms associated with hypoglycorrhachia and a history of contact with mice or hamsters further suggest the diagnosis. The definitive diagnosis is established by LCM virus isolation from blood or cerebrospinal fluid until early in the second week of illness. Because of the impracticality of viral isolation (in experimental animals), the indirect immunofluorescent antibody test is the optimum serologic procedure for the diagnosis of acute LCM because of the rapid appearance of these antibodies and the sensitivity and specificity of this test. The complement-fixation antibody test is too insensitive, and the test for neutralizing antibody is impractical for other than epidemiologic investigations.

There is no specific therapy for LCM virus infection. Prevention of this disease relies on public education about the risks associated with pet hamsters. No vaccine is available.

Lassa fever

Since its first description in 1969, Lassa fever has been seen in many countries of West Africa, and the prevalence of seropositivity extends into Central Africa. The reservoir, a multimammate rat, is widespread throughout the African continent. This rodent remains infected for life and excretes large quantities of virus in the urine. In addition to primary human infection transmitted through direct contact and contamination of food with rodent excreta, nosocomial and community human-to-human transmission are believed to occur via close unprotected contact. In Sierra Leone, where 8% to 52% of the population is seropositive, Lassa fever has been well studied. The ratio of clinical to subclinical disease in Sierra Leone is believed to be as low as 1:4 to 1:10; this ratio may be much higher in other settings. Up to 25% of populations studied undergo seroconversion per year; however, some of these seroconversions are suspected to be reinfections, because 6% of some populations revert to seronegativity each year. Laboratory-acquired infection has also been reported. Clusters of Lassa fever cases have occurred throughout the year; illness occurs more frequently between February and May in Sierra Leone. All ages are affected, but pregnant women seem prone to severe disease, especially during the third trimester. Furthermore, Lassa fever is a common cause of septic abortion.

The pathogenesis of Lassa fever is incompletely understood. Viremia has been documented for up to 16 days after the onset of clinical disease, and its magnitude has been directly associated with fatality rates. Pathologically, the most marked findings include eosinophilic necrosis of hepatocytes without an inflammatory response; Lassa virions are found within hepatocytes. Despite these findings, the degree of hepatic necrosis is insufficient to account for death in fatal cases. Similar necrosis occurs in the spleen surrounding depleted lymphoid follicles and in the adrenal gland. Involvement of other organs is reflected by edema and variably by hemorrhage and perivascular cuffing with round cells, as well as by parenchymal inflammation.

Disseminated intravascular coagulation (DIC) is not observed commonly during Lassa fever and does not contribute to death. An inhibitor of platelet aggregation in the plasma of patients with Lassa fever has been defined between days 1 and 10 of illness; the amount of platelet inhibition is proportional to disease severity. In addition, deficient in vitro prostacyclin production by endothelial cells from infected moribund primates has been demonstrated. These reversible platelet and endothelial defects are believed to account for microcirculatory dysfunction leading to the fluid and solute loss from the intravascular compartment seen during severe Lassa fever. Plasma from patients with Lassa fever has been shown to inhibit neutrophil function during the same period of illness when platelet aggregation is also abnormal. A role for global disarray of cellular function accounting for illness severity has therefore been suggested during Lassa fever.

The severity of Lassa fever ranges from subclinical disease to a severe and progressively fatal illness. After an incubation period of 7 to 18 days, the onset of Lassa fever is insidious, with fever (peak of 39° to 41° C) and malaise present universally; these complaints are often accompanied by headache, which is predominantly frontal but persistent, and myalgias, which are frequently worse in the lumbar area. The frequency and timing of these and other signs and symptoms that develop as the disease worsens are shown in Table 248-2. Sore throat may be so severe as to cause dysphagia. Physical findings may include hypotension (80%), pharyngitis (70%) with a white patchy exudate (40%), facial and neck swelling (30%), abdominal tenderness (45%), rales, conjunctival edema and injection, a macular rash, and, less commonly, abnormal bleeding with petechiae. In mild and moderately severe cases, recovery occurs during the second and third weeks; in more severe cases associated with fatalities, the disease progresses to the development of an altered sensorium; pulmonary and peripheral edema; the accumulation of pleural, pericardial, and ascitic fluid; and hypovolemia and shock, probably as a result of diffuse capillary breakdown. During a case control study of Lassa fever in Sierra Leone, the best clinical predictor of fatality was bleeding, usually from mucosal surfaces and from the respiratory, gastrointestinal, and genitourinary tracts. Symptoms and signs may be similar in children, but in endemic areas the disease is usually mild in this age group; the most common manifestations are fever, hepatosplenomegaly, malaise, cough, and abdominal complaints. Lassa virus infection has been associated with hearing deficits of sudden onset in approximately one third of acutely ill hospitalized patients; the presence of residua after Lassa infection has been suggested by the 18% prevalence of sensorineural hearing deficits among seropositive residents of West Africa.

Laboratory findings include an early leukopenia (40%), elevated hematocrit level (due to dehydration), proteinuria (67%, often massive), azotemia, and elevated serum enzyme levels (AST, creatinine kinase). Chest radiographs have revealed patchy infiltrates or pleural effusions. Electrocardiogram findings may be consistent with myocarditis.

Table 248-2. Approximate day of onset and frequency of signs and symptoms during acute Lassa fever

Sign or symptom	Day of onset	Frequency (%)
Arthralgia (large joints)	3-4	50
Myalgia	3-4	35-65
Cough (nonproductive)	3-4	65
Headache	4-5	75
Sore throat	4-5	70
Chest pain (retrosternal, sharp)	3-4	70
Abdominal pain (crampy)	4-5	65
Vomiting	4-5	75
Diarrhea	4-5	75
Dizziness	7-21	75
Dysuria	—	35
Hearing loss	10-15	5-18

Recovery from Lassa fever is usually complete, although unilateral or bilateral deafness may be permanent. Oculogyric crisis is an occasional distinctive feature of convalescence. Many patients experience alopecia during convalescence. Although mortality rate was first reported to be 40% to 50%, more recent estimates among hospitalized patients range from 9% to 38%, suggesting a geographic variation of virulence of Lassa virus strains; the exceptions to these mortality figures are individuals who have nosocomial infections and pregnant women, who seem to be at high risk and have experienced fatality rates of 52% and 67%, respectively. The overall mortality rate among all infected patients is estimated at 1% to 2%. A useful predictor of mortality is an AST value above 150 IU per liter (55%); viremia levels greater than $10^{3.6}$ tissue culture infectious doses per milliliter have also been associated with a fatal outcome (76%).

The diagnosis of Lassa fever is suggested in a patient who has high fever, prostration, erosions or a membranous exudate in the pharynx, marked myalgias of the limbs or back, retrosternal pain, proteinuria, and a history of recent travel to West Africa; these findings in a person caring for a similarly ill patient with a history of such travel would also suggest this diagnosis. Definitive diagnosis is accomplished by isolation of Lassa virus from serum or throat washings; isolation can be attempted up to 15 days after onset of illness, but throat washings are unreliable for diagnosis. Viruria is detectable in only 3% of patients. However, attempts to isolate the virus should be made only in maximum-containment laboratories because of the high risk of working with this agent. The polymerase chain reaction has successfully been applied to both serum and urine to detect Lassa viral RNA during acute infection. Lassa antigen detection in serum by enzyme-linked immunosorbent assay (ELISA) is a rapid method for early diagnosis during acute disease. Serologic diagnosis is best performed with IgM- and IgG-specific indirect immunofluorescent or ELISA antibody testing as early as 1 to 2 weeks into the illness. The presence of IgM antibody at more than 1:4 dilution of serum or a four- to eightfold rise in IgG antibody titer level comparing acute and convalescent serum specimens would be diagnostic.

The therapy of Lassa fever is largely supportive and symptomatic; attention should be directed to careful fluid and electrolyte management. For patients with moderate or severe Lassa fever, intravenous ribavirin (or oral, though less effective) should be given for 10 days. The mortality rate is reduced in these patients from 61% to 75% if untreated to 5% to 9% with intravenous ribavirin given within 6 days of onset of fever. The treatment regimen is given in the box on p. 2020. Adverse effects are limited to a reversible anemia. Lassa immune globulin or plasma has been shown to have minimum or no effect on mortality and is not recommended. In severe Lassa fever, exchange transfusion has anecdotally been reported to reverse platelet dysfunction (apparently by removing platelet inhibitors in plasma) and to result in clinical improvement. Maintenance of strict patient isolation and scrupulous specimen-handling procedures are vital to the prevention of secondary nosoco-

Ribavirin treatment and prophylaxis for Lassa fever*

Treatment regimen (total of 10 days)
30 mg/kg iv as a loading dose, followed by
16 mg/kg iv q6h for 4 days, and
8 mg/kg iv q8h for 6 days
Prophylaxis
500 mg orally q6h for 7 days

*Centers for Disease Control phone numbers for managing patients with Lassa fever: (404) 639-1344 or (404) 639-3308.

mial cases of Lassa fever. Patients should be kept in strict isolation for 3 weeks, and known contacts should be observed for a similar period. Persons with percutaneous or mucosal exposure to materials likely to contain Lassa virus should be considered for prophylactic oral ribavirin (see the box above). Recombinant vaccinia virus vaccines containing the Lassa virus glycoprotein genome are being tested, but the persistence of Lassa viremia during clinical illness despite the presence of antibody raises concern about the potential efficacy of traditional vaccine approaches against this infection. Rodent control in dwellings is most important for prevention of Lassa fever in Africa.

Hemorrhagic fevers

Argentinian hemorrhagic fever (AHF) occurs in a progressively expanding area radiating from Buenos Aires and now covering 120,000 km^2. This enzootic infection is continuing to spread northward, involving previously unimplicated rodent species. Infection occurs primarily in male farm workers between February and August when a wound is contaminated with urine from a chronically infected field mouse. Mucosal contamination with virus-contaminated airborne dust is another potential mechanism for acquisition. Transmission via contaminated foods also seems likely. Approximately 12% of the population in the endemic area is seropositive, with one of every three infections being subclinical. Thus almost 90% of the population remains susceptible. A mean of 360 cases per year has been seen for the last 5 years. Although Bolivian hemorrhagic fever (BHF) is less common in recent years because of improved rodent control, a few cases occur annually. The likely routes of transmission of BHF are similar to those of AHF.

The pathogenesis of both AHF and BHF is poorly understood. Initial viral replication in tissue phagocyte organs, especially in monocytes (macrophages), with a secondary viremia and ensuing capillary lesions, is believed to be important in AHF. Complement activation is involved in the early stages of AHF, but consistent evidence for involvement of immune complexes in its pathogenesis has been lacking. Other documented abnormalities include thrombocytopenia, presence of a concomitant plasma inhibitor of platelet aggregation (possibly interrelating with observed perturbations of the membrane calcium and sodium/potassium adenosine triphosphate (ATP)–dependent pumps), prolonged partial thromboplastin time, and low factor VIII:C activity without evidence of DIC. Endogenous alpha-interferon levels have been directly associated with fever, chills, and backache during AHF and inversely correlated with recovery. Generalized vasocongestion with hemorrhage is noted as a pathologic finding with bone marrow depletion in severe cases.

The clinical features of AHF and BHF are similar. After an incubation period of 5 to 19 days, AHF (or BHF) appears with gradual onset of fever, chills, malaise, severe myalgia, headache, dizziness, retro-ocular pain, anorexia, nausea and vomiting, and cutaneous hypoesthesia. The physical findings include toxicity, conjunctival injection, cutaneous and mucosal rashes, adenopathy, and mucosal petechiae. In BHF, nosebleed and gastrointestinal bleeding occur early in the disease. Toward the end of the first week of the illness, clinical findings worsen, with the development of hypotension, relative bradycardia, and oliguria. In severe cases, shock, neurologic abnormalities, hypothermia, a bleeding diathesis, and, in fatal cases, a capillary leak syndrome supervene. In individual cases, the findings are primarily either hemorrhagic or neurologic. Convalescence in either disease begins at 10 to 15 days of illness and is often marked by alopecia. Fatality rates vary from 5% to 30%, averaging 16% in AHF.

Laboratory findings include leukopenia (neutropenia with AHF), thrombocytopenia, proteinuria, and depressed levels of selected complement components and some clotting factors. Diminished plasminogen activity has been detected during AHF. Absolute numbers of B and T lymphocytes, as well as T helper and T suppressor cells, are decreased; mononuclear leukocyte mitogen responses are also depressed during acute illness. Humoral antibody is not detected until as late as 3 weeks after onset. Possibly related to these immunologic changes and neutropenia are secondary bacterial pulmonary infections, which have been noted during AHF. There is no evidence of DIC or immune complex disease during either illness. Electrocardiographic findings are consistent with myocarditis.

The diagnosis of AHF or BHF is suggested by the epidemiologic and clinical history. Viral isolation from blood, throat washings, or urine during the acute illness establishes the diagnosis. In up to 96% of patients with AHF, Junin virus has been isolated from peripheral blood mononuclear cells by cocultivation with vero cells. A fourfold rise of the neutralizing, indirect immunofluorescent, or complement-fixation antibody titer against Junin or Machupo virus also supports the diagnosis of AHF or BHF, respectively.

The therapy of AHF and BHF is supportive. The mortality rate is reduced to 2% or less when immune plasma is given within 8 days of disease onset; the dose of immune plasma should provide more than 3000 therapeutic units of neutralizing antibody per kilogram. However, although these reports of therapeutic benefit are promising, in an alarming 10% of treated patients cerebellar dysfunction developed 4 to 6 weeks after recovery. This postimmunotherapy neurologic syndrome is manifested by fever, dizziness, ataxia, nystagmus, diplopia, headache, dysarthria, and vomiting; it resolves in 1 to 3 months, but mild, permanent abnormalities of auditory-evoked responses have recently been described. Preliminary results of therapy for late, severe AHF with ribavirin are encouraging.

Prevention of both AHF and BHF is presently limited to improved rodent control. However, the 90% seronegativity to Junin virus among the Argentine population underscores the need for an effective vaccine for AHF. Optimism can be derived from the success of a candidate glycoprotein subunit vaccine for AHF in guinea pigs. A live, attenuated Junin virus vaccine (Candid 1) is currently undergoing clinical tests. Tacaribe virus, a nonpathogen for humans, has also been proposed as a human vaccine candidate agent because of its broad cross reactivity with Junin virus.

COLORADO TICK FEVER

Colorado tick fever (CTF) is a benign viral infection transmitted by ticks that occurs primarily in the western mountainous regions of the United States and Canada. Because the early clinical syndromes of CTF and the rickettsial disease Rocky Mountain spotted fever (North American tick typhus) are similar, the two diseases are often confused (Chapter 256).

Classification and characteristics

Colorado tick fever virus, a double-stranded RNA virus, is a member of the family Reoviridae and the *Orbivirus* genus because of its biochemical, serologic, and electron microscopic properties. Its taxonomic status as an orbivirus has recently been questioned because of the number of segments (12) in its RNA genome. The virus is stable at 4° C for up to 16 months in clotted blood. It is usually isolated from human plasma or erythrocytes by subinoculation into suckling mice.

Epidemiology

The geographic occurrence of CTF is determined by the presence of its primary vector, the hardshelled wood tick *Dermacentor andersoni,* and its definitive hosts and reservoirs, including the golden-mantled ground squirrel, the chipmunk, and other mammals. The virus has been identified in Colorado, Idaho, Nevada, Utah, Wyoming, and Montana; in the eastern sections of Washington, Oregon, and California; in the northern portions of Arizona and New Mexico; and in Alberta and British Columbia. Reports of CTF virus isolation from ticks on Long Island remain unconfirmed. Antibody to CTF virus (or a CTF-like virus) has recently been demonstrated in mammals from western California, where a viral isolate similar or identical to CTF virus has also been recovered from a rabbit. This area is outside the known distribution of *D. andersoni* and the common mammalian hosts of CTF virus. Therefore CTF may be a more widespread zoonosis than was previously suspected. Furthermore, because a few documented human infections from western California have occurred, additional possible vectors and/or mechanisms of transmission of CTF to humans are now being considered.

During the spring and summer months, viral replication results from transmission between larval or nymphal ticks and small rodents during the life cycle of the virus. These rodents also serve as reservoirs because of their protracted viremia, which lasts up to several months. In this way, they may contribute to overwintering of the virus. After molting to the adult stage, ticks feed on large mammals, including humans, who become incidental "dead-end" hosts. The virus is carried transstadially (not transovarially), and, after hibernation, infected nymphs reinitiate the cycle during the following spring.

Most cases of CTF occur between April and August, with the peak incidence in May and June. The several hundred cases reported annually probably represent a significant underestimate of true disease incidence. Although up to 90% of patients relate tick exposure, only 50% may report an actual tick bite. Because of occupational exposure outdoors, most cases occur in males less than 60 years of age.

Pathogenesis

After human inoculation via tick bite, CTF virus causes no local cutaneous reaction, and the mechanism and site(s) of early replication are unknown. Virus can be detected free in serum or plasma, usually during the first week of illness and occasionally during the second week. Intraerythrocytic viremia then appears, and peak titers are achieved during the second and third week of illness. The virus has been occasionally isolated from erythrocytes for up to 101 days after the onset of clinical illness, and viral antigen has been shown to persist in circulating erythrocytes for up to 135 days. Prolonged viremia is believed to be related to viral replication within infected erythropoietic precursors as they differentiate, resulting in protection of intraerythrocytic virus from humoral antibody. Transfusion-associated CTF has been documented.

Symptoms of central nervous system, pulmonary, pericardial, testicular, dermal, and ocular involvement during CTF suggest the potential for pantropism (ability to infect any tissue) of this virus in humans. Some of these manifestations may be immunologically mediated. Recent work does document a relationship of serum interferon levels to body temperature elevation. Despite evidence for murine teratogenicity, CTF has not been clearly related to human fetal abnormalities.

Clinical disease

Asymptomatic illness is infrequent. In 3 to 6 days after a tick bite, most patients experience a sudden onset of fever, with chills, lethargy, headache (usually retrobulbar), and myalgias, which primarily affect the extremities and back. Although these complaints are nonspecific, other complaints are less common and more variable: vomiting, abdominal pain, diarrhea, stiff neck, vertigo, and sore throat. The acute illness often lasts 7 to 10 days. After 2 to 3 days, fever often remits, leaving the patient very weak, only to recur within another 2 to 3 days. This biphasic, "saddle-back" fever pattern occurs in 50% of patients and is virtually diagnostic of CTF in the correct epidemiologic setting. Rash, when present, is commonly macular or maculopapular and is usually located on the trunk. When the rash is petechial, it is often peripherally located. Conjunctival injection may accompany fever. Palpable splenomegaly may occur. Unusual but potentially severe complications in children include encephalitis, meningitis, and meningoencephalitis. Pericarditis, pleuritis, myocarditis, orchitis, and bleeding diathesis are rare.

Leukopenia (fewer than 4500 white blood cells/mm^3 and often 2000 to 3000 white blood cells/mm^3) is the most consistent and diagnostically helpful laboratory finding, occurring in two thirds of patients with confirmed disease early in the course. Lymphocytes and granulocytes are usually equally affected. Mild to marked thrombocytopenia may be seen. Neurologic involvement is often associated with cerebrospinal fluid lymphocytosis (fewer than 500 white blood cells/mm^3).

Recovery from CTF is eventually complete, with resultant lifelong immunity. Fifty percent or more of the patients, especially adults over 30 years old, experience a prolonged convalescence, with asthenia that is unrelated to persistent viremia. Occasional residua have been reported after CTF accompanied by neurologic syndromes. Infection during pregnancy is usually benign.

Diagnosis

The differential diagnostic considerations include dengue fever, Rocky Mountain spotted fever, ehrlichiosis, and viral meningitides, arboviral encephalitides, and tick paralysis when neurologic involvement is evident. Because of the nonspecificity of the clinical manifestations of CTF, a specific diagnosis requires isolation of the virus from serum (or plasma), blood clot, or cerebrospinal fluid. In addition to viral isolation, viral antigen may be demonstrated in erythrocytes with a direct fluorescent antibody test for prolonged periods into convalescence. The direct fluorescent antibody test is not usually positive before the sixth day of illness. The indirect fluorescent antibody method for detecting antibodies to CTF virus becomes positive earliest and is the most sensitive serologic test for the diagnosis of this disease. Neutralizing antibodies are delayed in appearance. Complement-fixing antibodies also appear slowly and are present in only 75% of patients.

Treatment and prevention

The therapy of CTF is symptomatic. Prevention relies on public education concerning avoidance of tick-infested areas and use of protective clothing and insect repellents. The use of experimental inactivated and live attenuated vaccines is limited because of the small number of persons routinely exposed. Patients should be restricted from serving as blood donors for 5 to 6 months after the illness. Avoidance of aspirin for symptomatic therapy in children seems advisable because of the bleeding tendencies seen among patients with CTF in this age group.

PARVOVIRUS INFECTIONS

The parvoviruses are one of three genera in the family Parvoviridae, which includes the dependoviruses (including human adeno-associated virus) and densoviruses (of insects). The parvoviruses were thought to be pathogens of a broad range of nonhuman vertebrate hosts until 1975, when Cossart identified a parvovirus-like structure in the sera of persons being screened for hepatitis B antigen. One of these sera was identified as B19, a designation that remains for this virus, subsequently identified by French, British, and Japanese investigators. B19 was first associated with symptomatic human infection in 1980. Subsequently it was linked with aplastic crises in patients with sickle cell disease in 1981, with erythema infectiosum and stillbirths in 1984, and with arthritis in 1985. Its clinical relevance is now well established.

Parvovirus B19 is a small, nonenveloped single-stranded deoxyribonucleic acid (DNA) virus with a host range limited to humans. It is difficult to propagate in culture, requiring human erythroid bone marrow cells and exogenous erythroprotein. The major source of viral antigen for antibody assays is the serum of infected patients with hemolytic disorders or immunocompromise. B19 inhibits erythroid colony formation by infecting progenitor cells of the erythroid series. The virus probably also replicates in other tissues, including fetal myocardial cells and possibly peripheral blood leukocytes.

The most common clinical forms of B19 infection, erythema infectiosum (EI) and aplastic crisis (AC), occur in school-age children (see box below). The age distribution of cases in one outbreak is depicted in Table 248-3. Although there is no gender bias among primary cases, previously uninfected mothers within households more frequently acquire secondary cases of EI than fathers, presum-

Clinical and hematologic sequellae of parvovirus B19 infection

1. Acute infection
   - Erythema infectiosum (with reticulocytopenia, lymphopenia, neutropenia, and/or thrombocytopenia)
   - Aplastic crisis (in patients with an abnormality of erythrocytes resulting in increased turnover)
   - Fetal infection and anemia leading to hydrops fetalis and spontaneous abortion (low risk)
2. Postinfectious complications
   - Arthritis/arthralgia
   - Purpura
3. Chronic syndrome
   - Chronic bone marrow suppression in immune compromised hosts
   - ?Fibromyalgia

Table 248-3. Age distribution of cases of erythema infectiosum during an outbreak

Age groups (years)	Percentage of cases
<5	10%
5 to <15	70%
≥15	20%

Modified from Lauer BA et al: Am J Dis Child 130:252, 1976.

ably as a result of closer contact with an infected child. The risk of secondary case acquisition within households ranges from 15% to 50%; the inverse relationship of risk for secondary cases to their age suggests a protective role for antibody, because 40% to 60% of adults over 20 years of age are seropositive. When arthritis is part of the clinical presentation, adult women are most often affected.

Additional epidemiologic settings for B19 transmission, other than child-to-child contact in schools and play settings, include pediatric wards, day care centers, and classrooms when several adults and children may be exposed in the same setting. In each of these circumstances, susceptible adults (up to 50%) may be exposed, leading to the potential for more consequential infection, especially in the pregnant female. B19 transmission and infection have also been documented by transfusion of pooled coagulation factor concentrates but rarely after single donor transfusion.

Parvovirus B19 is believed to be spread by respiratory droplets. During volunteer studies, B19 DNA has been detected in respiratory secretions from 7 to 11 days after intranasal inoculation, with concomitant viremia, fever, malaise, and pruritis.

During the second week of experimental infection, IgM antibody appears, when no peripheral reticulocytes are detected and mild neutropenia, lymphopenia, and thrombocytopenia are found. The subsequent rash develops on days 17 or 18, after secretions have become negative for viral DNA. Hematologic abnormalities resolve by the third week after infection. It is presumed, therefore, that B19 infection, after respiratory exposure, results in the rash of EI at a time when the patient is briefly or no longer infectious by the respiratory route. If arthritis develops, it often accompanies the rash during the third week after infection, as the IgG antibody response appears, suggesting an immune complex mechanism for the arthropathy.

Erythema infectiosum (or fifth disease) was recognized as a distinct entity in 1896 among a group of pediatric exanthems that had been numbered, including rubeola, scarlet fever, rubella, and roseola; its cause remained unrecognized until 1983-84. EI usually occurs in outbreaks during late winter and spring. After exposure the incubation period for EI is 4 to 14 days, followed by the sudden onset of a "slapped cheek" appearance (50% to 100% of cases of EI during outbreaks), with evolution to a lacy generalized maculopapular rash on extremities and trunk. A prodrome of fever, coryza, malaise, and sore throat may precede the rash in 20% to 60% of cases. The generalized rash typically waxes and wanes with varied stimuli, including irritation, bathing, stress, sunlight, and temperature change. This rash persists or recurs over less than 10 days in 55% of patients, for more than 20 days in 15%, and for more than 80 days in 1% or less of patients. The truncal rash may be varied in appearance: morbilliform, circinate, confluent, papular, vesicular, or purpuric. Despite the rash, most children with EI feel well and have only a low-grade fever; pruritis may also complicate the course.

Results of most laboratory studies during acute EI are normal, with the exception of the previously mentioned hematologic abnormalities. In up to 80% of adults with EI arthralgias/arthritis develops, more commonly in women, usually after the rash; the peripheral joints, especially the small joints of the hands, the knees, wrists, ankles, feet, and elbows, are primarily affected symmetrically. The pain is moderately severe but typically resolves in 2 to 4 weeks, occasionally lasting several months or years. The syndrome may mimic seronegative rheumatoid arthritis or Lyme disease. B19 infection may cause some cases of fibromyalgia.

By using IgG antibody seroconversion or development of an acute IgM antibody to define infection, studies have demonstrated that in over half of those infected rash does not develop; 17% to 25% are asymptomatic; and the remainder of those without rash experience systemic, gastrointestinal, or respiratory symptoms.

After the initial descriptions of the association of B19 with AC, a number of subsequent studies have concluded that B19 is the cause of 90% or more of AC in patients with increased red blood cell turnover (Chapter 90).

These settings include hemolytic anemias caused by hemoglobinopathies, pyruvate kinase deficiency, hereditary spherocytosis and stomatocytosis, and various acquired hemolytic disorders. Chronic bone marrow suppression may also occur in B19-infected patients with acquired immunodeficient states produced by hematologic malignancy, connective tissue disorders, and human immunodeficiency virus 1 (HIV-1), as well as in apparently normal individuals. Most of these patients relate a viral prodrome, followed by development of weakness and pallor. The severity of the anemia parallels the hemolytic process; the mechanism is presumed to involve B19 infection and inhibition of erythroid precursors. Children and presumably adults with AC may be particularly infectious because of the absence of rash during viral excretion at, before, or for 1 week or more after onset of disease. Virus appears to be present in large quantities in both blood and respiratory secretions.

B19 infection of pregnant women has become a concern since reports of fetal hydrops and death after maternal infection appeared. The virus seems to cause fetal anemia, resulting in heart failure in the fetus. However, no fetal anomalies after maternal B19 infection have been documented. Overall, B19 is an infrequent cause of fetal infection or spontaneous abortion. The risk of B19-related fetal death has been estimated at 1% to 2% for an exposure of a woman without known serologic status within the first 20 weeks of gestation in the household setting; this risk in the occupational setting is estimated at less than 1%. There is no risk estimate for women exposed after 20 weeks of gestation. The American Academy of Pediatrics has recommended that a pregnant (seronegative) women not care for a patient with AC, because such patients may be very contagious.

The diagnosis of parvovirus B19 infection is complicated by the lack of a ready source of viral antigen. However, an enzyme immunoassay (EIA) and a radioimmunoassay (RIA) have been adapted using antibody capture techniques with amplification to detect both IgM and IgG antibodies and viral antigen. The EIA has been shown to be both sensitive and specific (Table 248-4). The IgM assay is the most sensitive for detection of recent infection, but IgM antibody may persist for up to 6 months. Newer EIAs have utilized synthetic viral peptides as antigen with promising results.

Successful use of very sensitive assays for viral DNA has been recently reported. These assays use hybridization of viral DNA probes and the polymerase chain reaction. Viral DNA may persist for up to 2 months after the onset of clinical illness. B19 may be identified in tissues by detection of intranuclear inclusions in formalin-fixed tissues, which are not evident in routinely processed, air-dried preparations. Electron microscopic examination of infected tissues may reveal parvovirus-like particles for diagnostic purposes.

There is no treatment for acute EI, other than symptomatic management. In the adult with arthralgias/arthritis, nonsteroidal anti-inflammatory agents are of value. For patients with AC or chronic B19 infection, immune serum globulin has been of value in some cases.

Currently there is no vaccine to prevent B19 infection. Because most patients with acute B19 infection are no longer infectious when clinical symptoms occur, prevention of transmission is not feasible. Patients with AC or chronic B19 infection may be infectious and should be managed in the hospital setting with respiratory isolation (in addition to universal blood and body fluid precautions). Pregnant women should be educated about the potential risks of caring for such patients and about preventive measures; they can be given the option of not providing care for such patients. Immunoglobulin prophylaxis after exposure of a pregnant women to a patient with EI or AC has been suggested as a possible course of action without data for efficacy.

Table 248-4. IgM and IgG antibody responses to parvovirus B19 infection detected by enzyme immunoassay according to day after onset of illness

Day after onset	Percentage of patients positive	
	IgM	IgG
0-2	78	42
3-7	93	90
8-28	93	100
29-56	74	94
57-112	74	91
>112	67	100

Modified from Anderson RD et al: Pediatr Infect Dis 2:243, 1983.

REFERENCES

Arenavirus Infections

Carballal G et al: Tacaribe virus: a new alternative for Argentine hemorrhagic fever vaccine. J Med Virol 23:257, 1987.

Centers for Disease Control: Management of patients with suspected viral hemorrhagic fever. MMWR 37(suppl S3):1, 1988.

Cummins D: Acute sensorineural deafness in Lassa fever. JAMA 264:2093, 1990.

Enria DA et al: Importance of dose of neutralizing antibodies in treatment of Argentine hemorrhagic fever with immune plasma. Lancet 2:255, 1984.

Enria DA et al: Current status of the treatment of Argentine hemorrhagic fever. Med Microbiol Immunol 175:173, 1986.

Enria DA et al: Preliminary report—tolerance and antiviral effect of ribavirin in patients with Argentine hemorrhagic fever. Antiviral Res 7:353, 1987.

Frame JD: Clinical features of Lassa fever in Liberia. Rev Infect Dis 11(suppl 4):S783, 1989.

Helmick CG et al: No evidence for increased risk of Lassa fever infection in hospital staff. Lancet 2:1202, 1986.

Huggins JW: Prospects for treatment of viral hemorrhagic fevers with ribavirin, a broad-spectrum antiviral drug. Rev Infect Dis 11(suppl 4):S750, 1989.

Johnson KM et al: Clinical virology of Lassa fever in hospitalized patients. J Infect Dis 155:456, 1987.

Levis SC et al: Endogenous interferon in Argentine hemorrhagic fever. J Infect Dis 149(3):428, 1984.

McCormick JB et al: Lassa fever—effective therapy with ribavirin. N Engl J Med 134(1):20, 1986.

McCormick JB et al: A case-control study of the clinical diagnosis and course of Lassa fever. J Infect Dis 155:455, 1987.

McCormick JB et al: A prospective study of the epidemiology and ecology of Lassa fever. J Infect Dis 155:437, 1987.

Molinas FC et al: Hemostasis and the complement system in Argentine hemorrhagic fever. Rev Infect Dis 11(suppl 4):S762, 1989.

Peters CJ et al: Pathogenesis of viral hemorrhagic fevers: Rift Valley fever and Lassa fever contrasted. Rev Infect Dis 11(suppl 4):S743, 1989.

Vanzee BE et al: Lymphocytic choriomeningitis in university hospital personnel—clinical features. Am J Med 58:803, 1975.

Walker DH et al: Pathologic and virologic study of fatal Lassa fever in man. Am J Pathol 107(3):349, 1982.

Weissenbacher MC et al: Argentine hemorrhagic fever. Curr Top Microbiol Immunol 134:79, 1987.

Colorado Tick Fever

Andersen RD: Colorado tick fever and tick paralysis in a young child. Pediatr Infect Dis 2:243, 1983.

Ater JL et al: Circulating interferon and clinical symptoms in Colorado tick fever. J Infect Dis 151(5):966, 1985.

Ellison RT III: Colorado tick fever or ehrlichiosis. JAMA 258:1731, 1987.

Emmons RW: Ecology of Colorado tick fever. Annu Rev Microbiol 42:49, 1988.

Goodpasture HC et al: Colorado tick fever: clinical, epidemiologic, and laboratory aspects of 228 cases in Colorado in 1973. Ann Intern Med 88:303, 1978.

Lane RS et al: Survey for evidence of Colorado tick fever virus outside of the known endemic area in California. Am J Trop Med Hyg 31:837, 1982.

Spruance SL and Bailey A: Colorado tick fever—a review of 115 laboratory confirmed cases. Arch Intern Med 131:288, 1973.

Parvovirus Infection

Anderson LJ: Human parvoviruses. J Infect Dis 161:603, 1990.

Anderson LJ et al: Detection of antibodies and antigens of human parvovirus B19 by enzyme-linked immunosorbent assay. J Clin Microbiol 24:522, 1986.

Cartter ML et al: Occupational risk factors for infection with parvovirus B19 among pregnant women. J Infect Dis 163:282, 1991.
Centers for Disease Control: Risks associated with human parvovirus B19 infection. MMWR 38:81, 1989.
Erdman DD et al: Human parvovirus B19 specific IgG, IgA, and IgM antibodies and DNA in serum specimens from persons with erythema infectiosum. J Med Virol 35:110, 1991.
Frickhofen N et al: Persistent B19 parvovirus infection in patients infected with human immunodeficiency virus type I (HIV-1): a treatable cause of anemia in AIDS. Ann Intern Med 113:926, 1990.
Gillespie SM et al: Occupational risk of human parvovirus B19 infection for school and day-care personnel during an outbreak of erythema infectiosum. JAMA 263:2061, 1990.
Harris JW: Parvovirus B19 for the hematologist. Am J Hematol 39:119, 1992.
Koch WC et al: Manifestations and treatment of human parvovirus B19 infection in immunocompromised patients. J Pediatr 116:355, 1990.
Kurtzman G et al: Pure red-cell aplasia of 10 years' duration due to persistent parvovirus B19 infection and its cure with immunoglobulin therapy. N Engl J Med 321:519, 1989.
Lauer BA et al: Erythema infectiosum: an elementary school outbreak. Am J Dis Child 130:252, 1976.
Naides SJ et al: Rheumatologic manifestations of human parvovirus B19 infection in adults. Arthritis Rheum 33:1297, 1990.
Plotkin SA et al: Parvovirus, erythema infectiosum and pregnancy. Pediatrics 85:131, 1990.
Plummer FA et al: An erythema infectiosum–like illness caused by human parvovirus infection. N Engl J Med 313:74, 1985.

CHAPTER

249 Bunyavirus and Togavirus Infections (Viral Encephalitis and Dengue and Yellow Fever)

Jerome F. Hruska

The arthropod-borne animal viruses (arboviruses) have been taxonomically classified into several families. The majority belong to either the Togaviridae or Bunyaviridae families and cause such clinical disease syndromes as viral encephalitis, yellow fever, dengue fever, and hemorrhagic fever.

CLASSIFICATION

The *International Catalogue of Arboviruses* lists over 350 candidates. Ten genus-level taxa are required for classification, although most arboviruses belong to three genera in either the Togaviridae (alphavirus and flavivirus) or Bunyaviridae families. The major viruses responsible for human disease, which are discussed in this chapter, are shown in Table 249-1, according to both the new and old classifications.

Table 249-1. Classification of selected arboviruses

Family	Genus	Old arbovirus group	Species
Togaviridae	Alphavirus	A	Eastern equine encephalitis
			Western equine encephalitis
			Venezuelan equine encephalitis
			Chikungunya
			O'Nyong-nyong
			Sindbis
	Flavivirus	B	Dengue fever types 1-4
			St. Louis encephalitis
			Yellow fever
			Powassan encephalitis
			Russian spring-summer encephalitis
			West Nile encephalitis
			Japanese B encephalitis
Bunyaviridae	Bunyavirus	C	California encephalitis viruses
			Subtypes: California encephalitis La-Crosse, Tahyna
			Rift Valley fever

CHARACTERISTICS

The togaviruses and bunyaviruses are spherical particles bound by a host-derived lipoprotein envelope with virus-specified glycoprotein projections from their surfaces. Each family contains more than 70 members, each slightly variable one from the other. All possess hemagglutinins and are destroyed by lipid solvents such as ether. The togaviruses are relatively heat-unstable, losing most of their infectivity if incubated at 60° C for half an hour. Although a great deal of size variation occurs, the bunyaviruses are larger (90 to 100 nm) than the togaviruses (40 to 70 nm).

The nucleic acids of both families of viruses are ribonucleic acid (RNA), but the genome of the togaviruses consists of a continuous single strand (42S) that is infectious when extracted from the virion. The bunyaviruses, however, have a segmented genome composed of single strands of RNA (32S, 26S, and 16S) that are not infectious after extraction. An RNA polymerase has been reported in the virions of the bunyaviruses, which synthesize messenger RNA using the virion RNA as template.

The morphogenesis of the arboviruses is not uniform even within genera, but all mature in the cytoplasm. For example, in the Togaviridae family, the alphaviruses form nucleocapsids intracellularly and usually acquire a peripheral coat by budding through the cell membrane. Flaviviruses mature on internal cytoplasmic membranes. Bunyaviruses also form by budding into intracellular vesicles, especially those of the Golgi complex. Release of flaviviruses and bunyaviruses from the cell is believed to occur by either exocytosis or cell lysis.

EPIDEMIOLOGY

Mosquitoes are the predominant arthropod vector for most arbovirus infections, with the exception of Powassan and Russian spring-summer encephalitides, which are caused by ticks. Table 249-2 lists the common vectors, hosts, and geographic areas of arbovirus infection. The mosquito acquires the infection by ingesting the blood of a viremic host. The virus rapidly infects most tissues of the mosquito, eventually multiplying in the salivary glands. The mosquito's bite remains infectious for the lifetime of the insect in many instances. The time from the initial blood meal until virus is produced in the salivary glands is called the extrinsic incubation period; during this period, the arthropod cannot transmit the infection by bite. The mosquito subsequently

Table 249-2. Epidemiology of selected arboviruses

Virus	Vector*	Normal host	Geographic range	Vector habitat
Group A				
Eastern equine encephalitis	Culiseta melanura and various Aëdes species	Birds	Eastern United States; rarely, Caribbean	Coastal freshwater hardwood swamps
Western equine encephalitis	Culex tarsalis (western United States)	Birds	Predominantly western United States	Agricultural irrigation projects among others
	Culiseta melanura (Eastern United States	Birds		
Venezuelan equine encephalitis	Culex	Water birds, rodents, equine	Southern United States (Everglades), Central America, South America	Freshwater swamps and slow-moving bodies of water
Group B				
Dengue	Aëdes aegypti	Humans	Caribbean and Central America, Mexico, South Pacific, Australia, Southeast Asia, Hawaii	Tropical-subtropical urban areas
Japanese B encephalitis	Culex tritaeniorhyncus	Birds (pigs)	Eastern Asia, Japan, Korea, Siberia, Taiwan	
Murray Valley encephalitis	Culex annulirostris and others	Birds	Australia	
Powassan encephalitis	Ixodes cookei	Rodents	Northern United States, Canada	
Russian spring-summer encephalitis	Ixodes ricinus and I. persulcatus	Forest mammals (occasionally birds)	Northern Europe, Russia	Forest regions
St. Louis encephalitis	Culex tarsalis, Culex pipiens, Culex nigripalps, and others	Birds	Western Hemisphere	
Yellow fever				
Urban	Aëdes aegypti	Humans	South America, Caribbean islands, Africa	Urban areas predominantly, although A. aegypti in Africa can be both domestic and wild
Sylvan	Aëdes species	Simian species	South America, Africa	Jungle canopy, ground-level clearings, and jungle residence
Group C				
Bunyavirus				
California encephalitis	Aëdes melanimon	Ground squirrels	United States	
LaCrosse subtype	Aëdes triseriatus	Chipmunks, squirrels	North central and northeastern United States	Tree holes or breeding sites
Hantaan	Aerosolized excreta	Fieldmouse	Eastern Asia Eastern Europe	Farmers and military in fields
Phlebotomus fever viruses	Phlebotomus sandfly species	Not identified	Mediterranean, Middle East, India, Pakistan	Sandy areas near ground level

Modified from Downs WG: In Evans AS, editor: Viral infections of humans. New York, 1979, Plenum.
*All are mosquito vectors except the tick ixodes.

bites another vertebrate, and a second round of infection is established. In many cases, the vertebrate hosts appear healthy and unaffected (e.g., birds in western equine encephalitis [WEE]), whereas in others, illness and death result (e.g., simian species in sylvan yellow fever; horses in Venezuelan equine encephalitis [VEE]).

Except for dengue and urban yellow fever, most of these viruses cause zoonoses among wild animals, and humans are incidental rather than primary hosts.

Yellow fever has two epidemiologic patterns: (1) the sylvan (endemic or enzootic) cycle, in which several mosquito species spread the disease among forest-dwelling primates and humans are only incidentally infected, and (2) the urban (epidemic) cycle, in which spread occurs from human to human via an infected Aëdes aegypti mosquito after an 8 to 12 day extrinsic incubation period. Dengue is transmitted exclusively from human to human by Aëdes mosquitoes.

Summer is the main period of activity of arboviruses in temperate regions. The incidence of reported encephalitis cases and that of arthropod-borne encephalitis is highest in the summer months, although in a large number of encephalitis cases, no etiologic diagnosis is made. The higher level of activity in the summer corresponds to the increased mosquito population. Elimination of the mosquito vector by either insect control or cold weather terminates an epidemic. In tropical zones, the disease may occur endemically year round, with increased activity in the rainy season, when mosquito numbers increase.

The demographic distribution of disease caused by these viruses is shown in Table 249-2. It should be noted that several indigenous cases of dengue fever have been reported in Texas. In addition, a newly introduced A. albopictus mosquito vector has established itself in northern as well as southern states; thus the potential for more indigenous transmission by both the A. aegypti and A. albopictus vectors exists.

PATHOPHYSIOLOGY

Encephalitis viruses

The lesions produced by St. Louis encephalitis, WEE, eastern equine encephalitis (EEE), and VEE are sufficiently similar that morphologic examination cannot be used for identification. The experimental model of VEE in mice is cited to generalize the events that follow infection with the arboviruses that cause encephalitis.

Within 24 hours, virus is detected in the blood and peripheral tissues, such as lymph nodes, bone marrow, spleen, lung, liver, and most other organs. Whether or not some of these sites represent accumulation of virus by filtration in blood-rich organs is unknown. At 2 days, marked lymphocyte destruction and lymph node necrosis are observed. On the fourth day, the lymph nodes are extensively destroyed and replaced by macrophages, the bone marrow is depleted, and megakaryocyte nuclei and cytoplasm are degenerating, yet minimum encephalitis is seen. As the virus titer level in the peripheral tissues decreases, the titer in the brain increases, eventually surpassing levels in other tissues. At 6 days, the brain (predominantly the gray matter), spinal cord, and meninges are extensively involved with severe lymphocytic perivascular cuffing, marked gliosis, and neuronal necrosis.

Primary dengue fever

After an incubation period of 5 to 8 days after a bite by infected mosquitoes, a fever and viremia with as many as 10^6 human infectious doses per milliliter develop. A maculopapular rash appears 3 to 4 days later. A skin biopsy shows endothelial cell swelling, perivascular edema, and mononuclear cell infiltrates. Type-specific antibody to the infecting dengue type develops, conferring long-term autologous protection; reinfection with another serotype can occur.

Dengue hemorrhagic fever and dengue shock syndrome

Dengue hemorrhagic fever and dengue shock syndrome are primarily seen in south and southeast Asia in children, most of whom are between 3 and 6 years of age and have been infected a second time with dengue virus. These diseases are also seen in children 7 to 8 months of age born to mothers who have pre-existing dengue antibodies. Most geographic areas where these syndromes are seen have endemic disease with two or more serotypes of dengue. These data suggest, but do not prove, that dengue hemorrhagic fever and dengue shock syndrome may be due to an immune complex disease that occurs after a second infection with a different dengue serotype. Various complement components, fibrinogen, and platelet counts are depressed, suggesting complement activation and consumptive coagulopathy.

Petechial hemorrhages in many tissues are seen in fatal cases, along with vasodilatation, congestion, and edema. Gastrointestinal hemorrhages may produce hematemesis and melena.

Yellow fever virus

In yellow fever, the greatest damage is found in the liver, kidney, heart, and gastrointestinal tract. The highest concentration of virus is in the liver and bone marrow, with lesser amounts in the kidney and mesenteric lymph nodes, according to measurements done in rhesus monkeys.

The liver demonstrates a characteristic lack of inflammatory cells, even in severe cases, in which there may be acute coagulative necrosis of the midzonal portion of the liver lobule, with formation of intracellular hyaline deposits called Councilman bodies. Liver function tests and prolonged prothrombin time are abnormal. The kidney also lacks inflammatory cells. The proximal tubules exhibit cloudy swelling and fatty degeneration and are filled with granular debris. The renal failure in yellow fever has been attributed to hemoglobinuric nephrosis. The heart, when involved, is flabby and pale with scattered pericardial petechial hemorrhages. Myocardial fiber degeneration is seen microscopically. Clinically these patients have vascular collapse. Gastrointestinal hemorrhage is such a frequent event in yellow fever that the disease was often known as "black vomit" because of the hematemesis from many oozing gastrointestinal petechiae. Hemorrhages may also be found in the mucous membranes and skin.

CLINICAL MANIFESTATIONS

The patterns of clinical syndromes in arbovirus infection are shown in Tables 249-3 and 249-4. Arbovirus infections in most cases are asymptomatic; seroconversion is the only evidence of contact (Table 249-5).

Encephalitis viruses

Few distinguishing characteristics allow an etiologic diagnosis of an arbovirus infection on clinical grounds alone. Clinical presentations may include a mild, undifferentiated febrile illness or a syndrome indistinguishable from influenza. The common clinical signs and symptoms of encephalitis include fever, headache, vomiting, nuchal rigidity, alteration in consciousness, lethargy, and convulsions (Chapter 233). Physical findings include neck stiffness, with a positive Kernig's sign. Pathologic reflexes, generalized muscular weakness, and paralysis may be variably present. Lumbar puncture usually reveals a pleocytosis with less than 200 cells per cubic millimeter and rarely more than 1000. Mononuclear cells predominate, but polymorphonuclear leukocytes may be seen in the early phases (days 1 and 2) of EEE and Japanese B encephalitis. The protein level may be mildly elevated, but the glucose level is normal.

Most patients seek medical care within the first 3 days of the onset of symptoms; recovery, when it occurs, is in 5 to 10 days. The mortality rate in symptomatic cases varies according to the etiologic agent (Table 249-4). The incidence of EEE in the general population is low because of the swamp-breeding characteristic of its vector, but the mortality rate is high. By contrast, the incidence of the bunyavirus infections (LaCrosse, California, Tahyna viruses) is very high in exposed populations although the sequelae are few and mortality rate is relatively low. The incidence of sequelae is predominantly age-dependent. For example, in EEE and WEE, most sequelae are found among the young, whereas in St. Louis encephalitis, severe disease occurs more frequently in the elderly. The reported sequelae range from such nonspecific complaints as persistent headaches and nervousness to severe impairments in speech or visual and gait disturbances, paralysis of extremities, and convulsions.

Table 249-3. Patterns of host response to arbovirus infections in humans

Response	Examples*
Asymptomatic infection	WEE, SLE, CE
Mild febrile illness	WEE, SLE, CE, yellow fever
Influenza-like illness with aching and joint pains	Dengue, chikungunya, Hantaan, phlebotomus fever
Encephalitis, mild	CE, WEE, SLE
Encephalitis, severe	SLE, EEE, WEE, tick-borne encephalitis
Jaundice, proteinuria	Yellow fever
Rash, sometimes with hemorrhagic manifestations	Dengue (chikungunya?) Hantaan
Shock syndrome	Dengue (after secondary infection with a different dengue serotype)

From Downs WG: In Evans AS editor: Viral infections of humans. New York, 1979, Plenum.

WEE, western equine encephalitis; SLE, St. Louis encephalitis; CE, California encephalitis; EEE, eastern equine encephalitis.

*Certain viruses have been selected for this list particularly to illustrate the range of symptoms that may be seen in populations infected with a single virus.

Dengue fever

There are two clinical patterns in dengue fever: primary classic dengue fever and secondary dengue hemorrhagic fever, often associated with shock syndrome.

Classic dengue fever starts after a 5 to 8 day incubation period with nonspecific flu-like symptoms of headache, backache, stiffness, general malaise, and flushed skin. The onset is sudden, with a rapid rise in temperature to 102.2° to 104° F (39 to 40° C). The fever lasts for 5 to 6 days and can be associated with a temporary remission after the third day, hence the name *saddleback fever*. The fever is accompanied by retro-orbital pain on eye movement, photophobia, backache, and joint pain so severe that the disease is often called *bone break fever*. During the later days of the fever, a maculopapular morbilliform or scarlatiniform rash develops over the thorax and spreads to the extremities and face. Scattered petechiae may be present during resolution of the illness. Lymphadenopathy, a relative bradycardia, and leukopenia are common during the second febrile phase.

Dengue hemorrhagic fever

Dengue hemorrhagic fever is characterized by a worsening of illness 2 or more days after the onset of dengue fever, with hypoproteinemia and one or more bleeding abnormalities (thrombocytopenia [$<100,000/mm^3$], prolonged bleeding time [>5 minutes], or an elevated prothrombin time). Dengue shock syndrome refers to a subgroup of dengue hemorrhagic fever characterized by hypotension and hemoconcentration, usually with elevated serum transaminase levels. Patients may have melena or hematemesis. Physical findings include petechiae, purpura, ecchymosis, epistaxis, and a positive tourniquet sign. As mentioned earlier, laboratory values may show a reduction in serum complement level and signs of a consumptive coagulopathy (decreased fibrinogin, increased fibrin split products, decreased platelets). Mortality rate in some epidemics has been 10% (30.5% in those with the shock syndrome); death usually occurs on the fourth or fifth day of illness. Children who survive improve rapidly.

Table 249-4. Prognosis and sequelae in arbovirus infections

Virus	Inapparent/ apparent cases	Serologic incidence in endemic area	Approximate mortality rate in symptomatic cases (%)	Age of affected population and sequelae
Alphavirus				
Eastern equine encephalitis		Rare	50-80	Children: severe disease with sequelae Adults: few sequelae if recovery occurs
Western equine encephalitis			5-15	Sequelae occur in children
Venezuelan equine encephalitis		Frequent in areas of epidemic equine disease	1	Most deaths in children
Flavivirus				
St. Louis encephalitis	64:1	10%-70% in epidemic area	2-20	Greater severity in elderly
Dengue classic		High in endemic area	Rare	All ages
Dengue hemorrhagic fever and dengue shock syndrome			30-50	Children almost exclusively
Yellow fever	9:1	Rare	Up to 50 in severe cases	All ages
Bunyavirus				
California encephalitis	High	11%-60%	<5	Sequelae uncommon; disease mostly in children <15 yr of age

Other aspects of the spectrum of illness in dengue fever include asymptomatic disease, fever without symptoms and fever with coryza, pharyngeal inflammation, and cough.

Yellow fever

The classic syndrome of yellow fever starts after a 3 to 6 day incubation period with the sudden onset of fever and chills. Headache, backache, generalized pain, nausea and vomiting, flushed face, conjunctival injection, and leukopenia are common. After 3 days of symptoms, the fever typically remits. In the classic syndrome, the fever reappears after several days, along with jaundice, punctate soft-palate hemorrhages, epistaxis, gingival bleeding, and hematemesis (black vomit). In up to 50% of patients, Faget's sign develops. It is a relative bradycardia inappropriate for the fever (but not below 60) and may be due to direct cardiac involvement. Shock may occur if cardiac damage is extensive. Coma and death occur in 10% to 60% of patients within 6 to 8 days of onset.

Yellow fever may also appear as a mild illness of less than 1 week's duration, simulating dengue fever, influenza, malaria, or typhoid. The classic syndrome may mimic viral hepatitis, leptospirosis, or carbon tetrachloride poisoning.

The epidemiology of yellow fever was elucidated by the Yellow Fever Commission headed by Dr. Walter Reed in Cuba. Initially using themselves as subjects, commission members discovered that the *A. aegypti* mosquito was necessary for transmission and that contact with patients' clothing or other fomites does not spread the disease. Later, another member of this group, Dr. James Carroll, showed that the causative agent is filterable but smaller than bacteria. By use of mosquito control, yellow fever was shortly thereafter eliminated from Havana and later from many other parts of the world. However, *A. aegypti* mosquitoes have subsequently repopulated many of these areas, and the specter of the return of yellow fever to urban centers by reintroduction from the enzootic jungle cycle is ever-present.

DIAGNOSIS

The diagnosis of most togavirus and bunyavirus infections is most often established by examining acute and convalescent sera for neutralization (the most specific), hemagglutination inhibition, complement-fixing antibodies, or immunoglobulin M enzyme-linked immunosorbent assay (IgM-ELISA). Because of the high cross-reactivity of hemagglutination inhibition, and complement-fixing antibodies within genera, other indigenous arboviruses are often simultaneously included in the tests.

In some instances, the diagnosis may be established by isolation of the virus from blood, cerebrospinal fluid, throat swabs, or necropsy specimens of brain (encephalitis) or liver (yellow fever) (Table 249-5). Liver biopsy for the antemortem diagnosis of yellow fever is not recommended because of the high complication rate.

The histologic changes in the liver are pathognomonic of yellow fever and include acidophilic necrosis of hepatocytes, with formation of Councilman bodies. Routine postmortem liver biopsies have been used to monitor the incidence of disease in South America. The lesions of encephalitis caused by arboviruses are not specific enough to allow identification of the various agents.

Table 249-5. Diagnosis, prevention, and vaccination in arbovirus infection

Virus	Isolation of virus	Serology	Treatment	Prevention	Vaccine
Alphaviruses					
Eastern equine encephalitis	Brain Blood and CSF (poor)	HI, CF, N, ELISA	Supportive	Equine vaccine and mosquito control in epizootic disease	Equine use only; experimental in humans
Western equine encephalitis	Brain Blood and CSF (difficult)	HI, CF N, ELISA	Supportive	Mosquito control in epizootic disease or in epidemics	Equine use only; experimental in humans
Venezuelan equine encephalitis	Blood (easy) Throat swab (easy)	HI, CF, N, ELISA	Supportive	Equine vaccine	TC-83 live attenuated vaccine, predominantly for horses (occasionally used for laboratory personnel)
Flaviviruses					
Dengue fever	Blood	HI, CF, N, ELISA		Mosquito control	Experimental
St. Louis encephalitis	Brain Blood and CSF	CF, N, ELISA	Supportive	Mosquito control in epidemics	None
Yellow fever	Blood Liver (biopsy not recommended due to bleeding)	HI, CF, N, ELISA	Supportive	Vaccine, mosquito control	Chick embryo vaccine 17D (live attenuated) Revaccinate every 10 yr
Bunyaviruses					
California encephalitis	None reported	HI, CF, N, ELISA	Supportive	Protective clothing, mosquito repellent	None

HI, hemagglutination inhibition; CF, complement fixation; N, neutralization; IgM-ELISA, enzyme-linked immunosorbent assay.

TREATMENT AND PREVENTION

The treatment of patients with any of the arbovirus encephalitides, dengue fever, or yellow fever is symptomatic. Patients with dengue hemorrhagic fever and yellow fever must be carefully observed for signs of shock and disseminated intravascular coagulopathy and treated appropriately. There is no antiviral therapy for these viruses.

Prevention of infection is achieved primarily by mosquito control: vaccination is useful in some cases (Table 249-5). The live yellow fever vaccine is the only vaccine regularly used for humans. Although two vaccines for yellow fever have been developed, the 17D chick embryo vaccine developed by Theiler in 1937 is used exclusively because it produces less postvaccination encephalitis than the French neurotropic vaccine. The 17D vaccine is much more heat-labile. It should be used within 1 hour of reconstitution and kept out of direct sunlight to prevent inactivation.

Vaccines for equine use have been developed for EEE, WEE, and VEE. Vaccination of horses against VEE may help to terminate an epidemic in humans. Human epidemics of VEE often follow the first observation of equine disease by several weeks. The horse-mosquito transmission cycle is probably important, because in the horse, the high levels of viremia that develop are capable of reinfecting more mosquitoes. Interruption of the equine-mosquito cycle by horse vaccination generally leads to a gradual decrease in human disease. By contrast, in equines (or humans), the levels of viremia in WEE and EEE do not become high enough to infect mosquitoes. Thus immunization of equines has little effect on interrupting the natural transmission cycle in WEE or EEE.

Mosquito control and prevention of mosquito bites are valuable preventive measures in all the arbovirus infections. Various means have been used, including removal of mosquito breeding areas in city areas, use of persistent organophosphorus larvicides, and spraying of organophosphorus insecticides in ultra-low volumes from aircraft. Some mosquitoes, such as *A. aegypti,* in the Americas, exist primarily as domestic species, and eradication stops the epidemic. On the other hand, other mosquitoes exist as both domestic and wild species (e.g., *A. aegypti* in Africa), or live in vast territories in the wild; as a result eradication is impractical. The surveillance program to detect infected mosquitoes has been successful in monitoring disease prevalence to help decide when to practice mosquito control. Finally, mosquito repellents, netting, and protective clothing are individual measures useful for decreasing the chances of being bitten by an infected mosquito.

REFERENCES

Casals J and Clark DH: Arboviruses; group A and arboviruses other than groups A and B. In Horsfall FL, and Tamm I, editors: Viral and rickettsial infections of man ed 4. Philadelphia, 1986, Lippincott.

Centers for Disease Control: Imported dengue—United States, 1987, MMWR 38:463, 1989.

Centers for Disease Control: Leads from the MMWR: yellow fever vaccine. JAMA 251:442, 1984.

Centers for Disease Control: Leads from MMWR: dengue and dengue hemorhagic fever in the Americas, 1986. JAMA 59:1781, 1988.

Downs WG: Arboviruses. In Evans AS, editor: Viral infections of humans. New York, 1979, Plenum.

Gonzalez-Scarano N and Nathanson N: Bunyavirus. In Fields BN et al, editors: Virology. ed 2. New York, 1990, Raven Press.

Halstead SB: Selective primary health care: strategies for control of disease in the developing world. XI. Dengue. Rev Infect Dis 6(2):251, 1984.

Hammon WM and Ho M: Viral encephalitis. Dis Mon, February 1973.

Henderson BE and Coleman PH: The growing importance of California arboviruses in the etiology of human disease. Prog Med Virol 13:404, 1971.

Kappus KD et al: Human arboviral infections in the United States in 1980. J Infect Dis 145(2):283, 1982.

Luby JP: St. Louis encephalitis. Epidemiol Rev 1:55, 1979.

Monath TP: Alphavirus (eastern, western, and equine encephalitis). In Mandell GL, Douglas RG Jr, and Bennett JE, editors: Principles and practice of infectious diseases. New York, 1990, Churchill Livingstone.

Monath TP: Flaviviruses. In Fields BN et al, editors: Virology. ed 2. New York, 1990, Raven Press.

Monath TP: Flavivirus (yellow fever, dengue, and St. Louis encephalitis). In Mandell GL, Douglas RG Jr, and Bennett JE, editors: Principles and practice of infectious diseases. New York, 1990, Churchill Livingstone.

Peters CJ and Dalrymple JM: Alphaviruses. In Fields BN et al, editors: Virology. ed 2. New York, 1990, Raven Press.

Sanford JP: Arbovirus infections. In Wilson JD et al, editors: Principles of internal medicine, ed 12. New York, 1991, McGraw-Hill.

Woodall JP: Summary of the symposium on yellow fever. J Infect Dis 144(1):87, 1981.

CHAPTER

250 Rotavirus and Norwalk-Like Virus Infections

Suzanne M. Matsui

Acute infectious gastroenteritis is an extremely common disease worldwide and has a significant public health impact. Its most devastating effects are seen in developing countries in Asia, Africa, and Latin America, where 3 to 5 billion cases of diarrhea occur each year and lead to death in 5 to 10 million individuals. Approximately 40% of these deaths are linked to rotavirus infections that primarily affect children below the age of 2 years. In developed nations, the effect of infectious gastroenteritis on morbidity and mortality rates is less pronounced, but not trivial. For example, acute gastroenteritis is the second most common illness encountered in American families, with an incidence in the range of 10% to 15%. In American children, epidemiologic studies indicate that gastroenteritis is responsible for approximately 800,000 to 1 million hospital admissions and approximately 250 deaths per year. Elderly patients (>74 years old), particularly those residing in long-term care facilities, are also at higher risk of dying of diarrhea or its associated complications. In younger adults, acute gastroenteritis tends to run a self-limited course, but its economic impact, as measured in days lost from work, may be substantial (Chapter 236).

It is currently estimated that viruses account for 30% to 40% of the cases of infectious gastroenteritis in the United States. This exceeds the number of cases that can be attributed to bacterial and parasitic pathogens. These estimates are sure to require adjustment in the future, because the cause of gastroenteritis cannot be determined in approximately 40% of cases with current diagnostic tests.

Five major groups of viruses have been identified in association with acute gastroenteritis. This chapter focuses on the two groups that are the most important from a medical and public health standpoint: the human rotaviruses and Norwalk-like viruses. Detailed discussion of enteric adenovirus, astroviruses, and classic caliciviruses is beyond the scope of this chapter, and the reader is referred to recent reviews for more information.

ROTAVIRUS INFECTIONS

Characteristics

Rotaviruses are members of the family Reoviridae. The viral genome is composed of 11 segments of double-stranded ribonucleic acid (RNA) and is enclosed in a double-shelled, icosahedral capsid that measures approximately 75 nm in diameter. With one exception, each of the gene segments encodes a single viral protein. Classification of rotaviruses has depended on the serologic characteristics of three structural proteins. Viral protein (VP) 6, a major component of the inner capsid, is a determinant of group (A to G) and subgroup (I or II for group A rotaviruses) specificity. Commercial immunoassays are based on reactivity with antigenic regions of VP6. The two proteins that the outer capsid comprises, VP4 and VP7, are the primary targets to which neutralizing antibodies are directed. Viral serotype is determined by VP7, the viral surface glycoprotein. At least eight serotypes of human rotavirus have been identified to date. Most infections, however, appear to be caused by only four of these (types 1 to 4).

The genome of rotavirus, like that of influenza virus, is segmented. This means that during mixed infection with two parental strains of rotavirus, each gene segment of the progeny viruses is contributed by one parent or the other. Thus gene reassortment has the potential to produce a wide array of progeny viruses with different combinations of parental genes. Although this feature has been useful in the laboratory setting to determine the gene(s) responsible for a specific viral phenotype, it has not been shown conclusively that new or more virulent strains of rotavirus have evolved in nature by this mechanism.

Epidemiology

Group A rotaviruses are the most important cause of severe, dehydrating diarrhea in infants throughout the world. (Unless otherwise specified, the term *rotavirus[es]* is used to indicate group A rotavirus[es]). Recently, two antigenically distinct groups of rotaviruses (groups B and C) have been linked with human disease. Group B rotaviruses have caused large outbreaks of waterborne diarrhea among adults in China; group C rotaviruses have been found in association with sporadic cases of childhood diarrhea in various parts of the world. Rotaviruses of groups D and E appear to be strictly animal pathogens.

Group A rotavirus is primarily a pathogen of childhood. By age 3 nearly every child throughout the world will have had at least one rotavirus infection and will have developed antibodies to rotavirus. Symptomatic infections appear to occur most frequently in young children between the ages of 6 and 24 months. Of hospitalizations for childhood diarrhea 30% to 50% are due to group A rotavirus. In adults, group A rotavirus infection is generally milder or asymptomatic, but severe or prolonged infections have been reported among elderly, institutionalized patients and immunocompromised individuals. Rotavirus is also a minor cause of traveler's diarrhea.

Rotavirus infection tends to occur in the cooler winter months in temperate climates. In the United States, for example, the rotavirus "season" begins in November in the Southwest and gradually moves eastward, peaking on the East Coast in February and March. In warmer, tropical climates, infection occurs year round, but some increase in incidence is observed during the cooler, rainy season.

Infected patients shed large numbers of viral particles in the feces (10^7 to 10^{10} or more virions/gram) and the infectious dose is low. Rotavirus is most likely transmitted by the fecal-oral route. There is little evidence to suggest that aerosols or fomites are important vehicles of transmission. Rotaviruses are heat- and acid-stable and can remain infectious on environmental surfaces for hours to days. They are resistant to a variety of antiseptic agents, although 95% ethanol is an effective disinfectant. Therefore improved hygienic and socioeconomic conditions may not be sufficient to reduce the incidence of rotavirus diarrhea but may result in a more favorable outcome for infected individuals.

Pathophysiology

Rotavirus infects and replicates in the mature, columnar, epithelial cells of small intestinal villous tips. Infection begins in the proximal small bowel and may spread to involve the entire small bowel. Diarrhea and dehydration result from the loss of these mature absorptive cells during infection. Abnormalities in D-xylose absorption, disaccharidase levels, and lactose tolerance have been observed but may not be clinically significant in all cases. Adenylate cyclase stimulation, a feature of enterotoxin-induced diarrhea, is not seen with rotavirus-induced illness. Pathologic features indicated by light microscopy include shortening and blunting of the villi, infiltration of the lamina propria by mononuclear cells, and elongation of the villous crypts. Electron microscopic analysis shows swelling of mitochondria, dilatation of the endoplasmic reticulum, and destruction of microvilli. Rotavirus particles have been visualized in the dilated endoplasmic reticulum and lysosomes of columnar epithelial cells.

Rotavirus-induced diarrhea in immunocompetent individuals is usually self-limited. Pathologic features and their functional correlates return to normal as virus is cleared from the intestinal tract and diarrhea ceases. Prolonged or chronic symptomatic infection may be seen in immunocompromised individuals.

In most children serum antibodies develop by 2 to 3 years of age. The level of one's pre-existing serum antibody does not accurately predict susceptibility or resistance to disease. Local immunity, measured by the level of immunoglobulin A (IgA) antibodies in intestinal fluids, appears to correlate more reliably with protection. IgA in human colostrum and breast milk may be responsible for the observation that rotavirus-infected breast-fed infants appear to shed smaller quantities of rotavirus in feces.

Clinical disease

Rotavirus infection can result in a wide range of manifestations from no symptoms, to mild diarrhea, to severe diarrhea with dehydration, and occasional fatalities. As mentioned previously, children in the 6 to 24 month age group appear to be most susceptible to symptomatic infection and may require hospitalization or aggressive fluid resuscitation. In natural infections, the incubation period averages 1 to 3 days. Fever and vomiting, and in some cases, respiratory symptoms, may precede the onset of diarrhea. Vomiting usually resolves in 2 to 3 days with proper fluid replacement. Diarrhea is watery and nonbloody and lacks fecal leukocytes. Diarrhea generally begins later than the other symptoms and lasts 5 to 6 days. Viral shedding may persist for up to 10 days. Full clinical recovery is seen in most patients. Laboratory abnormalities, such as elevated urine specific gravity, elevated blood urea nitrogen level, and hyperchloremic metabolic acidosis, indicate the level of dehydration in the patient.

Adult volunteers given a rotavirus inoculum had an incubation period of 1 to 4 days. Vomiting and fever began as early as 1 day after inoculation; the diarrhea phase generally began 2 to 4 days after inoculation and lasted up to 7 days. Associated symptoms included anorexia and abdominal discomfort. In general, illness in adults tended to be milder than symptomatic childhood infection.

Immunocompromised individuals are at risk for prolonged or chronic infections. Rotaviruses with genome rearrangements and other abnormalities have been identified in rotavirus-infected immunocompromised patients.

Diagnosis

Although the clinical presentation combined with the epidemiologic pattern frequently suggests the diagnosis, it may be necessary to confirm the diagnosis by detection of virus or viral antigens and/or demonstration of a serologic response. Because rotaviruses are shed in large quantity in infected stools and the viral particles have characteristic surface features, they can be easily and accurately identified by electron microscopy of an unconcentrated, negatively stained specimen. Electron microscopy has the added advantage of recognizing not only group A rotaviruses but other rotavirus groups as well. Rotavirus antigen can also be detected by a number of commercially available enzyme immunoassays (EIA) or latex agglutination tests that recognize VP6, the inner capsid protein that is a determinant of group specificity. These tests are sensitive, specific, relatively inexpensive, and rapid. In addition, the presence of rotavirus in fecal samples may be determined by extraction of viral RNA from these specimens and subsequent analysis by polyacrylamide gel electrophoresis. Molecular techniques, such as dot blot hybridization and polymerase chain reaction, have recently been adapted to the identification of rotaviruses, but their efficacy and usefulness in evaluating large numbers of specimens remain to be established. Serologic response can be evaluated in several ways, including EIA, neutralization, inhibition of hemagglutination, immune electron microscopy, and complement fixation.

Treatment and prevention

The primary goal of therapy is to prevent or reverse dehydration and to correct electrolyte abnormalities. In most cases, this can be accomplished with glucose-based oral rehydration solutions (ORS) tailored to the severity of fluid or electrolyte imbalance. According to recommendations from the American Academy of Pediatrics, solutions used for rehydration should contain 75 to 90 mEq/L of sodium (as found in WHO-ORS).For patients in whom maintenance of hydration status or prevention of dehydration is the goal, solutions lower in sodium (40 to 60 mEq/L, as found in Pedialyte or Ricelyte) may be used. Administration of these glucose-based ORS does not decrease the duration of diarrheal illness. Thus early feeding and adequate caloric intake are important adjuncts to ORS in promoting recovery in these patients. Intravenous fluid resuscitation is rarely needed and reserved for advanced cases of dehydration or hypovolemic shock.

Antiviral chemotherapy is not likely to help much in the treatment of rotavirus diarrhea, because viral replication and intestinal damage precede the onset of diarrhea. In immunocompromised children, passive immunotherapy with human milk containing rotavirus antibodies has been shown to shorten the course of rotavirus infection.

Prevention and control of rotavirus infection can occur if fecal-oral transmission is interrupted. As noted, improved hygienic and socioeconomic conditions alone may not affect the incidence of rotavirus diarrhea but may decrease the numbers of severe and fatal cases. Parents, hospital/institutional workers, and child care providers must be educated in proper disinfection techniques, isolation strategies, and appropriate use of gloves and handwashing. Another approach to prevention of rotavirus infection is immunoprophylaxis. The efficacy of immunoprophylaxis with live, attenuated vaccines is currently being tested. The ideal vaccine is one that is safe and can be administered orally to stimulate local protective immune responses to all serotypes of human rotavirus.

NORWALK-LIKE VIRUS INFECTIONS

Characteristics

Norwalk virus is the prototype strain of a group of small (27 to 40 nm), round, icosahedral viruses with relatively amorphous surface features revealed by electron microscopy. Viruses in this group cause outbreaks of gastroenteritis in older children and adults. Because they have not been fully characterized, most of these viruses bear the names of the outbreak locations such as Norwalk (Ohio), Hawaii, Snow Mountain (Colorado), Montgomery County (Maryland), and Taunton (United Kingdom). The Marin County (California) virus was originally thought to be yet another Norwalk-like virus but has now been classified as an astrovirus.

The Norwalk virus was identified by immune electron microscopy in 1972, but progress in characterizing the Norwalk-like viruses has been hampered by the inability to cultivate these viruses in vitro, inability to cause productive infection in animal models, and the small amount of virus ($< 10^6$ virions per gram feces) that is shed for brief periods during infection. Much of the currently available information and diagnostic reagents have been derived from human volunteers who were administered a safety-tested viral inoculum from the original Norwalk outbreak.

Norwalk and Snow Mountain viruses, although antigenically distinct, share a protein structure similar to that of caliciviruses. Recent molecular analysis of Norwalk virus indicates that its genome is composed of single-stranded, positive-sense RNA, like that of caliciviruses. In addition, it appears that the genome organization resembles that of caliciviruses. Caliciviruses, however, display a much more striking surface structure on electron microscopy and tend to cause gastroenteritis in younger children.

Epidemiology

Norwalk and Norwalk-like viruses are a major cause of epidemic gastroenteritis. At least 30% to 40% of the outbreaks examined in two separate studies were due to Norwalk and serologically related viruses, as determined by the presence of viral antigen in clinical samples or serum immune responses. It has been estimated that serologically distinct viruses with similar electron micrographic features may be the etiologic agents of an additional 20% to 25% of such outbreaks.

In the United States, serum antibodies to Norwalk virus are rarely detected in childhood, increase in incidence during the teenage years and early adulthood, and are found in approximately 60% of 40 to 60 year old adults. In contrast, antibodies to Norwalk virus are acquired early in childhood in developing nations. These observations support the hypothesis that transmission of Norwalk virus occurs by the fecal-oral route. The association of serum antibody levels and protection from illness is less well understood. A paradoxic relationship between serum antibody response and long-term (>2 years) protection from illness has been observed in adult volunteers in the United States. This suggests that immune response is not the only determinant of susceptibility to infection.

Exposure to Norwalk virus can occur year-round in a variety of settings. Outbreaks of gastroenteritis have been reported aboard cruise ships, at family gatherings, and in nursing homes, summer camps, and schools. Contaminated food and/or water has been responsible for many of these outbreaks. Transmission through infected food handlers and from person to person has also been reported. Some of the largest epidemics of Norwalk gastroenteritis have involved the ingestions of contaminated clams and oysters. Standards for shellfish safety are typically based on fecal coliform counts. It has been shown, however, that the absence of fecal coliforms in shellfish may not accurately reflect the level of viral contamination in the shellfish.

Norwalk virus is also a minor cause of traveler's diarrhea, as evidenced by the outbreak of gastroenteritis in a military unit in Operation Desert Shield in which serum immune responses to Norwalk virus were demonstrated. In immunocompromised patients, the importance of Norwalk-like viruses has not been clearly established. Two independent studies failed to agree on the incidence of Norwalk virus–induced diarrhea in acquired immunodeficiency syndrome (AIDS) patients.

Pathophysiology

Experimental infection of adult volunteers with Norwalk or Hawaii viruses resulted in histologic changes in the small intestine. More specifically, during the symptomatic phase of infection, intestinal villi were broadened and flattened and epithelial lining cells appeared vacuolated and disorganized. Mononuclear and polymorphonuclear cell infiltrates in the lamina propria and crypt cell hyperplasia were also observed. Effects of viral infection indicated by electron micrographs included dilatation of the endoplasmic reticulum, multivesiculate bodies, widened intercellular space, and shortened microvilli. No viral particles were identified within these cells. Some of the asymptomatic, infected patients also demonstrated a few of these histologic changes on biopsy. In general, however, more severe biopsy lesions were seen in the more symptomatic volunteers. Repeat biopsy during recovery (a few weeks after the acute phase of infection) indicated complete resolution of these abnormalities.

Functional abnormalities observed during symptomatic infection included transient malabsorption of fat, D-xyose, and lactose and decrease in brush border enzyme levels compared to individual baseline values. Although histologic abnormalities were not found in the stomach or colon, gastric motility was decreased during infection. This may account for the nausea and vomiting that are prominent features of this illness. Altered adenylate cyclase levels were not observed.

Clinical disease

The clinical features of Norwalk virus–induced illness have been investigated in a controlled manner in adult volunteers. In a typical study, volunteers were given a safety-tested oral inoculum derived from a secondary case of the original Norwalk epidemic. In approximately 50% of the infected volunteers clinical disease developed after an average incubation period of approximately 24 hours. Nausea was reported by nearly all of the ill volunteers and vomiting was experienced by >90%. Diarrhea was reported by more than 50% of the volunteers. Some volunteers also complained of fever, headache, myalgias, and abdominal cramps. Mild leukocytosis was occasionally detected. Symptoms generally resolved within 72 hours of onset. Experimental infection with Snow Mountain and Hawaii viruses caused illness that was clinically indistinguishable from Norwalk virus illness.

Gastroenteritis associated with Norwalk-like viruses in the field is characterized by the sudden onset of nausea and vomiting, with or without diarrhea. The clinical course resembles that of the ill volunteers. The illness is generally self-limited, lasting 12 to 60 hours. Although vomiting is a frequently reported symptom, severe dehydration is only occasionally seen and rarely does the patient require hospitalization or aggressive fluid resuscitation. Elderly, debilitated patients may be more susceptible to severe dehydration and occasional deaths related to complications of Norwalk gastroenteritis have been reported in this group.

Diagnosis

Immune electron microscopy (IEM), radioimmunoassays (RIA), and enzyme immunoassay (EIA) have been used in research laboratories to identify Norwalk antigen–containing fecal samples and to detect changes in the level of Norwalk antibody in paired (acute and convalescent) serum samples. These tests are not widely available because they rely on reagents that are in short supply and have not been standardized from laboratory to laboratory. Diagnostic tests, such as PCR assays, based on recent advances in studying the molecular biologic characteristics of Norwalk virus, should soon be developed and make simpler the detection of this elusive virus.

Treatment and prevention

Because this illness is generally self-limited, specific treatment is usually not necessary. If significant dehydration develops, oral or intravenous fluid resuscitation should be administered. No antiviral chemotherapy is available for these viruses.

Large epidemics have been associated with the consumption of raw or undercooked shellfish. Until adequate seafood safety standards regarding virus contamination are established, it is prudent to advise the public of the risks of eating raw shellfish and the proper way to ensure that shellfish is fully cooked. For example, clams open after 1 minute of steaming, but 4 to 6 minutes of steaming are necessary to ensure that the internal temperature of the clam reaches that required to inactivate viruses (100° C).

The role for immunoprophylaxis is not clear, given the paradoxic association between the level of immune response and protection from disease. Further research in this area is needed before vaccine development can begin.

REFERENCES

Blacklow NR and Greenberg HB: Viral gastroenteritis. N Engl J Med 325:252, 1991.

Duggan C et al: The management of acute diarrhea in children: oral rehydration, maintenance, and nutritional therapy. MMWR 41 (RR-16):1, 1992

Greenberg HB et al: Role of Norwalk virus in outbreaks of nonbacterial gastroenteritis. J Infect Dis 139:564, 1979.

Greenberg HB and Matsui SM: Astroviruses and caliciviruses: emerging enteric pathogens. Infect Agents and Dis 1:71, 1992.

Hirschhorn N and Greenough WB III: Progress in oral rehydration therapy. Sci Am 264:50, 1991.

Hyams KC et al: Diarrheal disease during Operation Desert Shield. N Engl J Med 325:1423, 1991.

Kapikian AZ and Chanock RM: Norwalk group of viruses. In Fields B, editor: Virology, New York, 1990, Raven Press.

Kapikian AZ and Chanock RM: Rotaviruses. In Fields B, editor: Virology, New York, 1990, Raven Press.

Kaplan JE et al: Epidemiology of Norwalk gastroenteritis and the role of Norwalk virus in outbreaks of acute nonbacterial gastroenteritis. Ann Intern Med 96:756, 1982.

LeBaron CW et al: Viral agents of gastroenteritis: public health importance and outbreak management. MMWR 39:1, 1990.

Lew JF et al: Diarrheal deaths in the United States 1979 through 1987: a special problem for the elderly. JAMA 265:3280, 1991.

Morse DL et al: Widespread outbreaks of clam- and oyster-associated gastroenteritis: role of Norwalk virus. N Engl J Med 314:678, 1986.

Parrino TA et al: Clinical immunity in acute gastroenteritis caused by Norwalk agent. N Engl J Med 297:86, 1977.

Wadell G et al: Enteric adenoviruses. In Bock G and Whelan J, editors: Novel diarrhoea viruses. Ciba Foundation Symposium 128, Chichester, 1987, John Wiley and Sons.

CHAPTER

251 Herpesvirus Infections (Herpes Simplex Virus, Varicella-Zoster Virus, Cytomegalovirus, Epstein-Barr Virus)

David A. Katzenstein
M. Colin Jordan

CHARACTERISTICS

The five herpesviruses that infect humans are herpes simplex virus (HSV-1 and HSV-2), varicella-zoster virus (VZV), cytomegalovirus (CMV), Epstein-Barr virus (EBV), and the newly described human B cell lymphotropic virus (HBLV) or human herpesvirus 6 (HHV-6). All are symmetric icosahedral enveloped viruses containing a DNA genomic core that is 30 to 45 nm in diameter. An electron-dense capsid consisting of 162 capsomers surrounds the deoxyribonucleic acid (DNA) core. The entire virion, including the envelope, ranges between 120 and 250 nm in diameter; the nucleic acid has a molecular weight of approximately 150×10^6 daltons. Although the clinical manifestations produced by each virus are diverse, several common features are shared. The herpesviruses are among the most ubiquitous human pathogens. In general, infection is more frequent and occurs in younger age groups in populations of lower socioeconomic status. With the exception of VZV, the vast majority of infections are asymptomatic. Once infection is established in the host, the virus persists indefinitely in a nonreplicating, dormant state in specific cells and tissues. Under certain conditions, the virus may be induced to replicate, producing either secondary disease or asymptomatic viral shedding. In the severely immunocompromised host, life-threatening disease may result from local viral invasion or widespread dissemination.

HERPES SIMPLEX VIRUS

The two strains of HSV that cause human disease, HSV-1 and HSV-2, are closely related antigenically and share nearly 50% DNA homology. HSV-1 is the more common cause of orolabial lesions (cold sores or fever blisters), whereas the majority of genital infections are caused by HSV-2. With certain exceptions, notably herpetic encephalitis, which is nearly always the result of HSV-1 infection, and meningitis, which is usually caused by HSV-2, the two HSVs may cause identical lesions and disease.

Epidemiology

HSV-1 infection is frequently acquired in the first decade of life. By adulthood as many as 85% of the population have been infected as determined by serologic surveys. Nevertheless, only 15% to 25% of individuals suffer from recurrent orolabial herpetic infection. Between symptomatic episodes, HSV may be present in oral secretions in as many as 5% of healthy adults with a history of cold sores. Such asymptomatic shedding of HSV presumably plays an important role in the spread of viral infection in the normal population. HSV-2 infection is more closely linked to sexual activity in that the prevalence of antibody rises rapidly after puberty and is related to the age of first intercourse and the number of sexual partners. In women, asymptomatic shedding of HSV-2 in cervicovaginal secretions can be detected between episodes of clinically apparent genital infection. Asymptomatic HSV shedding from the urethra may occur in men.

Pathogenesis

The pathogenesis of infections with herpesviruses is summarized in Table 251-1. Vesicular lesions caused by HSV are the result of lytic infection of epithelial cells of the skin

Table 251-1. Clinical manifestations of uncomplicated infection with herpesviruses

Virus	Primary infection	Chronic infection	Latent infection	Reactivation
HSV	Often asymptomatic Mucocutaneous lesions	Intermittent shedding in saliva, vagina, and tears	Neurons in sensory ganglia	Shedding; mucocutaneous lesions; neuropathy
VZV	Varicella in 95%	Hyperkeratotic lesions in AIDS	Sensory ganglia	Zoster
CMV	Usually asymptomatic; mononucleosis	Shedding in urine, saliva, vagina, semen, breast milk	Peripheral leukocytes ?Other tissues	Shedding; dissemination
EBV	Usually asymptomatic; mononucleosis	Shedding in pharynx	B lymphocytes	Shedding; B cell lymphoma

and mucous membranes. Typically, lesions begin in crops of painful small, fluid-filled vesicles. On the mucous membranes of the mouth, vagina, or rectum, the vesicular stage may not be appreciated, and shallow circular ulcers develop. On the epidermis, vesicles may contain clear fluid or appear pustular; they ulcerate, form crusting lesions after 3 to 5 days, and usually heal without scarring. In the course of primary infection HSV enters the sensory nerve endings in the skin or mucous membrane and then migrates to the sensory nerve ganglia that innervate the affected area. In the neuron, the virus establishes a nonreplicating latent infection. An "antisense" messenger ribonucleic acid (RNA) transcribed from a region of the viral genome encoding a regulatory protein (ICP-O) has been detected in latently infected neurons; no later gene products have been found, suggesting that HSV replication is restricted at a very early phase. Virus within neurons is capable of repeated reactivation, causing recurrent lesions or asymptomatic viral shedding. Frequently, prodromal dysesthesias or paresthesias are produced by migration of the virus down the nerve axon to the skin or mucous membrane. At the level of the vesicular lesion, cell-mediated immunity appears to play a crucial role in containment of the lytic infection. There is some experimental evidence to suggest that specific antiviral antibody is important in modulation of the latent HSV infection of neurons. During primary infection or in immunosuppressed patients, bloodborne virus may be carried to visceral organs.

Disease states

Orolabial infection. Orolabial HSV-1 infection is usually acquired during childhood when infectious virus comes in contact with skin or mucous membranes. Primary infection is most often asymptomatic or results in only a few scattered vesicular lesions on the lips. In a small number of children and adults, primary oral infection results in a severe gingivostomatitis characterized by confluent vesicles or ulcers on the tongue, buccal and sublingual mucosa, pharynx, and submandibular lymphadenopathy with fever.

Recurrent orolabial lesions (fever blisters or cold sores) are usually limited to the vermillion border of the lip and do not involve the oral mucosa. In a given individual, vesicles tend to recur in the same location, and often the appearance of lesions is preceded by hyperesthesia in the affected area and local lymphadenopathy. Recurrences are associated with exposure to intense sunlight, fever, stress, or injury to the trigeminal ganglion. In severely stressed patients, the rate of shedding of oral virus may be as high as 20%.

Genital infection. Genital herpes is more commonly caused by HSV-2 and is acquired through contact with oral or genital secretions that contain infectious virus (Chapter 238). Rarely, genital infection results from autoinoculation in patients with oral or digital lesions. The incubation period after sexual contact ranges from 2 to 7 days. In most patients, the primary acquisition of genital herpes is asymptomatic, and the infection is manifested only by recurrent disease months or years later. In women, herpes lesions occur on the labia, vaginal mucosa, cervix, or the skin of the perineum. Occasionally crops of lesions may appear on the buttocks or thighs. In men, lesions most frequently involve the shaft of the penis, the foreskin, and, less often, the scrotum, thighs and buttocks. Lesions on the glans penis frequently appear macular and fail to vesiculate. Male homosexuals often have perianal or rectal lesions.

Morbidity associated with primary and recurrent genital infection is widely variable. The initial primary genital infection may result in widespread lesions and a systemic illness with fever and malaise persisting for weeks. In some individuals, frequent recurrences may occur for years; in others there are no further episodes. Recurrent lesions are preceded by prodromal hyperesthesia and frequently occur in association with menstruation or after vigorous sexual activity. In some women, recurrent cervical HSV infection may be manifested only as a watery vaginal discharge. In general, recurrent episodes of genital herpes become less frequent and severe over months to years. However, genital infection tends to recur more frequently than does orolabial disease; this greater relative frequency appears to be due to HSV-2 per se, because HSV-1 genital infection recurs much less often. Shedding of HSV in cervical secretions has been demonstrated during symptom-free periods in a small percentage of women. Complications of genital infection include urinary retention and cystitis, proctocolitis, and aseptic meningitis. Any of these may become a recurrent process. Transverse myelitis with irreversible neurologic deficits has also been reported.

Herpes encephalitis. HSV-1 is an important cause of sporadic necrotizing encephalitis in all age groups. It may occur in patients with or without a clinical history or serologic evidence of previous infection. The predominant clinical manifestations relate to the focal nature of the disease in most cases, characteristically involving the temporoparietal or frontotemporal region of one cerebral hemisphere. Thus differential diagnosis includes focal suppurative lesions such as brain abscess or subdural empyema, mycotic aneurysm, brain tumors, vascular lesions, cysts, and granulomas. Initial symptoms of HSV-1 encephalitis are usually fever, headache, olfactory hallucinations, personality changes, and alterations of consciousness. These are frequently followed rapidly by the onset of focal hemispheric signs such as hemiparesis, focal or major motor seizures, and unilateral cranial nerve palsies. Profound coma may develop and is a very grave prognostic sign. In addition, the intensity of the necrotizing inflammation and cerebral edema may lead to increased intracranial pressure, producing papilledema and, in some instances, cerebral herniation. Spinal fluid examination usually demonstrates a mononuclear pleocytosis with an elevated protein concentration, a normal glucose level, and the presence of red blood cells. Initial lumbar puncture findings are normal in about 10% of cases, however. Because HSV-1 cannot be recovered from the spinal fluid, definitive diagnosis depends on isolation of virus from brain tissue after surgical biopsy or at autopsy. Fluorescence staining for HSV antigens in brain tissue yields a positive result in 70% of cases. Electroencephalography, technetium brain scans, and computed tomography usually demonstrate focal cerebral abnormalities with surrounding edema. Because approximately 50% of cases of suspected herpes encephalitis are found to have a variety of other infectious, malignant, or vascular lesions at brain biopsy, the procedure is recommended for definitive diagnosis. However, if recent reports of detection of HSV DNA in spinal fluid by the polymerase chain reaction are confirmed, biopsy will no longer be necessary.

Herpetic whitlow. Periungual inoculation of HSV results in recurrent infection of the pulp of the finger, or herpetic whitlow. This disease occurs most often in medical and dental personnel after direct contact with herpes lesions or secretions containing HSV. Occasionally, whitlow results from autoinoculation in patients with oral or genital HSV infection. The appearance of vesicles or pustules is preceded by pain, redness, and swelling of the affected finger, and lesions may be accompanied by lymphangitis and regional lymphadenopathy. Some individuals have repeated bouts of herpetic whitlow. The primary value in diagnosis is the prevention of repeated attempts at incision and drainage and needless antibiotic therapy.

Herpes keratitis. Corneal epithelium can be a site of primary as well as recurrent HSV infection. Herpes keratitis begins with small punctate vacuoles in the cornea that coalesce to form dendritic lesions. In advanced disease, after frequent recurrences, corneal ulcers and scarring may result. The signs of infection are a foreign body sensation followed by follicular conjunctivitis and preauricular lymphadenopathy. It is important to avoid the use of corticosteroid-containing ophthalmic solutions in patients suspected of ocular herpes infection.

Infection in compromised hosts. Oral and genital HSV infection may cause life-threatening disease in severely immunosuppressed patients. Reactivation of endogenous virus frequently occurs in patients with hematologic malignancies, bone marrow and organ transplants, and acquired immunodeficiency syndrome (AIDS). In these patients, herpetic lesions involve extensive areas of epidermis, the oropharynx, and the esophagus. Occasionally, hematogenous dissemination of HSV in compromised hosts produces extensive skin lesions resembling varicella. In patients with extensive skin damage from burns, pemphigus, Sézary syndrome, and eczema, HSV infection can involve large areas of denuded and intact epithelium and can be disseminated to visceral organs. In compromised patients subjected to endotracheal intubation, tracheobronchitis and pneumonitis caused by HSV may develop. Rarely, systemic dissemination of HSV with lethal, fulminant hepatitis in pregnant women and transplant recipients has been observed (Table 251-2).

Congenital and neonatal infection. Transmission of virus to the fetus in utero is a rare complication of HSV infection in pregnancy. The clinical manifestations are similar to those of other congenital infections in which microcephaly, jaundice, hepatosplenomegaly, chorioretinitis, and thrombocytopenia are present at birth. Acquisition of HSV by the infant during passage through an infected birth canal is much more common, especially after recent primary infection of the mother. Clinical manifestations develop within 2 to 10 days after birth and include fever, cranial nerve palsies, seizures, and lethargy progressing to coma. Because characteristic herpetic skin lesions occur in only 60% of infected infants, the disease is frequently mistaken for neonatal sepsis. When it is untreated, the mortality rate is 50% to 60%, usually as a result of necrotizing encephalitis and hepatic necrosis (Table 251-2).

Diagnosis

In most cases of HSV infection, the diagnosis is apparent on clinical examination. Examination of stained cells from the base of an ulcer (Tzanck preparation) often demonstrates characteristic multinucleate giant cells and intranuclear inclusions (see Plate V-13). The clinical diagnosis can be confirmed by culture of vesicle fluid or cells scraped from the base of an ulcer. HSV produces distinct cytopathic effects in a variety of cell cultures within 24 to 96 hours, and culture remains the most sensitive and specific means of diagnosis (Chapter 226). Because most neonatal HSV infections occur in children born of mothers with no history of symptomatic genital lesions, routine screening cultures of pregnant women with a history of genital herpes are of no value. New diagnostic reagents, biotin and fluorescein-labeled monoclonal antibodies, have been developed that

Table 251-2. Complications of herpesvirus infection

Virus	Congenital infection	Peripartum infection	Primary infection	Recurrent infection	Associated neoplasma
HSV	Microcephaly Hepatosplenomegaly Thrombocytopenia	Disseminated visceral and cutaneous disease	Encephalitis Keratitis Stomatitis Proctitis Whitlow Hepatic necrosis Aseptic meningitis Tracheobronchitis	Erythema multiforme Aseptic meningitis Whitlow Sensory and autonomic neuralgia	Cervical carcinoma
VZV	Limb atrophy Skin lesions Eye lesions Nervous system abnormalities	Varicella	Pneumonitis Meningoencephalitis Hepatitis Reye's syndrome	Disseminated zoster	None
CMV	Cytomegalic inclusion disease Asymptomatic infection	Interstitial pneumonitis	Hepatitis Guillain-Barré syndrome Interstitial pneumonitis Encephalitis Pancreatitis Chorioretinitis Colitis	Same as primary	Kaposi's sarcoma
EBV	None known	None known	Polyclonal B cell proliferation Complications of mononucleosis	Poorly defined	Nasopharyngeal carcinoma Burkitt's lymphoma B cell lymphoma

may provide rapid diagnosis based on antibody binding to infected cells. Currently, the ability of these tests to exclude HSV infection is not resolved. In the case of brain biopsy for suspected herpes encephalitis, fluorescein-labeled antibody staining appears to be a useful adjunct to histopathologic evaluation and culture of biopsied materials. Serologic detection of neutralizing or complement-fixing antibodies against HSV has little role in clinical diagnosis. However, it has been useful as a means of distinguishing "true primary" HSV infection from "recurrent primary" infection. In the former case, serum antibody is absent at the time of the first clinical episode of HSV, and antibody titers are present 2 to 4 weeks later. In "recurrent primary" infection, antibody is present, indicating antecedent infection before the initial clinical presentation. Diagnosis of HSV infection by serologic testing is further complicated by cross reactivity between HSV-1 and HSV-2 antibodies and fluctuations in titers caused by other diseases.

Treatment

The recent development of antiviral compounds that specifically inhibit the replication of HSV has greatly altered the approach to management (Table 251-3). Topical use of such drugs is effective in herpetic keratitis, in which application of idoxuridine (IUdR), adenine arabinoside (vidarabine [ara-A]), trifluridine, and acycloguanosine (acyclovir [ACV]) has been shown to speed resolution and prevent corneal ulceration and visual impairment. In genital herpetic infection, topical ACV has modest efficacy for primary episodes but none for recurrent bouts. Treatment does not appear to alter the frequency of subsequent recurrent episodes. Recent studies indicate that oral ACV is effective for treatment of primary herpes genitalis and prevention of recurrent episodes and is indicated for treatment of severe orolabial HSV-1 disease in immunocompromised patients. Again, however, the frequency of recurrence of lesions is not altered by therapy once treatment is stopped. HSV mutants resistant to ACV have been recovered particularly from AIDS patients undergoing multiple courses of therapy. In HSV-1 encephalitis, intravenous therapy with ACV or ara-A significantly reduces mortality rate, particularly if treatment is begun before coma supervenes. However, many survivors of herpetic encephalitis have moderate to severe neurologic impairment. Acyclovir has fewer side-effects and greater efficacy than ara-A. In disseminated herpetic infection of the newborn, intravenous treatment with ACV or ara-A substantially reduces mortality rate. HSV infections resistant to ACV can be effectively treated with foscarnet.

VARICELLA-ZOSTER VIRUS

Epidemiology

Varicella is a very common childhood disease with a peak incidence in late winter and early spring. Approximately two thirds of the cases occur in the 5 to 9 year age group. Despite the fact that chickenpox is a highly communicable

Table 251-3. Chemotherapy of herpesvirus infections

Virus	Host	Disease	Drug	Route	Treatment vs. prophylaxis	Approx. response to drug*: Virus shedding	Approx. response to drug*: Clinical response	Comments
Herpes simplex	Normal or immunocompromised	Initial genital, orofacial, or other mucocutaneous infection	Acyclovir	Topical	Treatment	++	+	Excellent documentation for genital infection; poor for other sites of infection. Oral or intravenous therapy should be employed in every case of initial infection
			Acyclovir	IV	Treatment	++++	+++	
			Acyclovir	Oral	Treatment	+++	+++	
		Recurrent genital, orofacial, or other	Acyclovir	Topical	Treatment	+/0	0	Excellent documentation for genital infection; fair for recurrences at other sites
			Acyclovir	Oral	Treatment	++	++	
			Acyclovir	Oral	Prophylaxis	N/A	+++	
		Encephalitis	Vidarabine	IV	Treatment	N/A	++	Acyclovir has been shown to be superior to vidarabine in two comparative clinical trials
			Acyclovir	IV	Treatment	N/A	+++	
		Disseminated infection in the neonate	Vidarabine	IV	Treatment	+++	+++	Acyclovir and vidarabine are comparable
			Acyclovir	IV	Treatment	+++	+++	
		Keratitis	Idoxuridine Vidarabine Trifluorothymidine Acyclovir	Topical	Treatment	+++	+++	Activity of these drugs topically is approximately equivalent
	Immunocompromised	Resistant to acyclovir	Acyclovir	Continuous infusion	Treatment	++	+++	Acyclovir-resistant virus often relapses after foscarnet therapy
			Foscarnet	IV	Treatment	+++	+++	
			Vidarabine	IV	Treatment	+	+	
Varicella zoster	Normal	Chickenpox (initial infection)	Acyclovir	Oral	Treatment	++	++	Reduces severity when begun within 24 hours
		Zoster	Acyclovir	IV	Treatment	+++	+++	No effect on postherpetic neuralgia. High dose resulted in significant toxicity. Most experts recommend no treatment
			Acyclovir	Oral	Treatment	+++	+++	
	Immunocompromised	Chickenpox	Vidarabine	IV	Treatment	+++	++	Acyclovir is more effective
			Acyclovir	IV	Treatment	++++	+++	
		Zoster	Vidarabine	IV	Treatment	+++	++	No comparative studies; most authorities prefer acyclovir (less toxic; possibly more effective)
			Interferon	IV/IM	Treatment	+++	++	
			Acyclovir	IV	Treatment	+++	++	
			Foscarnet	IV	Treatment	+++	+++	Foscarnet used for acyclovir resistant virus
Epstein-Barr virus	Immunocompromised	Lymphoma or progressive infection	Acyclovir	IV	Treatment	+/0	+/0	Documentation of clinical efficacy is poor
Cytomegalovirus	Immunocompromised	Various (retinitis, colitis, esophagitis, pneumonitis, etc.)	Acyclovir	IV/Oral	Prophylaxis	++	++	IV or high dose oral acyclovir reduces rate of CMV disease in transplant recipients
			Ganciclovir	IV	Treatment	++	+++	Ganciclovir treatment reduces rate of pneumonia in marrow recipients with CMV in bronchial lavage; ganciclovir and foscarnet equally effective in controlled trials for retinitis; ganciclovir probably effective for other forms of CMV disease
			Foscarnet	IV	Treatment	++	+++	

*0, no effect; ++++, maximum effect.

disease, demonstration of infectious VZV in respiratory secretions is difficult. Nevertheless, airborne droplet spread is presumed to be the mode of transmission. In contrast to other herpesvirus infections in the vast majority of cases, VZV infections are clinically apparent and only 5% occur silently. The incubation period of chickenpox ranges from 10 to 21 days. Shingles or zoster is a nonseasonal infection that occurs most often in older age groups and in immunosuppressed patients. In nonimmune individuals chickenpox may develop after contact with individuals who have zoster.

Pathogenesis

Varicella-zoster virus causes varicella (chickenpox) as a primary infection, generally in childhood, and then may cause recurrent disease later in life in the form of zoster (shingles). A relationship between the two diseases was recognized nearly a century ago when it was observed that children could acquire chickenpox after exposure to adults with zoster. More recently, characterization of the viruses has provided convincing evidence that the same agent causes both diseases. In the case of varicella, the virus is probably introduced into the host via the respiratory tract or oropharyngeal mucosa. After local virus replication, a viremia ensues during which VZV is carried to mucosal and cutaneous sites elsewhere in the body. The viremia is most likely cyclic in nature, because cutaneous vesicles tend to develop in crops. Within a few days, specific humoral and cell-mediated immune responses appear, and interferon concentrations in the vesicle fluids rise. Virus eventually disappears from the lesions as the cellular inflammatory infiltrate heightens. The mechanism by which the sensory ganglia are infected with VZV is not clear (i.e., whether virus seeds the ganglia hematogenously or is carried to the ganglia via sensory nerves). Shingles, which may occur decades after varicella, results when dormant virus in the sensory ganglia begins to replicate and migrates down the sensory nerve axon to the skin. In the vast majority of cases, cutaneous lesions are distributed in the area of a single dermatome. Although the precise immune deficit allowing activation of virus in the ganglia has not been identified, waning cell-mediated immunity associated with advancing age is probably an important factor. Dissemination of VZV via the bloodstream may occur in some patients, particularly those with impaired immune mechanisms caused by underlying lymphoma, leukemia, AIDS, or chemotherapy.

Disease states

Varicella. Chickenpox results from primary infection with VZV in an immunologically naive host and characteristically presents as widely disseminated cutaneous disease. Varicella is communicated by close, but not necessarily intimate, contact, probably by shedding of infectious virus in oropharyngeal secretions for 2 to 4 days before the clinical illness. Direct contact with vesicle fluid of either varicella or zoster may also result in acquisition of the virus. The first symptom of varicella in children is usually the characteristic exanthem. Small, irregular erythematous macules appear in a centripetal distribution, with lesions more prominent on the trunk, head, and proximal extremities. Within individual lesions, tiny vesicles (1 to 4 mm) containing clear fluid appear. These either rupture or, if left undisturbed, become cloudy. Within hours to days, the vesicles burst to form dry crusted lesions on an erythematous base. New crops of lesions appear for 2 to 4 days, and, characteristically, all three stages of lesions, macular, vesicular, and crusted, are present simultaneously.

Clinical disease in varicella varies from mild illness in which only a few vesicles are present to widespread infection covering the entire body with lesions. Fever may occur for 1 to 2 days before the onset of skin lesions and during the first 2 to 3 days of illness in children. In adults, varicella is a more severe illness with prolonged fever, malaise, arthralgias, and frequently pulmonary involvement (varicella pneumonia). The pneumonia may be micronodular, interstitial, or even lobar in distribution and has a high mortality rate in pregnant women. After convalescence, pulmonary diffusion capacity may remain abnormal for several months. Less common complications include cerebritis, encephalitis, Guillain-Barré syndrome, and myocarditis. Especially in patients with poor hygiene, the skin lesions of varicella may become superinfected by bacteria (usually streptococci or staphylococci).

Congenital and neonatal varicella. On rare occasions, in utero infection of the fetus occurs when the varicella develops in the mother in the first or second trimester. Afflicted children may have atrophy of a limb, cicatricial skin lesions, various ocular disorders, cortical atrophy, and seizure disorders (Table 251-2). Maternal varicella near the end of pregnancy may result in chickenpox in the newborn. If the maternal illness occurs within 2 weeks before delivery, the risk of varicella in the infant is approximately 25%. Mortality rate approaches 30% when the onset of varicella in the newborn is between 5 and 10 days after delivery. Overall, the mortality rate is approximately 10%.

Zoster. Herpes zoster (shingles) is the result of the reactivation of dormant VZV in the sensory ganglia in an individual who has had varicella previously. The incidence of zoster increases with age from less than 0.1% per year in the first decade of life to more than 1.0% per year above the age of 80. Most patients who have shingles do not have underlying malignancy. However, drugs and diseases that impair cell-mediated immunity may trigger the development of zoster, leading to the conclusion that cellular mechanisms are more important than humoral in the suppression of latent VZV infection. Herpes zoster characteristically causes pain and paresthesias that precede the development of a vesicular eruption in a single dermatomal distribution. Thoracic dermatomes are most commonly involved, followed by disease in the distribution of a single cervical, facial, lumbar, or sacral ganglion. The prodromal neuralgic symptoms may include pruritis, tingling, exquisite tenderness, and deep pain in an affected area for 1 to 2 days before skin lesions develop. The rash begins as maculopapules, which rapidly develop into crops of vesicles on an erythematous base. New lesions continue to appear for 3 to 5 days as the older ones ulcerate and crust. Crusting lesions and pain in the affected area may persist for several weeks, however. In the absence of bacterial superinfection, there is complete healing without scarring.

The most prominent complication (Table 251-2) of herpes zoster is the occurrence of persistent or intermittent pain in the affected area for months to years after resolution of acute zoster infection (postherpetic neuralgia). Postherpetic neuralgia is common in patients above the age of 60 and is rare in children. Involvement of motor and sympathetic nerves adjacent to the involved sensory ganglion also may complicate zoster. Sacral lesions may be accompanied by bowel or bladder dysfunction. Zoster in the distribution of the second or third cervical dermatome can cause facial muscle paralysis with or without involvement of cranial nerve VIII (Ramsay Hunt syndrome). Involvement of the ophthalmic branch of the trigeminal ganglion may result in conjunctivitis and rarely, infection of the eye with keratitis and iritis. Disseminated zoster can develop in both normal and immunocompromised patients, although this is much more common in patients with impaired immunity (see later discussion).

Zoster in immunocompromised patients. The increased incidence of zoster in the setting of certain disease states (AIDS, lymphoma, Hodgkin's disease, lupus erythematosus) and in association with immunosuppressive therapy (steroids and antineoplastic drugs) has served to demonstrate the importance of the immune system in maintenance of VZV in a latent state. Of patients with various malignancies, approximately 13% to 15% eventually have shingles. In addition, immunosuppressed patients and transplant recipients may have a risk of dissemination of virus approaching 25% to 30% if zoster develops. Generalization of the vesicular exanthem usually occurs 7 to 10 days after onset of the localized eruption. Virus may also invade the lungs, central nervous system, pancreas, or liver.

Treatment and prevention

Ordinarily, varicella and zoster do not require specific therapy. In older patients with shingles, two studies have indicated that a short course of corticosteroids given early in the illness may reduce the risk of postherpetic neuralgia. No deleterious effects have been described in the normal host. However, corticosteroids should not be given to immunocompromised patients with zoster because of the risk of dissemination. Adenine arabinoside at an intravenous dose of 10 mg/kg/day or ACV at 20 mg/kg/day appears to accelerate healing of lesions and to diminish the rate of dissemination if given early in immunocompromised patients (Table 251-3). It is ineffective, however, once dissemination has begun. In one study, early administration of acyclovir appeared to halt further progression even after dissemination had begun. Vidarabine, acyclovir, and interferon have all been shown to have a modestly beneficial effect in chickenpox occurring in immunocompromised children if therapy is started early. In patients with AIDS who have received multiple courses of ACV, a new syndrome of chronic zoster has been described. Painful hyperkeratotic papules or ulcers continue to yield VZV on culture despite high-dose oral or intravenous ACV. The VZV strains recovered are highly resistant to ACV but susceptible to foscarnet.

Studies of a live, attenuated vaccine against VZV have been ongoing in Japan for a number of years and have been initiated recently in the United States. Passive immunization with VZV immune globulin (VZIG) is available for certain high-risk patients who are exposed to cases of chickenpox or shingles. It should be administered within 72 hours of exposure to patients with leukemia or lymphoma, or congenital or acquired immunodeficiency, patients receiving immunosuppressive drugs or high-dose steroids, and newborn infants whose mothers had varicella within 5 days before delivery.

CYTOMEGALOVIRUS INFECTION

Epidemiology

CMV infections, most of which are subclinical, are extremely common throughout the world. The prevalence of CMV infection in a given population is directly related to lower socioeconomic status, crowded living conditions, and poor hygiene. Although little is known about the means of virus spread among individuals, the risk of acquisition of CMV infection is partially understood for certain age groups. In the newborn infant, infection may be acquired during passage through the birth canal, where cervicovaginal secretions may contain infectious virus. CMV may also be transmitted during the neonatal period by breast milk. Subsequently, shedding of CMV in urine or saliva is common in healthy young children, particularly in day care centers, where as many as 60% have viruria. It is likely that widespread infection among asymptomatic children plays an important role in the spread of virus to other children and adults. Although the risk of infection appears to be low from any given encounter with an asymptomatic virus shedder, the virus is so ubiquitous that repeated opportunities for exposure undoubtedly occur. There is evidence that suggests that in adolescence and adulthood, infectious CMV in vaginal secretions, semen, and saliva may also be spread by sexual activity. Finally, it is important to note that in any age group virus may be transferred from donor to recipient by blood transfusion and organ transplantation (kidney, heart, lung, and liver).

In the United States, approximately 2% of all newborn infants are infected with CMV in utero as evidenced by the detection of virus in urine at birth. Most of these children appear normal and do not have obvious cytomegalic inclusion disease. Two studies have indicated, however, that in a small percentage psychomotor retardation, sensorineural hearing loss, and/or deficiency of intelligence quotient subsequently develops. Overt cytomegalic inclusion disease is present at birth in approximately 10% of infants infected in utero.

Pathogenesis

Four different types of virus-host interaction are recognized with respect to CMV (Tables 251-1 and 251-2): (1) Primary infection in which initial acquisition of virus occurs. The vast majority of these infections are asymptomatic in the normal host, although transplacental passage of the virus during pregnancy may produce cytomegalic inclusion disease of the fetus. Mononucleosis is the most common clinical manifestation of CMV infection in previously healthy adults. In immunocompromised individuals, primary infection may result in widespread CMV disease, particularly interstitial pneumonitis, hepatitis, colitis, and central nervous system involvement. (2) Chronic or persistent infection in which asymptomatic viral shedding occurs in various sites (urine, saliva, semen, cervicovaginal secretions) for months or years despite a specific humoral and cell-mediated host immune response. This type of infection probably has special significance with respect to spread of CMV in the normal population. (3) Latent infection or persistence of CMV in a nonreplicating form in host cells or tissues. Although the cellular repository of the dormant virus has not yet been identified definitively, CMV in this state can be transmitted by blood transfusion or organ transplantation. The clinical consequences of virus transfer are more severe when the recipient has not previously been infected with CMV. (4) Reactivation or recurrent infection in which CMV reappears in a replicating form. Reactivation may result in asymptomatic viral shedding or in severe disseminated disease, particularly in the immunocompromised host (e.g., the patient with AIDS). In addition to reactivation by immunosuppression, latent CMV may be activated in pregnancy or during lactation.

In congenital infection, recent studies indicate that reactivation of endogenous CMV in the mother is the most common mechanism of fetal infection. However, symptomatic cytomegalic inclusion disease in the infant results predominantly, if not exclusively, when the mother acquires the virus as an exogenous primary infection. The vast majority of maternal infections in this setting are not associated with symptomatic maternal disease, although a few cases of CMV mononucleosis with transplacental passage of the virus have been described. Primary maternal CMV infection in the first trimester of pregnancy may be more likely to result in congenital disease.

In virtually all cases of congenital or acquired CMV disease, viremia can be detected by recovery of virus from peripheral blood leukocytes in tissue culture. Frequently, the viremia antedates the development of tissue injury, particularly interstitial pneumonitis. CMV can be recovered primarily with the polymorphonuclear leukocyte population of blood cells during viremic infection.

Disease states

Congenital infection. As noted, 85% to 90% of infants infected with CMV in utero appear normal at birth, whereas cytomegalic inclusion disease is apparent in 10% to 15%. Manifestations include jaundice, hepatosplenomegaly, thrombocytopenia, petechiae, and various neurologic conditions. Microcephaly, motor disability, chorioretinitis, cerebral calcifications, and seizure disorders have also been described. Subsequently, mental retardation and hearing loss may become apparent in children who survive. In general, neurologic manifestations persist or worsen, whereas hepatosplenomegaly, jaundice, and hemorrhagic phenomena may subside eventually.

Cytomegalovirus mononucleosis

CMV is responsible for approximately two thirds of the cases of heterophil-negative infectious mononucleosis that meet conventional hematologic and clinical criteria. The disease may occur spontaneously in previously healthy individuals or within 3 to 8 weeks after blood transfusion. In spontaneous illness, the age of the individuals afflicted (18 to 30 years) is somewhat higher than in EBV infectious mononucleosis. Clinically, CMV mononucleosis is characterized by less impressive tonsillopharyngitis and lymphadenopathy than EBV disease, although considerable overlap has been reported. Exudative pharyngitis is particularly rare in CMV mononucleosis. Although the heterophil test result is always negative, other evidence of disordered immunoregulation seen in CMV disease includes positive rheumatoid factor tests findings, cryoglobulinemia, high-titered cold agglutinins, positive results for antinuclear antibody, and false-positive syphilis serologic findings. As in EBV mononucleosis, complications such as Bell's palsy, Guillain-Barré syndrome, and a maculopapular rash after administration of ampicillin may be seen. Rare complications include thrombocytopenia, hemolytic anemia, myopericarditis, pneumonitis, and meningoencephalitis.

Infection in the compromised host

CMV infection is most likely to be life-threatening when it occurs in the host whose defense mechanisms are impaired by underlying disease or superimposed immunosuppressive therapy. Patients with hematologic malignancies, recipients of organ transplants, and individuals with AIDS are particularly susceptible to disseminated CMV infection. In this setting, the virus may involve the liver, pancreas, colon, adrenals, ocular structures, and the central nervous system. However, the major threat to life results from interstitial pneumonitis with progressive hypoxemia, which is now the most common cause of death in recipients of marrow transplants. In the latter, CMV infection is closely associated with graft-versus-host disease. In the case of CMV-seronegative renal and cardiac transplant recipients, the highest risk of CMV disease is in patients who receive an organ from a CMV-seropositive donor. On the other hand, marrow transplant recipients appear to experience CMV disease after reactivation of endogenous latent virus. CMV infection of homosexual men and patients with AIDS is extremely common. Symptomatic CMV disease usually occurs late in the progression of AIDS. Chorioretinitis is the most common initial manifestation. CMV esophagitis and colitis also occur frequently. At autopsy, CMV involvement of the central and peripheral nervous system, pneumonitis, hepatitis, and necrotizing adrenalitis are common findings in patients who died of AIDS.

Diagnosis

CMV infection can be diagnosed by recovery of the virus in human diploid cell cultures. Specimens appropriate for virus culture include urine, saliva, breast milk, semen, cervicovaginal secretions, peripheral blood leukocytes, intraocular fluids, and tissues obtained by biopsy or at autopsy. Depending on the amount of infectious virus present in the sample, 7 to 30 days is usually required for recovery of CMV. Although culture is specific for CMV infection, it does not distinguish between asymptomatic shedding and invasive disease in a given patient. As previously noted, however, recovery of virus from peripheral blood leukocytes is a valuable correlate of active or impending CMV disease. Positive "buffy coat" culture results have been reported in patients with congenital disease, or CMV mononucleosis, and in immunocompromised patients with disseminating infection. More rapid methods for detection of CMV in clinical specimens using centrifugal "shell vial" assays and monoclonal antibodies are now available. For diagnosis of CMV interstitial pneumonitis, open lung biopsy may be necessary to provide tissue for histologic examination and virus culture. Occasionally characteristic inclusion-bearing cells indicating CMV infection can be detected in bronchial washings or lavage.

A variety of serologic tests are now available for detection of CMV antibody in serum, including complement fixation, immunofluorescence, anticomplementary immunofluorescence, indirect hemagglutination, and enzyme-linked immunosorbent assay (ELISA) (Chapter 226). In these tests, a seroconversion from negative to positive or a fourfold or greater rise in titer in paired sera is necessary to confirm the presence of active CMV infection. CMV-specific IgM antibody can be demonstrated by either immunofluorescence or ELISA methods. Its detection suggests recent or active infection as opposed to more remote CMV infection. CMV-IgM antibody can be detected in approximately 75% of cord blood specimens from infants infected in utero; however, rheumatoid factor may cause a false-positive result.

Prevention and treatment

Field trials of an attenuated CMV vaccine are in progress. The risk of serious CMV disease can be reduced in transplant recipients by use of CMV-seronegative donors and blood transfusions and by administration of prophylactic acyclovir; CMV-immunoglobulin, or ganciclovir (the latter in marrow recipients). Ganciclovir (5 mg/kg twice daily intravenously) has proven efficacy for treatment of CMV retinitis in AIDS and probably in other forms of CMV disease. However, indefinite maintenance therapy with single daily infusions of 5 to 6 mg/kg of ganciclovir is virtually always necessary to prevent symptomatic relapse. Unfortunately, CMV may become resistant to ganciclovir after multiple courses. Efficacy of ganciclovir for treatment of interstitial pneumonitis in marrow recipients is enhanced when it is combined with immunoglobulin. The main side-effect of ganciclovir therapy is neutropenia. Foscarnet has recently been approved for use in treatment of CMV retinitis in AIDS and is active against ganciclovir-resistant strains of CMV. Its main side-effects are nephrotoxicity, hypocalcemia, and seizures.

EPSTEIN-BARR VIRUS

Epidemiology

Infections with EBV as measured by the presence of serum viral capsid antibody are extremely common throughout the world. In general, infection occurs early in life among individuals in lower socioeconomic groups and in developing countries. In some parts of the world, virtually 100% of the population has had EBV infection by the age of 10 years. The vast majority of these infections are asymptomatic or perhaps associated with mild nonspecific respiratory symptoms. Infectious mononucleosis occurs most often in older children or in young adults from the upper socioeconomic groups. The incidence is highest among university students and military cadets, where the rate of EBV infection among susceptible persons ranges from 12% to 30% per year. Infectious mononucleosis develops in approximately one half of infected individuals. Presently, the exact means of transmission of EBV is not well defined. On the basis of protracted shedding of virus in the oropharyngeal secretions of individuals recently infected, it appears likely that EBV is spread via the respiratory route. Relatively intimate contact (e.g., kissing) appears to be necessary. The incubation period of infectious mononucleosis appears to be 4 to 7 weeks. EBV may also be transmitted by blood transfusion, although transfusion-associated infections are much less common with EBV than with CMV.

Pathogenesis

Among the herpesviruses, EBV is unique in several respects. The virus cannot be propagated in conventional tissue culture cells. It does replicate in vitro in human B lymphocytes, although most of these cells are abortively infected (i.e., progeny virus is not produced and the cells are not lysed by EBV). The infected B cells are "immortalized" by the viral infection and proliferate indefinitely in vitro. In general, EBV infection of lymphocytes is a prerequisite for the immortalization response. Several new antigens appear on the membranes of EBV-infected B cells, including the nuclear antigen, the viral capsid antigen, and the lymphocyte-determined membrane antigen. EBV genetic material persists indefinitely in the form of an extrachromosomal plasmid, many copies of which are present in infected B lymphocytes.

The pathogenesis of infectious mononucleosis induced by infection with EBV is now understood to an extent, although several aspects remain to be defined. The virus is introduced into the susceptible host as a result of close contact (e.g., kissing) with another individual who is shedding

EBV in the oropharynx. Initial virus replication occurs in the epithelial cells of the oropharynx and the salivary glands. A localized inflammatory response produces the pharyngeal exudate. Subsequently, virus is carried via the lymphatics to local lymph nodes, and a viremia ensues. Local and generalized lymphadenopathy as well as splenomegaly then develop. Whether proliferation of lymphoid cells in these sites involves EBV-infected B cells themselves or is caused indirectly by "reactive" T cells is not yet clear. In the peripheral blood, EBV infection can be demonstrated in only a very small percentage of B cells. The vast majority of atypical lymphocytes, which are the hallmark of infectious mononucleosis, are T cells. These cells are apparently produced in response to infected B lymphocytes that express novel viral antigens on their surfaces. Initially, suppressor or cytotoxic T cells predominate in association with cutaneous anergy. Later, helper or inducer T cells are produced and correlate with eventual recovery. Secretion of the heterophil agglutinin, which is a macroglobulin, and several other aberrant antibodies results from polyclonal activation of infected B cells. Characteristically, EBV is shed in the oropharynx for many months after recovery from the clinical illness.

After initial subclinical infection or after infectious mononucleosis, EBV is permanently established in its latent form in B lymphocytes. In contrast to the other herpesviruses, in EBV infection no disease syndromes are clearly associated with reactivation of the dormant virus. EBV infection is strongly associated, however, with several malignant disorders, including Burkitt's African lymphoma and nasopharyngeal carcinoma. High titers of EBV antibody are found in individuals with these diseases, and large quantities of viral DNA have been detected in the tumor cells. Non-Hodgkin's lymphomas in recipients of kidney, bone marrow, and heart transplants who receive immunosuppressive drugs on a long-term basis appear to be induced by EBV. Finally, a diffuse polyclonal lymphoma of the B cell type has been described repeatedly in immunodeficient hosts, including recipients of organ transplants, patients with severe combined immunodeficiency and ataxia-telangiectasia, and patients with AIDS. An X-linked lymphoproliferative syndrome has also been reported in males.

Disease states

Infectious mononucleosis. The hallmark symptoms of infectious mononucleosis caused by EBV (EBV mononucleosis) include fever, fatigue, cervical adenopathy, and sore throat. The onset is often insidious with the gradual development of increasing malaise, fever, and chills for less than a week, followed by the onset of pharyngitis. The pharyngitis may be mistaken for streptococcal infection. However, administration of ampicillin (and to a lesser extent other penicillins) results in the rapid appearance of a generalized maculopapular rash in the majority of patients with infectious mononucleosis (IM). Findings on physical examination often include periorbital edema; palatal petechiae; cervical, axillary, and epitrochlear lymphadenopathy; splenomegaly and hepatomegaly; and a variety of skin rashes. Rarely, IM caused by EBV may present as an aseptic meningitis or meningoencephalitis with a normal CSF glucose level and a mononuclear pleocytosis. Neurologic manifestations of EBV infection, which occur in approximately 1% of patients, include Guillain-Barré syndrome, transverse myelitis, Bell's and other cranial nerve palsies, and mononeuritis multiplex. Hematologic complications include a Coombs positive hemolytic anemia result and profound thrombocytopenia in less than 4% of cases. The acute splenic congestion and subcapsular hemorrhages in IM place patients at risk for splenic rupture caused by relatively minor trauma or exertion. The acute symptoms of EBV mononucleosis usually last from 2 to 4 weeks, although malaise, fatigue, and depression can be protracted and may be exacerbated by injudicious exercise. Splenomegaly and enlarged lymph nodes may persist for several months after the abatement of symptoms. In older adults EBV infection is more likely to be manifested as a typhoidal illness with fever and malaise without splenomegaly or lymphadenopathy.

Laboratory features. The hallmark laboratory features of IM produced by EBV are the presence of heterophil antibodies, atypical lymphocytosis, and mildly elevated hepatic enzymes (SGOT and SGPT) levels. Heterophil antibodies are IgM antibodies, which selectively agglutinate erythrocytes of other species, including sheep RBC (the Paul Bunnell test) and the horse RBC (the basis for the rapid agglutination or "monospot" test). Although these antibodies are usually detected at the time of presentation in more than 85% of patients with EBV infection, in a small number of patients the heterophil antibody test result may not be positive until 3 to 4 weeks after the onset of the illness. IM caused by EBV usually is characterized by leukocytosis ($>10^9$/L) and relative and absolute lymphocytosis, and at least 10% of the lymphocytes have the characteristics of activated lymphocytes. The atypical lymphocytes characteristic of IM, "Downey cells," are T lymphocytes with surface marker phenotypes of suppressor/cytotoxic T cells.

Diagnosis

Although the diagnosis presents little difficulty in most instances, there are several diagnostic pitfalls of which to be aware: (1) A diagnosis of streptococcal pharyngitis may be made if the systemic nature of the illness is not appreciated. (2) The heterophil agglutinin may take 3 to 4 weeks to appear. (3) Polymorphonuclear leukocytosis may be present initially although many of the lymphocytes present are atypical. (4) Tonsillopharyngeal involvement, lymphadenopathy, and splenomegaly may be minimal or absent ("typhoidal" presentation). (5) The characteristic findings may be overshadowed by complicating features (neurologic manifestations, jaundice, thrombocytopenia with hemorrhage, hemolytic anemia, or splenic rupture).

In most cases the diagnosis of EBV mononucleosis is confirmed by the presence of heterophil antibody and atypical lymphocytosis. However, in heterophil negative mononucleosis or in the absence of atypical lymphocytosis, EBV-specific serologic evaluation may be helpful. In these cases, the presence of IgM antibodies against EBV is virtually diagnostic of acute infection, as is the development of antibody against the EBV nuclear antigen (EBNA) in paired sera. The absence of antibody against the viral capsid antigen (VCA) of EBV after 2 weeks of illness excludes EBV infection.

CMV mononucleosis may closely mimic EBV-induced disease in terms of the hematologic manifestations, neurologic complications, production of aberrant antibodies, and ampicillin-induced rash. However, the heterophil test result is always negative. Clinically, CMV mononucleosis is characterized by less intense tonsillopharyngeal involvement (exudate is extremely uncommon) and lymphadenopathy. Other disorders that may present some features similar to those of infectious mononucleosis include toxoplasmosis, hepatitis A, adenovirus or herpes simplex, pharyngitis, enteroviral infections, Hodgkin's disease, angioimmunoblastic lymphadenopathy, and drug reactions (allopurinol, diphenylhydantoin, para-aminosalicylic acid, hydralazine, and methyldopa). In these entities, however, the atypical lymphocytosis is less intense and of much shorter duration.

Prevention and treatment

There is currently no effective means of preventing EBV infection. EBV mononucleosis is usually a benign, self-limited illness disease in which treatment is confined to the relief of symptoms. Headache, fever, and painful pharyngitis should be treated with acetaminophen, and the use of aspirin should be avoided in EBV mononucleosis because of the risk of subcapsular splenic hemorrhage. Patients with EBV mononucleosis who have skin rashes after inadvertent administration of ampicillin should be reassured that the reaction is not a specific drug allergy and will not occur on rechallenge.

Treatment with corticosteroids (prednisone, 40 mg/day for 5 to 7 days) is indicated for patients with severe tonsillar enlargement that may result in upper airway obstruction. Parenteral administration of prednisone may be necessary if swallowing is difficult. Other indications for a brief course of steroids are severe hemolytic anemia or thrombocytopenia and possibly aseptic meningitis or encephalitis. Steroids do not benefit patients with protracted fatigue and malaise caused by EBV mononucleosis. Patients should be cautioned to avoid exertion during the acute illness and during convalescence. Relapses of fever and malaise commonly occur in patients who prematurely return to their customary level of activity.

HUMAN HERPESVIRUS 6

Human herpesvirus 6 (HHV-6) was recently isolated from lymphocytes of patients with lymphoproliferative disorders and human immunodeficiency virus infection. Infection with HHV-6 appears to be relatively common among the normal population, where antibody prevalences of 20% to 40% have been detected. The virus has also been recovered from saliva of normal individuals. At the present time, no disease states have been definitively associated with the infection, except exanthem subitum (roseola infantum).

REFERENCES

Balfour H et al: Acyclovir halts progression of herpes zoster in immunocompromised patients. N Engl J Med 308:1448, 1983.

Brown ZA et al: Effects on infants of a first episode of genital herpes during pregnancy. N Engl J Med 317:1246, 1987.

Corey L and Spear PG: Infections with herpes simplex viruses. N Engl J Med 314:686, 749, 1986.

Erice A et al: Progressive cytomegalovirus disease due to ganciclovir-resistant virus in immunocompromised patients. N Engl J Med 320:289, 1989.

Evans AS, Niederman JC, and McCollum RW: Seroepidemiological studies of infectious mononucleosis with EB virus. N Engl J Med 279:1121, 1968.

Ho M: Cytomegalovirus: biology and infection, ed 2. New York, 1991, Plenum.

Jacobson MA et al: Acyclovir-resistant varicella-zoster virus infection after chronic oral acyclovir therapy in patients with the acquired immunodeficiency syndrome. Ann Intern Med 112:187, 1990.

Jacobson MA and Mills J: Serious cytomegalovirus disease in the acquired immunodeficiency syndrome (AIDS). Ann Intern Med 108:585, 1988.

Jones JF et al: T-cell lymphomas containing Epstein-Barr virus DNA in patients with chronic Epstein-Barr virus infections. N Engl J Med 318:733, 1988.

Jordan MC et al: Latent herpesviruses of humans. Ann Intern Med 100:866, 1984.

Meyers JD, Fluornoy N, and Thomas ED: Nonbacterial pneumonia after allogenic marrow transplantation: a review of ten years experience. Rev Infect Dis 4:1119, 1982.

Prober CG et al: Use of routine viral cultures at delivery to identify neonates exposed to herpes simplex virus. N Engl J Med 318:887, 1988.

Stagno S et al: Congenital cytomegalovirus infection: the relative importance of primary and recurrent maternal infection. N Engl J Med 306:945, 1982.

Straus SE et al: Suppression of frequently recurring genital herpes: a placebo-controlled double-blind trial of oral acyclovir. N Engl J Med 310:1545, 1984.

Weller TH: Varicella and herpes zoster: changing concepts of the natural history, control, and importance of a not-so-benign virus. N Engl J Med 309:1362, 1434, 1983.

Whitley RJ et al: Vidarabine versus acyclovir therapy in herpes simplex encephalitis. N Engl J Med 314:144, 1986.

CHAPTER

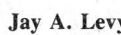

252 Human Retrovirus Infections

Jay A. Levy

Retroviruses have been found associated with three different pathologic conditions in humans: adult T cell leukemia (ATL), tropical spastic paraparesis (TSP), and acquired immunodeficiency syndrome (AIDS). A retrovirus of an oncovirus type has been recovered from ATL patients, who are found primarily in southwestern Japan, the Caribbean basin, and certain areas of the southwestern United States. A similar agent isolated from patients with TSP has been frequently found in the Caribbean islands and Japan. A retrovirus with the biologic, morphologic, and molecular features of a lentivirus has been isolated from AIDS patients. Both of these human viruses preferentially replicate in human T cells. The virus associated with ATL induces the cells to divide continuously; the virus associated with AIDS causes cytopathic changes leading to cell death.

CHARACTERISTICS

A retrovirus is a 100 nm lipid-enveloped, single-stranded ribonucleic acid (RNA) virus. Its genome consists of regions responsible for its assembly, including the gag (core region), pol (polymerase), env (envelope), and other portions coding for proteins that may be involved in replication and transformation (e.g., onc). Retroviruses derive their name from the presence of an enzyme (RNA-dependent deoxyribonucleic acid [DNA] polymerase or reverse transcriptase) that enables these viruses to make a copy DNA (cDNA) of their genomic RNA. This cDNA duplicates itself, circularizes, and subsequently integrates into the host cell chromosome. The virus then exists as a provirus in the cell and can be passed with the host genome to future cell generations.

By morphologic, biologic, and genetic properties, the retrovirus family has been recently divided into seven genera, which include the oncoviruses, the spumaviruses, and the lentiviruses. The human retroviruses consist of the oncovirus associated with ATL, the retroviruses resembling a lentivirus found in AIDS, and the human foamy virus, a spumavirus. The last-mentioned, the first human retrovirus identified (in 1971), has not been associated with any diseases in humans. Thus each of the three previously recognized subfamilies of animal retroviruses has a human counterpart.

The ATL-associated retrovirus is characterized by its morphologic features when budding from the cell surface. An incomplete core is formed at the cell membrane, and the full virion develops by budding into immature and mature forms containing a nucleoid of about 92 nm (Fig. 252-1, *A, B*). The AIDS-associated lentivirus is characterized by a similar budding process, but the core can be complete before budding, and the nucleoid in the mature form is cylindrical (Fig. 252-1, *C, D*). Thus on cross section by electron microscopy, a lentivirus has a 42 nm core, but on tangential section, it has a bar-shaped nucleoid (Fig. 252-1, *D*). Because of their lipid envelope, retroviruses are sensitive to polar solvents and heating in liquid form. However,

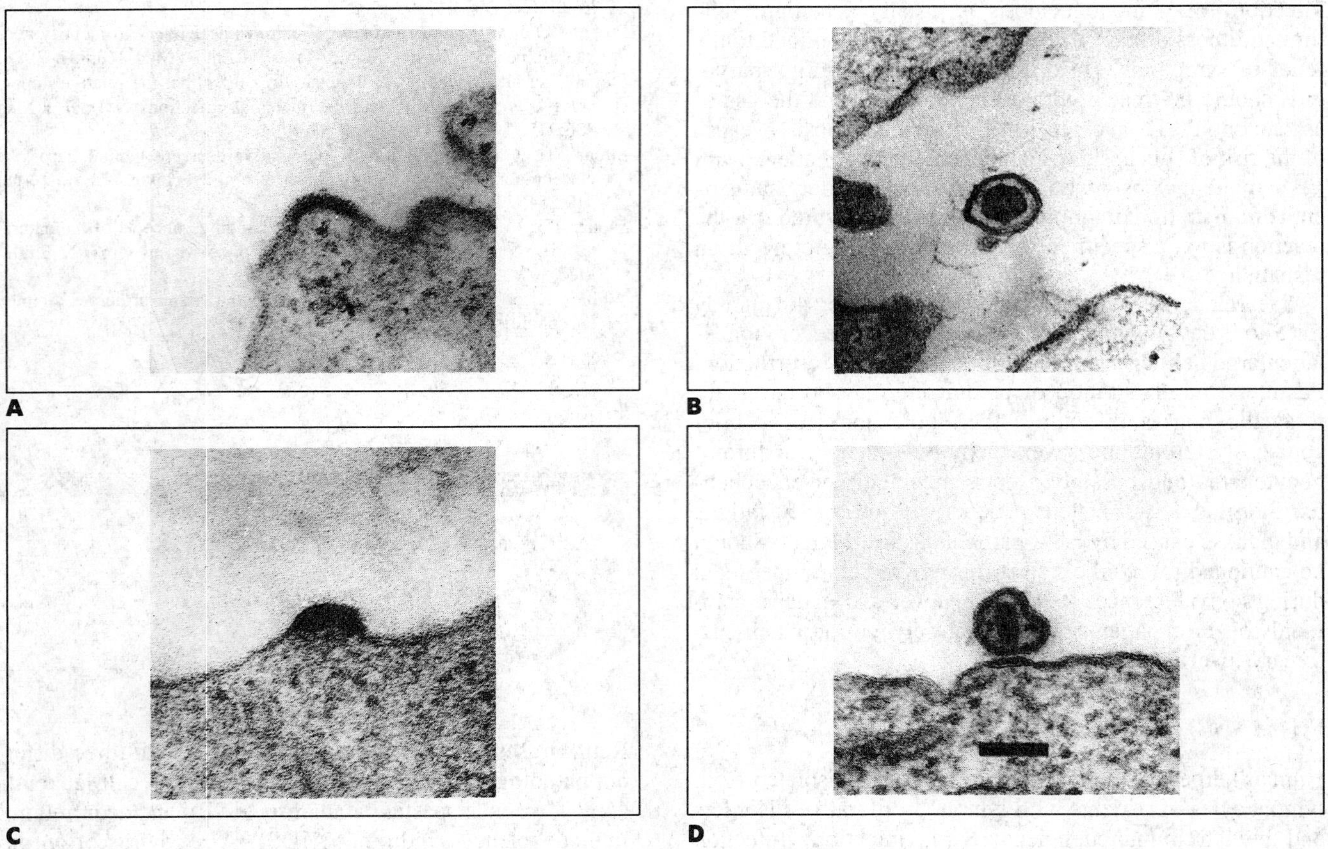

Fig. 252-1. Electron micrograph examination of the human T cell leukemia virus type I (HTLV-I) and the human immunodeficiency virus (HIV). **A,** Budding HTLV-I. **B,** Mature HTLV-I. **C,** Budding HIV-1. **D,** Mature HIV-1. Note cone-shaped core. Marker, 100 nm. (Photos provided by Dr. Lyndon S. Oshiro, California State Public Health Laboratory, Berkeley.)

when dried down in the presence of proteins, they can withstand heating up to 68° C for several hours.

The retroviruses associated with human disease preferentially infect helper T cells but can infect other cells of the immune system. The AIDS retroviruses can also infect cells of the neurologic and gastrointestinal systems.

The human C retrovirus associated with ATL has been called human T cell leukemia virus type I (HTLV-I). It is also known as adult T cell leukemia virus (ATLV) for the original isolate found in Japan. HTLV-II, which resembles HTLV-I, was recovered from a cell line established from a patient with hairy cell leukemia. This virus, however, has not yet been found associated with any human disease.

The retroviruses recovered from AIDS patients were initially named differently by the groups responsible for their isolation: lymphadenopathy-associated virus (LAV), human T cell lymphotropic virus type III (HTLV-III), and the AIDS-associated retrovirus (ARV). Molecular, serologic, and epidemiologic data suggest that these AIDS viruses now called human immunodeficiency virus (HIV) are part of the same lentivirus genus of human retroviruses. The HIV differ in morphologic characteristics, biologic properties, and molecular structure from the viruses responsible for ATL, which, as noted, are a separate group of human retroviruses.

ADULT T CELL LEUKEMIA

Epidemiology and clinical disease

Adult T cell leukemia (ATL) has been a recognized disease entity since 1977. It occurs primarily in clusters in southern Japan, namely, the islands of Kyushu, Shikoku, and Okinawa (Chapter 93). The disease also is present with some frequency in blacks in the Caribbean basin and in individuals in the southeastern United States. By clinical and pathologic criteria, ATL encompasses human T cell leukemias characterized by (1) onset in adulthood, (2) usually acute but somewhat chronic course, (3) leukemic cells with T cell properties and pleiomorphic features (indented and lobulated nuclei are also frequently found), (4) lymphadenopathy and hepatosplenomegaly, (5) absence of mediastinal lymph node involvement, (6) frequent lytic changes in bone with hypercalcemia, and (7) in some cases, leukemic cell infiltration of the skin. The disease generally can be distinguished from cutaneous T cell lymphoma by (1) absence of typical Sézary cells, (2) absence of leukemic cell infiltration of the epidermis despite infiltration into the dermis or subcutaneous tissue, (3) bone marrow and pulmonary involvement, and (4) shorter survival time. The median survival with ATL is usually 1 year or less.

HTLV-I antibodies are measured by an indirect immunofluorescence assay (IFA) or enzyme-linked immunosorbent assay (ELISA) using virus-infected T cells or purified viral antigens. Virus can be detected in peripheral lymphocytes by monoclonal antibodies to specific viral proteins. Antibodies to the virus have been found highly prevalent in ATL patients; populations at risk for development of this leukemia, particularly those individuals living in endemic areas in Japan; and family members of individuals with ATL. Evidence of exposure to the virus is also found in areas of Haiti and other islands of the Caribbean and in Central Africa. Recently, antibodies to the virus, particularly the HTLV II subtype, have been found in increasing frequency in intravenous drug users in the United States. Antibodies to the virus are not detected in patients with the typical cutaneous T cell leukemia/lymphoma found distributed throughout the world.

Pathophysiology

HTLV-I causes its disease by infecting primarily the helper subset of human T cells and establishing a chronic infection in which T cells are induced to grow continuously. In this manner, the infection of T cells by HTLV-I resembles the effect of EBV on human B cells (Chapter 251). The mechanism for this immortalization is not yet known. It may involve proteins made by the virus acting at a distance from the viral genome and turning on certain genes in the virus or the cell to induce continuous replication. The leukemic cells then spread through the body and invade certain lymphoid areas. The bone lesions in this disease may result from circulating humoral substances that induce osteoclastic activity rather than from invasion by malignant cells.

HTLV-I also causes fusion of cells in tissue culture. It may use this mechanism for entering and spreading among lymphocytes and other cells in the body. The virus appears to be passed in the infected individual by cell-to-cell contact, because cell-free transmission is a rare event in the laboratory. The T cells infected by the virus generally do not show evidence of this infection by expression of viral proteins in vivo. Virus is detected only after the cells are placed in culture. From experimental studies it is clear that many different T cells are initially infected, but eventually one autonomous clone grows out into the leukemic line. The route of transmission of the virus between individuals is unknown, but it may be passed via blood and body secretions (seminal fluid) containing infected T cells. It can also be passed by the intrauterine route or by milk from mother to child. The virus has been reported in mothers and their children, and in spouses. It appears that many individuals are infected with the virus and antibodies to it develop without causing leukemia. These antibodies can be of the virus-neutralizing type. In some individuals, antibodies to the virus have appeared 10 to 30 years before the development of leukemia. Because other types of T cell leukemias are not associated with HTLV-I infection, the virus may act not as an initiator but as a cofactor in promoting the emergence of autonomous clones of malignant T cells.

Treatment

No specific therapy is available. Standard chemotherapy can lead to a prompt reduction in tumor cell mass, but long-term survival of patients is rare. Hypercalcemia can be managed with oral phosphates, calcitonin, or mithramycin.

TROPICAL SPASTIC PARAPARESIS

Epidemiology

The distribution of cases of tropical spastic paraparesis (TSP) suggests that it occurs in a rather restricted area that favors its development. Most cases have been reported from tropical islands (e.g., Seychelles, Jamaica, Dominican Republic, and Martinique), but the disease has also been described in Central and South America, Africa, and India. A similar or related form of chronic spastic myelopathy has been noted in Japan in areas of high ATL prevalence. Because of the association with HTLV-I, it has been called HTLV-associated myelopathy (HAM). Both TSP and HAM occur more frequently in females than males, and their neuropathologic picture and clinical findings strongly suggest they are identical syndromes.

Clinical features and pathogenesis

Generally, the onset of TSP is gradual, but occasionally acute cases have been described, suggesting transverse myelopathy. In some cases, TSP has developed as early as 3 years after receipt of an HTLV-containing blood transfusion. In most patients with TSP, one leg is primarily affected. The progression is slow and may take several years to reach the most severe level of disease. Generalized symptoms include weakness of the legs, back pain, leg numbness, and dysesthesia of the feet. Also, bladder dysfunction, constipation, and penile impotence may occur. On neurologic examination, patients with TSP have spastic paraparesis or paraplegia, increased reflexes in the legs, as well as other signs of involvement of the pyramidal tracts. Many have brisk reflexes in the upper limbs as well. Mental function is usually normal as is cranial nerve function. Cerebral spinal fluid (CSF) examination generally yields normal findings with little or no pleocytosis. CD4/CD8 ratios are usually in the normal range but can show an elevated CD4 lymphocyte number.

Recent reports have now confirmed that individuals with TSP have a high prevalence of antibody to HTLV-I in both the serum and CSF. The virus has been recovered as well from CSF and serum of some patients, and the isolates are very similar to the HTLV-I associated with ATL. All this information emphasizes the potential neuropathic effects of HTLV-I. The pathogenesis involved in the disease is not known. Perivascular cuffing of some small vessels by lymphocytes penetrating the central nervous system has been reported as well as demyelination of the spinal cord and brain. The disease may result from direct infection of nerve cells by the virus, secondary effects of autoimmune responses, or inflammation caused by infiltrating HTLV-I–containing cells present in the spinal cord. Because high levels of antibodies to HTLV are associated with TSP, a hypothesized autoimmune or immunologic mechanism has been favored. Neurologic cases with antibodies to HTLV-1 are being classified as a separate group to follow their prognosis and potentially specific clinical features.

Treatment

Some patients with TSP have shown improvement with prednisone, but whether steroids or other immunosuppressive agents can be helpful is not clear. Other drugs being considered are antiretroviral agents such as 3-azidothymidine (Zidovudine).

ACQUIRED IMMUNODEFICIENCY SYNDROME

Epidemiology

Acquired immunodeficiency syndrome (AIDS) was first recognized in the United States in 1981, when *Pneumocystis carinii* pneumonia, and/or Kaposi's sarcoma was identified in an unusually large number of homosexual men (Chapter 242). Subsequently, these conditions as well as B cell lymphomas in some patients were found to be associated with an acquired immunodeficiency state that epidemiologically appeared to be spread by a virus. Retrospective studies identified AIDS cases initially in New York and Haiti as well as Africa as early as 1978. Individuals at risk in Western countries are primarily homosexual and bisexual men (73%) and intravenous drug abusers (17%). The disease has also been found in recipients of blood transfusions and blood products (hemophilia A and B patients), in heterosexual contacts of infected individuals, as well as in infants born of mothers who are in one of the risk groups (Chapter 242). In Africa, heterosexual activity is the primary source of virus transmission, most likely because of the concomitant presence of venereal diseases.

Pathophysiology

The human immunodeficiency virus (HIV) has a host range that involves preferential infection and replication in human T cells with the helper cell phenotype. However, the virus can also infect other T cells, macrophages, and B lymphocytes, particularly if they carry the helper cell (OKT4A, Leu 3) marker. This CD4 protein may be a major receptor for attachment of the virus to cells. Other cellular receptors for HIV are probably present because CD4-negative cells (e.g., fibroblasts, glial cells) can be infected by the virus. The virus causes a cytopathic effect in lymphocytes, leading to fusion and formation of mononucleated cells, which eventually die. This preferential infection of certain helper T cells contributes to a gradual reduction in the helper T cell number and a reversal of helper/suppressor T cell ratios (normally 2:1) to less than 1.0 as observed in AIDS patients. Autoantibodies to helper T cells may also have a role in this disorder. This deficit in immune function leads to the opportunistic infections and cancers (B cell lymphomas, Kaposi's sarcoma) characteristic of AIDS. Cofactors, such as infection with Epstein-Barr virus (EBV) and cytomegalovirus (CMV), also appear important in depressing the helper/suppressor T cell ratios in AIDS. These viruses alone can cause these changes in T cell ratios (Chapter 242). The AIDS retrovirus can also infect the central nervous system, where it gives rise to neurologic syndromes, including headaches, dementia, global encephalopathy, and sensory neuropathy. Cerebrospinal fluids contain the AIDS virus and show generally elevated protein levels without pleocytosis. Vacuolating myelopathy in the spinal cord of some patients has been described and appears to be caused directly by the virus.

Chronic diarrhea is another common symptom in individuals infected with HIV. In Africa it has been termed slim disease. Recent studies indicate direct infection of crypt cells of the bowel (including enterochromaffin cells) by the virus. This finding may explain the malabsorption and fluid loss observed in some infected individuals.

Transmission of HIV occurs via blood and body secretions, particularly seminal fluid. Unlike HTLV-I, the AIDS retrovirus can be transferred in a cell-free state, but the virus-infected cell also appears to be the major source of transmission. The virus has been isolated in very small amounts from saliva, but epidemiologic evidence does not suggest this route as a mechanism for its spread. Because of the relatively low incidence of heterosexual spread of HIV, the virus appears to pass preferentially through the mucosal membrane barrier of the anal canal rather than the squamous cell epithelium of the vagina, although some cases of heterosexual spread through conventional sexual contact have been reported. Studies in Africa strongly suggest that a major cofactor for heterosexual transmission is venereal disease, particularly genital ulcers caused by herpes virus or by Haemophilus ducreyi (chancroid) as well as the increased number of virus-infected cells in genital fluids associated with the inflammation.

Antibodies to HIV develop days to weeks after the infection, and rarely clinically healthy individuals without anti-HIV antibodies can be found with virus in their lymphocytes and plasma. Most individuals experience seroconversion within 1 to 3 months after infection, and it is generally agreed that by 1 year all infected individuals show antibodies to the virus. Asymptomatic individuals probably handle HIV infection by four different mechanisms: (1) On very rare occasions, they ward off the infection and eliminate the virus. (2) They keep the virus latent in the system, as with EBV infection of B lymphocytes. (3) They are "carriers" of the virus and can pass it to others through seminal (and vaginal) fluid and blood. (4) They are healthy except for a persistent lymphadenopathy, which reflects infection with the virus and perhaps a host response to the agent. The lymphadenopathy syndrome may represent an immunologic response of the individual against the virus, because those individuals who have shown no lymphadenopathy and then go on to have AIDS often have a much more contracted course.

Neutralizing antibodies are produced against the virus in some individuals, but the virus envelope may change sufficiently rapidly to escape their protective effect. Antibodies to other viral proteins are present in nearly all individuals with AIDS and can be detected by IFA, ELISA, Western blot, and radioimmune precipitation tests using virus-infected cells or purified viral antigens. Antibody levels decrease with severity of disease and may be extremely low at death, when most of the antibody-producing cells have been reduced by the overwhelming virus and opportunistic infections. Like HTLV-I, the AIDS retrovirus can remain with minimal expression in clinically healthy individuals, but then gradually (or suddenly) replicate to high levels and induce the immune abnormalities and clinical findings characteristic of AIDS. The CD8+ lymphocyte may be an important cell involved in suppressing this virus replication and preventing the subsequent induction of disease. Thus variations in the virus (e.g., its pathogenic potential) and the host (e.g., immunologic response) determine progression to disease. Kaposi's sarcoma could result from the release by normal cells of immune modulating factors with angiogenesis-promoting activity. These factors may induce endothelial cell proliferation leading to Kaposi's sarcoma. Similarly, the B cell lymphomas may be caused by hyperresponsive immune cells with cytokine production that results from the compromise of T cell function that generally controls B cell growth.

Clinical disease

AIDS is characterized by a deficit in the cellular immune system, including T cells, B cells, and macrophages. The T cells involved are primarily those of the helper subset. The pathologic features of AIDS (as outlined previously) involve a destruction of immune mechanisms, which permits the superinfection of individuals with a variety of organisms normally not pathogenic to humans, including *Pneumocystis carinii,* CMV mycobacteria, toxoplasma, and certain intestinal parasites. Malignancies, as noted, also can appear in infected individuals. In some individuals, neurologic symptoms such as encephalopathy and dementia can appear without major abnormalities observed in the immune system. Moreover, some patients have primarily gastrointestinal problems caused in some by direct infection of the bowel by HIV. Most recent studies suggest that it takes at least 10 years for 50% of infected individuals to develop AIDS; 25% will have symptoms, and the rest will still be clinically healthy.

Diagnosis

Epidemiologic, clinical, pathologic, and sociologic factors are important in making the diagnosis of AIDS. AIDS as defined by the Centers for Disease Control includes the presence of specific opportunistic infections and cancer (Chapter 242). Definitive proof of retrovirus infection can be obtained through the study of antibodies to HIV or isolation of the virus from blood. However, as with HTLV-I, antibodies to the agent in clinically healthy individuals cannot yet be interpreted in terms of the chance of developing AIDS.

Treatment and prevention

There is no curative treatment yet for AIDS. Several attempts with antiretrovirus compounds have met with some success in reducing symptoms and prolonging life. New drugs and approaches against the opportunistic infections have been particularly helpful. The antireverse transcriptase drug azidothymidine (Zidovudine) has shown promise in patients with disease. Its use has also been recommended for individuals whose CD4+ cell count drops to less than 500 CD4+ cells/ml as a preventive approach to AIDS. Nevertheless, the appropriate time to introduce this therapy is still under study. Immune-modulating factors (e.g., interferon and interleukin 2) have not been universally helpful. Prevention has been recommended through selection of blood and blood products that are free of the virus and avoidance of contact with body fluids from virus-infected individuals. Studies have shown that heating (68° C) lyophilized factor VIII and factor IX products for several hours eliminates infectious virus. No vaccine is yet available.

REFERENCES

Blattner WA, Takatsuki K, and Gallo RC: Human T-cell leukemia-lymphoma virus and adult T-cell leukemia. JAMA 250:1074, 1983.

Bunn PA Jr et al: Clinical course of retrovirus-associated adult T-cell lymphoma in the United States. N Engl J Med 309:257, 1983.

Levy JA et al: Isolation of lymphocytopathic retroviruses from San Francisco patients with AIDS. Science 225:840, 1984.

Levy JA: The multifaceted retrovirus. Cancer Res 46:5457, 1986.

Levy JA: Human immunodeficiency viruses and the pathogenesis of AIDS. JAMA 261:2997, 1989.

Roman GC: The neuroepidemiology of tropical spastic paraparesis. Ann Neurol 23:S113, 1988.

Yamamoto N and Hinuma Y: Viral aetiology of adult T-cell leukaemia. J Gen Virol 66:1641, 1985.

Yoshida M et al: Viruses detected in HTLV-1–associated myelopathy and adult T-cell leukaemia are identical on DNA blotting assay. Lancet 1:1085, 1987.

CHAPTER

253 Adenovirus Infections

John Mills

CHARACTERISTICS

Adenoviruses are nonenveloped viruses that contain double-stranded deoxyribonucleic acid (DNA) as their genetic material. The virus particle is approximately 70 nm in diameter and is therefore intermediate in size for a nonenveloped virus. The surface of the virus is relatively complex and consists of three types of capsomers (subunits): hexons, pentons, and rod-like structures that project from the penton base, known as fibers. The arrangement of these structures is shown in Fig. 253-1. The capsomer types differ from each other morphologically, antigenically, and functionally. The hexon and penton bases contain group antigens that are common to all human adenovirus types, whereas the fibers have primarily type-specific antigens.

Over 40 types of human adenoviruses have been recognized, and other adenoviruses are important pathogens of animals. Adenoviruses can be identified serologically on the basis of a group antigen, which is detected by complement-fixation techniques, or group-specific fluorescein-labeled antisera. The type-specific antigen is detected by either neutralization or hemagglutination inhibition. The adenoviruses most important for human disease are the lower serotypes (types 1 to 8, 11, 14, and 21). With the exception of the enteric adenoviruses, types 40 and 41, other serotypes usually are associated with asymptomatic colonization.

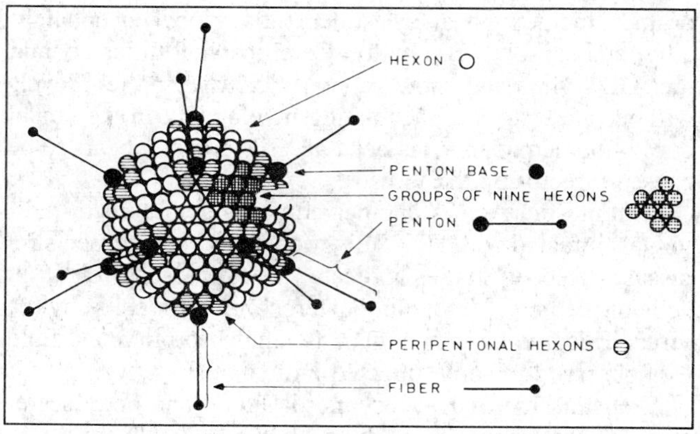

Fig. 253-1. Structure of adenovirus virion. (From Phillipson L et al: Molecular biology of adenoviruses: virology monographs 14. New York, 1975, Spring-Verlag.)

Some adenoviruses are oncogenic for tissue culture and newborn animals, but the highly oncogenic types (12, 18, and 31) are isolated infrequently from humans. There is abundant evidence that adenoviruses are not a cause of human cancer. Adenoviruses are capable of forming hybrids with the oncogenic simian virus SV40 in vitro. In these virus particles, SV40 genetic material is covalently linked with the adenovirus genome. Although human infection with these viruses occurred during trials with adenovirus vaccines produced in monkey kidney tissue culture, there has been no evidence of long-term sequelae.

Adenoviruses are regularly accompanied by a small defective DNA virus known as adenoassociated virus, or adenosatellite virus. These viruses cannot undergo productive replication in tissue culture or in animals without the association of adenoviruses (cytomegalovirus also can provide this helper function), although latent infection may occur. Adenovirus infection in humans is commonly accompanied by infection with adenoassociated virus, although the latter does not produce any unique disease syndrome. Most persons have antibodies to at least one of the four adenoassociated virus serotypes by 10 years of age.

EPIDEMIOLOGY

Adenoviruses, like the enteroviruses and many other nonenveloped viruses, are hardy agents and capable of transmission by a number of routes. Transmission within families and among children seems to be primarily via fecal–oral spread. Asymptomatic fecal excretion of adenoviruses may continue for years after initial infection, especially in children. Respiratory transmission by aerosols has been found in military populations and may also occur in civilian adults. Transmission by fomites or direct contact has been associated with swimming pools and physicians' offices where sterilization or hand washing has been inadequate. Asymptomatic infection and a chronic carrier state are common with adenoviruses.

Infection with the lower serotypes tends to occur very early in life, particularly in developing countries. Infection in children results in disease approximately half the time and is associated almost exclusively with isolation of the virus from the upper respiratory tract. Adenovirus infections appear to account for between 5% and 20% of cases of respiratory disease in children and for approximately 5% of cases of pneumonia and bronchitis. Adenovirus infections in adults tend to be sporadic, involve primarily the upper respiratory tract, and are strongly associated with contact with children. Adenovirus rarely produces pneumonia in civilian adults.

Epidemics of pneumonia and febrile lower respiratory tract infections in military recruits were noted as early as the Civil War. It was later demonstrated that a significant proportion of these illnesses could be ascribed to adenoviruses, particularly type 4 and, to a lesser extent, types 7 and 21. Despite the high incidence of infection in recruits (infection rates as high as 4 cases/100 recruits/week of training), little spread to dependents was seen. An attenuated vaccine for adenovirus type 4 that was effective in preventing adenovirus 4 infection and disease in small-scale field trials was developed. When immunization was applied to entire recruit populations, the incidence of adenovirus 4 infection decreased markedly, but the incidence of adenovirus 7 and 21 infection and illness increased substantially. This is one of the few examples in which immunization against one infectious agent created an ecologic vacuum that was promptly filled by another pathogen. Later immunization with adenovirus 7 and 21 vaccines did not result in the appearance of additional adenovirus serotypes.

Epidemic keratoconjunctivitis, also known as "shipyard eye," is also due to adenovirus infection. This disease is usually caused by adenovirus type 8 and was originally described in shipyard workers during World War II. The disease was spread by ocular tonometers that were inadequately sterilized between uses and by physicians' unwashed hands.

Pharyngoconjunctival fever (an illness characterized by fever, pharyngitis that is often exudative, and conjunctivitis or keratoconjunctivitis) is also commonly due to adenovirus infection. This illness is usually caused by adenoviruses types 3 and 7, may be epidemic or endemic, and is primarily seen in young children during the summer months. Epidemics have been associated with swimming pool water contaminated with adenoviruses, usually occurring because of inadequate chlorination or failure of the filtration system. Adenovirus conjunctivitis without pharyngitis also has been seen in this setting. Nosocomial epidemics of pharyngoconjunctival fever also have occurred.

Enteric adenoviruses (types 40 and 41) are common causes of endemic and epidemic viral gastroenteritis. However, disease is seen primarily in children, and unusually in adults.

PATHOPHYSIOLOGY

Adenoviruses may infect the respiratory tract, ocular mucosa, intestinal tract, and genitourinary tract. Little is known about the pathophysiology of infections in humans. In the case of respiratory tract disease, adenovirus infection is associated with cytopathology and necrosis of cells of the respiratory tract. Presumably, this is a direct effect of the virus, because complete virus as well as isolated virus components, primarily the penton base, may cause identical cytopathologic changes in tissue culture. Tissue invasion with viremia may occur and may result in disseminated infection in a susceptible host. Most infections result in a brisk serum antibody response. Serum neutralizing antibody is protective against subsequent illness and, to a lesser extent, against asymptomatic reinfection.

Latent infection is common with these agents but appears to occur by a mechanism of low-level replication on mucosal surfaces or in lymphoid tissue rather than by integration of the viral genome into the host's DNA. Latent infections lasting months to years have been described in the respiratory tract (human tonsils) and in the gastrointestinal tract. Latent infections are probably important in maintenance of the virus in populations, but there is no evidence that ill health results from the carrier state.

CLINICAL SYNDROMES

Respiratory disease produced by adenovirus may involve all parts of the respiratory tract and is most frequently caused by adenoviruses types 1 to 7, 14, and 21. Pharyngitis is a common manifestation of adenovirus infection and may be associated with fever, pharyngeal exudate, and anterior cervical adenopathy, thus closely mimicking streptococcal pharyngitis. Pneumonia occurs commonly in infants and in military recruits and has also been reported in immunocompromised patients. Adenovirus infection also has been associated with a whooping cough syndrome, which may result occasionally from isolated adenovirus infection but is more frequent during dual adenovirus–*Bordetella pertussis* infection.

Conjunctivitis or keratoconjunctivitis is usually caused by adenovirus type 3, 7, or 8. Conjunctivitis is usually relatively mild and may be associated with pharyngitis. Keratoconjunctivitis may follow corneal trauma. Although adenovirus conjunctivitis is usually self-limited, keratoconjunctivitis may cause lasting impairment of vision.

Hemorrhagic cystitis may occur with infection of the bladder; adenovirus 11 is the type most commonly involved. This illness occurs primarily in children and may be either epidemic or endemic. In contrast to bacterial cystitis, adenovirus cystitis tends to affect males three times as often as females. The symptoms are similar to those seen in patients with bacterial cystitis. The illness is self-limited, with the hematuria clearing within 1 or 2 days and the other manifestations clearing within a week. Asymptomatic urinary shedding of adenoviruses (usually type 34 or 35) is common in patients with AIDS.

Adenovirus has been isolated from the cerebrospinal fluid in patients with meningoencephalitis. The infection is mild and self-limited, with primarily meningeal manifestations. A possible exception to this rule is bone marrow transplant recipients, where fatal adenovirus meningoencephalitis has been reported.

Gastrointestinal infection with adenoviruses is usually asymptomatic. Although epidemics of gastrointestinal disease secondary to adenoviruses have been described in the past, the studies were conducted before the intestinal parvoviruses and rotaviruses were described. Recently, however, studies employing immune electron microscopy have demonstrated that adenovirus types 40 and 41 are an important cause of infantile diarrhea. Adenovirus infection of the gastrointestinal tract has been associated with an intussusception in infants and children, but pathogenetic relationship is unproven.

Disseminated infections with adenoviruses have been described in infants and very young children and in patients with immunodeficiencies. In some cases, the adenoviruses have been associated with circulating leukocytes. All organ systems may be affected, but pneumonia, hepatitis, myocarditis, encephalitis, and nephritis are clinically prominent. Children who have had liver transplantation appear to be particularly susceptible, and hepatitis is common.

DIAGNOSIS

Adenovirus infections may be diagnosed by detecting the virus or viral antibodies. Adenoviruses can be identified in clinical specimens by culture, detection of viral antigens (e.g., by immunofluorescence or enzyme-linked immunoassay), or detection of viral DNA. Viral DNA in patient material may be detected directly by hybridization with an adenovirus-specific labeled probe or after amplification by polymerase chain reaction. Culture is satisfactory for many clinical situations except enteric infections (because of the less easily cultured adenovirus types 40 and 41), where antigen detection by immunoassay and detection of viral DNA after polymerase chain reaction amplification are the preferred diagnostic methods. Both group-specific and type-specific antibodies are produced by adenovirus infection. Paired acute and convalescent serum specimens may be screened for adenovirus infection using group-specific antigens and then tested for type-specific antibodies if necessary. Serologic testing for group-specific antibody alone detects 80% to 90% of symptomatic adenovirus infections, particularly in adults.

In patients with respiratory or ocular disease, culture of an adenovirus, especially one of the lower serotypes (types 1 to 15), strongly suggests an etiologic relationship to the illness. However, asymptomatic infections with prolonged virus shedding are common, particularly with higher serotypes (types 22 to 39) and in the gastrointestinal tract; if there is doubt, the relationship between the virus isolated and the clinical findings can be reinforced by showing a rise in antibody titer between acute and convalescent serum specimens.

TREATMENT AND PREVENTION

At the present time, there are no effective chemotherapeutic agents for adenovirus infection. Drugs that are effective against other DNA viruses (e.g., adenine arabinoside and cytosine arabinoside) do not appear to be effective in adenovirus infections. Although associated with significant morbidity, adenovirus infections are uncommonly associated with mortality or permanent sequelae.

Immunity to adenovirus infection is due to the presence of type-specific neutralizing antibody. Protection is afforded against both illness and infection. Heterotypic immunity (cross immunity between serotypes) does not occur. The degree of illness may be inversely proportional to the amount of secretory immunoglobulin A (IgA) present in nasal secretions, suggesting a moderating role for local antibody. Ocular infections may occur even in the presence of significant levels of serum antibody, and a role for local antibody in protection against these infections is suspected as well.

A live attenuated vaccine has been developed by the novel technique of packaging wild-type (nonattenuated) live adenovirus in enteric-coated capsules. This ensured enteric infection without infection of the respiratory tree. The enteric infection in adults is asymptomatic but results in the production of protective serum antibody. Although no difficulties have been associated with the use of the enteric-coated vaccines in military populations, there is significant transmission of these viruses within families by the fecal-oral route. Intrafamilial spread could conceivably produce significant disease, particularly in children. Enteric-coated adenovirus vaccines types 4, 7, and 21 have been developed and used in the military with good success and little evidence of any morbidity.

Environmental manipulation also may be important for the control of adenovirus infections. Disease in military recruit populations may be minimized by not mixing incoming recruits with recruits who have already been in training for several weeks or by reducing the size of the recruit training groups. Unfortunately, tightly sealed, energy-efficient buildings also appear to favor transmission of adenoviruses. Immunization with nonrespiratory vaccines (typhoid, tetanus toxoid, diphtheria, pertussis) during the first week of recruit training may also increase the risk of adenovirus infection and disease. As adenovirus infections may spread through improperly sterilized tonometers, through contact with physicians' hands, and through swimming pool water, proper environmental controls must be applied in these areas as well. Swimming pool chlorination and filtration should be carefully monitored, particularly during periods of heavy use. Ophthalmologists and other physicians who examine patients with ineffective conjunctivitis should either wear gloves or scrupulously wash their hands between patients. Materials placed in patients' eyes, particularly tonometers, should be sterilized between examinations by a method known to be effective against adenoviruses.

REFERENCES

Allard A et al: Polymerase chain reaction for detection of adenoviruses in stool samples. J Clin Microbiol 29:2683, 1991.

Davis D et al: Fatal adenovirus meningoencephalitis in a bone marrow transplant patient. Ann Neurol 23(4):385, 1988.
Horowitz MS: Adenoviruses. In Fields BN and Knipe DM, editors: Virology. ed. 2. New York, 1990, Raven Press.
Michaels MG et al: Adenovirus infection in pediatric liver transplant recipients. J Infect Dis 165:170, 1992.
McMinn PC et al: A community outbreak of epidemic keratoconjunctivitis in central Australia due to adenovirus type 8. J Infect Dis 164:1113, 1991.
Mufson MA and Belshe RB: A review of adenoviruses in the etiology of acute hemorrhagic cystitis. J Urol 115:191, 1976.
Wood DJ: Adenovirus gastroenteritis. Br Med J 296:229, 1988.
Zahradnik JM: Adenovirus pneumonia. Semin Respir Infect 2:104, 1987 (review).

CHLAMYDIAL DISEASES

CHAPTER

254 Chlamydial Infections

Julius Schachter

CLASSIFICATION

The chlamydiae are members of a genus of obligate, intracellular, gram-negative bacteria that are distinguished from all other bacteria by a unique growth cycle. They are placed in their own order, Chlamydiales, in the family Chlamydiaceae, with a single genus, *Chlamydia,* having three species, *psittaci, trachomatis,* and *pneumoniae*. These species are differentiated on the basis of inclusion type and susceptibility to sulfonamides. *Chlamydia trachomatis* is sensitive to sulfonamides, produces inclusions that stain with iodine because they contain a glycogen-like material, and causes trachoma, conjunctivitis, and pneumonia in infants and several sexually transmitted diseases in adults. *Chlamydia psittaci,* on the other hand, is resistant to sulfonamides, its inclusions do not contain enough glycogen to stain with iodine, and it causes psittacosis in humans. What were called the TWAR strains of *C. psittaci* have been placed in a new species, *C. pneumoniae,* based on morphology and lack of DNA relatedness.

CHARACTERISTICS

The chlamydial infectious particle is a coccal elementary body that is approximately 250 to 400 nm in diameter. TWAR elementary bodies are pear shaped. It attaches to the host cells in a process that may involve specific receptor sites. The coccal elementary body is then ingested by the susceptible host cell. This uptake process is selective and is induced by the chlamydiae. The chlamydiae remain within an endosome throughout their developmental cycle. Chlamydiae suppress phagolysosomal fusion. The entire growth cycle of the chlamydia takes approximately 48 hours. During the first 8 hours the infecting particle changes into a larger (approximately 1 μm in diameter), ribonucleic acid– (RNA)-rich reticulate particle that is metabolically active and divides by binary fission. The reticulate particles are noninfectious. Metabolic processes of the chlamydiae peak between 8 and 24 hours. At approximately 24 hours the reticulate bodies (also called initial bodies) begin to condense into infectious elementary bodies. At approximately 48 hours the inclusion bursts and releases the infectious coccal elementary body progeny.

Chlamydia psittaci contains many serologic types and biotypes. Unfortunately, there are no convenient laboratory methods for identifying these types, and thus their relevance in different disease conditions in humans or animals cannot be determined. Only one *C. pneumoniae* serovar has been identified. With *C. trachomatis,* however, serovars have been identified by two tests: a mouse toxicity prevention test and a microimmunofluorescence test. It has been found that four of the *C. trachomatis* serovars (A, B, Ba, and C) are associated with endemic trachoma. Three of the serovars (L-1, L-2, and L-3) are the causative agents of lymphogranuloma venereum (LGV) and represent a separate biovar (in terms of pathogenicity and receptor sites) within *C. trachomatis*. The other serovars of *C. trachomatis* (D through K) are usually transmitted sexually. Monoclonal antibodies to most of the serovars are available.

ECOLOGIC NICHE—EPIDEMIOLOGY

Chlamydia psittaci

Chlamydia psittaci is a common pathogen of domestic and feral mammals, in which it causes a wide variety of diseases. Most chlamydiae are transmitted by a fecal-oral or respiratory route. In their infectious cycles, they often colonize the gastrointestinal tract. These mammalian chlamydiae, although economically significant because of the morbidity they produce in domestic mammals, are of little significance in terms of human health.

Chlamydia psittaci is virtually ubiquitous among avian species: more than 130 different avian species have been identified as hosts. Although the respiratory tract of birds may be infected, the infections are usually gastrointestinal. Inapparent or latent infections are common in birds or mammals. Stress, such as caused by crowding, aging, nutritional deficits, or breeding, may activate the inapparent infection, resulting in clinical disease. Healthy carriers or diseased birds may shed *C. psittaci* in feces. Because *C. psittaci* is highly stable, this shedding may result in environmental contamination.

Chlamydia psittaci strains of avian origin are highly infectious for humans, in whom they produce the disease psittacosis. Human respiratory tract infection usually results from exposure to aerosols of infective feces. The term psittacosis has been used historically to refer to *C. psittaci* infection in human or psittacine species, whereas the term ornithosis has been used to designate this infection in extrapsittacine birds. Exotic pet birds are often the reservoir for human infections. Poultry, particularly turkeys in the United States and ducks in eastern Europe, have also been important sources of human infection with *C. psittaci*. This infection may be considered an occupational hazard, particularly important to those working in poultry processing plants.

Chlamydia pneumoniae

The TWAR strain appears to have no animal reservoir. It is apparently exclusively a human pathogen. Seroepidemiologic studies indicate infections are acquired relatively early in childhood. Seroprevalence rates reach 30% to 45% in many communities, indicating that exposure to this organism is common in most parts of the world.

Chlamydia trachomatis

Chlamydia trachomatis is almost exclusively a human pathogen. With the exception of a single rodent strain, no other natural hosts are known. The agent is spread by close personal contact. In trachoma endemic areas, *C. trachomatis* is spread from child to child or within families in households. Moisture-seeking flies that feed on ocular discharges may act as mechanical vectors. In adults (particularly in industrialized societies), *C. trachomatis* is largely transmitted by sexual activity and is one of the most common of the sexually transmitted pathogens. In the United States, the current estimate is that 4.5 million infections occur each year.

Vertical transmission of *C. trachomatis* also occurs. An infant born through an infected birth canal may acquire the infection. In the infant, the eye, upper and lower respiratory tracts, gastrointestinal tract, and vagina may be infected.

Although chlamydial infections may cause severe disease, clinically inapparent infections are common. In adults, inapparent infection occurs in both the male urethra and the female cervix. In infants, clinically inapparent nasopharyngeal infections appear to be common, as do, to a lesser extent, gastrointestinal tract infections.

PATHOPHYSIOLOGY

Although some virulence factors are associated with the chlamydiae (i.e., surface antigens that appear to induce phagocytosis and prevent phagolysosomal fusion), there is no clear understanding of the pathogenesis of human chlamydial disease. *Chlamydia psittaci* strains appear to have a broad host cell spectrum in vivo and are often found replicating within mononuclear phagocytic cells. *Chlamydia trachomatis* (with the exception of LGV strains) appears to be restricted to columnar epithelial cells for replication. Both chlamydial species are cytocidal in that they kill cells as part of their growth cycle. It is probable that much of the disease associated with *C. trachomatis* represents the host's inflammatory reaction to this lethal effect of chlamydial infection on some of its cells. *Chlamydia psittaci* strains are more destructive than *C. trachomatis* strains. LGV strains cause far more damage and are far more invasive than the other *C. trachomatis* strains.

There is an abundant immune response to chlamydial infection, although immunity to these infections is poor and highly specific. Challenge infection with heterologous serotypes may actually result in more severe disease (as may homologous reinfection when immunity wanes). Animal experiments suggest that the hypersensitivity or hyperreactivity seen in second infections is a response to a genus-specific antigen. A heat shock protein, related to the gro-el antigens, has been identified as a sensitizing antigen.

DISEASES PRODUCED IN HUMANS

Chlamydia psittaci

Human infection with *C. psittaci,* called psittacosis, has two clinical forms. The one most commonly recognized is a form of atypical pneumonia, which is often termed flu-like and is characterized by fever, severe headache, nonproductive cough, and a protracted course (Chapter 231). The second form of human psittacosis is often referred to as a typhoidal or toxic disease. It lacks the respiratory component and is characterized by severe headache, a protracted course, fever, and chills. In either instance, the pulse may be slow relative to the fever. Hepatosplenomegaly is common. Hepatitis, myocarditis, endocarditis, and meningitis are among the many complications known to occur.

Chlamydia pneumoniae

The TWAR strain appears to cause a respiratory disease in young adults that is clinically indistinguishable from atypical pneumonia, caused by Mycoplasma pneumoniae (Chapter 255). The symptoms may include a severe pharyngitis. Severe and even fatal pneumonias may occur in older individuals with underlying disease. The potential role of *C. pneumoniae* in inducing asthma is being actively investigated. Because the organism is such a common pathogen many studies have suggested a broader clinical spectrum, including coronary disease and pneumonia in acquired immunodeficiency syndrome (AIDS) cases. Further studies are needed to define a chlamydial role, if any, in these conditions.

Chlamydia trachomatis

Lymphogranuloma venereum. Lymphogranuloma venereum is a systemic, sexually transmitted infection (Chapter 238). In males, the disease usually presents as inguinal lymphadenopathy. The male/female ratio for inguinal buboes is often as high as 20:1. Systemic signs, such as fever, shaking chills, and severe headache, are often associated with the inguinal lymphadenopathy. The disease is often described in stages: A primary lesion (a shallow ulcer or vesicle on the penis) is the first sign of the infection. The appearance of a bubo is the secondary stage, and the late sequelae, such as proctitis, rectal strictures, and proctocolitis, represent the tertiary stage. In the female, the vaginal tract's lymphoid drainage is retroperitoneal, so inguinal lymphadenopathy does not usually develop in women. Women are seen with late complications of LGV, such as perirectal strictures or the anogenital syndrome, which may involve stricture, proctitis, or rectovaginal fistula. These conditions result from a combination of inflammation, tissue destruction and fibrosis. Although proctocolitis is generally considered one of the later lesions, a relatively severe form (often associated with weight loss and fever) may be seen as an early form of LGV in homosexual males.

Such complications as hepatitis and joint and central nervous system involvement are known. Lymphadenopathy may occur at many sites. For example, ocular infection may result in a diagnosis of Parinaud's oculoglandular syndrome. Respiratory tract infection has been a common result of accidental exposure produced by laboratory accident.

Trachoma. Trachoma is a chronic follicular conjunctivitis that may afflict all members of a community or household in hyperendemic areas. Active disease is seen in young children, and virtually all of them will be infected before they are 2 years old (this pattern changes; as living conditions improve, the age of onset of disease increases). The infection is chronic, and reinfections may follow spontaneous clearance. The natural tendency of chlamydial infections to decrease in severity is interfered with by the secondary bacterial infections (pneumococci, *Haemophilus influenzae, H. aegyptius,* and *Moraxella* species) that are often common and may be seasonal in trachoma endemic regions. As a result of severe trachoma, there may be necrosis that will produce conjunctival scarring. Although the active disease occurs in young children, blindness occurs in adults. It takes many years for the shrinkage of scars to turn the upper lid inward, so that the eyelashes abrade the cornea. These lesions, trichiasis and entropion, are the blinding lesions of trachoma.

Chlamydia trachomatis in the male genital tract. The most common disease resulting from *C. trachomatis* infection in men is nongonococcal urethritis (Chapter 238). This condition may be clinically indistinguishable from gonorrhea, although there is a tendency for the discharge to be scanty and mucoid rather than frankly purulent. *Chlamydia trachomatis* is the major cause of acute epididymitis in young men. Rectal infection may result in proctitis.

Many men with gonorrhea have concomitant chlamydial infection. If these men are treated with penicillin, which is not active against chlamydiae, postgonococcal urethritis, a specific subset of nongonococcal urethritis, will usually develop.

Chlamydia trachomatis in the female genital tract. The cervix is the most common site of chlamydial infection in women. There are no pathognomonic findings to indicate the presence of the infection, and inapparent infections occur. When disease develops, it is an endocervicitis, and *C. trachomatis* may be significantly associated with a mucopurulent endocervical discharge and hypertrophic cervical erosions. Many women with chlamydial infections have involvement of the urethra, and dysuria is a common symptom. Chlamydia may cause bartholinitis. *C. trachomatis* is also a cause of infection in the upper female genital tract. The organism clearly causes endometritis, although data concerning the frequency of this condition are not available. *Chlamydia trachomatis,* however, is a major cause of acute salpingitis and appears to be the leading cause of perihepatitis (Fitz-Hugh–Curtis syndrome). Chlamydial salpingitis is usually clinically milder than salpingitis caused by gonococci or anaerobes, but the risk of infertility appears to be approximately the same for chlamydial salpingitis as for other forms. Chlamydial salpingitis can be clinically inapparent. Many women suffering from tubal factor infertility or ectopic pregnancy have no history of acute salpingitis but show serologic evidence of previous chlamydial infection. Because of the inability to make an early diagnosis and because the condition is of polymicrobial origin, therapy for salpingitis should include antibiotics active against chlamydiae as well as the other causative agents.

Inclusion conjunctivitis. Inclusion conjunctivitis occurs in infants or adults who are exposed to infected genital tract discharges. An acute mucopurulent conjunctivitis develops in the infant approximately 5 to 14 days after birth. If the infection is untreated, it tends to be self-limited, usually resolving within 2 months. In some infants, however, chronic infections that may threaten sight develop. In infants who are not treated early, some scarring of the conjunctiva and a micropannus may develop, although there is usually no deleterious effect on vision.

Acute follicular conjunctivitis develops in adults (infants usually do not have follicular conjunctivitis until they are 1 to 2 months of age) and persists for months. Keratitis and micropannus are common. In severe cases, the disease is clinically indistinguishable from acute trachoma.

Extraocular infection in infants. The most severe chlamydial disease in infants is a characteristic pneumonia syndrome, which can develop between the ages of 2 weeks and 4 months. The infants are afebrile, have a protracted course, suffer from tachypnea (occasionally apnea), and have a dry, hacking cough. Many of the infants have conjunctivitis indicated either by history or by examination. Some of these pneumonias are associated with an acute serous otitis media. Radiographs show a diffuse interstitial pneumonia with hyperinflation. Elevated levels of immunoglobulins are usually found (particularly immunoglobulin M (IgM), and a relative eosinophilia is common. Although chlamydial pneumonia is not a life-threatening disease, affected infants may suffer from permanent lung damage. Rhinitis and bronchiolitis are part of the spectrum of chlamydial infections of the respiratory tract in infants, but the incidence of these conditions is not known. Rectal and vaginal infections occur but have not been clearly associated with disease at these sites.

Respiratory tract infections in adults

Serologic studies have implicated *C. trachomatis* as a cause of acute pharyngitis or pneumonia in adults. It is probable that most of these studies were actually detecting cross-reacting genus-specific antibodies to the TWAR organism, *C. pneumoniae,* which is now recognized as a common respiratory tract pathogen. *C. trachomatis* has been occasionally isolated from lungs of patients with pneumonia and the acquired immunodeficiency syndrome.

PERTINENT DIAGNOSTIC TESTS

Methods of diagnosing chlamydial infection are essentially the same as those used for diagnosing other bacterial diseases. The agent may be demonstrated directly in tissue samples. This does not apply to human psittacosis, but some of the infections with *C. trachomatis* may be diagnosed by appropriate staining of epithelial cell scrapings (Plate V-11). It is imperative that an adequate sample of epithelial cells be obtained to demonstrate the characteristic intracytoplasmic inclusions. Giemsa stain can be of particular use in identifying inclusion conjunctivitis in infants and in adults. Acute trachoma may also be diagnosed cytologically. Cytologic procedures are not routinely useful for diagnosing genital tract infections; isolation is much more sensitive. A number of nonculture diagnostic tests are available. The most commonly used tests are based on antigen detection and include enzyme immunoassay for genus-specific LPS, and use of fluorescein-conjugated monoclonal antibodies against a *Chlamydia* species–specific antigen to detect elementary bodies in clinical specimens. These tests have a sensitivity of 80% to 90% and specificity of about 97%, as compared to culture for diagnosis of genital tract infections. They offer the possibility of placing chlamydial diagnosis in laboratories that currently cannot do tissue culture work. Antigen detection methods seem best suited for use in high-risk populations. Because of potential false-positive results, these antigen detection methods should not be used in low-prevalence settings, where the results may have medicolegal implications. In moderate-risk and low-risk populations the positive nonculture test results should be considered presumptive and should be confirmed by either a confirmatory assay or another test based on a different principle. In high-prevalence settings, such as sexually transmitted disease (STD) clinics, the results of the initial test may be accepted.

Serologic tests are usually useful in diagnosing psittacosis, TWAR infection, and LGV in which exuberant antibody responses are seen. Paired acute and convalescent sera usually show a fourfold rise in complement-fixing antibodies when the patient has psittacosis. In LGV, very high titer levels are seen, but it is difficult to demonstrate rising titer levels because patients are usually examined well into the course of the disease. Genital tract infections with *C. trachomatis* are seldom diagnosed serologically because of the high prevalence of antibodies in sexually active populations and the chronic nature of the disease. This makes it difficult to time the collection of paired serum specimens appropriately. In patients having their first bouts of the disease, seroconversion is usually demonstrated, but microimmunofluorescence techniques must be used, because the complement-fixation procedure is too insensitive. Serodiagnosis may be better for the systemic complications of *C. trachomatis* infections (epididymitis in men, salpingitis in women, pneumonia in infants) than for the more common mucous membrane infections. The systemic infections result in higher levels of IgG or IgM antibodies, and, in infants, IgM antibody titers are particularly useful. Infants with *Chlamydia* pneumonia may show relative eosinophilia and virtually always have elevated serum globulin levels, particularly of the IgM class.

Isolation of the infectious agent is seldom accomplished with *C. psittaci*. The TWAR agent is particularly difficult to isolate although use of HL cells improves recovery. Because of superficial localization, *C. trachomatis* agents may be readily isolated. Inoculation of the collected specimens into McCoy cells treated with cycloheximide enhances chlamydial replication. Specimens containing epithelial cells must be collected directly from the involved site. Culture of discharges is less than optimum. Sensitivity of cultures probably varies by the site and the disease involved. It is probably as high as 95% for inclusion conjunctivitis of newborns but is more likely between 70% and 80% for uncomplicated genital tract infections; because of sampling problems, it certainly would be less than that for some of the systemic complications of *C. trachomatis* infections.

TREATMENT

The treatment of choice for any chlamydial infection of adults is considered to be tetracycline (Table 254-1). The regimen may vary somewhat with the disease. Thus human psittacosis should be treated for 3 weeks with 1 g of tetracycline per day (250 mg, four times a day). Shorter courses may result in relapse. No controlled treatment trials for TWAR infection exist. Published experience indicates that erythromycin at 1 g per day for 3 weeks is effective. Tetracyclines at equivalent dosage would also be expected to be active. *Chlamydia trachomatis* infections are usually more responsive to chemotherapy; LGV, however, does not respond rapidly to the antibiotic. In treating LGV, it is common to obtain a rapid response in terms of constitutional signs; thus the fever and chills may disappear quickly, but the buboes may take months to resolve. Adults with genital tract disease caused by non-LGV *C. trachomatis* respond to treatment with tetracycline (1 g/day for 14 days, or 2 g/day for 7 days). Erythromycin at equivalent doses is considered to be the alternative drug of choice. It is the drug that should be used in treating infants. Erythromycin succinate (40 mg/kg in four divided doses daily) for 2 weeks should be given to infants with chlamydial pneumonia or inclusion conjunctivitis of the newborn. Topical treatment is inadequate for this conjunctivitis. Failure rates as high as 50% have been observed for infants receiving topical therapy with sulfonamides or tetracycline. It is clear that most of these children have nasopharyngeal infections and will often reinfect themselves after topical treatment.

Topical treatment is the standard for mass therapy of trachoma in developing countries. By analogy with chlamydial infection in infants in industrialized societies, it is easy to see that this regimen would fail if the children in trachoma endemic areas also had extraocular infections. This is known to occur, and it is likely that some form of systemic treatment will be required to ensure a cure.

Sulfonamides (sulfisoxazole, 4 g/day for 7 to 14 days) is effective in treating most *C. trachomatis* infections. This is not considered a treatment of choice for the chlamydial infections of the genital tract because many of these infec-

Table 254-1. Treatment of chlamydial infections

Organism and condition	First choice Drug	First choice Dose	Second choice Drug	Second choice Dose
C. psittaci				
Psittacosis	Tetracycline	250 mg qid × 3 wk	Erythromycin	250 mg qid × 3 wk
C. trachomatis				
LGV strains	Tetracycline	500 mg qid × 3 wk	Sulfamethoxazole	1 g bid × 3 wk
Non-LGV strains				
Genital tract infections (e.g., urethritis, cervicitis)	Tetracycline	500 mg qid × 1 wk	Erythromycin	500 mg qid × 1 wk
Pregnant women	Erythromycin	500 mg qid × 1 wk	Amoxicillin	500 mg tid × 1 wk
Infant pneumonia	Erythromycin	10 mg/kg qid × 2 wk	Sulfsoxazole	37.5 mg/kg qid × 2 wk
Inclusion conjunctivitis (infants)	Erythromycin	10 mg/kg qid × 2 wk	Sulfisoxazole	37.5 mg/kg qid × 2 wk
Inclusion conjunctivitis (adults)	Tetracycline	250 mg qid × 3 wk	Erythromycin	250 mg qid × 3 wk

tions are not specifically diagnosed as a result of lack of laboratory facilities and thus must be treated empirically. With nongonococcal urethritis, for example, the standard procedure would be to determine the presence of urethritis, rule out gonorrhea, and treat with tetracyclines, because they are effective against both *C. trachomatis* and a putative cause of this disease. Ureaplasma urealyticum (which is resistant to sulfonamides).

Treatment of gonorrhea with tetracycline for a week (as recommended for nongonococcal urethritis) after immediate treatment with amoxicillin or ampicillin plus probenecid (Benemid) reduces the incidence of postgonococcal urethritis in men and postgonococcal cervicitis and salpingitis in women.

In 1992, azithromycin was approved for treatment of uncomplicated lower genital tract infections with *Chlamydia trachomatis*. The standard treatment regimen is 1 g given as a single dose. Thus this antibiotic presents the promise of minimizing the compliance problems inherent in the longer terms of therapy that have been previously required. In clinical trials, a single 1 g dose of azithromycin was found equal to a 1 week course of doxycycline in treating uncomplicated lower genital tract infections with *C. trachomatis*.

PREVENTION

There are no effective vaccines available for human chlamydial infection. Control of sexually transmitted diseases also requires identification and treatment of contacts. A chlamydial infection in an infant, such as conjunctivitis or pneumonia, is an indicator of genital tract infection in the mother, and she and her sexual contact(s) should receive treatment. Adults with inclusion conjunctivitis require systemic treatment, because they invariably have genital tract infections. Their sex partners should also be treated. Neonatal ocular prophylaxis is not effective. In high-prevalence settings pregnant women should be screened for chlamydial infection and treated as needed.

Prevention of the serious consequences of sexually transmitted *C. trachomatis* infection require more than simple treatment of the symptoms. Because of the high prevalence of asymptomatic infections in both sexes, screening of high-risk male and female populations is needed to identify the infected and reduce the reservoir.

REFERENCES

Beem MO and Saxon EM: Respiratory-tract colonization and a distinctive pneumonia syndrome in infants with *Chlamydia trachomatis*. N Engl J Med 296:306, 1977.

Chernesky MA et al: Detection of *Chlamydia trachomatis* antigens by enzyme immunoassay and immunofluorescence in genital specimens from symptomatic and asymptomatic men and women. J Infect Dis 154(1):141, 1986.

Grayston JT et al: A new *Chlamydia psittaci* strain, TWAR, isolated in acute respiratory tract infections. N Engl J Med 315(3):161, 1986.

Holmes KK et al, editors: Sexually Transmitted Diseases, ed 2. New York, 1990, McGraw-Hill.

Mardh PA et al: *Chlamydia trachomatis* infection in patients with acute salpingitis. N Engl J Med 296:1377, 1977.

Mardh PA et al: Chlamydial infection of the female genital tract with emphasis on pelvic inflammatory disease: a review of Scandinavian studies. Sex Transm Dis 8(suppl 2):140, 1981.

Moulder JW: Looking at chlamydiae without looking at their hosts. ASM News 50(8):353, 1984.

Oriel JD and Ridgway GL: Genital infection by *Chlamydia trachomatis*. London, 1982, Edward Arnold.

Schachter J: Chlamydial infections. N Engl J Med 298:428, 490, 540, 1978.

Schachter J and Dawson CR: Human Chlamydial infections. Littleton, MA, 1978, Publishing Sciences Group.

Schachter J and Grossman M: Chlamydial infections. Annu Rev Med 32:45, 1981.

Sweet RL et al: Failure of beta lactam antibiotics to eradicate *Chlamydia trachomatis* in the endometrium despite apparent clinical cure of acute salpingitis. JAMA 250(19):2641, 1983.

Westrom L: Incidence, prevalence, and trends of acute pelvic inflammatory disease and its consequences in industrialized countries. Am J Obstet Gynecol 138:880, 1980.

Mycoplasmal Diseases

CHAPTER

255 Mycoplasmal Infections

John Mills

The first mycoplasma was discovered by Nocard and Roux in 1898. This organism, now known as *Mycoplasma mycoides,* caused bovine pleuropneumonia and thus was originally termed pleuropneumonia-like organism (PPLO). The clinical syndrome of cold agglutinin–positive primary atypical pneumonia, distinct from bacterial pneumonias, was delineated between 1938 and 1943. In 1944, Eaton showed that tissue suspensions and allantoic fluid from eggs inoculated with sputum filtrates from patients with atypical pneumonia produced a similar pneumonia in cotton rats. A similarity of the Eaton agent to the PPLO was noted, and sensitivity of the Eaton agent to several antibiotics was demonstrated, raising doubts as to the presumed viral cause of the disease. In 1962, Chanock, Hayflick, and Barile cultured the Eaton agent on cell-free medium and showed it to be a *Mycoplasma,* later named *Mycoplasma pneumoniae*. Koch's postulates were satisfied when *M. pneumoniae* isolated from patients caused pneumonia when inoculated into volunteers.

MICROBIOLOGY

Mycoplasma and *Ureaplasma* belong to the family Mycoplasmataceae. They are considered to be bacteria on the basis of nucleic acid homology and their intracellular organization and metabolism. However, unlike bacteria, these organisms lack a cell wall, and, unlike bacterial spheroplasts (which also lack a cell wall), they cannot synthesize cell wall precursors. Seven species of *Mycoplasma* and one *Ureaplasma* species have been recovered from humans. Many other species pathogenic for other animals and plants are known. The only species that cause disease in humans are *M. pneumoniae, M. hominis,* and *Ureaplasma urealyticum,* the latter two often referred to together as the genital mycoplasmas. Only one serotype of *M. pneumoniae* is known, whereas there are at least 7 serotypes of *M. hominis* and 11 of *U. urealyticum*. The mycoplasmas are the smallest free-living organisms known, varying between 125 and 150 nm in diameter. The organisms are pleomorphic, are bound by a triple-layer cell membrane, and lack a cell wall. Growth of wild-type strains of mycoplasma and ureaplasma is slow (this is particularly true of *M. pneumoniae*), and 1 to 3 weeks may elapse before colonies are detected. *Mycoplasma pneumoniae* is unique in the ability to produce hemolysis of sheep and guinea pig erythrocytes. *Ureaplasma* is regarded as a separate genus because of its small size and its ability to hydrolyze urea to ammonia and carbon dioxide.

As shown in Table 255-1, the other *Mycoplasma* species are commonly recovered from the oropharynx or urogenital tract but, with the exception of the genital mycoplasmas (*M. hominis* and *U. urealyticum*), are not associated with any disease processes. On the other hand, recovery of *M. pneumoniae* from patients is almost invariably associated with disease.

EPIDEMIOLOGY

Mycoplasma pneumoniae is transmitted most commonly by means of aerosols, although occasional contact transmission may occur. Spread of disease is slow even among family members, although the ultimate risk of infection to exposed, susceptible persons within a family is over 90%. Epidemics are occasionally reported, especially in closed and crowded populations, such as military camps and chronic care facilities. Two well-documented point-source outbreaks have also been described: among persons attending a college fraternity pledge initiation ceremony that "degenerated into a gross bachanal" and among employees of a dental prosthodontics laboratory involved in the construction and alteration of dental prostheses using abrasive drills and grinding wheels. The presumed mode of transmission of *M. pneumoniae* in both instances was via heavily infective aerosols from a single individual.

Infection occurs throughout the year, although the incidence of disease is usually increased during the fall. Infection rates vary widely from year to year. *Mycoplasma pneumoniae* appears to be a common cause of pneumonia in all parts of the world, accounting for up to 10% to 20% of all pneumonic illnesses (Chapter 231). People of age groups except neonates may be affected, although the disease is most commonly seen from age 5 through the third decade. Prolonged carriage in the pharynx of those infected may occur even after antibiotic therapy and may account for persistence of the infection in large populations.

PATHOGENESIS AND PATHOPHYSIOLOGY

Mycoplasma pneumoniae is almost exclusively a pulmonary pathogen. Information on the lesions caused by this organism is sparse because the disease is rarely fatal. Interstitial pneumonia and acute bronchiolitis with peribronchial lymphocytic infiltrates and edema of the bronchiolar wall have

Table 255-1. Common mycoplasmataceae recovered from humans

Species	Usual location
M. pneumoniae	Oropharynx, lung
M. salivarium	Oropharynx
M. orale 1-3	Oropharynx
M. fermentans	Urogenital tract
M. hominis	Oropharynx, urogenital tract
U. urealyticum	Urogenital tract

been described in the few patients coming to autopsy. Transbronchial clearance of small particles is impaired, presumably as a result of alterations in the respiratory epithelium and ciliostasis. Bacterial superinfection, however, is rare, although an increased risk of meningococcal meningitis was noted in one study in Africa.

Virulence factors of *M. pneumoniae* have not been well characterized. The organism attaches to specific glycoprotein receptors on the cell membrane of respiratory epithelium by a specialized surface protein. After attachment, there is interruption of host cell RNA and protein synthesis, leading to ciliostasis and cell death. Because *M. pneumoniae* does not invade lung parenchyma, the pulmonary infiltrates in mycoplasmal pneumonia may partly result from the host's immune response. Infection early in life (<3 years of age) is rarely associated with pneumonia, whereas infection occurring after 4 or 5 years of age, by which time the vast majority of the population has sensitized lymphocytes, is often associated with pulmonary infiltrates. The pathogenesis of the extrapulmonary disease caused by *M. pneumoniae* is unclear. Both direct cytopathic effects and immunologic injury have been postulated as mechanisms of production of disease.

Persons with high antibody titers from previous exposure to the organism are relatively protected from illness, although such exposure may still result in infection, with shedding from the oropharynx. Immunity acquired after natural infection apparently lasts about 1 to 5 years, although reinfection with production of illness (i.e., second attacks) has been documented as early as 1 year after the previous exposure. Patients with defective humoral immunity have had more prolonged, more severe disease than do normal hosts, although these patients have not had pulmonary infiltrates as part of the disease process.

Table 255-2. Symptoms and findings in patients with documented *Mycoplasma pneumoniae* pneumonia

Symptom	Percentage of patients
Cough	99
Fever ≥ 100° F (37.8° C)	94
Fever ≥ 102° F (38.9° C)	77
Family size four or more persons	91
Malaise	89
Headache	66
Chills	58
Sore throat	54
Sputum production	45
Hoarseness	37
Earache (subjective)	31
Ear infection (objective)	21
Nausea and/or vomiting	29
Coryza	29
WBC ≥ 10,000/mm^3	27
WBC ≥ 15,000/mm^3	5
Recurrent pneumonia	22
Skin rash	17
Diarrhea	15
Pre-existing disease	14
Pleuritis	2
Hospitalization	2

From Foy HM et al: JAMA 214:1666, 1970.

CLINICAL SYNDROMES

Disease in humans is usually localized to the respiratory tract. Pneumonia, the best known clinical manifestation of infection, occurs in only 10% to 30% of those infected during endemic disease. Most *M. pneumoniae* infections cause rhinitis, pharyngitis, and tracheobronchitis that are clinically indistinguishable from acute respiratory tract infection produced by other agents.

After an average incubation period of 2 to 3 weeks, *Mycoplasma* pneumonia presents with the gradual onset of fever, cough, malaise, and headache (Table 255-2). Cough is usually distressing but nonproductive; pleurisy and hemoptysis are rare. Upper respiratory tract symptoms often accompany or precede the pneumonic manifestations. Frequently, other family members have had recent respiratory illness. The patient usually appears only mildly ill, and hospitalization is seldom required. Cyanosis, dyspnea, and tachypnea are rare. Fever, which is proportional to the severity of the pneumonia, seldom exceeds 104° F (40° C). The pulse usually rises with the fever, although fever-pulse dissociation may be present. Physical examination reveals tympanic membrane inflammation in up to 20% of patients. The incidence of true bullous myringitis is less. This condition may not develop until late in the course of mycoplasmal pneumonia and may occur in the absence of pneumonia. Conjunctivitis and pharyngitis, occasionally with a tonsillar exudate, and cervical adenopathy may be present. The chest findings may be normal in the presence of radiographically defined pulmonary infiltrates, but localized rales and rhonchi without signs of consolidation or effusion are usually present.

The importance of *Mycoplasma* pneumonia in patients with impaired immune responses has not been established. The disease in patients with sickle cell anemia may be severe and require hospitalization. Prolonged fever, respiratory distress, severe pleuritic chest pain, large pleural effusions, and pneumonia involving more than one lobe seem to be much more common in this population. In patients with impaired humoral immunity, the disease may result in moderate weight loss, prolonged fever, and cough, without pulmonary infiltrates.

The white blood cell count may be slightly elevated but is usually less than 15,000 per cubic millimeter. The differential is often normal but may show polymorphonuclear predominance. Gram-stained sputum reveals inflammatory cells and alveolar macrophages without significant bacteria; cultures show no growth or scant normal oral flora.

The radiographic appearance of *Mycoplasma* pneumonia is variable and cannot be distinguished reliably from that of other causes of pneumonia. Reticular and interstitial infiltrates are usually unilateral and involve one of the lower lobe segments. Bilateral disease has been reported in 10%

to 40% of cases. Upper lobe disease, multiple segmental infiltrates, lobar infiltrates, consolidation, pneumatoceles, abscesses, coin lesions, hilar adenopathy, and significant pleural effusions are unusual.

The erythrocyte sedimentation rate is frequently elevated, and occasional positive Coombs test results and false-positive serologic test results for syphilis have been noted.

Patients with untreated mycoplasmal pneumonia gradually recover over a period of 2 to 6 weeks. Headache and fever resolve in 10 to 14 days, but the cough and pulmonary infiltrates are slower in resolving, lasting an average of 3 to 4 weeks and sometimes longer. Death caused by respiratory insufficiency is rare.

Mycoplasma pneumoniae may affect organ systems other than the respiratory tract (refer to the box below). When this occurs, it is most commonly a complication of primary respiratory disease, although primary nonpulmonary involvement has also been described. The pathogenetic relationship between *M. pneumoniae* infection and bullous myringitis, skin rashes, and hemolytic anemia is well established. Polyarthritis is very rare, but *M. pneumoniae* has been isolated from the joint fluid in one case. Likewise, the organism has been recovered from cerebrospinal fluid in a few cases of meningoencephalitis, confirming a pathogenetic relationship. The other extrarespiratory complications have not been firmly established as related to *Mycoplasma* infection.

The hemolytic anemia found with mycoplasmal pneumonia is uncommon but may be severe, with up to 70% reduction in hemoglobin levels. Hemolysis usually occurs during the second or third week of illness when titers of cold agglutinins are highest (≥1:512). The cold agglutinins in these patients exhibit a high thermal maximum (>25° C). Hemolysis may follow cooling in these patients, as during bathing or alcohol sponging. The hemolysis is transient and is followed in a few days by recovery, manifested as a reticulocytosis with gradual restoration of normal hemoglobin levels. Mild hemolysis without reductions in hemoglobin may be common in patients with *M. pneumoniae* infection because 83% in one series had a positive direct Coombs test result and 64% had reticulocytosis above 2%.

Nonrespiratory manifestations of *Mycoplasma pneumoniae* infection

- Dermatologic
  - Maculopapular rashes
  - Vesicular rashes
  - Urticaria
  - Erythema multiforme minor
  - Erythema multiforme major (Stevens-Johnson syndrome)
  - Erythema nodosum
- Neurologic
  - Meningoencephalitis
  - Toxic psychosis
  - Peripheral neuropathy
  - Guillain-Barré syndrome
  - Cerebellar ataxia
- Cardiovascular
  - Myocarditis
  - Pericarditis
- Gastrointestinal
  - Hepatitis
  - Pancreatitis
  - Gastroenteritis
- Hematologic
  - Hemolytic anemia
  - Thrombocytopenic purpura
- Musculoskeletal
  - Polyarthritis

DIAGNOSIS

Because of the technical difficulties encountered in culturing *Mycoplasma pneumoniae* from patient specimens, diagnosis of *M. pneumoniae* infection has traditionally relied on detection of antibodies. *M. pneumoniae* infection results in the production of autoantibodies that agglutinate erythrocytes at 4° C. Cold agglutinins are immunoglobulin M (IgM) antibodies that bind to the erythrocyte I antigen, and may be induced because of cross-reactive antigens between the organism and the red blood cell membrane. Agglutination is reversible and is favored by low temperature. The presence of cold agglutinins, especially in low titer, is nonspecific and can be found in other conditions, including approximately 20% of patients with adenovirus pneumonia, some patients with *Legionella pneumophila,* and many nonmycoplasmal respiratory diseases affecting children. Titers of 1:64 or greater are present in 40% to 70% of cases of *Mycoplasma* pneumonia. In general, the height of the response is directly proportional to the severity of the disease.

A simple bedside test for cold agglutinins can be performed by adding 0.4 ml of blood to a tube containing 0.2 ml of 3.8% sodium citrate solution and then placing the tube in ice water for 30 seconds. Floccular agglutination of red blood cells can be observed by tilting the tube on its side. This positive result corresponds to a quantitative titer of 1:64 or greater, and the incidence of false-negative results for this method is less than 1%. Glass tubes containing sodium citrate solution are commonly used to collect blood samples for prothrombin time determinations.

Antibodies to *M. pneumoniae* have been measured by using complement fixation, indirect hemagglutination, growth inhibition, and other methods. The most widely used of these is the complement-fixation test. A fourfold rise in the complement-fixing antibody titer from acute to convalescent serum is considered to be diagnostic of recent infection. A rise in titer is demonstrated in about 75% of cases. If the first titer value is not obtained within the first week of illness, a fourfold rise may not be demonstrated, because the complement-fixing antibody response may peak during the first several weeks of the disease. A single high titer level (≥1:32) of complement-fixing antibody is also highly suggestive of recent infection, because complement-fixing antibodies are usually short-lived. An enzyme-linked immunoassay has been developed that permits separate measurement of IgG and IgM antibody; this test is supplanting the complement-fixation test.

Recently, *M. pneumoniae* antigens and DNA have been detected in respiratory secretions. Mycoplasmal antigens were demonstrated on desquamated respiratory epithelial cells by immunofluorescence, and the test was sensitive and specific. Mycoplasmal DNA was detected in respiratory secretions, either directly or after polymerase chain reaction amplification; these tests also had good sensitivity and specificity. These results suggest that clinically useful rapid tests for diagnosis of *M. pneumoniae* infection may be available soon.

TREATMENT AND PREVENTION

Mycoplasma pneumoniae shows in vitro sensitivity to macrolides, such as erythromycin, and to the tetracyclines. Because the organisms lack a cell wall, they are resistant to beta-lactam antibiotics. Erythromycin shows greater in vitro activity against *M. pneumoniae* than does tetracycline, but these two antibiotics are equally effective in shortening the duration of symptoms. Treatment should be with 1.5 to 2.0 g per day for 10 to 14 days, or up to 3 weeks in cases of severe disease. Doxycycline, 100 mg twice a day, has equivalent activity.

Antimicrobial treatment of a patient with mycoplasmal pneumonia reduces the duration of fever by an average of 4 days and the duration of cough and pulmonary infiltrates by about 6 days. *Mycoplasma pneumoniae* can still be recovered from many patients during therapy and for up to 3 months after treatment. Rare instances of tetracycline-resistant *M. pneumoniae* have been reported.

Patients with *Mycoplasma* pneumonia should be instructed to cough into a handkerchief to limit infectious droplet spread. Respiratory isolation of the rare patient requiring hospitalization is not necessary, because transmission requires prolonged close contact. Ten days of tetracycline prophylaxis for family members of an index case was effective in prevention of illness, although colonization still occurred. Vaccines are not available.

GENITAL MYCOPLASMAS

Mycoplasma hominis and *U. urealyticum* are referred to as the genital mycoplasmas. Both organisms are found commonly in the urogenital tract of healthy adults, and this high incidence of colonization in persons without evidence of disease has been the cause of considerable difficulty in assigning genital mycoplasmas a pathogenic role (Chapter 238). *Mycoplasma hominis* and *U. urealyticum* can be isolated from one third and one half, respectively, of sexually active adults. Colonization occurs by sexual contact, and thus the rate increases with increasing promiscuity. Heterosexual men are more likely to be colonized with *U. urealyticum* than are homosexual men. Women are more readily colonized with genital mycoplasmas than men. The relative virulence of different serotypes of genital mycoplasmas is not known.

Ureaplasma urealyticum is one cause of nongonococcal urethritis in men, although its role in this syndrome is questioned by some authorities (Chapter 238). *Ureaplasma urealyticum* may be more important in the first episode of urethritis in males, because a significant difference in isolation rates can be shown between men with urethritis and those without it. In these same two groups of men, quantitative cultures have shown that there are more organisms in the presence of urethritis. Additional evidence of the pathogenicity of *U. urealyticum* in nongonococcal urethritis comes from studies in which men treated with antibiotics active only against *Chlamydia* were not cured if both *Ureaplasma* and *Chlamydia* were initially present. Of three investigators inoculated intraurethrally with a pure culture of *U. urealyticum,* urethritis developed in two. *Mycoplasma hominis,* on the other hand, is not a cause of urethritis.

Mycoplasma hominis has been isolated from the fallopian tubes of women with salpingitis, and, in addition, these patients usually exhibit a rise in serum antibody titers to the organism. The overall importance of *M. hominis* as an etiologic agent in pelvic inflammatory disease is unclear, although it is probably insignificant in comparison with that of the gonococci, anaerobic and aerobic enteric bacteria, and *Chlamydia*. *Ureaplasma urealyticum* probably plays an even lesser role. *Mycoplasma hominis* is also the cause of some cases of postpartum and postabortal fever or sepsis, and a rare cause of pyelonephritis, septic arthritis, and peritonitis.

Recently, S-C Lo and his collaborators have isolated a novel strain of mycoplasma, GTU-54, from a patient with HIV infection. These same investigators and others have shown that AIDS patients have a high prevalence of active *M. fermentans* infection. However, the relationship between infection by these mycoplasmas and disease in HIV-infected patients remains unclear.

REFERENCES

Bayer AS et al: Neurologic disease associated with *Mycoplasma pneumoniae* pneumonitis: demonstration of viable *Mycoplasma pneumoniae* in cerebrospinal fluid and blood by radioisotopic and immunofluorescent tissue culture techniques. Ann Intern Med 94:15, 1987.

Bernet C et al: Detection of *Mycoplasma pneumoniae* by using the polymerase chain reaction. J Clin Microbiol 27:2492, 1989.

Blanco JD et al: A controlled study of genital mycoplasmas in amniotic fluid from patients with intra-amniotic infection. J Infect Dis 147:650, 1983.

Burdge DR et al: Septic arthritis due to dual infection with *Mycoplasma hominis* and *Ureaplasma urealyticum*. J Rheumatol 15(2):336-338, 1988.

Cassell GH and Cole BC: Mycoplasmas as agents of human disease. N Engl J Med 304:80, 1981.

Cassell GH et al: Pathogenesis and significance of urogenital mycoplasmal infections. Adv Exp Med Biol 224:93, 1987.

Couch RB: *Mycoplasma pneumoniae* (primary atypical pneumonia). In Mandell GL, Douglas RG Jr, and Bennett JE, editors: Principles and practice of infectious diseases. ed 3. New York, 1989, Churchill Livingstone.

Harai Y et al: Application of an indirect immunofluorescence test for detection of *Mycoplasma pneumoniae* in respiratory exudates. J Clin Microbiol 29:2007, 1991.

Harris R et al: Laboratory diagnosis of *Mycoplasma pneumoniae* infection. 2. Comparison of methods for the direct detection of specific antigen or nucleic acid sequences in respiratory exudates. Epidemiol Inf 101:685, 1988.

Kenny GE et al: Diagnosis of *Mycoplasma pneumoniae* pneumonia: sensitivities and specificities of serology with lipid antigen and isolation of the organism on soy peptone medium for identification of infections. J Clin Microbiol 28:2087, 1990.

Kleemola SR et al: Rapid diagnosis of *Mycoplasma pneumoniae* infection: clinical evaluation of a commercial probe test. J Infect Dis 162:70, 1990.

Kraus VB et al: *Ureaplasma urealyticum* septic arthritis in hypogammaglobulinemia. J Rheumatol 15(2):369, 1988.

Kundsin RB: The definite diagnosis of *Mycoplasma* infections. Adv Exp Med Biol 224:85, 1987.

Lo S-C et al: Newly discovered mycoplasma from patients infected with HIV. Lancet 2:1415, 1991.

Madoff S and Hooper DC: Nongenitourinary infections caused by *Mycoplasma hominis* in adults. Rev Infect Dis 10(3):602, 1988 (review).

Mokhbat JE: Peritonitis due to *Mycoplasma hominis* in a renal transplant recipient. J Infect Dis 146:713, 1982.

Moore PS et al: Respiratory viruses and mycoplasma as cofactors for epidemic group A meningococcal meningitis. JAMA 264:1271, 1990.

Taylor-Robinson D and McCormack WM: The genital mycoplasmas. N Engl J Med 302:1003, 1063, 1980.

RICKETTSIAL DISEASES

CHAPTER 256 Rickettsial Infections

David T. Durack
David H. Walker

The genus *Rickettsia* comprises a heterogeneous group of microorganisms whose definitive hosts are arthropods or small mammals. Some nine species in this genus can cause disease in humans. Electron microscopy reveals that rickettsiae are actually bacteria, with a structure very similar to that of gram-negative bacilli. They are obligate intracellular parasites and therefore cannot be cultured on standard laboratory media. Typically, these organisms cause disease by proliferating inside the endothelial cells of small blood vessels, producing vascular injury. In this chapter, Rocky Mountain spotted fever (RMSF) is described in some detail, being the paradigm of rickettsial infections and the most important rickettsiosis in the United States. Other rickettsial diseases are mentioned briefly.

HISTORICAL NOTE

Louse-borne epidemic typhus fever has been important throughout human history. The disease, which was endemic in Europe and Asia, flared periodically into major epidemics during periods of war, poverty, and social upheaval. For example, notable epidemics occurred during the Thirty Years War, the Napoleonic Wars, and World War I. During these conflicts, deaths related to illness, especially typhus fever, usually greatly outnumbered deaths in battle. Many thousands of cases occurred in Germany, Poland, and Egypt during World War II.

Ricketts's classic studies in western Montana from 1906 to 1909, which led to his discovery of the etiologic agent and vector for RMSF, were the scientific basis for our understanding of this disease. The introduction of chloramphenicol in 1947 provided the first effective treatment for rickettsial diseases. In recent years new species of rickettsiae and new vectors have been discovered and their ecologic relationships have been better defined.

EPIDEMIOLOGY

Within the United States, RMSF is the most prevalent rickettsial disease. The number of reported cases appears to show cyclic variations. A 10 year decline began in 1950, followed by a 20 year resurgence; from 1977 to 1983 more than 1000 cases were reported in the United States each year. This peak has been succeeded by another downward cycle, with approximately 600 cases reported annually from 1988 to 1991. North Carolina and Oklahoma usually report more cases than any other state. Paradoxically, the disease has become distinctly uncommon in the Rocky Mountain states, probably as a result of declining populations of infected ticks in that area.

Of the other rickettsial diseases that occur in the United States, ehrlichiosis, imported boutonneuse fever, murine typhus, and Q fever are uncommon, and typhus, recrudescent typhus (Brill-Zinsser disease), and rickettsial pox are rare. Some facts regarding geographic distribution of rickettsial diseases are given in Table 256-1, but a discussion of their worldwide epidemiology is beyond the scope of this chapter.

All the rickettsioses are zoonoses. They may be accidentally transmitted to humans by arthropod vectors (Table 256-1), but humans do not play an important role in the natural life cycle of these organisms, except in the case of epidemic typhus. It is possible that mammalian hosts serve as a reservoir or as a mechanism for amplification of the infected tick population, but transovarial transmission of rickettsiae from one generation of female ticks to the next appears to be the most important mechanism for maintenance of *Rickettsia rickettsii* in nature. In any case, the infected tick is the primary means by which *R. rickettsii* is introduced into humans. Activities that bring humans into contact with infected arthropods favor the development of disease. These relationships are clearly illustrated by the epidemiology of RMSF. When adult ticks of the species *Dermacentor variabilis* (the common dog tick), *Dermacentor andersoni* (the wood tick), or *Rhipicephalus sanguineus* that are infected with *R. rickettsii* feed on a human for several hours, inoculation of organisms from the ticks' salivary glands into the dermal blood vessels can occur. Persons who spend time outdoors in areas where active, infected ticks abound are most likely to contract RMSF. Therefore the disease occurs most frequently in male children in South Atlantic and South Central states between April and September.

Table 256-1. Characteristics of the major rickettsioses

Disease	Organisms	Vector	Vertebrate host	Means of transmission to humans	Geographic distribution	Mortality rate (%)	
						Untreated	Treated
Spotted fever group							
Rocky Mountain spotted fever	*R. rickettsii*	Ticks, e.g., *Dermacentor variabilis, D. andersoni*	Rodents	Tick bite	North, Central, and South America	20-25	3
Boutonneuse fever	*R. conorii*	Ticks	Rodents	Tick bite	Africa, Asia, and Mediterranean basin	?	1-3†
North Asian tick typhus	*R. sibirica*	Ticks	Rodents	Tick bite	Asia	0	0
Queensland tick typhus	*R. australis*	Ticks	Rodents, marsupials	Tick bite	Eastern Australia	2	0
Rickettsial pox	*R. akari*	Mite	Mice	Mouse to mite to human	USA, USSR, possibly worldwide	0	0
Oriental spotted fever	*R. japonica*	Unknown	Unknown	Presumed tick bite	Japan	0	0
Typhus group							
Epidemic typhus	*R. prowazekii*	Body louse	Humans	Human to louse to human	Worldwide	15-30*	5*
Murine typhus	*R. typhi (mooseri)*	Rat flea	Rats	Rat to rat flea to human	Worldwide	1	0-1†
Scrub typhus group							
Scrub typhus	*R. tsutsugamushi*	Larvae of mites (chiggers)	Rats, other rodents, birds	Mite to human	Asia, Pacific islands, and Australia	5	1
Other genera							
Q fever	*Coxiella burnetii*	Tick (but usually by aerosol)	Cattle, goats, sheep, other mammals	Livestock to human, by aerosol	Worldwide	5	0‡
Ehrlichiosis	*E. chaffeensis*	Ticks	Unknown	Tick bite	North America and Europe, possibly worldwide	2	?

*Mortality can be high in debilitated, malnourished patients; otherwise, it is lower than that for RMSF.

†In hospitalized patients.

‡Excluding Q fever endocarditis, which causes significant mortality.

PATHOPHYSIOLOGY

The hallmark of infections by members of the genus *Rickettsia* is vascular damage. Rickettsiae are first introduced into dermal tissue by feeding ticks (RMSF, boutonneuse fever, and other spotted fevers), by mites (scrub typhus, rickettsial pox), or by scratching when the skin is contaminated with infected feces of the human body louse (epidemic typhus) or the rat flea (murine typhus). Then rickettsiae spread via the bloodstream to infect vascular endothelial cells. *Rickettsia rickettsii* infects vascular smooth muscle cells as well. The organisms multiply intracellularly, achieving large numbers; they damage the host cells and cause foci of vasculitis (Plates V-49 and V-50). The inflammatory infiltrate consists primarily of mononuclear cells, with a few polymorphonuclear leukocytes. These foci are the direct cause of the rash, encephalitis, interstitial pneumonia, portal triaditis, interstitial nephritis, myocarditis, and presumably the vasculopathic consumption coagulopathy that may occur.

Disseminated infection of the cells lining the blood vessels has two important pathophysiologic consequences: increased vascular permeability and multifocal vasculitis at sites where injury induced by rickettsiae is most intense. Altered vascular permeability is manifested by edema and focal hemorrhages, not only in the skin and subcutaneous tissues (Plate V-50) but in the viscera. Noncardiogenic pulmonary edema, hypovolemia, and acute renal failure can result. Focal vasculitis is more common than frank thrombosis of involved vessels. Intravascular thrombi are usually eccentric and nonocclusive (Plate V-49), seldom resulting in infarction. The combined effects of increased vascular permeability, multifocal vasculitis, and associated coagulopathy account for the clinical features of these diseases. Any organ may be affected, but involvement of the skin (Plate V-50), lung, and brain usually is most prominent.

Vasculitis is not a typical manifestation of *Coxiella burnetii* infection, called Q fever. This species of rickettsia can cause mild or severe, acute, subacute, or chronic systemic infection with fever, pneumonia, granulomatous hepatitis, and occasionally infective endocarditis, osteomyelitis, or central nervous system (CNS) involvement. Q fever may be transmitted by tick bite but is most often acquired by rural aerosols of *C. burnetii* shed into the air by infected livestock or animal products.

CLINICAL MANIFESTATIONS

The cardinal features of RMSF are fever, headache, rash, and history of tick bite or exposure. However, only a small minority of RMSF patients have the full syndrome at presentation. This explains why the correct diagnosis is made in only about half of RMSF cases at first contact with a physician, the time when treatment is most likely to be effective.

The incubation period of RMSF after inoculation by an infected tick ranges from 2 to 12 days, with a median of 7 days. The onset of illness is often abrupt, entailing severe headaches and moderately high, continuous fever. Myalgias and muscle tenderness are common, as are mild or moderate conjunctival injection and photophobia. Chills occur, but true rigors are uncommon.

The rash usually develops after the patient has already been ill for 3 to 5 days, but it may appear earlier or much later and is absent entirely in up to 10% of patients—Rocky Mountain "spotless" fever. It may be overlooked easily in dark-skinned persons. Mortality rate is higher in patients without a rash, because the diagnosis is often delayed in these cases. The rash itself consists of maculopapular pink or purplish spots, 1 to 5 mm in diameter. These usually appear first on the extremities, especially around the ankles and wrists. Over the next 1 to 2 days the rash spreads centripetally, sometimes involving the entire body. The palms and soles are frequently involved, but the face is often spared. In about 50% of cases, the lesions become petechial or ecchymotic (Plates V-18 and V-50), but usually only after the fifth day of illness. Frank purpura may develop, especially in patients with thrombocytopenia (see Plate V-19). Necrosis of the skin and peripheral gangrene occur in about 5% of hospitalized patients with RMSF. These are due to extensive small vessel thrombosis in response to vasculitis, rather than to occlusion of large arteries or fully developed disseminated intravascular coagulation, which is uncommon in RMSF.

Gastrointestinal symptoms are common. Nausea, vomiting, diarrhea, and/or abdominal pain occurs in about two thirds of patients, often early in the illness. Therefore the initial diagnosis is often "gastroenteritis."

Involvement of vessels in the lung is evidenced by cough, interstitial and alveolar infiltrates, and development of noncardiogenic pulmonary edema in severe cases.

Central nervous system manifestations are common and important. Most patients have headache, which often is severe. This symptom is useful in evaluation of adults and older children but not in very young children, who cannot describe headache. Signs of central nervous system involvement range from lethargy, confusion, and delirium to focal deficits, papilledema, seizures, and coma. About one fourth of patients have a stiff neck, which can be due to myalgia or to meningismus. Cranial and peripheral nerve lesions are rare.

As the disease progresses, diffuse edema develops in many patients because of leakage of plasma from damaged vessels. Attempts to correct hypotension with infusion of saline or colloid solutions may lead to worsening of the edema, which persists until the vasculitis resolves. Acute renal failure, which occurs in 10% to 15% of patients, is secondary to hypovolemia produced by damaged, leaking vessels rather than to rickettsial vasculitis of the kidney itself.

Most clinical reports of RMSF have described hospitalized patients, who are more likely to have severe disease and complications than are outpatients. However, some patients with RMSF have mild disease and may be managed safely as outpatients. Because some patients undoubtedly recover spontaneously, remaining undiagnosed and untreated, the true incidence of subclinical or mild forms of RMSF is not yet known. Serologic surveys suggest that subclinical infection is common in endemic areas.

DIFFERENTIAL DIAGNOSIS

The diagnosis of RMSF poses a serious problem for the physician of first contact, because symptoms and signs are nonspecific, early treatment is needed to reduce mortality, and no laboratory test is available to confirm the diagnosis immediately except direct demonstration of *R. rickettsii* in skin lesions by immunofluorescence or immunoperoxidase. Rickettsemia can be detected by the polymerase chain reaction, but this technique is not yet applicable in routine diagnosis.

In the United States, meningococcemia (Chapter 263) and enteroviral (Chapter 244) infections are the most common alternative diagnoses in patients who have a syndrome compatible with RMSF, and vice versa. Other initial diagnoses sometimes made in patients with RMSF include pneumonia, scarlet fever, Henoch-Schönlein purpura, and various vasculitides, viral encephalitides, rubella, mononucleosis, typhoid fever, and hepatitis. Atypical measles in a partially immune host also should be considered (Chapter 246). In developing countries measles, malaria, dengue, hemorrhagic fevers, other rickettsial infections, and many other locally endemic, acute febrile syndromes may be included in the extensive differential diagnosis.

The detection of purulent meningitis in a patient from an endemic area for RMSF who exhibits fever, headache, and rash strongly suggests meningococcal infection, but in patients whose spinal fluid is normal or nearly normal, it may be impossible to decide on clinical grounds whether the patient has RMSF or meningococcemia. Such patients should be treated with chloramphenicol, the only antimicrobial agent that is fully effective in both diseases.

LABORATORY DIAGNOSIS AND IMMUNE RESPONSE

Only one fourth of patients with RMSF have leukocytosis, despite their toxic clinical appearance. The majority have normal or low white blood cell counts in peripheral blood. However, about three fourths show an increased proportion of band forms, often with toxic granulation of neutrophils. Sometimes band forms outnumber segmented neutrophils. The combination of a low or low-normal white blood cell count with striking left shift in a febrile patient in an endemic area should raise the possibility of rickettsial infection. The platelet count is less than 150,000 per microliter in about half the patients, and less than 100,000 per microliter in 10% to 20%.

Significant hyponatremia occurs in about half the patients. The serum albumin concentration falls below 3 g per deciliter in about one third of severe cases. Elevations of serum transaminases, alkaline phosphatase, and/or bilirubin occur in 10% to 20%. Striking elevations of creatine phosphokinase serum concentrations have been reported, confirming the presence of myositis.

Thus when a patient from an endemic area has fever and headache in spring or summer, the combination of a low or low-normal total leukocyte count in peripheral blood with a striking left shift indicated on smear, hyponatremia, and thrombocytopenia strongly suggests the diagnosis of RMSF. However, these abnormal laboratory findings are nonspecific and not present in all patients; their absence does not exclude RMSF.

Cerebrospinal fluid (CSF), which usually is obtained to help differentiate RMSF from meningococcal meningitis, is abnormal in up to two thirds of RMSF patients. In these cases, the CSF profile is consistent with a mild aseptic meningitis; from 5 to 200 leukocytes may be present, with a predominance of either mononuclear or polymorphonuclear cells. The protein concentration may be slightly or moderately elevated. The glucose concentration usually is normal, but occasionally mildly reduced. The finding of more extreme abnormalities in the CSF during RMSF is unusual.

The etiologic diagnosis of any infectious disease is best achieved by isolation of the causative organism. Unfortunately, rickettsiae are highly biohazardous agents that have caused laboratory-acquired infections and deaths, especially in the preantibiotic era. Isolation of rickettsiae still requires complex systems such as inoculation of embryonated hens' eggs, cell cultures, or laboratory animals. These cumbersome, prolonged, and somewhat hazardous procedures are rarely useful in the care of an individual patient, but isolation and identification in research laboratories are necessary if we are to learn whether the numerous other species of rickettsiae found in insects and animals in the United States (e.g., *R. montana, R. canada, R. rhipicephali, R. bellii*) cause human disease. Recently, the shell vial centrifugation enhanced cell culture technique, which has proved useful in isolation of some viruses from blood, has been adapted to isolate *R. conorii* in a timely manner.

The diagnosis of rickettsial disease usually can be confirmed by measurement of an immune response in survivors. Unfortunately, the inherent delay in the appearance of a detectable immunologic response to infection means that most patients require evaluation and treatment before a positive result is available. Eventual serologic confirmation is important, not only for epidemiologic and public health reasons but also for the individual patient, who may expect immunity after a confirmed attack, and for the primary physician, who needs to know whether his or her clinical diagnoses are accurate.

The Weil-Felix test, using agglutination of cross-reacting *Proteus* OX-19, OX-2, and OX-K antigens, has been the main diagnostic test for rickettsial infection in the United States for many years. A fourfold rise in titer after an illness compatible with RMSF or murine typhus is confirmatory. Unfortunately, the test's lack of specificity and sensitivity is a major drawback. Diverse other conditions, including *Proteus* urinary tract infections, leptospirosis, and various liver diseases, can cause false-positive test results. Single titers in the range of 1:160 are equivocal. The standard spotted fever complement-fixation test has proved more specific than the Weil-Felix test, but it is relatively insensitive, giving false-negative results in as many as 50% of tests. Recently developed tests that yield both sensitive and specific results are indirect fluorescent antibody, passive hemagglutination, microagglutination, and latex agglutination. For routine diagnostic purposes, the Weil-Felix test should now be replaced by the latex agglutination test.

Rapid, specific diagnosis of RMSF has been achieved by use of immunofluorescence or immunoperoxidase to demonstrate *R. rickettsii* in biopsy specimens from skin lesions. Although success requires the presence of a rash and selection of an appropriate biopsy site, the procedure is moderately sensitive and highly specific. Positive results can be expected in about 75% of cases; the sensitivity falls if the patient has been treated with active antibiotics for 1 day or more. A positive test result indicates the need for specific treatment, alerts the physician to possible complications, and eliminates the need for isolation and treatment for possible meningococcemia.

In nonimmune hosts, virulent rickettsiae taken up by macrophages can escape from phagosomes into the cytoplasm, where multiplication proceeds unhindered until the host cell lyses. When specific antibody is present, the rickettsiae remain within macrophage phagolysosomes and are killed. However, these same antibodies do not prevent rickettsiae from multiplying inside their endothelial target cells. Thus effective in vivo immunity requires the interaction of both cellular and humoral responses.

Specific cell-mediated immune responses have been documented in humans, and experimental studies in animal models indicate that such responses are of major importance in providing immunity to rickettsial diseases. T lymphocytes, gamma interferon, and tumor necrosis factor appear to be important components of the normal host immune response, which achieves clearance of rickettsiae and provides long-term immunity in most patients who have recovered from rickettsial infection.

TREATMENT

Rickettsiae are generally susceptible to chloramphenicol and the tetracyclines. Treatment of RMSF and typhus fever with these drugs is usually effective, reducing mortality rate 5- to 10-fold (Table 256-1). The morbidity of rickettsial infections that seldom cause death, such as rickettsial pox or murine typhus, can also be reduced by antibiotic treatment. Rocky Mountain spotted fever should be treated with tetracycline 25 to 50 mg/kg/day orally or chloramphenicol 30 to 50 mg/kg/day orally in four divided doses, or doxycycline 200 mg/day in two divided doses, continuing for 2 to 3 days after resolution of fever. For practical purposes, all these regimens are equally effective. In severely ill patients, the initial doses should be given parenterally.

Most cases of louse-borne typhus and scrub typhus can be cured with a single dose of 200 mg of doxycycline. Occasional relapses occur, requiring retreatment. Boutonneuse fever responds to treatment with fluoroquinolone drugs such as ciprofloxacin and ofloxacin, which would probably also be effective against other rickettsioses.

Corticosteroids probably do not affect the infectious process itself but can provide symptomatic improvement in patients with typhus fever. Their value in RMSF is unproved. Likewise, no proof exists that heparin is useful in severe cases, even in those few in whom true disseminated intravascular coagulation develops.

The child living in an area where RMSF is endemic who has a febrile illness during the summer presents a special problem. Most have minor or self-limited infections requiring no specific treatment. However, it is evident that those few children who have RMSF must be treated early to reduce morbidity and mortality rates. In practice, it is reasonable to treat potentially exposed children who have persistent fever for more than 2 days with tetracycline 25 mg/kg/day orally for 5 days. This is especially appropriate for those with prominent headache (after consideration of the possibility of bacterial meningitis and the indications for a spinal tap), while remembering that young children do not describe headache in the same way as older children and adults. The danger of inducing tooth discoloration with such a short course of tetracycline is low and is even lower with doxycycline; it is negligible in children above 6 years of age. Because most of these children actually have self-limited diseases other than RMSF, it is undesirable to expose them to even a small risk of drug-induced marrow aplasia by using chloramphenicol too freely. Prophylactic antibiotic treatment of patients after tick bite is not indicated, because less than 1% of the ticks carry virulent *R. rickettsii*. Moreover, chloramphenicol and tetracycline are rickettsiostatic, not rickettsiocidal drugs. Therefore attempted prophylaxis with antibiotics after exposure to ticks, mites, or fleas is not recommended; this might merely prolong the incubation period until the rickettsiostatic drug is discontinued.

Good nursing care is needed for severe cases of rickettsial disease. Hypovolemic shock, respiratory failure, or renal failure, which often coexist in patients with severe disease, requires management in an intensive care unit. Surgery is occasionally needed in the unfortunate patients who have extensive cutaneous necrosis or gangrene of the extremities.

OTHER RICKETTSIAL DISEASES

Louse-borne epidemic typhus

Louse-borne epidemic typhus fever ranks with RMSF as the most virulent of the rickettsioses. The human body louse, which is responsible for transferring typhus from human to human, is itself infected and eventually killed by *Rickettsia prowazekii*. Humans are considered to be the principal reservoir; if so, this feature would be unique among the rickettsioses. However, in the eastern United States, natural infection occurs among flying squirrels and can be the source of human infection. These squirrels, and possibly other mammals not yet identified, may constitute reservoirs for *R. prowazekii* other than humans. Stupor and inanition are even more marked in typhus than in RMSF, and the typhus rash usually spares the palms and soles; otherwise, these diseases share many clinical features. Late recrudescences many years after the original infection result in a milder form of typhus known as Brill-Zinsser disease. Fully virulent *R. prowazekii* can be recovered from the blood of such patients, perhaps explaining how typhus can reemerge in epidemic form after long periods of quiescence if social conditions favor proliferation of lice.

Murine typhus

Murine typhus *(R. typhi, R. mooseri)* is transmitted from rats to humans by the rat flea. *R. typhi* can cause serious illness, but usually the disease is much milder than epidemic typhus, with less than 1% mortality rate.

Rickettsial pox begins with a localized papule that develops 7 to 10 days after inoculation via the bite of an infected mite. This papule grows into a fluid-filled vesicle on an inflamed base, forms a black eschar, and finally heals with scarring. Systemic symptoms, including fever, headache, myalgia, and generalized maculopapular rash, appear a few days after the primary lesion. Rickettsial pox is not a fatal disease, but it should be treated because its symptoms, which can be severe, respond well to tetracycline. The Weil-Felix reaction remains negative in this disease, but serologic diagnosis can be provided by a complement-fixation test.

Scrub typhus

Scrub typhus is common in Asia and the western Pacific region, in both local populations and transients, such as soldiers who served in Vietnam. An eschar forms at the site of a chigger bite during a 7 to 14 day incubation period, with associated lymphadenopathy. Systemic disease follows, with fever, rash, and splenomegaly. Central nervous system involvement and/or pneumonitis is frequently prominent. The eschar may be absent in many patients with scrub typhus.

Boutonneuse fever

Boutonneuse fever is characterized by development of a local eschar at the site of inoculation by *Rhiplicephalus sanguineus* and possibly other ticks, with associated lymphadenopathy in approximately 50% of cases. This is followed a few days later by fever and generalized rash. This infection occurs in Africa, in Asia, and in the Mediterranean basin. In the United States, imported cases occur in tourists returning from Europe and Africa.

Q fever

Q fever is unique among rickettsial diseases in that it is usually transmitted by inhalation rather than by an arthropod vector, is not associated with a rash, does not cause a rise in Weil-Felix agglutinins, and may cause granulomatous hepatitis and infective endocarditis.

Q fever occurs worldwide and is strongly associated with exposure to animals, especially farm livestock. Veterinarians and laboratory workers are at high risk. Epidemics have arisen from exposure to infected parturient cats and wild rabbits.

The disease can consist of an acute, self-limited fever with or without atypical pneumonia, or can linger on in subacute or chronic forms. It has been reported to be a common cause of atypical pneumonia in France, and most cases undoubtedly are undiagnosed in North America. Patients with Q fever endocarditis have a high mortality rate but sometimes can be cured by valve replacement and long-term antibiotic therapy. Late relapses, even after years, can occur in this form of the infection.

The antibody response to natural infection is complex, involving the immunoglobulin M (IgM), IgG, and IgA titers to phase 1 and phase 2 antigens of *C. burnetti*. High IgG and IgA titers to phase 1 antigen suggest chronic Q fever infection with endocarditis.

Ehrlichiosis

Ehrlichiosis is a newly described disease of humans caused by *Ehrlichia chaffeensis*. A closely related intraleukocytic rickettsia, *E. canis,* was known previously to cause infection in dogs. The only previously known human disease caused by this genus is an infectious mononucleosis-like disease observed in Japan and Malaysia, caused by *E. sennetsu*.

Seven to twenty-one days after a tick bite, fever, chills and rigors, headache, myalgias, and anorexia develop. Only 20% of patients have a rash. Leukopenia, thrombocytopenia, and elevated liver enzymes in serum are typical. The disease can be severe: more than 250 cases have been reported and the majority required hospitalization. Fatalities have been documented. Tetracycline appears to provide effective therapy. Serologic confirmation of *E. chaffeensis* infection is provided by fourfold or greater rise in immunofluorescent antibody titer. Retrospective studies indicate that 10% to 14% of patients with RMSF-like illnesses and negative serologic results for RMSF may have ehrlichiosis.

More rickettsial diseases may remain to be recognized, for example, a novel spotted fever–group rickettsia was recently isolated from patients with oriental spotted fever in Japan, and Israeli spotted fever appears to be caused by another distinct spotted fever group of rickettsia.

PREVENTION

Louse-borne epidemic typhus disappeared from the United States more than 50 years ago as a result of improving social and economic conditions. However, effective prevention of other rickettsial diseases in the United States has not yet been achieved. The use of environmental acaricides, tick repellents, and protective clothing has had no permanent impact on the incidence of RMSF. Eradication of the infected tick population is probably not feasible. Thus the single effective preventive measure presently available is to search the body and remove ticks several times daily when ticks are active, with special attention to the scalp, axillae, and pubic regions. Attached ticks should be removed with care, to prevent inoculation of rickettsiae during removal.

Scrub typhus can be prevented by taking doxycycline once weekly while in endemic areas.

No licensed RMSF vaccine is available. Previously available vaccines made from whole killed rickettsiae were only marginally effective; they have been withdrawn from use. There is no need for a vaccine against typhus fever in the United States, and none is available.

REFERENCES

Dumler JS, Taylor JP, and Walker DH: Clinical and laboratory features of murine typhus in South Texas, 1980 through 1987. JAMA 266:1365, 1991.

Dumler JS and Walker DH: Human ehrlichiosis. Curr Opin Infect Dis 4:597, 1991.

Eng TR et al: Epidemiologic, clinical, and laboratory findings of human ehrlichiosis in the United States. JAMA 264:2251, 1990.

Hattwick MA, O'Brien RJ, and Hanson B: Rocky Mountain spotted fever: epidemiology of an increasing problem. Ann Intern Med 84:732, 1976.

Hechemy KE et al, editors: Rickettsiology: current issues and perspectives. Ann NY Acad Sci 590:1, 1990.

Helmick CG, Bernard KW, and D'Angelo LJ: Rocky Mountain spotted fever: clinical, laboratory, and epidemiologic features of 262 cases. J Infect Dis 150:480, 1984.

Kaplowitz LG, Fischer JJ, and Sparling PF: Rocky Mountain spotted fever—a clinical dilemma. Curr Clin Top Infect Dis 2:89, 1980.

Kirk JL et al: Rocky Mountain spotted fever: a clinical review based on 48 confirmed cases, 1943-1986. Medicine 69:35, 1990.

McDade JE, and Newhouse VF: Natural history of *Rickettsia rickettsii*. Am Rev Microbiol 40:287, 1986.

Sexton DJ and Corey GR: Rocky Mountain spotless and almost spotless fever: a wolf in sheep's clothing. Clin Infect Dis 15:439, 1992.

Walker DH, editor: Biology of rickettsial diseases. Boca Raton, FL, 1988, CRC Press.

Walker DH: Rocky Mountain spotted fever: a disease in need of microbiological concern. Clin Microbiol Rev 2:222, 1989.

BACTERIAL DISEASES

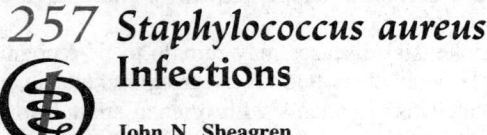

CHAPTER

257 *Staphylococcus aureus* Infections

John N. Sheagren

THE ORGANISM

Staphylococcus aureus continues to be one of the most important bacterial pathogens of humans. It usually produces localized disease but can be rapidly invasive, spreading through the tissues, invading bone, and seeding the bloodstream to produce a fulminant picture of septic shock, disseminated intravascular coagulation, and rapid demise. It can persist deep within tissues, being carried asymptomatically for years without causing disease. The balance between host and parasite that results in these kinds of relationships is only partially understood. *S. aureus* is a member of the family Micrococcaceae. There are only a few other clinically important species in this family, of which *S. epidermidis* and *S. saprophyticus* are notable.

Characteristics

Staphylococcus aureus (the species designation *aureus* meaning "gold") is a gram-positive coccus that grows in clusters in liquid or semisolid media or within tissues when causing infection (Plate IV-19). It grows well on blood agar plates, producing small, shiny, (ultimately) golden-yellow colonies that usually are surrounded by a clear zone of beta hemolysis. Although the colonies may initially look dull gray or even white, they rapidly turn a golden-yellow when the plates are exposed to air. The organisms grow well anaerobically or aerobically; in blood culture media, both bottles of a single set usually yield positive results.

There are no reproducible serologic typing schemes available to classify subtypes of *S. aureus;* however, bacteriophage typing has been useful in identifying strain characteristics and providing epidemiologic data on organism spread. Bacteriophages are viruses that attach to the mucopeptide–teichoic acid complex of the cell wall. Five major groups of organisms that have generally similar characteristics (phage groups I to V) have been designated. For example, some phage groups of staphylococci are more likely to produce certain toxins than are others. Recently plasmid profiles and immunoblotting techniques have produced staphylococcal "fingerprints," which have been useful epidemiologically. As increasing numbers of strains of *S. aureus* have not been phage-typable, plasmid-profile typing has increased in usefulness. Plasmid-profile analysis is carried out by separating plasmid contents from other *S. aureus* cell components and characterizing the isolated plasmids with restriction endonucleases. The resultant deoxyribonucleic acid (DNA) fragments can be separated by electrophoretic techniques, and the pattern produced by a given strain of *S. aureus* can be compared with others (Fig. 257-1). Plasmid-profile typing seems most reliable during focused outbreaks of infection, for the plasmid content of a given *S. aureus* strain may not be stable over a prolonged period.

Coagulase production, the most important classification method, is detected by incubating a small volume of a broth culture (or a colony from a plate suspended in broth) with an equal volume of citrated rabbit plasma; a clot must form within a 3 hour incubation period. This simple test permits the relatively rapid separation of coagulase-positive from coagulase-negative organisms, date critical to decision making when positive blood culture findings are reported. Other methods of rapidly detecting *S. aureus* are now available.

Epidemiology

Staphylococci may colonize almost all animal species. However, certain strains of *S. aureus* are limited to humans, whereas others are found in cattle, swine, and other ani-

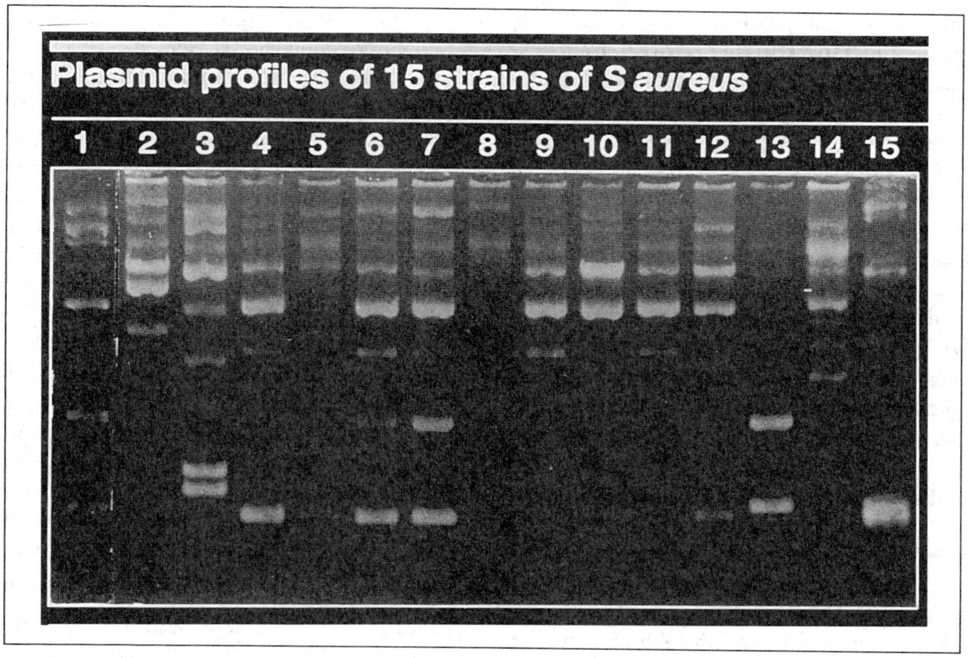

Fig. 257-1. Plasmid profiles of 15 strains of *S. aureus,* showing the differences and similarities of plasmid DNA fragments from the various strains. Plasmids are isolated and treated with restriction endonucleases, and the resulting DNA fragments are separated by electrophoresis to reveal the profile. (Reproduced with permission from Herwaldt LA: Coagulase-negative staphylococci; the surprise of the 1980s. In Doebbeling BN et al: Current concepts: hospital-acquired infections: new challenges. Kalamazoo, Mich, 1991, The Upjohn Co.)

mals. Humans carry *S. aureus* primarily in the nasopharynx, and heavily colonized individuals may become a source of recurrent infections both to themselves and to others. Most humans probably carry a few *S. aureus* organisms among the normal flora of every body site but in such low numbers that routine cultures rarely reveal the organism. Individuals regularly or intermittently using needles to inject substances either intravenously (such as drug addicts or patients on hemodialysis) or subcutaneously (such as insulin-dependent diabetics or patients receiving allergy shots) have a higher than normal rate of carriage of *S. aureus* in the nose and throat. Patients with chronic, especially exudative skin diseases also are heavily colonized.

In newborn nurseries, the rate of colonization increases rapidly after birth. In most nurseries, it is not uncommon to see colonization rates of about 25%, with most infants remaining asymptomatic. Yet outbreaks of disease within nurseries may be traced to more "virulent" strains of *S. aureus,* sometimes traceable to a common carrier among the personnel. Colonization of hospitalized adults increases throughout hospitalization. Once an individual is a carrier, spread may occur to other areas of patient's own body as well as to clothing and other items and to individuals with whom the individual comes in contact. The most effective single technique of stopping transmission from person to person in a hospital setting is simple. *Physicians should meticulously wash their hands immediately before and immediately after examining a patient.* This is particularly important when one is examining patients with obvious staphylococcal lesions and/or chronic exudative dermatoses. Some strains of staphylococci not only are more virulent than others but seem to spread more aggressively in a hospital environment. Outbreaks may occur, during which 20% to 30% of hospital personnel and patients entering the hospital may acquire the epidemic strain; subsequent multiple individual infections may occur.

Pathophysiology

Staphylococcus aureus is a ubiquitous and highly pathogenic organism. It produces a large number of enzymes that, together with its surface and cell wall components, contribute to its pathogenicity.

Any strain of *S. aureus* from either an environmental or a personal culture is almost inevitably more virulent than non-coagulase-producing staphylococci; however, there is substantial strain-to-strain variation in pathogenicity among *S. aureus* strains. Virulence is probably related to the sum of enzyme production that permits the organism to resist degradation by environmental substances, resist phagocytosis by polymorphonuclear leukocytes (PMNs), produce specific exotoxins that may directly cause damage to tissues or cells, or possess surface receptors that permit it to adhere to inflamed or traumatized tissues. Most strains of *S. aureus* release a multitude of such toxins, including hemolysins, toxins that cause hemolysis and injure leukocytes as well as other tissues. Another enzyme, leukocidin, is particularly toxic to white blood cells.

Surface receptors for a variety of tissue ligands (such as fibronectin and laminen) permit the organism to adhere to inflamed and/or traumatized tissues. Only *S. aureus* seems to possess such receptors, this explains why *S. aureus* so commonly seeds into sites of chronic inflammation such as healing, traumatized tissues and osteoarthritic joints. The staphylococci are catalase-positive and thus interfere with hydrogen peroxide production; when hydrogen peroxide is produced in suboptimum amounts (as in the leukocytes of patients with chronic granulomatous disease of childhood), the presence of catalase helps the organism avoid being killed.

S. aureus also produces a number of toxins that can cause disease in organs distant from the site of production. The best-described of these is the exfoliative toxin (epidermolysin or exfoliatin) responsible for the staphylococcal scalded skin syndrome (SSSS). There may, in fact, be two such toxins, which produce skin denudation by causing skin lysis at two different layers within the epidermis. The new syndrome that is clearly related to *S. aureus* toxin production is the toxic shock syndrome (TSS) (refer to the box below).

Enterotoxins are produced by a large number of strains of *S. aureus;* enterotoxin-producing strains growing in high-carbohydrate-containing food products (such as banana cream pies) produce staphylococcal gastroenteritis.

The primary host-defense systems against *S. aureus* are nonspecific. *S. aureus* gains access to tissues by rapidly colonizing and proliferating in breaks in the barrier systems (skin and mucous membranes). Thus barrier system defects are major predisposing factors to infection. Once the dermal and/or mucosal barriers are breached, the organism begins to proliferate rapidly through tissues, aided in its spread by the multitude of enzymes it produces; the PMN then becomes the primary host-defense cell responsible for constraining the organism. The PMN does not "automatically" arrive at the site to interact with the organism but is attracted into the infected area primarily via the complement system. Thus activation of the complement system (either by the organism itself or by tissue breakdown products), primarily via the alternative pathway, produces chemotactic factors that attract the PMN and activate it to phagocytize and kill the invading microbes more avidly. Antibody to cell wall components may enhance phagocytosis and killing of *S. aureus,* but in experimental system, passive antibody administration or active immunization of animals generally does not lead to demonstrable protection against staphylococcal infections. The cellular immune system does not seem to play a major host-defense role.

Diseases produced by *Staphylococcus aureus*

Toxin production

Gastroenteritis
Staphylococcal scalded skin syndrome (SSSS)
Toxic shock syndrome (TSS)

Direct invasion

Cutaneous infections (paronychiae, cellulitis, boils, furuncles, carbuncles, surgical wound)
Pyomyositis
Osteomyelitis and septic arthritis (hematogenous or contiguous spread)
Pneumonia
Meningitis, cerebritis
Endocarditis

Primary staphylococcal bacteremia

Transient
Complicated (associated with metastatic abscess formation)

DISEASES PRODUCED IN HUMANS

Diseases related to toxin production

The syndrome of gastroenteritis is produced by enterotoxin ingestion (Chapter 236). The ingestion of the preformed enterotoxin in foodstuffs causes acute gastroenteritis without requiring the presence of living organisms. Another gastroenteric syndrome caused by *S. aureus* is known as acute staphylococcal enterocolitis. This disease occurs in patients on broad-spectrum antibiotics and is characterized by fever, tachycardia, abdominal cramps, diarrhea (not infrequently with blood), and, in some cases, nausea and vomiting. Pseudomembrane formation may be demonstrable on sigmoidoscopy. The stool Gram stain predominantly shows masses of *S. aureus*. The organism must be present in the gut along with the production of an enterotoxin. Undoubtedly, many cases diagnosed as staphylococcal enteritis in the past were actually cases of antibiotic-associated colitis, now known to be caused by *Clostridium difficile*.

The SSSS is also produced solely by the systemic effect of a toxin. This syndrome occurs mainly in infants and young children but may rarely be seen in adults, especially those who are immunosuppressed (patients with chronic renal failure who are on dialysis, who have had kidney transplantation, or are on cytotoxic or steroid therapy). The patient usually has a primary focus of infection, which may not be apparent; infection of the umbilicus in the neonate, conjunctivitis, or an earlier staphylococcal infection may have been minor and completely localized and may have been unnoticed. Patients first experience tender skin and a bright red rash, either diffuse (as in scarlet fever) or macular. Blisters and bullae form as the upper epidermis splits off in large sheets (a positive Nikolsky sign). This phenomenon results from the action of exfoliative toxin, which attacks the skin in the middle layers of the epidermis. The finding of an intraepidermal lesion on skin biopsy differentiates this condition from the more severe, drug-related disease called toxic epidermal necrolysis (TEN), a variant of the erythema multiforme–Stevens-Johnson syndrome.

Staphylococci producing the exfoliative toxin are usually classified by phage typing as phage group II organisms.

The TSS described recently has emerged as various strains of *S. aureus* have acquired the genetic capability to produce a new protein toxin. It is now known that the genetic material to produce the toxin is acquired by lysogeny (carried into the staphylococcus by a temperate bacteriophage). Two groups of investigators have described an immunologically identical toxin called either staphylococcal pyrogenic exotoxin C or enterotoxin F. It is now named toxic-shock syndrome toxin-1 (TSST-1). How it works is still unclear, but it appears (either directly or indirectly) to be a very powerful cytotoxin that injures literally any cell surface with which it comes in contact. Two theories presently attempt to explain how TSST-1 produces the septic shock/multiple organ system failure syndrome. First, TSST-1 may enhance the effect of subtoxic amounts of bacterial endotoxin. Second, TSST-1 may (at least in part because of its ability to be a superantigen) stimulate the production of one or more cell-damaging mediators, the most important of which seems to be tumor necrosis factor (cachectin), now known to play a central role in bacteremic septic shock. Individuals colonized with one of these toxin-producing strains may have a low-grade, localized infection (e.g., vaginitis during menstruation, especially if a superabsorbent tampon is used, or a small, peripheral abscess or wound infection). The toxin is produced at the site of the low-grade infection and, when absorbed systemically, causes a dramatic, multisystem disease characterized by all or most of the following: high fever, headache, confusion, myalgias, scarlatiniform rash followed by desquamation, conjunctival suffusion, subcutaneous edema, vomiting, profuse watery diarrhea, oliguria, a propensity to acute renal failure, hypocalcemia, liver function abnormalities, disseminated intravascular coagulation, and often severe, prolonged shock. In contrast to the group of patients with bacteremic (endotoxin-like) shock, these patients are rarely bacteremic with the causative organism. Yet, as noted, the substances mediating this variety of septic shock may be the same as those mediating bacteremic shock syndromes. Therapy is directed at drainage and eradication of the peripheral focus of infection using antistaphylococcal antibiotics, surgery, and meticulous supportive care of the patient in shock. Approximately 10% of patients severely ill with TSS die. Patients with menstrually associated TSS should not use tampons during subsequent menstrual cycles; the recurrence rate is 70% without antibiotic therapy and only 20% if antibiotics are used during the initial episode and tampon use is subsequently discontinued. Nonmenstrual cases of TSS now account for about one third of all patients.

Diseases related to direct invasion by *S. aureus*

Dermal infections. Most minor skin infections are due either to *S. aureus* or to group A streptococci. Infections around nails (paronychiae) occur with great frequency, as do boils. Cellulitis may develop around sites of a minor abrasion or cut and progress rapidly to lymphangitis. Clinically, there is no way to differentiate between group A beta-hemolytic streptococcal infections and those caused by *S. aureus:* this is a point of therapeutic import. *S. aureus,* together with group A beta-hemolytic streptococci, may cause classic impetigo in children. Larger localized skin infections are called furuncles and carbuncles. When a patient with a localized *S. aureus* skin infection manifests fever and chills, bacteremia must be considered; prompt diagnostic and therapeutic intervention must be initiated (see Primary Staphylococcal Bacteremia).

Bone and joint infections. *Staphylococcus aureus* has a definite predilection for seeding to bones or joints (see Osteomyelitis [Chapter 237] and Septic Arthritis [Chapter 315]). This seeding can result from direct inoculation, as in trauma or penetrating wounds, or from a transient bacteremic episode. The latter event usually stems from cutaneous infections. As noted, because of the presence of surface receptors, the circulating bacteria tend to lodge in areas of recent trauma, or chronic inflammation or around a foreign body. Thus the syndrome tends to occur in children with a bruised or bumped extremity and is particularly common in teenage athletes (wrestlers or football players). The traumatized area, usually on the ankle, knee, or shin, becomes acutely red, warm, and swollen and may appear to be a primary cellulitis. Fever, shaking chills, and positive blood culture results are common. Hematogenous osteomyelitis or arthritis in adults is usually less acute. The syndrome of vertebral osteomyelitis often occurs in elderly patients who are often diabetic, and manifests itself as chronic back pain and low-grade fever; *S. aureus* may be cultured either from the blood or from an aspirate of the bone. Patients on hemodialysis may have osteomyelitis related to bacteremia (often asymptomatic) from infected shunts. Drug addicts may have primary osteomyelitis almost anywhere; this is related to the injection of their nasally carried strain of *S. aureus* along with the narcotics. Isolated staphylococcal septic arthritis often occurs as a complication of chronic underlying arthritis (such as rheumatoid or osteoarthritis) and also results from asymptomatic bacteremia seeding to one of the previously inflamed joints. Increasing symptoms develop in one joint, together with fever; joint aspiration reveals a purulent effusion containing the organism.

Staphylococcal pneumonia. Many cases of staphylococcal pneumonia follow viral infections of the lower respiratory tract (Chapter 231). The disease is most common in children, especially infants, and should be considered when the patient has a high fever in the course of a lower respiratory tract infection. The chest radiograph usually reveals patchy infiltrates, which may excavate rapidly to produce pneumatoceles. Rapid development of pleural effusions and empyema and/or pneumothorax may occur. A large number of such children are bacteremic. Staphylococcal bronchitis and pneumonia also are seen in children with cystic fibrosis. Adult patients with influenza have an increased incidence of *S. aureus* pneumonia. The patient usually has typical symptoms of influenza, begins to improve, but then fever and chills with chest pain develop rapidly. Gram stain of the sputum reveals large clumps of gram-positive cocci. Mortality rate in this syndrome is high; it is related to serious, localized, rapidly progressive pulmonary disease and the bacteremia that often accompanies it.

Staphylococcal meningitis-cerebritis. Staphylococcal meningitis unassociated with endocarditis usually develops as a complication of a diagnostic or surgical procedure (Chapter 233). Occasionally, spontaneous *S. aureus* meningitis occurs in patients with endocarditis. Thus, the features of this syndrome are similar to those in patients bacteremic with *Streptococcus pneumoniae* in whom meningitis develops. An occasional patient has purpura and vascular collapse in which differentiation from meningococcal meningitis is difficult. The cerebrospinal fluid from patients with staphylococcal meningitis or cerebritis is typically purulent, with pleocytosis and elevated protein level, and low to normal glucose level, but a Gram stain usually reveals no organisms, and culture results may be negative.

Staphylococcal endocarditis. *Staphylococcus aureus* causes the majority of cases of acute bacterial endocarditis but may also produce the syndrome of subacute bacterial endocarditis (Chapter 15). Endocarditis may occur in any bacteremic patient, but most cases occur in individuals with previously damaged valves. Typically, an individual with a history of heart murmur has fever, chills, and systemic toxicity; *S. aureus* grows out of almost all blood cultures. Over the next several days, the murmur may change, and multiple embolic phenomena (Janeway lesions, cutaneous infarcts, petechiae, etc.) occur, substantiating the diagnosis of the valvular infection. Parenteral drug users have a high incidence of tricuspid valve endocarditis, often do not have a history of previous valvular lesions, and may not have murmurs on admission to the hospital (Chapter 241). Septic pulmonary emboli are common. The syndrome of spontaneous staphylococcal bacteremia is suspected when a young, otherwise healthy person without any sign of a portal of entry spontaneously has high fever and chills and *S. aureus* in all blood cultures. The majority of these patients actually have endocarditis and a changing murmur, usually aortic insufficiency develops. A recent review by Bayer and colleagues of patients with *S. aureus* bacteremia with and without endocarditis identified four parameters that predicted endocarditis: (1) absence of an obvious primary site of infection, (2) community acquisition of infection, (3) metastatic sequelae, and (4) echocardiographically demonstrable vegetations. The *absence* of an obvious primary focus of infection in a patient bacteremic with *S. aureus* is very strong evidence favoring the presence of endocarditis. The mortality rate in endocarditis produced by *S. aureus* is still very high and is related to age and underlying physical condition. In chronic disease in elderly patients and in left-sided endocarditis, the mortality rate, even with therapy, exceeds 50%; in the young drug user, however, it is less than 10%.

Primary staphylococcal bacteremia

Occasionally, young persons have staphylococcal bacteremia even though evidence of a peripheral site of infection is absent and the site of seeding is not clear. It is presumed that the organism is disseminated from minor skin infections (acne or follicular lesion) or from the nose or pharynx in carriers who have mild viral upper respiratory tract infections. Hospital-associated staphylococcal bacteremias are common in patients suffering long, complicated medical and surgical illnesses in whom a peripheral intravenous site becomes infected. Organisms may seed to several peripheral sites, including the aortic or mitral heart valve, and may cause endocarditis. *S. aureus* is now the most common single organism isolated from hospital-acquired bacteremic episodes. Hospitalized patients are more likely to have impaired host-defense mechanisms, either from underlying disease or from therapy, and bacteremia may have disastrous results. In otherwise healthy persons without underlying organic valvular lesions, endocarditis or metastatic infection of any other organ is unusual; thus the majority of patients who have staphylococcal bacteremia in the hospital require only brief treatment (2 weeks of parenteral antibiotics). The standard approach to such patients should be the following:

1. Over the 10 to 14 day period after the episode of bacteremia-septicemia, the patient should be examined daily for new or changing heart murmurs, evidence of embolic phenomena, and signs of metastatic infection in bones, joints, kidneys (positive urine culture finding), meninges, lungs, or other deep organs.
2. If metastatic abscess formation is discovered, appropriate local drainage and more prolonged course of antibiotic therapy (e.g., 4 weeks) are required. In this subgroup of patients, a two-dimensional echocardiographic study may contribute to the diagnosis of endocarditis.
3. If no evidence of metastatic seeding is found clinically at the end of 14 days, the decision regarding the need for further therapy can be helped by the antibody titer to *S. aureus* teichoic acids (discussed later). If the titer of antibodies has increased fourfold, the infection is very likely to have seeded to some organ, and more prolonged therapy, either intravenous or oral, should be given. At that point, deep foci of infection should be sought with computed tomography and radionuclide scans. If, as occurs in the vast majority of patients, the titer of teichoic acid antibodies does not rise, the infection probably has not seeded, and antibiotics can be discontinued. The negative predictive value of the test result is probably its most valuable aspect.

DIAGNOSTIC TESTS

Staphylococcus aureus readily grows in both aerobic and anaerobic cultural conditions. Microbiology laboratories are usually readily able to identify the organism in culture media. The clinician usually is informed that the gram-positive cocci present in the blood cultures over the next 24 to 48 hours are coagulase-positive staphylococci. *S. aureus* is an uncommon contaminant in blood cultures, and, when present, it is usually in several blood cultures. Even a single blood culture positive for *S. aureus* is usually significant. Presence of *S. aureus* in the urine is difficult to interpret; it usually indicates a significant infection of the upper or lower urinary tract and may have resulted from a previously unrecognized bacteremic episode. Diagnosis of the organism as the cause of a variety of deep infections depends on how aggressively material is obtained for Gram stain and culture. Patients with chronic bone or joint infections should promptly undergo deep aspiration or operative culture of the involved area.

Teichoic acid antibody assay

In bacteremia, diagnostic assistance may be obtained from the assay for antibodies to staphylococcal cell wall teichoic acids. In a high percentage of patients with endocarditis, when studied with serial titers, such antibodies develop, as in most complicated *S. aureus* bacteremias. Complicated bacteremias are those in which the patient does not have endocarditis but shows evidence of seeding to bones, joints, meninges, or other deep organs. The variability of the assay among different laboratories has diminished its usefulness, and most therapeutic decisions are now made on purely clinical grounds.

TREATMENT

The vast majority (about 90%) of both community-acquired and hospital-acquired *S. aureus* strains are resistant to penicillin. Thus patients suspected of having an infection that could be caused by *S. aureus* require a penicillinase-resistant antibiotic. In the patient who is not allergic to penicillin, dicloxacillin, orally, or nafcillin or oxacillin, parenterally, is the drug of choice (Chapter 224). One can treat localized dermal and soft tissue infections orally for 10 to 14 days after drainage has been completed. Systemic infections require parenteral therapy. Four weeks of therapy should suffice in the uncomplicated case of endocarditis. In adult patients with osteomyelitis, 4 to 6 weeks of therapy usually should be combined with wide surgical débridement and drainage. After discharge, oral therapy for 3 to 6 months may prevent late relapses.

A rise in methicillin-resistant, better termed beta-lactam antibiotic resistant, *S. aureus* organisms is becoming a significant problem. All *S. aureus* organisms that show in vitro resistance to methicillin should be considered resistant to all beta-lactam antibiotics (i.e., both penicillins and cephalosporins and probably even the newer beta lactam–like agents such as imipenem). Over the last 5 to 10 years, large university hospitals across the country have been reporting an increasing number of infections with these organisms. Also, in the Detroit metropolitan area, parenteral drug users are now regularly entering the hospital with serious infections caused by this organism. These bacteria are also resistant to the cephalosporins and carbapenems whether or not in vitro reports show resistance. Thus far, all beta-lactam antibiotic resistant organisms have remained sensitive to vancomycin, and many are sensitive to trimethoprim-sulfamethoxazole. The newly available quinolone group of antibiotics may also be effective. Ciprofloxacin is the most recently released quinolone, and it is orally well absorbed, making it an option for outpatient therapy of a variety of deep staphylococcal infections, even those produced by beta-lactam antibiotic resistant strains; however, increasing resistance of *S. aureus* strains to the quinolones is now being reported.

An important issue in the treatment of staphylococcal infections is whether vancomycin is as effective as a semisynthetic penicillin for the treatment of infections caused by beta-lactam antibiotic *sensitive* strains. Vancomycin is certainly the drug of choice for beta-lactam resistant strains, as few alternatives are available. Several studies evaluating efficacy of vancomycin versus that of semisynthetic penicillin (usually nafcillin) suggest that *S. aureus* bacteremia is terminated less rapidly with vancomycin. Thus a consensus is emerging that therapy of beta-lactam sensitive staphylococci should employ nafcillin or oxacillin rather than vancomycin.

The organism may produce a chronic infection when prosthetic devices are present, and the standard approach to the treatment of *S. aureus* infection of any type of implanted prosthetic device is to initiate antibiotic therapy and remove the prosthesis. If the involved prosthesis is critical to life function (e.g., a prosthetic heart valve), suppressive therapy may be tried. In such instances, if the patient is otherwise doing well, prolonged (possibly permanent) suppressive therapy should be administered, first parenterally and then orally. In *S. aureus* infection of prosthetic heart valves, early operative intervention is mandatory in the patient showing signs of progressive valvular malfunction. Approximately half the patients do well even if the operation has been carried out in the presence of active infection. In the patient allergic to penicillin, vancomycin is the drug of choice. Cephalosporins also may be used. Clindamycin is acceptable for bone and soft tissue infections but should not be used in bacteremic patients or in those with endocarditis because of a high relapse rate.

A particularly difficult problem for the internist is recurrent skin and soft tissue infections. Such patients initially may respond to antibiotics plus incision and drainage; however, relapse is common. Most such patients are found to be carrying the infecting organism in the nose and throat. In such instances, cultures of all family members should be made to make sure that the organism is not being passed back and forth. Staphylococcus carriers can then be treated with a combination of intensive cleansing (hand washing, nasal disinfectant soaps, and antibiotic creams) and a 5 day course of mupirocin calcium ointment intranasally BID. Intranasal mypirocin has been shown to eradicate nasal *S. aureus* carriage, subsequently reducing hand and skin colonization and, in at least one recent study, decreasing incidence of *S. aureus* bacteremias in hemodialysis patients. Other approaches to decreasing nasal carriage include the use of combined oral rifampin and dicloxacillin. By suppressing the nasal *S. aureus* carrier state, the episodes of recurrent superficial skin infections usually are terminated.

In the hospital setting, physicians, nurses, and others involved in patient care must wash their hands before and after examination of every patient to reduce the likelihood of both patient-to-patient and physician-or nurse-to-patient transfer of carried organisms. Recalcitrant nasal carriers also respond to brief courses of mupirocin therapy, decreasing nasal carriage and subsequent hand contamination.

PREVENTION

Measures for the prevention of *S. aureus* infections should focus primarily on the hospital environment and should be based on meticulous infection control techniques (Chapter 225). Hospital personnel must be educated as to how the organism is transmitted among individuals, and hand washing must be emphasized for all patient care team members. Meticulous attention must be paid to the use of medical devices that breach mucosal or dermal barriers. The placement of both routine and long-term intravenous lines (e.g., for hyperalimentation) should be done according to specific protocols developed by the hospital's infection control committee. No effective vaccines are available for *S. aureus*. Prophylactic antibiotics have been shown to reduce postoperative infections with *S. aureus,* especially those complicating implantation of prosthetic devices. Such regimens usually use a cephalosporin or vancomycin (to cover *S. epidermidis* as well as *S. aureus*), and the drug should be given 30 to 60 minutes before the procedure to produce good blood and tissue levels during operation. The drug should not be continued for more than 48 hours.

REFERENCES

Bayer AS et al: *Staphylococcus aureus* bacteremia: clinical, serological, and echocardiographic findings in patients with and without endocarditis. Arch Intern Med. 147:457, 1987.

Brumfitt W and Hamilton-Miller J: Methicillin-resistant *Staphylococcus aureus*. N Engl J Med 320:1188, 1989.

Easmon CSF and Adlam C, editors: Staphylococci and staphylococcal infections: clinical and epidemiological aspects (vol 1). The organism in vivo and in vitro (vol 2). London, 1983, Academic Press.

Haley RW: Methicillin-resistant *Staphylococcus aureus:* do we just have to live with it? Ann Intern Med 114:162, 1991.

Korzeniowski O, Sande MA, and the National Collaborative Endocarditis Study Group: Combination antimicrobial therapy for *Staphylococcus aureus* endocarditis in patients addicted to parenteral drugs and in nonaddicts: a prospective study. Ann Intern Med 97:496, 1982.

Marrack P and Kappler J: The Staphylococcal enterotoxins and their relatives. Science 248:705, 1990.

Sande MA: The use of rifampin in the treatment of nontuberculous infections: an overview. J Infect Dis 5(suppl 3):S399, 1983.

Scully BE et al: Mupirocin treatment of nasal staphylococcal colonization. Arch Intern Med 152:353, 1992.

Sheagren JN: Endocarditis complicating drug abuse. In Remington JS and Swartz MN, editors: Current clinical topics in infectious diseases. New York, 1981, McGraw-Hill.

Sheagren JN: *Staphylococcus aureus:* the persistent pathogen. N Engl J Med 310:1368, 1437, 1984.

Sheagren JN: Inflammation induced by *Staphylococcus aureus*. In Gallin JI, Goldstein IM, and Snyderman R, editors: Inflammation: basic principles and clinical correlates. New York, 1988, Raven Press.

Sheagren JN and Schaberg DR: Staphylococcal infections: a current concepts monograph. Kalamazoo MI, 1992, Upjohn.

Smith IM and Vickers AB: Natural history of 338 treated and untreated patients with staphylococcal septicaemia (1936-1955). Lancet 1:1318, 1960.

CHAPTER

258 *Staphylococcus epidermidis* and Other Coagulase-Negative Staphylococcal Infections

Gordon L. Archer

THE ORGANISM

Classification and characteristics

Staphylococcus epidermidis is a gram-positive coccus, 0.5 to 1.5 μm in diameter, of the family Micrococcaceae. The two genera of clinical significance in this family are *Micrococcus* and *Staphylococcus*. Both produce catalase, but micrococci are differentiated from staphylococci by the inability of micrococci to produce acid anaerobically from glucose. The differentiation of *S. aureus* from other staphylococci is accomplished in the clinical laboratory by two tests: *S. aureus* coagulates rabbit plasma, whereas other staphylococci do not; and *S. aureus* produces acid anaerobically from mannitol, whereas other staphylococci do not. Coagulase-negative staphylococci found on human skin have been divided into more than 20 species by DNA-DNA homology studies and biochemical testing. However, the majority of coagulase-negative staphylococci isolated from clinical specimens are *S. epidermidis*.

Epidemiology

Staphylococcus epidermidis is found on the skin and mucous membranes of all warm-blooded mammals and is the most numerous aerobic component of normal skin flora. It rarely is responsible for infection in normal hosts outside the hospital. In the hospital, it is the most common organism cultured from air and wounds during surgery, but it rarely causes disease. Infections have resulted from operative contamination but are usually associated with the insertion of indwelling foreign devices. Hospital-associated *S. epidermidis* infections are caused by organisms usually resistant to multiple antibiotics, including penicillin, semisynthetic penicillinase-resistant penicillins, cephalosporins, and aminoglycosides; infections acquired outside the hospital are due to antibiotic-susceptible organisms. Hospital personnel and patients appear to be reservoirs for these resistant organisms.

The identification of epidemiologically related strains of

S. epidermidis has been facilitated in recent years by using the tools of molecular biology (molecular epidemiology). Restriction endonuclease digestion of plasmid and chromosomal deoxyribonucleic acid (DNA), DNA-DNA hybridization using specific and nonspecific probes, generation of DNA fragments using the polymerase chain reaction, and identification of proteins using specific and nonspecific antibody all generate patterns unique to closely related organisms. These techniques can conceivably be used to associate epidemiologically linked isolates or to separate infecting from contaminating organisms. The latter is a major problem with coagulase-negative staphylococci recovered from clinical material.

Pathophysiology

Staphylococcus epidermidis is relatively avirulent for humans and laboratory animals. The failure of *S. epidermidis* to produce coagulase and lethal toxins, the absence of protein A in the cell wall to inhibit opsonization, and the absence of surface ligands that bind human proteins such as fibronectin and fibrinogen may all contribute to the lesser virulence of this organism as compared with *S. aureus*. This lack of virulence probably contributes to the indolent nature of *S. epidermidis* infections and the capacity of the organism to lie dormant in tissue for a year or more after surgical contamination before causing symptomatic disease. *S. epidermidis* commonly persists only in areas where local host defense mechanisms are impaired. These include endocarditic vegetations and tissues surrounding prosthetic devices, shunts, catheters, and sternal surgical incisions. Antibiotic therapy is often ineffective until foreign material is removed from the area of infection.

The virulence of *S. epidermidis* is related to its ability to adhere to foreign material and to produce abundant quantities of exopolysaccharide or "slime" that impede removal by host defense systems and allow organisms to remain fixed to an inanimate surface. The production of adhesins and exopolysaccharide seems to be unique to the species *S. epidermidis* and may account for its frequent involvement in foreign body infections.

DISEASES PRODUCED IN HUMANS

Because it is part of normal skin flora, *S. epidermidis* frequently contaminates cultures obtained by crossing skin. Therefore it can be implicated as a cause of disease only when the organism is cultured from a site at which there is clinical evidence of infection, when it is the only organism recovered, and when it is cultured on more than one occasion. Ideally, clusters of gram-positive cocci should also be identified in stained smears of infected material.

Bacteremia

Coagulase-negative staphylococci are the most common organisms causing nosocomial bacteremia. The source of the bacteremia is usually chronic indwelling intravenous catheters; the highest incidence is in neonatal intensive care units and hematology-oncology wards. Because coagulase-negative staphylococci are also the most common cause of blood culture contamination, care should be taken in interpreting blood cultures growing these organisms.

Endocarditis

Native valve endocarditis. Coagulase-negative staphylococci cause less than 5% of cases of endocarditis on native cardiac valves. Coagulase-negative species other than *S. epidermidis* account for 50% of this group. In contrast to the increase in the number of cases of coagulase-negative staphylococcal prosthetic valve endocarditis in recent years, the incidence of native valve endocarditis has remained constant in the antibiotic era. Native valve endocarditis caused by coagulase-negative staphylococci manifests itself as classic subacute to chronic bacterial endocarditis with nonspecific symptoms of fever, weight loss, and anorexia for many months (Chapter 15). There is little to distinguish its presentation, clinical findings, and laboratory values from those of viridans streptococcal endocarditis. Endocarditis is virtually always seen on rheumatic or previously abnormal valves.

Prosthetic valve endocarditis. One of the major changes in the sources of endocarditis in the antibiotic era has been the emergence of *S. epidermidis* as one of the most common organisms infecting prosthetic heart valves. In contrast to native valve endocarditis, this species accounts for more than 95% of infecting coagulase-negative staphylococci. *S. epidermidis* and non–group A streptococci are responsible for 60% to 70% of the cases of prosthetic valve endocarditis (PVE). Streptococcal PVE occurs more than 1 year after surgery, can usually be treated with antibiotics alone, and causes little mortality; however, *S. epidermidis* PVE occurs within the first year after valve surgery, is caused by an antibiotic-resistant organism, and has a mortality rate of up to 60%. *S. epidermidis* is probably inoculated into the area of the rigid sewing ring of the prosthesis at the time of surgery; organisms are hospital-associated (and thus antibiotic-resistant) and are in an avascular area protected from antibiotics. The high mortality rate is largely due to hemodynamic factors caused by valve dehiscence, obstruction of the valve orifice by large vegetations that grow over the valve orifice from the valve ring, or conduction disturbances resulting from spread of infection out to the conduction system.

Even though *S. epidermidis* is acquired at the time of surgery, PVE may not appear for months to more than a year. This slow incubation period probably reflects the lack of virulence of the organism and its propensity for causing indolent infections associated with minimum symptoms. One half of the cases of *S. epidermidis* PVE have classic symptoms of endocarditis, whereas the other half have few signs or symptoms and no peripheral embolic phenomena. Patients instead show acute hemodynamic decompensation caused by valve dysfunction or conduction abnormalities.

Diagnosis depends on detecting bacteremia; all patients with prosthetic cardiac valves who have fever, new murmurs, or any new valve dysfunction, regardless of the absence of signs or symptoms of classic endocarditis, should have blood cultures obtained. It is essential to obtain several blood specimens, drawn at different times through separate venipunctures to eliminate contamination. Once positive blood culture results establish the diagnosis of *S. epidermidis* PVE, prognosis depends on documenting the degree of valve dysfunction through echocardiography, serial electrocardiograms, and cineangiography.

Infection of cerebrospinal fluid shunts

Staphylococcus epidermidis causes 60% or more of the infections of ventriculoatrial and ventriculoperitoneal shunts used in the treatment of hydrocephalus. Meningitis and bacteremia are associated with infections of ventriculoatrial shunts, whereas meningitis and peritonitis are seen with ventriculoperitoneal shunt infections. One third of infections begin as wound infections in the early postoperative period, whereas the remaining two thirds are seen from 1 month to more than 1 year after surgery. Fever and evidence of shunt malfunction are the most common manifestations of infection. Organisms occasionally can be cultured repeatedly from shunt tubing when there is little evidence of infection and only minimum cerebrospinal fluid pleocytosis. It is not clear whether this represents colonization or early infection. Organisms probably also gain access to the central nervous system by contamination at the time of surgery. The majority of organisms are resistant to multiple antibiotics and resemble strains isolated from patients with prosthetic valve endocarditis. Mortality rate directly related to infection varies from 6% to 35%, depending on the series being reviewed. Related devices, such as reservoirs used for instillation of chemotherapy and ventriculostomy catheters used to decompress acutely increased intracerebral pressure, also commonly become infected with *S. epidermidis*.

Infection of prosthetic joints

Infections of total hip and knee arthroplasties are uncommon, occurring in only 1% of implanted prostheses (Chapter 315). However, they usually require surgical replacement and often result in loss of ambulation. *S. epidermidis* accounts for approximately 40% of infections and is second only to *S. aureus* in this regard. As with infections of other prosthetic devices, in prosthetic joint infection *S. epidermidis* is implanted into the wound at the time of surgery, may not produce symptoms of fever and pain for years, and is antibiotic resistant. Diagnosis is often difficult, as radiographs do not show changes of osteomyelitis until late in the infection. Bacteremia is uncommon.

Infections of indwelling catheters, vascular shunts, and vascular grafts

Chronic indwelling plastic catheters used for hyperalimentation, chemotherapy, or peritoneal dialysis; vascular shunts used as access for hemodialysis; and vascular grafts can become infected with *S. epidermidis*. Infection of vascular catheters and shunts is manifested as fever with positive blood culture findings (discussed earlier); infections of peritoneal dialysis catheters, as fever and abdominal pain with positive culture results of dialysis fluid; infections of vascular grafts, as fever, local wound purulence, and graft malfunction.

Infections in immunosuppressed patients

Coagulase-negative staphylococci are becoming important causes of bacteremia in immunosuppressed, neutropenic patients undergoing therapy for malignancy. The pathogenesis of bacteremia has been variously attributed to gut colonization with *S. epidermidis* after the use of oral antibiotics for gut sterilization and infection of long-term, indwelling plastic catheters used for administration of chemotherapy.

Sternal osteomyelitis after cardiac surgery

Staphylococcus epidermidis causes approximately 30% to 50% of cases of sternal osteomyelitis and costochondritis that occur in the median sternotomy wound after cardiac surgery (Chapter 237). Together, *S. aureus* and *S. epidermidis* cause 50% to 60% of these infections, which occur in 1% to 2% of patients who undergo cardiac surgery. Outbreaks have taken place, however, in which *S. epidermidis* sternal wound infections occurred in a much higher percentage of patients. Such factors as improper placement of wire suture, hemodynamic instability during bypass, overuse of bone wax, and faulty skin antisepsis have all been thought to be important in the pathogenesis of these infections. Diagnosis is often difficult in the immediate postoperative period because fever and chest pain can be due to many other factors. Organisms are antibiotic resistant, and medical therapy alone is rarely successful. Surgical débridement is essential to cure.

Urinary tract infections

Although urinary tract infections with *S. epidermidis* are very uncommon, one species of coagulase-negative staphylococcus, *S. saprophyticus,* has been found to be the second most common cause (next to *Escherichia coli*) of urinary tract infections in otherwise healthy young women seen as outpatients. Symptoms are indistinguishable from those experienced during urinary tract infections caused by *E. coli* (Chapter 240). *S. saprophyticus* has been differentiated from *S. epidermidis* in the laboratory by its resistance to the antibiotic novobiocin. Infections respond readily to usual urinary tract antimicrobials, and relapse is uncommon. Because they grow slowly, there may be fewer of these organisms in infected urine than the number ($>10^5$ CFU/ml) seen with gram-negative bacteria. *S. epidermidis* occasionally causes infections in urinary tracts of the elderly, in those with indwelling catheters, and in patients undergoing genitourinary surgery.

TREATMENT

Most infections with coagulase-negative staphylococci are hospital-acquired, and therefore these isolates should be considered resistant to the usual antistaphylococcal antibiotics. Many clinical laboratories report *S. epidermidis* isolates to be susceptible to semisynthetic penicillinase-resistant penicillins (particularly nafcillin) and cephalosporins when these isolates are actually resistant. Susceptibility testing using modified methods has revealed that this heteroresistant (methicillin-resistant) phenotype can be detected in more than 80% of *S. epidermidis* from such hospital-acquired infections as intravenous catheter–associated bacteremia, PVE, and infections of cerebrospinal fluid shunts.

Heteroresistant *S. epidermidis* is susceptible to vancomycin, but *S. hemolyticus,* a coagulase-negative staphylococcus occasionally isolated from patients with nosocomial infections, may be resistant. Both rifampin and gentamicin are extremely active in vitro against most isolates. However, the emergence of rifampin-resistant mutants after brief exposure of isolates to the drug, the rapid increase in plasmid-mediated gentamicin resistance among staphylococci in some hospitals, and the nephrotoxicity of gentamicin have somewhat limited the utility of these two antibiotics in the treatment of coagulase-negative staphylococcal infections. Although both methicillin-resistant and methicillin-susceptible coagulase-negative staphylococci appear to be moderately susceptible to quinolones (ciprofloxacin, ofloxacin, and temofloxacin) in vitro, there are few data on the role of these antimicrobial agents in treating documented infections caused by coagulase-negative staphylococci. However, on the basis of data showing rapid emergence of ciprofloxacin-resistant coagulase-negative staphylococci in areas where use of the drug is high and of the poor record of ciprofloxacin in therapy of methicillin-resistant *S. aureus* infections, quinolones should probably not be used to treat coagulase-negative staphylococcal foreign body infections until studies documenting their efficacy are available. Likewise, up to one half of nosocomial coagulase-negative staphylococci are susceptible to sulfamethoxasole-trimethoprim, but the role of this antimicrobial in foreign body infections is unknown. The high rate of resistance of nosocomial isolates to clindamycin (more than 60% are resistant) generally limits the use of this antibiotic in treating infections.

All patients who have infections caused by hospital-acquired *S. epidermidis* or other coagulase-negative staphylococci should be treated with vancomycin, 1 g IV q12h or 500 mg q6h, until appropriate laboratory tests accurately define the susceptibility of the infections isolates. Rifampin 300 mg PO q8h or 600 mg q12h, and/or gentamicin, 1 mg/kg IV or IM q8h, may be added to vancomycin to increase serum bactericidal activity. Rifampin-resistant mutants have been recovered from patients with prosthetic valve endocarditis receiving only vancomycin and rifampin. The addition of gentamicin as a third drug for the first 2 weeks of treatment prevented the emergence of rifampin resistance but led to increased nephrotoxicity. In most cases, it is impossible to eradicate infections of indwelling foreign devices with antibiotics alone without surgical removal of the devices. This is particularly true of prosthetic cardiac valves and prosthetic joints. However, in some cases cure of long-term indwelling intravenous catheter and peritoneal dialysis catheter infections has been achieved without catheter removal. Similarly, occasional cerebrospinal fluid shunt infections have responded to intraventricular vancomycin (10 to 20 mg/day for adults) and/or gentamicin (5 to

Table 258-1. Therapy for coagulase-negative staphylococcal infections

	ANTIMICROBIAL AGENT*		
Site of Infection	**Methicillin-susceptible**	**Methicillin-resistant**	**Duration**
Infected prosthetic cardiac valve, joint, or vascular graft; osteomyelitis	Nafcillin or oxacillin; ± gentamicin for 2 weeks (vancomycin or cefazolin if penicillin allergic)	Vancomycin ± rifampin; ± gentamicin for 2 weeks†	6 Weeks
Native valve endocarditis	Same	Vancomycin; ± gentamicin for 2 weeks	4 Weeks
Catheter infection	Nafcillin or oxacillin	Vancomycin	2 Weeks
Urinary tract infection	Amoxicillin or sulfamethoxasole/ trimethoprim *(S. saprophyticus)*	Vancomycin	3 Days (lower UTI) or 2 weeks (upper UTI)
CSF shunt	Systemic nafcillin or oxacillin and intraventricular methicillin and/or gentamicin	Systemic rifampin and intraventricular vancomycin and/or gentamicin	2 Weeks

*See text for exact dosage. CSF, cerebrospinal fluid; UTI, urinary tract infection.

†It may be possible to use a quinolone or trimethoprim/sulfamethoxasole in place of gentamicin for gentamicin-resistant organisms, but there are scant data in human infections to support this regimen.

8 mg/day for adults) administration and systemic rifampin without shunt removal. The rare methicillin-susceptible organism can be treated with systemic nafcillin or oxacillin (discussed later) and intraventricular methicillin (1 to 2 mg/kg twice a day). The latter beta-lactam is considered by some to be less epileptogenic than other beta lactams for intraventricular administration.

Coagulase-negative staphylococcal infections that routinely respond to conventional antistaphylococcal antibiotics are native valve endocarditis and outpatient *(S. saprophyticus)* urinary tract infections. Isolates from patients with native valve endocarditis who did not acquire their infections in the hospital are virtually always susceptible to semisynthetic penicillinase-resistant penicillins, but most produce penicillinase and are resistant to penicillin G. Nafcillin or oxacillin should be given in dosages of 8 to 12 g per day for 4 weeks. Cephalosporins may be given to penicillin-allergic patients who do not have a history of anaphylactic shock, and vancomycin may be given to those who do (Chapter 224). A compilation of therapeutic recommendations is shown in Table 258-1.

PREVENTION

Antibiotic prophylaxis is given to most patients undergoing surgery for the implantation of foreign devices. These antibiotics are directed primarily against staphylococci. Cephalosporins and semisynthetic penicillinase-resistant penicillins are the antibiotics most commonly administered and are probably effective in preventing infection of foreign devices with susceptible organisms. However, antibiotic prophylaxis has the following deleterious effects: (1) Coagulase-negative staphylococci resistant to the antibiotics used as prophylaxis cause most of the infections of implanted devices. (2) Prophylactic antibiotics select antibiotic-resistant skin flora. These antibiotic-resistant coagulase-negative staphylococci are spread from patients to hospital staff and thus increase the hospital reservoir for these organisms. Minimizing the duration of prophylaxis may ease some of the selective pressure for colonization with resistant organisms and decrease this reservoir.

Although clean-air systems (i.e., laminar air flow) reduce the number of airborne bacteria during surgery, there has been no clear demonstration that these systems are important in reducing the number of infections of implanted foreign devices. Meticulous surgical technique and appropriate barrier precautions during surgery remain the most important factors in the prevention of postsurgical infections.

REFERENCES

Archer GL: Antibiotic resistance in coagulase-negative staphylococci. In Mårdh P-A and Schleifer KH, editors: Coagulase-Negative Staphylococci, Stockholm, 1986, Almquist and Wiksell.

Archer GL and Armstrong BC: Alteration of staphylococcal flora in cardiac surgery patients receiving antibiotic prophylaxis. J Infect Dis. 147:642, 1983.

Caputo GM et al: Native valve endocarditis due to coagulase-negative staphylococci: clinical and microbiologic features. Am J Med 83:619, 1987.

Christensen GD et al: Nosocomial septicemia due to multiple antibiotic-resistant *Staphylococcus epidermidis*. Ann Intern Med. 96:1, 1982.

Jordan PA et al: Urinary tract infection caused by *Staphylococcus saprophyticus*. J Infect Dis 142:510, 1980.

Karchmer AW: Treatment of prosthetic valve endocarditis. In Sande MA, Kaye D, and Root RK, editors: Contemporary issues in infectious diseases. Vol. 2. Endocarditis. New York, 1984, Churchill Livingstone.

Karchmer AW, Archer GL, and Dismukes WE: Staphylococcus epidermidis prosthetic valve endocarditis: microbiologic and clinical observations as guides to therapy. Ann Intern Med 98:447, 1983.

Kotilainen P, Nikoskelainen J, and Huovinen P: Emergence of ciprofloxacin-resistant coagulase-negative staphylococcal skin flora in immunocompromised patients receiving ciprofloxacin. J Infect Dis 161:41, 1990.

Lowy FD and Hammer SM: *Staphylococcus epidermidis* infections. Ann Intern Med 99:834, 1983.

Quie PG and Belani KK: Coagulase-negative staphylococcal adherence and persistence. J Infect Dis 156:543, 1987.

Schaberg DR, Culver DH, and Gaynes RP: Major trends in the microbial etiology of nosocomial infection. Am J Med 91(3B):72, 1991.

Schoenbaum SC, Gardner P, and Shillito J: Infections of cerebrospinal fluid shunts: epidemiology, clinical manifestations, and therapy. J Infect Dis 131:543, 1975.

Wade JC et al: *Staphylococcus epidermidis:* an increasing cause of infections in patients with granulocytopenia. Ann Intern Med 97:503, 1982.

Winston DJ et al: Coagulase-negative staphylococcal bacteremia in patients receiving immunosuppressive therapy. Arch Intern Med 143:32, 1983.

CHAPTER

259 *Streptococcus pyogenes* Infections

Dennis L. Stevens

Streptococcus pyogenes (group A streptococcus [GAS]) perhaps more than any other pathogen has developed an intimate relationship with the human host. In some acute infections and certainly in the well-known postinfectious sequelae, it is the host response elicited by this unique relationship that accounts for the morbidity and mortality. This chapter emphasizes these host-microbe relationships to explain the unique epidemiologic and pathogenic features of *Streptococcus pyogenes*.

EPIDEMIOLOGY

The declining prevalence of both rheumatic fever and serious infection caused by group A streptococci throughout the twentieth century in much of the Western world has been attributed to improved socioeconomic conditions, timely antibiotic treatment of streptococcal pharyngitis, and secondary prophylaxis for rheumatic fever. Some have argued that this decline is due to cyclical virulence changes in the organism. The recent outbreaks of pharyngitis, acute rheumatic fever, and the newly recognized streptococcal toxic shock syndrome support this concept.

The greatest reservoirs of *S. pyogenes* are the skin and mucous membranes of humans, and nearly 5% of all people, regardless of age, carry the organism in their throats.

BACTERIAL CELL STRUCTURE AND EXTRACELLULAR PRODUCTS

Capsule

Some strains of GAS possess luxuriant capsules of hyaluronic acid resulting in large mucoid colonies on blood agar. M protein, especially M type 18, may also impart a mucoid phenotype.

M proteins

Over 80 different serotypes of GAS based on the M protein expressed are currently recognized. The protein is a coiled-coil consisting of four regions of repeating amino acids (A-D), a proline/glycine-rich region that serves to intercalate the protein into the bacterial cell wall, and a hydrophobic region that acts as a membrane anchor (Fig. 259-1). Region A near the N terminus is highly variable, and antibodies to this region confer type-specific protection. Within the more conserved B-D regions lies an area that binds one of the complement regulatory proteins (factor H), stearically inhibiting antibody binding and complement-derived opsonin deposition, and effectively camouflaging the organism against immune surveillance. M protein inhibits the phagocytosis of *S. pyogenes* by polymorphonuclear leukocytes (PMNL), though this property can be overcome by type-specific antisera. Kotb has shown that fragments of M protein can also act as superantigens. The regulation of M-protein synthesis is not firmly established but may be controlled by genetic elements of a vir gene composed of an upstream control sequence coupled to gene segments coding for M protein, immunoglobulin binding proteins, and C5a peptidase. Observations by Lancefield suggest that the quantity of M protein produced decreases with passage on artificial media and conversely increases rapidly with passage through mice. During untreated pharyngitis, the quantity of M protein produced by an infecting strain progressively decreases during convalescence.

Cell wall

The cell wall comprises a peptidoglycan backbone with integral lipoteicoic acid (LTA) components. The function of LTA is not well known; however, both peptidoglycan and LTA have important interactions with the host (Table 259-1).

Cytoplasmic membrane

Little is known about the function and composition of the cytoplasmic membrane, though it is clear that the membrane does serve as a site of cell wall synthesis. This process is orchestrated by five different penicillin binding proteins (PBPs) found within membrane fragments. The regulation of autolysis and cell wall synthesis during chain elongation is a dynamic process whose control is a reflection of the metabolic activity of the cell, which becomes dysregulated in the presence of cell wall active antibiotics. All PBPs are expressed during log phase growth of GAS, and it is at this stage that penicillin's effects are greatest.

Group carbohydrate

Rebecca Lancefield is credited with providing a classification scheme for streptococci based on carbohydrate antigen obtained by acid extraction of cell wall material. Currently, groups of streptococci from A to O have been defined by such typing. The role of carbohydrate antigen in pathogenesis is vague and probably not as important as other factors. Streptococcal typing has been simplified with the development of commercially available rapid latex agglutination schemes. Although the bacitracin susceptibility test has proved very reliable as a presumptive marker for group A, both false negative and false positive results are problematic.

Streptolysin O

Streptolysin O belongs to a family of oxygen-labile, thiol-activated cytolysins (TACs) and causes the broad zone of beta hemolysis surrounding colonies of GAS on blood agar plates. TAC toxins bind to cholesterol moieties on eucaryotic cell membranes, creating toxin-cholesterol aggregates that contribute to cell lysis via a colloid-osmotic mechanism. Exogenous cholesterol inhibits hemolysis both in vitro and in situations where serum cholesterol is high (e.g., nephrotic syndrome); thus elevated ASO titers occur because either cholesterol or anti-ASO antibody "neutralize SLO." Several TAC toxins including SLO have been cloned and sequenced and there exists striking homology among SLO, perfringolysin O, and pneumolysin in a 13 to 15 amino acid sequence upstream from the cysteine residue. The significance of SLO in pathogenesis is discussed later in this chapter.

Deoxyribonucleases A, B, C, and D

Expression of deoxyribonucleases (DNases) in vivo elicits production of anti-DNase antibody during and after infection. Antibodies to DNase A and DNase B have proved useful in the serologic diagnosis of pharyngeal and skin infections. The importance of these enzymes in the pathogenesis of GAS infections has not been proved.

Hyaluronidase

The extracellular enzyme hyaluronidase hydrolyzes the hyaluronic acid in deeper tissues and may facilitate the spread of GAS infections along fascial planes. Its clinical importance is unknown; however, a rise in antihyaluronidase titers follows GAS infections in general, especially those involving the skin.

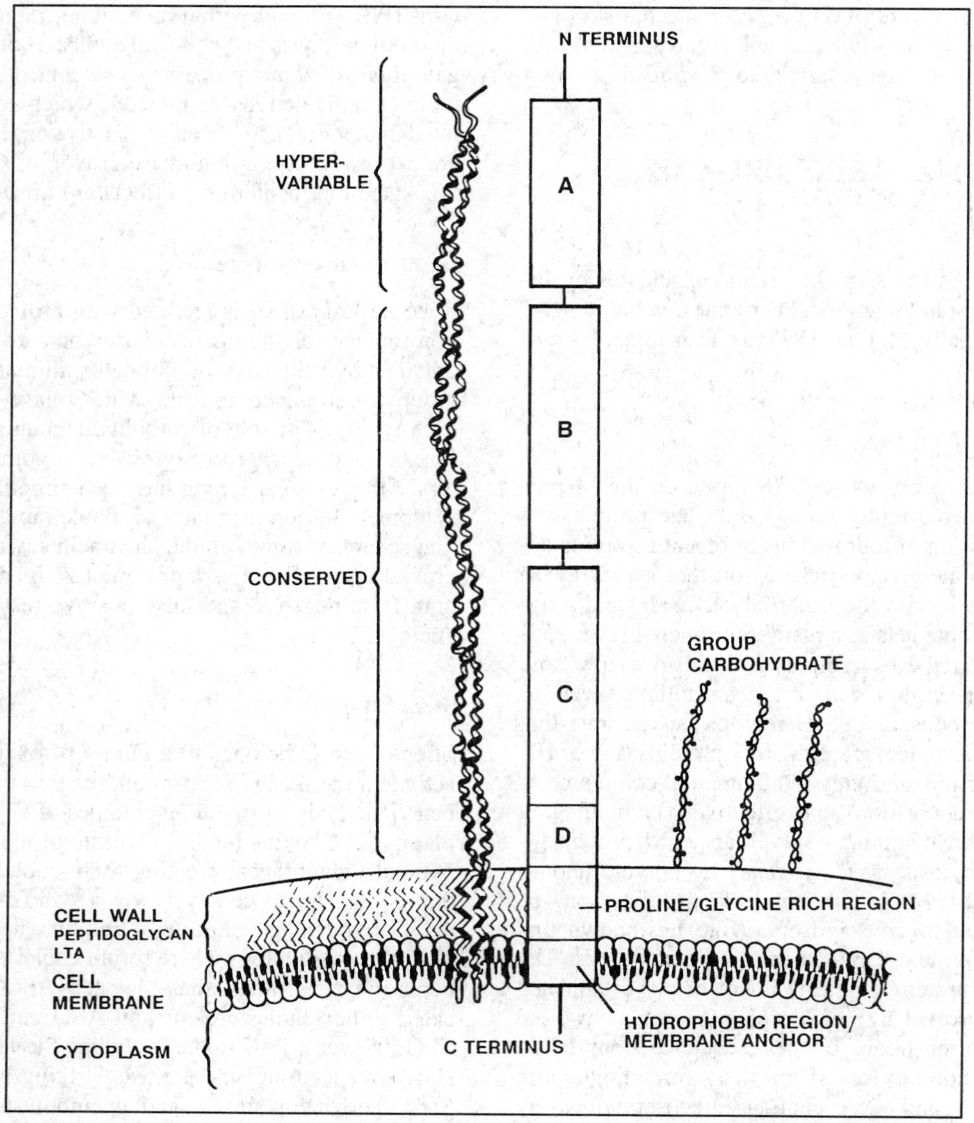

Fig. 259-1. Structural components of M protein. M protein is a coiled-coil consisting of four regions of repeating amino acids (A-D), a proline/glycine-rich region that serves to intercalate the protein into the bacterial cell wall, and a hydrophobic region that acts as a membrane anchor. (From Fischetti VA: Sci Am 264:58, 1991.)

Pyrogenic exotoxins A, B, and C

The pyrogenic exotoxins A, B, and C, also called scarlatina toxin and erythrogenic toxins, function to induce lymphocyte blastogenesis, potentiate endotoxin-induced shock, induce fever, suppress antibody synthesis, and act as superantigens.

The gene for pyrogenic exotoxin A (speA) is transmitted by bacteriophage, and stable toxin production depends on lysogenic conversion in a manner analogous to diphtheria toxin production by *Corynebacterium diphtheria*. Control of SPEA production is not yet understood, though the quantity of SPEA produced can vary dramatically from decade to decade. Historically, SPEA–producing strains have been associated with severe cases of scarlet fever and more recently, with the streptococcal toxic shock syndrome.

Although all strains of GAS are endowed with genes for SPEB (speB), like SPEA, the quantity of toxin produced varies greatly. SPEB is related to the proteinase precursor and the role of each in pathogenesis has only recently been investigated.

Pyrogenic exotoxin C (SPEC), like SPEA, is bacteriophage mediated and its expression is likewise highly variable. Recently Gaworzewska and Colman demonstrated that mild cases of scarlet fever in England have been associated with strains of GAS producing SPEC.

CLINICAL INFECTIONS

Pharyngitis and the asymptomatic carrier

Streptococcus carriage rate may rise from 5% to 15% to above 50% in school age children during epidemics of GAS

Table 259-1. The interplay between *Streptococcus pyogenes* and the human immune system

STREPTOCOCCAL

Host factor	Component	Pathogenic mechanism
Fibronectin	Fimbriae	Adherence to epithelium
Complement (C3)	Streptokinase	Inactivation of C3
Complement (C5a)	C5 peptidase	Destruction of chemotactic factor
Plasminogen	Streptokinase	Production of unregulatable form of plasmin
IgG	M-like protein	Binding or inactivation of IgG
Fibrin	Streptokinase	Dissolution of clot
PMNL	M-protein	Prevention of phagocytosis
	SLO	Degranulation Increased expression of adherence glycoprotein Cytolysis Generation of oxygen radicals
Monocytes	SPEA	Induction of TNF, IL-1*, IL-6
	SPEB	
	SLO	
	Cell wall	Induction of TNF
	LTA	
	Peptidoglycan	
Lymphocytes	SPEA	Action as a superantigen Induction of lymphocyte production of TNF
NK cells	SPEA	Induction of natural killer activity

*SLO and SPEA interact synergistically to induce IL-1-beta. IgG, immunoglobulin G; PMNL, polymorphonuclear leukocyte; SLO, streptolysin O; SPEA, pyrogenic exotoxin A; SPEB, pyrogenic exotoxin B; LTA, lipoteichoic acid; TNF, tumor necrosis factor; IL-1, interleukin-1; NK, natural killer.

pharyngitis. Transmission occurs via aerosolized droplets from the upper airway of one host to another. Patients with GAS pharyngitis (most frequently children 5 to 15 years of age) have sore throat, submandibular adenopathy, fever, and pharyngeal erythema with exudates. Acute pharyngitis is sufficient to induce antibody against M protein, SLO, DNase and hyaluronidase, and, if present, pyrogenic exotoxins. GAS pharyngitis may proceed to scarlet fever, bacteremia, suppurative head and neck infections, streptococcal toxic shock syndrome, carrier state, rheumatic fever, or poststreptococcal glomerulonephritis. Thus the outcomes depend on the interaction between streptococcal virulence factors and the host (Fig. 259-2).

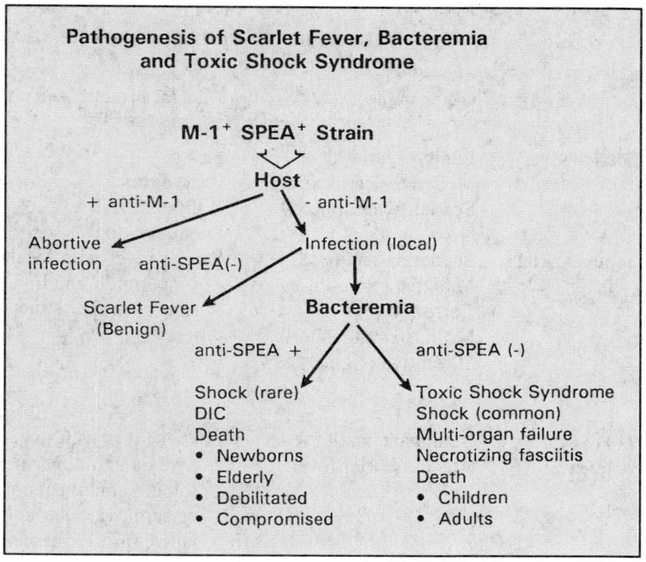

Fig. 259-2. Pathogenesis of scarlet fever, bacteremia, and streptococcal toxic shock syndrome. M-1$^+$ SPEA$^+$, a GAS strain that contains M protein type 1 and pyrogenic exotoxin A (SPEA); +anti-M1, presence of antibody of M protein type 1; −anti-M1, absence of antibody to M protein type 1; anti-SPEA+, antibody to SPEA; DIC, disseminated intravascular coagulation; GAS, group A streptococcus. (From Stevens DL: Invasive Group A Streptococcus Infections, Clin Infect Dis 14:2, 1992.)

During GAS epidemics, particularly where rheumatic fever or a poststreptococcal glomerulonephritis are prevalent, treatment of asymptomatic carriers may be necessary, and at times, programs that use monthly injection of benzathine penicillin have greatly reduced the incidence of GAS pharyngitis as well as rheumatic fever.

Scarlet fever

In the last decade, outbreaks of scarlet fever in the United States have often been associated with M 18 strains of GAS. The cases have been notably mild and the illness has been referred to as "pharyngitis with rash." Historically, this form was known as benign scarlet fever, though scarlet fever has not always been a mild disease: around the turn of the century mortality rates of 25% were common.

Scarlet fever has been divided into the following groups: mild, moderate, toxic, and septic (Table 259-2). Thus benign scarlet fever may be either mild or moderate, and the fatal or malignant form may be either septic or toxic. The toxic cases invariably began with a severe sore throat, marked fever, delirium, skin rash, and painful cervical lymph nodes. In severe toxic cases, fulminating fevers of 107° F, pulse rates of 130 to 160, severe headache, delirium, convulsions, little if any skin rash, and death within 24 hours were the usual findings. These cases occurred before the advent of antibiotics, antipyretics, and anticonvulsants, and deaths were the result of uncontrolled seizures and hyperpyrexia. The term *septic scarlet fever* refers to the form characterized by local invasion of the soft tissues of the neck and complications such as upper-airway ob-

Table 259-2. Comparison of the clinical characteristics of types of scarlet fever

	Other names	Clinical presentation	Complications*	Age (years)	Predisposing factors
Scarlet fever	Benign scarlet fever Moderate-scarlet fever Scarlet fever simplex	Fever Pharyngitis Scarlatina rash Desquamation	Late ARF or AGN Death rare	<10 (90%)	None
Septic scarlet fever	Scarlatina anginosa Malignant sore throat Garrotillo Morbus strangulatoris Ulcerative angina	Scarlet fever with local suppuration and invasion of deeper structures	Otitis Sinusitis Meningitis Airway obstruction Bacteremia Cavernous vein thrombosis	<10 (90%)	Before antibiotic era
Toxic scarlet fever	Malignant scarlet fever Atactic scarlet fever	Scarlet fever with hyperpyrexia and either neurologic complications or cardiovascular collapse; rash evanescent or absent	Convulsions Coma Sudden death	<10 (90%)	Before antibiotics, anticonvulsants, intravenous fluids

*ARF, acute rheumatic fever; AGN, acute glomerulonephritis.

struction, otitis media with perforation, profuse mucopurulent drainage from the nose, bronchopneumonia, and death. Note that necrotizing fasciitis and myositis were not observed in association with scarlet fever; the only exception was locally invasive infection of the soft tissues of the neck as a complication of pharyngitis.

Soft-tissue infection (also see Chapter 235)

Erysipelas. Erysipelas is caused exclusively by *S. pyogenes* and is characterized by an abrupt onset of fiery red swelling of the face or extremities. Distinctive features are well-defined margins, particularly along the nasolabial fold; scarlet or salmon red color, rapid progression; and intense pain. Flaccid bullae may develop during the 2nd to 3rd day of illness yet extension to deeper soft tissues is rare. Surgical débridement is not necessary and treatment with penicillin is very effective. Swelling may progress despite treatment, though fever, pain, and intense redness diminish. Desquamation of the involved skin occurs 5 to 10 days into the illness. Infants and elderly adults are most commonly afflicted and erysipelas was more severe before the turn of the century.

Streptococcal pyoderma (impetigo contagiosa). The thick, crusted skin lesions of streptococcal pyoderma frequently have a golden brown color resembling that of dried serum. Children between 2 and 5 years of age are most commonly infected. Epidemics occur throughout the year in tropical areas or during the summer months in more temperate climates and are usually associated with poor hygiene. Initially colonization of the unbroken skin occurs either exogenously from infected persons or endogenously by oropharyngeal organisms. Development of impetiginous lesions requires 10 to 14 days and likely is initiated by minor abrasions, insect bites, and so on, all of which serve as a means of intradermal inoculation. Patients should receive penicillin, though unlike treatment of rheumatic fever, penicillin may not prevent poststreptococcal glomerulonephritis.

Cellulitis. GAS may invade the epidermis and subcutaneous tissues, resulting in local swelling, erythema, and pain. The skin becomes indurated and, unlike erysipelas, is a pinkish color. Patients with lymphedema secondary to lymphoma, filariasis, or surgical node dissection (mastectomy, carcinoma of the prostate, etc.) are predisposed to development of GAS cellulitis, as are those with chronic venous stasis. Saphenous donor site cellulitis may be due to group A, C, or G streptococci. In such patients there may not be a site of inoculation. Cellulitis associated with a primary focus (e.g., an abscess or boil) is more likely caused by *Staphylococcus aureus*. Aspiration of the leading edge or punch biopsy yields a causative organism in 15% and 40% of cases, respectively. Patients respond quickly to penicillin, though in some cases where staphylococcus is of concern, nafcillin or oxacillin may be a better choice. If bluish or violet discoloration develop or if bullae become apparent, a deeper infection such as necrotizing fasciitis or myositis should be considered (see Necrotizing Fasciitis). In such cases, systemic toxicity is usually present. A serum (CPK) level should be obtained and if elevated, prompt surgical inspection and débridement should be performed.

Lymphangitis. Cutaneous infection with bright red streaks ascending proximally is invariably due to GAS. Prompt antibiotic treatment is mandatory because bacteremia and systemic toxicity develop rapidly.

Necrotizing fasciitis. Necrotizing fasciitis, originally called streptococcal gangrene, is a deep-seated infection of the subcutaneous tissue that results in progressive destruction of fascia and fat but may spare the skin itself. *Necro-*

tizing fasciitis is now the preferred term for the entity because *Clostridium perfringens, Clostridium septicum,* and *Staphylococcus aureus* can produce a similar pathologic process (Chapter 262). Infection may begin at the site of trivial or inapparent trauma. Within the first 24 hours, swelling, heat, erythema, and tenderness develop and rapidly spread proximally and distally from the original focus. During the next 24 to 48 hours, the erythema darkens, changing from red to purple and then to blue, and blisters and bullae that contain clear yellow fluid form. On the fourth or fifth day, the purple areas become frankly gangrenous. From the seventh to the tenth day, the line of demarcation becomes sharply defined, and the dead skin begins to reveal extensive necrosis of the subcutaneous tissue. Patients become increasingly prostrated and emaciated and may become unresponsive, mentally cloudy, or even delirious. Aggressive fasciotomy and débridement and Dakan's solution irrigation achieved mortality rates as low as 20% even before antibiotics were available. The increased severity of necrotizing fasciitis that has occurred among recent cases of streptococcal toxic shock syndrome (strep TSS) relative to shock, multiorgan failure, and mortality could be due to the emergence of increased virulence of GAS itself.

Myositis. Historically, streptococcal myositis has been an extremely uncommon GAS infection, and only 21 cases were documented from 1900 to 1985. Recently, an increased prevalence of GAS myositis has been reported in the United States, Norway, and Sweden. Translocation of GAS from the pharynx to the muscle site must occur hematogenously because penetrating trauma is usually not sustained. Further, most patients have not reported symptomatic pharyngitis or tonsillitis. Severe pain may be the only presenting symptom, swelling and erythema may be the only signs of infection, and muscle compartment syndromes may develop rapidly. In most cases a single muscle group is involved; however, because patients frequently have bacteremia, there may be several sites of myositis or abscess. Distinguishing streptococcal myositis from spontaneous gas gangrene caused by *C. perfringens* or *C. septicum* may be difficult, although the presence of crepitus or gas in the tissue would favor a diagnosis of clostridial infection. Myositis is easily distinguished from necrotizing fasciitis anatomically by means of surgical exploration or incisional biopsy, though clinical features of both conditions overlap. In published reports the case-fatality rate of necrotizing fasciitis is between 20% and 50%, whereas that of GAS myositis is between 80% and 100%. Aggressive surgical débridement is of extreme importance because of the poor efficacy of penicillin described in human cases as well as in experimental streptococcal models of myositis (see Antibiotic Efficacy).

STREPTOCOCCAL TOXIC SHOCK SYNDROME (Strep TSS)

In the late 1980s, reports of invasive GAS infections associated with bacteremia, deep soft-tissue infection, shock, and multiorgan failure began to appear in North America and Europe. Previously healthy individuals between the ages of 20 and 50 years have been most commonly afflicted, and overall 30% of patients die in spite of aggressive modern treatment.

Acquisition of GAS and predisposing factors

The portal of entry of streptococci could not be ascertained in 45% of cases, and preceding symptomatic pharyngitis was rare. Most infections occurred sporadically, though minor epidemics have been reported. Most commonly, the streptococcal infection occurred at a site of minor local trauma that frequently did not result in a break in the skin. Surgical procedures and viral infections such as varicella and influenza provided portals of entry in other cases.

A virus-like prodrome suggestive of influenza preceded the onset of streptococcal TSS by several days in adults. The use of nonsteroidal anti-inflammatory agents to treat pain may mask the presenting symptoms or predispose the patient to more severe complications such as shock.

Symptoms of streptococcal TSS

Pain is a common initial symptom of streptococcal TSS, is abrupt in onset and severe, and may not be associated with tenderness or physical findings. The pain most commonly involves an extremity, but may also mimic peritonitis, pelvic inflammatory disease, acute myocardial infarction, or pericarditis.

Physical findings of streptococcal TSS

Fever is the most common presenting sign, although on admission to the hospital, 10% of patients in one report had profound hypothermia secondary to shock. Confusion may be present in over half of the patients, and in some, it progresses to coma or combativeness. In our report, on admission 80% of patients had tachycardia and 55% had systolic blood pressure of less than 110 mm Hg. Although 45% of patients had normal blood pressure (systolic pressure, >110 mm Hg) on admission, in all of these patients hypotension developed within the subsequent 4 hours. Soft-tissue infection evolved to necrotizing fasciitis or myositis in 70% of cases, and in these cases surgical débridement, fasciotomy, or amputation was required. An ominous sign was the progression of soft-tissue swelling to formation of vesicles and then bullae, which took on a violaceous or bluish coloration. Among patients with no soft-tissue infection on admission, a variety of clinical presentations were observed; these included endophthalmitis, myositis, perihepatitis, peritonitis, myocarditis, and overwhelming sepsis. Patients who experience shock and multiorgan failure without clinical evidence of local infection have a worse prognosis because definitive diagnosis and surgical débridement may be delayed.

Laboratory test results for patients with streptococcal TSS

Evidence of renal involvement was apparent at the time of admission by the presence of hemoglobinuria and elevated serum creatinine level. The serum albumin level was moderately low (3.3 g/dl) on admission and dropped further (2.3 g/dl) by 48 hours. Hypocalcemia, including ionized hypocalcemia, was detectable early in the hospital course. The serum creatine kinase level is a useful test to detect deeper soft-tissue infections, such as necrotizing fasciitis or myositis.

The initial laboratory studies demonstrated only mild leukocytosis, but a dramatic left shift (43% of white blood cells were band forms, metamyelocytes, and myelocytes) (see Table 259-3). The mean platelet count was normal on admission but dropped to approximately 120,000 cells/mm^3 within 48 hours, frequently in the absence of criteria for disseminated intravascular coagulopathy.

Bacteriologic cultures

GAS was isolated from blood in 60% of cases, and from deep tissue specimens in 95%.

Clinical course

Shock was apparent early in the course and management was complicated by profound capillary leak. Adult respiratory distress syndrome (ARDS) occurred frequently (55%) and complicated fluid resuscitation. Renal dysfunction preceded hypotension in many patients and progressed or persisted 48 to 72 hours in spite of treatment. In all patients who survived, serum creatinine levels returned to normal within 4 to 6 weeks. Overall 30% of patients died in spite of aggressive treatment, including administration of intravenous fluids, colloid, pressors, and mechanical ventilation; and surgical intervention including fasciotomy and débridement, exploratory laparotomy, intraocular aspiration, amputation, and hysterectomy.

Characteristics of clinical isolates of GAS

M types 1, 3, 12, and 28 of GAS have been the most common isolates from patients with shock and multiorgan failure in studies made worldwide. Pyrogenic exotoxin A and/or B has been found in isolates from the majority of patients with severe infection. Infections in Norway, Sweden, and Great Britain have been primarily due to M type 1 strains of GAS that produce pyrogenic exotoxin B.

POSTINFECTIOUS SEQUELAE

Rheumatic fever

The prevalence of acute rheumatic fever (ARF) in the Western world decreased dramatically after World War II (0.5 to 1.88 cases/100,000 school age children/yr). In contrast, in India and Sri Lanka the prevalence of ARF has remained 140/100,000 for children between 5 and 19 years of age. Socioeconomic factors seem to be important because the highest rates in all countries has been among the impoverished in large cities. Although improved living conditions and the development of penicillin have had important roles in reducing the prevalence of ARF in the United States, the decreases had actually begun before antibiotics were available. In addition, a resurgence of ARF has occurred among U.S. military recruits and predominantly among white middle-class civilians. A particularly frightening aspect of these recent civilian cases was the low incidence of symptomatic pharyngitis (24% to 78%). Thus our modern primary prevention strategy (diagnosis of acute GAS pharyngitis with penicillin treatment within 10 days) would not have prevented ARF in these cases.

Variations in the expression of virulence factors of "rheumatogenic strains" of *S. pyogenes* may best explain these fluctuations in ARF. M types associated with rheumatogenic strains (i.e., M-1, 3, 5, 6, 14, 18, 19, and 24) have a common antigenic domain, which is immunologically cross-reactive with human heart tissue. Understanding this molecular mimicry holds great promise in the elucidation of the immune mechanisms resulting in clinical ARF. One other marker for rheumatogenicity is the mucoid appearance of fresh pharyngeal isolates from patients with ARF.

Although certain M types are strongly associated with ARF, such strains may cause other GAS infections as well. For example, M types 1 and 3 have also been associated with poststreptococcal glomerulonephritis and the streptococcal toxic shock syndrome. Further, epidemics of pharyngitis caused by M 1 are not invariably associated with epidemics of rheumatic fever. That host factors determine the clinical outcome of GAS is suggested by the observation that individuals with certain human leukocyte antigen (HLA) class II antigens are predisposed to development of ARF. Further, Stollerman suggests that a gradual acquisition of susceptibility to ARF by schoolchildren occurs after repeated infections. This is supported by the observations of Ayoub et al. that ARF is uncommon in children less than 2 years old and that antibody response to streptococcal antigens is exaggerated in children with ARF compared to those with GAS pharyngitis alone. In addition, Zabriski has shown that patients with ARF demonstrate increased expression of the B cell alloantigen D8/17 in comparison to unaffected family members, including identical twins. That some strains of GAS can cause ARF in any individual is suggested by the observation that the attack rate of ARF can vary from 388 cases/100,000 soldiers in World War II to 1/100,000 today. Such fluctuations among relatively homogenous populations separated in time suggest changes in relative rheumatogenicity of GAS and not unique host factors.

The clinical manifestations of acute rheumatic fever are multiple and because each is not specific for ARF, several criteria must be met to establish a definitive diagnosis. Simply put, two major manifestations or one major and two minor manifestations plus, in either case, evidence of an antecedent GAS infection are required for definitive diagnosis. The major manifestations and the frequency with which they occur during first attacks of ARF are as follows: arthritis (75%), carditis (40% to 50%), chorea (15%), and subcutaneous nodules (<10%). The minor manifestations are fever, arthralgia, heart block, presence of acute-phase reactants in the blood (C-reactive protein, leukocytosis, and elevated erythrocyte sedimentation rate), and prior history of ARF or rheumatic heart disease. Carditis, when present, occurs during the first 3 weeks of illness and may involve pericardium, myocardium, and endocardium. Patients with pericarditis may have chest pain or pericardial effusion, whereas those with myocarditis may have intractable heart failure. Manifestations of acute endocarditis involve the development of new murmurs of mitral regurgitation, or aortic regurgitation, the latter being sometimes associated with a low-pitched apical middiastolic flow murmur (Carey Coombs murmur). Murmurs of mitral stenosis and aortic stenosis are not detected acutely during first attacks of ARF but are chronic manifestations of rheumatic heart disease. Migratory arthritis involves several joints, most frequently the knees, ankles, elbows, and wrists, in more than 50% of patients. Each involved joint has evidence of inflammation that characteristically resolves within 2 to 3 weeks with no progression to chronic arthritis or articular damage. Subcutaneous nodules occur several weeks into the course of ARF and are found over bony surfaces or tendons. They last only 1 to 2 weeks and have in some cases been associated with severe carditis. Erythema marginatum is an evanescent, nonpainful erythematous eruption occurring on the trunk or proximal extremities. Individual lesions can develop and disappear within minutes, but the process may wax and wane over several weeks or months. Sydenham's chorea often occurs later in the course than other manifestations of ARF and is characterized by rapid nonpurposeful choreiform movements of the face, hands, and feet. Attacks usually disappear during sleep but may persist for 2 to 4 months.

Poststreptococcal glomerulonephritis

Acute glomerulonephritis (AGN) can follow either pharyngeal or skin infection and is associated with GAS strains possessing M types 12 and 49, respectively. During epidemics of skin or pharyngeal infection produced by a nephritogenic strain, attack rates of 10% to 15% have been documented with latent periods of 10 days after pharyngitis and 3 weeks after pyoderma. Nonspecific symptoms include lethargy, malaise, headache, anorexia, and dull back pain. The classic signs of AGN are all related to fluid overload and are manifested initially by edema, both dependent and periorbital. Hypertension develops in most patients and is usually mild. Severe cases may be characterized by ascites, pleural effusion, encephalopathy, and pulmonary edema though evidence of heart failure per se is lacking. Evidence of glomerular damage by renal biopsy has been documented in nearly 50% of contacts of siblings with AGN, suggesting that as in ARF, subclinical disease is not uncommon after infection with certain strains of GAS. Unlike rheumatic fever, but similar to scarlet fever, glomerulonephritis occurs most commonly in children between 2 and 6 years of age. Like ARF and scarlet fever, AGN may affect several members of the same family. Recurrences or secondary attacks occur only rarely and there is little to suggest that AGN progresses to chronic renal failure.

The differential diagnosis of poststreptococcal AGN must include Henoch-Schönlein disease, polyarteritis nodosa, idiopathic nephrotic syndrome, leptospirosis, hemolytic uremic syndrome (*Escherichia coli* 0157:H7), and malignant hypertension. The diagnosis is simpler if there is a recent history of symptomatic GAS pharyngitis, impetigo, or scarlet fever. Elevated or rising antibody titers to streptococcal antigens such as ASO, anti-DNase A or B, and/or antihyaluronidase are helpful, though ASO concentration may be low in patients with pyoderma. A careful urinalysis to document proteinuria and hematuria should be performed, but it is mandatory to demonstrate red blood cell casts because the latter is the hallmark of glomerular injury. The blood urea nitrogen and creatinine values are elevated and if nephrotic syndrome is present the serum cholesterol level is elevated and serum albumin concentration is low. Twenty four hour excretion of protein is usually less than 3 g and total hemolytic complement and C3 levels are markedly reduced.

Pathogenesis

Streptococcus pyogenes has great adaptive capacity for survival in the human host. Table 259-1 depicts some streptococcal components that interact with human host factors to facilitate invasion and contribute to pathogenesis.

Adherence of cocci to the mucosal epithelium occurs via the interaction of GAS fimbriae and host fibronectin. How GAS penetrate cells or cell junctions to reach the deeper tissue is not understood. Once within the tissues, the organisms evade the host's inflammatory defenses by destroying or inactivating complement-derived chemoattractants and opsonins, and by binding or inactivation of immunoglobulin. Expression of M protein, in the absence of type-specific antibody, protects the GAS from phagocytosis by polymorphonuclear leukocytes (PMNL) and monocytes, and secretion of SLO in high concentration destroys approaching phagocytes. Distal to the focus of infection, lower concentrations of SLO stimulate PMNL adhesion to endothelial cells, effectively preventing continued granulocyte migration. A unique feature of the pyrogenic exotoxins and some M-protein fragments is their ability to interact with certain V_{beta} regions of the T cell receptor in the absence of classical antigen processing by antigen presenting cells. In the nonimmune host, SLO, SPEA, and other streptococcal components stimulate host cells to produce tumor necrosis factor (TNF) and interleukin-1 (IL-1), cytokines that mediate hypotension and stimulate leukostasis, resulting in shock, microvascular injury, multiorgan failure, and, if excessive, death.

TREATMENT

The emergence of erythromycin resistance

The first erythromycin-resistant strain of *Streptococcus pyogenes* (GAS) was isolated in Great Britain in 1959, and by 1975, resistant strains had also been isolated in the United States, Canada, and Japan. Although the prevalence of erythromycin resistance among GAS has remained low (3.6% to 4.0%) in most Western countries, in Japan resistance increased from 8.5% to 72% between 1971 and 1974. Similarly, erythromycin resistance had been a rare finding in Sweden; however, in 1984 an epidemic of pharyngitis (294 cases) caused by erythromycin-resistant GAS was reported. Erythromycin resistance has also been documented in Finland, Australia, and Spain.

Sulfonamide resistance

Sulfonamide resistance currently is reported in less than 1% of GAS isolates.

Therapeutic failure of penicillin

The recommended antibiotic therapies for GAS diseases are shown in Table 259-3. The major problem in the treatment of GAS infections with penicillin is a lack of in vivo efficacy in spite of in vitro susceptibility to penicillin. Penicillin failure in pharyngitis, tonsillitis, or mixed infections has been attributed to inactivation of penicillin in situ by beta lactamases produced by cocolonizing organisms such as *Bacteroides fragilis* or *Staphylococcus aureus*. Further, active selection of these beta-lactamase-producing organisms may follow several courses of penicillin and may lead to treatment failures. For example, the failure rate of penicillin treatment of GAS pharyngitis may approach 25% and, with a second treatment with penicillin, increase to 40% to 80%. Smith and Kaplan described cures of 90% of such failures if the second treatment consisted of amoxacillin plus clavulanate compared to only 29% cure with a second regimen of penicillin. In addition, antibiotics that are unaffected by beta-lactamase activity (e.g., amoxicillin clavulanate or clindamycin) have a greater efficacy than penicillin in patients with recurrent GAS tonsillitis.

Genotypic penicillin tolerance could also explain penicillin's lack of efficacy in tonsillitis or pharyngitis. Tolerant strains demonstrate a slower rate of growth, a slower rate of bacterial killing by penicillin, and an absence of beta-lactam-induced cell lysis. Penicillin-tolerant GAS strains have been isolated from 11/18 cases of penicillin treatment failures of acute tonsillitis compared to 0/15 from successfully treated patients. Penicillin tolerant strains have also caused epidemics of pharyngitis.

Recently, reports that describe penicillin's reduced efficacy in the treatment of severe streptococcal infections in humans (i.e., streptococcal bacteremia, pneumonia, myositis, and streptococcal toxic shock syndrome) have surfaced. This phenomenon has not been comprehensively studied and no comparative clinical studies have been performed. However, studies made in animals demonstrated that penicillin was effective if given early, or if small numbers of GAS were used to initiate infection. With larger inocula, or if treatment was delayed, penicillin was no longer effective. Thus penicillin's efficacy was lost as the infection became more severe. In contrast, clindamycin had much greater efficacy even if treatment was delayed up to 16 hours. Clindamycin's greater efficacy could be due to its ability to suppress M-protein synthesis, its longer post-antibiotic effect, its indifference to in vivo inoculum effect, or its effects on the host's immune system.

Table 259-3. Antibiotic therapy of group A streptococcal disease

	Route	Dosage
Pharyngitis and impetigo		
Benzathine penicillin	im	1.2 million units (> 27 kg)
Penicillin G (or V)	po	200,000 units qid for 10 days
Erythromycin	po	40 mg/kg/day (up to 1 g/day)
Rheumatic fever prophylaxis		
Benzathine penicillin	im	1.2 million units every 28 days
Penicillin G	po	200,000 units bid
Sulfadiazine	po	1 g/day (> 27 kg)
		500 mg/day (< 27 kg)
Erythromycin*	po	250 mg bid

Modified from Kaplan EL et al: Circulation 55:S1, 1977.
*For use only in patients with sensitivity to both penicillin and sulfonamides.

REFERENCES

Bisno AL: Group A streptococcal infections and acute rheumatic fever. N Engl J Med 325(11):783-793, 1991.

Cleary R et al: A virulence regulon in *Streptococcus pyogenes,* Third International ASM conference on Streptococcal Genetics, American Society for Microbiology (ASM). Minneapolis, MN, Abstract 19, 1990.

Fischetti VA: Streptococcal M protein. Sci Amer 264(6):58-65, 1991.

Harris RW, Sims PJ, Tweten RK: Evidence that *Clostridium perfringens* theta-toxin induces colloid-osmotic lysis of erythrocytes. Infect Immun 59(7):2499, 1991.

Johnson LP, Tomai MA, Schlievert PM: Bacteriophage involvement in group A streptococcal pyrogenic exotoxin A production. J Bacteriol 166:623, 1986.

Kehoe MA et al: Nucleotide sequence of the streptolysin O (SLO) gene: structural homologies between SLO and other membrane-damaging, thiol-activated toxins. Infect Immun 55:3228, 1987.

Kohler W, Gerlach D, Knoll HL: Streptococcal outbreaks and erythrogenic toxin type A. Zentralbl Bakteriol Hyg 266:104, 1987.

Lancefield RC: Current knowledge of type specific M antigens of group A streptococci. J Immunol 89:307, 1962.

Nida SK, Ferretti JJ: Phage influence on the synthesis of extracellular toxins in group A streptococci. Infect Immun 36(2):745, 1982.

Smith TD et al: Efficacy of beta-lactamase-resistant penicillin and influence of penicillin tolerance in eradicating streptococci from pharynx after failure of penicillin therapy for group A streptococcal pharyngitis. J Pediatr 6:601, 1987.

Stevens DL: Invasive group A streptococcus infections. Clin Infect Dis 14:2, 1992.

Stevens DL et al: Reappearance of scarlet fever toxin A among streptococci in the Rocky Mountain West: severe group A streptococcal infections associated with a toxic shock-like syndrome. N Engl J Med 321(1):1, 1989.

Stollerman GH: Rheumatic fever and streptococcal infection. New York, 1975, Grune & Stratton.

Tweten RK: Nucleotide sequence of the gene for perfringolysin O (theta-toxin) from *Clostridium perfringens:* significant homology with the genes for streptolysin O and pneumolysin. Infect Immun 56:3235, 1988.

Wannamaker LW et al: Prophylaxis of acute rheumatic fever by treatment of the preceding streptococcal infection with various amounts of depot penicillin, Am J Med 10:673, 1951.

Watson DW and Kim YB: Erythrogenic toxins. In Montie TC, Kadis S, Ajl SJ, editors: Microbial toxins, vol 3. Orlando, FL, 1970, Academic Press.

CHAPTER

260 Enterococcal and Other Non–Group A Streptococcal Infections

Larry J. Strausbaugh

ENTEROCOCCI

Characteristics and classification

Enterococci are gram-positive, facultatively anaerobic bacteria that are ovoid in shape and appear on smears as short chains, as pairs, or as single cells. Their colonies are 1 to 2 mm in size and appear somewhat "buttery" in consistency. On blood agar plates they exhibit no hemolysis most frequently, alpha hemolysis occasionally, and beta hemolysis rarely. Enterococci usually possess the Lancefield group D antigen, an intracellular glycerol teichoic acid associated with the cytoplasmic membrane. Other distinguishing features include the ability to hydrolyze esculin, to grow in media containing 40% bile, to grow in 6.5% sodium chloride, to hydrolyze L-pyrrolidonyl-beta-naphthylamide (PYR), and to grow at both 10° and 45° Celsius. In addition, most enterococci do not produce gas from glucose and most (discussed later) show a zone of inhibition around a 30 μg vancomycin disk.

For many years enterococci were classified in the genus *Streptococcus,* but on the basis of nucleic acid hybridization studies they have recently been assigned to a new genus designated *Enterococcus*. From a medical viewpoint the most important species are *E. faecalis* and *E. faecium*. The 10 other proposed enterococcal species are rarely isolated from human specimens.

Epidemiology

Enterococci reside in the gastrointestinal tract of most normal adults. They are present in small numbers in the upper gastrointestinal tract but may achieve concentrations of 10^7 colony forming units per gram in feces. As a rule, *E. faecalis* is recovered more frequently and in higher numbers than *E. faecium,* but age, diet, and geography affect this finding. Enterococci, especially *E. faecalis,* have also been isolated from the oropharynx, the hepatobiliary tract, the vagina, the anterior urethra, and the skin of 5% to 25% of healthy individuals. Soft tissue wounds and cutaneous ulcers in hospitalized patients may yield enterococci in up to 60% of cases.

Enterococci are common causes of human disease (Table 260-1). Their role in community-acquired infections such as endocarditis has long been recognized. In the last decade they have also been recognized as nosocomial pathogens. Data from the Centers for Disease Control's National Nosocomial Infection Study indicate that enterococci are the third most frequently isolated pathogen. Moreover, data from several medical centers have indicated that the incidence of nosocomial enterococcal urinary tract infections and bacteremias has increased steadily during the last 15 years. *E. faecalis* is responsible for 80% to 85% of all enterococcal infections and *E. faecium* for the majority of the remainder.

Until recently most enterococcal infections were thought to arise from the patient's own endogenous flora, and this is probably true for patients with community-acquired infections. Recent studies, however, suggest that nosocomial infections may arise more frequently from exogenous strains acquired in hospital as a result of person-to-person spread. Transient carriage of enterococci on the hands of medical personnel has been an important mode of transmission in several hospital outbreaks and one interhospital outbreak, suggesting that enterococci behave as resistant staphylococci and gram-negative bacilli do in this regard.

Pathogenesis

The pathogenicity of enterococci has traditionally been ascribed to their place of residence. When disease or injury breaches the integrity of the bowel or the lower urogenital tract, enterococci find their opportunity to invade. Even so, they have often been viewed as reluctant pathogens, and debates about their pathogenic potential in the abdomen and pelvis persist. These debates notwithstanding, the rising incidence of enterococcal bloodstream infections and their attendant 30% to 65% case fatality rates have bolstered the enterococcus's reputation as a pathogen.

Antimicrobial resistance appears to account for much of

Table 260-1. Principal human diseases associated with enterococci

Type of infection	Frequency of enterococcal isolation (%)
Community-acquired	
Endocarditis	5-15
Intra-abdominal and pelvic*	25
Urinary tract	<5
Hospital-acquired	
Urinary tract	15
Surgical wound*	12
Other cutaneous*	9
Bacteremia*	7

*Enterococci often isolated with other bacterial pathogens.

Intrinsic antimicrobial resistance of enterococci

Resistance to

Antistaphylococcal penicillins
Cephalosporins
Clindamycin
Aminoglycosides
Polymyxin
Aztreonam
Trimethoprim-sulfamethoxazole*

Higher MICs of penicillin G, ampicillin, mezlocillin, and piperacillin than those of other streptococci.

Tolerance to bactericidal effect of virtually all antimicrobial agents.

Low-level production of aminoglycoside 6′-acetyltransferase by strains of *E. faecium* renders them more resistant to tobramycin, netilmicin, and sisomicin.

*May appear active against enterococci in vitro but clinical treatment failures and lack of efficacy in animal models have been reported. MIC, minimum inhibitory concentration.

the enterococcus's virulence. This property provides a selective advantage in the hospital environment and may explain the enterococcus's expanding role as a nosocomial pathogen. Its resistance is of two types: intrinsic and acquired. Intrinsic resistance, a species characteristic present in all or most enterococci and presumably derived from chromosomal genes, has a number of important therapeutic consequences, (refer to the box above). It limits therapeutic options; it necessitates the use of high dosages of penicillin G or other penicillin derivatives for the treatment of serious infections; it necessitates the use of synergistic combinations (e.g., ampicillin and gentamicin) for the treatment of endocarditis when bactericidal activity is required (Chapter 15); and it limits the number of aminoglycoside combinations available for *E. faecium* infections: ampicillin or vancomycin combinations with tobramycin, netilmicin, and sisomicin do not demonstrate a synergistic bactericidal effect against this species.

The transfer of plasmids or transposons during conjugation appears to be responsible for most of the enterococcus's acquired resistance. The list of acquired resistances in the enterococcus is growing (Table 260-2), and the appearance of penicillin G, ampicillin, vancomycin, and high-level aminoglycoside resistance in the last decade has alarmed the medical community. As indicated in Table 260-2, most acquired resistance in the enterococcus depends on either production of enzymes that inactivate the antimicrobial agent or changes in the molecular target of the antimicrobial agent (Chapter 224).

Most clinical isolates possess several different forms of resistance. Those with high-level resistance to all commercially available aminoglycoside antibiotics are most troublesome. Strains with high-level aminoglycoside resistance are not killed by beta lactam–aminoglycoside or vancomycin–aminoglycoside combinations; hence, these combinations do not provide the bactericidal therapy necessary for the cure of endocarditis caused by these strains. High-level aminoglycoside resistance and either penicillinase production or vancomycin resistance have been found together in some clinical isolates, but these strains are not yet widespread.

The prevalence of acquired resistance to various antimicrobial agents varies considerably. Resistance to chloramphenicol, erythromycin, tetracycline, and streptomycin has been common for several decades. High-level resistance to gentamicin and all other aminoglycosides appeared in *E. faecalis* during the early 1980s and has disseminated widely since then. It has subsequently been recognized in *E. faecium* but with lesser frequency so far. Penicillinase-

Table 260-2. Acquired antimicrobial resistance of enterococci*

Antimicrobial agent	Mechanism of resistance
Aminoglycoside (high-level)	
Streptomycin	Induction of ribosomal resistance Production of adenyltransferase
Kanamycin	Production of phosphotransferase
Gentamicin, kanamycin, tobramycin, amikacin, and netilmicin	Production of fusion protein with phosphotransferase and acetyltransferase activity
Beta lactams	
Penicillin G, ampicillin, piperacillin, and mezlocillin	Production of beta lactamase
Penicillin, ampicillin, and imipenem	Altered penicillin binding protein 5 in *E. faecium*
Glycopeptides	
Vancomycin, teicoplanin, and others	Production of membrane associated protein that may prevent drug access to its target site
Vancomycin alone	Unknown but associated with production of a different membrane protein (nontransferable)
Miscellaneous	
Chloramphenicol	Production of chloramphenicol acetyltransferase
Erythromycin	Methylation of ribosomal RNA (also confers high-level clindamycin resistance)
Tetracyclines	Protection of ribosome from tetracycline inhibition Induction of active transport system to remove tetracycline from cell

*Also see Chapter 224.

producing strains of *E. faecalis* and vancomycin–resistant strains of enterococci have appeared in various parts of the world during the last few years; the former remain rare, whereas the latter are increasingly prevalent. Resistance of *E. faecium* to penicillin G, ampicillin, and imipenem, which is not mediated by beta lactamases, also appears to be increasing. Approximately one third of clinical isolates in several centers currently exhibit this resistance.

Clinical manifestations

Endocarditis. Enterococcal endocarditis almost always occurs on previously damaged aortic or mitral valves even in intravenous drug addicts. It usually presents in a subacute manner though acute presentations are not unknown. In most case series men outnumber women 2:1. Male patients are generally in their fifth or sixth decade and often describe antecedent genitourinary tract procedures or infections. Woman patients are generally in their childbearing years and often relate histories of gynecologic or obstetric events that may have induced bacteremia. Features of this illness are described in Chapter 15.

Bacteremia without endocarditis. Overall enterococci are isolated from 5% of all positive blood cultures. Approximately 25% to 35% of bacteremias occur in patients with community-acquired infections, principally endocarditis, biliary tract or other intra-abdominal infections, and urinary tract infections.

Of enterococcal bacteremias 65% to 75% are nosocomial. As a rule, these occur in men and women above 50 years of age with serious underlying diseases (e.g., malignancies, traumatic injuries, or complicated surgeries). They often occur more than 3 weeks after admission to the hospital and after prolonged antimicrobial therapy, especially broad-spectrum cephalosporin therapy. Common sources of nosocomial enterococcal bacteremias include biliary, other intra-abdominal, or surgical wound infections (15% to 40% of cases); urinary tract infections (15% to 40%); burn wounds and other cutaneous infections (15% to 30%); and intravenous catheter infections (5% to 20%). The source of the bacteremia remains obscure in 15% to 20% of patients.

Of enterococcal bacteremias 25% to 45% are polymicrobial; gram-negative bacilli and staphylococci are isolated in association with enterococci most frequently. Patients with polymicrobial enterococcemia generally have more severe signs and symptoms of infection including hypotension and disseminated intravascular coagulation. In contrast, those with only enterococci in the blood tend to have more indolent disease characterized mainly by fever and signs referable to the primary site of infection.

Urinary tract infections. Enterococci account for approximately 2% of urinary tract infections in young, healthy women. They play a larger role in elderly men with prostatic disease and achieve prominence as a cause of nosocomial urinary tract infections, especially in patients undergoing urologic procedures and in those with genitourinary structural abnormalities or indwelling urinary catheters. The clinical manifestations of enterococcal infections are similar to those caused by other bacteria (Chapter 240).

Intra-abdominal and pelvic infections. Enterococci are frequently isolated from patients with secondary peritonitis, intra-abdominal or pelvic abscesses, biliary tract disease, and other infections that derive from bowel or vaginal flora. They are usually isolated in association with other members of the normal flora from these sites, but in patients who have received broad-spectrum antimicrobial therapy, they may be the sole isolate. Controversy surrounds the clinical significance of enterococci in these mixed infections, but the frequency of bacteremia that arises from such infections has generated some appreciation of their importance, especially in immunocompromised patients. Clinical features are discussed in Chapters 62, 65 and 232.

Skin and soft tissue infections. Enterococci are commonly isolated in mixed cultures from burns, decubitus ulcers, diabetic foot infections, and wounds associated with abdominal surgery. They are clearly opportunists in this setting, only affecting previously damaged tissue. Here again, it is difficult to assess the enterococcus's contribution in these conditions, but the frequency of bacteremia that arises from these sources suggests that their involvement is not always benign. Clinical features are discussed in Chapter 235.

Miscellaneous infections. Enterococci are rare causes of meningitis, pneumonia, and empyema. They are occasionally isolated from patients with infected medical devices such as orthopedic prostheses, central nervous system shunts, and peritoneal dialysis catheters.

Diagnosis

Although finding chains of gram-positive cocci on gram stains of unspun urine or pus from an intra-abdominal abscess strongly suggests enterococcal involvement, a definitive diagnosis is established by culture. Because enterococci rarely contaminate specimens from normally sterile body fluids, their isolation from blood, cerebrospinal fluid (CSF), synovial fluid, and so on, indicates infection. Their isolation from mucosal surface exudates, however, is more difficult to interpret.

Once enterococci are isolated from clinical specimens, speciated, and subjected to standard susceptibility tests, special susceptibility tests may also be needed. Isolates from patients with endocarditis require tests for high-level resistance (minimum inhibitory concentrations) [MICs] > 2000 mg/L) to streptomycin and gentamicin. Nitrocefin testing of blood and CSF isolates appears warranted to detect penicillinase-producing strains of *E. faecalis* because routine susceptibility tests do not detect this property. All blood and CSF isolates of enterococci require testing against vancomycin in some form of dilution assay because disk diffusion assays may not detect resistant strains. Enterococci from infections that persist or recur despite ap-

Table 260-3. Therapy of noncardiac enterococcal infections

Type of infection	First choices	Alternatives
Severe: with sepsis syndrome (e.g., bacteremia or cholecystitis)	Ampicillin 2 g IV q4h or Vancomycin 1.0 g IV q12h or Ampicillin 2 g and sulbactam 1 g IV q6h*	Mezlocillin 5 g IV q6h or Piperacillin 3 g IV q4h or Imipenem 0.5-1.0 g IV q6h or Ciprofloxacin 0.4 g IV q12h*
Mild: little systemic toxicity (e.g., uncomplicated urinary tract infection)	Amoxicillin 500 mg PO tid or Ampicillin 500 mg PO qid or Ciprofloxacin 250-500 mg PO q12h	Nitrofurantoin† 100 mg PO q6h Norfloxacin† 400 mg PO bid

*See text.
†Urinary tract infection only.

propriate therapy also merit special susceptibility tests to look for occult resistance.

Treatment

Enterococcal endocarditis requires bactericidal therapy with synergistic combinations of antimicrobial agents (Chapter 15). Ampicillin or vancomycin therapy alone suffices for other serious enterococcal infections (Table 260-3). Cephalosporins are not effective. Before the identity and susceptibility pattern of the infecting organism are known, three considerations influence the choice of antibiotics: the likelihood of encountering an ampicillin- or vancomycin-resistant strain; the patient's drug allergy history; and the concurrent need to treat other bacteria involved in a polymicrobial infection, for example, the necessity for covering gram-negative bacilli and anaerobes in a patient with a diverticular abscess (Chapter 232).

Ampicillin and sulbactam provide an alternative to vancomycin for treating penicillinase-producing strains of *E. faecalis* but offer no help for treating ampicillin-resistant strains of *E. faecium*. Although parenteral ciprofloxacin therapy is listed as an alternative, clinical experience is extremely limited and certain strains of *E. faecium* are clearly resistant. Nevertheless, it may be the principal choice for treating a severe infection caused by a vancomycin-resistant strain in patients with life-threatening penicillin allergies.

OTHER NON-GROUP A STREPTOCOCCI

Table 260-4 delineates the principal characteristics of four additional groups of medically important streptococci. Diagnosis rests on culture results from appropriate specimens. When they are isolated from blood, CSF, or other normally sterile body fluid, the diagnosis is definitive. When they are recovered from other specimens (e.g., swabs of wound exudates), assigning an etiologic role to these streptococci with precision may be difficult. Regardless, the availability of commercial reagents for Lancefield typing has facilitated detection of these organisms. During the past 15 years their role in human disease has been more clearly defined and recognized with increasing frequency.

Most of these streptococci are normal flora or pathogens of various mammals; all are, to a greater or lesser extent, colonizers of humans. Some infections result from animal contact. Most, however, derive from colonizing organisms that become invasive when trauma or disease provides opportunities to evade host defenses of the skin, respiratory tract, gastrointestinal tract, or genitourinary tract. Infection may be localized to the site of invasion or disseminated via blood or lymph to distant sites.

Penicillin G is the drug of choice for virtually all of the nonenterococcal streptococci. Dosages as high as 20 to 30 million units per day are employed for severe infections. An aminoglycoside antibiotic is often added for its synergistic bactericidal effect in the treatment of patients with endocarditis. Various cephalosporin antibiotics, erythromycin, vancomycin, and clindamycin are used for the nonenterococcal infections in patients who are allergic to penicillin.

Nonenterococcal group D streptococci

Streptococcus bovis, the principal member of this group, accounts for approximately 5% of infective endocarditis cases and occasional cases of bacteremia in older adults. Both endocarditis and bacteremia commonly arise from a colonic source; in fact, the association of either condition with unrecognized colonic neoplasms is sufficiently strong to justify a thorough examination of the colon whenever *S. bovis* is isolated from blood. Unlike enterococci, *S. bovis* is highly susceptible to penicillin G, and therapy for endocarditis conforms to that recommended for the viridans streptococci (Chapter 15).

Group B streptococci

S. agalactiae, the only species of group B streptococci, was initially recognized as a cause of meningitis and other serious infections in the newborn. More recently, it has been recognized as a cause of gynecologic, opportunistic, and nosocomial infections in adults. The annual incidence of group B streptococcal infections in adults has recently been calculated to be 2.4 infections per 100,000 population in metropolitan Atlanta. These organisms account for 8% of nonneonatal streptococcal bacteremias. Endomyometritis and occasionally urinary tract infections occur in postpartum women, whereas wound infections and pelvic cellulitis occur after gynecologic surgery. These infections are often polymicrobial and may give rise to bacteremia in up to one third of cases; in fact, *S. agalactiae* accounts for 10%

Table 260-4. Characteristics and ecology of nonenterococcal, non–group A streptococcal pathogens

Category and species	Microbiologic properties	Animal sources	Human colonization*
Nonenterococcal group D *S. bovis*	Usually alpha hemolysis; hydrolyze esculin; grow in 40% bile; do *not* grow in 6.5% NaCl	Commonly isolated from feces of cattle, swine, and sheep	Oropharynx rare Colon 5% to 15%
Group B *S. agalactiae*	Narrow-zone beta hemolysis; six serotypes on basis of polysaccharide capsular and protein antigens	Pathogen of cattle	Oropharynx <1% to 20% Vagina 5% to 40% Rectal up to 50%
Group C and G *Pyogenes*-like *S. equi* *S. equisimilis* *S. canis*	Large colonies with a broad band of beta hemolysis	*S. equi* pathogen of horses; *S. canis* pathogen of dogs; some group members isolated from cattle, swine, sheep, and other mammals	Skin transient but probably frequent Oropharynx <1% to 20% Vagina <1% to 5% Colon <1% to 13%
S. milleri group or *S. intermedius* group or *S. anginosus*	Minute, slow-growing colonies; microaerophilic or carboxyphilic; variable types of hemolysis; variable Lancefield groups none, G, or F common, A and C uncommon; positive Voges Proskauer test result	Not established	Skin—probably rare Oropharynx 1% to 11% Vagina 3% to 18% Colon 16% to 67%

*Site of colonization in humans and estimates or ranges of recovery from healthy adults.

to 20% of positive blood culture findings on obstetric services.

In older adults with major underlying diseases, especially malignancies, diabetes mellitus, and neurologic impairments, *S. agalactiae* infections are more diverse and involve a number of different organ systems. Skin and soft tissue infections such as cellulitis, infected decubitus ulcers, and postoperative wound infections predominate in most case series. Urinary tract infections, pneumonias, endocarditis, and primary bacteremias also occur. In some series a substantial number of infections involve intravenous or intra-arterial access devices. Bacteremia has been common in published cases, and secondary infections at distant sites have not been unusual. Case fatality rates in older adults usually exceed 40%.

Group C and G pyogenes-like streptococci

Group C and G pyogenes-like streptococcal bacteria, which closely resemble *S. pyogenes* (Chapter 259), cause a wide variety of suppurative infections: pharyngitis, pneumonia, cellulitis, and other skin and wound infections. Bacteremia may ensue and lead to endocarditis, meningitis, arthritis, osteomyelitis, and other infections at sites far removed from the portal of entry. Group G streptococci account for approximately 10% and group C for approximately 1% of all beta-hemolytic streptococcal bacteremias. Foodborne outbreaks of pharyngitis caused by group C and G streptococci have been reported, and poststreptococcal glomerulonephritis has been observed to follow a few cases of group C streptococcal pharyngitis.

Serious group C and G streptococcal infections often occur in older adults with significant underlying disease such as cancer, diabetes mellitus, and alcoholism. They may produce substantial mortality and morbidity rates in this population: endocarditis has a case fatality rate greater than 30%, and many survivors require valve replacement; pneumonia frequently leads to empyema; and approximately one half of the reported patients with meningitis have died.

Streptococcus milleri group

Despite confusing and unresolved taxonomy issues, the diverse group of *S. milleri* streptococci have increasingly been recognized to cause a variety of serious human infections. They are most frequently associated with abscesses, especially hepatic, dental, appendiceal, and brain abscesses (Chapters 232 and 234). In some case series the *S. milleri* group have been isolated from up to 80% of patients with liver abscesses, more than 50% of patients with appendiceal abscesses, and more than 50% of patients with brain abscesses. They are recovered less frequently from patients with pneumonia, empyema, primary bacteremia, endocarditis, arthritis, wound infections, and so on. In approximately half of the cases *S. milleri* group organisms are recovered in association with other bacterial pathogens.

REFERENCES

Chenoweth C and Schaberg D: The epidemiology of enterococci. Eur J. Clin Microbiol Infect Dis 9:80, 1990.

Chua D, Reinhart HH, and Sobel JD: Liver abscess caused by *Streptococcus milleri*. Rev Infect Dis 11:197, 1989.

Eliopoulos GM and Eliopoulos CT: Therapy of enterococcal infections. Eur J Clin Microbiol Infect Dis 9:118, 1990.

Gaunt PN and Seal DV: Group G streptococcal infections. J Infect 15:5, 1987.

Gossling J: Occurrence and pathogenecity of the *Streptococcus milleri* group. Rev Infect Dis 10:257, 1988.

Herman DJ and Gerding DN: Antimicrobial resistance among enterococci. Antimicrob Agents Chemother 35:1, 1991.
Herman DJ and Gerding DN: Screening and treatment of infections caused by resistant enterococci. Antimicrob Agents Chemother 35:215, 1991.
Hoge CW et al: Enterococcal bacteremia: to treat or not to treat, a reappraisal. Rev Infect Dis 13:600, 1991.
Lewis CM and Zervos MJ: Clinical manifestations of enterococcal infection. Eur J Clin Microbiol Infect Dis 9:111, 1990.
Maki DG and Agger WA: Enterococcal bacteremia: clinical features, the risk of endocarditis, and management. Medicine 67:248, 1988.
Murray BE: The life and times of the enterococcus. Clin Microbiol Rev 3:46, 1990.
Opal SM et al: Group B streptococcal sepsis in adults and infants. Arch Intern Med 148:641, 1988.
Salata RA et al: Infections due to Lancefield group C streptococci. Medicine 68:225, 1989.
Schwartz B et al: Invasive group B streptococcal disease in adults. JAMA 266:1112, 1991.
Singh KP et al: Clinically; significant *Streptococcus anginosus (Streptococcus milleri)* infections: a review of 186 cases. NZ Med J 101:813, 1988.

CHAPTER

261 Gram-Positive Aerobic Bacillary Infections: *Corynebacterium* and *Listeria*

John L. Ho
Warren D. Johnson, Jr.

CORYNEBACTERIUM

Classification and characteristics

The family Corynebacteriaceae includes genera *Corynebacterium, Listeria,* and *Erysipelothrix*. They are gram-positive, non-spore-forming, aerobic bacilli that exhibit a marked degree of pleomorphism, both in terms of biochemical characteristics and in the clinical diseases they produce. *Corynebacterium diphtheriae* is the type species of its genus and causes the disease diphtheria. Other corynebacteria, often referred to as diphtheroids, have traditionally been considered to be nonpathogenic for humans, although they may occasionally cause severe infections (*C. ulcerans, C. ovis, C. equi, C. pyogenes, C. bovis,* and *C. vaginale*).

Corynebacteria are aerobic, nonmotile, catalase-positive, pleomorphic rods with irregularly stained segments. They are part of the normal flora of skin, mucous membranes, and intestine. In stained smears, *C. diphtheriae* organisms exhibit a club-shaped appearance and are arranged in palisades. Three distinct colony types of *C. diphtheriae* (*gravis, mitis,* and *intermedius*) can be identified from their appearance on tellurite agar and their ability to ferment glycogen and starch. All three are capable of producing diphtheria toxin and clinical disease.

Epidemiology

Humans are the only significant reservoir of *C. diphtheriae*. Transmission between persons is usually via aerosolized droplets. In some tropical areas where skin infections with *C. diphtheriae* are common, the organisms may be spread by direct contact. Fomites, dust, and milk rarely have been implicated as disease vectors. Conditions that favor crowding are associated with increased transmission, and this explains the higher prevalence of disease in cold weather.

The Centers for Disease Control has been charting the cumulative incidence of diphtheria, a disease in which reporting is mandated. The improvement of health conditions and the introduction of diphtheria toxoid immunization have significantly reduced the number of cases in the United States (Fig. 261-1). By 1979 and 1980, there were 59 and 83 diphtheria cases, respectively with a total of two fatalities. A dramatic reduction was noted with only 23 cases with 2 fatalities from 1981 to 1989. Because 77% of the recent diphtheria cases occurred in persons above the age of 15 compared to the period between 1971 to 1981, when the rate in children below 15 years of age was four times that of adults, a loss of immunity may account for this shift to an older age group. Attack rates of diphtheria in Native Americans, Mexican Americans, and blacks are 10 times higher than in the rest of the population. Seventy-five percent of these cases occur in nonimmunized persons. Diphtheria remains a worldwide problem, particularly in developing countries. Outbreaks of diphtheria in developed countries have been reported in lower social economic groups as a result of crowding and increased opportunities for aerosol transmission. Diphtheria in immunized persons is usually mild and without either membrane formation or toxemia. Although a serum antitoxin level above 0.01 IU/ml is protective against disease acquisition, such individuals may serve as asymptomatic carriers of the organism.

Pathogenesis

Corynebacterium diphtheriae colonizes and multiplies on mucosal and epithelial surfaces. These organisms most commonly invade the upper respiratory tract. The serious manifestations of diphtheria are due to a potent toxin elaborated by the bacilli; however, the probability for disease acquisition may be influenced by genetic factors controlling virulence.

Diphtheria toxin is a heat-labile polypeptide with a molecular weight of about 62,000. It is produced only by strains of *C. diphtheriae* infected with a lysogenic bacteriophage. The toxin contains two fragments, A and B, which carry out different functions. Fragment B has no intrinsic toxicity but is responsible for the transport of the toxin into cells. Fragment A is the toxic portion and it inhibits polypeptide chain elongation in the presence of nicotinamide adenine dinucleotide by inactivation of elongation factor within cells. Elongation factor is necessary for the translocation of polypeptide transfer ribonucleic acid (RNA) from acceptor to donor site on the eukaryotic ribosome. Thus additional amino acids are prevented from join-

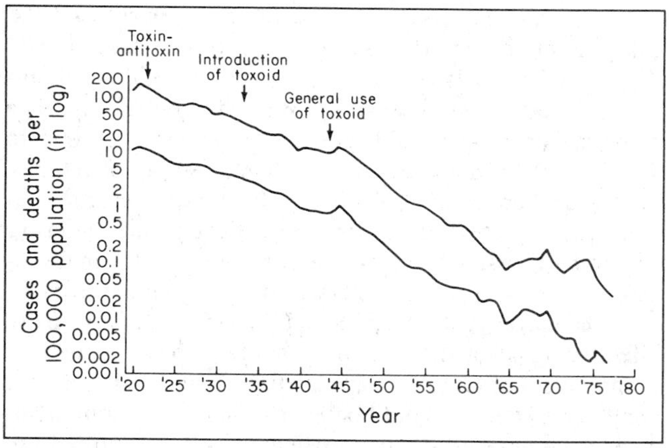

Fig. 261-1. Diphtheria case and death rates in the United States. 1920 to 1978.

ing the peptide chain, and this results in an arrest of protein synthesis.

Nontoxigenic strains of diphtheria also may produce a polypeptide that is similar to diphtheria toxin but has no biologic activity. Both toxigenic and nontoxigenic strains of diphtheria produce other biologically active substances, such as hyaluronidase, that contribute to the local inflammatory reaction.

Clinical disease

The incubation period of diphtheria is usually 2 to 4 days (range 1 to 7 days). The clinical manifestations depend on the immune status of the host, the location of the infection, and the toxigenic capacity of the microorganism. The first manifestation of disease is a marked local inflammatory response. This lesion may be transformed into a tough membrane composed of fibrin, cellular debris, and white and red blood cells. As the toxin gains access to the circulation, symptoms related to myocarditis and neuritis develop.

Types of diphtheria

Anterior nasal and cutaneous diphtheria. Cutaneous diphtheria is most common in tropical areas. Lesions appear as chronic, nonhealing ulcers over the face and upper extremities. The presence of bacterial superinfection may influence the clinical expression of cutaneous diphtheria. Constitutional symptoms and cardiac and neurologic complications are rare. Diphtheria involving the nasal area manifests itself in a serosanguineous nasal discharge, which may become crusted around the external nares and upper lip. Diphtheria conjunctivitis and corneal ulcers may develop. Primary diphtheria otitis media has been reported.

Tonsillar diphtheria. The onset of tonsillar diphtheria is usually sudden. A thin, patchy, readily removable exudate forms over one or both tonsils but is replaced within hours by a greenish-gray, firmly adherent, thick membrane. A sore throat is present in almost all cases and, in one series, was the chief complaint in 71% of patients. Cough, hoarseness, and dysphagia are present in 25% of patients.

Pharyngeal and laryngeal diphtheria. The membrane may extend to adjacent structures such as the faucial pillars, uvula, soft palate, and pharyngeal wall. Cervical lymphadenopathy and soft tissue swelling may develop and give the appearance of a "bull neck."

Extension of the diphtheria lesion into the larynx occurs in about 25% of patients. The membrane usually involves the epiglottis and, less commonly, the glottis and supraglottic structures. Hoarseness is common. Dyspnea, tachycardia, fever, and leukocytosis are poor prognostic signs.

Complications

Respiratory failure may result from severe pharyngeal or laryngeal involvement accompanied by airway obstruction. Myocarditis and polyneuritis are the major complications that result from the absorption of diphtheria toxin.

Myocarditis accounts for one half of diphtheria deaths. The incidence of myocarditis is highest in pharyngeal and laryngeal diphtheria, and circulatory failure results in up to 9%. The onset of myocarditis is usually insidious. Electrocardiographic abnormalities develop during the first week of illness and are characterized by atrial and ventricular arrhythmias. Atrioventricular block and left bundle branch block are associated with 70% to 100% mortality rates.

Nervous system involvement is a late complication that may occur up to a month or longer after the onset of illness. Paralysis of cranial nerves IX and X occurs in 50% of patients with neurologic involvement. This can result in aspiration and nasal regurgitation of liquids. Paralysis of the oculomotor and ciliary nerves is common. Rarely, multiple cranial nerves may be involved. One third of the patients with neurologic complications have peripheral neuritis. The upper extremities are as commonly affected as the lower. In a large number of cases, there is both cranial and peripheral nerve involvement. Fortunately, almost all neuropathies resolve without sequelae within 2 weeks of onset of neurologic symptoms.

Bacteremia with *C. diphtheriae* is a rare event; *C. diphtheriae* endocarditis has been reported. Toxigenicity and invasiveness are independent properties, and immunization eliminates only the effect of the toxin and does not prevent bloodstream invasion by the organism.

Infections due to other corynebacteria (diphtheroids)

Diphtheroids have traditionally been considered to be nonpathogenic for humans. These ubiquitous organisms frequently contaminate blood cultures but may also produce significant disease. Endocarditis is the most common serious infection produced by these organisms. Although diphtheroid endocarditis can occur on natural valves, it is most frequently associated with cardiac prostheses and, in that setting, has a 50% to 70% mortality rate. Other nondiphtheria corynebacteria *(C. equi, C. pyogenes)* have been reported to cause meningitis, pneumonia, osteomyelitis, and abscesses of brain and liver, Endocarditis of natural or prosthetic valves have been reported for *C. equi, C, pyogenes, C. pilosum* and *C. pseudodiphtheriticum*. *C. pseudotuberculosis* is a cause of subacute or chronic lymphadenitis. *C. ulcerans* may cause an illness similar to that produced by *C. diphtheria*. *C. jeikeium* (former JK strains) causes sepsis and other infections in severely neutropenic patients and in those with prosthetic devices. The more recently recognized *Corynebacterium* group D2 causes nosocomial infections, particularly of the urinary tract. *C. jeikeium* and *Corynebacterium* group D2 colonize skin of hospitalized patients and exhibit a female gender preference for group D2 and the opposite for *C. jeikeium*. Unlike most other corynebacteria, *C. jeikeium* and group D2 are usually resistant to penicillins, cephalosporins, and aminoglycosides. Vancomycin is the preferred treatment for *C. jeikeium* and ciprofloxacin and ofloxacin are the treatment of choice for group D2.

Diagnostic tests

A definitive diagnosis of diphtheria requires culture of the organism and the demonstration of toxin production. In patients with oropharyngeal diphtheria, however, it is often necessary to initiate therapy on the basis of the clinical diagnosis. Methylene blue stains of exudate material may be confused with other organisms (diphtheroids, actinomyces) that have similar morphologic characteristics. In the proper clinical setting, however, the presence of metachromatic granules (granules that stain deeply with methylene blue) is very suggestive of *C. diphtheriae*. Material from the lesion or, preferably, a piece of membrane, should be cultured on Loeffler's medium, a tellurite plate, and a blood agar plate before antibiotics are given. The recovery of beta-hemolytic streptococci should not rule out the diagnosis of diphtheria, because these organisms are recovered from the pharynx in 20% to 30% of cases of confirmed diphtheria.

Diphtheria-like organisms must be studied further for a determination of toxin production. Guinea pig inoculation or the more popular gel diffusion test (Elek plate method) is used to determine toxigenicity. The latter technique consists in placing a filter paper soaked in antitoxin on an agar plate and streaking a heavy inoculum of the organism at a right angle to the filter paper. If diphtheria toxin is elaborated, a precipitin line is formed by the toxin and the antitoxin.

Treatment

In suspected cases, diphtheria antitoxin should be administered promptly after cultures are obtained. Because up to 10% of the population may have allergic reactions to horse serum, a skin or conjunctival test should be performed by using 0.1 ml of a 1:20 saline dilution of the antitoxin. A positive reaction requires desensitization with increasing doses of the antiserum. Antitoxin is active only against free toxin and has no effect once the toxin has penetrated the cell. The minimum effective dose of antitoxin has not been determined. The dose of antitoxin and the route of administration depend on the severity of the disease. For mild or moderate pharyngeal and laryngeal diphtheria, 30,000 to 40,000 units of antitoxin given intramuscularly or intravenously is recommended. Patients with severe disease should receive 80,000 to 120,000 units of antitoxin intravenously.

Antibiotics should be administered to prevent multiplication of the organism at the site of infection and to eliminate the carrier state. Both penicillin and erythromycin are effective agents and should be given for 7 days in diphtheria carriers and 12 to 14 days if clinical disease is present. Diphtheria patients should be isolated until antibiotic treatment is completed and three negative culture results from the lesion are obtained.

Bed rest and care to prevent aspiration pneumonia are important in the management of diphtheria. Patients suspected of having myocarditis should be transferred to intensive care units for cardiac monitoring. Indirect laryngoscopy is recommended by some authorities, because laryngeal involvement may not be suspected clinically. Tracheostomy should be considered whenever laryngeal disease is present, because progression of the infection may be rapid and lead to airway obstruction.

The prognosis in diphtheria varies with the age of the patient, the severity of the disease, and the promptness with which antitoxin is administered. Laryngeal edema has a grave prognosis. The case/fatality ratio in one series was 0.27% when antitoxin was injected on the first day of illness, and it increased to 1.67%, 2.77%, and 11.39% when antitoxin was administered on the second, third, and fourth days of illness, respectively; however, in recent reports the case fatality rate of clinical diphtheria was between 10% and 17%. Reversible paralysis was observed in as many as 35% of the cases.

Prevention

The decline of diphtheria in industrialized countries is due largely to effective immunization programs. Children should receive five doses of diphtheria toxoid as part of the combined diphtheria-pertussis-tetanus vaccine (DPT) at 2, 4, 6, and 18 months, with a booster at 4 to 6 years of age. For continued protection booster immunizations are recommended every 10 years. In a recent randomized, stratified sample of urban adults, the overall protective level of antitoxin (greater than or equal to 0.01 IU/ml) was demonstrated in 26% of men and 21% of women. Other serosurveys have confirmed that at least 50% of adults are susceptible to diphtheria. Particular attention should be also be directed at revaccinating adults and particularly travelers to countries with higher endemic disease. For continued protection, booster immunizations are recommended at 25 years of age and every 10 years thereafter. For children 6 to 12 years of age, primary immunization consists of two doses of pediatric diphtheria-tetanus (DT) 6 weeks apart, with a booster 6 to 12 months later. For persons above 12 years of age, a smaller dose of diphtheria-tetanus toxoid should be used with the same schedule. The larger doses of diphtheria toxoid in DPT and DT may cause systemic reactions in older persons who have become sensitized by previous exposure to products of *C. diphtheriae*.

LISTERIA

Classification and characteristics

Listeria are small, nonsporulating, nonencapsulated gram-positive aerobic bacilli. *Listeria monocytogenes* was first recognized as a cause of disease in humans in 1929. It is the only important pathogen of humans of this genus.

Because of its coccoid appearance and uneven staining, *L. monocytogenes* may be confused with pneumococci, *Haemophilus influenzae,* and diphtheroids in stained smears of clinical specimens. *Listeria* are distinguished from other members of the family Corynebacteriaceae by their motility and their ability to hydrolyze esculin and to produce beta hemolysis. *Listeria* may be serotyped by their somatic (O) and flagellar (H) antigens.

Epidemiology

L. monocytogenes is worldwide in distribution. The organism is found in soil, water, and dust and has been isolated from a great variety of domestic and wild animals. Human fecal excretion of listeria occurs in about 1% of the normal population, in 4.8% of abattoir workers, and in 26% of contacts of patients with listeriosis. Listeria have been cultured from the human vagina and the male urethra. Transplacental and vaginal transmission of listeria are responsible for fetal and neonatal infection. There have been documented instances of listeriosis after the ingestion of contaminated cabbage, milk, cheese, and meat (turkey franks). In California in 1985, nearly 200 cases with more than 80 deaths were attributed to a single source of contaminated cheese. It is likely that listeria is enterically acquired in most cases and invasive systemic listeriosis occurs in a small percentage of these individuals.

In the United States, the incidence of listeriosis is not known because limited surveillance was started only in 1988. On the basis of active surveillance of 19 million persons in four states in the United States, the aggregate incidence was 7.4 per million. In pregnant women the incidence of listeriosis is 223 per million. Listeriosis is manifested as a wide spectrum of diseases in risk groups, such as pregnant women, infants, elderly adults, and immunocompromised hosts. It is rarely seen in persons with intact immunity. Pregnancy related infection accounts for approximately one third of the sporadic cases of listeriosis.

Pathogenesis

The pathogenesis of listeriosis is not well understood. Listeria has the ability to invade and propel itself through intestinal epithelial cells, allowing entry into the circulation. The association of human listeriosis and compromised host-defense mechanisms, as well as experimental animal studies, indicate that intact cellular and humoral immunity is important in the prevention of clinical disease. Gastric neutralization predisposes acquisition of listerial enteritis and bacteremia. Immunosuppression by corticosteroids may increase the risk of meningitis.

Clinical disease

The spectrum of disease caused by *L. monocytogenes* ranges from a transient asymptomatic carrier state to an acute fulminant septicemic illness. The different syndromes of human listeriosis are pregnancy infections, granulomatous infantiseptica, sepsis, meningoencephalitis, and localized infections.

Listeriosis of pregnancy may be asymptomatic or may manifest itself as an acute febrile illness. Back pain may be the only complaint and may suggest a diagnosis of pyelonephritis. The diagnosis is established only by obtaining a positive blood culture result, because there are no characteristic clinical findings. The infection most commonly occurs during the last trimester of pregnancy and may seriously affect the fetus. There are documented cases of bacteremic infections without fetal damage.

Granulomatous infantiseptica results from transplacental infection and is characterized by disseminated visceral abscesses and granulomas. Infants should be treated promptly if the diagnosis is suspected. Cultures of blood, spinal fluid, and meconium should be obtained, as well as cultures of the maternal vagina and lochia.

Listeria sepsis may occur in infants infected during vaginal delivery or in immunosuppressed adults. There are no characteristic clinical findings, and the diagnosis must be established by blood culture. The presentation may be similar to that of gram-negative sepsis with associated hypotension and a consumptive coagulopathy. Meningitis, and, rarely, endocarditis may result from the bacteremia.

Meningoencephalitis is usually a disease of immunosuppressed patients and neonates (Chapter 233). The infection also occurs in patients with cirrhosis of the liver and, occasionally, in normal individuals. The clinical illness may be insidious in onset, with anorexia, lethargy, behavioral changes, and low-grade fever; or it may be acute and fulminant. Pharyngitis, otitis media, and cranial nerve palsies may be present together with signs of meningitis and encephalitis. The cerebrospinal fluid (CSF) glucose level is usually low, but it may be normal. CSF cell counts range from 10.0 to 12,000 per cubic millimeter, and mononuclear cells may predominate. CSF protein concentrations usually are elevated. The CSF findings alone do not distinguish listeria infection from other forms of pyogenic meningitis but may mimic aseptic (viral) meningitis.

Localized listeria infection may follow direct contact with the organism (skin, conjunctiva) or may result from a bacteremia (arthritis, osteomyelitis, endocarditis, peritonitis, pleurisy). Skin and eye infections may be associated with granulomatous infantiseptica. Culture of the organism is necessary to establish an etiologic diagnosis, because there are no characteristic clinical findings.

Diagnostic tests

The protean manifestations of listeriosis and the lack of pathognomonic findings preclude diagnosis on clinical features alone. Isolation of the organism from either blood or infected tissues and secretions is required. If the clinical setting suggests listeriosis, the laboratory should be alerted to its possibility and should carefully evaluate all diphtheroid-like isolates.

Treatment

Most *L. monocytogenes* isolates are sensitive in vitro to the penicillins, ureidopenicillins, imipenem, and chloramphenicol. Most isolates are resistant to cephalothin, and third-generation cephalosporins have even less activity. Synergism between penicillin or ampicillin and the aminoglycosides has been demonstrated. Penicillin G (300,000 units/kg/day iv) or ampicillin (200 mg/kg/day) is the recommended therapy, with the addition of an aminoglycoside in the most seriously ill patients. There have been treatment failures with single-drug therapy (penicillin, ampicillin), and relative in vitro resistance to penicillin has been demonstrated.

The optimum duration of antimicrobial therapy is not established and varies with the type and severity of the infection and with the patient's underlying disease. Two weeks of therapy may be adequate in uncomplicated listeriosis in most patients. Granulomatous infantiseptica, endocarditis, and infections in severely immunosuppressed patients should probably be treated for 3 to 6 weeks.

Prevention

Although the current understanding of the epidemiology and pathogenesis of listeriosis is incomplete, it is prudent to advise persons at high risk for listeriosis that they should eat only thoroughly cooked foods. Prevention of exposure to the organism is not practical, because *L. monocytogenes* has been isolated from virtually every animal species cultured, as well as from soil, water, sewage, and dust. Prompt recognition of disease, particularly in high-risk persons, and early therapy reduce morbidity and mortality rates.

REFERENCES

Dobie RA and Tobey DN: Clinical features of diphtheria in the respiratory tract. JAMA 242:2197, 1979.

Gellin BG and Broome CV: Listeriosis. JAMA 261:1313, 1989.

Hande KP et al: Sepsis with a new species of *Corynebacterium*. Ann Intern Med 85:423, 1976.

Ho JL et al: Nosocomial *Listeria monocytogenes* infection in eight Boston hospitals. Arch Intern Med 146:520, 1986.

Hodes HL: Diphtheria (symposium on unusual infections). Pediatr Clin North Am 26:445, 1979.

Karzon DT and Edwards KM: Diphtheria outbreaks in immunized populations. N Engl J Med 318:41, 1988.

Linnan MJ et al: Epidemic listeriosis associated with Mexican-style cheese. N Engl J Med 319:823, 1988.

Lipsky BA et al: Infections caused by non-diphtheria corynebacteria. Rev Infect Dis 4:1220, 1982.

Louria DB et al: Listeriosis complicating malignant disease, a new association. Ann Intern Med 67:261, 1967.

McCloskey RV et al: Treatment of diphtheria carriers: benzathine penicillin, erythromycin, and clindamycin. Ann Intern Med 81:788, 1974.

Pappenheimer AM Jr: Diphtheria: studies on the biology of an infectious disease. Harvey Lect 76:45, 1982.

Rappuoli R et al: Molecular epidemiology of the 1984–1986 outbreak of diphtheria in Sweden. N Engl J Med 318:12, 1988.

Schuchat A et al: Epidemiology of listeriosis in the United States. In Proceedings of the International Conference on Listeria and Food Safety. Laval, France, ASEPT Editeur, June 13-14, 1991.

Soriano F and Fernandez-Roblas R: Infections caused by antibiotic-resistant *Corynebacterium* group O2. Eur J Clin Microbiol Infect Dis. 7:337, 1988.

Soriano F et al: Skin colonization by *Corynebacterium* groups D2 and JK in hospitalized patients. J Clin Microbiol 26:1878, 1988.

CHAPTER

262 Clostridial Infections

David N. Gilbert

BACTERIOLOGY

Clostridia are gram-positive, spore-forming anaerobic bacteria found in soil and as part of the normal flora of the intestinal tract of humans and animals. Over 80 species have been recognized, and approximately 30 species have been associated with human infections. All species grow better under anaerobic conditions, but some, such as *Clostridium perfringens*, can survive exposure to oxygen for as long as 72 hours. Spore formation is characteristic but not universal with standard laboratory culture conditions.

Clostridia have been found in the intestinal tract of virtually all animals studied. In 70% of humans, clostridia are found in concentrations of 10^8 to 10^9 per gram of stool. Less often, clostridia can be isolated from the normal flora of the female genital tract, oral cavity, and skin. *C. perfringens* is the most common clinical isolate and the most frequent clostridial constituent of human fecal flora.

The major virulence factor of clostridia is toxin production. Often, the target of toxin activity explains the clinical pattern of illness (Table 262-1). The neurotoxins of *C. botulinum* and *C. tetanus* are the most potent microbial poisons known: the lethal dose for humans is estimated at 10^{-9} mg/kg body weight.

GASTROINTESTINAL ILLNESS

Clostridia cause three distinctly different gastrointestinal illnesses: food poisoning (*C. perfringens*, type A), *C. difficile* toxin–induced antibiotic-associated diarrhea, and en-

Table 262-1. Summary of disease patterns, etiologic organisms, toxin production, and toxin target for major illnesses due to clostridial species

Disease pattern	Clostridia	Toxin	Toxin target
Gastrointestinal illness			
Food poisoning	*C. perfringens*, type A	Enterotoxin	Mucosal cells of the ileum
Enteritis necroticans	*C. perfringens*, type C	Beta toxin	Mucosal cells of the small bowel
Antibiotic-associated diarrhea/colitis	*C. difficile*	Toxin A-enterotoxin Toxin B-cytotoxin	Mucosal cells of the colon
Neurologic syndromes			
Botulism	*C. botulinum*	Botulinal toxins A, B, E, and F	Peripheral cholinergic synapses
Tetanus	*C. tetanus*	Tetanospasmin	Inhibitory neuro-transmitters
Skin/soft tissue			
Necrotizing fasciitis	*C. perfringens* *C. ramosum*	Multiple toxins especially alpha toxin (lecithinase) of *C. perfringens*	Multiple cell membranes; e.g., capillary endothelial cells, erythrocytes, platelets
Myonecrosis	*C. bifermentans* *C. septicum* *C. novyi* *C. histolyticum* *C. fallax*		

teritis necroticans (*C. perfringens,* type C). The same clostridia that cause gastrointestinal illness may cause extraintestinal disease (e.g., *C. perfringens* is the most common cause of gas gangrene [myonecrosis]). Other clostridia may use the gastrointestinal tract as a portal of entry, but the manifestations of their toxin activity are extraintestinal (e.g., the neurotoxicity of *C. botulinum* in patients with foodborne botulism).

FOODBORNE DISEASE CAUSED BY CLOSTRIDIAL SPECIES

C. perfringens food poisoning

Incidence, etiology, and epidemiology. *C. perfringens* is the second or third most common cause of food poisoning in the United States. Because symptoms are mild and the illness self-limited, many outbreaks, especially those resulting from home food preparation, are probably not reported.

Disease results from the production of an extracellular 35kD enterotoxin by type A *C. perfringens*. The same type A strains can cause gas gangrene.

Meat, meat products, and poultry are the suspected foods in most outbreaks. Identified epidemics are usually associated with commercial food production (e.g., restaurants, institutions, hospitals, factories, schools, and caterers). In the latter settings, it is necessary often to prepare food well in advance of serving.

Pathogenesis. *C. perfringens* is found in 30% to 80% of the carcasses of chicken and cattle in slaughterhouses. Contaminating organisms survive cooking by forming spores if the maximum temperature or duration of cooking is inadequate. It is necessary to ingest 10^8 to 10^9 viable bacteria to cause disease. This can occur either by prolonged warming of initially cooked foods at 43° to 47° C, or, more often, a by rewarming of leftover foods. It is believed the organism is ingested in the vegetative state and the toxin is elaborated in the intestinal tract.

The enterotoxin is a protein with molecular weight of about 35 kD. There is not enough enterotoxin preformed in foods to cause clinical illness; toxin is elaborated in the intestinal tract. The toxin binds to receptors on the mucosal cells of the ileum, inhibits glucose transport, and causes protein loss and promotes sodium secretion. Further, cellular macromolecular synthesis is inhibited, there is an influx of calcium into the cell, the cell's cytoskeleton collapses, and cell death ensues.

Clinical features and therapy. After an incubation period of 8 to 24 hours, the patient has diarrhea (90% of cases) and moderate to severe cramping, with midepigastric pain (80%); additional findings include nausea (25%) and infrequently vomiting (9%) and fever (24%). The illness is self-limiting and resolves in less than 24 hours.

Therapy is supportive with adequate fluid replacement as the major objective. There is no indication for use of an antimicrobial agent. In theory, drugs that inhibit peristaltic activity may prolong illness.

Laboratory diagnosis. The laboratory diagnosis require demonstration of more than 10^5 *C. perfringens* organisms per gram of suspect infected food, presence of more than 10^6 *C. perfringens* spores per gram of stool of ill person(s), and isolation of the same serotype of *C. perfringens* from the stool of infected person(s) and from the suspect contaminated food. The latter criterion is difficult. More than 90 serotypes of type A *C. perfringens* are recognized; of all strains isolated from patients, only 40% are typable. Hence, serotyping is best employed in epidemic situations only. Alternative methods of detecting the enterotoxin have been described (e.g., an enzyme-linked immunosorbent assay and a reverse passive latex agglutination test).

Prevention. To prevent *C. perfringens* food poisoning, cooked foods must be maintained above 60° C or cooled to below 10° C within 2 to 3 hours. Previously cooked and then refrigerated foods should be reheated to a minimum internal temperature of 75° C immediately before serving to ensure destruction of vegetative bacteria.

Enteritis necroticans

Enteritis necroticans, a serious disease of the small intestine, is caused by the beta toxin of *C. perfringens,* type C. Epidemics of disease, called *darmbrand,* occurred in malnourished individuals from Norway and Germany at the end of World War II. The same disease is endemic in the highlands of New Guinea, where it is called *pigbel* because of the association with pig feasts.

The target of the toxin is the mucosal cell of the small bowel; this feature explains the clinical picture. Patients have acute abdominal pain, bloody diarrhea, vomiting, shock, and peritonitis. The mortality rate is 15% to 40%. Pathologic examination demonstrates an acute segmental ulcerative process of the small bowel mucosa. The mucosa lifts off the submucosa, leaving a large denuded area; the partially sloughed epithelium may form pseudomembranes.

It is believed that the disease results from the absence, or a deficiency of, intestinal proteolytic enzymes specific for the type C toxin. The source of the organism is undercooked pork. The low level of protease activity may result from some combination of factors: (1) a low-protein diet and hence, a low level of intestinal proteases such as trypsin; (2) the simultaneous consumption of pork and sweet potatoes, which contain trypsin inhibitors; and/or (3) the parasitization of some individuals by Ascaris worms that secrete trypsin inhibitors. Antitoxin titers are demonstrable in patients who survive the disease; hence, the apparent predilection for children may reflect absence of protective antibody.

Medical therapy includes nasogastric suction, administration of penicillin or clindamycin, support with intravenous fluids, and use, if available, of antitoxin against the beta toxin. Resectional surgery is necessary in about half the patients. In the endemic area, a beta-toxoid vaccine is recommended for prevention in children.

A beta toxoid vaccine was successful in reducing hospital admissions caused by enteritis necroticans in New Guinea. This inexpensive vaccine should find use in Sri Lanka, Vietnam, Thailand, and other countries where the disease occurs.

Clostridium difficile toxin–mediated diarrhea and colitis

History of nomenclature. Selected time points in the history leading to the recognition of *C. difficile* toxin (CDT) as a cause of diarrhea and colitis are summarized in Table 262-2. Of interest, pseudomembranous colitis (PMC), albeit rare, was a recognized pathologic entity many years before the availability of antibiotics. In retrospect, it is likely that many of the patients with "staphylococcal pseudomembranous colitis" had *C. difficile* toxin–mediated enterocolitis. Perhaps because of the drug's antistaphylococcal activity, *S. aureus* was not isolated from the stool of any patient with "clindamycin" colitis. Within a short period, the pathogenetic role of CDT was recognized, and a specific sensitive biologic assay to detect the toxin became available. Presently, CDT is accepted as the cause of antibiotic-associated PMC in roughly 20% of patients.

Table 262-2. Historical evolution of the recognition of *Clostridium difficile* toxin as a cause of antibiotic-associated diarrhea/colitis

Year	Event
1893	Pathologic description of idiopathic pseudomembranous colitis (PMC)
1950	Increased incidence of PMC attributed to *S. aureus*
1970	Recognition and investigation of "clindamycin" colitis
1974	Description of pathogenetic role of *C. difficile* toxin
1979	Report of cytotoxicity assay for *C. difficile* toxin
1992	*C. difficile* toxin recognized as usual cause of PMC and of 15% to 30% of cases of antibiotic-associated diarrhea

Pathophysiology

***C. difficile* acquisition.** The occurrence of CDT-mediated diarrhea or PMC requires the presence of the organism, production of toxin A and toxin B, and presence of toxin receptors on the intestinal mucosal cells.

C. difficile has been isolated from sand, soil, mud, and feces of domestic animals. The organism is found as part of the fecal flora of only 2% to 3% of asymptomatic adults. Toxigenic *C. difficile* is found in the stool of 50% or more of healthy infants. High colonization rates have also been observed in patients with cystic fibrosis. In a Swedish study, the asymptomatic presence of *C. difficile* and CDT was 20 to 100 times greater after age 60. Hence, depending on toxin production and other host factors, such as presence of toxin receptors and/or specific intestinal human antibody, acquisition of *C. difficile* can result in a spectrum of host responses ranging from asymptomatic carriage to PMC.

Toxin production. The factors that stimulate toxin production in patients are unclear. In vitro, some strains increase toxin production in the presence of clindamycin. Constituents of the culture medium can influence toxin production. Sporulation and presence or absence of plasmids do not correlate with toxin production. In the hamster animal model and in human patients, administration of antimicrobial agents directly or indirectly stimulates an increase in the number of intestinal *C. difficile* and CDT production.

Toxin receptors. There is a paucity of information. A mucosal cell surface receptor for toxin A has been identified. It is theorized that infants may be resistant to toxin A because of the absence of receptors. Binding to receptors may be impeded by specific antibody in the intestinal lumen; breast milk antibody may be another mechanism to protect newborns from CDT.

Toxin A and toxin B. *C. difficile* can produce two toxins, designated toxin A and toxin B. Both are large proteins synthesized during rapid bacterial growth. Toxin B is a cytotoxin 1000 times more potent that toxin A; toxin A has the laboratory characteristics of an enterotoxin. Toxin A (enterotoxin) is believed responsible for clinical symptoms and pathologic findings. The gene for toxin A has been cloned. Gnotobiotic mice passively immunized with intravenous (IV) monoclonal antibody to CDT A were protected when subsequently challenged via gastric tube with toxin-producing *C. difficile*.

The clinical assay of stool filtrate for cytotoxicity is designed to detect toxin B. Toxin B is more potent and easier to detect; further, no toxin A positive–toxin B negative isolates have been reported.

The cellular mechanism of toxicity of toxin A is incompletely understood. In vivo studies suggest mediation by activation of neutrophils or damage to microcirculation. In vitro studies suggest mediation by activation of neutrophils or damage to microcirculation. In vitro studies demonstrate toxin mediated changes in intestinal epithelial cell permeability and structure with increased chloride secretion. The toxin-altered chloride secretion may explain the absence of toxic symptoms in patients with cystic fibrosis colonized with toxigenic strains of *C. difficile;* chloride secretion is abnormal in cystic fibrosis patients.

Pathology. The characteristic lesion induced by CDT is the pseudomembrane. In patients with PMC, the membranes appear as several elevated yellow-white plaques that vary from 5 to 10 mm in diameter. In mild or early disease, individual puncture lesions are seen; in late severe disease, the lesions coalesce and ultimately the mucosa may slough, leaving large denuded areas. There is a strong correlation between the presence of definite pseudomembranes and a positive test result of stool filtrate for CDT.

On microscopic examination, the pseudomembrane consists of inflammatory cells, mucin, fibrin, and sloughed mucosal epithelial cells. No bacteria are found in the pseudomembrane or invading the deeper layers of the bowel mucosa.

Epidemiology. The true incidence of CDC-induced diarrhea is unknown. The reported frequency varies with the type of antibiotic exposure and perhaps unexplained geographic factors. The disease is more common in the elderly and is infrequent in infants and young children. There is no predilection by sex. The vast majority of patients have received oral, intramuscular, intravenous, or topical antibiotic therapy.

Virtually all antimicrobial agents have been described as a factor in the genesis of CDT-mediated diarrhea/colitis. In general, drugs with the greatest influence on the bacterial flora of the colon are most often implicated: that is, ampicillin or amoxicillin, clindamycin, and cephalosporins. Other penicillins, quinolones, erythromycin, and trimethoprim-sulfamethoxazole are involved less often; aminoglycosides, sulfonamides, and tetracycline are seldom implicated. Even though they are used in treatment, both metronidazole and rarely vancomycin have been described as offending drugs.

Several hospital outbreaks of CDT-associated diarrhea and PMC have been described. In one prospective study in the absence of epidemic disease, asymptomatic carriage of *C. difficile*. was correlated with the prescription of stool softeners and antacids. The hands of health care workers have been shown to be contaminated with *C. difficile* and represent a mode of patient-to-patient disease transmission.

Clinical manifestations. Diarrhea can occur as early as 4 to 9 days after onset of antibiotic therapy to as long as 1 to 3 weeks after cessation of exposure to the antimicrobial agent. The severity of illness is variable (Chapter 41). Mild cases have only watery diarrhea; the stool contains no leukocytes or blood; and no pseudomembranes are seen at sigmoidoscopy. At the opposite end of the spectrum, patients have watery diarrhea with many fecal leukocytes, visible pseudomembranes, abdominal cramps, fever, leukocytosis, hypoalbuminemia, metabolic acidosis, and evidence of dehydration. Rare complications include toxic megacolon with colonic perforation. Without specific treatment, the illness can last 1 to 3 weeks after discontinuing the responsible drug.

Even in cases of mild CDT-mediated diarrhea, patients have more than just one or two loose stools; in one study, all patients with a positive CDT result had five or more loose stools per day.

Particularly difficult are patients in whom CDT-mediated PMC develops after abdominal surgery as they may have fever and leukocytosis and postoperative ileus rather than diarrhea. The disease may be limited to the cecum.

Rarely, *C. difficile* can invade and cause noncolonic disease. The organism has been implicated as etiologic in case reports of wound infections, peritonitis, abscesses, empyema, and bacteremia.

Diagnosis. A presumptive clinical diagnosis is justified in any patient who develops watery diarrhea while receiving, or shortly after receiving, an antibiotic. Classically, the stool contains fecal leukocytes, and endoscopy demonstrates raised, punctate, yellow-white 2 to 10 mm wide plaques (pseudomembranes). These findings are present only in the severe form of CDT diarrhea, and they are all nonspecific; a similar picture could occur in a patient with ulcerative colitis, regional enteritis of the colon, or rarely staphylococcal enterocolitis. Pseudomembranes are helpful when present, but they may be absent or limited to the right side of the colon.

Definitive diagnosis requires demonstration of CDT in the patient's stool. Selective media allow isolation of *C. difficile* from stool, but the need to demonstrate toxin production limits the clinical utility of finding the organism. The tissue culture assay for the presence of toxin B in stool filtrates is the accepted standard test. Stool filtrates can contain other toxins, and hence, the specificity of the cytotoxicity to cell culture monolayers must be confirmed in neutralization tests with specific CDT antisera. The tissue culture assay is very sensitive, but it is expensive and requires several days to complete.

Enzyme-linked immunosorbent assays (ELISAs) have the requisite specificity for toxins A and B; their sensitivity is satisfactory; and the test can be completed in 4 to 5 hours, as compared to 24 to 48 hours for the tissue culture assay. With further development, ELISA tests may obviate the need for tissue culture assays for CDT.

The Culturette Brand Rapid Latex Test for CDT is simple and takes only a few minutes but is apparently flawed. The test was designed to detect toxin A with latex particles coated with immunoglobulin G (IgG) antisera to toxin A. The test result was found to be positive in some patients with CDT-associated diarrhea but exhibited no reaction to purified preparations of toxin A. Furthermore, the result was positive in the presence of nontoxigenic strains of *C. difficile*. It is postulated that the toxin A used to prepare the "specific" antiserum was contaminated with another highly antigenic *C. difficile* protein. Until this problem is resolved, this test is not recommended.

Diagnostic tests based on the presence of the nucleic acid (gene) that codes for toxin A are in development and offer the promise of specificity and sensitivity. Both gene probe and polymerase chain reaction methods have been described.

Treatment of initial episode. The primary goal of therapy is cessation of the diarrhea/colitis with a drug that has minimal risk of causing an adverse reaction. To this end, virtually all patients respond to therapy with vancomycin or metronidazole. Ideally, the therapy employed would eradicate the toxin producing *C. difficile* and/or promote restoration of "normal" colonic microbial flora. Vancomycin and metronidazole frequently are unsuccessful as indicated by relapse rates reported to vary between 5% and 55%.

General principles of therapy include cessation of the antimicrobial therapy implicated as perturbing colonic flora, initiation of therapy active against *C. difficile* or use of a toxin-binding drug, and infusion of parenteral fluids, as needed for hydration. For some patients with mild disease, cessation of use of the offending antimicrobial agent may be the only therapy necessary. Antiperistalsis drugs, such as diphenoxylate with atropine (Lomotil), should be avoided as they are reported to increase the frequency or severity of symptoms.

Vancomycin. Drugs commonly prescribed are summarized in Table 262-3. Vancomycin taken orally is not absorbed to any substantial degree even from an inflamed gastrointestinal tract. Initially, a dose of 500 mg qid was employed; subsequently, the dose was reduced to 125 mg qid, with a response rate of nearly 100%. Even with the reduced dosage, fecal concentrations approximate 1000 μg/ml. Despite the high concentrations, spores of *C. difficile* survive vancomycin therapy and are recoverable from feces during and after therapy; the posttreatment strains remain vancomycin-susceptible in vitro. When *C. difficile.* is incubated in vitro with the concentrations of vancomycin found in feces, vancomycin is bacteriostatic. Resolution of diarrhea/colitis may result from the combination of vancomycin inhibition of *C. difficile,* peristalsis-induced washout of colonic content, and perhaps some reconstitution of the inhibitory influence of "normal flora." Relapse after vancomycin administration may result from toxin production by *C. difficile* spores and/or vegetative cells that were only inhibited by vancomycin. In addition, subinhibitory concentrations of vancomycin are reported to stimulate toxin production. Perhaps there is a transient period of subinhibitory colonic concentration of vancomycin that stimulates toxin production in vivo.

Oral vancomycin is expensive. The lower dosage of 125 mg qid for 10 days costs the pharmacist $145 to $160.

Metronidazole. Metronidazole provides effective therapy, with reported response rates varying from 95% to 100%. Metronidazole is absorbed rapidly from normal bowel; the drug is less well absorbed in the presence of colitis. Mean fecal concentrations of 10 μg/ml were reported in patients with PMC given 500 mg orally qid. Similar fe-

Table 262-3. Alternative therapies for *Clostridium difficile* toxin–mediated antibiotic-associated diarrhea or pseudomembranous colitis*

Treatment options:

Drug	Mechanism of action	Treatment regimen (po)	Fecal concentration (μg/ml)	Response rate (%)	Relapse rate (%)	Expense for 10 days†
Vancomycin	Inhibits *C. difficile*	125 mg qid × 7-10 days	1000	97	5-55	$110-160
Metronidazole	Cidal for *C. difficile*	500 mg tid × 7-10 days	10	95-100	5-32	$1
Bacitracin	Anti–*C. difficile*	25,000 U qid × 7-10 days	NA‡	80-100	33-344	$44
Cholestyramine	Binds *C. difficile* toxin A and B, and vancomycin	4 g qid × 7-10 days	NA	50-95	?	$29-40

*For all patients: (1) if possible, discontinue all antimicrobial therapy; (2) avoid drugs with antiperistaltic actions, e.g., diphenoxylate with atropine (Lomotil).
†Cost to pharmacist as of March, 1993.
‡NA, not available.

cal concentrations are reported after the intravenous administration of metronidazole. No reported clinical trials compare the efficacy of different dosage regimens. Response rates are similar with 500 mg tid or qid.

Of interest, the in vitro activity of metronidazole is bactericidal with a dose dependency to the cidal activity. At concentrations similar to those found in feces, a 99.99% reduction of *C. difficile* occurred; surviving organisms were a mixture of spores and vegetative forms. The reported relapse rate with metronidazole varies from 5% to 32%. The mechanism of relapse with metronidazole may relate to improved drug absorptions as the CDT-mediated colitis resolves. Lower fecal levels of metronidazole are reported in patients with CDT-mediated diarrhea as opposed to the levels found in patients with PMC. Hence, during or after a course of metronidazole therapy, colonic levels may fall sufficiently to allow germination of spores, toxin production, and relapse of diarrhea. Generic oral metronidazole is relatively inexpensive. With the regimen of 500 mg tid for 10 days, the approximate cost to the pharmacist is $1.

Other therapy. Alternative therapies employ bacitracin and cholestyramine. These drugs are used less often and data on fecal concentrations are not available.

Oral bacitracin is given as 25,000 units (approximately 500 mg) four times per day for 7 to 10 days. The drug is bitter and must be specially prepared in capsule form to prevent nausea. Systemic absorption across inflamed mucosa and frequency of relapse need study.

Cholestyramine is an anion exchange resin that was used to treat pseudomembranous colitis before the cause of the disease was known. It is now known that cholestyramine binds CDT A and B; the resin also binds vancomycin, precluding combination therapy. The oral adult dose is 4 g three to four times daily. Reported response rates vary from as low as 50% to 95%.

Treatment of PMC in patients with adynamic ileus. Drug delivery to the lumen of the colon is difficult in patients with gastrointestinal ileus of any cause. The absence of peristalsis may promote more toxin-induced injury with an increased risk of complications (e.g., bowel perforation and toxic megacolon).

There is no standardized treatment regimen as individual circumstances vary. An example of a recommended aggressive treatment regimen is vancomycin 125 mg via nasogastric tube four times a day plus vancomycin 125 mg via enema twice a day, plus vancomycin 1.0 g (if renal function normal) IV every 12 hours plus metronidazole 1 g IV every 12 hours. The patient is switched to a standard single-drug oral regimen once gastrointestinal continuity is reestablished.

Treatment of relapse. The reported frequency of relapse varies from 5% to 55% of patients treated. The accumulated data indicate that relapses are due to CDT production by the original strain of *C. difficile;* the organisms do not display in vitro resistance to the commonly prescribed drugs.

Typically, all symptoms of diarrhea/PMC subside during therapy only to recur 3 to 10 days after completion of metronidazole or vancomycin administration. There is no uniform recommendation for relapse management. Patients and physicians become frustrated frequently as 10% of patients may have two or more relapses and 5% may have three or more relapses. Conceptually, without availability of a drug to eradicate fecal vegetative or spore forms of *C. difficile,* giving repeated courses of therapy is an attempt to control toxin production until such time as "normal" fecal flora is re-established with concomitant cessation of toxin production.

Relapses are initially managed by repeated 7 to 10 courses of vancomycin or metronidazole in the same regimen employed for the initial episode. If a second course of therapy fails, repeat therapy with the combination of vancomycin in the initial dosage and rifampin 600 mg bid for 7 to 10 days is suggested.

Prevention. There is increasing consensus that *C. difficile* is acquired in the hospital environment. Numerous hospital outbreaks and case clusters have been described. The prevalence of asymptomatic fecal carriage of *C. difficile* is high in patient populations, whereas the carriage rate is low in the general adult population.

Mode of transmission in the hospital is unclear. *C. difficile* spores survive on inanimate objects in the immediate environment of the patient, but the significance is not known. Spread by the hands of hospital personnel is postulated. Reduction in incidence of *C. difficile* diarrhea was accomplished by mandated glove use by hospital personnel in one report. More aggressive control measures, such as treatment of all carriers with vancomycin or metronidazole, are expensive but might be considered in a true epidemic. Mainstays of prevention are judicious use of antimicrobial agents and implementation of universal precautions, especially use of gloves and hand washing, in patient care.

NEUROLOGIC SYNDROMES

Botulism

Definition. Botulism is a life-threatening neuroparalytic disease caused by toxins produced by *C. botulinum.* The disease is categorized by the circumstances under which it occurs: (1) foodborne botulism, (2) infant botulism, (3) wound botulism, and (4) unclassified cases.

History. The name of the disease derives from the Latin word for sausage, *botulus.* Outbreaks of "sausage poisoning" were common in the nineteenth century. In 1895, Van Ermengem isolated an anaerobic, spore-forming bacillus from a ham suspected to have caused illness; subsequently, he demonstrated that both the ham and a toxin from the organism could cause a paralytic illness in cats. Shortly after World War I, the rapid increase in both commercial and home canning resulted in many epidemics of botulism. Most of the recent cases of foodborne botulism are the result of improper home-canning procedures. Infant botulism was not recognized until 1976.

Etiology and pathogenesis. *C. botulinum* is an anaerobic spore-forming rod that synthesizes and releases a potent exotoxin during growth and autolysis. In young cultures, the organism stains gram-positive; after 18 hours of incubation, the organism may stain gram-negative. Each strain produces one of several antigenically distinct toxins, which are designated as types A through G. Types A, B, E, and rarely F cause human disease. Over the last 20 years, type A has been the most frequent cause of foodborne outbreaks. Types B and E follow in frequency. In 15% of outbreaks, the toxin type is not determined. Types C and D cause disease in a variety of animals. Type G toxin was isolated in 1977 to 1978 from autopsy material of five patients in Switzerland.

On a weight basis, botulinus toxins are the most potent poisons known. They are polypeptides with a molecular weight of approximately 150,000 daltons. The toxins are hematogenously disseminated and block neuromuscular transmission in cholinergic nerve fibers. They either inhibit acetylcholine release or bind to acetylcholine at its site of release in presynaptic clefts. The motor-end-plate responds to the direct application of acetylcholine. In humans, central nervous system cholinergic pathways and adrenergic fibers are not affected. The result is hypotonia with a descending symmetric flaccid paralysis.

Spores of organisms producing type A or B toxins are widely distributed in soil throughout the world. Strains that produce type A toxin are most common in the western United States, whereas type B toxin producers are most common in the eastern United States and in Europe. Type E toxin is found in organisms from water samples from northern latitudes, possibly accounting for the high incidence of type E strains in fish-borne botulism.

Spores of *C. botulinum* can withstand temperatures of 100° C for hours while the toxins are relatively heat-labile; boiling for 10 minutes or heating at 80° C for 30 minutes inactivates the toxins. Hence, terminal heating of toxin-containing food can prevent illness. Strict anaerobic conditions are not always necessary for toxin production. Toxin synthesis is optimal at 30° C but can occur at refrigerator temperatures. With some exceptions, home-canned acidic foods, such as tomatoes, are safer than alkaline foods because a low pH retards spore germination and toxin production.

Toxins are absorbed from the stomach and small intestine. Digestive enzymes do not denature toxin, and pancreatic trypsin may enhance the toxicity of type E toxin. Slow toxin absorption may occur from the colon. If *C. botulinum* organisms or spores are ingested and reach the colon, toxin production can occur in the human gastrointestinal tract. The latter may explain the presence of toxin in the bloodstream days after the ingestion of contaminated food.

Foodborne botulism

Epidemiology. Foodborne botulism results from the ingestion of preformed toxin in inadequately prepared food. An average of 15 "outbreaks" occurs each year in the United States, but usually only a single case is involved per outbreak. Home-canned foods with a putrefactive odor are the most often implicated vehicle. However, some contaminated food may look and taste normal.

Botulism can occur when the following conditions are met: (1) a food product contains viable *C. botulinum* bacilli or spores; (2) conditions allow spore germination; (3) time and conditions permit production of toxin before ingestion; (4) food is heated insufficiently to destroy toxin; and (5) the toxin-containing food is ingested by a susceptible host.

High-risk foods include home-canned or home-processed low-acid fruits and vegetables, fish and fish products, and condiments such as relish and chili peppers. Commercially processed foods and improperly handled fresh foods have been implicated in outbreaks of botulism. In addition, native traditional food preparation practices may perpetuate the problem. In Alaska, an area of one of the highest rates of foodborne botulism in the world, some beneficial changes in traditional fermentation food preparation were implemented, only to have new outbreaks from the improper preparation of nontraditional food.

Impaired function of cholinergic autonomic pathways may result in reduced salivation and lacrimation, constipation, and urinary retention. Nausea and vomiting may occur.

Physical examination finds an alert, oriented, and afebrile patient. Ptosis and weakness of the extraocular muscles are frequent findings; failure of accommodation occurs in some patients. Neuromuscular blockage results in symmetric weakness of the facial muscles, tongue, palate, larynx, diaphragm and intercostal muscles, and the extremities. Mild degrees of asymmetric muscle weakness may be encountered. Ileus of the intestinal tract and distention of the bladder may be present. Deep tendon reflexes vary with the severity of the illness; there are no pathologic reflexes. The sensory examination finding is always normal. Gait disturbances and incoordination are due to generalized weakness.

From the onset of symptoms, the disease progresses quickly over several days. The magnitude of neuromuscular impairment can progress hourly. Stabilization then occurs with subsequent recovery over days to months. The mechanisms of recovery is not well understood. As in tetanus, recovery from botulism does not confirm long-term immunity. Rare examples of a second episode in the same patient are described.

Laboratory diagnosis and neurologic tests. Routine laboratory tests are not helpful in the diagnosis. The most sensitive test remains injection of patient serum and stool and extracts of suspected food intraperitoneally into mice. Simultaneously, some mice are given polyvalent and type-specific monovalent botulinum antitoxins. In a positive test result, all mice expire within 24 to 48 hours, except those protected by the polyvalent and type-specific antisera. The isolation of *C. botulinum* from the stool of an ill person is considered confirmatory as the organism is rarely encountered in the intestinal flora of normal individuals. These tests are generally conducted in the laboratories of health departments or the Centers for Disease Control. Mouse bioassay and culture isolation have an overall case recognition rate of approximately 85%.

Except for occasional mild elevations in protein concentration, the spinal fluid is normal. Mild nonspecific electrocardiogram abnormalities may occur. Results of nerve conduction studies are normal; however, electromyography of involved muscle groups frequently reveals decreased amplitude of the muscle action potential and facilitation during rapid repetitive or posttetanic stimulation. These results are similar to the abnormalities found in patients with the Eaton-Lambert syndrome.

Differential diagnosis. The disease most frequently confused with botulism are those that produce generalized weakness. Patients with the Guillain-Barré syndrome almost always have mild sensory abnormalities and an increase in the spinal fluid protein concentration. A variant of Guillain-Barré, Fisher's syndrome, is characterized by ophthalmoplegia, ataxia, and reflexia: again, elevation of the spinal fluid protein concentration assists in diagnosis. The course of myasthenia gravis is more insidious, and the deep tendon reflexes and pupils are normal. An edrophonium chloride (Tensilon) test may help exclude myasthenia gravis; however, patients with botulism may have transient partial test responses. In tick paralysis, the weakness has an ascending pattern, paresthesias may be present, and a tick is found. Patients with diphtheria frequently have a prior history of pharyngitis with subsequent weakness of the palate. Patients with poliomyelitis have asymmetric weakness, sparing of the ocular muscles, and cerebrospinal fluid pleocytosis. Cerebrovascular disease of the brainstem causes associated cerebellar or corticospinal tract abnormalities. Atropine or scopolamine poisoning produces toxic delirium and marked pupils dilatation. In contrast, organophosphate insecticide poisoning causes cholinergic excess with miotic pupils. Other entities to consider include shellfish poisoning, familial periodic paralysis, and aminoglycoside antibiotic-induced neuromuscular blockade.

Treatment. Respiratory failure is the most important threat to the survival of patients with botulism. For this reason, patients with symptoms or known exposure should be hospitalized and observed closely, and sequential determinations of vital capacity should be made. Many patients require intubation and ventilatory support for days to months. Tracheostomy may prove necessary to manage secretions.

If bowel sounds are present, cathartics and enemas are given to remove unabsorbed botulinum toxin from the intestine. Magnesium salts (citrate or sulfate) should not be given as the magnesium can potentiate the toxin-induced neuromuscular blockade.

Other supportive care includes nasogastric suction and intravenous hyperalimentation if a severe ileus is present, use of a Foley catheter or bladder atonia, meticulous skin care, physical therapy, and close observation for hospital-acquired pneumonia or urinary tract infection.

As soon as the diagnosis is suspected, public health authorities* should be contacted, the case reported, and arrangements made to acquire trivalent ABE antitoxin (Connaught Laboratories). Retrospective data suggest that type-specific antitoxin is beneficial in patients with type E intoxication. The value in type A and B disease is less certain, especially if paralysis has already occurred. Because the toxin binds irreversibly to nerve endings and only circulating toxin is neutralized, antitoxin should be given as early in the course of the illness as possible. The antitoxin is of equine origin, and patients should be tested for hypersensitivity to horse serum. One can test for immediate hypersensitivity with either a skin test or instillation into the conjunctival sac; the latter method is preferred. Nonfatal hypersensitivity reactions occur in 15% to 20% of patients who receive the antitoxin. Those patients who react to a test dose must be desensitized.

In the absence of infectious complications, antibiotic therapy has no role in foodborne botulism. Antibiotics in other forms of botulism are discussed later.

Guanidine hydrochloride may produce some improvement in cranial nerve palsies or extremity muscle strength. However, improvement in vital capacity rarely, if ever, occurs, and hence, the use of guanidine is not recommended.

Prognosis. In the United States, the mortality rate of foodborne botulism is approximately 10% with higher mortality rates with type A than type B or E. Hospital deaths are due to complications such as mechanical failure of the respirator or pneumonia. The time for recovery ranges from 30 to 100 days. Full neurologic recovery is usual.

Prevention. Promptly notifying public health authorities of a suspected case may prevent further consumption of a contaminated home-canned or commercial food product. The disease is best prevented by adherence to recommended home-canning techniques. High-temperature pressure cooking is necessary to ensure spore elimination from low-acid fruits and vegetables. The toxin itself is heat labile and is destroyed by boiling food. Laboratory-acquired botulism has been reported from other countries. Laboratory workers who routinely work with *C. botulinum,* or its toxin, should receive the pentavalent botulinum toxoid vaccine.

Wound botulism

First recognized in 1943, over 30 cases of wound botulism have been reported in the United States. The typical patient is a young, previously healthy adult male who sustained severe trauma with open fractures contaminated by soil. Fewer than 10 cases have occurred in individuals who abuse parenteral drugs. Disease caused by toxin A and toxin B has been documented.

The disease is similar to foodborne botulism, except that

*Centers for Disease Control, 24 hour phone numbers:(404) 329-3753 (weekdays), (404) 329-2888 (nights and weekends).

nausea, vomiting, and diarrhea usually do not occur; fever generated by wound infection may be present; and the incubation period is longer, with a median of 7 days (range 4 to 18 days). The case fatality rate is approximately 17%. The clinical picture should cause little diagnostic confusion. Tetanus is often considered, but the differences in muscle tone in the two diseases are distinctive.

After serum is obtained for bioassay for toxin, botulinum antitoxin is administered as for foodborne botulism, and the wound is débrided even if it appears grossly normal. Anaerobic cultures of the wound should be performed to attempt to isolate *C. botulinum*. High-dose penicillin therapy, 10 to 20 million units intravenously per day if renal function is normal, is usually administered although its efficacy is not proved. The disease is best prevented by prompt, thorough débridement of contaminated wounds. Prophylactic use of antimicrobial agents after trauma cannot be relied on to prevent the disease.

Infant botulism

This disease was not recognized until 1976. It is now the most common form of botulism in the United States, with 30 to 80 cases documented annually.

Age appears to be an important factor in pathogenesis; 90% of recognized cases have occurred in children less than 6 months of age. In animals, the illness can be reproduced only during a few days of early life. In distinction to foodborne botulism, it is believed that the intestinal tract of infants first becomes colonized with *C. botulinum,* and then toxin is produced and absorbed, producing a slowly progressive disease. Quantitative studies demonstrated 10^3 to 10^8 *C. botulinum* organisms per gram of feces. Studies that compare the fecal flora of infants with botulism to those of infants without the syndrome suggest three possible factors in colonization of the intestine with *C. botulinum:* delay in establishment of a normal fecal flora, presence of other bacterial flora that inhibit or promote colonization, and/or altered intestinal function that promotes germination and growth of ingested spores.

Diet plays a role in the pathogenesis of infant botulism. Spores of *C. botulinum,* but not the toxin, are found in approximately 10% of honey samples. As a result, it is recommended that children less than 12 months not ingest honey. Honey does not contain botulinum toxin, and hence, it is safe for older children and adults. Honey exposure is associated with approximately one third of cases. In the majority of cases, no definite source of the *C. botulinum* spores is identified. Breast-feeding may be relatively protective, and iron supplementation may increase susceptibility to the disease.

Clinical illness. The earliest sign is constipation, which often appears 1 to 3 weeks before neurologic signs. Lethargy, listlessness, and anorexia then appear, accompanied by a weak cry, a decreased gag reflex, decreased sucking and drooling. The child may have difficulty holding his or her head erect, ptosis may develop, and the child may become floppy. This dramatic picture is typical of hospitalized patients. The full disease spectrum runs from mild constipation to sudden death. The disease is reversible. Complete recovery requires several weeks to months. The mortality rate is 3%.

Other diseases that produce hypotonia in infants must be considered: sepsis, poliomyelitis, Epstein-Barr virus infections, and diphtheria. Tick paralysis and congenital myasthenia gravis can cause hypotonia. Guillain-Barré syndrome is rare in infants less than 6 months of age.

Diagnosis. Diagnosis is by demonstration of presence of *C. botulinum* or botulinum toxin in stool specimens. Organisms and toxin may persist in stool after recovery has begun. In contrast to adults, infants rarely have detectable toxin in the serum. Electromyography demonstrates characteristic brief, small, abundant motor unit action potentials; posttetanic facilitation may be present.

Treatment. Meticulous supportive care is the mainstay of therapy. Because toxin is rarely detected in serum and because of risk of hypersensitivity reactions, botulinum antitoxin is usually not given. However, human-derived botulism immune globulin is available on a trial basis in some areas. Oral or parenteral penicillin therapy has no role. In contrast to adults, with respiratory failure who often require a tracheostomy, many infants are managed successfully with endotracheal intubation. No evidence shows that cathartics or enemas influence the course of the disease; however, this approach may be tried cautiously if no ileus is present. The mortality rate for hospitalized patients is 2%.

Unclassified botulism

Some patients above the age of 12 months have typical symptoms and signs of botulism, but no clear exposure is identified. It is possible that some cases result from production of toxin in vivo in a fashion analogous to that described for infant botulism.

TETANUS

Definition

Tetanus is an acute neurologic syndrome, often fatal, caused by a neuroexotoxin produced at the site of injury by *Clostridium tetani*. Tetanus is characterized by increased rigidity and convulsive spasms of the patient's skeletal musculature.

Etiology

Clostridium tetani is a strictly anaerobic, gram-positive, motile bacillus. The vegetative form of the organism forms a single, spherical, terminal endospore that swells the end of the organism with a resulting drumstick or tennis racket shape. The vegetative forms of the organism are very susceptible to heat, disinfectants, and other adverse conditions, whereas the spores can survive in soil for months to years, are highly resistant to antiseptics, and are moderately resistant to heat. Killing of spores requires boiling for a minimum of 4 hours or exposure to an autoclave for 12 minutes at 121° C.

It is possible to separate *C. tetani* into 10 types, based on their flagellar antigens. All 10 types produce the major toxin, tetanospasmin. Because the tetanospasmins produced are nearly identical antigenically, only one antitoxin is needed to neutralize the tetanus toxins produced by all strains. Tetanospasmin has a molecular weight of approximately 150,000. Along with botulism toxin, tetanospasmin is one of the most potent microbial toxins. One milligram of tetanospasmin can kill 50 to 70 million mice.

Epidemiology

The tetanus bacillus can be found in 20% to 65% of soil samples and as part of the normal flora of the intestinal tract of certain animals and humans. The highest yields of the organism are found in cultivated land; in hot, damp climates; in densely populated regions; and in soil rich in organic matter. The organism has also been found in house dust, operating rooms, and contaminated heroin.

Tetanus in the United States decreased from 560 reported cases in 1947 to 53 reported cases in 1988. Tetanus in the United States is a disease of older adults. Of the 109 tetanus patients reported to the CDC in 1989-90, 59% were above 50 years of age and 6% were below 20 years of age. There was one case of neonatal tetanus.

The age distribution suggests inadequate immunity of older adults. Serologic surveys since 1977 indicate inadequate circulating tetanus antitoxin levels in 6% to 11% of adults 18 to 39 years of age and 49% to 66% of adults above 60 years. Clinical tetanus occurs exclusively among unvaccinated or inadequately vaccinated persons or in individuals whose vaccination histories are unknown or uncertain.

Tetanus has occurred after surgery and seemingly harmless procedures such as skin testing or intramuscular injections of medication. Drug addicts represent another risk group. "Skin poppers" who injected drugs subcutaneously appear at particularly high risk. Of interest, heroin is often diluted with quinine, which lowers oxygen tensions at the site of injection and hence favors the growth of *C. tetani*.

A large problem exists in underdeveloped countries as a result of poor immunization standards and low levels of hygiene. One example is the practice of applying local dried clay to the umbilical stump of babies born of immunized mothers. Tetanus neonatorum is a major cause of infant mortality in economically deprived countries.

Pathogenesis

Because *C. tetani* is noninvasive, clinical tetanus can only occur when local tissue conditions allow toxin production and the host has no circulating antitoxin. Common portals of entry of the organism are puncture wounds and lacerations, surgical wounds, subcutaneous injection sites, chronic skin ulcers, otitis media, burns, infected umbilical cords, otitis media with tympanic membrane perforation, abortion, and pregnancy. Neonatal tetanus usually follows infection of the umbilical stump. In the United States, most cases result from cut or puncture wound incurred while working, gardening, or handling animals. The injuries are often trivial. In 10% to 20% of cases, no history of injury or portal of entry is identified. Because the spores are ubiquitous in the environment, most cases result from contamination from an exogenous source. Endogenous infection is possible in those rare cases that follow surgery on the intestinal tract.

Spores of *C. tetani* undoubtedly contaminate wounds frequently, but tetanus develops rarely because sporulation to the vegetative state requires an oxygen tension below that normally encountered in tissue. Occasionally, spores survive in a wound for months to years and ultimately produce disease after subsequent trauma that alters local conditions. Wound toxin production occurs under those conditions that reduce the local oxidation-reduction potential (Eh). Examples include the presence of suppuration, foreign body, necrotic tissue, and calcium salts. After conversion to the vegetative form, the tetanus bacillus stays localized, but the tetanospasmin enters peripheral nerve terminals and is carried within axons in membrane-bound vesicles toward the spinal cord at a rate of 250 mm per day. In the central nervous system, the toxin reaches presynaptic terminals, where it blocks release of neurotransmitter used by inhibitory afferent motor neurons. Loss of inhibition results in unrestrained action potentials and sustained muscle contraction. The result is muscle rigidity from uninhibited afferent stimuli entering the central nervous system from the periphery. Spasms result from more vigorous stimuli; even emotional and visual stimuli can result in muscle spasm. Tetanus toxin has other targets. Peripherally, it can produce neuromuscular blockades similar to that of the toxin of botulinum. Tetanus toxin can act directly on muscles to produce contraction. Some of the clinical manifestations suggest that the toxin has an effect on the sympathetic nervous system.

Tetanus toxin produces no permanent damage to the nervous system. Patients who recover have no detectable residual defects. A histopathologic change in the brainstem of patients who die of tetanus has been reported, and a toxic myocarditis has been described.

Clinical illness

The incubation period is 7 to 21 days, but cases can appear as early as 2 days or as late as 56 days after time of injury. The short incubation period indicates severe disease, usually after trauma. In general, the length of the incubation period reflects the distance of the site of injury from the central nervous system.

Regardless of severity, the patient usually has nonspecific symptoms such as restlessness, headache, and irritability. The most common presenting complaints are pain and stiffness in the jaw, abdomen, or back with associated difficulty swallowing; as the disease evolves, muscle stiffness becomes muscle rigidity and patients often complain of difficulty opening their mouth (trismus). Trismus is the most common sign of tetanus and is given the familiar descriptive name "lockjaw." As more muscles become involved, rigidity becomes generalized and the sustained contractions of the facial musculature result in a characteristic expression called *risus sardonicus*. Reflex muscle spasms develop within 24 to 72 hours of the first symptoms; the interval between first symptoms and reflex spasm is referred to as the onset time. A short onset time is associated with a poor prognosis. Any sudden increase in intensity of afferent stimuli arising in the periphery can cause painful and dangerous spasms. The spasms can interfere with respiration either by tonic contraction of the respiratory muscles or by production of laryngospasm. The resulting hypoxia can lead to irreversible central nervous system damage and death.

Clinical tetanus can be generalized or localized (to include cephalic tetanus and tetanus neonatorum). Patients with local tetanus complain of pain and stiffness in the area of the wound. Localized increases in muscle tone are often present. Cephalic tetanus is a rare form of local tetanus that results from contamination of wounds of the head or neck and may complicate otitis media or a head injury. Cephalic tetanus is manifested by ocular muscle palsies and evidence of facial nerve dysfunction. In some patients, progression to generalized tetanus is manifested initially by abdominal and back pain, stiffness of the neck and jaw, and dysphasia. Spontaneous muscle contractions (spasms) may occur. Physical examination reveals an alert, restless patient with trismus, rigid abdominal wall, and increased deep tendon reflexes. Low-grade fever is often present. Spasm of the facial muscles may result in risus sardonicus. Generalized tetanus may be mild, moderately severe, or severe. Mild cases have an incubation period of 10 days or longer and symptoms and signs develop over 4 to 7 days. Paroxysmal spasms and dysphasia are absent. Patients with moderately severe tetanus have an incubation period of less than 10 days, and symptoms and signs develop over 3 to 6 days. In addition to generalized muscle rigidity, these patients have dysphasia. Spasms occur but do not result in respiratory impairment. Patients with severe tetanus have incubation periods less than 7 days, and symptoms evolve over 3 days or less. Frequent severe spasms result in respiratory impairment and opisthotonos. Patients with severe tetanus may manifest autonomic instability and paroxysmal hypertension and hypotension, tachycardia, arrhythmias, high fever, and profuse sweating. The usual duration of disease, regardless of severity, is 3 to 4 weeks.

Tetanus neonatorum is generalized tetanus that results from infection in neonates within 10 days of birth. The child demonstrates irritability, facial grimacing, difficulty sucking, excessive crying, flexion of the arms, clenched fists, extension of the legs, plantar flexion of the toes, and intense rigidity, which may produce opisthotonos. The mortality rate usually is greater than 70%.

Complications

Some of the complications of tetanus derive from overly vigorous therapy and protracted bed rest, whereas other complications result from the action of the tetanus toxin itself. Respiratory complications include hypoxia from inadequate ventilation, atelectasis due to retained secretions, and the ever-present threat of aspiration of oropharyngeal content as a consequence of difficulty in swallowing. Protracted bed rest can lead to phlebothrombosis and pulmonary embolism. Involvement of the sympathetic nervous system can result in severe vasoconstriction, hypertension, tachycardia, and arrhythmias. Myocarditis can produce pulmonary edema and hypotension. Patients generally do not have a high fever; high fever usually indicates the presence of a secondary infection. Common secondary infections include pneumonia, infection of the original wound, infected decubiti, and infections of the urinary tract in patients with indwelling bladder catheters. Midthoracic vertebral fractures can occur as a result of severe muscle spasms and occur more often among children and adolescents. Gastrointestinal complications include paralytic ileus, constipation, and acute peptic ulceration.

Laboratory findings and diagnosis

The laboratory findings in patients with tetanus are nonspecific. One third of patients demonstrate a granulocytosis. Anemia is unusual. Results of blood chemistry panels are almost always normal initially. Electrocardiogram shows nonspecific changes only. The spinal fluid evaluation finding is normal. The electroencephalogram is consistent with a sleep pattern.

The diagnosis of tetanus is made on the basis of clinical criteria. Isolation of *C. tetani* in the absence of an appropriate clinical setting is confusing because the organism is frequently isolated from patients who do not have tetanus. The organism is identified in the laboratory with standard culture and morphologic characteristics plus the demonstration of toxin production in mice.

No other disease is easily confused with full-blown tetanus. In the early stages, the differential diagnosis includes oculogyric crisis secondary to phenothiazine toxicity, subarachnoid hemorrhage, severe hypocalcemia with tetani or severe alkalosis with tetani, meningitis, and strychnine poisoning. Strychnine poisoning produces symptoms similar to those of tetanus, but, in contrast to tetanus, patients with strychnine poisoning recover after 24 to 48 hours once exposure to the drug has ceased. The possibility of meningitis can be excluded by lumbar puncture.

Treatment

General measures. All patients are hospitalized after initial evaluation. Any recognized wound should be débrided. Abscesses require drainage. Patients should be placed in a quiet environment where they can be observed closely for the development of complications. It is necessary to monitor vital signs because of the autonomic nervous system instability. The patient requires careful positioning in bed to minimize the risk of aspiration. The usual steps should be taken to prevent development of contractures and decubitus ulcers. Routine nursing activities are best omitted because of the possible precipitation of dangerous and uncomfortable muscle spasms.

Antitoxin. Therapy is directed toward removing the source of the toxin and neutralizing circulating toxin. Circulating tetanospasmin is neutralized by the intramuscular administration of human tetanus immunoglobulin (TIG) in a dose of 3000 to 6000 units intramuscularly. No evidence shows that local infiltration at the site of the suspected wound or injury is of value. TIG has a half-life of 25 days, which results in substantial antitoxin levels for up to 16 weeks.

If human antitoxin is not available, equine tetanus immunoglobulin in the dosage of 50,000 to 100,000 units intramuscularly is equally effective. Because of the equine source of the antisera, the rate of reactions is high. Aqueous epinephrine in 1:1000 dilution should be readily available. Equine immunoglobulin is less expensive than TIG, and hence, is used extensively in underdeveloped countries.

Subsequent to recovery, patients require active immunization. The disease does not confer natural immunity.

Muscle spasms. Mild sedation is beneficial to diminish the effect of sensory stimuli and provide some degree of muscle relaxation. A variety of drugs have been used for this purpose. Mild tetanus is often treated with phenobarbital in adult doses of 50 to 100 mg every 3 to 6 hours. A more rapid effect can be achieved with the use of intravenous amylbarbital or pentobarbital in a dose of 50 to 200 mg. Barbiturates cannot be used for severe and frequent spasms because the doses required may lead to loss of consciousness and suppression of respiration. It is suggested that muscle relaxants be used alone or in combination with barbiturates for patients with moderate or severe disease. Chlorpromazine 200 to 300 mg per day, meprobamate, up to 2400 mg per day in adults, and diazepam, in adult doses of 40 to 120 mg per day, help control muscle spasms. Diazepam acts quickly, relieves muscle rigidity, and has a sedative effect without depressing respiration. When used alone in patients with moderately severe disease, diazepam has been demonstrated to lower oxygen consumption from levels that are three to five times normal to near-normal levels.

When muscle spasms are severe or interfere with ventilation, neuromuscular blocking agents such as pancuronium or tubocurare can be used. Great care must be used to ensure that paralyzed patients are provided controlled mechanical ventilation and close observation. Paralysis is best reserved for the treatment of severe tetanus not adequately controlled by other measures.

Tracheostomy. Tracheostomy must be considered in the management of patients with tetanus. Tracheostomy prevents hypoxemia caused by laryngospasm, reduces the risk of aspiration of oropharyngeal secretions, and facilitates the use of mechanical ventilators. If tracheal secretions are copious, tracheostomy should be performed early in the patient's course. Tracheostomy should be performed electively rather than as an emergency.

Other measures. Antibiotics are usually administered although no data indicate that they reduce the morbidity or mortality rate of the disease. It is theorized that the antibiotics assist in the elimination of the toxin-producing organism from an infected wound. Penicillin G is given parenterally in doses of 1 to 10 million units per day for 10 days. In the penicillin-allergic patient, tetracycline or erythromycin is a reasonable alternative.

If dysphasia is present, a nasogastric tube must be placed. Careful attention to fluid balance is necessary because large fluid losses can occur and are difficult to measure because of profuse sweating and unswallowed saliva.

Prevention

Nearly all cases of tetanus occur in unimmunized or inadequately immunized individuals. Immunization of children should begin at 6 to 8 weeks of age. The alum-adsorbed toxoid is preferred. Diphtheria-pertussis-tetanus (DPT) vaccine is the preferred preparation for administration to infants and children less than 7 years of age, unless contraindications exist, whereas the diphtheria-tetanus toxoid is used in older children and adults.

DPT is given to children at 2 months, 4 months, 6 months, 15 months, and 4 to 6 years. Protective levels of serum antitoxin persist for at least 10 years in individuals who complete the primary injection series. Tetanus and diphtheria (Td) toxoids adsorbed for adult use are recommended every 10 years at approximately ages 15 years, 25 years, and so on. The primary immunization schedule for unimmunized individuals above 7 years of age is Td initially, after 4 to 8 weeks, at 6 to 12 months after the second dose, and then every 10 years. Approximately 95% of the cases in the United States occur in persons who have not received the primary series of tetanus toxoid. Immunized mothers confer protection to their infants via transplacental maternal antibodies.

Of all individuals who receive emergency medical care for injuries known to predispose to tetanus, 1% to 6% receive less than the recommended prophylaxis. In 1987-1988, 58% of tetanus patients reported did not seek medical care for their injuries; of those who sought care, 81% did not receive the prophylaxis recommended by the CDC.

Postinjury tetanus prophylaxis requires good wound management, insistence on adequate immunity, and perhaps antibiotic prophylaxis. Surgical débridement removes purulent collections, foreign bodies, and necrotic tissues and hence reduces the risk of environmental conditions that promote spore germination. Chemoprophylaxis is neither practical nor useful. The need for tetanus toxoid (active immunization), with or without tetanus immune globulin as passive immunization, depends on the nature of the wound and the tetanus immunization history of the patient (Table 262-4). Tetanus has occurred rarely among individuals with documented receipt of the recommended primary immunization series.

For passive immunization, human TIG is recommended strongly; protection is longer than that provided with antitoxin of animal origin and produces fewer adverse reactions. The dose of TIG is 250 units IM; if it is given with

Table 262-4. Guide to tetanus prophylaxis in routine wound management, 1991

History of absorbed tetanus toxoid (doses)	Clean, minor wounds		All other wounds*	
	Td†	TIG	Td†	TIG
Unknown or <3 doses	Yes	No	Yes	Yes
Three or more doses‡	No§	No	No‖	No

Modified from MMWR 1991; 40(No. RR-10).
*Wounds contaminated with dirt, feces, soil, and saliva; puncture wounds; avulsions; and wounds resulting from missiles, crushing, burns, and frostbite.
†For children <7 years old; DTP (DT, if pertussis vaccine is contraindicated) is preferred to tetanus toxoid alone. For persons ≥7 years of age, Td is preferred to tetanus toxoid alone. Td, combined tetanus-diphtheria toxoid.
‡If only three doses of fluid toxoid have been received, then a fourth dose of toxoid, preferably an adsorbed toxoid, should be given.
§Yes, if >10 years since last dose
‖Yes, if >5 years since last dose. (More frequent boosters are not needed and can accentuate side-effects).

tetanus toxoid, the two should be prepared in separate syringes and administered at separate sites.

MYONECROSIS AND OTHER CLOSTRIDIAL INFECTIONS

The isolation of *Clostridium* species from a clinical specimen is not diagnostic of tissue invasion and infection. The spectrum of situations resulting in isolation of the organism run the gamut from simple contamination to massive muscle necrosis. An outline of infections, other than intestinal disorders, botulism, and tetanus, wherein the clostridia play a role is presented in the box at upper right.

Clostridia are part of the intestinal flora of 70% of humans and many animal species with fecal concentrations as high as 10^8 to 10^9 organism per gram of stool. Thirty or more species are present in the intestine; *C. ramosum* and *C. perfringens* are the most frequent clinical isolates. Clostridia can be isolated from the skin of the perineum and occasionally from other skin sites. Often clothing harbors large numbers of clostridial spores. Soil samples consistently contain *Clostridium* species in concentrations up to 10^4 bacteriam per gram.

The organism most often incriminated in producing tissue damage is *C. perfringens*. *C. perfringens* is relatively aerotolerant, causes "stormy fermentation" in milk, and is known to produce 12 toxins, as well as an enterotoxin. *C. perfringens* is divided into five types (A through E), based on the production of four major toxins: alpha, beta, epsilon, and iota. The alpha toxin is incriminated as causing the most tissue damage. Alpha toxin is a phospholipase C, a lecithinase, that hydrolyzes lecithin into phosphorylcholine and diglyceride. Alpha toxin is hemolytic, lyses platelets, and causes widespread capillary damage. When given intravenously, the toxin causes massive intravascular hemolysis and damages hepatic mitochondria. In experimental animals, the higher the concentration of alpha toxin in culture supernatant fluid, the smaller the inoculum necessary to cause tissue damage. The protective value of antiserum to the toxins of *C. perfringens* is proportional to the antiserum content of alpha antitoxin. Although beta, epsilon, and iota toxins can cause increases in capillary permeability, they do not have the histotoxic potential of alpha toxin.

Clostridium infections other than intestinal disorders, botulism, and tetanus

Simple contamination

Focal suppurative infection
Intra-abdominal
Cholangitis
Tubo-ovarian and pelvic abscess
Empyema

Skin and subcutaneous tissue
Localized infection
Anaerobic "cellulitis"
Perirectal abscess
Foot ulcers in diabetics
Amputation stump infections in diabetics and patients with severe peripheral vascular atherosclerotic disease
Suppurative myositis in heroin addicts

Diffuse spreading "cellulitis" and fasciitis

Myonecrosis (gas gangrene)
Extremities
Uterus
Spontaneous

Bacteremia

Simple contamination

Most culture isolations of clostridial species represent simple contamination. In the preantibiotic era, clostridia were cultured from 10% to 30% of the posttraumatic wounds in civilians and from 80% of combat injuries. In the Korean conflict, 27% of the war wounds were contaminated by clostridia without evidence of suppuration. In posttraumatic wounds, there is no difference in the frequency of culture isolation of clostridia from well-healing open wounds versus suppurative wounds. Because of the ubiquitous nature of clostridia, the diagnosis of a clostridial infection is made on clinical, not bacteriologic, grounds.

Focal suppurative infections

From both internal and surface sites of clostridial infection, the clostridia are most often part of a polymicrobic infection. In one study of soft tissue infection harboring clostridia, 84% of the cultures contained other pathogenic bacteria. *C. perfringens* is the most common clostridial species isolated although *C. ramosum* is nearly as frequent. Clostridia species can be isolated from severe localized suppurative processes without any clinical evidence of local or systemic damage caused by clostridial toxins.

Intra-abdominal infections. Infections complicating bowel perforation have a high likelihood of harboring clostridia. Gas gangrene is generally absent, and the flora is mixed aerobic/anaerobic organism; hence, it is not possible to distinguish clinically which infections will be culture-positive for clostridia. A clostridial intra-abdominal infection, especially *C. septicum,* has been associated with underlying carcinoma (e.g., silent perforation of a colon carcinoma, occult carcinoma of the pancreas, and leukemia/lymphoma).

Cholangitis. *C. perfringens* is found in 10% to 20% of diseased gallbladders cultured at surgery. *Emphysematous cholecystitis* refers to a severe cholangitis with gas formation in the biliary tract radicals and in the wall of the gallbladder; clostridial species are isolated in 50% of cases. There is a clinical association with the presence of diabetes mellitus. There is no evidence of muscle invasion or of systemic signs of clostridial toxin.

Tuboovarian and pelvic abscess. In 200 patients with pelvic infections, clostridia were isolated in 6%. Clostridia were encountered, most frequently, in patients with pelvic or tubo-ovarian abscess. Before the availability of antibiotics, *C. perfringens* was isolated so frequently from patients with mild endometritis after septic abortion that one author referred to the organisms as a "harmless saprophyte." Rarely, uterine gas gangrene can occur even in an uncomplicated delivery (discussed later).

Empyema. Clostridia have been isolated from a variety of pulmonary infections; however, clostridia have been noted most often in patients with empyema as a complication of chest trauma or, less often, in association with underlying aspiration pneumonia. Usually, there is no sign of local or systemic toxin production, and hence, the clinical presentation is indistinguishable from that of other microbial causes of empyema or aspiration pneumonia.

Skin and subcutaneous tissue

Localized infection. Although the word cellulitis is used frequently to describe soft tissue infections, it is often confusing because a cellule does not correspond to any specific anatomic structure of the skin or subcutaneous tissue. As used later, the term cellulitis is meant to connote inflammation of skin and subcutaneous tissue with sparing of underlying fascia and muscle.

Cellulitis, perirectal abscesses, foot ulcers in diabetic patients, and infections of inadequately perfused amputation stumps are examples of localized clostridial infections. If inadequately treated, any of the latter can extend to fascial planes and muscles with concomitant severe systemic disease and signs of toxemia.

Clostridial infections of the skin and soft tissue are indolent with slow spread to contiguous areas. Clostridia may be present in pure or mixed culture. No systemic signs of toxicity are evident. Minimal pain and edema occur; perhaps because of the lack of edema, tissue gas may be more evident than in patients with myonecrosis. By definition, there is no necrosis of, or gas in, muscle tissue.

Heroin addicts may develop a localized form of suppurative myositis. Local pain and tenderness develop in discrete areas, often on the thigh or forearm with the subsequent evolution of crepitance and fluctuation that requires surgical drainage. The process is unusual in that the local suppuration does not necessarily develop at sites of trauma or heroin injection, and the abscesses remain localized without systemic signs of toxicity. Histologic examination demonstrates the presence of subcutaneous abscesses, and purulent myositis-fasciitis from which clostridia can be recovered in pure culture.

Diffuse spreading "cellulitis" and fasciitis. In contrast to the focal processes, spreading cellulitis and fasciitis are associated with systemic signs of clostridial toxemia and death within 48 to 72 hours of onset. The disease may appear suddenly and spread through fascial planes, producing suppuration and diffuse crepitance. On examination, the involved area is only slightly painful, presumably because of necrosis of the dermal nerves, and diffuse subcutaneous crepitance is present. The crepitance is often palpable and can be detected with the diaphragm of a stethoscope. The extent of crepitance may be documented with soft tissue radiographs. Shock, renal failure, and intravascular hemolysis develop. Microscopic examination demonstrates intense inflammation of subcutaneous tissue and fascial planes with only minimal muscle inflammation. None of the muscle necrosis that typifies gas gangrene is evident; hence, there is no gangrenous muscle to be surgically removed. Bedside surgical incision may be useful for diagnostic purposes.

Myonecrosis (gas gangrene). Clostridial myonecrosis results from bacterial invasion of healthy muscle from adjacent traumatized muscle or soft tissue that has been contaminated with clostridia. This disease is uncommon after through-and-through bullet wounds but develops after penetration of shrapnel fragments, which cause necrosis of deep muscles. Any trauma with muscle necrosis and absent exposure to atmospheric oxygen favors germination of clostridial spores.

The incubation period is short. Symptoms can begin less than 24 hours after the initiating trauma or surgery. The average incubation period is 4 days with a range of 8 hours to 20 days. The patient suffers the sudden onset of pain in the wound, and over a few hours, the pain spreads beyond the wound margins. On examination, the skin is edematous with a color that is initially pale and then evolves into a reddish-blue hue. Large hemorrhagic bullae often develop. At this early stage, crepitance may be detected. The wound develops a thin, sweet-smelling, watery discharge that, on microscopic examination, demonstrates the presence of few inflammatory cells and many large gram-positive bacilli. Approximately 15% of patients have associated clostridial bacteremia.

A tachycardia develops that is disproportionate to the minimal elevations in temperature. Subsequently, shock and renal failure develop. Despite the gravity of the illness, the patient remains alert and oriented. Often, patients verbalize their sense of doom in a fashion unnerving to the physician. Just before death, toxic delirium and then coma ensure.

Definitive diagnosis and treatment require surgical intervention. In the early stages, the muscle is pale, is edematous, and does not contract when probed with instruments. In latter stages, the muscle turns beefy red and ultimately appears black and friable. If the stage of the disease is in doubt, a frozen section may help.

The differential diagnosis includes at least two other entities that present with rapidly spreading soft tissue infection. Group A streptococci can cause the clinical picture of necrotizing fasciitis (streptococcal gangrene of the skin) with, or without, myonecrosis. Similarly, mixtures of aerobic and anaerobic bacteria can produce synergistic infections, sometimes with gas formation that mimic necrotizing fasciitis and myonecrosis.

The pathophysiologic mechanism of gas gangrene requires initial necrosis of muscle in the presence of impairment of blood supply as a consequence of either the initial injury or associated peripheral vascular disease. The milieu for toxin production requires a low Eh potential, anoxia, and the availability of amino acids, peptides, and calcium. The toxins synthesized then produce necrosis of adjacent tissue, and the process becomes self-perpetuating.

In 80% of myonecrosis cases, *C. perfringens* is isolated. Most of the other 20% of cases are caused by *C. novyi, C. septicum,* or *C. bifermentans*. The initial trauma wounds are often contaminated with other miscellaneous aerobic and anaerobic bacteria. The mortality rate of gas gangrene is 40% to 60%. The highest mortality rate is in cases involving the abdominal wall; the lowest rate is in cases involving a single extremity.

Uterine myonecrosis. Clostridial destruction of the myometrium starts 2 to 3 days after a septic abortion or rarely after an uncomplicated normal delivery. Jaundice caused by massive alpha toxin–induced hemolysis develops rapidly. Renal failure occurs as a consequence of hemoglobinuria. Findings on pelvic examination may be minimal, but radiographs demonstrate gas in the wall of the uterus and adjacent tissues. Hypotension is usually present.

Milder forms of the disease result from toxin generation by organisms in small foci of residual placental tissue; this process is often successfully addressed with simple curettage. In severe cases, there is invasion of, and necrosis of, uterine muscles with spread into adjacent pelvic structures. Even with total hysterectomy and débridement, the prognosis is grave.

Spontaneous clostridial myonecrosis. An interesting variant is the patient in whom the classic picture of clostridial myonecrosis, usually on an extremity, develops without preceding trauma and without an apparent source. *C. septicum* has been implicated in the majority of reported cases. Most patients have an underlying intestinal abnormality, such as silent colon carcinoma, bowel wall infiltration by leukemia or lymphoma, or mucosal damage produced by cancer chemotherapy. The underlying bowel processes allow clostridial bacteremia. However, it is unclear how the anoxic conditions necessary for bacterial replication and toxin production are provided in nontraumatized muscle. This variant often follows a fulminant course, with hemolysis, hypotension, and renal failure eventuating in death within the first 24 to 48 hours of illness.

CLOSTRIDIAL BACTEREMIA

Up to 3% of all positive blood culture results are due to clostridia species. *C. perfringens* accounts for 50% to 60% of the isolates. A positive blood culture finding for clostridia does not correlate with a predictably stormy clinical course. In patients with septic abortion, positive blood culture results occurred in up to 27% of cases, and yet, the syndrome of uterine gas gangrene was rare. Most patients with clostridial bacteremia have a variety of associated conditions, and the significance of the clostridia is enigmatic. Occasionally, the patient has an associated mixed flora infection (e.g., aspiration pneumonia, decubitus ulcer, or intra-abdominal abscess), which represents the presumed portal of entry. Associated gas gangrene is rare. *C. perfringens* accounts for approximately 60% of positive blood isolate findings. Isolation of *C. septicum* from blood cultures suggests an underlying hematologic malignancy, neutropenia, or colonic carcinoma.

Diagnosis

The diagnosis of clostridial disease is primarily clinical. Clostridia are present in many wounds, and their presence at any site, including blood, does not necessarily indicate the presence of severe disease. Gram stains of exudates at sites of clostridial invasion demonstrate many large gram-positive bacilli as well as other organisms. Samples for culture require an appropriate anaerobic transport mechanism. Specimens are cultured in an anaerobic environment in selective media.

Patients with severe clostridial disease have protein and casts in their urine. The presence of hemolytic anemia results in hemoglobinemia and hemoglobinuria; muscle necrosis causes myoglobinuria. Renal failure often results. In severe disease, disseminated intravascular coagulation may occur. The clostridia may be visible on stains of peripheral blood or buffy coat.

Radiographic demonstration of gas in muscles, subcutaneous tissue, or the wall of the uterus or gallbladder is consistent with the diagnosis. However, atmospheric gas may enter traumatized wounds. Also, other bacteria, especially other anaerobic bacteria, mixed with aerobic organisms, may produce gas.

Treatment

Surgical débridement. The combination of surgical débridement and antibiotic therapy is the mainstay of therapy. The use of polyvalent gas gangrene antitoxin and hyperbaric oxygen is controversial. Simple wound contamination requires only mechanical cleansing. Localized infection of the skin and soft tissue, without evidence of extension to adjacent tissue or associated fever, can be managed primarily with débridement without systemic antibiotics. Fasciitis and myonecrosis require extensive débridement with excision or amputation of all necrotic tissue. In severe cases, amputation, hysterectomy, or excision of the entire anterior abdominal wall may prove necessary. Because the extent of tissue necrosis is difficult to judge at surgery, it is reasonable to return the patient to the operating room within a few hours for repeat débridement to ensure excision of all necrotic tissue.

Antimicrobial therapy. The use of antibiotics depends on the clinical situation. No antibiotic therapy is necessary for simple contamination or even for clostridial bacteremia if there are no concomitant signs or symptoms consistent with active infection. Localized skin and soft tissue infection may, or may not, require administration of antibiotics in addition to surgical débridement.

For fasciitis or myonecrosis, intravenous penicillin G, is the drug of choice. With normal renal function, the recommended dose is in the range of 20 million units per day. In the penicillin-allergic patient, alternative agents include chloramphenicol, clindamycin, and cefoxitin.

In severe clostridial disease, some thought should be given to patterns of antibiotic resistance. Virtually all *C. perfringens,* and 95% of other clostridia, are susceptible to penicillin G in vitro. In contrast, 15% to 20% of clostridia strains may be resistant to clindamycin. This is unfortunate because animal experiments indicate greater efficacy of clindamycin than of penicillin when the infecting organism is susceptible to both drugs. *C. ramosum, C. tertium, C. sporogenes,* and some strains of *C. perfringens* may demonstrate in vitro resistance to clindamycin and even penicillin G. Up to 25% of *C. perfringens* strains are resistant, in vitro, to metronidazole. Combination therapy is necessary for mixed aerobic/anaerobic infections.

Hyperbaric oxygen. Controlled rate experiments in animals indicate an increase in survival of approximately 10% in animals who were débrided, treated with penicillin, and exposed to hyperbaric oxygen as compared with animals managed with combined penicillin therapy and surgical débridement. No controlled human studies have been conducted. At present, the use of hyperbaric oxygen should be considered adjunctive only and should not be a reason to delay surgical débridement or antibiotic therapy.

Antitoxin. Some authorities still recommend polyvalent gas gangrene antitoxin. However, the antitoxin is not produced in the United States, and those products available are prepared in horses. Because of questionable efficacy and risk of hypersensitivity to horse serum, most centers have discontinued the use of antitoxin.

REFERENCES

General

Bartlett JG: Clostridial diseases. In Wyngaarden J and Smith L, editors: Cecil textbook of medicine. Philadelphia, 1988, Saunders.

Food Poisoning and Enteritis Necroticans

Lawrence G and Walker PD: Pathogenesis of enteritis necroticans in Papua New Guinea. Lancet 1:125, 1976.

Lawrence GW et al: Impact of active immunization against enteritis necroticans in Papua New Guinea. Lancet 336:1165, 1990.

Lund BM: Food-borne disease due to *Bacillus* and *Clostridium*. Lancet 336:982, 1990.

Murrell TGC: et al: The ecology and epidemiology of the pig-bel syndrome in man in New Guinea. J Hyg 64:375, 1965.

Shaudera WX et al: Food poisoning due to *Clostridium perfringens* in the U.S. J Infect Dis 147:167, 1983.

Clostridium difficile Toxin-Mediated Antibiotic-Associated Diarrhea and/or Colitis

Bartlett JG: Antibiotic-associated diarrhea. Clin Infect Dis 15:573, 1992.

Berry PR: Evaluation of ELISA, RTPLA, and Vero cell assays for detecting *Clostridium perfringens* enterotoxin in faecal specimens. J Clin Pathol 41:458, 1988.

Buggy BP et al: Therapy of relapsing *Clostridium difficile*–associated diarrhea and colitis with the combination of vancomycin and rifampin. J Clin Gastroenterol 9:155, 1987.

Burke GW: Absence of diarrhea in toxic megacolon complicating *Clostridium difficile* pseudomembranous colitis. Am J Gastroenterol 83:304, 1988.

Chang TW et al: Cytotoxicity assay in antibiotic-associated colitis. J Infect Dis 140:765, 1979.

Carthier G et al: Protection against experimental pseudomembranous colitis in gnotobiotic mice by use of monoclonal antibodies against *Clostridium difficile* toxin A. Infect Immun 59:1192, 1991.

Fekety R: Antibiotic-associated colitis. In Mandell GL et al, editors: Principles and practice of infectious diseases, ed 3. New York, 1989, Churchill Livingstone.

Finney JMT: Gastroenterostomy for cicatrizing ulcer of pylorus. Bull Johns Hopkins Hosp 4:53, 1893.

Johnson S et al: Nosocomial *Clostridium difficile* colonization and disease. Lancet 336:97, 1990.

Johnson S et al: Prospective controlled study of vinyl glove use to interrupt *Clostridium difficile* nosocomial transmission. Am J Med 88:137, 1990.

Kato N et al: Identification of toxigenic *Clostridium difficile* by the polymerase chain reaction. J Clin Microbiol 29:33, 1991.

Krentzer EW and Milligan FD: Treatment of antibiotic-associated pseudomembranous colitis with cholestyramine resin. Johns Hopkins Med J 143:67, 1978.

Levett PN: Time-dependent killing of *Clostridium difficile* by metronidazole and vancomycin. J Antimicrob Chemother 27:55, 1991.

Lyerly DM et al: *Clostridium difficile:* its disease and toxins. Clin Microbiol Rev 1:1, 1988.

McFarland LV et al: Risk factors for *Clostridium difficile* carriage and *C. difficile* associated diarrhea in a cohort of hospitalized patients. J Infect Dis 162:678, 1990.

Moore R et al: *C. difficile* toxin A increases intestinal permeability and induces Cl-secretion. Am J Physiol 259 (Gastrointest Liver Physiol 22):G165, 1990.

Price AB and Davis DR: Pseudomembranous colitis. J Clin Pathol 30:1, 1977.

Tedesco FJ, Barton RW, Alpers DH: Clindamycin-associated colitis: a prospective study. Ann Intern Med 81:429, 1974.

Tedesco FJ et al: Therapy of antibiotic-associated pseudomembranous colitis. J Clin Gastroenterol 1:51, 1979.

Van Ness MM: Fulminant colitis complicating antibiotic-associated pseudomembranous colitis: case report and review of the clinical manifestations and treatment. Am J Gastroenterol 82:374, 1987.

Walker RC et al: Comparison of culture, cytotoxicity assays, and enzyme-linked immunosorbent assay for toxin A and toxin B in the diagnosis of *Clostridium difficile*–related enteric disease. Diagn Microbiol Infect Dis 5:61, 1986.

Wren BW: Identification of toxigenic *Clostridium difficile* strains by using a toxin A gene-specific probe. J Clin Microbiol 28:1808, 1990.

Botulism

Chia JK et al: Botulism in an adult associated with foodborne intestinal infection with *Clostridium botulinum*. N Engl J Med 315:239, 1986.

Hughes JM et al: Clinical features of types A and B foodborne botulism. Ann Intern Med 95:442, 1981.

Lecour H et al: Food-borne botulism. Arch Intern Med 148:578, 1988.

McCarthy JD et al: Fever, dyspnea, and slurred speech following lower extremity trauma. Rev Infect Dis 13:172, 1991.

McDonald KL et al: Botulism and botulism-like illness in chronic drug users. Ann Intern Med 102:616, 1985.

MacDonald KL et al: The changing epidemiology of adult botulism in the United States. Am J Epidemiol 124:794, 1986.

Mills DC and Arnon SS: The large intestine as the site of *Clostridium botulinum* colonization in human infant botulism. J Infect Dis 156:997, 1987.

Schaffner W: *Clostridium botulinum* (botulism). In Mandell et al, editors: Principles and practice of infectious diseases, ed 3. New York, 1989; Churchill Livingstone.

Schreiner MS et al: Infant botulism: a review of 12 years' experience at the Children's Hospital of Philadelphia. Pediatrics 87:159, 1991.

Shaffer N et al: Botulism among Alaska natives: the role of changing food preparation and consumption practices. West J Med 153:390, 1990.

Simpson LL: Molecular pharmacology of botulinum toxin and tetanus toxin. Ann Rev Pharmacol Toxicol 26:427, 1986.

Tetanus

Armitage P and Clifford R: Prognosis in tetanus: use of data from therapeutic trials. J Infect Dis 138:1, 1978.

Brand DA et al: Adequacy of antitetanus prophylaxis in six hospital emergency rooms. N Engl J Med 309:636, 1983.

CDC: Summary of notifiable diseases, United States, 1991. MMWR 40(53):57, 1992.

CDC: Diphtheria, tetanus, and pertussis: recommendations for vaccine use and other preventive measures: recommendations of the Immunization Practices Advisory Committee. MMWR 40(No. RR-10):1, 1991.

CDC: Tetanus surveillance, United States, 1989-1990. MMWR 41:1, 1992.

Fairweather NF and Lyness VA: The complete amino acid sequence of tetanus toxin. Nucleic Acids Res 14:7809, 1986.

Faust RA et al: Tetanus: 2449 cases in 68 years at Charity Hospital. J Trauma 16:704, 1976.

Giangrosso J and Smith RK: Misuse of tetanus immunoprophylaxis in wound care. Ann Emerg Med 14:573, 1985.

Griffin JW: Local tetanus. Johns Hopkins Med J 149:84, 1981.

Halpern JL et al: Sequence homology between tetanus and botulinum toxins detected by an antipeptide antibody. Infect Immun 57:18, 1989.

Martin RR: *Clostridium tetani* (tetanus). In Mandell GL et al, editors: Principles and practice of infectious diseases, ed 3. New York, 1989, Churchill Livingstone.

Trujillo MJ et al: Tetanus in the adult: intensive care and management experience with 233 cases. Crit Care Med 8:419, 1980.

Bacteremia, Myonecrosis, and Other Clostridial Infections

Baxter CR: Surgical management of soft tissue infections. Surg Clin North Am 52:1483, 1972.

Bretzke ML et al: Diffuse spreading *Clostridium septicum* infection, malignant disease and immune suppression. Surg Gynecol Obstet 166:197, 1988.

Dellinger EP: Severe necrotizing soft tissue infections. JAMA 246:1717, 1981.

Dernello FJ et al: Comparative study of experimental *Clostridium perfringens* infection in dogs treated with antibiotics, surgery, and hyperbaric oxygen. Surgery 73:936, 1973.

Dornbusch K et al: Antibiotic susceptibility of *Clostridium* species isolated from human infections. Scand J Infect Dis 7:127, 1975.

Galandiuk S and Fazio VW: *Pneumatosis cystoides intestinalis:* a review of the literature. Dis Colon Rectum 29:358, 1986.

Gorbach SL: Other *Clostridium* species (including gas gangrene). In Mandell GL et al, editors: Principles and practice of infectious diseases, ed 3. New York, 1989, Churchill Livingstone.

Gorbach SL and Thadepalli H: Isolation of *Clostridium* in human infections: evaluation of 114 cases. J Infect Dis 131:S81, 1975.

Heimbach RD: Gas gangrene: review and update. HBO Rev 1:41, 1980.

Jendrzejewski JW et al: Nontraumatic clostridial myonecrosis. Am J Med 65:542, 1978.

Koransky JR et al: *Clostridium septicum* bacteremia. Am J Med 66:63, 1979.

Meleney FL: Bacterial synergism in disease processes with a confirmation of the synergistic bacterial etiology of a certain type of progressive gangrene of the abdominal wall. Am Surg 94:961, 1931.

NHLBI Workshop Summary: Hyperbaric oxygen therapy. Am Rev Respir Dis 144:1414, 1991.

Ramsay AM: The significance of *Clostridium welchii* in the cervical swab and blood stream in postpartum and postabortum sepsis. J Obstet Gynecol Br Commonwealth 56:247, 1949.

Stevens DL et al: Comparison of clindamycin, rifampin, tetracycline, metronidazole, and penicillin for efficacy in prevention of experimental gas gangrene due to *Clostridium perfringens*. J Infect Dis 155:220, 1987.

Stevens DL: Lethal effects and cardiovascular effects of purified alpha and theta-toxins from *Clostridium perfringens*. J Infect Dis 157:272, 1988.

Stevens DL et al: Spontaneous, nontraumatic gangrene due to *Clostridium septicum*. Rev Infect Dis 12:286, 1990.

Sutter VL and Finegold SM: Susceptibility of anaerobic bacteria to 23 antimicrobial agents. Antimicrob Agents Chemother 10:736, 1976.

Thadepalli H: Isolation of *Clostridium* in human infections: evaluation of 114 cases. J Infect Dis 131:S81, 1975.

Weinstein L and Barza M: Gas gangrene. N Engl J Med 289:1129, 1972.

Wilkins TD and Thiel T: Resistance of some species of *Clostridium* to clindamycin. Antimicrob Agents Chemother 3:136, 1972.

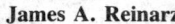

CHAPTER

263 *Neisseria meningitidis* Infections

James A. Reinarz

THE ORGANISM

Characteristics

Neisseria meningitidis (meningococcus) is a gram-negative, nonmotile, nonsporeforming, oxidase-positive, encapsulated coccus. The organism is fastidious and usually requires chocolate blood agar or other enriched media (e.g., Mueller-Hinton) for primary isolation. It is aerobic and grows best on surface plates or in agitated liquid media under 5% to 10% supplemental carbon dioxide at 37° C. Differentiation from *Neisseria gonorrhoeae* and other members of the family Neisseriaceae is based on glucose and maltose metabolism; *N. gonorrhoeae* does not use maltose. Separation of *N. meningitidis* from "nonpathogenic" *Neisseria* sp. requires immunologic (serologic) testing.

Meningococci are divided into subgroups on the basis of their capsular polysaccharide immunogenicity. Most human diseases are caused by *N. meningitidis* groups A, B, and C, although groups X, Y, Z, 29E, and W135 may cause severe and fatal illness.

Virulence factors for meningococci are incompletely understood. The capsular polysaccharide inhibits phagocytosis by polymorphonuclear leukocytes and may be important to intravascular replication. The meningococcal cell wall contains a lipopolysaccharide complex (endotoxin) considered to be one of the primary mediators of tissue injury.

Epidemiology

Serious outbreaks of spinal meningitis have been reported since the 1800s. Epidemic meningococcal disease has been documented in the United States at 7 to 10 year intervals during this century (Chapter 263). Major epidemics occurred during World War I, World War II, the Korean War, and the Vietnam conflict. Meningococcal disease remains a worldwide problem, and major outbreaks are reported regularly from Africa and South America. These epidemics involve thousands of individuals and have high morbidity and mortality rates. Group A *N. meningitidis* remains the primary cause in these areas. Most meningococcal disease in the United States occurs in two populations: young infants and military recruits. Sporadic cases occur in any age group without regard to social status or geographic location.

Until the 1960s most epidemic disease in the United States was caused by group A *N. meningitidis*. In the early 1960s group B emerged as the predominant serogroup. In 1967 to 1968, group C succeeded as the predominant cause of both sporadic and epidemic disease in closed populations, especially military training centers. In the 1980s and early 1990s groups B and C remained predominant, although groups Y and W135 recently have been reported with increasing frequency in Western Europe and the United States. Group Y is commonly associated with pneumonia.

Meningococci are confined entirely to human beings. No animal vectors have been detected. Spread presumably occurs from person to person by aerosol droplets, with subsequent colonization of the nasopharynx. In nonepidemic periods, nasopharyngeal carriage is approximately 5% to 15% but it may approach 60% to 80% in closed populations with or without coexistent meningococcal disease. Nasopharyngeal carriage is almost always asymptomatic. Carriage usually persists for several weeks, although chronic carriers are not uncommon. Nasopharyngeal acquisition is followed in 7 to 10 days by a highly specific serologic response (usually immunoglobulin M [IgM]) to the group-specific polysaccharide of the colonizing strain. Evidence strongly suggests that invasive meningococcal disease is most likely to occur within days of acquisition of a new strain of *N. meningitidis,* that is, before the development of a specific antibody.

Virtually all strains of *N. meningitidis* were once extremely sensitive to commonly employed antimicrobials, including sulfa drugs (sulfadiazine). However, within an extremely short interval during the early 1960s, most group B and group C *N. meningitidis* strains became resistant to sulfa. Unlike in the gonococcus, beta-lactamase production by *N. meningitidis* has been rare, and penicillin-resistant strains are not a clinical problem. However, relatively resistant strains are being documented in Europe and may be a harbinger of future problems.

Pathophysiology

Although acquisition of the organism is an essential antecedent to invasive meningococcal disease, host factors also appear to be extremely important. Invasive or disseminated meningococcal disease occurs almost exclusively in persons who have no measurable specific antimeningococcal bactericidal antibody to the colonizing group of *N. meningitidis*. The importance of this specific antibody-complement bactericidal system is further supported by the occurrence of multiple episodes of group-identical meningococcal disease in persons congenitally lacking terminal complement components C5 to C9, whose serum is thus incapable of complement-mediated bacteriolysis (Chapter 223). Recently an inordinate frequency of meningococcal disease has been described in several kindred with congenital deficiencies in the alternative complement pathway. In addition, susceptible individuals frequently experience a viral or mycoplasmal respiratory illness in the several days preceding bloodstream invasion. In some manner, perhaps secondarily to virus-induced defects in polymorphonuclear leukocyte function, antecedent viral illnesses may predispose to invasive meningococcal disease.

Once bloodstream invasion has occurred, the organism may replicate at an astonishing rate. The resulting disease varies from a transient, benign, almost asymptomatic bacteremia to a devastating, rapidly fatal illness. Few clinical diseases rival the fulminance of meningococcemia; within hours, a patient may deteriorate from good health to irreversible shock, obtundation, marked hemorrhagic diathesis, and death. *N. meningitidis* exhibits marked tropism for the central nervous system, especially the meninges, and skin. Tropism is also apparent for synovial joints, serosal surfaces, and adrenal glands. The most common clinical presentation is a composite of septicemic and meningitic features. Rarely, a relatively benign chronic meningococcemia may result.

Factors determining the clinical expression are poorly understood. Endotoxin is thought to play a role in more fulminant forms. Although endotoxin is difficult to detect and quantitate in vivo, the severity of clinical disease correlates with concentrations of circulating capsular polysaccharide, which is closely bound to the cell wall lipopolysaccharide (endotoxin). Endotoxin activates the clotting and complement cascades and produces extensive endothelial damage, both directly and indirectly (Chapter 233). Circulating tumor necrosis factor has been demonstrated in meningococcemia and may be a major factor in mortality.

Although adrenal involvement occurs frequently with meningococcemia, adrenal insufficiency does not explain the clinical syndromes, the profound shock, or the Waterhouse-Friderichsen syndrome. In fact, serum cortisol concentrations are usually markedly elevated during the illness, and adrenal function remains normal in most patients who recover. Additionally, in some patients who die of the Waterhouse-Friderichsen syndrome, the adrenal glands have been normal morphologically.

CLINICAL SYNDROMES

Nasopharyngeal involvement

Primary meningococcal infections, almost always in the nasopharynx, are usually asymptomatic or indistinguishable from viral coryzal syndromes. Diagnosis is rarely made unless frequent nasopharyngeal cultures are made of individuals at risk during epidemic periods. In most cases, nasopharyngeal colonization is entirely benign and is beneficial because it results in the production of protective bactericidal antibodies. Recently urethritis has been reported and is easily confused with *N. gonorrhea* urethritis.

Meningococcemia

Meningococcemia (alone or in association with meningitis) is the most frequently encountered clinical presentation. Early clinical features are protean, nonspecific, and difficult to distinguish from those of a viral respiratory disease or influenza syndrome (Chapter 245). However, fever (usually in excess of 102° F), chilliness, shaking chills, myalgias, and other systemic symptoms of toxicity appear rapidly.

Skin manifestations are the hallmark of meningococcal disease. A migratory evanescent macular rash, especially over the trunk, is indistinguishable from the "rose spots" associated with typhoid fever. Skin eruptions also may be papular or maculopapular. The macular eruption is subtle and is frequently overlooked by the inexperienced observer. Petechiae, almost universally present, can occur over the entire skin surface but are particularly prominent on the lower extremities, trunk, wrists, and palpebral and bulbar conjunctivae (Plate IV-2). Petechiae may rapidly increase in number and may coalesce to form ecchymoses. Subungual petechiae are unusual, but palmar and plantar petechiae and pustules are common. Unfortunately, the diagnostic value of petechiae is diminished by their frequency in active persons, such as military recruits, and in many other diseases.

Headache, neck soreness, nuchal rigidity, confusion, lethargy, obtundation, and other features of meningeal involvement may be presenting symptoms or may not be manifested for hours or days, if at all (Chapter 233). Alternatively, meningitis may be the predominant clinical expression, with few or subtle suggestions of meningococcemia. In adolescents and adults, purulent meningitis and a petechial rash must be considered to be caused by *N. meningitidis,* although *Haemophilus influenzae* may produce similar clinical features in young children (Chapter 265).

An extensive or progressive petechial or ecchymotic eruption, hypotension, peripheral cyanosis, tachypnea, confusion, and obtundation, especially if present on initial evaluation or developing rapidly, strongly suggests fulminant meningococcemia (Waterhouse-Friderichsen syndrome). Disseminated intravascular coagulation with resultant consumptive coagulopathy produces a marked bleeding diathesis from mucosal surfaces and skin puncture sites. The illness, progressing with astonishing rapidity, may end in death within hours.

Septic arthritis

Migratory arthralgias are common during meningococcemia. Occasionally an isolated septic arthritis may be manifested during or after meningococcemia (Chapter 315). The joint (usually a large joint) becomes erythematous, painful, and tender and develops an effusion. Tenosynovitis, commonly associated with gonococcemia, is unusual.

Myocarditis

Myocardial involvement is frequent in meningococcal disease. A majority of persons who die of meningococcal disease have extensive focal myocarditis. Decreased cardiac output, cardiac dilatation, and electrocardiographic changes occur with sufficient frequency to suggest that myocarditis is common among those destined to survive. Pericardial friction rubs and pericardial effusions may occur during the active disease or during convalescence; during the latter period they probably represent an immunologic reaction. Purulent pericarditis may occur.

Pneumonia

Pulmonary infiltrates are common in meningococcemia produced by the major serogroups, although clinical pneumonia is infrequent. However, with increasing frequency, meningococcal pneumonia is being recognized as a distinct syndrome. The clinical syndrome is similar to other bacterial pneumonias, with fever, chills, cough, pleuritic chest pain, tachypnea, bloody sputum, and occasionally, pleural effusion (Chapter 230). No features are pathognomonic. Group Y *N. meningitidis* is the most frequently implicated serogroup.

Chronic meningococcemia

Chronic meningococcemia is a rare condition of recurrent febrile episodes with petechiae. This entity is often confused with immunologically induced purpuric vasculitides. Blood culture findings are positive during bacteremic episodes, and the disease is promptly eradicated by treatment. Occasionally chronic meningococcemia may suddenly deteriorate into a syndrome similar to acute meningococcemia.

DIAGNOSIS

Definitive diagnosis of meningococcal diseases is made by recovery of *N. meningitidis* from a normally sterile site, such as blood, cerebrospinal fluid (CSF), joint fluid, petechial aspirate, or transtracheal aspirate. A presumptive diagnosis may be made by demonstrating group-specific polysaccharide in serum, CSF, or joint fluid by counterimmunoelectrophoresis (CIE) or by demonstrating gram-negative diplococci in CSF or petechial or buffy-coat smears. Antisera are available commercially for groups A, C, D, and Y. Reliable antiserum is not available for group B, which is responsible for a large percentage of cases in the United States. A positive CIE finding is supportive of the diagnosis; a negative CIE finding has little value. A specific antibody response may be diagnostic during convalescence.

In most cases, treatment must be based on a presumptive clinical diagnosis; to await confirmatory cultures is hazardous. A highly probably diagnosis is reasonably simple in a febrile patient with fulminant meningococcemia or with extensive petechial eruption, nuchal rigidity, and purulent CSF. With more subtle clinical presentations, however, the diagnosis may be extremely difficult. The principal clue is a skin rash, especially if petechiae are prominent. If there is any doubt, the individual should be hospitalized and further evaluated. A progressive petechial eruption is very suggestive. It must be emphasized, however, that not all individuals manifest cutaneous lesions, even with rapidly progressive illness. In these circumstances, the clinician is laboring under a great disadvantage. If meningococcal disease is suspected, cultures should be obtained and therapy started. The polymerase chain reaction (PCR) may permit retrospective diagnosis.

Gram-stained smears of petechial aspirates may be very helpful. These smears are obtained by slightly puncturing or excoriating a fresh petechia with the point of a sterile scalpel blade or a large-bore needle. Care must be taken not to incise deeply into the dermis and produce overt bleeding. The transudate of clear or slightly bloody fluid should be smeared on a glass slide (and applied onto a warmed chocolate blood agar plate for culture) (Chapter 226). Numerous leukocytes and intracellular and extracellular gram-negative diplococci may be seen. Such a finding is strong presumptive evidence of meningococcemia. Negative smear results should be interpreted with caution.

Two or three blood cultures should be obtained at short intervals before treatment. To minimize temperature shock, which might kill the organism, the medium optimally should be at body temperature before culturing. Air should be added to the culture bottle, because *N. meningitidis* is aerobic. Recovery of the organism may be enhanced if the bottle is agitated during incubation and the contents are subcultured to solid media within 12 to 24 hours.

Lumbar puncture is indicated in most, if not all, suspected cases of meningococcemia and all suspected cases of meningitis. If the diagnosis seems highly probable on clinical grounds, however, therapy should not be delayed for results of CSF analysis or lengthy study of petechial or buffy-coat smears. Indeed, in some patients with fulminant disease, institution of therapy should take precedence even over performance of the lumbar puncture.

Other laboratory data offer little support in diagnosis. A leukocytosis with a left shift is common, but normal hemogram findings are not unusual. Neutropenia may occur during fulminant disease. Thrombocytopenia is common and suggests disseminated intravascular coagulation. Decreased PCO^2 and metabolic acidosis secondary to tissue hypoperfusion are frequent. Prolonged prothrombin and partial thromboplastin times and decreased serum fibrinogen level are noted only in severe disease and suggest a poor prognosis.

Differential diagnosis requires one to discriminate among a wide array of viral, bacterial, and rickettsial infections. The more commonly confused entities include the viral exanthemata (rubeola, rubella, ECHO viruses), arthropod-borne encephalitides, Rocky Mountain spotted fever (Chapter 256), endemic typhus, and other forms of pyogenic meningitis.

TREATMENT

Penicillin G administration is the treatment of choice for all forms of meningococcal disease. For adults 10 to 20 million units should be administered intravenously daily; high doses are required to ensure adequate CSF and joint fluid concentrations. For children the dosage of penicillin is 100,000 to 250,000 units/kg/day. Strains of all serogroups are universally sensitive to very low concentrations of penicillin. Therapy should be continued for 7 to 10 days or until the patient has been afebrile for 5 days. For individuals with a known serious allergic reaction to penicillin, 4 g of intravenous chloramphenicol daily is a reasonable alternative. Meningococci are sensitive to first-generation cephalosporins. However, these agents cannot be relied on to yield adequate CSF concentrations. Cefuroxime and several third-generation cephalosporins are effective and achieve high CSF concentrations. Clinical experience with these antimicrobials is very limited. Because of unpredictable sensitivity, sulfonamides should not be considered for treatment. There is no advantage to using combined regimens, and some data suggest that chloramphenicol and penicillin together are less effective than either alone.

Supportive treatment is extremely important (Chapter 239). Adequate replacement of intravascular volume deficits and correction of acidosis and hypoxemia are essential.

Data are contradictory regarding the efficacy of heparin used either prophylactically or in treatment of documented disseminated intravascular coagulation (DIC). Glucocorticoids have no proven value.

Generally, replacement of clotting factors and platelets or the administration of E-aminocaproic acid (EACA) is contraindicated. However, a serious consumptive coagulopathy should be managed in consultation with a hematologist.

Clinical studies to assess the value of high-titer immunoglobulins with antibody to core antigen and to tumor necrosis factor have begun. However, commercially available intravenous immunoglobulin has no documented value in clinical disease. Monoclonal antiendotcxin has been reported to be effective in uncontrolled studies.

PROPHYLAXIS

Family contacts of patients with active meningococcal disease probably are at significant risk of nasopharyngeal colonization and development of meningococcemia. These individuals should receive prophylactic antimicrobial agents that achieve effective concentrations in the nasopharynx. Rifampin is the drug of choice, and 600 mg should be administered every 12 hours for 2 days (for children, 10 mg/kg every 12 hours for 2 days). For pregnant women, ceftriaxone, 125 mg intramusculary administered as a single dose, should be used rather than rifampin. Minocycline is effective, but a high incidence of vertigo is attendant on its use. Even large doses of penicillin, erythromycin, and the various tetracyclines are incapable of eradicating the organism from the nasopharynx and are useless for prophylaxis. Sulfonamides are very effective if the isolate is sensitive; however, sensitivity data may be unavailable when most needed. Several quinolones produce good mucosal concentrations and may emerge as useful prophylactic antibiotics in adults. The value of chemoprophylaxis for persons other than family contacts (e.g., coworkers) is much less certain. Population prophylaxis (e.g., of military personnel) with rifampin rapidly induces rifampin-resistant strains of *N. meningitidis* and cannot be recommended. Prophylaxis of hospital personnel is not indicated unless extensive contact (e.g., through mouth-to-mouth resuscitation) has occurred. The data regarding prophylaxis of school, classroom, and dormitory contacts and coworkers are equivocal. In general, such prophylaxis should be discouraged.

Immunoprophylaxis is a very valuable adjunct in high-risk populations. Purified tetravalent polysaccharide vaccines are available for groups A, C, Y, and W-135. A single injection of 50 μg rapidly induces protective antibody. Until very recently, the vaccine has produced only limited immunogenicity in infants; however, recent modifications offer hope of active immunization of infants who are at highest risk naturally. At present no passive prophylaxis is available, and intramuscular gamma globulin is ineffective. Vaccine should be offered to individuals with splenectomy.

Adult meningococcal disease should stimulate a careful history for meningococcal infection or other fulminating infections in family members. A positive family history or repeated episodes of meningococcal disease mandates an evaluation of both the classic and alternative complement pathways. The hemolytic complement assay (CH_{50}) detects most complement deficiencies and is recommended for screening adults with sporadic infections. Immunization is strongly recommended for those with complement deficiencies.

REFERENCES

Apicella MA: *Neisseria meningitidis*. In Mandell GL, Douglas RG Jr, and Bennett JE, editors: Principles and practice of infectious diseases. New York, 1985, Wiley.

Densen P et al: Familial properdin deficiency and fatal meningococcemia: correction of the bactericidal defect by vaccination. N Engl J Med 316(15):922, 1987.

Ellison RT et al: Meningococcemia and acquired complement deficiency: association in patients with hepatic failure. Arch Intern Med 146(8):1539, 1986.

Gaebler J et al: Prophylaxis of contacts of patients with meningococcal infection. J Indiana State Med Assoc 76(12):828, 1983.

Gardlund B: Prognostic evaluation in meningococcal disease: a retrospective study of 115 cases. Intensive Care Med 12(4):302, 1986.

Giraud T et al: Adult overwhelming meningococcal purpura: a study of 35 cases, 1977-1989. Arch Intern Med 151:310, 1991.

Goldschneider I, Gotschlich EC, and Artenstein MS: Human immunity to the meningococcus. I. The role of humoral antibiotics. J Exp Med 129(6):1307, 1969.

Goldschneider I, Gotschlich EC, and Artenstein MS: Human immunity to the meningococcus. II. Development of natural immunity. J Exp Med 129(6):1327, 1969.

Greenwood BM: Selective primary health care: strategies for control of disease in the developing world. XIII. Acute bacterial meningitis. Rev Infect Dis 6(3):374, 1984.

Halstensen A et al: Antimicrobial therapy and case fatality in meningococcal disease. Scand J Infect Dis 19:403, 1987.

Koppes GM, Ellenbogen C, and Gebhart RJ: Group Y meningococcal disease in United States Air Force recruits. Am J Med 62(5):661, 1977.

Kristiansen BE et al: Rapid diagnosis of meningococcal meningitis by polymerase chain reaction. Lancet 337:1568, 1991.

Lepow ML and Gold R: Editorial retrospective: meningococcal A and other polysaccharide vaccines: a five-year progress report. N Engl J Med 308(19):1158, 1983.

Mellado MC et al: Endotoxin liberation by strains of *N. meningitidis* isolated from patients and healthy carriers. Epidemiol Infect 106:289, 1991.

Moore PS et al: Respiratory viruses and *Mycoplasma* as cofactors for epidemic group A meningococcal meningitis. JAMA 264:1271, 1990.

Paterson PY: *Neisseria meningitidis* and meningococcal disease. In The biologic and clinical basis of infectious diseases. Philadelphia, 1986, Saunders.

Pinner RW et al: Meningococcal disease in the United States—1986. J Infect Dis 164:368, 1991.

Waage A, Halstensen A, and Espevik T: Association between tumour necrosis factor in serum and fatal outcome in patients with meningococcal disease. Lancet 1(8529):355, 1987.

CHAPTER

264 *Neisseria gonorrhoeae* Infections

Edward W. Hook III

THE ORGANISM

Characteristics

Neisseria gonorrhoeae is a gram-negative, oxidase-positive, nonsporeforming coccus; it usually is seen in pairs and causes infection of human mucosal surfaces. The organism is aerobic, grows best at 35° to 37° C and has growth facilitated in 5% carbon dioxide. It may be differentiated from *N. meningitidis* and other *Neisseria* species on the basis of the ability to utilize glucose but not maltose, lactose, or sucrose for growth or by using monoclonal antibody reagents specific for the organism's major outer membrane protein, protein I. Gonococci grow well on supplemented chocolate agar. For isolation from mucosal surfaces colonized by mixed bacterial flora, Thayer-Martin or an alternative medium containing antimicrobials to inhibit growth of other microorganisms is preferred.

On artificial media, gonococcal colonies may take one of three morphologic forms, designated P^+, P^{++}, or P^-

(formerly designated T_1 and T_2, T_3 or T_4, respectively). Forms P^+ and P^{++} are small colonies obtained from patients on primary isolation and contain gonococcal cells covered by surface pili, which enhance attachment to epithelial cells and block phagocytosis by polymorphonuclear leukocytes. The P^- colonial forms are larger and contain less virulent, nonpiliated organisms. P^+ or P^{++} gonococci may give P^- progeny during serial culture.

Gonococcal colonies of each type (P^+, P^{++}, or P^-) may also differ in opacity. Organisms in opaque colonies contain outer membrane proteins, termed *Opa (opacity) proteins,* whereas transparent colonies do not. Opa proteins promote aggregation of gonococci as well as mediating adherence of organisms to mammalian cells. Although opaque and transparent colonies are usually present in the same culture, opaque colonies predominate in men with gonococcal urethritis and in women midway through the menstrual cycle (day 15). Transparent colonies predominate in isolates from women at times other than midcycle and in isolates from blood, synovial fluid, and fallopian tubes in patients with complicated gonococcal infection. Transparent colonies are more resistant than opaque colonies to killing by normal human serum.

Several methods of distinguishing different strains of gonococci have been developed. An auxotyping system that differentiates organisms according to their ability to grow on media lacking nutrients (e.g., certain amino acids and pyrimidines) is widely used and differentiates over 30 different gonococcal strains. There are correlations between (1) auxotypes and differences in cell-surface antigens, and between (2) susceptibility to the bactericidal activity of human serum and the propensity to cause disseminated or asymptomatic disease. More recently, typing systems have been based on antigenic variability of protein I, the major outer membrane of the gonococcus. Early protein I typing systems based on the specificity of absorbed polyvalent antisera have been supplanted by monoclonal antibody–based typing systems, which facilitate use of gonococcal typing for epidemiologic and pathophysiologic studies. Other methods that differentiate gonococci by using pilus and lipopolysaccharide antigens have been developed but are not yet as widely used as the auxotyping and protein I–based systems for epidemiologic studies.

Epidemiology

The true incidence of gonorrhea is unknown because of incomplete reporting, treatment of the disease by nonmedical personnel, and presence of undetected carriers. The reported figures, however, represent less than one half the true incidence of gonorrhea infections.

In the United States, gonorrhea rates peaked in the mid-1970s when more than one million cases per year were reported. Since then, gonorrhea incidence plateaued and subsequently has declined. Infection rates initially fell as a result of factors such as changes in the proportion of the population aged 16 to 24 (the ages at which risk for gonorrhea acquisition is greatest) and the success of national gonorrhea control efforts by the U.S. Public Health Service. Nationwide changes in contraceptive practices away from the oral contraceptive pill (which may slightly increase risk for gonorrhea acquisition) in favor of barrier methods such as diaphragms, spermicidal preparations, and condoms (which reduce risk for gonorrhea) may likewise have contributed to falling rates. More recently, behavioral changes among both heterosexuals and homosexually active men in response to the threat of human immunodeficiency virus infection have probably also contributed to declining gonorrhea rates. From 1981 to 1991 the number of cases of gonorrhea reported fell nearly 37% from 990,864 to 620,478. The impressive decline in gonorrhea rates has not occurred uniformly throughout the population. For instance, gonorrhea rates among adolescents aged 15 to 19 years were unchanged at 1060/100,000 population during both 1981 and 1990.

The disease is almost exclusively transmitted by sexual contact, although perinatal transmission to infants occurs, and transmission by fomites has been described in children under conditions of crowding and poor hygiene. In the United States the highest incidence is in the 16 to 25 year age group, with 85% of patients less than 30 years old. Military personnel, urban dwellers, members of lower socioeconomic classes, homosexual males, and prostitutes all tend to have higher frequencies of gonococcal infections.

The spread of gonococcal disease occurs largely through contact with individuals with asymptomatic or ignored symptomatic infection. It is estimated that one fifth of infected men acquired infection after a single sexual exposure to a female with gonococcal cervicitis. The risk of transmission from infected male to female has not been well studied, but it is probably higher. The proportion of new infections that are asymptomatic probably varies, depending on regional differences in virulence of prevalent strains of gonococci.

Pathophysiology

Primary gonococcal infection in adults occurs almost entirely at sites lined with columnar or transitional epithelium, the mucous membranes of the urethra, cervix, rectum, and pharynx. Although the mode of transmission dictates these areas as primary sites of infection, the gonococcus has a number of characteristics that may facilitate initiation of infection.

Attachment of gonococci to cell surfaces is important in the pathogenesis of gonococcal infection. The presence of extracellular pili appears to be a virulence factor for initiation of gonococcal infections. Pili present on the surface of P^+ and P^{++} colonial variants facilitate attachment to human mucosal cells. Piliated gonococci have a much higher affinity for attachment to mucosal cells than to other human cells (e.g., leukocytes, erythrocytes, or fibroblasts). At least one other class of surface proteins (the Opa proteins) also mediates attachment to mucosal cells. In addition, gonococci produce an extracellular immunoglobulin A1 (IgA1) protease that cleaves secretory IgA1. Secretory IgA has been demonstrated to inhibit adherence of the organism to human mucosal cells. The pathogenetic significance of IgA1 protease production by the gonococcus, however, remains unclear because other types of secretory IgA are produced by patients with gonococcal infection, and the duration of local antibody production is relatively short lived.

Local gonococcal infection elicits an inflammatory response, which, if untreated, leads to formation of fibrous deposits and adhesions. This fibrous scarring is subsequently responsible for many complications, such as urethral stricture or tubal abnormalities, which, in turn, lead to tubal pregnancy and infertility.

Most gonococci that cause disseminated infection display resistance to complement-mediated bactericidal activity of human serum; this differentiates these organisms from the majority of gonococcal strains. Approximately 90% of serum-resistant strains isolated from patients with disseminated infection share the same major outer membrane protein (termed protein I) serotype and auxotype. Thus certain strains, through their resistance to serum bactericidal effects, are more likely to cause disseminated disease.

Under the selective pressure of therapy for gonococcal infections, the organisms have developed two distinct types of antimicrobial resistance. Since the mid-1950s most gonococci causing local disease have demonstrated a stepwise increase in resistance to penicillin. In 1954, 300,000 units of procaine penicillin G reliably cured gonococcal urethritis. Gradually increasing resistance necessitated stepwise increments in dosage up to 1 g of probenecid plus 4.8 million units of procaine penicillin G. In 1989, continued increases in resistance resulted in the decision that penicillin could not be recommended for routine therapy of gonorrhea for the first time since its introduction. This gradually increasing, low-level resistance (most gonococcal isolates in the United States continue to have minimal inhibitory concentrations for penicillin of less than 1 μg/ml) is the result of at least five separate chromosomal mutations resulting in altered susceptibility of the gonococcus to penicillin G. *N. gonorrhoeae* with clinically significant chromosomally mediated resistance to penicillin G are usually also less susceptible to other antimicrobials including tetracycline, erythromycin, and occasionally even spectinomycin.

The second form of gonococcal antimicrobial resistance is plasmid mediated. Gonococci have now been recognized with plasmids mediating high-level resistance to either penicillin or tetracycline. Organisms with plasmids for high-level penicillin resistance produce a beta lactamase that inactivates penicillin. A number of different beta-lactamase plasmids that vary in molecular weight have been described. Several different beta-lactamase plasmids may be found in a single community at the same time. The prevalence of penicillinase-producing gonococci varies from one area of the globe to another. In parts of Southeast Asia, 30% to 60% of gonococcal isolates produce beta lactamase. In the United States, the incidence of infection with beta lactamase–producing gonococci now exceeds 9% of all reported gonorrhea and shows substantial regional variation.

In 1985 gonococci were recognized with minimal inhibitory concentrations of tetracycline equal to or more than 16 μg per milliliter, which contained a conjugative plasmid carrying the tet M gene first described as found in streptococci. These organisms are essentially impervious to clinically attainable serum levels of tetracycline. An increased number of gonococcal isolates throughout the United States have plasmids both for penicillin and for tetracycline resistance.

In 1987, to monitor national trends and geographic patterns of antimicrobial resistance in *N. gonorrhoeae,* the Centers for Disease Control initiated nationwide sentinel surveillance of gonococcal susceptibility. This surveillance program now provides data that allow anticipatory adjustment of gonorrhea treatment recommendations based on laboratory results rather than on observed treatment failures, as was previously the case.

CLINICAL SYNDROMES (See Chapter 238)

Asymptomatic carrier

Although the prevalence of asymptomatic infection varies, asymptomatic carriers are a major source of new gonococcal infections. The belief, however, that gonococcal infection is usually asymptomatic in females and rarely asymptomatic in males is probably incorrect. The symptoms of genital gonococcal infection in women—dysuria, urinary frequency, increased vaginal discharge, and abnormal menses—are often transient and attributed to other causes such as "cystitis" and treated without confirmation. Both *N. gonorrhoeae* and *Chlamydia trachomatis* have been established as important causes of urethritis in young women. Tracing and treating asymptomatic contacts of men or women who have symptomatic, recently acquired gonorrhea is currently the mainstay of control. Routine screening cultures also are recommended during pregnancy and in certain high-risk populations. However, awareness of the symptoms of gonococcal genital infections in women and proper use of diagnostic testing when clinically indicated in patients with characteristic symptoms are equally important.

Gonococcal urethritis in males (See Chapter 238)

In males, the rarity of other urinary tract infections before age 40 justifies the assumption that dysuria in young, sexually active men usually represents sexually transmitted infection. Non-gonococcal urethritis is two to three times as common as gonococcal urethritis in men in the United States. Gonococcal urethritis represents the bulk of gonococcal disease seen in male patients. Clinical disease usually is manifested after a 2 to 7 day incubation period as urethritis with urethral discharge. The discharge is usually purulent but may be clear. Discharge and/or dysuria usually prompt males to seek evaluation and therapy. Untreated, discharge may persist an average of 8 weeks before remitting. Complications such as epididymitis (previously occurring in 5% to 10% of untreated males), prostatitis, and urethral stricture are now uncommon as the result of increased awareness and availability of appropriate therapy.

Gonococcal proctitis in homosexual men

Although many homosexually active men have modified their behavior in response to the epidemic of human immunodeficiency virus, homosexual men with multiple sex partners remain at a significant risk for development of gonococcal proctitis. Gonococcal anorectal infection results from receptive anal intercourse with men who have urethral infection. Anorectal gonorrhea may be asymptomatic or may cause symptomatic proctitis with tenesmus, anorectal pain, bloody rectal discharge, and constipation. Patients with symptomatic proctitis should be evaluated for other sexually transmitted organisms, including syphilis, amebiasis, and *Chlamydia, Campylobacter, Shigella,* and herpes simplex virus infections, as well as for gonorrhea. About 40% of homosexual males with proctitis have anorectal gonorrhea, but it is not unusual to discover several pathogens in patients with symptomatic proctitis. Men who have had receptive rectal intercourse with sex partners who have urethral gonococcal infection should be treated and have cultures made for gonorrhea, irrespective of the presence of symptoms.

Gonococcal infection in females

The usual primary site of gonococcal infection in the female is the endocervix, although organisms also are recovered frequently from the vagina, the urethra, and the rectum. Endocervical infection with *N. gonorrhoeae* or *C. trachomatis* either may be associated with no signs or symptoms or may cause mucopurulent cervicitis, which is manifested by purulent cervical secretions and friability of the cervix. Symptoms in females are often nonspecific and mild; most women with uncomplicated infection probably do note dysuria, frequency, abnormal menstruation, or change in vaginal discharge. About 40% of women with cervical gonorrhea have coexistent *C. trachomatis* infection; concomitant infection with *Trichomonas vaginalis* occurs in about 20% of women with gonorrhea.

Gonococcal salpingitis

The major complication of gonorrhea in women is contiguous spread of infection, which gives rise to salpingitis. This complication occurs in 10% to 15% of untreated women and may result in infertility caused by bilateral tubal obstruction or an increased likelihood of tubal pregnancy. Gonococcal pelvic inflammatory disease (PID) often manifests itself during menses or a few days after the onset of menstruation; clinically, it tends to be more acute than nongonococcal PID. In the United States, about 40% or more of cases of PID are associated with gonococcal infection. Other pathogens implicated as causes of PID include *C. trachomatis, Mycoplasma hominis,* and mixed aerobic-anaerobic infections. The most common presenting symptom of gonococcal salpingitis is relatively acute onset of lower abdominal pain, which is usually bilateral. Other findings may be history of recent dysuria, abnormal vaginal discharge, or abnormal menstruation. Physical examination may show bilateral adnexal tenderness that is worsened by movement of the cervix, and cervicitis, with increased leukocytes in cervical and vaginal secretions. Fever, localized rebound, guarding, and lower abdominal tenderness are also frequently present. The clinical diagnosis of PID is imprecise at best; however, given its sequelae (e.g., sterility, ectopic pregnancy), it is an important consideration in evaluating lower abdominal pain and pelvic tenderness in young women. Fever, leukocytosis, and elevated erythrocyte sedimentation rate, when present with adnexal tenderness and cervicitis, increase the likelihood of PID but need not be present. Infrequently, PID may cause the so-called Fitz-Hugh–Curtis syndrome, a perihepatitis that manifests itself with fever and subacute, pleuritic right upper quadrant pain and tenderness. Chronic right upper quadrant pain may result from "violin-string" adhesions between the liver and the abdominal wall. Both *N. gonorrhoeae* and *C. trachomatis* have been implicated as causes of perihepatitis complicating PID.

Acute gonococcal infection may lead to other local complications as well, the most common of which is acute Bartholin's gland inflammation or abscess. These are manifested as pain and swelling along the posterior third of the labia minora. Chronic Bartholin's gland cysts rarely involve active gonococcal infection. Similar, albeit less frequent, infections may involve the Skene's gland.

Gonococcal pharyngeal infection

Pharyngeal infection occurs in about 20% of persons engaging in fellatio with males with urethral gonococcal infection. Although pharyngeal infection is usually asymptomatic, it may be associated with exudative pharyngitis and cervical adenitis. Pharyngeal gonococcal infection is less common after cunnilingus with infected females.

Disseminated gonococcal infection

Only a very small percentage of gonococcal infections become hematogenously disseminated. Nonetheless, gonococcal arthritis is the most common cause of septic arthritis seen in young persons in the United States. Individuals with disseminated gonococcal infection (DGI) are often unaware of primary genital, oral, or rectal infection and discover their illness with the onset of polyarthritis or skin rash. Unlike patients with other bacteremic illnesses, patients with DGI rarely have high fever, dramatic leukocytosis, or other signs of clinical toxicity; most patients with DGI have temperatures of less than 38° C by mouth and peripheral leukocyte counts of less than $10{,}800/mm^3$. The arthritic component of the syndrome, present in over 75% of DGI, includes tenosynovitis, arthralgia, or purulent arthritis. Joints most commonly involved are knees, ankles, and wrists, but any joint may be involved. Skin rash is frequently seen with gonococcemia as well (Chapter 228). The rash is characteristically described as between 5 and 30 pustules on erythematous bases and located primarily on extremities (Plate IV-3). The rash may present as petechiae, papules, hemorrhagic bullae, or necrotic papules, as well as pustules. Disseminated gonococcal infection may follow an acute or subacute course. The onset in women often occurs with the initiation of menses. Gonococcal endocarditis and meningitis are rare, albeit devastating, complications of gonococcemia.

It is of interest that a single auxotype (requiring arginine, hypoxanthine, and uracil for growth) is associated with the majority of disseminated gonococcal infections in Caucasians and a disproportionate percentage of asymptomatic infections of males. This strain of gonococcus is usually resistant to the complement-mediated bactericidal activity of human serum and is significantly more susceptible to penicillin and tetracycline than are strains isolated from patients with symptomatic uncomplicated genital infection. Recently a number of cases of DGI caused by beta lactamase–producing gonococci (PPNG) or gonococci with chromosomally mediated antibiotic resistance have been reported.

Individuals with inherited deficiency of C5, C6, C7, or C8 components of complement are uniquely predisposed to dissemination of gonococcal and other neisserial infections (Chapter 222). These patients' sera lack bactericidal activity against gonococci, even against those normally sensitive to serum. Although less than 5% of patients with DGI have complement deficiency syndromes, individuals who have multiple systemic gonococcal or meningococcal infections should have serum hemolytic complement activity (CH_{50}) tested to screen for complement deficiency.

GONORRHEA IN PREGNANCY

Retrospective studies show that pregnant women with gonorrhea detected at term are more likely to have premature delivery, a low birth weight infant, delayed delivery after rupture of membranes, and chorioamnionitis.

Gonorrhea in children

During childbirth, infants passing through the birth canal may be infected with gonorrhea. The chief sites of infection in neonates are conjunctiva, pharynx, and anal canal. Gonococcal ophthalmia neonatorum is now largely prevented by routine screening for gonorrhea during pregnancy, by treatment of infected women, and by silver nitrate instillation in eyes of infants at birth. *Chlamydia trachomatis* has replaced the gonococcus as the leading cause of neonatal conjunctival infection and is not prevented by silver nitrate prophylaxis.

Between one year of age and puberty, gonococcal infection is unusual; most cases in this age group are vulvovaginitis in females sexually molested by a household member. For medicolegal as well as diagnostic purposes, complete bacteriologic evaluation is important.

DIAGNOSIS

In males, the diagnosis of gonococcal urethritis often can be made on the basis of Gram stain alone. Gram-negative intracellular diplococci in urethral exudate are virtually diagnostic. The diagnosis of symptomatic gonococcal urethritis by Gram stain can provide 95% sensitivity and 98% specificity. Urethral culture is confirmatory in Gram stain–positive patients and significantly increases diagnostic yield in patients without demonstrable discharge.

In homosexual males, rectal culture should be part of screening procedures. In homosexual males with proctitis, Gram stain is useful for detection of leukocytes (indicative of proctitis or colitis) and may show gonococci or *Campylobacter*. However, anorectal Gram stain smears often are hard to interpret, are not highly sensitive for detection of gonococci, and always should be supplemented by culture for *N. gonorrhoeae*. Patients with symptomatic proctitis should always undergo anoscopy, a simple office procedure. Those without gonorrhea should be investigated for *Chlamydia, Salmonella, Shigella,* and *Campylobacter* species; herpes simplex virus; and amebae, any of which may be present (Chapters 251, 254, 266, 268, and 280).

Pharyngeal cultures for *N. gonorrhoeae* are most useful in patients with DGI or symptomatic pharyngitis incurred as a result of practicing fellatio. The need for routine pharyngeal cultures in other settings is debatable, because most asymptomatic gonococcal infections subside spontaneously without therapy and without complication or further spread.

In testing women patients for gonococcal infection, one cervical culture provides the diagnosis in 80% to 90% of cases. Culture of the rectum and urethra increase yield by less than 5% each. Gram stain of cervical specimens showing gram-negative intracellular diplococci provides 60% diagnostic sensitivity, with over 90% specificity in high-risk populations, but staining alone cannot be relied on in diagnosing genital gonorrhea in women.

Although PID is often a clinical diagnosis, microbiologic studies may support the diagnosis. In women with lower abdominal pain and adnexal tenderness, isolation of *N. gonorrhoeae* and/or *C. trachomatis* from the cervix supports the diagnosis of salpingitis. The clinical value and cost-effectiveness of routine hospitalization and laparoscopy for the diagnosis of salpingitis are debated. Certainly, hospitalization and laparoscopy should be strongly considered in women with suspected PID who have atypical presentation, early pregnancy, or poor response to therapy.

Disseminated gonococcal infection is often a clinical diagnosis as well, with only 50% of patients with suspected DGI having positive blood, joint fluid, skin, or cerebrospinal fluid cultures. A presumptive diagnosis can be made on the basis of appropriate clinical presentation, positive culture for *N. gonorrhoeae* from genital sites, pharynx, or rectum, and significant clinical improvement within 48 hours of beginning therapy. The probability of isolating the organism from blood is highest during the first 48 hours after onset of symptoms. Synovial fluid cultures are more often positive later in the course or when synovial fluid leukocyte counts are in excess of 20,000 per cubic millimeter.

Careful culture techniques significantly increase the likelihood of positive culture findings. Small urethrogenital calcium alginate or dacron swabs on wire shafts are preferred for intraurethral culture in males. Specimens should be inoculated directly onto culture media at the time of collection. Commercially available modified Thayer-Martin medium packaged in small plastic bags to retain carbon dioxide generated after inoculation are cheap and efficient. Biplates containing Thayer-Martin medium and chocolate agar medium without antibiotics are increasingly popular because a variable percentage of gonococci are inhibited by the vancomycin in Thayer-Martin medium (vancomycin concentration should not exceed 3 μg/ml). Blood, synovial fluid, or cerebrospinal fluid should be inoculated into broth medium, but many gonococcal isolates are inhibited by the sodium polyanethol sulfonate (SPS) present in standard blood culture media. This inhibitory effect may be counteracted by addition of 1% gelatin to this medium.

At the present time, nonculture alternatives for diagnosis of gonorrhea based on detection of gonococcal antigens or metabolic products lack the specificity to be useful for diagnosis of cervical or rectal infection. Recently marketed diagnostic tests based on detection of gonococcal nucleic acids have not been fully evaluated but represent a promising alternative to culture for situations in which culture diagnosis is logistically complex.

Serologic tests currently being marketed for gonococcal screening have not been useful because of the inability to determine whether antibodies present represent previous or current infection, because of cross reaction with meningococcal infection, and because of low sensitivity. The predictive value of a positive test result with the serologic tests marketed in the United States up to 1982 was only 5% to 10%. Thus 90% to 95% of patients with "reactive" serologic findings indicated by these tests do not have gonorrhea.

In areas where beta lactamase–producing gonococci or gonococci with high-level, chromosomally mediated antimicrobial resistance are prevalent, culture diagnosis (rather than Gram-stain diagnosis) should be encouraged, and gonococcal isolates should be tested for antimicrobial resistance and for beta-lactamase production.

TREATMENT

Although many gonococci remain sensitive to a variety of antibiotics, including penicillin G, ampicillin, spectinomycin, cefoxitin, trimethoprim-sulfamethoxazole, and several third-generation cephalosporins, the continued development of antimicrobial resistance has resulted in deletion of penicillins from the list of drugs recommended for gonorrhea therapy. Treatment of gonococcal infection should be approached with consideration of efficacy, ease of administration, potential side-effects, and cost. Single-dose therapy is preferable for patients in whom compliance with several days of therapy may be a problem.

In 1989 the Centers for Disease Control issued new guidelines for gonorrhea therapy recommending ceftriaxone 125 to 250 mg for uncomplicated gonorrhea. These regimens have the advantages of proven efficacy for infections caused by gonococci with all currently recognized forms of antibiotic resistance at genital, rectal, and pharyngeal sites. Limited data also suggest that, particularly when given with doxycycline for coexistent chlamydial infection, this regimen is likely to be effective for incubating syphilis.

For patients who cannot receive ceftriaxone, a number of alternative regimens are listed. Although high-level spectinomycin resistance in gonococci has reduced the utility of this drug for gonorrhea treatment in the Far East, only a few infections caused by spectinomycin resistant gonococci have been reported across the United States to date. Other alternative single-dose regimens recommended for treatment of uncomplicated gonorrhea include ciprofloxacin 500 mg po; ofloxacin 400 mg po; norfloxacin 800 mg po; cefotaxime 1.0 g im; ceftizoxime 500 mg im; or cefuroxime axetil 1.0 g plus probenecid 1.0 g, both given orally. Single 400 or 800 mg oral doses of cefixime, an orally active third-generation cephalosporin, are reported to be as effective as ceftriaxone for gonorrhea therapy. Neither spectinomycin nor the quinolones (ciprofloxacin, ofloxacin, or norfloxacin) are active against *Treponema pallidum,* and experience with each of the cephalosporin regimens currently recommended is limited. Therefore repeat serologic testing for syphilis 1 month after treatment is recommended for all patients with gonorrhea. Similarly, none of the currently recommended regimens is effective for coexistent *C. trachomatis* infections. Concomitant treatment for chlamydia of all gonorrhea patients using a single 1 g dose of azithromycin or 7 days of doxycycline, tetracycline, or erythromycin is recommended. As a result of increasing numbers of treatment failures and antibiotic resistance, doxycycline, 100 mg, or tetracycline, 0.5 g, four times daily for 7 days, can no longer be considered as effective for treatment of genital gonococcal infection. However, these drugs are effective in eradicating concomitant *C. trachomatis* infection, which is present in 20% of men and 40% of women with gonorrhea. Treatment of heterosexual patients with uncomplicated gonorrhea using single-dose therapy plus 7 days of doxycycline, tetracycline, or erythromycin for possible *C. trachomatis* coinfection reduces the risk of complications due to chlamydia and is preferred to single-dose therapy alone. Patients with penicillin allergy may be preferred to single-dose therapy alone. Patients with penicillin allergy may be treated with spectinomycin, 2 g im once.

Men with anorectal gonorrhea should receive ceftriaxone or spectinomycin.

All patients treated for acute gonococcal infection should be advised to return in 7 to 14 days for a repeat culture, although the treatment failure rates for patients receiving currently recommended, dual therapy is unknown. In women, rectal as well as cervical culture is important, because 25% of female treatment failures will have only a positive rectal culture. Although the most common cause of recurrent infection is reinfection resulting from failure to locate and treat contacts of the initial case, any gonococci isolated on reculture should be tested for beta-lactamase production.

The therapy of acute gonococcal PID should be directed against gonococci, chlamydiae, facultative gram-negative bacilli, and the anaerobic bacteria associated with the illness, unless differentiation of etiologic agents has been carried out. Although efficacy is unproved, removal of intrauterine devices from women with acute PID is recommended. Patients in whom the diagnosis is unclear, who are unable to comply with outpatient therapy, who are suspected to have pelvic abscess, or who are not responding to outpatient management should be re-evaluated and hospitalized. Hospitalization of all women with PID is desirable to confirm the diagnosis, initiate parenteral therapy, ensure compliance, and monitor the clinical response. Although firm therapy guidelines for PID are not warranted on the basis of available data, the use of antibiotic combinations active against the major pathogens seems reasonable (e.g., cefoxitin plus doxycycline for initial parenteral therapy, until clear-cut clinical improvement occurs, followed by doxycycline 100 mg po twice daily to complete a 10 to 14 day total duration of therapy. Sex partners of all patients with PID should be screened and treated for sexually transmitted diseases.

In general, the organisms causing disseminated gonococcal infection are significantly more sensitive to penicillin and tetracycline than most strains causing symptomatic urethritis. Recently however, DGI caused by gonococci with both chromosomally and plasmid-mediated antimicrobial resistance has been reported. In addition, because of the risk of meningitis, endocarditis, and septic arthritis, patients with disseminated infection should initially be hospitalized and observed. Initial therapy should be 10 to 20 million units of aqueous penicillin G, iv or 3.5 g of oral ampicillin with probenecid, followed by 0.5 g of ampicillin four times daily (Table 264-1). Significant clinical response should occur within 48 hours of initiation of therapy. After clinical improvement, the patient may be followed as an outpatient while he or she is completing a 7 to 10 day course of ampicillin 2 g per day in four divided doses. Patients with high synovial fluid white blood cell counts may require repeated joint aspiration and irrigation to reduce inflammation. Painful joints may be ameliorated in some cases by a brief period of immobilization. As with all gonococcal infections, examination and treatment of the patient's contacts are of great epidemiologic importance.

Table 264-1. Therapy of gonococcal infections in hospitalized patients

Disease	Therapy
Acute salpingitis* (pelvic inflammatory disease)	Optimal therapy for acute salpingitis has not been established. Initial therapy should ideally include agents active against gonococci, chlamydiae, genital anaerobes, *Mycoplasma hominis,* and facultative gram-negative rods
Disseminated gonococcal infection	Ceftriaxone, 1 g im or iv every 24 hr daily until improvement occurs, followed by oral cefuroxime axetil, 500 mg twice daily, or amoxicillin, 500 mg with clavulanic acid three times a day, to complete 7 days of therapy
	or
	Ceftizoxime 1 g iv every 8 h daily until improvement occurs, followed by oral cefuroxime axetil, 500 mg twice daily, or amoxicillin, 500 mg with clavulanic acid three times a day, to complete 7 days of therapy
	or
	Ceftizoxime, 1 g iv every 8 hr daily until improvement occurs, followed by oral cefuroxime axetil, 500 mg twice daily, or amoxicillin, 500 mg with clavulanic acid three times a day, to complete 7 days of therapy
	or
	Spectinomycin 2.0 g im twice daily for 3 days (treatment of choice for disseminated infections caused by penicillinase-producing *N. gonorrhoeae,* or PPNG)

*Certain third-generation cephalosporins (e.g., ceftriaxone, cefotaxime, and cefuroxime) and cefoxitin, which are highly active in vitro against PPNG, are currently being evaluated and will probably prove effective for complicated gonococcal infections caused by PPNG, as well as for penicillin-allergic patients with complicated gonococcal infections.

PREVENTION

At present, useful preventive measures for reducing spread of gonococcal disease are treatment of acute infection, patient education, and careful tracing and treatment of contacts of patients with gonococcal disease. Use of condoms can prevent passage of infection between partners. Vaccines are not available. Prophylactic antibiotics, although effective, are expensive and carry the risk of increasing resistance of gonococci to antibiotics presently in use.

REFERENCES

Boslego JW et al: Effect of spectinomycin use on the prevalence of spectinomycin-resistant and of penicillinase-producing *Neisseria gonorrhoeae.* N Engl J Med 317:272, 1987.

Centers for Disease Control: 1989 Sexually transmitted diseases treatment guidelines. MMWR (Suppl)38:i, 1, 1989.

Centers for Disease Control: Antibiotic-resistant strains of *Neisseria gonorrhoeae:* policy guidelines for detection, management, and control. MMWR 36(Suppl 5): 1987.

Cohen MS and Sparling PF: Mucosal infection with *Neisseria gonorrhoeae:* bacterial adaptation and mucosal defenses. J Clin Invest 89:1699, 1992.

Dallabetta G and Hook EW III: Gonococcal infections. Infect Dis Clin North Am 1:25, 1987.

Eschenbach DA et al: Polymicrobial etiology of acute pelvic inflammatory disease. N Engl J Med 293:166, 1975.

Faruki H et al: A community-based outbreak of infection with penicillin-resistant *Neisseria gonorrhoeae* not producing penicillinase (chromosomally mediated resistance). N Engl J Med 313:607, 1985.

Handsfield HH et al: Epidemiology of penicillinase–producing *Neisseria gonorrhoeae* infections: analysis by auxotyping and serogrouping. N Engl J Med 306:950, 1982.

Handsfield HH et al: Treatment of the gonococcal arthritis dermatitis syndrome. Ann Intern Med 84:661, 1976.

Handsfield HH et al: A comparison of single dose cefixime with ceftriaxone as treatment for uncomplicated gonorrhea. N Engl J Med 325:1337, 1991.

Knapp JS et al: Serologic classification of *Neisseria gonorrhoeae* using monoclonal antibodies directed against gonococcal outer membrane protein I. J Infect Dis 150:44, 1984.

McGee ZA, Johnson AP, and Taylor-Robinson D: Pathogenic mechanisms of *Neisseria gonorrhoeae:* Observations on damage to human fallopian tubes in organ culture by gonococci of colony type 1 or type 4. J Infect Dis 143:413, 1981.

Quinn TC et al: The polymicrobial origin of intestinal infections in homosexual men. N Engl J Med 309:576, 1983.

Upchurch DM et al: Behavioral contributions to acquisition of gonorrhea in patients attending an inner city sexually transmitted disease clinic. J Infect Dis 161:938, 1990.

CHAPTER

265 Infections Caused by *Haemophilus* Species

David T. Durack
John R. Perfect

THE ORGANISMS

Classification

Haemophilus is a genus of small, pleomorphic, nonmotile, facultatively anaerobic coccobacillary gram-negative bacteria, several species of which are commonly present in the normal flora of humans. Encapsulated strains are important human pathogens, especially for young children and some immunocompromised adults.

The major pathogen in this group of organisms is *Haemophilus influenzae* type b, which causes a wide range of infections including pneumonia, bacteremia, meningitis, and cellulitis. This pathogen was isolated and described in 1892 by Richard Pfeiffer, who found it in the upper respiratory secretions of many patients with influenza, hence the name of the species. This led to the erroneous belief that this bacterium caused influenza, which persisted until influenza A virus was identified in the 1930s.

Characteristics

Haemophilus species require accessory growth factors, including heat-stable factor X (derived from hemoglobin) and heat-labile factor V (nicotinamide-adenine dinucleotide [NAD]), for successful cultivation in vitro. These requirements are supplied by special media, such as rabbit blood, Levinthal medium, Fildes enrichment, or chocolate agar. Some species have an absolute or relative requirement for carbon dioxide. These special nutritional requirements, together with the ability of some species to hemolyze blood, are used routinely to identify and speciate *Haemophilus* in the laboratory. Strains can be further subdivided into five biotypes by biochemical tests for indole production, urease, and ornithine decarboxylase. Proper collection of specimens, prompt inoculation into suitable media, and correct decolorization of Gram stains are necessary for isolation and identification of these relatively fastidious organisms. Standard antisera are used to determine whether strains of *H. influenzae* recovered from clinical specimens are type b (discussed later).

Epidemiology

Haemophilus influenzae. Members of the species *H. influenzae* reside only on living hosts, are not found free in the environment, and cause disease only in humans. Strains of *H. influenzae* are present in the normal flora of the nasopharynx of a majority of healthy children and adults. Most of these strains are unencapsulated, and therefore untypable. Of the encapsulated strains, about half are type b. The colonization rate with this type is very low in neonates, rising to approximately 5% in 5-year-olds. Nasopharyngeal colonization itself usually does not cause symptoms, but it provides the source for most cases of invasive disease.

Strains of *H. influenzae* can be found in the vaginal flora of normal women. From this site invasive infection can arise, sometimes as a complication during pregnancy.

The relative frequency of the various kinds of infection at different ages is summarized in Table 265-1. *H. influenzae* has a special predilection for children less than 5 years old, in whom type b strains cause more than 95% of systemic *Haemophilus* infections. Before the introduction of the first of three currently licensed polysaccharide protein conjugate vaccines in 1987, approximately 1 in every 1000 children in the United States less than 5 years of age had systemic *Haemophilus* infection each year. Rates are higher among blacks, native Americans, Eskimos, and children of low socioeconomic status groups. Factors that increase exposure include crowding, presence of young siblings, and attendance at day care centers. Other factors that influence susceptibility of individual children are duration of breast-feeding, parental smoking, and history of recurrent respiratory infections.

In older children and adults, a variety of conditions, including sickle cell anemia, asplenia, agammaglobulinemia, alcoholism, Hodgkin's disease, and acquired immunodeficiency syndrome (AIDS), predisposes to *H. influenzae* infection. The incidence of systemic disease caused by *H. influenzae* in adults in the United States seems to have increased during the past two decades. In one recent study, nearly one quarter of isolates from patients with invasive *Haemophilus* infection were from patients older than 18 years. Whether the overall incidence of systemic infections in all age groups has increased significantly remains controversial because apparent increases may be due more to variable reporting patterns and geographic differences than to real changes. Since the recent introduction of the new conjugate vaccines, the number of invasive infections in young children already has fallen sharply. Definitive assess-

Table 265-1. Relationship between age and the frequency* of major infections caused by *Haemophilus influenzae*

Infection	3 to 24 months	2 to 5 years	5 years and older
Otitis, sinusitis mastoiditis	+++	+++	++
Meningitis	+++	++	+
Bacteremia	+++	++	+
Pneumonia	++	+++	+
Cellulitis	+++	+	Rare
Epiglottitis	+	+++	Rare
Pyarthrosis	++	+	Rare
Endocarditis	Rare	Rare	Rare

*+++, most common; ++, less common; +, occasional.

ment of the long-term impact of these vaccines will have to await the results of prospective studies.

Other species of *Haemophilus*

Renewed interest in isolation and identification of the other species of the genus *Haemophilus* has expanded our knowledge of their ecology and pathogenicity for humans. Many of these species reside in the upper respiratory tract, forming part of the normal flora. *H. parainfluenzae* can be recovered from 10% to 25% of normal children. *H. haemolyticus* and *H. parahaemolyticus* are also commonly present in the upper respiratory tract. *H. aphrophilus* has been recovered from one third of healthy persons, and *H. paraphrophilus* also has been found in the mouths and throats of healthy individuals. These species can be recovered from a wide variety of clinical specimens and sites, and all occasionally may cause invasive infection (Table 265-2). For example, *H. parainfluenzae* can be found in the flora of the throat, vagina, and urethra of adults (2% to 13%) and can be sexually transmitted. When *Haemophilus* species are isolated from infections in soft tissue or bone, or infections related to the genitourinary or gastrointestinal tracts, polymicrobial infection with other bacteria is common.

CLINICAL DISEASES

Pathophysiology and immune responses

The pathogenicity of *H. influenzae* and the host's immune responses to infection with this important pathogen have been studied for nearly a century, but our understanding is not yet complete. The most important determinant of pathogenicity is the outer capsule of these organisms, which is composed of complex carbohydrate polymers. There are six antigenically distinct capsular types (designated a to f), each containing different sugars. Strains possessing the type b capsule, which contains polymers of ribose and ribitol phosphate (PRP), are strikingly more virulent than strains with other capsular types or nonencapsulated (untypable) strains. Nonencapsulated strains often are associated with sinusitis, otitis media, and bronchitis, but they seldom produce invasive, systemic disease such as bacteremia or meningitis except in neonates. Why the great majority of systemic infections are caused by strains with the type b capsule is not fully understood. The proven ability of the polysaccharide capsule to impede phagocytosis by leukocytes presumably is a key factor. Possession of the PRP capsule also favors intravascular survival of this organism.

It can be shown experimentally that the genes that control production of the type b capsule confer greater invasive potential than genes for other capsular types. For example, the gene for PRP, which is located within two 17 kilobase direct repeats in the chromosome of *H. influenzae* type b, can be inserted into a nonvirulent, capsule-deficient type d strain. The transformed type d strain produces capsule, survives better in the bloodstream, and becomes virulent. Genetic studies have also suggested that the lipopolysaccharide is important in enhancing the efficiency of *H. influenzae* translocation from the nasopharynx into the bloodstream. The precise mechanisms governing virulence currently are being studied by molecular techniques.

Infection with *H. influenzae* can result in production of specific bactericidal and anticapsular antibodies. Concentrations of 0.15 μg per milliliter are considered to be protective, whereas 1.0 μg per milliliter indicates long-term protection. Unfortunately, most children less than 2 years of age and a few apparently normal older children fail to produce protective quantities of antibody even after recovering from a major, invasive *Haemophilus* infection such as meningitis. Infants possess some maternal immunoglobulin G (IgG) antibody before 3 months of age and usually develop adult levels of bactericidal and anticapsular antibodies by 3 to 5 years of age. These antibodies are low or absent in the serum of most normal children between 3 months and 3 years of age, the period of greatest susceptibility to invasive *Haemophilus* disease. These observations indicate that bactericidal and anticapsular antibodies play a crucial role in normal host resistance to *H. influenzae*. However, susceptibility cannot always be predicted solely

Table 265-2. Relative frequency* with which *Haemophilus* species are isolated from various sites and clinical specimens

Organism	Blood and/or CSF	Throat† sinuses, ears	Sputum	Pus‡	Endocarditis	Conjunctivitis	Chancroid
H. influenzae (encapsulated)	+++	+	++	++	Rare	−	−
H. influenzae (untypable)	Rare	+++	+++	+	−	−	−
H. parainfluenzae	+	+	+	+	+	−	−
H. haemolyticus and *parahaemolyticus*	+	++	++	Rare	Rare	−	−
H. aphrophilus	Rare	+	+	+	+	−	−
H. paraphrophilus	Rare	+	+	+	+	−	−
H. aegyptius	+§	−	−	−	−	+	−
H. ducreyi	−	−	−	−	−	−	+

*+++, most common; ++, least common; +, occasional; −, does not occur.
†Including epiglottis.
‡Empyema, septic arthritis, pericarditis, ostemyelitis.
§ Brazilian purpuric fever.

on the basis of presence or absence of these antibodies; it is presently believed that other antibodies to nonencapsulated protein antigens, termed antisomatic antibodies, also may contribute to immunity. Another important defense mechanism that matures during the first few years of life is the ability of fixed macrophages of the reticuloendothelial system to clear circulating microorganisms. Notably, patients with anatomic or functional asplenia are several times more susceptible to *Haemophilus* infection, as are patients with human immunodeficiency virus (HIV) infection. The relative importance of cellular immunity and of genetic predispositions (such as IgG subclass II deficiency) to *Haemophilus* infections remains to be defined.

Clinical syndromes

The spectrum of *H. influenzae* infections is wide, and characteristically different at various ages (Table 265-1). Localized lumenal infections of the ears, paranasal sinuses, and bronchi occur in patients of all ages, but invasive infection is overwhelmingly more common in young children than in adults. The median age of children with pneumonia or epigottitis is between 2 and 5 years, which is older than the median age for meningitis and bacteremia.

Meningitis. *H. influenzae* type b is the most common cause of bacterial meningitis in young children (Chapter 233). The organisms originate in the nasopharynx, usually reaching the meninges by way of the bloodstream through the choroid plexus. In some cases, they invade locally, directly from colonized or infected paranasal sinuses or mastoids to the meninges. Cranial trauma with resulting cerebrospinal fluid leak can lead to *Haemophilus* meningitis, although pneumococcal meningitis is more common in this setting. Very young children manifest nonspecific symptoms including fever, vomiting, irritability, lethargy, and anorexia. Signs include somnolence, convulsions, coma, pain on handling or movement, hyperreflexia, cranial nerve pareses, and bulging fontanelles. In older patients, headache and meningismus are more prominent. These manifestations are indistinguishable from those of meningitis caused by *Neisseria meningitidis* or *Streptococcus pneumoniae*.

With modern antibiotic and supportive therapy, overall mortality can be reduced to about 1%. Mortality rate is higher in infants and in those in whom treatment is delayed until coma and/or cardiovascular collapse supervenes. Most patients who survive the first 2 days in the hospital recover, but up to one third suffer permanent sequelae including deafness or reduced intelligence, of varying degree. These defects may not be recognized until long after the acute illness has resolved. In some children, long-term sequelae improve slowly with the passage of time. Children are commonly treated with dexamethasone in addition to antibiotic during the first 2 or 3 days; this appears to reduce the frequency and severity of sequelae in children by mitigating inflammation, edema, and damage mediated by bacteria and cytokines. The value of dexamethasone for treatment of meningitis in adults is unproved.

H. influenzae meningitis is much less common in adults than in children. In contrast to the high frequency of hematogenous seeding in children, in adults the bacteria often reach the meninges by spread from a contiguous focus of infection or site of trauma involving the paranasal sinuses or mastoids. The clinical picture is similar to that found in other common forms of bacterial meningitis.

Bacteremia. In children, bacteremia occurs most often in association with invasive localized disease, such as pneumonia, meningitis, or cellulitis. However, children less than 2 years of age who have fever and leukocytosis may have positive blood culture results for *H. influenzae* despite the lack of any sign of localized infection. These children must be treated and watched closely for later-developing signs of a focus of infection. Although presence of a rash is unusual, in a few children with *H. influenzae* bacteremia a syndrome indistinguishable from acute meningococcemia, including a petechial or purpuric rash, develops.

In adults, *H. influenzae* bacteremia occurs most commonly in association with pneumonia, in patients who are compromised by alcoholism, hypogammaglobulinemia, bronchiectasis, chronic obstructive pulmonary disease, or HIV infection. In asplenic patients, *H. influenzae* can cause fulminant septicemia. Although pneumococci are the most common cause of this syndrome in both children and adults, patients known to be asplenic who have signs of fulminant septicemia should be treated initially for *H. influenzae* as well as *S. pneumoniae* infection until the cause is known (Chapter 260).

Otitis, sinusitis, mastoiditis. Otitis media in children is commonly caused by *H. influenzae*. These usually are untypable strains that may be isolated in mixed culture together with pneumococci (3% of cases) and/or other potential bacterial pathogens, including *Staphylococcus aureus* and anaerobes. In adults, acute maxillary sinusitis and mastoiditis often are caused by nonencapsulated strains of *H. influenzae* together with pneumococci (Chapter 230).

Lower respiratory tract infection. *H. influenzae* type b causes 20% to 30% of bacterial pneumonias in children, and 3% to 5% of those in adults. *Haemophilus* pneumonia cannot be distinguished clinically or radiologically from other bacterial lobar or bronchopneumonias (Chapter 231). Bacteremia occurs in about 20% of patients with *H. influenzae* pneumonia. The prognosis is good for treated cases, except when the patient has serious underlying disease such as chronic obstructive airways disease, or when a complication, for example, empyema, develops. Resolution is usually complete, without abscess formation or parenchymal scarring. The sputum of patients with chronic bronchitis usually contains *H. influenzae, Moraxella,* and pneumococci, but because these potential pathogens colonize the nasopharynx as well as abnormal bronchi, their potential role in pathogenesis or persistence of chronic bronchitis is difficult to confirm. Certainly, antibiotics given for treatment of chronic bronchitis or prevention of recurrences should be active against *Haemophilus* species (Chapter 230).

Cellulitis. Cellulitis of the head or neck in young children is commonly caused by *H. influenzae* (Chapter 235). Buccal, orbital, or periorbital cellulitis may represent a primary infection or may be associated with underlying ear or sinus disease. A characteristic bluish purple color may be present when the cheek is involved. *H. influenzae* type b cellulitis is an invasive infection that may progress to form an abscess or may spread to the meninges. *H. influenzae* rarely causes cellulitis in adults but should be considered in the differential diagnosis of cellulitis of the head, neck, and chest.

Epiglottitis. Epiglottitis is a serious illness that generally has an abrupt onset. Fever, sore throat, and dysphagia with drooling develop, usually in a child aged 2 to 5 years. Stridor with respiratory distress may soon follow, so this condition must be treated as an emergency (Chapter 230). When acute epiglottitis is suspected, the child should be taken quickly to an operating room. There a lateral radiograph of the neck to demonstrate swelling of the epiglottis may be performed to confirm the diagnosis, followed by direct visualization under conditions in which intubation or tracheotomy to secure the airway can be performed at once if necessary. If examination confirms the diagnosis of acute epiglottitis, immediate elective intubation is preferable to observation. Tracheotomy is not needed in most cases because the endotracheal tube can be left in place for several days until the soft tissue swelling resolves during antibiotic treatment. Epiglottitis may occur in adults but is much less common than in children and usually less severe.

Pyarthrosis. Although septic arthritis is less common than the other forms of invasive infection discussed, *H. influenzae* was the leading cause of pyarthrosis in children from 6 months to 2 years of age, before the recent introduction of the conjugate vaccine (Chapter 315). Involvement of a single large, weight-bearing joint is typical. Associated osteomyelitis is rare.

Infection at other sites. Pyogenic local infections (e.g., cholecystitis and osteomyelitis) occasionally are caused by *H. influenzae*. Such infections are clinically indistinguishable from those caused by more common bacterial pathogens. *H. influenzae* is found occasionally in the vaginal flora, giving rise to cases of endometritis, salpingitis, postpartum bacteremia, or neonatal infection. Despite the high frequency of bacteremias caused by this organism, *H. influenzae* endocarditis is rare.

Diagnosis

Recovery of the organism by culture from the blood or cerebrospinal fluid, or from a normally sterile body site such as the pleural cavity or a joint, provides definite evidence of infection. The possible significance of respiratory isolates must be evaluated in light of clinical findings. When *H. influenzae* is isolated from purulent sputum, it should be regarded as a potential rather than a proven pathogen; the natural history of the disease and the response to antibiotic treatment may indicate its significance in individual patients.

Gram stain of the cerebrospinal fluid (Plate V-8) correlates with culture results in about 70% of meningitis cases; the other 30% consist of false-negative and false-positive results in roughly equal numbers. Soluble type b capsular antigen can be detected in body fluids by latex agglutination or staphylococcal coagglutination tests. Detection of *H. influenzae* type b by one of these means may be diagnostically useful in cases of meningitis in which the Gram stain result is inconclusive, or in which antibiotics were started before cultures were taken. However, even these modern tests yield approximately 25% false-negative results, and occasional false-positive findings.

Treatment

H. influenzae is likely to be sensitive in vitro to a variety of antimicrobial agents, including beta lactams, chloramphenicol, tetracyclines, rifampin, sulfonamides, and trimethoprim-sulfamethoxazole (Chapter 224). Ampicillin was reliably effective until 1974, when plasmid-mediated resistance appeared. Since then, these beta lactamase–producing strains have proliferated worldwide. Although wide local variations exist, the overall incidence of ampicillin resistance in the United States has risen to about one third, with a range from 20% to 40%. Type b strains are about twice as likely to be resistant as non–type b isolates. Chloramphenicol, cefamandole, cefuroxime, cefotaxime, ceftriaxone, tetracycline, rifampin, and trimethoprim-sulfamethoxazole usually remain effective, but up to 2% of clinical isolates show resistance to one or more of these first-line drugs. Erythromycin, cephalexin, and sulfisoxazole are less active.

These findings have important implications for treatment. The rate of resistance is high enough in all areas that ampicillin alone should not be used for treatment of serious *Haemophilus* infections. Current practice favors use of a third-generation cephalosporin such as cefotaxime or ceftriaxone as first-line treatment for invasive *Haemophilus* infections in the United States (Chapter 233). The combination of ampicillin 200 to 400 mg/kg/day plus chloramphenicol 100 mg/kg/day remains appropriate as an alternative, but clinicians and microbiologists must be alert for possible multidrug-resistant strains that could cause treatment failure.

For localized infections such as otitis, sinusitis, or mastoiditis, the beta-lactam agents ampicillin, amoxicillin, or amoxicillin plus clavulanic acid usually provide safe and effective treatment. For patients allergic to penicillins or not responding to treatment, alternatives are available in trimethoprim-sulfamethoxazole, cefaclor, or erythromycin plus sulfonamide. These drugs are usually effective against both beta lactamase negative and positive strains. Some failures must be expected with any antibiotic regimen.

Patients with meningitis who remain febrile or suffer a recurrence of fever during treatment may have a complication such as a subdural effusion, drug fever, or nosocomial infection. Provided the organism does not possess primary resistance to the antibiotic used, persistent fever is usually due to causes other than antibiotic failure.

Prevention

Vaccination. Because *H. influenzae* infection is very common in infants and young children, much effort has been expended to develop an effective vaccine. Unfortunately, various earlier PRP vaccines failed to induce protective antibody levels reliably in children less than 18 months of age, the very group that most needs protection. The strategy of conjugating PRP to a protein such as tetanus or diphtheria toxoid has been more successful, conferring 80% to 90% protection against invasive *H. influenzae* disease. Three conjugate vaccines have been licensed in the United States. The Public Health Service Immunization Practices Advisory Committee presently recommends that all children receive conjugate vaccine at 2, 4, and 6 months of age, with a booster dose at 12 to 15 months. Conjugate vaccines should not be considered to double as an immunization against either tetanus or diphtheria, even though they contain toxoids; the normal schedule for diphtheria and tetanus immunization should be followed (see Appendix—Adult Immunization in the United States, p. 2861).

The new polysaccharide-protein conjugate vaccines are immunogenic for patients with Hodgkin's disease and HIV infection. Therefore vaccination of adults known to be at higher-than-normal risk of infection should be considered, although formal recommendations have not yet been issued.

Chemoprophylaxis. Children less than 5 years old who live in the same house or attend the same day care center as an individual who has an index case of invasive *H. influenzae* type b infection are at somewhat increased risk of developing this disease during the next few days (coprimary cases) or weeks (secondary cases). The attack rate in this age group was as high as 5% before the advent of effective vaccines, which is actually higher than the known risk for development of meningococcal infection in contacts of a patient with meningococcal disease. A short course of rifampin may protect these children and may eradicate the carrier state, but the available evidence is not conclusive and the effect of prior vaccination in this setting has not been determined. Prophylaxis with rifampin 600 mg orally twice daily for 2 days is nonetheless recommended for both child and adult family members if there are any children less than 4 years old living in the same household, or less than 2 years old attending day care, in the exposed group. This form of attempted prophylaxis may also be given to children exposed to actual cases (not carriers) in day care centers.

INFECTIONS CAUSED BY OTHER *HAEMOPHILUS* SPECIES

Little is known about specific host defense mechanisms against *Haemophilus* species other than *H. influenzae*. Under most circumstances these species appear to be much less virulent, yet paradoxically they cause infective endocarditis more commonly than either typable or untypable *H. influenzae*. They are sometimes involved in polymicrobial infections arising from oral, respiratory, gut, or genitourinary flora and can act as opportunistic pathogens in compromised hosts.

Haemophilus parainfluenzae

Bacteremia with the *H. parainfluenzae* organism has been associated with endocarditis, pneumonia, epiglottitis, meningitis, pharyngitis, and arthritis. It has been recovered from dental and brain abscesses. *H. parainfluenzae* causes the subacute form of endocarditis; patients may have no history of underlying heart disease. A significant feature of these cases is development of large vegetations, giving rise to a fairly high frequency of major arterial embolization.

Haemophilus aphrophilus and *Haemophilus paraphrophilus*

These species *H. aphrophilus* and *H. paraphrophilus* have been recovered in a variety of infections, including endocarditis, otitis media, sinusitis, laryngoepiglottitis, arthritis, peritonitis, meningitis, pneumonia, empyema, bacteremia, and osteomyelitis. They also have been isolated from brain abscesses and wound infections. An association with malignancy has been noted in approximately one fourth of the reported cases of *H. aphrophilus* infection.

Haemophilus aegyptius

The name *H. aegyptius* is applied to strains of *H. influenzae* isolated from the conjunctival sac, where they may cause an acute contagious conjunctivitis. They are indistinguishable from *H. influenzae* by routine microbiologic tests; special biochemical tests show that they belong in biotype III.

The syndrome of epidemic purpura fulminans in Brazilian children, associated with antecedent purulent conjunctivitis, has been named Brazilian purpuric fever. *H. aegyptius* was isolated from the blood of a high proportion of cases; these strains carried a plasmid not found in isolates from the conjunctivae of children who did not have the septicemia syndrome. A Brazilian study group has concluded that *H. aegyptius* probably causes this syndrome. The onset of *Haemophilus* septicemia follows 3 to 15 days after onset of conjunctivitis, by which time the ocular finding may have resolved. The disease carries a very high fatality rate.

Haemophilus ducreyi

Chancroid is a sexually transmitted disease characterized by painful, sharply demarcated, nonindurated genital ulceration (Chapters 238 and 264). Clinical disease usually appears 2 to 5 days after exposure. Initially, a tender papule forms; this lesion then becomes pustular and ulcerates. A single ulcer is most common, but several lesions may occur. Regional lymphadenitis that is usually unilateral and painful and sometimes involves the overlying skin is common. Chancroid easily can be confused with primary syphilis, herpes genitalis, or lymphogranuloma venereum. The diagnosis is confirmed by demonstration of *H. ducreyi* on smear and culture from the primary lesion or the secondary bubo. Gram-stained preparations should show gram-negative coccobacilli in chains or in a "school of fish" pattern. Culture of material taken from the ulcer or aspirated from the bubo should be placed in freshly clotted blood from the patient or on supplemented chocolate agar, incubated for 14 to 21 days, and subcultured at intervals. Because patients may contract syphilis simultaneously with chancroid, serologic characteristics should be checked after treatment. Genital ulcers promote transmission of HIV; thus chancroid may play a significant role in the epidemiology of AIDS in high-prevalence areas.

Treatment

Ampicillin has been used more than any other antibiotic for treatment of these infections, usually with good results despite the fact that ampicillin-resistant strains of *H. aphrophilus* and *H. paraphrophilus* are common. For endocarditis caused by one of these species, treatment with high-dose ampicillin for 3 to 4 weeks is usually effective, but some cases can be cured only by longer courses and/or valve replacement. Ceftriaxone appears to provide an excellent alternative. Overall mortality rate for endocarditis caused by these organisms is presently about 15%. Addition of an aminoglycoside could result in synergistic antibacterial action, but the potential benefit of combined therapy has not been validated in clinical practice. Unfortunately, it is technically difficult to perform antibiotic sensitivity tests and bactericidal assays on these fastidious, slow-growing organisms. Ampicillin-resistant strains producing meningitis can be treated with chloramphenicol or a third-generation cephalosporin; management of other resistant strains should be guided by in vitro sensitivities. Chancroid is effectively treated with ceftriaxone 250 mg IM in a single dose or erythromycin 500 mg PO qid × 7 days or ciprofloxacin 500 mg bid PO × 3 days. Alternatives are trimethoprim-sulfamethoxazole or amoxicillin/clavulanic acid. Aspiration of a bubo may be therapeutically useful in that it prevents spontaneous rupture and drainage.

Prevention

Most *Haemophilus* species other than *H. influenzae* cause human infection too infrequently to require any specific preventive measures. Identification and treatment of infections with potentially invasive strains may help to limit their spread. Use of a condom should prevent transmission of *H. ducreyi*.

REFERENCES

Bieger RC, Brewer NS, and Washington JA II: *Haemophilus aphrophilus*: a microbiologic and clinical review and report of 42 cases. Medicine 57:345, 1978.

Brazilian Purpuric Fever Study Group: *Haemophilus aegyptius* bacteremia in Brazilian purpuric fever. Lancet 2:757, 1987.

Casadevall A et al: *Haemophilus influenzae* type b bacteremia in adults with AIDS and at risk for AIDS. Am J Med 92:587, 1992.

Chunn CJ et al: Haemophilus parainfluenzae infective endocarditis. Medicine 56:99, 1977.

Dajani AS, Asmar BI and Thirumoorthi MC: Systemic *Haemophilus influenzae* disease: an overview. J Pediatr 94:355, 1979.

Daum RS et al: Epidemiology, pathogenesis, and prevention of *Haemophilus influenzae* disease. J Infect Dis 165(suppl 1):1, 1992.

Doern GV: National collaborative study of the prevalence of antimicrobial resistance among clinical isolates of *Haemophilus influenzae*. Antimicrob Agents Chemother 32:180, 1988.

Eskola J: Efficacy of *Haemophilus influenzae* type b polysaccharide-diphtheria toxoid conjugate vaccine in infancy. New Engl J Med 317:717, 1987.

Granoff DM: *Haemophilus influenzae* type b in a day care center: relationship of nasopharyngeal carriage to development of anticapsular antibody. Pediatrics 65:65, 1980.

Farley MM et al: Invasive *Haemophilus influenzae* disease in adults: a prospective, population-based surveillance. Ann Intern Med 116:806, 1992.

Hand WL: *Haemophilus* species. In Mandell GL, Douglas RG Jr and Bennett JE, editors: Principles and practice of infectious diseases, ed 3. New York, 1990, Wiley.

Istre GR: Risk factors for primary invasive *Haemophilus influenzae* disease: increased risk from day care attendance and school-aged household members. J Pediatr 106:190, 1985.

Morbidity and Mortality Weekly Reports: Recommendations of the Immunization Practices Advisory Committee (ACIP). 40: No. RR-1 and No. RR-12, 1991.

Moxon ER: *Haemophilus influenzae*. In Mandell GL, Douglas RG Jr, and Bennett JE, editors: Principles and practice of infectious diseases, ed 3. New York, 1990, Wiley.

Moxon ER and Kroll JS: Type b capsular polysaccharide as a virulence factor of *Haemophilus influenzae*. Vaccine 6:113, 1988.

Schlamm HT and Yancovitz SR: *Haemophilus influenzae* pneumonia in young adults with AIDS, ARC, or risk of AIDS. Am J Med 86:11, 1989.

Spagnuolo PJ: *Haemophilus influenzae* meningitis: the spectrum of diseases in adults. Medicine 61:74, 1982.

CHAPTER 266 Infections Caused by *Campylobacter* and *Helicobacter* Species

Jean-Paul Butzler

In the last decade certain members of the genus *Campylobacter* have emerged as a cause of human disease. Frequent in animals, particularly in ovines and bovines, campylobacteriosis has been known for more than 40 years as a veterinary disease. The first cases in humans, in a milk-borne outbreak, were described in 1946 by Levy, and organisms resembling *Campylobacter jejuni* were seen in blood cultures from several of the victims. *Campylobacter fetus* ssp. *fetus* was first found in humans by Vinzent, who isolated it from the blood of three pregnant women hospitalized because of fever of unknown origin. In 1957, King was the first to link *Campylobacter jejuni* with enteritis in humans, but her observations were based on only a few cases. The reason for this paucity of reports was that the selective culturing techniques necessary for the isolation of *Campylobacter* were not known at that time. It was not until 1972 that the first successful fecal isolations were reported in Belgium. This was the breakthrough that led to the discovery that *C. jejuni* enteritis is a common disease. The pathology caused by *C. fetus* ssp. *fetus* differs from that caused by *C. jejuni*. *Campylobacter fetus* ssp. *fetus* nearly always attacks debilitated individuals; *C. jejuni* is the most common cause of bacterial diarrhea.

Six *Campylobacter* species of clinical importance have now been described. *C. jejuni* and *C. coli* are by far the most frequently isolated from humans, mostly with enteric disease. These species will therefore be discussed in this review. Since they are almost identical in behavior and epidemiology, wherever the name *C. jejuni* is used in this review the enteric *Campylobacter* species are implicated as well.

Table 266-1. Campylobacter species of clinical importance

Approved name	Site isolated	Pathogenicity
Campylobacter fetus subsp. *fetus*	Blood, various other body fluids	Systemic campylobacteriosis in immunocompromised patients
Campylobacter jejuni	Feces	Acute enterocolitis
Campylobacter coli	Feces	Acute enterocolitis
Campylobacter lari	Feces	Acute enterocolitis
Campylobacter upsaliensis	Feces	Acute enterocolitis
*Campylobacter butzleri**	Feces	Acute enterocolitis

*This species has been shown to belong to the genus *Arcobacter*.

CLASSIFICATION

Campylobacters were originally referred to as "microaerophilic vibrios." It was not until 1963 that their proper taxonomic status was recognized and the genus *Campylobacter* (meaning "curved rod" in Greek) was established. Campylobacters classified in the family Spirillaceae are small, nonsporulating, gram-negative bacteria characterized by a curved, S-shaped, or spiral morphology. They grow only under conditions of reduced oxygen tension, which for different species vary from almost anaerobic to microaerophilic. The cells are highly motile, with a characteristic rapid, darting, corkscrewlike motility. The guanosine-plus-cytosine (G+C) content of the genus *Campylobacter* ranges from 29 to 38 moles percent, which is among the lowest known for bacteria. The *Campylobacter* species important in human pathology are listed in Table 266-1.

EPIDEMIOLOGY

The minimum infective oral dose of *C. jejuni* is approximately 10^3 organisms. In one study the dose needed to initiate illness was only 500 organisms (in milk). Outbreaks do result from contaminated food vehicles (milk, poultry, water) despite the fact that the organism does not grow in such vehicles at ambient temperatures and atmosphere. Campylobacter enteritis is a zoonosis of worldwide distribution, and there may be many pathways by which humans can become infected. *C. jejuni* can be found in the intestines of many animal species, and any raw meat from animals grown for consumption may be contaminated. Most sporadic infections are acquired through the consumption of foods contaminated from raw animal products. Humans may be sources of infection, although spread usually involves young children. Almost all parts of poultry carcasses—whether fresh, chilled, or frozen—can be contaminated with *C. jejuni*. Poultry constitutes the largest potential source of food-borne infection in humans. Infection can be acquired by handling the raw product in the kitchen or by consuming it raw or undercooked. Raw or undercooked beef hamburgers, sausages, and clams, as well as poultry, have been implicated in outbreaks of campylobacter enteritis. Massive outbreaks affecting several thousand persons have been caused by the distribution of raw or inadequately pasteurized milk or inadequately treated water.

CAMPYLOBACTER JEJUNI INFECTIONS

Clinical presentations

Acute enterocolitis, the most common presentation of *C. jejuni* infection, can affect persons of all ages (Chapter 236). *C. jejuni* has been found in virtually every country where it has been sought. Not all campylobacter infections produce symptoms. Asymptomatic excreters commonly occur among the close contacts of infected patients, although their incidence in the total population is less than 1%. The signs and symptoms of a *C. jejuni* infection are not distinct, and it is not possible to differentiate infection by this pathogen from illnesses caused by other pathogens. Symptoms may last for only 24 hours and may be indistinguishable from those associated with viral gastroenteritis. The incubation period is commonly 2 to 5 days, but estimates have extended up to 10 days. In about half of the patients, diarrhea is preceded by a febrile period with malaise, headache, myalgias, and abdominal pain; fever of 104° F (40° C) associated with confusion or delirium may be present. The stools rapidly become liquid and foul-smelling, then watery; fresh blood may appear by the third day. Fecal samples examined microscopically show an inflammatory exudate with leukocytes, and it is usually possible to see numerous campylobacters, owing to their characteristic morphology. Vomiting is rare. The diarrhea persists about 2 or 3 days, but abdominal pain and discomfort may persist after the diarrhea has stopped.

In a significant proportion of patients the infection is manifested as an acute colitis. Sigmoidoscopy usually reveals abnormalities ranging from mucosal edema and hyperemia, either with or without petechial hemorrhage, to mucosal friability. The disease may mimic acute ulcerative colitis. Since treatment with steroids can have serious consequences, it is imperative that the correct diagnosis be established. Severe abdominal pain may mimic acute peritonitis. Occasionally these patients, especially teenagers or young adults, develop peritonitis from acute appendicitis, but in most patients there is actually inflammation of some part of the ileum and jejunum with associated mesenteric adenitis. In young infants diarrhea is commonly mild, but blood may appear in the stools and mimic an intussusception. *C. jejuni* has also been shown to cause infectious proctitis in homosexual men. Erythema nodosum or a reactive arthritis may also complicate *Campylobacter* enteritis. *C. jejuni* meningitis rarely occurs. Urinary tract infection, Reiter's syndrome, and the Guillain-Barré syndrome caused by *C. jejuni* have been reported. Fever mimicking that associated with typhoid is sometimes the sole manifestation of *C. jejuni* infection. The mechanisms by which *C. jejuni* causes disease are not yet known, but the presence of bacteremia and the finding of dysenteric stools suggest that mucosal damage resulting from an invasive process analogous to that seen in shigellosis is important in the pathogenesis of the infection. Preliminary studies have shown that *C. jejuni* produces toxins that are cytotoxic for tissue culture cells, but the role of these toxins as virulence factors is not yet established.

Diagnosis

Campylobacter enteritis can be readily diagnosed by direct microscopic examination of fresh feces. With either a darkfield examination or phase-contrast optical system, campylobacters can be seen and distinguished from other organisms by virtue of their extremely rapid darting and spinning motions. The introduction of selective media has made the diagnosis of campylobacter enteritis a simple procedure for a clinical microbiologist. It is essential to incubate the cultures under conditions of reduced oxygen tension, ideally 5%. The thermophilic nature of *C. jejuni* means that cultures can be incubated to best advantage at 42° C. Although they may also grow well at 37° C, incubation at the higher temperature provides increased selection and quicker results. Campylobacter plates should be examined at 24 to 48 hours for small or mucoid, gray, nonhemolytic colonies. If a suspicious colony is seen, identification begins with a Gram stain. *C. jejuni* is a gram-negative bacillus, which can appear as short curves, S shapes, gull-wing shapes, and long spirals. When the Gram stain appears to be *Campylobacter*-positive, oxidase and catalase tests should be used to confirm the diagnosis; biotyping and serotyping complete further identification.

The disease can also be diagnosed serologically. The great majority of patients develop antibody to Campylobacter during the first few days of illness; the antibody level quickly reaches a maximum titer and then declines during the ensuing few months. In culture-negative cases of *C. jejuni* infection, for example in reactive arthritis and erythema nodosum, serologic diagnosis is useful. A complement-fixation test is commercially available.

Therapy

In general, campylobacter enteritis carries a good prognosis, and the isolation of campylobacters from stools does not warrant chemotherapy. By the time a bacteriologic diagnosis is made, the patient is usually recovering. In the absence of chemotherapy the feces of patients remain positive for about 2 to 7 weeks after the illness. Patients with mild cases excrete the organism for only a few days; occasionally, patients may excrete the organism for longer periods.

If patients are caught in the early stages of the disease or if they are distressed, appropriate chemotherapy is justifiable. Erythromycin has been advocated as the agent of choice for the treatment of campylobacter enteritis. It has excellent in vitro activity, low toxicity, a fairly narrow antibacterial spectrum, and relatively low cost. Resistant strains are on the whole rare and almost confined to *C. coli*. It probably matters little what preparation of erythromycin is given (other than enteric-coated pills). There are theoretical reasons for favoring the stearate, at least for adults. Apart from being acid-resistant and stable, it is incompletely absorbed, so there is the chance of a contact action in the bowel lumen as well as a systemic action in the blood. A dosage of 500 mg twice daily for 5 days has proved satisfactory in practice; higher doses of the stearate are liable to cause acute abdominal pain. Erythromycin ethylsuccinate at 40 mg/kg/d in divided doses is recommended for children. The newer macrolides (roxithromycin, rokitamycin, and clarithromycin) may have a future because of their pharmacologic advantages. Several clinical trials have shown that ciprofloxacin (and other fluoroquinolones) is an efficient treatment for *Campylobacter* enteritis. These drugs are also active against other causes of dysentery and constitute a sensible treatment for enteritis of unknown etiology, as well as for cases in which cultural confirmation of the causative agent is pending. Sensitivity tests should be conducted because erythromycin and tetracycline resistance have been described. In the industrialized countries dehydration caused by *C. jejuni* is infrequent, but fluid and electrolyte replacement are sometimes necessary in infected infants. The best treatment for *C. jejuni* infections in developing countries could well prove to be different.

Factors such as low socioeconomic status and malnutrition may determine the severity of a *C. jejuni* infection and its great prevalence in very young children. Vomiting and watery diarrhea are frequent, and sometimes oral rehydration is required in children. Antibiotics should be reserved for very severe cases. It is certain that education and better hygiene have far greater roles in reducing infections than do antibiotics.

CAMPYLOBACTER FETUS INFECTIONS

Clinical presentation

Since Vinzent described the first case of *C. fetus* infection in 1947, descriptions of 154 additional cases have been published. The most common form of this infection is a pure septicemia without dissemination and splenomegaly. Fever is a constant feature and explains why the organism was isolated from the blood in almost all cases. The pathology is extremely varied and includes pyogenic meningitis and meningoencephalitis, abortion, endocarditis, thrombophlebitis, septic arthritis, and icterus associated with hepatomegaly. *C. fetus* has been isolated from a pustule, pericardial fluid, cerebrospinal fluid, the brain, placental tissue, and the uterus. Bejot, reviewing the literature, distinguished five clinical groups: carditis, meningitis, arthritis, other pyogenic processes, and abortion. The clinical data from the described cases argue for a nonspecific pathology: all syndromes described are a result of bacteremia. *C. fetus* is an opportunistic organism, and its pathogenicity is directly related to its site of action. It chiefly attacks debilitated patients with impaired defenses against infection. A variety of underlying pathologic conditions are described in the literature, including cirrhosis, diabetes, gastrectomy, aplasia of the bone marrow, leukemia, neoplasms, immunosuppression, cardiopathy, Crohn's disease, alcoholism, and tuberculosis. Pregnant women and infants are especially susceptible to *C. fetus* infection.

Therapy

Anecdotal information about the effectiveness of antimicrobial therapy is provided by case reports of campylobacteriosis. In general, chloramphenicol, aminoglycosides, and tetracyclines have seemed to be effective. There are many reports available on temporary therapeutic failures with penicillins, followed by clinical and bacteriologic cures with alternate antibiotics. Death of infected patients is generally caused by aggravation of the underlying pathologic condition. The mortality is higher in patients with meningitis or endocarditis than in those with nonlocalized sepsis.

Epidemiology

The epidemiology of *C. fetus* infection is not well known. *C. fetus* is considered to be zoonosis, but this hypothesis has never been clearly demonstrated. *C. fetus* is an intestinal commensal in cattle, sheep, and poultry, and the possibility that humans are infected by eating contaminated food cannot be excluded.

HELICOBACTER PYLORI INFECTION

Today, there is overwhelming evidence that *Helicobacter pylori* is the major etiologic agent of chronic active (type B) gastritis and that it may further predispose to peptic ulceration. This includes histologic observations, the effect of therapeutic eradication of the organism on the underlying inflammation, challenge studies in human volunteers, experimental models, and possible pathogenetic mechanisms.

Clinical presentation

Studies from Australia, Canada, the United States, and Europe have shown a close correlation between *H. pylori* colonization of the gastric mucosa and clinical histologic gastritis. Evidence exists that *H. pylori* causes the gastritis and is not simply an opportunist harmlessly occupying a favorable ecologic niche. In infected patients the bacteria colonize the surface gastric epithelium (protected by gastric mucus) in enormous numbers. Colonization is associated with thinning of the epithelium and the presence of polymorphonuclear leukocytes. *H. pylori* grows in a near-neutral environment, in close contact with the mucosa, protected from the bactericidal gastric juice. *H. pylori* has a very high urease activity, permitting it to produce ammonium and carbon dioxide ions from urea. Sections of gastric biopsy material show that the organisms lie in the mucus layers covering the epithelium and on the epithelial surface at the intracellular junctions of the mucus-secreting cells. This observation has led to the hypothesis that *H. pylori* has a spiral morphology that enables it to move efficiently in a viscous environment and that the bacteria are attracted to the epithelial surface by the chemotactic influence of preferred metabolites diffusing from the tissue. Colonization of the stomach by *H. pylori* and the presence of gastritis may alter gastric permeability thus enhancing bacterial growth, which in turn could lead to the bulk diffusion of the hydrogen ions necessary for gastric and duodenal ulceration.

Diagnosis

The diagnosis of *H. pylori*–associated gastritis can be made either by histologic or microbiologic examination of gastric biopsy specimens. Several staining methods (Warthin-starry silver stain, hematoxylin-eosin, Gram stain, Giemsa, or fluorescent labeling with acridine orange) have been investigated and found effective for identifying campylobacters. Isolation and identification of *H. pylori* by culture methods are easily achieved, providing that appropriate transport and incubation conditions are respected. Sufficient decontamination of the endoscopes and the biopsy channels must absolutely be obtained to avoid bacterial outgrowth by contaminants. Three to 6 days are necessary for culture because of the slow growth rate of this bacterium. *H. pylori* is a gram-negative, oxidase- and catalase-positive curved or spiral rod that requires a microaerophilic environment for growth. The most peculiar characteristic of this organism is its ability to produce a large amount of urease. This property can be exploited as a rapid presumptive test for diagnosis and may be proposed as a reliable alternative test to culture and direct examination when laboratory facilities are not available. Since endoscopies consume considerable resources, serodiagnostic assays could provide an alternative, or at least a confirmatory, means of diagnosis. Current enzyme-linked immunosorbent assay (ELISA) techniques are sufficiently sensitive and specific to monitor patients presenting at gastroenterology clinics and to eliminate antibody-negative patients from endoscopal investigation, unless they are receiving nonsteroidal antiinflammatory drug therapy or have symptoms of reflux.

Epidemiology

There is still some controversy about the possible intrafamilial spread of *H. pylori*. Drumm et al documented familial clustering of seropositivity for *H. pylori*. They suggested that *H. pylori* is spread by close family contact, but whether this is fecal-oral, oral-oral, or by another route is unclear. In a recent study, Schembri et al compared the prevalence of *H. pylori* in gastroenterologists and gastroenterology nurses with general physicians and the normal population and drew the following conclusion: (1) the prevalence of *H. pylori* antibodies was significantly higher in gastroenterologists when compared with other population groups; (2) the prevalence of *H. pylori* increased significantly with number of years of practice in gastroenterology; and (3) the low incidence of *H. pylori* infection in gastroenterology nurses may be a reflection of their more thorough safety precautions (e.g., the wearing of gowns and gloves, washing of hands). Similar data reported by Mitchell et al lend support to the hypothesis that *H. pylori* is acquired by either fecal-oral or oral-oral transmission.

Therapy

In vitro antimicrobial work continues to be essential in the search for the most appropriate treatment. In vitro *H. pylori* is susceptible to a wide range of antimicrobial agents, including beta-lactams, quinolones, erythromycin, tetracycline, and metronidazole. Vancomycin, sulfamethoxazole, and trimethoprim are not inhibitory. *H. pylori* is susceptible to bismuth but not to cimetidine, sucralfate, or carbenoxolone. Obviously, antagonists of the histamine H_2 receptor are effective in promoting ulcer healing. However, this therapy does not promote healing of the antral gastritis or eradication of *H. pylori*. Residual organisms and the associated gastritis or duodenitis are thought to be responsible for recurrence of the ulcer. Several studies have shown that *H. pylori* was cleared by bismuth salts in 50% to 70% of patients; however, relapse was extremely common, and long-term clearance was achieved in only 30% of patients. Relapse usually occurred within 3 months. The most effective current therapy for *H. pylori* eradication is the combination of a bismuth salt (colloidal bismuth subcitrate or bismuth subsalicylate) with metronidazole (200 to 500 mg three times daily) or tinidazole (500 mg twice daily) in conjunction with either amoxicillin (500 mg three times daily) or tetracycline (250 to 500 mg four times daily). Despite different formulations, doses, and durations of therapy, eradication rates of 65% to 95% have been reported. The duration of bismuth administration is 2 to 4 weeks and of antibiotics 1 to 4 weeks. The optimal formulation of drugs as well as the daily dose and the number of administration times are presently not known and need to be further defined in controlled studies. Factors associated with failed eradication have included poor patient compliance, side effects, and metronidazole-tinidazole resistance of the organism. In such situations, retreatment by multiple-drug regimens, including metronidazole, may fail, and newer therapeutic alternatives are thus needed. Association of omeprazole with amoxicillin and metronidazole was evaluated in France in a group of 20 patients with duodenal ulcer and resulted in eradication of *H. pylori* in 90% of patients 6 weeks after the end of treatment. The use of omeprazole in association with amoxicillin alone or with amoxicillin and metronidazole might be proposed in countries where bismuth salts are not licensed, or perhaps after failure of triple-drug therapy. Controlled studies using well-defined methodology for diagnosis and assessment of follow-up are needed, however, before such therapy is recommended.

REFERENCES

Butzler JP and Oosterom J: *Campylobacter:* pathogenicity and significance in foods. Int J Food Microbiol 12:1, 1991.

Butzler JP et al: *Campylobacter* and *Helicobacter* infections. Curr Opin Infect Dis 5:80, 1992.

George LL et al: Cure of duodenal ulcer after eradication of *Helicobacter pylori*. Med J Aust 153:145, 1990.

Glupczynski Y and Burette A: Drug therapy for *Helicobacter pylori* infection: problems and pitfalls. Am J Gastroenterol 85:1545, 1990.

Goossens H et al: Evaluation of a commercially available second generation immunoglobulin G enzyme immunoassay for the detection of *Helicobacter pylori* infection. J Clin Microbiol 30:176, 1992.

Graham DY et al: The who's and when's of therapy for *Helicobacter pylori*. Am J Gastroenterol 85:1552, 1990.

Lamouliatte H et al: Controlled study of omeprazole-amoxicillin-timidazole versus ranitidine-amoxicillin-tinidazole in *Helicobacter pylori*–associated duodenal ulcers. Rev Esp Enferm Dige 78(suppl I):101, 1990.

Mitchell HM et al: Increased incidence of *Helicobacter pylori* infection in gastroenterologists: further evidence to support person-to-person transmission of *H. pylori*. Scand J Gastroenterol 24:396, 1991.

Rauws EA et al: Cure of duodenal ulcer associated with eradication of *Helicobacter pylori*. Lancet 335:1233, 1990.

Schrembi MA et al: *Helicobacter pylori* prevalence in endoscopy staff. Microb Ecol Health Dis 4:194, 1991.

CHAPTER

267 Infections Caused by *Vibrio* Species

Mary E. Wilson
Richard L. Guerrant

INTRODUCTION

With the re-emergence of cholera in the Americas for the first time in nearly 100 years, this most-feared epidemic disease of the nineteenth century has awakened new concerns about diagnosis, epidemiology, and control of "infections caused by vibrios." After its abrupt appearance in Peru in January, 1991, 391,000 cases and nearly 4000 deaths were reported in 1991 to the Pan American Health Organization, more than the total number reported worldwide over the last 5 years. Cholera has since become a concern throughout the Americas, with cases occurring in most countries in North and South America (including Mexico and the United States). In addition to epidemic cholera, there are other potentially life-threatening *Vibrio* infections associated with seafood or seacoast exposure. The alert physician and knowledgeable microbiologist must sustain a high index of suspicion to promptly treat vibrio infections, as is often required before the microbiologic diagnosis is available (Chapter 236).

THE ORGANISMS

Classification and characteristics

Members of the genus *Vibrio* are short, curved, gram-negative bacilli found commonly in seawater and in salt-water shellfish, fish, and crustaceans in many parts of the world. Historically, *Vibrio cholerae* O1, the organism that causes cholera, has been of primary interest to clinicians and epidemiologists, while other members of the genus were referred to as "noncholera vibrios" (NCV) or "nonagglutinable vibrios" (NAG). Subsequently, many of the NCV group were found also to be pathogenic for humans. Other members of the family Vibrionaceae include *Aeromonas* and *Plesiomonas,* which are also associated with human enteric disease.

Of the 35 recognized *Vibrio* species, at least 13 have been associated with disease in humans. In the laboratory, *Vibrio* species grow on usual media such as blood, chocolate, and Mueller-Hinton agars. They can be differentiated from Enteriobacteriaceae, *Aeromonas,* and *Plesiomonas* because all pathogenic *Vibrio* species are oxidase-positive and all tolerate relatively high salt concentrations and can therefore grow on thiosulfate citrate bile salts sucrose (TCBS) agar. Growth on TCBS agar for culture is recommended whenever *Vibrio* infection is suspected. The potential human pathogens listed in Table 267-1 can be further differentiated by the ability of some species (*V. cholerae* and *V. mimicus)* to grow in only trace concentrations of salt (nonhalophilic), whereas the remaining (halophilic) organisms require at least 0.5% sodium chloride to support their growth.

As one would predict from their growth requirements in vitro, *Vibrio* species are most often isolated from environmental sources in coastal waters, although they have been found in nearly all geographic locations in the United States. Inland the organisms can survive in brackish waters. Infections caused by *Vibrio* species are more common in the warmer months of the year, when aquatic bacterial counts are highest and when people increase their exposure to seawater through recreational habits. The organisms adhere to plankton, and since mollusks and crustaceans filter seawater and retain plankton along with their associated vibrios, vibrio-induced gastroenteritis is commonly associated with a history of ingestion of raw or undercooked shellfish. The seafood most commonly associated with vibrio infection in the United States is raw oysters. Similarly, wound infections caused by vibrios are often associated with a history of exposure of wounds to seawater or of handling sea fish or shellfish. An increased awareness of these infections by physicians, improved isolation techniques, and an in-

Table 267-1. Clinical syndromes seen with *Vibrio* infections

	Watery diarrhea	Dysentery	Septicemia	Wound infection	Otitis
Nonhalophilic					
V. cholerae (O1)	++				
V. cholerae (non-O1)[a]	+	+	±	+	±
V. mimicus[a]	+	+			+
V. albensis[b]				(±)	
Halophilic					
V. parahaemolyticus	+	+	(±)	+	+
V. vulnificus (L+)[a]			++	+	±
V. alginolyticus				+	+
V. fluvialis (EF6)	+	+			
V. furnisii[c]	+				
V. damsela				+	
V. hollisae[a]	+	(±)			
V. metschnikovii			(±)		
V. cincinnatiensis[d]			(±)		
V. carchariae[e]				(±)	

++ = commonly causes life-threatening disease; ± = rarely reported; (±) = one reported case.
[a]Disease is associated with the consumption of raw oysters.
[b]A single case of postoperative endophthalmitis caused by this organism is reported.
[c]Isolated from human stool specimens but not proven to be a pathogen.
[d]Associated meningitis is reported.
[e]Isolated from an infected shark bite wound.

crease in exposure to these aquatic organisms through foreign travel, consumption of raw shellfish, and water-based recreational activities have resulted in an increase in reported *Vibrio* infections over recent years. Additionally, the enlarging population of immunocompromised patients, either undergoing treatment for malignancies or infected with the human immunodeficiency virus, has increased the population of individuals at risk.

Clinical manifestations of *Vibrio* infections fall into one of five categories. *V. cholerae* serogroup O1 is the cause of cholera, the profuse watery diarrheal disease that can rapidly lead to severe dehydration, shock, and death if not promptly treated with adequate rehydration (Chapter 236). The stool characteristically has few or no polymorphonuclear leukocytes and no erythrocytes. Other vibrios may also cause diarrhea, which may mimic the watery diarrhea of cholera or which may present as dysentery with bloody diarrhea and fecal leukocytes on microscopic examination. Extraintestinal syndromes caused by vibrios include primary septicemia (often bacteremia), wound infections, and otitis (media or externa). As outlined in Table 267-1, infections with the different *Vibrio* species tend to manifest characteristic disease patterns. In some cases, pathogenic factors that may account for these differences in clinical manifestations have been identified. For instance, *V. cholerae* O1 is able to adhere to small-intestinal luminal cells and elaborate a potent secretion-inducing enterotoxin, whereas some strains of *V. parahaemolyticus* are more likely to adhere to the colonic mucosa, produce a cytotoxin, and cause local cell destruction and dysentery. The peculiar ability of *V. vulnificus* to cause septicemia may be related to its ability to survive in human serum, in contrast to other *Vibrio* species. The aggressive nature of *V. vulnificus* wound infections may relate to its potent extracellular toxins and enzymes, which cause profuse local cellular destruction. Recognition of characteristic clinical syndromes in the appropriate setting may result in earlier diagnosis and more effective treatment of the various types of *Vibrio* infections.

CHOLERA

Epidemiology

Cholera has been recognized as the cause of epidemic and endemic disease for several centuries, and as the cause of seven multinational pandemics. In the 1850s John Snow linked the development of cholera to the consumption of fecally contaminated water. The etiologic agent *(Vibrio cholerae)* was discovered by Robert Koch in 1884 in Calcutta. Since then *V. cholerae* has been recognized as the cause of endemic disease in Bengal and of several near-global pandemics. Like other vibrios, *V. cholerae* displays flagellar (H) and somatic (O) antigens; *V. cholerae* O group 1 is the cause of cholera. This group can exist as two biotypes, classical and El Tor, both of which can be further divided into three serotypes reflecting differences in O antigens: Ogawa (which expresses the O antigens A and B), Inaba (A and C), and Hikojima (A, B, and C). The Hikojima serotype is rare, but the other two are frequently isolated from infected humans. The two biotypes, El Tor and classical (each of which may include all three serotypes), correspond historically and clinically to human disease syndromes.

The first recognized cholera pandemic began in 1817 in India and Russia. Subsequently there were six major pandemics in the eighteenth and early nineteenth centuries. From 1883 through 1960 the classic biotype of *V. cholerae* dominated both endemic and epidemic disease. After its discovery in 1905, the El Tor biotype caused four outbreaks between 1937 and 1958, which were confined to Indonesia. In 1961 and 1962 the current outbreak of El Tor cholera began in the Celebes Islands and subsequently spread across Asia, the Middle East, Africa, and parts of Europe, constituting the seventh cholera pandemic. The El Tor biotype actually displaced the classic biotype from the endemic regions of cholera along the Ganges River and in Bangladesh. Factors favoring the spread of the El Tor biotype were a lower ratio of cases to carriers and longer viability of the organism in the environment. The classic biotype returned to Bangladesh in 1982 and has replaced El Tor as the predominant endemic strain in that area. However, the El Tor biotype continues to spread with the current pandemic. In 1991, epidemic cholera was reported in Peru, the first occurrence of the disease in South America in over 100 years. Over 320,000 cases have since been reported in Peru, and the disease has spread to other countries in the Americas including Ecuador, Columbia, Brazil, Bolivia, Chile, Venezuela, Mexico, Guatemala, El Salvador, Panama, Honduras, and the United States, among others. Vehicles responsible for spread of the disease have included public water supplies and sewage systems, water used for irrigation with resultant contamination of vegetables, sea water used for bathing, and fresh water crustaceans and shellfish. The nonhemolytic El Tor, Inaba *V. cholerae,* is closely related to the seventh pandemic isolates from Asia and Africa, and is quite different from the *V. cholerae* O1 isolates from the U.S. Gulf Coast noted below.

During the nineteenth century approximately 250,000 Americans died during three cholera epidemics. This was followed by a long disease-free period beginning in 1911 during which cholera was thought to be eradicated from the United States. In 1973, a sporadic case occurred in Texas from an unknown source. Between 1974 and 1985 there were three sporadic cases and 27 outbreak-related cases, including a 1978 outbreak of 11 cases in Louisiana that was attributed to the ingestion of locally harvested crabs. In 1981 there was an outbreak in Texas caused by the ingestion of contaminated rice. This was followed in 1986 by the largest recent outbreak in Louisiana, involving 18 persons and resulting in one fatality. Many of the infected individuals had recently consumed either crabs, raw oysters, or cooked shrimp.

Since 1973, the *V. cholerae* strain implicated in U.S. cholera cases has been a hemolytic toxigenic *V. cholerae* O1 serotype Inaba strain, which contains the phage VcA-3. This strain is identical to *V. cholerae* O1 strains isolated from the Gulf Coast waters; thus it is designated as the Gulf Coast strain. In 1991, however, U.S. Food and Drug Administration researchers isolated from the coastal waters in Mobile Bay, Alabama, a *V. cholerae* O1 serotype Inaba biotype El Tor that does not contain VcA-3. This strain is identical to the seventh pandemic strain by phage type, enzyme electrophoresis, and pulse field gel electrophoresis. Although the strain has not been implicated as a cause of autocthonous cholera in the United States, the isolation from the environment indicates that the potential for spread of cholera within the United States exists. To date, cases of cholera caused by the pandemic strain have been imported by travelers or in seafood either served on airplanes or imported into the United States from countries affected by the pandemic.

The question of a reservoir for cholera between outbreaks is obscure, since no animal reservoir is known. Chronic human carriers of the disease have been described but are rare. *V. cholerae* may actually be able to survive and multiply in the environment and may not require human transmission. Nontoxigenic O1 *V. cholerae* has been isolated from sea water and shellfish, and it may be that *V. cholerae* survives in association with marine life or in seawater sludge. *V. cholerae* O1 produces a chitinase that may facilitate its attachment to the exoskeletons of crabs and shrimp, which contain chitin. Similar to other vibrio infections, cholera is manifested primarily in the summer and early fall months, when environmental water is at its warmest. During outbreaks, water-borne fecal-oral spread is the dominant mode of transmission. Contaminated seafood (crabs, shrimp, raw oysters, and fish) and food contaminated with sea water have been implicated as well.

Pathophysiology

Establishment of cholera involves the ability of *V. cholerae* to pass beyond the acid environment of the stomach, to colonize the small intestine, and to produce its characteristic toxin. A pH of less than 2.4 is vibriocidal, and raising the gastric pH increases an individual's susceptibility to cholera. Thus the ingestion of *V. cholerae* with food, the use of antacids or H_2 blockers, achlorhydria for any reason, or partial gastrectomy decreases the required infective inoculum from 10^8 to 10^3 organisms.

Once past the stomach, *V. cholerae* penetrates the intestinal mucus and actively moves to the small intestinal mucosa, where it adheres and multiplies. On the brush border, the organism produces cholera toxin, which binds via its B subunit to the ganglioside GM_1 present on intestinal cells. Binding of the B subunit to GM_1 is facilitated also by the production of a neuraminidase by the organism, which catalyzes the conversion of higher-order sialo gangliosides to GM_1 and facilitates the binding of cholera toxin. Thus the neuraminidase increases the activity of cholera toxin in vivo. The A subunit is then translocated into the cell, where, by ADP-ribosylating the stimulating G_s-protein, it stimulates the cellular adenylate cyclase to produce cyclic adenosine monophosphate. Cyclic adenosine monophosphate stimulates the net secretion of chloride and decreases absorption of sodium chloride by the mucosal epithelium. Prostaglandin synthesis is also stimulated by choleratoxin and probably also contributes to fluid and electrolyte secretion. The result is the loss of massive amounts of electrolytes and water into the gut lumen, leading to hypovolemic shock, acidosis, and total body potassium depletion. Hypoglycemia may occur, particularly in children, despite the fact that the mechanism for glucose absorption in the gut remains intact. Manifestations of the disease are attributable to severe dehydration and electrolyte imbalance. Stool is isotonic, with sodium and chloride levels slightly lower and potassium concentrations slightly higher than those of serum.

The virulence of *V. cholerae* depends on both its ability to bind to intestinal mucosa and its ability to produce the enterotoxin. Antigens expressed by *Vibrio cholerae* thought to be important for its virulence include the cholera toxin, a secreted hemolysin, and the pilus TcpA, among others. TcpA has been found to facilitate attachment of the organism to intestinal mucosa, an important component of colonization. Furthermore, the ability of strains to produce cholera toxin A subunit, encoded by the gene *ctxA,* and the pilus encoded by *tcpA* are coregulated by the same protein, ToxR. Thus *toxR* expression is probably critical for the expression of virulence.

Natural infection with *V. cholerae* induces some immunity to the disease, as evidenced by the fact that in endemic regions, cholera is most common in children under 5 years, whereas epidemics affect all age groups. Patients who have had cholera develop circulating antibodies to H and O antigens as well as to the cholera toxin, although the presence of antitoxin antibodies is not well correlated with clinical immune status. The development of local immunity in the gut, with the production of *Vibrio*-specific secretory IgA by Peyer's patch lymphocytes, is more likely to be associated with protective immunity than systemic antibodies. Indeed, the importance of local gut immunity provides the basis for recent attempts to develop an oral vaccine that protects humans against challenge with the organism.

Clinical manifestations

Symptoms of cholera may range from an asymptomatic infection or mild diarrhea to a severe dehydrating illness, with death often occurring within hours to several days after the onset of diarrhea. Death resulting from massive fluid loss into the bowel has even occurred before the first watery stool. The syndrome usually begins as painless watery diarrhea, which soon becomes clear and odorless, with a typical "rice water" appearance (Chapter 236). Vomiting may be present, but typically there is little abdominal pain. Symptoms progress quickly because of rapid fluid losses and dehydration. Patients experience thirst and muscle cramps, and their mental status is detached or otherwise depressed. They may progress to shock within hours of the onset of symptoms. Laboratory data often reveal hyperchloremic acidosis and hemoconcentration. Hypoglycemia may occur, especially in children, and may lead to coma or seizures. Finally, either hypokalemia or hyperkalemia may be present; the former may lead to ileus or arrhythmias, and the latter is usually associated with severe acidosis and dehydration. Serious complications of cholera include renal failure secondary to hypoperfusion with acute tubular necrosis, or aspiration of vomitus.

The diagnosis of cholera can often be made on the basis of examination of the stool. Generally, few or no fecal leukocytes or erythrocytes are present, and *V. cholerae* can be detected by dark-field examination in 80% of cases. The organism has a characteristic "shooting star" motility, and it can be immobilized by specific *V. cholerae* antiserum. The sensitivity of the dark-field examination can be enhanced by first incubating stool in bile peptone broth for 8 to 18 hours at 37° C, increasing the yield to 95% of cases. Culture of the stool on selective TCBS media usually yields results within 48 hours. Rapid diagnosis has also been achieved with fluorescent antibody-labeling techniques. Serology is reserved for epidemiologic studies, since a rise in titer occurs too late for practical use in any individual case. Vibriocidal antibodies usually show a fourfold rise by the fourteenth day after the onset of illness, and may remain elevated for up to 2 to 3 months after symptoms subside.

Prevention

The mode of transmission of *Vibrio cholerae* O1 has been shown to be fecal-oral, usually in contaminated water or through the consumption of inadequately cooked or contaminated seafoods. The organism survives in food held at 55–60° C, indicating that great care must be taken in preparation to avoid contamination of foods after cooking. Thus the mainstay of prevention of cholera involves adequate sanitation. In regions where cholera is endemic and municipal water supplies are not adequately chlorinated, avoidance of contaminated water, ice, fruits, and raw vegetables or seafood greatly decreases the risk of disease.

Treatment

Prompt replacement of fluid and electrolytes is essential for the management of patients with cholera. In many instances this can be accomplished orally. The World Health Organization recommends an oral solution containing 3.5 g sodium chloride, 2.5 g sodium bicarbonate, 1.5 g potassium, and 20 g glucose (or 40 g sucrose) per liter of water. If these reagents are unavailable, a solution containing 5 g of sodium chloride and 20 g of glucose (or 40 g of sucrose, or 30 to 80 g of rice powder) per liter has also been shown to be effective. For patients with severe diarrhea (more than 100 ml/kg/day), abnormal mental status, or vomiting, intravenous replacement is advisable. Correction of hypoglycemia may be necessary, and glucose should be administered as an emergency measure if seizures or abnormal mental status are observed.

A historical perspective underscores the effectiveness of adequate oral replacement of fluids in the treatment of cholera. Mortality rates during the six major cholera pandemics of the nineteenth century exceeded 50% in major cities. In regions where recommended treatment with catharsis and blood-letting were practiced, mortality rates rose to over 90%. However, when I.V. fluids were utilized the mortality decreased to 33%, and the inclusion of bicarbonate in I.V. fluids decreased this mortality rate to 15%. The discovery that glucose and sodium transport are coupled in the small intestine, so that glucose accelerates the absorption of salt and water, led to the development of oral rehydration solution by researchers working in Dhaka and Calcutta in the 1960s. Widespread distribution of instructions for oral rehydration and packets of salts and sugar reduced the mortality rate to under 4%, when over 4000 patients were treated for cholera during the Bangladesh War of Independence. Finally, the exemplary response of Peruvian physicians, led by the pediatrician Eduardo Salazar-Lindo, largely averted a potentially disastrous outcome of the current epidemic of cholera in that country. Through the widespread use of oral and I.V. rehydration as well as appropriate use of antibiotics, the mortality rate during the epidemic has been <0.5% in Lima, the epicenter of the epidemic. Mortality rates of less than 5% have been achieved even in remote regions of the jungle in Peru.

Antibiotics have been shown to shorten the duration of diarrhea and to decrease stool output in patients with cholera. A combination of antibiotic therapy with I.V. or oral hydration greatly decreases the duration of disease, and thus the expense of treatment. *Vibrio cholerae* are often resistant to beta lactam antibiotics, and either tetracycline (250 mg orally every 6 hours) or doxycycline (300 mg once or 100 mg b.i.d. for 3 days) is considered the drug of choice in older children and adults. Other agents are also effective, including trimethoprim-sulfamethoxazole and chloramphenicol. Outbreaks of cholera caused by strains resistant to doxycycline, chloramphenicol, gentamicin, and trimethoprim-sulfamethoxazole have been identified in Bangladesh and parts of Africa, sometimes by a plasmid-borne resistance factor. For this reason, antibiotic susceptibility should be tested when possible. The quinolone antibiotics (e.g., ciprofloxacin) may be useful in treatment of resistant strains.

Vaccine development

A vaccine of killed *V. cholerae* in suspension is currently available for intramuscular, subcutaneous, or intradermal administration, but it affords protective immunity in only approximately 50% to 70% of cases and requires a booster every 3 to 6 months. It was previously administered to meet international immunization requirements, but most countries no longer require the administration of this vaccine. Because natural disease confers protection, researchers are concentrating on the development of a vaccine that can be administered orally and stimulate an immune response similar to that in natural infection. Several oral vaccines have recently been tested. One consists of a whole-cell vaccine of killed *V. cholerae* of both biotypes, along with the cholera toxin B subunit. A trial of the latter in Bangladesh revealed 85% efficacy in preventing cholera, but this declined to 50% after 36 months. More recently, genetically engineered live cholera vaccines containing deletions to render them nonpathogenic have also been tested. The *Salmonella typhi* Ty21a vaccine strain expressing *V. cholerae* O antigens was only 25% protective against cholera. In contrast, immunization studies with a *V. cholerae* O1 strain with the toxin subunit deleted resulted in higher levels of protection. However the latter resulted in an unacceptable rate of side effects with mild diarrhea and cramps, and therefore was abandoned. Finally, a vaccine strain in which both the enterotoxin and accessory toxins are deleted (CVD 103) is well tolerated, immunogenic, and protective in preliminary trials. Further studies of this strain for vaccination of populations at risk, including young children, are under way.

As the pandemic of cholera spreads to new areas in the Caribbean and South America, the need to educate peoples in diverse regions on treatment with oral rehydration therapy and antibiotics increases, as does the need to develop an effective vaccine. History teaches us that the pandemic is likely to continue because of contamination of environmental sources such as sea water, seafood, human water supplies, and sewage. An organized and unified approach to the treatment of this disease, such as was effected in Peru, will have tremendous impact in preventing mortality from this disease.

OTHER PATHOGENIC VIBRIOS

Non-O1 *Vibrio cholerae*

Much more common than cholera as a cause of gastroenteritis in the United States is a group of organisms that are genetically identical to *V. cholerae* but do not agglutinate in O group 1 antisera. Called *non-O1 V. cholerae,* these bacteria were previously referred to as *noncholera vibrios* or as *nonagglutinable vibrios,* a misnomer because they do agglutinate in their own specific antisera. A typical disease syndrome is difficult to describe because of a marked variability in the pattern of illness. More than one half of the cases in the literature involve a diarrheal illness, although extraintestinal manifestations also occur. Several outbreaks as well as many sporadic cases have been reported. The spectrum of illness ranges from severe watery cholera-like diarrhea to a dysentery-like syndrome with fever, abdominal pain, bloody diarrhea, and fecal leukocytes (Chapter 236). The severity of the clinical presentation is probably determined by whether an isolate possesses one of a number of virulence factors. Some non-O1 *V. cholerae* produce a cholera toxin–like enterotoxin. Other putative virulence factors include an El Tor–like hemolysin, Kanagawa hemolysin, shigalike toxin, hemagglutinin, and heat-stable enterotoxins. Furthermore the non-O1 *V. cholerae* produce two colony types on agar plates: opaque and translucent. The opaque morphology has been found to be correlated with increased virulence, an increased polysaccharide coat, and resistance to serum bactericidal activity. Some non-O1 *V. cholerae* have been noted to have invasive properties, unlike O1 *V. cholerae*. Treatment of non-O1 *V. cholerae* gastroenteritis consists primarily of fluid replacement. Whether antibiotics are of benefit is unclear. However, invasive disease with bacteremia clearly warrants antibiotic therapy.

Non-O1 *V. cholerae* organisms have been isolated from several extraintestinal sites, including bile, gallbladder, blood, wounds, ear drainage, sputum, and cerebrospinal fluid. Patients infected at these sites frequently are afflicted with an underlying disease such as cirrhosis, malignancy, diabetes, peripheral vascular disease, or conditions resulting in achlorhydria. These organisms are widely distributed in the environment in sea water, sewage, and brackish surface waters, with an increase in environmental isolates and disease prevalence during the warmer months. Non-O1 *V. cholerae* enteritis has been noted in association with the ingestion of undercooked shellfish or untreated surface water. In addition, the organism has been implicated as a cause of diarrhea in travelers to coastal areas such as Cancun, Mexico.

Vibrio parahaemolyticus

Vibrio parahaemolyticus has been recognized since the 1950s as the agent causing 70% of gastroenteritis cases in Japan, and is probably related to the common practice of consuming raw fish. It has also been noted since the 1950s as the cause of numerous outbreaks and sporadic cases of diarrhea and extraintestinal disease along the Pacific, Gulf, and Atlantic coasts in the United States and elsewhere. The organism has been isolated from sea waters during the warmer months and from sediment out of Chesapeake Bay during the winter. Its reservoir is believed to be saltwater fish and shellfish. It has been isolated from environmental samples associated with salt water or sewage in the Pacific Northwest, particularly when the ambient temperature exceeds 20° C. Because of this temperature variation, disease caused by *V. parahaemolyticus* tends to occur in the summer months in temperate climates and the dry season in equatorial regions. Outbreaks are often noted in association with consumption of raw seafood (e.g., raw oysters) or undercooked or poorly handled shellfish, in which the organism is able to multiply as rapidly as every 9 minutes. In addition, *V. parahaemolyticus* has been implicated as a cause of travelers' diarrhea.

Although both severe cholera-like illness and severe dysentery have been reported, *V. parahaemolyticus* gastroenteritis is more often mild and self-limited. Diarrhea, abdominal cramps, nausea, vomiting, headache, and fever are the most common manifestations, with temperatures rarely exceeding 102.5° F (38.9° C). Extraintestinal isolates have most often come from infected wounds, although one case each from blood, ear, and synovial fluid has been reported. Pathogenicity in strains of *V. parahaemolyticus* has been associated with the Kanagawa phenomenon, the ability to produce a hemolysin that can lyse blood in high salt-mannitol agar containing human erythrocytes (Wagatsuma agar). The majority of clinical isolates (96.5%) but very few environmental isolates (1%) exhibit the Kanagawa phenomenon. Virulence depends not only on the production of toxins, but also on the ability to colonize human intestine. There is evidence that *V. parahaemolyticus* pili facilitate binding of the bacteria to human intestinal mucosa. Up to 70% of clinical *V. parahaemolyticus* isolates have recently been found to possess a urease, which may prove to be yet another disease-associated biotype marker.

Vibrio vulnificus

V. vulnificus, also referred to as *lactose-positive (L+) vibrio,* is associated with a higher mortality rate than other *Vibrio* species. In contrast to *V. cholerae* and *V. parahaemolyticus, V. vulnificus* infections are usually extraintestinal. Two distinct clinical syndromes have been noted: primary sepsis and wound infection. The latter may or may not be associated with bacteremia. Primary sepsis occurs almost exclusively in patients with underlying disease, especially hepatic disease (present in 75% in one series), or disorders associated with increased serum iron such as hemochromatosis, hepatitis, or thalassemia major. Less often the syndrome occurs in patients with malignancy or after gastrectomy. The route of acquisition of the organism is usually through ingestion of contaminated food, often raw oysters or raw fish (sushi). These patients are bacteremic with *V. vulnificus,* and in a large portion hypotension is either found on presentation or develops subsequently. Early in the illness metastatic cutaneous lesions are common (75% of cases). Typically, the lesions develop bullae or vesicles and sometimes necrosis; microscopic examination reveals a necrotizing vasculitis. Osteomyelis, peritonitis with associated sepsis, and secondary massive rhabdomyolysis caused by *V. vulnificus* have been reported. Surgery may be required to eradicate localized peripheral lesions. However primary *V. vulnificus* sepsis is associated with a high mortality of around 50% in published series.

In contrast to patients with primary sepsis, wound infections with *V. vulnificus* most often occur in patients without underlying disease. These usually arise in conjunction with a history of exposure of a wound to sea water, or in an injury occurring in the sea. Wounds often progress to vesicles, bullae, and necrosis, and may extend to adjacent areas or cause secondary bacteremia. Surgical debridement is often required to arrest the progressive infection. Many *V. vulnificus* isolates are susceptible to the penicillins, cephalosporins, chloramphenicol, gentamicin, tetracycline, rifampin, and sulfisoxazole. Animal and human studies suggest that tetracycline and an aminoglycoside may be the drug combination of choice, although there are many examples of successful therapy with other agents. Mortality from *V. vulnificus* wound infections is approximately 16% and is closely correlated with the presence or absence of underlying disease.

Although the evidence for gastroenteritis from *V. vulnificus* is limited, the organism has also been isolated from patients with gastrointestinal illness, and many patients with primary septicemia develop diarrhea, nausea, and vomiting before their bacteremic disease. There are also cases that suggest that asymptomatic gastrointestinal *V. vulnificus* infection may serve as the route of entry for primary septicemia. As further evidence for this, almost all patients with primary septicemia have a history of consumption of raw oysters within 24 hours of admission. Alcohol abuse and the consumption of antacids or H-2-blockers may predispose to the development of *V. vulnificus* gastrointestinal infection.

In some studies, over 50% of oyster lots sampled during selected months have been culture-positive for *V. vulnificus*. However, not all individuals ingesting these oysters become infected, illustrating that both bacterial virulence factors and host immune defenses must contribute to the development of symptomatic *V. vulnificus* disease. The extreme pathogenicity of *V. vulnificus* is related to a number of bacterial virulence factors. The organism produces a cytotoxin-hemolysin, an elastolytic protease, a collagenase, and various phospholipases, all of which have been hypothesized to aid in the invasion of this organism into a host. Virulent strains of *V. vulnificus* are surrounded by a capsule that is associated with the production of opaque colonies on culture plates, as opposed to nonvirulent translucent colonies. The capsular antigen in opaque variants enables the organism to resist phagocytosis by neutrophils and to evade the bactericidal activity of human serum, both of which predispose to the development of bacteremia. Finally, the propensity of some patients with liver disease or hemochromatosis to develop primary sepsis probably relates to the ability of encapsulated isolates to use transferrin-bound iron for growth if the transferrin is 100% saturated. The bacteria require high concentrations of iron, and the increased iron load in patients with cirrhosis or hemochromatosis facilitates the growth of the organism in their serum.

Vibrio alginolyticus

The pathogenicity of this organism in humans was not recognized until 1973. Since that time there have been a number of case reports of extraintestinal infections with *V. alginolyticus*. Most commonly reported are wound infections, infected cutaneous ulcers, or otitis. Rare cases of *V. alginolyticus* conjunctivitis and bacteremia in compromised hosts have been reported as well. The majority of wound infections occur after exposure to sea water, and cases of otitis media have been reported in patients with perforated tympanic membranes. In most cases, the infected individuals do not have underlying diseases and are not seriously ill. As with other vibrios, the organism can be cultured from sea water during the warm summer and early fall months.

Vibrio mimicus

Vibrio mimicus is a nonhalophilic species previously classified as biochemically atypical non-O1 *V. cholerae*. It was subsequently found by DNA analysis to constitute a separate species. *V. mimicus* has been isolated primarily from patients with diarrhea, but 13% of clinical isolates are derived from patients with internal or external otitis. The diarrhea is often associated with abdominal cramps, vomiting, and fever. Inflammatory diarrhea occurs in fewer than half of cases. Epidemiologically *V. mimicus* gastroenteritis has been linked to consumption of raw oysters, and otitis usually occurs after exposure to sea water.

Investigators have found a toxin immunologically and biologically similar to cholera toxin elaborated by *V. mimicus,* but this is rare (10% of clinical, 1% of environmental isolates). Examination of *V. mimicus* strains from Bangladesh revealed that 75% of whole cell cultures of patient isolates were cytotoxic according to two assays, but this was not caused by an elaborated enterotoxin. In the same study, 25% of environmental isolates exhibited cytotoxicity as well. Finally, the production of a metalloprotease by *V. mimicus* has been associated with fluid secretion into rabbit intestines. The clinical significance of these cytotoxic and proteolytic activities is as yet unclear.

Vibrio fluvialis and other species

Between 1976 and 1977, 4.9% of patients with diarrhea in Bangladesh (constituting over 500 cases) were found to harbor *V. fluvialis*. These patients often had a severe watery diarrhea with dehydration mimicking cholera, but some were observed to have bloody diarrhea. Seventy-five percent of the patients were proved to have fecal leukocytes, demonstrating its ability to invade the intestinal mucosa. Consistent with this finding, *V. fluvialis* isolates have been found to elaborate enterotoxins. The organism is widely distributed in marine environments in Great Britain as well, and it has been reported in association with wound infections, in addition to gastroenteritis. Other *Vibrio* species (*V. furnisii, V. damsela, V. hollisae, V. metschnikovii, V. cincinnatiensis, V. carchariae,* and *V. albensis*) have also been associated with human disease (see Table 267-1).

Treatment

Most cases of gastroenteritis caused by vibrios other than *V. cholera* O1 are self-limited, and treatment other than fluid and electrolyte replacement is not usually required. Extraintestinal disease such as otitis, conjunctivitis, cellulitis, and bacteremia, however, often require specific antibacterial therapy. Antibiotics effective against most *Vibrio* organisms include tetracycline, doxycycline, chloramphenicol, and the aminoglycosides. The beta lactams may or may not be effective, as indicated by in vitro drug susceptibilities. The quinolones such as ciprofloxacin and norfloxacin are very active in vitro against *Vibrio* organisms, and although there are not many clinical studies to date, it is likely that quinolones will have a role in the treatment of infections caused by these organisms. Whether antibiotics are administered enterally or parenterally should be determined by the severity of the disease. Finally, some cases of wound infection in normal hosts (e.g., caused by *V. damsela*) can be effectively treated with surgical debridement alone and do not require specific antibiotic therapy.

REFERENCES

General

Janda JM et al: Current perspectives on the epidemiology and pathogenesis of clinically significant *Vibrio* spp. Clin Microbiol Rev 1:245, 1988.

Cholera

Almeida RM et al: Vibriophage VcA-3 as an epidemic strain marker for the U.S. Gulf Coast *Vibrio cholerae* O1 clone. J Clin Microb 30:300, 1992.

Attridge S: Oral immunization with *Salmonella typhi* Ty21a-based clones expressing *Vibrio cholerae* O-antigen: serum bactericidal antibody responses in man in relation to preimmunization antibody levels. Vaccine 9:877, 1991.

Carpenter CCJ: The treatment of cholera: clinical science at the bedside. J Infect Dis 166:2, 1992.

Clemens JD et al: Field trial of oral cholera vaccines in Bangladesh: results from three-year follow-up. Lancet 335:270, 1990.

DePaolo A et al: Isolation of Latin American epidemic strain of *Vibrio cholerae* O1 from US Gulf Coast. And McCarthy SA. Toxigenic *Vibrio cholerae* O1 and cargo ships entering Gulf of Mexico. Lancet 339:624, 1992.

Finch MJ et al: Epidemiology of antimicrobial resistant cholera in Kenya and East Africa. Am J Trop Med Hyg 39:484, 1988.

Galen JE et al: Role of *Vibrio cholerae* neuraminidase in the function of cholera toxin. Infect Immun 60:406, 1992.

Glass RI, Libel M, and Brandling-Bennett AD: Epidemic cholera in the Americas. Science 256:1524, 1992.

Herrington DA et al: Toxin, toxin-coregulated pili, and the *toxR* regulon are essential for *Vibrio cholerae* pathogenesis in humans. J Exp Med 168:1487, 1988.

Holmgren J: Pathogenesis and prevention of cholera. Scand J Infect Dis 36(suppl):58, 1982.

Johnston JM et al: Cholera on a Gulf Coast oil rig. N Engl J Med 308:523, 1983.

Khin-Maung-U, and Greenough WB III: Cereal-based oral rehydration therapy. I. Clinical studies. J Ped 118:S72, 1991.

Levine MM: Modern vaccines: enteric infections. Lancet 335:958, 1990.

Lowry PW et al: Cholera in Louisiana. Arch Intern Med 149:2079, 1989.

Migasena S et al: Preliminary assessment of the safety and immunogenicity of live oral cholera vaccine strain CVD 103-HgR in healthy Thai adults. Infect Immun 57:3261, 1989.

Samadi AR et al: Classical *Vibrio cholerae* biotype displaces El Tor in Bangladesh. Lancet 1:805, 1983.

Winner L III et al: New model for analysis of mucosyl immunity: intestinal secretion of specific monoclonal immunoglobulin A from hybridoma tumors protects against *Vibrio cholerae* infection. Infect Immun 59:977, 1991.

Other Pathogenic Vibrios

Arita M et al: Purification and characterization of a new heat-stable enterotoxin produced by *Vibrio cholerae* non-O1 serogroup Hakata. Infect Immun 59:2186, 1991.

Barker WH: *Vibrio parahaemolyticus* outbreaks in the United States. Lancet 1:551, 1974.

Bode RB et al: A new *Vibrio* species, *Vibrio cincinnatiensis,* causing meningitis: successful treatment in an adult. Ann Inter Med 104:55, 1986.

Bonner JR et al: Spectrum of vibrio infections in a Gulf Coast community. Ann Intern Med 99:464, 1983.

Brennt CE et al: Growth of *Vibrio vulnificus* in serum from alcoholics: association with high transferrin iron saturation. J Infect Dis 164:1030, 1991.

Chowdhury MAR, Miyoshi S-I, and Shinoda S: Role of *Vibrio mimicus* protease in enterotoxigenicity. J Diarrhoeal Dis Res 9:332, 1991.

Chowdhury MAR et al: Toxin production by *Vibrio mimicus* strains isolated from human and environmental sources in Bangladesh. J Clin Microbial 25:2200, 1987.

Finch MJ et al: Non-O1 *Vibrio cholerae* infections in Cancun, Mexico. Am J Trop Med Hyg 36:393, 1987.

Gray LD and Kreger AS: Mouse skin damage caused by cytolysin from *Vibrio vulnificus* and by *V. vulnificus* infection. J Infect Dis 155:236, 1987.

Hughes JM et al: Non-cholera vibrio infections in the United States. Ann Intern Med 88:602, 1978.

Ichinose Y et al: Enterotoxicity of El Tor–like hemolysin of non-O1 *Vibrio cholerae*. Infect Immun 55:1090, 1987.

Johnson JA, Panigrahi P, and Morris JG Jr: Non-O1 *Vibrio cholerae* NRT36S produces a polysaccharide capsule that determines colony morphology, serum resistance, and virulence in mice. Infect Immun 60:864, 1992.

Kelly MT and Stroh EMD: Temporal relationship of *Vibrio parahae-*

molyticus in patients and the environment. J Clin Microbiol 26:1754, 1988.

Klontz KC et al: Syndromes of *Vibrio vulnificus* infections. Clinical and epidemiologic features in Florida cases, 1981-1987. Ann Intern Med 109:318, 1988.

Kothary MH and Richardson SH: Fluid accumulation in infant mice caused by *Vibrio hollisae* and its extracellular enterotoxin. Infect Immun 55:626, 1987.

Morris JG: *Vibrio vulnificus*—a new monster of the deep? Ann Intern Med 109:261, 1988.

Morris JG et al: Non-O group 1 *Vibrio cholerae* gastroenteritis in the United States. Ann Intern Med 94:656, 1987.

Nakasone N and Iwanaga M: Pili of a *Vibrio parahaemolyticus* strain as a possible colonization factor. Infect Immun 58:61, 1990.

Pavia AT et al: *Vibrio carchariae* infection after a shark bite. Ann Intern Med 111:85, 1989.

Shandera WX et al: Disease from infection with *Vibrio mimicus*, a newly recognized *Vibrio* species. Ann Intern Med 99:169, 1983.

Shinoda S et al: Inhibitory effect of capsular antigen of *Vibrio vulnificus* on bactericidal activity of human serum. Microbiol Immunol 31:393, 1987.

Spiratanaban A, and Reinprayoon S: *Vibrio parahaemolyticus:* a major cause of travelers' diarrhea in Bangkok. Am J Trop Med Hyg 31:128, 1982.

Tacket CO, Brennen F, and Blake PA: Clinical features and an epidemiological study of *Vibrio vulnificus* infections. J Infect Dis 149:558, 1984.

Tendolkar UM and Deodhar LP: *Vibrio albensis* as a cause of postoperative endophthalmitis. J Infect 20:261, 1990.

Wachsmuth IK et al: Difference between toxigenic *Vibrio cholerae* O1 from South America and U.S. Gulf Coast. Lancet 337:1097, 1991.

CHAPTER

268 Infections Caused by *Salmonella* and *Shigella* Species

Lee W. Riley
Jean W. Pape
Warren D. Johnson, Jr.

SALMONELLA

Classification and characteristics

Salmonellae are gram-negative, nonsporeforming bacilli that belong to the family Enterobacteriaceae. They are distinguished from other members of the family by their biochemical characteristics. Salmonellae are motile, do not ferment lactose or sucrose, but do ferment glucose and mannitol, producing acid and gas. Major exceptions are *S. typhi,* which does not produce gas, and *S. enteritidis,* serotype *gallinarum-pullorum,* which is nonmotile. Salmonella strains, including *S. typhi,* that do ferment lactose have been reported.

Salmonellae have undergone several taxonomical classifications. The Kauffmann-White schema classified salmonellae according to their serologic reactions against polyvalent antisera against their somatic (O) and flagellar (H) antigens. The O-antigens determined their serogroup, which was divided into serogroups A through I. The strains that cause human disease were predominantly in serogroups A through E. These serogroups were divided into more than 2000 serotypes, according to their H antigens. The most recent classification divides salmonellae by their DNA-DNA hybridization patterns into six groups, with most strains that cause human disease in subgroup 1. In this classification, the group Arizona is included in the *Salmonella* genus. Another classification schema divided the genus *Salmonella* into three primary species, *S. typhi, S. cholerasuis,* and *S. enteritidis; S. enteritidis* was divided into over 2000 serotypes. Under this schema, a serotype may be formally designated as *S. enteritidis* serotype *heidelberg,* but by convention and convenience, the strain is named *S. heidelberg*. This latter classification system is still widely used for epidemiological and clinical purposes.

Epidemiology

The salmonella infection incidence data in the United States are derived from a national surveillance program conducted jointly by the U.S. Public Health Service, the U.S. Department of Agriculture, the U.S. Food and Drug Administration, the Association of State and Territorial Epidemiologists, and State Public Health Laboratory Directors. Over 40,000 isolations of salmonellae from humans are reported to the Centers for Disease Control (CDC) each year. However, it has been estimated that these reported isolations represent only 1%-5% of salmonella infections that occur each year. The annual incidence increased by nearly 30% from 15.6/100,000 during 1976-1980 to 20.1/100,000 during 1986-1990 (Fig. 268-1). The peak in 1985 represents a multistate outbreak of *S. typhimurium* from contaminated pasteurized milk. Salmonellosis has a seasonal distribution, with a peak in the summer and fall. There are geographic variations in the distribution of serotypes. In the Northeast and Middle Atlantic states, *S. enteritidis* is more frequently isolated than is *S. typhimurium,* the most commonly isolated serotype nationwide. The age-specific isolation rate is highest during the second month of life (>180/100,000). The ten most commonly isolated *Salmonella* serotypes in 1989 (Table 268-1) accounted for over 70% of the reported cases.

The major reservoirs of salmonella in the United States include poultry (chickens, turkeys, ducks), domestic animals (cattle, swine, sheep, dogs), and wild animals, including reptiles (turtle, lizards, snakes), and insects. Humans are the only natural reservoir for *S. typhi*, the etiologic agent of typhoid fever. Salmonellae are the most common cause of food-borne disease outbreaks in the United States. Massive outbreaks caused by contaminated milk and eggs have been recently reported. Techniques to subtype *Salmonella* strains by their plasmid profiles have shown that a single clone can be disseminated in disparate geographic areas by a limited number of food vehicles, and such clones may not be detected as part of any recognized outbreaks. Nosocomial outbreaks of salmonellosis have become rare in the United States, but are a major problem in large urban cen-

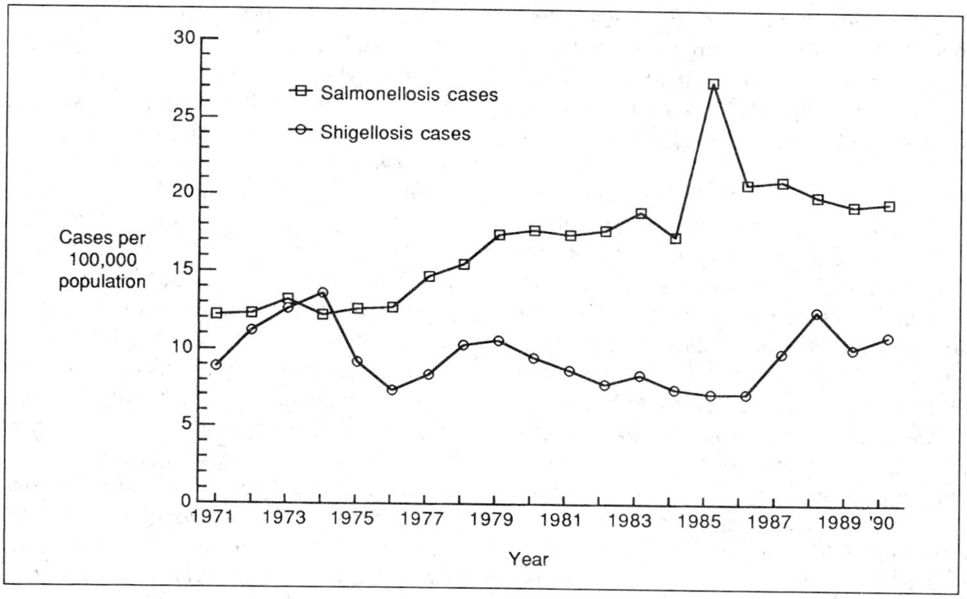

Fig. 268-1. Reported cases of salmonellosis and shigellosis per 100,000 population in the United States, 1971-1990. (Centers for Disease Control: Summary of notifiable diseases, 1990. MMWR 39:55, 1991.)

ters of developing countries. Salmonellae can be transmitted person to person, by fomites, from pets (turtles), and, rarely, by blood products and instrumentation (endoscopy).

Pathophysiology

The consequences of ingesting viable salmonella organisms are determined by host and microbial factors. The determinants of symptomatic infection include the serotype or strain of salmonella, type of vehicle, route of transmission, inoculum, and health status of the host. A large inoculum is usually required to produce disease in healthy subjects. Ingestion of 10^7 *S. typhi* caused typhoid fever in 50% of exposed persons. Volunteer studies have shown that an inoculum of 10^5 organisms produced disease in 28% of subjects, whereas 10^9 organisms produced disease in 95%. However, a smaller inoculum can cause disease if the organism is ingested with foods that buffer the gastric acid (e.g., milk) or if the host has had a gastrectomy or is achlorhydric.

Table 268-1. The ten most frequently reported *Salmonella* serotypes isolated from human sources in the United States, 1989

Rank	Serotype	Number	Percentage
1	*S. typhimurium**	8549	20.5
2	*S. enteritidis*	8340	20.0
3	*S. heidelberg*	4479	10.7
4	*S. newport*	1988	4.8
5	*S. hadar*	1904	4.6
6	*S. thompson*	906	2.2
7	*S. agona*	870	2.1
8	*S. infantis*	842	2.0
9	*S. montevideo*	755	1.8
10	*S. braenderup*	712	1.7
SUBTOTAL		29,345	70.4
TOTAL		41,730	

U.S. Public Health Service: Salmonella surveillance. Annual summary, Atlanta, Georgia, 1989, Centers for Disease Control.
*Includes *S. typhimurium*, var. copenhagen.

Intestinal motility and normal flora are intrinsic defenses of the small intestine. The administration of antimicrobial agents may reduce the inoculum required to produce disease, in part because changes in the normal flora favor multiplication of salmonellae within the intestine. It has also been suggested that a decrease in intestinal motility and a reduced transit time prolong the period of illness and the convalescent carrier state.

Salmonellae produce a wide spectrum of disease. Most strains cause either an asymptomatic infection or self-limited diarrheal illness. However, certain serotypes, such as *S. typhi*, *S. cholerasuis*, and *S. paratyphi* A are frequently associated with bacteremic illness. It is not known what characteristics of the organisms account for these varied clinical manifestations.

Salmonellae are invasive pathogens. The organisms are believed to enter the M-cells in the intestinal mucosa, elicit a polymorphonuclear leukocyte response, and in severe cases, enter the lymphatic system to cause a systemic infection. Although enterotoxin and cytotoxin production in some strains of salmonellae has been reported, the role of a toxin in the pathogenesis of diarrhea has not been definitively demonstrated. The genetic determinants of the virulence factors responsible for penetration of mammalian cells and the inflammatory response elicited by salmonellae have been identified and localized to both chromosomal and plasmid DNA.

The initial events after ingestion of *S. typhi* appear to be similar. However, *S. typhi* evokes a mononuclear cell inflammatory response, and the organisms penetrate to intestinal lymph follicles, mesenteric lymph nodes, and eventually the systemic circulation via the thoracic duct. They are cleared in the bloodstream by mononuclear phagocytes, principally in the liver and spleen. The organism possesses a surface antigen that impedes phagocytosis and killing by serum factors. This antigen has been termed Vi antigen (virulence), and it contributes to the ability of *S. typhi* to survive normal host-defense mechanisms.

Impairment of cellular and humoral immunity predisposes to the development of salmonella bacteremia. The specific mechanisms have not been determined, but it has been shown that patients with salmonella bacteremia have an increased incidence of underlying diseases, including lymphoma, leukemia, and sickle cell disease. There is also an increased incidence of salmonella infection and bacteremia in patients with hemolysis caused by bartonellosis and malaria. Nontyphoidal salmonellosis is one of the most important bacterial infections in patients with acquired immunodeficiency syndrome (AIDS) in salmonella endemic areas.

Clinical disease

The clinical manifestations of salmonella infection are quite varied. Asymptomatic infection is the most common sequela of ingesting salmonellae. When clinical disease develops, it usually takes the form of one of the following syndromes: enterocolitis, enteric or typhoid fever, bacteremia, localized infection, or a chronic carrier state.

Enterocolitis. Gastrointestinal symptoms predominate in two thirds of symptomatic salmonella infections (Chapter 236). *S. typhimurium* is the most common serotype causing intestinal infection in animals and humans. The usual incubation period is 12 to 72 hours, but it varies with the size of the inoculum. Incubation periods of up to 2 weeks have been reported. Nausea, vomiting, and chills are common initial symptoms. They are rapidly followed by colicky abdominal pain, diarrhea, and fever. The severity of the diarrhea ranges from a few loose stools to up to 30 bowel movements daily. The stools are characteristically watery, green, with offensive odor, and have variable amounts of mucus. Depending on the degree of colonic involvement, there may be a dysenteric presentation, with high fever and blood-tinged or frankly bloody mucoid stools. Symptoms usually subside within 5 days but may persist for as long as 2 weeks. The median duration of salmonella fecal excretion is about 5 weeks, with children less than 5 years old having a more prolonged excretion period.

Typhoid or enteric fever. There about 33 million cases of typhoid fever worldwide each year. Enteric fever is a clinical syndrome characterized by fever, headache, prostration, cough, splenomegaly, and leukopenia. Without therapy, the illness is prolonged and associated with serious complications. The classic syndrome is produced by *S. typhi,* and less commonly, by *S. paratyphi* A, B, and C. It is uncommon for other *Salmonella* species to produce this syndrome. The term *typhoid fever* has been applied when the causative organism is *S. typhi,* and the term *paratyphoid fever* is used when *S. paratyphi* is implicated.

The incubation period of typhoid is usually 7 to 14 days. There is an inverse relationship between the inoculum size and the incubation period, with the latter ranging from 3 to 60 days. The onset of illness is usually insidious. Fever is the earliest indication of disease. The temperature usually remains elevated, but a remittent pattern may occur. Rigors and sweats are uncommon before initiation of antibiotic therapy. A dull headache invariably accompanies the fever. Right lower quadrant or diffuse lower abdominal pain is frequent. Relative bradycardia is present in up to 75% of patients during the first 2 weeks of illness. Erythematous maculopapular lesions 2 to 4 mm in diameter that blanch on pressure and are referred to as *rose spots* may appear on the upper abdomen and lower thorax during the first or second week of illness. Rose spots usually appear in crops of 10 or fewer lesions and resolve in hours or days. They are present in less than one half of typhoid fever patients and may not be visible in dark-skinned individuals. Hepatomegaly and splenomegaly are detectable in one third and one half of patients, respectively. Cough is present in one third of patients, and nausea, vomiting, and diarrhea occur in up to one half of patients. Some patients may have constipation as their most prominent gastrointestinal complaint.

In the preantibiotic era, patients either slowly recovered or developed serious complications during the third and fourth week of illness. Mortality rates were 10% to 15%, with intestinal hemorrhage (5% to 20%) or perforation (2% to 5%) as the most serious complications. Other significant complications include myocarditis, hepatitis, bone marrow suppression, and localized infection (meningitis, osteomyelitis, endocarditis, arthritis). The mortality rate in typhoid fever is now less than 1% with appropriate antimicrobial therapy and supportive care. The incidence of hemorrhage and perforation is about 1%.

Relapse occurs in 5% to 10% of untreated patients and in 15% to 20% of patients receiving chloramphenicol. The symptoms in relapse are usually milder than those of the initial illness and begin about 2 weeks after discontinuation of the antimicrobial therapy. The incidence of relapse does not appear to be increased in patients treated with either ampicillin or trimethoprim-sufamethoxazole. The mechanism by which chloramphenicol therapy increases the relapse rate is not known.

A chronic intestinal carrier state, defined as documented fecal excretion of *S. typhi* for a minimum period of 1 year, is observed in 1% to 3% of typhoid fever patients. The gallbladder is the site of persistent intestinal infection, and this carrier state is asymptomatic.

Bacteremia. Bacteremia is a constant feature of *S. typhi* infection, and blood cultures are positive in at least 90% of typhoid fever patients. *S. cholerasuis* infections are associated with bacteremia in 50% of cases. In contrast, less than 5% of patients with infection caused by other *Salmonella* organisms have positive blood cultures. Salmonella infection in these patients may be manifested only by fever and positive blood cultures, and not by the usual gastrointestinal symptoms. When bacteremia does occur in this group, it is most common in very young or elderly persons and in patients with underlying diseases such as cirrhosis, hemolysis, and hematological malignancy. Recurrent salmonella bacteremia after appropriate antibiotic therapy has been documented in AIDS patients (Chapter 242).

Localized infection. During a salmonella bacteremia, localized infection may develop. In some patients, the infection develops in sites of preexisting disease such as vascular aneurysms, bone infarcts, congenital cysts, injection sites, and calculous gallbladders. Salmonella is the most common cause of osteomyelitis in patients with sickle cell anemia. The infection appears to localize in previously infarcted or ischemic areas of bone. Meningitis occurs primarily in neonates, whereas pneumonia and empyema are most common in elderly persons and in patients with underlying disease. Abscesses of the spleen, liver, and soft tissue rarely are encountered. Endocarditis may develop on natural or prosthetic valves.

Chronic carrier state. The fecal excretion of nontyphoidal salmonella organism for periods of days, or even months, after infection is not uncommon. Positive stool cultures are obtained in 10% to 15% of enterocolitis patients for 1 to 2 months after the illness. These patients have been termed *convalescent carriers*. Outbreaks in which convalescent carrier food handlers or hospital workers are implicated are extremely rare, and it suggests that these persons pose a minimal public health hazard. They invariably stop excreting the organism without antimicrobial therapy; thus, follow-up cultures are rarely necessary.

Persons who excrete salmonellae for a minimum period of 1 year are designated *chronic* or *persistent carriers*. The organism excreted by almost all of these individuals is *S. typhi*. Two thirds of the patients have a history of previous typhoid fever, and many have biliary tract disease. *S. typhi* is excreted in the bile, and stool contains 10^6 to 10^9 organisms per gram of feces. They are asymptomatic but serve as the natural reservoir for *S. typhi*. The chronic carrier state may persist for the lifetime of an individual if antibiotic therapy and/or biliary tract surgery are not undertaken.

Patients with urinary tract abnormalities caused by *Schistosoma haematobium* may chronically excrete salmonellae in their urine. Prolonged salmonella bacteremia also is associated with *Schistosoma mansoni* infection and hepatosplenic schistosomiasis. Fever may be the only manifestation of the salmonella bacteremia. Eradication of the adult schistosomes and correction of the urinary tract anatomic abnormalities *(S. haematobium)* eliminates the salmonella infection.

Diagnostic tests

The diagnosis of salmonella infection is established by isolating the organism from stool, urine, blood, or other infected secretions and tissues. Specimens that are ordinarily sterile, for example, blood, can be cultured on simple media. Stool should be cultured on selective or differential media (salmonella-shigella agar, MacConkey agar, eosin-methylene blue agar) and in enrichment broth (selenite or tetrathionate broth) to suppress the growth of other organisms present in the specimen. Microscopic examination of methylene blue–stained stool specimens reveals moderate numbers of polymorphonuclear leukocytes in salmonella enterocolitis and predominantly mononuclear cells in typhoid fever.

Blood cultures yield *S. typhi* in 90% of typhoid fever patients during the first week of illness. Stool and urine cultures may be negative at this time. After 3 to 4 weeks of untreated illness, the incidence of positive cultures of blood, stool, and urine is 50%, 85%, and 25%, respectively. *S. typhi* may also be recovered from cultures of bone marrow and rose spots.

Serologic tests are of no value in establishing a diagnosis early in the illness but may be useful retrospectively. Their greatest value is in epidemiologic investigations. Agglutinins against salmonella somatic and flagellar antigens are determined in the Widal test. Peak agglutinin titers occur during the third week of the disease. Fourfold or greater increases in titer are suggestive of salmonella infection. Single titers, even if elevated, are not very useful, because of cross-reactions with other Enterobactericeae and persistently increased titers after typhoid immunization. Chronic *S. typhi* carriers can now be identified by a simple passive hemagglutination test using highly purified Vi antigen. The test was 75% sensitive and 92% specific when used in an endemic area.

Therapy

The therapy of salmonella infections is influenced by the type of infecting organism, the site of infection, and the state of host-defense mechanisms. The selection of an antimicrobial agent is based on in vitro sensitivity testing, documented efficacy of the agent in clinical trials, and knowledge of the local epidemiology of drug-resistant isolates. Chloramphenicol, ampicillin, amoxicillin, trimethoprim-sulfamethoxazole, and the new fluoroquinolones are effective antimicrobial agents. The widespread distribution of R-plasmid-carrying strains affects the patterns of drug resistance. The worldwide use of antimicrobial agents in animal feed has contributed to the widespread distribution and maintenance of drug-resistant salmonellae in the human food chain (especially poultry and cattle). A recent exposure to antimicrobial agents, especially penicillins, is a risk factor for the subsequent acquisition of multidrug-resistant salmonella infection.

Enterocolitis is a self-limited illness that should be treated only with symptomatic therapy (fluid, electrolytes, antiperistaltics), unless there is evidence or suspicion of either an associated bacteremia or a localized infection. Antimicrobial therapy might also be given to a patient with impaired host-defense mechanisms (lymphoma, sickle cell disease, AIDS) for whom an increased risk of bacteremia is known to exist. Uncomplicated enterocolitis should not be treated with antibiotics. Antibiotics may prolong the period of convalescent excretion of the organism. The need to eradicate the organism in convalescent carriers who are health care workers is often raised, but nosocomial outbreaks of salmonellosis are quite rare in the United States, despite the high frequency of prolonged convalescent carriage. Hence, attempts to eradicate the organism in such persons are not justified and may not be effective. A recent randomized, placebo-controlled study showed that ciprofloxacin, a fluoroquinolone with a very high in-vitro activity against salmonellae, failed to eradicate salmonella in 64% of convalescent carriers, and actually prolonged the carriage state in some of the treated patients.

Typhoid and enteric fever should be treated with antimicrobial agents. They have been successfully treated with chloramphenicol I.V. or P.O. (50 mg/kg/day); ampicillin I.V. or P.O. (100 mg/kg/day); amoxicillin P.O. (4 g/day); trimethoprim-sulfamethoxazole (320 to 640 mg; 1600 to 3200 mg respectively), daily; and ciprofloxacin (1000–1500 mg) daily. Ciprofloxacin has excellent activity against *S. typhi* (MIC = 0.01-0.1 mg/ml). It is active against intracellular organisms and is concentrated in the biliary tract. Chloramphenicol, ampicillin, and amoxicillin are given in four divided doses, and trimethoprim-sulfamethoxazole and ciprofloxacin in two divided doses. The recommended duration of therapy is 2 weeks. The clinical response of typhoid fever patients is slow, regardless of the antibiotic used. Most patients require 3 to 5 days of therapy to become afebrile. Because ciprofloxacin is expensive and is not approved for use in children, chloramphenicol remains the drug of choice in most parts of the world. Ampicillin-resistant *S. typhi* has been reported from Mexico, France, South Asia, and Southeast Asia. Chloramphenicol-resistant *S. typhi* has been reported from these areas as well as West Africa, the Middle East, and India. Initial therapy with both chloramphenicol and ampicillin has been recommended in areas where resistance to these agents has been reported. If the organism is sensitive to both drugs, chloramphenicol is continued; if it is resistant to one antibiotic, the other antibiotic is continued alone. Fortunately, it is quite rare for *S. typhi* to acquire resistance to both ampicillin and chloramphenicol; in that situation, trimethoprim-sulfamethoxazole or a fluoroquinolone would be indicated. Corticosteroid therapy is recommended for all patients with suspected typhoid fever who are delirious, obtunded, stuporous, comatose, or in shock. In one study, dexamethasone 3 mg/kg body weight as an initial dose, followed by eight doses of 1 mg/kg every 6 hours significantly reduced the case-fatality rate.

Intestinal perforation complicating typhoid fever traditionally has been treated conservatively. Recently, early laparotomy with primary closure or resection has been advocated.

Bacteremia and localized infections usually are treated with either chloramphenicol, ampicillin, or a fluoroquinolone. If the organism is susceptible, ampicillin is preferred for localized disease, for example, osteomyelitis and intravascular infections, in which therapy should be continued for 6 or more weeks. Uncomplicated bacteremia without localized infection may be treated with either chloramphenicol, ampicillin, or a fluoroquinolone for 10 to 14 days. Extraintestinal salmonellosis resistant to ampicillin and chloramphenicol is usually treated with trimethoprim-sulfamethoxazole, which may be particularly useful for prostatic and urinary tract infections. Ciprofloxacin has been successfully used to suppress salmonella bacteremia in AIDS patients who had recurrent bacteremia after treatment with other antimicrobial agents.

Chronic carriers are usually treated with oral ampicillin 4 to 6 g daily and probenicid 2 g daily, each in four divided doses for 6 weeks. Relapses occur in 30% to 50% of these patients. Relapsing patients usually have biliary tract disease, and cure is achieved only if a cholecystectomy is performed. Ciprofloxacin, 750 mg twice daily for 3 weeks, has been recently used to successfully eliminate the chronic carriage state of *S. typhi*.

Prevention

Adequate protection of water supplies, vaccination of persons at risk, pasteurization of milk products, sanitary disposal of human excreta, and identification, isolation, and treatment of chronic typhoid carriers are the primary measures for control of typhoid fever. Since humans are the only natural reservoir for *S. typhi,* these measures have been very successful in developed countries. The situation is more difficult with nontyphoidal salmonellosis. Although the incidence of typhoid fever has declined in most of the world, the incidence of nontyphoidal salmonellosis has increased. Control of nontyphoidal salmonellosis also requires prevention of spread of salmonellae among animals and from animals to humans. Typhoid fever can be prevented by vaccines. The parenterally administered, heat-inactivated whole-cell preparations have efficacies of 50% to 90%, but they are associated with frequent local and systemic side effects. The vaccine is given in two doses, 4 weeks apart. An orally administered vaccine made from an attenuated, nonpathogenic strain of *S. typhi* (Ty21a) has been licensed in the United States. It is administered in four doses over a 7-day period. Studies of oral typhoid vaccines in Egypt, Chile, and Indonesia have found an efficacy comparable to that of the parenteral vaccines. The decision on whether to use an oral live vaccine or a killed parenteral vaccine must therefore be based on other considerations. Adverse reactions are rare with the oral vaccine and the immunization series is completed within 1 week. The cost of the oral vaccine is considerably more than that of the parenteral vaccine, but patient compliance in completing the series is not guaranteed. However, the discomfort and expense of injections is avoided. Finally, the protection afforded by both vaccines is relative and can be overcome by ingesting a larger inoculum of *S. typhi*.

SHIGELLA

Classification and characteristics

Shigellae are gram-negative, nonsporeforming bacilli that belong to the family Enterobactericeae. They are aerobic, nonmotile, and nonencapsulated. They ferment glucose without the production of gas but do not ferment lactose or produce hydrogen sulfide. *S. sonnei* ferments lactose after prolonged cultivation, and *S. boydii* serotypes 13 and 14 and some *S. flexneri* serotype 6 produce gas.

Shigellae are classified according to their somatic (O) antigens. The genus is divided into four species, *S. dysenteriae, S. flexneri, S. boydii,* and *S. sonnei,* which include over 40 serotypes. These species frequently are referred to as subgroups A, B, C, and D, respectively.

Epidemiology

Shigellosis occurs throughout the world and is responsible for over 576,000 deaths each year among children less than 5 years of age. There were over 27,000 isolations of shigella reported to the Centers for Disease Control in 1990. During the 5-year period between 1986 and 1990, there was an increase of nearly 20% in the average annual reported incidence compared to the 5-year period a decade earlier (see Fig. 268-1). *S. sonnei* is the most common species in the United States and Western Europe, whereas *S. flexneri* predominates in most developing countries. *S. dysenteriae,* the cause of dysentery pandemics, was the most common species isolated during the early 1900s. It virtually disappeared, only to emerge as the cause of pandemics in Central America (1969-1973), Bangladesh (1972-1977), southern India (1972-1978), central Africa (1979-1986), eastern India (1984), and Thailand and Myanmar (1984-1986).

Shigellosis is most common in late summer and is primarily a disease of children less than 4 years of age. Humans are the only known reservoir of the organism. Transmission is predominantly from direct person-to-person contact, rather than from ingestion of contaminated food or water. However, in 1988 over 3000 women attending an outdoor music festival in Michigan developed shigellosis after eating contaminated tofu salad. Fecal-oral transmission results in high attack rates in crowded, unsanitary custodial institutions; among homosexuals; and in environments lacking adequate sanitary facilities. The low bacterial inoculum required to produce disease makes it possible for fomites to serve as vectors. Intrafamilial spread is common, particularly when the index case is a young child. Family attack rates range up to 60%.

Fecal excretion of shigellae may continue for up to 6 weeks in untreated patients. Long-term carriage is very rare. When it occurs, there is persistence of organisms in the colon, rather than in the biliary tract as in cholera and salmonellosis.

Pathophysiology

The inoculum of *Shigella* organisms required to produce disease is the lowest of any of the enteric bacterial pathogens. Ten *S. dysenteriae* bacilli produce illness in 10% to 20% of healthy adults, and 200 *S. flexneri* or *S. sonnei* bacilli cause disease in 40% of subjects. Shigellae are more resistant to acid than are salmonellae or *Vibrio cholerae* organisms. Shigellae multiply within the small intestine and usually produce watery diarrhea initially. *S. dysenteriae* and certain strains of *S. flexneri* and *S. sonnei* elaborate an enterotoxin, which may be responsible for the early phase of the diarrhea.

Shigella organism's principal virulence property is its ability to invade the colonic mucosal cells. The bacilli penetrate and multiply within epithelial cells, and spread to adjacent cells and to the lamina propria to elicit an inflammatory reaction. These events result in the formation of microabscesses and ulcerations. The stool contains many polymorphonuclear leukocytes. These pathologic processes in the colon remain superficial, and hence bacteremia is uncommon.

The ability of virulent shigella to invade cells is attributed to five independent loci on a 220 kilodalton plasmid. Plasmid genes also encode for the intracellular multiplication of the bacteria, which is related to the production of a hemolysin that lyses the phagocytic membrane surrounding the intracellular bacterium. The role of the Shiga toxin in these pathologic processes has not been determined.

Clinical disease

Shigellosis is usually abrupt in onset, with an incubation period of 1 to 3 days. Watery diarrhea, crampy abdominal pain, and fever up to 104° F (40° C) are the most common early symptoms (Chapter 236). This phase of the illness lasts for several days in most patients. It is followed by the development of tenesmus, fecal urgency, and the passage of bloody, mucoid stools. Fever becomes less prominent, and the volume of the stools is decreased. This second phase of illness may last for 2 to 3 weeks without antimicrobial therapy.

Shigella bacteremia is a rare event. Almost 95% of reported bacteremic cases are in pediatric patients under 16 years old, particularly those under 5 years of age. Elderly and immunocompromised adults may also develop shigella bacteremia.

The severity of shigellosis is related to the infecting organism. *S. sonnei* produces the mildest illness, *S. flexneri* is intermediate, and *S. dysenteriae* type 1 causes the most serious illness. Many patients infected with *S. sonnei* are asymptomatic or have only a brief episode of watery diarrhea. In contrast, gross blood and mucus are present in the stool of a majority of patients infected with *S. dysenteriae*. Strain differences also are reflected in mortality rates. Shigellosis caused by *S. sonnei* is fatal in less than 1% of patients in most areas, whereas *S. dysenteriae* outbreaks have a mortality as high as 20% to 30%. Geographic differences also influence mortality figures. In Bangladesh, the case-fatality rates among hospitalized children were highest (10%) in those infected with *S. sonnei* in 1974-1988.

Convulsions are common in children less than 4 years of age. In one series, seizures developed in 25% of children with temperature exceeding 103° F (39.4° C). The incidence of seizures in children with a temperature of less than 103° F was about 6%. Hyperpyrexia may not be an independent variable, since dehydration and electrolyte abnormalities may be more severe in infants with higher temperatures. Complications of shigellosis that can lead to death have been identified in a recent 15-year study in Bangladesh and include intestinal perforation, toxic megacolon, dehydration, sepsis, hyponatremia, hypoglycemia, seizures, hemolytic-uremic syndrome, and pneumonia. Sepsis and hypoglycemia were found to be the most common causes of death.

Diagnostic tests

A definitive diagnosis of shigellosis is established by isolation of shigellae from stool or a swab of colonic lesions. Shigellae survive for only a short time in stool so fresh specimens should be inoculated promptly on appropriate culture media. The nutritional requirements of shigella are simple, and isolation is facilitated by the use of special media such as MacConkey, Hektoen, or deoxycholate agar. It is recommended that stool be cultured on 3 successive days, since a single culture may be negative in one third of patients with shigellosis. In severe dysenteric cases, it is very important to test a suspected shigella colony on a plate with a panel of group antisera to rapidly rule out *S. dysenteriae* type 1 because of this organism's tendency to cause widespread epidemics.

Microscopic examination of methylene blue–stained stool preparations is useful in distinguishing shigellosis from toxigenic or viral diarrheal syndromes. Numerous fecal polymorphonuclear leukocytes are usually found in shigellosis whereas fecal leukocytes are absent in toxin-induced or viral diarrhea. Sigmoidoscopy reveals diffuse mucosal inflammation, often with multiple shallow ulcers 3 to 7 mm in diameter.

Treatment

The correction of fluid, electrolyte, and glucose abnormalities is particularly important in elderly and very young patients. Although the use of antibiotics in adults with shigellosis is controversial, therapy does shorten the period of symptomatic illness and decreases the duration of fecal excretion of shigellae. Fever and diarrhea usually respond within 1 to 2 days of initiating effective therapy, and the mortality is reduced to less than 0.1%, even in severe shigellosis. The principal indications for *not* treating a known shigella infection are as follows: the patient is asymptomatic at the time of the diagnosis; the age, vocation, and personal habits of the patient make transmission to other individuals very unlikely; and the antibiotic sensitivity pattern of the organism precludes the use of relatively nontoxic drugs. Organisms resistant to multiple antibiotics are common, especially in Africa and Asia. In a recent study by the CDC, 32% and 7% of United States *Shigella* isolates were resistant to ampicillin and to trimethoprim-sulfamethoxazole, respectively. Isolates associated with foreign travel were resistant to trimethoprim-sulfamethoxazole in 20% of cases; no quinolone resistance was encountered.

Trimethoprim-sulfamethoxazole (160 mg and 800 mg, respectively) every 12 hours for 5 days is the treatment of choice for shigellosis not associated with foreign travel. Children may be given trimethoprim-sulfamethoxazole (10 mg/kg/day and 50 mg/kg/day, respectively) in two divided doses for 5 days. Ampicillin (500 mg P.O. q.i.d. for 5 days) is effective for sensitive organisms, as is a single oral dose of tetracycline (2.5 g). Fluoroquinolones such as norfloxacin and ciprofloxacin are effective drugs, especially for foreign travel–related shigellosis, but these drugs are not approved for pediatric use. Amoxicillin is not effective.

Antiperistaltic agents such as diphenoxylate hydrochloride with atropine sulfate (Lomotil) should be avoided because of the possibility that they will exacerbate symptoms and prolong fecal excretion of organisms.

Prevention

The most important control measures are the institution of proper sanitary and hygienic measures. Hand washing is extremely important in decreasing direct transmission of organisms. Asymptomatic and convalescent carriers should also be excluded from involvement in food preparation and handling. Effective vaccines are not available.

REFERENCES

Aserkoff B and Bennett JV: Effect of therapy in acute salmonellosis on salmonellae in feces. N Engl J Med 281:236, 1969.

Bennish ML: Potentially lethal complications of shigellosis. Rev Infect Dis 13(suppl 4):S319, 1991.

Butler T, Rumans L, and Arnold K: Response of typhoid fever caused by chloramphenicol-susceptible and chloramphenicol-resistant strains of *Salmonella typhi* to treatment with trimethoprim-sulfamethoxazole. Rev Infect Dis 4:551, 1982.

Chalker RB, and Blaser MJ: A review of human salmonellosis: III. Magnitude of salmonella infection in the United States. Rev Infect Dis 10:111, 1988.

Cohen JI, Bartlett JS, and Corey RG: Extraintestinal manifestations of salmonella infections. Medicine (Baltimore) 66:349, 1987.

Cohen ML and Tauxe RV: Drug-resistant *Salmonella* in the United States: an epidemiologic perspective. Science 234:964, 1986.

Hoffman SL et al: Reduction of mortality in chloramphenicol-treated severe typhoid fever by high-dose dexamethasone. N Engl J Med 310:82, 1984.

Hornick RB et al: Typhoid fever: pathogenesis and immunological control. N Engl J Med 283:686, 1970.

Jacobson MA et al: Ciprofloxacin for salmonella bacteremia in the acquired immunodeficiency syndrome (AIDS). Ann Int Med 110:1027, 1989.

Keush GT: Antimicrobial therapy for enteric infections and typhoid fever: state of the art. Rev Infect Dis 10:S199, 1988.

Lee LA et al: An outbreak of shigellosis at an outdoor music festival. Am J Epidemiol 133:608, 1991.
Levine MM: Bacillary dysentery: mechanisms and treatment. Med Clin North Am 66:623, 1982.
Neill MA et al: Failure of ciprofloxacin to eradicate convalescent fecal excretion after acute salmonellosis: experience during an outbreak in health care workers. Ann Int Med 114:195, 1991.
Riley LW et al: Evaluation of isolated cases of salmonellosis by plasmid profile analysis: introduction and transmission of a bacterial clone by precooked roast beef. J Infect Dis 148:12, 1983.
Ryan CA et al: Massive outbreak of antimicrobial-resistant salmonellosis traced to pasteurized milk. JAMA 258:3269, 1987.
Salam MA and Bennish ML: Antimicrobial therapy for shigellosis. Rev Infect Dis 13(suppl 4):S332, 1991.
Sansonetti PJ: Genetic and molecular basis of epithelial cell invasion by *Shigella* species. Rev Infect Dis 13(suppl 4):S285, 1991.
Simanjuntak CH et al: Oral immunisation against typhoid fever in Indonesia with Ty21a vaccine. Lancet 338:1055, 1991.
St. Louis ME et al: The emergence of grade A eggs as a major source of *Salmonella entiritidis* infections: new implications for the control of salmonellosis. JAMA 259:2103, 1988.
Tauxe RV et al: Antimicrobial resistance of *Shigella* isolates in the USA: the importance of international travelers. J Infect Dis 162:1107, 1990.

CHAPTER

269 Infections Caused by *Brucella, Francisella tularensis, Pasteurella,* and *Yersinia* Species

Nancy K. Henry
Walter R. Wilson

BRUCELLOSIS

Brucellosis (undulant fever; Malta fever; Mediterranean fever) is an infection that causes abortion in domestic animals and may be transmitted incidentally to humans. In humans, the acute form is characterized by fever without localizing findings. Chronic infection causes fever, weakness, and vague symptoms that may persist for months to years.

Classification and characteristics

Marston, in 1863, provided the first description of the clinical presentation in humans; the etiologic agent was isolated by Bruce in 1886. In 1897, Bang reported that *Brucella abortus* was the cause of contagious abortion in cattle. There are at least six species of the genus *Brucella*. Three of these, *B. melitensis* (goats), *B. abortus* (cattle), and *B. suis* (pigs), are responsible for the majority of infections in humans. Rarely, a fourth species, *B. canis* (dogs, especially beagles), has been isolated from infected humans.

The Brucellae are small, nonsporeforming, nonencapsulated, gram-negative coccobacilli. Growth is best at 37° C in trypticase soy broth or tryptose phosphate broth at a pH of 6.7 in an atmosphere containing 10% carbon dioxide. Brucellae do not ferment carbohydrates, and the species may be distinguished from each other by their requirements for carbon dioxide atmosphere for growth, growth in the presence of dyes, production of hydrogen sulfide and urease, and specific agglutination in antisera. On solid media, the colonies are usually slow-growing; small; smooth; translucent; and blue-, white-, or amber-colored; and require at least 2 days to demonstrate growth.

Epidemiology

The natural reservoir of brucellosis in the United States is domestic animals, especially cattle, sheep, goats, and swine. The disease is transmitted to humans primarily by contact with infected animals. The organisms may invade through the conjunctivae, nasopharynx, gastrointestinal tract, or genitourinary tract, or through abraded skin or inadvertent subcutaneous inoculation. Human-to-human transmission probably does not occur.

Brucellosis is primarily an occupational disease involving meat-packing plant employees, veterinarians, laboratory personnel, farmers, and ranchers. Less commonly, brucellosis may be acquired by ingestion of unpasteurized dairy products. The enactment of local and state ordinances for animal surveillance and for pasteurization of dairy products has resulted in a steady decline in the reported number of cases of human brucellosis from the 1940s to 1980s.

The usual male-female ratio is 6:1, with the peak incidence in 20- to 50-year-old males.

Currently, *B. abortus* and *B. suis* are the species most frequently isolated from human infections in the United States. On a worldwide basis, *B. melitensis* is the most common cause of brucellosis.

Pathophysiology

After invasion of the human host, the brucellae localize intracellularly in such tissues of the reticuloendothelial system as lymph nodes, bone marrow, liver, spleen, and kidneys. The bacilli are engulfed by macrophages, where they may be killed rapidly, or the organisms may replicate and destroy the phagocytic cells, releasing more bacteria into the environment. This results in proliferation of the reticuloendothelial system and a characteristic but nonspecific reaction of these tissues. Granuloma formation occurs with the appearance of epithelioid cells, giant cells of the foreign body or Langhans' types, lymphocytes, and plasma cells. Although the granulomas typically are noncaseating, caseous necrosis may occur, especially with *B. suis* infections. Brucellae may reside intracellularly in phagocytes, in which they are relatively protected from antibody and from antimicrobial agents. In most instances, the granulomas undergo a process of healing, with fibrosis, death of the organisms, and frequently, calcification. Uncommonly, suppuration and caseation of the granulomas may occur, and brucellae may survive for months to years, with periodic episodes of fever and nonspecific symptoms; or abscesses may develop in the reticuloendothelial system, testes, epididymides, ovaries, kidneys, brain, and other organs.

In animals, brucellae proliferate in the cytoplasm of the chorionic epithelial cells of the placenta as a consequence of the presence of high concentrations of erythritol, a carbohydrate that stimulates growth of brucellae. Erythritol is plentiful in the placentas of cattle, swine, goats, and sheep, but not humans. Possibly for this reason, brucellosis is a common cause of abortion in animals, but human abortion occurs no more frequently with this disease than with bacteremias caused by other microorganisms.

Clinical manifestations

The four species of *Brucella* that affect humans differ in their virulence for humans. *B. abortus* infection is mild and usually self-limited; severe complications are uncommon. *B. suis* infection is characterized by a destructive, suppurative disease often associated with a prolonged chronic localized infection. *B. melitensis* is the most virulent species and is associated with severe acute infection and the highest mortality rate. *B. canis* infection is similar to that caused by *B. abortus*.

Asymptomatic brucellosis. Asymptomatic infections may be the most common form of brucellosis. Approximately 50% of meat-packing plant employees and 33% of veterinarians who had positive serologic titers for brucellosis were unaware of a previous acute infection. Infection in children is also frequently asymptomatic (see Table 269-1).

Acute brucellosis. The incubation period is usually from 5 to 14 days, although many months may elapse between the time of infection and the first appearance of symptoms. Bacteremia occurs without specific localizing signs. Most patients complain of malaise, fever, lethargy, weakness, weight loss, and anorexia. Fever from 38° to 40° C is characteristically prominent in the afternoon or evening and is frequently associated with shaking chills and profuse sweats. Myalgias, headache, and backache occur frequently and are often severe. Approximately 20% of patients de-

Table 269-1. Syndromes and treatment of disorders caused by *Brucella, Francisella, Pasteurella, Yersinia,* and cat-scratch disease

Organism	Syndromes	Antimicrobial therapy
Brucella *B. abortus* *B. melitensis* *B. suis* *B. canis*	Acute	Doxycycline 200 mg/day plus rifampin 600-900 mg/day for 6 weeks *or* tetracycline 2 gm/day for 6 weeks plus streptomycin* 1 gm/day *or* gentamicin 5 mg/kg/day for 2 weeks.
	Endocarditis	Antibiotics as above plus cardiac valve replacement.
	Central nervous system	Third-generation cephalosporin plus rifampin for 6 weeks.
Francisella tularensis	Ulcerglandular Oculoglandular Pulmonary Typhoidal	Streptomycin 15-20 mg/kg/day *or* gentamicin 3-5 mg/kg/day for 7-14 days *or* doxycycline 200 mg/day *or* tetracycline 2 gm/day *or* chloramphenicol 2 gm/day for 14 days.
Pasteurella multocida	Soft tissue Respiratory	Penicillin V 2 gm/day *or* doxycyline 200 mg/day *or* TMP/SMX 1 DS tablet for 7-10 days.
	Endocarditis Osteomyelitis Bacteremia	Aqueous penicillin G 10-20 $\times$ 10^6 units/day *or* parenteral cephalosporin for 2-4 weeks.
Yersinia pestis	Bubonic Pneumonic Septicemic	Streptomycin 2 gm/day *or* gentamicin 5-7 mg/kg/day *or* tetracycline 2 gm/day for 10 days.
	Meningitis	Chloramphenicol 2 gm/day for 10 days.
Y. enterocolitica	Diarrhea Mesenteric adenitis	TMP/SMX—1 DS† twice daily *or* ciprofloxacin 500 mg-1 g/day *or* doxycyline 200 mg/day for 7-10 days.
	Bacteremia	Gentamicin 5 mg/kg/day *or* parenteral TMP/SMX, ciprofloxacin, *or* doxycycline as above.
Y. pseudotuberculosis	Mesenteric adenitis	Drug therapy controversial and includes aminoglycoside, chloramphenicol, tetracycline, or TMP/SMX.
Cat-scratch disease	Normal host	None
	Lymphadenopathy	None
	Immunocompromised host	Erythromycin, doxycline, ciprofloxacin, TMP/SMX, or gentamicin. Dosage and duration therapy not established.

*Streptomycin is no longer manufactured by United States pharmaceutical companies. It may be difficult to obtain. Gentamicin therapy may be substituted for streptomycin if streptomycin is unavailable.
†DS, double strength.

velop a monoarticular arthralgia affecting the large joints, especially the knee, shoulder, ankle, or elbow.

Abnormal physical findings, aside from tachycardia and fever, are often few or absent. Diffuse nontender lymphadenopathy and splenomegaly occur in 10% to 20% of patients, and hepatomegaly in 5% to 10%. Occasionally, patients develop tender testicles and, infrequently, acute epididymitis.

Localized brucellosis. Localized brucellosis occurs uncommonly, and less than 33% of these patients have fever, chills, malaise, and weight loss. Because the serologic titers in these patients may be low or absent, diagnosis is usually made by biopsy and isolation of the organism from culture. The most common sites of involvement of localized brucellosis (roughly in decreasing order of frequency) are bone and joint, spleen, endocardium, lung, genitourinary tract, and nervous system.

Bone and joint. Arthralgias and myalgias occur frequently in acute brucellosis, but these symptoms usually are self-limited or disappear with antimicrobial therapy. When localized disease occurs, the most frequent sites involved are the spine and knee. Spondylitis involves the intervertebral disk and adjacent structures. Localized pain and nerve root irritation are prominent complaints. Osteoporosis, periosteal thickening, or paravertebral abscess may occur. With healing, dense sclerosis results in the formation of a characteristic x-ray appearance of "parrot-beak" osteophytes. Differential diagnosis includes tuberculosis and *Staphylococcus aureus* osteomyelitis (Chapter 237).

Gastrointestinal. Multiple or single splenic abscesses of various sizes may occur. The characteristic x-ray appearance of splenic brucellosis is one of splenomegaly with multiple calcific lesions or concentric "bull's-eye" calcifications. Splenic brucellosis may be associated with sporadic febrile episodes of irregular periodicity. The episodes may occur frequently or may recur after 20 or more years of quiescence. Approximately 30% to 50% of patients with brucellosis develop abnormal liver function tests. Granulomatous hepatitis may occur especially with *B. abortus* infection.

Infective endocarditis. Brucellar endocarditis is an acute ulcerative process usually involving the aortic valve. Since most available antibiotics are bacteriostatic against brucellae, relapse rates have been reported to be high. Cardiac valve replacement is usually necessary to eradicate the infection.

Respiratory tract. Hilar adenopathy, often bilateral, and peribronchial and perihilar pulmonary infiltrates characterize the pulmonary form of brucellosis. Pleural effusion or empyema also may occur. Pulmonary nodules may be indistinguishable from carcinoma. Healed pulmonary brucellosis may be associated with multiple calcified granulomas that resemble histoplasmosis on chest x-ray.

Genitourinary tract. *B. suis* is the most common cause of renal brucellosis. Perinephric abscess or chronic granulomatous pyelonephritis may occur. Brucellae may be isolated from urine culture in these patients. Brucellosis and renal tuberculosis should be considered in the differential diagnosis of pyuria with negative routine microbiologic urine cultures. Testicular swelling and tenderness occur in at least 5% of cases, and *B. suis* is more commonly associated with testicular abnormalities than are other species. Sterility in the male occurs rarely. In females, tubo-ovarian and pelvic abscess with chronic endometritis and cervicitis have been described.

Nervous system. Rarely, brucellosis may cause meningoencephalitis, peripheral neuropathy, myelitis, or myelopathy. In chronic meningitis, pleocytosis is present, but cerebrospinal fluid cultures for brucellae are rarely positive.

Strain 19 vaccine disease. Strain 19 vaccine is a live brucella vaccine used by veterinarians to immunize cattle against *B. abortus*. Inadvertent self-inoculation of veterinarians, either through the skin or by conjunctival spray or ingestion, is relatively common. Vaccine-associated disease is usually milder than the naturally acquired form and is manifested by fever, chills, headache, fatigue, and myalgia. Multiple episodes of inadvertent inoculations are not uncommon. The condition is self-limited.

Chronic brucellosis. Chronic brucellosis is a poorly understood condition in which a small percentage of patients with acute brucellosis develop a chronic state of ill health that may persist for months or years. These patients complain of weakness, fatigue, mental depression, vague pains, and intermittent fever; they usually have no abnormal physical findings referable to brucellosis, except splenomegaly. These patients should be evaluated for possible sites of chronic suppuration, especially in the spleen, liver, or kidneys. Blood cultures are negative and serologic tests are of little value in the diagnosis of chronic brucellosis.

Diagnosis

Brucellosis should be suspected in patients who have been febrile for a week or more and who have a history of occupational or other exposure. Although the physical examination is usually normal, generalized lymphadenopathy or hepatosplenomegaly may be present. Routine laboratory tests are of minimal value in the diagnosis. Leukopenia or a normal white blood cell count occurs more commonly than does leukocytosis. The organism may be isolated from blood, urine, bone marrow, or tissue cultures. Bone marrow cultures are more often positive than blood cultures. It is important to notify the microbiology laboratory that brucellosis is suspected. Cultures must be kept for at least 3 to 4 weeks, and the use of biphasic trypticase soy broth and agar (Casteneda's medium) with a carbon dioxide atmosphere facilitates the isolation of brucellae from culture.

Serum antibody titer measured by the standard agglutination test primarily measures circulating IgM antibody. Within the first few weeks of acute infection, the standard agglutination titer increases fourfold to eightfold. A titer equal to or greater than 1:160 is considered significant. Despite appropriate antimicrobial therapy, the standard agglutination titer may remain persistently elevated for a prolonged period of time (up to 2 years) in 5% to 7% of patients. Consequently, the standard agglutination titer may not be useful in differentiating acute infection or acute relapse of a chronic infection from other causes of fever in patients with chronic brucellosis. A false-positive standard agglutination titer may occur as a result of immunologic cross-reactivity in patients with tularemia, *Yersinia* infection, or cholera, or with vaccination against these infections.

The 2-mercaptoethanol agglutination test destroys IgM antibody and measures IgG antibody. Although this test is not as sensitive as the standard agglutination test, a significantly elevated titer ($\geq$1:60) correlates better with activation of infection in patients with chronic brucellosis. Moreover, the 2-mercaptoethanol test is more often useful in predicting recovery from brucella infection. Titers usually disappear within 6 months after appropriate antimicrobial therapy. Radioimmunoassay or enzyme-linked immunosorbent assay detects IgM and IgG antibody and may be useful in distinguishing acute from chronic infection as well as acute exacerbation of chronic infection. The brucella skin-test antigen is of little diagnostic use and is probably best avoided.

Treatment

Many patients with brucellosis recover spontaneously, and patients should be reassured that recovery from infection with appropriate therapy is anticipated. Adequate rest, nutrition, hydration, and other supportive measures are important in managing patients with active infections.

Antimicrobial therapy shortens the duration and reduces the frequency of complications of acute brucellosis (Table 269-1). The use of a single antimicrobial agent for the treatment of patients with brucellosis is associated with a higher relapse rate than the use of combination therapy. Previously, the World Health Organization recommended the use of tetracycline for 6 weeks together with streptomycin for the first 3 weeks of therapy. Streptomycin must be administered intramuscularly, a factor that complicates therapy. Presumably, gentamicin may be substituted for streptomycin but limited clinical data are published with the use of gentamicin therapy for brucellosis. Currently, the World Health Organization recommends the use of doxycycline together with rifampin for 6 weeks (Table 269-1) and this regimen is probably the treatment of choice for patients with brucellosis. Patients unable to tolerate doxycycline, such as pregnant women or children, may be treated with a combination of trimethoprim-sulfamethoxazole and rifampin. More seriously ill patients should be treated with tetracycline for 4 to 6 weeks, together with streptomycin for 2 to 3 weeks, or cotrimoxazole together with streptomycin. Therapy with rifampin may be added to either regimen for 4 to 6 weeks. Patients with infective endocarditis or central nervous system infection should be treated with a combination of antimicrobial agents as above, but the duration of therapy should be at least 3 to 6 months. The large majority of patients with brucella endocarditis require cardiac valve replacement in addition to antimicrobial therapy.

Relapse occurs frequently after completion of treatment and may be treated with another course of antimicrobials. Relapse occurs less frequently after combined tetracycline-streptomycin therapy than with tetracycline alone. Approximately 5% of patients receiving antimicrobial therapy experience a Jarisch-Herxheimer reaction. Severe reactions may be treated with prednisone, 20 mg per day for 3 to 4 days.

The therapy of localized brucellosis depends on the site involved and the nature of the infection. All patients should receive appropriate antimicrobial therapy. Abscesses should be excised and drained; spondylitis may be treated with antimicrobials and immobilization. Splenectomy may be necessary in patients with splenic brucellosis associated with multiple relapses, splenomegaly, or large, calcific splenic granulomata.

The treatment of chronic relapsing brucellosis is frustrating. Localized areas of suppuration should be treated surgically. Antimicrobial therapy in these patients is usually ineffective, and psychotherapy, good nutrition, and reassurance are often more important than the use of antibiotics. Occasionally, the use of short-term (3 to 4 days) corticosteroid therapy is necessary for control of debilitating, episodic symptoms.

The mortality in untreated cases of brucellosis is small (3% to 5%). Deaths are most often associated with infective endocarditis. With appropriate antimicrobial therapy, the mortality rate is less than 1%. Complications occur in approximately 1% to 2% of patients. With adequate therapy, patients are able to return to work in 6 weeks or less.

Reinfection may occur. Immunity induced by one attack is only relative, and multiple reinfections may occur in individuals who have high risk of exposure. Some individuals who have recovered from one or more infections acquire hypersensitivity to brucella antigen. Veterinarians are especially susceptible to this problem, and accidental exposure to strain 19 may result in brief, violent local and systemic reactions.

Prevention

The only practical means of eliminating brucellosis is to eliminate the animal reservoir of the disease. A federally funded eradication program in the United States has drastically reduced the number of bovine cases. Porcine brucellosis remains a serious problem for individuals working in pork-processing plants. There is no entirely sure means of eliminating exposure to brucellosis for meat-packing plant workers, veterinarians, laboratory workers, or livestock workers. Employees should use protective gloves, eyeglasses, and clothing. Cuts or other skin abrasions should be dressed carefully. Ingestion of unpasteurized dairy products should be avoided. An active educational program should be instituted for high-risk individuals. No satisfactory vaccine for human use is available.

FRANCISELLA TULARENSIS

Classification and characteristics

Francisella tularensis causes tularemia (rabbit fever, deerfly fever), an infectious disease of animals that may be transmitted to humans by direct contact or by insect vector. In humans, infections are characterized by the presence of a cutaneous or mucocutaneous lesion, lymphadenopathy, high fever, and severe constitutional symptoms, which, if untreated, may persist for weeks to several months.

Francisella (Pasteurella) tularensis is a small, gram-negative, nonmotile, aerobic, pleomorphic coccobacillus. Special culture media, for example, glucose-cysteine blood agar, thioglycolate broth, or other cysteine-supplemented media, are required for growth. Growth is optimum at 37° C, and small, smooth, opaque colonies appear after 24 to 48 hours of incubation. The organism may be identified on the basis of its morphology, growth requirements, fluorescent staining, and agglutinins with specific antisera.

F. tularensis is related antigenically to the causative organisms of brucellosis and plague, and cross-reactions with serum agglutinins may occur among these organisms.

Epidemiology

F. tularensis has been isolated from more than 100 wild mammals; from amphibians, fish, birds, ticks, deerflies, and mosquitoes; and from water samples. In the United States, the most important reservoirs are rabbits and ticks.

Humans are highly susceptible to tularemia. Infection is most commonly acquired through the bite of an infected arthropod, through dermal or mucosal contact, or through inhalation of aerosolized organisms from tissue or body fluids of an infected animal. The gastrointestinal tract is relatively resistant to *F. tularensis* and, uncommonly, the infection may be acquired by ingestion of contaminated water or undercooked meat. The organism is highly infectious for laboratory personnel, and microbiologic cultures and infected animals should be processed with caution. Laboratory personnel who process these specimens should always be warned when tularemia is suspected. Culture plates should be handled in vented hoods to avoid inhalation of aerosolized organisms. Tularemia occasionally is transmitted by occupational exposure: veterinarians, trappers, meat-packing plant employees, and livestock workers are at risk.

Cases usually occur sporadically, but clusters and small epidemics have been reported. An epidemic in Vermont was attributed to infected muskrats. Human-to-human transmission probably does not occur.

The incidence of human tularemia in the United States reached a peak in the late 1930s and has declined steadily to levels of 0.6 to 0.7 per million population. The disease is most common in Texas, Arkansas, Illinois, Tennessee, Missouri, and Virginia. Most cases occur during the spring and summer months in areas where tick-borne cases predominate. During winter months, rabbit-associated cases are more common. Attack rates are highest among adult males.

Pathophysiology

In humans, as few as 50 organisms can cause infection if injected intradermally or inhaled, whereas at least 10^8 organisms are required when ingested orally. The most common portals of entry in humans are the skin and mucous membranes. *F. tularensis* is capable of penetrating intact skin, but more often the organisms are inoculated by insect bite or enter inapparent abrasions or anatomic openings such as hair follicles. Approximately 48 hours after the bacilli gain entry into the skin, a macular erythematous lesion develops and becomes papular. The papule is pruritic; it enlarges, and ulceration occurs, usually within 4 to 7 days after initial contact. The evolution of the cutaneous lesions is associated with fever, chills, regional lymphadenopathy, and bacteremia. The organisms are engulfed by cells of the reticuloendothelial system, in which they may survive intracellularly for long periods.

Evisceration of animals infected with tularemia may cause aerosolization of organisms, and in humans, inhalation results in the pneumonic form of tularemia. Bacteremia after cutaneous infection may also cause tularemic pneumonia. Ingestion of a large number of *F. tularemia* organisms may cause pharyngitis and cervical lymphadenopathy of a nonspecific febrile illness with no localized findings. The gastrointestinal form of tularemia occurs uncommonly, and a greater hazard associated with the ingestion of contaminated food may be aerosolization and inhalation of organisms during mastication.

Early lesions are characterized histopathologically by focal necrosis occurring especially in organs of the reticuloendothelial system. Subsequently, the necrotic areas may undergo granulomatous reactions with multinucleated giant cells and, occasionally, with caseation. Healing is associated with fibrosis and calcification of the granulomata.

Clinical manifestations

After an incubation period of 2 to 7 days, the large majority of patients with tularemia have an abrupt onset of fever and chills. Fever 39° to 40.6° C is continuous or mildly intermittent. Severe generalized headache and myalgias occur commonly. In untreated cases, fever may persist for a month or longer. Hepatosplenomegaly is common, especially in untreated cases. A generalized maculopapular rash occurs in approximately 25% of cases.

Patients with tularemia present one of the following clinical syndromes.

Ulceroglandular. The ulceroglandular form of tularemia (75% to 85% of cases) is characterized by the development of an indurated skin lesion at the portal of entry and by regional lymphadenopathy. The involved lymph nodes are exquisitely tender, warm, erythematous, and fluctuant. Drainage may occur spontaneously. Regional lymphadenopathy in patients with tularemia is usually more prominent and painful than that accompanying infections caused by other organisms. Generalized adenopathy may occur, but the regional lymph nodes are involved most prominently. In 10% of cases, the skin lesion may be inapparent (glandular form). In rabbit-associated cases, the skin lesion is located on the finger or hand in more than 90% of cases; in tick-borne cases, the ulcer is usually located on the lower extremity, perineum, or trunk. The location of the skin lesion accounts for the higher frequency of axillary or epitrochlear lymphadenopathy in rabbit-associated cases and for inguinal and femoral adenopathy characteristic of infections transmitted by tick bite.

Typhoidal. The typhoidal form (5% to 15% of cases) may occur after intradermal, respiratory, or gastrointestinal tract entry. Fever, chills, weight loss, and hepatosplenomegaly without localized findings occur. Skin lesions and regional lymphadenopathy are absent, and the only clue to the diagnosis may be a history of possible exposure.

The mortality among patients with typhoidal tularemia is higher than in patients with ulceroglandular disease. Factors associated with a higher mortality are delayed diagnosis and antimicrobial therapy, pneumonia, and abnormal renal function.

Oculoglandular. The conjunctiva is the portal of entry for oculoglandular tularemia (1% to 2% of cases), and patients have unilateral painful purulent conjunctivitis together with preauricular or cervical lymphadenopathy. Small nodular lesions or ulcerations of the conjunctiva may be present in some patients.

Oropharyngeal. Rarely, after gastrointestinal challenge, an acute exudative or membranous pharyngitis with cervical lymphadenopathy may occur (in less than 1% of cases).

Pulmonary. Pleuropulmonary complications occur in approximately 10% to 15% of ulceroglandular, and in as many as 80% of typhoidal, cases of tularemia. Cough is usually nonproductive. Physical examination of the chest is frequently normal. Bilateral patchy infiltrates or, occasionally, lobar pneumonia are visible on x-ray (Fig. 269-1). Pleural effusion may occur.

Complications. Meningitis, osteomyelitis, endocarditis, pericarditis, and peritonitis are rare complications of tularemia.

Diagnosis

Ulceroglandular tularemia must be distinguished from other conditions and infections associated with the clinical syndrome of fever, a cutaneous ulcer, and regional lymphadenopathy.

A thorough history is important in the diagnosis of tularemia. Contact with wild animals, ticks, or deerflies, or exposure in the case of veterinarians or laboratory personnel, should alert one to the diagnosis of tularemia in a patient with an acute febrile illness, especially if such factors are associated with a cutaneous lesion and lymphadenopathy. The typical features of ulceroglandular infection are often so characteristic of tularemia that this diagnosis is self-evident. Tularemia may be unsuspected in atypical cases or in the typhoidal form. As many as 80% of patients with the typhoidal form reportedly do not have a history of vector contact. Often, a high index of suspicion for tularemia in endemic areas is necessary to establish a diagnosis.

Gram-stained smears of sputum or exudate from ulcers or lymph nodes only rarely demonstrate *F. tularensis*. Special culture media are necessary to isolate the microorganism. Because of the high risk to laboratory personnel, most laboratories are reluctant to attempt isolation of *F. tularensis* from clinical specimens or animals. Preferably, only those laboratories with experienced personnel and adequate facilities for processing specimens and cultures should attempt microbiologic studies of *F. tularensis*. The agglutination test is a reliable, standard, and safe method for diagnosing tularemia. A fourfold increase in titer is diagnostic of infection; a single convalescent titer of 1:160 or greater is highly suggestive of recent or current infection. Agglutination titers are usually negative during the first week of illness and become positive in 50% of patients during the second week. Titers reach a maximum after 4 to 8 weeks and may remain elevated for months to years after an acute infection. Agglutinins for brucellosis may appear and increase during tularemia infection, but the antibody is present in low titer.

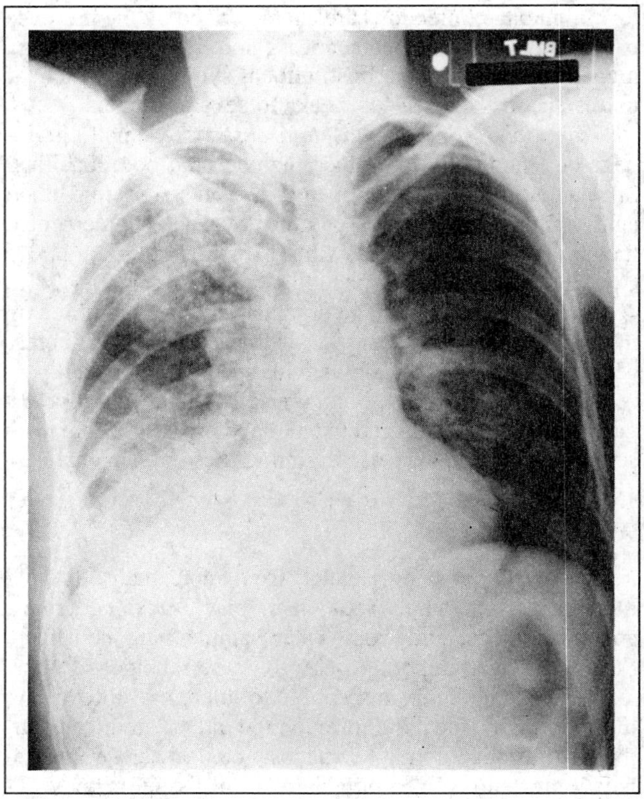

Fig. 269-1. Tularemia pneumonia.

Treatment

Streptomycin or gentamicin administered alone is the drug of choice for the treatment of patients with all forms of tularemia. Streptomycin 7 to 14 days is highly effective. Gentamicin therapy may be preferable in patients with preexisting vestibular dysfunction or in patients older than 65 years of age. Adjustments of streptomycin or gentamicin dosage must be made in patients with abnormal renal function (Chapter 224). For patients unable to tolerate streptomycin or gentamicin, therapy with tetracycline or chloramphenicol administered for 14 days may be employed. Relapse is not caused by resistant microorganisms and should be treated with another course of the same antimicrobial.

The mortality among untreated patients is 5% to 15%; the typhoidal form is associated with the higher figure. With appropriate antimicrobial therapy, mortality is less than 1%. Immunity after acute infection with *F. tularensis* is lifelong.

Prevention

Avoidance of contact with possible sources of infection is the most effective means of prevention. A live attenuated tularemia vaccine is available for high-risk individuals from the Centers for Disease Control in Atlanta, Georgia. The vaccine is administered intradermally by multiple-puncture techniques like those for vaccinia; it is effective but does not provide complete protection. The attack rate and severity of the infection are markedly reduced in vaccinated individuals.

Antibiotic prophylaxis with streptomycin or gentamicin after exposure to *F. tularensis* protects against infection. The use of tetracycline or chloramphenicol prophylactically, however, does not protect against infection and simply prolongs the incubation period.

PASTEURELLA SPECIES

Classification and characteristics

Pasteurellae are primarily animal pathogens, but they occasionally produce infection in humans; these infections range from small localized cutaneous abscesses to septicemia, osteomyelitis, and endocarditis. *Pasteurella multocida* is the species most often associated with disease in humans. Very rarely, human infections have been caused by other pasteurellae *(P. haemolytica, P. pneumotropica, P. ureae)*.

Pasteurellae are small, nonsporeforming, nonmotile, bipolar, gram-negative coccobacilli. Growth occurs in aerobic or facultatively anaerobic conditions at 37° C on ordinary culture media and is enhanced by blood- or serum-enriched agar under carbon dioxide atmosphere. The different species of *Pasteurella* may be distinguished by their ability to cause hemolysis on blood agar and pathogenicity in laboratory animals. Four serotypes of *P. multocida* have been identified.

Epidemiology

Pasteurella multocida has been isolated from a large number of wild and domestic animals. The highest carriage occurs in cats (50% to 90%), dogs or swine (50%), and rats (15%). The majority of human infections are associated with animal bites or scratches, especially those of cats and dogs. Human infection may also occur in association with animal exposure other than bites. These infections occur in persons who have frequent contact with animals and usually involve the upper respiratory tract, extremities, or intra-abdominal organs. Some patients with *P. multocida* infection (approximately 15%) have no known animal contact. Infection in these patients usually involves the upper respiratory tract or occurs intra-abdominally. *P. multocida* has been isolated from the nasopharynx of apparently normal individuals exposed to animals.

Pathophysiology

After cutaneous or subcutaneous inoculation, a local inflammatory reaction occurs; this is followed by necrosis and, in some cases, by abscess formation. Cellulitis and, infrequently, lymphangitis may occur. The oropharyngeal form is characterized by exudative pharyngitis, occasionally with the formation of tonsillar or peritonsillar abscess. Rarely, bacteremia occurs, and microabscesses may develop in multiple organs such as bone, brain, lung, or endocardium. The virulence of *P. multocida* is related to the degree of encapsulation; strains with large capsules are more resistant to phagocytosis and are more aggressive than those with small or absent capsules.

Clinical manifestations

The most common manifestation in humans is a localized soft tissue infection (usually on an extremity) that develops after direct animal contact, especially dog or cat bite. Within hours to several days after exposure, patients complain of pain of acute onset, erythema, and swelling at the site of inoculation. Serosanguineous drainage of the cutaneous lesion often occurs 1 to 2 days after onset of symptoms. A low-grade fever and regional lymphadenopathy occur commonly. Abscesses may form, and, rarely, osteomyelitis complicates local infection of the extremity.

P. multocida has been isolated, alone or in combination with other microorganisms, from the nasopharynx or sputum of patients with chronic obstructive pulmonary disease or with no apparent underlying condition. Many of these patients have no history of recent animal exposure. Rarely, *P. multocida* has been isolated from patients with sinusitis, pharyngitis, pharyngeal abscess, otitis, bronchiectasis, empyema, peritonitis, or pyelonephritis. *P. multocida* is a rare cause of infective endocarditis.

Diagnosis

P. multocida infection should be suspected in patients with a history of animal exposure and a cutaneous infection, especially that following a cat or dog bite. Gram-negative bipolar bacilli may be visualized on gram-stained smears of pus, exudate, or other specimens. Confirmation of this diagnosis requires isolation of *P. multocida* from culture.

Treatment

Penicillin is the drug of choice for the treatment of *P. multocida* and other *Pasteurella* species infections. Localized cutaneous infection without osteomyelitis may be treated successfully with penicillin V or amoxicillin/clavulanate potassium (Augmentin) administered orally for 7 to 10 days. Severe infections, for example, bacteremia, endocarditis, or meningitis, should be treated with intravenous penicillin for 2 to 4 weeks or longer, depending on the nature of the infection. Patients unable to tolerate the penicillins may be treated with parenteral cephalosporin, tetracycline, cotrimoxazole, or chloramphenicol. Orally administered cephalosporins such as cephalexin, cefaclor, and cefadroxil are less active than penicillin in vitro and should not be administered to patients with *P. multocida* infection. Ciprofloxacin is quite active in vitro against *P. multocida* but few data are published concerning the efficacy of ciprofloxacin therapy in humans. Appropriate surgical drainage or debridement is important in treating abscess, osteomyelitis, and other deep-seated infections. Death occurs very rarely in patients with *P. multocida* infections and is usually associated with endocarditis or meningitis.

Prevention

Avoidance of contact with wild and domestic animals is probably the only means of preventing human *P. multocida* infections. Animal bites, scratches, or other wounds should be cleaned, debrided, and dressed adequately.

YERSINIA SPECIES

The genus *Yersinia* includes *Y. pestis, Y. enterocolitica,* and *Y. pseudotuberculosis*. These organisms cause disease primarily in animals; humans most often acquire infection as a result of direct contact with infected animals or animal products. In humans, *Y. pestis* causes plague; mesenteric lymphadenitis and enterocolitis are caused by *Y. enterocolitis* or *Y. pseudotuberculosis*.

Yersinia pestis

Classification and characteristics. Throughout history, plague has been a source of dread and fascination. Pandemics of plague have caused human suffering and death unequaled by that of any other infectious disease. At least three great pandemics of plague have occurred in the last 1500 years. The first authentic pandemic was recorded in the sixth century A.D. The second pandemic, known as the "black death," swept through Europe, Asia, and Africa during the fourteenth century, killing an estimated one fourth of the world's population (60 million deaths). The last major pandemic originated in China in 1894 and reached the United States in 1900.

Y. pestis is a gram-negative, nonmotile, nonsporeforming, bipolar-staining, pleomorphic bacillus. The organism is an aerobe or facultative anaerobe that grows well at 37° C on many routine culture media. Growth is somewhat slow, and cultures should be held a minimum of 48 to 72 hours before being discarded as negative. The colonies are small and transparent and have the appearance of beaten copper.

Virulence is related to the production of endotoxin, exotoxin, and a substance called fraction 1. Fraction 1 is a soluble protein that makes the organism relatively resistant to phagocytosis. A lipopolysaccharide endotoxin is responsible for most of the clinical manifestations of plague.

Epidemiology. Plague occurs worldwide as an enzootic disease affecting more than 200 species of mammals, notably rodents. Disease in wild rodents (sylvatic plague) serves as a reservoir for infection for domestic rats (murine or rat plague), which, along with their ectoparasites (fleas), often live in close association with humans. The principal murine hosts, which have worldwide distribution, are the domestic rat *(Rattus rattus)* and the ectoparasite vector, the oriental rat flea *Xenopsylla cheopis*. Infection of the flea occurs by ingestion of blood from a bacteremic animal. The organisms multiply in the gastrointestinal tract of the flea and are regurgitated when the flea ingests another blood meal. Rat fleas will attack humans, especially during periods when the population of rats declines because of plague-associated deaths. Humans acquire the disease as a direct result of the flea bite or by scratching the regurgitated gastrointestinal contents of the flea into the bite.

Infection may also be acquired by direct contact with infected animals during evisceration, skinning, or, rarely, by animal bite. Human-to-human transmission may occur by inhalation of droplet nuclei from patients with the pneumonic form of plague. Airborne infection is highly contagious to individuals caring for patients with pneumonic plague, and such patients should be placed in strict isolation.

In the United States, the majority of cases occur in the southwestern states, especially New Mexico and Arizona. Males predominate, and two thirds of patients are less than 20 years old. In New Mexico, the majority of cases occur among native Americans living in rural areas.

Pathophysiology. After the flea-borne *Y. pestis* organisms gain access to a human host, the bacilli are phagocytized quickly by polymorphonuclear leukocytes and macrophages. The flea-borne bacilli are relatively resistant to intracellular killing and replicate rapidly, with the production of capsular antigen (factor 1) and other toxins. Lysis of phagocytes releases a large number of virulent microorganisms that are resistant to phagocytosis. A marked inflammatory response usually occurs in regional lymph nodes. Bacteremia results in metastatic foci of infection in the lungs, other lymph nodes, and viscera. A marked hemorrhagic diathesis develops as a result of a direct effect of plague toxin on blood vessels or as consequence of disseminated intravascular coagulation. Profound toxemia ensues, and even patients treated with appropriate antimicrobial therapy may die of fulminant toxemia despite eradication of the microorganism. The precise mechanisms of the severe tissue damage and toxemia caused by *Y. pestis* are not understood fully.

Clinical manifestations. Human plague usually presents three clinical forms: bubonic, pneumonic, or septicemic. These forms may appear singly or in combination.

Bubonic plague. Bubonic plague is the most common form of plague (90% to 95% of cases). After an incubation period of 1 to 12 days (usually 2 to 4 days), patients develop an acute, often fulminant illness. Symptoms begin abruptly with fever (39° to 41° C), shaking chills, nausea, vomiting, headache, delirium, and marked prostration. The flea bite portal of entry is rarely visible. If present, it is a vesiculopapular lesion that becomes pustular. More than two thirds of patients develop painful regional lymphadenopathy in the first 2 days of illness. Lymphadenopathy occurs most commonly in the inguinal area and (in decreasing order of frequency) in the axillary, cervical, and epitrochlear areas. Generalized lymphadenopathy occurs in approximately 15% of cases. Lymph nodes (buboes) are matted, tender, 2 to 5 cm in diameter, and surrounded by a zone of boggy hemorrhagic edema. Suppuration and drainage occur after 1 to 2 weeks of illness. Petechiae and large ecchymotic skin lesions occur, and hemorrhage into a serous cavity or viscus or into the gastrointestinal tract, respiratory tract, nasopharynx, or genitourinary tract is common. Occasionally, patients with disseminated intravascular coagulation develop gangrene of the fingers, toes, nose, or penis. The term "black death," used to describe cases of plague during the Middle Ages, is derived from the appearance of the hemorrhagic complications.

The course of bubonic plague is characterized by an irregular fever that often declines with the appearance of buboes and then increases again. In favorable outcomes, the fever decreases gradually, concomitantly with generalized improvement. In fatal cases, a precipitous increase or decrease in fever, often to a subnormal level, occurs just before death. Most fatalities occur during the first week of illness.

Pneumonic plague. Approximately 5% of patients with bubonic plague develop bacteremic pneumonia. Primary pneumonic plague occurs as a result of inhalation of droplet nuclei from a patient with pneumonic plague or as a result of laboratory-acquired infection. A large amount of blood-streaked, mucoid sputum is produced, which contains an enormous number of *Y. pestis* bacilli. Pneumonic plague is a fulminant illness accompanied by marked prostration, dyspnea, cyanosis, and death within 1 to 5 days in virtually 100% of untreated patients.

Septicemic plague. In approximately 5% to 10% of patients, an acute, prostrating febrile illness occurs without detectable lymphadenopathy. Manifestations are otherwise identical to those of bubonic plague. Untreated patients die as a result of endotoxemic shock and disseminated intravascular coagulation, usually within 3 to 5 days from onset of symptoms (Chapter 239).

Diagnosis. The diagnosis of plague should be suspected in individuals with fever and painful lymphadenopathy who reside in or travel to endemic areas. Bubonic plague mimics many diseases, including tularemia, severe staphylococcal or streptococcal infection, lymphogranuloma venereum, and cat-scratch fever. The septicemic form, or the early stage of infection before the appearance of localized signs, resembles typhoid fever, rickettsial infection, or malaria. *Y. pestis* may be isolated from blood culture or aspirate of buboes in at least 80 percent of patients with bubonic plague. Virtually all patients with the septicemic form have positive blood cultures and the bacteremia often reaches very high levels (10^4 to 10^6/mL). Gram-stained smears of bubo aspirates, or sputum from patients with pneumonic plague, demonstrate gram-negative bacilli. The classic bipolar staining is best demonstrated by Wright-Giemsa stains of aspirates or peripheral blood. Serologic diagnosis is helpful for retrospective confirmation.

Treatment. Strict isolation of patients with plague in hospital is mandatory until the completion of several days of antimicrobial therapy. High-dose streptomycin is administered for 2 to 3 days and followed by lower dosages to complete a total of 10 days of treatment is effective therapy. While streptomycin remains the drug of choice for the treatment of plague, gentamicin may be substituted for streptomycin. Tetracycline administered orally or intravenously in divided doses for 10 days is also effective. Patients with plague meningitis should be treated with chloramphenicol for 10 days of therapy.

The mortality in untreated bubonic plague is estimated to be 50% to 90%. Virtually all untreated patients with the septicemic or pneumonic plague die. With appropriate treatment, mortality in cases acquired in the United States has been reduced to 10% to 15%.

Prevention

Individuals in endemic areas should avoid contact with wild animals, particularly rodents. A formalin-killed plague vaccine is available for persons with high risk of exposure in plague-endemic areas and for laboratory personnel who work with *Y. pestis*.

Chemoprophylaxis should be administered to individuals who have had close contact with patients with suspected or confirmed plague pneumonia and for household contact of flea-borne plague cases. Tetracycline 30 mg/kg/day or sulfonamide 30 to 60 mg/kg/day administered orally in divided doses for 7 days is an effective chemoprophylactic agent.

Yersinia species

Classification and characteristics. *Y. enterocolitica* and *Y. pseudotuberculosis* are microorganisms that primarily inhabit a large variety of wild and domestic animals. *Y. enterocolitica* is a relatively common cause of enterocolitis and mesenteric lymphadenitis in Scandinavia. *Y. pseudotuberculosis* has been isolated from cases of mesenteric adenitis and septicemia.

Y. enterocolitica and *Y. pseudotuberculosis* are gram-negative, pleomorphic bacilli that do not ferment lactose, are urease-positive, and can be distinguished from each other and from *Y. pestis* by serologic and biochemical tests, pathogenicity in animals, and bacteriophage sensitivity patterns. *Y. enterocolitica* and *Y. pseudotuberculosis* grow well on conventional culture media at 37° C and in buffered saline at 4° C. Both are motile at 22° to 25° C but nonmotile at 37° C. At least 34 serotypes of *Y. enterocolitica* and 5 serotypes of *Y. pseudotuberculosis* have been identified. *Y. enterocolitica* produces a heat-stable enterotoxin and lipopolysaccharide endotoxin similar to that produced by other gram-negative bacilli. The virulence of *Y. pseudotuberculosis* appears to be related to the production of lipopolysaccharide endotoxin and to its ability to survive intracellularly.

Epidemiology. The incidence of *Y. enterocolitica* infections is highest in Scandinavia; sporadic cases have been reported in the United States. The means of transmission is unclear. The organism has been isolated from a large variety of wild and domestic animals, from fresh water, and from a number of foods, including meat, shellfish, tofu, and dairy products. Presumably, transmission from animals to humans occurs. Food-borne transmission to humans has been documented among school children. Infections occur most frequently in children and adolescents during the winter months.

Y. pseudotuberculosis has been isolated from many species of wild and domestic animals and from food, water, and environmental sources. Humans probably acquire infection as a result of contact with animals or through ingestion of contaminated food or water. The highest incidence occurs among Scandinavian children and adolescents during the winter months. Sporadic cases have been reported in the United States.

Pathophysiology. The presumed portal of entry for human cases of *Y. enterocolitica* and *Y. pseudotuberculosis* infections is the gastrointestinal tract. Human pathogenic strains of *Y. enterocolitica* cause mucosal ulcerations in the terminal ileum, necrosis of Peyer's patches, and mesenteric adenitis. Bacteremia occurs rarely and may be associated with metastatic abscess formation. Polyarthritis has been reported in association with *Y. enterocolitica* infection, especially among persons with histocompatibility antigen HLA-B27.

Y. pseudotuberculosis causes ulcerative lesions in the terminal ileum; it also causes mesenteric adenitis. Bactermia may occur rarely. Histopathologically, suppurative granulomatous lesions occur, and, in bacteremic cases, the liver, spleen, and other organs may be involved.

Clinical manifestations. Enterocolitis is the most common clinical manifestation of *Y. enterocolitica* infection (Chapter 236). Most patients are less than 5 years old and exhibit fever, abdominal pain, and diarrhea usually lasting 1 to 3 weeks. Fecal leukocytes are present on stool examination, and, occasionally, patients have bloody diarrhea. Mesenteric adenitis or terminal ileitis occurs in older children and adolescents and presents a syndrome that is clinically indistinguishable from acute appendicitis.

Polyarthritis involving the knees, ankles, wrists, fingers, and toes occurs in 10% to 30% of Scandinavian adults with *Y. enterocolitica* infection. Typically, arthritis begins a few days to a month after the onset of diarrhea. Symptoms often persist from 1 to 4 months. Erythema nodosum occurs in approximately 20% to 30% of cases. The presence of HLA-B27 antigen in patients with *Y. enterocolitica* infection has been related to Reiter's syndrome and in Scandinavia to arthritis and sacroiliitis.

Diagnosis. *Yersinia* organisms may be isolated from specimens of stool, mesenteric lymph nodes, blood, or abscess material. Inoculation of duplicate sets of cultures for incubation at 37° C and 25° C, respectively, enhances isolation of the microorganism. Serologic tests are helpful in the retrospective diagnosis of *Yersinia* infection.

Therapy. Patients hospitalized with *Yersinia* infection should be placed in enteric isolation. Cases of mesenteric lymphadenitis and terminal ileitis are usually self-limited, and the efficacy of antimicrobial therapy in these patients is unclear. The mortality associated with bacteremia caused by *Y. enterocolitica* or *Y. pseudotuberculosis* is high—50% to 75%—and these patients require prompt antimicrobial therapy. *Y. enterocolitica* is usually susceptible in vitro to aminoglycosides, chloramphenicol, tetracycline, co-trimoxazole, cefuroxime, fluoroquinolones, and third-generation cephalosporins. These microorganisms are usually resistant in vitro to penicillin, ampicillin, and first- and second-generation cephalosporins (other than cefuroxime). *Y. pseudotuberculosis* is usually susceptible in vitro to ampicillin, co-trimoxazole, tetracycline, chloramphenicol, cephalosporins, and aminoglycosides. The optimum antimicrobial therapy for patients with bacteremia caused by *Y. enterocolitica* or *Y. pseudotuberculosis* is not yet established. Empiric therapy with a parenterally administered aminoglycoside in combination with co-trimoxazole, a third-generation cephalosporin, or chloramphenicol is suggested. Antimicrobial therapy may be adjusted once the results of in vitro susceptibility tests are known.

Prevention. No specific preventive measures are known. General measures include those aimed at preventing ingestion of food or water contaminated with animal excreta.

CAT-SCRATCH DISEASE (CSD)

Cat-scratch disease or bacillary angiomatosis is a relatively common cause of benign regional lymphadenopathy in children and adolescents. Rarely, disseminated lesions occur in normal hosts. Disseminated CSD involving the liver, spleen, skeletal system, and other sites may occur in patients with acquired immunodeficiency syndrome (AIDS) or other immunocompromised conditions.

Classification and characteristics

In 1889, Parinaud described patients with oculoglandular fever associated with conjunctivitis or regional lymphadenitis with low-grade fever that persisted for weeks. Parinaud believed that these conditions were related to animal exposure. Debré in the 1930s described regional lymphadenopathy in young children and adolescents after cat scratches. Hanger and Rose prepared a skin test antigen from aspirated pus obtained from a patient with suppurative CSD that demonstrated a positive intradermal reaction in patients with CSD.

The etiology of CSD remained obscure until Wear and colleagues described a small gram-negative bacillus identified by Warthin-Starry stain in 34 of 39 lymph nodes from patients with CSD. Since that report, Wear et al. have identified this organism in hundreds of lymph nodes from patients with CSD and conjunctival or cutaneous lesions. In 1988, English et al. recovered a gram-negative bacterium or its cell wall deficient variants from lymph nodes of ten patients with CSD. It has been termed *Atypia felis*. They were able to demonstrate a fourfold or greater increase in antibody titer against this bacteria. These microorganisms produced lesions in the skin of an armadillo identical to the lesions in human skin.

Epidemiology

At least 90% of patients have a history of exposure to cats and a cat scratch or bite has been reported in at least 75% of these patients. Most often, the exposure is to a kitten, suggesting that CSD is transmitted from cat to human for a limited period of time. Cats show no evidence of illness and thus far the microorganism has not been demonstrated in stain or culture from cats implicated in transmission of CSD. Rarely, exposure to other animals, including monkeys or dogs, has been implicated in CSD. Over 80% of patients with CSD are less than 21 years old and males are slightly more commonly affected than females.

Pathophysiology

After invasion of the human host through the skin or conjunctiva, regional lymphadenopathy occurs. The histopathology of the lymph nodes demonstrates an early lymphoid hyperplasia or a progressive necrotizing granulomatous lymphadenitis. In a normal host, dissemination may occur rarely with the appearance of nectrotizing noncaseating granulomas in the liver, spleen, bone, and other tissue. As the process progresses, adjacent areas of necrosis coalesce to form abscesses. If the lymph node capsule ruptures, suppurative drainage occurs.

Clinical manifestations

Normal host. A primary skin papule or pustule forms as a primary lesion 3 to 10 days after a scratch or cat contact. Most primary lesions persist for about 1 to 3 weeks. Within 1 to 2 weeks, regional, usually solitary, lymphadenopathy occurs, which may persist for weeks to months. Systemic symptoms are usually mild and nonspecific and include malaise, fatigue, headache, sore throat, and low-grade fever. Lymphadenopathy is typically tender and most commonly involves the head, neck, or axillary nodes. Less commonly, epitrochlear, inguinal, or superclavicular nodes are involved. Solitary lymphadenopathy occurs in approximately 50% of patients. About one third of patients have lymphadenopathy involving multiple sites. Lymph node enlargement usually persists for 1 to 4 months but may last as long as 2 years. Suppuration occurs in approximately 10% of patients. Transient maculopapular, petechial, or erythema multiforme or erythema nodosum eruptions may occur. The oculoglandular form of CSD presents as an ocular granuloma or conjunctivitis with preauricular lymphadenopathy.

Most patients with CSD are only mildly ill and recover spontaneously without any residual effects. In 1% to 2% of patients, severe or systemic CSD occurs. Although approximately 90% of patients with CSD are less than 18 years of age, adults are disproportionately affected with severe disease. Most patients with severe CSD have persistent prolonged or severe symptoms. Rarely, extralymphocutaneous disease has been reported with central nervous system involvement, encephalopathy, lytic bone lesions, granulomatous hepatitis, pulmonary involvement, or hemolytic anemia. Children with central nervous system involvement usually experience sudden onset of fever and neurologic symptoms, which may progress to coma. Gradual, usually complete recovery occurs within 1 to 6 months.

Diagnosis

The diagnosis of CSD is usually suggested by the typical appearance of tender chronic regional lymphadenopathy that develops slowly over 2 to 3 weeks in a patient with a history of cat scratch or exposure. Diagnosis is confirmed by the demonstration of gram-negative bacilli using Warthin-Starry stain or recovery of the organism from culture. The CSD skin test antigen is positive in up to 90% of patients with CSD. However, the skin test reflects only previous exposure.

Treatment

The large majority of normal hosts with CSD recover spontaneously within several months without specific treatment. Needle aspiration or incision and drainage is necessary if suppuration of lymph nodes occurs. Normal hosts with disseminated CSD may respond to erythromycin, doxycycline, or trimethoprim-sulfamethoxazole therapy. However, in the majority of normal hosts with CSD, no antimicrobial therapy is recommended at this time.

Prevention

The only known effective means of prevention is avoidance of exposure to cats.

BACILLARY ANGIOMATOSIS

Another infection that appears to be transmitted by cats may produce cutaneous angiomas and peliosis of the liver or spleen in AIDS patients. It was initially confused with CSD (see Chapter 242) and was caused by *Rochalimaea quintana* and *R. henselae*.

Classification and characteristics

These bacilli produce an unusual vascular proliferation referred to as *bacillary epithelioid angiomatosis,* which occurs in immunocompromised hosts, especially patients with AIDS. These single or multiple skin lesions resemble proliferating angiomas (Plate V-42). Histologically, lobular capillary proliferation with edema and a mixture of acute and chronic inflammatory cells is present. Bacillary epithelioid angiomatosis may also involve the liver (peliosis hepatis), spleen, bone, and other tissues. Warthin-Starry stain may demonstrate numerous bacillary organisms in lymph node biopsy or in biopsy specimens of the cutaneous bacillary epithelioid angiomatosis.

Clinical manifestations

Typically, AIDS patients infected with *R. quintana* or *R. henselae* develop systemic symptoms of fever, chills, and night sweats. In some cases, a syndrome resembling septic shock occurs. Characteristically these patients also develop the single or multiple 0.5-6.0 cm exophytic nodules of bacillary angiomatosis. The nodules are friable, may be tender, and tend to bleed with minor trauma, whereas bleeding is less common with Kaposi's sarcoma. A second type of skin lesion may present as a deep subcutaneous mass with overlying skin changes resembling cellulitis. Disseminated bacillary epithelioid angiomatosis may involve the bone, spleen, liver, lung, and other tissues.

Treatment

Immunocompromised patients, including AIDS patients, with bacillary epithelioid angiomatosis have responded dramatically to erythromycin or doxycycline therapy, with complete resolution of cutaneous and osseous lesions. Therapy with ciprofloxacin or gentamicin has also reportedly been effective.

REFERENCES

Ariza J et al: Brucellar spondylitis: a detailed analysis based on current findings. Rev Infect Dis 7:656, 1985.

Boyce JM: Recent trends in the epidemiology of tularemia in the United States. J Infect Dis 131:197, 1975.

Brooks GF and Buchanan TM: Tularemia in the United States: epidemiologic aspects in the 1960s and follow-up of the outbreak of tularemia in Vermont. J Infect Dis 121:357, 1970.

Buchanan TM et al: Brucellosis in the United States, 1960–1972. An abattoir associated disease. I. II. III. Medicine (Baltimore) 53:403, 1974.

Butler T, Mahmoud AEF, and Warren KS: Algorithms in the diagnosis and management of exotic diseases. XXV. Plague. J Infect Dis 136:317, 1977.

Evans ME et al: Tularemia: a 30-year experience with 88 cases. Medicine (Baltimore) 64:251, 1985.

Fox MD and Kaufmann AF: Brucellosis in the United States 1965–1974. J Infect Dis 135:312, 1977.

Hoogkamp-Korstanje JA: Antibiotics in *Yersinia enterocolitica* infections. J Antimicrob Chemother 20:123, 1987.

Kaufmann AF, Boyce JM, and Martone WJ: Trends in human plague in the United States. J Infect Dis 141:522, 1980.

Koehler JE et al: Cutaneous vascular lesions and disseminated cat-scratch disease in patients with the acquired immunodeficiency syndrome (AIDS) and AIDS-related complex. Ann Intern Med 109:449, 1988.

Mann JM et al: Endemic human plague in New Mexico: risk factors associated with infection. J Infect Dis 140:397, 1979.

Marks MI et al: *Yersinia enterocolitica* gastroenteritis: a prospective study of clinical, bacteriologic, and epidemiologic features. J Pediatr 96:26, 1980.

Mason WL et al: Treatment of tularemia, including pulmonary tularemia, with gentamicin. Am Rev Respir Dis 121:39, 1980.

Mousa AR et al: The nature of human brucellosis in Kuwait: study of 379 cases. Rev Infect Dis 10:211, 1988.

Penn RL and Kinasewitz GT: Factors associated with a poor outcome in tularemia. Arch Intern Med 147:265, 1987.

Scribner RK et al: *Yersinia enterocolitica:* comparative in vitro activities of seven new beta-lactam antibiotics. Antimicrob Agents Chemother 22:140, 1982.

Wear DJ et al: Cat scratch disease: a bacterial infection. Science 221:1403, 1983.

Weber DJ et al: *Pasteurella multocida* infections. Report of 34 cases and review of the literature. Medicine (Baltimore) 63:133, 1984.

Wise RI: Brucellosis in the United States. Past, present, and future. JAMA 244:2318, 1980.

Young EJ: Human brucellosis. Rev Infect Dis 5:821, 1983.

CHAPTER

270 Infections Caused by *Bacteroides* and Other Mixed Nonsporulating Anaerobes

Anthony W. Chow

THE ORGANISMS

Classification and characteristics

Obligate anaerobes are a heterogeneous group of bacteria that require reduced oxygen tension for growth. By convention, they are defined as microorganisms that are unable to survive on the surface of solid media with less than 10% carbon dioxide in air (18% oxygen). In contrast, facultative bacteria can grow either in the presence or the absence of air, while microaerophilic or capnophilic bacteria grow poorly or not at all in air but grow better in less than 10% carbon dioxide in air or anaerobically. Within this broad definition, obligate anaerobes vary greatly in their sensitivity to oxygen. Extremely oxygen-sensitive anaerobes, for example, spirochetes and certain strains of *Clostridium,* cannot tolerate even 5 minutes of exposure to low concentrations of oxygen. As a general rule, obligate anaerobes commonly associated with infective processes are relatively aerotolerant and can survive for as long as 72 hours (but not replicate) in this environment.

Obligate anaerobes are part of the indigenous microflora on mucocutaneous surfaces, especially the oropharynx, skin, gastrointestinal tract, and genital tract. Infections involving these microbes, therefore, are primarily acquired endogenously. Such infections characteristically entail multiple organisms (polymicrobial), both anaerobic and facultative (mixed), reflecting the combined influence of the complex commensal flora and the unique microbiota of the underlying conditions. Clostridia (sporulating anaerobes) and actinomycetes are considered elsewhere (Chapters 262 and 277).

Taxonomic considerations. The generic classification of currently recognized, clinically important anaerobic bacteria, with their prevalence as normal flora or in infection, is presented in simplified form in Table 270-1. In the past, confusion over the nomenclature and taxonomy of obligate anaerobes was a major deterrent to recognition of the clinical significance of these microorganisms. More recently, aided by gas-liquid chromatographic analysis of acid end products, carbohydrate fermentation patterns, and other biochemical tests, clinically important anaerobes can be readily identified to species. The routine adoption of vastly improved culture techniques to achieve anaerobiosis; the introduction of prereduced, anaerobically sterilized media; and careful attention to specimen collection and transport have greatly enhanced the recovery of even very fastidious anaerobes from clinical material. This improved recovery has resulted in greater appreciation for the significance of these microorganisms. In addition, the unique association of specific nonsporulating anaerobes with certain clinical syndromes (e.g., *Bacteroides intermedius* and *B. gingivalis* in periodontal infections, and *B. bivius* and *B. disiens* in female genital infections) is being increasingly recognized. Such taxonomic differentiation clearly has important implications, not only in diagnostic and therapeutic considerations, but also in studies of the pathogenesis of these infections. In this regard, the not infrequent practice of referring to any gram-negative obligately anaerobic bacillus as a "bacteroides" and to those resistant to ampicillin and penicillin as *"B. fragilis"* without further bacterial speciation is not to be condoned.

Ecologic and host-parasite considerations

Indigenous microflora. Quantitatively, obligate anaerobes are the predominant bacteria present as normal microflora on mucocutaneous surfaces. They outnumber facultative bacteria by a factor of 10 to 1000 at several body sites, particularly the oropharynx, colon, and vagina (Table 270-2). Despite the complexity of the microbial composition, it is important to recognize the unique ecologic niches asso-

Table 270-1. Generic classification and prevalence of major anaerobic bacteria in normal flora and infection

Anaerobic bacteria	Genera	Normal flora: Skin	Oropharynx	Intestine	Genitalia	Common clinical isolates
Sporulating bacilli	*Clostridium*	0	±	2	±	*C. perfringens, C. difficile, C. ramosum, C. septicum, C. novyi*
Nonsporulating bacilli						
Gram-negative	*Bacteroides*	0	2	2	1	*B. fragilis, B. vulgatus, B. thetaiotaomicron, B. distasonis, B. melaninogenicus, B. asaccharolyticus, B. gingivalis, B. intermedius, B. bivius, B. disiens, B. capillosus*
	Fusobacterium	0	2	±	1	*F. nucleatum, F. necrophorum, F. varium, F. mortiferum*
Gram-positive	*Actinomyces*	0	1	±	0	*A. israelii, A. naeslundii, A. viscosus*
	Bifidobacterium	0	±	2	±	*B. eriksonii, B. breve*
	Eubacterium	±	1	2	±	*E. lentum, E. limosum*
	Lactobacillus	0	±	1	2	*L. casei, L. plantarum, L. acidophillus*
	Propionibacterium and *Arachnia*	2	±	±	1	*P. acnes, P. granulosum, A. propionica*
Cocci						
Gram-negative	*Veillonella* and *Acidaminococcus*	0	2	1	1	*V. parvula, A. fermentans*
Gram-positive	*Peptostreptococcus*	1	2	2	1	*P. asaccharolyticus, P. prevotii, P. magnus, P. variabilis, P. anaerobius, P. micros, P. parvulus, P. productus*
Spirochetes	*Treponema*	0	1	±	±	*T. vincentii, T. denticola*

0 = absent or rare; ± = irregularly present; 1 = usually present; 2 = predominant.

Table 270-2. Concentrations and distribution of major normal microflora at various body sites

Sites	Anaerobes		Aerobes	
	Bacterial concentration	Predominant genera	Bacterial concentration	Predominant genera
Skin	10^4-10^5/cm^2	*Propionibacterium*	10^2-10^3/cm^2	*Staphylococcus* *Micrococcus* "Diphtheroids"
Oropharynx	10^6-10^{11}/ml	*Peptostreptococcus* *Veillonella* *Actinomyces* *Bacteroides* *Fusobacterium*	10^4-10^6/ml	*Streptococcus*
Intestine				
Stomach and upper small bowel	10^1-10^4/ml	*Peptostreptococcus* *Veillonella*	10^1-10^4/ml	*Streptococcus* *Lactobacillus*
Lower small bowel	10^4-10^7/ml	*Bacteroides* *Bifidobacterium*	10^4-10^7/ml	"Coliforms"
Colon	10^{11}-10^{12}/ml	*Bacteroides* *Bifidobacterium* *Eubacterium* *Clostridium* *Peptostreptococcus* *Veillonella*	10^8-10^9/ml	*Escherichia* "Enterococci" *Lactobacillus*
Genitalia				
Vagina and endocervix	10^8-10^{10}/g	*Peptostreptococcus* *Lactobacillus* *Bacteroides*	10^7-10^9/g	*Lactobacillus* *Streptococcus* *Staphylococcus*

ciated with these indigenous bacteria. For example, in the oral cavity, *Streptococcus sanguis, S. mutans,* and *S. mitis,* as well as *Actinomyces viscosus,* preferentially colonize the tooth surface; in contrast, *S. salivarius* and *Veillonella parvula* have a predilection for the tongue and buccal mucosa. *B. vulgatus, B. thetaiotaomicron, B. fragilis,* and *B. distasonis* are primarily indigenous in the colon; *B. bivius* and *B. disiens* are primarily resident in the female genital tract.

The precise role of the indigenous microflora remains controversial. A prevailing view is that the presence of the indigenous flora provides a mucosal defense against colonization and subsequent invasion by organisms more traditionally associated with disease ("colonization resistance"). To accomplish this, these microbes must overcome many adverse host conditions to successfully colonize selective human mucosal surfaces. Some of these host conditions are mechanical, such as the flow of fluids over the epithelium, mucociliary clearance, and epithelial cell turnover. Some pertain to local environmental conditions, such as supply of essential nutrients, pH, oxidation-reduction potential (Eh), and oxygen tension. Still others relate to local immune factors that involve both specific and nonspecific antimicrobial systems. Thus, the mere introduction of an organism to a site does not ensure its establishment in the stable resident flora. It is likely that a highly specific microbe-host interaction ("adherence") is necessary for the indigenous flora to gain a selective advantage to be retained at a particular site, where the rate of microbial proliferation exceeds the rate of removal. It is curious that although the normal flora plays an important role in the mucosal host defenses, these same organisms have the potential to cause invasive disease under certain clinical conditions.

Although the microbial composition of the indigenous microflora at a given site in a specific individual appears to be relatively constant, this ecosystem is readily influenced by a variety of host and environmental factors. Thus, physiologic conditions such as pregnancy, menses, and age, underlying processes such as malignancy, and host factors such as diet, hospitalization, antimicrobial therapy, and recent surgery may all affect the indigenous microflora (Table 270-3). Knowledge of the anatomic location of the primary source of infection and the underlying condition of the host, therefore, is essential in predicting the probable organisms implicated in anaerobic and mixed infections associated with the indigenous microflora.

Pathophysiology

Obligate anaerobes implicated in mixed infections are generally of poor pathogenicity. However, under special circumstances that lead to either structural alterations in the normal mucosal barrier or tissue ischemia and lowered oxidation-reduction potential, these opportunistic organisms can proliferate and invade surrounding healthy tissues. Therefore, conditions that predispose to anaerobic infections are those that cause local ischemia or tissue necrosis, such as trauma, bite, foreign body, surgical manipulation, irradiation, or neoplasm.

Apart from impairment of local host defenses, certain microbial virulence factors may be particularly important for disease potential among some obligate anaerobes. This

Table 270-3. Effect of host conditions on indigenous microflora at various body sites

Site	Host factor	Change of flora
Gingiva	Dental caries and periodontal disease	Increased motile anaerobic gram-negative bacilli and spirochetes
Oropharynx	Hospitalization, antibiotics, or serious illness	Increased aerobic gram-negative bacilli
Upper small bowel	Achlorhydria, vagotomy, and pyloroplasty	Increased *E. coli, B. fragilis,* and *Bifidobacterium*
Small bowel	Regional enteritis, decreased motility, or stasis secondary to blind loop, obstruction, diverticula, irradiation, etc.	Colonic flora
	Disrupted anatomic continuity after bowel resection or bypass	Colonic flora
Large bowel	Colonic resection with ileostomy	Decreased anaerobes and some aerobes
Vagina	Parturition, hysterectomy, or irradiation	Increased *E. coli* and *B. fragilis*

concept is supported by the observation that the anaerobic pathogens commonly isolated in clinical infection often are not the organisms that are numerically dominant in the indigenous microflora. For example, in intra-abdominal infection after colonic perforation, *B. fragilis* is almost always present whereas *B. distasonis* and *B. vulgatus* are not, even though the latter organisms are more predominant in the normal colonic flora. It was later found that only *B. fragilis* is encapsulated, which accounts for its enhanced virulence, whereas the other members of the group are not.

Microbial factors considered important in the pathogenesis of anaerobic infections are summarized in Table 270-4. Obligate anaerobes are known to possess a number of extracellular or membrane-bound enzymes that may promote tissue destruction, provide nutrients, or allow microbial survival in a hostile environment. These enzymes include lipases, proteases, nucleases, and heparinases. Membrane-bound enzymes, for example, superoxide dismutase and beta-lactamases, may be important for protecting virulent organisms from the toxic effects of oxygen and beta-lactam antibiotics, respectively. Catalase may serve a function similar to that of superoxide dismutase. Organisms lacking these enzymes are susceptible to killing by toxic oxygen radicals and common antibiotics in the environment, and thus are less effective as pathogens.

Table 270-4. Microbial virulence factors important in mixed anaerobic infections

Microbial factors	Pathogenic effect
Histolytic enzymes (e.g., collagenase, fibrinolysin, hyaluronidase, protease, lipase, ribonuclease, deoxyribonuclease, etc.)	Tissue destruction
Oxygen-scavenging enzymes (e.g., superoxide dismutase, catalase, peroxidase)	Survival in aerobic environment
Endotoxin	Direct toxicity Hageman factor and complement activation
Capsular polysaccharide	Inhibition of phagocytosis Abscess formation
Surface ligands and charge	Adherence and bacterial interaggregation
IgA protease	Impairment of secretory and mucosal immunity
Heparinase	Promotion of coagulation and tissue ischemia
Beta-lactamase	Resistance to beta-lactam antibiotics
Bacteriocin and metabolites (e.g., fatty acids, H_2S, NH_3, etc.)	Inhibition of normal flora

B. fragilis and other anaerobes produce various short-chain fatty acids in vitro and in vivo. These fatty acids have been shown in several model systems to be deleterious to mammalian and bacterial cell function. Infections associated with *B. fragilis* are associated with production of high concentrations of succinic acid, which impairs the generation of the respiratory burst and profoundly reduces phagocytic killing and chemotactic responses of neutrophils. This effect is most evident at low pH and low Eh, and conditions present in abscesses and mixed infections. It has been suggested that succinic acid production may represent an important virulence mechanism by *Bacteroides* species in the pathogenesis of synergistic mixed infections.

B. fragilis, B. melaninogenicus, and a number of anaerobic gram-positive cocci are encapsulated. Possession of a capsule by these organisms is associated with increased virulence, as evidenced by their enhanced ability for abscess formation and systemic invasion. Interestingly, although nonencapsulated organisms by themselves may be unable to induce abscesses during experimental infection, many such strains become heavily encapsulated after a mixed infection with other aerobic and anaerobic bacteria. These heavily encapsulated strains are able to induce abscesses thereafter when inoculated alone. The selection of encapsulated anaerobes occurs in the presence of other encapsulated, or unencapsulated, but abscess-forming aerobic or anaerobic organisms. This phenomenon may help to explain how nonpathogenic organisms that are part of the normal host flora can become pathogens. It should be noted that although encapsulated anaerobes are more virulent than their nonencapsulated variants during experimental infection, and that encapsulated strains are more prevalent than nonencapsulated organisms at clinically infected sites, encapsulation is clearly not the only virulence factor important in the pathogenicity of polymicrobial infections containing obligate anaerobes. The capsular materials of *B. fragilis* and *B. melaninogenicus* have been extracted and purified. These large-molecular-weight polysaccharides have been demonstrated to inhibit phagocytosis in vitro and promote abscess formation in several animal models in vivo. In addition, several oral anaerobes, for example, *B. melaninogenicus, B. gingivalis,* and *B. intermedius,* are found to secrete IgA proteases that may impair secretory and local mucosal immunity.

Anaerobic gram-negative bacteria also possess lipopolysaccharides (LPS) in their outer cell membrane similar to their aerobic counterparts. However, the structure and biologic activity of LPSs from several anaerobic bacteria are distinctly different from those of the classic LPS of Enterobacteriaceae. For example, LPSs of *B. fragilis* and *B. intermedius* lack 2-keto-3-deoxyoctanoic acid and L-glycero-D-mannoheptose, and they have little endotoxic potency. The LPSs of *Fusobacterium nucleatum* and *V. parvula,* on the other hand, have biochemical and biologic properties similar to those of classic endotoxin.

Microbial synergy. Two thirds of infections in which obligate anaerobes can be isolated are mixed infections involving both anaerobes and facultative bacteria. The infectivity of obligate anaerobes in these instances is often facilitated by the coexistence of facultative organisms. Such examples of bacterial synergy are well demonstrated in periodontal infection, in progressive synergistic gangrene of Meleney, and in various animal models of intraabdominal and subcutaneous abscesses. A synergistic potential has been demonstrated between *Bacteroides* species and several aerobic bacteria, between *Bacteroides* species and most anaerobic gram-positive cocci, and between most anaerobic gram-positive cocci and *Pseudomonas aeruginosa* or *Staphylococcus aureus*. Participation by symbiotic facultative bacteria may be essential for the anaerobes by providing necessary growth factors, by lowering the oxidation-reduction potential of the environment, or by impairing local host defenses. Conversely, the presence of obligate anaerobes may benefit coexisting facultative bacteria either by growth enhancement, by protection from phagocytosis (e.g., succinic acid production by *Bacteroides* spp.) or by protection from beta-lactam antibiotics (e.g., beta-lactamase production). Microbial synergy for infection between an anaerobe and a facultative bacteria is best demonstrated within tissues where bacterial clearance is normally slow (e.g., subcutaneous abscesses, or fibrin clot in intraperitoneal infection) or is hampered by underlying disease. An understanding of the dynamic interactions between different components of a complex flora in mixed infections has important therapeutic implications. Microorganisms in mixed infections may handle antimicrobial agents differently from those in monomicrobial infections, and it may not be necessary to eradicate every bacterial species in mixed culture to achieve a cure. For example, in cases of pleuropulmonary infections associated with aspiration, penicillin therapy is often effective despite isolation of penicillin-resistant *B. fragilis* as part of a mixed flora. In this setting, the conventional sensitivity testing of every pathogen isolated as a guide to antimicrobial therapy may be obsolete.

CLINICAL PRESENTATIONS OF ANAEROBIC INFECTIONS

Anaerobic infections may involve any tissue or organ. Prospective studies utilizing modern anaerobic culture techniques indicate that anaerobic bacteria are particularly prevalent in infections of the head and neck, lung and pleural space, intra-abdominal organs, the female genital tract, and necrotic skin and soft tissues (Table 270-5). Salient clinical features of these infections are highlighted below.

Head and neck infections

Anaerobic infections of the head and neck most commonly involve the oral cavity and are odontogenic in origin (Chapter 230). These include dentoalveolar and periodontal infections and orofacial space abscesses. Anaerobes are also commonly present in chronic otitis media and mastoiditis and in tonsillar and peritonsillar abscesses. Acute sinusitis is seldom caused by anaerobic organisms unless it is associated with a dental infection. The clinical manifestations of these infections are largely dictated by the anatomic location and the extent and predetermined routes of spread (Fig. 270-1). Mandibular osteomyelitis may also result from infection complicating tooth extraction, from open fractures, or in association with debilitation, diabetes mellitus, radiation therapy, and malnutrition. Such infections not only may produce significant local symptoms but on rare occasions may also result in life-threatening complications, for example, mediastinal or intracranial extension,

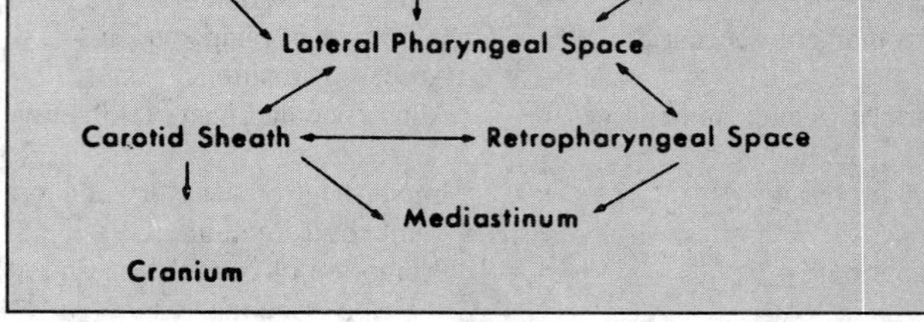

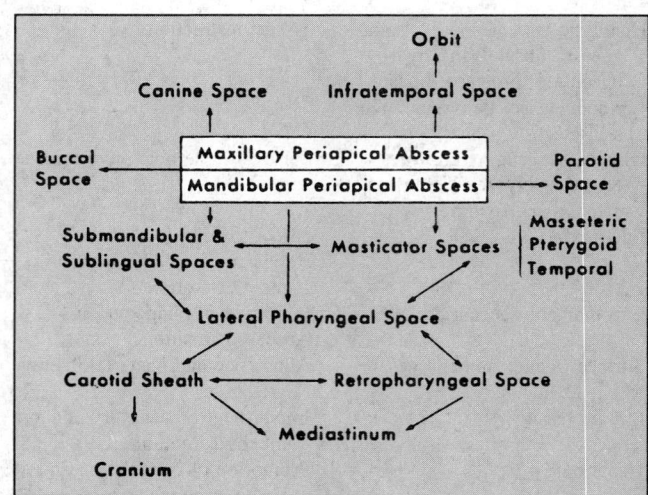

Fig. 270-1. Potential routes of spread of deep fascial space infections. (Reproduced with permission from Chow AW: Infections of the oral cavity, neck, and head. In Mandell GL, Douglas RG Jr, and Bennett JE, editors: Principles and practice of infectious diseases, ed 2. New York, 1985, Wiley.)

Table 270-5. Infections commonly or rarely associated with anaerobes

Site	Infections likely to involve anaerobes	Percentage with anaerobes	Infections unlikely to involve anaerobes
Head and neck	Periodontal and apical abscess	100	Acute infections of
	Fascial space infections	85	Sinuses
	Chronic sinusitis	50	Nasopharynx
	Chronic otitis media	50	Middle ear
Central nervous system	Brain abscess (not traumatic)	85	Meningitis
	Subdural empyema	(≅50)*	
Pleuropulmonary	Aspiration pneumonia	85	Bronchitis
	Necrotizing pneumonitis	85	Lobar pneumonia
	Abscess	90	
	Empyema	75	
Intra-abdominal	Peritonitis and abscess	95	Primary and "spontaneous" peritonitis
	Hepatic abscess	50	Cholecystitis or ascending cholangitis
			Pancreatitis
Female genital tract	Vulvovaginal abscess	75	Cystourethritis
	Salpingitis and pelvic peritonitis	50	Pyelonephritis
	Tubo-ovarian abscess	90	
	Posthysterectomy wound infection	70	
	Septic abortion and postpartum endometritis	75	
Skin, soft tissue, and bone	Crepitant cellulitis	(High)*	Septic arthritis
	Myonecrosis	100	Osteomyelitis of long bones
	Necrotizing fasciitis	(High)*	
	Synergistic cellulitis	(High)*	

*Percentages unavailable.

retropharyngeal spread with airway obstruction, pleuropulmonary suppuration, and hematogenous dissemination.

The concept of microbial specificity in odontogenic and other head and neck infections has been appreciated only recently. In the healthy periodontium, the microflora is sparse, consisting mainly of gram-positive organisms such as *S. sanguis* and *Actinomyces* species. In the presence of gingivitis, the subgingival flora shifts to a predominantly anaerobic gram-negative flora with *B. intermedius* as the most common isolate. In advanced periodontitis, the flora further increases in complexity, with a preponderance of anaerobic gram-negative motile bacilli and spirochetes; *B. gingivalis* is then most commonly isolated. Overall, the *B. melaninogenicus* strains (particularly *B. asaccharolyticus, B. gingivalis, B. intermedius,* and *B. melaninogenicus*), *F. nucleatum, Peptostreptococcus* species, *Actinomyces* species, and streptococci are the most prevalent isolates in pyogenic orofacial infections arising from odontogenic sources. *Fusobacterium, Bacteroides,* and anaerobic gram-positive cocci are also commonly isolated in chronic or recurrent maxillary sinusitis. *Fusobacterium necrophorum* and *B. melaninogenicus* are most frequently recovered from tonsillar and peritonsillar abscesses. Although the anaerobes associated with orofacial and upper respiratory infections were considered to be universally susceptible to penicillin in the past, recent data indicate that beta-lactamase–producing strains, particularly members of the *B. melaninogenicus* group and *B. oralis,* have become increasingly prevalent. Furthermore, rapid emergence of beta-lactamase–producing anaerobes as well as aerobes has been documented after a single course of penicillin therapy for acute tonsillitis. Such organisms not only can survive penicillin therapy, they may also protect other penicillin-susceptible bacteria by release of beta-lactamase in infected tissue. The selection of beta-lactamase–producing aerobes and anaerobes during therapy may account for suboptimal responses to penicillin in some cases of head and neck infections. Except in selected patients with serious underlying illness, aerobic gram-negative bacilli and staphylococci are not commonly involved in head and neck infections.

Central nervous system infections

Anaerobic bacteria are frequent pathogens in intracranial infections, particularly those caused by contiguous spread from chronic otitis media, mastoiditis, or sinusitis (Chapter 238). Intracranial extension may result in brain abscess, subdural empyema, epidural abscess, or suppurative thrombophlebitis of cortical vessels or venous sinuses. Anaerobic intracranial infections may also occur by hematogenous dissemination, particularly from chronic and suppurative pulmonary foci, or in the presence of cyanotic congenital heart disease. Purulent meningitis, except in the newborn, seldom involves anaerobic bacteria. Cerebral abscesses of sinus or dental origin are more probably caused by *Streptococcus milleri,* either alone or in mixed culture with other oropharyngeal aerobes and anaerobes. Otogenic cerebral abscesses, on the other hand, frequently involve *B. fragilis, Proteus* spp. and streptococci.

Pleuropulmonary infections

Anaerobic bacteria are important pulmonary pathogens, particularly after aspiration of oropharyngeal secretions (Chapter 230). Anaerobic pleuropulmonary infections include aspiration pneumonitis, putrid lung abscess, necrotizing pneumonia, and empyema. Pneumonitis is usually the initial lesion, and related symptoms in the early phases may be indistinguishable from other causes of acute bacterial pneumonia. However, if untreated, pulmonary abscess may occur after 8 to 14 days. Approximately one half of patients with lung abscess develop putrid-smelling expectorations. The subsequent clinical course depends largely on the nature of the underlying pulmonary pathologic condition. About 10% of patients with anaerobic infections of the lung parenchyma develop empyema. Necrotizing pneumonia is characterized by multiple small cavities within a pulmonary segment or lobe. The course is often fulminant, with rapid extension into adjacent segments.

Anaerobic pleuropulmonary infections are typically polymicrobial in nature. Predominant anaerobic isolates include *Peptostreptococcus* species, *F. nucleatum,* and the saccharolytic black-pigmented *Bacteroides (B. melaninogenicus* and *B. intermedius).* Aerobic and microaerophilic streptococci (e.g., *Streptococcus intermedius*) are also frequently isolated. Hospital-acquired infections have a higher co-isolation rate of aerobes such as *S. aureus, Escherichia coli, Klebsiella pneumoniae,* and *P. aeruginosa* than does community-acquired aspiration pneumonia.

Intra-abdominal infections

Intra-abdominal sepsis most commonly results from bacterial contamination of intraperitoneal or retroperitoneal spaces after intestinal perforation (Chapter 232). The initial event is peritonitis, either generalized or localized, with subsequent abscess formation. Common predisposing conditions include penetrating trauma, perforated appendicitis or diverticulitis, inflammatory bowel disease, intestinal malignancy with strangulation or obstruction, and anastomotic leak following intestinal surgery. Although a multiplicity of anaerobic and facultative bacteria may be isolated in intra-abdominal infections—particularly *B. fragilis, Peptostreptococcus* spp., *Clostridium* spp., Enterobacteriaceae, and *Streptococcus faecalis*—it is not always clear which components are the primary pathogens and which are merely symbionts or commensals. Animal studies of experimental peritonitis simulating intestinal perforation have further elucidated the pathogenesis of such infections and suggest a biphasic process. Early peritonitis and bacteremia are related to aerobic coliform bacteria, whereas late abscesses are caused by anaerobes, often in synergy with facultative bacteria. Apart from the causative agents in abscess formation, other intestinal bacteria not involved initially may subsequently translocate into the abscess. The most common translocating intestinal bacteria include enterococci and *E. coli*. The exact mechanism for this translocation, whether by hematogenous or lymphatic channels, by transmural migration from the intestinal lumen, or by phagocytic transport, is presently unknown. The presence of fibrin in the peritoneal cavity during peritonitis also appears to predispose to abscess formation. Fibrin appears to inhibit phagocytic function by entrapment of bacteria and neutrophils, impairing phagocytosis. The therapeutic implications of these studies are clear: both microbial components of intra-abdominal sepsis should receive appropriate antimicrobial attention. Early surgical debridement of fibrinous exudate and necrotic debris is critical. Use of fibrinolytic agents (e.g., trypsin) may be a useful adjunct in preventing abscess formation postoperatively.

Obstetric and gynecologic infections

Most female genital tract infections including the classic sexually transmitted diseases (STDs) are polymicrobial in nature and frequently involve both facultative and anaerobic bacteria. In general, three major classes of microorganisms have been implicated: (1) those considered to be exogenous STD pathogens (e.g., *Neisseria gonorrhoeae, Chlamydia trachomatis,* herpes simplex, *Trichomonas vaginalis*); (2) mixed aerobes and anaerobes indigenous to the cervicovaginal normal flora; and (3) genital mycoplasmas (e.g., *Mycoplasma hominis* and *Ureaplasma urealyticum*) (Table 270-6). Mixed aerobes and anaerobes are particularly important in closed-space infections such as vulvovaginal, adnexal, or tubo-ovarian abscesses, and in postsurgical and postpartum infections. Other common gynecologic and obstetric infections involving a mixed aerobic and anaerobic flora include acute and chronic salpingitis, infections associated with contraceptive intrauterine devices, postpartum or postcesarean section wound infections, endometritis, and amnionitis. The most common anaerobes found include *Bacteroides* spp. (especially *B. bivius, B. disiens,* and *B. melaninogenicus*), *Peptostreptococcus* spp., and *Actinomyces* spp. The most common facultative pathogens are Enterobacteriaceae (especially *E. coli*), and aerobic or microaerophilic streptococci. *B. fragilis* is not a common organism in the normal vagina, but its prevalence is increased in posthysterectomy and postcesarean section infections, and in pelvic infections associated with malignancy and immunosuppressive therapy. The entity of "nonspecific vaginitis" or bacterial vaginosis also appears to be a polymicrobial infection involving both aerobes and anaerobes. Apart from *Gardnerella vaginalis,* high concentrations of *Bacteroides* spp., *Peptostreptococcus* spp. and *Mobiluncus* spp. (a motile anaerobic curved gram-negative bacillus) can be regularly isolated from vaginal secretions compared with uninfected control specimens.

Necrotic skin and soft tissue infections

Necrotic wound and soft tissue infections are particularly prone to develop in areas that have been injured by trauma,

Table 270-6. Predominant microorganisms in female genital tract infections

Type of infection	Major pathogens implicated		
	Exogenous STD agents	Endogenous mixed aerobes and anaerobes	Genital mycoplasmas
Periurethral and labial pyrogenic infections	+	++	±
Vulvovaginitis	±	++	±
Cervicitis, endometritis, and salpingitis	++	++	+
Tubo-ovarian abscess	±	++	
Posthysterectomy and other pelvic infections		++	
Postpartum and postcesarean section infections		++	+

STD, sexually transmitted disease. + = less common; ++ = most common; ± = not present.

ischemia, or surgery (Chapter 235). Anatomic sites regularly exposed to fecal or oral contamination are particularly at risk, such as wounds associated with intestinal surgery, decubitus and diabetic ulcers, human bites, and infected pilonidal cysts. Clinical manifestations include crepitant cellulitis, synergistic necrotizing cellulitis or gangrene, myonecrosis, and necrotizing fascitis. The range of bacterial isolates in such infections is enormous. Anaerobes, including *Bacteroides* spp., anaerobic cocci, and clostridia, are almost universally present in mixed culture.

Anaerobic bacteremia and endocarditis

Obligate anaerobes account for 9% to 14% of all significant positive blood cultures from a general hospital population (Table 270-7). *Bacteroides* spp. are the predominant isolates, followed by *Peptostreptococcus* and *Clostridium* spp. *B. fragilis* has been reported as the third most common cause of gram-negative bacillary bacteremia, surpassed only by *E. coli* and *K. pneumoniae*. The clinical manifestations of anaerobic bacteremia and the specific organisms involved depend to a large extent on the portal of entry and the nature of the underlying disease. For example, *B. fragilis* is most common in bacteremia of gastrointestinal and necrotic soft tissue origin. Bacteroidaceae bacteremia of the female genital tract and odontogenic origin rarely involves *B. fragilis;* more commonly, *Peptostreptococcus* spp. is isolated. The latter is also associated with bacteremia related to necrotic soft tissue infections, and occasionally in necrotizing pneumonia and empyema. *Fusobacterium* spp., when isolated, are usually oropulmonary or pelvic in origin. Several clinical features are particularly distinctive in anaerobic bacteremia. Excessive jaundice with hyperbilirubinemia has been noted in 10% to 40% of cases. Suppurative thrombophlebitis may be present in 5% to 12% of cases, primarily involving the pelvic, hepatic, mesenteric, and portal veins. Polymicrobial bacteremia is particularly prevalent in infections of gastrointestinal, female genital, and odontogenic origin. Anaerobic bacteremia of female genital and odontogenic sources tends to be transient and self-limited. In contrast, anaerobic bacteremia of gastrointestinal and necrotic soft tissue sources tends to be recurrent and persistent in the absence of surgical drainage. Although anaerobic bacteria can cause endocarditis, such infections appear to be exceedingly rare.

Table 270-7. Prevalence of anaerobes in bacteremia

	Harbor-UCLA Medical Center	Vancouver General Hospital
Total number of patients with bacteremia	1348	686
Number with anaerobes (%)*	185 (14)	62 (9)
Number polymicrobial (%)*	42 (23)	12 (19)
Major isolates (%)*		
Bacteroides	46	61
Peptostreptococcus	16	13
Clostridium	10	22
Fusobacterium	4	2

*Percentage of cases with anaerobic bacteremia.

DIAGNOSIS

Clinical clues to anaerobic infections

Apart from actinomycosis and clostridial myonecrosis, infections involving obligate anaerobes are generally indistinguishable from other causes of sepsis. Clinical manifestations are largely determined by the organ system involved and by the extent and chronicity of the infection. The clinical setting of infection suggestive of local tissue ischemia or necrosis and the proximity of infection to mucosal surfaces where obligate anaerobes normally reside are the two most helpful clues. The presence of putrid, foul-smelling discharge is virtually diagnostic of infection involving anaerobes, although the absence of foul odor does not rule out this possibility. Similarly, the finding of crepitus or black discoloration of affected tissue is only suggestive evidence. A well-performed Gram stain of appropriately collected clinical material is a very useful diagnostic tool. Anaerobic infections are typically polymicrobial, and the characteristic cellular morphology of certain anaerobic pathogens may be recognized by an accomplished microscopist. The finding of "sterile" pus by conventional culture methods in the face of a positive Gram stain should be considered presumptive evidence of an anaerobic infection. In the final analysis, however, the accurate diagnosis of anaerobic infection depends on the ability of the laboratory to isolate these fastidious organisms from clinical material likely to yield meaningful bacteriologic data.

Specimen collection and transport

One of the major handicaps in the recovery of anaerobic bacteria is improper specimen collection and transport (Chapter 226). Care must be taken to avoid specimens that may be potentially contaminated by commensal flora of mucocutaneous surfaces where anaerobes normally reside (e.g., throat swabs, expectorated sputum, voided urine, bronchoscopic and nasotracheal aspirates, vaginal secretions, feces, colostomy effluent, or superficial wound swabs). Blood and other body fluids that are normally sterile and aseptically obtained should be routinely cultured for anaerobic bacteria. Other clinical materials and special procedures likely to yield meaningful bacteriologic data for anaerobic infections are summarized in Table 270-8.

Apart from judicious selection of appropriate specimens for culture, proper specimen transport to preclude aeration and adequate anaerobic culture techniques are equally important for documentation of an anaerobic infection. Many fastidious organisms are extremely oxygen-sensitive and cannot withstand even a brief moment of exposure to air. Fluid transport media such as thioglycolate broth or Stuart's medium support growth of aerobes as well as anaerobes. In the presence of a mixed infection, facultative organisms, which grow faster than anaerobes, frequently preclude recovery of the latter. An ideal transport system, therefore, should be nonselective and nonbactericidal, and have sufficiently low oxidation-reduction potential and minimum susceptibility to oxidation. Such an ideal system is costly and not readily available commercially. The closest substitute consists of gas-filled containers, usually flushed with carbon dioxide. Specimens are collected with a sterile needle and syringe, and care is taken to expel the air in the syringe before instillation of the specimen into the transport vial. If commercial anaerobic transport vials are not available, specimens should be retained within the needle and syringe, capped to minimize aeration, and delivered immediately to the clinical laboratory. If swabs are to be used, it is recommended that they be prepared, stored, and transported in gas-filled containers under anaerobic conditions. Immediate processing of specimens by the laboratory also improves recovery, but in practice, this is often not feasible.

Table 270-8. Recommended procedure for specimen collection for anaerobic culture

Source	Procedure
Pulmonary	Percutaneous transtracheal aspiration or bronchoscopic aspiration with protected catheter or brush
Pleural	Thoracentesis
Odontogenic space infections	Extraoral aspiration of abscess
Female genital	Culdocentesis or dilation and curettage per cervical os
Sinus tract or draining wounds	Needle and syringe aspiration of wound edge through intact skin; specimen obtained by tissue biopsy or curettage, or at surgery from depths of wound always preferred

Radiologic and imaging studies

Noninvasive tests such as computed tomography, ultrasonography, and gallium, technetium, or indium scanning are most useful for localization of suppurative infections in the central nervous system, and in intra-abdominal and pelvic organs. The sensitivity and specificity of these tests in detection of abscess and differentiation from tumor, hematoma, and other noninflammatory space-occupying lesions in various sites remain to be determined by careful prospective study. In general, it may be said that a positive scan is highly suggestive, particularly when supported by the clinical picture; however, a negative scan is much less useful in ruling out infection.

THERAPY

Antimicrobial susceptibility and empiric therapy

Successful treatment of anaerobic infections requires rational antibiotic selection in conjunction with judicial surgical resection and drainage. Choice of appropriate antibiotics should be guided by culture results and antibiotic susceptibility data on the specific organisms involved (Chapter 224). Unfortunately, there is considerable method-related variability in susceptibility results, and as yet there is no general agreement as to the "gold standard" method that should be followed in the clinical laboratory. For these reasons, and because certain drugs are essentially always active against certain anaerobes, it has been accepted that not all clinical anaerobic isolates require in vitro susceptibility testing. Susceptibility testing is important, however, particularly in clinical settings where there has been persistence of infection or suboptimal response to empiric antibiotic regimens. Which specific anaerobic isolate to test when several are present and which drugs to be included remain somewhat controversial issues. Certainly, organisms that are recognized as virulent and are frequently resistant and antibiotics that are frequently used as empiric therapy should be considered for testing. The former includes some members of the *B. fragilis* group, pigmented *Bacteroides* species, *B. bivius, B. disiens,* certain *Fusobacterium* species, and *Clostridium* species. The latter includes penicillin G, certain broad-spectrum antipseudomonal penicillins (e.g., ticarcillin, piperacillin, mezlocillin) and carbapenems (e.g., imipenem), clindamycin, and certain cephalosporins (e.g., cefoxitin, ceftriaxone, cefotetan, cefotaxime, ceftizoxime, ceftazidime, etc.).

In the absence of specific culture or susceptibility data,

initial antibiotic therapy requires empiric choices based on knowledge of the pathogens most likely to be present in a particular clinical setting, predicted in vitro susceptibility patterns (Table 270-9), and the toxicologic and pharmacokinetic characteristics of the agents being considered.

Although penicillin G has been considered the agent of choice for a number of mixed aerobic-anaerobic infections at various sites above the diaphragm (particularly in oropulmonary and head and neck infections), recent experience suggests that this general recommendation may no longer be tenable. This concern has arisen based on the following findings: (1) beta-lactamase production has been observed with increasing frequency among clinical isolates of anaerobic bacteria besides *B. fragilis* (particularly *B. bivius, B. disiens, B. gracilis,* and pigmented *Bacteroides* species); (2) beta-lactamase production is increasingly found among aerobic isolates, which may protect co-isolated penicillin-sensitive anaerobes (e.g., *Branhamella catarrhalis, Haemophilus influenzae, Staphylococcus* species); (3) beta-lactamase activity can be detected directly in clinical specimens; and (4) failure of penicillin therapy has been well documented. These data highlight the need to reassess the role of beta-lactamase production both as a virulence mechanism and as a cause for therapeutic failure in mixed infections. It remains to be seen whether routine use of a beta-lactamase inhibitor (such as clavulanic acid or sulbactam) in combination with penicillin will resolve these current concerns. Among the beta-lactams, susceptibility of obligate anaerobes to ampicillin is comparable to that of penicillin G, whereas penicillin V and semisynthetic penicillins (e.g., methicillin and cloxacillin) are distinctly less active. Among the cephalosporins, only cefoxitin, cefotetan, and ceftizoxime have enhanced antianaerobic spectrum. These agents appear to have comparable activity against *B. fragilis,* with resistance rates ranging from 3% to 17%, and none is as active as clindamycin or metronidazole. Other cephalosporins (e.g., cefazolin, cephalexin, cefamandole, cefuroxime, ceftriaxone, cefoperazone, ceftazidime, etc.) are much less active. Among the penems, imipenem-cilastatin is the most broadly active. It has the added advantage of excellent antipseudomonal and antistaphylococcal spectrum. The monobactam, aztreonam, is inactive against anaerobes as well as gram-positive aerobes.

Clindamycin remains highly active against *B. fragilis* and other anaerobes, although emerging resistance has been noted in some centers. Erythromycin is not considered useful for anaerobic infections because of relative resistance by *B. fragilis* and some strains of *Fusobacterium.* It is difficult to administer parenterally, and only low blood levels are achieved by the oral route. The role of newer macrolides (e.g., roxithromycin, azithromycin, clarithromycin) remains to be determined.

Metronidazole has excellent activity, particularly against *B. fragilis, Fusobacterium* spp., and *Clostridium perfringens.* However, *Peptostreptococcus* and *Bacteroides* species other than *B. fragilis* are only moderately sensitive, whereas nonsporulating gram-positive bacilli are relatively resistant to therapeutic levels of metronidazole. Metronidazole lacks activity against aerobic bacteria and should not be used as a single agent during empiric therapy, since most infections involving anaerobic bacteria are in fact mixed infections. Importantly, metronidazole is the only agent with consistent bactericidal activity against *B. fragilis,* and it crosses the blood-brain barrier well. For these

Table 270-9. Comparative in vitro antibiotic activity against major anaerobes

	Above diaphragm		Above/below diaphragm		Below diaphragm	
Antibiotic	***Fusobacterium***	***Bacteroides melaninogenicus* group**	***Peptostreptococcus***	***Actinomyces***	***Bacteroides fragilis* group**	***Clostridium***
Penicillin	S	S-R	S	S	R	S*
Ampicillin-sulbactam†	S	S	S	S	S	S
Piperacillin, ticarcillin, mezlocillin	S	S	S	S	S-R	S
Piperacillin-tazobactam	S	S	S	S	S	S
Imipenem	S	S	S	S	S	S
Cefazolin	S	S-R	S	S	R	S
Cefoxitin	S	S	S	S	S	S-R
Cefotetan	S	S	S	S	S-R	S
Ceftizoxime	S	S	S	S	S	S-R
Cefotaxime	S	S	S	S	S-R	S
Ceftriaxone	S	S-R	S	S	S-R	S
Cefoperazone	S	S	S	S	S-R	S
Ceftazidime	S	S-R	S	S	S-R	S
Clindamycin	S*	S	S*	S	S	S-R
Chloramphenicol	S	S	S	S	S*	S
Metronidazole	S	S	S-R	R	S	S
Tetracycline	S	S-R	S-R	S	S-R	S-R

S, >80% strains sensitive; S-R, 30%-80% strains sensitive; R, <30% strains sensitive.
*Emerging resistance noted.
†Similar combinations currently available are amoxicillin-clavulanic acid and ticarcillin-clavulanic acid; they have comparable activities against anaerobes.

reasons, it is particularly useful for treating anaerobic brain abscess or endocarditis.

Chloramphenicol is active against a wide range of anaerobic bacteria, including *B. fragilis,* and like metronidazole, no resistance to it by these strains has been noted. Because of its myelotoxic properties, it should be reserved for treating selected patients with anaerobic infections involving the central nervous system.

Tetracycline and its analogs can no longer be recommended as empiric treatment of anaerobic infections because of the substantial resistance acquired by *B. fragilis* and virtually all classes of other anaerobic bacteria. Tetracycline, however, remains useful in the treatment of actinomycosis.

Trimethoprim-sulfamethoxazole, vancomycin, and the fluoroquinolones have only limited activity against anaerobic bacteria. Vancomycin is effective against some gram-positive anaerobes (particularly *Clostridium difficile*) but has no activity against gram-negative anaerobes. Similarly, among the quinolones, ciprofloxacin is more active than enoxacin, ofloxacin, or norfloxacin, but none are reliable as single-agent therapy for anaerobic or mixed infections.

Aminoglycoside antibiotics are uniformly inactive against obligate anaerobes. These drugs are often included in antimicrobial regimens directed at facultative gram-negative bacilli for therapy of mixed infections.

The recommended regimens for empiric therapy of various anaerobic or mixed infections at different sites are summarized in Table 270-10. In general, therapy should be directed at both the aerobic and anaerobic components of the suspected microflora. Although a broad-spectrum single agent (e.g., cefoxitin, ceftizoxine, cefotetan, ampicillin-sulbactam, piperacillin-tazobactom, ticarcillin-clavulanic acid, imipenem-cilastatin) may be used to minimize toxicity and reduce cost, combination therapy is sometimes preferred to achieve synergistic activity (e.g., penicillin, clindamycin, metronidazole, or enhanced cephalosporins, each plus an aminoglycoside). A parenteral route for administration, relatively high dosages, and prolonged duration of treatment (3 to 6 weeks) are usually required because of the extent of tissue necrosis and tendency for relapse with these infections.

Surgical drainage of abscesses

Although surgical resection and drainage may be the decisive therapeutic modality for most suppurative anaerobic infections, several exceptions are noteworthy. In lung abscess, nonsurgical treatment alone is often effective, perhaps because of spontaneous drainage and expectoration of abscess contents through the tracheobronchial tree. Recent experience indicates, however, that certain cerebral abscesses may also respond to antibiotics alone even when well encapsulated. A similar experience has been noted with hepatic and tubo-ovarian abscesses. These data indicate that abscesses do not always require drainage, although it is not clear what factors are reliable predictors of a favorable response to antibiotics alone.

Adjunctive measures

Apart from surgical and antimicrobial therapy, adjunctive measures such as topical wound irrigations with hydrogen peroxide solution and hyperbaric oxygen treatment may further hasten eradication of infection and promote healing. Although data from well-controlled studies are lacking, hyperbaric oxygen therapy has been recommended for selected cases of necrotic soft tissue infections, and for recalcitrant anaerobic osteomyelitis involving the maxilla or mandible.

PREVENTION

Anaerobic infections can be prevented by avoiding conditions that predispose to invasion by surface microflora. In traumatic wounds, the most effective prophylaxis is thorough debridement and cleansing of the wound, elimination of foreign bodies and dead space, and reestablishment of good circulation. The complex gastrointestinal or vaginal flora can be numerically reduced before surgery. Mechanical cleansing of the bowel with a low-residue or liquid diet followed by cathartics, enemas, and luminal antibiotics effectively reduces the bacterial concentration in the colon preoperatively. Parenteral perioperative antibiotics also have been used prophylactically in gastrointestinal and gy-

Table 270-10. Empiric antimicrobial regimens for suspected anaerobic or mixed infections

Site	Treatment of choice	Alternate regimens
Pleuropulmonary, odontogenic, or human bite infections	Penicillin G IV, 1-4 MU q4h or ampicillin-sulbactam IV, 1-2 g q6h	Clindamycin IV, 600 mg q6h Cefoxitin IV, 1-2 g q6h Cefotaxime IV, 2 g q6h
Brain abscess or subdural empyema	Penicillin G IV, 4 MU q4h + metronidazole IV, 500 mg q6h	Penicillin G IV, 4 MU q4h + chloramphenicol 500 mg q6h
Intra-abdominal, pelvic, or necrotic soft tissue infections	Clindamycin IV, 600 mg q6h or metronidazole IV, 500 mg q6h; each + tobramycin IV, q8h or ciprofloxacin IV, 200 mg q12h	Cefoxitin IV, 2 g q6h, cefotetan IV, 2 g q12h, ceftizoxime IV, 3 g q8h, piperacillin IV, 3 g q4h, imipenem IV, 500 mg q6h, or piperacillin-tazobactam IV, 2-4 g q4-6h; each ± tobramycin IV, q8h or ciprofloxacin IV, q12h

necologic surgery when there is possibility of contamination with normal microflora at the operative site. Those operations that may benefit from prophylactic antibiotics include elective colorectal surgery, gastroduodenal surgery when intraluminal bacterial overgrowth is anticipated, cesarean section after rupture of the membranes and labor, vaginal hysterectomy in the premenopausal woman, and radical pelvic or head and neck surgery for malignancy. Several studies have shown significant reduction in the frequency of postoperative infections from about 20% to 30% to 4% to 8% after prophylactic administration of antibiotics in clean, uncontaminated surgery. Cephalosporins have been particularly useful in prophylactic regimens for head and neck, pelvic, and gastrointestinal surgery. Comparative studies have indicated that for surgical prophylaxis involving colorectal or pelvic procedures, a first-generation cephalosporin, such as cefazolin, may be as effective as some second- or third-generation cephalosporins, including cefonicid, cefoxitin, cefotetan, ceftizoxime, or cefotaxime. In contaminated or "dirty" surgery, early *treatment* rather than prophylaxis is essential for reduction of postoperative morbidity.

REFERENCES

Aldridge KE et al: Discordant results between the broth disk elution and broth microdilution susceptibility tests with *Bacteroides fragilis* group isolates. J Clin Microbiol 28:375, 1990.

Appleman MD, Heseltine PNR, and Cherubin CE: Epidemiology, antimicrobial susceptibility, pathogenicity, and significance of *Bacteroides fragilis* group organisms isolated at Los Angeles County–University of Southern California Medical Center. Rev Infect Dis 13:12, 1991.

Bartlett JG: Anaerobic bacterial infections of the lung. Chest 91:901, 1987.

Bennion RS et al: Gangrenous and perforated appendicitis with peritonitis—treatment and bacteriology. Clin Therapeut 12(suppl B):1, 1990.

Brook I: A 12 year study of aerobic and anaerobic bacteria in intra-abdominal and postsurgical abdominal wound infections. Surg Gynecol Obstet 169:387, 1989.

Browder W et al: Nonperforative appendicitis—a continuing surgical dilemma. J Infect Dis 159:1088, 1989.

Chow AW: Life-threatening infections of the head and neck. Clin Infect Dis 14:991, 1992.

Cuchural GJ Jr et al: Comparative activities of newer Ã-lactam agents against members of the *Bacteroides fragilis* group. Antimicrob Ag Chemother 34:479, 1990.

DiPiro JT and May JR: Use of cephalosporins with enchanced antianaerobic activity for treatment and prevention of anaerobic and mixed infections. Clin Pharm 7:285, 1988.

Finegold SM: Anaerobes—problems and controversies in bacteriology, infections, and susceptibility testing. Rev Infect Dis 12(suppl 2):s223, 1990.

Finegold SM and Wexler HM: Therapeutic implications of bacteriologic findings in mixed aerobic-anaerobic infections. Antimicrob Ag Chemother 32:611, 1988.

Garber GE and Chow AW: Female genital tract infections. In George WL and Finegold SM, eds: Anaerobic infections in humans. New York, 1989, Academic Press.

Garcia-Sabrido JL et al: Treatment of severe intra-abdominal sepsis and/or necrotic foci by an "open-abdomen" approach. Arch Surg 123:152, 1988.

Hackford AW et al: Prospective study comparing imipenem-cilastatin with clindamycin and gentamicin for the treatment of serious surgical infections. Arch Surg 123:322, 1988.

Kurtesz D and Chow AW: Infected pressure and diabetic ulcers. Clin Geriat Med 8:835, 1992.

Rotstein OD, Pruett TL, and Simmons RL: Mechanisms of microbial synergy in polymicrobial surgical infections. Rev Infect Dis 7:151, 1985.

CHAPTER

271 *Bordetella pertussis* Infection (Whooping Cough)

J. Owen Hendley

Pertussis (whooping cough) is an acute contagious disease of all age groups and is caused by *Bordetella pertussis,* a strictly human pathogen. In children, infection of the ciliated epithelium of the respiratory tract with *B. pertussis* results in the pathognomonic symptom complex of paroxysmal cough followed by an inspiratory whoop. In contrast, infection in adults characteristically causes a mild illness that mimics prolonged bronchitis.

THE ORGANISM

Classification

B. pertussis is a nonmotile, gram-negative coccobacillus approximately 0.5 × 1.0 μm in size; it produces beta hemolysis on Bordet-Gengou (B-G) agar. The genus *Bordetella* can be distinguished from *Haemophilus,* with which it was formerly classified, by the lack of growth requirements for factors X and V and lack of production of nitrate or indole. In addition to *B. pertussis,* the genus *Bordetella* includes *B. parapertussis* and the enzootic *B. bronchiseptica. B. parapertussis* infrequently produces mild disease in humans, in spite of the fact that immunity to *B. pertussis* does not protect against infection with *B. parapertussis.*

B. pertussis, like other gram-negative bacteria, has a wide array of antigens. Several are of interest because of the effort to produce an effective acellular vaccine to replace the vaccine containing whole organisms. Antigens elaborated by the organisms include filamentous hemagglutinin (FHA) and lymphocytosis promoting factor (LPF), also called *pertussis toxin.* Absorbed LPF may cause systemic effects such as the lymphocytosis in patients with pertussis. Serotyping of *B. pertussis,* begun in the 1950s, was based on demonstrating agglutinogens on the bacteria. Serotyping was simplified during the 1980s as workers in England established that *B. pertussis* has fimbriae of two antigenically distinct types, which correspond to agglutinogens 2 and 3 under the old scheme. Agglutinogen 1 is not fimbrial and is present on all strains of *B. pertussis.* Isolates can now be typed as having agglutinogen 1 plus none, one, or both types of fimbrial agglutinogens.

Epidemiology

Pertussis occurs worldwide with little seasonal variation. After widespread pertussis vaccination of infants in the late 1940s, the incidence of pertussis in children decreased by over 50%. In North America, the age-specific attack rate of pertussis has shifted from a peak in preschool and school-age children to higher attack rates in infants and adolescents. The shift to the older age group is consistent with the loss of vaccine-induced immunity after 10 to 12 years.

Pertussis is most severe in infants less than 6 months of age, and mortality is greatest in this age group. The occurrence of disease in young infants emphasizes the unusual lack of immunity in the newborn. Low levels of antibody in women of childbearing age may contribute to an absence of transplacentally acquired protective antibody.

Humans are the only known source of *B. pertussis* in nature. In spite of this, asymptomatic carriage is extremely uncommon; this distinguishes *Bordetella* from the majority of bacterial respiratory pathogens. Transmission occurs from case to case, usually within families. Unimmunized household contacts of patients with pertussis may have an attack rate of up to 100%. Adults with undiagnosed disease are an important source of infection for children and other adults within a household.

Pathophysiology

B. pertussis is found exclusively in association with ciliated respiratory epithelial cells (Fig. 271-1), which emphasizes the unique capability of the organism to attach to cilia. *B. pertussis* does not invade the respiratory epithelium. The characteristic lymphocytosis of pertussis can be attributed to absorption of pertussis toxin from the respiratory tract, but the pathophysiology of the prolonged paroxysmal cough remains unknown.

Adenoviruses have been associated with pertussis by seroconversion and viral isolation from the nasopharynx. An independent role for adenovirus in causing this disease is unlikely, however.

CLINICAL DISEASE

The clinical picture of pertussis varies with the age of the affected patient. In children, the hallmark of pertussis is the paroxysmal cough. After an incubation period of 7 to 10 days, the typical illness progresses through three stages, each of about 2 weeks' duration (Fig. 271-2). The catarrhal phase is initiated by rhinorrhea and low-grade fever. The disease is most contagious during this stage, yet it is difficult to recognize clinically because symptoms resemble those of the "common cold." Late in the catarrhal stage, a cough appears that becomes paroxysmal. During the paroxysmal stage, exhausting paroxysms of coughing may occur two to three times per hour. The relentless, repetitive cough leads to facial plethora and expectoration of viscid, tenacious mucus. Long paroxysms may terminate with cyanosis, apnea, vomiting, or a gasping inspiratory whoop. Pertussis is commonly called *whooping cough,* but the inspiratory whoop is by no means a constant feature of the disease. During the convalescent phase, the frequency and severity of paroxysms gradually diminish. Convalescence, however, may be punctuated by relapses of paroxysmal coughing.

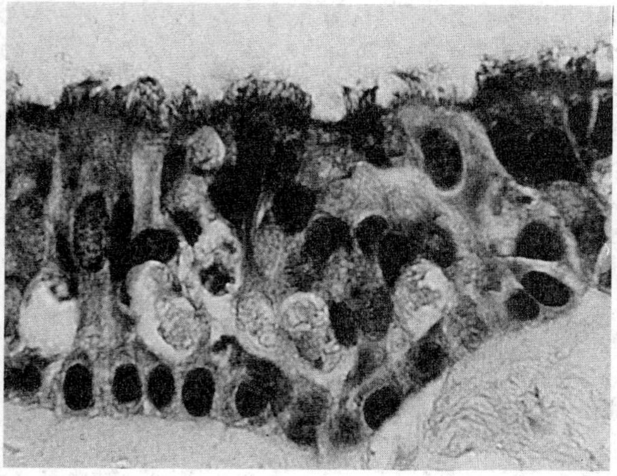

Fig. 271-1. *Bordetella pertussis* enmeshed in the cilia of respiratory epithelium (human nose). (Courtesy of Dr. Per Larsen, Gentofte Hospital, Copenhagen, Denmark.)

Peripheral lymphocytosis, often exceeding 30,000 cells per cubic millimeter, develops late in the catarrhal phase and continues into the paroxysmal phase. This characteristic finding is often the only laboratory data supporting the clinical impression of pertussis. Perihilar infiltrates may be seen on chest radiographs.

Clinical manifestations in adults may be similar to those in infants. More commonly, however, adults suffer only a nonspecific prolonged "bronchitis" and do not develop the characteristic paroxysmal cough. Lymphocytosis rarely accompanies adult disease.

The complications of pertussis have diminished significantly since the advent of antibiotics and improved supportive care. Secondary bacterial pneumonia, which is uncommon but may contribute to mortality, may be heralded by consolidation on chest x-ray and a shift from lymphocytosis to leukocytosis. Atelectasis and pneumothorax are infrequent, and long-term pulmonary sequelae are now rare. Convulsions and central nervous system damage (pertussis encephalopathy) may result from hypoxia and increased venous pressure accompanying cough paroxysms or from an undefined neurotoxin produced by the organisms.

Diagnosis

Recovery of *B. pertussis* from respiratory secretions provides a definitive diagnosis of pertussis. Obstacles to laboratory diagnosis by isolation of the organisms include culturing too late in the illness for organisms to be present, nonviable organisms resulting from antibiotic therapy prior to culture, and laboratory inexperience in growing the organisms. B-G agar, which was developed in 1900 with the use of secretions from Bordet's son who had pertussis, is the standard medium for isolation of *B. pertussis*. Inclusion of charcoal in the agar may improve performance. B-G agar, which has potato extract as its base, must be made with fresh animal blood. Tiny white colonies surrounded by a small zone of beta hemolysis appear after 3 to 5 days of incubation at 36° C. Inclusion of a penicillin or cephalosporin in the agar prevents overgrowth of normal respi-

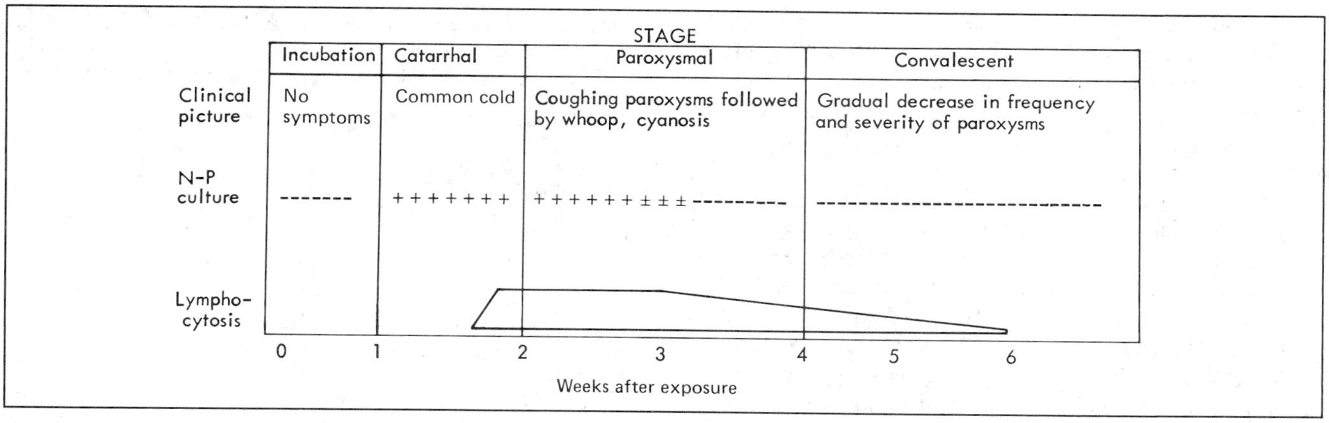

Fig. 271-2. Clinical course of pertussis. N-P, nasopharyngeal.

ratory tract flora, which obscures the recognition of the slowly growing *B. pertussis*.

Nasopharyngeal (not oropharyngeal) secretions should be obtained with a calcium alginate swab during the first 3 weeks of infection (see Fig. 271-2) and inoculated directly onto B-G or Regan-Lowe charcoal agar at the bedside. If this is not feasible, a semisolid agar transport medium containing charcoal and defibrinated horse blood may be used. Fluorescent antibody staining of respiratory secretions in experienced laboratories correlates well with positive cultures.

Serologic diagnosis of infection has not been reliable in the past, but an enzyme-linked immunosorbent assay (ELISA) for IgG, IgM, and IgA antibodies to *B. pertussis* developed in Finland is a promising tool for accurate serologic diagnosis. Workers have employed either an extract of whole organisms or specific antigens such as FHA or LPF as the antigen in ELISA testing of acute and convalescent sera. Interpretation of serologic findings is complicated by the fact that both IgG and IgM antibodies are generated after vaccination as well as infection. The IgG antibodies persist for years. On the other hand, IgA antibodies are produced only by infection (not vaccination), and IgM antibodies have a short half-life. Serologic evidence of infection is provided by either a fourfold rise in IgG antibody titer to *B. pertussis* antigen(s) or elevated IgM and/or IgA titers during or after illness. Studies utilizing ELISA serology in addition to culture have demonstrated that culture is positive in less than half of the cases of pertussis infection diagnosed with serology.

Therapy

The therapy of pertussis is largely supportive, although erythromycin therapy rapidly eliminates viable organisms. Nursing care and adequate nutrition are essential. In the acute paroxysmal stage, unnecessary manipulation of the child should be discouraged, since stimulation, particularly suctioning of the upper respiratory tract, may precipitate additional paroxysms of coughing.

Antibiotic therapy renders the patient noncontagious and may abort disease if administered during the incubation period or the catarrhal stage. However, once the paroxysmal stage is reached, antibiotics are not thought to alter the course of pertussis disease. *B. pertussis* is sensitive in vitro to ampicillin, erythromycin, chloramphenicol, tetracycline, and trimethoprim-sulfamethoxazole. Ampicillin does not reliably eradicate the organism from the nasopharynx. Nasopharyngeal shedding of the organism can be eradicated within 3 days with oral erythromycin (40 to 50 mg/kg/day in four divided doses; 1 g/day in adults). Therapy should be continued 14 days to prevent the reappearance of shedding seen after shorter antibiotic courses.

Pertussis immune globulin is of no benefit in treatment of pertussis. Corticosteroids in conjunction with erythromycin reduced the frequency of paroxysms of coughing in one controlled trial. Since complicating infections might be potentiated by this therapeutic regimen, however, additional study is needed before it can be recommended for routine use in pertussis. Albuterol (salbutamol) in a dose of 0.1/mg/kg t.i.d. by mouth is commonly employed as adjunctive therapy in Europe.

Prevention

Erythromycin prophylaxis (40 to 50 mg/kg/day for 14 days) of household contacts of a case of pertussis has been advocated as a means of preventing or attenuating disease in the contacts. Although it is not of proved efficacy, prophylaxis should be provided to infants and small children in view of the severity of disease in this age group.

Active immunization with pertussis vaccine is the only effective method of disease control. The specific protective antigen(s) of the whole cell vaccine has not been defined. Use of the vaccine is based on efficacy trials conducted in the late 1940s. Pertussis vaccine is not given to persons over six years of age, despite evidence that individuals vaccinated over 12 years before exposure are again susceptible to disease. The side effects of the whole cell pertussis vaccine have been a source of great controversy, although the protective efficacy of 70% to 90% is established. Concern over vaccine side effects in Japan and England led to a reduction in vaccine use with a resultant resurgence in incidence of pertussis. In studies in the United States, local reactions and fever have been associated with vaccine administration in approximately one half of the recipients. More serious, but transient, adverse effects (shocklike state, seizure) were observed in 1 in every 1750 doses of vaccine. Encephalopathy with residual neurologic deficits occurs rarely, if at all, after vaccine.

The antigens of *B. pertussis* in the whole cell vaccine that are responsible for stimulating vaccine-induced immunity have not been defined. This has made rational design and testing of acellular vaccines problematic. Proposed protective antigens include LPF (pertussis toxin), FHA, fimbrial agglutinogens 2 and 3, and a 69-kilodalton outer membrane protein. Other undefined antigens may also be important. Acellular vaccine containing LPF and FHA is used routinely in Japan. Recently, acellular vaccine containing either LPF or LPF plus FHA were field tested in infants in Sweden, where whole cell vaccine is not in use. The protective efficacy of both vaccines was lower than expected, and postvaccination levels of antibody to the two antigens did not correlate with protection against disease. Additional acellular vaccines containing two or more components of the organism are under development for prevention of this serious disease in young infants.

REFERENCES

Ad Hoc Group for the Study of Pertussis Vaccines. Placebo-controlled trial of two acellular pertussis vaccines in Sweden—protective efficacy and adverse events. Lancet 1:955, 1988.

Bass JW: Erythromycin for treatment and prevention of pertussis. Pediatr Infect Dis 5:154, 1986.

Broome CV et al: Epidemiology of pertussis, Atlanta, 1977. J Pediatr 93:362, 1981.

Cherry JD et al: Report on the Task Force on Pertussis and Pertussis Immunization—1988. Pediatrics 81(suppl):939, 1988.

Cody CL et al: Nature and rates of adverse reactions associated with DTP and DT immunizations in infants and children. Pediatrics 68:650, 1981.

Halperin SA et al: Evaluation of culture, immunofluorescence, and serology for the diagnosis of pertussis. J Clin Microbiol 27:752, 1989.

Halperin SA and Marrie TJ: Pertussis encephalopathy in an adult: case report and review. Rev Infect Dis 13:1043, 1991.

Mertsola J et al: Intrafamilial spread of pertussis. J Pediatr 103:359, 1983.

Olson LC: Pertussis. Medicine (Baltimore)54:427, 1985.

Robinson A et al: Pertussis vaccine: present status and future prospects. Vaccine 3:11, 1985.

Robinson A et al: Serotyping *Bordetella pertussis* strains. Vaccine 7:491, 1989.

Trollfors B and Rabo E: Whooping cough in adults. Br Med J 283:696, 1981.

CHAPTER

272 Infections Caused by Legionellae

Washington C. Winn, Jr.
Christopher J. Grace

THE ORGANISM

Classification and characteristics

Legionella pneumophila, the most important member of the family Legionellaceae, is an aerobic gram-negative bacillus that produces sporadic and epidemic respiratory illness ranging from a self-limited flulike syndrome to severe pneumonia and occasionally disseminated disease. Although this bacterium was identified first as an important human pathogen after an outbreak of respiratory disease at an American Legion convention in 1976, it was isolated from the blood of a patient with pneumonia in 1947. On the basis of cell wall composition, physiology, and DNA hybridization studies, the bacillus is unrelated to any previously recognized human pathogen.

Subsequently, a group of related bacteria that are distinct from *L. pneumophila* has been identified. The classification of the Legionellaceae is detailed in Table 272-1. *Legionella micdadei,* originally designated Pittsburgh pneumonia agent, was the first member of the genus to be isolated; it was recovered in 1943 from the blood of a soldier who had a nonfatal illness that was included in the designation *Fort Bragg fever*. Approximately 90% of reported

Table 272-1. Classification of Legionellaceae

Species isolated from humans	Species isolated from environment only
L. pneumophila (14 serogroups)	*L. steigerwaltii*
L. micdadei	*L. santicrusis*
L. bozemanii (2 serogroups)	*L. israelensis*
L. dumoffii	*L. gratiana*
L. gormanii	*L. fairfieldensis*
L. longbeachae (2 serogroups)	*L. moravica*
L. jordanis	*L. brunensis*
L. wadsworthii	*L. quinlivanii*
L. feeleii (2 serogroups)	*L. adelaidensis*
L. hackeliae (2 serogroups)	*L. spiritensis*
L. maceachernii	*L. jamestowniensis*
L. cincinnatiensis	"*L. londiniensis*"
L. birminghamensis	"*L. geestiae*"
L. oakridgensis	"*L. quarteiraensis*"
L. sainthelensi (2 serogroups)	"*L. nautarum*"
L. anisa	"*L. worsleiensis*"
L. parisiensis	
L. tucsonensis	
L. cherrii	
L. rubrilucens	

Legionella infections have been caused by *L. pneumophila* and *L. micdadei*.

L. pneumophila is a short, gram-negative bacillus, measuring 0.5 to 0.7 μm by 2 to 4 μm, with occasional filamentous forms up to 20 μm in length. Slightly tapered ends and central constrictions are present frequently. Gram stain detects the bacterium if large numbers of organisms are present, as in lung biopsy specimens. Prolonged staining with safranin or addition of carbolfuchsin to the counterstain improves the sensitivity of the Gram stain. Crystal violet (the "half Gram stain"), the Gimenez stain, and the Giemsa stain also demonstrate the bacilli. In tissue, one of the silver impregnation stains, for example, the Dieterle stain, is useful. None of these stains is specific for legionellae. They are, however, useful for screening specimens in which bacteria have not been demonstrated by conventional means or in which legionellae have not been detected by available fluorescent conjugates.

Fourteen serogroups of *L. pneumophila* are recognized currently. Antigens that are serogroup-specific and more broadly cross-reactive have been described. The majority of clinical isolates of *L. pneumophila* (at least 60%) have been serogroup 1 strains.

L. pneumophila is non-spore-forming, non-acid-fast, and requires the addition of cysteine to media for growth. Biochemical characterization is not useful for identification. Definitive identification may require genetic analysis of an isolate. For practical purposes, serologic characterization of an isolate that requires cysteine for growth and resembles *Legionella* morphologically is sufficient. If such an isolate does not react with available sera, it should be sent to a reference laboratory.

Epidemiology

Infection with *L. pneumophila* is widespread in the United States and elsewhere. Although infection with these organisms is clearly not restricted in its geographic distribution, serosurveys indicate that exposure to the organism varies widely from one location to another. In some populations, up to one third of individuals have serologic evidence of previous infection with *L. pneumophila* or related organisms. In other areas, only 1% of sample groups are seropositive. Studies from several centers have shown that as many as 5% of pneumonias are caused by these organisms (see Chapter 231). Thus, *L. pneumophila* appears to be a common respiratory pathogen with a wide distribution.

Legionella pneumonia has been described principally as an epidemic infection, with many cases related to a common source of exposure. Sporadic cases also occur in areas that have not experienced epidemic disease. *L. pneumophila* has been isolated from a variety of fresh water sources, including drinking water. A cloud of droplets generated by cooling towers and evaporative condensers has produced *L. pneumophila* infection. Other types of equipment that generate aqueous aerosols, for example, contaminated shower heads, humidifiers, and nebulizers, also have been implicated as sources of infection. Home heating systems may be a source for sporadic cases. Application of contaminated tap water to healing surgical wounds has caused nosocomial *L. dumoffii* infection. It is important to realize, however, that recovery of *L. pneumophila* from environmental sources has usually not been associated with disease. *L. pneumophila* infection occurs most commonly in the summer and early fall. Both epidemic and sporadic cases follow the same seasonal pattern. Nevertheless, infections have been seen year-round.

Legionella pneumophila pneumonia has been reported in all age groups, although most patients are over 50 years of age. A striking male predominance is seen. Patients with underlying chronic diseases and immune suppression are at increased risk for severe *Legionella* infection. A high index of suspicion is warranted for patients with chronic heart, lung, or renal disease; diabetes mellitus; solid organ or bone marrow transplantation; infection with human immunodeficiency virus; or chronic alcoholism. Patients who smoke cigarettes, recipients of antineoplastic chemotherapy, and particularly those who receive high doses of corticosteroids are also at increased risk.

Legionella pneumonia may be acquired in the community or in the hospital. Despite the fact that it is a respiratory tract disease that is transmitted by aerosols, person-to-person spread has not been documented.

The attack rate of the epidemic form of pneumonic illness is less than 5%, and the incubation period is usually between 2 and 10 days. In contrast, a nonpneumonic type of illness, known as *Pontiac fever,* has a very high attack rate and a very short incubation period. The explanation for the differing clinical and epidemiologic presentations is as yet unknown.

Pathophysiology

The only documented source of infection is water, and the predominant mode of transmission is by inhalation of a contaminated aerosol. An additional mode of transmission is direct transfer of bacteria in tap water to fresh surgical wounds.

Pathologically, the major finding is a lobular pneumonia, which may become so extensive that most of the lobe is involved. The infiltrate spreads in the lung through bronchioles and by direct alveolar extension. Nodular consolidation occurs, and abscesses are present in as many as 20% of cases. Fibrinous or fibrinopurulent pleural effusions occur frequently, but empyema is rare. Microscopically, the alveolar infiltrate consists of neutrophils and, frequently, a large component of macrophages. Innumerable short bacilli can be demonstrated by the Dieterle stain in a typical case, both extracellularly and in phagocytic cells. Most of the bacteria are in the alveolar infiltrate. Some are present in the interstitium, and bacilli have been demonstrated in regional lymph nodes, Kupffer's cells of the liver, and sinusoidal cells of the spleen. In addition, a variety of other extrapulmonary inflammatory lesions, including intravascular infections, have been documented, but these are unusual complications.

Legionella pneumophila is a facultative intracellular bacterium. Alveolar macrophages and later blood macrophages that enter the air spaces serve as the initial site for bacterial replication. Complement receptors on alveolar macrophages serve as binding sites for *Legionella,* and enhanced opsonization occurs in the presence of specific antibody. Once phagocytized, *Legionella* evades phagolysosomal fusion and grows within the phagocytic vesicles of the macrophage. Cell-mediated immunity is the primary host defense against *Legionella* infection. Macrophages that have been activated by specifically sensitized T-lymphocytes inhibit intracellular growth, although significant bactericidal activity has been difficult to demonstrate in vitro. Immunoprotective antigens have been identified experimentally, but no single dominant virulence factor has been uncovered. Polymorphonuclear neutrophils do not support the growth of *Legionella* in vitro. Experimental studies suggest a protective role for neutrophils and for antibody, but they are secondary to cellular immunity in importance.

The participation of toxins in the pathogenesis of disease has been suggested because of the prominence of extrapulmonary symptoms and because of extensive cytolysis of the pulmonary inflammatory infiltrate in some cases. At least two cytotoxins, an endotoxin-like substance, and numerous extracellular enzymes have been described, but their roles in the production of disease are not yet clear.

CLINICAL DISEASE

Legionella pneumophila

Legionella pneumophila produces two distinct syndromes (Chapter 231): Pontiac fever and Legionnaires' disease. Pontiac fever is a self-limited illness characterized by chills, fever, myalgias, and headache. The disease lasts 2 to 5 days, resolves without therapy, and leaves no sequelae. Pneumonia has not been associated with this syndrome.

Legionnaires' disease, the most common syndrome, is a pneumonic process that can be acquired in the community or the hospital (see Chapter 231). After an incubation period of 2 to 10 days, Legionnaires' disease begins with a prodrome of malaise, headache, and myalgia that lasts 1 to 2 days. The patient then becomes more acutely ill with chills, rigors, and prostration. Fever exceeds 40° C in 20% of patients. A more indolent onset is less common. The cough is initially dry or productive of only small amounts of mucoid sputum, but purulent sputum is eventually produced by 50% of patients. Dyspnea is common and 30%-40% of patients report chest pain. Hemoptysis is rare, but blood-tinged sputum is not uncommon. Extrapulmonary symptoms may be dramatic, including nausea, vomiting, and abdominal pain in 10%-20% and diarrhea in 50% of patients. One third of patients may have alterations in mental status, such as lethargy, confusion, agitation, and, less commonly, seizures, coma, or disturbances of gait.

On physical examination patients are usually moderately to severely ill. Relative bradycardia is present in 50% of patients. Physical examination of the chest reveals inspiratory rales. Signs of consolidation may be present, especially late in the course of illness.

In 70% of patients chest radiographs reveal a unilateral patchy alveolar infiltrate, usually in the lower lobes. Expansion of the infiltrate is common, more often to lobar consolidation or to adjacent lobes than to the contralateral lung. Pleural effusions occur in one third of patients. Hilar lymphadenopathy is unusual and abscesses are rarely demonstrated radiographically, although necrotizing inflammation and microabscesses are commonly demonstrated at postmortem examination. Other radiographic patterns include interstitial infiltrates and poorly defined rounded opacities that occur predominantly in the lower lobes and may suggest septic emboli. The chest radiograph may reveal a more extensive inflammatory process than would be suggested from physical examination. None of the above symptoms, signs, or radiographic patterns absolutely distinguishes *Legionella pneumophila* pneumonia from other causes of community- or hospital-acquired pneumonia.

Extrapulmonary inflammatory disease has been well documented but appears to be uncommon. Most dissemination probably occurs hematogenously, but direct extension could account for cases of pericarditis.

L. pneumophila has been reported as a cause of prosthetic and native valve endocarditis, myocarditis, pericarditis, hemodialysis fistula infection, sinusitis, pyelonephritis, pancreatitis, peritonitis, hepatic abscess, and postoperative wound infection. A leukocytosis of 10,000-20,000/mm^3 is common, but the white blood cell count may be normal. Leukopenia is a poor prognostic sign.

Hyponatremia (serum sodium < 130 meq/L), which occurs in 50% of patients, is probably caused by salt and water loss rather than by inappropriate secretion of antidiuretic hormone as originally hypothesized. Hyponatremia occurs significantly more often in Legionnaires' disease than in other community-acquired pneumonias. Other less common laboratory abnormalities, which do not differentiate *Legionella* infections from other pneumonias, include hypophosphatemia, hematuria, proteinuria, myoglobinuria, thrombocytopenia, hemolytic anemia, and elevations of serum aspartate aminotransferase, alkaline phosphatase, bilirubin, and serum creatine kinase.

Sputum frequently contains alveolar macrophages and polymorphonuclear leukocytes. The presence of many neutrophils and absence of bacteria in routine Gram stains of sputum is a useful clue to the possibility of Legionnaires' disease.

A specific diagnosis can be made by culture of the organism from clinical specimens, by detection of a serological response to *Legionella,* or by detection of bacterial antigen in body tissues or fluids. Recovery of the bacterium in culture is most definitive and should be attempted whenever possible. It is essential that the microbiology laboratory be notified that *Legionella* infection is suspected so that appropriate stains and media may be used when the specimens are processed. Sputum and other clinical specimens should be cultured on buffered charcoal yeast extract agar supplemented with alpha ketoglutarate (BCYE-α). Inoculation of an additional agar containing selective antimicrobial agents and brief acidification of the specimen may increase the yield from sputum to 70%, but a nonselective agar must be included. Growth is usually detected within 3 to 5 days. Dual infections occur with other pathogens, including other *Legionella* species.

Blood can be cultured for *Legionella* using techniques that include inoculation of material onto BCYE-α agar. The lysis centrifugation system (Isolator, DuPont), broth systems with subculture including the BACTEC system (Johnston Laboratories), and biphasic BCYE bottles have been inoculated successfully, but the sensitivity is not known.

Serum antibody to *Legionella* may be measured by microagglutination assays, by enzyme-linked immunoassays, or by indirect immunofluorescence (IFA) tests. The IFA test is the most readily available and the best studied serologic procedure for diagnosis of *Legionella* infections (Chapter 226).

A definitive diagnosis requires seroconversion, defined as a fourfold or greater increase in antibody titer to a minimum level of 1:128. A stable titer of 1:256 by IFA has been used to make a presumptive diagnosis when a compatible illness occurred in an epidemic setting. Most patients show seroconversion within 3 weeks of illness; some do not develop antibody until 6 weeks or later, and a few individuals never produce detectable antibody. Serum antibody may be measured by microagglutination or microenzyme-linked immunoassay procedures.

Antigen detection in clinical specimens has the advantage of providing prompt diagnosis. Organisms can be detected by direct immunofluorescence (DFA) examination of respiratory secretions. Positive tests may be obtained as late as 1 week after initiation of therapy. The sensitivity of DFA is approximately 50%. Cross-reactions have been demonstrated with *Pseudomonas* species, *Bacteroides fragilis*, and *Mycobacterium tuberculosis*. Cross-reactions are greatly diminished by use of a fluorescein-conjugated monoclonal antibody. In addition, contamination of reagents or specimens with environmental legionellae has produced falsely positive reactions. In areas that have a low incidence of *Legionella* infections, the positive and negative predictive values of direct immunofluorescence are unacceptable.

A sensitive and specific radioimmunoassay for serogroup 1 *Legionella pneumophila* antigen in urine is commercially available. The worth of commercial versions of enzyme immunoassays, latex agglutination tests, and genetic probes for bacterial RNA is not yet proved.

The response to therapy is variable. Some patients defervesce soon after treatment is initiated and experience an increased sense of well-being within 24 to 36 hours. Others remain febrile and clinically ill for several days and then begin to improve slowly. The disease may progress radiographically in spite of overall clinical improvement.

The principal complication of Legionnaires' disease is respiratory failure, which may be associated with hypotension, shock, and renal failure. Thus, appropriate antibiotic therapy often must be accompanied by aggressive, supportive care.

The prognosis of Legionnaires' disease is directly related to the presence or absence of underlying illness and to the use of appropriate or inappropriate antibiotics. Hospitalized patients who are otherwise in good health and who receive prompt erythromycin therapy have a mortality rate of less than 10%. On the other hand, the course of Legionnaires' disease has been fatal in more than three fourths of patients with significant underlying disease who did not receive erythromycin. Radiographic resolution of successfully treated *L. pneumophila* pneumonia often requires several months.

An approach to diagnosis and treatment of *Legionella* infections is outlined in Fig. 272-1. A high index of suspicion must be maintained for those patients with chronic underlying disease, immunosuppression, or advanced age, whether the infection is nosocomial or community-acquired. Clinical clues should further raise suspicion, although there are no pathognomonic findings. The diagnostic evaluation should include culture of respiratory secretions, including sputum, and blood for *Legionella* and collection of acute and convalescent serum specimens for serologic testing. The radioimmunoassay for serogroup 1 *Legionella pneumophila* antigen in urine should be used if available. Therapy with erythromycin should be started promptly after collection of diagnostic specimens and continued for 3 weeks. Initial therapy should be intravenous and rifampin should be added for severe disease or extremely compromised patients. If erythromycin is not tolerated, alternative treatments may be used if the clinical response is monitored carefully.

Two important points must be considered when assess-

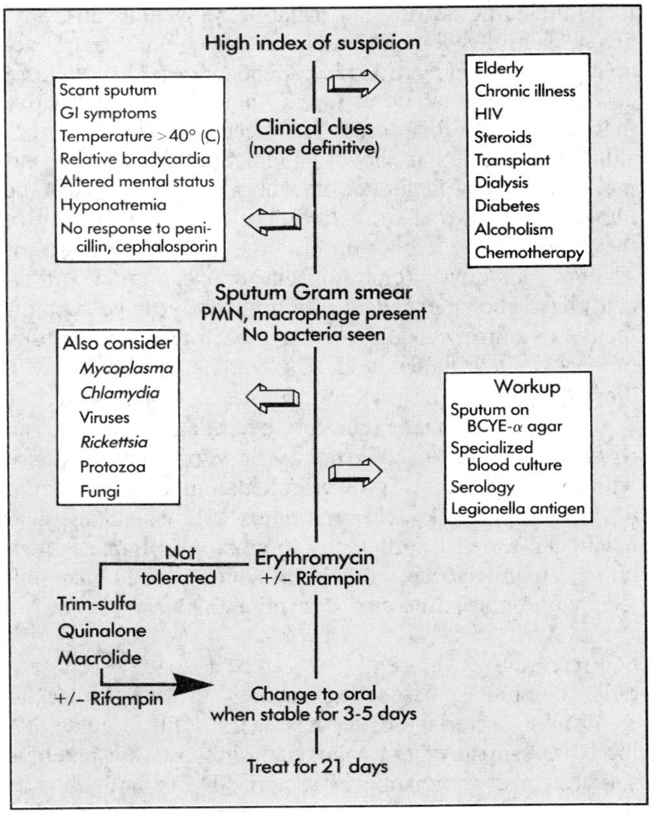

Fig. 272-1. Diagnostic and therapeutic algorithm for *Legionella* pneumonia.

ing antimicrobial efficacy against *L. pneumophila*. First, the bacterium lives and replicates intracellularly in macrophages. Second, it produces a beta lactamase that inactivates many beta lactam antibiotics. Effective antibiotics must resist enzymatic degradation and penetrate well into the cytoplasmic vacuoles where *Legionella* resides. Some antibiotics, such as aminoglycosides and cephalosporins, are active in vitro but are ineffective in vivo. Cell culture and animal models bring the testing process closer to in vivo reality, but ultimately clinical documentation of antimicrobial efficacy is required.

Erythromycin remains the antibiotic of choice for *Legionella* infections, based on in-vitro, cell culture, animal model, and uncontrolled human studies. Erythromycin is concentrated within macrophages at 24 times the extracellular level and can kill phagocytized *Legionella*. The dose is 500-1000 mg every 6 hours (7.5-12.0 mg/kg for children other than neonates). The higher dose and the intravenous form should be used for moderate to severe infection and for immune-compromised hosts. Once the patient's clinical condition has stabilized for 3-5 days, oral erythromycin therapy (500 mg P.O. q.i.d.) can be substituted. Therapy should be continued for a combined duration of 3 weeks. Rifampin (600 mg P.O. b.i.d.) should be added for documented *Legionella* pneumonia or for severe pneumonia if *Legionella* is a very likely etiologic agent. Rifampin should not be used alone, because of the likelihood that resistance will develop.

Erythromycin can cause several troublesome side effects, including hearing loss if large intravenous doses are given, painful venous sclerosis that may require central venous access, fluid overload in patients with cardiac disease, and gastrointestinal upset (see Chapter 224). Alternative therapy may, therefore, be needed. Trimethoprim-sulfamethoxazole has shown good activity in vitro, in animal studies, and in limited uncontrolled clinical use. The intravenous and oral forms are dosed at 10 mg/kg/day of the trimethoprim component in two to three divided doses. The new quinolones (ciprofloxacin, ofloxacin, and perfloxacin) have shown excellent in-vitro activity, have been effective in animal models, and have been used successfully in very limited human studies. Combination therapy with these quinolones and erythromycin needs further study.

The new macrolides (clarithromycin, azithromycin, and roxithromycin) also show promise in vitro, but experience with human infection is very limited. Imipenim-cilastatin, ticarcillin-clavulanic acid, and amoxicillin-clavulanic acid have been tested insufficiently to employ in human infections. Variable success has been achieved in human subjects with tetracycline or doxycycline therapy.

Prevention. At present, little can be done to prevent sporadic, community-based Legionnaires' disease. Molecular analysis of bacterial isolates has been useful in epidemiologic assessment of environmental sites that are potential sources for dissemination of bacteria. Decontamination of these sources may abort epidemic or hyperendemic infection. In particular, chlorination or heat treatment of potable water systems has been associated with cessation of ongoing nosocomial outbreaks on several occasions. Epidemiologic and clinical surveillance should focus on the presence of human disease rather than environmental colonization because of the widespread distribution of these bacteria. All means of environmental decontamination identified to date have potential adverse effects on the physical integrity of the plumbing systems or on the safety of the individuals who use the system. Common-sense measures, such as using sterile water for wound care and for filling nebulizers and other aerosol generators, are cheap and should be instituted in all hospitals.

Legionella micdadei (Pittsburgh pneumonia agent)

Pittsburgh pneumonia agent was recognized initially as a cause of severe pneumonia in immunosuppressed patients. Pathologically, the pneumonia resembles that produced by *L. pneumophila,* but the bacilli may be partially or totally acid-fast in tissue. The bacterium is more fastidious than *L. pneumophila* but has been cultivated on BCYE medium. It is not acid-fast when grown on agar. *L. micdadei* is differentiated from its relatives by cell wall analysis, antigenic composition, and acid-fastness in tissue scrapings or sections. An identical bacterium (Tatlock bacillus) was isolated from the blood of a patient with Fort Bragg fever in 1943. The other cases of this nonfatal illness could not be linked to the bacterium, and the significance of the isolate remains unclear. Pontiac fever has been associated with *L. micdadei*. The bacterium has been isolated from tap water in respiratory therapy nebulizers.

Other *Legionella* species

Infections with other species have been recognized infrequently or not at all. Pontiac fever has been caused by *L. feeleii* and *L. anisa*. *L. dumoffii* has produced clusters of nosocomial infection, including prosthetic valve endocarditis. Only *L. pneumophila,* however, has been responsible for large, explosive outbreaks. Most patients infected by nonpneumophila species have had serious underlying diseases; all species of *Legionella* should be considered potentially pathogenic, given a sufficiently debilitated host. From the limited data available, the clinical disease, pathologic lesions, treatment, and prognosis do not appear to differ substantially from infections caused by *L. pneumophila*. Serologic documentation of these infections necessitates the demonstration of seroconversion in acute and convalescent specimens. Species other than *L. pneumophila* may be inhibited by antibiotics in selective media, so a nonselective agar must be inoculated.

REFERENCES

Balows A and Fraser DW, editors: International symposium on Legionnaires' disease. Ann Intern Med 90:491, 1979.

Blander SJ and Horwitz MA: Vaccination with the major secretory protein of *Legionella* induces humoral and cell-mediated immune responses and protective immunity across different serogroups of *Legionella pneumophila* and different species of *Legionella*. J Immunol 147:285, 1991.

England AC III et al: Sporadic legionellosis in the United States: the first thousand cases. Ann Intern Med 94:164, 1981.
Fang GD, Yu VL, and Vickers RM: Disease due to the *Legionellaceae* (other than *Legionella pneumophila*). Historical, microbiological, clinical, and epidemiological review. Medicine (Baltimore) 68:116, 1989.
Muder RR, Yu VL, and Zuravleff JJ: Pneumonia due to the Pittsburgh pneumonia agent: new clinical perspective with a review of the literature. Medicine (Baltimore) 62:120, 1983.
Nash TW, Libby DM, and Horwitz MA: IFN-gamma-activated human alveolar macrophages inhibit the intracellular multiplication of *Legionella pneumophila*. J Immunol 140:3978, 1988.
Payne NR and Horwitz MA: Phagocytosis of *Legionella pneumophila* is mediated by human monocyte complement receptors. J Exp Med 166:1377, 1987.
Reingold AL: Role of legionellae in acute infections of the lower respiratory tract. Rev Infect Dis 10:1018, 1988.
States SJ et al: Chlorine, pH, and control of *Legionella* in hospital plumbing systems. JAMA 261:1882, 1989.
Tompkins LS et al: *Legionella* prosthetic-valve endocarditis. N Engl J Med 318:530, 1988.
Winn WC Jr: Legionnaires' disease: historical perspective. Clin Microbiol Rev 1:60, 1988.
Winn WC Jr and Myerowitz RL: The pathology of the *Legionella pneumonias*. A review of 74 cases and the literature. Hum Pathol 12:401, 1981.

CHAPTER

273 Infections Caused by *Treponema* Species (Syphilis, Yaws, Pinta, Bejel)

Michael F. Rein

The genus *Treponema* includes a number of species that reside in the gastrointestinal and genital tracts of humans. These organisms are culturable and frequently are isolated from mixed anaerobic (fusospirochetal) infections of the mucous membranes, but their specific pathogenic role is controversial. On the other hand, *T. pallidum, T. pertenue,* and *T. carateum* are human pathogens responsible for significant worldwide morbidity. These major pathogens are not cultivable by current techniques, and the diagnosis of a specific infection depends on clinical skills, pathologic specimens, and serologic tests.

The pathogenic treponemes are fine, spiral organisms approximately 0.15 μm wide and 6 to 15 μm long (Plate V-2). They have a trilaminar outer membrane similar to that of the gram-negative bacteria, but they have not been shown to possess a biologically active endotoxin.

The pathogenic treponemes are microaerophilic and survive poorly in atmospheric oxygen. They are sensitive to drying and to extremes of temperature, and they are therefore transmitted almost uniformly by direct contact. Thus syphilis is a venereal disease, and the nonvenereal treponematoses are most prevalent in situations of overcrowding and poor hygiene.

SYPHILIS

Syphilis is a specific infection with *T. pallidum* and manifests as a chronic disease with subacute symptomatic periods separated by asymptomatic intervals, during which the diagnosis can be made serologically.

Epidemiology

The venereal nature of syphilis was recognized in the earliest descriptions of the disease. Infection develops in 30% to 50% of the sexual partners of patients with syphilitic lesions, but the risk of acquiring syphilis from a single sexual exposure to an infected partner is unknown. The average prevalence among sexual partners is so high that all patients presenting themselves for treatment because of such sexual contact within the past 90 days (the maximum incubation period for syphilis) should be treated, even in the absence of clinical or serologic evidence of disease. Such *epidemiologic treatment* is an important element of syphilis control.

Since 1985, the incidence of primary and secondary syphilis has been increasing, with 50,000 cases reported in 1990, up 9% from 1989. The reported incidence of 20 cases per 100,000 persons is up 75% since 1985 and is the highest incidence reported in the United States since 1949. The association of syphilis with HIV infection is striking, with HIV infection found in one quarter of syphilitics in some STD clinic populations.

Syphilis is most prevalent in sexually active populations and age groups, and the highest age-adjusted rates for reported early syphilis are found among 20- to 24-year-old men and women, although syphilis is also prevalent among 24- to 34-year-old men. The incidence in homosexual groups has decreased because of changes in behavior in response to the acquired immunodeficiency syndrome (AIDS). Recently, the incidence of syphilis has dramatically increased in heterosexual, drug-abusing populations, even in some groups in which the incidence of gonorrhea has decreased. Patients diagnosed as having syphilis should be carefully evaluated for the presence of other sexually transmitted diseases, including HIV infection (Chapter 242).

Syphilis can be acquired by kissing a person with active oral lesions. Acquisition of syphilis by transfusion is no longer a significant problem, because serologic tests for syphilis are routinely performed on donated blood, and because *T. pallidum* does not survive many current methods of prolonged blood storage. Sexual abuse must be considered in any child with early syphilis. Syphilis may be transmitted transplacentally to the fetus, and the risk of congenital syphilis is increased if syphilis is acquired during pregnancy. Women with multiple sexual partners should be screened for syphilis several times during pregnancy.

Pathophysiology

T. pallidum can penetrate intact mucous membranes or infect via tiny defects in cornified epithelium. Spirochetemia occurs very early in infection, even before the first lesions have appeared or the blood test becomes reactive. This is particularly important in pregnancy, since pregnant women acquiring syphilis late in the third trimester may transmit the infection to the fetus but not manifest evidence of syphilis themselves until after delivery.

Syphilitic infection generally is characterized by an obliterative endarteritis resulting in impaired blood flow. The typical late manifestations of syphilis of the central nervous and cardiovascular systems largely result from vascular involvement in these areas.

Immune mechanisms contribute to the pathophysiology of syphilis. Late infection may elicit a granulomatous reaction called a *gumma*. The histopathology is nonspecific, and gummas may occur in any organ. Some experimental work suggests that the gumma results from delayed hypersensitivity in the immune host. The manifestations of congenital syphilis apparently result in part from an immune inflammatory reaction. Antigen-antibody complexes have been detected in the blood of patients with secondary syphilis and are responsible for the glomerulonephritis that may accompany this stage. At the same time, suppression of various aspects of cell-mediated immunity has been noted in syphilis and may contribute to the prolonged survival of *T. pallidum*.

Clinical manifestations

The natural history of syphilis is generally divided into stages. After acquiring the organism, but before clinical or serologic manifestations develop, patients are said to have "incubating syphilis." The incubation period usually lasts about 3 weeks but can range from 10 to 90 days. During this interval, the diagnosis of syphilis cannot be made on clinical or serologic grounds. Therefore, a patient who has had sexual exposure within the past 90 days to a person with infectious syphilis may have an undetectable infection. Such patients routinely should be treated.

Primary syphilis. At the end of the incubation period, the patient develops a lesion, called a *chancre,* at the point of initial inoculation and multiplication of the spirochete. Chancres are commonly located around the genitalia (Plate V-36) but may appear almost anywhere else on the body. Chancres of the gum, throat and tonsil, lip, nipple, and hand are well described, and syphilis should be considered as part of the differential diagnosis of ulcerated lesions at any anatomic site. The chancre begins as a papule that erodes to form a gradually enlarging ulcer with a clean base and an indurated edge; generally it is relatively painless. Although the chancre usually occurs as a single lesion, multiple chancres are not rare; and the observation of multiple lesions, particularly around the genitalia, should not dissuade the clinician from considering syphilis.

Of patients with primary syphilis of the external genitalia, 50% to 70% subsequently develop relatively painless, usually bilateral, inguinal adenopathy (satellite bubo). Inguinal adenopathy is less common with the chancres involving the glans, the cervix, or the proximal portion of the vagina because these sites are drained by the iliac nodes. Regional adenopathy results from primary inoculation at other sites; for example, cervical adenopathy may accompany a syphilitic lesion of the oral cavity. Affected nodes usually are manifested in a chain and are discrete, firm, and fairly movable.

Even without treatment, the chancre heals completely within about 4 to 6 weeks, and the regional adenopathy resolves.

Secondary syphilis. Two to eight weeks (but occasionally as long as 6 months) after the appearance of the chancre, the patient may develop the manifestations of secondary syphilis. Sometimes, primary and secondary syphilis overlap, and the chancre is still obvious. On the other hand, some patients never notice the primary lesion and initially have the manifestations of secondary syphilis. The stage is a generalized illness that usually begins with symptoms suggesting a viral infection: headache, sore throat, low-grade fever, and, occasionally, a nasal discharge. Moderate leukocytosis and relative lymphocytosis are common, but atypical lymphocytes are not seen.

The disease progresses with development of lymphadenopathy and lesions of the skin and mucous membranes. Adenopathy is recognized in 75% of affected patients and is often generalized. Nodes most commonly involved include the inguinal, suboccipital, posterior auricular, and cervical. Epitrochlear adenopathy is common and should raise suspicions of secondary syphilis. The affected nodes are usually discrete, relatively nontender, firm, and freely movable. Suppuration, periadenitis, and lymphangitis are rare. Generalized lymphadenopathy in sexually active individuals should also raise the question of HIV infection.

Skin lesions are manifested by 80% of the infected patients, but they are highly variable and often closely imitate other conditions. Macular lesions (Plate V-51) are most common and are usually observed over the thighs, abdomen, and trunk, where they are generally bilaterally symmetric, tend to follow lines of skin cleavage, and have a coppery or "boiled ham" color. The lesions are sometimes *mildly* pruritic. The rash almost invariably involves the genitalia and often is prominent on the palms (Plate V-52) and soles, a distribution in itself highly suggestive of syphilis. Maculopapular lesions are also common, and follicular lesions may be present. Vesicles or bullae are distinctly rare in secondary syphilis in adults, although they may accompany congenital syphilis.

The mucous membranes are involved in more than half of cases, but the lesions may be subtle, and limited, for example, to the undersurface of the tongue. About one third of patients develop mucous patches (painless, oval ulcerations usually covered with a gray or yellow membrane).

Condylomata lata are flat, hypertrophic lesions resembling warts. They develop in moist areas; frequently found around the anus or vagina, they do not reflect areas of inoculation but appear as a result of hematogenous dissemination of spirochetes.

Patchy, nonpruritic alopecia involving the scalp, beard, or eyebrows suggests secondary syphilis.

The central nervous system (CNS) is asymptomatically involved in about one third of patients with secondary syphilis, but CNS symptoms accompany only about 2% of the cases, which usually manifest themselves as acute syphilitic meningitis. In these cases, the cerebrospinal fluid (CSF) may contain up to 500 white blood cells per cubic millimeter, primarily mononuclear, and protein is frequently in excess of 100 μg per milliliter. The symptoms are those of a basilar meningitis and often include meningeal and cranial nerve signs. Such early involvement of the CNS may in some cases eventually progress to neurosyphilis even in the face of standard treatment for early syphilis. Until this is better established, one can still maintain that the CSF need not be examined in patients with secondary syphilis who do not have symptoms referable to the CNS. It may, however, be advisable to examine the CSF of *all* patients 1 year after they have been treated for early syphilis to detect those with persistent CNS infection.

Hepatitis and immune complex glomerulonephritis occasionally accompany secondary syphilis. Uveitis and osteitis are rarely observed. Ulceronodular gastritis is reported.

Secondary syphilis usually resolves within 2 to 6 weeks, even in the absence of therapy. Some of the lesions may heal with scarring.

Latent syphilis. After resolution of untreated secondary syphilis, the disease enters a latent stage, in which the diagnosis can be made only serologically. During the first 2 to 4 years of infection, but most commonly during the first year, at least 25% of patients have one or more mucocutaneous relapses in which the manifestations of secondary syphilis reappear. During these intervals, patients are once again contagious to sexual partners, and the underlying spirochetemia may result in transplacental transmission to the fetus. Such relapses are extremely rare after 4 years of latency.

About one third of patients entering latency are eventually spontaneously cured of their disease, with a gradual return of nontreponemal serologic tests toward nonreactive. Another third of patients remain infected but never develop further clinical manifestations of disease. The remaining third of patients eventually develop manifestations of late syphilis. Antibiotics administered for other infections may reduce the incidence of late syphilis.

Late syphilis. About 15% of untreated syphilitics eventually develop late benign syphilis. The disease is manifested by destructive granulomas that typically involve the skin and the bones. These granulomas, or gummas, may produce lesions resembling segments of circles. Skin lesions characteristically heal at one edge and advance at others (serpiginous lesions). Gummas often heal with atrophic, superficial scarring. Bones are frequently affected, with periostitis characterized by localized increases in bone density or destructive lesions surrounded by sclerosis. The tibia is involved in about half of such patients, and the clavicle, skull, and fibula in about one fourth each. Biopsies are nonspecific and reveal granulomas. Organisms are rarely seen, and the pathogenesis of this stage may be largely hyperimmune.

About 10% of untreated patients eventually develop cardiovascular manifestations (see Chapter 16). *T. pallidum* may directly affect the aortic endothelium, yielding an irregular intima reminiscent of tree bark. Involvement of the aortic valve cusps results in rolling and thickening and may lead to aortic insufficiency. The coronary ostia may also participate in the endarteritis leading to coronary occlusion. Involvement of the vasa vasora weakens the aortic media, and the aorta may then develop an aneurysm. About half of syphilitic aneurysms occur in the arch, and another 40% involve other parts of the thoracic aorta. Aneurysm of the abdominal aorta is relatively rare.

Early evidence of cardiovascular involvement includes a localized aortic bulging on chest radiograph, an altered aortic second sound sometimes described as having a tambour quality, or precordial chest pain in a young person without other predisposing factors (see Chapter 16). Later on, symptoms of aortic insufficiency develop. An aortic diastolic murmur in a young person without hypertension or a history of rheumatic heart disease should suggest syphilis. Aortic insufficiency murmurs having a peak intensity at the third or fourth intercostal space at the right sternal border are associated with syphilitic disease. Later, patients often develop symptoms of congestive heart failure or angina, but dissection of a syphilitic aneurysm is uncommon. Antisyphilitic therapy does not reverse existing cardiac damage, but appropriate therapy may slow the progression of the disease.

In about 8% of untreated patients, late syphilis involves the CNS. Mild CNS involvement affects 15% to 40% of patients with cardiovascular syphilis. Initially CNS disease is asymptomatic and can be detected only by examination of the CSF. The CSF should be examined in any patient with clinical or serological evidence of syphilis and neurological signs or symptoms. Ideally, the CSF should also be examined in all patients being treated for syphilis of unknown duration or who have had syphilis for more than 1 year. This is particularly important for patients with a serum nontreponemal antibody titre of more than 1:16; who have other clinical evidence of active, late syphilis (e.g., aortitis, gumma, iritis); or for whom one is planning to administer therapy with an antibiotic other than a beta-lactam. Examination of the CSF is also indicated for all patients with syphilis who have a positive HIV antibody test. Finally, the CSF should be evaluated in patients who have had a suboptimum response to therapy for early syphilis, because unsuspected asymptomatic neurosyphilis may account for some small percentage of apparent treatment failures. Indeed, observations on CNS involvement in early syphilis support the recommendation that all patients with early syphilis undergo examination of the CSF at least 1 year after completing therapy.

Meningovascular syphilis results from endarteritis and

usually manifests itself as seizures or cerebrovascular accident. A stroke in a young person with no history of hypertension should prompt evaluation for meningovascular syphilis. Some patients exhibit a syndrome suggesting a basilar meningitis, and such persons usually have a lymphocytic pleocytosis and increased protein in the CSF.

Spirochetes also may involve the brain substance directly, producing general paresis, which usually manifests as a disorder of higher cerebral functions. Affected individuals undergo personality changes, and dementia and delusional states are common. One sometimes notes the Argyll Robertson pupil, which is small and further constricts with accommodation but does not react to light, a finding highly suggestive of neurosyphilis.

Tabes dorsalis results from involvement of the posterior columns and dorsal roots of the spinal cord. The disease manifests as a loss of vibration sense and proprioception that results in a characteristic broad-based gait. Affected patients also may note severe, sharp pains in any part of the body. Impotence and bladder dysfunction are relatively common. Optic atrophy is observed in one fourth of infected patients, and Argyll Robertson pupils are more common than in general paresis. Some patients with tabes have normal CSF and nonreactive nontreponemal tests for syphilis on serum and CSF.

Syphilis and human immunodeficiency virus infection. Anecdotal observations have suggested that immunodeficiency in AIDS may accelerate the course of syphilis, resulting in early manifestations of CNS disease. Patients with syphilis and human immunodeficiency virus (HIV) infection should be treated with regimens effective against CNS disease. Concurrent syphilis might, in theory, activate lymphocytes and promote expression of HIV. The immunocompromise induced by HIV infection may make the diagnosis of syphilis more difficult by reducing the sensitivity of serologic tests. After treatment for syphilis, the treponemal tests are more likely to revert to nonreactive in the presence of HIV infection than in otherwise normal hosts.

Congenital syphilis. Congenital syphilis follows maternal spirochetemia and transplacental transmission of the organism. Since spirochetemia is more common in early syphilis, babies born to women actually acquiring syphilis during pregnancy are more likely to have congenital syphilis than those whose mothers acquired syphilis before becoming pregnant. Consequent to the rise in early syphilis among heterosexuals, there has been a dramatic increase in congenital syphilis in some areas.

About three fourths of reported cases of congenital syphilis are diagnosed in patients over 10 years of age. Sometimes, the manifestations of congenital syphilis are recognized first by the internist.

Patients with late congenital syphilis may manifest the hutchinsonian triad, which includes Hutchinson's teeth: short, narrow, barrel-shaped incisors displaying a central notch. A second element of the triad is interstitial keratitis, which usually appears in patients between 5 and 20 years of age. The inflammation is expressed as photophobia, eye pain, blurred vision, and tearing. Nerve deafness completes the triad. Other late manifestations of congenital syphilis include fissuring around the mouth and anus (rhagades) and skeletal lesions that include anterior bowing of the tibia (sabre shin), enlargement of the medial end of the clavicle, perforation of the palate, and collapse of the nasal bones to produce a saddle-nose deformity.

Laboratory diagnosis

Dark-field microscopy. The moist lesions of syphilis, including the chancre, mucous patches, and condylomata lata, usually contain sufficient numbers of spirochetes to permit their direct observation. The surface of a suitable lesion is cleaned with a gauze pad and is then lightly abraded. Resulting blood is blotted away, and tissue fluid is expressed by squeezing the edges of the lesion. A small amount of fluid is transferred to a microscope slide and examined with the aid of a dark-field microscope. The dark-field condenser angles light through the specimen so that it does not directly enter the microscope objective. Thus the background appears dark. Objects in the fluid are visualized because light reflecting from them enters the objective. *T. pallidum* is recognized by its characteristic morphology and movement (Plate V-2). Six to fourteen regular spirals are maintained during its movements, and the organism is seen to rotate in corkscrew fashion around its long axis, to move forward and backward along this axis, and to bend at its midpoint. Dark-field examination of specimens from oral or intravaginal lesions is difficult because nonpathogenic spirochetes may closely resemble *T. pallidum*. The dry lesions of secondary syphilis are usually negative by dark-field examination.

Serologic diagnosis. A diagnosis of syphilis should be made or ruled out only after carefully considering all historical, epidemiologic, and clinical features of the case, and not on the basis of serologic results alone. The serology of syphilis is a far from perfect science. It has flowered because the organism cannot be cultured, and the disease has long intervals devoid of clinical manifestations. All serologic tests can be nonreactive in patients with certain stages of active syphilis. In the setting of low prevalence, the number of false-positive results increases relative to the number of true positives. All serologic tests for syphilis can be positive in patients without syphilis, and clinical judgment must enter into a decision to treat patients solely on the basis of serologic evidence of syphilis.

Patients with syphilis usually develop antibodies directed against a poorly defined lipid that may be a component of the spirochete. Cross-reacting lipids are found in a variety of normal tissues and serve as the basis of the nontreponemal tests for syphilis, which employ a lipid extracted from beef heart (cardiolipin) as an antigen. Nontreponemal tests are easy to perform and inexpensive; they include the Venereal Disease Research Laboratory (VDRL) test, the rapid plasma reagin (RPR) test, and the automated reagin test (ART). Unfortunately, similar antibodies are produced in a variety of diseases other than syphilis. These include acute viral illnesses (e.g., varicella, hepatitis, and infectious mononucleosis); bacterial infections (e.g., leprosy, tuberculosis, and leptospirosis); and diseases associated with the formation of unusual immunoglobulins (e.g., intravenous drug abuse and collagen vascular diseases).

Nontreponemal tests may be quantitated, and results are usually expressed as the highest dilution of serum yielding a positive reaction. The RPR and ART may yield titers two to eight times as high as those obtained with the VDRL on the same serum. Since rising or falling titers have considerable clinical significance, patients followed over time should be studied with the same nontreponemal tests.

The titer of a nontreponemal test generally is expected to fall by a factor of at least four after adequate therapy of syphilis. This fourfold drop in VDRL titer generally occurs about 3 months following treatment of early syphilis, and an eightfold drop is observed in 6 months. After adequate treatment for primary syphilis (Table 273-1), three quarters of patients have a nonreactive VDRL test result within 1 year, and 97% are seronegative within 2 years. With the RPR, however, the fraction of patients reverting to nonreactive after adequate treatment for primary syphilis is only 44% after 1 year and 60% after 2 years. After treatment for secondary syphilis, 42% of patients have a nonreactive VDRL test result within 1 year, and three fourths are seronegative within 2 years. Again, the percentage of patients seroreverting with the RPR is lower, being 22% after 1 year and 42% after 2 years. Patients having untreated syphilis for more than 2 years are unlikely to become nonreactive with the nontreponemal tests but should still show a fourfold drop in titer. Subsequent rises in titer suggest relapse or reinfection, and such patients should be reevaluated.

Patients with syphilis also develop antitreponemal antibodies, which can be detected by a variety of procedures that use *T. pallidum* as the antigen. In the fluorescent treponemal antibody-absorption (FTA-ABS) test, antitreponemal antibody is detected by indirect fluorescence of spirochetes. The microhemagglutination test for *Treponema pallidum* (MHATP) uses treponemal antigens attached to the surface of erythrocytes, which agglutinate when mixed with the serum from patients with syphilis. The MHATP is less sensitive than the FTA-ABS in primary syphilis (Table 273-2). Treponemal tests are generally used to confirm the diagnosis of syphilis in patients with reactive nontreponemal tests. They are not routinely quantitated and usually remain reactive even many years after adequate treatment. False-positive treponemal but, surprisingly, not nontreponemal tests are seen in about 40% of patients with Lyme disease and some cases of rat-bite fever.

Table 273-1. Percentage of patients with seroreversions of serologic tests after treatment of syphilis*

	Months				
	3	6	12	24	36
Microhemagglutination test for antibody to *T. pallidum* (MHATP)	3	5	8	9	13
Fluorescent treponemal antibody–absorbed (FTA-ABS)	3	7	11	15	24
Rapid plasma reagin (RPR)					
Primary	13	30	44	60	72
Secondary	1	6	22	42	56
Early latent	3	7	13	13	26
Venereal disease research lab (VDRL)					
Primary			67	85	
Secondary			42	75	

*Based on data from Romanowski B et al.

The interpretation of serologic tests for syphilis has resulted in some confusion. Certain facts should be borne in mind. Both treponemal and nontreponemal tests may be nonreactive in the patient who has just developed a chancre. A nonreactive test for syphilis therefore does not rule out the diagnosis in the patient whose lesion has just appeared. In this setting, up to 10% of patients have a nonreactive nontreponemal test and a reactive treponemal test for syphilis.

In secondary syphilis, all the serologic tests are reactive. Therefore a negative treponemal or nontreponemal serologic test for syphilis essentially rules out secondary syphilis. This is particularly useful because the clinical diagnosis of secondary syphilis may be difficult. Rarely, antibody levels in secondary syphilis are so high that nontreponemal tests performed on undiluted serum may be falsely negative. This so-called prozone phenomenon occurs when antigen-antibody lattice formation, which is necessary for the test to appear reactive, is inhibited by massive antibody excess. Quantitative tests, in which the serum is run at several dilutions, are reactive. The prozone phenomenon is not observed with the treponemal tests. Thus, the clinician suspecting secondary syphilis should request either a quantitative nontreponemal test or a treponemal test even if the undiluted nontreponemal test is nonreactive.

Unfortunately, nontreponemal tests for syphilis frequently become nonreactive in patients with late syphilis. Fully 50% of patients diagnosed as having tabes dorsalis have a nonreactive nontreponemal test for syphilis. Patients being worked up for late syphilis should have a treponemal test performed even if the nontreponemal tests are nonreactive, because many of these patients are diagnosed only by one of the more sensitive treponemal tests.

Although patients adequately treated for syphilis should show a drop in titer of the nontreponemal tests and may, in fact, revert to seronegativity, the treponemal tests remain positive for many years (possibly for life), even after adequate treatment for syphilis. Thus a persistently positive FTA-ABS test result is not an indication for re-treating patients with a history of adequate therapy. An outline of the interpretation of serologic tests is given in Table 273-2.

Evaluation of cerebrospinal fluid (CSF). The laboratory diagnosis of neurosyphilis may be difficult. Evaluation should include a cell count, protein, and VDRL (not RPR). All of these tests have relatively low sensitivity, and nega-

Table 273-2. Interpretation of serologic tests for syphilis*

Finding		
Nontreponemal tests	**Treponemal tests**	**Interpretation of finding: is syphilis present?***
Nonreactive	Nonreactive	*Early primary syphilis is not ruled out by negative serologic tests.* *Early syphilis* is present in 13%-30% of patients who have a negative MHATP test; in about 30% of patients who present with chancre but have a nonreactive reagin test; and in about 10% of patients who have a negative FTA-ABS test. *Late syphilis* is present in a very small fraction of patients. *Adequately treated syphilis in remote past* may produce these results, but treponemal tests usually remain reactive.
	Reactive	Observed in about 10% of patients with chancre. The treponemal tests may turn positive shortly before the reagin tests. Reagin tests repeated after several days are generally positive. *In adequately treated early syphilis,* the reagin test may return to nonreactive within 1-2 years, whereas the treponemal tests generally do not. *Late syphilis* is not ruled out by a negative reagin test. The sensitivity of the reagin tests is lower than that of treponemal tests in untreated late syphilis. In *secondary syphilis,* rarely, a highly reactive serum appears negative when tested undiluted with a reagin test because flocculation is inhibited by relative antibody excess. Not reported to occur with treponemal tests. Quantitative reagin test are positive. False-positive treponemal tests occur in 40% of patients with Lyme disease.
Reactive	Nonreactive	Finding is not diagnostic of syphilis but constitutes a classic biologic false-positive reaction.
	Borderline (FTA-ABS)	Not diagnostic of syphilis: most patients (90%) with this pattern do not develop clinical or serologic evidence of syphilis. Repeat test is indicated. Chronic borderline results are associated with a variety of conditions other than syphilis.
	Beaded (FTA-ABS)	Not diagnostic of syphilis. Seen with collagen vascular disease.
	Reactive	Findings diagnostic of syphilis or other treponemal disease. In *adequately treated syphilis,* one would expect (1) a sustained fourfold drop in titer of reagin test, although reagin test may remain positive after adequate therapy; (2) treponemal tests remain positive after adequate therapy. Concurrent false-positive results on both nontreponemal and treponemal tests could occur in rare instances. It may be impossible to rule out syphilis in an individual with this test profile.

*Serologic data must always be interpreted in the light of a total clinical evaluation. Diagnosis based on serologic criteria alone is fraught with error. Serologic tests apparently in conflict with clinical diagnosis should be confirmed by repetition or possibly referral to a reference laboratory.

tive results on any do not rule out the disease. Most patients with active neurosyphilis, however, have more than 5 white blood cells, usually lymphocytes, per mm^3 of CSF, although the counts are often less than 30. Protein may be slightly elevated. A reactive CSF-VDRL is considered diagnostic of neurosyphilis. Based on very few data, one might perform a CSF-FTA-ABS, recognizing that although the sensitivity for neurosyphilis is apparently very high, the specificity is low. The test may be positive because a small amount of antitreponemal antibody has leaked into CSF from the systemic circulation. A negative test probably rules out neurosyphilis to the extent possible by current means.

Therapy

Recommendations for the treatment of syphilis are summarized in Table 273-3. There is no evidence that *T. pallidum* has developed any resistance to penicillin. Recent work suggests that some strains are highly resistant to erythromycin, which should be used only if no alternative can be found. Patients with syphilis and HIV infection should be treated with regimens effective against neurosyphilis. Doxycycline yields higher CSF levels than does tetracycline. More than one half of the patients treated for early syphilis with penicillin experience a Jarisch-Herxheimer reaction. Usually beginning within 6 hours of treatment, the reaction consists of fever, a transient exacerbation of skin lesions or adenopathy, occasional arthralgias, and, rarely, transient hypotension. The reaction is usually mild and abates in less than 24 hours. It is thought to result from the release of treponemal antigens on destruction of the organisms by penicillin or other antibiotics, and it can usually be managed with aspirin and reassurance.

The recommended treatment of early syphilis in patients with HIV infection is the same as for other patients. Careful follow-up is critical. One should probably examine CSF in patients with any stage of syphilis and HIV infection, but it must be remembered that the spinal fluid formula in neurosyphilis may be identical with that in HIV infection. A reactive CSF VDRL mandates treatment for neurosyphilis, but the presence of a low-level lymphocytic pleocytosis or low-grade elevation in the CSF protein is often difficult to interpret. The conservative approach favors treat-

Table 273-3. Treatment of syphilis

Diagnosis	Recommended treatment	Alternative penicillin treatment	In penicillin allergy
Sexual contact to infectious syphilis (primary, secondary, early latent)	Benzathine penicillin G, 2.4 million U I.M. at a single treatment session	Procaine penicillin G, 600,000 U I.M. daily for 8 days	Tetracycline hydrochloride, 500 mg orally 4 times daily for 15 days or Doxycycline, 200 mg orally twice daily for 15 days or Ceftriaxone, 250 mg I.M. once*†
Early syphilis (primary, secondary, or latent of less than 1 year duration)	Benzathine penicillin G, 2.4 million U I.M. at a single treatment session	Procaine penicillin G, 600,000 U I.M. daily for 8 days	Tetracycline hydrochloride, 500 mg orally 4 times daily for 15 days or Doxycycline, 200 mg orally twice daily for 15 days or Ceftriaxone, 250 mg I.M. once daily for 10 days*
Syphilis of more than 1 year duration including latent, late benign, and cardiovascular	Benzathine penicillin G, 2.4 million U I.M. at weekly intervals for three doses	Procaine penicillin G, 600,000 U I.M. daily for 15 days	Doxycycline, 200 mg orally twice daily for 21 days or Ceftriaxone, 250 mg I.M. once daily for 14 days*
Neurosyphilis (asymptomatic paresis, tabes)	Aqueous crystalline penicillin G, 20 million U daily I.V. by continuous infusion or in divided doses, q4h for 15 d‡	Procaine penicillin G, 600,000 U I.M. daily for 15 days	Doxycycline, 200 mg orally twice daily for 21 days or Ceftriaxone, 1 g I.V. once daily for 14 days*
Pregnancy	Regimen appropriate for stage of maternal syphilis	Regimen appropriate for stage of maternal syphilis	Ceftriaxone*,§ or Erythromycin† regimen appropriate for stage of maternal syphilis

*Ceftriaxone should not be used if there is a history of anaphylaxis to penicillin.
†This regimen appears to abort most but not all cases of incubating syphilis.
‡Some experts have suggested following this regimen with benzathine penicillin G as administered for syphilis of more than one year's duration.
§The treatment of syphilis in the penicillin-allergic pregnant patient is very difficult, and desensitization may be required. Consultation with an expert is recommended.

ment of all patients with CSF abnormalities with regimens effective for neurosyphilis. The use of doxycycline for the treatment of syphilis in the HIV-infected patient has been criticized on the theoretical ground that the drug is bacteriostatic rather than bactericidal and may fail in the setting of impaired host defenses.

NONVENEREAL TREPONEMATOSES

Spirochetes closely related to *T. pallidum* cause three nonvenereal infections that rarely are seen in the United States but are of great significance in other parts of the world. In these infections, the skin or oral lesions contain large numbers of organisms that may be transmitted by personal, but not necessarily venereal, contact. As one might therefore expect, the diseases are most common in areas of poverty, poor hygiene, and overcrowding. Unlike venereal syphilis, these infections are generally acquired during childhood. Since the initial infection and spirochetemia occur before the childbearing years, congenital infection is essentially unknown. One theory holds that pinta is the oldest of the treponemal diseases, and that the ancestral spirochete subsequently evolved to produce yaws, then bejel, and, finally, venereal syphilis. The organisms producing these diseases are morphologically identical to *T. pallidum,* and each infection elicits antibodies reactive in the nontreponemal and treponemal tests for syphilis. Thus, a reactive serologic test for syphilis in a patient from an area endemic for any of these diseases should raise the possibility of the alternative diagnosis. All are treated successfully with long-acting penicillins.

Yaws

Yaws is common in the Caribbean, Latin America, Central Africa, and the Far East. In these tropical areas, climate may contribute to dissemination by reducing the need for clothing. Three to four weeks after infection with *T.*

pertenue, the patient develops a papule that enlarges to form a raised, crusted lesion known as the *mother yaw.* As in syphilis, nontender regional adenopathy is common. Spirochetemia occurs, and 3 to 12 weeks later, the patient develops a diffuse papular eruption, with moist, raised, yellowish lesions that persist for 2 to 3 years and eventually become crusted. Involvement of the soles may make walking painful (crab yaws). In some colder climes, attenuated yaws may manifest as only a few lesions or even a single lesion. The skeletal system often is involved, and the resulting osteitis or periostitis may contribute to the pain. Late yaws is quite similar to late benign syphilis, with granulomatous lesions involving the skin and bones.

Pinta

Unlike the other treponematoses, pinta (infection with *T. carateum*) is limited to the skin. It is found only in Latin America and was initially confused with leprosy by early European explorers—a misdiagnosis that resulted in killing or driving away large numbers of infected Indians. The initial, papular lesion appears 1 to 3 weeks after exposure and extends to become a scaly, flat, mildly pruritic patch accompanied by regional lymphadenopathy. Three to nine months later, the patient develops a generalized, scaly rash that may progress through a variety of changes of color including blue, violet, brown, and, finally, white. After 1 to 3 years, depigmentation appears, usually on the extremities. Although the early lesions contain spirochetes, organisms rarely are demonstrated in the late lesions.

Bejel

The spirochete of bejel is considered to be a variant of *T. pallidum.* It is found in saliva, and the infection is thought to be transmissible by kissing or by sharing eating utensils. Bejel is found in the eastern Mediterranean, the Balkans, and the cooler areas of northern Africa. Three weeks after infection, a transient, painless oral lesion is occasionally recognized but often goes unnoticed. Spirochetemia occurs, and the usual initial presentation of bejel resembles that of secondary syphilis. Patients develop mucous patches, condylomata lata, and adenopathy. Unlike secondary syphilis, however, generalized rash and alopecia are quite rare. The late lesions of bejel resemble those of late benign syphilis, and serpiginous skin lesions and bone pain are common.

Treatment of nonvenereal treponematoses

The nonvenereal treponematoses can be treated with a single injection of 1.2 million units of benzathine penicillin G. As with the spirochete of syphilis, there is no evidence of increasing resistance to the penicillins on the part of other *Treponema* species. Penicillin-allergic patients presumably can be treated with tetracycline or erythromycin, but experience is limited.

REFERENCES

Adler MW: ABC of sexually transmitted diseases. Syphilis: clinical features. Br Med J 288:468, 1984.

Brown ST et al: Serological response to syphilis treatment: new analysis of old data. JAMA 253:1296, 1985.

Centers for Disease Control: Sexually transmitted diseases: treatment guidelines 1989. MMWR 38(suppl 8):S1, 1989.

Centers for Disease Control: Primary and secondary syphilis—United States, 1981-1990. MMWR 40:314, 1991.

Drusin LM: Syphilis: clinical manifestations, diagnosis, and treatment. Urol Clin North Am 11:121, 1984.

Hook EW III: Treatment of syphilis: current recommendations, alternatives, and continuing problems. Rev Infect Dis 11(suppl 6):S1511, 1989.

Hume J et al: International symposium on yaws and other endemic treponematoses. Rev Infect Dis 7(suppl 2):S217, 1985.

Hutchinson CM et al: Characteristics of patients with syphilis attending Baltimore STD clinics. Multiple high-risk subgroups and interactions with human immunodeficiency virus. Arch Intern Med 151:511, 1991.

Jaffe HW et al: Examination of the cerebrospinal fluid in patients with syphilis. Rev Infect Dis 4(suppl):S842, 1982.

Musher DM: Syphilis, neurosyphilis, penicillin, and AIDS. J Infect Dis 163:1201, 1991.

Musher DM et al: Effect of human immunodeficiency virus (HIV) infection on the course of syphilis and on response to treatment. Ann Intern Med 113:872, 1990.

Rein MF: Syphilis. In Rakel R, editor: Conn's current therapy—1993. Philadelphia, 1993, WB Saunders.

Romanowski B et al: Serologic response to treatment of infectious syphilis. Ann Intern Med 114:1005, 1991.

WHO Expert Committee on Venereal Diseases and Treponematoses: Sixth report. WHO Tech Rep Ser 736:1, 1986.

CHAPTER

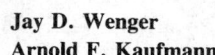

274 Infections Caused by Leptospires (Leptospirosis)

Jay D. Wenger
Arnold F. Kaufmann

CHARACTERISTICS

Leptospires are members of the family Spirochaetaceae. The genus *Leptospira* has only two species, *L. biflexa,* a free-living saprophyte, and *L. interrogans,* a parasitic pathogen. Recent studies of deoxyribonucleic acid relatedness and other characteristics of leptospires indicate that the leptospires are actually members of two different genera (*Leptospira* and *Leptonema*) and that the genus *Leptospira* comprises at least eleven species. For the purposes of this section, the established nomenclature will be followed. Leptospires are slender, threadlike organisms 0.1 μm wide and 6 to 12 μm long. They are tightly coiled, with an amplitude of 0.2 to 0.5 μm. With dark-field microscopy, leptospires appear actively motile, spinning rapidly about their long axis. Electron microscopy reveals an outer sheath and an axial filament, which runs the entire length of the organism.

Leptospira interrogans is a serologically diverse organism, having more than 200 serotypes (serovars). Some serotypes share common antigens and thus cross-agglutinate in immune serum. For convenience, these cross-reacting serotypes are referred to collectively as *serogroups*. For example, serogroup Icterohaemorrhagiae is composed of serotypes *icterohaemorrhagiae, copenhageni, mankarso,* and others. There are presently 19 serogroups, the most common of which in the United States are Icterohaemorrhagiae, Canicola, Autumnalis, Grippotyphosa, Hebdomidis, Australis, Pomona, and Ballum.

EPIDEMIOLOGY

Leptospira interrogans is present worldwide but is more common in the tropics. In the United States, approximately 100 cases of leptospirosis are reported annually. Leptospirosis is more common in the southern and Pacific tiers of states. In contrast to many infectious diseases, leptospirosis has been reported with increasing frequency over the past 50 years with a strong summer predominance. From 1974 to 1978, over half of the reported cases had their onset in the months July through October.

The reservoir for leptospirosis is wild, peridomestic, and domestic animals. Once an animal has acquired leptospirosis, it may become an asymptomatic renal carrier. To some extent, certain serotypes have become adapted to specific animals. For example, *canicola* is most often associated with dogs, *pomona* with cattle and swine, *hardjo* with cattle, *ballum* with mice, and *icterohaemorrhagiae* with rats.

Infection in humans is usually the result of direct or indirect exposure to urine of leptospiruric animals. Direct exposure is common for pet owners and certain occupational groups such as farm workers and veterinarians. Indirect exposure through contaminated soil and water accounts for most sporadic cases, common-source outbreaks, and cases in certain occupational groups such as rice field and sugarcane workers.

Humans are dead-end hosts in the chain of transmission. Person-to-person transmission of leptospirosis rarely occurs; hospitalized patients require no isolation, but care should be exercised when handling body fluids (i.e., blood/body fluid precautions).

CLINICAL MANIFESTATIONS

Human infection begins with penetration of the skin or mucous membranes by the leptospire. Scratches, abrasions, and prolonged immersion in water apparently favor penetration. After an incubation period of 2 to 20 days (mean, 10 days), the onset of illness is usually abrupt. Initial symptoms are nonspecific and include fever, chills, intense headache, myalgia, nausea, vomiting, and anorexia. Conjunctival suffusion, often in association with photophobia, occurs in 30% of cases and may be a valuable diagnostic clue.

In general, human leptospirosis can be divided into two distinct clinical syndromes—anicteric leptospirosis and icteric leptospirosis (Weil's syndrome). Anicteric leptospirosis is the milder illness and engenders only limited liver and kidney involvement. In icteric leptospirosis, severe liver and kidney involvement predominate, although incomplete syndromes occur. Both anicteric and icteric leptospirosis may follow a biphasic course. The first, or septicemic, phase, associated with leptospiremia, lasts approximately 7 days and is followed by a 2- to 3-day period of decreased fever intensity. Recurrence of high fever marks the onset of the second, or immune, phase, and it is temporally related to the appearance of IgM antibody. Complications such as meningitis and uveitis are more common in the immune phase. In icteric leptospirosis, continuing high fever and jaundice may obscure the two phases.

Infection with certain leptospiral serotypes (or serogroups) may be associated with specific syndromes or symptom complexes. For example, *icterohaemorrhagiae* infections are frequently associated with icteric disease; *grippotyphosa* infections, with a predominance of gastrointestinal complaints; and *canicola* infections with aseptic meningitis.

Liver, renal, and central nervous system (CNS) involvement may be present in any combination and are hallmarks of leptospiral infection. Liver involvement may be mild or severe, with bilirubin levels reaching 60 to 80 mg per deciliter in extreme cases. Although direct and indirect bilirubin may be elevated, the direct fraction accounts for most of the increase. Hepatomegaly is more common in icteric disease but occurs in up to 15% of anicteric cases. The alkaline phosphatase, lactic dehydrogenase, serum aspartate aminotransferase (AST[SGOT]), and serum alanine aminotransferase (ALT[SGPT]) may all be elevated, usually two to three times normal and infrequently to the higher ranges typical of acute viral hepatitis. The hepatic lesions of leptospirosis are completely reversible.

Pyuria, hematuria, and proteinuria are common findings in leptospirosis, even in the absence of functional renal impairment. Renal compromise primarily is a result of tubular damage. Dehydration may play a role in the subsequent development of renal insufficiency. Anuria augurs a poor outcome, and although the renal defect is usually reversible, it is still a leading contributing cause of death in leptospirosis.

CNS involvement in leptospirosis most commonly takes the form of aseptic meningitis (Chapter 233). Although abnormal cerebrospinal fluid (CSF) findings are reported in up to 80% of leptospirosis cases, only half are symptomatic. Conversely, it has been estimated that 10% of all cases of aseptic meningitis in the United States are caused by leptospirosis. Early in the course of the meningitis, neutrophils may predominate in the CSF, but later, lymphocytes predominate. The CSF protein may be elevated, but glucose is normal.

The white blood cell count may be depressed, normal, or elevated, but is usually associated with a left shift. Mild anemia is common; hemolytic anemia and disseminated intravascular coagulation have been described in severe cases.

Skeletal muscle involvement in leptospirosis occurs early in the course of the disease. Myalgia is reported in 70% to 80% of cases, with muscle tenderness being most common in the calves and thighs. Pathologic changes in skeletal muscle correlate clinically with myalgia and muscle tenderness. Early (within the first week of onset) elevations of creatine phosphokinase substantiate the above findings, and, when such increases are associated with mild elevations of liver enzymes, they should serve to heighten suspicion of leptospirosis.

Other, less common manifestations of leptospirosis are rash, generalized lymphadenopathy, pharyngitis, gastrointestinal hemorrhage, acalculous cholecystitis, adult respiratory distress syndrome, hemorrhagic pneumonia, and myocarditis.

LABORATORY TESTS

Leptospirosis can be diagnosed definitively by culture. However, leptospires are fastidious organisms and do not grow in ordinary blood culture broth or on routine agar plates. Organisms can be cultured from blood or CSF in the first 1 to 2 weeks after onset by inoculating specialized media, for example, Fletcher, Stuart, or Ellinghausen. After 1 to 2 weeks of illness, urine provides the highest yield of positive cultures.

Cultures are rarely obtained, since very few laboratories have facilities for culture of leptospires. Thus, infection is usually documented serologically. The microscopic agglutination test (MAT) evaluates the acute phase (within the first week) and convalescent phase (2 to 3 weeks after onset) serum specimens, which are tested against a battery of live leptospiral antigens. A fourfold rise in titer is confirmatory, and stable titers greater than or equal to 1:2000 are suggestive of leptospirosis. Delayed seroconversion (a month or more after onset) may occur. The macroscopic agglutination or slide test is more easily performed than the MAT but is less sensitive and specific. Newer serologic assays, such as enzyme-linked immunoassay tests, are being developed, but their diagnostic utility remains unclear.

Direct dark-field microscopy of urine or CSF specimens can sometimes be of value in the tentative diagnosis of leptospirosis; however, artifacts are common. Other techniques, for example, direct fluorescent antibody staining of fluids and tissues, may be of value in individual cases. The Dieterle stain demonstrates leptospires in tissues.

TREATMENT

The effectiveness of antibiotic therapy in human leptospirosis is controversial, but recent studies suggest therapy is of value if started within 3 to 4 days of onset. In a randomized, placebo-controlled study among military trainees with mild leptospirosis in Panama, doxycycline therapy significantly reduced duration of fever, headache, and myalgias in anicteric leptospirosis and prevented leptospiruria. In this study, patients were started on therapy early after onset (mean, 45 hours). In another recent placebo-controlled trial, patients receiving a 7-day course of intravenous penicillin (6 million units/day) had significantly reduced systemic, renal, and hepatic complications of leptospirosis compared with placebo recipients, even in the subgroup of patients with severe, advanced leptospirosis. These patients were ill an average of 9 days prior to initiation of therapy.

Penicillin is the antibiotic of choice, and a dose of 1 million units intravenously q6h has been recommended. Alternatively, tetracycline (250 to 500 mg P.O. q6h) or doxycycline (100 mg P.O. b.i.d.) may be given. Therapy should be initiated within 4 days of onset and continued for 7 to 10 days. In-vitro and experimental animal studies suggest that newer penicillins and cephalosporins may be useful; however, further clinical studies are needed to confirm the utility of these antibiotics in human disease.

Jarisch-Herxheimer reactions have been reported in leptospirosis but do not appear as regularly as in *Borrelia* infections. The overall mortality of leptospirosis in the United States is 5%, but it is higher for persons 60 years of age or older (19.5%).

PREVENTION

Prevention of leptospirosis largely depends on personal protective measures, environmental sanitation, and vector control. Doxycycline, 200 mg orally once per week, prevented disease when given prophylactically to military trainees in Panama. The efficacy of prophylaxis on a prolonged basis and among individuals with potential exposures to an expanded range of serotypes requires further evaluation.

Each case of leptospirosis should be reported to local and state health authorities, since subsequent epidemiologic investigations often have led to the discovery of large common-source outbreaks. Immunity to leptospirosis is probably serotype- and serogroup-specific. Repeated infection with members of different serogroups is thus possible.

REFERENCES

Anderson DC et al: Leptospirosis: a common-source outbreak due to leptospires of the Grippotyphosa serogroup. Am J Epidemiol 107:538, 1978.

Feigin RD and Anderson DC: Human leptospirosis. Crit Rev Clin Lab Sci 5:413, 1975.

Heath CW, Alexander AD, and Galton MM: Leptospirosis in the United States. Analysis of 483 cases in man, 1949-1961. N Engl J Med 273:1, 1965.

Martone WJ and Kaufmann AF: Leptospirosis in humans in the United States, 1974-78. J Infect Dis 140:1020, 1979.

McClain JBL et al: Doxycycline therapy for leptospirosis. Ann Intern Med 100:696, 1984.

Takafuji ET et al: An efficacy trial of doxycycline chemoprophylaxis against leptospirosis. N Engl J Med 310:497, 1984.

Watt G et al: Placebo-controlled trial of intravenous penicillin for severe and late leptospirosis. Lancet 1:433, 1988.

Yasuda PH et al: Deoxyribonucleic acid relatedness between serogroups and serovars in the family *Leptospiraceae* with proposals for seven new *Leptospira* species. Intern J Syst Bacteriol 37:407, 1987.

CHAPTER

275 Infections Caused by *Borrelia* (Relapsing Fever and Lyme Disease)

David T. Dennis
Grant L. Campbell
George P. Schmid

Borreliae are the causative agents of relapsing fever and Lyme disease, and the genus *Borrelia* is differentiated from the other five genera of the order Spirochaetales by morphologic, biologic, and ultrastructural characteristics. Borreliae are difficult to grow, and only limited phenotypic and genotypic work has been done to categorize them. Existing research is sufficient, however, to grossly categorize the borreliae that cause human illness into approximately 13 species that cause relapsing fever and one that causes Lyme disease.

RELAPSING FEVER

Classification and characteristics

Relapsing fever borreliae are typically 10 to 25 μm long and 0.2 to 0.5 μm wide, are less tightly coiled than leptospires, and have 3 to 10 (usually 5 to 7) uneven coils. The active, undulating motility of borreliae is caused by 15 to 22 fibrils inserted at each end of the cell that rotate about the cell body between an outer envelope, carrying specific antigen, and an inner cytoplasmic membrane. The biochemical properties of borreliae remain poorly defined, and not all species have been grown in artificial media. Borreliae are microaerophilic, require long-chain fatty acids, and ferment selected carbohydrates. Division is by transverse fission, with a generation time of 12 to 18 hours in vitro but about 3 hours in mice.

It is difficult to identify species among relapsing fever borreliae because they have similar morphology, are difficult to grow in vitro, and undergo marked antigenic phase variations during the clinical course of a patient's illness. The difficulty in identifying *Borrelia* species by usual bacteriologic methods has led to a categorization by agent-vector relationship. A high degree of DNA homology has been found between the three species of *Borrelia* that cause tick-borne relapsing fever (TBRF) in North America, which suggests that this categorization may soon be challenged.

Epidemiology

All relapsing fever *Borrelia* species except *B. recurrentis,* the agent of epidemic or louse-borne relapsing fever (LBRF), are transmitted by soft (argasid) ticks of the genus *Ornithodoros*.

Although TBRF occurs in all the inhabited continents except Australia, the individual *Borrelia* species and their associated tick vectors have restricted geographic distributions. In the United States and Canada, three species of ticks transmit borreliae to humans (Table 275-1) (*O. parkeri,* found in the Great Basin area of the United States, is rarely, if ever, the vector). Ticks that transmit borreliae to humans normally parasitize rodents and are mostly found in remote, natural settings in Western states. Infected ticks transmit infection to animals and man through salivary secretions at the time of feeding, pass borreliae to their progeny by transovarial transmission, and can remain infective for many years without feeding. These ticks attach briefly (10 to 20 minutes) and painlessly; hence, the bite is often unnoticed. Cases of TBRF in the United States typically arise from exposure to infected ticks in cabins and caves where there are rodent nests. Two recent outbreaks have occurred among visitors staying in cabins at the north rim of the Grand Canyon.

Although LBRF has been reported from all the inhabited continents except Australia, the only current major focus of LBRF is in Africa, primarily in the highlands of Ethiopia and the Central African Republic. Indigenous LBRF has not been reported in the United States in this century. LBRF often occurs in epidemic fashion in the wake of natural disasters and wars. The disease poses almost no risk to tourists abroad or to indigenous persons with good hygiene. The only host for *B. recurrentis* is humans. When the louse feeds on an infected human, the organisms pass into its midgut and thence into the hemolymph. Since lice are delicate, they are easily damaged when a bitten person scratches himself or herself. This breakage allows the escape of infected louse hemolymph into broken skin.

Table 275-1. *Borrelia* species causing relapsing fever in the United States and Canada and characteristics of their vectors

Species	Tick	Range	Habitat
B. hermsii	*Ornithodoros hermsi*	Western United States, Canada	Areas forested with ponderosa pine or Douglas fir: in decaying logs, cabins
B. turicatae	*O. turicata*	Western United States, Canada, Mexico	Caves, livestock barns, burrows of rodents, snakes, owls
B. parkeri	*O. parkeri*	Western United States, Canada	Caves, burrows (commonly of ground squirrels and prairie dogs)

Pathophysiology

Relapses are caused by the unusual ability of borreliae (like that of trypanosomes) to change antigenic composition (form new serotypes) and escape lysis by antibody and phagocytosis by leukocytes, which are responsible for clearing spirochetes from the blood and consequent clinical improvement between relapses. Traditionally, it has been thought that these new serotypes were sequestered in the liver, spleen, nervous system, or bone marrow until they enter the blood, but recent animal research suggests that spirochetemia may be constant, that conversion to different serotypes is continually occurring, and that a clinical relapse occurs when spirochetemia with a new serotype reaches a certain level. The clinical crises coincide with the appearance of antibody; leukocytic pyrogen and thromboplastin produced by mononuclear cells appear to be important mediators. Reinfection may occur.

Clinical disease

Differences in clinical illness caused by the various *Borrelia* species, particularly those between LBRF and TBRF, are primarily differences in degree; LBRF tends to be a severer illness than TBRF. After an incubation period of usually 5 to 9 days (range 2 to 29) the spirochetes invade the bloodstream, and clinical illness begins suddenly with fever (commonly ≥ 40° C), rigors, headache, myalgia, pain in small and large joints, nausea or vomiting, prostration, and, often, delirium. Eye pain, epistaxis, neck stiffness, nonproductive cough, and abdominal pain occur less commonly. Tachycardia and tachypnea are almost always present, whereas the frequency of other physical findings varies. Jaundice, meningismus, upper-quadrant abdominal tenderness with or without hepatomegaly or splenomegaly, nosebleed, and a petechial rash (usually truncal) occur in up to half of the patients (or more in LBRF). Neurologic manifestations, notably meningitis or encephalitis, may be prominent. An S_3 heart gallop and a macular rash (usually occurring at the end of the first attack) have been described; abnormal chest findings are unusual. The first attack lasts an average of 5 to 6 days in LBRF and 3 days in TBRF. Untreated, it ends by crisis characterized by an abrupt drop in temperature and sweating, followed by hypotension and prostration. If death occurs, it generally does so in the first attack of LBRF, but it may occur in subsequent relapses in TBRF. If untreated, zero to three relapses typically occur in LBRF, and three to five in TBRF. Between relapses, patients usually feel weak. The interval between the first attack and the subsequent relapse is 5 to 6 days in LBRF and slightly longer in TBRF. Successive relapses become shorter and milder.

During pregnancy, spontaneous abortion occurring as a result of crises is a recognized hazard. Transplacental transmission with resultant neonatal infection may also occur.

Borreliae may be found in the brain, heart, liver, spleen, kidney, skin, and bone marrow. Common causes of death, which occurs in 5% or less of treated patients, are myocarditis, hemorrhage (including intracranial), and shock.

Laboratory findings are nonspecific. The white blood cell count is usually normal but may be high or low; a left shift is common. Thrombocytopenia is common, particularly in patients with petechiae. Clotting studies are often abnormal, but disseminated intravascular coagulation is rare. The erythrocyte sedimentation rate is usually increased (often ≥ 60 mm per hour). The aspartate aminotransferase and bilirubin levels are usually mildly to moderately elevated. Proteus OX-K and syphilis reagin tests are occasionally positive. With central nervous system involvement, the cerebrospinal fluid (CSF) contains mostly mononuclear cells.

Laboratory tests

Diagnosis depends on demonstration of borreliae in the blood or, rarely, CSF or urine. The spirochetes can be visualized in fresh specimens by dark-field microscopy or, in stained smears, by light microscopy at 400 to 1000 magnification. With dark-field illumination, artifacts may be confused with borreliae. Borreliae are the only spirochetes in the blood that are stainable with aniline dyes (Giemsa or Wright); thin and thick (Giemsa requires no dehemoglobinization) smears are diagnostic in 70% of initial smears, and additional smears may increase this yield (Fig. 275-1). The *Borrelia* index (number of spirochetes per white blood cell in a thick smear) provides a clue to the severity of illness; indices greater than two are associated with more severe complications. *Borrelia* organisms are rarely visualized in the blood between relapses and become increasingly difficult to find during subsequent relapses. A microhematocrit technique may be more sensitive than smears; organisms are seen within the tube in, or just above, the buffy coat. Similarly, staining of blood smears with the nuclear stain acridine orange may be more sensitive than the use of aniline dyes. If microscopy does not demonstrate borreliae, citrated blood from TBRF patients can be injected into weanling mice or embryonated eggs. All clinical specimens

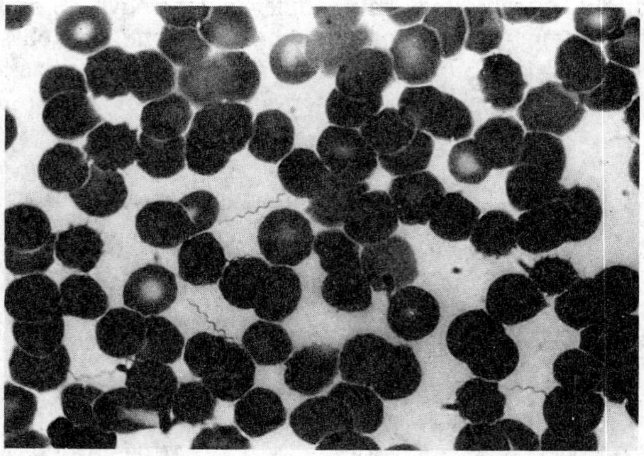

Fig. 275-1. Giemsa stain of thin blood smear shows *Borrelia* spirochetes.

should be handled with caution, since laboratory-acquired infections have occurred.

Because of *Borrelia's* unique ability to change antigenic composition and because of serologic cross-reactivity among spirochete genera, serology is difficult to perform and interpret. Although a variety of tests have been developed, none is readily available. Proteus OX-K, and OX-19, and syphilis reagin tests are occasionally positive. Cross-reactivity in Lyme disease serologic tests occurs. The organisms can be cultured in Kelly's medium or a modified Kelly's medium, such as the Barbour-Stoenner-Kelly (BSK) medium used for isolating *B. burgdorferi,* the agent of Lyme disease. Silver stains demonstrate borreliae in tissues.

Treatment

Erythromycin, tetracycline, doxycycline, chloramphenicol, and penicillin are commonly used in treatment, but no uniform recommendations exist. A Jarisch-Herxheimer reaction, sometimes life-threatening, may occur with all effective antimicrobials. It occurs regularly in the treatment of LBRF, with a highly predictive course of pathophysiologic events. Penicillin does not clear the blood of borreliae as quickly as the other antimicrobials listed above (in one study, 9.0 hours versus 3.1 hours) and produces a clinically less severe Jarisch-Herxheimer reaction, although physiologic measurements show that it is no less stressful. For TBRF, 500 mg of oral tetracycline every 6 hours for 5 to 10 days is recommended for adults. For LBRF a single oral dose of 500 mg of tetracycline or erythromycin, or 100 mg of doxycycline, has proved highly effective, although longer courses may be prudent. Short courses (e.g., 1 day) of penicillin do not prevent relapses in all cases.

All patients with LBRF should, if possible, be hospitalized and monitored for at least 24 hours after treatment for hypotension or cardiac failure; an intravenous line should be established before therapy. Intravascular volume needs to be carefully monitored and effective circulation maintained; digitalis glycosides may be required to improve cardiac output during the hypotensive phase of the posttreatment reaction. Less severely ill patients with TBRF may be managed as outpatients (although a brief hospitalization may be prudent), but they should be warned about the potential complications of a Jarisch-Herxheimer reaction. Acetaminophen, 650 mg P.O., or hydrocortisone, 500 mg I.V., 2 hours before and 2 hours after the administration of antimicrobials, may lessen the drop in systolic, but not diastolic, blood pressure occurring with the Jarisch-Herxheimer reaction.

Prevention

Prevention of LBRF depends on eliminating the poor hygienic conditions that favor the maintenance and spread of body lice. LBRF is a disease of the socioeconomically disadvantaged and usually occurs among groups of homeless, displaced persons who are unable to wash their clothing regularly. Emergency measures among groups at high risk, such as refugees, include providing a change of clothing and washing facilities, and treating clothes with insecticidal agents. TBRF can be prevented by avoiding known habitats of *Ornithodoros* ticks, such as rodent-infested caves and cabins, removing rodent nests from dwellings, and rodent-proofing and applying acaricidal agents to known infested dwellings. Chemicals containing N, N-diethyl-meta-toluamide (DEET) can be applied as tick repellents to skin and clothing, and permethrin-based acaricides can be applied to clothes and outer bedding in situations of high risk of exposure to infected ticks.

LYME DISEASE

Lyme disease is named after Lyme, Connecticut, where it was first studied in 1975. The disease is most commonly recognized by a characteristic skin lesion, erythema migrans (EM) (Fig. 275-2), which is often followed by arthritic, neurologic, and/or cardiac symptoms. EM was first reported in 1910 in Europe, where neurologic symptoms after EM were subsequently recognized (tick-borne meningopolyneuritis, Bannwarth's syndrome). The first reported case of EM acquired in the United States occurred in 1969, and the full clinical spectrum of Lyme disease was recognized in 1975 by Steere and associates.

Classification and characteristics

In 1981, the causative spirochete, *Borrelia burgdorferi,* was first identified in *Ixodes dammini* ticks (the deer tick), the principal vector of Lyme disease in the United States. Results of recent DNA relatedness studies on strains from the United States, Europe, and Asia suggest that *B. burgdorferi* will soon be split taxonomically into two or three separate but closely related species. Some European strains and all strains from the United States would continue to be classified as *B. burgdorferi*.

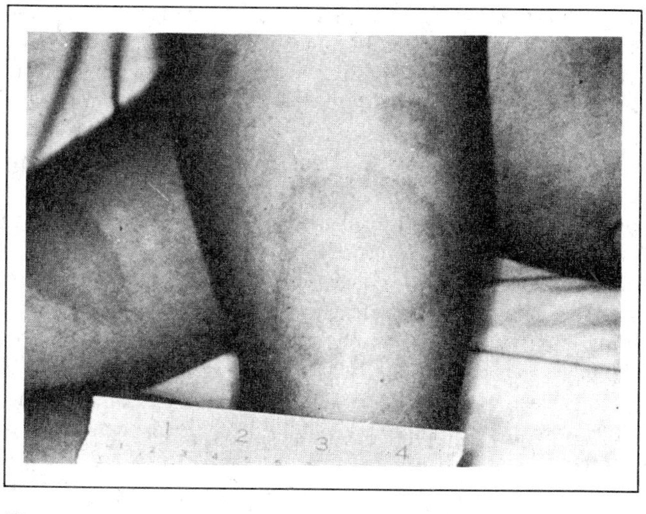

Fig. 275-2. Multiple erythema migrans skin lesions. (From AC Steere et al: Erythema chronicum migrans and Lyme arthritis: the enlarging clinical spectrum. Ann Intern Med 86:685, 1977.)

B. burgdorferi is 4 to 30 μm in length and 0.18 to 0.25 μm in diameter with looser coils and fewer fibrils (four to eleven) than other *Borrelia* species have. The organism is cultivable in Barbour-Stoenner-Kelly (BSK) modifications of Kelly's medium.

Epidemiology

Unlike tick-borne relapsing fever borreliae, which are transmitted by soft ticks, *B. burgdorferi* is carried by hard ticks of the genus *Ixodes*. Different species have been described as vectors in each continent where Lyme disease has been reported, and the complete range of tick vectors has not been determined.

In the United States, Lyme disease occurs at highest incidence in three broad geographic areas: northeast coastal states from Massachusetts to Virginia, the upper Midwest (especially Wisconsin and Minnesota), and northern California. *I. dammini,* the deer tick, is the most important vector in the United States, and its range parallels that of the distribution of Lyme disease cases in the Northeast and Midwest. *Ixodes pacificus,* the western black-legged tick, is the vector in the far West. *Ixodes scapularis,* the black-legged tick, is a potential vector in many southeastern and south-central states. *Ixodes* ticks may transport more than one organism pathogenic for humans, and coexistent cases of Lyme disease and babesiosis have occurred.

Ixodes ricinus (the sheep tick) is the vector of Lyme disease in the British Isles and throughout much of Europe, including states of the former Soviet Union. *Ixodes persulcatus* has been identified as the principal vector in central and eastern Russia, from the Urals to the Pacific Coast, in northern China, and in Japan. *Ixodes ricinus* and *I. persulcatus* are the principal vectors also of the virus causing tick-borne encephalitis. Persons with illness fitting the description of Lyme disease have been reported from Australia, South America, and Africa, but the occurrence of *B. burgdorferi* in these areas has not been established.

Lyme disease is a zoonosis in which humans are incidental hosts of *B. burgdorferi*. The life cycle of this parasite in the United States involves small rodents (especially the white-footed mouse in the East and the wood rat in California) as reservoirs of *B. burgdorferi* infection; transstadial transmission from larva to nymph; and maintenance of adult tick populations by deer, which serve as mating ground for ticks and as a source of the blood meal needed by ticks for the development of eggs. Humans mostly acquire Lyme disease from the bite of infective nymphs, usually in the late spring and early summer, and infrequently from adult ticks, which feed preferentially in the fall and winter, but also in early spring. The rates of infection of *I. dammini* nymphs and adults with *B. burgdorferi* in endemic northeastern and upper midwestern areas of the United States are in the range of 25% and 50%, respectively. In contrast, only 1% to 2% of *I. pacificus* ticks are usually found to be infected with *B. burgdorferi* in endemic foci in the western United States.

Lyme disease has become the most frequently reported arthropod-borne disease in the United States. More than 9300 cases were reported by 47 states in 1991; this represents a more than eighteenfold increase over the 497 cases reported by 11 states in 1982, and a 17% increase over the number reported in 1990. The national incidence was 3.97 per 100,000 population in 1991, ranging from 0 in several western states, Alaska, and Hawaii to 37.4 per 100,000 in Connecticut. More than 90% of cases were reported from the 23 states where populations of *I. dammini* and *I. pacificus* have been found; sources of human infection elsewhere are not well known, but it is likely that *I. scapularis* is responsible for sporadic transmission in southeastern and south-central states. Most cases have onset of illness in the months of May to August, reflecting times of greatest human outdoor activity and nymphal tick activity. The principal risk of exposure in the northeastern United States appears to be in wooded suburban residential settings; while persons living in endemic midwestern and Pacific coastal areas are most likely to be bitten by infected ticks in natural, forested sites frequented by persons seeking outdoor recreation.

Pathophysiology

Relatively little is known concerning the pathogenesis of Lyme disease. Both direct tissue invasion by *B. burgdorferi* and host immunologic response are thought to interact in the production of the various clinical manifestations of the disease. The organism widely disseminates from the site of tick inoculation in some patients with early Lyme disease. Viable *B. burgdorferi* apparently persist in some tissues throughout the course of the untreated disease, as evidenced by the occasional isolation of spirochetes from patients in later stages of illness. Intracellular sequestration of this organism may occur in some cells, for example, endothelial cells and fibroblasts. Transplacental transmission of *B. burgdorferi* has been reported but appears to be rare.

Immunoglobulin M (IgM) antibodies to *B. burgdorferi* generally develop within 2 to 4 weeks after the onset of EM, peak after 6 to 8 weeks of illness, and disappear after 4 to 6 months of illness in most cases, but can remain elevated for many months or reappear late in the illness. Immunoglobulin G (IgG) antibodies to *B. burgdorferi* are usually detectable within 6 to 8 weeks after the onset of EM, peak at 4 to 6 months after onset, and remain elevated indefinitely in patients with persistent infection. Antibiotic treatment of early Lyme disease can abort a detectable antibody response. Infection with *B. burgdorferi* may generate only transient immunity in at least some cases, since reinfections have been reported.

Circulating immune complexes can be found in most patients with EM, and high levels are maintained in the blood of those patients who subsequently develop neurologic or cardiac complications of Lyme disease. Patients who never develop these complications or who develop arthritis lose immune complexes from the blood, although high titers exist in the synovial fluid of patients with arthritis. Interleukin-1, released in response to *B. burgdorferi* or its constituents, may be responsible for triggering an inflammatory response that causes Lyme arthritis.

The virulence factors of *B. burgdorferi* are unknown. Antigens shared with *Treponema pallidum* and *B. hermsii* exist but their pathogenic role, if any, is unknown. Plasmids that encode for outer-surface protein antigens occur. Human monocytes and neutrophils phagocytize *B. burgdorferi* in vitro, but the roles that humoral and cellular immunity play in natural infection are unclear.

The recent development of a nonhuman primate model of early Lyme disease should lead to a better understanding of the pathophysiology of the disease.

Clinical disease

Lyme disease is an acute and chronic, multisystemic inflammatory disease with protean manifestations. The disease has been divided into early and late stages, the manifestations of which often overlap but may also occur independently. Most patients do not develop all of the major manifestations, and asymptomatic infections may occur. The earliest stage is usually characterized by the appearance of a distinctive rash at the site of the tick attachment, erythema migrans (EM), and accompanying constitutional symptoms. Untreated, the early signs and symptoms may be followed in days, weeks or months by neurologic, cardiac, and arthritic abnormalities. These later manifestations of disseminated disease may be acute and intermittent or chronic in nature.

In the majority of cases, Lyme disease begins with the appearance of erythema at the site of the tick bite occurring 3 to 32 days (median, 7 days) after the bite; however, less than 25% of patients remember a tick bite. Over days to weeks, spirochetes migrate outward in the skin, producing the characteristic large, expanding, annular ring of EM. In up to one half of cases, secondary skin lesions occur elsewhere within a few days of the first, suggesting blood-borne dissemination of spirochetes early in the course of infection. Most patients with EM experience constitutional symptoms of low-grade fever, fatigue, myalgia, arthralgia, headache (occasionally excruciating), and stiff neck. About 10% of patients develop symptoms of transient hepatitis. Lymphadenopathy, either regional or generalized, occurs in about one third of cases. Some patients develop signs of aseptic meningitis and meningoencephalitis. Conjunctivitis and endophthalmitis with impairment of vision may occur.

Untreated EM and associated early symptoms last about 3 weeks, but occasionally longer, before spontaneous resolution occurs. Neurologic abnormalities occur in about 10% to 15% of patients with EM not treated with antibiotics. Four neurologic syndromes occur with acute dissemination of the spirochete: meningitis, cranial neuritis, radiculoneuropathy, and meningoencephalitis. Facial palsy (which may be bilateral) occurs frequently. The most common neurologic symptom is headache, sometimes accompanied by signs of meningeal irritation and, less frequently, encephalitis (especially somnolence, mood disturbances, inability to concentrate, and memory loss). Patients with meningitic symptoms often have lymphocytic pleocytosis in cerebrospinal fluid, and *B. burgdorferi* has been cultured from the fluid. Peripheral nervous system involvement is most often manifest as motor and sensory radiculoneuritis, mononeuritis multiplex, or diffuse peripheral sensorimotor neuropathy in various combinations. Cardiac abnormalities occur less frequently than neurologic abnormalities. Varying degrees of atrioventricular block are the most frequently encountered sign of cardiac involvement, although left ventricular dysfunction can occur. Prolonged first-degree block (more than 0.30 millisecond) appears particularly likely to progress, often precipitously, to higher degrees of heart block.

Arthritis usually begins somewhat later (median 4 weeks after onset of EM) than neurologic and cardiac manifestations. Initially, brief attacks (median 8 days) of pain and/or swelling occur, usually in the large joints, separated by months of remission. Systemic symptoms, for example, fever and malaise, may recur with arthritis attacks. About 10% of these patients develop chronic arthritis, which clinically and pathologically resembles rheumatoid arthritis; alloantigen DRw2 occurs with increased frequency in patients with chronic Lyme arthritis. Months to years after the initial infection with *B. burgdorferi,* patients with Lyme disease may have chronic encephalopathy, polyneuropathy, or less commonly, leukoencephalitis. Memory, mood, and sleep disturbances commonly occur in persons with encephalopathy, and it is possible that infection with *B. burgdorferi,* as with *Treponema pallidum,* may occasionally cause severe cognitive deficits. Patients with encephalopathy usually produce intrathecal antibodies to the spirochete, may have evidence of continuing active infection, and usually improve with antibiotic therapy. Many of these patients also have peripheral nervous symptoms, either distal paresthesias or spinal or radicular pain. Electrophysiologic testing may reveal an axonal polyneuropathy. Chronic neurologic Lyme disease may be difficult to distinguish from multiple sclerosis and Alzheimer's syndrome. Intrathecal antibody production, the presence of lesions in the periventricular white matter, and the absence of myelin basic protein or oligoclonal bands in cerebrospinal fluid argue against a diagnosis of multiple sclerosis.

Diagnostic tests

A diagnosis of Lyme disease should be based on compatible symptoms and signs in a patient with a reasonable probability of previous contact with ticks in an endemic area. Current laboratory tests (with the exception of a positive culture for *B. burgdorferi*) are imperfect adjuncts only. In areas endemic for Lyme disease, the diagnosis can be made on clinical grounds alone in the presence of classic EM. Diagnostic difficulty occurs with early or atypical EM, or when compatible systemic symptoms or signs occur in the absence of EM.

Culture of *B. burgdorferi* from infected tissues is the only highly specific means of diagnosing Lyme disease. The limited sensitivity of culture, as well as technical requirements (e.g., the need for specialized medium), limit its use in routine diagnosis. The organism can be isolated from punch biopsies of EM lesions in 50%-80% of clinically diagnosed cases. However, the sensitivity of culture of blood, cerebrospinal fluid, synovial fluid, and other tissues appears to be much lower.

The most commonly used tests for Lyme disease are serologic, including enzyme-linked immunosorbent assays, immunofluorescent assays, and Western immunoblots. Unfortunately, none of these tests has been standardized with serum from a large group of culture-positive patients. Most use whole cell sonicate antigen preparations, which give poor precision and limited accuracy. A reliable and specific serologic test for Lyme disease is urgently needed. Nevertheless, current tests can be supportive of a diagnosis of Lyme disease in an appropriate clinical and epidemiologic setting. They are not recommended for screening purposes. Reasons for false-positive tests include cross-reactions with other spirochetes (e.g., *T. pallidum,* relapsing fever *Borrelia,* and possibly normal oral flora). Conversely, the fluorescent treponemal antibody absorption (FTA-ABS) test for syphilis can be positive in patients infected with *B. burgdorferi,* although reaginic tests and the microhemagglutination test for *T. pallidum* (MHA-TP) are negative. False-negative tests are common in early Lyme disease.

Clinical suspicion of CNS Lyme disease is an indication for lumbar puncture. Patients with CNS Lyme disease commonly have a lymphocytic pleocytosis, and many have evidence of intrathecal production of antibodies to *B. burgdorferi,* as evidenced by higher titers in CSF than in serum.

A variety of histologic and immunohistologic stains have been used to visualize *B. burgdorferi* in tissues, including EM lesions. These techniques are limited, however, by their apparent low sensitivity (a result of the apparent paucity of organisms in tissues), as well as by concerns about specificity. The use of the polymerase chain reaction to detect the *B. burgdorferi* genome in clinical specimens remains experimental. Other experimental approaches include detection of antigens in urine or CSF, and in-vitro measurement of specific cell-mediated immune responses to *B. burgdorferi*.

Treatment

For early Lyme disease with EM and without evidence of CNS involvement, the current drugs of choice are doxycycline, 100 mg twice per day, or amoxicillin, 250 to 500 mg three or four times per day (with or without probenecid 500 mg three or four times per day), given orally for 10 to 21 days. Erythromycin, 250 mg four times per day orally, can be used in penicillin-allergic patients for whom tetracyclines are contraindicated (e.g., pregnant or lactating women). Other oral antibiotics, including cephalosporins and azithromycin, are undergoing evaluation.

Therapy for later and more severe manifestations of Lyme disease continues to be controversial. Few controlled clinical studies have been reported. For Lyme arthritis without evidence of CNS involvement, oral doxycycline or amoxicillin with probenecid for 1 month appears to be effective. Ceftriaxone, 2 g daily, and penicillin G, 20 million units daily, for 2 to 3 weeks intravenously have also been used. Joint rest is indicated and joint aspiration may have therapeutic benefit. Concurrent intra-articular corticosteroids may increase risk of antibiotic failure. Inflammation may persist for variable periods after successful antibiotic treatment of Lyme arthritis. If joint inflammation has not resolved after 1 month of antibiotic therapy, then anti-inflammatory agents and a waiting period of 3 months before retreatment may be warranted. Arthroscopic synovectomy may be of value in patients with persistent chronic arthritis not responsive to repeated courses of antibiotics.

Lyme disease of the CNS should be treated with intravenous antibiotics for at least 2 weeks. Ceftriaxone is preferred, but penicillin G has also been used. Lyme facial palsy without pleocytosis or evidence of intrathecal production of antibodies to *B. burgdorferi,* however, can be treated successfully with oral antibiotics (doxycycline alone, or amoxicillin with probenecid).

Lyme carditis is generally a self-limited condition. Mild manifestations (e.g., first-degree AV block) may respond to oral antibiotics. Intravenous ceftriaxone or penicillin G has been used for more severe cardiac manifestations. Insertion of a temporary pacemaker may be necessary for some patients with complete heart block.

In general, therapy of Lyme disease in pregnant and lactating women is the same as in other adults. Tetracyclines, however, should not be used and the safety of probenecid in pregnancy is unknown. Intravenous penicillin should be considered when there is evidence of disseminated disease.

Persistent levels of IgG and IgM antibodies to *B. burgdorferi* do not necessarily indicate persistent infection. Therefore, the efficacy of antibiotic treatment should be judged on clinical response.

Prevention

Personal protection from bites of infective ticks is the principal prevention measure. The chances of being bitten by a tick can be decreased with a few precautions. Persons should avoid tick-infested areas, especially in spring and summer. Many health departments and park or agricultural extension services have information on the distribution of ticks in an area; in general, ticks prefer wooded, brushy, and grassy habitats where there is shade and moisture. When in tick-infested areas, persons should wear light-colored clothing so that ticks can be spotted more easily, and tuck pant legs into socks or boot tops. Insect repellents containing DEET can be applied to clothes and exposed skin other than the face, and permethrin compounds, which kill ticks on contact, can be sprayed on clothing. In endemic residential areas of the northeastern United States, wood lots, stone fences, and unkempt edges of yards pose a significantly greater risk than lawns and ornamental shrubby areas. Removing leaves and clearing brush around houses and at the edges of gardens may reduce the numbers of ticks that transmit Lyme disease. Application of acaricides to gardens, lawns, and the edge of woodlands near homes is being used to suppress vector ticks in some areas, as is the distribution of acaricide-impregnated cotton used by mice for nest building. One of the most important preventive measures is the early detection and proper removal by tweezers of ticks from the skin. Studies have shown that transmission of *B. burgdorferi* from an infected tick is unlikely to occur before 36 hours of attachment. Studies in areas endemic for Lyme disease show that the risk of infection with *B. burgdorferi* to persons who find and remove an attached deer tick is low, in the range of 1% to 3%. Therefore treatment of asymptomatic tick bites is not routinely indicated.

REFERENCES

Benach L and Bosier EM, editors: Lyme disease and related disorders. Ann NY Acad Sci 539:1, 1988.

Berger BW et al: Cultivation of *Borrelia burgdorferi* from erythema migrans lesions and perilesional skin. J Clin Microbiol 30:359, 1992.

Bryceson ADM et al: Louse-borne relapsing fever. A clinical and laboratory study of 62 cases in Ethiopia and a reconsideration of the literature. Quart J Med 39:129, 1970.

Cartter ML, editor: Lyme disease. Connecticut Med 53:319, 1989.

Centers for Disease Control: Lyme disease surveillance—United States, 1989-1990. Morbid Mortal Weekly Rep 40:417, 1991.

Dattwyler RL et al: Treatment of late Lyme borreliosis—randomized comparison of ceftriaxone and penicillin. Lancet 1:1194, 1988.

Horton JM and Blaser MJ: The spectrum of relapsing fever in the Rocky Mountains. Arch Intern Med 145:871, 1985.

Lane RS, Piesman J, and Burgdorfer W: Lyme borreliosis: relation of its causative agent to its vector and hosts in North America and Europe. Annu Rev Entomol 36:587, 1991.

Lastavica CC et al: Rapid emergence of a focal epidemic of Lyme disease in coastal Massachusetts. N Engl J Med 320:133, 1989.

Logigian EL, Kaplan RF, and Steere AC: Chronic neurologic manifestations of Lyme disesase. N Engl J Med 323:1438, 1990.

Maupin GO et al: Landscape ecology of Lyme disease in a residential area of Westchester County, New York. AM J Epidemiol 133:1105, 1991.

National Institutes of Health: Diagnosis and treatment of Lyme disease. Clin Courier 9:1, 1991.

Pachner AR and Steere AC: The triad of neurologic manifestations of Lyme disease: meningitis, cranial neuritis and radiculoneuritis. Neurology 35:47, 1985.

CHAPTER

276 Tuberculosis and Nontuberculous Mycobacterial Infections

Philip C. Hopewell
Peter M. Small

Three major categories of mycobacterial pathogens affect humans: the tuberculosis complex (*Mycobacterium tuberculosis, M. bovis, M. africanum,* and *M. microti*), the nontuberculous mycobacteria, and *M. leprae*. These bacteria are members of the family Mycobacteriaceae, order Actinomycetales, and share important characteristics: (1) After staining with certain dyes, they resist decolorization with an acid-alcohol mixture ("acid-fastness"); (2) their rates of growth are relatively slow; (3) they are obligate aerobes; and (4) under usual circumstances, they induce a granulomatous response in tissues of a susceptible host. In spite of these similarities, the organisms differ markedly in their ability to cause human disease and in the types of disease they may produce. Because *M. bovis, M. africanum,* and *M. microti* cause little human disease, they will not be considered. *M. leprae* is discussed in Chapter 276.

TUBERCULOSIS

Characteristics of *M. tuberculosis*

Mycobacterium tuberculosis is an acid-fast rod that typically is beaded or unevenly stained, is somewhat curved, and is approximately 0.3 to 0.6 μm in width and 1 to 4 μm in length. The acid-fast property is produced primarily by the lipid constituents of the mycobacterial cell wall and is usually demonstrated by the Ziehl-Neelsen staining procedure or a modification of this technique. The cell wall also has an affinity for the fluorescent dye, auramine O. Stains incorporating this reagent are used routinely by many laboratories. In Gram-stained preparations, *M. tuberculosis* may appear as gram-positive, although the staining is usually weak and varied. These staining characteristics are shared by all mycobacteria; thus, one cannot distinguish among *M. tuberculosis,* the nontuberculous mycobacteria, and *M. leprae* on a stained specimen. In addition, some *Nocardia* and *Actinomyces* species may be weakly acid-fast, and on rare occasions, be confused with mycobacteria.

Cultivation of the organism with examination of colonial appearance and determination of biochemical characteristics allows separation of *M. tuberculosis* from nontuberculous mycobacteria. The major categories of mycobacteria that may be pathogenic for humans are shown in the box on p. 2194). Mycobacteria typically are slow-growing. Under optimum conditions, laboratory strains of *M. tuberculosis* undergo one replication in approximately 18 hours; this compares with 20 to 60 minutes for most other bacteria. Colonies are visible on agar-based (Middlebrook 7H10) medium by 2 weeks, and on egg-based medium (Löwenstein-Jensen) by 3 weeks. Rarely do colonies appear after 6 weeks of incubation. By using a liquid culture medium such as Middlebrook 7H11 and a radiometric detection system, mycobacterial growth can be detected in as short a time as 7 to 10 days.

Colonies of *M. tuberculosis* are buff-colored and rough-surfaced. Exposure to light causes no change in their pigmentation. The lack of pigment production and the rate of growth enable *M. tuberculosis* to be distinguished from most nontuberculous mycobacteria. The niacin test, a procedure in which niacin production by the organism is measured, usually enables distinction between *M. tuberculosis* and the nonpigmented, slow-growing mycobacteria, particularly *M. avium* complex, with *M. tuberculosis* nearly always showing a positive result. The finding of a strongly positive nitrate reduction test confirms the identification in the occasional niacin test–negative isolate of *M. tuberculosis*.

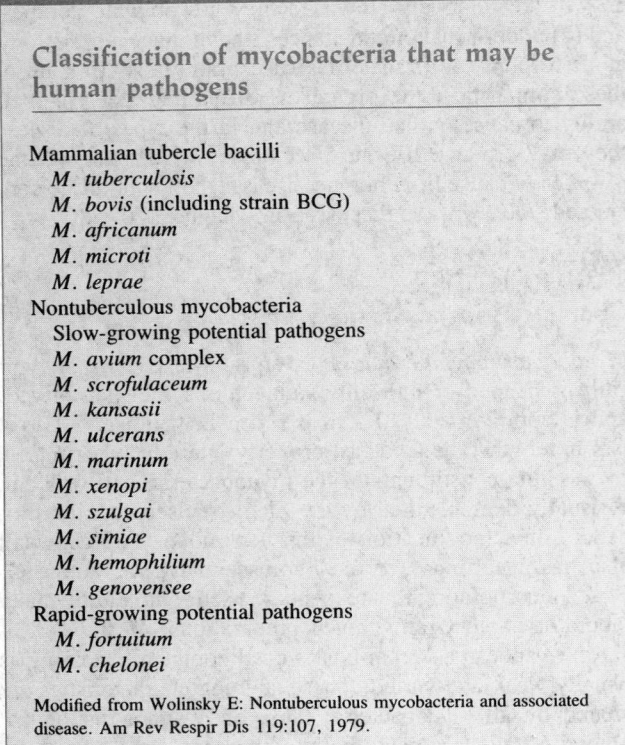

Classification of mycobacteria that may be human pathogens

Mammalian tubercle bacilli
- *M. tuberculosis*
- *M. bovis* (including strain BCG)
- *M. africanum*
- *M. microti*
- *M. leprae*

Nontuberculous mycobacteria
- Slow-growing potential pathogens
  - *M. avium* complex
  - *M. scrofulaceum*
  - *M. kansasii*
  - *M. ulcerans*
  - *M. marinum*
  - *M. xenopi*
  - *M. szulgai*
  - *M. simiae*
  - *M. hemophilium*
  - *M. genovensee*
- Rapid-growing potential pathogens
  - *M. fortuitum*
  - *M. chelonei*

Modified from Wolinsky E: Nontuberculous mycobacteria and associated disease. Am Rev Respir Dis 119:107, 1979.

Epidemiology

Among infectious diseases, tuberculosis is the leading cause of death worldwide. The World Health Organization estimates that approximately one third of the world's population is infected with *M. tuberculosis,* resulting in 8 million new cases of tuberculosis each year. The 2.9 million annual deaths from tuberculosis account for 6.7% of all deaths in developing countries and 26% of avoidable adult deaths. Though not yet quantified, it is feared that these numbers are increasing because of the HIV pandemic.

Tuberculosis is on the rise in the United States. After decades of steady declines in the annual incidence of new cases of tuberculosis, the number of cases began increasing in 1985, and between then and 1991 the number of cases increased 18% nationwide (Fig. 276-1). Had the previous trend of declining numbers continued through 1991, it is estimated by the Centers for Disease Control that 39,000 fewer cases would have occurred. The increase in cases was noted mainly within groups and in geographic areas where infection with HIV is prevalent, suggesting that a large proportion of these "excess cases" are occurring in HIV-infected individuals. However, other social factors such as homelessness, illicit drug use, and deteriorating public health infrastructures have also contributed significantly to the increase. Although composite data from the United States show low tuberculosis case rates, rates are high among specific groups. Case rates are particularly high among recent immigrants to the United States from countries having a high prevalence of tuberculosis, inner-city dwellers, men, and minority populations.

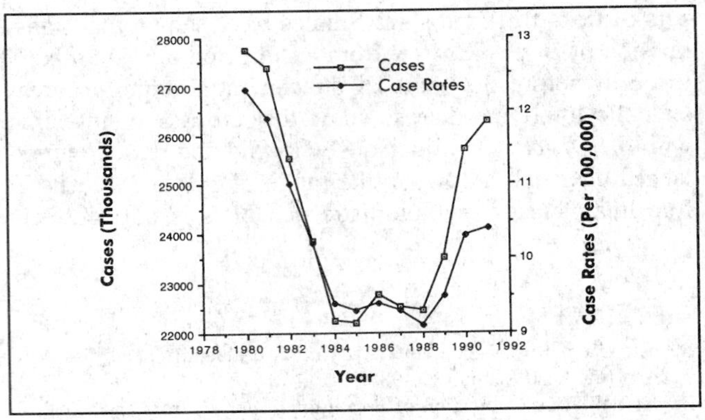

Fig. 276-1. Numbers and rates of new cases of tuberculosis annually in the United States 1980 to 1991.

In addition to increasing case rates, tuberculosis caused by organisms resistant to antimicrobial agents is also increasingly problematic. This has been particularly marked in certain urban areas, such as New York City, where one third of all cases are resistant to at least one agent.

A sensitive indicator of the seriousness of tuberculosis in a population is the age-specific prevalence of tuberculous infection as measured by tuberculin reactivity. According to the World Health Organization, in much of Asia and Africa, 40% to 80% of children are infected by the age of 14 years. By comparing the age-specific infection prevalence during different time periods, the effectiveness of tuberculosis control measures can be assessed precisely. For example, the infection prevalence data summarized in Fig. 276-2 clearly demonstrate the effectiveness of control measures in sharply reducing the amount of infectious tuberculosis present in an area of Alaska; corresponding case rates (all ages combined) dropped from 1854 per 100,000 in 1950 to 141 per 100,000 in 1970.

Transmission of tuberculous infection. The transmission of the tubercle bacillus from a communicable source to a potential new host nearly always takes place through the air. This route of transmission accounts for many epidemiologic features of the disease and is influenced by factors relating to the source of infection, the environment through which the infectious particle must travel, and the potential new host.

The vehicle for transmission of the tubercle bacillus is the droplet nucleus. Any exhalation of air from the lungs also expels water droplets. Once the droplet is outside the mouth, its water content quickly evaporates, leaving a solid nucleus. In persons whose respiratory secretions contain tubercle bacilli, the organism may be a part of this nucleus. Thus, the determinants of droplet formation and expulsion in the respiratory tract greatly influence the potential for transmission of the organism. Coughing is the most efficient means of generating droplet nuclei; therefore, the more symptomatic the person with pulmonary tuberculosis, the greater the infectious potential. Droplets are also generated by vocalization, sneezing, and normal breathing. The

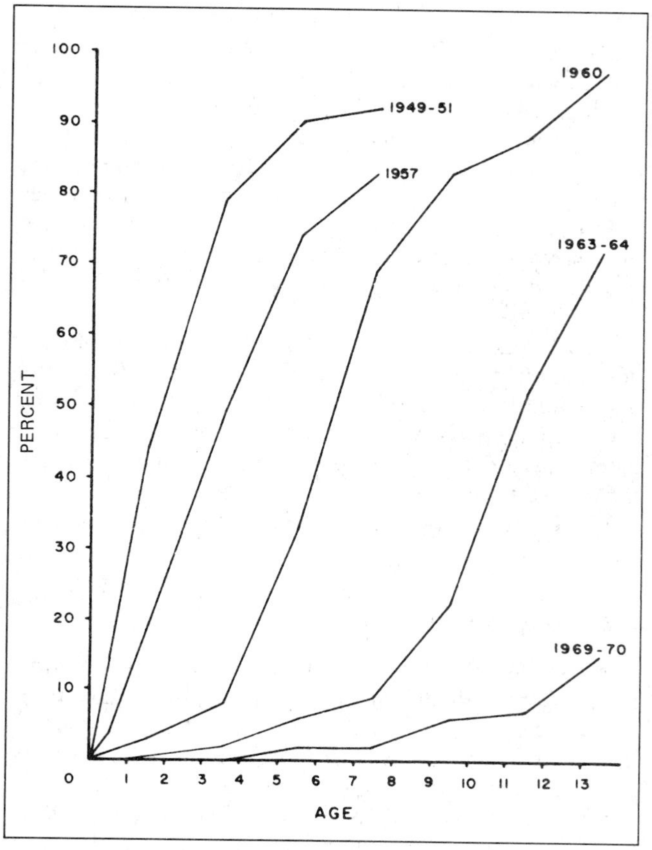

Fig. 276-2. Prevalence of tuberculin sensitivity among Eskimo children from the Yukon-Kuskokwin delta of Alaska in five successive surveys. (From Kaplan GJ, Fraser RI, and Comstock GW: Tuberculosis in Alaska, 1970. Am Rev Respir Dis 105:920, 1972. Reproduced with permission.)

volume and viscosity of the pulmonary secretions also influence droplet formation, with a greater number of droplets being formed from thinner, more voluminous secretions.

The infectious potential of a given person also varies with the numbers of organisms that have access to the airway and are subject to aerosolization. The numbers of organisms being excreted can be quantified roughly by examination of an acid-fast stained sputum smear. Persons with organisms visible on a smear are shedding more bacilli than persons who have a negative smear and a positive culture. Persons with negative smears but positive cultures have a larger number of organisms than do those whose bacteriologic evaluation (smear and culture) does not demonstrate bacilli.

The radiographic severity of pulmonary tuberculosis correlates with both the number of organisms in the lung and the degree of infectivity. Cavitary lesions usually contain large numbers of organisms and, thus, usually are associated with positive sputum smears and high infectivity. At the other end of the spectrum, negative sputum smears and cultures occur quite commonly with solitary nodular lesions in the lung.

Extrapulmonary tuberculosis is generally not infectious: transmission of *M. tuberculosis* occurs only under unusual circumstances from extrapulmonary sites.

Effective antituberculosis drug therapy promptly reduces infectiousness, although patients may continue to have positive sputum smears and cultures. This phenomenon was noted initially in animal studies and subsequently has been confirmed in several clinical studies.

Environmental factors also exert considerable influence on transmissibility. The concentration of organisms in the air is determined not only by the number of organisms being expelled but also by the volume of the air into which the bacilli are dispersed. Thus, exposures occurring in small, closed spaces are more likely to result in transmission than are those that take place in more open areas. Aerial transport of infectious particles is also dependent on particle size. Droplets produced from heavy, viscous mucus-containing debris and clumps of bacilli settle out of the air quite rapidly; however, particles of 1 to 5 μm in diameter have little settling tendency and disperse throughout the air into which they are expelled. The majority of organisms do not survive more than a few minutes beyond the time of their expulsion, even though the particle remains suspended. Viability of the organisms is greatly reduced by exposure to ultraviolet light, either from the sun or from artificial sources. Ultraviolet lights that are correctly installed and maintained can effectively sterilize large volumes of air.

Removal of droplet nuclei from a closed environment by venting air to the outside likewise greatly reduces the concentration of organisms in a given volume of air. Present hospital isolation standards specify a minimum of six air changes per hour and no cross-circulation or recirculation of potentially contaminated air. Filters capable of screening out particles the size of droplet nuclei may be employed in air-cleaning systems but are impractical for large-volume uses. A time-honored, though unproven, application of air filtration to decrease transmission is the use of masks. While most masks are constructed from materials capable of excluding 1- to 5-micrometer particles, their loose fit permits the entrainment of unfiltered air between the mask and face. This problem may be reduced with well-fitted disposable particulate respirators, but their long-term acceptability to patients or to persons in the patients' environment is limited.

There are also factors intrinsic to the potential recipient that influence his or her likelihood of acquiring a new tuberculous infection. The numbers of bacilli possibly inhaled by contact with a communicable source are determined by the duration of exposure as well as by the concentration of organisms in the air. Because tuberculous infection results in a specific cell-mediated immune response, further exposures to the tubercle bacillus are far less likely to cause new infections. Thus, tuberculin-positive persons are at lower risk of acquiring a new tuberculous infection than are tuberculin-negative persons. There have been, however, documented instances of exogenous reinfection of a previously infected person.

In immunocompromised persons, such as those with

HIV infection, the protection afforded by prior infection with *M. tuberculosis* may not be sufficient to prevent a new infection, and reinfection may be more likely in this group.

The transmission of tuberculosis can be minimized by adherence to basic principles. These include measures to promptly detect and treat persons with active tuberculosis and reduce microbial contamination of indoor air. Active surveillance for tuberculosis transmission is also needed. Compliance with these measures is particularly important in settings where tuberculosis is likely to be caused by organisms resistant to antimicrobial agents.

Pathogenesis

The fate of inhaled tubercle bacilli depends on a large number of factors, including the size of the inhaled particle (Chapter 231). Large droplets that are inhaled encounter a series of barriers in the nasal cavity and nasopharynx. Most particles larger than 8 to 10 μm in diameter are trapped in the upper airway. Particles between 5 and 10 μm enter the conducting airways, land on the mucociliary blanket that extends to the level of the terminal bronchiole, and are swept into the oropharynx. A substantial number of particles smaller than 5 μm in diameter penetrate beyond the ciliated epithelium and thus are retained in the lung.

Once in the alveolus, the tubercle bacillus encounters the second line of defense, the alveolar macrophage. Tubercle bacilli are chemotactic and attract macrophages, which ingest them. However, before the development of specific cellular immunity, the macrophage has only limited ability to kill the organism, and the bacillus proliferates within the cell. Depending on the number of infectious organisms inhaled and their rate of multiplication, an inflammatory response is generated in the area of implantation. At the same time, systemic hematogenous dissemination of the organisms occurs. The bacillemia usually does not cause symptoms but results in the seeding of other portions of the lungs and other organs with tubercle bacilli. Sufficient proliferation of organisms in either pulmonary or extrapulmonary sites may cause a clinically evident illness at this time. Immunosuppressed persons such as those with HIV infection are much more likely to develop tuberculosis soon after infection has occurred. In the vast majority of instances, however, the multiplication of organisms is held in check by nonspecific mechanisms until cellular immunity develops, usually 30 to 50 days after implantation. This is marked by the appearance of cutaneous reactivity to tuberculin. With the development of cellular immunity, sensitized T lymphocytes produce and release lymphokines on exposure to the antigens of the tubercle bacillus. These lymphokines attract and activate macrophages, which in turn become much more potent in killing the organism. This specific defense mechanism is usually successful in halting the proliferation of organisms and in greatly reducing the numbers of, but not eliminating, viable bacilli.

Artificial infection by vaccination with bacille Calmette-Guérin (BCG) stimulates host defenses, although less specifically, and also reduces the proliferation of implanted organisms.

It is estimated that in general, 3% to 5% of persons who acquire tuberculous infections develop clinically evident disease within 1 year after infection has taken place. In the remaining 95% to 97% of infected persons, the tuberculous infection is indicated only by a positive tuberculin skin test. Of this group of infected persons, approximately 5% develop clinically evident tuberculosis during their lifetimes. This risk varies considerably within the group, however. For example, tuberculin-positive persons who are also infected with HIV develop tuberculosis at a rate of 7% per year.

The factors responsible for endogenous reactivation of dormant tuberculous foci are largely unknown. Although it is possible to identify conditions that depress delayed hypersensitivity in most instances, these conditions are not evident in persons who develop tuberculosis. Thus, it is nearly impossible to predict who among the estimated 15 million infected persons in the United States will develop tuberculosis.

Clinical spectrum

The clinical manifestations of tuberculosis span a broad range, from a subtle, indolent process that is only fortuitously detected to an explosive, life-threatening or fatal illness. The symptoms produced may be both systemic and local in nature. The systemic manifestations are generally those of an infectious process, are often chronic, and include fever, weight loss, and fatigue. More specific symptoms are related to the location of the process.

While pulmonary disease accounts for the majority of cases of tuberculosis, extrapulmonary involvement (including lymphatic, pleural, genitourinary, bone, miliary, meningeal, and peritoneal tuberculosis) is increasingly common, particularly in HIV-infected individuals (Chapter 242).

Pulmonary tuberculosis

Clinical features. The majority of newly discovered cases of tuberculosis involve the lungs. Thus, strictly from a numerical standpoint, pulmonary tuberculosis is the most important form of the disease. Moreover, because tuberculosis is an airborne infection, pulmonary lesions are nearly the only source of new infections.

Cough is the most common nonsystemic symptom of pulmonary tuberculosis. Although the cough may be nonproductive early in the process, as the lesions become more extensive and involve airways more directly, sputum is produced. Hemoptysis of significant amounts is generally uncommon as an early symptom but may occur when there is necrosis of lung parenchyma. Hemoptysis may also result from residual bronchiectasis or cavities from previous tuberculous disease (with or without mycetoma formation), and less commonly from calcified hilar lymph nodes eroding into the airway *(broncholithiasis)*. Pleuritic chest pain may result from subpleural parenchymal inflammation with contiguous pleural membrane involvement or from tuberculous pleuritis without pulmonary parenchymal disease.

Abnormalities of respiratory function that are sufficiently severe to cause dyspnea are not common in tuberculosis. It should be emphasized, however, that extensive pulmonary tuberculosis may be the cause of acute respiratory failure that is occasionally accompanied by hypotension and disseminated intravascular coagulation (Fig. 276-3).

Laboratory studies. Patients with pulmonary tuberculosis may have abnormalities in routine laboratory studies, but these are not specific. Anemia is common in association with pulmonary tuberculosis but generally is caused by factors other than the lung infection itself. The syndrome of inappropriate secretion of antidiuretic hormone may account for the hyponatremia seen in some patients with pulmonary tuberculosis. Hyponatremia that does not promptly respond to water restriction should be evaluated further with tests of adrenal function.

Radiographic findings. Pulmonary tuberculosis nearly always produces an abnormality on the chest radiograph. Rarely, an endobronchial lesion may be present without radiographically evident parenchymal involvement. In this situation and in recently infected persons, tubercle bacilli may be present in the sputum, but no detectable abnormalities will be present on the chest film.

The typical radiographic pattern of pulmonary tuberculosis in adults is that of an upper lobe process that may be accompanied by cavitation. Most commonly, the site of involvement is the apical or posterior portions of the upper lobes (Fig. 276-4, *A, B*). From these sites, infected material may spread within the airways to involve any other portion of the lungs and may cause pneumonic or cavitary lesions. Adults or children who have been infected recently and in whom clinically evident primary tuberculosis develops (Fig. 276-5) often have a lower lobe pneumonic process that nearly always in children and occasionally in adults is accompanied by hilar adenopathy. Atypical presentations occur commonly in patients with associated diseases that may alter host responsiveness. This has been noted especially in patients who have HIV infection. In

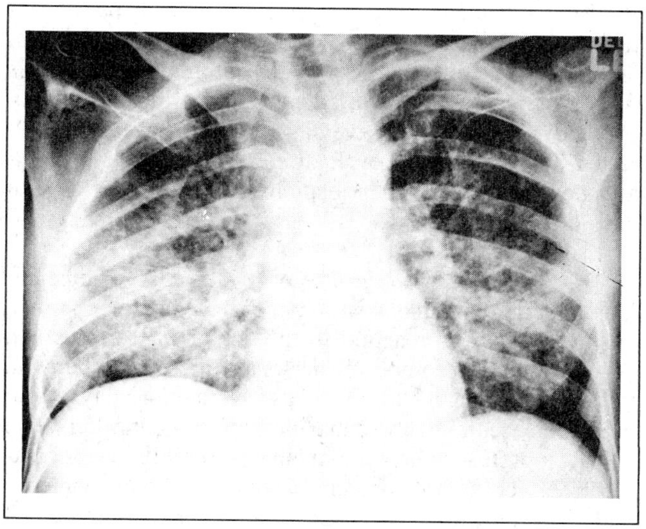

Fig. 276-3. Chest radiograph showing diffuse pulmonary infiltration caused by tuberculosis in a 38-year-old alcoholic man. In this patient, the process was rapidly progressive and caused severe respiratory failure, disseminated intravascular coagulation, and death.

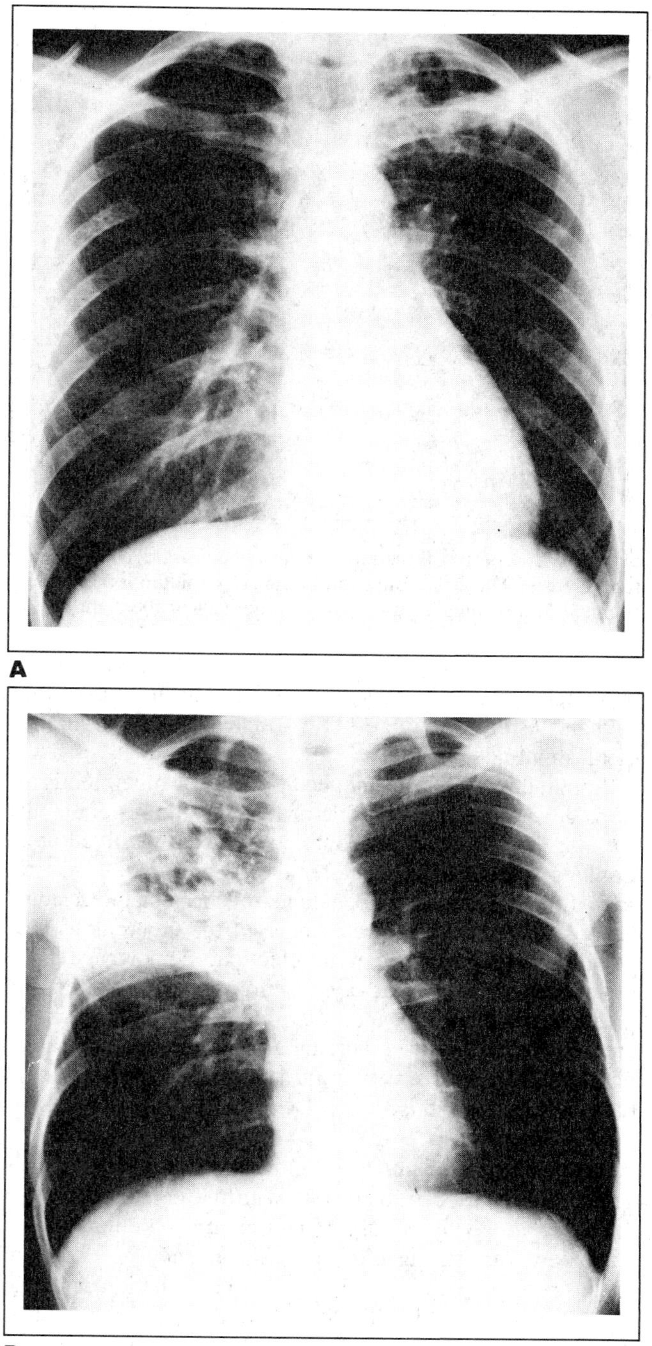

A

B

Fig. 276-4. Typical chest radiographs showing pulmonary tuberculosis. **A,** Cavitary lesion with adjacent infiltration in the apical posterior segment of the left upper lobe. **B,** Extensive destruction with cavitation involving all segments of the right upper lobe.

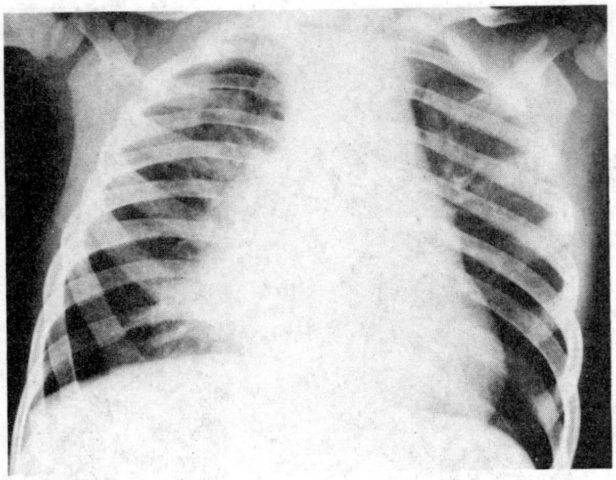

Fig. 276-5. Chest radiograph of a 1-year-old child with primary tuberculosis. There is infiltration in the right middle lobe with associated loss of lung volume and enlargement of the right hilum.

these patients tuberculosis is less likely to cause upper lobe cavitary lesions and more likely to have associated hilar or mediastinal adenopathy.

Spontaneous or drug-induced healing of tuberculous lesions generally leaves fibrotic or fibrocalcific residuals that are often associated with contraction of the involved area. Cavities also may persist after the active process has resolved. Changes in the appearance of these stable residual lesions may result from recurrence of the tuberculous process, superimposed bacterial infection, hemorrhage from old cavities or ectatic airways, or mycetoma formation in a preexisting cavity. In addition, there seems to be an increased frequency of carcinoma arising from scarred areas within the lung; thus, new infiltrates or mass lesions should be evaluated with this in mind.

Bacteriologic evaluation. Confirmation of the diagnosis of pulmonary tuberculosis rests with the demonstration of *M. tuberculosis* by culture of pulmonary secretions or tissue. However, strong clinical evidence may be sufficient for a presumptive diagnosis, and in combination with the finding of acid-fast bacilli on a stained smear of sputum is highly predictive of tuberculosis. Nonetheless, confirmation by culture is essential because of the identical clinical picture that may be caused by nontuberculous mycobacteria and the lack of features on the smear that allow *M. tuberculosis* to be distinguished from nontuberculous mycobacteria.

The best source of material for bacteriologic evaluation is spontaneously expectorated sputum. The rate of positivity is usually greater and contamination with other bacteria is usually less when specimens are collected during a 1- to 2-hour period after the patient arises (as opposed to a 24-hour collection). Bacilli are likely to be seen on the smear when there are more than 10,000 organisms per milliliter of sputum. False-negative smears are caused by intermittent shedding of organisms or by errors in preparation or examination of the specimen. For this reason, multiple specimens should be collected. The optimum number of specimens for the organism to be isolated appears to be a minimum of three and a maximum of six; collecting more specimens does not increase the yield. False-positive smears may be produced by nontuberculous mycobacteria, although the capability of certain of these organisms to cause disease cannot be dismissed. Smears stained with the fluorescent auramine or rhodamine dyes are more likely to be false positive because of staining artifacts and because of staining of nonviable bacilli. Positive fluorescent-stained smears therefore should be restained by the Ziehl-Neelsen technique or a related method. Because of the slow growth rate of *M. tuberculosis,* identification of the organism in culture using conventional methodologies may require up to 6 weeks. Sensitive radiometric techniques, which detect the liberation of radio-labeled by-products of growing bacteria, can currently be combined with species-specific DNA probes to provide results within 10 to 14 days. The time required to detect and identify mycobacteria may soon be reduced to a few days using highly sensitive polymerase chain reaction (PCR) DNA amplification–based assays.

There are several means of obtaining pulmonary secretions from persons who are not producing sputum. Sputum production may be induced by inhalation of hypertonic saline. Because these specimens look like saliva, they should be properly labeled so that they will not be discarded by the laboratory. Gastric lavage with saline also yields pulmonary secretions for examination. To be worthwhile this must be done early in the morning, before the patient has arisen. Once collected, the specimen should be processed promptly. The yield is less with gastric lavage than with induced sputum. Material also may be obtained by bronchoscopy with bronchial washing, bronchoalveolar lavage, and transbronchial biopsy.

Usually, patients who are severely ill with pulmonary tuberculosis have organisms present in their sputum smears, and therapy therefore can be started promptly. In patients who present more difficult diagnostic problems, therapy may be withheld until several specimens have been collected for bacteriologic evaluation. However, therapy usually does not reduce the isolation rate in the first several days of treatment.

Tuberculin skin testing. The only indication of tuberculous infection in persons who do not have tuberculosis is a positive cutaneous reaction to the tuberculin skin test. In immunologically competent persons, a positive tuberculin test can be elicited 2 to 10 weeks (average, 40 days) after infection occurs. Tuberculin purified protein derivative (PPD), a protein precipitate obtained from filtrates of heat-sterilized cultures of tubercle bacilli. PPD is available on multiple-puncture devices and in solution for intradermal injection (Mantoux method). The activity of this material is measured in tuberculin units (TU) and is determined by comparison with a standard batch of PPD. Although multiple-puncture methods often are used for testing children, the Mantoux method, which uses 5 TU of PPD ("intermediate" strength), is the best way to identify tuberculous infection. Test strengths of PPD containing 1 TU per 0.1 ml ("first" test strength) and 250 TU per 0.1 ml ("second" test strength) are available but have no demonstrable usefulness in ordinary practice. The tuberculin test is administered by using a 26- or 27-gauge needle to inject 0.1 ml PPD into the skin on the volar surface of the forearm, (although other sites may be used as well). The result is determined by measuring the diameter of induration 48 to 72 hours after injection. Most positive reactions remain positive for up to 7 days, however. The box below lists the American Thoracic Society/CDC classification for tuberculin skin test interpretations. Under most clinical circumstances, a reaction size of 10 mm or more in diameter to a 5-TU test is considered indicative of tuberculosis infection. However, 5 mm is considered positive in certain high-risk individuals, such as foreign-born persons, or those likely to have suppressed immunity, such as HIV-infected persons. Because of the marked propensity of HIV-infected individuals exposed to tuberculosis to progress rapidly to active tuberculosis, it is important to know the HIV status of contacts to infectious cases and to begin INH prophylaxis immediately in HIV-seropositive contacts who have had significant exposure.

False-positive reactions may result from infections with nontuberculous mycobacteria, causing a lower-grade tuberculin sensitization that usually produces reactions smaller than 10 mm. Vaccination with BCG also causes a reaction to the tuberculin test.

In persons who were infected some years in the past, tuberculin reactivity may diminish, causing the tuberculin test to become negative. However, the test itself may recall the sensitization and thus produce a subsequent positive test. This "boosted" reaction might be interpreted as being the result of a tuberculous infection that took place between the two tests, when in fact the infection predated the first tuberculin test. This misinterpretation can be avoided if a so-called two-step test is performed. This approach is necessary only in persons who are likely to be retested at regular intervals, for example, hospital employees. In the two-step tuberculin test, the test is applied in the usual fashion but is read 7 days rather than the usual 2 to 3 days later. If the test is negative, a second test is applied at that time and is read in 2 or 3 days. A positive response to the second test would be the result of boosting, not of a new infection, and would reflect accurately the person's previous infection.

When the tuberculin test is used in the evaluation of patients suspected of having tuberculosis, the major concern is not with false-positive but with false-negative results. The possible causes of a false-negative tuberculin test are listed in the box below.

The determination of true versus false negativity may be aided by administering, at the time of the second test, a battery of antigens to which most persons react. These include antigens made from mumps virus, *Candida,* tetanus toxoid, streptokinase-streptodornase, and, depending on geographic considerations, *Histoplasma capsulatum* or *Coccidioides* immitis. Detectable induration in response to any of these antigens indicates that cellular immune mechanisms are intact and, thus, that the tuberculin test is probably truly negative; however, selective tuberculin anergy may occur. If there is no reaction to any of these antigens, the tuberculin test cannot be interpreted as either truly or falsely negative.

Chemotherapy

The development and application of specific antituberculosis chemotherapy in the late 1940s and early 1950s revolutionized the care of patients with tuberculosis. In theory,

Criteria for defining tuberculin skin test reactions as positive

- >5 mm induration
  - Close contacts to infectious cases
  - Persons with abnormal chest radiograph
  - Persons with known or suspected HIV infection
- >10 mm induration
  - Residents of long-term-care facilities
  - Parenteral drug users
  - Foreign-born persons
  - High-risk minorities (especially African-Americans, Hispanics, and Native Americans)
- >15 mm induration
  - All other persons

Factors associated with false-negative tuberculin tests

- Technical errors
  - Improper administration
  - Inaccurate reading
  - Loss of potency of antigen
- Patient-related factors
  - Age
  - Nutritional status
  - Medications—corticosteroids, immunosuppressive agents
  - Severe tuberculosis
  - Coexisting diseases
    - HIV infection
    - Viral illness or vaccination
    - Lymphoreticular malignancies
    - Sarcoidosis
    - Solid tumors
    - Lepromatous leprosy
    - Sjögren's syndrome
    - Ataxia telangiectasia
    - Uremia
    - Primary biliary cirrhosis
    - Systemic lupus erythematosus
    - Severe systemic disease of any etiology

the initial treatment of tuberculosis should now be nearly uniformly successful. In practice, however, this is not the case. Success of therapy may be measured by the rates of sputum conversion and relapse after conversion. Data compiled by the Centers for Disease Control from tuberculosis control programs in the United States show that approximately 70% to 75% of persons with initially positive sputum had converted to negative within 6 months. Of patients not documented to have negative sputum, approximately 15% to 20% have not had sputum examined, 4% are lost to follow-up, and 4% are known to have positive sputum. The rate of relapse after sputum conversion has been achieved is not well documented but is probably no greater than 3% to 5%.

All these data indicate that in spite of our knowledge of what constitutes adequate chemotherapy, the overall success rate is not 100%. By far the most important reason for the failure of initial antituberculosis chemotherapy is the failure of the patient to comply with the prescribed regimen. At least three features of tuberculosis cause its treatment to be less well accepted than is usually the case with other infectious diseases: (1) the process is an indolent one and may produce few symptoms; (2) the disease must be treated with at least two drugs; and (3) the duration of treatment is lengthy. Thus, much of the recent investigation of drug regimens has been directed toward providing treatment options that are better suited to patients' different lifestyles. These data indicate that although rates of successful therapy are high, not all patients are promptly cured. Under current circumstances with the HIV epidemic and social conditions, such as homelessness, creating potentially hazardous environments, even a small number of poorly treated patients who continue to be infectious can have a major adverse effect on tuberculosis control efforts. For this reason, it is especially important that the details of therapy be carefully managed. In many instances directly observed therapy in which every dose of the drug is administered under direct supervision is necessary to ensure effectiveness.

The necessity for two drugs and for lengthy treatment reflects the microbiologic characteristics of the tubercle bacilli. First, in every group of tubercle bacilli there are naturally occurring drug-resistant mutants. Thus, to kill all the organisms, more than one drug must always be used. Second, because the multiplication time for tubercle bacilli is 18 to 24 hours and because the organisms may have periods of dormancy interspersed with spurts of growth, it is necessary that drugs be administered for long periods.

Concurrent administration of agents with different antimicrobial mechanisms is also beneficial because bacilli reside in a variety of different microenvironments, such as within macrophages, where different antimicrobials have variable effects. These factors combine to make treatment a much more difficult and tiresome process for the patient. Fortunately, with the advent of rifampin, the total duration of therapy necessary for successful treatment has been shortened substantially. In addition, twice-weekly regimens, both with and without rifampin, may be administered under direct observation to ensure that the patient receives the necessary amount of drug.

Antituberculosis drugs. Currently, there are 13 agents available in the United States for the treatment of tuberculosis (Table 276-1). The drugs are divided into two categories, primary and secondary. Agents in the primary group are those used in the initial treatment of tuberculosis. They represent the first choice because of their effectiveness, relatively low toxicity, and relatively low cost. The secondary agents are generally reserved for use in treating disease caused by organisms that are resistant to one or more of the primary drugs or in cases in which hypersensitivity or toxicity is caused by the primary drug. In general, the second-line drugs are less effective, more toxic, and more expensive than the primary agents.

Primary drugs. Isoniazid (INH) is the major drug in any initial treatment regimen. It is bactericidal and rapidly decreases the bacillary population in any lesion produced by tubercle bacilli that are susceptible to the drug. For this reason, it is probably the most important means of diminishing or abolishing the infectious potential of the patient with newly diagnosed tuberculosis. Because INH penetrates well into body tissues and fluids, it is equally effective in pulmonary and extrapulmonary disease. The drug is available in parenteral form and, thus, may be used in combination with an aminoglycoside antibiotic, usually streptomycin, in treating patients who cannot take oral medications.

Rifampin is also a potent bactericidal agent and is especially effective in eradicating organisms that grow in spurts. Rifampin is the agent that always should be used in patients who have INH-resistant organisms or have developed documented untoward effects from INH. In addition, as described below, the INH-rifampin combination forms the core of current treatment regimens. Rifampin penetrates well into body fluids, including cerebrospinal fluid.

Both streptomycin and pyrazinamide are bactericidal under the proper pH conditions (streptomycin, alkaline; pyrazinamide, acid). Streptomycin is probably most effective in its early effect on rapidly proliferating organisms, but it is less effective in this regard than INH. On the other hand, pyrazinamide, because it is most efficient in an acid environment, is thought to inhibit or kill organisms that are contained within macrophages.

Ethambutol is not a particularly potent agent but is effective as a companion to the more potent agents because it diminishes the likelihood of proliferation of drug-resistant strains.

Secondary drugs. The other oral agents, ethionamide, cycloserine, and p-aminosalicylic acid, are bacteriostatic and are less efficacious than the first-line agents, and, in addition, are associated with frequent and serious toxic effects that greatly limit their use. The antibiotics kanamycin, capreomycin, and amikacin have properties similar to those of streptomycin; however, they tend to be more toxic (to kidneys and to the auditory component of the VIIIth cranial nerve) and are more expensive. Fluoroquinolones are another class of promising agents that have minimal toxicities.

Drug regimens for initial treatment. A number of effective regimens can be fashioned using the primary agents de-

Table 276-1. Drugs used in the treatment of mycobacterial disease

Antituberculosis drugs	Adult dosage: Daily	Adult dosage: Twice weekly	Most common side effects	Tests for side effects
Primary				
Isoniazid	5-10 mg/kg, up to 300 mg P.O. or I.M.	15 mg/kg P.O. or I.M.	Peripheral neuritis, hepatitis, hypersensitivity	AST-ALT
Ethambutol	15-25 mg/kg P.O.	50 mg/kg P.O.	Optic neuritis (reversible with discontinuation of drugs: very rare at 15 mg/kg), skin rash	Red-green color discrimination and visual acuity*
Rifampin	10-15 mg/kg, up to 600 mg P.O.	600 mg P.O.	Hepatitis, febrile reaction, purpura (rare), drug interactions	AST-ALT
Streptomycin	15 mg/kg, up to 1 g I.M.	15-25 mg/kg I.M.	VIIIth nerve damage (vestibular), nephrotoxicity	Vestibular function, audiograms,* BUN, and creatinine
Pyrazinamide	25 mg/kg, up to 2 g P.O.		Hyperuricemia, hepatotoxicity	Uric acid, AST-ALT
Secondary				
Capreomycin	12-15 mg/kg, up to 1 g I.M.		VIIIth nerve damage (auditory), nephrotoxicity, vestibular toxicity (rare)	Vestibular function, audiograms,* BUN, and creatinine
Kanamycin	12-15 mg/kg, up to 1 g I.M.		VIIIth nerve damage (auditory), nephrotoxicity, vestibular toxicity (rare)	Vestibular function, audiograms,* BUN, and creatinine
Amikacin	15 mg/kg		Auditory, vestibulary, renal	Same as other aminoglycosides
Ethionamide	15 mg/kg, up to 1 g P.O.		GI disturbance, hepatotoxicity, hypersensitivity	AST-ALT
p-Aminosalicylic acid (aminosalicylic acid)	150 mg/kg, up to 12 g P.O.		GI disturbance, hypersensitivity, hepatotoxicity, sodium load	AST-ALT
Cycloserine	15 mg/kg, up to 1 g P.O.		Psychosis, personality changes, convulsions, rash	
Ofloxacin	600 mg		Rash, GI	
Ciprofloxacin	500-700 mg		GI, CNS	

BUN, blood urea nitrogen; AST, serum aspartate aminotransferase; ALT, serum alanine aminotransferase.
*Determine at the start of treatment.

scribed above. The overall goal is to use a regimen that combines optimal effectiveness with the shortest possible duration of administration. It is presumed that shorter durations of treatment foster patient compliance and thus allow resources to be focused on ensuring completion of treatment. Since the early 1950s, when truly effective treatment first became available, the necessary duration of therapy has been reduced from 24 months to 6 months. This reduction was largely brought about through the use of rifampin and, to a lesser extent, pyrazinamide. The regimen most widely used in the United States currently consists of INH, rifampin, pyrazinamide, sometimes supplemented ethambutol for 2 months, followed by INH and rifampin for 4 months. Regimens shorter than 6 months have had an unacceptably high rate of unfavorable outcome and should not be used. If pyrazinamide is not used, INH and rifampin must be given for at least 9 months.

As discussed subsequently, regimens of 6 to 9 months should be used only when susceptibility to INH and rifampin is proved or is highly likely. When there is resistance to one or both agents, regimens must be modified and given for a minimum of 12 months.

Special considerations in choosing a drug regimen. The important factors to be taken into account in deciding on an antituberculosis drug regimen are listed in the box on p. 2202.

History of previous therapy. Persons who have been treated previously with non-rifampin-containing regimens and have had subsequent recurrence of disease have a greater probability of having organisms that are resistant to the drugs they received previously. In a Public Health Service survey of 4017 patients who had received previous antituberculosis therapy and developed a subsequent recurrence of tuberculosis, 41% had organisms that were resistant to INH, streptomycin, or *p*-aminosalicylic acid, either

Considerations in choosing an antituberculosis drug regimen

History of previous therapy
Probability of primary isoniazid resistance
Assessment of patient compliance
Presence of coexisting diseases
Results of drug susceptibility studies
History of untoward reactions to antituberculosis drugs

alone or in combination. Previous therapy for tuberculosis in which a single agent, usually INH, was used was associated with a much greater frequency of resistance. In addition, the greater the length of therapy, the greater the likelihood of resistance. Patients who had received INH combined with one or more other agents for 1 to 6 months had a 23% incidence of resistance to INH. This increased to 53% with 1 to 2 years and to 72% with more than 2 years of therapy. Because of the likelihood of drug resistance, patients who have received previous therapy should be treated with at least two drugs that they have not been given in the past, preferably with at least one of the bactericidal agents. When the results of drug susceptibility testing are available, the regimen can be modified if necessary. In patients with INH-resistant organisms, a regimen of rifampin and ethambutol given for 12 months should be effective. If a rifampin-containing regimen was used, then it is likely that the organism will retain susceptibility to both INH and rifampin.

Probability of primary drug resistance. The frequency of resistance to INH occurring in patients who have not had previous INH therapy (i.e., primary resistance) has not appreciably increased in the United States during the past 15 to 20 years. There are, however, specific circumstances in which primary resistance is more common. In many parts of the world, the prevalence of primary INH resistance is much higher than in the United States. Persons likely to have acquired tuberculous infection in Southeast Asia, Korea, the Philippines, Hong Kong, Central America, Mexico, and Africa should have their initial chemotherapeutic regimens selected as if the organisms were resistant to INH. An appropriate regimen would consist of INH, rifampin, pyrazinamide, and ethambutol. Drug susceptibility studies should be obtained and the results used to modify the regimen. The same approach should be taken for patients thought to have acquired tuberculous infection from a person known to be excreting drug-resistant bacilli. Success rates with appropriate therapy for extended periods of time approximate those of tuberculosis that is sensitive to all agents.

Tuberculosis that is caused by organisms resistant to two or more primary agents (multidrug-resistant [MDR]) has become a major problem in areas such as New York City, where 19% of isolates from a 1 month period in mid-1992 were resistant to both INH and rifampin. MDR tuberculosis should be suspected in all patients who may have recently acquired their infections in the urban eastern United States, particularly if they are infected with HIV or have been treated previously for tuberculosis. Empiric therapy should be tailored to match the local drug resistance patterns. Generally regimens should include isoniazid and rifampin unless resistance to these agents is documented. Treatment should be based on in-vitro drug susceptibilities of the isolate and should include three agents to which the isolate is sensitive. Even with optimal therapy, including judicious use of surgical resection of involved lung, treatment failure rates approach 50% in immunocompetent patients and are significantly higher in HIV-infected patients.

Patient compliance. The major reason for treatment failure in tuberculosis is failure of the patient to take medications as prescribed. This problem cuts across many demographic variables such as education, social class, occupation, age, and sex, making identification of patients who will be noncompliant a difficult task. For this reason, intensive efforts should be made at the outset of treatment to educate the patient about the disease and its treatment and to monitor compliance closely. If the patient shows a tendency toward noncompliance, close supervision should be maintained for the duration of the treatment program, or directly observed biweekly therapy should be used.

Coexisting diseases. When possible, drugs having toxicities that may add to the effects of coexisting diseases should not be used. For example, the aminoglycoside antibiotics and capreomycin should be avoided in patients who have significant renal disease and in patients with impaired hearing or vestibular dysfunction. Ethambutol should not be given to patients with significant loss of vision.

An exception to the general rule stated above is the use of INH and rifampin in patients with liver disease. Because of the central importance of these agents, they should not be considered to be contraindicated in the presence of liver disease. In general, in this situation they do not contribute to the further impairment of liver function. Although in this setting careful monitoring of liver function should be performed, it may be difficult to determine whether changes are caused by the underlying disease or the drugs.

Rifampin is a rather potent inducer of hepatic microsomal enzymes, which may accelerate the metabolism of certain drugs and thus decrease their effectiveness. Such interactions have been documented for oral contraceptives, cyclosporin, dapsone, corticosteroids, warfarin, methadone, oral hypoglycemic agents, and digoxin. The management of disorders for which these drugs are being used may be made more difficult by the use of rifampin but can be compensated for by adjusting their doses.

Drug susceptibility studies. The results of drug sensitivity testing may not be available until 8 to 12 weeks after submission of the specimen; thus, initial therapy should be based on the considerations mentioned above. Subsequently, however, the results of such susceptibility studies can be used to modify the regimen. Susceptibility studies should be obtained for all previously treated patients and for patients with a high probability of primary-drug resistance.

History of drug toxicity or hypersensitivity. If there is a clear history of a toxic reaction or an allergic reaction to a previously administered drug, the drug should be avoided and another agent substituted. It may be necessary to challenge the patient with the suspected drug under close observation to confirm the untoward effect. This is particularly true with INH and rifampin because of their central importance.

Management. Successful drug therapy using a combination of INH and rifampin should eradicate tubercle bacilli from the sputum of 90% of patients within 3 months, and of nearly 100% within 6 months. Patients whose sputum still contains organisms after 3 months of treatment should be carefully reevaluated to determine whether they are taking the drugs as prescribed and whether the organisms are susceptible to the agents being used. If the organisms are not resistant, strong consideration should be given to institution of a directly observed drug regimen. Patients who complete a 6-month regimen should have a follow-up evaluation approximately 6 months after completion of therapy. The relapse rate after therapy is completed is 1% to 2% and nearly all occur during the first 6 months after termination of treatment. Further routine follow-up evaluations are not necessary, but patients should be instructed to have any new respiratory symptoms evaluated promptly. Patients infected with HIV, who have tuberculosis caused by drug-sensitive *M. tuberculosis,* and who comply with therapy respond well to conventional therapy, although they do have a high incidence of adverse drug reactions.

In a patient who is receiving adequate chemotherapy, nonspecific factors such as rest, nutrition, and occupation have no effect on outcome. Activity should be regulated by symptoms, and diet by appetite. Patients whose symptoms allow it may resume working after adequate chemotherapy has been established.

Before the development of effective drug therapy, resectional surgery and collapse procedures were important in the treatment of pulmonary tuberculosis. Currently, however, surgical treatment has a very limited role. Resection may be considered when the tuberculosis is caused by organisms that are resistant to multiple drugs and there is a localized area of involvement. In addition, resection may be necessary because of massive hemoptysis originating either in an area of active tuberculous disease or in residual cavities or bronchiectasis left by previous tuberculosis.

The use of corticosteroid treatment in patients with pulmonary tuberculosis should be reserved for those who have extensive parenchymal infiltration with significant effects on respiratory gas exchange. Corticosteroids, by reducing the inflammatory response, may considerably improve arterial oxygen tension. Doses of 40 to 60 mg of prednisone or the equivalent of other corticosteroid preparations should be used, with the amount given being gradually reduced during a 1-week period before cessation, to decrease the likelihood of a sudden, "rebound" effect. Corticosteroids should not be used if the patient is not on effective chemotherapy.

Extrapulmonary tuberculosis

The relative frequency of extrapulmonary tuberculosis was increasing prior to the HIV epidemic but has gone up considerably in association with HIV. In patients with advanced HIV infection and tuberculosis approximately 60% have extrapulmonary involvement with or without pulmonary disease. Extrapulmonary tuberculosis presents several important problems that differ from those presented by pulmonary disease.

1. Extrapulmonary tuberculosis is often a much more obscure process that is more difficult to diagnose than pulmonary tuberculosis.
2. Bacteriologic confirmation of the tuberculous nature of the process usually requires an invasive procedure.
3. Guidelines for chemotherapy and need for adjunctive measures are not as clear as with pulmonary tuberculosis.
4. Several forms of extrapulmonary tuberculosis may be life-threatening and if cured, may leave significant residual effects (disseminated, meningitis, pericarditis).

Compared with pulmonary tuberculosis, extrapulmonary disease is more common among younger persons, among ethnic groups other than blacks or whites, and among women. As with pulmonary tuberculosis, however, there is a progressive increase in case rates with increasing age. Exceptions to this trend include lymphatic and meningeal tuberculosis, for which the case rates are highest in the 0- to 4-year-old age group.

The pathogenesis of most forms of extrapulmonary tuberculosis is the same as that of pulmonary tuberculosis. The sites are seeded at the time of initial dissemination, and organisms tend to persist in areas where the environment is favorable, probably where the oxygen tension is relatively high. Subsequently, because of some usually unidentifiable shift in the host-parasite relationship, the organism begins to proliferate, and clinical disease ensues. In some instances, direct invasion from contiguous sites may produce new foci of disease—pleuritis from subadjacent parenchymal involvement, pericarditis from rupture of adjacent lymph nodes. Distant sites may also be involved via spread through tubular structures—bladder, from renal foci; peritoneum, from female genital involvement; or gastrointestinal tract, from swallowed organisms originating in the lungs.

The definitive diagnosis of extrapulmonary tuberculosis depends on isolation of the organism. This is much more difficult than in pulmonary tuberculosis because there often is no ready source of specimens and, in addition, the numbers of organisms in extrapulmonary lesions are generally small. Of the 3850 cases of extrapulmonary tuberculosis reported in 1983, 92% had bacteriologic results, of which 77% (71% of the total) were positive. Ancillary diagnostic studies, for example, as body fluid examination and histologic examination of biopsy specimens, provide important clues to the diagnosis of extrapulmonary tuberculosis. The tuberculin skin test has the same diagnostic value for extrapulmonary as for pulmonary disease. As previously stated, a negative tuberculin test does *not* exclude active tuberculosis. In patients with disseminated tuberculosis, because of the frequent severe systemic effects, the tuberculin test may be negative in as many as 50% of patients.

The basic principles of chemotherapy apply equally to extrapulmonary and pulmonary tuberculosis. Although few carefully designed studies that define optimum drug regimens and duration of treatment have been done, increasing experience has provided good evidence that 6- to 9-month regimens are equally effective in extrapulmonary tuberculosis. Thus, the same regimens recommended for initial treatment of pulmonary tuberculosis can be recommended for extrapulmonary forms. In contrast to pulmonary tuberculosis, however, corticosteroid treatment and surgical interventions may play an important role in managing extrapulmonary tuberculosis.

Lymphatic tuberculosis. The presenting manifestations of lymph node tuberculosis depend, in part, on the location of the involved nodes. By far the most frequent site of involvement is the neck, with mediastinal involvement being second; however, any lymph node in the body may be affected. Typically, the process is first noted as a painless enlargement of one or more of a group of nodes. Although initially discrete and firm, they tend to become matted, inflamed, and fluctuant and subsequently drain spontaneously if they are not treated. Mediastinal nodes may compress airways, causing cough, whereas abdominal adenitis may be associated with abdominal pain. Systemic symptoms are generally absent unless there is other involvement. The differential diagnosis can be extensive, ranging from cat-scratch disease to lymphoma. However, in a young, otherwise healthy patient with a positive tuberculin test, the diagnosis is usually apparent. When there is doubt, excisional biopsy or aspiration may be necessary. Cultures are positive in only 50% to 60% of cases thought to be tuberculous. In children, because of the greater frequency of adenitis caused by nontuberculous mycobacteria, culture of the organism is essential.

Chemotherapy is nearly always successful. However, resolution of the clinical findings is slow, and nodal enlargement and inflammation persist for many months. During the initial months of chemotherapy, the response is considered adequate if the condition does not worsen. Surgery rarely is needed, except to provide diagnostic material. If a fluctuant node appears to be ready to erode through the skin, however, aspiration is indicated. This minimizes the risk of chronic draining of sinus tracts that may result from spontaneous rupture.

Pleural tuberculosis. Tuberculous pleuritis may present as a subacute or acute process with pleuritic pain and fever. As pleural fluid increases, the pain tends to decrease, and, in the majority of cases, the process resolves spontaneously. This form of pleural involvement is thought to be caused by rupture of an inapparent pulmonary parenchymal focus into the pleural space, with a subsequent hypersensitivity response to the tuberculoprotein of the organisms.

The fluid in a tuberculous effusion is serous and exudative, and typically has a white blood cell count of 1000 to 5000 per microliter, of which more than 80% are mononuclear cells. Very early in the course, however, the cells may be predominantly polymorphonuclear leukocytes. Only rarely are acid-fast bacilli seen on smears of pleural fluid. Cultures of the fluid yield the organism in approximately 40% to 50% of specimens. Closed-needle biopsy of the pleura, with culture of the biopsy specimen in addition to histologic examination, provides the diagnosis in 75% to 80% of cases. In spite of the relatively low yield of the standard bacteriologic procedures, the diagnosis can be established presumptively in the presence of compatible pleural fluid findings and a positive tuberculin test result. In this setting, even in the absence of bacteriologic confirmation, the patient should be treated for tuberculous pleuritis. Corticosteroids may cause more rapid resolution of the effusion and less residual pleural scarring, but such scarring only rarely presents a problem in any event.

Tuberculous empyema is a much less common form of pleural involvement. This is a more chronic, indolent process that is usually associated with evident pulmonary parenchymal tuberculosis. The empyema is produced by discharge of a large number of organisms into the pleural space, often via a bronchopleural fistula. The fluid produced is thick and frankly purulent and contains easily demonstrable acid-fast bacilli. Antituberculous chemotherapy alone is rarely successful in eradicating the infection, and surgical drainage procedures generally are required. If not drained, the empyema may erode directly through the chest wall (empyema necessitatis).

Genitourinary tuberculosis. The symptoms produced by genitourinary tuberculosis depend, in large part, on the specific site of involvement. Typically, urinary symptoms predominate over systemic symptoms, and dysuria, urinary frequency, hematuria, and, occasionally, flank pain are the most frequent complaints. In males with lower urinary tract involvement, epididymitis, orchitis, or prostatitis may be the causes of the initial manifestations. In women, infertility, pelvic pain, and menstrual irregularity may be presenting complaints. In women, involvement of the reproductive organs without concomitant renal tuberculosis is more common than in men. Constitutional symptoms also may occur but are more common when there is extragenitourinary involvement. In view of the indolent nature of tuberculosis, it is not surprising that the diagnosis is made in many cases by evaluating incidental findings such as an abnormal routine urinalysis in asymptomatic patients.

The urinalysis shows abnormalities in the vast majority of patients with genitourinary tuberculosis. The combination of pyuria in an acid urine without detection of pyogenic bacteria in culture is highly suggestive of tuberculosis. The results of urinalysis may be normal, however, in association with isolated genital lesions, especially in women, or when the drainage from a tuberculous kidney is blocked. When there is bladder involvement, pyogenic organisms also may be present and mask the tuberculous nature of the process.

When genitourinary tuberculosis is suspected, at least three first-voided morning urine specimens should be obtained. Smears of urine specimens from men occasionally show saprophytic acid-fast organisms and therefore should be interpreted cautiously. Cultures may be negative under the conditions described above, with normal urinalysis results. Conversely, in patients with tuberculosis in other sites, especially the lung, urine cultures may grow *M. tuberculosis* in the absence of any evidence of genitourinary involvement. The diagnosis of isolated involvement of reproductive organs may require biopsy of the suspected site and culture of the tissue.

In most series of patients with genitourinary tuberculosis, 50% to 75% have chest radiographs indicative of old or current pulmonary tuberculosis. Other extrapulmonary sites may be involved as well.

Renal tuberculosis originates in the cortex of the kidney. Parenchymal destruction may occur, causing spread into the medulla and associated papillary necrosis or cavitation. The inflammation and scarring also may involve the collecting system and ureters, with subsequent stricture formation and hydronephrosis. Involvement of the bladder can cause marked scarring and contraction. The involved kidney or bladder may become nonfunctional. All these changes may be visualized on an intravenous pyelogram, retrograde pyelogram, or renal arteriogram. Calcified lesions may be seen on plain films and suggest the diagnosis.

As in other forms of tuberculosis, chemotherapy is highly successful in the genitourinary type. Rarely, nephrectomy may be indicated because of intractable pain, chronic pyogenic infection in a nonfunctioning kidney, massive hematuria, or persistent tuberculous disease caused by organisms resistant to multiple drugs. Surgery also may be required, to relieve symptomatic obstruction caused by ureteral stricture or to create an ileal bladder when the urinary bladder is nonfunctional. Patients who have evidence of ureteral stricture or extensive renal destruction should have repeat intravenous pyelograms at 4- to 6-month intervals during treatment, and annually for 5 years after completion of therapy. Performance of routine follow-up radiographic evaluation in uncomplicated cases is controversial and probably is unnecessary if there are no symptoms and the results of urinalysis are normal.

Bone and joint tuberculosis. Skeletal tuberculosis most frequently involves the spine or weight-bearing joints, although any bone or joint in the body may be affected (Chapter 315). In most series of patients with skeletal tuberculosis, the spine is involved in 50% to 70%. Multiple lesions also may occur and may be difficult to distinguish from metastatic neoplasm solely by clinical or radiographic criteria. Pain is the usual presenting complaint, although the process is usually more indolent than is septic arthritis or osteomyelitis. Soft tissue swelling may also occur but usually fits the pattern of a "cold abscess" without apparent erythema or tenderness. In most instances, bone involvement occurs together with joint space invasion; thus, arthritic symptoms may predominate. Spinal tuberculosis also may be associated with abscess formation in the paraspinous tissues and within the confines of the spinal canal. The latter occurrence can cause nerve root or spinal cord compression, sometimes with severe neurologic sequelae, including paraplegia.

Radiographically, skeletal tuberculosis cannot be distinguished with certainty from other chronic infectious processes and, as was noted earlier, it may occasionally mimic metastatic neoplastic lesions. Typically, the radiographic picture is one of concurrent lysis and sclerosis of bone, with articular cartilage destruction indicated by narrowing of the joint space. In the spine, this is most commonly seen in the lower thoracic or upper lumbar vertebrae in adults, and in the thoracic vertebrae in children (Fig. 276-6). With progressive bone destruction, the anterior portions of adjacent vertebrae collapse, producing a gibbous deformity. A paraspinous abscess may be seen adjacent to the abnormality in the spine and is usually a spindle-shaped mass on anteroposterior views. Computed tomographic scanning of the spine is a more sensitive means of detecting both bone lesions and paraspinous abscesses than is conventional radiographic examination.

Although a strong presumptive diagnosis of skeletal tuberculosis may be made on the basis of radiographic findings, final diagnosis usually requires a positive tuberculin skin test, evident tuberculosis elsewhere, or biopsy confirmation. Aspiration of joint fluid and needle or open biopsy of bone lesions or synovium usually provides histologic and bacteriologic confirmation of the diagnosis.

The basic principles of chemotherapy for pulmonary tuberculosis apply to skeletal disease. Surgical intervention is usually unnecessary. Surgical decompression and debridement, sometimes accompanied by vertebral fusion, may be essential in spinal tuberculosis that is causing progressive neurologic abnormalities. Other involved joints should be immobilized and prevented from bearing weight.

Disseminated tuberculosis. Disseminated (miliary) tuberculosis is a multisystem process producing a complex of usually nonspecific symptoms including fever, anorexia, weight loss, weakness, and fatigue. More specific symptoms occur, depending on the sites of involvement. In children and immunosuppressed patients, disseminated tuberculosis is a direct result of progressive primary infection. In older persons, however, the pathogenesis is that of bloodstream seeding during recrudescence of previously dormant foci, usually within the lungs.

Physical findings are often nonspecific. Fever is documented in 75% to 80% of cases, with pulmonary findings, hepatomegaly, lymphadenopathy, and splenomegaly found in descending order of frequency. Neurologic findings and meningismus may dominate when there is meningeal involvement, and there may be detectable ascites when peritonitis is present. The only specific physical finding consists of tubercles in the choroidal coat of the retina, which are visible through an ophthalmoscope. The choroidal tubercles are usually multiple; about one fourth the diameter of the disk; gray, gray-white, or yellow in color; and most easily detected when the pupil is dilated.

Because of the nonspecific nature of presenting manifestations, disseminated tuberculosis often poses a difficult diagnostic problem. Although usually abnormal, the chest film may show no abnormalities until well after the onset of symptoms. The typical abnormality consists of uniformly distributed small nodular densities (Fig. 276-7). Additional findings suggestive of endogenous reactivation of tuberculosis may also be present, and pleural effusion may be seen.

Presumably because of more severe systemic effects of the disease, the tuberculin skin test is less frequently positive in miliary tuberculosis than in other forms of the disease. Most series report 50% to 55% of patients with an initial positive reaction to 5 TU of PPD.

Because the miliary lesions in the lungs are predominantly interstitial in location, sputum smears and cultures are less likely to demonstrate tubercle bacilli than in usual pulmonary tuberculosis. Acid-fast stains show organisms in 25% to 30% of patients, and *M. tuberculosis* is isolated in 50% to 70%. When sputum smears are negative, other sources of diagnostic material should be sought. Bronchoscopy with transbronchial biopsy has a high yield and in most instances should be the next step. In addition, joint, pleural, or peritoneal fluid should be aspirated, with subsequent biopsies as indicated; lumbar puncture should be performed if there are neurologic signs or symptoms. Biopsy of liver or bone marrow, with histologic examinations and culture, each has a 30% to 40% positive yield. Unfortunately, biopsies from both of these sources, particularly the liver, may show noncaseating granulomas and be bacteriologically negative, thus not substantiating the diagnosis.

Disseminated tuberculosis has been associated with a wide range of hematologic abnormalities. In some instances these are unusual enough to obscure the diagnosis. Anemia

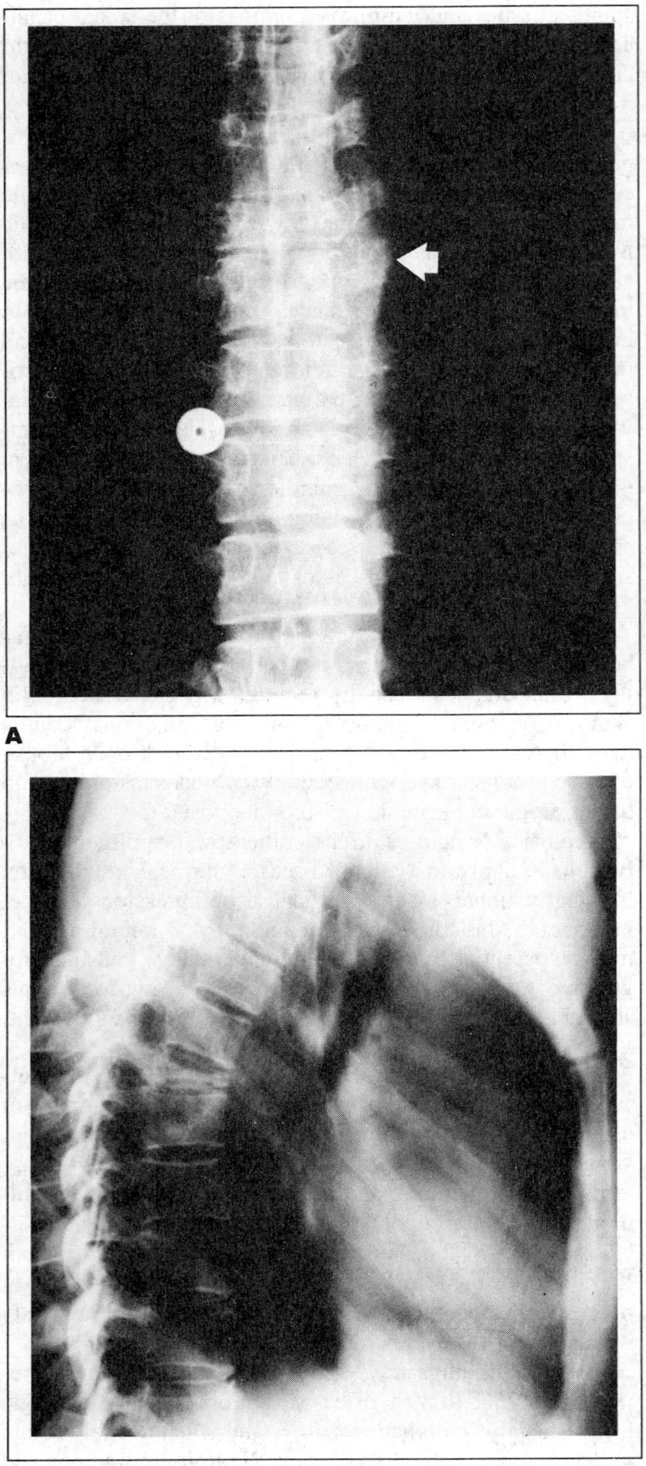

A

B

Fig. 276-6. Anteroposterior *(A)* and lateral *(B)* views of the thoracic spine, showing total collapse of the sixth thoracic vertebra, narrowing of the intervertebral space, and early destructive changes in the seventh thoracic vertebra. In addition, there is a rounded density *(arrow)* on either side of the vertebral column at the level of the affected vertebrae, indicating a paraspinous abscess. This patient's complaints were back pain for 1 month and rapidly progressive weakness of the lower extremities.

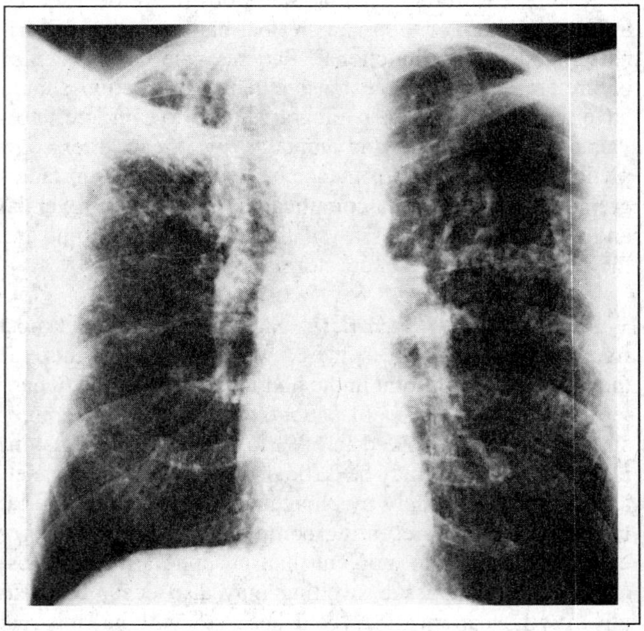

Fig. 276-7. Chest radiograph showing diffuse pulmonary infiltration in a miliary pattern. There is also a cavitary process in the right upper lobe, from which the hematogenous spread probably occurred.

has been noted in 50% to 60% of patients with disseminated tuberculosis but is severe (hematocrit less than 30%) only in about 15%. The pattern is usually that of an anemia of chronic disease but may resemble aplastic anemia or myelofibrosis with pancytopenia. Abnormalities of the white blood cells also are encountered, and leukemoid reactions, agranulocytosis, and leukopenia are reported. In recent years, there have been several reports of disseminated intravascular coagulation, often accompanied by the adult respiratory distress syndrome, occurring in association with disseminated tuberculosis.

After the diagnosis has been established or strongly presumed, therapy should be based on previously described principles. Before the advent of chemotherapy, the prognosis was regarded as uniformly hopeless. With chemotherapy, mortality rates are very low unless meningitis is present. Without meningitis, the prognosis is determined mainly by patient age and co-existing diseases.

Central nervous system tuberculosis. In spite of the effectiveness of antituberculosis chemotherapy, tuberculous meningitis remains a highly lethal condition, and mortality rates in modern series range from 25% to 50% (Chapter 233). The poor prognosis is caused in part by the long duration of the process before therapy is started. The symptoms usually evolve over a period of several weeks to months and include at the outset fever, malaise, and anorexia; these progress to include headaches, behavioral changes, stiff neck, photophobia, and, finally, seizures and coma. Physical findings may consist of fever, nuchal rigidity, papilledema, choroidal tubercles, and focal neurologic signs. Because of the predilection for the inflammation to be most marked at the base of the brain, cranial nerve palsies are fairly common. Focal neurologic signs also may be present in patients with isolated tuberculomas without meningitis. Tuberculomas may also involve any area of the spinal cord, producing symptoms relating to the site of the lesion. More than 50% of patients with tuberculous meningitis have evidence of tuberculosis elsewhere, whereas those with tuberculomas usually have no other evident sites of disease.

Lumbar puncture in patients with meningitis typically shows an increase in cerebrospinal fluid pressure. The fluid itself usually contains 10 to 1000 white blood cells per microliter that are predominantly mononuclear leukocytes, an increased protein concentration, and a decreased glucose concentration. Protein concentrations may be extremely high, depending on the intensity and duration of the illness. Acid-fast staining of cerebrospinal fluid smears shows organisms in only a small number of patients, and the organism is isolated in cultures in 30% to 50%. The differential diagnosis of these clinical, neurologic, and cerebrospinal fluid findings is extensive. Often, however, the diagnosis can be strongly inferred if there is evidence of tuberculosis elsewhere.

There are no specific radiographic findings associated with tuberculosis of the central nervous system. In children, however, there may be radiologic evidence of intracranial hypertension. Rarely, the skull itself may be involved. Computed tomographic examination of the head is a sensitive means of detecting tuberculomas.

Treatment should be started promptly in all patients in whom central nervous system tuberculosis is proved or strongly suspected. Isoniazid and rifampin, and to a lesser extent streptomycin, ethambutol, and pyrazinamide, all penetrate inflamed meninges sufficiently to provide adequate cerebrospinal fluid concentrations. Intrathecal therapy is not necessary. Corticosteroids are especially beneficial in patients with more severe neurologic impairment, especially those with cerebral edema or high CSF protein concentration.

Surgical intervention in tuberculosis of the central nervous system is limited to two indications: (1) insertion of shunts to manage hydrocephalus as a sequela of meningitis, and (2) diagnosis of a tuberculoma and resection of the lesion if it is causing either intracranial hypertension or specific neurologic deficits because of compression of adjacent structures.

A poor prognosis in tuberculous meningitis correlates with increasing age, with the presence of coma or confusion at the time of diagnosis, and with increasing protein concentrations in the cerebrospinal fluid. The effects of these factors are reflected in both death rates and frequency of neurologic residua. Mortality continues to be 25% to 50%, and the frequency of persisting neurologic findings in survivors is 15% to 20%.

Gastrointestinal tuberculosis. Although rarely encountered, tuberculosis of the gastrointestinal tract, abdominal organs, and peritoneum are forms of the disease that often are especially perplexing. Any portion of the alimentary tract from mouth to anus may be involved, although lesions proximal to the terminal ileum are extremely unusual. The sites of most common occurrence are the terminal ileum, cecum, and rectum. In the ileum and cecum, presenting manifestations are usually pain and/or intestinal obstruction, whereas rectal lesions may be manifested as fistulas, fissures, or abscesses. Radiographically, the lesion may be impossible to distinguish from neoplasm or inflammatory bowel disease, and in most patients, the diagnosis is made during surgery.

Tuberculous involvement of the peritoneum is manifested most frequently with abdominal pain, which often is accompanied by abdominal swelling. Fever, weight loss, and anorexia are also common. Some combination of these symptoms is usually present several months before the diagnosis is made. Radiographic evidence of pulmonary tuberculosis (current or old) varies in reported series from 6% to 80% but, when present, can lend weight to the diagnostic suspicion.

Ascitic fluid from patients with tuberculous peritonitis typically is exudative. It should be kept in mind, however, that when hypoalbuminemia is present, the protein content of the fluid may be less than 3.5 g per deciliter and yet be an exudate. White blood cell counts in the fluid range from as low as 50 to 10,000 per microliter and are predominantly lymphocytes, although polymorphonuclear lymphocytes occasionally predominate. Acid-fast organisms are seen rarely on stained smears of ascitic fluid. The frequency with which the organism is recovered in cultures varies in reported series from less than 10% to 83% and greater yields are obtained from large amounts of fluid (1 liter or more).

Histologic examination and culture of peritoneal tissue provide the best diagnostic yield. Laparoscopy or limited laparotomy is the preferred technique and allows directed biopsies. Because of abdominal pain or mass, laparotomy often is performed for diagnostic purposes. It should be emphasized that when findings compatible with tuberculosis are encountered during laparotomy, specimens should be obtained for both histologic and bacteriologic evaluations.

Antituberculosis chemotherapy is quite successful in treating any form of gastrointestinal tuberculosis. The frequency with which fibrotic residua cause bowel obstruction is not established. Although corticosteroids have been recommended for prevention of severe scarring, documentation of benefit is lacking.

Pericardial tuberculosis. Tuberculous involvement of the pericardium is an uncommon (but potentially lethal and therefore important) form of extrapulmonary tuberculosis (Chapter 18). The symptoms, physical findings, and laboratory abnormalities associated with tuberculous pericarditis may be the result of the infectious process itself or of the pericardial inflammation causing pain, effusion, and eventually hemodynamic effects. The systemic symptoms produced by the infection are nonspecific. Fever, weight loss, and night sweats are common in reported series. Symptoms of cardiopulmonary origin tend to occur later and include cough, dyspnea, orthopnea, ankle swelling, and chest pain that occasionally mimics angina but is described as a dull ache; often it is affected by position and worsens on inspiration.

Apart from fever, the most common physical findings are those caused by the pericardial fluid and/or fibrosis, that is, the physical findings of some degree of either cardiac tamponade or constriction.

Definitive diagnosis of tuberculous pericarditis requires identification of the tubercle bacillus in pericardial fluid or tissue. Although not absolutely conclusive, demonstration of caseating granulomas in the pericardium in the presence of consistent clinical circumstances provides convincing evidence of a tuberculous etiology. Less conclusive, but still persuasive, evidence is the finding of another form of tuberculosis in a patient with pericarditis of undetermined etiology. Still less direct and more circumstantial evidence of a tuberculous etiology is the combination of a positive intermediate-strength tuberculin reaction and pericarditis of unproved etiology.

Tubercle bacilli are identified in pericardial fluid in less than 25% to 30% (smear and culture combined). Biopsy of the pericardium with both histologic and bacteriologic evaluation is much more likely to provide a diagnosis, although a nonspecific histologic pattern and failure to recover the organisms do not exclude a tuberculous etiology. Approximately 25% to 30% of patients with tuberculous pericarditis have evidence of other organ involvement when the pericarditis is diagnosed.

Because of the potentially life-threatening nature of pericardial tuberculosis, treatment with antituberculosis agents should be instituted as soon as the diagnosis is made or strongly suggested. The likelihood of cardiac constriction is greater in patients who have had symptoms longer; thus, early therapy may reduce the incidence of this complication.

Current data indicate that corticosteroids are valuable in treating tuberculous pericarditis. In a prospective randomized study, South African and British investigators reported a significantly lower mortality rate and need for subsequent surgical treatment in patients treated with corticosteroids. The benefits were seen both in patients with effusion and in those with constrictive pericarditis.

The doses have been in the range of 60 to 80 mg of prednisolone or prednisone given daily for the first 4 weeks with a gradually decreasing dose during the next 6 to 8 weeks.

If hemodynamic compromise occurs, pericardiectomy may be necessary. Although pericardiocentesis generally improves the circulatory status, the improvement is usually temporary. Pericardial windows with drainage into the left pleural space often provide only temporary relief. The selection of patients for pericardiectomy is not clear cut except for those who have severe hemodynamic compromise. Persisting effusion, even with evidence of venous hypertension for as long as 6 months, has eventually responded to medical therapy alone. On the other hand, the longer the effusion persists, the thicker and more adherent is the pericardium, and the more difficult the procedure. In general, if venous hypertension persists beyond 6 months because of pericardial disease, pericardiectomy is indicated. Surgery also is indicated when there is decreasing heart size associated with increasing venous pressure, which indicates increasing constriction.

With proper therapy, mortality is probably in the range of 15% to 20%, and constriction occurs in about 15%. Constriction, if it is going to occur, is most likely to be apparent within 2 years and certainly within 5 years.

Prevention of tuberculosis

Isoniazid (INH) preventive therapy. There is now a large body of data to substantiate the effectiveness of INH in preventing the progression of tuberculous infection to tuberculous disease. Presumably, INH decreases the number of tubercle bacilli in (usually) inapparent foci formed at the time of the primary infection; the drug thereby decreases the likelihood that clinically evident disease will emerge from these foci. In a large series of studies of preventive therapy conducted by the Public Health Service involving some 70,000 participants, the case rate during the treatment year for those given INH was reduced by 84% compared with those given placebo. During subsequent years, there continued to be a greater number of cases in those who had received placebo. Overall, during a 10-year period of observation, INH preventive therapy resulted in a 61% reduction in tuberculosis cases.

Hepatitis is the major toxic effect of INH and must be balanced against the benefit of preventive therapy. The risk of INH-associated hepatitis increases with age: it is rare among persons under 20 years of age but occurs in approximately 2.3% of persons older than 49 years. Daily use of alcohol also increases the risk of hepatitis. Asymptomatic increases in serum transaminase levels are much more frequent than symptomatic hepatitis and occur in nearly 10% of all persons taking INH.

The indications for the use of INH preventive therapy are listed in Table 276-2. With each of these indications, the beneficial effect of INH in prevention of tuberculosis clearly outweighs the risk of hepatitis. It should be kept in mind, too, that the protective effect of INH is of extended (perhaps lifelong) duration, whereas the risk of hepatitis applies only during the medication year. Conversely, the risk of hepatitis during the treatment year may outweigh the risk of tuberculosis.

For preventive therapy in adults, a standard daily dose of 300 mg of INH should be given. For children, the dose is 10 mg per kilogram of body weight, up to a dose of 300 mg per day. The recommended minimum duration of INH administration is 6 months; however, persons with radiographic abnormalities suggestive of previous tuberculosis should be treated with INH for 12 months.

Persons receiving INH preventive therapy should be interviewed at monthly intervals to detect symptoms that may be caused by drug-related hepatitis. These symptoms are nonspecific in nature and include anorexia, gastrointestinal complaints, fever, and myalgia. Complaints more specifically related to the liver, such as jaundice, dark urine, and abdominal discomfort in the right upper quadrant are relatively uncommon. Patients having these or other suggestive symptoms of hepatitis should have tests of liver function performed, and if they are abnormal, the drug should be discontinued. Routine measurement of liver function is not indicated except in persons who are at increased risk of hepatitis—those older than 35 years, alcohol users, and persons with preexisting, but stable, liver disease. Preventive therapy with INH should not be administered to persons with current unstable liver disease or to pregnant women. Persons with radiographically visible lesions or symptoms that could be tuberculous in origin must be fully evaluated, and current tuberculosis excluded before preventive therapy is started.

Table 276-2. Indications for use of isoniazid preventive therapy

Group	Risk of tuberculosis
HIV-infected contact of infectious case	May exceed 30% with significant exposure
Recently infected persons (tuberculin convertors)	3%-5% during first yr after infection
Positive tuberculin test associated with chest radiographic abnormalities suggestive of previous tuberculosis	1% per yr for life
Tuberculin-positive close contact of newly discovered case	3.3% during first yr after discovery
Household contacts who are tuberculin-negative at the time of initial evaluation	0.5% during first yr after discovery
Tuberculin-positive adolescents	0.2% per yr for 2-3 yr
Tuberculin reactors in special clinical situations	Risk is not quantified
Prolonged corticosteroid or immunosuppressive therapy	
Hematologic or reticuloendothelial malignancies	
Insulin-requiring diabetes mellitus	
Pneumoconiosis	
After gastrectomy	
HIV infection	

Preventive therapy in persons who have been exposed to INH-resistant organisms is an issue of increasing concern. Unfortunately, no other agents have been evaluated for use in this situation. Given the lack of data, the choice of treatment should be based on a case-by-case assessment that takes into account (1) the probability that infection with an INH-resistant organism has occurred, an analysis that can be derived in part from an evaluation of the previously listed factors that influence transmission, and (2) an estimation of the possible consequences of the infection—the probability of tuberculous disease and its severity. When the probability that transmission has occurred is thought to be small and the consequences not severe, INH may be used according to the usual criteria. When the risk of transmission is great and the consequences are possibly grave, rifampin is the agent of choice.

If the index case is also resistant to rifampin, multidrug preventive therapy should be strongly considered.

Immunization. The BCG vaccine was derived from a strain of *M. bovis* and attenuated through serial passage in culture. Artificial infection with the organism stimulates the immunologic response that was described above as occurring with natural tuberculous infection. The effect of this nonspecific response is to improve the ability of a person who has recently been infected with *M. tuberculosis* to contain the infection thereby preventing early dissemination of the organism. No protection is provided for persons who are already infected when BCG is given. The reported effectiveness of BCG vaccination varies widely, probably because of variations in the potency of different strains of the organism and differing conditions and methods of administration of the vaccine. Indications for the use of BCG in developed countries are limited. Current recommendations in the United States state that BCG should be considered only for tuberculin-negative persons who are repeatedly exposed to untreated or ineffectively treated tuberculosis. Vaccination also may be considered for identified groups within the population that demonstrate an excessive rate of new infections (usually more than 1% per year) and in which the usual approaches to tuberculosis control have failed or have been shown not to be applicable.

In addition to the lack of consistent effectiveness of BCG immunization, administration of the vaccine usually produces a positive tuberculin skin test; the test therefore can no longer be used to identify tuberculous infection. This is a particular problem in immigrants to the United States from areas where BCG is commonly used. Because it is not possible to separate a BCG-induced tuberculin reaction from true infection, the history of BCG immunization is generally ignored, and the tuberculin reaction is interpreted and acted on according to standard criteria.

Public health considerations

Appropriate management of patients with tuberculosis must include attention to the public health aspects of this disease. Reporting of new cases of tuberculosis to public health authorities is generally mandatory. This ensures that cases are promptly and effectively treated, that the appropriate epidemiologic investigations are conducted, and that accurate data are collected. The most effective means of reducing the spread of tuberculous infection is prompt diagnosis and treatment of a patient with tuberculosis, which, as discussed previously, rapidly renders the person noninfectious. Thus, tuberculosis is one of the few diseases in which treatment of the disease itself benefits not only the health of the patient but the health of the public as well.

These ends are served not only by instituting proper therapy but by monitoring the effects of therapy to ascertain that the response to treatment is as predicted and that the patient is not encountering adverse effects of the drug. Patients should be seen and evaluated at least at monthly intervals. Sputum specimens should be evaluated after 2 to 3 months of treatment to determine if sputum conversion has occurred. If conversion has not occurred, the use of public health personnel to directly supervise therapy should be considered. Sputum smear and culture should also be performed after 6 months of treatment to document the bacteriologic negativity. These examinations at 3 and 6 months should be regarded as part of the basic public health management of the patient.

The most effective tool for finding previously undetected cases of tuberculosis is the evaluation of contacts of newly identified cases. By incorporating an understanding of the factors that govern transmission of infection into the epidemiologic investigation, the investigation can be conducted in a prompt and efficient manner. Contacts should be evaluated using a "concentric circle" approach, starting with those persons in closest contact with the index case and working in progressively widening circles with decreasing levels of contact. Because tuberculosis can spread rapidly in populations that have a high incidence of HIV infection, special efforts must be made to rapidly investigate contacts in such settings. Contacts should receive a tuberculin test usually soon after being identified. Those with positive tests should have a chest film taken, and if there are radiographic abnormalities, a sputum examination should be performed. Children younger than 6 years of age should have a chest film taken even if the tuberculin test is negative because of the more severe nature of untreated tuberculosis in this age group. Contacts whose initial tuberculin test is negative should be retested approximately 8 weeks after contact is broken or the index case becomes noninfectious. This period allows sufficient time for tuberculin reactivity to develop if the contact was infected shortly before the index case was identified. As indicated previously, INH preventive therapy should be given to all household or other close contacts, particularly those infected with HIV. INH can be discontinued in those who remain tuberculin-negative on the 8-week tuberculin test.

The other major public health function with regard to tuberculosis is the collection and analysis of epidemiologic and program management data. Accurate information allows for proper priority assignment for tuberculosis control activities, identification of areas and groups in need of special attention, and evaluation of the effectiveness of control measures.

NONTUBERCULOUS MYCOBACTERIAL INFECTIONS

Although types of mycobacteria other than *M. tuberculosis* and *M. bovis* were recognized before the end of the nineteenth century, the potential pathogenic role of these organisms was not clearly appreciated until the early 1950s. Since that time, there has been increasing awareness of the spectrum of disease produced by these types of mycobacteria. Similarly, with advances in techniques for studying mycobacteria, their classification and taxonomy have become increasingly precise. Several important generalizations can be made regarding the nontuberculous mycobacteria.

1. They may produce pulmonary disease that is clinically, radiographically, and pathologically indistinguishable from tuberculosis, or they may exist as saprophytes in the lungs and cause no disease.
2. With the exception of *M. kansasii,* they are usually resistant to antituberculosis agents.
3. Their epidemiology is largely unknown, but there are no proved instances of person-to-person transmission.

Characteristics of nontuberculous mycobacteria

As was stated previously, the nontuberculous mycobacteria share many of the properties of the tubercle bacilli. They are nearly identical among themselves and to *M. tuberculosis* in their staining characteristics and in the tissue reaction produced. The major differences are in their cultural, biochemical, and antigenic features. Several classification schemes have been developed to allow grouping of like organisms; none has proved entirely satisfactory. The box on p. 2194 is a classification of potentially pathogenic mycobacteria that separates the nontuberculous mycobacteria only on the basis of their growth rates and emphasizes the need for species identification rather than grouping of the organisms.

The most frequently encountered mycobacteria are those of the *M. avium complex, M. kansasii,* and *M. scrofulaceum.* The *M. avium* complex contains a large number of serotypically distinct strains that are otherwise difficult to separate. Colonies of these organisms are usually buff-colored and may resemble *M. tuberculosis*. *Mycobacterium kansasii* generally produces colonies that acquire a yellow-orange color after exposure to light, whereas *M. scrofulaceum* colonies produce pigment without being exposed to light. These characteristics form the basis of the Runyon classification, which is as follows: group I, photochromogens *(M. kansasii);* group II, scotochromogens *(M. scrofulaceum);* group III, nonchromogens *(M. avium complex);* and group IV, rapid growers *(M. fortuitum).*

Epidemiology. The epidemiology of the nontuberculous mycobacteria is largely unknown. There are, however, well-documented and striking foci of endemicity indicated by geographic distribution of reactors to skin tests with specific antigens and the distribution of disease. *M. avium* complex is highly endemic in the southeastern United States and is also found in western Australia and Japan, whereas *M. kansasii* is predominant in the westernmost midwestern states (Kansas and Nebraska), and in New Orleans, Dallas, and Chicago. Infection and disease caused by both organisms are found throughout the Midwest, and scattered pockets of disease caused by either *M. avium* complex or *M. kansasii* have been found throughout the United States.

In spite of the strikingly high prevalence of nontuberculous mycobacterial infection in many areas, the frequency with which clinically evident disease develops is much less than occurs after infection with *M. tuberculosis*.

Nontuberculous mycobacteria have been found in soil, seawater foam, tap water, pond water, milk, and bird feces. However, none of these sources or animals seems to serve as a reservoir.

The frequent occurrence of disease caused by *M. avium* complex in patients with AIDS does not fit with the pattern of distribution of organisms just described. Studies of the cumulative incidence of *M. avium* complex indicate that infection occurs in up to 24% of AIDS patients.

Clinical features of nontuberculous mycobacterial disease

In immunocompetent persons the nontuberculosis mycobacterial diseases are similar to tuberculosis in many ways, but they differ in several important respects: (1) the diseases tend to remain localized and progress extremely slowly; (2) constitutional symptoms are less prominent; (3) isolation of a nontuberculous mycobacterium from pulmonary secretions does not always confirm a diagnosis; (4) skin testing with tuberculins made from these organisms is of little value in making a diagnosis of disease resulting from a nontuberculous organism; and (5) with the exception of *M. kansasii,* response to chemotherapy is generally poor.

Pulmonary disease. The lungs are the most frequent site of involvement for *M. kansasii* and *M. avium* complex; however, all the organisms (see box, p. 2194) have been associated with pulmonary disease. Disease occurs more commonly in men, and there is a definite association with preexisting lung disease, such as silicosis, bronchiectasis, or old tuberculosis. The following criteria must be met before pulmonary disease can be ascribed to a nontuberculous mycobacterium: (1) there must be a compatible pulmonary process visible on the chest radiograph; (2) colonies of the same organism must be isolated from several sputum specimens, or the organism must be isolated from biopsied lung tissue; and (3) tuberculosis must be excluded.

Treatment of pulmonary *M. kansasii* disease with a regimen of INH, rifampin, and ethambutol for 2 years is successful in more than 90% of patients, and surgery is indicated only rarely. *M. avium* complex and the other nontuberculous organisms that may cause lung disease are much more difficult to treat. Regimens containing four, five, or six drugs sometimes supplemented by resectional surgery have been successful in only 41% to 77% of patients. Because of the potential toxicity and discomfort of regimens containing so many agents, the decision to treat disease caused by *M. avium* complex should not be made lightly and should take into account the disease's tendency to stabilize without treatment or to progress very slowly.

Lymphatic disease. Disease of the lymph nodes is most commonly caused by *M. scrofulaceum*. In contrast, more than 90% of culture proven mycobacterial lymphadenitis in adults is caused by *M. tuberculosis,* although *M. kansasii* and *M. avium* complex also cause adenitis.

When the diagnosis is suspected, excisional biopsy is the diagnostic procedure of choice. The major differential diagnosis is tuberculosis. The distinction can usually be made from epidemiologic features and the tuberculin skin test. Drug therapy is usually not indicated, and even partial excision of involved nodes is often successful.

Disseminated disease in immunocompromised patients. Another indication of the low virulence of the nontuberculous mycobacteria is the infrequency with which disseminated disease occurs. The majority of patients who have had disseminated disease have also had serious hematologic or immunologic disorders. The mortality rate in these patients is extremely high.

The clinical manifestations of disease caused by the nontuberculous mycobacteria deserve special mention. As mentioned previously, a large proportion of patients with AIDS have disease caused by *M. avium* complex when their CD4 cell counts fall below 50. The involvement is largely extrapulmonary, with lymph node, blood, bone marrow, and a variety of viscera being the sources of positive cultures. Striking features of the illness are the nearly total absence of any granulomatous response to the organisms and the enormous numbers of bacilli present (Fig. 276-8).

The severity of systemic illness and the effects on organ function caused by *M. avium* complex are not clear. Patients commonly have a number of other infections that obscure the features of illness caused by any single organism. Weight loss of greater than 20 pounds, anorexia, abdominal pain, and diarrhea have been suggested as more common in patients with *M. avium* infection than in patients with other complications of HIV infection. Diagnosis is made by culturing the organism, usually from the blood.

Although early reports on the response to treatment of

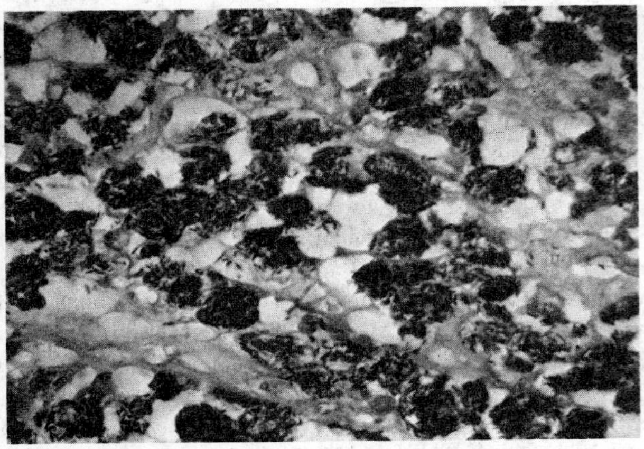

Fig. 276-8. Photomicrograph of acid-fast stain of lymph node biopsy from patient with AIDS and disseminated *Mycobacterium avium* complex disease. Specimen is noteworthy for the large number of organisms present (more darkly staining areas) and the absence of an inflammatory response.

M. avium complex were discouraging, recent trials of multidrug regimens including ciprofloxacin, clofazimine, ethambutol, rifampin, and amikacin show symptomatic relief and improvement in microbiologic indicators.

Soft tissue and skeletal disease. Soft tissue and skeletal sites of disease have been identified in association with a variety of nontuberculous mycobacteria. Common causes of these are cutaneous granulomas and ulcers from *M. marinum*. The lesions usually are the result of a break in the skin contacting contaminated water, which is often, but not necessarily, inhabited by fish. Such infection may heal spontaneously, but if treatment is necessary, the lesion may respond to treatment with rifampin and ethambutol as well as other agents.

Injection-site abscesses caused by *M. chelonei* have been reported in several large groups. More recently, *M. chelonei* has been reported as the etiologic agent in several cases of sternal osteomyelitis and mediastinitis after open heart surgery. *M. chelonei* does not respond to standard antituberculosis drugs but is susceptible to tetracyclines, cephalosporins, and sulfonamides. These agents plus debridement and drainage, with removal of infected tissue, are the only forms of treatment likely to succeed.

REFERENCES

American Thoracic Society/Centers for Disease Control: Treatment of tuberculosis and tuberculosis infection in adults and children. Am Rev Respir Dis 1993 (in press).

Barksdale L and Kim K: Mycobacterium. Bacteriol Rev 41:217, 1977.

Barnes PF et al: Tuberculosis in patients with human immunodeficiency virus infection. N Eng J Med 324:1644, 1991.

Bloom BR and Murray CJL: Tuberculosis: commentary on a reemergent killer. Science 257:1055, 1992.

Dooley SW et al: Multidrug-resistant tuberculosis (editorial). Ann Int Med 117:257, 1992.

Hopewell PC: Factors influencing the transmission and pathogenicity of *Mycobacterium tuberculosis:* implications for clinical and public health management of tuberculosis. In Sande MA, Hudson LD, and Root RK, editors: Contemporary issues in infectious diseases. vol 5, Respiratory infections. New York, 1986 Churchill Livingstone.

Horsburgh CR: *Mycobacterium avium* complex infection in the acquired immunodeficiency syndrome. N Engl J Med 324:1332, 1991.

Rieder HL et al: Epidemiology of tuberculosis in the United States. Am J Epi 11:79, 1989.

Wallace RJ et al: Diagnosis and treatment of disease caused by nontuberculous mycobacteria. Am Rev Respir Dis 142:940, 1990.

Wolinsky E: Nontuberculous mycobacteria and associated disease. Am Rev Respir Dis 119:107, 1979.

FUNGAL DISEASES

CHAPTER

277 Infections Caused by Fungi

John R. Graybill

Pathogenic fungi are eukaryotic, nonmotile cells that possess a cell wall made up of chitin and polysaccharides. Within the cell wall is an ergosterol-containing cell membrane, the site of action of amphotericin B. Fungi in tissue may be identified by Gomori's methenamine silver stain for cell walls. Most also stain with periodic acid Schiff stain. Beyond these few similarities, there is a considerable variability among fungi and the diseases they produce.

Some fungal pathogens, such as the dermatophytes and *Candida* species, are present in a worldwide distribution, whereas others are found within a geographically defined area. The latter are considered the "major endemic mycoses" and include *Coccidioides immitis, Histoplasma capsulatum, Blastomyces dermatitidis,* and *Paracoccidioides brasiliensis*. While each occupies a different geographic niche, all are dimorphic: they have a free-living mycelial form that produces infectious conidia; these are inhaled and convert to yeastlike pathogenic forms that produce disease but are not transmissible from human to human. Under certain in-vitro culture conditions, yeastlike forms recovered from culture specimens revert to the mycelial form. Spores tend to produce asymptomatic infections in many persons; in a much smaller number, they cause mild, influenzalike disease; widespread dissemination results in a very few. Host cell–mediated immunity (CMI) is critical to successful resistance, and depressed CMI may be associated with activation of quiescent disease or conversion from a chronic to a fulminating course.

Other fungal pathogens, for example *Sporothrix schenkii* and the agents of chromoblastomycosis, are also dimorphic and may infect healthy persons after traumatic inoculation through the skin. They are far less common, however, and cause sporadic rather than endemic disease. Still others, for example *Candida, Aspergillus* and *Zygomycetes,* have an almost ubiquitous distribution and commonly colonize humans. In the presence of severely depressed host defenses, these fungi are able to disseminate widely and with consequently high mortality.

Nocardia and *Actinomyces* are higher bacteria, closely related to the mycobacteria taxonomically. They are traditionally, but mistakenly, grouped with the fungi by the clinician. Among their distinguishing features are the absence of the ergosterol-containing cell membrane and, thus, resistance to the polyene antibiotics, for example, amphotericin B and nystatin.

HISTOPLASMOSIS

Microbiology and epidemiology

Histoplasma capsulatum exists in nature as a mycelium that includes 2- to 4-μm microconidia and larger macroconidia, the latter bearing rather characteristic tuberculate chlamydospores. The mycelial phase of *H. capsulatum* has exacting nutritional requirements, most of which are met by the excreta of chickens, certain other birds, and bats. At 37° C, with cysteine-enriched culture media, the mycelial form converts in vitro to the pathogenic yeast form, a characteristic that aids in identification. The organism grows slowly; cultures of human material first convert back to the mycelial phase (at 25° C) and then take up to 6 weeks to grow out into visible colonies. In tissues, the yeast forms are usually found within giant cells or macrophages (Fig. 277-1). However, in histoplasmoma and chronic pulmonary histoplasmosis, they may be scattered centrally in areas of caseating necrosis.

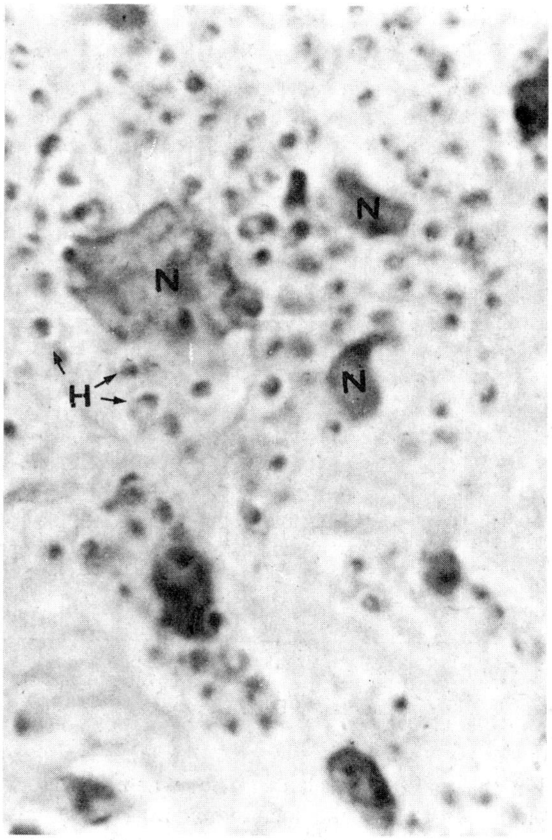

Fig. 277-1. Morphology of *H. capsulatum.* Parasitic form, with many small yeast cells *(H)* found with histiocytic cells, whose nuclei are indicated by *(N).*

Growth requirements of *H. capsulatum* contribute to its concentration in areas of bird roosts and bat-infested caves, and the association of epidemics with disturbances of nesting sites or spelunking. Many residents of the central United States have been infected with *H. capsulatum,* as manifested by a positive skin test; initial infection occurs in childhood and is frequently asymptomatic. Outbreaks of histoplasmosis often occur on the periphery of the endemic areas, where there are more susceptible individuals during a point-source exposure. What further limits the distribution of *H. capsulatum* to the Mississippi River Valley region in the central United States or the smaller foci in South America is not known precisely. With this organism and *C. immitis,* the intensity of exposure and the immune status of the host are inextricably entwined in the clinical outcome of infection. A notable exception has been the 1978 Indianapolis outbreak. This has caused exposure of several hundred thousand persons.

Beginning in the early 1980s, there were increasingly frequent scattered reports of disseminated histoplasmosis in residents of New York and the west coast of the United States. These patients were usually Caribbean immigrants, who were infected by HIV and late in the course of AIDS developed disseminated histoplasmosis. The Caribbean islands are endemic for *H. capsulatum* but New York is not, and it was presumed that in these patients the infection was an endogenous reactivation of foci latent for many years (Fig. 277-2). Later in the 1980s, patients who acquired HIV infection in cities on the east or west coast of the United States later moved to cities in the endemic zone and then most likely developed primary disseminated histoplasmosis. In either case the disease appeared at a time of severely deficient cell-mediated immunity and took the course of widespread, sometimes fulminating disease. The Indianapolis outbreak of 1978 has in effect continued, but with a dramatic shift of new cases to HIV-infected patients. In the *H. capsulatum* endemic area of the United States, at present more than 20% of patients with AIDS develop histoplasmosis, and it is a more frequent threat to them than cryptococcosis. AIDS is now by far the most common setting for histoplasmosis, and disseminated disease is the usual manifestation.

Pathophysiology

Infection occurs by inhalation of the microconidia, which are small enough to reach the alveolar spaces. These microconidia convert into yeast cells, the tissue phase of histoplasma. The organisms proliferate locally and are carried

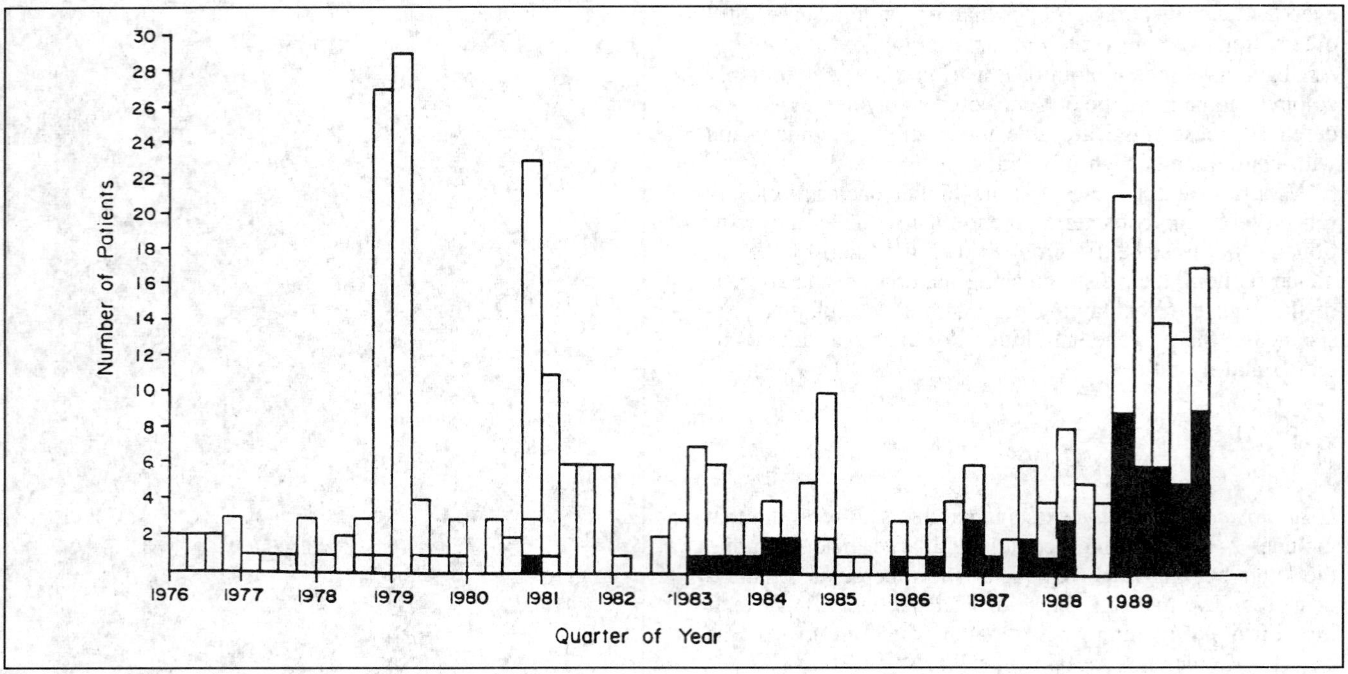

Fig. 277-2. Probable development of histoplasmosis in patients with AIDS, showing two distinct patterns. (From Wheat LJ et al: Medicine 69:361, 1990.)

via lymphatics into the bloodstream, where hematogenous dissemination to the reticuloendothelial organs is universal (Fig. 277-3). The onset of clinical symptoms of primary histoplasmosis is associated with the conversion of the histoplasmin skin test to positive and a granulomatous response at each focus of organisms. These foci may later calcify. If there is failure of CMI, the organisms proliferate unchecked in macrophages and produce diffuse reticuloendothelial organ hyperplasia, which they cause by literally stuffing the cells with fungi (Fig. 277-1). Histoplasma tend to induce a strong host inflammatory response, and excessive or aberrant response to primary or reinfection histoplasmosis probably contributes to the syndromes of fibrosing mediastinitis, broncholithiasis, histoplasmoma, and, possibly, chronic pulmonary histoplasmosis. Massive reinfection of an "immune" individual may produce an acute hypersensitivity pneumonitis. Chronic recurrent endogenous exposure from breakdown of encapsulated old foci may cause the recurrent episodes of chronic pulmonary histoplasmosis.

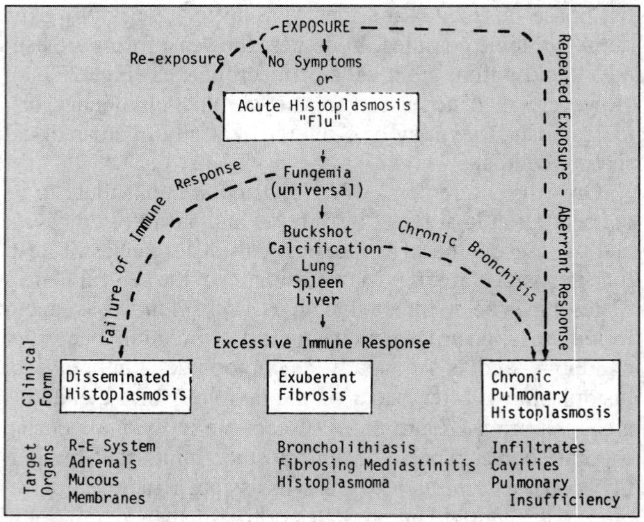

Fig. 277-3. Diagram suggesting pathogenetic interrelationships of various clinical forms of histoplasmosis.

Clinical manifestations

In the normal host, inhalation of small numbers of histoplasma microconidia is followed either by no symptoms or, a few weeks later, by an illness that may be passed off as a "viral" respiratory infection. These symptoms of primary histoplasmosis are not specific and consist of cough, fever, myalgias, and, sometimes, pleuritic chest pain. After more intense exposure, severe pulmonary illness can occur, with diffuse infiltrates, dyspnea, hypoxia, and acute respiratory distress. Pericarditis, arthritis, and widespread dissemination may also occur, as was the case in some victims of the Indianapolis outbreak. Primary histoplasmosis usually subsides within 10 days, leaving an individual either no residua or punctate calcifications scattered throughout the lungs and/or spleen. A massive exposure produces severe symptoms and greater likelihood of disseminated disease.

Disseminated histoplasmosis results from failure of CMI. It may manifest itself as a fulminating illness, especially in infants and patients on immunosuppressive medication, and, more recently, in patients with the acquired immunodeficiency syndrome (AIDS). Reactivation histoplasmosis may occur in patients who have long since left the endemic region. Histoplasmosis may occur as a primary illness or as endogenous reactivation in patients who have left the endemic areas.

The most fulminate form of disseminated histoplasmosis occurs in the setting of severe immunosuppression, particularly in the HIV-infected patient. Histoplasmosis is an AIDS-defining condition, and typically does not develop until the CD4 lymphocyte count is well below 200. The most common presentation is a febrile "failure to thrive" illness. Weight loss, nausea, vomiting, diarrhea, and anorexia are among the most common features (Table 277-1). Given the similarity to other AIDS-related problems such as infection with various mycobacterial species, chronic salmonellosis, lymphoma and other malignancies, and concurrent other infections or tumors, histoplasmosis may not be readily apparent. Evidence of lymph node enlargement, hepatosplenomegaly, oral mucosal ulcers, hypoadrenalism, or colonic masses should raise suspicion for this disease. Meningitis may occur in up to 20% of patients. Leukopenia and thrombocytopenia may reflect the often intense marrow infiltration with *H. capsulatum*. In its most aggressive form histoplasmosis may also present as a fulminating syndrome similar to bacterial sepsis, with death in days to weeks. AIDS-related histoplasmosis is now far the most common form of this disease.

Subacute and chronic disseminated histoplasmosis have somewhat similar manifestations but run a slower course. In addition, there is a greater frequency of focal lesions. Marrow involvement is much less prominent, and duration of untreated illness before death is longer, averaging 10 months in one series.

The most chronic forms of disseminated histoplasmosis occur in adults, without underlying immunosuppression. Focal lesions predominate, and constitutional symptoms of fever and weight loss are minimal. Most patients have local lesions, for example, oropharyngeal ulcers, which are frequently mistaken for carcinoma. Meningitis, Addison's disease, and other locally invasive manifestations also may occur. Hepatomegaly occurs in only one half of patients and splenomegaly in one third. Anemia, leukopenia, and thrombocytopenia are rare. The course of the illness is slow, and death may result from hypoadrenalism.

In marked contrast are forms of histoplasmosis that result from excessive host inflammatory response. These appear as either constrictive or mass lesions. The histoplasmoma is usually noticed as an asymptomatic "coin" lesion on radiographic examination. It is characterized by concentric "onion skin" calcified rings. Bronchopulmonary lithiasis is caused by erosion of a calcified granuloma into the airways, where it may become a focus for obstruction and distal infection. Fibrosing mediastinitis presumably is caused by strong fibrotic reaction to histoplasmal antigens. This produces a variety of entrapment syndromes involving superior vena cava, major airways, and the aorta.

Chronic pulmonary histoplasmosis has a striking predilection for males with chronic obstructive pulmonary disease. Histoplasma antigens probably elicit an acute inflammatory response. There is infarctlike necrosis at the center, and intense lymphocyte, plasma cell, and macrophage accumulation around the periphery. Symptoms begin abruptly and include cough, malaise, chilliness, fever, and pleuritic chest pain. These symptoms may last from a week to as long as 4 months. Radiographic patterns may include infiltrates, cavities, and, often, a characteristic fibronodular streaking from a peripheral lesion to the hilum. Episodes may be single or recurrent. Dissemination to extrapulmonary sites is rare. Death is from respiratory failure.

Table 277-1. Manifestations of histoplasmosis occurring in 78 Texas patients with concurrent HIV infection

Symptoms		Signs	
Fever	69	Splenomegaly	33
Weight loss	50	Lymphadenopathy	24
Abdominal pain	4	Hepatomegaly	15
Malaise	5	Skin lesions	15
Headache	1	Colitis	3
Arthralgia	1	Abdominal mass	1

Modified from Table 1, Graybill JR et al: The major endemic mycoses in the setting of AIDS. In Vanden Bossche H et al, editors: Mycoses in AIDS patients. New York, 1990, Plenum Press.

Diagnostic tests

Histoplasmosis may mimic a broad variety of illness, from influenza through lymphoma to tuberculosis, and diagnosis is often difficult (Table 277-2). Cultures of sputum, urine, lymph node, liver, and bone marrow are frequently positive in disseminated disease, but, since the organism grows slowly, results may be delayed for weeks. In patients with AIDS and histoplasmosis, more than half will have positive peripheral blood and/or bone marrow stains for *H. capsulatum*.

The infection is so intense that cytocentrifuged specimens of peripheral blood show *H. capsulatum* yeasts in monocytes in up to 70% of patients.

The standard tests for histoplasmosis have been the complement fixation test and the immunodiffusion test (Table 277-1). The complement fixation test is nonspecific at titers less than 1:8, is cross-reactive with other fungal pathogens, and may be negative in patients with disseminated disease. The immunodiffusion test to H and M antigens is positive in up to 90% of patients (probably less commonly with AIDS) and specific. However, the most useful test is a radioimmunoassay recently developed at the University of Indiana. The test is highly sensitive and specific in both urine and blood. In addition to being valuable in diagnosis, a declining titer of antigen is associated with response to therapy, while a rising titer may predict progression or relapse (Fig 277-4).

Table 277-2. Serologic tests for diagnosis of fungal disease

Disease	Test	Comment
Histoplasmosis	Complement fixation	Titer <1:8 is nonspecific.
	Immunodiffusion complement fixation	May be negative in up to one third of disseminated histoplasmosis patients.
		Tends to level off at 1:32 maximum titer, though may be higher.
		With yeast phase antigen, is higher in disease.
		With mycelial antigen, may be boosted by positive skin test to histoplasmin.
		Extensive cross-reaction with *B. dermatitidis*.
		Low-grade cross-reaction with *C. immitis*.
	Immunodiffusion	H band and M bands are specific, and one or both are positive in up to 90% of patients.
	Radioimmunoassay for antigen	Investigational in serum and urine. Highly useful in rapid diagnosis and monitoring treatment response in disseminated histoplasmosis. Available from Dr. J. Wheat, University of Indiana, Indianapolis.
Coccidioidomycosis	Complement fixation or immunodiffusion complement fixation	Specific, with only minimal cross-reaction in histoplasmosis.
		Highest titers occur in most severely ill patients (titer ≥ 1:6 associated with serious disease). Titer rises more slowly and is more sustained than in the precipitin test. Any titer in cerebrospinal fluid is diagnostic of meningitis. May be used to follow the course of disease; that is a declining titer is a good prognostic sign.
	Tube precipitin or immunodiffusion tube precipitin	Highly specific. Converts to positive in over 85% of patients, usually within weeks of infection. Cannot be titrated.
		Usually reverts to negative quickly, even though active disease persists.
	Radioimmunoassay for antigen	Investigational (J. Galgiani, University of Arizona, Tucson).
Blastomycosis	Complement fixation	Positive in only 50%-70% of patients. Highly cross-reactive with *H. capsulatum*.
Paracoccidioidomycosis	Immunodiffusion for bands 1 and 2	Specific, but is not titrated. Not helpful in assessing activity of disease.
	Complement fixation	As in coccidioidomycosis, higher titers occur with more severe disease.
		Cross-reacts with *H. capsulatum*.
Sporotrichosis	Complement fixation	No widespread serologic tests.
Aspergillosis	Immunodiffusion	Helpful in confirming diagnosis of allergic bronchopulmonary and mycetoma forms. Often negative in widespread dissemination.
	Immunoassay for circulating antigen	Specific but not sensitive. May be useful in disseminated disease. Investigational and not widely available. (V. Andriole, Yale University, New Haven, Conn.).
Candidiasis	Immunodiffusion	Antibodies present in many normal persons. Not especially helpful in diagnosis of disease.
	Multiple-antigen tests	Variable in sensitivity and specificity for *Candida* antigen and intermittently promising. None have survived beyond initial efforts at marketing. The lack of *Candida* and *Aspergillus* antigen testing is a great impediment to rapid diagnosis of mycosis in the leukopenic host and is a primary driving force perpetuating empiric use of antifungal agents.
Zygomycosis	No serologic tests available	
Nocardiosis	No serologic tests available	
Actinomycosis	No serologic tests available	
Chromomycosis	No serologic tests available	
Phaeohyphomycosis	No serologic tests available	
Fusarium	No serologic tests available	
Trichosporonosis	No serologic tests available	May see a "false positive" test for cryptococcal capsulatum polysaccharide.

Treatment

Treatment depends on the form of the disease and the immunologic status of the host (Table 277-3). Primary histoplasmosis need be treated only if a patient is severely symptomatic or hypoxic from a massive exposure. Although itraconazole has not been evaluated specifically for primary histoplasmosis, a course of 400 mg per day for 3 to 6 months may be as effective and less toxic than amphotericin B. Corticosteroids may be used to reduce the inflammatory response but should not be given in the absence of antifungal therapy. Antifungal therapy is not indicated

Table 277-3. Treatment of histoplasmosis

Form of disease	Antifungal chemotherapy	Other
Primary histoplasmosis		
Mild symptoms	No treatment	
Severe symptoms	Amphotericin B, up to total of 500 mg I.V. or ketoconazole 400 mg/day for several months	If hypoxic, may add short course (1 week) of corticosteroids.
Sequelae of healed primary histoplasmosis		
Broncholithiasis	None	Resection if there is distal bronchiectasis or abscess.
Histoplasmoma	None	Resection if diagnosis is in doubt.
Fibrosing mediastinitis	None	Surgical decompression of vital structures.
Chronic pulmonary histoplasmosis		
Small cavities, mild symptoms	None	Stop smoking (all forms of pulmonary histoplasmosis).
Large cavities, severe symptoms	Itraconazole, 200 mg twice daily for 6 months or more, or amphotericin B up to 50 mg qd I.V. (or 1 mg/kg if less than 50 kg), up to a total dose of 25 to 35 mg/kg I.V.	Surgical resection of cavity when feasible.
Disseminated histoplasmosis	Itraconazole at doses of 200 mg twice daily, P.O., for 6 months, is the drug of choice in nonfulminating disease. Ketoconazole, 400 mg/day, or amphotericin B up to 50 mg qd I.V. (or 1 mg/kg if less than 50 kg), up to a total dose of 25 to 35 mg/kg I.V.	Corticosteroid replacement is warranted if adrenal insufficiency is confirmed.

Table 277-4. Comparison of azole antifungal drugs now available

	Ketoconazole	Fluconazole	Itraconazole
Route administered	Oral	Oral/I.V.	Oral only
Achlorhydric effect	Marked	Minimal	Significant
Half-life	5-9 hrs	24-30 hrs	30-42 hrs
Clearance	Hepatic	Renal, largely unchanged	Hepatic, with active metabolite
Usual highest dose*	400 mg/D	400 mg/D	400 mg/D
Drug interactions:			
Phenytoin	+++	++	+++
Rifampin	+++	++	+++
H_2 blockers	+++	+	+++
Cyclosporine A	+++	+	++
Differences in spectrum (estimate of overall efficacy, based on noncomparative studies)			
Histoplasma	++	++	+++
Coccidioides	+	++	+++
Blastomyces	+++	++	+++
Paracoccidioides	++	++	+++
Sporothrix	+	++	+++
Aspergillus	0	0	+++
Chromomycosis	Unk	Unk	+++
Dematiaceous	Unk	Unk	++
Candida			
Mucosal	++	+++	+++
Dissem.	+	++	Unk
"Meningitis"	+	+++	+++
Toxicity:			
Nausea/vomit	+++	+	+
Hepatic	++	+	+
Endocrine	+++	0	0†

* = All three drugs have been used at more than 1 gram/D, with ketoconazole showing marked gastrointestinal and endocrine effects above 400 mg per day, and fluconazole showing no clear toxic effects at up to 2 grams per day. Loading doses of 600-800 mg per day can be used for 2-3 days to accelerate achieving steady state.

† = Infrequently seen side effects include edema, hypertension, and hypokalemia, which may be endocrine in cause, although unpublished investigations have not identified an endocrine cause (Graybill JR et al).

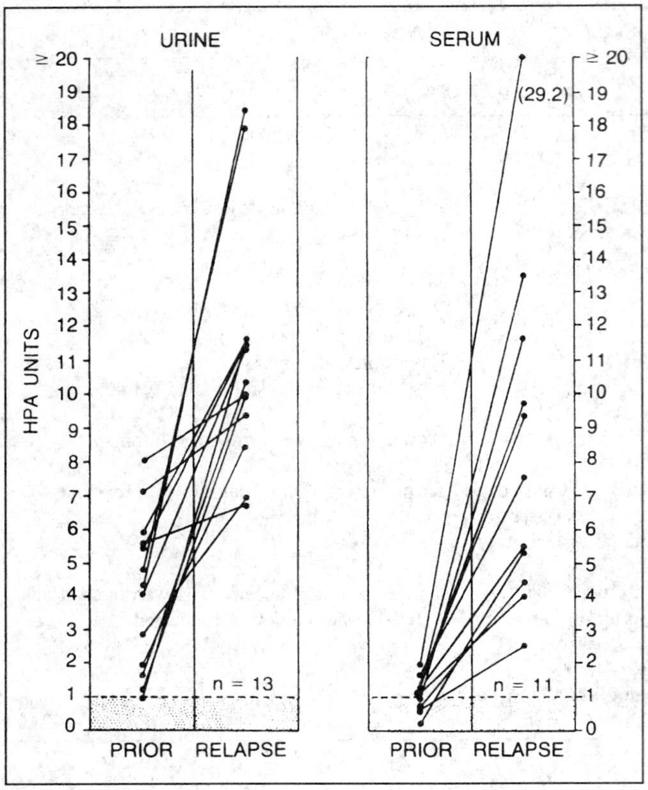

Fig. 277-4. Pre- and postrelapse antigen titers in patients with histoplasmosis in the setting of AIDS. (From Wheat LJ et al: Ann Int Med 115:936, 1991.)

for broncholithiasis, histoplasmoma, or mediastinitis. Mediastinitis may require surgical decompression of vital mediastinal structures.

Optimal treatment of chronic pulmonary histoplasmosis has been well defined. Azole antifungal therapy may be of value. Resection of large cavities may be of value in severely ill patients whose pulmonary function will tolerate surgery.

General comment on antifungal therapy. Until the mid-1980s, amphotericin B was the primary drug for most of the systemic mycoses. The Mycoses Study Group then reported that ketoconazole, in doses of 400 mg per day for 6 months, was as effective as amphotericin B in histoplasmosis and blastomycosis, and a reasonable alternative to amphotericin B for coccidioidomycosis. However, irregular absorption, gastrointestinal side effects, dose-dependent suppression of testosterone and cortisol synthesis, hepatotoxicity, and adverse drug interactions with rifampicin, phenytoin, cyclosporine, and other drugs all made ketoconazole a less-than-ideal-drug. Additionally, the drug was useful in fungal meningitis only at high doses that were poorly tolerated by patients.

Recently developed alternatives have included two triazole antifungals, fluconazole and itraconazole. Both of these have longer half-lives than ketoconazole, at 24-30 hours for fluconazole and 40+ hours for itraconazole. However, as shown in Table 277-4, other characteristics are quite different. In general, both drugs are markedly less toxic than ketoconazole, and neither has clear endocrine-mediated effects. Hepatotoxicity may be less with itraconazole than fluconazole, though both are thought to be less hepatotoxic than ketoconazole. Although fluconazole penetrates the cerebrospinal fluid readily and itraconazole does not, both are effective in cryptococcal meningitis.

The status of antifungal therapy is presently in great flux. Itraconazole has been licensed only for histoplasmosis and blastomycosis, though it is highly efficacious in many other mycoses, including sporotrichosis, aspergillosis, phaeohyphomycosis, paracoccidioidomycosis, chromomycosis, and coccidioidomycosis. Fluconazole is licensed at present for candidosis and cryptococcosis, though it is effective in coccidioidomycosis, paracoccidioidmycosis, blastomycosis, and sporotrichosis. Direct comparative studies of these drugs are in process for some of these mycoses, and pending results of these studies, the drug of choice is selected based on assessment of open studies.

A major use for triazoles, particularly fluconazole, is for prophylaxis of infections in the neutropenic patient. Recent studies have found that a dose of 400 mg per day, initiated at the time of conditioning for a bone marrow transplant, is associated with significantly fewer systemic fungal infections than in controls. However, one potentially significant and increasing problem in fluconazole recipients appears to be the development of fungemia from fluconazole-resistant fungi such as *Candida kruzei*. Also, prolonged use of fluconazole to suppress *C. albicans* (thrush) in patients with HIV infection is being done commonly. This is associated with increasing fluconazole resistance of *C. albicans*.

The place for amphotericin B, while shrinking, is still solid as initial therapy for patients whose condition is so grave that they might not survive for a week or two (i.e., long enough for azoles to show effect). The ability to give amphotericin B intravenously and the generally slower onset of action of the azoles favor use of amphotericin B in the most desperately ill patients. Specific management suggestions are given in the box at right. There are presently in clinical trials several lipid-associated forms of amphotericin B. Their purpose is to deliver a high dose of amphotericin B, up to 5+ mg/Kg, without untoward toxicity. Although high doses of amphotericin B are tolerated reasonably well, superior efficacy has not yet been demonstrated.

Specific management of histoplasmosis. In the noncompromised host, primary histoplasmosis is usually a self-limiting disease that is undiagnosed and therefore untreated. In the case of very heavy exposure (i.e., spelunking, digging up bird roosts), a short course of amphotericin B, possibly combined with corticosteroids to reduce inflammatory response, may be required. A role for azoles is not clearly established, though they may be effective. Histoplasmoma is often diagnosed inadvertently at resection for presumed pulmonary neoplasm. Broncholithiasis and fibrosing mediastinitis may require surgical therapy, but neither these nor histoplasmoma need antifungal chemotherapy. Adrenal in-

Guidelines for parenteral administration of amphotericin B

Preparation

1. Add 50 ml of sterile water to 50 mg vial.
2. Shake vigorously.
3. For I.V. use, add up to 50 mg to 500 ml of 5% dextrose in water. To minimize nephrotoxicity, precede amphotericin B with 1000 ml saline I.V.
4. For intrathecal use, add 0.5 to 2.0 mg to 10 ml of 5% or 10% dextrose in water and 10 to 20 mg of hydrocortisone.

Administration

1. Infuse 1 mg "test dose" over 1-4 hours (if hypotension occurs [rare] another antifungal may be needed).
2. If well tolerated, follow test dose with 20 to 50 mg dose given over 1-4 hours and continue on daily basis or doubled doses three times weekly. There is disagreement over whether rapid infusion is better tolerated than slow infusion. Rapid infusion may be associated with acute hyperkalemia and cardiac arrhythmia, especially in the presence of renal failure. If this occurs, administer over 12-18 hours.
3. Premedication with 600 mg aspirin or diphenhydramine (50 mg) or meperidine may reduce nausea, fever, vomiting.
4. Heparin and corticosteroids are of uncertain value against thrombophlebitis.
5. If serum creatinine reaches 3 mg/dl, stop amphotericin B and resume cautiously after several days.
6. For intrathecal dose, start with 0.1 mg, increasing to 0.2 mg, 0.3 mg, and 0.5 mg on alternate days. Corticosteroid reduces arachnoiditis and headache. Up to 2 mg per dose in coccidioidomycosis.

Examples of use in specific diseases

1. Histoplasmosis: total dose in primary disease, 250-500 mg. In more serious diseases, 35 mg/kg.
2. Coccidioidomycosis: total dose 35 mg/kg I.V. May be much higher, depending on clinical response. For meningeal disease, may give 1 g I.V. as well as variable dose intrathecally. As meningitis improves, space out doses to twice per week, then twice per month, then once per month until cerebrospinal fluid is essentially normal for 1 year.
3. Blastomycosis: 25 to 35 mg/kg total dose.
4. Candidiasis: 30 to 50 mg/day for 1 to 2 weeks for disseminated disease; for up to 6 weeks for endocarditis, but even then it may fail. For chronic mucocutaneous disease, systemic use is rarely indicated.
5. Sporotrichosis: for chronic pulmonary or disseminated disease, up to 35 mg/kg total dose.

sufficiency may be a late complication of scarring of adrenal glands, and requires specific replacement therapy.

Chronic pulmonary histoplasmosis and disseminated histoplasmosis both respond very well to azole antifungals. Ketoconazole is effective in both forms of disease in non-HIV-infected patients. However, both fluconazole and itraconazole are as effective as and better tolerated than ketoconazole and are recommended at 400 mg per day for 6 months.

The most common form of histoplasmosis is now aggressive disseminated disease associated with AIDS. In the moribund patient amphotericin B at 50 mg per day should be used until the patient is clearly improving, usually 1-2 weeks. Then therapy should be switched to an azole antifungal. Perhaps because of poor oral absorption, ketoconazole has not been very effective in AIDS-associated histoplasmosis. Informal reports have suggested that fluconazole is effective, but the largest reported experience is with itraconazole, as evaluated by the ACTG. Itraconazole has proven effective in 80% of patients as both chronic maintenance therapy (200-400 mg/D) and as primary treatment in all but the most desperately ill patients (800 mg per day loading dose for several days, then 400 mg per day). Clinical improvement is usually evident within 2 weeks. Treatment should be continued for lifetime. Recrudescence has been uncommon and is often associated with noncompliance.

COCCIDIOIDOMYCOSIS

Microbiology and epidemiology

Like *H. capsulatum, C. immitis* has two distinct forms (Fig. 277-5). The free-living form is a fragile mycelium made up of intercalating arthroconidia and "ghost cells." This form can easily disperse in wind, and spores can be carried for miles. Once inhaled by humans or animals, these spores convert to spherules, which are progressively enlarging, round, chitinous structures, up to 60 μm in diameter at maturity. These spherules spontaneously rupture, releasing many endospores, which repeat this parasitic cycle. *C. immitis* thrives on most culture media, appearing a week after culture.

C. immitis is an organism that is very well adapted to its habitat, the Lower Sonoran life zone and the desert regions of the tropical Americas. The mycelium survives the arid summer months in protected locations below the soil surface, where temperatures are relatively cool. With the onset of spring rains, the mycelium grows up to the soil surface. In the desert, a breeze disrupts it into a cloud of flying arthroconidia. Major outbreaks have followed desert storms.

Pathophysiology

Like histoplasmosis, the course of primary coccidioidomycosis depends largely on the immune status of the host. Once inhaled, arthroconidia convert to spherules. These spherules repeatedly cycle through rupture and discharge of endospores, which are ingested, but not killed, by neutrophils. The neutrophils in turn die, releasing endospores that mature into other spherules. If the host fails to develop an adequate cell-mediated immune response, the infection may produce fulminating coccidioidal pneumonia and widespread extrapulmonary abscesses. In a satisfactory host response, *C. immitis* stimulates formation of granulomas at each focus of infection. The granulomas ultimately resolve,

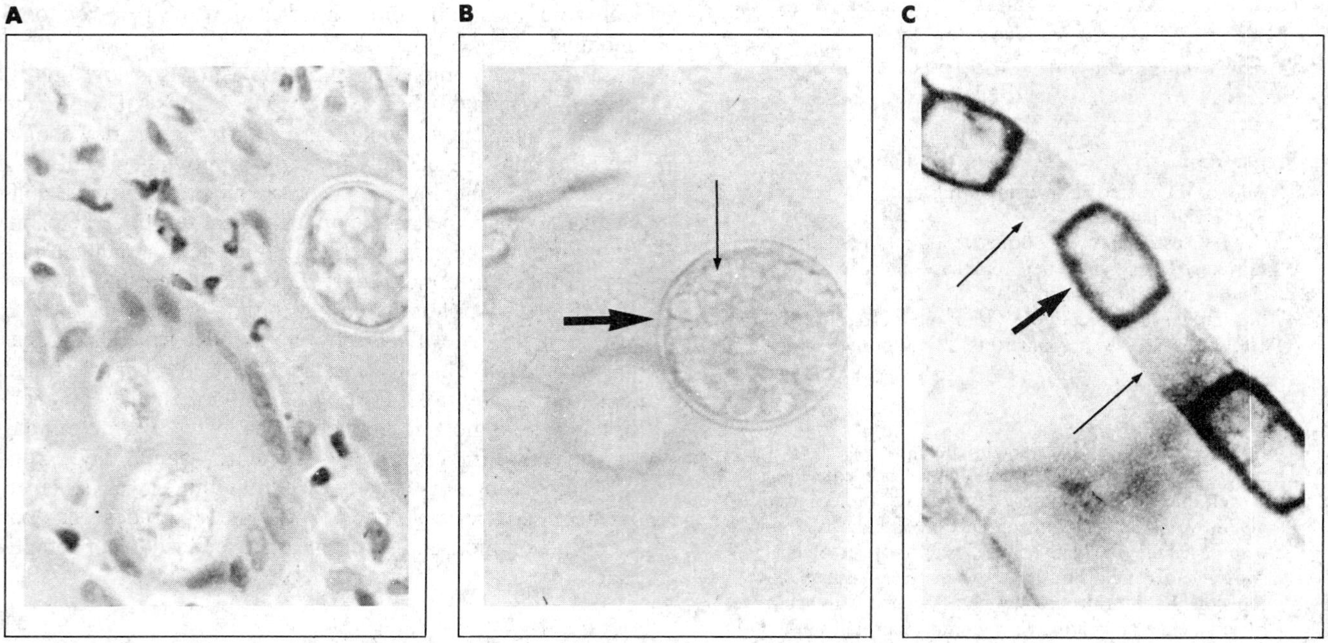

Fig. 277-5. Morphology of *C. immitis*. **A,** Spherules within Langhans' giant cells, shown by hematoxylin and eosin stain. **B,** Spherule, shown in unstained potassium hydroxide preparation. Note the endospores within spherule *(small arrow)* and the clearly defined double wall of spherule *(large arrow)*. **C,** Free-living form, with barrel-shaped arthroconidia *(large arrow)* spaced between intercalating "ghost cells" *(small arrows)*.

with less intense fibrotic reactions than *H. capsulatum*. Factors such as intensity of exposure, racial susceptibility (heightened in blacks, Mexican Indians, and Filipinos), immunosuppressive medications, and pregnancy adversely affect the course.

Coccidioidomycosis occurs uncommonly in AIDS patients. It may take a more fulminating disseminated form in these individuals. Most patients appear ultimately to succumb from this infection, and there is no clearly established therapy.

Between the uneventful resolution of illness and the fulminating dissemination, there is a broad spectrum of presentations. The organism often targets (hematogenously) one organ system, for example, the skin, a joint, or the meninges, and produce a chronic granulomatous infection that may wax and wane for years. Pulmonary infiltrates may persist or rapidly cavitate. Cavities may remain stable, enlarge, or disappear spontaneously. Erosion of blood vessels occasionally may produce severe hemoptysis. Coinfection by *Aspergillus* or *Mycobacterium tuberculosis* may occur in coccidioidal cavities.

Clinical manifestations

Primary coccidioidomycosis commences after an asymptomatic period of 1 to 2 weeks and produces an influenzalike syndrome in about one half of the patients. A number of features, thought to be allergic, distinguish primary coccidioidomycosis. These features have generated some of its common names, for example, "desert rheumatism" (migratory polyarthralgias and nondeforming arthritis) and "the bumps" (erythema nodosum or erythema multiforme, and other rashes), both of which occur more commonly in women. Pulmonary infiltrates, pleural effusions, and peripheral blood eosinophilia are commonly associated with primary coccidioidomycosis and resolve with subsidence of the illness. Primary coccidioidomycosis may resolve uneventfully (up to 90% of patients), rapidly progress to fulminating disease, or stabilize, resulting in cavities, persistent infiltrates, or persistent hilar adenopathy. Cavitary disease is more frequent in diabetics.

Patients with AIDS may develop focal pulmonary disease or diffuse pulmonary disease. The latter occurs in a setting of more profound immune deficiency and is associated with extrapulmonary dissemination and poor response to chemotherapy.

Chronic pulmonary coccidioidomycosis includes disease limited to the thoracic cavity and persisting more than 3 months after the onset of primary coccidioidomycosis. It is manifested by cough, hemoptysis, and dyspnea, particularly if there is underlying chronic pulmonary disease. Coccidioidal pulmonary lesions do not calcify like those of histoplasmosis; a characteristic large, thin-walled cavity has been described but is not always present. Many cavities resolve spontaneously over 2 years without any specific treatment.

Disseminated coccidioidomycosis primarily affects the skin and subcutaneous tissues, and the lymph nodes, bones, joints, and meninges. Cutaneous lesions may be nodular, ulcerative, or nondescript pigmented scars that irregularly break down and discharge small amounts of pus (Fig. 277-6). These lesions may be local or may represent extension of fistulous tracts from deep sites in muscles or viscera. They are not commonly painful. A common site for soft tissue invasion is the lymphatic system. Suppuration of bubos commonly occurs. Large paraspinous abscesses may produce radiculopathies and may be associated with vertebral osteomyelitis (Fig. 277-7). Coccidioidal osteomyelitis occurs in up to 20% of patients with disseminated disease. Arthritis tends to involve the spine and weight-bearing joints. The process is chronic, with thickened synovium and little bone destruction. The most common form of nervous system involvement is basilar meningitis. Untreated, coccidioidal meningitis progresses to involve cranial nerves and produce obstructive hydrocephalus caused by blocking of the aqueduct of Sylvius. Alternately, communicating hydrocephalus may occur. Patients with meningitis may have no other manifestations of coccidioidomycosis. The course is often chronic rather than acute. Patients develop cranial nerve impairments, personality changes, headaches, dulled mentation, and coma. Even with the most vigorous management, the mortality is 20% to 50%. Relapses are common.

Diagnostic tests

C. immitis can be cultured readily from sputum or infected tissues. Biopsy is usually necessary in establishing a diagnosis of coccidioidal arthritis, since the joint fluid is often culture-negative. The culture may take a week to grow. The

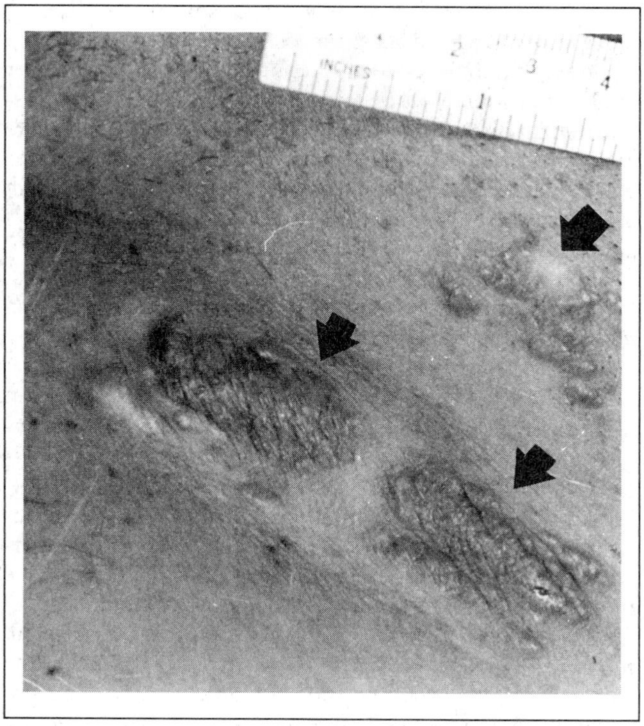

Fig. 277-6. Nodular coccidioidal skin lesions that had persisted for more than 6 years on the neck of this man.

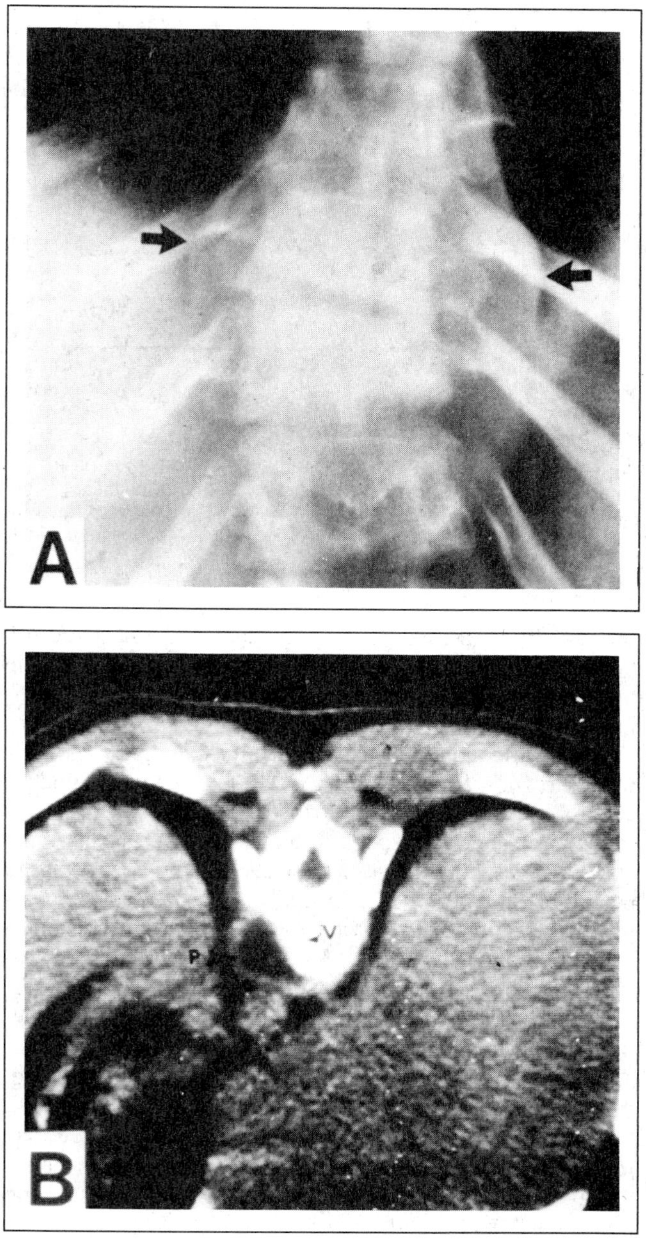

Fig. 277-7. **A,** Radiograph outlining paraspinous mass caused by *C. immitis*. **B,** Same patient with CT scan showing paravertebral mass *(P)*, and vertebral lytic lesions *(V)*. (From Graybill JR et al: Rev Infect Dis 2:661, 1981.)

morphology of the spherule is so characteristic that it can be easily seen on hematoxylin and eosin stains and may also be readily identified in potassium hydroxide preparations of purulent exudates. A positive histologic diagnosis is as reliable as culture of the organism.

In coccidioidomycosis, host immunity strongly influences the outcome. The same tests may be used for immunologic diagnosis and prognosis. The skin test with coccidioidin or spherulin is positive in many healthy persons living in endemic areas and converts to positive in most patients with primary coccidioidomycosis (Fig. 277-8). Un-

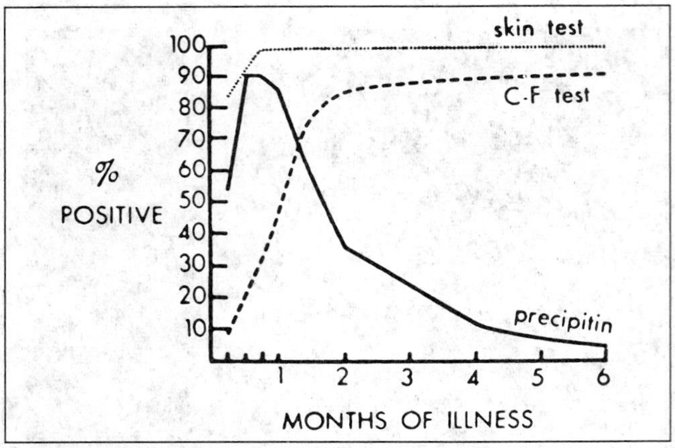

Fig. 277-8. Time course to conversion of skin test, precipitin, and complement fixation tests in primary coccidioidomycosis. (From Huppert M: Serology of coccidioidomycosis. Mycopathol Mycol Appl 41:1, 1970).

fortunately, a positive skin test indicates previous exposure but not active disease. Thus, the skin test has limited value in endemic areas, where up to 90% of residents are positive. Serologic tests are more helpful; within the first few weeks of infection, IgM antibody tests (precipitin test, immunodiffusion tube precipitin (IDTP), or counterimmunoelectrophoresis) convert to positive. These tests are not titrated and are highly specific. However, even in the presence of continuing disease, the tests may revert quickly to negative. The titer of IgG antibody, measured by the complement fixation test, correlates with prognosis. In experienced laboratories, a titer of 1:16 or higher is associated with the more serious forms of disseminated disease. This test also has been modified for immunodiffusion complement fixation (IDCF), which makes it technically simpler. A rising titer by the IDCF test indicates worsening disease, whereas a falling titer indicates improvement. Serologic titers tend to change less in chronic pulmonary disease than in disseminated disease. Skin tests do not interfere with serology, so both tests may be serially repeated to assess immune status and prognosis.

The diagnosis of coccidioidal meningitis is more difficult, since *C. immitis* is cultured from cerebrospinal fluid (CSF) in fewer than half of specimens. Lymphocytic pleocytosis and a depressed glucose level are found in about half of the initial CSF specimens. The presence of meningitis should be presumed if the CSF is abnormal and *C. immitis* is isolated from a nonmeningeal site. The precipitin test and latex agglutination tests are not of value in CSF testing, but a positive CSF complement fixation test is diagnostic of coccidioidal meningitis.

Treatment

Of the major endemic mycoses, coccidioidomycosis has traditionally been the most refractory to amphotericin B and the most likely to relapse, sometimes years after completion of "successful" therapy. Commonly amphotericin B has been used intravenously at 50 mg three times weekly up to a cumulative dose of 2.5 to 3 grams, or 35 mg/Kg. Intralesional injections have also been used, but these are poorly tolerated because they produce an intense inflammatory response. Assessment of clinical response to amphotericin B has been complicated by the frequent fluctuations in clinical course.

At the time ketoconazole entered clinical trials, the Mycoses Study Group first devised uniform response criteria that incorporated the variables of lesion severity and location, changes in serologic titers, and cultures. The first use of this was in a large study comparing ketoconazole at 400 mg per day versus 800 mg per day. While there was clearly dose-related drug intolerance, there was little difference in clinical response, fewer than 40% of patients achieving clinical remission. Further, more than one third of those who did achieve remission later relapsed during posttreatment observation.

For later studies with itraconazole and fluconazole, criteria were expanded to include symptoms. Serologic scoring and lesion size and location were redefined, and remission was defined as reduction of the total pretreatment disease score by at least 50% and negative follow-up cultures if they were done. Most patients received 400 mg itraconazole per day for 6 months after they achieved remission. Although the scoring system was different for the triazoles, almost 60% of itraconazole recipients entered remission with itraconazole therapy, and fewer than 20% relapsed in a median of a year posttreatment follow-up. A comparable study with fluconazole at 400 mg per day has had similar response rates, but the posttreatment follow-up for relapses is still ongoing.

In all three studies patients with soft tissue disease, chronic pulmonary disease, or osteoarticular disease fared equally well. Independently conducted studies by Tucker et al found somewhat better responses in patients with osteoarticular disease. Both itraconazole and fluconazole were remarkably better tolerated than ketoconazole, which was better tolerated than amphotericin B. Therefore at present amphotericin B is warranted only for failures to the triazoles or for acute life-threatening situations. There are few treatment data for AIDS patients with coccidioidomycosis. Experience with the triazoles is still small, but there is an impression that nothing reliably induces sustained remissions.

Nowhere have developments in antifungal therapy been more dramatic than in the treatment of coccidioidal meningitis. Intrathecal amphotericin B has been used in many regimens, but never without toxicity from this highly irritating drug. Therapy was ultimately limited by meningeal inflammation, and relapses were common. Fluconazole therapy, at 400 mg per day, is a benign and highly effective treatment that can be sustained indefinitely, and induces remission in more than 75% of patients. Because of frequent remissions, when treatment is interrupted, fluconazole should probably be continued for lifetime duration. Itraconazole is also efficacious, but experience is more limited.

Coccidioidomycosis is the only fungal infection in which systematic trials of human vaccine have been conducted.

Despite immune conversion, a large clinical trial indicated that there is no protection conferred by vaccination.

BLASTOMYCOSIS

Microbiology and epidemiology

Blastomyces dermatitidis is a biphasic yeast that grows freely at room temperature as a mycelium, and at 37° C in the parasitic yeast form. The yeast is distinguished from *Cryptococcus neoformans* by the absence of a capsule and thick-walled buds to daughter cells, and from *P. brasiliensis* by single buds, which remain attached to the mother cell until almost mature. Also, *B. dermatitidis* characteristically forms complex inflammatory lesions with both pyogenic and granulomatous components.

A natural reservoir has been found in the soil of riverbanks. Persons who engage in outdoor occupations such as highway construction and farming are more likely than city dwellers to get blastomycosis. The range of *B. dermatitidis* is roughly comparable to that of *H. capsulatum*.

Pathophysiology

Infection is thought to occur by inhalation of spores; these spores convert to yeast forms and produce a primary flu-like infection manifested by fever, cough, and chest pain. Lung infiltrates may clear or persist as fibrocavitary lesions. Hematogenous dissemination occurred to the skin and bones in two thirds of patients in one large series, and to the prostate, liver, spleen, and kidney in one half. Less frequent are central nervous system and lymph node involvement. The adrenals are involved only occasionally.

Clinical manifestations and treatment

The characteristic clinical presentation is subacute or chronic, with fever, cough, weight loss, and an associated skin lesion. The skin lesions are often found to be several in number when carefully searched for and may range from small acneiform pustules to large nodular or papulopustular lesions with heaped-up edges and small, black (pepper-like), pinpoint lesions in the central eschar (Plate V-53). They often are mistaken for carcinomas. They appear on exposed surfaces of the body and infrequently involve mucosal surfaces. Such lesions are accompanied by pulmonary and skeletal lesions in up to 40% of patients. Blastomycosis is rarely associated with AIDS.

Diagnosis of blastomycosis requires demonstration of the fungus by biopsy or potassium hydroxide preparation of a lesion specimen, with confirmation by culture. Urine and prostatic secretions are rewarding sites for fungal culture material, even in the absence of symptoms. Serologic and skin tests cross-react with histoplasma antigens, but newly licensed tests are increasingly specific indicators of disease.

Treatment is for systemic disease, even when the patient has only a skin lesion as evidence of disease. Itraconazole is the drug of choice in non-life threatening disease with over 90% responses. A dosage of 200 mg twice daily for at least 6 months is recommended. Ketoconazole 400 mg/day for at least 6 months is also effective. Fluconazole appears to be somewhat less effective. Alternatively, one may use amphotericin B. The usual course of amphotericin B is a total of 2 to 3 g for an adult.

PARACOCCIDIOIDOMYCOSIS

Microbiology and epidemiology

Paracoccidioides brasiliensis is dimorphic, with a presumably free-living mycelial form, which produces arthrospores and chlamydospores. The parasitic form is an oval or round yeast cell up to 40 μm in diameter, which is surrounded by multiple daughter buds, giving a "pilot wheel" appearance. This fungus is geographically restricted to the area from Mexico south through Argentina. Appearance of disease in humans occurs many years after presumed inhalation exposure. There have been no epidemics to yield information on primary disease or natural reservoirs. The disease occurs sporadically. Men, particularly those engaged in outdoor occupations, are affected far more frequently than women, possibly because estrogen inhibits the organism.

Clinical manifestations

Patients may present with pulmonary disease or with the sequelae of hematogenous dissemination. The illness clinically resembles chronic coccidioidomycosis, with a predominance of respiratory symptoms. Central and basal infiltrates are common, whereas cavities are uncommon, and the apices are frequently spared. The lesions heal (under the influence of therapy) with bullae and fibrosis, which may produce right ventricular failure. Mucosal or cutaneous ulcerated or nodular lesions can occur. Lymph node involvement is frequent, often leading to spontaneous drainage of purulent material. These lesions contain epithelioid cells, Langhans' giant cells, and neutrophils on biopsy. The genitourinary tract and adrenal glands may be involved. Both coccidioidomycosis and paracoccidioidomycosis may co-exist with tuberculosis. This is an exceedingly rare disease in the AIDS setting.

Diagnostic tests

The diagnosis is established by demonstration of the characteristic mother-daughter cell complex on potassium hydroxide preparation or fungal strains and culture of the organism from tissue. The skin test is unreliable, owing to the occurrence of false-negative reactions. The diagnosis also can be established with serologic tests. The immunodiffusion test is positive in 95% of patients and is highly specific. The complement fixation test also is specific.

Treatment

Itraconazole, 100 mg per day for 6 months, is the drug of choice. An alternative is ketoconazole, which can be given at 200 mg per day or 400 mg per day for prolonged periods without toxicity. Clinical response is prompt. At least 1 year of therapy is recommended. *P. brasiliensis,* like *H. capsulatum,* targets the adrenal glands. Tests of adrenal reserve are recommended, especially if ketoconazole is to be used. Sulfa drugs are commonly used in South America, because of low cost. Responses are less frequent and relapses may occur.

SPOROTRICHOSIS

Microbiology and epidemiology

Sporothrix schenkii grows at room temperature as a mycelium and at 37° C as a yeast. In nature, *S. schenkii* may be cultured from the soil and a variety of vegetations; there is no endemic region. Traumatic inoculation of contaminated materials selects both the victims of cutaneous sporotrichosis (those who work in farming, plant nurseries, gardening) and the most common sites of primary lesions (extremities in adults, trunk and face in children).

Pathophysiology

More than three fourths of patients have locally inoculated lymphocutaneous disease. Disease develops weeks after inoculation and consists of a papular or ulcerated painless lesion. Over succeeding weeks, satellite lesions appear along the lymphatics draining the primary site (Plate V-25). *Sporothrix* rarely disseminates; when it does, it produces osteomyelitis and arthritis. It is uncertain whether pulmonary involvement is primary or secondary to hematogenous dissemination. There is evidence from immunologic studies in humans and from challenge studies in animals that CMI is important in host defense against sporotrichosis. (Also see Plate V-54.)

Clinical manifestations

The clinical manifestations of sporotrichosis are mild and chronic. An appropriate history together with the finding of the typical cutaneous lesion should provide strong suggestive evidence. The peripheral lesion can be mimicked by mycobacterial infection *(Mycobacterium marinum, M. chelonei, M. fortuitum),* nocardiosis, actinomycosis, or leishmaniasis. Bone and joint lesions must be distinguished from other forms of granulomatous osteomyelitis and arthritis. Pulmonary infiltrates and cavities may mimic coccidioidomycosis or tuberculosis.

Diagnosis

The diagnosis is most readily made by biopsies of infected tissues or sputum. The organism is often difficult to find by histologic methods, so culture is the best test.

Treatment

The least expensive form of treatment is saturated solution of potassium iodide, begun at 5 drops three times per day and progressively increased to 120 drops per day. This is often poorly tolerated and is reliable only for lymphocutaneous disease. Therefore, itraconazole has become the drug of choice for sporotrichosis. It may be given at 100 to 400 mg per day for 3 to 6 months, with the lower dose and shorter time for lymphocutaneous disease and the more intense courses for disseminated disease. Itraconazole is effective in more than 90% of patients with lymphocutaneous disease and about 75% of patients with extracutaneous disease. Fluconazole has also been used, but the response of lymphocutaneous disease, even at doses of 400 mg per day, appears to be less than with itraconazole.

CHROMOBLASTOMYCOSIS AND MYCETOMA

Chromoblastomycosis

Chromoblastomycosis is a disease with many pathogens, mainly species of the genera *Fonsecaea* and *Cladosporium*. Infection is established after traumatic inoculation, usually into the extremities of barefoot farm workers of tropical countries. Lesions begin with papules and spread to nodules or large cauliflower-like excrescences (Fig. 277-9). The disease is chronic and it rarely disseminates. The diagnosis is made by histologic and cultural demonstration of pigmented fungi in biopsies. These organisms may be saprophytes or colonizers, so deep sampling of tissue is important.

The definitive treatment is surgical, with excision of local lesions; amputation may be required. The drug of choice is itraconazole, 200 to 400 mg per day for "years." Response is excellent in modest disease. Treatment with am-

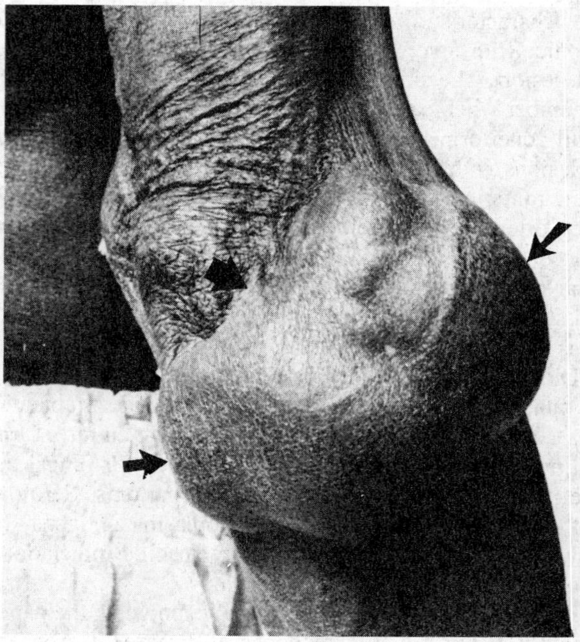

Fig. 277-9. Chromoblastomycotic lesion of elbow.

photericin B and flucytosine has been successful in selected cases.

Mycetoma

Mycetoma is the name given to the destructive soft tissue and bone lesions caused by many fungi, including organisms of *Pseudoallescheria (Petriellidium), Phialophora, Aspergillus, Streptomyces,* and *Nocardia* species. This disease was first described in India, hence the name *madura foot*. It occurs in the southern United States and tropical countries. Mycetoma commences after traumatic inoculation and progresses by formation of nodular granulomas and progressive destruction of tissues. Histologic and cultural studies of involved tissues yield the pathogens. Definitive treatment is surgical. Itraconazole is of limited value in some patients.

PHAEOHYPHOMYCOSIS

This is a chronic necrotizing infection caused by any of a number of mycelial fungal species characterized by the presence of dark melanin pigment. The genera *Exserohilum, Alternaria,* and *Bipolaris* are commonly involved, among others. Disease may follow traumatic inoculation (soft tissue, osteoarticular foci) or inhalation of candida (sinusitis, chronic pneumonia. Disease is characteristically slowly progressive, destroying tissue over many months. An allergic form of sinusitis may occur, and is characterized by the absence of tissue destruction and eosinophil-containing debris in sinus contents. Diagnosis is by direct demonstration of fungal hyphae and culture of the specific pathogen.

Treatment options are varied. The fungal pathogens are often but not always susceptible to amphotericin B, and this has been successful, as has ketoconazole. However, failures have prompted the search for other alternatives, and among these itraconazole appears to be quite effective. In one survey of patients treated with 50-400 mg per day, 11 of 17 patients had stabilization or improvement of disease with chronic itraconazole therapy.

ASPERGILLUS

Microbiology and epidemiology

Aspergillus species are widespread throughout the world and are cultivable only in the mycelial form. Hyphae are bamboo-shaped, with septate branching at 45°-angles. The fungus grows rapidly in vitro, and colonies appear in 3 to 7 days on most bacteriologic media. *Aspergillus* is ubiquitous, and exposure most commonly occurs through inhalation of the spores.

Pathophysiology and clinical manifestations

Aspergillus species produce three common pulmonary illnesses, whose expression depends in large part on the status of the host. The first, bronchopulmonary allergic aspergillosis, occurs in atopic persons with preexisting asthma or cystic fibrosis. The disease is caused by the host response to the organism, with eosinophilia, pulmonary infiltrates, and bronchial plugging by secretions containing eosinophils and aspergillus organisms. The condition may lead to bronchiectasis, but widespread invasion almost never occurs.

The second common manifestation of aspergillosis is pulmonary fungus ball. This usually results from aspergillus colonization of a preexisting cavity produced by tuberculosis, histoplasmosis, or coccidioidomycosis. A central fungus ball is often freely movable within the cavity (Fig. 277-10) and gives rise to the "movable crescent" that can be seen on chest x-ray. This form of aspergillosis is rarely invasive.

The third form of pulmonary aspergillosis is a fulminating disease associated with widespread dissemination to vital organs, especially in the gastrointestinal tract and the central nervous system. Disseminated aspergillosis usually begins in the setting of severe leukopenia, thrombocytopenia, and corticosteroid therapy. The disease progresses from local tissue invasion to a vasculitis caused by the mycelia. This vasculitis and plugging of pulmonary vessels may produce a clinical syndrome quite similar to that of pulmonary embolus, with similar radiographic changes. Sputum smears and cultures are occasionally positive for *Aspergillus*. Mortality is high in leukopenic patients and correlates closely with delays in initiation of treatment and with persistent leukopenia. Patients with persistent leukopenia have a diffuse aggressive disease, whereas those whose leukocytes return tend to develop pulmonary fungal balls that slowly resolve. In those of the latter group with cavitary disease, there is a danger of severe hemoptysis.

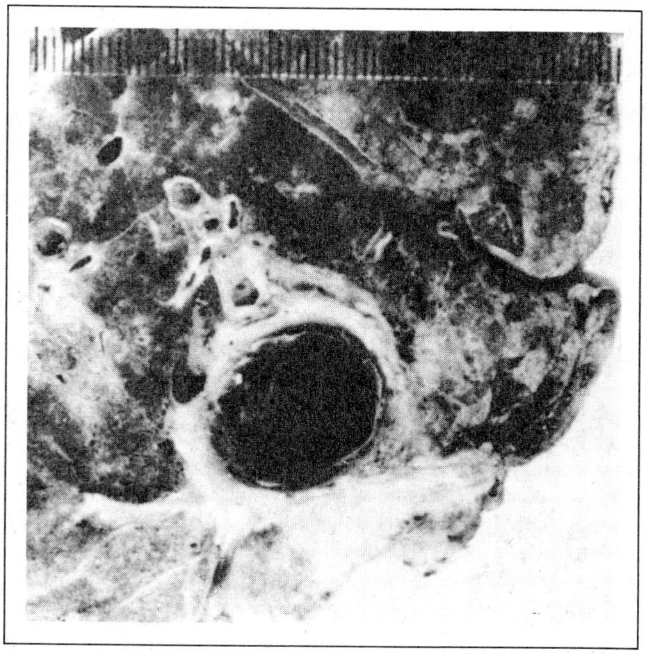

Fig. 277-10. Pulmonary fungus ball. (From Mandell GL, Douglas RG Jr, and Bennett JE, editors: Principles and practice of infectious diseases. New York, 1980, Wiley.)

Uncommon forms of aspergillosis include endocarditis, locally invasive disease, and madura foot. Endocarditis usually occurs on a prosthetic heart valve, possibly owing to contamination of the operative field by spores. Like candida, the organisms tend to form very large vegetations, with frequent emboli to large vessels. Diagnosis is especially difficult, since blood cultures are almost always negative. The only clue to diagnosis may be obtained from histologic examination of embolus. Locally invasive disease may occur after traumatic inoculation of an otherwise healthy person. Necrotizing cutaneous ulcers may occur in leukopenic patients. Madura foot, or mycetoma, may have *Aspergillus* species contributing to the pathology. Aspergilli may also form a mycetoma of the paranasal sinuses and chronic infiltrative pulmonary disease.

Diagnosis

Diagnosis of aspergillosis may be made presumptively from the characteristic septate hyphae seen in biopsied tissues stained with Gomori's methenamine silver (Fig. 277-11). Because invasive procedures are often required, there has been a search for serologic tests for diagnosis. Tests for precipitating antibodies are almost always strongly positive in bronchopulmonary allergic aspergillosis, are usually positive in pulmonary mycetoma, and usually are negative in patients with disseminated disease. As with candida, attention has been turned to antigen detection systems using radioimmunoassay. Aspergillus antigen may be detected in blood and bronchoalveolar lavage of patients with disseminated disease. The test is highly specific and does not cross-react with other fungi. The slow development of these procedures has been discouraging.

Treatment

Treatment of aspergillosis depends on the site of disease and the form it takes. Bronchopulmonary aspergillosis is effectively treated with corticosteroids. The goal is to reduce the host response (which produces most of the symptoms) without rendering the host severely immunosuppressed. Itraconazole may also be useful in reducing the fungal (antigen) burden.

If progression of disease is documented, it may be necessary to treat local fungus balls of sinus and lung with excision. Because underlying cavitary disease is often so severe as to preclude surgery, one usually does little unless hemoptysis forces intervention. Amphotericin B penetrates poorly into the mass of fungus in the mycetoma, and systemic treatment is rarely successful alone.

Disseminated disease should be treated promptly and aggressively with amphotericin B (1 mg/kg/day). Duration of treatment is uncertain but should continue at least until manifestations appear to be subsiding. Aspergillus endocarditis requires surgery, and mortality is high. Dual therapy with flucytosine may be helpful. There is no place for ketoconazole. Itraconazole is useful in disseminated or pulmonary invasive aspergillosis, with response rates above 50% (Mycoses Study Group, unpublished studies). of aspergillosis; the availability of an intravenous form in the future will increase its usefulness.

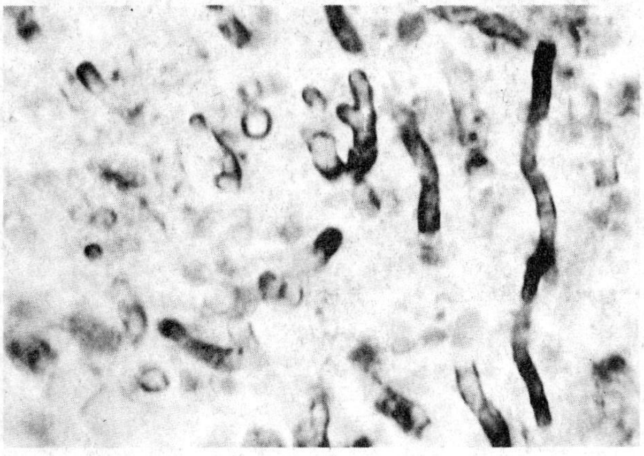

Fig. 277-11. Photomicrograph of vegetation on an aortic valve showing the characteristic regular, septate branching hyphae of *Aspergillus flavus*. Gomori's methenamine silver stain. Original magnification × 1000.

ZYGOMYCETES

Microbiology and epidemiology

The three genera *Absidia, Mucor,* and *Rhizopus* account for most cases of zygomycosis. They can be readily distinguished from *Aspergillus* species by the pleomorphic, nonseptate hyphae, good staining with hematoxylin and eosin, and right-angle branching.

Pathophysiology

Zygomycetes are found abundantly in nature and are common sources of bread mold contamination. Inhalation of the spores probably occurs repeatedly for most humans, and there must be some host alteration to permit establishment of a pathogenic process. Both acidosis and hyperglycemia are important predisposing factors, and uncontrolled diabetics thus are especially susceptible to invasive zygomycosis. Polymorphonuclear leukocytes readily kill the hyphae, and severe leukopenia is associated with lethal pulmonary disease.

Clinical manifestations

The most common manifestation of zygomycosis is rhinocerebral disease. The fungus produces a necrotizing locally invasive process of the palate or sinuses that directly invades and destroys adjoining structures. Vasculitis is frequent, with fungi invading and occluding arteries and veins. The clinical manifestations of zygomycosis directly reflect this pattern. The illness begins with headache, eye irritation, and nasal stuffiness, sometimes with bloody discharge. There may be a fluffy, black coating to the turbinates, and distinguishing this from blood clots may be difficult. Erosion into the orbit is associated with infraorbital numbness, proptosis, loss of vision, and both internal and external ophthalmoplegia. Ultimately, the fungi reach the brain, usually through the cribriform plate, and cause epidural and cerebral abscess, often complicated by cavernous sinus thrombosis. The course may be slow or fulminating.

Zygomycosis of the lungs may occur alone or as part of widely disseminated disease. This disease is similar to fulminating aspergillosis, with the "pulmonary infarct" syndrome in thrombocytopenic patients caused by masses of fungi occluding blood vessels. The mortality is high. Like that of aspergillosis, the diagnosis is difficult to make antemortem.

In addition, zygomycetes may invade denuded surfaces, especially burn wounds or operative wounds. Outbreaks have been associated with contaminated dressings.

Diagnosis and treatment

There are no serologic methods for diagnosis. Biopsies of deep specimens for histologic examination and culture are critically important.

The treatment is amphotericin B, coupled with repeated vigorous surgical debridement. One must rapidly accelerate the dose to as high as 1.0 to 1.5 mg/kg/day and maintain this until the patient is clinically well. Another treatment factor is control of the underlying process, particularly diabetes mellitus or leukopenia.

REFERENCES

Dismukes WE et al: Treatment of blastomycosis and histoplasmosis with ketoconazole. Ann Intern Med 103:861, 1985.

Dismukes WE: Cryptococcal meningitis in patients with AIDS. Infect Dis 157:624-632, 1988.

Fish DG et al: Coccidioidomycosis during human immunodeficiency virus infection: a review of 77 patients. Medicine 69:384, 1990.

Goodwin RA Jr et al: Chronic pulmonary histoplasmosis. Medicine (Baltimore) 55:413, 1976.

Graybill JR: Future directions of antifungal chemotherapy. Clin Infect Dis 14:S17-181, 1992.

Graybill JR et al: Itraconazole treatment of coccidioidomycosis. Am J Med 89:282, 1990.

Graybill JR et al: The major endemic mycoses in the setting of AIDS: clinical manifestations. Mycoses in AIDS patients, H Vanden Bossche, ED179-190, 1990.

Hay RJ, DuPont B, and Graybill JR, editors: First International Symposium on itraconazole. Rev Infect Dis 9(suppl 1):S1, 1987.

Laine L et al: Fluconazole compared with ketoconazole for the treatment of *Candida esophagitis* in AIDS. Am Coll Phys 655-660, 1992.

Powderly WG et al: A controlled trial of fluconazole or amphotericin B to prevent relapse of cryptococcal meningitis in patients with the acquired immunodeficiency syndrome. NEJM 326:793-798, 1992.

Restrepo A et al: Itraconazole therapy in lymphangitic and cutaneous sporotrichosis. Arch Dermatol 122:413, 1986.

Rosenberg M et al: Clinical and immunologic criteria for the diagnosis of allergic bronchopulmonary aspergillosis. Ann Intern Med 86:405, 1977.

Saag MS et al: Comparison of amphotericin B with fluconazole in the treatment of acute AIDS-associated cryptococcal meningitis. NEJM 326:83-89, 1989.

Saag MS and Dismukes WE: Minireview. Azole antifungal agents: emphasis on new triazoles. Antimicrob Agents Chemother 32:1, 1988.

Sarosi GA and Davies SF: Blastomycosis. State of the art. Am Rev Respir Dis 120:911, 1979.

Sharkey PK et al: Itraconazole therapy of phaeohyphomycosis. J Am Acad Dermatol 23:577, 1990.

Tucker RM et al: Treatment of coccidioidal meningitis with fluconazole. Rev Infect Dis 12(suppl 3)S380-389, 1990.

Wheat LJ et al: Effect of successful treatment with amphotericin B on *Histoplasma capsulatum* variety capsulatum. Polysaccharide antigen levels in patients with AIDS and histoplasmosis. Am J Med 92:153-160, 1992.

Wheat LJ et al: Disseminated histoplasmosis in the acquired immune deficiency syndrome: clinical findings, diagnosis and treatment, and review of the literature. Medicine 69:361, 1990.

Wheat LJ et al: Histoplasmosis relapse in patients with AIDS: detection using *Histoplasma capsulatum* variety capsulatum antigen levels. Ann Int Med 115:936, 1991.

Wheat LJ et al: A large urban outbreak of histoplasmosis: clinical features. Ann Intern Med 94:331-337, 1981.

CHAPTER

278 Infections Caused by *Candida, Actinomyces,* and *Nocardia* Species

John E. Edwards, Jr.

CANDIDA

Microbiology and epidemiology

Candida species are small (4 to 6 μm), oval, thin-walled cells that reproduce by budding. Three morphologic forms are found in tissue: yeast, pseudohyphae, and hyphae. They can be identified in clinical specimens with warm 10% potassium hydroxide or Gram stain. The organism is ubiquitous in nature and is a common human saprophyte. It grows well on most media used for routine recovery of microbial pathogens. Culturing from blood is facilitated with the lysis centrifugation technique. While there are over 100 species of *Candida,* those infecting man are limited predominately to *C. albicans, C. tropicalis, C. krusei, C. parapsilosis, C. guilliermondii, C. stellatoidea, C. pseudotropicalis, C. lusitaniae,* and *C. glabrata* (formerly *Torulopsis glabrata*). These species vary in their pathogenicity, epidemiology, organ predilections, and sensitivity to antifungal drugs.

Candida species have risen in importance to become among the most common nosocomial pathogens. They constitute 10% of isolates from blood cultures of hospitalized patients. Their emergence to this high level of prominence is a consequence of the introduction of modern therapeutic modalities into the treatment armamentarium of patients who are seriously ill and require intensive therapy and monitoring for life support. Mucocutaneous candidal infections are among the most common opportunistic infections of patients with AIDS.

Pathophysiology

Most frequently, candidal infections result from some form of compromise in the host defense mechanisms normally

Table 278-1. Treatment of candidiasis

Form of disease	Treatment regimen	Comments
Uncomplicated mucosal disease	For thrush, clotrimazole troches or nystatin. For esophagitis, ketoconazole or fluconazole. For intertriginous disease or vaginal disease, topical miconazole, clotrimazole.	Fluconazole and ketoconazole are effective but should be reserved for severe or refractory infections. In AIDS patients, fluconazole has been more effective than ketoconazole.
Chronic mucocutaneous candidiasis	Ketoconazole 200 to 600 mg/day, P.O. Fluconazole 200 mg/day, P.O.	For control, intermittent I.V. amphotericin B may be necessary.
Upper urinary tract infection	Intraveous amphotericin B, 0.3-0.6 mg/kg/day until evidence of resolution. Fluconazole is under investigation.	
Cystitis	Remove catheter, amphotericin B bladder washout. 5-FC, 50-75 mg/kg/day, P.O. Fluconzole under investigation. For severe cases, amphotericin B, I.V.	Resistance to 5-FC may be present and also may develop during therapy.
Disseminated candidiasis and candidemia	Amphotericin B, 0.3-0.6 mg/kg/day for 1 to 3 weeks depending on severity. Flucytosine, 100 to 150 mg/kg/day, P.O., may be added depending on severity. Patients with catheter-associated candidemia and a low probability of having disseminated candidiasis should receive fluconazole, 200 to 400 mg/day. All patients with candidemia, whether or not it is associated with a catheter, should be treated with an antifungal unless there is a contraindication.	A large, multicenter clinical trial comparing amphotericin B with fluconazole in candidemia is in progress. It will clarify the role of fluconazole when completed.
Candida endophthalmitis	Amphotericin B at 0.3 to 0.6 mg/kg/day until evidence of resolution occurs. In severe cases or in cases where the macula is involved, 5-FC, 100-150 mg/kg/day, P.O., should be added. Fluconazole is under investigation.	Partial vitrectomy should be considered with ophthalmological consultation.
Candida endocarditis	Infected valve should be removed as soon as possible. After surgery, amphotericin B and 5-FC should be given for 6 weeks or more.	There are reports of rare cases of cure with amphotericin B therapy. They are the exception and the valve should be removed whenever possible.
Prosthetic implants infected with *Candida*	Removal of implant is almost always necessary. Amphotericin B should be given after removal.	The role of fluconazole is not yet known.

active against this saprophytic organism. Candidal infections that do not result from compromised host defenses include infections of the chorioretina and heart valves in heroin addicts, who inject the organism directly into their blood stream. Also included is candidal vaginitis resulting mainly from local overgrowth of the organism after suppression of bacterial flora from antibiotic use.

In most circumstances, candidal infections result from either local (mucocutaneous) or systemic immunocompromise. Precisely what components of the normal host defense mechanisms are responsible for defense against the organism have not been defined. Clinical and in-vitro observations suggest that cell-mediated immunity (CMI) (particularly lymphocyte function) is important in maintaining mucosal defense. For instance, patients with certain congenital abnormalities of the lymphocytic component of their CMI are prone to have chronic mucocutaneous candidiasis. Additionally, patients with AIDS are also prone to candidal mucocutaneous infections, presumably as a result of their lymphocyte deficiency. Invasive candidiasis of the deep organs, usually initiated by hematogenous seeding, is considered to result from deficiencies in phagocytic mechanisms. Neutrophils and monocytes kill *Candida* in vitro; neutropenia in patients treated with cytotoxic chemotherapeutic drugs for cancer is correlated with candidal infections. Complement and antibodies are opsonins for *Candida*. The role of antibody in defense against *Candida* is not clear; IgG anticandidal antibodies are present in nearly all normals. Noncellular serum constituents other than complement and antibody may also have anticandidal properties.

While *Candida* species are saprophytic, they have certain microbial characteristics that are likely to facilitate invasion once normal defense mechanisms are compromised. The organisms adhere to vaginal and oral epithelial cells, fibronectin, platelet-fibrin clots, acrylic, endothelium, plastics, and subendothelial matrix. They secrete proteases and phospholipases. *C. albicans* may be able to mechanically invade tissue with its tubular structures that form during germination. Certain *Candida* species have receptors on their surface that mimic human receptors and may facilitate their ability to invade tissue or escape host defense mechanisms.

Although the precise interactions between these potential pathogenicity factors and the specific defects in host defense mechanisms are not yet known, certain clinical circumstances are particularly prone to result in severe candidal infections. Generally, these clinical circumstances are characterized by iatrogenic compromise of the defense mechanisms. Therefore, these organisms have evolved predominantly as a consequence of the advancement of medical therapeutics. The specific factors associated with severe candidal infections are the use of antibiotics, implantation of plastic indwelling intravascular catheters, cytotoxic chemotherapeutics for treatment of neoplastic diseases, steroids, and immunosuppressive drugs for preventing transplanted organ rejection. The populations most often subjected to these factors are patients with cancer, patients undergoing complex surgical procedures (usually abdominal surgery), patients receiving transplants, patients having prosthetic material implants, and low-birth-weight neonates requiring intensive support for life maintenance. The susceptibility of such a broad range of patients is why *Candida* species have emerged as such common nosocomial pathogens during the last 2 decades.

Clinical manifestations

The term *thrush* refers to a form of candidiasis characterized by creamy white, curdlike patches on mucous membranes. When removed by scraping they leave a raw, bleeding, ulcerative, painful surface. Thrush may occur in the mouth, esophagus, gastrointestinal tract, vagina, or bladder. The patches are pseudomembranes consisting of desquamated epithelial cells, leukocytes, bacteria, keratin, and necrotic tissue. The *Candida* can be visualized with 10% potassium hydroxide or Gram stain. Simply culturing a plaque for *Candida* is not sufficient to make a diagnosis, since the organisms may be present in the mouth without causing thrush. A specific diagnosis is necessary, since the patches of thrush are not distinctive in appearance and can be confused with other white lesions on mucous membranes such as hairy leukoplakia in the mouth and the white plaques caused by gastric acid reflux in the esophagus. Thrush occurs most commonly in neutropenic patients, patients with diabetes, patients who have received antibiotics, patients with mucosal disruption from dentures, and patients who are generally severely debilitated by generalized illnesses or malnutrition. In patients who are neutropenic, cytomegalovirus and herpes viruses may cause lesions resembling thrush or may be present in thrush lesions concomitantly with the *Candida*. Esophagitis frequently occurs without obvious oral thrush. Candidal esophagitis may cause severe phagodynia. In its later stages, it may become asymptomatic as a result of extensive involvement of the esophageal nerves. Identifying lesions consistent with candidal esophagitis, from which *Candida* species are recovered on plaque brushings, is sufficient reason to initiate therapy. To exclude other causes of the plaque or concomitant pathogens, biopsy is necessary. However, the safety of biopsy is unclear, particularly with respect to dissemination. So biopsy should be reserved for special circumstances. Dissemination may occur from the esophagus in severe cases, and perforation may rarely occur. The presence of thrush of the mouth or esophagus, in the absence of an obvious reason for its occurrence, is a signal for a thorough evaluation for AIDS.

In addition to infecting the oral and esophageal mucosa, *Candida* species may infect the remainder of the intestinal tract. Gastric involvement may occur in patients with gastric ulcers that have become colonized and eventually infected with the organism, and in patients who are neutropenic from cancer chemotherapy. Infection of the mucous membranes of the gastrointestinal tract (including the stomach) occurs most commonly in neutropenic patients. The forms of infections are plaques of thrush, superficial erosions, ulcerations, and pseudomembrane formation. Perforation and presumably dissemination may occur. Diarrhea may be a consequence. Other organs within the abdomen that may become infected with *Candida* species are the gallbladder, liver, spleen, and pancreas. In the gallbladder, a generalized cholecystitis may occur, or fungus balls that obstruct drainage may form. The extent of infection in the liver, spleen, and pancreas may range from small micro and macro abscesses to large abscesses that cause extensive necrosis and organ failure. Hepatosplenic candidiasis or chronic disseminated candidiasis has emerged as an important problem in neutropenic patients. The latter term is preferable for describing this syndrome, since organs other than the spleen and liver are frequently involved, such as kidney. Usually, multiple micro and macro lesions are distributed throughout the involved organs from hematogenous seeding. The infection usually persists for many months and is generally refractory to therapy with the standard antifungals.

Candidal peritonitis has emerged as a serious problem in patients undergoing gastrointestinal tract surgery or sustaining trauma to the abdomen. Its diagnosis is difficult without biopsy of the involved peritoneum. Frequently, *Candida* species are isolated from drainage of the peritoneum along with bacteria, so determining the precise role of the *Candida* is problematic.

Another important mucous membrane infection caused by *Candida* is vaginitis. This infection is exceedingly common. It occurs after a course of antibiotic treatment in the majority of patients. Either a thick, curdlike discharge or a scanty discharge may occur. Pruritus is almost always present. The urethra and the endometrium may become infected secondarily. Some patients have frequent recurrences. Masses of hyphae, pseudohyphae, and leukocytes are present in the discharge.

A rather large number of common cutaneous syndromes are caused by *Candida* species. Diaper rash in infants is frequently caused by *Candida*. It usually starts in the perianal area and spreads over the distribution of the diaper. Wet diapers predispose to the infection. *Candida* species are frequent causes of paronychia, especially in individuals who often immerse their hands in wash water. The lesion is a focal infection adjacent to the nail that becomes warm, glistening, and tense. It may extend under the nail. Candidal intertrigo is a common condition that begins as vesicopustules, which enlarge and rupture to cause maceration and fissures. It occurs in warm and moist areas of the skin surface that are in juxtaposition, such as under the breasts or in the inguinal areas. Satellite lesions may be present. It is associated with diabetes and obesity. Numerous organisms have been associated with pruritus ani; *Candida* species are commonly recovered when this condition is present. Marked erythema of the perianal skin occurs, maceration develops, and severe pruritus is present. The condition may spread extensively over the perineum or deep within the anal canal.

In addition to these common cutaneous conditions, a variety of less common conditions are caused by *Candida* species. Generalized cutaneous candidiasis is a widespread eruption of the trunk, thorax, and extremities. It is usually more pronounced in the genitocrural folds, anal region, axillae, hands, and feet. Both children and adults may be affected. *Erosio interdigitalis blastomycetica* is a term applied to the red-based, painful infection occurring in macerated skin between the toes and fingers. Candidal folliculitis is another cutaneous infection that occurs rarely. Candidal balanitis begins as vesicles on the distal end of the penis and frequently develops into patches. It may become extensive and spread beyond the genital area and is frequently associated with severe burning and itching. Chronic mucocutaneous candidiasis is a condition characterized by refractory infection of the skin, mucous membranes, and nails that is associated with a heterogenous group of immunological abnormalities (Chapter 223). The major immune defect is failure of T cell lymphocytes (thymus-derived) to respond to stimulation in vitro with candidal antigen. Cutaneous anergy occurs in half the patients. Patients are heterogenous in their deficiency of antigenic response both in vitro and cutaneously. Their immune deficiency is considered to be congenital. However, certain patients do not show evidence of the condition until their adult years. Whether the disease may be acquired in these patients, rather than congenital, remains unknown. Approximately half the patients have an associated endocrinopathy such as hypoparathyroidism, Addison's disease, hypothyroidism, or diabetes. Approximately half the patients have autoantibodies to renal, thyroid, and gastric tissues also. Additional associations with the syndrome are thymoma, dermatophytosis, dental dysplasia, vitiligo, polyglandular autoimmune disease, and autoantibodies to melanin-producing cells. Most patients survive for prolonged periods. However, the disease may become very severe and disfiguring. Death usually results from bacterial sepsis rather than disseminated candidiasis.

Infection of the deep organs with *Candida* species is responsible for the substantial increase in frequency of nosocomial candidal infections and is the central problem of concern. The deep-organ infection usually occurs as a result of widespread hematogenous dissemination during conditions of relative immunocompromise. The populations usually acquiring widespread hematogenous infections are patients treated with cytotoxic chemotherapy for cancer, patients on immunosuppressive therapy after organ transplantation, patients sustaining burns, severely ill neonates with low birth weights, and patients having protracted postoperative courses (most frequently after gastrointestinal tract surgery). Iatrogenic factors common to these patients, other than cytotoxic immunosuppressives and steroids, are general debilitation, the use of antibiotics, the use of indwelling intravascular catheters for intravenous infusions or for monitoring cardiovascular status, and the use of hyperalimentation fluids for nutritional support. Precisely how the organism enters the blood stream is not clear. In some patients it may enter through intravenous access catheters. In others, probably the majority, it enters through the gastrointestinal tract, after it has proliferated to large numbers from iatrogenic factors promoting its growth. Once the vascular compartment has been invaded, the organism can disseminate to nearly any organ of the body. Those most commonly infected are the kidney, brain, heart, liver, spleen, skin, and eye. Those less commonly involved are skeletal muscle, bone marrow, spine, joints, and lung. Within these organs, micro and small macro abscesses develop that are generally diffusely spread throughout the organ. Except in the case of hepatosplenic involvement, the lesions rarely attain a size identifiable by currently available radiographic or radionucleotide imaging techniques.

After the organism has entered the intravascular compartment, it may trigger a shock syndrome in some patients. This syndrome is clinically indistinguishable from shock caused by gram-negative organisms. *Candida* species do not have an endotoxin that closely resembles that of the gram-negative organisms and the syndrome is probably a result of cytokine production by the host. After infecting the deep organs, generalized organ failure may develop. Either extensive, diffuse cerebral infection or meningitis may develop from the central nervous system involvement. Heart failure and arrhythmias may be a consequence of the diffuse myocardial involvement and invasion of the cardiac conduction system. Liver failure and elevated hepatic enzymes may develop. Diminished renal function may be manifested by an elevation in blood urea nitrogen or serum creatinine, and the glomerular filtration rate may decrease. Blindness may result from hematogenous candidal endophthalmitis. A miliary pattern may be present on chest x-ray in a small number of patients during the preterminal phase of their illness. Pain frequently accompanies the skeletal muscle infection. Small, macronodular skin lesions that contain the organisms on biopsy may develop. In rare instances, bone marrow failure may be a consequence of severe marrow infection.

Management of patients with candidemia, who are predisposed by the iatrogenic factors associated with disseminated candidiasis, is highly challenging. No method exists to separate patients who have transient, catheter-associated candidemia from those with candidemia who have foci of infection in the deep organs. In the general hospitalized patient population, patients with candidemia have an overall mortality rate of approximately 50%. The mortality is attributable to *Candida* species in approximately 40%. An unknown number of patients have a delayed complication of the candidemia, such as hematogenous ocular, renal, or bone infection, that may become clinically overt anywhere from days to years after the initial candidemia. While extensive investigations have focused on the role of certain serodiagnostic techniques for separating patients with transient candidemia from those with visceral organ infection, there are none available currently for practical use. The situation is complicated even more by the fact that approximately 40% of patients with widespread hematogenous infection do not have positive blood cultures. Therefore, even blood cultures are relatively insensitive in detecting visceral organ infection. Because of the high mortality rates associated with candidemia, the lack of ability to distinguish those patients with transient candidemia from those with deep organ infection, and the possibility of late complications of the candidemia, there is a consensus among certain clinical mycologists working in the field that all patients with candidemia should receive antifungal therapy, unless there is a contraindication to antifungal drugs. Until national cooperative studies are completed comparing amphotericin B with fluconazole, patients with a high probability of deep organ involvement (the majority) should receive amphotericin B.

Two forms of candidal infection, associated with the candidemia–hematogenous-dissemination syndrome, deserve emphasis. They are hematogenous candidal endophthalmitis and the macronodular skin lesions resulting from dissemination to the skin. Both the skin lesions and the ocular infection are important to establish the diagnosis of widespread hematogenous candidiasis, since they are both strongly correlated with involvement of multiple deep organs. Hematogenous candidal endophthalmitis is important not only for signalling the presence of infection in other deep organs, but also because the lesions may cause permanent blindness. Furthermore, in patients who are not neutropenic, involvement of the chorioretina may be a relatively common complication of candidemia caused by *Candida albicans*. One prospective study has defined an incidence of 27% for the occurrence of hematogenous endophthalmitis in patients with candidemia. The lesions of hematogenous candidal endophthalmitis are round, cotton ball–like lesions associated with vitreous haze. They may expand into a severe generalized endophthalmitis and may necessitate enucleation in some cases.

Several deep-organ candidal infections occur that are not complications of the candidemia-disseminated candidiasis syndrome. Candidal meningitis may occur as a complication of brain surgery or as a result of the implantation of prosthetic materials into the central nervous system. Rarely, candidal meningitis may occur de novo. Nearly all patients have a pleocytosis; in 50% it is predominately lymphocytic. Hypoglycorrhachia and elevated protein are present frequently, and the organism is seen on Gram stain or wet preparation of the cerebral spinal fluid in 40% of patients. Two forms of candidal pneumonia exist. One is the diffuse miliary pattern associated with widespread hematogenous dissemination. It is almost always a preterminal event. The other form is that of a necrotic bronchopneumonia. It is rare and considered to be a result of a candidal superinfection of a bacterial pneumonic process. Care must be taken to avoid diagnosing candidal pneumonia in patients with a pulmonary infiltrate on chest x-ray and recovery of candida from the sputum. Biopsy evidence of candidal invasion of the pulmonary parenchyma is necessary to definitively establish this diagnosis. *Candida* may infect prosthetic cardiac valves and the cardiac valves of drug addicts.

Candidal infection of the cardiovascular system. Rarely, native valves may become infected, especially in patients who have had a long-term intravenous catheter for parenteral fluid administration. Eradication of the infection from heart valves is exceptionally difficult; surgery is almost always required. In addition to occurring in the setting of widespread disseminated candidiasis, candidal pericarditis can complicate cardiac surgery, and candidal sternal osteomyelitis may occur at the surgical site. Candidal arthritis may occur as a result of joint trauma, surgery, intraarticular injections of steroids, and heroin injection. Candidal vascular infections occur most commonly at the site of intravascular catheter insertion. Thrombosis and infection caused by *Candida* have been growing problems in recent years. Extensive infection of the thrombophlebitis caused by the catheter may develop, necessitating surgical removal of the clot. Fungus balls in the right atrium have been reported from indwelling subclavian catheters. Septic arterial emboli may also occur and cause mycotic aneurysms. They are usually a complication of candidal endocarditis.

Candidal infections that have been reported but will not be elaborated upon include middle-ear infections, nasal ulcers, keratitis, lymphadenitis, sinusitis, laryngeal infection, diarrhea, the "drunken disease" (a syndrome described in Japan considered to be caused by alcohol absorption from fermentation by *Candida* of carbohydrates in the gastrointestinal tract), and the yeast connection (fatigue and immune suppression postulated to result from overgrowth of *Candida* on skin and mucous membranes).

Diagnostic tests

Despite extensive investigations into antigen and antibody detection systems and detection of products secreted by the organism, there are no commercially available serodiagnostic tests for diagnosing candidal infection of the deep organs that are considered to have acceptable true positive and true negative detection rates. With current techniques there is still approximately a 40% false negative rate in culturing *Candida* from the blood. The lysis-centrifugation technique both increases the sensitivity of blood cultures and reduces the time necessary for the organisms to grow. It is likely that a panel of serodiagnostic tests will be developed in the future to derive a probability for deep organ infection based on the number of positive tests and perhaps on quantitative aspects of their positivity.

Currently the only method to definitively diagnose deep

organ involvement is to demonstrate tissue invasion by *Candida* on biopsy specimens. In certain clinical situations, however, a decision to initiate treatment may be made without definitive diagnosis. The two best examples are hematogenous candidal endophthalmitis and chronic hepatosplenic candidiasis. For instance, in a patient who is candidemic, who is known to have had a normal ocular fundus prior to the candidemia, and who develops lesions clinically compatible with the ocular lesions caused by *Candida* seeding, empiric therapy is initiated for treatment of the ocular disease. Similarly, in neutropenic patients who are candidemic and develop lesions in the liver compatible with hepatosplenic candidiasis, therapy may be initiated without biopsy of the lesions. Alternatively, an example for which a specific diagnosis is desirable is candidal pulmonary infection. A patient who has a pulmonary infiltrate on chest x-ray and has *Candida* in the sputum may not have candidal pneumonia. Biopsy evidence of *Candida* invading the pulmonary parenchyma is necessary to definitely establish the diagnosis of candidal pneumonia.

Treatment

The treatment of candidal infections must be directed at the specific form of infection, because of their varied nature and severity (see Table 278-1). The majority of the cutaneous syndromes, such as candidal intertrigo, can be treated with topical imidazoles, such as miconazole or clotrimazole. More severe cutaneous syndromes, such as chronic mucocutaneous candidiasis, require oral imidazoles such as ketoconazole or fluconazole for eradication. In especially severe circumstances, brief courses of amphotericin B may be necessary. Candidal vaginitis is usually responsive to topical imidazoles. In refractory cases, oral ketoconazole or fluconazole may be necessary, but care should be taken to avoid its use in pregnancy. Neither drug is approved by the Federal Drug Administration for candidal vaginitis. For thrush, nystatin has been used for decades. However, it is being replaced by clotrimazole troches, which are considered more palatable by most patients. In refractory cases either ketoconazole or fluconazole may be necessary. Candidal esophagitis can be treated successfully with oral ketoconazole or fluconazole. Recent studies in patients with AIDS have shown fluconazole to be more effective. It has the advantage of not requiring gastric acid for absorption; many patients with AIDS are relatively achlorhydric. In refractory cases, brief courses of intravenous amphotericin B may be effective. Candidal infection of the gallbladder associated with obstruction usually requires surgery. Candidal peritonitis should be treated with intravenous amphotericin B in severely ill patients. Patients undergoing chronic peritoneal dialysis may benefit from fluconazole, although the data are limited at present. Whether removal of the dialysis catheter is necessary remains controversial; both successes and failures have been reported. In general, infection of the deep organs such as the lung, heart, kidney, brain, bone, liver, spleen, and joints requires amphotericin B. (The role of fluconazole in these deep infections has not been clarified to date.) When comparative studies are performed, fluconazole may be found to be an effective alternative to amphotericin B. Of particular interest will be the brain and the kidneys because of the excellent penetration of fluconazole into the brain and its high level of excretion into the urine. Currently, candidal cystitis is treated successfully by removal of an indwelling urinary bladder catheter, if present. If postcatherization candiduria persists in asymptomatic patients, it may resolve spontaneously. If not, amphotericin B bladder washout may be an alternative. 5-fluorocytosine has been used successfully. However, de novo resistance to 5-FC may be present and resistance may develop during therapy. Fluconazole may be an effective alternative. Data on its effectiveness are limited at this time. Candidal endophthalmitis should be treated with intravenous amphotericin B. In patients whose lesions continue to progress under therapy or who have lesions in proximity to the macula, 5-FC should be added. The role of partial vitrectomy is highly important and ophthalmological consultation should be obtained for consideration of this procedure. The role of intravitreal antifungals remains controversial. Although fluconazole penetrates the intraocular structures, its use in patients with hematogenous candidal endophthalmitis is limited and preliminary studies in animal models have shown it to be less effective than amphotericin B. More experience in humans is necessary to clarify its role.

The treatment of patients with candidemia deserves special emphasis. Because of the high mortality rate associated with candidemia, the high rates of attributable mortality to candidal infections complicating the candidemia, and the current lack of reliable methods to distinguish patients at high risk for widespread disseminated candidiasis from those with low probability, all patients with candidemia should be treated with antifungal agents unless there is a contraindication to the drugs. Amphotericin B should be used for those with a high probability (the majority) and fluconazole reserved for those with a low probability. How successful fluconazole will be as an alternative to amphotericin B has not been determined. However, national cooperative studies are underway to compare amphotericin B and fluconazole. If possible, if the candidemia is related to an intravascular catheter, the catheter should be removed. Certain clinical situations exist in which catheter removal is problematic and adjustments are necessary.

ACTINOMYCOSIS

Microbiology and epidemiology

The organisms of the genus *Actinomyces* are true prokaryotic bacteria that cause diseases that are indolent and resemble fungal infection. These bacteria are gram-positive, filamentous (1 μm diameter), and branching. They are either microaerophilic or anaerobic. Failure to culture clinical specimens in anaerobic conditions has caused serious delays in diagnosing actinomycosis. A hallmark of the species is its ability to form "sulfur" granules in tissue. These granules are amorphous masses of organisms that can become large enough to be seen without microscopy. Characteristic "bread crumb" colonies form in thioglycollate broth. On solid media, early colonies are delicately branched. As they mature, they become large and heaped up with a lobulated surface. They resemble a molar tooth standing up from the agar's surface. The most important species causing human infections are *Actinomycetes israelii, A. naeslundii, A. viscosus,* and *A. odontalyticus*. A related organism, *Arachnia propionica,* is capable of causing classical lesions of actinomycosis. These organisms are human commensals found most commonly on the oral and pharyngeal mucosa.

Pathogenesis

Actinomyces organisms are saprophytes with a low level of virulence. Apparently normal host defense mechanisms are highly efficient in protecting against them, since they are not common pathogens, even in the setting of severe iatrogenic immunosuppression. Generally, tissue trauma is necessary to provide a milieu conducive for invasion. Once established in a focus, the organisms proliferate to form the classic "sulfur" granules. Induration of the infected tissues is common. Another characteristic is the presence of other bacteria in addition to the *Actinomyces* species. These accompanying organisms are usually actinobacilli, Haemophilus species, and/or various oral anaerobes. These accompanying bacteria may facilitate the tissue invasion by the weakly pathogenic *Actinomyces*.

The histopathology of the lesions is characterized by numerous foamy macrophages, eosinophils, and giant cells, unlike the classic polymorphonuclear response seen with pyogenic bacteria. As chronicity increases, plasma cells appear, granules form, and extensive induration develops. A hallmark of the infection is its ability to cross anatomical barriers and to form sinus tracts extending to other organs or to the skin. When the sulfur granules become large enough to be visible without microscopy, they are yellow or dull white, hard, gritty structures that may be as large as 2 mm.

Clinical manifestations

The most common infections of actinomycosis are cervicofacial, thoracic, abdominal, pelvic, and disseminated. Cervicofacial disease almost invariably begins as an extension from a peridental origin (Plate V-55). Frequently, minor trauma initiates the process. Although the most common form is an indolent, slowly evolving disease, a more rapidly progressive form occurs rarely. The disease process crosses anatomical boundaries and causes lumpy swelling of the face that may develop sinus tracts. The mandible is a much more frequent site of origin compared to the maxilla. However, almost any facial or cervical structure may become involved including the tongue, sinuses, or thyroid. Rare complications are direct extension into the brain and hematogenous dissemination. The development of "cold" abscesses and draining sinus along the ramus of the mandible is the condition referred to classically as "lumpy jaw."

Thoracic actinomycosis is usually aspiration pneumonia, but it may result from extension into the thorax from adjacent anatomical sites such as the neck or abdomen. Rarely, it may be a result of hematogenous dissemination. The forms of pulmonary parenchymal involvement are nonspecific and include a bronchopneumonia or, rarely, a mass lesion. Empyema may develop. Extension through the lung parenchyma and pleural space into and through the chest wall may occur, resulting in a pulmonic-cutaneous sinus tract. An osteomyelitis of the rib may develop as the infection invades through the chest wall. The process may extend to the mediastinum or cross the boundary formed by the diaphragm into the abdominal cavity. Characteristic of actinomycotic infections in general, the infection is indolent and may be relatively asymptomatic. Thoracic x-ray findings are not specific. Thoracic disease may resemble tuberculosis.

Abdominal actinomycosis is usually a complication of a primary nonactinomycotic process, such as inflammatory bowel disease or surgery, and occasionally complicates blunt trauma. *Actinomyces* may cause a chronic ileocecal inflammation resembling Crohn's disease or ileocecal tuberculosis. Virtually any portion of the gastrointestinal tract may be involved; gastric actinomycosis may resemble gastric ulcer disease. When the bowel is infected, secondary infection of the liver is relatively common. Sinus tracts may form and the process may extend directly into the thoracic or pelvic cavities. Because of the indolent nature of the infection, diagnosis is invariably delayed.

Pelvic actinomycosis usually originates as an extension from an abdominal source. Virtually any pelvic organ may be involved. The ovaries and fallopian tubes are infected most commonly, although rare pelvic infection may result from the use of indwelling intrauterine contraceptive devices. In either case, the process may become extensive and involve nearly all the pelvic structures, including the urinary tract, by direct extension. Central nervous system actinomycosis occurs most commonly as a result of hematogenous spread from an abdominal or thoracic focus. Usually solitary mass lesions occur. Meningitis or meningoencephalitis occurs less commonly. Extensive intracerebral infection may result from direct extension of a facial or cervical focus.

Osseous actinomycosis occurs either from direct extension or from hematogenous spread. Radiographic findings are nonspecific. Occasionally, trauma may be the etiology.

Diagnosis

Demonstration of invasion by the characteristic branched gram-positive filamentous structures on Gram-stain, with confirmation by culture, is necessary for definitive diagnosis. Proper processing of the specimen for anaerobic culturing is essential. Because of the similarities in the forms of clinical infection and similar appearance of the organisms on Gram stain, it is desirable to distinguish actinomycosis from nocardiosis. The two diseases are treated with different antibacterials, so identifying the infecting agent facilitates early administration of the proper therapy. In contrast to *Nocardia,* the *Actinomyces* are not acid-fast. They form sulfur granules in tissues, a characteristic that *Nocar-*

dia does not have except in exceptionally rare circumstance. Infection with the *Actinomyces* usually is accompanied by additional bacteria. The presence of the bread-crumb colonies in thioglycolate broth and the molar tooth colonies of *Actinomyces* facilitates the early laboratory confirmation of the clinical and Gram-stain findings. There are no helpful skin or serodiagnostic tests.

Treatment

Nearly all cases respond to high-dose intravenous aqueous penicillin given for 4 to 6 weeks and followed with oral penicillin for months. In refractory cases, surgery may be necessary. Surgery may be especially advantageous if the initial presentation is complicated by involvement of large masses of tissue. Alternatives to penicillin are tetracycline, erythromycin, and clindamycin. First-generation cephalosporins, ampicillin, and amoxacillin are also substitutes. There is no significant species variation in susceptibility to the agents.

NOCARDIOSIS

Microbiology and epidemiology

The *Nocardia* species are classified in the family Actinomycetaceae. They are differentiated from organisms causing actinomycosis by being acid-fast and growing aerobically. They are related to mycobacteria. A special acid-fast stain is necessary using an aqueous sulfuric acid as the decolorizer rather than the acid alcohol used in the classic Ziehl-Neelsen stain, which will decolorize *Nocardia* species. The organisms are branched, filamentous, and gram-positive. *Nocardia* species are slow-growing; in suspected cases, culturing specimens for a prolonged period may be helpful.

Nocardia are ubiquitous saprophytes found in a large number of animal species and in decaying organic matter. They have been isolated from respiratory tract secretions of patients with chronic obstructive pulmonary airways disease, who have no evidence of a *Nocardia* infection.

Pathophysiology and clinical manifestations

The most common species of *Nocardia* infecting man are *N. asteroides, N. brasiliensis,* and *N. otitidism-caviarum.* Other species rarely cause infection.

Nocardiosis is usually an opportunistic infection, although a significant number of infected patients have no recognizable immunocompromise. The most commonly infected immunocompromised patients are those treated with steroids, patients with malignancies (especially lymphoreticular and chronic malignancy in general), patients treated with cytotoxic chemotherapy, and transplanted patients on immunosuppressives. Patients with primary alveolar proteinosis have a particularly high propensity for nocardial infections, probably as a result of inadequately functioning pulmonary macrophages. Some *Nocardia* species can invade and replicate within macrophages. Acquisition of the disease is usually through inhalation of spores. Human-to-human transmission is possible and outbreaks have been reported in transplant units. Cutaneous forms of nocardial infection usually result from inoculation of soil harboring the organism.

The most common nocardial infection is pulmonary. After inhalation and establishment of infection, a necrotizing pneumonia develops that is usually not associated with an extensive inflammatory response of leukocytes. Once the necrotizing pneumonia begins, tissue destruction may occur, and the process becomes chronic. Like actinomycosis, patients with nocardiosis may develop sinus tracts extending through the chest wall onto the skin. Virtually any intrathoracic structure may become involved by direct extension. Hematogenous extension to the brain is not uncommon. Any patient with pulmonary nocardosis, whether or not they may be immunocompromised, should be evaluated carefully for the possibility of hematogenous dissemination to the brain. Hematogenous extension to nearly any organ is possible and a myriad of hematogenous infections have been reported, including infections of the liver, spleen, kidney, adrenal gland, thyroid gland, prostate gland, and eye. X-ray and other radiologic findings are nonspecific. Hematogenous nocardial endophthalmitis has been specifically diagnosed with fine-needle retinal biopsy. In recent years *Nocardia* has been one of many of the pathogens found in patients with AIDS. Infection in a variety of organs, including the lungs, brain, and esophagus, has been reported in addition to suprarenal and paraspinal abscesses.

Diagnosis

There are no diagnostic blood or skin tests. Blood cultures are not helpful. Diagnosis requires biopsy showing the characteristic organisms infecting tissue, and positive cultures are confirmatory. Differentiation from actinomycosis is accomplished by demonstrating the acid-fast properties of *Nocardia,* the lack of sulfur granules or other accompanying pathogens, aerobic growth, and the lack of molar tooth colony formation in cultures.

Treatment

Long-term therapy is necessary for virtually all forms of nocardiosis. Sulfonamides, most commonly sulfadiazine, are the first-line agents. Surgical intervention may be necessary, especially in central nervous system infection. Certain investigators consider trimethoprim-sulfamethoxazole (TMP-SMX) as the first-line agent in preference to sulfadiazine. The problems for TMP-SMP are treatment failure in some cases, lack of synergistic activity in approximately one third of species, and more toxicity in general than sulfadiazine alone. The increased toxicity is a particular problem in AIDS patients. Cycloserine has been advocated as an adjunctive therapy to the sulfadiazine. Additional agents that have been advocated include amikacin, cefotaxime, imipenim, ceftriaxone, and cefuroxime. Imipenim-cefotaxime, amikacin-TMP-SMX, and imipenim-TMP-SMX have all shown synergistic activity in vitro. Since the species of *Nocardia* vary in sensitivity it is advisable to obtain sensitivity testing on clinical isolates for selection of the most effective therapeutic agent or combination of agents.

Most forms of nocardiosis require 4-6 weeks of treatment. In many instances even more prolonged therapy is necessary. Clinical response to treatment does not occur early and an initial delay of clinical response should be expected.

REFERENCES

Anaissie E: Opportunistic mycoses in the immunocompromised host: experience at a cancer center and review, Clin Infect Dis 14(suppl 1):S43, 1992.

Bodey GP: Azole antifungal agents, Clin Infect Dis 14(suppl 1):S161, 1992.

Bross JE and Gordon G: Nocardial meningitis: case reports and review, Rev Infect Dis 13:160, 1991.

Budren P: Actinomycosis, J Infect 19:95, 1989.

Edwards JE Jr and Filler SG: Current strategies for treating invasive candidiasis: emphasis on infections in nonneutropenic patients, Clin Infect Dis 14(suppl 1):S106, 1992.

Fife TD, Finegold SM, and Grennan T: Pericardial actinomycosis: case report and review, Rev Infect Dis 13:120, 1991.

Goodman HM and Centeno BA: A 41-year-old woman with a swollen left leg, pelvic mass, and bilateral hydronephrosis. Case records of the Massachusetts General Hospital, New Eng J Med 326:692, 1992.

Kim J, Minamoto GY, and Grieco MH: Nocardial infection as a complication of AIDS: report of six cases and review, Rev Infect Dis 13:624, 1991.

Krone A et al: Nocardial cerebral abscess cured with imipenem/amikacin and enucleation, Neurosurg Rev 12:333, 1989.

Kwong JS et al: Thoracic actinomycosis: CT findings in eight patients, Radiology 183:189, 1992.

Lecciones JA et al: Vascular catheter-associated fungemia in patients with cancer: analysis of 155 episodes, Clin Infect Dis 14:875, 1992.

Meunier F, Aoun M, and Bitar N: Candidemia in immunocompromised patients, Clin Infect Dis 14(suppl 1):S120, 1992.

Perelow JH et al: Disseminated pelvic actinomycosis presenting as metastatic carcinoma: association with the progesteasert intrauterine device, Rev Infect Dis 13:1115, 1991.

Poland GA, Jorgensen CR, and Sarosi GA: *Nocardia asteroides* pericarditis: report of a case and review of the literature, Mayo Clin Proc 65:819, 1990.

Walsh TJ et al: Experimental antifungal chemotherapy in granulocytopenic animal models of disseminated candidiasis: approaches to understanding investigational antifungal compounds for patients with neoplastic diseases, Clin Infect Dis 14(suppl 1):S139, 1992.

Yew WW et al: Two cases of *Nocardia asteroides* sternotomy infection treated with ofloxacin and a review of other active antimicrobial agents, J Infect 23:297, 1991.

CHAPTER

279 *Cryptococcus neoformans* Infections

Michael S. Saag

Cryptococcosis, caused by *Cryptococcus neoformans,* is an indolent fungal infection acquired through the respiratory route. It primarily causes disease in the lungs, skin, and central nervous system (CNS) and is the leading cause of fungal meningitis in humans.

THE ORGANISM

Characteristics

C. neoformans exists as round or ellipsoid yeasts 4 to 6 μm in diameter, surrounded by a thick-walled polysaccharide capsule that is present in both tissue and cultural forms. Grown under aerobic conditions at room temperature on solid media such as Sabouraud glucose agar, the organism appears as smooth yellow or tan colonies, usually within 1 week of inoculation.

All species of cryptococci reproduce by budding, usually through one or two narrow-based buds from the parent cell. A sexual state, termed *Filobasidiella neoformans,* has recently been described. Since this phase produces filaments and terminal spores when reproducing sexually, the organism could technically be considered dimorphic. However, *C. neoformans* exists as a yeast both in infected tissue at 37° C and in culture at room temperature.

Four serotypes of *C. neoformans* are recognized: *C. neoformans* var. *neoformans* (serotypes A and D) and *C. neoformans* var. *gattii* (serotypes B and C). Serotypes differ in the size of their capsules, their biochemical properties, and their virulence in animal models of infection. Serotypes also differ in geographic distribution and frequency of isolation from pigeon droppings. Serotype A is the most common strain among both natural and clinical isolates and is found chiefly in the eastern and central United States. Interestingly, *C. neoformans* var. *neoformans* has been recovered almost exclusively from patients with cryptococcosis related to acquired immunodeficiency syndrome (AIDS), including those residing in areas such as southern California, Central Africa, and Australia, where var. *gattii* is endemic. In contrast to *C. neoformans,* nonpathogenic cryptococci do not grow at 37° C and are further distinguished from the pathogenic variety by specific biochemical tests.

Epidemiology

C. neoformans is widely distributed around the world, especially in soil enriched by pigeon droppings. Roosts and nests are also rich sources of the organism, although birds themselves are highly resistant to infection. Disease caused by *C. neoformans* has been described in warm-blooded feral animals as well as cattle, horses, cats, dogs, and dolphins. Humans acquire infection through inhalation of aerosolized yeasts; animal-to-human or human-to-human transmission has not been documented except in a single case of a corneal transplant recipient. Similarly, clusters of cases or mini-outbreaks suggesting a common source of infection have rarely been reported. No occupations are known to predispose to cryptococcosis; specifically, mycologists and other laboratory workers are not at increased risk, despite exposure to aerosols of the organism.

C. neoformans is not part of the normal pharyngeal flora, although it may colonize damaged respiratory tissue. Aside from the occasional patient who harbors *C. neoformans* in the sputum as a saprophyte, humans do not carry the organism chronically in an asymptomatic state. Cryptococcosis occurs at any age and has no obvious sex or occupational predilection. Most patients with cryptococcosis are immunocompromised, although 30% have no identifiable factor that predisposes them to infection. Many patients are receiving corticosteroids and/or immunosuppressive agents after renal transplantation or for therapy of lymphoreticular malignancies or chronic inflammatory diseases. Sarcoidosis and diabetes mellitus are less clearly established as predisposing factors. In addition, cryptococcosis is one of the opportunistic infections that occurs with increased frequency in persons with advanced human immunodeficiency virus type 1 (HIV-1) infection. As the most common cause of meningitis in this population, cryptococcal disease occurs in 7% of HIV-1–infected patients and is the initial AIDS-defining illness in 45% of those with cryptococcosis.

Pathophysiology

The polysaccharide capsule is an important virulence factor of *C. neoformans*. The capsule inhibits phagocytosis, impairs leukocyte migration, and induces T suppressor cell activity. Conversely, it also activates the alternate complement pathway, which results in production of opsonic and chemotactic factors necessary for an effective host response. Cellular immunity is the most important host defense. As a result, patients with defective T cell immunity, such as those with HIV-1 disease, are more likely to develop disseminated infection with *C. neoformans*. Neutrophils initially clear most of the cryptococci, whereas monocytes are prominent in the later inflammatory reaction. Within neutrophils and macrophages, myeloperoxidase-peroxide-halide activity, release of lysosomal hydrolases, and the presence of specific anticryptococcal antibody all play a role in the ingestion and killing of the organism.

After inhalation of aerosolized spores, most infections with *C. neoformans* begin as asymptomatic pulmonary foci from which hematogenous dissemination follows. Meningoencephalitis is the most common clinical expression of cryptococcosis. The preferential involvement of the CNS may be explained partially by the absence of complement and soluble anticryptococcal factors (which are present in plasma) in cerebrospinal fluid (CSF) and by a decreased or absent inflammatory response to cryptococci in brain tissue. The typical lesion of cryptococcal meningoencephalitis is a basilar arachnoiditis, which is often accompanied by clusters of yeasts scattered diffusely within the cerebral cortex and basal ganglia, frequently surrounded by little or no inflammation. Tissue damage results from physical displacement or compression caused by multiplying foci of organisms; no exotoxins are produced. Organ dysfunction is believed to be a function of fungal burden.

DISEASES PRODUCED IN HUMANS

Meningoencephalitis

The onset of CNS cryptococcosis is usually gradual, with symptoms waxing and waning over weeks to months. Headache is the most common symptom and occurs in more than three quarters of patients. Impairment of memory or judgment and alterations of personality are typical. Nausea or vomiting is present in one third of patients. Altered level of consciousness occurs less frequently but, when present, is associated with a poorer response to therapy (see later discussion). Blurred vision, dizziness, and clumsiness may be other complaints. Constitutional symptoms such as weight loss and malaise may occur, although chills and sweats are rare.

Fever, up to 102° F, is present in more than one half of patients and is the most common physical finding. Nuchal rigidity occurs in only 20% of patients and is less frequent in AIDS patients. Lethargy occurs in a third; more profound depression of consciousness is noted in about 15% of patients. Less common findings are papilledema, cranial nerve palsies, decreased visual acuity (occasionally from invasion of the optic nerve), diplopia, facial hypesthesia or paresis, and signs of focal motor tract involvement, including paresis, hyperreflexia, clonus, or extensor plantar response. Seizures occur in less than 5% of patients.

Among patients with AIDS, CNS disease occurs in 85% of those with cryptococcal disease. In this population, fever is present in 80% to 90%, and decreased levels of consciousness are noted in up to one third of patients; otherwise, symptoms and signs occur as described previously. Unexplained, protracted malaise and fever in a person with HIV infection should raise suspicion of cryptococcosis.

Untreated, cryptococcal meningoencephalitis is universally fatal; death may occur in as little as 2 weeks or may be delayed for several years. The illness may be more acute in patients receiving corticosteroids or other immunosuppressive agents. In contrast, AIDS patients with CNS cryptococcosis may have a more indolent course, often with symptoms present over weeks to months. A recrudescence of symptoms, especially altered mental status, after completion of treatment may signify relapse or the development of communicating hydrocephalus.

Intracranial mass lesions, or cryptococcomas, may or may not be associated with clinical meningitis. Lesions may be single or multiple. Headache is the most common symptom. Papilledema occurs in one third of patients, and focal neurologic findings, (e.g., hemiparesis, hemianopsia, seizures) are seen in two thirds.

Respiratory disease

The lungs are the only site of cryptococcal disease in up to 20% of patients. Saprophytic colonization of the respiratory tract is more common than cryptococcal pneumonia. Typically, patients have no symptoms or signs of pneumonia. Similarly, in patients with meningoencephalitis who also have a concomitant pulmonary cryptococcoma, the lung lesion is usually asymptomatic. Patients with chronic obstructive pulmonary disease, inactive tuberculosis, and lung cancer appear to be at increased risk. In symptomatic patients the most common complaints are dry cough, occasionally productive of scant sputum, dyspnea, dull chest pain, and rarely hemoptysis. Pleuritic disease occurs infrequently. With illness of longer duration, constitutional symptoms such as low-grade fever, sweats, and weight loss may occur. In patients with AIDS, fever and weight loss are common findings.

Spontaneous regression of clinical and radiographic manifestations occurs often, especially among immunocompetent patients. However, pulmonary disease occurring in an immunocompromised patient requires antifungal therapy. All patients with pulmonary cryptococcosis require an evaluation to rule out occult CNS disease.

Other disease manifestations

From 10% to 15% of patients with disseminated cryptococcosis have one or more cutaneous lesions. Skin lesions present as painless erythematous papules, pustules, or subcutaneous nodules that gradually enlarge, ulcerate, and eventually drain pus. The face and scalp are the most frequent sites of involvement.

Mucosal lesions, regional lymphadenopathy, and bone disease occur in less than 5% of patients. Infrequent manifestations of disseminated cryptococcosis include endophthalmitis, pericarditis, endocarditis, hepatitis, peritonitis, renal abscess, prostatitis, orchitis, myositis, arthritis, and bursitis.

DIAGNOSIS

Meningoencephalitis

A lumbar puncture or other procedure to obtain CSF is essential in the diagnosis of cryptococcal meningoencephalitis. The opening pressure is elevated in one third of patients and may be one of the most important signs predictive of poor outcome. Among non-AIDS patients the white blood cell count (WBC) ranges from 10 to 500 leukocytes/mm^3, predominantly consisting of lymphocytes and mononuclear cells. WBCs of 10 or fewer cells/mm^3 may be seen in as many as 25% of patients, especially among those with AIDS or other immunocompromised conditions. The glucose level is depressed to less than 50 mg/dl in two thirds of non-AIDS patients; HIV-infected patients usually have a normal glucose level. The protein level is increased in approximately 75% of patients, typically in the 50 to 300 mg/dl range. India ink preparations are positive in one half of non-AIDS patients (Fig. 279-1). The sensitivity of the

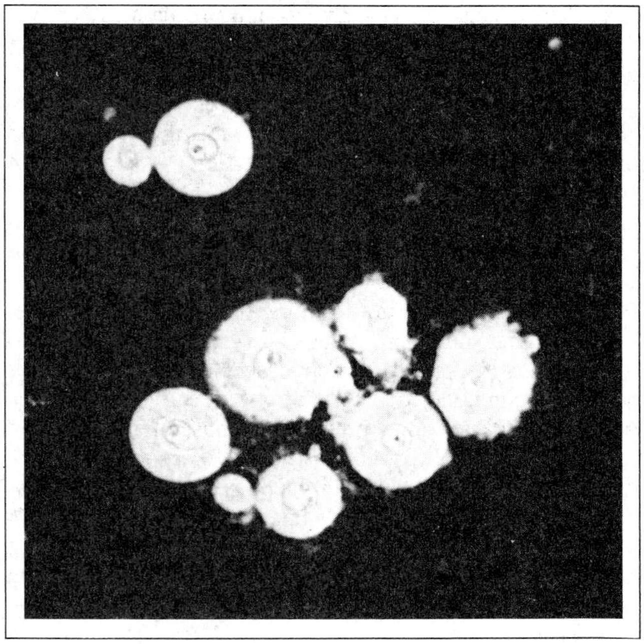

Fig. 279-1. India ink preparation showing *Cryptococcus neoformans* in cerebrospinal fluid. Note varying sizes of the cells and the characteristic budding, sharply demarcated capsules, and doubly refractile cell walls. (×1000.)

test is increased by centrifugation of large volumes of CSF and repeated examinations. In patients with AIDS, India ink preparations are positive in 75% and are often loaded with organisms; capsule-deficient yeasts have been observed. Because the CSF formula is often normal or only slightly abnormal in patients with AIDS, greater diagnostic reliance should be placed on the results of tests such as India ink preparation, culture, and CSF cryptococcal antigen titer.

The latex agglutination test to detect cryptococcal polysaccharide capsular antigen is a very useful, rapid diagnostic test of cryptococcal disease. CSF is positive at a titer of 1:8 or greater in more than 90% of non-AIDS patients; in AIDS patients the antigen titer is almost invariably positive, with median titers of 1:1024 or greater. Cryptococcal antigen, in varying titers, is present in the serum in more than 80% of non-AIDS patients and more than 95% of those with AIDS. The possibility of a prozone effect should be suspected when negative cryptococcal antigen titers are observed in AIDS patients with documented cryptococcosis. False-positive tests are infrequent but may be caused by high titers of rheumatoid factor. Serologic evaluation of anticryptococcal antibodies and skin testing with cryptococcal antigen are not helpful diagnostically.

Cultures on appropriate media (e.g., Sabouraud glucose agar) are the "gold standard" in establishing a diagnosis. For best sensitivity, cultures should be made from the centrifuged sediment of at least 3 ml of CSF. Cultures are usually positive within 7 days but should be held for 4 to 6 weeks before being reported as negative. Other possible sources of viable cryptococci include the blood (in 25% of non-AIDS patients, 67% of those with AIDS), urine, sputum, skin lesions, bone marrow, and prostatic secretions. AIDS patients with cryptococcal meningitis frequently have positive cultures from multiple sites.

Although sophisticated diagnostic procedures are not indicated routinely, most patients, especially those with AIDS or with altered sensorium at presentation, should undergo computed tomography (CT) of the head before their initial lumbar puncture. CT scans are abnormal in up to 30% of patients with *C. neoformans* disease; imaging studies also help rule out other concomitant processes such as CNS lymphoma or toxoplasmosis. Scanning or imaging is also useful in patients failing to respond to chemotherapy and to demonstrate the presence of hydrocephalus. Remarkably, normal to small-sized ventricles are usually noted, even when the CSF opening pressure is substantially elevated (especially in AIDS patients). The incidence of CNS cryptococcomas in patients with meningoencephalitis is unknown. Cryptococcomas are imaged on CT as isodense or lucent tumors that are enhanced homogeneously by contrast and may be surrounded by a small amount of edema, with or without mass effects.

Respiratory disease

Chest radiography usually reveals either a single, well-circumscribed mass lesion or multiple mass lesions that vary in size from small (1 to 3 cm) nodules to larger densities (5 to 10 cm in diameter). Segmental pneumonia, cavitation, hilar adenopathy, pleural effusion, and a diffuse interstitial pattern are less often seen. Calcification does not occur. Cryptococcal antigen is detectable in the serum of only one third of patients with lung disease alone. Expectorated sputum yields a positive culture in 10% to 30% of patients with invasive disease. Since saprophytic colonization of the respiratory tract may result in positive sputum cultures, a lung biopsy via bronchoscopy or thoracotomy is often required to establish a diagnosis of tissue-invading disease. *C. neoformans* appears as yeast cells with narrow-based buds, best seen with periodic acid–Schiff, methenamine silver, or mucicarmine stains. All lung biopsy specimens should be cultured on appropriate media.

Other tests

Skin, bone, and other cryptococcal lesions require biopsy for diagnosis. Organisms are usually present in abundance and easily demonstrated in wet-mount preparations, by special histologic stains, and by culture. Radiographs of bony lesions typically appear as cold abscesses with round, lytic foci and little or no sclerosis at the margins.

TREATMENT

Meningoencephalitis

Standard treatment of cryptococcosis in non-AIDS patients consists of amphotericin B (AMB), 0.3 mg/kg/day by intravenous (IV) infusion over 4 to 6 hours, plus flucytosine (5-FC), 100 to 150 mg/kg/day given in divided doses every 6 hours orally. Combination therapy usually permits the use of lower doses of AMB; however, higher doses of AMB, up to 0.5 to 0.8 mg/kg/day, should be considered for selected patients with severe cryptococcal disease or greatly impaired host defenses, such as those with HIV disease. Although a few reports of *C. neoformans* resistant to AMB have recently appeared, most cryptococci are sensitive to the drug. Less than 5% of cryptococcal isolates are initially resistant to 5-FC, but most isolates rapidly become resistant when 5-FC is used as monotherapy. However, the emergence of resistance during therapy is infrequent when 5-FC is combined with AMB. Diarrhea, nausea, vomiting, leukopenia, thrombocytopenia, and hepatitis are common toxicities of 5-FC that may require reduction in dosage or discontinuation of the drug. Because the drug is excreted by the kidneys, dosage should also be adjusted in patients with renal insufficiency. 5-FC doses are reduced by 50% when the creatinine clearance is 25 to 50 ml/min and by 75% when the clearance is 10 to 25 ml/min. With severe renal impairment and/or dialysis, use of 5-FC should be avoided or dosages should be adjusted to maintain a serum level of 50 to 100 μg/ml 2 hours after an oral dose. During combination therapy the serum creatinine level should be monitored twice weekly and the creatinine clearance and serum 5-FC level measured weekly in all patients.

Cultures of CSF usually become sterile within 10 to 14 days with the combination regimen in non-AIDS patients. If blood and CSF cultures become negative within the first 2 weeks of therapy and the patient regains his or her baseline neurologic status, treatment can usually be stopped after a total of 6 weeks. Nonimmunosuppressed patients who have no neurologic complications and have pretreatment serum cryptococcal antigen titers less than 1:32 and CSF leukocyte counts of 20 cells/mm^3 or greater may be successfully treated with 4 weeks of combination AMB/5-FC therapy. By the end of the fourth week of treatment, serum and CSF titers should be less than 1:8 and CSF India ink preparation should be negative for the patient to be eligible for this short course of therapy. The overall rate of cure when these criteria are met is about 90%. All transplant recipients and patients with AIDS must be treated for at least 6 weeks. Serial lumbar punctures with CSF cultures are indicated at least at weeks 2, 4, and 6. In patients with persistently positive CSF cultures, treatment must be continued for 8 to 12 weeks.

An initial course of combination therapy cures two thirds of non-AIDS patients; one sixth die during the first few weeks, and one sixth relapse after the conclusion of seemingly successful therapy. Among the patients who relapse after therapy, more than 90% do so within 6 months. Relapsed patients are cured by retreatment with the same regimen in half the cases. Even among patients who are initially cured, up to 40% may have a persistent neurologic deficit, such as loss of visual acuity, cranial nerve palsy, localized paresis, or personality change.

Among non-AIDS patients, favorable pretreatment prognostic factors for successful therapy are normal mental status, headache, and CSF leukocyte count greater than 20 cells/mm^3. A serum cryptococcal antigen titer of 1:32 or greater decreases the likelihood of cure. Favorable factors during antifungal treatment are lack of immunosuppressive therapy, return to normal or baseline neurologic status, sterile CSF culture after 2 weeks, and negative India ink preparation after 4 weeks. A serum or CSF cryptococcal antigen titer of less than 1:8 at the end of treatment also favors cure. On the other hand, a serum or CSF titer of 1:8 or greater at 1, 3, or 6 months after the completion of therapy increases the likelihood of relapse. Susceptibility of the patient's cryptococcal isolate to 5-FC does not correlate with outcome.

Single-drug therapy with IV AMB, 0.4 to 0.8 mg/kg/day, is an acceptable alternative to combination therapy for those patients unable to take 5-FC. Usually, 8 to 12 weeks of treatment are needed to obtain results similar to those with combination therapy. The use of intrathecal AMB generally is not required; however, it may be helpful in those patients who have failed conventional treatment or in those who have renal insufficiency that would be further impaired by additional IV AMB. Miconazole appears to offer no advantage over established regimens; however, in selected patients with refractory cryptococcosis, miconazole given IV and intrathecally may be curative. Ketoconazole does not provide adequate CSF concentrations or adequate anticryptococcal activity to treat meningoencephalitis effectively.

Fluconazole, a novel bistriazole antifungal agent, has recently been shown to be effective in the treatment of AIDS-associated cryptococcal meningitis. In a comparative study of oral fluconazole (200 mg/day) versus IV AMB (0.4 to 0.5 mg/kg/day) conducted by the National Institutes of Health Mycoses Study Group and the AIDS Clinical Trials Group, successful outcome, defined as two consecutive negative CSF cultures within a 10-week period, was noted in 40% of AMB recipients and 34% of fluconazole recipients ($p = 0.40$). A remarkable number of patients in each group (27% and 26% in AMB and fluconazole groups, respectively) had so-called quiescent disease, defined as clinical improvement or resolution of symptoms with persistently positive or only one negative culture within the 10-week study period. Therefore overall clinical response to either AMB or fluconazole was 67% versus 60% ($p = 0.39$), respectively. Toxicity requiring discontinuation of drug occurred more often in AMB than in fluconazole recipients (8% versus 2%, $p = 0.02$). Mortality from cryptococcal disease was no different between the two groups (14% AMB versus 18% fluconazole), although most deaths in the fluconazole group occurred within the first 2 weeks of treatment. The most important presenting factor predictive of mortality was abnormal mental status; other pretreatment factors that were less strongly predictive included CSF cryptococcal antigen titer greater than 1:1024 and a CSF WBC less than 20 cells/mm^3. Overall, time to the first negative CSF culture was similar in each group; however, a trend toward earlier conversion of CSF cultures was noted in the AMB group (Fig. 279-2). Taken together, the later conversion of CSF cultures and the trend toward more early deaths in the fluconazole group suggest that initial treatment with oral triazole therapy is best reserved for those patients with normal mental status at baseline.

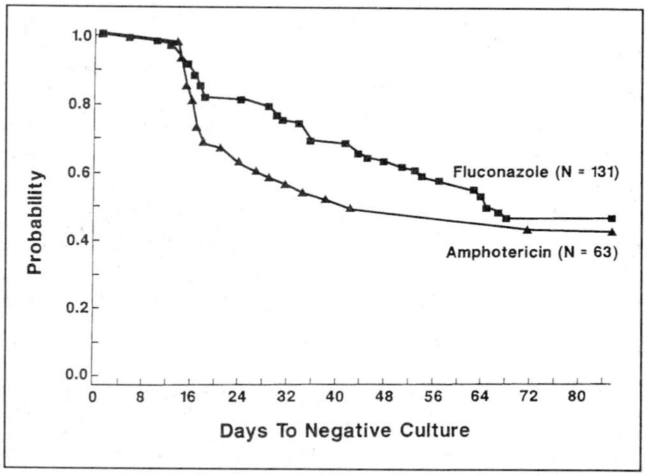

Fig. 279-2. Kaplan-Meier estimates of length of time to first negative CSF culture when comparing intravenous amphotericin B (0.4 mg/kg/d) with fluconazole (200 mg/day orally) as treatment for acute cryptococcal meningitis in AIDS patients. (Reproduced with permission from NEJM 326:83, 1992.)

Optimum therapy for those patients with baseline presenting factors indicative of poor outcome remains to be defined. Clinical trials of small numbers of patients suggest higher doses of AMB (0.7 mg/kg/day for the first 2 weeks), with or without 5-FC, may be more effective than standard doses of AMB. The use of 5-FC in AIDS patients remains controversial; excessive toxicity has been noted in some reports, whereas other reports imply superior outcome. Careful clinical monitoring is required whenever 5-FC is administered to patients with HIV disease.

In contrast to the 15% relapse rate among non-AIDS patients, more than 80% of AIDS patients will develop recurrent disease unless long-term suppressive therapy is administered. A recently conducted trial has demonstrated superior outcome in patients receiving daily oral fluconazole (200 mg/day) compared with once weekly IV therapy with AMB (1 mg/kg/wk). In that study, 2 of 111 (2%) fluconazole patients relapsed compared with 14 of 78 (18%) AMB recipients ($p < 0.001$). All patients in this study had negative cultures at initial evaluation. Estimates of the proportion of patients remaining relapse free at 1 year are shown in Fig. 279-3. Toxicity also occurred more frequently in AMB recipients, with more than two thirds of AMB patients having an adverse experience compared with one third of fluconazole recipients. Daily fluconazole is now the treatment of choice as maintenance therapy in AIDS-associated cryptococcal disease.

The role of fluconazole as primary prophylaxis for cryptococcal disease, and fungal infection in general, is poorly established. Routine prophylaxis of all patients with advanced HIV disease is not recommended at this time because of the possibility of establishing triazole-resistant organisms. No information exists regarding the use of fluconazole as primary treatment of cryptococcosis in non-AIDS patients. Moreover, routine maintenance therapy to prevent relapse of cryptococcal infection in the non-AIDS population is usually not required.

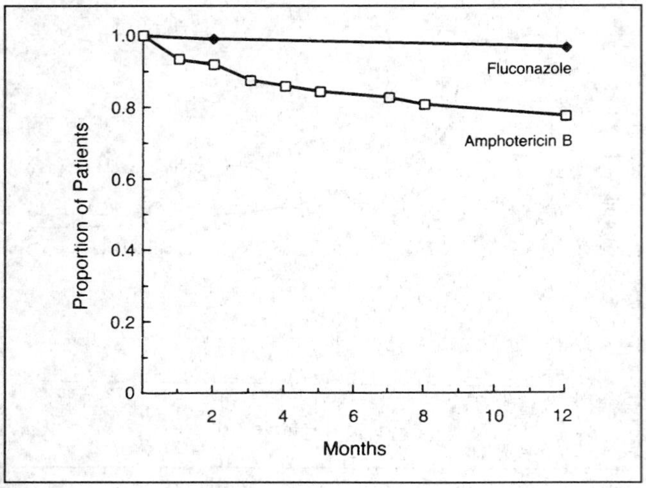

Fig. 279-3. Kaplan-Meier estimates of the proportion of patients remaining free of cryptococcal disease after receiving maintenance therapy with either amphotericin B (1.0 mg/kg/week) or fluconazole (200 mg/day) for 1 year. (Reprinted with permission from NEJM 326:793, 1992).

Respiratory disease

In all patients with pulmonary cryptococcosis, evidence of extrapulmonary disease should be carefully sought. CSF evaluation should be performed in all patients with pulmonary disease, even if no CNS symptoms or signs are present. In normal hosts with no evidence of extrapulmonary involvement, 2 or 3 months of observation without therapy is indicated for pulmonary lesions that are small and not increasing in size or number. During this time, chest radiography, serum cryptococcal antigen titer, and sputum culture should be repeated at monthly intervals until the lesions resolve, the antigen titer significantly falls or becomes negative, and cultures are persistently negative. Treatment, as previously outlined for meningeal disease, is indicated if the patient's clinical status deteriorates, the chest radiograph worsens, or evidence of CNS involvement develops. All immunocompromised patients with pulmonary cryptococcosis require treatment to prevent dissemination. The duration of therapy depends on clinical response and results of chest radiographs, cryptococcal antigen titers, and cultures. The role of fluconazole therapy for isolated pulmonary disease remains to be established. Surgery generally is not indicated, but resection of a single nodule in a normal host is curative.

Other disease

The presence of skin, bone, or other lesions indicates that hematogenous dissemination has occurred; consequently, chemotherapy is always necessary. A lumbar puncture to rule out CNS disease is required. Debridement may be helpful in patients with osseous disease. AMB, with or without 5-FC, is administered until there has been clinical, serologic, cultural, and radiographic resolution of all lesions. The roles of ketoconazole, fluconazole, and itraconazole, another investigational orally administered triazole compound, remain to be determined for treatment of patients with non-CNS cryptococcal disease.

REFERENCES

Bennett JE et al: A comparison of amphotericin B alone and combined with flucytosine in the treatment of cryptococcal meningitis. N Engl J Med 301:126, 1979.

Chuck SL and Sande MA: Infections with *Cryptococcus neoformans* in the acquired immunodeficiency syndrome. N Engl J Med 321:794, 1989.

de Wytt CN et al: Cryptococcal meningitis: a review of 32 years' experience. J Neurol Sci 53:283, 1982.

Dismukes WE: Cryptococcal meningitis in patients with AIDS. J Infect Dis 157:624, 1988.

Dismukes WE et al: Treatment of cryptococcal meningitis with combination amphotericin B and flucytosine for four as compared with six weeks. N Engl J Med 317:334, 1987.

Fromtling RA and Shadomy HJ: Immunity in cryptococcosis: an overview. Mycopathologia 77:183, 1982.

Fujita NK et al: Cryptococcal intracerebral mass lesions: the role of computed tomography and nonsurgical management. Ann Intern Med 94:382, 1981.

Kerkering TM et al: The evolution of pulmonary cryptococcosis: clinical implications from a study of 41 patients with and without compromising host factors. Ann Intern Med 94:611, 1981.

Kovacs JA et al: Cryptococcosis in the acquired immunodeficiency syndrome. Ann Intern Med 103:533, 1985.

Larsen RA et al: Fluconazole compared with amphotericin B plus flucytosine for cryptococcal meningitis in AIDS: a randomized trial. Ann Intern Med 113:183, 1990.

Liss HP and Rimland D: Asymptomatic cryptococcal meningitis. Am Rev Respir Dis 124:88, 1981.

Perfect JR et al: Cryptococcemia. Medicine (Baltimore) 62:98, 1983.

Powderly WG et al: A controlled trial of fluconazole or amphotericin B to prevent relapse of cryptococcal meningitis in patients with the acquired immunodeficiency syndrome. N Engl J Med 326:793, 1992.

Saag MS et al: Comparison of amphotericin B with fluconazole in the treatment of acute AIDS associated cryptococcal meningitis. N Engl J Med 326:83, 1992.

Stamm AM et al: Toxicity of amphotericin B plus flucytosine in 194 patients with cryptococcal meningitis. Am J Med 83:236, 1987.

PROTOZOAL DISEASES

CHAPTER

280 Infections Caused by Protozoa

James H. Leech
Carolyn Petersen

Protozoa are unicellular organisms that have the basic cellular organization of eukaryotes; that is, the cellular contents are delineated into many membrane-bound organelles (nuclei, mitochondria, Golgi complexes, lysosomes, food vacuoles). Most protozoa that infect humans are obligatory parasites, meaning they are obliged to live in or on host cells and derive protection and nutrition from the host. However, not all the pathogenic protozoa are obligatory parasites. For example, *Naegleria* and *Acanthamoeba* are free-living amebae that can invade the human nervous system. Conversely, some parasitic protozoa may infect humans but rarely, if ever, cause disease. These organisms are able to live in apparent harmony with the host and are considered to be commensals. Examples of parasitic protoza that are usually commensals are *Dientamoeba fragilis* and *Blastocystis hominis*.

The classification of the protoza that infect humans is currently based on differences in morphology and life cycle (Table 280-1). All share the ability to multiply in the human host to virtually unlimited numbers, except when limited by innate resistance or acquired immunity. Many parasitic protozoa have developed mechanisms for evading the host's immune response, leading to persistent and repeated infections.

Clinicians and public health workers need to have a broad general knowledge of protozoology for two reasons. First, some parasitic protozoa have worldwide distributions and can pose clinical and public health problems anywhere. For example, infections with *Toxoplasma, Isospora,* and *Cryptosporidium* typically occur in patients with acquired immunodeficiency syndrome (AIDS) and are being seen with increasing frequency in the United States (Chapter 242). Second, international travelers and refugees may bring protozoa ordinarily limited to the tropics to the notice of clinicians in developed countries. It is thus essential that clinicians recognize when protozoan diseases should be considered in the differential diagnosis.

Table 280-1. Classification of parasitic protozoa

Classification	Characteristics	Examples
Phylum Sarcomastigophora		
Subphylum Mastigophora	Trophozoites have one or more flagella; asexual reproduction	*Leishmania* *Trypanosoma* *Giardia* *Dientamoeba* *Trichomonas*
Subphylum Sarcodina	Locomotion by pseudopods	*Entamoeba* *Acanthamoeba* (free living) *Naegleria* (free living)
Phylum Apicomplexa	Invasive stages have apical organelles	
Class Sporozoa (Sporozoea)	Asexual (schizogony) and sexual (sporogony) reproductive cycles	*Isospora* *Toxoplasma* *Plasmodium* *Babesia* *Cryptosporidium* *Sarcocystis*
Phylum Microspora	Released into a cell from a spore by ejection from a long coiled polar tube	*Encephalitozoon* *Enterocytozoon* *Nosema* *Pleistophora*
Phylum Ciliophora	Simple cilia or compound ciliary organelles; asexual (binary) fission and sexual (conjugation) multiplication	*Balantidium*

MALARIA

Human malaria is caused by four species of *Plasmodium: P. falciparum, P. vivax, P. ovale,* and *P. malariae*. Each species has its own characteristic epidemiology, biology, morphology, and clinical manifestations. *P. falciparum* causes most of the morbidity and virtually all the mortality resulting from malaria and also presents the problem of drug resistance. The occurrence of *P. falciparum* in a nonimmune host, such as a traveler, is a medical emergency that demands hospitalization and prompt treatment with appropriate drugs. In some imported cases, death from falciparum malaria has resulted from delay in diagnosis or failure to institute proper treatment. *P. vivax, P. ovale,* and *P. malariae* can cause significant morbidity but rarely cause death and are generally sensitive to the most frequently used antimalarial drug, chloroquine. In the tropics and subtropics, malaria continues to be one of the most prevalent of all infectious diseases despite the use of insecticides against the vector and antimalarial drugs for the treatment and prophylaxis of disease. The failure of these methods to eradicate malaria has led scientists to study other approaches to the control of malaria, including new approaches to treatment, malaria vaccines, and the biologic control of mosquitoes. Research on the molecular biology of malaria parasites has accelerated in the past decade and is yielding new insights into the pathogenesis of malaria.

Biology and life cycle

About 100 species of plasmodia infect a variety of vertebrates, including birds, reptiles, monkeys, apes, and humans. Each species of plasmodia exhibits remarkable host specificity, which is probably based on the parasite's recognition of specific receptor molecules on the surface of the host's cells. Except for some laboratory infections, virtually no exchange of plasmodia occurs between humans and animals. This means that no animal reservoir of human malaria exists and that the parasite is maintained in nature by alternating between a sexual life cycle in mosquitoes and an asexual life cycle in humans.

Female anopheline mosquitoes are the only insect vectors of human malaria. Among the approximately 400 species of *Anopheles,* 25 to 30 are associated with a significant degree of malaria transmission. The capacity of a particular species to be a vector is determined by the efficiency with which malaria parasites infect and complete their life cycle in the mosquito, by the preference of the mosquito for human blood rather than animal blood, and by the longevity of the mosquito. During a blood meal, female anopheline mosquitoes inoculate sporozoites into the subcutaneous capillaries of the human host. The sporozoites circulate in peripheral blood for less than an hour. They rapidly invade hepatic parenchymal cells, where they proliferate into thousands of intracellular merozoites. The parasites within hepatic cells are called *exoerythrocytic forms*. Between 1 and 2 weeks after the initial mosquito bite, the merozoites rupture the hepatic cell and are released into the circulation, where they immediately invade erythrocytes to begin the erythrocytic stage of the infection. All the exoerythrocytic forms of *P. falciparum* and *P. malariae* rupture at the same time; none persist in the liver. With *P. vivax* and *P. ovale,* however, not all the exoerythrocytic forms rupture initially. Some remain dormant for months or years before they rupture and produce relapses of erythrocytic infection. The dormant exoerythrocytic forms are called *hypnozoites*. Erythrocytic parasites never reinvade the liver. Therefore only *P. vivax* and *P. ovale* that are transmitted by mosquitoes can produce relapses.

After the merozoites invade the host's erythrocytes, most of the parasites develop asexually from young ring forms into larger, more cytoplasmic trophozoites. They then undergo asexual division and become schizonts, which contain 6 to 24 merozoites, the number varying with the species of plasmodia. When mature, the schizont ruptures the host erythrocyte and releases the merozoites, which rapidly invade fresh erythrocytes and begin the asexual life cycle again. The duration of the erythrocytic life cycle is 48 hours with *P. falciparum, P. vivax,* and *P. ovale* and 72 hours with *P. malariae*.

Some intraerythrocytic parasites do not develop asexually but differentiate into sexual parasites, the gametocytes. Gametocytes (male and female) can be distinguished morphologically from asexual parasites, and the gametocytes of different *Plasmodium* species can also be distinguished from each other. Once ingested by a mosquito, the gametocytes lyse the erythrocyte and become extracellular in the gut of the mosquito. The male gametocyte releases eight spermlike gametes, one of which fertilizes the female gamete to produce a zygote. The zygote rapidly transforms into an ookinete, which penetrates the wall of the mosquito's midgut and forms an oocyst. Within the oocyst, thousands of sporozoites develop over 9 to 14 days, depending on the ambient temperature. This process (sporogony) is more rapid at warm temperatures and ceases altogether at temperatures below 20° C for *P. falciparum* and 16° C for *P. vivax*. Sporogony culminates with rupture of the oocyst and release of the sporozoites. The sporozoites migrate to the mosquito's salivary glands and are injected into a human or animal during the next blood meal.

The invasion of hepatocytes by sporozoites and of erythrocytes by merozoites is mediated by specific receptors on the parasite surface that recognize determinants on the surface of the host cell. A major protein on the surface of the sporozoite has been identified, and its gene has been cloned and sequenced. Monoclonal antibodies to this protein inhibit the invasion of hepatocytes by sporozoites, and vaccines that produce immunity to the sporozoite surface protein are currently being tested. Candidate receptor molecules on the surface of merozites have also been identified. In addition, much has been learned recently about determinants on the erythrocyte surface that are involved in invasion. The Duffy blood group system appears to be required for invasion of erythrocytes by *P. vivax*. Blacks who are Duffy blood group negative (FyFy) are refractory to erythrocytic infection by *P. vivax*. The sialoglycoproteins (glycophorin and band 3) on the erythrocyte surface appear to be involved in invasion by *P. falciparum*. *P. vivax* and *P. ovale* can invade only reticulocytes, which limits the parasitemia to the number of circulating reticulocytes. *P. falciparum* invades reticulocytes preferentially but can infect erythrocytes of all ages, thereby producing infections with high parasitemias. *P. malariae* infects only mature erythrocytes.

Intraerythrocytic malaria parasites derive their energy from the anaerobic metabolism of glucose to lactic acid. Infected erythrocytes consume much more glucose than uninfected erythrocytes, and in some patients with very high parasitemias, this consumption of glucose may contribute to hypoglycemia. Malarial parasites obtain most of their amino acids for protein synthesis by ingesting hemoglobin from the host erythrocyte and digesting it within a food vacuole. Compounds that inhibit hemoglobin degradation by the parasite provide a promising new approach to treatment for malaria. A by-product of the hemoglobin digestion is malarial pigment (hemozoin), which consists of ferriprotoporphyrin IX, methemoglobin, and some malarial proteins. The parasites synthesize pyrimidines de novo but obtain purines from the host erythrocyte or from the blood plasma.

Malarial parasites produce morphologic and functional changes in the membranes of infected erythrocytes. *P. falciparum* produces protrusions, called *knobs,* on the surface of erythrocytes containing trophozoites and schizonts. Knobs mediate attachment to venular endothelium. The parasites are thereby sequestered in the postcapillary venules of many organs. Because of sequestration, only ring forms of *P. falciparum* circulate in peripheral blood, a property that is helpful in distinguishing *P. falciparum* from other species of plasmodia. The mature parasites that are sequestered avoid circulating through the spleen, which is a major site of parasite destruction in malaria. In addition, the sequestered parasites may obstruct blood flow in cerebral vessels, leading to cerebral malaria. *P. vivax* and *P. ovale* produce indentations in the erythrocyte membrane, called *caveolar-vesicle junctions,* which on Giemsa-stained blood smears produce the characteristic Schüffner's dots. The function of the caveolar-vesicle junctions is not known. The membrane of schizont-infected erythrocytes is more permeable to some small molecules than is the membrane of uninfected erythrocytes. This partial permeability may contribute to the increased uptake of glucose by infected erythrocytes and also leads to an increase in the intraerythrocytic sodium concentration and a decrease in the intraerythrocytic potassium concentration of infected erythrocytes. An excessive loss of potassium occurs with the *P. falciparum*–infected erythrocytes of individuals with hemoglobin S/A (Hb S/A) at low oxygen tensions. This loss of intracellular potassium is detrimental to the parasite and may be the mechanism for the protective effect of Hb S/A in falciparum malaria, since sequestration in postcapillary venules exposes the infected erythrocytes to low oxygen tension for 24 hours or longer.

Epidemiology

Accurate data on the worldwide occurrence of malaria and the number of deaths from malaria are not available. However, most authorities estimate that there are more than 100 million cases per year worldwide and more than 1 million deaths from malaria each year in Africa alone. Endemic malaria is largely a tropical disease, since mosquito transmission requires high relative humidity (> 35%) for mosquito longevity and high ambient temperature (> 16° C) for the sporogonic cycle of the parasite in mosquitoes. The degree to which *P. falciparum* is endemic within an area is determined by the intensity of mosquito transmission and by host immunity. Intense, year-round transmission results in a high prevalence (> 75%) of infection and disease in young children, but those who survive to adulthood have acquired immunity and generally have few or no symptoms. With intense seasonal transmission, adults as well as children have symptomatic infections because immunity wanes during the seasons when no transmission occurs. With less intense transmission, the prevalence of infection falls, but the infections that occur often produce severe disease in children and adults.

Tropical Africa south of the Sahara is the major focus of malaria in the world (see the box at right). *P. falciparum* is the predominant malarial parasite and causes high mortality in children. Those who survive to adulthood usually have a high degree of acquired immunity. *P. falciparum* is also prevalent in India, Southeast Asia, Haiti, New Guinea, Mexico, Central America, and South America. *P. vivax* can be transmitted at lower ambient temperatures than *P. falciparum* and thus has a range that extends further into the temperate zone countries. *P. vivax* is the predominant malarial parasite in India, Sri Lanka, Pakistan, Bangladesh, and Central America and is also quite prevalent in Southeast Asia, South America, and Oceania. *P. ovale* has replaced *P. vivax* in West Africa and much of East Africa because most blacks in these areas have the Duffy blood group–negative phenotype and are resistant to *P. vivax*. *P. malariae* is cosmopolitan.

Most patients who are seen with malaria in Europe and the United States are refugees, travelers, or military personnel who acquired their infections in endemic areas (imported cases). Other causes of malaria in nonendemic areas include congenital malaria, blood transfusion, and the sharing of needles by drug addicts. A relatively new phenomenon is the occurrence of malaria among individuals residing near international airports because of the accidental importation of infected mosquitoes ("airport malaria"). In the central valley of California, occasional outbreaks of *P. vivax* malaria are transmitted by local *Anopheles* mosquitoes, which become infected by feeding on immigrants or migrant farm workers with malaria. Congenital malaria is transmitted at birth and should be considered in any infant born to a mother who has recently emigrated from an endemic area. The incidence of transfusion malaria has been greatly reduced by the exclusion of donors for 3 years after travel to or residence in an endemic area. However, since *P. vivax* and *P. ovale* may persist in the human host for 3 to 5 years and *P. malariae* for 50 years or more, an occasional case of transfusion malaria can still be expected to occur.

Geographic distribution of malaria*

P. falciparum
Sub-Saharan Africa
Southeast Asia
Haiti
New Guinea, Oceania
India, Pakistan
South America
Central America
Mexico
Middle East

P. vivax
India
Sri Lanka
Pakistan
Bangladesh
Southeast Asia
South America
Central America
Mexico
Asia
New Guinea
Oceania
Middle East

P. ovale
Africa

P. malariae
All malarious areas

*Areas where particular species of malaria are predominant. However, malaria must be considered as a potential cause of disease in travelers to all areas of the tropics and subtropics.

Pathogenesis and immunity

The clinical manifestations of malaria are caused entirely by asexual, erythrocytic parasites. Symptoms, as well as morbidity and mortality, generally occur at lower parasitemias in nonimmune hosts. The fundamental processes in the pathogenesis of malaria are (1) the rupture of schizont-infected erythrocytes, with release of merozoites plus pyrogens and toxins; (2) destruction of host erythrocytes by the rupturing parasites; (3) changes in rheology produced by decreased deformability of infected erythrocytes and by the adherence of *P. falciparum*–infected erythrocytes to the endothelium of postcapillary venules; and (4) response of the host's immune and reticuloendothelial systems to malaria.

Malaria characteristically causes paroxysms of fever.

These paroxysms occur at the time of rupture of schizonts and are probably caused by unidentified pyrogens and other toxins released by the rupturing schizonts. The fever pattern is determined by the degree to which the erythrocytic parasites are synchronized and rupture together. Thus highly synchronized infections produce a regular, intermittent fever pattern that occurs every 48 or 72 hours, depending on the species of plasmodia. However, infections are frequently asynchronous, especially with *P. falciparum*. When the erythrocytic parasites are not synchronized, the fever pattern may be irregular or even continuous. The fever of malaria is associated with peripheral vasodilatation and a reduced effective intravascular volume.

Anemia is a common manifestation of malaria caused by all four species of plasmodia. The predominant mechanism is hemolysis secondary to the rupture of infected erythrocytes, although some children with chronic malaria may also have a dyserythropoietic state with low reticulocyte counts and recovery after treatment with antimalarials. Hemolysis may also be secondary to a Coombs-positive hemolytic anemia induced by quinine or may be produced by the administration of oxidant drugs, (e.g., primaquine) to patients with glucose-6-phosphate dehydrogenase (G6PD) deficiency. With *P. falciparum,* high parasitemias or drug-induced hemolysis may produce marked intravascular hemolysis and hemoglobinuric renal failure ("blackwater fever").

The consequences of rheologic changes occur predominantly with *P. falciparum*. Erythrocytes containing trophozoites and schizonts have reduced deformability, which may lead to sluggish blood flow through the capillaries. In addition, infected erythrocytes adhere specifically to venular endothelium through parasite-induced knobs on the erythrocyte membrane. Blood flow therefore may be obstructed, with resultant tissue anoxia, and changes also may occur in the permeability of the venular and capillary endothelium, allowing blood to extravasate into surrounding tissues. The principal target organs are the brain and intestines. A variety of cerebral symptoms may be produced in *P. falciparum* infections (cerebral malaria; see next section). Pathologically the capillaries and venules of the gray matter of the cortex are filled with infected erythrocytes, ring hemorrhages develop around capillaries, and the brain is edematous. Sequestration and sludging in the intestinal capillaries and venules may lead to diarrhea and malabsorption.

Renal failure in *P. falciparum* malaria may result from hemoglobinuria, acute tubular necrosis, or ischemia of the renal cortex, perhaps related to splanchnic vasoconstriction. Pulmonary edema occurs in *P. falciparum* malaria, often as a terminal event. Increased permeability of the pulmonary-capillary membrane appears to occur, but the pathogenesis of this complication is not known.

The host's immune response also contributes to the pathogenesis of some manifestations of malaria. Elevated levels of tumor necrosis factor have been correlated with severe falciparum malaria. Thrombocytopenia occurs frequently with all four species of plasmodia, but its cause is unknown. A chronic, immune complex glomerulonephritis occurs with *P. malariae*. The immune complexes contain antibody specific for *P. malariae* antigens as well as complement. This complication does not respond to treatment with antimalarials. It is not known why immune complex disease does not occur with the other species of plasmodia. Splenomegaly and occasionally hypersplenism are caused by hyperplasia of the reticuloendothelial system. Some patients who reside in endemic areas of Africa, Indonesia, and New Guinea develop chronic, massive splenomegaly and a lymphocytic infiltrate in the sinusoids of the liver (tropical splenomegaly). Often these patients have high levels of antimalarial antibodies and no detectable parasites in their peripheral blood, but they respond to chronic antimalarial chemoprophylaxis. The pathogenesis of this syndrome is unknown. Malaria may prevent the host from developing a normal immune response to antigenic challenge, causing reduced response to some vaccines and a greater chance of intercurrent infection during malaria.

Acquired immunity to malaria develops only after repeated or prolonged infection and is predominantly directed against erythrocytic parasites. Immunity is usually not sterile, and individuals can be infected and may have circulating parasites, but the infection produces no symptoms. Immunity to malaria is species specific. With *P. falciparum* malaria, immunity has been shown to be strain specific, indicating that antigenic diversity exists among parasites. Although the passive transfer of antibody from immune individuals to nonimmune individuals protects against the symptoms of malaria, the renewed induction of immunity requires helper T cells. The spleen is the major site of parasite destruction in malaria and is of primary importance in the host's survival. The mechanisms of parasite killing in the spleen are not known. Splenectomy may lead to a recurrence of disease or may render a previously immune individual susceptible to severe disease.

Besides acquired immunity, several genetically determined host factors influence host susceptibility to malaria. Hb S, thalassemia, and G6PD deficiency are associated geographically with the distribution of *P. falciparum* malaria. Direct evidence indicates that individuals who are heterozygous for the Hb S gene (Hb A/S) have a selective advantage against *P. falciparum* malaria compared with either homozygote (Hb A/A or Hb S/S). This has led to the persistence of the gene for Hb S as a balanced polymorphism in endemic areas. The mechanism of protection by Hb S appears to be the inhibition of parasite growth in Hb A/S erythrocytes at the low oxygen tensions that occur during sequestration in postcapillary venules. Other forms of genetically determined resistance include the Duffy blood group–negative phenotype (FyFy), which confers resistance to *P. vivax,* and ovalocytosis, which results in reduced invasion of erythrocytes by *P. falciparum*. The mutations that have been selected by malaria are an important legacy of the disease that will persist long after the disease is eradicated.

Clinical manifestations

Patients infected by mosquito bite have an incubation period of 8 to 30 days before the onset of symptoms. However, chemoprophylaxis may prolong the incubation period to several months (all four species) or several years (*P. vivax, P. ovale.*) Before the onset of fever, many patients have a prodrome consisting of malaise, myalgia, cough, and headache that is often mistaken for a viral illness. The most characteristic symptom of malaria caused by all four species of plasmodia is the paroxysm of a shaking chill followed by fever and then sweating. The fever typically lasts for several hours and may reach 40° C or higher. With *P. falciparum,* the fever may last longer or may be continuous. Many patients also have nausea, vomiting, diarrhea, headache, backache, abdominal pain, or delirium during the fever. Resolution of the fever is often accompanied by drenching sweats.

Periodicity of the fever is produced by synchronized infections in which all the schizonts rupture at the same time. Synchronized infections occur most often with *P. malariae* (paroxysms every 72 hours) and with relapses of *P. vivax* and *P. ovale* (paroxysms every 48 hours). Some patients may be quite asymptomatic between paroxysms. Fever is less likely to be periodic in *P. falciparum* infections or in the initial attack of *P. vivax.*

On physical examination, many patients have splenomegaly and liver tenderness. Vigorous palpation of the spleen should be avoided because of the risk of splenic rupture. Scleral icterus, jaundice, and herpes labialis sometimes occur. During the rigor that initiates the malaria paroxysm, patients may have cold skin because of vasoconstriction. During the febrile stage, the skin is warm and postural hypotension may be caused by peripheral vasodilatation.

Patients usually have a normochromic, normocytic anemia from hemolysis, a moderate leukopenia, and thrombocytopenia. The thrombocytopenia is rarely sufficient to cause bleeding. The peripheral smear may show monocytes containing malarial pigment. Malaria does not cause eosinophilia. Hyponatremia is common in *P. falciparum* malaria and is probably caused by sodium depletion and water retention. The urine should be examined for the presence of hemoglobinuria or evidence of acute tubular necrosis. The serum bilirubin level may be mildly elevated because of hemolysis, and there may be transaminase elevations to three to four times the normal values. More marked rise in the transaminase levels should raise the question of centrilobular necrosis (seen in severe malaria) or the possibility of another disease (e.g., viral hepatitis). The serum glucose level should be checked in patients with *P. falciparum* malaria, since hypoglycemia resulting from high parasitemia or from quinine-induced insulin secretion sometimes occurs.

Complications in malaria are most common with *P. falciparum* because of the high parasitemias that occur. Patients with more than 100,000 parasitized erythrocytes/mm^3 of blood are at great risk for severe hemolytic anemia and renal failure from hemoglobinuria (blackwater fever). Hemolysis and hemoglobinuric renal failure may also be produced by quinine sensitivity or by the treatment of G6PD-deficient patients with oxidant drugs. Renal failure in patients with malaria may also be caused by hypovolemia and acute tubular necrosis. Patients with malaria are extremely catabolic, and uremia may progress very rapidly.

Cerebral malaria occurs with *P. falciparum* and may present as alterations in the level of consciousness, organic psychosis, major motor seizures, or rarely as hemiparesis or a movement disorder. The cerebrospinal fluid (CSF) is usually normal, although a mild pleocytosis may occur. It must be emphasized that cerebral malaria is a diagnosis of exclusion, and it is imperative that other diseases (e.g., encephalitis, meningitis, brain abscess) be considered, even if the patient has circulating parasites. Pulmonary edema is usually a terminal event and is probably caused by increased capillary permeability. Rehydration is usually necessary because of fever and sweating, but it should be done with great care in patients with high parasitemias.

Malaria in pregnancy may increase the chances of abortion or a low-birth-weight infant, especially in primiparous women. Malaria in children may be more indolent and chronic, presenting as a wasting disease with anemia and hepatosplenomegaly. Tropical splenomegaly with hypersplenism and Burkitt's lymphoma are two diseases associated with *P. falciparum* malaria.

Complications from nonfalciparum malaria occur infrequently. *P. vivax* produces rapid splenic enlargement and sometimes splenic rupture even after treatment has been started. *P. malariae* in children may cause a chronic, progressive glomerulonephritis that responds poorly to treatment with antimalarial drugs.

The duration of erythrocytic infection in untreated or inadequately treated patients with malaria varies with the species of *Plasmodium.* The mean duration of *P. falciparum* infection is about 100 days, and most infections are eliminated within 1 year. However, a few untreated or inadequately treated infections have lasted for 3 to 4 years. Acquired immunity or partial treatment reduces parasitemia and symptoms. Periodic rises in parasitemia can produce recurrent symptoms (recrudescence). *P. malariae* infections that are not treated persist for the life of the host. Patients with chronic *P. malariae* infection are usually asymptomatic, but they may have a recrudescence associated with surgery, splenectomy, or immunosuppressive therapy. *P. vivax* and *P. ovale* persist as latent forms in the hepatic parenchymal cells. Recurrences from hepatic forms are called *relapses.* Latent hepatic forms may persist for 3 to 5 years.

Diagnosis

Malaria should be suspected in any febrile patient who has traveled in an endemic area, who has abused intravenous drugs, or who has had a recent blood transfusion. In addition, the diagnosis of malaria should be considered in individuals with unexplained fevers who reside near international airports or in the central valley of California. Diagnosis requires demonstration of malarial parasites on Giemsa-stained blood smears. Blood smears should be examined immediately and every 12 hours until the diagnosis is confirmed or rejected because nonimmune patients may have symptoms at very low parasitemias and because parasitemias (especially in *P. falciparum* malaria) may fluctuate. Thick smears permit more blood to be screened in less time but require greater experience on the part of the examiner. Once malarial parasites have been identified on the blood smear, the next step is to determine whether the patient has *P. falciparum* malaria because the species influences treatment. Patients with malaria who have recently returned from Africa or Haiti are very likely to have falciparum malaria, since *P. falciparum* is the predominant malaria parasite in these areas. The following morphologic criteria suggest falciparum malaria: the predominance of small ring forms and the occurrence of multiply infected erythrocytes; appliqué forms in which the ring parasite appears to be adjacent to the erythrocyte membrane; rings with two nuclei; and crescent-shaped gametocytes (Color Plate V-14). *P. falciparum* is also very likely if 5% or more of erythrocytes are infected. Morphologic criteria for *P. vivax* and *P. ovale* include the presence of trophozoites and schizonts as well as rings on the peripheral smear; enlargement of the infected erythrocytes (reticulocytes); and pink stippling of infected erythrocytes (Schüffner's dots) (Color Plate V-15). Other distinguishing characteristics are listed in Table 280-2. Serologic tests are not useful in the diagnosis of acute malaria.

Treatment

Patients with acute attacks of *P. vivax, P. ovale,* and *P. malariae* can be treated with chloroquine (Table 280-3). Outpatient therapy is appropriate if the patient does not vomit the medicine. With *P. vivax* and *P. ovale* the eradication of persistent hepatic forms (hypnozoites) requires treatment with primaquine phosphate, 26.3 mg daily for 14

Table 280-3. Chemotherapy for patients with malaria

Clinical setting	Drug treatment
P. vivax, P. ovale, P. malariae, and chloroquine-sensitive *P. falciparum*	Chloroquine phosphate, 1 g PO followed by 500 mg in 6 hours and 500 mg daily for 2 days. For *P. vivax* and *P. ovale,* primaquine phosphate, 26.3 mg daily for 14 days, to eradicate persistent hepatic forms. Check G6PD level before treating with primaquine.
Chloroquine-resistant *P. falciparum*	Quinine sulfate, 650 mg PO q8h for 3 days, and tetracycline, 250 mg q6h for 7 days, or clindamycin, 900 mg tid for 3 days.
Severe or complicated *P. falciparum* (parasitemia > 100,000/mm^3; hematocrit < 30; renal failure; cerebral malaria; severe vomiting or diarrhea)	Quinidine, 10 mg/kg loading dose over 1 hour, then continuous infusion of 0.02 mg/kg/min for 3 days. Give slowly (over 4 hours) with continuous electrocardiographic monitoring. Begin oral medication with tetracycline or clindamycin when the patient is stable.

Table 280-2. Clinical and diagnostic features in human malaria

	P. falciparum	*P. vivax*	*P. ovale*	*P. malariae*
Incubation period (days)*	8-25 (avg. 12)	8-27 (avg. 14)	9-17 (avg. 15)	15-30
Clinical features and complications	Fever often asynchronous, severe hemolysis, renal failure, pulmonary edema, cerebral malaria, thrombocytopenia, hypoglycemia	Anemia, thrombocytopenia, splenic rupture	Similar to *P. vivax*	Glomerulonephritis; erythrocytic infection persisting for years
Duration of erythrocytic cycle (hours)	48	48	48	72
Chloroquine resistance	Yes, widespread	Rare	No	No
Relapses from liver	No	Yes	Yes	No
Sequestration of trophozoites and schizonts	Yes	No	No	No
Morphologic characteristics	Rings predominate, thin cytoplasm, double nuclei, appliqué forms, multiply infected erythrocytes, crescent-shaped gametocytes	Enlarged erythrocytes, trophozoites with ameboid cytoplasm, Schüffner's dots	Oval erythrocytes, compact cytoplasm, Schüffner's dots	Erythrocytes not enlarged, compact cytoplasm (band forms)

*Incubation period may be prolonged by prophylactic medication. The incubation period of *P. vivax, P. ovale,* and *P. malariae* is occasionally months to years.

days. The patient should first be checked for G6PD deficiency. Severe G6PD deficiency is a contraindication to primaquine, and such patients should be followed and any erythrocytic relapses treated with chloroquine. Patients with mild G6PD deficiency can be treated with primaquine at a reduced dosage of 45 mg weekly for 8 weeks. Primaquine is not indicated in patients with malaria acquired by transfusion or with congenital malaria, since erythrocytic parasites do not infect the liver.

The management of patients with *P. falciparum* malaria is more complicated because of the life-threatening nature of the infection and the possibility of drug resistance. Early diagnosis and rapid initiation of appropriate treatment are essential, and patients must be monitored closely to assess the response to treatment and to identify complications. The choice of initial treatment should be based on the severity of the infection and the possibility of drug resistance. Resistance to chloroquine is widespread and increasing, and there are only a few areas of the world from which chloroquine resistance has not been reported. Resistance to the combination of pyrimethamine plus sulfadoxine (Fansidar) has also been reported in Southeast Asia, Panama, South America, and East Africa. Fansidar has also been associated with severe allergic reactions (Stevens-Johnson syndrome, toxic epidermal necrolysis), with death occurring in approximately 1 in 20,000 persons taking the drug.

Patients with uncomplicated, chloroquine-sensitive *P. falciparum* malaria can be treated with chloroquine (Table 280-3). Areas with chloroquine-sensitive *P. falciparum* are listed in the box at upper right. However, the reader is cautioned that resistance is spreading rapidly. Patients who have uncomplicated falciparum malaria acquired in an area of known chloroquine resistance or who have transfusion malaria (source unknown) should be treated with quinine sulfate plus tetracycline or clindamycin (children, pregnant women) (Table 280-3). Quinidine can be substituted for quinine.

Patients with severe or complicated *P. falciparum* malaria (parasitemia > 100,000 organisms/mm^3, hematocrit < 30%, cerebral symptoms, or renal failure) or who have severe and repeated vomiting or diarrhea should be treated with intravenous (IV) quinidine (Table 280-3). Vital signs should be monitored frequently, and the electrocardiogram (ECG) should be monitored continuously during IV quinidine administration. The maintenance dose of quinidine should be reduced in patients with renal failure. When the patient can take oral medication, quinine sulfate should be substituted and tetracycline or clindamycin added. All patients with cerebral symptoms should have a blood sample drawn for glucose assay, and 100 ml of 50% dextrose should be administered IV. Exchange transfusion has been reported to be efficacious in some patients with severe malaria and should be strongly considered as an adjunct to antimalarial chemotherapy in patients with high parasitemias (> 10%) or end-organ failure (renal failure, cerebral symptoms, pulmonary edema). Corticosteroids (dexamethasone) are not effective in the treatment of cerebral malaria and have been associated with a higher risk of complications, such as pneumonia and gastrointestinal bleeding.

Areas with chloroquine-sensitive *P. falciparum* (as of April 1992)*

Mexico
Central America north of Panama
Haiti
Dominican Republic
Middle East (including Egypt but not Pakistan)

*Patients with malaria caused by *P. falciparum* acquired anywhere else in the world should be presumed to have chloroquine-resistant parasites. The reader must be aware that chloroquine-resistant *P. falciparum* continues to spread and is a possibility with infection acquired anywhere, including the countries listed above.

Patients being treated for *P. falciparum* should be monitored for at least 72 hours, since complications can occur even after therapy has been initiated. It is also important to demonstrate a decline in the parasitemia within 24 to 48 hours. The asexual parasitemia should be completely resolved in 4 to 5 days. Gametocytes are not affected by most antimalarials, and their continued presence in the blood is not indicative of treatment failure. Patients must be warned about the possibility of a recrudescence 4 to 5 weeks (rarely several months) after treatment.

Chloroquine has minimum toxicity. Its major toxicity occurs in Africans, who frequently experience itching. Quinine or quinidine may produce symptoms resembling cinchonism (nausea, vomiting, tinnitus, vertigo), but this is not an indication to alter or discontinue treatment. Rarely, quinine causes severe Coombs-positive hemolytic anemia or an immune thrombocytopenia, requiring that the drug be stopped immediately.

Prevention in travelers

Prevention of malaria in travelers is increasingly difficult because of the spread of chloroquine-resistant *P. falciparum* and the toxicity of some antimalarial drugs (Chapter 241). Physicians should warn travelers that fever occurring during or after travel in an endemic area may be caused by malaria even if chemoprophylactic drugs were used. Current recommendations are listed in Table 280-4. *P. vivax, P. ovale, P. malariae,* and chloroquine-sensitive *P. falciparum* can usually be prevented with chloroquine phosphate, 500 mg weekly. The drug should be continued for 4 weeks after leaving the endemic area. Travelers can minimize their exposure to infectious mosquitoes by avoiding outdoor nocturnal activities, by using netting over the bed, and by applying mosquito repellents. If the traveler was heavily exposed to *P. vivax* or *P. ovale,* hepatic forms can be eliminated about 80% of the time with primaquine, 26.3 mg daily for 14 days. Prophylactic primaquine should not be given during travel or to G6PD-deficient patients. Alternative prophylactic regimens have considerably more toxicity than chloroquine.

For travelers visiting areas with chloroquine-resistant *P.*

falciparum, the risks of exposure must be balanced against the risks of the drugs.

Mefloquine is recommended for persons traveling to areas with chloroquine-resistant *P. falciparum* (Table 280-4), but the physician must be aware that sporadic resistance to mefloquine has been reported despite the relatively recent introduction of the drug. Although mefloquine at prophylactic dosages (250 mg weekly) appears to be generally well tolerated, higher dosages have been associated with nausea, diarrhea, dizziness, seizures, ataxia, and psychosis. Mefloquine should not be given to children weighing less than 15 kg or pregnant women or persons with hypersensitivity. In addition, mefloquine should probably be avoided in individuals with histories of seizures or psychiatric disorders. Mefloquine should be used with caution in patients taking beta blockers, calcium channel blockers, and other drugs that may prolong cardiac conduction and in patients whose occupations require fine motor control. Doxycycline is an alternative, but it may cause severe sun sensitivity and should not be given to children less than 8 years of age.

As mentioned, malaria, especially chloroquine-resistant *P. falciparum* malaria, may occur despite chemoprophylaxis. Therefore it is recommended that travelers planning trips that will include extensive travel in rural areas without access to medical care should carry medication for emergency self-treatment of resistant *P. falciparum* in case of a persistent fever. Two alternative regimens include quinine sulfate (see Table 280-3 for dosages) or Fansidar (pyrimethamine plus sulfadoxine) (3 tablets as a single dose). However, the toxicity of Fansidar is too severe (potentially lethal Stevens-Johnson syndrome) and too frequent (1 in 20,000) to justify its use as a routine, weekly prophylactic medication. Physicians should consult with the Centers for Disease Control (CDC) in Atlanta (tel. no. 404-488-4046), when advising travelers planning to visit areas with resistant *P. falciparum*.

Pregnant women who travel to the tropics will encounter a variety of infectious risks, including malaria. Chloroquine is the only antimalarial that is generally safe during pregnancy. Chemoprophylaxis with other drugs carries a risk for the fetus. For the pregnant woman with acute malaria, however, the disease is a grave risk to mother and child. Severe hypoglycemia is a common complication of *P. falciparum* infection during pregnancy. Treatment is the same as outlined in Table 280-3.

Table 280-4. Prevention of malaria in travelers

Chemoprophylaxis	
Travel to areas with *P. vivax, P. ovale,* or *P. malariae* and/or chloroquine-sensitive *P. falciparum* (see box on p. 2247).	Chloroquine phosphate, 500 mg weekly, beginning 1 week before travel and continuing for 4 weeks after return. Travel to areas with *P. vivax* or *P. ovale* (see box on p. 2243) should be followed by treatment with primaquine phosphate,* 26.3 mg daily for 14 days, to eradicate persistent liver stages.
Travel to areas with chloroquine-resistant *P. falciparum* (including areas that also have *P. vivax* or *P. ovale*).	Mefloquine,† 250 mg weekly beginning 1 week before travel and continuing for 4 weeks after return. Primaquine (as above) should be given if person exposed to *P. vivax* or *P. ovale*. Individuals who cannot take mefloquine (see text) may substitute doxycycline,‡ 100 mg daily (if > 8 years old).
Advice to the traveler	
Avoid nocturnal outdoor activities as much as possible.	
Cover skin and use insect repellents in the evening.	
Use insecticide-impregnated bed nets for outdoor sleeping.	

*Check G6PD level before administering primaquine.
†Resistance to mefloquine occurs infrequently but has been reported sporadically from several countries. (See text.)
‡Doxycycline may cause severe sun sensitivity, a significant problem during travel in the tropics.

BABESIOSIS

Human babesiosis is a zoonotic, tickborne infection of erythrocytes that is caused by two species of *Babesia: B. microti* and *B. divergens*. Babesiosis in cattle (Texas fever) was the first disease shown to be transmitted by an arthropod vector (1893).

Biology and life cycle

Babesia organisms are transmitted by *Ixodes* (hard-bodied) ticks during the course of a blood meal that must last for approximately 12 hours for transmission to occur. *Ixodes* ticks also transmit the spirochete that causes Lyme disease, and cotransmission of the two organisms may occur. *Babesia* infection may also be acquired by blood transfusion from an infected donor. In the vertebrate host, organisms invade erythrocytes and have an asexual, erythrocytic life cycle similar to that of *Plasmodium*. There is no exoerythrocytic cycle. *Babesia* species have a wide host range, which includes a variety of wild and domestic animals. Humans are infected when they intrude on the habitat of the tick and the animal reservoir.

Epidemiology

Symptomatic human babesiosis occurs infrequently. Most reported cases have been caused by *B. microti* acquired along the northeastern coast of the United States (Nantucket Island, Martha's Vineyard, Long Island, Shelter Island). However, the range of the tick vector appears to be increasing, and human babesiosis may become more widespread. *B. divergens* infections have occurred only in individuals without spleens and have been reported from Europe and North America.

Pathogenesis and immunity

Clinical consequences are produced by multiplication of organisms within erythrocytes and rupture of the infected erythrocytes. Infection may persist for months, perhaps because of antigenic variation by the parasite. Symptoms are more severe in elderly and splenectomized individuals. It is not known whether infection confers immunity.

Clinical manifestations

B. microti infections may be asymptomatic or may produce clinical manifestations from mild to severe. The incubation period with *B. microti* is 1 to 4 weeks in patients who can remember a tick bite. There is usually a gradual onset of fever, chills, myalgias, and fatigue. Fever is irregular and not periodic. Physical examination may show hepatosplenomegaly. Patients usually have a moderate anemia, leukopenia, and elevated liver enzymes. All the reported patients with *B. microti* infection have recovered, although malaise and fatigue often persist for several months.

B. divergens causes rapid onset of fever, chills, nausea, vomiting, and severe hemolysis in patients without spleens. Hemoglobinuria and renal failure are common. Most reported cases have been fatal.

Diagnosis

Babesiosis should be suspected in patients with fever and history of a tick bite, especially if the patient has been in the endemic area of the northeastern United States or if the patient lacks a spleen. Babesiosis should also be considered in patients who become ill following a blood transfusion. Diagnosis is made by microscopic examination of Giemsa-stained blood smears. Repeat examinations may be required. *Babesia* organisms are morphologically similar to *P. falciparum,* but experienced microscopists can distinguish between the two. Inoculation of gerbils or hamsters has also been used to establish the diagnosis.

Treatment and prevention

Infection with *B. microti* is usually self-limited, but if symptoms are severe or persistent, treatment with a combination of quinine and clindamycin has been reported to reduce symptoms but not to eradicate parasitemia. Chemotherapy for patients with *B. divergens* has not been shown to be successful, but empiric treatment with quinine and clindamycin or with pentamidine is reasonable. Exchange blood transfusion may reduce parasitemia and is a reasonable therapeutic maneuver in severely ill patients.

Infection can be prevented by avoiding exposure to ticks or by searching for and removing ticks, since prolonged feeding is required for transmission.

TOXOPLASMOSIS

Toxoplasmosis is caused by the sporozoan parasite *Toxoplasma gondii*. The organism is ubiquitous in nature and infects more than 50% of individuals in some populations. Infection is often asymptomatic but may cause severe clinical consequences in immunocompromised hosts or if infection is acquired in utero. Central nervous system (CNS) toxoplasmosis is a common opportunistic infection in patients with AIDS (Chapter 242). Effective treatment is available for some forms of toxoplasmosis, but it may be impossible to eradicate the infection completely in patients with AIDS. In patients with congenital toxoplasmosis, irreversible sequelae may have occurred before therapy is initiated.

Biology and life cycle

T. gondii is an obligate intracellular parasite. The organism has a sexual cycle in the intestinal epithelium of cats (the definitive host) and an asexual extraintestinal cycle in the tissues of humans, most mammals, and birds (incidental hosts). Toxoplasma exist in three forms: trophozoites (or tachyzoites), cysts (which contain bradyzoites), and oocysts. *Trophozoites* invade cells and multiply intracellularly by asexual division. *Cysts* contain latent but viable trophozoites and are responsible for chronic infection. *Oocysts* are produced by sexual reproduction of toxoplasma in cats and, except for transmission, have no role in the pathogenesis of human disease. Human infection is acquired by five different routes: ingestion of oocysts in material contaminated by cat feces; ingestion of tissue cysts in raw or undercooked meat; transplacental passage of trophozoites from an acutely infected pregnant woman to her fetus; transfusion of blood containing infected leukocytes; and transplantation of an infected organ.

The life cycle in humans is as follows. Ingested tissue cysts or oocysts are disrupted by digestive enzymes, and viable organisms are released. The organisms invade intestinal epithelium, multiply intracellularly to produce trophozoites, then disseminate throughout the body. Trophozoites are ovoid or crescent shaped and are stained by Giemsa. They can invade virtually any nucleated mammalian cell by endocytosis and multiply within the endocytic vesicle. Their intracellular survival in phagocytic cells is enhanced by the ability to prevent fusion of the host lysosomes with the endocytic vesicles containing trophozoites. In immunocompetent hosts the acute infection is terminated by a combination of humoral and cellular immunity, and the organisms form tissue cysts, which are resistant to destruction and are the hallmark of chronic infection. Tissue cysts may occur in any organ but are most often found in brain, heart, and skeletal muscle (especially the diaphragm). Trophozoites within cysts divide slowly (bradyzoites), producing about 300 viable organisms per cyst. Tissue cysts evoke minimum inflammatory response despite the presence of parasite antigens in the cyst wall. The cyst wall can be stained with silver and the bradyzoites stain strongly with periodic acid–Schiff. In immunodeficient hosts, it is postulated that tissue cysts rupture, releasing trophozoites, which multiply rapidly (tachyzoites), disseminate, and produce disease.

Cats are also infected by the ingestion of oocysts or tissue cysts. The organisms released into the intestine may either develop asexually as just described or, alternatively, may differentiate into male and female gametocytes. Fertilization occurs within the intestinal epithelial cells, and an oocyst is produced. The oocyst is released into the intestinal lumen and is excreted with the feces. Cats begin to excrete oocysts about 1 to 2 weeks after they are infected by eating tissue cysts or about 3 weeks after eating oocysts. Cats excrete 10 million oocysts per day for about 3 weeks, and then their feces are no longer infectious. Although cats can be reinfected, oocyst excretion rarely occurs with the reinfections. Excreted oocysts must sporulate in the environment before they are infectious for other animals. Sporulation requires 1 to 21 days, depending on environmental factors. Infectious oocysts may survive in moist soil for more than 1 year and may contaminate fruits and vegetables.

Epidemiology

T. gondii is a zoonosis with a worldwide distribution, but the organism is more prevalent in areas with a warm, moist climate than in areas that are cold or arid. Serologic studies have demonstrated a high prevalence of antibody to toxoplasma in many populations. The antibody persists for life, and the prevalence of seropositivity increases with age. In many countries, more than 50% of individuals are seropositive by the fourth decade of life. In most areas, cats are the major source of transmission, but where raw or undercooked meat (especially mutton and pork) is eaten, infectious tissue cysts can transmit disease. Slaughterhouse workers may be at increased risk of infection.

The incidence of congenital toxoplasmosis is about the same in countries with high and low prevalence of seropositivity. Congenital infection occurs only if there is an acute infection during pregnancy, and only seronegative women are at risk of acute infection. Populations with a high prevalence of seropositivity contain a small group of seronegative women who are at high risk of acquiring infection during pregnancy. Populations with a low prevalence of seropositivity contain a large group of seronegative women at low risk of acquiring infection during pregnancy. Thus, for both populations, the proportion of women who acquire toxoplasmosis during pregnancy and transmit it to the fetus is about the same. The greatest risk of congenital infection probably occurs when a pregnant woman from a low-prevalence area travels to a high-prevalence area (e.g., El Salvador, Tahiti, France).

Pathogenesis and immunity

Most manifestations of toxoplasmosis are caused by replicating trophozoites that disseminate throughout the body, destroying host cells and producing necrotic foci. Antibody and complement can kill extracellular trophozoites, but cell-mediated immunity and an effective oxidative burst by mononuclear phagocytes are required to stop the proliferation of intracellular organisms. Tissue cysts are not destroyed by the immune system but appear to persist in a latent but potentially infectious form for the life of the host. If the immune system is disturbed by intercurrent illness (e.g., AIDS, lymphoreticular malignancy) or by immunosuppressive therapy, tissue cysts may rupture and produce disseminated disease.

The pathologic changes of toxoplasmosis vary with the host's immune status. Most data on disease in immunocompetent hosts come from lymph node biopsies. *Toxoplasma* lymphadenitis produces a characteristic picture of follicular hyperplasia with clusters of epithelioid histiocytes invading the germinal centers. Trophozoites or tissue cysts are rarely seen. Toxoplasmosis in neonates and in patients with immunodeficiency may affect many organs, but the CNS is most often involved. The lesions in infants and adults are similar. Typically a meningoencephalitis occurs, which may be focal or diffuse and is characterized by necrosis and reactive microglial nodules. Trophozoites may invade the endothelium of blood vessels, producing ischemia and coagulation necrosis in the area supplied by the affected blood vessel. Lesions are usually multiple and may occur anywhere in the brain, although there is a predilection for the gray matter of the cortex and the basal ganglia. Patients with AIDS typically exhibit a mass lesion or lesions suggestive of a brain abscess. Trophozoites and tissue cysts can usually be identified histologically. Infected infants often have a periventricular and periaqueductal vasculitis, which may lead to obstructive hydrocephalus and is responsible for the periventricular calcifications often seen on radiographs. Myocarditis, interstitial pneumonitis, pancreatitis, and skeletal myositis also occur frequently.

Ocular toxoplasmosis is usually a late manifestation of congenital infection. Tissue cysts that develop in the retina during acute infection release invasive trophozoites, which produce a necrotizing retinitis. Granulomatous inflammation of the choroid often follows, and with increasing tissue destruction there may be iridocyclitis, glaucoma, or cataracts.

Clinical manifestations

In the normal adult, most infections with *T. gondii* are asymptomatic. When symptoms occur (10% to 20% of infections), the most common manifestation is cervical lymphadenopathy, but any or all lymph node groups can be affected. The nodes are typically discrete, not matted together, and no overlying erythema or warmth and no suppuration occur. Retroperitoneal or mesenteric lymphadenopathy may produce abdominal pain. In addition to lymphadenopathy, some patients have headache, fever, malaise, myalgias, sore throat, or a maculopapular rash. Hepatosplenomegaly occurs occasionally, but the existence of a true *Toxoplasma* hepatitis has not been proved. Atypical lymphocytosis has been described, but toxoplasmosis is an infrequent cause of the infectious mononucleosis syndrome.

In the immunodeficient host, disseminated toxoplasmosis occurs most often by relapse of a chronic infection. CNS manifestations are the most frequent and occur in 10% to 25% of AIDS patients in the developed world. Manifestations include focal neurologic signs of subacute onset and signs of generalized cerebral dysfunction (e.g., confusion, lethargy). Some patients have seizures, which may be generalized or focal. Fever is sometimes present. The manifestations of cerebral toxoplasmosis are not pathognomonic. The differential diagnosis includes chronic meningitis (especially from fungi or syphilis), herpes simplex encephalitis, encephalitis caused by human immunodeficiency virus (HIV) infections, drug toxicity, progressive multifocal leukoencephalopathy, and CNS malignancy. In patients with focal findings, the possibility of cerebrovascular accident must also be considered. CSF abnormalities seen with toxoplasmosis are nonspecific and include mild mononuclear pleocytosis and elevated protein content with normal glucose level, but in some patients the CSF is entirely normal. Computed tomography (CT) of the brain frequently shows abnormalities. Multiple contrast-enhancing lesions with either a homogeneous density or ring enhancement are most common. Occasionally, only a single lesion is seen, or the lesions are of low density and are not enhanced by contrast. Double-dose contrast administration appears to be superior to standard CT scanning. Some patients with normal CT scans have had focal abnormalities demonstrated by magnetic resonance imaging (MRI) scans. Although CNS findings predominate in immunocompromised patients, *Toxoplasma* interstitial pneumonitis is increasing in incidence in AIDS patients, perhaps because of improved diagnosis or increasing longevity of AIDS patients. The diagnosis is made by detection of *Toxoplasma* organisms in bronchoalveolar lavage fluid or lung biopsy specimens. Toxoplasmosis in the immunocompromised person may also present as fever of unknown origin or as a necrotizing myocarditis.

Congenital toxoplasmosis may occur when a previously uninfected (seronegative) woman is acutely infected during pregnancy. The infection in the mother is usually asymptomatic but may produce fever and lymphadenopathy. Risk of fetal infection is lowest during the first trimester but results in the most severe disease. The risk of fetal infection is highest during the third trimester, but disease is less severe.

Toxoplasma infection during pregnancy may produce a variety of consequences. Spontaneous abortions occur, but their frequency is unknown. If the neonate has clinical evidence of infection at birth, sequelae are usually severe. Involvement of the CNS is always present and may include microcephaly, hydrocephalus, convulsions, deafness, and mental retardation. Intracranial calcifications may be apparent on radiographs after several months. Evidence of generalized infection may be present but is variable. Manifestations include lymphadenopathy, hepatosplenomegaly, jaundice, thrombocytopenia, anemia, fever, pneumonitis, and a rash. The differential diagnosis in neonates includes cytomegalovirus, rubella, and herpes encephalitis.

If congenital infection is subclinical at birth, clinical manifestations will develop in most children observed into adolescence. Chorioretinitis is the most common late manifestation of congenital toxoplasmosis. The course of the disease consists of remissions and relapses. Patients may have intermittent unilateral blindness or pain in the eye. Microphthalmia, cataracts, and glaucoma also occur. During the initial stages, funduscopy reveals clusters of elevated, yellowish white patches. Later the lesions may be pale and contain black pigment. Other late sequelae of congenital infection include psychomotor retardation, seizures, cerebellar signs, and deafness.

Diagnosis

Two primary methods exist for the diagnosis of toxoplasmosis: histopathologic identification of the organism in biopsy material and serologic tests for antibodies to *Toxoplasma*. In addition, the histology of *Toxoplasma* lymphadenitis is very characteristic and in some hands diagnostic. Various serologic tests are available. The Sabin-Feldman dye test is very specific and detects immunoglobulin G (IgG) antibodies that fix complement and lyse trophozoites. These antibodies appear 1 to 2 weeks after infection and are usually present at high titer (>1:1000) within 6 to 8 weeks. The titer then slowly declines over months to years, but generally the test remains positive at titers of 1:16 to 1:64 for the life of the host. Indirect fluorescent antibody (IFA) tests detect IgG or IgM antibodies to *Toxoplasma*. IFA tests are easier to perform and more readily available than the dye test, but they are less reliable. Rheumatoid factors may cause false-positive results. IgM is detectable within a week of infection, rises rapidly to high titers (>1:160), then disappears within a few months. The IgG detected by IFA follows a pattern similar to that described for the dye test. An enzyme-linked immunosorbent assay (ELISA) that detects IgM antibodies is more sensitive than the IFA test and eliminates the false-positive results caused by rheumatoid factor, but this test is not routinely available. Other tests, including indirect hemagglutination, complement fixation, and direct agglutination, have been developed but are not in general use.

The approach to diagnosis should be determined by the clinical setting. In the immunocompetent host the diagnosis of acute acquired toxoplasmosis is confirmed by seroconversion from a negative to a positive dye test or IFA test or by a rise in titer of IgG antibody of two or more dilutions in sera drawn at 3-week intervals. A single high-titer dye test or IFA test is suggestive but not diagnostic of acute infection. An IgM antibody titer of 1:160 or higher by the ELISA test or by IFA is also diagnostic of acute infection.

Diagnosis of toxoplasmosis in immunocompromised patients is difficult because antibody responses are depressed. Serum IgG antibody is usually detectable, since most cases of toxoplasmosis in immunocompromised hosts are caused by relapses or reactivation of chronic infection. However, 3% of AIDS patients with CNS disease do not have antibodies to *Toxoplasma*. Diagnostic changes in the titer of IgG antibody occur infrequently, even in biopsy-proven disease, and tests for IgM antibody are usually negative. The diagnosis can be definitively made by demonstrating organisms in biopsy specimens from accessible lesions. However, if the CNS toxoplasmosis is strongly suspected on clinical grounds, it is reasonable to institute a therapeutic trial and observe an immunocompromised patient closely for evidence of a response consistent with the diagnosis. This is particularly true for the patient with AIDS and a positive *Toxoplasma* titer who has single or multiple ring-enhancing cerebral mass lesions. Since CNS toxoplasmosis is by far the most likely diagnosis, a 2-week trial of sulfadiazine and pyrimethamine with follow-up CT scanning is a common approach. If the patient does not have a positive *Toxoplasma* titer or lesions fail to improve, brain biopsy is recommended. If clinical or radiographic improvement is seen, chronic therapy (see next section) is indicated.

The serologic diagnosis of congenital infection is complicated by the transplacental transfer of maternal IgG, which may persist in the infant for 6 to 12 months, and by the inability of infants to make antibodies to *Toxoplasma* until the second or third month of life. Serologic diagnosis of congenital toxoplasmosis requires persistent or rising titers of IgG antibody or the demonstration of IgM antibodies to *Toxoplasma*. Repeat tests should be performed monthly.

The diagnosis of ocular toxoplasmosis is based on the observation of typical retinal lesions. A positive dye test or IFA test for IgG antibody is consistent with the diagnosis, and a negative IgG test probably excludes the diagnosis. However, no characteristic changes occur in antibody titer because the acute infection is usually remote. Lesions that are not typical of toxoplasmosis should not be presumed to be caused by toxoplasmosis on the basis of a positive serologic finding.

Table 280-5. Treatment of patients with toxoplasmosis

Clinical setting	Suggested treatment
Acute infection in immunocompetent patients	
Mild	No treatment
Severe or prolonged symptoms	Pyrimethamine, 200 mg loading dose in two divided doses followed by 25-75 mg/day, plus sulfadiazine, 100 mg/kg/day in three divided doses, plus folinic acid, 10 mg/day, for 3-4 weeks
Toxoplasmosis in immunodeficient patients	
Acute	Pyrimethamine, 200 mg loading dose followed by 75 mg/day, plus sulfadiazine, 100 mg/kg/day (to 8 g/day) in three divided doses, plus folinic acid, 10 mg/day, for 6 weeks (with clinical or radiologic response)
Acute, sulfa allergic	Pyrimethamine, 200 mg loading dose followed by 75 mg/day, plus clindamycin, 600-1200 mg IV every 6 hours or 600 mg PO every 6 hours, plus folinic acid, 10 mg/day, for 6 weeks (with clinical or radiologic response)
Maintenance	Pyrimethamine, 25 mg PO daily, plus sulfadiazine, 500 mg PO four times a day, or clindamycin, 1200 mg PO daily in divided doses
Ocular, congenital, and pregnancy associated	See text

IV, Intravenously; PO, orally.

Treatment and prevention

Acute toxoplasmosis in the normal host is usually self-limited, and treatment should not be given unless symptoms are severe or persistent or the patient is pregnant.

Treatment is indicated for immunocompetent patients with severe or prolonged symptoms, for pregnant women, for immunocompromised individuals with disseminated toxoplasmosis, for patients with chorioretinitis caused by toxoplasmosis, and for those with congenital toxoplasmosis. The choice of drugs and the duration of treatment are determined by the clinical setting. Recommendations are given in Table 280-5.

Pyrimethamine and sulfadiazine are active against *T. gondii* and are synergistic when given together. It is recommended that this combination be the regimen of first choice except during the first trimester of pregnancy, when pyrimethamine may be teratogenic. Some studies of toxoplasmosis in patients with AIDS suggest that higher daily doses of pyrimethamine (75 to 100 mg/day) may be beneficial. However, therapeutic recommendations for treatment of toxoplasmosis in AIDS patients have developed on the basis of consensus rather than clear-cut results of clinical studies and are frequently varied in patients with drug intolerance.

Recommendations for treatment of toxoplasmosis may be expected to change as new data become available. Folinic acid should generally be added because pyrimethamine is a folic acid antagonist. Blood counts should be checked frequently. Alternative drugs are needed, since 50% of AIDS patients who take pyrimethamine and sulfadiazine for CNS toxoplasmosis develop toxicity that necessitates discontinuation of the drugs and some do not respond to this regimen. Clindamycin has been found to be effective in combination with pyrimethamine for the treatment of CNS toxoplasmosis in humans and can replace sulfadiazine in patients who are allergic to sulfa drugs. However, clindamycin maintenance therapy may result in unacceptable toxicity. Newer drugs, including atovaquone and three macrolides (azithromycin, roxithromycin, clarithromycin), show promise in the treatment of CNS toxoplasmosis. Gamma interferon as an adjunct to antibiotic therapy may also prove helpful in persons with AIDS.

Immunologically normal individuals with severe symptoms caused by acute toxoplasmosis should be treated for 3 to 4 weeks. The treatment of immunocompromised patients with disseminated (usually CNS) toxoplasmosis appears to result in improvement in about 80% of patients. Information from AIDS patients indicates that it is necessary to continue maintenance therapy indefinitely after clinical remission or improvement. In other immunocompromised patients, maintenance therapy should be continued as long as the immunocompromised state continues. Infants with congenital toxoplasmosis should be treated for 1 year. Various regimens have been suggested, and the reader is referred to specialty texts for details. Treatment of acute infection in pregnant women has the goal of preventing congenital disease. One recommended regimen is to treat the patient with pyrimethamine plus sulfadiazine in 5-week cycles consisting of daily treatment for 2 weeks followed by no treatment for 3 weeks; the cycle is continued until term. Pyrimethamine should be omitted during the first trimester, and sulfadiazine should be omitted near term because it increases the risk of kernicterus in neonates with hyperbilirubinemia. In a study from France, spiramycin (3 g/day) was used to treat maternal infections from the time of diagnosis until the end of the pregnancy, with some evidence of decreased sequelae in neonates. Ocular toxoplasmosis is treated for 1 month. A clinical response occurs in about 70% of patients.

Prevention is most important for seronegative women during pregnancy and for seronegative patients who are immunodeficient. Tissue cysts in meat are killed by temperatures over 66° C. Hands should be washed after handling raw meat. Cat feces should be avoided, gloves should be worn while gardening, and fruits and vegetables should be washed thoroughly. If a seronegative individual requires transfusion of leukocyte-rich blood products or an organ transplant, seropositive donors should be excluded if possible.

Twenty-six percent of HIV-infected patients in the United States with antibody to toxoplasmosis will develop CNS toxoplasmosis. Thus this group is at high risk for disease and will benefit from prophylaxis when appropriate regimens have been determined.

OTHER COCCIDIAN PARASITIC DISEASES

The coccidia have life cycles similar to that of *T. gondii,* with a sexual stage in the intestinal epithelium of the definitive host and an asexual stage in the gastrointestinal tract or the tissues. *Isospora* and *Cryptosporidium* have both sexual and asexual stages confined to the intestinal mucosa of a single host. *Sarcocystis* has sexual and asexual cycles in different hosts and may involve the gastrointestinal tract or skeletal muscles of humans.

Cryptosporidiosis

Infection with *Cryptosporidium* in the immunocompetent as well as the immunodeficient host has been documented with increasing frequency since 1982, when it was recognized as a pathogen in AIDS patients. From 10% to 15% of AIDS patients in the United States and up to 50% in developing countries are estimated to develop cryptosporidiosis during the course of AIDS.

Biology and life cycle. Cryptosporidiosis is a zoonotic disease that frequently infects the young of many species, including calves, lambs, piglets, and children. *Cryptosporidium parvum,* the species that infects humans, has no host specificity among mammals and is thus readily passed between them. Asexual and sexual cycles of *C. parvum* occur in the epithelial cells of the small or large intestine, resulting in the development of fully sporulated oocysts that are shed into the environment. Infection occurs when oocysts are ingested and excystation occurs in the small bowel, releasing four motile sporozoites that invade the epithelial cells of the gastrointestinal tract and differentiate into merozoites. Merozoites may be released and reinvade adjacent cells to continue the asexual cycle or may develop into sexual forms that combine to form an oocyst. The oocyst may undergo excystation in the host of origin and repeat the cycle, or it may be excreted in an environmentally resistant form to continue the cycle in another host.

Epidemiology. Infection is most common in children, animal care workers, travelers, hospital personnel, and immunocompromised persons, especially transplant recipients and AIDS patients. Transmission is by the fecal-oral route, and person-to-person transmission of *Cryptosporidium* has been documented. Studies with infant macaques indicate that very small inocula of oocysts, less than 100, are needed for infection; the infectious dose for infant or adult humans is not known. Contaminated water has been implicated in many outbreaks and is the suspected mode of transmission to travelers. Oocysts, the infecting stage, are difficult to remove by filtration because of their small size and are resistant to many disinfectants. Household pets or other domestic animals may constitute a reservoir for human infection.

Pathology and immunity. Histologic changes in the human small intestine associated with cryptosporidiosis have been described most thoroughly in patients with AIDS. They include villus atrophy and blunting, epithelial flattening, and inflammation of the lamina propria characterized by infiltration of plasma cells, lymphocytes, and macrophages. When infected, the pancreatic ducts, biliary tree, and gallbladder show moderate to severe epithelial hyperplasia and mural thickening. The cause of these histopathologic changes has not been determined; a toxin has not been identified. Lactose intolerance and fat malabsorption have been well documented in patients with cryptosporidiosis. Rarely, immunocompromised hosts may develop cryptosporidiosis of the bronchial epithelium or sinuses associated with gastrointestinal disease.

Both the humoral and the cellular immune responses appear to be important in the control of cryptosporidiosis, but their relative importance and the mechanism by which they do so have not been established.

Clinical manifestations. Infection with *C. parvum* may be asymptomatic or may produce acute, self-limited, watery diarrhea in normal hosts. Low-grade fever may occur. Immunodeficient patients may have severe diarrhea with malabsorption, weight loss, and dehydration (Chapter 242). Profuse, watery diarrhea exceeding 20 L/day has been described. Severe, progressive disease occurs frequently in patients with AIDS, who may also have involvement of the biliary tract with symptoms of nausea, right upper quadrant abdominal pain, and elevated serum alkaline phosphatase.

Diagnosis. The diagnosis of cryptosporidiosis is often difficult because the oocysts in stool are very small and may be difficult to distinguish from yeast. It may be helpful to concentrate the organisms by sucrose flotation. Oocysts are not stained by periodic acid–Schiff or iodine but are acid fast and can be stained with a modified Kinyoun or Ziehl-Neelsen stain (Color Plate V-35). A sensitive and specific fluorescein-labeled IgG monoclonal antibody is commercially available.

Treatment and prevention. No effective treatment for cryptosporidiosis exists. Enteric precautions should be taken with infected individuals, especially in a hospital setting.

Isosporiasis

Species of the genus *Isospora* have a single host, and all stages of the life cycle occur in the epithelium of the small intestine. Human disease is caused by *I. belli*. Infection is acquired by the ingestion of oocysts present in the feces of infected humans. Isosporiasis occurs infrequently in the United States but is endemic in some areas of Indochina, South America, and islands of the southwestern Pacific. Infection may be asymptomatic or may cause watery diarrhea, abdominal cramping, nausea, and vomiting. Disease is usually self-limited and lasts 4 to 6 weeks but may be chronic and produce malabsorption and weight loss. Rarely, disseminated extraintestinal disease has been reported in patients with AIDS.

Symptoms of *Isospora* infection are more severe in immunocompromised individuals, especially those with AIDS (Chapter 242). Isosporiasis has been an infrequent pathogen among AIDS patients in the United States but has been reported to occur in 15% of patients in Haiti. A leukocytosis with moderate eosinophilia (7% to 15%) is common. The diagnosis is made by identifying oocysts in stool samples (Color Plate V-1) or by identifying intracellular forms in small-bowel biopsies. Trimethoprim (160 mg)/sulfamethoxazole (800 mg) orally four times a day for 10 days then twice a day for 3 weeks is an effective regimen. Pyrimethamine plus a sulfonamide is also effective. Pyrimethamine alone at doses of 50 to 75 mg/day has been used in persons who are allergic to sulfonamides. Relapses are common in immunodeficient patients, and indefinite maintenance therapy may be necessary.

Sarcocystosis

Species of *Sarcocystis* have life cycles involving two hosts. Humans may be infected as definitive hosts by ingesting *S. hominis*–infected tissue from cattle or *S. suihominis*–infected tissue from swine. Infection is confined to the epithelium of the intestinal tract and may produce abdominal cramping, nausea, vomiting, and diarrhea of several days' duration. A relapse may occur several weeks later, during the peak of oocyst shedding. Spontaneous recovery follows. Diagnosis is made by identifying oocysts in the stool.

Humans probably can also be infected as incidental hosts by ingestion of oocysts of various species of *Sarcocystis*. Such infections are usually asymptomatic, but muscle involvement with swelling and weakness, fever, leukocytosis, and eosinophilia have been reported. Bronchospasm can occur. Diagnosis can be made only by biopsy of affected tissue, usually muscle. Antifolate drugs (e.g., sulfonamides, trimethoprim, pyrimethamine) appear to be effective.

MICROSPORIDIOSIS

Protozoan parasites of the phylum Microspora infect insects and a variety of wild and domesticated animals. They are small, sporeforming, obligate intracellular parasites that are found in the intestine, liver, kidney, cornea, brain, nerves, and muscles of their animal hosts. Recently, microsporidiosis has been recognized as a cause of gastrointestinal disease and keratitis in AIDS patients. Microsporidia have not been studied extensively as agents of disease because they are small, stain poorly, evoke little inflammation, and are difficult to diagnose in the absence of electron microscopy.

Biology and life cycle

Microsporidia multiply in the cytoplasm of host cells. Four genera, *Nosema, Enterocytozoon, Encephalitozoon,* and *Pleistophora,* have been associated with human disease. Members of these genera have variable and complex structural relationships with the host cell cytoplasm. However, all are released into a cell from a spore by ejection from a long coiled polar tubule, a characteristic microsporidian feature. Within the host cell, development into schizonts (meronts), sporonts, sporoblasts, and spores occurs.

Epidemiology

The source of human infections is unknown, but both vertebrates and invertebrates may serve as reservoirs of infection. For example, *Encephalitozoon* infects birds and mammals, and *Nosema* infects insects. Spores, ingested after release from the gastrointestinal tract or in the urine of other infected animals, are thought to be the mode of transmission of disease. Serologic studies suggest that antibodies to *Encephalitozoon cuniculi* are widespread in animals and humans and are more frequently found in persons who have traveled to the tropics. Recently, *Enterocytozoon* infection of AIDS patients has been described. It has been suggested that *Enterocytozoon bieneusi* may be as common as *Cryptosporidium* as a cause of diarrhea in AIDS patients, but definitive studies have not been reported.

Pathology and immunity

Parasites may not evoke an inflammatory response in tissues, especially in immunocompromised patients, or may elicit moderate granulomatous inflammation with a mononuclear cell infiltrate. It is not known whether microsporidiosis in immunocompromised patients reflects activation of a latent infection.

Enterocytozoon bieneusi infection of the intestinal epithelium is confined to enterocytes covering the villi, especially those at the tip, and is associated with villous atrophy, cell degeneration, necrosis, and sloughing. The jejunum appears to be the preferred site of infection, the duodenum is less frequently infected, and the large intestine is relatively spared. *Encephalitozoon cuniculi* infection may involve the kidneys and CNS in a wide range of mammals, including humans.

Clinical manifestations

Although there are scattered reports of microsporidiosis in immunocompetent patients, disease caused by microsporidia is more widespread in immunocompromised hosts, especially those with AIDS. Infection of the intestinal epithelium with *Enterocytozoon bieneusi* is by far the most common manifestation of microsporidiosis in AIDS patients. Clinical manifestations of disease include wasting and chronic diarrhea and are indistinguishable from the manifestations of isosporiasis and cryptosporidioisis in AIDS patients. Diarrheal stools are watery and are not accompanied by blood or fever. Routine laboratory tests are normal, with occasional hypokalemia and hypomagnesemia. Carbohydrate and fat malabsorption are present.

Encephalitozoon has been reported in the cornea, peritoneum, and liver of AIDS patients; *Pleistophora* has been reported in skeletal muscle of one patient. These genera and sites of infection do not appear to occur frequently.

Diagnosis

Encephalitozoon spores are gram positive and some are acid fast, but spores of other genera stain unpredictably with these stains, and electron micrography may be required for identification. *Enterocytozoon bieneusi* may be identified on light microscopy of plastic sections of intestinal biopsy material stained with metheylene blue–azure II, basic fuchsin stain, or hematoxylin-eosin. Several groups have recently reported success with the use of Giemsa-stained stool specimens for diagnosis of *Enterocytozoon bieneusi* diarrhea, but these techniques have not come into common use. Giemsa-stained spores in the stool are oval, with the cytoplasm staining light gray-blue and the nucleus staining intensely purple.

Treatment

No established therapy exists for microsporidiosis.

AMEBIASIS

Amebiasis is the disease caused by infection with the sarcodinian parasite *Entamoeba histolytica*. Infection is often asymptomatic but may cause diarrhea, severe colitis, a colonic mass, or extraintestinal disease, particularly abscess of the liver. The overall prevalence of amebiasis in the United States is low, but significant endemic foci exist, and infection is common in homosexual men, immigrants, travelers, and refugees (Chapter 241). A major problem is the frequent failure of clinicians to consider the diagnosis of amebiasis. When the diagnosis is considered, many clinical laboratories lack expertise at identifying *E. histolytica* in the stool, leading to diagnostic errors. Serologic tests can detect antibodies to *E. histolytica,* but interpretation depends on the clinical setting. Effective therapy is available for most forms of amebiasis.

Biology and life cycle

The genus *Entamoeba* contains several species of human parasites *(E. histolytica, E. coli, E. hartmanni)* that may reside in the human colon. Identification of *Entamoeba* species is based on the number of nuclei in the cyst stage, the presence of erythrophagocytosis, and the size of the organisms. *E. histolytica* and *E. hartmanni* cysts contain four nuclei; *E. coli* cysts usually contain eight nuclei. *E. histolytica* produces larger cysts than *E. hartmanni* and phagocytizes erythrocytes. The presence of any of these organisms in stool indicates fecal-oral contamination, but only *E. histolytica* is able to invade the colonic mucosa. *E. hartmanni* and *E. coli* are generally considered to be nonpathogenic commensals.

E. histolytica is a species complex that includes strains that differ in virulence, isoenzyme type, size, and in vitro growth characteristics. Strains have been separated into pathogenic and nonpathogenic *E. histolytica* on the basis of isoenzyme pattern. Recently, surface antigens, deoxyribonucleic acid (DNA) markers to antigens, and ribosomal ribonucleic acid (rRNA) have been shown to differ between pathogenic and nonpathogenic strains. Virulence properties of pathogenic strains, including resistance to complement-mediated lysis, and production of specific extracellular proteases and a galactose-binding lectin have also been identified. These observations suggest that pathogenic and nonpathogenic *E. histolytica* are two distinct species. Invasive disease caused by pathogenic strains is prevalent only in certain geographic areas, principally the tropics, despite the organism's worldwide distribution.

E. histolytica has two stages (cyst, trophozoite) and multiplies asexually by binary fission. No sexual stage exists, and humans are the only hosts. Infection is usually transmitted by the ingestion of cysts present in feces or contaminated water or on fruits and vegetables. Trophozoites are killed by gastric acid and are not infectious when ingested orally. However, trophozoites inoculated into the rectum can transmit infection, and this may be one mechanism of transmission in male homosexuals.

Ingested cysts are disrupted in the ileum, and trophozoites are released. Trophozoites are microaerophilic and localize in areas where enteric bacteria have created anaerobic conditions. They colonize the cecum first and then move distally through the colon, residing in the lumen or the glandular crypts. Trophozoites within the lumen of the intestine are protected from the host's immune system and may persist there for years. Pathogenic strains may penetrate the mucosal epithelium and invade the wall of the colon.

Cysts are produced in the lumen of the colon as the stool

dehydrates. Therefore cysts are more frequently found in formed stools and trophozoites in diarrheal stools. After evacuation, cysts can survive refrigeration but not prolonged freezing, and they can survive in cool water for weeks. They are not killed by chlorination of water at the concentrations used by most municipalities. Cysts can also survive passage through the gastrointestinal tracts of flies. Cysts may be killed by dessication, boiling, or iodination. Most epidemics of amebiasis can be traced to contaminated water supplies, but where crowding or poor sanitation exists, direct fecal-oral transmission may occur.

Epidemiology

E. histolytica occurs in all climates throughout the world. The prevalence of infection may reach 50% in areas where there is contamination of drinking water or food crops with human feces. The prevalence of infection in most industrialized countries is 1% to 3%. In the United States, endemic foci have been identified on some native American reservations with poor sanitation and in mental institutions, where fecal-oral transmission probably occurs. Some urban populations of homosexual males have a high prevalence of infection (20% or more) that is maintained by sexual transmission.

Pathogenesis and immunity

E. histolytica within the lumen of the colon may provoke an increase in mucus secretion, a shortening of transit time for stool in the colon, or edema of the colonic mucosa. In general, however, the consequences of luminal infection are minimal.

Invasive disease requires a virulent strain of *E. histolytica*. Invasion usually begins in the glandular crypts of the cecum, appendix, or colon. Invasive amebae have a cytopathic effect on epithelial cells, leading to lytic necrosis. The organisms penetrate the epithelial layer and burrow to the muscularis mucosa. They may then spread laterally and produce a superficial ulceration or penetrate the muscularis and reach the submucosa, where there is little resistance to lateral spread. This process produces a flask-shaped lesion with a narrow neck at the portal of entry through the epithelium and a wide base in the submucosa. Histologically, lytic necrosis of host cells occurs, but little or no inflammatory cellular reaction. Amebae in the submucosa may coalesce and undermine the mucosa, producing shaggy ulcers with a diameter of several centimeters. Secondary bacterial invasion often occurs at this stage and is followed by infiltration of polymorphonuclear leukocytes. Trophozoites may continue to burrow through the wall of the colon, eventually penetrating the serosa and perforating the colon. Penetration of the intestinal wall is mediated by a proteolytic enzyme secreted by the parasite. Antibody to the protease appears to be predictive of invasive disease.

Amebomas are tumorlike lesions of the colon that are produced by an inflammatory reaction to the amebae and bacteria. Histologically, granulation tissue and fibrosis develop. Amebomas produce a localized thickening of the wall of the colon that may be mistaken for a malignant tumor on barium enema examination or on gross inspection at surgery.

Extraintestinal amebiasis is produced by perforation of the colon, by extension to the perianal skin, or by dissemination to the liver or other organs via the blood. Trophozoites in the wall of the colon penetrate mesenteric venules, enter the portal circulation, and are deposited in hepatic sinusoids, where they produce necrosis of the hepatic parenchyma and eventually an abscess. Amebic liver abscesses usually have a thin fibrous wall and contain necrotic debris. Viable organisms are located at the periphery of the abscess cavity. Neutrophils are generally absent unless secondary bacterial invasion occurs, but most amebic liver abscesses are bacteriologically sterile. Liver abscesses may rupture into the peritoneum, the pleura, or the pericardium. Rarely, amebae gain access via the blood to other organs (e.g., the brain). The presence and the extent of extraintestinal amebiasis are not related to the severity of intestinal disease, and most patients with liver abscesses do not have parasites identified on stool examination.

Invasive amebiasis produces high levels of precipitating, agglutinating, and complement-fixing antibodies, some of which persist for years after infection. Cell-mediated immune responses have been demonstrated in some patients with amebic liver abscesses. The role of these immune responses in protecting the host is unclear. Recurrences of liver abscesses after successful treatment are extremely rare, however, suggesting that this form of disease produces at least partial resistance.

Clinical manifestations

Intestinal amebiasis may be asymptomatic or may produce a spectrum of symptoms, from a slight loosening of the stool to severe colitis and dysentery. *E. histolytica* acquired in temperate countries is usually caused by nonpathogenic strains. Thus invasive colonic disease and liver abscess are rare in these areas. Acute infection with nonpathogenic strains does not result in morbidity, even in patients with AIDS.

The incubation period from infection to the appearance of organisms in the stool is 1 to 5 days. The clinical incubation period may be as short as 4 days or as long as several years. When amebae are limited to the lumen of the colon, patients may have intermittent increases in the frequency of stools and occasional mild abdominal cramping, and stools may fall apart more easily. Invasive amebiasis that is limited to the rectosigmoid colon produces rectal tenesmus, crampy lower abdominal pain, and bloody mucoid stools. Patients usually have no fever. The liver may be diffusely enlarged, and liver function tests may be abnormal. In the absence of an abscess, however, there is no evidence of invasion of the liver by trophozoites. Symptoms may resolve spontaneously. Severe colonic involvement causes 20 or more bloody stools per day and constant, intense rectal tenesmus. Patients with extensive involvement of the colon are more likely to have vomiting, fever, intravascular volume depletion, and shock. Toxic megacolon or perforation of the colon may occur. The abdomen may be distended, and bowel sounds may be absent. A plain film of the abdomen should be obtained and examined for evidence of perforation, cecal dilatation, or toxic megacolon.

The presentation of a patient with ameboma may be more subtle, although the stools are usually bloody and abdominal pain is present. A colonic lesion can often be palpated, or the lesion may be identified on barium enema examination. Involvement of the cecum or appendix by *E. histolytica* produces right lower quadrant pain and rigidity and may be mistaken for appendicitis.

Amebic abscess of the liver is the most common extraintestinal manifestation of *E. histolytica* (Chapter 62). The abscess is usually solitary and in 80% of patients is located in the right lobe of the liver. Typically, abrupt onset of pain in the right upper quadrant and fever occur. Pain may be referred to the scapula or shoulder and is exacerbated by pressure or coughing; 50% of patients have a cough. On physical examination the liver is enlarged and tender; some patients are jaundiced. There is often respiratory splinting on the right and dullness to percussion and decreased breath sounds at the base of the right lung field. A pleural or hepatic friction rub may be present. Abscesses in the left lobe of the liver produce epigastric or left shoulder pain. Some patients may have fever as the major symptom or may have a chronic course with anorexia and weight loss. Jaundice is present in about one third of patients. Patients usually have a neutrophilic leukocytosis; normochromic, normocytic anemia; and abnormal liver function tests. Amebiasis does not cause eosinophilia. Chest radiographs often show elevation of the right diaphragm, and a small, reactive pleural effusion may be seen if the abscess is superficial and near the diaphragm.

Complications of amebic liver abscesses include rupture and secondary bacterial invasion. Rupture from the right lobe of the liver may produce peritonitis or empyema. Amebae in the pleural space usually burrow into the bronchi, and trophozoites may be seen in the sputum. Abscesses in the left lobe of the liver may rupture into the pericardium and produce fulminant pericarditis or pericardial tamponade. Bacterial superinfection of an amebic abscess occurs in fewer than 5% of patients and is usually manifested by rigors, spiking fever, positive blood cultures, and failure to respond to antiamebic chemotherapy.

Rarely, *E. histolytica* spreads hematogenously to the brain. Brain abscesses are usually solitary and in the cerebral cortex. Symptoms include fever, headache, and altered mental status. More than 90% of patients also have amebic liver abscesses. The course is rapidly progressive. Most of these cases have been diagnosed on postmortem examination.

Diagnosis

Amebiasis should be considered in the differential diagnosis of any patient with colonic disease, especially if there is chronic diarrhea with blood or blood-streaked mucus in the stool (Chapter 236). Compared with bacillary dysentery produced by *Shigella* or *Campylobacter,* intestinal amebiasis has a more gradual onset and rarely produces vomiting, chills, or high fever (unless fulminant), and the stool contains few leukocytes. *Salmonella* enteritis is also more likely to cause fever and fecal leukocytes. Viral gastroenteritis tends to occur in seasonal epidemics and produces extraintestinal symptoms (e.g., coryza, myalgia, fever, headache). The distinction between inflammatory bowel disease (ulcerative colitis, regional enteritis) and amebic colitis may be difficult on clinical grounds. All patients in whom the diagnosis of inflammatory bowel disease is considered should have stool examined for *E. histolytica,* and a serologic test for amebiasis should be performed. Patients from endemic areas may have colonic disease of another etiology despite the presence of *E. histolytica* in the stool.

The diagnosis of amebiasis can be made in two ways: (1) by identification of trophozoites or cysts in feces or exudates and (2) by a positive serologic test in a patient with clinical manifestations of invasive amebiasis. Intestinal amebiasis must usually be diagnosed by stool examination or by examination of aspirates obtained during sigmoidoscopy. Serologic tests are usually negative with mild intestinal disease but may be positive in patients with invasive amebiasis. The appearance of organisms in the stool follows a cyclic pattern, and the diagnostic yield is increased by examining multiple stool samples over several days. Examination of three stools will yield the diagnosis in approximately 85% of infected individuals. Examination of a single stool may yield the diagnosis in only 40%. Amebae are more likely to be found in blood-tinged mucus than in fecal matter. A direct smear, examined while the stool is still warm, may reveal motile trophozoites. A direct smear should also be fixed and stained with iron hematoxylin or trichrome, and a concentrate (zinc-sulfate or formalin-ether) should be made (Color Plate V-56). The combination of these three procedures on three stool specimens gives the most accurate results. *E. histolytica* can also be identified histologically in colonic mucosa. Biopsies should be taken from the edge of an ulcer. False-negative stool examinations may occur if the microscopist is inexperienced or if interfering substances are present. Interfering substances include antibiotics, mineral oil, magnesium hydroxide, bismuth, kaolin, and barium. Tap water, saline, or soapsuds enemas may also interfere with diagnosis. False-positive results may occur if fecal leukocytes are misidentified as *E. histolytica*.

Diagnosis of extraintestinal amebiasis usually requires the combination of a compatible clinical syndrome and a positive serologic test. Liver abscess is usually detected by radioisotope liver scanning, ultrasonography, or CT. A gallium scan may be of value in differentiating amebic liver abscess from pyogenic liver abscess. Fewer than 20% of patients with extraintestinal amebiasis have organisms in the stool. Various serologic tests are available, most frequently agar gel diffusion-precipitation or counterimmunoelectrophoresis. These tests are positive only if invasive disease is present. Ninety-five percent of patients with liver abscess have positive serologic tests, and 80% to 90% of patients with severe intestinal disease have positive tests. Gel diffusion-precipitation and counterimmunoelectrophoresis become negative several months after cure of the liver abscess, and therefore these tests are useful in the assessment of treatment and the diagnosis of reinfection. Indirect hemagglutination is more sensitive, but the test remains positive for years and is therefore more useful in patients from nonendemic areas.

Treatment and prevention

The drugs that are effective against *E. histolytica* can be classified according to their site of action. Those that act primarily in the lumen of the bowel include iodoquinol, diloxanide furoate, tetracycline, and paromomycin. Drugs that act primarily in tissues include dehydroemetine and chloroquine. Metronidazole is active both within the lumen of the bowel and in tissues. The choice of a drug or drugs should be based on the clinical setting and the potential toxicities of the drugs. Table 280-6 presents treatment recommendations for patients with asymptomatic infection, mild intestinal disease, severe intestinal disease, and hepatic abscess.

Mild disease is defined as loose stool or diarrhea without blood. Severe disease means that there is evidence of tissue invasion (i.e., bloody stool or positive serologic finding). The regimen of metronidazole plus iodoquinol has proved effective in more than 90% of patients with intestinal disease. Occasional patients with extraintestinal amebiasis have not responded to metronidazole for unknown reasons. However, they have usually responded to subsequent treatment with chloroquine or dehydroemetine. The vast majority of patients with amebic liver abscess respond to metronidazole therapy alone. Therapeutic needle aspiration of amebic liver abscesses is controversial. No data from controlled studies suggest that this procedure accelerates healing. However, some experienced clinicians recommend aspiration if concern exists about an impending rupture.

Table 280-6. Treatment of patients with amebiasis

Clinical setting	Recommended treatment
Asymptomatic (cysts in stool)	Paromomycin, 10 mg/kg tid for 7 days, or iodoquinol, 650 mg tid for 20 days
Mild intestinal disease (no evidence of invasion)	Metronidazole, 750 mg PO tid for 7 days, followed by iodoquinol, 650 mg tid for 20 days, or paromomycin, 10 mg/kg tid for 7 days
Severe intestinal disease (evidence of invasion)	Metronidazole, 750 mg tid for 7 days (IV or PO), followed by iodoquinol, 650 mg tid for 20 days, or paromomycin, 10 mg/kg tid for 7 days; alternative regimen: dehydroemetine, 1 mg/kg IM daily for 10 days, followed by tetracycline, 500 mg four times a day for 10 days, plus iodoquinol, 650 mg tid for 20 days
Liver abscess	Metronidazole, 750 mg tid for 7 days (IV or PO), plus iodoquinol, 650 mg tid for 20 days; alternative regimen: dehydroemetine, 1 mg/kg IM daily for 10 days, followed by chloroquine phosphate, 1000 mg daily for 2 days then 500 mg daily for 21 days, plus iodoquinol, 650 mg tid for 20 days

PO, Orally; IV, intravenously; IM, intramuscularly; tid, three times a day.

After treatment of intestinal disease, follow-up stool examinations should be performed at 1 month and at 6 months to ensure eradication. For patients with liver abscess, a follow-up liver scan should be performed 2 to 4 months after treatment, by which time most lesions should have resolved. Occasionally, however, adequately treated liver abscesses may not resolve radiographically for 12 months. Metronidazole is usually tolerated well but may cause nausea and abdominal fullness. Alcohol should be avoided because a disulfiram-like reaction may occur. Metronidazole is carcinogenic in rodents and mutagenic in bacteria; however, women inadvertently treated for trichomoniasis during pregnancy with metronidazole have not been shown to have adverse fetal effects. Thus pregnant women with severe disease should be treated with metronidazole because the risks to the fetus and mother from untreated severe disease are great. Iodoquinol has been associated with subacute myelo-optic neuropathy in Japan, but its relation to this syndrome is unclear. The drug is usually well tolerated. However, it may interfere with thyroid function tests for months.

The treatment of patients with amebiasis does little to interrupt transmission of infection, since reinfection can occur and most carriers are asymptomatic. In nonendemic areas it is useful to evaluate the household and sexual contacts of patients by performing three stool examinations. However, homosexual males who are sexually promiscuous are likely to become reinfected. Prevention in endemic areas is difficult. Travelers may protect themselves by drinking only boiled or iodinated water. Fruits and vegetables must be washed with a strong detergent and rinsed with a dilute acid (e.g., vinegar) to eradicate infectious cysts.

INFECTIONS CAUSED BY FREE-LIVING AMEBAE *(NAEGLERIA, ACANTHAMOEBA)*

In contrast to the other protozoans that infect humans, the free-living amebae are not obligatory parasites; that is, they are able to survive and multiply in the environment in the absence of a host animal. Infection with the free-living ameba *Naegleria fowleri* causes an acute, primary meningoencephalitis that closely resembles bacterial meningitis clinically, usually in persons who are immunologically normal. Several species of *Acanthamoeba* can also cause an acute primary meningoencephalitis, but subacute or chronic disease, resembling a bacterial brain abscess, is more common. *Acanthamoeba* infection is more likely to occur in individuals who are immunosuppressed or who have diabetes, but otherwise healthy individuals may also be infected. AIDS may be a risk factor. *E. histolytica* may also cause amebic meningoencephalitis, but only after secondary spread from other foci of disease, such as liver abscess or pulmonary disease. Species of *Acanthamoeba* are also responsible for some cases of corneal ulceration.

Free-living amebae exist as trophozoites or cysts in fresh

water or soil. Human infection usually occurs when there is contact with fresh water in aquariums, hydrotherapy pools, freshwater springs, lakes, ponds, or swimming pools.

Naegleria species invade the CNS by penetrating the nasal mucosa of the cribriform plate and then spreading through the fila olfactoria. *Acanthamoeba* species usually invade the CNS hematogenously after primary infection of the eye, skin, lung, prostate, or uterus. *Naegleria* organisms multiply rapidly and produce hemorrhagic necrosis of the gray matter of the cerebral cortex and then of the white matter and cerebellum. The subarachnoid space is also invaded. Most patients have a neutrophilic pleocytosis, and organisms can be identified in CSF. Some patients also have an inflammatory myocarditis, but *Naegleria* organisms are not usually identified in the myocardium.

Acanthamoeba may produce a pathologic and clinical picture identical to that of *Naegleria* or, more frequently, a chronic encephalitis with multiple brain abscesses. Whereas the cellular response to *Naegleria* involves primarily polymorphonuclear leukocytes, the response to *Acanthamoeba* usually involves lymphocytes, monocytes, and plasma cells. Invasion of the subarachnoid space occurs less frequently with *Acanthamoeba,* and organisms are rarely found in CSF.

The incubation period of acute amebic meningoencephalitis is 5 to 7 days. There is usually sudden onset of severe headache, fever, and meningismus. The diagnosis of *Naegleria* infection may be suggested by abnormal sensations of taste and smell because of olfactory involvement and by the presence of myocarditis. Examination of the CSF in acute disease usually reveals a high white blood cell count with a predominance of neutrophils. The concentration of glucose is usually low. Amebae may be identified in the CSF as highly motile trophozoites.

Subacute or chronic disease caused by *Acanthamoeba* usually has a gradual onset. Headache, seizures, and focal findings on neurologic examination are common. MRI or CT of the brain may reveal multiple lesions, particularly in the white matter of the deep midline and midbrain structures. Examination of the CSF reveals an elevated white blood cell count with predominance of mononuclear cells but no organisms. The glucose level is usually normal.

The diagnosis of acute amebic meningoencephalitis is made by identifying trophozoites in the CSF in a patient with a history of exposure to fresh water (usually swimming or diving in a lake or pond). The diagnosis of chronic disease is more difficult. Brain biopsy will usually reveal trophozoites and cysts. Several serologic tests are available. They may be helpful in patients with a compatible history and CSF abnormalities but with lesions not readily accessible for biopsy.

Most cases of amebic meningoencephalitis are fatal. *N. fowleri* is sensitive to amphotericin B, and after test doses, a dose of 1 mg/kg/day should be reached as soon as possible. Intrathecal amphotericin B is recommended by some authorities. Miconazole and rifampin may also be active against the organism. There have been few survivors of cerebral disease caused by *Acanthamoeba*. In vitro data suggest that polymyxin B and flucytosine may be useful and that they may act synergistically if given together. Pentamidine and ketoconazole have also been reported to possess in vitro activity.

Corneal ulcerations caused by *Acanthamoeba* are associated with soft contact lenses or local trauma. Symptoms usually begin as a foreign body sensation, followed by pain, photophobia, conjunctivitis, and blurred vision. Spontaneous remissions and relapses may occur as part of the natural history of the disease. The ulcers are shaggy, have an irregular border, and may resemble herpes. Other findings include iritis, a corneal ring infiltrate, cataracts, and breakdown of the corneal epithelium. Complete destruction of the cornea may occur. Diagnosis is made by histologic examination and culture of corneal scrapings. Treatment of corneal disease has been more successful than treatment of cerebral disease. The cornea should be surgically debrided and treated topically for 3 to 4 weeks with 1% miconazole nitrate, 0.1% propamidine isethionate, and neosporin. Frequent application of propamidine isethionate (every 15 to 60 minutes for the first 3 days) has been recommended.

GIARDIASIS

Giardiasis is caused by the luminal flagellate *Giardia lamblia*. The organism was discovered by van Leeuwenhoek, the inventor of the microscope, who identified it in his own stool. Infection is frequently asymptomatic but may cause endemic or epidemic diarrhea. Effective treatment is available.

Biology and life cycle

The organism has two stages, trophozoite and cyst. Infection is acquired by the ingestion of as few as 10 cysts, which may be present in feces or contaminated water or food. Cysts rupture in the stomach and release trophozoites, which use their flagella to migrate to the duodenum and jejunum and attach to the brush border of intestinal epithelial cells. The parasite does not invade cells. To complete the life cycle, cysts are produced in the lumen of the intestine and excreted in the feces. Cysts may survive in cold water for several months. There may be animal reservoirs of giardiasis. Cysts from beavers are infectious for humans.

Epidemiology

G. lamblia has a worldwide distribution. It is a common pathogen in epidemics of waterborne infectious diarrhea. Hikers may be infected by cysts in mountain streams. Person-to-person and foodborne transmission also occur. Epidemics have occurred in day-care centers and in custodial institutions. Some urban populations of homosexual men have a high prevalence of infection (20% or more) that is probably maintained by sexual transmission.

Pathogenesis and immunity

The clinical consequences of infection are probably produced by heavy colonization of intestinal epithelium, disruption of the brush border, and interference with the bowel's absorptive capacity. Disaccharidase deficiencies, especially of lactase, occur. The parasite is not known to produce any toxins.

Repeated or prolonged exposure may produce a degree of protection, since residents of endemic areas seem to have a lower incidence of disease than nonimmune visitors. Hypogammaglobulinemia may predispose patients to more severe disease.

Clinical manifestations

Infection with *G. lamblia* may be asymptomatic or may cause a spectrum of manifestations, from acute, self-limited diarrhea to chronic diarrhea with malabsorption and weight loss (Chapter 236). Epigastric cramping, anorexia, nausea, flatulence, and vomiting also occur. The acute illness usually lasts 3 to 4 days, but patients may have mild symptoms of epigastric fullness, flatulence, and loose stools for several weeks. Infection probably resolves spontaneously in many patients. Patients with chronic infection may have intermittent bouts of diarrhea and malaise or severe persistent diarrhea with steatorrhea. Extraintestinal disease does not occur.

Few laboratory abnormalities are found. Blood counts, differential white cell count, and erythrocyte sedimentation rate are normal. Mild anemia may be present, more frequently in children than adults. Giardiasis does not cause fecal leukocytes, and usually no blood is seen in the stool. An upper gastrointestinal series may show mild dilatation, reduced transit time, and thickening of mucosal folds. Patients with hypogammaglobulinemia and giardiasis may have small-bowel lymphoid nodules.

Diagnosis

Giardiasis should be suspected in all patients with diarrhea lasting more than a few days, especially if no fever and no fecal leukocytes are present. The diagnosis should also be considered in patients with malabsorption, especially if the patient is immunodeficient. The diagnosis can often be made by stool examination (Color Plate V-57). The yield is increased by examination of three stools in three forms (fresh wet mount for motile trophozoites, stained smear, and zinc-sulfate concentration on each stool).

As with *E. histolytica,* false-negative results may occur in the presence of interfering substances, such as barium, antibiotics, or antidiarrheal compounds (kaolin, bismuth). If stool examination results are negative, the diagnosis may be made using commercial kits for detecting *G. lamblia* antigen in stools, a sensitive and specific method for diagnosis of giardiasis. The stool antigen test may ultimately replace other invasive tests, such as examination of duodenal material obtained by aspiration, string test (Enterotest, Hedeco, Palo Alto, Calif.), or biopsy. If performed, biopsies should be stained with Giemsa.

Serologic tests are available on a research basis.

Treatment and prevention

Quinacrine is the drug of choice for giardiasis. Nausea, vomiting, and mild diarrhea are the most common side effects. Exfoliative dermatitis and delirium have occurred rarely. Metronidazole is not approved for use in giardiasis in the United States but is usually effective at the recommended dose. Recommendations for treatment are given in Table 280-7.

The most important factor in preventing giardiasis is the proper treatment of water. Routine chlorination may not kill cysts; sedimentation, flocculation, and filtration should also be performed. Hikers can prevent giardiasis by boiling water for at least 1 minute or by adding halazone (5 tablets/L for 30 minutes) or iodine. Travelers to areas with contaminated water should drink only boiled or treated water and should not consume uncooked fruit or vegetables. Household and sexual contacts of infected individuals should have three stool examinations.

LEISHMANIASIS

Leishmaniasis is a general term for human disease caused by species of the genus *Leishmania*. Most human infections with *Leishmania* are transmitted by sand flies from mammalian reservoirs (i.e., the disease is a zoonosis). Leishmaniasis usually takes one of three clinical forms: cutaneous, mucocutaneous, or visceral (kala-azar). The form is determined principally by the species of parasite, although the host's immune status and genetic background may also affect clinical manifestations. The taxonomy of the *Leishmania* is unsettled and is changing because new criteria are being proposed for the identification of species and subspecies. The classification of species in this chapter is based on clinical manifestations and epidemiology. *L. tropica* causes cutaneous disease in the Old World; *L. mexicana* and some subspecies of *L. braziliensis* cause cutaneous disease in the New World; other subspecies of *L. braziliensis* cause mucocutaneous disease; *L. donovani* causes visceral leishmaniasis. Molecular research on *Leishmania* parasites promises to yield new approaches to taxonomy, diagnosis, and treatment.

Leishmaniasis is transmitted rarely in the southwestern United States, but most cases seen in the United States occur in travelers, immigrants, and refugees. The incubation period for mucocutaneous leishmaniasis may be months or

Table 280-7. Treatment of patients with giardiasis

Clinical setting	Recommended treatment
Immunocompetent or immunocompromised patients	Quinacrine, 100 mg tid for 5 to 7 days, or metronidazole, 250 mg tid for 5 to 7 days, or paromomycin, 10 mg/kg tid for 7 days
Pregnant women	Paromomycin, 10 mg/kg tid for 7 days

Tid, Three times a day.

years, and physicians must therefore have a high degree of suspicion and inquire about travel over preceding years if the diagnosis is to be made. Diagnosis is made by identifying organisms in Giemsa-stained impression smears or biopsies or by isolating the organism from infected tissues. A delayed hypersensitivity skin test and serologic tests may be helpful in some patients, and DNA hybridization probes have been developed. Effective chemotherapy is available for most clinical forms of leishmaniasis, but the drugs are toxic, and they are often difficult to administer in less developed countries.

Biology and life cycle

Leishmania have two forms: flagellated extracellular promastigotes in the sand fly vector and unflagellated intracellular amastigotes in mammalian hosts. All species of *Leishmania* are morphologically indistinguishable. The parasites multiply by asexual binary fission, and there is no sexual stage. *Leishmania* (and *Trypanosoma*) organisms have a DNA-containing organelle called the *kinetoplast* that stains intensely with Giemsa stain.

Leishmaniasis is transmitted to humans by the bite of infected female *Phlebotomus* sand flies or rarely by direct contact with infected cutaneous lesions. Promastigotes in the fly's proboscis are injected subcutaneously, where they bind to the surface of local tissue macrophages and are engulfed by phagocytosis. Recent studies indicate that the binding of promastigotes to macrophages is mediated by an intriguing example of molecular mimicry in which the promastigote becomes coated with the third component of complement, which then mediates binding of the promastigote to the C3 receptor on the macrophage. Once intracellular, the organisms transform into amastigotes, which multiply within phagolysosomes (Color Plate V-12). The biochemical basis for the parasite's ability to survive in the presence of lysosomal enzymes is unknown. After local proliferation at the site of inoculation, the organisms may remain localized or may metastasize to nasal mucous membranes or to the reticuloendothelial system, depending on the species of parasite. *L. tropica* and *L. mexicana* remain localized in the original site, the nearby skin, and the draining lymph nodes. *L. braziliensis* may metastasize to mucous membranes, but not to the viscera. *L. donovani* may spread through the blood to the reticuloendothelial system of multiple organs.

Sand flies that feed on infected humans or other mammals ingest dermal macrophages containing amastigotes. In the fly's gut the amastigotes exit from the macrophages and transform into flagellated promastigotes. The promastigotes multiply, migrate to the proboscis, and are injected into a human or animal at the fly's next feeding.

Epidemiology

Leishmaniasis is primarily a disease of the tropics and subtropics because sand flies require a habitat with high humidity and high temperature. Sand flies breed in cracks of building walls, in rodent burrows, in piles of rubbish, and in shaded vegetation. With the exception of *L. donovani* in India, the disease is a zoonosis. The sand flies feed on human and animal blood, and dogs, rats, gerbils, and a variety of other mammals form a reservoir for human infection. In India, *L. donovani* is transmitted from person to person by anthrophilic (human-biting) sand flies. The geographic locations of disease and the local animal reservoirs are listed in Table 280-8. The epidemiology of mucocutaneous leishmaniasis is of practical importance, since the risk of subsequent mucous membrane involvement is affected by the locale where the primary infection occurred.

Pathogenesis and immunity

The specific consequences of infection with *Leishmania* are determined by the tissue tropism of different species and by the host's immune response. The species that cause cutaneous or mucocutaneous disease may be limited in spread by temperature. With *L. tropica* and *L. mexicana,* amastigotes proliferate within macrophages at the site of the sand fly bite. An initial granulomatous reaction produces a papule that eventually breaks down and ulcerates. Cutaneous disease is usually self-limited and heals without chemotherapy. Antibody to leishmanial antigens is difficult to detect in patients with cutaneous disease and probably has little role in healing. Recovery depends on the development of cell-mediated immunity, which stops the intracellular multiplication of amastigotes and is manifested histologically as a lymphocytic infiltrate at the lesion. A delayed hypersensitivity skin test (Montenegro test) is positive. Healing leaves a flat, atrophic scar and results in resistance to reinfection with the homologous parasite species. Some patients have an exuberant granulomatous reaction that produces persistent nodules at the edge of the primary lesion (leishmaniasis recidivans). In the absence of cell-mediated immunity, no lymphocytic infiltrate occurs, and parasites proliferate in the skin, producing diffuse cutaneous leishmaniasis. It is not known whether immunosuppression is caused by a parasite product or by an abnormality of the host immune system.

With some subspecies of *L. braziliensis,* lesions develop in the cartilage and mucous membranes of the nose months to years after the primary skin lesion has healed. Although patients usually have intact cell-mediated immune responses to leishmanial antigens, the lesions progress and may be very destructive. Spontaneous recovery has not been reported.

L. donovani does not remain limited to the skin, but disseminates and multiplies within the macrophages of the spleen, liver, bone marrow, and lymph nodes. Cell-mediated immune responses to leishmanial antigens are depressed, but high levels of antileishmanial antibodies can usually be detected. Cell-mediated immune responses develop after successful treatment, and patients who recover are usually immune to reinfection. It is postulated that suppressor cells or circulating immune complexes may have a role in the immunosuppression observed with visceral disease. Massive splenomegaly occurs frequently and is accompanied by sequestration of erythrocytes, leukocytes,

Table 280-8. Leishmaniasis: summary of epidemiology, clinical features, and treatment

Species	Geographic location	Reservoir	Clinical features	Treatment
L. tropica				
L. tropica major	Desert areas of Central Asia, North Africa, Middle East	Desert rodents	Cutaneous: acute, wet, ulcerated lesions on extremities	Pentostam,* 20 mg/kg/day IV or IM for 20 days; repeated courses may be needed; alternative drugs: amphotericin B, ketoconazole, or pentamidine
L. tropica minor	Urban areas of Middle East, Mediterranean littoral areas, India, Pakistan, Africa	Dogs	Cutaneous: chronic, dry lesion that rarely ulcerates	Pentostam as for *L. tropica major*
L. mexicana	Yucatan peninsula, Belize, Guatemala, Venezuela, Dominican Republic, southern United States (rare)	Forest rodents	Cutaneous: chiclero ulcer; single or limited number of skin lesions; may cause diffuse cutaneous leishmaniasis or rarely, mucocutaneous leishmaniasis	Pentostam as for *L. tropica major;* most cases resolve spontaneously; if needed, Pentostam or amphotericin B in various doses for various lengths of time
L. braziliensis	Panama, Costa Rica, South America, including Brazil, Venezuela, Boliva, Peru, northern Argentina	Forest rodents and dogs	Cutaneous and mucocutaneous (especially Brazil)	Pentostam as for *L. tropica major*. Addition of allopurinol, 20 mg/kg/day in four divided doses for 15 days increased cure rates compared with pentostam alone. Allopurinol alone at the same dose was also effective.
L. donovani	Mediterranean littoral areas, Middle East, India, Pakistan, China, South and Central America *(L. chagasi),* Asia, Africa	Dogs, foxes, rodents; no animal reservoir in India	Visceral leishmaniasis	Pentostam as for *L. tropica major*

*Dosage of Pentostam is calculated as mg of sb/kg. In the United States, Pentostam is available from the Drug Service of the Centers for Disease Control (tel. no. 404-639-3670 or 404-639-2888).

and platelets in the spleen, leading to pancytopenia, which is compounded by decreased production by the infiltrated bone marrow. A polyclonal activation of B cells and hypergammaglobulinemia occur. Circulating immune complexes and rheumatoid factor can usually be detected, but their role in pathogenesis is not known. Many patients have a subclinical immune complex glomerulonephritis. After successful treatment, some patients develop disseminated skin lesions that contain *L. donovani* (post–kala-azar dermal leishmaniasis).

Clinical manifestations

Infections with *Leishmania* can be acquired from a single sand fly bite, so only brief residence in an endemic area is needed. In addition, infection can be acquired by direct contact with infected skin lesions or rarely by blood transfusion. The incubation period for leishmaniasis varies from a few weeks to several years, but with *L. tropica* and *L. mexicana* it is usually 2 weeks to 3 months and with *L. donovani,* 3 to 8 months. *L. braziliensis* usually has an incubation period of 2 to 8 weeks for the cutaneous lesions. The time between the primary skin lesion and mucous membrane involvement is usually several years, although it may be as short as 1 month and as long as 25 years.

Cutaneous leishmaniasis may have some variation in clinical manifestations, depending on the parasite species and the geographic location where infection was acquired (Table 280-8). Typically, there is first a papule, which enlarges, becomes crusted, and then (in *L. tropica major, L. mexicana,* and *L. braziliensis*) ulcerates. Ulcers have a diameter of about 2 cm and an indurated border. Satellite lesions may be adjacent to the primary skin lesion and along the draining lymphatics. Regional lymphadenopathy is common. Patients usually have no fever, and the lesions are painless unless secondarily infected by bacteria. Healing leaves a flat or depressed depigmented scar. Cutaneous lesions associated with particular geographic areas include chronic, dry, scaly solitary nodules on the face in *L. tropica minor* acquired in urban settings; acute, wet, ulcerated lesions on the extremities with *L. tropica major* acquired in rural locales; ulceration of the pinna of the ear (chiclero ulcer) with *L. mexicana* acquired by workers harvesting gum from chicle plants in Mexico, Belize, and Guatemala; hyperkeratotic or papillomatous lesions similar to yaws in Guyana, Surinam, and northern Brazil (forest yaws); and nodular lesions occurring in individuals residing in the Peruvian highlands (uta).

Diffuse cutaneous leishmaniasis has been observed in Ethiopia, Venezuela, Brazil, and the Dominican Republic. The lesions are widespread and typically remain as macules or papules without ulceration. The mucous membranes may be involved, but not the viscera. Lesions contain sparse lymphocytes, and there is cutaneous anergy to leishmanial antigens.

Mucocutaneous leishmaniasis (espundia) is caused by subspecies of *L. braziliensis* and is especially prevalent in Brazil south of the Amazon. In patients with cutaneous lesions the likelihood of subsequent mucous membrane involvement is about 80% if the infection was acquired in Brazil, 5% if acquired in Panama or Guyana, and less than 1% if acquired in Mexico. More than 90% of patients with espundia have scars of previous cutaneous involvement. Nasal lesions tend to destroy the cartilage of the septum and spread to the buccal mucosa, pharynx, and larynx. Isolated laryngeal involvement may occur. The initial manifestation of nasal involvement is usually nasal stuffiness. The disease is not self-limited and may progress to severe facial deformities. Complications include CSF leaks, meningitis, and cavernous sinus thrombosis.

Visceral leishmaniasis has similar clinical manifestations wherever it occurs. The onset of disease may be gradual or acute. There is usually fever, malaise, anorexia, cough, and weight loss. The liver and spleen are greatly enlarged, and some patients have diffuse lymphadenopathy. Pancytopenia secondary to hypersplenism and marrow infiltration is the most lethal complication of the disease. Light-skinned patients may be seen to develop a grayish discoloration of the skin, which led to the Indian name for the disease, *kala-azar,* which means "black fever." Death is usually caused by intercurrent bacterial infection, bleeding, or severe anemia. About 20% of Indian patients and 3% of African patients develop disseminated cutaneous lesions after treatment for visceral disease. The skin lesions may be nodular or flat and depigmented.

Diagnosis

A history of travel to or residence in an endemic area should lead to consideration of leishmaniasis in patients with skin lesions, nasal or oropharyngeal disease, or hepatosplenomegaly and pancytopenia. The potential for long incubation periods, especially in mucocutaneous disease, must be remembered. Cutaneous disease must be differentiated from leprosy, atypical mycobacterial infection *(Mycobacterium marinum),* blastomycosis, histoplasmosis, sporotrichosis, nocardiosis, syphilis, and yaws. The differential diagnosis of mucocutaneous disease includes leprosy, syphilis, Wegener's granulomatosis, midline granuloma, paracoccidioidomycosis, and nasopharyngeal carcinoma. Visceral leishmaniasis must be differentiated from malaria (especially the tropical splenomegaly syndrome), schistosomiasis, and lymphoma. The diagnosis of leishmaniasis can be made by identifying organisms in Giemsa-stained impression smears or biopsies or by culture of the organism in NNN or Schneider's *Drosophila* medium. In cutaneous disease, organisms are most abundant at the periphery of ulcerated lesions or in nodular lesions. In mucocutaneous disease, organisms may be obtained from scrapings or biopsy from the nasal mucosa, but usually, few organisms are seen. In visceral leishmaniasis, bone marrow examination and culture are positive in 90% of patients, and liver biopsy is positive in 70%. Some clinicians perform splenic aspiration, but this procedure may be complicated by splenic rupture and death. An antigen for skin testing is available from the World Health Organization Leishmaniasis Reference Center, Hadassah Medical Center, Jerusalem, Israel, and serologic tests for antileishmanial antibodies are performed at the Centers for Disease Control. Neither test is well standardized. Patients with cutaneous and mucocutaneous disease have positive delayed hypersensitivity skin tests. Patients with disseminated cutaneous leishmaniasis and visceral disease are anergic on the skin test but have high levels of circulating antibodies to leishmanial antigens. Some patients with mucocutaneous disease have positive serologic results.

Treatment and prevention

The pentavalent antimonial drug sodium stibogluconate (Pentostam) is active against all species of *Leishmania* and is available from the Centers for Disease Control (Table 280-8). Recent studies have helped to determine optimum doses and the duration of treatment. The dose of Pentostam now recommended for all clinical forms of leishmanial disease is 20 mg/kg/day for 20 days. The maximum daily dose should not exceed 850 mg of pentavalent antimony. If clinical response has not occurred, longer treatment may be given. These large doses of Pentostam generally require IV administration. Recent clinical experience suggests that Pentostam causes few side effects: principally weakness, anorexia, mild reversible liver function abnormalities, and transient abnormalities of the T wave on electrocardiogram testing. With longer periods of treatment, leukopenia and thrombocytopenia may occur.

Repeated courses of Pentostam are often required for cure of mucocutaneous and visceral leishmaniasis. Evidence indicates that cutaneous or visceral disease acquired in East Africa may be more resistant to treatment. Alternative drugs include amphotericin B and pentamidine isothionate. Scientists are attempting to develop new drugs based on metabolic differences between the parasite and the host. Results with purine analogs and ketoconazole are promising. Allopurinol alone or in combination with Pentostam was recently shown to be more effective than Pentostam alone in curing American cutaneous leishmaniasis. Whether or not allopurinol will prove to be effective against the other clinical forms of leishmaniasis remains to be determined.

Leishmaniasis is difficult to prevent. No vaccine and no

effective chemoprophylaxis are available. Control of animal reservoirs is difficult. The prospects for a vaccine appear to be good, since cutaneous infection produces lifelong species-specific immunity. Travelers can obtain partial protection by the use of insect repellents and netting.

AFRICAN TRYPANOSOMIASIS

African trypanosomiasis is a zoonotic disease that is caused by two subspecies of *Trypanosoma brucei: T. b. gambiense* and *T. b. rhodesiense,* which differ in clinical manifestations, epidemiology, and vector habitat. Infection is transmitted by members of the genus *Glossina* (tsetse flies). A third subspecies, *T. b. brucei,* is not infectious for humans but causes disease in livestock and has an important economic impact in Africa. Scientists have recently made rapid progress in understanding the biochemistry and molecular genetics of *Trypanosoma,* but so far with little impact on the disease. Drug treatment is toxic and often ineffective; immunoprophylaxis has been frustrated by the parasite's capacity for antigenic variation; and vector control is extremely expensive for governments in endemic areas.

Biology and life cycle

T. b. gambiense and *T. b. rhodesiense* are morphologically identical, and the two subspecies are differentiated on the basis of epidemiology, vector habitat, and disease manifestations (Table 280-9). They are flagellated, extracellular organisms that multiply in the blood, tissue spaces, and CSF of mammalian hosts. They are ingested by the tsetse fly vector during a blood meal. Within the fly's midgut, they shed their protective surface coat and transform into procyclic trypanosomes, which multiply and migrate to the salivary glands. Salivary gland organisms (called *epimastigotes*) multiply, then transform into nondividing metacyclic trypanosomes, which acquire a surface coat and are injected into a mammalian host during a fly's next blood meal. In the mammalian host, the parasites transform into slender, blood-stage forms that circulate in the blood and divide rapidly by binary fission. Some of the blood parasites develop into short, stumpy forms that are adapted for uptake by the tsetse fly.

Trypanosomes can be stained with Giemsa stain. They have a central nucleus and, as with *Leishmania,* a densely stained kinetoplast at the base of the flagellum. The surface coat of blood-stage forms is composed of a single glycoprotein, the *variable surface glycoprotein* (VSG). The genome of African trypanosomes contains a multiplicity of genes for VSGs of different antigenic structure. The gene that is to be expressed is duplicated and transposed to a different region of the chromosome in such a way that cells usually express only one VSG at a time. The dividing organism can displace the VSG gene that was expressed and replace it with a new gene so that a VSG of different antigenic type is expressed. This process of gene switching results in antigenic variation. As the host makes antibody to a VSG of one type, trypanosomes bearing a different VSG appear. The number of VSGs that can be produced appears to be unlimited.

Epidemiology

It is estimated that 45 million persons are at risk for infection with African trypanosomiasis and that about 10,000 new infections occur each year. Transmission by tsetse fly is limited to sub-Saharan Africa. *T. b. gambiense* occurs in West and Central Africa, *T. b. rhodesiense* in East Africa (Table 280-9). Infection can also be transmitted mechanically by blood-sucking insects, by blood transfusion, and congenitally from mother to child around the time of delivery.

Pathogenesis and immunity

At the site of the tsetse fly's bite, a mononuclear cell infiltrate produces a nodule (trypanosomal chancre). A systemic phase begins weeks to months after the tsetse bite and is characterized by recurrent waves of parasitemia, each consisting of serologically distinct parasites produced by antigenic variation of the VSG. Parasites eventually invade the CNS and produce a chronic meningoencephalitis. Histologically, perivascular infiltration by lymphocytes, monocytes, and plasma cells occurs. The plasma cells may be responsible for the high levels of IgM that occur in CSF. With *T. b. rhodesiense,* the systemic phase is usually fulminant. Cardiac involvement dominates the pathologic and clinical picture, and the pathologic changes in the CNS may not occur.

The mechanisms by which the extracellular organisms produce disease are unknown. Patients typically have very high levels of serum and CSF immunoglobulins caused by

Table 280-9. African trypanosomiasis: clinical and epidemiologic features

Trypanosoma subspecies	Geographic location	Animal reservoirs	Clinical features
T. b. gambiense	Forested areas of West and Central Africa south of the Sahara	Possibly pigs, dogs, hartebeest, sheep, cattle	Acute systemic illness followed by chronic meningoencephalitic illness
T. b. rhodesiense	Groups of trees in savanna areas of East Africa from Ethiopia and Uganda to Zambia and Zimbabwe	Antelopes, hogs, cattle, sheep, goats, dogs, hartebeest, lions, hyenas	Acute systemic illness with early invasion of the CNS and prominent myocarditis

polyclonal B cell activation. These immunoglobulins do not produce immunity, and it has been proposed that the proliferating B cells may infiltrate tissues and produce disease.

Clinical manifestations

The clinical manifestations of African trypanosomiasis are determined by the subspecies of parasite and may be different in travelers and expatriates compared with residents of the parasite's endemic area. With both subspecies the trypanosomal chancre is the first manifestation of disease. The chancre is typically on an exposed part of the body, is hard, red, and painful, and usually lasts 1 to 2 weeks. The systemic phase of illness is characterized by fever with a relapsing pattern, severe headache, and lymphadenopathy. Episodes of fever last 1 to 6 days. Afebrile remissions may last for several weeks. Posterior cervical nodes are classically enlarged (Winterbottom's sign). A nonpruritic, erythematous, macular rash may develop on the trunk. With West African trypanosomiasis *(T. b. gambiense),* neurologic manifestations include changes in personality early in the course of disease, progressing to lassitude, indifference, and an uncontrollable urge to sleep during the day. Some patients may develop a frank psychosis. Hypertonicity, cerebellar ataxia, and movement disorders (most often chorea and athetosis) may occur. Patients eventually become comatose. Splenomegaly is usually present during the later stages of disease. Death is often caused by intercurrent bacterial infection.

With East African trypanosomiasis *(T. b. rhodesiense),* the disease is more acute. Neurologic manifestations are less prominent, and myocarditis or pericarditis is more frequently the cause of death.

Laboratory examination usually shows anemia, monocytosis, and hypergammaglobulinemia. The level of CSF protein (especially IgM) is elevated, and a lymphocytic pleocytosis occurs. The CSF glucose level is normal. Large, vacuolated plasma cells are occasionally observed in the CSF.

Diagnosis

Physicians in the United States are most likely to see African trypanosomiasis in travelers, returning expatriates, immigrants, and refugees. The possibility of congenital transmission should be kept in mind; the mother may be relatively asymptomatic. A careful travel history is essential and should elicit the type of terrain as well as the countries visited to determine the probability of exposure to the vector. Most travelers will remember the painful trypanosomal chancre, even if it is no longer present. East African trypanosomiasis should be considered in individuals who develop fever, headache, myocarditis, or lymphadenopathy within a month after returning from an endemic area. West African trypanosomiasis is more indolent and requires a high index of suspicion if the diagnosis is to be made. The differential diagnosis includes malaria, tickborne or louseborne relapsing fever, typhoid fever, lymphoma, and other causes of chronic meningitis, encephalitis, or myocarditis.

The diagnosis is made by identifying organisms in Giemsa-stained blood smears, CSF, or lymph node aspirate (Color Plate V-16). The level of parasitemia in the blood varies with relapses and remissions, and multiple blood samples should be examined. With high parasitemias, organisms may be observed on thick blood smears, but diagnosis at lower parasitemias requires concentration techniques, such as examination of buffy-coat smears or filtration of blood through an ion-exchange column. A large volume of CSF (5 to 10 ml) should be centrifuged and stained if CNS disease is suspected. DNA hybridization probes and the polymerase chain reaction are being investigated for use in diagnosis.

Treatment and prevention

Chemotherapy of African trypanosomiasis requires prolonged administration of toxic drugs and is complicated by the emerging resistance of some strains. Suramin is used to treat blood-stage disease. A test dose of 100 mg is given IV, followed by 1 g on days 1, 3, 7, 14, and 21. Toxicities include proteinuria (frequent) and hypotension, fever, and desquamative dermatitis (infrequent). Suramin is not effective against parasites in the CNS. Alternative drugs include eflornithine or pentamidine (Table 280-10).

Table 280-10. Treatment of patients with African trypanosomiasis

Clinical setting	Treatment
Early (hemolymphatic stage) without meningeal involvement	Suramin, 100 mg test dose IV, then 1 g IV on days 1, 3, 7, 14, and 21; alternative regimens: eflornithine,* 400 mg/kg/day IV in four divided doses for 14 days followed by 400 mg/kg/day PO for 4 weeks, or pentamidine isethionate,* 4 mg/kg IV or IM daily for 10-14 days
Late stage with central nervous system (CNS) involvement	Melarsoprol,† 3.6 mg/kg/day IV for 3 days, repeated after 7-day rest period and again after 10-day to 14-day rest period; alternative regimens for patients who cannot tolerate melarsoprol: eflornithine as above or a combination of tryparsamide, 30 mg/kg IV (maximum, 2 g) every 5 days to a total of 12 injections, plus suramin, 10 mg/kg IV every 5 days to a total of 12 injections (regimen may be repeated after 1 month)

IV, Intravenously; IM, intramuscularly; PO, orally.
*Treatment with eflornithine is more effective against *T. b. gambiense* than against *T. b. rhodesiense*. Pentamidine is effective *only* against *T. b. gambiense*.
†Melarsoprol is a highly toxic arsenical drug that frequently causes a reactive encephalopathy. It is available in the United States from the Drug Service of the Centers for Disease Control (tel. no. 404-639-3670 or 404-639-2888). The addition of corticosteroids to melarsoprol may prevent or reduce the symptoms of arsenical encephalopathy.

Disease of the CNS is treated with arsenicals (melarsoprol or tryparsamide)) given IV (Table 280-10). Toxicities of arsenicals include encephalitis, exfoliative dermatitis, and peripheral neuropathy. Encephalopathy is more common in patients with heavy parasite burdens at the time of treatment. Adjunctive therapy with corticosteroids has been reported to prevent or ameliorate the symptoms of encephalopathy associated with arsenical treatment. Although it has generally been recommended that melarsoprol be given only if CNS disease is present, some authorities believe that CNS invasion occurs early in the disease and therefore recommend that a drug active in the CNS be given to all patients. Pentamidine has been effective in some cases of West African trypanosomiasis, and eflornithine has also been used successfully in a few patients.

Prevention of African trypanosomiasis is difficult. The most widely used approaches are vector control and the prospective searching for and treatment of infected individuals. However, the presence of animal reservoirs and the underground location of the tsetse pupal stage complicate control measures. The prospects for a vaccine are poor. An urgent need exists for development of new drugs. Travelers can partially protect themselves with insecticides, repellents, and netting and by keeping arms and legs covered while in endemic areas.

CHAGAS' DISEASE (AMERICAN TRYPANOSOMIASIS)

Chagas' disease is caused by *Trypanosoma cruzi,* a zoonotic organism that is transmitted between mammals and humans by triatomid insects (reduviid bugs.) The disease typically has an acute phase, which may be asymptomatic, followed years or decades later by a chronic phase, in which the heart and the gastrointestinal tract are affected. The available drugs have low efficacy or high toxicity. No immediate prospect exists for a vaccine. The recent influx of Central American immigrants into the United States may result in more cases of Chagas' disease.

Biology and life cycle

T. cruzi is transmitted to humans by insects of the genera *Triatoma, Rhodnius,* and *Panstrongylus*. The most effective vectors have adapted to human dwellings, where they live in thatched roofs and in the crevices between bricks and maintain a cycle between humans and domestic animals. Infectious metacyclic trypomastigotes are excreted in the insect's feces during or immediately after a blood meal, and the organisms invade through the damaged skin or through mucous membranes. Although triatomids in the United States are infected with *T. cruzi,* transmission to humans rarely occurs because the U.S. insects do not defecate during or after their blood meal. Infection can also be transmitted by blood transfusion and congenitally. Several accidental laboratory-acquired infections have occurred among investigators studying Chagas' disease.

After invasion the *T. cruzi* organisms attach to macrophages and are internalized by phagocytosis. Once intracellular, they transform into amastigotes (no flagellum), lyse the phagosome, and multiply within the cytoplasm (Color Plate V-17). Intracellularly, some amastigotes differentiate into trypomastigotes (flagellated), which are released into the blood and disseminate to all host tissues. Triatomids feeding on infected animals or humans ingest trypomastigotes, which in the bug's intestinal tract transform into epimastigotes and multiply by asexual division. Within approximately 2 weeks, they transform into metacyclic forms, which are excreted in the bug's feces.

As with *T. brucei* and the *Leishmania* species, *T. cruzi* has a DNA-rich kinetoplast that stains densely with Giemsa. No evidence indicates antigenic variation, and the chronicity of infection appears to result from the organisms' adaptation to intracellular life and their ability to evade the immune system.

Epidemiology

In 1970, 12 million persons in the Americas were estimated to be infected with *T. cruzi*. Approximately 50% of the infected individuals resided in Brazil. The distribution of the infection corresponds to areas where the triatomid insects live close to humans. Proximity to humans occurs frequently when rural areas are opened up for agricultural development and the habitat of the vector and the animal reservoir is disrupted. In Latin America, Chagas' disease is primarily a problem of poor persons in rural areas. Acute infection usually occurs in children, and the cardiac and gastrointestinal manifestations of chronic disease usually occur between ages 35 and 45 years. Both cardiac and gastrointestinal disease are common in Brazil, but gastrointestinal disease rarely occurs in Venezuela, Colombia, and Panama. Recent studies indicate that 2% to 5% of Central American immigrants may be infected with *T. cruzi* and are at risk for developing Chagas' disease or for transmitting the parasite by blood transfusion.

Pathogenesis and immunity

T. cruzi is not known to produce any toxins or cytotoxic factors; it is likely that many of the consequences of infection result from the host's immune response. Frequently a local inflammatory response occurs at the site of infection, producing a painful nodule (chagoma). Trypomastigotes can be detected in the blood during the acute disease. With chronic Chagas' disease the heart is most often affected. There are foci of fibrosis, which may be small or large and dense. When fibrosis is extensive, the heart is enlarged, the ventricular wall is thinned, and the fibrotic plaques may serve as the nidus for thrombosis. Fibrosis of the conducting system also occurs. The esophagus and colon may be greatly dilated and have hypertrophy of smooth muscle. Histologically, involved tissues contain a mononuclear cell infiltrate. In the heart, myocardial fibers degenerate and fibrosis occurs. The number of neurons in the myenteric plexus may be reduced, which may contribute to the muscular hypertrophy and dilatation of the esophagus and colon. Organisms are usually not apparent in the tissues in chronic disease, although they may be isolated from the blood by xenodiagnosis (see later discussion).

Clinical manifestations

The incubation period between infection and the onset of disease is not known but is probably longer than 1 week. The initial manifestation is usually the *chagoma,* a painful, red nodule at the site of infection. Conjunctival inoculation produces unilateral conjunctivitis and edema of the eyelids (Romaña's sign). The acute, intravascular stage of infection is usually asymptomatic, but fever, lymphadenopathy, hepatosplenomegaly, meningoencephalitis, myocarditis, or an erythematous rash may occur, especially in children. Some young patients may die with acute congestive heart failure during this stage of the illness, but most recover in 2 to 3 months and enter the prolonged, indeterminant stage of infection.

With chronic infection, patients may remain asymptomatic or may develop disease years or decades later. The most frequent and most serious manifestation is Chagas' cardiomyopathy (Chapter 17). Patients usually have palpitations and may have symptoms of heart failure. The most common abnormalities are electrocardiographic: right bundle branch block in more than 60% of patients, left anterior hemiblock, atrioventricular block, premature ventricular contractions, and T wave abnormalities. Atrial arrhythmias occur, but are less common. ECG changes mimicking acute myocardial infarction have been reported. Fibrotic involvement of the myocardium produces biventricular failure, but the heart is usually not enlarged until late in the course of the disease. When cardiac involvement is extensive, mural thrombi and emboli typically occur.

Megaesophagus causes dysphagia, regurgitation, odynophagia, chest pain, cough, and frequent pulmonary aspiration. Barium swallow examination shows a spectrum of abnormalities, from retention of barium in the lower esophagus without dilatation to a bulky, elongated, atonic esophagus. Megacolon causes constipation that may be extraordinarily severe, chronic abdominal distention, and pain. In patients with advanced disease, barium enema examination may show dilatation, but in the initial stages of disease, no abnormalities may be seen on radiographic examination. Colonic obstruction and perforation may occur.

Diagnosis

The most important consideration in the diagnosis of Chagas' disease is a history of travel to or residence in an endemic area. Transmission of *T. cruzi* in the United States has been reported but is exceedingly rare. The rapid diagnosis of acute Chagas' disease is best accomplished by identifying organisms in the blood, either by direct microscopic examination for motile trypomastigotes in the buffy coat or by Giemsa-stained blood smears. Organisms can be cultured on NNN medium in 1 to 2 weeks. Blood can be fed to reduviid bugs in the laboratory and the intestinal contents of the bugs examined later for parasites *(xenodiagnosis).* Xenodiagnosis is very sensitive but requires 30 days. An immunofluorescence test that detects IgM antibodies to *T. cruzi* is available, but serologic testing has limited usefulness in the diagnosis of acute Chagas' disease because seroconversion often requires 3 to 4 weeks.

Patients in the indeterminant stage of infection have antibodies to *T. cruzi,* and parasites can be isolated by xenodiagnosis. Chronic Chagas' disease is diagnosed by identifying antibodies to *T. cruzi* in the serum of a patient with compatible clinical manifestations. Organisms are sparse and are not usually identified in tissue or isolated except by xenodiagnosis. Several serologic tests are available for the detection of antibody. False-positive results may occur with serum from patients with leishmaniasis or syphilis.

Treatment and prevention

Nitrofurtimox (Lampit) is the only drug available in the United States for the treatment of Chagas' disease and can be obtained from the CDC (tel. no. 404-639-3670 or 404-639-2888). The drug reduces the duration of parasitemia and clinical manifestations in acute Chagas' disease, prevents seroconversion, and may occasionally cure infection. It is not known, however, whether cure of infection prevents chronic disease. No evidence indicates that nitrofurtimox will reverse the manifestations of chronic disease. Use of the drug in the indeterminant stage of infection is controversial. The recommended dose is 8 to 10 mg/kg/day in four divided doses for 90 to 120 days. Side effects include nausea, vomiting, peripheral neuropathy, dermatitis, leukopenia, and delirium. As many as 50% of patients may have to discontinue the drug before completing the course. An alternative drug, benzimidazole, is widely used in South America, but it does not appear to offer advantages over nitrofurtimox. Scientists are attempting to identify and develop other drugs for the treatment of Chagas' disease.

The treatment of patients with chronic Chagas' disease is supportive. Pacemakers may prolong the lives of patients with cardiac disease and conduction disturbances, but those with congestive heart failure respond poorly to inotropic agents. Megaesophagus can be treated by pneumatic dilatation of the cardia of the stomach. Megacolon may respond to laxatives or enemas, or, if severe, to resection of the rectosigmoid and descending colon.

Strategies to prevent Chagas' disease include vector control with insecticides and improved housing in rural areas. To prevent transmission by transfusion, seropositive donors should be excluded. If this is not feasible, gentian violet can be added to blood and will inactivate the organism. Travelers should avoid sleeping in dwellings with thatched roofs or in dilapidated buildings.

BALANTIDIASIS

Balantidiasis is a colonic disease caused by infection with the ciliated protozoon *Balantidium coli.* The disease is a zoonosis that affects a variety of domestic animals, especially pigs. Human infection is unusual but may occur with close contact with infected animals.

Biology and life cycle

Infection is transmitted by the ingestion of cysts in feces or contaminated food or water. Cysts rupture in the small intestine, and trophozoites localize in the colon. Trophozoites multiply asexually by binary fission and sexually by conjugation. The trophozoites use their cilia to invade the mucosal epithelium and may penetrate to all layers of the bowel wall. Some trophozoites undergo excystation in the lumen of the colon and are excreted in the feces.

Pathogenesis and immunity

Trophozoite invasion of the colonic mucosa produces ulcerated lesions, most often in the rectosigmoid colon. The organism may penetrate the entire colon wall and cause perforation. Despite the invasion of blood vessels in the wall of the colon, extraintestinal disease does not occur.

Clinical manifestations

Most infections are asymptomatic. Symptoms are more common in undernourished individuals. Patients may have recurrent episodes of diarrhea, which may be watery or may contain mucus and blood. Sigmoidoscopy reveals mucosal ulcerations with diameters of 1 to 2 cm.

Diagnosis

The diagnosis of balantidiasis should be suspected in individuals with colitis and a history of exposure to swine or other wild or domestic animals. Organisms can be identified in stool or in scrapings from ulcerations obtained during sigmoidoscopy. *B. coli* is a large organism (up to 150 μm long) and may be mistaken for debris.

Treatment and prevention

Untreated balantidiasis may be fatal in malnourished or immunocompromised individuals. Tetracycline in a dose of 500 mg four times a day is effective in most cases. The combination of iodoquinol (650 mg three times a day for 20 days) plus metronidazole (750 mg three times a day for 5 days) is also effective. Prevention requires reducing the contact between humans and infected animals and avoiding the contamination of food and water.

BLASTOCYSTIS HOMINIS

Blastocystis hominis is considered by most authorities to be a protozoan organism that can infect the human gastrointestinal tract, but its ability to cause disease is uncertain. The mechanism of transmission is unknown. Although *B. hominis* is frequently identified in fecal samples, its pathogenicity is controversial. No strong correlation has been found between *B. hominis* and gastrointestinal symptoms, and some patients have had resolution of symptoms despite the continued presence of *B. hominis*. Most patients with *B. hominis* in their feces have another etiology for their symptoms. The organism is probably a commensal ("benign fellow traveler") in most persons, and other causes of intestinal disease, both infectious and noninfectious, should be sought despite the identification of *B. hominis*. Patients with persistent diarrhea, repeated identification of *B. hominis* in the feces, and no other identifiable etiology of disease, may be treated with metronidazole (750 mg three times a day for 10 days) with or without the addition of iodoquinol (650 mg three times a day for 20 days). However, it is most important to conduct a thorough search for other etiologies of disease.

TRICHOMONIASIS

Biology and life cycle

Trichomoniasis is a genitourinary disease caused by the flagellate protozoon *Trichomonas vaginalis*. The organism has only a trophozoite stage and requires anaerobic, alkaline conditions for growth. It is transmitted only by direct contact, usually during sexual intercourse. Humans are the only hosts.

Epidemiology

T. vaginalis has a worldwide distribution. The prevalence of infection ranges from 5% to more than 50% in different populations. The factors associated with high prevalence include multiple sexual partners, poor personal hygiene, and low socioeconomic status. From 30% to 50% of women with gonorrhea have coexisting infection with *T. vaginalis*. From 66% to 100% of the female sexual partners of infected males become infected, and 30% to 80% of the male sexual partners of infected females become infected. Experimental data suggest that *T. vaginalis* can be transmitted by contaminated objects as well as by sexual intercourse.

Pathogenesis and immunity

Infection may be chronic and asymptomatic or may produce vaginitis. Clinical manifestations in infected women may be produced by factors that raise vaginal pH (pregnancy, menses, anaerobic infection). With symptomatic infection, inflammation of the epithelium and submucosa of the vagina and cervix occurs. The cervix may have multiple petechiae (strawberry cervix). Desquamation of squamous epithelial cells plus an inflammatory exudate combine to produce a yellow-green discharge. Infection in men is more likely to be asymptomatic and to resolve spontaneously. Urethritis is the most common manifestation in men.

Clinical manifestations

In women, symptoms usually begin or worsen during the menstrual periods. The most common symptom is acute vaginal discharge (Chapter 238). Some women may have dysuria, vaginal itching, painful intercourse, and rarely abdominal pain. The severity of the symptoms correlates with the number of polymorphonuclear leukocytes in the discharge. Physical examination reveals a vaginal discharge. The vulva is usually erythematous and edematous and may be excoriated. The vaginal mucosa and cervix are red, and small punctate hemorrhages or ulcers may be seen. A few patients have cervical tenderness. Most infected males are asymptomatic. Men with symptoms most often have dysuria and a scant penile discharge. However, *T. vaginalis* is an infrequent cause of nongonococcal urethritis, and the identification of *T. vaginalis* in urethral smears does not prove that *T. vaginalis* is the cause of the urethritis. Other potential causes should be pursued (Chapter 238). Unusual complications include epididymitis and prostatitis.

Diagnosis

T. vaginalis infection should be considered in women with a vaginal discharge or with dysuria and a negative urine culture and in men with nongonococcal urethritis, prostatitis, or epididymitis that does not respond to standard therapy. Diagnosis is made by identifying *T. vaginalis* in wet mounts or Pap smears. The organism can be readily identified on fresh wet mounts by virtue of its motility. Wet mounts are more likely to be positive if the patient is symptomatic. Culture, if available, is the most sensitive diagnostic test. In men a swab of anterior urethral exudate should be examined for motile trophozoites, preferably in the morning before urination. Individuals (men or women) with *T. vaginalis* infection should be screened for the presence of other venereal diseases.

Treatment and prevention

Most strains of *T. vaginalis* are sensitive to metronidazole, which can be given as a single oral dose of 2 g. The patients' sexual partners should also be treated. During the first trimester of pregnancy, metronidazole should not be given. Twice-weekly vinegar douches or local application of clotrimazole may be effective. Women who remain infected should be treated with metronidazole before delivery to prevent transmission to the newborn.

DIENTAMOEBA FRAGILIS

Dientamoeba fragilis is a flagellate related to the trichomonads. Its pathogenicity has been controversial for years, but improvement in gastrointestinal symptoms has been reported with treatment. In one study of a semicommunal group, 56% of the adults carried the parasite, and 85% of those infected had gastrointestinal symptoms, especially pain and flatus. Diarrhea occurred less frequently. Eosinophilia has been associated with infection. Treatment with iodoquinol at a dosage of 650 mg three times a day for 20 days eliminated the parasite in more than 80% of those treated, but the number treated was small and no control group was reported. Tetracycline (500 mg four times a day for 10 days) and paromomycin (10 mg/kg/day for 7 days) also appear to be effective against *D. fragilis* infection.

NONPATHOGENIC PROTOZOA

Nonpathogenic protozoa, such as *Entamoeba hartmanni, Entamoeba coli, Endolimax nana,* and *Iodamoeba bütschlii,* have been reported to produce diarrheal disease in immunocompromised patients with AIDS and to respond to treatment. However, these reports do not contain control groups, and relapse often occurs. Thus it is likely that these patients have diarrhea secondary to HIV infection of enterocytes, microsporidiosis, or as yet unrecognized pathogens. Nonetheless, appearance of any of the nonpathogenic protozoa in the stool is evidence of fecal-oral contamination and should alert the clinician to the possibility of undetected protozoan pathogens (e.g., *Giardia*) that may respond to empiric treatment.

REFERENCES

Adams EP and MacLeod IN: Invasive amebiasis. II. Amebic liver abscess and its complications. Medicine (Baltimore) 56:325, 1977.

Allason-Jones E et al: *Entamoeba histolytica* as a commensal parasite in homosexual men. N Engl J Med 315:353, 1986.

Daffos F et al: Prenatal management of 746 pregnancies at risk for congenital toxoplasmosis. N Engl J Med 318:271, 1988.

Dannemann B et al: Treatment of toxoplasmic encephalitis in patients with AIDS: a randomized trial comparing pyrimethamine plus clindamycin to pyrimethamine plus sulfadiazine. Ann Intern Med 116: 33, 1992.

DeHovitz JA et al: Clinical manifestations and therapy of *Isospora belli* infection in patients with the acquired immunodeficiency syndrome. N Engl J Med 315:87, 1986.

Drugs for parasitic infections. Med Lett Drugs Ther 34:17, 1992.

Gardner P: Immunizations, medications, and common sense for the international traveler. Infect Dis Clin North Am 4:179, 1990.

Godwin TA: Cryptosporidiosis in the acquired immunodeficiency syndrome: a study of 15 autopsy cases. Hum Pathol 22:1215, 1991.

Hagar JM and Rahimtoola SH: Chagas' heart disease in the United States. N Engl J Med 325:763, 1991.

Jacobson MA et al: Toxicity of clindamycin as prophylaxis for AIDS-associated toxoplasmic encephalitis. Lancet 339:333, 1992.

Kirchoff LV, Gam AB, and Gilliam F: American trypanosomiasis (Chagas' disease) in Central American immigrants. Am J Med 82:915, 1987.

Leech JH, Sande MA, and Root RK, editors: Contemporary issues in infectious diseases. Vol 7. Parasitic infections. New York, 1988, Churchill Livingstone.

Leport C et al: Treatment of central nervous system toxoplasmosis with pyrimethamine/sulfadiazine combination in 35 patients with the acquired immunodeficiency syndrome: efficacy of long-term continuous therapy. Am J Med 84:94, 1988.

Lobel HO et al: Recent trends in the importation of malaria caused by *Plasmodium falciparum* into the United States from Africa. J Infect Dis 152:613, 1985.

Looareesuwan S et al: *Plasmodium falciparum* hyperparasitemia: use of exchange transfusion in seven patients and a review of the literature. Q J Med 277:471, 1990.

Ma P et al: *Naegleria* and *Acanthamoeba* infections: review. Rev Infect Dis 12:490, 1990.

Mahmoud AAF: The challenge of intracellular pathogens. N Engl J Med 326:761, 1992.

Marsden PD, editor: Intestinal parasites. Clin Gastroenterol 7:1, 1978.

Martinez S and Marr JJ: Allopurinol in the treatment of American cutaneous leishmaniasis. N Engl J Med 326:741, 1992.

McCabe RE et al: Clinical spectrum in 107 cases of toxoplasmic lymphadenopathy. Rev Infect Dis 9:754, 1987.

McCue JD: Evaluation and management of vaginitis: an update for primary care practitioners. Arch Intern Med 149:565, 1989.

Miller KD, Greenberg CC, and Campbell CC: Treatment of severe malaria in the United States with a continuous infusion of quinidine gluconate and exchange transfusion. N Engl J Med 321:65, 1989.

Miller LH: Strategies for malaria control: realities, magic, and science. Ann NY Acad Sci 569:118, 1989.

Miller LH et al: Research toward malaria vaccines. Science 234:1349, 1986.

Miller RA and Minshew BH: *Blastocystis hominis:* an organism in search of a disease. Rev Infect Dis 10:930, 1988.

Millet V et al: *Dientamoeba fragilis,* a protozoan parasite in adult members of a semi-communal group. Dig Dis Sci 28:335, 1983.

Orenstein JM et al: Intestinal microsporidiosis as a cause of diarrhea in human immunodeficiency virus–infected patients: a report of 20 cases. Hum Pathol 21:475, 1990.

Panisko DM and Keystone JS: Treatment of malaria—1990. Drugs 39:160, 1990.

Pomeroy C and Filice GA: Pulmonary toxoplasmosis: a review. Clin Infect Dis 14:863, 1992.

Porter SB and Sande MA: Toxoplasmosis of the central nervous system in the acquired immunodeficiency syndrome. N Engl J Med 327:1643, 1992.

Recommendations for prevention of malaria among travelers. MMWR 39:1, 1990. (See also MMWR 40:72, 1991, for change in prophylactic mefloquine dosing to weekly instead of every other week.)

Reed SL: Amebiasis: an update. Clin Infect Dis 14:385, 1992.

Remington JS and Vildé JL: Clindamycin for toxoplasma encephalitis in AIDS. Lancet 338:1142, 1991.

Shadduck JA: Human microsporidiosis and AIDS. Rev Infect Dis 11:203, 1989.

Soave R and Johnson WD: *Cryptosporidium* and *Isospora belli* infections. J Infect Dis 157:225, 1988.

Warren KS and Mahmoud AAF: Protozoan diseases. In Warren KS and Mahmoud AAF, editors: Tropical and geographical medicine. New York, 1984 McGraw-Hill.

White NJ et al: Severe hypoglycemia and hyperinsulinemia in falciparum malaria. N Engl J Med 309:61, 1983.

Wong B et al: Central nervous system toxoplasmosis in homosexual men and parenteral drug abusers. Ann Intern Med 100:36, 1984.

CHAPTER

281 *Pneumocystis carinii* Infection

Sharon Safrin

THE ORGANISM

Despite the initial identification of the *Pneumocystis* organism in 1906 by Chagas and its recognition as a cause of pneumonia in humans in 1942, the inability to culture *Pneumocystis carinii* reliably in vitro has hindered our full understanding of its taxonomy and infected patients' optimum treatment.

Although classified as a protozoan for many decades, recent evidence indicates that *P. carinii* would more appropriately be considered a fungus. Specifically, the greater than 90% homology of its 16S ribosomal ribonucleic acid (rRNA) with *Saccharomyces* and the properties of its dihydrofolate reductase enzyme (i.e., low molecular weight, absence of thymidylate synthetase activity) suggest a phylogenetic link with fungi. To date, however, this organism's susceptibility to antifungal agents has been poor.

EPIDEMIOLOGY

Pneumocystis appears to have an extraordinarily wide host range and has been found in the lungs of many higher primates, including humans and domestic and wild animals (e.g., rats, guinea pigs, mice, rabbits). Although the organisms found in animals and humans are morphologically identical, antigenic differences revealed by immunoblotting studies suggest heterogeneity among species.

Infection in humans is ubiquitous and occurs early in life. Serologic studies reveal the absence of serum antibody before the age of 1 year, with a rapid rise in seroprevalence rates to greater than 80% by 4 years of age in the general population. Given that serum antibody tends to persist throughout life, most cases of *Pneumocystis* pneumonia appear to represent reactivation of latent infection occurring during periods of immunosuppression rather than newly acquired infection. However, small clusters of outbreaks in groups of individuals and data from animal studies suggest that airborne transmission of the organism may occasionally result in acute disease.

Studies have identified discrete characteristics of persons at risk for the development of *Pneumocystis* pneumonia, including those receiving intensive cytotoxic chemotherapy for malignancy, transplant recipients undergoing immunosuppressive therapy, and children and adults infected with the human immunodeficiency virus (HIV) (see the box on p. 2271). Interestingly, although a CD4 cell count less than 200/mm^3 is a strong marker in adults of risk for pneumocystosis, children may frequently manifest higher CD4 cell counts at the time of acute *Pneumocystis* infection.

PNEUMOCYSTOSIS

Pathophysiology

Both humoral and cell-mediated immunity appear to be important in the development of resistance to active *P. carinii* infection, since well-documented infections have occurred both in patients with isolated congenital immunoglobulin deficiencies and in patients with defective cell-mediated immunity who have normal immunoglobulin levels. However, the greater proportion of patients with pneumocystosis have defects primarily in cell-mediated immunity.

Proliferation of organisms contained within the alveolar space is facilitated by diminished cell-mediated and humoral host defenses. Fibronectin-mediated attachment of

Portions of this material have appeared in slightly altered form in Safrin S: New developments in the management of *Pneumocystis carinii* disease. In Volberding PA and Jacobson MA, editors: AIDS clinical review. New York, 1993, Marcel Dekker.

Common predisposing factors to development of pneumocystosis

Primary immunodeficiency
Congenital: humoral and/or cellular
Acquired

Secondary immunodeficiency
Prematurity
Malnutrition and/or starvation
Acquired immunodeficiency syndrome (AIDS)
Diseases often associated with corticosteroid and/or immunosuppressive drug therapy
Lymphoreticular malignancy
Organ transplantation
Collagen vascular disease
Nephrotic syndrome

Pneumocystis organisms to type 1 alveolar epithelial cells occurs by interdigitation of cell membranes; impaired replication of type 1 alveolar cells ultimately results in degeneration. The subsequent increase in alveolar capillary membrane permeability is associated with exudation of fluid into the alveolar space, decrease in surfactant levels, intrapulmonary shunting of blood with decreased lung compliance, and hypoxemia.

On pathologic examination, hematoxylin-eosin staining shows the alveoli to be filled with masses of eosinophilic material; these contain *Pneumocystis* cysts and trophozoites. Inflammatory cells in the alveoli are few, whereas the interstitial spaces contain variable numbers of plasma and mononuclear cells.

Clinical features

P. carinii pneumonia is generally manifested by fever, nonproductive cough, and progressive shortness of breath (Chapter 229). Although the onset of pneumocystosis in oncology patients is generally abrupt and rapidly progressive, it is often insidious and of prolonged duration in patients with the acquired immunodeficiency syndrome (AIDS), worsening slowly over weeks to months. Fever, although usually present, is seldom high; shaking chills are distinctly infrequent. Cough is typically nonproductive, although superimposed infection with bacteria or other organisms may result in the production of mucus. Findings on auscultation of the lungs are relatively unremarkable. Initially the chest radiograph may show symmetric, diffuse infiltrates with an interstitial and alveolar pattern. Subsequent progression may result in extensive consolidation (Fig. 281-1). Pleural effusion and mediastinal adenopathy are not typically present and should prompt consideration of alternative or additional diagnoses. Atypical radiographic findings have been described in patients with *Pneumocystis* infection, including coin lesions, focal consolidation, and cavitation. In addition, the chest radiograph may occasionally be within normal limits. Patients who have unsuccessfully received aerosolized pentamidine prophylaxis against *Pneumocystis* infection may exhibit atypical, apical infiltrates rather than diffuse opacities; the burden of organisms tends to be lower in such patients.

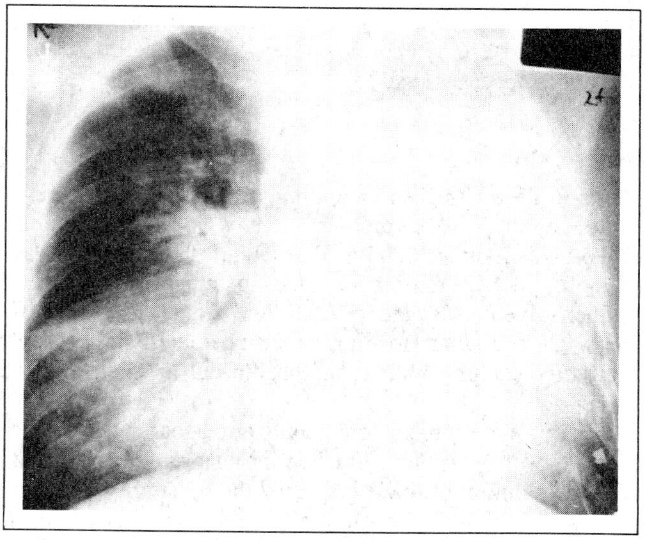

Fig. 281-1. Young woman with cadaveric renal transplant and extensive *Pneumocystis carinii* pneumonitis.

Laboratory studies (e.g., complete blood count, liver function studies) do not show abnormalities that are characteristic of pneumocystosis; however, parameters such as white blood cell count and serum albumin may be lowered as a reflection of underlying disease. The serum lactate dehydrogenase is elevated in more than 90% of patients with *P. carinii* pneumonia. In addition, studies suggest that the degree of elevation in serum lactate dehydrogenase (LDH) at initial evaluation correlates with prognosis, with patients having the highest levels demonstrating a poorer outcome. Those in whom serum LDH rises rather than falls during therapy for *P. carinii* pneumonia tend to have a decreased survival. Significant hypoxemia, manifested by a decreased arterial oxygen tension and/or an elevated arterial-alveolar oxygen gradient, is the rule, although abnormalities may be less pronounced in patients with early disease and minimum radiographic abnormalities. The degree of hypoxemia at initial presentation correlates with response to therapy. The diffusing capacity for carbon monoxide is also abnormal in virtually every patient and may serve as a useful marker of disease with which to determine the need for further evaluation in patients who have equivocal findings on the chest radiograph. Ancillary tests include the gallium radionuclide scan, a sensitive but nonspecific indicator of the propensity of persons with pneumocystosis to concentrate gallium in their lungs selectively.

Most *P. carinii* infections are confined to the lungs. However, an increasing number of extrapulmonary foci of infection have been described in the recent literature, particularly in HIV-infected patients who are receiving prophylactic aerosolized pentamidine. Organs involved to date include the lymph nodes, spleen, liver, bone and bone marrow, skin, thyroid, choroid, adrenal gland, intestine, ear, meninges, and pancreas.

Diagnosis

Tests to detect antigen or antibody in serum have been of little diagnostic value thus far, as have attempts to culture the organism on artificial media. Diagnosis is generally accomplished by examination of a specimen of sputum or bronchoalveolar lavage (BAL) fluid under light microscopy. Cysts and trophozoites have a characteristic morphology after staining with toluidine blue O or Giemsa (Fig. 281-2).

Use of hypertonic saline nebulization for sputum induction, as well as sputum liquefaction using reducing agents such as dithioreitol, have increased the sensitivity of the diagnosis of *P. carinii* pneumonia by examination of an induced sputum specimen to approximately 77%. Sensitivity can be further increased by using monoclonal antibodies directed against cyst wall and trophozoite antigens, available commercially as kits using either direct fluorescent or indirect fluorescent techniques. Deoxyribonucleic acid (DNA) amplification techniques are also currently under study. However, such methods carry the disadvantages of increased expense, increased technician labor, and risk of false-positive results. Most importantly, failure to detect *Pneumocystis* organisms in a specimen of induced sputum does not exclude the diagnosis (negative predictive value, approximately 60%).

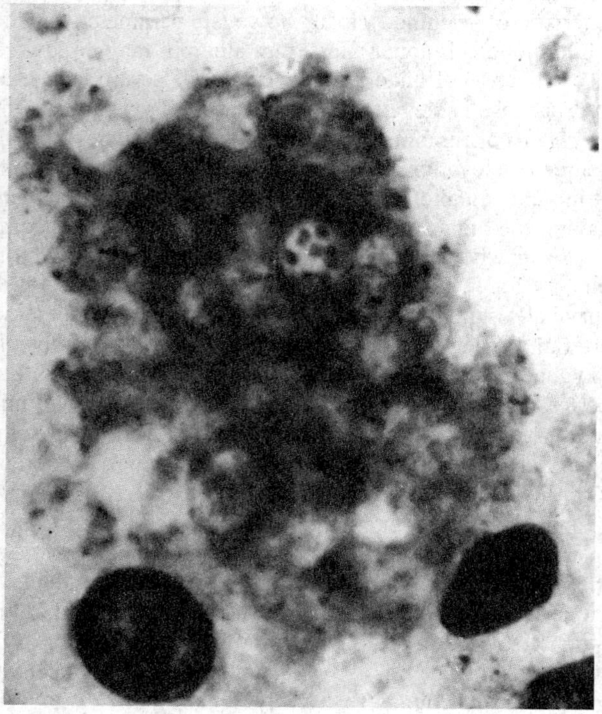

Fig. 281-2. *Pneumocystis carinii*. Giemsa-stained touch preparation of a transbronchial lung biopsy from a patient with AIDS. A clump of eosinophilic proteinaceous material contains numerous cysts of *P. carinii*, including one with eight sporozoites.

Use of BAL alone has a sensitivity of 86% to 97% and is most often employed to investigate further the possibility of *P. carinii* pneumonia when induced sputum specimens are nondiagnostic. Transbronchoscopic biopsy is generally reserved for patients in whom the diagnosis remains in question after preliminary studies.

Treatment

Our lack of ability to test the susceptibility of *P. carinii* against antimicrobial agents in vitro has forced us to rely on results from animal studies in the development of treatment and prophylactic regimens for pneumocystosis. Two treatment regimens, trimethoprim/sulfamethoxazole (TMP/SMX) and pentamidine isethionate, have long been recommended for treatment of *P. carinii* pneumonia. However, several other treatment regimens are either in clinical use or actively under investigation (Table 281-1).

Most comparative trials performed to date have found TMP/SMX and parenteral pentamidine to be equivalent therapies for the treatment of *P. carinii* pneumonia; comparing the efficacies of these therapies is difficult because of the high rate of changes in therapy necessitated by adverse reactions. Estimates of mortality in patients with *P. carinii* pneumonia range from 2% to 39%; the success of therapy depends on both the severity of infection at presentation and the presence of underlying pulmonary dysfunction. Oral or intravenous (IV) TMP/SMX therapy may be associated with rash in up to 50% of patients with AIDS; neutropenia, nausea, azotemia, elevation of liver function tests, and anemia are other potential side effects. Parenteral pentamidine may cause renal dysfunction, neutropenia, orthostatic hypotension, hypoglycemia, nausea, elevation of liver function tests, and acute or chronic hyperglycemia.

Several other agents have been proposed for treatment of *P. carinii* infection, based primarily on their efficacy in animal models. A randomized, controlled, double-blind study of 60 patients demonstrated equivalent success rates with the combination of dapsone (100 mg daily) and oral TMP (20 mg/kg/day) when compared with oral TMP/SMX in patients who had arterial oxygen tensions of 60 mm Hg or greater at initial evaluation. The dapsone/TMP regimen was associated with significantly fewer dose-limiting side effects. However, dapsone therapy is associated with a dose-dependent methemoglobinemia and hemolytic anemia, and its use is contraindicated in patients with a glucose-6-phosphate dehydrogenase (G6PD) deficiency.

Several investigators have assessed the treatment of patients with mild to moderate *P. carinii* pneumonia using a combination of clindamycin and primaquine. Although the earliest studies used IV clindamycin, investigators recently reported the successful treatment of 92% of 38 patients with oral clindamycin (600 mg every 8 hours) and primaquine (30 mg base daily). Side effects were dose limiting in 13% of patients, consisting of rash (three patients), diarrhea (one patient), and neutropenia (one patient). Primaquine, as with

Table 281-1. Drug regimens for treatment of patients with *P. carinii* infections

Regimen	Adult total daily dosage	Route	Interval	Dose-limiting side effects
Recommended regimens				
Trimethoprim (TMP)/ sulfamethoxazole (SMX)	15-20 mg/kg (TMP) 75-100 mg/kg (SMX)	PO or IV	q6-8h	Rash, nausea, neutropenia, anemia, hepatitis, azotemia, decreased platelet count
Pentamidine isethionate	3-4 mg/kg	IV or IM	q24h	Azotemia, neutropenia, hypoglycemia, hepatitis, orthostasis, diabetes mellitus
Atovaquone	2250mg	PO	q8h	Rash, hepatitis, neutropenia, nausea
Regimens under study				
Dapsone plus TMP	100 mg	PO	q24h	Rash, nausea, methemoglobinemia, anemia, hepatitis, neutropenia
	12-15 mg/kg	PO	q6-8h	
Clindamycin plus primaquine	1800 mg	PO or IV	q8h	Rash, diarrhea, neutropenia, nausea
	30 mg (base)	PO	q24h	
Pentamidine isethionate	600 mg	Aerosolized	q24h	Bronchospasm
Trimetrexate	45 mg/m^2	IV	q24h	Neutropenia, decreased platelet count, anemia, hepatitis
plus				
folinic acid	80 mg/m^2	PO or IV	q24h	

PO, Oral; IV, intravenous; IM, intramuscular; q, every; h, hours.
*Indicated for treatment of TMP/SMX–intolerant patients.

dapsone, may cause methemoglobinemia or hemolytic anemia; its use is contraindicated in patients with G6PD deficiency. Controlled studies of this combination are currently underway.

A trial comparing oral therapy with the experimental agent atovaquone (BW 566C80) with oral TMP/SMX showed lesser efficacy but fewer dose-limiting adverse reactions in patients with acute *P. carinii* pneumonia receiving the former drug. Oral atovaquone has recently been licensed for the treatment of acute PCP in patients with an intolerance to TMP/SMX. A randomized, controlled, double-blind study comparing aerosolized pentamidine therapy (600 mg daily) with TMP/SMX showed lesser efficacy but better tolerability with the pentamidine therapy.

A comparative study showed that the combination of the dihydrofolate reductase inhibitor trimetrexate (45 mg/m^2/day) plus folinic acid (80 mg/m^2/day) was inferior to IV TMP/SMX as a first-line therapy for patients with severe *P. carinii* pneumonia. Nevertheless, this new regimen may have benefit when used in patients who have failed to respond to standard regimens or are unable to tolerate them.

Regimens for which data are too scanty to make recommendations regarding use in treatment include pyrimethamine with sulfadiazine, pyrimethamine with sulfadoxine, eflornithine, and adjunctive interferon-gamma.

Response to therapy generally occurs within 5 to 7 days, whereas dose-limiting side effects most often appear in the second week of therapy. Recovery is complete in most patients, although a minority may develop interstitial fibrosis.

A series of recent studies demonstrated adjunctive corticosteroid therapy to be beneficial in patients with moderate or severe *P. carinii* pneumonia (i.e., oxygen tension $<$ 70 mm Hg or arterial-alveolar oxygen gradient $>$ 35). Such patients should receive prednisone (40 mg twice daily for 5 days, then 40 mg daily for 5 days, then 20 mg/day until completion of therapy) in conjunction with anti-*Pneumocystis* therapy. Corticosteroid therapy should be initiated as soon as the diagnosis is suspected in patients meeting the criteria just listed.

Prevention

Anti-*Pneumocystis* chemoprophylaxis should be initiated in patients at highest risk for infection, that is, those undergoing intensive immunosuppressive therapy, AIDS patients who have had an episode of pneumocystosis, and HIV-infected patients age 6 or older in whom the CD4 cell count has fallen below 200/mm^3. In patients who have had an episode of pneumocystosis, the risk of recurrent infection is high, approaching 35% in 6 months and 60% at 1 year after the acute episode. Therefore prophylaxis should be initiated immediately after completion of acute therapy. Guidelines for anti-*Pneumocystis* prophylaxis in children is shown in Table 281-2.

TMP/SMX, dapsone, and aerosolized pentamidine are the three agents most frequently used in prophylaxis, al-

Table 281-2. Recommendations for initiation of anti-*Pneumocystis* prophylaxis in HIV-infected children

Age	Recommendation
	Begin prophylaxis when CD4 cell count less than:
1-11 mo	1500/mm^3
12-23 mo	750/mm^3
25 mo-5 yr	500/mm^3
≥ 6 yr	200/mm^3

though direct comparison of efficacy and optimum dosing are not available. A placebo-controlled study of TMP/SMX (160/800 mg twice daily) documented the efficacy of this regimen in the prevention of pneumocystosis in patients with AIDS. The dosage of 300 mg monthly of aerosolized pentamidine was shown to be optimum in a three-arm, randomized multicenter trial. Two recent randomized multicenter comparisons of TMP/SMX (80-160/400-800 mg daily) and aerosolized pentamidine (300 mg monthly) with zidovudine showed TMP/SMX to be superior in efficacy but less well tolerated in primary and secondary *P. carinii* pneumonia. Aerosolized pentamidine prophylaxis, however, has been associated with a higher frequency of both extrapulmonary foci of infection and spontaneous pneumothorax. The possibility of further reduction in the dosage of TMP/SMX administered for prophylaxis has been suggested by noncomparative studies of thrice-weekly administration, showing preserved efficacy with a lower frequency of toxicity.

Uncontrolled studies of dapsone have used dosages ranging from 50 mg once daily to 200 mg once weekly. A recent randomized trial comparing TMP/SMX (160/800 mg) to dapsone (100 mg daily) for primary prophylaxis showed similar efficacy as well as high rates of toxicity for both drugs. A randomized trial comparing dapsone, TMP/SMX, and aerosolized pentamidine for primary prophylaxis of pneumocystosis is currently underway through the AIDS Clinical Trials Group of the National Institutes for Allergy and Infectious Diseases.

REFERENCES

Allegra CJ et al: Trimetrexate for the treatment of *Pneumocystis carinii* pneumonia in patients with the acquired immunodeficiency syndrome. N Engl J Med 317:978, 1987.

Black JR et al: Oral clindamycin plus primaquine therapy for *Pneumocystis carinii* pneumonia in AIDS patients. Abstract ThB42, VII International Conference for AIDS, Florence, Italy, 1991.

Blum RN et al: Comparative trial of dapsone versus trimethoprim/sulfamethoxazole for primary prophylaxis of *Pneumocystis carinii* pneumonia. J Acq Imm Defic Synd 5:341, 1992.

Centers for Disease Control: Guidelines for prophylaxis against *Pneumocystis carinii* pneumonia for children infected with human immunodeficiency virus. MMWR 40:1, 1991.

Edman JC et al: Ribosomal RNA sequence shows *Pneumocystis carinii* to be a member of the fungi. Nature 334:519, 1988.

Fischl MA, Dickinson GM, and LaVole L: Safety and efficacy of sulfamethoxazole and trimethoprim chemoprophylaxis for *Pneumocystis carinii* pneumonia in AIDS. JAMA 259:1185, 1988.

Gajdusek DC: *Pneumocystis carinii*—etiologic agent of interstitial plasma cell pneumonia of premature and young infants. Pediatrics 19:543, 1957.

Hardy WD et al: A controlled trial of trimethoprim-sulfamethoxazole for secondary prophylaxis of *Pneumocystis carinii* pneumonia in patients with the acquired immunodeficiency syndrome, N Engl J Med 327:1842, 1992.

Jules-Elysee KM et al: Aerosolized pentamidine: effect on diagnosis and presentation of *Pneumocystis carinii* pneumonia. Ann Intern Med 112:750, 1990.

Kovacs JA, Ng VS, and Masur H: Diagnosis of *Pneumocystis carinii* pneumonia: improved detection in sputum with use of monoclonal antibodies. N Engl J Med 318:589, 1988.

Leoung GS et al: Aerosolized pentamidine for prophylaxis against *Pneumocystis carinii* pneumonia. N Engl J Med 323:769, 1990.

Medina I et al: Oral therapy for *Pneumocystis carinii* pneumonia in the acquired immunodeficiency syndrome. N Engl J Med 323:776, 1990.

Montgomery AB et al: Aerosolized pentamidine vs. trimethoprim-sulfamethoxazole for acute *Pneumocystis carinii* pneumonia: a randomized double blind trial. Abstract ThB395, VI International Conference on AIDS, San Francisco, 1990.

The National Institutes of Health–University of California Expert Panel for Corticosteroids as Adjunctive Therapy for *Pneumocystis* Pneumonia: Consensus statement on the use of corticosteroids as adjunctive therapy for *Pneumocystis* pneumonia in the acquired immunodeficiency syndrome. N Engl J Med 323:1500, 1990.

Peglow SL et al: Serologic responses to *Pneumocystis carinii* antigens in health and disease. J Infect Dis 161:296, 1990.

Phair J et al: The risk of *Pneumocystis carinii* pneumonia among men infected with human immunodeficiency virus type 1. N Engl J Med 322:161, 1990.

Sattler FR et al: Trimethoprim-sulfamethoxazole compared with pentamidine for treatment of *Pneumocystis carinii* pneumonia in the acquired immunodeficiency syndrome: a prospective, noncrossover study. Ann Intern Med 109:280, 1988.

Schneider ME et al: A controlled trial of aerosolized pentamidine or trimethoprim-sulfamethoxazole as primary prophylaxis against *Pneumocystis carinii* pneumonia in patients with human immunodeficiency virus infection, N Engl J Med 327:1836, 1992.

Zaman MK and White DA: Serum lactate dehydrogenase levels and *Pneumocystis carinii* pneumonia: diagnostic and prognostic significance. Am Rev Respir Dis 137:796, 1988.

HELMINTHIC DISEASES

CHAPTER

282 Infections Caused by Helminths

G. Richard Olds

Worms, or helminths, are the most common parasites of humans, with almost half the world's population infected. Worms differ from other classes of infectious organisms in that they are large and multicellular and generally visible to the naked eye. Helminths have complex life cycles, often having several morphologically distinct forms (eggs, microfilaria, adult worms, migrating larvae) within the infected host. Intermediate hosts (freshwater snails) or insect vectors (mosquitoes) are common. In general, helminths do not multiply in humans. Host immunity is directed toward the invasive larval forms of the parasite, whereas adult worms are resistant to the host's immune attack. Pathologic immune responses are often directed toward the progeny of adult worms (microfilaria or eggs). Helminths also distinguish themselves from other infectious agents of humans by their unique association with eosinophilic staining polymorphonuclear leukocytes. Eosinophilia, however, is not universal among the helminth infections and is observed only when worms are present within host tissues. The mere presence of adult worms within the lumen of the intestine is not generally associated with peripheral blood eosinophilia. Clinically, most infected individuals are asymptomatic, with disease associated with either heavy infections or an abnormal immune response to one or more stages of the parasite. Reinfections are common, if not the rule. Treatment has vastly improved over the last decade, but the treatment of some tissue helminths remains complicated, occasionally even toxic.

Taxonomists traditionally divide the helminths into *nematodes* (roundworms), *trematodes* (flukes), and *cestodes* (tapeworms). For the clinician, helminths may be divided into three major groups based on the life cycle and the severity of illness induced in humans. In this chapter, worms whose entire life cycle in humans is confined to the gastrointestinal tract are discussed separately from those with a tissue-migrating phase or those that reside entirely within host tissues.

STRICTLY INTESTINAL HELMINTHS

Intestinal nematodes

Several species of nematodes never invade host tissue. Using the analogy of a doughnut, these worms live their entire life within the doughnut hole, that is, the human alimentary tract. They therefore never cause eosinophilia. These parasites are common even in industrially developed countries. More than 60 million Americans, for example, have pinworms. Such infections are rarely associated with serious clinical disease and are simple to treat medically. Reinfection remains the major obstacle to eradication.

Enterobiasis. Pinworms *(Enterobius* species, especially *vermicularis)* are typically found in families with small children or in individuals confined to institutions where fecal-oral contamination is difficult to control. Adult worms reside in the large intestines and migrate to the rectal orifice at night. The female then deposits her eggs on the perirectal mucosa. Ova are quite irritative, leading to rectal and perineal pruritus. Intensive pruritus also helps the eggs to gain access to the fingers and fingernails, aiding human-to-human transmission and autoinfection. Pinworm eggs remain viable for extended periods in the environment. Persons are easily reinfected and thus require repeated chemotherapy. Adult worms rarely cause more serious complications, although mechanical obstruction of the appendix has been reported. The diagnosis of enterobiasis is made by applying cellophane tape to the perianal skin and then examining the tape for characteristic eggs under the microscope. Treatment with mebendazole is always curative. Since reinfection frequently occurs, it is often advisable to treat all family members at the same time and repeat treatment 2 weeks later. Environmental manipulation (e.g., washing clothes in hot water) is best reserved for documented recurrent cases.

Trichuris tichiura. Whipworm *(T. trichiura)* is transmitted primarily in young children through fecal-oral contamination. Adult worms live in the colon, where they attach to the colonic mucosa. Most individuals are asymptomatic. Rarely, very heavy infections are associated with bloody diarrhea and rectal prolapse. Children with minimum iron stores may become anemic, but this occurs infrequently in well-nourished children. Whipworm is easily diagnosed by finding the characteristic football-shaped ova in the stool. Treatment with mebendazole for 3 days is generally curative. Albendazole is quite effective when given in a single dose but is currently unavailable in the United States.

Intestinal cestodes

Three species of cestodes, or multisegmental flatworms, never invade beyond the intestinal mucosa. In general, disease is associated only with nutritional deprivation of the host or irritation of the intestinal mucosa. Infection is established through the ingestion of raw or undercooked meat that contains encysted larvae. After ingestion, the head or scolex of the tapeworm attaches to the intestinal mucosa. The worm elongates, eventually producing egg-filled proglottids (individual segments) or free ova. A single worm infection is the rule. Because the larvae never penetrate tissue (the doughnut in the previous analogy), eosinophilia usually is not observed. Eosinophilia may be seen, however, with *Hymenolepsis nana,* which invades the mucosa only. The pork tapeworm, *Taenia solium,* can cause both luminal infection and direct tissue invasion. This cestode is therefore discussed both here and in a later section on tissue-invasive parasites (cysticercosis).

Taenia saginata. The beef tapeworm *(T. saginata)* is seen infrequently in industrial countries. Humans become infected by ingesting meat containing cysticerci (encysted larvae of cestodes). The adult worm can grow up to 7 m (23 feet) long and generally lives in the upper small intestines. Most infected individuals are asymptomatic. Patients usually become aware of infection by passing proglottids in the stool. The diagnosis can be confirmed by direct examination of the stool for eggs and proglottids or by adhesive tape examination for ova similar to that performed for pinworms. Unfortunately the specific species cannot be determined by the appearance of the ova. A closely related species, *Taenia solium,* can only be reliably differentiated from *T. saginata* by examination of passed proglottids, not by eggs. Since the treatment of all luminal tapeworms is niclosamide or praziquantel, determination of the specific species is now less important than in the past.

Taenia solium. The pork tapeworm *(T. solium)* causes two distinct diseases in humans. Luminal parasitism is caused by the ingestion of raw or undercooked pork. Adult *T. solium* worms cause few symptoms and are clinically indistinguishable from *T. saginata* infection. Unfortunately, ingestion of viable ova (rather than raw pork) can lead to tissue infections through direct invasion by infective larvae. This causes a much more severe disease known as *cysticercosis*. These two clinical diseases do not generally occur in the same individual, and thus cysticercosis is discussed in a later section. As with *T. saginata,* the diagnosis of intestinal infection is made by finding proglottids or eggs in the stool. Treatment with either niclosamide or praziquantel is curative, but praziquantel is preferred because it is effective against both the adults and the larvae.

Diphyllobothrium latum. The fish tapeworm *(D. latum)* is the largest of the human cestodes, reaching a length of 10 m (33 feet). Humans are infected through the ingestion of raw or undercooked freshwater fish, particularly perch and pike. Because of unique ethnic dietary habits, infection is typically found in individuals of Scandinavian, Japanese, Eskimo, and Jewish extraction. The life cycle in humans is similar to that of *T. saginata,* except the proglottids generally disintegrate in the small intestine. As a result, eggs rather than proglottids are passed in the stool in large numbers. Most infected individuals never develop symptoms as a direct result of parasitism. Unfortunately, *D. latum* has a unique affinity for vitamin B_{12}, leading to deprivation in the host. Therefore megaloblastic anemia, indistinguishable from that observed from other causes, is occasionally found. The diagnosis can be easily made by examination of the stool for ova. Both niclosamide and praziquantel are curative.

Hymenolepis nana. With dwarf tapeworms *(H. mana),* humans can be either the definitive host (intestinal infection) or the intermediate host (tissue infection). In contrast to *T. solium,* however, tissue infection is confined to the intestinal wall, and thus serious disease almost never occurs. The proglottids of *H. nana* autodigest in the small intestines, releasing viable ova that pass into the stool, where they are transmitted from person to person by fecal-oral contamination. Children are frequently infected.

The life cycle of *H. nana* is unique among the helminths and shares with *Strongyloides* the ability to cause internal autoinfection. This can lead to a large worm burden and clinical disease without the need for repeated reinfections. Although most infected individuals are asymptomatic, they have diarrhea and abdominal complaints during autoinfection. Occasionally, dizziness and even seizures occur. These symptoms are the result of absorbed neurotoxic products of the parasite. The diagnosis is made by examination of the stool for ova. Niclosamide is effective, but praziquantel is the drug of choice because it can kill both the adult worm and the larval phases of infection.

Intestinal trematodes

Several trematodes that infect humans live their entire life cycle confined to the intestinal lumen. All have snail intermediate hosts, and infection occurs through the ingestion of raw food. As with *H. nana,* these helminths all cause injury to the columnar epithelium and are therefore associated with significant eosinophilia. Infections are diagnosed by stool examination for ova and are easily treated with praziquantel.

Fasciolopsis buski. This infection is common in Southeast Asia, China, and India and involves freshwater snails as an intermediate host. Humans become infected by ingesting raw water chestnuts or bamboo contaminated with cercariae. The fluke develops in the intestines of humans and feeds on the columnar epithelial cells. Diarrhea may occur, and rarely, adult worms may obstruct the common bile duct or intestines, similar to ascariasis. Characteristic ova are found in the stool. Treatment with praziquantel or niclosamide is curative; oral hexylresorcinol and tetrachloroethylene have also been used. Infection can be prevented by proper sanitation.

Heterophyes heterophyes. This small intestinal fluke is common in the Orient, Africa, and the Middle East. Freshwater snails are the intermediate host and release cercariae into water. These organisms penetrate the skin of various species of fish, forming a resting stage of the parasite. Humans become infected by ingestion of the raw or undercooked fish. Adult worms can cause diarrhea and abdominal pain. Rarely, tissue invasion by eggs can occur. The diagnosis is made by stool examination for ova. Praziquantel is the only effective drug.

Metagonimus yokogawai. This parasite has a similar life cycle and causes the same clinical disease as *H. heterophyes. M. yokogawai* is found in the Orient, Russia, and Southern Europe.

Echinostoma ilocanum. Infection is found primarily in the Philippines and Indonesia. Snails are the intermediate hosts, with ingestion of raw freshwater mollusks leading to infection in humans. Diarrhea is the most common clinical sign and is easily diagnosed on stool examination for ova. Praziquantel is the drug of choice.

• • •

Table 282-1 lists the strictly intestinal helminths and their characteristic features.

INTESTINAL HELMINTHS WITH TISSUE MIGRATORY PHASES

This class of parasites has a typical life cycle in humans: a larval stage, during which the parasite migrates through host tissues, and an intestinal luminal phase, during which the adult worm resides in the intestine. During migration (often through the lungs) these nematodes may cause fever and transient pulmonary infiltrates and eosinophilia (PIE) syndrome. During this stage the diagnosis cannot be made by examining the stool for ova and parasites because the symptoms are produced by immature larvae. Serology is the only reliable way of making the correct diagnosis. Symptoms are transient and normally do not require specific therapy (with the exception of *Strongyloides* hyperinfection). The diagnosis and treatment of the adult intestinal stage is similar to that outlined for the strictly intestinal nematodes.

Table 282-2 lists intestinal helminths with a tissue migratory phase and their associated features.

Ascaris lumbricoides

The *A. lumbricoides* roundworms are among the most common helminth infections of humans, with more than a billion persons infected worldwide. Infection is found in individuals of all ages but occurs more often in children. In-

Table 282-1. Strictly intestinal helminths

Family	Species	Transmission	Major clinical presentation	Eosinophilia	Diagnosis (adults)	Treatment
Nematode	*Enterobius vermicularis* (pinworm)	Fecal-oral	Perianal pruritus	No	Cellophane tape applied to rectum	Mebendazole, 100 mg once (repeat in 2 weeks), or pyrantel pamoate 11 mg/kg (max, 1 g), or albendazole, 400 mg/kg once
Nematode	*Trichuris trichiura* (whipworm)	Fecal-oral	Diarrhea, rectal prolapse	No	Stool O&P	Mebendazole, 100 mg bid for 3 days, or albendazole,* 400 μg/kg once
Cestode	*Taenia saginata* (beef tapeworm)	Ingestion of raw beef	Passage of proglottids	No	Proglottid in stool	Niclosamide, 2 g once, or praziquantel,† 15-20 mg/kg once
Cestode	*Taenia solium* (pork tapeworm)	Ingestion of raw pork (see cysticercosis in text)	Passage of proglottids	No (yes in cysticercosis)	Stool O&P for intestinal infection	Praziquantel, 15-20 mg/kg once for intestinal infection
Cestode	*Diphyllobothrium latum* (fish tapeworm)	Ingestion of raw fish	Vitamin B_{12} deficiency	No	Stool O&P	Same as for *T. saginata*
Cestode	*Hymenolepsis nana* (dwarf tapeworm)	Fecal-oral	Diarrhea, dizziness in children	Yes	Stool O&P	Praziquantel, 25 mg/kg once
Trematode	*Fasciolopsis buski*	Ingestion of raw water chestnuts or bamboo	Diarrhea, intestinal or biliary obstruction	Yes	Stool O&P	Praziquantel, 25 mg/kg tid for 1 day or Niclosamide, 2 g once
Trematode	*Heterophyes heterophyes*	Ingestion of raw fish	Diarrhea, abdominal pain	Yes	Stool O&P	Praziquantel, 25 mg/kg tid for 1 day
Trematode	*Metagonimus yokogawai*	Ingestion of raw fish	Diarrhea	Yes	Stool O&P	Praziquantel, 25 mg/kg tid for 1 day
Trematode	*Echinostoma ilocanum*	Ingestion of raw fish	Diarrhea	Yes	Stool O&P	Praziquantel, 25 mg/kg tid for 1 day

*Not available in the United States.
†Considered an investigative drug by the U.S. Food and Drug Administration.
O&P, Ova and parasites; bid, Twice a day; tid, three times a day.

fection occurs from the ingestion of eggs through fecal-oral contamination. Ingested ova hatch in the intestine, and the larvae penetrate the intestinal mucosa. Larvae then migrate through the tissues to the lungs, penetrate into the alveolar spaces, migrate up the trachea, are swallowed, and finally arrive again in the intestinal lumen. Pulmonary symptoms (severe cough, allergic pneumonitis) are generally transient. Once the adult intestinal phase is reached, individuals are asymptomatic, but heavily infected small children may be nutritionally impaired. Rarely, adult worms obstruct the common bile duct or appendix, or masses of worms lead to small bowel obstruction in small children. The diagnosis is easily made by examining the stool for ova. Mebendazole and piperazine citrate are very effective but require 2 to 3 days of treatment. Pyrantel pamoate and albendazole are both effective as single-dose drugs, but pyrantel may be associated with gastrointestinal disturbances, dizziness, headache, and other systemic reactions, and albendazole is not available in the United States.

Necator americanus, Ancylostoma duodenale

Hookworms infect half a billion individuals worldwide. Two species, *N. americanus* (New World hookworms) and *A. duodenale* (Old World hookworms) cause identical clinical symptoms in humans but differ slightly in their re-

Table 282-2. Intestinal helminths with a tissue migratory phase

Family	Species	Transmission	Major clinical presentation	Eosinophilia	Diagnosis (adults)	Treatment
Nematode	*Ascaris lumbricoides* (giant roundworm)	Fecal-oral	PIE,* intestinal or biliary	During migration, obstruction	Stool O&P	Mebendazole, 100 mg PO bid for 3 days, or albendazole,† 400 μg/kg once
Nematode	*Ancylostoma duodenale* (hookworm)	Skin penetration	PIE, iron deficiency anemia, dermatitis	During migration	Stool O&P	Mebendazole, 100 mg PO bid for 3 days, or albendazole, 400 μg/kg once, or pyrantel pamoate,‡ 11 mg/kg (max, 1 g) for 3 days
Nematode	*Necator americanus* (hookworm)	Skin penetration	PIE, iron deficiency anemia, dermatitis	During migration	Stool O&P	Same as for *A. duodenale*
Nematode	*Strongyloides stercoralis*	Skin penetration	PIE, diarrhea, malabsorption Hyperinfection syndrome	Yes	Stool O&P	Thiabendazole, 25 mg/kg bid for 2 days, 5 days for disseminated infection, or albendazole,‡,§ 400 mg daily for 3 days, or ivermectin,‡,§ 200 μg/kg/day for 1-2 days

*Pulmonary infiltrates with eosinophilia.
†Not available in the United States.
‡Considered an investigational drug by the U.S. Food and Drug Administration.
§Should be considered experimental treatment.
O&P, Ova and parasites; PO, orally; bid, twice a day.

sponse to antihelminthic drugs. Hookworm larvae penetrate directly through intact skin on contact with contaminated soil. Clinically, this can lead to a pruritic rash or ground itch. Maturing larvae have identical migratory patterns as ascariasis larvae and cause the same transient eosinophilic pneumonitis. Adult worms ultimately reside in the small intestine by attaching to the mucosa. Numerous ova are passed in the stool to complete the life cycle. Most individuals are asymptomatic. Since each adult worm ingests about 0.2 ml of blood/day, iron deficiency anemia may develop in heavily infected children. The diagnosis of the intestinal phase of infection is easily made through examination of the stool for ova. Infection can be treated with pyrantel pamoate or mebendazole for 3 days or albendazole (not available in the United States) for 1 day.

Strongyloides stercoralis

Strongyloides species have a similar life cycle to hookworms. Larvae live in fecally contaminated soil, penetrate through unbroken skin (ground itch), migrate through the lungs (PIE syndrome), and ultimately reside in the small intestines. One unique feature of the life cycle important to clinicians is that eggs released by adults may hatch in the small intestines, and larvae can again penetrate the mucosa, causing autoinfection. Thus *Strongyloides* can multiply in humans without the requirement of reinfection from the environment. This allows individuals to remain infected for life. Eosinophilia is frequently found during both the migratory and the autoinfection phases of infection. Clinically, symptoms are rare but can be associated with diarrhea and vague abdominal complaints.

Unfortunately, severe, even fatal dissemination of *S. stercoralis* can be found in immunocompromised hosts. These include patients taking high doses of steroids, patients with lymphoma and other malignancies, those with severe malnutrition, and recently a patient with acquired immunodeficiency syndrome (AIDS). Disseminated *Strongyloides* infection (hyperinfection) normally presents with multiple gram-negative bacteremias and multiorgan involvement (renal, hepatic, pulmonary, and cardiac dysfunctions). Unfortunately, eosinophilia is frequently found in infected normal persons but is almost never observed in these patients because of their profound immunodepression. This makes diagnosis often difficult. Mortality rates are high even with appropriate therapy. Because of the severe and fatal nature of this complication, the diagnosis should be sought in patients with unexplained eosinophilia before initiation of immunosuppressive therapy.

The diagnosis of *S. stercoralis* may be difficult, since larvae may be found in the stool in small numbers. The Baermann technique of stool concentration is not currently performed by most clinical laboratories. Other concentration techniques are of questionable value at increasing the diagnostic yield. Thus multiple stool examinations may be necessary to diagnose *Strongyloides*. An alternate strategy is duodenal aspiration. Recently a specific serologic test has been developed that is clinically useful, particularly in the workup of patients with unexplained eosinophilia.

Because of the risk of dissemination, infected patients should always be treated. Thiabendazole is administered for 2 days for intestinal infections and is the drug of choice. Therapy is extended to 5 days when hyperinfection or dissemination is suspected. Unfortunately, thiabendazole may not kill tissue-stage larvae, and repeat treatment may be necessary. Recently, albendazole and ivermectin have been shown to be effective.

TISSUE HELMINTH INFECTIONS

Helminths that penetrate and live within human tissue are clearly the most important clinically and the most difficult of the worm infections to diagnose and treat. The diagnosis is difficult because examination of the stool for ova and parasites often does not suggest the diagnosis (trematodes are exceptions). Clinical manifestations are related to the infection's intensity and the host's immune response to various stages in the parasite's life cycle. Diseases are typically chronic, with symptoms developing months and usually years after a primary infection. All these tissue infections are associated with eosinophilia, which often suggests to the clinician the correct diagnosis. Recent drug developments (praziquantel, ivermectin, albendazole) make several previously untreatable infections curable.

Tissue nematodes

Filariasis. Almost half a billion people are infected with the Filarioidea family of tissue nematodes, mostly in tropical countries. Filariasis is transmitted by the bites of bloodsucking insects. During a blood meal the insect vector injects larvae into the definitive host (humans). Adult male and female worms mate, and the female releases *microfilariae,* which migrate through the blood or tissues. These larvae are picked up by the insect vector during a blood meal to complete the life cycle. Migration of microfilariae is often timed to maximize uptake of the parasite by the insect vector (nocturnal or diurnal). Clinical disease is generally related to an overexuberant host response to dead or dying adult worms or microfilariae (live worms are generally resistant to the host's immune attack). The location and severity of this inflammation gives rise to the clinical syndromes unique to each species of filariae. In general, eosinophilia is prominent in all patients with filariasis. In fact, filariasis is the most common cause of eosinophilia in Caucasians returning from sub-Saharan Africa. However, the specific diagnosis of filariasis is difficult and often requires the aid of a specialist. The treatment of infection with most forms of filariae still remains less than satisfactory, but promising studies are underway using either ivermectin to kill microfilariae or high-dose albendazole to kill adult worms.

Wuchereria bancrofti, Brugia malayi. In *lymphatic filariasis, W. brancrofti* or *B. malayi* infections are transmitted to humans by mosquitoes. Infections are typically found in tropical regions of Africa, South America, Southeast Asia, and several Pacific islands. Mature male and female worms reside in the lymphatics of the legs, scrota, arms, and thorax. Females release microfilariae into the bloodstream with a pronounced nocturnal periodicity (11 PM to 1 AM). In some strains found in the South Pacific, maximum microfilarial blood concentrations are found at noon.

Adult worms are resistant to the host's immune attack but secrete metabolic products that can cause local inflammation and induce thickening of the lymphatic walls. Some infected individuals are asymptomatic for years, and others never develop symptoms despite years of documented microfilaremia. When adult worms die, they become highly antigenic and evoke a sudden, severe local inflammatory reaction. Lymphangitis and lymphadenitis are usually the first clinical symptoms of infection and last several days to weeks (a single episode normally resolves without sequelae). Inflammation is usually associated with fever, adenopathy, and eosinophilia. Repeated episodes of lymphangitis lead to permanent obstructions to lymph drainage and chronic lymphedema. Hydrocele, chylous ascites, elephantiasis, and megascrotum are common chronic sequelae. Microfilariae, whether dead or alive, do not elicit any immunologic response, except in the unusual syndrome, tropical pulmonary eosinophilia (see later).

The diagnosis of lymphatic filariasis can be difficult. The definitive diagnosis is made by finding the characteristic microfilariae *(W. brancrofti, B. malayi)* in the blood. The highest yields occur in blood obtained between 11 PM and 1 AM. Circulation of microfilariae can also be induced by administering diethylcarbamazine (DEC) and collecting blood 1 hour later. Serologic tests may be suggestive but cross-react with all human and animal filariae and even with many other helminth infections. Recently, better serologic tests have been developed that may allow improved diagnosis and even quantification of the adult worm burden.

Treatment remains unsatisfactory. DEC kills microfilariae but requires daily therapy and can induce significant toxicity (e.g., fever, severe pruritus, postural hypotension, nausea, vomiting) in infected individuals. This results from host immune reactions to dead and dying microfilariae rather than a direct drug toxicity. Gradually increased doses of DEC are often required in an attempt to limit this toxicity. DEC is then continued for 3 weeks. DEC does not kill adult worms, and the microfilarial levels may return to pretreatment values several months later. Ivermectin will probably soon be the drug of choice for filiariasis. Ivermectin appears in preliminary trials to be quite effective when used in higher doses than those currently used in onchocerciasis (400 μg/kg) and may kill adult worms with repeated doses. In preliminary studies, treatment with albendazole (400 mg daily for 3 weeks) also appears to kill adult worms. Both these treatments, however, should still be considered investigational. Treatment of chronic lymphedema is largely unsuccessful but occasionally is correctable by surgery.

Onchocerca volvulus. *River blindness* is caused by the filiarial worm endemic in Central and South America and tropical Africa. Infection *(onchocerciasis)* is spread by the bite of a blackfly of the genus *Simulium*. Since the vector breeds in fast-flowing water, transmission is often seasonal and generally confined to the proximity to rivers and streams. Adult *O. volvulus* worms live in subcutaneous nodules. The female releases microfilariae, which migrate through connective tissues and skin.

Although both adult worms and microfilariae can evoke an immunologic response from the host, microfilariae are primarily responsible for the morbid sequelae of infection. Microfilariae in the skin or eye induce a low-grade inflammation, leading to chronic pathologic sequelae. Most individuals are asymptomatic early in infection. Painless subcutaneous nodules can be palpated over bony prominences. These are usually found in the patient's lower extremities and buttocks in Africa and around the head and neck in South and Central America. Recurrent pruritic rash or conjunctivitis is the first clinical manifestation of disease. During the chronic stages of infection the skin may become thickened and lichenified ("crocodile skin"). Blindness may ultimately occur because of recurrent punctate keratitis, corneal fibrosis, and chorioretinitis with or without glaucoma. Retinal involvement, including optic neuritis, may also occur.

The diagnosis of onchocerciasis is often suspected by a high level of eosinophilia and a history of travel to an endemic area. The definitive diagnosis is made by direct identification of microfilariae in skin snips (two to four square-millimeter, bloodless, superficial pieces of skin incubated in saline) or by visualization of microfilariae during a slit-lamp examination of the eye. Excision of the characteristic subcutaneous nodules may also provide the diagnosis. Occasionally the diagnosis can be made by observing the rapid development of a severe pruritic rash after a single test dose of DEC (Mazzotti test). A specific serologic test is currently available from the Centers for Disease Control (CDC) in Atlanta and is helpful in making the diagnosis.

DEC has been used for many years to treat onchocerciasis but is often associated with severe reactions in infected patients (see previous discussion on lymphatic filariasis) and must be administered daily for 14 days. Furthermore, DEC does not kill adult worms and may accelerate blindness. Treatment with suramin intravenously (IV) is necessary to eradicate adult worms but is quite toxic and now is almost never used. Therefore it is no longer acceptable to use these medications with the availability of newer drugs. Ivermectin is currently the drug of choice for onchocerciasis and can be obtained from the CDC. (Ivermectin has not been approved by the U.S. Food and Drug Administration) A single 150 μg/kg oral dose is used. This will eradicate microfilariae for almost a year, with a marked reduction in adverse side effects. Minor side effects include rash, pruritus, and fever and are a manifestation of dying microfilariae. A complete ophthalmologic examination should be performed before treatment. The dose of ivermectin is repeated every 6 to 12 months. Recent studies suggest that treatment with ivermectin every 3 to 4 months results in a slow reduction in the viability of adult worms, but this more aggressive use of ivermectin is still investigational.

Loa loa. *Loiasis* is endemic in eastern and central tropical Africa. Infection is transmitted by the bite of deerflies and horseflies. Adult worms migrate through subcutaneous tissues, releasing microfilariae into the bloodstream.

With *L. loa,* only the adults are involved in the pathology. Adult worms release antigenic secretions as they pass over bony prominences or joints, particularly the wrists. These antigens evoke intense local reactions called *Calabar swellings*. Localized areas of inflammation are intensely pruritic and generally bring the patient to the physician's attention. In industrialized countries this condition is often misdiagnosed as chronic urticaria or a pyogenic infection. Eosinophilia is very prominent. Rarely an adult worm is seen migrating across the conjunctiva or sclera of the eye, producing intense inflammation.

The diagnosis of *loiasis* is largely made on clinical grounds, since the patient may have Calabar swellings and intense eosinophilia months before microfilariae can be found in the blood. Since microfilariae are released with a diurnal periodicity, blood specimens can be collected at noon and midnight. No serologic tests are completely reliable but may suggest the proper diagnosis to the clinician.

DEC kills microfilariae and often adult worms in *L. loa* infection. However, treatment may precipitate Calabar swellings in locations where adult worms are migrating. When worms are present in the eye, surgical excision is advised. Preliminary studies suggest that both high-dose ivermectin and albendazole can be effective but are still investigational.

Other human filariases. Various other filariases affecting humans have been described but have limited pathogenicity. These include infections with *Dipetalonema perstans, D. streptocerca,* and *Mansonella ozzardi*. Normally these filariases are of importance only because they can be confused with other, more serious filarial pathogens of humans. These infections are treated with either DEC or ivermectin.

Nonhuman filarial infections. Various filariae with nonhuman hosts can occasionally infect people, but the life cycle is not completed. The most common helminths are *Dirofilaria immitis* and *D. tenuis* in North America. Dogs are the normal definitive host. Infected humans are almost always asymptomatic but have isolated pulmonary or subcutaneous nodules. Treatment is by excision.

Tropical pulmonary eosinophilia. Tropical pulmonary eosinophilia (TPE) is a syndrome that includes cough, dyspnea, and pulmonary infiltrates associated with intense eosinophilia in patients from areas endemic for lymphatic filariasis.

The exact pathogenic mechanism of TPE is unknown but is believed to be an overexuberant host response to microfilariae. Microfilariae are not found in the blood but have occasionally been found in lymph node or lung biopsy specimens. Adult worms have not been identified.

The syndrome is typically seen in young men. Initial symptoms include a dry cough, wheezing, dyspnea, low-grade fever, and occasionally diffuse lymphadenopathy and hepatosplenomegaly. The chest radiograph generally suggests diffuse, patchy infiltrates. Occasionally, hemoptysis occurs. Pathologic specimens of the lung demonstrate an intense eosinophilic bronchopneumonia. In untreated patients the syndrome can be quite prolonged, with frequent exacerbations and remissions. Pulmonary fibrosis can be a late complication.

The diagnosis depends on the correct combination of symptoms in an individual from an area endemic for lymphatic filariasis and exclusion of other likely diagnoses (generally tissue migration of other helminths, which is usually transient). Eosinophil counts are often quite high, as are serum immunoglobulin E (IgE) levels. Patients generally have elevated antibody titers to a variety of filarial antigens.

Patients with TPE normally respond to DEC (3 mg/kg three times a day for 14 days) without recurrence. Treatment with albendazole or high-dose ivermectin is still experimental.

Dracunculiasis. Also called *guinea worm disease,* dracunculiasis is an infection now found almost exclusively in Africa and is maintained in locations where humans must walk or step into their sources of drinking water.

Dracunculus medinensis larvae infect microscopic crustaceans that contaminate drinking water. After copepods are ingested, infective larvae are released into the small intestine. Parasites penetrate the intestinal wall and migrate through subcutaneous tissue to the lower extremities. A painful boil develops over the gravid female helminths. On immersion of the limb in water, the boil ruptures. The female's uterus is prolapsed through this ulceration, releasing larvae into the water, where they complete the life cycle.

The first symptoms of *D. medinensis* infection are usually an intense pruritus associated with formation of a painful papule. Multiple papules may develop and are typically found on the legs and feet. Occasionally, ulcers are found on the upper extremities and trunk. Diarrhea and urticaria may occur before ulceration.

The diagnosis can be made by immersion of the ulcer into water. This usually allows visualization of the adult female or demonstration of the larvae in the water after centrifugation.

Patients with dracunculiasis are treated with niridazole, followed by the mechanical removal of the worm. Infection can be prevented by sieving of drinking water or the elimination of open step-in wells.

Trichinella spiralis. *Trichinosis* (infection with *T. spiralis*) is distributed worldwide. Humans become infected by the ingestion of viable larvae encysted in raw or undercooked meat. After passage through the stomach, larvae mature into adult worms in the small intestine. Females produce larvae that penetrate the intestinal wall and migrate throughout the body, eventually undergoing encystation within striated muscle.

When the adult worms are in the intestine (first 2 to 3 weeks), they may cause enteritis. During the migrating phase, larvae attempt to penetrate a variety of host cells, generally leading to cell death. This is a particular problem when larvae penetrate into the brain, heart, or eye. Successful penetration occurs only in striated muscle tissue where encystation occurs. Penetration, however, still results in edema and myositis for 7 to 14 days.

Early symptoms of trichinosis are often mistaken for nonspecific gastroenteritis or flu. In the intestinal phase of infection, diarrhea, vomiting, and abdominal pain typically occur. The penetration of larvae can rarely be associated with gram-negative bacteremia (similar to disseminated *Strongyloides*). Classically, 1 to 2 weeks after ingestion of undercooked meat, patients have periorbital edema, petechial hemorrhages, fever, myalgias, and a prominent eosinophilia. The severity of symptoms usually relates to the size of the inoculation dose. Deaths (2% of patients) generally occur from cardiac, central nervous system (CNS), or pulmonary involvement.

The diagnosis of trichinosis can be aided by a recent history of ingestion of undercooked meat. Various meats have been implicated, including beef and pork as well as meat from wild animals. The total eosinophil count is very high, as are serum levels of creatine phosphokinase (CPK) and aspartate aminotransferase (AST, SGOT) from damaged muscles. Several serologic tests exist but may be negative early. Skeletal muscle biopsy of the deltoid or gastrocnemius allows for definitive diagnosis.

The therapy of trichinosis is less than satisfactory. Thiabendazole kills adult worms but has little effect on migrating larvae. Mebendazole and albendazole have also been used. Mild antipyretics and analgesics help with symptoms. Corticosteroids should be reserved for patients with severe or life-threatening infections.

Fortunately, it is easier to prevent than treat trichinosis. Cooking (59° C for 10 minutes) or freezing (−20° C for 3 days) kills *T. spiralis* larvae. Most infections occur as a result of ingestion of smoked, salted, or dried raw meat, particularly pork.

Angiostrongylus cantonensis, A. costaricensis. These parasites cause eosinophilic meningitis and abdominal pain in individuals from Southeast Asia and the Pacific islands *(A. cantonensis)* or Central America *(A. costaricensis).* Infection is acquired by the ingestion of raw or undercooked mollusks and crustaceans. The disease is generally self-limited, but rare fatalities do occur. No specific diagnostic test or therapy is available, although some suggest the clinical course is shortened by thiabendazole. Albendazole, levamisole, and ivermectin have all been effective in animals.

Gnathostoma spinigerum. *Gnathostomiasis* (infection with *G. spinigerum*) occurs in Thailand and Japan through the ingestion of raw fish. In humans, larvae penetrate the wall of the intestines and migrate through the body until they die. Although migratory subcutaneous swellings and occasionally eosinophilic meningitis can occur, illness is normally self-limiting. No specific therapy exists.

Anisakiasis. Infection with a variety of *Ascaris*-like marine nematodes can cause disease in humans after ingestion of raw fish. Anisakiasis (infection with *Anisakis marina*) therefore occurs frequently in Japan, Thailand, and Scandinavia. Larvae attempt to penetrate the intestinal mucosa but die. Inflammation around dead larvae produce an intense granulomatous reaction, which can resemble carcinoma of the stomach. The definitive diagnosis is made on endoscopic biopsy. No specific therapy exists.

Visceral larva migrans. Visceral larva migrans is caused by the accidental ingestion of dog or cat *Ascaris* eggs. Typically, small children ingest contaminated soil (pica). The larvae penetrate the intestinal mucosa and migrate through the liver, brain, eyes, and lungs. Eventually the larvae die, leading to massive inflammation with eosinophilic granulomatous reactions.

Patients have a variety of symptoms, from minor abdominal complaints to multiorgan involvement with high fever and eosinophilia. Hepatic and pulmonary involvement is quite common. Involvement of the eye causes endophthalmitis and is typically seen in children 5 to 8 years of age. The diagnosis can be made serologically. Illness is usually self-limited. Corticosteroids and thiabendazole have been used, but clinical studies on their efficacy are lacking. Ivermectin and albendazole may be effective in the future.

Cutaneous larva migrans. Cutaneous larva migrans is caused by the skin penetration of canine or feline hookworms or *Strongyloides* infection. The condition is most frequently found along the U.S. southern coast. The migrating larvae are unable to penetrate below the stratum germinativum of the skin and cause pruritic, serpentine, inflammatory lesions in the skin, particularly in areas in direct contact with the ground. Eventually the larvae die, but thiabendazole is often used either topically or systemically. Recently, albendazole (200 mg twice a day for 3 days) has been reported to be effective.

• • •

Table 282-3 lists nematodes infecting tissue and their characteristic features.

Tissue trematodes

Tissue trematodes are among the most important of the helminths that cause infection in humans. Freshwater snails,

Table 282-3. Tissue nematode infections

Species	Epidemiology	Transmission	Major clinical presentation	Diagnosis	Treatment
Filariae					
Wuchereria bancrofti (lymphatic filariasis)	Tropics, subtropics	Mosquito	Lymphatic obstruction	Night blood	Diethylcarbamazine (DEC),* 50 mg 1st day, 50 mg tid 2nd day, 100 mg tid 3rd day, 2 mg/kg tid for 20 days; or ivermectin,†,‡,§ 400 μg/kg; or albendazole,†,‡,§ 400 mg for 21 days
Brugia malayi (lymphatic filariasis)	South and Southeast Asia	Mosquito	Lymphatic obstruction	Night blood	Same as for *W. bancrofti*
Onchocerca volvulus (river blindness)	Central and South America	Blackfly	Dermatitis blindness	Skin snips	Ivermectin,†,‡ 150 μg/kg once every 6 to 12 months or every 4 months,§ or albendazole, 400 mg for 21 days§
Loa loa (Eyeworm)	West and Central Africa	Deerfly, horsefly	Calabar swellings	Day or night blood samples	DEC as for *W. bancrofti* or ivermectin
Tropical pulmonary eosinophilia (TPE)	All the above areas	Unknown	Eosinophilia pneumonitis	Serology and clinical picture	DEC, 2 mg/kg tid for 7-10 days; ivermectin or albendazole†,‡,§ as for *W. bancrofti*

Table 282-3. Tissue nematode infections—cont'd

Species	Epidemiology	Transmission	Major clinical presentation	Diagnosis	Treatment
Dracunculiasis medinensis (guinea worm)	Africa	Step-in wells	Painful boil in legs	Visualization of worm	Niridazole,† 25 mg/kg for 10 days, or metronidazole,† 250 mg tid for 10 days
Trichinella spiralis	Worldwide	Raw meat	Fever, myalgias, periorbital edema	Serology, muscle biopsy	Thiabendazole,‡ 25 mg/kg for 5 days (max, 3 g/day), and ?steroids
Angiostrongylus cantonensis	Southeast Asia, Pacific islands	Raw mollusks or crustaceans	Eosinophilia, meningitis	Clinical picture	Surgical removal
Angiostrongylus costaricensis	Same as above	Same as above	Same as above	Same as above	Surgical removal; mebendazole, 100 mg bid for 5 days, or ?thiabendazole, 25 mg/kg tid for 3 days
Gnathostoma spinigerum	Thailand, Japan	Raw fish	Eosinophilia, meningitis, subcutaneous swellings	Serology	Surgical removal; mebendazole,‡ 200 mg every 3 hours for 6 days
Anisakis species	Japan, Scandinavia	Raw fish	Benign stomach "tumor"	Endoscopy with biopsy, serology	Surgical removal
Visceral larva migrans	Worldwide	Ingestion of soil (pica)	Fever, abdominal pain, optic involvement, diarrhea	Serology	Thiabendazole, 25 mg/kg bid for 5 days (max, 3 g/day), or DEC,† 2 mg/kg bid for 10 days, and ?steroids‡
Cutaneous larva migrans	Worldwide	Skin penetration	Creeping eruption	Clinical picture	Thiabendazole, topically or 50 mg/kg/day (max, 3 g/day) for 2-5 days, or albendazole, 200 mg bid for 3 days
Strongyloidosis	Worldwide, immunosuppressor	Fecal-oral	Gram-negative bacteremia, multiple organ involvement	Stool ova and parasites, tissue biopsy	Thiabendazole, 25 mg/kg bid for 2 days, 5 days for dissemination; or albendazole, 400 mg/day for 3 days,†,§ or ivermectin, 200 μg/kg/day for 1-2 days†,§

*May precipitate severe reactions in infected individuals.
†Considered an investigational drug by the U.S. Food and Drug Administration.
‡Effectiveness not clearly established.
§Not available in the United States.
Tid, Three times a day; bid, twice a day

the intermediate hosts for all trematode infections, and the geographic distribution of the specific snail species generally determine the location of human disease. In the past, many trematode infections in tissue were either untreatable or cured only through the use of very toxic drugs. The recent development of praziquantel has allowed safe, effective treatment of all these infections (*Fasciola hepatica* is an exception).

Table 282-4 lists trematodes infecting tissue and their characteristic features.

Schistosomiasis (bilharziasis). An estimated 300 million

Table 282-4. Tissue trematode infections

Species	Epidemiology	Transmission	Location of adult worms	Major clinical presentation	Diagnosis	Treatment
Schistosomes (Schistosoma)						
S. mansoni	Africa, South America, Middle East, Caribbean	Contact with fresh water	Mesenteric vasculature	Portal hypertension hepatosplenomegaly	Stool O&P, rectal snips	Praziquantel, 20 mg/kg tid for 1 day, or oxamniquine, 10 mg/kg bid for 1 day
S. japonicum	China, Philippines, Indonesia	Contact with fresh water	Mesenteric vasculature	Same as for *S. mansoni* plus seizures	Same as for *S. mansoni*	Praziquantel, 20 mg/kg tid for 1 day
S. mekongi	Thailand, Laos, Cambodia	Contact with fresh water	Mesenteric vasculature	Same as for *S. japonicum*	Same as for *S. mansoni*	Praziquantel, 20 mg/kg tid for 1 day
S. haematobium	Africa, Middle East	Contact with fresh water	Vesical venules	Hematuria, hydronephrosis, carcinoma of bladder	Urine O&P	Praziquantel, 20 mg/kg tid for 1 day
Clonorchis sinensis	Japan, China, Korea	Raw fish	Biliary tree	Cholangitis, portal hypertension, cholangiocarcinoma	Stool O&P	Praziquantel,* 25 mg/kg tid for 2 days
Fasciola hepatica	Worldwide where sheep and cattle are raised	Raw watercress	Bile ducts, liver tissue	Right upper quadrant pain, fever, biliary obstruction, hepatic fibrosis	Stool O&P serology	Bithionol,† 30-50 mg/kg every other day for 15 days; ?albendazole‡,§
Paragonimus westermani	Orient, India, Central Africa	Raw crab	Lungs	Cough, sputum production; resembling tuberculosis	Sputum, stool O&P	Praziquantel,* 25 mg/kg tid for 2 days, or bithionol† as for *F. hepatica*
Opisthorchis viverrini, O. felineus	Europe, Asia, Southeast Asia	Raw freshwater fish	Biliary tree	Same as for *C. sinensis*	Stool O&P	Praziquantel,* 25 mg/kg tid for 1 week

*Considered an investigational drug by the U.S. Food and Drug Administration.
†Available only from the Centers for Disease Control.
‡Not available in the United States.
§Effectiveness not clearly established.
Tid, Three times a day; bid, twice a day; O&P, ova and parasites.

people throughout the world are infected with one of the four species of *Schistosoma*. *S. mansoni* is endemic in Africa, the Middle East, South America, and the Caribbean (including Puerto Rico). *S. haematobium* is typically found throughout Africa and the Middle East. The Far Eastern strain, *S. japonicum,* is endemic in China, the Philippines, and Indonesia, whereas *S. mekongi* is found in Southeast Asia and the Middle East.

Infected freshwater snails release cercariae, which penetrate human skin on contact with fresh water. Larvae migrate through the body, including the lungs, and mature into adult male and female worms. The precise location of adult worm pairs varies with the species. Adult *S. mansoni, S. japonicum,* and *S. mekongi* worms live on the mesenteric venules, whereas *S. haematobium* worms reside in the vesical venules. Female adult worms release 200 to 300 eggs daily, most of which pass out of the body in the urine or stool (depending on the species) to complete the life cycle.

Clinically, initial contact with cercariae can induce an intensely pruritic dermatitis (swimmers' itch). During migration of the larvae, symptoms include fever and PIE syndrome. Individuals with a heavy inoculum can develop a serum sickness–like syndrome termed *Katayama fever,* which is occasionally fatal.

Most individuals are chronically infected with schistosomes, and the pathology depends on the specific species. In *S. mansoni, S. japonicum,* and *S. mekongi,* eggs are passed in the stool. Chronic intestinal infections can lead to intermittent diarrhea and dysentery and vague somatic complaints. Unfortunately, some eggs are carried upstream with the portal blood flow, where they become lodged in the presinusoidal spaces of the liver. There they evoke granulomatous inflammatory reactions that result in enlargement of the liver and spleen. Hepatic fibrosis and a permanent obstruction to portal blood flow are late sequelae. The hepatic fibrosis induced by schistosomiasis is unique. Early fibrosis is confined to the portal tracts, hepatic architecture is preserved, and normal hepatocellular functions are maintained until very late in infection. Bleeding esophageal varices is the leading cause of death in intestinal schistosomes. Intestinal schistosomiasis may predispose to both hepatocellular carcinoma and carcinoma of the colon, but this association remains controversial.

The eggs of *S. haematobium* helminths are passed in the urine. Chronic granulomatous inflammation of infected organs leads to hematuria, hydronephrosis, and subsequent renal failure. Longstanding infection with urinary schistosomiasis is a documented risk factor in the development of carcinoma of the bladder.

Schistosomiasis can also cause several other clinical syndromes. Erratic migration of adult *S. japonicum* worms (and rarely *S. mansoni*) can lead to deposition of ova in the brain or spinal cord, leading to focal epilepsy or transverse myelitis. *Salmonella* can also live within the adult worms. This may lead to recurrent bouts of salmonellosis, including typhoid fever.

The diagnosis of schistosomiasis is generally made by finding schistosome ova in the stool or urine. Biopsy of the rectal mucosa (rectal snips) are often positive in light intestinal infections. Serology is available and may be of value with CNS involvement. The liver fibrosis induced by schistosomiasis gives a characteristic pattern on ultrasound and computed tomographic (CT) scans. The bladder frequently calcifies late in *S. haematobium* infection.

Treatment is now greatly simplified because praziquantel is very effective for all schistosome species infecting humans. Oxamniquine is also effective against *S. mansoni,* whereas metrifonate is effective against *S. haematobium*. Praziquantel is useful in the treatment of CNS infection.

Clonorchis sinensis (Opisthorchis sinensis). Chinese liver fluke *(C. sinensis)* infection is common in individuals from China, Japan, and Southeast Asia, as well as Hawaii. Humans become infected by ingestion of infected raw freshwater fish, causing *clonorchiasis*.

Larvae undergo encystation in the intestine and migrate up the biliary tract, where they mature into adult worms. Migration of these larvae is associated with fever, eosinophilia, liver enlargement, and occasionally cholangitis. The chronic presence of adult worms causes dilatation and inflammation along the biliary tree. Tissue damage with subsequent fibrosis can also occur in the liver parenchyma. Patients with light infections are generally asymptomatic, but longstanding infections can lead to periportal fibrosis, cirrhosis, and obstruction of portal blood flow. Chronically infected patients are also at risk for the development of cholangiocarcinoma.

The diagnosis of *C. sinesis* infection is made by examining the stool for ova or inspecting biliary aspirates in patients with light infection. Praziquantel is the drug of choice. Care must be taken during treatment, however, since dead worms may precipitate biliary obstruction, leading to suppurative cholangitis.

Fasciola hepatica. The liver fluke *F. hepatica* causes a disease known as sheep liver rot. This disease is found in sheep-raising and cattle-raising areas of the world. Infection is maintained in the environment by sheep and freshwater snails. Humans become accidentally infected through the ingestion of watercress contaminated with metacercariae. Larvae penetrate the small intestine into the peritoneum and migrate toward the liver. This acute phase of infection is associated with fever, pain in the right upper quadrant, myalgias, and occasionally urticaria. Adult worms live in the bile ducts and within the liver parenchyma. Eggs leave the liver through the common bile duct to be passed in the stool. Chronic infection may lead to fibrosis or necrosis of the liver. Adult worms may also obstruct bile ducts.

A unique clinical syndrome is caused by an unusual migration of the adult *F. hepatica* worms to the oral pharynx. This condition, known as *halzoun,* causes intense pain in the throat, edema, and occasionally laryngeal obstruction and death. Other ectopic migrations of the helminths can cause focal neurologic symptoms.

The diagnosis is generally made by finding the characteristic eggs in the stool. However, stool examinations will be negative if adults are present only in ectopic locations. Abdominal CT scans are very helpful in visualizing fascioliasis in the liver, and serologies are available to diagnose ectopic infections. *F. hepatica* is unique among the flukes in that infection does not respond to praziquantel. Bithionol (available through the CDC Drug Service, tel. no. 404-639-3670) is the drug of choice. In patients with halzoun, surgical removal of the fluke is indicated.

Paragonimus westermani. This lung fluke is typically found throughout the Orient but rarely may occur in the United States. Humans become infected by the ingestion of raw freshwater crabs or crayfish. Larvae undergo encystation in the duodenum, penetrate the intestinal wall, and migrate to the lungs. Adult worms live in fibrotic cysts located near the periphery of the lungs. Female worms deposit eggs, which penetrate through the bronchioles and are coughed up with sputum.

Clinically, most individuals are asymptomatic during this migration. Chronic *P. westermani* infection is characterized by persistent cough, intermittent hemoptysis, and pleuritic chest pain. The clinical symptoms and chest radiographs are similar to and often confused with those associated with tuberculosis. *Paragonimiasis* can rarely be complicated by bacterial infection, pleural effusions, and clubbing of the fingers and toes. Ectopic foci of adult worms in the brain can be confused with tumors.

The diagnosis of paragonimiasis can be made by finding eggs in the sputum or stool (ova are frequently swallowed). Eosinophilia is normally present. Serologic tests are available but cannot distinguish present from past infection. Praziquantel is effective in treatment.

Opisthorchis viverrini, O. felineus. In Southeast Asia these two species infect humans and cause *opisthorchiasis*. This disease is indistinguishable from clonorchiasis and responds to praziquantel.

Tissue cestodes

Tapeworms confined to the intestines of humans cause relatively minimum morbidity and almost no mortality (see earlier section). In contrast, significant clinical disease and mortality are observed when cestodes invade tissues. Patients are frequently asymptomatic during dissemination of the larvae. The diagnosis is difficult, since eosinophilia occurs infrequently, and negative serologies are seen in early infection. With death or rupture of the larval stage, an inflammatory response occurs, resulting in clinical disease.

Table 282-5 lists cestodes infecting tissue and their characteristic features.

Cysticercosis. Cysticercosis is the disseminated larval stage of the pork tapeworm, *T. solium*. It occurs frequently worldwide and is the world's leading cause of seizures. Humans become infected by ingestion of eggs of the adult tapeworm. This is in contrast to intestinal infection (pork tapeworm), which is caused by ingestion of raw pork. Autoinfection (infection caused by a person's own tapeworm) can occur. In general, most people with cysticercosis do not harbor adult tapeworms in their intestines.

After ingestion the larvae migrate throughout the body and form fluid-filled cysts that are 0.5 to 1.0 cm in diameter. Cysticerci remain viable for 3 to 5 years and evoke little or no host response. Cysticerci can develop in almost any tissue in the body, with the CNS frequently being infected. When they degenerate, cysticerci evoke a massive eosinophilic reaction. Calcified lesions are a late sequela. Clinically, headache, seizures, focal neurologic symptoms, and alterations in mental states are seen. Untreated, symptoms subside in weeks to months, then recur when another cysticercus dies.

The diagnosis of cysticercosis should be suspected in any individual with new onset of seizures. Characteristically, a contrast-enhanced CT scan of the head shows multiple-ring or single-ring enhancing lesions. Nuclear magnetic resonance imaging (MRI) scans are superior and may reveal cysticerci not apparent on CT. Radiographs of the skull and extremities may show calcified cysticerci. Cerebrospinal fluid (CSF) and serum indirect hemagglutination assays are not helpful because significant false-positive and false-negative results are obtained. The test of choice is an immunoblot assay available through the CDC and from some commercial laboratories. This test is almost 100% specific and 98% sensitive. Rare patients have a negative test early in the natural history of the disease. In these patients a therapeutic trial with praziquantel is probably more advisable than a craniotomy.

Praziquantel (50 mg/kg/day in three divided doses for 15 to 30 days) effectively kills the cysticerci but can also exacerbate neurologic symptoms by killing other cysticerci. This can be used diagnostically during therapeutic trials,

Table 282-5. Tissue cestode infections

Species	Epidemiology	Transmission	Major clinical presentation	Diagnosis	Treatment
Taenia solium (cysticercosis)	Worldwide	Ingestion of eggs or autoinfection from tapeworm	Seizures, focal neurologic symptoms, hydrocephalus	Serology, characteristic CT scan of head, radiograph of soft tissues	Praziquantel, 20 mg/kg tid for 5-30 days, or albendazole,*,† 5 mg/kg tid for 1 week, or albendazole 20 mg/kg/day in 3 divided doses for 21 days,*,† or all three with or without steroids
Echinococcus granulosus (hydatid disease)	Sheep and cattle areas of world	Association with dogs, ingestion of contaminated dog excreta	Single mass in liver or lungs, anaphylactic shock after blunt trauma	Characteristic abdominal CT scan, serology	Surgery; albendazole, 400 mg bid for 28 days; ?albendazole plus praziquantel*,‡
Echinococcus multilocularis	Northern latitudes; North America, Europe, and Asia contaminated with dog excreta	Associated with infected animals or ingestion of food	Alveolar mass in liver	Characteristic abdominal CT scan, serology	Same as for *E. granulosus* but surgery usually not feasible

*Considered an investigational drug by the U.S. Food and Drug Administration.
†Not available in the United States.
‡Effectiveness not clearly established.
CT, Computed tomography; tid, three times a day; bid, twice a day.

since treatment can reveal new lesions on CT and MRI brain scans. When the diagnosis is known, however, the concurrent use of steroids is strongly advised (prednisone, 10 mg three times a day, started 1 day before and taken through 3 days after praziquantel therapy). Concurrent steroid use does reduce the blood levels of praziquantel, but it is unknown whether this reduces the cure rate. Albendazole appears to be equally effective but is currently not approved for use in the United States; a dose of 15 mg/kg/day in three divided doses for 10 days has been used successfully. A recent report from Brazil suggests that higher doses of albendazole (20 mg/kg) for longer (21 days) result in more effective resolution of multiple cysts than 3 weeks of praziquantel. Albendazole can be obtained in the United States through the manufacturer for compassionate use. Steroids do not appear to decrease blood levels of albendazole.

***Echinococcus granulosus* (hydatid disease).** *E. granulosus* is a tapeworm of dogs and occurs frequently in the cattle-raising and sheep-raising areas of the world. Humans become infected by ingestion of the eggs, generally from intimate contact with dogs. Larvae undergo encystation in the small intestine, where they penetrate the intestinal wall and are carried by the mesenteric vasculature to various sites within the body, including the liver, lung, and rarely the brain. A single fluid-filled cyst forms and contains multiple protoscoleces (one protoscoleus is capable of forming a new cyst). Over the next several years, cysts slowly enlarge. Symptoms develop when the cyst becomes a large, space-occupying mass. The liver is the most common location, and abdominal pain and signs of cholestasis may develop. In the lungs, pleuritic pain and cough frequently occur. Rupture of the cyst may occur spontaneously or after blunt trauma, precipitating an anaphylactic reaction. The spillage of protoscoleces into the abdominal cavity also leads to multiple daughter cysts, which develop months to years later.

The diagnosis of hydatid disease is generally suspected on physical examination, when the cyst is felt as a large, nontender, intrahepatic mass. Abdominal CT scans show the cystic nature of the lesion, with the characteristic hydatid "sand" in dependent areas. Longer-term cysts may calcify and may be visible on plain radiographs. Several serologic tests are helpful in confirming the diagnosis.

Surgical removal of the cyst is curative, but spillage during the procedure may cause either an anaphylactic reaction or dissemination of daughter cysts. The cyst can be sterilized during surgery by instilling hypertonic saline into it. Medical treatment with mebendazole has been disappointing, although some cures have been documented. Albendazole appears to be the current drug of choice (400 mg twice a day for 28 days). Blood levels can be increased by giving the medication with a fatty meal. The combination of praziquantel and albendazole kills protoscoleces and should be tried if rupture or spillage occurs and if the regimen has been advocated preoperatively.

***Echinococcus multilocularis*.** *E. multilocularis* is similar to *E. granulosus* in its pathogenesis, but usually it infects wild canines such as foxes or wolves. Domestic dogs are occasionally infected. Humans become infected by association with canines or fecally contaminated foods. Infection occurs often in Alaska, Canada, Siberia, and northern parts of the continental United States and Europe. The cysts of *E. multilocularis* are alveolar and invade adjacent tissue. No clear limiting capsule is found, and infection may spread to adjacent sites. The cyst grows similar to a malignant tumor dissecting into the liver parenchyma. As a result, surgical removal is difficult, if not impossible. Mebendazole is occasionally effective. Albendazole appears to be the best clinical choice in inoperative patients, particularly if combined with praziquantel.

PARASITE-INDUCED EOSINOPHILIA

The preceding sections have presented specific helminthic infections. Unfortunately the clinician is often confronted with a patient who has unexplained eosinophilia associated with a strong clinical suspicion of a parasitic etiology. These patients include recent immigrants or visitors from developing countries, returning travelers from extended stays overseas, or indigenous patients in whom other etiologies (e.g., drug reactions, connective tissue diseases, malignancies, fungal infections) seem very unlikely or have been ruled out.

It is important to confirm that eosinophilia is actually present. Since the eosinophil is a relatively rare cell in the peripheral smear, significant errors can be made using the differential to estimate eosinophilia. An absolute eosinophil count should therefore always be performed (normal range, up to 0.45×10^9 cells/L). This number is also useful to confirm a therapeutic response to empiric trials with antiparasitic drugs.

An initial evaluation should include at least three stool examinations for ova and parasites. These results, however, may be misleading. Note that a few helminths do not cause eosinophilia (see Table 282-1) but are frequently found in the stool. In addition, except for trematodes, adult worms that produce eggs in the stool are not the stage of the life cycle responsible for esoniphilia; generally the migrating larvae stimulate eosinophilia. Since *Ascaris* or hookworm ova can be found in a fourth of the world's population, one should be careful to consider other possible etiologies.

Total IgE levels are generally elevated in parasitic infections. Other useful laboratory tests include a serum AST (SGOT), alkaline phosphatase, CPK, and erythrocyte sedimentation rate, as well as chest and thigh radiographs. An accurate travel history can generally suggest or exclude many potential pathogens.

A knowledge of the likely parasitic etiologies of eosinophilia is often helpful in directing further diagnostic tests. For example, in returning Caucasians from Africa, filariasis is the most likely etiology, whereas among Southeast Asian immigrants, *Strongyloides* is typically the causative infection. If three stool examinations do not reveal a pathogen, day and night blood samples and skin snips for microfilariae or rectal snips for schistosome ova are indicated (depending on the appropriate travel history). Serologies may also be useful; among the most useful are serologies for *Strongyloides stercoralis,* since it is frequently missed in the stool. Newer culture techniques will increase the diagnostic yield but are not generally available. A *Dirofilaria immitis* (dog heartworm) serology is positive in a variety of human filarial infections, including TPE. Although not diagnostic of any specific disease, if the titer is high, *D. immitis* serology can help direct further investigation. Other more specific serologies, such as the new serology for onchocerciasis and cysticercosis available from the CDC, the U.S. National Institutes of Health, and a variety of private laboratories, are helpful when used in the proper clinical setting.

Unfortunately a specific diagnosis will not be found in up to 40% of patients with eosinophilia of presumed parasitic etiology. Therapeutic trials with mebendazole, thiabendazole, praziquantel, or DEC are therefore often indicated. An immediate response to DEC is pathognomonic for filarial infection. When ivermectin and albendazole become available in the United States, these drugs would appear to be useful in empiric trials as well. Generally, 2 to 3 months are required to document a decrease in the patient's total eosinophil count in response to empiric drug treatment.

If eosinophilia persists despite these empiric trials, serious consideration should be given to the diagnosis of hypereosinophilic syndrome.

REFERENCES

Campbell WC: The chemotherapy of parasitic infections. J Parasitol 72:45, 1986.

Coulared JP and Rossignol JF: Albendazole, a new single dose antihelminthic: study in 1455 patients. Acta Trop (Basel) 41:87, 1984.

Drugs for parasitic infections. Med Lett 34:865, 1992.

Greene BM et al: Comparison of ivermectin and diethylcarbamazine in the treatment of onchocerciasis. N Engl J Med 313:133, 1985.

Harries AD, Myers B, and Chattacharrya D: Eosinophilia in Caucasians returning from the tropics. Trans R Soc Trop Med Hyg 80:327, 1986.

Jones SK et al: Oral albendazole for the treatment of cutaneous larva migrans. Br J Dermatol 122:99, 1990.

Kumaraswami U et al: Ivermectin for the treatment of *Wuchereria bancrofti* filariasis: efficacy and adverse reactions. JAMA 259:3150, 1988.

Mahmoud AAF, editor: Praziquantel for the treatment of helminthic infections. Adv Intern Med 32:193, 1987.

Norman RM and Kapadia C: Cerebral cysticercosis: treatment with praziquantel. Pediatrics 78:291, 1986.

Nutman TB et al: Eosinophilia in Southeast Asian refugees: evaluation at a referral center. J Infect Dis 155:309, 1987.

Peterson PK and Verhoef J, editors: Diethylcarbamazine and ivermectin. In Antimicrobial agents annual 2. New York, 1987, Elsevier.

Pinkston P et al: Acute tropical pulmonary eosinophilia: characterization of the liver respiratory tract inflammation and its response to therapy. J Clin Invest 80:216, 1987.

Seidel JS, editor: Symposium on parasitic infections. Pediatr Clin North Am 32(4), 1985.

Sturchler D et al: Thiabendazole vs. albendazole in treatment of toxocariasis: clinical trial. Ann Trop Med Parasitol 83:473, 1989.

Takayanagui OM and Jardin E: Therapy for neurocysticercosis: comparison between albendazole and praziquantel. Arch Neurol 49:290, 1992.

Tompkins RK: Management of echinococcal cysts of the liver. Mayo Clin Proc 66:1281, 1991 (editorial).

VanDellen RG, Ottesen EA, and Gocke TM: *Loa loa:* an unusual case of urticaria and angioedema in the United States. JAMA 253:1924, 1985.

Warren KS and Mahmoud AAF, editors: Tropical and geographic medicine, ed 2. New York, 1990, McGraw-Hill.

Wilson JF et al: Albendazole therapy in alveolar hydatid disease: a report of favorable results in two patients after short-term therapy. Am J Trop Med Hyg 37:162, 1987.

Wilson ME: A world guide to infections. New York, 1991, Oxford University.

PART EIGHT

Clinical Immunology, Rheumatology, and Dermatology

I PRINCIPLES OF IMMUNOLOGY

The immune response has developed through evolution to protect against environmental pathogens ("nonself"), while at the same time discriminating against the host's own tissues (noninfectious "self"). The two main phases of the response are an initial recognition event, followed by an effector phase. Immune recognition is critical in the normal functioning of the system and is accomplished by three sets of antigen-binding molecules: the T cell antigen receptor, the class I and class II molecules of the major histocompatibility complex (MHC), and the B cell antigen receptor (immunoglobulin). The effector phase is designed to block, isolate, or eliminate environmental pathogens and is mediated by a variety of cells and soluble factors. Occasionally the immune response is defective. Failure in "self" recognition can result in autoimmune diseases, whereas misdirected effector systems can induce tissue injury and hypersensitivity diseases. Chapter 283 is an excellent starting point for the uninitiated or those wishing an overview of the human immune response. The subsequent chapters detail the various elements of the recognition and effector systems.

CHAPTER

283 Human Immune Response

Robert R. Rich

IMMUNE FUNCTION AND SELF/NONSELF DISCRIMINATION

The vertebrate immune system is a complex, sophisticated mechanism of defense against invasion by infectious organisms. The system is multidispersed with cellular elements resident in or accessible to virtually every organ system. Organized tissues specialized for immune function are designated as primary or secondary. The *primary* lymphoid organs (bone marrow, thymus) are the sites of differentiation of lymphoid progenitors; the *secondary* lymphoid organs (lymph nodes, spleen, submucosal lymphoid tissues) are sites from which immune responses are mounted. The cells and tissues of the immune system are interconnected by a complex vascular system of lymphatic and blood vessels. This system delivers lymphoid cells and antigen from peripheral sites and transports cells between organs of the immune system and to inflammatory loci.

Microbial targets of an immune response include the entire range of infectious agents, from viruses to multicellular parasites. The specific defense may differ, however, based on the nature of the infecting organism and its physical location within the body. For example, defense against infections with intracellular organisms often depends predominantly on cytolytic T cell responses, whereas antibodies and granulocytes more frequently have principal roles as effectors against extracellular microbes. Regardless, one consequence of immune recognition is an inflammatory response, which attacks the invading organism, leading to its destruction. A secondary consequence of this attack may be significant damage to host cells, either as sites of microbial residence or as "innocent bystanders" that do not express the inducing antigen. Depending on the reaction's site and severity, it may be accompanied by the classic local and systemic symptoms and signs of inflammation.

The essence of immune system function is its capacity for molecular discrimination between "self" and "nonself." Such discrimination is entirely the responsibility of T lymphocytes. It reflects the selection within the thymus of those thymocytes that have generated antigen receptors with binding specificity for nonself. In simplest terms, T lymphocytes recognize antigens as short linear peptides (8 to 18 amino acids) that are bound to major histocompatibility complex (MHC) molecules on the surface of antigen-presenting cells. With the exception noted in the following discussion, T cells do not bind antigen in native configuration. Furthermore, they do not recognize antigen in soluble form and do not recognize nonpeptide antigens. This is in marked contrast to antigen recognition by antibody molecules. B cells are not selected for self/nonself discrimination. On the other hand, antibodies, unlike T cells, can bind specifically to complex macromolecules, which are encountered either at cell surfaces or in solution. Moreover, antigens reactive with antibodies include not only proteins, but also carbohydrates, nucleic acids, and lipids.

An essential element of self/nonself discrimination is the clonal specificity of recognition that targets potential invaders. Although the immune system can recognize a vast array of distinct antigens, all the receptors of a single T cell or B cell have identical antigen-binding sites and thus a particular specificity. An additional feature that enhances the effectiveness of the response is antigen-driven *immunologic memory*. This memory derives from the fact that, after an initial encounter with antigen, those clones of lymphocytes of appropriate specificity replicate, resulting in a greater and more rapid response on a subsequent antigen encounter. These features, clonal specificity and immunologic memory, provide a conceptual foundation for use of vaccines in the prevention of infectious diseases. Immunologic memory involves not only the T cells charged with initial discrimination between self and nonself, but also those effector cells that mediate the efferent limb of an inflammatory response. These include both T cells and B cells. On the efferent side the immune response may display exquisite *specificity,* such as the lysis of virus-infected target cells by cytolytic T cells, or *nonspecificity,* such as the response of macrophages to inflammatory mediators.

Implications for disease pathogenesis

The features of the immune system just described are important to understanding pathogenetic mechanisms of immunologic diseases. Four distinct pathways to pathogenesis can be identified (see the box below). First, immunologic disease may represent a failure or deficiency of the immune system. This mechanism is similar to that which accounts for most diseases of other organ systems. Failure may be congenital (e.g., x-linked agammaglobulinemia) or acquired (e.g., acquired immunodeficiency syndrome [AIDS]). It may be global (e.g., severe combined immunodeficiency) or quite specific, involving only a particular component of the immune system (e.g., selective immunoglobulin A [IgA] deficiency). Such failures are usually identified by increased susceptibility to infection, which may range from subtle to profound.

Dysregulation of an essentially intact immune system provides a second pathway to immune pathogenesis. Features of an optimum immune response include antigen recognition and elimination with little if any adverse consequence to the host. Both initiation and termination of the response involve complex regulatory interactions that may go awry when challenged by antigens of a particular structure or in a particular mode of presentation. Diseases of immune dysregulation typically reflect a combination of genetic and environmental factors that, acting together, subverts a normal immune response to some pathologic end. The acute allergic diseases are typical of these disorders. For example, the pathogenesis of allergic asthma may involve a genetically determined excessive response to some environmental antigen, such as the immunoglobulin E (IgE) response to animal danders, as well as an abnormality in effector responses to inflammatory signals.

The third and fourth pathways to pathogenesis are more specific to the immune system. The third lies at the heart of specific immune system function, that is, the molecular discrimination between self and nonself. An untoward consequence of ambiguity in this discrimination is the development of autoimmune tissue damage. Although such damage may be mediated either by antibodies or T cells, the basic pathogenesis of autoimmune diseases represents a failure of T cell function because of these cells' central responsibility for self/nonself discrimination. Failures may be general, leading to development of systemic autoimmune diseases, such as lupus erythematosus, or local, as in organ-specific autoimmune diseases. With local failure the attack is directed against specific cells and usually particular cell surface molecules expressed by such cells. Most often, pathology is a consequence of target tissue destruction (e.g., multiple sclerosis, rheumatoid arthritis, insulin-dependent diabetes mellitus). However, it may also reflect hormone receptor blockade (e.g., type B insulin-resistant diabetes) or hormone receptor stimulation (e.g., Graves' disease). Autoimmune disease may represent the consequence of an ambiguity in self/nonself discrimination resulting from an encounter with an infectious organism. In most cases the infectious episode is unidentified and merely postulated; in some cases, however, it may be associated with a clearly identified infectious event (e.g., rheumatic fever, Reiter's disease). The result in either case may be secondary autoimmune attack on a particular cell type, based on cross-reactivity of antigenic determinants between the infectious agent and the target tissue.

A fourth important pathogenetic mechanism is disease development as a consequence of physiologic rather than pathologic function. These are diseases in which the development of an inflammatory lesion represents nothing more than normal functioning of the system. Typical of such diseases is contact dermatitis to such potent skin sensitizers as urushiol, the causative agent of poison ivy dermatitis. These diseases may also have an iatrogenic etiology; they may range from benign (e.g., delayed hypersensitivity skin test reactions) to life-threatening (e.g., graft-versus-host disease, in which the physiologic immune function of an engrafting bone marrow threatens the viability of an immunologically incompetent host). Furthermore, studies in experimental animals have shown that diseases resulting from an encounter with certain infectious agents may reflect secondary consequences of a physiologic immune response to the infectious organism. Classic examples with probable implications for human diseases include coxsackie myocarditis and lymphocytic choriomeningitis in mice.

Pathogenetic processes in immunologic diseases

- Immunologic deficiencies (congenital or acquired)
- Immunologic dysregulation
- Ambiguity of self/nonself discrimination
- Inflammatory consequences of normal immune function

CONSTITUENTS OF IMMUNE SYSTEM

Immune responses are traditionally categorized as *humoral* or *cellular*. The first refer to those carried out by circulating antibodies and the latter those mediated by specifically sensitized T lymphocytes. The system actually is far more complex; it includes cellular interactions that control the development of antibody responses and the effects of short-range soluble mediators, termed *cytokines,* in the induction and regulation of both T cell–mediated and B cell–mediated immune responses.

Cellular components

The cellular constituents of the immune system are leukocytes and related cells with common precursors resident in solid organs. These cells arise from pluripotent stem cells present throughout life in the bone marrow. Components not derived from bone marrow include stromal elements of the solid lymphoid organs and certain specialized epithelial cells that are important in antigen presentation and lymphocyte differentiation, such as in the thymus.

The lymphocytes capable of specific immune recognition, based on their clonally specific cell surface display of antigen receptors, are T cells and B cells. Arising from bone marrow precursors, *T cells* are selected in the thymus based on the expression of T cell receptors (TCRs) useful in self/

nonself discrimination. Mature T cells emerging from this differentiative process are found in T cell–dependent areas of solid lymphoid organs and normally constitute 60% to 85% of the lymphocyte population in the peripheral blood of adults. *B cells* mature in the bone marrow. On emigration, they reside within lymphoid follicles and germinal centers of solid lymphoid organs; they represent 7% to 20% of lymphocytes in peripheral blood. When stimulated with antigen, B cells undergo terminal differentiation to nondividing, antibody-producing plasma cells. Plasma cells are resident within lymphoid tissues but do not normally circulate in the peripheral blood.

A third class of lymphocytes is comprised of those identified morphologically as *large granular lymphocytes* (LGLs) and functionally as *natural killer* (NK) *cells*. Such cells, representing 10% to 30% of circulating lymphocytes, are clearly distinct from T cells and B cells because they do not rearrange the genes encoding the antigen receptors of either. They are nevertheless capable of a less specific type of recognition that is likely important during primary encounter with certain cell-associated antigens, such as those expressed on tumor cells or virus-infected cells. The molecular basis of this recognition has not been defined.

The remaining mononuclear cell type present in peripheral blood is the *monocyte,* normally constituting 4% to 15% of total leukocytes. Monocytes and their relatives are important in antigen processing and presentation, particularly to T cells. Although apparently derived from a common monocytoid precursor in the bone marrow, such cells may exhibit a wide variety of morphologic features and specialized functions within solid organs, where they include macrophages and dendritic cells in lymph nodes, Kupffer's cells in the liver, Langerhans cells in skin, and microglial cells in brain.

Discussions of the specific immune system often overlook the *polymorphonuclear leukocytes* (PMNs). Nevertheless, these cells are essential to most antibody-mediated defenses. Derived from granulocyte precursors in the bone marrow, PMNs undergo terminal differentiation along three general pathways, as neutrophils (35% to 75% of total leukocytes in the circulation of adults), eosinophils (0% to 5%), and basophils (0% to 1%). *Neutrophils* are the principal effectors of responses to pyogenic infections. They phagocytose foreign particles coated (opsonized) with antibodies and/or complement components based on their cell surface display of immunoglobulin (Ig) Fc receptors and receptors for complement components, particularly C3b. Phagocytized particles are degraded within granules of PMNs; living organisms are killed by various cellular mechanisms, including generation of oxygen radicals and halogenation. In addition to their central importance in phagocytosis and killing of microorganisms, recent data point to a role for neutrophils as immunoregulators capable of synthesis and release of cytokines such as interleukin 1 (IL-1), IL-6, and tumor necrosis factor alpha (TNF-α).

Eosinophils and *basophils,* identified by the morphology and staining properties of their intracellular granules, are particularly important in host defenses to multicellular parasites. *Mast cells* are fixed tissue relatives of basophils; they are further divided into subtypes, mucosal and epithelial mast cells, based on tissue location and differences in morphology and function. Eosinophils, basophils, and mast cells are also prominent participants in acute allergic reactions, a secondary reflection of the shared role of IgE molecules in parasite defenses and the immune reactions of immediate hypersensitivity.

Soluble factors

Immunoglobulins, (ig) or antibodies, produced by plasma cells, are the soluble effectors of immune responses with specific antigen-binding activity. As such, they differ importantly from the other humoral constituents of immunity, which may be critical to genesis of an inflammatory response, but do not bind antigen. The five major Ig classes (isotypes) are IgM, IgG, IgA, IgD, and IgE. The IgG class is further divided into four subclasses and the IgA class into two subclasses. Antibody molecules are comprised of heavy and light chains, each of which has a *variable region* of 108 to 120 amino acids at the amino-terminal end connected to a carboxy-terminal *constant region* of approximately equal length for light chains and threefold or fourfold longer for heavy chains. The chains are connected to one another by interchain disulfide bonds. The major classes of antibody *(isotypes)* are defined by the heavy chain, the genes for which map to human chromosome 14q32.

During the course of an antibody response, a given B cell may change the class of antibody that it synthesizes *(isotype switching)* without affecting the antigen specificity. This is accomplished by differential ribonucleic acid (RNA) splicing or deoxyribonucleic acid (DNA) rearrangements, both of which have the effect of bringing the gene segments encoding a particular variable region into immediate proximity with one or another of the genes encoding constant region segments of the heavy chain (Chapter 285). Light chains are of two types, kappa (κ) and lambda (λ), encoded on chromosomes 2 and 22, respectively. Either light chain can associate with heavy chains of any class, but any particular B cell or plasma cell synthesizes antibody molecules of a single light chain isotype. All the antibodies synthesized by a particular cell have identical variable regions, a feature that is essential to the principle of clonal specificity of an immune response. This reflects that the genes on only one member of the pair of chromosomes encoding a heavy chain and only one of the pairs of either κ or λ light chain genes are active in any B cell. This process, termed *allelic exclusion,* also applies to the synthesis of T cell receptors.

Although the isotype of an antibody molecule does not affect its antigen-binding specificity, it largely determines the particular biologic activity and physical characteristics of the molecule. Serum IgM is a pentameric structure, each subunit of which is comprised of two mu (μ) heavy chains and two light chains (either κ or λ). It is the principal antibody of a primary immune response. Because of its large molecular mass (about 900 kilodaltons [kd]), IgM distribution is essentially limited to the vascular compartment. Monomeric IgM molecules are expressed as antigen receptors on the surface of B cells; RNA encoding the carboxy-terminal segment of the μ chains is differentially spliced to provide the transmembrane and intracytoplasmic domains absent from the secreted form of the molecule. IgG antibodies are the most abundant in the serum and are the principal antibodies of a memory (secondary) response. IgG is comprised of two light chains and two γ heavy chains. It is the only antibody isotype that is transported by an active process across the placenta from mother to fetus. IgA molecules are the principal antibodies in secretions across mucous membranes. In secretions, IgA is present as dimers connected by a joining chain; secretion is an active process promoted by the addition of *secretory component,* an epithelial cell product. Appropriate to its function, secretory IgA is relatively resistant to digestion by proteolytic enzymes. IgA is found in serum in monomeric or dimeric form, but without secretory component attached. IgD molecules are primarily expressed as antigen receptors on B cells, particularly memory B cells, either with or without cell surface IgM molecules of the same antigen-binding specificity. Only small amounts of IgD are found in serum, and the biologic function of soluble IgD is unknown. IgE is present in the serum in the lowest concentration of the five isotypes (about 1/120,000 of the IgG concentration). IgE molecules, however, may have profound biologic effects based on their specific binding to the surfaces of mast cells and basophils, which are induced to degranulate on cross-linking of surface IgE by antigen. This process is important in defenses against parasitic infestation and is also a critical pathogenetic event in the diseases of immediate hypersensitivity.

It is the variable portion of an Ig molecule, termed the *Fab fragment,* that contains the antigen-binding site. The biologic effector functions, on the other hand, are provided by distinct sites on the constant region of the heavy chains *(Fc fragment).* These include sites that bind and activate the first component of complement (IgM, IgG), that bind to the surface of phagocytic cells (IgM, IgG) or mast cells and basophils (IgE), and that account for the active transport of IgG across the placenta.

The biologic functions of IgG and IgM are largely reflections of their capacities to activate the complement cascade (Chapter 287). Through a series of sequential substrate-enzyme interactions, the 11 principal components of the complement system (C1q, C1r, C1s, C2 to C9) effect many of the principal consequences of an antigen-antibody interaction. These include the establishment of pores in a target membrane by the terminal components (C5 to C9), leading to osmotic lysis; opsonization by C3b, promoting phagocytosis; the production of factors with chemotactic activity (C5a); and the ability to induce mast cell degranulation (C3a, C4a, C5a). It is important to recognize that although complement activation is accomplished by the interaction between IgG or IgM and C1q (the *classic pathway*), many substances, including certain bacterial products, can directly activate the cascade through the central C3 component. This bypasses involvement of C1, C4, and C2 but leads to all the biologic consequences of C3 to C9 activation. Nonantibody-induced activation of C3 is referred to as the *alternative,* or *properdin, pathway.*

In contrast to the abundance of Ig molecules (up to 15 mg/ml or 0.1 M for IgG), the soluble products of T cells and antigen-presenting cells (APCs) are present at the sites of an immune response in extremely low concentration (e.g., approximately 10^{-10} M). These factors are a diverse group of generally small protein hormones (8 to 35 kd) that do not bind antigen and are collectively referred to as cytokines (Chapter 286). Among others, they include IL-1 through IL-13, interferon gamma (IFN-γ), TNF, transforming growth factor beta (TGF-β), and the colony-stimulating factors (CSFs). Some cytokines are produced predominantly by T cells (or T cells and mast cells). Others are produced by many cell types, including APCs and cells of other organ systems. A characteristic feature of cytokines is their pleiotropy of function. Within the immune system this can include promotion of proliferation of specific subsets, control of the differentiation of B cell and T cell effector functions and the regulation of immunoglobulin production and isotype switching. Certain cytokines, particularly IL-10, IL-13, and TGF-β are particularly important in downregulation of immunologic responses. Others, such as IL-3, IL-5, and the CSFs, are important as regulators of the differentiation of hematopoietic cells in the bone marrow. It is through the action of cytokines produced by T cells that their capacity for self/nonself discrimination is translated to control of antibody responses.

MOLECULAR IMMUNOLOGY AND IMMUNOGLOBULIN SUPERFAMILY

Many of the principal molecules involved in activation, regulation, cell-to-cell contact, and effector function in immune responses share structural features indicative of a common evolutionary origin. These molecules and the genes that encode them are collectively referred to as the Ig superfamily. The family includes more than 25 distinct members that exhibit significant sequence homology to one another. An essential feature is a *domain* subunit structure of approximately 100 amino acids, usually including a single intrachain disulfide bond. Protein organization generally correlates well with genomic structure, with separate protein domains typically encoded by distinct exons. Functions of the Ig superfamily are related principally to antigen binding (Ig, TCR, MHC molecules) and to cell-cell interaction and recognition (e.g., CD4,* CD8, lymphocyte function–associated [LFA] molecules, intercellular adhesion molecules [ICAMs]). A frequent feature of Ig superfamily interactions is that different members expressed on different cells function as ligand-receptor pairs for one another, often to increase adhesiveness of a cell-cell interaction (e.g., CD2 and LFA-3; LFA-1 and ICAM-1; CD8 and MHC class I; CD4 and MHC class II).

An understanding of molecular specificity of an immune response requires some appreciation of the structural basis

*CD designates *cluster of differentiation,* an official international nomenclature for designation of cell surface molecules expressed on leukocyte surfaces that vary with cell type. Thus they are useful in characterization of phenotypic subpopulations.

of antigen binding. The three types of molecules with this capability, MHC, Ig, and TCR, all construct an antigen-binding groove, with side chains and pockets that accommodate specific structural features of the ligand. For Ig molecules the ligand (an antigenic determinant, or *epitope*) may be present as a specific chemical moiety or conformational site on the surface of a molecule that varies in complexity from a simple substituted aromatic ring to a macromolecule. Binding by antibody is of relatively high specificity and high affinity. The TCR antigen-binding site is also of high specificity but probably of relatively low affinity, reflecting the process by which it is selected for self/nonself discrimination. The TCR binds, within a single complex site, both to a foreign peptide and the surrounding alpha helices of the MHC molecule that presents it. MHC molecules are the third members of the antigen-binding team. They bind short peptides, derived from either self or nonself proteins, with low specificity and medium to high affinity. Ig and TCR share a strategy for achieving specificity of the antigen-binding pocket that differs fundamentally from that of MHC molecules. Ig and TCR use families of rearranging gene segments to construct variable regions particular to specific T cells or B cells and their clonal progeny. MHC molecules, on the other hand, do not rearrange; they do not undergo allelic exclusion and are codominantly expressed. Thus a particular APC may display a full complement of MHC molecules, with capacity to bind numerous distinct antigen peptides in a nonclonally specific manner.

Immunoglobulin and T cell receptor diversity

Antigen-binding specificity of both Ig and TCR reflects the random joining by DNA rearrangement and splicing of two or three segments selected from a "gene library" encoding each chain of the variable domain of the molecule. For Ig heavy chains this involves the joining of one particular V segment (of more than 100 available) to one D segment (of at least 20) and a J segment (of six) (Chapter 285). The particular V-D-J unit is then joined (by RNA splicing or DNA rearrangement) to a C region, one of a series of tandemly arrayed genes encoding isotype-specific heavy chain constant regions, leading to transcription of a specific Ig heavy chain. For κ and λ light chains, only two segments, V and J, are used to encode the variable portion of the molecule.

The structure of TCR is highly homologous to that of Ig molecules. Four distinct rearranging gene families have been identified: α, β, γ, and δ. Two isoforms of TCR are expressed; both are heterodimers of integral membrane proteins, comprised of α and β chains or γ and δ chains. In the circulation, 97% or more of T cells display the αβ receptor, whereas in some tissue sites, such as the intestinal mucosa, γδ-bearing T cells may predominate. The αβ heterodimer is invariably bonded by an interchain disulfide link; γδ TCR may be disulfide linked or unlinked. Functional differences between T cells expressing αβ and γδ receptors are a matter of current study; they may reflect responses to antigens of differing origin or the use of distinct subsets of MHC class I molecules for presentation. Both TCR isotypes are associated with a multimeric structure, CD3, that is required for TCR cell surface expression and for signal transduction. In contrast to the TCR heterodimer, the CD3 components do not rearrange and do not exhibit clonal variability. The general strategy for assembly of TCR variable regions is the same as that for Ig, with some differences in gene organization that allow additional variability in rearrangement. The variable segments of β and δ chains are assembled from V, D, and J segments randomly selected and joined to the C region gene; α and γ chains, as with Ig light chains, are assembled only from V and J segments. Interestingly, genes for δ chains are imbedded within the chromosomal segment encoding α chains, between the Vα and Jα regions.

Extraordinary diversity is achieved, both for TCR and Ig molecules by the random selection of segments encoding the variable regions plus the additional "combinatorial" diversification accomplished by the pairing of particular chains with one another in construction of the complete Ig or TCR molecule. Further diversification is achieved by a mechanism termed *N-nucleotide addition,* in which one or more individual nucleotides, not encoded within the genome, are frequently added concomitantly, with gene rearrangement at the junctions between variable region segments. The addition of nucleotides results in a high likelihood of frame-shift mutations and increases the probability that any given rearrangement will be nonproductive.

One molecular mechanism in antigen receptor construction is unique to Ig genes. This is a process of somatic mutation that continues within the rearranged V-D-J gene throughout the lifetime of a particular B cell and its clonal progeny. Because clonal proliferation of lymphocytes is driven by contact with antigen, a B cell expressing surface Ig molecules that have higher affinity for a particular antigen than its parent or sibling cells will be preferentially selected and stimulated to divide. Consequently, over generations of the B cell response to antigen, antibodies of progressively higher affinity are produced. This process, termed *affinity maturation,* contributes significantly to the much higher antigen-binding affinity of Ig than TCR molecules. The difference, however, is at the core of the capacity for self/nonself discrimination uniquely possessed by T cells. Such discrimination requires that TCR affinity be fixed within the thymus before an encounter with foreign antigen. Thus somatic mutation of TCR does not occur during antigen-driven T cell clonal proliferation.

The third family of antigen-binding molecules is the product of the MHC. The MHC, termed *human lymphocyte antigen* (HLA) in humans and encoded on chromosome 6, represents a highly duplicated system of genes of two basic types, class I and class II. Products of the three principal MHC class I genes, designated HLA-A, HLA-B and HLA-C, are involved in antigen presentation. An as yet unknown number of additional "nonclassic" class I gene products may have more specialized roles in antigen presentation or cell-cell interaction. Three principal class II genes and gene products also exist, HLA-DR, HLA-DQ, and HLA-DP. Both class I and class II molecules possess a peptide-binding (antigen-binding) groove with walls of α helices and a floor of antiparallel β-pleated strands. The class I groove accommodates peptides 8 to 10 amino acids in length; the class II groove allows peptides of 12 to 18 amino acids. Although highly homologous to one another, the class I and class II molecules have substantial structural differences. Class I molecules are comprised of a polymorphic HLA-A, HLA-B, or HLA-C heavy chain of approximately 45 kd that is noncovalently associated with a nonpolymorphic non-MHC product, β_2 microglobulin (β_2m). The class I heavy chain is an integral membrane protein; β_2m is not. In contrast, both chains of class II molecules are encoded within the MHC, and both are integral membrane proteins. The class II polypeptides are of similar molecular size (28 to 32 kd). For HLA-DQ, both chains, designated α and β, are polymorphic, whereas for HLA-DR, polymorphism is essentially limited to the β chain. Because the MHC genes do not rearrange, they are far less diverse within an individual than the Ig and TCR products. Nevertheless, this lack of diversity does not greatly compromise their capacity for antigen binding because of their specificity. Moreover, the multiplicity of MHC genes coupled with their extraordinary population polymorphism ensures that an array of different MHC molecules are expressed on the surface of an APC.

ANTIGENS AND ANTIGEN PROCESSING

As noted earlier, T cells generally recognize antigen as short peptides located within the antigen-binding groove of MHC molecules. The process by which proteins are partially digested and re-presented to T cells as oligopeptides in an appropriate MHC context is termed *antigen processing*. Two distinct pathways can be distinguished, depending on the source of the antigen (Fig. 283-1). Antigens that are synthesized within the antigen-presenting cell (APC) itself (termed *endogenous* antigens, e.g., viral and tumor antigens) undergo hydrolysis to peptides of 8 to 10 amino acids within the cytoplasm. Components of the proteosomes that mediate this digestion and the transporter (TAP) proteins with which the peptide fragments are then associated are also encoded within the MHC. TAP-associated antigen peptides are then transported into the lumen of the endoplasmic reticulum, where they are loaded into the binding groove of newly synthesized MHC class I proteins. It is this complex of peptide, class I heavy chain, and β_2m that is then expressed at the cell surface, where it can be recognized by T cells of the CD8$^+$ subset. In contrast, antigens synthesized outside the APC (termed *exogenous* antigens) enter the cell by phagocytosis (e.g., monocytes, macrophages) or receptor-mediated endocytosis (e.g., B cells functioning as APCs). They are then hydrolyzed by lysosomal enzymes and, within endosomes, peptides of 12 to 18 amino acids are loaded into binding grooves of MHC class II molecules. Class II–peptide complexes are then transported to the cell surface for recognition by T cells of the CD4$^+$ subpopulation.

It is important to appreciate that the tissue distributions of class I and class II MHC molecules differ significantly.

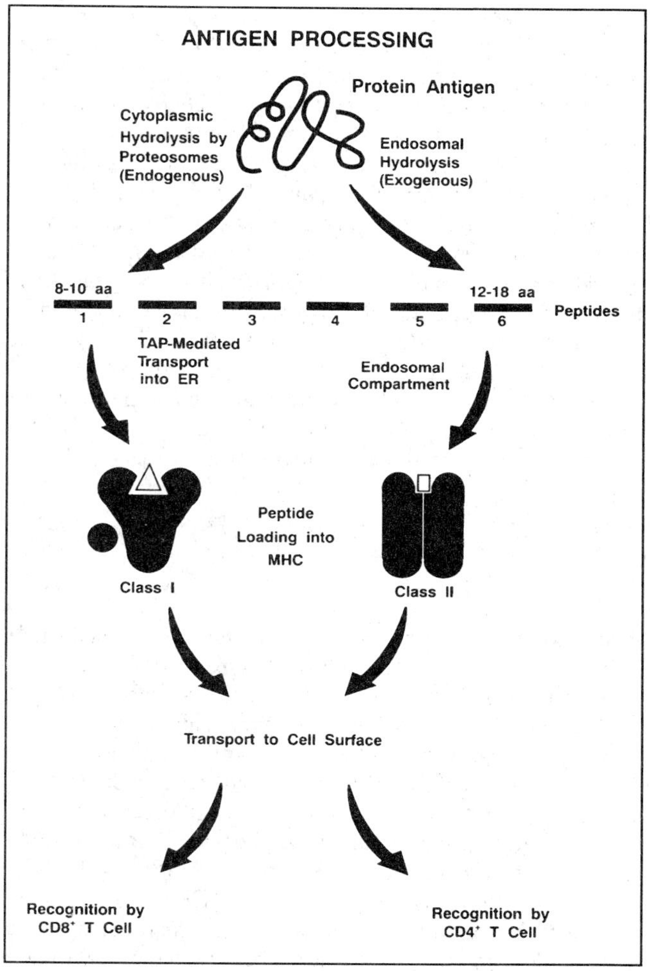

Fig. 283-1. Distinct pathways for processing (hydrolytic digestion) of endogenous and exogenous protein antigens and peptide loading into antigen-binding clefts of major histocompatibility complex (MHC) class I and class II molecules, respectively.

Class I molecules are expressed on almost all nucleated cells. Consequently, many cells that are not components of the immune system may be capable of presenting an endogenous antigen and may serve as targets of a CD8$^+$ T cell immune attack. In contrast, the tissue distribution of MHC class II molecules is quite restricted, being limited primarily to those cells of the immune system that have differentiated specifically to function as APCs. Because the initial activation of an immune response is controlled by CD4$^+$ T cells, it consequently depends on appropriate processing and presentation of antigen by MHC class II–expressing cells.

Recently recognized exceptions to these principles of antigen presentation and recognition are the so-called superantigens. They are exemplified by the staphylococcal enterotoxins and related exotoxins produced by gram-positive cocci. The superantigens are proteins of about 30 kd that do not require processing but bind in native form to class II MHC molecules outside the antigen-binding groove. Moreover, they activate both CD4$^+$ and CD8$^+$ T cells when bound to class II molecules. Superantigens' capacity to stimulate T cells is determined primarily by the V segment of the TCR β chain; it is largely independent of the other TCR components that define binding specificity for conventional peptide antigens. This results in a much higher frequency of T cells responsive to superantigens than to conventional antigens, thus their name. In the mouse, not only bacterial exotoxins but also certain retroviral products have been shown to exhibit superantigen properties, indicating considerable diversity in the origin of such antigens. Bacterial superantigens are etiologic agents of various important diseases, including staphylococcal food poisoning, toxic shock syndrome, and scarlet fever. Superantigens of undetermined origin have also been implicated indirectly in the pathogenesis of several autoimmune diseases, including rheumatoid arthritis and Kawasaki disease.

LYMPHOCYTE DIFFERENTIATION AND ACTIVATION

Thymocyte education

The extraordinary process of T cell education for self/nonself discrimination occurs during differentiation in the thymus; it reflects selection based on contact with self MHC molecules (plus peptide) in the thymic microenvironment. Prothymocytes, which enter the thymic cortex from the bone marrow, display CD2 (sheep erythrocyte receptor) and CD7; CD4 and CD8 have not yet been expressed, and TCR genes are in a germline (unrearranged) configuration. Soon thereafter the early thymocytes begin rearrangement of TCR genes and coexpress CD4 and CD8. TCR with randomly generated V regions, either αβ or γδ, are then coexpressed with CD3 at the thymocyte surface, where they encounter an array of self MHC class I and class II molecules on the surfaces of cortical epithelial cells. For most thymocytes the nascent TCR does not have appreciable affinity for any available self MHC molecule. In such cases, in the absence of TCR activation, the cell undergoes programmed death by a process termed *apoptosis* involving DNA fragmentation.

A few cells display appreciable affinity for one particular self MHC class I or class II molecule and are *positively selected* for further differentiation based on this property (Fig. 283-2, *A*). If the MHC molecule chosen is class II, the thymocyte downregulates its expression of CD8 and increases expression of CD4, becoming a *single-positive* $CD4^+$ thymocyte. Similarly, binding to a class I MHC molecule leads to development of a single-positive $CD8^+$ thymocyte. At this stage, those thymocytes that have survived the round of positive selection undergo a second round of *negative selection* (Fig. 283-2, *B*). The objective of negative selection is the opposite of the first round, that is, to eliminate those thymocytes that possess receptors of very high affinity for self MHC plus the self peptide (derived from autologous proteins) within the MHC antigen-binding groove. Elimination of such cells is essential to the process of self/nonself discrimination, since their emigration from the thymus would permit terminal differentiation of cells capable of autoimmune attack. Thus clones of cells with

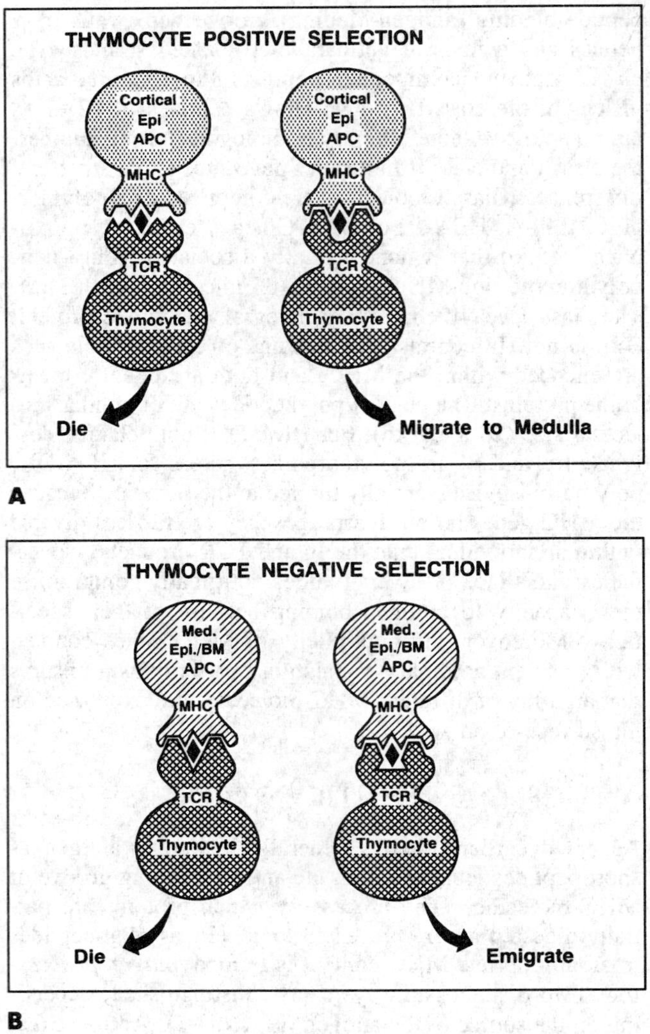

Fig. 283-2. Two-stage selection of thymocytes based on binding characteristics of randomly generated T cell responses (TCRs). **A,** Positive selection. *Double-positive* ($CD4^+$, $CD8^+$) thymocytes with TCR capable of *low* affinity binding to some specific "self" MHC molecule (either class I or class II) expressed by thymic cortical epithelial cells are positively selected; all other thymocytes die by apoptosis. The solid diamond represents a self peptide derived from hydrolysis of an autologous protein present in the thymus microenvironment or synthesized within the thymic antigen-processing cell (APC) itself. **B,** Negative selection. *Single-positive* ($CD4^+$ or $CD8^+$) thymocytes, positively selected in stage one, that display TCR with *high* affinity for the combination of self MHC plus some self (autologous) peptide present in the thymus are negatively selected (i.e., die). Those few thymocytes that have survived both positive and negative selection emigrate as mature T cells to the secondary lymphoid tissues.

high-affinity receptors for self MHC plus peptide are similarly deleted by an apoptotic process. In the end, fewer than 5% of the prothymocytes that enter survive the education/selection process to emerge several days later as mature T cells for distribution in the periphery. Such cells have low-affinity receptors for self MHC plus self peptide but may have increased affinity for the complex of MHC plus some undefined nonself peptide that may be subsequently encountered.

CD4 and CD8

Throughout the differentiative process, as well as in the peripheral tissues, CD4 and CD8 molecules are importantly involved in T cell activation. CD4 is a monomeric integral membrane protein with four extracellular domains, three of which share membership in the Ig superfamily. In contrast, CD8 is a dimeric structure, either a homodimer or heterodimer, both chains of which are transmembrane and both of which have a single Ig-like external domain. The contributions of CD4 and CD8 to T cell differentiation and function are twofold. First, CD8 molecules display a specific contact point for binding to a nonpolymorphic site on MHC class I molecules, thereby increasing the avidity of the $CD8^+$ T cell–APC interaction. Similarly, CD4 molecules bind to MHC class II molecules, enhancing the adhesiveness of that interaction. Because the TCR was specifically selected for its relatively low affinity for self MHC, the development of adhesion-strengthening interactions of this type is important to effective engagement of T cell and APC; other non-TCR-associated interactions, such as CD2 and LFA-1 on T cells with LFA-3 and ICAM-1 on APC, respectively, also contribute significantly in this respect. A second function of CD4 or CD8 is in signal transduction. These molecules interact with other membrane constituents (members of the *src* family of cellular oncogenes), resulting in protein phosphorylation associated with cell activation. Because the intracytoplasmic tail of the TCR heterodimer lacks sites for phosphorylation, perturbations of TCR-associated molecules, including CD3 and CD4 or CD8, are essential in transmitting the signal of antigen interaction to the cell's interior.

B cell differentiation

Progenitors of B cells are derived from lymphoid stem cells and are first identified by rearrangement of Ig heavy chain genes. As these cells differentiate into pre-B cells, they are distinguished by the expression of isolated μ chains within the cytoplasm. These represent the protein products of one of the two Ig heavy chain gene complexes that have undergone a productive genetic rearrangement. At the pre-B cell stage, the cells are devoid of surface Ig (sIg). As they differentiate into immature B cells, light chain genes are also rearranged, and their products (κ or λ chains) are combined with cytoplasmic μ chains, leading to the cell surface expression of monomeric sIgM. The B cell–specific differentiation markers CD19, C20 and CD21 are also sequentially expressed during the pre-B and immature B cell stages of differentiation. By a process of differential RNA splicing, immature B cells undergo their first Ig isotype switch, leading to the coexpression of IgM and IgD as antigen receptors at the B cell surface. On expression of sIg, B cells may emigrate from the bone marrow to the peripheral and the solid lymphoid organs, where they undergo further antigen-driven differentiation. On encounter with antigen in the periphery, B cell clones proliferate; this leads to development of memory B cells or to terminal differentiation into nondividing, Ig-secreting plasma cells. Reflecting secondary DNA rearrangements, memory B cells may lose expression of surface IgD and acquire instead sIgG, sIgA, or sIgE. On antigen stimulation, plasma cells cease cell surface expression of sIg as synthesis of Ig molecules switches from the membrane-bound to the secreted form. A notable distinction between the processes of B cell and thymocyte differentiation is that whereas both undergo random rearrangements of receptor genes to generate lymphocyte clones of diverse specificity, only thymocytes have imposed on them a selective process that results from antigen encounter within the primary lymphoid organ. Thus only T cells have been "educated" for self/nonself discrimination.

Lymphocyte activation

For both T cells and B cells, activation is a two-signal process. In both cases the first signal is supplied by antigen and the second by a cytokine or by engagement of an accessory cell surface molecule (e.g., CD28 for T cells) with its cellular ligand (i.e., B7). For T cells, cytokines such as IL-1 or IL-6 are provided by the APC. With B cells the second signal is generally a T cell product (e.g., IL-4), thereby establishing T cell control over B cell activation. If cells are stimulated only with signal one, in the absence of signal two the effect may be to render the cell tolerant *(anergic)* and refractory to subsequent activation. Cells stimulated in this manner may subsequently undergo apoptosis, which, in the intact animal, may lead to long-term unresponsiveness to a particular antigen and may be important as a secondary mechanism for self-tolerance.

On encounter with an APC, perturbations of the TCR stimulate membrane phospholipase C to hydrolyze phosphatidylinositol 4,5-bisphophate, leading to generation of diacylglycerol and inositol 1,4,5-triphosphate. Diacylglycerol secondarily activates protein kinase C, which catalyzes phosphorylation of several proteins. This process initiates transcription of genes associated with T cell activation. As already suggested, perturbation of TCR conformation is translated through interaction between charged amino acids within the cell membrane to CD3 and CD4 or CD8. This initiates the biochemical cascade that leads to cellular activation.

An exception to the generalization regarding two-signal activation of lymphocytes is seen with antigens with multiple repeating subunit structure that can directly stimulate B cells. Such antigens, the prototype of which are complex carbohydrates, can cause extensive cross-linking of sIg, leading to "thymus-independent" B cell activation by hydrolysis of phosphatidylinositol 4,5-bisphosphate and subsequent protein kinase C activation. Although stimulation by thymus-independent antigen stimulates B cell IgM production, it does not induce clonal proliferation or isotype switching, since these depend greatly on T cell–derived cytokines. Therefore antibody responses to thymus-independent antigens are generally limited to the IgM class and do not stimulate development of immunologic memory.

T CELL SUBSETS AND IMMUNOREGULATION

The essence of an immune response is defense and homeostasis. Several phenotypically distinct subpopulations of T cells have roles as the effectors and regulators of these processes. $CD8^+$ T cells, approximately one third of T cells normally present in peripheral blood, include the primary effectors of cytotoxic T lymphocyte (CTL) responses. Recognizing foreign peptide bound to class I MHC cells, CTLs directly transmit a unidirectional lethal signal to target cells. Neither the CTLs themselves nor any non-antigen-expressing "innocent" bystander cells are damaged in the process. In an experimental setting, $CD4^+$ T cells are also capable of differentiating into CTLs; in this case, however, target cell recognition is in the context of a class II MHC molecule.

Two subsets of $CD4^+$ T cells can be distinguished based on the pattern of cytokines that they elaborate when appropriately stimulated. Since both subsets exhibit helper function for B cells and other T cells, they have been designated TH_1 and TH_2 cells. The pattern of cytokine production of TH_1 cells is skewed to so-called inflammatory cytokines such as IL-2 and IFN-γ. IL-2 is the major growth factor for both $CD4^+$ and $CD8^+$ cells. IFN-γ is an inflammatory mediator that is a potent activator of APC and contributes to the differentiation of cytolytic activity by $CD8^+$ T cells; it also has reciprocal effects with IL-4 in regulation of Ig isotype synthesis. TH_2 T cells produce cytokines (e.g., IL-4) that are essential to proliferation and differentiation of B cells to antibody-producing cells. Some cytokines (e.g., IL-3) are produced in approximately equal quantity by TH_1 and TH_2 cells.

An important element of immune homeostasis is the production of cytokines that downregulate the response when appropriate. Two cytokines are particularly important in this regard. IL-10 inhibits production of IL-2 and IL-4; TGF-β, also inhibits production of IL-2 and IL-4, as well as the synthesis of antibodies, the proliferation of B cells and $CD4^+$ T cells, and the differentiation of $CD8^+$ cytotoxic T lymphocytes. Interestingly, TGF-β does act as a costimulator to promote the proliferation of a specific subset of $CD8^+$ T cells, possibly with suppressor cell function. A postulated role for suppressor T cells in control of physiologic immune responses and prevention of undesired responses has been controversial because of difficulties in in vitro growth of such cells and in the molecular definition of their antigen receptors. Nevertheless, substantial evidence suggests that a subset of T cells, designated Ts, is important in preventing synthesis of autoantibodies and in controlling the magnitude and duration of an immune response. Such cells are generally thought to be $CD8^+$ but are lacking in cytolytic activity. It is not clear whether they recognize antigen bound by class I MHC molecules or in another mode. Failure of $CD8^+$ immunoregulatory activity may be important in the pathogenesis of autoimmune diseases such as systemic lupus erythematosus.

Regulation of physiologic immune responses may also involve the generation of anti-idiotypic networks, both of antibodies and of T cells. The uniqueness of structure of the variable portions of Ig molecules and TCR implies that they may be recognized by other antibodies or T cells as antigenic determinants. Such antigenic determinants within the variable region of an Ig or TCR molecule are termed *idiotopes;* the complete molecules expressing them (Ig or TCR) are *idiotypes*. An immune response induced by and specific for variable region idiotopes is termed an *anti-idiotypic response*. The phenomenology of such complex and potentially endless circuitry is well established. Thus successive waves of antibody (or T cells) with specificities as idiotype, anti-idiotype, anti-anti-idiotype, and so on may result in a progressive network of mirrored reflections between antigenic image and complementary anti-image. The capacity of such networks to modulate an antibody response has also been clearly demonstrated. Their physiologic role in homeostasis, however, is a matter of continuing discussion.

SUMMARY

The human immune response represents a finely orchestrated interaction of leukocytes and their products that is highly differentiated for two principal purposes: (1) the molecular discrimination between self and nonself and (2) the destruction, through development of an inflammatory response, of those molecules, cells, and organisms identified as nonself. The process of self/nonself discrimination requires the differentiation within the thymus of T cells that express surface receptors with simultaneous binding affinity for self MHC and an antigenic peptide. Activation of T cells can lead directly to target cell destruction or, through the elaboration of cytokines, can stimulate (or suppress) antigen-driven B cell activation. Antibodies, the products of antigen-activated B cells, enhance the phagocytosis and digestion of antigenic particles (or cells) by exposure of binding sites to surface receptors on phagocytes and/or activation of the complement cascade. Damage to host tissues may be a secondary consequence of the inflammatory response that follows from T cell or B cell activation. This may result in local and/or systemic signs and symptoms of inflammation and may cause damage to host tissues that is disproportionate to that induced by the microbe (i.e., antigen) itself. Finally, the very sophistication of the immune response offers considerable opportunity for error. Those errors that lead to disease are primarily of two types, dysregulation and ambiguity in self/nonself discrimination, the consequences of which are a pathologically excessive immune response or autoimmunity.

REFERENCES

Altman A et al: T lymphocyte activation: a biological model of signal transduction. Crit Rev Immunol 10:347, 1990.

Balkwill FR and Burke F: The cytokine network. Immunol Today 10:299, 1989.

Brodsky FB and Guagliardi L: The cell biology of antigen processing and presentation. Annu Rev Immunol 9:707, 1991.

Drake CG and Kotzin BL: Superantigens: biology, immunology and potential role in disease. J Clin Immunol 12:149, 1992.

Janeway CA Jr: The immune system evolved to discriminate infectious nonself from noninfectious self. Immunol Today 13:11, 1992.

Matis LA: The molecular basis of T cell specificity. Annu Rev Immunol 8:65, 1990.

Mosmann TR and Coffmann RL: TH1 and TH2 cells: different patterns of lymphokine secretion lead to different functional properties. Annu Rev Immunol 7:145, 1989.

Rothbard JB and Geften ML: Interactions between immunogenic peptides and MHC proteins. Annu Rev Immunol 9:527, 1991.

Schwartz RH: Acquisition of immunologic self tolerance. Cell 57:1073, 1989.

Sinha AA et al: Autoimmune diseases: the failure of self tolerance. Science 248:1380, 1990.

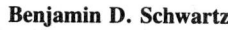

CHAPTER

284 Human Leukocyte Antigen Complex

Benjamin D. Schwartz

The human leukocyte antigen (HLA) complex is the major histocompatibility complex of humans. It was originally discovered as a result of the analysis of reactions of antibodies found in the sera of multiply transfused patients and multiparous women. Subsequently the complex became the object of study because of its roles in the rejection of tissue and organ transplants and in predisposition to certain diseases. The molecules determined by the HLA complex are now known to be critical to the regulation of several aspects of the immune response.

HLA GENETICS

The HLA complex is located on the short arm of chromosome 6 and contains multiple loci that determine several different types of molecules. The HLA-A, HLA-B, and HLA-C loci encode the class I, or classic histocompatibility molecules. The HLA-DR, HLA-DQ, and HLA-DP loci are within the HLA-D subregion and encode the class II molecules. The BF, C2, C4A, and C4B loci determine the second, fourth, and factor B components of the complement system. Several additional loci have been mapped to the HLA complex in the past several years, including the loci for 21-hydroxylase A and B, tumor necrosis factor alpha (TNF-α), tumor necrosis factor beta (TNF-β), heat shock protein-70, and molecules involved in proteolysis of antigens and transport of antigenic peptides. The relative location of these loci within the HLA complex is shown in Fig. 284-1.

The HLA complex is one of the most polymorphic genetic complexes known. Multiple alleles (alternative forms of a gene) at each locus have been identified in population studies. For example, 32 distinct alleles are present at the HLA-B locus. A complete listing of the currently recognized class I and class II alleles and the antigenic determinants they encode is given in Tables 284-1 to 284-4. Each allele is designated by the letter of the locus at which it is found and a four-digit number, for example, HLA-B*2701. The first two digits in the number (27) indicate the antigenic determinant expressed on the HLA molecule determined by that allele. The next two digits (01) constitute the allele designation. In some cases, several alleles encode distinct molecules, each of which nonetheless expresses the same antigenic determinant. Thus, for example, six alleles, designated HLA-B*2701 through HLA-B*2706, determine distinct HLA molecules, all of which express the HLA-B27 antigenic determinant.

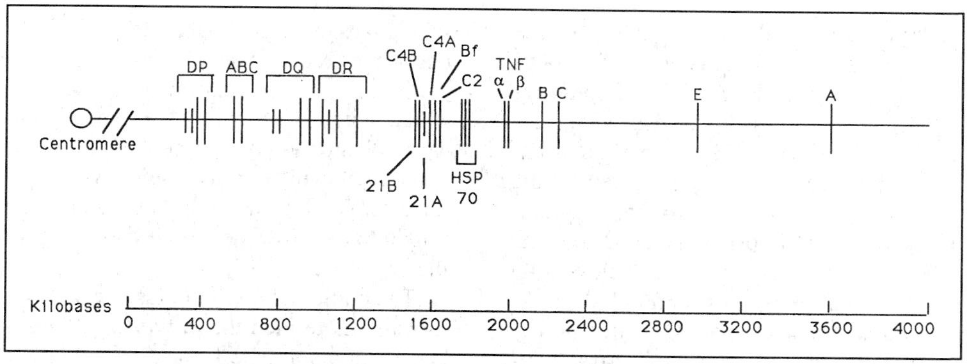

Fig. 284-1. HLA complex. The locations of genes within the HLA complex have been mapped by molecular biologic techniques. Distances are given in kilobases. *A, B, C,* and *E* are the HLA class I loci. *DR, DQ,* and *DP* are the HLA class II subregions, each of which contains multiple loci. *ABC* indicates the transporter associated with antigen-processing loci, Also in this region are two of the LMP, or low molecular mass polypeptide complex loci; *21A* and *21B* are the 21-hydroxylase loci; *C4A* and *C4B* are the duplicated loci encoding the fourth component of complement; and *Bf* and *C2* are the loci for properdin factor B and the second component of complement, respectively. *HSP-70* indicates the heat shock protein-70 loci. *TNF*-α and *TNF*-β are the tumor necrosis factor loci. Longer marks indicate the locus of a functional gene; shorter marks indicate the locus of a pseudogene (nonfunctional gene).

Table 284-1. Recognized HLA class I alleles and antigenic determinants

HLA allele	HLA antigenic determinant	HLA allele	HLA antigenic determinant	HLA allele	HLA antigenic determinant
A*0101	A1	B*0701	B7	Cw*0101	Cw1
A*0201	A2	B*0702	B7	Cw*0201	Cw2
A*0202	A2	B*0801	B8	Cw*02021	Cw2
A*0203	A2	B*1301	B13	Cw*02022	Cw2
A*0204	A2	B*1302	B13	Cw*0301	Cw3
A*0205	A2	B*1401	B14	Cw*0501	Cw5
A*0206	A2	B*1402	Bw65(14)	Cw*0601	Cw6
A*0207	A2	B*1501	Bw62(15)	Cw*0701	Cw7
A*0208	A2	B*1801	B18	Cw*0702	Cw7
A*0209	A2	B*2701	B27	Cw*1101	Cw11
A*0210	A2	B*2702	B27	Cw*1201	—
A*0301	A3	B*2703	B27	Cw*1202	—
A*0302	A3	B*2704	B27	Cw*1301	—
A*1101	A11	B*2705	B27	Cw*1401	—
A*1102	A11	B*2706	B27		
A*2401	A24(9)	B*3501	B35	E*0101	—
A*2501	A25(10)	B*3502	B35	E*0102	—
A*2601	A26(10)	B*3701	B37	E*0103	—
A*2901	A29(w19)	B*3801	B38(16)	E*0104	—
A*3001	A30(w19)	B*3901	B39(16)		
A*3101	A31(w19)	B*4001	Bw60(40)		
A*3201	A32(w19)	B*4002	B40		
A*3301	Aw33(w19)	B*4101	Bw41		
A*6801	Aw68(28)	B*4201	Bw42		
A*6802	Aw68(28)	B*4401	B44(12)		
A*6901	Aw69(28)	B*4402	B44(12)		
		B*4601	Bw46		
		B*4701	Bw47		
		B*4901	B49(21)		
		B*5101	B51(5)		
		B*5201	Bw52(5)		
		B*5301	Bw53		
		B*5701	Bw57(17)		
		B*5801	Bw58(17)		
		B*7801	—		

The antigenic determinants on the HLA molecules are recognized by antibodies, and are designated by the locus letter and a number, for example, HLA-B27. In some instances the number is preceded by a lowercase *w;* for example, HLA-Bw41. The *w* indicates that the particular antigenic determinant has not been officially accepted by the nomenclature committee of the World Health Organization. When the antigenic determinant is officially accepted, the *w* is dropped. In other instances the number is followed by a second number in parentheses, for example, HLA-A25(10). This designation indicates that the antigenic determinant given by the first number is a "split" of the antigenic determinant designated in parentheses. In our example, HLA-A10 was originally thought to be a single antigenic entity, but subsequent analysis indicated that HLA-A10 is a determinant present on two distinct molecules, which bear the distinct antigenic determinants HLA-A25 and HLA-A26. Thus HLA-A25 and A26 are said to be splits of HLA-A10.

Because of the presumed extensive interbreeding that has occurred throughout the existence of the human species, the chance of finding a particular allele at one locus together with a particular allele at a second locus should be the product of the frequencies of each of the alleles in a given population. However, particular combinations of alleles are found with an observed frequency greater than expected. This phenomenon, termed *linkage disequilibrium,* has been attributed both to a selective advantage of a particular combination of alleles and to the admixture of inbred populations. However, both these hypotheses remain speculative.

The combination of alleles at each locus on a given chromosome is termed the *haplotype*. Thus each individual inherits one haplotype from the mother and one from the father. Haplotypes are inherited in a simple mendelian fashion. Two siblings from the same parents have a 25% chance of being HLA identical, a 50% chance of being HLA haploidentical (i.e., sharing one haplotype), and a 25% chance of being totally HLA nonidentical. HLA molecules are expressed codominantly; that is, the HLA molecules determined by both maternal and paternal haplotypes are expressed in each individual. For example, each individual expresses two HLA-A molecules, one determined by each haplotype.

Table 284-2. Recognized HLA-DR alleles and antigenic determinants

HLA-DR allele	HLA-DR antigenic determinant	HLA-D-associated (T-cell-defined) determinant
DRB1*0101	DR1	Dw1
DRB1*0102	DR1	Dw20
DRB1*0103	DR'BR'	Dw'BON'
DRB1*1501	DRw15(2)	Dw2
DRB1*1502	DRw15(2)	Dw12
DRB1*1601	DRw16(2)	Dw21
DRB1*1602	DRw16(2)	Dw22
DRB1*0301	DRw17(3)	Dw3
DRB1*0302	DRw18(3)	Dw'RSH'
DRB1*0401	DR4	Dw4
DRB1*0402	DR4	Dw10
DRB1*0403	DR4	Dw13
DRB1*0404	DR4	Dw14
DRB1*0405	DR4	Dw15
DRB1*0406	DR4	Dw'KT2'
DRB1*0407	DR4	Dw13
DRB1*0408	DR4	Dw14
DRB1*0409	DR4	—
DRB1*0410	DR4	—
DRB1*0411	DR4	—
DRB1*1101	DRw11(5)	Dw5
DRB1*1102	DRw11(5)	Dw'JVM'
DRB1*1103	DRw11(5)	—
DRB1*1104	DRw11(5)	Dw'FS'
DRB1*1201	DRw12(5)	Dw"DB6'
DRB1*1202	DRw12(5)	
DRB1*1301	DRw13(w6)	Dw18
DRB1*1302	DRw13(w6)	Dw19
DRB1*1303	DRw13(w6)	Dw'HAG'
DRB1*1304	DRw13(w6)	—
DRB1*1305	DRw13(w6)	—
DRB1*1401	DRw14(w6)	Dw9
DRB1*1402	DRw14(w6)	Dw16
DRB1*1403	DRw14(w6)	—
DRB1*1404	—	—
DRB1*1405	DRw14(w6)	—
DRB1*0701	DR7	Dw17
DRB1*0702	DR7	Dw'DB1'
DRB1*0801	DRw8	Dw8.1
DRB1*08021	DRw8	Dw8.2
DRB1*08022	DRw8	Dw8.2
DRB1*08031	DRw8	Dw8.3
DRB1*08032	DRw8	Dw8.3
DRB1*0804	DRw8	—
DRB1*09011	DR9	Dw23
DRB1*09012	DR9	Dw23
DRB1*1001	DRw10	—
DRB3*0101	DRw52a	Dw24
DRB3*0201	DRw52b	Dw25
DRB3*0202	DRw52b	Dw25
DRB3*0301	DRw52c	Dw26
DRB4*0101	DRw53	Dw4, Dw10, Dw13, Dw14, Dw15, Dw17, Dw23
DRB5*0101	DRw15(2)	Dw2
DRB5*0102	DRw15(2)	Dw12
DRB5*0201	DRw16(2)	Dw21
DRB5*0202	DRw16(2)	Dw22

Table 284-3. Recognized HLA-DQ alleles and antigenic determinants

HLA-DQ allele	HLA-DQ antigenic determinant	HLA-D-associated (T-cell-defined) determinant
DQA1*0101	—	Dw1, w9
DQA1*0102	—	Dw2, w21, w19
DQA1*0103	—	Dw18, w12, w8, Dw'FS'
DQA1*0201	—	Dw7, w11
DQA1*03011	—	Dw4, w10, w13, w14, w15
DQA1*03012	—	Dw23
DQA1*0302	—	Dw23
DQA1*0401	—	Dw8, Dw'RSH'
DQA1*0501	—	Dw3, w5, w22
DQA1*05011	—	Dw3
DQA1*05012	—	Dw5
DQA1*05013	—	Dw22
DQA1*0601	—	Dw8
DQB1*0501	DQw5(w1)	Dw1
DQB1*0502	DQw5(w1)	Dw21
DQB1*05031	DQw5(w1)	Dw9
DQB1*05032	DQw5(w1)	Dw9
DQB1*0504	—	—
DQB1*0601	DQw6(w1)	Dw12, w8
DQB1*0602	DQw6(w1)	Dw2
DQB1*0603	DQw6(w1)	Dw18, Dw'FS'
DQB1*0604	DQw6(w1)	Dw19
DQB1*0605	DQw6(w1)	Dw19
DQB1*0201	DQw2	Dw3, w7
DQB1*0301	DQw7(w3)	Dw4, w5, w8, w13
DQB1*0302	DQw8(w3)	Dw4, w10, w13, w14
DQB1*03031	DQw9(w3)	Dw23
DQB1*03032	DQw9(w3)	Dw23, w11
DQB1*0401	DQw4	Dw15
DQB1*0402	DQw4	Dw8, Dw'RSH'

TISSUE DISTRIBUTION, STRUCTURE, AND FUNCTION

HLA class I molecules

The HLA-A, HLA-B, HLA-C (class I) molecules are found on virtually every cell. This wide tissue distribution befits their physiologic role. For a cell infected with virus to be killed by a cytotoxic CD8$^+$ T cell, the T cell must recognize a processed viral antigenic peptide in conjunction with a class I molecule. This phenomenon is known as *HLA restriction of T cell recognition* and is thought to be important in the distinction of nonself from self. A given T cell, specific for a given viral antigenic peptide, can recognize this peptide only when the peptide is associated with a particular class I molecule. It cannot recognize this viral antigenic peptide associated with a different class I molecule, it cannot recognize a different antigenic peptide associated with the same class I molecule, and it cannot recognize the class I molecule by itself.

This restriction phenomenon can perhaps best be appreciated through an understanding of the structure of the class

Table 284-4. Recognized HLA-DP alleles and antigenic determinants

HLA-DP allele	HLA-DP antigenic determinant
DPA1*0101	—
DPA1*0102	—
DPA1*0103	—
DPA1*0201	—
DPB1*0101	DPw1
DPB1*0201	DPw2
DPB1*02011	DPw2
DPB1*02012	DPw2
DPB1*0202	DPw2
DPB1*0301	DPw3
DPB1*0401	DPw4
DPB1*0402	DPw4
DPB1*0501	DPw5
DPB1*0601	DPw6
DPB1*0801	—
DPB1*0901	DP'Cp63'
DPB1*1001	—
DPB1*1101	—
DPB1*1301	—
DPB1*1401	—
DPB1*1501	—
DPB1*1601	—
DPB1*1701	—
DPB1*1801	—
DPB1*1901	—

I molecule (Fig. 284-2). The class I molecule consists of a 44,000-dalton glycoprotein chain designated the heavy chain, or alpha (α) chain, determined by an HLA class I allele, in noncovalent association with the 12,000-dalton β_2 microglobulin (β_2m) determined by a nonpolymorphic gene on chromosome 15. The HLA class I heavy chain consists of several domains. Three extracellular domains exist, designated α_1, α_2, and α_3, each consisting of approximately 90 amino acids, a transmembrane domain, and an intracytoplasmic domain. β_2m and the α_3 domain of the heavy chain have structural homology to the constant regions of the immunoglobulin (Ig) molecule, making the class I molecule a member of the Ig supergene family, and are essentially nonpolymorphic. In contrast, the α_1 and α_2 domains contain most of the polymorphism of the HLA molecule. X-ray crystallographic analysis has recently elucidated the structure of the class I molecule (Fig. 284-3). The α_3 domain and β_2m form a base that supports an interactive structure formed by the α_1 and α_2 domains. This structure is composed of a platform consisting of a β-pleated sheet (formed by eight β strands), on which rest two α helices that form a cleft into which a foreign (viral) antigenic peptide can fit. (The α helix should not be confused with the α chain or α_1 or α_2 domains, and the β sheet and the β strands should not be confused with β_2m.) These two α helices and the foreign antigenic peptide make up the ligand that is recognized by the T cell receptor on the CD8$^+$ T cells.

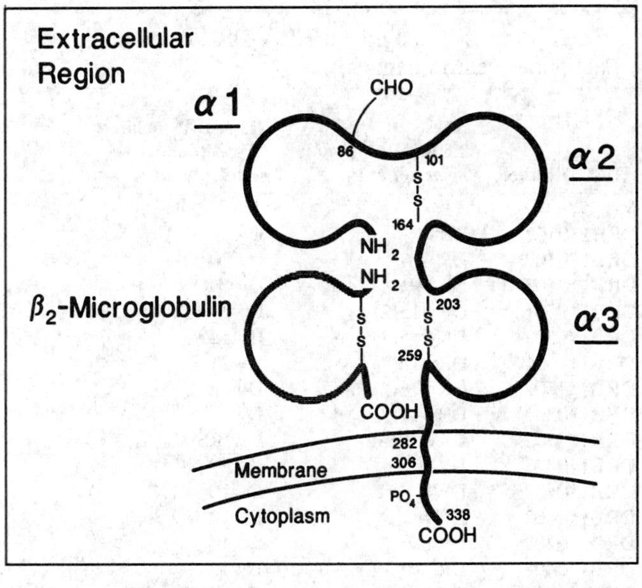

Fig. 284-2. Schematic representation of an HLA class I molecule. The molecule consists of a transmembrane glycoprotein termed the *heavy,* or α chain in noncovalent association with a protein termed β_2 *microglobulin.* The α chain has three extracellular domains, α_1, α_2, and α_3. *NH_2,* Amino terminus; *COOH,* carboxy terminus; *PO_4,* phosphate. Numbers indicate amino acid residues where certain features are found.

HLA class II molecules

In contrast to the class I molecules, the class II molecules have a restricted tissue distribution. They are found predominantly on immunocompetent cells, including B lymphocytes, activated T lymphocytes, and antigen-presenting cells (macrophages and dendritic cells). In addition, class II molecules can be induced on cells that do not normally express them. It has been speculated that this anomalous expression may contribute to the predisposition to certain autoimmune diseases (see following discussion). Foreign antigenic peptide is thought to be recognized in association with class II molecules by CD4$^+$ (predominantly helper) T lymphocytes, just as it is recognized in association with class I molecules by CD8$^+$ cytotoxic T cells.

HLA class II molecules are composed of two glycoprotein transmembrane chains, both encoded by the HLA complex (Fig. 284-4). The α chain is approximately 34,000 daltons, and the β chain is approximately 29,000 daltons. Each of these chains contains two extracellular domains, designated α_1 and α_2 or β_1 and β_2, respectively, a transmembrane domain, and an intracytoplasmic domain. The α_2 and β_2 domains have homology to the constant region domains of Ig, indicating class II molecules are also members of the Ig supergene family. Extrapolation from the class I crystallographic structure suggests that the α_2 and β_2 domains are closest to the cell membrane. The α_1 and particularly the β_1 domains are responsible for most polymorphism seen within the class II system. Recently obtained x-ray crystallographic data for the class II molecule indicate that the structure is extremely similar to that of the class I molecule. Thus the α_2 and β_2 domains form a base for the interactive structure formed by the α_1 and β_1 domains. This

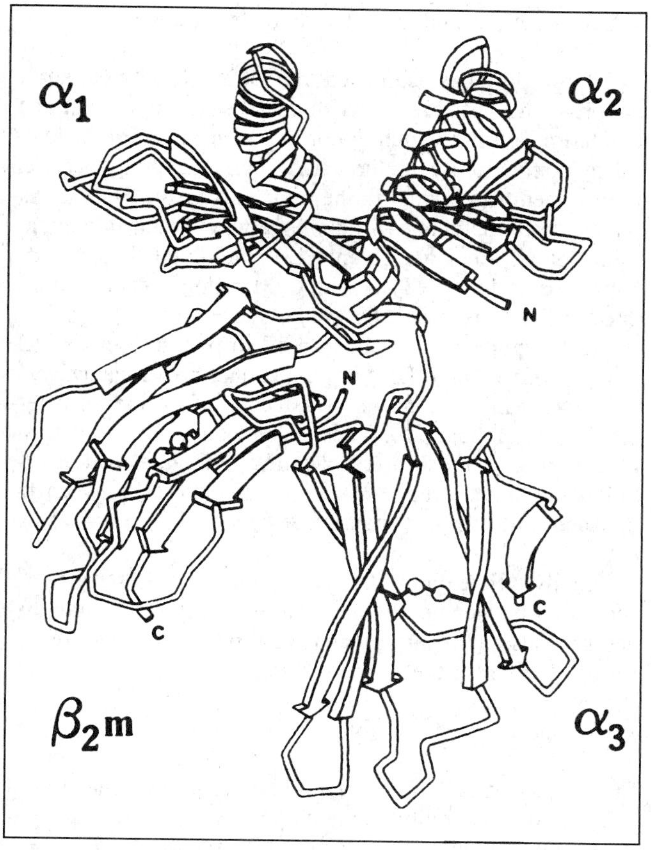

Fig. 284-3. Crystal structure of an HLA class I molecule. The extracellular portion of the molecule is depicted in side view, with the distal end on top and the proximal end at the bottom. The transmembrane and intracytoplasmic domains are not shown. The α_1, α_2, and α_3 domains are labeled, as is the β_2 microglobulin *(β_2m)*. β_2m and the α_3 domain form a base supporting the interactive structure formed by the α_1 and α_2 domains. This interactive structure consists of a platform of a β-pleated sheet supporting two α helices that form a cleft that binds foreign antigenic fragments. *N*, Amino terminus; *C*, carboxy terminus. (Reprinted by permission from Nature 329:506. Copyright © 1987 Macmillan Journals Limited.)

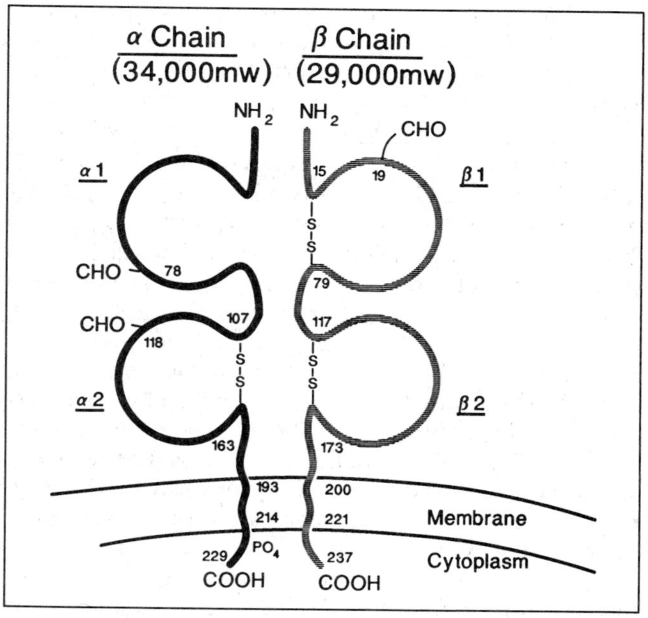

Fig. 284-4. Schematic representation of an HLA class II molecule. The molecule consists of two transmembrane glycoproteins, α and β, which are noncovalently associated. The α_1, α_2, β_1, and β_2 domains are labeled. *NH_2,* Amino terminus; *COOH,* carboxy terminus; *PO_4,* phosphate. Numbers indicate amino acid residues where certain features are found. The crystal structure of class II molecules closely resembles that of a class I molecule.

latter structure also consists of a platform of a β-pleated sheet, on which rest two α helices forming a cleft for foreign antigenic peptide.

HLA class II genes

As already indicated, three distinct sets of HLA class II molecules exist: DR, DQ, and DP. Although each consists of the αβ-chain structural unit just described, the organization and polymorphism of the genes determining this unit vary for each type of class II molecule (Fig. 284-5). The HLA-DR subregion contains one α-chain locus, designated DRA. The DRA gene is essentially nonpolymorphic. The DR subregion also usually contains three β-chain loci, designated DRB1, DRB2, and DRB3 (or DRB4 or DRB5). The DRB genes are highly polymorphic and encode the DRβ chains, which are responsible for the different DR types. Alleles at the DRB1 locus encode the DRβ1 chains responsible for DR types DR1 through DRw18. DRB2 is a pseudogene; that is, it is not expressed. The DRB3 gene encodes the DRβ3 chain bearing DRw52, the DRB4 gene encodes the DRβ4 chain bearing DRw53, and DRB5 alleles encode the DRβ5 chains bearing DRw15 or DRw16. DRB3, DRB4, and DRB5 appear to be mutually exclusive within a single haplotype. Both the DRβ1 chain and the

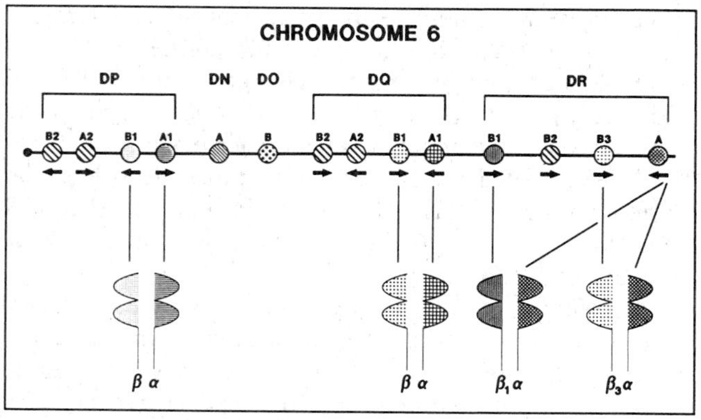

Fig. 284-5. HLA-D region. The organization of the genes within each of the three defined subregions, DP, DQ, and DR, is shown. The number of DRB genes varies with the DR type. DRB2, DQA2, DQB2, DPA2, and DPB2 are pseudogenes. Pairs of class II genes, which determine class II molecules, are shown. DNA and DOB are not currently known to be transcribed in vivo. The direction of transcription (5' to 3') is given below the genes.

DRβ3 (or DRβ4 or DRβ5) chains can combine with the DRα chain to form a DRαβ molecule. Thus, in most haplotypes, there are two distinct DR molecules: DRαβ1 and DRαβ3 (or DRαβ4 or DRαβ5).

The HLA-DQ subregion contains two pairs of α-chain and β-chain genes. One pair, designated DQA2 and DQB2, is a pair of pseudogenes and is not expressed. The other pair, DQA1 and DQB1, encodes the DQα and DQβ chains. In contrast to the DR molecules, in which the α chain shows no polymorphism, both the DQα and DQβ chains are polymorphic. This polymorphism may be important, in that the DQα chain encoded by one chromosome can combine not only with the DQβ chain encoded by the same chromosome, but also with the DQβ chain encoded by the second chromosome. If this proves to be true, HLA heterozygotes may have DQ "hybrid" molecules that would be unique to the heterozygotes and not found in either parent. These hybrid molecules could conceivably be important in terms of predisposition to disease (see following discussion).

As with the DQ subregion, the DP subregion also contains two pairs of α-chain and β-chain genes. One pair, designated DPA2 and DPB2, is a set of pseudogenes, wherein the expressed pair is designated DPA1 and DPB1. The DPα chain displays limited polymorphism, whereas the DPβ chain displays moderate polymorphism.

HLA TYPING

The HLA-A, HLA-B, HLA-C, HLA-DR, and HLA-DQ molecules are conventionally detected serologically by the microlymphocytotoxicity assay, which determines the HLA type by the ability of a given cell to by lysed by an antibody of known specificity. Although HLA-DP molecules can also be recognized by certain antibodies, HLA-DP typing is done by a methodology termed *primed lymphocyte testing* (PLT). In essence, this is a cellular assay that measures the ability of T cells primed against a given DP antigen to proliferate when they recognize the same DP antigen a second time. HLA-D antigens are also typed by a cellular assay, the *mixed lymphocyte reaction* (MLR). This typing assay measures the ability of nonprimed T lymphocytes to proliferate when they recognize nonself HLA-D determinants on foreign lymphocytes. There are no HLA-D molecules per se; MLR typing for HLA-D antigens actually measures the recognition of determinants found on HLA-DR, HLA-DQ, and HLA-DP molecules. The best correlation of the HLA-D antigens is with the HLA-DR molecules, which are thought to bear most epitopes recognized in an MLR.

Although most HLA typing is still done by the standard techniques outlined, newer techniques using molecular biology have recently been introduced. These techniques include the *polymerase chain reaction* (PCR), which selectively amplifies a region of the gene of interest; detection of a given HLA allele by hybridization of genomic deoxyribonucleic acid (DNA) with allele-specific oligonucleotide probes; and identification of allele-specific restriction endonuclease fragment length polymorphism patterns. These typing techniques are used predominantly in limited research situations and have not yet been used widely in clinical situations.

HLA typing has been used in a variety of clinical applications. The best known is that of tissue or organ transplantation, during which donor and host are typed to maximize compatibility at the HLA loci. Matching between family members results in the most successful tissue transplants. Such matching will almost always result in compatibility at all loci of a given HLA haplotype, because the haplotype is inherited as a unit. Matching between unrelated individuals is usually not so successful.

HLA typing has also been used in paternity cases. Although conventional HLA typing cannot prove paternity, it is accepted in most courts as a means of excluding paternity. The application of newer molecular biologic techniques may establish a test yielding individual patterns as unique as fingerprints, and identity of patterns between father and child may eventually be accepted as proof of paternity.

Finally, HLA typing has also been used to establish associations between particular HLA antigens and certain diseases. These associations and their possible basis are described further in the following section.

HLA AND DISEASE

In 1973, HLA-B27 was found to be highly associated with ankylosing spondylitis. Ninety percent of Caucasian patients with ankylosing spondylitis were found to possess HLA-B27, compared with only 8% of the normal Caucasian population. HLA disease associations within a population are quantitated by an entity termed the *relative risk* (RR), which indicates the strength of the association. The higher the relative risk greater than 1, the greater is the association of the given HLA antigen with disease. A relative risk between 0 and 1 indicates a negative association between the given HLA and a disease and suggests the given HLA antigen may be protective. For ankylosing spondylitis the relative risk is approximately 80; that is, an individual who possesses HLA-B27 is 80 times as likely to develop ankylosing spondylitis as is an individual who lacks HLA-B27. However, the absence of HLA-B27 does not guarantee that an individual will not develop the disease, and the presence of HLA-B27 does not suggest that an individual will definitely contract the disease. In fact, the absolute risk of developing ankylosing spondylitis if an individual possesses HLA-B27 is only 4%; that is, of 100 individuals who possess HLA-B27, only four will develop clinically significant and apparent ankylosing spondylitis.

Only a few diseases are associated with HLA class I antigens, but most HLA-associated diseases are associated with HLA class II antigens (Table 284-5). This association may well reflect the physiologic role of class II molecules in initiating the immune response by presenting processed antigenic peptide to helper $CD4^+$ T cells. Indeed, it has been proposed that anomalous expression of class II molecules on certain tissues, such as thyroid, pancreas, synovium, and others, may allow the presentation of otherwise nonimmunogenic tissue-specific antigens to helper T cells,

Table 284-5. Selected HLA and disease associations in Caucasian patients

Disease	Antigen	Approximate relative risk
Ankylosing spondylitis	B27	81.8
Reiter's syndrome	B27	40.4
Acute anterior uveitis	B27	7.98
Rheumatoid arthritis	DR4	6.4
Juvenile rheumatoid arthritis		
Seropositive	DR4	7.2
	Dw4	25.8
	Dw14	47
	Dw4/Dw14	116
Pauciarticular	DR5	2.9
Systemic lupus erythematosus	DR3	2.7
Behçet's disease	B5	3.3
Sjögren's syndrome	DR3	5.6
Graves' disease	DR3	3.8
Insulin-dependent diabetes mellitus	DR4	5.5
	DR3	6.3
	DR3/4	25.4
	DR2	0.3
	DQw8	31.8
	DQβAsp^{57}/ DQβAsp^{57}	0.1
Celiac disease	DR3	13.3
	DQw2	12.0
Psoriasis vulgaris	B13	4.5
	B17	3.1
	Cw6	7.2
Pemphigus vulgaris	DR4	21.4
Dermatitis herpetiformis	DR3	18.2
Idiopathic hemochromatosis	A3	6.6
	B14	3.7
Goodpasture's syndrome	DR2	19.8
Multiple sclerosis	DR2	2.8
Myasthenia gravis (without thymoma)	B8	3.3
Narcolepsy	DR2	129

resulting in an autoimmune response. In this context it should be noted that most HLA-associated diseases do show some manifestation of autoimmunity.

Comparisons of the HLA-DQ molecules possessed by normal and insulin-dependent diabetic individuals have allowed specific correlations to be established for predisposition to insulin-dependent diabetes mellitus. It appears as if the presence of a non–aspartic acid residue at amino acid position number 57 of the DQβ chain (as in DQw8) predisposes an individual to diabetes, whereas the presence of aspartic acid in this position protects an individual from this disease. For example, if both the HLA-DQβ chains possessed by an individual have an aspartic acid at position 57, the individual is highly protected from insulin-dependent diabetes mellitus (RR, 0.1).

In certain diseases, it appears as if gene complementation between two different class II genes may play a role in disease predisposition. In insulin-dependent diabetes, for example, the DR3/DR4 (RR, 25) and more recently the DQA1*0301-DQB1*0302/DQA1*0501-DQB*201 (RR, 35) heterozygous states occur more frequently than any antigen or allele in the homozygous state. Similarly, the antibody response to Ro (SS-A) and La (SS-B) antigens in Sjögren's syndrome and systemic lupus erythematosus is highest in patients who are DQw1/DQw2 heterozygotes. The molecular basis for these phenomena has not yet been clearly delineated, but may involve "hybrid" DQ molecules formed by the α chain encoded by one haplotype and the β chain encoded by the opposite haplotype, which cannot occur in DQ homozygotes.

Proposed mechanisms for HLA disease associations

Several hypotheses have been put forth to explain HLA disease associations. First, HLA molecules may serve as specific receptors for putative etiologic agents. If only a certain HLA antigen can act as such a receptor for an agent that causes a particular disease, the HLA disease association would be seen. The second hypothesis, designated the *molecular mimicry hypothesis,* suggests that a particular HLA antigen is immunologically similar to the etiologic agent that causes the disease and further suggests one of two alternatives. First, because of the similarity of the etiologic agent and the HLA antigen, the etiologic agent is not recognized as foreign, no immune response is elicited, and the disease caused by the etiologic agent proceeds without interference. The second alternative postulates that the etiologic agent is recognized as foreign, and a vigorous immune response is elicited. Because of the immunologic similarities between the etiologic agent and the HLA antigen, the HLA antigen becomes the target of the immune response, and an autoimmune disease is eventually manifest.

The third hypothesis states that the actual disease-susceptibility genes are not the HLA genes per se, but rather the T cell receptor α-chain and β-chain genes. This hypothesis holds that a particular T cell receptor α-chain and β-chain combination that predisposes to disease can only recognize a particular HLA antigen, or a processed foreign antigenic peptide in association with that particular HLA antigen. Because of this constraint on T cell receptor recognition, an apparent association with the HLA antigen is observed. The fourth hypothesis is based on the physiologic role of the class I and class II molecules in presenting foreign antigenic peptides to cytotoxic and helper T cells, respectively. This hypothesis holds that only certain class I and class II molecules can bind and present particular processed antigenic peptides. Depending on the pathogenesis of disease, the ability or inability of a given HLA molecule to bind and present a particular antigenic peptide may either predispose to or protect from disease.

Other mechanisms besides these have also been postulated. It should be noted that different mechanisms may apply in the predisposition to different diseases and that more than one mechanism may operate concurrently to predispose to a given disease.

As our understanding of the structure and function of the

HLA complex increases, the role of the HLA molecules in predisposing to disease will become elucidated and eventually may allow therapeutic intervention.

REFERENCES

Bjorkman PJ et al: Structure of the human class I histocompatibility antigen HLA-A2. Nature 329:506, 1987.

Bodmer JG et al: Nomenclature for factors of the HLA system, 1990. Hum Immunol 31:186, 1991.

Dalton TA and Bennett JC: Autoimmune disease and the major histocompatibility complex: therapeutic implications. Am J Med 92:183, 1992.

Heimberg H et al: Complementation of HLA-DQA and DQB genes confers susceptibility and protection to insulin-dependent diabetes mellitus. Hum Immunol 33:10, 1992.

Schwartz BD: Infectious agents, immunity, and rheumatic diseases. Arthritis Rheum 33:457, 1990.

Tiwari JL and Terasaki PI, editors: HLA and disease associations. New York, 1985 Springer-Verlag.

Todd JA, Bell JI, and McDevitt HO: HLA-DQβ gene contributes to susceptibility and resistance to insulin-dependent diabetes mellitus. Nature 329:599, 1987.

Trowsdale J, Ragoussis J, and Campbell RD: Map of the human MHC. Immunol Today 12:443, 1991.

CHAPTER

285 Antibodies: Structure and Genetics

Roger M. Perlmutter

The antibodies constitute an extremely diverse set of closely related serum glycoproteins (immunoglobulins) that mediate humoral immunity. During the past decade, advances in molecular biology have provided a detailed description of mechanisms that permit the somatic generation of more than 10^8 chemically distinct antibody molecules from a germline repertoire of fewer than 1000 genetic elements. Defects in this diversification process result in heightened susceptibility to infection and may also predispose to autoimmune disease.

STRUCTURE OF ANTIBODIES

Antibodies are polymeric molecules composed of paired disulfide-bonded heavy and light polypeptide chains in the general form $[(HL)_2]_n$. A typical serum antibody (immunoglobulin G, or IgG) consists of two identical heavy and two identical light chains (Fig. 285-1). The heavy and light chains are composed of a series of Ig domains, or *homology units,* each of which is about 110 amino acids in length and contains a centrally placed intrachain disulfide bond. The light chain contains two such domains, an amino-terminal variable domain (V_L) that participates in antigen binding and a carboxy-terminal constant domain (C_L) that assists in interactions with the heavy chain. Similarly, each heavy chain contains an amino-terminal variable domain (V_H) joined by a "hinge" region to a series of three constant domains designated C_H1, C_H2, and C_H3 (Fig. 285-1). The hinge region can be cleaved by enzymatic digestion to yield two antigen-binding, or *Fab,* fragments, containing the V_L and C_L domains of the light chain and the V_H and C_H1 domains of the heavy chain, and a third fragment, the *Fc* fragment, containing the remaining heavy-chain constant domains. Although all antigen-binding activity resides in the Fab fragments, the Fc fragment mediates important effector functions of antibody molecules, such as complement fixation and mast cell sensitization. Moreover, these functions can be localized to specific domains; for example, the C_H3 domain is principally responsible for binding to Fc receptors on macrophages and monocytes, and the C_H2 domain interacts with the C1q component of complement. Thus Ig domains are the structural and functional (and genetic) subunits of antibody molecules. Binding of antigen near the amino terminus of an antibody can alter the properties of the carboxy-terminal effector region, thus transducing a recognition signal.

In humans, as in all mammalian species, five classes of immunoglobulins exist: IgA, IgD, IgE, IgG, and IgM. There are also two subclasses of IgA (IgA1, IgA2) and four subclasses of IgG (IgG1, IgG2, IgG3, IgG4). These distinctions reflect variation in the structures of the constant domains and hinge regions of the heavy chains. Thus nine

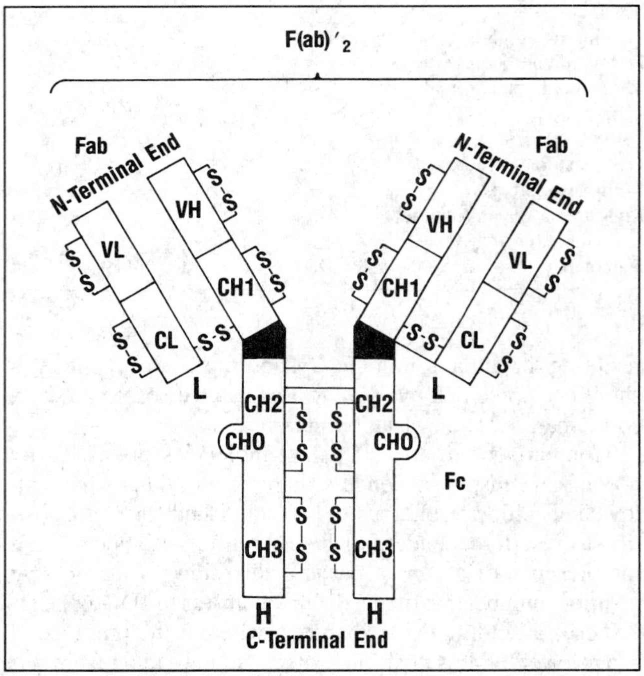

Fig. 285-1. Schematic diagram of immunoglobulin G1 (IgG1) molecule. *H* and *L* designate heavy and light polypeptide chains. Disulfide bonds are indicated by S-S links. The principal site of asparagine-linked carbohydrate is designated *CHO.* See text for descriptions of the domain organization and the Fc and Fab fragments.

different heavy chain types exist, which are identified using Greek letters: α1, α2, δ, ϵ, γ1, γ2, γ3, γ4, and μ. Each of these heavy chains mediates slightly different functions after antigen binding. In addition, there are two classes of light chains, kappa and lambda (κ, λ). About 70% of human antibodies contain κ light chains.

The classes and subclasses of immunoglobulins can be defined serologically and are collectively referred to as *isotypes*. All normal individuals are capable of generating antibodies of all isotypes. Serologic methods also permit the definition of determinants that are present on the antibody molecules of some individuals but not on those of others. These *allotypic* determinants are usually localized within the constant domains and behave as mendelian genetic markers. Finally, some serologic determinants are found in the variable regions and thus are associated with a specific antigen-binding structure. These are the *idiotypic* determinants of the antibody.

Importance of antibody class

The structural and functional properties of each antibody (Ig) class are summarized in Table 285-1 and are discussed next.

IgG. More than 70% of serum immunoglobulin is IgG, the dominant species induced by secondary immunization. IgG is always a four-chain molecule (Fig. 285-1), containing variable amounts of carbohydrate linked to the C_H2 domain. The human IgG subclasses are named in order of relative serum abundance, with IgG1 typically comprising about three fourths of the total serum IgG. Although functionally distinguishable, the γ1, γ2, γ3, and γ4 heavy chains are more than 90% identical in structure. The principal differences between the subclasses are found in the hinge regions and probably affect the flexibility of the molecule and its susceptibility to proteolysis. Certain immunogens recruit antibodies of particular subclasses; for example, bacterial carbohydrates elicit predominantly IgG2 responses. This fact may explain the heightened susceptibility to pyogenic infection seen in individuals with selective IgG2 or combined IgG2 and IgG4 deficiency. The Fc portions of IgG molecules, particularly IgG1 and IgG3, bear the determinants recognized by rheumatoid factors.

IgM. Primary immunization initially elicits an IgM response. IgM is the first antibody formed in the neonate and is the most evolutionarily conserved Ig class. The μ chain contains an additional C_H4 domain that appears to assist in complement fixation. In serum, IgM consists of five disulfide-linked μ_2L_2 units that form a circular array, with the 10 antigen-binding sites oriented outward. Another B lymphocyte product, the J chain, is required for the initiation of IgM polymerization. The J chain is 129 amino acids in length and joins two of the μ heavy chains through their carboxy-terminal cystine residues. Circulating IgM molecules are particularly important as rheumatoid factors, cold agglutinins, and isoagglutinins. IgM is also produced as a membrane-associated μ_2L_2 monomer in B lymphocytes, and this form serves as an antigen receptor (see following discussion).

IgA. Only about 10% of circulating immunoglobulin is IgA; however, it is the predominant Ig class in extravascular secretions, such as mucus, prostatic fluid, saliva, tears, and milk. Although IgA may circulate as an α_2L_2 monomer, it is most frequently encountered as a polymer of two or three such units joined with one molecule of J chain. Secretory IgA is a dimer associated with one molecule of J chain and a second polypeptide called the *secretory component* that is synthesized by epithelial cells. The secretory component is a fragment of the epithelial cell IgA receptor that permits the uptake of dimerized IgA from the serum and its subsequent transport and secretion. In humans, IgA1 is the principal subclass found in serum, whereas IgA2 is slightly more abundant than IgA1 in secretions. IgA in milk is extremely important in providing maternal immunity to the neonate postpartum. It is also extremely important in maintaining local immune defense in adults. Selective IgA deficiency occurs in about 1 in 700 persons and in some is associated with an increased frequency of autoimmune disorders, infections, and malabsorption syndromes.

Table 285-1. Properties of immunoglobulin (Ig) classes

Isotype	H chain designation	Molecular formula	Molecular weight (× 10^3 daltons)	No. of domains in H chains	Normal serum concentration (mg/ml)	Half-life (days)	Complement fixation	Placental transfer
IgG1	γ1	$(\gamma_1)_2L_2$	145	4	9	21	++	+
IgG2	γ2	$(\gamma_2)_2L_2$	145	4	3	20	+	+/−
IgG3	γ3	$(\gamma_3)_2L_2$	165	4	1	7	+++	+
IgG4	γ4	$(\gamma_4)_2L_2$	145	4	0.5	21	+/−	+
IgM	μ	$(\mu_2L_2)_5$-J	970	5	1.2	5	++++	—
IgA1	α1	$[(\alpha_1)_2L_2]_n$	160	4	2.0	6	—	—
IgA2	α2	$[(\alpha_2)_2L_2]_n$	160	4	0.5	?	—	—
sIgA	α1 or α2	$[(\alpha_1 \text{ or } \alpha_2)_2L_2]_2$-J-SC	400	4	0-0.05	—	—	—
IgD	δ	δ_2L_2	170	4	0.06	3	—	—
IgE	ϵ	ϵ_2L_2	190	5	0.0002	2.5-4.0	—	—

H chain, Heavy chain; SC, secretory component; sIgA, secretory IgA.

IgE. Although only a minor component of serum immunoglobulin, IgE is the principal Ig class involved in allergic reactions. IgE exists only in a monomer ϵ_2L_2 form. The ϵ heavy chain, as with μ, contains an extra constant domain but lacks the cystine involved in polymerization. After secretion by B lymphocytes, IgE adheres to mast cells and basophils through their high-affinity ϵ-specific Fc receptors. Binding of antigen by IgE provokes the release of vasoactive amines from these cells. IgE production is stimulated by parasitic infection, and it is believed that IgE antibodies assist in protection against parasitic disease.

IgD. Little is known about the function of IgD, which is principally a cell surface immunoglobulin. It exists only in the monomer form and is present at quite low levels in normal serum. B lymphocytes able to be stimulated usually possess both IgM and IgD antigen receptors. IgD does not fix complement and is not known to sensitize any phagocytic cell populations.

Immunoglobulins as B cell receptors

Although all antibody classes are secreted by B lymphocytes into the serum to some extent, they also serve as cell surface receptors. Each B lymphocyte synthesizes 7S antibody of a single specificity and displays this antibody on its surface. Interaction of antigen with the membrane-bound antibody triggers proliferation of the B lymphocyte and also induces increased secretion of the antibody. Thus antigen selectively expands individual clones of B lymphocytes by triggering B cell proliferation. The difference between the membrane-bound and secreted forms of antibodies lies at the carboxy-terminal end of the heavy chain. The membrane form terminates in a series of hydrophobic residues that anchor the entire protein in the lipid bilayer.

ANTIBODY GENES

The existence of variable and constant regions on the same polypeptide poses a genetic paradox: how is it possible to maintain hundreds of different heavy chain genes with identical constant regions? Over evolutionary time, these constant regions would be expected to accumulate mutations. Worse yet, individual variable regions are found associated with more than one type of constant region. How can this be explained? Dreyer and Bennett were the first to propose that some type of deoxyribonucleic acid (DNA) rearrangement mechanism might be responsible for the juxtaposition of variable and constant regions. Almost 10 years later, Tonegawa demonstrated that the variable region and constant region genes undergo specific gene rearrangements in lymphocytes. The organization and reorganization of antibody genes is now understood in considerable detail.

Light chain genes assembled from three gene segments

Antibodies are encoded by three unlinked gene tamilies, κ (chromosome 2), λ (chromosome 22), and heavy (chromosome 14). In each gene family, multiple gene segments positioned discontinuously on germline DNA are juxtaposed through DNA rearrangement events during B cell development. Fig. 285-2 diagrams the organization and reorganization of the κ locus. About 50 germline κ–variable region gene segments (V_κ) exist, all of which include a first exon encoding 5′ untranslated region and leader peptide sequences, a single intron of about 100 base pairs (bp), and a 300 bp second exon encoding most of the variable region. Immediately 3′ to this variable region are short sequences that are recognition sites for the DNA recombinase that catalyzes Ig gene rearrangement. In all, these variable region segments span more than 2 million bp of germline DNA. About 23 kilobases (kb) 3′ to the last V_κ gene segment is a series of five J_κ (for joining region) gene segments arrayed in a region of 2 kb. Each of these extremely short (13 codons) gene segments is preceded by rearrangement recognition sequences and ends in a typical eukaryotic splice donor sequence. The C_κ gene segment is represented on a single exon that is separated by a 2 kb intron from the J_κ gene segments. The intron contains an *immunoglobulin enhancer* sequence that is necessary for appropriate lymphocyte-specific transcription of the rearranged κ–light chain gene.

During B lymphocyte development, which occurs in the bone marrow in adults, a germline V_κ gene segment is juxtaposed to one of the five J_κ gene segments. This rearrangement is imperfect and may delete one or a few bases at the 3′ end of the V and at the 5′ end of the J. Although the enzymatic machinery responsible for catalyzing rearrangement of antibody gene segments remains incompletely characterized, details of the process have recently emerged. First, the same "recombinase" appears to regulate assembly of both heavy chain and light chain variable regions, as well as catalyzing rearrangment of the analogous gene segments that encode T cell receptor variable regions. In almost all cases, formation of a complete variable region–encoding sequence is achieved through somatic deletion of intervening DNA, even when many hundreds of kilobases of DNA must be excised. Two genes that encode components of the recombination machinery, called *RAG-1* and *RAG-2,* have been identified on human chromosome 11p13. Expression of these closely linked genes can confer antibody gene recombinase activity on fibroblasts and other nonlymphoid cells. In all cases, juxtaposition of antibody gene segments requires recognition of the recombination signal sequences positioned adjacent to each gene segment. Although it is believed that the RAG-1 and RAG-2 genes may themselves encode components of the recombinase, these genes may simply regulate expression of a quite different set of structural genes. The activity of a third gene, referred to as *SCID,* is required for satisfactory antibody gene recombinase activity, since mice bearing a homozygous defect in this gene fail to generate either T cell antigen receptors or antibodies and thus have a form of *s*evere *c*ombined *i*mmuno*d*eficiency. Detailed analysis of these genes should permit resolution of the molecular mechanism underlying the assembly of antibody variable region gene sequences.

Gene rearrangement permits formation of a complete transcriptional unit, since a promoter located upstream of

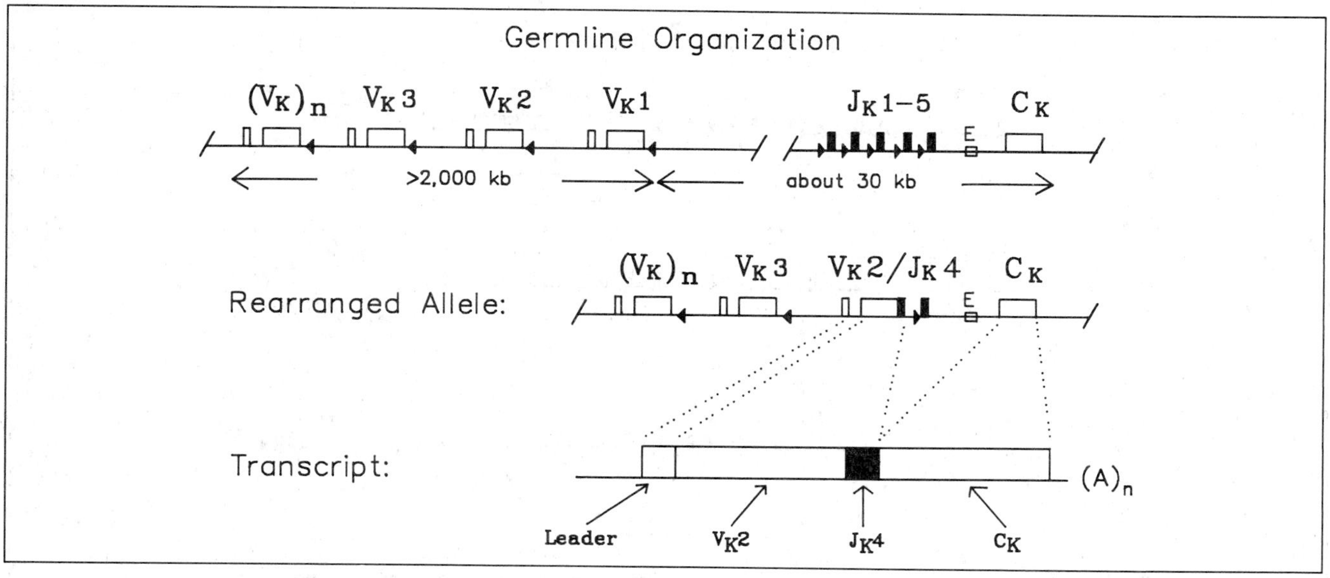

Fig. 285-2. Germline organization and reorganization of the κ–light chain locus in humans. Boxes represent coding exons. The J gene segments are shaded for emphasis. The box designated *E* represents the transcriptional enhancer. Shaded triangles denote recognition sequences for the antibody gene recombinase. The middle diagram shows the structure of the locus after joining of V and J (arbitrarily $V_\kappa 2$ and $J_\kappa 4$) gene segments. The bottom diagram illustrates the configuration of the mature messenger ribonucleic acid (mRNA) encoding the light chain polypeptide. See text for details.

the V gene segment is now in proximity with the enhancer element located within the intron between J and C. The primary transcript from this rearranged gene is spliced to produce mature κ–light chain messenger ribonucleic acid (mRNA). These events are diagrammed in Fig. 285-2.

Assembly of heavy chain gene from two rearrangement events

Rearrangements in the heavy chain locus resemble those in the light chain locus except an additional gene segment, the *diversity* (D) gene segment, contributes to the formation of the variable region. Probably more than 200 V_H gene segments span several million base pairs of germline DNA near the telomere of chromosome 14. Each has a leader exon and a 300 bp variable region exon, followed by rearrangement recognition sequences. More than 50 D_H gene segments may be present, varying in length from as few as 9 to perhaps 30 bp, positioned at some distance from the V elements. Each of these D gene segments is flanked by recombination recognition sequences. In humans, six functional J_H gene segments are positioned 70 kb 3′ to the first V_H gene segment and about 3 kb 5′ to the first exon of the C_μ gene. The pattern of rearrangement of these elements is diagrammed in Fig. 285-3. As with the κ light chain, important transcriptional regulatory elements are located in the intron between the J_H and C_μ sequences. During B cell development, heavy chain rearrangement precedes light chain rearrangement and usually occurs on both alleles. Once again, rearrangement is often imperfect. With the heavy chain, bases may be truncated from the sites of V-D or D-J joining. In addition, bases are frequently added at the sites of joining by an independent template mechanism. These added bases are called *N regions* and are less frequently seen in rearranged light chain genes. It is believed that the enzyme terminal transferase is responsible for N region addition.

Alternative processing producing membrane-bound antibodies

Each domain of the heavy chain constant region is encoded by a separate exon. This observation is in accord with the view that the Ig domain is the principal functional and thus selective unit in antibody molecules. In addition, differential processing of the heavy chain mRNA can produce mature proteins that have either a secreted type or a membrane type of carboxy terminus. The membrane exon is positioned 3′ to the constant region gene (Fig. 285-3). Alternative polyadenylation yields a product that either is spliced to include the membrane exon or lacks the membrane exon entirely. The ratio of membrane-type to secreted-type heavy chain mRNA can be altered in response to stimulation. Thus cross-linking of surface Ig triggers increased expression of the antibody's secreted form in B lymphocytes.

Isotype switching with both alternative splicing and gene rearrangement events

Different antibody heavy chain classes are encoded by linked genes on chromosome 14. This arrangement explains how a single variable region sequence can be associated with many different constant region sequences. Immediately after rearrangement, B lymphocytes first express IgM

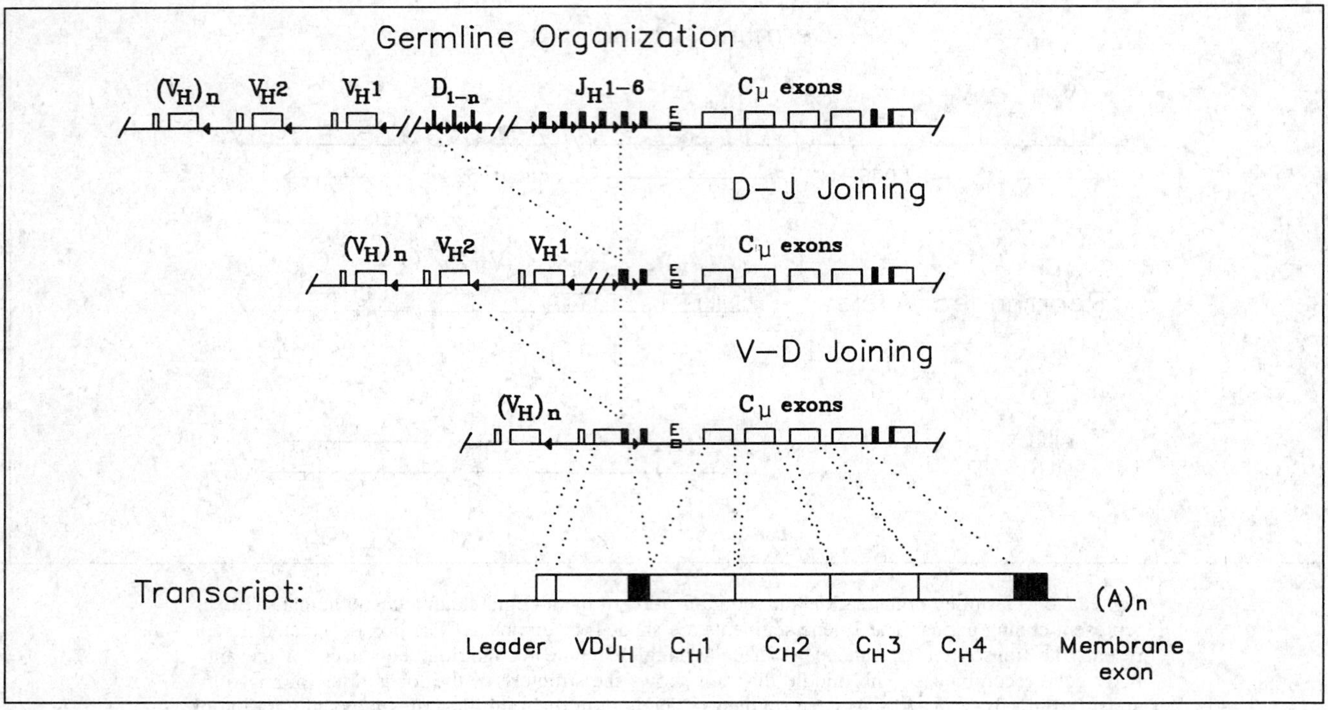

Fig. 285-3. Germline organization and reorganization of the human heavy chain locus. The D and J gene segments and the membrane exons are shaded for emphasis. V-D joining follows D-J joining and yields a functional transcriptional unit, the mature product of which encodes a membrane-associated μ chain. See legend to Fig. 285-2 for additional description.

and later both IgM and IgD. This dual expression is achieved by alternative splicing of a long primary transcript. The δ constant region sequences are positioned adjacent to the μ constant region exons. Subsequent expression of other isotypes may occasionally occur by differential processing of an exceedingly long (more than 250 kb) primary transcript but more frequently results from a second type of gene rearrangement event called *isotype switching*. As shown in Fig. 285-4, the isotype switching process occurs through the juxtaposition of specialized "switch" regions located 5′ to each constant region gene and results in the deletion of intervening constant region exons. This process permits the expression of an already rearranged V_H gene segment with a different constant region isotype.

Five mechanisms contributing to antibody diversity

Detailed characterization of antibody molecules produced in response to immunization has delineated five important mechanisms responsible for antibody diversification.

1. The germline repertoire includes hundreds of tandemly linked variable region gene segments. (The actual complement of variable regions inherited by each individual varies somewhat, which may contribute to susceptibility to both infectious and autoimmune diseases.)

2. "Combinatorial" joining of germline V, D, and J gene segments produces a repertoire of more than 10,000 different heavy chains. Joining of V and J gene sequences yields at least 1000 different κ light chains. The human λ–light chain repertoire includes four different constant region gene segments, each with its own J and at least 30 different V_λ gene segments.

3. Flexibility in the joining process adds increased variability at the sites of joining. Although two thirds of the

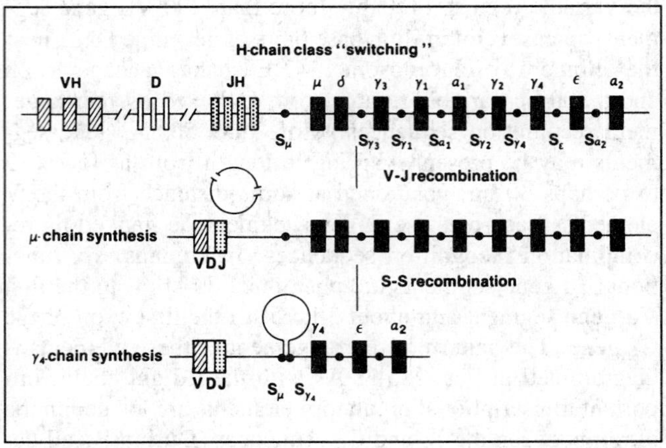

Fig. 285-4. Mechanism of isotype switching. V-D-J recombination permits μ chain synthesis. Juxtaposition of the γ4 gene is achieved through a deletion mechanism involving recombination at specialized "switch" sequences *(S)*. See text for description.

flexibility at the site of J region joining will yield out-of-frame (and thus nontranslatable) antibody chains, flexibility in joining probably increases the overall size of the repertoire by at least a factor of 10. Included in this description of flexibility is the phenomenon of N region addition by terminal transferase.

4. Combinatorial association of heavy and light chains yields many different combining sites. Thus, if 10,000 different heavy chains pair randomly with 1000 different light chains, 10^7 different antibodies are produced. If flexibility in the joining process increases the potential repertoire of heavy and light chains by 10-fold, at least 10^8 different binding sites can be generated through gene rearrangement.

5. Superimposed on these combinatorial mechanisms is a process of somatic hypermutation that introduces deletions, insertions, and substitutions into the rearranged V gene segment. Hypermutation is quite specific in that it targets only a region of about 1000 bases centered around the rearranged V element and operates only during a limited time during the life of an individual B lymphocyte. The hypermutation process is partially responsible for the phenomenon of *affinity maturation:* antibodies synthesized late in a response have higher overall affinity for antigen than do antibodies synthesized early in the response. The rate of hypermutation is extremely high, greater than 10^{-3}/bp/generation (at least four orders of magnitude higher than rates for other non-Ig genes). Thus the extent of antibody diversity may be essentially unlimited.

Developmental order of antibody gene rearrangements

The rearrangement of antibody genes follows a precisely regulated developmental sequence. Although the mechanism responsible for this regulation is still speculative, it is nevertheless clear that in B lymphoid progenitors, joining of D_H to J_H gene segments occurs first and typically on both alleles. This is followed by V_H-D_H joining to produce a functional heavy chain transcript. If a first rearrangement yields a nonfunctional product, a second rearrangement event occurs. This developmental program appears to be responsible for the phenomenon of *allelic exclusion:* individual B lymphocytes express products of only one set of antibody gene alleles. B-lineage cells that have rearranged heavy chain but not light chain sequences are designated *pre-B cells.* Often these pre-B cells have a C_μ heavy chain detectable by cytoplasmic staining. Light chain rearrangement occurs next and also follows a specific order. The κ genes rearrange first, one allele at a time, until a functional product is obtained. If neither allele yields a functional product, λ–light chain gene rearrangement occurs. Thus λ-secreting B lymphocytes contain rearranged (or in some cases deleted) κ loci, whereas κ-secreting B lymphocytes generally retain their λ genes in germline configuration. Somatic hypermutation occurs to the greatest extent in mature B lymphocytes. Isotype switching occurs last and is often associated with terminal differentiation into plasma cells. Some IgG B lymphocytes differentiate into *memory cells,* which may remain in the peripheral lymphoid organs for many years. This explains the long-lasting serologic immunity achieved by vaccination.

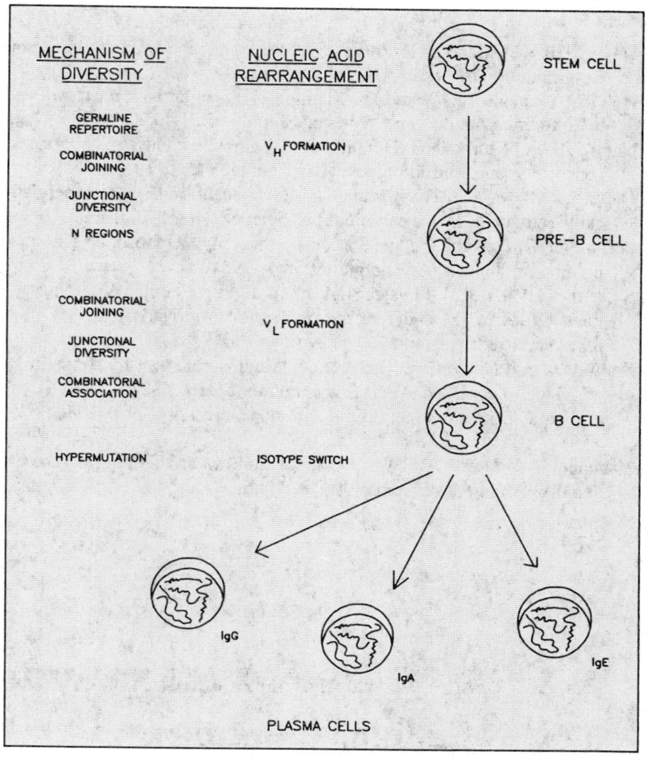

Fig. 285-5. Generation of antibody diversity. Each of the mechanisms of antibody diversification *(left)* is associated with specific nucleic acid rearrangements *(center)* and occurs at defined points along the time line of B cell development *(right).* (Reproduced from Perlmutter RM et al: Adv Immunol 35:1, 1984.)

Fig. 285-5 outlines the major events in B cell differentiation from the perspective of antibody genes.

Pathologic gene rearrangements in lymphoid cells

Rearrangement of antibody genes (and of T cell antigen receptor genes, which are similarly organized) occurs uniquely in lymphoid cells. This rearrangement process occasionally operates on inappropriate substrates, resulting in pathologic changes in DNA content. For example, virtually all examples of Burkitt's lymphoma in humans contain an 8;14 chromosomal translocation that juxtaposes antibody heavy chain genes with the proto-oncogene c-*myc.* Similarly, a large percentage of follicular B cell lymphomas contain a 14;18 translocation, resulting in juxtaposion of the antibody genes with the proto-oncogene *bcl*-2. In each case, good reason exists to believe that activation of the translocated oncogene contributes importantly to the expansion of the malignant clone. Thus the process of gene rearrangement, although a spectacularly effective mechanism for diversifying the repertoire of antigen receptors, represents a form of mutagenesis that can predispose persons to the development of neoplastic disease.

REFERENCES

Davies DR and Metzger H: Structural basis of antibody function. Annu Rev Immunol 1:87, 1983.

Hood L, Kronenberg M, and Hunkapiller T: T cell antigen receptors and the immunoglobulin gene supergene family. Cell 40:225, 1985.

Natvig JB and Kunkel HG: Human immunoglobulins: classes, subclasses, genetic variants and idiotypes. Adv Immunol 16:1, 1973.

Oettinger MA et al: RAG-1 and RAG-2, adjacent genes that synergistically activate V(D)J recombination. Science 248:1517, 1990.

Perlmutter RM et al: The generation of diversity in phosphorylcholine-binding antibodies. Adv Immunol 35:1, 1984.

Schroeder HW Jr et al: Physical linkage of a unique human V_H gene segment (V_H6) to D_H and J_H gene segments. Proc Natl Acad Sci USA 85:8196, 1988.

Showe LC and Croce CM: The role of chromosomal translocations in B- and T-cell neoplasia. Annu Rev Immunol 5:253, 1987.

Tonegawa S: Somatic generation of antibody diversity. Nature 302:575, 1983.

Yancopoulos GD and Alt FW: The regulation of variable region gene assembly. Annu Rev Immunol 4:339, 1986.

CHAPTER

286 Cellular Immunity

Thomas D. Geppert
Peter E. Lipsky

Cell-mediated immunity is the major defense against obligate intracellular pathogens such as viruses, certain bacteria, fungi, and protozoa. It also plays a major role in the defense against neoplasia and mediates graft rejection. As opposed to the humoral immune system, which generates specific antibodies as the effector limb of the response, the effectors in the cellular immune response are the antigen-specific thymus-derived lymphocytes (T lymphocytes); various cell types that are not antigen-specific, including mononuclear phagocytes and natural killer cells; and a variety of soluble factors, termed *cytokines,* that are produced by these cells. The activity of the cellular immune system is largely controlled by T lymphocytes that confer antigen specificity to the response. The importance of the T lymphocyte and the cellular immune response in general is evident in the current epidemic of acquired immunodeficiency syndrome (AIDS), in which the loss of a functionally important subset of T cells, the $CD4^+$ T cells, results in profound defects in the cellular immune response and the development of a variety of infectious and neoplastic disorders.

DELAYED-TYPE HYPERSENSITIVITY

Delayed-type hypersensitivity refers to the inflammatory reaction that occurs locally at the site of antigenic challenge as a result of the activation of immune T cells. It serves as a good model of the events involved in cell-mediated immune responses. When antigen is administered intradermally, the delayed-type hypersensitivity reaction (erythema and induration) can first be detected within 6 to 8 hours and reaches its peak 24 to 48 hours after the antigen's introduction. This delayed reaction can be contrasted with antibody-mediated reactions, which are more rapid. The classic example of delayed-type hypersensitivity in humans is the response of sensitized individuals to the intradermal injection of tuberculin or purified protein derivative (PPD), a soluble product of *Mycobacterium tuberculosis*. Similar responses are observed after intradermal injection of various recall antigens, including soluble extracts of fungi, viruses, and bacterial products. Delayed-type hypersensitivity can also be elicited as a result of skin sensitization to chemical haptens such as picryl chloride (chlorotrinitrobenzene).

Histologically, delayed-type hypersensitivity reactions differ from species to species. In some laboratory animals the predominant cells in the infiltrates are polymorphonuclear leukocytes (PMNs), whereas in humans the most numerous cells infiltrating such inflammatory reactions are blood-derived mononuclear phagocytes. Since macrophages lack the ability to recognize antigens in a specific manner, their predominance in delayed-type hypersensitivity infiltrates indicates that most cells that participate in these reactions are not antigen specific. In addition to mononuclear phagocytes, in humans both CD4 (helper-inducer) and CD8 (suppressor-cytotoxic) T cells have been shown to infiltrate delayed-type hypersensitivity lesions, although CD4 cells predominate in the responses elicited by PPD. Besides macrophages and T cells, small numbers of other cell types, including PMNs, basophils, and eosinophils, are also found.

The initial events in delayed-type hypersensitivity involve the entry of mononuclear phagocytes into the site. Although basophils and neutrophils may precede monocytes, the appearance of monocytes as a result of emigration through postcapillary venules signals initiation of the response's immunologically mediated phase. In the tissue, monocytes ingest foreign material, degrade this material, and present it to blood-derived antigen-specific T cells. It has been shown in mice that two different populations of T cells are involved in the development of such responses. After recognizing specific antigen, the first T cell subpopulation secretes a soluble factor that induces histamine and serotonin release by mast cells. These mediators cause additional vascular gaps that permit access of a second population of T cells, including the effectors of a later phase of delayed-type hypersensitivity. This phase results from the antigen-stimulated release of a series of soluble factors, including a migration inhibition factor (MIF), which inhibits migration of monocytes from the inflammatory sites, and a macrophage-activating factor (MAF; interferon gamma [IFN-γ]), which induces profound functional changes in mononuclear phagocytes. The result of these factors' activity is the localized accumulation of mononuclear phagocytes with enhanced functional activity directed toward elimination of the foreign material.

The scope of delayed-type hypersensitivity reactions is

limited by a series of antigen-specific and antigen-nonspecific suppressor T cells. In general, suppressors of delayed-type hypersensitivity can be classified into two types. *Afferent suppressors* inhibit the stimulation of antigen-specific T cells and therefore are active at the initial immunization. By contrast, *efferent suppressors* inhibit the expression of primed T cell activity and therefore are effective at the secondary challenge. Immunosuppression may be achieved by the production either of antigen-specific suppressive molecules or of factors that inhibit responses nonspecifically. In humans, most suppressor T cells express the CD8 phenotype, although the induction of antigen-specific suppressor T cell activity requires the participation of a CD4 suppressor-inducer cell. As a result of the activity of suppressor T cells, the scope of delayed-type hypersensitivity reactions is limited to avoid potential tissue damage.

The chronic equivalent of delayed-type hypersensitivity is the formation of a granuloma. A *granuloma* is a localized inflammatory response composed predominantly of mononuclear cells. Although macrophages are the major cell constituents, variable numbers of other cells, including lymphocytes, plasma cells, neutrophils, and eosinophils, may also be found. Granulomas arise after chronic stimulation with foreign materials or living cells. The factors that cause an acute lesion to evolve into a granuloma are not completely understood, although it appears to be an active process governed by chronic local stimulation of antigen-reactive T lymphocytes by persistent nondigestible materials or living cells. In granulomas, macrophages differentiate into epithelioid cells and fuse, giving rise to multinucleated giant cells.

CELLS INVOLVED IN CELL-MEDIATED IMMUNITY

Mononuclear phagocyte system

The mononuclear phagocyte system comprises a family of lineally related cells scattered throughout the body that function as the major effectors of cell-mediated immunity (Table 286-1). Mononuclear phagocytes not only function as effector cells of inflammation, but also constitute the major defense against a number of intracellular pathogens. In addition, they function as antigen-presenting cells for the induction of immune responses, dispose of damaged or senescent cells, and play a role in tumor resistance.

The mononuclear phagocyte system consists of bone marrow precursors, blood monocytes, and tissue macrophages. The cells of this system are characterized by a common lineage, accentuated phagocytic capacity, long life span in tissues, and capacity to differentiate or develop enhanced activity in response to local stimuli.

Table 286-1. Cells of mononuclear phagocyte system

Cell type	Location	Designation
Monoblast	Bone marrow	
Promonocyte	Bone marrow	
Monocyte	Bone marrow, peripheral blood	
Macrophage	Connective tissue	Histiocytes
	Liver	Kupffer cells
	Lung	Alveolar macrophages
	Lymph nodes	Macrophages
	Spleen	Macrophages
	Serous cavities	Pleural and peritoneal macrophages
	Central nervous system	Microglial cells
	Bone	Osteoclasts
	Synovium	Type A cells
	Inflammatory tissues	Inflammatory macrophages, multinucleated giant cells, epithelioid cells

Maturation. The maturation of mononuclear phagocytes from pluripotent stem cells is regulated by several cytokines. Interleukins 1, 3, 6, and 7 (IL-1, IL-3, IL-6, IL-7) and stem cell factor act on pluripotent stem cells to generate cells that are able to respond to additional factors that direct their subsequent differentiation. The importance of stem cell factor in this process is evidenced by the severe deficiency in hematopoiesis in animals with defects in its production or with defects in the production of its receptor. In the presence of IL-3, granulocyte-macrophage colony-stimulating factor (GM-CSF) stimulates the development of stem cells into bipotential cells with the capacity to develop into either granulocytes or monocytes. These cells are then directed to develop into either granulocytes or monocytes by granulocyte colony-stimulating factor (G-CSF) or macrophage colony-stimulating factor (M-CSF). IL-1 also promotes the development of pluripotent stem cells into mature cell types by stimulating them to become responsive to other CSFs.

Phagocytosis. Mononuclear phagocytes are able to ingest and degrade a variety of foreign materials, as well as senescent autologous cells and tissue debris. Despite their great phagocytic capacity, they lack the ability to bind and ingest many particles. After such particles are opsonized with immunoglobulin G (IgG, or IgM) and complement, however, they can be recognized by means of Fc and C3 receptors on cells of the mononuclear phagocyte system. As a result of the activity of these receptors, opsonized particles are ingested at a greatly accelerated rate.

Cytokines. Mononuclear phagocytes secrete several cytokines, including IL-1, IL-8, macrophage inflammatory protein 1 (MIP-1), tumor necrosis factor alpha (TNF-α), G-CSF, M-CSF, GM-CSF, and IL-6. The release of these cytokines can be stimulated by a variety of agents, including bacterial endotoxin, immune complexes, and sodium urate crystals. The production and release of these cytokines are not limited, however, to mononuclear phagocytes, since various other cell types also release these cytokines. Each cytokine has pleiotropic effects on a variety of cell types. Thus, for example, IL-1 amplifies the B and T cell response to antigen, promotes T cell IL-2 production, stimulates hypothalamic cells to produce fever, stimulates the adrenohypothalamic axis, induces the release of prostaglandin E_2 (PGE_2) by a variety of cells, stimulates fibroblast collagenase production, promotes the production of acute phase reactants from the liver, and induces the release of proteolytic enzymes from chondrocytes. In addition, IL-1 promotes the release of IL-6 from fibroblasts and hepatocytes. IL-6 also stimulates the production of acute phase reactants by the liver and promotes B and T cell responses. TNF-α has been found to share many biologic activities of IL-1 and also appears to be the mediator responsible for the clinical signs and symptoms of shock. Moreover, TNF-α is a potent inducer of IL-1 production by mononuclear phagocytes. IL-8 and MIP-1 share a capacity to attract and activate PMNs, but each has several unique properties. For example, IL-8 is a chemoattractant for basophils and T cells and can inhibit polymorphonuclear adherence to endothelial cells and migration into inflammatory sites. MIP-1 can induce fever that is not blocked by inhibitors of PGE synthesis and functions to enhance the ability of M-CSF or GM-CSF to stimulate the development of stem cells into bipotential cells with the capacity to develop into either granulocytes or monocytes. Thus many systemic manifestations of inflammatory disease may be accounted for by the action of these secretory products of mononuclear phagocytes.

Secretion. In addition to the production of various cytokines, macrophages secrete enzymes such as lysosomal hydrolases, lysozyme, and neutral proteases (e.g., collagenase, plasminogen activator, elastase). They also secrete enzyme inhibitors such as $alpha_2$ macroglobulin, complement components (C1, C4, C2, C3, C5, factor B, factor D, properdin, C3b inactivator, β_1H), biologically active molecules (e.g., interferon alpha [IFN-α], CSFs, IL-1), and oxygen metabolites such as hydrogen peroxide. Moreover, mononuclear phagocytes secrete various arachidonic acid metabolites, including prostaglandins, thromboxanes, and the leukotrienes. Other secretion products of mononuclear phagocytes include tissue factor (procoagulant), fibronectin, angiotensin-converting enzyme, and apoprotein E. Various stimuli trigger macrophages to release their secretory products. Secretion of several products is stimulated by phagocytic challenges, bacterial endotoxin, or T cell lymphokines, whereas other products such as lysozyme are released constitutively.

Activation. Mononuclear phagocytes are the major effector cells in cell-mediated immune responses. At inflammatory sites, macrophages are stimulated to become "activated." Although macrophages may be activated by several nonspecific stimuli, such as bacterial endotoxin and immune complexes, the most effective trigger for macrophage activation appears to be the T cell lymphokine IFN-γ.

Activated macrophages differ functionally from their nonactivated precursors. The former have increased phagocytic activity, acquiring the capacity to ingest particles opsonized by C3b in addition to those bound by the Fc receptor. Several other characteristics of macrophages change after activation, including their capacity to kill intracellular pathogens. Much acquired microbial resistance characteristic of cell-mediated immunity can be accounted for by the accentuated capacity of activated macrophages to kill various pathogens. Before activation, many intracellular pathogens, such as *Salmonella, Brucella, Toxoplasma,* and *Trypanosoma cruzi,* are able to bypass the normal killing mechanisms of mononuclear phagocytes and propagate within these cells. Activated macrophages, however, do not permit the growth of such pathogens and are able to kill many of them. Of importance, the enhanced antimicrobial effects of macrophages activated by IFN-γ is nonspecific in that a variety of unrelated pathogens can be killed, whereas production of IFN-γ by the primed T cell is highly specific because only the immunizing antigen will stimulate the release of this lymphokine.

Intracellular killing of pathogens by activated macrophages results mainly from production of reactive oxygen metabolites such as hydrogen peroxide and hydroxyl radicals. The generation of such products from the "respiratory burst" of oxidative metabolism is unique to phagocytic cells (mononuclear phagocytes, eosinophils, neutrophils). Macrophages also use reactive oxygen metabolites to kill organisms too large to be ingested (e.g., *Schistosoma mansoni*). In these situations, macrophages actively secrete oxygen metabolites, which results in killing of the pathogen but which may also cause damage to the surrounding tissues. Despite the importance of the respiratory burst, mononuclear phagocytes appear to have additional mechanisms for killing intracellular pathogens, since macrophages from patients with chronic granulomatous disease that are unable to generate the respiratory burst of oxidative metabolism are still able to kill some microorganisms, such as *Chlamydia* and *Toxoplasma*.

Several other functions change as macrophages become activated, including an increase in (1) the content of lysosomal hydrolases, (2) the number of Fc receptors, and (3) the ability to accomplish antibody-dependent cellular cytotoxicity (see following discussion). Activated macrophages also have an increased ability to bind and subsequently kill neoplastic cells. Although the mechanism of tumor cell lysis is not completely defined, several secretory products of macrophages appear to participate in this activity. These include reactive oxygen metabolites such as hydrogen peroxide, nitric oxide, and a cytolytic protein (CP), a serine protease with lytic capacity preferentially, although not exclusively, directed toward neoplastic cells. Recent evidence suggests that macrophage lytic capacity may depend on the production of nitric oxide generated from L-arginine. Finally, after activation, macrophages have an increase in the capacity to synthesize and secrete arachidonic acid metabolites. Secretion of products of both the cyclo-oxygenase pathway (e.g., PGE_2) and the lipoxygenase pathway (e.g., hydroxy- and hydroperoxyeicosatetraenoic acids, leukotrienes) may be increased in activated macrophages. Different stimuli may increase activity in one or another of these pathways preferentially. Thus, for example, bacterial endotoxin increases secretion of cyclo-oxygenase pathway products in macrophages, whereas zymosan, a phagocytic stimulus, increases secretion of both cyclo-oxygenase and lipoxygenase pathway products. By contrast, IFN-γ inhibits the release of prostaglandins from macrophages. Mononuclear phagocytes also play an important role in the presentation of antigens to antigen-specific T cells (Chapter 283).

T cells

T cells are lymphoid cells that originate in the bone marrow. During embryonic life the T cell precursors leave the marrow and migrate to the thymus. In the thymic microenvironment, T cells differentiate and become functionally mature. The mechanisms controlling T cell differentiation within the thymus remain largely unknown.

It appears that several cytokines, including IL-1, IL-2, IL-4, and IL-7, are involved. Various soluble thymic mediators have also been described, including thymosin, thymopoietin, and serum thymic factor *(facteur thymique serique)*. The precise nature and role of each of these thymic factors have not been completely defined. During ontogeny in the thymus, T cells acquire immunocompetence. After their maturation the functionally mature T cells leave the thymus and migrate to the paracortical areas of the lymph nodes and to the white pulp of the spleen. T cells can be divided into two distinct subsets based on the structure of their receptor for antigen (TCR). Most T cells express a 90-kilodalton (kd) disulfide-linked dimer composed of 45 kd α and β chains (TCR2). A few T cells express an 80 kd dimeric T cell antigen receptor composed of 45 kd and 35 kd γ and δ chains (TCR1). The function of this latter subset of T cell is unclear at present, but the cells are enriched at several epithelial surfaces, including the skin and gastrointestinal and genitourinary tracts.

Maturation. The thymic maturation of T cells expressing the αβ-chain T cell antigen receptor (TCR2) has been divided into three stages. The first two stages of maturation occur in the cortex of the thymus, whereas the third takes place in the thymic medulla. Precursor T lymphocytes expressing the CD7 surface molecule enter the thymus, where they acquire the T cell–specific marker (CD2), the receptor for the lymphocyte function–associated antigen 3 (LFA-3) found on a variety of human cell types, including thymic epithelium. CD2 is also the receptor for sheep erythrocytes. In addition, immature thymocytes express the CD38 molecule and the transferrin receptor CD71, (stage I: $CD2^+$, CD38, $T10^+$). As they mature, the cells acquire a surface molecule with characteristics in common with class I major histocompatibility complex (MHC) molecules (CD1), lose transferrin receptors, and acquire both the T cell–subset–specific cell surface molecules CD4 and CD8 (stage II: $CD1^+$, $CD2^+$, $CD4^+$, $CD8^+$, CD38). Afterward, thymocytes migrate to the medulla of the thymus, where they undergo the next step of maturation, which involves the loss of CD1 and the division of thymocytes into two nonoverlapping subsets. One of these subsets loses CD8 but retains CD4, whereas the other loses CD4 but retains CD8. At the same time, thymocytes acquire the CD3 complex and the T cell receptor for antigen (stage III: $CD2^+$, $CD3^+$, $CD4^+$, CD38; or $CD2^+$, $CD3^+$, $CD8^+$, CD38). The development of T cells expressing functional T cell receptors and either CD4 or CD8 depends on the recognition of class I or II MHC molecules. T cells that recognize "self" class I or II MHC molecules in a manner that might initiate an autoimmune response are deleted by a process of programmed death called *apoptosis*. T cells that express $CD4^+$ and T cell receptors with the capacity to recognize foreign antigen in the context of self class II MHC molecules and T cells that express CD8 and T cell receptors with the capacity to recognize antigen in the context of self class I MHC molecules are expanded. In the absence of MHC antigen expression, mature T cells do not develop. The mechanisms mediating this positive and negative selection are discussed in Chapter 283.) T cell receptors bearing T cells subsequently lose the CD38 molecule and leave the thymus as mature T cells (mature T cell: $CD2^+$, $CD3^+$, $CD4^+$; or $CD2^+$, $CD3^+$, $CD8^+$).

The steps involved in the maturation of T cells expressing the γδ-chain T cell receptor for antigen are not known. However, most of these cells appear to lack both CD8 and CD4. In peripheral blood, 55% to 70% of T cells express CD4, whereas 25% to 40% express CD8. One to five percent of peripheral blood T cells express the γδ T cell receptor for antigen. Functionally, CD4 and CD8 cells appear to be different. Thus CD4 cells are the major helper-inducer population in addition to being the only T cells that proliferate in response to soluble antigens. CD8 cells contain the major suppressor T cell population. Both T cell populations contain cytotoxic T cells and cells that proliferate when stimulated with nonspecific mitogens or alloantigens in the mixed lymphocyte reaction. Whereas the function of T cells that express the γδ T cell receptor for antigen is not known, it has been demonstrated that they can function as antigen-nonspecific and antigen-specific cytotoxic cells and also produce a variety of soluble cytokines.

Emigration. To initiate and maintain an immune response, T cells must first emigrate to the site of inflammation. Emigration through endothelium involves several interactions between T cells and endothelium that both stabilize the adhesion of lymphocytes to endothelium and are involved in migration of T cells through the endothelium and into tissues. The expression of these molecules and their ability to participate in interactions is controlled by cytokines such as IL-1 and TNF released at the inflammatory site. By inducing receptor expression and triggering their ability to interact with ligands, TNF and IL-1 promote the accumulation of lymphocytes at the inflammatory site. The interactions involved in lymphocyte binding and emigration through endothelium include the following T cell/endothelial cell surface molecules: lymphocyte function–associated antigen (LFA)–1/intercellular adhesion molecule (ICAM-1), LFA-1/ICAM-2, very late antigen (VLA)–4/vascular cell adhesion molecule (VCAM)–1, CD2/LFA-3, cutaneous lymphocyte–associated antigen (CLA)/E-selectin, and L-selectin and CD44 on T cells with unidentified receptors on endothelial cells.

Antigen recognition. Both the αβ and the γδ T cell antigen receptors have extensive homology to immunoglobulin. The receptors are expressed clonally on T cells. During maturation of T cells, rearrangements of the genes that encode the T cell receptor occurs, such that distinct elements are brought together in a manner that permits each T cell to express a unique T cell receptor gene product. Since this process of gene rearrangement is largely random and occurs uniquely in each T cell, the number of different antigens that can be recognized by T cells is very great. CD3 is a molecular complex made up of at least six chains that are noncovalently linked to either the αβ or the γδ T cell antigen receptor. CD3 is expressed by all functionally mature T cells, and although it is not directly involved in recognition of antigen, CD3 plays a necessary role in the activation of T cell function by antigen. The expression of both the antigen receptor and the T3 molecule indicates that the T cell has become immunocompetent.

In contrast to B cells, which use surface immunoglobulin molecules as antigen receptors and thus can recognize antigen in its native form, the T cell receptor for antigen does not recognize antigen directly. For T cell recognition, the antigen must be processed to small peptides and presented on the surface of an antigen-presenting cell in the context of class I (HLA-A, HLA-B, and HLA-C in humans) or class II (HLA-D region antigens in humans) MHC molecules. This latter requirement imposes genetic restriction on T cell responsiveness in that T cells recognize antigen only in the context of autologous or syngeneic but not allogeneic antigen-presenting cells. The pathways for processing antigens are detailed in Chapter 283.

It is now clear that the antigen-binding site within class II MHC molecules is made up of amino acids within the hypervariable regions of class I and II MHC molecules. Thus the capacity of each MHC molecule to bind a particular peptide is determined by the hypervariable region. The nature of the hypervariable region therefore controls the nature of the antigenic peptide and the specificity of the immune response. This finding may explain the link between MHC phenotype and various immune-mediated diseases.

Normally, expression of class II MHC molecules is limited to monocytes, B cells, dendritic cells, and Langerhans cells of the skin. Thus antigen presentation in the context of class II MHC molecules is limited to these cell types. At inflammatory sites, however, several other cell types are induced to express class II MHC molecules, including fibroblasts and endothelial cells. The cytokine responsible for inducing class II MHC molecules under these conditions appears to be IFN-γ. The role of such cells in the immune response is not clear. In contrast, class I MHC molecules are expressed by all cell types; therefore, it is likely that all cell types can present class I MHC–restricted antigens.

Cytotoxic T cells. A subset of T cells differentiate into cytotoxic T cells. For these cells, antigen recognition activates cytotoxic machinery that lyses the target cell. Both $CD4^+$ and $CD8^+$ T cells can develop into cytotoxic cells, but the predominant cytotoxic effector cells are $CD8^+$. The predilection for $CD8^+$ T cells to develop into cytotoxic T cells may facilitate their ability to control disorders caused by agents (e.g., viruses) that synthesize antigens intracellularly.

In some circumstances the differentiation of cytotoxic lymphocytes requires the interplay of a series of functionally and phenotypically distinct T cells. Cytotoxic T lymphocyte precursors may be activated by interaction with the appropriate antigen but fail to proliferate or differentiate into cytotoxic effector cells. The activated cells, however, express receptors for IL-2. When a second helper-inducer T cell is also stimulated and produces IL-2, proliferation and differentiation of cytotoxic T cells can occur. Since resting precursors of cytotoxic T cells do not express IL-2 receptors, only those cells specifically activated by antigen will be stimulated to expand and differentiate into cytotoxic effector cells. In the systems studied the precursor of the cytotoxic cell is usually a $CD8^+$ T cell, the activation of which is restricted by class I MHC molecules, whereas the helper-inducer is a $CD4^+$ T cell activated by antigen in the context of class II MHC determinants.

Soluble mediators. Many lymphokine genes have been cloned using recombinant deoxyribonucleic acid (DNA) technology. This has dramatically increased our understanding of the structure of these molecules and has made it possible to obtain pure preparations of the various lymphokines. The availability of pure lymphokine preparation has greatly facilitated a delineation of the function of these molecules. It is clear from this work that all lymphokines studied have pleiotropic effects on a variety of cell types. Thus, for example, T cells produce a cytokine designated *IL-2* that not only is an autocrine growth factor for T cells, but also plays a role in natural killer (NK) cell and B cell proliferation, macrophage activation, and the differentiation of cytotoxic effector T cells. In addition, T cells produce IL-6, which upregulates class I MHC antigen expression on a variety of cell types, promotes T cell IL-2 production and B cell differentiation into Ig-secreting cells, and stimulates liver cells to produce acute phase reactants and monocytes to release IL-1 and TNF-α. Multiple effects have been noted for the T cell lymphokines IFN-γ, lymphotoxin, IL-3, IL-4, IL-5, IL-8, IL-9, IL-10, and MIP-1 (see Table 286-2). Lymphokines are produced by T cells after activation with antigen, mitogen, or alloantigen. It has been demonstrated that the biologic activities of IL-2, IL-3, IL-4, IL-6, lymphotoxin, and IFN-γ are mediated by specific receptors. It appears that all T cells have the capacity to produce all lymphokines when stimulated maximally with mitogens in vitro. However, the possibility that T cells produce a more limited spectrum of lymphokines when stimulated by antigen in vivo has been suggested. Thus it has been shown that antigen-specific T cell clones in the mouse can be divided into cells that produce IL-2, IFN-γ, and lymphotoxin and mediate delayed-type hypersensitivity (TH_1 cells) and those that produce IL-4 and IL-5 and serve as helper cells

Table 286-2. Lymphokines produced by activated T cells

Lymphokine	Other nomenclature	MW (kd)*	Target cell	Effect
Interleukin 2	T cell growth factor	15	T cells	Promotes growth of activated T cells and differentiation of cytotoxic T cells
			B cells	Promotes growth and differentiation of B cells into Ig-secreting cells
			Natural killer (NK) cells	Promotes growth and activation of NK cells
			Macrophages	Activates macrophages
Interleukin 3	IL-3, multicolony-stimulating factor	15	Mast cells	Promotes mast cell growth
			T cells	Stimulates T cell maturation (i.e., 20-hydroxysteroid dehydrogenase expression)
			Hematopoietic stem cells	Stimulates proliferation of early pluripotent stem cells
Interleukin 4	T cell growth factor 2, B cell–stimulating factor 1, B cell differentiation factor γ, mast cell growth factor 2	20	T cells	Promotes growth of at least some T cells and promotes T cell IL-2 production
			B cells	Induces class II MHC molecule expression and IgE Fc receptors on resting B cells and promotes growth of activated B cells; promotes IgE and IgG1 production by activated B cells
			Macrophages	Enhances tumoricidal activity; enhances expression of class II MHC molecules; enhances antigen-presenting cell capacity; induces multinucleated giant cell formation
			Hematopoietic stem cells	Costimulates growth of murine erythroid, macrophage, granulocyte, and mast cell colonies
			Mast cells	Supports proliferation of murine mast cells
Interleukin 5	T cell–replacing factor, B cell growth factor II, eosinophil differentiation factor	13	Macrophages	Activates macrophages
			Eosinophils	Promotes differentiation of eosinophils
			B cells	Stimulates B cell growth and IL-2 receptor expression; promotes activated B cell IgA production
			Thymocytes	Induces thymocyte IL-2 receptor expression
			Cytotoxic T cells	Promotes differentiation of cytotoxic T lymphocytes
Interleukin 6	IL-6, interferon β_2, B cell–stimulating factor 2	26	General	Stimulates increase in class I MHC antigen expression
			T cells	Promotes T cell IL-2 production
			B cells	Promotes B cell differentiation into Ig-secreting cells
			Liver	Stimulates production of acute phase reactants by liver cells
			Mononuclear phagocytes	Stimulates mononuclear phagocyte IL-1 and release of tumor necrosis factor
			Hematopoietic stem cells	Stimulates growth of granulocyte-macrophage progenitors; stimulates growth of multipotential hematopoietic progenitors
Interleukin 8	IL-8, neutrophil attractant/activating protein, T lymphocyte chemoattractant factor	8	Polymorphonuclear leukocytes (PMNs)	Chemoattracts and activates PMNs; enhances expression of adhesion molecules on PMNs
			Basophils	Chemotactic for basophils
			T cells	Chemotactic for T cells
Interleukin 9	IL-9, T cell growth factor III, mast cell growth-enhancing factor	14.1	Mast cells	Enhances IL-3-induced proliferation of bone marrow–derived mast cells; promotes mast cell IL-6 production
			Thymocytes	Promotes IL-2-induced thymocyte growth
			Hematopoietic stem cells	Supports erythroid colony formation with erythropoietin

Continued.

Table 286-2. Lymphokines produced by activated T cells—cont'd

Lymphokine	Other nomenclature	MW (kd)*	Target cell	Effect
Interleukin 10	IL-10, cytokine synthesis inhibitor factor	18.7	Macrophages	Inhibits macrophage accessory cell function and IL-1, IL-6, and TNF-α production
Macrophage inflammatory protein 1	MIP-1	8	PMNs	Chemoattractants and activates PMNs
			Hypothalamus	Induces fever
			Hematopoietic stem cells	Enhances M-CSF–induced and GM-CSF–induced granulocyte and macrophage colony formation
Lymphotoxin/tumor necrosis factor β	LT/TNF-β	18	Various nonlymphoid cells	Causes growth inhibition and lysis of various cells other than lymphocytes
			PMNs	Activates PMNs
			Adipocytes	Induces lipoprotein lipase
			General	Induces shock when injected into mice
			T cells	Enhances T cell proliferation
			Monocytes and many other cells	Synergizes with gamma interferon to upregulate class II MHC antigen expression
			Fibroblasts and endothelial cells	Enhances growth of fibroblasts and endothelial cells; enhances adherence of endothelial cells for PMNs, lymphocytes, and monocytes
			NK cells	Activates killing by NK cells
			B cells	Facilitates B cell proliferation and differentiation into Ig-secreting cells
Granulocyte-macrophage colony-stimulating factor	GM-CSF, pluripoietin, colony-stimulating factor 2 (CSF-2)	22	Hematopoietic stem cells	Stimulates growth and differentiation of early pluripotent stem cell into bipotential granulocyte/monocyte precursor
Gamma inteferon	Interferon gamma (IFN-γ)	17	Monocytes and many others	Activates monocytes; upregulates class I and class II MHC antigen expression
			NK cells	Activates NK cells
			B cells	Promotes B cell differentiation into Ig-secreting cells
			General	Stimulates antiviral activity
Transforming growth factor β	TGF-β	25	Connective tissue	Promotes collagen synthesis
			T cells	Inhibits IL-2-dependent T cell proliferation
			B cells	Inhibits differentiation of antibody-forming cells
			Tumor cells	Inhibits growth of some neoplastic cell lines
Tumor necrosis factor α	TNF-α	17	T cells	Enhances proliferation and IL-2 receptor expression
			B cells	Enhances proliferation and differentiation of activated B cells into antibody-forming cells
			NK cells	Enhances cytolytic potential; synergizes with IL-2
			Hepatocytes	Increases production of complement factors B and C3 and αantichymotrypsin
			Hematopoietic stem cells	Inhibits proliferation and differentiation
			Tumor cells	Cytotoxic for some tumors
			Macrophages	Induces production of IL-1, PGE_2, and PAF
			Osteoclasts	Increases bone resorption
			Fibroblasts	Stimulates production of PGE_2, GM-CSF, G-CSF, collagenase, membrane IL-1, and IL-6
			Adipocytes	Inhibits lipoprotein lipase
			Endothelial cells	Enhances production of IL-1, GM-CSF, G-CSF, PAF, and procoagulant activity; increases neutrophil adherence

*Molecular weight of cloned protein in kilodaltons.

Ig, Immunoglobulin; MHC, major histocompatibility complex; M-CSF, G-CSF, macrophage, granulocyte colony-stimulating factor; PGE_2, prostaglandin E_2; PAF, platelet-activating factor.

for B cell differentiation (TH_2 cells). A functional dichotomy of T cells may occur in humans in certain circumstances when there is persistent stimulation with antigen, as may occur in patients with certain allergic conditions.

Natural killer cells

By definition, NK cells are effector cells with spontaneous cytotoxic activity against a variety of target cells, including neoplastic cells, fetal cells, virally infected cells, and some normal lymphoid or hematopoietic cells. NK-mediated cell lysis lacks MHC restriction and can be observed across species barriers. In addition, NK cells lack markers of monocytes, granulocytes, or cytotoxic T lymphocytes. Morphologically, NK cells are lymphoid in appearance but contain large cytoplasmic azurophilic granules and therefore are referred to as *large granular lymphocytes* (LGLs). Phenotypically, human NK cells have some distinctive characteristics, such as the expression of IgG Fc receptors (CD16), that are similar to those of granulocytes. In addition, all LGLs express a surface glycoprotein known as *asialo GM1*, which is also expressed by granulocytes and monocytes, but not by lymphoid cells. Additional markers are expressed by some but not all LGLs. For example, 40% to 60% express a myelin-associated glycoprotein, most express receptors for C3b inactivated, and approximately 50% have receptors for sheep erythrocytes.

Although most NK cell activity in human peripheral blood can be ascribed to LGLs, several reports have shown that other cell types can also accomplish NK-like functions after stimulation with lectins, allogeneic cells, or lymphokines. These cells are called lymphokine-activated killer cells (LAK cells). Although it is clear that T cells can mediate LAK activity, NK cells whose function has been upregulated by IL-2 also account for some LAK activity. LAK cells have recently been used in the treatment of various malignancies, including colon carcinoma, melanoma, and renal cell carcinoma, because of their enhanced capacity to mediate cytotoxic effector function. These treatments have been effective in a small subset of patients but are accompanied by significant toxicity.

In addition to IL2, several lymphokines upregulate NK cell activity, including IFN-α, IFN-γ, TNF-α, and IL-1. The mechanism whereby these cytokines upregulate NK cell function is not known, but it has been suggested that some LGLs are precursors for functional NK cells and require additional signals from these cytokines for maturation.

The nature of the target structure for NK-mediated lysis remains a matter of controversy. Since only dividing cells are targets of NK cells, it has been suggested that an activation-associated surface molecule might be the structure recognized by NK cells. The mechanisms of NK-mediated killing seem to be similar to those of cytotoxic T cells. Although the initial step of adhesion of the cytotoxic cell to the target is mediated by a different recognition structure, the lytic protein–containing granules appear to be very similar, if not identical.

Antibody-dependent cellular cytotoxicity (ADCC) is another mechanism of cell killing that can be accomplished by a variety of effector cells, including monocytes, some T cells, NK cells, PMNs, eosinophils, and a cell that lacks phenotypic characteristics of the other cells and is called a K (killer) cell. A common feature of all cells mediating ADCC is the presence of receptors for the FC fragment of IgG. ADCC can be distinguished from typical cytotoxic T lymphocyte activity or NK-mediated killing by the requirement for antibody of the IgG class directed against structures on the target cell. Such IgG molecules constitute a bridge between effector cells and their targets. ADCC may be important in host defense against neoplasia and infection with some viruses. In addition, eosinophil-mediated ADCC appears to play an important role in the defense against various helminths.

FUNCTIONS OF CELL-MEDIATED IMMUNITY

Cell-mediated immunity is the primary defense mechanism against infections with a variety of intracellular pathogens. These infections include viral diseases and infections with other obligate intracellular bacterial pathogens. Cell-mediated immunity also appears to have an important role in the defense against tumors. Since neoplastic cells express tumor-specific antigens on their surface, these cells can be recognized by tumor antigen–committed cytotoxic T cells. In addition, nonspecific cytotoxic NK cells or macrophages are also thought to play a role in host defense against the emergence of neoplastic cells.

Cell-mediated immunity also plays a major role in graft rejection. Allospecific T cells recognizing determinants on the graft are responsible for this process. Both T8 and T4 cells may participate in graft rejection, although the rejecting organ is usually infiltrated predominantly with T8 cells. Cell-mediated immunity also plays a major role in graft-versus-host disease, in which the immunocompetent T cells contained in bone marrow grafts are able to generate an immune response against host tissues they recognize as allogeneic. T8 cells appear to be the major population mediating graft-versus-host disease.

DERANGEMENTS OF CELL-MEDIATED IMMUNITY

Various primary immunodeficiency diseases exist in which the defect is mainly at the level of cell-mediated immunity (Chapter 289). Of the congenital syndromes, the most extreme example is severe combined immunodeficiency, in which both cell-mediated and humoral immunity are abnormal. These patients develop chronic infections caused by fungi (e.g., *Candida albicans)* or protozoa (e.g., *Pneumonitis carinii*) and also have an increased susceptibility to viral infections. Smallpox vaccination results in disseminated vaccinia, and bacillus Calmette-Guérin vaccination may result in overwhelming mycobacterial infection. The nature of the primary defect is unknown, but thymic function is abnormal in these patients. Other conditions also lead to severe deficiencies of cell-mediated immunity, including inborn errors of metabolism such as adenosine deaminase deficiency and purine nucleoside phosphorylase deficiency. Other primary T cell deficiencies include the Wiskott-Aldrich syndrome, which is an inherited defect in the expression of a cell surface molecule, CD43, normally expressed on all circulating blood cells. Although the function of this molecule is not known, it appears to be important for the survival of blood cells and may function during cell-to-cell interactions by virtue of its capacity to bind ICAM-1. DiGeorge syndrome (thymic aplasia with hypoparathyroidism resulting from the congenital absence of the third and fourth pharyngeal arches) is manifested by a variable defect in cell-mediated immunity. Another disease with a rather selective lack of T cell responsiveness against the antigens of *C. albicans* is chronic mucocutaneous candidiasis, in which patients are unable to mount an effective immune response against this fungal pathogen.

Among the acquired defects of cell-mediated immunity, the most striking one is AIDS, which is caused by a human immunodeficiency virus (HIV) that infects and kills CD4 cells. The wide spectrum of clinical and immunologic abnormalities in AIDS patients clearly reflects the role of CD4 cells in the immune response and emphasizes the role of cell-mediated immunity in host defense against a variety of intracellular pathogens. In addition, AIDS patients frequently develop Kaposi's sarcoma and lymphomas of B lymphocyte origin, indicating the important role of cell-mediated immunity in the defense against neoplastic disease.

REFERENCES

Adams DO and Hamilton TA: The cell biology of macrophage activation. Annu Rev Immunol 2:283, 1984.

Dinarello CA and Mier JW: Lymphokines. N Engl J Med 317:940, 1987.

Geppert TD and Lipsky PE: Antigen presentation at the inflammatory site. CRC Crit Rev Immunol 2:6071, 1989.

Gillis S: Interleukin-2: biology and biochemistry. J Clin Immunol 3:1, 1983.

Mizel SB: Interleukin-1 and T cell activation. Immunol Rev 63:51, 1982.

Nathan CF et al: Identification of interferon gamma as the lymphokine that activates human macrophage oxidative metabolism and microbial activity. J Exp Med 158:670, 1983.

Oettgen HC and Terhorst C: A review of the structure and function of the T-cell receptor–T3 complex. CRC Crit Rev Immunol 7:131, 1987.

Ortaldo JR and Herberman RB: Heterogeneity of natural killer cells. Annu Rev Immunol 2:359, 1984.

Paul WE: Fundamental immunology. New York, 1989, Raven.

Reinherz EL et al: The human T cell receptor: analysis with cytotoxic T cell clones. Immunol Rev 74:83, 1983.

Romain PL and Schlossman SF: Human T lymphocyte subsets: functional heterogeneity and surface recognition structures. J Clin Invest 74:1559, 1984.

Rosen FS, Cooper MD, and Wedgwood RJP: The primary immunodeficiencies (parts 1 and 2). N Engl J Med 311:235, 300, 1984.

Thomas R and Lipsky PE: Monocytes and macrophages. In Kelley WN et al, editors: Textbook of rheumatology. Philadelphia, 1993, WB Saunders.

Van Voorhis WC, Witmer MD, and Steinman RM: The phenotype of dendritic cells and macrophages. Fed Proc 42:3114, 1983.

CHAPTER

287 Complement System and Immune Complex Diseases

M. Kathryn Liszewski
John P. Atkinson

The complement system consists of plasma and membrane proteins that play a major role in host defense against microbes (Tables 287-1 and 287-2). Complement proteins of plasma are synthesized in the liver, but cells that accumulate at sites of inflammation and tissue injury, such as monocytes, macrophages, and fibroblasts, also synthesize many components.

Complement functions in two major ways:

1. *Modification of the membranes of infectious agents.* Complement proteins bind to the membranes of microbes and thereby facilitate phagocytosis (opsonization) or membrane disruption (lysis). The process of opsonization is complement's most important role.
2. *Promotion of the inflammatory response.* Low-molecular-weight peptide fragments of complement

Table 287-1. Complement serum (plasma) proteins

Component	Molecular weight (daltons)	Serum concentration (μg/ml)
Classic		
C1q	410,000	150
C1r	90,000	100
C1s	85,000	50
C4	206,000	300
C2	117,000	15
Alternative		
Factor B	90,000	225
Factor D	25,000	3
Properdin	110,000-220,000	25
Both pathways		
C3	190,000	1200
Terminal components		
C5	185,000	85
C6	128,000	60
C7	120,000	55
C8	150,000	55
C9	79,000	60
Regulators		
C1 inhibitor	105,000	275
Factor I	88,000	35
Factor H	150,000	500
C4-binding protein	560,000	250
S protein	84,000	500
Anaphylatoxin inactivator	310,000	35
SP-40,40	80,000	50

Table 287-2. Complement membrane proteins

	Molecular weight (daltons)	Tissue distribution
Regulators		
DAF	70,000	All peripheral blood cells, epithelial and secretory cells, fibroblasts, endothelial cells
MCP	45,000-70,000	Same as DAF (but not on erythrocytes)
CD59	18,000	Same as for DAF
Receptors		
CR1	190,000-280,000	Erythrocytes, monocytes/macrophages, B cells, some T cells, granulocytes, kidney podocytes
CR2	140,000	B cells
CR3	150,000/90,000	Monocytes/macrophages, neutrophils, some lymphocytes
C3aR	?	Mast cells, basophils
C5aR	?	Granulocytes, monocytes

DAF, Decay-accelerating factor; MCP, membrane cofactor protein.

components alter vascular permeability and attract leukocytes to an area of inflammation.

Anomalies of the complement system, whether genetic or acquired, impair host defenses and immune complex processing, resulting in a predisposition to infectious diseases and autoimmune conditions. Complement measurements are also useful in establishing a diagnosis and monitoring the course of immune complex–mediated and autoimmune illnesses, especially systemic lupus erythematosus (Chapter 290).

NOMENCLATURE AND REACTION MECHANISMS

The complement reaction sequence behaves as a biologic cascade in which one component activates the next. The complement system consists of two independently triggered pathways that merge in a common series of events designed to opsonize or lyse a foreign cell. The *classic pathway,* discovered first, becomes activated when antibody complexes with antigen. The second route of activation is the *alternative pathway*. This system does not require the presence of antibody, but rather plays a protective, surveillance role by providing a natural, immediately available line of defense. This results because of a constant "trickle" of an activated component, which is always "on guard" to commence the cascade on an appropriate surface.

Components of the classic pathway and the terminal sequence are indicated by the letter *C* followed by a number (e.g., C1, C2). Proteins of the alternative pathway as well as certain regulatory components are termed *factors* and symbolized by letters (e.g., B, P, D, I). Constituents cleaved from the precursor protein are designated with the suffixes *a, b,* and so forth (e.g., C3a, C3b). Usually the "a" fragment is a smaller, released peptide that can promote the inflammatory response, whereas the "b" component represents the remaining, larger portion of the precursor that binds with the target and continues the cascade.

CLASSIC PATHWAY

The classic pathway serves primarily as a self-assembling series of components activated by antibody complexed to antigen (Fig. 287-1). When bound to antigen, immunoglobulins M (IgM) and G (IgG, subclasses 1 and 3) efficiently activate the classic pathway.

Four functional concepts describe the sequence of events in the classic pathway: attachment, activation, amplification, and attack.

Attachment

The classic pathway is initiated when the C1 component binds to the Fc portion of an antibody molecule that has attached to an antigen. C1 is present in serum as a noncovalently linked complex consisting of a single element called C1q and the calcium-dependent tetramer C1s-C1r-C1r-C1s. This large unit has a molecular weight of approximately 750,000 daltons.

C1q consists of an aggregate of 18 polypeptide chains of three distinct types that are organized into a complex re-

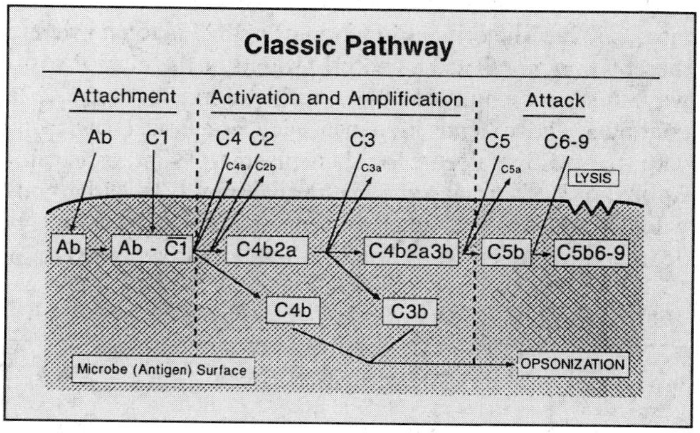

Fig. 287-1. Binding of antibody to antigen—in this case, on the membrane of a microbe—initiates the classic pathway, which consists of four functional steps. (1) *Attachment*. Binding of the C1 complex, via C1q, to the Fc portion of antibody initiates the cascade. (2 and 3) *Activation and amplification*. Activated C1 cleaves C4 and then C2. A single C1 can activate many C4 and C2 molecules. C4b attaches covalently to the membrane. Although most act as opsonins, some bind C2a and thereby form the C3 convertase, C4b2a, which in turn activates C3 by proteolysis. C3b, the larger activation fragment of C3, covalently binds to the membrane and promotes microbial destruction by serving as an opsonin while a few molecules form the C5 convertase (C4b2a3b). During the activation process, low-molecular-weight proinflammatory peptides, C4a, C3a and C5a, are produced by proteolytic cleavage. (4) *Attack*. The complement-coated microbe is "attacked" (a) by host cells that possess complement receptors that bind and ingest complexes via the C4b and C3b fragments (opsonization) or (b) by the membrane attack complex, which causes lysis.

sembling a bouquet of flowers (Fig. 287-2). The six globular heads possess sites for attaching the Fc portion of an immunoglobulin molecule. This interaction activates C1s-C1r-C1r-C1s.

Activation

In this step, complement components with protease (esterase) activity are produced. These subsequently activate other complement proteins through proteolytic cleavage to continue the cascade. The binding of C1q to antibody activates C1r, which then cleaves C1s. C1s cleaves C4 to remove a smaller fragment, C4a, which drifts away and is a weak anaphylatoxin (i.e., a peptide that produces contraction of smooth muscle and dilatation of blood vessels). The remaining larger fragment, C4b, may attach covalently to a nearby surface. In addition to cleaving C4, C1s also activates C2 after it attaches to C4b. This removes a peptide, C2b, which diffuses away. The larger C2a fragment remains bound to C4b to produce the enzymatic complex C4b2a, termed the *C3 convertase*. This enzyme cleaves C3.

Amplification

After activation, the next series of reactions produces a rapid increase in the cascading of the classic pathway. Amplification begins during the activation process when each activated C1 can generate many C4b components. Some of these serve as opsonins; others participate in the convertase, C4b2a. The critical function of C4b2a is to cleave and thereby *activate* C3, the central protein of the classic pathway. Just as C1 initiates the amplification process, C4b2a continues and extends it, since each convertase can activate many C3 molecules. When plasma C3 interacts with C4b2a, C3a is released. The remaining C3b either covalently attaches to the cell surface or diffuses away and is degraded. The deposition of C3b is the major objective of the complement system because C3b serves an important role as an opsonin. *Opsonization* is the process whereby cellular receptors bind deposited C3b or C4b and subsequently internalize and digest the particles. Additionally, surface-bound C3b possesses a site to which C5 attaches to continue the sequence of reactions leading to cell lysis.

Attack

In addition to opsonization, a second method of destroying a foreign target is the assembly of the membrane attack complex (MAC), which involves C5 to C9. C3b provides a binding site for C5 and makes it susceptible to cleavage by either the classic pathway or the alternative pathway convertases. The products of this reaction are the 11,000-dalton peptide C5a and the major fragment C5b. Activated C5b has a metastable binding site for C6 and combines with it to form C5b6, which in turn reacts with C7. Binding of the nascent C5b67 complex to cell membranes is the first step in assembly of the MAC (Fig. 287-3). The attachment of C8 initiates membrane damage, but formation of the stable transmembrane channel requires the addition of multiple molecules of C9. The C5b-9 complex is inserted through the lipid bilayer of the cell membrane with hydrophobic residues on its exterior in contact with the lipid bilayer and a hydrophilic interior, which allows the passage of ions and water. This loss of control dooms the cell to the intake of water, with eventual swelling and rupture. Such reactions occur on the membranes of bacteria and nucleated cells, as well as on the sheep erythrocytes often used in model systems to study this lysis step.

ALTERNATIVE PATHWAY

Although discovered many years after the classic pathway, the alternative pathway apparently developed much earlier in evolution and provides a natural, immediate line of defense that *does not require specific antibodies*. It is both a

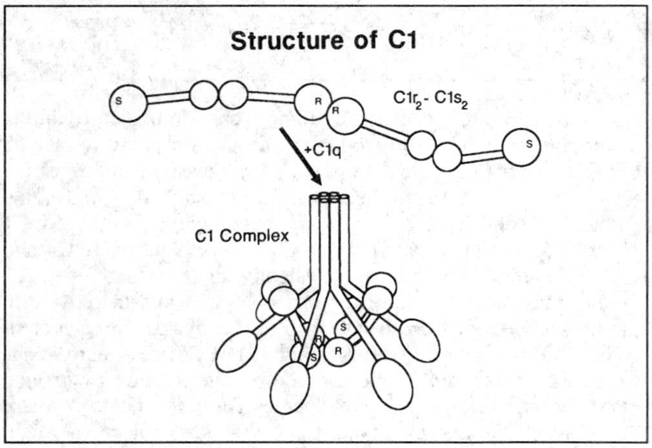

Fig. 287-2. Model proposed for the C1 complex. The top portion shows the linear structure of the $C1r_2$-$C1s_2$ subunit. The bottom part demonstrates the manner in which the catalytic domains of C1r and C1s may be brought into close contact. (Modified from M. Columb M et al: Philos Trans R Soc Lond Biol 306:283, 1984).

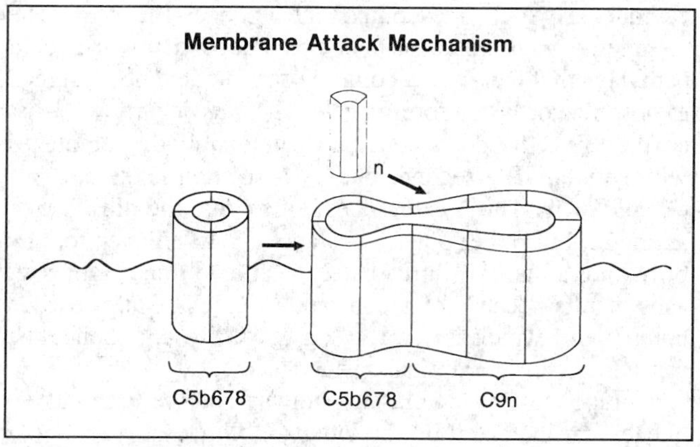

Fig. 287-3. Mechanism of action of the membrane attack complex. When C8 joins C5b67, a small pore or channel is formed in the membrane. Binding of multiple C9 components accelerates lysis. (Modified from Frank MM. In Samter M, editor: Immunological diseases, vol I. Boston, 1988, Little, Brown.)

recognition and an effector pathway and thus functions as an independent immune system. The following proteins constitute the alternative pathway: C3, factor B, factor D, and properdin (factor P).

C3 is a critical and pivotal component of both the classic and the alternative pathways. A highly reactive thioester bond that C3 possesses (Fig. 287-4) allows for its covalent attachment to reactive substrates. Since this bond is unstable, some C3 is constantly becoming activated in plasma and binds to a water or protein molecule or to a cell membrane. Such a continual "ticking over" of activated C3, although constituting a small percentage of total plasma C3, provides a constant sentry for the presence of foreign particles, on the surfaces of which the system amplifies.

Whether initially provided by the "ticking over" of C3 or by the C3 convertase of the classic pathway (Fig. 287-5), the C3b so formed can bind plasma factor B to form C3bB. The complex becomes activated when a single arg-lys bond is cleaved in B by factor D, a serine protease of plasma.

The critical role of the resulting C3bBb is to split more C3 to C3b, which quickly amplifies the cycle by binding more factor B. Thus this alternative pathway convertase parallels the function of the convertase of the classic pathway (C4b2a) and sets in motion an amplification loop that deposits large amounts of C3b on foreign particles. However, C3bBb is extremely labile unless stabilized by the binding of a plasma protein called *properdin*.

The subsequent processing of the particle by opsonization or by reaction with components of the MAC complex is identical to that of the classic pathway.

ANAPHYLATOXINS

Anaphylactic-like reactions are produced by certain peptide fragments cleaved during complement activation. The most potent is C5a, followed by C3a, and, to a much lesser degree, C4a. Receptors for C3a and C5a are found on basophils and mast cells. Binding of the fragment to its receptor causes release of mediators, such as histamine. This produces biologic effects of increased vascular permeability, contraction of smooth muscle, and local edema. The actions of the anaphylatoxins are regulated by carboxypeptidase N (anaphylatoxin inactivator), which splits a terminal arginine residue to inactivate the peptides. C5a is also a major chemotactic factor. It binds to receptors on neutrophils and monocytes that cause directed cell movement.

REGULATION OF COMPLEMENT SYSTEM

Considering the proinflammatory and destructive capabilities of the complement pathways, precise control of this potent effector system is necessary (Table 287-3). As evidence of this fact, deficiencies of control proteins can lead to excessive complement activation and disease. The system is regulated at the critical steps of initiation, C3 cleavage, and MAC insertion. This inhibitory system is designed to prevent activation both in the fluid phase and on "self" tissue. Consequently, overlapping activities exist between the plasma and membrane inhibitory proteins. Such an arrangement evolved because of the requirement for unimpeded activation on microbial targets but for endogenous control designed to limit the activation process in both time and space. The *time* of activation must be finite to avoid using excessive quantities of complement components for one reaction. Restriction of activation in *space* is needed because the reaction must be focused on the target and not be allowed to spread into the fluid phase or to self tissue.

Initiation of classic pathway

The classic pathway is triggered by the interaction of IgM or IgG with antigen to form immune complexes (ICs). The

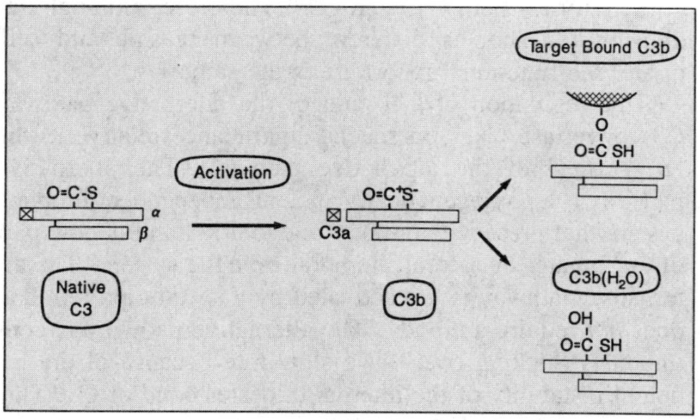

Fig. 287-4. Activation of C3. Native C3 contains a highly reactive thioester bond (S − C = 0) in its α chain. Activation of C3 by the C3 convertase liberates C3a and C3b. In this process the thioester bond within C3b is also broken, which allows metastable (a transiently reactive species) C3b to attach covalently to target surfaces or become inactive through an interaction with small molecules such as water.

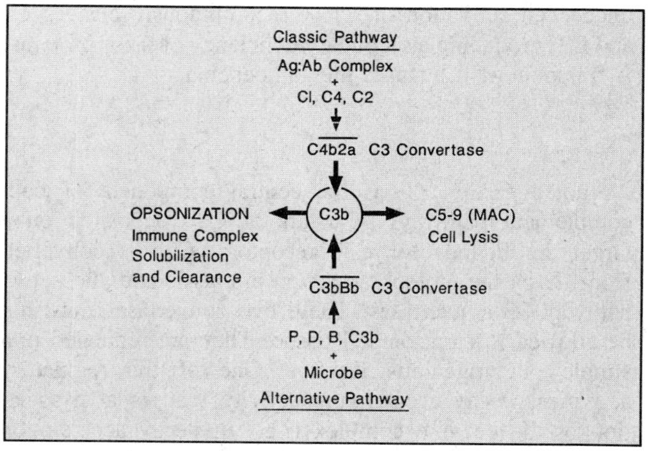

Fig. 287-5. Simplified scheme of complement pathways. C3 is the central component of both classic and alternative pathways. Its reaction product, C3b, promotes the opsonization of the foreign particle to which it is attached, or it may interact with C5. The latter reaction produces lysis by the membrane attack complex *(MAC)*. *Ag:Ab,* Antigen:antibody.

Table 287-3. Regulatory proteins of complement

	Molecular weight (daltons)	Serum concentration (μg/ml)	Action
Fluid phase			
Activation step			
C1 inhibitor	105,000	275	Inactivates C1r and C1s
Amplification step			
C4-binding protein	560,000	250	Binds C4b alone or in convertase and serves as cofactor for C4b degradation by factor I
Factor H	150,000	500	Binds C3b alone or in convertase and acts as cofactor for C3b proteolysis by factor I
Decay-accelerating factor (DAF)	70,000	Membrane	Accelerates decay of C3 convertases
Membrane cofactor protein (MCP)	45,000-70,000	Membrane	Cofactor for factor I–mediated proteolysis of C4b and C3b
Complement receptor one (CR1)	190,000-280,000	Membrane	Receptor; inhibitory profile similar to DAF and MCP
Factor I	88,000	35	Inactivates C4b or C3b
Membrane attack			
Vitronectin	84,000	500	Blocks fluid phase of MAC
CD59	18,000	Membrane	Blocks MAC on host cells
SP-40,40	80,000	50	Modulates MAC
Other			
Anaphylatoxin inactivator	305,000	35	Inactivates C4a, C3a, C5a

MAC, Membrane attack complex.

plasma protein *C1 inhibitor* (C1-INH), a serpin, regulates the serine protease subcomponents, C1r and C1s, of C1. This occurs rapidly if C1 is activated in the fluid phase by nonimmunologic means and after a few minutes if C1 is activated by an IC. A delicate balance exists in that C1-INH must not prevent appropriate activation but also must not allow excessive consumption of complement components. A disruption of such a balance is seen in the disease hereditary angioedema. A deficiency of C1-INH allows the unchecked activation of C1. C1 continuously cleaves C4 and C2, producing a secondary deficiency of these proteins. A fragment of C2 causes the angioedema.

C3 cleavage

As noted earlier, C3 is the central component of both complement pathways. Clusters of C3b deposited on a target are ligands for C3b receptors. C3b is converted from C3 by the proteolytic action of classic and alternative pathway C3 convertases. These two convertases must not be allowed to form on self tissue. They are regulated in a simple but ingenious fashion. One of the regulatory activities, decay accelerating activity, causes a dissociation of the enzyme complex (i.e., in decay acceleration the protease component is dissociated from C4b or C3b). However, the remaining C4b or C3b still has hemolytic potential because it can bind C2 or factor B. Consequently, further modification is necessary. To accomplish this, C4b and C3b are degraded by a serine protease of plasma, *factor I,* but only in the presence of a cofactor protein. The cofactor activity may be mediated by the same protein that serves as a decay accelerator or by an entirely different protein. In plasma, *C4-binding protein* binds C4b, and another protein, *factor H,* binds C3b. These two proteins each have decay-accelerating activity and cofactor activity for their respective substrate. In contrast, self tissue employs a different system. One protein (decay-accelerating factor, DAF) has decay-accelerating activity for both convertases, whereas a second protein (membrane cofactor protein, MCP) has cofactor activity for both C4b and C3b. Therefore, although the division of labor is different between plasma and self tissue, the functional repertoire is the same.

This regulation of C3b and of the alternative pathway C3 convertase takes on special significance relative to the "triggering" of the alternative pathway. The alternative pathway is a phylogenetically ancient, independent immune system that preceded antibody in evolution and is now part of our innate, or natural, humoral immune system. The alternative pathway is *not* activated by a specific protein and does *not* require antibody. The alternative pathway is continuously "ticking over" at a slow rate because of the inherent instability of the internal thioester bond of C3. This state is analogous to an idling automobile or to a sentry guarding a gate. The C3 that is ticking over while idling stays in the fluid phase or occasionally binds to self tissue. In either location, this C3b is inactivated through cofactor activity. If a microbe is present, the "ticked over" C3 will also land on it. Having no regulatory proteins, microbe-bound C3b will bind factor B, thereby forming the alternative pathway C3 convertase. This in turn results in a feedback loop leading to amplification of the alternative pathway and C3b, as well as MAC deposition on the microbe. As a result, host tissue is protected while foreign particles are attacked,

Membrane attack complex

Regulation of the MAC also occurs in the fluid phase and on cells. Cleavage of C5 produces C5b, which can bind C6 and C7. This C5b67 complex can insert into biologic membranes. To prevent the C5b67 complex from binding to self membranes, a plasma protein, *vitronectin,* combines with the complex and thereby blocks the ability of the C5b67 complex to attach to biologic membranes. If C5b67 does manage to attach to self, another regulatory protein, *CD59,* prevents the further assembly of the MAC. This is analogous to regulation of the C3 and the C5 convertases in that inhibitory proteins with a similar overall functional capacity, one in plasma and the other on self-tissue, mediate the desired protective effect.

To summarize, the complement system is tightly regulated at key steps in its pathways. Inhibitory activity is aimed at initiation and the membrane-modifying steps of C3b deposition and MAC formation. The goal is to allow rapid, unimpeded activation on microbes while at the same time blocking undesired fluid phase activation and potentially destructive activation on self tissue. Expression of a set of regulatory proteins provides a simple means for the complement system to distinguish self from nonself.

COMPLEMENT RECEPTORS

Many host cells possess receptors for complement components. These promote IC clearance and induce cellular responses.

Complement receptor type 1 (CR1)

Most blood cells possess CR1, which binds C3b-coated and/or C4b-coated particles.

CR1 plays a critical role in the clearance of C3b-coated particles and ICs from plasma and tissue. Erythrocyte (E) CR1 binds intravascular ICs and serves as a vehicle to transport them to the liver and spleen. Macrophages then "clear" such ICs by stripping them from the E, which subsequently returns to circulation. Within tissues, CR1 on neutrophils and monocytes targets ICs for destruction. When the receptor binds C3b- or C4b-bearing ICs, a cellular response may be initiated that promotes internalization and digestion.

Complement receptor type 2 (CR2)

Most mature B lymphocytes possess this 140,000-dalton membrane glycoprotein. The specificity of CR2 for the C3 degradation products (C3d, C3dg) helps localize antigen-bearing, complement-coated ICs to B cell–rich areas in the spleen and lymph nodes. Within CR2 is a binding site for the Epstein-Barr virus, which uses this receptor to gain entrance to the cell.

Complement receptor type 3 (CR3)

CR3 also binds and promotes the opsonization of particles bearing fragments of C3, especially C3bi. CR3 is present on macrophages/monocytes and certain lymphocytes and is part of the integrin family of adherence-promoting molecules involved in host defense. Deficiency of this receptor is associated with severe childhood infections. CR3 promotes ingestion more efficiently than does CR1. ICs possess varying quantities of C3b, C3bi, and C3dg, and these ligands in turn interact with their specific receptors. The biologic advantage may be that receptors cooperate to clear IC and facilitate immune responses to antigens.

Receptors for C3a, C4a, and C5a

Binding by the C5a receptor to its ligand activates neutrophils, macrophages, mast cells, or basophils. In addition, this binding has a spasmogenic effect on various tissues by a direct action on smooth muscle cells or secondarily by the release of mediators such as histamine. The C5a receptor recently has been cloned and shown to belong to the G superfamily of transmembrane proteins. It is expected that C3a will belong to this group as well. Less is known about the C4a receptor.

Other receptors

Recently, receptors for C1q and factor H have been found on such cells as neutrophils, monocytes, and B cells. Their function is not known.

METABOLISM OF COMPLEMENT PROTEINS

The liver synthesizes the complement components of plasma. Thus after hepatic allografting, for example, the electrophoretic polymorphic types of C3 and C6 change from those of the recipient to those of the donor. In normal individuals the rate of synthesis is the major determinant of plasma concentration. Most complement components are acute phase proteins that are elevated up to twofold in response to cytokines such as interleukins 1 and 6 (IL-1, IL-6). Local synthesis of complement proteins in areas of inflammation may serve to initiate responses in the microenvironment.

IMMUNE COMPLEX DISEASES

This section focuses on the diseases caused by ICs, but the reader should appreciate the beneficial nature of IC formation. When the body is assaulted by a foreign antigen (Ag), the normal and expected response is to bind, inactivate, and destroy the material evoking the response. Consequently, the formation of IC facilitates the removal of the antigenic substance.

The components of the immune system that accomplish

this goal are the plasma elements of antibody (Ab), complement (C), and anti-immunoglobulins (i.e., rheumatoid factors [RFs]), and cellular elements that include tissue monocytes and peripheral blood cells. Since IC normally do not accumulate, this system correctly and consistently accomplishes its task.

Immune complex formation and processing

After Ag penetrates body barriers, Ab are formed that can bind and eliminate the Ag in conjunction with other effector systems such as C and RFs. If Ab already exist, binding to the foreign target in the immune host occurs immediately; otherwise, Ab will be synthesized by the nonimmune host. IgM and IgG binding to Ag activates the classic C pathway. C activation produces both low-molecular-weight fragments that promote the inflammatory response through their vasodilatory and chemotactic properties and large C fragments that become bound to the Ag and Ab in the IC. When antigens are "coated" by Ab, C, or both, these attached molecules serve as ligands for Fc and C receptor-bearing cells, which in turn bind and dispose of the IC. For Ab the "constant" or Fc portion of the immunoglobulin (Ig) molecule serves as the ligand for Fc gamma receptors. The principal ligands for C receptors are C3b and C4b, which, in association with C activation, become covalently bound to the Ag and the Ab. Peripheral blood cells and tissue macrophages interact with IC through both C and Fc receptors. The combination of IgG and C3b attached to an antigen particularly enhances Ag clearance. C3b promotes the initial attachment of an IC to a cell, whereas IgG more efficiently signals internalization. Further, the deposition of C3b onto the IC enhances its solubility (i.e., keeps IC in solution so it can be bound by cells). RF facilitates this removal process by binding to the IC and by fixing more C. Most likely, this type of scavenging system evolved to rid the host of potentially damaging immune aggregates, such as those that contain an infectious particle, and to prevent the deposition of this material in inappropriate locations.

Erythrocyte processing of immune complexes

A specialized metabolic pathway for IC processing has been elucidated in primates. The primary cellular element of this system is the erythrocyte (E). Most IgM- or IgG-containing ICs activate C. C3b and C4b attached to the IC serve as ligands for C receptors. More than 85% of the C3b/C4b receptors (complement receptor type one, or CR1) in peripheral blood are on the surface of E. Consequently, complement-fixing ICs rapidly become bound to E. CR1, along with a serum protease known as factor I, degrade some of the C3b to C3bi and C3dg. These degradative fragments of C3b in turn may interact with other types of C receptors, particularly those found on various leukocytes. The E transports the IC to the liver or spleen, where the IC is transferred to hepatic mononuclear phagocytes (Kupffer's cells) while the E returns to circulation. Thus the E, through its C3b receptor, serves as a "sump," "processing station," and "taxi" for ICs (Fig. 287-6).

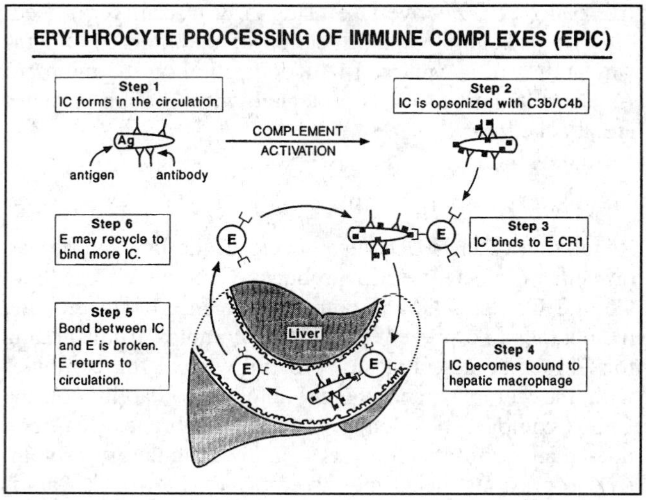

Fig. 287-6. Schematic representation of erythrocyte *(E)* processing of immune complex *(IC)* mechanism. (Modified from Hebert LA and Cosio FG: Kidney Int 31:877, 1987.)

Pathologic formation of immune complexes

Based on an analysis of this model, inappropriate handling or deposition of ICs might occur in the following situations.

1. *Excessive IC formation*. Clearance mechanisms are overwhelmed, as may occur in systemic lupus erythematosus (SLE), chronic viral syndromes, or mixed cryoglobulinemia.
2. *Deficient Ab response*. Synthesis of insufficient amounts of Ab results in poor C activation, or the humoral response is largely of the IgA isotype, which does not activate the classic C pathway. (Henoch-Schönlein purpura may be an example of the latter.)
3. *Deficiency of a component in the classic C pathway up to and including C3*. Such a defect would result in inefficient deposition of C3b. Examples include inherited deficiencies of C1, C4, C2, or C3. Interestingly, syndromes of IC excess, most often SLE, develop in individuals with these inherited deficiencies.
4. *Quantitative or qualitative abnormalities of C and Ig receptors*. Receptors could be synthesized in reduced numbers, qualitatively altered, or blocked by an autoantibody or IC.

In one particularly well-studied primate model, formation of IgA-containing IC rather than IgG-containing IC, presence of inhibitors that block the activation of the classic C pathway, and receptor blockade all led to the same consequences: more rapid removal of IC from the blood but less binding to E and, most importantly, increased deposition of the IC in inappropriate locations (e.g., kidney, lung). When C3b is not efficiently bound to the IC or the receptors are blocked, other factors play a role in IC deposition. Research largely performed on nonprimates has shown the charge of the Ag and/or Ab, RFs, vasoactive modulators, and other host factors to be important. In some cases, the Ag may be deposited before it is bound by Ab.

Localization of immune complexes

Diseases result when ICs form in excessive amounts or are not properly cleared. Three basic categories of tissue damage have been defined, based on the anatomic site at which the ICs form.

Immune complex formation in tissue. In this category, Ab react with locally produced Ag. Examples include infections of the ear, throat, and lung and certain forms of vasculitis. The *Arthus reaction* represents the classic model for this type of tissue injury. Rabbits subcutaneously inoculated with horse serum at weekly intervals developed a marked localized inflammatory reaction. Further studies determined that this response was not limited to the skin but also occurred if Ag was injected almost anywhere (e.g., pericardium, joints). Ab made by the host to various components of the horse serum reacted after reinjection of the "antigen."

Local tissue injury from the Arthus reaction proceeds from the following sequence of events. *Immune aggregates form* in tissue at sites proximal to blood vessels, where IgG and Ag come into contact. *Complement is activated* and chemotactic and vasodilatory factors are liberated, causing cells such as neutrophils to move into the area. Moreover, C4b and C3b are deposited not only on the Ag and Ab, but also on tissue in which the ICs are deposited. Neutrophils then accumulate and, through their Fc and C3b receptors, bind and ingest the IC. In this process, lysosomal enzymes, oxygen radicals, and other potentially toxic metabolites are released as the neutrophil attempts to phagocytose the particulate ICs. *Tissue damage* follows. If the ICs lodge in blood vessels, the pathologic process produces a vasculitis. Normally the reaction subsides quickly because ICs are processed with only minimum tissue injury. However, continued exposure to the Ag or injection of larger amounts of Ag on even one occasion can result in severe damage.

Clinically an Arthus-type reaction is observed in humans after the excessive repetitive administration of tetanus toxoid, in serum sickness, in some forms of thyroiditis, in certain synovial inflammatory reactions (e.g., rheumatoid arthritis), and in a variety of vasculitic syndromes. Additionally, individuals possessing high levels of IgG Ab to certain molds may develop inflammatory lung lesions after inhaling such fungi or spores (e.g., farmer's lung, cheese maker's lung, pigeon breeder's lung).

Immune complex formation in circulation. ICs that form in the circulation tend to deposit in areas of high blood flow, such as the kidney, lung, and skin. In these conditions, Ag present in the circulation, as occurs in chronic viral hepatitis and many parasitic infections, combines with Ab. For ICs to persist, some defect in the immune response or in the IC clearance mechanism is presumably present.

When ICs form in the circulation, severe consequences may result if they lodge in vessels of organs other than the liver and spleen. The glomerulus, choroid plexus, synovium, and uveal tract all possess a high degree of blood flow per unit mass of tissue and are particularly prone to IC deposition. Also, the dermal-epidermal junction of the skin is a frequent site of IC deposition. Further, among skin sites the lateral aspects of the lower legs are particularly prone to such a problem, possibly related to hydrostatic factors.

Serum sickness. The study of serum sickness in rabbits and humans has contributed much to our understanding of the pathophysiology of diseases associated with the presence of circulating ICs. Serum sickness may be either acute or chronic. The acute form was noted soon after the introduction of heterologous hyperimmune sera for the treatment of bacterial infections. A clearly documented syndrome, termed *serum sickness,* was observed in some patients 8 to 12 days after the injections and consisted of fever, cutaneous eruptions, arthralgias/arthritis, and lymphadenopathy. In humans the illness resolved spontaneously within 1 to 2 weeks, usually without permanent tissue damage. The discovery and use of vaccines and antibiotics lessened the need for heterologous antisera, except for the immediate treatment of tetanus, rabies, botulism, and snakebites, and to reduce immune cell populations from bone marrow transplants. As a result, acute serum sickness occurs less from the use of heterologous serum and more from the administration of antibiotics such as penicillins.

When intravascular ICs are formed as a result of the intermittent or continuous presence of Ag, a chronic form of serum sickness may develop. Chronic serum sickness–like reactions may occur in diseases such as SLE and some forms of chronic glomerulonephritis and with systemic manifestations of infectious illnesses, as in chronic viral hepatitis.

Serum sickness, whether acute or chronic, possesses features of the Arthus reaction (see earlier) with similar pathogenic steps. ICs form in the circulation and activate the C system. At the point of slight Ag excess, ICs tend to precipitate in blood vessels of joints, skin, and kidney. Complement fragments C4a, C3a, and C5a are released and activate mast cells, basophils, and neutrophils. These cells in turn discharge their reactive contents, such as histamine and lysosomal enzymes. These cause increased vascular permeability, contraction of smooth muscle, local edema, attraction of more neutrophils, and tissue destruction, all components of a local and potentially inflammatory reaction.

Thus, as ICs lodge in blood vessel walls, neutrophils migrate to these areas and try to ingest the complex. Neutrophils release enzymes and other toxic metabolites that have the ability to damage vessel walls, surrounding tissue, and cells. If vessels are seriously damaged, the blockage of blood flow may cause tissue necrosis.

In acute (one-shot) serum sickness, the lesions abate as ICs are cleared (Ab excess is attained). For the chronic form, however, the continuous or intermittent presence of Ag fuels the disease state.

Immune complex formation against structural components of host. If autoimmune Ab bind to Ag on the surface of cells, the resultant complex may cause such cells to be disrupted, ingested, or lysed. Attachment of Ab to E or to platelets produces the syndromes of autoimmune hemolytic anemia and immune thrombocytopenia, respectively. Certain drugs may combine with E or platelet membrane components and thereby elicit an Ab response. The presence of Ab and C destroys host cells just as if they were microbes.

An example of a structurally based autoimmune illness is myasthenia gravis. Ab binds to the acetylcholine receptor at the muscle end-plate. The ICs so formed activate C, and a local inflammatory reaction ensues. The results are fewer available acetylcholine receptors and a disorganized receptor region (Chapter 289).

Another example is Goodpasture's syndrome, which is a rare form of human glomerulonephritis and pneumonitis that results from autoantibodies to a protein component of basement membrane of the kidney and lung. C activation occurs, and damage ensues to the basement membrane and adjoining structures.

REFERENCES

Complement System

Frank MM: Complement in the pathophysiology of human disease. N Engl J Med 316:1525, 1987.

Hourcade D, Holers VM, and Atkinson JP: The regulators of complement activation (RCA) gene cluster. Adv Immunol 45:381, 1989.

Joiner KA, Brown EJ, and Frank MM: The role of complement in infectious diseases. Annu Rev Immunol 2:461, 1984.

Kahl LE and Atkinson JP: Autoimmune aspects of complement deficiency. In Tan M, editor: Clinical aspects of autoimmunity, vol 2. New York, 1988, F&M Projects.

Morgan P: Complement—clinical aspects and relevance to disease. San Diego, 1990, Academic.

Reid KBM: Activation and control of the complement system. Essays Biochem 22:69, 1986.

Ross GD, editor: Immunobiology of the complement system: an introduction for research and clinical medicine. Orlando, Fla, 1986, Academic.

Ross SC and Densen P: Complement deficiency states and infection, epidemiology, pathogenesis, and consequences of neisserial and other infections in an immune deficiency. Medicine (Baltimore) 63:243, 1984.

Immune Complex Diseases

Hebert LA and Cosio FG: The erythrocyte–immune complex–glomerulonephritis connection in man. Kidney Int 31:877, 1987.

Lawley TJ et al: A prospective clinical and immunologic analysis of patients with serum sickness. N Engl J Med 311;1407, 1984.

Liszewski MK and Atkinson JP: The role of complement in autoimmunity. In Bigazzi P and Reichlin M, editors: Systemic autoimmunity. New York, 1991, Marcel Dekker.

Mannik M: Immune complexes and immune complex–mediated diseases. In Tan M, editor: Clinical aspects of autoimmunity, vol 2. New York, 1987, F&M Projects.

Schifferli JA, Ng YC, and Peters DK: The role of complement and its receptor in the elimination of immune complexes. N Engl J Med 315:488, 1986.

Schifferli JA and Taylor RP: Physiological and pathological aspects of circulating immune complexes. Kidney Int 35:993, 1989.

CHAPTER

288 Immediate Hypersensitivity

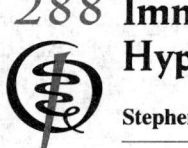

Stephen I. Wasserman

In humans the term *immediate-type hypersensitivity reaction* refers to a collection of signs and symptoms comprised of respiratory, cutaneous, cardiovascular, gastrointestinal, and systemic responses to a variety of pharmacologically active proinflammatory substances called *mediators*. These reactions require the concerted interaction of three major components: sensitizing antibody, specific target cells, and the mediators themselves. The most compelling evidence for the role of these three factors in human disease, both acute and subacute, has been derived from observations in the skin and lung. Studies of patients with allergic asthma demonstrated that inhalation of a specific antigen induced both immediate and delayed (4 to 12 hours) airway dysfunction. Both early and late responses were independent of immunoglobulin G (IgG) antibody and could be abolished by pretreatment with disodium cromoglycate, a drug that can prevent mast cell–mediator release.

More elaborate experiments in the skin have demonstrated that intracutaneous administration of specific antigen to sensitized individuals or of antibody to human IgE can induce both early wheal-and-flare reactions and late inflammatory responses. Passive transfer of purified IgE antibody can prepare the skin of unsensitized hosts for antigen-induced early and late reactions. The early skin lesion is a classic pruritic wheal and flare, whereas the later response is inflammatory and tender and manifested as a poorly demarcated erythematous swelling that persists for 4 to 24 hours. Assessment of the early lesion reveals superficial edema formation with mast cell degranulation. The later inflammatory lesion consists of these elements and also a profound tissue infiltration comprised of neutrophils, eosinophils, basophils, mononuclear leukocytes, and lymphocytes. In addition, vascular damage and even frank necrotizing vasculitis may ensue. In the lung, early responses are manifested by hyperemia, edema, and release of mucus. Later, infiltration by CD4-bearing T lymphocytes and eosinophils is prominent. Any formulation of immediate-type hypersensitivity reactions therefore must also explain these late reactions.

Both the severity and the type of manifestations of either immediate or late reactions may reflect the concentration of the responsible reactants, the complex regulatory interactions involving target tissue sensitivities, or the availability and degradation of mediators. Although several mechanisms exist for generation of individual mediators, this does not diminish their importance in immediate hypersensitivity reactions but rather extends their potential contribution to non-IgE-mediated inflammatory disorders.

ANTIBODIES RESPONSIBLE FOR IMMEDIATE HYPERSENSITIVITY

Antibodies responsible for immediate hypersensitivity reactions (termed *reagins*) first were described by Prausnitz and Küstner in 1921, but protein purification was not accomplished until more than 40 years later. Only IgE reaginic antibody has been conclusively demonstrated in humans. This unique antibody is composed of two light chains, kappa or lambda (κ or λ), and two epsilon (ϵ) heavy chains linked by disulfide bridges. IgE is a glycoprotein (190,000 daltons, 8 S sedimentation coefficient) digested by papain into two Fab' fragments possessing the antigen-binding sites and an Fc fragment responsible for the special cell-binding characteristics of this immunoglobulin (Ig) class. As little as 4×10^{-5} μg antibody nitrogen/ml of human IgE can sensitize human tissues for a reversed passive anaphylactic reaction. This sensitization is caused by the ability of the Fc portion of IgE to bind tightly and persistently (half-life, 8 to 14 days) to specific high-affinity receptors. A second, lower-affinity receptor for the Fc portion of IgE, FcϵRII, has been identified on lymphocytes (CD23).

The production of IgE antibody is under complex regulatory control. Genetic influences are important. Most humans have less than 100 units IgE/ml of serum, but IgE levels are higher in atopic individuals and their families. In animals, IgE synthesis requires both T and B lymphocytes. Neonatal thymectomy abolishes and T lymphocyte transfer restores IgE responses in mice. Moreover, subclasses of T lymphocytes that have helper and suppressor effects on IgE B cells have been demonstrated. Thus removal of T suppressor cells by cytotoxic drugs or irradiation enhances IgE response. Human T lymphocytes secrete two important regulatory factors for IgE synthesis. Interleukin 4 (IL-4) promotes and interferon gamma (IFN-γ) inhibits B cell production of IgE. IgE-rich responses are thought to result from a specific helper T cell population (TH_2) that generates IL-4 but not IFN-γ, whereas TH_1 lymphocytes produce INF-γ but not IL-4 and inhibit IgE production. The precise regulatory relationships of these and perhaps other cytokines are currently under active investigation.

CELLS RESPONSIBLE FOR IMMEDIATE HYPERSENSITIVITY

Mast cells and basophils

The *mast cell* (Fig. 288-1) is a tissue cell of uncertain origin that is present in humans at concentrations of 1 to 10 $\times 10^6$ cells/g of tissue. It is prominent in submucosal loose connective tissue, particularly around blood vessels. Mast cells also are in the mucosa of the upper and lower respiratory tract, in the gastrointestinal and genitourinary systems, and in skin; they also have been found free in the bronchial lumen. Mast cell production, migration, and life span in humans are unknown.

Two types of mast cells have been identified in humans. A *connective tissue* subset of mast cells has its precursor in the bone marrow, but its growth and differentiation are not understood. The second, a *mucosal* subtype, is rich in gastrointestinal mucosa, and its precursor matures under the influence of the T lymphocytes. In rodents, IL-3 is the most important mast cell growth factor. In humans a more complex mix of growth factors, including IL-3, IL-4, IL-9, and IL-10, as well as nerve growth factor and mast cell growth factor (kit ligand, stem cell factor), have been described. Factors produced by fibroblasts have been suggested to stimulate connective tissue mast cell phenotype expression. The connective tissue mast cell contains tryptic and chymotryptic proteases, a cathepsin G–like enzyme, and carboxypeptidase A and is the predominant form in skin and loose connective tissue. The mucosal mast cell predominates in the gut mucosa and alveolar walls and lacks chymase. Individual mast cells contain several hundred metachromatically staining granules with a distinctive subgranular architecture. The mast cell plasma membrane is reduplicated, and within it reside 50,000 to 300,000 receptors for the Fc portion of IgE, functionally defined receptors for the anaphylatoxins (C3a, C5a), and growth factors.

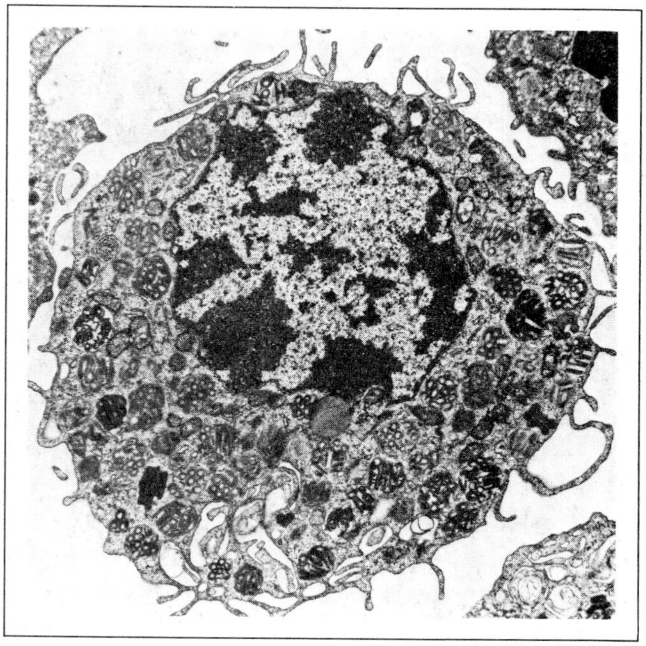

Fig. 288-1. Electron micrograph of a human mast cell. Note numerous membrane projections and presence of intragranular structures of mast cell. (Reprinted from Caulfield JP et al: J Cell Biol 85:299, 1980. With permission of author and publisher.)

Basophils are bone marrow–derived polymorphonuclear leukocytes (PMNs) and are most closely related to eosinophils. Basophils and mast cells originate and develop independently. Basophils possess numerous metachromatically staining granules, but the granules are amorphous in appearance and lack tryptase and chymase. Receptors for the Fc portion of IgE, as well as for C3a and C5a, are present.

The antigen activation of mast cells and basophils requires cross-linking of two adjacent IgE molecules, which

Table 288-1. Vasoactive mediators

Mediator	Structural characteristics	Function	Inhibition	Inactivation	Disease association
Histamine (mast cells)	β-Imidazolyl-ethylamine (111 daltons)	Contracts smooth muscle Increases vascular permeability Stimulates suppressor T lymphocytes (H_2) Generates prostaglandins Enhances (H_1) or inhibits (H_2) chemotaxis Elevates AMP (H_2) and GMP (H_1) Increases mucus production	H_1 and H_2 antihistamines	Histamine (diamine oxidase) or histamine *N*-methyltransferase	Asthma Allergic rhinitis Urticaria Anaphylaxis Mastocytosis
Slow-reacting substance of anaphylaxis, or SRS-A (mast cells, monocytes, eosinophils)	Leukotrienes C = 5 (*S*)-OH-6(*R*)-*S*-glutathionyl-7,9-*trans*,11, 14-*cis*-eicosatetraenoic acid D = 5(*S*)OH-6(*R*)-*S*-cysteinylglycyl-7,9-*trans*,11,14-*cis*-eicosatetraenoic acid E = 5(*S*)-OH-6(*R*)-*S*-cysteinyl-7,9-*trans*,11,14-*cis*-eicosatetraenoic acid	Contracts smooth muscle Increases vascular permeability Synergistic with histamine Generates prostaglandins Vasodepressor Cutaneous Vasoconstriction (C) Vasodilatation (D, E) Increases mucus production Depresses cardiac performance	FPL-55712	Peroxidases Lipoxygenase Peroxides Peptidases Hypochlorous acid	Anaphylaxis
Platelet-activating factor, or PAF (neutrophils, monocytes, mast cells, eosinophils)	1-*O*-2-acetyl-*sn*-glyceryl-3-phosporylcholine	Release of platelet amines Platelet and neutrophil aggregation Sequestration of platelets	Unknown	Phospholipases Acetylhydrolase	Anaphylaxis Physical urticaria

		Decrease in blood pressure; Bronchospasm; Increased vasopermeability			
Prostaglandins					
D_2 (mast cells)	C_{20} fatty acids	Contracts smooth muscle; Vasodepressor; Elevates AMP	Synthesis blocked by nonsteroidal anti-inflammatory agents	Specific dehydrogenases	Asthma; Allergic rhinitis; Mastocytosis
E_2 (many cell types)		Relaxes smooth muscle, elevates AMP			
$F_{2\alpha}$ (many cell types)		Lowers AMP, contracts smooth muscle			
I_2 (many cell types)		Elevates AMP, inhibits platelet aggregation, contracts smooth muscle			
Thromboxane A_2 (many cell types)		Contracts smooth muscle; Stimulates platelet aggregation			
Endoperoxides (G_2, H_2) (many cell types)		Contract smooth muscle			
Prostaglandin-generating factor	Peptide (about 1400 daltons)	Induces prostaglandin production from surrounding cells			
Adenosine	Nucleoside	Inhibits platelet aggregation; Enhances mast cell preformed-mediator release; Constricts bronchial smooth muscle in asthmatic persons; Coronary vasodilatation	Xanthines	Adenosine deaminase	Asthma

cAMP, Cyclic adenosine monophosphate; cGMP, cyclic guanosine monophosphate.

translates through the membrane receptor a signal that initiates degranulation. The sequence of noncytolytic secretory events that result in degranulation includes adenyl cyclase activation, lipid metabolism, phospholipase activation, arachidonic acid liberation, calcium influx, cyclic adenosine monophosphate (cAMP) generation, protein kinase utilization, granule dissolution, granule-to-granule membrane fusion, granule–plasma membrane fusion, and finally, discharge of granule constituents to the external milieu. After antigen activation of sensitized mast cells, this entire sequence is completed in less than 5 minutes, but it requires 10 to 30 minutes in basophils. In addition to being degranulated by antigen and anaphylatoxin, connective tissue–type mast cells may be degranulated by such nonimmunologic stimuli as highly charged antibiotics, radiocontrast media, opiates, various neuropeptides, and adenosine triphosphate (ATP).

MEDIATORS

The activation and degranulation of mast cells and basophils cause the release of preformed, granule-associated *(primary)* mediators and the generation and release of unstored *(secondary)* mediators. Table 288-1 lists these mediators in terms of function. Such mediator functions include smooth muscle reactivity, chemotactic potential, enzymatic activity, structural properties, as well as a group of cytokines. The mediators have been defined best for the rodent mast cell, but it is presumed that the human mast cell has similar properties.

Smooth muscle–reactive mediators

Histamine, the decarboxylation product of histidine, is ionically bound to the proteoglycan-protein backbones of mast cell and basophil granules. Histamine is displaced by sodium exchange in the extracellular fluid. Histamine is catabolized either by oxidative deamination (histaminase) or by combined demethylation and oxidative deamination (histamine *N*-methyltransferase plus monoamine oxidase). The effects of histamine are expressed as a constriction of smooth muscle and an increase in the distance between endothelial cells of venules, which thus increases the potential for transudation of serum and extravasation of leukocytes. The biologic activities of histamine follow its interaction with three specific classes of receptors on target cells. Receptors designated H_1 predominate in skin and smooth muscle and are inhibited by classic antihistamines, whereas H_2 receptors are selectively blocked by ranitidine and cimetidine. H_3 receptors are defined by selective agonists and regulate histamine production and release, particularly in the nervous system. Pulmonary bronchoconstriction, vasodilatation, and increased cyclic guanosine monophosphate (GMP) are H_1 effects, whereas H_2 effects include elevations in gastric acid secretion and AMP and inhibition of human lymphocyte–mediated cytotoxicity. The wheal-and-flare response to histamine in the skin, adverse effects on the heart, and headache are caused by a combined effect on H_1 and H_2 receptors.

Products of arachidonic acid oxidation

Arachidonic acid is mobilized from cell membrane phospholipids by the action of phospholipase A_2 or by the concerted action of phospholipase C and diacylglycerol lipase. Arachidonic acid then may be converted through a cyclo-oxygenase–dependent pathway to prostaglandins (PGs) and thromboxanes or by a lipoxygenase enzyme to hydroperoxyeicosatetraenoic acid (HPETE) and then to monohydroxy fatty acids or leukotrienes (LTs). *Prostaglandin D_2* (PGD_2) has been identified as the major cyclo-oxygenase product produced after immunologic activation of human cutaneous mast cells, whereas lesser amounts are generated by mucosal mast cells. Other metabolites have been demonstrated after IgE-dependent activation of chopped human lung and may reflect the action of histamine or a peptide termed *prostaglandin-generating factor*. Both animal and human smooth muscle is constricted by PGD_2, and it causes intense bronchoconstriction in asthmatic persons. PGD_2 is a potent inhibitor of platelet activation and is thought to be responsible for flushing and hypotensive episodes in patients with mastocytosis. It can cause wheal-and-flare reactions in skin and potentiates chemotactic responses induced by other mediators (see following discussion).

The action of a 5-lipoxygenase enzyme found in mast cells, eosinophils, neutrophils, and mononuclear leukocytes generates 5-HPETE, which then is further metabolized to a monohydroxy fatty acid (5-HETE) or to leukotriene A_4 (LTA_4). LTA_4 is further metabolized to the chemoattractant dihydroxy fatty acid LTB_4 (mast cells, neutrophils) or, by the addition of the tripeptide glutathione (cys-gly-glu), to LTC_4 (eosinophils, mast cells). Further metabolism of LTC_4 by γ-glutamyl transpeptidase to LTD_4 and by other peptidases, including a neutrophil dipeptidase to LTE_4, occurs and varies in different tissues. Thus LTE_4 is a prominent product in the intestine, and LTC_4 is prominent in the nose. Three molecules (LTC_4, LTD_4, LTE_4) make up the *slow-reacting substance of anaphylaxis* (SRS-A).

These LTs are prominent products of human mast cells. They interact with a specific receptor, and the sulfidopeptide and carbonyl domains appear most important to their function. LTs are degraded by oxidant reactions. The sulfidopeptide LTs are important constrictors of smooth muscle and induce bronchospasm, wheal-and-flare vasopermeability reactions, increases in mucus release, and decreased cardiac performance, whereas LTB_4 depresses lymphocyte function. In most assays, LTD_4 is the most potent and LTE_4 the least active leukotriene. LTE_4 is thought to induce prolonged, nonspecific bronchial hyperreactivity.

Platelet-activating factor (PAF) is a unique phospholipid generated from mast cells by IgE-dependent mechanisms. Human macrophages, neutrophils, and eosinophils can also generate this molecule. Its structure is 1-*O*-acyl-2-acetyl-*sn*-glycerol-3-phosphorylcholine. The molecule is most active when the acyl group is C16 or C18; removal of the acetyl group or the choline moiety totally inactivates PAF. Thus PAF can be degraded by an acid-labile serum acetylhydrolase or by several phospholipases. PAF is capable of inducing aggregation of human platelets and secretion of their serotonin. In animals, PAF causes sequestration of platelets in the lung or skin and is a potent hypotensive agent. In humans, PAF is a strong bronchoconstrictor and can induce wheal-and-flare vasopermeability responses. Inhalation of PAF also induces long-lasting bronchial hyperreactivity to nonspecific irritants. In animals, PAF also produces neutrophil activation and aggregation, hypotension, and vascular collapse, as well as adverse effects on cardiac performance. Pulmonary mechanical changes depend on platelet activation, whereas the other effects of PAF do not.

The nucleoside *adenosine* is released from activated mast cells in vitro and is increased in the blood of humans after antigen-provoked bronchospasm. Adenosine is a potent inhibitor of platelet activation, enhances IgE-mediated mast cell responses, induces bronchospasm in asthmatic persons (but not in normal individuals), is a potent coronary vasodilator, and can alter lymphocyte function. It is removed by its active uptake into cells or by destruction via adenosine deaminase. Adenosine interacts with cell surface receptors to increase (A_2) or decrease (A_1) intracellular cAMP concentration. In mast cells, A_2 receptors predominate. Adenosine interaction with receptors is prevented by xanthines, and its uptake is inhibited by dipyridamole.

Chemotactic mediators

Eosinophil chemotactic factors. A low-molecular-weight peptide (300 to 500 daltons) has been identified in anaphylactic supernatants of challenged human lung, in isolated human lung mast cells, and in the circulations of patients with experimentally induced physical urticaria and antigen-induced bronchospasm. Also, human mast cells contain preformed, immunologically releasable, chemotactic factors (1500 to 3000 daltons) with specificity for eosinophilic PMNs. Factors of similar molecular weight and chemotactic specificity have been identified in the circulation of patients after experimental induction of physical urticaria or antigen-provoked bronchospasm.

High-molecular-weight neutrophil chemotactic factor. HMW-NCF has been described in human lung fragments, in leukemic basophils, and in the sera of patients with physical urticaria or asthma after physical or antigen challenge. HMW-NCF is a 660,000-dalton, neutral protein that attracts and deactivates neutrophils.

Other chemotactic factors. Chemotactic factors with specificity for both neutrophilic and eosinophilic PMNs can be generated by the lipoxygenase-dependent pathway of arachidonic acid metabolism. PAF is also a potent leukoattractant, particularly for eosinophils. Less well characterized are factors chemotactic for T and B lymphocytes, monocytes, and basophils.

MAST CELL ENZYMES AND PROTEOGLYCANS

Tryptase

A preformed enzyme called tryptase is released subsequent to antigen challenge of IgE-sensitized human mast cells. This enzyme has a tryptic specificity and can cleave kininogen, C3, and other proteins susceptible to tryptic proteases. Tryptase is not inhibited by serum antitrypsins and is stabilized by its ionic binding to heparin. It is present in all human mast cells. A captopril-insensitive, chymotryptic protease capable of generating angiotensin is present in connective tissue–type human mast cells. A cathepsin G–like protease and a carboxypeptidase are also present in connective tissue mast cells.

Lysosomal enzymes

Myeloperoxidase, superoxide dismutase, arylsulfatases A and B, β-glucuronidase, hexosaminidases, and amino peptidase have been identified in isolated human or rat mast cells. These lysosomal enzymes can degrade ground substance proteoglycans.

Heparin

This sulfated, metachromatic mucopolysaccharide has been identified in the mast cells of human lung and skin. Human heparin interacts with human antithrombin to accelerate anticoagulation. Heparin may interfere with several complement functions, liberates lipoprotein lipase, binds to platelet factor IV and to tryptase to prevent its inactivation, and is a potent endothelial growth factor.

Chondroitin 4-sulfate and 6-sulfate proteoglycans

These proteoglycans predominate in human basophils. In mucosal mast cells, highly sulfated varieties of chondroitin sulfate also are present.

Cytokines

Rodent mast cells have been demonstrated to synthesize and release a variety of cytokines and growth factors, including tumor necrosis factor alpha (TNF-α); interleukins 3, 4, 5, and 6; and granulocyte-macrophage colony-stimulating factor (GM-CSF). IL-4 has also been identified in human lung mast cells. A role for these cytokines has been postulated in mast cell growth and differentiation; in eosinophil growth, maintenance, recruitment, and activation; in IgE synthesis; and in fibrosis. The pattern of mast cell cytokine synthesis is similar to that of TH_2 helper T lymphocytes and may be an important contributor to allergic inflammation, such as that noted in asthma (Chapter 300).

SUMMARY

The relevance of the preformed and newly generated mediators released by IgE-dependent and IgE-independent activation of mast cells and basophils to human immediate hypersensitivity reactions has been shown (1) by analysis of their varied and potent biologic effects using purified mediators, (2) by identification of mediators in blood or tissue in human allergic disorders, and (3) by the known pathophysiology of allergic disease.

Mediators have the ability to induce both immediate-onset, short-lived and delayed-onset, prolonged inflammatory events. The former, presumably caused by the smooth muscle–reactive mediators, are exemplified by wheal-and-flare reactions, acute decrease in blood pressure, and smooth muscle contraction of the type noted in gastrointestinal disturbances or airway dysfunction. The more persistent inflammatory reactions represent a response to the concerted effect of enhanced permeability, activation of other amplification mediators (complement, clotting, fibrinolytic, and kinin-generating systems), leukocyte infiltration resulting from chemotactic mediators, and cytokine release and tissue destruction by active enzymes. A good example is late-onset bronchospasm. The prolonged effect of antigen may explain the chronic abnormalities seen in patients with asthma (bronchial hyperreactivity, mucus formation, smooth muscle hypertrophy, cellular infiltration, subepithelial fibrosis, epithelial damage) and also may explain the lack of immediate correlation between antigen exposure and asthmatic response noted in many patients.

REFERENCES

Irani A and Schwartz LB: Mast cell heterogeneity. Clin Exp Allergy 19:143, 1989.

Ishizaka K: Control of IgE synthesis. In Middleton EE et al, editors: Allergy: principles and practice, ed 4. St Louis, 1992, Mosby–Year Book.

Ishizaka T: Mechanisms of IgE-mediated hypersensitivity. In Middleton EE et al, editors: Allergy: principles and practice, ed 4. St Louis, 1992, Mosby–Year Book.

Plaut M et al: Mast cell lines produce lymphokines in response to crosslinkage of FcERI or to calcium ionophore. Nature 339:64, 1989.

Solley GO et al: The late phase of the immediate wheal and flare skin reaction: its dependence on IgE antibodies. J Clin Invest 58:408, 1978.

Wasserman SI: Mediators of immediate hypersensitivity. J Allergy Clin Immunol 72:101, 1983.

CHAPTER

289 Tolerance and Autoimmunity

Alfred D. Steinberg

Autoimmune diseases are manifested by immune responses against self antigens (autoantigens). One such disease, systemic lupus erythematosus (SLE), is an organ-nonspecific disease characterized by the production of antibodies reactive with many different self antigens, including many nuclear antigens. A related disorder, polymyositis, is characterized by a more limited autoantibody repertoire, as well as by cell-mediated immunity against muscle cells. Certain autoimmune diseases are caused by antibodies reacting with specific receptors: Graves' disease, the thyroid-stimulating hormone receptor, and myasthenia gravis, the acetylcholine receptor. In others a cell-mediated immune reaction may occur against the target organ, such as the pancreatic islet cell in juvenile diabetes. In all these autoimmune diseases, an apparent loss of self tolerance occurs, in that there are immune responses "against" self antigens.

Not all of the anti–self-immunity is induced by self antigens. Some autoimmunity originates as immune responses to foreign agents. A severe infection with particular strains of group-A beta-hemolytic streptococci (especially if the organisms have thick capsules, which make them unusually virulent and immunogenic) may induce a vigorous immune response against streptococcal antigens; some of the antibodies induced also react with human heart antigens. Thus infection with a group-A beta-hemolytic streptococcus and the resultant immune response leads to the disease acute rheumatic fever. However, many individuals colonized by such apparently pathogenic streptococci do not develop autoimmunity. Therefore, in dealing with other diseases in which the causes are less well understood, one should recognize that although autoimmunity might be induced by exogenous agents, additional factors may be critical to the outcome. Loss of self-tolerance appears to play a primary role in some diseases and a critical role in the others. Studies of experimental tolerance have helped us to understand mechanisms by which such tolerance might be lost in association with disease.

EXPERIMENTAL TOLERANCE

Experimental tolerance may be induced in many different ways. One example, drug-induced tolerance, provides a simple framework for conceptualization. In this form of tolerance, many of the lymphocytes reactive with a given antigen are eliminated by sequential administration of the antigen and the killing of the reactive lymphocytes with a cytotoxic drug such as cyclophosphamide. A mouse is given an antigen, such as sheep erythrocytes. The antigen administration causes specific proliferation of T and B cells stimulated by the various antigenic determinants on the foreign erythrocytes. Next, cyclophosphamide is administered to selectively kill proliferating cells. Subsequent immunization with sheep erythrocytes leads to a blunted response relative to a control mouse given another antigen plus cyclophosphamide.

Several additional methods have been used to induce tolerance in animals: (1) giving an antigen to a very young animal, (2) deaggregating an antigen to make it less immunogenic and more toleragenic, (3) giving very small or very large doses of an antigen, (4) attaching an antigen or hapten to a molecule that tends to induce tolerance rather than immunity, (5) binding the antigen to an autologous lymphocyte, (6) placing the antigen directly in the thymus, (7) giving multiple injections of an antigen, and (8) feeding the antigen. All these methods are designed to perturb the immune system so as to predispose to the induction of a hyporesponsive state with regard to the particular antigen, by either reducing the immunogenicity of the antigen in question or limiting the animal's ability to mount a full (normal) immune response to a subsequent immunizing dose of that antigen.

Giving antigen to a very young animal allows antigen to be presented to an immune system skewed toward suppression and away from immunity. As a result, there is not only impaired immunity, but also induction of a memory for hyporesponsiveness to that antigen (rather than of the hyperresponsiveness that might have occurred had the recipient been an adult). Deaggregation allows the antigen to interact with specific receptors on lymphocytes without immunogenic presentation of antigen by potent antigen-presenting cells. Very small doses of antigen may induce antigen-specific suppressor cells to function without sufficient stimulation of helper T cells and B cells. This mechanism may be important for induction of tolerance to certain self antigens present in low concentrations. Feeding antigen and coupling antigen to immunocytes induce suppressor function preferentially relative to helper function.

The relevance of tolerance to autoimmune diseases is intuitively obvious. Moreover, strains of mice that develop spontaneously a generalized autoimmune disease resembling human SLE (NZB, [NZB × NZW] F1, BXSB, MRL-1pr/1pr mice) are defective in that they normally fail to be made tolerant to many tolerogens. It appears that both the tolerance defect and the autoimmune process may be part of an immune abnormality that underlies autoimmunity.

Mice injected with deaggregated bovine gamma globulin (BGG) and later challenged with aggregated (immunogenic) BGG normally fail to make a good antibody response to the subsequent challenge with aggregated BGG. Tolerance occurs if either the T cell population or the B cell population is made tolerant. Although both B and T cells normally are made tolerant, the time courses and strengths of tolerance in those two populations differ. Tolerance in the T cell population can be induced with very small doses of tolerogen, occurs very fast, and lasts a long time. B cells require much larger doses of tolerogen and take longer for induction, and the period of being completely tolerant is much shorter. For most of the period of tolerance, therefore, the T cell population is responsible.

Since the tolerance is maintained primarily by the T cell population, one can overcome it by bypassing the T cell tolerance so as to stimulate B cells directly to produce antibody. Thus administration of bacterial lipopolysaccharide (endotoxin), 8-substituted guanosines, or other polyclonal B cell activators at the time of administration of tolerogen prevents tolerance, since the early tolerance is entirely T cell mediated. Similarly, many weeks after tolerance induction, when B cell tolerance has waned, such agents are able to break tolerance.

When NZB and other mice with lupus-type disease are injected systemically with tolerogenic gamma globulin, they fail to be made tolerant. As a result, when subsequently challenged with immunogenic gamma globulin, they produce substantial amounts of antibody (as if no tolerogen had been given). Since androgens tend to counteract the tolerance defect, this may help to explain the relative increase of SLE in females (Table 289-1). The NZB tolerance defect resides in the bone marrow stem cells, which give rise to mature T lymphocytes.

A similar tolerance defect is observed when NZB mice are given the tolerogen by mouth. For most mice, such oral administration results in tolerance, even if antigen is not deaggregated. NZB mice fail to be made tolerant. In normal mice the tolerance is mediated by suppressor cells; in the NZB mice, however, suppressor cells are only transiently induced, and within 3 days suppressor function is lost.

Table 289-1. Defective tolerance induction in NZB mice: studies of tolerance to bovine gamma globulin (BGG) in (NZB × DBA/2) F1 radiation chimeras

Recipients*	Thymus donor	Marrow donor	Response to challenge
Male or female	DBA	DBA	+
Male or female	DBA	NZB	+
Male	NZB	DBA	+
Female	NZB	DBA	+++
Castrated male	NZB	DBA	+++
Female plus androgens	NZB	DBA	+
Male or female	NZB	NZB	+++

*All animals shown were given the tolerogenic ultracentrifuged BGG and later were challenged with immunogenic BGG in adjuvant, and the antibody response was measured. Additional control animals (not shown) were challenged without receiving the ultracentrifuged BGG.

Defective systemic and oral tolerance in the NZB mice could result from either the lack of adequate suppressor function or some interference with such suppressor function. The data indicate that these mice have T cells that prevent suppressor cells from functioning. If there is an expansion in lupus mice of T cells that produce factors that drive B cells to proliferate and differentiate, such T cells would act as exogenously administered lipopolysaccharide to bypass T cell tolerance and directly stimulate B cells to produce antibody. This may be the explanation for the defect in experimental tolerance to BGG in NZB mice. The same mechanism also may explain loss of self-tolerance to a variety of self antigens, the production of large amounts of antibodies reactive with self T cells and deoxyribonucleic acid (DNA), and a systemic autoimmune disease (Fig. 289-1).

One mechanism by which self-reactive cells are rendered inoperative is called *apoptosis,* programmed cell death. It is believed that certain self-reactive cells will undergo apoptosis during selection in the thymus. In addition, peripheral apoptosis accounts for postthymic deletion. Researchers have been searching for defects in apoptosis as a cause of autoimmunity. One candidate has been the *fas* gene product, a cell surface protein that is critical to apoptosis. Recent studies of lupus-prone MRL–*1pr*/*1pr* mice suggest that the autoimmunity-associated *1pr* gene encodes a defective *fas* protein. This finding provides a mechanism for widespread loss of tolerance, giving rise to generalized autoimmunity.

Studies of transgenic mice

Transgenic mice carry an introduced gene or genes that may be expressed from very early in development. Such mice

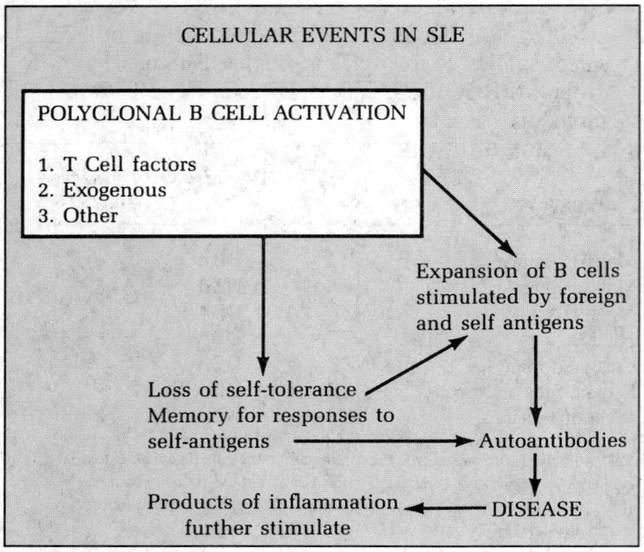

Fig. 289-1. Polyclonal B cell activation serves as the initial abnormality in systemic lupus erythematosus (SLE). Polyclonal immune stimulation may be caused by genetic elements that lead to increased production of endogenous factors able to augment B cell proliferation/differentiation or exogenous activators (e.g., viral or bacterial). Such factors also serve to break self-tolerance mechanisms. These processes are largely antigen independent. In the absence of adequate downregulating control elements, autoimmune reactions progress without inhibition. These are largely antigen dependent and give rise to pathogenic autoantibodies. The resulting inflammation leads to the release of self antigens (autoantigens) which further stimulate the process.

allow studies of the interaction between gene expression and the immune system, a new approach to tolerance. Mice expressing the lysozyme transgene and others carrying both an antilysozyme immunoglobulin (Ig) transgene and a lysozyme transgene have been analyzed. In the double-transgenic mice, tolerance occurs to lysozyme: antilysozyme B cells do not produce antibody. This tolerance is not caused by deletion of lysozyme-reactive (self-reactive) B cells, since transfer of those B cells to nontransgenic mice allows them to produce antilysozyme antibody when stimulated by antigen and helper T cells. In contrast, when the B cells are transferred to lysozyme single-transgenic mice, the continuous production of high concentrations of lysozyme maintains tolerance. In vitro studies of B cells from double-transgenic mice show that bacterial lipopolysaccharide is able to induce both proliferation and antibody production by previously tolerant B cells. These studies suggest that certain forms of tolerance may involve downregulation (anergy) rather than deletion of "self-reactive" B cells. Moreover, a loss of such tolerance may be induced by polyclonal immune activators such as bacterial lipopolysaccharide. Thus an endogenous immune stimulatory environment (equivalent in effect to exogenous lipopolysaccharide) or excessive sensitivity to environmental stimulators may contribute to loss of self-tolerance.

In contrast to this transgenic tolerance model, relevant especially to humoral autoimmunity, other transgenic experiments point to deletion of self-reactive B cells. Thus a mouse bearing the anti–major histocompatibility complex (MHC) class I Ig transgene demonstrates deletion of self-reactive B cells. Such a mechanism may be especially important for avoiding organ-specific autoimmune diseases.

INDUCTION OF ORGAN-SPECIFIC AUTOIMMUNITY

Induction of organ-specific autoimmunity is somewhat more straightforward than that of organ-nonspecific autoimmunity. If one prepares transgenic mice such that they express the transgene product on cell surfaces after the neonatal period, one has a model for neoantigen expression. When such a neoantigen is expressed on an endocrine or exocrine gland, an immune response against that tissue occurs; if the response is sufficiently intense, destruction of the gland may occur. This same destructive process is induced by viral infection of a gland and expression of viral antigens on the cell surfaces. A similar destructive process may be brought about by induction of class II MHC gene products (Ia molecules) on glandular cell surfaces, so that self antigens are presented to the immune system in a manner analogous to foreign antigen presentation by Ia-bearing antigen-presenting cells. Destruction of the pancreatic islets in juvenile-onset diabetes may result from such a process.

Induction of Ia molecules on gland cell surfaces may occur through several different mechanisms; however, viral infection is likely to be one of the most important. If a viral infection causes an inflammatory response in a gland, local production of interferon (IFN) or tumor necrosis factor (TNF) induces Ia expression on cells in the gland. The Ia molecules could then serve to target adjacent self antigens to autoreactive T cells, which would then initiate an immune response against the gland. This process can lead to autoimmune thyroiditis. An unusual expression of Ia molecules has been demonstrated on the thyroid glands of patients with autoimmune thyroiditis.

A person's ability to mount an immune response against a self antigen by the mere induction of a class II MHC product on the cell surface indicates the fragile balance between health and disease. However, other factors appear necessary for disease. One important factor is the extent of the immune response. People with the genotype HLA-A1,B8,DR3 tend to be especially predisposed to autoimmune phenomena and make especially strong antibody responses to a variety of antigens. Such individuals probably manifest a shift in the immune thermostat toward increased immunity. Such a shift may have adaptive value in guarding against infections; however, the trade-off is increased predisposition to loss of self-tolerance and the development of autoimmune diseases.

MOLECULAR MIMICRY

By adaptive evolution, structure-function–dictated coevolution, or purely random processes, many bacteria and viruses share striking structural homologies with mammals.

The presence on viruses or bacteria of structures with strong homology to host self antigens leads to the possibility of antiself responses being commingled with normal defensive immunity. Moreover, the mimicry involved in such situations often is a critical adaptation to allow the foreign invader to enter cells or otherwise facilitate its life cycle. For example, a virus with a structure homologous to a hormone would be able to interact with the receptor for that hormone to facilitate entry into the cell. However, an immune response against such a virus might include an autoimmune component.

IDIOTYPY AS MECHANISM OF AUTOREACTIVITY

A process similar to molecular mimicry also may induce autoimmunity. This process involves not homology but a lock-and-key structural relationship. For example, some organisms have evolved so as to use receptors on mammalian cells for entry. An antibody response may be induced against the portion of the organism that serves as a ligand for the receptor. Such a response includes a population of antibodies (called *Ab 1*) having antibody with combining sites with structures *(idiotopes)* closely related structurally to portions of the original receptor. The structures or idiotopes are able to induce an antibody response: the resulting antibodies (*Ab 2,* or second antibody in the series) are called *anti-idiotype antibodies* because they recognize the relatively unique structures (idiotopes) on a population of antibodies made by the body. However, the anti-idiotype antibodies (Ab 2), by virtue of recognizing the idiotope, also recognize the closely related structure on the original receptor. Such antibodies may be observed as antireceptor antibodies.

Just as idiotypy may be found for antibody molecules, in an analogous fashion, idiotypy occurs for T cell receptors for antigen critical for cell-mediated immunity. A variety of autoimmune diseases may result partly or completely from such a T cell response. In addition, skewing of the T cell repertoire toward T cells that recognize Ia molecules might generally increase T cell activation and lead to autoimmunity.

IMPLICATIONS FOR THERAPY

Understanding the mechanisms of tolerance induction and interference could lead to strategies for preventing or treating patients with autoimmune diseases. For many years, studies of experimental tolerance appeared to bear little relationship to human disease. A breakthrough came with the application of human immunology to Rh factor mismatches. An Rh (D)-negative woman married to an Rh (D)-positive man is subject to being immunized by fetal Rh (D)-positive erythrocytes (Rh [D]positive inherited from the father) that enter the maternal circulation at delivery. When such immunization occurs, maternal antibodies develop that, in subsequent pregnancies, enter the fetal circulation and react with fetal erythrocytes to produce erythroblastosis fetalis. Once it is produced, the maternal antibody cannot easily be inhibited. However, the antibody can be prevented by injecting the mother with antibodies to Rh (D) within 3 days of delivery. By extension, many possible manipulations of the immune system seem possible for dealing with a great variety of autoimmune diseases. For example, there are trials of oral tolerance with a self-antigen in patients with cell-mediated autoimmune disorders.

REFERENCES

Bottazzo GF, Pujol-Borrell R, and Hanafusa T: Role of aberrant HLA-DR expression and antigen presentation in induction of endocrine autoimmunity. Lancet 2:1115, 1983.

Claman HN: Immunological tolerance. In Samter M, editor: Immunological diseases. Boston, 1988, Little, Brown.

Fuchs EJ and Matzinger P: B cells turn off virgin but not memory T cells. Science 258:1156, 1992.

Karjalainen J et al: A bovine albumin peptide as a possible trigger of insulin-dependent diabetes mellitus. N Engl J Med 327:302, 1992.

Lehmann PV et al: Spreading of T-cell autoimmunity to cryptic determinants of an autoantigen. Nature 358:155, 1992.

Marrack P and Kappler J: The staphylococcal enterotoxins and their relatives. Science 248:705, 1990.

Posselt AM et al: Prevention of autoimmune diabetes in the BB rat by intrathymic islet transplantation at birth. Science 256:1321, 1992.

Steinberg AD et al: Systemic lupus erythematosus. Ann Intern Med 115:548, 1991.

Steinberg AD et al: Theoretical and experimental approaches to generalized autoimmunity. Immunol Rev 118:129, 1990.

Watanabe-Fukunga R et al: Lymphoproliferation disorder in mice explained by defects in Fas antigen that mediates apoptosis, Nature 356:314, 1992.

Webb S, Morris C, and Sprent C: Extrathymic tolerance of mature T cells: clonal elimination as a consequence of immunity, Cell 63:1249, 1990.

Weigle WO: The effect of lipopolysaccharide desensitization on the regulation of in vivo induction of immunologic tolerance and antibody production and in vitro release of IL-1. J Immunol 142:1107, 1989.

Weiner HL et al: Double-blind pilot trial of oral tolerization with myelin antigens in multiple sclerosis. Science 259:1321, 1993.

LABORATORY AND DIAGNOSTIC TESTS II

CHAPTER

290 Complement Measurements

M. Kathryn Liszewski
John P. Atkinson

The proteolytic reactions characterizing the complement system are irreversible and result in cleaved proteins that are rapidly cleared from the circulation. Thus an ongoing immunologic event that is activating the complement system in vivo may produce a decrease in plasma levels of these proteins if catabolism outstrips synthesis. Conversely, the abatement of the complement-activating stimulus may be paralleled by a return of the complement levels toward normal. Localized infectious processes, such as pneumonia, or immune-complex–mediated syndromes, such as certain forms of arthritis, are usually not associated with a change in static levels. A chronic systemic illness with circulating high levels of immune complexes, such as systemic lupus erythematosus (SLE) or cryoglobulinemia, is most frequently associated with hypocomplementemia.

METHODS OF MEASUREMENT

Complement can be assessed either by its activity in immune hemolysis or by its reactivity in antigenic assays. Functional assays have been devised to measure either groups of components (e.g., classic pathway, alternative pathway, terminal sequence) or individual components (e.g., C1, C4, C2, C3). The total hemolytic complement (THC, or CH_{50}), which measures activation of the entire classic pathway, and immunoassays are generally used in clinical practice. Assays for C4 and C3 are the most widely available. Radial immunodiffusion, which measures the size of a precipitin ring formed in an agarose gel containing specific antibody to an individual complement protein, and nephelometric immunoassays, which detect changes in the intensity of light scatter as complement proteins interact with their specific antibodies, are often used. The detection of activation or cleavage products such as the anaphylatoxins (C3a, C5a), the cleavage peptides released from C4 (C4d), C3 (C3d), and factor B (Bb) or of neoantigens resulting from activation fragments are also becoming more available. Their clinical usefulness remains to be determined.

INTERPRETATION OF TEST RESULTS

Several of the complement proteins (C1, C2, D) are heat labile. Consequently, THC assays require careful collection, processing, and storage of specimens. A common cause of a depressed serum THC is improper specimen handling. The THC provides a functional assessment of the classic pathway based on the ability of the test serum to lyse sheep erythrocytes (E) optimally sensitized with rabbit antibody. All nine components of the classic pathway (C1 to C9) are required to give a normal THC. A THC of 200 means that at a dilution of 1:200 the tested serum lysed 50% of the antibody-coated sheep E in the standard assay system (Table 290-1).

The most common indication for ordering a THC is in the initial evaluation of a patient with a rheumatic disease or unexplained recurrent pyogenic (especially neisserial) infection. For an SLE patient, a THC of 0 most likely indicates a severe depletion of the early components of the classic pathway or a deficiency of C2. However, for those with recurrent neisserial infections, a 0 value suggests a deficiency of C5, C6, C7, or C8 (Chapter 298).

The range of normal complement protein concentrations is quite broad, usually approximating ±50% of the normal population mean. Complement proteins are acute phase reactants, and levels tend to increase, even with minor intercurrent illnesses, thereby increasing the scatter in the "normal" population. Thus the interpretation of an isolated static value from an individual may be difficult. Serial changes in levels for a given patient over a period of time are generally more informative than is comparison with an absolute range of normal. Low values usually suggest ongoing disease, whereas normal or high values are less helpful.

ALTERATIONS IN DISEASE

Complement proteins are acute phase reactants and, as with several other proteins such as fibrinogen and C-reactive protein, tend to be elevated in many inflammatory conditions. Such elevations are common and nonspecific and therefore of little clinical usefulness. In most infectious diseases, complement values are normal or elevated. Depressions associated with in vivo complement activation are more informative. Virtually any disease that gives rise to circulating immune complexes can cause hypocomplementemia, provided the complexes contain immunoglobulin G or M (IgG, IgM) antibodies capable of activating complement (see the box at lower right).

In SLE, THC levels are depressed at some time in more than 50% of patients, whereas levels are generally normal in patients with discoid lupus. As a rule, complement depressions are associated with increased severity of disease, especially renal disease. Component analyses have demonstrated low levels of C1, C4, C2, and C3. Serial observations often reveal decreased levels preceding clinical exacerbations; reduction in C4 tends to occur before reduction in C3, THC, and other components. As attacks subside, levels return toward normal in reverse order, with C4 tending to remain depressed longest. However, certain considerations must be taken into account when interpreting the result of clinical assays. Normally, C4 and factor B are present in concentrations of one-fourth to one-sixth that of C3. For C3 to drop below normal, a substantial activation of either the classic or alternative pathway must be ongoing. Additionally, the quoted normal levels represent ±2 standard deviations, and individual baseline (predisease) levels of C3 or C4 are usually not available. Since normal C4 levels are 16 to 48 mg/dl, it would require less classic pathway activation to depress C4 values from 20 than from 40. Such considerations must be taken into account when interpreting the results of these clinical assays.

Serum levels of THC, C3, and C4 are usually normal or elevated in patients with rheumatoid arthritis. Depressed levels are associated with extra-articular manifestations of the disease, particularly vasculitis. Such patients usually also have high titers of rheumatoid factor and immune complexes in their serum. Synovial fluid complement levels are usually low in patients with rheumatoid arthritis when measured by activity determinations but may be normal when measured by immunoassay. The presence of antigenic fragments that are nonfunctional (which have not been cleared from the joint space and remain reactive in the immunoassay) may account for these findings. Because measurement

Table 290-1. Interpretation of results of complement determinations

Case	Test results*				Interpretation
	THC (units/ml)	C4 (mg/dl)	B (mg/dl)	C3 (mg/dl)	
1	300	45	50	200	Acute phase protein response; any type of inflammatory condition may produce this set of values
2	125	12	30	120	Classic pathway activation (mild)
3	100	8	30	80	Classic pathway activation (moderate)
4	50	4 or <8†	30	50	Classic pathway activation (marked)
5	<10	24	30	140	Congenital deficiency or in vitro activation‡
6	75	8	10	50	Classic pathway plus engagement of feedback loop or activation of both classic and alternative pathways
7	75	24	5	50	Alternative pathway activation

From Ross G, editor: Immunobiology of the complement system. Orlando, 1986, Academic.
*Normal values: THC (total hemolytic complement), 150-250 units/ml (will vary depending on the assay system used); C4, 16-48 mg/dl; factor B, 20-40 mg/dl; C3, 100-180 mg/dl.
†The sensitivity of some assays is only to about 8 mg/dl. Therefore a value of <8 only implies this fact and cannot be interpreted to mean C4 deficiency.
‡In vitro (in the test tube) activation is suggested (and is much more common than a congenital deficiency) by the normal antigenic levels of C4 and B; that is, by protein analysis, neither pathway is being activated, but no functional activity is detectable. During in vitro activation antigenic material is still present, so the protein levels are normal.

Diseases associated with immune complexes

- Autoimmune diseases
  - Rheumatoid arthritis, Felty's syndrome, SLE, Sjögren's syndrome, MCTD, periartertitis nodosa, systemic sclerosis
- Glomerulonephritis
  - Exogenous and endogenous antigens
- Neoplastic diseases
  - Solid and lymphoid tumors
- Infectious diseases
  - Bacterial
    - Infective endocarditis, meningococcal infections, disseminated gonorrheal infection, children with recurrent infections, infected ventriculoatrial shunt, streptococcal infections, leprosy, syphilis
  - Viral
    - Dengue hemorrhagic fever, cytomegalovirus infections, viral hepatitis, infectious mononucleosis, SSPE
  - Parasitic
    - Malaria, trypanosomiasis, schistosomiasis, filariasis, toxoplasmosis
- Other conditions
  - Dermatitis herpetiformis and celiac disease; ulcerative colitis and Crohn's disease; myocardial infarcts; idiopathic interstitial pneumonia; cystic fibrosis; sarcoidosis; multiple sclerosis; amyotrophic lateral sclerosis; myasthenia gravis; uveitis; otitis media; atopic diseases; arthritis associated with intestinal bypass procedure for morbid obesity; sickle cell anemia; TTP; primary biliary cirrhosis; kidney and bone marrow transplantation; pregnancy, pre-eclamptic and eclamptic syndrome; Lyme arthritis; steroid-responsive nephrotic syndrome; xanthomatosis; vasectomy; oral ulceration and Behçet's syndrome; pemphigus and bullous pemphigoid; IgA deficiency; thyroid disorders; ankylosing spondylitis; iatrogenic diseases

SLE, Systemic lupus erythematosus; MCTD, mixed connective tissue disease; SSPE, subacute sclerosing panencephalitis; TTP, thrombotic thrombocytopenic purpura.

of complement levels in joint, pleural, spinal, and pericardial fluids is complicated technically and difficult to interpret, such determinations are seldom helpful in clinical decision making.

Any cause of chronic antigenemia that is associated with an antibody response may lead to acquired hypocomplementemia, including subacute bacterial endocarditis; hepatitis B surface antigenemia; gram-negative sepsis; viremias, such as measles; or recurrent parasitemias, such as malaria. Essential mixed cryoglobulinemia, a disease characterized by arthritis or arthralgias, cutaneous vasculitis, and nephritis, is often accompanied by profound hypocomplementemia resulting from classic pathway activation by the cold-precipitating immune complexes that occur in this disease.

Most immune complex diseases show evidence of classic pathway activation, but type II membranoproliferative glomerulonephritis is associated with hypocomplementemia, a normal C4, and low C3; this combination of findings indicates activation of the alternative pathway. The responsible mechanism in some patients involves a circulating C3 nephritic factor, an autoantibody directed against the alternative pathway C3-cleaving enzyme. It combines with and stabilizes this enzyme, then promotes positive feedback through the amplification loop.

Certain inherited deficiencies of control proteins lead to uncontrolled cycling of the activation pathway to which they belong and to secondary consumption of complement protein with resulting hypocomplementemia. C1 inhibitor deficiency permits the unopposed cleavage of C4 and C2 by C1 and is associated with the clinical syndrome of hereditary angioedema. Deficiency of either of the control proteins, I or H, leads to uncontrolled cycling of the amplification loop with secondary depletion of C3 and other alternative pathway proteins. Clinically the deficiencies of H and I associated with recurrent pyogenic infections are presumably caused by impaired opsonization of the bacteria consequent to the low C3 levels (Chapter 298).

Paroxysmal nocturnal hemoglobinuria (PNH) is an acquired clonal disorder of hematopoietic stem cells. Such cells are unable to add glycolipid anchors to proteins. As a result, these proteins are deficient. Decay-accelerating factor (DAF) and CD59 are glycolipid-anchored membrane proteins. Their deficiency produces PNH because of complement-mediated damage to the cell. THC, C3, and C4 levels, however, are normal because the amount of complement required for lysis is small.

MEASUREMENT OF IMMUNE COMPLEXES

Circulating immune complexes (ICs) play an immunopathologic role in a wide variety of diseases, including autoimmune disorders, vasculitic syndromes, infectious illnesses, and malignancies (see the box on p. 2339). Consequently, the demonstration of ICs in tissues and biologic fluids can be of aid in elucidating the pathophysiology of certain conditions (Chapter 287).

Detection of immune complexes

In tissues, ICs are demonstrable by histologic, histochemical, and light and electron microscopic methods. Histologically the patterns of tissue injury resemble those in experimental animals induced to develop "IC disease." Electron-dense accumulations of IC may be observed in subepithelial or subendothelial locations of kidney glomerular vessels. Scattered subepithelial deposits are characteristic of poststreptococcal glomerulonephritis, whereas extensive subepithelial deposits are the hallmark of membranous glomerulopathy. In lupus nephritis, electron-dense deposits are often observed in a subendothelial position. Of the immunohistochemical techniques available, the most widely used is immunofluorescence, which uses fluorochrome-labeled antibodies for detecting immunoglobulins (Ig) and complement (C) fragments within tissue specimens. The two major antibody-induced forms of glomerular injury (antiglomerular basement membrane, or GBM; glomerulonephritis; IC glomerulonephritis) display different patterns of Ig deposition under immunofluorescence. Anti-GBM antibodies react with antigen distributed throughout the GBM and deposit evenly to produce a smooth, linear pattern, whereas ICs that randomly deposit from the circulation into the glomerular filter are detected as granular, interrupted deposits.

More than 30 different tests have been described for the measurement of IC in blood, yet no *one* test is particularly satisfactory for routine clinical use. Procedures for detecting ICs containing unknown antigens in biologic fluids are based on (1) physical properties of IC; (2) interactions of IC with certain serum factors, such as complement or rheumatoid factors (RFs); and (3) interactions with cells bearing Fc and C receptors, such as B lymphocytes, macrophages, platelets, and erythrocytes.

The Raji cell assay, a frequently used IC test, demonstrates some of the difficulties in this area. First, the assay is not only technically complex but also requires a tissue culture system to grow this human pre-B lymphocyte tumor cell line. The Raji cell possesses complement receptor type II (CR2), which primarily binds the C3 breakdown product, C3dg, but does not contain CR1, which primarily binds C3b. Thus the assay detects only ICs with C3dg. Non–complement-fixing ICs either are not detected at all or are inefficiently measured by this assay. Finally, antilymphocyte antibodies are common in rheumatic diseases and give a false-positive test, since the Raji cell is a human B cell tumor line.

Currently, no universal and absolutely specific reagent is available for IC detection and quantitation. Most assays detect only complement-fixing, large-size complexes and do not differentiate between specific complexes and nonspecific aggregates. Moreover, the complement-dependent techniques may give false-positive results because of the presence of interfering substances in the serum sample, such as deoxyribonucleic acid (DNA) or endotoxin. The RF-based tests may be influenced by the presence of endogenous RF in the serum sample and high levels of serum IgG. Cellular techniques may give false-positive results because of the presence of anticellular antibodies frequently found in sera of patients with autoimmune disorders. Even in experienced hands, therefore, the screening for ICs in human sera may require the use of several tests, and considerable caution in their interpretation is necessary.

Finally, it should be emphasized that detection of ICs in biologic fluids does not necessarily indicate that the pathology of the disease under study results from these complexes. The most direct test would be one that demonstrates IC in the affected tissue itself. More importantly, however, experience over the past 10 years has pointed to the limited usefulness of IC measurements for decision making in clinical medicine. ICs are typically present in infectious diseases; malignancies; idiopathic chronic inflammatory conditions involving the lung, kidney, or liver; and most inflammatory rheumatic diseases.

Two clinical tests that are more frequently used than IC assays to provide useful information regarding the presence of ICs are those for complement and cryoglobulin.

1. *Complement assays*. The reduction in circulating components of the classic pathway of complement (i.e., C1, C4, C2, C3) is usually related to IC formation, since ICs activate this cascade (Chapter 287).
2. *Cryoglobulins*. Mixed cryoglobulins are special types of ICs: ones that precipitate from serum in the cold. Such complexes usually consist of IgG, a C3 fragment, RF (IgM), and antigen. This test provides a direct and quantitative measurement of an important IC (Chapter 314).

On the more positive side, a correlation exists between levels of circulating IC and disease activity in patients with SLE. Several investigators, using different techniques, have found a relationship between IC levels, antibodies to DNA, low complement levels, and clinical manifestations. Also, in patients with bacterial endocarditis, a correlation has been found between circulating IC levels, duration of disease, and extravalvular manifestations.

REFERENCES

Complement Measurements

Alexander RL Jr: Comparison of radial immunodiffusion and laser nephelometry for quantitating some serum proteins. Clin Chem 26:314, 1980.

Guiguet M et al: Laser nephelometric measurement of seven serum proteins compared with radial immunodiffusion. J Clin Chem Clin Biochem 21:217, 1983.

Schur PH: Complement studies of sera and other biologic fluids. Hum Pathol 14:338, 1983.

van Es L et al: International collaborative study of four candidate reference preparations for the antigenetic hemolytic measurement of human serum complement components. J Biol Stand 9:91, 1981.

Weinstein A et al: Antibodies to native DNA and serum complement (C3) levels: application to diagnosis and classification of systemic lupus erythematosus. Am J Med 74:206, 1983.

Whaley K: Methods in complement for clinical immunologists. New York, 1985, Churchill Livingstone.

Measurement of Immune Complexes

Brouet JC et al: Biological and clinical significance of cryoglobulinemia: report of 86 cases. Am J Med 57:775, 1974.

Dixon FJ, Cochrane CC, and Theofilopoulos AN: Immune complex injury. In Samter M et al, editors: Immunological diseases, vol 2. Boston, 1988, Little, Brown.

Gorevic PD: Cryopathies: cryoglobulins and cryofibrinogenemia. In Samter M et al, editors: Immunological diseases, vol 2. Boston, 1988, Little, Brown.

CHAPTER

291 Evaluation of Cellular Immune Function

Thomas D. Geppert
Peter E. Lipsky

The initiation and regulation of an immune response is dependent on the tightly orchestrated activities of a variety of specialized cells. Increases in our understanding of the complex interactions regulating the immune response have led to the development of new methodologies to assess various aspects of the immune system. Thus, for example, advances in molecular biology have greatly increased our knowledge of the structure of various soluble factors that regulate the immune response and have provided pure preparations of these factors for study. These studies have led to the development of in-vitro techniques to assess the capacity of various cell types both to produce and to respond to these cytokines. Application of these new methodologies to study normal and disease-associated aberrant immune responses has greatly expanded our understanding of the normal immune response and is beginning to provide new insights into derangements of immune function characteristic of disease states. This chapter reviews the assays currently available to assess quantitative and functional aspects of the various lymphoid populations.

DELAYED-TYPE HYPERSENSITIVITY

Despite many recent technical advances in assessing the cellular immune response, the intradermal skin test remains the most effective screening procedure for evaluating cell-mediated immunity. A positive skin test requires a complex series of interactions involving most of the components of the cellular immune system, and thus implies intact delayed-type hypersensitivity and, with few exceptions, cell-mediated immunity. Failure to respond is termed *cutaneous anergy* and implies a defect in this process, but does not localize this defect further. In addition to evaluating cellular immune function in the aggregate, skin testing can also be used to determine specific prior sensitization to various viral, bacterial, and fungal antigens, and this information can be useful diagnostically.

The skin test is performed by injecting an antigenic preparation intradermally. At 24, 48, and 72 hours, the degree of induration is assessed clinically. Induration of more than 5 mm is commonly considered a positive result. When evaluating the tuberculin test, however, induration of 10 mm in diameter or greater indicates probable exposure to *Mycobacterium tuberculosis,* while induration of 5 to 10 mm suggests that specific sensitization is doubtful, and 0 to 4 mm is a negative test. Patients who develop 5 to 10 mm of induration may have had a previous bacillus Calmette-Guérin (BCG) vaccination or have been exposed to one of the atypical *Mycobacteria*. Skin testing to assess established delayed-type hypersensitivity is done with a battery of recall antigens including mumps, *Candida,* trichophytin, and tuberculin. When such a battery of antigens is used, it is unlikely that an individual will have failed to encounter one of them. More than 97% of normal persons develop at least one positive reaction when three or more antigens are used.

If there is no reaction to any of the recall antigens utilized, delayed-type hypersensitivity can be tested by attempting to sensitize the individual with dinitrochlorobenzene (DNCB), a very reactive hapten that binds to skin proteins and becomes highly immunogenic. This procedure tests both the ability to be sensitized to an antigen (afferent limb) and the ability to respond to the antigen (efferent limb of immunity). Ninety percent of the population can be sensitized to DNCB. The procedure involves painting 2000 μg of DNCB dissolved in acetone on the volar forearm and examining the site for a flare response 14 to 16 days later. If no response is observed, a challenge dose of 50 μg of DNCB is applied, and the response is assessed 24 and 48 hours later. The DNCB response tests both the ability to generate specific memory T cells and the ability to mount a delayed-type hypersensitivity response. Certain patients (e.g., some individuals with solid tumors) have been described who are able to respond to common microbial antigens, but not DNCB, suggesting a defect in the afferent limb of cell-mediated immunity. Recently, it has become clear that a small percentage of individuals, especially the elderly, may show no reaction when tested initially yet show a significant reaction if tested a week later with the same dose of antigen; this effect has been called the *booster response*. This finding has led to the suggestion that negative tuberculin skin tests be followed 7 or more days later by a second skin test, to detect those persons who develop a positive response related to the booster effect. This procedure may help avoid the unnecessary evaluation and treatment of those individuals whose subsequent skin tests are positive. It has also been suggested that the size of the increase in skin-test positivity can be used to discriminate between individuals exhibiting a booster effect and those individuals with a positive skin test related to a new infection with *Mycobacterium* tuberculosis. An increase in the skin test response of 12 mm or more has been found to be related to a new infection, whereas smaller increases in the response resulted from the booster effect.

A variety of nonimmunologic and immunologic conditions are associated with cutaneous anergy (see box to the right). Many of the nonimmunologic causes may have similar etiologies. For instance, zinc deficiency appears to play a role in the anergy seen in surgical patients, sickle cell anemia, and malnutrition. Immunologic causes include inadequate numbers of helper cells, intrinsic T cell defects, lack of lymphokine production, suppressive serum factors, lymphocytotoxic antibodies, and hyperactive suppressor T cells. In addition, defects in macrophage function that have not yet been well defined may also play a role.

Causes of cutaneous anergy

I. Immunologic
   A. Acquired
      1. Acquired immunodeficiency syndrome (AIDS)
      2. Acute leukemia
      3. Carcinoma
      4. Chronic lymphocytic leukemia
      5. Hodgkin's disease
      6. Non-Hodgkin's lymphoma
   B. Congenital
      1. Ataxia telangiectasia
      2. Di George's syndrome
      3. Nezelof's syndrome
      4. Severe combined immunodeficiency
      5. Wiskott-Aldrich syndrome
II. Infections
   A. Bacterial
      1. Bacterial pneumonia
      2. Brucellosis
   B. Disseminated mycotic infections
   C. Mycobacterial
      1. Lepromatous leprosy
      2. Miliary and active tuberculosis
   D. Viral
      1. Varicella
      2. Hepatitis
      3. Influenza
      4. Infectious mononucleosis
      5. Measles
      6. Mumps
III. Immunosuppressive medications
   A. Cyclophosphamide
   B. Methotrexate
   C. Rifampin
   D. Systemic corticosteroids
IV. Other
   A. Alcoholic cirrhosis
   B. Anemia
   C. Biliary cirrhosis
   D. Burns
   E. Crohn's disease
   F. Diabetes
   G. Malnutrition
   H. Old age
   I. Pregnancy
   J. Pyridoxine deficiency
   K. Rheumatic diseases
   L. Sarcoidosis
   M. Sickle cell anemia
   N. Surgery
   O. Uremia

QUANTITATIVE ASSESSMENT OF HUMAN MONONUCLEAR CELLS

The first step in evaluating a suspected defect in cell-mediated immunity is to determine whether the defect is caused by an insufficient number of one of the cells involved. A complete blood count and differential identify gross abnormalities in the number of circulating lymphocytes, such as found in chronic lymphocytic leukemia, systemic lupus erythematosus, or the acquired immunodeficiency syndrome (AIDS), but they are not sufficient to identify more subtle defects. Since the circulating lymphocyte pool is composed of several subpopulations, including B lymphocytes, T helper–inducer cells, T suppressor–cytotoxic cells, and natural killer (NK) cells, a total lymphocyte count does not identify a deficiency in a specific population. Moreover, a deficiency in any one subset of lymphocytes could be obscured by the others.

A number of techniques have been developed to obtain a better quantitative assessment of the various lymphocyte subpopulations. For example, T lymphocytes bind sheep erythrocytes, forming rosettes with the bound red cells, termed *erythrocyte* (E) *rosettes,* which can be enumerated with a light microscope. This technique is a widely accepted means of identifying T cells. Sixty percent to 70% of peripheral blood mononuclear cells form E rosettes. T cells and T cell subsets can be further identified by using monoclonal antibodies (see next page).

B lymphocytes can also be quantitated, since they express certain unique markers on their surfaces. For example, B cells contain surface membrane–associated immunoglobulin that can be detected by reacting the cells with an anti-immunoglobulin antibody. Since most B cells express surface IgM and many also have surface IgD, reagents directed against these immunoglobulin isotypes detect B cells with the greatest degree of specificity. Although some B cells also express surface IgG, other cell types may have IgG bound onto their Fc receptors; therefore detection of

IgG-bearing cells may not uniquely identify B cells. B cell subsets can also be further defined with use of monoclonal antibodies.

Monocytes can be identified by a number of characteristics, including their phagocytic capacity as tested by challenge with latex particles or their nonspecific esterase activity.

CELL ANALYSIS USING MONOCLONAL ANTIBODIES

The use of murine monoclonal antibodies directed at specific cell surface proteins has become the standard way to identify lymphocyte populations and subpopulations. A list of a number of cell surface molecules used to identify cell types is included in Table 291-1. These antibodies can be used to stain individual cells in suspension or cells in tissue sections. By directly labeling these antibodies with a fluorescent dye or by using a labeled secondary antibody directed at the monoclonal antibody, it is possible to delineate the various lymphocyte populations using either a fluorescence microscope or the fluorescence-activated cell sorter. The fluorescence-activated cell sorter has several advantages including objectivity and speed, permitting the analysis of thousands of cells per sample. Fluorescence microscopy, however, is also an effective technique with most of the commonly employed monoclonal antibodies. Through this technique the expression of various lymphocyte cell surface molecules can be assessed. Thus, patients with a syndrome characterized by recurrent bacterial and fungal infections, progressive periodontitis, and/or delayed umbilical cord separation that is associated with a defect in the expression of LFA-1 (CD11a/18), a surface molecule involved in cellular adhesion, can be identified. Similarly, patients with Wiskott-Aldrich syndrome can be detected by a defect in CD43 expression. In addition, this technique can be used to evaluate the number of circulating T cells, T cell subsets, B cells, monocytes, and NK cells.

The clinical value of careful enumeration of mononuclear cell subsets is expanding. These tools have been used in characterizing various hematologic malignancies and have led to specific therapies based on the phenotype of the malignant cell. In addition, many of the congenital or acquired immunodeficiency states are characterized by gross deficiencies in particular subgroups.

Quantifying the number of $CD4^+$ cells in patients with AIDS can be a useful indicator of prognosis, as those with fewer than 400 $CD4^+$ cells per mm^3 have a poor prognosis. Finally, some patients with autoimmune disease have been found to have increased numbers of a B cell subset expressing the CD5 determinant. This subset appears to include precursors of autoantibody producing cells. Other patients with autoimmune disease have been reported to manifest a deficiency in a $CD4^+$T cell subset identified by the 2H4 monoclonal antibody that recognizes the CD45R determinant. This subset of suppressor inducer cells appears to be responsible for inducing suppressor effector T cell function from $CD8^+$T cells.

DELINEATION OF LYMPHOID POPULATIONS ON TISSUE SECTION

Although it is useful to delineate the various subpopulations of lymphoid cells in the peripheral blood, abnormalities observed may not be representative of events occurring at the tissue level. Histochemical and immunohistologic evaluation of tissue sections permits the direct examination of lymphoid subpopulations in the tissue. Examination of lymph node morphology has been used for many years to help assess immunocompetence. Since the lymph node is divided into a paracortical area that contains T cells and germinal centers and primary follicles that contain B cells, routine histologic evaluation can identify various gross deficiencies. Thus, isolated T cell deficiencies result in either sparsely populated paracortical areas or paracortical areas in which T cells are replaced by non–T cells such as histiocytes or eosinophils. Isolated B cell deficiencies are characterized by absence of germinal centers and plasma cells.

The development of monoclonal antibodies specific for the various lymphoid subpopulations has led to the use of immunohistologic techniques to examine tissue sections. These techniques have recently been applied to study the tissue obtained from several different inflammatory sites including skin test sites, various infectious processes, allograft rejection, sites of graft-versus-host disease, and malignancies. From these studies it has become clear that the predominant cell infiltrating sites of delayed-type hypersensitivity is the helper-inducer $CD4^+$ T cell. In contrast, suppressor-cytotoxic $CD8^+$ cells predominate during graft-versus-host disease, allograft rejection, and lepromatous leprosy.

FUNCTIONAL ASSESSMENT OF CELLULAR IMMUNITY

The assays described previously quantitate lymphocyte subpopulations but do not evaluate the functional capacity of these cells. Moreover, delayed-type hypersensitivity skin tests measure activity of the entire system, but cannot assess specific functional capabilities of the various cells involved in cell-mediated immunity. Several in-vitro assays have been developed to assess more specific functional aspects of these cells.

One in-vitro correlate of cell-mediated immunity is the assay of T cell proliferation. This method evaluates the capacity of T lymphocytes that have been primed in vivo to respond in vitro after culture with the appropriate antigen. The first step in this response is the interaction of antigen-specific T cells with antigen-presenting cells. After recognition of the specific antigenic moiety, the T cell undergoes a series of physiologic changes resulting in its transformation to a lymphoblast and culminating in cell division. Although a variety of changes can be measured, because of ease and tradition lymphocyte responsiveness is most commonly assessed by measuring DNA synthesis as determined by the incorporation of radiolabeled thymidine. Measurements of T cell DNA synthesis stimulated by specific

Table 291-1. Cell surface molecules used to identify cell types

CD designation	Molecular/functional characteristics	Primary reactivity
CD1 (a-c)	Transmembrane 49 kd (CD1a), 45 kd (CD1b), and 43 kd (CD1c) glycoproteins. Associated with β_2 microglobulin.	Thymocytes B cell subset Langerhans cells Dendritic cells
CD2	Transmembrane 50 kd glycoprotein. Receptor for LFA-3.	T cells
CD3	Transmembrane complex of at least 5 distinct molecules (δ, ϵ, γ, ζ, η). Noncovalently associated with the T cell receptor for antigen.	T cells
CD4	Transmembrane 59 kd glycoprotein. Binds class II MHC molecules.	Class II restricted T cells Monocytes
CD5	Transmembrane 67 kDa glycoprotein.	T cells and a subset of B cells
CD6	Transmembrane 100 kDa glycoprotein.	T cells and a subset of B cells
CD7	40 kDa glycoprotein.	T cells
CD8	Transmembrane $\alpha\beta$ hetero or $\alpha\alpha$ homo dimers. α and β chains are 32 kDa glycoproteins. Binds to class I MHC molecules.	Class I restricted T cells
CD13	150 kDa glycoprotein.	Monocytes Granulocytes
CD14	55 kDa phosphoinositol-linked glycoprotein. Receptor for complexes of LPS and an LPS binding protein.	Monocytes
CD16	50-65 kDa single-chain glycoprotein. Low-affinity receptor for complex IgG (Fc γ R III).	NK cells Activated monocytes Granulocytes
CD18	Transmembrane 95 kDa glycoprotein noncovalently linked to CD11a,b,c.	Leukocytes
CD19	Transmembrane 90 kDa glycoprotein.	B cells
CD20	Transmembrane phosphoprotein expressed in two forms (35 and 37 kDa).	B cells
CD25	Transmembrane glycoprotein. Low-affinity receptor for IL2.	Activated T and B cells Monocytes
CD28	Homodimeric transmembrane glycoprotein. Each subunit is 44 kDa.	T cell subsets
CD34	Transmembrane 105-120 kDa glycoprotein.	Hemopoietic progenitor cells
CD43	95 kDa glycoprotein. Deficient in patients with Wiscott-Aldrich syndrome.	T cells Granulocytes Brain Some B cells
CD45RA	220 kDa isoform of CD45 a transmembrane tyrosine phosphatase.	T cell subsets B cells Granulocytes Monocytes
CD45RB	190-220 kDa isoform of CD45.	T cell subsets B cells Granulocytes Monocytes
CD45RO	180 kDa isoform of CD45.	T cell subsets B cells Granulocytes Monocytes
CD64	Transmembrane 75 kDa glycoprotein.	Monocytes Activated granulocytes
CD68	Transmembrane 110 kDa glycoprotein.	Macrophages

antigens occasionally suggest a specific defect in antigen responsiveness or a lack of antecedent sensitization. However, a poor response to a single antigen does not necessarily imply a more global dysfunction of cell-mediated immunity.

Besides specific antigen, a variety of nonspecific stimuli can be used to activate T cells in vitro. Mitogens, such as phytohemagglutinin or concanavalin A, are part of a group of substances that stimulate T cells nonspecifically. This activation is dependent on an accessory cell such as the monocyte. Thus, activation by mitogens can be used to test the integrity of T cell–monocyte interaction and the ability of the T cells to proliferate. Recently, several systems have been developed to study T cell activation in the absence of accessory cells. One system involves culturing T cells with antibodies to the T cell antigen receptor complex that have been immobilized onto plastic microtiter plates. These systems have the capacity to examine intrinsic T cell function independent of accessory cell function. Since mitogens activate cells irrespective of their antigen specificity, no previous sensitization is required.

Altered lymphocyte function can result in abnormal responses to mitogens, manifested as diminished peak responses or as shifts in either the dose-response curve or the kinetics of the response. Results from studies comparing delayed-type hypersensitivity skin testing and in-vitro mitogen responses suggest there is a good correlation between the two. Anergic patients usually do not mount normal mitogen responses in vitro. Since delayed-type hypersensitivity requires activities not tested by the in-vitro analysis of mitogen responsiveness, such as chemotaxis of monocytes and lymphocytes, an occasional anergic patient responds to mitogens in vitro.

In addition to antigen and mitogen responses, T cells also respond to allogeneic cells. This response, which is known as the *mixed lymphocyte reaction* (MLR), does not require prior sensitization and is directed primarily at human leukocyte antigen, locus D (HLA-D)–region antigens on the stimulator cells. A similar although less intense response is observed when autologous cells are used. This response is called the *autologous mixed lymphocyte reaction* (AMLR). The in-vivo significance of the AMLR is unknown, but it appears to be deficient in a variety of autoimmune diseases, such as systemic lupus erythematosus, Sjögren's syndrome, active rheumatoid arthritis, multiple sclerosis, and several neoplastic disorders including Hodgkin's disease and chronic lymphocytic lymphoma.

T CELL HELP OF B CELL IMMUNOGLOBULIN PRODUCTION

B cell immunoglobulin production is dependent on T cell–B cell contact and T cell cytokine production. A number of assays of the ability of T cells to support B cell immunoglobulin production are now available. The most straightforward assay of T cell help is to culture resting B cells with activated T cells and assess B cell proliferation and immunoglobulin production. The ability of T cells to proliferate and produce IL-2 is not necessarily correlated with their ability to promote B cell immunoglobulin production. For example, T cells isolated from the rheumatoid joint are unable to proliferate or produce IL-2 but they are very effective helper T cells. Whether the enhanced ability of these cells to provide help is responsible for the autoimmune manifestation of this disorder is not yet clear.

T CELL–MEDIATED CYTOTOXICITY

Cytotoxic T cells are specifically committed effector T cells that have the capacity to lyse target cells bearing antigens to which the cytotoxic cells have been primed. Cytotoxic T cells primed to the major histocompatibility complex (MHC)–encoded antigens of the stimulator cells can be generated during the MLR. Cytotoxic T cells directed as class I MHC antigens are usually of the $CD8^+$ phenotype, whereas those directed at class II MHC antigens are usually $CD4^+$ cells. The function of cytotoxic T lymphocytes can be assayed by their capacity to lyse target cells labeled with radioactive chromium. The amount of released label is a measure of cytotoxicity. In general, T cell–mediated cytotoxicity plays a role in the host's defense against viral infection and may play a role in preventing neoplasia. There are a number of diseases, such as polymyositis, Vogt-Koyanagi-Harada disease, and hepatitis B–related chronic active hepatitis, in which tissue pathology may be mediated by these cells. Finally, a defect in the generation of influenza-specific cytotoxic cells has been reported in ataxia-telangiectasia.

CYTOKINE PRODUCTION

T cells activated by a variety of stimuli produce a number of biologically active mediators called *lymphokines*. The genes for many of the lymphokines have been cloned using recombinant DNA technology. This advance has led to a dramatic increase in our knowledge about the structure and function of these molecules. It is clear from these studies that lymphokines have pleiotropic effects on a variety of cells types. The function of the various lymphokines is depicted in Table 286-2 (p. 2317). Monocytes also synthesize and secrete a variety of biologically active mediators, including interleukin-1, tumor necrosis factor α, interleukin 6, platelet-derived growth factor, alpha interferon, and various colony-stimulating factors. Like lymphokines, monocyte-derived cytokines also have pleiotropic effects on a variety of cell types.

The capacity of various cells to produce these factors can now be assessed. For some lymphokines, such as interleukin-2 (IL-2), production can be assessed using radioimmunoassays, whereas measurements of other lymphokines rely on cumbersome and inexact biologic assays. Recently, techniques have also been developed to determine the production of specific messenger RNA molecules for each lymphokine. These studies have greatly expanded our understanding of the regulation of lymphokine production in normal lymphocytes and may someday provide insight into the mechanisms underlying abnormal lymphokine production in such disorders as systemic lupus erythematosus (SLE).

Several studies have examined cytokine production in various clinical states. For instance, it has been demonstrated that surgical patients and patients with SLE do not produce IL-2 normally. In addition, it has been suggested that deficiencies in specific cytokines may play a role in certain disease states. For instance, T cells from patients with lepromatous leprosy have a selective inability to produce interleukin-2 in response to *Mycobacterium leprae*. In addition, in response to *M. leprae,* mononuclear cells from these patients fail to produce cytokines that activate monocytes to kill intracellular pathogens, whereas mononuclear cells from patients with tuberculoid leprosy produce such cytokines normally.

SUPPRESSOR ASSAYS

The discovery of separate subsets of helper and suppressor T cells has led to the development of several assays to measure their function. In general, suppression is measured by examining the effect of adding one population of cells to a reference culture. Peripheral blood mononuclear cells that are stimulated by any one of a variety of stimuli, including mitogens, antigens, or alloantigens, can be used as reference cultures. Besides suppressor T cells, monocytes also produce several nonspecific suppressive factors, including prostaglandins and hydrogen peroxide. The effect of suppressor cells on either T cell proliferation or B cell immunoglobulin synthesis can be measured. Defects in suppressor cell function can now be further analyzed by examining the production of the factors thought responsible for the generation and function of suppressor cells, including gamma interferon, transforming growth factor β, IL-2, and prostaglandin E_2. Clinical studies comparing patients with SLE with normal controls have revealed an inability to generate suppressor cells in SLE patients. In addition, hyperactive suppressor T cells have been described in patients with common variable hypogammaglobulinemia, fungal infections, Hodgkin's disease, IgA deficiency, and multiple myeloma. Enhanced suppressor cell function has also been described in patients with sarcoidosis and in some patients with multiple myeloma, tuberculosis, and schistosomiasis, but this function appears to reside in the monocyte population.

MONOCYTE-MACROPHAGE ASSAYS

Mononuclear phagocytes perform several important and necessary functions for immune responses. One function is antigen presentation, which is necessary to initiate cell-mediated immunity. Antigen presentation involves taking up native antigen, processing it, and presenting it to relevant T cells. For activation, T cells must see antigen in the context of class II products encoded by genes of the major histocompatibility locus on the antigen-presenting monocyte. An inability to express class II molecules has been described in several patients with severe immunodeficiency.

Functional tests of monocyte activity include assays of chemotaxis, bacterial killing, and cytotoxicity. Patients with lepromatous leprosy or neoplasia have been described with defects in chemotaxis and cytotoxicity, respectively. In addition, it has been suggested that patients with malacoplakia have a defect in monocyte killing of *Escherichia coli* organisms.

NATURAL KILLER CELL ASSAYS

Natural killer (NK) cells recognize and kill targets without the need for antecedent sensitization, and thus play a role in the "natural resistance" of the host. They are thought to play an important role in resistance to malignancies and viral infections. NK function is assessed by culturing effector cells (from peripheral blood, spleen, or inflammatory exudates or tissue) with labeled targets. Target-cell lysis is then assessed by measuring the release of the label. In addition to assessing lysis, the ability of the effector cells to bind with the target can also be assessed. Target cells are usually malignant cell lines such as the erythroleukemia cell line, K562. Since interferons enhance normal NK function, most studies examining NK function also assess the ability of interferons to enhance the function of NK cells.

A variety of abnormalities in NK function have been described in different disease states. For instance, it has been reported that 50% of patients with metastatic epithelial carcinomas have deficient NK function. Patients with SLE have been shown to have antibodies directed at NK cells that inhibit NK killing without affecting target cell–effector cell binding. In addition, patients with Chédiak-Higashi syndrome, the later stages of syphilis, juvenile rheumatoid arthritis, paroxysmal nocturnal hemoglobinuria, Sjögren's syndrome, and AIDS have been shown to have depressed NK activity compared with normal controls. The ability of interferons to normalize depressed NK function is variable. For example, patients with either premalignant cervical intraepithelial neoplasia or invasive cervical carcinoma have deficient NK function; however, interferon can enhance NK function only in the premalignant condition. Finally, several conditions have been described with increased NK cell–mediated killing, including syphilis (before antilipoidal antibodies appear) and pulmonary tuberculosis.

REFERENCES

Ahmed AR and Blose DA: Delayed-type hypersensitivity skin testing: a review. Arch Dermatol 119:934, 1983.

Coligan JE et al: Current protocols in immunology. New York, 1991, John Wiley & Sons.

Lachman PJ and Peters DK: Clinical aspects of immunology. Oxford, England, 1980, Blackwell Scientific.

Morimoto C et al: The isolation and characterization of the human suppressor inducer T cell subset. J Immunol 134:1508, 1985.

Morimoto C et al: The isolation and characterization of the human helper inducer T cell subset. J Immunol 134:3762, 1985.

Palmer OL and Reed WP: Delayed hypersensitivity skin testing. Clinical correlates and anergy. J Infect Dis 130:138, 1974.

Romain P and Schlossman SF: Human T lymphocyte subsets: functional heterogeneity and surface recognition structures. J Clin Invest 74:1559, 1984.

Stites DP et al, editors: Basic and clinical immunology. Los Altos, 1984, Lange Medical.

Todd RF and Schlossman SF: Utilization of monoclonal antibodies in the characterization of macrophage-monocyte differentiation antigens. In Bellanti JA and Herscowitz HB, editors: The reticuloendothelial system: a comprehensive treatise, vol 6. Immunology. New York, 1986, Plenum.

CHAPTER

292 Laboratory Methods in Immediate Hypersensitivity

Stephen I. Wasserman

Traditionally, the laboratory assessment of immediate hypersensitivity disease has been based on the ability to reproduce in a controlled and localized fashion in-vivo anaphylactic reactions to suspected antigenic substances. These in-vivo techniques have been supplemented in recent years by precise and sensitive in-vitro tests capable of measuring the amounts and antigenic specificity of individual immunoglobulins.

IN-VIVO TECHNIQUES

Skin tests

Testing of antigens in the skin can be performed by intradermal and prick-puncture methods. The latter route is favored because of its reproducibility, low incidence of false-positive reactions, lesser risk of systemic (anaphylactic) reactions, better accuracy (particularly regarding food antigens), and better patient acceptance. Skin-test sites (back and forearm) are cleansed, and a single drop of antigen solution is placed on the skin. A needle or commercial prick-puncture device is inserted into the skin through the antigen. Only superficial penetration is made, and no bleeding should occur. The antigen is removed by blotting 30 to 60 seconds after skin puncture, and the test site is measured for erythema (flare) and edema (wheal) 15 minutes later. Intradermal testing should be reserved for antigens that are of suspected clinical relevance but are nonreactive by prick-puncture techniques. Twenty to 50 microliters (0.02 to 0.05 ml) of antigen solution is injected intracutaneously, and the area of wheal and flare determined 15 minutes later. Various grading systems have been employed to describe the wheal-and-flare reaction and any associated pseudopodia. For both prick-puncture and intradermal techniques, appropriate controls are required to exclude unreported antihistamine ingestion, to verify skin reactivity, and to rule out dermographism. Use of diluent, histamine (0.01% intradermal, 1% prick-puncture), and codeine (a nonspecific mast cell degranulator) provides negative and positive controls. Interpretation of skin tests, either prick-puncture or intradermal, requires that the response to diluent be absent or minimal (0 to 2 mm), and the response to histamine or codeine, or both, be present (8 to 10 mm intradermal, 5 to 6 mm prick-puncture). Because false-positive as well as false-negative reactions occur, it is essential that reactions be interpreted in light of the clinical history. In addition, the antigens employed must be fresh and must have antigenic reactivity, and the tests must have been properly administered. Since intradermal administration of concentrated antigens may cause wheal-and-flare reactions in a very high proportion of nonsensitive individuals, the more dilute the solution causing a positive response, the more likely the antigen is to be clinically relevant.

The skin also may be used for another form of testing—the P-K (Prausnitz-Küstner) reaction. Rarely performed because of the risk of introducing viral infection, this test employs sera from an individual in whom IgE antigenic sensitivity is suspected. A volunteer (nonallergic) is injected with 0.05 to 0.10 ml of the patient's serum intradermally, and this site and a control area are challenged with antigen (0.02 ml) 24 to 48 hours later. The test is read as for intradermal skin testing. This procedure was employed for research purposes and, occasionally, to evaluate food or drug sensitivity, but now should be abandoned.

In rare cases, bronchial or nasal allergen challenge may be performed to assess allergic reactivity. These techniques, however, generally lack sensitivity and/or precision, more readily induce systemic reactions, are expensive, and may be confounded by nonspecific hyperirritability, which makes their interpretation more difficult. They should be reserved for unique situations. Since skin-test reactivity to an antigen is highly correlated with bronchial reactivity to the same antigen, such testing generally is redundant.

IN-VITRO ASSAYS

IgE measurement

Total serum IgE concentrations are too low to permit assessment by immunodiffusion techniques, therefore various radioimmunologic or enzymatic assays have been developed. The most commonly used test is the PRIST (paper disc radioimmunoassay technique, Fig. 292-1), in which the patient's serum is reacted with antibody to human IgE bound to a paper disc. After incubation, the disc is washed, and a radiolabeled antibody to human IgE is added; the disc is again washed. The amount of radioactivity bound to the paper disc correlates directly with the serum level of IgE. This technique is capable of measuring IgE in picogram quantities. IgE is reported as units or nanograms per milliliter. One unit is equivalent to 2.4 ng.

Antigen-specific IgE may be measured directly by the radioallergosorbent test (RAST, Fig. 292-1) or by measuring the antigen-induced release of histamine from basophil leukocytes. The RAST is similar in principle to the PRIST. In this test, specific antigens, rather than IgE molecules, are bound to a solid matrix and exposed to the patient's serum. The matrix is washed and reacted with radiolabeled antibody to human IgE. The amount of radiolabel bound to

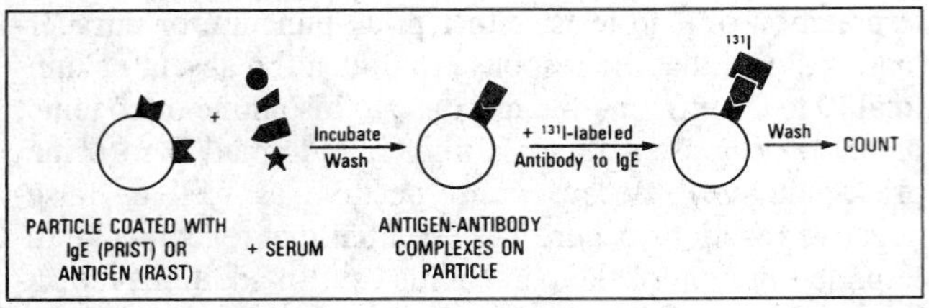

Fig. 292-1. Principle of the radioimmunoassays (RAST and PRIST) used in the measurement of IgE or antigen-specific IgE.

the solid phase is directly proportional to amounts of IgE in serum with specificity to the test antigen. The results are semiquantitative and are reported in comparison to a serum known to contain antigen-specific IgE. Modifications of this test employing fluorescence or luminescence are available. This test also can be modified to assess antigen-specific IgG antibodies. Such *in-vitro* tests of specific IgE correlate well with other in-vitro and in-vivo tests of IgE reactivity, including skin testing, bronchial provocation, and leukocyte histamine release. Controversy exists over the relative utility of in-vitro measurement of specific IgE compared with in-vivo skin testing. The advantages and disadvantages (see Tables 292-1 and 292-2) must be weighed before either is utilized. At present, however, it appears that skin testing performed by a skilled individual with appropriate experience in interpretation is the cost-effective method of choice for assessing antigen-specific IgE in most clinical situations.

The release of histamine from peripheral blood basophils also can be used to define the presence and specificity of IgE in patients. Patient leukocytes, in whole blood or after washing to remove serum constituents, are interacted with various quantities of antigen, and the amount of histamine released is measured. This test requires fresh leukocytes in large numbers from patients not taking inhibitory drugs. Moreover, histamine measurements are laborious and expensive. Patient serum can be used to passively sensitize donor leukocytes, but this procedure suffers from the same difficulties as the direct test and is generally reserved for research purposes.

IMMUNOTHERAPY

Although not specifically a test or a diagnostic procedure, immunotherapy is directly linked to the proper interpretation of the demonstration of antigen-specific IgE. Allergen injection therapy, or immunotherapy, as it is generally known, has been utilized since the early 1900s, but at present is generally reserved for patients with IgE-dependent allergic diseases whose symptoms are not controlled by environmental manipulation or medications, or in whom such medications are contraindicated or not tolerated. Immunotherapy is efficacious in the treatment of allergic rhinitis, venom hypersensitivity, and asthma. Antigens that have been employed successfully include pollens, molds, danders, and insect and mite antigens. Foods are not used. Immunotherapy is complicated in patients receiving β-adrenergic blocking agents because of difficulty in treating anaphylaxis in this setting.

Table 292-1. Skin testing

Advantages	Disadvantages
Inexpensive	Requires discontinuation of antihistamines
Antigens are available	Can cause anaphylaxis
Rapid	Dermographism precludes testing
Precise	Extensive skin disease may preclude testing
Sensitive	Difficult to perform and/or interpret in some elderly patients

Table 292-2. RAST testing

Advantages	Disadvantages
No risk of anaphylaxis	Expensive and slow
No risk of sensitization	Most tests use radioactivity
No need to interrupt antihistamines	Fewer antigens available
Dermographism or skin disease irrelevant	Lower sensitivity
	Lack of quantification
	Requires known positive serum
	High levels of antigen-specific IgG may interfere
	Does not directly measure clinical severity

Immunotherapy is performed by the sequential (generally, weekly) subcutaneous injections of gradually increasing amounts of antigen to which the patient has been shown to be sensitive by clinical and laboratory assessment. Initial dosage generally consists of 0.02 to 0.05 ml of a 1:100,000 concentration (weight: volume) or 100 protein nitrogen units (pnu) per milliliter of each antigen. Standardized (by RAST inhibition) allergens are increasingly available, are preferable, and are in A.U. (allergy units). Aqueous extracts of antigen generally are employed, but alum-precipitated antigen or polymerized antigens have been reported to be even more efficacious and/or safer. Weekly incremental doses of 0.05 to 0.10 ml are administered until, after 4 to 6 months, the patient is receiving 0.5 to 0.7 ml of a 1:100 w:v or 10,000 pnu per milliliter of solution. Forms of immunotherapy that do not advance to high doses of antigen are ineffective. The skin site should be observed 15 to 30 minutes after each injection, and any erythema, edema, or tenderness noted. The rate of increase in concentrations of antigen may be slowed if large local reactions develop. Systemic reactions (wheezing, generalized pruritus, urticaria, hypotension) require a twofold to tenfold reduction in antigen dose and a slower schedule of advancement. A 2- to 3-year course of immunotherapy is associated with improvement in symptoms of allergic rhinitis in 60% to 75% of well-selected patients, and good results may be noted within the first year. The mechanism whereby immunotherapy provides relief remains elusive. Patients receiving immunotherapy initially experience a rise in serum antigen–specific IgE and IgG concentrations, but with time, the IgE falls and IgG elevation persists. Postseasonal IgE rises are blunted or absent after immunotherapy and a diminished release of histamine from basophils, both to specific antigen and spontaneously, is observed. Finally, increases in antigen-specific CD8 lymphocyte reactivity, decreases in antigen-specific CD4 reactivity, and generation by macrophages of an inhibitor of histamine release have been reported to accompany clinically successful immunotherapy. Skin tests, which reflect mast cell sensitivity, generally do not change greatly with immunotherapy; however, successful immunotherapy with hymenoptera venom is associated in some patients with loss of skin reactivity. A more rapid procedure to initiate immunotherapy (RUSH) is used for hymenoptera venoms.

REFERENCES

Adkinson NF, Platts-Mills TAE: IgE and atopic disease. In Samter M et al, editors: Immunologic disease, ed 4. Boston, 1988, Little, Brown.

Bousquet J and Michel FB: In vivo methods for study of allergy: skin tests, techniques, and interpretation. In Middleton EE et al, editors: Allergy: principles and practice, ed 4. St. Louis, 1993, Mosby.

Bryant DM, Burnes MW, and Lazarus L: The correlation between skin tests, bronchial provocation tests, and the serum level of IgE specific for common allergies in patients with asthma. Clin Allergy 5:145, 1975.

Goodnow CC, Brink R, and Adams E: Breakdown of self-tolerance in anergic B lymphocytes. Nature 352:532, 1991.

Hamburger HA and Katzaren JA: Methods in laboratory immunology: principles and interpretation of laboratory tests for allergy. In Middleton EE et al, editors: Allergy: principles and practice, ed 4. St. Louis, 1993, Mosby.

Rocklin RE: Clinical and immunological aspects of allergen-specific immunotherapy in patients with seasonal allergic rhinitis and/or allergic asthma. J Allergy Clin Immunol 72:323, 1983.

Van Metre TE et al: A comparative study of the effectiveness of the Rinkel method and the current standard method of immunotherapy for ragweed pollen hay fever. J Allergy Clin Immunol 66:500, 1980.

CHAPTER

293 Autoantibodies

Liam Martin
Marvin J. Fritzler

Diseases associated with autoimmune phenomena tend to distribute themselves along a spectrum with organ-specific diseases at one end and non–organ-specific diseases at the other (Table 293-1). The organ-specific diseases, typified by Hashimoto's thyroiditis, are characterized by antibodies directed to, and inflammatory lesions within, a single organ. At the other end of the spectrum, typified by systemic lupus erythematosus (SLE), autoantibodies are directed against multiple organs and the inflammatory lesions are widely disseminated. Common organs affected in organ-specific disease include thyroid, stomach, pancreas, and ad-

Table 293-1. Spectrum of autoimmune diseases and related autoantibodies

Disease	Autoantibody target
Organ-specific diseases	
Graves' disease	TSH receptor
Hashimoto's thyroiditis	Thyroglobulin
	Thyroid peroxidase)
	Thyroid microsomes
	Thyrotrophin receptor
Myasthenia gravis	Acetylcholine receptors
	Striational skeletal muscle and cardiac muscle
Insulin-dependent diabetes	Pancreatic islet cells
	Insulin
	Glutamate acid decarboxylase
Insulin-resistant diabetes	Insulin receptor
Pernicious anemia	Gastric parietal cells (proton pump)
	Vitamin B_{12} binding site of intrinsic factor
Addison's disease	Adrenal cortex
Idiopathic hypoparathyroidism	Parathyroid cells
Pemphigus vulgaris	Cell adhesion molecules (cadherins)
Bullous pemphigoid	Basement membrane zone of skin and mucosa
Non–organ-specific diseases	
Idiopathic thrombocytopenic purpura	Platelets
Autoimmune hemolytic anemia	Erythrocytes
Primary biliary cirrhosis	Mitochondria (pyruvate dehydrogenase complex), PBC 95K
Chronic active hepatitis	Nuclear lamina
Goodpasture's syndrome	Glomerular and alveolar basement membrane
Rheumatoid arthritis	Gamma globulin
	Types II and III collagen
Sjögren's syndrome	SS-A/Ro; SS-B/La
	Salivary duct
	Gamma globulin
Scleroderma	Scl-70 (topoisomerase I)
	Nucleolar antigens
CREST-variant scleroderma	Centromere/kinetochore
Polymyositis	Jo-1 (histidyl tRNA synthetase)
	PM/Scl (Pm-1)
	Other tRNA synthetases
Polymyositis/scleroderma overlap	Pm/Scl (Pm-1)
	Ku
Mixed connective tissue disease	Nuclear (U1) RNP
Systemic lupus erythematosus	dsDNA
	Sm
	Histones
	RNP
	Cyclin (PCNA)
Vasculitis (Wegener's granulomatosis, microscopic and classic polyarteritis)	Neutrophil cytoplasmic antigen (myeloperoxidase, proteinase 3)

renal, whereas in non–organ-specific diseases, the kidneys, nervous tissue, skin, joints, and muscle are commonly involved. In organ-specific diseases, the lesions are relatively restricted, because the antigen in the organ serves as a target for the immune and inflammatory response. In non–organ-specific diseases, circulating immune complexes deposit, systemically giving rise to a widespread inflammatory response.

Interestingly, there are overlaps at each end of the spectrum. For example, thyroid antibodies are very prevalent in pernicious anemia patients, and these patients have a higher prevalence of autoimmune thyroid disease than is seen in the normal population. Similarly, patients with autoimmune thyroid disease have a high prevalence of parietal cell antibodies and, to a lesser extent, pernicious anemia. The systemic rheumatic diseases at the opposite end of the spectrum show considerable overlap. For example, features of scleroderma and polymyositis, or rheumatoid arthritis and SLE, are frequently seen in individual patients.

LABORATORY TESTS FOR SERUM ANTIBODIES IN AUTOIMMUNE DISEASE

The detection of autoantibodies in serum and other biological fluids is carried out in the clinical laboratory primarily through (1) immunohistochemical techniques, such as immunofluorescence and enzyme-labeled antibody techniques; and (2) serologic techniques, such as complement fixation, hemagglutination, latex particle aggregation, immunodiffusion, radioimmunoassay (RIA), enzyme-linked immunosorbent assay (ELISA), and Western immunoblotting (IB). The production of highly purified reagents in the form of monoclonal antibodies and recombinant antigens is now changing the laboratory approach to the investigation of autoimmune diseases.

Immunohistochemical techniques, RIA, and ELISA detect the presence of antibody through use of labeled molecules: for example, fluorescein-labeled molecules, enzyme-labeled (e.g., peroxidase) molecules, or radioisotope-labeled molecules. These techniques are highly sensitive for the identification of antibody binding to antigens. Tests involving secondary antigen-antibody reactions, such as agglutination (aggregation) or agar precipitation (immunodiffusion), are not so sensitive as the other techniques but are nevertheless quite suitable for the detection of certain antibodies.

The indirect immunofluorescence test is the most widely used immunohistochemical test to screen for serum autoantibodies (Fig. 293-1). Indirect immunofluorescence assays are performed by placing a test serum on antigen localized in tissue sections on a glass slide. The excess antibody is removed by washing and the bound antibody is detected by applying a "second" antibody—for example, a fluorescein-labeled antihuman immunoglobulin reagent—that has been raised in animals such as goats or rabbits. After the excess "second" antibody has been washed away, the slide is viewed in a microscope fitted with an ultraviolet light source. This procedure allows the technician to determine the antibody binding site in the cell and also, through grading the intensity of fluorescence, provides a semiquantitative measurement of the antibody concentration in the serum.

The technique of Western immunoblotting has proven useful in identifying target antigens in different substrates. IB is performed by reacting patients' sera with cellular antigens that have been separated on polyacrylamide gels and electrophoretically transferred onto nitrocellulose sheets. Reactive antigens are visualized by applying horseradish peroxidase–conjugated second antibody to the strip and reacting with a hydrogen peroxide. This technique is extremely sensitive and is useful in determining the specificity of antibodies, which on IIF, for example, give a speckled pattern.

The investigation of organ-specific autoimmune diseases dictates the use of slides that contain a variety of endocrine tissues, such as human thyroid, mouse stomach, or adrenal tissue. The detection of autoantibodies in non–organ-specific diseases has traditionally relied on the use of cryopreserved sections of rodent liver or kidney, but more recently the use of tissue culture cells as a tissue substrate has shown advantages of increased sensitivity and reliability. The pattern of immunofluorescence (e.g., homogeneous, speckled, nucleolar, mitochondrial, or microsomal) can provide important information if it is interpreted in light of the antibody titer and the patient's clinical history.

INTERPRETATION OF TESTS FOR AUTOANTIBODIES

After a specific pattern of staining of the tissue substrate is detected, the titer of the antibody is the next most important component of the laboratory result. A high titer of autoantibody is significant, but a low, or even absent, autoantibody titer does not rule out a particular disorder. As examples of the latter, thyroid antibodies are present in low titer even in the presence of significant disease, and antibodies to some nuclear antigens in SLE (e.g., Ro antigen) may not be detected by standard autoantibody screening, such as the antinuclear antibody (ANA) test. In the case of low titers of thyroid antibodies, it is believed that the thyroid may serve as an in-vivo immunosorbent of the antibody. It is important to note that changing titers of some autoantibodies may relate to the severity, progression, or successful treatment of the disease, whereas other autoantibodies may not vary at all with disease course.

In addition to the false-negative results referred to above, the presence of autoantibodies in the patient's serum does not necessarily establish the diagnosis or the immunopathogenic origin of the disease. It should be remembered that many normal individuals have detectable titers of autoantibodies. Therefore, when clinicians interpret the autoantibody test results, they must recognize the potential for false-positive results, especially when present in low titer. In many of these individuals the antibodies may persist through their lifetime with no apparent pathologic sequelae. False-positive results are particularly common in women, in patients on certain drugs (e.g., procainamide, hydralazine), in the first-degree relatives of patients with con-

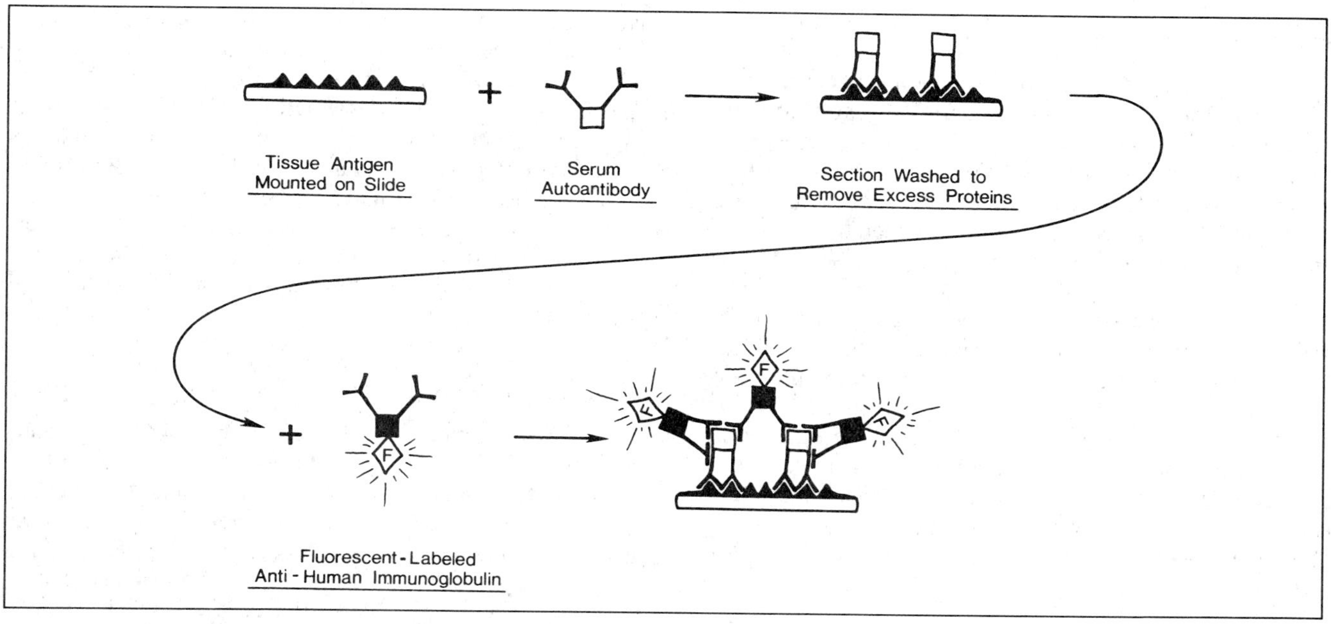

Fig. 293-1. Indirect fluorescent-labeled antibody method for the detection of autoimmune antibody.

firmed autoimmune disease, in acute viral or bacterial infections, in certain malignancies, and in the older (>60 years) population. The frequency and titer of antinuclear antibodies, for instance, rises in each decade after age 45.

SIGNIFICANCE OF COMMONLY ENCOUNTERED AUTOANTIBODIES

Thyroid antibodies

Three types of thyroid autoantigens have been characterized that bind to antibodies in the sera of patients with Graves' disease or Hashimoto's throiditis: thyroglobulin, thyroid microsomal antigen, and the thyrotrophin receptor. Patients with Hashimoto's thyroiditis have autoantibodies to thyroglobulin and/or thyroid microsomal antigen in 95% of cases. A negative test with both antigens virtually rules out the diagnosis. Low to moderate titers of thyroglobulin antibody are present in myxedema, thyrotoxicosis, adenomatous hyperplasia, thyroid carcinoma, rheumatoid arthritis (RA), and SLE. Twenty percent of normal middle-aged women have antibodies to thyroglobulin. Two percent of healthy men and 6% of women have antibodies to thyroid microsomal antigen.

The thyroid microsomal antigen has been identified as thyroid peroxidase, the enzyme oxidizes iodine to a free radical form during the formation of thyroid hormones. Whether thyroid microsomal antibodies block in-vivo production of thyroid hormones is unknown.

In Graves' disease, antibodies that react against the thyrotrophin receptor have been found. These antibodies are divided into stimulatory, thyroid-stimulating antibody (TSAb), and thyrotropin binding-inhibiting immunoglobulin (TBII). The TSAb includes the long-acting thyroid stimulator (LATS) and an antibody that prevents LATS binding, called *LATS protector*. Thyroid receptor-binding antibodies are measured by a radioreceptor assay.

Gastric antibodies

Antibodies to gastric parietal cells are present in the sera of 90% of patients with pernicious anemia. These antibodies inhibit the activity of the proton pump in in-vitro experiments, suggesting that they have a major role in the development of hypo/achylia in pernicious anemia. The antibody is detected in many patients with atrophic gastritis, is occasionally found in iron-deficient anemia, and is noted in thyroiditis and hyperthyroidism. Parietal cell antibodies, which increase with age, are present in Addison's disease (30%) and juvenile diabetes. Antibody to intrinsic factor is found in 50% to 70% of patients with pernicious anemia. Two types of intrinsic factor antibody exist: one prevents vitamin B_{12} binding to intrinsic factor, and the other binds to the intrinsic factor–B_{12} complex. Patients with smooth-muscle antibody also demonstrate gastric parietal cell–antibody activity; the cross-reacting antigen is related to F-actin.

Adrenocortical antibodies

Fifty percent of patients with primary Addison's disease display antibodies to the cytoplasm of adrenocortical cells in an indirect immunofluorescence assay. The antibodies react with cells in all three cortical layers of the adrenal gland. These antibodies are only rarely seen in secondary adrenal insufficiency, in other autoimmune diseases, and in inflammatory or neoplastic diseases.

Striated-muscle antibodies

These antibodies, detected by immunofluorescence, react with both skeletal and cardiac muscle. Fifty percent of patients with myasthenia gravis and 95% of myasthenia patients with a thymoma have antibodies that bind striated skeletal muscle. High titers of antibodies have been correlated with more severe disease, and generally, a titer of greater than 1:60 is specific for myasthenia. Some normal subjects also have the antibody, but the titers are usually less than 1:30. Patients with postpericardiotomy syndrome and occasional patients with dermatomyositis also display the antibody, but it is not found in patients with SLE or RA.

Cardiac muscle antibodies are found in one third of patients with rheumatic fever, as well as patients with recent streptococcal infections, or acute glomerulonephritis. These antibodies are also observed in patients after cardiac surgery or trauma and in certain patients with ischemic heart disease.

Acetylcholine receptor antibody

Acetylcholine receptor (AChR) antibody is thought to be directly involved in producing the weakness in myasthenia gravis. Antibody may attach directly to the receptor or immediately adjacent to it, causing an increased turnover of the receptor. Patients with rheumatoid arthritis treated with penicillamine can develop AChR antibodies and myasthenia gravis. Antibodies to AChR are detected by radioimmunoassay.

Smooth-muscle antibodies

High titers of antibodies to smooth muscle are found in up to 70% of patients with chronic active hepatitis. These antibodies are also found in some patients with viral hepatitis, infectious mononucleosis, asthma, chronic bronchitis, chronic renal disease, and mycoplasmal pneumonia. Of normal individuals, 5% to 6% also have the antibody in their blood in low titer. The smooth-muscle antigen against which these antibodies react is F-actin. Moreover, smooth-muscle antibody titers in chronic active hepatitis may be higher (>1:80) and relatively more persistent than those seen in the other disorders. Primary biliary cirrhosis may be associated with smooth-muscle antibody titers of 1:10 to 1:40. There may be a decrease in titer of the antibodies during remission of chronic active hepatitis.

Mitochondrial antibodies

Ninety percent of patients with primary biliary cirrhosis (PBC) have antibodies to mitochondria. A high titer of mitochondrial antibodies (1:160 or greater) is consistent with PBC, although from 5% to 15% of patients may show low or trace amounts of the antibody. The titer of the antibody does not correlate with the severity or treatment of the disease. Several other diseases, including SLE, are accompanied by the presence of mitochondrial antibodies, but the titers are usually lower than those observed in PBC. Other conditions associated with mitochondrial antibodies include bile stasis, chronic active hepatitis, cryptogenic cirrhosis, and extrahepatic biliary obstruction. The reactive antigen is present on the inner mitochondrial membrane and has been characterized as a subunit of the pyruvate dehydrogenase complex (PDC), a major mitochondrial enzyme. Other related mitochondrial enzymes have also been identified as antigenic targets. In in-vitro studies, mitchondrial antibodies can inactivate the catalytic activity of PDC and related enzymes.

Reticulin antibodies

Antibodies to reticulin are present in up to 78% of patients with celiac disease. They tend to occur more frequently in pediatric than in adult patients and are usually of the IgA class. These antibodies are not specific for celiac disease and occur in adult patients with Crohn's disease, RA, and Sjögren's syndrome and in normal individuals. The incidence of the antibody in dermatitis herpetiformis is between 12% and 68%. High titers of the antibody are suggestive of celiac disease. In patients treated with a gluten-free diet the titer of reticulin antibodies falls. Reticulin antibodies are also useful predictors of disease relapse in patients who have undergone gluten challenge.

Myelin antibodies

Multiple sclerosis or amyotrophic lateral sclerosis patients demonstrate IgA and IgM antibodies to myelin of rabbit spinal cord. IgA and IgM antibodies are found in approximately 70% of these patients; when IgG myelin antibody is present, it is suggestive but not diagnostic of these diseases. IgG antibodies are found in 80% of normal individuals but at titers of 1:4 or less. Recent studies have suggested that myelin basic protein may be one of the antigens recognized by antibodies from multiple sclerosis patients. Antibodies to peripheral nerve myelin have been described in Guillain-Barré syndrome. A reduction in antibody levels after plasmapheresis was associated with clinical improvement. A rise in antibody titer after treatment was associated with clinical relapse.

Islet-cell antibodies

Juvenile diabetics have pancreatic islet cell antibodies (ICA) in 80% of cases. The ICA gives a weak staining pattern, and a high concentration of antigen is required in the substrate. Four kinds of ICA have been described. The first two react with islet-cell cytoplasm, and one of them fixes complement (CF-ICA); the third antibody is cytotoxic to islet cells; and the fourth one reacts with islet-cell-surface antigens (ICSA). First-degree relatives of patients with juvenile diabetes, particularly those with CF-ICA in their serum, have an increased risk of developing diabetes. This risk is increased if they share one or two HLA-haplotypes with the affected sibling. Cytotoxic ICA and ICSA have also been recorded in the sera of patients for years prior to the development of diabetes. A subgroup of type II diabetics with no other endocrine disease who have ICA and an increased prevalence of HLA DR3 have been shown to become insulin-dependent.

Skin antibodies

Antibodies to skin are found in some of the bullous diseases (see Chapter 325). These antibodies are useful adjuncts to diagnosis, and the antibody titers are often related to disease activity. Antibodies to a keratinocyte cell surface glycoprotein have been identified in pemphigus vulgaris. This protein is a member of the cadherin family of cell adhesion molecules. In skin organ cultures these cadherin antibodies can cause loss of cell-cell adhesion. Antibodies to the basement membrane at the dermal-epidermal junction are seen in pemphigoid.

Cytoskeletal antibodies

Antibodies to components of the cytoskeleton, particularly microfilaments, intermediate filaments, and microtubules, have been noted in many rheumatic and infectious diseases but they currently do not have any known disease specificity. There is also a high prevalence of these antibodies in low titer in the normal population.

Antinuclear antibodies

Antinuclear antibodies (ANAs) react with a variety of nuclear antigens, including native, or double-stranded (ds) DNA; denatured, or single-stranded (ss) DNA; histones (basic nuclear proteins); nonhistone nuclear proteins; the nucleoli; nuclear lamins; and the nuclear matrix. ANAs occur in high frequency in systemic rheumatic diseases such as SLE, progressive systemic sclerosis (PSS), mixed connective-tissue disease (MCTD), and RA (see Table 293-2). In situations in which the clinician is faced with a patient who has features of more than one autoimmune systemic disease, the diagnostic dilemma may be solved by knowing the specificity of the ANA.

Examples of commonly encountered ANA staining patterns observed by indirect immunofluorescence on tissue culture cells are shown in Fig. 293-2. The figure shows three staining patterns: (1) a homogeneous nuclear pattern, (2) a speckled nuclear pattern, and (3) a nucleolar pattern. Caution should be exercised in attempting to interpret immunologic specificities of ANA by pattern alone, as antibodies with different specificities may produce similar patterns. Further testing of sera by techniques such as immunodiffusion, ELISA, or immunoblotting is required to define the specificity of the antibodies. An approach to the use and interpretation of the ANA test in the setting of rheumatic diseases is shown in Fig. 293-3.

Table 293-2. ANA specificities and disease associations

Antibody to	Disease association
1. Double-stranded (native) DNA	Highly specific for SLE (40%-60% incidence) when in moderate to high titer
2. Single-stranded (denatured) DNA	Present in SLE and other rheumatic and nonrheumatic diseases
3. Individual histones, H1, H2A, H2B, H3, H4	SLE (70%) drug-induced LE (>95%), RA (15%)
4. Histone complexes H2A-H2B	Drug-induced LE (>60%)
5. Sm (proteins complexed with U-RNAs)	SLE (30%), highly specific
6. U1-RNP (proteins complexed with U1-RNA)	MCTD (>95%), SLE (35%)
7. SS-A/Ro (proteins with small RNAs)	SS (70%), SLE (50%), other other CTDs
8. SS-B/La (45K protein with RNA polymerase III transcripts)	SS (40%-50%), SLE (15%)
9. Proliferating cell nuclear antigen (PCNA/cyclin)	SLE (3%)
10. Ma antigen	SLE (20%)
11. Ki antigen	SLE (12%)
12. Scl-70 (topoisomerase I)	PSS (20%) highly specific
13. Centromere/kinetochore	CREST (70%-90%), diffuse scleroderma (10%-20%)
14. RANA (rheumatoid arthritis–associated nuclear antigen [EBV related])	RA (90%)
15. Mi-1	Dermatomyositis (11%)
16. Jo-1 (histidyl-tRNA synthetase)	Polymyositis (31%)
17. Ku	Polymyositis-scleroderma overlap (55%)
18. NuMa (nuclear mitotic apparatus) antigen	RA, Sjögren's syndrome, carpal tunnel syndrome
19. PM/Scl (PM-1)	Polymyositis-scleroderma overlap

EBV, Epstein-Barr virus; SLE, systemic lupus erythematosus; MCTD, mixed connective tissue disease; SS, Sjögren's syndrome; PSS, progressive systemic sclerosis; CREST, calcinosis, Raynaud's phenomenon, esophageal hypomotility, sclerodactyly, and telangiectasia; RA, rheumatoid arthritis.

Antibodies to DNA. High titers of dsDNA antibodies occur almost exclusively in patients with SLE, especially in patients with active nephritis or central nervous system disease. Low or absent titers are seen occasionally in other rheumatic diseases and in SLE in remission. Antibodies to ssDNA are seen in SLE, drug-induced SLE, and other rheumatic and nonrheumatic diseases. The antigenic determinants in dsDNA are felt to be present on the deoxyribose-phosphate backbone. Antibodies to ssDNA probably react with purine and pyrimidine bases that are accessible in the single-stranded conformation. By immunofluorescence, antibodies to dsDNA produce a homogeneous or rim pattern, but antibodies to ssDNA, when found in isolation, do not give a positive ANA. In certain patients the titer of antibodies to dsDNA may be used to monitor the patients' response to therapeutic measures.

Antibodies to centromere/kinetochore. Antibodies to the centromere/kinetochore region (ACA) of the chromosome

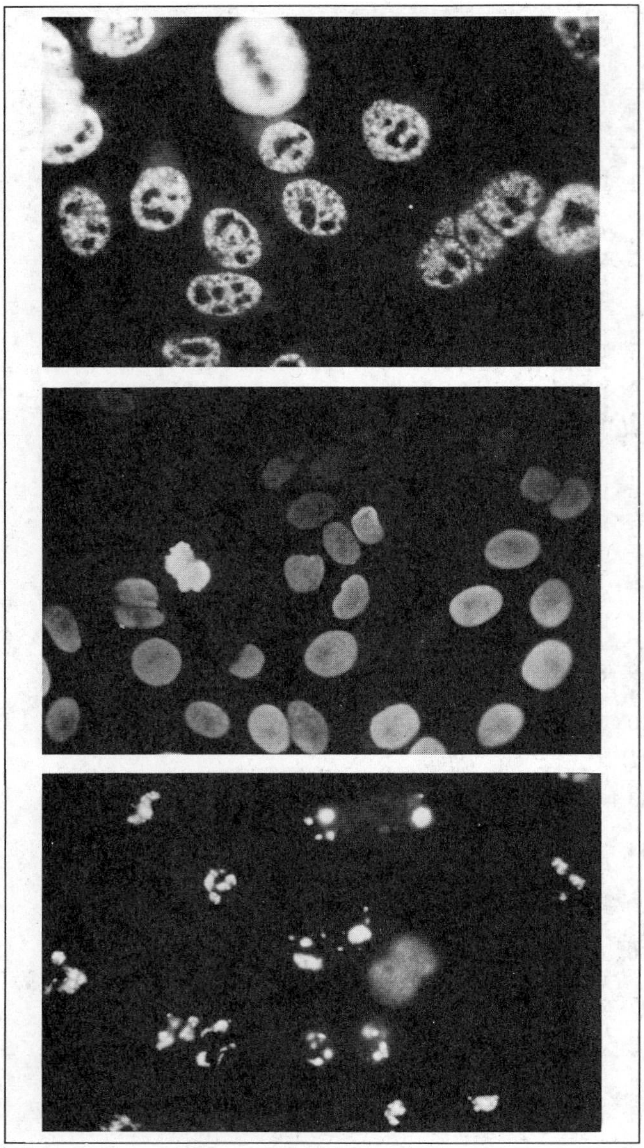

Fig. 293-2. Composite showing different patterns of nuclear staining produced by antinuclear antibodies. Speckled nuclear staining with the absence of nucleolar staining is shown in the figure on top. Homogeneous staining that includes the entire nucleus and nucleolus is shown in the middle figure. Nucleolar staining is demonstrated in the lower figure. The substrate was Hep-2 cells grown on microscopic slides. ×500.

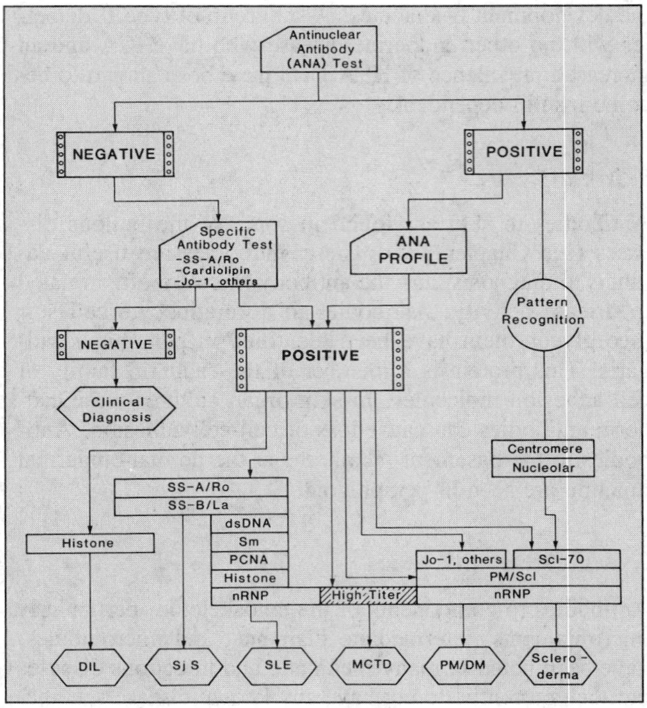

Fig. 293-3. An algorithm showing the diagnostic approach to the use of ANA in the clinical setting. ANA = antinuclear antibodies; DIL = drug-induced lupus; dsDNA = double-stranded DNA; MCTD = mixed connective tissue disease; nRNP = nuclear ribonucleoprotein; PCNA = proliferating cell nuclear antigen (cyclin); PM/DM = polymyositis/dermatomysitis; SjS = Sjögren's syndrome; SLE = systemic lupus erythematosus; SS-A, SS-B = Sjögren's syndrome antigens A,B. (Reprinted from the *Bulletin on the Rheumatic Diseases,* copyright © 1985. Used by permission of the Arthritis Foundation.)

display a characteristic speckled staining pattern on cultured cells by indirect immunofluorescence. These antibodies are most commonly associated with the scleroderma group of diseases, which includes systemic sclerosis, CREST syndrome, and Raynaud's phenomenon. The highest titer of ACA is found in the CREST syndrome, a less severe variant of systemic sclerosis.

Antibodies to histone. Antibodies that bind to histone are present in up to 70% of SLE patients and 15% of RA patients when sera are screened by ELISA. In drug-induced SLE (DIL) 95% to 100% of patients have histone antibodies. These antibodies react with all major classes of histone—H1, H2A, H2B, H3, and H4. Up to 75% of patients treated with procainamide or hydralazine develop histone antibodies. Of these patients, 15% develop overt clinical symptoms, including fever, malaise, myalgias, arthralgias, and pleural effusions. Other drugs associated with the development of histone antibodies include phenytoin and carbamazepine. Withdrawal of the offending drugs results in symptomatic relief and clearance of histone antibodies. By immunofluorescence on tissue culture cells, antibodies to histone produce a homogeneous staining pattern. The fact that antibodies to other nuclear proteins are absent in DIL may help to separate DIL from SLE, which is characterized by multiple autoantibody specificities.

Antibodies to nonhistone proteins. The other major class of ANAs in systemic autoimmune disease is characterized by reactivities with soluble nonhistone nuclear protein and protein-RNA complexes (Table 293-2). Most of these proteins are easily extractable in physiologic buffers and are called *extractable nuclear antigens* (ENAs). Double immunodiffusion or related techniques are used to detect antibodies to these proteins. Antibodies to Smith (Sm) antigen are highly specific for SLE and are present in the sera of 15% to 30% of SLE patients. High titers of antibody to nuclear ribonucleoprotein (nRNP) are characteristic of MCTD, but low titers of this antibody may be found in SLE, PSS, and other connective tissue diseases. Sm antibodies bind to nuclear proteins that are complexed to uridine-rich RNA (U1, U2, U4, U5, U6), and these complexes of nuclear protein and RNA are called *small nuclear ribonuclear particles* (SnRNP). Antibodies to nRNP bind to proteins containing U1-RNA.

Antibodies against two other nuclear antigens, SS-A/Ro and SS-B/La, have been detected in high frequency in Sjögren's syndrome. Antibodies to SS-A/Ro antigen are present in 70% of patients with primary Sjögren's syndrome, in 15% of patients with secondary Sjögren's syndrome and RA, and in 40% of patients with SLE. Almost all newborns with the neonatal lupus syndrome have antibodies to SS-A/Ro. This syndrome consists of congenital heart block and/or a skin rash similar to that seen in subacute cutaneous lupus. Almost half of the mothers of these children have connective tissue disease. The remaining mothers are asymptomatic at delivery, but follow-up studies have shown that many of them eventually develop a systemic rheumatic disease such as SLE. Antibodies to SS-B/La antigen are present in approximately 50% of patients with Sjögren's syndrome and in 15% of SLE patients, but rarely are seen in any other connective tissue disease. Both antigens have been characterized at the macromolecular level.

An antibody that is reactive with a nuclear protein restricted to proliferating cells is present in 3% of SLE patients. The reactive antigen, termed *proliferating cell nuclear antigen* (PCNA), has been characterized and is known as *cyclin*. Another ANA observed relatively frequently in sera from SLE patients is directed against the nuclear antigen named *Ma*.

Antibodies to the Jo-1 antigen have been noted in 30% to 50% of patients with polymyositis (PM), but they are uncommon in dermatomyositis and rare in other autoimmune disease. In PM the antibody to Jo-1 appears to be closely related to the development of pulmonary fibrosis. The Jo-1 antigen has been shown to be histidyl-tRNA synthetase. In patients with PM/PSS overlap and polymyositis an antibody against the PM/Scl antigen has been observed in high frequency.

Current studies of ANA in progressive systemic sclerosis (PSS) patients using tissue culture cells, such as HEp-2 cells, have demonstrated ANA in almost all scleroderma patients. Various patterns of nuclear staining are seen in PSS sera, including speckled, nucleolar, and homogeneous. One such antibody is directed against a nuclear antigen Scl-70 and is highly specific for PSS, although it is of low sensitivity, being present in less than 30% of patients. The antibody has not been found in other connective tissue diseases.

Antibodies to nucleolar antigens are present in up to 50% of PSS patients, and antibody titers in PSS are higher than those found in other connective tissue diseases. Three distinct patterns of nucleolar staining can be seen by immunofluorescence, speckled, homogeneous, and clumpy patterns. Antibodies with a speckled pattern were shown to immunoprecipitate RNA polymerase 1 complex, the enzyme transcribing ribosomal genes in the nucleolus. This antibody is restricted to scleroderma and is associated with the diffuse form of the disease. Antibodies with a clumpy staining pattern are also restricted to PSS and recognize a protein that is part of the U3-RNP complex in the nucleolus. Antibodies to the PM/Scl antigen display a homogeneous pattern of nucleolar staining.

Antibodies to phospholipids (anticardiolipin antibodies). These antibodies are found in up to 50% of patients with SLE but also occur in individuals without evidence of SLE. They are responsible for the in-vitro lupus anticoagulant test and for false-positive VDRL tests because of the inclusion of cardiolipin, a phospholipid, in the test substrate. Phospholipid antibodies are associated with a variety of clinical conditions, including recurrent fetal loss, recurrent venous and arterial thrombosis, thrombocytopenia, and labile hypertension. It has also been suggested that they are associated with cerebrovascular accidents and early myocardial infarcts. However, studies on unselected groups of patients have not confirmed these initial observations. Current opinion holds that IgG phospholipid antibodies are of greater pathologic significance than IgM antibodies.

Antibodies to neutrophil cytoplasm (ANCA). Antineutrophil cytoplasmic antibodies were intially described in patients with segmental necrotizing glomerulonephritis. Since that time, these antibodies have been identified in a number of vasculitic disorders, such as Wegener's granulomatosis, classic and microscopic polyarteritis, and necrotizing and crescentic glomerulonephritis. Two patterns of neutrophil staining can be recognized by IIF: (1) granular cytoplasmic (C-ANCA) and (2) perinuclear (P-ANCA). The P-ANCA pattern is caused by artifactual redistribution of certain proteins in a perinuclear fashion. In general, the C-ANCA pattern is caused by reactivity with PR3, an enzyme component of the primary granules, and the P-ANCA pattern is caused by reactivity with myeloperoxidase. C-ANCA is a very sensitive marker for classic Wegener's granulomatosis, characterized by necrotizing granulomas of the respiratory tract, necrotizing small vessel vasculitis, and segmental necrotizing glomerulonephritis. This sensitivity decreases when cases without the classic triad are included.

Current data suggest that ANCA are useful in the investigation of patients with vasculitis, but the presence of these antibodies alone without a tissue diagnosis, does not provide sufficient information on which to base treatment.

REFERENCES

Asherson RA and Cervera R: The antiphospholipid syndrome: a syndrome in evolution. Ann Rheum Dis 51:147, 1992.

Bergman DA: Thyroid physiology and immunology. Otolaryngol Clin North Am 23:231, 1990.

Bottazzo GF et al: Novel considerations on the antibody/autoantigen system in type 1 (insulin-dependent) diabetes mellitus. Ann Med 23:453, 1991.

Christian CL: Biology of autoimmunity: a review. Clin Exp Rheum 9:213, 1991.
Fritzler MJ and Salazar M: Diversity and origin of rheumatologic autoantibodies. Clin Microbiol Rev 4:256, 1991.
Reimer G: Autoantibodies against nuclear, nucleolar and mitochondrial antigens in systemic sclerosis (scleroderma). Rheum Dis Clin North Am 16:169, 1990.
Rowley MJ et al: Inhibitory autoantibody to a conformational epitope of the pyruvate dehydrogenase complex, the major autoantigen in primary biliary cirrhosis. Clin Immunol Immunopath 60:356, 1991.
Tan EM: Antinuclear antibodies: diagnostic markers for autoimmune disease and probes for cell biology. Adv Immunol 44:93, 1989.
Third International Workshop on Antineutrophil Cytoplasmic Antibodies. Am J Kidney Dis 18:145, 1991.
Worman HJ and Courvalin J-C: Autoantibodies against nuclear envelope proteins in liver disease. Hepatology 14:1269, 1991.

CHAPTER

294 Rheumatoid Factors

Dennis A. Carson

Autoantibodies against IgG, commonly termed *rheumatoid factors,* are characteristic of rheumatoid arthritis and Sjögren's syndrome and may contribute to immune complex formation and tissue damage. However, IgM rheumatoid factors are not specific for rheumatic disease but are found in many chronic inflammatory conditions (Table 294-1). The malignant B cells from patients with chronic lymphocytic leukemia and Waldenström's macroglobulinemia frequently express surface IgM with rheumatoid factor activity. Also, recent experiments have shown that normal humans and animals regularly synthesize rheumatoid factors during anamnestic immune responses. The rheumatoid factors probably are an integral component of the network that has been postulated to regulate humoral and cellular immunity. Indeed, the immunoglobulin genes encoding rheumatoid factor have been cloned and are prevalent in all normal people.

Because the specificity of IgM rheumatoid factor for rheumatoid arthritis increases with serum titer, all patients suspected of the diagnosis should have a quantitative assay performed. IgM rheumatoid factors are multivalent and agglutinate IgG-coated latex particles to produce a visible flocculation (Fig. 294-1). IgM rheumatoid factor titers are expressed as the highest dilution of serum yielding detectable agglutination. At a serum dilution that excludes 95% of the normal human population, more than 70% of rheumatoid arthritis patients are seropositive. Individuals with borderline titers should be retested after several weeks; only patients with IgM rheumatoid factor titers in the normal range on consecutive determinations should be considered seronegative.

Patients with very high IgM rheumatoid factor titers usually have more aggressive arthritis and more extra-articular rheumatoid disease than those with low titers. In some patients, but not all, a remission in disease activity is heralded by a reduction in IgM rheumatoid factor titers. Small variations in IgM rheumatoid factor titers, however, are of little clinical significance in monitoring the response to therapy.

Rheumatoid factors of the IgG class, when compared with IgM rheumatoid factors, are inefficient agglutinators. Hence, their measurement by latex agglutination is imprecise and requires the prior removal of IgM rheumatoid factors by chromatography, centrifugation, or enzymatic digestion. IgG rheumatoid factors characteristically form intermediate sedimenting immune complexes that are detectable in the analytic ultracentrifuge. While large amounts of such IgG rheumatoid factor–containing intermediate complexes are quite common in rheumatoid synovial fluids, their appearance in serum usually is associated with prominent extra-articular disease, such as vasculitis or Felty's syndrome, hyperglobulinemic purpura, or the hyperviscosity syndrome.

In the human infectious diseases associated with rheumatoid factor production, the autoantibody disappears from the circulation after removal of the inciting stimulus. The

Table 294-1. Diseases commonly associated with rheumatoid factor

Rheumatic diseases	Rheumatoid arthritis, Sjögren's syndrome, systemic lupus erythematosus, scleroderma, mixed connective tissue disease
Acute viral infections	Mononucleosis, hepatitis, influenza, and many others; after vaccination (may yield falsely elevated titers of antiviral or antibacterial antibodies)
Parasitic infections	Trypanosomiasis, kala-azar, malaria, schistosomiasis, filariasis, etc.
Chronic inflammatory disease	Tuberculosis, leprosy, yaws, syphilis, brucellosis, subacute bacterial endocarditis, salmonellosis
Other hyperglobulinemic states	Hypergammaglobulinemic purpura, cryoglobulinemia, chronic liver disease, sarcoid, other chronic pulmonary diseases

Modified from Kelley WN et al, editors: Textbook of rheumatology, ed 3. Philadelphia, 1991, Saunders.

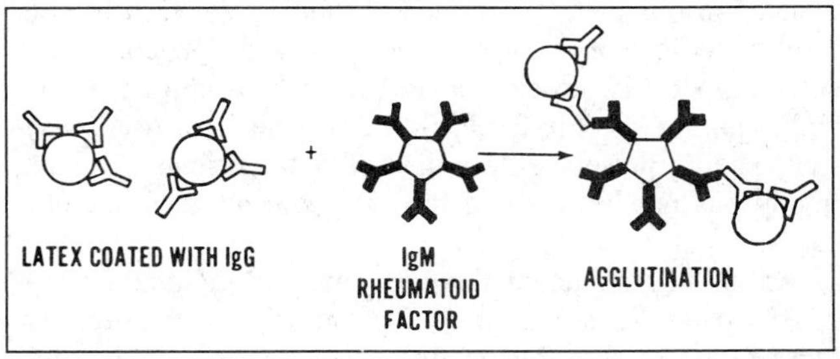

Fig. 294-1. Latex fixation test for IgM rheumatoid factor.

reasons for the persistence of rheumatoid factor in patients with rheumatoid arthritis are not known. Contributing factors probably include the localization of the rheumatoid factor–producing cells to the synovial membrane, the progressive accumulation of somatic mutations in the rheumatoid factor genes, a loss of regulation by T lymphocytes, an abnormality in B lymphocyte differentiation, and perhaps the repeated deposition of immune complexes.

Because of the occurrence of rheumatoid factor in some apparently normal individuals and the absence of significant titers of rheumatoid factor in some patients with definite rheumatoid arthritis, one can legitimately question the importance of the autoantibody in the pathogenesis of chronic synovitis. It must be remembered, however, that several characteristics distinguish the rheumatoid factors in patients with rheumatoid arthritis from those in normal subjects. In rheumatoid arthritis patients, rheumatoid factors are usually of high titer, are synthesized at least in part in the inflamed synovial membranes, and have a greater preponderance of IgG rheumatoid factors. The latter antibodies in high concentration have the unique ability to aggregate in the absence of exogenous antigen and can react with IgM rheumatoid factors.

Complement fixation by rheumatoid factor, as for other antibodies, depends on an exact stoichiometry between antigen and antibody. It may be that only in the rheumatoid factor–synthesizing synovial membrane is the concentration of normal IgG low enough, and rheumatoid factor high enough, to permit extensive lattice formation and efficient complement consumption. Indeed, hemolytic complement levels characteristically are depressed in seropositive rheumatoid synovial fluids but are near normal in companion sera.

REFERENCES

Carson DA: Rheumatoid factor. In Kelley WN et al, editors: Textbook of rheumatology, ed 3. Philadelphia, 1991, Saunders.

Carson DA et al: Rheumatoid factor and immune networks. Annu Rev Immunol 5:109, 1987.

Carson DA, Chen PP, and Kipps TJ: New roles for rheumatoid factor. J Clin Invest 87:379, 1991.

Carson DA: Genetic factors in the etiology and pathogenesis of autoimmunity. FASEB J 6:2800, 1992.

CHAPTER

295 Synovial Fluid Analysis

Nathan J. Zvaifler

Synovial fluid is readily obtained by aspiration from most joints, and its analysis is an essential evaluation of any patient with joint disease. Some disorders, such as gout, calcium pyrophosphate dihydrate (CPPD) deposition disease, and septic arthritis, can be diagnosed definitively by this procedure. Other diseases, including rheumatoid arthritis and systemic lupus erythematosus, may be considered or excluded. Indeed, synovial fluid analysis better reflects the events in the articular cavity than do abnormal blood tests, since antinuclear antibodies and increased erythrocyte sedimentation rate, elevated uric acid concentrations, or rheumatoid factors can be seen in normal individuals or in unrelated joint diseases.

NORMAL SYNOVIAL FLUID

Small quantities of a clear, pale-yellow or straw-colored, viscous, and slightly alkaline liquid are present in normal joints. The viscosity and mucinous characteristics of the synovial fluid depend on the integrity of hyaluronate, a large, highly polymerized mucopolysaccharide.

Synovial fluid is essentially a plasma dialysate, but because of the physical characteristics of the hyaluronate, certain molecules are preferentially excluded from the joint. Most electrolytes are present in amounts comparable to those in blood—including glucose, which approximates but is usually 10 mg/dl less than in blood. Proteins, particularly those with high molecular weight or asymmetrical shape, are preferentially excluded. Because fibrinogen and many of the clotting factors are missing, normal synovial fluid does not clot. The total protein content is usually less than 2.0 g per deciliter, with the smaller molecules, such as albumin, disproportionately represented.

Normal synovial fluid is relatively acellular, with only a few hundred cells per cubic millimeter, predominantly mononuclear. Occasionally, large synoviocytes are seen. Red blood cells and platelets are absent. The cellular characteristics of the synovial fluid are independent of the peripheral blood count.

ARTHROCENTESIS

There are no absolute contraindications to synovial fluid aspiration, although patients with sepsis or taking anticoagulation therapy require special care, and the aspirating needle should not be placed through areas of tissue infection or cellulitis. The skin should be cleansed and aseptically prepared; gloves and drapes are not necessary. A local anesthetic agent minimizes discomfort but should not be injected into the joint prior to fluid aspiration. The routes for arthrocentesis are varied, but sites of obvious bulging are most easily entered as long as vital anatomic structures are avoided. As much fluid as possible should be removed from the joint and allocated into containers appropriate for bacteriologic studies; a test tube with heparin for cell count and cytologic examination; a potassium oxylate–containing tube for glucose; and a clean, glass tube for special tests, such as complement or protein determination. When fluid is limited, the heparin-containing tube suffices for all studies. Simultaneous blood and serum samples for glucose, protein, and complement are advisable.

SYNOVIAL FLUID TESTS

Gross examination

Observing the fluid obtained at the bedside helps plan subsequent studies, particularly if only small volumes are available. Generally, the cloudier the fluid, the more cells it contains. Occasionally, an opacity results from crystalline materials, fibrin, or fragments of cartilage. As is seen in Table 295-1, fluids from degenerative, traumatic, or metabolic arthropathies and mechanical derangements of joints are usually colorless, in contrast to fluids from the inflammatory or septic rheumatic disorders. Streaks of blood can result from injury to small vessels during arthrocentesis, but grossly bloody fluids (hemarthrosis) are associated with a number of rheumatic disorders (see box to the right).

Viscosity can be estimated by observing the rate at which synovial fluid extrudes from the syringe. Normally, because of high viscosity, a drop forms but leaves reluctantly; as it does, a long thread develops. Unusually viscous fluids are obtained from ganglia and in hypothyroid effusions. With increasing inflammation, viscosity is generally decreased, especially in chronic processes.

Cytology

Leukocyte counts are an essential part of synovial fluid analysis and form the basis for classification of joint effusions (Table 295-1). Those with leukocyte counts from 200 to 2000 mm^3 are generally termed *noninflammatory*. Polymorphonuclear cells should constitute less than 25% of the total. As the count rises into the inflammatory and septic range, the proportion of polymorphonuclear leukocytes generally increases, not infrequently accounting for 90% of the total white blood cell population. Occasionally, however, in the early phases of rheumatoid arthritis or in certain infections such as tuberculosis, mononuclear cells may predominate. Leukocyte counts in excess of 100,000 mm^3 are generally, but not exclusively, associated with joint infection; marked elevations are uncommonly seen in rheumatic fever, crystal-induced arthritides, rheumatoid arthritis, and Reiter's syndrome. Conversely, early in infectious processes or in those incompletely treated, counts of less than 100,000 mm^3 are found. Gonococcal arthritis, tuberculosis, and certain fungal infections of joints regularly have lower counts (Fig. 295-1).

Conditions associated with hemarthrosis

Hereditary deficiency of clotting factors
Anticoagulation therapy
Sickle cell anemia
Thrombocytopenia
Pseudogout
Amyloidosis (xanthochromia only)
Pigmented villonodular synovitis
Synovial hemangioma
Rheumatoid arthritis
Infection
Trauma with or without fracture
Osteoarthritis
Neuropathic joints
Metallic joint prosthesis
Primary or metastatic neoplasm of joints
Myeloproliferative disease
Scurvy

In general, the synovial fluid white blood cell count can be anticipated from the clinical examination. Joint redness and tenderness are usually paralleled by elevated leukocyte counts, with two significant exceptions. Systemic lupus erythematosus (SLE) and hypertrophic osteoarthropathy characteristically have clinically inflamed joints but noninflammatory effusions. Both have elevated protein content, suggesting exudates; SLE fluids usually have very low hemolytic complement activity.

Wet preparations

Examination of a drop of fresh synovial fluid by light microscopy is often the single most important test of synovial fluid. The slides and cover glasses must be scrupulously cleaned prior to use because dirt, minute pieces of glass, and fibers from lens paper can be confused with crystalline and fibrillar materials. Red and white blood cells are easy to distinguish and their numbers estimated.

Lipid droplets free in the synovial fluid usually signify fractures or trauma to the joint, but they can be seen in avascular necrosis, fat embolism, and, rarely, inflammatory effusions. Irregular strands of fibrin or fibrillar fragments of

Table 295-1. Classification of synovial effusions

Gross examination	Normal	"Noninflammatory"	Inflammatory	Septic
Viscosity	High	High	Low	Variable
Color	Colorless to straw-colored	Straw-colored to yellow	Yellow	Variable
Clarity	Transparent	Transparent	Cloudy	Opaque
WBC (per mm^3)	<200	200 to 2000	2000 to 75,000	Often >100,000
PMN leukocytes (%)	<25	<25	Often >50	>75
Mucin clot	Firm	Firm	Friable	Friable
Glucose (A.M. fasting)	Nearly equal to blood	Nearly equal to blood	<25 mg/dl lower than in blood	>25 mg/dl lower than in blood

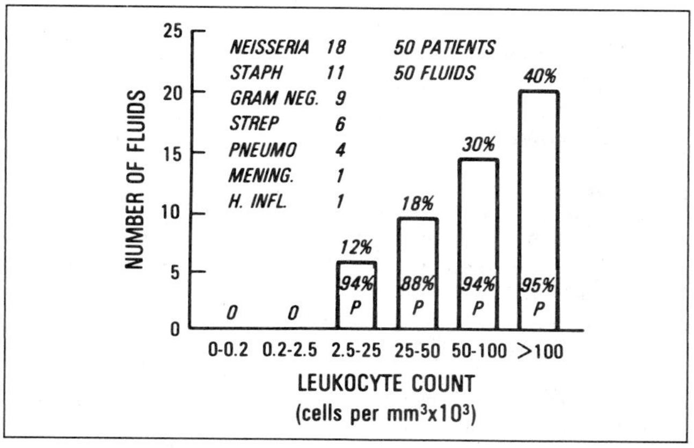

Fig. 295-1. The leukocyte counts in 50 synovial fluids with various forms of septic arthritis. The percentage of the total sample that was present in each range of the white cell count appears above the bar; the percentage of polymorphonuclear *(P)* cells within the bar. (Reprinted with permission from Krey PR and Bailen DA: Synovial fluid leukocytosis. Am J Med 67:436, 1979.

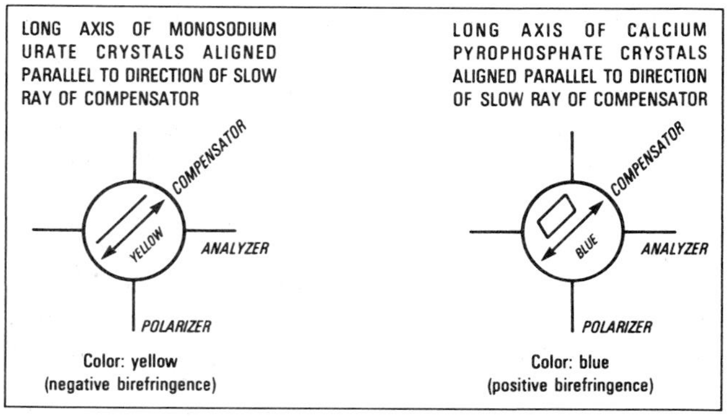

Fig. 295-2. Use of the first-order red compensator (retardation plate), demonstrating the principles of polarized light microscopy as applied to the analysis of crystals in synovial fluid. (From Cohen AS: Laboratory diagnostic precedures in the rheumatic diseases, ed 3. New York, 1985, Grune & Stratton.)

cartilage accompany degenerative arthritis. Both are faintly birefringent and should not be confused with crystalline materials.

All synovial fluids should be examined for crystals. Crystals of importance (as opposed to dust or debris) tend to have straight, parallel edges. Monosodium urate (MSU) appears as monotonously similar 8- to 10-μ needle- or rod-shaped crystals. In contrast, calcium pyrophosphate dihydrate (CPPD) crystals assume multiple three-dimensional forms; rods, rhomboids, and parallelepipeds occur simultaneously. It is important to note whether the crystalline material is intra- or extracellular. During acute attacks of gout and "pseudogout," crystals are engulfed by leukocytes; in the intercritical periods, the crystals may lie free in the fluid. Crystal identification is greatly enhanced by compensated polarized light microscopy. Most rheumatologic textbooks discuss the theory of polarization microscopy; the principle is shown in Fig. 295-2.

Monosodium urate crystals appear as brightly birefringent rods or needles that give a yellow color when the crystal axis is parallel to the slow ray compensator. This is termed *negative birefringence* (Plate VI-1). CPPD crystals are much less birefringent and, therefore, more difficult to identify. They have a *positive birefringence;* that is, their slow ray is in the long axis of the crystal, giving them a bluish appearance (Plate VI-1). MSU crystals are virtually pathognomonic for gouty arthritis, and CPPD crystals are associated with CPPD deposition disease. However, two rheumatic diseases may coexist. This is particularly true for CPPD, which is present in the articular cartilages of 5% of the population. It is not surprising, therefore, that CPPD crystals have been identified in effusions from a number of inflammatory joint diseases, particularly rheumatoid arthritis. Acute infections and crystal-induced arthritis may also occur together and should be considered in any patient with unusually high joint fluid leukocyte counts or in whom articular inflammation fails to subside with appropriate therapy for the crystal-induced disorder.

Basic calcium phosphate (BCP) crystals, including apatite, octacalcium phosphate, and tricalcium phosphate, are associated with subcutaneous calcification and calcific periarthritis and tendinitis. Recently BCP crystals have been found in both acute and chronic synovitis (see Chapter 320). Unfortunately, the size of BCP crystals is below the limits of resolution of optical microscopy. However, these crystals do have a tendency to aggregate, giving them the appearance of shiny laminated printed "coins" by light microscopy. This appearance may suggest the need for further studies, of which transmission electron microscopy is the most readily available.

MSU or CPPD can be confused with other birefringent materials, including crystalline anticoagulants, such as calcium oxalate and ethylenediaminetetraacetic acid or repository forms of certain corticosteroid preparations (betamethasone and prednisolone *tert*-butylacetate are negatively and positively birefringent rods, respectively). Cholesterol crystals, usually found in chronic effusions of rheumatoid arthritis, are easily distinguished because of their large size and flat, platelike shape with notched corners.

Cytology

Wright's staining for cellular morphology provides accurate differential leukocyte counts. Typical LE cells may be found in centrifuged specimens from SLE effusions and, occasionally, in patients with Felty's syndrome. Large mononuclear cells are derived from the synovial lining (synoviocytes).

Gram's and Ziehl-Nielsen stains

Smears, staining, and identification of organisms are performed in the usual manner on heparinized synovial fluid samples or specimens that have been concentrated by centrifugation. Interpretation is sometimes difficult because bacteria can be confused with precipitated hyaluronate (mucin).

Glucose

Generally, the intra-articular glucose concentration parallels the blood level, but the turnover in the joint differs; therefore, spurious results will be obtained if the sample is not obtained after prolonged fasting. Modest differences are not significant, particularly in the presence of large numbers (>50,000/mm^3) of granulocytes, but a synovial fluid glucose reduction of more than 50 mg per deciliter, as compared with a companion blood sample, is most compatible with a joint infection.

Serum proteins

Normally, most serum proteins are excluded from the articular cavity, but with increasing inflammation, large molecules gain access to the joint fluid. Thus, the protein content of fluids from acute and chronic inflammatory forms of arthritis exceeds the normal 1.5 to 2.0 g per deciliter and approach serum concentrations. In rheumatoid arthritis and certain other chronic inflammatory arthritides, there is also a small contribution from local production of immunoglobulins or complement components. Pathologic fluids occasionally clot, owing to the presence of coagulation factors in the effusion that are normally absent from the joint. Antinuclear antibodies and rheumatoid factors produced in the chronically inflamed synovium are rarely detected when they are not demonstrable in the serum.

Complement

In general, the total hemolytic activity of synovial fluid is proportional to the white cell count or the concentration of total protein. For most inflammatory effusions, the complement activity is 50% or more of serum values. Effusions from patients with Reiter's disease have very high values, reflecting the fact that complement responds as an acute-phase reactant and is often markedly increased in the serum of these patients. In contrast, the joint fluids from patients with rheumatoid arthritis or SLE show low complement values as a result of intra-articular utilization. To avoid confusion caused by low serum levels of hemolytic activity (as might occur in SLE), the fluid complement value can be expressed as a percentage of the expected value based on comparison with serum concentrations of other proteins or individual complement components. Total hemolytic activity is usually less than 30% of the expected value in rheumatoid and SLE effusions. Similar low values may also be seen in certain immune complex forms of arthritis, such as acute hepatitis. Synovial fluid must be centrifuged and the supernatant frozen at −70° C until tested to ensure correct total hemolytic complement determinations.

Measurements of complement components (e.g., C3, C4), although easier to perform, are less reliable because when activated they generate small-molecular-weight byproducts (see Chapter 290), that are retained in the joint and are still detectable by the immunodiffusion techniques employed for their measurement.

REFERENCES

Bunch TW et al: Synovial fluid complement: usefulness in diagnosis and classification of rheumatoid arthritis. Ann Intern Med 81:32, 1974.

McCarty DJ: Synovial fluid In McCarty DJ and Koopman W, editors: Arthritis and allied conditions, ed 12. Philadelphia, 1993, Lea & Febiger.

Pekin TJ and Zvaifler NJ: Synovial fluid findings in systemic lupus erythematosus (SLE). Arthritis Rheum 13:777, 1970.

Schumacher HR: Synovial fluid analysis. In Kelley WN et al, editors: Textbook of rheumatology, ed 3. Philadelphia, 1989, Saunders.

Wild JH and Zvaifler NJ: An office technique for identifying crystals in synovial fluid. Am Fam Prac 12:72, 1975.

Wild JH, and Zvaifler NJ: Hemarthrosis associated with sodium warfarin therapy. Arthritis Rheum 19:98, 1976.

CHAPTER

296 Imaging Evaluation of Patients with Arthritis

Donald Resnick
David J. Sartoris

The proper analysis and treatment of patients with articular disorders require careful radiographic examination. It can be used in some individuals whose clinical manifestations are confusing, allowing a specific diagnosis to be made. In other individuals in whom a clinical diagnosis is readily apparent, the radiographs document the extent and the severity of joint involvement. Furthermore, sequential radiographic examinations allow analysis of the efficacy of various therapeutic regimens.

Any summary of the radiographic evaluation of patients with arthritis must discuss the available imaging techniques and modalities, the cardinal roentgen signs of articular disease, and the peculiar predilection of certain disorders to affect specific "target areas" in the body.

IMAGING TECHNIQUES AND MODALITIES

Plain film examination

Initial plain film examination almost universally requires that more than one projection of a symptomatic joint be obtained. Reliance on a single projection frequently leads to misdiagnosis. For example, subtle osseous erosions in a hand or wrist of a patient with rheumatoid arthritis may not be detected on frontal or lateral views but are readily apparent on oblique projections.

In patients with polyarticular disease, it is impractical to obtain a survey of all joints. The radiographic examination should emphasize those articulations that are symptomatic and those that are common target sites of the disease in question. As an example, the patient with rheumatoid arthritis requires careful roentgen analysis of the hands, wrists, feet, knees, shoulders, and cervical spine, and the patient with calcium pyrophosphate dihydrate (CPPD) crystal deposition disease requires careful analysis of the hands, wrists, knees, and pelvis.

Additional radiographs are required of certain sites in the evaluation of patients with ankylosing spondylitis (thoracic and lumbar spine, sacroiliac joints), diffuse idiopathic skeletal hyperostosis (thoracic and lumbar spine), and hemophilia (ankles, elbows).

Weight-bearing, stress, and traction radiographs

In certain situations, radiographs obtained during weight-bearing, stress, or traction can supplement the plain film examination. In evaluating patients with osteoarthritis of the knee, radiographs obtained while the patient is standing on the affected leg can be extremely useful, allowing more precise documentation of the integrity of the articular cartilage. Furthermore, knee radiographs obtained during weight bearing allow analysis of the amount of displacement of the tibia on the femur and the degree of varus or valgus angulation. Slight flexion of the knees during the examination may be of added benefit. Weight-bearing radiography is less useful in the evaluation of other articulations.

Radiographs exposed during the application of stress across an articulation provide information regarding the integrity of surrounding ligaments and soft tissue structures. "Stress" radiographs are useful in the analysis of ligamentous injury of the knee, ankle, and first metacarpophalangeal joint. Analysis of the acromioclavicular joint after trauma may require the stress produced by tying a 5- or 10-lb weight to the wrist, while lateral radiographs of the lumbar spine obtained after prolonged standing with or without the application of additional weight may provide a more accurate assessment of any osseous defect in the neural arch (spondylolysis) and the presence of vertebral slippage (spondylolisthesis).

Conventional and computed tomography

In certain locations, such as the sternoclavicular and temporomandibular joints, it is difficult to obtain adequate plain films, so conventional tomography is often essential. In any location, conventional tomography can detect subchondral alterations such as transchondral fractures (osteochondritis dissecans), cysts, and neoplasms. It may allow differentiation of severe osteoporosis (reflex sympathetic dystrophy syndrome, transient osteoporosis) with thinning of the subchondral bone plate and infection with disruption of the bone plate.

Computed axial tomography has the ability to differentiate between areas that differ only slightly in density and to reconstruct the images in multiple planes. Computed axial tomography has been used to investigate such disorders of the musculoskeletal system as spinal stenosis, intervertebral disk displacement, soft tissue neoplasms, osteoporosis, and spinal and pelvic fractures, as well as sacroiliac joint disease. It is best applied to areas of complex anatomy that are difficult to evaluate with routine techniques.

Arthrography

Intra-articular injection of contrast media, air, or both has been used in investigating various articular problems. Knee arthrography is most frequently applied to an analysis of meniscal injuries, but it also may be used to outline collateral and cruciate ligament tears, articular cartilage alterations, synovial processes, masses, and periarticular synovial cysts (popliteal cysts). In the hip, arthrography is most commonly employed to evaluate for the presence of prosthetic loosening or infection. Glenohumeral joint arthrography is helpful in the evaluation of rotator cuff tears, adhesive capsulitis, previous dislocations, synovial processes, infection, and bicipital tendon abnormalities. It should be stressed, however, that the application of magnetic resonance imaging to analysis of the musculoskeletal system has lessened the need for arthrography.

Magnetic resonance imaging

This revolutionary technique demonstrates excellent contrast resolution and satisfactory spatial resolution, and it can be used to evaluate a variety of musculoskeletal processes. Important examples of such processes include intraspinal abnormalities, soft tissue infections and tumors, diseases leading to alterations in bone marrow, osteonecrosis, and intra-articular ligamentous and cartilage injuries. Magnetic resonance imaging has become the method of choice in evaluating internal derangements of the knee and shoulder, and it competes effectively with arthrography in assessing many wrist abnormalities. When combined with intravenous injection of certain contrast agents, magnetic resonance imaging allows differentiation of inflamed synovial tissue and joint effusion. Newer imaging sequences have showed promise in the analysis of cartilage integrity. Additional applications of magnetic resonance imaging include the evaluation of nerve entrapment syndromes, synovial cysts, and tendinitis.

CARDINAL ROENTGENOGRAPHIC SIGNS OF ARTICULAR DISEASE

The appendicular skeleton

Soft tissue swelling. Soft tissue prominence may reflect an accumulation of intra-articular fluid, capsular distention, soft tissue edema, or peri- or intra-articular masses. In rheumatoid arthritis, fusiform periarticular soft tissue swelling is characteristic (Fig. 296-1). A similar appearance may be identified in psoriatic arthritis, Reiter's syndrome (Fig. 296-2), juvenile chronic arthritis, and infection, as well as in hemophilia caused by the intra-articular accumulation of blood and the presence of synovial hypertrophy. In pigmented villonodular synovitis, the soft tissue swelling may appear more nodular, creating a lobulated, radiopaque shadow. Lobulated soft tissue swelling also is seen in gout (Fig. 296-3), xanthomatosis, and amyloidosis. In gouty ar-

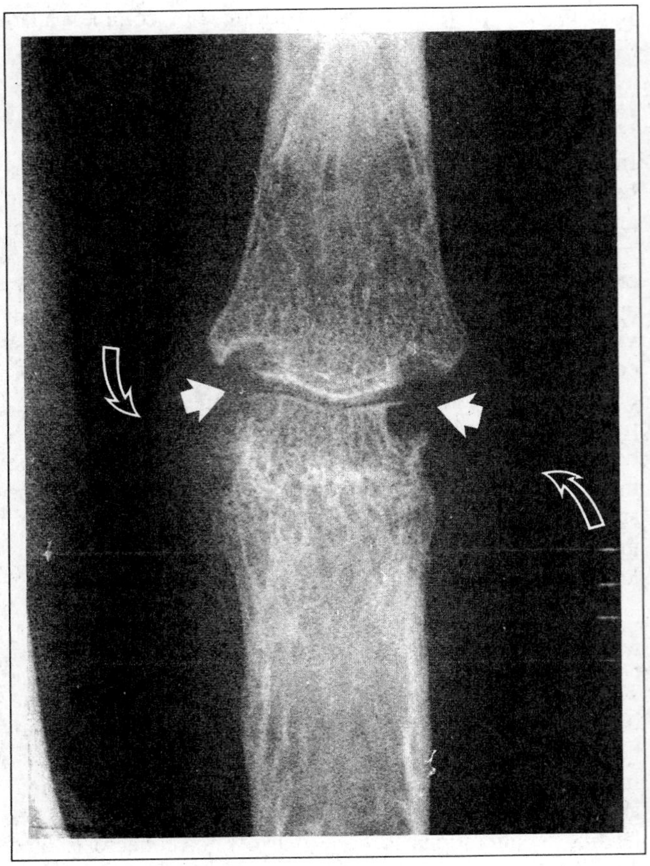

Fig. 296-1. Rheumatoid arthritis. Findings include fusiform soft tissue swelling about the proximal interphalangeal joint *(curved arrows)*, diffuse joint space loss, periarticular osteoporosis, and marginal erosions *(arrowheads)*.

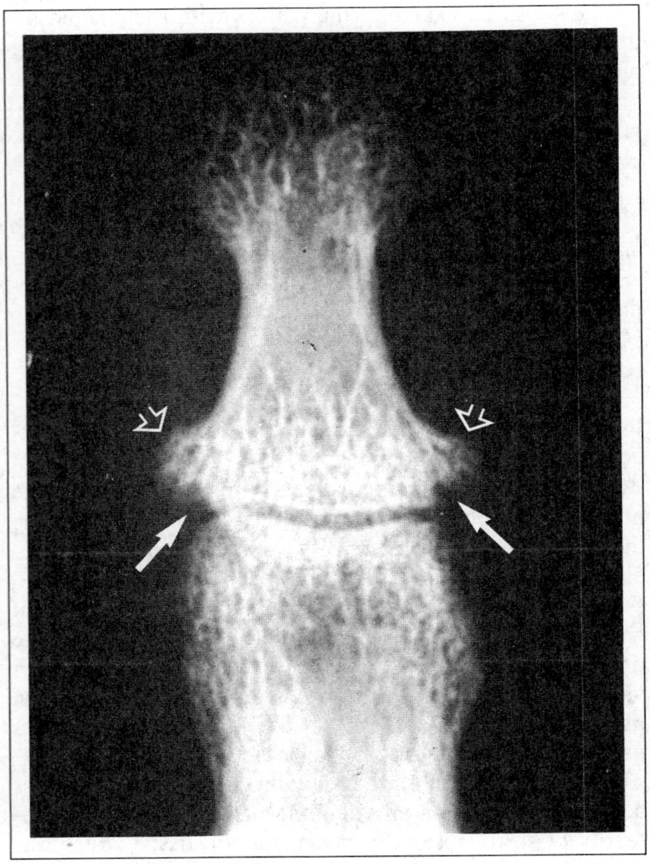

Fig. 296-2. Reiter's syndrome. Observe the marginal erosions *(arrows)*, most evident along the base of the distal phalanx, and a characteristic proliferative component creating an ill-defined osseous surface *(arrowheads)*. The joint space is mildly narrowed, and there is no evidence of periarticular osteoporosis. Fusiform soft tissue swelling is evident. These changes occurring in a distal interphalangeal joint are more typical of psoriasis than Reiter's syndrome.

thritis, the masses reflect the presence of tophi. Xanthomas are commonly encountered in tendinous structures such as the extensor tendons of the hand and the Achilles tendon. A peculiar prominence of the soft tissues of the shoulder, the "shoulder-pad" sign, is recognized in some cases of amyloidosis.

Reduction in bone density. Periarticular osteoporosis, an increased radiolucency of bone (osteopenia/porosis), is a well-recognized manifestation of certain articular disorders. In rheumatoid arthritis, synovitis with accompanying hyperemia leads to juxta-articular osteopenia, especially in the hands, wrists, and feet (Fig. 296-1). In this disease, similar osteopenia may occur about larger articulations such as the knee and the hip, although bony sclerosis or eburnation may be evident in these sites. During the acute inflammatory stage of certain of the seronegative spondyloarthropathies, periarticular osteopenia also may be evident, but it is more typical for these latter disorders to be unaccompanied by osteopenia, perhaps owing to the intermittent or episodic nature of the synovial inflammation (Fig. 296-2). Osteopenia is distinctly unusual in gouty arthritis and degenerative joint disease (osteoarthritis) and is infrequent in pigmented villonodular synovitis and idiopathic synovial osteochondromatosis. It may be apparent during acute episodes of pyogenic arthritis and during the course of tuberculosis and hemophilia.

Joint space narrowing. Cartilaginous destruction is accompanied by loss of the interosseous space *(joint space)*. In rheumatoid arthritis, early cartilaginous destruction is typical and leads to diffuse loss of interosseous space (Fig. 296-1). This finding is especially prominent in the proximal interphalangeal and metacarpophalangeal joints of the hand; all the compartments of the wrist (Fig. 296-4); and the metatarsophalangeal joints of the foot, the knee, and the hip. Diffuse joint space loss is also common in ankylosing spondylitis, psoriatic arthritis, and Reiter's syndrome.

In gouty arthritis, joint space diminution is a less constant manifestation of the disease. In fact, the recognition of significant osseous erosion in the presence of a normal joint space is an important clue to the diagnosis of gout. The integrity of the articular space in gout is apparently re-

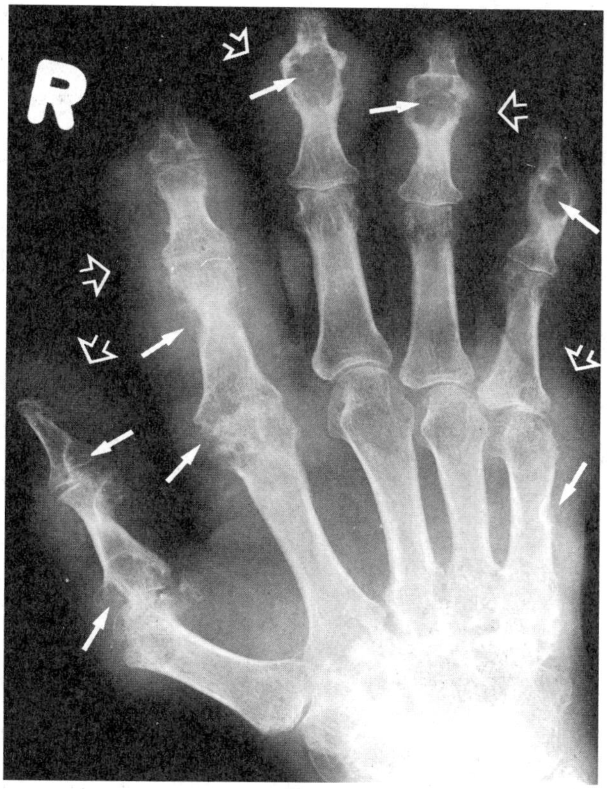

Fig. 296-3. Gouty arthritis. Extensive involvement of the wrist and hand can be seen. All the compartments of the wrist, the metacarpophalangeal joints, and the proximal and distal interphalangeal joints are affected. Extensive intra- and periarticular erosions are evident *(arrows),* without significant osteoporosis. Lobulated soft tissue swelling is apparent *(arrowheads).*

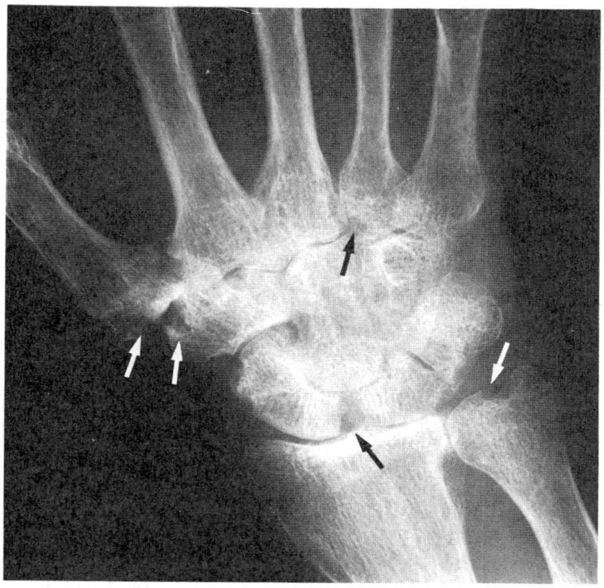

Fig. 296-4. Rheumatoid arthritis. Note the diffuse involvement of all the compartments of the wrist, including the radiocarpal compartment, inferior radioulnar compartment, midcarpal compartment, common carpometacarpal compartment, and first carpometacarpal compartment. Marginal erosions *(arrows),* soft tissue swelling, joint space narrowing, and mild osteoporosis are seen.

lated to the presence of relatively intact articular cartilage between areas of cartilaginous destruction.

Although joint space loss is also evident in degenerative joint disease (osteoarthritis), it involves limited areas of the articulation. The joint space narrows in the stressed area of the articulation. The hip joint space loss is usually maximum on the superolateral aspect of the joint (Fig. 296-5), whereas, in the knee, it is the medial femorotibial space that is characteristically narrowed. Osteoarthritis of the interphalangeal and metacarpophalangeal joints of the hand and the first metatarsophalangeal joint of the foot may be accompanied by more diffuse loss of articular space (Fig. 296-6).

Pyogenic arthritis also is associated with early and diffuse loss of joint space. In tuberculosis and fungal disorders, such loss is a later radiographic manifestation.

Osteonecrosis of epiphyses of tubular bones, such as the femoral and humeral heads, is associated with considerable subchondral bony abnormality in the form of osteolysis, osteosclerosis, and cyst formation, in the absence of joint space narrowing. This combination of findings reflects the integrity of the articular cartilage, which derives most of its nutrition from the adjacent synovial fluid and is therefore unaffected by disruption of blood supply to the subchondral bone. Cartilage atrophy related to disuse or immobilization, in which the synovial fluid may not effectively nourish the cartilage, is accompanied by diffuse loss of interosseous space.

Preservation of interosseous space is common in patients with pigmented villonodular synovitis and idiopathic synovial osteochondromatosis.

Intra-articular bone ankylosis. Intra-articular bone ankylosis occurs in certain disorders. In rheumatoid arthritis, this finding is usually limited to the carpal and tarsal areas. In psoriasis, such ankylosis can be evident in interphalangeal joints of the hands and feet (Fig. 296-7) and in metacarpophalangeal and metatarsophalangeal articulations. In ankylosing spondylitis, large joints such as the hip may fuse.

Intra-articular bone ankylosis also is well recognized in the interphalangeal joints of patients with inflammatory or erosive forms of osteoarthritis. Bone ankylosis of joints in patients with gout, neuroarthropathy, tuberculosis, pigmented villonodular synovitis, and idiopathic synovial osteochondromatosis is uncommon, but it may be seen following pyogenic arthritis and in juvenile chronic arthritis.

Bone erosion. In some diseases, osseous erosions are initially evident at marginal areas of the joint (marginal erosions), at sites where the synovium abuts bone that does not possess protective cartilage. Marginal erosions are early

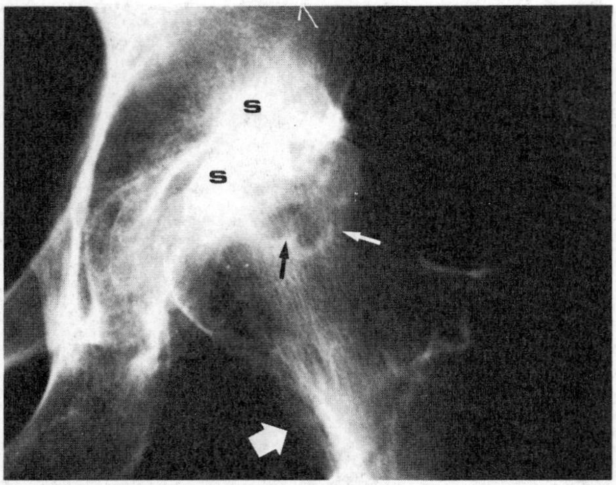

Fig. 296-5. Osteoarthritis. The maximum area of joint space loss involves the superior aspect of the articulation. There is superior migration of the femoral head with respect to the acetabulum. Note the asymmetric nature of the joint space loss and the sclerosis *(S)* and cyst formation *(arrows)* on the superior aspect of the femoral head and adjacent acetabulum. There is thickening, or buttressing, along the medial aspect of the femoral neck related to new bone formation *(arrowhead)*. In this example, osteophytosis is not prominent.

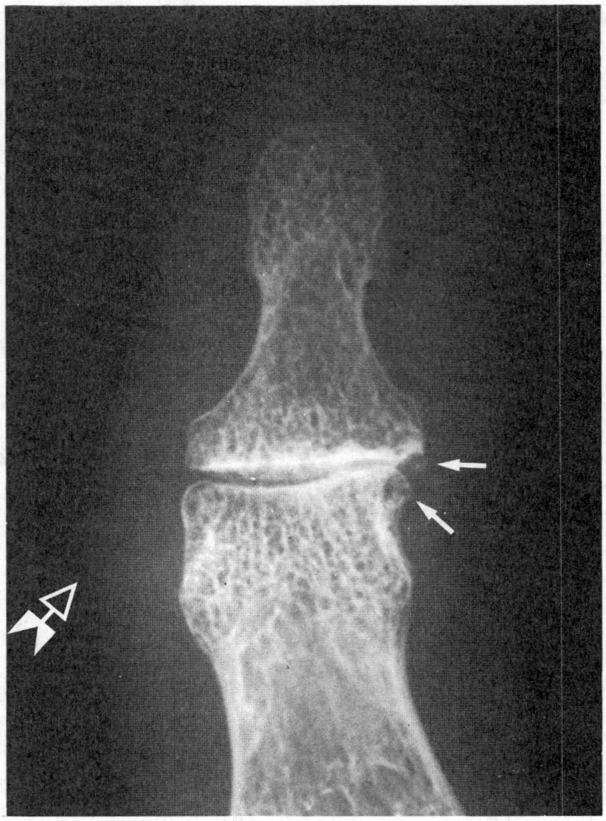

Fig. 296-6. Osteoarthritis. Mild involvement of a distal interphalangeal joint is characterized by articular space diminution, and minimal eburnation of bone. Osteophytosis *(small arrows)* is not prominent. Soft tissue swelling is evident *(large arrows)*.

features of rheumatoid arthritis (see Fig. 296-1) and other processes characterized by synovial inflammation such as psoriatic arthritis, Reiter's syndrome (see Fig. 296-2), ankylosing spondylitis, and infection. With progression of disease, synovial inflammation leads to destruction of portions of subchondral bone as well. Transchondral extension of inflammatory synovial tissue or pannus also can create cystic lesions that may appear enclosed on radiographic examination.

In inflammatory forms of osteoarthritis, central erosions may be identified within the interphalangeal joints of the hand. The distinctive central location of these osseous lesions may be related to the presence of bone collapse. Such erosions are accompanied by peripherally located osteophytes occurring at the attachment of the joint capsule, creating a "bird-wing" or "sea-gull" configuration.

Osseous erosions in gout occur in both intra-articular and extra-articular locations, frequently in relation to adjacent tophi (see Fig. 296-3). Eccentric erosions arise at the margins of affected joints and progress slowly. They are well circumscribed, of variable size, and are commonly associated with a sclerotic margin and an elevated osseous spicule, the "overhanging-edge" sign. These erosions can occur in the absence of joint space narrowing and are usually accompanied by lobulated soft tissue swelling. Central osseous erosions also appear in gout, related to extension of cartilaginous deposits of urate into subchondral bone. Extra-articular erosions can appear anywhere in the skeleton beneath tophaceous deposits.

Intra-articular bone erosions may be evident in pigmented villonodular synovitis and idiopathic synovial osteochondromatosis, especially in the hip, elbow, and wrist. Single or multiple well-defined osseous defects appear in association with soft tissue prominence and, in the case of idiopathic synovial osteochondromatosis, intra-articular calcification and ossification.

Bone sclerosis, osteophytosis, and proliferation. Sclerosis, or eburnation of subchondral bone, is a fundamental feature of osteoarthritis. It occurs in the stressed area of the affected articulation, in association with joint space narrowing and cyst formation. Sclerosis is especially prominent in osteoarthritis of the hip (see Fig. 296-5) and knee.

Extreme sclerosis is characteristic of neuropathic disease of the skeleton, especially that occurring in syphilis and syringomyelia (Fig. 296-8). Other disorders associated with bone eburnation include CPPD crystal deposition disease, osteonecrosis, and pyogenic arthritis.

Osteophytosis also is a well-recognized feature of osteoarthritis. Typically, the developing osteophyte is manifested as a ledge of bone at the margin of an articulation. Marginal osteophytes are especially characteristic along the medial aspect of the femoral head in association with osteoarthritis of the hip, and on the medial and lateral aspects of the distal femur and proximal tibia and posterior aspect of

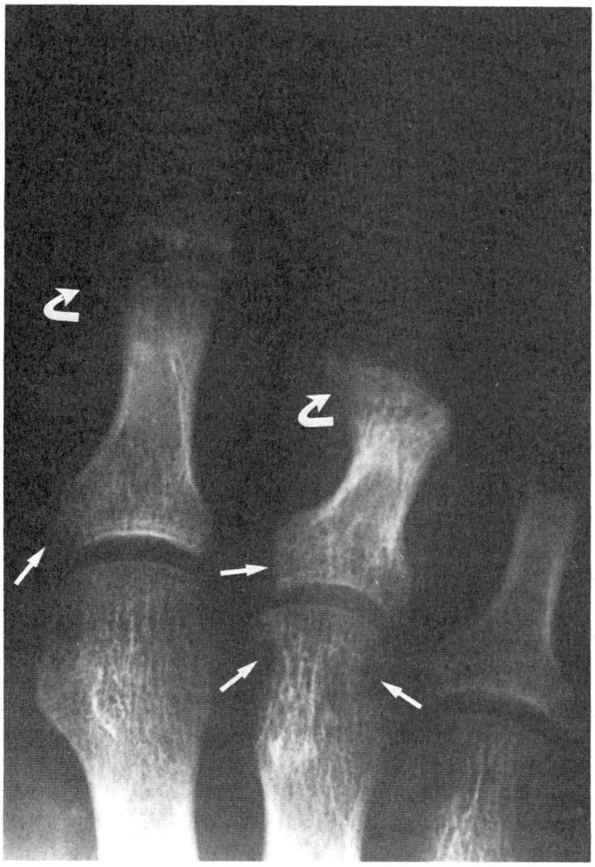

Fig. 296-7. Psoriatic arthritis. Observe bony ankylosis involving interphalangeal joints of two toes *(curved arrows),* accompanying soft tissue swelling, and marginal erosions of bone at the metatarsophalangeal joints *(straight arrows)*.

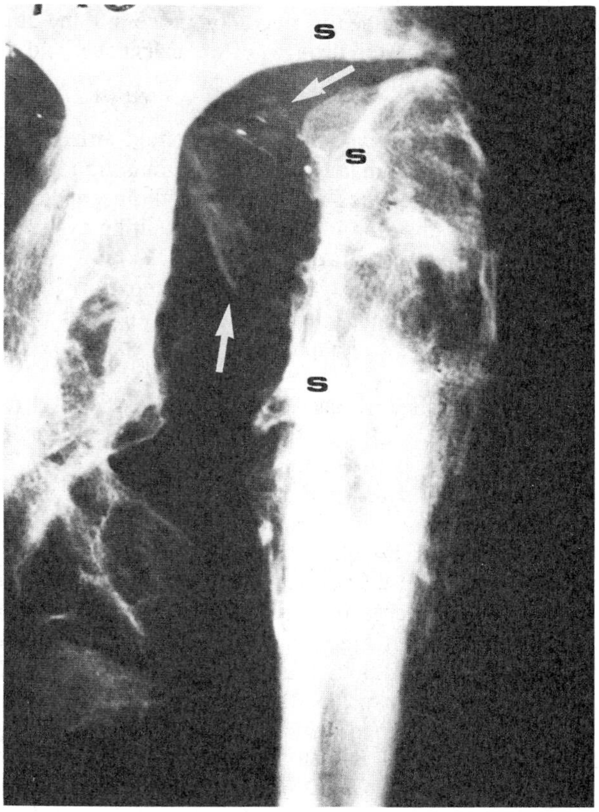

Fig. 296-8. Neuroarthropathy *(syphilis)*. Considerable sclerosis *(S)* and fragmentation *(arrows)* are seen. There is subluxation of the femoral head with respect to the acetabulum.

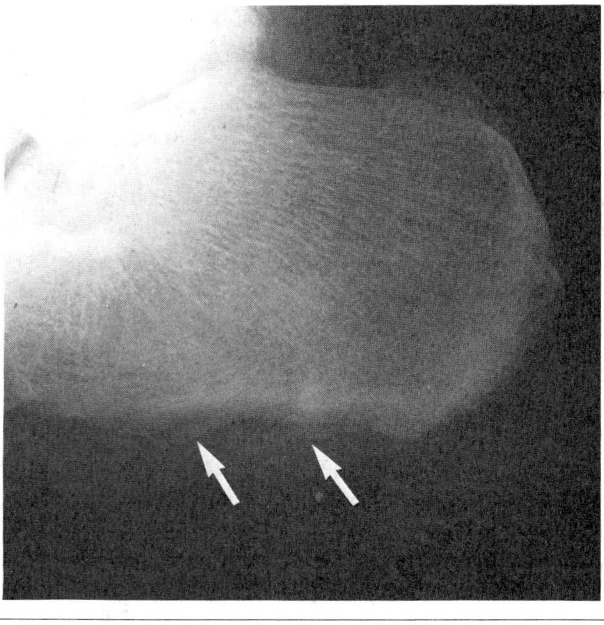

Fig. 296-9. Psoriatic arthritis. Note the ill-defined proliferative bony changes along the plantar aspect of the calcaneus *(arrows)*. These findings are compatible with psoriatic arthritis, Reiter's syndrome, or ankylosing spondylitis.

the patella in association with osteoarthritis of the knee. In the interphalangeal joints of the fingers, osteoarthritis is accompanied by capsular osteophytes related to outgrowths appearing at the osseous attachment of the joint capsule. One additional type of osteophyte that appears in osteoarthritis is related to bone irritation by the synovial membrane (the intra-articular counterpart of the periosteum). In the hip, these latter osteophytes extend across the femoral neck just inferior to the femoral head and are combined with proliferation along the medial aspect of the femoral neck, a phenomenon called *buttressing*.

Ill-defined osseous excrescences accompany bone erosions in the seronegative spondyloarthropathies, psoriatic arthritis, Reiter's syndrome, and ankylosing spondylitis. The affected bone appears "whiskered" because irregular outgrowths are seen about the sites of osseous erosion. Similar ill-defined osseous excrescences also appear at sites of tendinous and ligamentous attachment to bone. These sites include the femoral trochanters, humeral tuberosities, and plantar surface of the calcanei (Fig. 296-9).

In diffuse idiopathic skeletal hyperostosis (ankylosing hyperostosis of Forestier), well-defined bone outgrowths appear at osseous sites of tendinous and ligamentous attachment. These sites include the olecranon process of the ulna, the plantar and posterior surfaces of the calcaneus, and the anterior surface of the patella.

Subchondral cyst formation. In rheumatoid arthritis and other synovial inflammatory processes, transchondral extension of pannus creates subchondral radiolucent lesions of variable size. In some instances, the resulting cysts may lead to spontaneous fracture.

Cyst formation also is frequent in osteoarthritis. The cysts frequently are multiple, involving both sides of the articulation, and are accompanied by joint space loss and bone sclerosis.

In osteonecrosis, necrosis of bone and marrow is followed by osteoclastic resorption of dead trabeculae, with cyst formation. In contradistinction to the situation in osteoarthritis, these cysts may appear without loss of interosseous space.

Cyst formation is a recognized manifestation of the structural joint disease (pyrophosphate arthropathy) that accompanies CPPD crystal deposition disease. Additional structural changes include sclerosis, bone fragmentation, and osteophytosis. Although the resulting radiographic picture simulates that in osteoarthritis, the presence of cartilage calcification (chondrocalcinosis) and the involvement of unusual articular sites such as the wrist and elbow allow accurate diagnosis of CPPD crystal deposition disease in most instances.

Multiple subchondral cysts also can be seen in pigmented villonodular synovitis and hemophilia.

Bone fragmentation and collapse. Neuroarthropathy is the arthritic disorder that is associated with the most extensive fragmentation and collapse of apposing articular surfaces (see Fig. 296-8). Fragments of bone and cartilage may be displaced into the articular cavity, existing as "loose" bodies or becoming embedded in the synovial membrane at a distant site.

Pyrophosphate arthropathy can be associated with rapidly progressive fragmentation of bone. Other findings, such as chondrocalcinosis, provide helpful clues to the correct diagnosis. Fragmentation of subchondral bone is also evident in osteonecrosis and transchondral fractures (osteochondritis dissecans).

Intra-articular and periarticular calcification. Calcification of hyaline or fibrocartilage or both (chondrocalcinosis) is a fundamental radiographic sign of idiopathic CPPD crystal deposition disease (Fig. 296-10). The calcific deposits in fibrocartilage appear shaggy and are most commonly found in the menisci of the knee, triangular fibrocartilage of the wrist, and symphysis pubis. Hyaline cartilage calcification creates thin, curvilinear radiodensities that parallel the subchondral bone; any joint can be the site of such calcification. Synovial and capsular calcification also may be apparent.

Primary hyperparathyroidism and hemochromatosis can be associated with CPPD crystal deposition with chondrocalcinosis. Although cartilage calcification is occasionally observed in gout, the deposits are less extensive and usually are limited to one or two articulations.

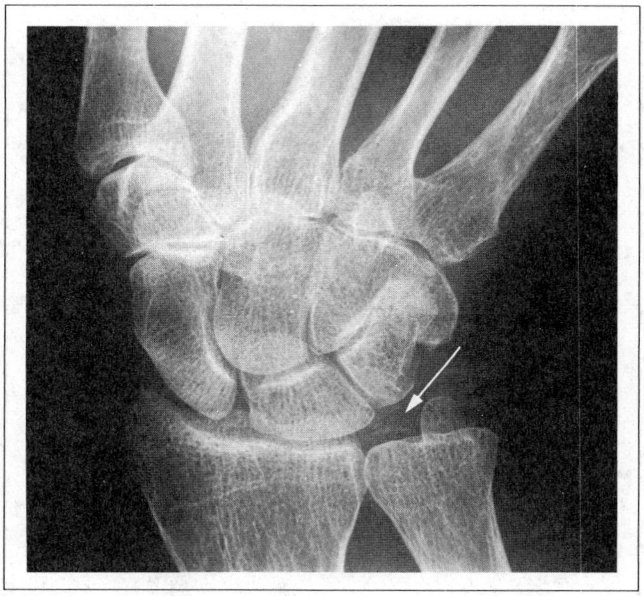

Fig. 296-10. Calcium pyrophosphate dihydrate crystal deposition disease. The radiographic finding in this case is cartilage calcification (chondrocalcinosis) involving principally the triangular fibrocartilage of the wrist, creating a density adjacent to the distal ulna *(arrow)*.

Tendon calcification sometimes is evident in CPPD crystal deposition disease, but such calcification is much more frequent in hydroxyapatite crystal deposition disease, in which case it may lead to symptoms and signs of tendinitis. Calcific tendinitis is most common in the shoulder, although it may also be observed about other articulations such as the wrist, hip, and elbow. The radiograph outlines linear radiodensities within the substance of the tendon.

Cloudlike tumoral deposits of calcification about one or more articulations are observed in renal osteodystrophy with secondary hyperparathyroidism, collagen vascular disorders such as scleroderma and systemic lupus erythematosus, milk-alkali syndrome, hypervitaminosis D, and sarcoidosis. Tuftal calcification with or without resorption of the terminal phalanges is a well-recognized manifestation of scleroderma, and linear calcification in subcutaneous and muscular tissue can be evident in scleroderma, dermatomyositis, and systemic lupus erythematosus.

The axial skeleton (Table 296-1)

Intervertebral disk space narrowing. Degenerative disease of the nucleus pulposus of the intervertebral disk leads to progressive narrowing of the disk space associated with intradiskal collections of gas (vacuum phenomena) and sclerosis of the adjacent vertebral bodies (Fig. 296-11). The sclerotic vertebrae usually possess a well-defined margin bordering on the intervertebral disk.

Osteomyelitis of the spine frequently begins within the

Table 296-1. Arthritis of the axial skeleton

	Intervertebral disk space narrowing	Vacuum phenomena	Intervertebral disk space calcification	Bone outgrowths	Apophyseal joint erosion	Apophyseal joint ankylosis	Atlantoaxial subluxation
Rheumatoid arthritis	+	–	–	–	+	±	+
Psoriatic arthritis, Reiter's syndrome	±	–	–	Paravertebral ossification	±	±	+
Ankylosing spondylitis	±	–	±	Syndesmophytes	+	+	+
Juvenile rheumatoid arthritis	+	–	±	–	+	+	+
Degenerative disease of the nucleus pulposus	+	+	–	–	–	–	–
Spondylosis deformans	–	–	–	Osteophytes	–	–	–
Diffuse idiopathic skeletal hyperostosis	–	–	±	Flowing anterolateral ossification	–	–	–
Alkaptonuria	+	+	+	Syndesmophytes (rare)	–	–	–
Infection	+	–	–	–	–	–	–

+ = common presentation; ± = uncommon; – = rare or absent.

vertebral body and spreads to the neighboring intervertebral disk. The resulting radiographic findings include osteolysis and osteosclerosis of the vertebra and intervertebral disk space narrowing. Eventually, the adjacent vertebra also is involved. The margins of the affected vertebrae usually are ill defined, and the intervertebral disk lacks a vacuum phenomenon. These radiographic features usually allow differentiation of infection and degenerative disease of the nucleus pulposus.

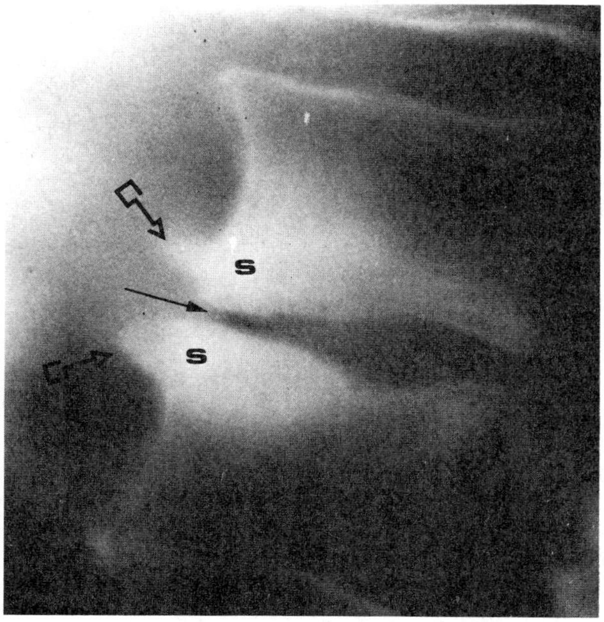

Fig. 296-11. Degenerative disease of the nucleus pulposus. The radiographic abnormalities include considerable loss of intervertebral disk space height, a vacuum phenomenon creating a small radiolucency overlying the anterior aspect of the intervertebral disk *(solid arrow)* and considerable reactive sclerosis *(S)* of the neighboring vertebral bodies. Triangular osteophytes are present along the anterior surface of the vertebrae *(open arrows)*.

Rheumatoid arthritis is associated with narrowing of the cervical intervertebral disks, with irregularity of the vertebral surface. Osteophytes are absent, but subluxation at one or more cervical levels (including the atlantoaxial junction) and apophyseal joint erosions can be seen.

Alkaptonuria (ochronosis) can be accompanied by diffuse calcification of intervertebral disks and disk space narrowing. Multiple vacuum phenomena are common.

Other causes of intervertebral disk space narrowing and irregularity of adjacent vertebral bodies include neuroarthropathy, intraosseous diskal herniation (cartilaginous or Schmorl's node), trauma, and crystal deposition diseases. Such narrowing also occurs in dialysis spondyloarthropathy and may be related to amyloid deposition.

Osteophytosis and other bone outgrowths. Degenerative changes in the anulus fibrosus of the intervertebral disk lead to spondylosis deformans, resulting in widespread spinal osteophytosis. The outgrowths are horizontally oriented and extend in an anterolateral direction.

Widespread spinal excrescences having a predilection for the lower thoracic and upper lumbar vertebrae are a fundamental feature of diffuse idiopathic skeletal hyperostosis (ankylosing hyperostosis) (Fig. 296-12). The radiographs reveal a flowing pattern of ossification along the anterolateral aspect of the spine, with a bumpy spinal contour and preservation of intervertebral disk height.

Ankylosing spondylitis is associated with thin vertical radiodense spicules (syndesmophytes) that extend from one vertebral body to its neighbor (Fig. 296-13). Syndesmophytes initially are evident at the thoracolumbar and lumbosacral junctions but soon extend to other portions of the

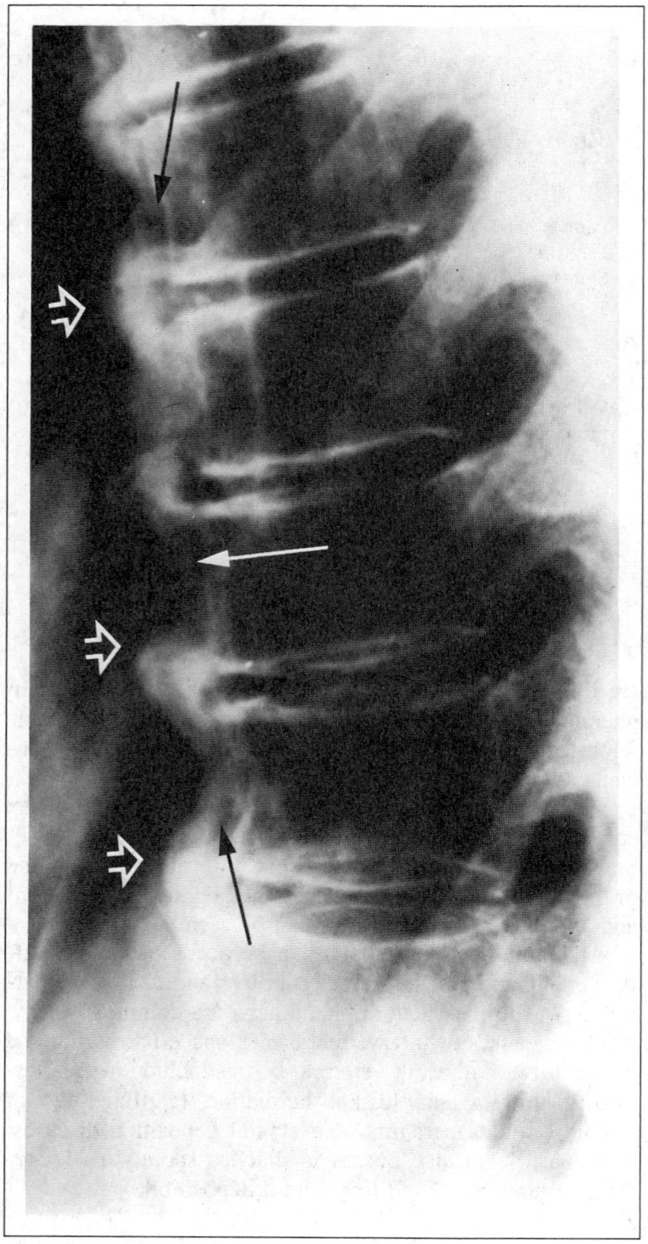

Fig. 296-12. Diffuse idiopathic skeletal hyperostosis. In this disorder, characteristic flowing ossification appears along the anterolateral aspect of the thoracolumbar spine. Note the bumpy spinal contour *(arrowheads)* and a radiolucency beneath the deposited bone, between it and the underlying vertebral body *(arrows)*.

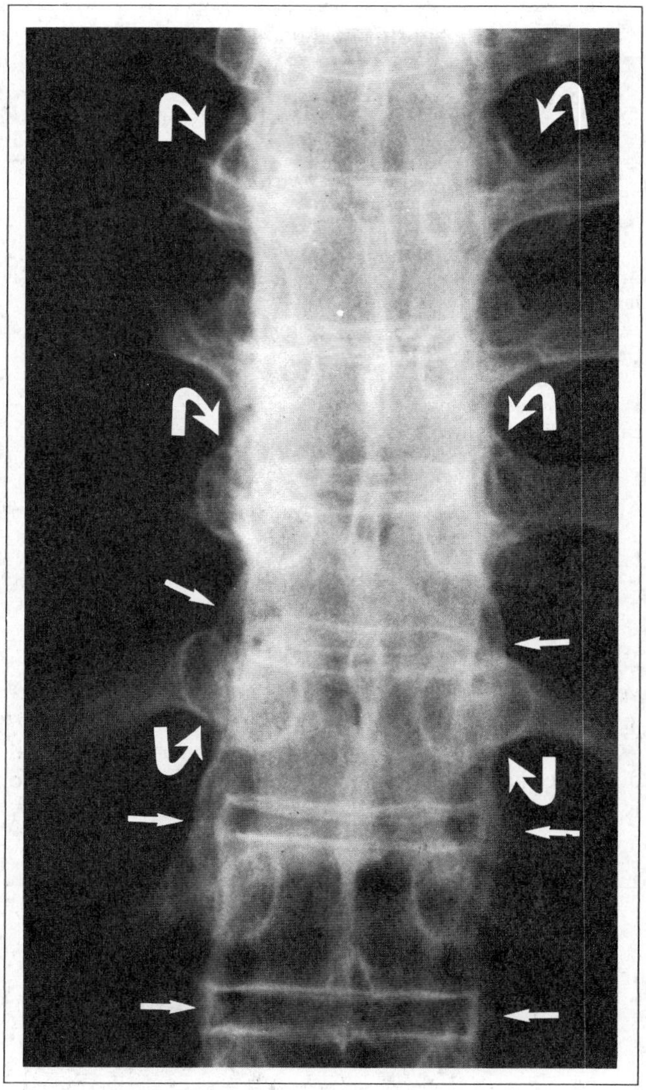

Fig. 296-13. Ankylosing spondylitis. Syndesmophytes extend as vertical radiodensities between vertebral bodies *(straight arrows)*, producing bony ankylosis of the spine. Also evident is costovertebral joint ankylosis *(curved arrows)*.

spine. Additional findings include reactive sclerosis of the corners of the vertebral bodies (osteitis), straightening or squaring of the anterior vertebral margins, and apophyseal and costovertebral joint ankylosis. Eventually, widespread bone formation produces a "bamboo spine." Many of these findings in ankylosing spondylitis also are evident in the spondylitis accompanying inflammatory bowel diseases, such as ulcerative colitis and Crohn's disease.

Paravertebral ossification is seen in psoriatic arthritis and Reiter's syndrome. Such ossification creates initially ill-defined radiodense shadows separated from the edges of the vertebral bodies and intervertebral disks, particularly at the thoracolumbar junction, and eventually larger better-defined excrescences that merge with the vertebrae and disks. It is their larger size and asymmetric distribution that distinguish these outgrowths from the syndesmophytes of ankylosing spondylitis and inflammatory bowel disorders.

Bone outgrowths of the spine also are seen in fluorosis, acromegaly, and hypoparathyroidism.

Intervertebral disk calcification. Extensive calcification of multiple intervertebral disks is virtually pathognomonic of alkaptonuria. Globular calcification of one or several intervertebral disks can occur on a dystrophic basis after injury or infection. In children, calcification of one or more cervical intervertebral disks can be associated with significant clinical findings (diskitis) that disappear in weeks or months. Calcification of the outer fibers of the anulus fibrosus may appear in CPPD crystal deposition disease. Diskal calcification also can occur in any disease that produces bone ankylosis between vertebral bodies or joint fusion in the corresponding apophyseal articulations.

Atlantoaxial subluxation. Inflammation of the synovial sac between the transverse ligament of the atlas and the posterior surface of the odontoid process produces atlantoaxial subluxation, manifested as increased distance between the anterior arch of the atlas and the odontoid process of the axis on lateral films of the cervical spine, especially those exposed during neck flexion (Fig. 296-14). Rheumatoid arthritis, psoriatic arthritis, Reiter's syndrome, and ankylosing spondylitis show atlantoaxial subluxation, and each also may produce odontoid erosions on the anterior or posterior surfaces, or both.

Paravertebral swelling. Fusiform soft tissue masses about the spine can occur in association with a psoas abscess, seen in pyogenic infection of the spine as well as in tuberculosis. In the latter disease, calcification of the psoas abscess may be identified. Paravertebral masses also can be evident, with posttraumatic hemorrhage, and with spinal neoplasms, indicating tumor extension.

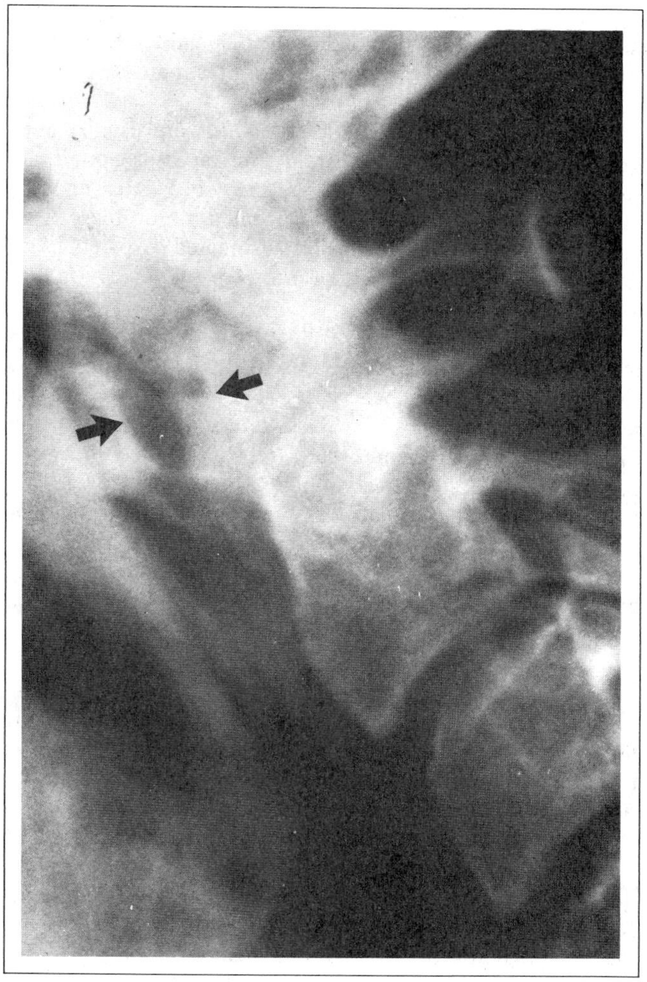

Fig. 296-14. Rheumatoid arthritis. In this example, prominent atlantoaxial subluxation is seen. This radiograph was exposed during flexion of the neck and demonstrates an increased distance between the anterior arch of the atlas and the odontoid process *(between arrows)*. Similar changes may be seen in other inflammatory synovial processes.

CHARACTERISTIC TARGET AREAS OF ARTICULAR DISEASE

In addition to the morphology of articular lesions, the distribution of these lesions within the appendicular and axial skeleton provides clues to accurate diagnosis.

Hand

The articulations of the digits of the hand include the metacarpophalangeal, proximal interphalangeal, and distal interphalangeal joints and the interphalangeal joint of the thumb. Rheumatoid arthritis produces alterations that predominate in the metacarpophalangeal and proximal interphalangeal joints and in the interphalangeal joint of the thumb (see Fig. 296-1). Although erosions may be apparent in distal interphalangeal joints, these are infrequent.

Osteoarthritis primarily involves the distal interphalangeal, proximal interphalangeal, and, less commonly, the metacarpophalangeal joints (see Fig. 296-6). Although changes may be isolated in distal interphalangeal or proximal interphalangeal joints, they are rarely isolated in the metacarpophalangeal joints. Extensive abnormalities in the last site should raise the possibility of CPPD crystal deposition disease.

Inflammatory or erosive osteoarthritis most frequently produces alterations in the distal interphalangeal and proximal interphalangeal joints. CPPD crystal deposition disease produces structural joint changes that predominate at the metacarpophalangeal joints. Gouty arthritis may affect any articulation of the digits (see Fig. 296-3). Psoriatic arthritis may be manifest as a destructive arthritis of distal interphalangeal and proximal interphalangeal joints.

Wrist

The wrist is not a single joint; rather, it consists of a series of compartments: the radiocarpal compartment between the distal radius and proximal carpal row, the midcarpal compartment between the proximal and distal carpal rows, the common carpometacarpal compartment between the distal carpal row and metacarpals of the four ulnar digits, the first carpometacarpal joint between the trapezium and the first metacarpal, and the inferior radioulnar compartment between the distal radius and ulna. The radial aspect of the midcarpal compartment is conveniently termed the *trapezioscaphoid* space.

Rheumatoid arthritis initially involves the radiocarpal,

midcarpal, inferior radioulnar, and pisiform-triquetral compartments, as well as the tendon sheaths and tendons of the wrists (see Fig. 296-4). Eventually, all compartments of the wrist are altered.

Osteoarthritis produces alterations that are usually confined to the first carpometacarpal and trapezioscaphoid areas. Without a history of trauma, any process that appears degenerative in nature but is not located within these typical compartments should not be designated as osteoarthritis until other possibilities, especially crystal deposition, are excluded.

Inflammatory osteoarthritis may result in abnormalities in the first carpometacarpal and trapezioscaphoid areas. Changes elsewhere in the wrist are unusual. Involvement in CPPD crystal deposition disease usually appears in the radiocarpal compartment. Gout can be associated with pancompartmental alterations although the most severe involvement may be noted in the common carpometacarpal compartment. The findings in juvenile rheumatoid arthritis may be noted throughout the wrist, but the radiocarpal compartment often is spared.

Foot

The articulations of the foot are the distal interphalangeal, proximal interphalangeal, and metatarsophalangeal joints, the interphalangeal joint of the great toe, and numerous articulations in the midfoot and hindfoot.

The major changes in rheumatoid arthritis are apparent in the metatarsophalangeal joints, interphalangeal joint of the great toe, and the articulations of the midfoot and hindfoot. The earliest changes in this disease may appear in the metatarsophalangeal articulations, especially in the fifth digit. Posterior calcaneal erosions and well-defined plantar calcaneal spurs are additional findings.

Gouty arthritis predominates in the first digit at both the metatarsophalangeal and interphalangeal joints, although any joint in the foot may be affected. Any articulation of the foot also may be altered in psoriasis and Reiter's syndrome, although sites of predilection include the metatarsophalangeal joints and interphalangeal joint of the great toe (see Fig. 296-7). In both disorders, proliferative erosions are noted on the plantar and posterior calcaneal surfaces (see Fig. 296-9). Osteoarthritis may produce changes at the first metatarsophalangeal joint.

CPPD crystal deposition disease may be associated with selective involvement of the talonavicular area. The same articulation is also involved in neuroarthropathy accompanying diabetes mellitus.

Knee

Three spaces or compartments in the knee joint are the medial femorotibial, lateral femorotibial, and patellofemoral spaces. Rheumatoid arthritis and related synovial diseases such as ankylosing spondylitis produce symmetric loss of joint space in the medial and lateral femorotibial compartments. This involvement may be combined with alterations of the patellofemoral space.

Osteoarthritis produces asymmetric joint space narrowing. More frequently, it is the medial femorotibial space that is affected. In addition, the patellofemoral compartment may be altered in osteoarthritis, although abnormality in this area usually is combined with changes in the medial femorotibial space. Joint space narrowing confined to the patellofemoral compartment is more typical of CPPD crystal deposition disease. A similar predilection for patellofemoral compartmental alteration is seen in hyperparathyroidism.

Hip

The hip can be considered as a single articulation, but it is helpful to identify which area of the joint is predominantly affected.

In rheumatoid arthritis, symmetric loss of joint space is the rule. This may eventually result in acetabular protrusion into the pelvis. A similar pattern may be noted in ankylosing spondylitis and in CPPD crystal deposition disease, although osteophytosis may accompany the loss of articular space in both disorders.

In osteoarthritis, joint space loss most characteristically occurs in the superior aspect of the joint (see Fig. 296-5). Eventually, large osteophytes appear along the medial aspect of the femoral head, and the resulting radiographic picture may resemble symmetric loss of space.

Sacroiliac joint

Many disorders are associated with erosion and sclerosis of the ilium and sacrum, and widening or narrowing of the sacroiliac joint with or without intra-articular bone ankylosis; therefore, it is the distribution of the changes that produces the most important clue to accurate diagnosis (Table 296-2). Changes may be bilateral and symmetric, as in ankylosing spondylitis (Fig. 296-15), or bilateral and asymmetric, as in Reiter's or psoriatic arthritis. Unilateral involvement always should suggest an infectious process, although this may be an early appearance in any of the spondyloarthropathies.

Table 296-2. Sacroiliac joint abnormalities

	Bilateral symmetric	Bilateral asymmetric	Unilateral
Ankylosing spondylitis	+		
Psoriatic arthritis	+	+	+
Reiter's syndrome	+	+	+
Inflammatory bowel disease	+		
Rheumatoid arthritis		+	+
Gout	+	+	+
Infection			+
Hyperparathyroidism	+		

+ = common presentation.

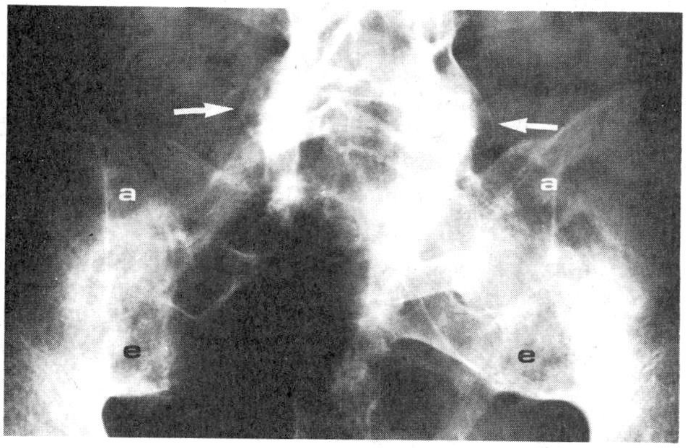

Fig. 296-15. Ankylosing spondylitis. Bilateral symmetric sacroiliac joint abnormalities consist of erosion *(e)*, predominantly on the ilium, and intra-articular bony ankylosis *(a)*. Syndesmophytosis of the lower lumbar spine is evident *(arrows)*.

ADVANCED IMAGING METHODS

It is difficult in a short chapter to detail the many applications of computed tomography and magnetic resonance with regard to the musculoskeletal system. Two major advantages of these methods are cross-sectional imaging capability and excellent contrast resolution. Also, magnetic resonance imaging does not produce radiation exposure. This last technique has invaded the territory once held firm by arthrography, and it allows excellent visualization of the menisci of the knee, wrist, and temporomandibular joint, the collateral and cruciate ligaments, the tendons, and the subchondral bone. The reported accuracy of magnetic resonance imaging in the depiction of abnormalities of some of these structures has reached 90% to 95% (Fig. 296-16).

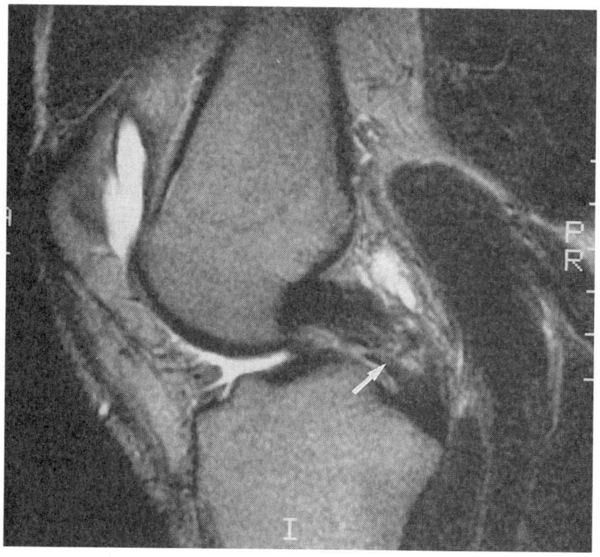

Fig. 296-16. Note tear of the posterior cruciate ligament *(arrow)* on this magnetic resonance image. In this sequence, fluid appears bright.

Although magnetic resonance possesses excellent sensitivity in the assessment of many musculoskeletal problems, its specificity has been somewhat disappointing to date. Many processes of soft tissue and bone marrow lead to similar changes, and, with regard to neoplastic diseases, it may be difficult at times to differentiate between benign and malignant lesions.

REFERENCES

Aisen AM et al: Cervical spine involvement in rheumatoid arthritis: MR imaging. Radiology 165:159, 1987.

Dalinka MK, Reginato AJ, and Golden DA: Calcium deposition diseases. Semin Roentgenol 17:39, 1982.

Edeiken J: Radiologic approach to arthritis. Semin Roentgenol 17:8, 1982.

Fam AG et al: Clinical and roentgenographic aspects of pseudogout: a study of 50 cases and a review. Can Med Assoc J 124:545, 1981.

Goldman AB: Some miscellaneous joint diseases. Semin Roentgenol 17:60, 1982.

Kursunoglu-Brahme S et al: Rheumatoid knee: role of gadopentetate-enhanced MR imaging. Radiology 176:831, 1990.

Lawson TL et al: The sacroiliac joints: anatomic, plain roentgenographic, and computed tomographic analysis. J Comput Assist Tomogr 6:307, 1982.

Martel W: Erosive osteoarthritis and psoriatic arthritis: a radiologic comparison in the hand, wrist, and foot. Am J Roentgenol 134:125, 1980.

Martel W et al: Radiologic features of Reiter disease. Radiology 132:1, 1979.

Mitchel DG et al: Avascular necrosis of the femoral head: morphologic assessment by MR imaging with CT correlation. Radiology 161:739, 1986.

Nance EP Jr and Kaye JJ: The rheumatoid variants. Semin Roentgenol 17:16, 1982.

Resnick D: Patterns of femoral head migration in osteoarthritis of the hip: roentgenographic-pathologic correlation and comparison with rheumatoid arthritis. Am J Roentgenol 124:62, 1975.

Resnick D: Rheumatoid arthritis of the wrist. The compartmental approach. Med Radiogr Photogr 52:50, 1976.

Resnick D: Infectious arthritis. Semin Roentgenol 17:49, 1982.

Resnick D: Shaul S and Robins J: Diffuse idiopathic skeletal hyperostosis: extraspinal manifestations of Forestier's disease. Radiology 115:513, 1975.

Resnick D et al: Clinical, radiographic, and pathologic abnormalities in calcium pyrophosphate dihydrate deposition disease (CPPD): pseudogout. Radiology 122:1, 1977.

Sanchez RB and Quinn SF: MRI of inflammatory synovial processes. Magn Reson Imaging 7:529, 1989.

Summers MN et al: Radiographic assessment and psychological variables as predictors of pain and functional impairment in osteoarthritis of the knee or hip. Arthritis Rheum 31:204, 1988.

Thomas RH et al: Compartmental evaluation of osteoarthritis of the knee: a comparative study of available diagnostic modalities. Radiology 116:585, 1975.

Weissman BN: Arthrography in arthritis. Radiol Clin North Am 19:379, 1981.

III Clinical Immunology

CHAPTER

297 Immunodeficiencies

Harry G. Bluestein

Specific immunologic responses result from complex interactions among the various lymphoid cell types that constitute the immune system. Advances in delineating the development and functional capacity of immunocompetent cells have been driven to a large extent by analysis of the immune deficiencies in patients with genetic abnormalities of the immune system. The cells of the immune system are derived from hematopoietic stem cells in the bone marrow (Fig. 297-1). Among the differentiated progeny of stem cells are common lymphoid precursor cells, which under the influence of the thymus or the human equivalent of the bursa of Fabricius, differentiate further into T and B lymphocytes, respectively. The immune process is activated when monocytoid cells, also derived from hematopoietic stem cells, present antigen to lymphocytes. Under the influence of T cell regulation providing helping and suppressing signals, B cells differentiate into class-specific immunoglobulin-producing cells. Many of the genetically determined immunodeficiency syndromes can be attributed to a cellular defect at one of those levels of lymphoid differentiation. A listing of some of the major illustrative primary forms of immunodeficiency selected from the World Health Organization 1986 classification is provided in Table 297-1.

INHERITED IMMUNODEFICIENCIES

Severe immunodeficiencies

Reticular dysgenesis. The progenitor stem cell that gives rise to lymphoid cells shares a precursor cell in common with the progenitors of myeloid and monocytoid cells. A defect in that relatively primitive hematopoietic stem cell would be expected to result in the absence of granulocytes and monocytes as well as the absence of T and B lymphocytes. A few such patients have been recognized, although they almost invariably die during the first weeks of life from overwhelming staphylococcal sepsis. Those patients have had severe neutropenia, lymphopenia, and lymphoid tissue depletion, including dysplasia of the thymus.

Combined cellular and humoral immunodeficiencies. The severe combined immunodeficiencies (SCID) are a group of primary genetic disorders characterized by profound T cell dysfunction and hypogammaglobulinemia. Awareness of clinical distinctions among members of the group, particularly in the phenotypic characterization of the patients' lymphoid cells, has led to advances in identification of the responsible genetic defects. It is useful to subgroup the combined immunodeficiencies into those lacking T and B cells, those with B cells but not T cells, and those with T and B cells. For instance, in "Swiss-type" immunodeficiency there is a striking alymphocytosis and hypoplasia of lymphoid organs because of developmental failure of both T and B cell lymphocyte lineages. Familial studies usually reveal an autosomal recessive mode of inheritance. There is growing evidence that the specific genetic defect leads to abnormal gene rearrangements in lymphocytes. In SCID mice, defective recombinations effecting both immunoglobulin and T cell receptor genes have been documented. Similar defects have been found in bone marrow B cell precursors from human SCID infants.

A more frequent form of SCID presents with normal or elevated numbers of immature B cells, but no T cells. The mode of inheritance is most often X-linked and the involved gene has been mapped to Xq1.3. Studies in cells from female carriers of X-linked SCID have shown a skewed pattern of X-chromosome inactivation, and the techniques involved can be used for carrier detection and prenatal diagnosis.

A smaller subset of SCID patients have T cells and B cells but they are functionally impaired. A variety of different defects have been identified in this heterogeneous group. Immunodeficiency associated with the absence of the major histocompatibility complex (MHC) class II molecules on cell surfaces appears to result from defective transcription of normal MHC class II structural genes. These individuals have less severe immunodeficiency, but rarely survive more than 2 decades. Mutations in the structural genes encoding CD3 T cell surface molecules also are associated with SCID in some cases. It is hypothesized that the normal aggregation of CD8 or CD4 with CD3 and the T cell receptor that is involved in T cell signaling is impaired by the structural changes induced by the CD3 mutations. Defects in postsignaling intracellular activation mechanisms have also been seen in cells from several patients with combined immunodeficiencies. Best documented is a structural abnormality in NF-AT (nuclear factor of activated T cells), a molecule that participates in the regulation of a group of cytokines including IL-2, -3, -4, -5, and gamma interferon.

Patients with SCID usually suffer devastating infections commencing before 6 months of age, and, as might be expected, they lack both cellular and humoral immunity. Viral, bacterial, fungal, and protozoal infections all occur. Treatment in the acute phase is dependent upon the use of appropriate antibiotics for the infecting agent and the administration of gamma globulin. Care must be taken to avoid immunization with live viruses, because of their infectious potential in the absence of T cell immunity; blood products should be irradiated prior to transfusion to eliminate any viable lymphocytes that could produce a graft-versus-host (GVH) reaction.

Transplantation of histocompatible bone marrow is the definitive treatment. The immunopotent stem cells in the bone marrow graft can restore immunologic competence to

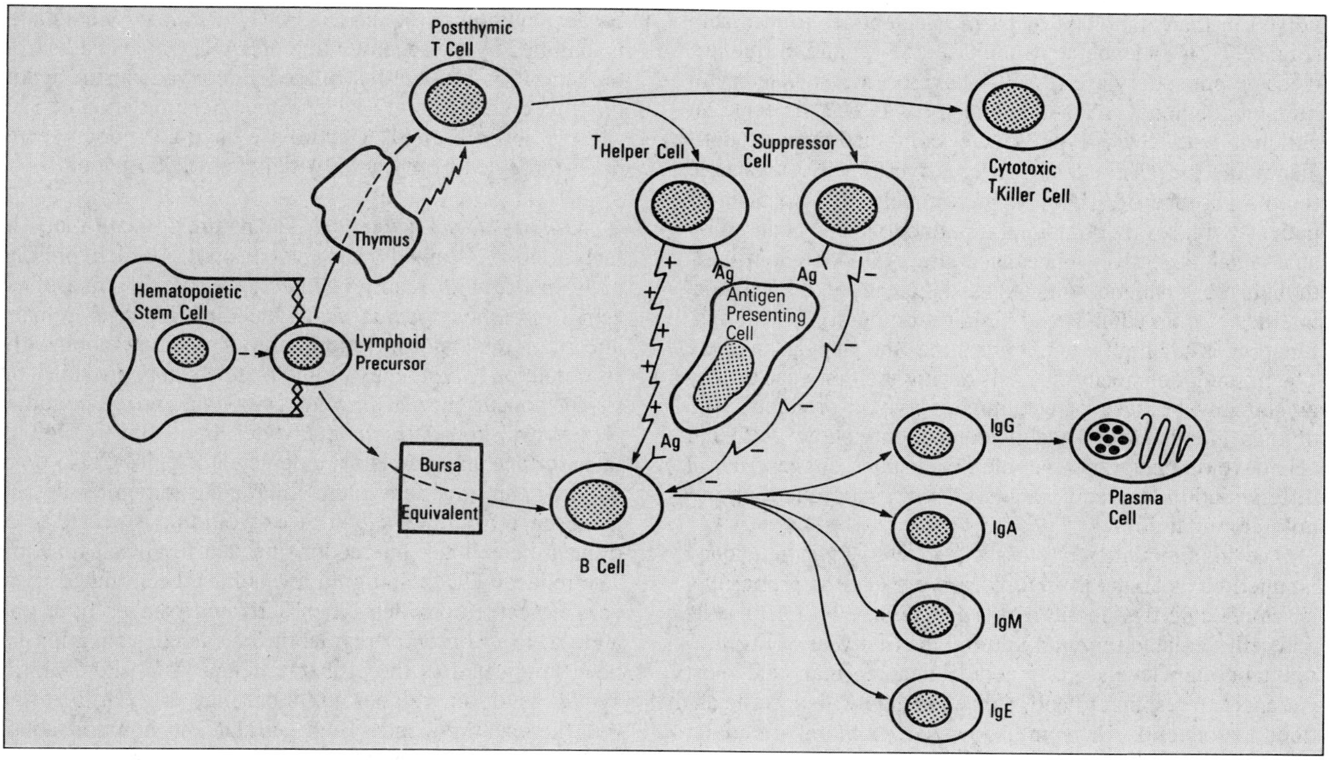

Fig. 297-1. Development of immunocompetent lymphoid cells.

these infants. In some instances successful marrow transplantation has been achieved with a match at the HLA-D but not the -A or -B locus. Transplantation of unmatched marrow produces a fatal GVH reaction. When a histocompatible marrow has not been available, human fetal liver hematopoietic cells and fetal thymus transplants have been used with some success.

Immunodeficiency associated with enzyme deficiencies in the purine metabolic pathway. Deficiencies of enzymes in-

Table 297-1. Primary immunodeficiency diseases with lymphocyte dysfunction*

Designation	Functional deficiency	Circulating lymphocytes	Presumed cellular defect	Inheritance
Severe combined immunodeficiency (reticular dysgenesis, Swiss-type, adenosine deaminase, purine nucleoside phosphorylase, HLA deficiency)	CMI and Ab	↓ T and B or ↓ T	Unknown; HSC?; T cell?	AR or XL
Wiskott-Aldrich syndrome	Ab, later CMI	Progressive ↓ T	Altered cell membrane molecules; HSC?	XL
Ataxia telangiectasia	CMI and Ab	↓ T	Unknown; abnormal DNA repair	AR
Di George syndrome	CMI	↓ T	Embryopathic thymic development	None or unknown
X-linked agammaglobulinemia	Ab	↓ B	Pre–B cell	XL
Selective Ig deficiencies (↓ IgA, ↓ IgM, ↓ IgG, ↓ Ig with ↑ IgM)	Partial Ab	Normal	B cell isotype switch or terminal differentiation defect	Various, AR, XL
Common variable immunodeficiency	Ab ± CMI	Normal or ↓ B or ↓ T	Intrinsic B cell defect; defective T cell help; active T cell suppression; lymphocytotoxic antibodies	AR, AD, unknown

*Selected from World Health Organization Classification (1986).
CMI, cell-mediated immunity; Ab, antibody; HSC, hematopoietic stem cell; AR, autosomal recessive; XL, X-linked; AD, autosomal dominant.

volved in the catabolism of purine nucleotides to uric acid (Fig. 297-2)—adenosine deaminase (ADA) and purine nucleoside phosphorylase (PNP)—have been associated with immunodeficiency. ADA deficiency was first detected in children with Swiss-type severe combined immunodeficiency disease. An autosomal recessive trait is responsible for the absence of ADA. Approximately 30% to 50% of patients with severe combined immunodeficiency caused by autosomal recessive inheritance are ADA-deficient. Although most patients with ADA deficiency exhibit abnormalities of both cellular and humoral immunity, T cell dysfunction is generally more profound and appears earlier. The immunodeficiency worsens during the first year of life, presumably because of accumulating toxic products. The thymus glands of ADA-deficient patients show epithelial cell development, and pathologic changes suggest initial differentiation of T cell precursors, with subsequent immunologic involution.

The immunodeficiency associated with PNP deficiency is inherited as an autosomal recessive trait. It is primarily a T lymphocyte dysfunction with progressive loss of T cells and cell-mediated immunity during the first year of life. Immunoglobulin levels are generally near normal, and most patients can respond to antigenic challenge with specific antibody production. In some, however, humoral immunity also diminishes with time.

ADA catalyzes the conversion of deoxyadenosine to deoxyinosine, and PNP abets the conversion of deoxyguanosine to guanine—both key steps in the catabolism of those deoxyribonucleosides. Deficiency of ADA or PNP leads to accumulation of the deoxynucleosides deoxyadenosine or deoxyguanosine, either of which can have profound effects on lymphocyte function. The phosphorylated deoxynucleosides dATP and dGTP are potent feedback inhibitors of the enzyme ribonucleotide reductase, which is required to generate the deoxynucleotide triphosphates (see Fig. 297-2) needed for DNA synthesis in rapidly proliferating cells such as those engaged in mounting an immune response. In addition, the accumulation of deoxyadenosine or adenosine that accompanies ADA deficiency can cause lymphotoxicity by interfering with methylation reactions derived from the conversion of S-adenosylmethionine to S-adenosyl homocysteine (SAH) (Fig. 297-3). Methylation is inhibited by the accumulation of SAH, which results from the inhibition of SAH-hydrolase by deoxyadenosine and by the high concentration of adenosine. Accumulation of SAH and the absence of SAH-hydrolase have been documented in erythrocytes from an ADA-deficient SCID patient.

Wiskott-Aldrich syndrome. The nature of the primary defect in this X-linked recessive disorder, which presents early in life with recurrent infections and the triad of eczema, thrombocytopenia, and a bleeding diathesis, remains uncertain. An abnormal expression of a cell membrane glycoprotein on T lymphocytes and platelets may provide a basis for concurrence of thrombocytopenia and immunodeficiency. Wiskott-Aldrich leukocytes have little CD43 on their surface and platelets are depleted of gplb. CD43 binds ICAM-1, an important intercellular adhesion molecule, and its absence from the cell surfaces would be expected to diminish the cell-cell interactions needed for T cell function. The reduced CD43 and gplb levels have been linked to the enzyme calpein, which when activated cleaves both gplb and CD43. Abnormal regulation of calpein activation has been implicated as the probable defect in Wiskott-Aldrich syndrome. If so, calpein inhibitors may prove to be effective therapeutic agents. Both cellular and humoral abnormalities have been identified. T cell dysfunction includes absent delayed hypersensitivity skin tests, retarded allograft rejection, and diminished numbers of E rosette–forming cells. Monocyte chemotaxis is impaired. Abnormalities of humoral immunity include diminished serum IgM levels together with markedly elevated concentrations of IgE and, often, increased IgA and IgD. These quantitative changes in serum immunoglobulin concentrations appear to result from increased catabolic rates of IgA, IgE, and IgM. Increased synthetic rates of IgE and IgA, which are elevated three- to fivefold in these patients, compensate for the enhanced catabolism, but the IgM synthetic rate is normal, hence the low serum level. Serum IgG levels are generally normal, as are the number of circulating B cells. Children with this disorder commonly die during the first decade of life from infection, usually with polysaccharide-containing organisms, or from cerebral hemorrhage. Those who sur-

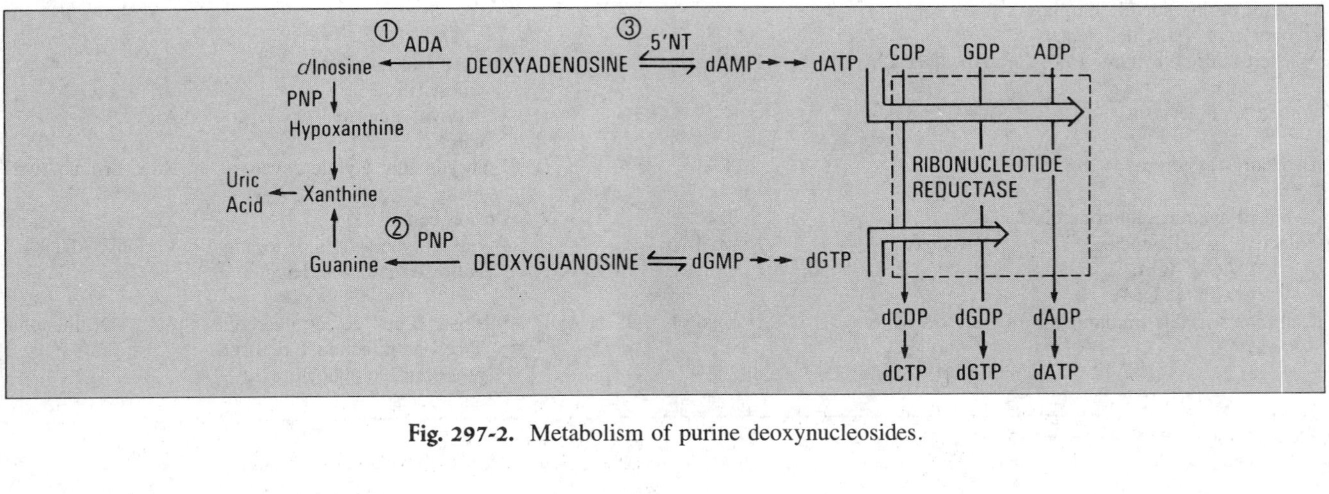

Fig. 297-2. Metabolism of purine deoxynucleosides.

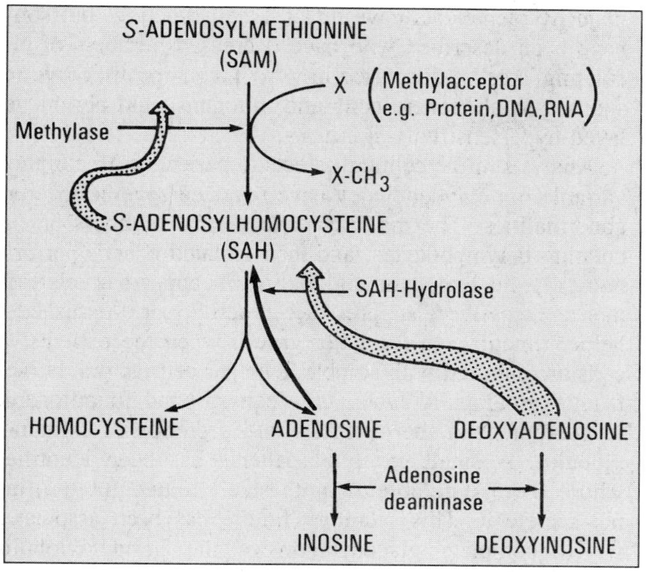

Fig. 297-3. Inhibition of methylation reactions derived during the conversion of S-adenosylmethionone (SAM) to SAH resulting from deoxyadenosine accumulation.

vive have an inordinately high incidence of lymphoreticular malignancies, perhaps because of the diminished capacity of T cells to provide immune surveillance. Bone marrow transplantation after ablation of the patient's own marrow can correct all of the Wiskott-Aldrich defects.

Ataxia telangiectasia. Recurrent susceptibility to infection is a relatively late development in children with ataxia telangiectasia, which is inherited as an autosomal recessive trait. Ataxia, initially truncal and subsequently involving extremities as well, appears in the first year of life, whereas the oculocutaneous telangiectasias may appear at any time from birth to several years of age. Increased susceptibility to sinopulmonary infections begins at about 3 years of age. Patients with ataxia telangiectasia also may have endocrine disturbance (e.g., insulin-resistant diabetes; testicular or ovarian dysgenesis; pigmentary changes; and progeric signs, including premature aging of the skin and graying hair). Patients generally die from infection during childhood, but some have survived into the fifth decade. The risk of the development of lymphoreticular malignancies increases with age.

Lymphoid tissue is diminished, but not absent. Only one third of the patients are lymphopenic, and their lymph nodes reveal a few lymphocytes in both T and B cell areas. Humoral abnormalities include markedly diminished serum and secretory IgA concentrations and, in many patients, the presence of monomeric 7S IgM. Cellular immunity becomes increasingly impaired with the passage of time and is manifested in these patients as absent delayed hypersensitivity skin reactions and delayed allograft rejections. The basis for this widespread systemic illness remains undefined.

The cells of patients with ataxia telangiectasia exhibit heightened sensitivity to ionizing radiation, leading to chromosomal breaks and translocations most commonly involving chromosomes 14 and 7. Similar anomalies of chromosome 14 have been associated with some lymphomas, suggesting that the high incidence of those malignancies in ataxia telangiectasia may be caused by the chromosomal defects rather than by diminished immune surveillance. There is some evidence that the enhanced radiation damage is related to defective DNA repair. However, no single defect can account for radiation sensitivity in all patients with ataxia telangiectasia. Cell fusion experiments combining fibroblasts from different patients have shown reciprocal correction of the radiation response defect. These fusion studies have revealed that there are at least five different complementation groups. Thus, a number of different genetic mutations may lead to ataxia telangiectasia. To date, there is no effective treatment for this disorder.

T-cell immunodeficiency

Congenital thymic hypoplasia (DiGeorge syndrome) is a relatively pure form of T cell immunodeficiency. Infants with the disorder do not develop T cells, and they lack any form of cell-mediated immunity. Immunoglobulin levels and T cell–independent humoral immunity, on the other hand, are usually normal. The hypoplastic thymus in these infants is unable to induce differentiation of lymphoid precursor cells into mature T cells. The thymus and parathyroid glands are derived from the floor of the third and fourth pharyngeal pouches and migrate to their normal locations during the twelfth week of gestation. During this same period, the philtrum of the lip and the ear tubercles become differentiated. DiGeorge syndrome results from a failure in embryogenesis, and the infant has abnormal facial features at birth, including low-set ears with notched pinnae, micrognathia, hypertelorism, and a fish-shaped mouth. Anomalies of the great blood vessels around the aortic arch are regularly present. Infants who survive the neonatal period develop the recurrent chronic infections characteristic of T cell deficiencies, with viral, fungal, and facultative intracellular bacterial agents. Fetal thymus transplants may reconstitute cellular immune function in some patients with the DiGeorge syndrome. The use of early fetal tissue assures that the thymic graft does not contain immunocompetent T cells and avoids a GVH reaction. Mature fetal grafts have been implanted, encased in plastic chambers sealed with filters that prevent cells from leaving but allow free passage of soluble molecules. The rapid reconstitution of T cell function in some patients indicates that they have adequate numbers of precursor cells, which are readily induced to differentiate into mature T cells by soluble thymic (hormone?) factors.

Humoral (B cell) immunodeficiency disorders

X-linked hypogammaglobulinemia. This disease of male infants, formerly called *Bruton's syndrome,* is first seen from 6 to 9 months of age and is manifested by severe bacterial infections, including recurrent pneumonias, otitis, sinusitis, and meningitis; the disease results from the lack of differentiation of pre–B cells into mature B cells. Peripheral blood B lymphocytes and plasma cells are completely absent, but there are normal numbers of pre–B cells in the marrow. Humoral immunity and serum immunoglobulin concentrations are markedly diminished. Peripheral blood lymphocyte numbers, however, are usually normal, since the majority of circulating lymphocytes are T cells. The cellular immune system is intact, with normal thymic development and normal formation of the thymic-dependent areas of peripheral lymphoid tissue. Treatment with gamma globulin injections effectively raises the level of circulating immunoglobulins and protects the patient from infections.

Selective immunoglobulin deficiencies. The absence of one or two of the immunoglobulin classes from serum is a common occurrence. Isolated IgA deficiency is the most frequent, occurring in approximately 1 in 500 in the general population. Most of these individuals are asymptomatic, but there is an increased incidence of immunopathogenetic disorders, especially rheumatoid arthritis, systemic lupus erythematosus (SLE), and atopy. There is no specific therapy. It must be recognized that these patients can develop antibody to IgA if given blood products, and life-threatening anaphylaxis may result.

The absence of IgA and IgG, with normal or elevated IgM levels, is a well-recognized partial immunoglobulin deficiency. Two forms of this syndrome have been identified; one, apparently inherited as an X-linked phenomenon, has been described in children, whereas an acquired form may be found in young adult females. Clinically, these patients have an increased incidence of pyogenic infections and associated autoimmune phenomena, including thrombocytopenia, aplastic or hemolytic anemia, and neutropenia.

Common variable immunodeficiency

Gathered under the rubric of common variable immunodeficiency is a heterogeneous group of disorders characterized by the development of hypogammaglobulinemia manifesting itself after childhood in previously healthy individuals. This form of idiopathic immunodeficiency syndrome generally is seen first as recurrent chronic sinopulmonary infections. Patients with chronic progressive bronchiectasis should be prime suspects for this diagnosis. The peak incidence is in young adulthood (15 to 35 years of age), but it may occur at any age. Males and females are affected equally, and although multiple cases within a family have been described, no clear genetic susceptibility has been documented.

Immunologic evaluation reveals hypogammaglobulinemia as a constant feature. Total serum immunoglobulins are usually less than 300 mg per deciliter, and IgG, less than 250 mg per deciliter. IgM and IgA levels generally are depressed and may be absent. In patients with borderline immunoglobulin values, the lack of normal antibody response after immunization establishes the diagnosis. Studies of cellular immunity provide more heterogeneous results. The majority of patients have intact T cell function, but some have been described who have decreased numbers of circulating T cells, decreased in vitro T cell–proliferative responses to allogeneic cells and mitogens, and absent delayed hypersensitivity skin tests.

Analysis of the cellular defects in patients with common variable immunodeficiency have revealed several different abnormalities. The majority have normal numbers of circulating B lymphocytes, and their isolated B cells perform normally; the hypogammaglobulinemia appears to relate either to excessive T suppressor cell activity or diminished T helper function. In the latter group, when the patients' B cells are cultured with soluble T helper cell factors derived from normal individuals, they can respond to mitogenic stimulation with the synthesis and secretion of immunoglobulin. A small group of patients has been identified whose B cells are able to synthesize immunoglobulin, but not secrete it. This secretory failure has been associated with incomplete glycosylation of the immunoglobulin heavy chain in those individuals.

Patients with common variable immunodeficiency frequently have other characteristic, associated clinical manifestations. Prominent among these is a spruelike intestinal disorder with diarrhea, steatorrhea, and, occasionally, protein-losing enteropathy. Intestinal biopsies may reveal nodular lymphoid hyperplasia, and *Giardia lamblia* infection is common. In many cases, however, intestinal biopsy discloses no abnormality. Treatment for giardia infection may reverse the malabsorption syndrome. Hepatosplenomegaly and lymphadenopathy are frequently present. Noncaseating granulomas of unknown etiology occur in liver, spleen, lung, and skin. Those manifestations respond to corticosteroid therapy.

Common variable immunodeficiency also is associated with an increased incidence of autoimmune disorders. Autoimmune hemolytic anemia and pernicious anemia occur frequently. T cell reactivity to intrinsic factor has been reported in some patients with pernicious anemia. In addition, a number of patients have been reported with features suggesting systemic lupus erythematosus, mixed connective tissue disease, dermatomyositis, or rheumatoid arthritis. Interestingly, there is a higher than expected incidence of SLE, hemolytic anemia, thrombocytopenic purpura, and positive tests for rheumatoid factor among family members of patients with common variable immunodeficiency.

Although the hypogammaglobulinemia in these individuals results from several different mechanisms, the therapeutic approach remains prophylactic gamma globulin injections.

ACQUIRED IMMUNODEFICIENCY SYNDROME

Acquired immunodeficiency syndrome (AIDS) is a clinical syndrome of opportunistic infections or unusual malignancies, or both, in individuals with a pattern of immunodeficiency characterized quantitatively by lymphopenia with selective depletion of the CD4 subset of T lymphocytes. In the United States and Europe, AIDS has been identified primarily in three at-risk groups: sexually active gay males, intravenous drug users, and hemophiliacs and other recipients of blood or blood products. However, the incidence of heterosexual transmission is increasing (see Chapter 242). AIDS is the consequence of an infection with the human immunodeficiency virus (HIV). HIV is an RNA retrovirus that has several structural and biologic characteristics in common with lenteviruses, and like them, it produces a slowly but relentlessly progressive fatal disease. HIV has been recovered from the blood, lymph nodes, and nervous system of AIDS patients. HIV binds specifically to the CD4 cell membrane molecule. There can be a long latency between HIV infection of CD4-bearing T cell helper cells and the appearance of immunodeficiency. During the latent period, however, there is a gradual decrease in the number of circulating CD4-bearing T cells, and there is evidence of blunted T cell responses because of HIV molecules synthesized in the T cells. The mechanisms involved in overcoming HIV's latency resulting in a high level of viral replication and cytopathic death of the CD4-bearing cells are poorly understood. Interestingly, the cytokines TNF-α, GM-CSF, and IL-6, which normally participate in intercellular signaling during immune responses can induce activation of HIV replication in latently infected monocytes and T cells. Thus, early in HIV infection, prior to the development of immunodeficiency, the immune system when stimulated may accelerate its own destruction by inducing active viral replication.

As a result of HIV cytopathicity, patients with AIDS are lymphopenic with selective depletion of CD4 cells. In-vitro immune reactions that require T cell activation, including responses to mitogens and recall antigens, are markedly reduced. In-vivo delayed-type hypersensitivity responses are lost.

B cell function is also affected in AIDS. Antibody production in response to specific immunization is reduced. Most important, especially for infants with AIDS, there is an inadequate IgM response on exposure to pathogenic bacterial organisms. Paradoxically, although specific antibody responses are reduced, there is increased spontaneous immunoglobulin production by B cells from AIDS patients and elevated serum immunoglobulin levels. The cause of the polyclonal B cell hyperactivity has not been fully defined but may result from a combination of diminished T cell regulatory signals and direct B cell stimulation by virus. Both HIV and Epstein-Barr virus, a frequent active infection in AIDS patients, induce polyclonal B cell activation in vitro.

HIV infection also appears to affect the monocyte/macrophage–derived cells that phagocytize infecting organisms and present their antigens to the immune system. The monocytes of AIDS patients are defective in a number of functions related to that role, including reduced chemotaxis and reduced intracellular killing. Those defects can be largely restored by treating the monocytes with gamma interferon, a lymphokine produced by normal CD4 cells. Thus, those monocyte defects may be another consequence of the depletion of CD4 cells by HIV infection.

In AIDS, as in other immunodeficient states with T cell abnormalities, patients typically present with a variety of opportunistic infections and/or malignancy. Kaposi's sarcoma, the neoplasm that is most strikingly apparent in AIDS, has not been associated with other immunodeficiency disorders, and the reason for its association with AIDS is unknown. AIDS does share with other T cell immunodeficiencies an unusually high frequency of B cell lymphomas. The infectious agents responsible for the opportunistic infections in AIDS are also typical of those expected in subjects with cell-mediated immunodeficiency—that is, viruses, fungi, and facultative intracellular parasites. *Pneumocystis carinii* pneumonia, *Candida albicans*–caused oral thrush, and cytomegalovirus infection are common in patients with AIDS, as they are in other patients with inherited or chemotherapy- or radiation-induced T cell deficiencies. In AIDS patients, there are also unusually high incidences of infection with *Mycobacterium avium intracellulare,* and the unicellular intestinal parasites *Isospora* and *Cryptosporidia*. Meningitis from *Cryptococcus neoformans,* other atypical mycobacterial infections, disseminated herpes virus infections, and toxoplasmosis also occur with appreciable frequency. The characteristics of those infections and approaches to therapy are described in Part Seven, Infectious Diseases.

REFERENCES

Arnaiz-Villena A: Human T cell activation deficiencies. Immunol Today 13:259, 1992.

Conley ME et al: X-linked severe combined immunodeficiency: diagnosis in males with sporadic severe combined immunodeficiency and clarification of clinical findings. J Clin Invest 85:1548, 1990.

Fauci AS et al: Immunopathogenic mechanisms in human immunodeficiency virus (HIV) infection. Ann Intern Med 114:678, 1991.

Fischer A: Severe combined immunodeficiencies. Immunodefic Rev 3:83, 1992.

Hirschhorn R: Inherited enzyme deficiencies and immunodeficiency; adenosine deaminase (ADA) and purine nucleoside phosphorylase (PNP) deficiencies. Clin Immunol Immunopathol 40:157, 1986.

McKinnon PJ: Ataxia-telangiectasia: an inherited disorder of ionizing-radiation sensitivity in man. Hum Genet 75:197, 1987.

Primary immunodeficiency diseases: Report of a World Health Organization Scientific Group. Clin Immunol Immunopathol 40:166, 1986.

CHAPTER

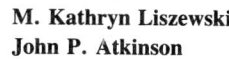

298 Inherited Complement Deficiencies

M. Kathryn Liszewski
John P. Atkinson

Inherited deficiencies of complement components are rare but instructive anomalies of nature. They predispose an individual to bacterial infections and/or immune-complex excess syndromes such as systemic lupus erythematosus (SLE) (Table 298-1). These conditions are inherited as au-

Table 298-1. Inherited complement deficiencies

Components	Associated illness
C1, C4, C2	SLE or lupuslike illness; glomerulonephritis
C3	Pyogenic infections; SLE
C5-8	*Neisseria* infections
D and properdin	*Neisseria meningitidis* infections
Regulators	
C1 inhibitor	Hereditary angioedema
DAF and CD59	Paroxysmal nocturnal hemoglobinuria
Factors H and I	Secondary deficiency of C3; *Urticaria*

tosomal codominant (recessive) traits except for C1 inhibitor deficiency (autosomal dominant) and properdin deficiency (sex-linked). Complement deficiency states are associated with predictable defects in complement-dependent functions. The activity of the individual protein is lost, as are the activities of the proteins that follow in the cascade.

CLASSIC PATHWAY

Deficiencies of the early components of the classic pathway (C1, C4, C2) are frequently associated with immune complex–mediated syndromes, especially systemic lupus erythematosus (SLE) or a lupuslike illness. The latter is characterized by a low or negative antinuclear antibody (ANA) test although antibodies to ribonuclear proteins, especially anti-Ro (SS-A), are present in most of these patients.

Approximately 90% of C1- and C4-deficient patients are afflicted with systemic lupus erythematosus (SLE). In addition, approximately 50% of individuals lacking C2 (the most common deficiency) develop SLE or a related illness. In some patients with these deficiencies there is an increased frequency of infections. Except for an increased frequency of skin lesions, those afflicted with classic pathway deficiency show similar clinical manifestations to those seen in other SLE patients.

Normally the early complement components effectively remove immune complexes. Without such processing, immune complexes may accumulate in excessive quantities in plasma and deposit in inappropriate locations. Immune complex deposition is a pathologic hallmark of SLE and is responsible for much of the tissue damage.

C4

C4 is a pivotal protein of the classic pathway. On activation, it becomes covalently bound to a particle surface and can function as an opsonin or continue the cascade. A deficiency in C4 predisposes to SLE or autoimmune disorders.

Plasma C4 is composed of two distinct but similar glycoproteins, termed *C4A* and *C4B*, coded for by two separate genes. C4A binds more efficiently to amino-containing (NH_2) substrates, whereas C4B binds more effectively to hydroxyl (OH) groups. This genetic diversity thus allows C4 to react with a larger variety of pathologic substrates—a selective advantage for a host defense system.

A partial deficiency of C4 also predisposes to SLE or related disorders. Of Caucasian SLE patients, 10% to 15% are null (no protein produced) for C4A. Additionally, C4A heterozygous deficiency (i.e., only one of the two C4A alleles abnormal) is increased among SLE patients. C4A or C4B deficiency has been associated with scleroderma, IgA nephropathy, Henoch-Schönlein purpura, childhood diabetes mellitus, chronic forms of hepatitis, and subacute sclerosing panencephalitis.

C3

Deficiency of C3, the component common to both the classic and alternative pathways, results in severe, recurrent infections with encapsulated bacteria that begin shortly after birth. The clinical course resembles that observed in congenital hypogammaglobulinemia. If they survive the infections, these patients are also plagued with problems associated with excess immune complexes, such as glomerulonephritis.

These clinical problems relate directly to the critical role played by C3 in opsonization/phagocytosis and in immune-complex handling.

MEMBRANE ATTACK COMPLEX (MAC)

Deficiency of components of the MAC (C5-8) is primarily associated with infection by *Neisseria* species. Otherwise, such affected individuals are surprisingly healthy. C9-deficient individuals appear to be normal.

ALTERNATIVE PATHWAY

Inherited defects of components of the alternative pathway (D and properdin) are exceedingly rare. Affected individuals usually develop recurrent and severe infections, especially with *Neisseria meningitidis*. Their serum demonstrates impaired complement activation in the absence of specific antibody.

COMPLEMENT RECEPTORS

Complete deficiencies of CR1 (C3b/C4b receptor) and CR2 (C3dg/Epstein-Barr virus receptor) have not been reported. A small, dysfunctional form of the CR1 is associated with SLE and an acquired reduction in the levels of CR1 occurs in immune complex–mediated syndromes. A deficiency of CR3, an integrin that has C3bi as one of its ligands, causes recurrent, severe bacterial *(Staphylococcus aureus/Pseudomonas)* infections. This condition, known as *leukocyte adhesion deficiency syndrome* (CD11-CD18 deficiency), may be suspected at birth if there is delayed separation of the umbilical cord and development of omphalitis. Most patients die in childhood of refractory infections involving soft tissue, mucosal surfaces, and the intestinal tract.

INHIBITOR DEFICIENCIES

C1 inhibitor (C1INH)

The illness produced by functional deficiency of the C1 inhibitor is hereditary angioedema (HAE), a familial tendency toward recurrent episodes of nonpainful, nonpruritic, nonerythematous angioedema. Facial and extremity involvement are primarily a cosmetic problem, but severe abdominal pain may result when swelling involves the bowel wall, and edema of the larynx can be fatal. The attacks usually develop in adolescence and continue throughout life. Precipitating factors, other than trauma, are not known. Swelling resolves spontaneously within 48 to 72 hours, leaving no residua. Unlike genetic deficiencies of other complement components, heterozygotes are afflicted. The C1INH levels are decreased 5% to 20% of normal.

A deficiency of C1 inhibitor prevents the proper regulation of activated C1. Consequently, plasma levels of C4 and C2, the substrates of C1, are chronically low. The diagnosis is suggested by the clinical history and the finding of low C4 levels. A normal C4 value, especially during an episode, excludes the diagnosis. Treatment usually involves the administration of nonmasculinizing androgens to stimulate increased hepatic synthesis of the C1 inhibitor. Attacks will subside as the C1 inhibitor rises above 25% to 30% of normal. An adequate physiologic level of the C1INH is indicated by the normalization of C4.

Factors H and I

Afflicted individuals develop recurrent infections, hemolytic anemia, and urticaria. Since factors H and I regulate C3, a deficiency of either allows the alternative pathway to fire to exhaustion and thereby consume C3. Infusion of plasma (source of H or I) can temporarily alleviate clinical symptoms as C3 levels normalize.

Decay accelerating factor (DAF) and CD59

These membrane-anchored proteins inhibit complement activation on host tissue. DAF inhibits the C3 convertases and CD59 blocks binding of C8 and C9 to MAC as it assembles. A deficiency of DAF and CD59 on erythrocytes predisposes these cells to lysis and produces the illness paroxysmal nocturnal hemoglobinuria (PNH). DAF and CD59 are anchored to the membrane by a glycolipid scaffold. PNH represents an acquired somatic stem-cell defect in the machinery for the attachment of this anchor to proteins.

NEPHRITIC FACTORS

A C3 deficiency state arises when an autoimmune antibody is made against the C3 convertase. The autoantibody against the alternative pathway convertase is called the *C3 nephritic factor,* while that against the classic pathway convertase is termed the *C4 nephritic factor*. The autoantibody stabilizes the convertase causing excessive C3 cleavage, which results in a secondary deficiency of C3.

These patients, predominantly children, may present with glomerulonephritis, partial lipodystrophy, or frequent infections with an encapsulated bacteria.

REFERENCES

Figueroa JE and Densen P: Infectious diseases associated with complement deficiencies. Clin Microbiol Rev 4:359, 1991.

Frank MM: Complement in the pathophysiology of human disease. N Engl J Med 316:1525, 1987.

Kahl LE and Atkinson JP: Autoimmune aspects of complement deficiency. Clin Aspect Autoimmun 2:8, 1988.

Ross SC and Densen P: Complement deficiency states and infection; epidemiology, pathogenesis and consequences of neisserial and other infections in an immune deficiency. Medicine (Baltimore). 63:243, 1984.

ATOPIC DISEASES AND RELATED SYNDROMES IV

CHAPTER

299 Rhinitis

Robert S. Zeiger
Michael Schatz

The term *rhinitis* is used to describe disorders of the nasal mucosa. These diseases, with their associated symptoms of nasal discharge or obstruction, sneezing, rhinorrhea, pain, and anosmia, cause more than 28 million restricted days, 6 million bedridden days, and loss of 3 million work days and 2 million school days each year, at a medical cost of $500 million. Although not life-threatening, rhinitis may substantially interfere with the quality and enjoyment of life. Simple diagnostic tests generally allow classification of the patient's problem and allow initiation of therapy programs that provide increased comfort and function.

APPLIED NASAL ANATOMY AND PHYSIOLOGY

The nose is composed of a 10-12 cm mucosal passage, extending from the nasal orifice to the nasopharynx and pharynx, that is occupied by three turbinates. The nasolacrimal duct opens beneath the inferior turbinate; the orifices of the frontal, anterior ethmoid, and maxillary sinuses extend from anterior to posterior in the order listed, beneath the middle turbinate, and together with the anterior ethmoid air cells make up the ostiomeatal complex. The openings of the posterior ethmoid and sphenoid sinuses empty into the superior meatus. Disruption, distortion, or swelling of the turbinates or meatal mucosal inflammation can occlude the orifices of the sinuses. In particular, disease of the ostiomeatal complex appears to predispose to chronic or recurrent maxillary, ethmoid, or frontal sinusitis. The vulnerable position of the eustachian tube orifice in the posterior nasopharynx is evidenced by the frequent auditory problems, serous otitis media, infection, or hearing loss associated with nasal mucosal and turbinate swelling.

Microscopically, the nasal mucosa is composed of stratified squamous epithelium in its anterior one third, and of ciliated pseudostratified columnar epithelium interspersed with mucus-secreting goblet cells in the remainder. The lamina propria contains seromucous glands, blood vessels, nerves, and ground substance. This structure provides the substrate for the main nonolfactory functions of the nose: warming, humidification, and filtration of inspired air. Humidification is accomplished by the transudation of fluid from the fenestrated capillaries to the mucosal surface. Sinusoids situated over the turbinates provide accumulations of pooled blood, which transfer heat. Filtration occurs by a variety of mechanisms. The architecture of the nasal airway creates turbulent airflow that fosters deposition of large particles (>10 μm) on the anterior nasal surfaces, and local immune responses permit inactivation or neutralization of inspired foreign material. Beating cilia transport mucus and trapped particles posteriorly toward the nasopharynx at an average rate of 5 mm per minute, leading to clearance of particles in 10 to 15 minutes. Structural or functional ciliary abnormalities increase nasopharyngeal and/or sinus infection. The nose also acts as a "gas mask" by retaining 99% of inhaled water-soluble gases, including common pollutants (SO_2, formaldehyde, and ozone).

Nasal structures are controlled by autonomic reflexes generated from mucosal afferent fibers. The vasomotor fibers innervating the vasculature are parasympathetic efferents that dilate, and sympathetic (primarily alpha-adrenergic) efferents that constrict, vessels. The secretomotor fibers that innervate the glands are parasympathetic. Glandular secretion is indirectly affected by sympathetic activity through alpha-adrenergic innervation of its vasculature; however, cholinergic influence predominates.

A normal cycle of alternating constriction and dilation of the turbinate sinusoids every 2.0 to 4.0 hours leads to continual differences in patency between the nostrils. This turbinate cycle usually can be detected only by rhinometric flow-volume measurements. Patients with nasal disorders experience an exaggerated turbinate cycle, described as alternating nasal congestion. Increased alpha-adrenergic activity, stimulated by normal homeostasis, exercise, or local or systemic sympathomimetics, leads to vasoconstriction and increased nasal patency, while its reduction because of drug administration (e.g., reserpine) or disease (hypothyroidism) results in vasodilatation and decreased patency. Parasympathetic (cholinergic) stimulation (cold, odors, irritants) causes vasodilatation and hypersecretion.

Nasal vasomotor instability can be best understood as a local autonomic imbalance with hyperresponsive cholinergic reactivity leading to exaggerated nasal turbinate swelling and hypersecretion. This vasomotor instability is characterized clinically by alternating nostril congestion and symptoms in response to recumbency, alcohol intake, temperature and humidity changes, and other nonspecific irritants (inert dust, smoke, fumes, aerosols, powders, and strong odors). Any inflammatory, noninflammatory, or structural cause of chronic rhinitis may lead to vasomotor instability. Its presence is not diagnostic of a specific disorder, but rather indicates a general nasal malfunction.

INCIDENCE

Chronic rhinitis is estimated to affect up to 20% of the population. Seasonal allergic rhinoconjunctivitis caused by pollen is most common in young adults and accounts for about half the cases; the various types of perennial rhinitis comprise the remainder. IgE-mediated reactivity against house dust mites, mold, and animal danders participates in the illnesses of about one third of patients with chronic perennial rhinitis; another one third is caused by chronic infections, either nasopharyngitis or sinusitis. The remainder comprises perennial eosinophilic, nonallergic rhinitis—ENR—(15%), structurally related rhinitis (5–10%), rhinitis medicamentosa (less than 5%), and nasal mastocytosis (rare). ENR occurs later than allergic rhinitis (age at diagnosis 38 versus 25 years), and nasal polyps occur in at least one third of patients with ENR. An undefined proportion of patients with ENR are exacerbated by aspirin and other nonsteroidal anti-inflammatory agents. The prevalence of nasal polyps in the population is about 1%; their occurrence increases with age and is associated with asthma (especially nonallergic) and aspirin idiosyncrasy.

PATHOPHYSIOLOGY

Allergic (seasonal) rhinitis

In the sensitized individual, inhaled allergen rapidly initiates release of chemical mediators from mast cells; these mediators cause variable degrees of vasodilation and edema (nasal congestion), increased mucus secretion and cellular recruitment (rhinorrhea), and increased capillary and mucosal permeability. The mediators probably also disturb the balanced nervous control of nasal function, leading to direct and reflex vascular dilation and hypersecretion. The sneezing threshold falls. After continued daily allergen exposure, lesser quantities of specific allergen cause severe nasal symptoms (priming). Similar mechanisms lead to the characteristic ocular symptoms of tearing and itching associated with allergic rhinitis. Nonspecific nasal mucosal hyperreactivity (i.e., enhancement of symptoms by physical stimuli, irritants, or emotions) is characteristically coincident with allergic reactivity of the nasal mucosa.

Nonallergic (perennial) rhinitis

Our understanding of the pathophysiology of most types of nonallergic inflammatory rhinitis is limited. In ENR, the specific stimulus for eosinophil attraction to nasal and sinus mucosa is unknown, but the presence of the eosinophils per se may lead to tenacious, viscid mucus, and release of eosinophil constituents such as major basic protein may produce mucosal damage. *Aspirin idiosyncrasy* refers to a clinical syndrome that, in its entirety, includes ENR, nasal polyps, hyperplastic and secondarily infected sinuses, and asthma. Respiratory and/or cutaneous manifestations, which are not immunologically mediated, follow ingestion of aspirin and nonsteroidal anti-inflammatory agents. In nasal mastocytosis, presumably increased "spontaneous" or nonspecific triggered mediator release from increased numbers of mucosal mast cells leads to nasal symptomatology. Although the pathophysiology of nasal/sinus infection may be straightforward, the factors that increase individual susceptibility to recurrent or chronic infectious rhinosinusitis (other than nasal or sinus obstruction) and the contributory role of noninfectious sinus mucosal inflammation are incompletely understood.

Noninflammatory (vasomotor) rhinitis

Vasomotor instability, present in patients with rhinitis medicamentosa, rhinitis associated with systemic autonomic states, high-output vascular conditions, endocrine disorders (typically hypo- or hyperthyroidism), or pregnancy, and idiopathic vasomotor rhinitis, are thought to result from a direct effect of medication or endocrine or neurologic factors on the nasal vasculature and/or the autonomic nervous system.

Structural rhinitis

Anatomic disturbances, such as nasal septal deviation, fractures, foreign bodies, or choanal atresia, produce rhinitis by physical mechanisms specific to the abnormality. Secondary nasal mucosal hyperreactivity may also result from the structurally induced abnormalities of nasal air flow.

PATIENT EVALUATION: HISTORY, PHYSICAL EXAMINATION, AND LABORATORY EVALUATION

A proper evaluation of patients with chronic rhinitis requires a correlation of historical data, physical findings, and nasal cytology (Table 299-1). In many clinical circumstances, the nose can be adequately examined physically by anterior rhinoscopy (using a nasal otoscope adapter or nasal speculum). Rhinopharyngeal endoscopy (flexible or rigid) in the hands of an experienced and skilled clinician allows better definition of mucosal edema, inflammation, pathologic drainage, or polyp formation in the entire nasal cavity, including accessible components of the ostiomeatal complex. Rigid endoscopy provides better image clarity than flexible endoscopy and allows sampling of purulent discharge from the middle meatus, the cultures of which have been shown to correlate with cultures of ipsilateral maxillary and ethmoid sinuses.

Nasal cytologic examination can be performed on expelled mucus but should preferably be done on materials obtained by scraping the nasal turbinates and mucosal surfaces with a flexible nasal probe (Rhinoprobe).

Sinus radiographs are particularly revealing in patients experiencing chronic, unremitting postnasal discharge in association with nasal neutrophilia, and such radiographs often demonstrate mucosal thickening, opacification, and/or air-fluid levels. Abnormal sinus radiographs also are observed in perennial nonallergic eosinophilic rhinitis and in aspirin hypersensitivity. More than 50% of children coming to allergy clinics with chronic rhinitis characterized by postnasal discharge and nasal neutrophilia demonstrate on sinus radiographs gross abnormalities that respond to antibiotics. For patients with clinical features of chronic or recurrent sinusitis, computed tomography scans of the sinuses in the coronal plain are the procedures of choice because they allow better definition of disease of the ostiomeatal complex.

Specific IgE should be determined by skin tests (preferable) or RAST tests in patients who have a clear history of allergy and in those with nasal eosinophilia and/or basophilia. Skin tests are performed to confirm the diagnosis, to direct specific environmental measures, and to select immunotherapeutic extracts (see Chapter 292). An adequate battery of skin-test antigens includes house-dust mites, clinically relevant danders, molds (of the genera *Alternaria, Hormodendrum, Penicillium, Aspergillus,* and *Helminthosporium*), and the prevalent local pollens.

Perennial allergens, like danders and dusts, are of particular importance in the winter months, when the home is closed and forced air circulates. Atmospheric and indoor molds are also perennial problems in climates not affected by frost or snow. Pollen allergens generally follow a characteristic seasonal pattern in temperate climates (trees in early spring, grasses in late spring, and weeds in the fall). Grasses may become perennial allergens in subtropical climates, pollinating from February through December; nevertheless, a peak seasonal worsening can be elicited in the spring.

Rhinomanometry can provide objective and quantitative measurement of nasal airway resistance. However, for routine clinical evaluation rhinomanometry may not be particularly useful because of considerable overlap of nasal airway resistance in normal subjects and those with rhinitis. Rhinomanometry may be useful, though, for serial measurements of changes in nasal patency after allergen or chemical challenges and drug therapy.

To evaluate for anosmia or hyposmia, the threshold for detecting inhaled pyridine may be determined. A saccharin test is a useful screening procedure for mucociliary dysfunction.

DIAGNOSIS

A practical diagnostic chart utilizing clinical symptomatology, physical findings, and nasal cytology is outlined in Table 299-1. It is important to note that nasal disorders, although classified as distinct entities, often coexist.

Table 299-1. Classification and therapy of chronic rhinitis

Diagnostic classification	Differential clinical findings	Nasal cytology	Allergy skin tests	Pharmacologic therapy	Nonpharmacologic therapy
I. Inflammatory rhinitis					
A. Eosinophilic allergic rhinitis	Onset typically in, but not limited to, childhood Sneezing, nasal itching clear rhinorrhea, ocular symptoms Pale swollen nasal mucosa Specific allergen precipitants (historically) Associated atopic disorders	↑ Eosinophils with or without ↑ basophils and/or mast cells	Positive and correlate with history	Antihistamines Antihistamine-decongestant combinations Intranasal corticosteroids Intranasal cromolyn	Antigen avoidance Immunotherapy
1. Seasonal	Hay fever Typically spring, summer, fall Extended asymptomatic intervals common				
2. Perennial	Typically daily Usually triggered by animals, dust mites, mold				
B. Eosinophilic nonallergic rhinitis	Onset in adulthood (usually) Perennial symptoms Prominent pale mucosal edema Aspirin may increase symptoms Anosmia common Frequent polyps and/or sinus disease	↑ Eosinophils with or without ↑ basophils and/or mast cells	Negative or coincidental (not correlated with history)	Antihistamine-decongestant combinations Intranasal corticosteroids Oral corticosteroids (for severe cases)	Saline lavage Exercise
C. Primary nasal mastocytosis	Onset adulthood (usually) Perennial rhinorrhea and congestion May be associated with migraine headaches or asthma Nonspecific precipitants frequent	↑ Mast cells	Negative or coincidental	Intranasal corticosteroids Intranasal cromolyn Systemic oral corticosteroids (for severe cases)	
D. Nasal polyps	Severe obstruction Anosmia Polyps on physical examination Sinus involvement common				Polypectomy with or without submucous resection Ethmoidectomy
1. Eosinophilic	Incidence, 85% Uncommon in children Seromucous secretion Associated with aspirin sensitivity, intrinsic asthma Role of allergy doubtful Steroid responsive	↑ Eosinophils with or without ↑ basophils and/or mast cells	Negative or coincidental	Intranasal corticosteroids Oral corticosteroids	

Table 299-1. Classification and therapy of chronic rhinitis—cont'd

Diagnostic classification	Differential clinical findings	Nasal cytology	Allergy skin tests	Pharmacologic therapy	Nonpharmacologic therapy
2. Neutrophilic	Incidence, 15% Purulent secretions Associated with cystic fibrosis, Kartagener's triad, ciliary disturbances, sinusitis, immune deficiency Steroid unresponsive	↑ Neutrophils with or without bacteria	Negative or coincidental	Antibiotics	
E. Neutrophilic nasopharyngitis or sinusitis	Prominent postnasal drip Frequent sinus pain or tenderness Purulent secretions in nose and throat Infection characteristic Sinus films frequently abnormal (sinusitis) May complicate eosinophilic rhinitis or polyps or occur with immune deficiencies, foreign bodies, or trauma or without demonstrable cause	↑ Neutrophils with prominent bacteria	Negative or when positive may be related to underlying allergic rhinitis	Control underlying rhinitis/polyps (if present) Topical decongestants (short courses) Antibiotic courses (2 to 3 weeks) Possibly oral decongestants Sometimes longer-term antibiotics Possibly mucoevacuants Sometimes oral corticosteroids, plus antibiotics	Saline lavage Sinus irrigation Sinus surgery (especially ethroidectomy with or without sphenoidectomy)
F. Atrophic rhinitis	Severe nasal obstruction Physiologically patent nasal passages Associated with aging, too extensive nasal tissue extirpation, Wegener's granulomatosis	Unremarkable unless infected	Unrelated	Antibiotics when appropriate	Saline lavage Lubricants (petrolatum) Surgical transplantation
II. Noninflammatory rhinitis					
A. Rhinitis medicamentosa	Obstruction (most prominent symptom)	Unremarkable (usually)	Negative or related to underlying disorder		Saline lavage Exercise
1. Topical	Associated with local sympathomimetic abuse			Discontinue topical decongestants Intranasal corticosteroid Oral corticosteroids (for severe cases)	
2. Systemic	Current antihypertensive therapy, oral decongestant (rare), beta agonist, birth control pills			Consider reducing dosage or discontinuing (if possible) or switching to alternate effective medication or therapy Intranasal corticosteroids	

(Continued.)

Table 299-1. Classification and therapy of chronic rhinitis—cont'd

Diagnostic classification	Differential clinical findings	Nasal cytology	Allergy skin tests	Pharmacologic therapy	Nonpharmacologic therapy
B. Vasomotor instability	Nonspecific hypersensitivity of nasal mucosal vasculature and glands apparently related to local autonomic nervous system imbalance	Unremarkable	Unrelated	Possibly oral decongestants Intranasal ipratropium for prominent rhinorrhea	Saline lavage Exercise Avoid precipitants
1. Associated with systemic conditions	Thyroid disorders Pregnancy			Correct disorder (if possible)	
2. Idiopathic vasomotor rhinitis (primary vasomotor instability)	Most common in young adult women				Exercise essential
III. Stucturally related rhinitis	Frequent history of nasal trauma Unilateral obstruction Abnormality diagnosed on physical examination	Unremarkable	Unrelated		Surgery (including laser)

TREATMENT

General measures

Vigorous exercise induces sympathetic discharge and redistribution of blood flow and is the body's most efficient homeostatic control for reducing nasal obstruction. Increased patency develops rapidly and persists for at least 15 to 30 minutes. The maintenance of a regular exercise program provides an effective regimen for patients with chronic rhinitis and may counteract vasomotor instability. Increased nasal airway resistance characteristically occurs in recumbency but may be counteracted, in part, by the patient's lying supine with the head elevated.

The annoyance caused by profuse rhinorrhea can be reduced somewhat by occluding the anterior nares with absorbent, nonshredding facial tissue, replacing the tissue when saturated. Forceful blowing of the nose must be avoided to prevent epistaxis and unnecessary irritation.

Nasal tissue appears to benefit greatly from warm irrigation with saline. Its use should be considered for all patients with chronic rhinitis; benefit appears maximal for topical rhinitis medicamentosa, atrophic rhinitis, nasopharyngitis, and sinusitis. The most effective method of saline irrigation is provided by an adaptation of the Water-Pik device. Warm saline is delivered in a pulsating stream at 20 pulses per second through a special right-angled rubber-tipped nasal adaptor placed loosely within one naris; the patient leans over a sink to perform the irrigation. Alternatively, a soft vinyl bulb syringe may be used for saline (8 oz water + ¼ tsp salt) irrigation.

Specific medications

Antihistamines and decongestants. The antihistamines used to treat rhinitis are chemically diverse. These agents competitively antagonize histamine at its H_1-receptor site and exert varying degrees of anticholinergic, local anesthetic, CNS-depressant, and ganglionic and adrenergic-blocking activities. In addition, a number of antihistamines, especially newer ones (e.g., ketotifen, azelastine), may inhibit mediator release from mast cells and basophils.

Antihistamines have been classified on the basis of their chemical structures. However, this classification appears to have limited value for predicting the efficacy or adverse effects of specific agents, and some of the newer agents do not fit readily into the traditional classification. Hydroxyzine appears to be the most potent of the first-generation antihistamines.

Use of first-generation antihistamines has been limited

by their sedative and anticholinergic side effects. Approaches to minimize the sedative side effects have included bedtime dosing, gradually increasing daytime dosing, and combining antihistamines with sympathomimetic agents (which may also enhance their therapeutic efficacy). Recently, second-generation antihistamines that do not cross the blood-brain barrier and are devoid of anticholinergic or demonstrable sedative effects have become available (terfenadine, astemizole) or may be available soon (loratadine, cetirizine). Of these newer agents, only astemizole appears to be as effective as hydroxyzine and more effective than traditional agents such as chlorpheniramine, and these second-generation antihistamines are generally considerably more expensive than older antihistamines.

In patients with daily symptoms, antihistamines should be taken regularly for best therapeutic results. Loss of clinical efficacy of a previously useful antihistamine may occasionally occur during continuous administration. Recent studies suggest that this is not generally caused by true tachyphylaxis but rather by the increased severity of the underlying disorder and/or secondary complications. When effective, antihistaminic agents may be used in rhinitis with coexisting asthma, except during status asthmaticus.

Oral sympathomimetic amines (decongestants) effectively reduce nasal congestion and are available singly or combined with antihistamines. Rebound rhinitis medicamentosa is rarely associated with chronic use of oral decongestants. These agents may cause insomnia and irritability and should be avoided in hypertensive patients and in those receiving MAO inhibitors.

Intranasal cromolyn. Disodium cromoglycate (cromolyn sodium as a 4% solution—Nasalcrom) is an effective medication in the treatment of allergic rhinitis and reduces the need for antihistamine medication. The usual dosage for patients 6 years old and older is one (5.2 mg) spray in each nostril three to four times a day. If needed, the dose may be doubled. Treatment with nasal cromolyn is more effective if started prior to contact with the offending allergen. Adverse reactions are minimal and have included sneezing, nasal stinging, headache, and bad taste.

Corticosteroids. The usefulness of corticosteroids in the treatment of inflammatory disorders has been recognized for many years. Highly potent, surface-active, rapidly metabolized corticosteroids, such as beclomethasone dipropionate (Vancenase or Beconase), flunisolide (Nasalide), and triamcinolone (Nasacort) have been introduced for intranasal use. Extensive clinical and toxicologic studies have documented their efficacy and safety in managing eosinophilic-associated rhinitis (seasonal or perennial allergic rhinitis, eosinophilic nonallergic rhinitis, and eosinophilic polyps). The usual recommended starting dosage is two sprays in each nostril two times per day. Higher doses may be necessary for more recalcitrant rhinitis. Clinical improvement should be achieved within 1 to 2 weeks, but may not be maximal for 4-6 weeks. After optimal improvement, the dosage should be tapered by one spray in each nostril each week until the minimally effective dose is determined. Patients with allergic rhinitis without polyp disease may require therapeutic doses of topical corticosteroids during peak allergy triggering, followed by a tapering to low-dose maintenance therapy. Patients with perennial nonallergic rhinitis with eosinophilia usually require a moderate maintenance dose, and those with eosinophilic polyps a larger maintenance dose. Side effects of these agents have been minimal and include mild nasal bleeding (5%), irritation in the form of stinging or burning (40% of patients using flunisolide), and transient episodes of sneezing. Intranasal *Candida* infection and septal perforation are rare.

Antibiotics. Acute sinusitis generally is caused by *Streptococcus pneumoniae, Moraxella catarrhalis* (especially in children), or *Haemophilus influenzae,* whereas chronic sinusitis is more often caused by anaerobic organisms (especially in adults). Thus, no antibiotic has a spectrum broad enough to cover all possibilities. Amoxicillin in doses of 500 mg t.i.d. in adults (50 mg/kg/24 hours in children) is the drug of choice in non-penicillin-allergic persons, since approximately 80% of the usual organisms are susceptible, tissue penetration is good, and dosing intervals are convenient. Ampicillin is less expensive but requires more frequent administration and does not penetrate sinus tissues as well. Beta-lactamase-producing *H. influenzae* and *Moraxella catarrhalis,* however, are resistant. Amoxicillin/clavulanate or cefuroxime is usually adequate for beta-lactamase-producing strains as well as the other usual organisms. In patients allergic to penicillin, doxycycline; trimethoprim and sulfamethoxazole; erythromycin and sulfisoxazole; or clindamycin may be alternatives. Coverage for anaerobes is generally provided by amoxicillin, clindamycin, erythromycin plus sulfonamides, cefuroxime, and metronidazole (which essentially only covers anaerobes).

Decreased postnasal discharge, pain, and clearing of nasal neutrophilia and bacteria usually occur within 3 to 4 days after starting therapy. Treatment should continue for at least 2 to 3 weeks, the exact duration depending on the chronicity of the condition. The use of prophylactic antibiotics, such as sulfisoxazole or tetracycline for 1 to 2 months, in a fashion analogous to that used in the treatment of frequent urinary tract infections, may be appropriate for patients with frequent relapses.

Other. Mucoevacuants, such as guaifenesin (600-1200 mg b.i.d.) or iodinated glycerol (2 tablets q.i.d.) are being increasingly recommended for patients with chronic nasopharyngitis/sinusitis, although proof of their efficacy is lacking. Intranasal ipratropium (two sprays in each nostril b.i.d. using a nipple adapter) may be useful for patients with vasomotor rhinitis associated with watery rhinorrhea or to prevent reflux rhinorrhea in response to spicy foods (gustatory rhinitis) or cold air.

Immunotherapy

Immunotherapy, frequently termed *desensitization* or *hyposensitization,* is reserved for rhinitis caused by IgE-mediated hypersensitivity. Immunotherapy is beneficial in IgE-mediated allergic rhinitis in children and adults when (1) strict diagnostic criteria for clinically significant IgE reactivity are met, and (2) administration of high doses of potent allergens is continued for a specified amount of time. The clinical benefit derived from immunotherapy can be measured in partial reduction in symptoms and/or medication usage, not in eradication or cure. Immunotherapy should be given a 12-month trial and, if effective, continued for 3 to 5 years, and then evaluated for trial discontinuation. Because of potential life-threatening side effects, it should be carried out only by specialists trained in its use, and it should be reserved for patients whose disease is not adequately controlled by other means.

TREATMENT OF SPECIFIC DISEASES

Pharmacologic and nonpharmacologic measures for treating the various causes of chronic rhinitis are listed in Table 299-1. A few additional points about common conditions follow.

Allergic rhinitis

Proper management begins with elimination or avoidance of the responsible allergen or allergens. Outdoor pollen exposure may be reduced by use of pollen masks and indoor pollen exposure by use of air-conditioners or air purifiers (containing HEPA filters). The most important aspects of mite environmental control are (1) encasing pillows and mattresses in plastic and (2) washing bed clothes in hot water every 7-10 days. Although maximal reduction of animal dander exposure entails elimination of pets from the home, recent studies suggest that regular bathing of the pet and use of air purifiers reduce animal dander antigen exposure. Finally, mold control is facilitated by reducing indoor humidity and use of a fungicide in areas where mold is growing.

Symptoms can usually be controlled using as-needed or regular antihistamines or antihistamine-decongestant combinations, intranasal cromolyn, or (most effectively in moderate or severe disease) intranasal corticosteroids. Occasionally, oral corticosteroids are required for severe episodes. If these medications fail, a trial of immunotherapy is indicated in properly selected patients.

Eosinophilic nonallergic rhinitis

Regular use of antihistamines and decongestants may provide acceptable control, but intranasal steroids frequently are required. An occasional patient needs episodic or even long-term alternate-day oral corticosteroid therapy. Surveillance for secondary nasopharyngitis-sinusitis and the development of nasal polyps is particularly important.

Eosinophilic rhinosinusitis with or without complicating nasal polyps often is associated with sinus abnormalities. It is frequently difficult to know whether infection or eosinophilic infiltration remains responsible for the sinus abnormalities. Cytology of a postnasal mucus specimen may reveal infectious (neutrophilic) or noninfectious (eosinophilic) inflammation. Frequently, a combination of appropriate antibiotic and short course of daily oral corticosteroid is necessary to ameliorate the condition. Radiologic as well as clinical improvement should be documented.

Nasopharyngitis-sinusitis

Chronic or acute bacterial infection of the nasopharynx or paranasal sinuses may complicate other forms of rhinitis or may occur alone. Proper management requires control of the underlying rhinitis, regular saline lavage, and intermittent courses of appropriate antibiotics supplemented for 3 to 5 days with topical decongestants. Oral decongestant medications and mucoevacuants (guaifenesin, iodinated glycerol) are often recommended, although proof of their value is lacking. Corticosteroids, in addition to antibiotics, are occasionally useful for relief of severe noninfectious sinus or nasal inflammation complicating the infectious process. Long-term antibiotics and surgical sinus therapy must be considered for particularly recalcitrant cases.

Nasal polyps

Long-term intranasal steroids are the mainstay of therapy. Intermittent courses of oral corticosteroids may be necessary to shrink the polyps to a size controllable by intranasal steroids. Some patients may require long-term alternate-day oral corticosteroid therapy. Appropriate treatment of secondary infection is essential. For patients requiring long-term corticosteroids or those who fail to respond, surgical therapy must be considered.

Rhinitis and pregnancy

Chronic rhinitis may be the most frequently occurring medical illness during pregnancy. The physiologic increase in turbinate congestion associated with the normal hormonal changes of pregnancy and the frequency of allergic rhinitis in women of child-bearing age contribute to this problem. Avoidance of allergens and nonspecific precipitants and the use of intranasal saline is the initial approach, supplemented by *intermittent* topical oxymetazoline. Nasal congestion not responding to short-term or intermittent topical therapy is usually effectively treated with oral decongestants (pseudoephedrine), whereas itching, sneezing, or rhinorrhea may require antihistamines (tripelennamine) or cromolyn. Intranasal steroids should be used for recalcitrant eosinophilic rhinitis or nasal polyps during pregnancy. Amoxicillin and erythromycin appear to be the drugs of choice for nasal or sinus infection during pregnancy; tetracycline is contraindicated. Cephalosporins are also generally considered safe during pregnancy and sulfonamides may be considered in early or midpregnancy.

REFERENCES

Bolger WE and Kennedy DW: Current perspectives on sinusitis in adults. J Resp Dis 13:421, 1992.

Jalowayski A and Zeiger RS: Examination of nasal and conjunctival epithelial specimens. In Lawlor CJ and Fischer TJ, editors: Manual of allergy and immunology: diagnosis and therapy, ed 2. Boston, 1987, Little, Brown.

Juniper EF et al: Comparison of beclomethasone diproprionate aqueous spray, astemizole and the combination in the prophylactic treatment of ragweed pollen–induced rhinoconjunctivitis. J All Clin Immunol 83:627, 1989.

Juniper EF et al: Comparison of the efficacy and side effects of aqueous steroid nasal spray (budesonide) and allergen-injection therapy (Pollinex R) in the treatment of seasonal allergic rhinoconjunctivitis. J All Clin Immunol 85:606, 1990.

Meltzer ED, Schatz M, and Zeiger RS: Evaluation and therapy of rhinitis. In Middleton E Jr et al, editors: Allergy: principles and practice, ed 3. St. Louis, 1988, Mosby.

Mikaelian AJ: Vasomotor rhinitis. Ear Nose Throat J 68:251, 1989.

Mullarkey MF: Eosinophilic non-allergic rhinitis. J All Clin Immunol 82:941, 1988.

Mygind N and Anggard A: Anatomy and physiology of the nose—pathophysiologic alternations in allergic rhinitis. Clin Rev All 2:173, 1984.

Naclerio RM: Allergic rhinitis. N Engl J Med 325:860, 1991.

Settipane GA: Nasal polyps: Epidemiology, pathology, immunology and treatment. Am J Rhinol 1:119, 1987.

Simons FER: H1-receptor antagonists: clinical pharmacology and therapeutics. J All Clin Immunol 84:845, 1989.

Slavin RG: Medical management of nasal polyps and sinusitis. J All Clin Immunol 88:141, 1991.

CHAPTER

300 Asthma

Timothy D. Bigby
Stephen I. Wasserman

Asthma is a common disorder long recognized by clinicians as reversible airway obstruction with cough and/or wheeze. Recent advances in our understanding of the pathophysiology of asthma have expanded this definition to also include airway inflammation and hyperresponsiveness to a broad range of physical, chemical, and pharmacological stimuli. An understanding of how inflammation is engendered, of the relationship between inflammation and hyperresponsiveness, and of the mechanism whereby hyperresponsiveness causes airway symptoms provides a variety of avenues for therapeutic intervention in this disorder. This chapter summarizes our basic understanding of these processes, places them in a clinical context, and provides a framework for understanding the modern approach to asthma therapy.

EPIDEMIOLOGY

Estimates indicate that asthma occurs in 4% to 6% of the population in the United States, the disorder being more common in urban than in rural populations and in African Americans than in whites. Some estimates also suggest that asthma is more common in Hispanics, Southeast Asians, and Pacific Islanders. In childhood, the male-to-female ratio is 2:1, but this ratio equalizes in adulthood. The age of onset of disease is widely distributed. One half of patients develop asthma by the age of 10, but onset into the sixth and seventh decades is common. With respect to duration of disease, 50% or fewer of childhood asthmatics continue to have asthma in adulthood; on the other hand, asthma that develops in adulthood rarely remits.

There is a trend in the United States and worldwide of increasing prevalence of asthma. The cause of this increase is unknown, but it may relate to increasingly urban living conditions with resulting greater exposure to environmental and occupational pollutants. There is also a strong association between passive exposure to smoke in childhood (i.e., parental smoking) and the development of asthma and atopy.

PATHOLOGY

The lungs in patients dying of fatal exacerbations of asthma reveal evidence of hyperinflation with thick, tenacious mucous plugging of airways. The content of these mucous plugs can have several characteristic appearances. Curschmann's spirals are spiral casts of the airways consisting of mucus and shed epithelial cells; Creola bodies are compact clusters of epithelial cells; and Charcot-Leyden crystals are crystals of eosinophil constituents. Microscopic examination of postmortem specimens of human airways show patchy denudation of the airway epithelium, airway edema, marked mucosal inflammatory cell infiltration, and some evidence of smooth muscle hypertrophy. The most readily apparent features of the inflammatory cell infiltrate in asthma are the presence of eosinophils, lymphocytes, and with special stains, mast cells. Neutrophils, monocytes, and macrophages are also present.

The pathology of asthma has also been investigated indirectly during life with sputum examination, bronchoalveolar lavage, and endobronchial biopsies. These studies have demonstrated increased numbers of inflammatory cells in asthmatic sputum. Eosinophils in the sputum have been suggested as a marker of asthma, but this has not proven to be either sensitive or specific for asthma. Bronchoalveolar lavage studies confirm these observations and also note a small increase in the number of mast cells in the lavage fluid. However, there is no specific profile of bronchoalveolar lavage cells in asthmatics and bronchoalveolar lavage has no clinical utility in the diagnosis or management of asthma. Endobronchial biopsies reveal inflammatory cell influx similar to that found in postmortem specimens of airways, even when disease is relatively quiescent. A subbasement membrane deposition of types III and V collagen is also apparent.

ETIOLOGY, PATHOGENESIS, PATHOPHYSIOLOGY

Numerous hypotheses have been put forth to explain the clinical syndrome of asthma. An initial focus was upon abnormalities in neural and humoral receptor control of airway smooth muscle. Although intriguing data regarding such a dysfunction has accumulated, these concepts have not provided a complete understanding of asthma. More recently, an appreciation of airway inflammation in asthma has led to a re-examination of the etiology, pathogenesis, and pathophysiology of asthma. The terms "intrinsic" and "extrinsic" no longer adequately reflect our current understanding. We now appreciate that asthma is a heterogeneous disorder, with multiple triggers initiating the development of airway hyperresponsiveness and the clinical endpoint of bronchoconstriction.

During the last decade, attention has been focused on the relationship between the inflammatory response in the airway and the development of airway hyperresponsiveness and clinical asthma (Fig. 300-1). Experimental work indicates that viral respiratory tract infection, oxidant pollutants, some chemicals, and exposure to antigen are associated with inflammatory cell infiltration into the airway. These agents are also associated with the development of airway hyperresponsiveness. Most data suggest that airway inflammation precedes the development of hyperresponsiveness and may therefore be the prerequisite feature necessary for the development of hyperresponsiveness and clinical bronchospasm. However, airway inflammation is not universally associated with hyperresponsiveness. For example, purulent bronchitis or the purulent sputum of pneumonia can be present without the development of airway hyperresponsiveness or clinical bronchospasm. Thus, airway inflammation may be a necessary but not sufficient reason for the development of asthma or, alternatively, there may be specific characteristics of the inflammatory response in this disorder.

The pathogenesis of allergic asthma has been studied extensively. A variety of in-vivo and in-vitro experiments suggest that, in susceptible hosts, a T cell–mediated immune response to inhaled antigen occurs. Human T helper cells can be divided into subsets, TH_1 and TH_2 based on the profile of lymphokines they produce (Chapter 283). In asthma the predominant CD4 helper cell in the lung produces an array of cytokines, including granulocyte-macrophage colony stimulating factor (GM-CSF) and interleukins (IL) 3, 4, 5, and 10. These are characteristic of the TH_2 subset. The spectrum of cytokines contributed by activated TH_2 cells could explain many features of allergic asthma, that is, mast cell growth (IL-3, 4, 10), IgE synthesis (IL-4), and eosinophilia (GM-CSF and IL-5). In addition, IL-4 upregulates adhesion molecules on eosinophils, basophils, and vascular endothelium. Immunostaining shows these lymphokines in the lung and skin of allergic individuals and in situ hybridization demonstrates the expression of their genes. In addition, the same cytokines have been found in fluid lavaged from the airways of symptomatic asthmatics and are generated acutely during antigen-provoked bronchospasm. However, no data available permit the extrapolation of this scenario for allergic inflammation of the airway to the setting of inflammatory responses induced by other asthma triggers, such as oxidant pollutants and viral respiratory tract infection.

Controversy exists regarding the relative importance of different inflammatory cell types in asthma. Mast cells and eosinophils are prominent and easily discernible features of the inflammatory response in asthmatic airways. Mast cells are effector cells of an IgE mediated allergic response. These cells are the source of vasoactive substances (Chapter 292) and a variety of cytokines including IL-4 and tumor necrosis factor-α (TNF-α). Thus, mast cells may complement the proinflammatory cascade of cytokines produced by TH_2 lymphocytes, which in turn contribute to the cellular and physiological changes observed in asthma. The re-

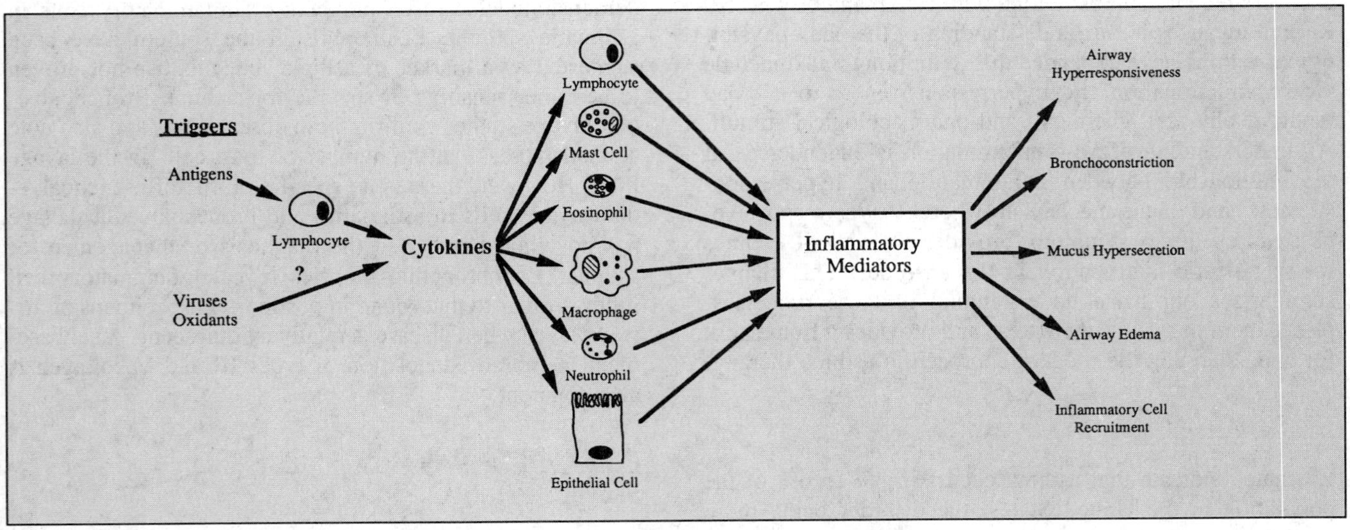

Fig. 300-1. Model of the pathogenesis of asthma. Antigen, oxidants, or viral respiratory tract infection trigger the release of cytokines that stimulate the recruitment of inflammatory cells to the airway and enhance their ability to release inflammatory mediators. These mediators, in turn, cause end-organ effects. Noninflammatory cells, such as epithelial cells, may participate in this process. In the case of antigens, lymphocytes seem to be the principal source of cytokines. With other triggers, the source of cytokines is unknown.

sponse to a specific antigen in the airway has been presumed to involve specific IgE on the surface of the mast cell and, furthermore, responses that involve the mast cell have often been thought to be stimulated by specific antigen. However, we now understand that allergic responses and mast cell function are more complex. For example, IgE not only binds to mast cells, but also to monocytes, macrophages, and platelets via specific receptors. Further, these cells can be stimulated by specific antigen. On the other hand, mast cells are not stimulated exclusively by antigen. Other biochemical mediators and changes in osmolality may induce mast cell mediator release. Therefore, some of the effects of antigen may not be mediated by mast cells and some of the effects of mast cells may not be caused by antigen.

There is substantial evidence that eosinophils play an important role in asthma. Increased numbers of eosinophils are found in the blood, sputum, and bronchoalveolar lavage of asthmatics. Eosinophil accumulation in the airway seems to be a prominent feature of the late asthmatic response to allergen challenge in allergic asthmatics as assessed by bronchoalveolar lavage and endobronchial biopsy. Eosinophils are attracted to the airway by the generation of IL-5 from TH_2 lymphocytes and by lipid or peptide chemoattractants. The eosinophil is prominent in the asthmatic airway, in submucosal tissue, in the epithelium, and in the airway lumen. They have been shown to release a variety of mediators that have effects in the airway. Likewise, recent studies suggest that the eosinophil may be a source of cytokines, including GM-CSF, transforming growth factor-β, and IL-5. These products may have autoregulatory effects on the eosinophil. Some of their other mediators include major basic protein, eosinophil cationic peptide, eosinophil peroxidase, and eosinophil-derived neurotoxin. These are highly basic molecules and are toxic to airway epithelial cells, causing desquamation of airway epithelium in vitro similar to that seen in clinical asthma. Eosinophils are also the source of a variety of other mediators with bronchoactive effects including leukotriene C_4 and platelet-activating factor. The stimulus for eosinophil recruitment to the airway is uncertain, but platelet-activating factor has been found to selectively stimulate eosinophil chemotaxis. The precise mechanism by which eosinophils are activated in asthma to generate lipid mediators or to degranulate remains uncertain, but IgG- and IgA-containing immune complexes are potent degranulation stimuli. In addition, GM-CSF, IL-5, and IL-3 prime the eosinophil to a more responsive state. When compared to peripheral blood eosinophils, those in the airway are hypodense and demonstrate granular dissolution, suggesting ongoing eosinophil activation in asthma.

Mast cells and eosinophils are not the only inflammatory cells present in asthmatic airways. Neutrophils and macrophages are also present. These cells are capable of releasing mediators with effects on smooth muscle tone, mucus secretion, and airway edema. Transient airway hyperresponsiveness has been induced in the laboratory with agents that recruit neutrophils and macrophages into the lung. These and other data have been used to argue that neutrophils or macrophages may be responsible for the development of airway hyperresponsiveness. A substantial body of evidence obtained in animal models and human studies supports this hypothesis. Macrophages also participate in regulating the airway inflammatory response, in part through the generation of specific cytokines, including IL-1, IL-6, IL-8, GM-CSF, TNF-α, and histamine-releasing factors.

The link between inflammation and airway hyperresponsiveness is thought to be provided by the ability of these inflammatory cells to synthesize and release a large number of potent chemical mediators (Table 300-1). A wide range of mediators, including histamine, prostaglandins, thromboxane A_2 leukotrienes, platelet-activating factor, proteases, neuropeptides, peptide chemotactic factors, and oxygen radicals have been shown to have effects on airway function (Table 300-1). Hyperresponsiveness can be induced with leukotriene E_4 and platelet-activating factor, mast cells and eosinophils being prominent sources of both of these compounds. Hyperresponsiveness has also been induced experimentally by mast cell tryptase. In addition, mast cells generate the vasoactive and spasmogenic compounds histamine, leukotriene C_4, prostaglandin D_2, and adenosine. A variety of chemoattractant molecules (some of which are specifically directed toward eosinophils), structural proteoglycans, heparin, tryptase, chymase, and cytokines are also products of mast cells, as previously noted. The concerted actions of these molecules can cause acute smooth muscle constriction, airway hyperemia, edema, and secretion of mucus. Some mediators released from inflammatory cells function primarily to amplify and extend the inflammatory response. The role of each mediator, however, has been difficult to determine without specific inhibitors. Thus far, histamine has not been demonstrated to play a major role because antihistamines have lit-

Table 300-1. Inflammatory mediators and asthma

Mediator	Effects
Histamine	Bronchoconstriction
Cyclo-oxygenase products	Bronchoconstriction
$PGF_{2\alpha}$, thromboxane, PGD_2	
Leukotrienes	
LTB_4	Chemotaxis
LTC_4, LTD_4	Bronchoconstriction, mucus hypersecretion, edema
Platelet-activating factor	Eosinophil recruitment, bronchoconstriction, airway hyperresponsiveness
Neuropeptides	
Substance P	Bronchoconstriction, airway edema, mucus hypersecretion
Oxygen radicals	Bronchoconstriction?
Peptide chemotactic factors	
IL-8	Inflammatory cell chemotaxis
Proteases	Hyperresponsiveness
Cytokines (GM-CSF, TNF-α, IL-3, 4, 5, and 10)	Modulation of immune and inflammatory cell function

tle long-term effect in asthma. Although platelet-activating factor has been shown to have significant effects on airway function and to recruit eosinophils to the lung, initial clinical trials with antagonists have been disappointing. Additional studies also suggest that many of the effects of platelet-activating factor are mediated secondarily by the cysteinyl leukotrienes. The relative importance of proteases, neuropeptides, and oxygen radicals in human asthma is poorly defined at this time and specific inhibitors do not exist for potential clinical use.

Slow-reacting substance of anaphylaxis (SRS-A) was demonstrated to induce sustained airway smooth muscle contraction more than 50 years ago. Since 1980, this mediator substance has been chemically characterized as the cysteinyl leukotrienes-leukotriene C_4 (LTC_4), leukotriene D_4 (LTD_4), and leukotriene E_4 (LTE_4). These compounds are part of a larger family of mediators derived from arachidonic acid via the 5-lipoxygenase pathway. LTC_4 and LTD_4 induce not only sustained smooth muscle contraction in the airway, but also mucus hypersecretion and airway edema. A related compound, leukotriene B_4 (LTB_4), is a potent chemotactic factor and is responsible, in part, for the recruitment of inflammatory cells to the airway and stimulation of inflammatory cell secretion. The effects of LTB_4 on airway smooth muscle are controversial. Some studies have suggested that LTB_4 may increase airway smooth muscle responsiveness to subsequent stimulation. However, these studies have not been reproduced in people. Clinical trials have begun to examine the effects of 5-lipoxygenase inhibitors and LTD_4 receptor antagonists on clinical asthma. Thus far, these compounds show promise with respect to clinical efficacy, indirectly providing further evidence that leukotrienes are important mediators in asthma.

Some specific triggers of asthma may also add to our fund of knowledge about the cause of asthma. Patients with exercise-induced asthma may have this as one of many triggers or as the sole trigger of their disease. The aspects of exercise that induce bronchoconstriction are not known with certainty, but seem to be related to cooling and drying of the airway. The mechanism of hyperresponsiveness and bronchoconstriction in this case may be via neurogenic reflexes, but this is unlikely to explain exercise-induced bronchoconstriction completely. Furthermore, studies with leukotriene receptor antagonists and 5-lipoxygenase inhibitors indicate that exercise-induced bronchoconstriction can be inhibited by these agents. These findings are consistent with the knowledge that increased osmolarity, as occurs in drying of the airway, is known to stimulate mast cell–mediator release.

Another unique form of asthma is associated with the use of nonsteroidal anti-inflammatory drugs (NSAIDs). Aspirin and other NSAIDs may provoke manifestations of hypersensitivity that include rhinorrhea, flushing, eosinophilia, and nasal polyps in association with asthma. The reaction is not immunologic, but the molecular mechanism responsible for this syndrome is not known. Nevertheless, increased production of leukotrienes after aspirin ingestion has been demonstrated in these patients by the identification of increased amounts of leukotriene E_4 in the urine. The ability to induce this reaction is shared by all NSAIDs that inhibit cyclo-oxygenase activity, while salicylates that do not inhibit cyclo-oxygenase do not elicit this response. However, why this syndrome occurs in only a small fraction of patients taking NSAIDs remains unexplained.

In summary, the association of inflammation with asthma is clear. Virtually all data support a causal role for airway inflammation in the development of airway hyperresponsiveness and bronchoconstriction. Considering the substantial redundancy of the inflammatory cells and mediators involved in asthma, a single cell or a single mediator is inadequate to explain the syndrome. The pathogenetic trigger for this process is best worked out for allergic asthma. In this case, the lymphocyte, specifically the TH_2 helper cell, seems to play a key role via release of cytokines that modulate cell function in the airway. In nonallergic asthma, inflammation also plays a major pathogenetic role, but the relative importance of specific inflammatory cells is less well known. Both allergic and nonallergic airway hyperresponsiveness can be mimicked in the laboratory over the short term. However, in both allergic and nonallergic asthma, the mechanism that sustains the inflammatory and hyperresponsive state of the airway over the long term, resulting in the chronic clinical disorder we call asthma, remains unknown.

CLINICAL MANIFESTATIONS

History

In general, the clinical hallmarks of asthma are episodic wheezing associated with dyspnea, cough, and sputum production. Between episodes of wheezing asthmatics have symptoms that at least improve and may completely remit. In describing the clinical manifestations of asthma, acute symptoms should be distinguished from chronic symptoms. However, the chronic symptoms of asthma are essentially the same as those observed acutely, but they usually lack severity and fluctuate over greater periods of time.

The symptoms of acute bronchospasm can range from subtle to dramatic (Table 300-2). A vague sense of chest tightness can be the sole manifestation, but more often this is accompanied by wheezing, dyspnea, and cough. Most patients note wheezing as the development of a musical sound in their chest associated with respiration, and they may be able to discern differences in severity. However, some patients are unable to detect their wheezing. Dyspnea may develop gradually or suddenly and may become severe during acute bronchospasm. Symptoms vary widely in intensity. Cough can occasionally be the only symptom of asthma, and in the evaluation of chronic cough, asthma should be included in the differential diagnosis. The cough associated with asthma can be dry, but it often produces thick, tenacious sputum, which may contain mucus plugs. The patient may also note that the sputum becomes purulent as symptoms worsen. This may represent secondary bacterial infection, but also can be caused by inflammatory cell infiltration in the lung without viral or bacterial suprainfection.

Related historical details are of benefit in the care of

Table 300-2. Asthma severity: clinical characteristics

Severity	Symptoms	Signs	Laboratory data
Mild	Wheezing, ± Dyspnea	Expiratory wheezes, I:E<1:3	FEV_1> 70% of predicted
Moderate	Wheezing, dyspnea, fatigue	Inspiratory wheezes, expiratory wheezes I:E≥1:3, Tachycardia	FEV_1<70% of predicted
Severe	Wheezing, profound dyspnea	Inspiratory wheezes only, I:E>1:3, + accessory muscles, retractions, tachycardia > 120 per minute, decreased breath sounds, pulsus paradoxus > 18 mm Hg	FEV_1<50% of predicted

asthmatics. The age of onset, frequency of episodes, severity of disease, requirements for medications, hospitalizations, and prior need for mechanical ventilation are all key features. The patient should be questioned about a history of travel, GI symptoms, and occupational or recreational exposure to dust, fumes, chemicals, and pets. A history of allergy, atopy, eczema, allergic rhinitis, or nasal polyps may be elicited. Medication allergies or symptoms associated with the use of nonsteroidal anti-inflammatory drugs may be associated with asthma. A seasonal component to symptoms or a temporal relationship associated with exposure to specific antigens is suggestive of allergy.

Physical examination

The hallmark of acute bronchospasm is wheezing. This finding may change with the severity of obstruction (Table 300-2). In general, less severe bronchospasm is associated with only expiratory wheezes. As severity increases, wheezing may be heard in inspiration and expiration. With profound bronchospasm, wheezing may be heard only on inspiration or may be absent with diminished air movement. However, the intensity and the phase of wheezing may not correlate well with the severity of obstruction. When wheezing is correlated with other physical examination findings, a more reliable assessment can be made of the severity of obstruction. For example, the expiratory phase of the respiratory cycle is prolonged by bronchospasm. Normally the inspiratory:expiratory ratio is less than 1:2, but this ratio increases in a graded fashion to 1:3 or 1:4 with increasing degrees of airway obstruction. When severe obstruction is present, the intensity of breath sounds also diminishes. During symptomatic episodes, respirations may become labored, the patient may begin to use the accessory muscles of respiration, and intercostal or supraclavicular retractions may be present. With severely labored respirations, the patient may become diaphoretic, anxious, and unable to speak in full sentences. A respiratory rate greater than 30 breaths per minute and a heart rate of 120 beats per minute suggest severe bronchospasm. A fall in systolic blood pressure of greater than 18 mm Hg with inspiration (pulsus paradoxus) also suggests a severe episode. Agitation, confusion, somnolence, and cyanosis are foreboding findings and suggest impending respiratory failure. Unilateral loss of breath sounds can be consistent with mucus plugging and secondary atelectasis, but these findings must raise the possibility that a pneumothorax has developed. Patients are at increased risk of barotrauma during a severe exacerbation of asthma. In addition to pneumothorax, pneumomediastinum may be a manifestation of barotrauma and is strongly suggested by the development of subcutaneous emphysema.

In the chronic setting, findings associated with asthma are essentially the same, but less severe. Furthermore, most patients have symptom-free intervals in which physical findings are essentially absent. The durations of these symptom-free intervals depend on the severity and the adequacy of control of the patient's disease. Exacerbating factors also play a role in the duration of these disease-free intervals. During symptom-free intervals, wheezing can very often be elicited by forced expiration. However, this finding is not specific for asthma.

LABORATORY FINDINGS

Hematology

Blood counts may reveal evidence of eosinophilia, which is usually mild, representing 5%-15% of the differential count. Profound eosinophilia (25% or greater, 3000 per μl or greater) should suggest another cause. In the setting of symptoms of asthma, transient pulmonary infiltrates, worldwide travel, and profound eosinophilia, tropical eosinophilia should be considered. Allergic bronchopulmonary aspergillosis and the hypereosinophilic syndrome are also causes of profound eosinophilia that may be confused with asthma.

Serology

Total IgE is frequently elevated in serum in asthmatics, but there is controversy regarding the frequency of this finding, the usefulness of this data clinically, and the implications of elevated IgE in the pathogenesis of asthma. Large population surveys demonstrating high frequencies of asthma in groups with elevated serum IgE and relative absence of asthma in groups with low serum IgE have been interpreted as indicating an allergic basis for all asthma, but other studies have failed to show such an association. In general, total serum IgE has little utility in the diagnosis and management of asthma. Antigen-specific IgE measurements may be of use in patients with a history compatible with specific allergy and asthmatic symptoms associated with that allergen. Very high elevations of IgE should suggest a disorder such as allergic bronchopulmonary aspergillosis.

Sputum examination

Wright stains usually reveal inflammatory cells, including neutrophils and eosinophils, in the sputum of asthmatics, although this finding is of little diagnostic value. Sputum cultures during an acute exacerbation may occasionally reveal a specific predominant pathogen associated with bacterial bronchitis, but these cultures more often reveal normal oral flora. The presence of mycoplasma in the sputum may be significant. Examination of bronchoalveolar lavage fluid, a powerful research tool, has no current value in clinical diagnosis or management.

Pulmonary function studies

During acute bronchospasm, spirometry reveals evidence of obstruction with decreased FEV_1 and midexpiratory flows. The FEV_1/FVC ratio is also reduced. With more severe obstruction, hyperinflation is evident, with an increased residual volume and functional residual capacity. The flow-volume loop often reveals evidence of obstruction with diminished flows and coving inward of the expiratory limb. One of the hallmarks of asthma is partial or complete reversal of airway obstruction after the administration of a bronchodilator. This response can also be used to gauge the adequacy of treatment. However, the lack of response to a one-time dose of bronchodilator does not preclude a reversible component to the patient's obstruction. The diffusing capacity of the lung for carbon monoxide, also termed *transfer factor* in Great Britain, is often increased in asthmatics who do not smoke. The exact mechanism of this increase is unknown, but it is thought to represent an increase in pulmonary capillary blood volume associated with obstruction. Peak flow measurements are also reduced. Peak flow meters are inexpensive simple devices that patients can use and interpret. These provide the patient with objective information about the severity of their airway obstruction.

Bronchial challenge testing can be used to establish the presence of airway hyperresponsiveness. Nonspecific bronchial hyperresponsiveness is demonstrated by exaggerated bronchoconstriction to inhaled histamine or methacholine. These techniques are widely available in most full-service pulmonary function laboratories. Nonspecific bronchial challenge is most useful to assist in the evaluation of cough or to establish the diagnosis of asthma when the patient presents with a compatible history, but physical examination and pulmonary function evidence of obstruction are lacking. It additionally has some utility during disability evaluations and medical-legal evaluations of pulmonary dysfunction. However, bronchial challenge can be a hazardous procedure and should not be performed when significant airway obstruction is present. A more reasonable diagnostic maneuver in the latter setting would be the administration of a bronchodilator to assess the degree of reversibility. Specific bronchial challenge has utility in selected cases. This can be performed to a broad range of provocative agents including exercise, cold air, specific antigen, dust, fumes, and oxidant pollutants. However, specific airway challenges should only be performed in specialized centers experienced with these procedures.

Arterial blood gases

Assessment of arterial blood gases is usually not necessary in the management of asthma in either the acute or chronic setting. However, during moderately severe exacerbations pulse oximetry may be of value. During severe exacerbations or in the setting of a serious complicating condition, arterial blood gases are indicated. Hypoxemia is a frequent finding in this setting and is caused by a mismatch of ventilation and perfusion associated with bronchoconstriction, with a resultant increase in the alveolar-arterial oxygen difference. Patients with mild to moderate obstruction hyperventilate, and thus the arterial P_{CO_2} is decreased. However, during prolonged and severe episodes of airway obstruction the patient may develop respiratory muscle fatigue and the P_{CO_2} may normalize or become elevated. A normal P_{CO_2} during a severe exacerbation of asthma is thought to be an ominous sign, suggesting impending respiratory failure. Some experts have recommended early intubation of such individuals to avoid profound respiratory muscle fatigue or respiratory arrest. However, clinical studies indicate that asthmatics with severe obstruction and normal or elevated P_{CO_2} do not necessarily require intubation and often improve with aggressive bronchodilator therapy, without mechanical ventilation.

Chest radiography

In the setting of chronic asthma and in the absence of another underlying condition, chest radiographs are normal. During an exacerbation, chest radiographs are not required unless fever, sputum production, chest pain, leukocytosis, or physical evidence of barotrauma are present. Hyperinflation of the lung may be present during severe exacerbations, but the remainder of radiographic abnormalities seen in asthmatics are complications of their disease such as pneumonia, pneumothorax, or pneumomediastinum. Infiltrates may be seen in allergic bronchopulmonary aspergillosis.

DIAGNOSIS AND DIFFERENTIAL DIAGNOSIS

The diagnosis of asthma is made principally on clinical grounds and laboratory data are utilized in a supplementary or confirmatory fashion. A history of episodic wheezing in a nonsmoking patient, with findings of wheezing on physical examination, is strongly suggestive of asthma. Other causes of wheezing should be reasonably excluded. The diagnosis is confirmed with spirometry, which demonstrates obstruction (an FEV_1 of 80% of predicted or less) that resolves or significantly improves with a bronchodilator. If pulmonary function is normal, spirometry should be repeated after a forced expiratory maneuver, which usually induces a fall in FEV_1 in asthmatics. If spirometry still remains normal, bronchial challenge testing should be considered. Alternatively, the patient can be followed over time with serial spirograms to demonstrate a variable obstructive ventilatory defect.

Not all patients who wheeze have asthma. Additional diagnoses should be considered in both the acute and chronic settings. Upper airway obstruction, tracheomalacia, and tracheal or bronchial masses can all masquerade as asthma. These disorders are usually distinguished by the presence of stridor on physical examination and flow limitation on a flow-volume loop. Laryngeal (vocal cord) dysfunction can be clinically indistinguishable from asthma. This disorder is caused by inappropriate aposition of the vocal cords during the respiratory cycle and can be very successfully treated by speech therapy. These patients with laryngeal dysfunction have often been misdiagnosed; when the dysfunction is severe, they have even been treated with systemic corticosteroids for presumed severe asthma. The clue to this diagnosis is inspiratory stridor on physical examination. Flow-volume loops demonstrate normal or near-normal expiratory flow with a flow-limited inspiratory limb. Vocal cord dysfunction is confirmed by direct laryngoscopy.

Patients with chronic fixed airway obstruction such as emphysema or chronic bronchitis may have acute wheezing episodes, which are most often associated with exacerbations of their disease. These patients often have airway hyperresponsiveness that is enhanced during their exacerbation. In the past, these patients have been labeled as having asthmatic bronchitis. Whether they have a "reactive component" to their disease and actually represent an overlap between fixed and reversible airway obstruction is not clear. Such patients are usually older with a later onset of disease and a history of smoking. They are differentiated from asthmatics by a history of smoking, a component of their disease that responds poorly to aggressive bronchodilator therapy, and pulmonary function findings of an obstructive defect that does not reverse over time. However, acute bronchitis can be associated with the development of airway hyperresponsiveness. The most common clinical setting for this is the development of wheezing with viral respiratory tract infection. In children, respiratory syncytial virus infection is frequently associated with the development of wheezing and an obstructive ventilatory defect. Most of them have transient symptoms that resolve spontaneously, but a small subgroup may develop sustained clinical asthma. Similarly, other viral respiratory tract infections are associated with transient wheezing, with some patients developing sustained asthma. The possibility that bacterial bronchitis might be associated with clinical wheezing in previously unaffected people is less certain. However, such an association has been suggested for mycoplasma and chlamydia.

Other disorders are associated with wheezing. Patients with left ventricular failure can wheeze during episodes of fluid overload and show nonspecific bronchial hyperactivity. These patients are usually easily differentiated from asthmatics by clinical evidence of left ventricular dysfunction with an S_3 gallop, rales, and jugular venous distention. However, the occasional patient may lack these clinical findings. The mechanism by which individuals with left heart failure wheeze is unknown, but airway edema is suspected.

Ten percent to 15% of patients with pulmonary embolus develop wheezing. Although the wheezing associated with pulmonary embolus is short-lived, consideration of pulmonary embolus must be included in the differential diagnosis of patients presenting for the first time with dyspnea and wheezing. In the more chronic setting, other diagnoses must also be considered. Patients with hypersensitivity pneumonitis, sarcoidosis, lymphangioleiomyomatosis, and pulmonary helminth infections can also have a component of wheezing and airway obstruction associated with their disease. The mechanisms by which these disorders result in wheezing is unknown.

THERAPY

The general goal for the treatment of asthma is maintenance of a normal or near-normal lifestyle without functional limitation. Other goals include the aggressive, early therapy of exacerbations to minimize or eliminate the need for emergency care. Nonpharmacologic interventions play a central role in optimal treatment. Most important among these interventions is patient education. Detailed understanding of asthma and its treatment allows patients to participate in their own care, to recognize potential problems, and to facilitate early treatment, thus avoiding severe exacerbations. Recognizing the stimuli that provoke bronchospasm, such as exercise, cold air, animal dander, dust, and perfumes, among others, allows the patient to plan for these eventualities or to avoid them. Patients should also avoid medications such as nonsteroidal anti-inflammatory drugs and β-blockers. Pretreatment prior to exercise or cold exposure as well as avoidance of antigens contributes significantly to improved care. Although not a cause of asthma, anxiety or fatigue can contribute indirectly to symptoms. Knowledgeable patients can be instructed to initiate specific therapies such as increased inhaled β_2-agonist treatment or oral corticosteroids if specific symptoms develop. This approach avoids the delay associated with contacting the primary physician and may prevent worsening symptoms that dictate emergency care. Obviously, such pharmacologic interventions by the patient must be followed by physician contact.

Aerosol medications

Inhaled bronchodilators are central in the management of both acute and chronic asthma. The determinants of aerosol deposition in the lung are (1) size of the particle (1-5 μm), (2) the flow rate at which the particle is inhaled (i.e., higher flow rates favor impaction in the upper airway), (3) the duration that the aerosol is in the lung, and (4) the device from which the aerosol is generated. Jet nebulizers and ultrasonic nebulizers have been suggested to have an advantage in patients with severe disease treated with inhaled bronchodilator. However, numerous studies show that inhalers are at least as effective as nebulizers in both chronic and acute settings, provided the metered-dose inhaler is used correctly. Proper use of a metered-dose inhaler is a major problem, however; as few as 20% of patients use this device correctly. The problem can be minimized by the use of spacing devices, which should be prescribed to all patients. Use of metered-dose inhalers in all clinical settings for the treatment of asthma would substantially reduce health care costs for these patients.

β_2 Adrenergic agonists

One of the most important consequences of stimulation of β_2 receptors in the lung is direct relaxation of airway smooth muscle. Metaproterenol, albuterol, and terbutaline are intermediate-acting β_2-selective agonists commonly used in the United States. Longer-acting agents are available in Europe. A current controversy surrounding β_2-agonist use focuses on the issues of drug tolerance, hyperresponsiveness, and mortality. It has been suggested that tolerance to β_2 agonists in the lung may develop and that frequent regular use of β_2 agonist may increase airway hyperresponsiveness. Recent studies have further suggested a link between the use of β_2 agonists and mortality from asthma. However, these observations do not distinguish between increased utilization of drug by patients with more severe disease, which may be fatal, and the possibility that β_2 agonists contribute to mortality by enhancing disease severity.

β_2 Agonists are also available for oral or parenteral administration. Oral preparations, especially long-acting forms, have been recommended for improved control of bronchospasm because they result in fewer fluctuations in drug levels throughout the day, but toxicity is greater with the oral route because of higher systemic levels of the drug. Furthermore, the maximal degree of bronchodilation achieved orally is less when compared to the inhaled route of administration. For these reasons, the oral route is not recommended for β_2 agonists. In severe acute exacerbations of asthma, the parenteral administration of adrenergic agonists has been recommended for many years. Epinephrine and terbutaline have been given subcutaneously for this purpose. However, toxicity is greater via this route and it does not offer any advantage in terms of bronchodilation. Thus, in the emergency-room setting the systemic administration of adrenergic agonists, especially epinephrine, should be discouraged. A selective β_2 agonist delivered via the inhaled route is preferred. If the clinical response is insufficient and if clinical signs of toxicity are absent, the drug may be readministered.

Theophylline

The mechanism of theophylline's action in asthma remains unclear. Theophylline is a phosphodiesterase inhibitor and therefore increases intracellular cyclic AMP levels, which in turn may relax smooth muscle. However, these effects occur at doses of theophylline that exceed the therapeutic range used in the treatment of asthma. Theophylline is also an adenosine-receptor antagonist, and this antagonism does occur in clinically relevant concentrations. Some related agents that are more potent adenosine receptor antagonists, however, have no bronchodilating effects. Theophylline also may have modest anti-inflammatory properties, but their relevance to clinical asthma is unknown.

Theophylline is an effective bronchodilator, about one fourth as potent as inhaled β_2 agonists. It enhances mucociliary clearance, increases diaphragmatic contractility, and can dilate pulmonary arteries and increase respiratory drive in the central nervous system. However, these additional effects are unlikely to be of great clinical importance in the treatment of asthma. Theophylline, given orally, is of proven benefit in the chronic management of asthma. The most convincing data pertain to asthmatics with relatively mild symptoms that occur primarily at night. With sustained-release preparations, these patients have improved control and are thus better able to sleep than with the intermediate-acting inhaled β_2 agonists. When theophylline is added to a regimen of inhaled β_2 agonists there is greater bronchodilation, but these effects are additive as opposed to synergistic.

In severe exacerbations, the standard of care has been to administer intravenous theophylline (as aminophylline). There is not good evidence, however, that adding intravenous aminophylline to inhaled β_2 agonists in the emergency room setting is of clinical benefit. Moreover, intravenous aminophylline has a low therapeutic index and the consequences of theophylline toxicity can be profound. Therefore, if used intravenously to treat acute exacerbations of asthma, aminophylline should be employed judiciously and with monitoring of serum levels.

The resurgence in theophylline use with the development of long-acting preparations has been associated with a significant increase in serious theophylline toxicity. Risk factors for theophylline toxicity include advanced age, congestive heart failure, liver disease, profound hypoalbuminemia, and coadministration of drugs that interfere with theophylline's metabolism such as cimetidine, erythromycin, allopurinol, and some quinilone antibiotics.

Glucocorticosteroids

Corticosteroids have the potential to modify the severity of disease in asthma as well as to treat bronchospasm. The mechanism of action of corticosteroids is still controversial, but with the recognition that inflammation of the airway is associated with asthma, the focus has been on their anti-inflammatory and immunomodulatory properties. These agents are known to limit inflammatory cell recruitment and inflammatory cell stimulation. They also inhibit the arachidonic acid cascade, including cyclo-oxygenase and lipoxygenase pathways, by inhibiting arachidonic acid release. In the acute setting, however, corticosteroids may increase the number and affinity of β_2 receptors in the lung before affecting the inflammatory and immunologic cascades. Corticosteroids have been shown to modify disease severity by decreasing airway hyperresponsiveness in the long term.

Corticosteroids have been underutilized and misused in the treatment of asthma. For example, systemic steroids have been employed in settings where inhaled steroids would be adequate. Chronic systemic administration of corticosteroids may be necessary for patients with severe disease not controlled with other agents, but extended treatment is accompanied by profound side effects. The most important are bone mineral loss with secondary fracture, avascular bone necrosis, cataract formation, hyperglycemia, psychiatric disturbance, and opportunistic infection. For patients requiring continual systemic corticosteroids for control of severe disease, alternate-day treatment should be attempted to minimize long-term side effects. Unfortunately, alternate-day therapy often fails in these patients. Short courses of systemic corticosteroids can be used with relative safety to gain control of acute exacerbations of chronic asthma. Most side effects associated with courses of less than 2 weeks are not life-threatening and include sleep disturbance, increased appetite, and mood alterations, although avascular bone necrosis has been attributed to such use. Patients treated with corticosteroids for less than 2 weeks can have these drugs abruptly reduced or stopped. Tapering the corticosteroids in patients treated with high doses for long periods or with frequent short courses is more difficult. Although it seems logical to reduce the dose of corticosteroids rapidly, too aggressive a taper often precipitates a second exacerbation and ultimately results in the patient receiving systemic corticosteroids for a longer period. The maximal dose, the duration of therapy, and frequency of courses should all be considered in determining the rate of tapering systemic steroids. Patients treated with large doses of systemic steroids for 1 month or longer can demonstrate biochemical and/or clinical evidence of pituitary-adrenal insufficiency. The risk of adrenal insufficiency is directly correlated with dose and duration of therapy.

Inhaled corticosteroids provide a relatively safe and effective alternative to systemic steroids. Recent trends, supported by numerous clinical studies, favor earlier and more aggressive use of inhaled corticosteroids. Adrenal-suppressive effects of inhaled steroids are not seen with standard doses and have not been found with doses as high as four times the dose recommended by the manufacturer. Although most inhaled corticosteroids are recommended for three or four daily administrations, they are effective when used twice per day. Inhaled corticosteroids should, in general, be stopped and systemic corticosteroids substituted during acute exacerbations of asthma because of the tendency of many inhaled agents to stimulate cough or bronchospasm. However, they should be restarted as systemic corticosteroids are reduced. The known side effects of inhaled steroids are relatively few. Dysphonia and vocal cord atrophy are uncommon complications, but do occur. Oral candidiasis develops in about 15% of patients, but can be easily minimized by the use of a spacing device and rinsing the mouth after inhalations; treatment with antifungal drugs is occasionally necessary. The long-term consequences of inhaled corticosteroids, especially at high doses, have not been examined with respect to effects on bone mineral metabolism, cataract formation, or other potential toxicities. Preliminary studies suggest that such long-term effects may be possible. Delayed long bone growth may result from the use of inhaled corticosteroids in children.

Cromolyn

Cromolyn is another agent that has been shown to modify the severity of asthma and decrease airway inflammation and hyperresponsiveness. The mechanism of action of cromolyn is unknown. The drug is thought to stabilize mast cells and to prevent mediator release from this cell type. Such effects have been demonstrated in nonhuman mast cells, but in humans this has proven more difficult to demonstrate. Cromolyn may also effect other cell types, including macrophages, neutrophils, and probably eosinophils by inhibiting secretion of mediators and blocking arachidonic acid metabolism. Another drug, nedocromil, has a different chemical structure but a similar pharmacologic profile. Nedocromil will probably become available in the United States in the near future. The proper role for cromolyn in the treatment of asthma remains unclear after 25-30 years of use. Cromolyn at clinical doses does not have direct bronchodilating effects and is used as a disease-modifying treatment and prophylactic agent. Predicting which patient will respond to cromolyn is difficult, but younger patients tend to respond more often than older patients. An allergic component to the patient's disease is not predictive of a clinical response. The significant advantage of cromolyn is its virtual lack of side effects, but its substantial expense and lack of a predictable clinical response should limit its use. Cromolyn has been found effective and is recommended for use in exercise-induced asthma, but β_2 agonists are also effective and less expensive.

Anticholinergics

Anticholinergics block reflex bronchoconstriction, but they have no direct relaxing effect on airway smooth muscle. The introduction of ipratropium bromide has allowed the administration of inhaled anticholinergics without significant systemic toxicity. The onset of action of ipratropium is delayed up to 30 minutes after an inhalation, although it is then sustained for up to 6 hours. Unfortunately, only a small fraction of asthmatics have a significant response to ipratropium, and the responses are usually modest. Predictors are lacking, although older patients are more likely to improve than younger patients. The effects of these medications should be determined with clinical or pulmonary function assessments.

Immunotherapy

Although specific immunotherapy has been advocated for patients with allergic asthma, allergen avoidance is the first line of treatment. The second line of therapy should be more conventional antiasthma drugs. If these fail and/or symptoms are severe, specific immunotherapy can be considered. Data are available suggesting that specific immunotherapy is of benefit in some instances of house dust mite, animal dander, and pollen-induced asthma. These benefits must be weighed, however, against the risk of a systemic reaction to allergen extract injections.

Antibiotics

Antibiotics are frequently used for treatment of purulent bronchitis in patients having an exacerbation of asthma, based on the assumption that purulent secretions are caused by a bacterial infection. However, most respiratory tract infections in asthmatics are viral. Furthermore, patients with asthma can develop purulent secretions during exacerbations as a result of inflammatory cell influx into the airway, rather than infection. Sputum cultures are difficult to interpret and are complicated by bacterial colonization of the respiratory tract in many patients and oropharyngeal contamination of collected specimens. Specific changes in the rate of improvement have been difficult to demonstrate in exacerbations of asthma treated with oral antibiotics.

Other therapies

Some other treatments of asthma are worthy of mention. Antihistamines have been evaluated at several times in the past as potential bronchodilators. The more sedating, less potent antihistamines such as chlorpheneramine have been shown to lack benefit in the treatment of asthma. More specific H_1 antagonists, including terfenadine, azelastine, and cetirizine may inhibit histamine or even antigen-induced acute bronchospasm acutely, but they have little if any proven benefit in the treatment of chronic asthma. Ketotifen, an antihistamine with other anti-inflammatory properties, is of questionable value in the treatment of asthma. Calcium channel blockers have been evaluated without convincing evidence of their efficacy. Intravenous or inhaled magnesium has been advocated in the treatment of acute bronchospasm in the emergency room setting based on limited clinical trials.

A variety of other treatments are investigational or are potential therapies of the future. Troleandomycin (TAO) has been used in corticosteroid-dependent asthmatics as a steroid-sparing drug. TAO is known to prolong the half-life of corticosteroids by slowing their metabolism in the liver. Direct effects of TAO in asthma have also been suggested, but never established. Clinical trials using TAO have reported conflicting results. Cytotoxic and immunosuppressive drugs have been tried in severe, steroid-dependent asthma. Methotrexate has been found by one group of investigators to have significant steroid-sparing effects in severe asthmatics, but substantial toxicity can be associated with its administration. Additional data are needed to evaluate the efficacy and long-term side effects of this drug before it can be recommended for treatment of severe asthma. Cyclosporin and gold are reported to be of value in the treatment of severe asthma, but further study is required.

A recent major focus of the pharmaceutical industry is the development of inhibitors of 5-lipoxygenase- and LTD_4-receptor antagonists. These appear to inhibit exercise-induced and possibly antigen-induced bronchospasm. This class of drugs is just now beginning clinical trials, and no results from intermediate or long-term studies have yet been reported. Despite initial excitement about platelet-activating-factor antagonists, the effect of these agents in clinical asthma has been disappointing.

Management strategies

The chronic management of asthma is changing (Table 300-3). Mild intermittent symptoms may be controlled by inhaled β_2 agonists as needed. If symptoms are uncontrolled by this treatment, inhaled β_2 agonists can be increased to regular dosing intervals of every 4 to 6 hours. However, concerns about the effects of β_2 agonists on severity of disease have discouraged the regular use of these drugs and instead have favored the addition of a second drug. In the past, theophylline was the major second-line agent; however, inhaled corticosteroids should now supplant theophylline. Inhaled steroids have also been championed as first-line therapy. If symptoms are not controlled by inhaled β_2 agonists and inhaled corticosteroids, theophylline is a logical third choice. Theophylline should be started at a low dose and gradually increased. A dose of 10 mg/kg/d should not be exceeded without theophylline blood levels. These levels should be monitored closely to guide adjustments in therapy and to assess symptoms that suggest toxicity. The therapeutic range is 5-15 μg/ml. The practice of increasing the theophylline level to the high therapeutic range adds little in terms of bronchodilation and should be discouraged because of the risk of toxicity. Cromolyn can be instituted early in this scheme, and its efficacy evaluated after several weeks of therapy. Ipratropium bromide can also be tried if symptoms are uncontrolled. Patients may be considered for immunotherapy if demonstrable specific allergy plays a role in their disease and asthma symptoms are not controlled by the first three lines of therapy. Chronic systemic administration of corticosteroids should be reserved for patients who have failed all other measures. Corticosteroid-sparing agents remain controversial at this time.

The management of acute exacerbations should rely heavily on inhaled β_2 agonists (Table 300-3). These should be delivered by metered-dose inhaler whenever possible. Systemic administration of these drugs should be avoided in the treatment of asthma. Furthermore, intravenous administration of aminophylline is controversial in the setting of an acute exacerbation and is not routinely recommended by the authors. Systemic corticosteroids are recommended if inhaled β_2 agonists do not rapidly result in clinical improvement. However, corticosteroids are relatively slow in their onset of action in the acute setting and may require 6-8 hours for beneficial effects to become evident. If the patient is well enough to return home but requires therapy in addition to inhaled β_2 agonists, 60 mg of prednisone by mouth followed by 60 mg daily for 7 days with a rapid taper is usually adequate. In severely ill patients, corticosteroids are usually administered intravenously in the acute setting at doses of 60-120 mg of methylprednisolone I.V. every 6 hours. However, there is no evidence that intravenous cor-

Table 300-3. Guidelines for management

	Therapy			
	First line	**Second line**	**Third line**	**Alternatives**
Chronic asthma				
Mild	Inhaled β_2 agonists p.r.n.	Inhaled corticosteroid b.i.d.-q.i.d.		
Moderate	Inhaled β_2 agonists p.r.n.	Inhaled corticosteroid b.i.d.-q.i.d. (high dose)	Sustained-release theophylline (5 mg/kg b.i.d.)	Cromolyn Ipratropium
Severe	Inhaled β_2 agonists p.r.n.	Corticosteroid (high-dose inhaled or systemic)	Sustained-release theophylline (5mg/kg bid)	Consider above ± systemic corticosteroids
Acute exacerbation				
Mild	Increased inhaled β_2 agonists			
Moderate	Increased inhaled β_2 agonists	0.5-1 mg/kg p.o. q.d. prednisone		
Severe	Increased inhaled β_2 agonists	1-2 mg/kg q6h of p.o. prednisone or I.V. methylprednisolone		Oxygen Antibiotics Mechanical ventilation

ticosteroids are superior to oral. Ipratropium bromide can be tried if symptoms are uncontrolled with inhaled β_2 agonists, but this is not often of benefit. Patients that develop overt respiratory failure require intubation and mechanical ventilation. In those who are difficult to ventilate because of high peak airway pressures and agitation, sedation and paralysis may be necessary to lower peak pressures and lessen the risk of barotrauma. Controlled hypoventilation is occasionally necessary for patients with profound respiratory failure.

PROGNOSIS

The long-term outlook for patients with asthma is age-dependent. Whereas 25% or more of childhood asthmatics continue to have symptoms as adults, more than 90% of asthmatics with the onset of symptoms as adults continue to have symptoms throughout their lives. On the other hand, little is known about the evolution of severity of disease and whether severity increases or decreases with age.

Although mortality rates from asthma in the United States declined during the 1970s, they have steadily increased in the 1980s and are currently in excess of 1.7 per 100,000 per year. Currently, estimates suggest that mortality exceeds 4500 deaths per year. Increases in asthma death rates have also been reported for New Zealand, Great Britain, Canada, France, Germany, and Denmark. A number of hypotheses have been put forward to explain these apparent increases. Some data suggest the increase in the prevalence of asthma is associated with oxidant pollutants. Other possibilities include a perceived rather than real increase resulting from diagnostic coding trends, shifts in physician diagnostic patterns, an increase in the ability of the physician to detect asthma, and changes in health care access. Another possible explanation for the increase in asthma mortality is that specific therapies for asthma contribute to the severity of disease. Specific therapy could increase airway responsiveness, induce tolerance to that specific drug, or facilitate abuse of medications with resulting toxic side effects. One transient increase in asthma mortality in Great Britain in the 1960s was associated with the clinical use of a high-potency isoproterenol metered-dose inhaler. The role that medications may play in the current rise in asthma mortality is being examined and suggests an association between the long-acting inhaled β_2 agonist, fenoterol, and the rise in mortality in locations such as New Zealand, Great Britain, and Canada.

Little is known about the long-term effects of asthma on the lung and lung function. Some studies suggest that fibrosis with narrowing of the airway and basement membrane thickening may be long-term consequences of asthma. The clinical correlate of these studies may be the development of fixed airway obstruction as a consequence of long-standing asthma. Recent data suggest that the normal age-related loss in FEV_1 is accelerated in asthmatic patients. These important issues warrant further investigation.

REFERENCES

Blake KV et al: Relative amount of albuterol delivered to lung receptors from a metered-dose inhaler and nebulizer solution. Chest 101:309, 1992.

Chan-Yeung M: Occupational asthma. Chest 98:148S, 1990.

Goldman J and Muers M: Vocal cord dysfunction and wheezing. Thorax 46:401, 1991.

McFadden ER: Methylxanthines in the treatment of asthma: the rise, the fall, and the possible rise again. Ann Int Med 115:323, 1991.

National Heart Lung and Blood Institute: Guidelines for the diagnosis and management of asthma. Bethesda, Md, 1991, U.S. Department of Health and Human Services.

Robinson DS et al: Predominant TH_2-like bronchoalveolar T-lymphocyte population in atopic asthma. N Engl J Med 326:298, 1992.

Sears MR et al: Regular inhaled beta-agonist treatment in bronchial asthma. Lancet 336:1391, 1990.

Sears MR et al: Relation between airway responsiveness and serum IgE in children with asthma and in apparently normal children. N Engl J Med 325:1067, 1991.

Spitzer WO et al: The use of beta-agonists and the risk of death and near death from asthma. N Engl J Med 326:501, 1992.
Weiss KB, Gergen PJ, and Hodgson TA: An economic evaluation of asthma in the United States. N Engl J Med 326:862, 1992.
Weiss KB and Wagener DK: Changing patterns of asthma mortality. Identifying target populations at high risk. JAMA 264:1683, 1990.
Young S et al: The influence of a family history of asthma and parental smoking on airway responsiveness in early infancy. N Engl J Med 324:1168, 1991.

CHAPTER

301 Anaphylaxis

Diana L. Marquardt

Clinical manifestations of anaphylaxis

Respiratory
- Bronchospasm
- Laryngeal edema
- Rhinorrhea

Cardiovascular
- Hypotension, syncope
- Dysrhythmias
- Shock
- Headache

Cutaneous
- Urticaria
- Angioedema
- Flushing
- Pruritus

Gastrointestinal
- Nausea, vomiting
- Diarrhea
- Abdominal cramping

Anaphylaxis is a sudden, untoward, often life-threatening event characterized by a constellation of signs and symptoms involving one or more organs or tissues. Classically, anaphylaxis constitutes a systemic immediate hypersensitivity reaction induced by specific antigen cross-linking immunoglobulin E (IgE) molecules on the surface of tissue mast cells, resulting in the release of vasoactive, chemotactic, and enzymatic mediators, including measurable amounts of histamine and tryptase. In practical terms the precise mechanism of a particular anaphylactic reaction may not be understood, and the syndrome is better defined by clinical manifestations than by the involvement of a defined immunologic reaction. Thus, the term *anaphylactoid,* used to describe non-IgE-mediated systemic, life-threatening reactions or reactions of unknown immunologic basis, has become outmoded.

The clinical presentation of anaphylaxis may include respiratory, cardiovascular, cutaneous, or gastrointestinal manifestations (see box above). Upper airway obstruction may be experienced as hoarseness, dysphonia, or a "lump in the throat" and may be evidenced as inspiratory stridor suggestive of laryngeal edema. The lower airway obstruction symptoms of chest tightness or wheezing may also ensue. In one large series of fatal anaphylaxis case reports, 70% of the deaths were attributed to respiratory causes, underscoring the importance of these findings. Primary cardiovascular events include hypotension, dysrhythmias, and circulatory collapse, and myocardial infarction may complicate anaphylaxis. Urticaria, angioedema, pruritus, and flushing are common dermatologic manifestations present in nearly 80% of anaphylaxis episodes and may precede more serious events. Abdominal cramping, nausea, vomiting, and diarrhea may occur as a result of gastrointestinal smooth-muscle spasm.

Although anaphylaxis caused by IgE-related mechanisms is perhaps best understood, immune complexes, agents that alter arachidonic acid metabolism, direct mast cell–degranulating drugs, and idiopathic mechanisms have been implicated in anaphylaxis. In IgE-mediated anaphylaxis a previous, sensitizing exposure to antigen is required to induce synthesis of specific IgE antibodies to sensitize mast cells and basophils. Reexposure to a specific antigen, generally a large polypeptide or protein or a small molecule combining as a hapten with human protein, may elicit an anaphylactic response. Penicillin, hymenoptera venom, and allergenic extracts used in skin testing and desensitization are among the common causes of anaphylaxis today, although intraoperative anaphylaxis to latex has been recognized as a problem of increasing frequency in recent years. The risk of anaphylaxis is increased with the length and frequency of antigenic exposures, and a parenteral exposure is more dangerous than an oral one. Mucocutaneous exposures may induce anaphylaxis as well. The administration of whole blood, immunoglobulin, or serum products may be associated with immune complex formation, complement activation, and anaphylaxis. This response is best illustrated by a patient lacking native IgA but possessing IgG or, less commonly, IgE antibodies to IgA by some prior exposure. Aspirin-induced anaphylaxis has been postulated to result from alterations in arachidonic acid metabolism, because the nonsteroidal anti-inflammatory drugs that similarly inhibit the cyclo-oxygenase enzyme also provoke the response. It has been reported that platelets obtained from aspirin-sensitive individuals may be activated by aspirin to produce inflammatory mediators, whereas those of normal individuals lack this response. A group of agents apparently capable of directly inducing mast cell degranulation includes radiocontrast media, plasma expanders, and opiates. These agents require no previous host sensitization, although reexposure to radiocontrast media in an individual with a history of a previous adverse reaction carries a markedly increased risk of anaphylaxis. Idiopathic anaphylaxis implies an unknown mechanism underlying a documented anaphylactic episode. Food or drug ingestion may account for some cases in this category, as new antigens, including psyllium, papain, latex, and some hormonal preparations, continue to be recognized. A small group of patients has been identified with exercise-induced anaphylaxis, and in others no precipitating factor can be determined.

Because the interval between antigenic exposure and life-threatening complications may be only a matter of minutes, the treatment of anaphylaxis is emergent. Subcutaneous epinephrine is the mainstay of therapy and is often sufficient to reverse the symptoms. In more severe reactions, airway patency is compromised and must be maintained, and intravenous fluids may be necessary to maintain blood pressure. Glucocorticoids may help to prevent a biphasic response or later recurrence of symptoms and should be administered early in all but mild cases. Antihistamines aid in symptomatic relief of pruritus or swelling and may assist in control of hypotension. With the possible exception of the perioperative period, both H_1 and H_2 blockers appear to be beneficial. Aminophylline, parenteral beta-adrenergic agonists, or oxygen may be required in selected circumstances. The symptoms of anaphylaxis usually respond to early appropriate therapeutic measures. However, patients receiving beta-adrenergic blocking drugs may be resistant to the beneficial effects of beta agonists and are at greater risk for a severe and protracted course of symptoms. Patients undergoing chronic angiotensin-converting enzyme inhibitor or calcium channel–blocker therapy also may be more susceptible to severe manifestations of anaphylaxis.

STINGING INSECT HYPERSENSITIVITY

Stings from insects of the order Hymenoptera result in anaphylaxis in an estimated 0.5% of the population. Sensitivity to honey bee or vespid (yellow jacket, yellow hornet, and bald-faced hornet) venoms are mediated by IgE and may be confirmed by skin testing or radioallergosorbent (RAST) testing with the specific venom extract. Adults who have had systemic allergic reactions to insect stings should be hymenoptera venom skin-tested. Patients with positive skin tests should receive venom immunotherapy, since up to 60% of these individuals develop anaphylaxis when re-stung. Those who have had only large local sting reactions do not require venom immunotherapy, since the risk of subsequent systemic sting reactions is less than 10%. Children less than 16 years of age with a history of strictly cutaneous sting reactions rarely develop serious reactions upon re-stinging and may not require immunotherapy.

Venom immunotherapy induces an increase in IgG-blocking antibodies to venom that correlate with clinical protection against serious sting reactions. Regular venom immunotherapy should be administered at 4- to 6-week intervals to maintain adequate IgG antibody levels. Current evidence indicates that the risk of systemic sting reactions may return within a year after immunotherapy is discontinued, especially in patients with more severe preimmunotherapy reactions and in those with less than 5 years of venom immunotherapy. Therefore, the duration of immunotherapy should be individualized. A general recommendation is for at least 2 to 5 years of immunotherapy or longer if sensitivity persists.

Patients with sting anaphylaxis but negative skin tests for IgE are not candidates for immunotherapy, and these and other patients with prior histories of systemic reactions to stings should be equipped with kits that allow self-treatment with subcutaneous epinephrine. Preloaded syringes or spring-loaded automatic injection syringes containing measured doses of epinephrine have shelf life of at least 18 months and should be immediately available. Patients given such syringes should be carefully instructed in their use and warned to seek medical treatment as soon as possible when symptoms require.

Although much less common than hymenoptera venom reactions, both fire ant venom and stings from insects of the genus *Triatoma* have been shown to induce anaphylaxis on an IgE-mediated basis in certain individuals. Immunotherapy has been effective in reducing the risk of serious reactions to these agents as well.

DRUG REACTIONS

In a general sense, drug reactions are relatively frequent, varied, and often poorly understood. However, some types of drug reactions have a well-defined immunologic basis, and a subset of these can be predicted and/or prevented. IgE-mediated drug reactions result in signs and symptoms of the type described above for anaphylaxis. Penicillin and other beta-lactam antibiotics account for the largest group of IgE-mediated reactions, including more than 400 deaths yearly in the United States. Penicillin-sensitive individuals can be identified by skin testing with the major and minor haptenic determinants. Patients identified as penicillin-allergic by skin testing who require penicillin therapy for a serious indication may be desensitized to penicillin under close supervision by a graded oral or parenteral regimen. Desensitization is effective but short-lived, and once a course of drug therapy has been discontinued, restarting therapy requires repeat skin testing and desensitization, if necessary. Penicillin allergy itself appears to be a dynamic process; patients receiving frequent, intermittent courses of antibiotic therapy develop a greater risk for reactions. Hypersensitivity often declines with time, and up to 80% of patients with documented penicillin allergy no longer exhibit positive skin tests 10 years after the last exposure. Therefore, penicillin therapy should be avoided in patients with a history of penicillin reactions, but previously sensitive patients requiring penicillin for a life-threatening indication should be skin-tested and desensitized if necessary. The entire procedure must be repeated each time penicillin therapy is considered.

Other drugs that may cause IgE-mediated reactions that can be predicted by testing include cephalosporins (which cross-react to some extent with penicillins), insulin, streptokinase, egg-related vaccines, and some local anesthetics and muscle relaxants. Some studies to predict reactivity to sulfa drugs have indicated some potential utility for skin

Prevention of drug reactions

1. Take a thorough medical history.
2. Avoid agents known to have caused previous reactions and educate the patient accordingly.
3. Require a clear indication for drug usage.
4. Observe the patient after injections and administer drugs orally when possible.
5. Test for drug allergy when feasible and desensitize if necessary.
6. Maintain current immunizations.

testing to these agents, but such tests are not yet in routine use.

Non–IgE-mediated drug reactions are generally unpredictable and often require symptomatic treatment rather than prophylaxis. An exception to this rule is the radiocontrast media reaction that may be prevented or limited by pretreatment of high-risk patients with antihistamines and glucocorticoids or by the use of nonionic low osmolality agents. Reactions to iodinated radiocontrast media, however, cannot be detected by skin testing, and an adverse reaction may occur on the first exposure to such agents. Other types of immunologic drug reactions include cytotoxic reactions in which drug antigen interacts with cell membranes, inducing IgG and IgM cytotoxic antibodies. Hemolytic anemia, thrombocytopenia, and leukopenia are common clinical sequelae of these reactions, and penicillin and quinine are two drugs likely to produce them. Immune complex drug reactions result from deposition of antigen–IgG immune complexes within vessel walls or basement membranes and complement fixation. Serum sickness is based primarily on this immune mechanism. Cell-mediated or delayed hypersensitivity reactions are best exemplified by allergic contact dermatitis, characterized by topical sensitization and a subsequent eczematous outbreak up to 48 hours later.

Unfortunately, many drug reactions, including fixed drug eruptions, drug fevers, and some organ toxicities, have no defined immunologic basis and thus cannot be predicted or prevented. Any previous untoward drug reaction calls for a careful consideration of alternate therapeutic approaches. Some other general methods of preventing severe drug reactions are noted in the box above.

REFERENCES

Gold M et al: Intraoperative anaphylaxis: an association with latex sensitivity. J Allergy Clin Immunol 87:662, 1991.

Golden DBK and Schwartz HJ: Guidelines for venom immunotherapy. J Allergy Clin Immunol 77:727, 1986.

Greenberger PA and Patterson R: The prevention of immediate generalized reactions to radiocontrast media in high-risk patients. J Allergy Clin Immunol 87:867, 1991.

Kivity S and Yarchovsky J: Relapsing anaphylaxis to bee sting in a patient treated with beta-blocker and calcium blocker. J Allergy Clin Immunol 85:669, 1990.

Lieberman P: The use of antihistamines in the prevention and treatment of anaphylaxis and anaphylactoid reactions. J Allergy Clin Immunol 86:684, 1990.

Marquardt DL and Wasserman SI: Anaphylaxis. In Middleton EE et al, editors: Allergy: principles and practice, ed 4. St. Louis, 1993, Mosby.

Reisman RE and Lantner R: Further observations of stopping venom immunotherapy: comparison of patients stopped because of a fall in serum venom-specific IgE to insignificant levels with patients who stopped prematurely by self-choice. J Allergy Clin Immunol 83:1049, 1989.

Saxon A et al: Immediate hypersensitivity reactions to beta-lactam antibiotics. Ann Intern Med 107:204, 1987.

Schwartz LB et al: Tryptase levels as an indicator of mast cell activation in systemic anaphylaxis and mastocytosis. N Engl J Med 316:1622, 1987.

Sheffler AL and Austen KF: Exercise-induced anaphylaxis. J Allergy Clin Immunol 73:699, 1984.

Sheffler AL and Pennoyer DS: Management of adverse drug reactions. J Allergy Clin Immunol 74:580, 1984.

Valentine MD and Lichtenstein LM: Anaphylaxis and stinging insect hypersensitivity. JAMA 258:2881, 1987.

RHEUMATIC DISORDERS V

CHAPTER

302 Periarticular Rheumatic Complaints

Harry G. Bluestein

Pain and stiffness of the soft tissues around joints occurs commonly after unaccustomed physical activities. Those acute symptoms are short-lived and generally resolve completely. Persistent subacute or chronic rheumatic complaints, however, require medical evaluation to differentiate symptoms caused by a variety of systemic illnesses from those caused by a primary rheumatic disorder. Recognition of the differences between arthritis, an intra-articular process, and periarthritis is essential (see Chapter 303—Evaluation of Joint Complaints). With periarticular involvement, physical examination shows that the pain is not localized to the articulation and passive range of motion of the joint is usually minimally affected. Thus, history and physical examination are generally sufficient to recognize most periarticular problem syndromes. Laboratory tests and radiographs contribute little, but they may play an important role in excluding alternative causes of the symptoms. Other imaging techniques, such as MRI, are more revealing, but usually not cost-effective. An exception may be evaluation of the rotator cuff of the shoulder.

As a group, the periarticular musculoskeletal conditions entail complaints of pain and stiffness on motion, which are generally most severe in the morning. Each condition, however, has a relatively unique anatomic distribution. Most are regional, affecting a single joint or extremity. Primary diffuse rheumatic symptoms affecting periarticular tissues are also common and are problematic because they must be differentiated from symptoms secondary to other systemic illnesses and because they tend to be more chronically persistent. In evaluating diffuse symptoms, it is especially important to exclude malignancies, the myopathy of hypothyroidism, other endocrinopathies, and systemic rheumatic disorders. Among the last-mentioned, polymyalgia rheumatica (Chapter 307) is most important because it causes profound stiffness and pain, often in the absence of physical findings.

FIBROMYALGIA

Fibromyalgia, the currently preferred name for the most common diffuse periarticular rheumatic syndrome, is characterized by musculoskeletal pain, chronic fatigue, and, often, disordered sleep. Typically the fibromyalgia patient is a middle-aged woman, although the disease can occur at any age and in both sexes. The etiopathogenesis is unknown, and the validity of fibromyalgia as a distinct nosologic entity remains controversial. To some, it is but one form of psychogenic rheumatism, the symptoms representing a somatization of psychologic stresses. In fact, many fibromyalgia patients do exhibit signs or symptoms of depressive anxiety. To others, the characteristic presentation of myofascial pain and stiffness with a bilateral distribution of tender-point sites that are reproducible from patient to patient marks a distinct entity. Those who believe it to be unique also point to the fact that many fibromyalgia patients are not depressed or anxious and that there is very little success in treating this condition with psychotherapy. Adherents to the notion of a fibromyalgia syndrome note the frequent occurrence of a disturbance in restorative non-REM sleep, which may play a pathogenic role since depriving normal healthy subjects of stage 4 non-REM sleep often results in myofascial pain and fatigue. Other hypotheses to explain the pain implicate subtle abnormalities at the neuromuscular junction or deficiencies in neurotransmitters such as serotonin or somatomedin.

Clinically, patients with fibromyalgia present to the physician with a history of chronic, widespread aching pain or burning, and stiffness with increased emphasis truncally. Most patients also have arthralgias involving the small joints of the hands and sometimes other joints. Examination reveals joint tenderness without other physical findings. Musculoskeletal trigger or tender points are common and localized to typical areas (Fig. 302-1). These are regularly elicited by firm digital palpation. Often the rheumatic complaints are accompanied by profound fatigue, which is present throughout the day and indistinguishable from that described by patients with chronic fatigue syndrome. Also

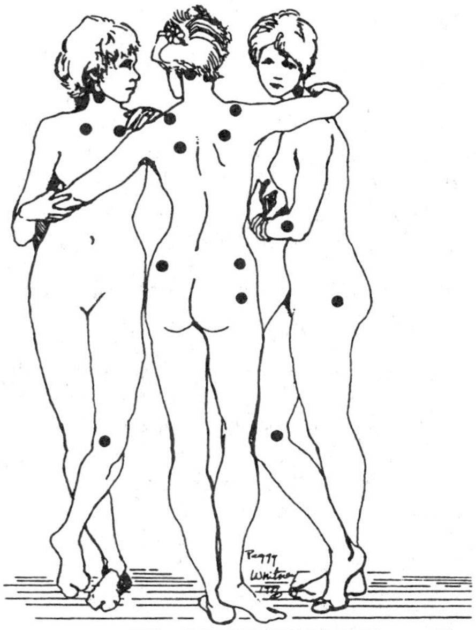

Fig. 302-1. Tender-point locations for the 1990 ACR classification criteria for fibromyalgia (*The Three Graces,* after Baron Jean-Baptiste Regnault, 1793, Louvre Museum, Paris). See the box on p. 2402 for details of the tender-point locations. (From Wolfe F et al: The American College of Rheumatology criteria for the classification of fibromyalgia: report of the Multicenter Criteria Committee. Arthritis Rheum 33:160, 1990.)

common are a variety of neurologic symptoms unmatched by abnormalities on neurophysiologic testing, including paresthesias, dizziness, and clumsiness. Tension headaches, irritable bowel syndrome, and symptoms of urethrocystitis in the absence of infection occur with a greater frequency in fibromyalgia patients than controls.

The diagnosis of fibromyalgia can only be made on clinical grounds since laboratory studies are normal, including the sedimentation rate and autoantibody profiles. Fibromyalgia needs to be considered in any patient with the characteristic complaints of musculoskeletal pains and stiffness plus the demonstration of typical tender points. Systemic illnesses that can produce diffuse musculoskeletal pain should be excluded.

The diagnostic criteria of the American College of Rheumatology (see box, p. 2402) perform well with a sensitivity of 88.4% and a specificity of 88.1%.

The natural history of fibromyalgia is not well defined, but it appears to be a chronic condition with fluctuating symptomatology. Although tissue damage does not occur, many patients become disabled by their inability to function with their pain. Treatment is generally unrewarding. Simple analgesics, muscle relaxants, and nonsteroidal anti-inflammatory drugs are regularly employed but provide only minimal benefit. Small doses of tricyclic antidepressants are used to help restore a normal sleep pattern, and a nonimpact exercise regimen working toward an aerobic level of conditioning may help to ameliorate the symptoms.

The American College of Rheumatology 1990 criteria for the classification of fibromyalgia*

1. History of widespread pain.
   Definition. Pain is considered widespread when all of the following are present: pain in the left side of the body, pain in the right side of the body, pain above the waist, and pain below the waist. In addition, axial skeletal pain (cervical spine or anterior chest or thoracic spine or low back) must be present. In this definition, shoulder and buttock pain is considered as pain for each involved side. "Low back" pain is considered lower segment pain.
2. Pain in 11 of 18 tender point sites on digital palpation.
   Definition. Pain, on digital palpation, must be present in at least 11 of the following 18 tender point sites:
   Occiput: bilateral, at the suboccipital muscle insertions.
   Low cervical: bilateral, at the anterior aspects of the intertransverse spaces at C5-C7.
   Trapezius: bilateral, at the midpoint of the upper border.
   Supraspinatus: bilateral, at origins, above the scapula spine near the medial border.
   Second rib: bilateral, at the second costochondral junctions, just lateral to the junctions on upper surfaces.
   Lateral epicondyle: bilateral, 2 cm distal to the epicondyles.
   Gluteal: bilateral, in upper outer quadrants of buttocks in anterior fold of muscle.
   Greater trochanter: bilateral, posterior to the trochanteric prominence.
   Knee: bilateral, at the medial fat pad proximal to the joint line.
   Digital palpation should be performed with an approximate force of 4 kg.
   For a tender point to be considered "positive" the subject must state that the palpation was painful. "Tender" is not to be considered "painful."

From Wolfe F et al: The American College of Rheumatology criteria for the classification of fibromyalgia: report of the Multicenter Criteria Committee. Arthritis Rheum 33:160, 1990.

*For classification purposes, patients will be said to have fibromyalgia if both criteria are satisfied. Widespread pain must have been present for at least 3 months. The presence of a second clinical disorder does not exclude the diagnosis of fibromyalgia.

Massage, acupuncture, and the injection of local anaesthetics into tender points may provide temporary relief. Perhaps most important is the physician's support and constant reassurance that fibromyalgia is a benign condition and physical damage to the body does not occur.

REGIONAL PERIARTICULAR SYNDROMES

Tendinitis, bursitis, and capsulitis are the major causes of pain around a single large or medium-sized joint. *Tendinitis* is usually caused by a mechanical stress to the involved tendon. Repeated injury to a tendon may result in calcium deposits, primarily in the form of calcium hydroxyapatite. *Calcific tendinitis,* as this condition is called, is hypothesized to result from the combination of diminished blood supply and recurrent trauma. *Bursitis* is an inflammation of a synovial-lined sac located at sites of maximum movement of tendons over bones. Like tendinitis, bursitis is often triggered by repetitive or excessive use. Often the process is indolent, but the bursa may become inflamed as part of a systemic inflammatory disorder. Gout and pseudogout as well as bacterial infection can produce a dramatic acute bursitis, while the chronic inflammatory arthritides may cause subacute bursitis. A swollen, inflamed bursa should always be aspirated and the fluid examined for monosodium urate or calcium pyrophosphate dihydrate crystals (see Chapter 295). Microbiologic studies are always advisable when large numbers of leukocytes are present.

The shoulder, because of its complex anatomy (Fig. 302-2), is particularly susceptible to multiple forms of periarthritis. *Bicipital tendinitis* is common and generally readily recognized. It is triggered by heavy lifting or repetitive movements effecting the long head of the biceps. Typically bicipital tendinitis presents as pain or aching over the anterior shoulder and upper arm. Examination reveals tenderness along the tendon, particularly as it passes through the bicipital groove. Speed's test, the sharp exacerbation of pain on anterior flexion of the shoulder against resistance with the arm outstretched in supination, is usually positive. *Rotator cuff tendinitis* is a more complex common cause of shoulder pain. It occurs after overuse of the shoulders, particularly with the arms over the head. The supraspinatus tendon, an essential part of the rotator cuff mechanism, is injured as a result of its impingement between the head of the humerus and the acromion, which occurs as the arm is abducted. With this form of tendinitis deep palpation elicits tenderness that is maximal on the lateral aspect of the shoulder over the greater tuberosity and below the acromion. The supraspinatus tendon is the most frequent site of calcific tendinitis. Deposits of calcium hydroxyapatite accumulate in the region of the tendon where there is maximal stress from the shoulder impingement syndrome.

The shoulder is also the site of the most common examples of bursal inflammation, namely *subacromial or subdeltoid bursitis*. Physical findings often mimic those of rotator cuff tendinitis and in fact bursitis and tendinitis tend to coexist. These subacute forms of inflammation in the periarticular tissues of the shoulder usually show no visible signs of inflammation. Indeed, if swelling, redness, and heat are detected, infection or crystal-induced disease is likely to be present. *Adhesive capsulitis* may be a sequela of unresolved tendinitis and bursitis at the shoulder. In this condition, there is thickening of the capsule with adhesion to the underlying humerus, producing a markedly restricted

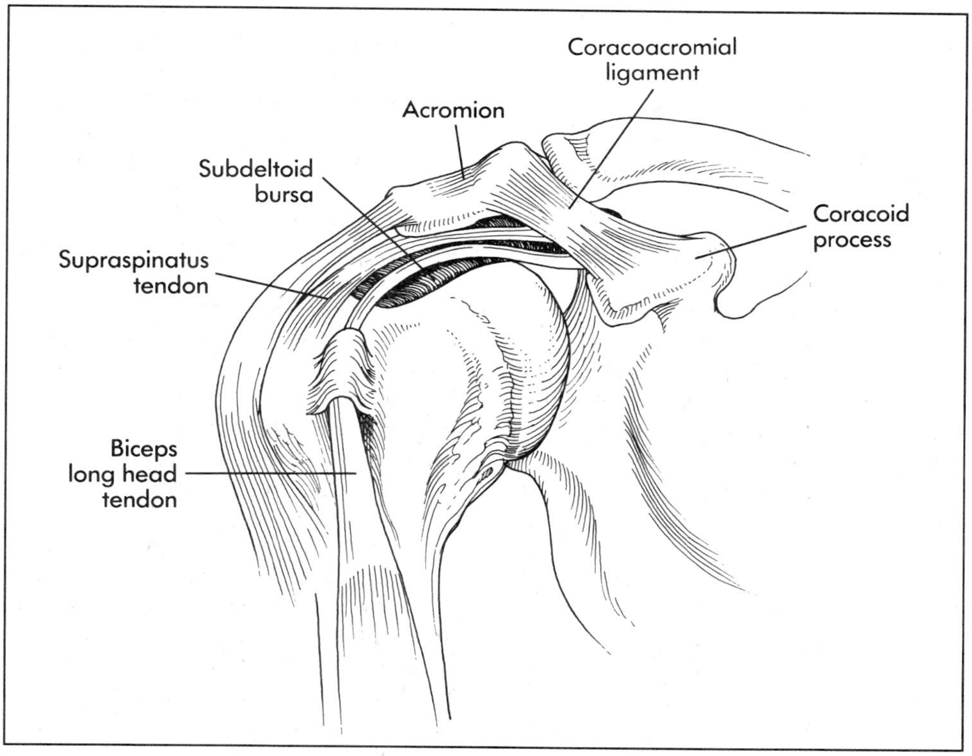

Fig. 302-2. Anatomic relationships among periarticular structures of the shoulder. Note the susceptibility of the subdeltoid bursa and supraspinatus tendon to impingement between the humerus and the acromion and coracoacromial ligament when the arm is raised over the head.

range of motion often called a "frozen shoulder." Adhesive capsulitis can result from any condition that leads to prolonged immobilization of the shoulder. In addition to markedly restricted active and passive range of motion, there is diffuse tenderness around the shoulder. Arthrography documents a constricted capsule and reduced volume of the joint space. Once developed, stretching the capsule with intraarticular injections of a local anesthetic and nonabsorbable corticosteroids may hasten improvement and permit gradually advancing range-of-motion exercises.

At the elbow, the olecranon bursa is susceptible to all of the potential pathogenic mechanisms that produce a bursitis. In many cases, a bland effusion is present, presumably secondary to trauma although the injury may be unrecognized by the patient. An inflammatory effusion in the bursa may occur in rheumatoid arthritis (particularly in patients with rheumatoid nodules), acute gout, and infection. Tendinitis at the elbow occurs directly at the site of attachment of tendons to the lateral or medial epicondyles; the extensor muscles to the hand insert laterally and the flexors medially. Tendinitis at the lateral epicondyle is more common. It is often called *tennis elbow* and results from repetitive forceful extension at the wrist. The opposite motion, forceful flexion, leads to *golfer's elbow* or tendinitis at the medial epicondyle.

A common form of tendinitis occurring near the wrist is called *De Quervain's tenosynovitis*. It is an inflammation of the abductor pollicis longus and extensor pollicis brevis tendons of the thumb at the site where they pass over the medial end of the radius. Finkelstein's test, which triggers exquisite pain by ulnar deviation of the wrist while the flexed thumb is gripped by the fingers, is an important diagnostic finding.

The hip is the site of *trochanteric bursitis* localized to the bursa that underlies the insertion of the gluteal muscles into the lateral and posterior portions of the greater trochanter. Often there is no clear precipitating event, but it can occur with chronic irritation to the region as a result of leg-length discrepancy, persistent running across a slope, or repetitive use of the hip to push doors or other objects. Trochanteric bursitis presents as pain on the lateral aspect of the hip, often radiating toward the knee. There is local tenderness at the edge of the greater trochanter and the pain is aggravated by lying on the affected side.

Two common types of bursitis occur in the knee region. Prepatellar bursitis, commonly called *housemaid's knee,* produces pain in the front of the knee aggravated by bending the knee. A fluid collection is usually apparent directly over the patella. *Anserine bursitis* causes pain below the tibia-femoral articulation on the medial aspect of the knee. The anserine bursa underlies the insertion of the gracilis, sartorius, and semitendinosus muscles into the anteromedial condyle of the tibia. Pain from anserine bursitis is aggravated when climbing stairs. Palpation over the region of the bursa produces pain.

The commonest periarticular problems about the ankle

relate to the Achilles tendon. Achilles tendinitis occurs in long-distance runners or as part of a systemic inflammatory disorder, particularly the spondyloarthropathies (Chapter 312). Less often, Achilles tendinitis may be a symptom of gout or pseudogout. The retrocalcaneal bursa, which underlies the insertion of the Achilles's tendon into the calcaneus, can also become inflamed. Retrocalcaneal bursitis can occur from pressure from tight shoes or as a part of the synovial involvement of rheumatoid arthritis and other chronic inflammatory arthropathies.

Treatment for all of the regional periarticular problems is similar. It includes rest of the affected area with only enough exercise to maintain range of motion, local heat or cold as preferred by the patient, and local injection of a mixture of a nonabsorbable corticosteroid preparation and a local anesthetic. For tendinitis the corticosteroid should be injected around, not into, the tendons. This treatment is not advised for Achilles tendinitis because of the risk of tendon rupture.

REFERENCES

Doherty M et al: Rheumatology examination and injection techniques. London, 1992, Saunders.

Guyton JM and Koopman WJ: Shoulder, hip, and extremity pain. In Ball GV and Koopman WJ, editors: Clinical rheumatology. Philadelphia, 1986, Saunders.

Wolfe F et al: The American College of Rheumatology criteria for the classification of fibromyalgia: report of the Multicenter Criteria Committee. Arthritis Rheum 33:160, 1990.

Yunus MB and Masi AT: Fibromyalgia, restless legs syndrome, periodic limb movement disorder, and psychogenic pain. In McCarty DJ and Koopman WJ, editors: Arthritis and allied conditions. Philadelphia, 1993, Lea & Febiger.

CHAPTER

303 Evaluation of Joint Complaints

Nathan J. Zvaifler

Arthritis is a symptom. Indeed, patients may develop joint complaints during the course of more than 100 different illnesses. The relevance of this symptom and recognition of its cause usually can be ascertained in the course of a careful history and physical examination. The scheme shown in Fig. 303-1 is an approach that the author has found useful. It categorizes musculoskeletal complaints in a manner that leads to a proper diagnosis in most instances when combined with appropriate observations of extra-articular manifestations, laboratory findings, and radiologic investigation. In the initial confrontation, the physician must determine whether the patient's rheumatic symptoms arise from involved joints or from periarticular tissues. In the former, the pain is primarily confined to the articulation and is aggravated by movement or use of the affected part. Examination often demonstrates distortion of the normal joint anatomy, signs of inflammation, or limitation in range of motion. In periarthritis, such as tendinitis, bursitis, or fibrositis, the symptoms can mimic arthritis, but physical examination usually places the problem beyond the articulation. Moreover, periarthritis tends to involve only one, or a few, of the larger joints but spares the wrists, hands, and feet, which so often participate in true arthritic disorders, (Chapter 302).

After establishing that the patient has arthritis, recognition of the *pattern* of arthritis is paramount. Several distinctions are necessary: is the process *monarticular* (one joint) or *polyarticular* (many joints)? (The terms *oligoarticular* or pauciarticular usually imply that two to four joints are affected.) Is the process involving the joint inflammatory (characterized by warmth, erythema, and boggy synovial swelling) or noninflammatory in nature? What is the actual distribution of joint involvement? Examples include symmetric versus asymmetric joint disease, axial (spinal) versus peripheral arthritis, or large versus small joints. The duration of the disease process also provides important diagnostic information. *Chronicity* is usually defined as 6 to 8 weeks of continuous disease in an articulation.

Employing this method, the examiner can develop a profile that allows immediate recognition of many rheumatic disorders. Thus, rheumatoid arthritis would be described as a chronic inflammatory polyarthritis that involves large and small joints in a symmetric fashion. In contrast, the arthritis that accompanies inflammatory bowel disease is characteristically short-lived, inflammatory, and oligo- or polyarticular, but asymmetric and with a propensity to involve the large joints of the lower extremities.

The scheme outlined in Fig. 303-1, which places particular emphasis on recognition of inflammatory joint disease and the distribution of involvement, is similar to the approach presented in the examination of synovial fluid (Chapter 295) and in the radiologic evaluation of arthritis described in Chapter 296. The reader is encouraged to refer to these chapters.

MONARTICULAR DISEASE

Monarthritis can be acute or chronic. It is essential, however, that all monarticular arthritis be considered to be infectious arthritis until proved otherwise, because failure to recognize a pyogenic arthritis may result in permanent joint injury. Furthermore, and perhaps more important, most bacterial infections of joints are derived from the blood stream; therefore, coexistent foci of infection and septicemia are usually present. Any very painful joint may be septic. Once infectious arthritis is suspected, the diagnosis is suggested by the finding of an inflammatory joint fluid, often with more than 50,000 polymorphonuclear leukocytes per cubic millimeter, and confirmed by positive Gram stain and/or culture. After infection the next most important condition to recognize is crystal-induced monarthritis. The diagnosis is easily made by microscopic examination of the synovial effusion and demonstration of the characteristic

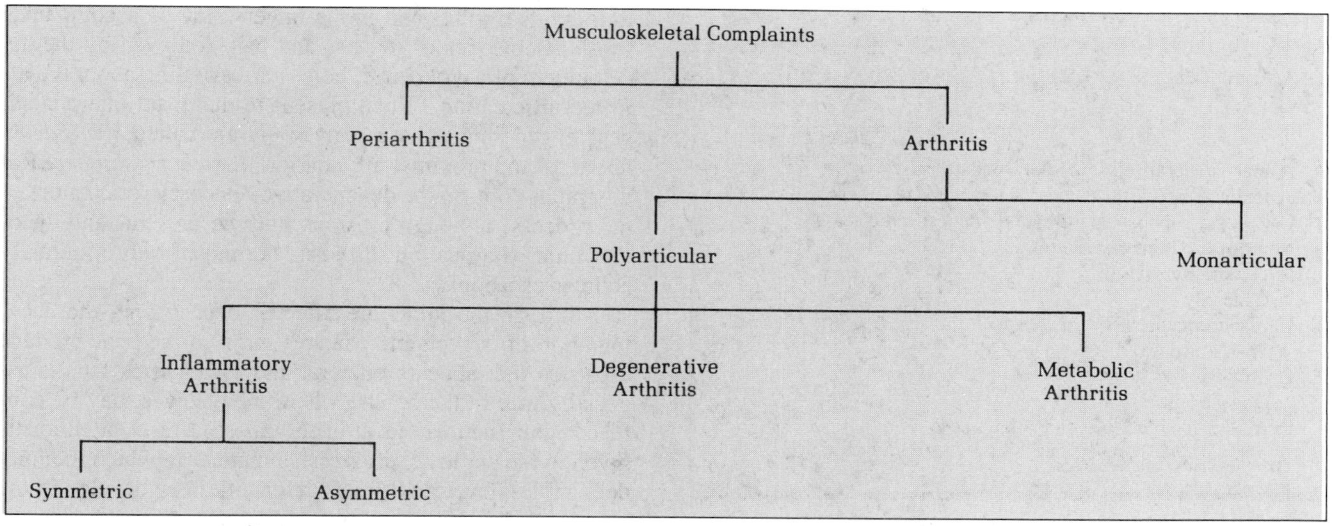

Fig. 303-1. Systematic evaluation of musculoskeletal complaints.

shape and birefringence of monosodium urate or calcium pyrophosphate dihydrate (CPPD) crystals. There are many other less common causes of acute and chronic monarthritis (see box below). It is also important to recognize that disorders normally characterized by polyarthritis may begin in a monarticular form. This is particularly true of rheumatoid arthritis, and, occasionally, observation for many months may be required before the disease assumes its typical appearance.

POLYARTICULAR DISEASES

Polyarthritis can be divided into arthritides that are degenerative (generally noninflammatory), inflammatory, or metabolic in origin. The last-mentioned (see box at right) are most diverse. For example, chronic tophaceous gout may involve large or small joints in an asymmetric (usual) or symmetric (less common) fashion, whereas CPPD deposition disease may mimic a severe form of osteoarthritis, often in unusual locations such as the wrist, or have a symmetric rheumatoid-like pattern, or appear as a degenerative process limited to one or a few weight-bearing joints. The joint symptoms of metabolic disease are usually caused by the deposition of materials in and around articulations; these deposits often give the joint an unusual configuration that is easily appreciated on physical examination. Thus, deposits of monosodium urate (tophi) or lipid in capsular structures or tendons tend to give the joint a lumpy, bumpy, asymmetric appearance, contrasting with the usually smooth contour produced by conventional inflammatory synovitis. Amyloid infiltration of the shoulders makes them seem unusually large and bulky (the shoulder-pad sign). In the rare destructive arthropathy known as *multicentric reticulohistiocytosis,* granulomas form about the nail beds or over the eyelids, where they may be confused with xanthelasma.

Causes of monarthritis

Infection*,†,or‡
Crystal-induced†
Trauma†
Hemarthrosis†,‡
Foreign body‡
Pigmented villonodular synovitis‡
Joint neoplasms‡
Aseptic necrosis‡
Osteochondritis dissecans‡
Mechanical internal derangement†,‡
Sarcoidosis‡
Neuropathic (Charcot's) joint†,‡
Onset of polyarthritis†,‡

*The most important diagnosis.
†Acute.
‡Chronic.

Causes of polyarthritis: metabolic (deposition) joint diseases

Gouty tophi*
Calcium pyrophosphate dihydrate deposition disease*
Hydroxyapatite crystalline arthritis
Amyloidosis
Hyperlipidemia
Multicentric reticulohistiocytosis

*The most important diagnoses.

Degenerative polyarthritis

The prototype of the degenerative form of polyarthritis is primary generalized osteoarthritis (see box, p. 2406). This

Causes of polyarthritis: degenerative joint diseases

Primary generalized (erosive) osteoarthritis*
Secondary osteoarthritis*
Calcium pyrophosphate dihydrate deposition disease
Neuropathic joint disease
Hyperparathyroidism
Acromegaly
Hemochromatosis
Wilson's disease
Ochronosis
Osteodystrophies
Heritable disorders of connective tissue

*The most important diagnoses.

disorder characteristically affects women around the time of menopause and involves the distal and proximal interphalangeal joints, the carpometacarpal articulation at the base of the thumb, and the hips, knees, lumbar spine, and first tarsometatarsal (bunion) joints. Symptoms are limited to individual joints and in the fingers may be accompanied by short episodes of redness and pain followed by the development of asymmetric, bony-hard swelling about the affected articulation. When present in the distal interphalangeal finger joints, these bony spurs are called *Heberden's nodes;* at the proximal articulation, *Bouchard's nodes*. Radiographs confirm the degenerative, osteosclerotic nature of the process, although erosions may be present, and synovial fluid examination discloses normal or only minimally cellular effusions.

Although the joints are affected one by one, the accumulation of irreversible changes may, in the end, produce a pattern that appears bilateral and symmetric. This is especially true in the hands, where the changes may be confused with rheumatoid arthritis unless careful attention is given to the additive, progressive manner in which the joint deformities develop. Similar deformities can develop in the absence of any inflammatory component. Secondary forms of osteoarthritis may be limited to a few joints when they are the result of trauma or may be widespread when they reflect metabolic abnormalities that influence the integrity of cartilage. The complicating joint injuries seen in athletes and industrial workers or the exaggerated degeneration that accompanies neurologic lesions are examples of the former; the arthropathy of acromegaly, hyperparathyroidism, hemo-

Table 303-1. Causes of polyarthritis: inflammatory joint diseases

	Course			Distribution	
Cause	Acute	Intermittent	Chronic	Symmetric	Asymmetric
Rheumatoid arthritis*		±	+	+	±
Systemic lupus erythematosus*		±	±	+	
Other connective tissue diseases		±	±	+	
Crystal deposition diseases		±	+	+	±
Neisserial infection	+			±	+
Hepatitis B	+		±	+	
Rubella	+			+	
Lyme arthritis	±	+	±		+
Bacterial endocarditis	+			+	±
Rheumatic fever	+			+	±
Erythema nodosum	+	±		+	±
Sarcoidosis	+	+	±	+	+
Hypersensitivity to serum or drugs	+	±		+	±
Henoch-Schönlein purpura	+			±	+
Relapsing polychondritis	±	+	±	+	+
Juvenile (rheumatoid) polyarthritis	±	±	+	+	+
Hypertrophic pulmonary osteoarthropathy	±		+	+	
Ankylosing spondylitis*		±	+	±	+
Reiter's disease*	±	±	±	±	+
Enteropathic arthropathy*	±	+	±	±	+
Psoriatic arthritis*		±	+	+	+
Reactive arthritis	+	±	±	±	+
Behçet's disease	±	+	±		+
Familial Mediterranean fever	±	+	±		+
Whipple's disease	±	+	±	±	+
Palindromic rheumatism	±	+		±	+

*The most important diagnoses.
+ = most common; ± = less common.

chromatosis, and ochronosis would be examples of the latter.

Inflammatory polyarthritis

The causes of inflammatory polyarthritis are many (Table 303-1). In some, arthritis is the dominant feature, whereas in others it is merely one manifestation of a systemic disorder. The proper distinction of this group of diseases is facilitated by recognition of the duration of the inflammatory polyarthritis as well as the typical distribution of involved joints. For example, both rubella and acute infectious hepatitis can present with symmetric, inflammatory swellings of the proximal and metacarpophalangeal joints in a picture indistinguishable from that of rheumatoid arthritis. One reaches a correct diagnosis by recognizing that neither rubella arthritis nor the articular manifestations of acute infectious hepatitis persist more than a few weeks. Indeed, although rheumatoid arthritis may be difficult to diagnose correctly, especially early in its course, chronicity is a primary feature. Finally, however, it is the development of an inflammatory, bilateral, symmetric polyarthritis affecting both the large and small joints that distinguishes rheumatoid arthritis from the other important group of inflammatory polyarticular diseases, the spondyloarthropathies (Table 303-1).

A number of other disorders may mimic the pattern of rheumatoid arthritis. Most prominent among these are the connective tissue diseases, especially systemic lupus erythematosus (SLE). In general, their less-destructive nature and their accompanying systemic features allow them to be recognized. Thus, the distinctive skin rashes, the polyserositis, and the hematologic, central nervous system, and renal abnormalities of SLE point the way to the correct diagnosis. So, too, do the thick skin, Raynaud's phenomenon, sclerodactylia, telangiectasia, calcinosis, and esophageal and gastrointestinal disturbances of scleroderma. Dermatomyositis is suggested by the typical edematous, dusky, violaceous, periorbital, and malar rash and by the symmetric weakness and occasional atrophy of the proximal muscles of the limb girdle, the neck, and the pharynx.

Other members of this group may have distinctive disease manifestations, such as the painful, necrotic pustules of gonococcemia, the palpable purpura of hypersensitivity angiitis or Henoch-Schönlein purpura, the tender pretibial erythematous nodules of erythema nodosum or erythema chronicum migrans, the hallmark of Lyme arthritis. The findings of clubbed fingers or floppy ears and saddlenose should alert the physician to hypertrophic osteoarthropathy and relapsing polychondritis, respectively.

The spondyloarthropathies, as the name implies, comprise a disparate group of diseases that share the features of an asymmetric, oligo- or polyarthritis that favors the large joints of the lower extremities. They affect men predominantly. Periostitis, a characteristic radiologic feature often seen along the shafts of the digits, has its counterpart in the beefy, swollen toes (dactylitis, or "sausage toes") noted in patients with Reiter's disease and psoriatic arthritis, and, less frequently, in the enteropathic or reactive joint diseases. Sacroiliitis and inflammatory disease of the apophyseal joints of the lumbar, thoracic, and cervical spine are regular features of ankylosing spondylitis; they affect many persons with Reiter's disease and a greater than expected (by chance alone) number of patients with psoriasis, reactive arthritis, and the various forms of inflammatory bowel disease. An association with the HLA haplotype B27 is seen in those who have spondylitis. Psoriatic arthritis may involve the distal joints of the fingers; almost invariably, however, the contiguous nail shows psoriatic changes, which facilitate the distinction from inflammatory (erosive) forms of generalized osteoarthritis.

REFERENCES

Agudelo C and Wise CM: Evaluation of the patient with symptoms of rheumatic disease. In Schumacher HR Jr, editor: Primer on the rheumatic diseases. Atlanta, 1988, Arthritis Foundation.

Arnett FC et al: The American Rheumatism Association 1987 revised criteria for the classification of rheumatoid arthritis. Arthritis Rheum 31:315, 1988.

Perkins GD: Bone, joint, muscle in clinical examination. In Epstein D et al, editors: London, 1992, Gower Medical.

CHAPTER

304 Rheumatoid Arthritis

Nathan J. Zvaifler

Rheumatoid arthritis (RA), a chronic, usually progressive inflammatory disorder of joints, occurs in a worldwide distribution and affects 1% to 2% of most populations studied. The disease is 2 to 3 times more common in women than in men; it can begin at any age, but has a peak incidence between 25 and 55 years. There is a significant concordance of disease in identical twins but an analysis of families with more than one affected member suggests that rheumatoid arthritis (RA) is polygenic. Moreover, since genetic susceptibility only accounts for about 30% of the risk, there must be other important environmental factors, including an infectious etiology. However, almost 80% of patients with seropositive RA carry specific class II major histocompatibility complex (MHC) molecules, either HLA-DR1 or HLA-DR4 (Dw4, Dw14, Dw15 haplotypes). Genes for the HLA-DR subregion encode one α chain but several polymorphic HLA-DR β chains. The β chains contain regions of remarkable hypervariability, particularly in the amino acid sequences surrounding position 70 of the first domain of the HLA-DR $\beta 1$ chain (corresponding to its third hypervariable region—HVR). Each of the haplotypes associated with susceptibility to RA has the same amino acids at positions 70-74 in the HVR. These shared epitopes imply an MHC-associated genetic predisposition to disease.

PATHOLOGY AND PATHOGENESIS

The pathology and pathogenesis of rheumatoid joint disease can be considered in three distinct stages: (1) the initiation of synovitis by the primary etiologic factor, (2) the subsequent immunologic events that perpetuate the initial inflammatory reaction, and (3) the transition of the inflammatory allergic reaction in the synovium to a proliferative, destructive granulation tissue (pannus).

The earliest events in RA are difficult to document, but the available evidence suggests that microvascular injury and mild synovial cell proliferation are the first lesions. The changes are probably nonspecific, since they are seen in other acute inflammatory joint diseases.

In established RA, the tissues that line the joint (synovium) appear edematous and protrude into the joint cavity as slender villous projections. Light microscope examination discloses a characteristic, but not pathognomonic, constellation of histologic changes, including (1) hyperplasia and hypertrophy of the synovial lining cells; (2) focal or segmental vascular changes; and (3) the connective tissue stroma of the synovial villous, which normally has few cells, is packed with mononuclear cells, some collected into aggregates, particularly around small blood vessels (Fig. 304-1). Lymphocytes predominate in these follicles, with a mantle of plasma cells about their periphery. Multinucleated giant cells, when present, are usually in areas of synovial lining–cell hyperplasia. Abundant fibrinlike material is deposited on the synovial cell surface and in the intracellular matrix.

The rheumatoid synovium contains large amounts of immunoglobulin when examined by immunofluorescent technique. Deposits of IgG and IgM, alone or in combination, are demonstrable in synovial lining cells, blood vessels, and the interstitial connective tissues. A significant number of the plasma cells in the rheumatoid synovium make an IgG rheumatoid factor that combines in the cytoplasm with similar IgG molecules ("self-associating IgG") and de novo immunoglobulin synthesis can be demonstrated in rheumatoid synovial explants or continuous cultures of lymphocytes from synovium.

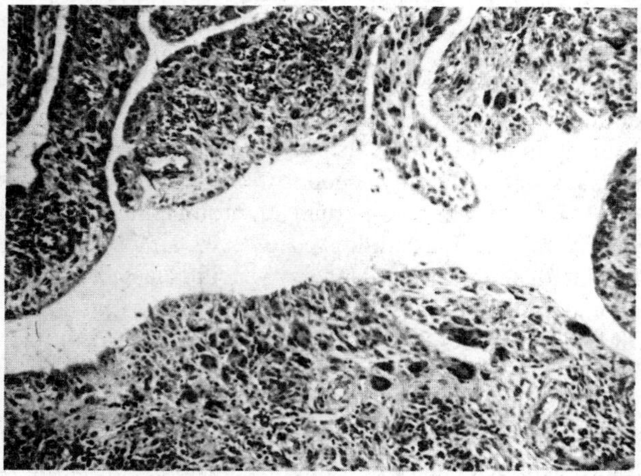

Fig. 304-1. Active rheumatoid synovitis from a patient with seropositive rheumatoid arthritis. The redundant hypertrophic villous structures contain a dense infiltration of lymphocytes and occasional giant cells. The synovial lining cells are hyperplastic.

Based on these findings, two pathogenetic mechanisms have been advanced to explain rheumatoid synovitis. The first—the "extravascular immune complex hypothesis"—proposes an interaction of antigens and antibodies in synovial tissues and fluid. The antibodies are, in general, locally produced, especially the self-associating dimers and higher multiples of the IgG–anti-IgG complex. Other potentially important complexes are those in which the antigens are constituents of articular tissues or by-products of the inflammatory process—collagen, cartilage proteoglycans, fibrinogen or fibrin, partially digested IgG, and soluble nucleoproteins. Immune complexes that form in joint tissues activate the complement system, generating a number of biologically active products, that increase vascular permeability and allow an influx of serum proteins and cellular blood elements into the site where the complexes reside. In the articular cavity, polymorphonuclear leukocytes attracted by complement-derived chemotactic factors ingest the complexes with subsequent release of large quantities of hydrolytic enzymes and production of toxic O_2 and OH radicals and arachidonic acid metabolites. Each may participate in the inflammation and tissue damage.

An alternative hypothesis is that rheumatic joint disease results from cell-mediated damage. Beneath the lining cells of the synovial membrane, CD4+ (helper/inducer) memory lymphocytes accumulate in perivascular areas. Dispersed among them are antigen-presenting cells, macrophages, and dendritic cells. An expected consequence of their interaction is the elaboration of soluble factors that cause T cell proliferation, differentiation of B cells into antibody producers, and the production of other cytokines. Despite the predominance of lymphocytes, the cytokines found in the RA synovium are mainly factors produced by fibroblast-like lining cells and macrophages, such as IL-1, TNFα, IL-6, and GM-CSF, with a paucity of interleukins made by activated T cells. Thus, although T lymphocytes appear to be critical for the initiation of synovitis, as the inflammation becomes chronic, they are anergized or downregulated by factors in the microenvironment such as transforming growth factor β, prostoglandins, or a naturally occurring antagonist to the IL-1 receptor on T cells. Macrophages and synoviocytes, however, remain unopposed and free to express their proinflammatory and destructive potential (see below). The continued accumulation of memory lymphocytes in the synovium might reflect either the presence of autoantigens within the joint (type II collagen, articular proteoglycans, and heat shock proteins are favorite candidates) or an increased binding of T cells to adhesion molecules induced on the endothelium of postcapillary venules by inflammatory cytokines. The ligands for such adhesion molecules are expressed on all T cells, but in significantly greater amounts or with greater avidity on mature CD4 cells. Thus, they preferentially accumulate and are also retained in the inflamed synovium by virtue of the expression of still other cell surface integrins, which are receptors for matrix proteins (see Chapter 286).

Chronic rheumatoid arthritis is characterized by destruction of articular cartilage, ligaments, tendons, and bone. The damage results from a dual attack—from without, by inflammatory molecules derived from phagocytic leukocytes in the synovial fluid, and from above and below, by granulation tissue (pannus). This vascular granulation tissue is composed of proliferating fibroblasts, numerous small blood vessels, and various numbers of mononuclear inflammatory cells. Cartilage matrix collagen and proteoglycans seem to be enzymatically digested in the region immediately surrounding the nests of cells. In other areas, a dense avascular, acellular, fibrous type of pannus acts as a mantle, interfering with cartilage nutrition.

Cultured explants of rheumatoid synovial fragments produce large quantities of proteinases, collagenase, and stromelysin, and prostaglandins capable of destroying the matrix proteins present in cartilage and bone. The responsible cells are synoviocytes, which produce these materials when stimulated by IL-1, TNF-α, and several mitogenic growth factors. The collagenase is released from isolated synovial cells in an inactive or latent form. Treatment with trypsin or plasmin (the latter is potentially important in vivo because plasminogen activator is demonstrated in cultured rheumatoid synovial cells) can activate the latent enzyme. Synoviocytes also produce metalloproteinase inhibitors, and inflammatory synovial fluid contains α_2 macroglobulins. These are potent inhibitors of collagenase, but these important regulatory mechanisms appear to be overwhelmed in RA. Chondrocytes also respond to cytokine stimulation by the production of proteinases and are probable participants in cartilage destruction. Some work suggests that chondrocytes can transform and become a fibrous type of pannus.

Using these observations the following scheme of joint destruction has been proposed. Inflammation of the synovium alters the display of adhesion molecules on the endothelium of small synovial blood vessels. These engage circulating blood cells, allowing them to accumulate in the joint. The lymphocytes and macrophage in the synovium, individually or in concert, release soluble products that cause tissue inflammation, further permeability of synovial blood vessels, and the production of proteinases and prostaglandins by synovial cells and chondrocytes. The proliferation and overgrowth of synoviocytes under the influence of these cytokines leads to irreversible damage of joint structures.

Extra-articular manifestations of rheumatoid arthritis

The cause of the various vascular and parenchymal lesions of RA and their relation to one another have not been defined. A number of observations suggest that the lesions result from injury induced by circulating immune complexes. Anti–gamma globulins of the IgG and IgM classes, as well as IgG, are integral parts of these complexes. Their presence correlates somewhat with the severity of articular and extra-articular manifestations, but whether they are responsible for these changes or are merely markers for severe rheumatoid disease remains a moot question.

Likewise, genetic factors are probably important because the most severe forms of RA, and those with extraarticular features, particularly Felty's syndrome (see below), occur in HLA-DR4–positive individuals, especially those homozygous for the RA susceptibility haplotype (see Chapter 284).

CLINICAL FEATURES

Rheumatoid arthritis is a highly variable disease, ranging from a mild pauciarticular illness of brief duration to a relentlessly progressive, destructive polyarthritis associated with a systemic vasculitis. The extent of articular involvement correlates poorly with constitutional symptoms and extra-articular manifestations, but both destructive arthritis and extra-articular features are more common in patients whose serum contains high titers of rheumatoid factors (see Chapter 294).

Joint disease

Rheumatoid arthritis often begins with prodromal symptoms such as fatigue, anorexia, and weakness, and generalized aching and stiffness that is not clearly localized to articular structures. Joint symptoms usually appear gradually over weeks to months. Occasionally, there are brief remittent episodes of articular involvement prior to the development of more persistent arthritis, and approximately 20% of patients have an abrupt onset, with rapid development of polyarthritis that is often accompanied by severe constitutional symptoms.

Articular involvement is manifested clinically by pain, stiffness, limitation of motion, and the signs of inflammation, that is, swelling, warmth, erythema, and tenderness. Difficulty in making a fist, poor grip strength, and morning stiffness lasting more than 30 minutes (and frequently several hours) are characteristic of RA. Joint swelling results from synovial hypertrophy, thickening of the joint capsule, and, frequently, from an increase in the volume of synovial fluid. Initially, pain limits motion, but later, capsular fibrosis, bony or fibrous ankylosis, and soft tissue contracture become responsible.

Rheumatoid arthritis can affect any diarthrodal joint; those most commonly involved initially are the small joints of the hands or feet, the wrists, and the knees. At the outset, there may be any pattern of joint disease, although usually it is bilateral and polyarticular. In a small percentage of patients, the disease remains unilateral or monarticular (commonly the knees) for periods of months to years. As the disease becomes established, the arthritis spreads to the elbows, shoulders, hips, ankles, and subtalar and sternoclavicular joints. Less often, the temporomandibular and cricoarytenoid joints are affected. Spinal involvement usually is limited to the upper cervical articulations.

Joint examination early in the disease reveals fusiform (spindle-shaped) swelling of the proximal interphalangeal

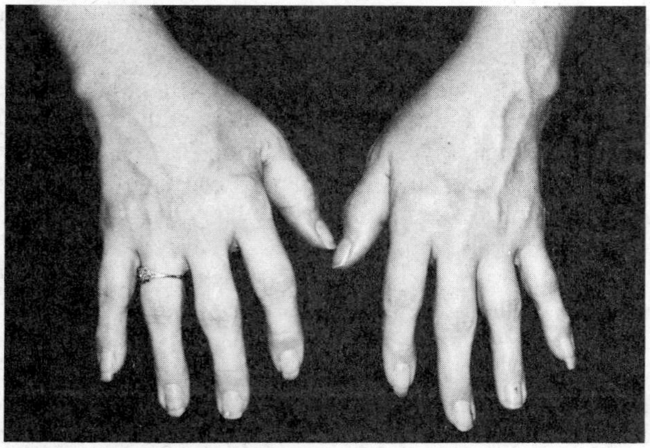

Fig. 304-2. Early changes of rheumatoid arthritis in the hands, showing swelling, mainly limited to the proximal interphalangeal joints.

(PIP) joints (Fig. 304-2). This swelling may clear after a few years. Bilateral and symmetric swelling of the metacarpophalangeal (MCP) joints, particularly the second and third, is very common and remains long after PIP joint inflammation has subsided (Fig. 304-3). The distal interphalangeal (DIP) joints more often are spared. As the disease progresses, characteristic hand deformities develop, including ulnar deviation of the digits, hyperextension at the PIP joints with flexion at the DIP joints ("swan's neck" deformity) or a flexion deformity of the PIP joints, with extension of the DIP joints ("boutonniere" deformity). Rheumatoid involvement of the thumb causes hyperextension at the interphalangeal joints and flexion of the MCP joints with a resultant loss of pinch. Tenosynovitis is a cardinal feature

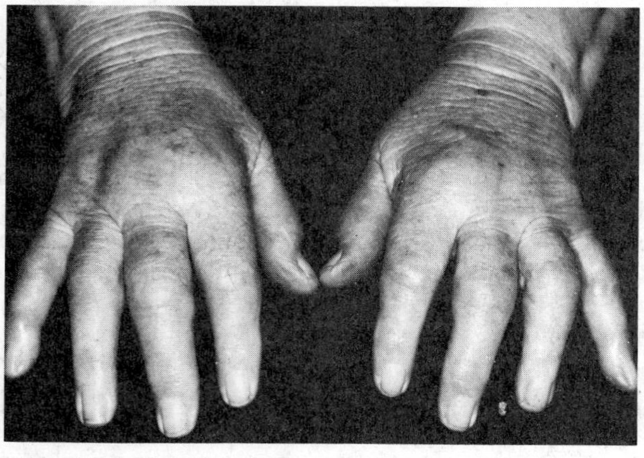

Fig. 304-3. Advanced changes in the hand. Swelling and synovial hypertrophy are predominantly in the metacarpophalangeal articulations, especially the second and third; note the early flexion contractures of the fingers.

of RA. A sudden loss of ability to extend the fingers—especially the third, fourth, and fifth digits—follows rupture of the extensor tendons or their dislocation into the intermetacarpal space.

Wrist disease is an almost invariable accompaniment of RA. Synovial hypertrophy and tenosynovitis on the volar aspect may compress the median nerve beneath the transverse carpal ligament, producing a "carpal tunnel syndrome," with paresthesia and dysesthesia of the thumb, the second and third digits, and the radial aspect of the fourth finger. Late in the disease, wrist immobility develops, and pronation and supination may be severely limited.

Flexion contractures of the elbow are frequent, even at an early stage of the disease. Shoulder involvement is not uncommon. Examination generally reveals limitation of motion together with tenderness just below and lateral to the coracoid process. Swelling is rarely seen.

Rheumatoid arthritis of the hip joints is less common, develops late in the illness, and is characterized by discomfort in the groin or buttocks. Hip disease may be recognized only because of gait abnormalities or limitation of joint motion. Aseptic necrosis of the femoral head, perhaps related to corticosteroid therapy, produces identical findings.

The knee joint is commonly affected, displaying synovial hypertrophy, chronic effusion, and, later, ligamentous laxity. A regular accompaniment of knee involvement is quadriceps atrophy, often of great severity. Pathologic enlargement of the normal gastrocnemius-semimembranosus bursa (Baker's cyst) may compress structures behind the knee, causing discomfort. Occasionally, the bursa dissects or ruptures, giving rise to symptoms and signs mimicking acute thrombophlebitis. Arthrography usually confirms the diagnosis (Fig. 304-4) and should be performed in any patient with RA who develops acute unilateral tenderness, warmth, or edema of the lower leg (pseudophlebitis).

Arthritis in the feet and ankles creates a number of vexing problems. Limited flexion and extension of the foot results from disease of the mortise joint, subtalar involvement impairs eversion and inversion, and pain on walking may result from bursitis beneath the insertion of the Achilles tendon into the calcaneus. In the foot proper, synovitis of the metatarsophalangeal joints is particularly common, whereas interphalangeal joint involvement is less usual. Subluxation of the metatarsal heads, hallux valgus, and lateral deviation and clawing of the toes develop with progression of the disease.

In RA, intermittent cervical spine pain and stiffness are frequent, whereas neurologic complications are rare. Symptoms may result from spinal cord compression by anterior dislocation of the first cervical vertebra, by vertical subluxation of the odontoid process of the second vertebra, or by torsion and compression of the vertebral arteries, which causes vertebrobasilar insufficiency and syncope on downward gaze. Headache, a frequent complaint, is most commonly occipital, but occasionally radiates over the top of the cranium. Neck examination discloses localized tenderness, muscle spasm, and limitation of rotary motion with retention of flexion and extension.

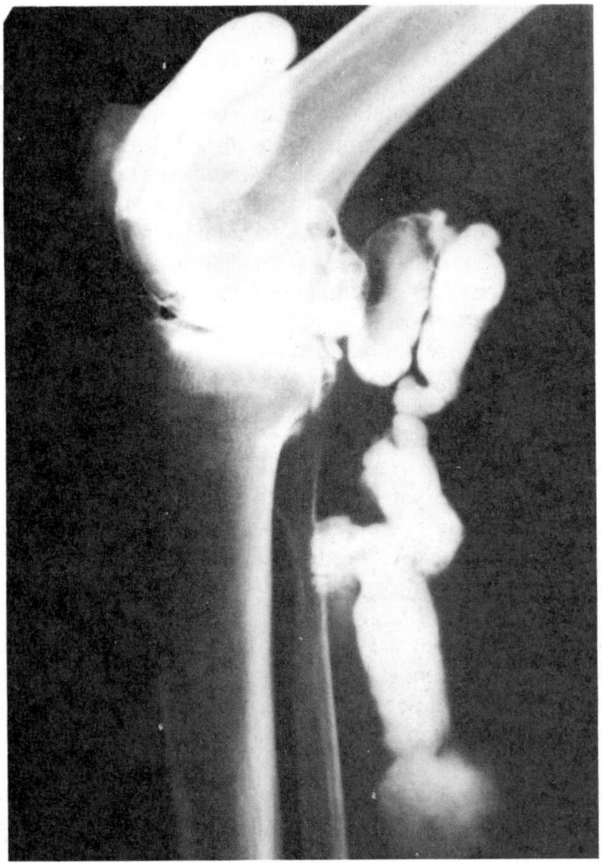

Fig. 304-4. Dissecting popliteal (Baker's) cyst. Arthrogram of the knee in lateral projection demonstrating dissection of radiocontrast material into the lower leg.

Extra-articular manifestations

Systemic features of RA (see the box) are frequent but usually occult and of limited clinical significance. Occasionally, however, they dominate the clinical picture.

Rheumatoid nodules. At some time, subcutaneous nodules appear in 15% to 20% of patients as firm, nontender, rounded, or oval masses in the subcutaneous or deeper connective tissues, varying in size from less than 0.5 cm to several centimeters in diameter. Areas subjected to mechanical pressure are common sites, especially the olecranon and extensor surface of the forearms and the Achilles tendon. Unusual locations include the pleura, meninges, ears, and bridge of the nose. Subcutaneous nodules seldom cause symptoms, but they occasionally break down or become infected and may be overlooked as portals for bacteremia and septic arthritis. Typically, they develop insidiously and persist, but regression is possible at any time. Because they are almost invariably found in patients with seropositive disease, rheumatoid nodules portend a severer and more destructive arthritis.

Extra-articular manifestations of rheumatoid arthritis

- Constitutional
  - Weight loss
  - Fever, sweats
  - Fatigue
- Lymphadenopathy and splenomegaly
- Nodules
  - Subcutaneous
  - Parenchymatous
- Ocular
  - Episcleritis
  - Scleritis
  - Scleromalacia
  - Sjögren's syndrome
- Cardiac
  - Pericarditis
  - Myocarditis and vasculitis
  - Endocardial and valvular granulomata
- Pulmonary
  - Pleuritis
  - Interstitial fibrosis
  - Nodules—Caplan's syndrome
  - Fibrosing alveolitis
  - Bronchiolitis obliterans
- Neurologic
  - Cord compression
  - Cerebral vasculitis
  - Entrapment neuropathies
  - Distal sensory neuropathy
  - Mononeuritis multiplex
- Vasculitis
  - Cutaneous necrotizing vasculitis
  - Dermal infarcts
  - Periunguinal infarcts
  - Digital gangrene
  - Leg ulcers
  - Polyarteritis
- Hematologic
  - Anemia
  - Eosinophilia
  - Felty's syndrome
- Miscellaneous
  - Myositis
  - Amyloid
  - Osteoporosis

Vasculitis. RA has a spectrum of vascular lesions: capillaritis and venulitis, which are thought to be important in the development of rheumatoid nodules and synovitis; a bland intimal proliferation commonly affecting digital and mesenteric vessels; subacute lesions of arterioles and venules in scattered locations; and finally, an acute, widespread, necrotizing ateritis of small- and medium-sized arteries that may be indistinguishable from polyarteritis nodosum. This most severe form of rheumatoid vasculitis, designated *rheumatoid arteritis,* characteristically produces polyneuropathy, skin necrosis and ulceration, digital gangrene, ulceration or perforation of the nasal septum, and visceral infarction. When present, the neuropathy takes the form of an acute sensorimotor mononeuritis (mononeuritis multiplex) with dropped foot or wrist and a patchy sensory loss in one or more extremities. Ischemic skin lesions appear in crops as small, brown spots (not unlike splinter hemorrhages) in the nail beds, nail folds, and digital pulp. Large ischemic ulcerations can develop in the lower extremities, particularly over the malleoli. Fatal intestinal and myocardial infarction have been reported. Fever, polymorphonuclear leukocytosis, and thrombocytosis are common. Many patients have concomitant episcleritis, scleromalacia, pleuritis, myocarditis, and/or pericarditis. The prognosis in the untreated, fulminant form of vasculitis is exceedingly poor. Fortunately, the full-blown picture is rare, and individual features can exist independently, persist for long periods, and pose little threat to life.

Neuropathy. Rheumatoid arthritis tends to spare the central nervous system, but causes a number of abnormalities in peripheral nerves, including the severe sensorimotor neuropathy (mononeuritis multiplex) accompanying vasculitis; entrapment neuropathies of the median, ulnar, or anterior tibial nerves; and a mild, generally benign, symmetric distal sensory or sensorimotor neuropathy.

Myopathy. Weakness and atrophy of skeletal muscle are commonly observed in the absence of neurologic abnormalities and are most pronounced in muscle groups that cross involved joints. The cause is unknown. Biopsies show nodular infiltrates of lymphocytes, reduction in skeletal muscle fiber number and circumference, and condensation of sarcolemmal nuclei. Electromyograms (EMGs) may display myopathic changes. Neither biopsy nor EMG correlate well with clinical observations. Muscle enzymes are usually normal. In rheumatoid patients with proximal muscle weakness, the possibility of steroid myopathy or chloroquine neuromyopathy should be considered.

Cardiac manifestations. The most common symptomatic lesion is acute pericarditis, which appears most often in males with seropositive disease. An associated pleural effusion is often detected. Characteristics of both pericardial and pleural fluids are a low glucose concentration, increased lactic dehydrogenase and gamma globulin levels, and low complement activity. The course of the pericarditis is variable, ranging from a mild, self-limited process to cardiac tamponade and death. A good response to steroid therapy can be expected, but chronic effusion or constriction may ensue and necessitate pericardiectomy. Recurrences are not uncommon. Less common are granulomatous lesions that are histologically similar to rheumatoid nodules and involve the epicardium, myocardium, and valves; also uncommon are focal interstitial myocarditis and arteritis of coronary vessels. Occasionally, valvular insufficiency or conduction abnormalities may be recognized during life, and, rarely, myocardial infarction occurs as a manifestation of coronary arteritis.

Pleuropulmonary manifestations. The respiratory symptoms encountered in most rheumatoid patients can usually be ascribed to more common disorders, but some pulmonary abnormalities seem to be intimately related to the rheumatoid process. They include (1) pleurisy with or without effusion, (2) nonpneumoconiotic intrapulmonary rheumatoid nodules, (3) rheumatoid pneumoconiosis (Caplan's syndrome), (4) diffuse interstitial fibrosis and pneumonitis, and (5) an involvement of the intima of small pulmonary arteries and arterioles that leads to pulmonary hypertension. Considerable overlap exists among these syndromes. Upper airway obstruction with hoarseness and stridor may result from cricoarytenoid arthritis, and bronchiolitis obliterans is a recognized complication.

The presence of numerous rheumatoid nodules in the lungs of patients with a history of pneumoconiotic exposure and in whom RA develops is referred to as *rheumatoid pneumoconiosis,* or *Caplan's syndrome*. First described in Welsh soft-coal miners, the same phenomenon occurs in asbestos and ceramic workers, gold and chalk miners, and others with arthritis and an appropriate industrial exposure. Radiographs reveal multiple, well-defined nodular opacities (0.5 to 5.0 cm in diameter) widely distributed throughout the lungs, or large numbers of smaller nodules that present a "snowstorm" appearance. Occasionally, nodules coalesce into large conglomerate masses, and cavitation has been observed. Typical lesions sometimes antedate the development of RA, occasionally by years. Although usually unexplained, diffuse pneumonitis may be caused by treatment with gold, penicillamine, or methotrexate.

Ocular manifestations. Rheumatoid disease uncommonly, but characteristically, is associated with inflammatory lesions of the episclera and sclera. Episcleritis is a relatively benign, transient condition that causes mild discomfort in the eyes but does not interfere with vision. Scleritis is more serious, can cause blindness, and may proceed as an indolent, slowly progressing process or as recurrent subacute episodes of ocular inflammation. Lesions usually originate in the superior sclerae, surrounded by hyperemia of the deep scleral vessels. Inflammation may spread to other coats of the eye, ciliary body, and retina, resulting in secondary complications. The histologic finding is that of a rheumatoid nodule, and the lesions are most often found in patients with high titers of rheumatoid factor and subcutaneous nodules.

The most common ocular abnormalities of RA (approximately 15% to 20% of patients) are the corneal and conjunctival lesions associated with Sjögren's syndrome. This syndrome, which is more properly viewed as a concomitant of, rather than as a manifestation of, rheumatoid disease, is presented in detail in Chapter 305.

Renal involvement. The kidneys are remarkably spared in RA, although unexplained, mild proteinuria and occasional red blood cells (RBCs) in the urine sediment may be found. More often, renal abnormalities are a consequence of drug therapy: that is, interstitial nephritis from nonsteroidal anti-inflammatory drugs (NSAIDs), gold nephropathy, or penicillamine glomerular nephritis. Complicating amyloidosis may produce a nephrotic syndrome.

Lymphadenopathy, splenomegaly, and Felty's syndrome. Lymph nodes may be enlarged proximal to inflamed joints or in areas remote from articular inflammation. Up to 10% of patients with RA have palpable splenomegaly. Felty's syndrome is a symptom complex of chronic RA associated with splenomegaly, leukopenia, skin hyperpigmentation, leg ulcers, lymphadenopathy, anemia, and thrombocytopenia. A rare finding is nodular regenerative hyperplasia of the liver. Commonly, patients have high titers of rheumatoid factor and antinuclear antibodies, subcutaneous nodules, and manifestations of systemic rheumatoid disease. The leukopenia is, in fact, a selective neutropenia and may be very profound; polymorphonuclear counts of less than 1000 per cubic millimeter are frequent. Marrow examination usually reveals moderate hypercellularity with a paucity of mature neutrophils. Multiple explanations for neutropenia have been proposed; including hypersplenism, but splenectomy often fails to correct the abnormality. The incidence of gram-positive infections can decline after splenectomy, however, even when the neutropenia remains unaltered. A portion of Felty's patients have lymphocytosis caused by an expansion of an unusual (T_γ) large granular lymphocyte subpopulation. Splenectomy is contraindicated in these patients.

Complications

An increased frequency of infections is observed in RA patients, particularly those with systemic rheumatoid disease. Infections may be local (pyarthrosis) (see Chapter 315) or extra-articular. Herpes zoster is more common. Mortality from septicemia, pneumonia, lung abscess, empyema, or pyelonephritis is well recognized.

Clinically significant amyloidosis is infrequent and is rarely a cause of death. Amyloidosis should be considered in rheumatoid patients who develop renal insufficiency (especially with a nephrotic syndrome) and in those with unexplained gastrointestinal hemorrhage.

Osteoporosis, either generalized or involving thoracic or lumbar vertebrae, may complicate RA. The etiology is probably multifactorial, with contributions from generalized malnutrition; the postmenopausal state; immobilization; steroid therapy; and perhaps the catabolic state imposed by chronic rheumatoid disease itself.

Rarely, a hyperviscosity syndrome occurs as a result of the intravascular interaction of large quantities of rheumatoid factor and circulating IgG. Symptoms may include a bleeding diathesis (with bruising, epistaxis, and gingival hemorrhage), confusion, vertigo, retinal hemorrhages, congestive heart failure, and intestinal ischemia.

LABORATORY FINDINGS

A normocytic, normo- or hypochromic anemia, usually associated with a low serum iron and a normal or low iron-binding capacity, is a common feature of RA. Large stores of unutilized iron are found in the bone marrow. The white blood cell count is usually normal, but a mild increase in polymorphonuclear leukocytes is not uncommon. Leukocytosis, in general, does not indicate enhanced disease activity; but eosinophilia, when present, is often associated with severe systemic rheumatoid disease. The erythrocyte sedimentation rate (ESR) is elevated to a variable degree in most patients and roughly parallels disease activity.

Serum protein analysis may reveal elevation in the alpha-2 and gamma globulin fractions and a mild to moderate diminution in serum albumin. The gamma globulin increase is polyclonal. Liver and renal function tests are usually normal, as is the urinary sediment.

Conventional IgM rheumatoid factor is demonstrable in approximately 70% of adults with RA but is not specific for this disease. The presence and amount of the autoantibody have important prognostic as well as diagnostic significance (Chapter 294). Five percent to 10% have false-positive tests for syphilis. At least 25% of seropositive rheumatoid patients have serum antinuclear antibodies, generally with a homogeneous pattern of nuclear immunofluorescence. Antibodies to native double-stranded DNA are very rare. Circulating immune complexes and cryoprecipitable proteins consisting of immunoglobulins, complement components, and rheumatoid factors are demonstrable in the serum of some patients with RA, especially those with vasculitis or Felty's syndrome. Normal serum complement values are the rule, but depressed values are seen in patients with systemic complications.

Synovial fluid analysis can be of value in establishing the diagnosis of RA, although no one finding is specific (Chapter 295). Characteristically, the fluid is exudative, with white blood cell counts ranging from 5000 to 20,000 per cubic millimeter; counts in excess of 50,000 are occasionally encountered. Polymorphonuclear leukocytes comprise at least two thirds of the cells, except very early in the disease. The synovial fluid is turbid in appearance, with reduced viscosity; it forms a loose, friable clot on addition of dilute acetic acid (the mucin clot test). The protein content, normally less than 2 g per deciliter, often is elevated to levels exceeding 3.5 g. Hemolytic complement is reduced to less than one third of the serum values, especially in patients with seropositive disease; C4 and C2 levels are most profoundly depressed. Glucose concentrations may be low or normal, similar to rheumatoid effusions in other body fluids.

RADIOLOGIC FINDINGS

No roentgenographic features are pathognomonic of RA, but the diagnosis frequently is suggested by a characteristic pattern of joint erosions. The tendency toward symmetry in established disease and the predilection for certain anatomic sites—notably the MCP and PIP joints of the hands, wrists, and knees and the MTP joints of the feet—are important in differentiating RA from degenerative joint disease and from other inflammatory arthritides. So, too, is the relative lack of bone formation in the presence of advanced joint destruction, a feature that contrasts with the exuberant new bone formation often seen in ankylosing spondylitis, Reiter's syndrome, and psoriatic arthritis. Specific roentgenographic abnormalities are detailed in Chapter 296.

COURSE AND PROGNOSIS

It is impossible to reliably predict the course that RA will follow when the patient is seen at the inception of the disease. The "natural history" of RA (i.e., in the absence of therapy) is not completely understood, but there are several valid impressions. Of any 100 rheumatoid arthritis patients studied, approximately 15% have a short-lived joint disease that remits without significant residua. In another 15% to 25%, the disease may persist for some period of time but then leaves with only mild to moderate damage to the joints. Fifty percent of patients have persistent activity of the arthritis punctuated by exacerbations and remissions but invariably leading to progressive deformity with a variable disability. The remaining 10% have a relentless disease that is unresponsive to therapy and eventuates in complete disability with the patient restricted to a bed or wheelchair existence (prior to the availability of joint replacement).

Some features that portend either a favorable or a dismal outcome have been identified (Table 304-1). In general, remissions are most likely to occur during the first year of disease, especially after an acute onset with systemic manifestations. Men do better than women, and disease beginning before age 45 seems to augur a better outcome. It is axiomatic that the longer an active progressive disease continues, the worse the outlook. The appearance of extra-articular disease is associated with a particularly poor prognosis, and patients developing such features have twice the mortality rate of conventional rheumatoid patients. Factors that presage a less favorable course are an insidious onset of disease; persistence beyond 1 year without remission; early appearance of bone erosions on radiologic examination of the joints; development of nodules; and, most important, the presence of serum rheumatoid factor, particularly in high titers. Patients who are HLA-DR4 (Dw4) do worse, as do those with a low socioeconomic status or lack of education.

Patients rarely die of RA, although systemic vasculitis and atlantoaxial subluxation can be lethal. Rheumatoid patients may succumb to overwhelming sepsis or complications of drug or surgical therapy, but the majority die of the same diseases as age-matched cohorts, except 5 to 10 years sooner.

Table 304-1. Prognostic features in rheumatoid arthritis

Good	Bad
Acute onset	Bone erosions
Disease of <1 year	Continuous disease activity
Age <40 years	Extra-articular manifestations
Male	Rheumatoid nodules
	Rheumatoid factor
	HLA-DR4, Dw4

DIAGNOSIS

Like most diseases, rheumatoid arthritis can be diagnosed easily in its advanced and characteristic form, but early in the course, the diagnosis is often obscured. Considerable diagnostic confusion results when the disease is manifested with only constitutional symptoms or when the initial joint disease is spotty or monarticular. The earliest features of the inflammatory synovitis usually appear in the wrists, knees, PIP and MCP joints of the hands, and the MTP joints of the feet. The joints are painful, often appearing swollen and sometimes red. In time, the disease spreads, finally assuming its typical form as a bilateral, symmetric polyarthritis involving small and large joints in both the upper and lower extremities. The axial skeleton is usually spared, except for the cervical spine. The demonstration of subcutaneous nodules is especially helpful confirmatory evidence. Additional findings that substantiate the diagnosis are positive tests for rheumatoid factor, an exudative synovial fluid analysis showing polymorphonuclear leukocytosis and depressed complement values, and radiographic findings of bone demineralization and erosions about the affected joints. In the majority of patients, the disease has assumed its more characteristic clinical features in 1 or 2 years.

The American Rheumatism Association criteria for the diagnosis of RA are outlined in the box on p. 2415. Any combination of four or more of this group of symptoms, signs, and laboratory findings in a patient whose disease has been continuous for at least 6 weeks is designated *rheumatoid arthritis*. It should be appreciated, however, that these criteria were not developed for the bedside diagnosis of rheumatoid arthritis, but rather to classify large groups of patients for inclusion in epidemiologic surveys, drug trials, and studies of the natural history of the disease. An individual's failure to meet an arbitrary set of criteria therefore should not preclude the diagnosis of RA, especially in its early stages.

DIFFERENTIAL DIAGNOSIS

Joint symptoms are common and have a multiplicity of etiologies (detailed in Chapter 303). Some diseases, however, have chronic polyarticular inflammation as a major component, and it is these diseases that most often have to be distinguished from RA. Two groups are particularly important: the connective tissue diseases and the seronegative spondyloarthropathies. In the former, distinctive skin rashes, typical organ system involvement, and the availability, in some instances, of definitive serum antibodies help one to make the correct diagnosis. The spondyloarthropathies, however, particularly when peripheral arthritis predominates, may prove more challenging. These disorders often have a chronic, destructive polyarthritis which, on examination, shows synovial hypertrophy and histologic features resem-

1987 Revised criteria for classification of rheumatoid arthritis

1. Morning stiffness in and around the joints lasting at least 1 hour before maximal improvement.
2. At least three joint areas with simultaneous soft-tissue swelling or fluid (not bony overgrowth alone) observed by a physician. The 14 possible joint areas are right or left PIP, MCP, wrist, elbow, knee, ankle, and MTP joints.
3. At least one joint area swollen as above in a wrist, MCP, or PIP.
4. Simultaneous involvement of the same joint areas (as in 2) on both sides of the body (bilateral involvement of PIP, MCP, or MTP is acceptable without absolute symmetry).
5. Subcutaneous nodules over bony prominences, or extensor surfaces, or in juxta-articular regions, observed by a physician.
6. Demonstration of abnormal amounts of serum "rheumatoid factor" by any method that has been positive in fewer than 5% of normal control subjects.
7. Radiographic changes typical of RA on posteroanterior wrist radiographs, including erosions or unequivocal bony decalcification localized to or most marked adjacent to the involved joints (osteoarthritic changes alone do not qualify).

Arnett FC et al: 1987 revised American Rheumatism Association for classification of rheumatoid arthritis. Arthritis Rheum 31:315, 1988.

bling those of RA. As a rule, the peripheral joint disease tends to be asymmetric, favoring the larger joints, and except for psoriatic arthritis, lower extremity involvement predominates. Psoriatic arthritis characteristically has a predilection for the distal interphalangeal joints of the hands, especially when there is disease of the associated fingernail. Reiter's disease, ankylosing spondylitis, and, less regularly, psoriatic and colitic arthritis produce remarkable erythema and swelling of individual proximal and distal joints of the toes, an uncommon location in RA. An important distinguishing feature is that sacroiliitis and spondylitis of the thoracic and lumbar articulations are common to the group, and iridocyclitis is a frequent accompaniment. The association with the HLA-B27 haplotype may be useful.

For the various other joint diseases that occasionally may be confused with rheumatoid arthritis, the reader is referred to the more extensive differential diagnosis of arthritis presented in Chapter 303.

MANAGEMENT

The natural course of RA is characterized by spontaneous remissions and exacerbations that make the evaluation of therapy difficult. Although there is a general agreement that certain treatment modalities are helpful in the short term, retrospective analysis of RA patients treated longer than 5 to 7 years shows that less than 25% are still taking their original medications. Since there is no known cure of RA, it follows that a variety of therapies have to be tried until an appropriate combination is found. An empathetic doctor-patient relationship, in which the physician devotes the time necessary to explain to the patient both the disease and the reasons for selecting one or another treatment, is an absolute prerequisite for success. A total management program requires the participation of a variety of medical and paramedical personnel: physiatrists, orthopedic surgeons, visiting nurses, and, when indicated, other medical specialists. No one physician's practice can encompass these many special areas; he or she must be willing to "orchestrate" this complex program.

Basic program

Rest and exercise. Rheumatoid arthritis has many of the manifestations of a constitutional disease. Fatigue is frequently a cause of considerable disability. Most patients recognize the need for rest but require specific directions as to when to rest and how much rest is necessary. There is disagreement about the importance of complete bed rest but the unwillingness of insurers to fund prolonged hospitalization makes the issue moot.

During periods of rest at home, individual inflamed joints should be supported with well-fitted splints or plastic shells. The mattress must be firm, and a bed board is useful. A bed cradle and a padded footrest to prevent deformities of the feet and ankles should be employed regularly. Positions that lead to contractures, such as pillows beneath the knees or lying on the side with the knees flexed, must be discouraged. Patients with hip disease ought to lie prone on a firm surface for 30 minutes twice daily to prevent hip flexion contractures.

As patients return to more regular activities, a rest period should be prescribed. For workers, the most practical approach is to recline for 30 to 60 minutes during the lunch period. Homemakers should lie down for a similar period during the nap time of young children. Thirty minutes of rest before dinner is helpful. Weekend activities may have to be curtailed to provide additional rest, and others in the family should be recruited to perform the duties of the member with RA.

Exercises to maintain joint mobility and regain muscle strength are an integral part of the basic treatment program. It takes only 10 to 15 minutes to put all the joints through a complete range of motion, and this should be done twice daily. Isometric exercises prevent quadriceps atrophy, but resistance exercises should be avoided. Heating pads or hot packs applied to affected joints for 15 to 20 minutes three times daily give good relief of pain and allow greater range of motion; occasionally, cold applications are efficacious. Paraffin baths and whirlpool units are available for home use, but their use should be taught to the patient by a physical therapist before their introduction into a home program. Soaking the hands or a hot shower in the morning before starting the exercise program usually decrease muscle spasm and stiffness and allow more effective participation.

Drugs

An array of new drugs has been added to those already available for treating RA. No single drug is specific or universally successful, but for most patients, some combination can be found that diminishes the articular disease. Several classes of such agents are recognized: analgesics; NSAIDs; glucocorticoids; remissive, slow-acting, or disease-modifying antirheumatic drugs (DMARDs); and immunomodulatory compounds. Early in the illness, patients are usually managed with NSAIDs only, but those with poor prognostic signs or more aggressive or chronic disease have one of the DMARDs added. Various combinations are possible, all have been tried, and none appears appreciably better; failure with one combination does not preclude success with another. Fortunately, there are very few drug interactions between NSAIDs and DMARDs. Usually, adrenocorticosteroids or immunosuppressive drugs are considered only after other modalities have been exhausted. A possible exception is methotrexate, which is increasingly used as the first drug in patients with features that portend a poor outcome (Table 304-1). The pharmacology, dosage schedules, and toxicity of the individual medications are considered in Chapter 317. Subsequent remarks in this chapter will be limited to their use in RA.

Analgesics. Acetaminophen (Tylenol), 300 to 600 mg, three to four times daily, or propoxyphene hydrochloride (Darvon), 32 or 65 mg, three or four times daily, may be used for pain relief, although neither substitutes for the antiinflammatory effects of aspirin or NSAIDs. Severe pain is occasionally managed with oral codeine, but its potential for addiction when employed in a chronic disorder such as rheumatoid arthritis precludes its regular use.

Nonsteroidal anti-inflammatory drugs. Aspirin remains an important drug for the treatment of rheumatoid arthritis. Its successful use depends on dosing at regular intervals and in large amounts, usually 3.6 to 5.4 g (12 to 18 tablets) per day. Administration immediately after meals or with food minimizes gastric irritation. The last dose is usually prescribed for bedtime. Some patients, particularly the elderly, cannot take these optimal amounts of aspirin. Tinnitus is a common side effect but is easily controlled by a slight reduction in dose. Gastric irritation is a frequent accompaniment of aspirin therapy. Buffered preparations, aspirin suspensions, or enteric-coated aspirin may be better tolerated. Other salicylate compounds may substitute for aspirin. Sodium salicylate, calcium salicylate, choline magnesium trisalicylate, benorylate, and diflunisal are all reported to produce significantly less gastrointestinal symptoms and blood loss. Chemical detection of small amounts of blood in the stool is not an indication to discontinue the medication. Other important toxicities include aspirin sensitivity and effects on platelet adhesiveness.

In spite of the increased cost, most patients prefer NSAIDs because of the less frequent dosing (see complete list in Table 317-1). No one NSAID is significantly better than another, but most patients find one that gives significant relief. Therefore, trials of each are indicated. Since their onset of action is rapid, trials need not exceed 2 to 3 weeks. There is no indication that combinations of NSAIDs and aspirin are better than either alone, with the possible exception that indomethacin in a slow-release form at a dose of 75 to 100 mg at bedtime is particularly effective in relieving night pain and the duration of morning stiffness.

Adrenocorticosteroids. Every attempt should be made to employ conservative measures and the disease-modifying agents listed below before instituting treatment with adrenocorticosteroids. Most rheumatologists, however, accept that in some patients this therapy is justified. Use of these drugs requires an intimate knowledge of their long-term toxicity (Chapter 317). Indications for the judicious use of corticosteroids for long periods are (1) as an aid in the rehabilitation of patients who otherwise might be invalided or remain housebound, (2) in treatment of disability resulting from acute systemic or febrile manifestations of the disease, and (3) in the presence of deterioration that has continued in spite of all other conservative forms of treatment (not including cytotoxic agents).

There is relatively little advantage of one synthetic steroid over another. Cortisone and hydrocortisone have limited usefulness because of their salt-retaining effects. Prednisone and prednisolone are preferred because they are least expensive. If a decision to employ long-term corticosteroid therapy is made, the smallest possible daily total dose should be selected. The patient must be informed that this dose will not be exceeded, except under unusual circumstances. Generally, the average daily prednisone dose for men should not be more than 7.5 mg and for women 5.0 mg daily. Smaller doses should be prescribed for children and postmenopausal females, two groups that are particularly susceptible to side effects. Divided doses may be more effective than single morning or evening administration but result in more side effects. Alternate-day corticosteroids are usually not successful in the management of RA, but may be worth a trial given the lower frequency of undesirable side effects. Initiating therapy with large priming doses followed by a stepwise decrease is not recommended. "Pulse therapy" with intravenous methylprednisolone (Medrol) in 1 g doses may have short-term benefits.

Even with small maintenance doses of prednisone, patients develop suppression of adrenal gland function. Therefore, the amount of corticosteroid must be sharply increased in situations of acute or overwhelming stress and prior to major surgery. Cortisone acetate or hydrocortisone sodium succinate (Solu-Cortef) (but not hydrocortisone acetate) should be administered intramuscularly in 50- to 100-mg doses 4 to 6 hours before operation, and continued intravenously or intramuscularly at those intervals for 24 to 48 hours after surgery or until the patient begins oral feeding. Thereafter, a rapid reduction to the maintenance dose is permissible. Aseptic necrosis, particularly in the hip joints, can develop from prolonged or intermittent steroid therapy. Continued use of corticosteroids to treat the pain and limitation of motion due to osteonecrosis can compound an already difficult situation.

Intra-articular corticosteroids. The intra-articular injection of microcrystalline suspensions of corticosteroids may be of use in patients with a limited number of involved joints or in whom a few joints are disproportionately inflamed. Joint aspiration to exclude infection is mandatory, and removing large effusions can decrease joint distention and reflex spasm of surrounding muscle groups. The dose employed depends on the size of the joint. In the knee, 20 to 40 mg of triamcinolone hexacetonide or a comparable, relatively nonabsorbable corticosteroid preparation is usually used. Lesser amounts are appropriate for smaller joints. Aside from pain and the potential for introducing infections, atrophy of the injection site is the only frequent complication. The response to intra-articular therapy is variable. Complete relief of inflammation and pain sometimes lasts many months. If it is short-lived, the risks outweigh the benefits, since joints that are repeatedly injected occasionally develop accelerated degenerative arthritis. Therefore, it is wise to limit intra-articular therapy in a single joint to two or three times a year.

Disease-modifying antirheumatic drugs. This group of compounds includes gold, D-penicillamine, the 4-aminoquinolines, and sulfasalazine (Azulfidine). A description of the individual drugs is presented in Chapter 317. Each should be used separately and continued for 3 to 6 months before a decision is made about its effectiveness, unless toxicity supervenes. Improvement is always gradual, and a rebound in disease activity is not observed after discontinuation.

Gold compounds. Most rheumatologists advocate the use of gold. The disadvantages of weekly visits to the physician, injections, and additional laboratory tests to avoid toxic side effects are offset by the occasional dramatic responses obtained with this treatment. In general, one patient in five has an excellent result; an additional two patients receive significant benefits. Gold is recommended early in the disease when there is active joint inflammation and before significant destructive changes have occurred, but control studies have shown benefits at every stage of rheumatoid arthritis.

Patients should be instructed to pay particular attention to pruritus, minor skin rashes, particularly in seborrheic areas, and a metallic taste in the mouth. These are all forerunners of more serious problems. There may be a long lag from the initiation of gold therapy until benefits are noted. Without this knowledge, patients may become discouraged and discontinue treatment. Either gold sodium thiomalate (Myochrysine) or gold thioglucose (Solganal) is given intramuscularly at weekly intervals: 10 mg the first week, 25 mg the second week, and 50 mg weekly thereafter. Usually by the tenth to fourteenth injection, the patient notices signs of improvement. At this time, 50 mg of the drug can be given every other week for the next four to eight injections; and, with continued improvement, 50 mg can be given every third or fourth week, for a minimum of 2 years (and possibly indefinitely). Should symptoms return, weekly injections of 50 mg can be reinstituted, sometimes with good results. If the patient has not improved by the time 1 g of drug has been given, another form of treatment is indicated.

Undesirable side effects include proteinuria, thrombocytopenia, leukopenia, and, rarely, anemia and pancytopenia. A urinalysis and complete blood count must be checked before each injection for the first 4 weeks and biweekly or monthly thereafter. The drug should be discontinued if leukopenia or proteinuria develops. When the white blood cell count or urinalysis returns to normal, gold can be reinstituted at one half the normal dose, and the effect observed. If there is no adverse reaction, the full treatment program can be continued. Similarly, when pruritus or dermatitis clears, therapy often can be reinstituted after a judicious trial at a smaller dose. Severe dermatologic complications may require antihistamines or steroids. Treatment with BAL (British anti-lewisite) should be reserved for patients with profound dermal, renal, or hematopoietic toxicity. Pneumonitis, hepatitis, peripheral neuritis, and enterocolitis are rare side effects of gold treatment.

An oral gold compound (auranofin) is now available. When prescribed at 3 mg twice a day, it is somewhat less effective than injectable gold but has less severe dermal, renal, and hematologic side effects. Diarrhea, however, can be a troublesome complication. Three months of treatment should be tried before abandoning this therapy.

D-Penicillamine. Although D-penicillamine is effective in patients with RA, its use is plagued with frequent and annoying, but generally reversible, side effects that limit its use. The percentages of good responses, type of toxicity, and delayed onset of improvement are similar to those with gold. Treatment is initiated at 250 mg daily and increased by that amount every 3 months until clinical improvement or toxicity intervenes, or a dose of 1.0 g daily is reached. Skin rash, transient loss of taste, stomatitis, gastric upset, leukopenia, thrombocytopenia, and proteinuria are common and often can be controlled by reduction in dose. The frequency of dermatitis may be greater in patients who developed a rash from gold, but allergy to penicillin is not a contraindication. Rare complications include glomerulonephritis, Goodpasture's syndrome, and myasthenia gravis. Blood counts and urinalyses are required at least monthly. Treatment is continued indefinitely; after months or years, tolerance sometimes develops.

Antimalarials (4-aminoquinolines). Chloroquine diphosphate is administered in a dose of 250 mg once daily, generally at bedtime; this tends to minimize complicating gastrointestinal or vasomotor symptoms. Hydroxychloroquine sulfate (Plaquenil) is taken in a dose of 200 mg twice daily. Patients who develop side effects of headache, nausea, abdominal cramping, diarrhea, or skin rash from one antimalarial may tolerate another. Improvement with these agents occurs slowly, seldom before 4 weeks; 3 to 6 months of drug administration are usually required before maximum benefits are achieved. If improvement occurs, the drug is continued, often at a reduced dose, but only if the patient has funduscopic examinations two or three times yearly by an ophthalmologist acquainted with the drug's rare but potentially severe ocular toxicity. Early detection of retinal abnormalities and immediate discontinuation of therapy may arrest or reverse the ocular damage.

Sulfasalazine. Sulfasalazine (Azulfidine) has some value in the treatment of RA with improvement occurring in 6 to 12 weeks. Enteric-coated tablets are given in an initial dose of 500 mg twice a day, and if tolerated increased to 1000 mg two to three times daily. Nausea or dyspepsia are the major side effects of the drug. Rashes occur infrequently and neutropenia is a rare serious complication. Hemolyses can occur in patients with underlying G6PD deficiency (see Chapter 90).

Methotrexate. The folic acid analog methotrexate is currently the most widely used disease-modifying agent for the treatment of rheumatoid arthritis. Though normally considered to be a cytotoxic drug, its rapid onset of action and the recurrence of disease soon after discontinuation suggests that it may be working in RA as a unique form of anti-inflammatory treatment. Initial therapy consists of one tablet (2.5 mg) given every 12 hours for 3 doses once a week. If a response is not observed in 3 to 6 weeks, subsequent adjustments upward to a total of 15 mg per week may be tried. Larger doses, either oral or intramuscular, are likely to produce side effects without additional benefits. Clinical improvement is seen in two thirds of patients often within a few weeks of starting methotrexate, but progression of bone erosions may be observed even in asymptomatic subjects. Adverse effects include nausea, vomiting, stomatitis, and diarrhea. Hematologic abnormalities are uncommon at the low doses used in RA, but monthly blood counts are advised. Other toxicities include an acute interstitial pneumonitis; skin rash; and the possibility of hepatotoxicity, which may be accompanied by mild elevations in liver enzymes. Currently, many clinicians are using methotrexate in combination with second-line drugs, although the benefits of such combination have not been proven in controlled studies. Additional information on methotrexate is provided in Chapter 317.

Cytotoxic (immunosuppressant) drugs. Cytotoxic drug therapy should be limited to the small number of rheumatoid patients for whom all other therapeutic modalities have failed or who have life-threatening systemic complications or have experienced unacceptable corticosteroid side effects. The patient and the prescribing physician must have full knowledge of the serious immediate and potential long-term complications. Specific agents are described in Chapter 317. Immunomodulatory agents (e.g., levamisole), lymphoplasmapheresis, and total lymphoid irradiation are controversial therapies.

Surgical management

Orthopedic surgery can be preventive or restorative. Synovectomy in joints unaffected by local or systemic therapy can improve function and eliminate swelling for a period of time. Soft-tissue damage such as tendon rupture can be minimized or repaired. Excision of subluxated, painful metatarsal phalangeal joints aids ambulation, and realignment of finger joints improves hand function. For predictable relief of pain and restoration of function, however, the procedure of choice is total joint replacement.

The availability of prosthetic joints, especially hips and knees, has revolutionized the care of rheumatoid patients with multiple joint involvement. Early consultation with orthopedic surgeons to plan appropriate interventions is an essential part of the management program.

REFERENCES

Firestein G and Zvaifler NJ: Rheumatoid arthritis. A disease of disordered immunity. In Gallin JI, Goldstein IM, and Snyderman R, editors: Inflammation: basic principles and clinical correlates, ed 2. New York, 1992, Raven Press.

Gordon DA, Stein JL, and Broder I: The extra-articular features of rheumatoid arthritis: a systemic analysis of 127 cases. Am J Med 54:445, 1973.

Harris ED Jr: Rheumatoid arthritis. Pathophysiology and implications for therapy. N Engl J Med 322:1277, 1990.

Pincus T: The paradox of effective therapies but poor long term outcomes in rheumatoid arthritis. Semin Arthritis Rheum 21(suppl 3):2, 1992.

Utsinger PD, Zvaifler NJ, and Ehrilich GE: Rheumatoid arthritis, etiology, diagnosis, management. Philadelphia, 1985, Lippincott.

Vollerstsen RS et al: Rheumatoid vasculitis: survival and associated risk factors. Medicine (Baltimore) 65:365, 1986.

Zvaifler NJ: Etiology and pathogenesis of rheumatoid arthritis. In McCarty DJ and Koopman W, editors: Arthritis and allied conditions, ed 12. Philadelphia, 1993, Lea & Febiger.

CHAPTER

305 Sjögren's Syndrome

Robert I. Fox

Sjögren's syndrome (SS) is a chronic autoimmune disorder characterized by lymphocytic infiltration of the lacrimal and salivary glands, leading to severe dryness of eyes (keratoconjunctivitis sicca) and mouth (xerostomia). SS may exist as a primary disorder (primary, 1° SS) or in association with other autoimmune diseases (termed 2° SS), including rheumatoid arthritis (RA), systemic lupus erythematosus (SLE), or progressive systemic sclerosis (scleroderma, PSS). Patients with primary SS frequently have extraglandular manifestation including rash, arthritis, pneumonitis, nephritis, and nervous system involvement.

CLASSIFICATION CRITERIA AND EPIDEMIOLOGY

There has been considerable debate about the diagnostic criteria for the diagnosis of SS, leading to confusion in clinical practice and in research studies. The specific criteria used for the diagnosis of SS at our institution are listed in the box on p. 2419. SS patients should have objective ev-

Criteria for diagnosis of primary and secondary SS

I. Primary Sjögren's syndrome
   A. Symptoms and objective signs of ocular dryness
      1. Schirmer's test less than 8 mm wetting per 5 minutes
      2. Positive rose bengal or fluorescein staining of cornea and conjunctiva to demonstrate keratoconjunctivitis sicca
   B. Symptoms and objective signs of dry mouth
      1. Decreased parotid flow rate using Lashley cups or other methods
      2. Abnormal biopsy of minor salivary gland (focus score of ≥2 based on average of four evaluable lobules)
   C. Evidence of a systemic autoimmune disorder
      1. Elevated titer of rheumatoid factor ≥1:320
      2. Elevated titer of antinuclear antibody ≥1:320
      3. Presence of anti-SS A [Ro] or anti-SS B [La] antibodies

II. Secondary Sjögren's syndrome
   Characteristic signs and symptoms of SS (described above) plus clinical features sufficient to allow a diagnosis of RA, SLE, polymyositis, or scleroderma

III. Exclusions: sarcoidosis, pre-existent lymphoma, acquired immunodeficiency disease, and other known causes of keratitis sicca or salivary gland enlargement

idence of dry eyes, as measured by Schirmer's test (paper strips placed in the lower conjunctival sac) and installation of rose bengal or fluorescein to demonstrate keratoconjunctivitis sicca. Dryness of the mouth is documented by measurement of saliva flow using either a Lashley cup (a suction cup fitting over the opening of Stensen's duct), a sponge placed under the tongue, or simple observation of the decreased weight of a sugarless candy placed in the mouth for 3 minutes. When objective dryness of eyes and mouth is documented, the critical question is whether these problems result from an "autoimmune" attack on the glands. The presence of circulating autoantibodies and a minor salivary gland biopsy with lymphocytic infiltration (described below) indicate SS as the cause of the sicca symptoms. Finally, other disease processes can result in lacrimal and salivary gland swelling and chronic dysfunction (see box, p. 2421). These include sarcoidosis, lymphoma, tuberculosis, and acquired immunodeficiency syndrome (AIDS).

Since there are no uniform diagnostic criteria for SS, the incidence and prevalence vary widely in the literature. Using the stringent criteria listed in the box above, the prevalence of primary SS is roughly 1/2500. The disease affects predominantly women, with a peak onset during the sixth decade of life and a less frequent onset during childhood or the third decade. Secondary SS is more common, since up to 20% of RA patients and up to 30% of SLE patients have significant sicca symptoms.

PATHOGENESIS

The initiating factors in SS remain unknown but genetic and environmental factors are likely to play a role. Among a small number of identical twins studied with first-degree SS, the disease shows concordance in approximately 20%. The failure of the other identical twin to develop SS indicates the important role of extragenetic factors. No single environmental factor has been found as a trigger in SS, but indirect evidence has suggested Epstein-Barr virus (EBV) as a potential cofactor. Recently, a potential role for a retrovirus has been suggested in patients and in animal models of SS.

Salivary glands exhibit focal lymphoid infiltrates (Fig. 305-1, *A*) that are not detected in normal biopsies *(B)*. Antibodies directed against salivary gland cells are not detected in most primary SS patients and immune complexes are not detected at the basement membrane around the blood vessels or salivary gland epithelial cells. Taken together, these results suggest a cell-mediated immune mechanism rather than a humoral mechanism for glandular destruction.

CLINICAL MANIFESTATIONS

The most common ocular symptom is a dry, gritty feeling caused by a decrease in the volume and alteration in the composition of the tear film. Dry mouth is another common complaint and often is accompanied by rampant periodontal problems. Many patients describe difficulty in swallowing food, problems in wearing dentures, change in their sense of taste, burning of the oral mucosa, intolerance of acidic or spicy foods, and inability to speak continuously for more than a few minutes because of dryness. Nutrition may be compromised and sleep disturbed by nocturia resulting from increased fluid intake.

Dryness of the skin has been attributed to a decrease in the secretory capacity of the sebaceous glands in some patients. Oral candidiasis, particularly angular cheilitis, is extremely common in these patients and an important contributing factor in their increased mouth pain and decreased sensation of taste.

Vasculitis in SS patients may present as leukocytoclastic vasculitis or as hypergammaglobulinemic purpura. Periungual telangiectasis may be detected in primary SS patients, but the presence of a large number of lesions suggests an increased chance of later development of scleroderma.

Involvement of exocrine glands in the upper respiratory tract leads to dryness of the nasal passages in approximately 50% of the patients. SS patients may develop pleurisy with and without effusion, and lymphoid interstitial pneumonitis. Mucus plug inspissation associated with bronchospasm and dyspnea is a relatively common problem. This often occurs after upper respiratory tract infection when tenacious secretions cannot be adequately mobilized, or in the postoperative setting. Clinically significant hypothyroidism develops in 10% to 15% of SS patients. Thus endocrine as

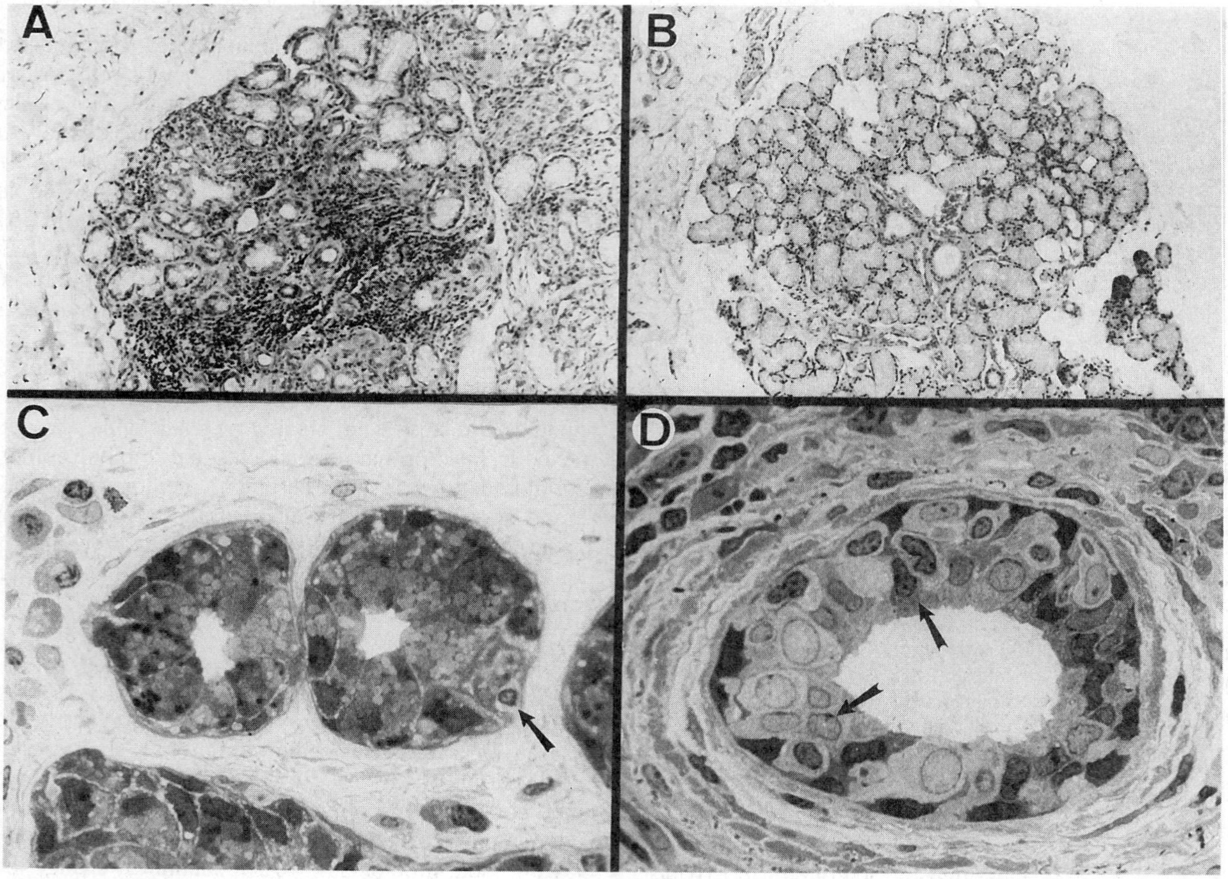

Fig. 305-1. Salivary gland (SG) biopsies from a patient with Sjögren's syndrome (SS) (**A**) and from a normal individual (**B**). **C** and **D** show higher magnification views of acini and ducts from the same SG as in **A**.

well as exocrine glandular cells may be targets for immune attack in primary SS.

The most common functional renal abnormality noted in SS patients is the inability to acidify the urine in response to an administered acid load, such as ammonium chloride. In rare SS patients with interstitial nephritis, hypokalemia may be severe enough to produce paralysis. Glomerulonephritis is uncommon in primary SS patients and generally suggests the development of SLE. However, glomerulonephritis may be associated with mixed cryoglobulemia or amyloidosis in the primary SS patient. SS patients can develop obstructive nephropathy resulting from enlarged lymph nodes, or renovascular hypertension caused by vasculitis.

Hematologic disorders in the primary SS patient include an anemia of chronic disease, iron deficiency related to medications, and occasionally hemolytic anemia. Neutropenia in SS is frequent but rarely reaches a level of clinical significance. An increased frequency of non-Hodgkin's lymphoma, especially involving the salivary glands and cervical lymph nodes, occurs in SS patients. There is no evidence to suggest that other solid tumors are increased in this patient population.

Central nervous system abnormalities, including vasculitis, transverse myelitis, and aseptic meningitis, may occur in primary SS patients in patterns similar to those seen in SLE patients. Peripheral sensory neuropathy affecting the lower extremities is relatively common, particularly in SS patients with hyperglobulinemic purpura. Mononeuritis multiplex caused by vasculitis occurs much less frequently.

LABORATORY FEATURES

SS patients generally have a positive antinuclear antibody (ANA) test because of the presence of anti-SS A and anti-SS B antibodies (see Chapter 293). The SS-A and SS-B antigens are identical to the "Ro" and "La" antigens, respectively. Although a sensitive indicator for SS, anti-SS A antibodies are not specific for SS since they also are present in SLE patients who lack SS symptoms. Anti-SS B antibodies are more consistently associated with sicca symptoms, but approximately half the primary SS patients lack this autoantibody.

Rheumatoid factor (RF) is an autoantibody directed against the Fc portion of IgG. The titers of RF are relatively low (1:320 to 1:640) in most primary SS patients, so a very high titer (>1:10,000) in an SS patient suggests a superimposed problem such as rheumatoid arthritis or a monoclonal RF paraprotein.

Elevated liver function tests are uncommon and, when present, suggest viral hepatitis or toxic side effects of medications. In some patients, SS coexists with biliary cirrhosis, which can be distinguished by antibodies against the mitochondrial enzyme 2-oxoacetic acid dehydrogenase. Finally, elevated liver function tests in some SS patients may result from elevated levels of type II mixed cryoglobulins.

DIFFERENTIAL DIAGNOSIS

Dryness of the eyes and mouth can accompany aging and therefore dryness does not necessarily indicate a disease process. Often, the symptoms of dryness become clinically apparent in the elderly when they take medications with anticholinergic side effects such as tricyclic antidepressants, muscle relaxants, diuretics, cardiac medications, and over-the-counter cold remedies. Also, anxiety can lead to increased symptoms of dryness, since stimulation of the sympathetic nervous system leads to decreased glandular flow. Thus, the vast majority of dry eye patients do not have evidence of an autoimmune disorder and it is important to reassure these individuals that they do not have a systemic disease.

In patients with significant dryness and salivary gland swelling, other processes such as retrovirus (HIV) infection, sarcoidosis, and lymphoma must be considered (see the box). Less common causes of chronic bilateral salivary gland swelling include mycobacterial and fungal infections, amyloidosis, and salivary gland tumors. Suppurative (bacterial) parotitis should be suspected in any patient with a sudden increase in salivary gland size, particularly older patients in the postoperative setting.

Causes of keratitis and salivary gland enlargement other than SS

Keratitis

1. Mucus membrane pemphigoid
2. Sarcoidosis
3. Infections: virus (adenovirus, herpes, vaccinia), bacteria, or chlamydia (i.e., trachoma)
4. Trauma (i.e., after contact lens) and environmental irritants including chemical burns, exposure to ultraviolet lights or roentgen rays
5. Neuropathy including neurotropic keratitis (i.e., damage to fifth cranial nerve) and familial dysautonomia (Rily-Day syndrome)
6. Hypovitaminosis A
7. Erythema multiforme (Stevens-Johnson syndrome)

Salivary gland enlargement

1. Sarcoidosis, amyloidosis
2. Bacterial (including gonococci and syphilis) and viral infections (i.e., infectious mononucleosis, mumps)
3. Tuberculosis, actinomycosis, histoplasmosis, trachoma, leprosy
4. Iodide, lead, or copper hypersensitivity
5. Hyperlipoproteinemia, especially types IV and V
6. Tumors (usually unilateral) including cysts (Warthin's tumor), epithelial (adenoma, adenocarcinoma), lymphoma, and mixed salivary gland tumors
7. Excessive alcohol consumption
8. Human immunodeficiency virus (HIV)

TREATMENT

Dry eyes (keratoconjunctivitis sicca) can range in severity from a mildly annoying complaint to a significant clinical problem that can lead to loss of employment and even blindness. The mainstay of therapy is topical treatment using artificial tears. Artificial tears containing corticosteroids are to be avoided when possible because of the significant complications, including subcapsular cataracts, increased ocular pressure, and risk of infection. A wide variety of artificial tears are commercially available; they differ in their preservatives and viscosity. Artificial tears must be used on a regular basis and their frequency of use increased in response to increased local dry environmental conditions. In some patients, a particular artificial tear may cause a burning sensation in the eyes. This may result from topical irritation caused by the preservative in the artificial tear. The recognition of this problem can lead to the choice of another artificial tear preparation with a different preservative. Also, several types of preservative-free artificial tears have been developed. It is worth emphasizing that SS patients are at increased risk for corneal abrasions during anesthesia, because of the use of anticholinergic agents and the low humidity of the operating room. Therefore, ocular lubricants are recommended for all SS patients during surgery and in the postoperative recovery room.

To help prevent progressive periodontal problems, intensive oral hygiene is required. Topical application of a neutral fluoride may help strengthen dental enamel and retard dental deterioration. A common problem in the SS patient is oral candidiasis, which may reflect the absence of naturally occurring antiyeast substances in saliva. Treatment with topical nystatin or clotrimazole for 4 to 6 weeks may be required to alleviate symptoms and prevent recurrences For arthralgias and myalgias, nonsteroidal antiinflammatory drugs (NSAIDS) may be used, but with particular caution since they may precipitate renal or liver abnormalities. In addition, these agents can provoke esophageal injury in SS patients because they adhere to the drier walls of the esophagus in the absence of the normal salivary flow.

Systemic corticosteroids are generally reserved for life-threatening vasculitis, hemolytic anemia, and pleuropericarditis resistant to NSAIDs. As in SLE patients, other drugs may be used to help lower the dosage of corticosteroids, including hydroxychloroquine and azathioprine. When cyclophosphamide has been necessary for vasculitis, intravenous pulse therapy at 1-3 month intervals is preferred over daily therapy to decrease risk of lymphoma.

REFERENCES

Block K et al: Sjögren's syndrome. Medicine 44:187, 1965.
Fox RI et al: Primary Sjögren's syndrome: clinical and immunopathologic features. Rheum Dis Clin North Am 18:517, 1992.
Itescu S et al: A diffuse infiltrative CD8 lymphocytosis syndrome in human immunodeficiency virus (HIV) infection: a host immune response associated with HLA-DR5. Ann Intern Med 112:3, 1990.
Schmid U, Helbron D, and Lennert K: Development of malignant lymphoma in myoepithelial sialadenitis (Sjögren's syndrome). Virchows Arch 395:11, 1982.
Talal N et al: Extrasalivary gland abnormalities in Sjögren's syndrome. Am J Med 43:50, 1967.

CHAPTER

306 Systemic Lupus Erythematosus

John H. Klippel
John L. Decker

Systemic lupus erythematosus (SLE) is a chronic relapsing and remitting inflammatory disease of unknown etiology. Antibodies reactive with nuclear and cytoplasmic antigens ("autoantibodies") are the hallmark of the disease. No single cause has yet been identified, although genetic, hormonal, and environmental factors are regarded as probable contributors to the altered immune state. The notable pathologic feature of the disease is the deposition of immunoglobulins, presumably in the form of antigen-antibody complexes, and complement along the vascular basement membranes of various target organs. Multiple organs may be affected, most commonly the skin, joints, serosal surfaces, kidneys, heart, lungs, and central nervous system. The modes of presentation and clinical manifestations are protean. The disease course is highly variable, with periods of exacerbations and remissions. Medical therapies are directed at suppression of local tissue inflammation as well as suppression of immune function.

INCIDENCE AND PREVALENCE

Recent epidemiologic studies have found a far greater frequency of disease than was revealed by surveys of previous decades. The incidence of SLE is currently estimated to be 50 to 70 new cases per year per million population with a prevalence of approximately 500 patients per million. It is unlikely that the disease frequency is actually increasing; greater physician awareness of the disease and the ready availability of sensitive serologic tests for diagnosis probably account for the differences.

The prevalence of SLE is markedly increased in several segments of the population. Females, particularly during the reproductive years, are at significantly greater risk than males; the female-to-male sex ratio is about 9:1. Although lupus may develop at any age, the highest incidence is observed in the age group 20 to 40 years. Finally, racial factors appear to be important with increases in the frequency of SLE reported in African Americans, Native Americans, Puerto Ricans, and Chinese.

ETIOLOGY

No single cause for SLE has yet been identified, but genetic, endocrine, and environmental factors are thought to be important. It is generally believed that these factors act synergistically to produce the disease. Moreover, depending on the relative contribution of these various factors, distinct serologic and clinical subsets may be produced.

Genetic factors

The importance of genetic factors is evident by the finding of clinical SLE in approximately one of ten first-degree relatives of SLE patients. Nonspecific immunologic abnormalities such as diffuse hypergammaglobulinemia, antinuclear antibodies, and false-positive tests for syphilis are even more common in otherwise completely asymptomatic relatives. A high degree of disease concordance in monozygotic, but not dizygotic, twin pairs implies a primary genetic, as opposed to environmental, explanation for the observations. Studies of HLA in SLE have found associations with HLA-DR3 and the linked specificities DR2 and DQw1, which confer a relative risk of approximately 3.

Inherited deficiencies of several complement components have been associated with lupuslike illnesses. The most common is a deficiency of the second component of complement (C2); deficiencies of other classic as well as alternate pathway components in patients with SLE have been noted. Some, but not all, are coded by autosomal recessive genes of the sixth chromosome, which are in linkage dysequilibrium with HLA-DRw2. Whether the association of complement deficiencies with SLE results simply from linkage to HLA-D–region genes or an inherent susceptibility induced by the complement deficiency itself is not known.

Environmental factors

Several environmental factors, including ultraviolet light, bacterial and viral infections, and drugs (see Drug-Induced Lupus Syndromes, below) appear to be capable of inducing or exacerbating lupus. It is thought that these may have in common the ability to alter immune function. For instance, the exposure of DNA to ultraviolet light in vitro causes the formation of thymine dimers. This significantly alters the antigenicity of DNA and could result in the formation of DNA antibodies. Similarly, bacterial lipopolysaccharides (potent polyclonal B-cell activators) administered to animals induce the formation of circulating immune complexes and, subsequently, antibodies to both single- and double-stranded DNA. Viruses are postulated to play a major role in both murine and canine models of SLE. Theoretically, the chronic infection of lymphocytes with a virus might account for many of the immunologic aberrations present in SLE. Indirect evidence for a persistent viral infection in SLE includes increases in antibodies to multiple DNA and RNA viruses; the presence of electron-dense paramyxovirus-like cytoplasmic inclusions, so-called tubuloreticular structures, along vascular endothelium and within circulating lymphocytes; and reports of type C oncornaviruses in involved renal and skin tissue. Recent studies have focused mainly on retroviruses. However, attempts to isolate retroviruses from SLE tissues by hybridization and cocultivation techniques have been largely unsuccessful. Thus, the proposed viral etiology of SLE remains an attractive, yet entirely unproved, hypothesis.

Endocrine factors

The disproportionate number of females with SLE and the propensity for the disease to worsen during pregnancy and in the immediate postpartum period underscore a potential harmful role for estrogens. SLE patients demonstrate alterations in sex hormone metabolism—in particular an increased hydroxylation of estrone, which may enhance estrogenic activity. Similarly, the increased frequency of SLE in patients with Klinefelter's syndrome suggests that androgens may serve a protective function. Opposing effects of sex hormones on both humoral and cellular immunity have been described and may eventually explain these clinical observations.

PATHOGENESIS

The regulation of antibody production of B lymphocytes, ordinarily a function of subpopulations of T lymphocytes termed *T-suppressor cells,* appears to be defective in SLE. Whether this results from a primary failure of the B lymphocytes to respond to suppressor signals, from defects in the T-regulatory lymphocytes, or from both is uncertain. The net result in lupus, however, is the development of a state of spontaneous B-lymphocyte hyperactivity with the uncontrolled production of a wide variety of antibodies to both host and exogenous antigens. Although, theoretically, an endless spectrum of antibodies should be produced there is for unexplained reasons some selectivity to the disordered immunity.

Antibodies to nucleic acids and nucleic acid–protein complexes such as the nucleosome made up of DNA and histones predominate. These antibodies are thought to combine with antigens to form circulating antigen-antibody complexes. The immune complexes become deposited in the subendothelial layers of vascular basement membranes of multiple organs. The sites of deposition and pathologic potential of immune complexes in skin, kidney, choroid plexus, or serosal surfaces are dictated in part by physicochemical properties of the antigen or antibody, such as size, charge, molecular configuration, immunoglobulin class, and complement-fixing properties (discussed in detail in Chapter 287). Finally, direct antibody-mediated injury may be associated with some manifestations of lupus, such as hemolytic anemia and thrombocytopenia. Once deposited, the immune complexes initiate a localized inflammatory response involving activation of complement, emigration of neutrophils, the release of kinins and prostaglandins, and, in all likelihood, antibody-dependent cell-mediated tissue injury.

PATHOLOGY

The earliest pathologic events demonstrable in SLE are those of an acute vasculitis. The periarteriolar supporting tissue becomes edematous and infiltrated, first with neutrophils and later with plasma cells and lymphocytes. The persistence of inflammation results in the local deposition of an acellular, homogenous eosinophilic material, histologically similar to fibrin and called *fibrinoid material*. In addition, nuclear debris from cellular necrosis reacts with antinuclear antibodies and coalesces to form intensely basophilic-staining material referred to as hematoxylin bodies.

When examined by indirect immunofluorescence, the vascular lesions can be shown to contain immunoglobulins, presumably complexed with antigen, complement components, and fibrin. These findings can be demonstrated along the basement membrane of skin, serosal surfaces, choroid plexus, pulmonary parenchyma, endocardial vegetations, splenic vessels, and renal glomeruli. Elution studies have revealed the predominant antibodies to be of IgG and IgM classes, directed primarily against DNA.

Involvement of the kidney results in several different forms of renal pathology (detailed in Chapter 354). The most common type is characterized by swelling and proliferation of glomerular, mesangial, endothelial, or epithelial cells (proliferative glomerulonephritis). The vascular tufts become infiltrated with neutrophils and lymphocytes. Adhesions form between the vascular tufts and the parietal layer of Bowman's membrane, leading to epithelial crescents. By electron microscopy, dense deposits can be demonstrated in the mesangium and between endothelial cells and the glomerular basement membrane. Cellular proliferation that is confined to the mesangium is termed *mesangial nephritis*. Proliferative changes of the glomerular capillaries are classified as focal or diffuse nephritis. The distinction between these forms of nephritis is made on the basis of both qualitative and quantitative features.

The other major form of lupus renal involvement is membranous nephritis. This is pathologically indistinguishable from idiopathic membranous disease. When studied by light microscopy, the glomerular basement membrane is uniformly thickened by an eosinophilic material. Thickening of the basement membrane may be accentuated in isolated glomerular tufts to produce a "wire-loop" appearance. By electron microscopy, dense deposits are seen in the subepithelial spaces (see Chapter 354).

There is no adequate explanation for the different types of renal pathology in SLE. It is speculated that physical properties of the immune complexes involved, dynamics of tissue deposition, or genetically determined differences in host reactivity may account for them.

CLINICAL FEATURES

The spectrum of clinical manifestations of SLE ranges from a mild systemic illness with a photosensitive facial rash and transient diffuse arthritis to a fulminant presentation with life-threatening involvement of the heart, lungs, kidneys, or central nervous system. Episodes of disease exacerbations, or flares, are of varying severity and often quite individualized for any particular patient.

The disease course is remarkably unpredictable. Flares of the disease are typically followed by periods of clinical remission. The duration of the cycles in this disease pattern are of various lengths, transitions occurring abruptly, unexpectedly, and without obvious cause. The survival after diagnosis is currently estimated to be greater than 90% at 10 years. The highest mortality is in patients with progressive renal involvement or central nervous system disease. The most frequent causes of death are primary organ failure (renal or central nervous system), infections, and cardiovascular disease.

The nonspecific systemic features of the illness are extremely common and may be striking in severity. Fatigue, anorexia, weight loss, and unexplained fever, occasionally with rigors and night sweats, may suggest the presence of an underlying infection. The increased susceptibility of SLE patients to both common and opportunistic infections demands careful evaluation for occult infectious processes in all patients with febrile systemic presentations.

Mucocutaneous features

The variability of mucocutaneous involvement in SLE is truly astounding. The acute erythematous, maculopapular eruption on the malar region of the face ("butterfly rash") (Fig. 306-1, *A*), arms, and trunk and the chronic scarring lesions of discoid lupus (Fig. 306-1, *B*) are easily recognized. An interesting subset of generalized, nonscarring cutaneous lupus, termed *subacute cutaneous lupus,* appears to be intermediate between these two common forms of lupus skin involvement. Both papulosquamous (psoriasiform) and annular (polycyclic) variants have been described. A broad spectrum of other skin manifestations including bullae, urticaria, verrucae, and angioedema have been noted. Most lupus rashes are worsened by exposure to ultraviolet light.

Superficial vasculitis of dermal vessels produces erythematous, tender areas on the fingertips and palms, splinter hemorrhages of the nailbeds, and periungual infarctions. Livedo reticularis and dependent nonthrombocytopenic purpura often are associated with increased levels of serum cryoglobulins. Peripheral vasomotor instability, often exacerbated by cold exposure or heightened emotions, leads to color changes of fingers and toes that are characteristic of Raynaud's phenomenon. Inflammation in the subcutaneous fat (lupus profundus) can cause extensive skin ulceration and calcifications on healing.

Hair loss results in either diffuse or patchy alopecia. In the absence of scarring of the scalp by discoid lesions, the alopecia generally is entirely reversible. The regrown hair in involved areas is often brittle, with a short, stubby appearance. Superficial ulcerations of oral and genital mucous membranes are typically painless and often go undetected. Deep ulcerations of the soft palate, often infected with *Candida* species, may be quite painful and may limit eating. Ulcerations of the nasal mucosa can lead to epistaxis and perforation of the nasal septum.

Musculoskeletal features

The arthritis of SLE is typically a transient peripheral polyarthritis with symmetric involvement of both small and large joints. In spite of complaints of joint pain, signs of intense joint inflammation with effusions and palpable synovial thickening are infrequent. The joint complaints are rarely chronic and essentially never associated with cartilage loss, subchondral cystic changes, or bony erosions. The development of persistent synovitis in a single joint suggests a superimposed complication such as osteonecrosis or septic arthritis. Periarticular structures, particularly tendon sheaths, may be involved, and can lead to acute rupture of the Achilles or patellar tendons.

Reducible, rheumatoidlike hand deformities with ulnar deviation of the phalanges and flexion and extension abnormalities of the small joints of the fingers develop in about 10% of patients. In contrast to rheumatoid arthritis, bony erosions of the wrist, metacarpal heads, or interphalangeal joints are not present on radiographs. The arthropathy is similar to the hand deformities described after rheumatic fever (Jaccoud's arthritis) and is thought to be caused by capsular and tendon laxity from recurrent chronic inflammation.

The major disabling chronic joint disease of SLE is the arthropathy of osteonecrosis, or avascular necrosis. This complication most commonly affects large weight-bearing joints such as the hips, knees, and ankles. Technetium bone scans and nuclear magnetic resonance imaging studies are sensitive methods of detecting this complication prior to the development of classic late radiographic findings (Fig. 306-2). Osteonecrosis is frequently seen following the use of high-dose corticosteroids; however, corticosteroids are not an essential requirement. Osteonecrosis may produce significant pain and disability, and orthopedic surgery with total joint replacement may be necessary.

Serositis

Inflammation of serosal surfaces leads to sterile pleuritis, pericarditis, or peritonitis. The pain produced is often very severe and may suggest myocardial infarction, pulmonary embolus, or acute abdominal crisis. Fluid accumulation is usually modest, although occasionally pericardial tamponade or massive ascites develops. Analysis of the fluid in patients with chronic serositis is necessary to exclude an underlying infection. Typically, the fluid has a white cell count of less than 3000 cells per cubic millimeter (predominantly monocytes and lymphocytes); reduced levels of complement as compared with serum levels; and, often, the finding of LE cells formed in vivo.

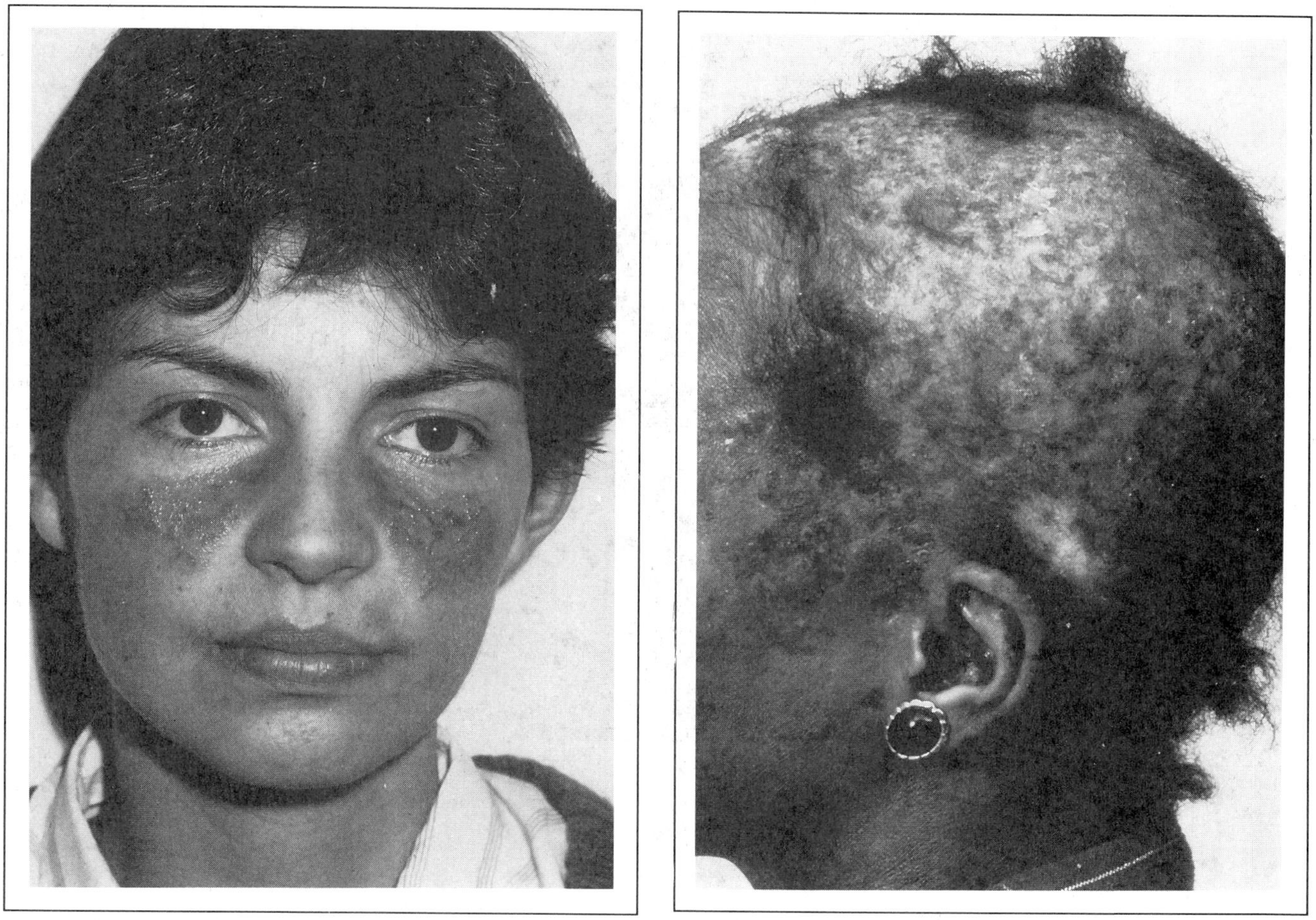

A B

Fig. 306-1. A, Erythematous malar ("butterfly") rash in patient with SLE. **B,** Scarring discoid rash of the scalp with extensive alopecia in patient with SLE. (From Dieppe PA et al, editors: Atlas of Clinical Rheumatology. London, 1986, Gower Medical.)

Cardiac features

An inflammatory process involving the myocardium can produce persistent tachycardia, ventricular arrhythmias, conduction abnormalities, and, occasionally, intractable congestive heart failure. It is often associated with a more generalized peripheral inflammatory myopathy. Chemistry studies reveal increased levels of muscle enzymes, particularly the MB isoenzyme of creatine phosphokinase.

Ischemic heart disease from coronary arteritis or, more commonly, atherosclerotic coronary disease may produce angina or myocardial infarction. Patients with severe nephrosis or those treated with prolonged courses of corticosteroids are at increased risk for atherosclerosis. Noninfectious vegetations of the ventricular surface of valvular leaflets (Libman-Sacks endocarditis) may develop on the mitral, aortic, and tricuspid valves. These endocardial lesions may produce valvular regurgitation and require valve replacement. The vegetations are a potential nidus of superimposed bacterial infection. In addition, endocardial fragments may break off to produce arterial emboli.

Pulmonary features

Although pulmonary function studies reveal minor diffusion and obstruction abnormalities in a high proportion of patients, clinical problems secondary to pulmonary involvement in SLE are distinctly unusual. Transient basilar pneumonic infiltrates ("lupus pneumonitis") with nonproductive cough, hypoxemia, and complaints of dyspnea must be distinguished from infection. Alveolar hemorrhage producing rapid obliteration of the lung fields may develop acutely, resulting in massive hemoptysis. Pulmonary hypertension is a rare complication also associated with an increased mortality.

Gastrointestinal symptoms

Abdominal complaints, typically from peritonitis, are frequent. Acute and chronic pancreatitis may develop secondary to active lupus or as a complication of drug therapy. Hepatic involvement is distinctly unusual. Hepatitis, when found, is typically secondary to the use of salicylates or other nonsteroidal drugs, fatty infiltration from corticosteroids, or other non-SLE-related causes. Primary biliary cir-

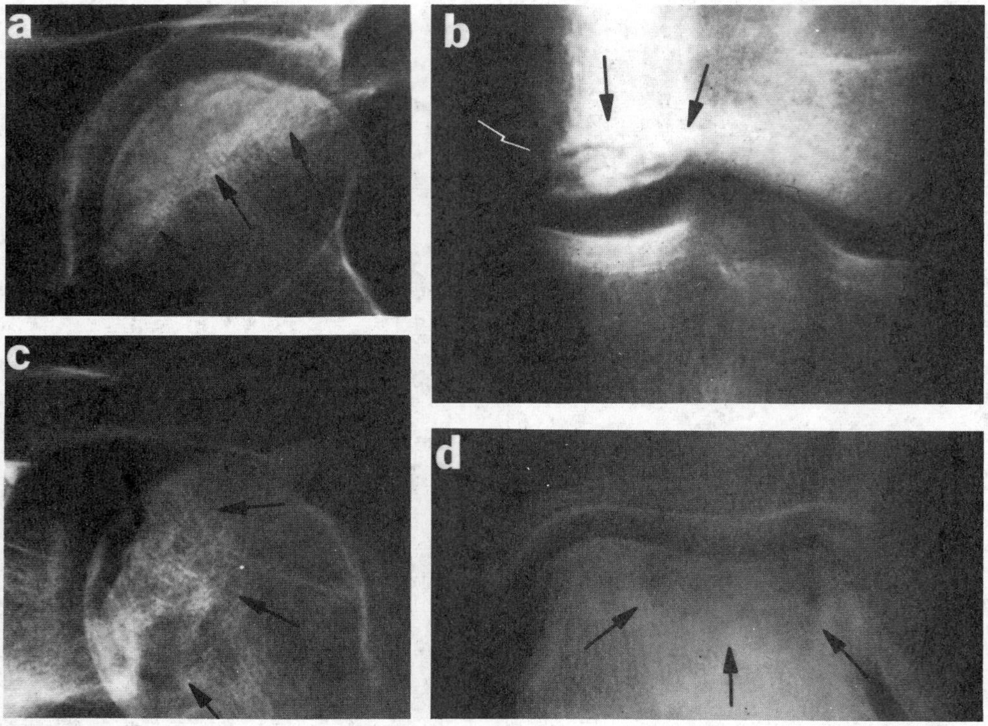

Fig. 306-2. Osteonecrosis of (**a**) femoral head, (**b**) medial femoral condyle, (**c**) humeral head, and (**d**) superior talus. The margins of the necrotic segment undergo sclerotic change *(arrows)*.

rhosis has been reported to be increased in lupus patients. Vasculitis of the mesentery and intra-abdominal organs may lead to acute abdominal crises requiring surgical exploration. Infarction and perforation of the bowel or viscera are associated with a high mortality.

Renal features

Active glomerulonephritis can be detected on urinalysis by the finding of red cells, white cells, and granular and red blood cell casts in the urine sediment. Proteinuria may lead to the nephrotic syndrome. The course of renal disease is highly unpredictable. Although progression is often associated with persistent clinical or serologic abnormalities, exceptions are sufficiently common to make these abnormalities unreliable monitors of renal inflammation. Loss of renal function may be acute, similar to that of rapidly progressive glomerulonephritis, or, more typically, chronic with a slowly progressive rise of serum creatinine over the course of many years. End-stage renal failure can be successfully managed with dialysis or transplantation.

The role of renal biopsy in the clinical management of SLE is controversial. By electron microscopy, virtually all patients have evidence of immune-mediated glomerulonephritis. Pathologic classification of light microscopy findings on renal biopsy are based on the extent and distribution of proliferative changes and membranous disease (see Chapter 354). These characteristics provide some estimate of renal outcome. Biopsy findings of mesangial nephritis are generally associated with a relatively benign future course, whereas diffuse proliferative or membranoproliferative nephritis indicates a much less favorable renal outcome. Recent studies have shown that individual so-called chronic biopsy features such as glomerular sclerosis, fibrous crescents, interstitial fibrosis, and tubular atrophy predict a poor outcome.

Neuropsychiatric features

Various forms of neurologic and psychiatric manifestations may develop. The most common abnormalities are disturbances of mental function. These range from states of mild confusion, with memory deficits and impairments of orientation and perception, to frank psychiatric disturbances of hypomania, delirium, and schizophrenia. Patients may become aphasic or lapse into unexplained coma. Seizures may be the presenting manifestation of SLE and may long antedate multisystem disease. These are usually of the grand mal type, although petit mal, focal, and temporal lobe epilepsy have been described. Severe headaches, often with scotomata typical of the fortification spectra of migraine, are increased in lupus patients. The sequelae of cerebrovascular accidents from hemorrhage or cerebral infarction are major causes of morbidity and mortality. Less common neurologic disturbances include cranial neuropathies, transverse myelopathy, aseptic meningitis, pseudotumor cerebri, chorea, hemiballismus, a parkinsonian picture, and both sensory and motor peripheral neuropathies.

Before attributing signs and symptoms of central nervous system dysfunction to active lupus it is important to consider other causes for the observed abnormality. Infections (meningitis, intracranial abscess); renal failure (azotemia, hypertension); drug effects (corticosteroids, antimalarials, anticonvulsants); mass lesions (tumors, subdural hematoma); structural defects (hydrocephalus, aneurysms); and arterial emboli from endocardial vegetations can all mimic CNS lupus.

Conventional studies done to evaluate the central nervous system are often of limited value in the assessment of patients. The cerebrospinal fluid may show mild elevations of protein and IgG, oligoclonal bands on electrophoresis, and pleocytosis, usually lymphocytes. On the other hand, the fluid is often normal, even in the presence of major clinical dysfunction. The electroencephalogram may be normal or show local or diffuse changes. Arteriographic studies rarely demonstrate evidence of vasculitis of small or large vessels. Abnormalities of static pertechnetate brain scans, computed tomography, and magnetic resonance imaging have been reported.

Pregnancy

Pregnant lupus patients are at increased risk of disease flares during the pregnancy, as well as in the immediate postpartum period, and need to be followed closely. In general, it is recommended that pregnancy be avoided during periods of disease activity involving major organs, particularly nephritis. Premature delivery, fetal wastage, and spontaneous abortion are all increased in systemic lupus. These complications are increased in mothers with high titers of anticardiolipin antibodies. The passive transfer of maternal antibodies across the placenta can produce transient abnormalities in the newborn (e.g., hepatosplenomegaly, cytopenias, and photosensitive rashes), which resolve as antibody titers decline. Congenital heart block and other cardiac abnormalities are increased, particularly in infants born of mothers with antibodies to Ro(SS-A) (see Chapter 293).

Lymphadenopathy

Enlargement of peripheral and axial lymph nodes and splenomegaly occur, but are usually transient. Biopsy of lymph nodes demonstrates hyperplasia with preservation of the normal architecture. Patients with SLE may be at increased risk of development of lymphoma, particularly if there is associated secondary Sjögren's syndrome.

LABORATORY FINDINGS

SLE patients display a host of serologic, chemical, and hematologic abnormalities reflecting the multisystem nature of the disease. Hematologic abnormalities occur frequently. Moderate anemia with normocytic, normochromic erythrocyte indices is a consistent feature. Although a positive Coombs test can be demonstrated in many patients, anemia from actual hemolysis is infrequent. Leukopenia, particularly lymphocytopenia, is common and often accurately reflects disease activity. Thrombocytopenia is usually low grade; counts of 50,000 to 100,000 per cubic millimeter are the rule. Lower platelet counts may be associated with bleeding and are an indication for aggressive treatment. Bone marrow aspirates are generally normal or hypercellular. Cellular destruction within the marrow may lead to the phagocytosis of nuclear debris and the formation of in vivo LE cells.

Prolongation of the partial thromboplastin time results from antiphospholipid antibodies, which inhibit activation of prothrombin. False-positive serologic tests for syphilis are commonly seen in these patients as a result of cross-reactivity of the antibody with other phospholipids. Paradoxically, these patients with the so-called lupus anticoagulant have an increased incidence of venous and arterial thromboses rather than bleeding. Other antibodies against coagulation factors VIII, IX, XI, and XII have been described.

The most distinctive laboratory feature of SLE is the development of antibodies to host antigens, especially to nuclear antigens, including single- and double-stranded DNA, nuclear histones, and specific soluble ribonuclear protein antigens, notably the antigen Sm. Antinuclear antibodies act as opsonins for nuclear antigens and are responsible for the LE cell. Routine screening studies to detect these antibodies use indirect immunofluorescent assays of cultured cell lines, fixed tissue sections, or the haemoflagellate *Crithidia luciliae*. Different specificities produce distinct patterns of immunofluorescence, commonly referred to as *homogeneous, speckled, nucleolar,* or *rim patterns* (see Chapter 293). Sera from SLE patients are capable of producing all patterns, although the rim pattern, produced by antibodies to double-stranded DNA, is the most specific for the disease. Antinuclear antibodies may produce a false-positive beaded pattern in the fluorescent treponemal antibody (FTA) assay.

The antigen specificities of many of the antinuclear antibodies found in lupus patients have been identified and assays developed to directly measure these antibodies (Table 306-1). Antibody to double-stranded DNA is commonly used to monitor the disease, particularly in patients with lupus nephritis. Antibodies to ribonuclear protein antigens are of interest; antibodies to the Sm (Smith) antigen are essentially diagnostic of lupus; antibodies to U1-RNP, Ro (SS-A), and La (SS-B) are characteristically seen in lupus overlap syndromes.

Serum levels of complement proteins generally are reduced, particularly during states of active disease. Reductions occur as a result of consumption of classic and alternate pathway components at the tissue sites of immune complex deposition and as a result of impaired synthesis. Levels of total hemolytic complement (CH_{50}), C3, and C4 often are used as monitors of disease activity. Persistent and markedly reduced levels of CH_{50} should suggest the possible presence of an inherited complement deficiency, most commonly a deficiency of C2 (see Chapter 228).

Nonspecific elevations in levels of immunoglobulins,

Table 306-1. Antibodies to nuclear antigens in SLE

Antibody specificity	% SLE patients with antibody	Clinical association
1. DNA		
Double-stranded	60	Highly specific. Titers parallel disease activity, particularly lupus nephritis
Single-stranded	60	Nonspecific, present in many other rheumatic diseases
2. Histones	70	Higher frequencies (90%) in patients with drug-induced forms of lupus
3. Ribonucleoproteins		
Sm	30	Found only in SLE (diagnostic)
U1 RNP	40	Common in lupus "overlap" syndromes
Ro (SS-A)	30	Common in lupus with Sjögren's syndrome or subacute cutaneous lupus. Related to neonatal lupus and congenital heart block
La (SS-B)	15	Common in lupus with Sjögren's syndrome
Ribosomal P	5	Associated with lupus psychosis

particularly IgG and IgM, are frequent. It is of interest that an actual deficiency of IgA appears to be more common in SLE than in normal persons. Monoclonal gammopathies occasionally have been described. Marked increases in gammaglobulins may result in a hyperviscosity syndrome or renal tubular acidosis. Serum cryoglobulins of the mixed IgG-IgM type are often found in patients with Raynaud's phenomenon, purpura, or renal involvement and hypocomplementemia. The finding of complement proteins in the cryoglobulins suggests that the antibodies may be precipitated complexed to antigens.

DIAGNOSIS

The diagnosis of SLE poses little problem if the clinical features are classic and evolve over a brief time period. The documentation of serologic abnormalities such as positive LE cells, positive antinuclear antibodies, antibodies to native DNA, and hypocomplementemia serves to confirm the clinical diagnosis. Frequently, however, clinical presentations are atypical or occur so sporadically as to make diagnosis quite difficult. Furthermore, the finding of serologic abnormalities in low titers, often with absent or nonspecific symptoms, further confuses diagnostic efforts. Under these circumstances, extended careful observation, often for months or years, is required before the diagnosis can be made with certainty.

Classification criteria for SLE have been proposed (Table 306-2). Although these criteria were developed principally for research studies and not for diagnostic purposes, any combination of four or more criteria over any time period has been found to be a sensitive and specific means of identifying patients with SLE. The high specificity of select laboratory studies such as antibodies to double-stranded DNA, antibodies to the ribonuclear protein antigen Sm, or hypocomplementemia in the setting of multisystem disease makes these serologic studies valuable in diagnosis.

TREATMENT

Patients should be educated as to the chronic and unpredictable nature of the illness and the need for periodic, routine evaluations to monitor the course of the disease. Factors associated with disease exacerbations, particularly ultraviolet light exposure and physical and emotional stresses, need to be identified and, if possible, minimized. Hypertension and infections, two complications prevalent in SLE patients, need to be aggressively treated. Female patients should be counseled concerning the importance of birth control and the potential adverse effects of pregnancy on the fetus and propensity for SLE exacerbation.

The drug treatment of SLE is largely empiric and is derived from current management concepts for an immune-mediated inflammatory condition. The concept of disease activity, which considers the type and severity of organ involvement, serves to guide therapy.

Moderate doses of salicylates (2.4 to 3.6 g daily) are of-

Table 306-2. The 1982 revised criteria for the classification of systemic lupus erythematosus

Criterion	Frequency in SLE (%)
1. Malar rash	57
2. Discoid rash	18
3. Photosensitivity	43
4. Oral or nasopharyngeal ulcers	27
5. Nonerosive arthritis	86
6. Pleuritis or	52
pericarditis	18
7. Persistent proteinuria or	50
urinary casts	36
8. Seizures or	12
psychosis	13
9. Hemolytic anemia or	18
leukopenia ($<4000/mm^3$) or	46
lymphopenia ($<1500/mm^3$) or	—
thrombocytopenia ($<100{,}000/mm^3$)	21
10. LE cells or	73
DNA antibody or	67
Sm antibody or	31
serologic test for syphilis	15
11. Antinuclear antibody	99

Tan E et al: Arthritis Rheum 25:1271, 1982.

ten used to treat musculoskeletal and other systemic features of the disease such as fever and mild pleurisy. These doses are generally well tolerated and produce minimal gastrointestinal disturbance. Interestingly, patients with lupus treated with salicylates (or other nonsteroidal drugs) seem prone to the development of hepatitis, with increases in SGOT and SGPT, as well as transient impairments of renal function. These two complications are readily reversible on discontinuing the drug.

Nonsteroidal anti-inflammatory drugs (NSAIDs) such as indomethacin, ibuprofen, naproxen, tolmetin, and fenoprofen should be considered as alternatives to salicylates. There is no evidence, however, that any of these drugs are actually superior to salicylates in treating symptoms produced by mild inflammation. Moreover, these drugs may have adverse side effects, including skin rashes, impairment of renal function, and aseptic meningitis, which can easily be confused with active lupus.

Adrenal corticosteroids should be reserved for patients with mild disease that is not responsive to salicylates or other NSAIDs or for patients with particularly severe disease. Daily corticosteroids, occasionally necessary in divided doses to suppress severe inflammatory states, are generally superior to alternate-day regimens. Manifestations such as fever, fatigue, polyarthritis, or serositis typically respond to treatment with low doses, 10 to 20 mg of prednisone daily. Severe and often life-threatening manifestations such as pericarditis, myocarditis, hemolytic anemia, thrombocytopenia, acute glomerulonephritis, and central nervous system disease are indications for higher doses (60 mg prednisone daily, or more). Bolus intravenous methylprednisolone (1 g or 15 mg/kg) offers an alternative to conventional high-dose oral corticosteroids in the treatment of acute, severe SLE.

The adrenal corticosteroid dosage should be kept constant until the inflammatory state is well under control. However, the numerous complications of corticosteroid vary directly with dosage and the duration of administration. Thus, a cautious reduction in corticosteroids, once inflammation has subsided, is critical in the prevention of corticosteroid toxicity. Patients who fail to respond to high-dose corticosteroids, relapse with dose reduction, or develop unacceptable toxicities are candidates for alternate forms of therapy. Topical or intralesional corticosteroids may be used in managing cutaneous disease.

The antimalarial drugs chloroquine, hydroxychloroquine, and quinacrine have a definite adjunctive role in the treatment of the mild systemic features of SLE, especially SLE with mucocutaneous manifestations. The mechanisms of action of this class of drug in SLE are unknown. The daily dose of antimalarials should not exceed 250 mg chloroquine, 400 mg hydroxychloroquine, or 100 mg quinacrine. At these doses, the risk of retinal toxicity is quite small; however, as a precaution, eye examinations for disturbances in color vision and retinal changes should be performed every 6 to 12 months during antimalarial drug treatment. Additional complications of antimalarial drugs include rashes, photosensitivity, and pigmentary changes of skin, mucous membranes, and hair.

Some manifestations of SLE are best treated with specific attention to the complication at hand and not directed to the underlying lupus. For instance, the initial therapy of seizure disorders should be with anticonvulsant medications. Similarly, hematologic cytopenias unresponsive to a trial of corticosteroids often are reversed by splenectomy.

Therapies directed at the suppression of the immune system are used in patients with life-threatening manifestations including lupus nephritis, central nervous system involvement, or hematologic complications such as thrombocytopenia or hemolytic anemia. Most commonly these approaches involve the use of cytotoxic or antimetabolite drugs such as cyclophosphamide (a nitrogen mustard alkylating agent) or azathioprine (a purine analogue). These drugs have been best studied in lupus nephritis and, in long-term controlled trials, have been shown to preserve renal function and reduce the likelihood of end-stage renal failure. Side effects of these drugs are potentially serious and it is recommended that they only be administered by physicians experienced in the use of these agents.

DRUG-INDUCED LUPUS SYNDROMES

A number of structurally diverse drugs (see box below) are capable of producing serologic abnormalities and, less frequently, clinical syndromes resembling SLE. Two drugs in particular, procainamide and hydralazine, are extremely potent inducers of antinuclear, antierythrocyte, and antilymphocyte antibodies. Approximately 60% of patients receiving these drugs develop such antibodies. The antibodies themselves appear to be harmless and do not necessitate

Drugs capable of producing serologic and clinical features of systemic lupus erythematosus

- Antihypertensive
  - Hydralazine
  - Methyldopa
- Antiarrhythmics
  - Procainamide
  - Practolol
- Anticonvulsants
  - Phenytoin
  - Mephenytoin trimethadione
  - Ethosuximide
  - Primidone
- Miscellaneous
  - Isoniazid
  - Penicillamine
  - Chlorpromazine
  - Propylthiouracil
  - Methylthiouracil
  - Chlorthalidone
  - Sulfonamides
  - Penicillin
  - Chlorprothixene

drug withdrawal. High antibody titers may persist for months without the development of any clinical symptom. Furthermore, antibody titers usually remain elevated for months and years, even after the drugs have been discontinued. However, in a small percentage of patients who develop the antibodies, a clinical syndrome with a predominance of pulmonary and polyserositic symptoms that resembles SLE may develop. Renal and neurologic disease are distinctly uncommon. The clinical syndrome is generally reversible on discontinuing the suspected medication although anti-inflammatory drugs, including corticosteroids, may be required to treat symptoms.

The pathologic mechanisms whereby drugs induce autoantibodies are unknown. The rate of drug metabolism, host genetic factors, and drug influences on immune regulation are considered to play a role in pathogenesis. It is of interest that the lupus-inducing drugs do not appear to exacerbate idiopathic SLE and thus can be used safely and as needed.

REFERENCES

Alarcón-Segovia D et al: Antiphospholipid antibodies and the antiphospholipid syndrome in systemic lupus erythematosus. A prospective analysis of 500 consecutive patients. Medicine 168:353, 1989.

The Canadian Hydroxychloroquine Study Group: A randomized study of the effect of withdrawing hydroxychloroquine sulfate in systemic lupus erythematosus. N Engl J Med 324:150, 1991.

Klippel JH: Systemic lupus erythematosus: treatment-related complications superimposed on chronic disease. JAMA 263:1812, 1990.

Lahita RG, editor: Systemic lupus erythematosus. New York, 1992, Churchhill Livingstone.

McLaughlin J et al: Kidney biopsy in systemic lupus erythematosus. II. Survival analysis according to biopsy results. Arthritis Rheum 34:1268, 1991.

Nossent HC et al: Systemic lupus erythematosus after renal transplantation: patient and graft survival and disease activity. Ann Intern Med 114:183, 1991.

Sibley JT et al: The incidence and prognosis of central nervous system disease in SLE. J Rheumatol 19:47, 1992.

Wallace DJ and Hahn BH, editors: Dubois' lupus erythematosus. Philadelphia, 1992, Lea & Febiger.

CHAPTER

307 Vasculitic Syndromes

Gene G. Hunder
J.T. Lie

This category includes a broad spectrum of diseases marked by inflammatory lesions of blood vessels. The inflammation produces variable injury or necrosis of the blood vessel wall that may result in narrowing, occlusion, or thrombosis of the lumen, or the formation of aneurysms or rupture.

The clinical course may be brief and self-limited or prolonged, progressive, and fatal. Arteries and veins of all sizes may be involved, leading to a great variety of symptoms and findings. The inflammatory lesions tend to be focal and scattered along the courses of vessels, but in some instances longer segments may be affected. Vasculitis occurs as a primary disease process or as a secondary manifestation of another disease, such as rheumatoid arthritis. Some forms of vasculitis occur infrequently, but in the aggregate, the vasculitides are not rare and are likely to be seen by most physicians.

Etiologies and disease mechanisms are not understood in most instances. These factors, plus the marked variability of cases of the same disease, have made it difficult to formulate criteria for a satisfactory classification of vasculitis. In addition, it appears that an etiologic classification (once etiologies are better known) will not simply define a set of clinical features including involved blood vessels and affected organs. This is suggested by the observation that one suspected etiologic agent, the hepatitis B virus (HBsAG), is related to at least two different vasculitic syndromes, polyarteritis nodosa and mixed cryoglobulinemia.

A classification that helps to understand the clinical manifestations of these diseases is simply to group them according to the predominant size of vessels involved. In such a scheme, three or four broad categories can be made. The categories include large arteries (aorta and its primary branches), large and medium-sized arteries, muscular arteries (medium-sized and small, grouped or separated), and small vessels (arterioles, capillaries, venules) (Table 307-1). This framework is used in this chapter to discuss specific clinical syndromes. It should be emphasized that clinical and morphologic distinctions frequently are blurred and that cases with overlapping features are often observed. Pathologic processes seldom stop abruptly when a certain caliber of blood vessel is reached! Infective arteritis (e.g., syphilitic, tuberculous, bacterial, and viral) and Buerger's disease (thromboangiitis obliterans) should be kept in mind when considering the differential diagnosis, but they are not discussed here.

PATHOGENESIS

Immunopathogenetic mechanisms, especially the deposition of circulating immune complexes, are considered directly or indirectly responsible for many forms of vasculitis. It is also possible, however, that circulating immune complexes in certain of the vasculitides are secondary or epiphenomena related to some other primary underlying mechanism of tissue damage and vascular injury. In most instances the composition of the putative immune complexes is unknown, and the frequency of their detection is variable. However, in some cases (as noted above) HBsAg and immunoglobulins have been identified in the arterial wall in an area of inflammation, along with the presence of circulating viral-antibody complexes and decreased serum complement. This combination of findings is strong evidence of an immune complex pathogenesis. Other viral infections, such as cytomegalovirus, infectious mononucleosis, and human immunodeficiency virus, have also been associated with vasculitis that may be caused by immune

Table 307-1. Classification of vasculitic syndromes

Clinical syndrome	Predominant vessels affected
Takayasu arteritis	Large arteries (aorta and primary branches)
Giant-cell (temporal) arteritis	Large and medium-sized arteries (aorta, primary and secondary branches)
Thromboangiitis obliterans (Buerger's disease)	Medium-sized and small muscular arteries (diverse distributions and locations)
Kawasaki disease	
Polyarteritis nodosa	
Allergic angiitis and granulomatosis (Churg-Strauss syndrome)	
Vasculitis in rheumatic disease (e.g., rheumatoid arthritis, Behçet's syndrome)	
Granulomatous angiitis of CNS	
Wegener granulomatosis	
Vasculitis associated with malignancy (e.g., hairy-cell leukemia)	
Hypersensitivity vasculitis (e.g., serum sickness, drug reactions)	Small vessels (arterioles, capillaries, venules)
Henoch-Schönlein purpura	
Mixed cryoglobulinemia	
Hypocomplementemic urticarial vasculitis	
Cutaneous vasculitis associated with other diseases (e.g., biliary cirrhosis, ulcerative colitis)	

complex mechanisms. Occasionally, herpes zoster ophthalmicus is followed by acute contralateral hemiparesis caused by direct invasion of the regional arteries rather than by a circulating immune complex-mediated process. Polyarteritis nodosa has been reported in patients with neoplasms in whom immune complexes composed of antibodies and tumor antigens may be important. Reports of vasculitis associated with congenital complement deficiency and alpha-1 antitrypsin deficiency suggest that the lack of certain components and enzyme inhibitors may in some way predispose patients to the development of arteritis. Polyarteritis nodosa has been observed in drug abusers, particularly users of amphetamines. Some of these patients may also have had HBsAg involvement.

In other diseases with lymphocytic or granulomatous inflammatory infiltrations, such as Takayasu arteritis, giant-cell arteritis, and Wegener granulomatosis, cell-mediated immune processes are likely to be operative.

TAKAYASU ARTERITIS (AORTIC ARCH SYNDROME)

Takayasu arteritis is a chronic vasculitis that affects the aorta and its primary branches. The onset is usually between the ages of 20 and 40 years, and it tends to be gradually progressive over subsequent years. Eighty percent to 90% of cases are in women. The highest incidence appears to be in the Orient, especially Japan. Many patients also have been reported from Mexico and India. The incidence rate in Caucasians in the United States has been estimated at 2.6 per million per year.

The etiology is unknown. An occasional association with disorders such as rheumatoid arthritis, ankylosing spondylitis, and ulcerative colitis has raised the question about a possible autoimmune process.

Pathology

Diffuse or patchy involvement of the aorta and its branches in the trunk, neck, and proximal extremities occurs. Although stenosis predominates, aneuryms occur in 20% of patients. The aortic valve and coronary ostia are affected in some cases. The pulmonary artery and branches may be affected.

Early histopathologic changes are observed predominantly in the adventitia and outer media. Later, a granulomatous panarteritis may develop with infiltration by lymphocytes, plasma cells, histiocytes, and variable numbers of polymorphonuclear leukocytes and multinucleated giant cells (Fig. 307-1). Elastic fibers and smooth muscles in the media undergo fragmentation and necrosis, and lymphocytes collect around the vasa vasorum. Extensive transmural fibrosis and dissipation of the inflammatory cell infiltrate signify the end-stage lesions. The thickened intima and the contraction of the fibrotic media and adventitia cause narrowing or obliteration of the arterial lumen. Formation of aneurysms and arterial dissection, with or without rupture, may also complicate Takayasu arteritis.

Clinical features

Involvement may be limited to a portion of the aorta and its branches, but most cases show more generalized involvement. In the early phase (prepulseless phase), nonlocalizing systemic symptoms include low-grade fever, arthralgias, or mild synovitis. Later, diminished pulses and/or bruits are found over large arteries (pulseless phase). The upper extremities become cool, and claudication or ischemic ulcers may develop. Collateral circulation may be noted about the shoulders or elsewhere, and narrowing of the aorta or renal arteries may cause hypertension. Blood pressure is sometimes difficult to assess because of arterial narrowing.

In advanced cases the arterial insufficiency may cause atrophy and ulcerations of the skin over the face and scalp, loss of hair and/or teeth, dementia, syncope, and diminished vision secondary to decreased cerebral blood flow, abdominal angina, and myocardial ischemia.

Laboratory tests

In the active phase of the disease, the erythrocyte sedimentation rate is increased, and moderate anemia is common. Serum gamma globulins are frequently increased. Chest ra-

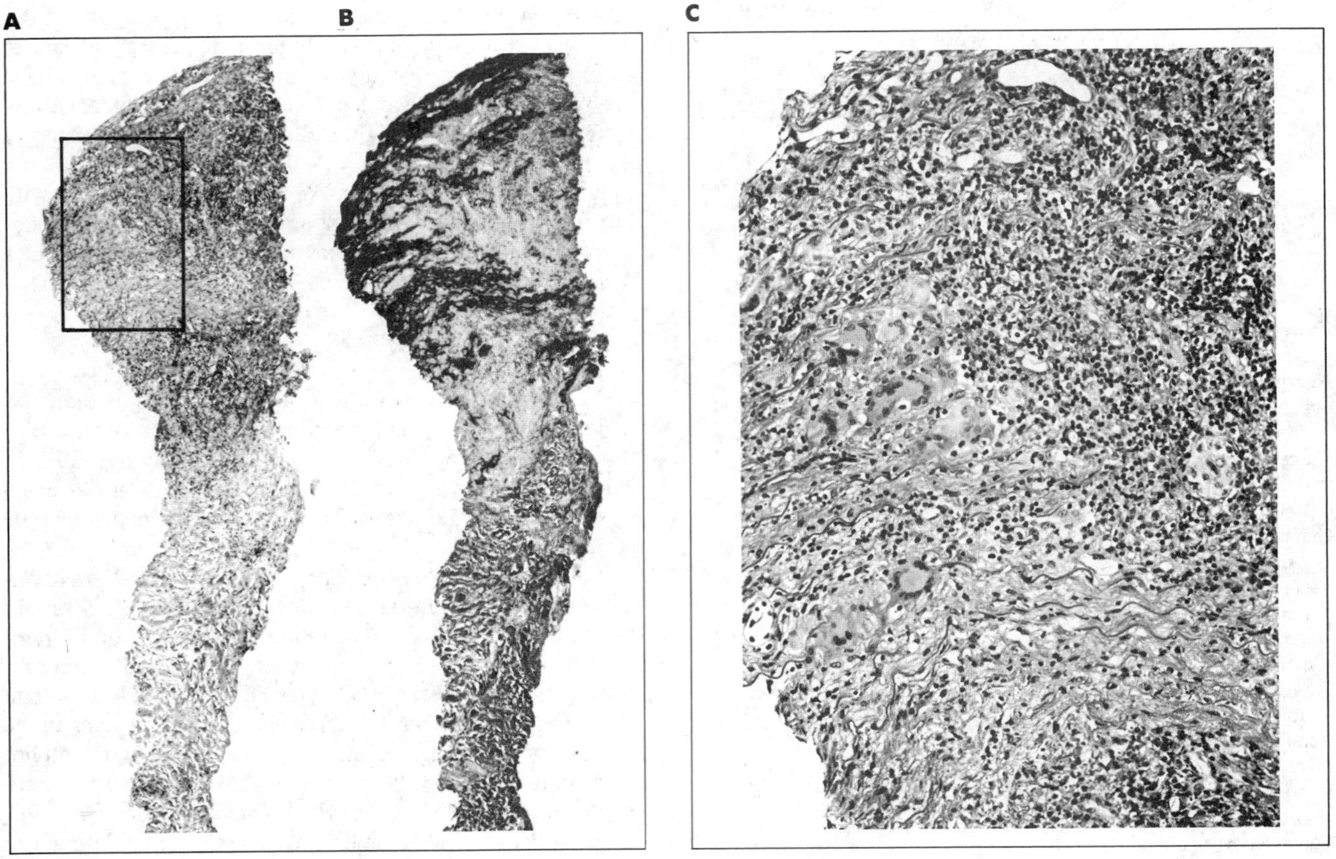

Fig. 307-1. Photomicrographs of biopsy of an aorta in Takayasu arteritis. **A** and **B,** Low-magnification views of granulomatous giant-cell aortitis involving the media with focal disruption of the elastic laminae. **C,** High-magnification view of the boxed area in **A,** showing a cluster of multinucleated giant cells within the predominantly lymphoplasmacytic inflammatory infiltrate. (Hematoxylin and eosin stain; A ×40, C ×160. Elastic stain; B ×40.)

diographs may show widening or irregularity of the aorta, and electrocardiographic changes of hypertension may be evident.

Diagnosis

Recognition of Takayasu arteritis depends on detecting bruits or decreased pulses over large arteries, and the diagnosis is confirmed by arteriography. Arteriograms show focal or lengthy narrowed vascular segments with smooth tapered walls and other areas of dilation in the aorta and branches. Involved arteries are generally too large to biopsy without risk of creating further vascular insufficiency, but any part of the lesion excised at the time of attempted surgical bypass should be examined for histologic confirmation of the disease (see Fig. 307-1).

Treatment

In the early part of the disease, adrenocorticosteroids suppress the systemic symptoms and may arrest the progression of arterial narrowing. After fibrotic changes or thrombi have developed, the response to corticosteroids is diminished. An initial daily dose of 45 to 60 mg prednisone, or an equivalent dose of a similar steroid, may be administered. Once the laboratory tests have reverted to normal and pulses have improved to the maximum, the corticosteroid dose can be reduced to the lowest amount that suppresses the inflammatory components of the disease. In late cases with ischemic symptoms not responding to corticosteroids, arterial bypass grafts or balloon dilation may be considered. Five-year survival was over 90% in one series of 32 North American patients.

POLYMYALGIA RHEUMATICA AND GIANT-CELL ARTERITIS

Etiology and incidence

Polymyalgia rheumatica is a syndrome that affects persons 50 years of age and older. It is characterized by the presence of aching and stiffness in the proximal extremities and torso together with evidence of a systemic process. The aching may be the result of inflammation of the synovial membranes of the proximal joints, tendons, and bursae and ligamentous structures. Giant-cell arteritis is a vasculitis that generally involves the arteries of the head and neck. It is also referred to as *temporal arteritis, cranial arteritis,* or *granulomatous arteritis*. Polymyalgia rheumatica and giant-cell arteritis are closely related to each other because they occur in the same patient population and often in the same person.

Polymyalgia rheumatica and giant-cell arteritis are relatively common, at least in Europe and the United States. In Minnesota a prevalence of active and remitted giant-cell arteritis of 223 per 100,000 population 50 years of age and older was found. A similar study on polymyalgia rheumatica in the same population showed a prevalence of 500 cases per 100,000 population, including active and remitted patients.

Pathology

In polymyalgia rheumatica, a mild lymphocytic synovitis has been found on biopsies of the knees, sternoclavicular joints, and shoulders. In giant-cell arteritis, granulomatous inflammatory infiltrates are found most often in vessels that originate from the arch of the aorta, but almost any artery of the body may be affected (Fig. 307-2). The arteries often are affected in a segmental or patchy fashion. Histopathologically, histiocytes, giant cells, monocytes, and lymphocytes are seen infiltrating the vessel walls. Lymphocytes are mainly T cells, and the majority are of the helper-inducer subset.

Clinical and laboratory findings

The mean age at onset of polymyalgia rheumatica and giant-cell arteritis is approximately 70 years. Constitutional symptoms are present in the majority of patients. In polymyalgia rheumatica, stiffness in the morning and after inactivity is characteristic. Muscle strength is usually unimpaired, although discomfort makes assessment of muscle strength difficult. Synovitis may be found on careful examination of the knees, sternoclavicular joints, and other joints.

Headache is the most common symptom in giant-cell arteritis and is present in two thirds of patients or more. Tender, swollen temporal or other cranial or cervical arteries may be present. Symptoms related to the eyes are the most common serious complication. Visual loss, either partial or complete, develops in about 20% of cases and is caused by ischemia of the optic nerve or tracts.

Intermittent claudication may occur in the muscles of mastication and the extremities and, occasionally, in the muscles of the tongue or those involved in swallowing. In the jaw muscles (jaw claudication) the patient notes discomfort, especially when chewing meat.

Large-artery involvement has been noted in 10% to 15% of cases. Findings include upper or lower extremity claudication, bruits or decreased pulses of the neck or extremity vessels, and, occasionally, aortic rupture. Less common symptoms include sore throat, cough, depression, hemiparesis, peripheral neuropathy, acute hearing loss, brainstem strokes, and myocardial infarction. Fever is present in about one half of the patients; some patients present with fever of unknown origin.

Polymyalgia rheumatica occurs in approximately 50% of patients with giant-cell arteritis. In patients with polymyalgia rheumatica who have no signs or symptoms of arteritis clinically, temporal artery biopsies show giant-cell arteritis in a frequency of 10% to 15%.

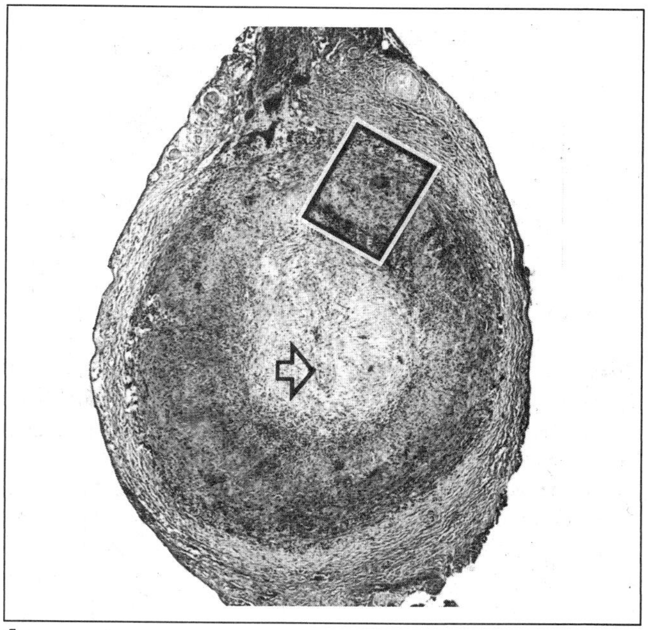

A

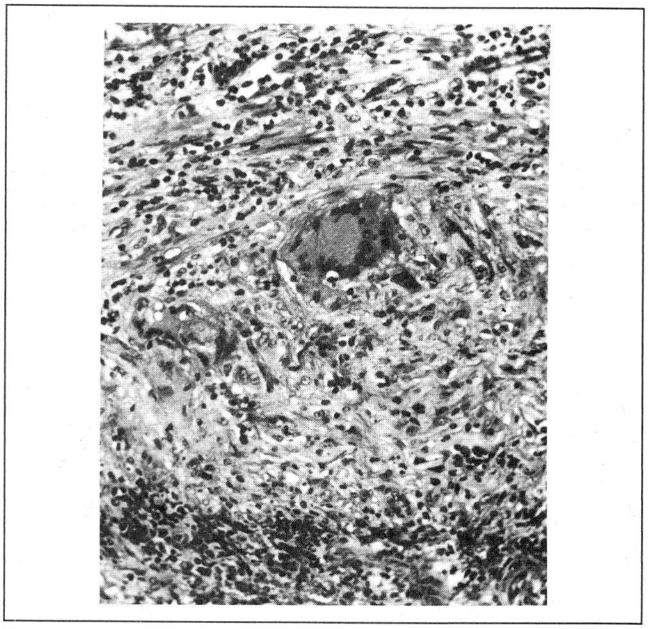

B

Fig. 307-2. Photomicrographs of typical giant-cell arteritis in a temporal artery biopsy. **A,** Low-magnification view of a cross section of the cordlike temporal artery, showing granulomatous inflammation of the media and luminal occlusion *(arrow)* caused by intimal proliferation. **B,** High-magnification view of the boxed area in **A,** showing multinucleated giant cells in a predominantly lymphomononuclear inflammatory cell infiltrate. (Hematoxylin and eosin stain; A ×40, B ×160.)

Laboratory results in polymyalgia rheumatica and giant-cell arteritis are similar. A mild to moderate normochromic anemia is present in both types of patients during the active phase of the disease. Platelet counts often are increased. A markedly elevated erythrocyte sedimentation rate is characteristic of both conditions. Levels over 100 mm in 1 hour (Westergren) are common. Liver function tests are mildly abnormal in approximately one third of patients with either syndrome.

Diagnosis

The diagnosis of polymyalgia rheumatica is based on the presence of aching and morning stiffness in two of the three commonly affected areas (neck, shoulder girdle, and hip girdle) of 4 weeks' duration, or longer, plus a Westergren erythrocyte sedimentation rate above 40 to 50 mm in 1 hour in the absence of any other disease. The diagnosis of giant-cell arteritis should be considered in any patient over the age of 50 years who has a new form of headache, transient or sudden loss of vision, polymyalgia rheumatica, unexplained prolonged fever or anemia, and high erythrocyte sedimentation rate. Diagnostic temporal artery biopsy is recommended in all patients suspected of having giant-cell arteritis. Because the involvement may be focal, a symptomatic or clinically abnormal segment of the artery should be chosen for biopsy. When the blood vessels are palpably normal, it is important to include in the biopsy a several-centimeter segment of one or both of the temporal arteries and to examine multiple histologic sections.

Other forms of vasculitis (e.g., polyarteritis nodosa) may affect the temporal artery, but the histologic features of acute necrotizing arteritis provide the necessary clues to the correct diagnosis.

Treatment

In patients with polymyalgia rheumatica without giant cell arteritis 5- to 15-mg daily doses of prednisone (or an equivalent amount of another corticosteroid preparation) may be started. These doses usually result in rapid improvement of the musculoskeletal aching and stiffness but may not suppress the underlying arteritis if it is present. In mild cases, nonsteroidal anti-inflammatory drugs may be tried.

Patients with temporal arteritis should be given corticosteroid treatment as soon as the diagnosis is made. The initial dose is 45 to 60 mg prednisone (or its equivalent) per day. After reversible clinical and laboratory findings have become normal, the dose can be reduced gradually by 2.5 to 5.0 mg each 1 to 2 weeks, according to the patient's symptoms and laboratory tests, especially the erythrocyte sedimentation rate. Both polymyalgia rheumatica and giant-cell arteritis tend to run self-limited courses over several months to several years, and, eventually, the corticosteroids can be reduced and discontinued in most patients. No effective corticosteroid-sparing drugs have been identified.

POLYARTERITIS NODOSA

Polyarteritis nodosa, periarteritis, and just *polyarteritis* are synonymous terms for a vasculitic syndrome that involves medium-sized and small muscular arteries. It is an uncommon condition, with an average annual incidence of about 1 per 100,000 population. Men are affected twice as often as women. The disease may begin at any age. Immunologic processes appear to be involved in some instances, but etiologies and pathogenetic mechanisms are likely to be diverse.

The relationship between specific antigen-antibody complexes and polyarteritis nodosa has been documented well only in the case of hepatitis B virus. HBsAg has been identified in blood of about 15% of patients with polyarteritis and thus does not appear to account for the majority of cases. Hepatitis C virus has also been found in some patients with polyarteritis nodosa. Vasculitis may be the first manifestation or it may become apparent simultaneously with or after clinical hepatitis.

Pathology

Necrotizing vasculitis with fibrinoid necrosis represents the early or active lesion and is observed in medium (up to 5 mm in diameter) and small (down to 50 μm in diameter) vessels. The necrotic vessel wall structures are replaced by the amorphous, eosinophilic, fibrinlike (fibrinoid necrosis) material (Fig. 307-3, *A*). An intense inflammatory infiltrate of predominantly polymorphonuclear cells is present. In some instances, necrotizing lesions are not completely circumferential and form a "blow-out" type of aneurysm; the remaining part of the vessel wall may look normal or only minimally involved (Fig. 307-3, *B*).

Fibrous intimal proliferation and scarring of the media represent the healed, or end-stage, vascular lesion. There is usually some periarterial (adventitial) fibrosis, with mononuclear cell infiltrate (Fig. 307-3, *C*), which may result in the cordlike or nodular thickening of the vessel. The coexistence of active and healed lesions in the same vessel or adjacent vessels is a unique morphologic feature of polyarteritis.

Clinical features

Polyarteritis ranges from a mild and transient process to fulminating and rapidly fatal disease. Virtually any organ can be affected as the initial manifestation or during the course of the disease. Typically, systemic symptoms are present, along with multisystem involvement such as nephritis, peripheral neuropathy, skin rash, asymmetric polyarthralgia, or arthritis.

Nerve lesions occur in 60% to 80% of cases. Both an abrupt peripheral sensory or motor neuropathy (mononeuritis multiplex or a peripheral polyneuropathy) occur. Central nervous system involvement is less common.

Kidney involvement occurs in about 75% of patients with polyarteritis. Glomerulonephritis is most frequent, with urinary findings of red cells, red cell casts, and proteinuria. Renal infarction and rupture of intrarenal arteries may occur. Renal insufficiency is the cause of death in about 50% of fatal cases. Hypertension may also develop.

Gastrointestinal symptoms are present in about 60% to 70% of patients. Ischemic changes secondary to narrowing

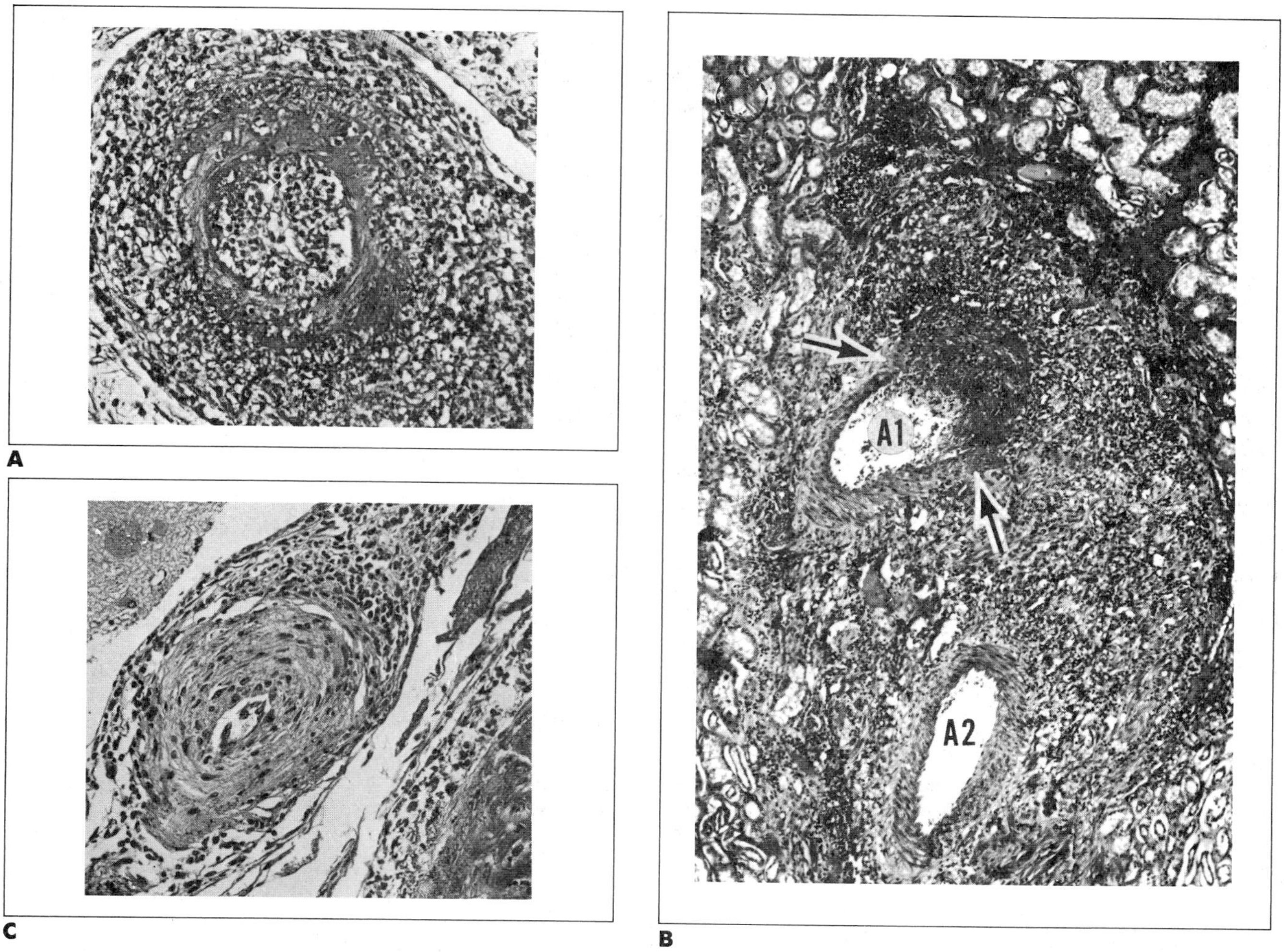

Fig. 307-3. Photomicrographs illustrating the histopathologic spectrum of classic polyarteritis. **A,** Necrotizing vasculitis with fibrinoid necrosis of an arteriole in muscle biopsy. **B,** Two small arteries of a kidney; the upper artery *(A1)* shows a segmental, aneurysmal, blow-out type necrosis of the vessel wall *(arrows)* while the adjacent lower artery *(A2)* appears uninvolved. **C,** An arteriole showing healing-phase lesion of polyarteritis with cellular proliferation and fibrosis of the vessel wall and perivascular lymphomononuclear cell infiltrate. (Hematoxylin and eosin stain; A and C ×160, B ×64.)

of mesenteric arteries cause abdominal pain, hematemesis, and hematochezia. In cases associated with HBsAg, the hepatitis is often mild. The vasculitis is similar in cases positive and negative for HBsAg.

Coronary arteritis may cause myocardial infarction or congestive heart failure.

Skin manifestations are seen in approximately 50% of patients. Depending on the size and extent of vessels involved, cutaneous lesions may include livedo reticularis, ulcerations, or ischemic changes of digits and tend to be more prominent over dependent areas such as the lower extremities and feet.

Arthralgias are common, and mild nonerosive asymmetric polyarthritis is seen occasionally in the large joints of the lower extremities. Skeletal muscle artery involvement may cause pain and, occasionally, intermittent claudication.

Ocular involvement may result in toxic retinopathy with hemorrhage and exudates.

Laboratory tests

Frequent abnormalities include increased erythrocyte sedimentation rate, normochromic anemia, and elevated platelet count. Neutrophilic leukocytosis and increased globulins may also be found. Mild to moderate eosinophilia may be encountered. Urinalysis shows protein and red cell casts.

Decreased concentration of serum complement and the presence of cryoglobulins and serum rheumatoid factor occur in some patients with diffuse cutaneous vasculitis, renal disease, or those with HBsAg. Intravascular coagulation may also develop.

Diagnosis

Polyarteritis should be suspected in a patient with a systemic "toxic" or febrile illness accompanied by fever, weight loss, and multisystem organ involvement. It should be remembered that similar findings may be present in infection, malignancy, and cardiac myxoma embolism.

Whenever possible, the diagnosis should be confirmed by a biopsy of involved tissue. An electromyogram may help document sural nerve compromise before clinical involvement is obvious. Renal biopsy usually reveals focal necrotizing glomerulonephritis and, less commonly, arteritis. Blind muscle biopsies are of less value. When there is no obvious involved tissue to biopsy, visceral arteriography may help by demonstrating aneurysms or other vascular irregularities (Fig. 307-4). In some patients with Cogan's syndrome (keratitis and nerve deafness), a systemic vasculitis similar to polyarteritis occurs.

Treatment

In active cases, prednisone, or an equivalent corticosteroid, should be started in a dose of 1 to 2 mg per kilogram body weight (approximately 60 mg/day). Higher doses may be required. Once the disease is controlled, the dose should be reduced gradually to the lowest level that suppresses the arteritis. In severe cases cytotoxic drugs are used along with corticosteroids. Cyclophosphamide, in a dose of 1 to 2 mg per kilogram body weight (usually 75 to 150 mg/day), has been used more often than other cytotoxics. The 5-year survival is 50% or better. Most deaths occur in the first year.

KAWASAKI DISEASE

Kawasaki disease, or mucocutaneous lymph node syndrome, is an acute febrile illness of young children, although adults with this illness have been reported. Early cases of Kawasaki disease were reported from Japan, but subsequently have been seen worldwide, including the United States. The incidence in males is two to three times that in females.

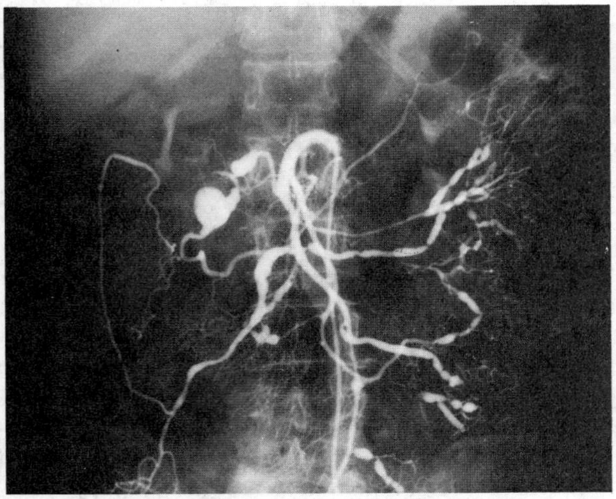

Fig. 307-4. Mesenteric angiogram in a patient with polyarteritis. Note the characteristic multiple small and large aneurysms, as well as focal constrictions between dilated arterial segments.

Clinical features

Fever usually is the initial symptom. After several days the skin of the distal fingers becomes edematous and firm, and an irregular erythematous eruption develops over the trunk. The conjunctivae become injected, the lips become reddened and dry, and the tongue becomes strawberry-colored. Pauciarticular arthritis develops in about 40% of cases. Lymphadenopathy is apparent early in the course. This syndrome subsides spontaneously in 3 to 6 weeks.

The vast majority of patients recover without apparent sequelae, but death occurs in 1% to 2% between the tenth and thirtieth day after onset from coronary arteritis. Autopsy studies suggest that a more widespread angiitis also may be common.

Laboratory tests

The laboratory findings include leukocytosis (with an increase in immature cells), mild anemia, and thrombocytosis. Urinalysis frequently shows white blood cells and proteinuria. The erythrocyte sedimentation rate and other acute-phase reactants are elevated. Transaminases may be increased. Antiendothelial cell antibodies are present during the active phase.

Diagnosis

The diagnosis in a febrile child can be made when four of the following five criteria are met: conjunctivitis, involvement of the mucous membranes of the upper respiratory tract, truncal rash, indurative rash of the palms and soles, and lymphadenopathy.

Treatment

There is no specific treatment, but large doses of intravenous gamma globulin appear to shorten the disease and reduce vasculitis complications. Aspirin may help symptomatically. Coronary bypass surgery has been performed in some patients.

VASCULITIS ASSOCIATED WITH RHEUMATIC DISEASES

In many instances, the underlying pathologic processes in connective tissue diseases involve blood vessels. Proliferation of the vascular intima (obliterative endarteritis) may become marked and cause tissue ischemia. For example, narrowing of digital arteries in rheumatoid arthritis causes small dermal infarctions at the edges of nailfolds and elsewhere. A similar process of bland intimal thickening is seen in scleroderma; this thickening results in ischemia or infarction of the distal finger pads. In a small proportion of cases of rheumatoid arthritis, systemic lupus erythematosus, and other connective tissue disorders, necrotizing vasculitis occurs. Medium-sized and small muscular arteries and arterioles may be involved. Histopathologically, the vascular lesions are indistinguishable from polyarteritis nodosa. Immune complex–related processes are considered important in the vasculitis of connective tissue diseases.

Clinical features

Patients with rheumatoid arthritis who develop necrotizing vasculitis are likely to have erosive articular disease, rheumatoid nodules, high titers of serum rheumatoid factor, and antinuclear antibodies. As the vasculitis develops, rheumatoid factor titers may rise further, serum complement levels diminish, and immune complex–like materials appear in the serum. Common clinical manifestations include cutaneous infarctions over the lower extremities, with ulceration, mononeuritis multiplex, and mesenteric ischemia. Renal disease rarely, if ever, occurs in rheumatoid vasculitis. Patients with lupus erythematosus who develop necrotizing vasculitis are not as readily identifiable, but they frequently have marked livedo reticularis, Raynaud's phenomenon, and digital gangrene. Precipitating antibodies to DNA may be more common in this group.

Treatment

Patients with necrotizing vasculitis may respond to corticosteroids in high doses. Cytotoxic drugs may be useful for corticosteroid-resistant patients.

CHURG-STRAUSS SYNDROME (ALLERGIC ANGIITIS AND GRANULOMATOSIS)

Churg-Strauss syndrome or allergic angiitis and granulomatosis is a less common form of vasculitis. It is characterized by the presence of vasculitis and extravascular granulomas. The age at onset varies from 15 to 70 years, with a mean of about 50 years. Men are affected twice as often as women.

Pathology

The granulomatous inflammation may be seen in practically any tissue of the body but occurs predominantly in the lungs, heart, gastrointestinal tract, and skin. Individual granulomas are usually of microscopic size, but by confluence may result in larger lesions. Histopathologically, there is necrosis and intense eosinophilic infiltration, accompanied by histiocytes (epithelioid cells) and a variable number of giant cells.

The vascular lesions usually involve small arteries and veins. Both necrotizing and eosinophilic granulomatous vasculitis may be observed (Fig. 307-5). Healing is by complete resolution or scar formation of the active lesions.

Clinical features

There is often a history of atopy. Asthma often precedes the onset of systemic vasculitis by several years but tends to subside as disseminated vasculitis begins. Pulmonary infiltrations, fever, and weight loss are frequent initial manifestations. The lung infiltrates may be transient (Loeffler's syndrome) or more persistent. Interstitial lung disease may also develop. Other than pulmonary involvement, the distribution of vasculitic and granulomatous lesions and thus the spectrum of manifestations is somewhat similar to those in polyarteritis nodosa.

Laboratory tests

Eosinophilia is the characteristic feature in Churg-Strauss syndrome. The eosinophil count frequently ranges from 5000 to 20,000 per cubic millimeter but may be higher. It usually drops as the patient improves or is treated. Anemia and an elevated erythrocyte sedimentation rate are found during active disease.

Diagnosis

The appearance of a multisystem disease in a patient with a history of asthma and presence of eosinophilia should suggest this diagnosis. This disease needs to be differentiated from polyarteritis nodosa. Wegener's granulomatosis, sarcoidosis, and bronchopulmonary aspergillosis.

Treatment and course

Corticosteroid treatment is similar to that used in polyarteritis nodosa, but little information concerning the effect of cytotoxic drugs is available.

WEGENER GRANULOMATOSIS

Wegener granulomatosis is characterized by the presence of vasculitis and necrotizing granulomatous lesions. In typical cases the upper airways, lungs, and kidneys are involved, but the disease may be limited to any combination of these or other organs. The incidence is less than that of polyarteritis nodosa. The mean age at onset is 40 years, and men are affected twice as commonly as women.

Pathology

Typical changes in biopsies of the upper respiratory tract consist of severe, nonspecific inflammation with dense infiltration by polymorphonuclear leukocytes, plasma cells, lymphocytes, and histiocytes. Necrosis and ulcerations supervene and are accompanied by granulomas (with palisading epithelioid cells and giant cells) and necrotizing inflammation of small arteries and veins (50 to 500 μm in diameter). Similar histologic features are seen throughout the lower respiratory tract (Fig. 307-6, *A*). The kidney typically shows a focal necrotizing glomerulonephritis (Fig. 307-6, *B*).

Clinical features

Initial symptoms usually are related to the respiratory tract, such as a productive cough, sinusitis, or secretions that have

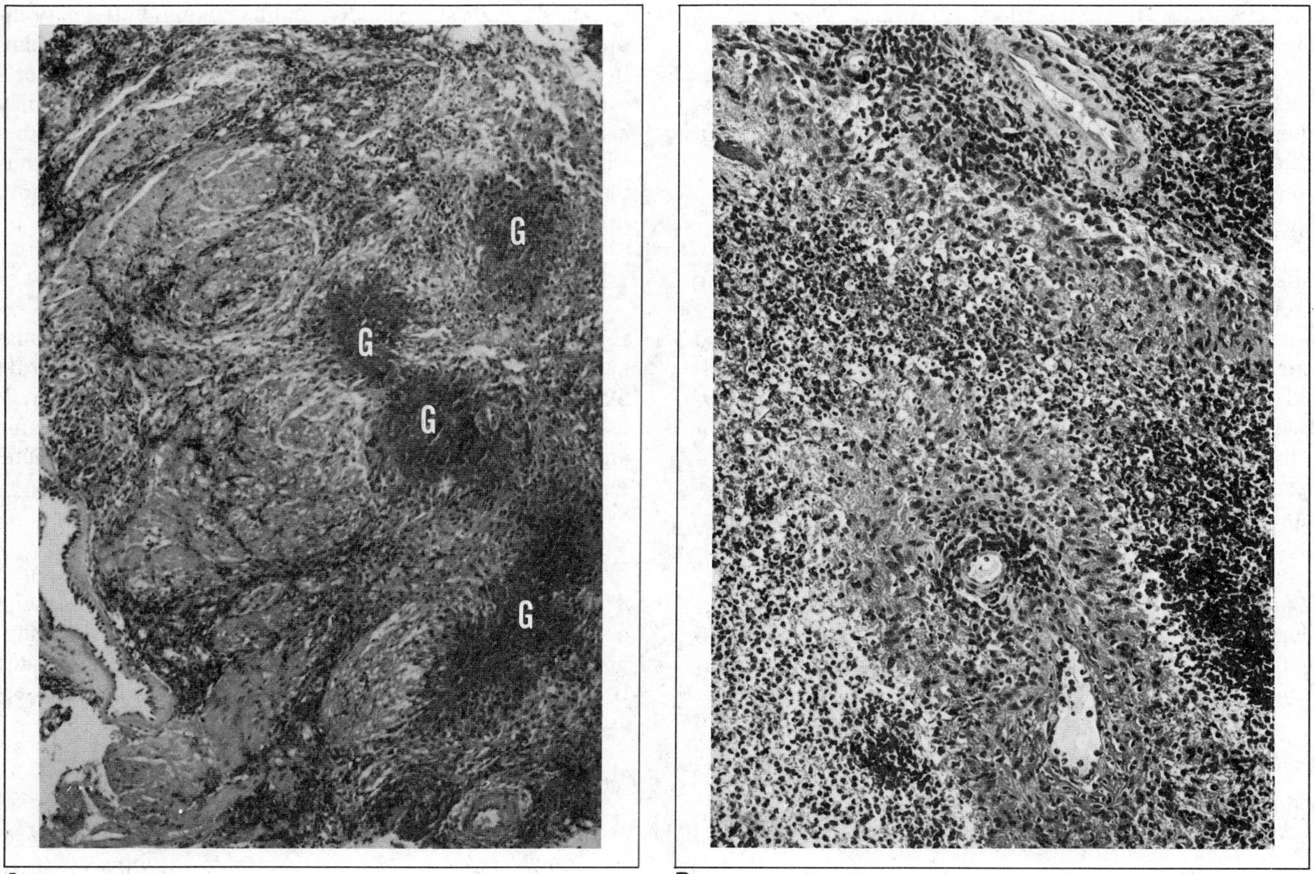

A B

Fig. 307-5. Photomicrographs of Churg-Strauss syndrome. **A,** Bronchial biopsy showing vasculitis and multiple eosinophilic necrotizing granulomas *(G)*. **B,** Lung biopsy showing granulomatous vasculitis with an eosinophil-rich inflammatory cell infiltrate. (Hematoxylin and eosin stain; A ×64, B ×160.)

responded incompletely to antibiotics. Fever, malaise, and weight loss often follow.

Examination often reveals ulcerations of the nasal mucosa. Destruction of the nasal cartilages leads to a saddle deformity of the nose. The inflammatory processes extend to the surrounding tissues and to the central nervous system to produce diabetes insipidus or cranial nerve lesions. Cerebrovasculitis has been reported. Serous otitis media may occur secondary to obstruction of the eustachian tubes.

Pulmonary infiltrations and nodules that cavitate are frequent radiographic changes. Renal involvement varies from focal glomerulonephritis to an acute necrotizing glomerulonephritis with rapidly deteriorating renal function. Urinalysis shows proteinuria, hematuria, and red cell casts.

Skin involvement is manifested as a purpuric rash, ulcers, nodules, or vesicles. Ocular findings include conjunctivitis, scleritis, episcleritis, corneal and scleral ulcers, uveitis, optic neuritis, pseudotumor of the orbit, orbital cellulitis, and retinal artery occlusion. Occasionally there is proptosis or cavernous sinus thrombosis.

Arthralgias are found in up to 50% of cases, but synovitis is less common. Nervous system lesions, occurring in 25%, include cranial nerve palsy, mononeuritis multiplex, and polyneuropathy. Cardiac manifestations include pericarditis, myocarditis, myocardial infarctions caused by coronary arteritis, and arrhythmias. Granulomatous lesions and vasculitis may also be found in other organs such as the gut or elsewhere, with symptoms that reflect the site and extent of involvement.

Laboratory tests

Common findings are normochromic anemia, moderate leukocytosis without eosinophilia, elevated erythrocyte sedimentation rate, increased platelet count, and hyperglobulinemia. Serum antibodies against antigens in the cytoplasm of neutrophils (ANCA) appear to be present in three fourths or more of cases with active disease. Two cytoplasmic staining patterns may be seen when the indirect immunoflourescent method is used employing alcohol-fixed neutrophils as substrate. A diffuse cytoplasmic pattern (C-ANCA) is characteristic for Wegener granulomatosis and a perinuclear pattern (P-ANCA) is more commonly found in necrotizing crescentic glomerulonephritis. The major antigen

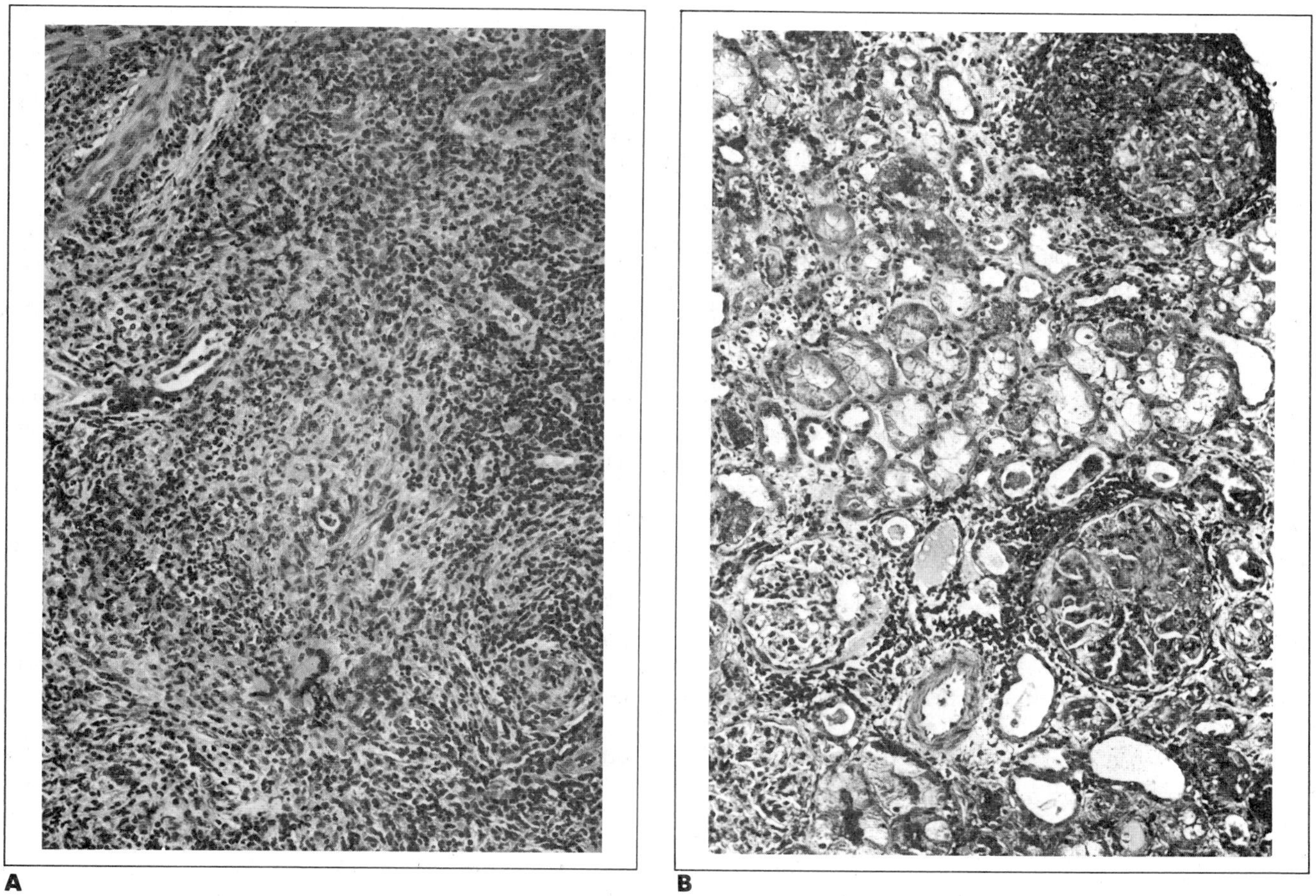

Fig. 307-6. Photomicrographs of typical lesions in Wegener's granulomatosis. **A,** Lung biopsy showing necrotizing vasculitis and extravascular granulomas. **B,** Renal biopsy showing focal necrotizing glomerulonephritis. (Hematoxylin and eosin stain; A and B ×160.)

producing the C-ANCA pattern is a serine proteinase. The major antigens producing the P-ANCA pattern are myeloperoxidase and elastase, which are solubilized during the fixation and diffuse and bind to the nucleus (see Chapter 293). Antinuclear antibody and cryoglobulins are usually absent, and complement levels are normal.

Diagnosis

Wegener granulomatosis should be considered in a patient with upper respiratory symptoms that are unresponsive to antibiotics. The presence of nasal mucosal ulcerations, lung infiltrations or cavitations, and renal findings should further suggest this diagnosis.

Biopsy of involved nasal mucosa or other respiratory tissues generally offers the best opportunity to confirm a histologic diagnosis of Wegener granulomatosis. Needle biopsy of the kidney usually shows glomerulonephritis, and in a patient with an otherwise compatible clinical picture, this finding is strong confirmatory evidence.

Diseases that need to be differentiated from Wegener granulomatosis include lymphomatoid granulomatosis (polymorphic reticulosis), which is characterized by an angiocentric infiltration of atypical lymphoid and plasma cells, nasopharyngeal carcinoma, lung tumors, and mycobacterial or fungal infections.

Treatment and course

Corticosteroids may be tried in patients with mild or limited disease, but cyclophosphamide needs to be added. The usual dose of cyclophosphamide is 1 to 2 mg per kilogram body weight (usually 100 to 150 mg) given orally in a single morning dose. Fluid intake must be generous to minimize the risk of hemorrhagic cystitis. The leukocyte count should be followed carefully and the drug temporarily discontinued if the white blood cell count drops below 3000 per mm.[3] The optimal duration of treatment with cyclophosphamide is unknown, but most physicians continue the drug for about a year after the patient has become asymptomatic. Even with the use of cyclophosphamide, the mortality remains up to 30 percent. Superimposed infections in the respiratory tract may occur before or during therapy. Relapses are not infrequent months or years after cyclophosphamide has been discontinued, necessitating another course of this drug.

VASCULITIS OF SMALL BLOOD VESSELS

This group includes a variety of conditions in which involvement of small blood vessels (arterioles, capillaries, venules) is predominant. *Hypersensitivity vasculitis* is the term sometimes used to describe this category. However, that designation should be reserved as a diagnosis of patients who have developed vasculitis after exposure to a substance, often a drug, that appears to have been the inciting agent. *Leukocytoclastic vasculitis* is a term used to describe the histopathologic picture of nectrotizing inflammation in most conditions in this group. It is characterized by infiltrations of the vessel walls and perivascular areas by polymorphonuclear leukocytes, with leukocytoclasis and fragmentation of nuclei ("nuclear dust"). Leukocytoclastic vasculitis is found in such diverse conditions as Henoch-Schönlein purpura, mixed cryoglobulinemia, hypocomplementemic urticarial vasculitis, bacterial endocarditis, benign hyperglobulinemic purpura, Sjögren's syndrome, chronic active hepatitis, ulcerative colitis, malignant lymphomas, retroperitoneal fibrosis, primary biliary cirrhosis, and Goodpasture's syndrome. In some instances of vasculitis of small vessels, the cell infiltration may be lymphocytic, and in others the infiltrates are indistinguishable from those of polyarteritis. As in other categories of vasculitis, the different syndromes appear to be related to a multiplicity of etiologies mediated by various pathogenetic mechanisms.

Because vasculitis of the skin is easily identified, it is frequently the first or even the only manifestation recognized in patients in this category. Patients with vasculitis confined to the skin generally have a good prognosis. Typical cutaneous lesions appear as flat, erythematous, purpuric macules that progress to papules of "palpable purpura." The palpable quality distinguishes these lesions from noninflammatory purpura. Such eruptions can occur on any part of the body, but when extensive are seen especially over dependent areas such as the lower extremities, back, gluteal region, extensor surface of the forearms, and hands. A "crop" of palpable purpura may develop as a single event or as episodes at irregular intervals. Individual lesions last from 1 to 4 weeks and frequently leave pigmented spots and sometimes atrophic scars. Lesions may become confluent and nodular; they extend several centimeters when purpura is confluent. In some instances, vasculitis produces urticaria or annular lesions resembling erythema multiforme. Vesicles and bullae may arise from a purpuric area in severe cases. Ulcers may develop in areas with many lesions.

CLINICAL APPROACH TO VASCULITIS: A SUMMARY

The vasculitides can be looked on as a disparate group of diseases linked together by the fact that they affect the same tissue—namely, blood vessels. Because of the great variability in the nature of these conditions, there is no simple or uniform method of evaluating patients suspected of having vasculitis. A detailed history, careful physical examination, and appropriate laboratory tests are needed to determine the type of onset, course of the illness, organ systems involved, and the extent of the involvement. Information regarding possible pathogenetic mechanisms (e.g., drug exposure) may also be obtained in this way. Similarly, conditions mimicking vasculitis may be identified or excluded (Table 307-2). It must be recognized that some patients cannot easily be assigned a diagnostic label because of insufficient or atypical findings or because of clinical data that include criteria of more than one type of vasculitis ("overlap syndrome").

Vasculitis should be considered in any patient with a febrile "toxic" multisystem illness; however, many cases do not present in such a fashion. Awareness of the variable nature of vasculitis is helpful in this regard.

In suspected cases of vasculitis, a pathologic confirmation of the clinical diagnosis is highly recommended to help clarify the nature of the disease and to aid in making decisions regarding treatment. The decision to begin therapy without biopsy sometimes seems easy, but difficulties may arise several months later when side effects of the medications become prominent and the clinical findings have become blurred. The better established the diagnosis was initially, the easier these later decisions become. Chances of obtaining a positive biopsy are greatest when a specimen is taken from an involved portion of an affected organ and when the tissue sample size is adequate. Common sites to biopsy are skin, sural nerve, muscle, and temporal artery. "Blind" biopsies of muscle, liver, kidney, or other asymptomatic tissue reveal vasculitis in a minority of cases. A specimen of adequate size that is thoroughly examined will afford the best chance of identifying an abnormal vessel if vasculitis is present. Histopathologic findings evolve as lesions progress from acute to healing stages and also under

Table 307-2. Common and uncommon conditions simulating vasculitis

Clinical syndrome	Predominant vessels affected
Fibromuscular dysplasia Radiation fibrosis Neurofibromatosis Congenital coarctation of aorta	Large arteries (aorta and primary branches)
Ergotism Cholesterol embolization Atrial myxoma Malignancies (e.g. lymphomatoid granulomatosis/polymorphic reticulosis)	Medium-sized and small muscular arteries
Mycotic aneurysm and embolization Bacteremia Infective endocarditis Thrombocytopenia and other processes causing purpura	Small vessels (arterioles, capillaries, venules)

the influence of treatment. Thus, "classic" or stereotypical changes may not be found. An awareness of the spectrum of pathologic changes may be helpful in confirming or refuting a suspected diagnosis when interpreted in the light of clinical findings.

In some forms of vasculitis, including polyarteritis nodosa, giant-cell arteritis, and Takayasu arteritis, angiograms can be used to aid in identifying, characterizing, and determining the extent of vasculitis. Angiographic changes are not necessarily pathognomonic in themselves but may provide enough information to make a diagnosis when added to other clinical data.

Proper treatment of vasculitis depends on characterizing the nature of the disease as well as possible in each patient. Decisions regarding therapy may be more difficult in patients with atypical or overlapping findings and in those who have suggestive clinical features but lack biopsy confirmation. Experience is useful in these instances. Focal and transient cases may require brief or no therapy, whereas systemic progressive cases may require prompt initiation of large doses of corticosteroids. In other patients, especially those with Wegener's granulomatosis, cytotoxic drugs may be life-saving.

REFERENCES

Caselli RJ et al: Peripheral neuropathic syndromes in giant cell (temporal) arteritis. Neurology 38:685, 1988.

Churg A and Churg J, editors: Systemic vasculitis. New York, 1991, Igahu-Shoin.

Conn DL and Hunder GG: Vasculitis and related disorders. In Kelley WN et al, editors: Textbook of rheumatology, ed 4. Philadelphia, 1993, Saunders.

Hall S et al: Takayasu arteritis. A study of 32 North American patients. Medicine (Baltimore) 64:89, 1985.

Hoffman GS et al: Wegener granulomatosis: an analysis of 158 patients. Ann Intern Med 116:488, 1992.

Hunder GG et al: The American College of Rheumatology 1990 criteria for the classification of vasculitis. Introduction Arthritis Rheum 33:1065, 1990.

Jennette JC and Falk RJ: Diagnostic classification of anti-neutrophil cytoplasmic autoantibody-associated diseases. Am J Kidney Dis 2:184, 1991.

Lanham JG et al: Systemic vasculitis with asthma and eosinophilia: a clinical approach to the Churg-Strauss syndrome. Medicine (Baltimore) 63:65, 1984.

Leung DYM: Immunologic aspects of Kawasaki syndrome. J Rheumatol 17(suppl 24):15, 1990.

Lie JT: Vasculitis simulators and vasculitis look-alikes. Curr Opin Rheumatol 4:47, 1992.

Machado EBV et al: Trends in incidence and clinical presentation of temporal arteritis in Olmsted County, Minnesota, 1980-1985. Arthritis Rheum 31:745, 1988.

Quint L et al: Hepatitis C virus in patients with polyarteritis nodosa: prevalence in 38 patients. Clin Exp Rheumatol 9:213, 1991.

Sanchez-Guerrero J et al: Vasculitis as a paraneoplastic syndrome: report of 11 cases and review of the literature. J Rheumatol 17:1458, 1990.

CHAPTER

308 Raynaud's Phenomenon

Richard M. Silver

Maurice Raynaud described the clinical syndrome of episodic digital ischemia provoked by cold or emotion. The classic attack of Raynaud's phenomenon (RP) is triphasic, that is, pallor followed by cyanosis, and then by hyperemia, often accompanied by numbness and discomfort. Actually, history of a tricolor response is not common, and RP will be underdiagnosed if all three phases, white, blue, and red, are required for diagnosis. Pallor is the most reliable sign of RP and erythema is the least reliable sign in subjects with cold-sensitive digits.

PREVALENCE

Reports of the prevalence of RP are variable and sometimes overestimated, depending upon the study population, the referral bias of the reporting center, and the method of assessment. In a carefully conducted population-based study, the prevalence of RP among adults living in the southern United States was estimated to be 4.6%. The prevalence may be higher in colder climates and in selected populations.

CLASSIFICATION

Raynaud's phenomenon may be a benign condition (Raynaud's disease, or primary RP), or it may be associated with an underlying disorder (secondary RP) (see box, p. 2442). It is important to evaluate patients having RP for the presence of an underlying condition, particularly connective tissue diseases such as systemic sclerosis in which RP may be the initial clinical manifestation (see box, p. 2442).

DIAGNOSIS

A history of a bicolor cold-induced response, particularly if it includes white fingers, is sufficient for a diagnosis of RP. Provocative tests, for example, immersion of the hands in iced water, are unnecessary, painful, and may be dangerous. The following clinical features are seen in secondary but not in primary RP: late age of onset, digital ulcers, and asymmetric distribution. If present, an underlying condition should be sought. Prospective studies of individuals having RP have revealed two readily available tests that are highly predictive of the presence or eventual development of a connective tissue disease: nailfold capillary microscopy and antinuclear antibodies (ANA).

The nailfold capillary bed at the edge of the cuticle can be visualized using in-vivo microscopy or a hand-held oph-

Conditions associated with Raynaud's phenomenon

Occupational/environmental exposures
- Vinyl chloride disease
- Vibration injury
- Cold injury
- Posttraumatic injuries, e.g. hypothenar-hammer syndrome

Drug exposures
- Beta blockers
- Ergotamines
- Bleomycin

Occlusive vascular diseases
- Arteriosclerosis obliterans
- Thromboangiitis obliterans (Buerger's disease)
- Thoracic outlet syndrome
- Thromboembolism
- Takayasu's disease
- Other vasculitic syndromes

Connective tissue diseases
- Systemic sclerosis (scleroderma)
- Systemic lupus erythematosus
- Polymyositis/dermatomyositis
- Rheumatoid arthritis
- Overlap syndromes or mixed connective tissue disease

Hematologic conditions
- Polycythemia
- Cryoglobulinemia
- Cold agglutinin disease
- Cryofibrinogenemia

Miscellaneous conditions
- Primary pulmonary hypertension
- Reflex sympathetic dystrophy
- Myxedema
- Carpal tunnel syndrome
- Ovarian cancer

thalmoscope. Distinctively abnormal nailfold capillaries are present in the majority of patients with systemic sclerosis (Fig. 308-1) and many patients with dermatomyositis. The presence of abnormal nailfold capillaries in a patient with RP is highly predictive of the eventual development of clinically apparent connective tissue disease, especially a scleroderma-spectrum disorder.

A positive test for ANA in a patient with RP may also be predictive of the presence of or evolution to a connective tissue disease. Certain types of ANA are specific and predictive of particular connective tissue diseases. For example, anticentromere antibodies are predictive of the CREST syndrome (limited cutaneous systemic sclerosis). Antibodies to topoisomerase I (anti-Scl-70) are specific for diffuse systemic sclerosis. All patients with RP should be screened with a complete history and physical examination searching for features of an underlying condition, and routine laboratory testing should include tests for ANA and nailfold capillary microscopy.

Other vascular processes that may mimic the cyanotic phase of RP include livedo reticularis, acrocyanosis, and chronic pernio. Each of these conditions lacks the episodic character of RP as well as the characteristic pallor. Livedo reticularis refers to a purplish appearance of the skin with a netlike pattern usually affecting the extremities. It is usually idiopathic and benign, but it may be associated with connective tissue diseases, vasculitis, cholesterol embolization, or blood dyscrasias. Acrocyanosis is a benign condition in which the hands and sometimes the feet are persistently cold and blue, regardless of ambient temperature. Pernio is a chronic vasospastic disorder in which hemorrhagic vesicles and ulcers occur on the toes, usually resolving in warm weather.

Diagnostic evaluation of the patient with Raynaud's phenomenon

History: including occupational and drug exposure, smoking, symptoms of connective tissue disease, frequency and duration of RP attacks

Physical examination: including skin examination, palpation of peripheral pulses, auscultation for bruits

Laboratory studies: complete blood count, ESR, thyroid function tests, cryoglobulins, ANA, nailfold capillary microscopy

Ancillary tests: anticentromere, anti-Scl-70 and anti-DNA antibodies if screening ANA positive or connective tissue disease suspected; arteriography only if peripheral pulses asymmetric or diminished

Modified from Maricq HR et al: Diagnostic potential of in vivo capillary microscopy in scleroderma and related disorders. Arthritis Rheum 23:183, 1980.

THERAPY

Treatment of RP per se depends on the severity (threshold, frequency, duration) and on the existence of any associated condition. Patients with mild primary or secondary RP may require no treatment other than modification of lifestyle to avoid undue exposure to cold or cigarette smoke. Biofeedback training is beneficial for some patients. Patients with more severe primary or secondary RP may require additional treatment. Calcium-channel blocking agents such as nifedipine are effective in many cases, more in primary than in secondary RP. Other vasodilator drugs that may be effective include prazosin, hydralazine, reserpine, and topical nitrates. The addition of antiplatelet agents may be beneficial for some patients.

Severe digital ischemia may progress to gangrene. Impending gangrene requires aggressive vasodilator therapy, and serial sympathetic ganglion blockade is sometimes beneficial. Surgical sympathectomy is not recommended because of the high rate of recurrence of RP. Prostacyclin infusion may be effective and is warranted in severe cases. Dry, gangrenous digits should be allowed to autoamputate. Surgical amputation is reserved for patients with intractable pain or superinfection.

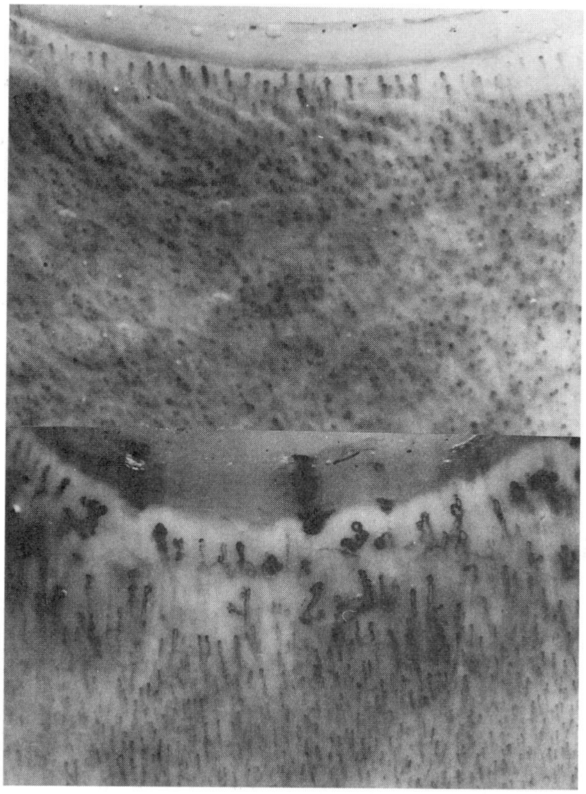

Fig. 308-1. Nailfold capillary bed in a normal subject *(top)* and in a patient with systemic sclerosis *(bottom)*. Enlarged capillaries as well as areas of avascularity are present in the patient with systemic sclerosis, as are capillary hemorrhages in the cuticle. (Reprinted with permission from Maricq HR: Nailfold biopsy in scleroderma and related disorders. Dermatologica 168:73, 1984.)

REFERENCES

Harper FE et al: A prospective study of Raynaud phenomenon and early connective tissue disease. A five-year report, Am J Med 72:883, 1982.

Kallenberg CGM, Wouda AA, The TE: Systemic involvement and immunological findings in patients presenting with Raynaud's phenomenon. Am J Med 69:675, 1980.

Maricq HR: Nailfold biopsy in scleroderma and related disorders. Dermatologica 168:73, 1984.

Maricq HR et al: Diagnostic potential of *in vivo* capillary microscopy in scleroderma and related disorders. Arthritis Rheum 23:183, 1980.

Maricq HR et al: Prevalence of Raynaud phenomenon in the general population. J Chron Dis 39:423, 1986.

Raynaud M: On local asphyxia and symmetrical gangrene of the extremities. Selected monographs, trans. Barlow T. London, 1888, New Sydenham Society.

Spencer-Green G: Raynaud phenomenon, Bull Rheum Dis 33:1, 1983.

CHAPTER

309 Systemic Sclerosis (Scleroderma)

Thomas A. Medsger, Jr.

Systemic sclerosis is a chronic multisystem disorder resulting in thickening of the skin (scleroderma) and involving other organ systems. A spectrum of disease exists (see box below). With *limited cutaneous* involvement, skin thickening is most often restricted to the fingers and/or face. This variant has been termed the CREST (*c*alcinosis, *R*aynaud's phenomenon, *e*sophageal hypomotility, *s*clerodactyly, and *t*elangiectasia) syndrome. With *diffuse cutaneous* involvement, in contrast, the skin of the distal and proximal extremities (above the elbows), face, and trunk (chest, abdomen) is affected. In both variants the dermis, internal organs, and blood vessels show increased deposition of connective tissue matrix (collagen, glycosaminoglycans), leading to organ dysfunction and ischemia. Distinctive serum autoantibodies are found in over 90% of cases. The cause is unknown, and no specific therapy is available.

EPIDEMIOLOGY

Annual incidence is approximately 20 cases per million population with a female-to-male ratio of 3:1. Incidence

Classification of scleroderma

I. Systemic sclerosis (progressive systemic sclerosis, systemic scleroderma)
   A. With diffuse cutaneous involvement: symmetrical widespread skin changes, affecting both distal and proximal extremities and often trunk and face; tendency to rapid progression of skin thickening and early appearance of visceral disease
   B. With limited cutaneous involvement: symmetrical restricted skin thickening, affecting distal extremities (often confined to fingers) and face; prolonged delay in appearance of distinctive internal manifestations (e.g., pulmonary arterial hypertension, biliary cirrhosis); prominence of calcinosis and telangiectasias
   C. With "overlap": having typical features of one or another connective tissue disease (e.g., polymyositis/dermatomyositis or systemic lupus erythematosus)
II. Localized scleroderma
   A. Morphea: single or multiple (generalized) plaques
   B. Linear scleroderma: with or without melorheostosis; includes scleroderma *en coup de sabre,* with or without facial hemiatrophy
III. Scleroderma-like
   A. Eosinophilic fasciitis
   B. Eosinophilia-myalgia syndrome
   C. Toxic oil syndrome

peaks over age 60, and the disease is rare in childhood. Familial systemic sclerosis is uncommon. Although there is no obvious precipitating event or exposure, certain environmental "triggers" to scleroderma-like illnesses are recognized, including exposure to vinyl chloride, other organic hydrocarbons, silica dust, and the tumoricidal drug bleomycin.

PATHOGENESIS

Scleroderma skin fibroblasts synthesize excessive quantities of collagen precursors. The reason for this abnormality is obscure, but vascular and immunologic hypotheses have been proposed.

Clinical and pathologic evidence of vascular disease is abundant. Endothelial cell antigens and the products of platelet aggregation are found in increased amounts in peripheral blood. Ischemia is believed to play a role in fibroblast stimulation. Subintimal fibroplasia leads to narrowing of the lumens of small arteries and arterioles and later to capillary obliteration (Fig. 309-1).

The immunologic hypothesis is supported by the early appearance of mononuclear cell (T cell) infiltration in the skin (Fig. 309-2), lung, and other affected tissues. Cytokines produced by peripheral blood mononuclear cells can cause dermal fibroblast proliferation and increased collagen production in tissue culture. The presence of disease-specific serum autoantibodies also suggests participation of the immune system, but these antibodies are not themselves found in involved blood vessel walls or other affected tissues.

ORGAN INVOLVEMENT
Skin

In the early or edematous phase, the fingers and hands are tight and puffy (Fig. 309-3, *A*). This stage may last indefinitely or be replaced gradually after several weeks or months by skin thickening (indurative phase). At this time, the most accurate method for establishing a diagnosis is careful palpation. In limited scleroderma (see box, p. 2443). skin thickening is generally restricted to the fingers, hands, and face, whereas diffuse scleroderma first affects the most distal parts of the extremities and then spreads at a variable rate to the forearms, upper arms, thighs, upper anterior chest, and abdomen. Hyperpigmentation with surrounding hypopigmentation leads to a "salt-and pepper" appearance of the skin (Fig. 309-3, *B*). The patient's face may become pinched, immobile, and expressionless, with thin, tightly pursed lips and reduced oral aperture (Fig. 309-3, *B*). In limited cutaneous disease, the most striking digital and facial finding is that of numerous telangiectasias (Fig. 309-4).

After several years, the dermis tends to soften considerably or actually become thin (atrophic phase). Skin overlying bony prominences (extensor surfaces of the proximal interphalangeal joints, elbows) is extremely vulnerable to trauma and may break down, leaving painful, slow-healing ulcerations. Skin healing in other locations is normal.

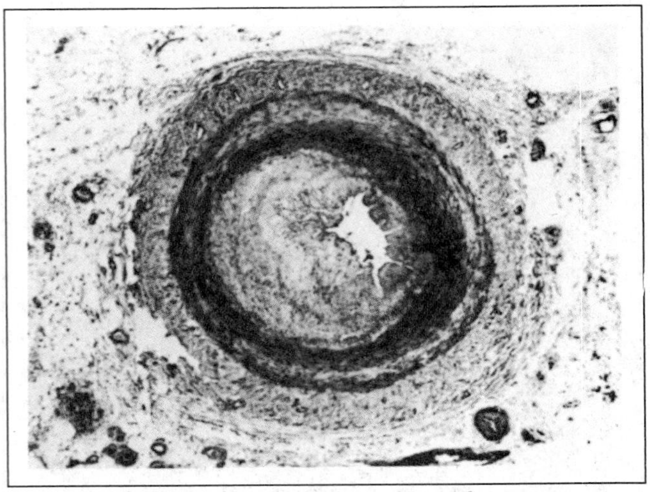

Fig. 309-1. Photomicrograph of a digital artery obtained at autopsy from a 45-year-old woman with diffuse cutaneous systemic sclerosis who had Raynaud's phenomenon for over 20 years prior to her death. There is near occlusion of the lumen, owing to striking subintimal proliferation. Periadventitial fibrosis is also present.

Especially in limited scleroderma, there is a tendency to develop intracutaneous and subcutaneous calcification, chiefly in the digital pads and periarticular tissues, along forearm extensor surfaces, in the olecranon bursae, and in the prepatellar areas. Overlying skin may ulcerate, with extrusion of calcareous material and secondary bacterial infection.

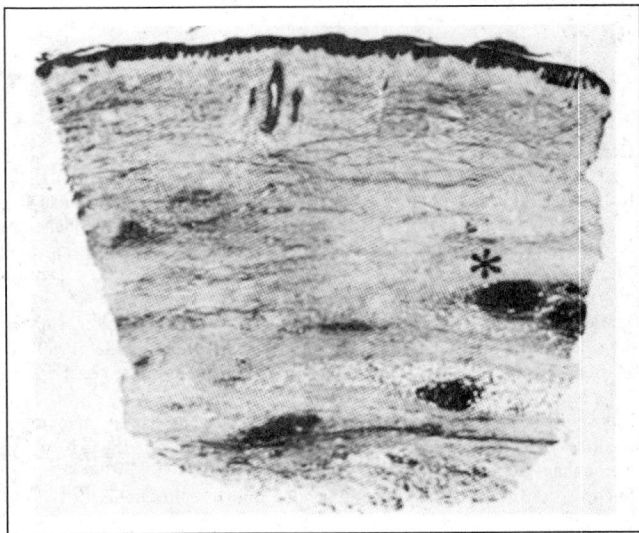

Fig. 309-2. Photomicrograph of a skin punch biopsy obtained from the dorsum of the forearm of a 53-year-old woman with diffuse cutaneous systemic sclerosis. Skin appendages are atrophic, and the dermis is markedly thickened by the deposition of dense collagenous connective tissue. Prominent collections of small round cells *(asterisk)* are present; they were identified as T-lymphocytes.

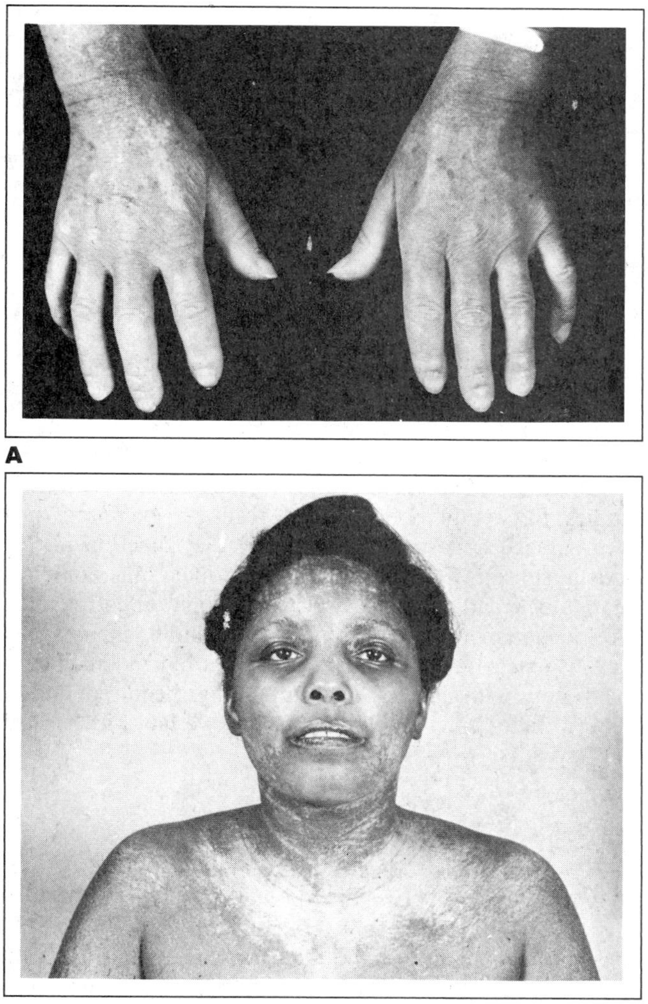

A

B

Fig. 309-3. The characteristic taut, thickened, shiny skin of scleroderma with pigmentary abnormalities. **A,** Hands, showing typical skin changes with flexion contractures of the fingers. **B,** Facial features of scleroderma showing pursed mouth, prominent teeth, pinched nose, and loss of skin folds.

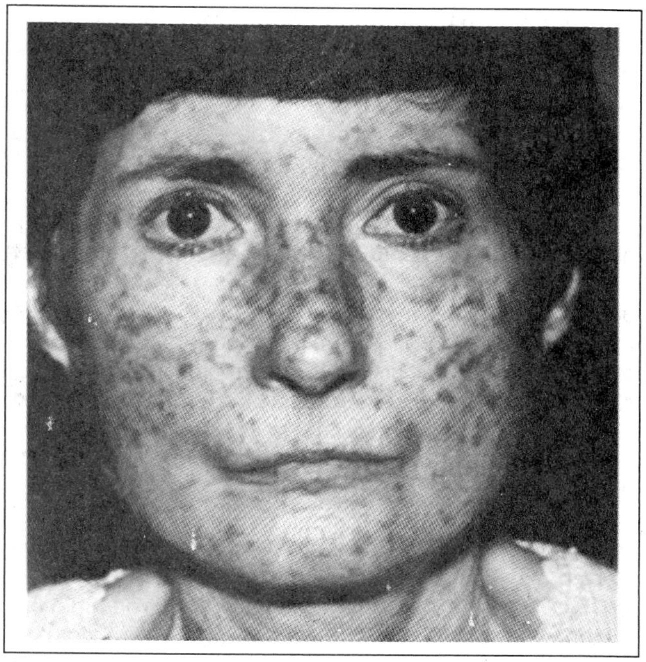

Fig. 309-4. Face of a 45-year-old woman with limited cutaneous systemic sclerosis showing multiple telangiectasias.

Peripheral vascular system

Raynaud's phenomenon is often the first symptom and occurs eventually in over 95% of patients. Small areas of ischemic necrosis or ulceration of the fingertips leave pitted scars, and, rarely, terminal phalangeal gangrene may ensue. Angiographic studies disclose narrowing and obstruction of the digital arteries, which histologically show prominent subintimal connective tissue proliferation, without inflammation, as well as adventitial fibrosis (see Fig. 309-1). Concomitantly, the capillary circulation is altered by the appearance of "giant loops" and, in diffuse scleroderma, a paucity of nailfold vessels on microscopy.

Joints, tendons, and bones

Symmetrical polyarthralgias, joint stiffness, and symptoms of median nerve compression are frequent initial or early complaints, but palpable synovitis is unusual. Coarse, leathery crepitus (tendon friction rubs) may be felt during joint motion over the elbows, wrists, fingers, knees, and ankles. These rubs are relatively specific for diffuse scleroderma and often antedate an explosive increase in skin thickening. Flexion contractures of the fingers (Fig. 309-3, *A*) and other, larger joints usually become apparent within several months in the diffuse cutaneous variant.

The most frequent bony radiographic abnormality is resorption of the tufts of the terminal phalanges of the digits. A few patients develop severe erosive changes of the finger joints. Other examples of bone resorption include "notching" of the posterior ribs and dissolution of the condyle and ramus of the mandible.

Skeletal muscle

In most instances, weakness and atrophy of skeletal muscle result from disuse caused by joint contractures or chronic disease. However, approximately 15% of patients have a primary myopathy. Of these, some have typical polymyositis, but the majority have a subtle, noninflammatory fibrous myopathy that tends to be nonprogressive.

Gastrointestinal tract

Esophagus. Esophageal dysfunction, the most common internal organ manifestation, eventually develops in nearly 90% of scleroderma patients. Dysphagia for solid foods and mild retrosternal burning pain, postprandial fullness, and regurgitation are frequent. Radiographic and manometric abnormalities are found initially in 75% of patients, including some who have no esophageal symptoms, and consist of reduced peristalsis in the distal esophagus and gastroesophageal reflux. In limited scleroderma, chronic peptic esophagitis is complicated by distal narrowing or stricture and, rarely, by serious bleeding from mucosal telangiectasias.

Small intestine. In a few patients, the illness is dominated by intestinal complaints, consisting of marked bloating, abdominal cramps, and episodic diarrhea. Severe bowel atony produces a functional ileus (pseudo-obstruction), which may simulate mechanical obstruction. Hypomotility favors bacterial overgrowth in the proximal small intestine and may lead to malabsorption with extreme wasting. These functional abnormalities are caused by atrophy of intestinal smooth muscle with collagenous replacement.

Colon. Constipation, either alone or alternating with diarrhea, may signal colonic involvement. Patchy atrophy of the muscularis leads to the development of wide-mouthed diverticula, which usually occur along the antimesenteric border of the transverse and descending colon. Rectal incontinence and prolapse are rare but disabling problems.

Lung

Lung involvement occurs in over 70% of scleroderma patients, and exertional dyspnea is present in nearly 50%. Cough and pleurisy are less common, and many patients are asymptomatic. Examination may reveal bibasilar "fibrotic" rales or pleural friction rubs but is most often normal.

In over one third of patients the chest radiograph discloses bilateral basilar interstitial fibrosis. Pulmonary function abnormalities (over 65% frequency) most commonly include restrictive defects (reduced vital capacity) and impaired gas exchange (reduced diffusing capacity for carbon monoxide). In most instances, deterioration of pulmonary function does not occur or evolves very slowly. A few patients, however, especially those with diffuse cutaneous involvement, develop progressive pulmonary dysfunction during the first several years, leading to respiratory failure. Early in disease, a prominent alveolar macrophage and/or lymphocyte inflammatory component is present, but later there is diffuse alveolar, interstitial, peribronchial, and pleural fibrosis. Modest secondary pulmonary hypertension, with relatively slow progression, may follow.

A very different entity, severe "isolated" pulmonary arterial hypertension, is encountered almost exclusively in patients with limited cutaneous scleroderma, typically after 15 to 30 years of observation. Rapidly worsening dyspnea on exertion (over the course of several months) is a clue to this diagnosis. The chest radiograph is typically normal and restrictive physiology absent, but the diffusing capacity is extremely low. Diagnosis is confirmed by echocardiogram or by right heart catheterization. Right-sided cardiac failure ultimately develops. This complication is uniformly fatal with a mean survival of only 2 years. Pathologic findings include severe narrowing and/or occlusion of small pulmonary arteries caused by subintimal proliferative changes and medial smooth muscle hypertrophy without evidence of vasculitis.

Lung cancer, independent of smoking, occurs with increased frequency in late-stage systemic sclerosis, usually in the setting of long-standing pulmonary fibrosis.

Heart

Primary cardiac problems include pericarditis with or without effusion, left ventricular or biventricular failure, or serious supraventricular or ventricular arrhythmias without other etiology. Cardiac tamponade is rare in systemic sclerosis. Clinically apparent congestive failure caused by myocardial fibrosis occurs in less than 10% of patients, nearly all of whom have diffuse skin thickening. Radionuclide studies frequently reveal subtle resting-, exercise-, and cold-induced abnormalities of ventricular function in this patient subset. Cardiac arrhythmias, including complete heart block and other electrocardiographic abnormalities, are encountered. The typical pathologic finding in advanced cases is extensive replacement of myocardium and conducting system with fibrosis. Myocarditis has been reported in several patients with scleroderma in overlap with typical polymyositis.

Kidney

"Scleroderma renal crisis" is encountered in 20% of persons with diffuse scleroderma, especially those with rapidly advancing cutaneous involvement of less than 4 years' duration. This complication is characterized by the abrupt onset of malignant hyperreninemic arterial hypertension followed promptly by acute oliguric renal insufficiency. Accompanying findings include severe headache, visual symptoms from hypertensive retinopathy, seizures, sudden left ventricular failure, microscopic hematuria, and proteinuria. On occasion blood pressure remains normal and azotemia and severe microangiopathic hemolytic anemia are the dominant features. Pathologic findings include subintimal proliferative changes of the intralobular arteries and fibrinoid necrosis of the walls of these vessels, afferent arterioles, and glomerular tufts. The pathogenesis of these renal circulatory abnormalities remains unclear.

Other organs

Primary biliary cirrhosis occurs in some women with limited cutaneous scleroderma, often coexisting with Sjögren's syndrome. These patients develop pruritus, jaundice, hepatomegaly, elevation of serum alkaline phosphatase, and serum antimitochondrial antibodies.

Hematologic studies are usually normal, although anemia is recognized and may be caused by blood loss (peptic esophagitis or intestinal telangiectasias), excessive red blood cell destruction (microangiopathic hemolysis), or metabolic causes (intestinal malabsorption). Leukopenia is often present when scleroderma exists in overlap with other connective tissue diseases.

Primary disorders of the nervous system are seldom encountered. When present, trigeminal sensory neuropathy is associated with serum anti-U1RNP antibodies. Vasculitis, with sensory neuropathy and/or mononeuritis multiplex, impotence, and autonomic neuropathy all have been described. The most common association of these features is Sjögren's syndrome, which is believed to be the underlying cause of neurologic findings. Secondary nerve compression—for example, carpal tunnel syndrome—is frequent.

Dry eyes and dry mouth are frequent complaints, and unequivocal Sjögren's syndrome (see Chapter 305) is present in at least 20% of patients. Lip biopsy shows fibrosis of minor salivary glands more often than lymphocytic infiltration.

Hypothyroidism, often clinically unrecognized, occurs in one fourth of patients and is frequently accompanied by serum antithyroid antibodies. As in the salivary glands, fibrosis is a prominent histologic finding and lymphocytic infiltration typical of Hashimoto's thyroiditis is less common.

COURSE

The natural history of systemic sclerosis is extremely variable and certainly not always "progressive." With limited cutaneous disease, skin thickening tends to remain minimal over many years. The most reliable early signs predicting diffuse skin involvement are the appearance of cutaneous thickening prior to the onset of Raynaud's phenomenon, rapid proximal progression of scleroderma, and the presence of palpable tendon friction rubs and serum anti–topoisomerase I antibody. The life span of patients with limited cutaneous disease is significantly longer than that of individuals with diffuse scleroderma, in part because the former rarely, if ever, develop myocardial or renal involvement. Cumulative survival 10 years after disease onset is approximately 75% in the limited cutaneous variant and 55% in the diffuse cutaneous subset.

LABORATORY TESTS

Routine laboratory tests are generally normal. The most consistent serologic abnormality is the presence of serum antinuclear antibodies, detected in nearly 95% of patients. During recent years several new autoantibodies have been identified that are relatively specific for systemic sclerosis (see Chapter 293). Seven different autoantibodies now identify approximately 85% of patients (Table 309-1). Of the antibodies found in patients with limited cutaneous involvement, anticentromere accounts for 60% and anti-Th (nucleolar staining) for 10% respectively. Anti–topoisomerase I (speckled and/or nucleolar staining) and anti-RNA polymerase III (speckled or nucleolar staining) together account for over 80% of patients with diffuse disease. Finally, anti-U3RNP (nucleolar), U1RNP (speckled), or anti-PMScl (nucleolar) antibodies are found in the majority of cases of systemic sclerosis in overlap.

Each of these autoantibodies has correlations with certain clinical and laboratory features (Table 309-1). Interestingly, it is rare to find two scleroderma-specific serum autoantibodies in a single patient. The production of several of these antibodies has been linked to genetic factors, for example, anti–topoisomerase I with HLA-DR5 and anti-PMScl with HLA-DR3.

DIFFERENTIAL DIAGNOSIS

The diagnosis of advanced systemic sclerosis is straightforward. Much more difficult is the identification of a specific connective tissue disease when only Raynaud's phenomenon is present. This symptom is relatively common in the general population and in most instances no systemic disease etiology is found. However most Raynaud's patients who develop an underlying connective tissue disorder do so within 2 years. Clues to such evolution include arthralgias or arthritis, tenosynovitis with tendon friction rubs, carpal tunnel syndrome, puffy or swollen digits, sclerodactyly, cutaneous hyperpigmentation, digital pitting scars, nailfold capillary changes, bibasilar rales, heartburn or distal esophageal dysphagia, and proximal muscle weakness. Unilateral and unidigital Raynaud's phenomenon are not often found in connective tissue disease. Other causes for Raynaud's to be considered are extrinsic vascular compression (thoracic outlet syndrome), occupational trauma (chainsaw and jackhammer use), and vasoconstricting drugs (ergot derivatives, beta blockers).

The several forms of localized scleroderma include morphea (patches of disease), generalized morphea (widespread confluent patches), and linear scleroderma (bandlike involvement, often in a dermatomal distribution). Lesions of these several morphologic types may occur alone or in com-

Table 309-1. Systemic sclerosis subsets according to serum autoantibodies

	Autoantibody subtype						
Clinical features	**ACA**	**Th**	**U1RNP**	**PMScl**	**U3RNP**	**RNA Pol III**	**Topo I**
ANA staining pattern	Centromere	Nucleolar	Speckled	Nucleolar	Nucleolar	Speckled/nucleolar	Speckled/nucleolar
Proportion of patients	25%	<5%	10%	<5%	<5%	25%	20%
Skin classification	←—limited		—→			←—	diffuse—→
Organ involvement	PHT	PHT small bowel	muscle	muscle	muscle PHT	kidney	lung (fibrosis) kidney

PHT = "primary" pulmonary hypertension

bination. Children and young women account for 80% of cases. In contrast to systemic sclerosis, localized scleroderma often involves the subcutaneous tissue, does not tend to symmetrically affect the digits, is often unilateral, and has no associated Raynaud's phenomenon or visceral disease. The individual lesions are ivory-colored centrally with an erythematous surrounding zone. They are usually located in the extremities, but truncal and facial involvement also may be seen. Laboratory abnormalities include peripheral blood eosinophilia and anti–single stranded DNA antibodies.

Eosinophilic fasciitis (Chapter 310) is distinguished from systemic sclerosis by a number of findings, including relative sparing of the digits; prominent involvement of the lower extremities (feet, lower legs); skin dimpling, signifying retraction of the subcutis; and absence of Raynaud's phenomenon, visceral involvement, and scleroderma-specific serum antinuclear antibodies. Two epidemic disorders, eosinophilia-myalgia syndrome caused by ingestion of contaminated L-tryptophan, and toxic oil syndrome attributed to ingestion of adulterated cooking oil, closely resemble eosinophilic fasciitis. However, they are more serious conditions that can result in pulmonary infiltration with hypoxia, pulmonary arterial hypertension, and severe ascending polyneuropathy, which may cause fatal respiratory muscle paralysis.

TREATMENT

The physician should take the time to discuss scleroderma with the patient and family, who are often unreasonably pessimistic. Such discussion helps to establish a strong patient-physician relationship, which is important in this chronic, demanding condition. When possible, classification as diffuse or limited cutaneous disease should be established since this distinction is helpful in predicting the future risk of visceral complications. Evaluation of the effectiveness of treatment has proved difficult because of variability in disease severity and rate of progression, failure to classify patients into the above subsets, limitations in the availability and application of objective criteria for ascertaining improvement (or deterioration), and the influence of psychological factors on symptoms.

Drugs

No drug or combination of drugs is of proved value in systemic sclerosis. In general, anti-inflammatory agents and corticosteroids have been disappointing, although relatively small doses of corticosteroids may be helpful in some patients with myositis, symptomatic serositis, and, on occasion, refractory arthritis or the "edematous" phase of skin involvement. High-dose corticosteroid therapy may precipitate renal crisis. Treatment with dipyridamole and aspirin, agents designed to protect injured endothelial cells, has resulted in laboratory but not clinical evidence of improvement.

In numerous uncontrolled studies D-penicillamine has been reported to reduce skin thickness and the frequency of new renal involvement and to improve pulmonary function and survival. Dosage recommended and toxicity encountered are similar to those in rheumatoid arthritis (see Chapter 304). Up to 20% of patients cannot tolerate the drug. Other unproven remedies include colchicine, cytotoxic drugs (azathioprine, methotrexate, cyclosporin A), and apheresis.

Supporting measures

Raynaud's phenomenon. Avoidance of cold exposure, dressing warmly, and abstinence from tobacco are helpful. Various vasodilating drugs have been used, the most promising of which are the calcium-channel blockers, for example, nifedipine. When large vessels are involved, such as radial and/or ulnar arteries, microvascular reconstruction should be considered. Digital tip amputation for gangrene may occasionally be required.

Calcinosis. Reliable treatment to eradicate calcinosis is not available. Surgical excision may be helpful in selected instances. Suppression of local inflammation surrounding calcinosis has been accomplished with colchicine.

Skin. Special lotions, soaps, and bath oils are used to relieve skin dryness. Excessive bathing and use of household detergents may aggravate this symptom. Noninfected ulcers respond to occlusive dressings, such as Duoderm, that are also protective. Superficial bacterial infections (almost always caused by staphylococci) are treated with half-strength hydrogen peroxide soaks, gentle local debridement, and, sometimes, oral antibiotics. Deeper infections, especially septic arthritis or osteomyelitis, must be approached aggressively with intravenous antibiotics, excision of infected and devitalized tissue, joint fusion, and, rarely, amputation.

Joints and muscles. Articular complaints may be treated with salicylates and other nonsteroidal anti-inflammatory drugs. Corticosteroids are seldom necessary, except for active polymyositis. Elective proximal interphalangeal joint replacement arthroplasties and fusions have been performed.

Gastrointestinal tract. Metoclopramide improves esophageal motility in some patients, whereas nifedipine, a smooth-muscle relaxant, may reduce it. Reflux esophagitis can be minimized by sitting upright during and after eating, avoiding food before bedtime, raising the head of the bed on blocks, antacids, histamine (H_2)–receptor blockade, and cytoprotection. Esophageal stricture may require periodic dilatation, or rarely, surgical correction.

Improvement in steatorrhea and other signs of malabsorption may follow the administration of tetracycline or other broad-spectrum antibiotics, but the underlying hypomotility is unaffected. Prokinetic drugs have not been successful in such advanced cases. Parenteral hyperalimentation may be necessary in this circumstance.

Lungs. In patients with pulmonary fibrosis, bacterial bronchitis or pneumonitis require prompt and vigorous antibiotic treatment. For inflammatory alveolitis caused by scleroderma, documented by bronchoalveolar lavage or open lung biopsy, corticosteroids alone or in combination with an immunosuppressive drug (cyclophosphamide or azathioprine) may be efficacious. D-penicillamine may limit progression in milder cases of interstitial fibrosis but apparently cannot alter the course of advanced involvement. When exercise results in hypoxia, supplemental oxygen is indicated. No effective vasodilator or other therapy is available for pulmonary arterial hypertension at present.

Heart. Symptomatic pericarditis should be treated with nonsteroidal drugs or corticosteroids. Hemodynamically significant pericardial effusion may have to be managed with pericardiocentesis or, if recurrent, an open pericardial window. If myocarditis is suspected, glucocorticoids should be tried. The typical progressive left ventricular failure caused by myocardial fibrosis is unaffected by any therapy and is generally fatal. Because digitalis intoxication is common, greater reliance is placed on diuretics. Serious arrhythmias often complicate this situation and respond inconsistently to antiarrhythmic drugs.

Kidneys. The most important aspect of therapy of renal involvement is early detection; at highest risk are patients with rapidly progressive diffuse cutaneous disease. A recent significant elevation of blood pressure is likely to signal the onset of "renal crisis." The early and aggressive use of angiotensin-converting enzyme inhibitors, other new potent antihypertensive agents, and improved dialysis procedures and care have dramatically reduced mortality. Survival with adequate renal function is the rule today. Some dialyzed patients continuing on captopril or one of the other ACE inhibitors have slow reversal of renal vascular damage and can be removed from dialysis after a number of months. Many instances of successful renal transplantation have been reported.

REFERENCES

Campbell PM and LeRoy EC: Raynaud's phenomenon. Semin Arthritis Rheum 16:92, 1986.

Cannon PJ et al: The relationship of hypertension and renal failure in scleroderma (progressive systemic sclerosis) to structural and functional abnormalities of the renal cortical circulation. Medicine 53:1, 1974.

Follansbee W: The cardiovascular manifestations of systemic sclerosis (scleroderma). Curr Publ Cardiol 11:242, 1986.

Jablonska S: Scleroderma-like conditions. In Jablonska S, editor: Scleroderma and pseudoscleroderma. Warsaw, 1975, Polish Medical Publishing.

Maricq HR: Widefield capillary microscopy: technique and rating scale for abnormalities seen in scleroderma related disorders. Arthritis Rheum 29:1159, 1981.

Owens GR et al: Pulmonary function in progressive systemic sclerosis: comparison of CREST syndrome variant with diffuse scleroderma. Chest 84:546, 1983.

Steen VD and Medsger TA Jr: Epidemiology and natural history of systemic sclerosis. Rheum Dis Clin N Amer 16:1, 1990.

Steen VD, Medsger TA Jr, and Rodnan GP: D-Penicillamine therapy in progressive systemic sclerosis (scleroderma). Ann Intern Med 97:652, 1982.

Steen VD, Powell DL, and Medsger TA Jr: Clinical correlations and prognosis based on serum autoantibodies in patients with systemic sclerosis. Arthritis Rheum 31:196, 1988.

Steen VD et al: Outcome of renal crisis in systemic sclerosis: relation to availability of angiotensin converting enzyme (ACE) inhibitors. Ann Intern Med 113:352, 1990.

Stupi A et al: Pulmonary hypertension (PHT) in the CREST syndrome variant of progressive systemic sclerosis (PSS). Arthritis Rheum 29:515, 1986.

CHAPTER

310 Diffuse Fasciitis with Eosinophilia

Richard M. Silver

Eosinophilic fasciitis (EF) (diffuse fasciitis with eosinophilia or Shulman's syndrome) was first described in 1974. Subsequently, more than 200 cases have been reported. It is a rare rheumatic disease that superficially may resemble systemic sclerosis (scleroderma), but whose treatment and course are quite different.

CLINICAL FEATURES

EF is characterized by the acute onset of aching stiffness in the extremities accompanied by cutaneous and subcutaneous edema and fibrosis. Increased numbers of eosinophils are present in the blood and usually in the affected tissues. In nearly half of all cases the onset occurs soon after strenuous exertion. Men and women are affected equally, usually between the third and seventh decades, but cases with childhood onset have been described.

Both upper and lower extremities may be affected by pain, swelling, and extreme tenderness. Asymmetric involvement is not uncommon, and the trunk may also be affected. Facial involvement is rare and, although the distal extremities (forearms and calves) may be severely affected, the fingers and toes are spared. The absence of acrosclerosis, as well as the general absence of Raynaud's phenomenon, antinuclear antibodies, and abnormal nailfold capillaries, serves to distinguish EF from systemic sclerosis (scleroderma).

The skin is edematous in the acute phase, and the extremities often exhibit pitting edema. Carpal tunnel syndrome may result from the edema, and it may be the presenting manifestation. As the acute phase subsides, the skin develops a woody induration, which may evolve to a hidebound state. Joint flexion contractures may result. Some patients have a peau d'orange appearance to the skin; others may have plaques resembling localized scleroderma (morphea).

Arthralgia and inflammatory polyarthritis may be present in the early phase. Tests for rheumatoid factor are generally negative, and erosive arthritis is rare. Hypergammaglobulinemia is common, and the ESR is often elevated. Hematologic abnormalities occur rarely, including thrombocytopenia, aplastic anemia, and leukemia.

PATHOLOGY AND ETIOLOGY

Histopathologic confirmation requires a full-thickness skin biopsy. The epidermis is normal or only mildly atrophic. The dermis may or may not be thickened because of edema, inflammation, and collagen deposition, but typically the most intense inflammation is present in the subcutis, including the fascia (Fig. 310-1). Eosinophils may be seen but are not always noticeable. The fascia is markedly thickened.

The etiology of EF is unknown. Rare cases have been associated with hematologic or solid tissue malignancy. Many recently reported cases were in fact manifestations of the eosinophilia-myalgia syndrome (EMS) associated with the ingestion of contaminated L-tryptophan. This essential amino acid was frequently used to treat insomnia, depression, fibromyalgia, and premenstrual symptoms. The syndrome now known as EMS reached epidemic proportions in the United States in the fall of 1989. Over 1500 cases were reported to have fulfilled the strict criteria of the Centers for Disease Control: (1) eosinophilia in excess of 1000 cells/mm^3; (2) myalgias severe enough to interfere with daily activities; and (3) exclusion of infection or malignancy that might also produce eosinophilia and myalgia. Common clinical manifestations of EMS that rarely occur in idiopathic EF include pneumonitis (eosinophilic) and neuropathy. The latter was sometimes severe, and many of the EMS-related deaths (2.5% of all reported EMS cases in the United States) were related to respiratory failure secondary to neuropathy.

EMS bears a striking resemblance clinically and histopathologically to the toxic oil syndrome (TOS) that occurred in Spain in 1981, affecting 20,000 individuals. In both syndromes, inflammation and fibrosis occurred in the panniculus and fascia, often extending to the perimyseal tissues. Serum aldolase levels were mildly elevated, but the creatine kinase was usually normal. Whereas EF tends to involve the subcutis alone, EMS and TOS tend to be pancutaneous and subcutaneous.

TOS was associated with the ingestion of adulterated rapeseed oil, but the precise etiologic agent was never identified. EMS has been associated with the ingestion of L-tryptophan containing trace amounts of a contaminant, 1′1-ethylidenebis[L-tryptophan] (EBT), as well as other trace contaminants. At this time it is not known whether EBT is the etiologic agent of EMS or merely a marker for another agent yet to be identified. It is conceivable that similar chemical compounds may have induced these remarkably similar fibrosing syndromes. Another possible link between the two syndromes is an alteration in the metabolism of L-tryptophan via the kynurenine pathway. High levels of L-kynurenine have also been described in the plasma of some patients with EF or idiopathic scleroderma.

THERAPY

Moderate- to high-dose corticosteroid therapy (30 to 60 mg prednisone daily) has been used to treat patients with EF. The majority have a partial or complete response. Blood eosinophil levels and the erythrocyte sedimentation rate return promptly to normal. Early-phase edema usually resolves, but softening of the skin happens only gradually. Relapses occur rarely. Hydroxychloroquine has been useful in some patients, with or without concomitant corticosteroid therapy. Spontaneous remission of EF has been noted.

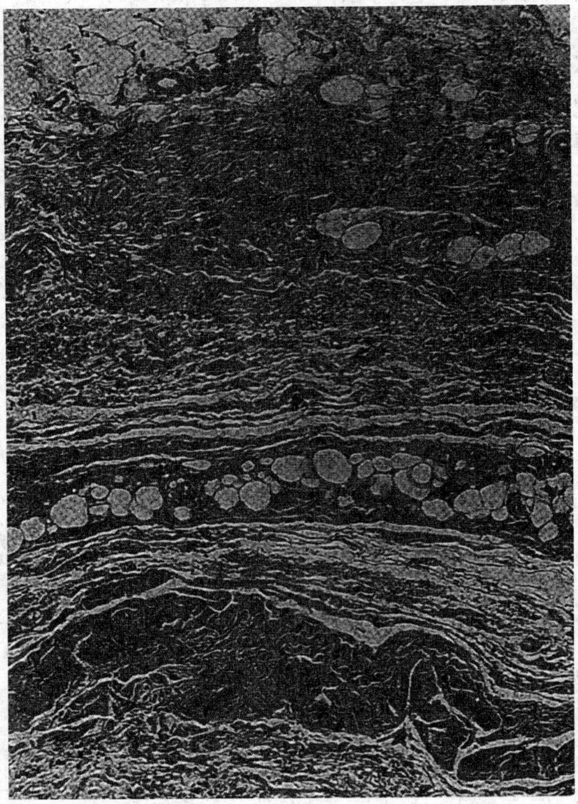

Fig. 310-1. Subcutaneous inflammation in eosinophilic fasciitis (EF). Inflammation tends to involve subcutaneous tissue and fascia. Plasma cells and eosinophils are often but not consistently present. (from Feldman SR, Silver RM, and Maize JC: A histopathologic comparison of Shulman's syndrome (diffuse fasciitis with eosinophilia) and the fasciitis associated with the eosinophilia-myalgia syndrome. J Amer Acad Dermatol 26:95, 1992.)

Patients with EMS also tended to respond to corticosteroid therapy if initiated in the acute phase, with prompt resolution of edema, dyspnea, and eosinophilia; myalgia improved but often recurred as corticosteroid doses were tapered. The metabolic alterations in L-tryptophan metabolism were reversed with corticosteroid therapy and remained normal after discontinuation of corticosteroids. It is uncertain whether corticosteroid therapy affected other aspects of the syndrome, such as cutaneous sclerosis and neuropathy. Follow-up is required to determine the long-term outlook for patients with EMS. Pulmonary hypertension, which was seen in a number of patients with TOS, has been reported in EMS, but it is not known whether this potentially fatal complication will develop later in the course of this illness.

REFERENCES

Blauvelt A and Falanga V: Idiopathic and L-tryptophan associated eosinophilic fasciitis before and after L-tryptophan contamination. Arch Dermatol 127:1159, 1991.

Feldman SR, Silver RM, and Maize JC: A histopathologic comparison of Shulman's syndrome (diffuse fasciitis with eosinophilia) and the fas-

ciitis associated with the eosinophilia-myalgia syndrome. J Amer Acad Dermatol 26:95, 1992.
Lakhanpal S et al: Eosinophilic fasciitis: clinical spectrum and therapeutic response in 52 cases. Sem Arthritis Rheum 17:221, 1988.
Mayeno AN et al: Characterization of "Peak E," a novel amino acid associated with eosinophilia-myalgia syndrome. Science 250:1707, 1990.
Shulman LE: Diffuse fasciitis with hypergamma-globulinemia and eosinophilia: a new syndrome? J Rheumatol 1(suppl):46, 1974.
Silver RM et al: Scleroderma, fasciitis, and eosinophilia associated with the ingestion of L-tryptophan. N Eng J Med 322:874, 1990.
Silver RM et al: Alterations in tryptophan metabolism in the toxic oil syndrome and in the eosinophilia-myalgia syndrome. J Rheumatol 19:69, 1992.
Slutsker L et al: Eosinophilia-myalgia syndrome associated with exposure to L-tryptophan from a single manufacturer. J Amer Med Assoc 264:213, 1990.

Classification of idiopathic inflammatory myopathies

- Primary idiopathic polymyositis
- Primary idiopathic dermatomyositis
- Dermatomyositis or polymyositis associated with malignancy
- Childhood dermatomyositis or polymyositis
- Polymyositis or dermatomyositis associated with another connective tissue disease
- Inclusion body myositis
- Miscellaneous—eosinophilic myositis, localized nodular myositis, and others

From Schumacher HR: Primer on the rheumatic diseases, ed 10. Arlington, Va, Arthritis Foundation (in press).

CHAPTER

311 Inflammatory Myopathies

Paul H. Plotz

INTRODUCTION

The inflammatory myopathies are a collection of uncommon diseases, primarily of skeletal muscle, that present most often as weakness (see box above). The two best-known variants—polymyositis and dermatomyositis—occur alone, as a part of a related connective tissue disease, or accompanied by a malignancy. There are less common variants—inclusion body myositis, eosinophilic myositis, focal nodular myositis, and orbital myositis—and there is a childhood variant that most closely resembles dermatomyositis. These diseases are classified as autoimmune connective tissue diseases because they are chronic idiopathic inflammatory diseases characterized by lymphocytic infiltration of affected tissue, and they are often accompanied by autoantibodies. Furthermore, the clinical manifestations overlap with those of other members of that disease family, and except for inclusion body myositis, they are more common in females. There are about ten new cases per million per year in the United States.

ETIOLOGY AND PATHOGENESIS

It is certain that immune mechanisms are important in the pathogenesis of the idiopathic inflammatory myopathies. The major evidences that the humoral immune system is involved are the presence of myositis-specific autoantibodies in many patients, the presence of other autoantibodies such as those found in systemic lupus in some patients, and the deposition of complement components in the muscle, especially in patients with dermatomyositis. The major evidence for the involvement of cellular immune system is the presence of an inflammatory infiltrate consisting largely of T cells in the muscle. The infiltrate may be perivascular, around the muscle fascicles, infiltrating the fascicles, and even within individual muscle cells. In polymyositis and inclusion body myositis, CD 8+ (cytotoxic) cells predominate, while in dermatomyositis, there are more CD 4+ (helper) cells.

Except for the few cases that can be ascribed to drugs or viruses (see box, p. 2452), the presumed etiologic agents in inflammatory myositis are unknown. Although viruses, especially picornaviruses, several of which can cause a myositis in humans and animals, are attractive candidates, there is little direct evidence that they play a role. A recent extensive search by sensitive molecular techniques in muscle biopsy specimens for all of the proposed candidate viruses was negative.

HISTORY, PHYSICAL EXAMINATION AND LABORATORY FINDINGS

Patients complain of the progressive onset of weakness affecting actions requiring proximal arm and leg muscles (shoulder and pelvic girdles). They have difficulty lifting things above their heads or combing their hair, climbing stairs, getting into or out of a car, or lifting their head off a pillow. Less often, muscle pain or tenderness is the dominant complaint. Patients may have difficulty in swallowing—either food gets stuck in the throat, pharynx, or upper esophagus, or liquids may regurgitate through the nose. Some patients note a change in their voice. There is great variation in the rapidity of disease onset. Some patients, usually with severe disease, can name a day when the symptoms began, and disability can progress with frightening speed. Others may fail to notice a gradual decline in function or accept it as part of an aging process and not seek medical attention for years. Most often, a patient has symptoms for several months before first complaining to a physician, and several more months then elapse before the diagnosis is established.

When a rash accompanies the muscle complaints, the disease is called *dermatomyositis,* and occasionally a typi-

Differential diagnosis of idiopathic inflammatory myopathy

Neuromuscular disorders
- Genetic muscular dystrophies
- Spinal muscular atrophies
- Neuropathies: Guillain-Barré and other autoimmune polyneuropathies, diabetes mellitus, porphyria
- Myasthenia gravis and Eaton-Lambert syndrome
- Amyotrophic lateral sclerosis
- Myotonic dystrophy and other myotonias

Endocrine and electrolyte disorders
- Hypokalemia, hyper- or hypocalcemia, hypomagnesemia
- Hypothyroidism, hyperthyroidism
- Cushing's syndrome, Addison's disease

Metabolic myopathies
- Familial periodic paralysis
- Disorders of carbohydrate metabolism—McArdle's disease, phosphofructokinase deficiency, adult acid maltase deficiency, and others
- Disorders of lipid metabolism—carnitine deficiency, carnitine palmitoyl transferase deficiency
- Disorders of purine metabolism—myoadenylate deaminase deficiency
- Mitochondrial myopathies

Toxic myopathies
- Alcohol
- Chloroquine and hydroxychloroquine
- Cocaine
- Colchicine
- Corticosteroids
- D-penicillamine
- Ipecac
- Lovastatin and other lipid-lowering agents
- Zidovudine

Infections
- Viral—influenza, EBV, HIV, coxsackievirus
- Bacterial—staphylococcus, streptococcus, clostridia
- Parasitic—toxoplasmosis, trichinosis, schistosomiasis, cysticercosis

Miscellaneous
- Polymyalgia rheumatica
- Vasculitis
- Eosinophilia myalgia syndrome
- Paraneoplastic syndromes

cal rash precedes the weakness by up to several months. The almost diagnostic rashes of dermatomyositis are a purplish (heliotrope) discoloration of the eyelids—sometimes only along the edge of the upper lid, but sometimes involving all of both lids to give an owl's eye appearance; a raised, plaquelike, sometimes scaly eruption over the interphalangeal joints, or just erythema of those knuckles, called Gottron's sign; a related flat or scaly erythema of the interphalangeal joints of the toes, knees, elbows, or malleoli; a flat or slightly raised facial rash that may be sun-sensitive, resembling the lupus butterfly rash (but often distinguished from it because in dermatomyositis the nasolabial folds may be involved); and a flat or slightly raised erythematous rash of the V region of the neck or over the upper back (shawl sign).

These diseases rarely affect the facial or extraocular muscles, and muscle atrophy or contractures are not common early. The distal muscles are not usually much affected except in inclusion body myositis, where distal weakness and a mild accompanying peripheral neuropathy including foot drop may confuse the picture. Except in inclusion body myositis, involvement is generally symmetrical.

Involvement outside the skeletal muscles may be very important in determining the outcome of the disease. Interstitial lung disease is the most common and threatening extraskeletal muscle manifestation, occurring mainly in patients with one of the myositis-specific autoantibodies, anti-Jo-1 (or the related autoantibodies anti-PL-7, anti-PL-12, anti-OJ, or anti-EJ). Cardiac involvement in the form of rhythm disturbances or, more rarely, frank myocarditis and cardiac failure is less frequent. Gastrointestinal involvement below the esophagus is uncommon but may cause diarrhea or even rectal incontinence.

The correct diagnosis of myositis depends upon the typical findings by history and on examination *and* upon several laboratory tests. The muscle-related enzymes, creatine kinase and aldolase, are most specific, but the transaminases and LDH are usually elevated, too. The creatine kinase is elevated in almost every patient with myositis, and if muscle disease is suspected, a serum creatine kinase should be obtained since an elevated level of the other enzymes alone may lead to an incorrect diagnosis of liver disease. The electromyogram helps rule out other neuromuscular diseases that may resemble myositis, such as myasthenia gravis or motor neuron disease. A muscle biopsy should be performed early in the course of every patient in whom the diagnosis of an inflammatory myopathy is thought likely to confirm the presence of the characteristic findings of degeneration and regeneration of muscle fibers and lymphocytic inflammation, to seek inclusion bodies (best seen on a snap-frozen specimen stained with trichrome), and to rule out the occasional surprise such as a dystrophy, sarcoidosis, amyloidosis, polyarteritis, or an unusual metabolic myopathy. A magnetic resonance image of muscles using the STIR technique is a sensitive way to locate muscle inflammation and may be useful to help select a site for biopsy.

DIFFERENTIAL DIAGNOSIS

The differential diagnosis of muscle weakness must take into account a broad range of conditions; the physician should consider diseases of the central and peripheral nervous system, genetic metabolic disorders of muscle, several endocrine diseases, electrolyte abnormalities, drug-induced myopathies, several infections, and a variety of other diseases such as polymyalgia rheumatica and the eosinophilia myalgia syndrome (see box at left). A careful history and physical examination suffice to point to or away from inflammatory muscle disease. The following items point away from myositis: a family history of a similar muscle disease; symptoms in an adult that began in childhood; weakness that develops during or after exercise; facial or extraocular muscle involvement; fasciculations or myotonia (difficulty relaxing a muscle after a prolonged contraction); involvement of only one muscle; significant hypertrophy or atrophy. A search for drugs or toxins that cause myopathy is essential, especially for those that may be hidden or denied at first such as alcohol, cocaine, ipecac, or zidovudine. Infections are not common as a cause of muscle weakness, but HIV infection—perhaps because it predisposes to other viruses or to bacterial pyomyositis—and Lyme disease and influenza may present as a myositis. Of the endocrine diseases, myxedema can mimic polymyositis closely.

IMPORTANT VARIANTS

Several of the variants of inflammatory myopathy deserve special mention. *Inclusion body myositis* is a slowly progressive disease closely resembling polymyositis found in older patients (rarely before age 40, except in a familial childhood type) in which distal weakness, asymmetric involvement, isolated muscle atrophy, a history of unexpected falling, and the absence of rash, interstitial lung disease, and myositis-specific autoantibodies are distinguishing features. Occasionally, however, other autoantibodies or features of another connective tissue disease such as Sjögren's syndrome are present. Inclusion body myositis responds relatively poorly to standard treatment although some investigators report that progression of weakness can be slowed or halted even if strength does not return. *Cancer-associated myositis* presents a difficult diagnostic problem. There is an increased incidence of cancer in the entire population of myositis patients. It is more likely to occur in older patients and those with dermatomyositis. A sensible approach to the freshly diagnosed patient with myositis is to perform a meticulous history and physical exam including pelvic and rectal exams, supplement it with a standard battery of lab tests including stools for occult blood and other tests such as a chest x-ray and mammography as dictated by good medical practice for a person of that age group. Any abnormality not clearly related to myositis should then be followed until a satisfactory explanation is obtained. *Connective tissue disease–associated myositis* is most often found in patients with lupus erythematosus, mixed connective tissue disease, or scleroderma, and it commonly responds very well to anti-inflammatory therapy.

TESTS FOR AUTOANTIBODIES

Antinuclear or antiextractable nuclear antigen (ENA) antibodies are often positive in patients with myositis, but these autoantibodies are found in many other diseases. Of great interest are a series of recently described autoantibodies that occur almost exclusively in myositis. Some patients have autoantibodies directed against a series of enzymes that join an amino acid to its proper transfer RNA—anti-Jo-1, anti-PL-7, anti-PL-12, anti-EJ, and anti-OJ. Some patients have autoantibodies to other intracellular proteins or particles such as the signal recognition particle (SRP), and Mi-2. Careful study of the clinical manifestations and the presence of serum autoantibodies has drawn attention to the fact that polymyositis and dermatomyositis may actually be a group of syndromes, some of which are characterized by a particular autoantibody. These differ from one another not only in their autoantibodies and clinical manifestations, but also in their extraskeletal muscle manifestations, racial predominance, HLA type, rapidity or even season of onset, and response to therapy and prognosis. Table 311-1 presents features of several of these syndromes.

TREATMENT

When the diagnosis of polymyositis or dermatomyositis has been established, corticosteroids are the preferred first treatment, usually prednisone, 1 mg/kg/day, in a single morning dose. This dose is maintained until the creatine kinase reaches normal and there is substantial symptomatic improvement, and it is then lowered slowly, by 10 mg/day each month. Few patients achieve a complete return to normal strength, and most require continuing low-dose corticosteroid therapy to maintain a remission. If a patient fails to respond to this regimen, if the disease recurs with tapering, or if steroid side effects are a major problem, a second agent should be considered—methotrexate at 7.5 to 25 mg once a week by mouth or up to 50 mg per week parenterally or azathioprine at up to 2.5 mg/kg/day. Alternative therapies for which there is anecdotal evidence of efficacy include pulse corticosteroids, chlorambucil, cyclophosphamide, cyclosporin A, and intravenous gamma globulin. Plasmapheresis and lymphapheresis are ineffective. In unremitting cases of well-established disease, other vigorous

Table 311-1. Some syndromes associated with myositis-specific autoantibodies

Autoantibodies	Gender HLA type	Characteristic clinical features
Anti-Jo-1 Anti-PL-7 Anti-PL-12 Anti-OJ Anti-EJ	♀:♂ = 2.7 HLA DR3	Relatively acute onset; frequent interstitial lung disease, fever, Raynaud's phenomenon, arthritis, and "mechanic's hands." Moderate response to therapy, but persistent disease.
Anti-SRP	♀:♂ > 6 HLA DR5	Very acute onset, often in fall, severe weakness, no rash, palpitations, ♀>♂, poor response to therapy.
Anti-Mi-2	♀:♂ = 1.2 HLA DR7	Relatively acute onset, classic dermatomyositis with V sign and shawl sign rashes, cuticular overgrowth, good response to therapy.

From Schumacher HR: Primer on the rheumatic diseases, ed 10. Arlington, Va, Arthritis Foundation (in press).

regimens such as a combination of two cytotoxic agents may be justified, but a repeat muscle biopsy ought to be considered to hunt for inclusion body myositis. Steroid-related myopathy frequently complicates treatment and should always be considered in a weak patient who fails to respond to increasing therapy or whose weakness is not accompanied by elevated muscle enzymes. The rash of dermatomyositis may respond well to hydroxychloroquine (200 mg bid). If the diagnosis of inclusion body myositis has been established the proper approach to therapy remains controversial. Unless there are contraindications to steroid and/or cytotoxic therapy, treatment should be undertaken, particularly if there is inflammation on the muscle biopsy and the creatine kinase is elevated. The goal is stabilization, not remission, and it may take a year or more of therapy and then a period off treatment to be sure that even this limited goal has been achieved.

Assessment of treatment should rest upon the triad of history, strength testing, and creatine kinase levels. Sole reliance upon only one, such as the creatine kinase, may well lead to improper or unnecessarily erratic therapy. Attentive physical therapy including active exercise after acute inflammation has subsided is important to preserve or even restore strength and range of motion.

REFERENCES

Engel AG and Arahata K: Mononuclear cells in myopathies: quantitation of functionally distinct subsets, recognition of antigen-specific cell-mediated cytotoxicity in some diseases, and implications for the pathogenesis of the different inflammatory myopathies. Hum Pathol 17:704, 1986.

Fraser DD et al: Magnetic resonance imaging in the idiopathic inflammatory myopathies. J Rheumatol 18:1693, 1991.

Leff RL et al: Viruses in idiopathic inflammatory myopathies: absence of candidate viral genomes in muscle. Lancet 339:1192, 1992.

Lotz BP et al: Inclusion body myositis. Observations in 40 patients. Brain 112:727, 1989.

Love LA et al: A new approach to the classification of idiopathic inflammatory myopathy: myositis-specific autoantibodies define useful homogeneous patient groups. Medicine (Baltimore) 70:360, 1991.

Oddis CV and Medsger TA: Current management of polymyositis and dermatomyositis. Drugs 37:382, 1989.

Oddis CV et al: Incidence of polymyositis-dermatomyositis: a 20-year study of hospital diagnosed cases in Allegheny County, PA 1963-1982. J Rheumatol 17:1329, 1990.

Plotz PH et al: Current concepts in the idiopathic inflammatory myopathies: polymyositis, dermatomyositis, and related disorders. Ann Intern Med 111:143, 1989.

Sigurgeirsson B et al: Risk of cancer in patients with dermatomyositis or polymyositis. A population-based study. N Engl J Med 326:363, 1992.

Zuckner J: Drug-induced myopathies. Semin Arthritis Rheuma 19:259, 1990.

CHAPTER

312 Spondyloarthropathies

Michael H. Weisman

Spondyloarthropathy is a term used to describe certain rheumatic diseases that have a characteristic involvement of the joints of the peripheral and axial skeleton. These include ankylosing spondylitis, Reiter's disease, reactive forms of arthritis, psoriatic arthritis, and the arthritis associated with chronic inflammatory bowel diseases (Chapter 43). Spondyloarthropathies are readily distinguished from rheumatoid arthritis (RA) on historic, geographic, epidemiologic, genetic, clinical, pathologic, and radiographic grounds, but separating one form of spondyloarthropathy from another often proves difficult (Table 312-1). All too often patients appear to "evolve" over time, losing features of one disease while adding new elements of another. In particular, the separation between Reiter's syndrome and reactive arthritis is arbitrary and historical, not substantive.

Hypertrophy of the synovial membrane with exudation of inflammatory synovial fluid limited to the confines of the joint capsule is a regular feature of rheumatoid arthritis. In contrast, although the spondyloarthropathies may also have synovitis, they characteristically produce inflammation in and around the entheses (the sites of ligament and tendon attachment into bone) or even in areas quite remote from joints, such as along the periosteal membrane of the pelvic brim, ischial tuberosity, or calcaneous. The distribution of articular involvement is unique and different from that found in RA. Patients with RA almost always have bilateral, symmetric polyarthritis of large as well as small joints, with equal frequency in the upper and lower extremities. The spondyloarthropathies typically involve large joints in an asymmetric fashion with a predilection toward joints in a lower extremity. When spondyloarthropathies involve small joints, they produce a characteristic picture—interphalangeal joints are affected out of proportion to metacarpal phalangeal joints of the hands or metatarsophalangeal joints of the toes.

Disease manifestations in extraskeletal sites and a variety of skin and mucous membrane lesions are commonly associated with the spondyloarthropathies. Sites of inflammation and clinical disease include the ciliary body of the eye, the intraventricular septum of the heart, the aortic root, the interstitial connective tissue surrounding the alveolar air spaces of the upper lung fields, the dura covering the lumbar nerve roots exiting from the spinal canal, the loose fibrous connective tissue of the prostate and seminal vesicles, and even the submucosa of the intestinal tract. The vascular channels that supply many of these sites have anastomotic connections with the plexus of veins (Batson's plexus) extending up and down the spine. These shared connections may in some way provide a clue to the unique lo-

Table 312-1. Characterization of the spondyloarthropathies as typified by a comparison of ankylosing spondylitis and rheumatoid arthritis

	Ankylosing spondylitis	Rheumatoid arthritis
Ancient history	Evidence in animals and humans dating from 3000 B.C.	Questionable evidence for existence in humans prior to the nineteenth century
Geographic distribution	Racial and genetic associations; following prevalence of HLA-B27	Worldwide in all populations
Prevalence	Estimated 0.1%	1%-2%
Etiology	Unknown	Unknown
Sex distribution	Male predominance	Female predominance
Age group	Peak at 20-30 years, rare after age 50	All ages
Joints involved	Oligoarthritis (four or fewer joints) asymmetric, large joints, lower limbs, interphalangeal articulations may predominate	Polyarthritis, symmetric, small and large joints, upper and lower limbs
Sacroiliac involvement	Always	Rare
Spinal involvement	Total (ascending)	Neck only
Eyes	Uveitis	Sicca syndrome; episcleritis, scleritis, scleromalacia perforans
Lungs	Rare upper lobe pulmonary fibrosis	Diffuse interstitial pulmonary fibrosis, effusions, nodules
Heart	Aortitis, aortic root dilatation, aortic regurgitation, atrioventricular conduction disturbances	Pericarditis; rare aortic and mitral valve involvement
Rheumatoid factor	No	Yes
HLA-B27	Yes	No
Pathology	Enthesopathy, reactive bone, and synovitis	Synovitis predominates
Radiology	Erosions, periosteal new bone formation, fibrous and bony ankylosis, fusion of joints, dense bones	Erosions, osteopenia, joint space loss, absence of new bone formation

calization of many of the features of the spondyloarthropathies.

Individuals compromised by human immunodeficiency virus (HIV) infection often develop more exaggerated, severe forms of Reiter's disease and psoriasis. The arthritis in RA patients may be ameliorated by the HIV infection, suggesting a key role for CD8 T cells in the pathogenesis of the former (spondyloarthropathies) and CD4 T cells in the latter (RA).

Maleness, familial aggregation, and apparent clinical "overlap" as these conditions evolve over time typify patients with spondyloarthropathies. There is a genetic predisposition to this group of diseases that is affixed to the B locus of the HLA chromosome region. The overwhelming majority of Caucasians with ankylosing spondylitis and Reiter's syndrome possess HLA-B27. Strong associations with HLA-B27 are found in patients with the other spondyloarthropathies, depending on the subset studied, race, degree of spinal involvement, and other clinical features.

The HLA-B27 molecule is undoubtedly important. Transfection of human B_{27} and B_2 microglobulin genes into susceptible strains of rats results in a disease of the integument and articulations indistinguishable from ankylosing spondylitis and psoriasis.

The strongest association to B27 is between Caucasian patients with ankylosing spondylitis (85% to 90%) compared with that of the entire population of North America and Europe (6% to 8%). The point prevalence of ankylosing spondylitis parallels the B27-antigen frequency in most worldwide populations. However, B27 is neither a necessary nor a sufficient cause of disease. Additional genetic and/or environmental factors seem to play a role. For example, black Americans have a low prevalence of HLA-B27 and a weak association between the disease and HLA status. In random B27-positive people, the risk of developing ankylosing spondylitis is 1% to 3%; however, the risk increases considerably (15% to 25%) if a B27-positive person is related to a B27-positive patient with known ankylosing spondylitis.

Reiter's syndrome and ankylosing spondylitis have been shown to "breed true" within families and within specific populations in which there is a high incidence of each, especially in certain native American groups. It is estimated that there is a 20% to 25% risk for development of Reiter's disease after a B27-positive individual is exposed to enteric pathogens and a 10% to 20% risk after contracting nongonococcal urethritis.

ANKYLOSING SPONDYLITIS

Incidence and prevalence

Ankylosing spondylitis has an insidious onset in most cases and incidence figures are difficult to interpret because of selection bias toward more advanced disease at academic medical centers. Depending on which criteria are used, most reports place the overall prevalence at 0.1% of the Caucasian population. Asymptomatic disease certainly occurs, and the diagnosis is made less often in women because the condition is probably milder in females and often presents with peripheral joint manifestations in advance of symptomatic sacroiliitis. The 10:1 male-to-female ratio frequently cited in textbooks most certainly is overstated, although the true ratio is unknown.

Pathology and radiology

Although frank arthritis (histologically similar to rheumatoid arthritis) may occur, the characteristic lesions of ankylosing spondylitis are periarticular and occur at insertions of ligaments and tendons (entheses) into bone. The earliest histologic changes appear to be infiltration of macrophages and lymphocytes, followed by a proliferative fibroblastic response that progressively replaces the inflammatory cells. There is a frank osteitis of the adjacent subchondral bone. Reactive new bone replaces the eroded and destroyed segments, and the process takes place progressively at ligamentous insertions along the superior iliac crest, the inferior rami of the pubis, and peripheral sites such as the calcanei. When the outer fibers of the anulus fibrosus are involved, this results in syndesmophyte formation and "squared" vertebral bodies. A similar process affects both the synovial-lined lower two thirds and the fibrous upper one third of the sacroiliac joints in a symmetric fashion, producing an initial erosion followed by sclerosis and replacement of cartilage by reactive bone. This results in complete obliteration of the joint in the later stages of disease. The zygoapophyseal joints of the lumbar spine appear to be particularly susceptible to this disease, and early involvement may produce significant limitation of motion in the absence of any radiographic changes surrounding the vertebral bodies themselves.

History

Bilateral low back pain that awakens the patient at night best differentiates ankylosing spondylitis from other causes of low back pain. Patients usually get out of bed in the early morning hours and try to find a comfortable position somewhere in the house; often, they lie down on a hard surface, such as the floor. Other features that point to ankylosing spondylitis are pain lasting longer than 3 months, morning stiffness, improvement of the pain with exercise, pain radiating to the buttocks, and disease onset before the age of 40 in males.

It is important to note that ankylosing spondylitis patients may present with transient sharp pains in the heels, pelvis, shoulders, ribs, or sternum in advance of back pain. Spine symptoms are often not noticed or dismissed in the presence of these peripheral manifestations.

Physical examination

The examiner should look for (1) paravertebral muscle spasm and loss of lumbar lordosis, (2) decreased lumbar spine mobility in anterior and lateral planes, (3) fixed and unbending movement of the low back when the patient leans forward, (4) diminished chest expansion, and (5) tenderness over thoracolumbar spinous processes, sacroiliac joints, and in other places where periostitis is likely to occur, such as the sternum, the clavicles, the iliac crests, or the heels. Three sensitive maneuvers reveal objective impairment in patients with early ankylosing spondylitis.

Mennell's sign. With the patient prone on the examination table, hyperextend the thigh while pressing on the ipsilateral sacroiliac joint. Pain in the sacroiliac joint after 10 degrees of hyperextension occurs in the presence of sacroiliitis.

Shober's test. The degree of restriction of forward flexion can be measured by the distraction of 2 points on the skin when the patient bends maximally forward in the upright position. The lower mark is chosen at the level of the lumbosacral junction: an upper point is placed 10 cm cephalad. This distance increases to 15 cm in normal subjects and is reduced to less than 13 mm in patients with spondylitis.

Observation of spontaneous movement. Ask the patient to change from a prone to a supine position on the examining table. Normal subjects coil and uncoil their bodies to perform this maneuver. Spondylitics move gingerly in a single unit, or en bloc.

Radiographic changes

At the present time the diagnosis of ankylosing spondylitis requires the presence of radiologic evidence of sacroiliitis. Clearly, some patients may have symptoms in advance of obvious x-ray changes; however, the search for additional imaging procedures for early disease has not led to improved accuracy in questionable cases. The frontal radiograph of the pelvis sooner or later shows the earliest changes of ankylosing spondylitis. These changes are (1) blurring or indistinctness of the margins of the lower two thirds of the joint, especially on the iliac side; (2) juxta-articular sclerosis; and (3) erosions plus adjacent sclerosis giving the appearance of a "pseudowidening" of the sacroiliac joint. In more advanced sacroiliitis there is progression of the sclerosis with erosions and joint space destruction, leading to total ankylosis and obliteration of the joint (Fig. 312-1). The severity of these changes is graded from 0 to 4, depending on the amount of joint destruction observed. In some patients, pelvic disease does not develop beyond grade 2 or 3 and remains limited to the pelvis. What determines the progression to ascending spinal disease is unknown. Early change in the lumbar spine is recognized by squaring of the superior and inferior margins of the vertebral body caused by inflammatory disease at the site of insertion of the outer fibers of the anulus fibrosus. This may progress to typical syndesmophyte formation (Fig. 312-2). More severe progressive changes result in the classic, although rare, "bamboo" spine. Other features seen are irregularity and sclerosis of the symphysis pubis; and whiskering, an almost frayed appearance to the iliac crests, ischial tuberosities, and greater tronchanters. For more details, see Chapter 294).

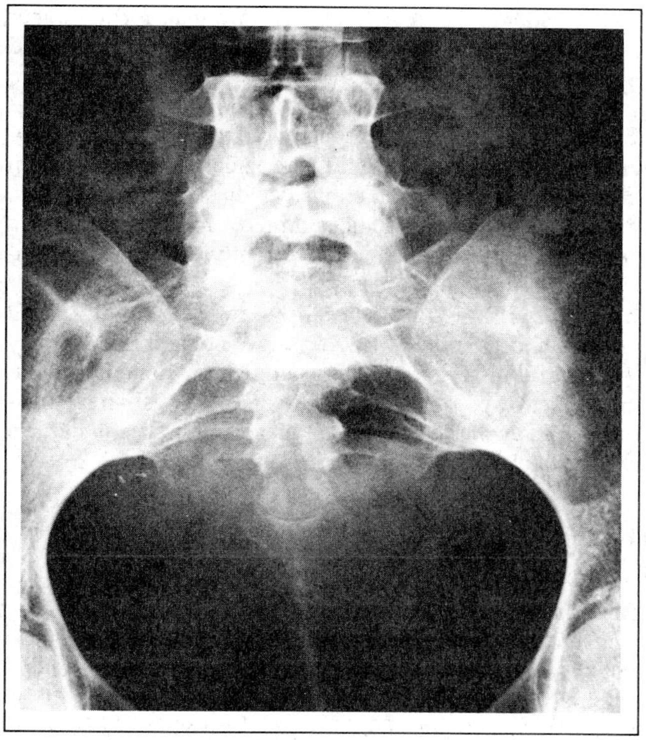

Fig. 312-1. Ankylosing spondylitis. Note the total ankylosis of right sacroiliac joint and moderate change in left joint. Juxta-articular sclerosis, joint space narrowing, and irregularity are seen, with partial fusion.

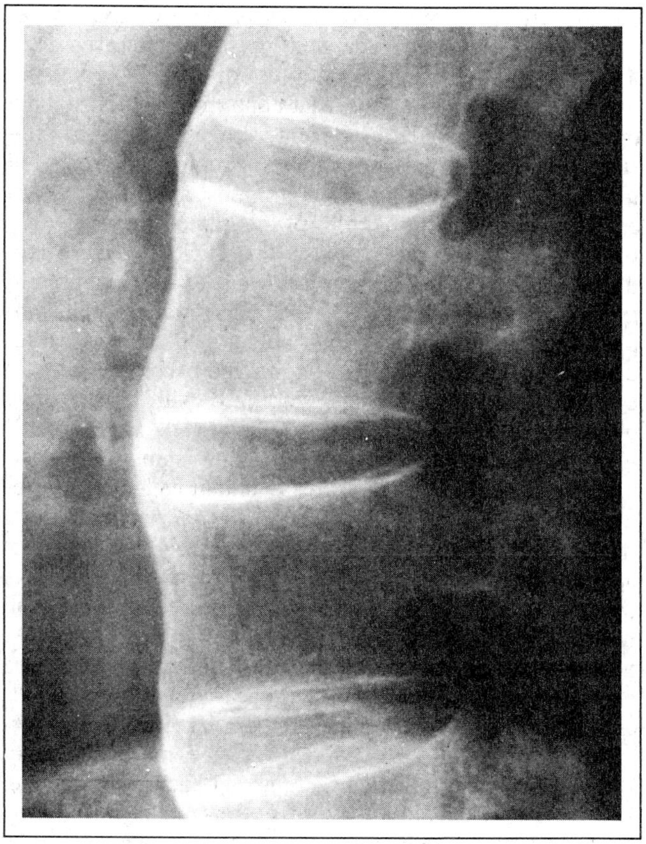

Fig. 312-2. Same patient as shown in Fig. 312-1. Note ossification in the anterior fibers of anulus fibrosus between the lumbar vertebrae.

Juvenile ankylosing spondylitis

Teenagers present with features of ankylosing spondylitis that may mimic other diseases, and the diagnosis is frequently delayed. In contrast to patients with juvenile chronic polyarthritis, these youngsters are older, are male, and display oligoarthritis of the lower extremities. Blood tests for rheumatoid factor and antinuclear antibody are negative. In an older male child, lower-extremity peripheral arthritis may evolve into ankylosing spondylitis at a later date. On occasion, children present with profound systemic features—such as fatigue, anemia, weight loss, high erythrocyte sedimentation rate, and severe spine pain—suggesting infection or neurologic disease. The major problem in confirming a diagnosis of juvenile ankylosing spondylitis concerns the pelvic radiograph; in teenagers, the sacroiliac joint margins are indistinct and appear widened in the normal state.

Extraskeletal manifestations

Inflammatory granulation tissue trapping the nerves exiting from the lower spinal canal may produce a cauda equina syndrome. Uveitis occurs in approximately 20% of patients during the course of the illness. Painful eye inflammation is acute; it begins unilaterally, but later episodes may be bilateral. If untreated, blindness may ensue. Chronic pulmonary infiltrates and fibrotic changes in the upper lung fields can mimic tuberculosis. Aortic incompetence, cardiomegaly, and persistent atrioventricular conduction defects develop in a small percentage of those with severe long-standing spinal disease.

Prognosis and treatment

The prognosis in ankylosing spondylitis is highly variable and difficult to predict in the individual patient. In general, patients tend to function well in spite of severe restriction of motion, and in progressive disease extraspinal involvement is often an important determinant of prognosis. Some epidemiologic surveys indicate that if only mild disease and mild loss of spinal motion occur within the first 10 years, the disease will not progress. Severe peripheral joint involvement at the onset is thought to convey the worst prognosis. Most patients with ankylosing spondylitis, however, have mild disease and manage to lead full social and professional lives. In general, women have less severe and less progressive spinal disease but may have more peripheral joint involvement. The bamboo spine is seen more frequently in men.

Two features of ankylosing spondylitis bear directly on morbidity, mortality, and prognosis. Both are thought to result from trauma—one unrecognized and inapparent, the other overt. The former is a discovertebral destructive lesion, usually occurring in a well-localized spinal segment, heralded by acute pain or acute loss of height. Bone scintigraphy and tomography reveal abnormalities across both the anterior and posterior elements. Infection must be considered in the differential diagnosis. Prompt and prolonged immobilization results in healing in most cases. The weakened biomechanical properties of the immobilized osteoporotic spine predisposes to these "insufficiency"-type fractures. A second complication follows severe or even minor trauma. Overt fractures can result in complete or incomplete spinal cord compression; the cervical spine is particularly vulnerable. Spinal fusion may be necessary to manage fractures that cannot be stabilized with conservative treatment.

The primary objectives of ankylosing spondylitis treatment are to relieve pain, decrease inflammation, begin remedial muscle-strengthening exercises, and maintain good posture and function. Although it is unlikely that any therapeutic program can alter the course of the disease, it is fairly certain that good posture and sense of well-being can be enhanced. Treatment for the spondylitic should apply 24 hours a day, every day of the year. The patient should be encouraged to sleep on his or her back with a firm mattress and a single, thin pillow; the use of a large pillow or several pillows should be avoided. In the morning, a hot shower should be followed by remedial back-strengthening and extension exercises. These exercises can be demonstrated by the physician or physical therapist and should be performed regularly by the patient at home. Assuming a prone position for several minutes a few times a day is an ideal way to maintain spinal extension. Exercises are necessary because the disease tends to produce progressive spinal flexion; therefore, the spinal extension musculature must be strengthened. Additional maneuvers include stretching, deep breathing, and isometric lumbar flexion. During the day, attention to posture must be stressed. Chairs with a hard back are preferable, but any opportunity to walk rather than sit should be taken. Swimming is the most appropriate sport, since the musculature can be strengthened in a position of extension. Spinal fusion, a frequent consequence of spondylitis, should take place in the best possible position of function, with avoidance of compensatory flexion contractures of the hips and knees. Patients should be advised to stand tall at all times, as if their heels, buttocks, shoulders, and occiput were always "against the wall."

Anti-inflammatory medications relieve pain, decrease inflammation, and enhance the patient's quality of life. Whether they actually increase mobility or retard progressive fusion is not known. Indomethacin (Indocin), 75 to 150 mg per day, has the best record of success. If patients are not able to tolerate gastric upset or central-nervous-system side effects of headache and dizziness, other nonsteroidal anti-inflammatory drugs may be tried in an empirical fashion (Chapter 317). For patients with disease not responsive to indomethacin or the newer nonsteroidal anti-inflammatory agents, phenylbutazone, 100 to 300 mg per day, may be tried. The incidence of agranulocytosis or aplastic anemia is greater for this drug than for any other nonsteroidal anti-inflammatory agent, and this issue should be discussed openly with the patient so that the risks are fully understood. Monitoring of blood cell and platelet count is mandatory. In patients with peripheral joint polyarthritis, agents such as gold and penicillamine have been used. Recently published clinical studies of sulfasalazine in ankylosing spondylitis indicate improvement in pain and in spinal mobility. This agent is currently undergoing extensive controlled clinical trials.

Is HLA-B27 testing clinically useful? Under almost all circumstances the HLA B27 test does not add substantially to a careful history, physical examination, spine or peripheral joint x-ray, joint fluid culture and analysis, and knowledge of a few basic differential diagnostic issues in clinical rheumatology.

REITER'S SYNDROME AND REACTIVE ARTHRITIS

Reiter's syndrome (reactive arthritis) is probably the most frequent cause of inflammatory arthritis in the young male population of North America and Europe. Pure Reiter's syndrome historically is rooted in the classic tetrad of arthritis, conjunctivitis, urethritis, and dermatitis. Many experts only accept all four criteria, and for that reason we often hear the term *classic Reiter's*. Clearly, incomplete forms of the same disease exist. A reactive arthritis has been described after *Salmonella, Shigella, Yersinia,* or *Campylobacter* enteric infections. These reactive arthritides have displayed classic Reiter's syndrome manifestations (the complete tetrad) or various combinations thereof. There is no reason to keep both of these terms *(Reiter's disease, reactive arthritis),* since both describe the same disease. There are differing clinical manifestations depending on race, gender, and genetic background, and these blends of clinical differences cross over into each previously described category. At present, it is commonly recognized that there are two initiating causes: venereal (sexually)-acquired arthritis, thought in some cases to be caused by infection with either *Chlamydia trachomatis* or *Ureaplasma urealyticum,* and postdysenteric (enteric)-acquired.

HLA-B27 is strongly associated with Reiter's syndrome (65% to 75%), either postdysenteric or postvenereal. B27-negative patients appear to have a milder course. Sacroiliitis may be silent and may occur early in the disease. Enteric infections in the United States are most commonly associated with Reiter's syndrome. The diarrhea portion of the illness may be clinically silent. Cases of Reiter's syndrome are now being described with increasing frequency in HIV-positive individuals and individuals with AIDS. In these situations, the arthropathy as well as the nonarticular features of Reiter's disease appear particularly severe and unremitting.

Incidence and prevalence

The prevalence of sporadic Reiter's syndrome is not known. Analysis of epidemics of enteritis causing Reiter's syndrome has led to prevalence figures ranging from 1% to 2% of infected persons, whereas 20% of individuals with HLA-B27 develop reactive arthritis. Reiter's syndrome has a worldwide distribution: the prevalence roughly follows the frequency of HLA-B27 and the presence of intestinal infections from *Shigella flexneri, Salmonella* of different groups, *Yersinia enterocolitica* of different serotypes, *Yersinia pseudotuberculosis,* and *Campylobacter jejuni/coli.*

Diagnosis and clinical features

Reiter's syndrome may begin with arthritis or with extra-articular features, usually 1 to 3 weeks after the diarrhea episode. The urethritis may be mild or suppressed and thus overlooked by the patient. Some patients may have only a cystitis manifest by sterile pyuria. Mouth and tongue ulcers are virtually never noted by the patient, since they are painless; the examiner must search diligently for these shallow erosions on the tongue or soft palate.

Dermatologic manifestations occur in 50% of patients and take two basic forms, depending on whether they are present on moist mucous membrane surfaces unexposed to outside air or on exposed surfaces where keratinization occurs (Color Plate VI-2). In the former situation, shallow painless erythematous ulcers occur on the uncircumcised glans of the penis and the oral mucous membranes. These lesions develop serpiginous gray borders, sometimes forming a circle, called *circinate balanitis.* In contrast to most other causes of genital ulcerations, especially herpes simplex, these lesions are painless. On surfaces exposed to the outside ambient air (e.g., circumcised glans of the penis, palms, soles) the Reiter's lesion evolves from a small macule to a vesicle followed by progressive thickening and hyperkeratinization. These scattered, crusted lesions develop insidiously and are called *keratodermia blennorhagica.* Patients may display a thickening and subsequent detachment at the nail base, lifting the nail from its foundation and resulting in loss of the entire nail.

The arthritis of Reiter's syndrome is indistinguishable from the peripheral arthritis of ankylosing spondylitis and predominantly involves the large joints of the lower extremities in an asymmetric manner. The feet, however, are the focal point for the diagnosis in most cases. Insertions of ligaments and tendons in the feet are favorite places for Reiter's syndrome to be manifest—plantar fasciitis at the plantar aponeurosis ("lovers heels"), Achilles tendinitis (Fig. 312-3), retrocalcaneal bursitis, and tendinitis along the tibialis posterior tendon sheath as it courses under the medial malleolus. On occasion the foot is diffusely swollen with a fine erythematous macular rash; in these cases it is often difficult to decide if arthritis, tenosynovitis, or periostitis is present. Patients with reactive arthritis often develop swelling and tenderness along the finger or toe, between the interphalangeal joints—particularly in the dorsum of the digits. This swelling is referred to as a *sausage digit,* but *dactylitis* is a more appropriate designation (Fig. 312-4). On occasion, a patient with Reiter's disease displays a toxic-appearing syndrome characterized by high fevers, weight loss, and anemia; these signs and symptoms occur at presentation of disease and dominate the clinical picture for days to weeks. The important differences between Reiter's syndrome and gonococcal arthritis when the patient presents with monarticular arthritis are displayed in Table 312-2.

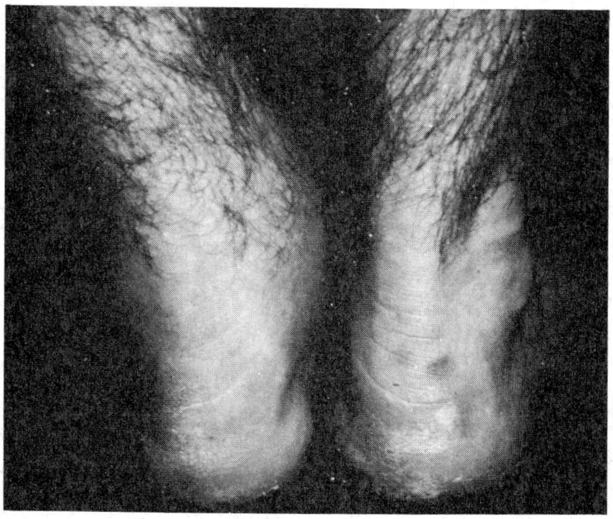

Fig. 312-3. Swelling of the Achilles tendon of the right foot in a patient with reactive arthritis.

Prognosis and management

The natural history of Reiter's syndrome is not known with certainty and is unpredictable for the individual patient. It is estimated that up to 50% of patients suffer a single self-limited episode, the remaining patients divided between

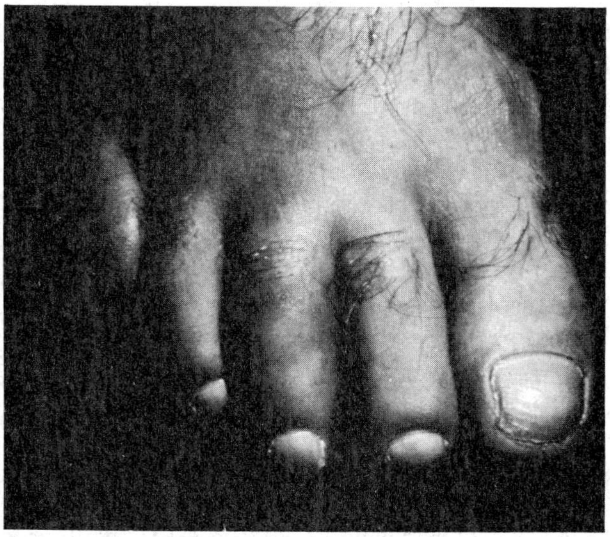

Fig. 312-4. "Sausage digit," or dactylitis of the third toe.

Table 312-2. Important differences between Reiter's syndrome and gonococcal arthritis when the patient presents with monarticular arthritis

	Reiter's disease	Gonococcal arthritis
History	Episode of enteritis preceding arthritis	Migratory tenosynovitis preceding overt arthritis
Arthritis	Large volume effusion compared to degree of pain	Small volume effusion compared to degree of pain
Skin lesions	Painless, must be looked for	Always painful
Spine	Search for symptomatic or asymptomatic sacroiliitis	Not involved

those who have a relapsing course separated by long symptom-free intervals and those who have chronic persistent arthritis and progressive spondylitis. There is no cure for Reiter's syndrome. Symptomatic management includes the use of nonsteroidal anti-inflammatory drugs as discussed earlier under Ankylosing Spondylitis. The role for antibiotics in the early stages of Reiter's syndrome remains controversial.

Intra-articular corticosteroids are very important adjuncts but should be used sparingly. Both methotrexate and azathioprine have been administered for relentlessly progressive disease. Special caution should be exercised when contemplating antimetabolite or cytotoxic therapy in Reiter's patients. The use of these agents has, according to anecdotal reports, accelerated the appearance of AIDS or a fatal outcome in those persons who already have the disease. Infection with HIV should therefore be considered a contraindication to the use of these agents.

Sacroiliitis and spondylitis of inflammatory bowel disease (IBD)

Arthritis in the axial skeleton indistinguishable from that of idiopathic ankylosing spondylitis is present in more than 5% of individuals with chronic ulcerative colitis or regional enteritis. That represents approximately a tenfold increase in incidence compared with that in the general population. Approximately 80% of individuals with the spondylitis of inflammatory bowel disease are HLA-B27 positive. In contrast to the situation in full-blown idiopathic ankylosing spondylitis, which is a predominantly male disorder, females may comprise as many as 40% of patients with spondylitis accompanying IBD.

The clinical manifestations and the course of spondylitis accompanying inflammatory bowel disease are indistinguishable from idiopathic ankylosing spondylitis. Unlike the peripheral joint manifestations, the activity of the spondylitis is generally independent of the activity of the underlying bowel disease, and it is not unusual for the spondylitis to antedate the appearance of IBD by many years. With the exception of inflammatory eye involvement, there appears to be little relationship between the development of spondylitis and other extraintestinal manifestations. Management of this form of spine disease should be the same as that outlined for idiopathic ankylosing spondylitis.

PSORIATIC ARTHRITIS

Several clinical observations suggest that psoriatic arthritis is a distinct entity, although this position is not universally accepted. Whereas rheumatoid arthritis patients without psoriasis usually test positive for rheumatoid factor, these serologic reactions are generally negative in patients with arthritis associated with psoriasis. Epidemiologic studies have established a high frequency of psoriasis (up to 20%) in association with seronegative arthritis; rheumatoid factor–positive arthritis patients have the same low frequency as the general population. Polyarthritis occurs in 7% of patients with psoriasis, as compared with a prevalence of 1% for rheumatoid arthritis in the general population. There are distinct morphologic/radiologic differences between the polyarthritis associated with psoriasis and classic rheumatoid arthritis. New bone formation (periostitis, enthesitis, ankylosis) predominates in the former, whereas bone atrophy without evidence of healing occurs in the latter. The interrelationships between psoriatic arthritis and the other spondyloarthropathies, including the HLA-B27 frequency in psoriatic arthritis patients with sacroiliitis, all point to psoriatic arthritis as a distinct entity quite separable from rheumatoid arthritis. Additional evidence for the association of psoriasis and arthritis comes from genetic and family studies. Females and males are equally affected by psoriatic arthritis, as opposed to a female-to-male ratio of 3:1 seen in rheumatoid arthritis and the male predominance noted in Reiter's syndrome and ankylosing spondylitis.

Physical findings

Arthritis and psoriasis generally begin about the same time—or at least within 1 to 2 years—but exceptions are frequent. The association between distal interphalangeal (DIP) joint involvement and psoriatic nail changes has been noted by many observers. However, although DIP disease occurs in 16% of psoriatic arthritis cases, the DIP joints are frequently affected in rheumatoid arthritis and osteoarthritis. Recognition of the pattern of joint disease and unique physical features of the DIP involvement can distinguish psoriatic arthritis from these two more common conditions affecting the hands (see below).

Five clinical categories of psoriatic arthritis have been described. These groupings reflect the disease as seen at a particular point in time (Table 312-3). There is little information about the natural evolution of the disease, but it is strongly suspected that the disease advances to involve additional joints. Therefore, strict boundaries should not be placed around the categories.

Table 312-3. Forms of psoriatic arthritis

Type	Appearance	Approximate frequency (%)
"Classic" psoriatic arthritis	Predominant involvement of distal interphalangeal joints and nail lesions	5-15
Symmetric "rheumatoid arthritis-like" arthritis	Bilateral symmetric large and small joint involvement	15-20
Oligoarticular arthritis	Asymmetric large or small joints; periostitis about the small joints leads to sausage digits and dactylitis	50-70
Ankylosing spondylitis	Sacroiliac or spinal joint disease; may be asymmetric; often associated with other types of peripheral joint involvement	5-20
Arthritis mutilans	Osteolysis of phalangeal and metacarpal joints; associated spondylitis	5

Differential diagnosis

Psoriatic arthritis should be recognized in three unique differential diagnostic settings and may resemble other articular conditions.

Acute gout. Acute monarticular arthritis with markedly inflammatory joint fluid occurs in the setting of psoriasis and hyperuricemia. The hyperuricemia is a reflection of the skin disease.

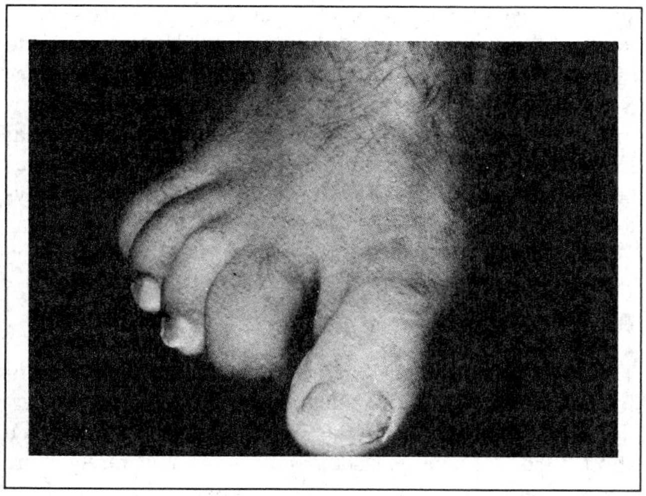

Fig. 312-5. Appearance of the feet in psoriatic arthritis, showing the changes in the interphalangeal joints and the digits produced by periostitis.

Rheumatoid arthritis. In classic RA the disease is generally limited to the structures within the capsule of the joint. Hence "fusiform," or side-to-side, swelling is observed in the hands of patients with RA. Psoriatic interphalangeal involvement extends beyond the joint capsule; large circumferential swellings are noted. In addition, the swelling may be quite firm, reflecting underlying periostitis and/or enthesitis (Fig. 312-5).

Mechanical derangement of the knee. In a young, otherwise healthy person the insidious development of monarticular arthritis of the knee is often ascribed to minor trauma. Psoriasis is usually not recognized or not diagnosed. In this setting, knee arthroscopies, meniscus repair, or synovectomies have been performed. Examination of the synovial fluid reveals true arthritis with a high protein content and inflammatory white blood cell counts, and a search for psoriasis should be made.

Extra-articular features

Nail pitting may be striking. Most commonly, onycholysis, crumbling, and hyperkeratosis represent psoriatic dystrophic nail changes (Fig. 312-6). There is no relationship between the extent of arthritis and the degree of psoriasis.

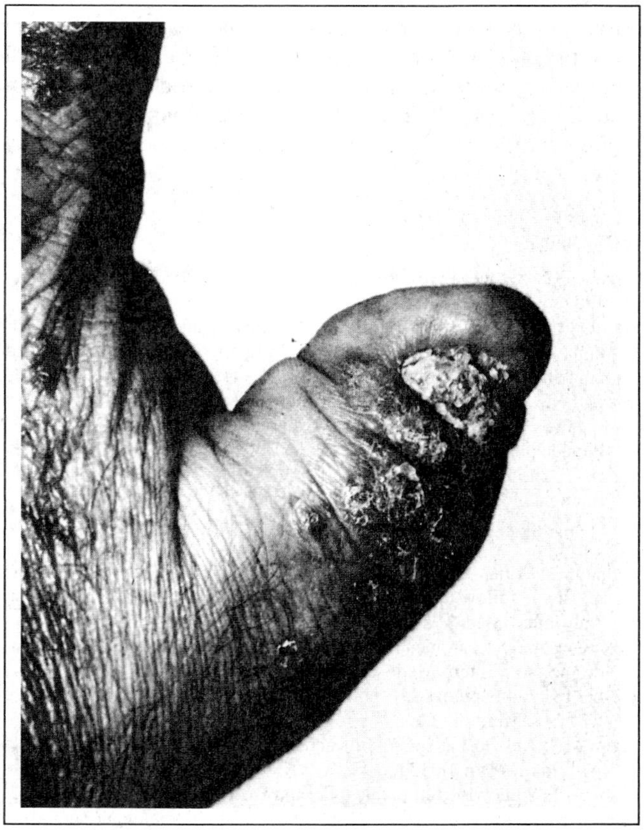

Fig. 312-6. Severe psoriatic nail disease with arthritis in the distal interphalangeal joint. The thumb is short because of severe bony resorption (osteolysis) in the area of the affected joint.

One should search, therefore, for areas of hidden psoriasis in the scalp, natal cleft, external auditory canal, and umbilicus, as well as in the nails.

Radiographic features are helpful because they are distinct from those of rheumatoid arthritis. The changes noted in psoriatic arthritis are no different from those described in Reiter's syndrome and/or ankylosing spondylitis.

Prognosis and management

It has been stated that most patients with psoriatic arthritis follow a benign, episodic course. However, a number of patients develop severe, progressive, destructive disease leading to total disability.

Treatment of the skin disease has been studied in relationship to improvement in the arthritis. Photochemotherapy using psoralens and ultraviolet light has been successful in treating the psoriasis as well as suppressing the associated arthritis. This occurred, however, in only those patients that did not have associated spine involvement. Traditionally, antimalarials, gold, and penicillamine have been considered contraindicated because of the possibility of exacerbating the skin component, but there are few data to support this assertion. All three agents have been used, but direct proof of their efficacy is lacking. Antimetabolite and cytotoxic agents, including methotrexate, have been shown to benefit patients with severe psoriatic arthritis. Sulfasalazine is an attractive alternative medication but has yet to be proven useful in controlled trials. Because of the small number of joints involved, as well as the absence of systemic or toxic features, the use of nonsteroidal anti-inflammatory drugs may provide sufficient benefit in most cases.

REFERENCES

Arnett FC: Seronegative spondylarthropathies. Bull Rheum Dis 37:1, 1987.

Ball GV: Ankylosing spondylitis. In McCarty DJ and Koopman WJ, editors: Arthritis and allied conditions. A textbook of rheumatology, ed 12. Philadelphia, 1993, Lea & Febiger.

Bennett RM: Psoriatic arthritis. In McCarty DJ and Koopman WJ, editor: Arthritis and allied conditions. A textbook of rheumatology, ed 12. Philadelphia, 1993, Lea & Febiger.

Calin A: The natural history and prognosis of ankylosing spondylitis. J Rheumatol 15:1054, 1988.

Calin A, editor: Spondyloarthropathies. New York, 1984, Grune & Stratton.

Calin A and Fries JF: An "experimental" epidemic of Reiter's syndrome revisited: follow-up evidence on genetic and environmental factors. Ann Intern Med 84:564, 1976.

Fox R et al: The chronicity of symptoms and disability in Reiter's syndrome. Ann Intern Med 91:190, 1979.

Gerber LH and Espinoza LR, editors: Psoriatic arthritis. New York, 1985, Grune & Stratton.

Kahn MA: Ankylosing spondylitis and heterogeneity of HLA-B27. Semin Arthritis Rheum 18:134, 1988.

Kahn MA: Spondyloarthropathies. Rheum Dis Clin North Am 18:1, 1992.

Kammer GM et al: Psoriatic arthritis: a clinical, immunologic and HLA study of 100 patients. Semin Arthritis Rheum 9:75, 1979.

Keat A: Reiter's syndrome and reactive arthritis in perspective. N Engl J Med 309:1606, 1983.

Moll JMH and Wright V: Psoriatic arthritis. Semin Arthritis Rheum 3:55, 1973.

Noer HR: An "experimental" epidemic of Reiter's syndrome. JAMA 197:693, 1966.

Paronen I: Reiter's disease: a study of 344 cases observed in Finland. Acta Med Scand 131(suppl 212):1, 1948.

Proceedings sulfasalazine in rheumatic diseases. J Rheumatol 15(suppl 16), 1988.

CHAPTER

313 Uncommon Arthropathies

Nathan J. Zvaifler

FAMILIAL MEDITERRANEAN FEVER (FMF)

Familial Mediterranean fever is a heritable disorder, the incidence of which is largely restricted to individuals of Eastern Mediterranean origin. Transmission is by an autosomal recessive gene; males are more frequently affected than females. FMF most commonly begins in the second decade of life and is marked by recurrent paroxysms of fever, serositis, and arthritis and by the subsequent insidious development of amyloidosis of the kidneys. The acute attacks usually last several days to weeks. Joint pain and swelling may occur independently and most commonly involve the large joints, particularly the knees, ankles, and hips. The arthritis is typically monarticular and lasts longer than the other features; it is associated with exquisite pain, synovial hypertrophy, and effusion, but few signs of inflammation. Occasionally, arthritis is protracted (more than 4 weeks' duration) and despite considerable disability, often disappears, leaving completely normal function. In the hip, this process may be complicated by avascular necrosis and residual incapacity. Radiographs usually show only osteoporosis, but after prolonged attacks (particularly in the knees), joint space narrowing, osteophyte formation, and a discrete radiolucent line beneath the femoral condyle may be seen. Synovial fluid analysis may be normal or show an inflammatory effusion containing primarily polymorphonuclear leukocytes. Colchicine can abort acute attacks; it also has been used prophylactically, and may prevent or retard amyloidosis.

OTHER INTERMITTENT ARTHRITIDES

Palindromic rheumatism

This disorder is characterized by recurrent attacks of painful swelling of joints associated with articular and periarticular inflammation. The attacks are abrupt in onset and short-lived, frequently lasting only hours and rarely more than a few days. The pattern is peculiar to individual patients, and the intervals between attacks vary from days to weeks to months. Once established, the pattern remains relatively unchanged for the duration of the illness, which may go on for decades. Any joint can be affected, and there is an unusual periarticular swelling of the heels, finger pads, and palms that resembles angioedema. Despite the chronicity, the joints are not damaged. In one third to one half of patients, the disorder progresses into typical rheumatoid arthritis. The remainder continue unchanged. Treatment with injectable gold may be effective in chronic cases.

Intermittent hydroarthrosis

This condition consists of recurrent attacks of unilateral, relatively painless, noninflammatory joint effusion (usually in the knee of women) that occur with a predictable periodicity. The disease occurs once or twice monthly, often in association with the menses. The fluid accumulates rapidly and is resorbed over a period of several days. Laboratory studies are unremarkable, and joint fluids appear benign, with few cells. There is no satisfactory treatment.

ERYTHEMA NODOSUM

Erythema nodosum (EN) is characterized by the presence of raised, warm, painful, erythematous nodules of various sizes, occurring typically over both shins and less commonly on the thighs and forearms (Plate V-7). Recognized causes include infection (tuberculous, fungal, or streptococcal); sarcoidosis; sensitivity to drugs, such as sulfonamides, iodides, and birth control medications; inflammatory bowel disease; and neoplasms, including leukemias and Hodgkin's disease. In many patients, however, no etiology is found. Biopsy of the lesion shows inflammation of the septum between fat lobules. Vasculitis of the veins or arteries in this region can be identified, together with occasional immunoglobulin deposits. EN can be confused with erythema induratum, which produces inflammation of the fat lobule, panniculitis, and nodular cutaneous periarteritis nodosa. Two thirds of EN patients have arthralgia. Arthritis develops in approximately one third and is benign, self-limited, and affects primarily the knees, wrists, and ankles. The latter show a brawny periarticular edema. The arthropathy may precede the skin lesions, and may persist for weeks or last several years, eventually clearing without deformity. Radiographs of the affected joints are normal; the erythrocyte sedimentation rate usually is elevated; tests for rheumatoid factor are generally negative, except with underlying chronic infections, sarcoid, or leprosy. Joint symptoms usually respond to salicylates given in full doses, but, in the rare persistent case, corticosteroids may be required. Recurrences of both the erythema nodosum and joint symptoms are not uncommon.

PANNICULITIS

Histologically, the subcutaneous fat is divided into lobules by fibrous septae through which course the arteries and veins. Panniculitis may originate as an inflammation of the blood vessels or as inflammation within the fat lobules. Vasculitis, primarily of venules, is responsible for the panniculitis accompanying several systemic illnesses and often takes the form of erythema nodosum; an immune complex–induced arteriolitis is responsible for lupus profundus, the panniculitis accompanying systemic lupus erythematosus. Inflammation originating within the fat lobules characterizes relapsing nodular panniculitis (Weber-Christian syndrome). Both vascular and primary fat-lobule inflammation have been implicated in nodular liquefying panniculitis, which accompanies pancreatic disease. Bone and/or joint pain and inflammation may result from intramedullary and periarticular fat necrosis, respectively.

Relapsing febrile nodular panniculitis (Weber-Christian syndrome)

This rare syndrome probably represents several different entities that share similar clinical and pathologic manifestations. As its name indicates, it is characterized by recurrent, indurated, and generally tender subcutaneous nodules that may be mobile initially but generally become adherent to the dermis and leave a dimple in the skin as the edema subsides. The nodules occur in crops, primarily on the trunk, but may involve the proximal extremities and are accompanied by constitutional symptoms, including fever, weight loss, and the anemia of chronic disease. Liquefaction of the fat tissue may cause chronic sinus tract drainage of an oily, viscous material. Panniculitis involving the pericardial fat, mesentery, and retroperitoneal tissue may accompany the subcutaneous lesions. Corticosteroid therapy may be useful during acute phases, but there is no definitive therapy.

Panniculitis of pancreatic diseases

Patients with acute and chronic pancreatitis and pancreatic neoplasms may develop a nodular liquefying panniculitis that is manifested as tender, red subcutaneous nodules occurring primarily on the lower extremities. Unlike those of erythema nodosum, these nodules generally are movable when they first appear. Typically, they occur on the posterior aspect of the legs and may leave a hyperpigmented, depressed scar. Serositis involving the synovium, pleura, mesentery, and pericardium can occur. An immune complex–induced vasculitis has been implicated in its pathogenesis.

ARTHRITIS OF IDIOPATHIC INFLAMMATORY BOWEL DISEASE (IBD)

Chronic ulcerative colitis and regional enteritis have many distinguishing pathologic and clinical features (see Chapter 43), but the inflammatory joint disorders that accompany them are essentially identical and are generally considered together. Two independent forms of inflammatory arthritis have been recognized. Peripheral joint disease with a rheumatoid variant pattern of involvement was recognized first and is called *colitic arthritis*. Subsequently, it became apparent that patients with inflammatory bowel disease also have a significantly greater than expected incidence of sacroiliitis and spondylitis that are indistinguishable from those seen in idiopathic ankylosing spondylitis (see Chapter 312).

Colitic arthritis

The *peripheral arthritis* of IBD characteristically manifests itself acutely as an asymmetric, predominantly lower extremity inflammation of knees, ankles, and, less commonly, small joints of the toes. It is often accompanied by periarticular inflammation and tendinitis, particularly involving the ankle and Achilles tendon. This form of joint disease generally appears after or concomitantly with the onset of inflammatory bowel disease and tends to parallel the activity of the bowel disease. Control of the latter usually results in remission of the "colitic arthritis."

Among the other extracolonic manifestations of IBD, peripheral arthritis is most closely correlated with erythema nodosum and oral mucous membrane ulceration. It may also be associated with uveitis, but not pyoderma gangrenosum.

Patients with colitic arthritis generally do not have detectable rheumatoid factor in their serum. The peripheral joint manifestations of inflammatory bowel disease are not associated with an increased incidence of HLA-B27 antigen. Synovial fluid analysis reveals an inflammatory effusion, with leukocyte counts ranging from a few thousand to 50,000 per cubic millimeter, predominantly polymorphonuclear. The protein concentration in the exudative fluid is usually about 50% of the serum protein level.

Because of its close relation to the underlying inflammatory bowel disease, and because it rarely produces joint deformity or bony destruction, treatment of colitic arthritis should be directed primarily at the underlying bowel disease. When necessary, joint symptoms may be treated with salicylates or other nonsteroidal anti-inflammatory drugs, although there are reports of exacerbation of the bowel disease by those agents. The arthritis is generally exquisitely sensitive to corticosteroid therapy when that is used for control of the colitis, but joint activity itself should generally not be considered an indication for the use of corticosteroids.

WHIPPLE'S DISEASE ARTHRITIS

Articular complaints occur in the majority of patients with Whipple's disease, a rare disorder characterized by diarrhea, malabsorption with steatorrhea, fever, anemia, and hyperpigmentation (Chapter 42). In more than one third of the patients, joint symptoms antedate apparent bowel involvement by 10 or more years. The joint involvement is generally episodic, inflammatory, and of abrupt onset; it involves predominantly the larger joints. It is often bilateral, however, and may involve the upper extremities as well, including the wrists and fingers. As the bowel disease progresses and steatorrhea becomes prominent, the arthritis often regresses.

Laboratory evaluation reveals negative rheumatoid factor studies and a mildly inflammatory joint fluid with a preponderance of mononuclear cells, but no findings are specific for this syndrome. Synovial biopsies have shown nonspecific mild inflammation and only infrequently show the PAS-positive inclusion bodies that characterize the small-bowel histopathology in this disorder. The diagnosis requires the demonstration of those bodies in macrophages in the small-intestinal mucosa. Treatment of the bowel disease with tetracycline generally leads to elimination of the arthritis within a few weeks.

BEHÇET'S DISEASE

Behçet's disease is a complex of inflammatory manifestations, the classic features of which are recurrent aphthous stomatitis, genital ulcers, and hypopyon iritis. The disease occurs worldwide, but with particularly high frequency in countries of the eastern Mediterranean and in Japan. The etiology of this inflammatory disorder is unknown. The histopathology of all involved sites is similar, showing edema and mononuclear cell infiltration.

Diagnostic criteria established by the Behçet Research Committee of Japan include characteristic skin lesions plus the classic triad as major criteria. Among the skin manifestations are erythema nodosum, subcutaneous thrombophlebitis, and a papulopustular eruption resembling acne vulgaris. Hyperirritability of the skin, with the development of a papular eruption at the site of an aseptic needle prick, is a characteristic and useful diagnostic sign occurring in the majority of patients.

Other important features of Behçet's disease, considered minor criteria because of their lower frequency of occurrence, include (1) arthritis that mimics colitic arthritis; (2) enterocolitis with mucosal ulcerations, occasionally perforating and sometimes complicated by the development of malabsorption; (3) epididymitis; (4) vascular lesions, inflammatory in origin, involving arteries and veins, which may produce aneurysms and arterial or venous occlusions; and (5) central nervous system involvement, with dementia, meningoencephalitis, or a brainstem syndrome with forced laughter, spontaneous crying, and swallowing disturbances that may progress to fatal bulbar paralysis.

A diagnosis of "complete" Behçet's syndrome requires that all four major symptoms occur during the course of the patient's illness. Any three major symptoms, or two major symptoms including typical eye involvement, warrants the diagnosis of "incomplete Behçet's syndrome," which is strengthened considerably if accompanied by any of the minor criteria. Blindness occurs in up to 50% of patients in Japan. The mortality is low (3% to 4%), but the prognosis is poor; central nervous system involvement and major vessel disease account for most of the deaths. There is no specific therapy for Behçet's disease. Colchicine may reduce the orogenital ulcers and iritis, and corticosteroids may be palliative for eye and central nervous system disease. In steroid-resistant cases, immunosuppressive therapy with azathioprine, chlorambucil, or cyclosporin A may be effective.

SARCOIDOSIS

Perhaps one quarter of patients with pulmonary sarcoidosis develop two distinct types of joint symptoms: (1) an acute transient polyarthritis associated with erythema nodosum and (2) a chronic, persistent variety. The first is migratory, involves especially the large joints of the extremities, is self-limited, and appears at the onset of sarcoidosis, often in association with bilateral hilar adenopathy. The disease usually begins before the age of 30 and is more common in women. Chronic arthritis, which is much less frequent, results from granulomatous involvement of the synovium or juxta-articular bone. When the phalanges are affected (dactylitis), there is diffuse swelling, which may be mistaken for rheumatoid arthritis. Granulomatous synovitis may manifest as chronic monarticular arthritis, and very rarely (almost exclusively in African Americans), as a destructive arthropathy. Radiographs may show the typical lacy cystic appearance of sarcoid bone disease. Synovial effusions are variably inflammatory, with either mononuclear or polymorphonuclear predominance. Treatment is symptomatic and is usually limited to nonsteroidal anti-inflammatory drugs (NSAIDs), but responses to chloroquine, colchicine, and corticosteroids have been reported.

RELAPSING POLYCHONDRITIS

Relapsing polychondritis is an intermittent, inflammatory, and sometimes destructive disease of cartilages throughout the body. Fever, iritis, episcleritis, aortic insufficiency, and rapidly progressive glomerulonephritis are recognized associations. Tracheal and bronchial collapse may lead to suffocation and death. Arthritis is widespread, including both cartilaginous (symphysis pubis and manubriosternal) and synovial joints. The pain, swelling, and effusion may resemble rheumatoid arthritis. Laboratory findings include an elevated erythrocyte sedimentation rate, a negative rheumatoid factor, hypergammaglobulinemia, anemia, and antibodies to type II collagen. Occasionally, polychondritis may complicate another rheumatic disease, such as rheumatoid arthritis or systemic lupus erythematosus. An association with Behçet's syndrome is also recognized. Corticosteroids are effective in controlling the cartilage inflammation and inflammatory eye disease, but may not influence the course of the disease. Dapsone, 50 to 200 mg per day, may be beneficial.

MULTICENTRIC RETICULOHISTIOCYTOSIS (LIPOID DERMATOARTHRITIS)

Multicentric reticulohistiocytosis is a rare, chronic, and often very destructive polyarthritis affecting primarily adult women. The disorder is accompanied by firm, yellowish brown or red nodules appearing at the base of the fingernail or scattered throughout the upper extremities, face, and scalp. The skin lesions, which may be confused with xanthelasmas, tend to wax and wane independently of the symmetric polyarthritis. The disease frequently masquerades as rheumatoid arthritis. Predominant involvement of the distal interphalangeal joints is a distinguishing feature. Spontaneous remissions occur, but the arthritis often progresses to a mutilating, severely deforming condition. Radiographs of the joints confirm the extensive destructive changes and show loss of cartilage and striking resorption of subchondral bone. The skin and synovium are infiltrated by foamy histiocytic cells and by multinucleated giant cells that contain an undefined lipid or glycoprotein material. Cyclophosphamide appears to be an effective treatment.

HYPERTROPHIC OSTEOARTHROPATHY

Hypertrophic osteoarthropathy (HOA) consists of clubbing of the fingers plus pain, swelling, tenderness, and stiffness of peripheral joints, especially the wrists, ankles and fingers. The adjacent long bones are often tender, with edema and erythema of the overlying skin as a result of periarticular and osseous proliferation (periostitis). Joint symptoms occasionally precede clubbing or radiologic evidence of periosteal change, although radionuclide bone scan identifies areas of increased uptake along the margins of the bone. The polyarthritis may be mistaken for rheumatoid arthritis, but the synovial fluid is characteristically noninflammatory.

Carcinoma of the lung is by far the most common cause of HOA, but numerous nonpulmonary etiologies are recognized. Resection of the primary neoplasm, sectioning of the vagus nerve supplying the affected lung, or eradication of other underlying causes occasionally produces dramatic relief of symptoms. NSAIDs or corticosteroids are effective treatments. A rare primary form (pachydermoperiostosis) also exists. The clubbing and bone changes occur in young boys, usually accompanied by a marked thickening of the skin of the face, forehead, and scalp, together with excessive sebaceous gland activity.

Arthritis and malignancy

Aside from HOA, there are a number of situations in which joint symptoms accompany neoplasm. Children with leukemias (especially those with early forms of the disease) may appear to have juvenile polyarthritis. Occult malignancy (breast in women, lung in men) is a rare cause of asymmetric polyarthritis. Rheumatoid factor tests are negative. Patients with leukemia and lymphoma, particularly children, develop osteoarticular pain. Lymphoma or metastatic disease to the vertebral bodies may produce confusing spinal complaints. Amyloid arthropathy can complicate multiple myeloma. Some patients with pancreatic cancer have a syndrome of synovitis, panniculitis, and nodular dermal infiltrates. Polymyositis associated with neoplasm may produce prominent articular complaints. Gouty arthritis occasionally occurs secondarily to hematologic malignancy.

Primary malignant tumors of the joints (synovioma and chondrosarcoma) are rare, but pigmented villonodular synovitis, a benign tumor composed of matted masses of villae and synovial nodules, is a more common source of complaints. The condition occurs primarily in young adults as a monarticular arthritis, most frequently in the knee but occasionally involving the hip, elbow, ankle, or foot. The principal symptoms are pain and swelling. Radiographic examination shows soft-tissue densities, diffuse rarefactions, and erosions. Joint aspiration typically reveals a serosanguineous effusion. Histologically, the synovium is infiltrated with lymphocytes, giant cells, and lipid-laden macrophages interspersed among areas of hemorrhage and synovial cell proliferation. Occasionally, the process can be quite destructive of underlying bone, particularly in joints with a tight capsule, such as the hip. Wide excision of the lesion is recommended, but recurrences are common.

HEMATOLOGIC DISORDERS

Coagulation disorders

Hemophilia and related coagulation disorders produce profound joint changes through recurrent hemorrhages into articulations and adjacent soft tissues. Hemarthrosis occurs in 80% to 90% of hemophiliacs and causes exquisitely painful, warm, swollen joints. This is treated with immobilization to prevent deformity, ice packs initially, and analgesics as required. Patients are often made aware of impending hemarthrosis by a deep, burning pain in the joint and treat themselves with appropriate plasma factors at home. Hemarthrosis occasionally requires aspiration after appropriate replacement therapy. The main aim of treatment is to avoid muscle wasting, contracture, and joint deformity. In children, repeated hemarthroses result in abnormalities of the epiphyseal plate and irregular bony overgrowth.

Sickle cell disease and related hemoglobinopathies

The crises of sickle cell disease often are associated with intense bone and joint pains and, occasionally, with effusions or inflammation resulting from small infarctions in the synovium and periarticular bone. In young children with sickle cell disease, acute swelling of the hands and feet may occur in association with marked periosteal reaction along the phalanges, metacarpals, and metatarsals. Joint hemorrhages, a susceptibility to osteomyelitis, and, in adults, the development of hyperuricemia and gouty arthritis all produce complicating articular complaints. Avascular necrosis of the femoral head and, less commonly, of the humerus, patella, and vertebral bodies (presumably caused by thrombosis in epiphyseal vessels) is a recognized complication in individuals with sickle cell trait, sickle cell–hemoglobin C disease, and sickle cell thalassemia, as well as SS hemoglobinopathy.

HYPERLIPOPROTEINEMIAS

Individuals with familial hypercholesterolemia (type II hyperbetalipoproteinemia) may develop tender tuberous and periosteal xanthomatosis and have repeated episodes of a migratory polyarthritis of the large peripheral joints. In children, the process may simulate rheumatic fever. Painful swelling of the Achilles tendon, either unilateral or bilateral, can be the presenting symptom of type II hyperbetalipoproteinemia and may recur throughout the life of the individual. An unproved association of arthralgia and transient synovitis has been claimed for type IV hyperlipoproteinemia. Subchondral collapse of bone resulting from infiltration with foam cells has been recorded in hyperlipoproteinemia, complicating biliary cirrhosis.

ENDOCRINE DISEASES

Endocrine and metabolic disorders frequently produce confusing joint complaints. Hypothyroidism can be complicated by joint pain, stiffness, myopathy, pyrophosphate arthropathy, and symptoms of median nerve compression. Effusions, when present, are bland and hyperviscous. Periarticular osteoporosis has been described. Thyroid acropachy (exophthalmus, pretibial myxedema, digital clubbing, and osteoarthropathy) is a rare syndrome seen in patients with treated hyperthyroidism.

Diabetes mellitus has a number of musculoskeletal consequences. Neuroarthropathy with osteolysis (Charcot's arthropathy) is seen in weight-bearing joints and in the forefoot of diabetics. Flexion contracture of the fingers, periarthritis of the shoulders, and waxy, thickened skin can be confused with scleroderma in young, type I diabetics. There is a reported increased incidence of gouty arthritis, pseudogout, and osteoarthritis with glucose intolerance.

Hyperparathyroidism has a recognized association with chondrocalcinosis and pyrophosphate arthropathy. Articular manifestations also result from bone demineralization, subchondral trabecular fractures, collapse of cysts, and small-joint erosions, all related to the underlying metabolic bone disease. Spontaneous rupture of tendons is a recognized complication.

Acromegaly, with its attendant increased levels of growth hormone, results in exaggerated growth of articular cartilage and bone. Hypertrophy of other structures, including the synovium, bursa, and tendon sheath, may result in effusions and symptoms of median nerve compression (carpal tunnel syndrome). Dorsal kyphosis of the spine and severe osteoarthritis of the hips may produce significant disability. Radiographs disclose thickening of the soft tissue and degenerative changes. Early in the process, particularly, there is a paradoxical widening of the cartilage space, especially prominent in the small joints of the hands and feet. Mottling of the metacarpal and metatarsal heads and thickening of the trabecular bone occur. The vertebral bodies have a typical appearance produced by marked bony overgrowth on their anterior aspects.

AVASCULAR NECROSIS

Although most bones have a highly developed vascular system, some areas of the skeletal system have a tenuous blood supply and are prone to develop avascular necrosis. The femoral and humeral heads, the navicular and lunate bones in the wrists, and the talus in the foot are all particularly susceptible. Many conditions produce avascular necrosis; among these are fracture and dislocation of the neck of the femur and diseases that interrupt the blood supply, such as caisson disease, hemoglobinopathy, and vasculitis from any cause. Alcoholism, corticosteroid use, and pancreatitis are all recognized precipitants, perhaps through altered fat metabolism and fat microemboli. In patients with systemic lupus erythematosus, collapse of multiple bones, even in some not treated with corticosteroids, frequently develops.

Diagnosis rests on the recognition of typical symptoms of pain and limitation of motion in the affected joint and radiographic findings. Unfortunately, the typical radiologic changes of subchondral rarefaction of bone followed by porosis and later compression of the articular surface are all absent in the early stages of the disease. Radionuclide scanning can be helpful at this stage. Scintigrams obtained within weeks of an avascular insult show as a cold area; later, when the reparative processes are under way, there is an increased uptake of the isotope. Nuclear magnetic resonance can detect defects even in advance of radionuclide scans and is the procedure of choice in the earliest stages of the disease. Bone decompression and grafting to enhance revascularization before the appearance of radiographic abnormalities may retard bone injury. Replacement arthroplasty is usually required in the chronic stage.

REFLEX SYMPATHETIC DYSTROPHY SYNDROME

Reflex sympathetic dystrophy, originally called the *shoulder-hand syndrome,* is manifested as pain and swelling in an extremity. In the arm, there is associated edema and trophic skin changes of the hand and forearm, remarkable vasomotor instability expressed as excessive perspiration and warmth of the hand, and pain and limitation of the ipsilateral shoulder. The symptom complex appears to be caused by an excessive, or abnormal, response of the sympathetic nervous system in an extremity to an injury or other insult, such as neurologic disease (stroke with hemiplegia, spinal cord lesions, radiculopathies, and/or postherpetic neuralgia) or atherosclerotic cardiovascular disease (myocardial infarction, severe angina pectoris, or coronary bypass surgery). Isoniazid and barbiturates also have been implicated. Similar findings may complicate arthroscopic surgery. A number of other trauma-related conditions such as causalgia, posttraumatic osteoporosis, traumatic vasospasm, and Sudek's atrophy are included under this designation. After the initial inflammatory edematous stage, patients develop dystrophic changes, with cool skin, loss of hair, loss of motion, and bone rarefaction. If spontaneous remission or response to treatment does not occur at this point, a superimposed atrophy of skin and soft tissue, contractures, osteopenia, and neuralgic pains with poor potential for reversibility occur. Early in the course, radiographs show patchy osteoporosis. Bone scans show increased uptake, often in a periarticular distribution, which is present prior to radiographic abnormalities. There are no specific laboratory diagnostic findings. Treatment consists of early mobilization, application of local heat, and performance of range-of-motion exercises. Reportedly, sympathetic nerve block and transcutaneous nerve stimulation have been used with some success. Corticosteroid treatment, initially in a dose of 60 mg per day for 1 to 2 weeks, followed by rapid reduction in dose, is claimed to interrupt the process in most patients, particularly in the acute stage.

NEUROPATHIC JOINT DISEASE (CHARCOT'S JOINTS)

The loss of sensation to a joint may result in a chronic, progressive, and destructive arthropathy. Ordinarily, there is a combination of joint instability, exaggerated degenerative changes, and florid new bone formation. Exceptions include the shoulder in syringomyelia and the tarsal and metatarsal joints in diabetic neuropathy, in which resorptive changes prevail. The prototype of the arthropathy was described by Charcot in relation to tabes dorsalis, in which loss of proprioception leads to relaxation of supporting structures, joint instability, and progressive damage by repeated unappreciated trauma. Similar changes have been seen in a variety of neurologic disorders, including meningomyelocele, leprosy, paraplegia, and congenital indifference to pain. The joint affected is determined by the neural lesion; in tabes dorsalis, the knees, hips, ankles, and vertebrae; in diabetic neuropathy, most commonly the forefoot and ankle; and in syringomyelia, the shoulder or elbow. The joint disease is usually progressive, with insidious swelling and instability of a single joint. Although said to be painless, Charcot's joints may be painful, but not in proportion to the joint destruction. Occasionally, the onset is abrupt, with associated inflammation of the surrounding soft tissues. Radiographs disclose only effusion initially, which is followed rapidly by cartilage loss, fragmentation, and resorption of subchondral bone, and development of large, bulky, osteophytic bony overgrowths. Pathologic fractures are common. Management is limited to immobilization and restriction of weight bearing. Surgical arthrodeses are often unsuccessful, as are prosthetic joints.

REFERENCES

Caldwell DS: Musculoskeletal syndromes associated with malignancy. Semin Arthritis Rheum 10:198, 1981.

Caughey DE and Bywaters EGL: The arthritis of Whipple's syndrome. Ann Rheum Dis 22:327, 1963.

Doherty M, Martin MF, and Dieppe PA: Multicentric reticulohistiocytosis associated with primary biliary cirrhosis. Successful treatment with cytotoxic agents. Arthritis Rheum 27:344, 1984.

Firestein GS et al: Mouth and genital ulcers with inflamed cartilage: MAGIC syndrome. Five patients with features of relapsing polychondritis and Behçet's disease. Am J Med 9:65, 1985.

Ginsburg WW et al: Multicentric reticulohistiocytosis: response to alkylating agents in six patients. Ann Intern Med 111:384, 1989.

Greenstein AJ et al: The extra-intestinal complications of Crohn's disease and ulcerative colitis: a study of 700 patients. Medicine (Baltimore) 55:401, 1976.

Hench PS and Rosenberg EF: Palindromic rheumatism: a "new," oft recurring disease of joints (arthritis, periarthritis, para-arthritis) apparently producing no articular residues: report of 34 cases; its relation to "angioneural arthrosis," "allergic rheumatism," and rheumatoid arthritis. Arch Intern Med 73:292, 1944.

Hickling P et al: A study of amyloid arthropathy in multiple myeloma. Q J Med 50:417, 1981.

Kozin F: The reflex sympathetic dystrophy syndrome. Bull Rheum Dis 36:1, 1986.

Mielants H et al: HLA antigens in seronegative spondyloarthropathies, reactive arthritis and arthritis in ankylosing spondylitis: relation to gut inflammation. J Rheumatol 14:466, 1987.

Myers BW, Masi AT, and Feigenbaum SL: Pigmented villonodular syno-

vitis and tenosynovitis: a clinical epidemiologic study of 166 cases and literature review. Medicine 59:223, 1980.
Panush RS et al: Weber-Christian disease: analysis of 15 cases and review of the literature. Medicine 64:181, 1985.
Shimizu S et al: Behçet's disease (Behçet syndrome). Semin Arthritis Rheum 8:223, 1979.
Weisman MH: Arthritis associated with hematologic disorders, storage diseases, disorders of lipid metabolism and dysproteinemias. In McCarty D, editor: Arthritis and allied conditions, ed 11. Philadelphia, 1989, Lea & Febiger.

CHAPTER

314 Cryoglobulinemia

Peter D. Gorevic

Cryoglobulins are immunoglobulins that have the property of precipitating reversibly at low temperatures. Although cryoproteinemia associated with severe Raynaud's phenomenon was first described by Wintrobe and Buell in 1933 as a concomitant of multiple myeloma, it is now recognized that cryoglobulins may occur in a variety of infectious, neoplastic, and autoimmune diseases, the most common of which are listed in Table 314-1.

Table 314-1. Types of cryoglobulins and their associated diseases

Type	Frequency (%)
I. Monoclonal	25-40
A. Multiple myeloma (IgG, IgA)	
B. Macroglobulinemia (IgM)	
C. Chronic lymphocytic leukemia and other lymphoproliferative disorders	
D. Angioimmunoblastic lymphadenopathy	
E. Idiopathic	
II. Mixed (most often IgM-IgG*)	60-75
A. Infections (often transient)	
1. Viral: hepatitis B; hepatitis C; infectious mononucleosis; cytomegalovirus	
2. Bacterial: subacute bacterial endocarditis, leprosy, poststreptococcal nephritis, intestinal bypass, syphilis	
3. Parasitic: schistosomiasis, toxoplasmosis, malaria, kala-azar, etc.	
B. "Autoimmune" diseases: systemic lupus erythematosus, rheumatoid arthritis, polyarteritis nodosa, Sjögren's syndrome; scleroderma, etc.	
C. Lymphoproliferative diseases: macroglobulinemia, various lymphomas, chronic lymphocytic leukemia, angioimmunoblastic lymphadenopathy, hairy cell leukemia	
D. Renal disease: proliferative glomerulonephritis	
E. Liver diseases: Laennec's cirrhosis, biliary cirrhosis, chronic hepatitis	
F. Familial	
G. Essential	

*The division into groups with a "monoclonal" or "polyclonal" IgM is arbitrary and reflects the predominance of IgM components with kappa light chains, many of which bear specific idiotypic determinants.

ETIOLOGY AND INCIDENCE

Monoclonal-type cryoglobulinemia is generally associated with multiple myeloma, macroglobulinemia, and other rarer neoplastic proliferations of plasma cells and lymphocytes. These cryoglobulins occur in large amounts (1 to 5 g/dl) and are readily detected as monoclonal components on electrophoresis of whole serum or the isolated cryoprecipitate. In many instances, production of these proteins does not cause clinical symptoms, and they are detected accidentally during a routine laboratory analysis when a precipitate is noted in a serum that has been stored in a refrigerator. On occasion, however, they cause symptoms of cold intolerance marked by Raynaud's phenomenon, vascular ulcers, purpura, livedo reticularis, and, in severe cases, ischemia and gangrene of the extremities. In several large series of patients with cryoglobulins, this type of protein constitutes approximately one third of those seen. As is the case with all immunoglobulin-producing tumors, IgG cryoglobulins are more common than IgM cryoglobulins, and these, in turn, are more common than IgA cryoglobulins. On occasion, Bence Jones proteins also are found to precipitate in the cold.

The second, and by far more common, kind of cryoglobulin, which constitutes about two thirds of the cryoglobulins seen in the Western world and is even more frequently associated with many of the infectious disease encountered in developing countries, is referred to as *mixed cryoglobulin* because it consists of more than one class of immunoglobulin. In general, mixed cryoglobulins contain an IgM molecule together with IgG, although other combinations—such as IgA and IgG or IgM, IgG, and IgA—occasionally are present in these complexes. Mixed cryoglobulins may be difficult to detect, may precipitate slowly, and tend to be present in small amounts (50 to 500 mg/dl). Nevertheless, since they appear to be immune complexes, they very frequently give rise to clinical symptoms of a systemic nature by causing vasculitis involving many different organ systems. Mixed cryoglobulins have been further subdivided into those in which one of the components, usually the IgM, appears to be monoclonal since it contains only one type of light chain, most often of the kappa type, and those in which all components are polyclonal. These monoclonal IgMs share variable region (i.e., idiotypic) antigenic determinants with similar molecules occurring in patients with known lymphoproliferative (e.g., chronic lymphocytic leukemia) or rheumatic (e.g., Sjögren's syndrome) diseases, reflecting in turn selective germ-line gene usage. However, though this subdivision is of obvious significance in individuals with malignancies of lymphocytes and plasma cells, it generally is of little importance in patients whose mixed cryoglobulins are associated with nonmalignant disorders such as hepatitis, systemic lupus erythematosus, rheumatoid arthritis, and other connective tissue diseases. Clinically and prognostically too, there is little difference between the apparently monoclonal and the polyclonal mixed cryoglobulins in the nonneoplastic diseases.

PATHOPHYSIOLOGY

Monoclonal cryoproteins are usually products of a malignant clone of cells and are structurally indistinguishable from their noncryoprecipitable counterparts. Symptoms caused by these proteins are vascular occlusive phenomena, probably caused by their precipitation at the lower temperatures encountered in toes and fingers. In addition to the purely physical obstructive process, they may also initiate an inflammatory response via the activation of complement or through their direct interaction with various inflammatory cells.

Little is known about the etiology of the mixed cryoglobulins. However, their frequent association with chronic viral and bacterial infectious diseases (including hepatitis B and C viruses, infectious mononucleosis, and subacute bacterial endocarditis) and the discovery in some instances of bacterial antigens or antibodies in the cryoprecipitates suggest that perhaps a viral or bacterial infection results in the production first of antibodies to the infectious agent and then of antibodies directed against the antibodies (Fig. 314-1).

Mixed cryoglobulins are cold-precipitable complexes consisting of IgM anti–gamma globulins and IgG antigens; they may contain other antigens, including hepatitis B virus, nuclear antigens, and on occasion, other viruses. It appears quite likely that these and other unidentified substances represent the inciting antigens that lead to the production of the antibodies that ultimately give rise to the unusual cryoprecipitable IgM anti–gamma G globulins. Patients with mixed cryoglobulins tend to be markedly hypocomplementemic and most often have a severe depression of the C4 and C2 components, with less involvement of C3 or late-reacting components. The presence in serum of cryoglobulins and other immune complexes associated with hypocomplementemia initiated a search for each of these components in the vasculitic lesions. Since by immunohistochemical techniques it is possible to localize IgM, IgM rheumatoid factor, IgG, complement components, and at times, viral antigens in tissue lesions, there can be little question that many of the lesions are a consequence of the deposition of immune complexes in small vessels and the resultant inflammatory response, which initiates a systemic vasculitis (Fig. 314-1). Why some patients with immune complexes have symptoms and others do not, and the reason for differences in organ involvement in those with the disease, remain to be elucidated. Determining factors may be related to the nature of the antigen, the nature of the antibody, the size of the complexes, the function of the reticuloendothelial system, or the ability of the complex to activate complement. The lesions in patients with monoclonal cryoglobulins are probably a consequence of the fact that they are cold-insoluble proteins that plug up the small vessels and initiate an inflammatory response and result in ischemia. Mixed cryoglobulins, on the other hand, resemble other types of immune complexes in that the vascular inflammation is a result of their deposition in the small vessels followed by activation of complement leading to an inflammatory response and vasculitis.

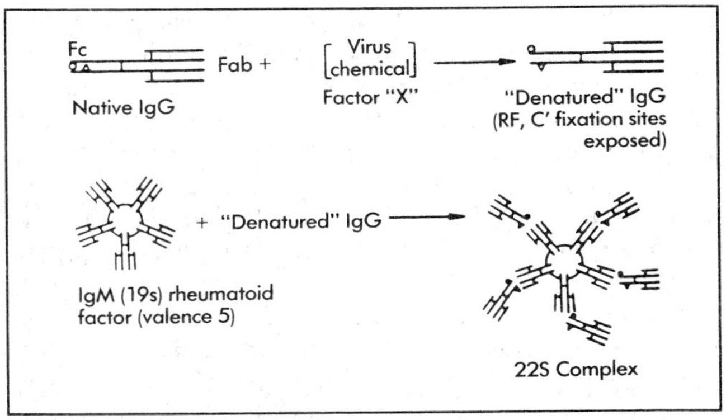

Fig. 314-1. Possible mechanism for the formation of circulating immune complexes and their conversion to a mixed cryoglobulin (MC) through the formation of an IgM-anti-IgG with unusual solubility properties. Activation of complement then leads to vasculitis and/or nephritis with deposition of immune complexes.

PATHOLOGY

Since cold insolubility may be rapid, especially if the protein is of high thermal amplitude and present in large amounts, care should be exercised in handling biopsy material to prevent ex vivo cryoprecipitation in tissue. The histological hallmark of monoclonal cryoglobulinemia is the vascular occlusive lesion that stains for the specific immunoglobulin isotype. However, necrotizing vasculitis and immune complex nephritis may also be seen. Conversely, patients with mixed cryoglobulins tend to have a vasculitic process involving small- and medium-sized vessels in many organs, most often the skin and kidneys and less often the heart, adrenals, gastrointestinal tract, pancreas, muscles, lungs, and other organs. In the skin the typical lesion is a leukocytoclastic vasculitis, whereas in the kidneys the lesions resemble an acute or subacute glomerulonephritis. Also characteristic in kidney are hyaline inclusions in glomeruli that also stain positively by indirect immunofluorescence for the components of the cryoglobulin.

CLINICAL AND LABORATORY FINDINGS

The most characteristic symptom complex associated with mixed cryoglobulinemia consists of arthralgias, dependent purpura, and one or more common manifestations, such as Raynaud's phenomenon, cutaneous ulcers, cold urticaria, pericarditis, thyroiditis, Sjögren's syndrome, and other symptoms seen in many of the connective tissue diseases. The severest manifestation of the presence of this type of cryoglobulin is the renal disease that develops as a consequence of an immune complex–type of nephritis and a peripheral neuropathy that may be caused by a vasculitis of the peripheral nerves. The renal disease can progress very rapidly, resulting in severe renal failure; in about 25% of patients, it can be arrested or halt spontaneously. Patients with mixed cryoglobulins often have hepatosplenomegaly, subclinical evidence of liver disease, and moderate lymphadenopathy.

Laboratory analysis reveals the cold-precipitable proteins and, often, an elevated erythrocyte sedimentation rate, moderate diffuse hypergammaglobulinemia, and the absence of a monoclonal spike on protein electrophoresis. A positive test for IgM rheumatoid factor is invariably found if sensitive assays are used.

The course of this disorder is variable and depends on the organs involved. In patients having only purpura and arthralgias, the course can be indolent and last for more than 20 years; in 40 patients, some of whom were followed over that long a period, the average length of follow-up was approximately 10 years, with only a small number of deaths in this group. Patients with renal disease, however, tend to have a poor prognosis, with an average follow-up of approximately 6 years and a much higher mortality. At autopsy, there are signs of systemic vasculitis involving the skin, kidneys, heart, adrenals, liver, pericardium, and many other organs. Overwhelming infections often contribute to death.

DIAGNOSIS

Serum containing cryoglobulins becomes opalescent and forms a visible precipitate when incubated at 0° to 4° C. The quantity of cold-insoluble protein can be determined either by means of a cryocrit or, better, by isolating the cryoglobulin and measuring the amount of protein precipitated. Further characterization of the type of protein in the precipitate is most readily carried out by immunoelectrophoresis or immunoglobulin quantitation. In searching for cryoglobulins, it is important to draw the blood in a warm syringe, to allow it to clot and to separate the serum at 37° C, and to incubate the serum in the cold for several days. It should be remembered that symptoms are not related to the amount of cryoglobulins and that small amounts are often as significant as large ones.

Monoclonal cryoglobulins or myeloma proteins with the property of precipitating in the cold show no unique structural features that can readily explain this phenomenon. Cryoprecipitability may represent the tendency of certain molecules to interact with themselves or to change their conformation at low temperatures. Mixed cryoglobulins generally consist of several immunoglobulins, the IgM component being the most important. It was demonstrated in the 1960s that cryoprecipitability is not intrinsic in either of these components but requires the patient's IgM and the addition of IgG from almost any source. Thus, mixed cryoglobulins appear to be anti-immunoglobulins with the IgM fraction behaving as a cold-insoluble rheumatoid factor.

TREATMENT

Since monoclonal cryoglobulins almost invariably accompany multiple myeloma and macroglobulinemia, treatment is directed toward the control of the underlying neoplasm. If the cryoglobulins produce no symptoms, no additional therapy is necessary. In the event that the cryoproteins result in severe cold intolerance or vascular insufficiency, plasmapheresis may be indicated to remove the cryoprotein until the disease can be brought under control by using other therapeutic agents.

The situation in patients with mixed cryoglobulins is different. Here again, treatment of the associated disease is indicated (e.g., interferon, especially for hepatitis-associated cryopathy). The idiopathic form of the disease, with manifestations limited to purpura and arthralgias, requires only symptomatic therapy. In the presence of systemic symptoms such as renal disease, neuropathy, or severe debilitating ulcers, more aggressive therapy is warranted. Because of the relative rarity of these disorders, no well-controlled studies have been carried out, and it should be remembered that spontaneous remissions may occur.

From the experience in several limited series, it appears that vigorous plasmapheresis (2 to 3 L/exchange) plus treatment with prednisone (up to 60 mg/day) and either chlorambucil or cyclophosphamide may hasten remission. Rapid improvement was seen in renal impairment, purpura, and ulcerating lesions of the skin, but little reversal of peripheral neuropathy. Although these modalities appear to be effective, there was a high incidence of infectious complications, which may limit their usefulness.

ACKNOWLEDGMENTS

This chapter is dedicated to my teacher, Dr. Edward Franklin, who made many seminal contributions to this field.

REFERENCES

Brouet JC et al: Biological and clinical significance of cryoglobulins. Am J Med 57:775, 1974.

Casato M et al: Long-term result of therapy with interferon-α for type II essential mixed cryoglobulinemia. Blood 78:3142, 1991.

Gorevic PD: Cryopathies: cryoglobulins and cryofibrinogenemia. In Samter M, editor: Immunologic diseases, ed 4. Boston, 1989, Little, Brown.

Gorevic PD and Frangione B: Mixed cryoglobulinemia cross-reactive idiotypes: implications for the relationship of MC to rheumatic and lymphoproliferative diseases. Semin Hematol 28:79, 1991.

Grey HM and Kohler PF: Cryoimmunoglobulins. Semin Hematol 10:87, 1973.

Lospalluto J et al: Cryoglobulinemia based on interaction between a macroglobulin and 7S gammaglobulin. Am J Med 32:142, 1962.

Wintrobe MM and Buell MV: Hyperproteinemia associated with multiple myeloma. With report of a case in which an extraordinary hyperproteinemia was associated with thrombosis of the retinal veins and symptoms suggesting Raynaud's disease. Bull Johns Hopkins Hosp 52:156, 1933.

CHAPTER

315 Infections of the Joints

Adolf W. Karchmer
Michael H. Weisman

SEPTIC ARTHRITIS

Arthritis caused by an infectious agent may come from (1) direct invasion by the microorganism, (2) a "reaction" to an organism that has invaded a site remote from the joints (rheumatic fever, Reiter's disease), or (3) unknown (as yet) mechanisms whereby certain agents such as viruses that are not recovered from the joints cause arthritis. This chapter focuses on arthritis caused by joint invasion with bacteria as the major cause. Almost every study evaluating management of bacteria-caused (septic) arthritis points to one essential fact: the rapidity with which the diagnosis is made and treatment initiated has the greatest bearing on outcome. If the infection remains unrecognized and untreated, permanent joint damage and even mortality may occur. Therefore, antibiotic therapy should be given empirically pending the results of initial studies. Likewise it is important to recognize that an infected joint is almost always the result of hematogenous seeding by bacteria originating from a primary focus of infection at a site removed from the joint itself. Exceptions to this rule are rare (i.e.,direct penetration into the joint may occur from foot puncture wounds, acupuncture, repeated intra-articular injections, human bites, and traumatic femoral venipunctures in neonates). Among adults, a variety of factors appear to predispose to acute nongonococcal bacterial arthritis. These include coexisting extra-articular infection; a preexisting destructive arthritis, particularly rheumatoid arthritis; serious underlying diseases, such as diabetes, cirrhosis, and malignancy; immunosuppression caused by corticosteroid or cytotoxic therapy; and parenteral narcotic abuse.

Clinical features

With the exception of arthritis caused by *Neisseria gonorrhoeae,* septic arthritis is typically monarticular. In more than 80% of patients with acute bacterial arthritis, a single joint is involved. Infection most commonly involves the knee, followed by the hip, shoulder, elbow, wrist, and ankle. The onset is abrupt, and fever is common. The infected joint is usually erythematous, warm, painful, and swollen, and it contains an effusion. Motion of the joint and weight bearing are markedly limited by pain. These signs of joint infection are the most reliable. Infection in more deeply situated joints, such as the sacroiliacs or hips, may be cryptic because of the lack of local inflammatory findings. With infection of the hip, pain may be referred to the anterior thigh or knee, whereas with infection of the sacroiliac joint, it often is noted in the buttocks, low back, or sciatic distribution. Polybacterial infection of the hip, especially if anaerobic bacteria and intra-articular gas are noted, suggests the dissection of infection from an intra-abdominal retroperitoneal site into the joint.

Polyarticular septic arthritis is uncommon except in the syndrome of disseminated gonococcal infection where multiple joint infection occurs frequently. Patients with this syndrome present with fever, a characteristic acral papulopustular erythematous rash (Plate V-22) and migratory polyathralgias and tenosynovitis. A monarthritis may subsequently become the dominant clinical picture. Disseminated gonococcal infection tends to occur in women with asymptomatic genital tract infection who are in the latter half of pregnancy, or at the onset of menstruation, or in asymptomatically infected men. Multiple joint involvement in nongonococcal septic arthritis is, in general, infrequent. Nevertheless, patients with rheumatoid arthritis, systemic lupus erythematosus, and significant immunodepression are particularly prone to a polyarticular infection caused by *Staphylococcus aureus* or gram-negative bacilli. In these patients the septic arthritis may be obscured by the more dramatic features of their primary illness.

In patients with rheumatoid arthritis, septic arthritis is an important cause of morbidity and mortality. These patients are typically elderly, have long-standing deforming arthritis, and are receiving oral or intra-articular corticosteroid therapy. Although patients are often febrile, hectic fever and chills are infrequent; the presentation is commonly an insidious worsening of symptoms in one or more joints. Infection involving a contiguous bursa or the development of a sinus tract from joint to skin should prompt an evaluation for joint infection. Prosthetic joint infection may arise through hematogenous seeding and be manifested as an acute, febrile purulent arthritis involving a previously well-functioning prosthesis. More indolent infection of prosthetic joints, with symptoms developing over months to years, may result from organisms that were introduced at the time of surgery. In this situation, severe pain or loosening of the prosthesis may be the only symptom of infection.

The arthritis caused by fungi and mycobacteria is usually monarticular and has a more insidious onset and indolent course. These chronically infected joints are painful, warm, and swollen. The inflammatory features, however, are muted, and the swelling has a doughlike consistency as a result of synovial thickening. The range of joint motion is restricted. Tenosynovitis and the carpal tunnel syndrome may be present.

Etiologic agents

The spectrum of bacteria that causes septic arthritis reflects the interplay of various factors: the unique vulnerability of patients to bacterial invasion at specific ages, increased susceptibility to infection caused by immunosuppressive therapy and underlying diseases, and the presence of primary infections serving as sites from which joints are seeded hematogenously. These factors, and consequently the frequency with which specific bacteria cause arthritis, vary with age (Table 315-1). *N. gonorrhoeae* is the most common cause of acute bacterial arthritis among sexually ac-

Table 315-1. Bacteriology of nongonococcal septic arthritis according to the age of the patient

	Percentage of cases		
	Children*		Adults†
Organism	≤5 years	6-15 years	>15 years
Gram-positive cocci			
Staphylococcus aureus	14	33	56
Streptococci	13	15	19
Other	3	2	2
Gram-negative bacteria			
Haemophilus influenzae	25	—	1
Escherichia coli	—	—	7
Pseudomonas aeruginosa	3	3	4
Other gram-negative bacilli	4	5	9
Others	3	5	2
Unknown	35	37	—

*Data from Pediatrics 50:437, 1972.
†Data from J Bone Joint Surg 52(A):1595, 1970; Arch Intern Med 139:1125, 1979; Am J Med 60:369, 1976; Arthritis Rheum 23:889, 1980.

tive young adults, accounting for 65% of cases in this group. In contrast, gram-positive cocci account for 75% of acute joint infections among older adults. *Staphylococcus aureus* causes almost 60% of acute nongonococcal bacterial arthritis and an even larger proportion (80%) of joint infections superimposed on rheumatoid arthritis. Among children from 1 month to 2 years of age, *Haemophilus influenzae* is the most frequent cause of septic arthritis, but this organism is a rare cause of arthritis after 5 years of age. In children less than 1 month of age, the most common bacteria to infect joints are group B streptococci, *S. aureus,* and gram-negative bacilli.

In adults, aerobic gram-negative bacilli are responsible for 10% to 20% of joint infections, especially in patients with coexisting extra-articular infection or significant underlying diseases. Septic arthritis associated with intravenous narcotic abuse may be caused by exotic organisms and affect unusual joints. Early studies revealed a high prevalence of gram-negative bacilli, including *Pseudomonas aeruginosa, Serratia marcescens,* and *Klebsiella* and *Enterobacter* species, as causes of arthritis in intravenous narcotic abusers. More recently, *Staphylococcus aureus,* particularly strains resistant to methicillin, and groups A and G streptococci have predominated. There is a predilection for involvement of the sternoclavicular, sternochondral, or sacroiliac joints in these patients.

Chronic infectious arthritis is usually caused by *Mycobacterium tuberculosis;* atypical mycobacteria, especially *M. kansasii* or *M. intracellulare;* or fungi (discussed below). Although rare causes of arthritis, any of the primary invasive fungi (*Sporothrix schenkii, Coccidioides immitis,* and *Blastomyces dermatitidis*) may be responsible for joint infection. *Cryptococcus neoformans* and *Candida* species are more likely to be pathogens in immunocompromised hosts.

The indolent arthritis associated with prosthetic joints is usually caused by contamination of the joint at surgery with relatively avirulent organisms such as *Staphylococcus epidermidis,* alpha-hemolytic streptococci, and diphtheroids. In contrast, late-onset acute hematogenous infection involving prosthetic joints is caused by invasive bacteria including *Staphylococcus aureus,* pneumococci, beta-hemolytic streptococci, and gram-negative bacilli.

Although arthritis has been reported as an atypical feature of infection by viruses of many types, it is a common event in infection by some viral agents including mumps, parvovirus, rubella, alpha viruses, and hepatitis B (see "Viral Arthritis").

Laboratory tests

An analysis of the synovial fluid is the most important diagnostic study. An acute bacterial arthritis is suggested by a synovial fluid leukocyte count of 50,000 or more per cubic millimeter with 90% polymorphonuclear leukocytes (Table 315-2). Synovial fluid leukocyte counts of greater than 100,000 strongly indicate sepsis; nevertheless, leukocyte counts below 50,000 or even in the 10,000-to-20,000 range are noted in some patients. Considerable overlap exists between leukocyte counts of gout, pseudogout, or rheumatoid synovial fluid and those of bacterial sepsis, and there is no single cutoff point between infectious and noninfectious fluids. Consequently, even when a noninfectious inflammatory arthritis is suspected clinically, the synovial fluid should be cultured. Patients with an untreated septic joint may show a striking increase in WBC count if the synovial fluid analysis is repeated in 12 to 48 hours, whereas stable or falling cell counts suggest a noninfected inflammatory condition, such as gout or rheumatoid arthritis. The difference in glucose concentration between simultaneously obtained specimens of blood and synovial fluid is not a helpful discriminator between infectious and noninfected fluids; both may show a low fluid-to-plasma ratio. In fact, chemistry studies of synovial fluid, including glucose, protein, and lactate dehydrogenase, do not discriminate effectively between infectious and noninfectious inflammatory arthritis and thus should not be ordered.

Gram stain and culture of the synovial fluid are positive in 65% and 90% of acute nongonococcal bacterial arthritis, respectively. In addition to the substantial false-negative rate (35%), the usefulness of the Gram stain is diminished by a variable but significant technical problem of false-positive staining caused by the mucopolysaccharide content of synovial fluid. In monarticular arthritis caused by *N. gonorrhoeae,* only 50% of synovial fluid cultures yield the organism, whereas in the polyarticular-dermatitis form of disseminated gonococcal infection the synovial fluid is usually sterile. Synovial fluid should be cultured on blood and chocolate agar media (not the antibiotic-containing selective medium for isolation of gonococci—e.g., Thayer-Martin) and in thioglycolate broth. Cultures should be incubated aerobically in a carbon dioxide–enriched environment. When gonococcal arthritis is suspected, specimens from all potential portals of entry—that is, the endocervix,

Table 315-2. Synovial fluid in untreated infectious arthritis

Organism	Leukocyte count	Polymorphonuclear leukocytes (%)	Positive stained smear (%)	Culture
Pyogenic bacteria	10,000->100,000	>90	65	+
Mycobacteria	10,000-25,000	50-70	20	+*
Fungi	3,000-25,000	>70	<20	+*

*Higher yield with additional culture of synovial tissue.

urethra, rectum, and pharynx—should be cultured on a selective medium. As a rule, in any patient with an infected joint, cultures of extra-articular sites of infection and blood should be obtained since they may suggest an etiologic diagnosis.

The synovial fluid from joints with chronic infection caused by mycobacteria or fungi is less inflammatory than that from pyogenic arthritis (Table 315-2). Occasionally, synovial fluid leukocyte counts are low, and mononuclear cells predominate. Specifically stained smears of the joint fluid may reveal the organism. Among patients with tuberculous arthritis, synovial fluid is positive by Ziehl-Neelsen–stained smears in 20% and by culture in 80%. An additional 10% yield may be obtained from culture and/or histopathologic examination of synovial tissue. In fungal arthritis, the specifically stained smears and cultures of synovial fluid are less frequently diagnostic than are those from mycobacterial arthritis. An open or closed biopsy of the synovial membrane, with appropriate histopathologic examination and culture, is more likely to yield a diagnosis.

Radiographs taken early in acute bacterial arthritis usually show only distention of the joint capsule and periarticular soft-tissue swelling. Occasionally, a pre-existing adjacent focus of osteomyelitis is recognized. Repeat radiographs obtained 3 to 4 weeks after treatment are useful in the assessment of joint damage; narrowing of the joint space, subchondral bone erosions, and complicating osteomyelitis may be seen. These radiographic changes and osteoporosis may be noted at the time of diagnosis in chronic infectious arthritis. In particular, destructive osteomyelitic lesions are often seen adjacent to joints infected by *C. immitis* or *B. dermatitidis*.

Special studies may help in recognizing and assessing infection of the sternoclavicular, sternochondral, symphysis pubis and sacroiliac joints. When pain is nonlocalizing, a ^{99m}Tc bone scan may identify infection in the hip, symphysis pubis, or sacroiliac joint. Tomography (computed or conventional) of the joint and adjacent bones is indicated for assessing bone destruction in sternoclavicular, symphysis pubis and sacroiliac pyogenic arthritis.

Differential diagnosis

An infectious etiology should be strongly considered for any monarticular or pauciarticular arthritis with an abrupt onset. Although noninfectious chronic forms of arthritis may begin in a manner similar to infectious forms, with identical synovial fluid WBC counts, the patient should be considered to have a septic joint until proved otherwise.

Gout or calcium pyrophosphate dihydrate deposition disease can mimic the clinical and laboratory features of septic arthritis, but these diagnoses can be established by identification of sodium urate or calcium pyrophosphate crystals, respectively, in the synovial fluid. Rarely, bacterial infection may coexist with crystal-induced arthritis. Hence, when very inflammatory synovial fluids are found to contain urate or pyrophosphate crystals, it is prudent to institute antibiotic therapy until culture results from the synovial fluid are available.

The acute onset of rheumatoid arthritis, seronegative spondylarthropathies, Reiter's syndrome, and acute rheumatic fever may resemble an acute bacterial arthritis. Various nonarticular clinical aspects of these entities or serologic tests may suggest the diagnosis; however, occasionally only the absence of organisms by Gram-stained smear and culture of the synovial fluid and the course of the illness eliminate an infectious etiology from consideration. An incomplete Reiter's syndrome, with only urethritis and arthritis, may resemble gonococcal infection and require antibiotic therapy until the diagnosis becomes apparent as the arthritis fails to respond to antibiotic treatment or as new features of the syndrome develop. Bacterial infection superimposed on rheumatoid arthritis is almost always caused by *Staphylococcus aureus,* may affect more than one joint and a contiguous bursa, and can present with spontaneous drainage. This complication must be considered when there is an abrupt increase in joint inflammation for one (or more) joints out of proportion to the others.

Although chronic inflammatory monarticular arthritis may be seen with rheumatoid arthritis, the spondylarthropathies, sarcoidosis, or Lyme disease, such a presentation strongly suggests infection by mycobacteria or fungi. In such patients, a synovial biopsy should be done, and the tissue examined for these organisms by appropriate culture and histologic techniques.

Treatment

Effective therapy of an infected joint must combine an appropriate antimicrobial agent and adequate drainage of the joint space. Adequate drainage is essential to remove collagenase and the neutral and acid proteases that are derived from polymorphonuclear leukocytes, synovial lining cells, and bacteria if the integrity and health of cartilage and joint function are to be maintained. In addition, the promptness with which therapy is initiated and the pre-existing status of the joint are major factors in the recovery of joint function after infection is eradicated. Delayed initiation of effective therapy is associated with poor recovery of function. Because of these prognostic factors, antibiotic therapy is initiated before the results of bacteriologic cultures are available. Antibiotics are selected to cover the pathogens most likely to be present. This choice is based on the age of the patient, clinical and epidemiologic information, the probable etiology of coexisting extra-articular infection, and the organisms suggested by the Gram stain of the synovial fluid (Table 315-3). For example, when no organisms are seen on Gram stain of the synovial fluid from a healthy, sexually active young adult, initial treatment should be directed against *Neisseria* species, as well as staphylococci and streptococci. However, when this situation pertains to an older patient with underlying diseases, treatment should be directed against both staphylococci and gram-negative bacilli. After identification of the bacterial pathogen, antibiotic therapy is revised (Table 315-4). The recommended antibiotics readily enter the joint fluid from the blood. With parenteral therapy as recommended, therapeutic levels in synovial fluid and serum are achieved. Intra-articular injection of antibiotics is unnecessary and may irritate the synovium. With the exception of gonococcal arthritis, oral antibiotics generally are not recommended as treatment for acute septic arthritis.

The in-vivo efficacy of a regimen may be evaluated by the serial analyses of the synovial fluid, which should become sterile within a few days. The synovial fluid volume and leukocyte count should fall gradually over the first week. The specific antibacterial activity in the synovial fluid can be assessed by exposing an inoculum of the infecting bacteria to serial dilutions of the synovial fluid and noting the growth inhibition and killing achieved.

Guidelines for empiric therapy in the setting of presumed septic arthritis will change from time to time; at present broad coverage is provided by imipenem, 500 mg every 6 hours, which will treat streptococci, staphylococci, gonococci, and most gram-negative organisms. If unusually resistant gram-negative bacilli are suspected, an aminoglycoside may be added. Certain aspects of the patient, the inflammatory response, or the pathogen may warrant modifications of the recommended regimens (Table 315-4). It is recommended that arthritis caused by gram-negative bacilli be treated with the combination of an aminoglycoside plus an effective beta-lactam antibiotic (a broad-spectrum, potent cephalosporin or penicillin agent). In some instances these combinations also exert synergistic antibiotic activity. Although experience is limited, it may be found that gram-negative bacillus arthritis (other than that caused by

Table 315-3. Suspected organisms causing septic arthritis based on Gram-stained smear of synovial fluid and age of the patient

	Suspected organisms			
	Gram-stained smear of synovial fluid			
Age of patient	**Gram-positive cocci**	**Gram-negative cocci**	**Gram-negative bacilli**	**No organism seen[a]**
Neonate	*Staphylococcus aureus*, group B or A streptococcus	*Neisseria gonorrhoeae*	Enterobacteriaceae	*S. aureus*, group B streptococcus, Enterobacteriaceae, *Candida*[b]
Child (2 mo-5 yr)	*S. aureus*, *Streptococcus pneumoniae*, group A streptococcus	*Haemophilus influenzae*[f]	Enterobacteriaceae *H. influenzae*	*H. influenzae*, *S. aureus*, group A streptococcus, *S. pneumoniae*, Enterobacteriaceae
Child (5-15 yr)	*S. aureus*, group A streptococcus, *S. pneumoniae*	*N. gonorrhoeae*,[c] *H. influenzae*	Enterobacteriaceae	*S. aureus*, group A streptococcus, *S. pneumoniae*, Enterobacteriaceae[b]
Adult (16-40 yr)	*S. aureus*, group A streptococcus	*N. gonorrhoeae*[c]	Enterobacteriaceae, *P. aeruginosa*[d]	*N. gonorrhoeae*,[c] *S. aureus*, group A streptococcus, Enterobacteriaceae,[b] *P. aeruginosa*[b,d]
Adult (>40 yr)	*S. aureus*, group A streptococcus, *S. pneumoniae*, *S. epidermidis*[e]	*N. gonorrhoeae*[c]	Enterobacteriaceae,[b] *P. aeruginosa*[b]	*S. aureus*, group A streptococcus, Enterobacteriaceae[b]

[a]Decreasing order of likelihood.
[b]Related to serious underlying disease or immunosuppressive conditions or hospital-acquired.
[c]Sexual activity; possible exposure to *N. gonorrhoeae*. Will occasionally be *Neisseria meningitidis*.
[d]Related to parenteral drug abuse.
[e]Prosthetic joint.
[f]*H. influenzae* are small rods or appear as coccobacilli; if true cocci, suspect gonococci (in the setting of sexual abuse) or meningococci.

Table 315-4. Antibiotic therapy of acute septic arthritis in adults*

Organism	Duration (days)	Drug of choice	Alternative drug/dose
Streptococci (nonenterococcal) or pneumococci	14	Penicillin G, 150,000 units/kg/d I.V. in q4h doses	Cephalothin,† 150 mg/kg/d I.V. in q4h doses
Enterococci	28	Penicillin G, 150,000 units/kg/d I.V. in q4h doses, *plus* gentamicin,‡ 3-5 mg/kg/d I.M. or I.V. in q8h doses	Vancomycin, 30 mg/kg/d I.V. in q6h doses, *plus* gentamicin,‡ in doses noted
Staphylococcus aureus	28-42	Nafcillin or oxacillin, 150 mg/kg/d I.V. in q4h doses	Vancomycin or cephalothin† in doses noted above
S. aureus or *Staphylococcus epidermidis* (methicillin-resistant)	28-42	Vancomycin, 30 mg/kg/d I.V. in q6h doses	—
Pseudomonas aeruginosa	42	Tobramycin,‡ 5-6 mg/kg/d I.M. or I.V. in q8h doses, *plus* ticarcillin, 250-300 mg/kg/d I.V. in q4h doses	An aminoglycoside‡ *plus* piperacillin, mezlocillin, or ceftazidine in full doses may be used if resistance encountered
Other facultative gram-negative bacilli (susceptibility permitting)	28-42	Gentamicin,‡ 5-6 mg/kg/d I.M. or I.V. in q8h doses, *plus* a broad-spectrum penicillin (mezlocillin or piperacillin) or a third-generation cephalosporin (cefotaxime, ceftizoxime, or ceftazidine) in doses for life-threatening infection	Tobramycin,‡ netilmicin,‡ or amikacin,‡ *plus* either a third-generation cephalosporin, piperacillin, or mezlocillin, each in doses for life-threatening infection

*Recommended doses assume normal renal function. Many agents require dose adjustments if renal function is reduced.
†An equivalent cephalosporin antibiotic and dose may be used.
‡Lean body weight used to calculate doses.

Pseudomonas aeruginosa) can be effectively treated with the potent new beta-lactam agents such as third-generation cephalosporins or imipenem. The efficacy of the new fluoroquinolones as single-agent therapy for arthritis caused by gram-negative bacilli has not been established; additionally, these agents should not be used to treat arthritis caused by staphylococci and streptococci. Avoiding prolonged courses of aminoglycosides reduces the risk of renal injury.

For patients with a nonimmediate type of penicillin hypersensitivity, cephalosporin antibiotics may be used to treat streptococcal (nonenterococcal), pneumococcal, and staphylococcal arthritis, whereas in the setting of immediate-type hypersensitivity, vancomycin should be used for these infections. Furthermore, vancomycin should be used in lieu of penicillin in all penicillin-allergic patients with enterococcal infection. Aminoglycoside and vancomycin doses must be adjusted for patients with reduced renal function, as should doses of some penicillin and cephalosporin drugs if renal dysfunction is severe. Extra-articular infection, osteomyelitis, or preexisting structural joint disease may warrant more prolonged parenteral therapy in some patients.

Among patients in the United States, the proportion of isolated *Neisseria gonorrhoeae* that is resistant to penicillins or tetracyclines has increased dramatically. Consequently, penicillins and tetracyclines are not recommended as therapy for gonococcal infections. Although gonococcal arthritis has been caused classically by uniquely penicillin-susceptible strains, arthritis caused by resistant strains, including those that produce beta-lactamase, is being encountered. Thus, unless a strain has been demonstrated to be penicillin-susceptible, acute gonococcal arthritis should be treated with ceftriaxone 1 g I.M. or I.V. daily (or ceftizoxime or cefotaxime 1 g I.V. every 8 hours) for 7 to 10 days. If the patient has improved after 2 to 3 days of parenteral therapy, treatment may be completed with cefixime 400 mg, ciprofloxacin 500 mg, or ofloxacin 400 mg given orally twice daily. In patients highly allergic to penicillins or cephalosporins, therapy may be initiated with spectinomycin 2 g I.M. twice daily, ciprofloxacin 400 mg I.V. twice daily, or ofloxacin 400 mg I.V. twice daily. After an adequate response has been obtained, therapy may be completed with ciprofloxacin or ofloxacin orally, as noted. *Chlamydia trachomatis,* which often simultaneously infects the genital tract of patients with gonorrhea, is eradicated only by the 7-day ofloxacin regimen; consideration should be given to treating this organism when therapy for gonococcal arthritis is provided (Chapter 264).

Adequate drainage of pyogenic joint infection to reduce intra-articular pressure and remove proteolytic enzymes is essential in protecting the articular cartilage. Furthermore, removal of purulent fluid enhances antibiotic efficacy. Acute gonococcal arthritis may respond adequately to the initial joint aspiration for diagnosis and appropriate antibiotic therapy, but most pyogenic arthritis requires repeated needle aspirations at least once or twice daily. Arthrocentesis should continue for as long as significant effusions reaccumulate. This may require 7 to 10 days but is equivalent to surgical drainage if the synovial fluid remains sterile and its volume, white count, and percentage of polymorphonuclear leukocytes are decreasing. In general, it is desirable to avoid the potential complications of an open wound and to be able to assess the results of therapy by repeated synovial fluid analyses, but any deviation from the anticipated course requires surgical intervention. Arthroscopic or open drainage is indicated if loculation of purulent fluid prevents adequate needle drainage or if synovial fluid culture, volume, and analysis indicate no improvement in the intra-articular inflammation despite repeated aspirations. In infants and small children, a rapid increase in hip joint pressure can compromise the blood supply to the capital femoral epiphysis, causing permanent damage or even dissolution of this important structure. Therefore, open surgical decompression and drainage is mandatory as soon as the diagnosis is made. Among older children and adults it is not clear that these joints must be drained. Nevertheless, many physicians prefer primary surgical drainage regardless of the patient's age when infection involves the shoulder or hip. Additionally, when there has been a delay in the diagnosis (> 3 days) or when infection is caused by a highly antibiotic-resistant organism, primary surgical drainage should be considered. Septic arthritis in the elderly, rheumatoid arthritis patients, and those who are immunocompromised may also benefit from early surgical drainage. Although comparative trials are not available, the ability to effectively decompress, debride, and lavage infected joints with minimal operative morbidity by using the arthroscope has prompted earlier drainage where this approach is technically feasible. In addition, early surgical drainage and debridement are recommended for sternoclavicular pyoarthrosis because of frequent adjacent osteomyelitis and the posterior extension of infection into the mediastinum. In joints with marked pre-existing structural damage—for example, caused by rheumatoid arthritis—or in joints severely damaged by infection, late synovectomy and arthrodesis may be required to control infection. Eradication of infection involving joint devices usually requires removal of the prosthesis and vigorous debridement. Reimplantation of a new prosthesis can be undertaken at a later date when it is clear that infection has been eradicated.

Although splinting of the infected joint is usually not necessary, the joint should be immobilized and placed at rest until inflammation and pain begin to subside. Passive range-of-motion exercises may be initiated after a few days of treatment, and active exercises begun as inflammation resolves. Weight bearing is prohibited until all signs of active inflammation have cleared.

LYME DISEASE

First noted in the United States in the area of Lyme, Connecticut, this multisystem illness occurs in stages, with remissions and exacerbations of symptoms if treatment is not initiated (see also Chapter 275). The disease is associated with infection by a tick-transmitted spirochete, *Borrelia burgdorferi*. Lyme disease has been acquired in areas of the United States, Europe, and Australia that are inhabited by ticks of the *Ixodes ricinus* complex. In the United States, nymphal and adult ticks of the species *Ixodes dammini* (Northeast and Midwest) and *Ixodes pacificus* (far West) are the predominant vectors.

Early clinical manifestations include a characteristic rash, erythema migrans (EM), which is noted in 75% of patients; approximately 30% of these patients recall a tick bite at the site of the EM lesion within the previous month. The EM lesion appears as a red macule often on the proximal extremity or trunk. The lesion then expands with central clearing and develops into a large ring with an intense red border that, while hot to the touch, is not painful (Fig. 315-1). There may be concentric erythematous rings and multiple, smaller annular lesions at sites that are not associated with prior tick bites. Malaise, fatigue, headaches, fever, regional lymphadenopathy, and migratory musculoskeletal pain are frequently experienced at this time. Although EM can recur, this complex of symptoms fades within a few months. Several weeks to months after the onset of illness, 15% of patients develop neurologic syndromes, including aseptic meningitis, cranial nerve palsies, and peripheral radiculoneuropathies. During this same period, cardiac abnormalities are detected in fewer than 10% of patients; these abnormalities primarily include fluctuating degrees of atrioventricular block, but occasionally include myopericarditis and cardiomegaly. In general, both neurologic and cardiac involvement clear spontaneously over a period of weeks to months.

Joint involvement, which occurs in more than 50% of patients with untreated infection, begins from months to years after the onset of illness. The natural course of the arthritis is highly variable; individual joints may be inflamed for weeks or months and then subside. Recurrences are common but are unpredictable in frequency or duration. Joints are commonly more swollen than painful and while warm are rarely erythematous. Fatigue is a common association with arthritis, but fever and other systemic symptoms are rare. Synovial fluid contains from 500 to 75,000 cells per cubic millimeter with 80% polymorphonuclear leukocytes. In approximately 10% of patients, particularly those with the B cell alloantigen DR2, chronic arthritis with destruction of cartilage develops in large joints.

Although the relative roles of direct infection and of the

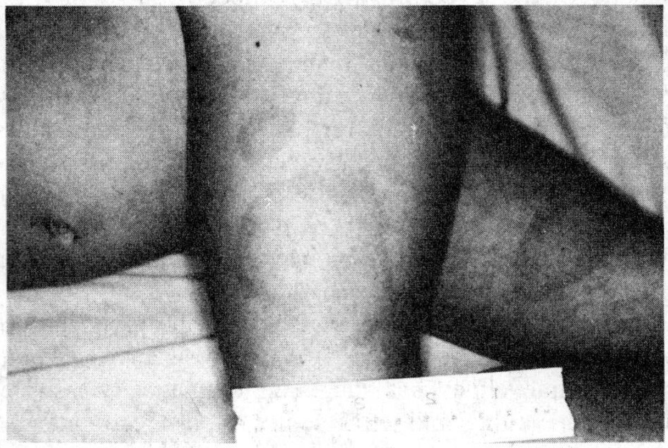

Fig. 315-1. Erythema chronicum migrans. Note the intense erythematous border with central clearing, as well as the multiple, smaller annular lesions. (From Steere AC: Erythema chronicum migrans and Lyme arthritis: the enlarging clinical spectrum. Ann Intern Med 86:685, 1977. With permission.)

immune reaction induced by the infecting spirochete in the pathogenesis of Lyme disease have not been clarified, this illness can be effectively treated with antibiotics. Early treatment with doxycycline or amoxicillin reduces EM and associated symptoms and often prevents development of major late complications, including myocarditis, meningoencephalitis, and recurrent arthritis. Erythromycin is less effective. The treatment of choice for adults with early disease (EM or mild carditis) is doxycycline 100 mg orally twice daily or amoxicillin 500 mg orally three times daily for 10 to 21 days. In patients with neurologic manifestations, severe carditis or arthritis, ceftriaxone 2 g I.V. or I.M. daily for 14 days is recommended. Although recovery proceeds slowly, 90% of patients with recurrent arthritis or neurologic symptoms respond to ceftriaxone. Doxycycline 100 mg twice daily or amoxicillin and probenecid, each 500 mg four times daily, have been used orally for 30 days to treat arthritis with response rates of 60% to 70%. Among patients with arthritis who fail these oral regimens, ceftriaxone cures 35% to 40%. Neither systemic nor intra-articular corticosteroids should be given because they may impair the response to antibiotics. Doxycycline should not be administered to women who are pregnant.

MYCOBACTERIAL AND FUNGAL ARTHRITIS

Tuberculosis and fungal infections are still commonly encountered, and the articular features of these diseases may dominate the clinical picture or may even be the presenting manifestation. There are basic principles common to joint involvement in these conditions that should be kept in mind at all times:

1. Certain clinical settings strongly suggest the diagnosis of mycobacterial or fungal etiology; these are (a) chronic monarticular arthritis, especially of large weight-bearing joints; (b) tenosynovitis about the hands or wrists; (c) erythema nodosum skin lesions; and (d) patients with significant immunodepressed states (e.g., AIDS).
2. Serologic studies may be helpful, but the diagnosis is always based on the identification of organisms from either synovial fluid or synovial tissues.
3. Both constitutional symptoms and other anatomic sites of infection may be absent despite the presence of fungal or mycobacterial arthritis.
4. Synovial fluid inflammation varies widely; the presence of either a bland or an inflammatory effusion does not rule out mycobacterial or fungal disease; neither does it enable one to discriminate between them and other causes of monarticular arthritis.

Tuberculosis

Tuberculous arthritis is usually the result of hematogenous spread of organisms to the vertebral bodies, the appendicular skeleton, or the synovium. The hip, knee, and ankle (and the tendons of the hand and wrist) are involved most commonly. The traditional view of the basic joint lesion is that it results from erosion of osseous disease into the joint space; however, synovial disease can occur primarily and without recognizable bone involvement.

Pulmonary findings may be absent in one half of the cases. The tuberculin skin test (PPD-S) is usually positive; but anergy may exist, or the skin test may be negative in a few healthy nonanergic patients. The diagnosis is made by identification of the organism from cultures of synovial fluid (80% of cases) or synovial tissues (90% of cases). The synovial fluid is variably inflammatory (see Table 315-2). Antituberculous chemotherapy is the cornerstone of management, and a combination of agents is recommended (Chapter 276).

Coccidioidomycosis

Coccidioidomycosis (see Chapter 277) occurs almost exclusively in the southwestern United States and causes arthritis in healthy individuals; certain ethnic groups, such as African Americans, Asians, and persons with AIDS are prone to much severer (disseminated) disease. The benign, self-limited primary infection, following inhalation of spores, is characterized by fever, cough, and erythema nodosum with or without polyarthritis. The disease disseminates in 0.2% of cases; bone infection can take place in multiple sites, especially over bony prominences. Arthritis is usually monarticular with the knee most commonly affected, then the ankle. In 40% to 80% of reported cases, bone or joint localization may be the *only* sign of disseminated disease. The diagnosis is made by identification of the organism in either synovial fluid or synovial tissues; the complement-fixation titer to *C. immitis* is usually positive in all forms of disseminated disease, including arthritis. Systemic administration of amphotericin B is required to eradicate the infection; synovectomy may be useful in selected cases.

Other fungal infections

Blastomycosis (Chapter 277) is endemic in the Ohio and Mississippi river basins, the Middle Atlantic states, and the Southeast and may occur as a primary joint infection via hematogenous spread. The disease is usually manifested as a monarticular arthritis of the lower extremities; in some patients the appearance resembles an acute septic joint. The diagnosis is made when the organism is grown from infected tissues. Although histoplasmosis may disseminate (and in these situations the prognosis is poor), arthritis is a very uncommon manifestation. Sporotrichosis occurs worldwide and is an occupational cutaneous and lymphatic infectious problem for people whose hands are commonly in soil. Systemic disseminated infection may occur in a healthy host without prior skin or lung disease and usually takes the form of a unifocal infection of a bone or joint. In debilitated individuals, the disease is more extensive and may be seen in multiple sites. *Candida* septic arthritis virtually always occurs in a compromised host (transplant patients, diabetics, immunosuppressed persons, etc.), frequently in the setting of clinically obvious, widespread disseminated candidiasis. Therapy is very difficult; intravenous amphotericin B and closed-needle drainage may be effective in some cases.

Patients with AIDS are at risk for disseminated fungal and mycobacterial infection; these infections may involve joints and should be considered in the differential diagnosis of an AIDS patient with articular signs or symptoms. Therapy for tuberculosis follows standard guidelines, but atypical or MAI organism infection requires complex multidrug regimens. Cryptococci may cause arthritis in patients with AIDS. In these patients cryptococcal capsular antigen is detectable in the synovial fluid and serum; infection may involve the meninges as well. Treatment similar to that given for cryptococcal meningitis should be considered and lifelong suppressive therapy is warranted.

VIRAL ARTHRITIS

Acute, self-limited episodes of joint inflammation sometimes are observed in association with what otherwise appear to be typical viral illnesses, yet only a few virus-associated syndromes have been studied in detail. Arthritis is a distinctly unusual manifestation of infection caused by some viruses: vaccinia, adenovirus, varicella, Epstein-Barr (infectious mononucleosis), herpes simplex, rubeola, influenza, echovirus, and lymphocytic choriomeningitis. During infection with some other viruses, arthritis may be a common aspect of the clinical illness: smallpox, mumps, alpha virus (chikungunya, O'nyong-nyong), rubella, parvovirus, and hepatitis B. An analysis of arthritis associated with viral illness has shown a heterogenous pattern of joint and periarticular inflammation, ranging from a symmetric polyarthritis of large and small joints to an oligoarthritis principally of the lower extremities. The inflammatory response in the synovium is also variable; cell counts ranging from 100 to 30,000 per cubic millimeter have been reported, with either polymorphonuclear leukocytes or mononuclear cells predominating. Different patterns may even be noted within patient groups infected by a single virus. There is evidence to suggest that immune complex–mediated mechanisms account for hepatitis B–associated arthritis; comparable studies have not been performed in other viral infections. Typically all of the virus-induced arthritides are of short duration and entirely reversible; however, some may be recurrent or persistent, and this leads to speculation that undiscovered viral infections may have an important role in the etiopathogenesis of chronic rheumatic diseases.

Hepatitis B virus infection gives rise to the most frequently diagnosed virus-associated arthritis (Chapter 57); besides being involved in a transient arthritis syndrome (see below) this virus has been implicated in three other more persistent systemic illnesses—a polyarteritis nodosa (PAN)–like necrotizing vasculitis, mixed cryoglobulinemia, and chronic glomerulonephritis. The arthritis begins abruptly, persists for 1 or 2 weeks, and then disappears with the development of jaundice. Joint involvement is typically a symmetric polyarthritis of large and small joints, especially the metacarpophalangeal and interphalangeal joints. The hands often appear to have prominent periarticular swelling. Preceding the arthritis, 50% of the patients have a rash that is usually urticarial, but may be macular, or even frankly vasculitic (palpable purpura). Hepatitis B surface antigen and circulating immune complexes containing complement are detectable during the articular phase; as the arthritis resolves, the immune complexes containing complement disappear. Synovial fluid white cell counts are highly variable but usually mildly inflammatory. Surprisingly (because the patients are often febrile and appear acutely ill), the Westergren ESR is usually normal, that is, below 15 mm per hour. The arthritis appears to be entirely self-limited.

Both the natural rubella infection and rubella vaccine may be associated with arthritis in a large number of subjects (estimated from 10% to 60%) (Chapter 246). Joint involvement is usually of sudden onset and short duration (less than 2 weeks), and is typically a symmetric polyarthritis of large and small joints. Postpubertal women appear more susceptible than men or children. Vaccine-induced rubella arthritis is similar to the natural disease, but in some patients, the arthritis is oligoarticular; that is, the knees alone may be involved. In addition, the vaccinated patients may have recurrent disease in the same joint for up to 3 years, especially those with knee involvement.

Arthralgias, polyarticular and migratory arthritis, and monarticular arthritis associated with mumps occur primarily in men. Large joints are involved most commonly. Joint symptoms have preceded parotitis but usually occur 1 to 3 weeks after the onset of parotitis or systemic viral symptoms. Joint symptoms resolve completely in several months and can be controlled by treatment with a nonsteroidal anti-inflammatory agent. Visceral complications are seen with increased frequency in patients with mumps arthritis.

Parvovirus B19 has been associated with aplastic crisis of hemolytic anemias, erythemia infectiosum (fifth disease) in school-age children, and arthritis/arthralgia in adults. Typically, polyarthritis occurs abruptly in association with flulike symptoms. Women are affected more often than men. In the majority of cases the arthritis clears in 1 to 2 weeks; in a small number it may persist for up to 2 years or recur at a later date. The diagnosis is confirmed by demonstrating an IgM antibody response to the B19 strain.

In addition to causing AIDS, infection with the human immunodeficiency virus (HIV) has been associated with arthritis. Many HIV-infected patients with arthritis have either Reiter's syndrome or a reactive arthritis. However, a painful subacute oligoarticular arthritis has been described in patients with AIDS who had no infections predisposing to reactive arthritis and who were HLA-B27–negative. The synovial fluid contained 50-2600 white blood cells/mm^3, predominantly lymphocytes, and synovial biopsies revealed mild chronic synovitis with mononuclear cell infiltration. Symptoms abated with nonsteroidal anti-inflammatory drugs or intra-articular corticosteroid treatment.

REFERENCES

Bayer AS et al: Gram-negative bacillary septic arthritis: clinical, radiographic, therapeutic, and prognostic features. Semin Arthritis Rheum 7:123, 1977.

Berney S, Goldstein M, and Bishko F: Clinical and diagnostic features of tuberculous arthritis. Am J Med 53:3, 1972.

Chandrasekar PH and Narula AP: Bone and joint infections in intravenous drug abusers. Rev Infect Dis 8:904, 1986.
Espinoza LR et al: Rheumatic manifestations associated with human immunodeficiency virus infection. Arthritis Rheum 32:1615, 1989.
Esterhai JL Jr and Gelb I: Adult septic arthritis. Orthoped Clin North Am 22:503, 1991.
Gardner GC and Weisman MH: Pyarthrosis in patients with rheumatoid arthritis: a report of 13 cases and a review of the literature from the past 40 years. Am J Med 88:503, 1990.
Goldenberg DL and Reed JI: Bacterial arthritis. N Engl J Med 312:764, 1985.
Inman RD et al: Clinical and microbial features of prosthetic joint infection. Am J Med 77:47, 1984.
Masi AJ and Eisenstein BI: Disseminated gonococcal infection (DGI) and gonococcal arthritis (GCA). II. Clinical manifestations, diagnosis, complications, treatment, and prevention. Semin Arthritis Rheum 10:173, 1981.
Rahn DW and Malawista SE: Lyme disease: recommendations for diagnosis and treatment. Ann Intern Med 114:472, 1991.
Rynes RI et al: Acquired immunodeficiency syndrome–associated arthritis. Amer J Med 84:810, 1988.
Shaw BA and Kasser JR: Acute septic arthritis in infancy and childhood. Clin Orthoped Rel Res 257:212, 1990.
Steigbigel NH: Diagnosis and management of septic arthritis. In Remington JS and Swartz MN, editors: Current clinical topics in infectious diseases, vol 4. New York, 1983, McGraw-Hill.
Sutker WL, Lankford LL, and Tompsett R: Granulomatous synovitis: the role of atypical mycobacteria. Rev Infect Dis 1:729, 1979.
Vincent GM and Amirault JD: Septic arthritis in the elderly. Clin Orthoped 251:241, 1990.

CHAPTER

316 Rheumatic Fever

Angelo Taranta

ETIOLOGY AND INCIDENCE

Rheumatic fever is an inflammatory syndrome that sometimes follows group A streptococcal infections of the throat (Chapter 259). Like the infections that lead to it, rheumatic fever affects mostly children of 5 to 15 years of age, but is seen also in young adults. Its incidence had been declining steadily in affluent countries, but very recently it may be staging a comeback.

Sore throats have long been known to precede attacks of rheumatic fever. In modern times, such "rheumatogenic" sore throats have been shown to be streptococcal, and rheumatic fever attacks not preceded by a sore throat have been shown to follow asymptomatic streptococcal infections by serologic techniques. Moreover, if streptococcal pharyngitis is treated so that streptococci are eradicated from the throat, rheumatic fever does not follow; if patients with previous attacks of rheumatic fever receive continual antibiotic prophylaxis, recurrences do not occur. In either case, the few failures of preventing rheumatic fever can be traced to failures to eradicate the streptococci from the throat or to prevent reinfection, respectively.

Although all attacks of rheumatic fever follow a streptococcal infection, only a few streptococcal infections are followed by rheumatic fever. Some streptococcal strains are more likely than others to cause rheumatic fever ("rheumatogenic streptococci"). Host factors may also be important, since the concordance rate for rheumatic fever is seven times higher in monozygotic twin pairs (18.7%) than in dizygotic twin pairs (2.5%).

PATHOPHYSIOLOGY

Although streptococci remain localized to the site of infection, their products diffuse out. Antibodies against these products (and T cells specifically sensitized to them) are demonstrable in the serum and in the skin (by tuberculin-type testing) or by in-vitro lymphocyte responses. Several streptococcal antigens cross-react immunologically with mammalian tissue antigens, including human myocardial sarcolemma. A circulating antibody response or a state of delayed hypersensitivity elicited by streptococcal membrane antigens may damage the myocardial cell membrane and mediate tissue damage in rheumatic carditis.

PATHOLOGY

In patients dying of acute rheumatic fever, a pancarditis is usually present, with exudative pericarditis, cardiac dilatation, and verrucous lesions on heart valves. Fibrin and serosanguineous fluid may be present in the pericardium. With healing, fibrosis and adhesions develop, but constrictive pericarditis is rare.

A diffuse myocardial interstitial infiltrate, predominantly lymphocytic, is usually present, in addition to Aschoff bodies. Myocytolysis and complete loss of fibers occur in some areas.

Endocarditis resulting from acute rheumatic fever consists of verrucous lesions at the base and edges of one or more cardiac valves. Initially, there is a mass of eosinophilic material staining as fibrin. With progression, granulation tissue develops, and vascularization and progressive fibrosis occur. Pathologic changes involve the annulus as well as the valve cusps, and the chordae tendineae often are shortened as a result of scarring and thickening (see Chapter 15).

CLINICAL FINDINGS

The natural history of rheumatic fever begins with the streptococcal infection that precedes it. The infection need not be symptomatic but must be localized in the throat and must evoke an antibody response. After a 2- to 3-week latent period, the patient develops one or more of the "major" clinical manifestations of rheumatic fever described below.

Arthritis

The most common manifestation, arthritis, is benign, although acutely painful. Usually several joints are affected, those of the legs more than the arms, and the knees most of all. The joints of the axial skeleton and the temporomandibular joints are almost always spared, and the small joints of the hands and feet are usually not involved, especially by themselves alone. Each joint is affected for a week or so, but the process shifts from joint to joint with some overlap in time, one joint improving as another becomes inflamed. Thus, the total duration of the arthritis may be 2 to 6 weeks if no treatment is given.

In any individual joint, the arthritis reaches its acme quickly, usually within a day or two. There is tenderness, often exquisite, swelling, local warmth, and redness, accompanied by inability to move, but often not much effusion; the pain is sometimes more than one would expect from the physical findings. Characteristically, the arthritis of rheumatic fever heals completely even without treatment. Arthritis tends to be more common, more severe, less migratory, and longer-lasting in adults than in children, but it still remains within the boundaries just described.

Carditis

Rheumatic carditis is the most important manifestation of acute rheumatic fever, and when severe, death may result from acute heart failure. More commonly, rheumatic carditis causes few or no symptoms and is diagnosed in the course of the examination of a patient who comes to medical attention because of arthritis or chorea. Patients with asymptomatic rheumatic carditis may later demonstrate rheumatic heart disease, despite the absence of a history of a recognized rheumatic attack (Chapter 16).

Patients with acute rheumatic fever may have endocarditis, myocarditis, and pericarditis, often in combination. Important criteria for the diagnosis of carditis include organic heart murmur(s) not previously present, enlargement of the heart, congestive heart failure, and pericardial friction rubs or signs of effusion.

Organic murmurs are almost invariably present in patients with acute rheumatic carditis. The mitral valve is most commonly involved; a high-pitched, usually loud, apical systolic murmur is a common finding and indicates acute mitral regurgitation (Chapter 16). Valvulitis may be manifested by cusp thickening or verrucae, and depending on its extent, the murmur of mitral regurgitation may persist after the acute rheumatic attack or disappear. A middiastolic murmur, usually following a third heart sound, is commonly heard in patients with rheumatic fever and acute mitral regurgitation.

The second most common valvular lesion during acute rheumatic fever is aortic regurgitation (Chapter 16). This lesion produces a soft, high-pitched decrescendo diastolic murmur that begins immediately after the second heart sound.

Congestive heart failure is the least common but most serious manifestation of rheumatic carditis. It usually develops in patients with combined severe valvular and myocardial inflammation. Congestive heart failure occurs in 5% to 10% of patients with first attacks of rheumatic carditis and is more common during recurrences. Pericarditis occurs in up to 10% of patients with rheumatic fever, but always together with valvular involvement. Cardiac tamponade is rare.

Delayed atrioventricular (AV) conduction is a common finding during acute rheumatic fever, but it does not necessarily indicate clinical carditis. Various dysrhythmias may occur, but atrial fibrillation is rare (in contrast to its frequency in patients with chronic mitral valve disease). In addition, the electrocardiogram (ECG) may show nonspecific ST-T changes consistent with myocarditis, diffuse S-T segment elevation or T-wave inversions caused by pericardial disease, or evidence of acute left atrial pressure elevation.

The chest radiograph is frequently normal but may indicate cardiac dilatation and/or pulmonary venous hypertension. An echocardiogram is useful in patients with acute rheumatic fever for detecting the presence of pericardial effusion, of chamber dilatation, or of valve abnormalities.

Chorea

Chorea is manifested by involuntary, abrupt, nonrepetitive limb movements and characteristic grimaces. The children so affected may cry or laugh inappropriately and may be extremely weak. Speech is often halting, jerky, or slurred. All of these symptoms disappear, without residua, in a few weeks or months.

Other major manifestations

Subcutaneous nodules are painless, roundish, firm lumps overlaid by normal skin. They range from a few millimeters to 1.5 cm in diameter, localize over bones and near joints, and rarely last longer than a month.

Erythema marginatum is a painless, evanescent, nonitching, macular, pink skin rash with the shape of smoke rings, but often festooned or circinate. It is limited to the skin of the trunk and proximal parts of the limbs, lasts for hours or days, and recurs.

Arthritis, carditis, and chorea may occur singly or in combination, but subcutaneous nodules and erythema marginatum are rarely, if ever, seen without carditis. Chorea typically occurs months, rather than weeks, after the provocative streptococcal infection.

In addition to these major clinical manifestations, patients with rheumatic fever have fever, malaise, and fatigue (especially when carditis and heart failure are present). The fever is usually moderate and without wide swings.

The long-term outlook depends on the presence and severity of carditis. Patients with no carditis during the acute attack have an excellent prognosis; those with carditis may lose all evidence of heart disease or may develop chronic, sometimes progressive, rheumatic heart disease. Whether the disease follows one course or the other depends primarily on the severity of the original carditis and on the effect of recurrences, if any.

LABORATORY FINDINGS

Antibody levels against one or more streptococcal extracellular products, such as streptolysin O, are regularly increased. Antistreptolysin O (ASO) is elevated in approximately 80% of cases; ASO levels of at least 250 units in adults and 333 units in children over 5 years of age are considered evidence of a recent streptococcal infection. In the remaining 20%, in whom ASO is low, elevations of antihyaluronidase, antistreptokinase, or anti-DNase B are found almost invariably.

The erythrocyte sedimentation rate (ESR) is markedly elevated, the C-reactive protein (CRP) test is positive, and the WBC count is moderately increased. None of these changes, of course, is specific for rheumatic fever.

DIAGNOSIS

Unlike pneumococcal pneumonia, which invariably affects the lungs, rheumatic fever has no obligate target organ. No single manifestation is diagnostic, but the greater the number of manifestations, the firmer the diagnosis. The most common presentation (also the least specific) is arthritis without carditis.

T. Duckett Jones proposed this empirical guide: the diagnosis is likely in the presence of two major manifestations or of one major and two minor manifestations (the minor being less specific than the major). Evidence of a preceding streptococcal infection was given a special status in the current revision (Table 316-1). In clinically questionable cases, exclusion of a previous streptococcal infection by repeated multiple streptococcal antibody determinations is helpful in ruling out rheumatic fever.

As noted earlier, not all streptococcal infections elicit an ASO response (only about 80% do); but all, by definition, elicit an antibody response to one or another streptococcal product.

Table 316-1. Jones criteria (revised)* for guidance in the diagnosis of rheumatic fever

Major manifestations	Minor manifestations
Carditis	Clinical
Polyarthritis	Fever
Chorea	Arthralgia
Erythema marginatum	Previous rheumatic fever or rheumatic heart disease
Subcutaneous nodules	
	Laboratory
	Markedly elevated erythrocyte sedimentation rate
	Positive C-reactive protein test
	Leukocytosis
	Prolonged P-R interval

PLUS

Supporting evidence of preceding streptococcal infection (increased ASO or other streptococcal antibodies; positive throat culture for group A streptococcus; recent scarlet fever)

*Courtesy of the American Heart Association.

NOTE: The presence of two major criteria, or of one major and two minor criteria, indicates a high probability of the presence of rheumatic fever if supported by evidence of a preceding streptococcal infection. The absence of the latter should make the diagnosis suspect, except in situations in which rheumatic fever is first discovered after a long latent period from the antecedent infection (e.g., Sydenham's chorea or low-grade carditis).

TREATMENT

Aspirin is very effective in suppressing the arthritis of rheumatic fever, and a prompt response of the arthritis to aspirin strengthens the diagnosis. More vigorous anti-inflammatory treatment, as with prednisone, is useful in controlling pericarditis and the congestive failure of acute carditis, but this treatment has no effect on the incidence of residual heart disease. Aspirin is administered to children in a dose of 80 mg per kilogram per day for the first 2 weeks, and 60 mg per kilogram per day for the following 6 weeks.

In patients with cardiomegaly, aspirin often is insufficient to control fever, discomfort, and tachycardia or does so only at toxic or near-toxic doses. These patients may then be treated with corticosteroids, as should all patients with definite evidence of heart failure. Prednisone may be started at a dose of 40 to 60 mg per day, to be increased if control of heart failure is not obtained. In extremely acute and severe cases, therapy may begin with intravenous administration of methylprednisolone (10 to 40 mg), followed by oral prednisone. After 2 or 3 weeks, prednisone should be slowly withdrawn, the daily dose being decreased at the rate of 5 mg every 2 to 3 days. When tapering is started, aspirin should be added at standard dose and continued for 3 or 4 weeks after prednisone is stopped. This "overlap" therapy reduces the incidence of posttherapeutic rebounds.

Patients who have had a definite attack of rheumatic fever should be protected from recurrences by the continual administration of antistreptococcal medication. Best results are obtained with the injection of 1.2 million units of benzathine penicillin G every 4 weeks.

In patients intolerant of benzathine penicillin prophylaxis because of pain at the site of injection, continual oral medication is prescribed. Sulfadiazine (0.5 g once daily in children weighing less than 30 kg, 1 g in others) and oral penicillin (200,000 to 250,000 units twice a day) are about equally effective. Patients taking sulfadiazine should have a blood count after 2 weeks and also whenever they develop a rash in association with fever or sore throat. The drug should be stopped if the white blood cell count falls below 4000 or the neutrophils below 35%. For the exceptional patient sensitive to both penicillin and sulfa, erythromycin may be prescribed (100 to 250 mg twice daily).

The risk of recurrence is greatest during the first 3 to 5 years after an attack, and every effort should be made to maintain prophylaxis during this critical period. For patients with no evidence of cardiac involvement, prophylaxis is recommended until 20 years of age or at least for a minimum of 5 years. In patients with rheumatic heart disease, medication should be continued well into adult life, past the years when school-age children are in the home.

An attempt should be made to prevent first attacks of rheumatic fever by accurately diagnosing and effectively treating streptococcal infections. The most effective treatment is benzathine penicillin by injection (0.6 million units in children weighing less than 30 kg, and 1.2 million units in others). Penicillin by mouth (200 to 250,000 units three or four times a day) is also effective, but compliance may be a problem.

REFERENCES

Bisno AL: Group A streptococcal infections and acute rheumatic fever. New Engl J Med 325:783, 1991.

Stollerman GH: Rheumatic fever and streptococcal infection. New York: Grune & Stratton, 1975.

Taranta A and Markowitz M: Rheumatic fever, ed 2. Dordrecht, Boston, London, 1989, Kluwer Academic Publishers.

Taranta A: Rheumatic fever. In McCarty DJ and Koopman WJ, editors: Arthritis, ed 12. Philadelphia, 1993, Lea & Febiger.

Veasy GL et al: Resurgence of acute rheumatic fever in the intermountain area of the United States. N Engl J Med 316:421, 1987.

CHAPTER

317 Antirheumatic Drugs

Philip J. Clements
Harold E. Paulus

Several distinct classes of drugs are used to treat patients with rheumatic diseases. In general, these drugs nonspecifically modify normally protective host defense mechanisms to diminish the harmful effects of misdirected inflammatory and immune responses, thus decreasing the manifestations of rheumatic diseases without eliminating their (usually unknown) causes. Nonsteroidal anti-inflammatory drugs, corticosteroids and disease-modifying antirheumatic drugs are discussed in this chapter. Drugs that decrease plasma uric acid concentrations, used to treat the hyperuricemia associated with gout, are discussed in Chapter 319.

NONSTEROIDAL ANTI-INFLAMMATORY DRUGS

Nonsteroidal anti-inflammatory drugs (NSAIDs) reduce, but do not eliminate completely, the signs and symptoms of established inflammation. They have a rapid onset of effect and their withdrawal is followed immediately by an exacerbation of signs and symptoms. NSAIDs have no effect on the underlying course of the disease process, nor do they protect against tissue or joint injury. NSAIDs inhibit cyclo-oxygenase, thus interfering with the transformation of arachidonic acid (via endoperoxides) to prostaglandins, prostacyclin, and thromboxanes. Arachidonic acid metabolites help to mediate inflammation, among myriad other activities. NSAIDs also suppress bradykinin release, decrease granulocyte and monocyte migration and phagocytosis, and alter lymphocyte responses under some laboratory conditions. In addition to their anti-inflammatory properties, the analgesic, antipyretic, and antiplatelet properties of NSAIDs contribute to their beneficial effects.

Salicylate

Aspirin is an acetylated salicylate. The acetyl group is responsible for certain unique characteristics of aspirin that are not shared by the other salicylates. Aspirin is a very effective inhibitor of cyclo-oxygenase, whereas the nonacetylated salicylates are only weak inhibitors. Aspirin irreversibly acetylates platelet cyclo-oxygenase and plasma proteins. The acetyl group also seems to be related to the inordinate gastric toxicity of aspirin.

Aspirin is rapidly hydrolysed to its active metabolite, salicylate. For an intense chronic inflammatory condition such as rheumatoid arthritis, aspirin doses should be adjusted to achieve a therapeutic serum salicylate level of 20 to 30 mg per deciliter. The metabolism of salicylate by humans consists of a complex combination of capacity-limited and first-order kinetics for its various metabolites. Because of this peculiar metabolism, the time for the serum salicylate level to decrease by one half (half-life) is not constant, as it is with most drugs, but increases as the serum salicylate level increases. At 8 mg per deciliter, the half-life is 4 hours, but at 25 mg per deciliter, the half-life is about 12 hours. Thus, it is not always necessary to give salicylates in q4h doses if the serum concentration is at a therapeutic level. The peculiarities of salicylate metabolism sometimes result in a nonlinear serum salicylate response to increasing the dose. Therefore, one must be particularly cautious about the rate of increase of salicylate doses as therapeutic levels are approached. A wait of 5 to 7 days is indicated between changes in doses to allow drug levels to stabilize. Salicylate induces its own metabolism. After 3 weeks of administration, salicylate levels are substantially lower than at the end of the first week. Because of these peculiarities and because of marked individual variations in salicylate metabolism, plasma levels should be monitored carefully during the first 4 weeks of therapy. Subsequently, plateau salicylate levels remain quite stable for a given dose in a particular individual.

Gastric intolerance of aspirin often prompts a search for alternative salicylate preparations. Modern enteric-coated aspirin preparations are well absorbed and produce stable steady-state salicylate levels. Large, carefully controlled comparison studies of equivalent doses of aspirin and choline magnesium salicylate or salicyl salicylate in the treatment of rheumatoid arthritis showed similar improvement in the number of painful joints and the number of swollen joints. Thus it would appear that nonacetylated salicylate is as effective as aspirin in rheumatoid arthritis.

There are inherent problems in the salicylate treatment of arthritis. Effective antirheumatic concentrations sometimes cause severe problems because of toxicity. Wide individual variability in the serum level–dose relationships necessitates careful dose titration to achieve therapeutic levels. At or near therapeutic levels, a small increase in dose may cause a large increase in serum level. A major problem is a widespread perception that aspirin is not a real medication; patients, physicians, and nurses therefore tend to become careless about its use.

NSAIDs

Because of the problems with aspirin, there has been a continuing search for less toxic NSAIDs that retain the effectiveness of aspirin. It is useful clinically to classify NSAIDs by their serum half-life (Table 317-1). The drugs with a serum half-life of at least 12 hours may be given once or twice daily, whereas those with shorter half-lives should be given more frequently.

NSAIDs tend to cause gastric irritation, to exacerbate peptic ulcers, and to make gastrointestinal bleeding worse by increasing acid production in the stomach and by decreasing platelet adhesiveness. Suppression of prostaglandins increases acid production and may decrease gastroesophageal sphincter tone, thus permitting acid regurgitation into the esophagus. NSAIDs also decrease the production of gastric mucus and the rate of cellular proliferation of the gastric mucosa. Further, indomethacin, sulindac, etodolac, and meclofenamate have an enterohepatic recirculation, which increases gastrointestinal exposure to these drugs and enhances their gastrointestinal toxicity.

The anticoagulant effects of NSAIDs are of two types. Salicylate in toxic concentrations may displace warfarin from plasma protein-binding sites, thus increasing its anticoagulant effect. Secondly, NSAIDs decrease platelet adhesiveness by inhibiting a prostaglandin-initiated sequence that is necessary for platelet activation. Acetylation of platelet cyclo-oxygenase by aspirin irreversibly inhibits platelet aggregation, and this effect persists until the acetylated platelets are replaced by newly produced platelets that have not been exposed to aspirin (10 to 12 days). For the other NSAIDs, the platelet effects are reversible and persist only so long as the drug is present. Therefore, it is safest to use a short half-life drug if one is worried about its possible effects on bleeding, as in a preoperative patient.

For acute inflammation, as seen in gout or acute bursitis, and for the spondylarthropathies, such as ankylosing spondylitis and Reiter's syndrome, the NSAIDs are usually more effective than the salicylates. Indomethacin often is remarkably effective when used in relatively high doses. The newer NSAIDs all appear to be effective in acute gout, except for tolmetin which, in one study, was reported not to control this disease.

For rheumatoid arthritis, aspirin is often tried first, although many physicians prefer to initiate therapy with one of the NSAIDs. The dose is adjusted to achieve a serum salicylate level of 20 to 30 mg per deciliter. If gastric side effects are unacceptable, enteric-coated aspirin, choline magnesium trisalicylate, or salicyl salicylate (salsalate) may be substituted. If salicylates are ineffective or toxic, they are discontinued, and one of the other NSAIDs is substituted. Its dose is cautiously increased and continued at the optimum tolerated level for at least 2 weeks before one decides that the drug is ineffective. Therapeutic trials of individual NSAIDs continue until the patient appears to have achieved adequate control of the inflammation with minimal side effects. Although the addition of an NSAID to a salicylate or to another NSAID is often attempted, there are

Table 317-1. Some nonsteroidal anti-inflammatory drugs

Drug	Dose range (mg/day)	Half-life (h)	Side effects: Dyspepsia, ulcer, etc.	Side effects: Others
Short serum half-life				
Diclofenac	75-200	1	++	Hepatotoxicity
Etodolac	600-1200	6-7	+	—
Fenoprofen	1200-3200	2	++	Nephrotoxicity
Flurbiprofen	200-400	3-4	+	—
Ibuprofen	1200-3200	2	++	—
Ketoprofen	100-400	2	++	—
Ketorolac	60-150 I.M. 10-60 oral	4-6	++	—
Meclofenamate sodium	200-400	2-3	++	Diarrhea
Tolmetin	800-2000	1	++	—
Long serum half-life				
Indomethacin	50-200	3-11	++++	Headache
Nabumetone	1000-2000	23-30	+	—
Naproxen	250-1500	13	+	—
Piroxicam	20	30-86	++	—
Sulindac	300-400	16	++	—
Oxaprozin	600-1800	21	+	—
Salicylate				
Aspirin	1000-6000	4-15	++++	Tinnitus
Choline magnesium salicylate	1500-4000	4-15	+	Tinnitus
Salicyl salicylate	1500-5000	4-15	+	Tinnitus
Diflunisal	500-1500	7-15	++	—

few data to support this practice, and it is likely that the addition of one NSAID to optimal doses of another merely increases the opportunities for adverse effects or drug interactions.

"Adequate control" of inflammation does not imply that all inflammation has been suppressed. If evidence of joint inflammation continues, particularly if radiographic evidence of bone erosions develops, a disease-modifying antirheumatic drug is added to the NSAID.

DISEASE-MODIFYING ANTIRHEUMATIC DRUGS

Disease-modifying antirheumatic drugs (DMARDs) are a diverse group of agents that share a common pattern of clinical response. In contrast to the NSAIDs, their administration does not produce any immediately discernible clinical benefit. After weeks or months of treatment, the subtle onset of clinical improvement may be recognized, and, with continued administration, complete suppression of some or all disease manifestations may occur in some patients. Laboratory evidence of disease suppression also may occur, but if drug administration is discontinued, disease manifestations gradually recur. Because their use may be associated with significant, and occasionally fatal, toxicity, they are usually reserved for patients with severe progressive or life-threatening disease manifestations. Background therapy with an NSAID is continued when a DMARD is started, and regular monitoring for adverse effects is mandatory.

Two recent studies employed different strategies but reached similar conclusions about the relative efficacy and tolerability of the different DMARDs for rheumatoid arthritis. Notably, the tolerability rankings were based on the relative frequency and severity of the commonly occurring adverse effects in controlled clinical trials and did not consider the impact of rare lethal side effects such as agranulocytosis with gold injections or acute drug-induced pulmonary failure with methotrexate (see the box below).

Relative ranking for efficacy and tolerability among the DMARDS*

Efficacy

Most efficacious: methotrexate = injectable gold
Less efficacious: penicillamine = azathioprine
Least efficacious: hydroxychloroquine = sulfasalazine = auranofin

Tolerability

Best tolerated hydroxychloroquine = azathioprine = methotrexate
Less well tolerated: auranofin = sulfasalazine
Least tolerated: penicillamine = injectable gold

*See Felson DJ et al, 1990, and Furst DE, 1990.

Gold compounds

Sulfhydryl-containing organic gold compounds were first used to treat chronic polyarthritis in the 1920s, and Forrestier's enthusiastic report in 1934 stimulated their widespread acceptance. It was not until 1960, however, that the value of gold therapy of rheumatoid arthritis was documented in a large, double-blind, carefully controlled trial. Additional controlled studies have led to the current standard methods of administration. Gold therapy is indicated in patients with adult and juvenile rheumatoid arthritis or psoriatic arthritis, whose disease has been poorly controlled by rest, physical modalities, and NSAIDs in full doses. Radiologic evidence of joint destruction reinforces, but is not essential to, the decision to initiate chrysotherapy.

Aurothiomalate (Myochrysine) and aurothioglucose (Solganal) are 50% gold by weight and are given by intramuscular injection. The oil-based suspension of aurothioglucose is less rapidly absorbed than the aqueous solution of aurothiomalate. The usual schedule includes test doses of 10 mg the first week and 25 mg the second week (to exclude idiosyncratic reactions), followed by injections of 50 mg weekly. The orally absorbed gold preparation auranofin is lipid-soluble and 30% gold by weight, but is incompletely absorbed. It is effective in a dose of 6 mg daily. Total body retention of gold is prolonged; 30% of an injected gold isotope was retained 4 months after a single dose of aurothiomalate. Steady-state plasma levels with auranofin are about 10% to 15% of those with the injectable preparations, reflecting its incomplete absorption, lower dose, and lower gold content. Gold is excreted predominantly in urine for the injectable preparations and in the stool for auranofin.

Gold compounds inhibit lysosomal enzymes either directly or by membrane stabilization. Human lymphocyte responses to mitogens and antigens are inhibited by gold added to culture conditions. Monocyte participation in cell-mediated in-vitro responses is impaired by gold. In patients receiving gold therapy, there is no evidence of generalized suppression of cellular or humoral immune responses or of inflammatory responses. Nevertheless, gold treatment reduces the progression of joint erosions and produces major improvement and, occasionally, remission in many patients with rheumatoid arthritis.

Toxicity occurs in 30% to 50% of patients. During the first year of treatment, 10% to 25% discontinue gold because of insufficient clinical benefit. Approximately 40% to 50% improve, and gold is continued indefinitely; however, the frequency of injections gradually may be decreased to every second, third, or fourth week. Improvement usually begins around 8 to 30 weeks; remissions become more frequent with increasing duration of treatment. However, despite a good response and continued gold therapy, arthritis often recurs or exacerbates, eventually prompting a change to another DMARD. Only 10% to 20% of patients continue to receive and benefit from gold for 5 years or longer. Important side effects include pruritic rashes (15% to 25%), proteinuria caused by an immune complex—mediated membranous glomerulonephritis (10%

to 20%), stomatitis (5% to 10%), and hematologic abnormalities (1% to 2%). Although rare, thrombocytopenia, aplastic anemia, or pancytopenia caused by gold may be fatal. Complete blood counts and urine protein determinations are done before each injection to monitor for toxicity.

Perhaps related to the lower absorbed dose of gold, auranofin appears to be slightly less effective and substantially less toxic than the injectable gold preparations. The rare fatal gold reactions also appear to be less frequent with auranofin.

D-Penicillamine

Penicillamine was introduced for the treatment of rheumatoid arthritis in the early 1960s, but until its efficacy was documented in a large, double-blind placebo-controlled trial in 1973 it was not generally accepted. Subsequently the recognition of frequent side effects required discontinuation of the drug in 30% to 60% of patients. These side effects included dermatitis (12% to 25% of patients); anorexia, stomatitis, nausea, vomiting, diarrhea (12% to 20%); dose-dependent thrombocytopenia (5% to 10%); neutropenia or aplastic anemia (rare); proteinuria (10% to 20%); and, rarely, autoimmune syndromes such as myasthenia gravis, polymyositis, Goodpasture's syndrome, pemphigus and pemphigoid, and systemic lupus erythematosus. These side effects have markedly limited its use.

Antimalarial drugs

Chloroquine and hydroxychloroquine may be used to treat discoid and systemic lupus erythematosus and rheumatoid arthritis. Placebo-controlled studies of more than 1 year's duration document its efficacy in rheumatoid arthritis and its delayed onset of effect. Usual doses are 250 mg daily of chloroquine or 200 to 400 mg daily of hydroxychloroquine, orally. The drugs are well absorbed, and peak plasma levels are rapidly reached. They are extensively distributed into the tissues, with very high concentrations in liver, lung, kidney, heart, and pigmented tissues. Excretion is very slow and may continue for as long as 5 years after discontinuation of the drug. Antimalarial compounds have been reported to interact with nucleic acids; inhibit DNA, RNA, and protein synthesis; interfere with antigen-antibody reactions; suppress lymphocyte responses to mitogens; inhibit chemotaxis and phagocytosis by neutrophils; and stabilize lysosomal membranes.

High concentrations of chloroquine and hydroxychloroquine in the pigment layers may lead to retinal damage, with destruction of rods and cones and migration of pigment to the nuclear layers. The incidence of visual acuity deterioration appears to be low in patients taking no more than 250 mg per day of chloroquine or 400 mg per day of hydroxychloroquine, but patients should be examined for retinal toxicity by an ophthalmologist every 3 to 6 months. Other side effects include dermatitis, nausea, diarrhea, hemolytic anemia, reversible drug deposition in the cornea and ciliary body of the eye, and, rarely, blood dyscrasias or neuromyopathy.

Sulfasalazine

Sulfasalazine (Azulfidine) is an acid azo compound of 5-amino-salicylic acid (5-ASA) and sulfapyridine (SP), first synthesized in the 1930s. Most of an ingested dose is split into 5-ASA and sulfapyridine by colonic bacteria. Sulfapyridine is absorbed and appears to be responsible for clinical benefit in RA, whereas most 5-ASA remains in the bowel and is the effective constituent for inflammatory bowel disease. Maximum serum concentrations of SP occur between 12 and 24 hours after ingestion; disposition half-life is 5.5 hours in fast acetylators and 15 hours in slow acetylators (who have a higher incidence of side effects).

Sulfasalazine may alter intestinal bacterial flora, inhibit folate absorption and metabolism, inhibit prostaglandin synthesis and degradation, decrease leukotriene production, and inhibit acute carrageenan-induced rat paw inflammation and rat adjuvant arthritis. Its efficacy in RA is comparable to that of gold, both in clinical use and in controlled clinical trials. Enteric-coated tablets are given in a dose of 2 or 3 g daily. Nausea, vomiting, or dyspepsia cause 20% of patients to stop the drug. Severe neutropenia is rare but has been fatal in a few cases. Rashes occur in 1% to 5% of patients. Reversible decreases in sperm count occur during therapy, but the overall toxicity appears to be less than that of gold and D-penicillamine.

Immunosuppressive (cytotoxic) drugs

A number of cytostatic or cytotoxic drugs alter various aspects of immune responses in in-vitro or animal systems, and the efficacy of some has been documented or suggested in various rheumatic diseases. This class of drugs affects the metabolism and proliferation of all cells; presumably these effects are more intense in the rapidly metabolizing and proliferating cellular participants in immune and inflammatory reactions. Clinical benefit may occur in the absence of demonstrable immunosuppression.

The alkylating agents cyclophosphamide and chlorambucil, the purine analog azathioprine, and the folic acid antagonist methotrexate have been used to treat rheumatic diseases. Because of their many significant, and sometimes lethal, side effects (Table 317-2), they are reserved for severe, life-threatening conditions; patients must be fully informed about potential problems and should be followed carefully. Benefit has been reported in controlled studies of rheumatoid arthritis (azathioprine, cyclophosphamide, methotrexate); psoriatic arthritis (azathioprine); Behçet's disease (azathioprine, chlorambucil); systemic lupus erythematosus (intravenous cyclophosphamide); and polymyositis (azathioprine). Uncontrolled series have also reported favorable results for chlorambucil in rheumatoid arthritis; for all four drugs in polymyositis; for azathioprine and cyclophosphamide in polyarteritis nodosa; and for methotrexate in Reiter's syndrome and psoriatic arthritis. Azathioprine has been widely used in systemic lupus erythematosus, but

Table 317-2. Adverse drug experiences associated with the use of the cytotoxic drugs (when used in the dosages commonly employed in the rheumatic diseases)

Adverse experience	Azathioprine	Cyclophosphamide	Chlorambucil	Methotrexate
Toxicity common to the cytotoxic agents				
Dose-related marrow suppression	++	++	++	++
Leukopenia	+ to ++	+ to ++	+ to ++	+
Thrombocytopenia	+	+	++	+ to ++
Susceptibility to infection	+	++	++	+ to ++
GI intolerance	++	++	+	++
Rash	+	++	++	+
Toxicity not shared by all drugs				
Hepatic damage	+	0	0	+ to ++ *(M)*
Oral ulcers	0	0	0	++
Hair loss	0	+++	+ to ++	++
Azospermia	0	+++	++	0
Anovulation	0	+++	++	0
Cystitis (hemorrhagic, fibrotic)	0	++ *(M)*	0	0
Teratogenesis	0	++ *(M)*	++ *(M)*	+++ *(M)*
Neoplasia	?	Probable *(M)*	Probable *(M)*	?

0 = considered not to occur; + = may occur, but usually in less than 5% of patients; ++ = occurs in more than 5% of patients; +++ = occurs very frequently (>30%-40%); *(M)* = adverse effect of major concern; ? = uncertain.

without unequivocal evidence of its efficacy. In contrast, cyclophosphamide appears to be life-saving in Wegener's granulomatosis and is part of the initial therapy of this disease. In other conditions, these drugs are generally employed only after other measures have failed.

Methotrexate

The folic acid antagonist methotrexate was introduced for clinical use in 1948, but it was not until 1964 that Black et al (in a blinded placebo-controlled study) demonstrated that methotrexate was effective (albeit toxic) in an arthritic disease (psoriasis). It was used sporadically thereafter in many rheumatic diseases. In the mid-1980s several blinded placebo-controlled trials demonstrated that methotrexate was effective in rheumatoid arthritis. In the few years since, it has become the most widely used disease-modifying agent in the United States for rheumatoid arthritis. Although the FDA has only approved its use for cutaneous psoriasis and rheumatoid arthritis, it is commonly employed in a number of other rheumatic diseases: polymyositis, and to a lesser extent Reiter's syndrome, polyarteritis nodosa, Wegener's granulomatosis, psoriatic arthritis, and sarcoidosis.

Bioavailability of methotrexate is nearly complete at the low oral doses usually employed in rheumatic diseases (i.e., 7.5-15.0 mg/week). As the oral dose increases, the bioavailability decreases. After oral or I.M. administration, it attains peak blood levels within 1-2 hours. Even though gut flora metabolize some methotrexate (especially when taken orally), the major route of elimination is by glomerular filtration and by active secretion by the renal tubule: 30%-80% of a dose is excreted in the urine within 24 hours. Lesser amounts are eliminated through the bile and feces. The active secretion of methotrexate by the renal tubules may be affected by competition for secretion by other medications, notably NSAIDs, aspirin, probenecid, and trimethoprim/sulfamethoxasole.

Methotrexate is an anti-metabolite that inhibits the synthesis of the pyrimidine and purine precursors of DNA, most notably by inhibiting the enzyme dihydrofolate reductase. Active metabolites of methotrexate are known to be retained within cells for days (intracellular polyglutamates of methotrexate) and as a result methotrexate's antimetabolite activity may remain clinically significant for several days after a single dose. Its ability to reduce the generation of leukotriene B4 by inhibition of the 5-lipoxygenase pathway may also be important to its anti-inflammatory action.

In treating rheumatoid arthritis methotrexate is usually administered once weekly in an initial dose of 7.5 mg either orally or by parenteral injection (bioavailability nearly equivalent). Clinical benefit (or relapse) tends to occur within 3 to 6 weeks. If the initial dose is ineffective, the amount of drug may be increased in 2.5-5.0 mg/wk increments every 3-6 weeks until one of the following occurs: the disease comes under control, the weekly dose reaches 20-25 mg, or toxicity supervenes. Once the disease is controlled, the dose may be continued as maintenance or reduced slowly. If the disease flares as the dose decreases, the dose can be raised to the lowest effective dose.

Toxicity remains the primary cause of permanent discontinuation of methotrexate (two to three times more common than loss of effectiveness) but 52%-86% of patients with rheumatoid arthritis continue to take methotrexate at 2 years and 31%-49% at 5 years. Hepatotoxicity is the most feared toxic reaction: elevated liver enzymes have been noted at some point in 70%-88% of patients treated for 4-5 years and hepatic fibrosis has been noted in about 17% (range: 0%-52%). Other toxicities include nausea, stomatitis, leukopenia, thrombocytopenia, alopecia, rash, acute pulmonary insufficiency, increased susceptibility to *H. zoster* and other infections, teratogenicity (in pregnant women), and oligospermia (Table 317-2). To minimize morbidity from methotrexate, patients should avoid drinking alcohol, and a complete blood count and quantitative platelet count should be obtained every 2-3 weeks with blood chemistries (including liver function tests) every 4-8 weeks. Some rheumatologists recommend liver biopsies after cumulative doses of 1500 mg of methotrexate.

Azathioprine

Azathioprine was introduced in 1961 for use in human organ transplantation. In the 1970s and early 1980s several well-controlled studies proved its efficacy in rheumatoid arthritis, for which it is now FDA-approved. Controlled trials have also supported its efficacy in psoriatic arthritis, polymyositis, and Behçet's disease. Azathioprine is also commonly used in systemic lupus erythematosus, polyarteritis nodosa, and Reiter's syndrome.

Bioavailability of orally administered azathioprine is at least 60%. Although azathioprine itself is inactive, it is rapidly metabolized to 6-mercaptopurine and other metabolites, two of which are cytotoxic (6-thioguanylic acid and 6-thioinosinic acid). Peak serum levels of azathioprine and 6-mercaptopurine occur within 2 hours of ingestion. Azathioprine and its active by-products are completely metabolized and excreted (largely in the urine) within 24 hours.

Azathioprine is an antimetabolite purine analogue that interferes with the synthesis of DNA by suppressing several steps in the synthesis of adenine and guanine, thereby inhibiting the first step of de novo purine biosynthesis. It also prevents the interconversion of purine bases via feedback inhibition.

In rheumatoid arthritis and most of the other rheumatic diseases, the effective azathioprine dose is generally between 1.5-3.0 mg/kg/day (i.e., usually 75-150 mg daily). Patients with psoriatic arthritis, however, often require (and tolerate) higher doses (up to 5 mg/kg/day). The initial dose of azathioprine is usually 75-100 mg daily, with incremental increases of 25-50 mg every 4-8 weeks until the disease comes under control or toxicity supervenes. Clinical benefit or relapse tends to occur within 3 to 9 months.

Between 36% and 81% of patients started on azathioprine continue it for 1 year, 48%-67% for 2 years, and about 50% continue it for 3 years. Withdrawals during the first 6 months of azathioprine therapy are usually for toxicity while later withdrawals are equally divided between toxicity and loss of efficacy. The most frequent side effects include nausea, vomiting, diarrhea, leukopenia, rash, and hepatitis (Table 317-2). The possibility of oncogenesis is variously estimated to be up to two times that of the general population. To minimize toxicity, a complete blood count and quantitative platelet count should be obtained every 2-4 weeks until the dose is stabilized and every 4-8 weeks thereafter. Blood chemistries (including liver function tests) should be obtained every 3-6 months (more often if the patient complains of severe nausea, vomiting, or abdominal discomfort).

Glucocorticoids

Low doses of glucocorticoids rapidly moderate established inflammation without preventing the progression of joint damage in rheumatoid arthritis. Very high doses have immunosuppressive effects on both humoral and cell-mediated immunity.

Hydrocortisone (cortisol) is the 17-hydroxycorticoid compound secreted by the adrenal cortex. Cortisol production is regulated by the anterior pituitary hormone ACTH (adrenocorticotropic hormone), which is regulated by the hypothalamic peptide, corticotropin-releasing factor. Chemical manipulation of the steroid structure has resulted in a number of synthetic glucocorticoids that vary in anti-inflammatory and sodium-retaining potency and in half-life. Cortisone and prednisone must be activated by liver metabolism. Biologic half-life is much longer than measurable plasma half-life. Hydrocortisone, cortisone, prednisolone, and methylprednisolone are considered short-acting (biologic half-life, 8 to 36 hours) while dexamethasone is long-acting (36 to 54 hours).

Corticosteroids exert their major effect on inflammation by decreasing leukocyte accumulation at an inflammatory site. They decrease granulocyte chemotaxis, adherence, and egress from the circulation; impair monocyte accumulation in inflammatory lesions and interfere with their function; decrease production of immunoglobulins; inhibit immune clearance of sensitized erythrocytes; and limit the passage of immune complexes across basement membranes. In humans, they cause a transient but profound lymphopenia and monocytopenia as a result of redistribution of circulating cells. Cell-mediated immune responses are suppressed by corticosteroids.

With this multiplicity of actions, corticosteroids are remarkably active in rheumatic diseases that involve inflammation and autoimmunity. Unfortunately, they have many serious side effects (see box, p. 2448). Thus, their use must be based on a careful balancing of the potential benefit in a particular rheumatic disease against probable side effects in the patient under consideration. High daily doses (60 mg or more) of prednisone frequently are life-saving therapy in dermatomyositis, systemic lupus erythematosus, polyarteritis, polychondritis, giant-cell arteritis, and some of the complications of rheumatoid arthritis; but prolonged administration inevitably leads to iatrogenic disability and, frequently, to decreased life span.

Toxicity and efficacy are greatest with prolonged administration of divided daily doses. Taking the entire dose in the morning is slightly less toxic and simulates the normal diurnal cortisol cycle. Administration of a short-acting preparation like prednisone every other morning as a single dose greatly decreases corticosteroid side effects, and may be used to maintain remission. Judicious injections of slowly absorbed corticosteroid preparations into joints may decrease local inflammation and will minimize most systemic toxicity. Intravenous infusion of 1000 mg doses of methylprednisolone is used in managing "crises" in systemic lupus erythematosus, Goodpasture's syndrome, and other rheumatic diseases.

Disadvantages of daily glucocorticosteroids in rheumatic disease

- Acne
- Aseptic necrosis of bone
- Carbohydrate intolerance
- Ecchymosis and petechiae
- Edema
- Electrolyte imbalance
- Fatty deposition
  - Facial rounding
  - Cervical fat pads
  - Supraclavicular fat pads
  - Increased abdominal girth
- Gastrointestinal ulceration
- Glaucoma
- Growth arrest
- Hirsutism
- Hyperlipidemia
- Hypertension
- Impaired wound healing
- Infections
- Menopausal symptom acceleration (sweats and hot flashes)
- Menstrual disorders
- Myopathy
- Osteoporosis and fracture
- Pancreatitis
- Perspiration increase
- Psychic disturbances
  - Insomnia
  - Restlessness, overstimulation
  - Euphoria
  - Depression
  - Agitation
  - Psychosis
- Striae
- Suppresses pituitary-adrenal axis
- Thromboembolic phenomena
- Withdrawal syndrome

In general, corticosteroid treatment should be limited to life-threatening manifestations of rheumatic diseases. Initially, high daily doses (60 mg or more) of prednisone may be employed to rapidly suppress the life-threatening manifestation. Once accomplished, the dose on the alternate day is gradually reduced stepwise, with careful monitoring for recurrence of disease activity, until a dose of 60 mg every other day is reached. This alternate-day dose is then gradually tapered unless recurrence of disease activity requires temporary increases. Inability to control the disease or serious drug side effects may prompt the addition of an immunosuppressive drug.

GENERAL CONSIDERATIONS

The practical application of drugs to the treatment of rheumatic diseases is an exercise in risk-benefit assessment. All the drugs discussed in this chapter have significant side effects; with many of them, some side effects may be fatal. The autoimmune rheumatic diseases may involve many organ systems. The degree to which the patient's life is threatened is largely determined, not by the diagnosis, but by the critical organ systems that are injured. Thus, the choice of drugs often depends on the organs affected, rather than on the name of the disease that has been diagnosed.

Salicylates or NSAIDs are the basic therapy for arthritis. If significant disability from arthritis appears probable, a DMARD is added to attempt to suppress disease progression. Systemic corticosteroids generally are not advisable because of the many devastating side effects associated with their prolonged use. However, high-dose corticosteroids are first-line drugs for nephritis, vasculitis, carditis, inflammatory myositis, and cerebritis, in which inadequate treatment frequently leads to a fatal outcome. In these situations, immunosuppressive drugs may be added if the disease cannot be controlled by corticosteroids or if steroid side effects themselves become life-threatening. After the acute organ inflammation has been suppressed, emphasis is placed on careful adjustment of drug and dosage regimens to minimize iatrogenic side effects while still maintaining suppression of the disease; continuing drug administration is required unless a spontaneous remission has occurred. These therapeutic problems continue as long as our therapies are broadly directed at entire processes of inflammation or immunity, rather than at the specific aberrations that are causing the disease.

REFERENCES

Avioli LV, Ginnari L, and Imbimbo B, editors: Glucocorticoids and their biological consequences. Adv Exp Med Biol 171:1, 1984.

Bax DE and Amos RS: Sulfasalazine: a safe, effective agent for prolonged control of rheumatoid arthritis. A comparison with sodium aurothiomalate. Ann Rheum Dis 44:194, 1985.

Black RL et al: Methotrexate therapy in psoriatic arthritis. Double-blind study on 21 patients. JAMA 189:743, 1964.

Bowles C et al: Colchicine prevents recurrent pseudogout: multicenter trial. Arthritis Rheum 29(suppl 4):S38, 1986 (abstract).

Brooks PM and Day RO: Plasma concentrations and therapeutic effects of antiinflammatory and antirheumatic drugs. In Lewis AJ and Furst DE, editors: Nonsteroidal antiinflammatory drugs: mechanisms and clinical use. New York, 1987, Marcel Dekker.

Clements PJ and Davis J: Cytotoxic drugs: their clinical application to the rheumatic diseases. Semin Arthritis Rheum 15:231, 1986.

Dudley Hart F and Huskisson EC: Nonsteroidal anti-inflammatory drugs: current status and rational therapeutic use. Drugs 27:232, 1984.

Felson DT, Anderson JJ, and Meenan RF: The comparative efficacy and toxicity of second-line drugs in rheumatoid arthritis. Arthritis Rheum 33:1449, 1990.

Fries JF et al: Impact of specific therapy upon rheumatoid arthritis. Arthritis Rheum 29:620, 1986.

Furst DE: Rational use of disease-modifying antirheumatic drugs. Drugs 39:19, 1990.

Heller CA, Ingelfinger JA, and Goldman P: Nonsteroidal antiinflammatory drugs and aspirin: analyzing the scores. Pharmacotherapy 5:30, 1985.

Jaffe IA: Penicillamine. In McCarty DJ Jr, editor: Arthritis and allied conditions, ed 11. Philadelphia, 1989, Lea & Febiger.

Lipsky PE: Remission-inducing therapy in rheumatoid arthritis. Am J Med 75(4B):40, 1983.

The Multicenter Salsate/Aspirin Comparison Study Group: Does the acetyl group of aspirin contribute to the efficacy of salicylic acid in the treatment of rheumatoid arthritis? J Rheumatol 16:321, 1989.

Paulus HE and Furst DE: Aspirin and other nonsteroidal antiinflammatory drugs. In McCarty DJ Jr and Koopman WJ, editors: Arthritis and allied conditions, ed 12. Philadelphia, 1993, Lea & Febiger.

Pullar T, Hunter JA, and Capell HA: Which component of sulfasalazine is active in rheumatoid arthritis? Brit Med J 290:1535, 1985.

Runge LA: Antimalarials. In McCarty DJ Jr and Koopman WJ, editors: Arthritis and allied conditions, ed 12. Philadelphia, 1993, Lea & Febiger.

Samuelsson B: An elucidation of the arachidonic acid cascade. Discovery of prostaglandins, thromboxane and leukotrienes. Drugs 33(suppl 1):2, 1987.

Schlegel S: General characteristics of nonsteroidal antiinflammatory drugs. In Paulus HE, Furst DE, and Dromgoole SH, editors: Drugs for rheumatic disease. New York, 1987, Churchill Livingstone.

Scully CJ, Anderson CJ, and Cannon GW: Long-term methotrexate therapy for rheumatoid arthritis. Semin Arthritis Rheum 20:317, 1991.
Skosey JL: Gold compounds and *d*-penicillamine. In McCarty DJ Jr and Koopman WJ, editors: Arthritis and allied conditions, ed 12. Philadelphia, 1993, Lea & Febiger.

VI Joint Diseases

CHAPTER

318 Osteoarthritis

Kenneth D. Brandt

Osteoarthritis (OA), also called *degenerative joint disease* and *osteoarthrosis,* is the most common of all joint diseases to affect mankind and is marked by progressive loss of articular cartilage, thickening of subchondral bone, bony remodeling, and development of bony spurs (osteophytes). The clinical features include joint pain and stiffness, swelling, crepitus, low-grade synovitis, and loss of mobility. OA represents failure of the diarthrodial joint. In primary (idiopathic) OA, no predisposing factor is recognizable. In secondary OA, an underlying insult to the joint is apparent.

Classification of osteoarthritis

I. Primary
   A. Idiopathic
   B. Generalized osteoarthritis
   C. Erosive osteoarthritis
II. Secondary
   A. Resulting from mechanical incongruity of joint
      1. Congenital or developmental defects, hip dysplasia, Legg-Calvé-Perthes disease, slipped femoral capital epiphysis, femoral neck abnormalities, protrusio acetabuli, multiple epiphyseal dysplasia, osteochondritis, Morquio's syndrome
      2. Posttraumatic
   B. Resulting from prior inflammatory joint disease—for example, rheumatoid arthritis and variants, chronic gouty arthritis, pseudogout, infectious arthritis
   C. Resulting from metabolic disorders—for example, hemochromatosis, ochronosis, Wilson's disease, chondrocalcinosis, Paget's disease
   D. Resulting from endocrinopathies—for example, diabetes mellitus, acromegaly, sex hormone abnormalities, iatrogenic hyperadrenocorticism
   E. Resulting from miscellaneous causes—for example, osteonecrosis, hemarthrosis associated with blood dyscrasias

EPIDEMIOLOGY

Of all of the specific joint diseases, OA is the single most frequent cause of rheumatic complaints. More than 80% of all people over the age of 55 have radiographic evidence of OA; while not all of these individuals are symptomatic, some 10%-30% of those affected have significant pain and disability. OA of the knee is the leading cause of chronic disability in the United States.

Aging

Age is the most powerful risk factor for OA. Only 21% of women under the age of 45, but 30% of those between 45 and 64 and 68% of those age 65 or older, have radiographic evidence of OA. The same trend was observed in men. When all age groups are considered, the prevalence of OA in men is comparable to that in women, although women are more likely to be symptomatic.

OA is often considered a *consequence* of "aging," that is, senescence of the articular cartilage chondrocyte, with "running down" of its metabolic machinery. However, since joints accumulate mechanical insults throughout a lifetime, the distinction between wear-and-tear and aging is blurred. In normal human joint cartilage, only a modest reduction in cellularity occurs after maturity and the cells remain metabolically active; indeed, the net rate of proteoglycan synthesis per cell is as high in normal cartilage from aged individuals as in that from younger adults. And, although age-related changes occur in the chemical composition of normal articular cartilage, they are very different from those in OA cartilage and have not been clearly shown to predispose to OA.

Race and genetics

Racial differences in the prevalence of OA are apparent. In the United States, OA is more common in Native Americans than in the general population. Hip and interphalangeal joint OA are much less prevalent in South African blacks than in whites in the same population. Chinese in Hong Kong have a lower prevalence of hip OA than Caucasians. Whether such variations are related to heredity or to cultural differences in joint usage is not known.

Other examples may be cited in which the etiologic role of genetic factors is less ambiguous. In some instances the genetic defect results in a change in the gross structure of the joint, affecting congruity (e.g., acetabular dysplasia). In others, it may lead to OA through systemic metabolic effects. Heberden's nodes (distal interphalangeal joint OA), clearly are inherited. Recently, a point mutation in the cDNA coding for articular cartilage collagen was identified in several generations of a family with mild chondrodysplasia and secondary OA involving multiple joints. In ochronosis, a heritable disorder characterized by a deficiency of homogentisic acid oxidase, accumulation of homogentisic acid polymers leads to stiffening of articular cartilage and decreased ability of the tissue to transmit load.

Joint distribution; relation of OA to joint overload and trauma

Under the age of 55 the pattern of joint involvement in men and women is similar. In older people, OA of interphalangeal joints and the base of the thumb is more common in women, whereas hip OA is more often seen in men.

In the normal joint, some incongruity of the surfaces during loading is important for "pumping" nutrients from the synovial fluid into the cartilage, and catabolites from the cartilage into the fluid. Alterations in congruity caused by congenital or developmental defects have been considered to underlie nearly all cases of idiopathic, or primary, OA of the hip in man. In such instances OA may be caused by mechanical "fatigue failure" of the matrix, increased contact stresses, or impaired nutrition of the chondrocyte.

Major joint trauma is an important risk factor for OA. Anterior cruciate ligament insufficiency, meniscus damage, and meniscectomy all lead to knee OA. Osteochondral fractures and fractures that heal with deformities that result in concentration of stress within the joint also predispose to OA.

The site of involvement is strongly influenced by prior usage of the joint. Thus, OA is common in ankles of ballet dancers, shoulders and elbows of professional tennis players, and metacarpophalangeal joints of boxers. Repeated overload of the joint by vocational or avocational use is an important—and potentially modifiable—cause of OA. Although jogging has been reported not to cause OA, selection bias (i.e., early cessation of the activity by those who incur joint damage) cannot be excluded in those studies.

Jobs requiring repeated knee bending and moderate physical demand appear to predispose to knee OA. The prevalence of hip OA is increased in farmers. Among groups of textile workers performing different repetitive manual tasks, OA was more prevalent in hand joints used repetitively for the task than in other hand joints.

Obesity

Obesity has long been associated with an increased prevalence of knee OA. Recent epidemiologic data indicate that obesity is not merely the result of decreased physical activity resulting from the painful knee, but may precede, and represent an important risk factor for, knee OA. In a strain of guinea pigs at risk for development of spontaneous knee OA, dietary restriction sufficient to decrease body weight by 28% decreased the severity of OA pathology by 40%. Furthermore, in obese women, weight loss reduced the risk of *symptomatic* knee OA. Whether metabolic factors as well as mechanical effects contribute to development of OA in obesity is unclear.

Risk factors for pain and disability in OA

In general, the association between the severity of pathologic changes of OA and joint pain is weak. Many subjects with advanced radiographic changes of OA are asymptomatic. The risk factors for pain and disability are poorly understood. However, psychosocial factors may be important determinants of who with OA becomes symptomatic and who does not; given comparable degrees of pathologic severity, women are more likely to be symptomatic than men, divorced individuals more likely than those who are married, and people on welfare more likely than those who are employed.

PATHOLOGY

Although loss of articular cartilage is the pathologic hallmark of OA, in the earlier stages of OA the cartilage is thicker than normal, in association with increases in both the water content and proteoglycan concentration of the matrix. Localized softening of the cartilage (chondromalacia) is present in load-bearing areas. With progression of the disease, the surface becomes disrupted and fissures develop (fibrillation). With joint motion the fibrillated cartilage is lost, exposing underlying bone that becomes thickened and eburnated. Microfractures of subchondral trabeculae may be seen. Bone cysts, reflecting localized osteonecrosis, form beneath the surface and weaken the osseous support for the overlying cartilage. New bone formation leads to osteophytes (spurs), which extend into the joint capsule and ligament attachments or into the joint space, where they may restrict joint movement.

Although mitosis of chondrocytes is never seen in normal adult articular cartilage, chondrocyte proliferation may be extensive in OA. Late in the disease, however, the cartilage becomes hypocellular. Capillaries from the underlying subchondral bone invade the tidemark and provide a basis for fibrocartilaginous outgrowths that may replace the defective hyaline cartilage. The repair cartilage, however, is inferior to the native cartilage in its ability to withstand mechanical stress. The synovium shows foci of inflammation, lining-cell hyperplasia, and villus hypertrophy. The capsule becomes thickened, further limiting joint motion. Periarticular muscle atrophy is common and may contribute significantly to disability. Notably, synovial and cartilage pathology may be as severe in those who are asymptomatic as in patients complaining of joint pain.

PATHOGENESIS

No single factor triggers the processes that result in cartilage destruction and new bone formation in OA. Most current theories of the pathogenesis of OA focus on the breakdown of the articular cartilage, which may be primary, or secondary to abnormalities in subchondral bone, synovium, or extra-articular structures (ligaments, neuromuscular apparatus) (see box, p. 2489).

The importance of articular cartilage lies in the fact that it fulfils two essential functions within the joint: first, it provides a remarkably smooth bearing surface, so that with joint movement one bone glides effortlessly over the other. Second, it prevents the concentration of stresses, so that the bones do not shatter with loading of the joint.

OA develops in either of two settings: (1) the biomaterial properties of the articular cartilage and subchondral bone are normal but excessive loads applied to the joint cause the tissues to fail, or (2) the applied load is physiologically reasonable but the material properties of the cartilage or bone are inferior.

Although mechanical "wear" is undoubtedly a factor in the loss of cartilage in OA, lysosomal and neutral metalloproteinases account for much of the loss of cartilage matrix. Whether their synthesis and secretion are stimulated by cytokines derived from the inflamed synovium (e.g., interleukin-1) or by other factors (e.g., mechanical stimuli), neutral metalloproteinases, plasmin, and cathepsins produced by the chondrocytes are central to the breakdown of articular cartilage in OA. Endogenous tissue inhibitors of these enzymes (e.g., tissue inhibitors of metalloproteinases [TIMP], plasminogen activator inhibitor) may stabilize the system, at least temporarily, and growth factors (e.g., IGF-1, TGF-β) drive repair processes that may heal the lesion or at least stabilize the damage. A stoichiometric imbalance has been shown to exist between levels of matrix-degrading enzymes, which may be several-fold higher than normal, while the level of TIMP is only modestly increased.

The chondrocytes in OA cartilage undergo active cell division and are very active metabolically, producing increased quantities of collagen (which provides cartilage with tensile strength) and proteoglycans (which are responsible for the stiffness of the tissue and its ability to resist compression). Prior to the loss of cartilage, this marked biosynthetic activity may lead to an increase in proteoglycan concentration, which may be associated with thickening of the cartilage and "compensated," stabilized OA. Indeed, these homeostatic mechanisms may maintain the joint in a reasonable functional state for many years. The repair tissue, however, does not hold up as well under mechanical stress as normal hyaline cartilage. Eventually, at least in some cases, the rate of proteoglycan synthesis declines and "end-stage" OA develops.

CLINICAL FEATURES

The joints most commonly involved in primary OA are the distal and proximal interphalangeal joints of the hands; the metacarpophalangeal joint of the thumb; the knees; hips; cervical and lumbar spine; and the metatarsophalangeal joint of the great toe. In primary OA most other joints are spared; if they are affected, secondary OA (Table 318-1) is probably present.

The predominant symptom of OA and the complaint that most often leads the patient to seek medical attention is joint pain. This may be caused by subchondral microfractures, irritation of periosteal nerve endings during remodeling or osteophyte formation, hemodynamic changes in subchondral bone resulting from distortion of the subchondral capillaries by thickened bony trabeculae, ligamentous strain, periarticular inflammation (bursitis or tendinitis), or low-grade synovitis.

The patient complains of a deep ache, which is usually localized to the involved joint but occasionally is referred. Typically, the pain occurs after joint usage and is relieved by rest, but in advanced OA it may be present also at rest. In severe hip OA, night pain is common. Brief gelling of the joint after disuse is characteristic. Morning stiffness usually lasts less than 30 minutes. Constitutional features, such as weight loss, anemia, fatigue, and fever, are not present in OA.

Physical findings include tenderness, bony crepitus, limitation of motion, and enlargement of the involved joint. Swelling may be caused by thickening of the synovium and capsule, effusion, or osteophytes. With progression of the disease, gross deformity occurs, with subluxation and marked bony enlargement.

When OA of the spine involves apophyseal joints, parasthesias, muscle weakness, and hyperreflexia may be caused by osteophytes, prolapse of the degenerated disk, or narrowing of neural foramina by apophyseal joint subluxation. In the cervical region, osteophytes may compress the spinal cord, producing long tract signs. Osteophytes in the joints of Luschka may alter the course of the vertebral artery, producing vertigo, diplopia, scotomata, nystagmus, or ataxia. Symptoms of vertebral insufficiency in cervical OA may be related to the position of the neck.

PRIMARY OA

Heberden's nodes

These represent bony, cartilaginous, synovial, and capsular enlargements of the distal interphalangeal joints of the hands (Fig. 318-1). Similar changes may occur in the proximal interphalangeal joints (Bouchard's nodes) and may be associated with flexion deformities and lateral deviation of the involved phalanges. Although they are usually associated with little discomfort, the nodes may present acutely with redness, swelling, and pain. Heberden's nodes are ten times more common in women than in men, and a strong hereditary tendency is apparent.

Table 318-1. Clinical features of primary osteoarthritis

Age	Usually elderly
Joint distribution	Mono- or oligoarthritis
Most frequent sites	Distal and proximal interphalangeal joints of fingers, first carpometacarpal joint, first metatarsophalangeal joint, hips, knees, cervical spine, lumbar spine
Joints usually spared	Metacarpophalangeal joints, wrists, elbows, glenohumeral joints, ankles
Systemic manifestations	Absent
Characteristics of joint discomfort	Aggravated by use and relieved by rest (but pain also at rest with severe disease); gelling sensation; morning stiffness absent or less than 30 minutes in duration
Joint examination	Local tenderness, bony and/or soft-tissue swelling, crepitus, effusion
Characteristics of synovial fluid	Normal viscosity, normal mucin test, mild leukocytosis (<2000 wbc/mm^3), predominantly mononuclear cells

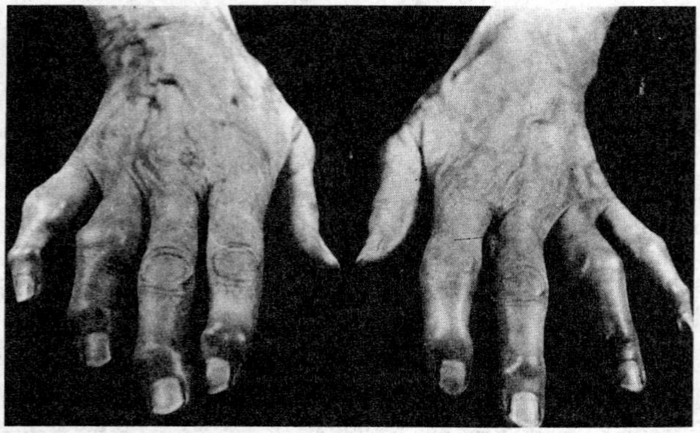

Fig. 318-1. Osteoarthritis of the distal interphalangeal joints. Note the bony enlargement and deformity (Heberden's nodes). The node on the right index finger is inflamed, and the overlying skin is erythematous. Bony enlargement is present also at several proximal interphalangeal joints (Bouchard's nodes).

Erosive osteoarthritis (EOA)

This disorder occurs particularly in postmenopausal women and affects distal and proximal interphalangeal joints and, occasionally, the metacarpophalangeal joints. Inflammation is generally much more marked than in the typical patient with Heberden's nodes. Recurrent acute painful flare-ups are typical. Radiographs show collapse of the subchondral plate and bony erosions in addition to the typical features of OA (see Chapter 296). Deformity may be severe, and ankylosis may develop. The synovium is infiltrated with lymphocytes and monocytes to a greater degree than usually seen in primary OA. Pannus, which is rare in other forms of OA, may develop. Some 15% of patients with EOA may eventually develop rheumatoid arthritis, although tests for rheumatoid factor are negative.

Primary generalized osteoarthritis (GOA)

GOA is marked by involvement of three or more joints or groups of joints and, like EOA, occurs predominantly in middle-aged postmenopausal women. Interphalangeal joints of the hands and the first carpometacarpal joint are involved most often, but GOA also affects knees, hips, big toe, and spine. The course is typically episodic, with intermittent bouts of pain in the involved joint(s), often accompanied by warmth and effusion.

Chondromalacia patellae

This clinical syndrome of patellofemoral pain occurs chiefly in young adults. Females are affected more than males. Softening of cartilage occurs where the patella comes in contact with the femur in midflexion of the knee. The changes are usually *not* progressive; in only a minority of cases does chondromalacia patellae seem to lead to OA.

Spondylosis deformans

This term refers to degenerative disease in the intervertebral disks, rather than in the synovial joints of the spine. Progressive changes in the nucleus pulposus are similar to those in articular cartilage in OA. The hyaline cartilage end plates fibrillate and disintegrate, leading to eburnation of subchondral bone. The nucleus pulposus may herniate into the vertebral body through the disrupted end plate (Schmorl's node). Vertebral osteophytes commonly develop.

SECONDARY OA

OA may occur as a sequel to a variety of diverse endocrine or metabolic disorders or to inflammatory joint disease (see box, p. 2489) when the capacity of the chondrocyte to maintain a normal matrix has been diminished, when joint congruity has been affected, or when the biomechanical properties of the cartilage or subchondral bone have been altered.

For example, secondary OA commonly develops in the wake of rheumatoid arthritis or infectious arthritis. In such cases the cartilage is damaged initially by enzymes released from inflammatory cells in the synovium or joint space. Interleukin-1 and tumor necrosis factor, which are produced by mononuclear cells in the inflamed joint, suppress PG synthesis by the chondrocyte and stimulate it to synthesize and release matrix-degrading proteases (e.g., stromelysin, collagenase, gelatinase), resulting in a matrix vulnerable to mechanical breakdown.

Hemochromatosis, Wilson's disease, ochronosis, gout, and calcium pyrophosphate dihydrate (CPPD) crystal deposition disease also may lead to secondary OA. In these instances, deposits of hemosiderin, copper, homogentisic acid polymers, crystals of monosodium urate, or crystals of CPPD, respectively, may damage the chondrocyte. In some cases they may exert a direct mechanical effect, increasing cartilage stiffness and altering load forces.

LABORATORY STUDIES

No specific clinical laboratory abnormality is present in primary OA. The sedimentation rate is normal for the age of the patient. The synovial fluid shows only a slight increase in cell count (<2000 cells/mm^3), with normal viscosity and normal mucin. Fragments of cartilage and/or bone ("wear particles") or crystals of calcium hydroxyapatite, calcium pyrophosphate dihydrate, or both, may be seen.

RADIOGRAPHIC EXAMINATION

The radiographic findings in OA are described in Chapter 296. A combination of joint space narrowing, sclerosis of subchondral bone, and bony outgrowths (osteophytosis) is typical. Notably, in some patients with joint pain caused by OA, joint radiographs may be normal even in the presence of full-thickness ulceration of the articular cartilage (as revealed by arthroscopy). Osteophytes alone, without joint space narrowing or bony changes, may be caused by aging and do not necessarily indicate underlying cartilage damage. They are thus not diagnostic of OA.

TREATMENT

The goals of treatment are to relieve pain, increase mobility, reduce disability, and prevent progression of the disease. Although many patients require only reassurance, a mild analgesic, and instruction about joint protection, cases of more severe OA warrant an aggressive, comprehensive approach utilizing drugs, physical measures, and surgery.

Drug therapy

In OA, drug therapy today is aimed at relief of pain; it does not influence the natural progression of joint breakdown. Salicylates and other nonsteroidal anti-inflammatory drugs (NSAIDs) often produce symptomatic relief. In many cases this may be a result of their analgesic properties rather than their anti-inflammatory effects. Thus, an anti-inflammatory dose of NSAID may be no more effective than a lower (essentially analgesic) dose of NSAID or than a pure analgesic, for example, acetaminophen. Furthermore, the presence of clinical evidence of joint inflammation (i.e., swelling, synovial tenderness) does not necessarily predict a better response to an anti-inflammatory drug than to an analgesic in OA.

Systemic corticosteroids have no place in treatment of OA. However, intra-articular injection of a glucocorticoid may provide pain relief and improve motion. The procedure should not be repeated more often than every 4 to 6 months, since frequent intra-articular steroid injections may lead to joint breakdown. Gold salts, antimalarials, penicillamine, and immunosuppressive drugs are not indicated in OA. Capsaicin cream, which depletes sensory nerve endings of substance P, a neuropeptide mediator of pain, may reduce joint pain when applied topically by patients with hand or knee OA.

Reduction of joint loading

OA may be caused or aggravated by poor body mechanics. For example, genu varum or valgum or pronated feet may create excessive loading on the knee. This can be corrected with orthotics or osteotomy. A wedged insole may reduce joint pain in patients with early knee OA. Use of a running shoe with a well-cushioned sole as primary daily footwear may also be helpful. Since the excessive load imposed by adiposity may accelerate cartilage breakdown in lumbar spine and lower-extremity joints, the obese patient should be encouraged to lose weight.

Activities that cause excessive loading of the damaged joint should be avoided. For the patient with OA of the hip or knee, the workplace may be modified to permit sitting instead of standing. Kneeling and squatting should be eliminated. Jogging and participation in racket sports should be discouraged. Swimming and biking are good alternatives. A cane (held in the contralateral hand) is helpful if hip or knee OA is unilateral; crutches or a walker are preferable if it is bilateral. For symptomatic OA of the first carpometacarpal joint, splinting may be effective.

For painful OA of the neck a cervical pillow may be useful. The patient should be instructed not to maintain prolonged neck flexion or extension (as when shampooing the hair, sitting in the front row of a theater, or viewing television while lying on a sofa). Repetitive cervical rotation (e.g., watching a tennis match from a midcourt seat) should also be discouraged.

Physical and occupational therapy

Local application of heat or cold and an exercise program are useful adjuncts in management of OA. Exercises should be designed to preserve or improve the range of motion and to strengthen involved muscles. Isometric rather than isotonic exercises are generally preferable. Transcutaneous electrical nerve stimulation may diminish pain that proves to be unresponsive to analgesics or NSAIDs and the above measures. Muscle relaxants or massage may reverse muscle spasm.

Orthopedic surgery

Total joint arthroplasty should be considered for patients with advanced OA with unremitting pain or severely impaired function who are unresponsive to an aggressive approach encompassing the above measures. Surgery may be remarkably effective in such cases, especially in patients with hip or knee OA. In the earlier stages of OA, osteotomy, which redistributes compressive stresses, may relieve pain and also prevent progression of the disease. Arthrodesis, which permanently eliminates joint motion, is used with some frequency for OA of the subtalar joint and first carpometacarpal joint.

Arthroscopic removal of loose cartilage fragments (joint mice) may prevent locking, eliminate pain, and reduce abrasive wear of the joint surfaces. Saline lavage of the OA knee, flushing out cartilage shards and other debris, may provide months of relief for patients whose joint pain has been refractory to pharmacologic measures, including intra-articular steroid injection.

REFERENCES

Bradley JD et al: Comparison of an anti-inflammatory dose of ibuprofen, an analgesic dose of ibuprofen, and acetaminophen in the treatment of patients with osteoarthritis of the knee. N Engl J Med 325:87, 1991.

Brandt KD: Management of osteoarthritis. In Kelley WN et al, editors: Textbook of rheumatology, ed 4. Philadelphia, 1993, Saunders.

Brandt KD and Mankin HJ: Pathogenesis of osteoarthritis. In Kelley WN et al, editors: Textbook of rheumatology, ed 4. Philadelphia, 1993, Saunders.

Brandt KD and Radin E: The physiology of articular stress: osteoarthrosis. Hosp Pract 22:103, 1987.

Mankin HJ and Brandt KD: Biochemistry and metabolism of cartilage in osteoarthritis. In Moskowitz RW et al, editors: Osteoarthritis—diagnosis and management, ed 2. Philadelphia, 1992, Saunders.

CHAPTER

319 Gout and Hyperuricemia

Robert A. Terkeltaub

The term *gout* denotes a heterogeneous group of disorders characterized by one or more of the following: (1) an increase in the serum concentration of uric acid (hyperuricemia); (2) recurrent attacks of a characteristic type of acute inflammatory arthritis, in which microcrystals of the physiologic salt of uric acid, monosodium urate monohydrate, are demonstrable in synovial fluid leukocytes (acute gouty arthritis); (3) deposition of aggregates of monosodium urate monohydrate crystals (tophi), chiefly in and around joints and in soft tissues; (4) renal impairment associated with interstitial deposition of monosodium urate crystals (gouty nephropathy); and (5) uric acid urolithiasis. Hyperuricemia reflects a variety of metabolic or physiologic derangements that predispose to the clinical events listed above via the deposition of crystals of monosodium urate monohydrate or uric acid from supersaturated extracellular fluids. Although hyperuricemia is necessary, it most often is not sufficient for expression of gout. Asymptomatic hyperuricemia therefore is not a disease state and should be distinguished clinically from gout.

ETIOLOGY AND INCIDENCE

As a result of the evolutionary absence of the enzyme uricase, humans are unable to oxidize uric acid to the soluble compound allantoin and must excrete uric acid as the end product of purine metabolism. This defect predisposes the entire human species to the hazards of hyperuricemia and tissue deposition of crystalline forms of this relatively insoluble substance. In addition, the sum of the complex array of renal mechanisms involved in uric acid excretion is net retention of more than 90% of urate filtered at the glomerulus. Although the biochemical and physiologic mechanisms governing uric acid metabolism are usually sufficient to assure clearance of the compound, this clearance is accomplished only at the expense of serum urate concentrations, which in normal adult males and females average nearly 6 mg and 5 mg per deciliter, respectively (as measured by the specific uricase method). The narrow margin of safety attained is underscored by the proximity of these values to the theoretical limit of solubility of monosodium urate in plasma (about 7 mg/dl).

These facts and the multiplicity of genetic and environmental influences on the chain of events governing uric acid formation, transport, and disposal (discussed later) indicate that superimposition of any one or a combination of potential degrangements in these processes can lead to hyperuricemia and gout. In fact, it appears likely that hyperuricemia (as defined by serum urate > 7 mg/dl in men and > 6 mg/dl in women) occurs in 5% to 10% of asymptomatic adult Americans. Evidence to date suggests that less than 20% of this group develops clinically apparent urate crystal deposition, supporting conservative management for asymptomatic hyperuricemic individuals. The incidences of gouty arthritis and of uric acid urolithiais among previously asymptomatic persons increase with the severity of hyperuricemia and become substantial when serum urate exceeds 9 mg per deciliter. However, recent data relevant to the long-term effects of hyperuricemia on renal function suggest that in most individuals higher degrees of hyperuricemia are tolerated with little apparent jeopardy to the kidney.

The prevalence of gout appears to have increased over the last few decades in the United States and in certain other countries that possess a high standard of living. Gout is predominantly a disease of adult men, with a peak incidence in the fifth decade. In 1986, the prevalence of self-reported gout in the United States was estimated at 13.6 per 1000 men and 6.4 per 1000 women. Gout is not only a common disease but also a significant public health problem because of its frequent association with short-term disability, occupational limitations, and the utilization of medical services.

Gout rarely occurs in males before adolescence or in females before menopause. These features correlate well with age-related patterns of serum urate concentration, which in men show a sharp increase during puberty, with a subsequent plateau. In contrast, serum urate concentrations during the reproductive period in women average nearly 1 mg per deciliter lower than those in age-matched males. The uricosuric effects of estrogens are believed to contribute to this phenomenon. Serum urate concentrations rise in women after menopause to levels comparable to those in males.

PATHOGENESIS

Purine metabolism

Uric acid is the physiologic end product of human purine metabolism (Fig. 319-1), and its remote sources are the ingestion of dietary purine-containing foods and the endogenous synthesis of purine nucleotides, which are building blocks in the synthesis of nucleic acids. Degradation of nucleic acids and free purine nucleotides to the purine bases xanthine and hypoxanthine and the sequential oxidation of these bases (mainly in the liver) to uric acid by the enzyme xanthine oxidase constitute the catabolic steps resulting in uric acid production. Urate circulates in the plasma predominantly in an unbound form. Renal excretion is the major route for uric acid disposal and accounts for about two thirds of the daily loss of this compound from the body. Extrarenal urate disposal is accomplished mainly by bacterial oxidation of urate secreted into the gut.

De-novo synthesis. The synthesis of purine nucleotides involves a complex interplay of two alternative biochemical pathways. In the pathway of purine synthesis de novo, small-molecule precursors of uric acid are incorporated into a purine ring synthesized in 10 sequential steps on a ribose-phosphate backbone donated by 5-phosphoribosyl-1-

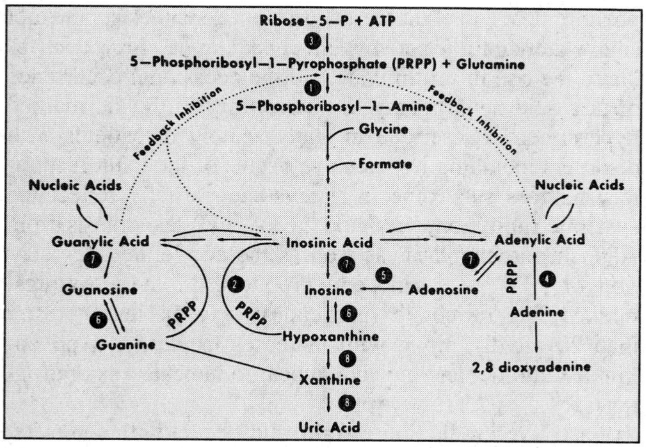

Fig. 319-1. Outline of purine metabolism: (1) amidophosphoribosyltransferase, (2) hypoxanthine-guanine phosphoribosyltransferase, (3) PRPP synthetase, (4) adenine phosphoribosyltransferase, (5) adenosine deaminase, (6) purine nucleoside phosphorylase, (7) 5′-nucleotidase, (8) xanthine oxidase. (Reproduced with permission of the Arthritis Foundation.)

pyrophosphate (PRPP) (Fig. 319-1). The first reaction committed to purine synthesis de novo is catalyzed by amidophosphoribosyltransferase, an enzyme with allosteric properties that correlate with a rate-determining role for this reaction in the pathway. Amidophosphoribosyltransferase activity is inhibited by purine nucleotide products of the pathway; feedback inhibition is reversed by PRPP, a substrate usually present in limiting concentration in the cell. The antagonistic interaction of purine nucleotides and PRPP at the level of activity of amidophos-phoribosyltransferase appears to be of paramount importance in regulating the rate of purine synthesis de novo. Additional controls on the rate of purine nucleotide synthesis are exerted at the level of synthesis of PRPP and at the more distal branch point, which determine proportions of adenylate and guanylate nucleotides synthesized.

Base-salvage synthesis. The second pathway of purine nucleotide synthesis involves the two enzymes adenine phosphoribosyltransferase and hypoxanthine-guanine phosphoribosyltransferase (HGPRT), which catalyze single-step synthesis of purine nucleotides from the respective purine base substrates by reactions with PRPP (Fig. 319-1). The relationship between the rates of the base salvage and de novo pathways is likely to be governed in part by availability of the common substrate PRPP and by concentrations of the nucleotide products common to the pathways. Since the cell requires considerably less energy for purine base salvage than for purine synthesis de novo, preferential utilization of PRPP for purine base salvage is likely.

Production, excretion, and accumulation of uric acid

Measurements of uric acid synthesis and disposal have shown that the readily miscible urate pool averages about 1200 mg (range 800 to 1600 mg) in normal men and is about half this value in normal women. Uric acid production averages about 750 mg per day in men; thus, about two thirds to three fourths of the urate pool is turned over daily. Urinary uric acid excretion in normal men receiving a purine-free diet, although somewhat variable, averages 426 ± 81 mg per day. The large discrepancy between daily urinary uric acid excretion and pool turnover is accounted for by extrarenal uric acid disposal.

From these considerations, a number of potential mechanisms for excessive uric acid accumulation, and thus hyperuricemia, emerge. However, only diminished fractional uric acid excretion by the kidney, increased uric acid production, or both of these mechanisms acting in concert have been demonstrated to contribute substantially to the hyperuricemia of patients with the various forms of gout (Table 319-1).

The majority of patients with gout excrete normal total quantities of uric acid in their daily urine. In the remaining individuals, urinary uric acid excretion is excessive. The latter constitutes overexcretion, which has been defined by different laboratories as more than 600-700 mg per day in adult males on a purine-free diet or more than 800-1000

Table 319-1. Working classification of hyperuricemia and gout

Uric acid overproduction

- Primary hyperuricemia and gout
  - Idiopathic
  - HGPRT deficiency (partial and complete)
  - PRPP synthetase superactivity
- Secondary hyperuricemia and gout
  - Excessive dietary purine intake
  - Accelerated ATP degradation
    - Ethanol abuse
    - Glycogen storage diseases (types I, III, V, VII)
    - Fructose ingestion, hereditary fructose intolerance
    - Hypoxemia and tissue hypoperfusion
    - Severe muscle exertion
  - Increased nucleotide turnover
    - For example, myeloproliferative or lymphoproliferative disorders, hemolytic diseases, psoriasis

Uric acid underexcretion

- Primary hyperuricemia and gout
  - Idiopathic
- Secondary hyperuricemia and gout
  - Diminished renal function
  - Inhibition of tubular urate secretion
    - Competitive anions (e.g., keto- and lactic acidosis)
  - Enhanced tubular urate reabsorption
    - Dehydration, diuretics
  - Mechanism incompletely defined
    - Lead nephropathy
    - Hypertension
    - Hyperparathyroidism
    - Certain drugs (e.g., cyclosporine, pyrazinamide, ethambutol, low-dose salicylates)

PRPP, 5-phosphoribosyl-1-pyrophosphate; HGPRT, hypoxanthine-guanine phosphoribosyltransferase.

mg per day on a typical American diet, in the presence of normal renal function. Importantly, increased rates of uric acid synthesis (overproduction) are almost invariably demonstrable by isotopic labeling studies in overexcreting subjects.

A working classification of hyperuricemia appears in Table 319-1. In this scheme, patients in whom manifestations of urate deposition are prominent components of the overall clinical picture can be classified as having primary hyperuricemia, in contrast to patients in whom hyperuricemia and gout are generally minor clinical features secondary to any of a number of genetic or acquired processes.

Overproduction of uric acid can be associated with a primary derangement in the mechanisms regulating de-novo purine nucleotide synthesis. Specific inherited enzyme aberrations can be identified in a small proportion of patients. In both the partial and virtually complete deficiencies of HGPRT, intracellular accumulation of PRPP resulting from diminished utilization of this regulatory substrate in purine base salvage drives purine synthesis de novo at an increased rate. In the case of variant forms of PRPP synthetase with excessive activity, increased PRPP availability for purine synthesis de novo results from increased synthesis of PRPP. Thus, aberrations of these X-linked enzymes yield an increased uric acid synthesis by altering the balance of control of purine synthesis de novo toward increased production.

An increase in the net degradation of the adenine nucleotide ATP has been proposed to be a factor in both the hyperuricemia of a subgroup of patients with primary gout and the hyperuricemia of a number of clinical disorders. First, the accelerated degradation of ATP to AMP via the conversion of acetate to acetyl CoA in the metabolism of ethanol may be an important mechanism in hyperuricemia associated with alcohol ingestion. Furthermore, excessive alcohol consumption is a frequent feature in many individuals with gout. Second, hyperuricemia and gout are strongly associated with type 1 glycogen storage disease (glucose 6-phosphatase deficiency). There is evidence that hypoglycemia, a central feature of this disorder, stimulates uric acid synthesis via elevated levels of glucagon. Glucagon activates glycogen phosphorylase, and it is believed that an unopposed accumulation of phosphorylated sugars in the liver in the presence of glucose 6-phosphatase deficiency causes hepatic ATP depletion and the accumulation of AMP (adenylic acid), which is degraded to uric acid (Fig. 319-1). Third, fructose infusion and certain inborn errors of fructose metabolism have been reported to increase hepatic concentrations of phosphorylated sugars, consume hepatic ATP, and induce hyperuricemia. Fourth, in glycogen storage disease of types III, V, or VII, in which enzyme defects impair the resynthesis of ATP from ADP in exercised muscle, moderate exercise provokes the enhanced release of uric acid precursors into the serum, resulting subsequently in hyperuricemia. In addition, the hyperuricemia known to occur with vigorous muscular exercise carried to exhaustion in normal individuals is associated with muscle ATP depletion and with marked elevations in plasma hypoxanthine. Thus, increased uric acid synthesis, and not solely dehydration and hyperlacticacidemia, may contribute to the rise in serum urate and the occasional occurrence of uric acid nephropathy in this setting. Fifth, the marked hyperuricemia described in many acutely ill patients with disorders including hypotensive events or the adult respiratory distress syndrome is believed to partially reflect the systemic inhibition, via hypoxia, of ATP resynthesis from ADP in mitochondria, as well as the accelerated degradation of ADP to purine end products. In these settings, marked hyperuricemia (particularly a peak level greater than 20 mg/dl), along with increases in plasma hypoxanthine, xanthine, and inosine, appear to indicate a poor prognosis.

Last, overproduction of uric acid occurs with some frequency in a variety of acquired disorders in which there are excessive rates of cell turnover or tissue destruction. These conditions include several benign and malignant proliferative diseases.

In patients with gout and normal total uric acid excretion, a relative deficit in the renal excretion of uric acid is the probable basis of hyperuricemia. That is, the excretion of normal amounts of uric acid is accomplished in these individuals only when serum urate concentrations are inappropriately high, a fact made apparent by the demonstration of decreased uric acid clearance in gouty normal excretors compared with normal individuals whose serum urate levels are experimentally made comparable by feeding of purine-rich diets. It is likely that virtually all plasma urate is filtered at the glomerulus, with more than 95% of the filtered load undergoing proximal tubular reabsorption. Subsequent tubular secretion contributes the major share to excreted uric acid, but the net urate excreted is modulated by substantial postsecretory tubular reabsorption.

There is no evidence that gouty "normal" excretors constitute a population with a single genetic or acquired renal defect. A diminished tubular secretory rate may contribute to hyperuricemia in some of these patients, and the possibility of increased tubular reabsorption in other patients with renal urate retention has not been dismissed. Whether such tubular abnormalities reflect primary defects in transport mechanisms or are caused by impairment of tubular processes by interfering metabolites that accumulate in the course of one or more genetic metabolic disorders is uncertain. A precedent for the latter possibility is the contribution of lactic acid–induced diminished renal urate secretion to the hyperuricemia of type I glycogen storage disease. That acquired, cryptic forms of renal impairment can be manifested initially by gouty arthritis alone has been demonstrated among chronically lead-intoxicated users of unbonded whiskey in the southeastern United States.

Gout patients as a group have a relatively high incidence of other diseases predisposing to diminished renal function, such as hypertension and diabetes mellitus. Another frequent factor in the occurrence of gout with normal total uric acid excretion is the administration of pharmacologic agents that alter renal tubular function either as a major action or as an unintended side effect. Among these agents are diuretics (thiazides, furosemide), cyclosporine, pyrazinamide, ethambutol, and low-dose salicylates. The diverse actions of therapeutic agents on renal uric acid handling point out the many sites for potential alteration of uric acid metabolism with the consequent nonspecific end point of hyperuricemia.

Genetics and gout

The familial occurrence of gout was first commented on nearly 2000 years ago, but an ordered approach to the genetics of gout became possible only when the biochemical basis of the disorder was understood. A.E. Garrod included gout among the inborn errors of metabolism in 1931, concluding that the disease reflected a dominantly inherited trait, incompletely expressed in women. He predicted that an even greater number of hyperuricemic, but asymptomatic, persons would be found. Although about 20% of gouty patients give family histories positive for the disease, and the incidence of hyperuricemia among close relatives of gouty individuals is 15% to 25%, pedigree analyses failed to confirm a unitary genetic aberration leading to hyperuricemia and gout. As a consequence, attention was turned toward the study of the individual steps of uric acid synthesis and excretion in gouty patients in the hope of finding groups of patients with well-defined specific abnormalities, the heredity of which could be determined. Inherited changes in the activities of a number of enzymes (as in Table 319-1), have been identified among patients with increased rates of purine synthesis and uric acid overproduction. However, alterations in the activities of the HGPRT and PRPP synthetase enzymes account for less than 10% of all patients with excessive purine nucleotide and uric acid production, and the relative contributions of the other genetic defects underlying uric acid overproduction to clinical hyperuricemia and gout remain to be quantified.

A number of kindreds with relatively early-onset gout and a markedly reduced fractional excretion of urate have been described, supporting the existence of specific inheritable defects in the renal excretion of uric acid. Inherited disorders of carbohydrate metabolism (e.g., type I glycogen storage disease) and amino acid metabolism (e.g., maple syrup urine disease) can induce hyperuricemia by means of inhibition of renal tubular urate secretion as a result of lacticacidemia and ketonemia, respectively; this finding indicates that even genetic aberrations primarily affecting other metabolic pathways are capable of altering uric acid metabolism with the end result of hyperuricemia.

In summary, hereditary influences appear to underlie the development of hyperuricemia in the majority of individuals with primary gout. In individual families, this influence may be under polygenic or monogenic control and may be manifested by disordered regulation of uric acid synthesis, inefficient uric acid excretion, or a combination of these mechanisms. The hereditary diathesis may be sufficient in magnitude for expression of the disease or may be insufficient, requiring the contribution of acquired factors before clinical symptoms result.

PATHOPHYSIOLOGY AND PATHOLOGY

Although hyperuricemia has been associated epidemiologically with a number of abnormal processes (hypertension, obesity, glucose intolerance, coronary occlusive disease), no pathogenetic relationships per se have been established. Similarly, a role for hyperuricemia per se as an isolated risk factor in the development of renal impairment is not proven. Rather, structural and functional kidney damage caused by uric acid excess from any cause is directly related to the physical deposition of crystals of monosodium urate at pH 7.4 or of crystals of undissociated uric acid in acidic urine (see also Chapter 349). Only a fraction (possibly one fifth) of individuals with sustained hyperuricemia develop tophi and gouty arthropathy. Currently, the factors that determine the predilection for urate crystal deposition are poorly understood. The diminished solubility of urate at the cooler temperatures of peripheral structures, such as the toes and ears, may help explain why urate crystals deposit in these areas. In addition, the propensity for marked urate crystal deposition in the first metatarsophalangeal joint may also relate to repetitive minor trauma there. The observations that urate crystals often deposit in relatively avascular and proteoglycan-rich areas such as articular cartilage, that hemiplegia appears to have a sparing effect on the development of tophi and acute gout on the paretic side, and that tophi and acute gout occur within interphalangeal joints at the location of established osteoarthritic disease, suggests the potential importance of both the structure and turnover of connective-tissue matrix in urate crystal deposition.

Macroscopic accumulations of urate can usually be visualized arthroscopically in the synovial membrane by the time of the first gouty attack. Urate crystals found in joint fluid at the time of the acute attack may derive from rupture of these preformed synovial deposits or may have precipitated de novo, as exemplified in certain instances by the recognition of urate spherulites. In some individuals with gout, urate crystals can be found in asymptomatic metatarsophalangeal and knee joints that have never been involved in an acute attack of gout confirming that gout can exist in an asymptomatic state.

Deposits of fine acicular monosodium urate crystals with a surrounding mononuclear cell inflammatory reaction and associated foreign body granuloma characterize the tophus, the pathognomonic lesions of chronic gout. Tophaceous deposits are common in cartilage (including articular cartilage), synovium, periarticular structures (including tendon sheaths and bursae), epiphyseal bone, and subcutaneous tissue; they can also occur in the renal interstitium. Tissue disruption and destruction proceed slowly, particularly as adjacent tophi coalesce, are joined by additional deposits, and provoke localized tissue responses such as pannus formation and osteoclasis in synovium and subchondral bone. The destructive effects of chronic tophaceous gout can progress even with antihyperuricemic therapy and are believed to be mediated by the ability of urate crystals to stimulate the release from mononuclear phagocytes and from synovial fibroblasts of inflammatory mediators implicated in bone and cartilage erosion and bone resorption. These mediators include interleukin-1, tumor necrosis factor-alpha (TNF), and prostaglandin E_2. Chronic multicentric urate deposition over a number of years can result in severe, deforming articular erosions, huge subcutaneous amorphous deposits, and localized tendon disruption or nerve entrapment. Tophi can appear rarely in visceral organs except for muscle, liver, spleen, and lung. They do not occur in the central nervous system because of the impermeability of the blood-brain barrier to uric acid and the inability of the central nervous system cells to generate uric acid as an end product of purine metabolism.

Interstitial deposition of monosodium urate in the kidney is associated with fibrotic and inflammatory changes in the renal medulla and pyramids resembling those of chronic pyelonephritis, with progressive damage in tubular epithelium of the loop of Henle and a peculiar form of glomerular sclerosis. The severity of gout correlates with vascular changes in the glomerular capillary bed and larger vessels.

At the usual acidic pH of urine, the equilibrium between uric acid and urate is shifted in favor of the undissociated acid, the solubility of which is only 15 mg per deciliter. Even under physiologic conditions, supersaturation of the urine with uric acid is required for excretion of the normal load of uric acid in a normal urine volume. With acutely increased loads, uric acid crystal deposition in the collecting tubules can result in acute renal failure. More often, in hyperuricemic individuals in whom renal uric acid loads are chronically increased (overproducers), precipitation of uric acid crystals within a protein matrix in the renal pelvis, ureters, or bladder can lead to uric acid urolithiasis.

By far the most common clinical consequence of urate deposition is acute gouty arthritis, in which monosodium urate crystals liberated from deposits in and about the joint space, or precipitated de novo, appear to activate several humoral and cellular inflammatory mediator cascades, characteristically resulting in a severe bout of joint inflammation with extension of the process into periarticular tissues.

Although the precise roles of the individual inflammatory mediator systems in acute gout remain to be defined, experimental evidence supports the belief that early vasodilation, enhanced vascular permeability, and pain are largely provoked by the effects of urate crystal–induced prostaglandin release from cells within the joint space and the crystal-induced cleavage of biologically active complement peptides and kinins from inactive precursors. The release of a variety of cellular mediators (including interleukin-1 [IL-1], TNF, and IL-8 from synovial mononuclear phagocytes and cartilage) and humoral mediators (including C5a) probably triggers initial neutrophil adhesion to endothelium and neutrophil ingress into joints. Subsequent neutrophil phagocytosis of intra-articular urate crystals is believed to be associated with (1) the secretion of potent low-molecular-weight peptide chemoattractants for neutrophils (including IL-8) and arachadonic acid-derived chemotaxins (including leukotriene B_4 [LTB_4]); (2) the release of lysosomal enzymes by secretion as well as by cell death via urate crystal–induced phagolysosome membrane lysis. These events have been proposed to help establish a cycle of further neutrophil ingress, neutrophil activation by exposure to crystals and soluble mediators, and the amplification of inflammation. Furthermore, the systemic release from the gouty joint into the venous circulation of IL-1, TNF, IL-6, and IL-8 appears to be responsible for systemic manifestations (e.g., fever, leukocytosis, hepatic acute phase protein response) in acute gouty arthritis, and may help explain the capacity of the acute gouty attack to affect joints in more than one region.

The demonstration that experimental urate crystal–induced synovitis is markedly diminished when neutrophils are depleted by cytotoxic drugs or antineutrophil antiserum supports the critical role of polymorphonuclear leukocytes as the effector arm of acute gouty inflammation. Furthermore, the efficacy of colchicine in the prophylaxis of acute gout and in the treatment of early acute gout (discussed below) is believed to reflect its ability to suppress the release from leukocytes exposed to urate crystals of chemoattractants for neutrophils.

The mechanism whereby acute gouty paroxysms terminate (often without specific therapy) is probably multifactorial. Factors other than urate crystal dissolution or sequestration must play a role, as free urate crystals are often found in synovial fluid for weeks after subsidence of an acute gouty attack. Such factors are thought to include changes in the balance between pro- and anti-inflammatory factors as well as modulation of crystal-phagocyte interaction via changes in the physical properties of the urate crystals. In addition, the limited functional lifespan (days) of normal neutrophils is believed to make continued ingress of neutrophils critical for the perpetuation of acute gouty inflammation.

CLINICAL FEATURES

Although it is presumed that patients with genetic gout possess from birth the underlying defects predisposing them to the disease, clinical expression is very infrequent in males prior to puberty and in females before menopause. However, uncommon exceptions to this observation exist, and include type I glycogen storage disease in both sexes, in which severe derangements in the control of uric acid synthesis or disposal result in early and severe hyperuricemia, and the X-linked inherited states of partial deficiency of HGPRT and milder forms of superactivity of PRPP synthetase, where early-adult-onset gout and a high incidence of uric acid urinary tract stones constitute the usual clinical phenotype in affected male children. Severe HGPRT deficiency is associated with spasticity, choreoathetosis, mental retardation, and compulsive self-mutilation (Lesch-Nyhan syndrome) in addition to clinical manifestations of hyperuricemia. Furthermore, in some individuals, regulatory defects in PRPP synthetase are accompanied by sensorineural deafness and neurodevelopment defects. Importantly, women carriers of HGPRT deficiency and PRPP synthetase superactivity are predisposed to develop symptomatic consequences of hyperuricemia in their postmenopausal years.

Clinical gout usually appears in men during middle life,

a time in which the contributions of environmental factors and the attenuation of renal uric acid excretory function perhaps combine with possible hereditary influences to elevate serum urate levels into the hyperuricemic range. In addition, the incidence of clinical gout appears to be increasing in both elderly men and women in North America, probably as a consequence not only of increased life span but also of the high rate of thiazide diuretic use in this population. The propensity of urate crystals to deposit in osteoarthritic joints may make gouty arthritis more difficult to recognize in the elderly.

Acute gouty arthritis

Acute gouty arthritis is characteristically (but not invariably) a disabling inflammatory process so dramatic in its onset and intensity as to have provoked numerous vivid literary descriptions. Often, the onset of exquisite pain and signs of inflammation occurs within minutes to hours, sometimes preceded by a few premonitory twinges in the affected area. Less frequently, the patient is warned of an impending attack by several days of slowly increasing discomfort, which eventuates in a full-blown episode. Typically, the patient, well upon retiring, is awakened from sleep. The pain of acute gouty arthritis is usually so severe as to preclude weight bearing, and the patient may be unable to tolerate even the weight of a sheet on the inflamed area.

A precipitating event such as an injury, a surgical operation, a bout of excessive alcohol ingestion, an unusually heavy meal, an emotional stress, or a period of unaccustomed physical exertion may be related to the acute attack. Early in the course of treatment for hyperuricemia with uricosuric drugs or allopurinol, repeated acute gouty attacks are not uncommon. The precise manner in which these changes relate to urate deposition is unclear.

Certain features of acute gouty arthritis are of value in establishing a specific diagnosis. These features include the pattern of joint involvement, the features of gouty inflammation, and the course of the attack. Monarticular arthritis is the most common presentation, and a particular predilection is shown for the larger peripheral joints in the lower extremities. Podagra, acute gout of the metatarsophalangeal joint of the great toe, was described by Hippocrates, and the great toe remains the most common site of initial involvement. Prior to the availability of effective treatment to reduce the frequency of gouty attacks, 90% of patients with gout experienced podagra at some point in the course of their disease. The ankle, midfoot (instep), and knee joints also are affected relatively frequently, upper extremity involvement in the wrists, elbows, and metacarpophalangeal joints occurs occasionally. Bursal inflammation, particularly of the olecranon bursae, is common. The hips, shoulders, and spine very rarely are involved, especially early in the course of clinical gout.

Gouty inflammation involves not only the joint but also periarticular structures and skin, often yielding heat, redness, swelling, and tenderness in a wide area beyond the joint. The resulting appearance may suggest cellulitis, septic arthritis, osteomyelitis, or (especially in the foot) polyarticular arthritis. The tense and shiny skin overlying the area of inflammation may undergo desquamation as the attack subsides. Fever, leukocytosis, and elevated erythrocyte sedimentation rate may suggest an infectious process. If untreated, acute gouty arthritis usually resolves gradually, but completely, in a period of 1 to 2 weeks. Occasionally, another attack in the same or another joint occurs during the recovery period.

After the initial attack, about 10% of patients experience no recurrence over many years, despite persistent hyperuricemia. More commonly, however, a symptom-free interval (intercritical gout) is terminated by a recurrent attack of arthritis, often during the first year after the initial episode. In the absence of treatment, the ultimate course of gouty paroxysms is extremely variable; the majority of patients experience an increase in the frequency of acute gouty attacks that may become more often polyarticular, more severe, and longer lasting. In other individuals, the annual frequency of attacks may remain constant or even diminish, but in some the interval between episodes may decrease to a point at which gouty inflammation is virtually always present. Finally, a few patients do not exhibit the usual episodic course of early gouty arthritis, and their disease may proceed, without obvious remission, to joint destruction and disability in a relatively short time. In these patients, gout occasionally may be confused with rheumatoid arthritis or other polyarticular inflammatory disorders.

Chronic tophaceous gout

In general, the interval between the initial attack of gout and the development of clinically visible tophi and crippling disease is prolonged, and tophi appear earlier and are more extensive in individuals with higher elevations in the serum urate concentration. However, great variability is shown in the development of structural changes in individuals at apparently comparable risk. Ten years after the initial attack, more than half of the patients in one large series had either no tophi or minimal deposits. After 20 years, however, over one half of the patients had tophi, and an appreciable proportion (24%) had deforming or disabling disease.

Clinically apparent tophi commonly appear as painless, firm deposits on the helix of the ear, less commonly on the antihelix. These tophi may be the sole urate deposits found or may be accompanied by irregular, occasionally large, and deforming tophi on the fingers, hands, or feet. The olecranon bursae, the ulnar surface of the forearms, the tibial surfaces, and the Achilles tendons may harbor lumpy tophaceous deposits. The disruption of articular structures by tophi may potentiate the effects of repeated acute episodes of gouty arthritis and lead to a chronic arthritis with irreversible erosion and deformity. Subcutaneous tophi may ulcerate through the skin and exude a white chalk or paste in which urate crystals are the major component. Such eroded tophi may drain for long periods and are susceptible to bacterial superinfection.

Uric acid urolithiasis

The incidence of uric acid urolithiasis in patients with primary gout is between 10% and 25% and appears to be related to the degree of hyperuricemia and hyperuricosuria. The mechanism of production, clinical symptoms, and management are discussed in Chapter 349.

Gouty renal disease

Urate crystal deposition and associated inflammation in the renal interstitium (urate nephropathy) and uric acid deposition in the collecting tubules (uric acid nephropathy) are relatively distinctive processes that can underlie the development of renal function abnormalities among gout patients. Nevertheless, the frequent concordance of gout and disorders such as hypertension and diabetes mellitus, both of which predispose to renal damage, and the association of lead poisoning with both nephropathy and hyperuricemia, often render speculative the attribution of chronic renal impairment to gout. These issues are discussed in greater detail in Chapter 346.

DIAGNOSIS

The diagnosis of acute gouty arthritis is usually not difficult to establish, particularly in the setting of an attack of podagra or of acute monarticular arthritis in a hyperuricemic individual. Hyperuricemia, however, is relatively frequent in the population and is sometimes absent at the time of an acute gouty attack; since other disorders (e.g., calcium pyrophosphate deposition disease, septic arthritis, rheumatoid arthritis) can present as acute monarticular arthritis, confirmation of the diagnosis should be sought by aspiration and examination of the synovial fluid from the affected joint. Demonstration by polarized microscopy of the needle-shaped, strongly negative birefringent urate crystals, free and within leukocytes, is pathognomonic for acute gout and can be achieved in over 95% of joint aspirates in this disease (see Chapter 295). The demonstration of typical crystals from tophaceous deposits is equally confirmatory, and recent studies indicate a high degree of success and specificity in establishing a diagnosis of gout between acute attacks by demonstrating urate crystals in aspirates from asymptomatic first metatarsophalangeal joints. The possibility of infection coexisting with gout (or substituting for it) should be excluded by Gram stain and culture of the fluid.

A prompt and dramatic response to colchicine of attacks of gouty arthritis treated within 24 hours of onset is relatively specific, since responses in sarcoid arthritis, pseudogout, and rheumatoid arthritis are less complete and less frequent. Radiographs are of little diagnostic value early in the disease but may show highly suggestive features once tophaceous deposits have developed, usually in areas of joints previously subjected to multiple acute attacks. Among typical radiographic features of gout are the presence of subcutaneous and periarticular masses adjacent to eroded bone, overall retention of bone density and joint spaces, asymmetric distribution of erosions (which may be periarticular or articular in location), and fine shelves of retained bone forming "overhanging edges" of erosions (Fig. 319-2).

Once a diagnosis of gout is established, it is important to ascertain whether the disease is primary or secondary (Table 319-1). A thorough history and physical examination, along with routine laboratory tests, can detect many diseases or environmental factors associated with hyperuricemia and gout, including (1) drug-induced hyperuricemia (e.g., diuretics, low-dose salicylates, cyclosporine, pyrazinamide, ethambutol, nicotinic acid); (2) chronic renal disease; (3) hematologic diseases (e.g., polycythemia vera, acute and chronic leukemias, sickle cell disease, hemolytic anemias) and other proliferative disorders (including psoriasis and Paget's disease of bone); (4) chronic lead intoxication; (5) alcoholism. In most patients, it is advisable to establish whether hyperuricemia is accompanied by excessive or normal uric acid excretion, since the determination can be used to guide the choice of hypouricemic therapy.

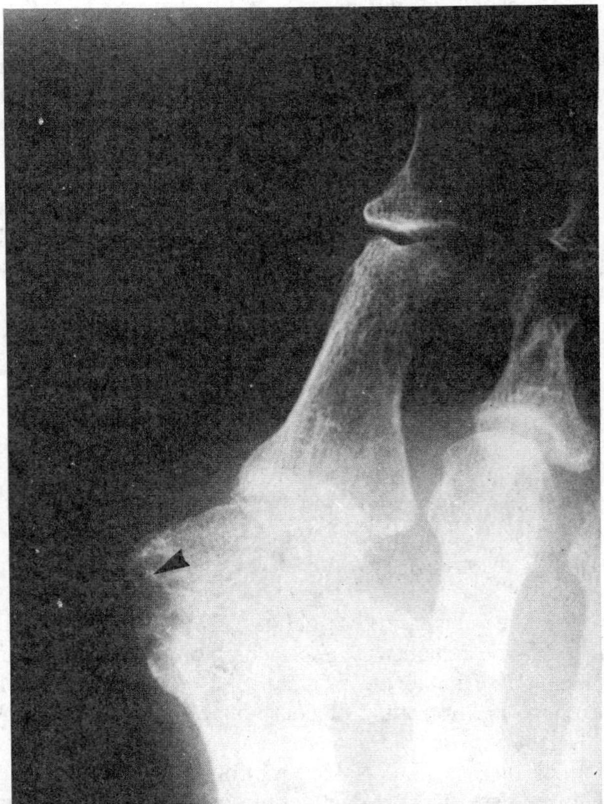

Fig. 319-2. Chronic tophaceous gout involving the distal metatarsal and metatarsophalangeal joint of the great toe. Note the overlying soft-tissue mass, the marginal and periarticular radiolucent bony defects (erosions) with a rim of cortical bone *(arrow)* forming an overhanging edge, and an area of stippled calcification within an erosion *(arrowhead)*. In this oblique view, joint spaces and bone density are maintained. (Courtesy of Dr. T. McDowell Anderson.)

In patients with intact renal function, this can be most readily ascertained by measuring the patient's urinary acid excretion during a 24-hour period. Overproduction is most reliably identified when patients are studied while maintained on a purine-free diet. Radiologic procedures employing contrast media and drugs that alter uric acid metabolism should be avoided in the midst of urine uric acid measurements.

MANAGEMENT

The aims of current therapeutic programs in gout and hyperuricemia are (1) to quickly resolve attacks of acute gouty arthritis with as few complications as possible; (2) to limit recurrences of acute gouty arthritis; (3) to prevent the disabling consequences of monosodium urate crystal deposition in articular, renal, and other tissues; (4) to prevent uric acid urolithiasis; and (5) to recognize and appropriately treat medical conditions commonly associated with gout, including hypertension, obesity, hyperlipidemia, chronic alcoholism, and chronic renal insufficiency. It is important to emphasize the distinctive rationale underlying use of antiinflammatory and antihyperuricemic drugs. Anti-inflammatory drugs are used to treat or, in the case of colchicine, to prevent gouty inflammation, but they do not alter the state of hyperuricemia leading to the inflammation. Similarly, the uricosuric drugs and allopurinol reduce serum urate levels but have no anti-inflammatory properties. In fact, their use in acute gouty arthritis is counterproductive.

Antihyperuricemic therapy in gout is expensive and potentially toxic, and it requires lifelong continuation. The therapeutic aims and the potential benefit/risk ratio of treatment should be weighed for each individual. As a general rule, one or more of the following serve as acceptable indications for antihyperuricemic therapy in patients with documented gout: (1) frequent attacks (more than three per year) of acute gouty arthritis, (2) the occurrence of acute polyarticular gout, (3) chronic joint changes, (4) tophi, (5) excessive urinary uric acid excretion, and (6) evidence of chronic renal damage. In addition, antihyperuricemic therapy is a rational measure for most patients with gout associated with persistent hyperuricemia of greater than 8 mg per deciliter, as such individuals usually experience future progression of the disease. It is important to recognize that in some individuals the serum urate concentration can be successfully normalized without antihyperuricemic drugs, by management of an associated condition or by removal of a specific etiologic factor (e.g., cessation of alcohol, or substitution of another class of antihypertensive agent for a thiazide in the treatment of hypertension).

Another important aspect of management relates to the issue of asymptomatic hyperuricemia. The great majority of individuals with this chemical aberration do not require drug treatment, although the adjunctive measures described below may be of value to the overall health of these people as well as patients with gout. The identification of which individuals with asymptomatic hyperuricemia are at highest risk and warrant specific therapeutic intervention is, however, an aim of management; conversely, avoidance of treatment in individuals in whom it is unnecessary is of equivalent importance.

Acute gouty arthritis

The severity of pain and disability associated with acute gouty arthritis demands prompt intervention despite the usual spontaneous resolution of the process within 1 to 2 weeks. In general, the earlier treatment is initiated, the more rapid and complete the response to anti-inflammatory agents. The involved joint should be placed at rest; on occasion, a narcotic analgesic may be required. Despite the impressive intensity of inflammation, gouty arthritis is usually quite successfully treated with any of a number of types of anti-inflammatory drugs including the nonsteroidal anti-inflammatory agents (NSAIDs) and colchicine.

At present, the NSAIDs are the preferred drugs in acute gouty arthritis. Indomethacin (50 mg three or four times daily for 2 to 3 days, with subsequent rapid tapering and discontinuation by 1 week) often leads to a prompt response, although headache and gastrointestinal side effects occasionally limit its use. Phenylbutazone, although effective, is limited by potential serious hematologic toxicity and is no longer recommended. Many of the newer NSAIDs (see Chapter 317) are being used successfully in gouty arthritis, reportedly with a lower incidence of side effects. Colchicine can also be used in low doses (0.5 or 0.6 mg by mouth twice daily) as an adjunct to NSAIDs for the therapy of more severe acute attacks.

There are several primary treatment options for acute gouty arthritis in individuals who cannot take NSAIDs. First, oral colchicine is usually rapidly effective when administered in the first 24 hours after onset of symptoms (usual dose 0.5 mg every hour until relief or side effects, most commonly diarrhea, occur or until a maximum total dose of about 5-6 mg (ten tablets) is reached). However, under most circumstances, colchicine has the poorest therapeutic benefit-to-toxicity ratio of drugs used to treat acute gout. In particular, the diarrhea almost always provoked by oral colchicine may be severe.

Intravenous colchicine has been employed under conditions where colchicine or NSAIDs can not be given orally (e.g., postoperative acute gout). In these instances, 1 mg of colchicine diluted in 20 ml of normal saline and administered slowly (over not less than 10 minutes) and given as a single dose has been adequate treatment for many attacks. It is important to note that a total intravenous dose of colchicine greater than 2 mg or repeated intravenous administration beyond 24 hours for one attack of gout are inadvisable. The risk of serious drug-induced morbidity (and mortality) for intravenous use of this potent antimitotic cell toxin is significant unless strict precautions are exercised. Care is necessary to avoid extravasation at the infection site because of the marked irritating properties of colchicine. Because colchicine is excreted in urine and bile, it is advisable that patients with oliguria, renal insufficiency, and biliary tract obstruction be treated with alternative agents. Bone marrow suppression is a particular risk in patients with renal insufficiency, preexisting marrow suppression, antecedent use of cytotoxic chemotherapy or of oral colchicine, and in the elderly, and marrow aplasia may occur even when clinicians judiously use lower than standard doses of intravenous colchicine in such patients.

A valuable alternative approach to the therapy of acute gout is the local intra-articular injection of a microcrystalline glucocorticosteroid ester. Such treatment is ideal and effective in a single large joint, regardless of the prior duration of the acute attack. Adrenocorticotrophic hormone (usual dose, 25 USP units by slow intravenous infusion with a repeat of this dose as often as q12 hours for 1-3 days in incomplete responders) or systemic anti-inflammatory corticosteroids (e.g., 30-60 mg prednisone per day or equivalent, tapering to less than 20 mg per day by 1 week, followed by continuing therapy for 1-3 weeks) may be effective in severe cases of acute polyarticular gout when the administration of other drugs is contraindicated. Acute gout can be observed in transplant patients taking small maintenance doses of prednisone, illustrating the low potency of systemic steroids in acute gout. In addition, rebound attacks of acute gout can be observed after cessation of therapy with systemic steroids. Thus, low-dose daily oral colchicine should generally be used as adjunctive therapy in patients with acute gout treated with ACTH or systemic corticosteroids.

Improvement with the treatment of acute gouty arthritis usually begins within 6 to 12 hours and is often complete within 3 days. In a small proportion of patients, particularly those in whom treatment has been delayed, improvement is minimal and resolution slow. In some gouty patients, attacks occur regularly after dietary excess, alcohol intake, or other identifiable precipitating events. When possible, avoidance of these circumstances can reduce the frequency of attacks. Patients should be encouraged to initiate therapy for recurrent attacks with either colchicine or an anti-inflammatory drug at the first premonition or symptom of an impending episode.

Intercritical therapy

Colchicine (0.5 or 0.6 mg once or twice daily) is an effective agent in the prophylaxis of recurrent attacks of acute gouty arthritis. If regular NSAID treatment is required for chronic joint symptoms or for other reasons, colchicine may usually be omitted since NSAIDs probably exert an adequate prophylactic effect. The propensity of gouty arthritis to occur repetitively in patients early in the course of antihyperuricemic therapy with either uricosuric agents or allopurinol is well established. (Such attacks should not, however, prompt discontinuation of the antihyperuricemic drug, even during treatment for the acute episode.) In these persons, colchicine should be given prophylactically until after the serum urate concentration has been reduced to a level of 6.0 mg per deciliter or less for a period of at least 3 to 6 months. In patients still experiencing recurrent attacks or in patients with chronic tophaceous gout, more prolonged use of prophylactic colchicine is indicated. It should be recognized that patients with diminished renal function taking customary prophylactic doses of colchicine over a prolonged period may develop a proximal myopathy, accompanied by a mild axonal polyneuropathy and elevations of serum creatine kinase. This condition is reversible on discontinuation of colchicine.

Tophaceous gout

In gout with or without evident tophi, the body pool of urate is expanded. Tophus formation represents crystal deposition from supersaturated extracellular fluids. Resolution of tophi, reduction of urate pool size to normal, and removal of the immediate source of further crystallization and clinical events are congruent aims that can be achieved by long-term reduction of serum urate concentration to below 6 mg per deciliter.

Dietary restriction of purine-containing foods, although capable of diminishing serum urate slightly (averaging 1 mg per deciliter in hyperuricemic patients), is seldom necessary because of the availability of two classes of potent antihyperuricemic agents—uricosurics and xanthine oxidase inhibitors. Uricosuric drugs increase renal clearance of uric acid; allopurinol, the xanthine oxidase inhibitor, blocks uric acid production and is used more often by clinicians than the uricosurics.

The uricosuric agents commonly used in the United States are probenecid and sulfinpyrazone. Both agents inhibit renal tubular uric acid reabsorption, thus increasing net uric acid excretion. It is essential to start uricosuric drugs at low doses to minimize the risk of uric acid urolithiasis. Adequate hydration via a daily fluid intake of 2 to 3 liters and alkalinization of the urine with sodium bicarbonate are also important measures for this purpose. In addition, prophylactic colchicine should be administered during the introduction of uricosuric agents and for a period after serum urate concentration is normalized and, in patients with tophi, until tophi are resolved.

The starting dose of probenecid is 0.25 g twice daily, with a gradual increase over 3 to 4 weeks to a usual maintenance level of 0.5 g two or three times daily. If serum urate concentration remains greater than 6.0 mg per deciliter, an increase in the dose to 2.5 or 3.0 g daily should be tried. Sulfinpyrazone is given in a starting dose of 50 mg daily, with a gradual increase to 100 mg three or four times a day.

Gastrointestinal symptoms and skin rash are the most common reactions to uricosuric agents; hepatic necrosis and bone marrow suppression occur very rarely. Aspirin and other salicylates are uricosuric at high blood levels; however, at lower levels, the major effect of salicylates is uric acid retention resulting from inhibition of tubular urate secretion. They also interfere with the action of uricosuric agents and should not be used in the treatment of gout. Uricosuric agents are very effective as first-line drugs for many patients with gout and normal urinary uric acid excretion. Uricosuric agents are not first-line drugs in patients with excessive uric acid excretion, with previous histories of uric acid stones, or with renal insufficiency (as defined by a creatinine clearance <80 ml per minute). These patients, and those in whom uricosuric drugs are ineffective, should receive allopurinol. Although tophi may be dissolved under uricosuric treatment, the rate of dissolution is usually faster with allopurinol, and most physicians consider the presence of tophi an indication for the latter drug.

Allopurinol is a hypoxanthine analog that undergoes oxidation to the metabolite, oxypurinol, a potent competitive inhibitor of xanthine oxidase. In this way, allopurinol reduces conversion of hypoxanthine to xanthine and xanthine to uric acid (see Fig. 319-1). Hypoxanthine and xanthine are cleared efficiently by the kidney and do not accumulate in significant concentrations in the serum. Allopurinol also decreases the rate of purine synthesis de novo. Thus, the reduced total purine load presented to the kidney, together with the redistribution of the purines into three compounds (hypoxanthine, xanthine, and uric acid) with independent solubilities, diminishes the likelihood of uric acid stone formation in patients with hyperuricemia and gout.

Allopurinol can be given in a single daily dose and initially should generally be administered with prophylactic oral colchicine or an NSAID. A dose of allopurinol of 300 mg per day is usually appropriate for an average-sized patient with normal renal function. The major active allopurinol metabolite, oxypurinol, is excreted by the kidneys, and its half-life is extended to beyond 24 hours in patients with renal insufficiency. Thus, to avoid the accumulation of oxypurinol and minimize certain allopurinol toxicities that correlate with daily dosage (discussed below), progressively smaller doses of allopurinol are used in patients with renal insufficiency. Thus, patients with a creatinine clearance of <30 ml/minute should receive 100 mg per day or less of allopurinol. Furthermore, the customary therapeutic target level for serum urate of ≤ 6.0 mg/dl should not be the goal in gout patients with substantial impairment of renal function.

Although uncommon, adverse effects with allopurinol are more severe and occur more often than with uricosuric drugs. These reactions include fever, eosinophilia, dermatitis, elevation of hepatic enzymes, renal failure, headache, diarrhea, and occasional vasculitis. The allopurinol hypersensitivity syndrome, consisting of some or all of these features, has a high mortality (20% to 30% of reported cases), dramatizing the importance of reserving the use of this agent for patients in whom it is clearly indicated. The risk of allopurinol hypersensitivity is greatly augmented in patients on thiazide diuretic therapy and in patients with diminished renal function who have received standard doses of allopurinol. In patients receiving allopurinol, the dose of the chemotherapeutic agents azathioprine and 6-mercaptopurine should be much lower than usual to avoid excessive accumulation of the cytotoxic agent. Allopurinol may also enhance the toxicity of cyclophosphamide.

Combined treatment with the two classes of antihyperuricemic drugs has been attempted. The greatest benefit of this combination may be to individuals whose serum urate levels are not satisfactorily controlled with either agent alone. In some patients with severe tophaceous gout, allopurinol and a uricosuric agent may hasten dissolution of trophi.

Asymptomatic hyperuricemia

Epidemiologic associations between hyperuricemia and a variety of disorders, including atherosclerosis, have been made. However, there is no evidence that increased serum urate concentration is a causative factor in these disorders. There is also no evidence that treatment of hyperuricemia alleviates these conditions. Furthermore, neither hyperuricemia nor gout is clearly related to the development of clinically significant renal disease. Finally, the great majority of asymptomatic individuals with hyperuricemia are likely to live their lives without the development of clinical manifestations of gout. These considerations suggest that treatment of all individuals with asymptomatic hyperuricemia is unnecessary. Even though the risk of gouty arthritis or of uric acid urolithiasis appears to increase substantially with increases in serum urate concentrations above 9.0 mg per deciliter, these manifestations are readily treatable if and when they occur and should then present no long-term danger to the patient. Use of hypouricemic agents to reduce urate levels in individuals with asymptomatic hyperuricemia appears to be warranted only when (1) evidence of uric acid overproduction or overexcretion exists, that is, when daily urinary urate excretion in the presence of normal renal function exceeds about 900 mg on a purine-free diet or 1100 mg on a routine diet; or (2) there is a strong family history of gout, nephrolithiasis, or renal failure.

Adjuncts to management

Although purine-restricted diets are infrequently advised in long-term management of gout, specific deletion of one or more purine-rich foods is sometimes advisable when identified as provocative agents in acute attacks. Weight reduction can contribute to lessening hyperuricemia and thus can lower the risk of gout through reduction in the rate of purine synthesis. Weight reduction to lean body mass, with special emphasis on reduced calorie and protein intake, is a general adjunctive measure especially likely to benefit the gouty population, in which obesity, hypertension, and hyperlipidemia are very common. Substitution of other antihypertensive therapies in the place of diuretics is sometimes sufficient to reduce hyperuricemia. Finally, reduction of alcohol consumption represents another approach applicable to the general population and is especially likely to benefit those gouty patients whose hyperuricemia is potentiated by the effects of alcohol on both production and urinary excretion of uric acid.

REFERENCES

Campion EW, Glynn RJ, and DeLabry LO: Asymptomatic hyperuricemia: risks and consequences in the normative aging study. Am J Med 82:421, 1987.

Fox IH, Palella TD, and Kelley WN: Hyperuricemia: a marker for cell energy crisis. N Engl J Med 317:111, 1987.

Hande KR, Noone RM, and Stone WJ: Severe allopurinol toxicity. Description and guidelines for prevention in patients with renal insufficiency. Am J Med 76:47, 1984.

Kuncl RW et al: Colchicine myopathy and neuropathy. N Engl J Med 316:1562, 1987.

Lin H et al: Cyclosporine-induced hyperuricemia and gout. N Engl J Med 321:287, 1989.

Roberts WN, Liang MH, and Stern SH: Colchicine in acute gout: reassessment of risks and benefits. JAMA 257:1920, 1987.

Terkeltaub R: Pathogenesis and treatment of crystal-induced inflammation.

In Koopman W and McCarty DJ, editors: Arthritis and allied conditions, ed 12. Philadelphia, 1993, Lea & Febiger.
Wilson JM et al: A molecular survey of hypoxanthine-guanine phosphoribosyltransferase deficiency in man. J Clin Invest 77:188, 1986.
Wortmann R: Management of hyperuricemia. In McCarty DJ and Koopman WT, editors: Arthritis and allied conditions, ed 12. Philadelphia, 1993, Lea & Febiger.

CHAPTER

320 Arthritis Associated with Calcium-Containing Crystals

Daniel J. McCarty

Monosodium urate monohydrate (MSU) crystals are easily identified in gouty joint fluid by compensated polarized light microscopy, as discussed in Chapter 295. Calcium pyrophosphate dihydrate ($Ca_2P_2O_7 \cdot 2H_2O$; CPPD) crystals were discovered in synovial fluid from patients with acute goutlike attacks (pseudogout) when this method was first applied as a diagnostic tool in 1960. The radiologic appearance of calcified cartilage is called *chondrocalcinosis*. Other types of radiodense crystals depositing in cartilage, such as calcium oxalates, are radiographically indistinguishable from CPPD deposits. Since joint degeneration often accompanies CPPD crystal deposition in joints and since these deposits occur in dense fibrous tissues such as joint capsules and ligaments, neither pseudogout nor chondrocalcinosis seemed appropriate terms for this condition. Therefore, the generic term *crystal deposition disease,* which embraces four specific, clinically polymorphic, metabolic arthropathies, was proposed. Thus, gout is MSU crystal deposition disease, and pseudogout is CPPD crystal deposition disease. Crystal aggregates composed of carbonate-substituted hydroxyapatite and octacalcium phosphate also occur in joint tissues and synovial fluid. Since these crystals are basic calcium phosphates (BCPs), the term *BCP crystal deposition disease* has been proposed. Lastly, calcium oxalate crystals deposit in cartilage, synovium, bone, skin, and other tissues in primary oxalosis and in azotemic patients treated with hemodialysis or peritoneal dialysis.

CPPD CRYSTAL DEPOSITION DISEASE

Etiology and incidence

Chondrocytes in all hyaline articular and fibrocartilages secrete inorganic pyrophosphate (PPi). Whether overproduction or underdestruction of PPi or some peculiarity of the local cartilage is responsible for nucleation and growth of the calcium salt of PPi is unknown. Cartilage is essentially a gel that contains cells. CPPD crystals have been grown in synthetic gels (e.g., gelatin) at an ambient pH 6.5 to 8.0, and the smallest CPPD crystal clusters in human cartilage are perilacunar in the midzone of hyaline articular cartilage. It is likely that PPi secreted by chondrocytes diffuses into surrounding gel and, under certain conditions, precipitates as its calcium salt, which is sparingly soluble at neutral pH.

PPi levels in urine and plasma are normal, but levels in cultured skin fibroblasts are elevated in many, but not all, patients with either the familial or the sporadic form of CPPD crystal deposition disease. Increased activity of the ectoenzyme nucleoside triphosphate pyrophosphohydrolase has been found both in cartilage extracts and in cultured fibroblasts of patients with sporadic but not familial CPPD crystal deposition. ATP levels in joint fluid are higher in patients with CPPD crystal deposits than in those with other types of joint disease. Chondrocyte PPi elaboration in vitro is stimulated by certain growth factors, such as TGF beta or by increased collagen synthesis. There appear to be multiple metabolic pathways of PPi elaboration by chondrocyte analogous to multiple pathways leading to hyperuricemia. In both gout and pseudogout, formation of a crystalline phase appears to be a final common etiologic pathway.

CPPD crystal deposits were found in the joints of about 5% of anatomical cadavers. Prevalence rates, judged radiographically, increase with age; nearly 30% of octagenarians are affected. The incidence of symptomatic disease is approximately equal to that of symptomatic MSU crystal deposition disease (gout).

Pathophysiology

All CPPD crystals found in joint fluid are probably derived from articular cartilage. Tophuslike masses of crystals of varying size, possibly formed by coalescence of the smaller perilacunar deposits, may eventually become contiguous to the joint space or are exposed to synovial fluid through cartilaginous fibrillation. These crystals are embedded in an organic matrix that stains differently than the normal cartilage.

Since the CPPD crystals are in equilibrium with joint fluid Ca^{2+} and $P_2O_7^{4-}$, a fall in the concentration of either ion increases their solubility and loosens the crystals from their organic "mold," resulting in crystal "shedding" into the joint fluid. Major surgery, especially parathyroidectomy, lowers serum calcium and, consequently, joint fluid calcium. Acute attacks of pseudogout occur typically after surgery on the second postoperative day, coincident with the nadir of the serum calcium fall, and have been induced in knee joints lavaged with magnesium-containing buffers. (Magnesium chelates PPi and is a CPPD crystal solubilizer.)

The PPi level in most arthritic joint fluids (2 to 20 μm) is higher than that of plasma (1 to 3 μm). The PPi levels in joint fluids in acute pseudogout are consistently lower than in chronically symptomatic joints. The intra-articular PPi pool turns over faster in inflamed joints; the lower PPi levels are caused by equilibration with plasma as a result of increased blood flow. Thus, once crystal shedding begins, the resultant inflammatory response causes joint fluid

PPi levels to fall, further increasing crystal solubility and accelerating the shedding process. The magnitude and duration of the inflammatory response may result from the number of crystals released and to the rate of release, respectively. Experimental crystal-induced joint inflammation is related to the amount and nature of crystals injected. Other mechanisms that may cause CPPD crystal shedding are (1) joint trauma, particularly microfracture of subchondral bone in weight-bearing joints; (2) digestion of the organic matrix holding the crystals in the cartilage by another cause of inflammation, such as sepsis or gout; and (3) metabolic perturbation of the composition of the organic matrix holding the crystals in cartilage. These mechanisms provide a conceptual framework for the finding of CPPD crystals in joint fluid after trauma, after joint inflammation resulting from other causes, and after treatment of myxedema with thyroid hormone.

CPPD crystals, like MSU, absorb various polypeptides, which are responsible for some of their biologic properties. Also like MSU, they are phagocytosed by neutrophils and release a glycopeptide that is chemotactic for neutrophils.

Almost no dissolution of CPPD occurs in the synovial fluid, and the crystals are phagocytosed avidly by fixed synovial macrophagelike cells. Even crystals that have been "processed" by neutrophils probably enter these cells eventually, together with the remnants of the neutrophils. CPPD crystals are slowly degraded in synovial cells, with a half-life of about 1 to 3 months. Thus, there appears to be a dynamic traffic of crystals in joints. The number of crystals in transit in joint fluid at a given time probably represents the net effects of release from cartilage and uptake by synovium.

Phagocytosis of CPPD crystals by synoviocytes in tissue culture stimulates the release of Prostaglandin E_2 via stimulation of phospholipase A_2 with generation of arachidonic acid products and of collagenase and stromelysin induction, phenomena that may be related both to the destructive arthropathy seen in some patients and to the shedding of more crystals. CPPD and other calcium-containing crystals are potent mitogens for fibroblasts, synovial cells, and chondrocytes. After endocytosis, they activate phospholipase C, with resultant activation of the phosphoinositol pathways. They also activate the proto-oncogenes C-*fos* and C-*myc*. Their mitogenic activity might relate to the synovial cell hyperplasia commonly noted clinically in patients with such crystal deposits.

Pathology

CPPD crystals deposit in hyaline articular cartilage but have a proclivity for deposition in fibrocartilages such as the menisci of the knee, the articular disk (triangular ligament) of the distal radioulnar joint, the glenoid and acetabular labra, the symphysis pubis, and the anulus fibrosus of the lumbar and dorsal intervertebral disks. In hyaline cartilage, the smallest deposits are perilacunar in the midzone. Crystals are seen in normal-appearing cartilage, in the tophuslike masses already described, and lining clefts caused by fibrillation of degenerative cartilage.

Clinical and laboratory findings

In our series of over 900 cases, men predominated in a 1.4:1.0 ratio. The mean age was 71.6 years (range, 36 to 98 years); the mean age at onset of symptoms of acute arthritis was 57 years (range, 30 to 90 years).

Cases of CPPD crystal deposition disease are classified as (1) familial; (2) associated with metabolic diseases or trauma, including joint surgery; or (3) sporadic. The absence of associated diseases (see box below) in the familial cases is noteworthy.

In many joints, CPPD crystal deposition appears innocuous, and neither joint inflammation nor cartilage degeneration occurs. In others, for unknown reasons, recurrent acute attacks, subacute inflammation, and/or progressive joint degeneration, sometimes very severe, occur.

Several patterns of arthritis can be distinguished clinically. CPPD deposition disease is a great mimic because it may resemble gout, rheumatoid arthritis, osteoarthritis, traumatic arthritis, or a neuroapathic joint; rarely, it even resembles ankylosing spondylitis, rheumatic fever, psychogenic arthritis, or generalized sepsis.

Radiographic features

CPPD crystals in fibrocartilaginous structures, hyaline (articular) cartilage, ligaments, and joint capsules present a characteristic appearance that is diagnostically helpful. Their typical location and appearance are shown in Fig. 320-1. Radiographic degenerative changes characteristic of CPPD crystal deposition are incorporated into the diagnostic criteria shown in the box on p. 2507 (see also Chapter 296).

An arthritic patient may be screened for CPPD with four suitably exposed radiographs: an anteroposterior (AP) view of each knee, an AP view of the pelvis, and a posteroanterior (PA) view of the wrists.

Diagnosis

Definite diagnosis rests on the specific identification of CPPD microcrystals (Chapter 295). The characteristic radiologic appearance of calcified cartilage and of certain degenerative changes is often helpful (Chapter 296). Symp-

Conditions associated with CPPD crystal deposition disease

Familial hypocalciuric hypercalcemia	Gout
Hyperparathyroidism	Neuropathic joints
Hemochromatosis	Aging
Hemosiderosis	Osteochondritis dissecans
Hypophosphatasia	Amyloidosis
Hypomagnesemia	Trauma (including joint surgery)
Hypothyroidism	

toms in such calcified joints can be caused by other types of arthritis, however, even if CPPD crystals are identified in joint fluid. The clinical picture is protean.

Therapy

Acute attacks may be treated by thorough aspiration of the joint, followed by injection of microcrystalline corticosteroid esters. Nonsteroidal anti-inflammatory drugs in large doses are usually effective. The response to oral colchicine is unpredictable, but intravenous colchicine (1 mg) dramatically suppresses inflammatory symptoms. Prophylactic daily doses of colchicine definitely reduce the number of acute attacks of pseudogout. Treatment of the associated chronic arthritis is the same as that for osteoarthritis (see Chapter 318). Removal of parathyroid adenomas, venesection for correction of iron overload in hemochromatosis, and correction of myxedema with thyroxine replacement do not result in resorption of the CPPD deposits.

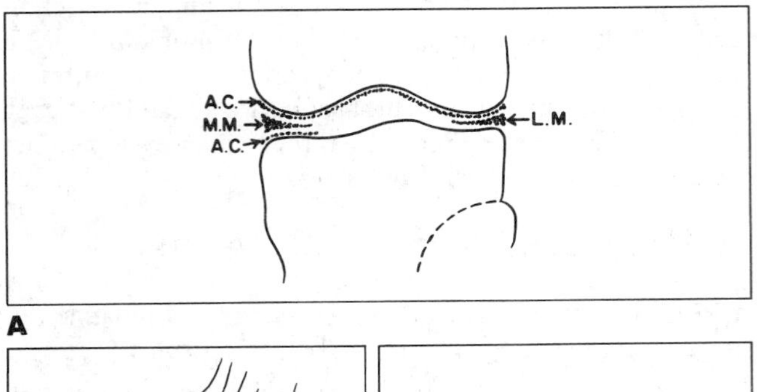

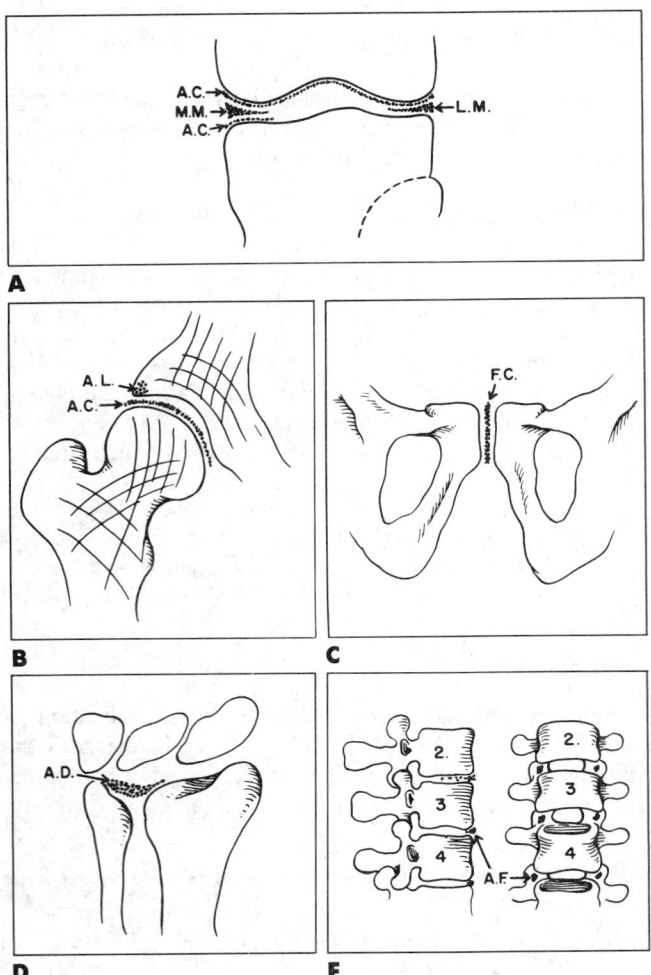

Fig. 320-1. Typical location and appearance of calcium pyrophosphate dihydrate (CPPD) crystals. **A,** Anteroposterior knee; calcification of medial meniscus *(M.M.),* lateral meniscus *(L.M.),* and articular cartilage *(A.C.).* **B,** Anteroposterior hip; calcification of acetabular labrum *(A.L.)* and articular cartilage *(A.C.).* **C,** Anteroposterior pelvis; calcification appears as vertical line in the symphysis pubis (fibrocartilage *[F.C.]*). **D,** Anteroposterior wrist; calcification of articular disk *(A.D.)* of distal radioulnar joint. **E,** Lateral and anteroposterior lumbar spine; calcification in anulus fibrosus *(A.F).*

Prognosis

Joint inflammation can be controlled in the great majority of patients with CPPD deposition disease, but joint degeneration, once established, often proceeds relentlessly and sometimes very rapidly to a severe destructive arthropathy.

TYPES OF CPPD DISEASE

Type A: pseudogout

This pattern is marked by inflammatory attacks of arthritis. Such episodes are self-limited and involve only one or a few joints. They can be severe, but less painful attacks occur and may outnumber full-blown attacks. About 25% of patients show this pattern.

Provocation of acute attacks by a surgical procedure or by medical illness is common in both gout and pseudogout. Trauma may provoke acute arthritis in either gout or pseudogout. Since both types of crystals are sometimes found in the same subject, joint aspiration and specific crystal identification are absolutely essential for precise diagnosis.

The knee joint is to pseudogout what the bunion joint is to gout and is the site of over half of all acute attacks. The patients are usually completely asymptomatic between attacks. Radiographic chondrocalcinosis is found in most patients who show this pattern.

Type B: pseudorheumatoid arthritis

Approximately 5% of patients have multiple joint involvement, with subacute attacks lasting 4 weeks to several months. Nonspecific symptoms, such as morning stiffness and systemic fatigue, are common. Synovial thickening, limitation of joint motion caused by inflammation and/or to flexion contractures, and elevated erythrocyte sedimentation rate are also found. About 10% of patients with CPPD-related arthritis have positive tests for rheumatoid factor, usually in low titer. CPPD deposits also have been described both histologically and radiographically in patients with bona fide rheumatoid arthritis.

A variant of type B often causes confusion clinically. The patient, usually elderly, has multiple acutely inflamed joints, marked leukocytosis, fever of 102° to 104° F (39° to 40° C), and disorientation. Systemic sepsis is suspected, and antibiotics are often prescribed, despite negative cultures. The entire picture reverses dramatically with anti-inflammatory drug therapy.

Types C and D: pseudoosteoarthritis

Approximately 50% of patients have shown progressive degeneration of multiple joints. The knees are most commonly affected, followed by the wrists, metacarpophalangeal

CPPD crystal deposition disease: diagnostic criteria

Criteria

I. Demonstration of CPPD crystals (obtained by biopsy, necropsy, or aspirated synovial fluid) by definitive means (e.g., characteristic "fingerprint" by x-ray diffraction powder pattern or by chemical analysis)

II. A. Identification of crystals showing either no birefringence or a weakly positive one by compensated polarized light microscopy

B. Presence of typical calcifications on radiographs*

III. A. Acute arthritis, especially of knees or other large joints, with or without concomitant hyperuricemia

B. Chronic arthritis, especially of knees, hips, wrists, carpus, elbow, shoulder, and metacarpophalangeal (MCP) joints, especially if accompanied by acute exacerbations. The following features are helpful in differentiating from primary osteoarthritis:

1. Uncommon site: for example, wrist, MCP, elbow, shoulder
2. Appearance of lesion radiologically: for example, radiocarpal or patellofemoral joint space narrowing, especially if isolated
3. Subchondral cyst formation
4. Severity of degeneration—progressive, with subchondral bony collapse (microfractures) and fragmentation, with formation of intra-articular radiodense bodies
5. Osteophyte formation—variable and inconstant
6. Tendon calcifications, especially Achilles, triceps, obturators

Diagnostic Categories

I. Definite: criteria I or IIA, plus B, must be fulfilled

II. Probable: criteria IIA or B must be fulfilled

III. Possible: criteria IIIA or B should alert the clinician to the possibility of underlying CPPD deposition

*Heavy punctate and linear calcifications in fibrocartilages, articular (hyaline) cartilages, and joint capsules, especially if bilaterally symmetric. Faint and/or atypical calcifications may be caused by DCPD ($CaHPO_4 \cdot 2H_2O$) deposits or to vascular calcifications. Both of these are often bilaterally symmetric also.

(MCP) joints, hips, shoulders, elbows, and ankles. Involvement is generally symmetric, although the degenerative process is often further advanced on one side, especially in joints that have been subjected to trauma. CPPD crystal deposition should be suspected in patients with bilateral varus deformities and/or flexion contractures of the knees, especially if accompanied by osteophytes and flexion contractures of other joints not affected by primary osteoarthritis (wrists, elbows, shoulders, and MCP joints).

About half of patients with joint degeneration have episodic superimposed attacks of acute arthritis and have been classified as type C. Those without a clinically apparent inflammatory component have been classified as type D.

CPPD crystals often are found in joints without radiographically detectable cartilage calcifications, especially those with extensive degenerative change. Squaring of bone ends, subchondral cystic changes, and hooklike osteophytes, particularly in the MCP joints, are characteristic (see Chapter 296).

Heberden's nodes and other stigmata of primary osteoarthritis often coexist with the pattern of joint involvement peculiar to CPPD crystal deposition, probably a chance association of two common conditions affecting elderly persons.

Type E: asymptomatic CPPD crystal deposition

Most joints with CPPD deposits plainly visible on radiographs are not symptomatic, even in patients with acute or chronic symptoms in other joints. Many patients with CPPD crystal deposits have neither acute attacks nor chronic joint symptoms.

Type F: pseudoneurotrophic joints

A destructive arthropathy may develop in some patients who have CPPD deposits and a normal neurologic examination.

Other patterns

In some familial cases, stiffening and straightening of the spine have been confused with ankylosing spondylitis. True bony ankylosis has also been described in familial cases and is occasionally seen in the hips or knees of elderly patients. Patients with CPPD deposition and transient acute attacks are sometimes misdiagnosed as having rheumatic fever or psychogenic arthritis. Hemarthrosis is not uncommon as a presenting feature. It is clear from the long-term observations of the natural history of CPPD joint deposition in familial cases that a given patient may show one pattern of arthritis early in the course of the disease and a different pattern later.

ASSOCIATED DISEASES

All putative disease associations are unproved; appropriately controlled comparisons either have not been done or, when done, have involved numbers so small as to make statistical application meaningless. The metabolic diseases listed in the box on p. 2505 affect connective tissue metabolism in some way. Since the prevalence of CPPD rises sharply with age, the question arises whether these metabolic conditions directly induce CPPD crystal deposition or cause a premature development of calcific deposits. CPPD crystal deposits associated with rare conditions such as hypophosphatasia and hypomagnesemia seem more likely to be "real" than do associations with glucose intolerance or hypertension. Although no causal relationships have been established, unsuspected metabolic abnormalities have been found repeatedly when appropriate laboratory studies are performed. Measurements of serum calcium, phosphorus, alkaline phosphatase, magnesium, serum iron, iron-binding capacity, ferritin, thyroxine, and TSH are indicated in all new cases of CPPD crystal deposition. Conversely, when arthritis supervenes in a patient with one of these metabolic conditions, the possibility of CPPD deposition disease should be considered.

Most series of patients with CPPD deposition show hyperparathyroidism in 5% to 15% of cases; about 20% of patients with hyperparathyroidism have radiologic evidence of chondrocalcinosis. Those with CPPD deposits are significantly older. The calcific deposits do not resorb after parathyroidectomy, and acute attacks often continue.

Nearly half the patients with hemochromatosis have arthritis, and half of these have radiologic chondrocalcinosis (usually the older patients in a series). CPPD-related joint complaints may be present in patients with asymptomatic hemochromatosis. That iron may be directly related to the development of calcific deposits is suggested by reports of CPPD deposition in patients with transfusion hemosiderosis.

Hypothyroidism has been reported as being associated with asymptomatic CPPD deposits; joint inflammation is sometimes observed after treatment with thyroid hormone. Hyperuricemia, often accompanying mild azotemia, is common in an elderly population. The coexistence of CPPD deposition disease and true gout with urate crystals has varied from 2% to 8% in most series.

BASIC CALCIUM PHOSPHATE (BCP) CRYSTAL ARTHROPATHIES: THE MILWAUKEE SHOULDER/KNEE SYNDROME

This syndrome is characterized by either stiff or hypermobile shoulders in elderly persons, mostly women. Glenohumeral degeneration and loss of the fibrous rotator cuff, often bilateral but most prominent on the dominant side, is accompanied by characteristic joint fluid findings including (1) BCP crystals (carbonate-substituted hydroxyapatite, octacalcium phosphate, and sometimes tricalcium phosphate) in microspheroidal aggregates; (2) particulate collagens (types I, II, and III); (3) collagenase and neutral protease activity; (4) low levels of alpha-1 antitrypsin and alpha-2 macroglobulin (the chief proteinase inhibitors found in serum or inflammatory joint fluid); and (5) leukocyte concentrations less than 500 per cubic millimeter. Symptoms occur late in the disease and are relatively mild. Pain after use and at night and decreased function of the affected arm are present most commonly, although the condition can be asymptomatic.

Histologic examination shows focal synovial cell hyperplasia associated with intracellular BCP crystal aggregates. Extracellular crystal aggregates are present, scattered among collagen fibers. Endocytosis of BCP crystals by cultured synovial cells stimulates secretion of collagenase and stromelysin, and incubation of tissues containing BCP crystals with collagenase in vitro results in release of the aggregates. If this process occurs in vivo, a cycle of crystal release, endocytosis, and protease release could account for the destructive arthropathy seen in these patients. BCP, like other calcium-containing crystals, is mitogenic to cultured synovial cells, which could account for the synovial hyperplasia found in patients.

A similar destructive process, associated with identical joint-fluid findings, occurs in the knees of patients with BCP crystal arthropathies, and the process is likely to involve the lateral tibiofemoral compartment, associated with a valgus deformity, rather than the medial tibiofemoral compartment producing a varus deformity, as in primary "nodal" osteoarthritis. A role for mechanical trauma is suggested by the greater involvement of the shoulder of the dominant extremity. Osteonecrosis of a femoral condyle or tibial plateau and osteochondromata are also prominent radiographic features. It is likely that other large joints, such as the elbow, hip, and ankle, can also be involved by a similar process, but synovial fluid findings have not been presented to support this idea.

Treatment is symptomatic. Rest of the affected joint and nonsteroidal anti-inflammatory drugs and/or analgesics are probably helpful. Surgical replacement arthroplasty has been used with fair to good results.

CALCIUM OXALATE ARTHROPATHY

Interstitial fluid is supersaturated with respect to calcium oxalate when serum creatinine exceeds about 8 mg per deciliter. These crystals have been associated with acute, subacute, or chronic joint symptoms in dialysis patients. They can also deposit in the skin, blood vessel walls, and other tissues. These crystals too are phagocytosed by neutrophils during acute attacks.

REFERENCES

Halverson PB and McCarty DJ: Arthritis associated with apatite and other calcium phosphate crystals. In McCarty DJ and Koopman WJ, editors: Arthritis and allied conditions, ed 12. Philadelphia, 1993, Lea & Febiger.

Reginato AJ et al: Arthropathy and cutaneous calcinosis in hemodialysis oxalosis. Arthritis Rheum 29:1387, 1986.

Ryan LM and McCarty DJ: Calcium pyrophosphate dihydrate crystal deposition disease. In McCarty DJ and Koopman WJ, editors: Arthritis and allied conditions, ed 12. Philadelphia, 1993, Lea & Febiger.

Terkeltaub R: Pathogenesis and treatment of crystal-induced inflammation. In McCarty DJ and Koopman WJ, editors: Arthritis and allied conditions, ed 12. Philadelphia, 1993, Lea & Febiger.

CHAPTER

321 Ochronosis and Alkaptonuria

J. Edwin Seegmiller

Etiology and incidence

Alkaptonuria results from a hereditary defect of tyrosine metabolism produced by a recessively inherited deficiency of the enzyme homogentisic acid oxidase. Consequently, instead of being oxidized in the tricarboxylic acid cycle, homogentisic acid becomes the end product of both tyrosine and phenylalanine metabolism and is excreted in large amounts in the urine throughout life (Fig. 321-1). Although this is a benign disorder during the first few decades of life, a black pigment derived from an oxidation product of homogentisic acid deposits progressively in the cartilage and connective tissue over the years, leading in the fifth or sixth decade of life to a severe degeneration of the cartilage of the spine and other major joints of the body. Upon microscopic examination of the black cartilage, Virchow in 1866 found a brownish ochre-appearing pigment, leading to the pathologic designation of *ochronotic arthritis*.

The disease is generally regarded as a very rare disorder. In Czechoslovakia, however, a simple screening test, applied to the urine of all newborns, showed a frequency of alkaptonuria of 1 in 25,000 births, and the same test applied in the area of Cardiff, Wales, showed a frequency of 1 in 45,000 births (a far higher frequency than most geneticists would have expected in a British population).

Historically, the disease has contributed substantially to our understanding of basic metabolic and genetic processes. The essential features of the one-gene, one-enzyme hypothesis were proposed in 1908 by Garrod as a result of studies of patients with alkaptonuria, a full 30 years before the more detailed development of this theory by microbiologists.

Pathophysiology

Characteristically, the urine turns dark on exposure to air, particularly if the urine is alkaline. Consequently, diapers of an affected child develop a brownish-black color if allowed to remain for any appreciable length of time in contact with urine. A similar darkening of clothing exposed to homogentisic acid in axillary perspiration and a darkening of axillary skin has been reported in some, but not all, patients. In occasional affected children, a lavender, or even red, color is found in diapers from conjugation of homogentisic acid with certain amino acids but does not persist beyond the first year of life.

The amount of homogentisic acid excreted in the urine is directly related to the dietary intake of tyrosine and phenylalanine. The pathway of metabolism in which the block occurs normally serves to oxidize, for energy production, the surplus quantities of tyrosine in excess of those needed for protein synthesis and other metabolic functions.

Homogentisic acid has a renal clearance rate essentially equal to that of blood flow. Consequently, the concentration of homogentisic acid in plasma of affected patients remains extremely low. No difference has been found in ability of alkaptonuric and nonalkaptonuric individuals to excrete homogentisic acid rapidly after oral administration. A copper-containing enzyme, homogentisic acid polyphenoloxidase, may be involved in oxidation of homogentisic acid by a single electron transfer to a free radical hydroquinone, which then receives a second electron to become benzoquinone acetic acid before it can be deposited in connective tissue. The presence of the hydroquinone intermediate suggests the possibility of a free radical mechanism being involved in the damage produced in cartilage. Recent studies have shown that the portion excreted in the urine as benzoquinone acetic acid is substantially greater in adult patients than in infants. Benzoquinone acetic acid was reduced to undetectable amounts in adult patients receiving ascorbic acid, a known free radical scavenger. The effect could also reflect the reducing action of ascorbic acid on preformed benzoquinone acetic acid. Also an inhibition of proliferation of both rabbit and human cartilage cells in culture has been induced by concentrations of homogentisic acid quite comparable to those encountered in the serum of affected individuals. Benzoquinone acetic acid and its further oxidation products can readily react with sulfhydryl and amino groups, and the binding of this compound to connective tissues could well produce alterations in tissue components that lead to the cartilage degeneration seen in ochronotic arthritis.

Pathology

Despite minimal superficial pigmentary changes, deposition of pigment in cartilage and connective tissue is most dramatic. At postmortem examination, dense pigmentation is found in cartilage of the larynx and in the costal cartilage in older alkaptonurics. Cartilage of the major joints of the body appears coal black. A similar pigmentation is also present throughout the body in fibrous tissue, tendons, ligaments, and fibrocartilage. Lesser degrees of pigment deposition are found in the intima of the large- and medium-sized arteries and arterioles, in arteriosclerotic plaques in the endocardium, in stenotic aortic valves, and in various organs (kidney and lung) and the epidermis. Pigment can

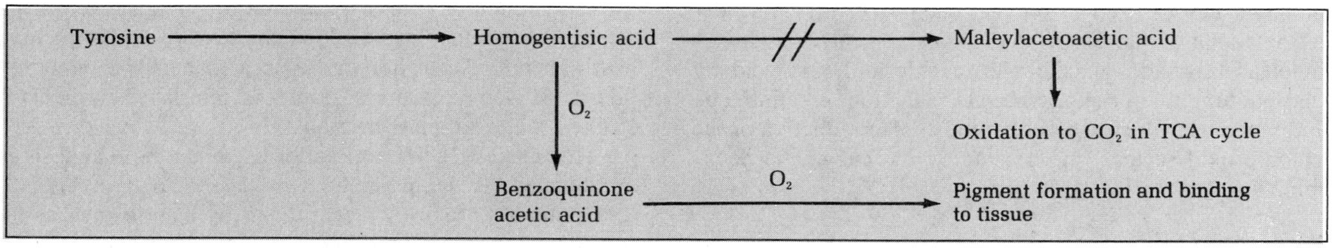

Fig. 321-1. Metabolic block in alkaptonuria and possible mechanism of pigment formation and deposition leading to ochronotic arthritis.

be both intracellular and extracellular and either granular or homogenous.

Clinical and laboratory findings

The first clinical evidence of pigment deposition in cartilage appears in adults between 20 and 30 years of age and consists of a slight slate-blue or grayish color showing through the skin overlying the cartilage areas of the ears and occasionally of the nose. The ear cartilage feels thickened and irregular and is calcified in advanced cases. A dusky discoloration sometimes can be seen over the area of tendons in the hands. Another, more obvious site of pigment deposition is in the sclera of the eyes, where it is usually found about midway between the cornea and the outer and inner canthi in the general region of insertion of the rectus muscles. In some patients, a more generalized pigmentation may also be detectable in the conjunctiva and cornea. With advanced disease, the pigmentation may be noticed around the perifollicular areas of the skin of the hands or malar area of the face.

The earliest clinical symptoms are attributable to ochronotic spondylitis. Patients complain of stiffness and discomfort in the lower back, and in 10% to 15% there is a herniation of a nucleus pulposus. Stiffness of the lower back proceeds to rigidity with loss of the normal lordosis. Rigidity progresses to involve the dorsal and later the cervical spine. The first diagnostic radiologic evidence of the disease is a wafer of calcification of the lumbar intervertebral disks. Subsequently, there is loss of joint space and development of small osteophytes on the vertebral bodies (Fig. 321-2). In contrast to ankylosing spondylitis, the sacroiliac joints are not fused.

The peripheral joints are involved later, with some degree of limitation of motion in the knee joint, hip, or, in some cases, the shoulders. Most patients have periods of acute joint inflammation that may resemble rheumatoid arthritis clinically. Later in the course of the disease, the joints show marked limitation of motion. Associated radiologic features include chondrocalcinosis and loose bodies in the joint space that may show calcification (see Chapter 296). NMR imaging holds promise for detection of the pigment deposits in vivo. In many patients the pigmentation is so slight as to be scarcely noticeable, and the first diagnosis of the disease frequently is made with the discovery of the typical black cartilage at surgery for removal of loose bodies from a joint. The strong reducing properties of homogentisic acid can interfere with a wide range of colorimetric reactions used in clinical chemistry, including determinations of protein by the biuret reagent, 5-hydroxyindoleacetic acid by acidic ferric chloride, uric acid by phosphotungstate or cupric acetate reduction, creatinine by Jaffe reaction, glucose by either the copper reduction or the glucose oxidase test, and oxalate by the enzymatic determination.

Diagnosis and treatment

Confirmation of the clinical or radiologic diagnosis is made by demonstrating the presence of homogentisic acid in the urine. A simple presumptive test consists of formation of a dark brown to black pigment on the surface layer of urine within 0.5 to 1.0 hour of its being made alkaline by addition of sodium or potassium hydroxide. Gentisic acid from aspirin and metabolites of dopa can give a similar positive test. Therefore, the homogentisic acid must be definitely identified. Paper chromatography or thin-layer chromatography are the simplest methods.

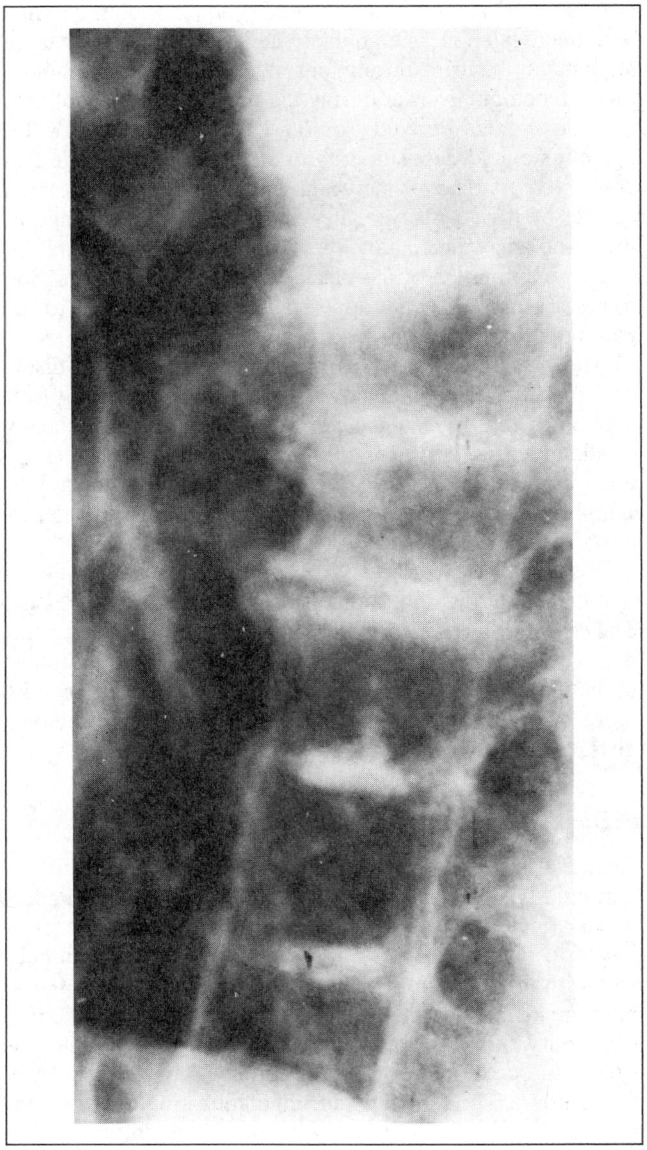

Fig. 321-2. Alkaptonuric (ochronotic) spondylitis with widespread loss of disk space and waferlike calcification of multiple intervertebral disks.

Treatment of ochronotic arthritis, once the diagnosis is established, is symptomatic with aspirin and other antiinflammatory drugs. A recent report by Konttinen et al describes the first successful noncemented total knee prosthesis in both knees of a patient with ochronotic arthropathy. Theoretically, at an early stage the disease could be prevented with rigid dietary restriction of phenylalanine and tyrosine intake to the minimal daily requirements. The possibility of preventing pigment deposition by use of large doses of ascorbic acid to prevent oxidation of homogentisic acid to the more reactive benzoquinone acetic acid has been considered. Unfortunately, no conclusive evidence of the clinical effectiveness of either approach has yet been obtained.

REFERENCES

Angeles AP et al: Chondrocyte growth inhibition induced by homogentisic acid and its partial prevention with ascorbic acid. J Rheumatol 16:512, 1989.

Feldman JM and Bowman J: Urinary homogentisic acid: determination by thin-layer chromatography. Clin Chem 19:459, 1973.

Konttinen YT et al: Ochronosis: a report of a case and a review of literature. Clin Exp Rheumatol 7:435, 1989.

Koska L: Artifacts produced by homogentisic acid in the examination of urine from alkaptonurics. Ann Clin Biochem 23:354, 1986.

LaDu BN et al: The nature of the defect in tyrosine metabolism in alcaptonuria. J Biol Chem 230:251, 1958.

Schumacher HR and Holdsworth DE: Ochronotic arthropathy. I. Clinical-pathologic studies. Semin Arthritis Rheum 6:207, 1977.

Srsen S et al: Screening for alkaptonuria in the newborn in Slovakia and in Wales. Lancet 2:576, 1978.

Wolff JA et al: Effects of ascorbic acid in alkaptonuria: alterations in benzoquinone acetic acid and an ontogenic effect in infancy. Pediatr Res 26:140, 1989.

Yamaguchi S, Koda N, and Ohashi T: Diagnosis of alkaptonuria by NMR urinalysis: rapid qualitative and quantitative analysis of homogentisic acid. Tohoku J Exp Med 150:227, 1986.

CHAPTER

322 The Amyloidoses

George G. Glenner

Amyloidosis is a disease complex encompassing over 20 distinct clinically defined syndromes, either hereditary or acquired, localized or systemic. Its incidence varies according to its related disorder, affecting as many as 4 million individuals with Alzheimer's disease. In the majority of the systemic cases it is a lethal, irreversible, inexorable process. Not until the early 1970s did the mystery of amyloidosis begin to unravel and its multiplastic nature become clear. *Amyloidosis* is, therefore, a generic term relating to specific chemical characteristics of the amyloid deposits unique to each of the wide variety of pathologic conditions in which it is found.

AMYLOID

The amorphous, eosinophilic material with the microscopic appearance of paraffin infiltrating between cells has been defined as an ordered structure with unique characteristics. After staining by the dye Congo red, amyloid affords a green color when viewed by polarization optics. It is birefringent and usually extracellular.

Electron microscopy reveals nonbranching fibrils, usually 7 to 10 nm in width. X-ray crystallography defines these structures as twisted β-pleated sheet fibrils identical to the egg stalk silk of the *Chrysopa flava* moth. The β-pleated sheet conformation of the fibrils explains their tinctorial and optical properties, as well as their determined insolubility and relative resistance to proteolytic digestion.

Chemical characterization

Once means were developed to concentrate the amyloid fibrils into homogenous preparations and to solubilize and fractionate them, their chemical nature became amenable to analysis. The results of these studies revealed that these fibrils were proteinaceous and that their chemical composition tended to be unique for each of the various syndromes defined clinically (Table 322-1). Amino acid sequence analyses of the amyloid fibril protein isolated from cases of B-lymphocyte and plasma-cell dyscrasias revealed the major fibrillar proteins were composed primarily of the amino-terminal variable region of the light polypeptide chain of an immunoglobulin protein (Chapter 285). Peptide digestion of a series of lambda light-chain proteins afforded, with some proteins, fibrils with the β-pleated sheet conformation. This study proved that amyloid fibrils could be produced by proteolysis of some, but not all, light-chain proteins and provided a pathogenetic mechanism for amyloid fibril formation. These findings also initiated the concept

Table 322-1. Chemically documented amyloidoses

Clinical association	Notation	Protein type
Acquired systemic amyloidosis		
Immunoglobulin light-chain (primary)	AL	Light chain, type and subtype
Multiple myeloma		
Reactive (secondary)	AA	Protein A
Hemodialysis amyloidosis	$A\beta_2M$	β_2 macroglobulin
Heredofamilial systemic		
Polyneuropathy	ATTR	Prealbumin, variant
Finnish	AGel	Gelsolin, variant
Familial Mediterranean fever	AA	Protein A
Organ-limited		
Alzheimer's disease	Aβ	β protein
Hereditary Icelandic congophilic angiopathy (CA)	ACys	Cystatin C, variant
Hereditary Dutch CA	Aβ	β protein, variant
Senile cardiac	ATTR	Prealbumin
Localized endocrine		
Pancreatic islet	AIAP	Islet amyloid protein
Medullary thyroid carcinoma	ACal	Precalcitonin

of the amyloidogenic protein. This concept helped to explain why "only" 10% of cases of multiple myeloma have an associated amyloidosis: that is, only this percentage of cases synthesized a free homogenous amyloidogenic light chain.

The amino acid sequences of other clinical types of amyloid proteins then began to be defined. In cases of rheumatoid arthritis and other chronic inflammatory conditions, the amyloid fibril protein was of a previously unknown type designated *protein A,* and the fibril type, AA. This protein apparently derives from a serum component, SAA, of 12,000 kD associated with high-density lipoproteins. Proteolytic cleavage is the most plausible mechanism for amyloid fibril formation. Based on the amyloidogenic protein concept, it was suggested that subtypes of SAA existed, one of which was amyloidogenic. This concept was conclusively demonstrated in the mouse, in which only one of two isotypes of SAA was found to compose the amyloid fibrils.

PATHOGENESIS

The fact that the majority of AL amyloid fibrils were composed of the amino-terminal variable half of a light chain and that fibrils having all the characteristics of amyloid fibrils could be created from some intact light chains by proteolytic cleavage suggested a proteolytic mechanism for amyloid fibril formation in the systemic amyloidoses. Proteolysis of an amyloidogenic serum protein by lysosomal or other enzymes in phagocytic cells would yield a fragment of the serum protein that rapidly converted into a β-pleated sheet fibril. However, insulin and glucagon can be converted into β-fibrils by physiochemical means other than proteolysis. Prealbumin (transthyretin, TTR) and β_2 microglobulin, both of which have over 50% β-structure, form amyloid fibers in the absence of proteolysis. Thus, although proteolysis of an amyloidogenic protein usually having significant intrinsic β-structure is probably the major mechanism for amyloid fibril formation, other physicochemical mechanisms exist.

CLASSIFICATION AND MANIFESTATIONS OF THE MAJOR AMYLOIDOSES

Systemic amyloidoses

Reactive amyloidosis. Reactive amyloidosis is an amyloidotic process usually associated with inflammatory disease, such as rheumatoid arthritis. It has also been reported in 50% of tuberculosis patients, as well as in ankylosing spondylitis, Reiter's syndrome, psoriatic arthritis, chronic rheumatic heart disease, dermatomyositis, scleroderma, Behçet's syndrome, and, rarely, systemic lupus erythematosus; also, it frequently complicates paraplegia. Other associations include familial Mediterranean fever, Hodgkin's disease, and hypernephroma. The organs most affected by amyloid deposits composed of AA protein are the spleen, kidney, and liver, with renal involvement producing the earliest manifestations.

Immunocytic amyloidosis. This category includes B-cell dyscrasias of a wide variety, including amyloidosis associated with plasma-cell myeloma, "light-chain" myeloma, idiopathic or "primary" amyloidosis, and nodular malignant lymphoma.

The presence of a monoclonal protein, especially a light-chain protein, in the serum or urine of a patient with amyloidosis suggests the existence of both an immunocytic amyloidotic process and AL amyloid fibrils.

The mean age at diagnosis of immunocytic amyloidosis is approximately 60 years. Virtually all patients with immunocytic amyloidosis have an excessive number of bone-marrow plasma cells with or without osteolytic lesions on radiographic survey. In nonosteolytic disease, random bone-marrow samples may fail to reveal plasmacytic abnormalities, but certain symptoms strongly suggest its presence.

The most relevant clinical manifestation is restrictive cardiomyopathy, which may be caused by amyloid infiltration of myocardial tissues. Second, an "idiopathic" peripheral neuropathy that closely resembles diabetic neuropathy may be a manifestation of the immunocytic amyloidoses. Neuropathy usually presents with painful sensory deficits in a "stocking-glove" distribution. Third, a relatively noninflammatory polyarthropathy occurring in a symmetrical distribution may be a sign of the immunocytic amyloidoses. Amyloid arthropathy has a predilection for large joints. Massive accumulation of amyloid material in the glenohumeral articulation presents the nearly pathognomonic "shoulder-pad" sign. Fourth, pinch purpura, postproctoscopic periorbital purpura, or waxy, cutaneous papules can be seen as dermatologic manifestations of the immunocytic amyloidoses. The fifth and sixth of the clinical conditions that may be the initial manifestation of immunocytic amyloidosis are macroglossia and idiopathic carpal tunnel syndrome (median nerve compression). The latter syndrome is uncommon in reactive amyloidosis.

Identification of any of these six symptom complexes with or without a detectable monoclonal immunoglobulin in the serum or urine warrants investigation for immunocytic dyscrasia associated with amyloidosis.

Heredofamilial amyloidosis

The first group of hereditary amyloidotic processes of autosomal-dominant inheritance that yielded to chemical definition were the familial polyneuropathies. Each is characterized by a specific substitution in a serum protein molecule. Most are TTR variants with the exception of the type III, which is an apolipoprotein A-1 variant, and the Finnish type IV, which is composed of a gelsolin variant. The familial polyneuropathies are listed in Table 322-2.

These findings provided a firm basis for categorizing this group of autosomal-dominant neuropathies and demonstrated the chemical validity of the older clinical classification of these diseases.

Hemodialysis amyloidosis

This amyloidotic syndrome is associated with chronic hemodialysis and by amyloid deposits of β_2-macroglobulin manifesting with carpal tunnel syndrome, lytic bone le-

Table 322-2. Heredofamilial amyloidotic polyneuropathies

Type	Ethnicity	Upper extremity	Lower extremity	Other	Nephropathy	Protein	Protein variant
I	Japanese Portuguese Swedish	3+ late	4+	Vitreous opacities Autonomic neuropathy	0	TTR*	Met 30
II	German Jewish Swiss	4+	3+ late	Vitreous opacities Carpal tunnel syndrome	0	TTR	His 58 Ile 33 Ser 84
III	English Irish Scottish	2+ late	4+	Peptic ulceration Autonomic neuropathy	4+	Apolipoprotein A-1	Arg 26
IV	Finnish	0	0	Lattice corneal dystrophy Cranial neuropathy Cutis laxa	0	Gelsolin	Asp 187
V	Appalachian	0	0	Cardiomyopathy Carpal tunnel syndrome Autonomic neuropathy	0	TTR	Ala 60

*Prealbumin—transthyretin

sions, pathologic fractures, spondyloarthropathy, or vascular involvement. The amyloidosis occurs in over 10% of patients with chronic renal disease maintained on hemodialysis for over 10 years. Hemodialysis does not lower the serum levels of β_2-microglobulin protein, and in fact, because of its failure to pass conventional cuprophan dialysis membranes, its serum concentration is increased and amyloid fibrils of this protein form spontaneously.

Localized amyloidoses

The cerebral amyloidoses. The observation that has recently thrust amyloidosis into the limelight is its association with Alzheimer's disease and Down's syndrome. Alzheimer's disease is diagnosed by the presence in the cortical gray matter of amyloid fibrils in neuritic plaques in the parenchyma, as well as by intraneuronal neurofibrillary tangles composed of paired helical filaments having a β-pleated sheet conformation. In addition, cerebrovascular amyloid deposits are also almost invariably present. Exactly the same lesions are seen in all Down's syndrome individuals over the age of 40. Previously denoted as "presenile dementia," this same pathologic process is found in 62% of demented individuals over age 65. Altogether, cerebral amyloidoses affect over 4 million individuals in the United States, making amyloidosis one of the most common lethal disease processes. Nonparalytic strokes occur in approximately 20% of patients as a result of rupture of amyloid-laden vessels with resulting hemorrhage. Recent chemical and biochemical data have proven that the vascular amyloid fibril protein, β protein, also composes the amyloid fibrils of the plaques. In addition, the gene encoding the β protein has been identified on chromosome 21, a finding consistent with the invariant presence of β protein in the cerebral lesions of Down syndrome. Mutations in the β protein precursor have been found in several cases of familial Alzheimer's disease.

Hereditary Icelandic Congophilic angiopathy (hereditary cerebral hemorrhage with amyloidosis) is an autosomal-dominant process with extensive cerebral cortical vascular amyloidosis. The cerebral amyloid fibrils have been found to be composed of a chemical variant of cystatin C (gamma trace), a cathepsin inhibitor. A Dutch variant has amyloid fibrils in the walls of cerebral vessels and preamyloid plaques. The amyloid fibrils are composed of a β protein variant.

Endocrine amyloidoses. The most common and perhaps most significant of the tissue-localized amyloidoses is that involving the islets of Langerhans of the pancreas and associated with type 2 diabetes mellitus. Fifty-nine percent of diabetics over the age of 50 have insular amyloid deposits. Recently, it has been shown that the insular amyloid fibril protein (IAP) has a 46% homology with the family of calcitonin gene-related proteins (α-CGRP and β-CGRP), and it has been found to exert a regulatory effect on insulin secretion and glucose metabolism.

DIAGNOSIS

The medical history, characteristic clinical features, and laboratory tests should distinguish the reactive, immunocytic, familial, and hemodialysis types of systemic amyloidosis. Rectal or gingival biopsies are positive in 80% and 60% of patients, respectively. Skin biopsy from either clinically involved or normal skin shows amyloid in over 50% of patients. Subcutaneous abdominal fat-pad biopsy is a simple, effective method of making the diagnosis. All tissues obtained are stained with Congo red and examined by polarization microscopy for the presence of a green polarization color and birefringence. Specific antibodies are available for immunohistochemical definition of the type of amyloidosis present. Some familial amyloidotic polyneuropathies can be diagnosed by both blood serum and genomic tests.

PROGNOSIS AND TREATMENT

In reactive amyloidosis, eradication of the predisposing disease slows, and can occasionally reverse, the progression of amyloid disease. Survival for 5 or 10 years after diagnosis is not uncommon. Patients with familial amyloidotic polyneuropathy have a prolonged course of severe incapacity and usually succumb to the illness 10 to 15 years after onset. Colchicine, 1.0 mg once or twice daily, can improve or prevent amyloid deposition when used prophylactically in individuals at risk for familial Mediterranean fever.

Patients with the immunocytic process who develop amyloidosis have the worst prognosis. Life expectancy is less than 1 year and often not more than a few months. Alkylating agents may be useful in a subset of cases and may induce temporary remissions. Now that newer dialysis membranes can pass β_2-microglobulin, these will undoubtedly be used in the future to prevent hemodialysis amyloidosis. Symptomatic therapy and supportive measures remain the mainstay of management of most of the amyloidoses. These may not significantly influence longevity, but they clearly improve the quality of life that may be attained by these patients.

REFERENCES

Benson MD and Dwulet FE: Identification of carriers of a variant plasma prealbumin (transthyretin) associated with familial amyloidotic polyneuropathy Type I. J Clin Invest 75:71, 1985.

Glenner GG: Amyloid deposits and amyloidosis: the β-fibriloses. N Engl J Med 302:1283, 1980.

Glenner GG and Wurtman RJ: Advancing frontiers in Alzheimer's disease research. Austin, Texas, 1987, University of Texas Press.

Glenner GG et al, editors: Amyloidosis, Fourth International Symposium. New York, 1986, Plenum.

Tanzi RE: Invited editorial. Gene mutations in inherited amyloidosis of the nervous system. Am J Hum Genet 49:507, 1991.

CHAPTER

323 Heritable and Developmental Disorders of Connective Tissue

Stephen M. Krane

Skeletal dysplasias result from growth abnormalities in utero or in infancy and childhood. Disturbances in the proportions and length of the fetus may be caused by disorders of chromosomes or by genetically determined abnormalities of morphogenesis, skeletal growth, and maturation. Some become manifest only after birth as short stature or disproportionate body habitus. Hydrocephalus, cranial synostosis, cleft lip and palate, and change in facial appearance may be accompaniments. In addition to shortened limbs, there may be other abnormalities, such as polydactyly, syndactyly, clubbing of fingers and toes, joint dislocations, and multiple fractures. The skeletal dysplasias can be divided into two groups: those caused primarily by abnormal growth of cartilage and/or bone (osteochondrodysplasias) and those that involve malformations of individual bones or combination of bones (dysostoses). The osteochondrodysplasias have been considered in three categories:

1. Chondrodystrophies, which result from defects in growth of bones (e.g., achondroplasia)
2. Disordered development of cartilaginous and fibrous components of the skeleton (e.g., multiple exostoses)
3. Abnormal structure of metaphyseal and diaphyseal bone caused by disordered modeling and remodeling (e.g., some forms of osteogenesis imperfecta)

Although in most of these disorders the fundamental defect is unknown, some (e.g., certain of the chondrodystrophies and forms of osteogenesis imperfecta) may be considered among the heritable disorders of connective tissue. As defined by McKusick, these are generalized defects that involve primarily one component of connective tissue—for example, collagen, elastin, or proteoglycan—and are transmissible in mendelian patterns. Many appear to be distinctive, although the clinical phenotype may vary considerably. It is possible that some of these disorders will turn out to be mutations in genes that are homologous to the homeobox genes in *Drosophilia*.

Traditionally, this variability had been ascribed to differences in penetrance and expression of single genes. It is likely, however, that genetic heterogeneity plays a major role in the differences in clinical manifestations. Since the group of heritable disorders of connective tissue comprises over 100 distinct disease entities, it is not possible to describe any in detail here. Many of the disorders do share common clinical and pathologic features, depending on which component of the connective tissue is involved predominantly.

The term *connective tissue* is usually applied to cartilage, bone, tendons, fascia, ligaments, and the walls of blood vessels. Connective tissue is also considered the extracellular matrix of many other tissues. The character of any connective tissue is determined by the function of the specific cells that comprise that tissue. Some components of the extracellular matrix are locally synthesized or modified by the component cells, whereas others are derived from the plasma.

The major fibrous proteins are collagen and elastin. The predominant nonfibrous (amorphous) components are the complex carbohydrates of the so-called ground substance, which include hyaluronic acid, the proteoglycans, and glycoproteins. Water and electrolytes derived from plasma are other important determinants of structure and function of many connective tissues. Finally, in bone, the presence of the calcium phosphate inorganic mineral phase contributes to its characteristics as a connective tissue. The particular organization of the cells and their extracellular matrices account for the mechanical properties of each tissue; included are such properties as ability to deform under load (articular cartilage), behavior as a rigid encasement to protect vital structures (bone of the skull), acting as levers for locomotion (long bones), or forming a flexible covering (dermis).

The heritable disorders of connective tissue may be considered either from the point of view of each of the components of the extracellular matrix or by the characteristic pattern of clinical manifestations, which mainly involves skin, bones, joints, blood vessels, and eyes. We focus on the major components, about which there are considerable chemical data regarding structure and biosynthesis. These major components are collagens, elastin, and the proteoglycans.

COLLAGENS AND POSSIBLE DISORDERS OF COLLAGEN STRUCTURE AND METABOLISM

Collagens are a class of proteins, members of which have chemical and structural features in common, but each of which is a product of a different gene. One property of collagen molecules is the unique triple helix, a particular conformation of three component polypeptide (α) chains. Each of the mature α chains of the most abundant collagens that form banded fibrils (types I to III) contains approximately 1000 amino acids. The conformation of the chains is determined by the amino acid content, with glycine constituting a third of the total and occurring at every third position in the amino acid sequence. Two major classes of collagens are recognized: those that form banded fibrils and fibers and those that do not (Table 323-1). Type I collagen is the major type in most connective tissues, including skin, bone, and parenchymal tissues and blood vessel walls; type II is the major type in articular cartilage and nucleus pulposus; type III is particularly abundant in skin, blood vessel walls, and parenchymal organs but is not found in bone matrix. Other collagens—such as type IV, the predominant type in basement membranes—have unique structures distinct from those that form fibrils, mainly because of interruptions by noncollagenous sequences of the characteristic collagen helical sequences. In tissues the fibers contain characteristic mixtures of different collagens: for example, types I and III in skin or types II and IX in articular cartilage. The collagen also interacts with other components of the extracellular matrix—for example, proteoglycans—in specific ways. Each of the polypeptide (α) chains of the collagens is a product controlled by different genes. At least 18 different gene products have been characterized as among the subunits of at least 13 collagen molecules. The genes for these collagens are complex and huge, and may contain as many as 50 intervening (noncoding) sequences. The genes for several of the collagens have been located on several different chromosomes. Even the genes coding for the two constituent chains of the most abundant collagen (type I) are present on separate chromosomes (α1 [I] on chromosome 17 and α2 [I] on chromosome 7). Biosynthesis of the collagen chains is a multistep process in which a precursor form (procollagen) is first synthesized, with peptide extensions at either end. During synthesis, several amino acids are uniquely modified posttranslationally (after incorporation into the polypeptide chains). These posttranslational modifications include hydroxylation of proline residues (hydroxyproline) and lysine residues (hydroxylysine) and addition of sugars (glucose and galactose) to the hydroxylysines, and formation of hydroxylysine and lysine aldehydes. Specific proteases act to cleave off the extensions of the procollagens to produce the processed collagen molecules, which can then polymerize to form fibrils and fibers.

Table 323-1. Major types of collagen and their tissue distributions*

Type	Tissue
Fibrillar	
Type I	Bone, skin, tendons, ligaments, and dentin (all >80%)†; also other tissues
Type II	Articular cartilage, fibrocartilage, vitreous gel (all 50% to 90%); many tissues in early development
Type III	Large blood vessels (30%), and other tissues in association with type I (except bone)
Type V	Large blood vessels (5%), cornea, bone, and a few others
Type XI	Articular cartilage (5% to 20%)
Basement membrane–associated	
Type IV	All basement membranes (95%)
Type VII	Anchoring fibrils of epidermal-dermal junction
Fiber-associated	
Type IX	Cartilage (5% to 20%)
Type XII	Small amounts with type I
Short chain	
Type VI	Aorta, cornea, skin, placenta, ligaments, cartilage
Type VIII	Endothelial cells
Type X	Hypertrophic cells of cartilage

*For more complete descriptions, see Prockop DJ, Williams CJ, and Vandenberg P: Collagen in normal and diseased connective tissue. In McCarty DJ and Koopman WJ, editors: Arthritis and allied conditions: a textbook of rheumatology, ed 12. Philadelphia, 1993, Lea & Febiger.

†Numbers in parentheses indicate approximate percentage of total collagen in the tissues indicated.

Given the enormous complexities of structure and biosynthesis, it is not surprising that abnormalities of collagen have been frequently identified in a few uncommon human diseases and in a limited number of cases of common disorders that affect connective tissues (Table 323-2).

Osteogenesis imperfecta

Osteogenesis imperfecta (OI) is the term used to describe clinical phenotypes with hereditary bone fragility (tendency to fracture with minimal trauma). There is extreme variability in the manifestations, however, indicating clinical as well as genetic heterogeneity. Thus, the OI syndrome has been subclassified using clinical and genetic criteria such as those shown in Table 323-3. Each of these types can be subclassified, and most are genetically and biochem-

Table 323-2. Diseases associated with mutations of collagen genes

Collagen	Frequency: Regular	Frequency: Occasional
Fibrillar		
Type I	Lethal osteogenesis imperfecta (type II)	Osteoporosis
Type II	Lethal chondrodysplasias	Osteoarthritis
Type III	Ehlers-Danlos syndrome (type IV)	Aortic aneurysms
Basement membrane–associated		
Type IV	Alport's syndrome	
Type VII	Epidermolysis bullosa (dystrophic form)	

ically heterogeneous. Some individuals with OI cannot be placed in any of these categories. For example, there are patients with moderately severe bone disease, with or without blue sclerae, in whom the inheritance pattern does not fit that of autosomal dominant.

The dominant form with blue sclerae is the most widely recognized. Nearly 100% of persons with this syndrome have abnormally thin sclerae, which take on a slate or blue-black hue. Bones fracture with minimal trauma, beginning in infancy or early childhood. Osteopenia may be detected radiologically prior to fracturing. Perinatal fractures and severe deformities are unusual. Other manifestations include joint laxity, scoliosis, and easy bruising. Dentinogenesis imperfecta, common in the severe deforming (type III) OI, is uncommon in type I. A hearing defect indistinguishable from that of otosclerosis usually begins in the second and third decades and occurs in about one third of patients with OI type I. Since the skeletal manifestations tend to diminish after puberty, the results of therapy are difficult to evaluate. The use of sex hormones (androgens in males and estrogens in females) has been advocated to induce early puberty; short stature may result from such treatment, however, because of premature closure of epiphyses. Sodium fluoride therapy also has been used, but with limited success. Bones of patients with OI type III usually begin to fracture shortly after birth or even prenatally and frequently continue to fracture with the development of severe skeletal deformities that are seemingly independent of fracturing; kyphoscoliosis also develops. These patients do not have an increased incidence of deafness, and their sclerae are not blue. This form of OI is probably genetically heterogeneous, although recessive patterns have been documented. Therapy has been ineffective.

The finding of woven bone and abnormal patterns of deposition of collagen fibers in bone from patients with OI is difficult to interpret because clinical and histopathologic correlations are generally poor. Recently, techniques of protein chemistry and molecular biology have made it possible to demonstrate the nature of the defects in type I collagen structure because of specific mutations in most affected individuals. A decreased content of type I collagen, and a relative increase in type III collagen have been found in the skin of patients with type I OI, particularly in those with the dominant form and blue sclerae. When compared with normal dermal fibroblasts, those cultured from such patients synthesize a higher ratio of type III/type I collagen. Since bone contains essentially only type I collagen, it is suggested that a decreased ability to synthesize this matrix component may be a basic defect.

Based on the results of recent studies, a considerable number of patients with OI have mutations in one or both structural genes of type I collagen. In some forms of OI—for example, the perinatal lethal form (type II)—most affected individuals have been shown to have such mutations. Many of the mutations are in different sites in the gene yet produce apparently identical phenotypes. The consequences of the mutations are substitutions or deletions of single amino acids, or deletion of whole exons (in phase) encoding multiple amino acids. Splicing mutations and others that produce frame-shifts have been described. In one example of the latter, a defect in the 3′ portion of the pro-α_2(I) gene resulted in the absence of secreted α_2 chains and deposition of α_1(I)-chain trimers. Despite this extraordinary defect the mutation was not lethal. In some instances, an abnormal chain resulting from a mutation in one allele produces devastating effects (resulting from so-called protein

Table 323-3. Osteogenesis imperfecta (OI)

Type	Name	Mode of inheritance	Major features
I	OI—Mild long-bone disease; trias fragilitas ossium	Autosomal dominant	Mild to moderate severity; blue sclerae; deafness; little progression after puberty
II	Lethal perinatal OI; lethal OI congenita	Autosomal recessive	Severe; often stillborn or death soon after birth; multiple fractures; crumpled bones (broad bones)
III	Progressively deforming with normal sclerae	Autosomal recessive	Normal birthweight; fractures of long bones and spine at birth or onset of walking; progressive severe deformity; ligamentous laxity; white sclerae; dentinogenesis imperfecta, common
IV	Dominant, with normal sclerae	Autosomal dominant	Variable severity at time of onset, with fractures of long bones and spine; some have dentinogenesis imperfecta

suicide), whereas some nonfunctioning alleles that result in formation of no protein at all may have mild consequences. A particularly common mutation results in substitution of cysteine for glycine within the helix. This disrupts the helix, but depending on the location of the substitution within the chain, the defects vary from mild to lethal. Another common feature is "overmodification" of the lysine residues (formation of glycosylated hydroxylysine), because of delays in helix formation. Most of the mutations are dominant, and many are new mutations. In some kindreds the defect has not yet been identified, but linkage of the disorder with the collagen genes can be shown by analysis of restriction length polymorphisms.

Ehlers-Danlos syndrome

A defect in collagen, particularly types I and III interstitial collagens, may be responsible for the Ehlers-Danlos syndrome. Clinical problems in this disorder include varying degrees of hyperextensible and soft, fragile skin, which may heal poorly when cut, leading to thin scars. Violaceous skin nodules (molluscoid pseudotumors), ecchymoses, and hyperpigmented skin may be found in areas subjected to repeated trauma. Calcified subcutaneous "spherules" may be palpated or detected radiologically. Some affected persons have hypermobile joints that display a tendency to dislocate recurrently. Other skeletal findings include intermittent joint pains, kyphoscoliosis, and deformities of the feet. Easy bruising is also common. In some people, sudden death results from rupture of a major blood vessel or viscera. Clinically and genetically, however, the Ehlers-Danlos syndrome is also heterogeneous, and it has been possible to subclassify the syndrome on these grounds.

Types of Ehlers-Danlos syndrome

Type I. In type I (gravis) syndrome, many of the clinical problems described previously may be present in the same affected person. Although a biochemical abnormality has not been identified, collagen fibers in skin and other tissues may be larger than normal and deposited in an irregular fashion.

Types II and III. In type II Ehlers-Danlos syndrome, all the manifestations are milder than in type I, and joint hypermobility is limited to the hands and feet. Cutaneous manifestations are mild or absent in type III Ehlers-Danlos syndrome, whereas hypermobility of joints is generalized and severe.

Type IV. Individuals with type IV syndrome (arterial, ecchymotic, or Sack's variety) have the poorest prognosis, with problems predominantly related to extensive bruising and fragility of arteries and veins. The skin, although not hyperextensible, is thin, particularly over acral parts, and the underlying venous network is prominent. There is a characteristic facies, with a pinched delicate nose, prominent eyes, and an appearance of premature aging. Vascular catastrophies or rupture of major viscera, such as the large intestine, occur in this group. Sudden death in the Ehlers-Danlos syndrome is a feature usually associated only with the type I and IV forms. The syndrome is also associated with mitral valve prolapse. The type IV syndrome is biochemically, and probably genetically, heterogeneous; in several instances defective deposition of type III collagen has been demonstrated. Abnormalities in production of type III collagen have also been described in otherwise normal individuals with ruptured cerebral aneurysms. In some affected individuals, type III collagen could not be found on analysis of skin, parenchyma, or walls of blood vessels. Furthermore, their skin fibroblasts do not synthesize detectable type III procollagen. In other subjects, type III procollagen is synthesized but is not normally secreted. Still other individuals with an indistinguishable clinical phenotype have type III collagen present, presumably in normal and sufficient amounts.

Types V and IX. Type V Ehlers-Danlos syndrome resembles type II; however, skin hyperextensibility may be striking, and the inheritance is X-linked. This syndrome may be related to cutis laxa, in that defective oxidation of lysine residues via the enzyme lysyl oxidase results in inadequate cross-linking of collagen molecules. Type IX Ehlers-Danlos syndrome includes individuals with such manifestations as urinary bladder diverticuli and spontaneous bladder rupture, inguinal hernias, slight skin laxity, and a number of skeletal abnormalities—a peculiar feature being occipital hornlike exostoses. Lysyl oxidase activity is low in fibroblast cultures from these individuals and may result from impaired synthesis of enzyme protein. It is not yet clear whether these abnormalities are fundamentally different from those reported in the type V Ehlers-Danlos syndrome.

Type VI. A form of Ehlers-Danlos syndrome (type VI) has been described in individuals with severe kyphoscoliosis, joint laxity, and recurrent joint dislocations; microcorneas; and soft, hyperextensible skin with a "velvety" feel and slow wound-healing ability. Analysis of dermal collagen from individuals in different kindreds has revealed a marked decrease in hydroxylysine content, a defect at the level of posttranslational modification, with insufficient activity of lysyl hydroxylase. The mutation is probably in the gene that codes for this enzyme that catalyzes the hydroxylation of specific lysyl residues after their incorporation into the growing (nascent) polypeptide chain. This syndrome is also biochemically heterogeneous. Inheritance is probably autosomal recessive. Clinical abnormalities may be accounted for by defective collagen cross-linking, which critically requires hydroxylysine residues. All interstitial collagens are not equally affected (e.g., skin is much more deficient than bone), and this suggests that there may be multiple forms of lysyl hydroxylase, only one of which is affected by a mutation that leads to this syndrome.

Type VII. Type VII Ehlers-Danlos syndrome is characterized by joint hypermobility and recurrent dislocations, moderate cutaneous hyperextensibility and bruisability, short stature, scoliosis, and a peculiar "scooped-out" facies with hypertelorism and epicanthal folds. Some have an abnormal collagen, the structure of which is consistent with partially processed procollagen. The incomplete processing of the procollagen is accounted for by abnormalities in the cleavage sites in the amino terminal portion of either procollagen chain caused by exon skipping and deletions of whole exons coding for 18 to 24 amino acids. A similar phenotype may also result from mutations in the enzyme responsible for the cleavage of the procollagen.

Type VIII. Type VIII Ehlers-Danlos syndrome represents a distinct entity characterized by moderate cutaneous fragility and severe generalized periodontitis, resulting in extensive alveolar bone resorption and premature loss of teeth. No biochemical defect has yet been identified.

Type X. A kindred has been described in which affected individuals had features of the Ehlers-Danlos syndrome with easy bruisability and a defect in platelet aggregation partially corrected by normal plasma or normal fibronectin. A defect in the structure of fibronectin might account for the bleeding abnormality as well as the connective tissue disorder, since fibronectin may function in adherence of cells to the extracellular, collagenous matrix.

Type XI. It has been suggested that the familial joint laxity syndrome be termed *type XI Ehlers-Danlos syndrome,* although no specific biochemical defect has been identified.

Fibrillin and Marfan syndrome

The Marfan syndrome includes a relatively common group of clinically heterogeneous heritable disorders of connective tissue. Initially felt to be a biochemical abnormality involving collagen, it has been recently shown that the defect resides in the fibrillin gene on human chromosome 15. Fibrillin, a (large 350 kD) connective tissue glycoprotein, is a component of microfibrils present in the connective tissue matrices of a variety of tissues, among which are the suspensory ligament of the lens, the wall of blood vessels, and the skin. Several point mutations in the gene segment 15q 15-21 plus abnormalities of fibrillin synthesis, extracellular transport, and incorporation into extracellular matrix have been reported in both familial and sporadic forms of Marfan syndrome.

The characteristic skeletal findings in the Marfan syndrome are dolichostenomelia (inappropriately long limbs compared with the trunk), arachnodactyly, pectus excavatum, and joint laxity. Scoliosis occurs at any level along the thoracolumbar spine; it is frequent and may worsen at the time of the pubertal growth spurt. Inguinal hernias are also common.

Over half of the Marfan cases have the classic ocular finding of ectopia lentis. The lens is usually displaced upward, but the zonules are intact and permit normal accommodation. In contrast, in homocystinuria, the lens is displaced downward; because the zonules are defective, accommodation is impaired. In addition, the globe is unusually long, and this contributes to a high frequency of myopia and an increased risk of retinal detachment.

Abnormalities of connective tissue may be found in the aortic wall and the heart. Histologic changes include disruption of elastic fibers in the blood vessel walls, increases in collagen deposition, and proliferation of smooth muscle cells. Such structural changes are manifested by enlargement of the aortic root, stretching of the aortic cusps, and progressive aortic regurgitation. The latter, if untreated, proceeds to left ventricular failure and death within a few years. Chest pain resembling angina pectoris may also develop. Aneurysms occur in the ascending and abdominal portions of the aorta. Aneurysms of the sinuses of Valsalva are common. Approximately a third of the patients have systolic clicks and murmurs, presumably of mitral origin. Echocardiographic abnormalities are detected in the majority of affected individuals. It would be unusual for a patient with strong clinical evidence of the Marfan syndrome not to have some cardiovascular finding that could be elicited either clinically or by echocardiography.

No therapy is available that can be directed against the fundamental defect or defects. Cardiovascular complications of the Marfan syndrome are managed like other forms of aortic and aortic valvular disease. Prophylactic repair of the ascending aorta prior to dilation is being investigated, as is the use of propranolol in patients who are unsuitable for surgery or in whom it is necessary to delay operation.

Cutis laxa

Cutis laxa, or dermatolysis, is another clinically and genetically heterogeneous disease characterized by loose hanging skin over all parts of the body. The condition is particularly noticeable over the face and around the eyes and produces a prematurely aged appearance. Although the skin is hyperextensible, it does not spring back into place. Easy bruisability is not apparent. Parenchymal involvement may occur in the lungs (emphysema) and in viscera with hernias, including diverticula of the gastrointestinal and genitourinary systems. The inheritance may be dominant, recessive, or X-linked. In one kindred in which the pattern has been X-linked, decreased activity of lysyl oxidase has been demonstrated.

Congenital contractural arachnodactyly (CCA)

An autosomal dominant disorder called CCA shares a number of musculoskeletal features with severe Marfan syndrome, but the patients have joint contractures rather than loose-jointedness. The eye and the aorta are not affected. CCA has been linked to a second fibrillin gene present on chromosome 5q 23-31.

ELASTIC TISSUE AND DISEASE

Elastic fibers interacting with collagens and other connective tissue components contribute to the distensible properties of structures such as arterial walls. The elastic fibers are comprised of two distinct proteins. The most abundant has an amorphous appearance by electron microscopy and the chemical composition of elastin. The other is a glycoprotein with a microfibrillar structure. Elastin consists of polypeptide chains rich in the amino acids glycine, alanine, and valine, but poor in polar amino acids. In mature elastin, these polypeptides are cross-linked through the side chains of lysines, some of which had been oxidized to aldehydes by the action of lysyl oxidase. In contrast, the microfibrillar component is rich in polar amino acids and does not contain these modified lysine residues and cross-links.

Pseudoxanthoma elasticum, a possible elastic tissue disease, is usually inherited in an autosomal recessive pattern, although a dominant pattern also has been described. Major manifestations occur in the skin and eye and the cardiovascular system. The skin shows thickened plaques and papules, most commonly localized to the face, neck, axillary and antecubital folds, lower abdomen, and thigh. The lesions may be 1 mm or less in diameter and barely visible, or they may be confluent yellowish plaques that tend to occur along skin creases. The typical ocular lesions are angioid streaks, which appear in the third or fourth decade, usually after the skin lesions. Angioid streaks result from cracks in Bruch's membrane, the structure located between the choroid and the retina. The vascular changes of pseudoxanthoma elasticum are usually confined to arteries, with occlusion of peripheral, coronary, and cerebral vessels. Bleeding may also occur, particularly into the gastrointestinal tract.

Histologically, in the skin, fibers accumulate that stain positively for elastic tissue, predominantly in the deeper dermis. The elastic fibers are swollen, irregularly clumped, and fragmented. These changes could result from a defect in elastin biosynthesis. The occurrence of calcium deposits and an increased content of proteoglycans are assumed to be secondary events.

COMPLEX CARBOHYDRATES OF THE GROUND SUBSTANCE AND THEIR DISEASES

The proteoglycans are composed of high-molecular-weight carbohydrates (glycosaminoglycans) attached covalently to a protein core. The glycosaminoglycans consist of repeating dimeric units of an amino sugar linked to a hexuronic acid or to galactose (as in keratan sulfate). The carbohydrate chains, in turn, are linked through xylose residues to the amino acids serine or threonine in the core protein. In articular cartilage, these proteoglycan subunits, containing many glycosaminoglycans, are attached, in association with a glycoprotein called *link protein,* to high-molecular-weight hyaluronic acid, the latter itself a glycosaminoglycan containing *N*-acetylglucosamine and glucuronic acid dimers.

The composition of the dimeric carbohydrate units of different glycosaminoglycans is unique; furthermore, the sugar residues may be sulfated at specific sites. For example, the dimeric unit of the chondroitin sulfate of cartilage consists of glucuronic acid and *N*-acetylgalactosamine, sulfated in the 4- or 6-position, whereas that of keratan sulfate consists of galactose and *N*-acetylglucosamine 6-sulfate. In dermatan sulfate, iduronic acid and acetylgalactosamine-6-sulfate make up the dimeric unit, whereas in heparan sulfate, glucuronic and iduronic acids are linked to either *N*-acetylglucosamine or glucosamine-*N*-sulfate.

In cartilage, the proteoglycans make up a significant portion of the extracellular matrix, although they are also found associated with the surfaces of cells in other tissues. Most diseases in which there has been a documented defect involving these substances, however, are due not to abnormal synthesis but to decreased degradation. The latter is ascribable to mutation in genes that code for the degradative enzymes or are responsible for some posttranslational modification. The secreted proteoglycans are taken up by cells through endocytosis, delivered to lysosomes, and then degraded by specific enzymes (endoglycosidases) that sequentially reduce the large carbohydrate chains to oligosaccharides. Thus, disorders of degradation are usually manifested by the intracellular accumulation of a polysaccharide modified no further than the site of defective enzymatic cleavage.

Clinical involvement is determined by the degree of enzymatic deficiency and tissue distribution relative to synthetic rates. The major organs most commonly involved are the skeleton, heart, nervous system, and eye. Although several of the disorders have their onset in infancy or early childhood with early death (e.g., Hurler syndrome), others may not be recognized until the second decade of life and are compatible with relatively long survival (e.g., Scheie syndrome). The consequences of lysosomal storage are enlargement and, occasionally, proliferation of cells, with-secondary deposition of other connective tissue components (e.g., collagen), resulting in the alteration and compression of surrounding structures.

Although the prognosis often is grave, in some instances, these diseases run a relatively mild course. Attempts are being made to replace the missing enzyme directly or by cell, tissue, or even gene transplantation.

REFERENCES

Akeson WH, Bornstein P, and Glimcher MJ, editors: Symposium on heritable disorders of connective tissue. St. Louis, 1982, Mosby.

Byers PH et al: Perinatal lethal osteogenesis imperfecta (OI Type II): a biochemically heterogeneous disorder usually due to new mutations in the genes for type I collagen. Am J Hum Genet 42:237, 1987.

Cole WG: Osteogenesis Imperfecta. In Martin TJ, editor: Bailliere's clinical endocrinology and metabolism. London, Philadelphia, 1988, Bailliere Tindall, Saunders.

Cole WG and Bateman JF: Regulation and organization of connective tissues. Aust NZ J Surg 58:263, 1988.

Dietz HC et al: Marfan syndrome caused by a recurrent de novo missense mutation in the fibrillin gene. Nature 352:337, 1991.

Kontusaari S et al: A mutation in the gene for type III procollagen (COL3 A1) in a family with aortic aneurysms. J Clin Invest 86:1465, 1990.

Krane SM: Genetic and acquired disorders of collagen deposition. In Piez KA and Reddi AH, editors: Extracellular matrix biochemistry. New York, 1984, Elsevier.

Kuivanieni H, Tromp G, and Prockop DJ: Mutations in collagen genes: causes of rare and some common diseases in humans. FASEB J 5:2052, 1991.

Lee B et al: Linkage of Marfan syndrome and a phenotypically related disorder to two different fibrillin genes. Nature 352:330, 1991.

Maslen CL et al: Partial sequence of a candidate gene for Marfan syndrome. Nature 352:334, 1991.

Neufeld EF and Muenzer J: Mucopolysaccharidoses. In Scriver CR et al, editors: The metabolic basis of inherited disease, ed 6. New York, 1989, McGraw-Hill.

Prockop DJ, Williams CJ, and Vandenberg P: Collagen in normal and diseased connective tissue. In McCarty DJ and Koopman WJ, editors: Arthritis and allied conditions: a textbook of rheumatology, ed 12. Philadelphia, 1993, Lea & Febiger.

Pyertiz RE: Heritable and developmental disorders of connective tissue and bone. In McCarty DJ and Koopman WS, editors: Arthritis and allied conditions: a textbook of rheumatology, ed 12. Philadelphia, 1993, Lea & Febiger.

Sakai LY, Keene DR, and Engvall E: Fibrillin, a new 350-kD glycoprotein, is a component of extracellular microfibrils. J Cell Biol 103:2499, 1986.

Spotila LD et al: Mutation in the gene for type I procollagen (COL1 A2) in a woman with postmenopausal osteoporosis; evidence for phenotypic and genotypic overlap with mild OI. Proc Natl Acad Sci USA 88:6624, 1991.

Uitto J et al: Elastin in diseases. J Invest Dermatol 79(suppl):160S, 1982.

Uitto J et al: Biochemistry of collagen diseases. Ann Intern Med 105:740, 1986.

VII DERMATOLOGY

CHAPTER

324 Cutaneous Manifestations of Connective Tissue Diseases

Thomas T. Provost
Eva Simmons-O'Brien
Michael D. Rader

> **Clinical features associated with subacute cutaneous (SCLE) and discoid lupus (DLE) erythematosus lesions**
>
> **SCLE**
>
> Nonscarring, minimal to moderate scale formation, no follicular plugging, very photosensitive.
>
> 30%-50% of SCLE patients satisfy diagnostic criteria for SLE.
>
> **DLE**
>
> Scarring lesion, prominent scale formation, follicular plugging, photosensitive but less than SCLE.
>
> 15%-20% of SLE patients have DLE lesions.

LUPUS ERYTHEMATOSUS

Cutaneous manifestations are common in lupus erythematosus. Only arthritis occurs more frequently. It has been estimated that approximately 15%-20% of patients with classic systemic lupus erythematosus (SLE) possess coin-shaped scarring lupus lesions (discoid lupus erythematosus, [DLE]). Furthermore, in the past it was estimated that approximately 60%-65% of SLE patients develop cutaneous manifestations during the course of their disease. With the increased use of systemic steroids and hydroxychloroquine, however, this frequency is probably less today.

The cutaneous manifestations of lupus erythematosus are divided into specific and nonspecific lesions. The specific lesions include the coin-shaped scarring (discoid) lesions as well as the generally nonscarring annular and psoriasiform erythematous lesions of subacute cutaneous lupus erythematosus (SCLE) (see box, above).

Discoid lupus

Discoid is a morphologic term meaning "coin- or disk-shaped" but unfortunately it has been employed incorrectly to differentiate cutaneous from systemic lupus erythematosus. Classic DLE lesions are round, annular, scarring lesions possessing an adherent scale and demonstrating telangiectasia. In addition, follicular plugging and hypo- and hyperpigmentation may be prominent. Most DLE lesions are found on light-exposed areas. In black patients, DLE lesions are frequently associated with prominent pigment alterations and can be extremely objectionable cosmetically.

The relationship between DLE lesions and systemic lupus erythematosus has intrigued physicians for years. In general, DLE lesions occur in the absence of systemic features and serologic abnormalities (antinuclear antibodies, etc.). DLE lesions can be viewed as one end of a spectrum of a multisystem disease. The other end of the continuum are those lupus patients with significant systemic disease (i.e., renal disease, etc.) without evidence of cutaneous disease. It is estimated that approximately 5%-10% of patients initially presenting with seronegative DLE lesions with time develop systemic disease.

It is important to emphasize that one cannot determine merely by examining the morphologic features of a discoid lupus lesion whether it is occurring in the presence or absence of systemic disease. This can only be determined by a history and physical exam and appropriate serologic tests.

Classic DLE lesions are seen in various forms. Discoid lupus lesions on the scalp produce a scarring, patchy alopecia. Over the malar eminences and the nose, they produce classic butterfly dermatitis. They may also occur as hyperkeratotic lesions, in which case the condition is termed *hypertrophic* or *hyperkeratotic lupus erythematosus*. Discoid lesions may also occur in association with tender or nontender nodular induration of the dermis and subcutaneous tissue. When these lesions occur the condition is termed *lupus profundus*. It has been determined that mucous membrane lesions characterized by ulceration and erosions have the same histopathologic features as classic discoid lupus lesions.

Discoid lupus lesions are characterized histologically by an inflammatory infiltrate composed predominantly of activated (HLA class II-positive) T lymphocytes (both CD4 and CD8).

Subacute cutaneous lupus erythematosus

The lesions of subacute cutaneous lupus erythematosus (SCLE) are annular, polycyclic, or psoriasiform with prominent scale formation. Unlike DLE lesions, those of SCLE generally do not scar and are not associated with follicular plugging or telangiectasia.

The serum of approximately 70% of these patients contains anti-Ro (SSA) antibody. Photosensitivity is a dominant feature of these patients; 90% of patients with anti-Ro (SSA) antibody are photosensitive. In fact, in many of these patients, skin disease is activated by long-wave ultraviolet light, and their skin will burn through window glass (see the box to the left).

Patients with distinctive SCLE cutaneous lesions have been described under a variety of headings, including antinuclear antibody–negative (ANA-negative) SLE; subacute cutaneous lupus erythematosus; late-onset lupus erythematosus; Sjögren's syndrome/lupus erythematosus overlap syndrome; and neonatal lupus mothers (Table 324-1). Identical lesions of SCLE have been seen in patients with homozygous C_2 and C_4 deficiency and in neonatal lupus infants. In addition to extreme photosensitivity, approximately 30%-50% of these patients satisfy the American College of Rheumatology minor criteria for the diagnosis of systemic lupus erythematosus. They lack, however, the increased frequency of severe renal disease associated with the presence of anti–double-stranded (native) DNA antibodies.

These annular polycyclic and psoriasiform lesions are most prominent in light-exposed areas and can involve widespread areas of the body. They may also involve the malar eminence and nose, producing classic butterfly dermatitis. Although SCLE lesions generally do not demonstrate the heavy lymphocytic infiltrate seen in the classic discoid lupus lesions, the inflammatory infiltrate is composed predominantly of $CD4^+$, $CD8^+$ activated T lymphocytes. Since these cutaneous lesions may be a prominent feature of neonatal lupus infants born of anti-Ro (SSA) mothers, it has been postulated that they arise, at least in part, by antibody-dependent cellular cytotoxicity mechanisms.

Prominent erythematous, edematous, "donutlike" lesions have been described in anti-Ro (SSA)-antibody–positive Asian patients, especially Japanese lupus patients. Approximately 50%-60% of Asian lupus patients are anti-Ro (SSA)-antibody positive (Table 324-1).

Table 324-1. Patient populations associated with anti-Ro (SSA) antibodies

Patient population	Frequency of anti-Ro (SSA) antibodies
Sjögren's syndrome	Variable; some cohorts by gel double diffusion ~ 30%-40% other cohorts by ELISA 80%-90%
Subacute cutaneous lupus erythematosus (SCLE)	~ 70%
Sjögren's syndrome/lupus erythematosus overlap syndrome (late-onset lupus erythematosus)	~ 80%-90%
Lupuslike disease associated with homozygous C_2 or C_4 deficiency	~ 50%-75%
Neonatal lupus infants' mothers	~ 95%
Japanese (All Asian?) lupus patients	~ 50%-60%

PHOTOSENSITIVITY

Photosensitivity is a major feature of lupus erythematosus; it has been noted in 40%-70% of SLE patients. As noted above, most DLE and SCLE lesions occur on light-exposed areas. Furthermore, recent studies have demonstrated that both UVB (280-320 nm) and UVA (320-400 nm) are capable of inducing the formation of lupus lesions in some DLE, SCLE, and SLE patients.

Nonspecific cutaneous lesions in systemic lupus erythematosus

In addition to the specific lesions listed above, lupus erythematosus patients frequently demonstrate a variety of nonspecific inflammatory and vascular lesions.

Alopecia is common in SLE (Plate VI-3). In addition to the scarring alopecia induced by DLE lesions, a diffuse alopecia may occur after flares of SLE. During these catabolic events, the normal growing hair bulbs (anagen) evolve prematurely into a resting phase (telogen). Approximately 3 months after induction of the telogen phase, the hair falls out (telogen effluvium) to be replaced by a normal (anagen) hair. This is a transient and diffuse alopecia.

In addition, the catabolic effect of an SLE flare may induce production of defective hair shafts that fracture a short distance above the scalp surface. This produces a characteristic thinning of the hair termed *lupus hair*. It is most prominent at the periphery of the scalp.

Inflammatory vascular disease in lupus erythematosus may manifest itself as short, linear telangiectasia in the cuticle nail folds; splinter hemorrhages; tender erythematous nodules on the tips of the fingers (Osler's nodes) and erythematous tender and nontender lesions on the thenar and hypothenar eminences (Janeway's spots). Urticaria-like lesions, livedo reticularis, and deep nodular lesions may also be manifestations of vasculitis. In addition, lupus patients may develop palpable and nonpalpable purpuric lesions over the lower extremities as manifestations of vasculitis; these lesions may or may not ulcerate. Histologically, most of these lesions demonstrate leukocytoclastic angiitis, but on occasion a mononuclear vasculopathy is seen.

Treatment. Cutaneous lesions of lupus erythematosus may be treated with a variety of preparations, including topical application and intralesional injection of corticosteroids and corticosteroid-impregnated tape. It must be stressed, however, that use of topical fluorinated corticosteroids, especially in the intertriginous areas of the groin, axillary regions, and the face, may produce atrophy and cosmetically objectionable telangiectasia.

Severe cutaneous lupus erythematosus may be successfully treated with a transient burst of parenteral corticosteroids (equivalent to 30-40 mg of prednisone daily and tapered over a period of 3 to 4 weeks). Pulse methylprednisolone therapy (1.0 gram intravenously on three successive days) is an additional option. Hydroxychloroquine, either alone or together with a burst of a methylprednisolone, may be used to control photosensitive lupus lesions. The patients are initially given 400 mg of hydroxychloroquine daily for 1 month and then 200 mg daily thereafter. Routine eye examinations are performed every 4 to 6 months to monitor for possible retinopathy. Quinacrine (Atabrine), 100 mg per day, has been effective in combination with hydroxychloroquine in controlling cutaneous lupus lesions. Quinacrine produces a characteristic yellow tint to the skin.

Recent studies have indicated that the skin lesions of some SCLE patients may respond to diaminodiphenylsulfone (Dapsone), 50-100 mg daily. This drug may be associated with a compensated hemolytic anemia, on unusual occasions with pancytopenia, and rarely with aplastic anemia. Glucose-6-phosphate dehydrogenase should be determined prior to initiating therapy, and at least monthly monitoring of a complete blood count is indicated in patients so treated.

In Europe, thalidomide has been reported to be effective in treating cutaneous lupus lesions. Also several reports indicate that retinoids (Etretinate) may be beneficial. In addition to these measures, lupus patients should be warned against excessive sun exposure. Protective clothing (i.e., long sleeved shirts and blouses, wide-brim hats, etc.) should be encouraged. Sunscreens protective against long- (UV-A) and short-wave ultraviolet light (UV-B; sunburn spectrum) should be judiciously applied. Sunscreens with a sun-protective factor rating of 15 are advisable.

Antiphospholipid syndrome (anticardiolipin, lupus anticoagulant)

In recent years, many reports have documented the existence of a syndrome characterized by multiple venous and arterial thrombosis, fetal wastage, thrombocytopenia, pulmonary and systemic hypertension, and livedo reticularis with or without ulcerations. This syndrome was first recognized 40 years ago in systemic lupus erythematosus patients who had a bleeding disorder and biological false-positive serologic test for syphilis. Since then, a group of antiphospholipid antibodies, including anticardiolipin antibodies, lupus anticoagulant, and others, has been described. Current figures estimate the prevalence of anticardiolipin antibodies in SLE patients to range between 30% and 50%. Most of these patients have low titer anticardiolipin antibodies by ELISA (less than five standard deviations); only 5%-10% of them have a history of a thrombotic episode.

The antiphospholipid antibodies (including lupus anticoagulant and the anticardiolipin antibody) are a group of related but distinct autoantibodies directed against negatively charged phospholipids (e.g., phosphotylcholine, phosphotylserine). Most recent experiments indicate that antiphospholipid antibodies require a cofactor present in normal sera. Several studies indicate that this cofactor is B_2-glycoprotein I (see also Chapter 293). The lupus anticoagulant interferes with the prothrombin activation complex (composed of activated factor X, factor V, platelet phospholipid, and calcium), prolonging the phospholipid-dependent coagulation tests, including the activated partial thromboplastin time, kaolin clotting time, Russell's viper venom time, and on occasion the prothrombin time. Mixing experiments with normal plasma fail to correct the prolonged coagulation times.

These autoantibodies produce in-vivo thrombosis and in vitro tests suggesting a defect in coagulation. The exact pathogenesis is unknown but may involve inhibition of prostacyclin, fibrinolysis, or protein C activation.

The antiphospholipid (APL) syndrome can occur in the presence or absence of SLE. In the absence of SLE the condition is termed the *primary APL syndrome*. In general, there is a gross direct correlation with the presence of clinical features of the APL syndrome and the titer of anticardiolipin antibodies. However, abnormal quantities of anticardiolipin antibodies in the absence of disease are seen in association with some medications (chlorpromazine, hydralazine), infections, carcinoma, human immune deficiency syndrome, and endocrinopathies.

The most common dermatologic association with APL is livedo reticularis, characterized by a violaceous netlike pattern involving the lower extremities. Stellate leg ulcers, tiny digital ulcers, or large deep suprainfected ulcerations may be present. In unusual instances, gangrene of digits may occur. Atrophie blanche (patches of ivory-white skin with telangiectasia surrounded by hyperpigmentation) indicative of a previous thrombotic event can be seen. Thrombophlebitis, ecchymoses, subungual splinter hemorrhages, and purpura are also observed. Prominent livedo reticularis of the lower extremities with central nervous system thrombosis (Sneddon's syndrome) is a manifestation of APL syndrome.

Treatment. At present, it is unclear what therapeutic modalities are effective in preventing this syndrome. Several therapeutic options exist. Anticoagulation with heparin and coumadin appear to inhibit the formation of new thrombi. However, complications arise, especially in patients with Sneddon's syndrome who have sustained strokes and are at risk for intracranial hemorrhage. Low-dose aspirin may also play a role in preventing the initiation of clot formation. Parenteral corticosteroids have been recommended (40 to 80 mg per day of prednisone). In fulminant cases, pulse intravenous methylprednisolone (1 gram infused over 4 hours daily for 3 successive days) may be indicated. Plasmapheresis has been employed to remove the circulating autoantibody. Cytotoxic agents have also met with some success. At present, however, no prospective control studies employing any of these treatments have been reported.

DERMATOMYOSITIS

Dermatomyositis is an inflammatory disease characterized by inflammation most prominently of proximal muscles and the skin (see Chapter 311). The amount or intensity of skin inflammation does not seem to be related to the degree of inflammation of the muscles. Rarely, the cutaneous manifestations of dermatomyositis can occur in the absence of muscle involvement (dermatomyositis sine myositis). In addition, it has been frequently noted that despite successful treatment of the myositis with immunosuppressive agents and/or corticosteroids, the skin disease fails to respond.

The cutaneous manifestations of dermatomyositis are characterized by erythematous, generally very pruritic lesions that may involve the trunk, extremities, and face. Photosensitivity is frequent. Lesions may appear as patchy, violaceous erythematous blotches or linear streaks. At times, the lesions may demonstrate atrophy, telangiectasia, and hypopigmentation, a condition termed *poikiloderma*. Facial lesions are characterized by periorbital edema and telangiectasia of the eyelids, giving a characteristic erythematous violaceous (heliotrope) appearance.

Involvement of the hands appears as erythematous, violaceous, slightly scaly papules over the extensor surfaces of the interphalangeal joints (Gottron's papules) (Plate VI-4). Similar violaceous erythematous papules can be found on the elbows and knees. Prominent cuticle nail fold telangiectasia is also frequently seen in dermatomyositis.

The pathologic features of the cutaneous lesions of dermatomyositis are quite similar to those of lupus erythematosus. The exact pathogenesis of these lesions is unknown, but there does not appear to be any relationship between cutaneous disease and the various autoantibodies associated with polymyositis and dermatomyositis (e.g., t-RNA synthetasis, [JO-1, PL-7, PL-12],and PM/Scl or Mi-2).

The presence of dermatomyositis, especially in patients over the age of 40, should stimulate a search for an underlying malignancy. These are most commonly adenocarcinomas of the gastrointestinal tract, but malignancies in other organs such as the breast and ovaries have also been detected. The presence of dermatomyositis may antedate by months or occur concurrently with the presence of the malignancy. Dermatomyositis may improve with the treatment of the malignancy and reappear with relapses.

Corticosteroids (equivalent to 60-80 mg of prednisone per day) and immunosuppressive drugs (e.g., methotrexate 25-50 mg I.M. once weekly) are effective in treating most patients with dermatomyositis, but as noted above the skin lesions may be resistant to this type of therapy. Chloroquine 250 mg daily or hydroxychloroquine 200-400 mg daily may control cutaneous manifestations. Antihistamines may also be needed to control the annoying pruritus so commonly associated with the cutaneous manifestations of dermatomyositis.

SCLERODERMA

There are three major forms of scleroderma: morphea, the acrosclerotic form, and progressive systemic sclerosis.

Morphea is a form of scleroderma characterized by sharply demarcated porcelain white plaques of indurated skin, with or without a surrounding halo of erythema occurring on all areas of the body. Plaques of morphea may be multiple and involve large areas of the body. This type of morphea has been termed *generalized localized morphea*. The white sclerotic portion of the lesion is thickened and demonstrates epidermal atrophy. At times, these lesions may be very superficial, failing to demonstrate induration. They are characterized by hyperpigmented patches, which frequently occur in a linear distribution. Classic morphea and this very superficial form of scleroderma are generally not associated with any features of systemic involvement. Raynaud's phenomenon, sclerodactyly, esophageal dysmotility, and pulmonary involvement are not features of this form of scleroderma.

Classic morphea lesions initially begin as erythematous edematous indurated plaques, which subsequently evolve into a sclerotic phase and finally an atrophic phase in which prominent hyperpigmentation may be present. The lesions may occur in a linear configuration producing depressed sclerotic deformities (coup de sabre).

The acrosclerotic form of scleroderma is characterized by sclerodactyly, Raynaud's phenomenon, facial and oral involvement, esophageal dysmotility, and pulmonary diffusion abnormalities (see Chapter 309). Cuticle nail fold injection is common. This is a chronic disease lasting many years or decades. The sclerodactyly leads to resorption of the terminal tufts of the phalanges; painful recalcitrant "ice-picked" ulcerations frequently occur. Secondary infection is common and may eventually lead to surgical amputation of the digit.

Facial involvement is prominent, leading to effacement of the normal wrinkles and a sharpening of facial features. Inability to wrinkle the forehead with upward gazing is common. Perioral tightening and contraction of the mouth is also common.

The CREST syndrome is a variant of this acrosclerotic form of scleroderma characterized by *c*alcinosis, *R*aynaud's phenomenon, *e*sophageal dysmotility, *s*clerodactyly, and *t*elangiectasia. The telangiectasia can be very prominent over the face. Unlike the telangiectasia of Osler-Weber-Rondu syndrome, from which it must be distinguished, the scleroderma telangiectasia generally do not involve mucous membranes. This form of acrosclerosis is associated with the anticentromere antibody.

The third form of scleroderma is characterized by a much more central onset with relatively rapid widespread dissemination and the rapid onset of pulmonary and other systemic involvement. Malignant hypertension is more frequent in this form of scleroderma. Anti–topoisomerase 1 antibodies (anti-Scl-70) are frequently found in this form of scleroderma.

The pathogenesis of the cutaneous lesions in scleroderma is unknown. A mononuclear inflammatory infiltrate occurs in the subcutaneous tissue beneath the dermis as the earliest change. Based upon in-vitro studies that demonstrate that gamma interferon and interleukin 1 (IL-1) are capable of inducing resting fibroblasts to synthesize collagen, it has been proposed that the sclerosis may be the result of the action of lymphokines released by these inflammatory cells. Currently there is no explanation for the small-vessel vasculopathy characterized by thickening of the intima of small arterioles and the Raynaud's phenomenon.

The treatment of all forms of scleroderma is unsatisfactory. Topical and parenteral steroids, azathioprine, and cyclophosphonide have all been tried with little or no effect. Recent studies, both retrospective and prospective, have suggested that D-penicillamine may produce beneficial effects in some scleroderma patients.

Scleroderma-like disease has been associated with various environmental exposures. For example, scleroderma has been associated with vinyl chloride exposure and more recently, sclerodermatous-like diseases have been associated with exposure to L-tryptophan and adulterated cooking oil (toxic oil syndrome) (discussed in Chapter 310).

VASCULITIS

Cutaneous lesions are commonly detected in patients with various forms of vasculitis. These include hypersensitivity vasculitis, Wegener granulomatosis, granulomatous vasculitis (Churg-Strauss syndrome), periarteritis nodosa, and giant cell arteritis (see Chapter 307). All these forms of vasculitis are putative immune complex–mediated diseases. The appearance of the vasculitis is determined by the intensity of the inflammatory insult and the level of blood vessel involvement in the skin. Inflammation of arterioles, venules, and capillaries high in the papillary portion of the dermis will probably produce petechial lesions. Involvement of the blood vessels in the reticular portion of the dermis most often produces erythematous, edematous lesions with or without induration. Vasculitis occurring in the subcutaneous tissue may cause tender or nontender nodular lesions, which may demonstrate varying degrees of erythema. If the inflammatory infiltrate is intense, tissue necrosis may be a prominent morphologic feature of the vasculitis. Tissue necrosis may take the form of small, shallow, or deep ulcerations, depending on the level of blood vessel involvement. Hemorrhagic necrosis resulting in bulla formation is also a variant of the tissue necrosis. The blisters may appear as sterile pustules because of the intense neutrophilic leukocyte infiltration into the vasculitic lesion. At times, the intensity of the inflammatory infiltrate may be very mild, producing plaquelike erythematous, edematous lesions or urticaria-like lesions. Some of these urticaria-like lesions may demonstrate petechiae and hyperpathia to light stimulation.

Of all the vasculitides with cutaneous manifestations, hypersensitivity vasculitis is by far the most common. Caused by inflammation of small blood vessels (postcapillary venules, capillaries, arterioles, and small arteries), this type of vasculitis is commonly seen in association with a drug-induced serum sickness, autoimmune connective tissue diseases such as lupus erythematosus and Sjögren's syndrome, and lymphoproliferative disorders. In addition, this form of vasculitis may be seen in association with infections (e.g., urticaria-like vasculitis associated with hepatitis B; the vasculitic lesions associated with subacute bacterial endocarditis, and the vasculitic lesions seen in the gonococcus arthritis-dermatitis syndrome).

Henoch-Schönlein purpura is a variant of hypersensitivity angiitis. It most frequently occurs in young children, but can also be seen in adults. It is characterized by purpuric lesions, with and without ulceration occurring most prominently over extensor surfaces of the skin (knees, elbows, and buttocks). In approximately 30% of cases, this form of vasculitis follows an upper respiratory infection. Besides the cutaneous manifestations, these patients frequently develop abdominal pain (secondary to vasculitic lesions of the serosal surface of the small intestine) or intersusception and arthritis. A small percentage of patients develop glomerulonephritis.

Erythema elevatum diutium is a chronic form of hypersensitivity angiitis characterized by erythematous, purplish, plaquelike lesions over the extensor surfaces of the skin (most commonly the dorsum of hands and knees). [Waldenström's benign hypergammaglobulemic purpura] is another form of hypersensitivity angiitis characterized by palpable and nonpalpable purpuric lesions occurring predominantly over the lower extremities. It is seen in association with hypergammaglobulemia and rheumatoid factor positivity. Hypocomplementemia may or may not be associated.

Approximately 10% of SLE patients develop urticaria. The urticaria-like lesions are cutaneous manifestations of a low-grade vasculitis and can be found anywhere, but they are most prominent on the lower extremities. These lesions are almost always seen in association with evidence of active SLE (i.e., hypercomplementemia and autoantibodies) and are not a feature of benign cutaneous lupus (discoid).

Another entity, hypocomplementemic urticarial vasculitis, has been described. Patients with this condition frequently have an autoantibody against C1q and present with widespread urticaria-like lesions which, on biopsy, demonstrate a leukocytoclastic vasculitis. They may also have an obstructive pulmonary disease.

Diagnosis

Suspicion of vasculitis should be confirmed by a biopsy. When appropriate, tissue from biopsies should be cultured and examined with Gram's stain to rule out septic embolization as a cause for the vasculitis.

It is important to remember that vasculitis is a systemic disease and other manifestations in other organs should be investigated. Many times the vasculitis is limited to small vessels and systemic involvement may be subclinical. With time, however, pulmonary disease, peripheral and central nervous system manifestations, or renal impairment may emerge and more aggressive therapy may be necessary to control the disease process.

Treatment

Treatment of hypersensitivity angiitis is complex. Obviously, if the vasculitis is secondary to a drug reaction, removal of the offending drug most often eliminates the vasculitis. Treatment of underlying infections, such as occur in subacute bacterial endocarditis and *Neisseria* gonorrhea, eliminates septic emboli as a cause of the vasculitis.

In cases of necrotizing vasculitis in which the etiology is unknown and suppression of the disease process is being considered, risk-benefit ratios must be taken into consideration. Corticosteroids and immunosuppressive drugs such as azathioprine and cyclophosamide suppress most cases of hypersensitivity angiitis. However, these agents are associated with significant side effects and treatment is often not necessary in patients with isolated hypersensitivity angiitis in whom there is no laboratory or clinical evidence of systemic involvement. Careful monitoring of these patients for evidence of systemic disease is warranted, however.

In some patients, dapsone (diaminodiphenylsulfone) may be effective, although this drug can be associated with the development of a compensated hemolytic anemia and, infrequently, with clinically symptomatic methemoglobinemia and sulfhemoglobinemia. On rare occasions, aplastic anemia has also been associated with dapsone use. Therefore, a complete blood count every 2 weeks for at least the first 4 to 6 months of therapy is recommended. Dapsone is most effective in treating the chronic form of hypersensitivity angiitis, erythema elevatum diutenum.

REFERENCES

Callen JP: Cutaneous lesions in connective tissue disorders. Clin Rheum Dis 7:325, 1982.

Dore N, Mogaveco H, and Provost TT: The cutaneous manifestations of connective tissue disease. In Mackie RM, editor: Immunodermatology, vol 11. New York, 1984, Churchill Livingstone.

Grob JJ and Bonderandi JJ: Thrombotic skin disease as a marker of the cardiolipin syndrome. J Am Acad Dermatol 20:1063, 1989.

Provost TT et al: The relationship between anti-Ro(SS-A) antibody–positive Sjögren's syndrome and anti-Ro(SS-A) antibody–positive lupus erythematosus. Arch Dermatol 124:63, 1988.

Sontheimer RD: The anticardiolipin syndrome. Arch Derm 123:590, 1987.

Sontheimer RD, Thomas JR, and Gilliam JN: Subacute cutaneous lupus erythematosus: a cutaneous marker for a distinct lupus erythematosus subset. Arch Dermatol 115:1409, 1979.

Soter NA: Two distinct cellular patterns in cutaneous necrotizing angiitis. J Invest Dermatol 66:344, 1976.

Soter NA, Austen FK, and Gigli I: Urticaria and arthralgias as manifestations of necrotizing angiitis (vasculitis) J Invest Dermatol 63:485, 1974.

Watson RM et al: Neonatal lupus erythematosus: a clinical serological and immunogenetic study with review of the literature. Medicine 63:362, 1984.

CHAPTER

325 Bullous Diseases

Diya F. Mutasim
Grant J. Anhalt

There are several skin diseases in which the primary lesion is a vesicle-bulla. The etiology of such diseases is variable. Some are infectious (bullous impetigo, herpes simplex, varicella). Others are caused by an inherited structural defect within the skin (the epidermolysis bullosa group of diseases), and some are caused by an allergic/hypersensitivity reaction to an antigen (allergic contact dermatitis, erythema multiforme). The above diseases are discussed under different chapters. This chapter addresses a group of diseases referred to as primary bullous diseases. These diseases, although distinct, share a putative and sometimes definite autoimmune etiopathogenesis.

PEMPHIGUS

The term *pemphigus* refers to a group of bullous diseases that share two distinctive features: acantholysis (detachment and rounding of adjacent epidermal cells from each other) and autoantibodies against specific antigens of what was formerly called the epidermal intercellular space. We now know that the autoantibodies do not bind to some amorphous space or substance, but to specific transmembrane cell adhesion molecules that belong to the family of adhesion molecules called *cadherins*—calcium-dependent adhesion molecules. The diseases vary with the level of acantholysis within the epidermis, and accordingly with the clinical appearance of the lesions, the epidemiology of cases, and finally, with the exact cadherin to which the autoantibodies bind.

Pemphigus vulgaris

Although this is a relatively rare disease, it is the most common form of pemphigus—hence the term *vulgaris*. It affects both sexes, predominantly during the fourth and fifth decades of life. The disease most often presents with painful oral erosions, which may last several months to a few years prior to diagnosis. Most patients ultimately develop skin lesions, which appear as flaccid bullae that rupture rapidly, leaving persistent erosions that become crusted and often infected. All mucous membranes with stratified squamous epithelium may become involved (mouth, pharynx, esophagus, nose, conjunctiva, glans, vagina, and anus). In extensive disease the scalp and upper trunk are consistently involved (Fig. 325-1, *A*). Pressure applied to an intact bulla leads to peripheral extension of the lesions, and shearing pressure applied to normal skin induces bulla formation (Nikolsky's sign). The course of the disease is marked by the continued appearance of new lesions, which heal very slowly. Data derived prior to the availability of oral corticosteroids showed the disease to be relentlessly progressive, with an ~ 50% mortality rate in the first 2 years and mortality approaching 100% by 5 years.

Histologic examination of an early lesion reveals acantholysis in a characteristic suprabasilar location. Basal cells remain attached to the basement membrane (Fig. 325-1, *B*). Ultrastructurally the initial site of separation of epidermal cells from each other is within nondesmosomal areas. Ultimately desmosomes split, resulting in complete acantholysis of epidermal cells.

Direct immunofluorescence (IF) performed on normal-appearing skin adjacent to a lesion consistently reveals deposition of IgG and to a lesser degree complement (C) components like C3 on epidermal cell surfaces. The majority of patients have circulating anti–cell surface IgG antibodies as detected by indirect IF using stratified squamous epithelium as substrate (Fig. 325-1, *C*). These antibodies bind

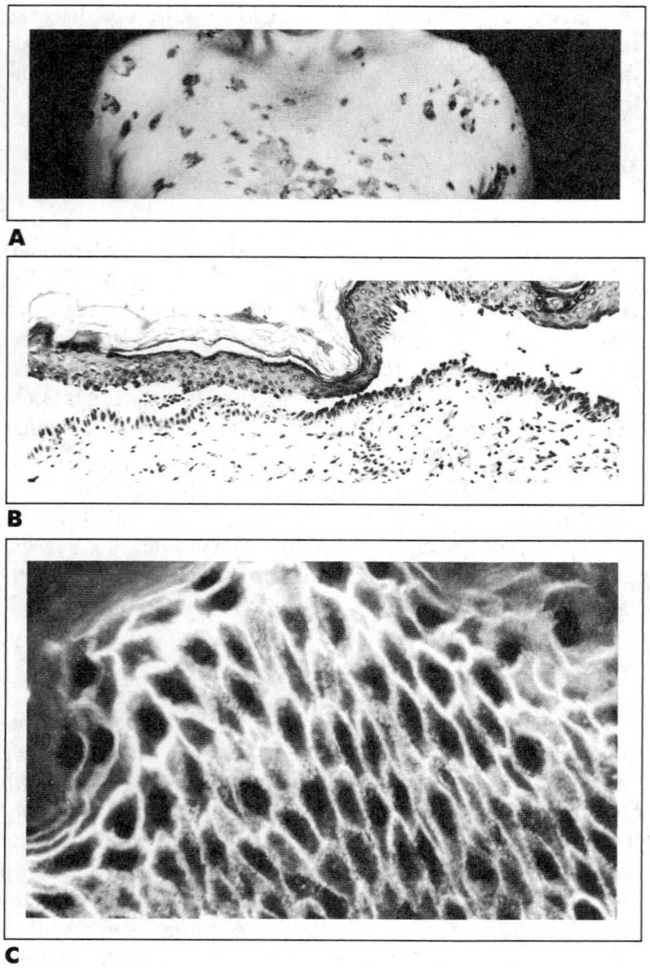

Fig. 325-1. Pemphigus vulgaris. **A,** Clinical presentation with erosions over the chest wall; intact blisters are seen less commonly because they rupture easily. **B,** Hematoxylin and eosin examination of a blister reveals intraepidermal splitting due to suprabasilar acantholysis. **C,** Indirect immunofluorescence performed on cryosections of normal human skin using the serum of a patient with pemphigus and fluorescein-labeled antihuman IgG. Note binding of antibodies to the intercellular space between epidermal cells.

the whole epidermal cell surface and identify a complex of epidermal proteins closely related to the desmosomes (M Wt. 210, 130, 85 kD). The 130 kD antigen is the pemphigus vulgaris antigen, an epithelial cadherin, the 85 kD band is a desmosomal plaque protein (plakoglobin) that is linked to the pemphigus antigen by reducible and nonreducible bonds, resulting in the detection of the lower M.Wt. band or the higher nonreducible complex at 210 kD. The autoantibodies are directed only against the 130 kD pemphigus antigen.

Pemphigus vulgaris is one of few diseases in which the autoantibodies have been proven to be pathogenic. When patients' IgG is injected intraperitoneally into neonatal mice, the animals develop a disease that is identical to the human disease. The mechanism by which the IgG induces acantholysis is not clear. There is in-vitro evidence that after IgG binds the epidermal cell surface, plasminogen activator is released from epidermal cells. This enzyme cleaves plasminogen into plasmin, which has proteolytic activity that may dissolve adhesion molecules of the cell surface and lead to acantholysis. On the contrary, there is also in-vitro evidence in other cells that antibodies binding to cadherins can cause cell-cell detachment in the absence of any other inflammatory event. The mechanism of cell dysadhesion in the human disease is probably quite complex.

Therapy must be aimed at clearing the pathogenic IgG autoantibodies. It is pointless to treat the target organ only (the skin), for the disease is a systemic autoimmune disease and disease activity is closely paralleled by rises and falls of the serum autoantibody levels. Reduction of autoantibody synthesis is often accomplished by long-term systemic corticosteroids such as prednisone in a 1-2 mg/kg/day dose. Pemphigus vulgaris has a chronic course and such long-term treatment with systemic steroids has potentially serious side effects. In addition, the disease may not be adequately controlled by corticosteroids alone. For these reasons, immunosuppressives such as azathioprine, cyclophosphamide, methotrexate, or cyclophosphamide plus plasmapheresis are required for their steroid-sparing effects in about one half of cases. Although patients with pemphigus vulgaris presently rarely die of their disease, some (approximately 5%) ultimately succumb to the side effects of therapy.

Pemphigus vegetans

This is a rare variant of pemphigus vulgaris in which the predominant site of lesions is the intertriginous areas (e.g., the axillae and groin). Lesions are persistent and characteristically thick and vegetating. This variant is believed to result from a peculiar host response to bullae in intertriginous areas or to chronic undertreatment of the disease.

Pemphigus foliaceus

Also referred to as "superficial pemphigus," this disease presents either in a sporadic form throughout the world or in an endemic form in South America (fogo selvagem).

The sporadic form most commonly affects the elderly. Lesions tend to appear and predominate over seborrheic areas such as the scalp, chest, and back. The primary lesion is a superficial vesicopustule, which may spread peripherally and then rupture, leading to the formation of scale-crust. Lesions may become secondarily infected. The severity of the eruption can be trivial, with only several persistent lesions, but may be life-threatening when a generalized exfoliative erythroderma develops. Unlike pemphigus vulgaris, mucosal lesions are extraordinarily rare and essentially "never" occur. This is a valuable clinical feature to differentiate pemphigus foliaceus from pemphigus vulgaris in which mucosal lesions predominate.

Histological examination of an early lesion reveals acantholysis within the granular cell layer with an occasional infiltration of neutrophils and/or eosinophils. Direct IF examination of normal-appearing skin adjacent to a lesion reveals deposition of IgG (predominantly IgG4) and occasionally C3 on the epidermal cell surfaces. Indirect IF reveals circulating anti–cell surface IgG antibodies in the majority of patients with active disease. These antibodies identify a complex of epidermal desmosomal proteins (M Wt. 160, 85 kD) by Western blotting and immunoprecipitation. The 160 kD target antigen of the autoantibodies is a cadherin called desmoglein I that is similarly complexed with plakoglobin to form the characteristic complex.

Like pemphigus vulgaris, pemphigus foliaceus is a tissue-specific autoimmune disease. Patients' IgG injected into neonatal mice induces characteristic cutaneous lesions in the animals. Remarkably, the epidermal lesions are superficial, as they are in affected humans. Again, it is thought that binding of IgG to the demoglein I abolishes the protein's physiologic function of epidermal cell adhesion, thus leading to acantholysis.

Most patients with pemphigus foliaceus can be controlled by a lower corticosteroid dose than is needed with pemphigus vulgaris. A dose in the range of 0.50 to 1.0 mg/kg/day of prednisone is usually sufficient. Most treated patients respond rapidly and the dose can be tapered over several months. The necessity to use steroid-sparing immunosuppressive agents in pemphigus foliaceus is uncommon.

Fogo selvagem (endemic pemphigus foliaceus)

This disease is similar to the sporadic variant of pemphigus foliaceous in its clinical presentation, histopathological and IF features, and immunochemical findings. It differs, however, in its geographical distribution (undeveloped areas near rivers in South America, especially Brazil) as well as its age of onset (both children and adults are affected). An insect vector is suspected of inducing the disease in South America.

Pemphigus erythematosus

This disease represents overlap of pemphigus foliaceus and lupus erythematosus. Patients exhibit a polymorphous eruption over the face and upper trunk that consists of vesicopustules and malar erythematous plaques that resemble lupus erythematosus. The histological findings are similar to those of pemphigus foliaceus, but IF reveals, in addition to IgG on the epidermal cell surfaces, multiple immunoglobulins and C3 at the basement membrane zone. Many patients have serologic abnormalities characteristic of lupus and some have clinical features of SLE. Some patients have an associated thymoma and occasionally myasthenia gravis. Therapy consists of corticosteroids and immunosuppressives.

Drug-induced pemphigus

Some patients using D-penicillamine, captopril, or rarely other medications develop a cutaneous disease that is indistinguishable from pemphigus foliaceus or, less commonly, pemphigus vulgaris. Such patients usually have autoantibodies against the cadherins that are recognized by sera from patients with idiopathic pemphigus foliaceus or vulgaris. These patients follow a course similar to the idiopathic disease variant.

Some patients taking the above medications develop a mild, transient variant of pemphigus that resolves shortly after discontinuation of the drug. These patients lack evidence of circulating or tissue-bound autoantibodies. There is evidence that D-penicillamine and captopril can directly induce acantholysis in skin explants in vitro, possibly by directly binding to the cadherins through their disulfide bond to plakoglobin and down-regulating their function.

Paraneoplastic pemphigus (PNP)

There are several reports of cases of pemphigus associated with cancer. These patients have been presumed to have PV in association with malignancy. This association has recently been investigated further, and a new variant of pemphigus has been reported. Patients with this disease have a malignancy, usually a lymphoreticular neoplasm, associated with a characteristic mucocutaneous eruption. The most commonly associated tumors include non-Hodgkin's lymphomas, chronic lymphocytic leukemia, thymomas, Castleman tumors, and poorly differentiated sarcomas. Lesions start within and around the oral and ocular mucosa as vesicles that rupture and develop into erythematous crusted erosions. At this stage the eruption is very similar to mucosal erythema multiforme/Stevens-Johnson syndrome. Later, generalized erythematous patches that undergo sloughing give the appearance of toxic epidermal necrolysis, or a more chronic, lichenoid eruption resembling a drug eruption can occur. Other mucosal epithelia can be affected. The course is rapidly progressive and often fatal within a few months when associated with a malignant neoplasm, but it usually resolves if a benign neoplasm (e.g., a thymoma or Castleman tumor) is found and removed completely.

Histologic examination of early lesions reveals features of PV (suprabasilar acantholysis) as well as features of erythema multiforme (lymphocytic infiltrate and keratinocyte necrosis). IF studies of perilesional normal-appearing skin reveal deposition of IgG and C3 both in the cell surfaces and occasionally in the basement membrane. Indirect IF reveals circulating antibodies against the cell surfaces of stratified squamous epithelia (like other pemphigus variants) as well as transitional epithelia, simple epithelia, and other tissues where desmosomes are present (hepatocytes and intercalated discs of myocardium). These antibodies identify a complex of epidermal proteins including desmoplakins I and II (M Wt. 250 and 210 kD) that are components of desmosomes, the 230 kD bullous pemphigoid antigen, found in the hemidesmosomes of the basement membrane zone, and a 190 kD antigen whose nature is unknown.

We suspect that the mucocutaneous disease results from a humoral and cellular immune response to anomalously expressed tumor antigens that cross-react with normal constitutive proteins of skin and other epithelia. A similar phenomenon is seen in paraneoplastic cerebellar degeneration syndrome and cancer-associated retinopathy.

PEMPHIGOID

The term *pemphigoid* is applied to a group of bullous diseases characterized by blistering at the dermal-epidermal junction (DEJ) and antibasement membrane zone (BMZ) antibodies that identify protein antigens of the hemidesmosome and lamina lucida. The different diseases are separated on the basis of their respective clinical presentations.

Bullous pemphigoid

Bullous pemphigoid (BP), the most common of this group of diseases, affects predominantly the elderly. The onset is frequently abrupt but occasionally may be insidious. Lesions tend to predominate over flexural areas but may be generalized. The initial lesions often appear as fixed urticarial plaques, which are later followed by tense, clear vesicles or bulla over inflamed as well as normal-appearing skin (Fig. 325-2, *A*). Bullae rupture, leading to crusted erosions that, unlike those of PV, heal within several days. Lesions continue to appear in crops and the disease usually follows a chronic course. Mucosal lesions occur only occasionally and are transient and trivial.

Histologic examination of an early lesion reveals separation of the epidermis from the underlying dermis and a variable infiltrate of eosinophils and lymphocytes in the upper dermis (Fig. 325-2, *B*). Ultrastructurally the separation occurs through the lamina lucida between the basal cell membrane and the lamina densa (basal lamina). Direct IF of perilesional skin consistently reveals intense deposition of C3 and relatively weak deposition of IgG (predominantly IgG4) at the DEJ. Electron microscopy shows these deposits to be within the lamina lucida in close proximity to the basal cell hemidesmosomes. Indirect IF reveals circulating anti-BMZ antibodies (predominantly IgG4) in 70% of patients (Fig. 325-2, *C*). These antibodies, like those of PV, bind only to stratified squamous epithelia, and specifically identify proteins of the hemidesmosomes (M Wt. 230 and 180 kD).

It is believed that after circulating BP antibodies bind the BMZ antigens, complement gets activated. Some complement components like C3a and C5a have the ability to attract polymorphonuclear leukocytes to the BMZ either directly or by an anaphylatoxin action on the mast cells with subsequent release of eosinophil chemotactic factors. The eosinophils then become activated and release proteolytic enzymes that digest the lamina lucida and lead to dermal-epidermal separation.

It is relatively easy to induce remission in most patients with BP. Corticosteroids in a dose of 0.5-1.0 mg/kg/day of prednisone are usually sufficient and can be tapered over 6-8 months. Infrequently, the addition of immunosuppressive medications such as azathioprine or cyclophosphamide is required for adequate control of the disease. Unlike PV, mortality from BP is rare.

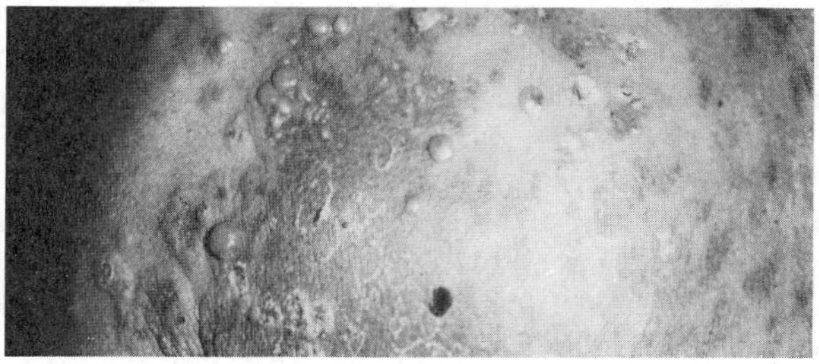

A

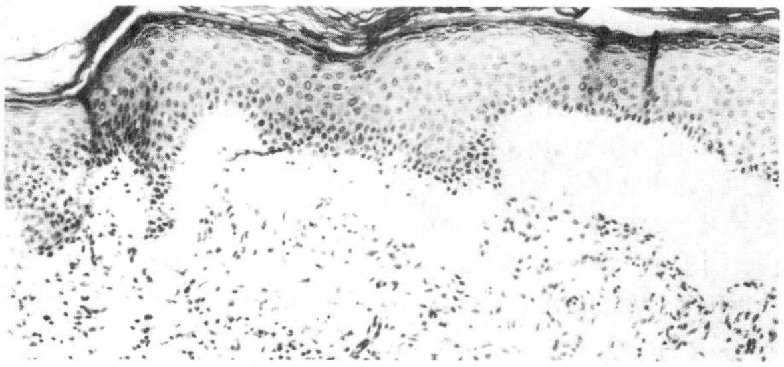

B

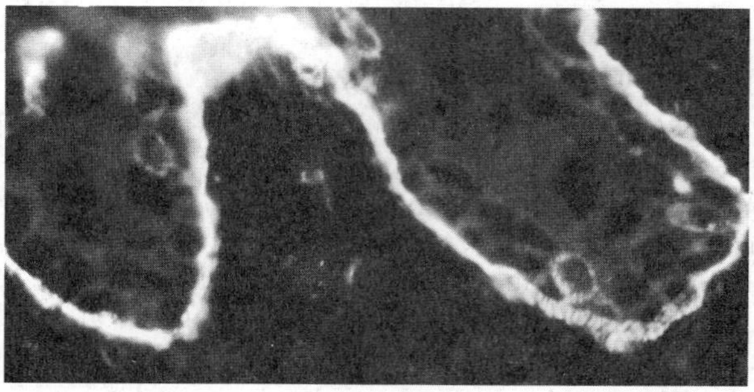

C

Fig. 325-2. Bullous pemphigoid. **A,** Clinical presentation with intact bullae as well as healing lesions. **B,** Hematoxylin and eosin examination of a blister reveals dermal-epidermal separation and a dermal inflammatory cell infiltrate. **C,** Indirect immunofluorescence performed on cryosections of rat tongue using serum for a patient with bullous pemphigoid, and fluorescein-labeled antihuman IgG. Note the binding of antibodies to the basement membrane zone in a linear and continuous pattern.

Cicatricial pemphigoid (CP)

Also known as benign mucous membrane pemphigoid, this disease involves exclusively or predominantly mucous membranes and consistently leads to scarring and dysfunction of the involved sites. The mucosal surfaces predominantly affected are the ocular and oral mucosae; less commonly the esophagus and nasopharyngeal and anogenital mucosae are involved. Lesions start as vesicles/bullae that rapidly rupture, leaving painful erosions that heal slowly with scar formation. In the eye, conjunctival scarring, entropion, and chronic inflammation of the ocular surface eventually lead to loss of vision if not adequately treated. In the esophagus, fibrosis and stenosis may lead to dysphagia or sudden death from choking on food. Similarly, laryngeal stenosis may require tracheostomy and result in asphyxiation.

The histological and IF features of CP are rather similar to those of BP except that only a minority of patients have circulating anti-BMZ antibodies.

Therapy is determined by the tissues affected and the anticipated morbidity. Oral lesions can be treated with topical and/or systemic corticosteroids. If the eye, esophagus, or larynx is involved, the anticipated morbidity or mortality requires treatment with systemic corticosteroids and cyclophosphamide. Dapsone and other immunosuppressives such as azathioprine have been used with some success.

Localized pemphigoid

Originally described by Brunsting and Perry, this is an uncommon disease that tends to involve most commonly the head and neck area, and occasionally the legs. Lesions tend to be limited to one area where recurrent vesicles-bullae heal with scarring. It is important to have a high index of suspicion for the disease, for the scarring can obscure any transient or infrequent blistering lesions. Histologic and direct IF findings are similar to those of BP. Only a few patients have circulating anti-BMZ antibodies.

Pemphigoid gestationis

More commonly known as herpes gestationis (HG), this is an uncommon disease that affects pregnant women and rarely women with ovarian tumors and secondary hormonal changes. The onset of the disease is during the late second or third trimester. Lesions appear first on the abdomen then spread to the rest of the trunk and proximal extremities and consist of urticarial papules and plaques followed by tense vesicles and bullae. Lesions cease to appear and the disease resolves within several days to a few weeks after delivery. The disease recurs during subsequent pregnancies and occasionally, in a mild degree, with menses and the intake of oral contraceptive hormones.

The histologic and direct IF findings are similar to those of BP. Sera of most patients have only trace amounts of an IgG anti-BMZ antibody (HG factor) that are undetectable by standard indirect IF testing. However, this IgG is avidly complement-fixing and is detectable by the in-vitro complement fixation IF on human skin substrate (HG factor test). The HG factor has the same ultrastructural binding site as BP IgG and it identifies most commonly the 180 kD and occasionally the 230 kD BP antigens. The pathogenesis of HG is believed to be similar to that of BP. The etiology remains uncertain and the importance of the underlying hormonal changes is unexplained.

Like BP, HG responds to moderate-dose systemic corticosteroid therapy. There may be a slightly increased risk of fetal morbidity and mortality, but this is controversial.

EPIDERMOLYSIS BULLOSA ACQUISITA

This disease was only recently identified, because it has clinical-pathologic features that in individual cases may closely resemble congenital epidermolysis bullosa, porphyria cutanea tarda, inflammatory BP, or cicatricial pemphigoid. It affects predominantly the elderly but has been reported in children as well. Lesions tend to start over the distal extremities and often are induced by trauma. Vesicles and bullae are usually followed by erosions that heal with superficial scarring and milia formation.

Oral, ocular, and other mucosal surfaces may be involved, mimicking a presentation similar to that of CP. The disease tends to be chronic with remissions and exacerbations. Histologically there is dermal-epidermal separation just beneath the lamina densa. There may be a dermal infiltrate of lymphocytes and neutrophils. Direct IF reveals IgG, IgM, IgA, and C3 at the BMZ of perilesional skin. Indirect IF reveals circulating anti-BMZ antibodies in only 50% of patients. These antibodies bind anchoring fibrils in the lower lamina densa and sublamina densa regions of the BMZ, and identify in SDS-PAGE a 290 kD subunit of collagen type VII, the major structural protein of dermal anchoring fibrils.

The pathogenesis of this disease is unknown but believed to involve antibody binding to the BMZ with subsequent activation of complement, chemoattraction of polymorphonuclear leukocytes, and finally proteolytic destruction of the subbasal lamina/anchoring fibril area that leads to blister formation.

Corticosteroids are of unpredictable benefit in this disease and are often effective only in very high doses. Most patients require the addition of other immunosuppressive drugs (azathioprine, cyclosporine, and others) for adequate control.

DERMATITIS HERPETIFORMIS

Dermatitis herpetiformis (DH) is an uncommon IgA-mediated bullous disease with a mean age of onset in the fourth decade. It is very rare in blacks and affects males more than females in a 3:2 proportion. Lesions classically involve the elbows, knees, buttocks, scalp, and face (Plate VI-5). The eruption is extremely pruritic. Primary lesions consist of grouped erythematous edematous papulovesicles and papulopustules that are only rarely seen intact because they are very rapidly excoriated. Occasionally, urticarial and bullous lesions are seen. Without therapy the disease is lifelong in almost all patients. DH is associated with thyroid disease as well as intestinal lymphoma. Of DH patients, 80% have histological evidence of gluten sensitive enteropathy (GSE) similar to that seen in celiac disease, that is, small-bowel villous atrophy and lamina propria lymphocytic infiltration. However, only 10%-15% of patients have symptomatic GSE. There is no correlation between the severity of DH and that of GSE.

The earliest histologic change is the appearance of neutrophilic microabscesses in dermal papillae that ultimately coalesce to form a subepidermal vesicopustule. Direct IF is diagnostic and reveals granular deposition of IgA in dermal papillae and to a lesser degree along the BMZ. Immunoelectron microscopy reveals the IgA to be deposited on microfibrillar components around fibers of elastin in the upper dermis. Indirect IF fails to reveal circulating antibodies against skin components. However, 40% of patients have IgA-containing circulating immune complexes. In addition, patients may have circulating antireticulin antibodies (40%), antigluten antibodies (80%), and antiendomysial antibodies (80%).

DH has a strong immunogenetic background. Most patients have the HLA B8, DR3, DQW2 phenotype. It is possible that an immune response–associated gene linked to the above phenotype is responsible for DH. However, the pathogenetic mechanisms responsible for IgA deposition in the skin are not clear. One theory proposes that gluten antigens gain access through the gut to the local lymphatics where sensitization takes place. Gluten proteins then bind dimeric IgA and complexes circulate in the serum until trapped by a specific antigen in the skin (possibly gluten receptor). Another theory proposes that GSE allows dietary (probably gluten) proteins to gain access to the circulation and induce the formation of antibodies that cross-react with skin antigens in the dermal papillae. Once IgA binds the skin, it is believed to fix complement via the alternate pathway. Some activated complement components (C3a, C5a) are potent chemoattractants for neutrophils that can digest the tips of dermal papillae, leading to blister formation.

DH responds dramatically to dapsone with cessation of pruritus within 24-48 hours. Most patients need lifelong therapy. A gluten-free diet may lead to clearance of lesions in 6-36 months, and may decrease or eliminate the dapsone requirement for disease control, but only if the diet is strictly observed.

REFERENCES

Anhalt GJ et al: Induction of pemphigus in neonatal mice by passive transfer of IgG from patients with the disease. N Engl J Med 306:1189, 1982.

Anhalt GJ et al: Paraneoplastic pemphigus. An autoimmune mucocutaneous disease associated with neoplasia. N Engl J Med 323:1729, 1990.

Jordon RE, Kawana S, and Fritz KA: Immunopathologic mechanisms in pemphigus and bullous pemphigoid. J Invest Dermatol 85:72S, 1985.

Katz SI and Strober W: The pathogenesis of dermatitis herpetiformis. J Invest Dermatol 70:63, 1978.

Mutasim DF and Diaz LA: The use of immunohistochemical techniques in the differentiation of subepidermal bullous diseases. Am J Dermatopath 13:77, 1991.

Mutasim DF et al: Definition of bullous pemphigoid antibody binding to intra- and extracellular antigen associated with hemidesmosomes. J Invest Dermatol 92:225, 1989.

Woodley DT et al: Identification of the skin basement membrane autoantigen in epidermolysis bullosa acquisita. N Engl J Med 310:1007, 1984.

CHAPTER

326 Cutaneous Malignancies

Renuka Diwan

A number of cutaneous malignancies arising from different constituent cells of the skin have been recognized. The commonest of these are basal and squamous cell carcinomas. Malignant melanoma is the most lethal of skin cancers. Other less commonly encountered cancers of the skin include verrucous carcinoma, microcytic adnexal carcinoma, Merkel cell carcinoma, dermatofibrosarcoma protuberans, leiomyosarcoma, carcinomas of the eccrine, apocrine, and sebaceous glands, and extramammary Paget's disease.

BASAL CELL CARCINOMA

Basal cell carcinoma (BCCA) is the commonest malignancy affecting humans. Its incidence exceeds 5 million cases per year in the United States. Predominantly a tumor of older age groups, its incidence continues to increase as the population ages. It is important that nondermatologists be able to recognize a BCCA because of its common occurrence.

The most frequent cause of BCCA is chronic exposure to ultraviolet B in the form of sunlight or artificial light sources used in tanning salons. Other less frequent situations in which BCCA arise include arsenic exposure, ionizing radiation, vaccination and chicken-pox scars, basal cell nevus syndrome, and xeroderma pigmentosum.

The typical patient with a BCCA is a fair-skinned elderly male engaged in outdoor work or recreation. The tumor typically occurs on sun-exposed skin. Most commonly a BCCA is an erythematous papule or nodule (Fig. 326-1), which may be ulcerated. On blanching a pearly appearance is visible. Prominent telangiectasias are often present on the tumor. A BCCA with this appearance is called *noduloulcerative* and is the most common clinical variety of BCCA. Other clinical types less frequently encountered are the morpheaform, superficial, and pigmented types. The morpheaform variety of BCCA is a whitish sclerotic plaque similar to a lesion of morphea (localized scleroderma). A superficial BCCA presents as an erythematous patch, often on a relatively non-sun-exposed area—the trunk, for example—and may be mistaken for a patch of eczema. A pigmented BCCA is a brown or black papule.

If a BCCA is encountered in a child or very young patient with a history of childhood BCCA, an underlying predisposing disorder such as the autosomal dominant basal cell nevus syndrome, xeroderma pigmentosum, or chronic arsenic exposure should be suspected.

The diagnosis of BCCA should be confirmed by a biopsy from the lesion. A biopsy also identifies the histologic subtype of BCCA and guides the selection of therapy. Histologic subtypes such as the morpheaform (which corre-

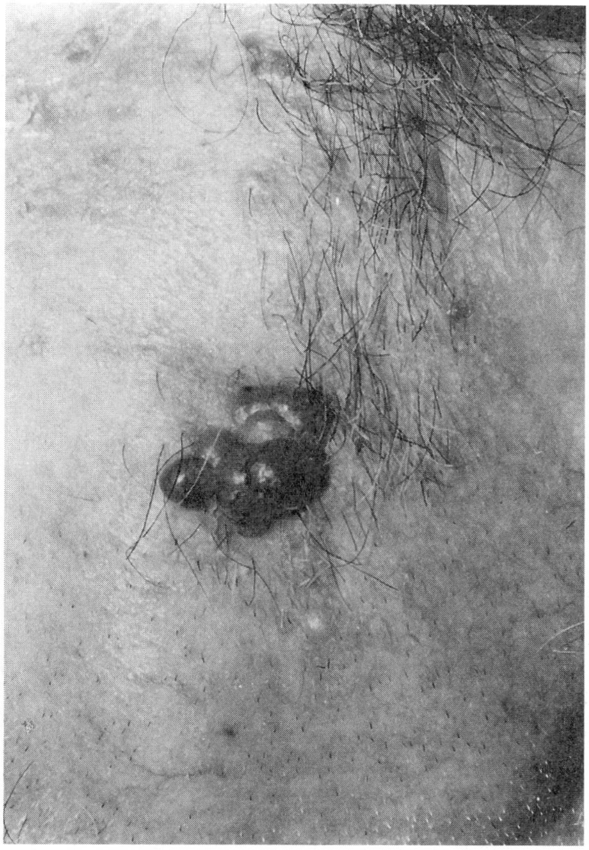

Fig. 326-1. Nodular basal cell carcinoma on the cheek presenting as an erythematous nodule with a pearly appearance and telangiectasias.

sponds with the clinical morpheaform type), micronodular, adenoid, and basosquamous forms tend to be more invasive and require special treatment to ensure complete eradication. The superficial type is amenable to a variety of superficial treatments.

There are many different methods of treating BCCAs. These include curettage and electrodessication, excisional surgery, cryotherapy, radiation therapy, topical 5-fluorouracil, and Mohs' micrographic surgery. The method chosen for a particular BCCA is determined by the risk of recurrence and the needs of the patient. Tumors likely to recur are those that are (1) recurrent after a prior treatment, (2) facial BCCAs larger than 2 cm in diameter, (3) BCCAs with morpheaform, micronodular, adenoid, or basosquamous histology, and (4) BCCAs located on the tip or alae of the nose or in the periorbital and periauricular areas. Tumors with any of these features, which make them difficult to cure, are best treated with Mohs' micrographic surgery to obtain the best possible cure rates of 97%–99%. Mohs' surgery also offers the additional advantage of being tissue-sparing. If a tumor with one of the above features is treated by one of the other methods, a cure rate of only 60%-80% can be expected. Tumors not at high risk for recurrence can be treated by any of the other alternatives to Mohs' surgery with cure rates of 90%-95%. Treatment with intralesional interferon is investigational at present.

Neglected BCCAs slowly cause extensive local tissue destruction (giving rise to the name "rodent ulcer"), but very rarely metastasize. Metastatic BCCA is fatal and there is very little data on its treatment, although chemotherapeutic agents have been tried with some success.

SQUAMOUS CELL CARCINOMA

Squamous cell carcinoma (SCCA) is the second most common malignancy of the skin and is most frequently caused by sun exposure (UVB). Other causative factors include exposure to ionizing radiation, arsenic exposure, products of coal combustion, oncogenic human papilloma viruses, chronic sinuses or ulcers, burn scars, and chronic heat exposure. An SCCA arising in a burn scar is also called *Marjolin's ulcer*. Immunosuppression associated with organ transplantation or diseases such as AIDS increases the incidence of squamous cell cancers.

An SCCA caused by sun exposure originates as atypical cells within the epidermis. Clinically, this alteration manifests as an actinic keratosis—a small, scaly or keratotic erythematous papule on a sun-exposed surface. An actinic keratosis is a precursor of an SCCA, which results from multiplication of the atypical cells that comprise the actinic keratosis.

The clinical appearance of an SCCA is variable. An SCCA in situ usually appears as as a scaly, erythematous patch or plaque, which may mimic eczema or a superficial BCCA. An invasive SCCA appears as a keratotic papule or plaque or, when the tumor has progressed further, a fungating mass (Fig. 326-2) or ulcer. An SCCA in situ located on the glans penis, also known as *erythroplasia of Queyrat,* appears as a solitary, well-defined erythematous plaque. The diagnosis of an SCCA must be confirmed by a

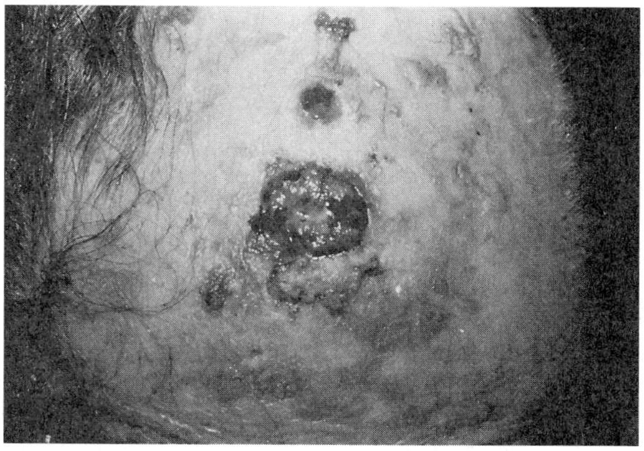

Fig. 326-2. Squamous cell carcinoma on a bald scalp presenting as a fungating friable tumor.

biopsy, which also provides other important histologic information, such as the degree of differentiation, that guides treatment.

The biologic behavior of an SCCA is influenced by its location, its etiology, the presence of immunosuppression, the degree of differentiation, and its size and depth of invasion. SCCAs arising from actinic keratoses are believed to be less likely to metastasize. Those on the lip have a much higher incidence of metastasis. This is also true for SCCAs arising in burn scars or chronic sinuses or in immunosuppressed patients. Poor differentiation, large size, and deeper invasion are associated with treatment failures and a greater likelihood of metastases.

Treatment of SCCA depends on the risk of recurrence of a particular lesion as described above. Small SCCAs on the extremities or trunk can be adequately treated by curettage and electrodessication, excision, or cryotherapy. SCCAs likely to metastasize are best treated with Mohs' surgery. Radiation therapy is usually reserved for inoperable tumors.

REFERENCES

Diwan R and Skouge JW: Basal cell carcinoma. Curr Probl Dermatol 2:70, 1990.

Dzubow L and Grossman D: Squamous cell carcinoma and verrucous carcinoma. In Friedman RJ et al, editors: Cancer of the skin. Philadelphia, 1991, Saunders.

Kwa RE, Campana K, and Moy RL: Biology of cutanoues squamous cell carcinoma. J Am Acad Dermatol 26:1, 1992.

Lang PG and Maize JC: Basal cell carcinoma. In Friedman RJ et al, editors: Cancer of the skin. Philadelphia, 1991, Saunders.

Rowe DE, Carroll RJ, and Day CL: Prognostic factors for local recurrence, metastasis and survival rates in squamous cell cancer of the skin, ear, and lip. J Am Acad Dermatol 26:976, 1992.

Swanson NA: Mohs surgery. Arch Dermatol 119:761, 1983.

CHAPTER

327 Psoriasis

Lisa A. Beck
Warwick L. Morison

Psoriasis is a chronic inflammatory skin disorder that affects 1%-2% of the world's population. It may be more common among Scandinavians and less common among American Indians and black Africans. Both sexes are affected equally.

GENETICS

A family history can be found in 5% to 10% of patients with psoriasis. Recent evidence from HLA antigen studies suggests a polygenic mode of inheritance. For example, certain class I MHC antigens (B13, B17, B37, B39, and Cw6) and class II MHC antigen DR7 occur with increased frequency in relatives of patients with psoriasis. A comparison of HLA haplotypes in 15 paired siblings with psoriasis revealed that 13 of the 15 pairs demonstrated identical HLA haplotypes, in contrast to the expected frequency of 4 identical HLA haplotypes. These results suggest that HLA-linked genes are in part responsible for the development of psoriasis. However, the fact that the concordance in homozygotic twins is only 66% suggests that environmental factors may also be important.

The onset of psoriasis is usually bimodal with the largest peak around the age of 16 to 20 years and a smaller peak from 50 to 60 years of age. Patients who develop psoriasis at an early age are more likely to have a positive family history, and approximately 85% are HLA-Cw6 positive. In contrast, patients with late onset usually do not have a family history and only 15% have the HLA-Cw6 haplotype. Patients with early onset often have more extensive disease and more nail involvement, and their course is often complicated by frequent relapses.

CLINICAL PRESENTATION

The diagnosis of psoriasis is usually made on the basis of the clinical exam only. With the exception of certain unusual variants of psoriasis, the presentation is one of symmetric, well-demarcated erythematous plaques with overlying silvery micaceous scales often with accompanying pruritus (Fig. 327-1). Removal of the scale typically demonstrates pinpoint bleeding, which is called the *Auspitz sign*. Although psoriasis may affect any part of the body, it has a predilection for the knees, elbows, scalp, intergluteal cleft, palms, and soles. Nail involvement occurs in up to 50% of patients. The nail changes are often nonspecific, but pinhead-sized pits, onycholysis, and a red-brown discoloration resembling a "drop of oil" are some of the more characteristic findings (Fig. 327-2). Oral psoriasis may be demonstrated histologically in less than 2% of patients. Clinically it may mimic a geographic tongue. A seronegative inflammatory arthritis is seen in approximately 7% of patients. Patients with psoriatic arthritis are more likely to have nail abnormalities and scalp psoriasis. A complete description of the characteristics of psoriatic arthritis are given in Chapter 312.

A common feature of psoriasis is its tendency to develop at sites of minor trauma. This occurrence, known as *Koebner's phenomenon,* is not unique to psoriasis and can be seen in other papulosquamous dermatoses such as lichen planus. For example, scratches, tattoo applications, and surgical incisions have all been known to elicit psoriatic lesions. Indeed, chronic trauma may be why psoriasis typically affects the skin over the knees and elbows. Other factors that may exacerbate psoriasis include psychosocial stress, antecedent infection (especially streptococcal), HIV infection, childbirth, and specific drugs. Several drugs that exacerbate psoriasis are beta blockers, lithium, nonsteroidal anti-inflammatory agents, interleukin-2, and, rarely, antimalarials. In addition, the use of systemic steroids, although helpful initially, may result in a dramatic flare or the development of a pustular variant of psoriasis when the

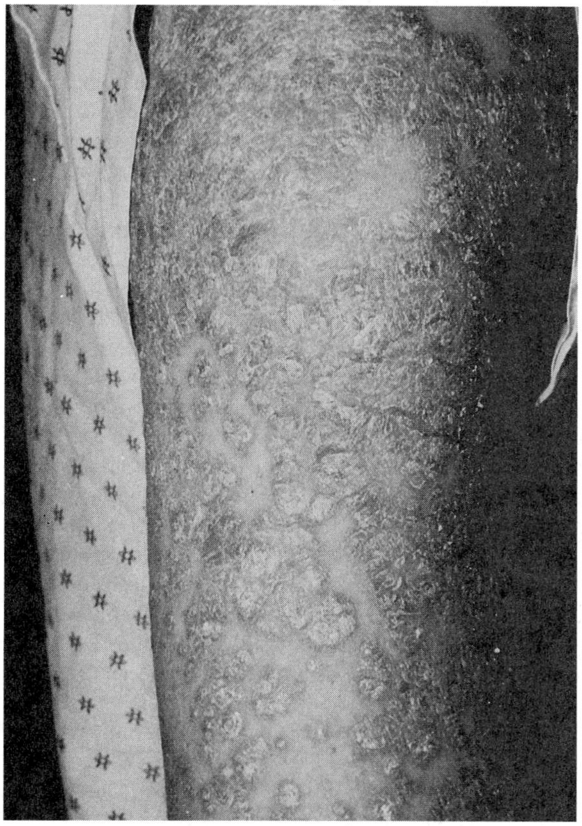

Fig. 327-1. Plaque-type psoriasis.

dose is reduced. Other dermatoses that might have a psoriasiform appearance include eczema, seborrhea, tinea, cutaneous T cell lymphoma, drug reactions, secondary syphilis, Reiter's syndrome, ichthyosis, and pityriasis rubra pilaris. When there is diagnostic confusion, a skin biopsy is often helpful. The histopathologic features of psoriasis are quite distinctive and are rarely confused with those of other dermatoses. Regular epidermal hyperplasia with focal parakeratosis, collection of neutrophils in the stratum corneum, and a mononuclear perivascular infiltrate are but a few of the characteristic changes.

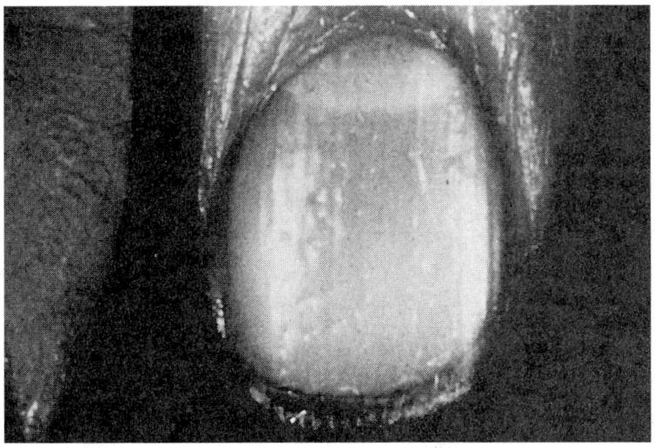

Fig. 327-2. Nail pitting seen in psoriasis.

There are five variants of psoriasis, which differ in their clinical appearance, severity, and response to treatment: guttate, plaque, inverse, pustular, and erythrodermic. *Plaque* type is the most frequently encountered variant. The lesions consist of indurated, sharply demarcated, oval to round plaques with the typical silvery scale (Plate VI-6). The lesions may be as small as a quarter or may expand to cover the entire presacral area. When lesions reach large sizes they may develop deep, painful fissures that make daily activities difficult. The *guttate* variety develops suddenly and often appears after a streptococcal infection. It consists of numerous small papules with slight scale. This variant may respond to oral antibiotics or remit spontaneously but may require traditional treatments to clear. *Inverse psoriasis* is often misdiagnosed as or coexists with a yeast or dermatophyte infection because of its location in the intertriginous areas. Psoriasis involving the axillary vault or inguinal region often lacks the characteristic scale because of the maceration that develops in such areas. *Pustular* psoriasis comes in three forms: plaques with a rim of pustules, palmoplantar pustules, and a rare generalized pustular eruption (Fig. 327-3). The latter form is the most severe with accompanying high fevers and leukocytosis. Ag-

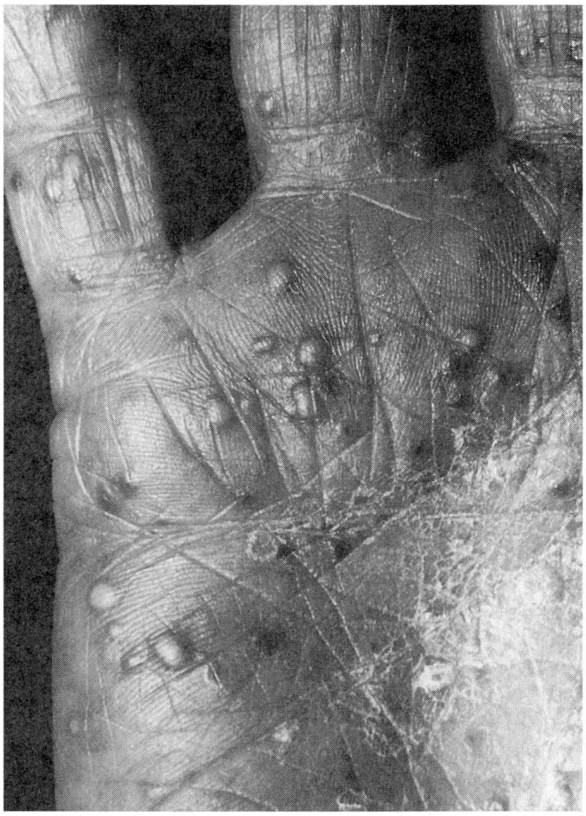

Fig. 327-3. Pustular psoriasis.

gressive treatment, often as an inpatient, including methotrexate or etretinate (Tegison), is often required. If psoriasis generalizes to involve the entire integument it is termed *erythroderma*. In this state, patients become hypermetabolic because of the water, protein, folic acid, and heat losses that develop as a consequence of a defective epidermal barrier. In patients with underlying coronary artery disease this hyperdynamic state may lead to high-output cardiac failure. A protein-losing enteropathy can also develop. Therefore, an erythrodermic patient must be treated aggressively and may often require in-hospital management.

PATHOGENESIS

Although psoriasis may vary widely in its clinical appearance, the tendency of the epidermis to hyperproliferate is common to all patients. Keratinocyte turnover is ten times more rapid and maturation is abnormal. Transplantation studies of human skin to nude mice have demonstrated that keratinocytes from both lesional and nonlesional psoriatic skin are hyperproliferative. What stimulates the epidermis to become psoriasiform has been the major focus of investigation for the last 20 years. Increased production of leukotrienes in the epidermis has been shown in some studies. The 5-lipoxygenase inhibitor benoxyprofen (taken off the market because of hepatotoxicity) produced remissions of psoriasis. The pattern of cytokine production from both perivascular T cells and keratincytes, as well the expression of adhesion molecules on endothelium have been the focus of more recent work. Tumor necrosis factor alpha (TNF-alpha) and interferon gamma (IFN-gamma) produced by mononuclear cells are probably responsible for stimulating keratinocytes to produce HLA-DR, intercellular adhesion molecule–1 (ICAM-1), interleukin-1 (IL-1), IL-6, IL-8, monocyte chemotactic activating factor (MCAF), and transforming growth factor alpha (TGF-alpha). Collectively these interactions result in keratinocyte activation and hyperproliferation, recruitment of inflammatory cells, and increased tortuosity of dermal papillary vessels, which are all characteristic of psoriasis. It remains unclear whether the primary defect in psoriasis resides in the inflammatory infiltrate or within the epidermis itself.

TREATMENT

Although there are no curative therapies for psoriasis, there are treatment options that adequately suppress the disease process and sometimes afford short periods of remission. The treatment is individualized based on the severity of a patient's disease, the patient's perception of his or her disease, accompanying medical problems, and the potential toxicities of each treatment. The treatments routinely offered fall in to five general categories: topical preparations, phototherapy, vitamin A analogs, antimetabolites, and 5-lipoxygenase inhibitors.

Topical therapeutic agents include corticosteroids, anthralin, and tar preparations. Corticosteroids are the most commonly prescribed therapy for psoriasis in North America, but it should be noted that the incidence of side effects has increased with the advent of the superpotent flourinated preparations. Only weak preparations, such as hydrocortisone, should be used on the face, perineum, and flexural areas. The major concerns with all corticosteroid preparations are dermal atrophy, skin fragility, fast relapse times, tachyphylaxis, and in rare cases, adrenal suppression resulting from systemic absorption.

Anthralin, a synthetic derivative of tree bark extract, has been used since 1916. It is used widely in Europe as part of the inpatient Ingram regimen. This regimen consists of a tar bath followed by exposure to ultraviolet B, which is followed in turn by an application of anthralin with salicylic acid. Repeating this sequence every 24 hours usually results in total clearing of extensive plaque-type psoriasis within 3 weeks. Anthralin can also be used as an Ingram regimen in patients with limited, thick, plaque-type psoriasis. The anthralin is administered in strengths up to 1% and applied directly to the psoriatic plaque for 10 minutes to 1 hour daily. Commonly experienced side effects are irritation of surrounding skin, brownish discoloration of treated areas, and purple discoloration of bathtubs and clothing or linen. It is not suitable for the head and neck, genitalia, or flexural areas, where it is too irritating.

One of the oldest remedies for psoriasis is crude coal tar, which is assumed to work by an antimitotic effect. Its use in psoriasis was popularized by Goeckerman in the 1930s, and the regimen now bears his name. This treatment consists of the daily application of 2% to 5% crude coal tar combined with a tar bath and ultraviolet light. Many modifications of this program have been put forth, the Ingram regimen being one of the more popular variants. Many psoriasis day care centers use a modification of the Goeckerman regimen for their patients. The criticisms of this treatment are the extended time commitments required of the patient and the associated mess. More recently, the use of liquor carbonis detergents (LCD) has replaced the use of crude coal tar.

Phototherapy refers to the use of sunburn-producing wavelengths (290-320 nm) of radiation or ultraviolet B for treating dermatoses. This therapy is administered three to five times per week and 20 to 30 treatments are required for clearing. Patients with erythrodermic or generalized pustular psoriasis usually do not respond to this therapy.

Photochemotherapy or PUVA refers to the combination of orally administered 8-methoxypsoralen, a photosensitizing drug, and exposure 1 to 1.5 hours later to ultraviolet A radiation (320-400 nanometers). In North America treatments are usually given three times per week, and 20 to 30 treatments are required for clearing. This form of phototherapy is more effective than ultraviolet B for thick plaque-type psoriasis, pustular psoriasis, and generalized erythroderma, but it also has more side effects. The major concerns are premature photoaging, nonmelanoma skin cancers, and premature cataract formation. A recent report identified 30 genital tumors in 14 men receiving PUVA therapy out of a cohort of 892. These risks may be minimized by having the patient wear ultraviolet A screening sunglasses, protecting the patient's skin for 12 hours after ingestion of the psoralen, providing genital protection during PUVA therapy, avoiding patients with prior arsenic or ionizing radiation exposure, and conducting regular skin and ophthalmologic exams. This therapy, like most systematic therapies for psoriasis, is contraindicated in pregnancy.

Etretinate (Tegison) is a vitamin A analogue that is particularly effective for acral or generalized pustular psoriasis. Etretinate is less effective in plaque-type psoriasis, in which other systemic therapies such as PUVA or methotrexate are preferred. Major side effects are mucocutaneous dryness, increased serum lipid concentration, and after prolonged treatment, skeletal changes. Etretinate is contraindicated in females capable of child-bearing except in exceptional circumstances because it can persist in the body for 2 years or more.

Methotrexate, a methyl analogue of folic acid, is the most commonly used antimetabolite for the treatment of psoriasis. Other antimitotic medications used less commonly include hydroxyurea and azathioprine. Methotrexate in doses of 2.5 to 25 mg per week is highly effective for extensive plaque-type psoriasis, pustular psoriasis, erythrodermic psoriasis, and psoriatic arthritis. It is thought to work by inhibiting DNA synthesis as well as neutrophil chemotaxis. Methotrexate is primarily used as a short-term treatment option to control psoriasis before switching to another therapy such as PUVA, UVB, or a topical regimen. Long-term methotrexate therapy is reserved for patients with severe psoriasis unresponsive to or intolerant of other less toxic treatments who have no contraindications to methotrexate as outlined by the American Academy of Dermatology in 1988. The major risks of long-term methotrexate treatment include hepatic fibrosis and cirrhosis, bone marrow suppression, and pulmonary toxicity. The most common side effects are nausea, loss of appetite, headaches, and alopecia. Conception must be avoided during treatment and for one menstrual cycle after completing treatment in women and 3 months after completing treatment in men.

A recent open study evaluating the benefit of an oral 5-lipoxygenase inhibitor, sulfasalazine (Azulfidine), found that 19 of 32 patients treated with 1.5 to 3.0 grams had a modest to marked improvement. Several trials are underway using similar preparations topically.

Cyclosporin, currently not licensed for use in psoriasis, has been shown in many studies to quickly clear 90% of psoriasis patients at a starting dose of 3 to 5 mg/kg a day orally. The risk of renal impairment and the consequences of immunosuppression have limited its use. Cyclosporin is most exciting because it may lead to a better understanding of the underlying immunologic mechanisms in psoriasis.

The treatment of each individual patient varies as dictated by the severity of the disease. Most patients experience both topical and systematic therapies during the course of their disease. It is not uncommon to combine therapies such as anthralin and PUVA, etretinate and PUVA, and methotrexate and PUVA to minimize the side effects of both treatment options and to shorten treatment times.

REFERENCES

Barker JNWN: The pathophysiology of psoriasis. Lancet 338:227, 1991.

Barker JNWN et al: Keratinocytes as initiators of inflammation. Lancet 337:211, 1991.

Henseler T and Christophers E: Psoriasis of early and late onset: Characterization of two types of psoriasis vulgaris. *J Amer Acad Dermatol* 13:450, 1985.

Morison W: Phototherapy and photochemotherapy of skin disease, ed 2. New York, 1991, Raven Press.

Nickoloff BJ: The cytokine network in psoriasis. Arch Dermatol 127:871, 1991.

Roenigk HH et al: Methotrexate in psoriasis: revised guidelines. J Amer Acad Dermatol 19:145, 1988.

Telfer NR et al: The role of streptococcal infections in the initiation of guttate psoriasis. Arch Dermatol 128:39, 1992.

CHAPTER

328 Dermatitis

S. Elizabeth Whitmore
James R. Nethercott

Dermatitis and eczema are interchangeable terms used to describe inflammation of the skin inclusive of the more superficial epidermal compartment. The histologic changes, which include edema and a mononuclear cell infiltrate in the epidermis, surface serous exudation, and a perivascular mononuclear cell infiltrate in the upper dermis, lead to the visible surface changes of edematous papules, vesicles, crusting, scaling, erythema, and edema. When the process becomes more chronic, the epidermis reacts by thickening or becoming acanthotic with the clinical appearance of a washboard; this change is termed *lichenification*. Dermatitis is a very broad term and for this reason different types of dermatitis have been defined. These definitions are based on frequently associated disorders, as in atopic dermatitis; cause, as in contact dermatitis; morphology, as in nummular dermatitis; and location, as in hand dermatitis. The different types of dermatitis may be caused by purely endogenous factors, exogenous factors, or a combination of the two.

ATOPIC DERMATITIS

Atopic dermatitis is usually seen in association with other manifestations of atopy, including allergic asthma or allergic rhinitis. Approximately 70% of patients give a history of atopy in the family. Although the etiology is not clear, it is considered to be a form of endogenous dermatitis and various immunologic alterations have been described in the majority of these patients. These include an elevated serum IgE antibody level, decreased delayed hypersensitivity responsiveness, decreased number of T suppressor lymphocytes, decreased number or activity of natural killer lymphocytes, and increased percentage of B lymphocytes with surface-bound IgE1. These immunologic abnormalities are probably involved in some way in atopic dermatitis, but it should be remembered that these changes are not present in all patients.

Atopic dermatitis is classically divided into three types depending on the time of onset. These include infantile, childhood, and adult atopic dermatitis. Key features of these subsets are outlined in Table 328-1.

It is frequently said that atopic dermatitis is the "itch that rashes," and therefore one of the fundamentals of treatment is reduction of pruritus. This is accomplished with avoidance of hot environments, sudden swings in environmental temperature, and large-fiber or stiff materials such as wools and starched clothing. The use of softened cotton clothing, gentle moisturizing cleansers, and frequent emollient lubrication is encouraged. Additionally, sedating antihistamines may be helpful purely because of their soporific effect. When clinical dermatitis is present, the first line of treatment is a topical corticosteroid. Not infrequently, patients also require oral antibiotics for recurrent infection or "dermatitis-aggravating" colonization with *Staphylococcus aureus*. When these treatments are ineffective, phototherapy with ultraviolet B radiation or photochemotherapy with ultraviolet A in combination with the oral photosensitizer, *psoralen,* may be quite effective. Immune-modulating therapies that have been used experimentally include interferon gamma, thymopoietin, and cyclosporin A.

Atopic dermatitis is clearly aggravated by irritants contacting the skin. Frequently, an adult patient who has a history of infantile or childhood atopic dermatitis experiences a recurrence of disease when exposed to irritants, particularly on the hands. It is for this reason that many dermatologists feel strongly that atopic individuals should be dissuaded from careers that involve a significant amount of wet work or frequent exposure to irritants.

NUMMULAR DERMATITIS

Nummular dermatitis is defined by its morphologic appearance of sharply circumscribed coin-shaped or discoid plaques of dermatitis. Although the etiology is not known, both patients and physicians have linked emotional stress to flares of disease. It seems likely that stress is not the primary cause, but instead an aggravating factor that causes patients to scratch more, thereby making the disease more persistent.

Patients affected by nummular dermatitis are usually adults. The typical presenting lesions are nummular plaques of coalescent papules and papulovesicles on an erythematous base. Early lesions usually have a moist surface as a result of a serous exudate that quickly becomes crusted. With time, the lesions become dry, scaly, and flattened. Al-

Table 328-1. Atopic dermatitis

	Onset	Characteristic localization of lesions	Lesion morphology	Typical topical corticosteroid treatment*	Natural history
Infantile atopic dermatitis	2 months-2 years	Face, extensor arms, legs	Localized areas of discrete and coalescing edematous papules with surface erosions, crusts, and scale	Hydrocortisone 1% ointment	Usual resolution within a few years
Childhood atopic dermatitis	2 years-adolescence	Flexural arms, legs, neck, wrists, ankles	Erythematous, slightly scaly papules coalescing into lichenified plaques; intermittent flares of more edematous, coalescing papules with surface erosions and crusts	Hydrocortisone 1% ointment up to midpotency fluorinated steroids†	Usual resolution by adulthood
Adult atopic dermatitis	Adulthood	Flexural sites as in childhood disease and/or hands and face	Erythematous, slightly scaly, papules coalescing into lichenified plaques; intermittent flares of more edematous, coalescing papules with surface erosions and crusts	Hydrocortisone 1% ointment up to midpotency fluorinated steroids†	Variable course

*Used adjunctively with the frequent application of emollients to protect and hydrate the skin.
†Midpotency fluorinated steroids should never be used on facial atopic dermatitis.

though the lesions are usually few in number, a generalized form with numerous nummular lesions may occur. Frequently, generalized nummular dermatitis becomes secondarily infected with *Staphylococcus aureus*.

Like atopic dermatitis, treatment includes avoidance of irritants and the use of emollients and topical corticosteroids. Secondary infection is treated with oral antibiotics.

ASTEATOTIC DERMATITIS

Asteatotic dermatitis is seen on a background of dry or xerotic skin. This dry skin is more vulnerable to irritants and it is this exposure that leads to subsequent inflammation or dermatitis of the skin.

Asteatotic dermatitis is seen most frequently in the winter months in older individuals exposed to environmental conditions that predispose to xerosis. These conditions include low ambient humidity and forced heat in the home, hot showers, and lack of emollient use. Once the skin becomes dry and develops microscopic cracks, it may sting, itch, and feel very tight. Patients begin to scratch, thereby causing more damage to the skin. Patients present with chapped-appearing, erythematous areas with a netlike pattern of fine scale, resembling tiny cracks in the skin. Lesions are usually seen on the legs, arms, and hands.

Treatment involves increasing the hydration of the skin and clearing the inflammation. For the former, warm showers or baths followed by oil-based emollients and avoidance of irritants is appropriate. For the latter, low- to midpotency topical corticosteroids are generally effective.

CONTACT DERMATITIS

Contact dermatitis is divided into two types: irritant and allergic contact dermatitis. The former is caused by an irritant contacting the skin. Susceptibility to irritants varies immensely among individuals. Patients having atopic dermatitis may develop irritant contact dermatitis from mild cleansers or even water, while "resistant" individuals may experience no visible skin changes with exposure to harsh detergents. Irritant contact dermatitis is most frequently seen on the hands, as this tends to be the area of greatest exposure. It is seen more commonly in individuals who are constantly wetting and drying their skin, exposed to cold outdoor winds or hot indoor forced heat, and exposed to any factors that dry the skin or strip away the outermost cells of the skin or surface water-holding substances. The most common irritants are alkaline solutions such as soaps and cleansers. These substances break down the protective keratin of the skin and allow penetration of substances into the skin.

If a harsh chemical has been encountered, the clinical change seen at the point of contact is that of a scalded, erythematous, moist area with peeling back of the overlying epidermis, leaving a fine, lacy scale at the border. In cases in which a mild irritant is encountered, the acute change is that of mild macular erythema. If exposure becomes chronic, secondary changes of scale and plaque formation occur, again localized to the area of contact. Treatment of irritant contact dermatitis involves eliminating the contactant(s) and the use of bland emollients and mild soap-free cleansing agents.

Allergic contact dermatitis is seen infrequently relative to irritant contact dermatitis. Unlike irritant contact dermatitis where a toxic effect occurs on the surface of the skin, allergic contact dermatitis involves an external antigen turning on an endogenous immune response of the delayed hypersensitivity type. The manifestation of this reaction requires an initial sensitization phase followed by a subsequent elicitation phase. A hapten is applied to the skin, binds to a cutaneous protein, and then encounters the immune cell of the epidermis, the Langerhans cell. If sensitization is to occur, the Langerhans cell moves into the dermis and travels through the lymphatics up to the regional lymph nodes where it stimulates production of a clone of T lymphocytes that recognize the antigen. Upon subsequent exposure to the hapten, Langerhans cells resident within the epidermis present the hapten to the circulating memory T helper cells that release interleukin-2 and interferon. These mediators recruit stimulated monocytes, which produce other cytokines. The resultant clinical reaction is that of an acute dermatitis.

The most common allergens clinically encountered are those of the *Rhus* genus including poison ivy, poison oak, and poison sumac. Exposure to the oil or oleoresin (containing urshiol) from these plants in sensitized individuals usually leads to an acute vesiculobullous eruption in the areas of contact. Other allergens tend to produce less dramatic reactions and sensitize a much smaller portion of the population. Such allergens include nickel, which is found in costume jewelry and various metal articles; neomycin, benzocaine, and merthiolate used as topical medicaments; fragrances found in most cosmetic and personal product items; and preservatives found in similar items, as well as dermatologic, ophthalmologic, and otic prescription and nonprescription formulations. Allergens that may be encountered in various occupations include potassium dichromate in persons working with cement, dyes, or textiles; epoxy resin in persons producing adhesives, product finishes, and casings for electrical devices; rosin in those working with or producing adhesive materials; thiuram and mercaptobenzothiazole in those working with or producing rubber products; glyceryl monothioglycolate and paraphenylenediamine in hairdressers applying permanent hair waves and dyes, respectively; and acrylates in production workers, orthopedic surgeons (from methylmethacrylate used in stabilizing implants), dentists, and manicurists and their patrons. Most often, persons having allergic contact dermatitis do not present with an acute dermatitis, but instead with a chronic dermatitis consisting of erythematous papules and lichenified plaques in the areas of contact. A meticulous history regarding both work and home exposures must be taken; if allergic contact dermatitis is then suspected, epicutaneous patch testing is performed in an attempt to reproduce the reaction. This involves applying a small amount of various suspected chemicals under occlusion for 48 hours; the sites are examined for localized reactions (erythema and edema, papules or vesicles) at 48 and 96 hours. Once the allergenic chemical(s) has been determined, avoidance of exposure is the cornerstone of treatment. Additionally, midpotency to high-potency topical corticosteroids clear the chronic dermatitis, while the extended use of emollients and avoidance of irritants protects the altered skin from further damage.

Contact urticaria

An important type of contact reaction that is not dermatitis is that of contact urticaria. This reaction is typically caused by a protein fraction of such things as latex, bacitracin, neomycin, benzocaine, lindane, and various metals, to name a few. The most frequent allergen seen causing immunologically mediated contact urticaria is latex. The incidence of this is thought to be increasing because of increased use of latex gloves, particularly in the medical profession. The immune reaction that occurs is an IgE-mediated response that clinically produces a localized hive (a sharply circumscribed area of erythema and edema that fades within minutes to hours). Much less frequently, the IgE reaction may become systemic, with generalized hives, and/or angioedema of the airway and hypotension causing anaphylactic shock. It is believed that individuals who are allergic to latex are at greater risk for an anaphylactic reaction when the antigen is encountered on mucosal surfaces such as the mouth, vagina, rectum, or internally as would occur with surgical procedures.

Recognition and diagnosis of this allergy with counseling on avoidance of latex exposures (latex gloves, balloons, condoms, etc.) and notification of these patients' physicians (patients require many specialized medical devices because latex tubing, endotracheal tubes, dental dams, surgical gloves, etc., all contain latex). Finally, patients must wear Medic Alert bracelets identifying their allergy and should carry an epinephrine-containing pen with them for emergencies.

HAND DERMATITIS

Hand dermatitis is a term frequently applied to any dermatitic reaction on the hands; the actual dermatosis that may be occurring may be atopic dermatitis, nummular dermatitis, contact dermatitis, or a primary "dyshidrotic hand dermatitis." This last-mentioned condition, unlike the first three, is always confined to the hands and has characteristic changes. The term is actually a misnomer in that there is no problem with hidrosis or sweating; the etiology is not known. The typical clinical presentation is that of deep seated, 1-2 mm vesicles primarily on the sides of the fingers, but also not infrequently over the palms. These are exquisitely pruritic and tend to cycle in waves. As the lesions clear, there is subsequent overlying desquamation and drying of the skin.

Treatment of this condition includes avoidance of irritants and application of emollients and topical corticosteroid creams or ointments for flares of disease. Additionally, it must be explained to the patient that this is a chronic relapsing disorder for which there is no cure.

INFECTIOUS ECZEMATOID DERMATITIS

This process of infection is a secondary change not infrequently seen in one of the previously discussed forms of dermatitis. It is marked by extensive serum crusting of the skin in the regions of dermatitis, and often, subsequent extension of the dermatitis and infection to areas not previously involved. The mainstay of treatment for this disorder includes antibiotics (covering for *Staphylococcus aureus,* the most common infectious agent), soaks, emollients, and topical corticosteroids as needed to control the primary dermatosis.

REFERENCES

Champion RH and Parish WE: Atopic dermatitis. In Rook A et al, editors: Textbook of dermatology, ed 5. Blackwell Scientific, 1992, Cambridge, Mass.

Domonkos AN, Arnold HL, and Odom RB: *Andrews' disease of the skin, ed 8. Philadelphia, 1990, Saunders.*

Fisher AA: Contact dermatitis, ed 3. Philadelphia, 1986, Lea and Febiger.

CHAPTER

329 Acne

Charlotte E. Modly

Acne vulgaris currently affects 80%-90% of young adults with sequelae that may persist indefinitely. Because of the physical and psychological impact, an understanding of the pathophysiology, clinical manifestations, and treatment modalities of acne vulgaris is essential.

EPIDEMIOLOGY

Although acne vulgaris is traditionally associated with adolescence, it can occur in the neonatal period and into the fourth decade of life. Under the influence of maternal androgens, the neonate's sebaceous glands are stimulated; this may account for the prevalence of acneiform lesions during the first weeks of life. Sebaceous glands become quiescent again until puberty, and the peak incidence of acne is in the mid to late teens. It is slightly more common in males than in females, and the severe forms of acne are much more common in males. Hormonal factors are probably responsible for the higher incidence of acne in postadolescent women than men.

PATHOGENESIS

The pathophysiologic events leading to the formation of an acne lesion occur within the microscopic structure known as the sebaceous follicle. The sebaceous follicle contains a small vellus hair and a large multilobulated sebaceous gland and is most concentrated on the face, back, chest, and shoulders. There are three principle components in the pathogenesis: (1) abnormal keratinization of follicular epithelium with the formation of the microcomedone (inspissated keratin, epithelial cells, sebum, and bacteria), (2) excess sebum production, and (3) enzymatic activity of *Proprionobacterium acnes* and *P. granulosum*. Host factors such as heredity, environment, and emotional state also contribute to the development of acne lesions.

The formation of the microcomedone is universal to all acne lesions. Abnormal follicular keratinization prevents the loss of epithelial cells normally carried out of the follicle by the flow of sebum. The epithelial cells adhere and trap sebum as well as bacteria in the infrainfundibular portion of the follicle. The microcomedone is not clinically apparent but is the precursor of all other lesions.

Sebum is extremely important in the development of acne. Sebum production is regulated by androgens of gonadal and adrenal origins through the conversion of testosterone to 5-dihydroxytestosterone by the sebaceous follicle. Individuals with severe acne produce more sebum, and those with low levels of androgens, such as castrated or adrenalectomized patients, do not develop acne. Sebum alters the environment in the follicle via three mechanisms: it accumulates behind the microcomedone causing follicular dilation, it provides a substrate for bacterial lipases that produce free fatty acids from the triglycerides in sebum, and it may contribute to abnormal follicular keratinization. The free fatty acids created are proinflammatory. In addition, the sebum from patients with severe acne is often deficient in linoleic acid, an essential fatty acid required for normal epithelial differentiation.

The anaerobic diphtheroids, *Proprionobacterium acnes* and *P. granulosum,* are primarily responsible for the inflammation seen in acne. Bacterial lipases produce free fatty acids, as mentioned above, but these are not as important as the recently identified low- and high-molecular-weight chemotactic peptides and proteolytic enzymes produced by the organisms. The peptides attract neutrophils, which in turn phagocytize the bacteria, thereby releasing proteolytic enzymes. These enzymes disrupt the follicular epithelium. Once the follicular contents contact serum in the dermis, complement is activated, and the inflammatory process continues.

CLINICAL MANIFESTATIONS

The lesions of acne vulgaris are heterogeneous. Localized primarily to the face and to a lesser degree to the back, chest, and shoulders, lesions can be inflamed or noninflamed. Erythematous papules, pustules, and large fluctuant nodules comprise the inflammatory subset. Open comedones ("blackheads") and closed comedones ("whiteheads") are the noninflammatory lesions. In patients with the severe form of acne known as *acne conglobata,* inflammatory cysts with sinus tracts are present.

The differential diagnosis of acneiform lesions includes acneiform drug eruptions, acne rosacea, chloracne, and chronic sun damage. Drugs such as lithium carbonate, dilantin, actinomycin D, bromide- or iodide-containing medications, and systemic corticosteroids can produce acneiform lesions, but usually they are more homogeneous than those of acne vulgaris. Recently, acneiform lesions have been recognized as a manifestation of anabolic steroid abuse. Acne rosacea, which can present with papules and pustules, also demonstrates telangiectases and sebaceous gland hyperplasia. Chloracne represents a reaction to chlorinated hydrocarbons and manifests itself as open comedones. The facial lesions of tuberous sclerosis can also mimic acne but upon close inspection are not follicular in distribution, are not heterogeneous or transient, and are associated with the neurologic, ophthalmologic, and cutaneous stigmata of tuberous sclerosis.

TREATMENT

Treatment of acne should be based on the pathogenic factors involved, that is, microcomedone formation, sebum production, and proliferation of *P. acnes*. Comedolytic agents include topical salicylic acid and topical tretinoin (transretinoic acid, Retin-A). Tretinoin is much more effective than salicylic acid, however, in preventing microcomedone formation and causing dissolution of mature comedones. Tretinoin normalizes epithelial differentiation and shedding, thereby preventing the cohesiveness that leads to microcomedone formation. It does not affect sebum production. Because the drug is now available in low-potency and less-irritating forms such as the 0.025% cream, tretinoin should be an essential part of the therapeutic regimen. Patients may experience some mild initial irritation and should be warned of enhanced photosensitivity while using tretinoin.

Sebaceous gland function can be altered through the use of hormonal therapy or isotretinoin. Estrogen and antiandrogen therapy is indicated in patients with evidence of ovarian androgen excess. Estrogens are usually prescribed in the form of oral contraceptives. Although it had been thought that at least 50 micrograms of estrogen per day are needed for a therapeutic response, recent evidence suggests that even 35 micrograms of estrogen, as is present in the newer triphasic contraceptives, may be sufficient to treat acne. Other antiandrogens, such as spironolactone, flutamide, and ciproterone acetate can be effective but usually require concomitant therapy with oral contraceptives to regulate menses. In patients with adrenal androgen excess, low-dose corticosteroids may be effective.

The most effective method of sebum suppression is through isotretinoin therapy. This systemically administered vitamin A derivative is reserved for severe cystic acne. It acts by markedly suppressing sebaceous gland function and abnormal keratinization and indirectly by decreasing bacterial growth. The impressive clinical performance of isotretinoin is tempered by the multitude of side effects, which range from universal drying of mucous membranes to hypertriglyceridemia and teratogenicity. Extreme caution should be used when prescribing isotretinoin to women of childbearing age. Concomitant contraceptive therapy is *mandatory*.

The anti-inflammatory armamentarium includes the benzoyl peroxides, topical and systemic antibiotics, and intralesional corticosteroids. The benzoyl peroxides are lipophilic, and antimicrobial without conferring resistance to the organisms. No significant clinical difference has been detected between 5% and 10% benzoyl peroxides. Topical erythromycin and clindamycin phosphate are equally effective in reducing acne lesions and are easily applied as solutions, gels, or ointments. The benefit of adding zinc to topical erythromycin solutions is currently being evaluated. Combining a topical antimicrobial with tretinoin enhances penetration of the antibacterial agent.

Systemic antibiotics used in acne include tetracycline, doxycycline, minocycline, erythromycin, and trimethoprim/sulfamethoxizole. Although tetracycline (1 gm/day) is used frequently and can be very effective, poor compliance can often interfere with therapeutic response. Doxycycline is also very effective but quite photosensitizing. Minocycline possesses better follicular penetrance and is very efficacious but expensive. Erythromycin (1 gm/day) is a cost-effective form of acne therapy, but *P. acnes* develops resistance to it more rapidly than to the tetracyclines. Long-term antibiotic therapy can sometimes lead to a secondary gram-negative folliculitis that may require therapy with antibiotics such as trimethoprim/sulfamethoxazole or isotretinoin.

Acutely inflamed lesions of acne often respond well to intralesional administration of triamcinolone acetonide. Systemic steroids are rarely used in the acute setting to treat a severe flare of nodulocystic acne. Surgical therapy, such as chemical peels, dermabrasion, scar revision, and soft tissue augmentation, is directed toward treating the disfiguring sequelae of acne.

In summary, a rational first approach to treating acne vulgaris includes comedolytic therapy with tretinoin and antibacterial therapy with benzoyl peroxides and/or topical antibiotics. A response requires 2-3 months of therapy, and if the response is inadequate, systemic antibiotics are necessary. Isotretinoin and hormonal therapy should be reserved for the specific situations outlined above.

REFERENCES

The American Academy of Dermatology: Guidelines of care for acne vulgaris. J Am Acad Derm 22:676, 1990.

Leyden JJ: The treatment and management of acne. J Int Postgrad Med 4:11, 1991.

Pochi PE: Guidelines for prescribing isotretinoin (Accutane) in the treatment of female acne patients of childbearing potential J Am Acad Derm 19:920, 1988.

Pochi PE: The pathogenesis and treatment of acne. Annu Rev Med 41:187, 1990.

Shalita AR: Pathogenesis of acne. J Int Postgrad Medicine 4:4, 1991.

Strauss JS: Biology of the sebaceous gland and the pathophysiology of acne vulgaris. In Soter NA and Baden HP, editors: Pathophysiology of dermatologic disease. New York, 1991, McGraw-Hill.

CHAPTER

330 Photodermatoses

Warwick L. Morison

Photodermatoses are disorders of the skin produced or exacerbated by exposure to sunlight or other sources of nonionizing radiation. Patients with these conditions are said to be photosensitive, and thus another name for these conditions is *photosensitivity disease*. Photodermatoses are common, and about 15% of people are photosensitive if exposed to a sufficient dose of sunlight. Fortunately, for most people the threshold of sensitivity is high. After one or two episodes these individuals usually appreciate their tolerance and subsequently avoid exposure of a duration sufficient to trigger the reaction. Thus, they rarely consult a physician. There are many different and distinct photodermatoses, but, fortunately for the clinician, five conditions account for almost all cases of photosensitivity: polymorphous light eruption (PMLE), solar urticaria, lupus erythematosus (LE), drug and chemical photosensitivity, and porphyria. Other disorders are very rare.

Ultraviolet (UV) radiation in sunlight is arbitrarily divided into the shorter UVB wave band (295 to 320 nm) and the longer UVA wave band (320 to 400 nm). UVB radiation is mainly responsible for a sunburn, a suntan, and other normal responses to sunlight. However, photodermatoses are often triggered by UVA radiation. An important practical point is that window glass filters out UVB radiation, so if a patient describes a reaction caused by sunlight through window glass, such a reaction is almost certainly abnormal.

Everyone shows some response to sunlight, and therefore the first step in diagnosing a photodermatosis is to determine whether the response of the patient is greater than normal. Photodermatoses take two forms: exaggeration of the normal responses to sunlight and the development of a separate and distinct rash from a normal exposure to sunlight.

EXAGGERATED NORMAL REACTIONS TO SOLAR RADIATION

Sunburn can appear as an extremely severe response in several situations. Skin that lacks normal pigmentation is obviously prone to severe sunburning. Thus, patients with albinism and vitiligo readily sunburn, and the underlying condition is usually quite evident. People with so-called type I skin, who always sunburn and never tan because they lack normal-functioning melanocytes, are also prone to develop severe sunburns. Freckling of the skin is a common added problem in these patients.

A severe sunburn in an otherwise normal person—that is, a severity out of proportion with the duration of exposure—is usually caused by drug or chemical phototoxic-ity. Compounds that commonly produce this reaction are listed in the box below. Systemic agents produce an exaggerated sunburn in all exposed areas, whereas topical agents produce a reaction limited to the area of contact exposed to sunlight. Phototoxic reactions may not follow the usual time course of a sunburn. They are often delayed in onset to 48 or 72 hours after exposure and may persist for a week or more. Dark pigmentation, often lasting for months, is a common sequela.

Several rare disorders should be considered in the diagnosis of a severe sunburn. In an infant or young child, repeated severe sunburns can be the first sign of xeroderma pigmentosum. Unfortunately, this early warning is usually not appreciated until the patient begins to develop multiple skin tumors as a teenager or young adult. Widespread freckling of exposed skin is another sign of this disorder and usually precedes malignancies. Erythropoietic protoporphyria (EPP) is another rare disorder that can present as an exaggerated sunburn. More commonly, however, the child or young adult with this condition complains of pain and tingling in the skin within minutes of exposure to sunlight, and the early onset of an exaggerated sunburn is only a minor consideration.

ERYTHEMATOUS MACULOPAPULAR REACTIONS

Rashes that are erythematous and either elevated above the skin (papular) or not elevated (macular) are the most common type of photodermatoses. Three conditions are in this category: PMLE, solar urticaria, and LE. Several points are important in the diagnosis. First, these eruptions are discontinuous; individual lesions are separated by normal skin, a feature that clearly distinguishes them from sunburn. Second, the eruption is confined to exposed skin but usually does not affect all exposed skin; a maximally exposed site such as the face might be spared while the eruption is confined to the minimally exposed lower limbs. Finally, the eruption is related to a specific exposure to sunlight. The patient is normal, goes out into sunlight, develops a rash minutes to days later, and recovers in hours to a week or more. These reactions do not usually persist throughout summer.

PMLE affects about 10% of Caucasians and is usually diagnosed as sun poisoning. The rash appears hours to a day or so after exposure to sunlight and persists for days or sometimes a week or more. Apart from macules and papules, vesicles may be present, plaques may form because of coalescence of lesions, and pruritus may change the lesions as a result of excoriations. LE can closely resemble PMLE, but the severity of the reaction, a history of burning through window glass, persistence beyond one week, scarring, and the presence of systemic symptoms help to warn that LE is the probable diagnosis (Chapter 306). Whenever in doubt, serologic tests, including an anti-Ro(SS-A) antibody determination to exclude a diagnosis of LE, are essential. Solar urticaria is a common skin condition in which hives appear after exposure to sunlight. This disorder is easily distinguished from PMLE and LE because it begins within minutes of exposure and resolves within hours.

Common phototoxic agents

- Psoralens (as medication and in plants and fruits)
- Coal tar derivatives (in medications and cosmetics)
- Vitamin A acid (Retin-A)
- Para-aminobenzoic acid esters
- Sulfonamides
- Nalidixic acid
- Demeclocycline
- Amiodarone

ECZEMATOUS REACTIONS

An eczematous reaction to sunlight may initially resemble a maculopapular reaction, but within a day the eruption becomes vesicular and continuous with no intervening normal skin. The rash eventually becomes scaly and crusted. Pruritus is a prominent symptom, whereas it is usually mild or absent with a maculopapular reaction.

There are several types of sun-induced eczema. The most common variety is photoallergy, and some of the common photoallergens are listed in the box on p. 3542. A usual sequence includes an acute episode related to topical application of the photoallergen, followed by exposure to sunlight. Provided further contact does not occur, the reaction clears within a week or two. Systemic photoallergy is usually caused by ingested drugs, and if use of the agent is continued without awareness of the causal relationship, the reaction persists and ceases to be related to specific exposures to sunlight. Thiazides are the most common cause of systemic photoallergy. Often the rash persists throughout summer and then subsides to some extent during winter. It is important to identify photoallergens, because repeated exposure to these agents can lead to a persistent light reaction that continues in the absence of the photoallergen and may become a lifetime problem.

BULLOUS REACTIONS

The most common bullous reaction to sunlight is porphyria cutanea tarda, and in this condition the lesions are usually confined to or are more prominent on the dorsum of the hands and forearms (Color Plate VI-7). The onset of lesions is usually related to minor trauma of the skin rather than sunlight. Thus, this is not a true photodermatosis, and the patient seldom complains of sunlight being a causal factor. Instead, the distribution of the rash suggests a photodermatosis.

Bullous pemphigoid and pemphigus can occasionally be triggered by exposure to sunlight, but this presentation is rare. More commonly, a bullous eruption caused by insect bites is confused with a photodermatosis because it occurs outdoors and is largely confined to exposed areas of skin.

Common photoallergens

Fragrances (musk ambrette and methyl coumarin)
Sunscreens
Halogenated salicylanilides (soaps and cosmetics)
Phenothiazines
Thiazides
Sulfonamides
Piroxicam

DIAGNOSIS OF PHOTODERMATOSES

The process of establishing the correct diagnosis of a photosensitivity disease often differs from that in other disorders of the skin because patients tend to present after the event, with normal skin and only a history of the reaction. However, it is still essential to see the reaction, which may require provocative exposure to either sunlight or an artificial source of light. The first step is to establish that the patient does have a photodermatosis. The history of the relationship between exposure to sunlight and appearance of the reaction, plus the distribution of the response, are the key indicators. Photodermatoses are usually confined to exposed areas, exhibit sharp cutoffs at the margin of clothing, and spare relatively nonexposed areas such as behind the ears, under the chin, and the inner aspect of the arms.

Provocative testing is very useful when the patient has already recovered from a reaction or to determine if a reaction is normal. Sunlight is a convenient source of radiation. The patient should be asked to expose a forearm to sunlight for a time sufficient to produce the response. In the case of a rash, this permits its examination and also a biopsy of skin for histologic evaluation. Other special tests such as urine and red cell porphyrins, patchtesting for photoallergens, and serology for LE may be required for diagnosis of some patients.

TREATMENT OF PHOTODERMATOSES

Specific treatment is available for a few photodermatoses, including phlebotomy for porphyria cutanea tarda, beta-carotene for EPP, and elimination of a phototoxin or photoallergen. The treatment of most photodermatoses, however, is nonspecific and consists of avoiding exposure to sunlight, use of protective clothing and sunscreens, and measures to decrease photosensitivity. A sunscreen with a high sun protective factor (SPF 15 or higher), broad-spectrum protection in both UVA and UVB, and good substantivity (labelled "waterproof") should be applied prior to any significant exposure to sunlight. Sunscreens are very effective in blocking UVB radiation but provide less protection against UVA radiation. Therefore, if a person is sensitive to these longer wavelengths, avoidance of exposure or physical protection with clothing is necessary. Patients who are markedly incapacitated by their photosensitivity can be desensitized by deliberate exposure to selected wavelengths of radiation, but this should be done only in specialized centers.

REFERENCES

Epstein JH: Polymorphous light eruption. J Am Acad Dermatol 3:329, 1980.
Frain-Bell W: Cutaneous photobiology. Oxford, 1985, Oxford University Press.
Harber LC and Bickers DR, editors: Photosensitivity disease, ed 2. Toronto, Philadelphia, 1989, BC Decker.
Jillson OF and Baughman RD: Contact photodermatitis from bithionol. Arch Dermatol 88:409, 1963.
Morison WL: Phototherapy and photochemotherapy of skin disease, ed 2. Raven Press, 1991, New York.
Parrish PA, Kripke ML, and Morison WL: Photoimmunology. New York and London, 1983, Plenum.

CHAPTER

331 Superficial Fungal Infections

Barbara Braunstein Wilson

Superficial fungal infections are those that involve the skin, hair, or nails. They are frequent in healthy individuals but are more common, more severe, and more resistant to therapy in immunocompromised hosts.

DERMATOPHYTE INFECTIONS

Dermatophyte infections (tinea) are acquired by contact with infected humans, animals, or soil. Although they are rarely life threatening, they are a cause of significant morbidity. The anthropophilic species *Trichophyton rubrum* is the most common cause of human infection. Zoophilic species such as *Microsporum canis, T. mentagrophytes,* and *T. verrucosum* can be acquired by humans from infected animals such as dogs, cats, and cattle. Dermatophyte infections manifest in several different ways, depending on the location of skin involvement.

Clinical presentations

Tinea corporis (Fig. 331-1) is a dermatophyte infection of the glabrous, or nonhairy, skin that begins as one or several small, pruritic, scaly patches that gradually enlarge to form annular lesions with erythematous, scaly, or vesicular borders and central clearing. New rings may form in the center and give rise to concentric rings.

Tinea cruris ("jock itch") is a dermatophyte infection of the groin seen most frequently in men. The eruption usually begins in the inguinal creases and may spread to the inner thighs and gluteal fold, but usually spares the scro-

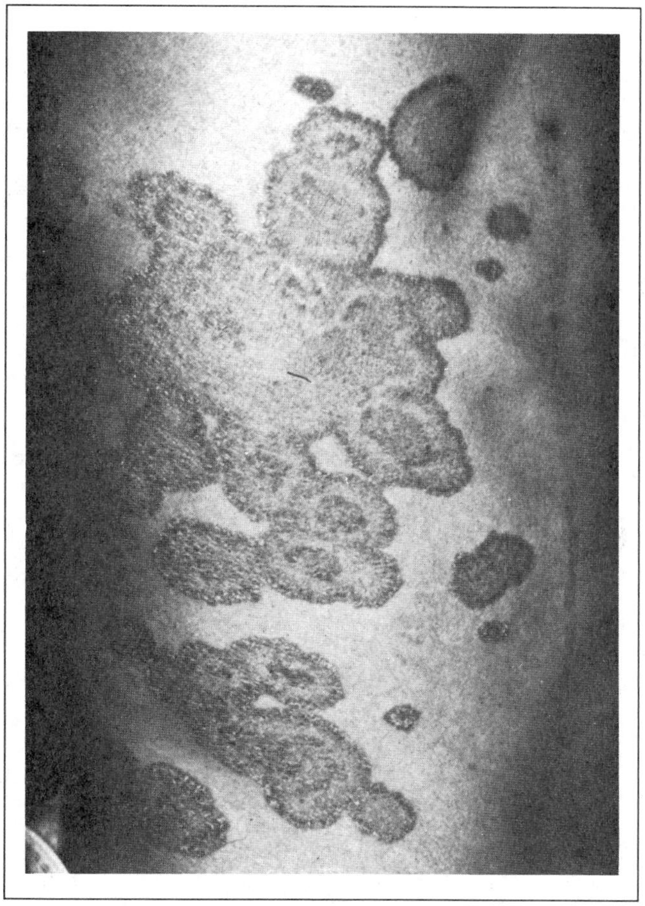

Fig. 331-1. Characteristic annular scaly erythematous lesions of tinea corporis.

tum. The eruption has a distinct, scaly, erythematous border and partial central clearing.

Tinea pedis (athlete's foot) is an extremely common affliction, especially of adult men. Tinea pedis is uncommon but does occur in children. Tinea pedis may present in three different ways. The most common presentation is infection of the toeweb spaces, especially the fourth, with mild to severe scaling, maceration, and fissuring of the interdigital skin. Another presentation is the so-called moccasin foot, in which the entire sole and sometimes the sides and dorsa of the feet are covered with fine scale and mild erythema. *T. Rubrum* is most often the causative organism. The toenails are also frequently infected. One or both hands *(tinea manus)* may show a similar eruption (Fig. 331-2). This clinical syndrome is chronic, extremely resistant to therapy, and frequently relapses after treatment. A third presentation is an acute inflammatory infection with vesicles and bullae on the feet.

Tinea capitis is seen primarily in children and usually presents as one or more localized, scaly patches on the scalp. The hair becomes lusterless and fragile and may eventually be lost. If the hairs are lost by breakage near the scalp, typical "black dots" are seen on the scalp. When marked inflammation is present, the patient may develop a tender, boggy, exudative plaque, called a *kerion* (Fig. 331-3). This inflammatory response is usually self-limited but may become secondarily infected with bacteria and can lead to significant scarring and permanent hair loss if left untreated.

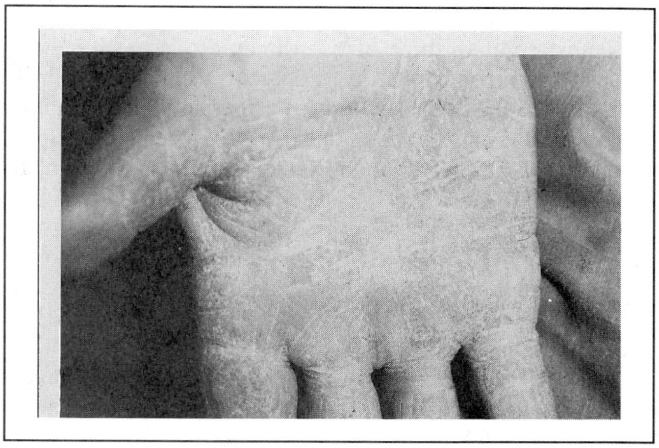

Fig. 331-2. Thickened, hyperkeratotic palmar skin in a patient with tinea manus caused by *Trichophyton rubrum*.

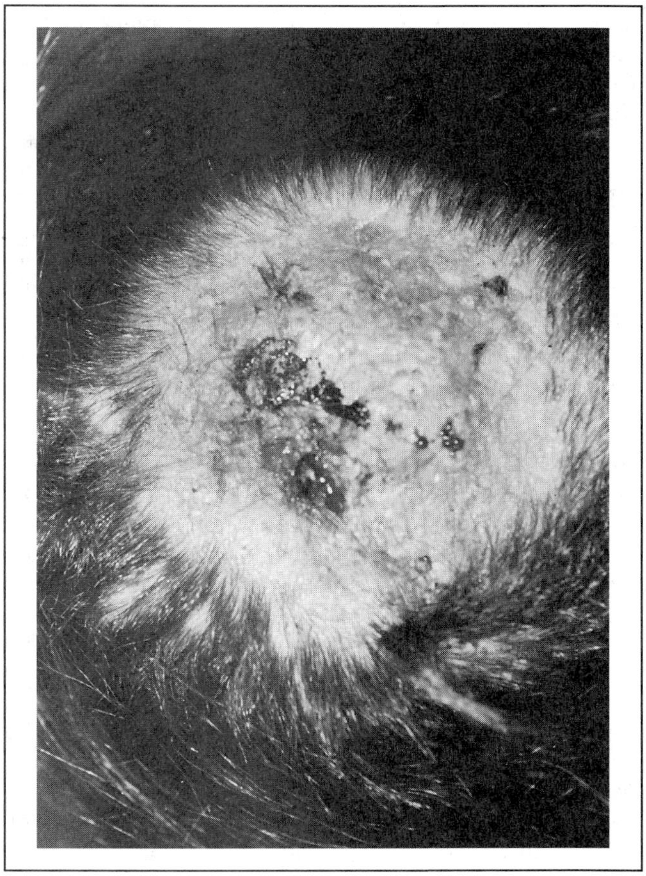

Fig. 331-3. Typical kerion of the scalp manifested as a tender, crusted, boggy plaque with overlying alopecia.

Tinea unguium is a dermatophyte infection of the nails. The most common type of tinea unguium is distal subungual infection manifested by yellow-white, thickened, brittle nails that may be lifted up from the nail bed by subungual debris. Proximal subungual disease presents as yellow-white discoloration that begins under the proximal nail plate and extends distally. This type of infection is rare in immunocompetent hosts. A third manifestation of tinea unguium, known as superficial white onychomycosis, presents as one or several chalky white spots on the surface of the nail. This is the only type of tinea unguium likely to respond to topical antifungal therapy.

It is not known why most people experience self-limited dermatophyte infections and others develop extensive, chronic, recalcitrant infections, usually caused by *T. rubrum*. Chronically infected persons frequently demonstrate decreased cell-mediated immunity to Trichophyton on skin testing. Host factors such as an atopic diathesis and genetic factors may predispose to chronic infection. *Trichophyton rubrum* has been shown to produce an immunoinhibitory factor that may suppress the host's cell-mediated immune response to infection.

Diagnostic procedures

Although a dermatophyte infection of the skin can be suspected clinically, the clinical impression should be confirmed with a potassium hydroxide (KOH) preparation of scale from an active border of a lesion. The presence of the characteristic fungal hyphae confirms the diagnosis (Fig. 331-4, *A*).

In the case of tinea capitis, several hairs should be removed from the affected scalp and the bulbs examined with a KOH preparation. A KOH preparation of subungual debris should be performed when evaluating tinea unguium.

A fungal culture using appropriate media such as Sabouraud's agar or Dermatophyte Test Media (DTM) should be performed if needed to confirm the diagnosis of tinea.

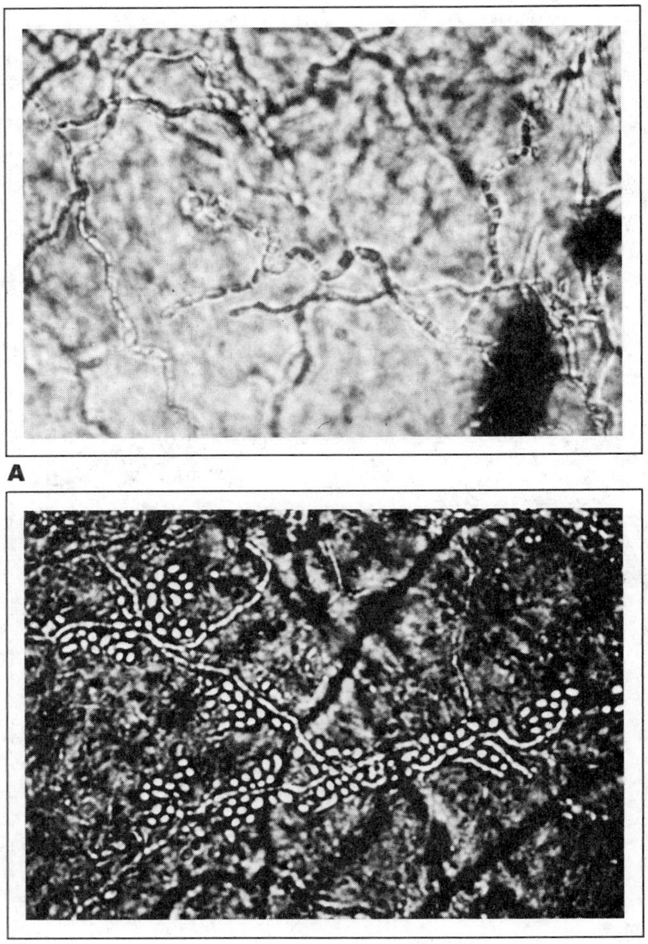

A

B

Fig. 331-4. Fungal hyphae can be seen on a potassium hydroxide preparation. **A**, Dermatophyte. **B**, *Candida*.

Therapy

There are many effective topical antifungal preparations including clotrimazole, miconazole, sulconazole nitrate, cyclopirox olamine, naftifine hydrochloride, ketoconazole, oxiconazole nitrate, and econazole nitrate. Mild, localized dermatophyte infections of the skin usually respond to a topical antifungal cream applied twice daily for 2 to 4 weeks.

Widespread, chronic, recalcitrant infections of the skin and virtually all cases of tinea capitis and tinea unguium require systemic antifungal therapy. Griseofulvin is the drug of choice for the therapy of dermatophytosis and is available in either a microsized or an ultramicrosized form. Most adult infections respond to 250 mg twice a day of the microsized griseofulvin or 125 mg twice a day of the ultramicrosized griseofulvin. Chronic, recalcitrant, cutaneous infections or nail infections may require twice the usual dose. Patients receiving long-term therapy should undergo periodic monitoring of their hepatic, renal, and hematopoietic systems.

Tinea capitis usually requires a 4- to 6-week course of griseofulvin, although longer periods of therapy may be necessary. When a kerion is present, therapy should include local application of wet compresses three times daily, and a broad-spectrum antibacterial antibiotic if secondary bacterial infection is suggested. A 2-week tapering course of oral prednisone may decrease inflammation and thereby minimize scarring.

Dermatophyte infections of the fingernails should be treated with griseofulvin for 6 to 9 months, and toenail infections for 9 to 18 months. Surgical or chemical avulsion of the nail before therapy may shorten treatment time and increase the likelihood of a cure; however, relapse rates remain high.

Ketoconazole is an effective, broad-spectrum, oral antifungal drug generally reserved for the therapy of dermatophytosis that is unresponsive to griseofulvin. The usual dose is 200 mg per day. Although most cases of tinea respond well to ketoconazole, relapse rates for tinea unguium and the chronic type of tinea pedis remain high. A rare but serious adverse reaction to ketoconazole is toxic hepatitis. Although terbinafine and itraconazole are not yet available in this country, studies indicate that they both are very effective in the treatment of dermatophyte infections.

TINEA VERSICOLOR

Tinea versicolor (TV) is a very common superficial fungal infection of the skin caused by the organism *Pityrosporum orbiculare (Malassezia furfur)*. Some predisposing factors are warm climate, pregnancy, corticosteroids, and immunoincompetence. Genetic factors may play a role.

Tinea versicolor is asymptomatic or mildly pruritic and most commonly involves the seborrheic areas of the skin, such as the neck, upper trunk, upper arms, and groin. The eruption consists of small hyperpigmented or hypopigmented, scaly patches that coalesce as they enlarge (Fig. 331-5). A KOH preparation of scale shows round budding spores and hyphae.

Pityrosporum also can cause a pruritic folliculitis on the upper trunk and shoulders. Although this eruption usually is seen in healthy persons, pityrosporum folliculitis has been described in bone marrow transplant recipients 2 weeks after transplantation.

Tinea versicolor can be treated with many different agents. Topical antifungal creams such as those used to treat dermatophytosis are effective but expensive when large areas of skin are involved. A mainstay of therapy is 2.5% selenium sulfide lotion, which is applied to affected skin for 10 minutes and then rinsed off. This is repeated for 10 consecutive days. No matter which agent is used, retreatment on 2 days of each month for 1 to 2 years often is required to prevent recurrence. Ketoconazole also has been used successfully in patients with extensive, recalcitrant TV. A recommended regimen is 200 mg daily for 5 days. This regimen is repeated monthly for 2 months. Selenium sulfide lotion can be used for maintenance therapy.

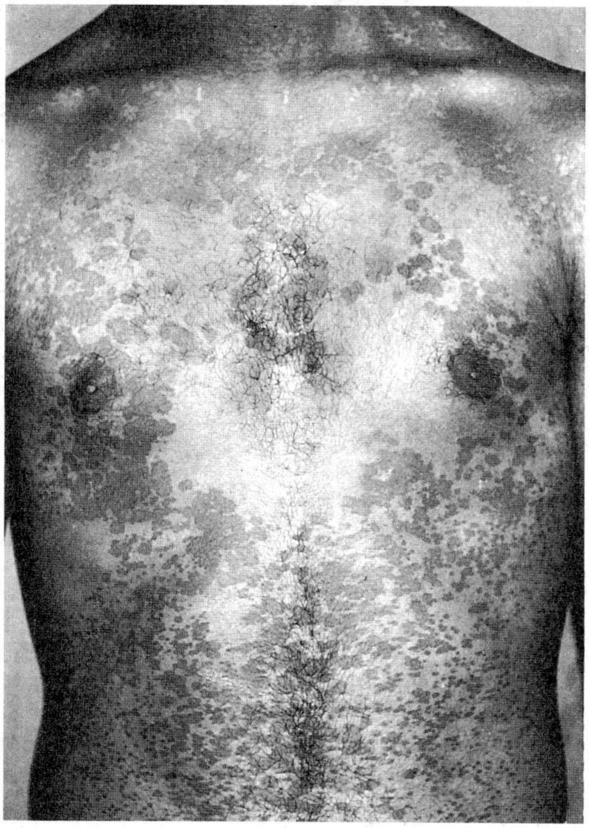

Fig. 331-5. Typical scaly hyperpigmented macules on the trunk of a patient with tinea versicolor.

CANDIDIASIS

Candidiasis is primarily an infection of skin and mucous membranes; under some circumstances, however, systemic involvement can occur. Predisposing factors for candidiasis are pregnancy, birth control pills, diabetes, antibiotics, corticosteroids, debilitation, and immunosuppression. Environmental conditions that encourage the growth of *Candida* are warmth, moisture, and occlusion.

Mucosal candidiasis

Oral candidiasis (thrush) presents as discrete, creamy white, friable patches on the oral mucous membranes. Removal of the patches with gentle scraping discloses an underlying inflamed mucosa.

Candidal vulvovaginitis causes vulvar pruritus and a cheesy vaginal discharge. Examination shows erythema and inflammation of the vaginal mucosa and vulvar area. Candidal balanitis is seen most frequently in uncircumcised males and usually presents as an erythematous papulopustular eruption near the coronal sulcus.

Cutaneous candidiasis

Candidal intertrigo involves skin folds such as the axillae, inframammary areas, groin, gluteal cleft, and interdigital skin. The affected skin is pruritic and intensely erythematous and may be macerated or eroded. The border of the eruption consists of papules and pustules that spread peripherally to form satellite lesions. In the male, candidiasis of the groin frequently involves the scrotum (Fig. 331-6). This finding helps differentiate candidiasis from dermatophytosis, in which the scrotum is seldom involved.

Candida can cause a chronic paronychia, which is manifested by erythema, edema, loss of the cuticle, mild tenderness, and occasionally by a purulent discharge from around the nail. Onycholysis (separation of the distal nail plate from the nail bed) is a frequent finding. Secondary *Pseudomonas* infection can cause a green discoloration under the nail.

Chronic mucocutaneous candidiasis

Chronic mucocutaneous candidiasis (CMC) is a progressive candidal infection seen in individuals with an underlying immune defect, usually of cell-mediated immunity. The disorder begins in infancy or childhood but also may be seen in adults with a thymoma and an associated immune deficiency. The infection begins as a typical, superficial

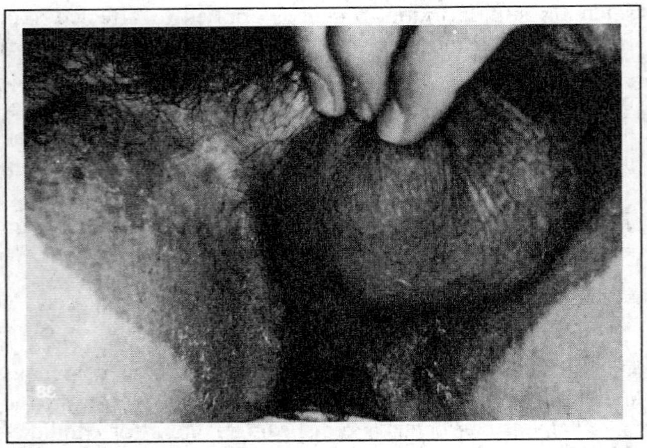

Fig. 331-6. Candidal intertrigo with characteristic scrotal involvement.

candidal infection but does not respond to conventional therapy. The eruption spreads to involve other areas of the skin, often becomes crusted and hyperkeratotic, and may lead to scarring and permanent hair loss.

Cutaneous manifestations of systemic candidiasis

Systemic candidiasis is seen most frequently in hospitalized patients who are debilitated and immunosuppressed. Other predisposing factors are indwelling intravenous lines, Foley catheters, and broad-spectrum antibiotics. The cutaneous eruption of candidemia consists of nonspecific erythematous macules and papules that may become hemorrhagic (Fig. 331-7).

Diagnostic procedures

The clinical diagnosis of cutaneous or mucosal candidiasis can be confirmed by performing a potassium hydroxide examination (see Fig. 331-4. *B*). Examination of the white patches of oral thrush, the vaginal discharge in vulvovaginitis, or a pustule from cutaneous candidiasis should disclose filaments as well as budding yeast forms. A skin biopsy of a lesion is needed to confirm the diagnosis of systemic candidiasis.

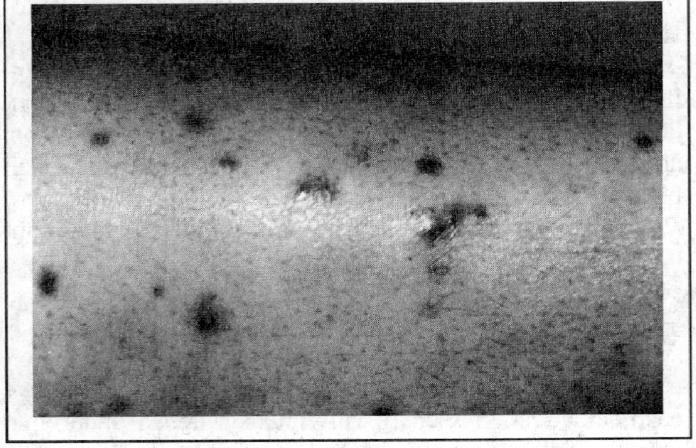

Fig. 331-7. Hemorrhagic papules in an immunosuppressed patient with candidemia.

Therapy

When possible, predisposing factors should be eliminated. Oral thrush responds well to nystatin suspension "swish and swallows" or clotrimazole troches, dissolved in the mouth several times daily. Candidal vulvovaginitis should be treated with intravaginal nystatin, miconazole, or clotrimazole cream or suppositories. A short course of oral fluconazole is also effective therapy against candidal vulvovaginitis. Candidal intertrigo should be treated with wet compresses, followed by air drying and the application of an antifungal cream, lotion, or powder three times daily. One percent hydrocortisone cream may be used concurrently to relieve itching and decrease inflammation. Recurrence is best prevented by keeping the area dry by using drying powders and wearing nonocclusive clothing.

Low-dose amphotericin B, oral ketoconazole, and more recently, fluconazole, are used to treat CMC, but the disease invariably recurs when medications are discontinued; therefore, maintenance therapy is required.

Amphotericin B remains the drug of choice for systemic candidiasis. Oral fluconazole also has been used successfully to treat systemic candidiasis.

REFERENCES

Allen HB and Rippon VW: Superficial and deep mycoses. In Moschella SL and Hurley HJ, editors: Dermatology. Philadelphia, 1985, Saunders.

Blake JS et al: An immunoinhibitory cell wall glycoprotein (Mannan) from *Trichophyton rubrum*. J Invest Dermatol 96:957, 1991.

Herbert AA: Tinea capitis: current concepts. Arch Dermatol 124:1554, 1988.

Jones HE: Cell mediated immunity in the immunopathogenesis of dermatophytosis. Acta Derm Venereol Suppl (Stockh) 121:73, 1986.

Roberts MM: Developments in the management of superficial fungal infections. J Antimicrob Chemother 28(suppl A):47, 1991.

Smith CB: Candidiasis: pathogenesis, host-resistance, and predisposing factors. In Bodey JB and Fainstein B, editors: Candidiasis. New York, 1985, Raven Press.

CHAPTER

332 Cutaneous Manifestations of Drug Reactions

Antoinette F. Hood

Drugs are ubiquitous in our society, and adverse reactions to drugs are common. These may occur in any organ and often are accompanied by a wide spectrum of signs, symptoms, and laboratory abnormalities. The Boston Collaborative Drug Surveillance Program reported drug-induced skin eruptions occurring in slightly more than 2% of all hospitalized patients. Although drug eruptions are only occasionally life threatening, they can produce significant morbidity, discomfort, and expense to the patient.

PATHOGENESIS

Drug eruptions can be produced by immunologic or nonimmunologic mechanisms. The basic pathogenic mechanisms involved in immunologic reactions are discussed in detail in Chapter 286 to 288 and discussed only briefly here.

Immunoglobulin E (IgE)–mediated drug *reactions* (immediate type hypersensitivity), as typified by penicillin allergy, are characterized by pruritus, urticaria, laryngeal edema, bronchospasm, and, occasionally, by anaphylactic shock. *Cytotoxic reactions* induced by drugs are generally manifested in the skin by purpura. *Immune complex–mediated drug reactions* are characterized by fever, arthritis, nephritis, neuritis, edema, and an urticarial or papular eruption. Serum sickness is the classic example of an immune complex–dependent reaction. Delayed hypersensitivity, or *T cell–mediated reaction,* as typified by contact drug hypersensitivity, appears as a papulovesicular eruption. Factors involved in the production of immunologically mediated drug reactions include the molecular characteristics of the drug, immunogenic load, and route of administration, as well as the patient's age and genetic ability to recognize antigenic determinants.

The pathogenesis of most cutaneous drug-induced reactions is not well understood. The terms *hypersensitivity* and *allergic* should be restricted to those reactions that are immunologically mediated or that can reasonably be presumed to be immunologically mediated. True allergic reactions affect a very small percentage of the population receiving a particular drug, and require prior exposure or a latent period for development of an immune response.

Numerous nonimmunologic mechanisms can be implicated in the production of cutaneous drug reactions. Anagen alopecia and mucositis are examples of *secondary side effects* of antimitotic chemotherapeutic agents. These drugs are unable to distinguish between rapidly dividing tumor cells and rapidly dividing normal cells and therefore inadvertently produce these effects. *Cumulative toxicity* occurs when there is a prolonged exposure to certain drugs. The blue-gray skin discoloration (argyria) due to prolonged silver ingestion is a striking example of chemical accumulation. Certain drugs may produce *exacerbation or precipitation of latent cutaneous disease* in genetically susceptible individuals. The administration of iodides may provoke lesions of dermatitis herpetiformis; porphyria cutanea tarda may be induced by the administration of barbiturates, oral contraceptives, or busulfan. *Alterations in normal flora* by antibiotics, corticosteroids, and immunosuppressive agents may result in the overgrowth of yeast such as *Candida albicans* or may facilitate the growth of cutaneous dermatophytes. Finally, there may be *nonimmunologic activation of effector pathways,* which may stimulate an allergic reaction but which are not antibody dependent. For example, certain drugs (e.g., codeine) can directly trigger the release of mast cell mediators and evoke an urticarial eruption.

CLINICAL MANIFESTATIONS

In this chapter, drug reactions are categorized by the clinical appearance of the eruption. However, several points should be emphasized. First, the morphology of the cutaneous eruption does not usually identify the drug causing a particular reaction because similar skin eruptions may be caused by widely disparate drugs. Second, although repeated administration of a given drug usually provokes the same reaction in an individual patient, this is not entirely predictable, and occasionally different reactions may be produced. And last, the same drug may produce markedly different reactions in different individuals. In the box below, the drugs commonly associated with various cutaneous reactions are listed. In terms of frequency, the exanthematous reaction occurs most commonly, followed by urticaria and erythema multiforme.

Acneiform eruptions

Drug-induced acneiform eruptions are generally more papulopustular and less comedonal than typical acne vulgaris (Fig. 332-1). The pathogenetic mechanisms producing acneiform eruptions are quite varied. Some drugs, such as oral contraceptives, act on the sebaceous gland and exacerbate pre-existing acne; other drugs, such as the halogens, lithium, and dactinomycin, induce pustular and inflammatory follicular lesions. Adrenocorticotropic hormone (ACTH) and corticosteroids produce comedonal lesions that are all in the same stage of development, presumably because of follicular occlusion.

Alopecia

Certain drugs, such as antimitotic agents, interfere with hair growth in the anagen or proliferative phase of the hair cycle, resulting in a so-called anagen effluvium. The mechanism of action for most of the other drugs that induce alopecia is not well understood, and therefore further classification is difficult. Diffuse alopecia may accompany administration of anticoagulants, antithyroid drugs, and vitamin A derivatives. Drug-induced alopecia is usually reversible on cessation of the offending agent.

Eczematous eruptions

Many drugs are used both externally and internally. An eczematous-type of drug eruption is similar in appearance to contact dermatitis and develops in patients who are already sensitized by topical exposure to a particular drug or to one chemically related to it. Subsequent systemic administration of the drug (by ingestion or injection) results in an acute papular and occasionally papulovesicular erythematous eruption. The reaction occurs within 2 days after the administration of the drug and is commonly localized to the site of previously existing allergic contact dermatitis. Patch testing may be used to demonstrate contact hypersensitivity to a suspected topical agent.

Agents present in topical preparations that frequently are associated with allergic contact dermatitis include neomycin, benzocaine, ethylenediamine diphenhydramine, and parabens.

Erythema multiforme

Erythema multiforme is characterized by discrete erythematous macules, papules, or plaques. Bullae may develop in the center of some of the lesions. The pathognomonic iris or target lesion may not be present in drug-induced erythema multiforme. The lesions are characteristically found on the distal extremities and face. Severe erythema multiforme with fever and mucosal involvement is also known as the *Stevens-Johnson syndrome* (Plate VI-8). Although many drugs have been incriminated in the production of erythema multiforme, the most common agents are sulfonamides, penicillins, hydantoins, and phenobarbitals. Erythema multiforme may be precipitated by a wide variety of agents in addition to drugs. Without actually rechallenging the patient with the suspected drug to reproduce the reaction, it may be difficult to prove or disprove a causal relationship between a particular medication and erythema multiforme.

Drug-induced cutaneous eruptions

Acneiform eruptions
- ACTH
- Bromides
- Corticosteroids
- Cyanocobalamin (vitamin B_{12})
- Dactinomycin
- Iodides
- Isoniazid (INH)
- Lithium
- Oral contraceptives
- Phenytoin

Alopecia
- Alkylating agents
- Allopurinol
- Amphetamines
- Anticoagulants (coumarin, heparin)
- Antimetabolites
- Antithyroid drugs (carbimazole, thiouracil)
- Cytotoxic agents
- Heavy metals
- Hypocholesterolemic drugs
- Levodopa
- Oral contraceptives
- Propranolol
- Retinoids
- Trimethadione
- Vinca alkaloids

Eczematous eruptions (topical sensitizer/systemic medication)
- Ampicillin
- Chlorbutanol/chloral hydrate
- Diphenhydramine (Caladryl/Benadryl)
- Ethylenediamine/aminophylline, antihistamines
- Iodine/iodides
- Neomycin sulfate/streptomycin, kanamycin
- Para-amino aromatic benzenes/para-aminobenzoic acid, sulfonamides, tolbutamide
- Penicillin
- Disulfiram (Antabuse)

Erythema multiforme
- Allopurinol
- Barbiturates
- Chlorpropamide
- Griseofulvin
- Hydantoins
- Nonsteroidal anti-inflammatory agents (meclofenamate, piroxicam, sulindac)
- Penicillin
- Phenothiazines
- Sulfonamides
- Thiazide diuretics

Erythema nodosum
- Bromides
- Codeine
- Iodides
- Oral contraceptives
- Penicillin
- Salicylates
- Sulfonamides

Exanthematous eruptions
- Allopurinol
- Antibiotics
- Anticonvulsants
- Barbiturates
- Benzodiazepines
- Captopril
- Gold salts
- Isoniazid
- Nonsteroidal anti-inflammatory agents (meclofenamate, naproxen, phenylbutazone, piroxicam)
- Para-aminosalicylic acid
- Penicillamine
- Phenothiazines
- Quinidine
- Thiazide diuretics
- Chlorpropamide
- Gold salts

Drug-induced cutaneous eruptions—*cont'd*

Exfoliative dermatitis
- Allopurinol
- Carbamazepine
- Gold salts
- Hydantoins
- Isoniazid
- Para-aminosalicylic acid
- Phenindione
- Phenylbutazone
- Sulfonamides
- Streptomycin

Fixed drug eruptions
- Allopurinol
- Barbiturates
- Chlordiazepoxide
- Nonsteroidal anti-inflammatory agents (naproxen, phenacetin, phenylbutazone, salicylates, sulindac, tolmatin)
- Phenolphthalein
- Sulfonamides
- Tetracycline

Leukocytoclastic vasculitis
- Allopurinol
- Cimetidine
- Gold salts
- Hydantoins
- Nonsteroidal anti-inflammatory agents (ibuprofen, meclofenamate, piroxicam)
- Phenothiazine
- Sulfonamides
- Thiazide diuretics
- Thiouracils

Lichenoid and lichen planus-like eruptions
- Antimalarials (chloroquine, hydroxychloroquine, quinacrine)
- Captopril
- Chlordiazepoxide
- Hydroxyurea
- Para-aminosalicylic acid
- Penicillamine
- Quinidine
- Thiazide diuretics

Photosensitivity eruptions
- Griseofulvin
- Indomethacin
- Nalidixic acid
- Phenothiazines
- Piroxicam
- Sulindac
- Sulfonamides
- Sulfonylureas
- Tetracycline
- Thiazide diuretics

Toxic epidermal necrolysis
- Allopurinol
- Barbiturates
- Hydantoins
- Nonsteroidal anti-inflammatory agents (phenylbutazone, sulindac)
- Penicillin
- Pentazocaine
- Sulfonamides
- Tetracycline

Urticaria
- Enzymes (L- asparaginase)
- Indomethacin
- Opiates
- Penicillin and related antibiotics
- Salicylates
- Sulfonamides
- X-ray contrast media

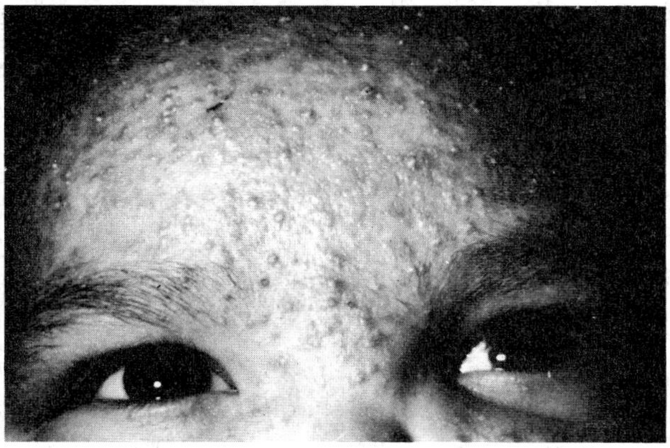

Fig. 332-1. Acneiform eruption following the administration of adrenocorticotrophic hormone (ACTH). The individual lesions are papules and pustules and characteristically appear to be in the same stage of development.

Erythema nodosum

Regardless of its cause, erythema nodosum is manifested clinically by the sudden appearance of painful contusiform nodules on the legs (Plate VI-9). Drugs most commonly associated with erythema nodosum are halides, sulfonamides, gold, and oral contraceptives. No clinical signs or symptoms distinguish drug-induced erythema nodosum from that induced by infectious agents.

Exanthematous eruption

This is the most commonly observed manifestation of a "drug rash." The pathogenesis of drug-induced exanthems is unknown (Plate VI-10). Exanthematous or morbilliform eruptions are characterized by bright red, blanchable macules and/or papules that may coalesce to form large confluent patches or plaques. The lesions are widespread and typically involve the palms and soles. Fever is usually present. Manifestations of an exanthematous reaction typically occur 2 to 3 days after the offending agent is begun; however, some antibiotics and allopurinol may induce eruptions that do not appear until 2 weeks after initial administration of the medication. Many drugs have been associated with the production of exanthematous eruptions, but those most frequently implicated are antibiotics, nonsteroidal anti-inflammatory drugs, thiazide diuretics, allopurinol, and gold salts. For reasons that are not known, exanthematous eruptions occur more commonly in certain populations: women have a higher incidence of this type of drug reaction than men; patients with infectious mononucleosis taking ampicillin and HIV-positive patients taking trimethoprim-sulfamethoxazole have unusually high reaction rates.

Exfoliative dermatitis

Exfoliative dermatitis or erythroderma caused by drugs is indistinguishable from exfoliative dermatitis caused by primary underlying skin disorders. The eruption characteristically begins with erythema, which spreads gradually to involve the entire body. Extensive and prolonged vasodilatation may result in abnormal temperature regulation, fluid imbalance, and right heart failure. The erythema is followed by diffuse desquamation. Gold salts and sulfonamides are frequently implicated offenders.

Fixed drug eruption

Fixed drug eruption is an uncommon reaction with a very characteristic clinical and histologic presentation. The skin lesions typically recur at the same sites with repetitive ingestion of the offending agent, hence the term *fixed eruption*. Initially there is an erythematous macule, which usually evolves to form a well-demarcated elevated lesion. Vesiculation and bullae formation may occur (Fig. 332-2). Resolution of the acute phase is usually accompanied by hyperpigmentation. The cause of fixed drug eruption is unknown. Drugs most frequently implicated in causing fixed drug reactions include phenolphthalein, tetracycline, and oxyphenbutazone.

Leukocytoclastic vasculitis

Drug-induced leukocytoclastic vasculitis presents as palpable purpura that is clinically indistinguishable from idiopathic leukocytoclastic vasculitis or leukocytoclastic vasculitis precipitated by infection or systemic disease (Plate VI-17). The eruption clears when the drug is discontinued. The presumed mechanism for leukocytoclastic vasculitis is an immune complex–mediated reaction. Penicillins, sulfonamides, and allopurinol frequently are implicated in drug-induced leukocytoclastic vasculitis.

Lichenoid and lichen planus–like eruptions

Drug eruptions clinically indistinguishable from idiopathic lichen planus (purple polygonal papules) have been described; however, lichenoid drug eruptions in general tend to be more scaly and eczematous in appearance than lichen planus, and may occur in a different distribution (i.e., sparing the mucous membranes and flexor surfaces). The accompanying pruritus is often intense. Irregular hyperpigmentation may be a disfiguring sequela.

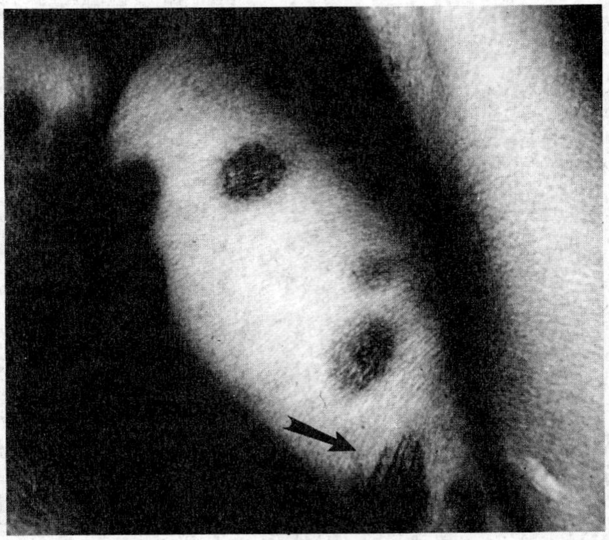

Fig. 332-2. Fixed drug eruption characterized by bullous (arrow) and hyperpigmented lesions that recur with subsequent administration of the offending agent.

Photosensitivity

Photosensitive drug-induced eruptions are discussed in Chapter 330 but some of the drugs associated with photosensitivity are listed in the box on p. 2548.

Toxic epidermal necrolysis

In toxic epidermal necrolysis, fever, and a diffuse, widespread macular erythema precede the formation of large flaccid bullae. Mucosal lesions such as stomatitis, pharyngitis, and conjunctivitis are common. Rupture of the blisters and loss of the overlying epidermis result in subsequent denudation of the skin (Plate VI-12). Fluid and electrolyte problems are similar to those occurring in a burn patient; secondary infection and sepsis are life-threatening complications. Mortality associated with toxic epidermal necrolysis varies from 15% to 60%. Drugs most frequently implicated in causing this reaction include antibiotics, nonsteroidal anti-inflammatory agents, barbiturates, phenytoin, and allopurinol. Survival of the acute episode is followed by healing, usually without scarring, in 2 to 4 weeks.

Urticaria

Urticarial lesions induced by drugs are second in frequency only to exanthematous eruptions. IgE-mediated urticarial reactions usually occur within minutes to hours of admin-

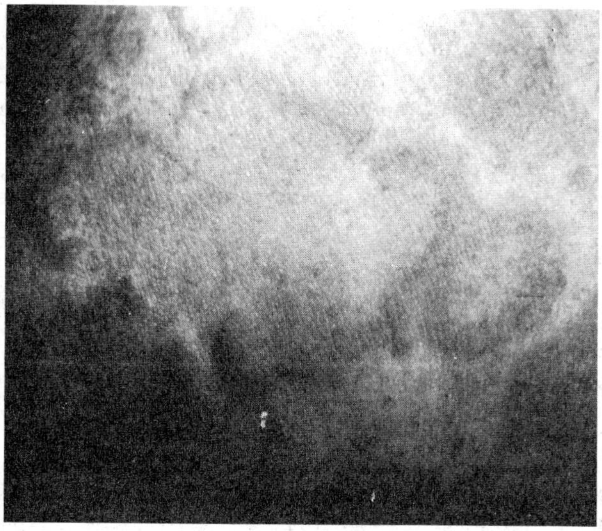

Fig. 332-3. Urticarial lesion with serpiginous elevated erythematous blanchable borders.

istration of the drug; urticarial lesions associated with serum sickness occur 7 to 10 days after administration of the drug. Some agents induce urticaria by nonimmunologic mechanisms such as local or systemic liberation of histamine from mast cells and basophils. Regardless of the pathogenic mechanism causing them, individual urticarial lesions should blanch, are usually pruritic, and should last less than 24 hours (Fig. 332-3). Agents most frequently implicated as a cause of urticaria are antibiotics, radiocontrast media, nonsteroidal anti-inflammatories, and opiates.

EVALUATION OF A PATIENT WITH A DRUG ERUPTION

The evaluation of a patient presumed to have a drug eruption is most challenging when the patient is receiving multiple medications. When attempting to determine the offending agent, it is wise to remember (1) most cutaneous drug reactions occur within 7 days of exposure to the medication, (2) certain drugs (e.g., antibiotics) have a higher incidence of cutaneous reactions than others, and (3) some drugs produce very characteristic reactions. A logical approach is to discontinue the most recently administered medication and/or drugs known to be frequent offenders.

REFERENCES

Bigby M et al: Drug-induced cutaneous reactions: a report from the Boston Collaborative Drug Surveillance Program on 15,438 consecutive inpatients, 1975-1982. JAMA 256:3358, 1986.

Bork K: Cutaneous side effects of drugs. Philadelphia, Saunders, 1988.

Bruinsma W: A guide to drug eruptions, ed 5. Amsterdam, Excerpta Medica, 1990.

CHAPTER

333 Cutaneous Manifestations of Internal Malignancy

Ellen B. Rest

Internal malignancies may manifest in the skin either with an infiltrate of malignant cells or as a paraneoplastic syndrome. In addition, certain syndromes with prominent cutaneous features identify patients predisposed to internal malignancy. This section reviews the cutaneous manifestations of each of these groups.

MALIGNANT INFILTRATES IN SKIN BIOPSY

Metastasis to the skin

Metastasis to the skin is not common and only occurs in a minority (0.6% to 9%) of patients with neoplastic diseases. In a retrospective study of more than 7000 patients, however, cutaneous metastasis was the presenting sign of malignancy in 1.8% of patients. Tumors that spread through the lymphatics tend to have local metastases, whereas hematogenous dissemination leads to distant recurrences. Women have cutaneous metastasis more frequently than do men because of their higher frequency of breast carcinoma, which metastasizes to skin in approximately 25% of cases. Skin metastases in men arise from lung and colon carcinoma, because these are their most common malignancies. Cutaneous metastases appear as nodules or ulcerated plaques. Breast carcinoma and, rarely, other tumors may present as inflammatory lesions. Skin biopsy is required to establish the diagnosis.

Lymphoma and leukemia

Cutaneous T cell lymphoma (CTCL) represents a heterogenous group of disorders that share early and prominent involvement of the skin but eventually involve the lymph nodes and viscera. Mycosis fungoides (MF), a term used to describe a classic form of CTCL, is described in detail in Chapter 154, but other primary CTCLs are now recognized.

Mycosis fungoides exists in three clinical stages: patch, plaque, and tumor, with disease progression roughly through the stages. Patch stage lesions are slightly raised, scaling, erythematous areas located on the trunk and extremities (Fig. 333-1). The patches often are mistaken for dermatitis; however, the lesions are refractory to standard therapy for dermatitis. Numerous skin biopsies may be required to establish the diagnosis, because nonspecific findings are often present at this early stage. Plaque stage lesions are well demarcated, indurated, elevated, and erythematous to violaceous in color. Arcuate or annular plaques are seen (Fig. 333-2). Patch and plaque lesions may coexist. Histopathologic confirmation is easier in plaque-

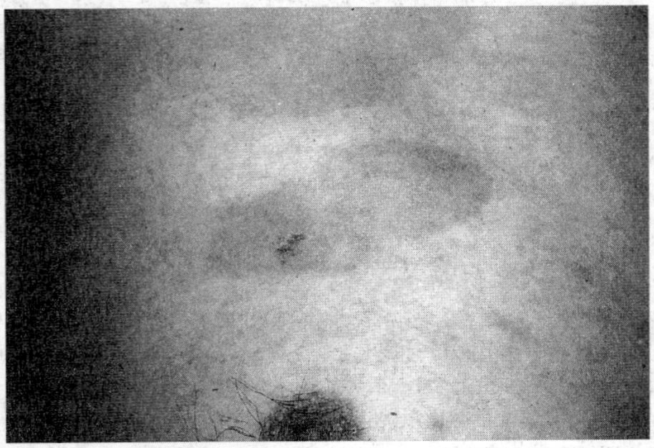

Fig. 333-1. Cutaneous T cell lymphoma. A patch stage lesion present on the chest.

stage lesions, and biopsies show infiltrations of the epidermis by atypical lymphoid cells (epidermotropism).

In progressive disease, tumors develop, especially on the face, scalp, and in body folds (Plate VI-13). Rarely, in the d'emblee variant, tumors are the initial manifestation of MF. Erosions, ulcers, and tumors are poor prognostic factors. There is eventual involvement of lymph nodes and viscera, although bone marrow involvement is minimal. In the Sezary syndrome, patients have diffuse erythema (erythroderma) and circulating atypical lymphocytes.

Other primary CTCLs are the large-cell-type, angiotropic T cell lymphoma, and HTLV-1–associated adult T cell lymphoma. Large-cell lymphoma, also known as Ki-1 lymphoma because a high percentage of infiltrating cells express the CD30 antigen or Ki-1, presents as a solitary plaque or as multiple nodules. Epidermotropism is minimal and tumor cells are large and atypical. In a large percentage of patients, the lymphoma is indolent. Angiotropic lymphoma is characterized by ulcerating plaques and nodules. Tumor cells are angiocentric and angiodestructive. Adult T cell lymphoma closely resembles MF, and patients have a leukemic phase resembling the Sezary syndrome. (See Table 81-2.) Prognosis is poor, and the disease runs a progressive and fatal course.

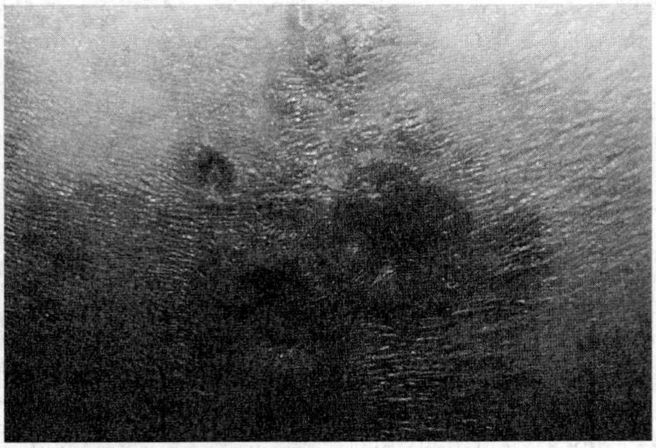

Fig. 333-2. Cutaneous T cell lymphoma. Plaque stage lesions in the groin show central ulceration.

Although most primary cutaneous lymphomas are T cell in origin, B cell lymphomas also may primarily affect the skin. These tumors are usually of the follicular center cell type and are generally low grade. Leukemic infiltration of the skin (leukemia cutis) occurs in approximately 3.1% of patients at the time of presentation and may precede appearance of tumor in the peripheral blood (Fig. 333-3). Nonspecific manifestations of lymphoma and leukemia include pruritus, petechiae, herpes zoster, or persistent warts.

NONMALIGNANT INFILTRATE ON SKIN BIOPSY

Acanthosis nigricans

Acanthosis nigricans (AN) is characterized by hyperpigmented, velvety areas in axillae and body folds. It is not specific for malignancy, because AN may be associated with endocrinopathies, obesity, medications, or heritable syndromes. In patients with malignancy, the AN tends to be more pruritic, to occur in older persons, and to involve the oral cavity. Acanthosis nigricans may precede, be concurrent with, or follow the discovery of a tumor. Associ-

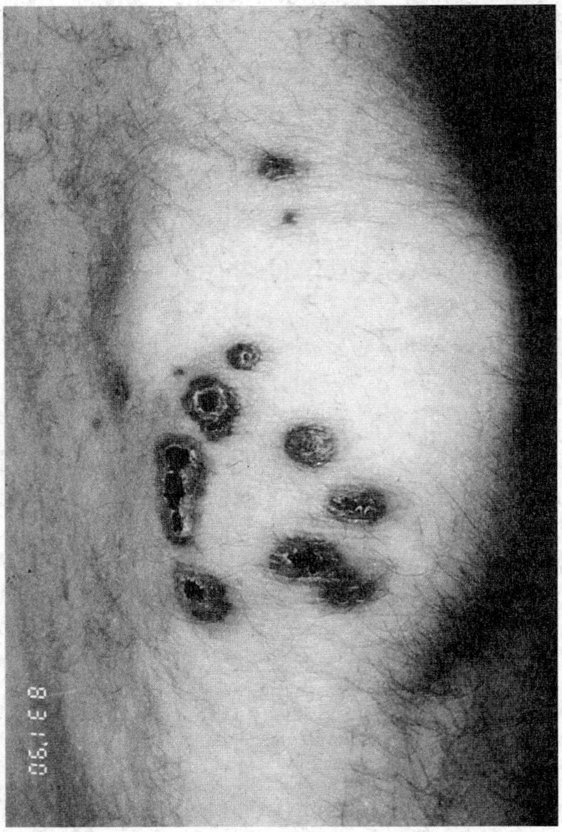

Fig. 333-3. Leukemia cutis. Hemorrhagic skin lesions as the presenting sign of leukemia.

ated malignancies are generally intra-abdominal adenocarcinomas, particularly gastric tumors. Numerous other tumors are reported, including squamous cell carcinoma and lymphoma.

Acrokeratosis paraneoplastica (Basex' syndrome)

Basex' syndrome is highly correlated with malignancy, which may follow the appearance of the skin eruption. The rash consists of erythematous, violaceous, hyperkeratotic plaques on the acral areas, always involving the nose and ears (Fig. 333-4). Associated malignancies are of the upper aerodigestive tract.

Dermatomyositis

Dermatomyositis is an uncommon disorder, occurring more frequently in women, characterized by heliotrope erythema of the face, periorbital edema, and erythema of the flexor surfaces of the upper extremities (Fig. 333-5). Dilated nail fold capillaries may be present and nail folds are erythematous and shiny. The cutaneous signs are accompanied by muscle weakness and inflammation. In adults, dermatomyositis seems to be associated with an increased risk of cancer, especially in women. Breast and ovarian carcinomas are commonly reported.

Erythema gyratum repens

A disorder highly correlated with malignancy, erythema gyratum repens often occurs shortly before the discovery of a tumor. Erythema gyratum repens is characterized by waves of erythema in parallel gyrate bands, resembling the grain of wood. Carcinoma of the lung is associated in most cases; other associated carcinomas include breast and cervix.

Hypertrichosis lanuginosa acquisita

Hypertrichosis lanuginosa acquisita refers to the sudden appearance of soft, nonpigmented, nonmedullated hair in a previously "hairless" area, sometimes associated with other symptoms such as glossodynia. Highly correlated with malignancy, this condition is more common in women and occurs in individuals with widespread disease.

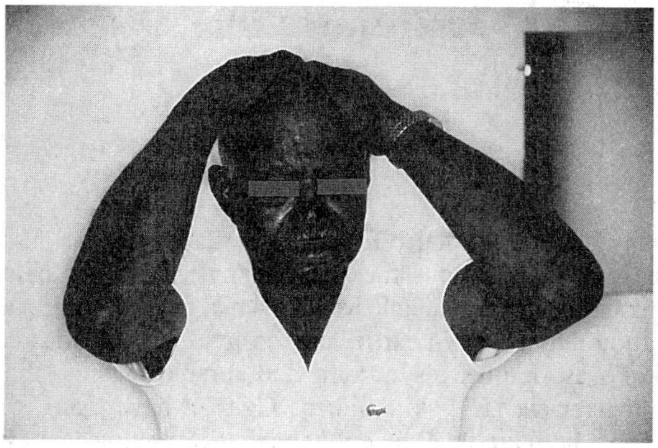

Fig. 333-4. Acrokeratosis paraneoplastica. Involvement of the skin of the nose, ear, and elbow is prominent.

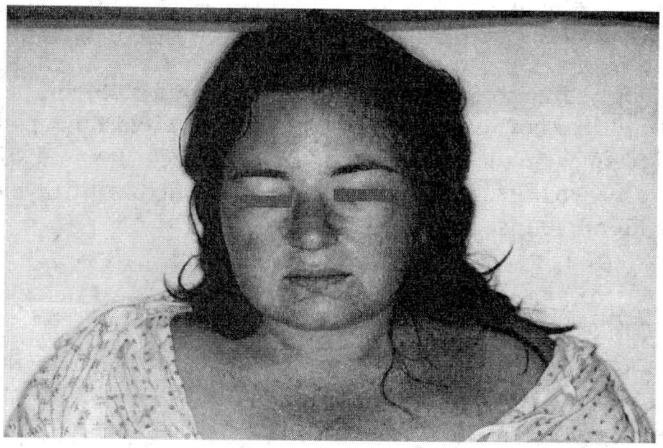

Fig. 333-5. Dermatomyositis. Erythema of the forehead, cheeks, and "V" of the neck and as mild periorbital edema.

Bullous disorders

There are occasional reports of bullous disorders such as pemphigus vulgaris or bullous pemphigoid associated with internal malignancy. Paraneoplastic pemphigus is a recently described, unique immunobullous disorder that always occurs in the setting of a tumor. Affected patients have severe mucocutaneous involvement and a unique set of circulating antiepidermal antibodies (see Chapter 325).

Pruritus

Pruritus (itching) is common and not specific for malignancy; however, malignancy should be considered when pruritus is persistent and unresponsive to therapy. Hodgkin's disease and other lymphomas are most commonly associated.

Ichthyosis

Acquired ichthyosis is associated with lymphoreticular malignancy and, less commonly, solid tumors. It is clinically indistinguishable from the autosomal dominant type and is characterized by roughened skin and coarse scaling, but unlike the heritable type, has an onset after the age of 20.

Sign of Leser-Trelat

The sign of Leser-Trelat refers to a sudden increase in the number or size of seborrheic keratoses, generally associated with adenocarcinoma of the stomach. Caution is advised in observing this sign, because seborrheic keratoses are very common and often present in large numbers. Suspicion is aroused by the new onset or explosive increase of such keratoses in a young person.

Acute febrile neutrophilic dermatosis (Sweet's syndrome)

Sweet's syndrome is a disorder characterized by fever, neutrophil leukocytosis, and erythematous to violaceous painful plaques on the extremities, face, and neck. It is not specific for malignancy, but may be associated with myeloproliferative diseases.

SYNDROMES WITH PROMINENT CUTANEOUS FINDINGS MARKING A PREDISPOSITION FOR DEVELOPMENT OF INTERNAL MALIGNANCY

Cowden's syndrome

Cowden's syndrome is characterized by adenoidal facies, high arched palate, scrotal tongue, oral papillomas, and verrucous facial, hand, and foot lesions. Associated malignancies include breast carcinoma and thyroid adenocarcinoma.

Gardner's syndrome

Gardner's syndrome is characterized by intestinal polyposis, osteomas, and cutaneous features such as epidermoid cysts (50% to 60% of patients) and desmoid tumors (9% of patients). It is inherited as an autosomal dominant disease with high penetrance and variable expressivity. The most commonly associated malignancy is colon carcinoma, occurring in almost all untreated patients. Other reported tumors include periampullary carcinoma, brain tumors, and endocrine adenomas.

Peutz-Jeghers syndrome

Peutz-Jeghers is inherited as an autosomal dominant trait and is characterized by gastrointestinal hamartomas, hyperpigmentation, gonadal tumors, and breast carcinoma. Cutaneous findings include hyperpigmented macules, most commonly on the lips and buccal mucosa, but also located elsewhere.

Cronkhite-Canada syndrome

This is a sporadic syndrome of adult onset, occurring most commonly in men. Clinical features include rapid and progressive alopecia, macular hyperpigmentation, and prominent onychodystrophy, which involves all digits. Affected nails show splitting, separation from the nail bed, and complete nail loss. Associated malignancies include carcinoma of the colon, stomach, and rectum.

Muir-Torre syndrome

Muir-Torre syndrome consists of sebaceous neoplasms and visceral carcinomas. Cutaneous findings are sebaceous adenomas, epitheliomas and carcinomas, and keratoacanthomas. There are colonic polyps and colon carcinomas, as well as other tumors.

Multiple mucosal neuroma syndrome

Affected patients have a marfanoid habitus and mucosal neuromas involving the tongue, lips, and eyelids. Associated tumors include medullary carcinoma of thyroid, parathyroid adenomas, and pheochromocytoma.

Ataxia telangiectasia

Ataxia telangiectasia is an autosomal recessive disorder characterized by progressive cerebellar ataxia, recurrent respiratory infections, and ocular and cutaneous telangiectasias. Immunologic defects and radiosensitivity are present. Malignancies are reported in both homozygotes and heterozygotes, especially breast carcinoma in women, with a five-fold greater risk than noncarriers.

REFERENCES

Anhalt GJ et al: Paraneoplastic pemphigus. N Engl J Med 323:1729, 1990.
Barron LA, Prendiville JS: The sign of Leser-Trelat in a young woman with osteogenic sarcoma. J Am Acad Dermatol 26:344, 1992.
Brown J, Winkelmann RK: Acanthosis nigricans: a study of 90 cases. Medicine (Baltimore) 47:33, 1986.
Brownstein MH, Helwig EB: Metastatic tumors of the skin. Cancer 29:1298, 1972.
Jemec GBE: Hypertrichosis languinosa acquisita. Arch Dermatol 122:805, 1986.
Lookingbill DP, Spangler N, Sexton FM: Skin involvement as the presenting sign of internal carcinoma. J Am Acad Dermatol 22:19, 1990.
Paul R, Paul R, Jansen CT: Itch and malignancy prognosis in generalized pruritus: a 6-year followup of 125 patients. J Am Acad Dermatol 16:1179, 1987.
Richard M, Giroux J-M: Acrokeratosis paraneoplastica (Basex' syndrome). J Am Acad Dermatol 16:178, 1987.

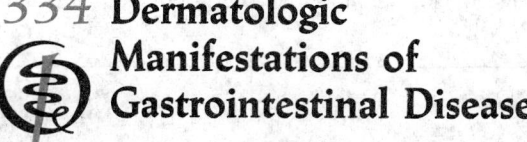

CHAPTER

334 Dermatologic Manifestations of Gastrointestinal Disease

Lisa A. Beck
Eva Simmons-O'Brien

Many gastrointestinal (GI) disorders have specific dermatologic manifestations that are either necessary or helpful in establishing the diagnosis. In fact, a careful skin examination may result in earlier diagnosis of such serious conditions as Gardner's syndrome and hereditary hemorrhagic telangiectasia. The skin and the GI tract have many similarities; both are lined by epithelia that communicate at mucosal surfaces, they are the body's major interface with the external environment, and they both play critical roles in immune surveillance. To completely cover all of the associated disorders of the GI tract and the skin is beyond the scope of this chapter. Instead the focus will be on the cutaneous manifestations of the polyposis syndromes, GI malignancies, various disorders associated with GI bleeding, and inflammatory bowel disease. Nutritional deficiencies, autoimmune blistering diseases, and rheumatologic diseases are covered elsewhere.

GASTROINTESTINAL POLYPOSIS SYNDROMES

The polyposis syndromes are a group of rare disorders characterized by proliferation of hyperplastic and adenomatous polyps throughout the GI tract. Risk of malignant transformation is variable, but is most common in Gardner's syndrome, in which the risk of colonic adenocarcinoma approaches 100% by 25 years of age. Several of these syndromes have distinctive cutaneous manifestations that often enable the clinician to make the diagnosis at an earlier state in the disease (Table 334-1).

Gardner's syndrome (a variant of familial adenomatous polyposis) has several characteristic clinical features: epidermoid cysts, desmoid tumors, osteomas, dental abnormalities, and congenital pigmented lesions of the ocular fundus. Regular examinations including upper and lower intestinal endoscopy are indicated and may lead to prophylactic total colectomy. Additionally, these patients also have a slightly increased risk of duodenal, thyroid, liver, and central nervous system malignancies.

The diagnosis of Cronkhite-Canada syndrome is based on a tetrad of manifestations: hamartomatous polyps found throughout the GI tract, numerous patches of cutaneous hyperpigmentation, partial or complete alopecia, and nail dystrophy. Although malignant degeneration of the polyps has been reported in approximately 14% of patients, most patients die of other complications of their disease, as listed in Table 334-1. The overall mortality is estimated to be 40% to 60%.

Cowden's syndrome is characterized by colonic polyps. The lesions are not associated with malignant degeneration.

Table 334-1. Cutaneous manifestations of gastrointestinal polyposis

Syndrome	Inheritance and onset	Cutaneous manifestations	GI manifestations	Other associated abnormalities
Cronkhite-Canada	Acquired Average age of 59 years	Hyperpigmentation of hands and arms > head, neck, and trunk Diffuse alopecia Nail dystrophy	Generalized polyposis (hamartomas) Risk of hemorrhage, intussusception, perforation, sepsis, and malignant degeneration (14%)	None
Familial adenomatous polyposis (Gardner's)	Autosomal dominant Age of presentation—mid-50s	Epidermal cysts, desmoid tumors, lipomas, osteomas (mandible, maxilla, calvarium)	Adenomatous polyps of colon and rectum. Lifetime risk of adenocarcinoma approaches 100%	Supernumarary teeth, dental cysts, or early loss of teeth Pigmentation of ocular fundus
Multiple hamartoma syndrome (Cowden's)	Autosomal dominant Onset in teens	Facial papules in 83% Usually trichilemmomas Less commonly fibromas Keratosis of hands and feet Mucosal papillomas Scrotal tongue Lipomas, hemangiomas, neuromas	Polyps mainly found in rectosigmoid area (hamartomas) in 33%	High arched palate Hyperplasia of mandible and maxilla <5% thyroid carcinoma >25% adenocarcinoma of the breast
Muir-Torre	Autosomal dominant Onset in late teens	Sebaceous tumors and hyperplasias Keratoacanthomas	Adenomatous polyposis in association with visceral carcinomas; usually of the colon, duodenum, kidney, lungs or uterus	None
Neurofibromatosis (Plate VI-14)	Autosomal dominant	Café-au-lait macules Axillary freckling Neurofibromas Giant pigmented hairy nevi	Neurofibromas of the stomach and duodenum Risk of hemorrhage, obstruction, and malignant degeneration	Lisch nodules Plexiform neurofibromas CNS, cardiac, and renal tumors Endocrine disorders
Peutz-Jeghers	Autosomal dominant Onset in childhood	Pigmented labial macules Melanotic macules of the hands and feet	Hamartomatous polyps of small bowel also may be found in the stomach or colon. Risk of GI malignancy is 2%-3% and intussusception is 47%	Increased risk of breast, ovarian, and testicular carcinoma

The diagnosis carries with it an increased risk of breast and thyroid malignancies.

The association of multiple skin tags (or acrochordons) and adenomatous polyps was first proposed in 1982, but several recent studies have failed to confirm this association. Most gastroenterologists currently recommend performing colonoscopy only on those patients with multiple acrochordons who have symptoms or signs suggestive of colonic polyps.

DISEASES OF CONNECTIVE TISSUE

Cutis laxa is a disorder resulting from the premature degeneration of elastic fibers that leads to the appearance of loose pendulous skin (Table 334-2). Although patients may experience GI bleeding from diverticula, hernias, or gastric ulcer, the major complication is usually pulmonary emphysema. Ehlers-Danlos syndrome encompasses a variety of inherited defects of collagen synthesis that differ in their mode of inheritance and phenotypic expression. Ehlers-Danlos type IV (ecchymotic form) is a rare but severe variant that usually results in death from colonic, arterial, or uterine rupture by the third or fourth decade. Pseudoxanthoma elasticum, or PXE, is another rare inherited disorder attributed to calcification of elastic tissue. Many patients die prematurely of cerebral hemorrhage, coronary artery occlusion, or massive GI bleeding. Treatment options are limited in these diseases and are generally restricted to supportive care, including strict control of blood pressure.

VASCULAR MALFORMATIONS

Osler-Weber-Rendu or hereditary hemorrhagic telangiectasia (HHT) is a disorder characterized by widely disseminated telangiectasias of both the skin, mucous membranes, and viscera. The telangiectasias resemble those seen in CREST or the limited form of scleroderma. The presence or absence of Raynaud's phenomenon, sclerodactyly, and subcutaneous calcification help to distinguish the two diseases. In HHT, perioral skin, fingers, and nasal and oral

Table 334-2. Diseases of connective tissue and vascular malformations

Syndrome	Inheritance and defect	Cutaneous manifestations	GI manifestations	Other associated abnormalities
Cutis laxa (generalized elastolysis)	Autosomal recessive and dominant pattern and acquired variant Deficiency and degeneration of elastic fibers	Pendulous folds around eyelids, cheeks, and abdomen	Esophogeal diverticula or dilation Gastric ulcers or rectocele Hiatal or ventral hernias	Tracheobronchomegaly Cardiomegaly Aortic dilation Uterine prolapse Ruptured patellar tendons
Ehlers-Danlos type IV	Autosomal recessive and dominant patterns Abnormal type III collagen synthesis and secretion	Fragility of the skin and blood vessels Impaired wound healing	GI bleeding and rupture	Large artery aneurysms Uterine hemorrhage
Pseudoxanthoma elasticum	Autosomal recessive and autosomal dominant types Degeneration and calcification of elastic fibers	Generally soft, lax skin with small yellow papules on lips, neck, flexures, buccal mucosa, and soft palate	Upper > lower GI bleeding Cobblestone-like lesions seen on radiography	Arterial occlusion Hypertension Angioid streaks in the eyes
Osler-Weber-Rendu (hereditary hemorrhagic telangiectasia)	Autosomal dominant 18%-46% occur without family history	Numerous well-demarcated telangiectasias on face, lips, hands, chest, feet, tongue and palate	Nodular angiomas found in the stomach and duodenum A-V malformations Aneurysms	Anemia due to hemorrhage; epistaxis, bleeding in the kidney, spleen, bladder, liver, lungs, and brain
Blue rubber bleb Nevus syndrome	Autosomal dominant	Cutaneous cavernous hemangiomas, predominately on the trunk and arms	Hemangiomas located throughout the large or small bowel; high incidence of bleeding	Iron deficiency anemia Hemangiomas of the liver, lung, eye, and CNS
Kaposi's sarcoma	Disorder of lymphoreticular and endothelial cell proliferation	Commonly presents as red-brown-blue macules, patches, nodules, or plaques sometimes with associated lymphedema; commonly appears on extremities, trunk, or oral mucosa	Sarcomatous lesions may involve GI tract diffusely Endoscopically may mimic ulcerative colitis Mesenteric adenopathy	Lungs, heart, liver, conjunctiva, adrenal glands
Degos disease (malignant atrophic papulosis)	Wedge-shaped necrosis of arterioles and small arteries	Pale pink, edematous, firm dome-shaped papules with porcelain-white centers	Anemic infarcts mainly in the small bowel, leading to bleeding, cramping, and occasionally perforation or peritonitis	Episcleritis CNS infarcts Serositis

mucosa are most commonly involved. The pathogenesis of HHT is unknown, but there is some evidence for a defect in the perivascular supportive tissue, which histologically appears as large gaps between endothelial cells. Gastrointestinal bleeding has been reported in as many as 40% of patients and is seen most commonly after the age of 50. Early detection followed by endoscopy with electrosurgery or laser therapy to the vascular lesions may reduce bleeding complications of the disease.

Blue rubber bleb nevus syndrome consists of soft, compressible, blue tumors involving the skin and GI tract. The cutaneous lesions are seen most commonly on the trunk and upper arms, and may be associated with localized pain or sweating. They vary from 1 mm to several centimeters in size. Histologically, the tumors resemble cavernous hemangiomas, which may explain their tendency to bleed. Hemodynamically significant bleeding rarely occurs, however.

Kaposi's sarcoma (KS) is a tumor of vascular and stromal components. When the disease occurs in elderly people of Mediterranean descent, it is only slightly symptomatic, with median survivals ranging from 8 to 13 years. Mortality in this "classic" form of KS is only attributable to the disease in 20% of the patients. Much more common is the aggressive variant seen in immunocompromised patients (Chapters 297 and 337). This "epidemic" form of KS is seen in approximately 30% of patients with the acquired immunodeficiency syndrome (AIDS). In this setting, 50% to 80% of the patients have cutaneous lesions, and 100% of the patients with oral lesions have GI involvement.

Malignant atrophic papulosis (Degos' disease) is a rare, acquired disorder affecting primarily the skin, GI tract, and central nervous system. The typical cutaneous lesion consists of a pink papule with an atrophic white center, usually on the trunk. The diagnosis is suggested if skin or small bowel biopsy demonstrates wedge-shaped areas of necrosis with an underlying lymphocytic necrotizing vasculitis. Prognosis is poor, with 50% of patients dying within 3 years of diagnosis, secondary to intestinal perforations or cerebral infarcts.

Cutaneous manifestations of gastrointestinal malignancy

Certain skin signs should arouse concern for an underlying malignancy (Table 334-3). Some of these syndromes are suggestive of specific tumors; such as tylosis (hyperkeratosis of palms and soles), which is typically seen in the setting of esophageal carcinoma, or may indicate malignant disease in general. Acanthosis nigricans (AN) and necrolytic migratory erythema may be noted in patients with no underlying malignancy. In fact, AN is typically seen in obese or diabetic patients. If the involvement is very sudden in onset and extensive, it is more indicative of an occult malignancy. Necrolytic migratory erythema is usually

Table 334-3. Cutaneous manifestations of gastrointestinal paraneoplastic disorders

Syndrome	Cutaneous presentation	GI malignancy	Other systemic associations or malignancies
Acanthosis nigricans (AN)	Dark, hyperkeratotic velvety plaques that affect body-fold sites such as the neck, axillae, breast, umbilicus, perianal area, and popliteal fossae. Rarely involves palms, soles, or oral mucosa	75% of all AN-associated tumors are adenocarcinomas primarily of the stomach. AN commonly resolves after surgical resection of the tumor	Obesity, endocrinopathies Squamous cell carcinomas Lymphomas Osteosarcomas
Acrokeratosis paraneoplastica (Basex' syndrome)	Violaceous erythema and scaling of fingers, toes, nose, and the helix of the ear Nail dystrophy Palmoplantar keratoderma	Esophageal malignancy with squamous differentiation	Upper respiratory tract carcinomas of squamous differentiation
Perianal extramammary Paget's disease	Well-defined, indurated eczematous plaques in the anogenital region	Occasional association with underlying rectal carcinoma	Vulva, penis, scrotum, and groin can be involved and associated with an underlying adenocarcinoma
Sign of Leser-Trélat	Acute onset or rapid increase in number and size of seborrheic keratosis	67% of cases are associated with GI adenocarcinoma. The lesions may disappear after surgical resection	33% of cases are seen in other malignancies such as lung, prostate, leukemia or mycosis fungoides
Tylosis (Howel-Evans syndrome)	Diffuse palmoplantar hyperkeratosis Oral leukoplakia	95% risk of esophageal carcinoma	Periodontitis
Necrolytic migratory erythema (glucagonoma syndrome)	Erythematous, scaly, crusted erosions or blisters with necrosis involving the perineum, lower abdomen, perioral, and flexural areas	Associated with a tumor of pancreatic alpha cells or adenocarcinoma of the jejunum	Glucose intolerance, anemia, weight loss, and venous thrombosis

associated with a pancreatic glucagonoma and appears as eroded, erythematous patches around orifices and in body folds. Unfortunately, these paraneoplastic syndromes do not often aid in earlier diagnosis of the underlying malignancy because they typically develop late in the course of the cancer. Treatment of the malignancy often results in improvement or total resolution of the cutaneous manifestations.

Inflammatory bowel disease

Inflammatory bowel disease (IBD) is characterized by inflammation of the large or small bowel with a tendency for relapse and recurrence (See Chapter 43.) There are many cutaneous manifestations associated with IBD, some of which may be the presenting feature, whereas others may occur with or postdate the intestinal disease process. Ulcerative colitis (UC) and Crohn's Disease (CD) are the two major forms of inflammatory bowel disease. Both diseases usually develop in adolescence or early adulthood and often present with a similar constellation of symptoms, including diarrhea, abdominal pain, fevers, anorexia, and weight loss.

It has been estimated that approximately 25% to 36% of patients with UC or CD have extraintestinal complications of the disease. Approximately 15% of these complications are cutaneous (Table 334-4). Erythema nodosum (EN) and pyoderma gangrenosum (PG) are two of the most frequently encountered conditions.

Erythema nodosum is characterized by the development of warm, tender, erythematous, subcutaneous nodules, most commonly seen on the lower extremities (Color Plate VI-9). It is estimated that 9% of UC patients and 15% of CD patients develop EN. In addition to the painful nodules, most patients also experience fever, chills, malaise, and arthralgias. Erythema nodosum may precede the diagnosis of inflammatory bowel disease, but more commonly it is seen in conjunction with a flare of the IBD. Erythema nodosum usually resolves with bed rest over 3 to 6 weeks; however, corticosteroids (systemic or intralesional), nonsteroidal anti-inflammatory agents, dapsone, colchicine and potassium iodide all have been tried with varied success. Erythema nodosum, in fact, is more commonly seen in the setting of streptococcal infections, sarcoidosis, tuberculosis, or drug reactions.

Pyoderma gangrenosum usually presents as small pustules, papules, or hemorrhagic blisters that enlarge and form ulcers with bluish undermined borders (Color Plate VI-15). These lesions commonly occur on the lower extremities, but may present anywhere on the skin. The pain associated with them is typically out of proportion to that predicted from the clinical appearance. Pyoderma gangrenosum is seen more commonly in UC patients (12%) than in CD patients (1% to 2%). One quarter of patients have noted that their lesions develop at sites of minor trauma such as surgical scars or ostomy sites. Most patients develop PG during flares of their GI disease. In turn, they note improvement with treatment of the inflammatory bowel disease. Management of PG may require aggressive treatment such as high-dose oral corticosteroids, pulse corticosteroids, dapsone, azathioprine, cyclosporine A, clofazimine, or even resection of the severely inflamed bowel.

Table 334-4. Cutaneous manifestations of inflammatory bowel disease

Crohn's disease (CD)	Ulcerative colitis (UC)
Erythema nodosum (15%) Pyoderma gangrenosum (1%-2%) Oral manifestations (8%-15%): aphthae, cobblestoning, cheilitis glandularis Nutritional deficiencies: Vitamin B_{12}, Folic acid, iron, zinc, essential fatty acids	Erythema nodosum (9%) Pyoderma gangrenosum (12%) Oral manifestations (6%): aphthae, glossitis, gingivitis Minimal nutritional deficiencies
Cutaneous polyarteritis nodosa (5%) Sweet's syndrome (2 case reports) Clubbing (58%)	Leukocytoclastic vasculitis (more common in UC than CD) Sweet's syndrome (4 case reports) Coagulation defects (1.2%)

Nutritional deficiencies are a rare complication of UC patients; however, zinc deficiency may occur in 35% to 45% of patients with longstanding CD. Zinc deficiency often presents as eczematous or vesiculobullous eruptions in the perioral, acral, or perineal areas. Laboratory findings suggestive of zinc deficiency, other than decreased plasma or serum zinc, include decreased retinal binding protein, serum testosterone, and alkaline phosphatase. In addition iron, ascorbate, and essential fatty acid deficiencies may develop in patients with DC. These deficiencies cause dry skin, angular stomatitis, poor oral hygiene, generalized pruritus, alopecia, and poor wound healing.

REFERENCES

Apgar JT: Newer aspects of inflammatory bowel disease and its cutaneous manifestations: a selective review. Seminars in Dermatology 10:138, 1991.

Burgdorf W: Cutaneous manifestations of Crohn's disease. J Am Acad Dermatol 5:689, 1981.

Golitz LE: Heritable cutaneous disorders which affect the gastrointestinal tract. Med Clin North Am 64:829, 1980.

Greenstein AJ, Janowitz HD, and Sachar DB: The extra-intestinal complications of Crohn's disease and ulcerative colitis: a study of 700 patients. Medicine 55:401, 1976.

Gregory B and Ho VC: Cutaneous manifestations of gastrointestinal disorders. Part I. J Am Acad Dermatol 26:153, 1992.

Gregory B and Ho VC: Cutaneous manifestations of gastrointestinal disorders. Part II. J Am Acad Dermatol 26:371, 1992.

Marks J: The relationship of gastrointestinal disease and the skin. Clin Gastroenterol 12:693, 1983.

Shum DT and Guenther L: Metastatic Crohn's disease. Arch Dermatol 126:645, 1990.

CHAPTER

335 Cutaneous Manifestations of Endocrine Disorders

Rosemarie M. Watson

The skin may be the presenting organ of involvement or may be affected later in the disease course of many endocrine disorders. Changes may be subtle or obvious. When they are subtle, early recognition can facilitate a prompt diagnosis.

PITUITARY GLAND

Excessive secretion of growth hormone and somatomedin produces typical features of acromegaly. These features include a generalized increase in skin thickness and mass, resulting in coarse facies with thick lips, large nose, and soft-tissue swelling of hands and feet. Additional features include prominent skin creases, hyperpigmentation, and sessile or pedunculated fibromas. The cutaneous manifestations of acromegaly often develop so slowly that changes are not recognized by the patient.

Panhypopituitarism is characterized by a generalized pallor and a decreased ability to tan due to an absence of melanocyte-stimulating hormone (MSH). The skin is typically dry and smooth, but in the presence of severe thyroid hormone deficiency, the skin may become coarse and show scaling. Loss of gonadotropic hormones (follicle-stimulating hormone [FSH] and luteinizing hormone [LH]) results in a loss of body hair, which is also a frequent finding in hypopituitarism.

Basophilic adenomas produce Cushing's disease. The clinical features of this disease are discussed in Chapter 160.

THYROID GLAND

The cutaneous manifestations of hyperthyroidism involve the skin, hair, or nails (Table 335-1).

Patients with hyperthyroidism demonstrate warm skin and palmar erythema secondary to increased cutaneous blood flow. Skin hyperpigmentation may be diffuse or patchy, but, paradoxically, vitiligo may be found in 20% of patients with Graves' disease.

Thyroid hormone plays a prominent role in hair and nail growth. In hyperthyroidism, the patient's hair may be fine and friable, and a variable degree of alopecia is common. Nail changes include onycholysis of the distal nail with an upward curve of the free edge (Plummer's nails) and thyroid acropachy, an apparent clubbing of the fingers caused by subperiosteal new bone formation.

Pretibial myxedema, an uncommon but well-recognized cutaneous sign of Graves' disease, is characterized by flesh-colored, erythematous or violaceous plaques and nodules with a *peau d'orange* appearance, commonly located on the

Table 335-1. The cutaneous features of thyroid dysfunction

	Hypothyroidism	Hyperthyroidism
Skin	Cool, dry	Warm, moist
	Pallor, yellow color (carotenemia)	Easy flushing
	Coarse texture with boggy nonpitting edema	Palmar erythema hyperpigmentation
	Characteristic facies (coarse with periorbital edema, large tongue)	Vitiligo (7%) Pruritus (uncommon)
	Decreased sweating	Increased sweating
	purpura/ecchymoses hyperkeratotic palms and soles (uncommon)	Pretibial myxedema (Graves' disease)
Hair	Coarse; brittle	Fine; friable
	Diffuse alopecia	Diffuse alopecia
Nails	Brittle	Onycholysis
	Slow growth	Thyroid acropachy
		Plummer's nails

shins (Fig. 335-1). The condition is caused by deposition of acid mucopolysaccharides, as in myxedema, and may precede or follow Graves' disease by months to years.

In hypothyroidism, the skin is cool, rough, and dry; the face is puffy and features are coarsened. Less commonly, the skin displays a generalized yellow discoloration due to hypercarotenemia. Hyperkeratosis of the palms and soles and xanthomas also are seen. The hair is coarse and brittle. Loss of hair is common, the characteristic location being the outer third of eyebrows.

PARATHYROID GLAND

Primary hyperparathyroidism is generally not associated with cutaneous manifestations. In contrast, secondary hyperparathyroidism in the setting of chronic renal failure is sometimes complicated by subcutaneous metastatic calcification and a refractory pruritus, which on occasion necessitates a subtotal parathyroidectomy.

Hypoparathyroidism is associated with various cutaneous features. In idiopathic hypoparathyroidism, mucocutaneous candidiasis develops in approximately 20% of patients and appears to be related to a concomitant defect of cell-mediated immunity. Additional features include a paucity of body hair and nail deformity due to increased friability. In postoperative hypoparathyroidism, hair and nail changes are also common. The skin is dry and may be pigmented; on occasion, eczematous patches are prominent.

ADRENAL GLANDS

Chronic hypersecretion or excess exogenous administration of glucocorticoids can produce Cushing's syndrome, the cutaneous manifestations of which are summarized in the box on p. 2560. Prominent hirsutism or acne vulgaris suggests excessive androgen secretion, as can be seen with adrenal

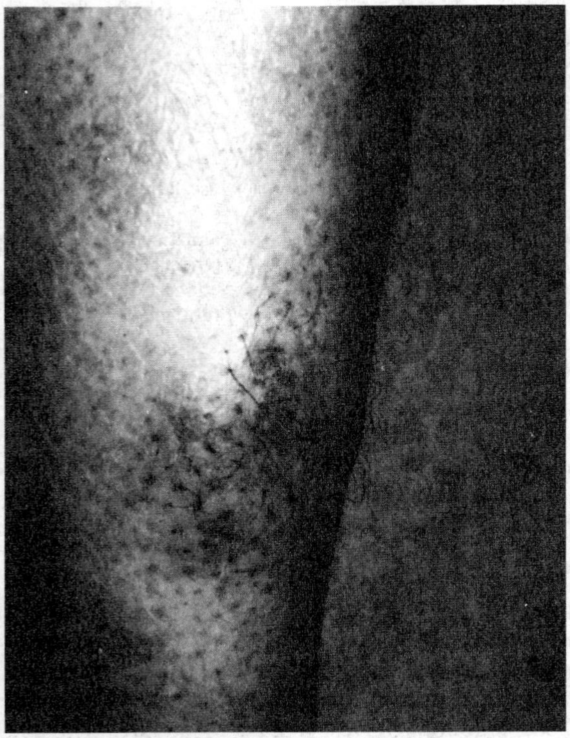

Fig. 335-1. Pretibial myxedema in a patient with Graves' disease.

The cutaneous features of Cushing's syndrome

Face
- Characteristic moon shape
- Telangiectasia
- Erythema
- Acne vulgaris
- Hirsutism
- Male pattern alopecia

Trunk
- Obesity
- Supraclavicular fat pads
- Buffalo hump
- Striae (intense purple color)
- Hyperpigmentation (Cushing's disease, neoplasia)
- Dermatophyte infection

adenoma, carcinoma, or congenital adrenal hyperplasia. Hypofunction of the adrenal gland (Addison's disease) is characterized by hyperpigmentation predominantly affecting the palmar creases, lips, gums, buccal mucosa, and areas of friction (Plates VI-16 and VI-17). A similar pattern of dermal pigmentation can be seen in patients with either active Cushing's disease or after bilateral adrenalectomy (Nelson's syndrome), indicating a pituitary origin of the pigmentary stimulus (excessive stimulation of skin melanocytes by MSH and adrenocorticotropic hormone [ACTH]). Vitiligo also occurs in a significant number of Addisonian patients (Plate VI-18).

DIABETES MELLITUS

Cutaneous findings are common in diabetes mellitus and are summarized in the box on p. 2561.

Bacterial or fungal infections of the skin are common. Bacterial infections are often difficult to eradicate, perhaps reflecting the intrinsic granulocyte dysfunction seen in this disorder. In diabetic ketoacidosis, a careful search for bacterial cellulitis as a potential cause of the acute loss of metabolic control should be sought. Rhinocerebral mucormycosis is a well-recognized complication of diabetic ketoacidosis, and because of the propensity of these fungi to hematogenous dissemination, widespread tissue infarction can develop rapidly. Other mycotic infections, (candidiasis, *Trichophyton*) also are seen, and glucose intolerance should be sought in individuals with recurrent candidal intertrigo, vaginitis, or vulvitis. Candidiasis is a common cause of vulvar pruritus in diabetic patients.

The vascular and neurologic changes of long-standing diabetes mellitus predispose to the development of neutrotrophic ulcers on the soles (malum perforans), which often require surgical intervention, including occasional amputation. Thus, careful instruction of the diabetic patient regarding care of the feet is a vital component of successful management (see Chapter 168).

Necrobiosis lipoidica diabeticorum (NLD) is a characteristic but uncommon cutaneous lesion occurring in 0.3% of diabetics. It is now recognized that 30% of patients with NLD do not have overt glucose intolerance at the time of diagnosis. Current data, however, suggest that most such patients ultimately develop diabetes mellitus. The lesion begins most frequently on the anterior shins as dusky red, elevated nodules with clearly demarcated borders; these nodules eventually increase in size to form plaquelike lesions with irregular margins (Plate VI-19). Plaques may develop a yellowish color, skin atrophy, telangiectasias, hyperpigmentation, and ulceration.

Histologically, an obliterative endarteritis may be seen with secondary necrosis of collagen. In early lesions, a granulomatous reaction with giant cells may simulate sarcoidosis. Occlusion of blood vessels probably also accounts for the lesions of diabetic dermopathy, which are characterized by atrophic, circumscribed brownish lesions typically distributed on the lower extremities.

An unusual bullous disease has been described in diabetes and termed *bullous diabeticorum*. The bullae range in size from several millimeters to centimeters. They are not related to trauma, although many patients do have an accompanying peripheral neuropathy. The typical location is on the fingers, toes, feet, or forearms, and they tend to be self-healing.

Cutaneous xanthomas, a characteristic feature of hyperlipidemic states, may be encountered in diabetes; indeed, diabetes mellitus is the most common cause of eruptive xan-

Classification of skin disorders associated with diabetes mellitus

- Cutaneous complications of diabetes mellitus
  - Infection
    - Furuncles
    - Carbuncles
    - Candida (paronychia, intertrigo, vaginitis, vulvitis)
    - Dermatophytosis
    - Mucormycosis
  - Diabetic foot
    - Ischemic ulcers
    - Gangrene
    - Trophic ulcers (malum perforans)
  - Xanthomatosis
    - Xanthelasma
    - Eruptive xanthomata
  - Necrobiosis lipoidica diabeticorum
  - Diabetic dermopathy
  - Bullous diabeticorum
  - Gustatory sweating
- Clinical associations
  - Vitiligo
  - Acanthosis nigricans
  - Granuloma annulare
  - Lichen planus
  - Werner's syndrome
  - Glucagonoma
  - Hemochromatosis
  - Scleredema
  - Porphyria
  - Lipodystrophies
  - Kyrle's disease
- Complications of treatment
  - Insulin lipoatrophy
  - Insulin lipohypertrophy

thomas. These lesions present as waxy papules varying in size from 2 to 4 mm and may be found on the trunk and limbs. Their occurrence and disappearance parallel the onset and resolution of the lipid disorder.

Of the additional skin lesions found in association with diabetes mellitus, acanthosis nigricans deserves special mention. Originally considered a harbinger of intra-abdominal carcinoma, acanthosis nigricans is now recognized in association with various endocrinopathies (refer to the box at upper right). Acanthosis nigricans may be a feature of insulin-resistant diabetes mellitus. It presents as a symmetric verrucous dermatosis with hyperpigmentation and a velvety texture, with a predilection for the flexor areas of the body (Plate VI-20). Particular sites of involvement are the back of the neck, the axillae, the dorsum of the fingers, and the belt line. Acanthosis nigricans is a disorder of unknown pathogenesis, although data indicate that its onset is related to secretion of a peptide of pituitary or tumor origin. Because most individuals with this lesion are overweight, obesity also appears to contribute to the fullest expression of the disease.

The clinical associations of acanthosis nigricans

- Endocrinopathies
  - Acromegaly
  - Gigantism
  - Cushing's syndrome
  - Stein-Leventhal syndrome
  - Hypothyroidism
  - Lipodystrophy
  - Diabetes mellitus
  - Insulin-resistant states
- Neoplasia
  - Adenocarcinoma
  - Lymphoma
- Obesity
- Congenital

The treatment of diabetes can result in cutaneous lesions; lipoatrophy or lipohypertrophy occasionally develops at the site of insulin injection, but can be avoided by varying the injection sites.

SUMMARY

Disorders of the endocrine system are frequently associated with skin changes. In certain instances, attention to the integument can provide valuable clues to the existence of a previously unrecognized serious metabolic abnormality. In others, recognition and treatment of such lesions are essential to overall management of the patient.

REFERENCES

Braun-Falco O et al: Dermatology. Berlin, 1991, Spring-Verlag.

Feingold KR and Elias PM: Endocrine-skin interactions: cutaneous manifestations of pituitary disease, thyroid disease, calcium disorders and diabetes. J Am Acad Dermatol 17:921, 1987.

Feingold KR and Elias PM: Endocrine-skin interactions: cutaneous manifestations of adrenal disease, pheochromocytomas, carcinoid syndrome, sex hormone excess and deficiency, polyglandular autoimmune syndromes, multiple endocrine neoplasia syndromes, and other miscellaneous disorders. J Am Acad Dermatol 19:1, 1988.

Flier JS: Metabolic importance of acanthosis nigricans. Arch Dermatol 121:93, 1985.

Freinkel RK and Freinkel N: Dermatologic manifestations of endocrine disorders. In Fitzpatrick TB et al, editors: Dermatology in general medicine. New York, 1981, McGraw-Hill.

Heymann WR: Cutaneous manifestations of thyroid disease. J Am Acad Dermatol 26:885, 1992.

Jelinek JE, editor: The skin in diabetes. Philadelphia, 1986, Lea & Febiger.

Moschella SL and Hurley HJ: Dermatology. Philadelphia, 1992, Saunders.

Muller SA and Winkelmann RK: Necrobiosis lipoidica diabeticorum: a clinical and pathological evaluation of 171 cases. Arch Dermatol 93:272, 1966.

CHAPTER

336 Cutaneous Manifestations of Sarcoidosis

Steven R. Feldman

The cutaneous manifestations of sarcoidosis are quite variable, sometimes isolated, but more often with associated pulmonary, ocular, and other systemic involvement (see Chapter 207). Both specific and nonspecific lesions (Table 336-1) can be seen. Specific lesions are characterized by granulomatous inflammation; nonspecific lesions do not have a granulomatous basis. The importance of cutaneous sarcoidosis rests in its usefulness as a marker of systemic involvement, its ready access for histologic diagnosis, and its ability to cause disfigurement.

CLINICAL FEATURES

Most inflammatory dermatoses exhibit a characteristic lesion morphology. In contrast, patients with cutaneous sarcoidosis may present with any one of a myriad of different morphologic patterns. Therefore, sarcoidosis must be considered in the differential diagnosis of many eruptions, particularly in high-risk populations (e.g., American blacks).

The most common morphology of the specific lesions of cutaneous sarcoidosis is a papular eruption (see Color Plate VI-21). The papules tend to be flesh colored to hypopigmented in blacks and reddish-orange to violaceous in whites. The eruption is often symmetric and nonpruritic, and areas of predilection include the central face, posterior neck, and trunk. An annular arrangement of the papules may be seen, and it is not uncommon for the lesions to develop in scars. On the trunk and extremities, the papules may be more lichenoid, that is, flat-topped and scaly. The papules and nodules tend to resolve with the formation of atrophic scars.

Plaques larger than 1 cm are common and may have a slightly scaly surface. The term *angiolupoid* is used to describe those plaques that have telangiectatic vessels on their surfaces. Chronic plaques present on the nose, ears, cheeks, and fingers are called *lupus pernio* (see Color Plate VI-22). Otolaryngologic examination may be of value in patients with this pattern to detect involvement of the upper respiratory tract.

Less common specific manifestations of sarcoidosis include subcutaneous nodules, hypopigmentation, ichthyosis, ulcerations, generalized or photodistributed eruptions, morpheaform lesions, pruritic papulonodules, scarring alopecia, and nail abnormalities. Mucous membranes also may be involved.

The nonspecific manifestations of sarcoidosis include erythema nodosum, calcinosis cutis, pruritus, and erythema multiforme. Of these, erythema nodosum is the most important. Clinically, it consists of erythematous, warm, and tender nodules of the anterior legs. Biopsy discloses a septal panniculitis. When the onset of sarcoidosis is acute and manifested by erythema nodosum in association with arthralgias, elevated sedimentation rate, and hilar adenopathy, there is often a good prognosis with spontaneous regression.

Table 336-1. The cutaneous manifestations of sarcoidosis

Specific lesions	Nonspecific lesions
Papules and nodules	Erythema nodosum
Lesions in scars	Pruritus
Annular patterns	Erythema multiforme
Lichenoid papules	Digital clubbing
Plaques	Calcinosis cutis
Angiolupoid plaques	
Lupus pernio	
Subcutaneous nodules	
Hypopigmentation	
Ichthyosis	
Ulcerations	
Generalized or photodistributed eruptions	
Morpheaform lesions	
Pruritic papulonodules	
Scarring alopecia	
Pterygium of the nail	
Mucous membrane lesions	

PATHOLOGY

The histopathologic hallmark of sarcoidosis is granulomatous inflammation. In the skin, aggregates of epithelioid mononuclear cells are present in the superficial dermis, extending into the deep dermis and occasionally the subcutis (see Color Plate VI-23). Multinucleated giant cells are often present, but in contrast to tuberculosis, there are few accompanying lymphocytes and no caseous necrosis. Asteroid bodies (stellate eosinophilic inclusions) and Schaumann bodies (lamellate round concretions) may be present in the giant cells, but are a nonspecific finding also present in other granulomatous processes.

Polarization microscopy should be performed to rule out foreign body reactions. Zirconium and beryllium can induce similar histologic patterns and should be excluded by history and special studies if needed.

Intradermal testing with heat-sterilized sarcoid tissue (the Kveim test) is of limited clinical utility but is a useful model for the immunopathology of sarcoidosis. By 6 hours after injection, the presence of helper T cells can be demonstrated. This is followed by infiltration with mononuclear cells, which is maximal after 48 hours. Granulomas are found after 12 days. Increased numbers of antigen-presenting cells also have been identified in the overlying epidermis and in the granulomas.

TREATMENT

The treatment of sarcoidosis must take into consideration its prognosis and severity. Acute involvement may resolve spontaneously and usually can be treated conservatively. At the other end of the spectrum, life-threatening internal organ involvement warrants aggressive attempts at management, including the use of systemic immunosuppressive agents. Generally, cutaneous disease falls between these extremes, rarely justifying extreme measures except to prevent severe disfigurement. Because treatment for cutaneous involvement is based solely on the risk of disfigurement, serum angiotensin-converting-enzyme levels and gallium scans, although useful in following the progression of systemic sarcoidosis, are rarely helpful for managing cutaneous manifestations.

When a patient presents with cutaneous sarcoidosis, a careful search for systemic involvement must be initiated. Of special concern is possible retinal and pulmonary involvement. The presence of systemic involvement may dictate treatment with systemic corticosteroids. With only limited cutaneous involvement, in which potential scarring and disfigurement are minimal, potent topical corticosteroids may be used. Unfortunately, these agents have only a limited ability to penetrate to the granulomatous inflammation in the deep dermis, and their use is limited by the complication of epidermal atrophy. Intralesional injection allows delivery of the corticosteroids the full thickness of the dermis. This is particularly of value in the treatment of localized plaques and nodules.

Systemic corticosteroids are used only when there is widespread disfigurement, scarring alopecia, or systemic disease (e.g., pulmonary or retinal involvement). For cutaneous disease, alternate-day regimens may be used, starting at 30 mg of prednisone and tapering to the minimal required dose. To avoid systemic corticosteroids or to reduce the dose, hydroxychloroquine therapy may be tried. Doses of 200 to 400 mg daily are employed. If there is a response to this therapy, after several months, the dose may be gradually reduced. For severe, treatment-resistant lesions, oral methotrexate also has been advocated. Using a low-dose regimen of 7.5 to 22.5 mg per week, a response may be seen in several weeks, although maximum effects require 6 to 9 months. Monitoring these patients for side effects of methotrexate is essential; it may be difficult to distinguish the pulmonary effects of methotrexate from pulmonary sarcoidosis.

REFERENCES

Elgart ML: Cutaneous sarcoidosis: definitions and types of lesions. In Izumi T, editor: Clinics in dermatology: sarcoidosis. Philadelphia, 1986, Lippincott.

Hanno R, Callen JP: Sarcoidosis. In Jordon RE, editor: Immunologic diseases of the skin. Norwalk, Conn, 1991, Appleton & Lange.

Hess SP et al: Ichthyosiform and morpheaform sarcoidosis. Clin Exp Rheum 8:171, 1990.

Jones E and Callen JP: Hydroxychloroquine is effective therapy for control of cutaneous sarcoidal granulomas. J Am Acad Dermatol 23:487, 1990.

Webster GF et al: Weekly low-dose methotrexate for cutaneous sarcoidosis. J Am Acad Dermatol 24:451, 1991.

White CR Jr: Predominantly mononuclear cell granulomas. In Farmer ER and Hood AF, editors: Pathology of the skin. Norwalk, Conn, 1990, Appleton & Lange.

CHAPTER

337 Cutaneous Features of Human Immunodeficiency Virus Infection

Thomas D. Horn
Kathryn A. O'Connell

Cutaneous signs of human immunodeficiency virus-1 (HIV-1) infection are divided into inflammatory, infectious, and neoplastic conditions (see the box on p. 2564). Skin disease in the HIV^+ individual is frequently the presenting feature of the progressive immunologic failure of the acquired immunodeficiency syndrome (AIDS). The eruptions may be mild and usually represent conditions ordinarily encountered in HIV^-, healthy persons, such as seborrheic dermatitis, folliculitis, and molluscum contagiosum. As the peripheral $CD4^+$ lymphocyte number decreases, cutaneous disease tends to become more severe, more resistant to treatment, and more HIV restricted (e.g., cryptococcosis, Kaposi's sarcoma, *Mycobacterium hemophilus*). Thus, clues that skin disease represent a manifestation of HIV infection include unusually wide distribution and large numbers of lesions, frequent recurrence, poor response to therapy, and identification of unusual infectious agents or neoplastic conditions (Table 337-1). Although cutaneous disease is rarely life threatening, successful treatment greatly improves the quality of life and gives the patient a measure of control over the most visible aspects of the disease.

INFLAMMATORY CONDITIONS

Papular eruption of HIV

Many individuals develop the rapid onset of skin-colored to erythematous papules on the trunk and extremities within several weeks to months of HIV infection. The eruption is asymptomatic or mildly pruritic and displays the nonspecific histologic findings of a predominantly lymphocytic perivascular inflammatory cell infiltrate with mild dermal edema and occasional eosinophils. This exanthem may be the first clinical manifestation of HIV infection. The cause is unknown. Treatment is symptomatic.

Cutaneous signs of HIV-1 infection

Infection

Viral infections
- Oral hairy leukoplakia
- Molluscum contagiosum
- Epstein-Barr virus
- Human papillomavirus
- Cytomegalovirus
- Herpesvirus infection (herpes simplex, herpes zoster-varicella)

Fungal infections
- Oral candidiasis
- Dermatophytosis
- *Pityrosporon ovale*
- Cutaneous manifestations of disseminated systemic infection
  - *Cryptococcus neoformans*
  - *Histoplasma capsulatum*
  - *Coccidioides immitis*
  - *Sporothrix schenckii*

Bacterial infections
- Pyoderma, folliculitis, secondary impetiginization
- Mycobacterium
- Syphilis
- Rickettsial-Bacillary angiomatosis

Protozoal infections
- *Acanthamoeba castellani*

Inflammatory dermatoses

Xerosis, ichthyosis
Granuloma annulare–like lesions
Exacerbation of pre–existing skin disease, especially psoriasis
Drug eruptions
Papular (pruritic) eruption
Seborrheic dermatitis

Neoplasm

Lymphoma
Kaposi's sarcoma
Other vascular proliferations
- Angiomas
- Telangiectasia

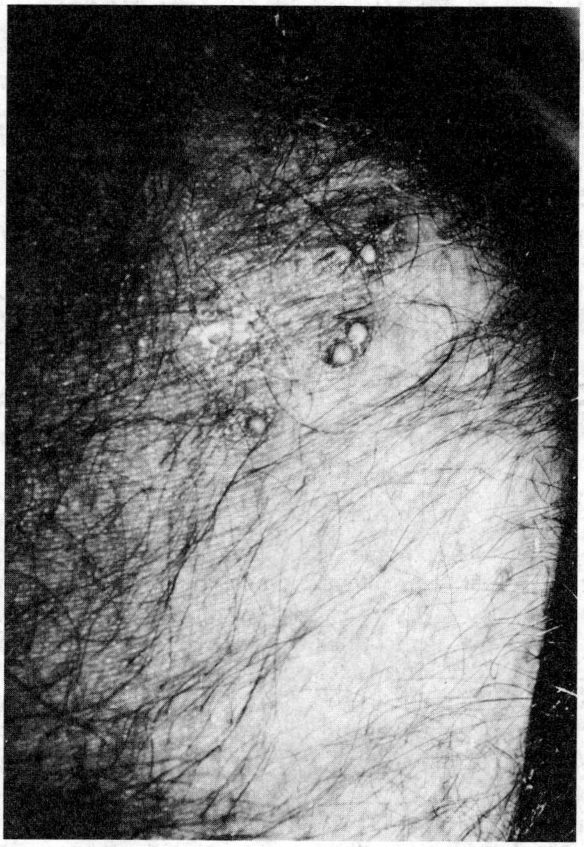

Fig. 337-1. Herpes simplex infection on the posterior thigh of an otherwise asymptomatic HIV$^+$ man.

Psoriasis

Psoriasis affects approximately 1% of the population in the United States. In some patients with pre-existing psoriasis, there is little change in disease severity with HIV infection, whereas in others, the erythematous, scaling plaques rapidly multiply and spread, often eventuating in erythroderma. Psoriasis may first appear during the course of HIV infection. Severely affected patients develop pustules and may experience fevers and arthralgias (Fig. 337-1). Skin biopsy specimens of HIV-associated psoriasis are more likely to contain high numbers of plasma cells and fewer T cells than tissue taken from HIV$^-$ patients. Mild disease may be treated with topical corticosteroid application, whereas more severe psoriasis requires therapy with ultraviolet B (UVB), psoralen plus ultraviolet A (PUVA), and/or systemic retinoid administration (etretinate). Methotroxate should be avoided. Remission of disease is rare; thus, treatment is often lifelong.

Reiter's syndrome

Reiter's syndrome may develop or worsen in association with HIV infection. The triad of arthritis, urethritis, and conjunctivitis is associated with lesions of psoriasis as well as discrete and confluent keratotic papules and pustules of the palms and soles (keratoderma blennorrhagica) as well as annular, scaling, erythematous patches on the penis (balanitis circinata). The individual manifestations of Reiter's syndrome in the HIV$^+$patient are often more severe and recalcitrant than the usual case.

Seborrheic dermatitis

Seborrheic dermatitis is a common and early manifestation of HIV infection, occurring in up to 80% of patients. The primary lesion is an erythematous, scaling papule or plaque, with an oily or dry surface. The usual distribution is in the midfacial region, with extension to cover the entire face and

Table 337-1. Frequency of cutaneous features of HIV infection

	Common	Less common	Rare
Infections	Oral candidiasis Molluscum contagiosum Warts Herpes virus infections	Oral hairy leukoplakia Pityrosporon folliculitis Syphilis	Disseminated fungal infection Bacillary angiomatosis
Inflammatory dermatoses	Seborrheic dermatitis Drug eruption	Psoriasis Papular eruption	Granuloma annulare
Neoplasms	Kaposi's sarcoma	Basal cell carcinoma Melanoma	Lymphoma

scalp (Fig. 337-2). Heavy concentration in the eyebrows and nasolabial folds is characteristic. Erythema is often more intense in the HIV^+ person, corresponding to the greater inflammatory cell infiltrate noted in biopsy specimens. The infiltrate is also deeper than usual, with scattered neutrophils and lymphocytoclasia. Therapy with topical corticosteroid and antifungal application is standard. The yeast, *Pityrosporon ovale,* is implicated in causing seborrheic dermatitis. The eruption often responds to topical or oral administration of ketoconazole.

Pruritus and xerosis

Itching and dry skin are two very common manifestations of HIV infection. Pruritus may occur without any visible change in the skin and may become incapacitating. Antihistamine medication and skin lubrication may provide some relief, but severe cases require therapy with ultraviolet light. Psoralen plus ultraviolet A treatment generally results in improvement within 10 to 15 exposures. Xerosis may become progressively severe leading to fish scale–like ichthyosis. Use of emollients such as petrolatum and decreased use of soap and exposure to hot water are usually beneficial.

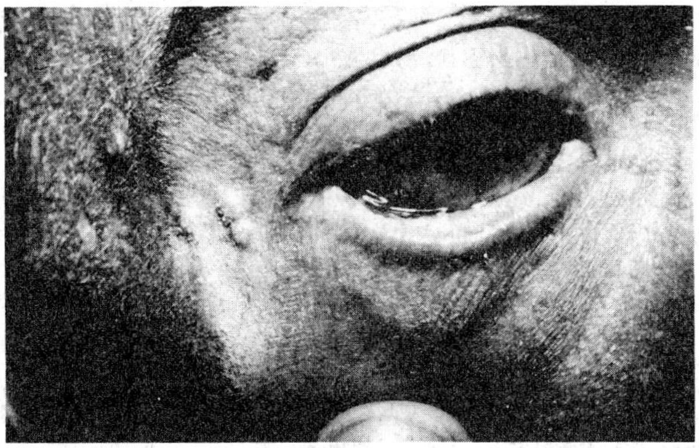

Fig. 337-2. Molluscum contagiosum lesions lateral to the eye. Small, bluish lesion on the lower lid is an example of the subtleness of some Kaposi's sarcoma lesions.

Prurigo nodularis

A prurigo lesion is a keratotic papule or nodule often with secondary erosion or ulceration. This lesion represents the skin's response to chronic trauma, such as picking or itching and from chronic folliculitis. Therapy directed against pruritus, as noted above, or against specific infectious causes of folliculitis is helpful. Interruption of the itching–picking cycle is the goal.

Drug reactions

Administration of trimethoprim–sulfamethoxazole is associated with a high incidence of cutaneous eruptions in HIV^+ individuals, consisting of widely distributed erythematous, often edematous macules and patches (Fig. 337-3). The T cells infiltrating the skin are often disproportionately $CD8^+$ compared with similar drug eruptions in HIV^- persons. Itching may be severe. Certain individuals may develop stigmata of erythema multiforme (target lesions, ocular and oral erythema and erosion) and rarely toxic epidermal necrolysis (widespread, full-thickness epidermal necrosis with denudation). Such drug reactions may progress despite discontinuation of the offending agent. Supportive care, including scrupulous skin care, is the best treatment.

Azure blue lunulae of the nails may develop and extend

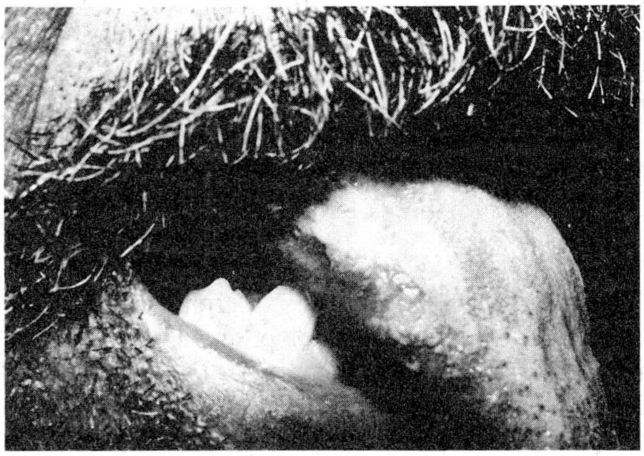

Fig. 337-3. Oral hairy leukoplakia. White papillomatous plaques on the lateral border of the tongue.

distally because of azidothymidine (AZT) administration. This discoloration is especially notable in more darkly pigmented persons.

Facial flushing

Uncommonly, HIV^+ patients manifest a diffusely erythematous face with occasional telangiectasia and mild scale. The appearance is that of a deep flush. Its cause is uncertain. There are similarities to acne rosacea, but a definite association is not established. Treatment with systemic tetracycline or topical metronidazole may be of benefit.

Granuloma annulare

Widespread papules and plaques with histologic features of granuloma annulare are reported in HIV^+ individuals. Biopsy specimens display the characteristic infiltrate of lymphocytes and histiocytes in a palisade around a subtly altered focus of collagen with increased mucin. The cause of granuloma annulare and the reason for an association with HIV infection are unknown.

INFECTIOUS CONDITIONS

In general, the microbes that infect the skin of HIV^- individuals are also the most frequently encountered in the HIV^+ patient. Infections tend to be more severe, more resistant to treatment, and more often recurrent. Skin infections with *Staphylococcus aureus,* herpes simplex virus, varicella-zoster virus, molluscum contagiosum, *Candida* sp., and dermatophytes are most common, but one must remain vigilant for unusual infectious agents in the skin. Cultures of the skin surface and skin biopsy specimens for histologic examination and tissue culture are very helpful in patient management. Cutaneous protozoal infections are reported in HIV^+ patients; however, this is exceedingly rare, and protozoal infections are not considered further.

Viral infections

Molluscum contagiosum is a pox virus that commonly infects HIV^+ homosexual patients. The typical lesion is a white, firm papule, often with a small central depression (Fig. 337-4). The papules frequently occur on the face and genitalia. Significantly larger lesions are referred to as giant molluscum. Progressive and recurrent disease is usual despite destruction with cryotherapy or curettage. Cutaneous cryptococcosis may mimic molluscum contagiosum; if in doubt, histologic confirmation is required (see below).

The manifestations of herpes simplex virus infection are protean. The typical presentation of grouped vesicles on an erythematous patch may develop in any location, commonly perioral or perineal (Fig. 337-5). Severe ulcers may ensue, frequently perianally, where they may be coinfected with cytomegalovirus. Methods of documenting the presence of herpes simplex (and varicella-zoster) include Tzanck smear, viral culture, and histologic examination. A Tzanck smear is properly performed by firmly scraping the

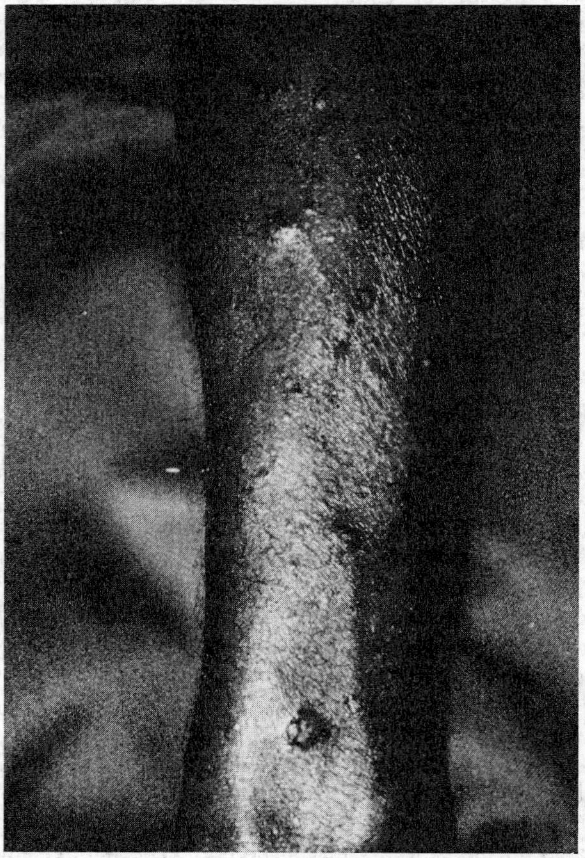

Fig. 337-4. Disseminated cryptococcus presenting with variably sized cutaneous nodules resembling molluscum contagiosum.

base of the vesicle/ulcer with a scalpel blade. The accumulated tissue is smeared on a glass slide, fixed, and stained with eosin and Wright's stain. Correctly executed, the Tzanck smear is a rapid and reliable test to establish the diagnosis of herpes simplex virus or varicella-zoster virus infection. A positive smear contains multinucleated keratinocytes with molded nuclei and surrounding pale cytoplasm. Acyclovir, administered orally or intravenously, is the best treatment. Route of administration and dosage depends on the degree of immunosuppression and drug resistance. Resistant strains may respond to high doses or ganciclovir administration.

Shingles, due to varicella-zoster virus reactivation, may be an early sign of immunosuppression in the HIV^+ person. As a rule, the eruption develops in the usual dermatomal patterns. Depending on the degree of immunosuppression, disseminated cutaneous disease (more than 10 lesions outside the dermatome of primary infection) may occur. Disseminated secondary disease as well as primary varicella infection may eventuate in varicella pneumonia. As with herpes simplex virus, the typical primary lesions may be missed; the patient may present with ulcers or disseminated lesions. Oral and intravenous acyclovir is first-line treatment for these infections.

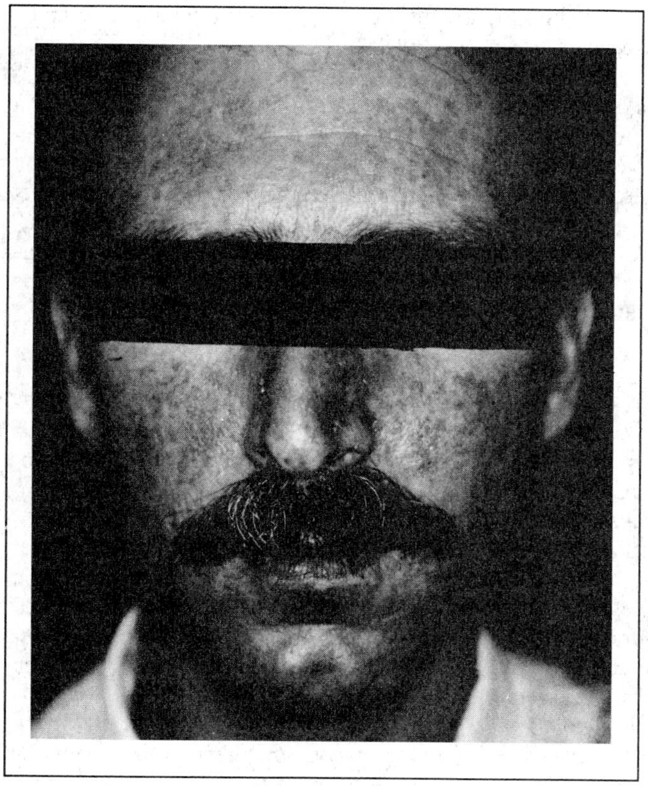

Fig. 337-5. Seborrheic dermatitis in an HIV^+ individual.

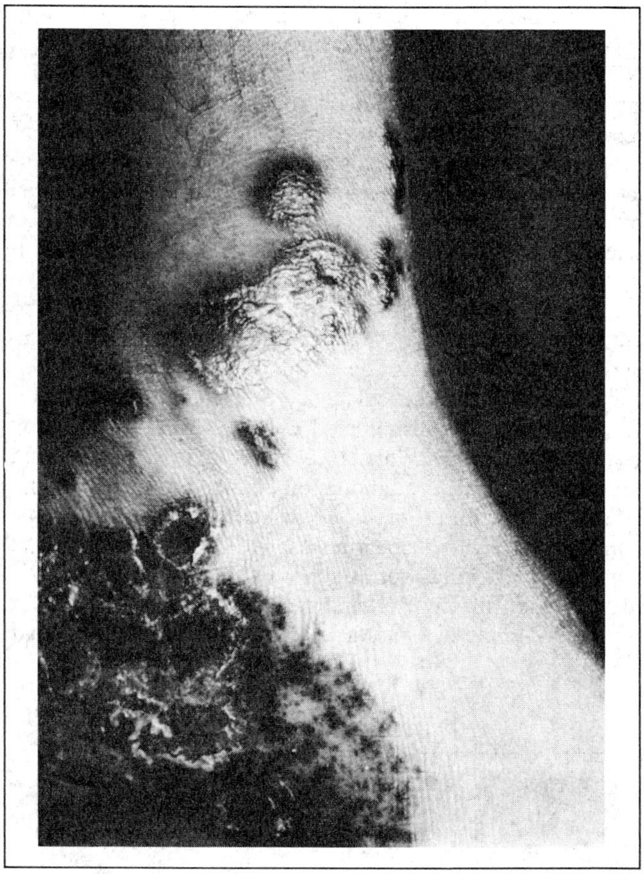

Fig. 337-6. A young intravenous drug user who presented with explosive onset of psoriasis and was found to be HIV^+.

Perianal ulcers are the only cutaneous lesions repeatedly demonstrated to contain cytomegalovirus (CMV). The cytopathic effect of CMV may be identified histologically in skin biopsy specimens from a wide range of clinical lesions. Cytomegalovirus is probably not the cause of the lesion examined through biopsy. Cutaneous lesions directly attributable to Epstein-Barr virus (EBV) infection do not exist, but EBV is implicated in the development of oral hairy leukoplakia (OHL)(Color Plate V-45). Oral hairy leukoplakia is a common manifestation of HIV infection and appears as white plaques with a warty surface, along the lateral margins of the tongue (Fig. 337-6). Other intraoral locations are described. Because OHL is mostly asymptomatic, treatment is not required. Human papillomavirus also may play a role in the cause of OHL.

Verruca vulgaris (wart) and condyloma are due to infection with the human papillomavirus (HPV). Warts proliferate with worsening immunosuppression. Usually the hands, feet, and perineum are most severely affected. Response to therapy is directly related to CD4 counts. In a large number of patients, treatment is palliative; the goal is to keep the size and distribution of lesions limited. Cryotherapy, podophyllum, and intralesional interferon injections are partially successful. Perianal condylomata are particularly recalcitrant; rectal lesions must be treated concomitantly if the goal is to clear the patient of lesions. Bowenoid papulosis may occur in HIV^+ individuals. This condition is HPV induced, and the lesion is a skin-colored or hyperpigmented papule with a verrucous surface. Histologic examination shows full-thickness epidermal dysplasia. Unlike the squamous cell carcinoma in situ of the genitalia, Bowenoid papulosis lacks metastatic potential.

Fungal infections

Superficial infections with *Candida albicans* most often involve the oropharyngeal mucosa and intertriginous surfaces of the skin. In the mouth, one finds adherent, white plaques of variable extent and distribution. Potassium hydroxide (KOH) examination readily shows pseudohyphae and spores. On the skin, candidiasis causes moist, eroded, erythematous plaques with peripheral pustules and erythematous papules. Potassium hydroxide examination and fungal culture confirmed the diagnosis. More severe involvement is manifested by esophageal disease and by widely distributed cutaneous disease. Oral candidiasis responds to nystatin oral suspension given several times each day. Oral or cutaneous disease may require treatment with oral ketoconazole or difluconazole. As a sole agent, a topical antifungal is of little benefit. Cutaneous septic emboli due to candidemia appear as violaceous, ulcerated nodules. This diagnosis is best established by skin biopsy and tissue culture.

Dermtophytosis is generally limited to the hands, feet,

and inguinal region, but invasive dermatophyte infection may occur. Generally, the dermatophyte infection antedates HIV infection, but the condition worsens despite appropriate therapy. Nail involvement (onychomycosis) is largely resistant to all forms of therapy. The choice of treatment of dermatophytosis depends on the extent of involvement and the degree of immunosuppression. Localized diseases of the feet may respond to topical antifungal agents. More widespread infection is best treated with oral griseofulvin or ketoconazole.

Disseminated fungal infections occur uncommonly. The cutaneous eruptions caused by such infections are protean and often nonspecific. The new onset of any widely distributed or generalized cutaneous eruption is an indication for skin biopsy. Disseminated *Cryptococcus neoformans, Histoplasma capsulation, Blastomyces dermatitidis,* and *Sporothrix schenckii,* among others, are reported in the HIV^+ population. Of these, cryptococcosis is perhaps most common, typically appearing as widely distributed white papules, mimicking molluscum contagiosum (Fig. 337-7). Identification of any disseminated fungal infection should prompt systemic evaluation. Examination of cerebrospinal fluid is important with the recognition of cutaneous cryptococcosis.

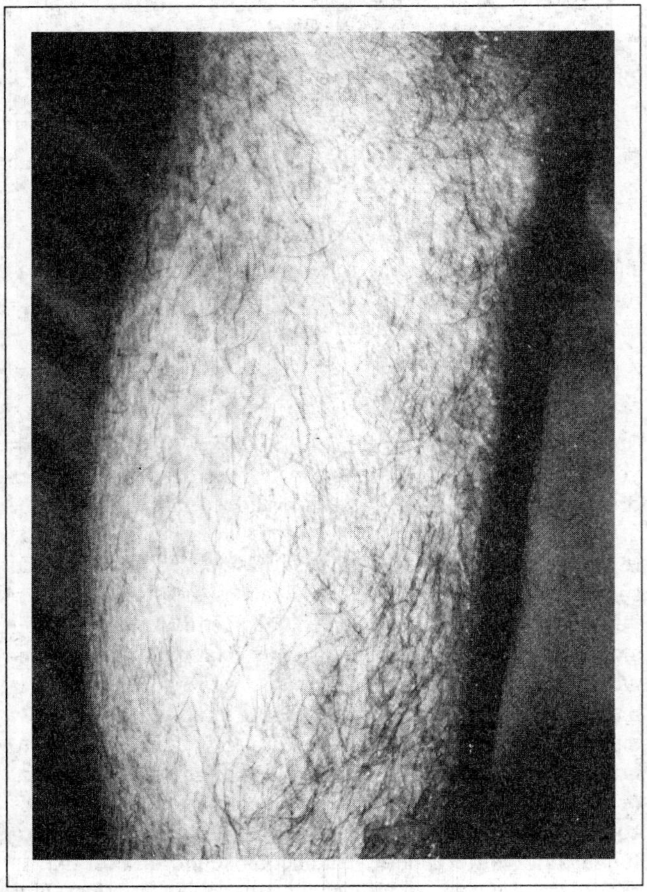

Fig. 337-7. Morbilliform eruption associated with trimethoprim-sulfamethoxazole sensitivity in an HIV^+ man.

Pityrosporon ovale (Malassezia furfur) causes tinea versicolor in humans. *P. ovale* is implicated in the cause of a modestly inflammatory folliculitis seen commonly in HIV^+ persons. Follicular pustules with minimal or no erythema are present on the trunk and proximal extremities. Patients frequently complain of itching. Oral ketoconazole gradually lessens the eruption and improves the pruritus. Topical sodium thiosulfate lotion or selenium sulfide lotion helps reduce the growth of *P. ovale*.

Bacterial infections

Folliculitis due to *Staphylococcus aureus* or *Streptococcus* sp. is the most common cutaneous bacterial infection associated with HIV infection. Deep-seated inflammation and abscess formation characterize the development of furuncles. Oral or intravenous antibiotics are generally helpful in conjunction with culture and determination of antibiotic sensitivities. In addition, furuncles may require incision and drainage. Use of an antibacterial soap helps to decrease recurrent disease. Other cutaneous bacterial infections such as *Haemophilus influenza* cellulitis and *Pseudomonas aeruginosa* ulcers are reported.

Any of the myriad cutaneous manifestations of syphilis may occur. The stigmata of secondary syphilis range from a few, isolated papules to the classic generalized erythematous exanthem involving palms and soles. Although serologic studies are less reliable than in HIV^- individuals, confirmatory tests include the rapid plasma reagin (RPR), Venereal Disease Research Laboratory (VDRL), fluorescent treponemal antibody absorption test (FTA-ABS), skin biopsy, and darkfield examination. Lesions of primary and secondary syphilis, especially condyloma lata, contain numerous spirochetes identifiable by correctly performed darkfield microscopy. The syphilitic chancre must be differentiated from chancroid and other causes of genital ulceration. Skin culture and biopsy are helpful when the diagnosis is uncertain. Appropriate therapy for syphilis is discussed in Chapter 238).

Mycobacterial infections primarily involving the skin are rare. Disseminated cutaneous tuberculosis and scrofuloderma are reported in HIV^+ individuals. Although systemic infection with *M. avians-intracellulare* is fairly frequent, a specific skin lesion attributable to this "atypical" mycobacterium is not recognized. *M. hemophilum* is reported to cause cutaneous ulceration in HIV^+ patients.

Bacillary angiomatosis (or epithelioid angiomatosis) is a rickettsial infection causing a dermal lobular capillary proliferation. Clinically, the lesions appear as erythematous to violaceous papules and nodules. The number and distribution of lesions are variable. The organisms are identified as clumps of pleomorphic bacilli staining with the Warthin-Starry silver stain. The organism appears closely related to *Rochalimaea quintana*. The lesions resolve with oral erythromycin.

NEOPLASIA

AIDS-associated Kaposi's sarcoma

One of the most striking dermatologic manifestations of AIDS is Kaposi's sarcoma. Classic Kaposi's sarcoma (originally described in 1872) manifests as a rare, benign, localized proliferation of mesenchymal cells, most commonly on the lower extremities of elderly men. The relationship between this classic form of Kaposi's sarcoma and the Kaposi's sarcoma associated with AIDS is unknown, as is the equally puzzling presentation of non–AIDS-associated Kaposi's sarcoma in Africa.

Kaposi's sarcoma was recognized as a common manifestation of AIDS very early in the epidemic; its incidence now, however, is decreasing in the homosexual male population. Several very striking features of its epidemiology provide clues to the underlying mechanism of the disease. Perhaps most surprising is that Kaposi's sarcoma is being reported in an enlarging cohort of HIV^- homosexual men. This is consistent with the observation that Kaposi's sarcoma is almost always associated with sexually acquired HIV infection, as opposed to HIV acquired through intravenous drug use or contaminated blood products. Moreover, HIV^+ women appear to be at risk for Kaposi's sarcoma when their infection is acquired by sexual contact with bisexual males. These clues have led many to suggest that AIDS-associated Kaposi's sarcoma is initiated by a sexually transmitted infectious agent other than HIV and that the severe presentation of Kaposi's sarcoma in the HIV-infected host reflects the inadequate immune response.

AIDS patients who present with Kaposi's sarcoma in the absence of other opportunistic diseases have a better prognosis than other HIV^+ individuals. It was thought initially that AIDS-associated Kaposi's sarcoma progressed from skin involvement to systemic disease, but more frequent use of bronchoscopy and endoscopy in the AIDS patient population has now challenged this view; skin involvement may be less frequent than gastrointestinal lesions. Cutaneous Kaposi's sarcoma in the AIDS patient is characterized by atypical lesions, increased severity, and refractoriness to routine therapies (Color Plates V-40, *B* and VI-24). Specifically, the most common sites are not the extremities but rather the face, especially the nose, the oral cavity, and the trunk. The lesions often follow natural skin lines in a symmetrical pattern, appearing as reddish-purple patches or plaques surrounded by a "halo" of brownish discoloration (Fig. 337-8). Advanced cutaneous lesions can cause functional impairment due to associated edema and infection. Lesions at any stage are often associated with significant psychological morbidity. Because AIDS-associated Kaposi's sarcoma often mimics other conditions and the lesions are usually multiple, patients presenting with a suspicious lesion should receive a complete skin and oral cavity examination and biopsy. Histologically confirmed Kaposi's sarcoma, of course, necessitates testing for HIV infection. There is as yet no consensus regarding the utility of invasive studies to identify gastrointestinal involvement, especially because these lesions are usually asymptomatic. A positive history of gastrointestinal or respiratory symptoms should prompt referral to an appropriate specialist; a chest roentgenogram can aid in identifying pulmonary involvement, which necessitates aggressive systemic chemotherapy.

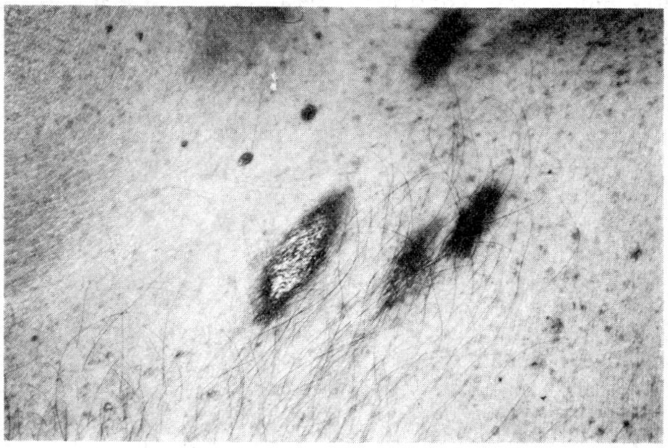

Fig. 337-8. Kaposi's sarcoma lesions. Typical, oval, reddish brown plaques following skin lines on the anterior chest.

Therapy for AIDS-associated Kaposi's sarcoma involving the skin is frustrating for both the patient and the physician. Early lesions are generally responsive to the traditional treatments such as local radiation therapy, cryosurgery, and simple excision, but the lesions usually recur, sometimes within weeks, and the number of lesions may render this approach impractical. More advanced nodular lesions are often refractory to treatment, although limited success has been reported with intralesional chemotherapy. Oral lesions are particularly problematic because the underlying immune deficiency renders patients susceptible to poor healing after destructive treatment modalities, and the functional impairment aggravates the already significant nutritional deficits in these patients. More aggressive regimens using systemic chemotherapy, such as vinblastine, vincristine, methotrexate, or interferon-α, have yielded variable and often disappointing results. Clearly, this disease requires innovative therapeutic options, a need to be met soon, it is hoped, by research into the molecular pathogenesis of Kaposi's sarcoma.

Lymphoma

Lymphoma cutis develops in approximately 10% to 20% of systemic lymphomas and may occur as part of the HIV-related spectrum of disease. Lymphoma cutis generally presents as erythematous to violaceous nodules. B cell origin for HIV-related lymphomas is common.

Carcinoma

Although rare, squamous cell carcinoma arising in anal and perianal tissues is reported in homosexual men. An association is postulated between perianal squamous cell carcinoma and human papillomavirus infection. Basal cell carcinoma, squamous cell carcinoma in other sites, and melanoma are relatively common tumors in HIV^- individuals. These cancers are reported in HIV^+ persons, but whether their incidences are higher than expected is unknown.

REFERENCES

Beral V et al: Kaposi's sarcoma among persons with AIDS: a sexually transmitted infection? Lancet 335:123, 1990.

Cockerell CS et al: Clinical, histologic, microbiologic, and biochemical characterization of the causative agent of bacillary (epitheliod) angiomatosis: a rickettsial illness with features of bartonellosis. J Invest Dermatol 97:812, 1991.

Friedman-kien AE et al: Kaposi's sarcoma and pneumocytosis pneumonia among homosexual men—New York and California. MMWR 30:250, 1981.

Goodman DS et al: Prevalence of cutaneous disease in patients with acquired immunodeficiency syndrome (AIDS) or AIDS related complex. J Am Acad Dermatol 17:210, 1987.

Horn TD, Herzberg GZ, and Hood AF: Characterization of the dermal infiltrate in HIV infected patients with psoriasis. Arch Dermatol 125:1462, 1990.

Horn TD and Hood AF: Cytomegalovirus is predictably present in perineal ulcers from immunosuppressed patients. Arch Dermatol 126:642, 1990.

Ziegler JL and Dorfman RF: Overview of Kaposi's sarcoma history, epidemiology, and biomedical features. In Kaposi's sarcoma: pathophysiology and clinical management. New York, 1988, Decker Publishers.

Part Nine

Renal and Electrolyte Disorders

I BASIC PHYSIOLOGY

CHAPTER

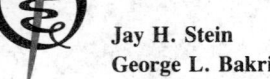

338 Principles of Renal Physiology

Jay H. Stein
George L. Bakris

RENAL PHYSIOLOGY

The kidney modulates sodium, water, hydrogen, and potassium balance. In a normal setting, sodium intake can be varied from negligible amounts to 500 mEq per day without the formation of edema or substantial changes in systemic hemodynamics. Urinary osmolality may be varied from 40 to 1200 mOsm per kilogram H_2O, whereas hydrogen ion excretion may be increased several fold after the ingestion of an acid load. A large exogenous potassium load, which potentially could cause life-threatening hyperkalemia, can be excreted rapidly by the normally functioning kidney.

In this section, we review the composition of body fluids and the factors that maintain their constancy, the determinants of glomerular filtration, and the renal functional events that are involved in the regulation of sodium, water, hydrogen, and potassium balance.

Composition of body fluids

Water and the major electrolytes are distributed among the various body fluid compartments on the basis of a complex series of transport and diffusional processes. Water accounts for 45% to 75% of total body weight, depending on the amount of adipose tissue, which is a function of the person's age and sex. Water is distributed between two basic compartments, extracellular and intracellular (Fig. 338-1), which are separated by the cellular membrane. Cell water accounts for approximately 60% of total body water. The extracellular compartment has been divided, somewhat artificially, into four subcompartments: plasma; interstitial fluid (including lymph); fluid within dense connective tissue, cartilage, and bone; and transcellular fluid (gastrointestinal secretions, urine, cerebrospinal fluid, sweat, etc.). Interstitial fluid makes up approximately half of the extracellular fluid (ECF).

Table 338-1 lists the electrolyte content of plasma, plasma water, interstitial fluid, and skeletal muscle intracellular water. As can be noted, sodium is the only major cation in ECF, whereas chloride and bicarbonate are the principal anions. In contrast, the intracellular concentration of sodium is one-tenth that in ECF, whereas the cellular potassium concentration is approximately 150 mEq/L. Further, intracellular chloride and bicarbonate are low, with the anionic content of cells consisting primarily of inorganic and organic phosphates and proteins.

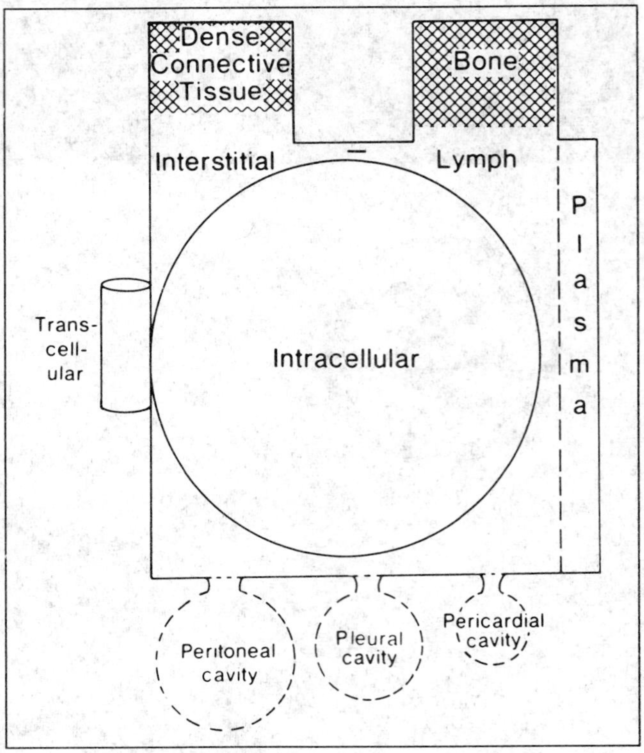

Fig. 338-1. Compartmentalization of body water. (From Maffly RH: The body fluids: volume, composition, and physical chemistry. In Brenner BM and Rector FC Jr, editors: The Kidney, ed 2. Philadelphia, 1981, Saunders.)

The differences between the composition of plasma and interstitial water are the consequence of the much higher concentration of proteins in plasma compared with that in

Table 338-1. Ionic composition of the body water compartments

Ion	Plasma (mEq/L)	Plasma water (mEq/L)	Interstitial fluid (mEq/L)	Skeletal muscle cell (mEq/L)
Cations				
Na^+	142.0	152.7	145.1	12.0
K^+	4.3	4.6	4.4	150.0
Ca^{2+}	2.5	2.7	2.4	4.0
Mg^{2+}	1.1	1.2	1.1	34.0
Total	149.9	161.2	153.0	200.0
Anions				
Cl^-	104.0	111.9	117.4	4.0
HCO_3^-	24.0	25.8	27.1	12.0
HPO_4^{2-}, $H_2PO_4^-$	2.0	2.2	2.3	40.0
Proteins	14.0	15.0	0.0	54.0
Other	5.9	6.3	6.2	90.0
Total	149.9	161.2	153.0	200.0

interstitial fluid. When a concentration difference exists for a given impermeable charged particle across a membrane, the ionic particles to which the membrane is permeable (e.g., sodium and chloride) are distributed in a mathematically predictable manner. This is the so-called Gibbs-Donnan effect.

The mechanisms responsible for the compositional differences between extracellular and intracellular fluid are more complex. The values listed in Table 338-1 for intracellular electrolyte content are taken from skeletal muscle. In addition, the complex structure of the cellular matrix may markedly alter the activity of these various electrolytes. For example, it has been proposed that the chemical activity of intracellular potassium is markedly reduced because of the attraction of the cation to cell protein anions.

The electrolyte content of the different transcellular fluids is also variable. The potassium concentration averages 4 mEq/L in biliary and pancreatic fluid, but may reach 20 mEq/L in saliva and cecal fluid. Further, the bicarbonate concentration is essentially zero in gastric juice and as high as 90 mEq/L in pancreatic secretions. Although the pH of most transcellular fluid is close to 7.4, gastric juice may have a pH as low as 1.0.

Osmotic equilibrium exists between the plasma and the interstitial and intracellular compartments. Thus, the size of each space is determined by the number of osmotically active particles present. Sodium and its attendant anions are the primary solutes in ECF, whereas potassium salts are the principal intracellular osmoles. A water load administered to a patient is rapidly distributed across all these major compartments until osmotic equilibrium is again reached. An isosmotic infusion of sodium chloride will be distributed only in ECF and will expand the extracellular volume without altering the tonicity. A solution of hypertonic sodium chloride also is distributed in ECF, but also causes a rapid loss of intracellular water until the osmotic pressure is the same in all compartments. After these initial alterations in body fluid dynamics, the renal excretion of salt or water, and changes in antidiuretic hormone release and in the thirst mechanism restore the previous steady-state condition.

The exchange of fluid between the plasma and interstitial compartments also is determined in great part by the Starling forces across the capillary wall. The net flow across the capillary is determined by the differences between the capillary and the interstitium in the oncotic and hydrostatic forces, or

$$\text{Net flow} = K_f[(P_{cap} + \pi_{IF}) - (\pi_{cap} + P_{IF})]$$

where K_f refers to the ultrafiltration coefficient across the capillary, P_{cap} and P_{IF} are the hydrostatic pressures in the capillary and interstitium, respectively, and π_{cap} and π_{IF} are the oncotic processes in the capillary and interstitium. Because π_{IF} and P_{IF} are substantially less than π_{cap} and P_{IF} and approximately equal, net filtration is determined by the difference between P_{cap} and π_{cap}. At the arterial end of the capillary, P_{cap} exceeds π_{cap} by about 7 mm Hg, and net filtration occurs. On the venous end of the capillary, the reverse is true ($\pi_{cap} > P_{cap}$), and reabsorption of fluid back into the capillary occurs. The pathophysiologic significance of this phenomenon is discussed in other sections.

Glomerular ultrafiltration

The production of an ultrafiltrate of plasma across the glomerulus occurs by a process entirely analogous to that discussed in the preceding section on transcapillary fluid movement. The net driving force affecting ultrafiltration of fluid across the glomerular capillary wall ($\bar{P}_{uf}$) is given by the difference between the transcapillary hydraulic pressure (ΔP) and the corresponding change in oncotic pressure ($\Delta\pi$). Thus, the rate of ultrafiltration along a glomerulus (GFR) is given by

$$\text{GFR} = K_f\bar{P}_{uf} \text{ or}$$
$$\text{GFR} = K_f(\Delta P - \Delta\pi)$$

where K_f is the ultrafiltration coefficient (the product of the hydraulic permeability coefficient and the surface area); ΔP is equal to the difference between the hydraulic pressure within the glomerular capillary ($\bar{P}_{GC}$) and the pressure in Bowman's space (P_T); and $\Delta\pi$ is the difference between the mean oncotic pressure within the glomerular capillary ($\bar{\pi}_{GC}$) and that in the glomerular ultrafiltrate.

Direct measurements of these variables have been obtained in the rat. Several points are worthy of note. First, the pressure drop between the aorta and glomerulus is much greater than had been believed, with $\bar{P}_{GC}$ averaging approximately 45 mmHg. Since the plasma oncotic pressure is approximately 25 mmHg and P_T is 10 mm Hg, $\bar{P}_{uf}$ at the afferent end of the glomerulus is only 10 mm Hg. As ultrafiltration occurs, $\bar{\pi}_{GC}$ increases substantially and may, in fact, equal ΔP. When ΔP and $\Delta\pi$ become equal, filtration ceases, and a state of filtration equilibrium is present. When filtration equilibrium is present, filtrate formation is markedly dependent on renal plasma flow. Thus, the various factors that affect renal resistance (intrinsic tone, sympathetic activity, humoral release of various vasoactive substances, renin-angiotensin system, prostaglandin release, kinin release, etc.) are major determinants of GFR in a setting in which filtration equilibrium exists at the end of the glomerulus. Whether this phenomenon occurs in humans is, of course, not known.

Finally, it should be emphasized that K_f may have a major effect on GFR. Recent work has demonstrated that angiotensin II, antidiuretic hormone, cyclic adenosine monophosphate (AMP), and other agents may decrease the K_f. Further, K_f has been shown to be reduced in various experimental models of acute glomerulonephritis and acute renal failure.

Sodium balance

Because sodium salts constitute more than 90% of the total solute content in the ECF, the net transport of these ions by the kidney is the primary determinant of the status of ECF volume. In the steady state, sodium intake and urinary excretion are approximately equal. If sodium intake is acutely increased, urinary sodium excretion increases, but it may take 3 to 5 days for a new steady state to be established (Fig. 338-2). In this interval, there will be a concomitant weight gain and a period of positive sodium balance until intake and output are again equivalent. It is assumed that the increase in sodium intake expands ECF volume, which in some manner leads to an increase in sodium excretion and the eventual attainment of a new steady state at a higher level of ECF volume. Although this concept seems simple, the components of the afferent and efferent limbs responsible for this critical homeostatic mechanism are still far from being clearly understood.

Afferent limb

The status of the ECF volume should be viewed in terms of the relationship between the volume of fluid contained in that compartment and the holding capacity of that compartment. The latter is determined by the capacity of the vascular tree and the compliance of the interstitial space. The vasodilatation that accompanies normal pregnancy results in sodium retention not because of an absolute deficit of ECF volume but because of the expanded ECF capacity. Cirrhosis, arteriovenous fistula, and assumption of the upright posture are other examples of conditions of relative volume depletion that result in sodium retention. Conversely, exposure to cold and immersion in water are instances in which relative increases in ECF volume occur, enhancing sodium excretion.

If the kidney is to respond appropriately to either absolute or relative changes in ECF volume, there must be some mechanism for sensing these changes. The possible components of the afferent limb are summarized in the box below. It seems likely that there is more than a single afferent receptor and that the kidney itself may be intimately involved in sensing the "fullness" of the ECF space.

Possible afferent components of extracellular fluid volume control

Intravascular receptors
  Cardiac atrial natriuretic hormone
  Arterial baroreceptors
Interstitial volume or pressure
Intrarenal hemodynamic and compositional receptors

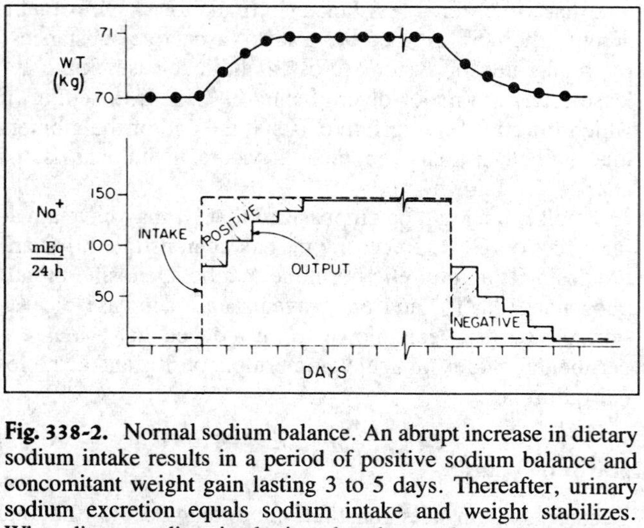

Fig. 338-2. Normal sodium balance. An abrupt increase in dietary sodium intake results in a period of positive sodium balance and concomitant weight gain lasting 3 to 5 days. Thereafter, urinary sodium excretion equals sodium intake and weight stabilizes. When dietary sodium intake is reduced, negative sodium balance occurs and body weight decreases until, after 3 to 5 days, a steady state is again achieved. (From Reineck HJ and Stein JH: Regulation of sodium balance. In Maxwell M and Kleeman CR, editors: Clinical disorders of fluid and electrolyte metabolism, ed 3. New York, 1980, McGraw-Hill.)

Efferent limb

Glomerular filtration rate. The urinary excretion of sodium is determined by the difference between the rates of filtration and tubular reabsorption. In normal humans, the filtered load of sodium equals approximately 14 mEq per minute. The urinary excretion rate is about 1% of this amount, or 0.14 mEq per minute, indicating that 99%, or 13.86 mEq per minute, is reabsorbed. If GFR increases by as little as 1% and reabsorption remains unchanged, urinary sodium excretion doubles.

Conversely, small decreases in GFR would be associated with a relatively large decrease in sodium excretion if there were not some type of coupling between filtration and sodium reabsorption. Yet, there is abundant evidence of a relationship between filtration and reabsorption. In other words, an increase in GFR is associated with a comparable increase in tubular sodium reabsorption. Conversely, a decrease in GFR leads to a parallel reduction in absolute sodium reabsorption.

Thus, under normal circumstances, there is a direct relationship between filtration rate and tubular sodium reabsorption, which would tend to minimize changes in sodium excretion as the filtered load is varied.

Aldosterone. The fact that aldosterone is necessary for the maintenance of normal sodium balance is illustrated by the observation of renal salt wasting in adrenal insufficiency. Because volume depletion stimulates aldosterone secretion and ECF expansion suppresses it, it has been attractive to credit this hormone with an important regulatory role in controlling urinary sodium excretion and ECF volume. Indeed, clearance, in vivo micropuncture, and in vitro microperfusion studies have demonstrated the importance of this hormone in the tubular reabsorption of sodium, especially along the distal nephron, where it affects potassium secretion as well. Several observations, however, indicate that aldosterone is not solely responsible for regulating sodium excretion. Most important, the chronic administration of mineralocorticoid causes only a transient period of salt retention, after which sodium balance is restored ("desoxycorticosterone [Doca] escape" phenomenon).

After mineralocorticoid is administered, a period of sodium and water retention ensues that lasts for 3 to 5 days. Then, in spite of continued mineralocorticoid administration, a natriuresis occurs, and balance is restored, albeit at a higher level of extracellular volume. This indicates that the sodium-retaining action of mineralocorticoid is overcome by a factor or factors that become operative as ECF volume is expanded.

Therefore, some factor or factors other than GFR and aldosterone play an important role in the regulation of sodium balance. In fact, it has been demonstrated that a natriuresis will occur after expansion of the ECF volume in spite of a reduction in GFR and maintenance of high levels of exogenous aldosterone. Renal physiologists have struggled diligently for several decades to understand this finding, and the mechanisms proposed to explain it are summarized in the box below.

Peritubular capillary forces. An increase in postglomerular capillary oncotic pressure or a decrease in hydrostatic pressure would increase the uptake of fluid from the interstitium into the capillary. Conversely, opposite changes in the Starling forces would lead to a net decrease in proximal tubular reabsorption. This mechanism has been suggested to be a regulator of sodium transport primarily in the proximal convoluted tubule and to be responsible, at least in part, for the alteration in sodium transport that occurs with expansion of ECF volume. Because these physical factors seem to operate only in the proximal tubule, it would appear that other mechanisms must affect sodium transport in more distal nephron segments.

Medullary blood flow. In addition to the alterations in net transport in the proximal tubule that may occur by purely passive means, hemodynamic alterations may change sodium transport in the distal nephron. An increase in medullary blood flow occurs during extracellular volume expansion, leading to a dissipation of the usual hypertonicity of the medullary interstitium. As a consequence of this change in the medullary environment, sodium excretion may increase in certain settings.

Redistribution of blood flow and/or filtrate. The anatomy of the kidney is complex, and various differences have been noted between nephrons in the outer and inner cortex and their vascular supply. Primarily because of these anatomic differences, many studies have been done to determine whether blood flow or filtrate redistribution occurs in various pathophysiologic states. In addition, microperfusion techniques have been used to compare various functional aspects of transport in superficial and juxtamedullary nephrons. Although many interesting findings have been noted in these studies, their relevance to the regulation of sodium balance is still not clear.

Atrial natiuretic peptide. Atrial natriuretic peptide (ANP) is produced mainly in the heart and released into the circulation in response to atrial stretch. The circulating peptide is 28 amino acids long, with a 17-member cystine-cystine ring. Exogenous administration of synthetic analogs of atrial natriuretic peptide increases the glomerular filtration rate through an increase in the glomerular capillary hydrostatic pressure and possibly an increase in the glomerular capillary permeability coefficient, K_f. The capability of ANP to increase the GFR together with its direct effects on the collecting tubule result in a profound natriuresis and diuresis.

In addition to its natriuretic-diuretic effect, atrial natriuretic peptide has been shown to inhibit almost all vasoconstrictors tested so far, including norepinephrine, angiotensin II, and vasopressin. It also has been shown to inhibit renin and aldosterone secretion both directly and indirectly. Circulating levels of this hormone are elevated in congestive heart failure, cirrhosis, and renal insufficiency and are normal or low in nephrotic syndrome, volume depletion, and possibly idiopathic edema.

Sympathetic activity. Altered adrenergic nervous activity can modify urinary sodium excretion by influencing the Starling forces in the peripheral capillary bed, by affecting the central blood volume and thus the distribution of ECF, or by changing renal hemodynamics. A more direct effect of autonomic nervous activity on increasing renal tubular sodium reabsorption also has been demonstrated. It should be noted, however, that patients with a renal transplant (i.e., a denervated kidney) seem to handle a sodium load normally. An increase in sympathetic tone and arterial pressure may also result in a "pressure natriuresis." This results from a decrease in sodium reabsorption in the deep nephrons of the Loop of Henle and questionably the proximal tubule. Thus, further studies are needed for a better understanding of the role of the renal nerves in the physiologic control of urinary sodium excretion.

Possible efferent components of extracellular fluid volume control other than glomerular filtration rate and aldosterone

Peritubular capillary forces:
  Hydrostatic and colloid osmotic pressures
Medullary blood flow
Redistribution of renal blood flow or glomerular filtrate
Humoral substances: "atrial natriuretic peptide"
Sympathetic nerve activity

Water metabolism

Normal persons possess a remarkable ability to maintain the tonicity of body fluids within very narrow limits, ranging from 285 to 295 mOsm per kilogram H_2O. This regulatory function requires the complex coordination of a variety of factors. When plasma osmolality begins to rise, mechanisms required to prevent further increases include stimulation and perception of thirst, release of antidiuretic hormone (ADH), and the renal expression of that hormone that permits maximum concentration of the urine. Conversely, small decreases in tonicity are corrected by suppression of thirst, inhibition of ADH release, and subsequent elaboration of a maximally dilute urine. The regulation of thirst and ADH release are discussed in Chapter 350. The following section describes the renal handling of water.

Renal concentrating and diluting mechanisms. Even in the presence of intact thirst and ADH-releasing mechanisms, maintenance of normal water balance requires that the kidney be capable of maximum dilution or concentration of the urine. The ability to concentrate and dilute the urine is indicated by maximum and minimum urine osmolality (U_{osm}), respectively. During water deprivation and maximum ADH release, U_{osm} approaches 1200 mOsm per kilogram H_2O; during water diuresis with total suppression of ADH, normal persons can lower U_{osm} to nearly 50 mOsm per kilogram H_2O. Although clinically useful, U_{osm} is a purely quantitative term and does not necessarily indicate a normal ability to excrete a water load or retain water. The former is determined by measurement of free water clearance (C_{H_2O}), which indicates the amount of solute-free water that the kidney can excrete per unit time. C_{H_2O} is calculated by the following formula:

(EQ. 1)

$$C_{H_2O} = V - C_{osm}$$

where V = urine volume and C_{osm} = osmolar clearance, calculated as follows:

(EQ. 2)

$$C_{osm} = \frac{U_{osm}}{P_{osm}} \times V$$

where U_{osm} = urine osmolality, and P_{osm} = plasma osmolality. Combining (EQ. 1) and (EQ. 2),

(EQ. 3)

$$C_{H_2O} = V \left[\frac{U_{osm}}{P_{osm}} \times V\right]$$

Several important points regarding C_{H_2O} deserve comment. First, from close scrutiny of this equation, it is apparent that the maximum amount of free water that can be excreted is dependent on solute load as well as on ADH suppression and minimum urine osmolality. For instance, if a person with a plasma osmolality of 300 mOsm per kilogram H_2O ingests and excretes 1500 mOsm of solute per day (U_{osm} V) and can reduce U_{osm} to 50 mOsm per kilogram H_2O, V is 30 liters per day, and C_{osm} is 5 liters per day. C_{H_2O} is, therefore, 25 liters per day, meaning the person can ingest 30 liters of water per day without dilutional hyponatremia developing. This quantity contrasts with the maximum fluid intake for a person ingesting and excreting 600 mOsm of solute per day. With the same dilute urine (50 mOsm per kilogram H_2O), V = 12 liters per day and C_{osm} = 2 liters per day; maximum C_{H_2O} is now only 10 liters per day. Hyponatremia results with a fluid intake in excess of 12 liters per day.

An important aspect of C_{H_2O} relates to the nephron site responsible for the generation of "free water." As is discussed in more detail later, urinary dilution involves removal of solute from the tubular fluid without extraction of water. In the mammalian kidney, this process begins along the ascending limb of Henle's loop at the point at which the osmolality of the tubular fluid becomes hypotonic relative to plasma. Distal to this point, further dilution of tubular fluid occurs and free water is generated. From this consideration, it is obvious that maximum C_{H_2O} depends on quantitative delivery of filtrate to this nephron site, where free water formation begins.

The ability to conserve water maximally is quantitatively expressed by the term *free water reabsorption* (T^CH_2O). This value is calculated by the following formula:

$$T^CH_2O = C_{osm} - V \text{ or}$$

$$T^CH_2O = \frac{U_{osm}V}{P_{osm}} - V$$

As can be seen, this expression is the opposite of free water clearance (C_{H_2O}) and is therefore sometimes termed *negative free water clearance*. The same principles that apply to maximum C_{H_2O} (i.e., dependence on maximum ADH release, solute excretion, and distal delivery) are also applicable to T^CH_2O. Maximum T^CH_2O is physiologically important in preventing the development of water deficits. It should be stressed that once a water deficit is incurred (e.g., by profuse sweating or diarrhea), the thirst mechanism also must be activated to replace these losses.

As was noted earlier, the maintenance of normal water balance requires that the kidney be capable of responding to the extremes of ADH exposure. Maximum dilution of the urine is relatively straightforward and, as previously alluded to, requires removal of solute without water. In the absence of ADH, the remainder of the nephron distal to this diluting segment is relatively impermeable to water, and, as a result, a dilute urine is excreted.

The process of urinary concentration is more complex and is schematically represented in Fig. 338-3, *A*. Perhaps paradoxically, it too is dependent on the removal of solute without water from the ascending limb of the loop of Henle. This dependence is because this process is the driving force necessary for establishing a hypertonic medullary interstitium. As tubular fluid leaves the thick ascending limb, it enters the distal convoluted tubule and cortical collecting tubule, which, in the presence of ADH, are permeable to water but not to urea. Thus, as the initially dilute fluid traverses these segments, in which interstitial tonicity is equal to that of plasma, water is removed and osmolality increases. The tubular fluid next enters the outer medullary collecting duct, which is also water permeable and urea impermeable. Because this segment lies in the hypertonic interstitium, as water is removed, the urea concentration and osmolality of the tubular fluid increase further. Finally, the fluid enters the inner medullary collecting duct, where further water extraction occurs. In addition, at the junction of the outer and inner medulla, the collecting duct epithelium becomes permeable to urea, which then diffuses passively down a concentration gradient, supplying solute to the inner medulla. The urea permeability of this segment is enhanced by ADH. As fluid enters the medulla from the proximal tubule, the characteristics of the thin descending limb allow for diffusion of water into the hypertonic interstitium without solute. As a result, the sodium chloride concentration at the bend of Henle's loop is high.

In addition to the loop of Henle and the collecting duct, the vasa recta play an important role in maintaining urinary concentrating ability. As is shown in Fig. 338-3, *B*, these vascular capillary loops serve a dual function: They remove water that enters the medullary interstitium from the descending limb of Henle's loop and the collecting duct, and by virtue of their permeability to sodium chloride and urea, they serve as countercurrent exchangers to maintain the hypertonicity of the medulla.

RENAL ACIDIFICATION

Under steady-state conditions, the excretion of acid by the kidney precisely balances the acid that enters the ECF. As a consequence of the renal excretion of acid, the extracellular bicarbonate concentration is stabilized, and the maintenance of systemic acid–base homeostasis is facilitated. The rate of nonvolatile acid production in the adult is estimated to be 1 mEq per kilogram body weight per day, or 70 mEq per 1.73 m^2. Because at the minimal urine pH only trivial amounts of hydrogen are present as the free ion, acid (hydrogen) excretion in the urine is buffered by ammonia or other buffers, particularly inorganic phosphate, which is measured as titratable acid. The excretion of acid as ammonium accounts for about two thirds of the acid present in urine, whereas approximately one third of the acid is excreted as titratable acid. The magnitude of titratable acid excretion depends on the rate of excretion of the buffer involved, its p*K*, and the urinary pH. Net acid excretion by the kidney may be expressed as the sum of the ammonium and titratable acid excreted minus any bicarbonate that may be present in the urine.

The hydrogen ions that enter the ECF are primarily formed through catabolism of ingested food or tissue stores. Sulfuric acid produced as the neutral sulfur in sulfur-containing amino acids is oxidized. Similarly, the incomplete oxidation of carbon foodstuffs produces organic acids such as pyruvic, lactic, citric, and acetoacetic acid. The hydrolysis of organic orthophosphate and pyrophosphate gives rise to phosphoric acid, and the metabolism of nucleoproteins gives rise to uric acid. As these various nonvolatile acids dissociate, the hydrogen ions react with the body buffers (e.g., bicarbonate, dibasic phosphate, protein) to yield a neutral sodium salt and carbonic acid (H_2CO_3). The H_2CO_3 is excreted as carbon dioxide by the lungs.

As previously indicated, the renal contribution to systemic acid–base homeostasis is to regulate plasma bicarbonate concentration. This regulation is achieved by the appropriate reabsorption of filtered bicarbonate and the regeneration of the bicarbonate decomposed by reaction with nonvolatile acids, as has been discussed. As the neutral salts of the nonvolatile acids are presented to the kidney in the glomerular filtrate, the anion is excreted with hydrogen, and the sodium, together with the newly formed bicarbonate, is returned to the ECF. The quantity of hydrogen excreted as titratable acid and ammonium is equivalent to the amount of bicarbonate regenerated.

As it is generally conceived, hydrogen ions are actively secreted at the luminal membrane into the tubular urine (Fig. 338-4). Associated with this secretion of hydrogen ions is the return of bicarbonate to the ECF. In the lumen, the hydrogen ions react either with filtered bicarbonate to

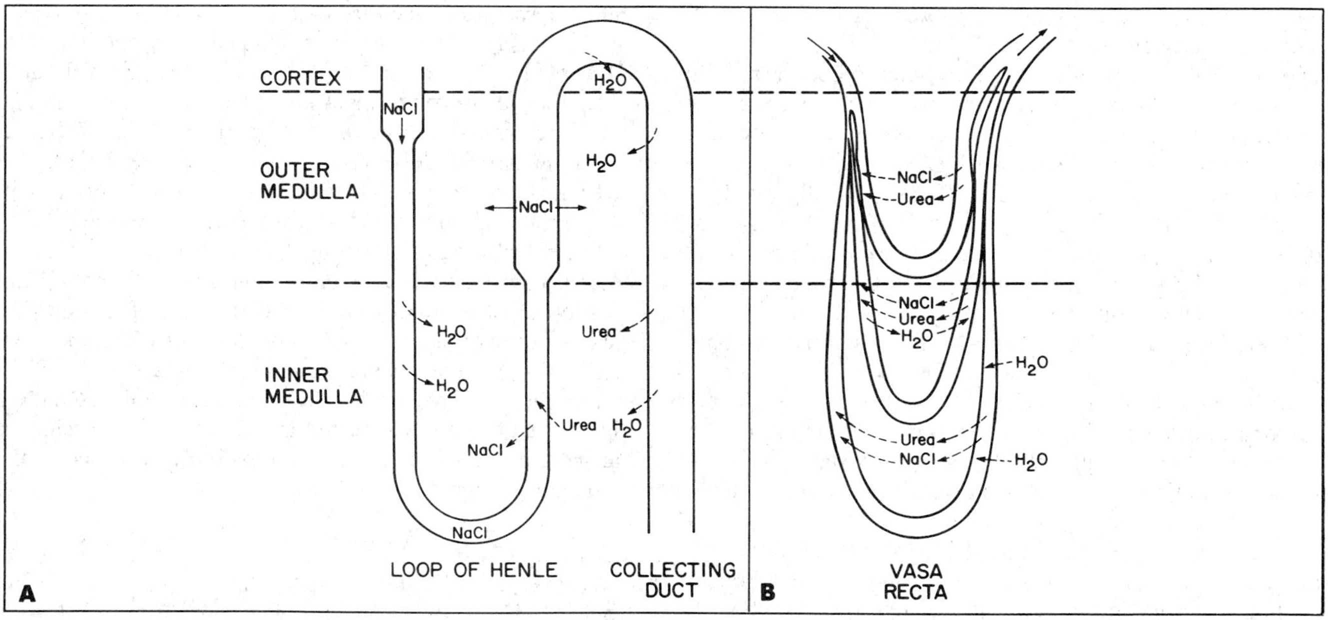

Fig. 338-3. Urinary-concentrating mechanisms. **A,** The loop of Henle and collecting duct serve as a source of solute (NaCl and urea) to provide a hypertonic interstitium (see text for detailed explanation). **B,** The complex of vasa recta entering and leaving the medulla provides a mechanism for removing water from and trapping solute within the medullary interstitium.

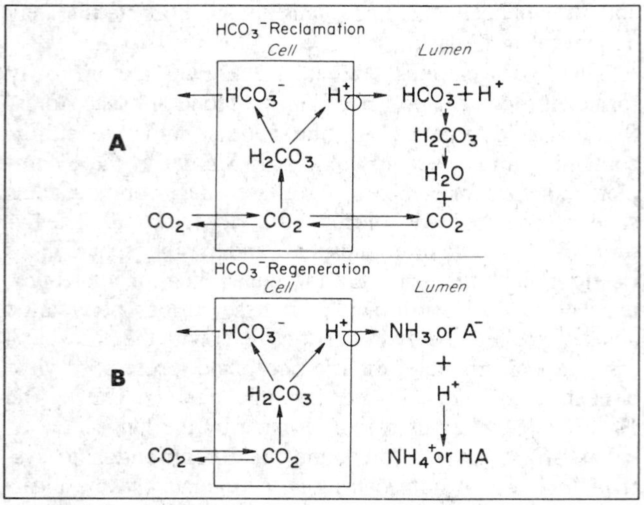

Fig. 338-4. Tubular acidification. Hydrogen ions secreted at the luminal border effect **(A)** bicarbonate reabsorption from the glomerular filtrate or **(B)** bicarbonate regeneration. The generation of hydrogen and bicarbonate ions may not occur precisely as shown, but the net effect is as illustrated.

form H_2CO_3, which dehydrates to water and carbon dioxide, or, as discussed previously, with certain salts to form the acid salt (HA) and with ammonia to form ammonium (NH_4^+). The relative distribution of the reaction of hydrogen ions between filtered bicarbonate and nonbicarbonate buffers depends on the pH of the tubular urine. In more proximal nephron segments, where the luminal bicarbonate concentration is high, most of the hydrogen ion secreted results in bicarbonate reabsorption. As bicarbonate reabsorption nears completion, the luminal bicarbonate concentration decreases, and an increasingly larger fraction of the secreted hydrogen reacts with the nonbicarbonate buffers. The enzyme carbonic anhydrase plays an important role in renal acid excretion in many portions of the nephron.

Renal acid excretion is influenced by a number of factors, some of which are capable of enhancing acidification, whereas others have the opposite effect. Clinically, the levels of ECF volume expansion, carbon dioxide tension, potassium, mineralocorticoids, and perhaps calcium, phosphorus, and parathyroid hormone, have the greatest influence on renal acidification.

Clearance studies have suggested that potential renal bicarbonate reabsorption is inversely related to the degree of effective ECF volume expansion. Thus, the addition of bicarbonate to the ECF in a patient with contraction of the effective volume results in a higher steady-state bicarbonate concentration than when it is given in the volume-replete state.

An acute increase in plasma PCO_2 stimulates renal hydrogen ion secretion. Because the quantity of bicarbonate in the glomerular filtrate is limited, however, bicarbonate reabsorption can only increase to the extent that tissue buffers are titrated, forming extra bicarbonate. More chronic (more than 24 hours) increments in the plasma PCO_2 result in increases in net acid excretion, adding new bicarbonate to the ECF. After a variable period, net acid excretion returns to normal as a new steady state is attained.

Mineralocorticoids and potassium have a complex and interrelated effect on renal hydrogen ion secretion. Current studies suggest that mineralocorticoid excess and potassium deficiency, when present as individual entities, have a very modest effect, if any, on net acid excretion and the extracellular bicarbonate concentration. Yet, the effect of combined potassium deficiency and mineralocorticoid excess in humans can lead to significant increases in net acid excretion and extracellular bicarbonate concentration. Mineralocorticoid deficiency results in a modest metabolic acidosis, as a consequence of a decrease in net acid excretion.

RENAL POTASSIUM TRANSPORT

In this section, we present a brief description of the characteristics of potassium transport within individual nephrons and between different nephron populations.

Most of the filtered potassium is reabsorbed in the proximal nephron, that is, the proximal tubule and the loop of Henle. More distal portions of the nephron, namely, the distal tubule, the collecting tubule, and the collecting duct, are the sites where the final regulation of renal potassium transport occurs.

Proximal nephron

Direct micropuncture study of the superficial proximal convoluted tubule of the mammalian kidney has shown that this segment reabsorbs filtered potassium in proportion to the amount of sodium and water reabsorbed. Under control circumstances, this is 50% to 60% of the filtered load. The intraluminal concentration of potassium in the proximal tubule approximates the plasma level.

At the superficial early distal tubule, only about 10% to 15% of the filtered load of potassium remains. This indicates that reabsorption must take place in at least one distinct anatomic segment in the superficial loop of Henle. When potassium delivery to the bend of Henle's loop of juxtamedullary nephrons was measured in control circumstances, the amount of potassium present represented 113% of the filtered load, indicating that a net addition of potassium occurred between the glomerulus and the bend of Henle's loop. If the proximal convoluted tubule of juxtamedullary nephrons reabsorbs potassium, as does its superficial cortical counterpart, then the addition of potassium must occur in the proximal straight tubule or the thin descending limb. Studies have suggested that the added potassium is derived, at least in part, from potassium reabsorbed in the collecting system.

Distal nephron

Micropuncture studies of the superficial distal tubule have indicated that this nephron site is a major contributor to urinary potassium and the site where a number of factors that influence renal potassium excretion express their effect.

The superficial distal tubule, like the loop of Henle, does

not consist of a single anatomic or functional unit but is composed of a number of different segments. The initial superficial distal tubule contains, for the most part, the distal convoluted tubule, but later segments may have cells typical of the cortical collecting tubule. Between these two may be a segment where both histologic types are seen. The distal tubule can demonstrate either net reabsorption or secretion of potassium, with secretion being restricted to the distal half of this tubular segment. Therefore, although 10% to 15% of the filtered potassium may arrive at the early distal tubule, at its most distal portion, the amount present may be less than, equal to, or more than the amount that arrived at the early distal site.

The cellular mechanisms responsible for such divergent transport properties have been the subject of extensive study. The late distal tubular cell is assumed to be asymmetrically polarized, with the electrical potential difference across the peritubular membrane exceeding that across the luminal membrane. Potassium secretion is envisioned as comprising active and passive components. The active component takes place on the peritubular border, where potassium is moved into the cell by a process coupled with extrusion of sodium from the cell and associated with (Na^+ + K^+)-ATPase. Potassium movement from cell to lumen is assumed to be passive, proceeding down a favorable electrochemical gradient. Viewed simply, the amount of potassium secreted depends on the rate of potassium uptake into the cell, the permeability of the luminal membrane, and the electrochemical gradient for potassium across the luminal membrane. Net potassium reabsorption also can be observed in the distal tubule when dietary potassium is restricted.

The collecting system comprises a number of different anatomic segments, including the cortical collecting tubule, the outer medullary collecting duct, and finally the papillary collecting duct. The cortical collecting tubule is capable of active potassium secretion but has not been observed to reabsorb potassium. The more terminal portions of the collecting duct have the potential to reabsorb or secrete potassium, depending on the experimental circumstance examined.

A number of factors—namely, potassium balance, mineralocorticoids, glucocorticoids, ADH, catecholamines, acid-base balance, and the delivery of sodium and water to distal nephron segments—appear to be capable of exerting profound effects on renal potassium transport.

Acute respiratory and metabolic alkalosis and potassium administration are known to increase the renal excretion of potassium. Conversely, both potassium deprivation and acute respiratory and metabolic acidosis may diminish the urinary excretion of potassium. The ability of mineralocorticoids to enhance potassium excretion may, at least in part, be mediated by their increasing the quantity of potassium incorporated into the cellular transport pool and thereby increasing the electrochemical gradient of potassium from cell to lumen. Mineralocorticoids also may increase the permeability of the luminal membrane to potassium. Glucocorticoids appear to affect potassium transport primarily by altering renal hemodynamics. Antidiuretic hormone directly stimulates distal potassium secretion. Epinephrine inhibits potassium secretion, an effect mediated by the $beta_1$-adrenergic receptor. The mechanism of this effect is still undergoing investigation. Finally, it has been known for some time that urinary potassium excretion may vary in parallel with the flow rate of urine and the delivery of sodium to the distal nephron. The potentiating effect of enhanced distal water and sodium delivery on potassium transport is also seemingly mediated through changes in the electrochemical gradient of potassium, although the precise nature of this relationship has yet to be clearly defined.

REFERENCES

Arendshorst W and Gottschalk CW: Glomerular ultrafiltration dynamics: historical perspective. Am J Physiol 248:F163, 1985.

Bakris GL and Stein JH: Sodium metabolism and maintenance of extracellular fluid volume. In DeFronzo R and Arieff A, editors: Fluids and Electrolytes, ed 2. New York, 1992, Churchill Livingstone.

Dibona GF: Neural regulation of renal tubular sodium reabsorption and renin secretion: integrative aspects. Clin Exp Hypertens 9(suppl I):151, 1987.

Eveloff JL and Warnock DG: Activation of ion transport systems during cell volume regulation. Am J Physiol 252:F1, 1987.

Gluck SL: Cellular and molecular aspects of renal [H^+] transport. Hosp Pract May 15:149, 1989.

Kurtzman NA: Disorders of distal acidification. Kidney Int 38:720, 1990.

Lassiter WE and Gottschalk CW: Regulation of water balance: urine concentration and dilution. In Schrier RW and Gottschalk CW, editors: Diseases of the Kidney, ed 4. Boston, 1988, Little, Brown.

Stanton BA: Electroneutral NaCl transport by distal tubule: evidence for Na^+/H^+-Cl^-/HCO_3^- exchange. Am J Physiol 254:F80, 1988.

Steinmetz PR: Cellular organization of urinary acidification. Am J Physiol 251:F173, 1986.

Wright FS: Renal potassium handling. Semin Nephrol 7:174, 1987.

LABORATORY TESTS AND DIAGNOSTIC METHODS II

CHAPTER

339 Urinalysis

Marvin Forland

The urinalysis is one of the oldest, simplest, and most useful laboratory tests in clinical medicine. Traditionally, it has been regarded as an extension of the physical examination, to be performed regularly as part of the periodic health evaluation and as an essential part of the evaluation of the sick patient. Despite its relatively low cost, it is a significant component of laboratory expenditures due to its widespread use. Extensive studies of its cost-effectiveness are being conducted to better determine its screening and preoperative usefulness as well as to evaluate the use of reagent strip testing as a screening procedure before performing the more labor-intensive microscopic examination.

ROUTINE URINALYSIS

The routine urinalysis usually consists of the following information:

1. Source of the specimen, indicating the means of collection
2. Description of the urine, including its color and appearance
3. pH
4. Specific gravity or osmolality
5. Protein concentration
6. Glucose concentration
7. Microscopic examination

With the availability of reagent strip techniques, semiquantitative measurement of concentrations of keto acids, bilirubin, urobilinogen, and heme-containing materials (erythrocytes, hemoglobin, myoglobin) are also usually included. Screening for leukocyturia and bacteriuria are additional options available with reagent strips.

Collection

Urine for examination must be freshly collected or refrigerated immediately if storage is necessary. If the examination is delayed, multiplication of bacteria will result in pH alteration, cells may degenerate, and casts will often dissolve in alkaline urine. A specimen collected immediately after arising in the morning ("first morning specimen") is usually preferred for examination; the urine is generally more concentrated, and has a lower pH, which provides a greater possibility for observing formed elements. The purpose of the examination determines the method of collection. For routine urinalysis, an unprepared specimen in a clean container is satisfactory; if observation for bacteria or a culture is desired, the patient must use cleansing techniques, and the specimen should be a clean-voided or, more rarely, a catheterized specimen. Suprapubic or transvaginal aspiration techniques have been described and are used under special circumstances.

Color

The color of the urine may provide a useful diagnostic clue. Many alterations are due to drug ingestions. Table 339-1 summarizes the conditions or drugs responsible for some of the more common color alterations of the urine.

Table 339-1. Urine color alterations

Color	Cause
Black	Melanoma
Brown	Bilirubin (to olive green on standing), blood, cascara, hemoglobin, homogentisic acid (to black on standing), myoglobin, phenacetin, quinine
Greenish blue	Biliverdin, indigo blue, methylene blue, tetrahydronaphthalen (Cuprex)
Orange	Salicylazosulfapyridine (Azulfidine), phenazopyridine (Pyridium), rifampin (Rifadin, Rimactane)
Purple	Porphyrin (on standing)
Red	Beets, free hemoglobin, fresh blood, phenolphthalein, phenytoin, vegetable dyes
Yellow	Quinacrine (Atabrine), riboflavin

Specific gravity and osmolality

Plasma osmolality is maintained in a narrow range of approximately 285 ± 5 mosm/kg H_2O because of the kidney's ability to reabsorb or excrete water as mediated by the tubular effect of antidiuretic hormone (ADH). Urinary specific gravity or osmolality reflects the activity of ADH and the sensitivity of the collecting tubule to its effects, except in situations in which abnormal solutes are excreted by the kidney, resulting in an osmotic diuresis.

Urinary specific gravity depends on the size and weight of urinary solutes. It represents the weight of 1 ml of urine, a mixture of water and solute, compared with the weight of 1 ml of pure water. The possible range is 1.001 to 1.040 (the approximate specific gravity of serum is 1.010). The normal range is 1.003 to 1.025. Specific gravity is usually determined by a hydrometer. High molecular weight particles present in abnormal quantities in the urine will significantly elevate specific gravity. The following are the most frequent corrections necessary: Reduce measured specific gravity by 0.003 for each g/dl of protein and by 0.004 for each g/dl of glucose.

Specific gravity may be measured with only a few drops of urine using a total solids meter. This very simple instrument measures refractive index and is calibrated to indicate specific gravity. However, the refractive index of urine is more closely related to osmolality. Osmolality indicates the total solute particle number per kilogram of urine water. It is the physiologically significant measurement of renal concentrating and diluting ability, because it is unaffected by particle size and weight. Osmolality is usually determined by measuring freezing point depression with an osmometer. It is based on the physical principle that a solute concentration of 1000 mosm/kg H_2O depresses the freezing point of water by 1.86° C.

A reagent strip is now available for determining urinary specific gravity based on a polyacid whose acidity is sensitive to the ionic concentration of the urine specimen. Correlation with pycnometry or a total solids meter determination is altered by urinary pH greater than 6.5, albumin concentration greater than 100 mg/dl, and glucose greater than 1000 mg/dl. The physiologic range of urinary osmolality achievable in humans is approximately 50 to 1200 mosm/kg. In the absence of extreme deprivation or unusual intake, the urinary range is 150 to 900 mosm/kg. Usually, the principal value of urine specific gravity measurement in routine urinalysis is to make certain the urine is not so markedly dilute as to permit false-negative values, particularly for proteinuria or formed elements. Urinary abnormalities should not be ruled out unless specific gravity of the specimen is greater than or equal to 1.015 or osmolality is greater than or equal to 600 mosm/kg H_2O.

URINARY pH

Because of the relatively high amount of sulfur-containing protein in the human diet, an adult must excrete in the urine approximately 1 mEq of hydrogen/kg body weight each day to maintain acid-base balance. Because maximum acidification of the urine can lower the urine pH only to 4.5 to 5.0, virtually all hydrogen ions are buffered by urinary ammonia and phosphate. However, normal urine is generally of acid pH except for the postprandial "alkaline tide," which may result in a transient rise in urinary pH. The upper physiologic limit of urinary pH is approximately 8.

The most common methodology used for measuring urine pH is color-sensitive dye impregnated on multipurpose reagent sticks. Nitrazine paper is frequently used for patients whose urinary pH is being regulated as a therapeutic maneuver; the color changes usually permit estimation of 0.5 pH units. The most accurate results are obtained through the use of the pH meter; the urine should be collected under oil to prevent diffusion of carbon dioxide and consequent elevation of urinary pH.

Persistently alkaline urine may indicate an infection with a urea-splitting organism such as *Proteus mirabilis,* the usual cause for urinary pH greater than or equal to 8. Urinary pH of 7 or more is also associated with a systemic alkalosis, as seen with hyperaldosteronism or severe vomiting. Distal-type renal tubular acidosis is characterized by an alkaline urine despite systemic acidosis.

PROTEINURIA

Persistent proteinuria provides one of our best clues to the presence of primary renal disease or renal involvement in systemic illness. Proteinuria is often an initial manifestation of a renal abnormality during an as yet asymptomatic phase and always requires further evaluation and clarification of its cause. Although approximately 180 liters of plasma containing over 12,000 g of plasma protein are filtered across the glomeruli each day, the glomerular filtration barrier permits the passage of only a very small amount of protein. Micropuncture data from experimental animals suggest that proximal tubular fluid may contain 1 to 10 mg of protein/dl. Because normal humans excrete only 50 to 150 mg of protein each day, the renal tubules consequently must reabsorb most of the approximately 2 to 20 g that may be filtered.

The 50 to 150 mg of protein found normally in the urine each day is made up of a variety of components. Some of these proteins are identical to serum proteins and presumably represent filtered plasma components that have escaped tubular reabsorption. Albumin is a major component of this fraction and represents 10% to 20% of the total excreted protein. The principal urinary protein components, representing approximately one third of the total weight, are high molecular weight glycoproteins believed to be secreted by the more distal segments of the renal tubule. The Tamm-Horsfall glycoprotein is the major component and also a primary constituent of hyaline casts. The remaining urinary proteins are a heterogeneous mixture of as many as 30 components, mainly demonstrating the electrophoretic mobility of globulins. In abnormal proteinuria, albumin usually is the predominant component because of its high serum concentration and relatively low molecular weight.

A number of methods are available to detect proteinuria on routine urinalysis. These range from the traditional semiquantitative heat-acid turbidity tests to the use of the simple and rapid reagent stick. Clear urine is used in the heat-acid test, following centrifugation if necessary; 10 ml of urine is placed in a test tube, and the upper portion of the urine is boiled over a Bunsen burner; if the urine becomes cloudy, three drops of concentrated acetic acid are added (this will redissolve phosphates but not protein). The urine is then heated to boiling. Persistent cloudiness indicates proteinuria and is reported on a scale of 0 to 4+.

The reagent stick test is based on the reaction of tetrabromophenol blue plus citrate buffer, resulting in a color change when the stick is dipped into protein-containing urine. A trace reaction indicates approximately 20 mg of protein/dl.

Most nephrologists prefer the sulfosalicylic acid method because test results are more clearly defined than on the reagent stick. Two to three drops of 20% sulfosalicylic acid are added to 3 to 5 ml of clear urine. The degree of turbidity is estimated. Slight turbidity is reported as trace proteinuria and indicates approximately 4 to 10 mg protein/dl; the presence of a flocculent precipitate indicates 4+ proteinuria and generally reflects in excess of 500 mg of protein/dl. The intermediate ranges of turbidity are scaled from 1+ to 3+. False-positive readings may occur in urines that contain radiologic contrast material, tolbutamide, sulfisoxazole metabolites, or massive doses of penicillin. Highly buffered alkaline urines may give a false-positive protein reading. The sulfosalicylic acid method will give a positive result with Bence Jones proteinuria, which may not be evident by the reagent stick method, because the latter technique detects principally the anionic proteins, with albumin predominating.

The availability of radioimmunoassays for the quantitation of urinary albumin excretion at levels not detectable by usual clinical methods has led to considerable investigation of the significance of "microalbuminuria." A series of studies have indicated the predictive value of the presence of microalbuminuria for the development of overt nephropathy in patients with both insulin-dependent and non-insulin-dependent diabetes mellitus. In normal subjects urine albumin excretion rates rarely exceed 15 μg/min, with a mean value of 5 μg/min. Normal 24-hour excretion is up to 20 mg. The albumin/creatinine ratio in single, untimed specimens found predictive of identifying diabetic subjects at risk of developing overt nephropathy is $\geq$ 30 mg/g. A urine test strip providing a semiquantitative immunoassay for microalbuminuria has been introduced. For orthostatic or postural proteinuria see Chapter 343.

GLUCOSE

Plasma glucose is freely filterable across the glomerulus and normally is virtually entirely reabsorbed in the proximal tubules. The transport maximum in normal males is approximately 375 mg/min and is somewhat lower in females. The renal threshold at which glucose will first appear in the urine is a plasma concentration of 160 to 180 mg/dl. Normal subjects excrete approximately 100 to 200 mg of reducing substances in the urine in 24 hours. These include glucose, lactose, levulose, pentose, and such nonsugars as ascorbic acid, which will reduce an alkaline-copper solution. These substances usually are not present in adequate quantities to cause a positive clinical laboratory test for urinary reducing substances. The presence of a positive test for urinary glucose indicates either that the normal renal threshold has been exceeded by the plasma level of glucose or that a reduction has occurred in the reabsorptive capacity of the kidney.

The traditional test for measuring urinary glucose has been a positive reduction test with Benedict's cupric sulfate solution. It must be remembered that sugars such as fructose and lactose will reduce the reagent, as will such non-sugar-reducing substances as salicylates, paraldehyde, and chloral hydrate. The semiquantitative Benedict's cupric sulfate reduction test is performed by adding eight drops of urine to 5 ml of Benedict's solution and heating the mixture to boiling. The color reactions range from green, indicating 250 to 500 mg glucose/dl, to orange, representing 2 g/dl.

Tablets for measuring sugar-reducing agents have been largely replaced by enzyme-impregnated reagent strips that produce a color reaction when moistened with a glucose solution. Because they contain glucose oxidase, they test specifically for glucose. They are more sensitive than Benedict's solution and Clinitest tablets and will detect glucose in concentrations of 100 mg/dl or less. After rapid dipping, comparison is made with color standards on the container. Attention to timing is critical.

KETONE BODIES

The ketone bodies include acetoacetic acid, β-hydroxybutyric acid, and acetone. They are normal intermediates in the oxidation of fatty acids formed in the liver and most other tissues and are completely metabolized with negligible excretion in the urine. Normal blood levels are 1.5 to 2.0 mg/dl, and urine excretion is less than 1 mg/24 hours. Elevation in blood levels is called *ketosis* or *ketonemia,* and increased urinary concentration is termed *ketonuria*.

Ketosis occurs with the excessive formation and accumulation of ketone bodies. Blood levels may reach 200 mg/dl with renal excretion of over 60 g/24 hours. The usual tests can detect less than 10 mg/dl. The increased concentration of ketone bodies results in an anion gap acidosis. The β-hydroxybutyric acid component normally constitutes 40% to 70% of the total ketone bodies, but the commonly used laboratory methods do not measure this component. When lactic acidosis is superimposed on diabetic ketoacidosis, almost all ketones are β-hydroxybutyric acid, and the diagnosis of ketoacidosis may be missed with dependence on ketone-body testing alone. A similar predominance of β-hydroxybutyric acid is seen in alcoholic ketoacidosis.

The traditional Lange test for ketones is performed by adding three crystals of sodium nitroprusside and three drops of glacial acetic acid to 5 ml of urine in a test tube. The mixture is shaken to dissolve the crystals and then overlaid with 2 ml of concentrated ammonium hydroxide. A purple ring at the zone of contact indicates a positive reaction for ketone bodies. The test is sensitive but difficult to quantitate. The essential ingredients of the Lange test have been incorporated in tablet form. Results are determined from a color standard chart after the placement of one drop of urine on the surface of the tablet. Reagent strips that are impregnated with nitroprusside and react when moistened with urine or serum-containing ketones are now widely used.

BLOOD PIGMENTS

Pigmenturia can be related to the abnormal presence of a number of heme-containing pigments; these may be derived from the presence of red cells in the urine *(hematuria)*. The presence of free hemoglobin *(hemoglobinuria)* is usually indicative of intravascular hemolysis. *Myoglobinuria* is the designation for free myoglobin in the urine resulting from muscle injury. All three forms of pigmenturia will give a positive orthotolidine test, and additional procedures are thus necessary to identify the specific type of heme pigment in the urine. Acrylamide-gel electrophoresis or immunodiffusion techniques provide the most definitive differentiation between hemoglobin and myoglobin. Examination of the patient's serum may facilitate the differentiation between myoglobin and hemoglobin; hemolysis results in a pink-tinged serum, whereas the serum maintains a more normal straw color with rhabdomyolysis.

Both tablet and reagent stick forms of test are available for determining heme pigments. The reaction is based on the catalyzation by hemoglobin of the oxidation of orthotolidine by peroxide, resulting in a blue color. This reaction occurs with red blood cells, hemoglobin, and myoglobin, but occurs more readily with free hemoglobin in the urine and may be negative with few red blood cells if none is lysed.

Bilirubin

To be present in the urine, bilirubin must be conjugated by the hepatic cell with glucuronic acid and excreted in the bile. The bilirubin appears in the urine when plasma-conjugated (direct-acting) bilirubin concentrations are elevated.

In the Harrison-Fouchet spot test, the traditional method for determining urinary bilirubin, 5 ml of 10% barium chloride is added to 10 ml of urine to precipitate the bilirubin.

The solution is filtered; two drops of Fouchet's reagent (25% trichloroacetic acid, 0.9% ferric chloride) is added to the filter paper. A greenish blue color (the Gmelin reaction) indicates the presence of urinary bilirubin. The test is sensitive, detecting bilirubin in a concentration of 1 mg/dl; however, salicylate may also give a positive reaction. Both tablet and reagent strip methods are available for determining urinary bilirubin and have widely replaced the multistep Harrison-Fouchet spot test.

Urobilinogen

Urobilinogen is a colorless chromogen derived from bilirubin by bacterial metabolism occurring in the bowel. It may become oxidized to urobilin, which can impart a light brown color to the urine. Urobilinogen is partially reabsorbed in the small bowel, with both renal and hepatic excretion. Normally, up to 4 mg is excreted in the urine daily. Urinary urobilinogen excretion is increased with increased turnover of bilirubin, as occurs with a hemolytic anemia, or with impaired hepatic excretion of bilirubin, as seen with parenchymal hepatic disease. Urobilinogen may be decreased or absent from the urine with complete bile duct obstruction or with the use of antibiotics that reduce intestinal bacteria capable of converting bilirubin to urobilinogen.

Urobilinogen gives a characteristic color with Ehrlich's benzaldehyde reagent that is similar to other chromogens such as porphobilinogen or *p*-aminosalicylic acid. This cumbersome colorometric technique has been largely replaced by a reagent strip containing 4-methoxybenzene-diazonium-tetrafluoride in an acid medium, which forms a red-azo dye when coupled with urobilinogen.

MICROSCOPIC EXAMINATION OF THE URINARY SEDIMENT

The urinary sediment may be considered an "exfoliative biopsy specimen" of the genitourinary tract. It contains formed elements that may be derived from the renal parenchyma or elsewhere in the course of the collecting system. Immediate examination of a concentrated first-voided morning urine specimen is most suitable for studying sediment.

A variety of techniques have been described for preparing the sediment for examination. The following is generally accepted: 15 ml of urine are placed in a clean conical tube and centrifuged at 2000 rpm for 5 minutes. The tube is inverted to allow the supernatant urine to run off, and the remaining urine is shaken gently to resuspend the sediment. A drop of the suspension is pipetted onto a clean slide, topped with a clean square cover glass, and examined while still wet. Using the subdued light of the microscope, the slide is examined under low power initially and then under high power. Quantitation of formed elements is accomplished by counting at least ten fields and averaging the number of casts per low power field and cells per high power field. Fat bodies are most readily detected by their cross pattée configuration under polarized light. Glitter cells are easily seen by phase microscopy. Microorganisms are best identified in a Gram stain preparation.

Red blood cells

Red blood cells normally appear as biconcave disks. Their form in urine is partially dependent on osmolality, and they may appear crenated, shrunken, or swollen. A few red blood cells may be found normally in the urine following passage across the glomerular filtration barrier or tubules by the process of diapedesis. Adults will often show an occasional red blood cell per high power field. More than two red blood cells per high power field is generally considered abnormal. Red blood cells must be differentiated from fat droplets, degenerated epithelial cells, yeast, and amorphous urates in acid urine. The lysis of red blood cells by 2% acetic acid is often a helpful differential feature.

The presence of red blood cells in the urine is usually indicative of renal parenchymal or genitourinary disease.

Recent studies indicate that urinary red blood cells of renal origin exhibit a wide range of morphologic variation, frequently with loss of hemoglobin. These "dysmorphic" changes contrast with the predominantly morphologically uniform "isomorphic" cells characteristic of nonrenal bleeding. Red cells in normal subjects are dysmorphic but few in number (less than 1000 cells/ml by centrifugation and phase contrast microscopy). Recognition of these distinctions is facilitated by use of phase microscopy.

White blood cells

Leukocytes in the urine must be differentiated from columnar epithelial cells from the tubules and squamous and transitional cells from lower in the genitourinary tract (Fig. 339-1). In a study of 24-hour urine excretory rates, Addis found up to 2 million white cells and nonsquamous epithelial cells excreted by normal subjects. Normally, two or fewer white cells are observed per high power field using centrifuged

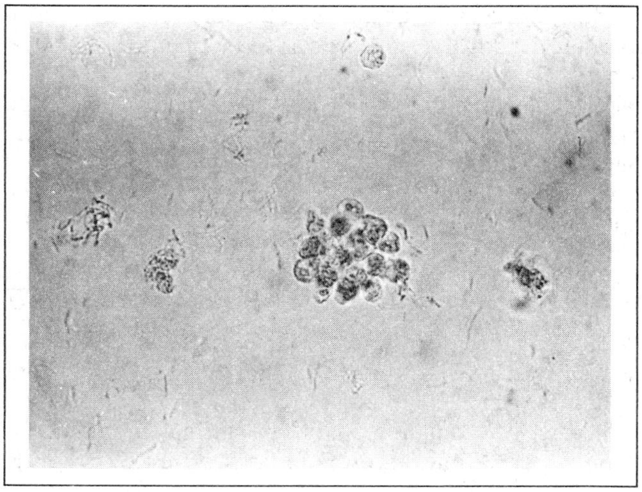

Fig. 339-1. A cluster of white cells in a field containing numerous bacteria. ×400.

urine. Women are more likely to have urinary leukocytes than are men because of vestibular contamination. It was suggested that leukocytes originating from the renal parenchyma tend to be larger, appear pale blue with Sternheimer-Malbin stain, and have granules exhibiting Brownian movement. These Schilling, or glitter, cells were subsequently found to be the result of a hypotonic medium, and their frequent observation in patients with pyelonephritis is related to the concurrence of pyuria and a urinary concentrating defect. Significant pyuria is most often associated with bacterial infection of the urinary tract. Its occurrence in the absence of bacteriuria on routine culture suggests the possibility of *Chlamydia* infection, renal tuberculosis, acute glomerulonephritis, or systemic lupus erythematosus. Techniques for quantitating white blood cells in uncentrifuged urine specimens using a hemocytometer have been reported as providing greater reliability and reproducibility in diagnosing urinary tract infection than routinely examined urinary sediments. Reagent strip testing for leukocyturia is based on the colorometric detection of granulocytic leukocyte esterase.

A variety of epithelial cells may be seen in the urine as a result of normal desquamation or contamination. Large, flat squamous epithelial cells have a single, small nucleus and may originate from the urethra or represent vaginal or vulvar contamination. Bladder or transitional epithelial cells are intermediate in size between squamous cells and leukocytes and have a moderate-sized, round nucleus. They often are flat or cuboidal. Renal tubular cells are round, slightly larger than leukocytes, and have a large, single nucleus. Eosinophiliuria comprising more than 5% of total urinary leukocytes is highly characteristic of drug-induced acute tubulointerstitial nephritis and is detected with preparation of Wright's or preferably Hansel's stained urinary sediments.

Casts

Casts are cylindrical masses of agglutinated material that represent a mold of a tubular lumen; they are usually formed in the distal convoluted tubule or the collecting tubule. Addis found normal cast excretion to be 5000 to 10,000/24 hours. The most simple type of cast is termed *hyaline cast* and is composed of the Tamm-Horsfall mucoprotein originating in the kidney. This is a low molecular weight protein whose precipitability is promoted by the presence of small quantities of urinary albumin and a low urinary sodium concentration. More recent studies using immunofluorescence techniques have demonstrated the inclusion of various immunoglobulins as well. Casts are best observed with subdued light and may be recognized by their parallel walls, squared ends, and faint pink staining with Sternheimer-Malbin stain. They may dissolve in alkaline solutions, hence the usefulness of attempting to collect an acid, first-voided morning urine specimen. Their excretion is increased with fever, exercise, and congestive heart failure.

Casts are often of critical diagnostic importance. White cell casts indicate the presence of a leukocytic response within the renal tubules. They are most commonly seen with renal parenchymal infection or glomerulonephritis. Bacterial casts have also been described with upper tract infection. Red cell casts usually indicate renal parenchymal disease, most commonly an acute glomerular inflammatory process (Fig. 339-2); however, they may be seen in patients with acute tubular necrosis. The red cells may be distinct or may lyse and become incorporated in a homogeneous mass characterized by a rust or orange-red color. These are termed *blood casts*. Broad casts are two to six times normal diameter and were observed by Addis to occur in situations of massively dilated and static collecting ducts and hence are also called *renal failure casts:* they often have a homogeneous waxy appearance (Fig. 339-3). The presence of pigmenturia, caused by myoglobin, hemoglobin, or bilirubin, may result in staining of the excreted casts. Degeneration of cellular inclusions may result in the frequently granular appearance of casts. Electron microscopy supports this sequence; however, some workers suggest that the granularity represents simply a modification of the basic fibrillar protein constituents (Figs. 339-4 and 339-5).

Urinary fat

Free-floating fat droplets may be present in the urine as an external contaminant or from seminal vesicle or vaginal secretions. When fat droplets are observed within cells or casts, they are usually associated with massive proteinuria and are characteristic of a renal process capable of causing nephrotic syndrome. This type of lipiduria apparently is of dual origin: it may represent increased filtration of lipid in association with the hyperlipoproteinemia of nephrotic syndrome. A second mechanism appears to be the increase in tubular reabsorption of protein associated with altered glomerular permeability, which results in tubular cell degeneration with the appearance of cholesterol esters in the tubules. These fatty droplets also may be shed and make their way into casts.

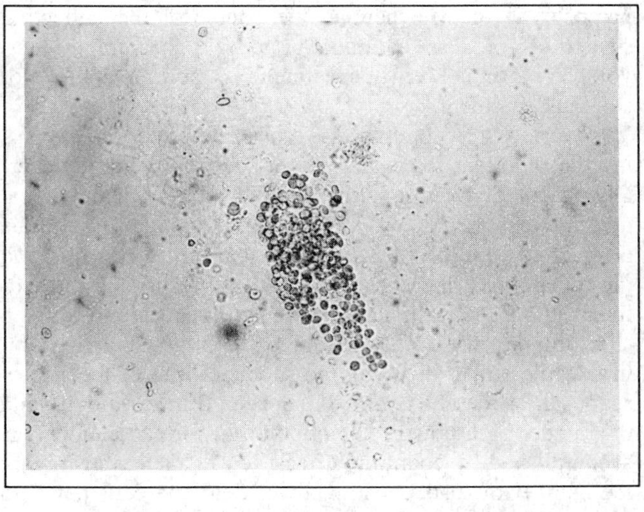

Fig. 339-2. A red blood cell cast with clearly defined cells within a more extensive hyaline matrix. ×400.

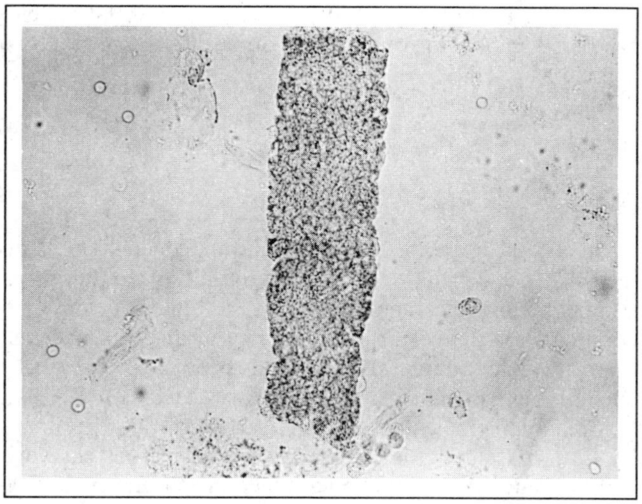

Fig. 339-3. A broad, or renal failure cast with a finely granular matrix. ×400.

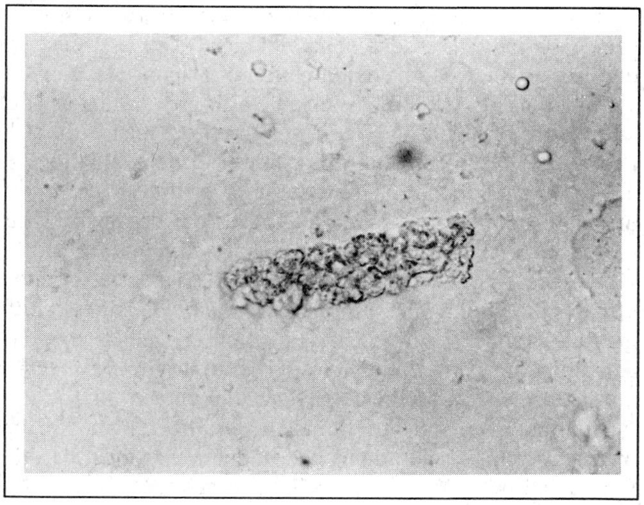

Fig. 339-5. A coarsely granular cast with still recognizable cellular elements. ×400.

Oval fat bodies are degenerated, swollen, fat-filled tubular cells that appear dark in subdued light but refractile in bright light (Fig. 339-6). The presence of urinary fat may be suggested by the highly refractile appearance of the droplet. It is best confirmed with the use of polarized light. The doubly refractile element then appears as a brilliant white color. This usually takes the characteristic shape of a Maltese cross or, more accurately, cross pattée (Fig. 339-6). Staining with Sudan III dye is also helpful for demonstrating fat particles.

Crystals

Crystals are often present in normal urine, particularly when pH is at the extremes of the normal range, and may give the urine a cloudy appearance. The nature of urinary crystals becomes significant in evaluating the patient with demonstrated or suspected renal calculous disease or in the now rare instances of obstruction due to crystalluria.

With alkaline urine, phosphates are precipitated and characteristically will redissolve with the addition of dilute acetic acid. Triple phosphates or ammonium calcium magnesium phosphates have a characteristic coffin-lid shape. Calcium phosphates may be amorphous or wedge shaped. Calcium carbonate and ammonium urate are also frequently present. With acid pH, uric acid may appear as red, rhombic prisms or as plates; sodium urate appears as amorphous brown clumps, needles, or fan shapes. Calcium oxalate has a characteristic envelope shape. Cystine is one of the most significant findings, because its presence is highly indicative of cystinuria. The crystals have a characteristic hexagonal or benzene-ring form.

A variety of elements may be observed on microscopic

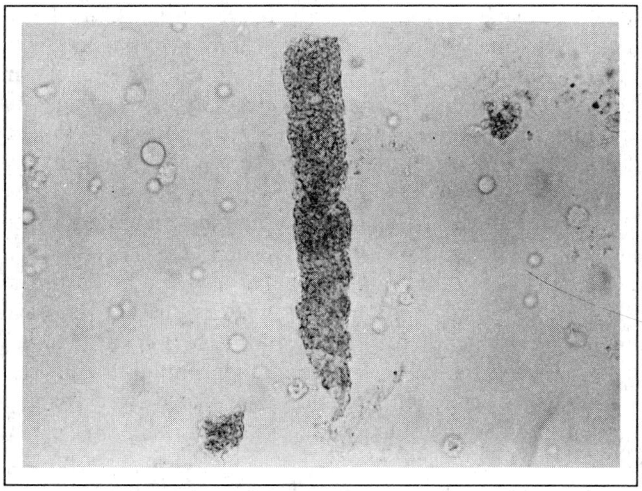

Fig. 339-4. A finely granular cast surrounded by red blood cells and white blood cells. ×400.

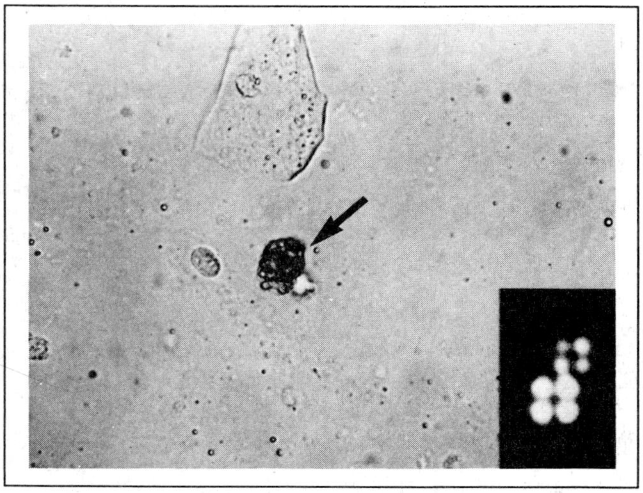

Fig. 339-6. An oval fat body beneath a large squamous epithelial cell. ×400. *Insert:* High power view of lipid droplets under polarized light demonstrating the characteristic cross pattée pattern.

examination that may be of pathogenic potential or significance or may represent contamination. The presence of bacteria on microscopic examination of a spun, clean-catch specimen using carefully cleansed glassware correlates well with culture growth of 100,000 or more organisms/ml and is a useful initial screening procedure in the evaluation of urinary tract infection. Gram staining facilitates detection of small numbers and identification of the organism. The presence of yeast forms, predominantly *Candida albicans,* may reflect vaginal contamination or may indicate genitourinary infection. The protozoan *Trichomonas vaginalis* may also reflect genitourinary infection or fecal or vaginal contamination. In endemic areas, urinary *Schistosoma haematobium* ova are of diagnostic importance.

Spermatozoa, mucous threads, hair, fibers, and oil or ointment droplets are among the findings that must be differentiated from organisms, cells, and casts.

REFERENCES

Corwin HL, Bray RA, and Haber MH: The detection and interpretation of urinary eosinophils, Arch Pathol Lab Med 113:1256, 1989.

Cushner HM and Copley JB: Back to basics: the urinalysis: a selected national survey and review, Am J Med Sci 297:193, 1989.

Guthrie RM et al: Does the dipstick meet medical needs for urine specific gravity? J Family Practice 25:512, 1987.

Is routine urinalysis worthwhile? (editorial) Lancet 1:747, 1988.

Kiel DP and Moskowitz MA: The urinalysis: a critical appraisal, Med Clin North Am 71:607, 1987.

Lawrence VA and Kroenke K: The unproven utility of preoperative urinalysis. Clinical use, Arch Intern Med 148:1370, 1988.

Mogensen CE et al: Microalbuminuria: studies in diabetes, essential hypertension, and renal diseases as compared with the background population, Adv Nephrol 20:191, 1991.

Nelson RG et al: Assessment of risk of overt nephropathy in diabetic patients from albumin excretion in untimed urine specimens, Arch Intern Med 151:1761, 1991.

Pollock C et al: Dysmorphism of urinary red blood cells—value in diagnosis, Kidney Int 36:1045, 1989.

Schumann GB and Schweitzer SL: Examination of urine. In Henry JB, editor: Clinical diagnosis and management by laboratory methods, Philadelphia, 1991, WB Saunders.

CHAPTER

340 Renal Function Tests

T. Dwight McKinney

GLOMERULAR FILTRATION RATE

The most useful index of overall renal function is the glomerular filtration rate (GFR). The GFR is the amount of plasma ultrafiltered across the glomeruli per unit of time and is expressed in milliliters per minute. GFR is measured indirectly by estimating the clearance from urine of a plasma-borne substance. If the substance is not bound to serum proteins, is freely filtered across the glomeruli, and is neither secreted nor reabsorbed by the renal tubules, its rate of urinary excretion will be proportional to GFR, and can be taken as a measure of it. Formally, clearance *(C)* is defined as

(EQ. 1)

$$C = \frac{U \times V}{P}$$

where *U* and *P* are the urine and plasma concentrations of the substance (mg/dl) and *V* is the urine flow rate (ml/min). Although inulin clearance represents the "gold standard" for determination of GFR, the complexity of this test makes it impractical for routine use. In clinical practice, the clearance of endogenous creatinine (Ccr) is usually used.

Creatinine (molecular weight 113) is produced primarily from muscle and is excreted in the urine at a relatively constant rate. With stable renal function, plasma creatinine concentrations are relatively constant, and Ccr reflects GFR. In an average size normal man (70 kg, 1.73 m^2), the GFR is approximately 125 mg/min/1.73 m^2, and the plasma creatinine concentrations range between 0.7 and 1.5 mg/dl. The corresponding values in normal women are somewhat less, 115 ml/min 1.73 m^2 and 0.5 to 1.3 mg/dl, respectively. Because creatinine production, urinary excretion, and plasma concentrations are higher in muscular individuals, their normal Ccr will also be somewhat higher; the opposite is true in asthenic individuals. Generally, the Ccr is determined by collecting all urine produced over a 24-hour period, obtaining a blood sample once during this interval, and calculating clearance by EQ. 1. To assess the adequacy of urine collection, the total amount of creatinine excreted should be determined; this total should be in the range of 20 to 26 mg/kg/day for men and 15 to 20 mg/kg/day for women.

The relationship between Ccr and plasma creatinine concentration is shown in Fig. 340-1. Creatinine clearance normally decreases with age beyond the fourth decade and decreases with progressive renal disease. Once Ccr falls to 10 to 15 ml/min, patients are usually in need of renal replacement therapy in the form of dialysis or renal transplantation (Chapter 348). Because a larger proportion of urinary creatinine is due to tubular secretion in patients with renal insufficiency, Ccr will overestimate GFR more in these patients than in normals. Conversely, some drugs, including cimetidine, trimethoprim, and probenecid, will inhibit creatinine secretion and raise serum creatinine and decrease Ccr without changing GFR.

Because of the difficulties in obtaining accurately timed urine collections for determination of Ccr, especially on a repeated basis, other methods have been used to estimate GFR. Once Ccr has been determined in the conventional manner described here, because of the reciprocal relationship between the serum creatinine concentration and Ccr, subsequent changes in Ccr can be estimated from changes in serum creatinine concentration alone (assuming no major changes in muscle mass). For example, if a serum creatinine concentration of 1 mg/dl is associated with a Ccr of 100 ml/min, then elevation of serum creatinine concentration to 2, 4, and 8 mg/dl will reflect a Ccr of 50, 25, and 12.5 ml/min, respectively. It is also possible to estimate Ccr

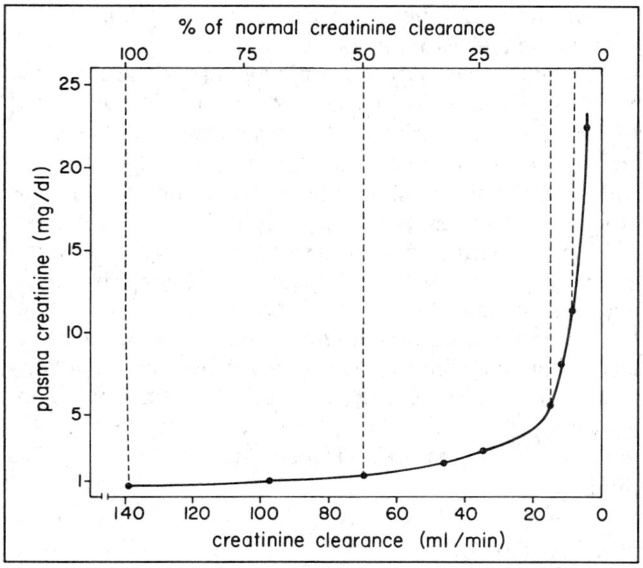

Fig. 340-1. Relationship between creatinine clearance and plasma creatinine concentration. Note that at low concentrations of plasma creatinine, small changes in plasma creatinine concentration are associated with major changes in creatinine clearance. For example, as plasma creatinine rises from 0.7 to 1.4 mg/dl, creatinine clearance falls from 139 to 69 ml/min (*dashed lines* at 100% and 50%). However, when levels are already elevated, large changes in plasma creatinine concentration are associated with only small changes in creatinine clearance. For example, as plasma creatinine rises from 5.6 to 11.2 mg/dl, creatinine clearance falls only from 17.4 to 8.7 ml/min (*dashed lines* at the right of the figure).

without the need for urine collection, by the following formula:

(EQ. 2)

$$\text{Creatinine clearance} = \frac{(140 - \text{age}) \times \text{weight (kg)}}{72 \times \text{plasma creatinine (mg/dl)}}$$

The result should be multiplied by 0.85 in women. This method is the least expensive manner of estimating GFR. Other methods occasionally used involve administration of tracer amounts of radioisotopes such as ^{125}I-iothalamate. Regardless of which method is used to estimate GFR, in patients with renal disease serial measurements are necessary to assess progression of their disease and their response to therapy.

In the past, the blood urea nitrogen concentration (BUN) and urea clearance have been used to estimate GFR. Normally, the ratio of BUN to plasma creatinine concentration is 10. Although the BUN generally increases with a decline in GFR, numerous factors besides changes in GFR will disproportionately elevate the BUN. These include tetracycline antibiotics, corticosteroids, gastrointestinal bleeding, urinary tract obstruction, high dietary protein intake, and prerenal azotemia. Conversely, liver disease and dietary protein restriction disproportionately lower the BUN. Consequently, the BUN per se is not a reliable index of renal function.

RENAL BLOOD FLOW

Renal blood flow (RBF) is not commonly measured in clinical medicine. However, when it is, para-aminohippurate (PAH) clearance is usually measured. Through glomerular filtration and tubular secretion, 70% to 90% of PAH is removed from the blood as it traverses the kidney. Renal plasma flow (RPF) is determined by infusing PAH to a constant plasma concentration and calculating PAH clearance by EQ. 1. RBF is calculated as follows:

(EQ. 3)

$$\text{RBF} = \frac{\text{RPF}}{1 - \text{hematocrit}}$$

Because PAH is secreted by an organic anion transport pathway in the proximal tubules, PAH clearance may be reduced by drugs that compete for this pathway (e.g., salicylates). RPF in normal individuals is around 600 to 650 ml/min/1.73 m^2, and RBF is around 1200 ml/min/1.73 m^2. RPF can also be estimated using clearance of ^{131}I-iodohippurate or other radionuclides.

FRACTIONAL EXCRETION OF SODIUM

Under normal steady-state conditions, urinary sodium excretion approximates intake. Determining the fraction of sodium undergoing glomerular filtration that is excreted in the urine is useful in evaluation of patients with an acute fall in urine output and/or rise in serum creatinine or BUN concentration. Fractional excretion of sodium (FE_{Na}) as a percentage of filtered sodium can be determined from single blood and urine samples as follows:

(EQ. 4)

$$FE_{Na} = \frac{\text{urine sodium conc.}}{\text{plasma sodium conc.}} \times \frac{\text{plasma creatinine conc.}}{\text{urine creatinine conc.}} \times 100$$

To accurately interpret FE_{Na}, patients should not have recently received diuretics. FE_{Na} is greater than 1% and usually greater than 3% with acute tubular necrosis and severe obstruction of the urinary drainage of both kidneys. It is generally less than 1% in patients with acute glomerulonephritis, hepatorenal syndrome, and states of prerenal azotemia such as congestive heart failure or dehydration. FE_{Na} may also be less than 1% with acute partial urinary tract obstruction.

A similar approach can be used to determine the fractional excretion of other substances in the urine and may be useful in evaluating patients with disorders of calcium, phosphorus, bicarbonate, potassium, and uric acid metabolism.

TESTS OF RENAL ACIDIFICATION

The kidneys normally maintain blood pH and bicarbonate concentrations within narrow ranges through tubular reabsorption of all bicarbonate from the glomerular filtrate and excretion of 1.0 to 1.5 mmol/kg/day of net acid in the form of titratable acid and ammonium. The majority of bicarbonate reabsorption occurs in the proximal tubule. Net acid excretion requires a steep pH gradient from blood to tubular fluid. This gradient is present only in the distal nephron segments (distal convoluted tubules and, especially, collecting ducts). Consequently, hyperchloremic metabolic acidosis, referred to as *renal tubular acidosis* (RTA), may result from incomplete bicarbonate reabsorption with bicarbonaturia or from decreased net acid excretion. The former is termed *proximal RTA* and the latter *distal RTA* (Chapter 353).

The ability to maximally acidify the urine is usually evaluated by an ammonium chloride loading test: 0.1 g ammonium chloride per kilogram body weight is ingested over 1 hour and urine samples are collected for the next 8 hours. Two hours after ammonium chloride ingestion, urine pH in normal individuals falls to 5.3 or less. Ability to lower urine pH to this level, either spontaneously or after ammonium chloride loading, excludes the diagnosis of classic distal (type I) RTA. In certain forms of distal RTA (type IV or hyperkalemic distal RTA), urine may be acidified normally while urinary ammonium and net acid excretion are diminished (Chapter 353). Determination of urinary ammonium may be useful in the differential diagnosis of these disorders. Whether or not ammonium is present in the urine can be estimated by calculation of the urine anion gap (UAG).

$$\text{UAG} = \text{urine } (\text{Na}^+ \text{ conc.} + \text{K}^+ \text{ conc.} - \text{Cl}^- \text{ conc.}) \qquad \textbf{(EQ. 5)}$$

Because ammonium (an unmeasured cation) in the urine is accompanied by an anion (predominantly Cl^-), when ammonium is present the UAG will be negative. Conversely, a positive UAG indicates the absence of urinary ammonium. A normal response to ammonium chloride loading does not rule out proximal forms of RTA. In proximal RTA, if significant metabolic acidosis is present (plasma bicarbonate concentrations below 15 to 18 mEq/L), urine pH will be low. Proximal and distal forms of RTA are generally differentiated by measuring the fractional excretion of bicarbonate ($FE_{HCO_3^-}$). With a normal plasma bicarbonate concentration (which will require administration of exogenous alkali in patients with RTA), $FE_{HCO_3^-}$, calculated by EQ. 4, in patients with proximal RTA exceeds 10%, whereas values of less than 3% to 5% are observed in distal forms of RTA. In addition to urinary bicarbonate wastage, some patients with proximal RTA excrete excessive amounts of other solutes normally reabsorbed in the proximal tubule, including glucose, phosphate, amino acids, and uric acid. This condition of multiple proximal tubule abnormalities is referred to as the *Fanconi syndrome*.

URINARY CONCENTRATION AND DILUTION

Normal individuals are able to vary urine osmolality between approximately 50 and 1000 mosm/kg H_2O under conditions of water loading and deprivation, respectively. This ability, which results in either water excretion or conservation and depends on proper renal and hypothalamic-pituitary function, allows for maintenance of plasma osmolality in the narrow range of 280 to 298 mosm/kg H_2O.

Maximum urinary concentrating ability is usually tested by measuring urine osmolality after overnight fluid deprivation. Urine osmolality under these conditions is considered normal if it is greater than 800 mosm/kg H_2O. Patients with marked polyuria should be observed carefully for signs of volume depletion during the period of water deprivation.

Urinary diluting ability is tested by administering water, 20 ml/kg body weight, orally over 30 minutes and collecting urine samples every 30 minutes for the next 4 hours. Normal individuals excrete greater than 80% of the water load during this time period and lower the urine osmolality to less than 100 mosm/kg H_2O. To avoid acute water intoxication, water loads should not be administered to individuals with serum sodium concentrations less than 130 mEq/L.

RENAL BIOPSY

Percutaneous needle biopsy of the kidney, and less commonly open surgical biopsy, may be useful in establishing diagnosis, determining prognosis, and directing therapy in a variety of renal diseases. These indications especially include the nephrotic syndrome, hematuria, clinical acute and chronic glomerulonephritis, acute renal insufficiency of uncertain etiology or prolonged duration, some cases of chronic renal insufficiency of uncertain etiology, and renal insufficiency in renal transplant recipients. Tissue is generally examined by light, electron, and immunofluorescence microscopy. Contraindications to renal biopsy include bleeding disorders, uncontrolled hypertension, urosepsis, hydronephrosis, and the presence of a solitary kidney. The only absolute contraindication to percutaneous biopsy is an uncooperative patient. Overall, renal biopsy is a safe procedure with less than 0.1% mortality. The most common complications are hematuria, which is gross in about 5% of patients, and perinephric hematoma. The latter complication is present on abdominal computed tomography study in up to 60% of patients but is clinically apparent in only about 1%. Clinically significant arteriovenous fistulas and laceration of adjacent organs are rare complications.

REFERENCES

Gault MH. Prediction of creatinine, Nephron 16:31, 1976.

Cogan MG and Rector FC Jr: Acid-base disorders. In Brenner BM and Rector FC, Jr, editors: The kidney, ed 4, Philadelphia, 1991, WB Saunders.

Kassirer JP and Harrington JT: Laboratory evaluation or renal function. In Schrier RW and Gottschalk CW, editors: Diseases of the kidney, ed 5, Boston, 1992, Little, Brown.

Lemann J Jr et al: Use of the serum creatinine to estimate glomerular filtration rate in health and early diabetic nephropathy, Am J Kidney Dis 16:236-243, 1990.

Levey AS: Measurement of renal function in chronic renal disease, Kidney Int 38:167-184, 1990.

Madaio MP: Renal biopsy, Kidney Int 38:529-543, 1990.

Perrone RD et al: Utility of radioisotopic filtration markers in chronic renal insufficiency: simultaneous comparison of ^{125}I-iothalamate, ^{169}Yb-DTPA, ^{99m}Tc-DTPA and inulin, Am J Kidney Dis 16:224-235, 1990.

Robertson GL and Berl T: Pathophysiology of water metabolism. In Brenner BM and Rector FC Jr, editors: The kidney, ed 4, Boston, 1991, Little, Brown.
Steiner RW: Interpreting the fractional excretion of sodium, Am J Med 77:699, 1984.

CHAPTER

341 Imaging of Renal Disorders

Abraham A. Ghiatas

Diagnostic radiology makes a significant contribution to the evaluation of the urinary system. Almost every available diagnostic modality has important applications in the evaluation of the kidneys and urinary tract providing excellent anatomic details as well as significant physiologic information. This chapter outlines the diagnostic methods available for evaluation of various urinary tract diseases and provides some diagnostic algorithms to use these imaging modalities.

METHODS OF EXAMINATION

Intravenous pyelography/urography

Intravenous pyelography (IVP) or urography (IVU) remains the most important imaging modality for evaluation of kidney and urinary tract pathology. Intravenous contrast medium (iodinated products) is administered, which is then concentrated and excreted by the kidney. This process produces opacification of the renal parenchyma, collecting system, ureter, and bladder.

A scout view of the abdomen (KUB) (Fig. 341-1) is an important part of the IVP. An IVP should not be performed nor interpreted without a scout view of the abdomen, which provides significant information regarding calcifications of the kidney and/or urinary tract (the presence of contrast media within the urinary tract may obscure calcifications). It also provides information regarding the bones (metastasis, fracture, etc.) and gas pattern. It is highly advisable to obtain a precontrast tomographic exposure of the kidneys for evaluation of the position, size, shape, etc.

After the intravenous administration of contrast media (bolus or drip infusion), several films of the abdomen and tomograms of the kidneys are obtained. Compression may be used to partially obstruct the ureters and achieve better visualization of the pyelocalyceal system (compression is contraindicated in urinary tract obstruction, abdominal aneurysms, and recent abdominal surgery).

The IVP has two phases. During the first phase, the nephrogram phase, the contrast media is in the tubular space, which provides information about the renal parenchyma. During this phase the kidney appears homogeneously dense (white). During the second phase, the pyelogram phase, the contrast media is in the pyelocalyceal system (Fig. 341-2). Approximately 3 minutes after the administration of contrast media, the ureters opacify and can

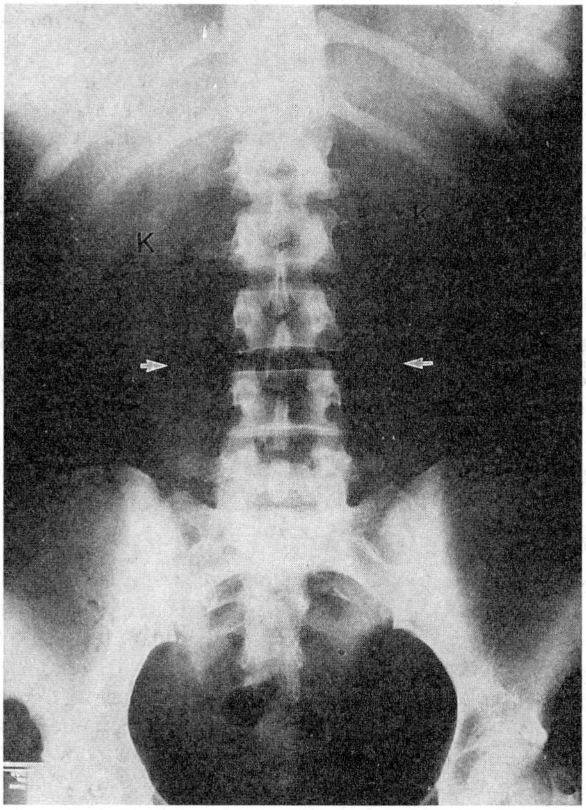

Fig. 341-1. Normal KUB. *K,* kidneys; *arrows,* psoas muscles.

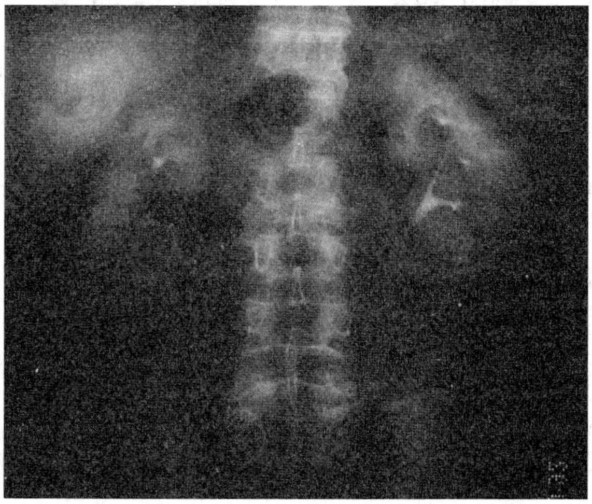

Fig. 341-2. Normal IVP: Nephrogram and pyelogram phases are well demonstrated.

be evaluated for defects indicating calculi, tumors, or blood clots. Their course and relationship to the psoas muscle and spine are also evaluated.

Abnormalities in the course of the ureters indicate the presence of extrinsic mass compressing on the ureters. In an IVP study dilatation of the mid-third of the ureter is a normal finding and is caused by compression of the ureter by the iliac vessels. In females there may be a vascular compression of the right ureter at the level L4-5 caused by the ovarian vein as it enters the inferior vena cava. The urinary bladder is evaluated (shape, position, contour, residual urine volume, filling defects) when filled with contrast media as well as when empty (on postvoid film). In females, compression of the dome of the bladder is usually caused by the uterus, whereas compression of the base of the bladder, in males, is caused by a hypertrophic prostatic gland.

Ultrasound

Diagnostic ultrasound (US) is an accurate, noninvasive, cost-efficient, and portable imaging modality that has become essential in the evaluation of the urinary system. Neither radiation nor contrast media is needed for imaging. In cases where renal insufficiency or allergy to contrast media precludes the use of IVP or CT, sonography assumes a primary role in the evaluation of renal pathology. US can accurately diagnose and grade hydronephrosis by detecting and grading the dilatation of the collecting system.

Renal masses are easily imaged by US, and differentiation of a cystic from solid mass is mainly made by sonography. Cysts less than 1 cm in diameter and solid masses of approximately 2 cm in diameter can easily be evaluated by sonography.

In a normal renal sonogram the kidney will appear as an ovoid (bean-shaped) solid structure with three distinct sonographic zones:

1. Central zone: renal sinus, fat, blood vessels and pyelocalyceal system of high echogenicity.
2. Peripheral zone: sonolucent and consisting of the renal pyramids of the renal medulla
3. Outer zone: represents the renal cortex (tubules, glomeruli, connective tissue) of medium level echogenicity (Fig. 341-3).

In medical renal disease, the echogenicity of the cortex is increased almost to the level as that of the liver (compare Fig. 341-4 with Fig. 341-3).

New dedicated sonographic probes (endorectal) have the ability to image the prostate in a very detailed manner. The use of Doppler analysis of blood flow is rapidly becoming an important noninvasive modality in accessing renal vascular pathology such as renovascular disease, thrombosis of renal vein, and renal transplant rejection.

Computed tomography

The introduction of computed tomography (CT) in the evaluation of the urinary system has been revolutionary. It is the examination of choice for detailed imaging of the

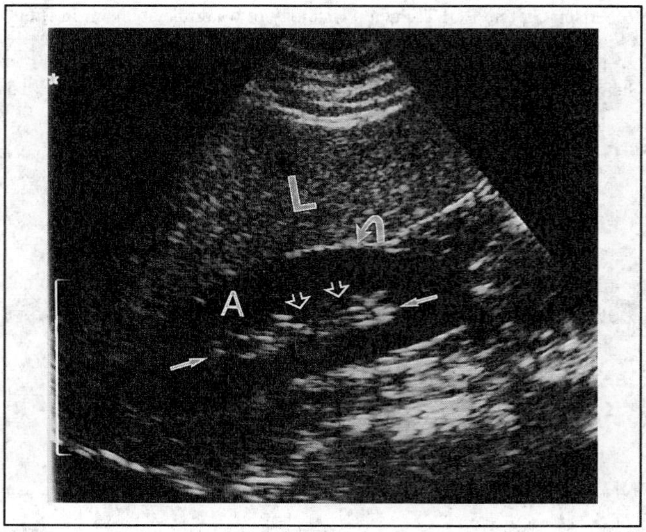

Fig. 341-3. Normal US of kidney. *Arrows,* renal sinus; *open arrows,* pyramids, *A,* cortex; *curved arrow,* retroperitoneal fat stripe. The renal cortex is of lower echogenicity when compared to the liver (L).

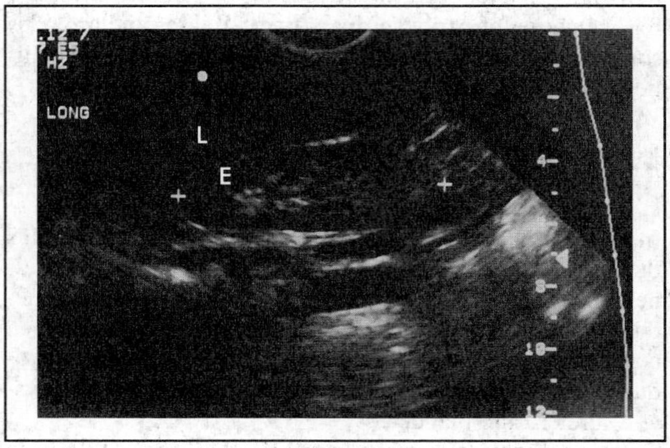

Fig. 341-4. Medical renal disease. *E,* cortex; *L,* liver.

kidneys, adrenals, perirenal spaces, and pararenal spaces (Fig. 341-5). Performance of CT and acquisition of diagnostic images of high quality require preparation and cooperation of the patient and specific protocols for the examination.

The kidneys are imaged before and during the intravenous administration of contrast media and 5 or 10 mm thick slices are obtained. Nonenhanced images provide information regarding calcifications involving the urinary system, which otherwise will be masked by contrast media.

Renal masses/malignancies are primarily evaluated by CT, which significantly has replaced angiography as the primary imaging modality for evaluation of renal mass/malignancy. The primary malignancy, possible vascular involvement and proximal as well as distant metastasis are accu-

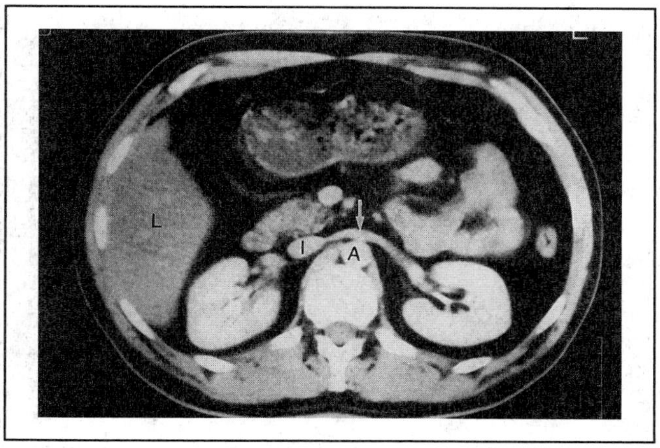

Fig. 341-5. Normal enhanced CT of kidneys. *I,* IVC; *A, aorta; arrow,* renal vein; *L,* liver.

rately evaluated by CT. CT adequately evaluates ureter and bladder pathology.

Nuclear medicine

Nuclear scintigraphy provides information about the function and anatomy of the kidney. It provides quantitative evaluation of the kidney, which cannot be provided by other radiographic techniques. The radiopharmaceutical agents used for renal evaluation/imaging are of low toxicity and low radiation. ^{99m}Tc-DTPA is an agent used for imaging and evaluation of glomerular filtration (Fig. 341-6, *A, B*). For imaging only, especially in patients with renal failure, ^{99m}Tc-DMSA or ^{99m}Tc-glucoheptonate (GHA) can be used. ^{131}I-orthoiodohippurate (OIH) is used for tubular function evaluation. Visualization of the kidney by nuclear medicine requires minimal renal function.

Imaging by nuclear medicine is useful for evaluation of the function of each kidney separately to follow up the progress of obstruction, to evaluate the presence or absence of functioning renal parenchyma, to search for ectopic kidney, and to evaluate renal hypertension.

Magnetic resonance imaging

Magnetic resonance imaging (MRI), the newest imaging modality, uses electromagnetic forces to generate images. The patient is placed into a strong magnetic field (0.2 to 1.5 T), which magnetizes the patient's protons (mainly the hydrogen protons). A radiofrequency pulse stimulates the protons in the area of interest (of the body) by altering their orientation in relation to the main magnetic field. When the radiofrequency pulse ceases the stimulated protons return to their baseline position by emitting a radiofrequency energy that generates the images.

MRI does not use ionizing radiation and has the capability of multiplanar imaging (coronal, axial, sagittal). At the present time the use of contrast media is not necessary, reducing the risk of allergic reactions. Contraindications for performing MRI include cardiac pacemaker, certain prosthetic heart valves, cerebrovascular clips, and cochlear stimulators. MRI is a well-established imaging modality for the nervous and musculoskeletal systems, whereas in the chest and abdomen, cardiac, respiratory, and bowel motion create some deterioration of the images. Advanced MRI techniques such as respiratory and cardiac gating, as well as specific coils, have improved the quality of the images.

In the genitourinary system, MRI provides adequate anatomic information. The corticomedullary differentiation is routinely seen on MRI. The renal artery, vein and inferior vena cava (IVC) are easily assessed by MRI, which is one

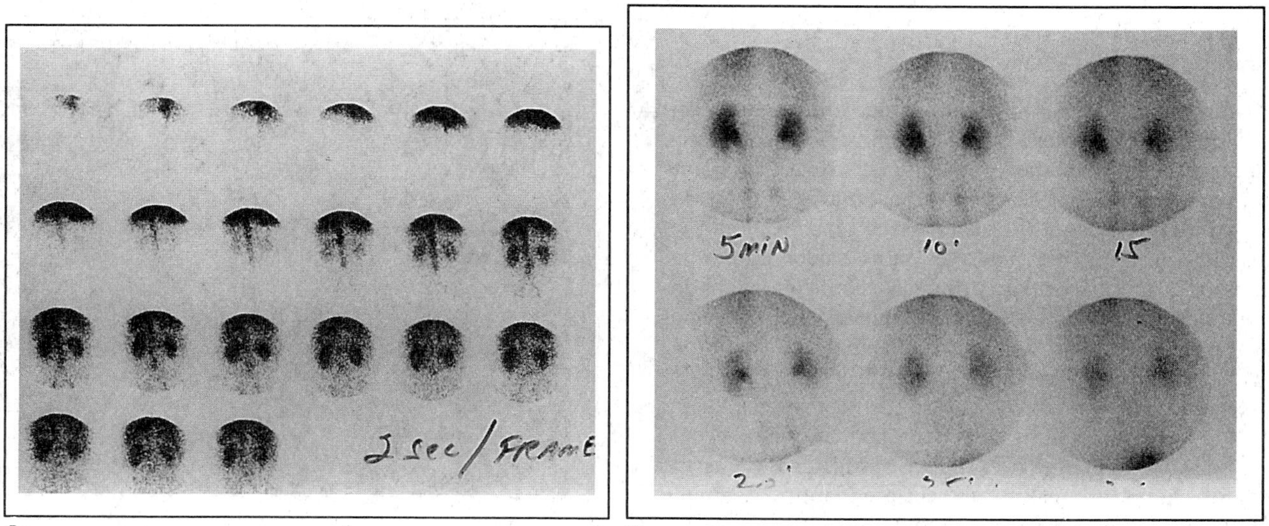

A **B**

Fig. 341-6. Normal radionuclide renal scan. **A,** Dynamic phase. **B,** Static phase.

of the imaging modalities of choice for evaluation of the vascular pedicle of the kidney in renal malignancies. Although MRI is inferior to CT in spatial resolution when compared to CT, it is equal and in some instances, superior to CT in the pelvis (bladder, prostate).

Angiography

The introduction of new imaging modalities such as CT and MRI has decreased the need for angiography in the evaluation of renal pathology. Renal angiography may be used for preoperative vascular "mapping" of a renal mass and for evaluation of renal vascular abnormalities. This most invasive imaging modality, it requires puncturing of the femoral artery and placing the tip of a catheter in the abdominal aorta above the orifices of renal arteries. Contrast media is injected at this area and information is gained for the aorta and renal arteries. Then the catheter is manipulated and placed into the orifice of each renal artery where contrast media is injected selectively, providing detailed vascular information of each kidney.

Besides its diagnostic role, angiography is gaining importance as a therapeutic modality for preoperative embolization of renal tumors, angioplasty of renal artery stenosis, and stenting of renal arteries.

Retrograde pyelography

Retrograde pyelography is an imaging modality in which the contrast medium is injected into the ureter in a retrograde fashion for visualization of the ureter and renal pelvis. This radiographic method is used for evaluation of the collecting systems and ureters in cases where IVP fails to optimally visualize these structures. It is also indicated for evaluation of filling defects in the ureter and/or pelvis.

Since the development of CT and US and improvement of IVP techniques, retrograde pyelography is performed less frequently.

PATHOLOGY

Renal mass

The work-up of a renal mass can include almost every imaging modality. Because IVP is the most frequently used imaging modality for the evaluation of urinary problems (i.e., flank pain, hematuria), most renal masses are first visualized by this modality. Renal masses have different presentations on IVP. They may present as a nephrogram defect, renal contour irregularity (bulge), calcifications, or abnormal position of the kidney. Involvement of the pelvicocalyceal system by a mass appears as distortion, amputation, invasion, clubbing, or displacement (Fig. 341-7). Renal carcinoma may narrow or obstruct the renal vein, resulting in hypofunctioning or nonfunctioning kidney.

A mass on IVP may be solid or cystic, and US is the study of choice for making the differentiation. A simple cyst will need no further evaluation because it is benign. A solid mass or a complex cyst requires further evaluation to determine whether it is benign or malignant. A simple cyst

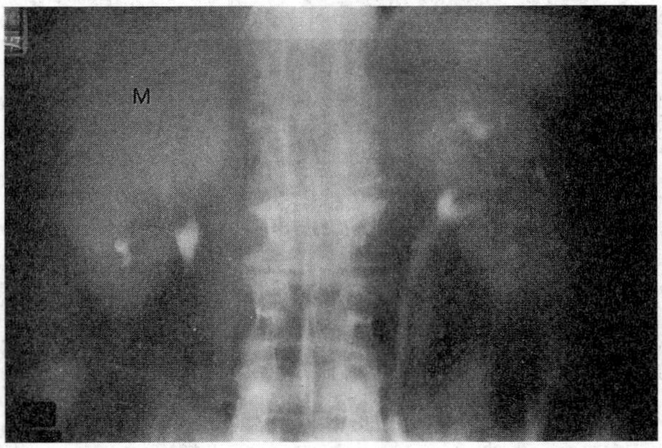

Fig. 341-7. Nephrotomogram demonstrating a large mass *(M)* involving the upper aspect of the right kidney with amputation of the collecting system.

must meet *all* the following sonographic criteria (Fig. 341-8):

1. Echo-free
2. Smooth wall with good through transmission of the sound
3. Enhanced back wall

If any of these criteria are not met, the cyst cannot be classified as simple. A complex cyst on sonography will demonstrate thick wall, calcifications, solid components, and/or mixed echogenicity (Fig. 341-9). Renal sonography for evaluation of a mass should always include the renal veins and IVC for the presence of thrombus.

Evaluation of a solid or complex cystic mass requires the use of CT. Renal cell carcinoma, the most common renal malignancy (83%), appears on CT as a mass of low density (as compared to the rest of renal parenchyma), which will enhance after the intravenous administration of contrast

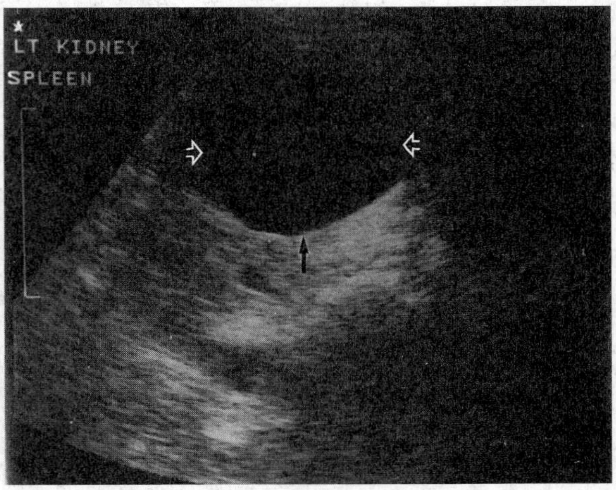

Fig. 341-8. Simple cyst. *Open white arrows,* smooth wall; *black arrow,* enhanced back wall.

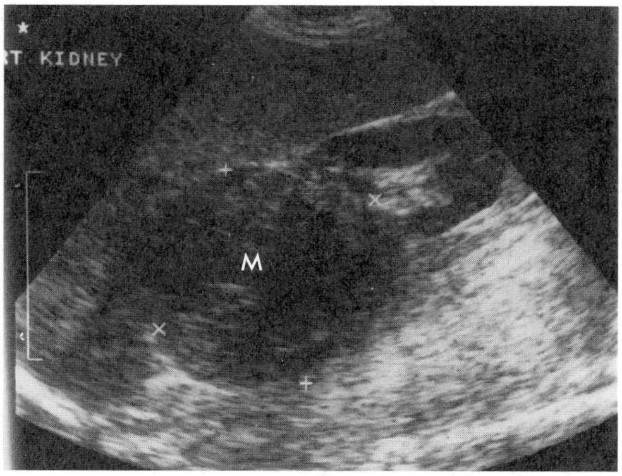

Fig. 341-9. Large renal cell carcinoma. Inhomogeneous mass *(M)* arising from the upper pole of the right kidney.

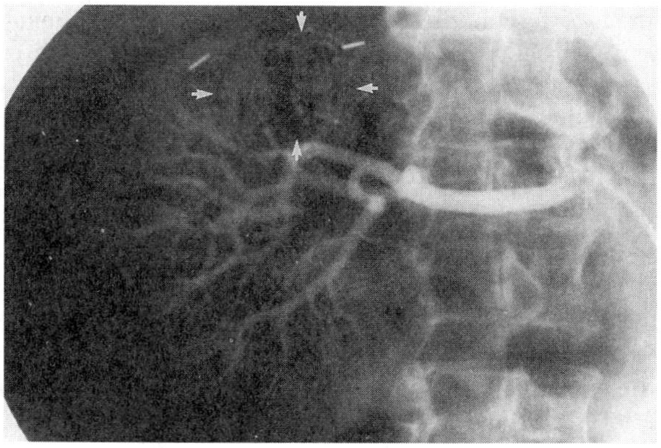

Fig. 341-11. Renal cell carcinoma: right renal angiography reveals a vascular mass *(arrows)* containing abnormal vessels and pooling of contrast media.

media but will still remain less dense than the rest of the enhanced renal parenchyma (Fig. 341-10).

Staging of renal carcinoma is primarily performed by CT because this method has the ability to provide a global (or panoramic) view of the abdomen. Local extension, lymphadenopathy, or distant metastases are easily delineated by CT.

The use of arteriography in evaluating renal masses and more specifically, renal cell carcinoma, has decreased since the introduction of cross-sectional imaging (CT, US, MRI). The main role of angiography in diagnosis is to provide a preoperative vascular mapping of the mass (Fig. 341-11). Angiography may also be of significant help in embolizing the tumor to decrease its vascularity and to facilitate surgical removal. Renal cell carcinoma appears as a hypervascular mass (80%) demonstrating capillary blush, vascular encasement, tortuosity of vessels, early venous filling, and pooling of the contrast media. Involvement of the renal vein is easily demonstrated (Fig. 341-12). Approximately 15% of renal cell carcinomas are hypovascular and 5% are avascular. Renal scintigraphy is limited in the evaluation of re-

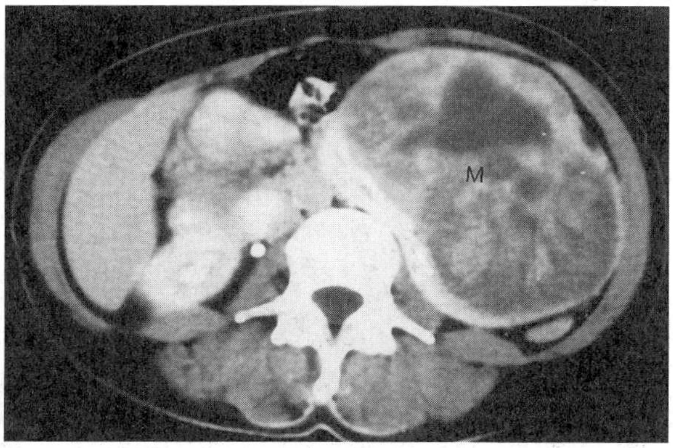

Fig. 341-10. Large renal cell carcinoma. Large mass *(M)* containing areas of high enhancement, low enhancement, and necrosis.

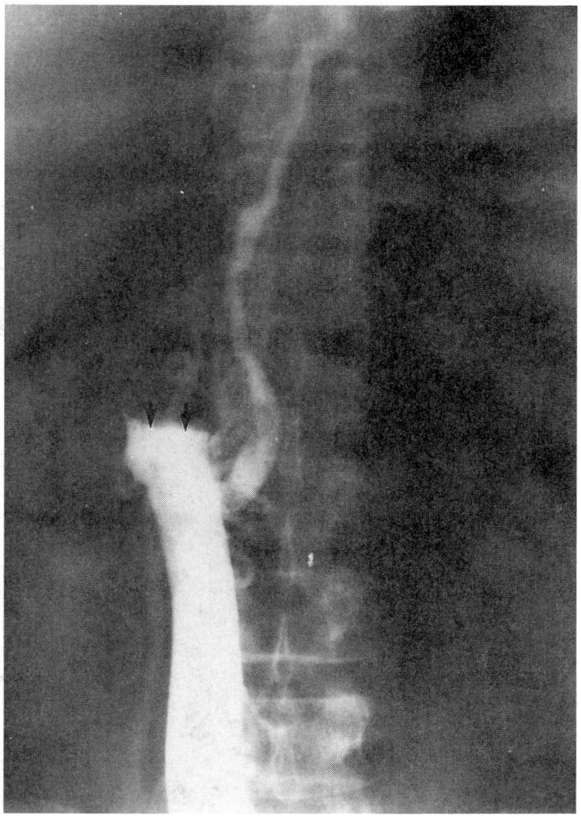

Fig. 341-12. Renal cell carcinoma with involvement of the IVC *(arrows)*.

nal mass because it will only demonstrate the renal defect without differentiating between a benign and malignant lesion. The role of MRI has not yet been completely defined. A renal mass will appear as an inhomogeneous mass of low signal intensity on T_1-weighted imaging and high signal intensity on T_2-weighted imaging (Fig. 341-13). A simple cyst will appear as a well-delineated homogeneous mass of low signal intensity on T_1-weighted imaging and high signal intensity on T_2-weighted imaging. The multiplanar imaging capabilities of MRI have increased the accuracy in staging renal malignancies. MRI is also helpful in assessing the patency of renal veins and IVC (Fig. 341-14).

Besides renal cell carcinomas, other tumors may involve the kidney. Benign neoplasm include the following:

1. Oncocytoma: on cross-sectional imaging will appear as a solid mass with a central scar. Angiography will demonstrate a hypervascular mass with a "spoke wheel" pattern. Despite its characteristic appearance malignancy cannot be totally excluded.
2. Adenoma: slow growing solid tumors that may exhibit cystic areas and calcifications. Adenomas larger than 3 cm are considered potentially malignant.
3. Angiomyolipomas: solid tumors containing fat, muscle, and blood vessels. CT will demonstrate fat as a low-density area (or mass); while on ultrasound, fat will appear echogenic (Fig. 341-15). The combination of CT and US findings of fat strongly suggests angiomyolipoma. (Fat on IVP will appear radiolucent; on MRI fat appears as high-signal intensity on T_1-weighted imaging and low signal intensity on T_2-weighted imaging.

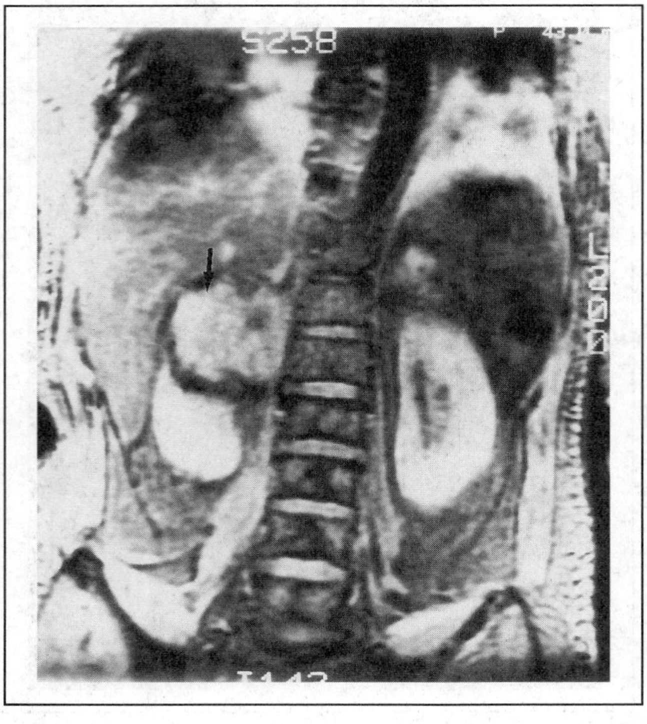

Fig. 341-13. Coronal view of renal MRI. *Arrow,* mass involving upper pole of right kidney.

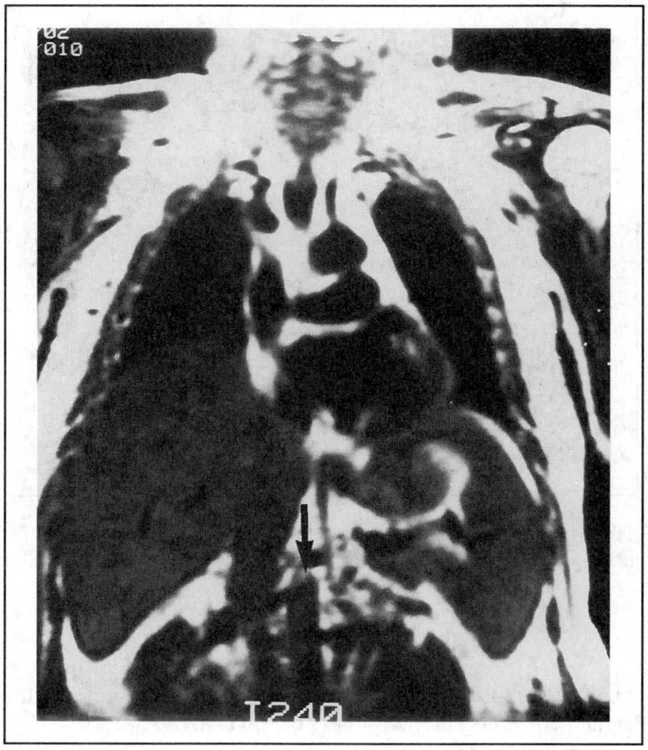

Fig. 341-14. Same patient as in Fig. 341-12 on coronal view of renal MRI demonstrating involvement of IVC *(arrow)*.

Other malignant tumors include metastases and lymphoma, which are difficult to differentiate from renal cell carcinoma. Transitional cell carcinoma is the most common malignancy involving the renal pelvis, ureters, and bladder. On IVP it will appear as an irregular filling defect destroying the pelvicocalyceal system. Hydronephrosis is frequently present. Similar findings are seen on the cross-sectional images. Fig. 341-16 provides a diagnostic algorithm for renal mass found on IVP.

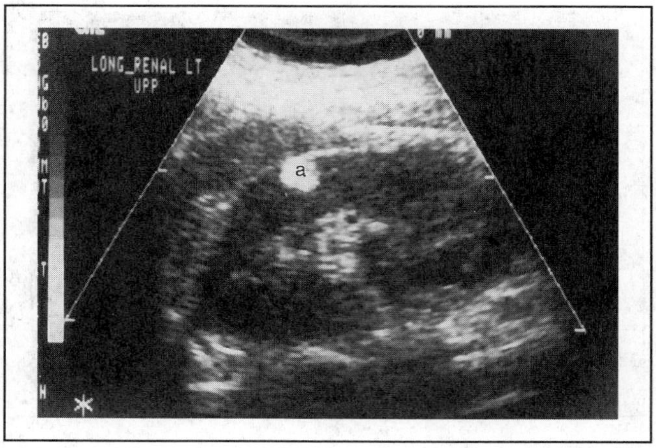

Fig. 341-15. Renal sonogram demonstrating an angiomyolipoma *(a)*.

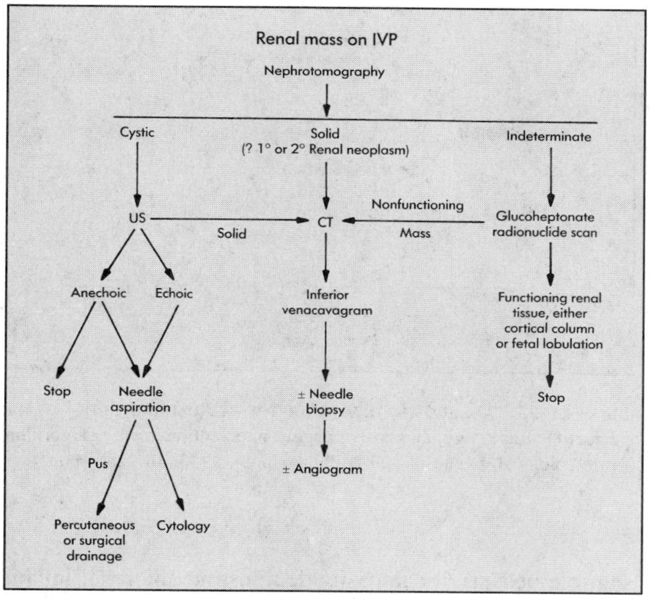

Fig. 341-16. Diagnostic algorithm for renal mass on IVP. (From Ferruci JT: Radiology, diagnosis-imaging-intervention imaging algorithms for radiological diagnosis, vol I, Philadelphia, 1986, JB Lippincott.)

Obstructive uropathy (hydronephrosis)

The radiologic evaluation of obstructive uropathy is clinically important because it provides significant information such as level and degree of obstruction and physiologic status of the involved kidney. The main imaging modalities involved in the evaluation of hydronephrosis include IVP, US, nuclear medicine, and CT.

On IVP, the KUB will frequently demonstrate the level of obstruction by delineating a calcified calculus. In the acute phase of obstruction, the kidney may be of normal size or enlarged. A delayed, dense, and persistent nephrogram appears, which is followed by a moderate distention of the collecting system. On delayed views the level of obstruction may be demonstrated by a columnized and dilated ureter down to the level of obstruction (Fig. 341-17). Complete obstruction may cause forniceal rupture of the calyces (acting as a safety valve) and extravasation of the contrast media. Chronic obstructive uropathy will be manifested by dilated collecting system filled by nonopacified urine, which appears lucent against the dense (by contrast media) renal parenchyma. This negative pyelogram sign will later become positive when contrast media enters the collecting system and displaces the nonopacified urine.

In long-standing and severe obstruction, the renal parenchyma will atrophy and will appear during the parenchymal phase of the IVP as a thin, dense rim (the rim sign). US is a sensitive modality demonstrating various degrees of hydronephrosis (Fig. 341-18). Sonography's ability to visualize the kidney does not depend on the renal function, making this modality ideal for evaluating obstruction in patients with renal failure. It is an important imaging modality in the follow-up of the progression of hydronephrosis because it is sensitive in delineating changes of the collecting system dilatation and does not require contrast media for imaging. The sensitivity of US is significantly reduced beyond the renal pelvis. Nuclear medicine provides more physiologic than morphologic information about the status of the obstructed kidney. Renal failure is not a significant obstacle and the radiation dose is minimal (Fig. 341-19).

Nuclear medicine provides estimation of the renal func-

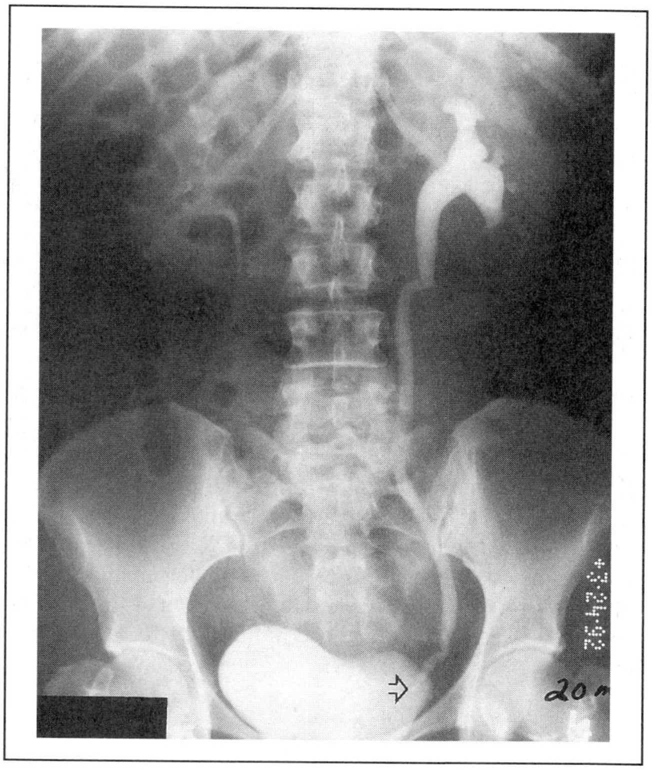

Fig. 341-17. Left obstruction demonstrating dense nephrogram-dilated collecting system and ureter. *Open arrow,* calculus of the ureterovesicle junction responsible for the obstruction.

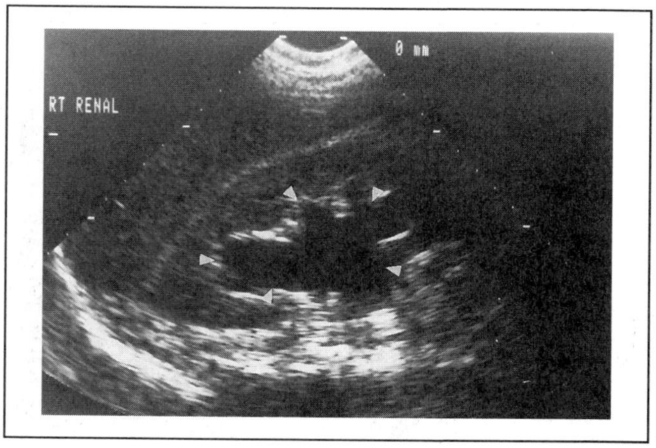

Fig. 341-18. Renal US demonstrating severe dilatation of the pelvis and collecting system *(arrowheads)* due to obstruction.

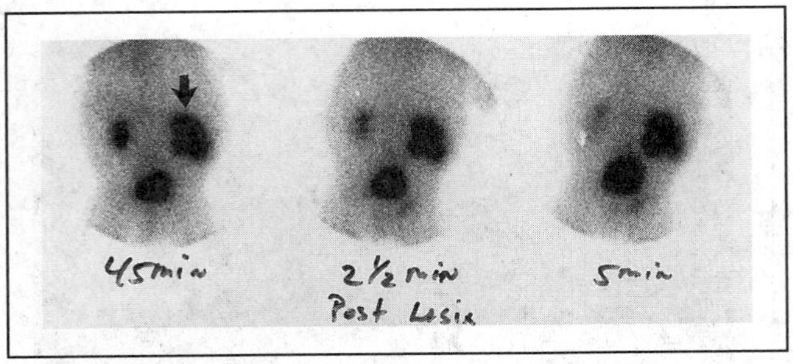

Fig. 341-19. Renal radionuclide scan: Right hydronephrosis *(arrow).*

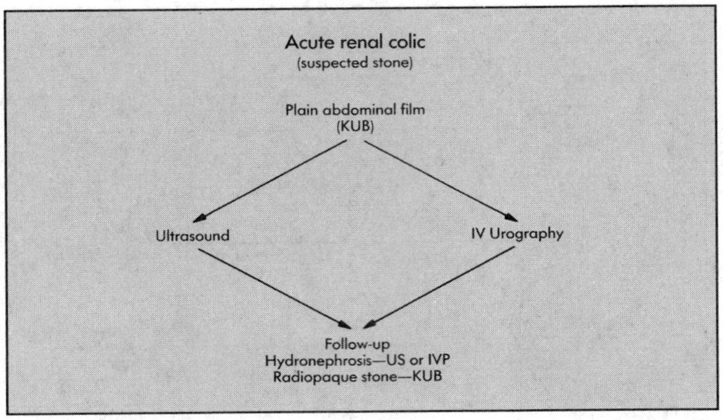

Fig. 341-21. Diagnostic algorithm for acute renal colic. (From Ferruci JT: Radiology, diagnosis-imaging-intervention imaging algorithms for radiological diagnosis, vol I, Philadelphia, 1986, JB Lippincott.)

tion and is used in the follow-up of the progression of hydronephrosis. CT demonstrates obstructed kidney and involved dilated ureter (Fig. 341-20). CT is not usually obtained for screening purposes but for determination of the etiology of hydronephrosis and the extension of the process. Fig. 341-21 provides diagnostic algorithm for acute renal colic.

Inflammation

Approximately 25% of patients with acute pyelonephritis or focal nephritis manifest no urographic abnormalities. Renal enlargement, diminished nephrogram, alteration of the collecting systems, and poorly defined renal outlines are some of the urographic abnormalities, which may be either focal or diffuse. Sonography is not sensitive for delineating abnormalities and in many instances is normal. Hypoechoic areas within the renal parenchyma indicate edema or inflammation. CT provides a better demonstration of the renal and pararenal inflammatory changes than IVP.

Renal abscess appears as an area of diminished contrast enhancement on IVP and CT. If there is gas formation, it will appear as small bubbles of air. CT has assumed a leading role because it can easily demonstrate the renal inflammatory process as well as its extension beyond the kidney (Fig. 341-22). US will easily demonstrate an abscess as an area of mixed echogenicity, with gas appearing as echogenic focus with some shadowing (Fig. 341-23).

Chronic

Chronic pyelonephritis is usually a focal disease manifested by alteration of the renal outlines due to the formation of scars. There is also dilatation of the calyx at the proximity of the scar. The kidney is small. These findings are easily seen on IVP and CT. Sonography reveals the same findings, as well as echogenic kidney due to the stiffness of the parenchyma (Fig. 341-24).

Xanthogranulomatous pyelonephritis is a chronic inflammatory disease characterized by the presence of lipid-containing histiocytes. The diffuse form of the disease (85% to 90%) is characterized as an enlarged nonfunctioning kidney containing a staghorn calculus or a calculus in the re-

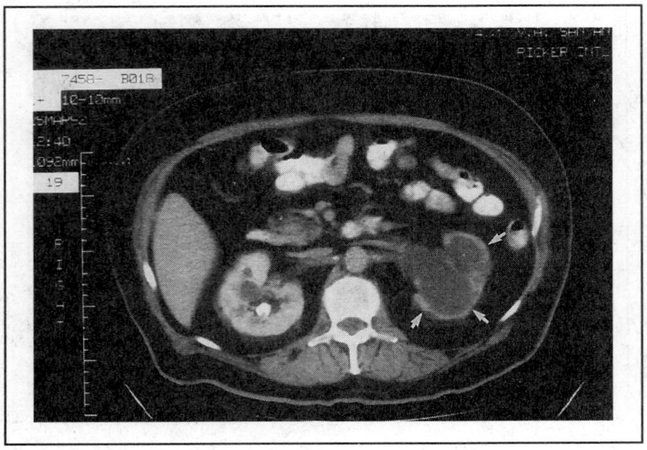

Fig. 341-20. The rim sign well demonstrated on CT *(arrows).*

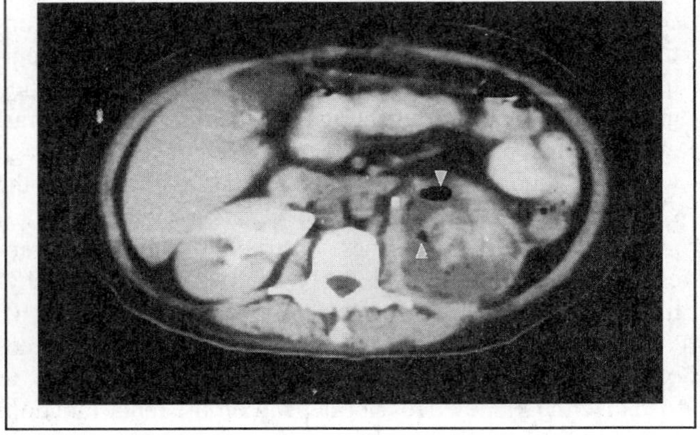

Fig. 341-22. Enhanced renal CT. Left renal abscess with pockets of gas *(arrowheads).*

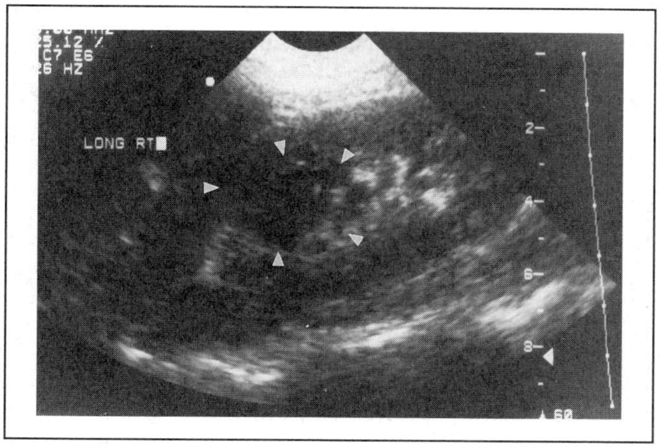

Fig. 341-23. Renal sonogram demonstrating an inflammatory mass as an area of mixed echogenicity *(arrowheads)*.

nal pelvis (Fig. 341-25). The focal form is manifested by a focal mass involving a functioning kidney.

Renovascular disease

Angiography is the main diagnostic modality for the evaluation of renovascular disease. Radionuclide renal scan offers a safe, easy, accurate screening method for evaluation of renovascular hypertension.

The most common vascular lesion is atherosclerosis, which involves the proximal aspect of the renal artery (usually 1 to 2 cm from its origin at the aorta). The lesions may be single or multiple (Fig. 341-26). Angiography accurately demonstrates the stenotic portion of the renal artery, collateral arteries in cases of severe stenosis, and poststenotic dilatation.

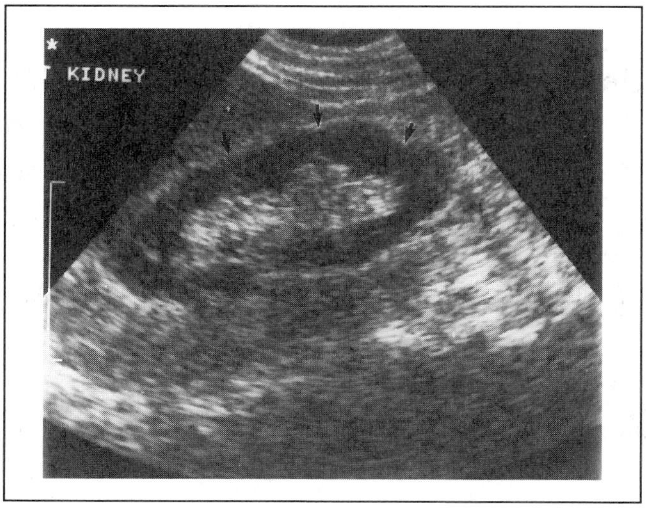

Fig. 341-24. Scarring *(arrows)* involving the kidney as a result of pyelonephritis.

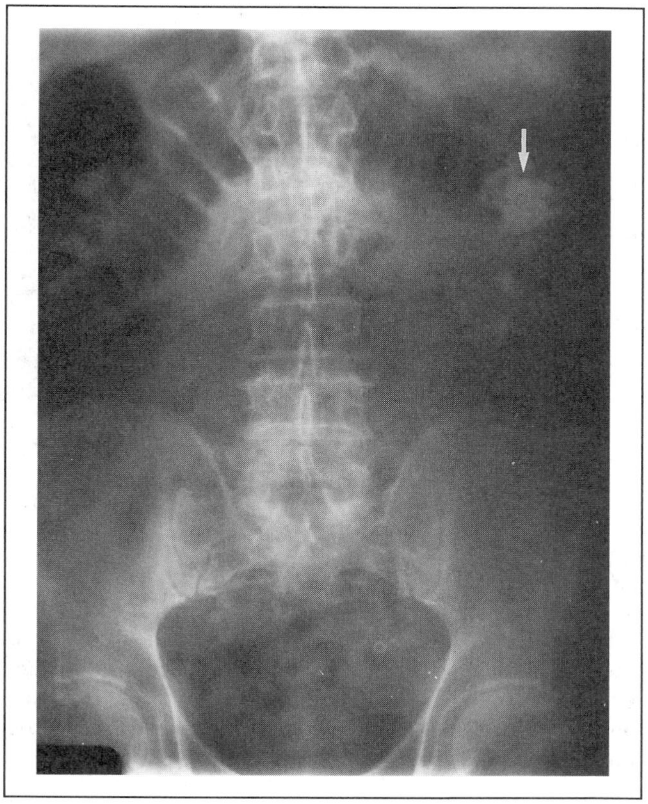

Fig. 341-25. KUB: Slaghorn calculus *(arrow)*.

Fibromuscular dysplasia, another cause of hypertension, occurs more frequently in women (80% of the cases). Bilateral lesions occur approximately 50% of the time; unilateral lesions more often occur in the right artery. Typically, the lesions appear as a string of beads in the middle and distal portions of the renal artery (Fig. 341-27).

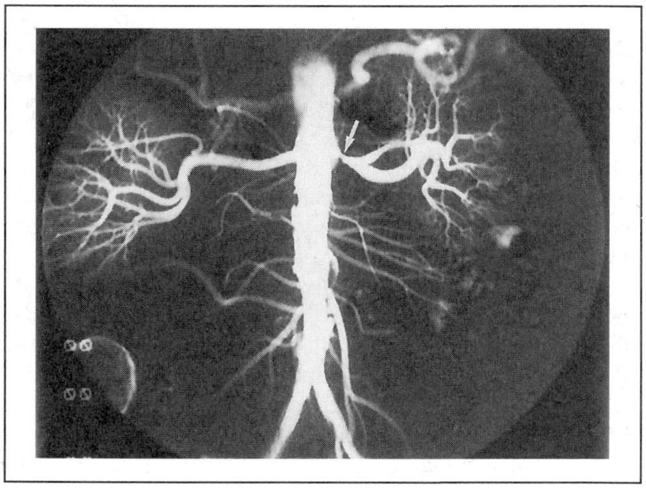

Fig. 341-26. Left renal artery stenosis *(arrow)*.

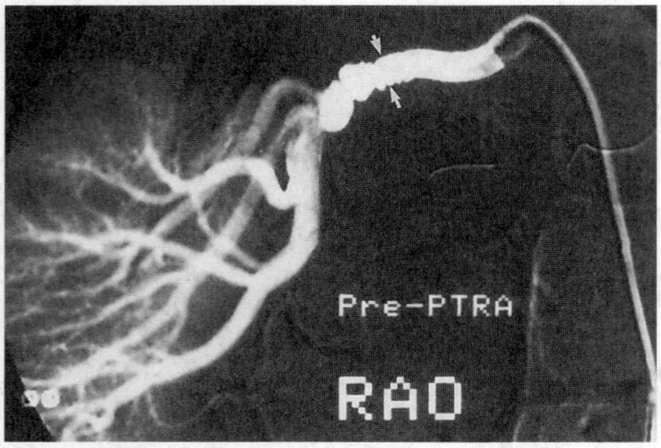

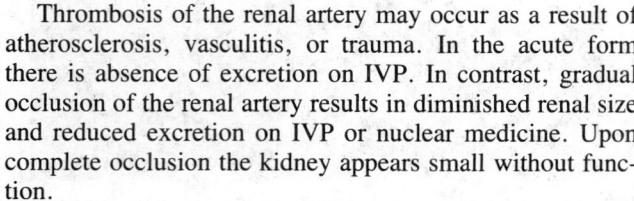

Fig. 341-27. Right fibromuscular dysplasia *(arrows)*.

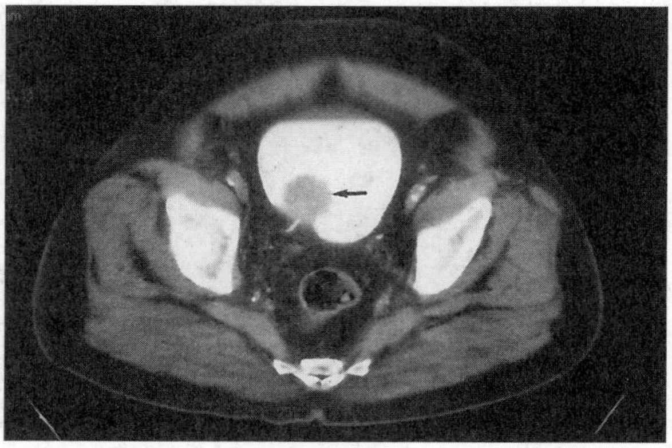

Fig. 341-28. Enhanced CT of pelvis. Tumor involving the urinary bladder *(arrow)*.

Thrombosis of the renal artery may occur as a result of atherosclerosis, vasculitis, or trauma. In the acute form there is absence of excretion on IVP. In contrast, gradual occlusion of the renal artery results in diminished renal size and reduced excretion on IVP or nuclear medicine. Upon complete occlusion the kidney appears small without function.

Emboli to the renal arteries may originate from the left atrium (in the case of atrial fibrillation), cardiac vegetations, aorta, etc. IVP will demonstrate absence of excretion with a normal-sized kidney and collecting system by retrograde pyelography or US, whereas arteriography demonstrates the obstruction of the renal artery or its branches.

Renal artery aneurysms may be diagnosed on plain radiography of the abdomen if they are calcified (approximately 30% of renal artery aneurysms are calcified). Arteriography demonstrates the size, shape, and location of the aneurysm. Other renal vascular abnormalities include renal infarct and renal and perirenal hematoma.

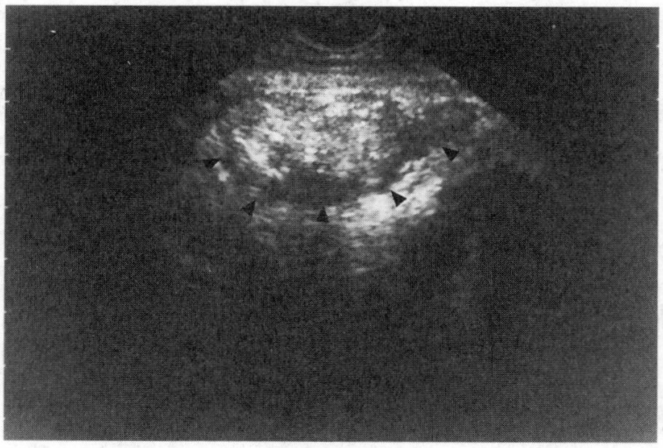

Fig. 341-29. Endorectal sonography demonstrating the prostate *(arrowheads)*.

Lower urinary tract/prostate

Bladder tumors can be visualized by IVP; however, CT and MRI are more sensitive because both imaging modalities evaluate the tumor from its extension within the wall of the bladder to the bowel and distant metastasis (Fig. 341-28). Diseases of the urethra are usually evaluated by cystourethrography or retrograde urethrography. Pathology of the prostate is best evaluated by prostatic sonography performed by endorectal probe and MRI of the prostate.

Prostatic sonography provides information about the prostate gland and seminal vesicles and the relationship of the prostate to the urinary bladder (Fig. 341-29). MRI of the prostate evaluates the gland itself as well as any metastatic disease involving the periprostatic region and distant to the prostate areas. MRI, with its ability to image in a multiplanal fashion, is an excellent imaging modality for outlining the relationship of the gland to the colon and bladder.

REFERENCES

Elkin M: Radiology of the urinary system, 2 vol, Boston, 1980, Little, Brown.

Kutcher R and Lautin EM: Genitourinary radiology: a multimodality approach, New York, 1990, Gower Medical Publishing.

Lee JT, Sagel SS, and Stanley RS: Computed body tomography with MRI correlation, ed 2, New York, 1989, Raven Press.

Pollack HM: Clinical urology, vol 1, Philadelphia, 1990, WB Saunders.

Rumak CM, Wilson CM, and Charboneau WJ: Diagnostic ultrasound vol 1, St Louis, 1991, Mosby–Year Book.

Taveras JM and Ferrucci JT: Radiology, diagnosis—imaging—intervention, vol 1 and 4, Philadelphia, 1986, JB Lippincott.

III Basic Clinical Syndromes

CHAPTER

342 Hematuria

B. S. Kasinath

Hematuria is encountered frequently in general practice. Often it is recognized for the first time during routine health screening procedures for employment or insurance purposes. It may occur in isolation or be associated with other abnormalities found on urinalysis such as proteinuria and cellular casts. It may be macroscopic or microscopic, intermittent or persistent.

DEFINITION

Since normally up to a million erythrocytes pass into the urine daily, it is not unusual to encounter some erythrocytes in the urine sediment. Most authorities agree that the presence of greater than three erythrocytes in a high-powered field in a centrifuged specimen of urine qualifies as significant microscopic hematuria. Red-colored urine does not always imply hematuria because several drugs (phenothiazines, phenazopyridine) and coloring agents in food (beets, rhubarb) may discolor the urine.

Hematuria is detected on urinalysis by dipstick or microscopic examination. Dipsticks rely on chemical detection of hemoglobin present in the urine. A positive reaction on the dipstick should always be confirmed by microscopic examination of the urine sediment to confirm the existence of hematuria as defined previously because dipsticks can react with myoglobin seen in rhabdomyolysis. False-negative reactions may be seen in patients taking large amounts of vitamin C (ascorbic acid). To gain maximum information, an early morning, freshly voided urine should be examined for hematuria and presence of red cell casts. Dysmorphic erythrocytes favor glomerular etiology of hematuria. It is important to avoid specimens obtained during menstruation or after recent instrumentation of the genitourinary tract.

ETIOLOGY

The etiology of hematuria may be considered in two categories: extrarenal and renal parenchymal (See the accompanying box). Extra-renal causes include postrenal genitourinary tract diseases such as calculi, tumors of renal pelvis, ureter, bladder, prostate, or urethra, infections of the genitourinary organs such as cystitis, prostatitis, and urethritis caused by bacterial, viral, fungal or parasitic organisms.

Common causes of hematuria

I. Extrarenal causes
- A. Genitourinary tract diseases
  - Calculi—renal pelvis, ureter, bladder, urethra
  - Neoplasms—renal pelvis, ureter, bladder, prostate, urethra
  - Infections—bladder, prostate, urethra, epididymis
  - Others—drugs (cyclophosphamide), foreign bodies, benign prostatic hypertrophy, endometriosis, trauma, strictures, vesicoureteral reflux
- B. Unrelated to genitourinary tract
  - Coagulopathies
  - Anticoagulation

II. Renal Parenchymal Causes
- A. Glomerular diseases
  - Mesangial proliferative glomerulonephritis (e.g., IgA nephritis)
  - Acute proliferative glomerulonephritis (e.g., post-streptococcal nephritis)
  - Glomerulonephritis due to systemic diseases (e.g., lupus)
  - Rapidly progressive glomerulonephritis (e.g., Goodpasture syndrome)
  - Membranoproliferative glomerulonephritis
  - Vascular (e.g., malignant hypertension, vasculitides)
  - Familial (e.g., Alport syndrome, thin glomerular basement membrane disease)
  - Miscellaneous (e.g., loin pain-hematuria syndrome)
- B. Tubulointerstitial diseases
  - Infections (e.g., pyelonephritis, tuberculosis)
  - Interstitial nephritis, acute (e.g., drugs) chronic (e.g., analgesic abuse)
  - Polycystic kidney disease
  - Vascular—renal infarction, cortical necrosis, renal vein thrombosis, malformations
  - Neoplasms—renal cell carcinoma
  - Others—papillary necrosis, trauma, hypercalciuria, hyperuricosuria

Although benign prostatic hypertrophy has been suggested to cause hematuria, another, independent cause should be considered. Chemical cystitis, for example, due to cyclophosphamide, can cause hematuria. Anticoagulants or coagulation abnormalities can result in hematuria, although underlying genitourinary tract pathology should be excluded in these cases. Renal parenchymal causes could involve glomerular or nonglomerular structures. Glomerular diseases could be primary (e.g., IgA nephropathy [Berger's disease]) or secondary to systemic diseases (e.g., systemic lupus erythematosus, vasculitis). Familial glomerular diseases such as Alport syndrome and thin glomerular basement membrane disease can cause hematuria. Nonglomerular renal parenchymal diseases (e.g., acute interstitial nephritis, polycystic kidney disease, renal cell carcinoma, and renal infarction) can be associated with hematuria. Recently, metabolic disorders such as hypercalciuria and hyperuricosuria have been implicated in hematuria. Strenuous exercise can lead to transient hematuria.

APPROACH TO DIAGNOSIS

The objective of investigation of hematuria is to uncover potentially serious diseases such as malignancies or severe glomerulonephritides in order to institute early therapeutic intervention where possible. Proper evaluation of hematuria requires detailed history including timing of hematuria during passage of urine, physical examination and a thorough urinalysis including examination of spun urine sediment by the physician, followed by appropriate investigations (Fig. 342-1). Urinalysis should exclude factitious hematuria (e.g., urine discoloration due to coloring agents in drugs and foods, myoglobinuria, porphyria).

The timing of hematuria during micturition may be helpful. Urethral diseases cause hematuria in the initial part of the stream, whereas terminal hematuria usually suggests bladder disease. Other etiologies usually cause hematuria throughout the stream.

Symptoms of dysuria, urgency, and increased frequency suggest infection of the urinary tract. Presence of symptoms of photosensitivity, rashes, arthritis, Raynaud's phenomenon point to collagen vascular diseases as possible etiology (e.g., systemic lupus erythematosus). A thorough history should include inquiries of drugs including over-the-counter formulations, family history of renal disease and stones, and foreign travel, especially to regions where infestation with *Schistosoma haematobium* is endemic. On physical examination, one should search for hypertension, edema (suggests glomerular etiology in the younger patient), and prostatic nodularity or enlargement; bimanual pelvic examination should be performed in women to search for invasive pelvic neoplasms. Signs of systemic diseases such as rashes, arthritis, and palpable purpura may point to collagen vascular disease and/or vasculitis.

Strategies for laboratory evaluation depend on whether one has uncovered clues to the presence of renal parenchymal or extrarenal causes during a thorough initial evaluation consisting of history, physical examination, and urinalysis. For instance, presence of proteinuria, especially greater than 3.5g/day, dysmorphic erythrocytes, erythrocyte casts, and renal insufficiency point to glomerular etiology. Dysuria, fever, chills, leukocyturia, and bacteriuria suggest infection of the urinary tract. If these clues are not present, it is wise to exclude asymptomatic urinary tract infection by urine culture. Hematuria associated with "sterile" pyuria should prompt a search for genitourinary tuberculosis and interstitial nephritis. A negative urine culture should be followed by intravenous pyelography (IVP), which may delineate neoplasms, calculi, anatomic abnormalities, or cystic diseases of the urinary tract. In patients who are sensitive to contrast media or in whom acute renal failure due to contrast media is considered a high probabil-

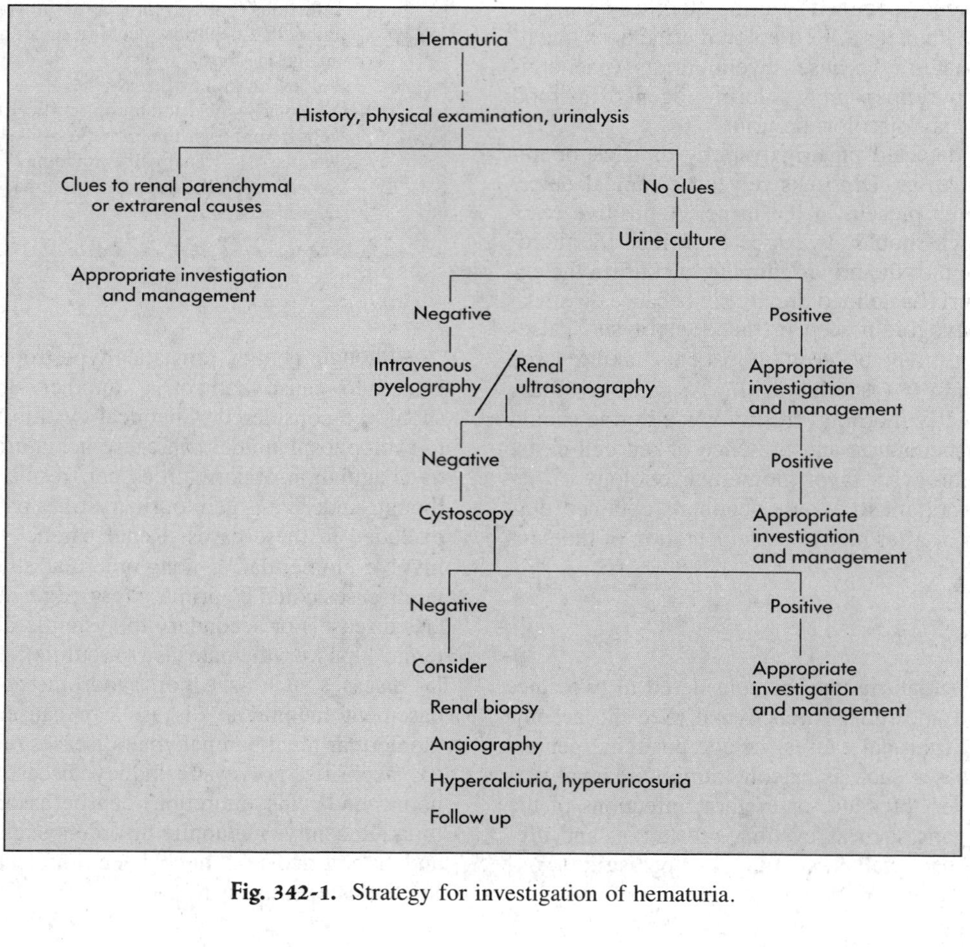

Fig. 342-1. Strategy for investigation of hematuria.

ity, ultrasonography of the genitourinary tract may be performed in the place of IVP.

If ultrasound or IVP is equivocal or normal, cystoscopy is generally performed, especially in the elderly, to detect lower urinary tract pathology, as well as to determine whether hematuria is originating from one or both kidneys. Retrograde pyelography may be needed to define ureteral lesions. A negative cystoscopic examination should lead to considerations of renal biopsy for renal parenchymal diseases, renal angiography to diagnose vascular malformations or neoplasms that are too small to be seen on IVP, or a search for hypercalciuria and hyperuricosuria. Computerized tomography has been used to delineate the anatomic structure of mass lesions found on IVP or ultrasound. Urinary cytology may help in the detection of malignant cells that suggest diagnosis of genitourinary malignancy.

Some caveats should be kept in mind. Significant pathology, particularly malignancies of the genitourinary tract, is more likely to be discovered in the elderly population, especially males. Although a thorough investigation may still not reveal an identifiable cause in up to 12% of patients, urologic disease may still be present, and periodic follow-up in such cases is recommended. Complications from radiation exposure, reactions to contrast media including acute renal failure in susceptible patients, untoward consequences of renal biopsy, patient's underlying illness and general condition, and expenses of work-up should be considered as factors that affect the investigation of individual cases of hematuria.

REFERENCES

Andres A et al: Hematuria due to hypercalciuria and hyperuricosuria in adult patients, Kidney Int 36:96-99, 1989.

Glassock RJ: Hematuria and pigmenturia. In Massry SG, Glassock RJ, editors: Textbook of nephrology, ed 2, Baltimore, 1989, Williams & Wilkins.

Mariani AJ et al: The significance of adult hematuria: 1000 hematuria evaluations including a risk-benefit and cost effectiveness analysis, J Urol 141:350-355, 1989.

Schoolwerth AC: Hematuria and proteinuria: their causes and consequences, Hosp Pract 22:45-62, 1987.

Spencer J, Lindsell D, Mastorakou I: Ultrasonography compared with intravenous pyelography in the investigation of adults with haematuria, Br Med J 301:1074-1076, 1990.

Tiebosch AT et al: Thin basement membrane nephropathy in adults with persistent hematuria, N Engl J Med 320:14-18, 1989.

CHAPTER

343 Proteinuria

B. S. Kasinath
Manjeri A. Venkatachalam

An abnormal urinary excretion of protein, commonly termed *proteinuria,* is often a sign of primary intrinsic renal disease but can also be found in a multitude of other disorders.

Normally, an average adult excretes approximately 80 mg of protein daily, and usually not more than 150 mg/day. The accepted normal value in adolescence and pregnancy is somewhat higher (up to 300 mg/day). In the healthy adult, the protein excretion consists of approximately 40% albumin, 40% tissue protein, 15% immunoglobulins (5% to 10% IgG or its fragments, 5% light chains, and 3% IgA), and 5% other filtered plasma proteins. A portion of the tissue protein is Tamm-Horsfall protein, a glycoprotein produced by cells of the thick ascending limb of the loop of Henle. The function of this negatively charged glycoprotein is not known. However, it constitutes more than 80% of the mass of "casts" that are found in the urine in disease states (Chapter 339).

Urinary protein excretion in normal individuals varies under different circumstances and is markedly influenced by posture and exercise, proteinuria being greater in the erect posture and after exercise. Change in protein excretion with position has also been demonstrated in patients with pathologic protein loss from disorders such as pyelonephritis or glomerulonephritis. Renal hemodynamic changes induced by change of posture and exercise may underlie the concomitant alterations in protein excretion (see later discussion).

MECHANISMS OF PROTEINURIA

Enhanced urinary protein loss can occur by any of five mechanisms (Fig. 343-1): (1) an increased delivery and filtration of low molecular weight proteins in the plasma, which overwhelms the reabsorptive capacity of the tubule to reclaim normally filtered proteins; (2) an increase in glomerular capillary permeability; (3) impaired capacity of the tubule to reabsorb normally filtered proteins; (4) hemodynamic alterations; and (5) extensive bleeding or severe infection in the urinary tract. Figure 343-1 illustrates the anatomic sites of these mechanisms and lists the most important conditions associated with each of them.

Increased protein delivery

Low molecular weight proteins are normally filtered across glomerular capillaries, but are readily reabsorbed by the tubules. If the delivery of a low molecular weight protein exceeds this reabsorptive capacity, proteinuria results. For proteinuria to occur, one of two situations must exist: Ei-

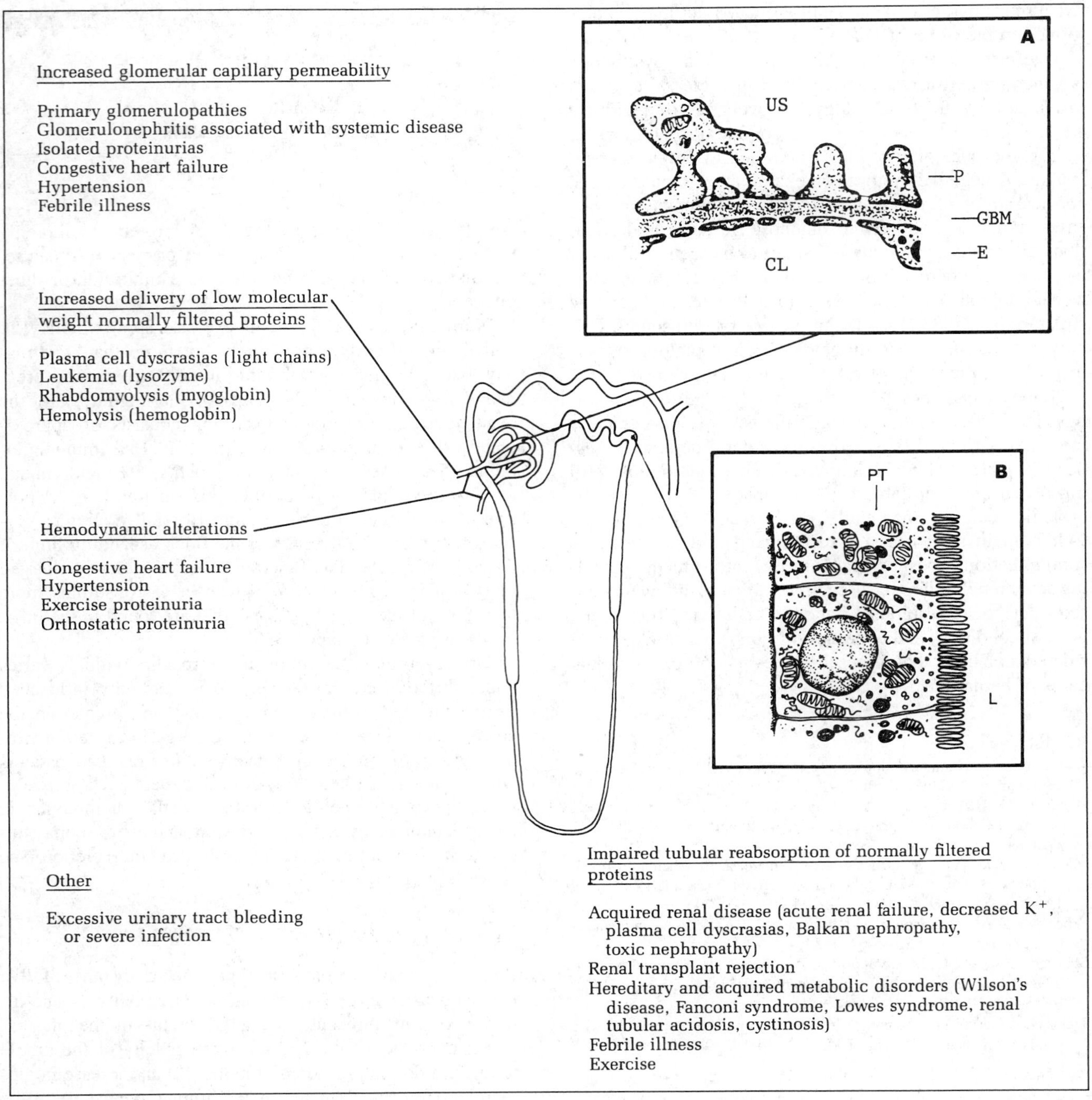

Fig. 343-1. Mechanisms of proteinuria. The glomerular capillary wall and proximal tubular cell are depicted in expanded views. The glomerular capillary wall *(inset A),* which separates the capillary lumen (CL) from the urinary space (US) consists of endothelial cell (E), glomerular basement membrane (GBM) and foot process (P) of the glomerular visceral epithelial cell. In the proximal tubule *(inset B),* protein is reabsorbed from fluid in the tubular lumen (L) by the proximal tubular epithelial cell (PT).

ther overproduction alone exceeds normal maximum reabsorptive capacity, or overproduction is associated with a reduced maximum reabsorptive capacity due to an effect of the disease on tubular function. Which of these mechanisms is more significant has not been studied in detail. Various types of leukemia, multiple myeloma, rhabdomyolysis, and hemolysis can cause proteinuria from protein overproduction. Such proteinuria is also referred to as *overflow proteinuria.*

In monocytic and myelomonocytic leukemia, lysozyme may be produced in large amounts by the leukemic cells. Lysozyme has an isoelectric point of 11 and a low molecular mass (14,000 daltons); both of these features facilitate filtration (see later discussion). When the renal absorptive threshold for lysozyme is exceeded, the filtered lysozyme is excreted in the urine, sometimes in very large amounts, up to 2.6 g/day. Although it is a feature of leukemia, lysozymuria can also be due to primary tubular damage or to tubular damage secondary to glomerular disease. In these instances, the lysozymuria is due to a reduced reabsorptive capacity, not to overproduction.

Immunoglobulin light chains (22,000 daltons) are normally filtered across glomeruli, reabsorbed by the tubules, and degraded. If they are produced and filtered in amounts greater than the tubular reabsorptive capacity, light chains will appear in the urine in pathologic amounts. Accordingly, the normal excretion rates of kappa and lambda chains are less than 2 and 1 mg/day, respectively, whereas amounts varying from 100 mg to 10 g may be excreted in diseases characterized by increased immunoglobulin production (e.g., multiple myeloma) (Chapter 356).

When released into the blood and filtered in sufficient quantity, both myoglobin and hemoglobin may lead to detectable proteinuria. Myoglobin can be released in excessive amounts due to a number of acquired or hereditary muscle disorders. Trauma is a frequent cause of myoglobinuria. In hemolytic states, the release and subsequent filtration of hemoglobin results in proteinuria.

Altered glomerular capillary permeability

Considering the large amounts of plasma proteins that are presented to the glomerular capillaries, very little appears in the urine normally (less than 150 mg/day). Normal glomeruli limit the filtration of molecules on the basis of their size, shape, and electrical charge. This selectivity has been shown to be responsible for the virtual exclusion from the filtrate of plasma proteins equal to or greater than the size of albumin molecules. On the other hand, proteins smaller than albumin are filterable. The components of the glomerular filter are shown in Fig. 343-1 (inset A). The capillary endothelium has fenestrations with pores of about 1000 A diameter that offer little resistance to protein diffusion. The glomerular basement membrane, which consists of negatively charged glycoproteins and proteoglycans as well as collagen, is the major structural barrier to the filtration of macromolecules. Importantly, the negative charges in the basement membrane pose an additional, electrical barrier to the passage of negatively charged proteins. Further, structures called *slit diaphragms,* which bridge adjacent foot processes of the glomerular visceral epithelial cells, offer additional resistance to any proteins that may have penetrated the basement membrane.

Alterations in the selective permeability properties of glomeruli lead to glomerular proteinuria. Structural defects in the filtration pathway that increase "porosity," or molecular defects that give rise to abnormal electrical charge interactions, or both, may account for glomerular protein leakage. Defects in structure and increased porosity, associated mostly with destructive and inflammatory processes, lead to loss of size discrimination. Therefore the filtrate and urine contain high molecular weight globulins and albumin in ratios that approach those of plasma. On the other hand, there are proteinuric glomerulopathies (such as lipoid nephrosis; see also Chapter 354) in which urinary protein is almost exclusively albumin. It would appear that the responsible glomerular defect in such cases is a decrease in the net negative charge of the filter, diminished repulsion of negatively charged albumin molecules, and therefore increased leakage of albumin. Although recent investigations have demonstrated increased urinary losses of large molecules of the size of immunoglobulin in these states, comparatively, the increase in fractional clearance of albumin is still greater than the increase in fractional clearance of immunoglobulin.

Many disorders result in proteinuria due to altered glomerular permeability (see Fig. 343-1). All primary glomerulopathies and glomerulopathies associated with systemic diseases have at least this mechanism responsible for proteinuria. Changes in glomerular permeability leading to proteinuria are also suggested, though not proved, in congestive heart failure, hypertension, and febrile illnesses. Isolated proteinuria may be at least partially due to a glomerular permeability mechanism and is discussed separately.

Impaired tubular reabsorption

Proteins filtered by glomeruli are reabsorbed and degraded by the renal tubules. The filtered load of protein in normal kidneys is not precisely known, but micropuncture studies in rats suggest an upper limit of 2.5 mg albumin/dl of filtrate. Almost all of this amount is reabsorbed by the tubules. These considerations immediately suggest that if tubular function is impaired, protein reabsorption will be decreased, resulting in proteinuria. Such tubular proteinuria is characterized by the presence of low molecular mass globulins (less than 60,000 daltons) in the urine in amounts equal to or greater than albumin. These globulins are normally present in the serum and are filtered relatively freely but are almost completely reabsorbed. The daily excretion of beta-2 microglobulin (the best studied globulin) is approximately 30 to 370 μg/day, but in tubular disease as much as 100 mg may be excreted. Similarly, lysozyme, which is normally filtered but reabsorbed, will appear in the urine during tubular proteinuria. This condition must be differentiated from lysozymuria, which may occur solely due to excessive production, and from saturation of tubular reabsorptive capacity. Tubular proteinuria occurs in diverse disease states (Fig. 343-1) and is sometimes used to monitor tubular function. In tubular proteinuria the total amount of protein excreted daily is rarely greater than 2 g/day and is usually much less.

Hemodynamic alterations

Glomerular filtration is affected by hemodynamic factors such as transcapillary hydrostatic and oncotic pressure gradients, plasma flow, and the filtration surface area and permeability (Chapter 338). One or more of these factors may be altered, giving rise to glomerular protein leakage and, potentially, proteinuria. For example, in congestive heart failure, there is an increase in the filtration fraction due to disproportionate reduction in glomerular plasma flow compared to the filtration rate. In this situation, complex changes occur in the Starling forces that govern filtration, causing protein leakage, rarely exceeding 1 to 1.5 g/day. Treatment of heart failure resolves or markedly diminishes the proteinuria.

Proteinuria may occur in situations in which glomerular blood flow and hydrostatic pressure rise (e.g., in some types of hypertension and during the adaptation that residual nephrons undergo after the destruction of substantial amounts of renal mass). These intrarenal circulatory abnormalities may damage glomeruli and increase protein leakage. Proteinuria is usually moderate, reaching daily excretions of 2 to 3 g only in severe hypertension or unusual cases. Control of hypertension diminishes the proteinuria, in line with its postulated hemodynamic basis. In this regard, angiotensin-converting enzyme inhibitors are thought to be effective not only as systemic antihypertensives but also as agents that specifically correct the altered glomerular hemodynamics that lead to proteinuria. Of note, proteinuria due to drug-induced glomerular damage has been reported as an uncommon side effect of some converting enzyme inhibitors. Chronic dietary restriction of protein intake is known to ameliorate proteinuria as well as retard the progression of nephron destruction in diverse renal diseases. It is thought that correction of altered glomerular hemodynamics underlies this protection also. The value of protein restriction therapy is currently the subject of intense scrutiny.

The other forms of proteinuria that may be hemodynamically mediated include orthostatic proteinuria and exercise-induced proteinuria. Orthostatic proteinuria is abnormal protein excretion that occurs during erect posture and subsides on assumption of recumbent position (see ISOLATED PROTEINURIA). Totally reversible marked proteinuria may occur after severe exercise and, if not recognized as such, may cause undue concern.

Other causes of proteinuria

Extensive bleeding or severe infection of the urinary tract can be associated with excretion of abnormal amounts of plasma proteins and therefore must be taken into account in the evaluation of urinary protein excretion.

LABORATORY DETERMINATION OF PROTEINURIA

Initial determination of proteinuria is accomplished either by a protein precipitation method (i.e., sulfosalicylic acid test) or a dipstick colorimetric method. The dipstick method has replaced precipitation methods in most clinical laboratories for initial screening because of its simplicity. Dipstick strips are sensitive to a protein concentration as low as 20 mg/dl. They react preferentially with albumin and are relatively insensitive to globulins and Bence Jones proteins. Protein precipitation methods flocculate all proteins and are useful in detecting nonalbumin proteins (e.g., in multiple myeloma).

Quantification of confirmed proteinuria is accomplished with a 24-hour urine collection. As mentioned, the upper limit in the average adult is approximately 150 mg of protein per day. Several studies have shown that protein-creatinine ratios in urine samples voided randomly during waking hours correlate well with 24-hour protein values.

Further characterization of the proteinuria as to the selectivity of protein loss is possible by urine protein electrophoresis, but this differentiation has limited clinical application. Urine protein electrophoresis along with immunodiffusion and immunoelectrophoresis (on concentrated urine) is required to characterize the immunoglobulins in proteinuria associated with plasma cell dyscrasias.

EVALUATION OF PROTEINURIA

Proteinuria can occur in several different clinical settings: (1) renal disease occurring as a part of acquired or hereditary systemic disorders (e.g., in systemic lupus erythematosus and Alport's syndrome); (2) primary renal disease (e.g., glomerulonephritis); (3) protein overproduction due to plasma cell dyscrasias, leukemia, rhabdomyolysis, or hemolysis; (4) proteinuria resulting from renal hemodynamic alterations, as in congestive heart failure; and (5) patients having no evidence of disease by history, physical examination, or laboratory examination and having normal renal function except for proteinuria with a normal urinary sediment. The last-mentioned category is referred to as *isolated proteinuria*. The likelihood of an underlying disease is high if quantitative proteinuria exceeds 2 g/day. Proteinuria in excess of 3.5 g/day, consisting mostly of albumin, is considered to be in the range usually seen in the nephrotic syndrome (Chapter 346). This amount of proteinuria (greater than 3.5 g/day) indicates glomerular disease at least as a component (assuming the proteinuria is not due to overproduction, as in multiple myeloma).

The first three categories of proteinuria are discussed in detail elsewhere (Chapters 346, 354, 355, and 356). Patients with proteinuria due to hemodynamic alterations will usually have a profound reduction in protein excretion with appropriate treatment of the underlying disease. Otherwise healthy individuals with isolated proteinuria deserve special consideration, as discussed below.

ISOLATED PROTEINURIA

Isolated proteinuria is not a rare finding in practice, with the incidence reported between 0.55% and 5.8% of young servicemen or college freshmen. The range of protein loss can vary from less than 1 g/day to the values associated with the nephrotic syndrome. When the proteinuria is greater than 1 g/day the likelihood of finding underlying glomerular disease increases, and a renal biopsy may be indicated. Isolated proteinurias can be further divided into transient, intermittent, constant, or orthostatic. These patterns do not represent specific disease and may occur in the same patient at different times.

Transient proteinuria is defined as proteinuria present on initial examination of apparently healthy individuals and absent on subsequent urinalysis. It is a common type of proteinuria in children and young adults. Transient proteinuria can also be seen during exercise and fever. There is no evidence of renal disease in these patients.

Intermittent proteinuria does not define a specific group of patients. In one group of individuals with intermittent proteinuria studied by biopsy, 30% demonstrated minimal or no change and 70% demonstrated either interstitial fibrosis or other glomerular pathology. Although a significant number of patients show some renal histologic changes, the prognosis for most patients in this group is good, and proteinuria disappears in a few years in most patients. Persons under 30 years of age have mortality rates similar to comparable age-matched controls. In general, infrequent follow-up is recommended, with evaluation of blood pressure, urine, and renal function.

The *constant* pattern of isolated proteinuria is associated with a higher mortality than the intermittent pattern and a greater risk of death due to renal disease. It should be distinguished from orthostatic proteinuria, which carries a very good prognosis. The constant pattern correlates with a variety of renal lesions on biopsy, and thus a uniform prognosis cannot be predicted. Renal biopsy may show a normal pattern or mild mesangial proliferation ($\approx$ 70%), definite glomerular lesions (20%), and/or interstitial nephritis ($\approx$ 5%). Up to 50% of these patients may develop hypertension over a 5-year period, and renal insufficiency has occurred in up to 20% of patients during 10 years of follow-up.

Orthostatic proteinuria must be distinguished from the constant pattern. Urine samples are obtained in the morning on awakening, while still supine, and after 2 hours of continuous walking or standing. Orthostatic proteinuria is defined as proteinuria present only in the urine samples obtained in an upright position. Patients with orthostatic proteinuria have a low risk of developing renal insufficiency. In a 20 year follow-up study of young men, none had developed any evidence of renal functional impairment, and only a few continued to be proteinuric.

REFERENCES

Anderson S, Garcia DL, and Brenner BM: Renal and systemic manifestations of glomerular disease. In Brenner BM and Rector FC Jr, editors: The kidney, ed 4, Philadelphia, 1991, WB Saunders.

Dennis VW and Robinson RR: Clinical proteinuria. In JT Lamont, JJ Leonard, and MD Siperstein, editors: Advances in internal medicine, Chicago, 1986, Year Book.

Glassock RJ: Focus on proteinuria, Am J Nephrol 10(Suppl 1):88-93, 1990.

Hostetter TH and Rosenberg ME: Hemodynamic effects on glomerular permselectivity, Am J Nephrol 10(Suppl 1):24-27, 1990.

Kanwar YS et al: Current status of the structural and functional basis of glomerular filtration and proteinuria, Semin Nephrol 11:390-413, 1991.

Poortmans JR: Post exercise proteinuria in humans. Facts and mechanisms, JAMA 253:236, 1985.

Scandling JD et al: Glomerular permselectivity in healthy and nephrotic humans, Adv Nephrol 21:159-176, 1992.

Schoolwerth AC: Hematuria and proteinuria: their causes and consequences, Hosp Pract 22:45-62, 1987.

Schwab SJ et al: Quantitation of proteinuria by the use of protein-to-creatinine ratios in single urine samples, Arch Intern Med 147:943-944, 1987.

CHAPTER

344 Dysuria

Marvin Forland

Dysuria literally means difficult urination, but in customary clinical usage it refers to the painful passage of urine, often accompanied by frequency, urgency, and a sense of incomplete bladder emptying. Although this symptom complex is characteristic of bacterial cystitis-urethritis, the differential diagnosis is broad (see accompanying box) but is usually readily narrowed by a careful history and physical examination, aided by a few easily obtainable laboratory data. Dysuria is a far more frequent complaint among women than among men, and we will consider the sexes separately.

DYSURIA IN WOMEN

Infectious causes

Urinary tract infection. The presence of costovertebral or flank pain or tenderness and fever in association with dysuria strongly suggests upper urinary tract infection. In less acutely ill women, a distinction has been made between *internal dysuria* —perceived by the patient as inside the body and experienced with urethritis—and *external dysuria*—pain felt in the inflamed vaginal labia, induced by the stream of urine, and characteristic of vaginitis.

Urinary tract infection is confirmed by the culture findings of 100,000 or more colonies per milliliter of urine obtained from a clean-voided midstream urine specimen. This widely used criterion was based largely on studies of women with acute pyelonephritis or asymptomatic bacteriuria. In a series of recent studies of symptomatic women, only one third to two thirds of the patients whose urine contained organisms on suprapubic aspiration or urethral catheterization met this standard. Finding 100 or more colonies per milliliter of urine was the diagnostic criterion providing the most useful sensitivity and specificity in this symptomatic population. The finding of pyuria is nonspecific, but in association with dysuria it strongly suggests an infectious origin. The presence of organisms on direct examination of the fresh, spun, preferably Gram-stained urine, is helpful, rapid confirmation.

The presence of pyuria in association with dysuria and in the absence of bacteriuria by standard techniques should alert the physician to the possibility of genitourinary tuber-

Differential diagnosis of dysuria

- I. Urinary tract infection
  - A. Enterobacteriaceae
  - B. Gram-positive organisms
  - C. *Chlamydia trachomatis*
  - D. *Mycobacterium tuberculosis*
- II. Vaginitis
  - A. Fungi *(Candida albicans)*
  - B. Bacterial
    1. *Gardnerella vaginalis (Haemophilus vaginalis)*
    2. *Neisseria gonorrhoeae*
    3. *Treponema pallidum* (endourethral chancre)
    4. *Chlamydia trachomatis*
  - C. Protozoa *(Trichomonas vaginalis)*
- III. Genital infection
  - A. Herpes simplex (genitalis)
  - B. Condyloma accuminatum
  - C. Paraurethral glands
- IV. Estrogen deficiency
- V. Interstitial cystitis (Hunner's ulcer)
- VI. Reiter's syndrome
- VII. Chemical irritants
  - A. Douches
  - B. Deodorant aerosols
  - C. Contraceptive jellies
  - D. Bubble bath
- VIII. Impedance to flow
  - A. Urethral caruncle or diverticula
  - B. Meatal stenosis or stricture
  - C. Transient urethral edema
  - D. Chronic fibrosis after trauma
  - E. Impaired synergy: bladder contraction and sphincter relaxation
- IX. Regional disease
  - A. Crohn's disease
  - B. Diverticulitis
  - C. Cervical radium implant
- X. Bladder tumor

culosis. Tuberculin skin testing is appropriate, and, if the findings are positive, a series of first morning urine specimens should be cultured for *Mycobacterium tuberculosis*. Dysuria has been reported as a prominent symptom in 20% to 34% of patients with renal tuberculosis.

An additional consideration is *Chlamydia trachomatis* infection. This organism was implicated in more than half the women with dysuria and frequency, sterile bladder urine, and pyuria in a study using cell culture techniques for isolation of the organism. Sexual transmission appears likely. Diagnosis has been facilitated by the availability of fluorescein-labeled monoclonal antibodies permitting immediate identification of characteristic chlamydial inclusions by fluorescence microscopy.

Vaginitis. Vaginitis assumes a major role when dysuria is described as external and particularly when it is accompanied by an unusual or malodorous vaginal discharge, dyspareunia, or vulvar itching or discomfort. Dysuria is a less common symptom with vaginitis than with urinary tract infection but may be more often attributable to vaginitis in young women because vaginitis occurs far more frequently than urinary tract infection. *Candida albicans* is the most common cause of symptomatic vaginitis, and the fungal growth may be sustained by elevated estrogen levels. Consequently, it occurs more frequently in pregnancy or with the use of oral contraceptives, and the patient may experience premenstrual exacerbations. Candidal discharge is characteristically white, thick, curd forming, and adherent, and organisms are readily identifiable on wet mount.

Trichomonas vaginalis infection is associated with dysuria or frequency in about 25% of infected women. The discharge is classically described as profuse, yellowish green, frothy, and malodorous; but it is highly variable. Identification of the organisms by wet mount is successful in 60% to 70% of infected women; culture provides a significantly higher yield.

Bacterial vaginosis is now the preferred term for the most prevalent vaginal infection in the reproductive years, previously called nonspecific vaginitis. The designation emphasizes its noninflammatory characteristics and its relationship to the interplay of several species of facultative anaerobic bacteria, genital mycoplasma, and suppression of the usually dominant *Lactobacillus*. A vaginal malodor, often described as fishy, is the major symptom. The discharge is small to moderate in amount, gray, malodorous, thin and adherent. While *Gardnerella vaginalis* may be a necessary pathogenic component, it is no longer considered the sole etiologic agent. However, its presence is an important diagnostic finding, evident on wet mount examination as tiny granules studding the vaginal epithelial cells, termed *clue cells*. Additional characteristic findings are a vaginal pH greater than 4.5 and a positive amine test, established by elicitation of a fishy odor upon addition of 10% KOH to vaginal secretions.

Gonorrhea continues to be a major consideration in the differential diagnosis of dysuria. This diagnosis was made in 8% to 29% of women with dysuria as an initial complaint and accounted for over 60% of those with "negative" urine cultures in one experience. The symptoms were similar to those in the group with urinary infection and sometimes included fever. Thus a preliminary diagnosis of acute pyelonephritis was not rare in those subsequently found to have gonorrheal infection. A complete pelvic examination and a Thayer-Martin culture of a cervical specimen must play an important role in initial evaluation in populations at risk of gonorrhea.

Less common infectious causes include the presence of an endourethral chancre, herpes simplex (genitalis) usually located on the labia, or condyloma accuminatum. Infection localized to the small Skene's glands that empty into the urethra has been suggested as analogous to male prostatitis. Exudate may be expressed from the glands for smear and culture.

Noninfectious causes

Atrophic vaginitis. In the postmenopausal woman, dysuria may be a consequence of estrogen deprivation, resulting in senile or atrophic vaginitis with associated urethral irritation. Vaginal discharge, itching, and dyspareunia are frequent accompanying symptoms. The vaginal mucosa appears thin, often inflamed, and bleeds easily. Infections occur with increased frequency. A wet smear of vaginal cells shows a marked predominance of parabasal cells. Response to estrogen administration is usually rapid.

Interstitial cystitis. Persistent dysuria with sterile cultures raises the possibility of interstitial cystitis, an uncommon bladder lesion of unknown etiology seen most often in women. The classic symptom complex includes continuous frequency and urgency and suprapubic pain relieved by voiding. Pyuria and hematuria are sometimes present but not uniformly, and the findings of exfoliative cytologic examination are negative. The diagnosis is made by cystoscopy, with the characteristic findings of reduced bladder capacity and the presence of superficial, often stellate Hunner's ulcers. In the earlier stages of the disease, however, only multiple petechiae-like hemorrhages (glomerulations) may be observed after second distention of the bladder on cystoscopy, and the capacity may be normal. Increased numbers of mast cells have been described on detrusor muscle biopsy of patients with presumed interstitial cystitis, but therapeutic results with mast cell stabilizing agents have been poor. An autoimmune response to Tamm-Horsfall protein has been suggested as a possible etiology and measurement of serum antibody to the protein as a potential noninvasive diagnostic test.

Urethral syndrome. The *urethral syndrome,* or *frequency and dysuria syndrome,* is a term that has been used to describe the approximately 50% of women presenting with these complaints who have either no growth or counts below 100,000 colonies per milliliter on repeated urine cultures. The majority of these symptomatic women with low colony counts on conventional cultures have been found to have pathogenic organisms present on cultures of suprapubic aspiration or urethral catheterization specimens. Response to antibacterial therapy is usually prompt.

A smaller subset of patients is defined by the presence of sterile urine and absence of correlation between symptoms and evidence of genitourinary tract inflammation. Measures effective for bacteriuric patients fail to relieve symptoms, among which frequency is often more prominent than dysuria. Diazepam (Valium) has been suggested as an effective agent for the symptomatic abacteriuric patient, the drug acting perhaps through a bladder mechanism rather than through its better-described psychopharmacologic effect.

The patient must be questioned concerning the possibility of a chemical irritant. These have included a variety of topical applicants such as douching agents, deodorant aerosols, and contraceptive jellies. Bathing preparations have also been implicated.

Impedance to urine flow may produce complaints of hesitancy, frequency, urinary straining, diminished caliber of the stream, and dribbling. The prominence of these symptoms, rather than burning pain, and the negative bacterial cultures suggest such an etiology. Meatal stenosis or stricture, urethral caruncle, or diverticula may be responsible. Transient edema may be related to sexual activity or straddle-position injury. Functional lesions related to impaired synergy between bladder contraction and sphincter relaxation have also been described. Less common causes include infiltrating bladder tumors or inflammation secondary to regional disease such as Crohn's ileocolitis or diverticulitis.

DYSURIA IN MALES

Presentation with dysuria raises the possibilities of cystitis-urethritis or pyelonephritis, as in women, and the additional consideration of prostatitis. Terminal dysuria, pyuria, or bacteriuria first evident or increased in expressed prostatic fluid or in a post-prostatic-massage voiding (third-glass collection) all suggest prostatic localization. This determination is of importance in deciding on the extent of diagnostic evaluation appropriate and in selecting antibacterial agents capable of concentrating within the prostatic parenchyma. Bacterial urinary tract infection is more likely to be associated with an underlying anatomic abnormality in the young male or with calculi or prostatic hypertrophy with obstruction in the older male, hence the need for thorough evaluation.

Dysuria as well as a urethral discharge is seen in approximately 80% of men presenting with gonorrhea; 10% may be symptomatic without a discharge. The diagnosis is made on the basis of the characteristic intracellular diplococci found on urethral smear in 95% of patients. Thayer-Martin cultures will confirm the diagnosis in the remaining few.

A number of organisms are suspected of playing a role in nonspecific urethritis. *C. trachomatis,* an obligate intracellular parasite, has been isolated in 30% to 50% of symptomatic males. It is found in only 3% of sexually active asymptomatic men. Its recovery from symptomatic women supports its pathogenicity. *Ureaplasma urealyticum* has been reported in up to 80% of men with nonspecific urethritis, but its presence in 60% of asymptomatic males has raised questions concerning its significance.

Trichomonas is seen in about 5% of men with nongonorrheal urethritis. It is best observed as well as cultured with a first morning urine specimen.

Dysuria may be related to balanitis-urethritis with Reiter's syndrome. The classic tetrad of this symptom complex also includes conjunctivitis, mucocutaneous lesions, and arthritis; however, more limited clinical expression is frequently observed.

REFERENCES

Fowler JE Jr: Urinary tract infection and inflammation, Chicago, 1989, Year Book.

Fairley KF and Birch DF: Detection of bladder bacteriuria in patients with acute urinary symptoms, J Infect Dis 159:226, 1989.

Johnson JR and Stamm WE: Urinary tract infections in women: diagnosis and treatment, Ann Intern Med 111:906, 1989.

Komaroff AL: Urinalysis and urine culture in women with dysuria, Ann Intern Med 104:212, 1986.

Lipsky BA: Urinary tract infections in men. Epidemiology, pathophysiology, diagnosis, and treatment, Ann Intern Med 110:138, 1989.

McCue JD: Evaluation and management of vaginitis, Arch Intern Med 149:565, 1989.

Neal DE Jr, Dilworth JP, and Kaack MB: Tamm-Horsfall autoantibodies in interstitial cystitis, J Urol 145:37, 1991.

Pappas PG: Laboratory in the diagnosis and management of urinary tract infections, Med Clin North Am 75:313, 1991.

Sobel JD: Vaginal infections in adult women, Med Clin North Am 74:1573, 1990.

Svanborg C, DeMan P, and Sandberg T: Renal involvement in urinary tract infection, Kidney Int 39:541, 1991.

CHAPTER

345 Acute Nephritic Syndrome

B. S. Kasinath

Glomerular diseases can present in the form of acute nephritis, nephrotic syndrome, or asymptomatic urinary abnormalities of hematuria and proteinuria. Acute nephritic syndrome is suggested by the sudden appearance of hematuria (gross or microscopic) often associated with erythrocyte casts with some or all of the following: variable degree of proteinuria (mild to nephrotic range), edema, hypertension, and renal insufficiency. A subset of these patients presents with rapidly progressive glomerulonephritis (RPGN) defined as 50% or greater loss of glomerular filtration rate in 3 months associated with extensive crescents usually involving 50% or more glomeruli as the principal finding on renal biopsy. The clinician should recognize acute nephritic syndrome, especially RPGN, without delay and assiduously pursue the underlying etiology, as timely intervention can save renal function in many cases.

ETIOLOGY AND PATHOLOGY

A large variety of glomerular diseases can present as acute glomerulonephritis; the more common causes are shown in the accompanying box. In primary renal disease, the original disease process first affects the kidney without involvement of other organ systems by the same process. Secondary renal diseases are characterized by multisystem organ involvement, including the kidneys, by a single disease process.

Renal pathology usually shows proliferation of glomerular mesangial or endothelial cells; "crescents" may be seen surrounding the glomeruli and are composed of proliferating glomerular epithelial cells and monocyte/macrophages. Evidence of focal or diffuse necrosis may be present. Vascular lesions may predominate in diseases such as hemolytic uremic syndrome. Immunofluorescence and electron microscopic examination may reveal evidence of immune reactants in mesangial, subendothelial, or subepithelial locations or in the glomerular basement membrane.

Common causes of acute glomerulonephritis

I. Hypocomplementemic glomerulonephritis
   - A. Primary renal diseases
     1. Acute poststreptococcal glomerulonephritis
     2. Membranoproliferative glomerulonephritis
   - B. Systemic diseases
     1. Systemic lupus erythematosus
     2. Infectious endocarditis
     3. Ventriculoatrial shunt infection associated nephritis
     4. Cryoglobulinemia

II. Normocomplementemic glomerulonephritis
   - A. Primary renal diseases
     1. IgA nephritis
     2. Idiopathic rapidly progressive glomerulonephritis
     3. Antiglomerular basement membrane disease
   - B. Systemic diseases
     1. Vasculitis (e.g., Wegener's granulomatosis, polyarteritis nodosa, hypersensitivity vasculitis)
     2. Goodpasture syndrome
     3. Henoch-Schönlein purpura
     4. Others (e.g., hemolytic-uremic syndrome, thrombotic thrombocytopenic purpura, visceral abscesses)

Modified from Madaio M and Harrington JT: N Engl J Med 309:1299-1302, 1983.

APPROACH TO DIAGNOSIS

A thorough history should include inquiry of recent or current infections, especially of the pharynx and skin, as poststreptococcal glomerulonephritis may occur after either pharyngitis (postpharyngitic) or cutaneous infection. An upper respiratory tract or gastrointestinal tract "infection" may be associated with acute presentation of IgA nephritis. Recurrent sinusitis and otitis resistant to therapy may be seen in Wegener's granulomatosis. Hemoptysis, dyspnea, and exposure to hydrocarbons may be relevant in pulmonary-renal syndromes (e.g., Goodpasture syndrome). Symptoms suggestive of collagen vascular disease such as rashes, photosensitivity, arthritis, and Raynaud's phenomena should be sought. On physical examination, one should focus on blood pressure, edema, evidence of congestive heart failure, and signs of collagen vascular diseases (e.g., arthritis, rashes). Roth spots, new cardiac murmurs, and splenomegaly may suggest infectious endocarditis. Necrotizing lesions of the nasal mucosa, sinusitis, and palpable purpura may lead to considerations of vasculitis.

The next step is careful evaluation of a freshly voided urine sample preferably obtained early in the morning. Dipstick and urine sediment microscopy should reveal presence of erythrocytes in significant numbers; dysmorphic red cells are suggestive of glomerular origin of hematuria (Chapter 342). Erythrocyte casts are highly suggestive of acute glomerulonephritis. Proteinuria may be mild or nephrotic. Nephrotic proteinuria (nephritic-nephrotic presentation) as revealed by greater than 3.5 g protein excretion in urine over

24 hours can be seen in lupus or membranoproliferative glomerulonephritis. Screening blood tests should include blood urea nitrogen (BUN) and serum creatinine to assess the extent of renal functional impairment, serum electrolytes, and complete blood count including platelet count. The peripheral blood smear may reveal schistocytes, suggesting a microangiopathic process (e.g., thrombotic thrombocytopenic purpura). Microcytic, hypochromic anemia may be seen in pulmonary-renal syndromes (e.g., Goodpasture syndrome) due to hemoptysis. Measurement of serum complement components C3, C4, and CH50 has been found to be of great assistance. Presence of hypocomplementemia suggests a short list of causes of acute glomerulonephritis (see the box). Serologic tests for antinuclear antibody including antibody against double stranded DNA, cryoglobulins, antibodies against streptococcal antigens (antistreptolysin-O, antihyaluronidase, antideoxyribonuclease-B), blood cultures, cultures of foci of infections (e.g., throat, skin) may be undertaken depending on the clues obtained, although patients with lupus may not always present with characteristic constellation of symptoms. Detection of antibodies against glomerular basement membrane in the serum point to Goodpasture syndrome as diagnosis.

Recently, presence of increased titers of antineutrophil cytoplasmic antibodies (ANCA) have been shown to correlate with the diagnosis of Wegener's gramulomatosis and idiopathic (pauci-immune) RPGN. The precise histologic diagnosis can be established only by a renal biopsy. Close, daily monitoring of renal function is essential. It should be emphasized that in the face of a rapidly deteriorating renal function (e.g., RPGN) one should perform renal biopsy as soon as it is safely possible. In severe glomerulonephritis (e.g., crescentic nephritis), if therapy is not instituted at an early stage, renal function may be irrevocably lost. The histologic information and the assessment of reversibility of a particular lesion on renal biopsy help the clinician to decide whether to treat and, if a decision is made to treat, which therapeutic modality to choose.

REFERENCES

Couser WG: Rapidly progressive glomerulonephritis: classification, pathogenic mechanisms and therapy, Am J Kidney Dis 11:449-464, 1988.

Falk RJ: ANCA—associated renal disease, Kidney Int 38:998-1010, 1990.

Madaio MP and Harrington JT: Current concepts: the diagnosis of acute glomerulonephritis, N Engl J Med 309:1299-1302, 1983.

Niles JL et al: Antigen specific radioimmunoassays for antineutrophil cytoplasmic antibodies in the diagnosis of rapidly progressive glomerulonephritis, J Am Soc Nephrol 2:27-36, 1991.

CHAPTER

346 Nephrotic Syndrome

Francisco Llach

The nephrotic syndrome is a clinical entity of diverse etiology characterized by the triad proteinuria, hypoalbuminemia, and edema. The quantity of proteinuria is usually greater than 3 g/1.73 m^2 body surface area/day, and the serum albumin concentration is decreased (usually less than 2.5 g/dl). In addition, other biochemical abnormalities are usually present, including hyperlipidemia and hypercoagulation. It must be emphasized, however, that there is no distinct boundary between persistent, significant, but asymptomatic proteinuria and the proteinuria of the nephrotic syndrome.

The nephrotic syndrome occurs in association with a wide variety of primary renal diseases and many systemic illnesses (see the accompanying box). Clinically, the nephrotic syndrome is associated with conditions that may be primary (idiopathic) or secondary. Idiopathic nephrotic syndrome occurs in association with a primary glomerular disease whose cause is unknown. Secondary nephrotic syndrome occurs in association with a systemic disease or after exposure to a specific, identifiable etiologic factor or physical agent (e.g., toxins, allergens, drugs).

The incidence of the nephrotic syndrome varies from country to country and among different age groups. Thus in Western Europe and North America, it is most commonly observed in patients with primary glomerular disorders and diabetes mellitus. In other parts of the world, where quartan malaria is endemic and uncontrolled, nephrotic syndrome secondary to malaria is common. In general, idiopathic nephrotic syndrome in children accounts for 90% of all the cases of nephrotic syndrome observed, with minimal change disease accounting for 70% of these patients and 20% due to proliferative or membranoproliferative glomerulonephritis, 5% to 10% due to focal glomerulosclerosis, and 5% due to membranous nephropathy. In the adult population, the remaining 10% of cases, 30% to 40% are secondary to a systemic process, most commonly diabetes mellitus. The remaining 70% include primary or idiopathic nephrotic syndrome in association with membranous nephropathy, 40%; membranoproliferative glomerulonephritis, 30%; minimal change disease, 15% to 20%; and focal sclerosis, 5% (Chapter 354). The frequency of these forms of primary glomerular disease is variable according to country and type of hospital.

PATHOPHYSIOLOGY

A schematic outline of the pathophysiologic abnormalities observed in the nephrotic syndrome is shown in Fig. 346-1.

Differential diagnosis of the nephrotic syndrome

Primary nephrotic syndrome (idiopathic)
- Minimal change disease (lipoid nephrosis)
- Membranous nephropathy
- Membranoproliferative glomerulonephritis
- Focal sclerosis
- IgA nephropathy (Berger's disease)
- Proliferative glomerulonephritis

Secondary nephrotic syndrome
- Systemic disease
  - Diabetes mellitus
  - Collagen vascular disease (e.g., systemic lupus erythematosus, polyarteritis, Sjögren's syndrome, Henoch-Schönlein purpura)
  - Amyloidosis
  - Sarcoidosis
- Malignancies
  - Soild tumors
  - Lymphoma and leukemia
  - Multiple myeloma
- Infections
  - Bacterial (poststreptococcal glomerulonephritis, endocarditis, shunt nephritis, syphilis)
  - Protozoal (malaria, toxoplasmosis)
  - Helminthic (schistosomiasis, trypanosomiasis)
  - Viral (hepatitis B, cytomegalovirus)
  - Specific toxins
    - Heavy metals
    - Drugs (probenecid, penicillamine, mercury, captopril, trimethadione, mephenytoin, organic gold, perchlorate)
    - "Allergens" (bee sting, poison ivy, poison oak, snake venom)

Hereditary disorder
- Alport's syndrome
- Congenital nephrotic syndrome
- Nail-patella syndrome

Miscellaneous
- Transplant rejection
- Eclampsia
- Thyroiditis
- Pregnancy?
- Congestive heart failure?
- Constrictive pericarditis?

Proteinuria (see also Chapter 343)

Proteinuria in the nephrotic syndrome is due to an increase in glomerular permeability and not to a decrease in tubular reabsorption of filtered plasma proteins. Albumin is the main constituent of urinary protein, but larger molecular weight proteins may also be excreted in excess in some patients. By definition, the urinary protein excretion exceeds 3 g/1.73 m^2/day, and it may be greater than 20 g/day. However, the magnitude of the proteinuria varies widely and is influenced considerably by the glomerular filtration rate, the plasma concentration of albumin, and dietary protein intake. For instance, a marked decrement in serum albumin may lead to a dramatic reduction of the proteinuria even though the fundamental deficit in glomerular capillary remains unchanged. Likewise, the dietary protein intake greatly influences both urinary protein excretion and hepatic synthesis of albumin. Thus a high protein intake in nephrotic patients leads to an increase in proteinuria and albumin synthesis. Recently, it has been shown that nonsteroidal anti-inflammatory agents as well as angiotensin-converting enzyme inhibitors reduce proteinuria by 40%. The effects are reversible and not fully understood, although a decline in glomerular filtration rate (GFR) may be an important factor. In addition, some other plasma proteins may be lost in the urine. These include peptide hormones, clotting inhibitors, transferrin, and hormone-carrying proteins.

Attention has been given to the selectivity of the proteinuria in patients with nephrotic syndrome. Highly selective proteinuria has been defined as clearance of molecules similar to albumin (66,000 daltons), transferrin (88,000 daltons), and small amounts of gamma globulins (150,000 daltons), and exclusion from urine of higher molecular weight plasma proteins. In patients with lesser degrees of selectivity, the clearances of larger globulins approach those of albumin and transferrin and include large plasma proteins such as alpha-2 macroglobulins. However, although originally such selectivity was thought to be a useful diagnostic and prognostic measure, subsequent application of this index has yielded disappointing results.

The magnitude of proteinuria usually underestimates the net loss of albumin from the body. It has been estimated that in normal humans 0.5 to 2.5 g of filtered protein per 24 hours is reabsorbed by the renal tubule. With increased glomerular permeability, the protein reabsorption by the renal tubule probably also increases and may exceed 10 g/day. Thus this protein digested within the renal tubule may account for further loss of protein from the body.

Hypoalbuminemia

As a consequence of the proteinuria, the serum albumin concentration falls. The normal liver has a synthetic capacity to increase the total albumin pool by approximately 25 g/day. In patients with the nephrotic syndrome, hepatic albumin synthesis has been reported to be normal or even slightly increased. In patients with severe hypoalbuminemia, however, hepatic synthesis of protein may be inadequate and insufficient for the levels of serum albumin. A good example is the patient undergoing continuous ambulatory peritoneal dialysis (CAPD). These patients have extrarenal losses of albumin from the peritoneum that result in markedly increased hepatic synthesis to compensate for the albumin losses. The result is maintenance of normal serum albumin levels in CAPD patients. Thus it is clear that the liver response to renal albumin losses is inadequate in nephrotic patients. This response may be due at least partially to protein deficiency because in nephrotic patients a high protein diet increases hepatic albumin synthesis and restores serum albumin levels toward normal. As noted, increased renal catabolism of protein may be another factor in the hypoalbuminemia of nephrotic patients. All of this

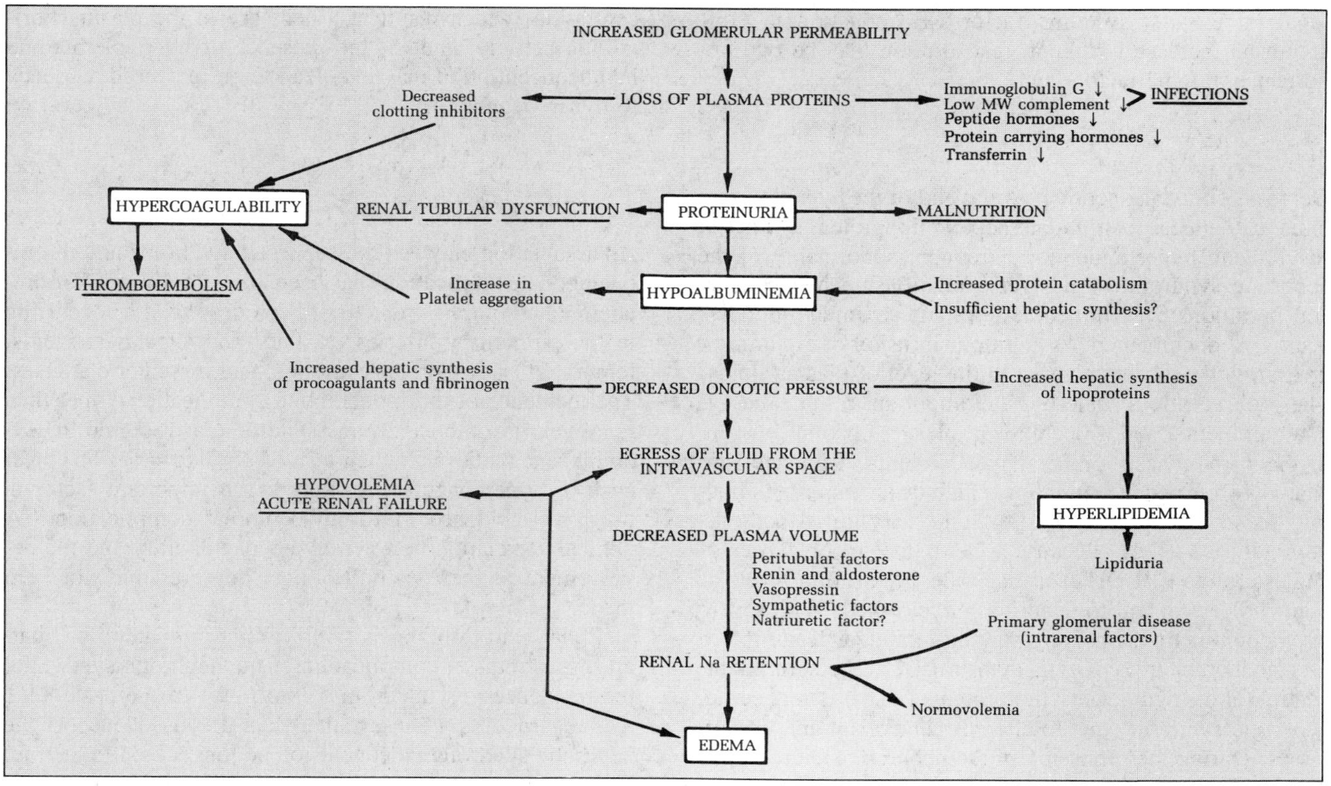

Fig. 346-1. The pathophysiology of the nephrotic syndrome. Capital letters represent the major pathophysiologic alterations; boxed capital letters are the major components of the syndrome; small letters represent major pathogenetic factors leading to clinical complications; underlined capital letters indicate the major complications of the nephrotic syndrome.

together may explain the occasional presence in the nephrotic patient of seemingly inappropriately low levels of serum albumin for the degree of proteinuria.

In addition to a decrease in the serum albumin concentrations, other low molecular weight plasma proteins, such as transferrin, ceruloplasmin, thyroid-binding globulin, immunoglobulin G, corticosteroid-binding globulin, and vitamin D-binding globulin, are also reduced.

Edema

The hypoalbuminemia leads to a decrease in plasma oncotic pressure, which results in an imbalance of Starling forces at the level of the peripheral capillaries. At the arteriolar end, the hydrostatic pressure within the capillary exceeds the oncotic pressure, leading to an egress of fluid into the interstitial space. As the egress of fluid occurs, plasma protein concentration increases until the flux of fluid is reversed at the venous end of the capillary. With the development of hypoalbuminemia, this process is altered so that interstitial volume increases and edema eventually results. Additional factors must be considered. These are detailed in Chapter 351.

Although the classic view of the nephrotic syndrome is defined as a state of low intravascular volume, systemic venous pressure, cardiac output, and elevated plasma aldosterone levels, many patients with nephrotic syndrome associated with various nephropathies display normal intravascular volume and low aldosterone levels. Thus two groups of patients have been identified. The first group has the classic form of disease, which, in keeping with the traditional view mentioned earlier, was observed in patients with minimal change disease. This form is characterized by a decrease in blood volume, high levels of plasma renin and aldosterone, and an increase in peripheral vasoconstriction and marked hypoalbuminemia. A second group of nephrotic patients presents primarily with chronic glomerulonephritis and renal insufficiency. These patients have a normal or even increased intravascular volume and low plasma levels of renin and aldosterone. Recent data, however, suggest that the mechanism of edema formation is more complex than is described in the above-mentioned groups. Thus various studies have failed to demonstrate consistently a reduction in blood volume in nephrotic patients. Furthermore, volume expansion produced by hyperoncotic plasma infusion in nephrotic patients does not result in a consistent diuresis in many patients, suggesting that volume alone is not responsible for the fluid retention. Available data suggest that renal sodium retention may be a primary initiating event and that this abnormality is the consequence of intrarenal rather than systemic factors. A reduction in GFR and/or an increase in tubular reabsorption may be two important intrarenal factors.

Hyperlipidemia

Decreased plasma oncotic pressure and/or the hypoalbuminemia also appear to stimulate hepatic lipoprotein synthesis, resulting in hyperlipidemia, a frequent abnormality of the nephrotic syndrome. An inverse relationship between the concentrations of serum cholesterol and serum albumin has been well documented. In addition, infusion of albumin or dextran will cause a decrease in the level of plasma lipids. These observations underline the important role of the hypoalbuminemia and a decrease in plasma oncotic pressure in the pathogenesis of the hyperlipidemia. Characteristic changes observed in serum lipids include an increase in both low-density lipoproteins (LDL) and very-low-density lipoproteins (VLDL). Because LDL is the major carrier of cholesterol and VLDL of triglycerides, the serum levels of both cholesterol and triglycerides are elevated. With severe hypoalbuminemia, lipolysis may be inhibited, leading to a greater increment in VLDL than in LDL. The serum concentration of high density lipoproteins (HDL) is reduced in nephrotic syndrome due to altered metabolism and urinary losses. During the remission of the nephrotic syndrome, as the proteinuria decreases and the levels of serum albumin return to normal, the serum levels of the lipoproteins return to normal.

Lipiduria is usually present in the nephrotic syndrome. Lipid-containing epithelial cells (oval fat bodies) are thought to be degenerated renal tubular epithelial cells containing cholesterol esters. Under polarized light, these oval fat bodies may have the appearance of a Maltese cross (Chapter 339). Lipiduria correlates with the magnitude of the proteinuria rather than with the level of the hyperlipidemia, suggesting that the filtered lipoproteins are engulfed by proximal tubular cells and eventually are desquamated into the urine.

Hypercoagulability

An enhanced coagulation is commonly observed in the nephrotic syndrome and may reflect the high incidence of thromboembolic complications encountered in this syndrome. This hypercoagulability has been attributed to several factors: (1) The decrease in plasma oncotic pressure leads to an increased hepatic synthesis of fibrinogen and procoagulant factors, which results in increased plasma levels of fibrinogen factors, V, VII, and X; (2) the hypoalbuminemia per se may increase platelet aggregation, and protein markers of platelet aggregation such as plasma β-thromboglobulin may be elevated; (3) urinary loss of clotting inhibitors such as the antithrombin III-heparin cofactor, which serves as an inhibitor to activated serum protease procoagulants; also, proteins C and S, two recently described, naturally occurring clotting inhibitors, have been found to be low in nephrotic patients, suggesting that they may play a role in enhanced coagulation; (4) a high alpha-2 macroglobulin concentration and a low plasminogen concentration, which result in a decrease in the plasma fibrinolytic activity; and (5) the presence of hypovolemia and hemoconcentration may also lead to an increased tendency to hypercoagulability.

COMPLICATIONS

Thromboembolic complications

An association between the nephrotic syndrome and thromboembolic complications has been known for years. Thromboembolic complications have been described as occurring in the pulmonary arteries, axillary and subclavian veins, femoral arteries, coronary arteries, and mesenteric arteries. The incidence of thromboembolic complications other than renal vein thrombosis in this syndrome as reported in several recent studies is in the range of 8.5% to 40%. The presence of hypercoagulability may be an important factor in the high incidence of thromboembolic complications. A clinical correlation between hypercoagulability and the development of these complications, however, has not been made.

Renal vein thrombosis (RVT), either unilateral or bilateral, is a frequent complication of the nephrotic syndrome, the incidence varying from 5% to 62%. In the past, RVT was regarded as a cause rather than a consequence of the nephrotic syndrome, a conclusion no longer held to be true. Certain glomerular lesions are more likely than others to be associated with RVT. These lesions include membranous nephropathy and membranoproliferative glomerulonephritis. RVT can present acutely or in chronic manner. Features suggestive of acute RVT include flank pain, gross hematuria, decrease in glomerular filtration rate, and asymmetry of renal size on x-ray study. Unfortunately, the majority of patients with RVT present in a chronic manner. These patients are usually asymptomatic, and the only suggestion of RVT may be scalloping of the ureters (due to the abundant collateral circulation) and episodes suggestive of pulmonary emboli. Renal vein thrombosis is best documented by selective renal venous angiography. Recently, both computed axial tomography and magnetic resonance imaging have been found to be good noninvasive techniques in the diagnosis of RVT.

Infections

Nephrotic patients are very susceptible to infections, from both common and opportunistic organisms. The reasons for this are not well defined, though the low levels of immunoglobulin G and low molecular weight complement may be important factors. Also, a decrease in serum levels of alternate complement factor B may play a role. This factor has been linked to defective opsonization of *Escherichia coli* in nephrotic patients. There seems to be a particular susceptibility to pneumococcal peritonitis and septicemia, especially in children with minimal change disease.

Established infections are also common in these patients, particularly cellulitis in the lower extremities; and they can be life-threatening. The infection may spread rapidly and progress to septic shock; there may be positive blood cultures.

Malnutrition

The nephrotic patient usually has a negative nitrogen balance secondary to massive proteinuria. In addition, anorexia and decreased dietary intake may worsen the already compromised nutritional status. The significance of urinary losses of other plasma proteins has not been completely evaluated; for example, losses of transferrin may lead to hypotransferrinemia, which could contribute to the anemia observed in nephrotic patients.

Miscellaneous

When proteinuria is massive, the serum albumin level is profoundly decreased, which will diminish circulating plasma volume and may even produce marked hypotension or circulatory collapse. In this setting, any superimposed renal injury may be conducive to acute renal failure. Although hypercholesterolemia is an acute risk factor for development of ischemic heart disease, the evidence regarding the occurrence of accelerated atherosclerosis in the nephrotic patient is conflicting. Further study must be carried out both in children and in adults with long-standing and responsive nephrotic syndrome.

Proximal tubular dysfunction has been noted in some nephrotic patients as manifested by glycosuria, aminoaciduria, phosphaturia, and renal tubular acidosis. The urinary loss of both cholecalciferol-binding protein and 25-hydroxycholecalciferol may lead to a vitamin D deficiency state and either osteomalacia or secondary hyperparathyroidism. A decrease in thyroxine-binding globulin may cause marked changes in various thyroid function tests, (e.g., low protein-bound iodine, decreased T_3 concentration, and increased T_3 resin uptake). Despite these abnormalities in thyroid hormone indices, however, patients with nephrotic syndrome do not have hypothyroidism and do not require thyroid hormone therapy.

Another potential complication is an increased drug toxicity that occurs when agents that are bound to protein are administered to nephrotic patients. Because these patients may have significant hypoalbuminemia, such drug administration may result in a decrease in the number of drug-binding sites, which in turn leads to an increase in the biologic action of some agents, resulting in toxicity.

GENERAL MANAGEMENT

Therapies for specific types of primary glomerular diseases are outlined in Chapter 354. Only the general management of the nephrotic patient is discussed in this section. The main therapeutic problem of these patients is the excessive retention of salt and water within the interstitial space. In general, the treatment of edema even in the asymptomatic patient is generally desirable from both emotional and physiologic points of view. Sodium intake should be limited to 2 to 3 g/day. Permanent correction of the hypoalbuminemia should be the ultimate goal; however, correction may depend on the specific therapy of the nephropathy. At present a high protein diet (1.5 to 2.0 g/kg/day) is advisable. Intravenous albumin may be of value in patients with symptomatic hypovolemia and hypotension or in patients with edema resistant to therapy with diuretic drugs. In this situation, the combined use of intravenous albumin and a loop diuretic may be useful, although it produces only a transient increase in plasma albumin concentration because most of the administered albumin is lost in the urine. Thus for long-term therapy, it is not a practical approach. However, an increase in dietary protein or intravenous albumin may ameliorate the hypoalbuminemia if either angiotensin-converting enzyme inhibitors or nonsteroidal anti-inflammatory agents are administered concomitantly. Thus small doses of these agents should be used simultaneously to decrease urinary protein excretion and to foster albumin synthesis.

Diuretics are the most important therapeutic agent in the treatment of edema; however, they should be used cautiously because vigorous diuresis may result in further lowering of effective plasma volume and GFR, leading to postural hypotension. On the other hand, in patients with normal or increased blood volume, removal of large volumes of fluid with diuretic therapy can be achieved while normal blood volume is maintained. The dose of diuretic should be reduced as edema diminishes, and the patient should be monitored for the presence of postural hypotension. An important guide for the evaluation of diuretic therapy in the nephrotic patient is the serial measurement of body weight. In patients with severe and refractory edema, a combination of furosemide and metolazone may be effective. Hyperoncotic salt-poor albumin infusion should be reserved for patients with orthostatic hypotension and hypovolemia in whom severe anasarca is usually a problem. Caution in the appropriate use of nonsteroidal anti-inflammatory agents is strongly advised because these agents may decrease renal function and aggravate edema formation.

Because thromboembolic complications are common in the nephrotic patient, the clinician should be aware of its presence. The documented presence of known thromboembolic complications should lead to serious consideration of long-term oral anticoagulation. Antithrombin III is the plasma factor required for the full expression of the heparin-induced anticoagulation. Thus the effectiveness of heparin may be impaired in the presence of low plasma antithrombin III levels. Simple prophylactic measures such as encouraging leg exercises, avoiding volume depletion, and immobilization should be applied.

Because of the protein malnutrition, a diet rich in biologic protein is advisable. Supplementation with vitamin D metabolites may be advisable if there is clinical evidence of osteomalacia or osteitis fibrosa cystica. On rare occasions, profound protein malnutrition or other complications of massive proteinuria may suggest obliteration of renal function by medical or surgical means.

Established infections should be treated promptly and urgently with appropriate antibiotic therapy. Patients taking steroid therapy for the nephropathy should receive hydrocortisone intravenously in the acute septic phase, because adrenal suppression may be present. The treatment of the hyperlipidemia is controversial; because few morbidity and mortality data are available, its value remains to be established.

REFERENCES

Bernard DB: Extrarenal complications of the nephrotic syndrome, Kidney Int 33:1184, 1988.

Kaysen GA, Kirkpatrick WG, and Couser WG. Albumin homeostasis in the nephrotic rat: Nutritional considerations, Am J Physiol 247:F192, 1984.

Levey AS, Madalo MP, and Perrone RD: Laboratory assessment of renal disease: clearances, urinalysis and renal biopsy. In Brenner BM and Rector FC Jr, editors: The kidney, ed 4, Philadelphia, 1991, Saunders.

Llach F: Nephrotic syndrome: hypercoagulability, renal vein thrombosis and other thromboembolic complications. In Brenner BM and Stein JH, editors: Contemporary issues in nephrology, vol. 9, nephrotic syndrome, New York, 1982, Churchill Livingstone.

Llach F: Acute renal vein thrombosis. In Schrier RW and Gottschalk GW, editors: Diseases of the kidney, ed 4, Boston, 1988, Little, Brown.

Llach F, Papper S, and Massry SG: The clinical spectrum of renal vein thrombosis: acute and chronic, Am J Med 69:819, 1980.

Mees EJD, Geers AB, and Koomans HA: Blood volume and sodium retention in the nephrotic syndrome: a controversial pathophysiological concept, Nephron 36:201, 1984.

Meltzer JL et al: Nephrotic syndrome: vasoconstriction and hypervolemic types indicated by renin-sodium profiling, Ann Intern Med 91:688, 1979.

Schieppati A et al: The metabolism of arachidonic acid by platelets in nephrotic syndrome, Kidney Int 25(4):660, 1984.

Schnaper HW and Robson AM: Nephrotic syndrome: minimal change disease, focal glomerulosclerosis, and related disorders. In Schrier RW and Gottschalk CW, editors: Diseases of the kidney, ed 4, Boston, 1988, Little, Brown.

Wagoner RD et al: Renal vein thrombosis in idiopathic membranous glomerulopathy and nephrotic syndrome: incidence significance, Kidney Int 23(2):368, 1983.

CHAPTER

347 Acute Renal Failure

Satish Kumar
Jay H. Stein

Acute renal failure can be defined as an abrupt reduction or cessation in renal function. Because of the importance of the kidney in the maintenance of the extracellular milieu, an acute decrease in renal function will affect many indeed, most organ systems. The presenting symptoms, clinical course, and complications are typically manifestations of these secondary effects.

ETIOLOGY

The majority of cases of acute renal failure (ARF) are seen in surgical patients, trauma victims, and patients with various acute medical illnesses. These account for 90% to 95% of all cases. Acute renal failure in the obstetric patient accounts for an additional 5% to 10%. The etiology of acute renal failure can be divided into three main categories: prerenal, postrenal, and intrinsic renal disease. The importance of prerenal and postrenal causes relates to the fact that they are relatively easily treated and, with definitive treatment, a rapid return of renal function may be expected.

Prerenal failure

Prerenal azotemia is the most common cause of a reversible increase in the creatinine and blood urea nitrogen (BUN) levels in hospitalized patients. The various factors listed in the box below will cause either a decrease in cardiac output or an increase in renal vascular resistance, or both. This will lead to a reduction in renal blood flow, an increase in salt and water reabsorption, oliguria, and azotemia. If the decrement in renal blood flow is severe and/or prolonged, ischemic damage to the tubules may occur and renal parenchymal damage ensue.

Postrenal causes

Postrenal failure is not as common as the prerenal entity, but because of the potential reversibility of this malady with the subsequent normalization of renal function, it is extremely important to consider the diagnosis in a patient with a rapid reduction in renal function. Postrenal causes include obstruction to the ureter(s), bladder, and/or urethra (see the box on p. 2615). These lesions may be clinically silent, though frequently the symptoms or physical findings will suggest the diagnosis. Obstruction must be excluded in every case of acute renal failure (see Chapter 361).

Intrinsic or parenchymal renal disease

A great variety of intrinsic renal lesions can be associated with the syndrome of ARF (see the box on p. 2615). They can be categorized as abnormalities of the vasculature, the glomeruli, interstitium, or tubules. Vascular lesions frequently accompany systemic diseases, for example, systemic lupus erythematosus (SLE), mixed cryoglobulinemia,

Prerenal causes of acute renal failure

I. Decreased cardiac output
   A. Myocardial infarction or contusion
   B. Severe congestive heart failure
   C. Arrhythmias
   D. Pericardial constriction (tamponade)
II. Hypovolemia
   A. Gastrointestinal losses (vomiting, diarrhea)
   B. Blood losses (peptic ulcer, gastritis, stress ulcer, phlebotomy)
   C. Renal losses (salt-losing nephritis, diuretics, mineralocorticoid deficiency, postobstructuve diuresis)
   D. Skin losses (burns)
III. Volume redistribution (decrease in effective blood volume)
   A. Hypoalbuminemic states (cirrhosis, nephrosis)
   B. Third space (ischemic bowel, peritonitis, pancreatitis, muscle trauma-rhabdomyolysis, surgery)
IV. Altered resistance
   A. Decrease in peripheral vascular resistance (sepsis, vasodilators, anaphylaxis)
   B. Increase in renal vascular resistance (renal artery stenosis, aortic or renal artery dissection)

Postrenal causes of acute renal failure

I. Ureteral and pelvic
  A. Intrinsic obstruction
    1. Blood clots
    2. Stones
    3. Sloughed papillae
    4. Fungus balls
  B. Extrinsic obstruction
    1. Malignancy
    2. Retroperitoneal fibrosis
    3. Iatrogenic: Inadvertent ligation
II. Bladder
  A. Stones
  B. Blood clots
  C. Prostatic hypertrophy or malignancy
  D. Bladder carcinoma
  E. Neuropathic
III. Urethral
  A. Strictures
  B. Phimosis

Henoch-Schönlein purpura, polyarteritis nodosa. These systemic diseases are often associated with glomerular and interstitial changes as well.

A second group, those associated with alterations in the glomeruli, include entities such as poststreptococcal glomerulonephritis, rapidly progressive glomerulonephritis, and systemic illnesses such as Goodpasture's syndrome. The pathologic changes typically reveal a marked proliferation of glomerular cells and, frequently, epithelial crescents.

A third group of intrinsic renal lesions are generally categorized under the term *acute interstitial nephritis* (AIN). Histologically, one notes peritubular and interstitial infiltration with polymorphonuclear cells, eosinophils, and occasionally plasma cells (see Chapter 362). Drugs and infections are the two main etiologic categories in this group. The most frequent causative drugs are the penicillins and the sulfonamide derivatives. Other antimicrobial agents, diuretics, anticonvulsants, nonsteroidal anti-inflammatory agents, hypouricemic drugs, phenobarbitol, and cimetidine may also be responsible for AIN. Infections associated with AIN include group A streptococci, malaria, toxoplasmosis, leptospirosis, and salmonellosis. Acute papillary necrosis is an extreme example of acute interstitial nephritis that is most commonly seen in analgesic abusers, diabetics, and patients with liver disease or sickle cell disease. Recently, it has been reported that various nonsteroidal anti-inflammatory agents may also cause papillary necrosis.

Primary intratubular obstruction may also cause acute renal failure. This category would include intratubular obstruction with uric acid, oxalate, and methotrexate crystals as well as obstruction by the intratubular deposition of myeloma proteins. Acute uric acid nephropathy is seen most frequently in association with hematologic malignancies and/or during the treatment of these conditions (see Chapter 362). Similarly, the intratubular deposition of calcium oxalate following ethylene glycol ingestion or methoxyflurane anesthesia may lead to acute renal failure. Methotrexate metabolites and sulfadiazine have also been associated with intratubular crystal deposition and tubular obstruction.

Finally, there is a group of entities frequently categorized under the term *acute tubular necrosis* (ATN). The two most common etiologies of ATN are ischemia and nephrotoxin exposure. Renal ischemia associated with severe hypovolemia, hemorrhagic shock, sepsis, severe cardiac failure, and postaortic or renal artery surgery is a frequent cause of ATN. In other words, prolonged or severe prere-

Causes of acute renal failure due to intrinsic or parenchymal kidney disease

I. Abnormalities of the vasculature
  A. Vasoconstrictive disease (malignant hypertension, scleroderma, hemolytic uremic syndrome, thrombotic thrombocytopenic purpura)
  B. Vasculitis (polyarteritis nodosa, hypersensitivity angiitis, serum sickness, Wegener's granulomatosis, giant cell arteritis, mixed cryoglobulinemia, Henoch-Schönlein purpura, systemic lupus erythematosus)
II. Abnormalities of the glomeruli
  A. Postinfectious (poststreptococcal, pneumococcal, gonococcal, staphylococcal, enterococcal, brucellosis, *Legionella, Listeria,* shunt nephritis, related to visceral abscesses, viral [hepatitis B and C, mumps, measles, Epstein-Barr], malaria, leprosy, leptospirosis)
  B. Noninfectious (rapidly progressive glomerulonephritis, membranoproliferative glomerulonephritis, Goodpasture's syndrome, systemic lupus erythematosus, Wegener's granulomatosis)
III. Acute interstitial nephritis
  A. Drug related (penicillins, sulfonamides, carbenicillin, cephalosporin, erythromycin, nafcillin, oxacillin, nonsteroidal anti-inflammatory agents, diuretics [furosemide, ethacrynic acid, thiazide, spironolactone, mercurials], phenytoin, phenobarbital, probenicid, allopurinol, cimetidine)
  B. Infection related (acute pyelonephritis, streptococcal, staphylococcal, leptospirosis, malaria, salmonellosis)
  C. Papillary necrosis (associated with diabetes mellitus, sickle cell diseases, analgesic abuse, alcoholism)
  D. Miscellaneous (sarcoidosis, leukemia, lymphoma)
IV. Intratubular obstruction
  A. Crystal deposition (uric acid, oxalate, methotrexate)
  B. Multiple myeloma and light chain disease
V. Acute tubular necrosis
  A. Nephrotoxins
    1. Antimicrobials (aminoglycosides, tetracyclines, amphotericin, polymyxin, cephalosporins)
    2. Heavy metals (mercury, lead, arsenic, gold salts, barium)
    3. Miscellaneous (cisplatin, doxorubicin, streptozocin, methoxyflurane, halothane, ethylene glycol, carbon tetrachloride)
  B. Ischemia (hemorrhage, hypotension, sepsis, burns, renal infarction, renal artery dissection, rhabdomyolysis, trauma)
  C. Miscellaneous (contrast agents, transfusion reactions, myoglobinemia, heat stroke, snake and spider bites)

nal events can and frequently do result in tubular necrosis and the syndrome of ATN. In addition, over the past two decades the recorded incidence of nephrotoxin-induced acute renal failure has markedly increased. This apparent increase is due at least in part to the more frequent recognition of elevated creatinine and BUN levels in automated laboratory determinations and in part to the greater use of potentially nephrotoxic antibiotics. The aminoglycoside antibiotics lead this category, but a number of other drugs are also listed as nephrotoxins in the box on p. 2615. Rhabdomyolysis, both following traumatic muscle injury and the nontraumatic type (secondary to hypokalemia, hypophosphatemia, drug overdose, heat stroke, or primary muscle disease), is also frequently associated with acute renal failure. Iodinated contrast dyes, transfusion reactions, heavy metals, or organic solvents may also lead to ATN.

PATHOPHYSIOLOGY

Prerenal failure

The usual common denominator in prerenal failure is a reduction in renal blood flow. Systemic hypotension is frequently present, and this may lead to the release of catecholamines, angiotensin, and/or vasopressin, which may further increase the renal vascular resistance. This will lead to a decrement in glomerular filtration pressure and thus a fall in glomerular filtration rate. These reactive substances may also decrease the permeability of the glomerulus, thereby reducing the glomerular filtration rate. If severe and prolonged, the decrease in renal blood flow may lead to a decrease in oxygen delivery to the kidney, ischemia to the tubules (especially those that have a high metabolic requirement), parenchymal damage, and the other manifestations of ATN.

Postrenal failure (see also Chapter 361)

During the early stages of obstruction, filtration rate may remain normal; however, as the ureteral and intratubular pressures progressively rise, renal vascular resistance increases (primarily as a result of afferent arteriolar vasoconstriction), and renal blood flow falls. The increase in tubular pressure, together with the decrease in renal blood flow, eventually may cause a decrease in the glomerular filtration rate. In addition, angiotensin II and thromboxane A_2 are increased and probably play an important role in the increase in renal vascular resistance and in the decrease in renal blood flow and glomerular filtration.

Intrinsic parenchymal disease

Though this group of diseases has a wide and varied number of etiologies, the pathophysiology can be considered together. Each of the five main categories listed in the box on p. 2615 demonstrates one or more of the following pathophysiologic abnormalities: hemodynamic alterations, tubular obstruction, back-leak of filtrate through damaged tubules, or a decrease in glomerular capillary permeability. For example, the decrement in glomerular filtration rate in glomerulonephritis is due primarily to a combination of altered glomerular permeability and decrement in glomerular blood flow. Similarly, renal vasculitis will frequently lead to a decrease in glomerular blood flow and possibly ischemic damage. Acute interstitial nephritis is associated with an inflammation of the interstitium, which may secondarily result in alterations in tubular and glomerular function. Intratubular obstruction caused by crystal deposition may lead to an increase in proximal tubular pressure that will impair filtration. In addition, intratubular obstruction leads to preglomerular vasoconstriction and thereby a decrease in glomerular blood flow. Acute tubular necrosis, resulting from either nephrotoxic or ischemic injury, causes a decrease in glomerular filtration rate through a combination of all four mechanisms (Fig. 347-1). Both nephrotoxic and ischemic insults may cause tubular necrosis. Multiple cellular mechanisms are involved, including inhibition and translocation of sodium pump and generation of oxygen free radicals. The sloughing of cells or cellular components into the tubular lumen will then result in intratubular obstruction. Additional obstruction is caused by precipitation of Tamm-Horsfall protein, a renal glycoprotein, in the form of tubular casts. The tubular obstruction leads to an increase in proximal tubular pressure and therefore a decrease in effective filtration pressure. In addition, intratubular obstruction is associated with mechanisms that result in an increase in afferent arteriolar resistance and a decrease in renal blood flow. The increase in proximal tubular pressure may also facilitate back-leak of filtrate through damaged tubular epithelium, thereby further decreasing the effective glomerular filtration rate. The importance of a decrease in glomerular capillary permeability in humans is not clear; it does appear to be important in at least some experimental models of acute renal failure.

DIAGNOSIS

The diagnostic approach to the patient with acute renal failure includes a careful history and physical examination, a thorough examination of a fresh urine specimen, appropri-

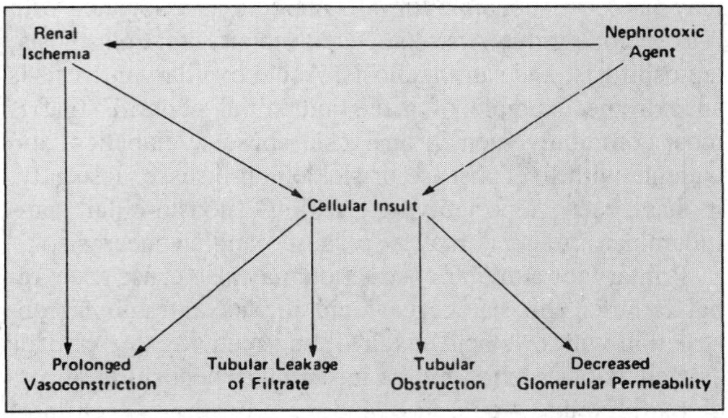

Fig. 347-1. Schematic of pathogenesis of acute renal failure. (Adapted from Stein JH, Lifschitz MD, and Barnes LD: Am J Physiol 234:F171, 1978.)

ate laboratory data, radiologic test(s), and under certain conditions, a renal biopsy.

Prerenal failure

The history and physical examination will under most circumstances strongly suggest the diagnosis. Indeed, in the face of an acute myocardial infarction, sepsis, or hemorrhagic hypotension, the diagnosis is usually readily apparent. In many cases more subtle clues must be searched for, such as an increase in diuretic dosage in a patient with decompensated cirrhosis or congestive heart failure.

The physical examination can contribute to the work-up by suggesting one of the etiologic categories (the box on p. 2615) or by demonstrating evidence of hypovolemia. Decreased skin turgor, dry mucous membranes or axillae, orthostasis, and tachycardia all suggest hypovolemia. Of these, orthostasis is the most useful sign and should be checked for in all patients with renal failure. At times, however, it may be extremely difficult to make a clinical diagnosis, and one must consider more invasive maneuvers such as central venous pressure or pulmonary capillary wedge pressure measurement for an accurate blood volume assessment.

The kidney's response to a decrease in blood flow is to avidly reabsorb salt and water. Thus in this setting, urine sodium concentration is typically less than 10 to 20 mEq per liter, the fractional excretion of sodium is less than 1 percent, as is the renal failure index (see below), and the urine osmolality is greater than 500 mOsm per liter. The fractional excretion (percent) of sodium (FE_{Na}) is calculated from:

$$FE_{Na} = \frac{\text{Sodium excreted}}{\text{Sodium filtered}} = \frac{U_{Na} \cdot V}{P_{Na} \cdot GFR}$$

where $GFR = U_{Cr} \cdot V/P_{Cr}$, and U_{Cr} and P_{Cr} are the urine and plasma creatinine concentrations, respectively. Thus

$$FE_{Na}(\%) = \frac{U_{Na} \cdot P_{Cr}}{P_{Na} \cdot U_{Cr}} \times 100$$

The renal failure index (RFI) is also simply calculated:

$$RFI = \frac{\text{Sodium excreted}}{GFR} = \frac{U_{Na} \cdot P_{Cr}}{U_{Cr}}$$

Since with prerenal azotemia there is no parenchymal damage, the urinalysis is typically normal; usually only finely granular casts and hyaline casts are present. Similarly, the amount of proteinuria is minimal. If significant numbers of red blood cells, white blood cells, or cellular casts are present, an alternate or additional abnormality must be considered. Creatinine is filtered at the glomerulus and is not reabsorbed. Therefore under conditions of avid water reabsorption, the urine creatinine concentration will rise, but its serum value will remain relatively constant, resulting in a high urine/plasma creatinine ratio (Table 347-1). Urea, on the other hand, is both filtered and reabsorbed.

Table 347-1. Urinary indices in acute renal failure

Index	Prerenal acute renal failure	Oliguric acute tubular necrosis
Urine osmolality (mOsm/L)	>500	<350
Urine sodium (mEq/L)	<20	>40
Urine/blood urea nitrogen ratio	>8	<3
Urine/plasma creatinine ratio	>40	<20
Renal failure index (percent) (see test)	<1	>1
Fractional excretion of sodium (percent)	<1	>1
Plasma urea nitrogen/creatinine ratio	>20	<10

Its reabsorption is flow dependent; thus during low flow conditions, more urea is reabsorbed, resulting in a high plasma urea/creatinine ratio. Water is, however, reabsorbed in excess of urea in this setting, and the urine/plasma ratio will still rise.

Postrenal failure

The history and physical examination may be helpful in delineating the duration of the symptoms and the location of the obstruction. Ureteral obstruction must either be bilateral or occur in a patient with only a single functioning kidney to result in ARF. The history may be suggestive when it includes an abrupt onset of ureteral colic or inability to void. Extrinsic compression of both ureters from retroperitoneal fibrosis or an intra-abdominal mass can lead to a slower development of obstruction and a less symptomatic onset. Similarly, acute bladder outlet obstruction is usually symptomatic, but if it develops slowly, the diagnosis may be suspected only by palpation of an enlarged bladder or by the demonstration of a large prostate gland. The urinalysis may be normal.

The urine flow rate may vary from anuria, as seen with complete obstruction, to polyuria, as may be seen in partial obstruction. Urine flow that fluctuates widely from day to day suggests the possibility of intermittent obstruction.

Laboratory findings are dependent on the time course and degree of obstruction. The renal response to acute obstruction is similar to that seen in prerenal azotemia, and similar laboratory indices are found, that is, high urine osmolality, low urine sodium, and low fractional excretion of sodium. After a few days of obstruction, the indices change and the urine becomes isotonic with a high fractional excretion of sodium.

A postvoiding residual urine measurement is a relatively simple and potentially revealing test that should be performed in any patient in whom obstruction is being considered. An intravenous pyelogram or renal sonogram will usually document obstruction and suggest the location of the obstruction. With the marked improvement in ultrasonography in the last few years, it has become the procedure of choice. If neither of these tests is helpful and a diagnosis of obstruction is still being considered, retrograde pyelography can be performed. This invasive test, which carries with it the potential for substantial complications, is rarely needed. If retrograde pyelography is done and one side reveals no obstruction, no further dye need be given. The complications of retrograde pyelography include a worsening of renal function secondary to edema of the ureter(s) following their manipulation. Additionally, the introduction of bacteria beyond the site of obstruction is a potential and very serious complication. If obstruction is diagnosed, it should be rapidly treated so as to prevent any secondary infection as well as any further parenchymal damage.

Parenchymal renal disease

Following the exclusion of prerenal and postrenal etiologies of acute renal failure, intrinsic or parenchymal causes must be considered. Pertinent aspects of the history may define the basis of the renal functional impairment. For example, it is not difficult to make the diagnosis of acute glomerulonephritis in a young patient with a recent sore throat who presents with hypertension, edema, and a dark-colored urine.

Acute glomerulonephritis of virtually any etiology can present as ARF. This includes systemic illnesses such as Goodpasture's syndrome or SLE. The diagnosis of glomerulonephritis is usually not difficult, though the delineation of the specific etiology may require an extensive laboratory investigation (see Chapter 354). Urinalysis usually reveals proteinuria. White blood cells, red blood cells, oval fat bodies, granular casts, and red blood cell casts are all frequently seen on microscopic examination of the urine. The specific diagnosis may require a multitude of blood tests including ASO titer, antinuclear antibodies, cryoglobulins, antiglomerular basement membrane antibodies, and serum complement levels. Indeed, a renal biopsy with electron microscopy and immunofluorescence is often required to make a definitive diagnosis.

The presentation of a vasculitic lesion has similarities to that of active glomerulonephritis. Indeed, it is not uncommon for a vasculitis to be associated with a glomerular lesion. In general, a renal vasculitis is also associated with systemic abnormalities such as skin lesions or lung abnormalities. Presence of antineutrophil cytoplasmic antibodies (ANCA) in serum suggests the diagnosis of Wegener's granulomatosis. A biopsy of either the kidney or another involved organ may be needed to make a definitive diagnosis.

Acute interstitial nephritis is a third category of intrinsic renal lesions that must be considered in the differential diagnosis (see Chapter 362). Antibiotics and other drugs are by far the most frequent causes. The renal lesion is commonly accompanied by fever, rash, and occasionally arthralgias. The patient may, however, be completely asymptomatic. The urine sediment reveals proteinuria, pyuria, hematuria, and in many cases eosinophiluria. Peripheral eosinophilia is also common. A renal biopsy is usually required for a definitive diagnosis.

The largest group of intrinsic renal lesions that cause acute renal failure is included under the heading of acute tubular necrosis. The diagnosis in these patients is made in part following the exclusion of prerenal and postrenal causes as well as the aforementioned intrinsic causes. Suggestive aspects of the history include the development of azotemia in the face of prolonged ischemia, severe trauma with myoglobinuria, major surgery, intravenous contrast medium exposure, and aminoglycoside or other nephrotoxic antibiotic administration. The physical examination may add support to the history. The urine flow rate depends in part on the underlying cause. Recent reviews of ATN have suggested that 30% to 50% of cases may have nonoliguric ARF (urine volume >400 ml/day). Oliguria is more frequent in patients with ischemic and pigment-related lesions, whereas nephrotoxin-induced ATN is more frequently nonoliguric.

The urinalysis is helpful and typically contains pigmented casts, renal tubular epithelial cells, renal tubular cell casts, and finely and coarsely granular casts. Red blood cell and white blood cell casts are usually not seen and suggest another diagnosis when present.

The urinalysis and laboratory values can help differentiate ATN from prerenal and postrenal causes of ARF (Table 347-1). Small amounts of protein are frequently present, but heavy proteinuria suggests another diagnosis. The urine is usually isotonic. The urine/plasma osmolality ratio in patients with ATN usually is less than 1.07. In addition, the urine sodium concentration is frequently 40 mEq per liter or greater. The fractional excretion of sodium and the renal failure index are also indicative of the kidney's inability to handle sodium appropriately; in most instances of ATN, values greater than 1% and frequently greater than 2% to 3% are encountered. One must be careful in interpreting urinary indices in the presence of recent diuretic use, however, as this may increase the urine sodium concentration and decrease the urine osmolality.

The creatinine and BUN levels in both urine and serum may help in the differential diagnosis of ARF. The urine/plasma creatinine, urine/plasma urea, and the plasma urea nitrogen/creatinine ratio can aid in differentiating prerenal from intrinsic causes of ARF (see Table 347-1). It should be realized that patients with nonoliguric ATN may have laboratory values that overlap both the prerenal and oliguric ATN ranges.

The laboratory can also be of help in the diagnosis of other causes of ARF. For example, oxalate crystals in the urine suggest ethylene glycol or methoxyflurane toxicity, and football-shaped uric acid crystals suggest uric acid nephropathy. The latter diagnosis is strengthened if the urine/plasma uric acid ratio is greater than 1.

CLINICAL COURSE AND COMPLICATIONS

The clinical course of acute renal failure depends in part on the underlying etiology. Prerenal and postrenal causes, if diagnosed and treated promptly, are rapidly reversed with a return to normal or near-normal renal function. Intrinsic causes of ARF are usually not as quickly reversed, and the clinical course of the largest group in this category, ATN, may span a number of weeks and be associated with a variety of complications. In the discussion to follow, we will primarily address this latter group of patients.

Approximately 30% to 50% of patients with ARF are nonoliguric (urine output >400 ml/day), with most of the remainder oliguric (<400 ml/day) and 3% to 10% anuric (<50 ml/day). Anuria and oliguria are associated with more prolonged courses and more frequent and serious complications than is the nonoliguric state. Typically, the BUN level will rise by 10 to 20 mg/dl/day. If the patient is hypercatabolic, as in association with trauma or sepsis, the rate of rise of the BUN may be even higher, exceeding 100 mg/dl/day in some reported cases. Similarly, if acute renal failure is complicated or occurs in association with gastrointestinal bleeding, the reabsorption of blood from the gastrointestinal tract may lead to greater increments in the BUN. The serum creatinine typically will increase by 0.5 to 1.0 mg/dl/day, though in the face of marked muscle breakdown, for example, with rhabdomyolysis or trauma, the rate of increase may be accelerated.

Metabolic acidosis is almost universally present in ARF unless the patient is on nasogastric suction. Only rarely, however, will the serum bicarbonate level fall to values less than 13 to 15 mM per liter. Normally, approximately 1 mEq per kilogram of hydrogen ions is generated and excreted each day. This production is considerably higher in catabolic states, resulting in the liberation of large amounts of hydrogen ions, mostly in the form of sulfuric and phosphoric acid, which cannot be excreted normally in ARF. The retention of these compounds results in a decrease in the serum bicarbonate concentration and an anion gap acidosis (see Chapter 353).

Hyperkalemia is a serious and life-threatening complication of ARF. It may be aggravated by exogenous potassium loads in the form of potassium-containing antibiotics, salt substitutes, and various drugs that impair renal or extrarenal potassium handling (beta blockers, converting enzyme inhibitors, heparin, potassium-sparing diuretics). Though the potassium level typically rises only slowly, it can quickly increase to life-threatening levels in patients with extensive tissue breakdown. Metabolic acidosis may aggravate and worsen the level of hyperkalemia. The most serious complication of hyperkalemia is cardiac arrhythmias. Fig. 347-2 illustrates ECG alterations that occur with hyperkalemia. The level at which a particular ECG change is seen is dependent on the rate of rise of the serum potassium level, the acid-base status, and other factors.

Hyponatremia and hypocalcemia are two other electrolyte disorders that are frequent in patients with acute renal failure. Hyponatremia is usually the result of excessive water ingestion either by oral or intravenous fluids. This can be readily avoided with appropriate attention to fluid management. In addition to the exogenous fluid intake, 300 to 500 ml of water is released from the endogenous catabolism of fat and protein each day. Furthermore, tissue breakdown may release substantial quantities of water into the extracellular space.

Hypocalcemia is often present though rarely clinically evident. There are a number of reasons why hypocalcemia may develop, including hypoalbuminemia, hyperphosphatemia, resistance to parathyroid hormone, and a reduction in the active component of vitamin D. Patients with rhabdomyolysis are at particular risk of severe hypocalcemia because of extensive deposition of calcium salts in necrotic tissue. These same patients may also develop frank hypercalcemia later in their course when blood returns to the severely damaged muscle and the calcium is reabsorbed back into the circulation. Hypermagnesemia is also frequent in patients with acute renal failure, though it is also rarely clinically significant. Hyperuricemia may accompany ATN, especially if extensive tissue breakdown is present. If the uric acid level reaches very high levels (>15 to 18 mg/dl), it may play an etiologic role in the maintenance of the renal functional impairment.

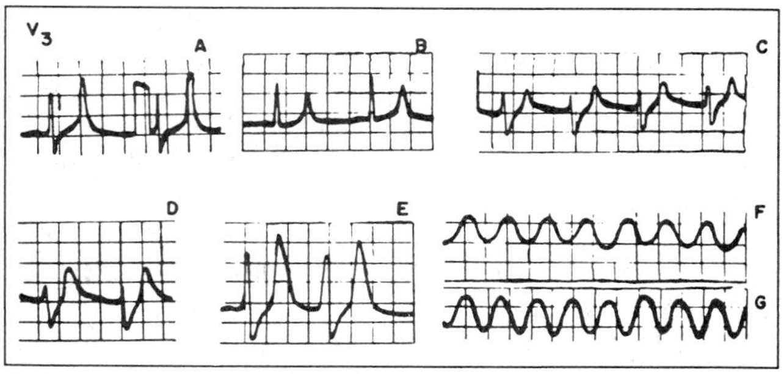

Fig. 347-2. Representative electrocardiograms in potassium intoxication. In general, the changes are sequential. The earliest change is the development of peaked T waves (**A** and **B**). The S wave may increase in depth and the S-T segment become depressed (**C**). The P wave disappears, and the QRS complex lengthens (**D** and **E**). Ventricular flutter or tachycardia supervenes (**F** and **G**). (From Merrill JP: The treatment of renal failure. New York, 1965, Grune & Stratton.)

In addition to the aforementioned electrolyte alterations, almost every organ system can be and frequently is involved in ATN. Alterations in the cardiovascular system occur mainly as the result of electrolyte and/or fluid alterations. Hypertension, edema, and congestive heart failure are all frequent complications of acute renal failure. They are the result of the retention of salt and water, which may be aggravated by therapy that necessitates the administration of large quantities of sodium. Life-threatening arrhythmias aggravated by or brought on by the electrolyte disorders do not occur as frequently as in the past. Similarly, pericarditis is now relatively rare, in part because of early institution of dialysis. Pericardial effusions in association with either pericarditis or congestive heart failure occur and may be asymptomatic. Pericardial tamponade can occur though this complication is at present uncommon.

A number of hematologic alterations complicate ARF. These include anemia, a bleeding diathesis, and alterations in the immune system. Anemia is frequent and results from a combination of factors, which include decreased erythropoiesis, hemolysis, shortened red blood cell survival, and blood loss. The etiology of the bleeding diathesis that occurs in ATN has not been completely determined. It appears to be the result, at least in part, of alterations in platelet aggregation and adhesiveness.

Alterations in the immune system are also common. Indeed, infection is the leading cause of death in patients with ARF. Defective chemotaxis, lymphopenia, and impaired cellular immunity contribute to the high incidence of infection. The lung is by far the most frequent site of infection, though the incidence of almost every type of infection is increased.

The gastrointestinal tract is commonly affected by ARF. Hiccups, nausea, vomiting, and/or anorexia are seen at some time in almost all patients. Ileus and/or gastrointestinal bleeding may occur in up to one-third of the patients. Gastrointestinal bleeding may be a consequence of altered hemostasis in the face of an increased incidence of gastrointestinal ulceration. Uremic colitis is a rare but ominous complication. Hyperamylasemia is almost always present and can be confused with acute pancreatitis. The serum lipase level may be helpful in the differential diagnosis.

In addition to the above manifestations, neurologic complications frequently accompany ARF. These include decreases in sensorium, disorientation, asterixis, seizures, and coma. Though subtle alterations are frequently seen, uremic encephalopathy is now uncommon, since dialysis is so often initiated early in the course of acute renal failure.

PROPHYLAXIS AND TREATMENT

Acute renal failure not only is more frequent in given clinical settings (cardiovascular surgery, trauma, shock, aminoglycoside treatment, rhabdomyolysis) but it is also more likely to occur in certain types of patients. The elderly, the diabetic, the patient with previous renal insufficiency, and the patient with heart or liver disease all are at greater risk. One must, therefore, be especially careful in these patients to avoid a situation that precipitates ARF. For example, dye-induced acute renal failure is more frequent in these groups of patients, and tests that expose these patients to iodinated contrast media should be undertaken only when absolutely necessary. Similarly, particular attention should be given to the fluid and electrolyte status of the elderly individual before, during, and after any surgical procedure.

The use of diuretics and/or mannitol in the prevention or reversal of ARF has been the subject of many experimental and clinical studies. These studies, however, have not been conclusive. These compounds are not without risk. In the patient with ARF, hearing loss is a major complication of both furosemide and ethacrynic acid. This complication though usually reversible can result in serious and irreversible deafness. Up to 50% of patients in some series have had at least transient hearing loss or tinnitus following treatment with intravenous furosemide. The toxicity of these agents seems to be related more to the rate at which they are given than to the actual dose, though this has not been completely substantiated by controlled trials. Mannitol can also be associated with side effects, including extracellular volume expansion, hyperosmolality, and hyperkalemia.

The loop diuretics and/or mannitol, when administered in high doses, increase the urine output in 25% to 30% of patients with ARF. Low-dose dopamine (1 to 5 μg/kg/min) has a renal vasodilatory effect and in combination with furosemide has also been shown to initiate diuresis in a few animal and uncontrolled human studies. However, the effect of these agents on reducing the duration of azotemia, hospitalization, or need for dialysis is not as clear. Advocates suggest that these agents do favorably affect the outcome and course of ARF and that, because of the enhancement of urine flow, the patient's fluid and electrolyte status is easier to manage. On the other hand, it may be that patients who respond to diuretics have less severe renal dysfunction initially and would have had a milder and perhaps shorter course of ARF if treated without pharmacologic intervention. No study to date has clearly shown any favorable effect of the diuretics on mortality. We do not advocate large doses or prolonged use of either mannitol or diuretics in the prophylaxis or treatment of ARF. If prerenal causes have been ruled out, an initial trial of 12.5 to 25 g of mannitol or 80 mg of furosemide intravenously (administered slowly) can be attempted, and if there is no response, a second, larger dose (approximately double) can be tried. Recently, data have become available that suggest that a 200 mg dose of furosemide intravenously has a maximal diuretic effect and that higher doses offer no additional benefit. Clinical studies are presently underway investigating the use of calcium channel blockers as well as atrial natriuretic peptides in acute renal failure.

Established acute renal failure

Despite much investigation into the pathophysiology of ARF, there is as yet no definitive treatment that will reverse its course. Therapy is aimed mainly at the prevention and/or treatment of the associated complications. The usefulness of growth factors and oxygen free radical scavengers remains under evaluation.

Dietary, fluid, and electrolyte management

Hyperkalemia was a frequent cause of death in the past but has become less frequent with greater access to dialysis and with development of rapid and accurate laboratory procedures to identify and monitor the clinical course. The restriction of potassium in the diet and the avoidance whenever possible of potassium-containing drugs is especially important. A diet containing no more than 40 mEq potassium per day is usually sufficient. Patients who are hypercatabolic may, however, have rapid increases in serum potassium level; hence rapid or emergent treatment of hyperkalemia may be needed. The therapy is dictated primarily by the changes in the ECG. These changes correlate more closely with the rapidity of the rise in potassium concentration than with the absolute value. The emergency treatment of hyperkalemia (also see Chapter 352 and Table 352-2) includes the use of intravenous calcium in an attempt to antagonize the effect of the hyperkalemia at the cell membrane level. In addition to this, the serum potassium level can be acutely lowered by driving potassium into cells with sodium bicarbonate and/or an infusion of glucose and insulin. One must also keep in mind that the emergency measures are only temporizing, since they do not remove potassium from the body but instead only counteract the effect of the high levels and/or cause intracellular shifts. One must in every case employ additional therapy directed toward the removal of potassium from the body. This can be accomplished with a sodium-potassium exchange resin such as Kayexalate. Kayexalate is administered by mouth (dose: 15 to 30 g in 50 ml of 20% sorbitol) or as a retention enema (50 g in 200 ml of 20% sorbitol). (Because Kayexalate alone causes constipation, sorbitol is added as a hyperosmotic cathartic.) Approximately 1 mEq of potassium is removed for each gram of Kayexalate. Alternatively, potassium can be removed from the body by dialysis. Dialysis provides a more rapid mode of removing potassium, though trained staff and appropriate equipment are required. The serum potassium level should be maintained below 5 mEq per liter in any patient with ARF to assure a safe margin for any unexpected alteration.

Abnormalities in water and sodium metabolism also occur in ARF. Insensible water losses approximate 400 to 800 ml per day. This is partially obviated by the 400 ml per day of water that is released from the metabolism of fat and protein. In hypercatabolic patients, the release of water from tissue breakdown and metabolism may far exceed 400 ml per day. It is wise to limit the oliguric patient's intake of fluid to approximately 400 ml per day plus an amount equal to the urinary output. Normally, a patient with ATN, if not receiving hyperalimentation, will lose 0.3 to 0.5 kg of weight per day. If this does not occur or if there is an actual weight gain, one must reevaluate fluid therapy. In association with the kidney's limited ability to excrete free water, hyponatremia may occur. More stringent fluid restriction should then be instituted.

Acidosis frequently occurs in ARF, though the serum bicarbonate level will usually remain above 12 to 15 mEq per liter except in the hypercatabolic patient. Modest amounts of sodium bicarbonate (either as sodium bicarbonate or as sodium citrate) may be administered if the serum bicarbonate level drops below 15 to 18 mEq per liter, though one should recognize the potential for volume overload. Hyperphosphatemia, if severe, should be treated with calcium carbonate or other phosphate binders. Hypermagnesemia, though relatively frequent, is only rarely clinically evident and usually only after large exogenous loads of magnesium-containing salts. If antacids need to be employed, those containing calcium or aluminum are preferable to those containing magnesium. If it is severe, the only available treatment for hypermagnesemia is dialysis.

Nutritional support is an important aspect of the treatment of acute renal failure. It should be designed to give the patient an adequate number of calories and protein but at the same time must avoid excessive volume. High biologic protein should be used to maintain a slightly positive nitrogen balance. The caloric requirements in ARF are considerably higher than under normal conditions and in the hypercatabolic state may exceed 5000 calories per day. A minimum of 100 g per day of carbohydrate should be administered with the intention of providing sufficient glucose to avoid endogenous breakdown of protein for glucose synthesis. The protein requirements also depend on the clinical status. With oral feedings, one can start with a diet of 40 g per day of high-quality protein and increase it as deemed necessary. Meeting the nutritional needs of the patient may not be possible without dialysis, which allows larger quantities to be given. Enteral or parenteral alimentation may be necessary in the postoperative patient or in those with anorexia, nausea, or vomiting. The use of essential amino acids or their keto analogs to favorably affect the outcome of ARF in the postoperative or trauma patient has been suggested in a number of recent clinical studies.

If conservative management fails, or if the patient is severely catabolic, dialysis must be considered (see the box below). Dialysis not only is helpful in the treatment of complications but also allows one to offer more extensive nutritional support. Early and intensive dialysis has been advocated to prevent or minimize the occurrence of complications. There are two main modes of dialysis, hemodialysis and peritoneal dialysis. The former is more efficient but is associated with more complications (hypotension, dysequilibrium syndrome, blood loss) and requires trained staff and sophisticated equipment (see Chapter 348). Peritoneal dialysis is associated with fewer complications, can be performed in almost any patient, and requires a minimum of staff and equipment. Unfortunately, it is considerably less efficient and may be inadequate in the treatment of the severely catabolic patient.

Indications for dialysis in acute renal failure

1. Hyperkalemia
2. Fluid overload
3. Pericarditis
4. Uremic symptoms
5. Blood urea nitrogen >100 mg/dl, creatinine >10 mg/dl (relative indication)
6. Certain toxins (ethylene glycol, methanol)
7. Acidosis

Continuous arteriovenous hemofiltration is an alternative to the above dialysis techniques. It uses a smaller blood filter than does hemodialysis, which is driven by the patient's blood pressure and can be used to remove excess fluid, that is, for ultrafiltration. It has the advantages of being hemodynamically safer and requiring less personnel and apparatus than hemodialysis, and it is considerably more efficient at fluid removal than is peritoneal dialysis. Its disadvantages are that it requires continuous use if clearance of substances other than water is required, and it requires systemic anticoagulation.

REFERENCES

Berkseth RO and Kjellstrand CM: Radiologic contrast-induced nephropathy. Med Clin North Am 68:351, 1984.

Better OS and Stein JH: Early management of shock and prophylaxis of acute renal failure in traumatic rhabdomyolysis. New Engl J Med 322:825, 1990.

Brenner BM and Stein JH, editors: In Contemporary issues in nephrology. New York, 1980, Churchill Livingstone.
Brezis M, Seymour R, and Epstein FH: Acute renal failure. In Brenner BM and Rector FC, editors: The kidney, ed 4. Philadelphia, 1991, Saunders, pp. 993-1061.
Fried TA and Stein JH: Experimental acute renal failure: pathophysiology and methods of protection. In Robinson RR, editor: Nephrology. New York, 1984, Springer-Verlag, pp. 731-747.
Grazianni G, Cantaluppi A, and Casati S et al: Dopamine and furosemide in oliguric acute renal failure. Nephron 37:39, 1984.
Kaplan AA, Longnecker RE, and Folkert VW: Continuous arteriovenous hemofiltration. Ann Intern Med 100:358, 1984.
Lazarus JM and Brenner BM, editors: Acute renal failure, ed 3. New York, 1993, Churchill Livingstone.
Myers BD and Moran SM: Hemodynamically mediated acute renal failure. N Engl J Med 314:97, 1986.
Solez K and Racusen LC: Acute renal failure. New York, 1991, Marcel Dekker.
Toback FG: Regeneration after acute tubular necrosis. Kidney International 41:226, 1992.
Weinberg JM: The cell biology of ischemic renal injury. Kidney International 39:476, 1991.

CHAPTER

348 Chronic Renal Failure

Robert G. Luke
Terry B. Strom

Chronic renal failure can be defined as a permanent and significant reduction in glomerular filtration rate (GFR). In nearly all patients, once GFR is reduced to about one-third of normal (GFR <30-40 ml/min, serum creatinine >3 mg/dl), progressive renal failure develops and leads eventually—but often slowly over as long as 20 to 30 years—to the *uremic syndrome* and *end-stage renal disease* (ESRD). *Chronic renal insufficiency* is present when the GFR is permanently and definitely reduced below normal, but progressive renal failure is not yet inevitable or established (serum creatinine in the range of 1.5 to 3 mg/dl). *Uremia* can be defined as the signs and symptoms associated with retention of the end products of nitrogen metabolism; in chronic renal failure it is eventually fatal unless *renal replacement therapy* (dialysis and/or renal transplantation) is introduced. The uremic syndrome is quite variable and unpredictable in its time of onset during the course of chronic renal failure, but it is unusual before the blood urea nitrogen (BUN) level reaches 60 mg/dl or the serum creatinine level 8 mg/dl (GFR <10 ml/min) and more commonly occurs at a BUN level of more than 100 mg/dl and a serum creatinine level of more than 12 mg/dl. It is good medical practice to initiate renal replacement therapy just before the onset of uremic symptoms, usually when the GFR is 5 to 10 ml/min. In making these assessments, it must be remembered that there is normally a reduction in GFR with aging; at age 85 to 90 years GFR is reduced about 50% of normal. This reduction may not be associated with an elevation in serum creatinine because muscle mass and consequently creatinine production also falls with aging.

Because all patients in whom no contraindication exists now receive renal replacement therapy, at least in the United States and most Western countries, it is useful to consider dialysis treatment as an extension of the natural history of chronic renal failure (Fig. 348-1). Importantly, dialysis treatment is equivalent to a GFR of only about 10 ml/min. Hence some problems of patients with chronic renal failure are not completely resolved by chronic dialysis. Nevertheless, virtually all patients on chronic dialysis would otherwise not survive for long.

Discussed in detail later (see PATHOPHYSIOLOGY) is the important concept that many patients with chronic renal failure progress along a final common path toward ESRD despite disappearance of the renal insult that initially led to the loss of some nephrons. If the pathogenetic mechanism for the loss of remaining nephrons can be elucidated and then prevented or modified, a substantial proportion of patients with chronic renal failure might be converted to nonprogressive chronic renal insufficiency, or at least progression toward ESRD might be slowed. Because development of ESRD is most frequent in older patients, even the latter benefit might avoid the need for renal replacement therapy.

ETIOLOGY AND INCIDENCE

To see the relative importance of the various causes of chronic renal failure, let us look at ESRD, for which data

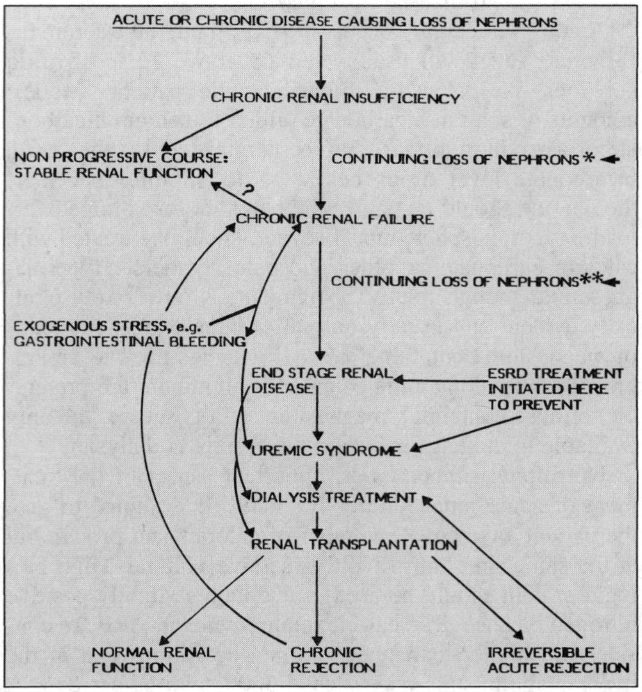

Fig. 348-1. Course of chronic renal failure due to progressive nephron loss from chronic renal insufficiency to end-stage renal disease (ESRD), including therapy for ESRD. Treatment at ★← may prevent progression and at ★★← may slow progression.

are best established, because the federal government assumes the heavy costs of such treatment. It should be noted, however, that because some diseases progress more slowly to ESRD than others, the data in Table 348-1 probably do not accurately reflect the relative prevalence of chronic renal insufficiency or of chronic renal failure in the community due to these diseases before ESRD.

It is striking that 60% of ESRD is now due to two systemic diseases—diabetes mellitus (diabetic glomerulosclerosis) and essential hypertension (hypertensive nephrosclerosis). One would assume that effective treatment of the primary disease would reduce the development of ESRD due to these renal complications, but to date, for reasons under intense study, this has not happened. The most common primary renal cause of ESRD is the glomerulonephritides.

There is an almost fourfold increase in ESRD (secondary to all causes except for congenital ones such as polycystic kidney disease) in blacks. The racial discrepancy is most marked for hypertensive nephrosclerosis in younger patients, for example, a black:white ratio of ESRD of 20:1 in the age group 25 to 45 years. Even after controlling for prevalence of primary and secondary causes before renal impairment, efficacy of treatment (e.g., glycemic or blood pressure control), and socioeconomic and demographic factors, the difference persists. The phenomenon is under current investigation, but it is possible that there is an increased renal susceptibility in blacks to primary or secondary hypertension. Approximately 600 patients per million population receive chronic dialysis in the United States and considerably more patients have less severe degrees of chronic renal failure. In summary, in a city of 100,000 people one might anticipate that each year 16 patients would develop ESRD, 60 patients would be on some form of chronic dialysis, and a greater but unknown number would have chronic renal failure or chronic renal insufficiency. Case finding in the latter groups will be essential if the final common path of nephron loss, referred to earlier and again in the next section, can be modified.

Table 348-1. Causes of annual incidence of new patients with ESRD ranked by percentage of total patients

Disease	%
Diabetic glomerulopathy	33
Hypertensive nephrosclerosis	29
Glomerulonephritis	15
Tubulo-interstitial*	6
Congenital†	5
Unknown	7
Total	100 (166)‡

From United States Renal Data System, Annual Data Report, Am J Kidney Dis 17:55:1-93, 1991.
*Mainly obstructive and analgesic nephropathy
†Mainly polycystic kidney disease
‡Patients per million US population

PATHOPHYSIOLOGY

The common clinical features of chronic renal failure and of the uremic syndrome relate to the diminishing number of nephrons that function relatively normally except for the increased excretion of solute per remaining nephron. This phenomenon is the *intact nephron hypothesis*. The process of chronic renal failure is essentially that of progressive loss of nephrons, irrespective of the primary site of attack (e.g., the glomerulus in glomerulonephritis and the medullary portions of the nephron in chronic pyelonephritis [reflux nephropathy]) on those nephrons. Ultimately, if damaged severely enough at any site, complete individual nephrons are destroyed. The site of primary damage, however, may be clinically evident and may help to indicate the type of disease process present: Nephrotic syndrome indicates a primary or secondary glomerular disease (e.g., glomerulonephritis), whereas severe impairment of the renal concentrating mechanism out of proportion to the reduction of GFR may suggest a primary tubulointerstitial disease process (e.g., hypercalcemic nephropathy). Nevertheless, chronic renal failure manifests many of the same signs and symptoms, irrespective of the specific primary cause of nephron loss (the "final common path").

As nephrons are lost, the remaining undamaged or less severely damaged nephrons (both glomeruli and tubules) undergo "compensatory hypertrophy." In human kidneys there are normally 1 million nephrons in each kidney and GFR of 120 ml/min. This would give a single nephron glomerular filtration rate (SNGFR) of 60 nl/min if the SNGFR is homogeneous. Animal models of chronic renal failure suggest that as nephrons are lost, the SNGFR in remaining "intact" nephrons tends to be increased. Thus normal GFR could, at least theoretically, be maintained despite the reduced number of nephrons until the limits of increase of SNGFR are reached. The alternative cause of reduced overall GFR, an asymmetric reduction in SNGFR in remaining nephrons, is not usually seen.

As nephrons are lost, if dietary intake remained the same, solutes such as sodium, chloride, potassium, and phosphate would accumulate in the body and cause symptoms if there were not *increased excretion of solute per remaining nephron*. Hyperkalemia, for example, is unusual until the GFR is reduced to less than 10 ml/min. We have already seen that there is increased GFR per remaining nephron; this process is supplemented by diminished fractional reabsorption of those substances normally reabsorbed (e.g., sodium, chloride, phosphate) and increased secretion per nephron for those substances normally secreted after filtration (e.g., potassium; in late chronic renal failure, potassium clearance may exceed inulin clearance). This process prevents solutes from increasing in concentration in the blood (e.g., phosphate) or in total amount in the body (e.g., sodium chloride) until much later in the course of disease—either until GFR is reduced to about 25% of normal (often, for substances reabsorbed but not secreted) or until even greater reductions in GFR take place (for substances secreted, e.g., as noted, potassium).

These *adaptations* in the function of remaining nephrons

are aided by humoral, hormonal, and paracrine changes that either decrease absorption of a solute (e.g., parathyroid hormone for phosphate) or increase its secretion (e.g., aldosterone for potassium). There is also evidence for accumulation of a natriuretic factor, which impairs tubular reabsorption of sodium chloride, perhaps due to inhibition of ($Na^+ + K^+$)-ATPase (sodium potassium activated adenosine triphosphatase) in response to minor degrees of sodium chloride retention and expansion of extracellular fluid (ECF) volume.

Although these adaptations of remaining nephron function maintain the constancy of the internal environment, they severely limit the capacity of these same remaining nephrons to cope with an additional acute task such as a sudden increase in potassium, water, or acid load. In a sense each remaining nephron has already used its reserve capacity. Thus the patient with chronic renal failure loses the capacity or flexibility to deal with alterations in solute intake in response to dietary changes or in solute production in response to metabolic changes, for example, in response to infection or trauma. To avoid unnecessary or even iatrogenic illness (e.g., excess water intake causing hyponatremia) in these circumstances, the physician must anticipate the limited renal capacity to deal with such changes.

These beneficial compensatory adaptations in residual nephron function and in systemic hormonal secretion may ultimately "trade off" for harmful renal (the adapted nephron) and systemic (e.g., renal bone disease due to secondary hyperparathyroidism) effects (Fig. 348-2). Indeed "nephron trade-off" secondary to the adapted nephron (Fig. 348-3) is responsible for some of the clinical similarities of the "final common path" of chronic renal failure irrespective of the primary cause of nephronal damage. Animal and some human studies suggest that important deleterious effects on the glomerulus relate to mechanical stress due to

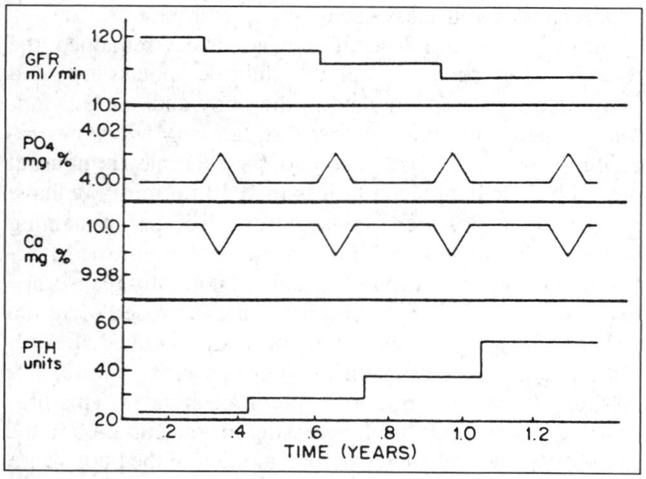

Fig. 348-2. As GFR falls, serum phosphate rises, especially after eating; this leads to a fall in serum calcium and thereby to an increase in parathyroid hormone (PTH) secretion, which reduces tubular reabsorption of phosphate and calcium to normal but at the expense of an ever-increasing PTH level. (From Arch Intern Med 123:543-553, 1969.)

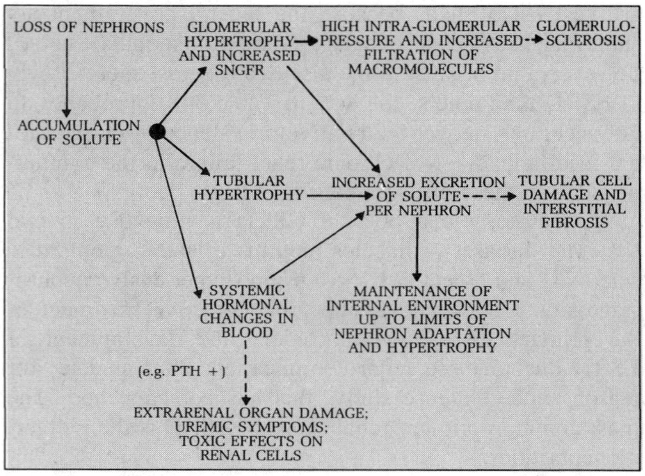

Fig. 348-3. Response to loss of nephrons. Originally constituting a beneficial response to allow increased excretion per remaining intact nephron, these changes ultimately lead to continuing nephron loss independent of the initial injury or disease (nephron trade-off). SNGFR, single nephron glomerular filtration rate. PTH, parathyroid hormone.

hypertension and hyperperfusion with increased glomerular permeability to macromolecules into the mesangium, cytokine and growth-factor-induced proliferative effects on mesangial, epithelial, and endothothelial cells with increased matrix protein and collagen formation, dyslipidemic endothelial and mesangial cell changes, and local coagulation abnormalities including platelet-endothelial interactions. Focal glomerulosclerosis is the prototypical glomerular lesion of nephron trade off and is best seen in nephrons initially damaged by a primary tubulointerstitial process such as reflux nephropathy (chronic pyelonephritis). The similarity of glomerulosclerosis to atherosclerosis is noteworthy; hypertension, hyperlipidemia, and coagulation abnormalities are risk factors. Nephron trade off also damages the tubules and interstitium by effects due to phosphate, urate, and ammonium excess per nephron and "hypermetabolic" effects in hyperperfused nephrons especially when accompanied by ischemia due to primary and secondary renal arteriolonephrosclerosis. Many therapeutic approaches in humans related to these pathogenetic mechanisms are being inspired by successful therapeutic interventions in various animal models of nephron loss. Specific examples of the limitations imposed by progressive nephron loss and nephron adaptation on renal handling of water, sodium, potassium, and acid-base balance are considered next.

Water excretion

With advancing renal disease, there is progressive impairment in the urinary concentrating ability. Whereas in health the maximum urine osmolality may be about four times greater than that of plasma, in progressive renal disease the maximum urine osmolality approaches that of plasma. If the total solute requiring excretion remains at about 600 mosm/day in uremia and the urine osmolality is fixed at slightly more than 300 mosm/kg water, about 1 L of water will have to be excreted with every 300 mosm of solute, and obligatory water excretion will approximate 2 L per day. This restricts the capacity of patients with chronic renal disease to lower water excretion during hydropenia to the levels seen in normal persons (500 ml/day at a urine osmolality of 1200 mosm/kg water). With a decrease in the nephron population, there is also a restriction on the upper limit of water excretion that can be achieved. Although diluting ability is well preserved in chronic renal disease, the total amount of free water that can be excreted decreases as the nephron population and GFR fall. For example, if 10% of GFR can be excreted as free water, the capacity to excrete free water in response to water excess is 0.4 ml/min (or 0.58 L/24 hr) in a patient with an inulin clearance of 4 ml/min, compared with 12 ml/min (or 17 L/24 hr) in a normal person.

The increased obligatory water excretion in chronic renal disease may lead to polyuria and nocturia. Occasionally, particularly when hypotonic fluids are administered, hyponatremia may result because of the diseased kidney's inability to increase water excretion appropriately. In conscious patients it is wiser to rely on the thirst mechanism, which is usually normal.

Sodium excretion

As renal disease progresses, fractional sodium excretion increases appropriately and external balance is maintained until late in the course of renal disease, hence ECF volume is relatively well preserved. With changes in sodium intake, the fractional excretion of sodium has to change substantially to maintain sodium balance. For example, in a normal person increasing sodium chloride intake from 3.5 to 7.0 g/24 hr, the fractional excretion of sodium has to change from 0.25% to 0.5% to maintain balance. The same increment in salt intake may require a change in fractional sodium excretion from 8% to 16% to remain in balance in a patient with a GFR of 4 ml/min. Hence, in renal failure, sodium excretion can be varied only over a restricted range, which progressively narrows as GFR declines.

With chronic renal disease, an upper and a lower limit of sodium excretion develop. At the lower limit, or "floor," the patient cannot conserve sodium maximally. Patients with renal disease fed a low-salt diet often cannot reduce sodium output over the usual time scale. A negative sodium balance ensues, and a corresponding volume of water is excreted. Plasma volume, ECF volume, and GFR fall. About 1% or 2% of patients with early chronic renal failure have a urine sodium leak, which causes sodium depletion even when salt intake is *normal*. Most of these patients have medullary cystic disease and analgesic nephropathy, but a few have obstructive uropathy, chronic interstitial nephritis, or polycystic kidney disease. They are typically normotensive and require a high sodium intake to maintain sodium balance.

Sodium retention is a more common problem than sodium depletion in chronic renal failure. It may occur due to associated nephrotic syndrome, cardiac failure or, in advanced chronic renal failure, due to lack of reduction of sodium chloride intake to match renal capacity to excrete those ions. The resulting positive balance in sodium chloride will expand ECF and plasma volume and may, in turn, lead to worsening hypertension and left ventricular or biventricular heart failure.

Potassium excretion

Normally, about 90% to 95% of ingested potassium is excreted in the urine, with the remainder being excreted in the stool. In chronic renal failure, a greater fraction of ingested potassium is excreted in the stool; 20% to 50% of the ingested amount may appear in the stool when the GFR falls below 5 ml/min.

There is also a marked increase in potassium excretion per nephron, and urinary potassium excretion approaches—and may even surpass—the filtered load of potassium. In chronic renal failure therefore, those adjustments in renal mechanisms that increase potassium excretion, together with the increased stool excretion of potassium, are enough to maintain a normal concentration of this cation in plasma, even on a normal intake of potassium (60 to 80 mEq/day), until the GFR falls below 10 ml/min.

In contrast to sodium, potassium excretion depends on tubular secretion to maintain balance. In health, aldosterone and the distal tubular flow rate are major mediators of potassium secretion in the distal nephron. In chronic renal failure, a rise in aldosterone levels and increased flow of fluid through the distal tubule may be important factors increasing potassium excretion per nephron. Care with prescription of converting enzyme inhibitors for hypertension is needed because they may reduce aldosterone levels and precipitate hyperkalemia. Increases in ($Na^+ + K^+$)-ATPase activity in the distal nephron may also underlie the greater capacity of the remaining nephrons to increase potassium excretion. Plasma potassium may rise in chronic renal disease due to redistribution of potassium between intracellular and extracellular compartments, usually as a consequence of progressive acidosis, or the use of beta-blocking drugs.

The maintenance of normal excretion of potassium by the kidney when the number of functioning nephrons is decreased depends on a large increase in the distal tubular capacity to secrete potassium. At very low GFRs, the secretory rate of potassium may be near maximum to maintain the steady state. Thus very little functional reserve remains to respond to sudden changes in potassium intake. Situations such as oliguria, a sudden increase in potassium intake, sudden metabolic acidosis, or catabolic states may result in life-threatening hyperkalemia in patients with far-advanced renal insufficiency. A circulating inhibitor of ($Na^+ + K^+$)-ATPase (a natriuretic factor) and other effects of uremia may lead to increased cellular sodium content, decreased transcellular potential, and a decrease in intracellular potassium levels; hence total body potassium may actually be decreased despite hyperkalemia.

Acid-base balance

The maintenance of acid-base balance in normal humans requires the renal reabsorption from the daily filtered load of approximately 4000 mEq of bicarbonate and the urinary excretion of 50 to 100 mEq of hydrogen ions in the form of ammonium and titratable acid (H^+ bound to phosphate and other buffer ions). Because of compensatory adaptations in acid excretion by the residual nephrons as renal function declines (except for a small group of patients with renal tubular acidosis associated with tubulointerstitial disease) most patients do not have significant acidemia due to renal disease until GFR falls below roughly 20% of normal.

Hydrogen ion excretion is impaired in chronic renal failure. Although ammonia excretion per residual nephron increases, total urinary ammonium excretion is lower than normal for the urinary pH. On the other hand, titratable acid excretion is normal or only slightly reduced, because the main buffers (phosphate and creatinine) are present in nearly normal amounts in the urine until very late in the course of renal disease. The result is decreased net acid excretion in the urine and a positive hydrogen ion balance.

A progressive fall in plasma bicarbonate below 15 mEq/L usually does not occur in chronic renal failure until GFR values are quite low, presumably because buffers such as the carbonate of bone are then being utilized in buffering the hydrogen ion retention (positive H^+ balance) that occurs in such patients. In some patients there is also a urinary bicarbonate leak when the plasma levels are restored toward normal by the infusion of bicarbonate. When the infusion is stopped, the renal excretion of bicarbonate continues until plasma bicarbonate falls back to its previous level. This bicarbonate leak may have several causes, including an effect of high parathyroid hormone levels or of occult volume expansion on bicarbonate reabsorption in the proximal tubule.

Two types of acidosis have been observed in chronic renal disease: (1) hyperchloremic acidosis (normal anion gap acidosis), which occurs relatively early in the course of renal insufficiency and is mild, and (2) metabolic acidosis with an increased anion gap, which is due to the accumulation of phosphate, sulfate, and other anions usually not measured during routine laboratory determinations. If the anion gap is greater than about 20 mEq/L other complicating events such as ketosis or lactic acidosis should be sought. In some patients with chronic renal disease and hyporeninemia, acidosis with hyperkalemia may occur (type IV renal tubular acidosis).

Magnesium

Most patients with chronic renal failure have normal or moderately elevated serum magnesium levels, which, however, seldom cause symptoms. The serum magnesium level rises further in response to acidosis, tissue trauma, and the administration of vitamin D and its analogs. Only in patients receiving occasional enemas or antacids containing magnesium are there marked increases in serum magnesium level. These elevations can lead to drowsiness, muscle weakness, and skin irritation. In patients with higher levels of magnesium, dramatic symptoms (muscle paralysis and respiratory failure) may occur.

Phosphate and calcium

Urinary phosphate excretion remains unchanged as GFR falls, due to a progressive decrease in phosphate reabsorption, the consequences of increased levels of parathyroid hormone in serum (see Fig. 348-2). When the GFR falls below 30 ml/min, however, even a marked decrease in phosphate reabsorption cannot compensate for the marked decrease in the filtered load of phosphate, and serum phosphate level rises. Hyperphosphatemia is therefore seen commonly in patients with a GFR of 25 ml/min or less on an unrestricted diet. It is also at this level of GFR that decreases in serum calcium concentrations occur.

The fall in calcium concentration is due to several factors (Fig. 348-4): The increase in serum phosphate leads to a reciprocal decrease in serum calcium and decreased serum levels of 1,25$(OH)_2$-vitamin D_3 which is also due to nephron loss. These changes, in turn, decrease calcium absorption from the gastrointestinal tract. In addition, the ability of parathyroid hormone to mobilize calcium from bone is impaired, and this "skeletal resistance" to the action of the hormone also contributes to the development of hypocalcemia. The metabolic acidosis present tends to increase the fraction of ionized calcium and prevents some of the clinical consequences of hypocalcemia. Rapid correction of the acidosis in patients with chronic renal disease may lead to a fall in ionized calcium and precipitate acute manifestations of hypocalcemia, including tetany and convulsions. A normal or elevated serum calcium in patients not receiving vitamin D derivatives suggests severe secondary hyperparathyroidism or the syndrome of aluminum-induced bone disease.

Uremic syndrome

The pathogenesis of the uremic syndrome is not precisely established but almost certainly has no single cause. Urea itself is relatively nontoxic, but measurement of blood urea (or blood urea nitrogen, BUN) offers the best single laboratory index of the likelihood of certain symptoms being "uremic" in origin. Restriction of dietary protein in association with maintenance of a caloric intake adequate to prevent gluconeogenesis frequently ameliorates uremic symptoms; likewise, a catabolic state often precipitates uremia at a GFR at which it would normally not occur (see Fig. 348-1). Hemodialysis, which most efficiently removes the many small molecular weight substances that are the end products of protein metabolism, also corrects the major manifestations of uremia, although there are some subtle persisting abnormalities, perhaps related to the less efficient clearance of "middle molecules" (molecular mass 300 to

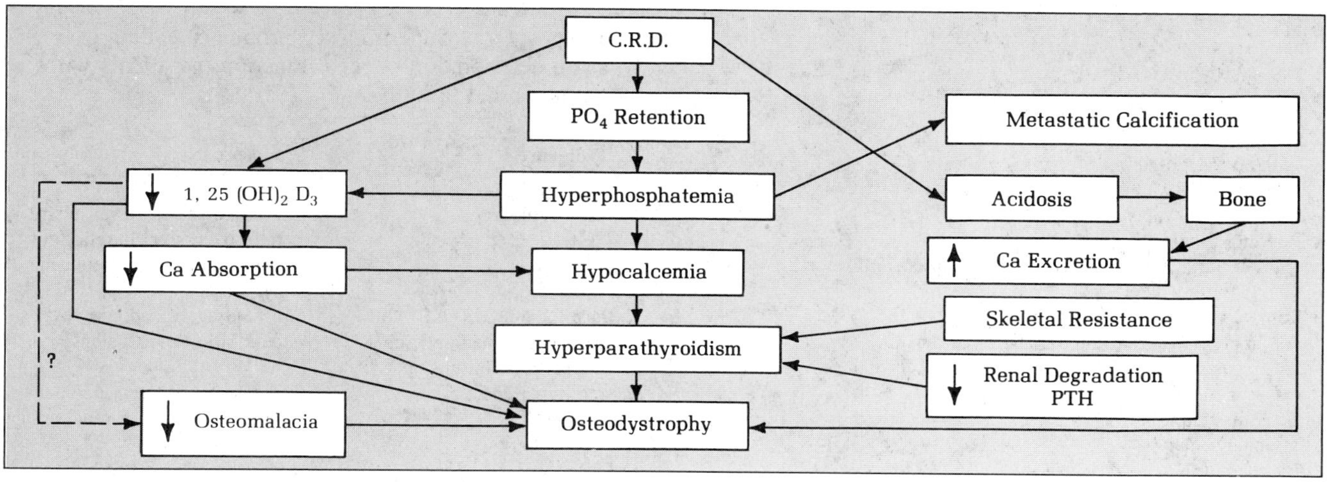

Fig. 348-4. Pathogenesis of osteodystrophy in patients with chronic renal disease (C.R.D.). The retention of phosphate leads to hyperphosphatemia and a decrease in serum calcium level (hypocalcemia). The hyperphosphatemia may also decrease the level of circulating $1{,}25(OH)_2$-vitamin D_3 by an effect on the renal 1-α-hydroxylase enzyme. The fall in the level of $1{,}25(OH)_2$-vitamin D_3 results in decreased gastrointestinal calcium absorption, which contributes to the hypocalcemia. The fall in serum calcium leads to increased secretion of parathyroid hormone (PTH) hyperparathyroidism. The level of PTH also increases as a consequence of decreased degradation by the kidney (as renal mass decreases) and skeletal resistance. The acidosis of chronic renal disease promotes the removal of calcium carbonate from bone and contributes to the osteodystrophy. Increase in PTH results in bone changes (osteitis fibrosa cystica). A negative calcium balance may result in osteomalacia. (From Slatopolsky E: Recommendation for the treatment of renal osteodystrophy in dialysis patients, Kidney Int 7:S253, 1975.)

2000 daltons). Likely major contributing mechanisms to the uremic state are the following:

1. Accumulation of "toxins"
   a. Small molecular weight substances (e.g., urea, urate, sulfate, phosphate, which result from failure to excrete the end products of nitrogen metabolism)
   b. A whole series of substances such as phenols, guanidines, and low molecular weight polypeptides (however, evidence linking accumulation of any single substance to a specific uremic manifestation or organ dysfunction is weak)
2. Extracellular and intracellular electrolyte and acid-base disturbances, including sodium, potassium, magnesium, and calcium. Inhibitors of Na, K, ATPase likely impair cell function.
3. Accumulation of various hormones due to
   a. Impaired renal degradation (growth hormone, glucagon)
   b. Responses to solute retention (natriuretic factor, parathyroid hormone)
   c. Impaired end-organ responses (follicle-stimulating hormone and luteinizing hormone)
4. Impaired production of renal hormones (e.g., erythropoietin, $1{,}25(OH)$-vitamin D_3).

Specific organ dysfunctions in patients with chronic renal failure, uremia, and ESRD are considered in the next section. However, it is likely that these various mechanisms lead to diffuse defects of cellular function and metabolism in general, including energy production, cell membrane function, and ion pumps.

It is important for the physician to remember that there are many other causes of acute symptomatic deterioration in patients with chronic renal failure than uremia per se. Water excess (hyponatremia), drug intoxication due to accumulation of a drug in the presence of impaired renal excretion, congestive heart failure, and hypertensive encephalopathy are examples of complications that may need specific treatment to avoid premature acceptance that the patient has reached ESRD and uremia.

CLINICAL PRESENTATION AND DIAGNOSIS

Manifestations

Chronic renal failure may present in a myriad of ways and stages from chronic renal insufficiency to the uremic syndrome. Its secondary manifestations are often mistaken for primary problems in the affected organ system; common examples are mistaking essential hypertension for renal hypertension, peptic ulcer disease for gastrointestinal symptoms of uremia, and various anemias for renal anemia. Failure of the renal regulatory mechanisms to maintain the constancy of the internal environment ultimately produces symptoms and signs in every organ system, often in varying degrees in different patients.

Major modes of presentation of chronic renal failure are listed in the box on p. 2628. Only a small minority of pa-

Presentations of chronic renal failure

- Renal symptoms
  - Nocturia, polyuria
  - Hematuria
  - Nephrotic syndrome
- Routine urinalysis
  - Proteinuria with or without urinary casts, RBCs, and WBCs
- Routine physical examination
  - Symptomatic or asymptomatic hypertension
  - Congestive heart failure
  - Cardiovascular disease
- General symptoms
  - General malaise
  - Lassitude
  - Anemia
  - Anorexia
  - Pruritus, bruising
  - Halitosis
- Specific extrarenal abnormalities
  - Impaired cognitive function
  - Peripheral neuropathy
  - Anemia
  - Renal bone disease
  - Gout or pseudogout
  - Pericarditis
  - Gastrointestinal bleeding

Table 348-2. Superimposed problems leading to acute deterioration of renal function in patients with chronic renal failure

Problem	Comment
Volume depletion	Extrarenal losses or salt restriction: excessive diuretic therapy, especially in nephrotic syndrome
Extracellular fluid (ECF) volume overexpansion ± congestive heart failure	Salt loading, vasodilators, excess blood transfusion
Severe hypertension	Can also result from ECF volume expansion or renal artery stenosis
Obstruction	Renal stone, prostatic hypertrophy
Urinary tract infection	Most likely to cause fall in GFR in abnormal urinary tract
Drug toxicity	Aminoglycosides, tetracycline, prostaglandin inhibitors, contrast media, cyclosporine converting enzyme inhibitors
Metabolic: hypercalcemia, acute, severe hyperuricemia	Volume depletion, vitamin D analogs
Endocrine deficiencies	Hypoadrenalism, hypothyroidism

tients present with specific renal complaints: conversely, the vast majority of patients with specific complaints related to the urinary tract do not have chronic renal disease but, rather, have problems such as urinary tract infection. Similarly, most patients with proteinuria do not have progressive renal disease (Chapter 343). However it is a rare patient with progressive renal disease who does not have proteinuric abnormalities, even though the proteinuria may be difficult to detect by dipstick methods in patients with polyuria and tubulointerstitial disease rather than glomerular disease, because the protein concentration in their urine is relatively low. An exception is medullary cystic disease, in which urinalysis may be completely normal.

By the time patients present with general symptoms and specific extrarenal abnormalities (Table 348-2), usually at least 75% of renal function has been lost because of the efficacy of the compensatory mechanisms already discussed.

Hypertension may occur early in some patients with progressive renal disease, even before the stage of chronic renal failure; this finding occurs in the more aggressive glomerulonephritides, in connective tissue disorders and vasculitides involving the kidney, in some patients with polycystic kidney disease, and in some with reflux nephropathy. Especially in white patients under the age of 30 years, the physician should remember to consider underlying renal parenchymal disease in patients presenting with even mild hypertension. Patients with evidence of hypertensive damage in brain, retina, or heart may also present with related symptoms and may have hypertension due to renal disease. At least two important risk factors for atherosclerosis are present in chronic renal failure—hypertension and hyperlipidemia; secondary hyperparathyroidism, with deposition of calcium in small blood vessels, may also contribute to the diffuse vascular disease that is not uncommonly found in patients presenting with chronic renal failure.

Common general presenting manifestations are listed in the box above left. Some, such as the alterations in cognitive function and lack of energy, develop so slowly that the patient often does not complain and, indeed, is not aware of them until improvement follows treatment. Sensory peripheral neuropathy is common and should be inquired for, as it may be the harbinger of motor neuropathy, which, unlike the sensory type, may not be reversible with therapy. Anorexia may be associated with vomiting and with negative nitrogen balance and malnutrition. A delayed presentation by the patient or a late diagnosis by the responsible physician prolongs treatment and inhibits rehabilitation, although almost all features of the uremic syndrome eventually respond.

Patients with a systemic illness causing chronic kidney disease most often come to attention because of the primary disease, such as diabetes mellitus, systemic lupus erythematosus, or scleroderma. Diabetic glomerulopathy (Chapter 355) is now the most common cause of ESRD. In insulin-dependent diabetes overt clinical renal disease with fixed proteinuria does not develop until 10 to 15 years after the onset of the disease. More patients, 60%, have diabetic renal disease in association with type II diabetes because it is a much more common variety, but the true duration of disease before the development of renal disease is often difficult to quantitate.

Differential diagnosis

When chronic renal failure is suspected, the physician should (1) rule out acute renal failure, especially that with a possibly reversible cause, (2) rule out reversible extrarenal or renal factors contributing to renal impairment independent of the underlying specific chronic renal disease (see Table 348-2), and (3) seek a specific diagnosis. Late in the course of chronic renal failure, differentiation may not always be possible because specific diagnostic histologic features may have been obscured by the general changes of ESRD (the final common path of nephron adaptation).

Especially when presentation occurs with acute uremia, differentiation between acute and chronic disease can be difficult. *Acute* disease is more often associated with potential reversibility and always indicates a vigorous search for a specific diagnosis.

A history of nocturia or polyuria, or of previous nephrotic or nephritic syndrome, or of long-standing symptoms suggestive of late chronic renal failure (e.g., pruritus), together with findings of bilaterally small or scarred kidneys, severe anemia, hyperphosphatemia, or evidence for some of the chronic systemic complications of chronic renal failure such as renal osteodystrophy, all favor a *chronic* over an acute disease process.

Likely causes of acute deterioration in renal function in patients with chronic renal failure—which may well lead to the initial physician contact—are listed in Table 348-2; a search for these reversible influences is important. They are often caused by the restricted compensatory flexibility of the kidney with a substantially reduced number of nephrons, as discussed earlier. A very careful assessment of vascular and ECF volume and of the potential nephrotoxicity of any ingested drugs is especially necessary.

After treatment of any remediable factors and determination that stable renal failure persists, an orderly approach to specific diagnosis should follow (see boxes on pp. 2629 and 2630). While specific diseases are discussed in various chapters, some salient diagnostic points helpful in differential diagnosis are commented on here. History may reveal a familial renal disease, including the need for renal replacement therapy in relatives, or of a systemic disease such as diabetes mellitus. Especially in the southeastern United States, a history of intake of illicit alcohol, gout, and long-standing hypertension is not infrequent, and lead nephropathy is often suspected though definitive proof is difficult. Initial and persistent denial of analgesic abuse is common. Most patients with chronic glomerulonephritis do not have a history of acute nephritic syndrome preceding it. Renal disease as a presenting feature of diabetes is rare. Most patients with glomerular-level proteinuria continue to excrete large amounts of protein until late in the course of chronic renal failure, but this usually diminishes considerably at the end stage. Patients with progressive primary tubulointerstitial renal disease, especially reflux nephropathy and analgesic abuse nephropathy, may develop a secondary focal glomerulosclerosis with associated glomerular-level proteinuria as part of the adapted nephron syndrome (see Fig. 348-3). Renal ultrasound is completely safe and should be the initial structural screening test. In some patients pelvocaliceal details are needed for specific diagnosis, which requires an excretory urogram, and the potential risks of the nephrotoxicity of radiopaque contrast media must be considered. In reflux nephropathy a voiding cystourethrogram may permit diagnosis and thus avoid intravenous contrast medium injection. Renal stones, including staghorn calculi, and nephrocalcinosis are usually detectable on an abdominal film or on ultrasonography. Tophaceous gout may contribute to, but rarely is a sole cause of, chronic renal failure.

Renovascular renal failure is increasingly being recognized in elderly patients with hypertension, diffuse atherosclerosis and renal impairment, and in some patients, further acute renal deterioration on converting enzyme inhibitors (CEI) even at acceptable blood pressure control levels. This CEI-induced abrupt but reversible drop in GFR can also be seen in severe nephrosclerosis or cardiac failure when GFR has become dependent on angiotensin-II maintained efferent arteriolar constriction. Renal arteriography should be reserved for carefully selected patients. Re-

Classification of causes of chronic renal failure

I. Hereditary
   A. Polycystic kidney disease
   B. Familial glomerulonephritis (Alport's syndrome)
   C. Medullary cystic disease
II. Systemic disease with potential for renal involvement
   A. Diabetes mellitus
   B. Connective tissue disorders
      1. Systemic lupus erythematosus
      2. Polyarteritis nodosa
      3. Scleroderma
      4. Wegener's granulomatosis
   C. Amyloidosis, myeloma kidney, gout
   D. Essential hypertension
III. Primary glomerulonephritis (major progressive types)
   A. Membranous
   B. Membranoproliferative
   C. Focal glomerulosclerosis
IV. Primary tubulointerstitial renal disease
   A. Reflux nephropathy
   B. Analgesic abuse nephropathy
   C. Renal stone disease and nephrocalcinosis
V. Primary vascular renal disease
   A. Hypertensive nephrosclerosis
   B. Bilateral renal artery disease
VI. Obstructive uropathy
   A. Congenital
   B. Stone disease
   C. Prostatic disease

An approach to diagnostic work-up

History
- Familial renal disease or systemic disease involving kidney
- History of analgesic intake
- Nephrotic or nephritic syndrome

Physical examination
- Large "knobby" (polycystic) kidney
- Evidence of systemic disease
- Enlarged bladder with incomplete emptying
- Rectal examination (prostate)
- Renal artery bruit

Urinalysis, 24-hour urine protein, and endogenous creatinine (Cr) clearance
- Proteinuria 3+ or 4+: glomerular disease
- Proteinuria 1+: tubulointerstitial disease
- Bence Jones proteinuria: myeloma kidney
- Red blood cell casts: glomerular disease
- White blood cell casts: tubulointerstitial disease
- Impaired concentrating ability *early* in tubulointerstitial disease (e.g., hypercalcemia)
- Proteinuria >5.0 g/dl: glomerular disease
- Proteinuria <1.5 g/dl: tubulointerstitial disease
- Urinary immunoelectrophoresis: myeloma kidney or light chain disease

Renal ultrasonography; excretory urogram (selected cases) for kidney size and symmetry

Obstruction, polycystic kidneys

Reflux nephropathy (chronic pyelonephritis)

Analgesic nephropathy (papillary necrosis)

Serology
- Complement abnormalities: membranoproliferative glomerulonephritis, systemic lupus erythematosus
- Antinuclear antibodies: systemic lupus erythematosus
- Antineutrophil cytoplasmic antibodies: Wegener's or polyarteritis nodosa
- Serum immunoelectrophoresis: myeloma
- Serum chemistries: hypercalcemia; severe hyperuricemia

Renal biopsy (selected cases)
- Evidence for glomerular disease: relatively well preserved kidney and symmetric kidney size are relative indications

Renal angiogram (highly selected cases)
- Suspected bilateral renal arterial disease

nal angioplasty or renovascular surgery may preserve function. Renal biopsy is occasionally indicated, especially if renal size is well maintained.

As should now be evident, the disease process is relatively slow and is silent unless the patient with chronic renal failure has an early acute event such as edema or hematuria, or an incidental urinalysis or measurement of BUN or serum creatinine level. Renal symptoms are usually absent, except for nocturia, until uremic symptoms develop. After discussing prevention of ESRD, next, we will review the signs and symptoms relevant to each organ system in patients with late renal failure both before and after dialysis treatment.

PREVENTION OR DELAY OF END-STAGE RENAL DISEASE

At present, if the diagnosis is made early enough, we have the ability to prevent progression in reflux nephropathy, analgesic nephropathy (if the patient discontinues intake), recurrent stone disease, and obstructive uropathy. It is certain that treatment of essential hypertension is protective for cardiovascular damage but not yet clear that it prevents, although it does slow, the development of chronic renal failure due to nephrosclerosis, especially in black patients. Similarly, euglycemic control of diabetes mellitus and careful blood pressure control with converting enzyme inhibitors, if used consistently before the onset of microangiopathy and fixed proteinuria, may forestall diabetic glomerulopathy. As discussed in Chapter 354, there is as yet little convincing evidence of the availability of specific, effective curative treatment for most of the glomerulonephritides.

An important question under intense current investigation is whether the development of nephron trade-off in the adapted nephron syndrome can be modified or slowed, especially when the primary disease process is no longer active. In polycystic kidney disease, for example, cysts continue to enlarge and compress remaining nephrons, and in some glomerulonephritides there is continuing immunologic attack. Nevertheless, when the inciting pathology is quiescent, it is a highly desirable goal to preserve the remaining nephrons; at any level of endogenous function above a GFR of 10 to 15 ml/min, this is far preferable to dialysis.

The major documented beneficial intervention is careful control of blood pressure. CEI and calcium channel blockers may offer additional advantages over other antihypertensives. Dietary protein restriction to around 0.6 g/kg body weight is indicated because of impressive animal and some clinical studies on the effects of protein restriction. Certainly a high protein diet should be avoided because of evidence that it increases intraglomerular flow and pressure. Control of serum phosphate and prevention of secondary hyperparathyroidism, and treatment of hyperlipidemia may all be indicated but specific benefit in human disease is not yet documented. Expert nutritional support is essential to maintain an appropriate caloric, phosphate, and nitrogen intake and avoid negative nitrogen balance.

ORGAN SYSTEM COMPLICATIONS OF CHRONIC AND END-STAGE RENAL DISEASE

Hematologic disorders

Anemia. A normochromic normocytic anemia is a consistent finding in chronic renal failure. As the GFR falls below 40 ml/min, the hematocrit decreases in proportion to the degree of renal insufficiency until a value of approximately 20% is reached with ESRD. Decreased or absent erythropoietin is the primary event underlying the anemia. As renal mass decreases, erythropoietin falls, leading to decreased red blood cell production by the bone marrow. Patients with polycystic kidney disease tend to have a higher hematocrit relative to the stage of renal failure, even while on dialysis. Recombinant human erythropoietin can now be used to treat renal anemia effectively and improve well-being in patients with chronic renal failure; however, it is expensive. Gastrointestinal bleeding is quite common and should be looked for especially if the response to erythropoietin is less than anticipated. Erythropoietin is now used routinely (intravenously or subcutaneously) in dialysis patients if hematocrit does not reach 30% to 35%. Lack of response to erythropoietin should suggest a search for iron-deficiency, aluminum-related or hyperparathyroid bone disease, inflammatory or neoplastic disease, or malnutrition. The availability of erythropoietin constitutes one of the largest advances in treatment for dialysis patients.

Coagulation abnormalities. A bleeding tendency manifested by epistaxis, menorrhagia, gastrointestinal bleeding, and prominent bruising after trauma is common in advanced renal failure. Patients with chronic renal failure have a qualitative defect in platelet function and abnormal factor VIII function. This condition is manifested as a prolonged bleeding time, although the partial thromboplastin time, prothrombin time, and clotting time are all within normal limits. The factors in uremic serum that induce the qualitative platelet defect are not well delineated, but dialysis does correct the defect; cryoprecipitate, DDAVP and conjugated estrogens may also help to alleviate uremic bleeding. The serum concentrations of the various proteins of the coagulation cascade are usually within normal limits unless the patient has the nephrotic syndrome in addition to chronic renal failure. However, plasma fibrinogen levels may be increased in renal failure, which may play a role in the increased erythrocyte sedimentation rate disproportionate to the anemia seen in uremia. Plasma fibrinolytic activity is decreased but improves after hemodialysis.

Hypertension

Hypertension may complicate chronic parenchymal renal disease even before azotemia develops, as in polycystic kidney disease or membranoproliferative glomerulonephritis. In most patients it develops later, and by end stage it occurs in 80% of patients. As noted, essential hypertension may also cause nephrosclerosis and progressive renal disease, especially in blacks. Even in such patients in whom hypertension appears to be primary, however, there is evidence for participation of a functional or structural renal abnormality in the pathogenesis of essential hypertension (Chapter 23).

The treatment of hypertension in patients with chronic renal failure at all stages is important. Otherwise, it is very likely to become more severe, accelerate loss of nephrons via nephrosclerosis, and likely also contribute to the high intraglomerular pressures thought to cause glomerular loss (nephron trade-off). CEI may offer some benefits for reducing intraglomerular pressure, especially in diabetic glomerulopathy.

Hypertension likely is due to elevated renin production in the kidneys and some sodium chloride retention even though overt edema may not be present. Plasma renin levels are high for the degree of ECF volume expansion. Accordingly, treatment usually begins with modest salt restriction and then, if needed, a loop diuretic such as furosemide (thiazides lose their effectiveness as the GFR falls below 40 ml/min). A third factor that may contribute to the hypertension is the failure of the diseased kidneys to produce physiologic vasodepressors (e.g., certain prostaglandins and a neutral lipid produced in the renal medulla).

At initiation of treatment, care must be taken not to superimpose prerenal azotemia, although a slight but usually reversible drop in GFR may occur early after blood pressure is restored to normal levels, especially in patients with more severe hypertension. In accelerated-phase or malignant hypertension, effective treatment of hypertension should be maintained, even though apparent ESRD develops and necessitates dialysis because the risk of developing hypertension-induced cerebrovascular and cardiovascular problems is otherwise too great. In such patients recovery of renal function after a few months occasionally occurs and allows cessation of dialysis treatment, for at least some months or even years. This recovery is thought to be due to healing of fibrinoid necrotic lesions in small arterioles as blood pressure control is maintained.

Once dialysis therapy is initiated, blood pressure usually can be regulated again by control of plasma volume with dialysis, ultrafiltration, and modest dietary restriction of salt. Hypertension in anephric dialysis patients is almost always due to excess volume.

Renal hypertension can be very severe and resistant to hypotensive drugs; formerly, bilateral nephrectomy was sometimes required for control of blood pressure but is now only used occasionally after successful renal transplantation. Fortunately, this is virtually never required now because of the efficacy of the converting enzyme inhibitors and the calcium channel blockers. If hypertension cannot be controlled by dialysis, hypotensive drugs can be used as in patients before dialysis. However, diuretic drugs have little or no place in patients on regular dialysis, and such patients may need to omit medications immediately before dialysis because of hypotension as ultrafiltration proceeds especially in patients with autonomic nerve insufficiency due to either chronic renal failure per se or diabetes.

A well-functioning renal allograft can cure hypertension; nevertheless, hypertension recurs in about 50% of renal transplant recipients on follow-up due to cyclosporine (which leads to renal vasoconstriction), chronic rejection, allograft renal artery stenosis, and renin effects of the native kidneys on the allograft.

Cardiopulmonary complications

Cardiovascular disease is the most important cause of death in patients on dialysis, and hypertension is the most important risk factor. Long-term survival (20 years) has now been demonstrated in chronic dialysis patients, and all of these long-term survivors have been maintained normotensive. Other risk factors for atherosclerosis are hyperlipidemia, smoking, hyperparathyroidism with vascular calcification, carbohydrate intolerance, and hyperuricemia. It is unlikely that the dialysis procedure itself causes accelerated atherosclerosis. Other common cardiovascular abnormalities seen are congestive heart failure, uremic pericarditis and effusion, in some cases with cardiac tamponade, and dysrhythmias, often associated with hyperkalemia.

The combination of hypertension, anemia, fluid overload, and acidosis all contribute to the uremic patient's increased tendency toward the development of congestive heart failure. Pulmonary edema may be the first manifestation of congestive heart failure in the patient with advanced renal disease, and this edema is often due to excess ECF volume. However, increased pulmonary capillary permeability, decreased oncotic pressure, and left ventricular dysfunction also may be present and contribute to the genesis of the disorder. Of course, cardiac disease of all types may coexist with renal failure and must be considered in patients with renal disease and congestive heart failure. The existence of a true uremic cardiomyopathy due to uremic toxins, independent of the above causes of ventricular failure, is not widely accepted. Metastatic calcification of the lungs and heart can be seen in far-advanced renal failure and may relate to secondary hyperparathyroidism, hyperphosphatemia, or vitamin D administration.

Pericarditis occurs in approximately half of undialyzed patients with chronic renal disease in whom terminal uremia develops. Before dialytic and transplantation therapy became available, pericarditis in the several days before death from uremia was a common event; aggressive dialytic therapy is usually effective in reversing the clinical manifestations of pericarditis. *Uremic serositis* includes pericarditis, ascites, and pleural effusion; and several, or only one, of these may manifest themselves in a single patient. These effusions are characteristically exudates and are made worse by fluid overload; other causes must be considered, for example, infection or malignant disease, especially if the effusions are not controlled by dialysis and fluid removal as indicated. The pathogenesis of uremic serositis is unknown but may relate to an effect of uremic toxins on capillary permeability. Serositis with or without effusion also occurs in chronic dialysis patients and indeed is now more commonly seen in these circumstances. The frequency of dialysis is often increased to daily, and the problem may then resolve. Because the pericardial effusion is most often hemorrhagic, heparin must be used with great caution. For increasing effusion and cardiac tamponade, the patient must be observed in the hospital. Tamponade requires pericardial stripping or pericardiocentesis and instillation of a nonreabsorbable steroid.

Uremic pneumonitis has been suggested as a diagnosis in certain patients with ESRD who show a characteristic radiographic appearance of perihilar vascular congestion with clear peripheral lung fields. Several authors have suggested that this characteristic is observed in uremic patients in the absence of circulatory overload. The concept of uremic pneumonitis as a separate entity, however, has not gained wide acceptance. Instead, the consensus is that the characteristic probably relates to circulatory overload in these patients.

Neuromuscular abnormalities

The central nervous system and peripheral nerves are affected, with diverse consequences. Nerve conduction time characteristically is prolonged; peripheral neuropathy may develop in advanced uremia; sleep patterns are disturbed; and asterixis, convulsions, and psychosis all may occur. The early changes of uremic encephalopathy are subtle. They consist of insomnia, inability to concentrate, lack of alertness, and slowing of cerebration. Ultimately, there may be loss of memory, confusion, hallucinations, and delirium or obtundation. Convulsions occur in about one third of the patients nearing terminal uremia. The electroencephalogram in uremia shows a "slow-wave pattern," which may be related to increased calcium in the brain, which in turn may be caused by high levels of circulating parathyroid hormone. Autonomic neuropathy occurs and can contribute to impotence in the male, absence of sweating, and dialysis hypotension. Cramps of various limb muscles, intermittent numbness and tingling of the hands and feet, and the "restless leg" syndrome (uncomfortable sensations in the legs occurring during rest and relieved by movement) are common in late chronic renal failure and during long-term hemodialysis. Shifts in water and electrolytes may in some way account for this syndrome and may also account for muscle cramps and distal limb paresthesias. With dialysis, overt clinical neuropathy is rare, and a subclinical form may be present in which only nerve conduction studies or special tests of cutaneous sensation are abnormal. Asymptomatic uremic neuropathy occurs in at least 50% of all patients who reach ESRD or who are on long-term hemodialysis.

Gastrointestinal disturbances

Gastrointestinal symptoms attributable to chronic renal failure usually do not appear until the GFR falls below 10 ml/min. Early symptoms include anorexia, nausea, and vomiting; the latter two symptoms are most prominent in the early morning, when vomiting may be a daily event. Early morning vomiting usually alleviates further nausea during the day, when appetite improves, allowing adequate oral intake.

Gastrointestinal bleeding is common in chronic renal failure. It may occur at any site, from the stomach to the rectum. The lesions found most commonly are shallow, small ulcers that bleed slowly. Mucosal ulcerations are a prominent feature of advanced uremia and occur along virtually the entire gastrointestinal tract. Superficial erosions of the buccal and gingival mucosa may occur; these lesions may also involve the tongue, lips, or larynx (uremic stomatitis). The stomach and the duodenum are also subject to superficial erosions and frequently are the site of chronic blood loss. More advanced peptic ulcerations are also observed in uremia, although gastric acid secretion is depressed in 40% of patients, while the other 60% have normal gastric acid secretion.

Immunoreactive plasma gastrin values increase progressively with renal failure. This increase may represent true gastrin or small peptides with gastrinlike antigen structure accumulating in plasma because of the inability of the diseased kidney to metabolize low molecular weight proteins.

Other gastrointestinal manifestations include colitis, ileus, parotitis, and, as already noted, ascites. Bloody diarrhea and abdominal cramps resulting from colonic ulcerations (uremic colitis) have been attributed to local irritation of the colonic mucosa by ammonia produced by the intestinal flora. Pancreatitis and parotitis occur with increased frequency in chronic uremia. However, the diagnosis is hampered by the frequent finding of elevated serum amylase in uremia as a result of decreased renal amylase clearance. Gastrointestinal-related hormones, such as cholecystokinin, gastric inhibitory polypeptide, and glucagon, all are elevated in the serum of patients with chronic renal failure. These elevations may be due to increased secretion and/or to failure of the diseased kidney to metabolize these hormones or their constituents. Small bowel and colonic bleeding in chronic dialysis patients is sometimes recurrent and due to angiodysplastic lesions, which are difficult to diagnose and treat. Heparinization during hemodialysis may precipitate bleeding.

After transplantation, two major life-threatening gastrointestinal complications occur. Upper gastrointestinal bleeding resulting from gastritis or peptic ulcer disease is seen in 5% to 10% of recipients, while bowel perforation due to ruptured diverticula is especially common in elderly patients. Symptoms may be masked by steroids.

Immunologic and infectious complications

Infection is a common cause of death in both acute renal failure and the terminal stages of chronic renal failure. Such patients are often malnourished or have other complications that predispose them to infection. Most infections in patients on dialysis are due to gram-positive organisms. Vascular and peritoneal accesses are common sites of infection. Pruritus may lead to skin infection by chronic scratching. The delayed wound healing seen in uremia probably plays a role in the increased incidence of postoperative and posttraumatic infections. However, additional factors that impair both cellular and humoral immunologic defenses likely underlie the increased incidence of infection in uremia.

Although granulocyte counts, total immunoglobulin, and complement levels are usually normal, polymorphonuclear leukocyte, T-cell, and B-cell functions are impaired in ESRD. Hence, some antibody responses and cell-mediated, immune, chemotactic, and phagocytic abnormalities are present.

As a general rule, diminished immunity has been associated with the predisposition to viral and fungal diseases. Exposure to serum hepatitis virus in hemodialysis units has provided a unique setting for comparing the responses to viral infections in normal and uremic subjects. The course of the disease in staff members who contract hepatitis in these units is characterized by acute liver damage, elevations of enzymes and bilirubin, and liver tenderness and enlargement, and is followed by recovery within 1 to 2 months. On the other hand, subacute hepatitis with mild to moderate, or no, clinical evidence of liver damage often develops in patients with uremia, but the course is protracted, and viremia persists for years.

These observations suggest impairment of host immune defenses. Uremic patients as a group have mild but not grossly impaired antibody responses, opsonic activity, and in vitro phagocytic capacity. Immunization for hepatitis B and influenza viruses is less effective than in normal persons but should still be offered.

By far the most dreaded complication of transplantation is infection, the leading early cause of death among allograft recipients. During the first posttransplant month, opportunistic infections are unusual, and the major infectious disease hazards are similar to those in other patients undergoing major urologic surgery (i.e., atelectasis with pulmonary wound, urinary tract, and intravenous line infections). The period between 1 and 6 months after transplantation, which coincides with attempts to reverse rejection episodes by high dose immunosuppressive therapy, is when the most dangerous opportunistic viral, fungal, and protozoan infections occur. Often, infection with cytomegalovirus precedes infection with other, potentially more dangerous microbes such as *Pneumocystis carinii*. Cytomegalovirus infection is especially common in patients lacking circulating anticytomegalovirus antibodies who have received a graft from a donor previously infected with cytomegalovirus. If this situation cannot be avoided, hyperimmune globulin and acyclovir may be given prophylactically. Acyclovir and bactrim are often also given prophylactically after transplant, especially for herpes simplex and *Pneumocystis*. The dire consequences of imprecise or delayed treatment in these immunosuppressed hosts dictate early antibiotic therapy and an aggressive and exacting approach to identifying the organism, its susceptibility to antimicrobial agents, and the site or sites of infection. For example, lung infection usually indicates urgent bronchoscopy.

Chronic progressive liver disease, likely related to chronic hepatitis B or C viral infection, is an important and eventually usually lethal late (3 to 10 years) complication of transplantation.

Renal osteodystrophy, hyperphosphatemia, hypocalcemia, bone and joint disease

For the reasons discussed earlier, progressive loss of renal mass ultimately leads to derangements in mineral and skeletal metabolism. Elevated levels of parathyroid hormone, a consequence of both increased secretion and decreased degradation, lead to increased bone reabsorption, especially subperiosteally, and reduced bone density may be found on x-ray examination. The serum levels of alkaline phosphatase are elevated. Decreased conversion of vitamin D to a more active form, $1,25(OH)_2$-vitamin D_3, results in decreased intestinal absorption of calcium and potentially in osteomalacia. Metabolic acidosis also contributes to bone disease by causing titration of the calcium carbonate salts of bone and leading to their dissolution.

Renal osteodystrophy is a common complication of chronic renal disease both before and after dialysis (see Fig. 348-4), is characterized histologically by several alterations in bone structure, including osteomalacia, secondary hyperparathyroidism, and, less commonly, osteosclerosis. Osteitis fibrosa cystica reflects the reabsorptive effect of increased osteoclastic activity due to secondary hyperparathyroidism, and osteomalacia a defect in bone mineralization that is secondary, at least in part, to alterations in the metabolism of vitamin D and is characterized by a widening of the osteoid seam and an absent or abnormal mineralization front. Less commonly, osteoporosis is seen in uremic patients.

These abnormalities of bone, calcium and phosphorus, vitamin D metabolism, and parathyroid hormone secretion can have devastating effects on patients. In children, there may be retardation of growth. In the adult, bone pain, fractures, collapse of vertebrae, necrosis of femoral heads, and skeletal deformities may occur. Along with osteitis fibrosa cystica, there may be metastatic calcification and medial calcification of arteries, with ischemic necrosis, calcification of soft tissues and skin, intractable pruritus, periarthritis from calcium hydroxyapatite precipitation, conjunctival calcification, and so on. This syndrome may necessitate subtotal parathyroidectomy (removal of three and a half glands).

Attempts to prevent renal osteodystrophy optimally now start early in the course of chronic renal failure. Recommended measures include dietary phosphate restriction, often usefully combined with protein restriction, prescription of calcitriol with careful follow-up of serum calcium and phosphorus to avoid hypercalcemia, and use of intestinal phosphate binders as necessary. Parathyroid levels are monitored to assess success in avoiding or minimizing secondary hyperparathyroidism. Ensuring near normal serum calcium and phosphorus levels also may help prevent progression of renal disease, as already discussed, as well as soft tissue and vascular calcification. Calcium carbonate or calcium acetate are preferred for phosphate-binding, because the use of aluminum-containing antacids as binders contributes to aluminum-related bone and muscle disease and microcytic hypochronic anemia.

Phosphate clearances on dialysis on an adequate protein and caloric intake are insufficient to control serum phosphate and binders must be continued. Aluminum-contained antacids should only be used for short periods to aid in controlling severe hyperphosphatemia, which should then be controlled by calcium carbonate or acetate, with monitoring of serum calcium to avoid hypercalcemia. If the latter remains a problem, dialysate calcium can be lowered and/or judicious amounts of magnesium-containing antacids can be used. Persistent hypocalcemia should be treated with calcitriol to avoid secondary hyperparathyroidism. These preventive measures have much reduced symptomatic renal osteodystrophy and the need for subtotal parathyroidectomy. The latter is still occasionally required for hypercalcemia or in a noncompliant patient with severe bone disease or extraosseous calcification.

Before virtual cessation of the chronic use of aluminum-containing antacids and efficient removal of aluminum from dialysate water, dialysis dementia, myopathy, anemia, osteodystrophy (unresponsive to calcitriol or measures to reduce parathormone levels and sometimes associated with hypercalcemia and severe bone pain and fractures) were seen quite frequently. When they occur now these consequences of aluminum intoxication can be treated with the chelating agent deferoxamine during hemodialysis. Calcium citrate must not be used as a phosphate-binding agent because it increases aluminum absorption from the gut.

After a successful renal transplantation, a phosphate diuresis promptly ensues. Usually, but not always, the transplanted organ promptly converts vitamin D to 1,25$(OH)_2$-vitamin D_3. In contrast, resolution of severe hyperparathyroidism is far more gradual. Posttransplantation osteodystrophy usually improves as normal vitamin D metabolism is restored, aluminum deposition secondary to intake of oral gels and hemodialysis reverses, and hyperparathyroidism resolves. In contrast, osteopenia secondary to steroid intake becomes manifest. A more feared complication, osteonecrosis, occurs in 5% of all patients; the head of the femur is the most common site.

Secondary gout may occur in chronic renal failure due to hyperuricemia, usually in those with a family history of gout. Allopurinol should not be used routinely for prophylaxis but only after gout has been firmly diagnosed (and it should be noted that the breakdown of azathioprine is much reduced in patients receiving allopurinol). Pseudogout mimics gout but joint aspiration does not reveal uric acid but rather calcium pyrophosphate crystals; associated chondrocalcinosis is common, and, like gout, it responds well to prostaglandin inhibitors such as indomethacin.

Another new form of bone and joint disease recognized in patients on dialysis for 5 to 10 years or more is due to the accumulation of an amyloid-like substance formed from beta-2 microglobulin (a normal protein of 11,800 daltons). The normal levels of the latter of 1 to 2 mg/L rise to 50 to 100 mg/L in late chronic dialysis patients because dialyzer clearance is inadequate. The clinical syndrome due to beta-2 amyloidosis include carpal tunnel, destructive osteoarthropathy of large joints, bone cysts, and pathologic fractures. Visceral deposition appears to be less common, and the reason for the atypical distribution of deposits is not known. There is no specific treatment except for surgery (e.g., for carpal tunnel syndrome), but prevalence may be less in those dialyzed by more permeable membranes (e.g., polysulphone).

Nutritional and metabolic alterations

Disorders of nitrogen metabolism. The occurrence of protein malnutrition in advanced uremia and the persistence of this disorder in some patients on long-term dialysis have stimulated the study of nitrogen, amino acid, and protein metabolism in chronic renal failure. The nutritional status of patients with uremia and those on dialysis has, no doubt, been greatly improved in recent years because of early initiation of dialysis and close attention to nutritional problems. Some observations indicate, however, that a lesser but significant degree of protein malnutrition may still be prevalent. Extravascular pools of albumin may be reduced, though serum albumin concentration is normal. Serum concentration of transferrin, possibly a better indicator of protein malnutrition, has been found to be low in many patients with moderate to advanced renal failure.

Although inadequate protein and/or caloric intake may well be the major cause of malnutrition in chronic renal failure, the possibility persists that one or more steps in the complex process of protein synthesis is disturbed by renal failure per se. The signs and symptoms of chronic malnutrition include loss of subcutaneous fat, dryness and scaling of the skin, and muscle atrophy and weakness. In children, modest to marked retardation of growth may be observed. Analysis of body composition may reveal a decrease in lean body mass and an increase in total body water, with an expanded ECF volume and a shrunken intracellular volume. The levels of certain amino acids are altered in plasma or muscle. A low serum albumin in dialysis patients is associated with a poorer prognosis.

Disorders of carbohydrate metabolism. Fasting blood glucose, when measured, is normal or slightly elevated in uremia. However, after oral or intravenous administration of glucose loads, carbohydrate tolerance is impaired in uremia. Several factors may be responsible for this abnormality. Skeletal muscle shows resistance to the action of insulin on glucose uptake and uremia reduces insulin release. Increased levels of growth hormone present in uremia may also contribute to the resistance of peripheral tissues to the action of insulin. Basal insulin levels in uremic patients are usually increased, presumably as a consequence of a decreased rate of renal removal of insulin. Although glucagon levels are elevated in uremia, their contribution to the glucose intolerance is not clear. In addition, increased gluconeogenesis and increased hepatic glucose release have also been proposed as mechanisms responsible for carbohydrate intolerance in uremic subjects. Other factors, such as acidosis, potassium depletion, hypermagnesemia, and increased levels of parathyroid hormone, may also play a role in the glucose intolerance of the uremic state.

It has been demonstrated that carbohydrate tolerance improves after hemodialysis and that the response of peripheral tissues to insulin is increased. Diabetic patients with progressive renal disease require diminishing doses of insulin as the disease progresses. Reduced caloric intake and weight loss, plus a reduced renal degradation of insulin, probably play a role in this decreased insulin requirement.

Steroid-induced diabetes mellitus occurs in 5% to 10% of all graft recipients. Ketoacidosis is rarely noted, and the steroid-induced diabetes may remit with reductions of steroid dosage.

Disorders of lipid metabolism. Uremic patients have elevated serum levels of triglycerides and lipoproteins. There is a decreased rate of removal of triglycerides from the plasma, as well as decreased activity of lipoprotein lipase and increased hepatic synthesis of very low density lipoproteins. The plasma levels of high-density, alpha-lipoprotein and low-density, cholesterol-rich lipoprotein are decreased. Plasma cholesterol levels are usually normal in uremia but elevated after renal transplantation. In renal failure, these abnormalities of carbohydrate and lipid metabolism presumably contribute to increased risk of atherogenesis, which may be troublesome in patients on chronic dialysis. Disturbances of lipid metabolism also occur in nephrotic patients (Chapter 171) with and without chronic renal insufficiency. A majority of patients with uremia and hyperlipidemia, however, are not nephrotic; moreover, their lipid profile differs from that of nephrotic patients who have increased cholesterol levels.

Abnormalities in endocrine function

Uremia alters virtually all hormones in the body, either in amount or in their effect. Not only are the hormones arising within the kidney affected by renal failure, but also those being produced elsewhere. The levels of calcitonin in plasma, as determined by radioimmunoassay, are elevated, probably as a result of a decreased rate of metabolic clearance by the kidney.

Patients with renal failure can appear hypothyroid and abnormalities in thyroid function tests are common; these abnormalities include normal free T4 but low free T3 levels (diminished T4 to T3 conversion in periphery) and diminished binding of T4 to thyroid-binding globulin. A sensitive thyroid-stimulating hormone (TSH) assay is the most helpful test for true hypothyroidism.

Gonadal dysfunction is characteristic of ESRD. Menstrual irregularities are very frequent; menstruation often ceases completely in ESRD, and amenorrhea may persist on dialysis. Menorrhagia occasionally occurs secondary to the hemostatic defect if menses recur. When GFR values fall below 20 ml/min, both conception and the ability to complete a pregnancy are severely impaired. Impotence and a diminished sperm count are common in men with chronic renal failure.

These abnormalities in both men and women are secondary to gonadal resistance to the effects of follicle-stimulating hormone and luteinizing hormone, to complex hypothalamic-pituitary disturbances, and to hyperprolactinemia. Men have diminished concentrations of testosterone in plasma, and both progesterone and estrogen are diminished in women. Gynecomastia is sometimes seen before, and despite, dialysis treatment. In men, administration of testosterone has been shown to suppress plasma luteinizing hormone, although with a slightly delayed response. Thus in the patient with chronic renal failure, gonadal resistance to the effect of pituitary trophic hormones is a major factor in sexual inadequacy. Depression is not uncommon in dialysis patients, and it may contribute, along with insomnia and poor nutritional intake, to sexual dysfunction.

TREATMENT

Treatment for chronic renal failure can be divided into *conservative treatment* and, for ESRD, *renal replacement therapy*. After general and comparative discussion of treatment here, the sections DIALYSIS and RENAL TRANSPLANTATION take up these topics in more detail.

Conservative treatment

Conservative treatment would include specific measures, if available, for the disease causing chronic renal failure. General measures, to prevent nephron trade-off have been discussed. All patients on conservative therapy should have renal function, serum electrolytes, calcium and phosphorus, and hematocrit monitored regularly after serum creatinine exceeds 2.5 to 3.0 mg/dl. Individual patients with chronic renal failure tend to deteriorate at a constant rate; this may best be seen when the reciprocal of the serum creatinine level is plotted serially. An accelerated rate of deterioration should engender a search for the remediable factors already discussed. Measures to prevent hyperphosphatemia and renal bone disease should be initiated. As discussed, even mild elevation of blood pressure should be treated; otherwise, it virtually always becomes more severe and leads to further deterioration of renal function. If serum bicarbonate falls below 20 mEq/L, exogenous bicarbonate in small amounts is indicated (each 650-mg tablet of sodium bicarbonate contains 8 mEq each of sodium and of bicarbonate). Each gram of protein in the diet leads to production of approximately 1 mEq of hydrogen ions. Usually, in the absence of renal tubular acidosis and frank bicarbonate wasting, 3 or 4 sodium bicarbonate tablets per day are adequate.

Chronic metabolic acidosis should be avoided for several reasons. First, hydrogen ions may be buffered, to some extent, by bone, which would worsen renal osteodystrophy. Second, chronic acidosis may cause symptoms such as malaise and dyspnea. Third, bicarbonate therapy should help to maintain plasma bicarbonate and prevent life-threatening acidemia, especially if an acute problem develops that leads to catabolism and increased production of hydrogen ions.

Care must be taken with all potentially nephrotoxic drugs and in determining the dosage of all drugs that are excreted substantially by the renal route. Several useful drug dosage lists are maintained and should be consulted regularly by physicians seeing patients with chronic renal failure. If no alternative is available, potentially nephrotoxic drugs such as the aminoglycosides can be used with appropriate modification in dosage or dosing intervals; but, whenever feasible, monitoring of serum levels is indicated. Digoxin dosage always has to be reduced below normal maintenance levels. Glycoside-induced anorexia and vomiting can be confused with uremia.

Dietary salt restriction should be instituted only for management of edema, hypertension, or congestive heart failure. However, most patients with GFR approaching 10 to 15 ml/min do require modest salt restriction (1 to 2 g sodium or 44 to 88 mEq Na^+ in the diet). Potassium restriction (40 to 50 mEq K^+) is usually not needed until GFR approaches 10 ml/min unless specific tubular defects are present. As noted, however, increased potassium intake is tolerated poorly, and potassium supplements with diuretics and "potassium sparing" diuretics such as spironolactone should generally be avoided. Beta-blockers, nonsteroidal anti-inflammatory drugs (NSAIDS), and converting enzyme inhibitors also increase the risk of hyperkalemia.

Restriction to 0.6 g/kg of dietary protein usually allows maintained nitrogen balance if there is an adequate caloric intake and controls or postpones uremic symptoms. Compliance with prescribed dietary protein restriction may be checked by observing the BUN/creatinine ratio, which should be less than the normal 10:1 in patients ingesting a low protein diet with adequate caloric intake, and by measuring urinary urea excretion. Reduction of protein intake for control of uremic symptoms should not be to levels below 0.6 g/kg body weight to avoid negative nitrogen balance and muscle wasting. Instead, renal replacement therapy should be started. A commonly used but never routinely prescribed diet in the later stages of conservative treatment is 0.8 g protein/kg body weight (plus an allowance for urinary protein losses if still high), 2 g Na^+ (88 mEq), and 40 mEq K^+. In some patients hyperkalemia also requires the oral administration of sodium-potassium exchange resins; 1 g of sodium polystyrene sulfonate (Kayexalate) will bind approximately 1 mEq of potassium. However, the sodium-potassium exchange process results in a net gain of sodium and dialysis needs to be instituted if hyperkalemia returns. Fluid restriction is not required unless there is significant hyponatremia, but fluid should not be pushed beyond what thirst dictates.

Planning for renal replacement therapy should begin well before ESRD has been reached; ESRD begins usually at a GFR of 5 to 10 ml/min (serum creatinine >7 to 8 mg/dl in women and >10 to 12 mg/dl in men). An arteriovenous fistula between radial artery and cephalic vein is constructed a few months before dialysis is required. If the vessels are unsuitable, a synthetic arteriovenous graft is inserted a few weeks before dialysis is to begin. These procedures are usually performed under local or regional anesthesia. Neither of these procedures offers immediately available access to the blood for dialysis and, in emergency, access is obtained via a subclavian or femoral venous catheter. The former can be maintained for a few weeks. A full explanation of the various treatment options available should be given to the patient. This procedure may require several visits to a renal treatment center. If live donor transplant is feasible, arrangements are made for tissue typing of family members. Proper planning and preparation of the patient allows efficient initiation of renal replacement therapy and avoids complications and catastrophes. Patients who present late with uremic symptoms often require long hospitalizations and experience delayed rehabilitation and even increased mortality rates.

Timing of initiation of renal replacement therapy requires careful and regular evaluation of patient well-being as well as of serum chemistries. The goal is to avoid, on the one hand, a uremic trough of illness, but, on the other hand, not to initiate expensive therapy prematurely. It is unusual for a patient not to need such treatment after serum creatinine is greater than 10 mg/dl in women and greater than 15 mg/dl in men. Congestive heart failure or fluid retention, severe anemia, severe hypertension, hyperkalemia, and sensory peripheral neuropathy all may indicate earlier initiation. Severe uremic complications (e.g., pericarditis) usually result from too long a delay in initiating renal replacement therapy. In patients with diabetic glomerulosclerosis, there is an increasing tendency to initiate replacement therapy earlier (serum creatinine 5 to 8 mg/dl) than in primary renal disease, because there is a compounding of many of the features of diabetic microangiopathy by uremia.

Renal replacement therapy

Although all patients with chronic renal failure nearing ESRD should be considered for renal replacement therapy, the obligation to the patient is not to provide such care uncritically but, rather, to determine if the patient will benefit from it. Patients with intractable, irremediable, severely disabling disease in other organ systems who would clearly not benefit from dialysis or transplantation should receive only conservative treatment. In cases of doubt as to benefit, and with the agreement of patient and family, a trial of dialysis can be initiated; later cessation of dialysis by mutual consent of physician, patient, and family is ethical. Chronic dialysis in patients with established AIDS and ESRD extends life in most patients by only a few weeks and is, in general, not indicated; however, each patient should be evaluated individually.

Chronic or acute dialysis in asymptomatic HIV carriers, but not renal transplantation, is usually indicated for acute or chronic renal failure. The various options for renal replacement therapy are summarized in Fig. 348-5. To date the number of patients on chronic dialysis (currently approximately 150,000) has not reached a plateau because the annual mortality (18% if all age groups are included) plus the annual successful transplantation rate (currently about 8,000 of the 10,000 performed) has not yet become equal to the annual influx of about 40,000 new patients with ESRD. Only 25% of patients developing ESRD are receiving transplanted kidneys; the fraction retaining such kidneys for many years is, of course, smaller. Thus until more kidneys are available and until the allograft survival rate for cadaveric transplantation improves further, most patients will require some form of dialysis to survive. The various forms of renal replacement should be highly integrated (Fig. 348-5); many patients will receive various forms at different times. Some patients who receive live donor kidneys now do so without preliminary dialysis. Forty percent of patients now entering ESRD treatment programs are over age 65, and most patients receiving a transplant are less than age 50; thus most patients under 50 years receive at least one renal transplant. The growth of continuous ambulatory peritoneal dialysis (CAPD) has been dramatic and is substantially responsible for the 20% of patients on dialysis outside a center. The patient should be fully informed about all appropriate options and involved in the choice of treatment. Important differences among the main treatment alternatives can be seen in Table 348-3.

Younger patients without major extrarenal disease fare very well, at least in the short term, with all three modes of renal replacement treatment. Children are best managed by CAPD first, then renal transplantation when feasible (the incidence of children reaching ESRD is relatively small (12 million/year). Live donor transplantation offers the best results in virtually all patients except the elderly, in the absence of contraindications to transplantation. There is now no specific age limit for transplantation, but most patients over 60 are still managed by dialysis.

Home dialysis and CAPD encourage patient interest, motivation, and self-help. Patient education for CAPD takes about 1 week compared with 6 weeks for home hemodialysis. CAPD allows more mobility and does not require a partner, in contrast to home hemodialysis. These methods are cheaper than in-center hemodialysis and are encouraged by the Medicare program by financial incentives

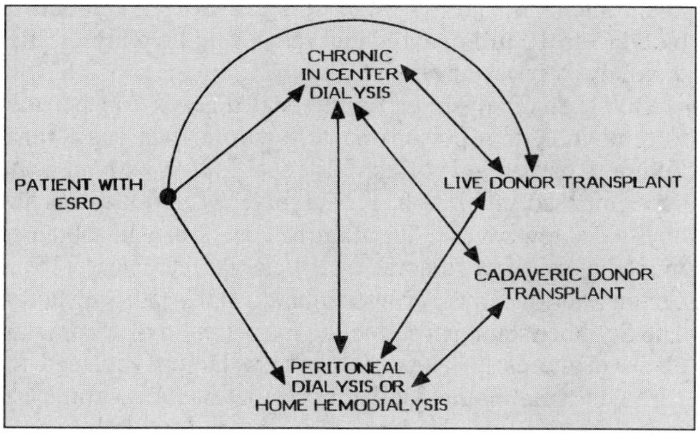

Fig. 348-5. Interrelationships between types of renal replacement therapy. The success of transplantation is aided by the ready availability of dialysis if the allograft fails.

Table 348-3. Renal replacement therapy: important clinical differences among major alternatives

	Hemodialysis	CAPD	Transplant
Dependence on machine	Yes	No	No
Excretory function	10% of normal	<10% of normal	May be normal
Endocrine function	No*	No	Yes
Major surgery	No	No	Yes
Immunosuppressive drugs	No	No	Yes
Vascular access problems	Yes	No	No
Peritoneal catheter problems and peritonitis	No	Yes	No
Regular exposure to heparin	Yes	No	No

CAPD, continuous ambulatory peritoneal dialysis.
Patients on continuous cycling (CCAD) do use an automatic cycler.
*Erythropoietin & calcitriol can be replaced.

to the patient and the dialysis center. CAPD and transplantation offer specific advantages to patients with type I diabetes: intraperitoneal insulin offers good glucose control and peritoneal dialysis avoids the need for vascular access in such patients, who often have peripheral vascular disease and may develop distal ischemia after a graft or fistula. In hemodialysis patients infection and thrombosis of the vascular access are the most common causes of admission to the hospital, whereas in CAPD patients the most common cause is peritonitis. Problems associated with prednisone and other long-term immunosuppressive drugs after transplantation are discussed in the section RENAL TRANSPLANTATION.

Rehabilitation after renal replacement therapy is negatively influenced by increasing age, presence of systemic diseases such as diabetes mellitus, and a poor work record before ESRD, and is best after successful renal transplantation at any age. This is counterbalanced, however, by some negative effects of failed renal transplants. Return to former social functioning is better with home dialysis and CAPD patients than with in-center dialysis patients, but this is at least in part due to a self-selection process: in general, the fitter, more self-reliant patients choose those treatment modalities. In one survey of rehabilitation in dialysis patients, as many as 40% to 50% were poorly rehabilitated.

The 1- and 5-year mortality rate for dialysis in all comers is 18% and 40%, respectively. It is markedly affected by age (e.g., 5-year survival rate is 90% in children and 20% in patients over 65 years). Another major factor adversely affecting mortality is diabetes mellitus as a cause of ESRD. There is a tendency after the first year of treatment for a lesser mortality rate in transplantation than in dialysis patients of the same age, but no strictly controlled prospective studies exist. The most important causes of mortality in dialysis patients are clearly cardiovascular (myocardial infarction, congestive heart failure, and stroke); collectively these causes are responsible for 65% of the deaths. Infection (15%) and hyperkalemia (3%) are also significant causes of mortality.

DIALYSIS

Principles of dialysis treatment

All forms of readily available dialysis depend on diffusion of small molecules across a semipermeable membrane, extracorporeal with a synthetic cellulose membrane in hemodialysis and intracorporeal with a biologic membrane in peritoneal dialysis. Dialysate must be sterile for peritoneal dialysis, but the semipermeable synthetic membranes exclude bacteria (though not endotoxin) and therefore the dialysate does not need to be sterile.

The principles of dialysis are outlined in Fig. 348-6. Solute can be removed from the blood (or as appropriate to the chemical gradient, can enter the blood) by diffusion or by convection when fluid is removed from the blood either by an osmotic gradient (e.g., high glucose in the peritoneal dialysate fluid) or by a hydrostatic gradient (e.g., by negative pressure on the dialysate side). A typical dialysate composition would be Na^{+}138, K^{+} 3 (variable), Cl^{-}105, HCO_3^{-}35 (or acetate or lactate, which results in equimolar HCO_3^{-} in the body), and Ca^{2+}3.5 mEq/L; because only the ionized fraction exchanges, calcium diffuses into the blood in most patients; a low calcium dialysate can be used to treat hypercalcemia. In hemodialysis patients, dialysate may contain no glucose or 100 mg/dl; in peritoneal dialysis patients, dialysate contains large amounts of glucose (1.5 to 4.25 g/dl) as an osmotic agent. Because the blood of dialysis patients is exposed to about 120 L of dialysate fluid per dialysis session, special preparation of the water is required to remove trace metals and other substances present in tap water. Reverse osmosis and deionization techniques are used to prepare dialysate water for chronic dialysis patients. Because this process has become routine, a syndrome of dialysis dementia due to aluminum intoxication has become very rare.

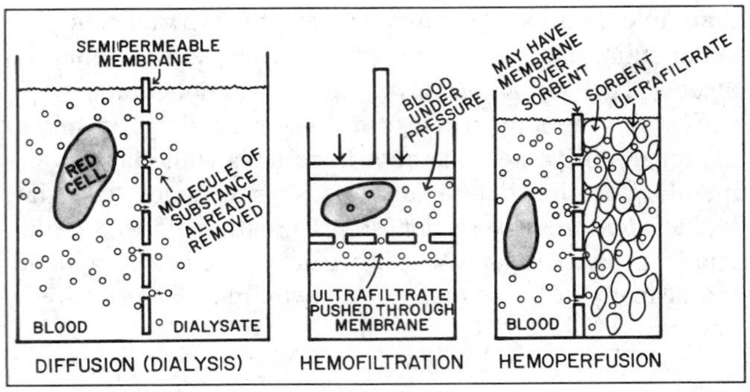

Fig. 348-6. Mechanisms for removing substances from blood include diffusion of solute across a semipermeable membrane into a dialysis solution, or dialysate *(left)*, and movement of solute along with the bulk flow of water. The fluid movement (ultrafiltration) may be initiated by hydraulic or osmotic pressure *(middle)* or by absorption of solute to a sorbent *(right)*. The blood may be separated from the sorbent by a membrane coating; solute and water cross the membrane by diffusion and ultrafiltration.

In all forms of dialysis, water-soluble vitamins may be lost from the blood. Routinely, dialysis patients should receive vitamin supplements, including B vitamins, vitamin C, and folate. Oral iron is usually also required, especially in chronic hemodialysis patients, because small amounts of blood (5 to 10 ml) unavoidably remain in the dialyser after the dialysis procedure.

Both hemodialysis and peritoneal dialysis can be used to remove certain poisons acutely and to treat acute renal failure (Chapter 347) or chronic renal failure with an acute superimposed problem (e.g., surgery) for periods of a few days to a few weeks. Temporary access can be obtained immediately by a femoral or subclavian catheter or by a Teflon arteriovenous Scribner shunt (usually radiocephalic). The Scribner shunt permitted the introduction of chronic dialysis in the early 1960s, but is now largely replaced for chronic access by the fistula or prosthetic graft. Acute peritoneal dialysis can also be used for acute renal failure or in ESRD, especially when the patient presents with late uremic symptoms, because there is clinical benefit in correcting severe uremia more slowly by the less efficient, peritoneal dialysis procedure. A temporary catheter can be inserted at the bedside and peritoneal dialysis performed by any of a number of techniques. Many nephrologists now prefer to use a Tenckhoff catheter from the beginning because of reduced risk of infection. Relative indications for peritoneal or hemodialysis in acute renal failure are discussed in Chapter 347.

Hemodialysis

A typical circuit for hemodialysis is shown in Fig. 348-7. An artificial kidney is made up of a dialysate delivery system, a blood pump to deliver blood at 150 to 300 ml/min from the arterial needle inserted in the cannula or fistula, various safety monitoring devices, and a dialyser, in which actual dialysis takes place. The two major dialysers now in use are the flat plate and the hollow fiber dialysers; in both, blood flow and dialysate flow (the latter usually at 500 ml/min) are countercurrent. Dialysers are now commonly reused by the same patient for economic reasons. Patients require small amounts of heparin (3000 to 10,000 units) either intermittently or by infusion during the procedure. In some patients with severe coagulopathy, it is possible with very careful monitoring to avoid the use of heparin. The usual duration of dialysis is 3.5 to 6.0 hours depending on patient size, level of persisting endogenous renal function, BUN level, creatinine level, etc., before dialysis, as well as on the amounts of ECF to be removed. The latter can be calculated from the ultrafiltration coefficient of the membrane and the net transmembrane hydraulic pressure; more than 1 L/hr can be removed. A physician's order for dialysis would normally indicate duration of dialysis, type of access, arterial flow rate, type of dialyser (several are available with different dialysis characteristics and extracorporeal volumes), anticoagulant dose, type of dialysate, and

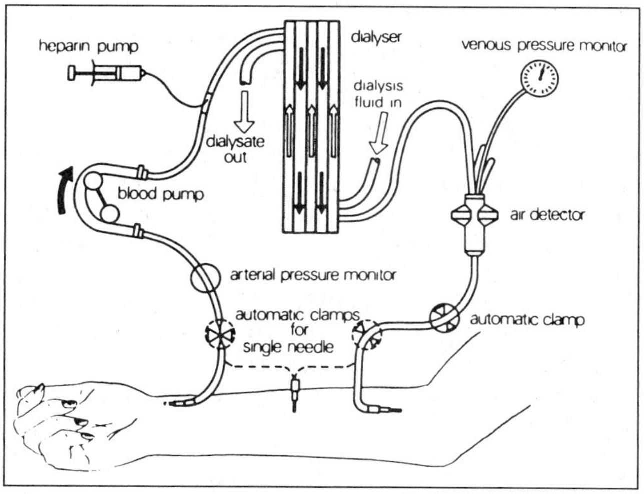

Fig. 348-7. Essential components of an artificial kidney in use for hemodialysis. The apparatus for using a single needle for inflow and outflow of blood from the patient is shown by a dashed line. From Drukker W, Parsons M, and Maher JF, editors: Replacement of renal function by dialysis, ed 2, Boston, 1983, Martinus Nijhoff.)

"dry weight" of the patient. The dry weight is an important concept in the chronic dialysis patient: It is the postdialysis weight at which the patient has an acceptable blood pressure and a plasma volume adequate for avoiding diminished cardiac output or lung congestion. Most patients on chronic hemodialysis need dialysis three times weekly, and the predialysis BUN in patients ingesting 1.0 g of protein/kg should be less than 90 mg/dl for optimum management.

High flux dialysis uses new membranes with increased solute clearances and hydraulic permeability and is increasingly used for selected patients with access blood flows of 300 ml/min or more, and interdialytic weight gains that are moderate (< 4 L). Its principal advantages are diminished time requirements (as little as 2 hours for smaller patients) and fewer hypotensive complications, but it does require more expensive equipment and monitoring devices and higher bloodflows from the vascular access. The new membrane, in contrast to the older cellulose membranes, are not only more permeable but are more biocompatible. There has been much recent interest in cell (lymphocytes, monocytes, polymorphonuclear leukocytes) membrane interactions during hemodialysis with resulting release of cytokines such as ILI, TNF (tumor necrosis factor) and activation of complement with subsequent leukocyte sequestration in the lungs, associated in the first hour of dialysis with leukopenia. These efforts may contribute to minor febrile episodes during dialysis, to slight hypoxia, and even to a modest catabolic effect of dialysis itself. The new membranes substantially diminish or avoid these cell-activating effects, but their increased permeability may allow backflux of small endotoxin molecules from dialysate. Bicarbonate rather than acetate must also be used as a source of base in the dialysate; this option is advantageous because acetate likely contributes to hypotension during dialysis.

Improved bioengineering now allows controlled rates of ultifiltration of excess fluid so that fluid removal is much more predictable, and again hypotension, nausea, and muscle cramps during the procedure are much reduced. As solutes are removed from plasma during hemodialysis, gradients are set up between, for example, muscle and brain cells and extracellular fluid, especially in too-rapid initial hemodialysis of a patient with chronic or acute renal failure with a high BUN. When this happens, a dialysis disequilibrium syndrome can develop, with headache and even seizures and focal central nervous system signs. This problem is avoided by initial slow daily dialysis for shorter periods and with lower blood flows. In chronic dialysis patients symptoms are much less but can be minimized by controlling dialysate sodium concentration ("sodium modeling") so that it is initially high and combats the cell-plasma gradient. Most dialyzers are now reused perhaps four to ten times for cost reasons. Careful interdialytic storage and sterilization is critical. Reuse has diminished patient side effects such as "first use syndrome" (urticaria, back pain, and hypotension), which relates to plasma protein membrane interactions with high Ig E levels in blood. This reaction is likely because reuse is associated with "lining" of the membrane by the patients own platelets and protein. Residual capacity of the dialyzer is tested before each use.

Together with erythropoietin, these upgrades in dialysis techniques have improved the dialysis patients' lives; there is less hypotension, nausea, and postdialysis "exhaustion," especially if the patient is compliant with minimizing interdialytic weight gain and maintains good nutrition.

With shorter dialysis times and an increase variety of dialyzers with different solute clearance and ultrafiltration capacities, more precise "prescription" of individualized dialysis for patients is necessary. It is now well established that adequate dialysis in patients dialyzed thrice weekly provides a Kt/v of at least 1.2 (where K = dialyzer clearance for urea [ml/min], t = dialysis time in minutes, and v = volume of distribution of urea—approximately the total body water in liters). It is also important that a low predialysis BUN and serum phosphate not automatically be regarded as "good," as it may reflect inadequate protein intake rather than excellent dialysis. Maintenance of a 1 g/kg protein intake and 35 calories/kg is vital for adequate nutrition.

Hemodialysis is now a remarkably safe procedure, and self-dialysis is feasible in motivated patients after about 6 to 8 weeks of careful training. Technical problems are rare but include air embolism, hemorrhage from accidental removal of the access needle, and dialysate that is too hot, too cold, or chemically inappropriate. Episodes of symptomatic hypotension (nausea and vomiting) and muscle cramps occur in part because fluid is removed rapidly from the vascular compartment but then has to be mobilized from the extracellular space (analogous to overrapid diuresis with diuretics). Muscle cramps can usually be treated by slowing ultrafiltration and by infusion of small amounts of hypertonic mannitol, saline, or glucose. Atypical hypotension should raise the consideration of pericarditis or other cardiac event, sepsis, or bleeding.

During dialysis, there is often an associated modest decrease in arterial oxygen levels. It has been shown that carbon dioxide is lost from the blood when acetate, and not bicarbonate with bubbled carbon dioxide, is used in the dialysis solution; hypocapnia may result in slowing of respiration and a decrease in arterial oxygen level of 10 to 20 mm Hg. In a few patients with cardiac or respiratory disease, oxygen administration during dialysis is indicated. As noted, pulmonary sequestration of leukocytes may also contribute to hypoxia.

When dialysis is terminated, the artificial kidney is usually rinsed with saline, and the blood is returned to the patient. However, a blood residue of up to 10 ml remains in the artificial kidney and so is lost to the patient. Over a prolonged period, total blood loss in the dialyser may be substantial.

Viral hepatitis can be transmitted by blood. Thus carriers of the hepatitis virus expose dialysis personnel and other patients to an increased risk of viral hepatitis, particularly if any drops of blood are allowed to contaminate the surrounding area during the process of initiating hemodialysis or at the end of dialysis. Although hepatitis epidemics have occurred among patients and personnel in some dialysis programs, an epidemic can usually be avoided if proper precautions are taken. These universal precautions are also effective against blood transmission of HIV, which is much less infective than the hepatitis B virus. HIV carriers do not need to be dialyzed in separate facilities, but hepatitis B carriers should be so dialyzed. Active immunization for hepatitis B should be given to all dialysis patients and staff who do not have immunity.

Hemodialysis can pose some risk to patients who have cardiovascular instability. During hemodialysis, blood pressure may fall (primarily due to rapid removal of sodium and water from the vascular space), even though the patient has expanded extravascular ECF spaces and often obvious edema. As noted, removal of fluid and sodium from the vascular space may not be accompanied by rapid mobilization of edema fluid into the vascular bed. Rapid and severe blood pressure decreases may compromise blood flow through diseased coronary arteries or the cerebral circulation and result in myocardial infarction, seizure, or stroke. Such patients may be better managed by peritoneal dialysis.

Peritoneal dialysis

The Tenckhoff catheter for chronic intermittent or continuous peritoneal dialysis is about 25 cm long and consists of intraperitoneal (pelvic), subcutaneous, and extracorporeal sections. Patients on chronic intermittent peritoneal dialysis use this catheter for instillation of fluid into, and drainage from, the abdominal cavity. CAPD patients usually perform 3 to 5 exchanges per day of 1.5 to 3.0 L of dialysate. Solution is instilled from plastic bags. A connecting tube allows the empty bag to remain attached to the chronic catheter, and the bag is used later for receiving drainage. The bag of drainage fluid is replaced with a fresh bag of solution and then is discarded. Y-shaped transfer sets have led to "bagless" CAPD. The bag is only needed for infusion and drainage. This technique provides essentially continuous slow dialysis, which has the advantage that it maintains essentially steady-state body fluid levels and thus avoids rapid fluctuations in body fluid solute concentrations and too-rapid shifts in body fluid compartments. On average, patients on CAPD suffer one episode of peritonitis per each 9 to 12 month of dialysis. Most of these episodes are mild, are due to gram-positive organisms from the skin, and respond to an increased rate of peritoneal exchange and to intraperitoneal or oral antibiotics. A modification of CAPD that uses an automatic cycling machine (cycler) at night during sleep with one CAPD exchange during the day (continuous cycling peritoneal dialysis, CCPD) is gaining in popularity, especially for those who wish to work or need help with their connections during exchanges.

CAPD, as compared to hemodialysis, has the additional advantages of avoiding the cardiovascular stress and eliminating the need for vascular access. Disadvantages include the high glucose load, which can cause obesity and aggravate hyperlipidemia, development of hernias, and the more likely eventual loss of peritoneal as compared to vascular access (one abdomen versus four limbs).

An increasing number of patients are remaining on this treatment modality for 10 years or more. Ultrafiltration failure sometimes occurs after many episodes of peritonitis due to a sclerosing peritonitis. This complication usually necessitates transfer to hemodialysis. Peritoneal function can be tested by measuring dialysate/plasma ratios over time for urea and creatinine, rate of fall of peritoneal glucose concentration, and fluid ultrafiltration rates.

Peritonitis is most often due to gram-positive skin organisms. The peritoneal dialysate fluid becomes cloudy and has a cell count of >100 cells/min^3 with >50% polymorphonuclear leukocytes. Multiple gram-negative or anaerobic organisms suggest a perforated viscus (but remember subphrenic free air may occur in PD patients "normally") or diverticulitis. Relapsing infections suggest a tunnel infection or catheter colonization. Fungal infection or relapsing infection usually requires catheter removal and a period of a few weeks of appropriate treatment on hemodialysis.

Patients on peritoneal dialysis also experience protein losses in the drainage, whereas protein losses during hemodialysis are minimal because proteins with molecular weight above 10,000 cross cellulose membranes to a minimal extent. With CAPD, average protein losses approach 12 g/day but increase considerably during episodes of peritonitis.

These protein losses can usually be overcome by an adequate dietary protein intake: protein intake should be 1.2 g/kg. Reduced blood loss may partly explain the tendency for anemia to be less severe in chronic peritoneal dialysis.

A comparison of solute clearances by hemodialysis, intermittent peritoneal dialysis, CAPD, and the normal kidney is given in Table 348-4.

Other forms of dialysis

Other forms of dialysis include isolated ultrafiltration, in which no dialysate is used, for patients with a marked need for fluid removal. This approach is especially important if hypotension and diminished cardiac output is a problem because hypotension is less when solute is not simultaneously removed by diffusion. Similarly, hemofiltration (see Fig. 348-6) occurs when fluid and solute are removed by ultrafiltration (not diffusion) across an unusually permeable synthetic membrane, similar to glomerular filtration in vivo. An arterial pump is not required, and this type of dialysis can be performed continuously at low rates in certain types of patients with acute renal failure, especially those with a very low cardiac output (continuous arteriovenous hemofiltration, CAVH). In a more complex type of hemofiltration, which can be used for chronic therapy, immediately before or after this ultrafiltration process the cellular and protein components of the blood are diluted with a replacement solution that ideally contains the essential substances and none of the undesirable ones. This technique is used in Europe but rarely in the United States. To date, it appears to offer no distinct advantage over hemodialysis. Hemoperfusion (see Fig. 348-6) is used especially for the treatment of certain lipid-soluble poisons: membrane-coated activated carbon is commonly used in the blood path of a dialysis cartridge.

RENAL TRANSPLANTATION

Successful transplantation often increases the quality of life for ESRD patients treated by dialysis, especially patients treated by hemodialysis. When successful, transplantation has allowed many patients to resume normal lives. Over the past decade, a striking improvement in renal transplant results has been obtained. Morbidity and mortality have declined. Mortality at the end of the first year, during which time most deaths occur, is less than 5% for live donor grafts and 5% to 10% for cadaveric grafts. In contrast, patients treated by dialysis are subject to a constant yearly death rate.

The only individuals with ESRD not considered for transplantation are the elderly, those with a recent history of malignancy, those with active glomerulonephritis or active sepsis (or those in whom chronic infection may be reactivated by treatment with steroids), and in some cases of sickle cell nephropathy and primary oxalosis, and in Fabry's disease.

Immunology (see Chapter 223)

In analyzing potential donors for kidney transplantation, presensitization to major human leukocyte antigens (HLA) and to certain minor, non-HLA antigens is important in tissue matching. It has long been known that compatibility for red cell ABO antigens between donor and recipient is of the utmost importance, since preformed natural anti-A and anti-B antibodies constitute a strong barrier to graft suc-

Table 348-4. Clearances by different dialysis methods, compared to normal kidney

	Weekly duration	Urea clearance (ml/min)	Inulin clearance (ml/min)
Normal kidney	Continuous	60	120
Hemodialysis	3 · 4 = 12 hours	11 (160)	0.3 (4)
Continuous ambulatory peritoneal dialysis	Continuous	7	3

Note: Clearances are time-averaged and are exclusive of residual renal function. Figures in parentheses are actual clearances during the procedure. Note that urea (60 daltons) is cleared better during hemodialysis while inulin (5200 daltons) is cleared relatively better by peritoneal dialysis, because of increased permeability of the peritoneal membrane to higher molecular weight solutes.

cess. Certain other preformed antibodies present at the time of transplantation portend an immediate vasculitic form of graft destruction (hyperacute rejection). It is clear that potential recipients harboring antibodies against HLA-A, -B, and -C class I, but not HLA-DR class II, antigens of the donor are at high risk for this process. Multiparous or frequently transfused women and patients, male or female, who previously have rejected an allograft are all at high risk of harboring such antibodies. Presensitization against a non-HLA antigen system shared between the endothelial surface of peritubular capillaries and monocytes also heralds accelerated rejection in the few patients who bear such antibodies.

Major histocompatibility antigens are highly polymorphic cell surface structures whose recognition by the host permits distinction between self and nonself. In humans, genes for the major histocompatibility complex are aligned in close proximity to each other on chromosome 6. The three well-defined class loci are the HLA-A, -B, and -C cell surface antigens, products of different gene loci but having an identical basic structure. Class I antigens usually are detected by a complement-dependent microlymphocytotoxicity assay, using anti-HLA antibodies of known specificity. The cell suspension is exposed to complement and eosin or trypan blue dye; cells bearing the target antigen sustain membrane damage, which is recognized by intracellular uptake of the dye.

Linked to the serologically defined HLA-A, -B, and -C antigens, but separate from them, is another genetic region, called HLA-D, which codes for glycoprotein class II HLA molecules that trigger the helper T-cell dependent proliferative response that occurs when lymphoid cells with mismatched HLA haplotypes are cultured together in a mixed lymphocyte culture.

The mixed lymphocyte culture is a 5- to 6-day test in which x-ray or mitomycin C inactivated mononuclear leukocytes obtained from a prospective graft donor are cultured together with mononuclear leukocytes from the prospective recipient. Responder cells react vigorously to test cells expressing foreign class II HLA antigens but weakly or not at all to cells that express antigens similar to their own. There are at least three class II HLA loci encoded within this region: DR, DQ, and DP. DR antigens are indeed potent stimulator antigens in the mixed lymphocyte culture; these antigens are not the only class II antigens that elicit primary or secondary mixed lymphocyte culture reactions. Class II antigens can be typed by complement-dependent microlymphocytotoxic techniques, using T cell depleted, B cell, and macrophage enriched mononuclear leukocytes.

Because chromosome 6 is paired, each individual inherits its genes for at least 12 HLA loci antigens (Chapter 223). Six antigens (HLA-A, -B, -C, -DR, -DQ, and -DP) are inherited from each parent. Tissue typing laboratories can readily define the phenotype of the HLA-A, -B, -C, and -DR antigens by serologic techniques; typing for the newly discovered DP and DQ loci is becoming well defined in clinical practice. By simple mendelian autosomal inheritance, any given pair of siblings of dissimilar parents will have a 25% chance of having identical haplotypes, a 50% chance of sharing one haplotype, and a 25% chance of being completely incompatible. By definition, a parent and child share one haplotype for each genetic trait. It has long been known that matching of HLA antigens is extremely valuable in choosing donor-recipient pairs for renal transplantation using closely related family members. A clear-cut gene-dose effect is observed when the rates of graft success are compared for recipients of familial grafts who are treated with traditional regimens of azathioprine plus corticosteroid and are matched for zero, one, or two haplotypes. Whereas 90% to 95% of HLA-identical sibling-donor renal grafts function at 1 year, the 1-year graft survivals for one-haplotype-matched donors (sibling or parent) and HLA-incompatible siblings are 75% and 60% respectively. Since the rate of graft success for first cadaveric renal allografts is now 80% in centers that are experienced with the use of cyclosporine, the routine use of living related donors is being challenged.

The HLA system is the most polymorphic genetic system known; hence, it is all but impossible to find perfectly matched cadaveric kidneys for prospective recipients. Nonetheless, it has been important to learn that matching for HLA, especially HLA-B and HLA-DR locus alleles, has a great impact on cadaveric renal graft success, even in transplantation performed following immunologic conditioning of the recipient with blood products and/or in recipients treated with cyclosporine.

Graft rejection

An oversimplified schema of graft rejection and the effect of immunosuppressive agents on these events is shown in Fig. 348-8. Activation of helper T cells by class II major histocompatibility complex antigens such as HLA-DR probably stimulates the release of a a macrophage stimulant and renders T cells sensitive to monokines such as interleukin-1 (IL-1) and interleukin-6 (IL-6). Antigen and monokine stimulated T cells express interleukin-2 (IL-2) receptors and release of IL-2 by helper T cells. IL-2 interacts with specific IL-2 receptors expressed on activated helper and cytotoxic T cells. This interaction stimulates the initiation of DNA synthesis and eventual clonal proliferation of IL-2 receptor-bearing cells. IL-2 in turn causes the release of gamma-interferon, which activates macrophages. IL-2 also stimulates the release of B-cell differentiation factors (e.g., IL-4 and IL-5) that are required for proliferation of antigen-activated B cells. The IL-2–dependent release of gamma-interferon by activated T cells may initiate a vicious circle as gamma-interferon induces the expression of class II molecules on endothelial cells as well as the expression of certain class II negative macrophages.

In brief, activation of helper T cells by alloantigen and monokines stimulates the release of a variety of lymphokines from helper T cells, which in turn activate macrophages, cytotoxic T cells, and antibody-releasing B cells, as well as increase the immunogenicity of the graft (see Fig. 348-8). These factors also support clonal expansion and viability of antigen-activated macrophages, and antibody.

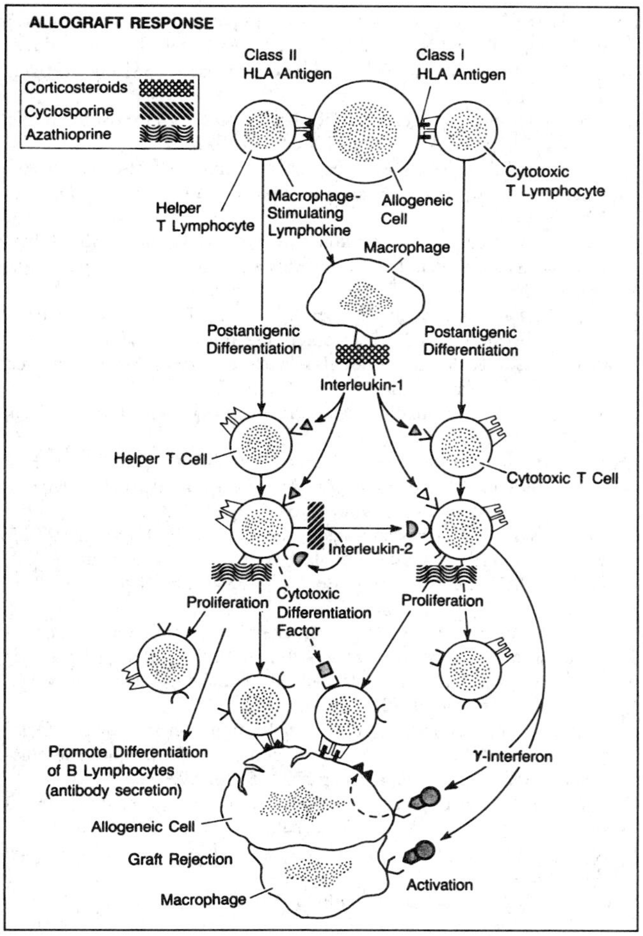

Fig. 348-8. The "allograft response": immunologic aspects of graft rejection and the site of action immunosuppressive drugs.

The immunosuppressive activities of each of the therapeutic agents used in clinical transplantation directly interferes with the "allograft response" (see Fig. 348-8). *Azathioprine,* an oral purine analog, one of whose in vivo metabolites is 6-mercaptopurine, has been the mainstay of antirejection therapy since it was introduced in 1961 as maintenance therapy for renal transplant recipients. This purine analog is an antimetabolite with multiple activities. Metabolites of azathioprine are incorporated into cellular DNA, inhibit purine nucleotide synthesis and metabolism, and alter the synthesis and function of RNA. As lymphocytic RNA synthesis, DNA synthesis, and proliferation result from antigenic stimulation, azathioprine acts at an early step in either B- or T-lymphocyte activation during the proliferative cycle of effector lymphocyte clones (see Fig. 348-8). Azathioprine is administered on a continuous basis; even temporary cessation of administration in the early posttransplant period results in a high rate of graft failure. Although azathioprine is a powerful inhibitor of primary immune responses, it has little or no effect on secondary responses. The drug is useful in preventing acute rejection, but it is not valuable in the therapy of ongoing rejection.

Corticosteroids were first used in transplantation to reverse acute rejection reactions in patients treated with maintenance doses of azathioprine. It is now customary to use modest doses of a corticosteroid in maintenance protocols that also utilize azathioprine or cyclosporine; high doses of corticosteroids are used to treat acute rejection. Through mechanisms quite distinct from the action of azathioprine, corticosteroids directly inhibit antigen-driven T cells proliferation. Steroids probably reverse in vivo rejection episodes by preventing the production of IL-2, thereby denying activated T cells an essential trophic factor. Steroids do not directly act on the IL-2–producing T cell, but they inhibit production of this lymphokine by preventing monocytes from releasing IL-1, thereby blocking IL-1 dependent release of IL-2 from antigen-activated T cells (see Fig. 348-8). Other effects of steroids on monocytes, such as inhibition of chemotaxis, also are likely to be important.

The fungal metabolite cyclosporine shares with corticosteroids the capacity to block the entry of activated T lymphocytes to the S phase of the cell cycle. Unlike corticosteroids, cyclosporine does not inhibit the capacity of all accessory cells to release IL-1. Cyclosporine does prevent activation of the IL-2 gene in activated helper T lymphocytes. The release of certain other lymphokines, such as gamma-interferon and B-cell growth and differentiation factors by activated T cells, also is inhibited by cyclosporine. Thus under the influence of cyclosporine, helper T cell–dependent B cells are not fully activated because of a lack of necessary helper T cell stimulants. Nonetheless, cyclosporine, in pharmacologic doses, does not grossly interfere with activation and proliferation of suppressor T lympocytes.

Cyclosporine is a neutral hydrophobic cyclic peptide consisting of 11 amino acids, including a previously unknown amino acid in position 9. The immunosuppressive activity depends on the presence of the carbon chains of the amino acids in position 1 and 11. For oral use, the drug is dissolved in olive oil. A galenic formulation is used for intravenous administration.

Cyclosporine levels in plasma or whole blood can be measured either by radioimmunoassay or high-pressure liquid chromatography. Although a strict relationship between drug levels and efficacy or toxicity is not found, assays have demonstrated that the rate and degree of drug absorption after oral administration are extremely variable. Many kidney transplant centers have adopted a policy of keeping plasma trough cyclosporine levels between 50 and 150 ng per milliliter. This policy may reduce, but certainly does not eliminate, episodes of cyclosporine nephrotoxicity. Many patients enjoy excellent graft function with "undetectable" plasma levels of cyclosporine.

Cyclosporine catabolism is hastened by rifampin, phenytoin, and other drugs by inducing production of degradative hepatic enzymes. Concurrent therapy with aminoglycosides, ketoconazole, amphotericin B, erythromycin, and possibly trimethoprim/sulfamethoxazole elevates plasma drug levels and results in increased nephrotoxicity.

The rate of graft success is invariably better by 10% to 20% in cadaveric kidney recipients treated with cyclosporine and prednisone than in patients receiving azathioprine and prednisone. Nonetheless, graft dysfunction is common among cyclosporine-treated patients. Trials in which patients are switched to conventional immunosuppression after an initial period of cyclosporine treatment show that improvements in graft function are frequently obtained with this approach. There can be no doubt that early nephrotoxicity is common and usually reversible, although a severe and irreversible form of nephrotoxicity marked by intense interstitial fibrosis occurs in heart graft recipients given high doses of cyclosporine. Nephrotoxicity may become manifest in the early postoperative course as acute renal failure or later in the course as an insidious decrease in glomerular filtration rate.

It is difficult to distinguish chronic drug nephrotoxicity from rejection. Both conditions usually become manifest only as an impairment of graft function without other clinical signs. Concurrent rejection and nephrotoxicity are common. Liberal use of graft biopsy to assess function in the early posttransplant period is useful, since cyclosporine nephrotoxicity, unlike rejection, does not cause interstitial nephritis.

The use of conventional (i.e., polyclonal) antilymphocyte antibody in preventing or reversing rejection episodes in renal allograft recipients is well established, although lot to lot variations and the presence of many non-lymphocyte-specific antibodies in such preparations have made standardization difficult. Hence, the use of pure anti–T cell monoclonal antibodies has been pursued as a possible safe mode of antirejection therapy. OKT3, an IgG monoclonal antibody, reacts with a 20-kd structure noncovalently associated with the T cell antigen receptor. T3 antigen is found on all mature postthymic T cells. OKT3 reverses almost all acute renal transplant rejection episodes. Although mild recurrent rejection is often noted after therapy is discontinued, this agent is superior to standard high-dose corticosteroid therapy for reversing allograft rejection (94% vs. 70% success).

Irradiation can produce profound immunosuppression. Remarkable tolerance to tissue and bone marrow grafts has been achieved in experimental animals following total lymphoid irradiation. Irradiated rodents became tolerant to marrow, skin, and cardiac allografts. Clinical trials using total lymphoid irradiation together with traditional immunosuppression in patients at high risk for allograft rejection have been completed. Side effects are commonplace. Preliminary results suggest at least adequate immunosuppression but a possible increased risk of lymphomas. More recent attempts to use total lymphoid irradiation together with low dose adjunctive immunosuppression for cadaveric renal transplants have produced dramatic results without causing the marked difficulties noted in the previous series.

REFERENCES

Ahmad S, Blagg CR, and Scribner BH: Center and home chronic hemodialysis. In Schrier RW and Gottschalk CW, editors: Diseases of the kidney, vol. 3. Management of end-stage renal failure. Boston, 1988, Little, Brown, pp. 3281-3322.

Bennett WM and Blyth WB: Use of drugs in patients with renal failure. In Schrier RW and Gottschalk CW, editors: Diseases of the kidney, vol. 3. Nutrition, drugs, and the kidney. Boston, 1988, Little, Brown, pp. 3437-3506.

Bricker NS: On the pathogenesis of the uremic state. An exposition of the "trade-off hypothesis." N Engl J Med 286:1093, 1972.

Delmez JA and Slatopolsky E: Hyperphosphatemia: its consequences and treatment in patients with chronic renal disease, Am J Kidney D, 19:303, 1992.

Diaz-Buxo JA: Technology of peritoneal dialysis. In Jacobson HR, Striker GE, and Klahr S, editors: The principles and practice of nephrology, Philadelphia, 1991, BC Decker.

Drukker W, Parsons FM, and Maher JF, editors: Replacement of renal function by dialysis, ed 2. Boston, 1983, Martinus Nijhoff.

Dumler F, Stalla K, Mohini R, et al: Clinical experience with short-time hemodialysis, Am J Kidney Dis 19:49, 1992.

Eschbach JW: Erythropoietin 1991—an overview, Am J Kidney Dis 18:S1:3, 1991.

Eschbach JW and Adamson JW: Anemia in renal disease. In Schrier RW and Gottschalk CW, editors: Diseases of the kidney, vol 3. Uremic syndrome. Boston, 1988, Little, Brown, pp 3019-3034.

Fraser CL and Arieff AI: Neurologic complications of chronic renal failure. In Schrier RW and Gottschalk CW, editors: Diseases of the kidney, vol 3. Uremic syndrome. Boston, 1988, Little, Brown, pp 3063-3092.

Hostetter TH and Mitch WE: Protein intake and prevention of chronic renal disease. In Schrier RW and Gottschalk CW, editors: Diseases of the kidney, vol 3. Nutrition, drugs, and the kidney. Boston, 1988, Little, Brown, pp 3347-3370.

Keshaviah P: Technology and clinical application of hemodialysis. In Jacobson HR, Striker GE, and Klahr S, editors: The principles and practice of nephrology, Philadelphia, 1991, BC Decker.

Kim KE and Swartz C: Cardiovascular complications of end-stage renal disease. In Schrier RW and Gottschalk CW, editors: Diseases of the kidney, vol 3. Uremic syndrome. Boston, 1988, Little, Brown, pp 3093-3126.

Koch KM: Dialysis-related amyloidosis, Kidney Int 41:1416, 1992.

Levey AS: Measurement of renal function in chronic renal disease, Kidney Int 38:167, 1990.

Milon CM: Chronic ambulatory peritoneal dialysis (CAPD) and chronic cycling peritoneal dialysis (CCPD). In Schrier RW and Gottschalk CW, editors: Diseases of the kidney, vol 3. Management of end-stage renal failure. Boston, 1988, Little, Brown, pp 3235-3279.

Morris P: Immunobiology and immunopharmacology of graft rejection. In Schrier RW and Gottschalk CW, editors: Diseases of the kidney, vol 3. Management of end-stage renal failure. Boston, 1988, Little, Brown, pp 3211-3234.

Ritz E and Bommer J: Endocrine and metabolic dysfunction in chronic renal failure. In Schrier RW and Gottschalk CW, editors: Diseases of the kidney, vol 3. Uremic syndrome. Boston, 1988, Little, Brown, pp 3127-3173.

Rostland SG et al: Racial differences in the incidence of treatment of end-stage renal disease. N Engl J Med 306:1276, 1982.

Rotellar C, Black J, Winchester JF, et al: Ten years' experience with continuous ambulatory peritoneal dialysis, Am J Kidney Dis 17:158, 1991.

Salehmoghaddam S et al: Pathophysiology and nephron adaptation in chronic renal failure. In Schrier RW and Gottschalk CW, editors: Diseases of the kidney, vol 3. Uremic syndrome. Boston, 1988, Little, Brown, pp 2985-3018.

Salusky IB et al: Aluminum accumulation during treatment with aluminum hydroxide and dialysis in children and young adults with chronic renal disease, N Engl J Med 324:527, 1991.

Sandler DP, Smith JC, Weinberg CR, et al: Analgesic use and chronic renal disease, N Engl J Med 320:1238, 1989.

Schoenfeld P and Feduska NJ: Acquired immunodeficiency syndrome and renal disease: report of the National Kidney Foundation-National Institutes of Health Task Force on AIDS and Kidney Disease, Am J Kidney Dis 16:14, 1990.

Schulman G and Hakim RM: Complications of hemodialysis. In Jacobson HR, Striker GE, and Klahr S, editors: The principles and practice of nephrology, Philadelphia, 1991, BC Decker.

Sherrard DJ and Andress DL: Renal osteodystrophy of chronic renal failure. In Schrier RW and Gottschalk CW, editors: Diseases of the kidney, vol 3. Uremic syndrome. Boston, 1988, Little, Brown, pp 3035-3061.

CHAPTER

349 Nephrolithiasis

Jacob Lemann, Jr.

Approximately one person per thousand in the United States receives hospital care each year for kidney stones. Moreover, the incidence of renal calculi, principally stones composed of calcium oxalate, appears to be increasing in industrialized nations. This increase is possibly related to changing dietary habits, particularly to increasing intake of animal protein. Bladder stones are uncommon in the United States, where they appear only as a consequence of urethral obstruction or of a neurogenic bladder complicated by urinary tract infection.

Because genetic factors are of pathogenetic importance, nephrolithiasis is frequently a recurrent malady among untreated patients, approximately 50% experiencing a second episode within 5 years of the first. Thus a systematic approach to the treatment of nephrolithiasis requires a correct diagnosis, determination of the composition of the stone, and assessment of possible abnormalities in the composition of the urine that led to crystallization of the constituents of the stone within the urinary tract, so that the risk of recurrence and the need for therapy to prevent recurrence can be assessed.

SYMPTOMS OF URINARY TRACT STONES

The symptoms of urinary stones vary widely. Some patients have no symptoms and are coincidentally found to have stones on plain abdominal radiographs, intravenous urograms, computed tomograms, or ultrasonograms obtained during the evaluation of other illnesses. The frequency of stone recurrence varies widely. Some patients pass only a single stone, never to have another, whereas others repetitively pass gravel or small stones every few days.

Typically, an obstructing or partially obstructing stone in the renal pelvis or upper ureter is associated with flank and abdominal pain that is often extremely severe and accompanied by nausea and vomiting. When the stone is present in the middle and lower segments of the ureter, the pain often radiates downward to the inguinal ligament and into the labia and urethra or testicle and penis. A stone located in the terminal segment of the ureter within the bladder wall may be accompanied by urinary frequency and dysuria. Because these symptoms are typical of cystitis and urethritis, the possibility of a stone located in the intravesical ureter should be considered in this setting.

Gross or microscopic hematuria may be associated with any of these patterns of pain. Gross painless hematuria occurs occasionally, and renal stones are occasionally discovered during the evaluation of patients found to have microscopic hematuria. Chills and fever, together with flank and back pain, are present only when obstructing or partially obstructing pelvic stones are the result of infection, or when the presence of stones of other types is complicated by secondary infection.

PRELIMINARY EVALUATION OF THE PATIENT WITH NEPHROLITHIASIS

The initial evaluation of patients suspected of having nephrolithiasis requires, in addition to a thorough history and physical examination, the administration of analgesics to relieve pain if present, a urinalysis, radiographic studies, and continuous efforts to recover small stones that may be spontaneously voided. The urinalysis, including a prompt search for crystals in the sediment obtained from a urine centrifuged immediately after voiding, may identify the type of stone present (Figs. 349-1 and 349-2) and should be performed promptly by the physician who is acquainted with the clinical history. Only the observation of crystals in the sediment from fresh, warm urine indicates crystallization within the urinary tract, because cooling (refrigeration) of concentrated urine from otherwise healthy subjects can result in the precipitation of crystals because of the reduction in the solubility of many compounds at reduced temperature. The urine should also be collected as a clean-voided midstream specimen or by catheterization, and a portion should be cultured for bacteria. Because 90% of all stones are radiodense, a plain radiograph of the abdomen will normally determine the location and site. An ultrasonogram or intravenous urogram is required to confirm the presence of radiolucent (mainly uric acid) stones and to determine whether or not partial or complete ureteral obstruction is present. These studies will also establish the presence of other structural abnormalities of the urinary tract that may predispose to stone formation (e.g., medullary sponge kidney, ureteropelvic junction obstruction).

Analysis of the composition of the stone is of vital importance in planning subsequently required studies and therapy (see Fig. 349-1). Thus efforts should be made to acquire the stone by collecting and sieving all the urine the patient voids from the moment the patient is first seen. Not uncommonly, small stones are passed spontaneously and are lost into the toilet during unsupervised voiding.

While these initial studies are in progress, intravenous fluids should be initiated to sustain an adequate urine flow rate.

Patients can be expected to pass spontaneously ureteral stones 6 mm or less in greatest diameter. Such patients are managed with analgesics and fluid. Large ureteral or pel-

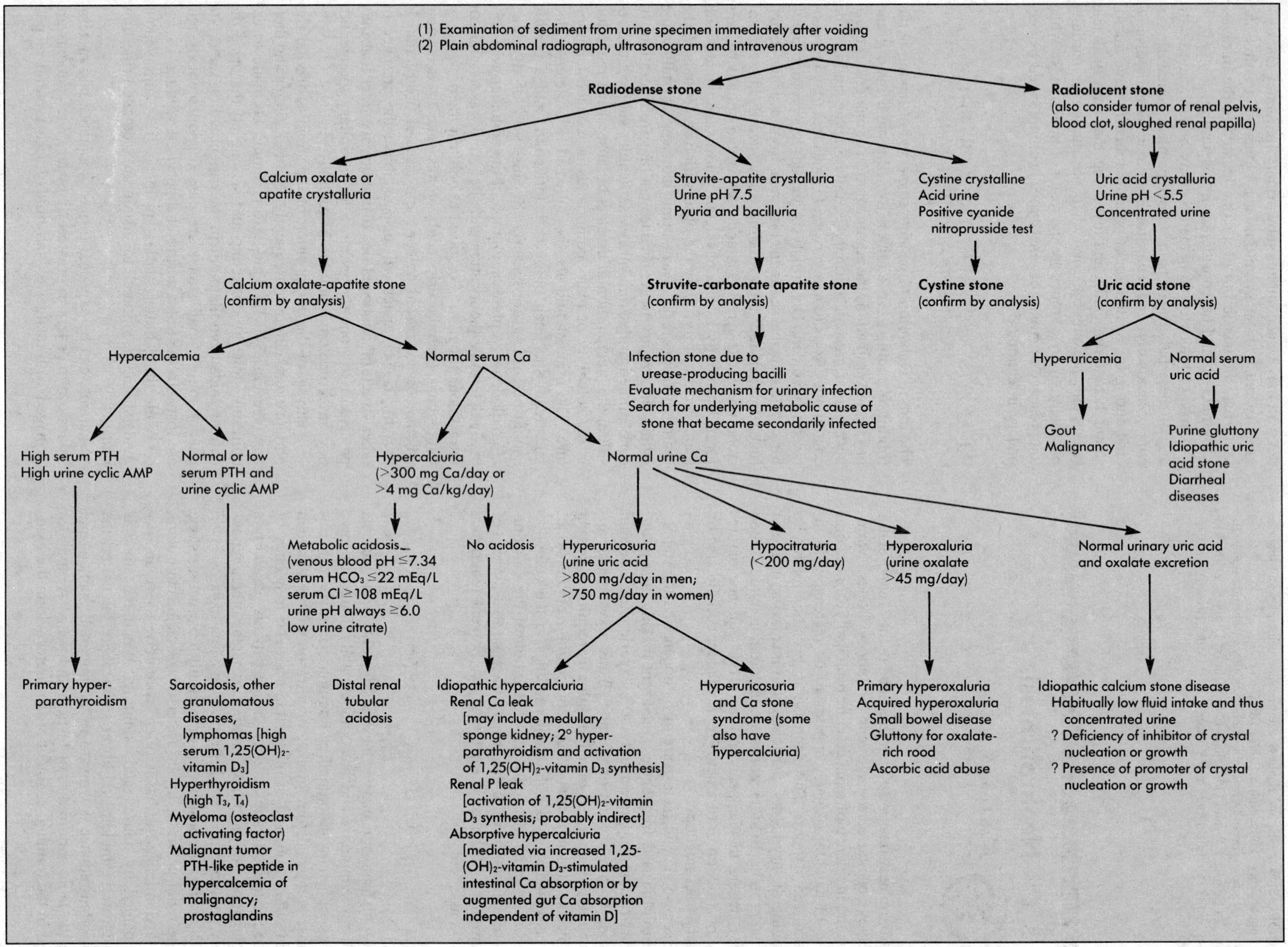

Fig. 349-1. Evaluation of patients with suspected nephrolithiasis (flank pain, ureteral colic, hematuria, fever).

vic stones (10 mm or more in greatest diameter) and obstructing stones of intermediate size (6 to 10 mm in greatest diameter) generally will require surgical removal. Thus patients with larger stones must be promptly evaluated and followed by urologic consultants. Extracorporeal shock wave lithotripsy (ESWL) is generally used to fragment stones less than 20 mm in diameter. Larger or infection stones are often treated by a combination of percutaneous nephrostolithotomy and ESWL. Generally, the type of stone present can be determined from the clinical setting, examination of the urine sediment, and the radiograph. Accurate analysis of a recovered stone, however, is required to confirm the diagnosis and should be performed by a laboratory experienced with optical crystallographic and x-ray diffraction techniques. Only these techniques will permit detection of stones of unusual composition. Chemical techniques do not generally provide accurate information regarding stone constituents.

Further studies are necessary to evaluate the presence of alterations in urine composition that can favor crystal nucleation and stone growth. Fig. 349-1 outlines a scheme for the systematic evaluation of patients with nephrolithiasis.

Abnormalities in the composition of the blood, such as hypercalcemia, hyperchloremic acidosis, and hyperuricemia, can be readily assessed during the initial evaluation of acutely ill patients. However, detailed evaluation of possible alterations in urine composition should generally be postponed until recovery from an acute episode of ureteral colic or a lithotomy procedure, when the patient is generally well, active, and eating normally.

COMPOSITION OF KIDNEY STONES

Approximately 75% of all stones are composed chiefly of calcium salts. Of these, about half are composed only of calcium oxalate, principally calcium oxalate monohydrate (whewellite), with variable amounts of calcium oxalate dihydrate (wedellite). The remaining half of these calcium stones are composed of calcium oxalate, together with apatite (hydroxyapatite) $[Ca_{10}(PO_4)_6(OH)_2]$ and carbonate apatite $[Ca_{10}(PO_4)_6CO_3]$ in small amounts, most often as the central nucleus. A small number of calcium stones are composed of apatite alone or calcium monohydrogen phosphate dihydrate alone (brushite, $CaHPO_4 \cdot 2H_2O$). The solubility of the latter compound is believed to govern the solubility of calcium phosphate in biologic fluids, and, after crystallization, it is rapidly transformed to apatite. About 10% of all stones are the result of urinary infection with urease-producing bacteria and are composed of magnesium ammonium phosphate hexahydrate (struvite, $MgNH_4PO_4 \cdot 6H_2O$), always together with carbonate apatite. An additional 10% of all stones are composed of uric acid, and about 2% are composed of cystine. Rare stones composed of other substances have also been observed. These substances include xanthine stones (xanthine oxidase deficiency; allopurinol therapy in patients with massive hyperuricosuria), 2,6-dihydroxyadenine stones (adenine phosphoribosyltransferase deficiency), and stones composed of several types of drugs, including allopurinol metabolites (allopurinol therapy) and triamterene (diuretic therapy).

CRYSTAL NUCLEATION AND STONE GROWTH IN THE URINARY TRACT

Several factors are currently recognized or thought to play a role in crystal formation, crystal growth and/or aggregation, and crystal attachment allowing stone growth within the urinary tract.

1. The average prevailing urinary concentration of solutes or substances capable of reacting with other urinary constituents to form insoluble salts may be elevated and increase the frequency of initial crystal formation. Hypercalcicuria, hyperoxaluria, hyperuricosuria, and cystinuria are examples of increased rates of solute excretion. Small daily urine volumes are observed during diarrheal diseases, with sweating or among patients who habitually drink only small quantities of fluid. Either or both of these circumstances raise the concentration of urinary solutes and may increase the frequency of crystal nucleation.
2. Alterations in normal diurnal variation in urinary pH (usually acid at night and in the early morning and relatively alkaline in the late morning and early afternoon) significantly affect the ionization of several sparingly soluble urinary constituents and thus their potential for crystallization. In only slightly acid urine of pH 6.8, about 50% of urinary phosphate is present as the HPO_4^{2-} ion ($H_2PO_4^- \leftrightarrows HPO_4^{2-}$, $pK_2 = 6.8$) that readily reacts with calcium to form sparingly soluble brushite ($CaHPO_4, \cdot 2H_2O$; solubility in water about 1.8 mmol/L). However, when the urine pH is 5.5, only about 5% of urinary phosphate is present as the HPO_4^{2-} ion. Because the solubility of $Ca(H_2PO_4)_2 \cdot H_2O$ (solubility in water about 7.1 mmol/L) is almost four times greater than that of brushite, the tendency for calcium phosphate precipitation is correspondingly reduced. On the other hand, the solubility of undissociated uric acid (pK_1 uric acid $\leftrightarrows$ urate $= 5.6$) in maximally acid urine of pH 4.5 to 5.0 is about 100 mg/L, whereas the solubility of (sodium) urate at pH 7 is about 16 times greater (1700 mg/L). Thus crystallization of uric acid is more likely to occur if the urine is persistently very acid.
3. Normal urine contains inhibitors of crystal nucleation that form complexes with potentially insoluble urinary constituents. Citrate can complex calcium and magnesium can form soluble complexes with oxalate. Hypocitraturia or hypomagnesuria may thus contribute to initial crystal nucleation.
4. Normal urine contains protein inhibitors of crystal growth. Two such proteins have now been identified: nephrocalcin, a glycoprotein containing gamma-carboxyglutamic acid and the bone protein, osteopontin. Both are potent inhibitors of calcium oxalate crystal growth. Presumably, genetically determined abnormalities in the structure of these protein inhib-

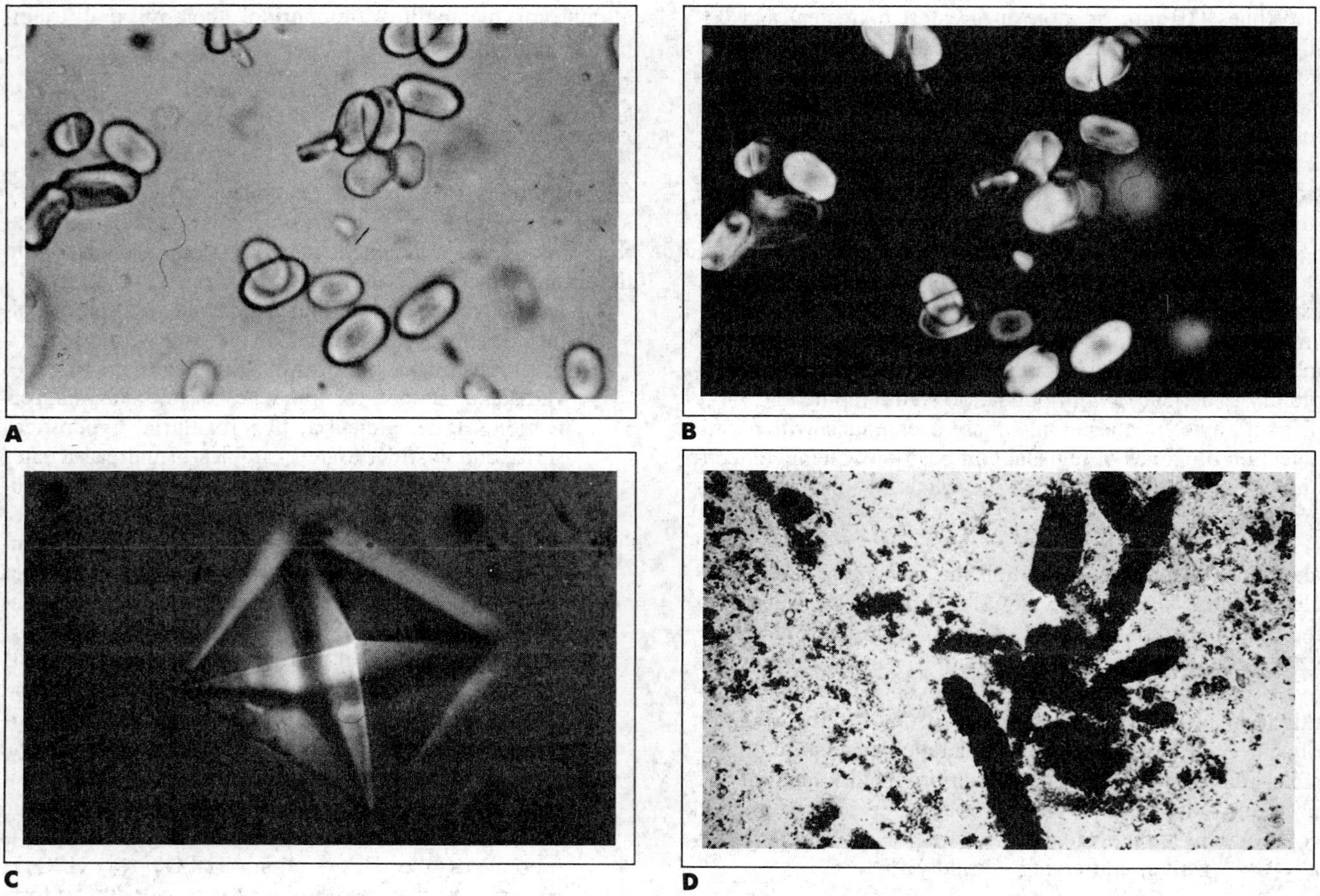

Fig. 349-2. Crystals that may be seen in the centrifuged sediment from fresh, warm urine in patients with nephrolithiasis and that reflect the composition of the patient's stone. **A,** Calcium oxalate monohydrate (whewellite). **B,** Same as in **A** under polarized light. **C,** Calcium oxalate dihydrate (wedellite). **D,** Calcium phosphate (amorphous apatite), single crystals, in clusters, and in casts. **E,** Magnesium ammonium phosphate hexahydrate (struvite). **F,** Cystine. **G,** Uric acid. **H,** Same as in **G** under polarized light.

itors that reduces their capacity to inhibit crystal growth contributes to the pathogenesis of stones. Urinary Tamm-Horsfall protein is an inhibitor of crystal aggregation. In a family with kidney stones, affected individuals have been shown to have an abnormal Tamm-Horsfall protein.

5. Crystals must attach to the papillary collecting duct or pelvic surfaces to provide sufficient time for growth to the size of a clinically relevant stone because rates of renal tubular fluid flow are too rapid to permit time for such crystal growth. Recent studies have demonstrated specific and inhibitable binding of calcium oxalate, apatite, and uric acid to papillary collecting duct cells in tissue culture at specific sites. These observations suggest that alternations in urothelial surfaces may play a role in the formation of kidney stones. In addition, most kidney stones contain a protein matrix that may initiate crystal nucleation or, in addition, attach small crystals as they form and thus allow time for their growth.
6. Crystals of one substance may be the nucleus for precipitation of another. For example, seeding of otherwise stable saturated solutions of calcium oxalate with apatite crystals leads to the removal of calcium and oxalate ions from solution and growth of calcium oxalate crystals upon the seed crystal of apatite. This effect is termed *heterogeneous nucleation* or secondary crystal growth because the molecular structure of calcium oxalate and apatite differ significantly. Uric acid seed crystals are similarly able to induce calcium oxalate crystal growth. Because calcium oxalate dihydrate and uric acid crystal lattices and surfaces are of similar dimensions on an atomic level, this effect is termed *epitaxial nucleation*.

The evaluation and therapy of patients with each of the major types of stones are considered in the subsequent paragraphs, following the scheme shown in Fig. 349-1. In general, patients who are discovered to have in blood or urine composition abnormalities that favor stone recurrence (e.g., primary hyperparathyroidism, distal renal tubular acidosis, hypercalciuria, hyperoxaluria, cystinuria, urinary infection) require specific or ongoing treatment to prevent further re-

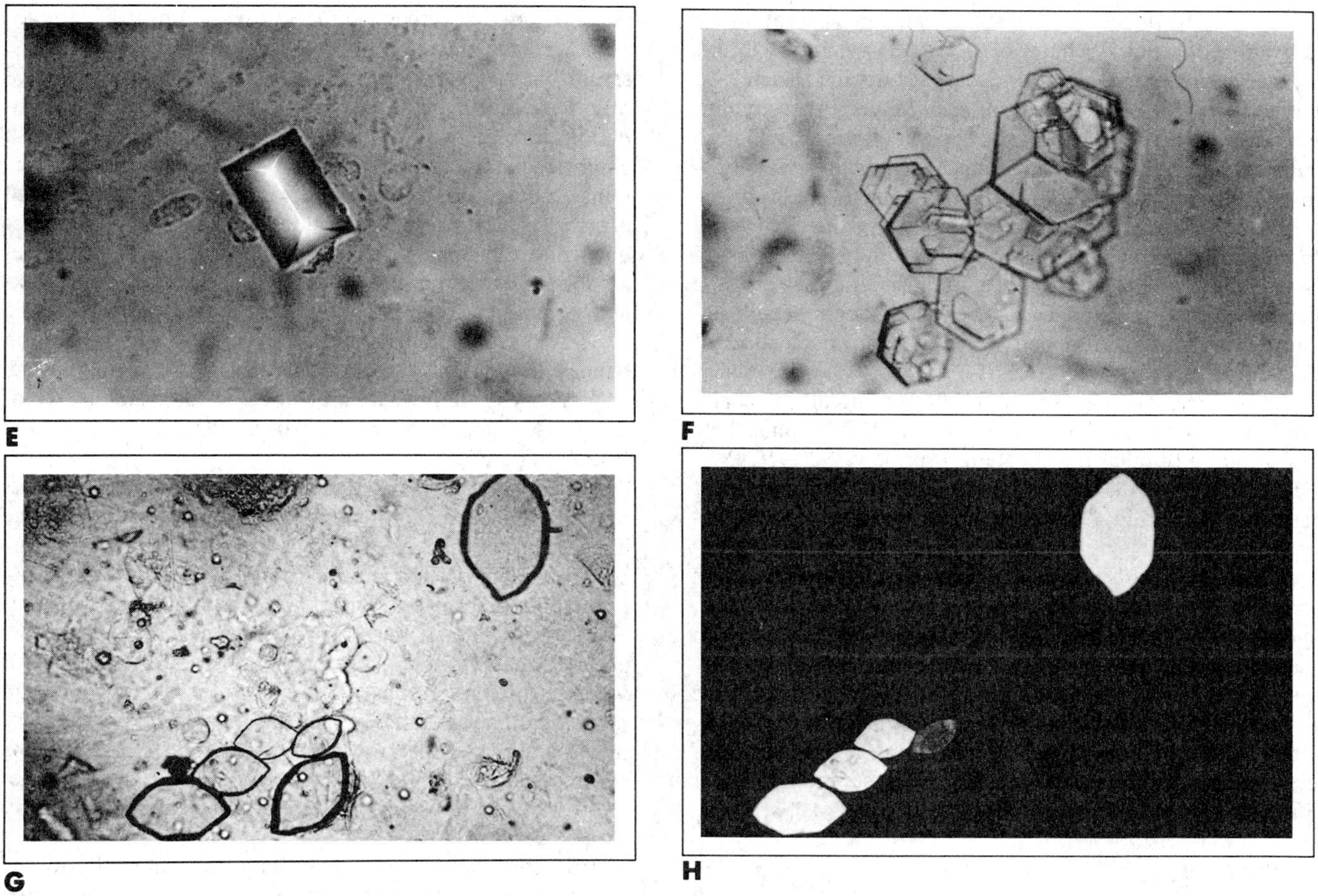

For legend see opposite page.

currences. On the other hand, patients with first stones that have been passed spontaneously and who have no currently detectable abnormality in urine composition (usually idiopathic calcium stone formers) may simply be advised to increase their water intake to avoid the burden and expense of lifelong drug therapy.

CALCIUM OXALATE AND APATITE STONES

Calcium oxalate alone and/or apatite account for about 75% of all renal stones. Thus the presence of a calcium stone is strongly suspected in all patients with radiodense stones simply because the stones are so common. The diagnosis is even more strongly suspected if calcium oxalate or apatite crystals are seen in the sediment of a fresh, warm urine (see Fig. 349-2, *A-D*) (1) that has a pH less than 7.5 and does not contain many neutrophils or bacilli, thus excluding struvite-apatite (infection) stones, and (2) in which the cyanide nitroprusside test is negative, thus excluding cystine. The diagnosis is established by stone analysis.

In general, increased rates of daily urinary calcium or oxalate excretion, low urine volumes, or deficiency in inhibitors of crystal nucleation and growth appear to be the major factors in calcium oxalate precipitation. Increased rates of calcium excretion, low urine volumes, and defective acidification of the urine appear to be the factors determining apatite precipitation. Genetic factors are also of importance. Calcium stones due to primary hyperoxaluria, a recessive trait, and distal renal tubular acidosis, a dominant trait in some families, may initially occur in children. Calcium stones associated with one of the idiopathic hypercalciuria syndromes or idiopathic calcium stone disease usually begin in the third or fourth decade of life, after growth is complete. Men outnumber women by about 3 : 1 among these patient groups, and more than one-half have a family history of stones, suggesting an X-modified polygenic inheritance pattern. In some families, a dominant pattern of inheritance is present.

CALCIUM STONES AND HYPERCALCEMIA

Primary hyperparathyroidism

Primary hyperparathyroidism is the most prominent underlying disorder in patients with calcium stones and hypercalcemia. It is defined as a fasting morning serum calcium concentration persistently higher than 10.4 mg/pdl in association with a serum parathyroid hormone (PTH) concentration >65 pg/ml. Primary increases in PTH secretion by a single adenoma in more than 90% of these patients, or by hyperplasia of all parathyroid glands in the remaining patients, lead to hypercalcemia by stimulating bone reabsorption, augmenting renal tubular calcium reabsorption, and indirectly increasing intestinal calcium absorption by activation of renal synthesis of 1,25$(OH)_2$-vitamin D_3. Increased serum calcium concentration results in an increased glomerular filtration of calcium that exceeds the simultaneous stimulation of renal tubular reabsorption of filtered calcium by PTH and thus results in hypercalciuria. Parathyroid hormone also inhibits proximal renal tubular bicarbonate reabsorption, thus tending to cause the final urine to be more alkaline. Apatite crystallization or stone growth is thus the consequence of hypercalciuria and the less acid urine, whereas calcium oxalate crystallization occurs because of hypercalciuria and heterogeneous nucleation of calcium oxalate by apatite.

Hypophosphatemia (serum PO_4 < 2.6 mg/dl) is usually present, because PTH also inhibits renal tubular phosphate reabsorption (tubular phosphate resorption < 80%; T_mPO_4/GFR < 2.6 mg/dl GFR). Hypercalciuria after overnight fasting (>0.12 mg Ca/mg creatinine) is also present because of persistent hypercalcemia due to ongoing bone resorption. Elevated serum alkaline phosphatase activity and radiographic evidence of hyperparathyroid bone disease, such as subperiosteal resorption and cortical tunneling in the phalanges, may be observed, depending on the severity and duration of hyperparathyroidism. Approximately one third of patients with hyperparathyroidism have kidney stones. Therapy consists in neck exploration and appropriate parathyroidectomy by an experienced surgeon (Chapter 360).

OTHER HYPERCALCEMIC DISORDERS

Hypercalciuria and, less often, hypercalcemia occur with several other specific disorders, although the formation of kidney stones in such patients is extremely unusual. These disorders include (1) hyperthyroidism as a consequence of direct stimulation of bone resorption by the thyroid hormones; (2) extrarenal synthesis of 1,25-$(OH)_2$-D_3 in macrophages in patients with sarcoidosis, tuberculosis and other granulomatous infections, foreign body granulomas, or occasional lymphomas; (3) as a consequence of bone resorption stimulated by metastatic tumors including multiple myeloma or because of more generalized stimulation of bone resorption by PTH-related peptide or other humoral factors produced by tumors; and (4) sudden immobilization because of fractures or paralytic disorders in patients with underlying rapid bone turnover as in rapidly growing adolescents or Paget's disease of bone.

HYPERCALCIURIA WITHOUT HYPERCALCEMIA

Although *distal renal tubular acidosis* is an infrequent cause of nephrolithiasis, screening studies for this disorder should be routinely carried out in patients with calcium stones, especially those with nephrocalcinosis whose stones are composed only of apatite. The diagnosis is established by the finding of a urine pH that is always 6.0 or higher, in the absence of urinary tract infection, when urine pH is measured at each voiding throughout the day with phenaphthazine paper, together with the observation of hyperchloremic metabolic acidosis (venous blood pH 7.34 or less, serum bicarbonate 24 mEq/L or less, serum chloride 108 mEq/L or higher). The acidosis is a consequence of a limitation in the capacity of the distal renal tubule to establish a normal and maximum hydrogen ion gradient between terminal tubular urine and blood (Chapter 353). Significant urinary bicarbonate wasting does not occur. As a consequence of the impaired acidification of the final urine, net renal acid excretion as titratable acid—and, to a less extent, as ammonium—is low relative to rates of endogenous fixed-acid production. A chronically positive hydrogen ion balance thus follows, accompanied by loss of bone mineral and usually by hypercalciuria. In addition, systemic acidosis is associated with low rates of urinary citrate excretion (<200 mg/day).

Increased bicarbonate delivery to distal tubule segments normally enhances net tubular calcium reabsorption, so the hypercalciuria may possibly be a result of reduced bicarbonate delivery when serum bicarbonate levels are below normal but the capacity for proximal tubular bicarbonate reabsorption is intact. Intestinal calcium absorption is apparently normal. Hypophosphatemia is also often present, but whether this is the consequence of an additional defect in renal tubular reabsorption or of compensatory secondary hyperparathyroidism in response to hypercalciuria remains controversial. Hypokalemia, occasionally of sufficient severity to cause muscular weakness or even paralysis, may also be present.

Effective therapy is achieved by the administration of sufficient base in divided doses throughout the day to sustain a normal morning serum bicarbonate concentration of 26 to 28 mEq/L; 1 to 3 mEq of alkali/kg body weight is usually required. As much of the alkali as possible should be administered as potassium citrate or a mixture of potassium citrate, acetate, bicarbonate because of frequent accompanying hypokalemia and because potassium has an additional effect to reduce urinary calcium excretion. Potassium supplements must be limited if kidney function is impaired. Potassium citrate or equivalent is generally begun at a dose of 20 mEq three times a day for a 60-kg patient. The dose is subsequently increased depending on serum bicarbonate and potassium concentration. Additional base can also be given as $NaHCO_3$ (1 650 mg tablet = 7.7 mEq) or Shohl's solution (sodium citrate and citric acid, 1 ml = 1 mEq). Relatively more alkali is required for children because of the acidifying effects of the deposition of alkaline bone salts during skeletal growth. These measures generally prevent the formation of new stones and progressive nephrocalcinosis despite a more alkaline urine. Moreover, bone disease, if present, may heal without the need for calcium or vitamin D supplements.

IDIOPATHIC HYPERCALCIURIA SYNDROMES

Several surveys of patients with calcium nephrolithiasis have shown that 30% to 60% exhibit hypercalciuria in the absence of fasting hypercalcemia, clinical evidence of a disorder causing accelerated bone turnover, or distal renal tubular acidosis. *Hypercalciuria* is defined as a urinary calcium excretion exceeding 300 mg/day or 4 mg/kg/day because metabolic studies of healthy adults without kidney stones or bone disease who are in calcium balance show urinary calcium excretion ranges from 55 to 285 mg/day while they are eating normal diets providing 600 to 1200 mg of calcium/day. Occasional patients with calcium stones and hypercalciuria give a history of gluttony for calcium-rich foods or the abuse of calcium carbonate-containing antacids, but dietary calcium intake of 2000 mg/day or more is generally required to produce urinary calcium excretion rates above 300 mg/day in healthy subjects. Thus factors other than high dietary calcium intake that produce elevated average calcium concentrations within the intestine and favor passive diffusion of calcium from the gut to the blood must be responsible for hypercalciuria in most patients.

Many studies have shown that patients with idiopathic hypercalciuria exhibit increased intestinal calcium absorption in comparison with normal subjects when both groups are eating diets containing normal amounts of calcium. Because such calcium stone formers do not have symptoms of bone disease or radiographic evidence of marked skeletal demineralization, the additional calcium appearing in their urine must ultimately be principally derived from the diet.

Recent studies have documented that serum 1,25$(OH)_2$-vitamin D_3 levels, the only currently known stimulus of intestinal calcium absorption, are elevated in many patients with idiopathic hypercalciuria. In a few patients, a renal calcium leak resulting in mild secondary hyperparathyroidism appears to be the basic defect. Parathyroid hormone stimulates 1,25$(OH)_2$-vitamin D_3 synthesis, elevates serum concentrations of this hormone, and thus stimulates the intestinal calcium absorption that compensates for the basic renal calcium wasting defect. This syndrome is manifested by hypercalciuria when the patients eat either a normal- or low-calcium diet (200 mg/day), hypercalciuria in the morning after overnight fasting (>0.12 mg Ca/mg creatinine), a tendency to low normal serum calcium level, high normal or slightly elevated serum PTH concentrations, and mild hypophosphatemia. Urinary hydroxyproline excretion is increased, and bone biopsies have indicated increased bone resorption and formation in response to the elevation of PTH.

Another subset of patients exhibit elevated serum 1,25$(OH)_2$-vitamin D_3 concentrations despite normal or low serum PTH concentrations in association with mild hypophosphatemia. The hypophosphatemia is present despite normal rates of urinary phosphate excretion, thus providing evidence of a renal phosphate leak. By analogy to studies showing that dietary phosphate deprivation increases renal 1,25$(OH)_2$-vitamin D_3 synthesis, it appears that an abnormality of phosphate metabolism in these idiopathic hypercalciuria patients is in some way responsible for the elevation of serum 1,25$(OH)_2$-vitamin D_3 concentrations, increased intestinal calcium absorption, and hypercalciuria. A third subset of idiopathic hypercalciuria patients with elevated serum 1,25$(OH)_2$-vitamin D_3 concentrations exhibit neither high serum PTH levels nor low serum phosphate concentrations, indicating that currently undefined factors may activate the vitamin D endocrine system in these patients. Finally, there have been studies showing that intestinal calcium absorption in some patients with idiopathic hypercalciuria may be increased independently of serum 1,25$(OH)_2$-vitamin D_3 concentrations.

Regardless of these uncertainties regarding the basic abnormality that leads to hypercalciuria among patients with the idiopathic form, there appears to be agreement regarding therapy. Long-term administration of an anti-calciuric diuretic (a thiazide, chlorthalidone, indapamide) in doses equivalent to 25 or 50 mg of hydrochlorothiazide twice a day, reduces urinary calcium excretion by 40% to 60% and effectively prevents stone recurrence. These drugs enhance distal renal tubular calcium reabsorption. The drugs are usually begun using a small dose and increasing the dose over several weeks to avoid symptomatic extracellular fluid volume depletion that may result from the sodium diuresis as treatment is initiated. Symptomatic hypokalemia seldom occurs during long-term therapy, and potassium supplements are not routinely prescribed. Supplementary phosphate may also be used and is given as neutral sodium and potassium phosphate in doses providing 1.5 to 2.0 g phosphorus/day. The patients are also advised to limit their intake of milk, cheese, or ice cream to one serving daily, limit their NaCl intake, and drink sufficient fluids to sustain urine volumes of 1500 ml/day or more.

HYPERURICOSURIA WITH OR WITHOUT HYPERCALCIURIA

A subset of calcium oxalate stone formers exhibit *hyperuricosuria,* defined as urinary excretion of uric acid >800 mg/day in men or >750 mg/day in women while the patients are eating their usual diets, selected by themselves. Many of these patients appear to eat a purine-rich diet habitually. Some are also mildly hyperuricemic and some may exhibit hypercalciuria. Hyperuricosuria may cause calcium oxalate stones because of epitaxial nucleation of calcium oxalate by uric acid, or reduction by uric acid of the activity of the inhibitors of calcium oxalate crystal growth. Therapeutic trials have shown that reduction of urinary uric acid excretion by the administration of allopurinol, 200 to 300 mg/day, effectively prevents stone recurrence. Patients with hypercalciuria should, in addition, be treated with a thiazide diuretic.

HYPEROXALURIA

Hyperoxaluria is a major risk factor in the pathogenesis of recurrent calcium oxalate stones. The possibility of primary hyperoxaluria should be considered when the onset of stone disease occurs before the age of 20 years, and acquired hyperoxaluria should be considered in patients with disease of the small intestine or with gluttony for oxalate-rich foods, in patients who have had intestinal bypass surgery, or in ascorbic acid abuse. Normal urinary oxalate in healthy adults eating normal diets ranges from 8 to 45 mg/day, so hyperoxaluria can be operationally defined as a urinary oxalate excretion exceeding 45 mg/day. Calcium oxalate monohydrate crystalluria appears to be common in these patients (see Fig. 349-2, *A* and *B*).

Primary hyperoxaluria is the result of a recessively inherited defect (type I: α-ketoglutarate:glyoxylate carboligase deficiency associated with increased urinary glyoxylate excretion; type II: D-glyceric dehydrogenase deficiency, associated with increased urinary L-glyceric acid excretion). The disorder usually begins in childhood in association with urinary oxalate excretion rates in the range of 90 to 270 mg/day and leads to renal failure because of nephrocalcinosis and repetitive episodes of ureteral obstruction that may be complicated by urinary infection. However, in some patients with less severe hyperoxaluria who habitually drink large amounts of water, the disorder may result in only periodic passage of stones and prolonged survival.

Supplementary pyridoxine, 25 to 200 mg/day, has been found to reduce oxalate excretion in some of these patients. Elimination of oxalate-rich foods from the diet is recommended. Other therapeutic efforts are directed toward minimizing calcium oxalate crystal nucleation and crystal growth by the following measures: (1) reduction of average urinary oxalate concentration by increasing water intake to ensure urine volumes greater than 2 L/day, with accompanying nocturia; (2) administration of a thiazide diuretic to reduce urinary calcium concentration; (3) administration of supplementary sodium-potassium phosphate in divided doses to provide 1.0 to 1.5 g of phosphorus/day in an attempt to increase urinary concentrations of pyrophosphate, a potent inhibitor of calcium oxalate crystal growth (bearing in mind that phosphate supplements can accelerate deterioration of renal function and potentially cause or aggravate secondary hyperparathyroidism so they must never be used in patients with even the slightest reductions in glomerular filtration rate).

Acquired hyperoxaluria among gluttons for oxalate-rich foods (rhubarb, spinach and other leafy vegetables, cashews, almonds, and strong tea) is managed by eliminating these foods from the diet. When acquired hyperoxaluria is related to abuse of ascorbic acid, which can be a precursor for endogenous oxalate synthesis (vitamin C use exceeding 500 mg/day), this supplement should be discontinued. Acquired hyperoxaluria in association with disease or resection or bypass of the small intestine is the result of increased colonic oxalate absorption. Treatment of these patients includes (1) a low oxalate diet; (2) water; (3) oral calcium carbonate, calcium gluconate, or calcium lactate supplements to provide 800 to 2000 mg calcium per day in divided doses in an attempt to precipitate calcium oxalate within the bowel and reduce oxalate absorption; and (4) the administration of the oxalate-binding anion exchange resin cholestyramine in a dose of 4 g three times a day, also to limit oxalate absorption.

HYPOCITRATURIA

Urinary citrate excretion ranges from approximately 350 to 1450 mg/day in health and, by complexing calcium, lowers urinary saturation with respect to calcium oxalate and apatite. Citrate excretion is higher in women than in men, and this may contribute to the lower incidence in women. Citrate excretion is low among some patients with calcium stones, regardless of hypercalciuria and in the absence of systemic acidosis. Urinary citrate excretion can be augmented by the administration of potassium citrate or $KHCO_3$, 20 mEq, 3 times daily and is effective in preventing stone recurrence.

IDIOPATHIC CALCIUM STONE DISEASE

Currently, about 25% of calcium stone formers have no quantifiable abnormality of urinary composition (e.g., hypercalciuria, hyperoxaluria, hyperuricosuria, hypocitraturia). A few of these patients appear by habit to drink very small amounts of fluid, so their daily urine volume is only 500 to 1000 ml, resulting in average prevailing urinary concentrations of calcium, oxalate, and phosphate that are higher than normal; hence, crystal nucleation and stone growth could occur even when daily excretion rates of these potentially insoluble urinary constituents are normal. Most idiopathic calcium stone formers, however, have normal urine volumes of 1500 to 2000 ml/day, so it appears likely that a deficiency of normal urinary inhibitors of crystal nucleation and crystal growth or the presence of promoters of crystal nucleation or growth accounts for stone formation. Therapy includes sufficient water intake to maintain urine volume above 1500 ml/day and the administration of a thiazide diuretic, as used in the treatment of hypercalciuric calcium stone formers.

INFECTION STONES

Stones related to urinary tract infection are composed of magnesium ammonium phosphate hexahydrate ($MgNH_4PO \cdot 6H_2O$), struvite (see Fig. 349-1, *E*), and variable amounts of carbonate apatite [$Ca_{10}(PO_4)_6CO_{3-}$], and are a consequence of infection of the kidney and/or bladder by bacteria that produce the enzyme urease. Struvite-apatite stones never form in persistently sterile urine and do not form as a consequence of urinary infection by organisms that do not produce urease. Urease-producing organisms cause hydrolysis of urea to ammonia and carbon dioxide. The immediate and subsequent reactions of ammonia either with water or with carbonic acid yield ammonium bicarbonate. Because the p*K* for the dissociation of ammonium to ammonia plus hydrogen ions is about 9, the urine becomes very alkaline (pH >7.5). Some carbonate ions are also formed because the p*K* for the dissociation of bicarbonate to carbonate is about 10. Moreover, because the p*K* for the reaction $HPO_4^{2-} \leftrightarrows PO_4^{3-}$ is about 11, small amounts of phosphate ions are also formed. Collectively, these reactions lead to marked elevations of urinary concentrations of NH_4^+, PO_4^{3-}, and CO_3^{3-}, which together with normal concentrations of urinary magnesium and calcium in these alkaline solutions cause precipitation of $MgNH_4PO_4 \cdot 6H_2O$ and $Ca_{10}(PO_4)_6CO_{3-}$.

Most patients who form infection stones exhibit abnormal urinary drainage and/or urinary obstruction that permits establishment and persistence of urinary infection. Predisposing abnormalities include congenital anomalies of the urinary tract (e.g., urethral valve, vesicoureteral reflux, exstrophy of the bladder), bladder dysfunction (urethral obstruction due to prostatism, intrinsic motor dysfunction, spinal cord injury or disease), chronic catheter drainage of the urinary tract (bladder, nephrostomy, ureterostomy), or ureteral diversion to an ileal or sigmoid conduit. Occasionally, infection stones complicate other metabolic derangements that cause kidney stones.

The symptoms of infection stones vary widely, depending on the circumstances leading to urinary tract infection. In some patients, stones in the renal pelvis or in the bladder may be present for long periods without symptoms. By contrast, in other patients, repeated episodes of flank pain together with bacteremia may occur as the result of local urinary obstruction associated with acute exacerbation of chronic infection.

Urinalysis generally demonstrates that the urine is persistently very alkaline, the pH being 7.5 or higher, with minor proteinuria (<1 g/day) and persistent pyuria and bacilluria. Cultures of the urine demonstrate significant growth of the bacteria that produce urease. These usually include *Proteus, Providencia, Klebsiella, Pseudomonas, Serratia, Enterobacter,* or *Staphylococcus* species. Plain radiographs of the abdomen demonstrate radiopaque kidney or bladder calculi that often exhibit a laminated structure. When large stones assume the shape of the renal pelvis and calices, they are termed *staghorn calculi.* Although most such large pelvic caliceal stones are related to urinary infection, cystine or uric acid stones may occasionally assume the staghorn configuration. Intravenous or retrograde urography is necessary to search for sites of urinary obstruction. Depending on the duration and severity of the urinary obstruction and infection, the glomerular filtration rate may be reduced and renal tubular function impaired, manifested by metabolic acidosis and loss of maximum renal concentrating capacity.

The natural history and progression of infection stones depends on whether or not the stones can be completely removed, the infection eradicated, the urinary obstruction relieved, and the abnormal portals of entry into the urinary tract for new bacterial pathogens closed. Appropriate antibiotic therapy may temporarily sterilize the urine. However, relapse of infection is frequent because organisms incorporated into the stones during their growth cannot be reached by adequate bactericidal drug concentrations, or because new infections result from urease-producing bacteria that enter the urinary tract in catheters. Treatment must be undertaken in collaboration with urologic consultants and aimed toward removal of all the residual stones, correction of obstruction, and restoration of normal urinary drainage. If infection stones can be removed, about half of such patients will be cured, although underlying structural abnormalities in the urinary tract or renal scarring often persist. In the remaining patients, infection persists and the formation of new stones is frequent. Because infection stones may complicate other types of calculous disease, underlying metabolic causes for urinary tract stone formation should be sought. If the urine can be sterilized, thus restoring normal urine acidity, struvite-apatite stones can theoretically be dissolved. Antibiotic therapy alone, however, seldom achieves this goal.

CYSTINURIA

The formation of kidney stones composed of the amino acid cystine

$$({}^{-}OOC{-}\underset{\displaystyle NH_3^+}{\underset{|}{CH}}{-}CH_2{-}S{-}S{-}CH_2{-}\underset{\displaystyle NH_3^+}{\underset{|}{CH}}{-}COO^{-})$$

is the result of a genetic abnormality of amino acid transport. Urinary excretion rates of cystine, together with the other dibasic amino acids lysine, arginine, and ornithine, are increased. Because cystine is only sparingly soluble, the excessive excretion rate leads to cystine crystallization within the renal pelvis and the formation of stones.

Cystinuria is an autosomal recessive trait resulting in defective renal tubular, as well as intestinal, transport of cystine, lysine, arginine, and ornithine.

Patients with cystinuria account for only about 1% to 3% of all patients with urolithiasis. Stone disease may begin at any age but appears most commonly in the second and third decades of life. The initial symptoms may be those of renal colic, with or without hematuria, but occasionally only vague backache is present, followed by the discovery of large pelvic staghorn calculi. The stones are radiopaque because of the sulfur contained in cystine, although they are not as radiodense as calcium-containing stones.

The diagnosis is suspected either when the typical hexagonal cystine crystals are observed in the urinary sediment (see Fig. 349-2, *F*) or when the results of the urinary cyanide nitroprusside screening test, which detects cystine in a concentration exceeding 75 μg/mg creatinine (normal less than 70 μg cystine/mg creatinine), are positive. The diagnosis is confirmed by the analysis of a stone or by quantitation of 24-hour urinary cystine excretion in the range of 425 μg/mg creatinine among cystinuric patients compared with less than 70 μg cystine/mg creatinine in healthy subjects. The urinary excretion of lysine, arginine, and ornithine is also observed to be elevated.

The frequency of stone recurrence and of complicating urinary obstruction tends to increase as urinary cystine excretion rates increase. As a consequence, ureteral obstruction requiring multiple lithotomies and complicating urinary infection can lead to progressive renal failure as a result of hydronephrosis and pyelonephritis. Thus the initial phase of therapy involves the education of the patient—and, in the case of a young child, the family—regarding the genetic basis for the cystinuria and the need for lifelong therapy. Treatment is aimed at both increasing the capacity of the urine to dissolve cystine and at reducing urinary cystine excretion. Because urinary cystine is derived from the sulfur-containing amino acids of dietary proteins, principally methionine, protein intake should probably be limited to 1 g/kg body weight/day. The solubility of cystine over the pH range 4.5 to 7.0 is limited to about 290 to 380 mg/L. Because 24-hour cystine excretion in cystinuric patients may be in the range of 700 to 1200 mg/day, they must learn to drink sufficient water to maintain a minimum urine volume of 3 L/day and to drink sufficient water at bedtime to induce nocturia. On arising to void, they should drink an additional 300 ml of water. Patients should collect and measure their own 24-hour urine volume on several occasions to ensure that their water intake is adequate.

The solubility of cystine in urine rises sharply to about 790 mg/L as urinary pH rises from 7.0 to 8.0. Thus sustained alkalinization of the urine, in addition to a large urine volume, will assist in maintaining cystine in solution. Approximately 2 mEq/kg body weight, or 150 mEq/day, of actual or potential bicarbonate, given in divided doses, is required to maintain the urine pH in the range of 7.5. This can generally be achieved by the administration of 35 to 50 mEq of sodium bicarbonate, or 40 to 60 ml of Shohl's solution, four times a day. Because dietary sodium chloride may enhance cystine excretion, dietary sodium chloride should be restricted and some of the needed base administered as potassium citrate or $KHCO_3$ rather than $NaHCO_3$. In addition, 250 mg of acetazolamide may be given at bedtime to inhibit proximal tubular bicarbonate reabsorption and induce a nocturnal alkaline diuresis. When acetazolamide is administered, an additional dose of sodium bicarbonate or Shohl's solution should be given during the night when the patient arises to void, to check the tendency for serum bicarbonate levels to fall and the urine to become more acid as the action of acetazolamide develops and then wanes. Patients should check their urine pH at each voiding for several days, using phenaphthazine paper to ensure that the pH is 7.5 or higher.

Daily cystine excretion can be reduced by the administration of the SH-containing drugs, D-penicillamine, mercaptoproprionylglycine (MPG) or captopril. These drugs can undergo a disulfide exchange reaction with cystine to form the mixed disulfide of cysteine and the drug. These mixed disulfides are very much more soluble than cystine. D-penicillamine may result in significant toxic side effects including fever, rash, leukopenia, thrombocytopenia, and the nephrotic syndrome. MPG appears to be less toxic. Captopril is effective but additional experience with its use is needed.

Collectively, these therapeutic measures may sometimes result in the dissolution of nonobstructing cystine stones, but more often they appear to be most useful in preventing further growth of existing stones and the formation of new stones.

URIC ACID STONES

Uric acid stones account for about 5% to 10% of all kidney stones and may be the consequence of increased daily urinary uric acid excretion, a persistently concentrated urine, or a persistently acid urine. Uric acid stones are radiolucent and should be differentiated from tumors of the renal pelvis, blood clots, sloughed renal papillae, and very rare xanthine stones. The diagnosis of uric acid urolithiasis may be suspected when uric acid crystals are observed in the urine sediment under bright field illumination and polarized light (see Fig. 349-2, *G* and *H*) and is confirmed by stone analysis.

The major determinants of uric acid crystalluria and stone formation are daily urinary uric acid excretion and urine volume, which determine the mean prevailing total urinary uric acid concentration and urinary pH, which in turn determines the concentration of free (undissociated) uric acid, the least soluble form of uric acid. Uric acid has two dissociable protons, the first having a p*K* of about 5.6 and the second a p*K* of about 11.0. Thus, at a minimum urinary pH of 4.5, approximately 95% of total urinary uric acid will exist as undissociated uric acid, whereas at a urinary pH of 7.0, approximately 95% of the total urinary uric acid will exist as urate ion. The solubility of undissociated uric acid in maximally acid urine is about 100 mg/L, whereas the solubility of (sodium) urate at pH 7.0 is about 1700 mg/L. Among healthy adults, who excrete approximately 500 mg of uric acid per day in a urine having a volume of 1 L and an average normal pH of 5.6, the estimated undissociated urinary uric acid concentration will be about 250 mg/L, a value clearly above the solubility of undissociated uric acid. Thus, normal urine would often appear to be supersaturated with respect to undissociated uric acid, and yet uric acid crystalluria and stones are not very common. Perhaps diurnal variation in urinary flow rate and the normal diurnal variation of urinary pH (alkaline at midday, acid at night and in the early morning) prevent uric acid crystal formation and growth. Whether or not normal urine contains inhibitors of uric acid crystallization or growth is not known. Clearly, therefore, when urinary uric acid excretion is greater than normal (>800 mg/day), or the urine volume is low (<1 L/day), or the urine is persistently acid (pH always <5.5), the urine may become more supersaturated with respect to undissociated uric acid, thus permitting the formation of uric acid stones.

Uric acid stones are common among patients with gout, increasing in frequency as urinary uric acid excretion increases among the subset of gouty patients who overproduce uric acid. Uric acid overproduction is a consequence of rapid cell turnover in myeloproliferative and other neoplastic diseases and may result in uric acid crystalluria and stones as an early symptom of the underlying malignancy. More frequently, however, crystalluria and stones are the preventable consequence of cytolytic chemotherapy. Purine gluttony resulting in hyperuricosuria may occasionally be a cause of uric acid stones, and the tendency toward crystal growth in this setting is probably contributed to by the concomitant high protein intake that increases fixed endogenous acid production and results in a persistently acid urine. Uric acid stones are also common among the majority of patients with gout who produce normal amounts of uric acid. In these patients, a persistently acid urine secondary to impaired renal tubular ammonium synthesis and the excretion of a persistently acid urine appear to be the causative factors.

A similar abnormality in renal ammonium excretion has been observed among idiopathic uric acid stone formers who do not exhibit hyperuricemia, hyperuricosuria, or gout. The defect is suspected on demonstrating that urinary pH is 5.5 or less at each voiding throughout the day and night for several days. Uric acid precipitation may be favored among patients with diarrheal diseases because of accelerated fecal bicarbonate losses and a tendency toward mild hyperchloremic metabolic acidosis and a persistently acid urine, as well as a persistently low urine volume as a consequence of accelerated fecal water losses. Similarly, accelerated cutaneous and pulmonary water losses in hot environments or during febrile illnesses may result in a persistently concentrated urine favoring uric acid crystallization and stone growth.

The therapy of uric acid nephrolithiasis is directed toward augmenting the solubility of uric acid in urine and reducing daily urinary uric acid excretion. Patients should be taught to drink sufficient quantities of water to maintain a urine volume of 2 L or more per day. If possible, the patient should drink sufficient water on retiring to cause nocturia and should also be asked to drink additional water on rising to void. Because maintenance of urinary pH in the vicinity of 6.5 markedly enhances uric acid solubility as urate, alkali therapy should also be utilized. Generally, about 1 mEq/kg body weight/day, or 70 mEq/day, of sodium bicarbonate or Shohl's solution is sufficient when administered in divided doses four times a day. In addition, 250 mg of acetazolamide can be given at bedtime to sustain a nocturnal alkaline diuresis. Patients should be taught to monitor urinary pH using phenaphthazine paper at each voiding for several days after the initiation of alkali therapy to ensure that the urine pH is maintained in the range of 6.0 to 6.5. Among patients who overproduce uric acid, dietary intake of purine-rich foods should be limited or avoided (liver, kidney, brains, sweetbreads; more than 200 g/day of meat, fish, or poultry; asparagus, spinach, peas, or beans).

In patients whose urinary uric acid excretion exceeds 800 mg/day or in whom such high rates of uric acid excretion can be anticipated when cytolytic drug therapy is initiated for a malignant disease, allopurinol therapy should be used. Allopurinol, an analog of hypoxanthine, is a competitive inhibitor of xanthine oxidase and thus blocks the synthesis of uric acid. The drug also inhibits purine biosynthesis. The more soluble compounds hypoxanthine and xanthine appear in the urine as predominant end products of purine metabolism. Customarily, 200 to 400 mg of allopurinol is administered in a single daily dose. Allopurinol occasionally causes skin rash, leukopenia, or cholestatic jaundice, which requires stopping the drug.

Increased fluid intake and alkali therapy are generally effective in preventing new uric acid stones and, together with allopurinol, may result in the dissolution of nonobstructing uric acid stones that are too large to be passed spontaneously.

REFERENCES

Coe FL and Favus MJ, editors: Disorders of bone and mineral metabolism, New York, 1992, Raven Press.

Coe FL and Parks JH: Nephrolithiasis: pathogenesis and treatment, ed 2, Chicago, 1988, Year Book.

Drach GW: Urinary lithiasis. In Walsh PC et al, editors: Campbell's urology, ed 6, Philadelphia, 1992, WB Saunders.

National Institutes of Health Consensus Statement on the Prevention and Treatment of Kidney Stones, JAMA 260:978-981, 1988.

National Institute of Health Consensus Development Conference on the Prevention and Treatment of Kidney Stones Proceedings, J Urol 141:705-803, 1989.

Pak CYC: Medical management of nephrolithiasis, J Urol 128:1157, 1982.

Segel S and Their SO: Cystinurias, In Scriver CS et al, editors: The metabolic basis of inherited disease, ed 6, New York, 1989, McGraw-Hill.

Smith LH and Khan SR, editors: The Finlayson Colloquium on urolithiasis, Am J Kidney Dis 17:386-457, 1991.

Walker VR et al, editors: Urolithiasis: Proceedings of the Sixth International Symposium, New York, 1988, Plenum Press.

DISORDERS OF ELECTROLYTE AND ACID-BASE BALANCE IV

CHAPTER

350 Disorders of Water Balance

Robert G. Narins
G. Gopal Krishna

Worsening weakness, lethargy, and nausea merge with progressive headache and obtundation to culminate in generalized seizures, coma, and, ultimately, death. This pernicious continuum of symptoms and signs describes equally well the deteriorating course of either hyponatremia or hypernatremia, the chemical hallmarks of disordered water balance. Disorders that spawn deranged water balance with its potentially lethal consequences are best understood in terms of the regulatory system that normally controls solute concentration *(osmoregulation)* with exquisite precision. Accordingly, after first outlining the chemical and physiologic principles that underlie the normal control of water balance, we develop a pathophysiologic approach to the classification, diagnosis, and therapy of the states of disordered osmoregulation. (See Chapter 338 for a more detailed discussion of solute and water balance.)

PRINCIPLES OF OSMOREGULATION

Definitions, water distribution, and solute concentration

Driven by osmotic forces, water moves freely across membranes from areas of low to areas of high solute concentration, thereby dissipating concentration gradients. Because all cell membranes (except renal medullary structures) are freely permeable to water, the solute concentration, or osmolality of intracellular fluid (ICF) always equals that of extracellular fluid (ECF).

Cell metabolism, membrane selectivity, and transport pumps create and sustain major qualitative differences in the solute composition of ICF and ECF (Fig. 350-1), whereas osmotic water movement ensures transcellular equality of concentration. In contrast to the low molecular weight, membrane-permeable anions in the ECF, intracellular anions are macromolecular and relatively nonpermeating. As defined by the *Gibbs-Donnan equilibrium* (Chapter 338), the compartment containing impermeable anions attracts more cations, which in turn leads to the osmotic attraction of more water. Cell swelling, dysfunction, and eventual rupture would occur if accrual of ions and water went unchecked. Membrane-associated cation pumps prevent cellular disruption by actively exporting sodium and importing potassium. Thus the (Na^+ + K^+)-ATPase (sodium-potassium activated adenosine triphosphatase) pump is responsible for potassium and sodium being the major cellular and extracellular solutes, respectively, and for negating passive cation and water entry into cells, thereby maintaining the stability of *cell volume*. The other prime determinant of cell volume is ECF osmolality. Dilution or concentration of ECF solute causes water to enter or leave cells, respectively, and thereby effects cell swelling or shrinkage (see later discussion). It follows therefore that osmoregulation is tantamount to control of cell volume. Indeed, most of hyponatremia's poisonous effect is secondary to brain cell swelling, whereas that of hypernatremia is due to brain cell shrinkage.

Addition of urea or ethanol, solutes that freely cross cell membranes, equally increases the solute concentration of the ECF and the ICF without provoking water movement. Urea and ethanol, therefore, are *ineffective osmols,* because their addition increases osmolality (solute concentration/kg water) without effecting water movement. Addition of sodium salts, which are largely restricted to the ECF, initially increases extracellular osmolality. This extracellular hypertonicity is minimized by solute-free water moving along osmotic gradients from the ICF to the ECF. Net water movement ceases when ECF and ICF osmolalities equalize at new, higher levels. Cell shrinkage resulting from this fluid redistribution can have disastrous effects (especially on the brain), but certain central receptor cells (see later discussion) respond by increasing thirst and the release of *arginine vasopressin* (AVP), the hormone that causes renal retention of acquired water. Retained exogenous water reexpands cells and normalizes the solute concentration of body fluid. Thus sodium salts are *effective osmols* because they increase osmolality and effect transfer of water. The term *tonicity* refers to the effective osmolality of serum. Hypertonic and hypotonic serums cause water to leave or enter cells, respectively. Addition of *ineffective* osmols (e.g., urea) to serum does not affect tonicity. Thus azotemic serum may be hyperosmolal without being hypertonic. Loss of sodium salts or the addition of water to the ECF transiently lowers ECF solute concentration, causing water to move into cells until ECF and ICF concentrations equalize at a new, lower value. Although resulting cellular expansion can be life-threatening, swelling of certain brain cells (see later discussion) diminishes thirst and water acquisition and suppresses AVP release, allowing the kidneys to excrete the excess water.

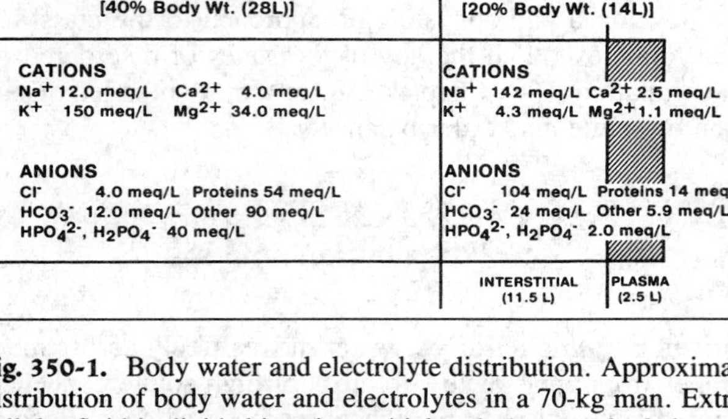

Fig. 350-1. Body water and electrolyte distribution. Approximate distribution of body water and electrolytes in a 70-kg man. Extracellular fluid is divided into interstitial and plasma *(shaded)* components.

Measurements of *osmolality* define the concentration of all plasma solutes (per kilogram of water), that is, electrolyte and nonelectrolyte solute and effective and ineffective osmols. The electrolyte component is almost entirely accounted for by sodium and its accompanying anions, and may be estimated by doubling the serum sodium concentration (Fig. 350-2). Urea and glucose account for virtually all of the normally occurring nonelectrolyte solute. The concentration of either may be converted from mass units (mg/dl) to mmols/L (which is equivalent to mosm/L), by dividing by its molecular weight. Because urea concentration is reported in terms of its nitrogen content (atomic weight 14) (i.e., blood urea nitrogen, or BUN), and because each mole of urea contains 2 moles of nitrogen, the osmolality of urea (mosm/L) from the mass of urea (mg/L or/dl) is found by dividing as follows:

(EQ. 1)

$$\text{BUN (mosm/L)} = \frac{\text{BUN (mg/L)}}{28} = \frac{\text{BUN (mg/dl)}}{2.8}$$

Because sodium, urea, and glucose are the principal contributors to plasma osmolality, it is logical to infer that calculated plasma osmolality should equal that measured in the laboratory. Indeed, under physiologic conditions the difference between measured and calculated osmolality, otherwise termed the *osmolal gap,* should equal 10 mosm/L (Fig. 350-2). Marked increases in plasma proteins and lipid levels cause underestimation of the plasma sodium concentration but do not interfere with the measured osmolality. Thus hyperlipidemia and hyperproteinemia spuriously increase the osmolal gap. A true increase in osmolal gap indicates the presence of an osmotically active solute not accounted for by sodium and its counterbalancing anions: urea, glucose, circulating ethanol, methanol, ethylene glycol, or other low-molecular weight toxins. Modest increases in

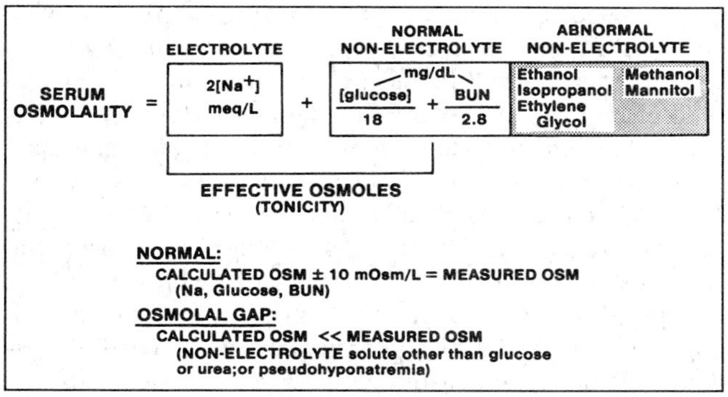

Fig. 350-2. Calculated and measured serum osmolality. Total serum osmolality comprises electrolyte and nonelectrolyte solute. The effective osmoles are largely restricted to the extracellular fluid. The common contributors to the pathologic accumulation of solute are shown in the shaded box.

the osmolal gap occur in nondialyzed patients with chronic renal failure and in patients with lactic and/or ketoacidosis. Therapeutic administration of osmotically active compounds such as mannitol, sorbitol, or glycine increase the measured but decrease the calculated osmolality by lowering serum sodium levels and thus increase the osmolal gap.

Sodium accounts for more than 95% of the ECF solute and potassium exerts an equivalent effect in the ICF. Thus because total body solute is virtually equivalent to the body content of exchangeable sodium (Na_e) and potassium (K_e) salts, it follows that the *concentration* of solute (i.e., the osmolality) is equal to the sum of these two salts, with their respective anions, divided by the volume of total body water (TBW):

(EQ. 2)

$$\text{ECF osmolality} = \text{ICF osmolality} = \frac{2\,(Na_e + K_e)}{\text{TBW}}$$

As discussed later, loss of Na_e or K_e at constant TBW causes hypotonicity. Water retention while body solute content remains constant has a similar effect. Solute gain or water loss causes hypertonicity. Because sodium is the major ECF solute, with rare exception (see later discussion), hypotonicity is equivalent to hyponatremia. However, because such effective osmols as glucose or mannitol may accumulate in the ECF and cause hypertonicity with or without changing sodium concentration, hypertonicity is *not* equivalent to hypernatremia (but hypernatremia always means that hypertonicity is present).

Proportionate accumulation of solute and water causes *isotonic expansion* of body fluid. States of solute and water depletion may be isotonic (normal serum sodium concentration) if solute and water are lost in proportion, hypotonic (hyponatremia) if proportionately more solute than water is lost, or hypertonic (hypernatremia) if proportionately more water is lost. It follows therefore that the serum sodium concentration only defines the ratio of sodium to water and should imply nothing about the state of body sodium content or ECF volume.

As influenced by the aforementioned forces, body water is distributed into cellular and extracellular compartments, the latter being further subdivided into interstitial and intravascular spaces (see Fig. 350-1). Transcellular fluid encompasses such epithelial cell secretions as sweat, gastrointestinal secretions, saliva, bile, and cerebrospinal, ocular, and joint fluids. These fluids, at any instant, do not constitute a large space, but because their turnover is great, their continued loss can eventually lead to severe fluid depletion. Capillary permeability characteristics cause entrapment of albumin and other large molecules in the vascular space, ensuring that interstitial fluid has little protein and that approximately 25% of ECF is retained in the vascular space because of the osmotic (oncotic) effect of protein.

Forces controlling fluid distribution are further illustrated by tracking the distribution of various parenteral fluids (Table 350-1). Rapid catabolism of administered dextrose allows remaining water to distribute throughout all fluid spaces. Thus of the liter of dextrose and water (Table 350-1), two thirds enters cells and only one fourth of the one third (i.e., 1⁄12, or 83 ml) remaining extracellularly is kept in the vascular space. Because sodium is restricted to the ECF, the entire liter of isotonic saline remains in this space, and, according to Starling forces (Chapter 338), 25% (250 ml) remains in the vascular space. It follows that for vol-

Table 350-1. Distribution of 1 L of infused fluid

Solution	Space of distribution	Change in volume*		
		ICW (ml)	ISF (ml)	Plasma (ml)
1000 ml 5% dextrose in water	Total body water	665	250	85
1000 ml normal saline	Only in extracellular water	0	750	250
1000 ml half normal saline				
500 ml water	Total body water	335	125	40
500 ml normal saline	Only in extracellular water	0	375	125
1000 ml plasma	Restricted to plasma	0	0	1000

ICW, intracellular water; ISF, interstitial fluid.
*Values rounded.

ume expansion saline is far superior to water but less effective than protein-containing solutions.

Osmoregulation: an integrated triarchy

Under control conditions normal humans can ingest and excrete up to 15 to 20 L of water daily with only a 1% to 3% reduction in serum osmolality. In this setting urine osmolality is reduced to 35 to 40 mosm. Under conditions of severe water restriction with continued evaporative losses, a 2% to 3% increase in serum osmolality causes urine volume to decrease to 0.4 to 0.5 L/day, whereas urine osmolality increases to 1200 to 1400 mosm. Thus, depending on the imposed demands for water conservation or excretion, urine volume can vary 50-fold and urine osmolality 35-fold (Fig. 350-3). Several important clinical points follow from these observations. The renal capacity for water excretion is enormous, making it extremely difficult to imbibe enough fluid to overwhelm a normally operating osmoregulatory system. Exceptions are discussed below. With total abstinence from water, the kidney can strikingly lower urine volume, but it continues to excrete an obligatory 400 to 500 ml of urine, which, along with continuing evaporative losses, causes serum hypertonicity to progressively worsen. Failure of maximal renal water retention would, of course, accelerate the progression of hypertonicity in thirsting subjects. Fig. 350-3 also emphasizes that the greatest water savings and reduction in urine volume occurs when urine osmolality is increased from maximal dilution to isotonicity. The additional water conserved in maximizing urine concentration is much less (Fig. 350-3).

The three key elements of the osmoregulatory system are *thirst, AVP,* and the *renal concentrating and diluting mechanism.* This system is exquisitely sensitive to small (1% to 2%) changes in effective ECF osmolality (tonicity) and is poised to maintain serum osmolality almost constant despite wide variations in water intake. Consequently, serum sodium concentration and cell volume are protected from disruptive and dangerously capricious changes in our daily water appetite. Contraction of intravascular volume requires that protective water retention occur to ensure vascular filling and continued perfusion of vital organs. Indeed, the osmoregulatory system also responds to volume demands, but is less sensitive to hypovolemia than to hypertonicity. Whereas a 1% to 2% change in serum osmolality provokes appropriate and salutary changes in the system, an 8% to 10% reduction in blood volume is required to stimulate AVP release and water retention. Thus regulation of solute concentration takes precedence over volume regulation when ECF volume contraction or expansion is modest. With severe contraction, however, water is retained, giving volume requirements precedence over osmoregulation. Thus in hypovolemic states water may be retained and tissue perfusion protected despite worsening hypotonicity.

Integrated overview of the osmoregulatory system (Fig. 350-4). Changes in ECF tonicity are translated into appropriate increments or decrements in plasma AVP levels by hypothalamic osmoreceptors, which signal neighboring nuclei and the neurohypophysis to alter AVP synthesis and release. Water acquisition or rejection is also provoked by

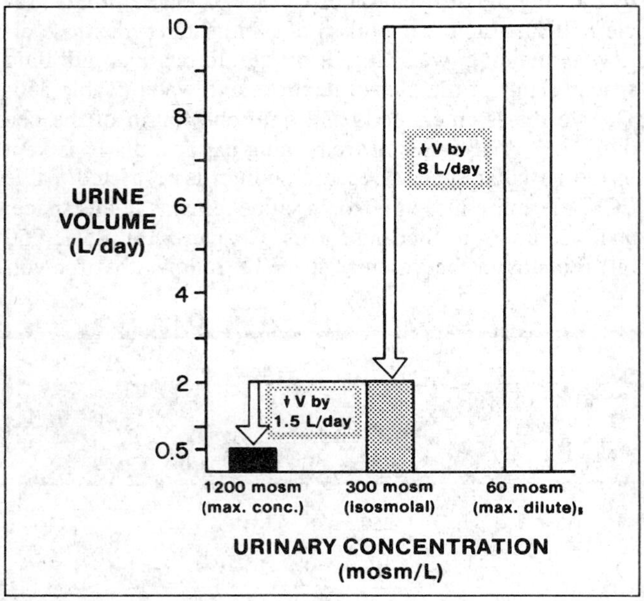

Fig. 350-3. Urine volume (V) in relation to urine osmolality. The figure illustrates the changes in urine volume that are seen as a subject excreting 600 mosm of solute daily concentrates his urine from maximum dilution to isosmolality to maximum concentration.

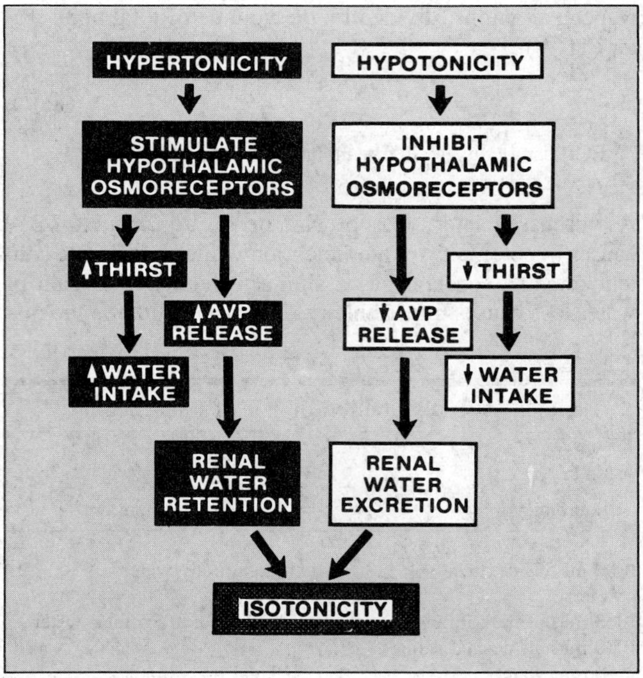

Fig. 350-4. Osmoregulation. The diagram illustrates the interaction of serum tonicity with hypothalamic centers for thirst and arginine vasopressin (AVP) release. Resulting renal retention or excretion of water restores serum isotonicity.

osmoreceptor signals to centrally located thirst-control centers. Thus *hypertonicity* elicits AVP release, which in turn stimulates renal retention of ingested water. Similarly, *hypotonicity* suppresses thirst and AVP release, enabling the kidney to excrete solute-free water. Renal retention of water in the former setting or excretion of water in the latter, re-establishes ECF isotonicity.

Control of arginine vasopressin (see also Chapter 161).

Osmotic stimulation. Rapid intracarotid injections of hypertonic solutions caused water-loaded, diuresing, conscious dogs to abruptly reduce urine volume and increase urinary tonicity. Failure of ineffective osmols to elicit a similar antidiuretic response led Verney in the 1940s to hypothesize that osmoreceptor cells contract or expand in response to altered ECF tonicity, and signal release or suppression of an antidiuretic principle. Since then, Verney's conclusions and hypotheses have been refined and extended but rarely challenged. The supraoptic and paraventricular nuclei of the hypothalamus synthesize the hormone that is transported with its carrier protein, *neurophysin,* intra-axonally to its storage site in the neurohypophysis.

When the ECF osmolality is less than or equal to 280 mosm, plasma AVP levels are undetectable, and the urinary osmolality is usually less than 150 mosm (Fig. 350-5). In this setting free-water excretion can be torrential, making 280 mosm the lower limit of achievable ECF osmolality, given a system that is operating normally. Exceptions are discussed below. Plasma AVP levels increase linearly as serum osmolality rises. When serum osmolality reaches 290 to 294 mosm, plasma AVP levels approximate 5 pg/ml and urinary osmolality approaches its upper limits of 1200 to 1400 mosm (see Fig. 350-5). Further increments in plasma AVP concentration are not translated into greater degrees of renal water retention. Thus the entire range of maximal renal concentration and dilution is realized over a plasma AVP concentration that spans from undetectable to 5 pg/ml. Indeed, AVP levels of 2.0 to 2.5 pg/ml convert maximally dilute urine to isotonicity, thereby effecting the greatest conservation of water over the range of dilution and concentration (see Fig. 350-5).

Nonosmotic stimulation. As noted earlier, *baroreceptors* located in the left atrium, aortic arch, and carotid sinus modify AVP release through signals carried by glossopharyngeal and vagal afferent nerves during periods of volume depletion and/or hypotension. In contrast to the linear relationship between osmolality and plasma AVP levels, the volume-AVP curve is exponential. Thus although relatively insensitive to changes in volume (see earlier discussion), the logarithmic increase in AVP levels allows for water retention and the establishment of the high concentrations required to achieve a pressor effect.

In addition to the osmotic and hemodynamic control of AVP levels, a variety of other modifying forces exist. Nausea, hypoglycemia, hypoxia, pain, and emotional stresses can dramatically increase AVP synthesis and release. These forces can sustain AVP secretion in several clinical circumstances in which hyponatremia commonly occurs (see later discussion).

During pregnancy, plasma osmolality, as well as the osmotic thresholds for the release of AVP and for thirst, decreases by approximately 10 mosm/L (i.e., AVP is released at lower levels of osmolality, and thirst is not extinguished until osmolality is below normal). These alterations in pregnancy appear to be independent of changes in effective plasma volume. Once hypotonicity reaches the new threshold level for thirst and AVP release, water intake and hormone secretion are extinguished, thereby establishing a new steady state. In addition to these changes in osmotic threshold, metabolic clearance of AVP is augmented from the

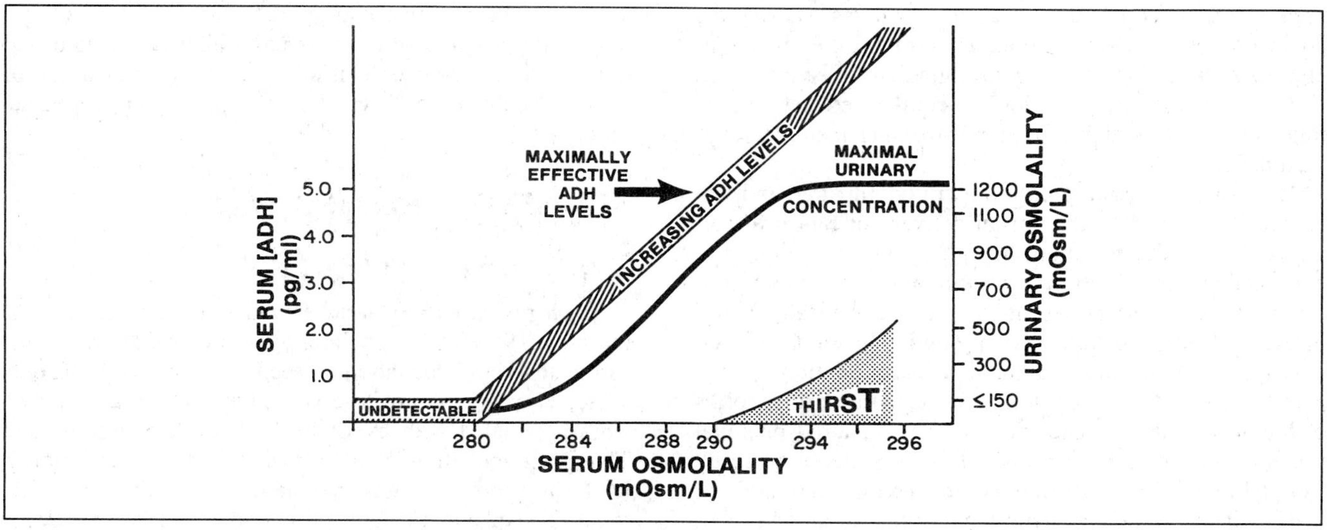

Fig. 350-5. Integration of osmoregulatory forces. The diagram suggests an approximate correlation between serum antidiuretic hormone (ADH) levels, urine and serum osmolality, and thirst. See text for details.

tenth week of gestation to midterm. The latter phenomenon has been attributed to an increase in the plasma concentration of a cystine aminopeptidase enzyme termed *vasopressinase*. Vasopressinase is elaborated by the placental tissue and inactivates both oxytocin and AVP. Enhanced release of vasopressinase may explain the unmasking of central diabetes insipidus during pregnancy.

Renal response to AVP. (See Chapter 338 for a more detailed discussion.) The volume of glomerular filtrate is reduced by approximately two thirds in the proximal convoluted tubule, but under all conditions remains isotonic through the last portion of this segment accessible to micropuncture analysis. The tonicity of fluid emerging from the thick ascending limb is always hypotonic, indicating that proportionately more solute than solvent is reabsorbed in Henle's loop. In the absence of AVP, the collecting tubules remain almost "waterproof," causing the final urine to be markedly hypotonic. The hormone's primary action is to increase the number of selective water channels in the luminal membrane of cortical and medullary collecting ducts, thereby effecting osmotic communication between dilute luminal fluid and the hypertonic medullary interstitium. Because medullary interstitial tonicity increases longitudinally, from the isotonic corticomedullary junction (300 mosm) to the hypertonic papillary tip (1200 mosm), collecting duct filtrate, in the presence of AVP, loses water and becomes progressively more concentrated.

Medullary hypertonicity is created and maintained by the interaction of several forces. The reabsorption of sodium and potassium chloride without water from the thick ascending limb of Henle's loop at once renders luminal fluid dilute and medullary interstitium, in receipt of salt, hypertonic. The countercurrent exchange mechanism in medullary vasa recta (Chapter 338 for details) prevents loss of medullary solute and allows for removal of reabsorbed water. In the presence of AVP, water is reabsorbed without urea in cortical and medullary collecting ducts, causing the concentration of unreabsorbed urea to progressively increase. A favorable concentration gradient is created such that urea diffuses from the inner medullary collecting duct fluid to the interstitium, further increasing medullary hypertonicity.

It follows that urinary dilution will be impaired and water retention favored when distal delivery of fluid and solute is reduced due to diminished glomerular filtration or to enhanced proximal reabsorption. Inhibition of salt reabsorption in the thick ascending limb and in more distal portions of the nephron, and failure to appropriately suppress AVP release will also limit maximal urinary dilution. These pathophysiologic forces find expression in the various forms of hyponatremia (see later discussion). Impaired maximal urinary concentration and loss of body water may result from inhibited salt reabsorption in the thick ascending limb, from reduced medullary hypertonicity due to altered medullary blood flow or intrinsic renal disease, and from lack of AVP secretion or failure of the tubules to normally respond to the hormone. These pathophysiologic forces find expression in the various clinical forms of hypernatremia (see later discussion).

Thirst. Although there are many qualitative similarities between the control of AVP secretion and thirst, important quantitative differences exist. Both processes are stimulated by hypertonicity and by ECF volume contraction. Although the AVP response to these stimuli has been defined with relative precision, the quantification of thirst has proved more elusive. Social and cultural forces play importantly on the "ebb and flow of body fluid," rendering difficult the development of standard tests for thirst in humans.

Whereas changes in plasma osmolality of 1% to 2% elicit a large outpouring of AVP and excretion of hypertonic urine, most humans do not experience thirst until the serum osmolality exceeds 295 mosm (see Fig. 350-5). Thus water ingestion is not stimulated until maximum renal water retention has developed. Speaking teleologically, thirst appears to function as a backup, or reserve, system for AVP-renal regulation of water balance. For a given increase in plasma osmolality, that caused by sodium stimulates thirst to a greater extent than does that caused by glucose.

It would also appear that thirst is less sensitive to hypovolemia than is AVP release, requiring a 20% reduction in blood volume for stimulation (compared with the 8% to 10% reduction needed for AVP release). Renal baroreceptors, located in the juxtaglomerular apparatus, seem to play a key role in stimulating thirst but do not significantly alter AVP secretion. Hypovolemia and reduced renal perfusion pressure activate the renin-angiotensin system, thereby generating angiotensin II, a central thirst stimulant. It is also true that angiotensin II is synthesized within the central nervous system and may play a more important role in controlling thirst than does peripheral angiotensin II.

In summary, the challenge of water excess is met primarily by suppression of AVP release with consequent renal excretion of solute-free water. Thirst is inhibited early in hypotonic states but seems to afford little protection above and beyond that contributed by the AVP-renal system. With progressive hypertonicity thirst comes into play only late in the course. This stimulation of water ingestion in severe dehydration is clearly an important protective addition.

STATES OF ABNORMAL WATER METABOLISM

Hyponatremic states (Fig. 350-6)

Etiology and pathogenesis. Because sodium accounts for more than 95% of ECF solute, hypotonic states are *always* associated with hyponatremia (see later discussion). The reverse, however, is not true (i.e., hyponatremia is not *always* associated with hypotonicity) (see later discussion). Thus the hyponatremias may be classified pathophysiologically into three variants: isotonic, hypertonic, and hypotonic. Tonicity is a calculated parameter; it is not directly measured (see Fig. 350-2). The serum concentrations of the common effective osmols, sodium and glucose, allow estimation of tonicity (see Fig. 350-2).

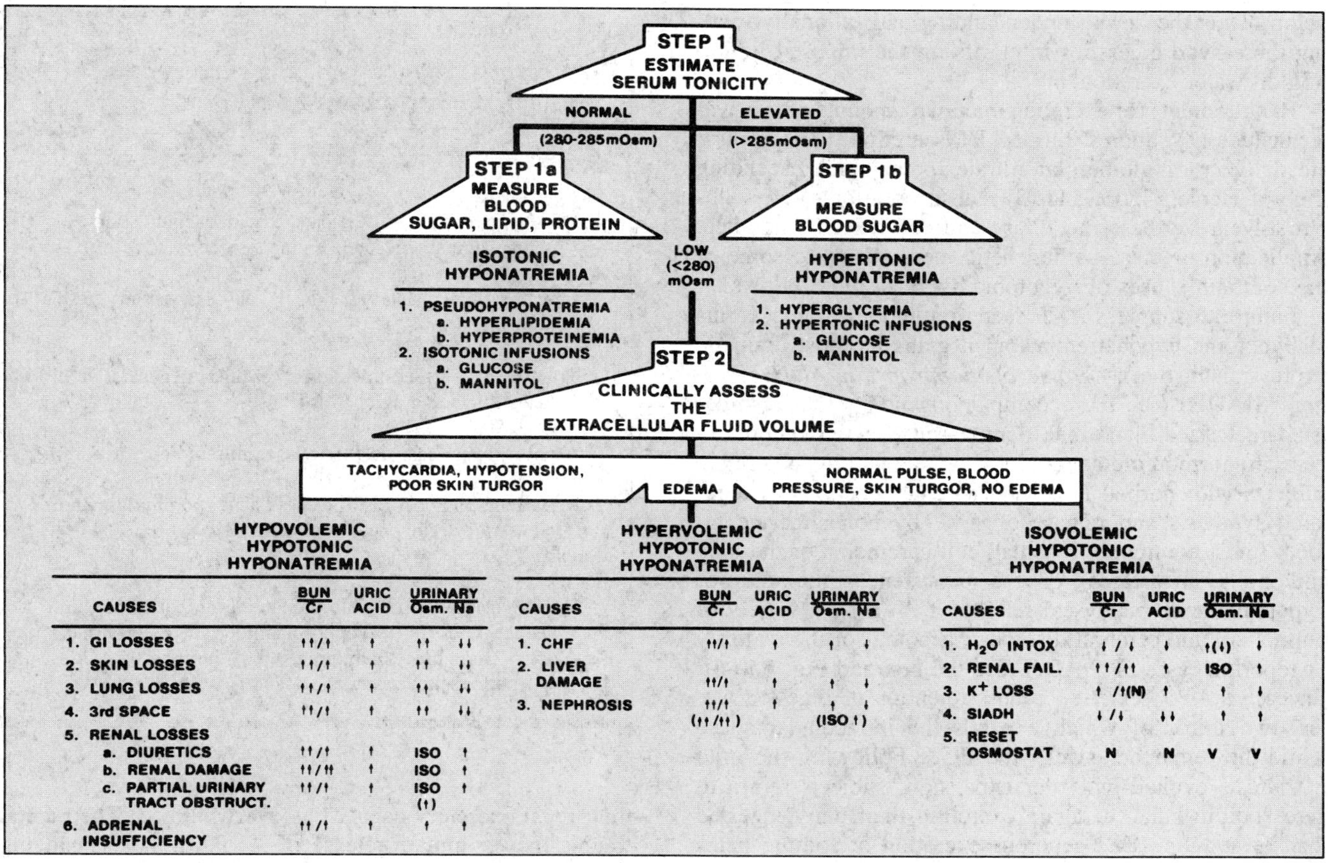

Fig. 350-6. Differential diagnosis of hyponatremia. The figure integrates the classification of the hyponatremias with a clinical and laboratory approach to their diagnosis. See text for details. CHF, congestive heart failure; ISO, isotonic; N, normal; V, variable. (Modified from Narins RG et al: Diagnostic strategies in disorders of fluid, electrolyte, and acid-base homeostasis, Am J Med 72:496, 1982.)

Isotonic hyponatremia. Isotonic hyponatremia occurs during the infusion of isotonic, sodium-free solutions or may be caused by a laboratory artifact. Administration of isotonic solutions of glucose (5%) or mannitol (5%) expands the ECF and dilutes serum sodium and the hexose prevents water movement into cells. Eventual entry of glucose into cells and its subsequent metabolism allow two thirds of the infused water to enter cells. The hyponatremia is thus transformed from isotonic to hypotonic as the sugar is oxidized. Renal excretion of mannitol has the same effect. Hyperlipidemia or hyperproteinemia (e.g., in myeloma or macroglobulinemia) displaces water from each liter of plasma. Because sodium salts only distribute in the water phase, each unit volume of plasma will contain less water and therefore less sodium. The sodium concentration in remaining plasma water, and therefore its osmolality, remain unchanged, but clinical laboratories expressing sodium concentration per liter of whole plasma report spuriously low values.

Hypertonic hyponatremia. Accumulation of effective osmols in the ECF dilutes serum sodium by causing the osmotic withdrawal of solute-free water from cells. Glucose and mannitol are the major clinically relevant osmols responsible for this effect. This solute-induced expansion of ECF volume may cause congestive heart failure in patients with marginal cardiac function. Accordingly, improvement in congestive symptoms may occasionally attend insulin therapy of severe hyperglycemia. Each 100 mg/dl increase in blood glucose reduces the serum sodium concentration by 1.6 mEq/L when the initial ECF volume is normal. In edematous states, the osmotic entry of the same amount of water into an expanded extracellular space will dilute sodium by a lesser amount. Conversely, entry of the same amount of cellular water into an osmotically enriched but contracted ECF compartment reduces the sodium concentration by more than 1.6 mEq/L.

Hypotonic hyponatremia. Hypotonic forms of hyponatremia are all characterized by a reduced ratio of body solute to water, which may be *clinically apparent or inapparent* (see Diagnosis) and may differ in terms of the underlying pathogenesis. Rarely, a deranged patient ingests such enormous amounts of water as to overwhelm the normal renal excretory capacity. All other hypotonic disorders are characterized by an absolute or relative impairment in free-water excretion; that is, if the kidney could normally excrete solute-free water, hypotonic hyponatremia could not develop. Thus the key to understanding and rationally treating these syndromes lies in clarifying the imposed limitation on water excretion.

Requirements for excreting maximal amounts of free water include (1) suppression of AVP secretion, (2) appropriate delivery of glomerular filtrate to the thick ascending limb of Henle's loop, and (3) reabsorption of solute without solvent by these medullary and cortical diluting sites. Application of these pathogenetic mechanisms to some of the common causes of hypotonic hyponatremia follows.

Failure to suppress AVP secretion underlies most forms of hypotonic hyponatremia, but it gains its most dramatic expression in the *syndrome of inappropriate ADH secretion* (SIADH) (see the accompanying box). This disorder is characterized by normal to increased effective blood volume in normoproteinemic, nonedematous, hyponatremic subjects with normal renal and adrenal function. Unregulated synthesis and release of AVP by nonendocrine tumors (most commonly by small cell carcinoma of the lung and/or its metastases) or the persistent stimulation of hypothalamic-hypophyseal release of AVP by a variety of pulmonary and cerebral disorders, account for the majority of reported cases of SIADH (see the box and Fig. 350-6). Excessive AVP secretion causes retention of ingested water, two thirds of which expands the intracellular space while the remainder swells the ECF. Following the mild natriuresis evoked by water expansion, subjects return to zero sodium balance, again excreting their daily ingested load of sodium. This generous excretion of sodium helps to distinguish these patients from hypervolemic and hypovolemic subjects with hyponatremia who are retaining sodium (see later discussion). Augmented renal clearances of urea and uric acid decrease their plasma concentrations to values that are often <10 mg/dl and <3.0 mg/dl, respectively. Impaired tubular reabsorption secondary to subtle degrees of volume expansion and enhanced tubular secretion contribute to the hypouricemia, which is so characteristic of this syndrome. Urine osmolality varies widely but is never maximally dilute (i.e., <100 mosm). Some patients excrete persistently hypertonic urine (>300 mosm), whereas others elaborate 150 to 300 mosm urine. Continued excessive water ingestion—in excess of reduced excretory capacity—is important in this latter group. A variety of drugs (see the box) can cause this syndrome by provoking sustained release of AVP or by sensitizing the distal nephron to even low circulating levels of the hormone or by directly mimicking the action of authentic AVP on the kidney. Adrenal insufficiency and hypothyroidism, presumably acting via baroreceptor-mediated mechanisms, are also associated with excess AVP release.

The postoperative setting is a virtual spawning ground for hyponatremia. Pain, narcotics, hypoxia, hypotension, and respirator therapy conspire to sustain the unregulated release of AVP. Renal water avidity prevents excretion of the dilute fluid these patients are often exposed to. Permanent neurologic damage may occur from the acute, severe hyponatremia that occurs in this setting. Psychopaths undergoing an acute exacerbation of disease are occasionally compelled to ingest such enormous quantities of water that their renal excretory capacity is overwhelmed. The mental trauma may stimulate release of AVP, further sensitizing them to acute hyponatremia.

Hyponatremic disorders associated with reduced effective blood volume stimulate AVP release via the previously discussed baroreceptor mechanisms. Reduction of circulating volume by hemorrhage, gastrointestinal, or renal fluid loss, or redistribution of plasma into the interstitial space, triggers baroreceptor-mediated release of AVP. Hypoproteinemic states (cirrhosis, nephrosis) and congestive heart failure similarly stimulate release of the hormone. It follows that these disorders limit the excretion of free water and thus sensitize these patients to hyponatremia.

Delivery of filtrate to the distal diluting segments is dependent on adequate glomerular filtration, normal proximal nephron reabsorption, and ingestion of adequate amounts of solute. As renal failure progresses and glomerular filtration rate declines, the absolute volume of filtrate reaching distal sites diminishes. With advanced disease, the maximum achievable volume of free water that can be generated and excreted is markedly reduced. Even modest increases in water intake may lead to hyponatremia in this setting. Disorders associated with diminished effective blood volume (see earlier discussion; Fig. 350-6) often reduce the glomerular filtration rate and, through various hormonal and physical changes that alter renal transport, stimulate proximal sodium and water reabsorption. The reduced volume of filtered blood, coupled with increased proximal capture of filtrate, compromises distal delivery and free-water generation. As noted earlier, these disorders also may provoke excessive release of AVP, which further sensitizes subjects to hyponatremia.

Differential diagnosis of the syndrome of inappropriate antidiuretic hormone (SIADH) secretion

Neoplasms
- Lung (small cell in 80%), pancreas, duodenum, lymphoma, ureter, prostate, Ewing's sarcoma

Pulmonary
- Infection (viral, bacterial, fungal), abscess, asthma, respirator therapy

Central nervous system
- Trauma, neoplasms, infections, vascular, degenerative diseases (including aging), psychoses

Cardiac
- Atrial tachycardias, post-mitral-commissurotomy syndrome

Metabolic
- Myxedema, adrenal insufficiency, acute porphyria, anterior pituitary insufficiency, angiotensin II

Stress

Drugs
- Hypoglycemic agents (chlorpropamide, tolbutamide), antineoplastic drugs (cyclophosphamide, vincristine), narcotics (morphine, barbiturates), psychotropics (phenothiazine derivatives)

Reduced solute ingestion will ultimately limit the volume of free water that can be excreted. For example, when a subject excreting 700 mosm of solute (ingested salts plus products of catabolism) in 24 hours undergoes a maximal water diuresis, urine osmolality may reach a nadir of 40 mosm/L. Thus excretion of 40 mosm of solute in each liter requires 17.5 L of urine. Reduction of solute excretion to 200 mosm/day, as can occur when beer, a solute-poor fluid, constitutes the entire daily fare, allows for excretion of only 5 L of maximally dilute urine (40 mosm/L). In this setting, ingestion of more than 5 L of solute-free water results in fluid retention and hyponatremia. "Beer-drinker's potomania" and hyponatremia are therefore due to limited water excretion coupled with excessive solute-free water intake. The virtue of pretzels, pizza, and potato chips in this setting should be apparent.

Even when filtration and distal delivery are well preserved, inhibition of sodium reabsorption in the thick ascending limb and cortical diluting site can strikingly limit free-water generation. The loop-active diuretics, furosemide, bumetanide, and ethacrynic acid, inhibit solute reabsorption in the thick ascending limb, thereby increasing salt and water losses but limiting solute-free water excretion. Some have argued that furosemide-stimulated synthesis of renal prostaglandins—peripheral antagonists of AVP—minimizes the incidence of hyponatremia in this setting. Thiazides and related diuretics inhibit solute reabsorption in the cortical diluting site and, like other diuretics, may provoke AVP secretion via baroreceptor mechanisms. Proximal reabsorption is eventually stimulated by diuretic-induced volume contraction, consequently limiting distal delivery and free-water generation. The greater incidence of hyponatremia from thiazides may relate to their inability to stimulate renal prostaglandin synthesis.

Symptoms (Fig. 350-7). The clinical manifestations of the hyponatremic syndromes are largely determined by the rate and magnitude of decline in plasma osmolality and by the nature of any associated disorders. Symptoms and signs of the *isotonic hyponatremias* relate to the effects of the hyperlipidemia, hyperproteinemia, or reason for treating with large volumes of isotonic glucose or mannitol. Likewise, the *hypertonic hyponatremias* owe their chemical and clinical features to the effects of hyperglycemia or reasons for administering hypertonic mannitol. Neurologic signs and symptoms are the primary manifestations of the *hypotonic hyponatremias*.

SERUM Na^+ (meq/liter)	SYMPTOMS	HYPOVOLEMIA	HYPERVOLEMIA
120-125	NAUSEA MALAISE	DIMINISHED BRAIN PERFUSION EXACERBATES SYMPTOMS	DIMINISHED EABV IN CHF, NEPHROSIS, CIRRHOSIS MAY REDUCE BRAIN PERFUSION AND EXACERBATE SYMPTOMS
115-120	HEADACHE LETHARGY OBTUNDATION		
<115	SEIZURES COMA		

Fig. 350-7. Symptoms of hypovolemic and hypervolemic forms of hyponatremia. CHF, congestive heart failure; EABV, effective arterial blood volume.

Acute hyponatremia, developing over hours, causes brain cell swelling, which results in confusion, lethargy, anorexia, and nausea and may progress to headache, stupor, and coma. In time (hours to days) brain cells effect remedial changes in cell volume by exporting solute (sodium, potassium, various organic acids) and inactivating retained osmols. This loss of effective intracellular osmols allows the brain to achieve the required level of hypotonicity without the added danger of imbibing extracellular water. Slowly developing hyponatremia is less likely to be symptomatic, presumably because the aforementioned brain cell compensations keep pace with the falling serum sodium concentration. Associated hepatic, renal, and cardiac disorders with coexisting but variable changes in effective blood volume and cerebral perfusion further modify the emerging clinical picture. Focal neurologic signs are unusual unless the patient has an underlying cerebral disorder.

Diagnosis. The exact etiology of hyponatremia can be extracted from its myriad possible causes by application of the principles outlined earlier. The algorithm illustrated in Fig. 350-6 classifies the hyponatremias in terms of the prevailing serum tonicity and then subclassifies hypotonic hyponatremia on the basis of the clinically apparent state of ECF volume.

The serum osmolality usually need not be measured, because the isotonic and hypertonic hyponatremias are most often recognized from the history, physical examination, or blood glucose levels. Lactescent serum, lipemia retinalis, and fatty deposits in the skin suggest that hyponatremia may be secondary to hyperlipidemia, whereas hyperproteinemic states are characterized by a typical history for multiple myeloma or macroglobulinemia. The use of hypertonic mannitol in acute renal failure or cerebral edema, or for continuous washing of the bladder during prostatic surgery, should alert the physician to the possibility of hypertonic hyponatremia. Once the likely isotonic or hypertonic causes have been excluded, one of the forms of hypotonic hyponatremia must be present.

Blood pressure, pulse, and their changes with posture, the presence or absence of edema, and normalcy of skin turgor provide the basis for assessing the state of ECF volume. A history of drug ingestion or the presence of ongoing diseases known to predispose to hypotonic hyponatremia is of obvious importance. On this basis, these syndromes may be sorted into the hypovolemic, hypervolemic, or the clinically apparent euvolemic hypotonic hyponatremias.

Patients with *hypovolemic hyponatremia* have reduced their effective blood volume through external loss of salt and water (renal or gastrointestinal losses or hemorrhage) or redistribution of plasma volume into an inflamed organ (e.g., pancreatitis, burns, trauma). Hypotension, tachycardia with postural accentuation, and diminished skin turgor characterize this group. Urinary losses are usually hypotonic when caused by diuretic excess, glycosuria, ketonuria, partial urinary tract obstruction or other interstitial nephritides, or adrenal insufficiency. Hyponatremia develops only because resulting volume contraction provokes retention of subsequently ingested or administered water. *Hyponatremia never occurs unless the patient is exposed to excess free water.* Gastrointestinal, blood, and redistributional losses are either hypotonic or isotonic. Urinary tonicity is relatively low and sodium concentration is high during renal fluid and solute-wasting (urinary sodium concentration is generally >20 mEq/L, fractional excretion >3.0%, and urine osmolality approximates that of serum), but with extrarenal losses tonicity is high and sodium excretion low (urine sodium concentration <20 mEq/L, fractional excretion <1%, and urine osmolality is greater than that of serum). Discontinuation of diuretics 12 or 24 hours before evaluation may cause the urine to assume the chemical characteristics of extrarenal sodium- and water-wasting syndromes. The history is key in the latter setting. Chemical screening of the urine for diuretics may be required in patients whose hyponatremia could be due to the surreptitious abuse of these drugs.

Edema is the hallmark of the *hypervolemic* syndromes. These hyponatremic disorders are characterized by reduced effective blood volume, which diminishes glomerular filtration rate, enhances proximal reabsorption, and stimulates the nonosmotic release of AVP. The synergy of these forces can markedly restrict free-water excretion. In general, however, a substantial degree of hyponatremia usually occurs late in the course of congestive heart failure and liver disease and suggests a poor prognosis. Hyponatremia is an unusual complication of untreated nephrotic syndrome; when present, it is usually associated with aggressive diuretic therapy. Urine in these sodium-avid states is characterized by increased osmolality and diminished volume and sodium concentration.

Typically, the *isovolemic* hyponatremias are associated with retention of 3 to 5 L of water, of which two thirds remains in cells. Thus the degree of ECF expansion is usually inadequate to detect edema. SIADH and the pathologic ingestion of excessive amounts of water were described earlier. As discussed, patients with acute or chronic renal failure have limited ability to generate and excrete free water, predisposing them to isovolemic hyponatremia. Another syndrome in this category has been variously termed the *reset osmostat,* or *sick-cell syndrome*. This functional disorder complicates a variety of chronic illnesses including pulmonary tuberculosis and cirrhosis. It is characterized by a lowering or resetting of the level of ECF osmolality that evokes release of AVP. Apart from this resetting, the osmoregulatory system apparently operates normally. Thus instead of being poised to protect a serum osmolality of 285 mosm (serum sodium concentration of 140 mEq/L), the system may now pathologically protect 250 mosm (i.e., a serum sodium concentration of 125 mEq/L). When challenged with an exogenous water load, patients with a reset osmostat, in contrast to those with SIADH, appropriately dilute their urine, eliminate the administered water load, and sustain a low but unchanged serum sodium concentration. With water deprivation, a concentrated urine is elaborated in pathologic protection of a fixed degree of hyponatremia.

Loss of 200 to 500 mEq of body potassium stores is commonly seen in various hypokalemic disorders. Because the total ECF content of this cation is normally less than 70 mEq, intracellular potassium stores obviously must contribute the bulk of lost electrolyte. Because potassium is the prime intracellular solute, its loss should cause transient intracellular hypotonicity, which in turn should simultaneously cause cell water to enter the ECF and extracellular sodium to enter cells in partial replacement of lost cation. Hyponatremia results from this diluting translocation of water and cation. Why the kidney retains the requisite quantity of water to sustain this hyponatremia is unclear. Disorders causing potassium wasting (e.g., diuretics, vomiting) and perhaps reduced cell volume resulting from potassium loss provoke sustained release of AVP.

Severe potassium depletion also impairs vasopressin's action on the distal nephron, thus facilitating water loss. Enhanced prostaglandin synthesis induced by potassium depletion may partially explain this effect. The change in plasma sodium concentration during potassium depletion therefore reflects the net balance attained between transcellular water and sodium fluxes, which tend to lower the sodium levels, and renal water losses, which tend to increase these levels.

In summary, the history, physical examination, and blood glucose level are usually sufficient to identify or exclude the isotonic and hypertonic hyponatremias. The hypotonic syndromes are classified through clinical assessment of ECF volume and urinary sodium excretion. Thus rapid clinical evaluation coupled with a few simple blood and urine tests allows one to quickly define the cause and develop a rational therapeutic approach to hypotonic hyponatremia.

Therapy. Fluid-electrolyte therapy is unnecessary in the *pseudohyponatremias* caused by hyperlipidemia and hyperproteinemia because serum tonicity remains normal in these disorders. Indeed, the inappropriate restriction of free water or administration of concentrated saline solutions could lead to dangerous degrees of hypertonicity. Therapy should be directed toward the abnormality of lipid or protein metabolism.

The *hypertonic hyponatremias* are best treated by eliminating the offending ECF osmol. Insulin therapy of hyperglycemia or the renal elimination of accumulated mannitol allows for the return to cells of water that had been osmotically displaced to the ECF. Resulting intravascular volume reduction should be buffered by administration of saline or colloid. Once intravascular volume has been stabilized, hypotonic solutions may be administered to replenish the loss of proportionately more water than sodium caused by glycosuria and mannitoluria (Chapter 168).

Glycine and sorbitol, used as irrigants for transurethral prostatic resection, may cause severe hyponatremia and neurologic symptoms (see earlier discussion). The component causes of the hyponatremia include the following. If a hypertonic irrigation solution is used, the induced hyperosmolality provokes movement of sodium-free cellular water into the ECF. If the irrigation fluid was hypotonic, electrolyte-free water is absorbed, and, of course, dilutes the serum sodium. Absorption of isotonic irrigation fluid does not immediately change serum osmolality but simply obligates the presence of absorbed water in the ECF. Glycine's eventual metabolism leaves free water behind. Acute hyperammonemia consequent to glycine metabolism may add to the neurologic deterioration in these patients.

Therapy of the *hypotonic hyponatremias* is dictated by the underlying pathophysiology. *Hypovolemic* disorders require re-expansion of ECF volume, which eliminates baroreceptor stimulation of AVP release and simultaneously restores glomerular filtration and the distal tubular delivery of filtrate. Normalization of renal free-water generation and excretion, coupled with sodium retention, re-establishes normonatremia. Attention to such precipitating causes as diuretic abuse, gastrointestinal fluid losses, and adrenal insufficiency (see Fig. 350-6) obviously must accompany fluid therapy.

Therapy of *hypervolemic* hypotonic hyponatremic syndromes usually entails water restriction and treatment of the precipitating heart, liver, or kidney disease (see Fig. 350-6, and earlier discussion). Addition of angiotensin-converting enzyme inhibitor (ACEI) to diuretic therapy of heart failure reverses associated hyponatremia more rapidly. The ACEI increases renal plasma flow and glomerular filtration, which simultaneously enhance the distal delivery of solute and diuretic. Cardiac output improves after afterload reduction and suppresses AVP secretion, further enhancing solute-free water excretion. It is instructive to calculate the time required to restore the normal serum sodium concentration from 120 mEq/L in a 70-kg man with 10 L of nephrotic edema. Assume daily evaporative losses of 500 ml and excretion of 1 L of urine containing 40 mEq of electrolyte (largely accounted for by sodium, potassium, and their accompanying anions). It is useful to divide the urine into its isotonic and free-water components. If the urinary electrolyte, 40 mEq/L, were suspended in only 0.33 L, its *concentration* would be 120 mEq/L (i.e., isotonic with existing plasma). The remaining 0.67 L of urine would then be electrolyte-free water. In this manner, 1170 ml of free water (500 ml from insensible loss plus 670 ml from urinary loss) and 330 ml of isotonic fluid are lost daily. If daily water intake were restricted to 500 ml and salt intake were limited to 40 mEq, isotonic electrolyte intake (330 ml) would equal its excretion, whereas subtraction of free-water intake (170 ml) from daily losses (1170 ml) defines a net water loss of 1000 ml daily. Since salt intake and excretion are identical, the body content remains unchanged. Apparent total body sodium, the product of total body water (60% body weight plus edema fluid) and serum sodium concentration (120 mEq/L) is 42 L ([70 kg × 0.6] + 10 L = 52 L). Thus the product of total body water (52 L) and serum sodium concentration (120 mEq/L) yields the apparent total body sodium content (6240 mEq). In what volume would these 6240 mEq have to be suspended to yield a concentration of 140 mEq/L (i.e., 6240 mEq/x L = 140 mEq/L)? These calculations indicate that with an unchanged body sodium content, the patient would have to reduce total body water by 7.4 L, from 52 L to 44.6 L (i.e., 6240 mEq of Na^+ in 44.6 L yields a concentration of 140 mEq/L). By losing 1 L of electrolyte-free water daily, slightly more than a week would be required to achieve normonatremia. Renal free-water excretion will improve as the associated heart, liver, or kidney disease is treated and thereby will reduce the time required for the shedding of retained water.

The *isovolemic* hypotonic hyponatremias are usually best treated by water restriction. An occasional patient with chronic hyponatremia may find water restriction too demanding, necessitating the addition of agents that enhance solute-free water excretion. This situation is seen most commonly in SIADH and usually when the syndrome is associated with a malignancy. Increasing sodium intake combined with furosemide may allow for an increase in water intake without compromising serum sodium concentration. Demeclocycline, a peripheral inhibitor of AVP action, induces enough free-water excretion to allow such patients to comfortably liberalize their daily water intake. Administration of this drug in cirrhotics may impair renal function. Lithium, another renal AVP-antagonist, is less often effective and is more likely to cause untoward reactions than is demeclocycline. These drugs take days to become effective and so are of no value in the emergency therapy of symptomatic hyponatremia.

Patients with symptomatic isovolemic hypotonic hyponatremia (see Fig. 350-6) occasionally require the emergency removal of body water to raise serum sodium to levels that reverse symptoms. Currently no drugs are available that can acutely and selectively increase renal free-water excretion. For now, the imperfect but effective loop-active diuretics may be used in this setting. These diuretics simultaneously cause both a water and a sodium diuresis. Return to the patient of shed sodium in small volumes of water (i.e., hypertonic solutions) allows for net water loss. For example, intravenous administration of 80 to 120 mg of furosemide every 1 to 2 hours causes loss of approximately 1000 ml of urine per hour with approximately 70 mEq of electrolyte. Return of these 70 mEq of NaCl in only 135 ml of water (i.e., as 3% saline) maintains body sodium content unchanged while allowing for net loss of 865 ml of water. In this manner, substantial volumes of solute-free water may be removed. Serum sodium concentration may be increased from 110 mEq/L to 120 mEq/L over 5 hours in a 70-kg man losing 865 ml of water hourly. When normal, this 70-kg man has a total body water of 42 L (60% body weight) and a serum sodium concentration of 140 mEq/L. His apparent total body sodium content is 140 mEq/L × 42 L, or 5880 mEq. What volume of body water must be present to dilute this sodium content to 110 mEq/L (i.e., 5880 mEq/x L = 110 mEq/L)? Solving this equation gives a volume of 53.5 Liters. Thus retention of 11.5 L of water reduced his serum sodium concentration from 140 mEq/L to 110 mEq/L. How much of this retained water must be removed to raise the sodium level to 120 mEq/L? Again, the calculation is based on the estimated normal sodium content and the volume of body water required to create the desired concentration: 5880 mEq/x L = 120 mEq/L. The volume required is 49 L; thus 4.5 L (53.5 − 49 = 4.5) must be removed to increase the serum sodium concentration from 110 mEq/L to 120 mEq/L. With loss of 865 ml of water hourly, it will take 5.2 hours to shed these 4.5 L. Care must be taken to assay urinary sodium and potassium losses and restore them. Administration of excessive amounts of electrolyte risks volume overload and pulmonary edema, whereas underreplacement results in potassium depletion and hypovolemia. Addition of furosemide not only prevents volume overload, due to infusions of hypertonic saline, but also enhances solute-free water clearance.

As discussed, brain cells adapt to hyponatremia by exporting solute and thereby avoid cerebral edema. Both the loss and eventual reconstitution of cell solute content takes 36 to 48 hours. If the rate of rise of serum sodium concentration exceeds the rate at which cell solute is replenished, cells will shrink, and this "osmotic shock" may cause permanent neurologic damage. Unduly rapid repair of hyponatremia may cause central pontine myelinolysis (CPM). If chronic hyponatremia is corrected too rapidly, seizures, coma, and demyelinating lesions in the central nervous system may occur. The latter seems to occur much more commonly in the pons. Women manifest these neurologic sequelae far more often than men. Although the pathogenesis of this disorder has yet to be clarified, many believe it is caused by adaptation of the brain to chronic hyponatremia, which sensitizes it to dehydration if the serum osmolality is corrected too rapidly. Survival depends on reducing brain cell swelling. Active export of cellular potassium and various amino acids with obligate amounts of water accomplish this life-saving effect. The resulting solute depletion then sensitizes cells to dehydration if the serum sodium level is raised too quickly.

Because the duration of hyponatremia is difficult to define in many patients, rapid correction, and certainly overcorrection, must be carefully avoided (see the accompanying box). On balance, the literature would suggest that the initial correction rates in symptomatic hyponatremic patients should not exceed 1 mEq/L/hr. As improvement is noted or if the serum sodium level has been increased by 4 to 5 mEq/L, the rate of correction should be reduced so that the increment in sodium concentration does not exceed 10 to 15 mEq/L/24 hr. Patients suffering from alcoholism, malnutrition, and liver disease are predisposed to demyelinating syndromes and deserve special attention during therapy. In all patients, serum sodium concentration must be monitored frequently as repair progresses. Current concepts suggest that if these guidelines are followed, the neurologic sequelae from rapid correction of hyponatremia can be avoided.

Treatment of hyponatremia

A. **Hypertonic hyponatremia:** Replace salt losses from the osmotic diuresis and treat the underlying disorder (e.g., hyperglycemia, exposure to mannitol, glycine)
B. **Isotonic hyponatremia:** Recognize the potential roles of hyperproteinemia and hyperlipidemia, or exposure to isotonic, sodium-free solutions (e.g., 5% dextrose)
C. **Hypotonic hyponatremia:**
   1. **Hypovolemic states:** Restore ECF volume status with isotonic saline and treat underlying gastrointestinal, adrenal, renal conditions
   2. **Hypervolemic states:** Water restriction and treatment of the underlying disorders (e.g., congestive heart failure, liver disease, nephrosis)
   3. **Isovolemic states:**
      a. **Asymptomatic:**
      Water restriction, increased sodium intake with furosemide, (demeclocycline, lithium, if antagonism of ADH is deemed necessary)
      b. **Symptomatic:**
      (i) Recognize predisposing causes for demyelination: women, elderly, alcoholism, liver disease, malnutrition.
      (ii) 3% saline with furosemide to achieve initial correction rates of 1.0 mEq/L/hr. Continue until symptoms abate or for 4 to 5 hours and then slow the rate of correction so as not to exceed increases of more than 10 to 15 mEq/L/24 hr.

Hypernatremic states (Fig. 350-8)

Because sodium is excluded from cells and is the major ECF solute, all hypernatremic states are at once *hyperosmolar* and *hypertonic* (see earlier discussion). Attraction of cellular water by ECF hypertonicity effects *ICF contraction* in all hypernatremic states regardless of whether ECF expansion or contraction coexists. Cerebral cells are unique exceptions to this rule by virtue of their ability to increase ICF osmolality by generating solute (idiogenic osmols) rather than by losing water.

Indeed the brain content of a variety of organic compounds such as glutamine, taurine, urea, myoinositol, betaine, glycerophosphorylcholine, and phosphocreatinine increase within several days after the onset of hypernatremia. Intracellular generation of these osmotically active particles by brain cells minimizes cell shrinkage and the neurologic consequences of this metabolic disorder. Within 2 days of correcting hypernatremia, the concentration of these solutes decreases.

In contrast to the constancy of ICF volume contraction, the *ECF volume* in hypernatremic states is quite variable (see later discussion). Indeed, these changes in ECF volume serve to classify the syndromes of hypernatremia (see later discussion).

Etiology and pathogenesis. The imbalance between body water and sodium content that characterizes all hypernatremic states may result from pure water loss or pure sodium retention. Since two thirds of body water resides intracellularly, pure water losses shrink both ICF and ECF, but reduction of the latter is usually clinically inapparent unless dehydration is severe (i.e., serum sodium concentrations in excess of 160 mEq/L). The hypernatremia caused by retention of salt without water simultaneously contracts the ICF and expands the ECF. The extracellular expansion is usually too modest to cause edema but may overload a previously compromised myocardium. The hypernatremia resulting from concomitant changes in sodium and water effect more striking changes in the ECF volume. Loss of hypotonic fluid (i.e., loss of proportionately more water than salt) reduces ECF volume in proportion to the loss of sodium, whereas a gain of hypertonic fluid (i.e., gain of proportionately more sodium than water) expands the ECF in proportion to the retained sodium.

As hypernatremia develops, thirst and AVP release are normally stimulated. The hormone AVP causes renal retention of ingested water, thereby re-establishing normal tonicity of body fluid. It follows that sustained hypernatremia could result from a defect in thirst, AVP synthesis or release, or failure of the kidney to respond to normally elaborated hormone. Net loss of hypotonic fluid by kidneys, gastrointestinal tract, skin, or lungs or net retention of sodium from massive exposure could also cause hypernatremia. These different syndromes are conveniently classified on the basis of the associated changes in ECF volume (see Fig. 350-8) and are discussed here.

Hypervolemic hypernatremia. Pure sodium retention as a cause of hypernatremia is usually iatrogenic, being restricted to specific clinical circumstances. Use of hypertonic sodium bicarbonate solutions (each 50-ml ampul contains approximately 1000 mEq/L) in various forms of severe metabolic acidosis will cause hypernatremia unless enough water is added to ensure isotonicity. Intra-amniotic injection of hypertonic saline (250 ml of a 25% solution), for a therapeutic abortion, is occasionally inadvertently misdirected into a vein, causing potentially catastrophic acute hypertonicity. Rarely, when infant feeding formula or dialysis solution is constituted with excess sodium, or when concentrated sodium salts are accidentally ingested in emetics or gargles, life-threatening hypernatremia results. Perhaps the most common iatrogenic form of hypernatremia occurs when patients dependent on parenteral fluids are given isotonic saline without free water to replace daily hypotonic insensible losses. In certain settings diuretics may cause hypernatremia. Hypotonic urine is generally excreted in response to vigorous diuretic therapy. Replacement of these losses with only free water commonly leads to hyponatremia, whereas replacement of sodium without free water results in hypernatremia. Indeed, most cases of edematous hypernatremia occur because incapacitated edematous patients receive diuretics while their access to water is restricted. The various syndromes of primary mineralocorticoid excess (Chapter 163) cause retention of sodium and water, and the resulting ECF volume expansion increases the threshold for AVP release. The latter provokes mild water loss, and a new steady state evolves that is characterized by mild hypernatremia. Potassium depletion and increased synthesis of prostaglandins may also contribute to the polyuria observed in these hypermineralocorticoid states. Prostaglandins, by antagonizing the effect of AVP on water reabsorption, impair the kidney's ability to elaborate a concentrated urine. (See earlier discussion.)

Hypovolemic hypernatremia. Loss of hypotonic solutions through the kidney, gastrointestinal, and respiratory tracts or the skin may result in hypernatremia (see Fig. 350-8). Such urinary losses are induced by pharmacologic and osmotic diuretics and by the obligatory relative polyuria that complicates acute or chronic renal failure. Glycosuria and the urea diuresis created by protein feeding in catabolic settings cause loss of sodium with large amounts of water. Failure to replace these losses results in hypovolemic hypernatremia. Partial urinary tract obstruction leads to distal tubular damage and a clinical syndrome characterized by polyuria, hyperkalemia, normal anion gap acidosis, and occasionally hypernatremia. Vomiting, diarrhea, lactulose therapy (for hepatic encephalopathy), and fistulous communications between the skin and gastrointestinal tract may cause hypotonic losses, which, when coupled with reduced free-water intake, provoke hypernatremia. Peritoneal dialysis removes hypotonic fluid and may increase the serum sodium concentration unless free water is returned in appropriate amounts.

Isovolemic hypernatremia (Fig. 350-8). The free-water losses underlying most cases of isovolemic hypernatremia occur through the skin or the kidney. Such renal losses are caused by either partial or complete failure to synthesize or release AVP (i.e., central diabetes insipidus) or from failure of the kidney to respond to normally elaborated AVP (i.e., nephrogenic diabetes insipidus) (Chapter 161).

Because the hypernatremia resulting from free-water loss stimulates thirst, most patients with diabetes insipidus have normal or only slightly increased serum sodium concentrations. It follows that hypothalamic lesions that concomitantly damage AVP synthesis and thirst provoke the worst degrees of hypernatremia.

Central diabetes insipidus (CDI) is discussed in Chapter 161.

Nephrogenic diabetes insipidus (NDI) occurs in two general forms. The first type is composed of acquired disorders causing structural renal damage that interferes with the generation of a properly functioning medullary countercurrent system. The second form is caused by familial and acquired disorders in the end-organ responsiveness to AVP. The forms of NDI caused by structural renal damage usually allow for excretion of isotonic urine and thus result in only mild polyuria (usually less than 8 L daily), whereas familial NDI often unleashes torrential volumes of urine.

The mild chronic polyuria and limited concentrating capacity attending most chronic renal diseases is well known. Rarely, *amyloidosis* and occasionally *partial urinary tract obstruction* cause enough selective distal nephron damage to effect substantial degrees of polyuria. *Potassium depletion* and *hypercalcemia* interfere with AVP's action, causing usually mild polyuria. *Lithium carbonate, demeclocycline,* and *methoxyflurane* also impair the cell's response to AVP. This interference is used to therapeutic advantage to treat SIADH.

The rare *congenital forms of NDI* are inherited as X-linked recessive or dominant disorders with partial pen-

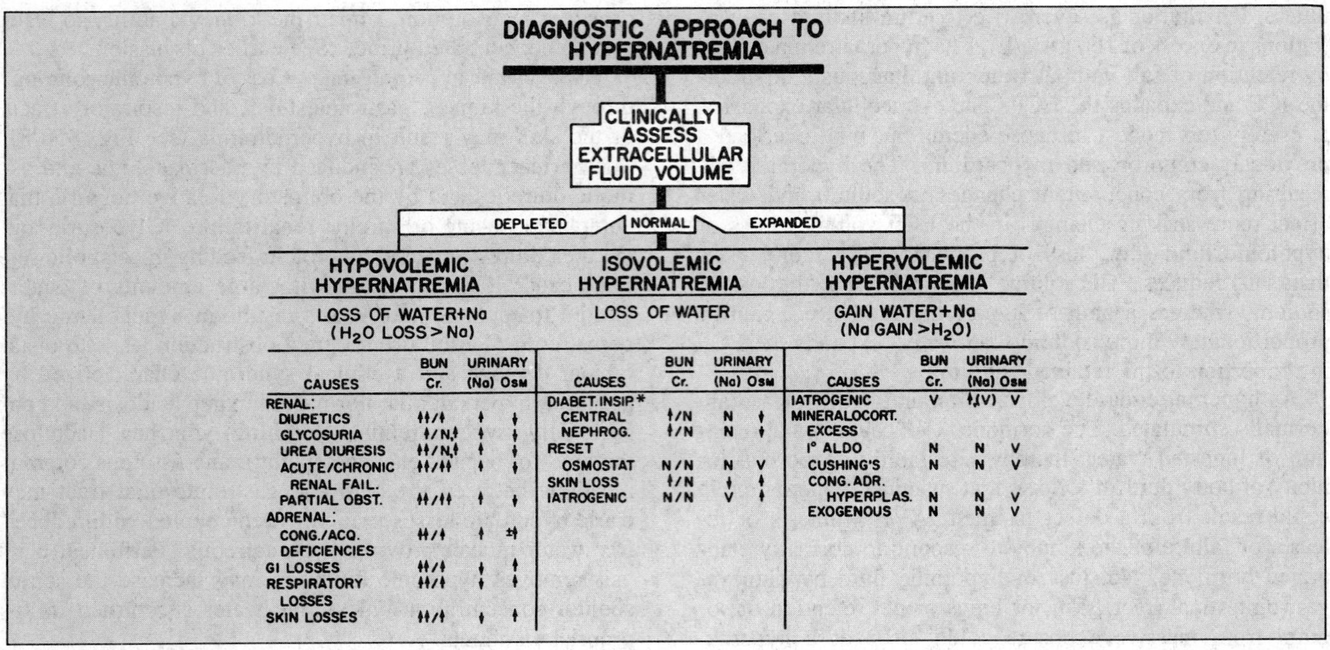

Fig. 350-8. Differential diagnosis of hypernatremia: the clinical and laboratory approach to the classification and diagnosis of the hypernatremic disorders is illustrated. See text for details. *, N, normal; V, variable; INSP, insipidus. (From Narins RG et al: Diagnostic strategies in disorders of fluid, electrolyte, and acid-base homeostasis, Am J Med 72:496, 1982.)

etrance in females. Thus males are most severely afflicted. Hypotonic polyuria that is unresponsive to AVP characterizes this syndrome. The inability of many such patients to increase their urinary cyclic AMP in response to supramaximum amounts of the hormone suggests that the defect resides at the AVP receptor or in the sustained generation of cyclic AMP.

Disorders of thirst and of the sensitivity of osmoreceptors to hypertonic stimuli may also spawn hypernatremic syndromes. Aging impairs thirst, thereby sensitizing elderly patients, whose access to water may be limited, to developing dehydration and hypernatremia. Because high serum sodium concentrations in the elderly usually complicate serious underlying disorders, hypernatremia augurs a poor prognosis. *Primary hypodipsia* may reduce water intake so severely as to allow normal insensible and urinary losses to increase serum sodium concentration. Appropriate renal water retention accompanying more mild thirst defects may simply result in reduced urine volume and relatively normal serum sodium concentrations. Hypothalamico-hypophyseal or cerebrocortical lesions that impair thirst are also the same disorders that can independently cause CDI. The reset *osmostat syndrome* (i.e., essential hypernatremia) results from simultaneous "upward resetting" of the osmostat and proportional insensitivity of thirst. As a result of the former defect, a greater degree of serum hypertonicity is required to elicit a given level of AVP secretion. Resulting water loss causes hypernatremia, which is sustained by the associated thirst defect. In some settings, AVP release is not stimulated until enough water has been lost to cause hypovolemia. These patients behave as if their osmoreceptors are totally defective while volume-dependent hormone release is intact.

Symptoms and signs. Irritability, lethargy, and weakness are early neurologic signs of acute hypernatremia. As serum sodium concentration climbs, cerebral dehydration worsens, soon provoking convulsive activity and eventuating in coma and death (Fig. 350-9). Contraction of brain cells stretches and distorts intra- and pericerebral veins, causing their rupture and eventually intracerebral and subarachnoid hemorrhage.

Within 24 to 36 hours of developing hypernatremia, idiogenic osmols form, causing water to return to and reexpand brain cells. Thus, patients with chronic hypernatremia may be relatively asymptomatic. It also follows that

SERUM Na^+ (meq/liter)	SYMPTOMS	HYPOVOLEMIA	HYPERVOLEMIA
150-155	WORSENING WEAKNESS, LETHARGY,	DIMINISHED BRAIN PERFUSION EXACERBATES SYMPTOMS	DIMINISHED EABV IN CHF, CIRRHOSIS, NEPHROSIS MAY REDUCE BRAIN PERFUSION AND EXACERBATE SYMPTOMS; PULMONARY SYMPTOMS MAY DOMINATE IN CHF
>160	TWITCHING, SEIZURES, COMA DEATH		

Fig. 350-9. Symptoms of hypovolemic and hypervolemic hypernatremia. CHF, congestive heart failure; EABV, effective arterial blood volume.

excessively rapid therapy with water, before the involution of cerebral idiogenic osmols, may lead to symptomatic and potentially fatal brain edema.

The clinical picture will, of course, also be colored by the disorder precipitating the hypernatremia. Hypovolemic and hypervolemic disorders tend to be more symptomatic, which is perhaps related to associated alterations in cerebral perfusion.

Diagnosis. Clinical clues suggesting the presence of hypernatremia should stimulate the physician to measure serum electrolytes, which establishes the diagnosis. Clinical assessment of the ECF volume serves as a useful basis for the differential diagnosis of hypernatremia (see Fig. 350-8). Hypovolemic disorders are characterized by postural accentuation of tachycardia and hypotension from hypotonic fluid losses. Renal and gastrointestinal losses account for most cases of hypovolemic hypernatremia. The presence of edema is required to clinically diagnose hypervolemic forms of hypernatremia. Previously edematous patients suffering hypotonic fluid losses from diuretics, gastrointestinal disorders, or underreplaced evaporative losses account for most of these cases. Excessive retention of hypertonic fluids can also cause this syndrome. The euvolemic disorders of hypernatremia may present primarily as polyuric, polydipsic disorders with varying degrees of hypernatremia or with few clinical signs associated with the serendipitous finding of an increased serum sodium concentration. An extensive discussion of the differential diagnosis of polyuria is beyond the intended scope of this chapter. Briefly, however, polyuric disorders are best classified by the character of the excreted urine, and on this basis they fall into the following three major groups: those caused by increased solute excretion, those in which excessive free-water excretion underlies the increased urinary volume, and those caused by combined solute and water excretory excesses. Measurement of osmolality in plasma and in timed urine specimens allows for calculation of osmolal (C_{osm}) and free-water clearances (C_{H_2O}) (Chapter 338). Solute diureses are caused by excessive excretion of urea, NaCl, $NaHCO_3$, glucose, or mannitol, and are characterized by isotonic urine and a C_{osm} that is generally greater than 3 ml/min. Water diureses are typified by hypotonic urine and C_{H_2O} usually in excess of 1 to 2 ml/min. Combined disorders manifest hypotonic urine in the face of increased C_{osm}. This mixed diuresis is seen, for example, when a patient with CDI is inappropriately treated with large amounts of saline.

As noted earlier (and in Chapter 161), free-water diureses are caused by compulsive water drinking and by CDI and NDI. Serum sodium concentration in the diabetes insipidus syndromes is normal to increased, whereas in the primary polydipsic syndromes it is normal to reduced. Careful restriction of water intake until body weight is reduced by 2% to 3%, or until the serum osmolality has increased to 290 to 295 mosm/L, increases urine osmolality to values in excess of plasma in compulsive water drinkers who manifest no further increase when 5 units of aqueous pitressin are given subcutaneously at the end of the period of thirsting. Patients with NDI sustain a constant level of hypotonic polyuria that is unresponsive to exogenous AVP. Those with complete CDI also continue to excrete a relatively constant volume of hypotonic urine during thirsting, but AVP administration elicits a striking decrease in volume and increase in tonicity of urine. With partial CDI, urine volume declines with thirsting, and urinary tonicity increases but plateaus at levels inappropriately low as compared with that seen in thirsting normal persons. Because their tubules are exposed to less than maximum concentrations of endogenous AVP, administration of the hormone at the end of the period of thirsting significantly increases the urine osmolality.

In summary, clinical assessment of the state of ECF volume expansion allows for the rapid classification of the hypernatremias. The urinary response to thirsting and to the administration of AVP provides a simple means for further subclassifying the euvolemic polyuric syndromes.

Therapy. Because poor tissue perfusion is most threatening, treatment of patients with hypovolemic hypernatremia who manifest prerenal azotemia and hypotension is best initiated with isotonic saline. Once hemodynamic stability and adequate urine volume are achieved, hypotonic solutions may be administered and serum sodium concentration normalized. Therapy of associated gastrointestinal and renal disorders that precipitated the hypernatremia must of course proceed in parallel with the administration of salt and water.

Therapy of hypervolemic hypernatremic syndromes requires removal of sodium in excess of water and is best achieved by replacing diuretic-induced sodium and water losses with only water. Oral or parenteral fluids may be used to replenish losses. Obviously, attention must also be paid to treating the underlying cause of the edema. Dialysis will be required to remove excess sodium in hypervolemic patients with hypernatremia who also have severe acute or chronic renal failure.

Chapter 161 thoroughly discusses treatment of CDI and NDI. Replacement of water losses in clinically euvolemic hypernatremic patients requires the following assumptions: that serum sodium behaves as if it is distributed in total body water; that total body water is 60% of normal body weight; and that the patient's body sodium content remains normal. Thus the amount of water required in a 70-kg man with isovolemic hypernatremia and a serum sodium level of 155 mEq/L is calculated as follows: Normal total body water $= 70$ kg $\times 0.6 = 42$ L. Normal total body sodium content $= 42$ L $\times$ 140 mEq/L $=$ 5880 mEq. In what reduced volume must the 5880 mEq be distributed to increase the serum sodium concentration to 155 mEq/L (i.e., 5880 mEq/x L $=$ 155 mEq/L)? Answer: 37.9 L. Thus loss of 4.1 L of water ($42 - 37.9 = 4.1$) accounts for the observed degree of hypernatremia. These 4.1 L should be replenished to restore normonatremia.

Some controversy exists as to how rapidly this fluid should be given. Most observers agree that the cerebral consequences from too rapid a rate of therapy can be avoided if the serum sodium concentration is reduced no faster than

1 to 2 mEq/L/hr. Ongoing water losses must be replenished along with deficits.

REFERENCES

Arief AI: Hyponatremia, convulsions, respiratory arrest, and permanent brain damage after elective surgery in healthy women, N Engl J Med 314:1529, 1986.

Ayus CL, Krothapalli RK, and Arief AI: Treatment of symptomatic hyponatremia and its relation to brain damage, N Engl J Med 317:1190, 1987.

Berl T: Treating hyponatremia: damned if we do and damned if we don't, Kidney Int 37:1006-1018, 1990.

Culpepper RM, Hebert SC, and Andreoli TE: Nephrogenic diabetes insipidus. In Stanbury JB et al, editors: The metabolic basis of inherited disease, ed 5, New York, 1983, McGraw-Hill.

Goldman MD, Luchins DJ, and Robertson GI: Mechanisms of altered water metabolism in psychotic patients with polydipsia and hyponatremia, N Engl J Med 318:397, 1988.

Howard RL, Bichet DG, and Schrier RW: Hypernatremic and polyuric states. In Seldin DW and Giebisch G, editors: The kidney: physiology and pathophysiology, ed 2, New York, 1992, Raven Press.

Jamison RL and Oliver RE: Disorders of urinary concentration and dilution, Am J Med 72:308, 1982.

Lindheimer MD, Barron WM, and Davision JM: Osmoregulation of thirst and vasopressin release in pregnancy, Am J Physiol 257:F159-F169, 1989.

Mattauer B et al: Sodium and water excretion abnormalities in congestive heart failure, Ann Intern Med 105:151, 1986.

Morrison G and Singer I: Hyperosmolal states. In Narins RG, editor: Clinical disorders of fluid and electrolyte metabolism. New York, 1993, (in press), McGraw-Hill.

Narins RG et al: Diagnostic strategies in disorders of fluid, electrolyte, and acid-base homeostasis, Am J Med 72:496, 1982.

Narins RG and Riley L: Polyuria: simple and mixed disorders, Am J Kidney Dis 17:237, 1991.

Sterns RH: Severe symptomatic hyponatremia: treatment and outcome. A study of 64 cases, Ann Intern Med 107:656, 1987.

Weisberg LS: Pseudohyponatremia, Am J Med 86:315-318, 1989.

CHAPTER

351 Disorders of Sodium Balance

Murray Epstein

The sodium content of a healthy 70-kg man ranges from 4400 to 5600 mEq. Of this pool, approximately 2800 mEq is contained within the extracellular fluid (ECF). Much of the remaining sodium exists in a poorly exchangeable pool bound to the crystalline structure of the bone and is thus not an osmotically active solute. As a consequence of an active transport mechanism that results in the extrusion of sodium from the intracellular fluid to the ECF, most of the sodium resides in the ECF. Therefore sodium, with its accompanying anions, chloride and bicarbonate, constitutes more than 90% of the total solute contained in the ECF. It follows that sodium is the major determinant of ECF volume.

Under normal circumstances, ECF volume is maintained relatively constant. The kidney compensates for either a deficit or excess of salt and water with great precision, thereby ensuring that ECF volume is maintained within narrow limits. The ECF volume deviates from these normal constraints when excess sodium is retained (edematous states) or when significant quantities of sodium are lost as a result of the loss or sequestration of body fluids containing substantial quantities of sodium (sodium depletion states).

EDEMATOUS STATES

Edema is an excessive accumulation of fluid within the interstitial space. Irrespective of its cause, generalized edema requires two events for its development. First, an imbalance of Starling forces favors outward movement of fluid across the capillary wall into the interstitial space. Such a perturbation of the Starling forces must be accompanied by the renal retention of sodium as the kidney attempts to refill the diminished vascular space. In the absence of renal sodium retention, edema formation would be largely self-limited because the imbalance of Starling forces would tend to correct itself as fluid accumulation progressed. Thus the clinical consequences of generalized edema derive from the fact that renal sodium retention maintains the edematous state.

The major edematous states differ one from the other with regard to both anatomic and functional abnormalities, but they have in common a deranged regulatory mechanism for maintaining sodium homeostasis. Thus in cirrhosis of the liver, the volume receptors appear to be intact and functioning normally, but circulating blood volume is maldistributed so that the kidney behaves as if it were underperfused. In another major edematous state, congestive heart failure, it has been proposed that sodium retention occurs because of damaged receptors that are incapable of adequately apprising the kidney that sodium excretion should be increased.

All the major edematous disease states are characterized by a continuing and unrelenting accumulation of salt and water. Even when the fluid retention has become massive, the kidney often continues to retain salt and water, behaving as though it were responding to a volume deficit. It has been proposed that the stimulus for sodium retention is a contraction of the "effective" blood volume, a feature common to all major edematous states. In this context, it is important to note that the term *effective plasma volume* refers to that part of the total circulating volume that is effective in stimulating volume receptors. The concept is somewhat elusive because the actual volume receptors remain incompletely defined. A diminished effective volume may reflect subtle alterations in systemic hemodynamic factors, such as decreased filling of the arterial tree, a diminished central blood volume, or both. In normal circumstances, effective blood volume correlates with total ECF volume; in contrast, in the major edematous states, it does not. Despite massive retention of salt and water, effective blood volume remains functionally contracted because of a disturbance in the Starling forces that govern the distribution of fluid within the ECF compartment.

In the light of this formulation, it is possible to understand why the retained fluid in major edematous states fails to modify the stimulus for continuing sodium and water retention. Despite a progressive increase in total ECF volume, fluid is sequestered into one or more of the other fluid compartments without succeeding in normalizing effective blood volume. Only a normalization of the disturbance in the forces governing fluid distribution will permit a reexpansion of effective blood volume to normal.

In summary, it is apparent that in two of the major edematous disorders (congestive heart failure and cirrhosis), the kidney is not the culprit in this situation but rather is best visualized as an innocent victim: The kidney's response is appropriate to the information it receives. What is inappropriate in this setting are the signals being transmitted to the kidney.

The accompanying box lists the conditions associated with generalized edema. This chapter does not cover the entire spectrum of edematous disorders. Rather, consideration will be given only to three of the four major disorders encountered frequently in clinical practice.

CONGESTIVE HEART FAILURE

In congestive heart failure (CHF), impaired cardiac emptying results in a rise in ventricular end-diastolic pressure. As depicted in Fig. 351-1, the consequent high venous pressure promotes transudation of fluid out of the vascular channel through several mechanisms. First, the mean capillary hydraulic pressure is increased. Because the resulting rate of fluid transfer from peripheral capillaries to the interstitial space exceeds the rate of return of interstitial fluid to the intravascular compartment, edema formation ensues. Furthermore, an increased peripheral venous pressure may cause a neurogenic resetting of precapillary and postcapillary resistances, leading to increased capillary hydraulic pressure and transudation of fluid from the intravascular to the interstitial space. Third, an increase in systemic venous pressure often leads to hepatic congestion, which may depress both plasma renin clearance and the hepatic metabolism of aldosterone. Fourth, there is reason to believe that an increase in systemic venous pressure per se may contribute to sodium retention via afferent pathways. There is supportive evidence for the existence of volume receptors in the low-pressure central venous portion of the circulation (referred to as *low-pressure volume receptors*). It is thus possible that an increased venous pressure activates such receptors, leading to sodium retention by the kidneys. Furthermore, salt and water retention in CHF leads to a mild decrease in systemic plasma protein concentration, with a decrease in the oncotic pressure gradient, thereby favoring edema formation. Finally, several lines of evidence suggest that the increase in central venous pressure in CHF retards lymph flow in the thoracic duct, with a resultant decrease in lymphatic drainage of peripheral interstitial spaces.

The decrease in cardiac output and sometimes in mean arterial pressure (MAP) characteristic of severe CHF may be associated with a reduction of the renal fraction of cardiac output and of both renal plasma flow (RPF) and glo-

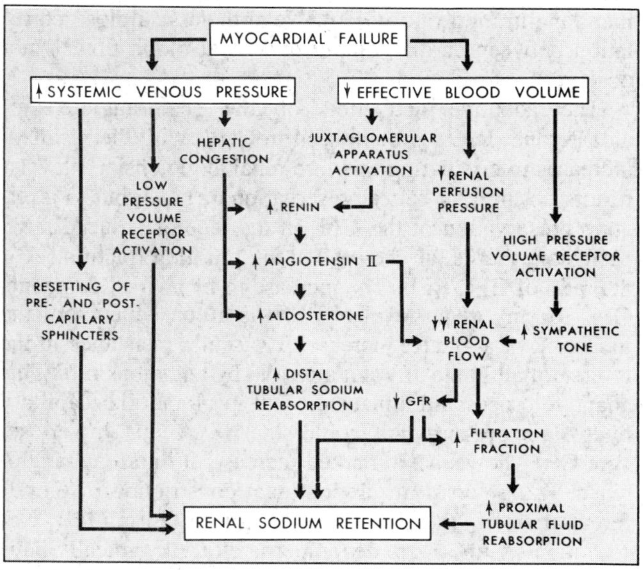

Fig. 351-1. The major pathophysiologic mechanisms leading to renal sodium retention in congestive heart failure. The increased systemic venous pressure promotes transudation of fluid out of the vascular channel by several mechanisms. Concomitantly, a diminution in "effective" blood volume promotes renal sodium retention through a number of hormonal, hemodynamic, and neural mechanisms. (Modified from Humes HD, Gottlieb MN, and Brenner BM: The kidney in congestive heart failure. In Brenner BM and Stein JH, editors: Sodium and water homeostasis, New York, 1978, Churchill Livingstone.)

Causes of generalized edema

I. Common causes
   - A. Congestive heart failure
   - B. Cirrhosis of the liver
   - C. Nephrotic syndrome
   - D. Acute "nephritic" syndrome
   - E. Pregnancy
     1. Normal pregnancy
     2. Toxemia of pregnancy
   - F. Idiopathic edema

II. Unusual causes
   - A. Arteriovenous fistulas
   - B. Hypothyroidism
   - C. Diabetes mellitus
     1. Associated with microangiopathy (rare)
     2. Associated with insulin treatment of ketoacidosis
   - D. Drugs
     1. Nonsteroidal anti-inflammatory drugs
     2. Estrogens
     3. Vasodilator antihypertensive drugs
     4. Hyperstimulation syndrome secondary to menotropins (Pergonal)

merular filtration rate (GFR). Nevertheless, a close correlation between cardiac output and renal blood flow is not observed.

The adaptive activation of the renin-angiotensin–aldosterone (RAA) system seen in CHF, with the resultant increases in circulating and intrarenal angiotensin II levels, results not only in better preservation of MAP but in a relative preservation of the GFR in the face of reduced renal perfusion, that is, an increase in the filtration fraction (FF), the ratio of GFR/RPF. The increase in FF, which augments GFR for any given level of RPF, is a consequence of the induction of a greater increase of vascular resistance in the efferent than in the afferent arteriole by angiotensin II. This adaptive process minimizes the fall in glomerular capillary hydrostatic pressure that would otherwise occur. In very severe CHF, however, a marked increase in intrarenal angiotensin II may result in predominant constriction of the afferent arteriole, thereby contributing to a fall in GFR.

Patients with severe decompensated CHF typically have marked, complex activation of several neurohumoral systems. These neurohumoral changes include those that produce systemic and renal microvascular vasoconstriction, tending to cause renal sodium and water retention, for example, activation of the RAA system, and the sympathetic nervous system, and increased release of arginine vasopressin (AVP). Neurohumoral activation not only reflects the magnitude of CHF, but probably directly contributes to functional impairment and poor long-term prognosis.

Because of the contraction of effective blood volume, the kidneys respond by retaining salt by several different mechanisms. The reduced effective blood volume activates the RAA system, with enhanced sodium reabsorption in the distal segments of the nephron. Concomitantly, there is a decrease in renal blood flow that is attributable to several mechanisms (see Fig. 351-1). The decline in renal perfusion is usually associated with little or no concurrent decline in glomerular GFR, thereby resulting in a rise in the ratio of GFR/RPF (i.e., the FF), which in turn is thought to play a fundamental role in promoting the sodium retention encountered (Chapter 338).

Concomitantly, there is activation of the sympathetic nervous system as well as stimulation of vasopressin release. These systems maintain systemic blood pressure and promote renal sodium and water retention during acute cardiac decompensation. In the chronic "compensated" phase of cardiac failure, which is associated with expansion of extracellular fluid volume and restoration of blood pressure, the plasma levels of the previously mentioned hormones generally return to normal.

Many patients with chronic severe (class III or IV) cardiac failure exhibit hyponatremia. Serum sodium concentration has been shown to be a useful predictor of the state of the renin-angiotensin and sympathetic nervous systems in cardiac failure. An inverse correlation has been reported between serum sodium concentration and plasma renin activity.

Finally, recent data have demonstrated that serum sodium concentration and plasma hormonal levels have prognostic value in predicting the survival of patients with CHF. Hyponatremic patients with CHF have a significantly shorter survival time than do normonatremic patients with cardiac failure. Patients with plasma norepinephrine levels greater than 800 pg/ml have a significantly worse prognosis than do those with plasma norepinephrine levels of 400 to 800 pg/ml. Patients whose plasma norepinephrine levels are nearly normal, that is, less than 400 pg/ml, have the best relative prognosis. These seemingly independent observations are clearly related: Patients with severely decompensated heart failure have elevated plasma vasoconstricting-sodium retentive hormones with consequent impairment of water excretion eventually resulting in hyponatremia.

Fluid restriction is generally not a useful measure to reverse CHF-associated hyponatremia. Similarly, discontinuation of furosemide alone rarely increases serum sodium level, although the withdrawal of thiazide-type diuretics may have this effect. The combined administration of an angiotensin-converting enzyme (ACE) inhibitor with furosemide (but usually not of either agent alone) usually reverses the hyponatremia, at least in part.

The reversal of hyponatremia in patients with CHF treated with both ACE inhibitor and diuretic probably results from the combined effects of the ACE inhibitor (e.g., decreased thirst, decreased proximal tubular resorption of sodium, interference with the hydro-osmotic effect of AVP) and the loop diuretic (increased distal delivery of glomerular filtrate, reduction in urine osmolality) acting to offset the pathophysiologic factors causing impaired excretion of water.

As discussed earlier, enhanced sodium reabsorption mediated by these several different mechanisms expands the *total* blood volume to values usually far in excess of normal. Despite such increases in ECF, effective blood volume remains contracted because the cardiac output remains low, and the central venous pressure remains elevated. Consequently, the stimulus for salt retention persists.

Successful therapy of CHF consists of interrupting this vicious circle. Improvement of the pumping action of the heart increases effective blood volume and lowers systemic venous pressure. Consequently, the two major afferent mechanisms leading to salt and water retention in CHF are interrupted. Traditional therapy of CHF has consisted mainly in measures to strengthen the force of contraction and to reduce elevated ventricular filling pressures. Accordingly, patients have been treated with a combination of an inotropic drug (one of the digitalis compounds) to stimulate myocardial contractility and a diuretic to increase renal excretion of salt and water.

Although such an approach is often successful in restoring adequate ventricular function in a setting of mild CHF, the more severe CHF affecting patients with ischemic heart disease or cardiomyopathy is often refractory to such therapy. More than a decade ago, a major change of approach in the management of heart failure began, with the demonstration that vasodilator drugs, which have no direct cardiac action, could dramatically improve left ventricular performance. The underlying concept of vasodilator therapy is to unburden the failing heart. Rather than stimulating contraction in a heart weakened by disease, it may be preferable to alter cardiac preload or afterload conditions with drugs that act in the periphery to lower vascular resistance or reduce venous return (Chapter 10).

CIRRHOSIS
(see also Chapter 56)

The clinical course in patients with decompensated Laenec's cirrhosis is often complicated by progressive impairment of renal sodium handling, leading to the formation of fluid in the peritoneal cavity (ascites) and peripheral edema. It should be underscored that cirrhotic patients who are unable to excrete sodium will continue to gain weight and accumulate fluid as long as dietary sodium content exceeds maximum urinary sodium excretion. If access to sodium is not curtailed, the relentless retention of sodium may lead to the accumulation of vast amounts of ascitic fluid (on occasion, up to 20 L). Weight gain and ascites formation promptly cease when sodium intake is limited. It should further be noted that the impairment of renal sodium handling in such patients is not a static and unalterable condition. Rather, cirrhotic patients may undergo a spontaneous diuresis followed by a return to avid salt retention.

Discussion of the pathogenetic events leading to the deranged sodium homeostasis of cirrhosis is simplified by considering the "afferent" and the "efferent" events that eventuate in this derangement.

Afferent events

Traditionally, it has been proposed that ascites formation in cirrhotic patients begins when a critical imbalance of Starling forces in the hepatic sinusoids and splanchnic capillaries causes an excessive amount of lymph formation, exceeding the capacity of the thoracic duct to return this excessive lymph to the circulation. Consequently, excess lymph accumulates in the peritoneal space, with a subsequent contraction of circulating plasma volume. Thus as ascites develops, there is a progressive redistribution of plasma volume. Although total plasma volume may be increased in this setting, the physiologic circumstance may mimic a reduction in plasma volume (a reduced effective plasma volume). The diminished effective volume is thought to constitute an afferent signal to the renal tubule to augment salt and water reabsorption.

Although an imbalance of Starling forces in the hepatosplanchnic microcirculation is thought to contribute importantly to the relative decrease in effective blood volume, it should be emphasized that this is not the sole mechanism. An additional determinant is total peripheral resistance, which is diminished significantly in most patients with cirrhosis who are retaining sodium and water. This decrease in peripheral vascular resistance is no doubt partially related to anatomic arteriovenous shunts, but it has also been proposed that some undefined vasodilator (either produced by or not inactivated by the diseased liver) plays a role. Thus despite an increase in *total* plasma volume, the relative "fullness" of the arteriovenous tree is diminished. Several hemodynamic events therefore act in concert to diminish the effective volume, thereby activating the mechanisms promoting sodium retention (Fig. 351-2). In sum, the traditional formulation suggests that the renal retention of sodium is a secondary rather than a primary event.

Recently, an alternative hypothesis, termed the *peripheral arterial vasodilatation hypothesis,* has been proposed to account for the initiation of sodium and water retention in cirrhosis. One may regard this theory as a revision of the underfill theory. The principal distinguishing feature of this newly proposed theory is that the decrease in effective blood volume is attributable primarily to an early increase in vascular capacitance. Thus peripheral vasodilatation is the initial determinant of intravascular underfilling, and an imbalance between the expanded capacitance and the available volume constitutes a diminished effective volume. This formulation recognizes that total peripheral resistance is diminished significantly in most edematous cirrhotic patients.

Both underfill theories possibly explain why fluid retention may fail to attenuate the stimulus for continuing sodium and water retention. Despite a progressive increase in total ECF volume, fluid is sequestered into one or more of the other fluid compartments without normalizing effective blood volume (EBV). Only correction of the disturbance in the forces governing fluid distribution will permit a re-expansion of EBV.

Over 2 decades ago, an alternative hypothesis was proposed. Lieberman and his associates postulated the "overflow" theory of ascites formation. In contrast to the traditional formulation, the overflow theory suggests that the primary event is the inappropriate retention of excessive sodium by the kidneys, with a resultant expansion of plasma volume. Studies in a canine model of cirrhosis have further supported this view. The mechanism(s) underlying a

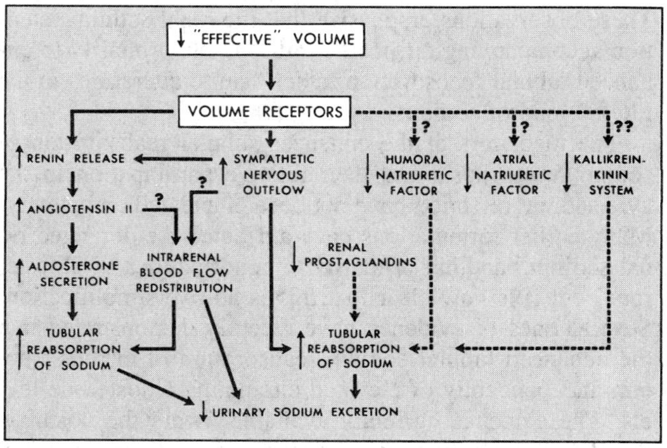

Fig. 351-2. Possible mechanisms by which a diminished "effective" volume results in sodium retention in cirrhosis. The heavy arrows indicate pathways for which evidence is available. The dashed lines represent proposed pathways, whose existence remains to be established. (Modified with permission from Epstein M: Renal sodium handling in liver disease. In Epstein M, editor: The kidney in liver disease, ed 3, Baltimore, 1988, Williams & Wilkins.)

primary retention of sodium by the kidney has not been elucidated. In the setting of abnormal Starling forces (both portal venous hypertension and a reduction in plasma colloid osmotic pressure) in the portal venous bed and hepatic sinusoids, the expanded plasma volume is sequestered preferentially in the peritoneal space, with ascites formation. Thus according to this formulation, renal sodium retention and plasma volume expansion precede rather than follow the formation of ascites.

Although we believe that the presently available evidence favors a prominent role for diminished *effective* plasma volume in mediating the avid sodium retention of many cirrhotic patients with established cirrhosis, it should be emphasized that these two theories may not be mutually exclusive. As noted earlier, cirrhosis is not a *static* disease but rather a constantly evolving clinical disorder. Yet virtually all the available clinical studies of deranged sodium homeostasis were carried out on a single state of the disease, at a time when decompensation was well established, with little information about the incipient stage of sodium retention. In contrast, the studies with the canine cirrhosis model deal with the relatively early stage of sodium retention. Any theory suggesting that the same antinatriuretic forces are operative throughout the evolution of sodium retention in a cirrhotic patient is probably a marked oversimplification. Rather, one should adopt a more global view of the pathogenesis of abnormal sodium retention in cirrhosis in which differing forces participate in varying degrees as the derangement in sodium homeostasis evolves.

Efferent events

Although initial attempts to explain the abnormalities of renal sodium handling focused on the decrement in GFR that occurs frequently in patients with advanced liver disease, it is clear that abnormalities of renal sodium handling occur despite preserved (and at times supranormal) GFR. These observations emphasize that the renal sodium retention accompanying cirrhosis is attributable primarily to enhanced tubular reabsorption rather than to alterations in the filtered load of sodium.

The mediators of the enhanced tubular reabsorption of sodium in cirrhosis and their relative participation in the avid sodium retention have not been elucidated completely. Many earlier formulations have attributed the deranged renal sodium handling primarily to abnormalities of aldosterone, but it is now clear that this is an oversimplification. Several lines of evidence have recently demonstrated that the enhanced tubular sodium reabsorption of cirrhosis occurs independently of elevated circulating aldosterone levels. The evidence currently available favors the postulate that the hyperaldosteronism of cirrhosis is a permissive factor only, and that the predominant component of the abnormal renal sodium handling is diminished distal delivery of filtrate. Only when distal filtrate delivery is enhanced by experimental or pharmacologic maneuvers does aldosterone play a major role in promoting sodium retention in cirrhosis.

The reappraisal of the role of aldosterone has prompted a search for additional effectors of sodium retention. Several hormonal, neural, and hemodynamic mechanisms have been implicated or suggested. The mechanisms, for which there is some evidence, and their interrelationships, are summarized schematically in Fig. 351-2. The diminution of effective volume results in activation of the renin-angiotensin system. As a consequence, aldosterone secretion is augmented, with a resultant increase in sodium reabsorption in the distal segments of the nephron. It is also possible that activation of the renin-angiotensin system may contribute to sodium retention by producing a redistribution of intrarenal blood flow.

Simultaneously, an increase in sympathetic nervous system activity may contribute to the sodium retention. Activation of the sympathetic nervous system is commonly present in patients with cirrhosis. Many investigators have shown that patients with cirrhosis have elevated plasma concentrations of the sympathetic neurotransmitter norepinephrine and higher rates of norepinephrine spillover to plasma from the body as a whole and from individual organs and vascular territories such as the kidneys and the hepatomesenteric circulation. That sympathetic nerve firing rates are elevated in patients with cirrhosis has been confirmed by a study in which sympathetic nerve discharge rates were recorded directly using clinical microneurography. Recently, Esler et al reported that acute sympathetic inhibition, achieved by intravenously administered clonidine, was accompanied by potentially clinically beneficial effects: the lowering of renal vascular resistance, elevation of glomerular filtration rate, and reduction of portal venous pressure. Such observations suggest an important pathophysiologic role for increased sympathetic nervous activity in mediating the sodium retention of cirrhosis. It is now well established that alterations of the input of cardiopulmonary receptors induce changes in renal sympathetic activity. Thus a decrease in blood volume could alter the afferent input from the cardiopulmonary region, with a resultant increase in sympathetic nerve activity. Such an increase could contribute to the antinatriuresis of cirrhosis by (1) effecting a redistribution of blood flow into the kidney that favors increased net reabsorption of filtrate, and (2) a direct tubular effect of the renal sympathetic nerves on renal sodium handling.

Additional evidence has been marshalled to support the possibility that a diminution in endogenous prostaglandin production contributes to the sodium retention. A large body of evidence demonstrates that nonsteroidal anti-inflammatory drugs (NSAIDs), which inhibit the endogenous production of prostaglandins, induce profound decrements of renal plasma flow, GFR, and sodium excretion in sodium-avid cirrhotic patients. Conversely, experimental manipulations that augment endogenous prostaglandins such as water immersion are associated with an increase in prostaglandin E and 6-keto prostaglandin $F_{1\alpha}$ excretion and a marked natriuresis and increase in creatinine clearance. In concert, these observations provide good evidence that renal prostanoid production contributes importantly to sodium retention. One can postulate that in the setting of cirrhosis, enhancement of prostaglandin synthesis is a compensatory or adaptive response to incipient renal ischemia. An important clinical corollary of this formulation is that the administration of agents inhibitory to prostaglandin synthesis may result in clinically important sodium retention and/or deterioration of renal function. Alterations in the kallikrein-kinin system, with diminished kinin formation, may contribute to the sodium retention encountered in liver disease.

Deficient production of endogenous natriuretic hormones has traditionally been suggested as another mechanism of sodium retention in cirrhosis. Two natriuretic hormones have been recognized: the atrial natriuretic peptide (ANP), mainly synthesized by atrial myocytes, and the so-called natriuretic hormone (NH), which is thought to be produced in the hypothalamus.

With the recent characterization of ANP and the demonstration that it participates in the regulation of volume homeostasis in both animals and humans, theoretical considerations suggest its possible role in the pathogenesis of sodium retention in cirrhosis. Nevertheless, recent evidence militates against an important role for ANF in mediating sodium retention. Experimental maneuvers such as water immersion have clearly demonstrated that cirrhotic patients augment plasma ANF to levels that either equal or exceed those of normal subjects studied under identical conditions, suggesting that sodium retention is not attributable to a diminished capacity to release ANF. Furthermore, recent studies during water immersion have demonstrated a striking dissociation between plasma ANF and the concomitant natriuretic response. In concert with data indicating that the natriuretic response to ANF infusion is markedly blunted or absent in approximately half of patients, these observations suggest that the sodium retention of cirrhosis may be related in part to a reduced renal responsiveness to ANF. It is conceivable that renal vasoconstriction mediated by diverse mechanisms including the observed activation of the renin-angiotensin and probably the sympathetic nervous systems impede the ability of ANF to promote natriuresis.

The role of NH in mediating the sodium retention of cirrhosis is controversial, primarily because it is difficult to measure this hormone. The chemical nature of NH has not been established and can only be evaluated indirectly by assessing its biologic activities, namely the ability to inhibit sodium and potassium-activated (Na-K-)ATPase and ouabain binding in vitro, cross-react with antidigoxin antibodies, and induce a natriuresis when infused into experimental animals. Initial studies using bioassay techniques suggested a defect in the release of NH. In contrast, more recent studies, in which NH was specifically investigated in plasma and urine from cirrhotic patients with and without ascites by assessing digoxin-like immunoreactivity (DLIA) and the inhibition of ouabain binding, suggest that this hormone is not reduced but rather increased in these patients. These preliminary results have suggested that sodium retention in cirrhotic patients cannot be attributed to a deficiency in this hormone. Alternatively, the increased activity of natriuretic hormone in patients with cirrhosis and ascites may represent a compensatory response that is insufficient to antagonize the renal effects of sodium-retaining forces.

Management

The rational management of excessive salt and water retention in the cirrhotic patient should be grounded on the realization that ascites, unless massive, may not require intervention with diuretic agents. The initial goal of any treatment program should be an attempt to obtain spontaneous diuresis by consistent and scrupulous adherence to a well-balanced diet with rigid dietary sodium restriction (250 mg/day). It should be emphasized that the sodium intake prescribed for cardiac patients (1200 to 1500 mg/day) is not sufficiently restrictive for the cirrhotic patient, who continues to gain weight on such a program.

When the response to dietary management is inadequate, or when the imposition of rigid dietary sodium restriction is not feasible due to the cost or unpalatability of the diet, the use of diuretic agents may be considered. When diuretics are used, the therapeutic aim is a slow and gradual diuresis not exceeding the capacity for mobilization of ascitic fluid. Shear and colleagues demonstrated that ascites absorption averages about 300 to 500 ml/day during spontaneous diuresis, with an upper limit of 700 to 900 ml/day. Thus any diuresis that exceeds 900 ml/day (in the ascitic patient without edema) must perforce be mobilized at the expense of the plasma compartment, with resultant volume contraction.

Because of the possible risk of hyponatremia, renal failure, and encephalopathy, therapeutic paracentesis has not enjoyed much popularity in the treatment of refractory ascites. Recently, several groups of investigators have evaluated the effects of large-volume paracentesis. They have suggested that therapeutic paracentesis, in the form of either repeated large-volume paracentesis or total paracentesis associated with an intravenous infusion of albumin (6 to 8 g/L of ascitic fluid removed), is a rapid, effective, and safe therapy for refractory ascites in patients with cirrhosis.

NEPHROTIC SYNDROME
(see also Chapter 346)

Normal adult humans excrete 100 to 150 mg of protein in the urine daily. In the setting of renal disease with involvement of the glomerulus, proteinuria ($>$150 mg/day) often supervenes. When the magnitude of proteinuria is great enough to exceed rates of albumin production by the liver, the concentration of albumin in plasma declines, and the complex of symptoms recognized as the nephrotic syndrome develops. The nephrotic syndrome may be defined as severe proteinuria (3.5 g or more), predominantly albuminuria, with concomitant hypoalbuminemia. Edema is the most prominent outward manifestation of the nephrotic syndrome and often provides the first evidence of disease noted by patients with some types of nephrotic syndrome.

Although the initiating event in these patients differs from that in patients with other edematous states, the overall pathogenetic cascade has many similarities. In contrast to patients with CHF and cirrhosis, patients with nephrotic syndrome frequently have a diminished total blood volume. The decrease in total blood volume (and thus in effective blood volume) is related to the hypoalbuminemia and diminished plasma oncotic pressure in the syndrome. Figure 351-3 summarizes the sequence of potential events that may contribute to the enhanced tubular reabsorption of sodium and edema formation. As a consequence of the diminished effective blood volume, the RAA system is activated, contributing to increased tubular reabsorption of sodium. As with cirrhotic patients, recent evidence suggests that the hyperaldosteronism of nephrotic syndrome is a permissive factor only and not the major determinant of the abnormal sodium retention. Concomitantly, several mechanisms act in concert to increase renal vascular resistance. Despite an increased renal vascular resistance, renal blood flow and GFR are not uniformly diminished, and in some instances GFR may actually be supranormal. The maintenance of the normal or increased GFR is thought to be related to the hypoalbuminemia, which decreases glomerular capillary oncotic pressure and therefore tends to increase net glomerular filtration pressure. In the presence of profound hypovolemia, however, the enhancement of GFR may be obscured by increased afferent arterial constriction, which diminishes glomerular capillary hydrostatic pressure.

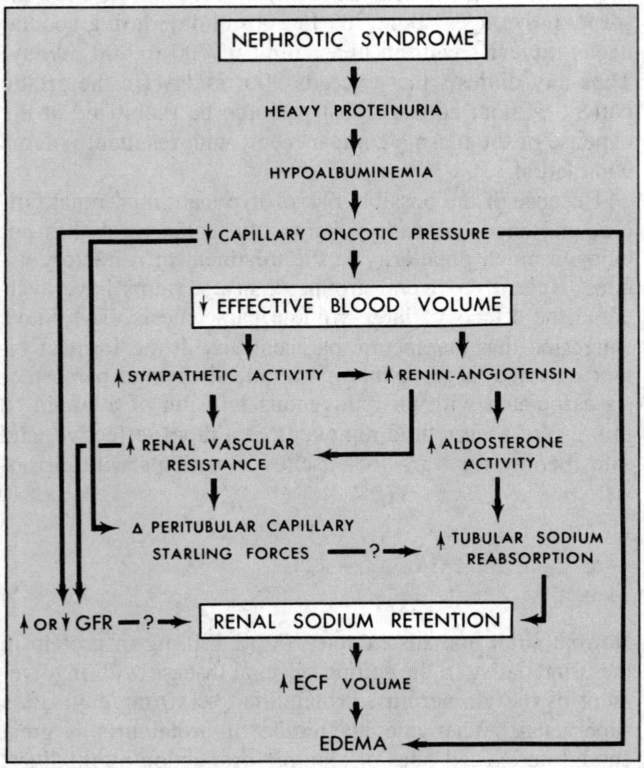

Fig. 351-3. The major pathophysiologic mechanisms leading to renal sodium retention in the nephrotic syndrome. As a result of the massive proteinuria, hypoalbuminemia and decreased plasma oncotic pressure ensue, with resultant diminution in total blood volume and effective blood volume. Depicted here are the sequence of potential hormonal, hemodynamic, and neural events that may be activated as a consequence thereof and the manner in which they may interact to promote sodium retention. (Modified from Schrier RW and Anderson RJ: Renal sodium excretion, edematous disorders, and diuretic use. In Schrier RW, editor: Renal and electrolyte disorders, ed 2, Boston, 1980, Little, Brown.)

The characteristics of the enhanced tubular reabsorption of sodium in patients with nephrotic syndrome may differ from those in CHF patients and patients with cirrhosis. It has been suggested that patients with nephrotic syndrome reabsorb less tubular sodium and water in the proximal tubule, perhaps due to the lowering of peritubular oncotic pressure with hypoalbuminemia. Accordingly, the main site for the enhanced sodium reabsorption in nephrotic syndrome might be localized to the distal nephron. Thus in the presence of blockade of distal reabsorption of sodium by large doses of ethacrynic acid and thiazide diuretics, nephrotic syndrome patients excrete a larger fraction of their filtered load of sodium than either cirrhotic patients or cardiac failure patients.

Aside from the administration of diuretics, several therapeutic considerations are unique to the nephrotic patient. Because the linchpin of the pathogenetic cascade responsible for sodium reabsorption is proteinuria, one may consider the administration of corticosteroids in an attempt to diminish or eliminate the proteinuria. Certain diseases causing the nephrotic syndrome, particularly lipoid nephrosis (nil disease), are amenable to such an approach (the diverse glomerulonephritides and their treatment are discussed in detail in Chapter 354). Although hypoalbuminemia is a salient feature of the nephrotic syndrome, the administration of albumin solutions is of little lasting value because the increase in plasma albumin concentration is only transient. In extremely severe hypoalbuminemia, however, an infusion of albumin may be a lifesaving maneuver in the management of a hypotensive episode.

ACUTE NEPHRITIC SYNDROME

The pathophysiology of sodium retention in the acute nephritic syndrome is discussed in detail in Chapter 345 and will not be considered further here.

IDIOPATHIC EDEMA

Idiopathic edema is a common disorder that occurs exclusively in women and is characterized by salt retention in the absence of cardiac, renal, or hepatic disease. Although the edema may be episodic and the disorder has been called cyclic edema, it can be persistent. In women afflicted with this disorder, edema of the face, hands, and feet develops rapidly, frequently accompanied by symptoms of headache, irritability, and depression. Some women can gain as much as 3 to 4 kg during a 24-hour period, with a concomitant decrease in urine output.

There is a significant postural component to the occurrence of edema. Although upright posture is associated with hyperaldosteronism and sodium retention in normal subjects, edema rarely occurs. In contrast, patients with idiopathic cyclical edema seem to have an exaggerated response to upright posture whereby the antinatriuresis of upright posture results in significant pitting edema of their lower extremities.

Another intriguing facet of the syndrome is its frequent association with *surreptitious* diuretic use. Many of the patients are obese women and there frequently is great anxiety about appearance and weight. Such concern can lead some women with idiopathic edema to take diuretics constantly and surreptitiously. The clinical presentation then may not be edema but rather unexplained hypokalemia, urinary potassium wasting, and elevated plasma renin activity, which can lead to the mistaken diagnosis of Bartter's syndrome.

In a similar vein, administration of potent diuretics in patients with idiopathic edema may have a deleterious effect by inducing ECF volume depletion, further exaggerating an already abnormal response to upright posture. The resultant hyperaldosteronism together with other mediators may induce sustained antinatriuresis for as long as 2 weeks after cessation of treatment. Furthermore, long-term diuretic therapy is associated with potassium depletion, which can potentiate the problem by producing symptoms of weakness, malaise, and irritability.

Despite much study, the mechanisms responsible for the sodium retention have not been established. Postulated mechanisms include a reduction in arterial blood pressure when standing, intermittent alteration in capillary permeability, increased aldosterone secretion, alteration in estrogen or progesterone secretion, and hypoproteinemia.

USE OF DIURETICS

When edema persists despite adequate treatment of the primary disease, diuretics may be required. It should be emphasized that the presence of edema alone is not a definite indication for diuretic treatment, and the physician must weigh any cosmetic value against the potential deleterious effect of the drug.

Once the decision is made to use diuretic agents to treat an edematous disorder, there are several guidelines for gauging the desired rate of diuresis. In general, it should approximate the rate of accumulation of the edema fluid. Thus acute pulmonary edema necessitates induction of a rapid diuresis, whereas less emergent edema formation is best treated with a more gradual diuresis. In either case, the rate of diuresis should be so limited that the potential rate of movement of interstitial fluid into the vascular compartment will not be exceeded to any large extent. If renal excretion does exceed the rate of mobilization of interstitial fluid, intravascular volume depletion and hypotension can result, even though ECF volume is still expanded. Intermittent diuretic therapy (e.g., alternate-day therapy) may be of value in avoiding intravascular volume depletion.

The rational basis of diuretic therapy lies in an understanding of the mechanism(s) and sites of action of the diuretic agent. The accompanying box summarizes the primary sites of action of the available diuretic agents. The loop diuretics ethacrynic acid, furosemide, and bumetanide are the most potent diuretic agents available. The very steep dose-response relationship they manifest has led to the label *high ceiling diuretics*. The inhibition of sodium and chloride reabsorption that these agents produce in the medullary ascending limb of the loop of Henle exceeds the rate-limited sodium reabsorption in the more distal nephron, and a maximal acute diuretic effect equivalent to 20% to 25% of the filtered load of sodium may be achieved. These drugs are effective immediately after intravenous administration and exert an effect within 1 hour of oral administration. In patients with pulmonary edema, the intravenous administration of furosemide not only induces a diuresis but also reduces the preload on the heart. The management of CHF is often complicated by an inability of orally administered furosemide to produce an effective diuresis, requiring intravenous furosemide to achieve the desired clinical response.

The distal tubular diuretics can be classified into two groups, namely, the potassium-losing and potassium-sparing diuretics. The thiazidelike diuretics chlorthalidone and metolazone, although chemically different, have diuretic effects similar to those of the thiazides. The diuretic effect of all of these compounds is attributable solely to the demonstrated inhibition of sodium and chloride reabsorption in the distal convoluted tubule. Consequently, these diuretics partially inhibit only urinary diluting capacity, not concentrating capacity. Thiazides are relatively safe and are the first-line drugs in patients with normal renal function. In contrast, they may exert little effect in patients with a GFR of less than 30 ml/min. The use of these diuretics, which act proximally to the distal site of potassium secretion, is associated not only with a natriuresis but also with an increase in urinary potassium excretion.

Classification of diuretics by site of action in the nephron

- Osmotic diuretics
  - Urea
  - Mannitol
- Proximal tubular diuretics
  - Mannitol
  - Acetazolamide
- Loop of Henle diuretics
  - Ethacrynic acid
  - Furosemide
  - Bumetanide
- Distal tubular diuretics
  - Potassium-losing diuretics
    - Thiazides
    - Chlorthalidone
    - Metolazone
    - Indapamide
  - Potassium-sparing diuretics
    - Triamterene
    - Spironolactone
    - Amiloride

The potassium-sparing diuretics act by blocking distal potassium-linked sodium reabsorption in the extreme distal tubule and collecting duct. Because these sites reabsorb relatively little sodium, these agents are weak diuretics, increasing fractional excretion of sodium to a lesser extent than thiazide-type diuretics. Consequently, their primary usefulness is in the prevention or treatment of hypokalemia caused by other diuretics.

Because the specific attributes and usage of the various diuretics used to mobilize ascites and edema in patients with liver disease are reviewed elsewhere (Chapter 56), it might be helpful at this point to consider the appropriate role of diuretics in the management of one of the prototypical edematous states—chronic liver disease. I suggest the following algorithm for management of cirrhotic ascites (Fig. 351-4). Approximately 10% of cirrhotic patients with ascites can be managed with bed rest and sodium restriction. The next step is the use of spironolactone in doses of up to 200 to 300 mg/day. If this is insufficient, a cautiously used combination of diuretic therapy using spironolactone and loop diuretics (with or without addition of metolazone) may induce a response in many additional patients. Simultaneous administration of colloid may help reduce the chance of hyponatremia and volume contraction. In some patients, especially those with peripheral edema, therapeutic paracentesis may be a reasonable alternative. For the patient who is truly refractory to these maneuvers, the therapeutic choices include extracorporeal techniques and the peritoneovenous shunt. The former include ascites reinfusion, dialytic ultrafiltration of ascites, or continuous arteriovenous hemofiltration (CAVH).

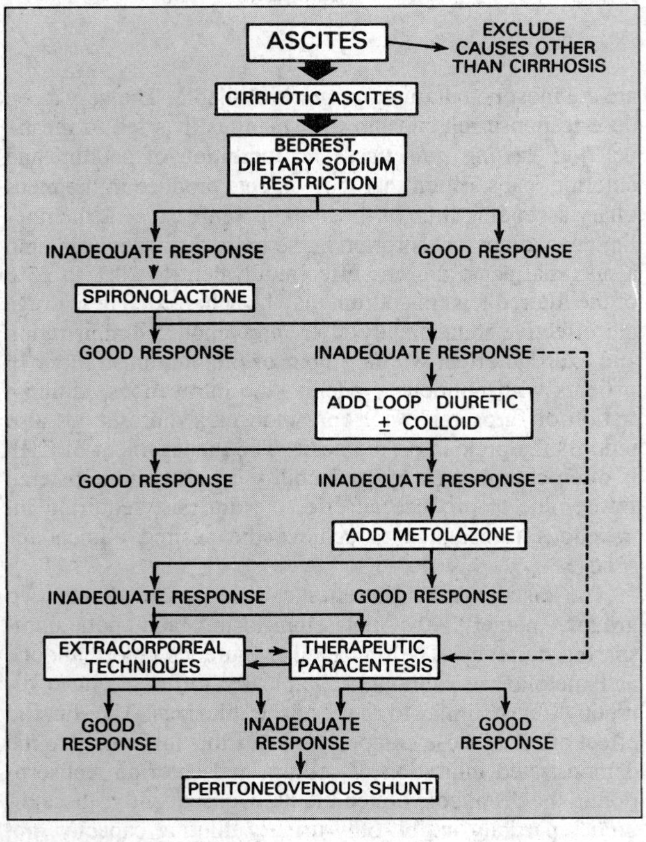

Fig. 351-4. Algorithm for the comprehensive management of cirrhotic ascites and edema. The solid lines represent therapeutic options and sequences that I believe are well established. The interrupted lines indicate uncertainty regarding the appropriate positioning of paracentesis in the therapeutic sequence. (Reproduced with permission from Epstein M: Diuretic therapy in liver disease. In Epstein M, editor: The kidney in liver disease, ed 3, Baltimore, 1988, Williams & Wilkins.)

SALT-WASTING STATES

As noted at the beginning of the chapter, ECF sodium constitutes the major determinant of ECF volume. It follows that an inordinate loss of sodium would result in a decrease in ECF solute, with a resultant contraction of ECF volume. The relentless progression of this process can result in circulatory collapse. The ultimate hemodynamic consequences of sodium depletion are dependent on both the magnitude and the rapidity of the development of sodium loss. Acute, profound sodium depletion that results in a 20% to 40% decrement in ECF volume results in marked decrements in mean arterial pressure and cardiac output. In contrast, a more gradual rate of sodium depletion (i.e., as much as 500 mEq over 10 days) is associated with only slight alterations in arterial pressure and pulse rate despite profound sodium deficits.

Sodium depletion results from the loss or sequestration of a variety of body fluids, ranging from gastrointestinal fluids to sweat, that contain substantial quantities of sodium. To afford a framework with which to approach this subject, it is worthwhile to classify these disorders of sodium depletion according to the source of the deficit (i.e., extrarenal sources and renal sources). Determining the urinary sodium concentration affords an easy means of classifying the source of sodium depletion. Urinary sodium concentrations of less than 10 mEq/L suggest an extrarenal source of sodium depletion (see the accompanying box), whereas urinary sodium concentrations greater than 20 mEq/L (and usually exceeding 40 mEq/L) suggest a renal cause (see the accompanying box).

EXTRARENAL SODIUM DEPLETION

Gastrointestinal origin of sodium loss

Because both the volume and sodium concentration of most gastrointestinal secretions are substantial, disturbances of the gastrointestinal tract have the potential for producing clinically significant sodium loss. In practice, gastrointestinal disturbances are responsible for extrarenal sodium depletion. As enumerated in the box, the mechanisms of gastrointestinal sodium loss are twofold: external loss of sodium and sequestration of sodium within the body.

Diarrhea is the most common gastrointestinal disturbance leading to sodium depletion through external losses. Any of the mechanisms that may result in diarrhea, including osmotic retardation of sodium and water reabsorption, abnormalities of sodium and water transport (as with *Vibrio*

Extrarenal causes of sodium depletion

I. Gastrointestinal sodium loss
  A. External loss of sodium
    1. Diarrhea
    2. Vomiting
    3. Small bowel suction
    4. Pancreatic, biliary, or intestinal fistula
  B. Sequestration of sodium
    1. Small bowel obstruction
    2. Pancreatitis
    3. Peritonitis
II. Skin sodium loss
  A. External loss of sodium
    1. Heat exposure
    2. Adrenal insufficiency
  B. Sequestration of sodium
    1. Burns
    2. Inflammatory disease
III. Miscellaneous sodium loss (external)
  A. Severe hemorrhage
  B. Central nervous system lesions (rare)
  C. Removal of large volumes of serous cavity fluid

Modified from Anderson RJ and Linas SL: Sodium depletion states. In Brenner BM and Stein JH, editors: Sodium and water homeostasis, New York, 1978, Churchill Livingstone.

cholera infection), and increased intestinal transport, can produce sodium depletion. Such losses can be marked, as exemplified by patients infected with *V. cholerae* who may manifest losses of up to 800 ml/hr of diarrhea fluid containing substantial concentrations of sodium. Sodium depletion can also occur from protracted vomiting and loss of gastrointestinal fluids through drainage of fistulas or ileostomies.

Another mechanism for gastrointestinal sodium loss is the sequestration of sodium-rich fluid within the gastrointestinal tract. Thus inflammatory diseases of the pancreas or peritoneum and mechanical small bowel obstruction can lead to sequestration of large volumes of sodium-containing fluid and resultant ECF volume depletion. Intra-abdominal sequestration of ECF volume may be difficult to detect clinically.

Loss of sodium through skin

It is not commonly appreciated that the skin may constitute an important source of sodium depletion. Physical labor at high ambient temperatures may be associated with as much as 5 L of sweat containing 60 to 70 mEq of sodium/L. Continuing loss of such a large quantity of sodium would be expected to result in volume depletion. In normal, acclimatized subjects, the volume and sodium concentration of sweat is reduced, diminishing the risk of volume depletion. In contrast, in unacclimatized subjects and patients with adrenal insufficiency, the volume and sodium concentration of sweat may fail to decrease, with resultant sodium depletion.

SODIUM DEPLETION OF RENAL ORIGIN

Because the kidney is the major organ that mediates sodium homeostasis, it is not altogether surprising that a failure of the kidney to conserve sodium will result in sodium depletion. Impaired renal sodium conservation is attributable to either intrinsic renal diseases or conditions extrinsic to the kidney (see the accompanying box).

Intrinsic renal diseases

Patients with chronic renal failure of diverse causes fail to conserve sodium as efficiently as normal volunteers in response to dietary sodium restriction. Although in many patients with chronic renal failure, urinary sodium excretion may eventually be lowered to equal intake, the interval required to attain sodium balance is markedly prolonged.

Aside from the mild sodium-wasting tendency of chronic renal failure, a relatively small number of patients with renal failure may manifest massive renal salt wasting characterized by urinary sodium excretion of 100 to 300 mEq/day despite negligible sodium intake. In general, the cause of the renal failure in these patients is either medullary cystic disease or interstitial renal diseases.

Several mechanisms have been postulated to explain the sodium wasting of intrinsic renal disease: anatomic damage to nephron segments involved in sodium reabsorption; an increased filtered load of solute per nephron, which could contribute to sodium wasting; hyperperfusion of re-

Renal causes of sodium depletion

I. Intrinsic renal processes
  A. Chronic renal failure
  B. Acute renal failure
    1. Nonoliguric acute renal failure
    2. Recovery from oliguric acute renal failure
  C. Salt-wasting nephropathy
    1. Relief of obstructive uropathy
    2. Nephrocalcinosis with interstitial nephritis
    3. Medullary cystic disease
    4. Polycystic kidney disease
    5. Proximal renal tubular acidosis
II. Extrinsic renal processes
  A. Solute diuresis/nonreabsorbable anion diuresis
    1. Endogenous (bicarbonate, urea, glucose)
    2. Exogenous (mannitol, dextran, urea, glycerol, radiocontrast media)
  B. Diuretic administration
  C. Mineralocorticoid deficiency
    1. Failure of steroidogenesis
    2. Failure of renin secretion
  D. Fasting
  E. Hypertensive hyponatremic syndrome
  F. Acute-phase vomiting

Modified from Anderson RJ and Linas SL: Sodium depletion states. In Brenner BM and Stein JH, editors: Sodium and water homeostasis, New York, 1978, Churchill Livingstone.

sidual nephrons, which could result in the delivery of sodium in amounts that exceed the capacity of the distal nephron to reabsorb sodium. Finally, it has recently been proposed that an adaptive process as yet undefined (perhaps mediated through a natriuretic hormone) contributes to the progressive natriuresis per nephron.

Although the exact mechanism(s) responsible for the sodium-wasting tendency of renal failure remain undetermined, this salt-wasting tendency can have serious consequences for the patient. The withdrawal of sodium from the diet or the induction of extrarenal sodium losses can result in marked volume contraction, with a dramatic deterioration in renal function. Implicit in this formulation is the clinical aphorism that an unexplained decline in renal function in patients with previously stable renal failure and in whom clinical evidence of volume overload is absent should prompt a trial of volume repletion.

Renal sodium loss due to conditions extrinsic to the kidney

Osmotic diuresis. An endogenous solute diuresis, such as that resulting from the glycosuria seen in patients with diabetic ketoacidosis or hyperosmolar, nonketotic coma, may result in significant renal sodium loss. Similarly, exogenous solutes, such as mannitol, dextran, glycerol, or radiopaque dye, may induce a solute diuresis, with the resultant loss of large volumes of urine containing as much as 70 mEq of sodium/L.

Mineralocorticoid deficiency. The failure of the kidney to conserve sodium is a prominent and well-recognized feature of primary adrenal insufficiency. A variety of adrenal insufficiency syndromes can produce sodium depletion, including primary adrenal insufficiency, adrenogenital syndromes, and isolated deficiencies in aldosterone biosynthesis. Although these syndromes differ in their biochemical defects, they share in common mineralocorticoid deficiency and thus are capable of inducing salt wasting.

Among the several variants of the syndrome of isolated hypoaldosteronism are specific adrenal enzymatic defects that result in impaired aldosterone biosynthesis in the setting of an intact renin-angiotensin axis and diminished aldosterone production secondary to diminished renin secretion (syndrome of hyporeninemic hypoaldosteronism). Patients with hyporeninemic hypoaldosteronism present with mild to moderate degrees of renal insufficiency and with acidemia and hyperkalemia disproportionate to their modest decrement in renal function.

It should be noted, however, that a large proportion of patients with isolated hypoaldosteronism are not actually volume depleted or salt wasting. On the contrary, many have hypertension and mild volume overload, and the latter may in fact be one of the causes of the suppressed plasma renin and aldosterone levels.

Treatment. The mainstay of treatment of sodium depletion includes prompt restoration of ECF volume and correction of the cause of the sodium loss.

The history and physical findings often provide significant clues in the assessment of patients with suspected volume depletion and prerenal azotemia. Table 351-1 summarizes the clinical signs of hypovolemia. As can be seen, ECF volume depletion will manifest itself by the following signs of increased sympathetic nerve activity: resting tachycardia worsened by sitting or standing, sustained cremasteric muscle contraction (testes held close to the perineum), and peripheral vasoconstriction with cool extremities. Sitting or standing blood pressure falls when intravascular volume is decreased by approximately 10%. Skin, axillae, and mucous membranes tend to be dry and skin turgor is diminished. Assessment of skin turgor is rather subjective and is influenced by loss of skin elasticity from aging and malnutrition. Nonetheless, with experience and by directing attention to the skin over the forehead and sternum (areas less influenced by age), one gains important insights into fluid status.

Because there is no reliable clinical method to determine the magnitude of sodium repletion necessary to achieve normovolemia, one may obtain a rough approximation of the underlying sodium deficit by computing the decrease in the patient's body weight (one may assume that each kilogram of body weight loss is equivalent to 1 L of 0.9% saline). If sodium depletion occurred in the absence of hemorrhage or hemolysis, one may calculate the sodium loss by utilizing the change in hematocrit.

Although alterations in the hematocrit and hemoglobin concentration may be helpful in approximating the degree of salt and water depletion, it should be emphasized that such computations constitute only a rough guide to management. A number of considerations should be borne in mind in the interpretation of such changes. First, it should be emphasized that red blood cell volume changes in accordance with changes in effective osmolality; hypo-osmolality increases and hyperosmolality decreases red cell

Table 351-1. Correlation of clinical signs with the magnitude of extracellular fluid volume contraction

Sign	Degree of dehydration		
	<5%	6%-10%	>10%
Skin			
Turgor	↓	↓ ↓	↓ ↓ ↓
Color	Pale	Dusky	Mottled
Mucosae	Dry	Very dry	Parchmentlike
Sympathetic overactivity			
Cremasteric contraction	+	++	++
Temperature of extremities	Cool	Cooler	Cold
Hemodynamics			
Pulse*	↑	↑ ↑	↑ ↑ ↑
Blood pressure*	± ↓	↓ ↓	↓ ↓ ↓

*Pulse and blood pressure changes augmented by posture.
Modified from Rudnick MR and Narins RG: The differential diagnosis of acute renal failure. In Brenner BM and Lazarus JM, editors: Acute renal failure, Philadelphia, 1983, WB Saunders.

size. Thus only in isotonic volume depletion, in which red cell volume remains normal, will the hematocrit properly reflect reduction in plasma volume. In hypertonic dehydration, a decrease in plasma volume is accompanied by a decrease in red cell volume, and therefore the hematocrit may remain close to normal. Conversely, in hypotonic dehydration, decrements in plasma volume are accompanied by increases in red cell volume, and the hematocrit tends to increase to a greater extent than one would anticipate from the degree of volume depletion. Because hemoglobin concentration does not change with alterations in osmolality, this variable should more accurately reflect alterations in intravascular volume. Finally, it is self-evident that hematocrit and hemoglobin levels are invalid indices of fluid loss when hemorrhage has occurred. From a practical standpoint, ECF volume repletion should be accomplished with careful and continuous clinical monitoring (preferably with central venous pressure determinations). A rapid or overly vigorous attempt at repletion may overcorrect, with resultant hypervolemia and cardiac failure. Finally, when hyponatremia coexists with volume depletion, consideration must be given to the rapidity with which serum sodium increases during therapy.

Although numerous reviews have suggested the use of a "fluid or diuretic challenge," their utility in the differentiation of prerenal and intrarenal azotemia is questionable. Not only does the use of diuretics provide minimal diagnostic insight, but their natriuretic effects worsen the condition of previously dehydrated patients.

REFERENCES

Anderson RJ and Linas SL: Sodium depletion states. In Brenner BM and Stein JH, editors: Sodium and water homeostasis, New York, 1978, Churchill Livingstone.

Atlas SA and Epstein M: Atrial natriuretic factor: implications in cirrhosis and other edematous disorders. In Epstein M, editor: The kidney in liver disease, ed 3, Baltimore, 1988, Williams & Wilkins.

Buckalew VA Jr: Natriuretic hormone. In Epstein M, editor: The kidney in liver disease, ed 3, Baltimore, 1988, Williams & Wilkins.

Cohn JN: Future directions in vasodilator therapy for heart failure, Am Heart J 121:969-973, 1991.

Cohn JN: Physiologic basis of vasodilator therapy for heart failure, Am J Med 71:135, 1981.

DeWardener HE: Idiopathic edema: role of diuretic abuse, Kidney Int 19:881, 1981.

Dorhout Mees EJ et al: Observations on edema formation in the nephrotic syndrome in adults with minimal lesions, Am J Med 67:378, 1979.

Dzau VJ: Renal and circulatory mechanisms in congestive heart failure, Kidney Int 31:1402-1415, 1987.

Epstein M: Atrial natriuretic factor in patients with liver disease, Am J Nephrol 9:89-100, 1989.

Epstein M: Diuretic therapy in liver disease. In Epstein M, editor: The kidney in liver disease, ed 3, Baltimore, 1988, Williams & Wilkins.

Epstein M: Renal sodium handling in cirrhosis. In Epstein M, editor: The kidney in liver disease, ed 3, Baltimore, 1988, Williams & Wilkins.

Epstein M: Role of the peritoneovenous shunt in the management of ascites and the hepatorenal syndrome. In Epstein M, editor: The kidney in liver disease, ed 3, Baltimore, 1988, Williams & Wilkins.

Esler M et al: Increased sympathetic activity and the effects of its inhibition with clonidine in alcoholic cirrhosis, Ann Intern Med 116:446-455, 1992.

Ginés P et al: Paracentesis with intravenous infusion of albumin as compared with peritoneovenous shunting in cirrhosis with refractory ascites, N Engl J Med 325:829-835, 1991.

Glassock RJ: Pathophysiology of acute glomerulonephritis, Hosp Pract 23:163-178, 1988.

La Villa G et al: Natriuretic hormone activity in the urine of cirrhotic patients, Hepatology 12:467-475, 1990.

Lieberman FL, Denison EK, and Reynolds TB: The relationship of plasma volume, portal hypertension, ascites and renal sodium retention in cirrhosis: the overflow theory of ascites formation, Ann NY Acad Sci 170:202, 1970.

Oster JR and Materson BJ: Renal and electrolyte complications of congestive heart failure and effects of therapy with angiotensin-converting enzyme inhibitors, Arch Intern Med 152:704-710, 1992.

Rodriguez-Iturbe B et al: Atrial natriuretic factor in the acute nephritic and nephrotic syndromes, Kidney Int 38:512-517, 1990.

Schrier RW: Pathogenesis of sodium and water retention in high-output and low-output cardiac failure, nephrotic syndrome, cirrhosis and pregnancy: part 1, N Engl J Med 319:1065, 1988.

Schrier RW: Pathogenesis of sodium and water retention in high-output and low-output cardiac failure, nephrotic syndrome, cirrhosis and pregnancy: part 2, N Engl J Med 319:1127, 1988.

Seifter J et al: Control of extracellular fluid volume and pathophysiology of edema formation. In Brenner BM and Rector FC Jr, editors: The kidney, ed 3, Philadelphia, 1986, WB Saunders.

Shear L, Ching S, and Gabuzda GJ: Compartmentalization of ascites and edema in patients with hepatic cirrhosis, N Engl J Med 282:1391, 1970.

Tulassay T et al: Atrial natriuretic peptide and other vasoactive hormones in nephrotic syndrome, Kidney Int 31:1391-1395, 1987.

CHAPTER

352 Disorders of Potassium Balance

Richard H. Sterns
Robert G. Narins

Potassium, the most prevalent intracellular cation, resides primarily in skeletal muscle (60%) and bone (18%). Although tissues vary, the mean intracellular potassium concentration approximates 150 mEq/L. The distribution of potassium between cellular and extracellular fluid is largely determined by cell membrane-associated (Na^+ + K^+)-ATPase (sodium potassium activated adenosine triphosphatase), which actively imports potassium in exchange for exported sodium. The extracellular fluid concentration of 4 to 5 mEq/L indicates that only 1% to 2% (70 mEq) of total body potassium resides outside cells. The cell's resting electrical potential difference is a function of the ratio of the concentrations of intracellular (Ki) to extracellular (Ke) potassium. Disturbances of potassium homeostasis alter this ratio because Ke changes proportionately more than Ki. Therefore hypokalemia tends to increase the ratio, thereby hyperpolarizing cell membranes, whereas hyperkalemia has the opposite effect (Fig. 352-1). These changes in membrane potential underlie many of the clinically important cardiac and neuromuscular manifestations of disordered potassium metabolism.

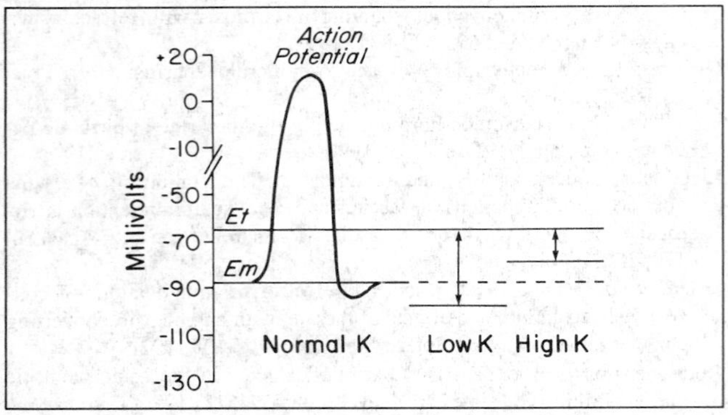

Fig. 352-1. The influence of hypokalemia and hyperkalemia on membrane excitability. Em, resting transmembrane electrical potential difference; Et, threshold potential. (Modified from Leaf A and Cotran R: Pathophysiology of potassium excess and deficiency. In Renal pathophysiology, ed 2, New York, 1980, Oxford University Press.)

EXTERNAL POTASSIUM BALANCE

Each day approximately 10% of the 50 to 100 mEq of dietary potassium normally escapes intestinal absorption, whereas the remaining 45 to 90 mEq enters the extracellular fluid. In the steady state, in the absence of net anabolism or net catabolism, the absorbed potassium is excreted in the urine (Fig. 352-2).

The kidneys regulate external potassium balance by matching the cation's excretion to the host's metabolic needs. Thus closely regulated renal excretion limits the risk of potassium surplus or deficit from largely unregulated dietary intake and absorption. Even small increases of the plasma potassium concentration markedly stimulate urinary potassium excretion. This response is amplified by aldosterone, a kaliuretic hormone secreted in response to hyperkalemia. Thus when renal function and aldosterone secretion are normal, accumulation of excess potassium is unlikely, even when intake of the cation is very large. Aldosterone secretion and renal potassium excretion are diminished by hypokalemia. However, potassium conservation in hypokalemia is less efficient than the excretion of excess potassium in hyperkalemia. Because potassium cannot be totally eliminated from the urine, severe dietary restriction of the cation can cause deficits.

Abnormalities in the renal regulation of external potassium balance may cause potassium surfeits or deficits. Impairment of this regulatory function may be caused by diseases of the kidneys themselves, by abnormalities in aldosterone secretion, by acid-base disturbances, and by pharmacologic agents.

INTERNAL POTASSIUM BALANCE

The distribution of potassium between extracellular and intracellular fluid compartments (internal balance) is a major determinant of the plasma potassium concentration. Extracellular leakage of only 70 mEq of the 4000 mEq of potassium contained in cells would result in lethal hyperkalemia (9 mEq/L), whereas intracellular translocation of only 45 mEq of the extracellular cation would cause severe hypokalemia (1.5 mEq/L). The membrane transport protein ($Na^+ + K^+$)-ATPase, is ultimately responsible for potassium's normal assymetric transcellular distribution. Both the number of transport molecules and their rate of transport are subject to regulation. Potassium itself plays a role in this regulation. For example, potassium depletion reduces the number of transporters, enabling cellular stores to replenish extracellular losses.

Insulin and *catecholamines* are the most important hormonal regulators of internal potassium balance. Both enhance cellular potassium uptake by stimulating the ($Na^+ + K^+$)-ATPase activity of skeletal muscle. Insulin's hypokalemic effect is dose-related, reaching a plateau at hormone levels many times greater than those required for maximum glucose utilization. Insulin deficiency impedes cellular uptake of excess potassium. The hypokalemic effect of catecholamines is mediated by cyclic-AMP and is promoted by beta$_2$-adrenergic agonists. Beta$_2$-adrenergic blockade can lead to hyperkalemia.

Acid-base disturbances are the most familiar modifiers of internal potassium balance. Acidemia provokes hyperkalemia by exchanging extracellular hydrogen ion for cellular potassium during tissue buffering. The reverse occurs in alkalemia or during correction of acidemia. In general, metabolic acid-base disturbances exert greater effects on potassium distribution than do respiratory disorders. However, the hyperkalemic effect of metabolic acidosis depends on the anion accompanying the accumulated hydrogen ion. If the anion is chloride (which does not readily enter cells), a transmembrane electrochemical gradient favoring potassium egress is created when protons are buffered intracellularly. By contrast, organic anions such as lactate and ketones are able to penetrate cells in the buffering process so that potassium exchange is not promoted. Thus organic acidoses by themselves have only a minimal effect on internal potassium balance.

Hypertonicity provokes potassium diffusion out of cells, presumably by increasing the intracellular potassium concentration as cells become dehydrated. Hyperglycemia in persons with diabetes with reduced renal potassium excretion is the most important example of this phenomenon. It also occurs when hypertonic mannitol or saline are infused into subjects with renal failure.

HYPOKALEMIA

Hypokalemia may result solely from disordered internal potassium balance, but more commonly it reflects potassium depletion from renal or extrarenal losses.

Spurious hypokalemia

This rare in vitro phenomenon can occur in acute myelogenous leukemia if the blood sample remains at room temperature before separation, allowing metabolically active leukemia cells to absorb potassium.

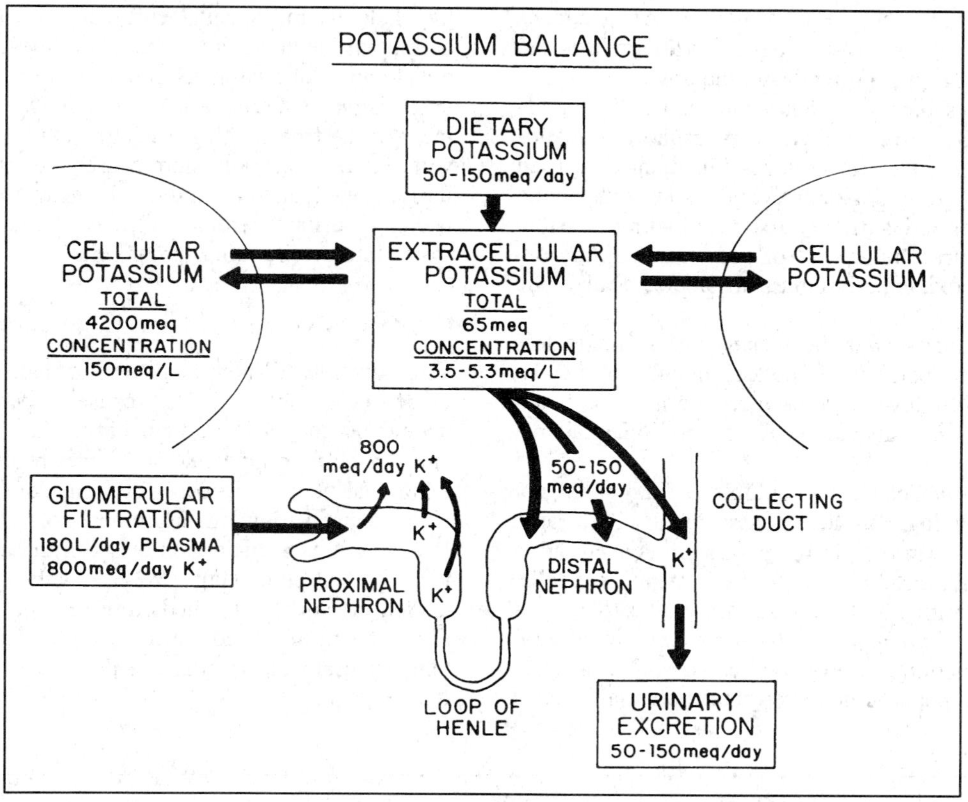

Fig. 352-2. Overview of potassium balance. The figure ignores fecal potassium excretion normally about 10% of dietary intake. See text for further details. (From Narins RG: Am J Cardiol 65:4E, 1990.)

True hypokalemia without potassium depletion

Transient hypokalemia may be caused by a shift of potassium into cells. This phenomenon should be suspected when hypokalemia resolves after little or no potassium replacement (Table 352-1).

Exogenous insulin can cause hypokalemia without potassium depletion (e.g., when excessive insulin is given with total parenteral nutrition). More commonly, however, insulin therapy unmasks or exacerbates hypokalemia in potassium-depleted patients with uncontrolled diabetes mellitus. Insulin-induced hypoglycemia reduces the plasma potassium concentration by virtue of the combined effects of insulin and the high levels of catecholamines released in response to the low blood sugar.

Endogenous catecholamines secreted in states of extreme stress (e.g., myocardial infarction, cerebral hemorrhage, and possibly delirium tremens) may cause transient hypokalemia. Exogenous catecholamines, particularly beta$_2$-adrenergic agonists used in the treatment of asthma (terbutaline, albuterol, and salbutamol) or premature labor (ritodrine) may cause marked, transient hypokalemia by shifting potassium into cells.

Hypokalemic periodic paralysis is a rare disorder characterized by intermittent episodes of muscle weakness associated with transient acute shifts of potassium into cells. Most cases are familial, but sporadic acquired cases may complicate thyrotoxicosis, especially in Asians. Thyroid hormone increases the number of (Na^+ + K^+)-ATPase pumps in the muscle cell membrane. Attacks may be precipitated by a carbohydrate-rich diet, glucose, insulin, and epinephrine, suggesting that the disease may result from enhanced sensitivity to the hormones that normally increase

Table 352-1. Factors that alter internal potassium balance

Increased cell K^+ uptake	Increased cell K^+ efflux
Insulin	Insulin deficiency
Endogenous catecholamines	Beta$_2$-adrenergic blockers
Beta$_2$-adrenergic agonists	Hypertonicity
Hypokalemic periodic paralysis	Hyperkalemic periodic paralysis
Alkalosis (metabolic $>$ respiratory)	Metabolic acidosis (mineral, not organic) and respiratory acidosis
Hypothermia	Vigorous exercise
Barium poisoning	Digitalis intoxication
Cell growth	Succinylcholine
	Arginine hydrochloride
	Cell lysis or catabolism

the rate of transport by $(Na^+ + K^+)$-ATPase. Acute attacks are treated with potassium, whereas acetazolamide is the most effective long-term prophylactic therapy.

Alkalosis favors potassium entry into cells, but the effect is small. Only extreme degrees of respiratory alkalosis, caused by improper respirator settings, have caused substantial degrees of hypokalemia. The effect of metabolic alkalosis is greater and is usually associated with potassium depletion. The intracellular shift of potassium slightly exacerbates the hypokalemia in potassium-depleted, alkalotic patients.

Hypothermia may lower the plasma potassium to less than 3.0 mEq/L by potentiating potassium entry into cells. The effect is rapidly reversed during rewarming, and if potassium has been administered, "overshoot" hyperkalemia may result.

Barium poisoning caused by soluble barium salts (not those used in radiologic studies) is associated with a rapid and severe decrease in the plasma potassium concentration that appears to be caused by a shift of potassium into cells. Complicating vomiting and diarrhea also play a role.

Vitamin B_{12} therapy of megaloblastic anemia rapidly increases net production of new blood cells, which incorporate extracellular potassium. Severe and potentially lethal hypokalemia may result. Thrombocytopenic patients with pernicious anemia seem especially prone to this form of hypokalemia. An analogous condition may occur during the *transfusion of frozen washed red blood cells*. Replenishment of the frozen cell's low intracellular potassium stores with extracellular potassium causes the hypokalemia. Similarly, acute leukemias and rapidly growing lymphomas (especially Burkitt's lymphoma) may also divert extracellular stores into proliferating tumor cells.

Hypokalemia with potassium depletion

Once disordered internal potassium balance has been excluded (see Table 352-1), a cause of potassium depletion should be sought. Although diminished intake can occasionally be incriminated, most cases result from excessive extrarenal potassium losses or from defective renal potassium conservation; measurement of urinary potassium losses permits a distinction between these two major diagnostic possibilities (Fig. 352-3). Daily urinary potassium excretion can be estimated from the potassium and creatinine content of a "spot" urine sample. The potassium content per gram of creatinine approximates the daily excretion level.

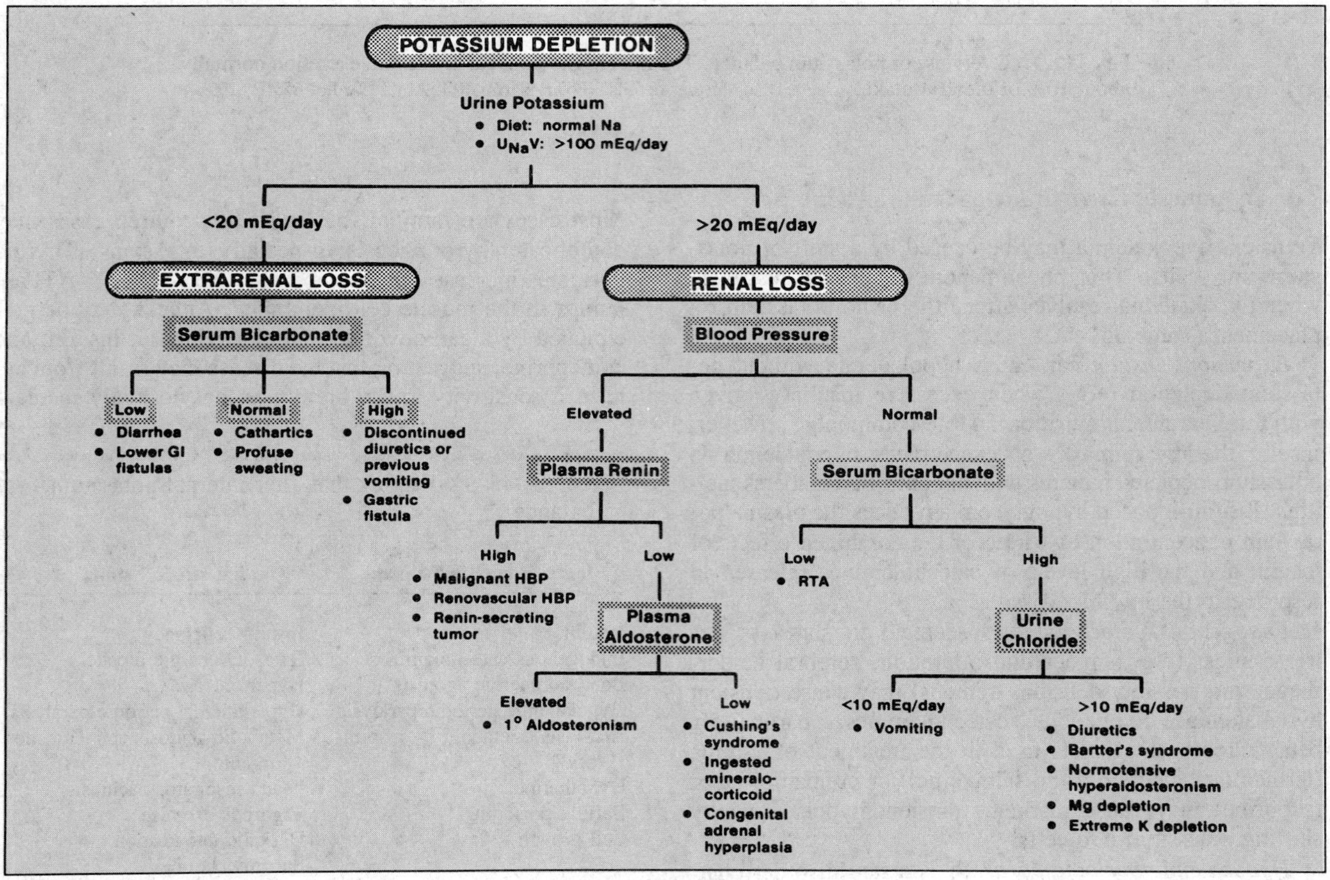

Fig. 352-3. Diagnostic approach to hypokalemia. Because renal potassium wasting may improve during sodium restriction, diminished potassium excretion is indicative of extrarenal loss only when the diet (and therefore the urine) is rich in sodium. See text for further details.

Decreased potassium intake

Renal conservation of potassium is imperfect, allowing deficits to develop when dietary intake is low, particularly if protein and calorie intake continues. Patients treated with total parenteral nutrition may develop profound potassium depletion if supplements are inappropriately withheld. In some areas of the southern United States, clay ingestion *(geophagia)* is inexplicably common. White clay binds dietary potassium, preventing its absorption from the gut; because protein intake is preserved, profound hypokalemia may result. Interestingly, red clay is rich in potassium and may actually be a cause of hyperkalemia in patients with renal failure.

Extrarenal potassium losses

Diarrhea from any cause can result in large potassium losses (see Fig. 352-3). Hypokalemia is particularly profound in patients with diarrhea caused by villous adenomas or non-beta-cell pancreatic islet cell tumors. When diarrhea causes hypokalemia, it is associated with a normal anion gap metabolic acidosis caused by fecal loss of alkali. Chronic laxative abusers may also develop severe potassium depletion. Inexplicably, many such patients are not acidotic and, indeed, sometimes a metabolic alkalosis actually develops. Coexistent self-induced vomiting or diuretic abuse may explain this finding in some patients. Lower intestinal potassium losses are associated with reduced urinary losses (<20 mEq/day). Loss of gastric fluid from vomiting or drainage also leads to potassium depletion despite the trivial amount of potassium lost in gastric fluid. Increased urinary potassium losses are the major cause of potassium depletion (see later discussion).

Renal potassium losses

Renal potassium wasting can be identified by the finding of "inappropriate" amounts in the urine in hypokalemic patients (see Fig. 352-3). When hypokalemia develops because of inadequate intake or lower intestinal or internal potassium losses, urinary potassium excretion usually diminishes to less than 20 mEq/day; a greater value indicates that renal potassium wasting underlies the hypokalemia. Renal potassium wasting occurs most commonly when high levels of mineralocorticoids are accompanied by a normal or increased distal tubular luminal flow rate. Causes of renal potassium wasting are best classified on the basis of the presence or absence of hypertension, associated acid-base disturbances, and the status of the renin-angiotensin-aldosterone axis.

Normotensive renal potassium wasting. Patients in this category can be further subdivided into those with metabolic acidosis and those with metabolic alkalosis.

Metabolic acidosis. Severe hypokalemia is usually present in patients with *distal renal tubular acidosis* and may cause quadriparesis. Alkali therapy diminishes the kaliuresis and renders chronic potassium replacement unnecessary as long as the acidosis is controlled. Hypokalemia is usually milder in patients with *proximal renal tubular acidosis,* and in this disorder renal potassium wasting is exacerbated by alkali therapy. The carbonic anhydrase inhibitor *acetazolamide* used in the treatment of glaucoma causes a similar phenomenon.

Metabolic alkalosis. *Active vomiting,* an important cause of hypokalemia and metabolic alkalosis, enhances renal excretion of potassium, sodium, and bicarbonate. Hypovolemic stimulation of NaCl reabsorption makes hypochloriduria a typical finding. With chronicity, $NaHCO_3$ reabsorption increases but the kaliuresis continues. Psychiatrically disturbed (bulimic) patients often deny self-induced vomiting. The finding of a urinary chloride concentration of less than 10 mEq/L in a persistently alkalotic patient is virtually diagnostic of gastric fluid loss, because it indicates that chloride (HCl) has been lost extrarenally.

Thiazide and loop diuretics (furosemide, bumetanide, and ethacrynic acid) are by far the most common cause of renal potassium wasting and alkalosis. Edematous conditions, although associated with high renin and aldosterone levels, do not by themselves cause potassium wasting. Increased proximal tubular reabsorption caused by the primary disorder reduces distal luminal flow, thereby limiting cation exchange. Diuretic therapy, however, by increasing distal sodium and fluid delivery, enables aldosterone to markedly increase urinary potassium losses. Surreptitious diuretic abuse must be excluded in all patients with normotensive renal potassium wasting of obscure etiology. Because diuretics may be taken intermittently, serial determinations of serum and urinary electrolytes may be helpful. While the diuretic is being taken, urinary chloride concentrations are high, but they decrease dramatically within hours after discontinuing the diuretic. Chromatography of the urine at the appropriate time will reveal the presence of the diuretic.

Bartter's syndrome should be considered in normotensive alkalotic patients with renal potassium wasting in whom surreptitious vomiting and diuretic abuse have been excluded. This rare disease, characterized by hyperreninemia, hyperaldosteronism, hyperplasia of the juxtaglomerular apparatus, increased prostaglandin secretion, and insensitivity to the pressor effect of exogenous angiotensin II, occurs more frequently in children than in adults but has been reported at all ages. Symptoms associated with hypokalemia are common (see later discussion), and affected children often have stunted growth. A defect in sodium chloride reabsorption in the loop of Henle and/or a distal nephron lesion that leads to enhanced potassium secretion are believed to be the underlying causes of the syndrome. Many features of the disease appear to be secondary complications of this primary defect. Overproduction of prostaglandins appears to be a nonspecific consequence of potassium depletion. Elevated levels of vasodilatory prostaglandins stimulate renin and thereby aldosterone release and also contribute to the resistance to the pressor effects of angiotensin II. Treatment with inhibitors of prostaglandin synthesis (e.g., indomethacin) has a slight effect on the biochemical and hemodynamic characteristics of the disease.

Acute myelocytic leukemias may be complicated by potassium wasting that is sometimes associated with increased urinary lysozyme excretion.

Magnesium depletion may be associated with hypokalemia that is resistant to potassium replacement therapy. Magnesium replacement corrects the kaliuresis and allows for repair of the potassium deficit. *Drugs* causing potassium (and usually magnesium) wasting include cisplatin, gentaminclude cisplatin, gentamicin, and levodopa. Carbenicillin, in large doses, may cause potassium wasting and alkalosis because it is excreted as a nonreabsorbable anion.

Hypertensive renal potassium wasting. Patients in this category usually have an associated hypochloremic, metabolic alkalosis with a urinary chloride excretion that matches dietary intake. These patients can be conveniently subclassified on the basis of plasma renin activity.

Low renin. *Primary hyperaldosteronism* should be suspected in hypertensives whose plasma renin levels remain low despite stimulation (a low salt diet or diuretics) and whose plasma aldosterone levels remain elevated despite suppressive maneuvers (acute saline loading or 5 to 7 days of a 200- to 300-mEq NaCl diet). A high sodium intake worsens hypokalemia by increasing the distal tubular luminal flow rate while hyperaldosteronemia persists. A single aldosterone-secreting adenoma (Conn's syndrome) is the most common cause of these findings, particularly in patients with clinically important hypokalemia. Patients with bilateral adrenal hyperplasia may also present with hypertension, but hypokalemia is usually milder. Elaboration of the recently described aldosterone-stimulating factor may be the underlying cause of the hyperplasia. Urinary excretion of this factor may differentiate the surgically incurable hyperplasia from the curable adenoma. Because of the wide range of "normal" for blood pressure, occasional hypokalemic patients with Conn's syndrome may be normotensive, mimicking Bartter's syndrome and other causes of normotensive renal potassium wasting.

Adrenogenital syndrome due to 11β-hydroxylase (masculinizing) or 17α-hydroxylase deficiency causes renal potassium wasting resulting from overproduction of deoxycorticosterone.

Liddle's syndrome is a rare familial disorder resembling Conn's syndrome except that plasma aldosterone levels are low. An as yet unidentified nonaldosterone mineralocorticoid may cause this syndrome.

Sodium glycyrrhizinate found in chewing tobacco, European licorice, and certain liquors, may cause low renin hypertension and hypokalemic renal potassium wasting. Although not a mineralocorticoid per se, sodium glycyrrhizinate inhibits 11 β-OH steroid dehydrogenase, which prolongs cortisol's half-life enabling this steroid to sustain its mineralocorticoid action.

High or normal renin. *Renovascular hypertension* is often complicated by mild degrees of hypokalemia, but this finding is not specific for the disorder because *malignant hypertension* and the *vasculitides* are also associated with high renin levels and may also cause hypokalemia. Rarely, *renin secreting tumors,* including Wilms' tumor and small renal juxtaglomerular cell tumors, produce hypertension and hypokalemia. The hypertension of *Cushing's syndrome* is associated with a normal or high plasma renin level. Most cases with severe hypokalemia occur in adrenal carcinoma or ectopic ACTH secretion, most commonly caused by small cell carcinoma of the lung.

Potassium depletion without hypokalemia

The osmotic diuresis and kaliuresis associated with *diabetic ketoacidosis* or *nonketotic hyperglycemia* result in large potassium deficits. In ketoacidosis the potassium losses are particularly large because acetoacetate and beta-hydroxybutyrate serve as nonreabsorbable anions, further enhancing renal potassium loss. Hypokalemia may be masked in these disorders because of abnormalities in internal potassium balance caused by insulin deficiency, hypertonicity, and catabolism. Ketoacidosis probably plays little role in masking the hypokalemia because organic acidoses do not appear to cause potassium exit from cells. Some patients may present with hyperkalemia despite potassium depletion. Because of changing internal balance, severe hypokalemia may emerge during insulin and fluid therapy.

CONSEQUENCES OF HYPOKALEMIA

The consequences of hypokalemia derive from potassium's role in regulating cellular metabolism and influencing the transmembrane electrical potential. In potassium depletion, the reduction in cellular potassium concentration is proportionally less than the reduction in extracellular potassium concentration, so that the ratio of intracellular to extracellular potassium concentration increases. Hypokalemia hyperpolarizes cell membranes, reducing membrane excitability, thereby provoking clinically important changes in the cardiac conducting system, skeletal and smooth muscle, and endocrine function.

Cardiac effects

In hypokalemia, potassium losses are less marked in cardiac than in skeletal muscle, causing striking hyperpolarization of cardiac conduction tissue. Characteristic electrocardiographic changes result (Fig. 352-4) and include S-T-segment depression, decreased amplitude or inversion of the T wave, and increased height of the U wave ($>$ 1 mm). These changes usually reflect a plasma potassium concentration of less than 3.0 mEq/L and are seen in the vast majority of cases with values below 2.7 mEq/L. With more severe hypokalemia, increased amplitude of the P wave, prolongation of the P-R interval, and widening of the QRS complex ensue. Severe hypokalemia may induce atrioventricular block and supraventricular and ventricular tachyarrhythmias, including ventricular fibrillation. The incidence of digitalis-induced dysrhythmias is increased in hypokalemia. Indeed, hypokalemia reduces renal excretion of digoxin and increases its binding to the heart, further predisposing patients to digitalis toxicity. In the absence of digitalis, there is disagreement as to whether mild hypokalemia (plasma potassium 3.0 to 3.5 mEq/L) causes dysrhyth-

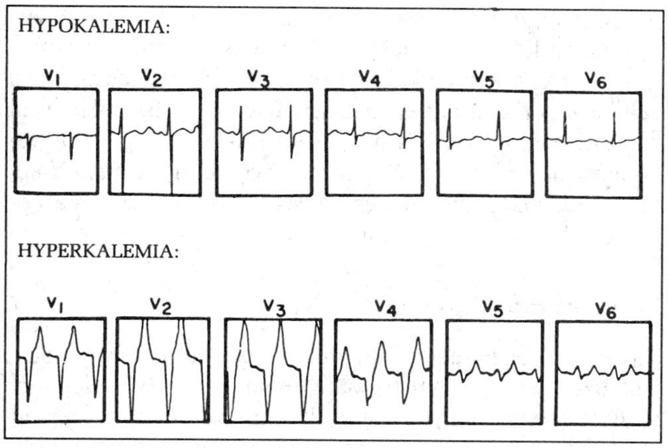

Fig. 352-4. Electrocardiographic changes induced by hypo- and hyperkalemia. Hypokalemic changes include flattened T waves and the presence of U waves. Hyperkalemic changes include peaked T waves, decreased R wave amplitude, and widened QRS complexes. (By permission from Gabow PA and Peterson LN. Disorders of potassium metabolism. In Schrier RW, editor: Renal electrolyte disorders, Boston, 1980, Little, Brown.)

mias. When patients with myocardial infarction present with hypokalemia, they are more prone to ventricular dysrhythmias. However, more severe infarctions may yield high levels of catecholamines, which may be the cause of both hypokalemia and dysrhythmias. Based on the available data, it appears prudent to treat hypokalemia in patients with underlying ischemic heart disease.

Muscle dysfunction

Patients with mild hypokalemia commonly complain of muscle cramps and may suffer mild muscle weakness. Impaired smooth muscle function may cause intestinal ileus. Severe hypokalemia (less than 2.5 mEq/L) may cause marked weakness or frank paralysis of skeletal muscles. The proximal muscles of the lower extremities are typically affected first, whereas in more severe cases the trunk and respiratory muscles can become involved, leading to respiratory failure. Severe potassium depletion may also lead to disruption of skeletal muscle cells, particularly during exercise. The normal hyperemic response to exercise depends on the local release of potassium from muscle. In potassium-depleted muscle, the lack of potassium-induced vasodilatation impairs muscle blood flow, leading to cramps, ischemic necrosis, and rhabdomyolysis.

Renal dysfunction

Renal blood flow and glomerular filtration rate are moderately and reversibly reduced in hypokalemia. The ability to excrete a sodium load is impaired, and edema may occur in potassium-depleted subjects on a high salt diet. Potassium depletion impairs the ability to maximally concentrate the urine and also directly stimulates thirst. Hence, polyuria and polydipsia are common symptoms of hypokalemia. Chronic, severe hypokalemia causes vacuolar lesions in the epithelial cells of the proximal and distal tubule and may increase the sensitivity to acute tubular necrosis during exposure to nephrotoxic antibiotics. Rhabdomyolysis caused by severe hypokalemia may produce myoglobinuric acute renal failure.

Endocrine dysfunction

Hypokalemia impairs the secretion of aldosterone, insulin, and possibly catecholamines. The impairment of insulin secretion may cause hyperglycemia even in patients without clinically apparent diabetes mellitus. Glucose intolerance is rapidly corrected by potassium replacement. Prostaglandin and renin synthesis are both increased in response to hypokalemia.

Metabolic alkalosis

Many of the disorders that cause hypokalemia also increase acid losses from the body (e.g., vomiting, hyperaldosteronism, diuretics). In addition, hypokalemia itself affects acid-base balance. Hydrogen ions shift into potassium-depleted cells, causing intracellular acidosis and a slight degree of extracellular alkalosis. The same intracellular acidification occurs in renal tubular cells, enhancing renal ammonia production and bicarbonate reabsorption by the proximal nephron; these effects favor the generation and maintenance of metabolic alkalosis. Because of enhanced renal ammonia production, potassium depletion may contribute to hepatic encephalopathy in cirrhotic patients.

Hyponatremia

Combined sodium and potassium depletion caused by diarrhea, vomiting, or diuretics may cause hyponatremia. Potassium lost from cells is partially replaced by sodium. By reversing this process, potassium repletion partially corrects hyponatremia in hypokalemic subjects.

TREATMENT OF HYPOKALEMIA

Preventive therapy

Although controversial, avoidance of diuretic-induced hypokalemia is by far the most common indication for potassium therapy in the United States. Routine administration of potassium or potassium-sparing diuretics should be discouraged in patients with renal disease, diabetes mellitus, or autonomic insufficiency, since the disordered external and internal potassium balances in these patients may predispose to life-threatening degrees of hyperkalemia. Only a small percentage of diuretic-treated patients develop severe hypokalemia (less than 3.0 mEq/L), and if the goal of potassium replacement were simply to avoid severe depletion, few patients would require therapy. A much larger percentage of diuretic-treated patients develop mild hypokalemia (3 to 3.5 mEq/L), the risk of which to nondigitalized patients is not clear. The incidence of hypokalemia can be reduced in hypertensive patients by using low doses of thiazide diuretics (the equivalent of 12.5 to 25 mg hydrochlorothiazide daily); higher doses cause greater kaliuresis with little additional antihypertensive effect. Hypokalemia can also be minimized by dietary sodium restriction (70 to 80 mEq/day), since high rates of sodium excretion promote urinary potassium losses. Encouraging intake of potassium-rich fruit is of dubious benefit. The calorie content is excessive, and since the potassium in fruit is associated not with chloride but with poorly reabsorbable anions, the cation is poorly retained. Effective therapy requires either high doses of KCl or a potassium-sparing diuretic (amiloride, triamterene, or spironolactone).

Correction of potassium depletion

When other variables affecting plasma potassium concentration have been avoided, metabolic balance studies show, deficits of 300 mEq/70 kg body weight (corrected for nitrogen) are required to lower the plasma potassium concentration by 1 mEq/L (Fig. 352-5). These estimates are valid only for chronic potassium depletion. When potassium is lost rapidly from the extracellular fluid (for example, by hemodialysis), loss of a mere 15 mEq can transiently lower the plasma concentration by 1 mEq/L. With time, cellular potassium partially replenishes extracellular fluid losses. The relationship between the potassium deficit and the plasma potassium concentration can be altered by factors that affect internal potassium balance. While it is difficult to quantify these effects, the presence of associated acid-base disorders, hormonal disturbances, etc., must be taken into account in planning therapy. Because the estimate of potassium deficits is crude, it is wise to remeasure the plasma potassium concentration frequently during the course of therapy. The administered dose should replace the patient's ongoing losses as well as correct the existing deficit. Once the deficit has been replaced, additional potassium may cause hyperkalemia, since the renal excretion and cellular uptake of excess potassium may not be efficient in chronically potassium-depleted subjects. Consequently, potassium therapy should be slowed once normokalemia is approached, and then frequent measurements of plasma potassium levels are essential.

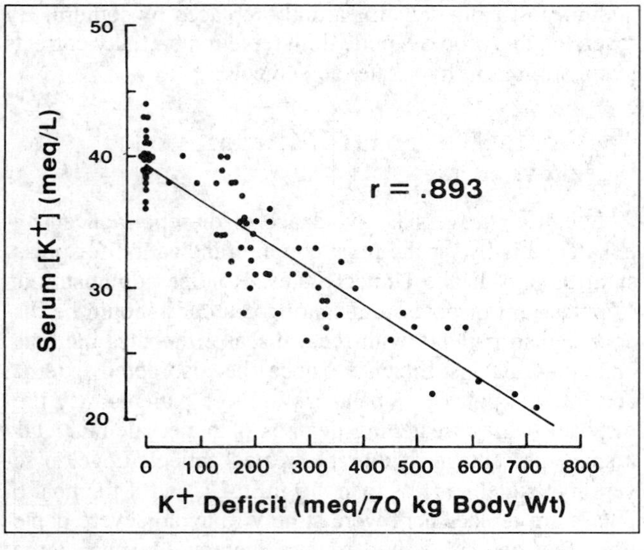

Fig. 352-5. The effect of uncomplicated potassium depletion on serum potassium concentration, as defined by published potassium balance studies. The decrease in serum potassium concentration equals 0.27 mEq/L for every 100 mEq of potassium deficit (r = .893). (By permission from Sterns RH et al: Internal potassium balance and the control of plasma potassium concentration, Medicine 60:339-354, 1981.)

Route of administration

Either oral or parenteral therapy is potentially dangerous, and treatment via either route requires careful attention. Oral potassium administration is more practical for repairing large deficits because intravenous therapy usually obligates the infusion of large amounts of fluid. Attempts to limit the fluid load by increasing the concentration of potassium in intravenous solutions create two problems: (1) the infusion must be carefully monitored to avoid the inadvertent infusion of large volumes of concentrated potassium and (2) potassium concentrations greater than 60 mEq/L are painful if infused into a peripheral vein unless the rate of administration is slow (5 to 10 mEq/hr). On rare occasions when rapid intravenous infusion of concentrated potassium is required, it can be safely infused into a central vein providing the patient is carefully monitored.

Rapid intravenous infusions of potassium are indicated only for the treatment of severe hypokalemia with such life-threatening complications as ventricular dysrhythmias or quadriparesis. When such rare emergencies occur, potassium can be infused for limited periods of time at a rate that exceeds the rate of ongoing external potassium losses by 20 to 60 mEq/hr. Infused potassium initially distributes in the extracellular fluid (20% of body weight), and with time most of the infused cation enters cells. Emergency therapy requires only that the plasma potassium concentration be raised to a safe level (usually an increase of approximately 1 mEq/L). This can be achieved by the infusion of only 15 mEq over a period of 15 minutes. Thereafter the deficit should be repaired more slowly. It is essential that the electrocardiogram be monitored for evidence of hyperkalemia and that the plasma potassium concentration be monitored at frequent intervals whenever it is administered aggressively.

HYPERKALEMIA

Hyperkalemic patients may be classified by the presence or absence of a potassium surfeit. It is important to note that patients with *chronic* hyperkalemia invariably suffer from a defect in renal potassium excretion. Extracellular translocation of potassium causes hyperkalemia only when it occurs suddenly or when there is an accompanying renal defect.

Spurious hyperkalemia

Local potassium release. Local release of potassium from ischemic exercising muscle can increase the serum potassium concentration by 1 mEq/L or more when the patient's fist is repeatedly clenched with a tourniquet in place during blood drawing. Use of a tourniquet without fist clenching does not cause spurious hyperkalemia.

In vitro hemolysis. Hemolysis extensive enough to visibly discolor the plasma can give the spurious impression of severe hyperkalemia. When whole blood is used for emergency potassium determinations by electrode, hemolysis will not be apparent; therefore the sample must be centrifuged to allow examination of the plasma.

Pseudohyperkalemia. Marked thrombocytosis (usually $> 1 \times 10^6/mm^3$) or leukocytosis (usually $> 250 \times 10^3/mm^3$) may falsely increase the potassium level because of in vitro release of cellular potassium during blood clotting. A simultaneously drawn plasma potassium concentration or whole blood potassium concentration will be normal. In chronic lymphocytic leukemia, loss of potassium from "fragile" leukemic cells may raise both the plasma and serum potassium concentrations if the blood sample is allowed to stand before separation.

True hyperkalemia without a potassium surfeit

Increased potassium loss from cells. Hyperkalemia may occur if potassium egress is rapid enough to overwhelm normal renal excretory function or if there is an associated defect in renal potassium excretion. *Tissue catabolism* after trauma, burns, ischemic muscle necrosis, or rapid lysis (particularly during chemotherapy of Burkitt's lymphoma) may rapidly release large amounts of potassium into the circulation. Hyperkalemia is more likely to be severe if acute renal failure develops.

Exercise causes release of potassium from skeletal muscle, and the plasma potassium concentration may increase transiently by more than 2 mEq/L after exhausting exercise. Nonselective beta-adrenergic blocking agents (e.g., propranolol) cause leakage of potassium out of cells and may contribute to hyperkalemia in patients with compromised potassium homeostasis. This problem can be avoided by the substitution of β_1-antagonists (e.g., metoprolol) in such patients.

Diabetic hyperglycemia may cause hyperkalemia in patients with impaired renal function. In nondiabetic subjects, glucose infusion lowers the plasma potassium concentration by stimulating insulin release. In the patient with diabetes, insulin fails to respond normally to administered glucose and the hypertonicity dehydrates cells, raises intracellular potassium concentration, thereby promoting diffusion of the cation out of the cell. Infusion of hypertonic mannitol to subjects with renal failure may cause a similar phenomenon. In patients with defects in renal potassium excretion (such as hypoaldosteronism), serious hyperkalemia may result.

Uremic metabolic acidosis and *hyperkalemic renal tubular acidosis* also induce potassium loss from cells, exacerbating the hyperkalemia caused by potassium retention in these conditions. *Acute respiratory acidosis* causes potassium loss from cells, which becomes maximal in about 4 hours, and may elevate the plasma potassium concentration, particularly in patients with renal failure. *Arginine hydrochloride* can cause severe hyperkalemia when used to treat metabolic alkalosis in patients with renal failure. The hyperkalemia does not appear to be related to the correction of the acid-base disturbance but rather to displacement of cellular potassium by this cationic amino acid. Patients with advanced liver disease are especially sensitive to this effect.

Digitalis poisoning causes severe hyperkalemia, a finding to be expected from the known inhibitory effect of cardiac glycosides on ($Na^+ + K^+$)-ATPase. *Succinylcholine,* a depolarizing muscle relaxant used in anesthesia, causes potassium loss from cells by increasing the ionic permeability of muscle. Patients with burns, muscle trauma, spinal injury, tetanus, and certain neuromuscular diseases are most sensitive to this effect and may develop severe hyperkalemia when given this agent.

Hyperkalemic periodic paralysis is a rare familial disorder characterized by recurrent attacks of hyperkalemia and muscle weakness or paralysis. Attacks are precipitated by the ingestion of small amounts of potassium or by a variety of other apparently unrelated stimuli (relaxation after exercise, excitement, cold, fasting, infections, and general anesthesia). The disease has been linked to an inherited defect in the sodium channel.

True hyperkalemia with a potassium surfeit
(see the accompanying box)

Body cells can function as a "sink" or as a source of potassium during periods of loading or depletion, respectively. Because cells are less able to take up potassium than to contribute it, hypokalemia is more effectively buffered than is hyperkalemia. Consequently, a much smaller change

Causes of sustained hyperkalemia

- Aldosterone deficiency
  - Addison's disease
  - Hyporeninemic hypoaldosteronism
  - Angiotensin-converting enzyme inhibitor therapy
  - Prostaglandin synthetase inhibitors
  - Corticosterone methyl oxidase deficiency
  - Heparin therapy
- Decreased response to aldosterone
  - Renal failure
    - Acute renal failure
    - Advanced chronic renal failure
    - Severe prerenal azotemia
  - Renal tubular disorders
    - Obstructive uropathy
    - Sickle cell disease
    - Renal transplantation
    - Amyloidosis
    - Systemic lupus erythematosus
    - Tubulointerstitial nephropathies
  - Potassium-sparing diuretics
  - Pseudohypoaldosteronism
  - Gordon's syndrome

in external potassium balance is required to raise the plasma potassium concentration above normal levels than to lower it below normal levels. It has been estimated that in a 70-kg man, only 100 mEq of excess potassium increases plasma potassium concentration from 4 to 5 mEq/L and even less may be required to increase the plasma potassium concentration further. Fortunately, normal renal potassium clearance is profound. Even a slight increase in plasma potassium concentration causes a brisk kaliuresis. Rarely, this large renal excretory capacity can be briefly overwhelmed by a large rapid potassium intake. Chronic hyperkalemia is almost always associated with reduced renal clearance of potassium. Although a steady state may be achieved, allowing daily potassium intake to match urinary removal, potassium excretion remains far less than appropriate for the degree of hyperkalemia. These disorders can be divided into those characterized by aldosterone deficiency and those in which renal resistance to the hormone causes hyperkalemia.

Combined aldosterone and glucocorticoid deficiency. Patients with combined mineralocorticoid and glucocorticoid deficiency present with the features of *Addison's disease*. Aldosterone deficiency causes renal sodium wasting and potassium retention, whereas glucocorticoid deficiency causes constitutional symptoms and water retention. These defects lead to hypotension, hyponatremia, and hyperkalemia. Plasma renin levels are elevated and plasma cortisol levels are low and unresponsive to ACTH stimulation. Addison's disease may result from destruction of the adrenals (by autoimmune disease, infection, or hemorrhage) or from bilateral adrenalectomy. Rarely, adrenal hormonal insufficiency results from congenital deficiency of 21-hydroxylase (congenital adrenal hyperplasia).

Selective aldosterone deficiency

Low renin. Hyporeninemic hypoaldosteronism is the most common cause of isolated aldosterone deficiency. Most patients have mild to moderate renal insufficiency secondary to tubular interstitial diseases (in 50%) or diabetic nephropathy. In contrast to addisonian patients, these patients are usually fluid overloaded; hyponatremia is unusual because cortisol levels are normal. Low aldosterone levels are associated with low levels of renin, which fail to increase with stimulatory maneuvers. The cause of renin deficiency may be multifactorial: suppression of renin secretion by extracellular volume expansion, sclerosis of the renin-secreting cells of the juxtaglomerular apparatus, secretion of inactive prorenin, autonomic insufficiency, and decreased prostaglandin synthesis have all been proposed as factors in its pathogenesis. Moreover, renin secretion decreases with age, possibly accounting for the increased prevalence of the disorder in elderly patients. Low renin levels reduce angiotensin II formation and may explain the diminished responsiveness of the adrenal gland to hyperkalemia (normally a potent stimulus to aldosterone secretion). Alternatively, a defect in aldosterone biosynthesis may coexist with renin deficiency in some patients. The hyperkalemia of hyporeninemic hypoaldosteronism is exacerbated by volume depletion, which, by reducing distal tubular luminal flow rate, worsens the potassium secretory defect. The majority of cases have an associated normal anion gap metabolic acidosis, termed *type 4 renal tubular acidosis* (RTA) (Chapter 353). The acidosis and hyperkalemia respond to treatment with fludrocortisone, a potent synthetic mineralocorticoid. Assessment of the response to fludrocortisone may be helpful diagnostically. The dose required is usually several times that needed in Addison's disease, implying that patients with hyporeninemic hypoaldosteronism have some degree of renal resistance. Alternatively, liberal salt intake, combined with such diuretics as furosemide or metolazone, increases potassium excretion by increasing the luminal flow rate in the distal nephron and prevents the sodium retention and hypertension that commonly complicate fludrocortisone therapy. *Prostaglandin synthetase inhibitors* (indomethacin, ibuprofen, naproxen) inhibit renin release and may cause reversible hyperkalemia and type 4 RTA, particularly in patients with renal insufficiency, in whom renin secretion may be marginal.

Normal renin, low angiotensin II. The angiotensin-converting enzyme inhibitors captopril, enalopril, and lisinopril inhibit the conversion of angiotensin I to angiotensin II, thereby reducing aldosterone levels. Although these drugs have caused a few cases of reversible frank hyperkalemia, in most patients only a slight increase in serum potassium (0.3 mEq/L) develops, but in patients with renal disease severe hyperkalemia may result.

Abnormal aldosterone biosynthesis. Rare congenital deficiencies of the enzymes required for the final steps in aldosterone biosynthesis (corticosterone methyl oxidase) result in a syndrome of isolated mineralocorticoid deficiency characterized by salt wasting, hyperkalemia, and metabolic acidosis in infancy. Some cases of acquired isolated aldosterone deficiency in adult diabetics have also been reported to result from defects in aldosterone biosynthesis. Heparin inhibits aldosterone secretion, probably by blocking the conversion of corticosterone to 18-hydroxycorticosterone; rare cases of hyperkalemia caused by heparin administration have been reported.

Decreased responsiveness to aldosterone

Renal failure. Patients with chronic renal failure are usually able to maintain potassium balance and normokalemia while on a normal diet until very late in their course. This adaptation appears to require increased aldosterone levels, implying that most patients with renal disease have some degree of "resistance" to mineralocorticoids. Relative hypoaldosteronism (i.e., when hyperkalemia fails to clearly increase plasma or urinary aldosterone levels) may respond to high doses of exogenous mineralocorticoids. Hyperkalemia is the rule in oliguric acute or chronic renal failure and may also be seen in oliguric patients with severe prerenal azotemia. In the latter circumstance, potassium excretion does not appreciably increase when exogenous mineralocorticoids are given.

Renal tubular disorders. A variety of disorders including lupus nephritis, allergic tubulointerstitial nephritis, and amyloidosis have been reported to cause mineralocorticoid-resistant potassium excretory defects with only mild azotemia. The plasma aldosterone level in these patients is usually high. Obstructive uropathy and sickle cell nephropathy may cause hyperkalemia and a normal anion gap metabolic acidosis. Although some patients with the aforementioned disorders have hyporeninemic hypoaldosteronism, others appear to have a mineralocorticoid resistant tubular defect analogous to that seen in patients treated with amiloride and have normal or elevated aldosterone levels. Mineralocorticoid-resistant hyperkalemia has been reported in transplanted kidneys, and hyperkalemia may be particularly prevalent when cyclosporine is used for immunosuppression.

Potassium-sparing diuretics. Spironolactone is a competitive inhibitor of aldosterone that impairs renal potassium excretion. Triamterene and amiloride also reduce potassium excretion but independently of aldosterone. Amiloride acts by blocking sodium channels in the distal luminal membrane; the transepithelial electrical potential is reduced, thereby impairing both potassium and hydrogen ion secretion. These agents are commonly combined with the thiazides or loop diuretics to avoid diuretic-induced hypokalemia. Administration of potassium supplements to patients receiving potassium-sparing diuretics is contraindicated.

Miscellaneous disorders. A number of rare disorders affecting renal potassium excretion have been reported. A syndrome known as *pseudohypoaldosteronism,* characterized by salt wasting, hyperkalemia, acidosis, and very high levels of renin and aldosterone, occurs in infants and improves with age. Another group of nonazotemic patients has been described in which hyperkalemia and acidosis are associated with hypertension and reduced renin and aldosterone levels. Renal potassium excretion in these patients does not respond to large doses of mineralocorticoids but does respond to thiazide diuretics (Gordon's syndrome). It has been proposed that the primary disturbance in these patients is an abnormally increased reabsorption of chloride in the distal nephron, which reduces the lumen's negative potential (thus decreasing potassium and hydrogen ion secretion) while at the same time augmenting distal sodium reabsorption, causing extracellular volume expansion, hypertension, and reduced levels of renin and aldosterone.

CONSEQUENCES OF HYPERKALEMIA

The most important effects of hyperkalemia derive from its action on cell membrane potentials. Because the intracellular potassium concentration increases minimally in hyperkalemia, the intracellular/extracellular potassium concentration ratio decreases, causing depolarization of the cell membrane; clinically important dysfunction of the heart and skeletal muscle results.

Cardiac effects

A characteristic progression of electrocardiographic changes (see Fig. 352-3) is seen with progressively more severe hyperkalemia. The earliest manifestation of hyperkalemia is a peaking and narrowing of the T wave, which usually becomes prominent once the plasma potassium concentration exceeds 6 mEq/L. With more severe hyperkalemia, the QRS complex is prolonged, followed by a decreased amplitude, prolongation, and ultimately disappearance of the P wave. With preterminal hyperkalemia, the markedly widened QRS complex merges with the T wave, giving the electrocardiogram a "sine wave" appearance. Soon thereafter, ventricular flutter, fibrillation, or standstill ensues.

Neuromuscular dysfunction

With severe hyperkalemia (usually when the plasma potassium concentration exceeds 8 mEq/L), muscle weakness develops, beginning in the lower extremities and usually sparing the respiratory muscles. Skeletal muscle weakness is sometimes accompanied by symptoms of distal paresthesias; both symptoms (which may mimic hysteria and hyperventilation syndrome) are important clues to the presence of life-threatening hyperkalemia.

Metabolic acidosis

Hyperkalemia is commonly associated with a normal anion gap metabolic acidosis. The uptake of excess potassium by cells displaces cellular hydrogen ions and causes a slight decrease in the plasma bicarbonate concentration. In addition, hyperkalemia impairs renal ammonia production, thereby reducing net acid excretion. Aldosterone deficiency also contributes to metabolic acidosis by impairing renal hydrogen ion secretion.

Hypertension

Partly by causing sodium retention, potassium depletion increases blood pressure in normotensive and hypertensive subjects. An increased dietary potassium intake may reduce the need for antihypertensive medications.

TREATMENT OF HYPERKALEMIA (Table 352-2)

A 12-lead electrocardiogram should be obtained in all hyperkalemic patients to assess the urgency of therapy. Severe hyperkalemia unaccompanied by electrocardiographic changes should suggest one of the causes of spurious hyperkalemia. Peaked T waves are usually seen when the plasma potassium concentration exceeds 6.5 mEq/L. This finding demands a prompt effort either to remove potassium from the body or to reverse factors responsible for potassium loss from cells (insulin deficiency or acidosis). Prolongation of the QRS interval and more advanced electrocardiographic changes usually appear once the plasma potassium concentration exceeds 7 to 8 mEq/L. These findings demand emergency administration of calcium (see later

Table 352-2. Emergency therapy of hyperkalemia

Therapeutic agent and mechanisms of action	Dose and administration	Onset	Duration
Antagonize cardiac effects			
Calcium gluconate 10%	10-30 ml IV	1 minute	30-60 minutes
Redistribution			
Glucose and insulin	50 g glucose IV hourly 5 units regular insulin q15min	5-10 minutes	2 hours
Sodium bicarbonate	50-100 mEq IV	2 hours	3-6 hours
Albuterol	10-20 mg by inhaler	30 minutes	2 hours
Removal			
Sodium polystyrene sulfonate (Kayexalate)	15-60 g with sorbitol orally or 50-100 g with retention enema (hold for 30-60 min)	1-2 hours	
Hemodialysis	Much more effective than peritoneal dialysis	Immediate	
Diuretics ("loop active")			
Furosemide	40-240 mg IV over 30 min	At onset of diuresis	
Ethacrynic acid	50-100 mg IV over 30 min		
Bumetanide	1-8 mg IV over 30 min		

discussion) as well as measures to lower the plasma potassium level.

Calcium

The administration of 10 ml of 10% calcium gluconate reverses the electrocardiographic findings of hyperkalemia rapidly (within seconds) and averts ventricular fibrillation or standstill. Calcium administration can also be helpful in determining whether the electrocardiographic abnormalities are caused by hyperkalemia. Calcium does not affect the plasma potassium concentration. An increased serum calcium concentration raises the threshold potential of neuromuscular tissue. In severe hyperkalemia the resting membrane potential falls below the threshold potential, rendering the cell unexcitable. By raising the threshold potential, calcium therapy re-establishes the difference between the resting and threshold potentials and restores cell excitability (see Fig. 352-1).

Insulin

Because the hypokalemic effect of insulin is dose related, insulin should be administered as an intravenous bolus to achieve high plasma levels. Repeated injections of 5 units every 15 minutes accompanied by the infusion of 50 g of glucose per hour can achieve a maximal effect, usually without hypoglycemia.

Sodium bicarbonate

Hyperkalemia is usually associated with a decreased plasma bicarbonate concentration. The administration of sodium bicarbonate promotes urinary potassium excretion and is also effective in driving potassium into cells even if used when the blood pH is normal. Doses in excess of the usual 50 to 100 mEq may be used in severely acidotic patients. Isotonic solutions are preferred and can be prepared by adding three ampules (50 mEq/ampule) to a liter of 5% dextrose in water. In anuric subjects the full hypokalemic effect of bicarbonate may not be seen for 2 to 3 hours. Thus bicarbonate infusion alone is inadequate in hyperkalemic emergencies.

Beta-2 adrenergic agonists

Inhaled beta-2 agonists have been used successfully to treat attacks of familial hyperkalemic periodic paralysis. There is also a limited experience in hyperkalemic patients with renal failure. Not all uremic patients respond however, and given the potential risk for cardiac toxicity and the effectiveness of glucose and insulin, these agents may not be appropriate for first-line therapy.

Measures to achieve negative potassium balance

Because the uptake of excess potassium by tissues is relatively limited, small potassium surfeits can cause marked hyperkalemia. It follows that the treatment of hyperkalemia does not usually require removal of large amounts of potassium.

Reduced intake. Potassium intake should be reduced, and "hidden" sources of potassium such as salt substitutes (10 to 13 mEq/g), potassium penicillin (1.7 mEq/million units), and stored blood should be sought.

Increased renal excretion. Potassium-sparing diuretics and (if the patient's cardiac condition permits) angiotensin-converting enzyme inhibitors should be discontinued. Negative potassium balance can be achieved by the administration of a loop diuretic (e.g., furosemide), replacing urine losses with NaCl or $NaHCO_3$.

Kayexalate (sodium polystyrene sulfonate). This cation exchange resin binds potassium secreted in the distal rectum. When given orally, it should be combined with sorbitol, an osmotic cathartic, to speed delivery to its site of action. Alternatively it can be given by retention enema. Each gram of the resin binds approximately 1 mEq of potassium while yielding approximately 2 mEq of sodium. The potential side effect of sodium overload can be offset by sorbitol-induced diarrhea. In high doses, however, the cathartic can cause negative water balance and hypernatremia.

Dialysis. Hyperkalemia can be corrected within minutes by hemodialysis. Peritoneal dialysis removes potassium more slowly than Kayexalate.

REFERENCES

Allon M, Dunlay R, and Copkney T: Nebulized albuterol for acute hyperkalemia in patients on hemodialysis, Ann Intern Med 110:426, 1989.

Blumbert A et al: Effect of various therapeutic approaches on plasma potassium and major regulating factors in terminal renal failure, Am J Med 85:507, 1988.

Giebisch G and Seldin DW, editors: The regulation of potassium balance, New York, 1989, Raven Press.

Knochel J: Neuromuscular manifestations of electrolyte disorders, Am J Med 72:521, 1982.

Krishna GG: Hypokalemic states: current clinical issues, Semin Nephrol 10:515, 1991.

Kruse JA and Carlson RW: Rapid correction of hypokalemia using concentrated intravenous potassium chloride infusions, Arch Intern Med 150:613, 1990.

Kupin W and Narins RW: The hyperkalemia of renal failure: diagnosis, pathophysiology, and therapy, Min Elect Metab (In press).

Narins RG et al: Diagnostic strategies in disorders of fluid, electrolyte and acid-base homeostasis, Am J Med 72:496, 1982.

Ponce SP et al: Drug-induced hyperkalemia, Medicine 64:357, 1985.

Schulman M and Narins RG: Hypokalemia and cardiovascular disease, Am J Cardiol 65:4E, 1990.

Stein JH: The pathogenetic spectrum of Bartter's syndrome, Kidney Int 28:85, 1985.

Sterns RH et al: Internal potassium balance and the control of the plasma potassium concentration, Medicine (Baltimore) 60:389, 1981.

Sterns RH and Spital A: Disorders of internal potassium balance, Semin Nephrol 7:206, 1987.

CHAPTER

353 Disorders of Acid-Base Balance

Melvin E. Laski
Neil A. Kurtzman

The high protein diet consumed by meat-eating people generates about 60 to 100 mEq of nonvolatile acid daily. To preserve homeostasis, this acid must be excreted by the kidney. When acid from metabolism *(HR)* is added to the circulation it is buffered according to the following reaction:

$$HR + NaHCO_3 \rightarrow NaR + H_2O + CO_2 \quad \text{(EQ. 1)}$$

The lung excretes the CO_2. The kidneys reverse this reaction so that HR is excreted in the urine and bicarbonate is regenerated and returned to the blood. The kidneys must also recapture most of the filtered bicarbonate.

If a person generates 100 mEq of acid per day the net acid excretion must be precisely 100 mEq. If more is excreted, metabolic alkalosis develops; if less is excreted, renal acidosis ensues. A total daily acid excretion of 100 mEq is not sufficient, however, if bicarbonate is lost in the urine. For example, if 100 mEq of acid and 100 mEq of bicarbonate are excreted, net acid excretion is zero.

Because the nephron cannot lower urine pH much below 4.5, acid must be excreted in buffered form. Buffers allow the urine to contain large amounts of acid at a relatively high pH. The two main urinary buffers are phosphate, the predominant component of titratable acid (TA), and ammonium. Net acid excretion = $(TA + NH_4) - HCO_3$.

This simple formula defines the kidney's role in acid-base homeostasis. It must reclaim the filtered bicarbonate while excreting appropriate amounts of buffered acid. Thus a subject generating a 100-mEq of acid per day might excrete 68 mEq of titratable acid, 34 mEq of ammonium, and 2 mEq of bicarbonate—a net acid excretion of precisely the required 100 mEq.

The glomerulus filters large amounts of bicarbonate (about 4000 mEq/day), virtually all of which must be reabsorbed by the tubules. The principal site of bicarbonate reabsorption is the proximal tubule. The main site of acid excretion, that is, where the nonbicarbonate buffers (TA and ammonia) are protonated, is the collecting duct.

Roughly two thirds of proximal tubule bicarbonate reabsorption is mediated by sodium-proton exchange at the luminal membrane; one third of the proton secretion is a result of the action of a proton ATPase pump. The energy for proton secretion mediated by the proton ATPase is the direct catalysis of ATP by this enzyme. The energy for sodium-proton exchange is provided by the sodium-potassium ATPase of the basolateral membrane, which transports sodium outward from the cytoplasm to the pericellular fluid. The pump lowers the cell sodium concentration and thus provides a driving gradient for sodium entry, which is directly linked to proton exit by the sodium-proton antiporter of the apical membrane. Secreted protons combine with filtered bicarbonate to form carbonic acid, which decomposes to carbon dioxide and water in a reaction that is greatly accelerated by the presence of luminal membrane carbonic anhydrase. The process generates intracellular bicarbonate. The net reaction $[CO_2 + H_2O \rightarrow H^+ + HCO_3^-]$ is catalyzed by cytoplasmic carbonic anhydrase. The intracellular bicarbonate exits the basolateral cell membrane to the blood via a sodium-bicarbonate co-transporter. The result is the transport of protons to the tubule lumen and bicarbonate to the blood, and the energy source for the entire process is the catalysis of ATP by the sodium-potassium ATPase.

Proximal tubule bicarbonate reabsorption is regulated by

several factors including the state of effective arterial blood volume, the blood potassium concentration, the partial pressure of CO_2, the presence of carbonic anhydrase, and the glomerular filtration rate (GFR).

Volume contraction stimulates proximal reabsorption; volume expansion depresses it. Proximal bicarbonate reabsorption is inversely proportional to the level of body potassium stores. In general, there is a reasonable correlation between potassium stores and serum potassium. Bicarbonate reabsorption correlates directly with the arterial P_{CO_2}. Carbonic anhydrase does not regulate bicarbonate reabsorption because it is always present in sufficient quantities to catalyze the hydration and dehydration of CO_2. Its clinical importance is that carbonic anhydrase-inhibiting diuretics, such as acetazolamide, exert their diuretic effect by inhibiting the enzyme. Obviously, bicarbonate excretion will be affected by the GFR. Under pathologic conditions, if the serum bicarbonate is high and the GFR is low, bicarbonate will be excreted with greater difficulty than if the GFR were normal.

Because the nonvolatile acids of protein metabolism titrate the blood buffers, the kidney must not only reclaim the filtered bicarbonate, but also excrete acid. Acid excretion occurs mainly in the collecting duct. Here protons are secreted into the urine by two types of proton pump: an electrogenic proton ATPase and an electroneutral proton-potassium ATPase similar to the gastric acid pump. These protons react with the major urinary buffers (phosphate and ammonia). Each mole of nonbicarbonate buffer titrated in the urine results in the formation and return to the blood of a mole of new bicarbonate (i.e., regenerated bicarbonate). The amount of acid that can be formed in this manner is limited by the strength of the proton pumps, which can generate a maximum pH gradient of three pH units, the impermeability of the duct to acid, and the amount of buffer in the urine.

The main filtered buffer is phosphate. When phosphate has been completely titrated, further acid excretion depends on the kidney's capacity to make ammonia. Ammonia is synthesized from glutamine, mainly in the proximal tubule. Its rate of formation is inversely related to the state of body potassium stores. It likely is also stimulated by aldosterone. Aldosterone stimulates cortical collecting duct sodium reabsorption, which generates a lumen-negative potential difference. This potential difference favors the secretion of protons. Aldosterone also directly stimulates the proton pump.

The proton-potassium ATPase pump does not appear to respond to aldosterone but is influenced by the state of potassium balance; activity increases in potassium deficiency and decreases in the presence of potassium excess. The net effect of potassium deficiency on distal renal acidification is difficult to predict because it stimulates the proton-potassium ATPase but depresses aldosterone levels and secondarily inhibits proton ATPase activity.

Distal proton secretion is also strongly influenced by the rate of distal sodium transport. Anything that inhibits distal sodium transport, such as a tubular defect or diminished distal sodium delivery, will also reduce distal acidification by the electrogenic proton ATPase. The nature of the anion delivered to the distal nephron will also affect acidification. Poorly reabsorbable anions such as sulfate will enhance the lumen negative potential difference and thus favor acid secretion.

In addition to the 100 mEq of nonvolatile acid produced daily, the body's metabolic machinery generates 10 to 12 mol of carbon dioxide, which is equivalent to the same amount of volatile acid. The lung returns it to the environment. Although the control of respiration lies in the central nervous system (the medulla), the sensory apparatus that provides information to it is located in the carotid body chemoreceptor. When the kidney and the lung function in concert, acid-base homeostasis is preserved.

EFFECTS OF pH ON ORGAN FUNCTION (Table 353-1)

Normally, arterial pH varies from 7.4 by less than 0.05. Even when the extremes of pH seen under pathologic conditions are considered (6.8 to 7.8), the variation of hydrogen ion concentration is remarkably small (15.8 to 158 nM). Thus it is not surprising that small variations in blood pH have profound consequences. It is also apparent that acidemia is better tolerated than alkalemia. The lowest pH consistent with survival is 0.6 pH units below normal; the highest is 0.4 above normal.

An arterial pH below 7.20 in experimental animals depresses myocardial metabolism and lowers intracellular calcium concentration. Both reduce myocardial contractility. Severe acidemia induces dysrhythmias, conduction defects, and ventricular fibrillation. It also depresses arterial vascular tone and reduces the response to catecholamines. In contrast, acidemia increases tone in venous capacitance vessels and in the pulmonary circuit. This combination produces cardiovascular decompensation and pulmonary edema.

Acidemia has major effects on electrolyte metabolism. It increases calcium solubility while decreasing protein binding. It favors the movement of phosphate out of cells. Its effect on transcellular potassium movement depends on the acid accumulated. Serum potassium rises when acidemia is caused by mineral acid, but organic acids have no effect on the serum potassium. The hyperkalemia typical of diabetic ketoacidosis is the result not of acidemia, but of insulin deficiency, glucagon excess, and hyperosmolarity.

The impact of acidemia on the central nervous system depends on whether pH has fallen because PCO_2 rises or because blood bicarbonate falls. The blood-brain barrier is relatively impermeable to bicarbonate, but CO_2 crosses easily. Thus respiratory acidosis will rapidly depress the pH of cerebrospinal fluid. The effect of metabolic acidosis on central nervous system function will take longer to manifest. Low pH in the cerebrospinal fluid depresses central nervous system function. Patients may suffer headache, lethargy, stupor, or coma.

Acidemia increases tissue oxygen delivery by decreasing the binding of oxygen to hemoglobin (the Bohr effect).

Table 353-1. Physiologic effects of pH change

	Alkalemia	Acidemia
Cardiovascular	↑ Dysrhythmias (multifocal AT, PVCs) ↓ Cerebral blood flow	Systemic vasodilatation Resistance to vasoconstrictors Pulmonary vasoconstriction ↓ Venous capacitance Myocardial depression ↑ Risk of ventricular fibrillation Conduction defects
Metabolic	↓ O_2 delivery (Bohr effect) ↑ Phosphofructokinase activity ↑ Glycolysis ↑ Lactate and pyruvate production	Acute ↑ Calcium solubility ↑ Serum phosphate ↑ Serum potassium (only if mineral acid or hyperosmolar state) ↑ O_2 delivery (Bohr effect) Chronic Loss of bone to buffering (metabolic acidosis) Loss of muscle protein
	METABOLIC pH SHIFTS	RESPIRATORY pH SHIFTS
Central nervous system	Little effect on CSF pH after acute or chronic changes	↑ PCO_2 induces CSF acidosis, CNS depression, and coma ↓ PCO_2 induces CSF alkalosis ↑ Seizure activity

AT, atrial tachycardia; PVC, premature ventricular contractions; CSF, cerebrospinal fluid; CNS, central nervous system.

It also decreases phosphofructokinase activity, which decreases the rate of glycolysis and, hence, lactate formation.

In many ways, the consequences of alkalemia mirror those of acidemia. Tissue oxygen delivery is reduced because of an increased affinity of hemoglobin for oxygen. This effect is important for only a short time because of the synthesis of 2,3-diphosphoglycerate, which opposes this effect on oxygen binding. Phosphofructokinase activity is increased causing increased glycolysis and, in turn, greater production of pyruvate and lactate. Alkalemia increases calcium binding to protein and lowers the solubility of calcium salts. The development of alkalemia in a borderline hypocalcemic patient can precipitate tetany. Alkalemia can trigger cardiac dysrhythmias, including multifocal atrial tachycardia and ventricular ectopy. Cerebral blood flow may fall substantially.

Chronic acidosis induces a variety of adaptive responses, many of which may be deleterious. Metabolic acidosis is buffered, in part, by the release of calcium salts from bone. Over time, clinically significant osteopenia may be produced. Conversely, chronic respiratory acidosis is associated with calcium deposition and increased bone density. Persistent acidosis also stimulates renal ammoniagenesis. This adaptation is mediated, in part, by protein catabolism, which may eventually produce muscle wasting. Patients with chronic renal failure may suffer significant muscle losses unless acidosis is appropriately treated.

The principal extracellular buffer is the bicarbonate/carbonic acid system. Clinically, acid-base disorders are defined by blood gas parameters. The Henderson-Hasselbalch equation relates the two components as follows:

(EQ. 2)

$$\text{pH} = \text{pK} + \log(\text{base/acid}) \text{ or pH} = 6.1 + \log(HCO_3/0.03 \times pCO_2)$$

The pK for the bicarbonate/carbonic acid buffer pair is 6.1. The solubility coefficient for CO_2 converts PCO_2 in mm Hg to carbonic acid in mM/L. Under clinical conditions the pH and PCO_2 of body fluids, usually blood, are measured, allowing calculation of the bicarbonate concentration. If one wishes to avoid the use of logarithms, the following formula gives a reasonable estimate of acid-base parameters:

(EQ. 3)

$$[H^+] \text{ (neq/1)} = (24 \times pCO_2)/\ [HCO_3]$$

These simple equations depict the dual role of the lungs and the kidneys in the regulation of acid-base homeostasis.

DIAGNOSIS OF ACID-BASE DISORDERS

The four acid-base disorders defined here may exist either alone or in combination with one or two others. When alone the disturbance is termed *simple*, when combined it is called *mixed*. The only prohibited combination is mixed respiratory acidosis and alkalosis. *Metabolic acidosis* is a primary fall in the bicarbonate concentration due to a gain of nonvolatile acid or a loss of bicarbonate. *Metabolic alkalosis* is a primary rise in the bicarbonate concentration due to a gain of bicarbonate or a loss of nonvolatile acid. *Respiratory acidosis* is a primary rise in the PCO_2 caused by a decrease in the rate of alveolar ventilation referable to CO_2

production. *Respiratory alkalosis* is a primary fall in the Pco_2 caused by an increase in the rate of alveolar ventilation referable to CO_2 production.

The terms *acidosis* and *alkalosis* differ from *acidemia* and *alkalemia* in that the latter two terms refer solely to changes in blood pH. The former terms refer to the processes defined here without regard to the blood pH. The presence of complicating disorders and/or compensatory mechanisms may result in a normal pH. A patient with metabolic acidosis may even be alkalemic if a second primary process (i.e., respiratory alkalosis) is also present.

Compensation is a secondary event that involves the component of acid-base regulation not primarily perturbed. Thus the lung mediates compensation of metabolic disorders, and the kidneys respond to respiratory derangements. It is never correct to speak of compensatory metabolic acidosis when metabolic compensation is intended.

The successful diagnosis of acid-base disorders requires more than a blood gas measurement or even the use of a blood gas nomogram. It is necessary to integrate the patient's history with appropriate laboratory data. These data may include not only blood gas measurements, but also serum electrolytes and anion gap, blood glucose, BUN and creatinine, serum osmolality and osmolar gap, urinalysis with careful measurement of urine pH, microscopic examination of the urine for crystals, and the calculation of the urine anion gap. In addition, a determination of serum ketones, lactate, methanol, or salicylates should be obtained if the clinical circumstances warrant it.

Anion gap

Although it is true that the total concentration of all the cations in a biologic fluid precisely equals that of all the anions, when one compares the total concentrations of easily measured cations and anions in serum an apparent "gap" is normally present.

$$(Na + K) - (Cl + HCO_3) = 16 \pm 4 \qquad \textbf{(EQ. 4)}$$

The newer chloride analysis devices provide a somewhat higher reading for chloride concentration with a consequent reduction in this gap by about 4. The anion gap occurs because there are more unmeasured anions than cations in serum. Albumin provides the great bulk of the unmeasured anion; the remainder is sulfate, phosphate, lactate, etc. The anion gap increases in patients with metabolic acidosis; it also rises during alkalemia.

Two types of metabolic acidosis are associated with an increase in the anion gap: acidosis of renal failure and acidosis associated with the accumulation of organic acids. In the former, the loss of renal mass causes the retention of phosphate-, sulfate-, and hippurate-containing acids. Examples of the latter are ketoacidosis and lactic acidosis.

The retention of these acids consumes bicarbonate without altering the chloride concentration; thus the apparent anion gap increase. If the acidosis results from the failure to excrete acid not associated with a major decrease in GFR (renal tubular acidosis), the loss of bicarbonate (e.g., diarrhea) or the addition of hydrochloric acid (e.g., ammonium chloride) bicarbonate will again be consumed; but there will be a corresponding increase in the chloride concentration, leaving the anion gap unchanged.

Alkalemia also increases the anion gap as a consequence of buffering by albumin. As the blood pH rises, the acidic side chain amino acids of albumin dissociate, exposing increased numbers of negative charges. In other words, the ratio of charged to uncharged albumin is directly proportional to the blood pH. This relationship should cause no confusion in patients with metabolic alkalosis, but in patients with acute respiratory alkalosis in whom blood electrolytes but not blood gases are available, care must be taken not to attribute an increased anion gap to metabolic acidosis. This problem is rare in chronic respiratory alkalosis because metabolic compensation usually brings the pH and the anion gap into the normal range.

The anion gap may also decrease. This change is commonly seen in patients with paraproteinemias. The abnormal immunoglobulins, such as IgG myeloma protein, are cationic. Thus a decreased anion gap should alert the clinician to the possibility of an undiagnosed monoclonal gammopathy.

Osmolar gap

The serum osmolar gap is the difference between the measured serum osmolality and calculated osmolality.

$$\text{Calculated osmolality} = 1.87\,([Na] + [K]) + BUN/2.8 + glucose/18 \qquad \textbf{(EQ. 5)}$$

This calculation yields results that agree closely with the measured osmolality unless other unmeasured osmoles are present, in which case the measured value will significantly exceed the calculated amount. Evaluation of the osmolar gap is useful in patients who have metabolic acidosis associated with methanol or ethanol ingestion. These low molecular weight compounds profoundly elevate the serum osmolality. Methanol ingestion is a medical emergency that requires prompt treatment as soon as the osmolar gap is discovered. One should not wait for the serum methanol measurement to become available before starting treatment.

Urine anion gap

The urine anion gap is the sum of the urine sodium and potassium concentrations minus the urine chloride. If this gap is large and the urine pH is high, the missing anion is bicarbonate. If the urine pH is low, a negative gap ($U[Na + K] < U[Cl]$) indicates that the urine is high in ammonium. If the patient is acidemic ($pH < 7.35$) the negative gap should exceed 80. Most clinical labs do not routinely measure urinary ammonium; the measurement of the urine anion gap is the easiest way to estimate urinary ammonium. In patients with aldosterone deficiency or resistance, or with hyperkalemic distal renal tubular acidosis, ammonia production and excretion is decreased.

The absence of a large urinary anion gap in a patient with systemic acidosis who has a normal serum anion gap denotes inadequate renal ammonia synthesis and/or excretion. A patient with anion gap acidosis, a low urine pH, and a decreased negative urinary anion gap likely has a high urinary concentration of an unmeasured anion, most probably either ketone bodies or lactate. Oxalate and formate are other possibilities.

CLINICAL DISORDERS OF ACID-BASE REGULATION

Metabolic alkalosis

Metabolic alkalosis has two phases, generation and maintenance (see accompanying box). It may be generated either by the loss of acid or by the addition of base. Clinical examples are the overuse of antacids, the administration of bicarbonate precursors such as citrate, and the administration of intravenous bicarbonate. The two organs that can lose acid under ordinary circumstances are the stomach and the kidney (Table 353-2).

Metabolic alkalosis

Generation

- Loss of acid
  - Gastrointestinal losses
  - Vomiting
  - Chloride-losing diarrhea of infancy
- Renal losses
  - Increased acid excretion due to aldosterone excess
    - Secondary hyperaldosteronism
      - All causes of volume loss, diuretics
    - Primary aldosteronism
      - Conn's syndrome
      - Cushing's syndrome
    - Pseudohyperaldosteronism
      - Liddle's syndrome
      - Bartter's syndrome
      - Licorice ingestion
- Ingestion of alkali
  - Absorbable antacids
    - "Milk alkali" syndrome
  - Absorbable bicarbonate precursors
    - Lactate, citrate, acetate
  - Intravenous alkali
    - Bicarbonate administration
    - Acetate in dialysis

Maintenance

- Volume depletion
  - Diminished filtered load of bicarbonate
  - Diminished distal delivery
- Role of potassium
- Role of chloride?

The loss of gastric juice, either by vomiting or by nasogastric suction, increases the plasma concentration of bicarbonate because of the high acid content of this fluid, about 90 mEq/L. Every mEq of acid lost is equivalent to a 1 mEq gain in bicarbonate. When the blood bicarbonate rises, the filtered load of bicarbonate also increases and urinary sodium bicarbonate increases as well. Thus the loss of HCl in gastric juice and $NaHCO_3$ in urine is the equivalent of the loss of NaCl, H_2O, and CO_2. The loss of salt and water contracts volume and increases proximal bicarbonate reabsorption, which then decreases bicarbonate excretion. Volume contraction also stimulates aldosterone release, which in turn increases potassium excretion. The ensuing hypokalemia further stimulates proximal bicarbonate reclamation and eventually suppresses aldosterone release. Note that early in the course of vomiting the urine pH and sodium concentration are high (the excretion of bicarbonate obligates sodium excretion). Later, the urine pH falls as does the sodium concentration; when the urine bicarbonate falls the urine sodium does likewise. The urine chloride, however, is always low. Thus in gastric alkalosis, the alkalosis is generated by acid loss from the stomach. It is maintained by accelerated renal bicarbonate reabsorption stimulated by volume contraction and hypokalemia. Any associated fall in GFR also helps maintain the disorder.

The other common form of metabolic alkalosis is caused by diuretic administration. Diuretics that act on the loop of Henle or distal tubule (e.g., furosemide, thiazide) contract volume and induce secondary hyperaldosteronism. The continued administration of the diuretic maintains the distal delivery of sodium even though volume is contracted. High distal sodium delivery in the presence of a high blood aldosterone level results in the renal loss of both acid and potassium. Hence the patient develops hypokalemic metabolic alkalosis. This form of metabolic alkalosis is generated by distal renal acid loss. It is maintained by increased proximal reabsorption stimulated by volume contraction and hypokalemia. Even if acid loss ceases, the metabolic alkalosis will not correct until volume and/or potassium have been restored. This is why the administration of salt and potassium chloride is the mainstay of the treatment of metabolic alkalosis.

In patients with primary steroid excess such as Conn's syndrome, metabolic alkalosis is generated by renal acid loss because of the stimulation of distal nephron proton ATPase by aldosterone. Sodium reabsorption is also stimulated and the patients are volume expanded rather than depleted. The alkalosis is maintained by potassium depletion and continued acid secretion. Potassium depletion may also stimulate the potassium-proton ATPase, resulting in even more distal acid secretion. Salt administration alone will not correct the alkalosis; potassium is required.

An interesting variety of metabolic alkalosis is seen in patients with chronic respiratory acidosis in whom hypercapnia is rapidly corrected. Because the blood bicarbonate is high in these patients due to metabolic compensation, the pH rises. When the Pco_2 falls the kidney should excrete sufficient bicarbonate over the next day so that the pH does not remain inappropriately high. If the patient's effective arterial blood volume is low because of salt depletion, heart failure, or another cause, bicarbonate will not be excreted in sufficient amounts to prevent or correct alkalemia and the patient will have posthypercapnic metabolic alkalosis. This disorder is prevented or corrected by maintaining a normal state of volume.

Compensation. Respiratory compensation of metabolic alkalosis requires that the patient hypoventilate to increase the PCO_2. Because hypoventilation also causes hypoxemia, the cure is worse than the disease. Thus it is not surprising that metabolic alkalosis is the least compensated acid-base disorder. A patient with chronic metabolic alkalosis with a PCO_2 greater than 50 and certainly greater than 55 should be suspected of having underlying pulmonary disease.

Treatment. Treatment has two aims. First, if possible, the process that generated the alkalosis should be reversed. If appropriate, nasogastric suction should be stopped and emesis treated. If there is primary mineralocorticoid excess, the oversecretion should be stopped or its effects blocked by spironolactone or amiloride. Second, the processes that maintain the alkalosis must be treated. Volume contraction should be reversed with saline infusion. If effective volume is contracted because of heart failure, salt should not be given; rather, the heart failure should be specifically treated. Potassium deficits should be corrected with potassium chloride. In patients with posthypercapnic metabolic alkalosis, treatment with the carbonic anhydrase inhibitor acetazolamide often helps. Patients with metabolic alkalosis and renal failure may require dialysis against a low bicarbonate bath.

Metabolic acidosis

Metabolic acidosis is usually divided into two types: anion gap and nonanion gap (or hyperchloremic) acidosis. A list of the various causes of metabolic acidosis arranged in this manner is presented in the accompanying box.

Metabolic acidosis

Anion gap present

- Ketoacidosis
  - Diabetic ketoacidosis
  - Alcoholic ketoacidosis
  - Starvation ketoacidosis
- Lactic acidosis
- Methanol ingestion
- Salicylate ingestion
- Paraldehyde ingestion
- Ethylene glycol ingestion
- Uremic acidosis

Anion gap not present

- Diarrhea
- Pancreato-cutaneous fistula
- Mineral acid ingestion
- Hyperalimentation
- Renal acidosis
  - Proximal renal tubular acidosis
  - Distal renal tubular acidosis
    - Hypokalemic
      - Pump failure
      - Acid backleak
    - Hyperkalemic
      - "Short-circuit acidosis" (voltage dependent)
      - Aldosterone deficiency or resistance
        - Addison's disease
        - Hyporeninemic-hypoaldosteronism
  - Renal failure with volume contraction

Metabolic acidosis with increased anion gap. The presence of an increased anion gap in a patient with metabolic acidosis indicates that an acid with an anion other than chloride has accumulated. Once anion gap acidosis has been diagnosed, the diagnostic possibilities are limited to a handful of disorders. The correct diagnosis is usually easy to make.

***Ketoacidosis* (Chapter 168).** The underlying problem in ketoacidosis is that a significant percentage of the body's cells cannot use glucose as a fuel. This occurs because insulin deficiency prevents cellular glucose entry or because starvation limits glucose availability. The ketones rise for two reasons. First, insulin deficiency induces an increase in fatty acid mobilization. Second, a rise in the ratio of glucagon to insulin results in increased oxidation of these fatty acids and the production of acetoacetate, acetone, and/or beta-hydroxybutyrate (i.e., ketone bodies) increases. Whether acetoacetate or beta-hydroxybutyrate predominates depends on the redox state of the cell. If the ratio of the reduced form of nicotinamide-adenine dinucleotide to its reduced form (NADH/NAD) is increased, the formation of beta-hydroxybutyrate will be favored. Acetoacetate will predominate when the ratio is decreased, which is important because the standard paper and tablet tests for ketone bodies do not detect beta-hydroxybutyrate. Thus patients with ketoacidosis and increased levels of NADH may test negative for ketone bodies even when they have severe ketoacidosis. Under these conditions, a specific test for beta-hydroxybutyrate should be used. Because ketone bodies are rapidly excreted in the urine, the urine may test positive before ketones are detected in the blood.

In diabetes, ketoacidosis is restricted to those patients in whom insulin is absent or nearly absent. In addition ketoacidosis only develops when glucagon excess is also present. The acidosis is invariably complicated by volume contraction resulting from the osmotic diuresis that follows hyperglycemia. Clinically, these patients present with evidence of central nervous system depression ranging from a clouded sensorium to coma. They may have abdominal pain. The acidemia stimulates hyperventilation in a pattern described as Kussmaul respiration. The presence of acetone on the breath causes the characteristic fruity odor.

Treatment requires prompt administration of insulin. Because these patients are both volume contracted and dehydrated they need appropriate amounts of salt and water. If renal function is good, the kidney will sort things out with respect to both salt and water balance. Thus isotonic saline administration is usually sufficient. When renal function is compromised, fluid replacement must be more exact. Salt with extra water is required. Some of the fluid given must be dilute, (i.e., some of it should be hypotonic saline). Careful attention must be paid to the blood osmolality to prevent hypotonicity.

Patients with diabetic ketoacidosis commonly present with hyperkalemia and hyperphosphatemia. With insulin replacement, however, hypokalemia and hypophosphatemia may rapidly develop. Thus blood potassium and phosphate should be closely monitored and replaced as soon as indicated.

Because both acetoacetate and beta-hydroxybutyrate are rapidly metabolized to bicarbonate when insulin and fluids are given, it is not usually necessary to treat these patients with bicarbonate. Severe acidemia (below 7.1), especially if accompanied by very high levels of potassium, may require judicious infusion of bicarbonate. If too much bicarbonate is given, the patient may develop metabolic alkalosis when the ketosis has been corrected. Further, the administration of highly concentrated sodium bicarbonate may induce hypertonicity.

The ketoacidosis that develops during starvation is generally less severe. Absent carbohydrate intake suppresses insulin release and stimulates glucagon secretion, hence the tendency to ketoacidosis. The obvious treatment is glucose administration. Because these patients are not diabetic, insulin treatment is not necessary. These patients do not develop the solute diuresis of glycosuria. Unless other losses are identified, vigorous volume repletion is not required.

Alcohol ketoacidosis is a third form of the disorder. Actually, it should be called alcohol withdrawal ketoacidosis. This disease is seen in heavy alcohol users who develop an acute gastrointestinal problem, which prevents further ethanol intake. The poor caloric intake typical of an alcoholic might be expected to cause ketosis, but ethanol inhibits ketogenesis. Thus ketoacidosis does not develop while the patient continues to drink. When alcohol intake stops because of a gastrointestinal disorder, adequate caloric intake, which might prevent ketosis, is precluded and ketoacidosis results. Treatment is administration of calories as intravenous glucose and the correction of any accompanying fluid deficits. One is cautioned to remember to provide thiamine to such patients.

Lactic acidosis. Lactic acidosis is also the product of abnormal metabolism. In this case, the problem is accelerated lactate production with decreased metabolism of lactate back to pyruvate. Normal glucose metabolism proceeds in two phases. First, cytoplasmic glycolysis generates two moles of pyruvate and two moles of ATP from one mole of glucose. Pyruvate then enters the intramitochondrial Krebs cycle where 36 moles of ATP are generated from the two moles of pyruvate. Alternate mitochondrial pathways may metabolize pyruvate to fat or amino acids. Before pyruvate enters the mitochondrion, it can be shunted to lactate, which is a metabolic dead end. Lactate can only be metabolized back to pyruvate. Pyruvate and lactate exist in free equilibrium. The ratio of the two depends on the redox state of the cell and thus is set by the NAD/NADH ratio. Under condition of tissue hypoxia there is an increase in NADH relative to NAD; the formation of lactate therefore is favored. The shunting of pyruvate to lactate prevents mitochondrial pyruvate metabolism. Metabolism is limited to anerobic glycolysis and the generation of two moles of ATP per mole glucose rather than the 38 generated during aerobic metabolism. Under anerobic conditions the metabolism of glucose is summarized thusly:

(EQ. 6)

$$\text{glucose} \rightarrow 2\text{ATP} + 2\text{ lactate} + 2\text{H}^+$$

Two moles of lactate are produced from each mole of glucose together with two moles of protons.

Accelerated lactate generation is not limited to pathologic states. Exercise increases muscle lactate formation, which causes the muscle fatigue characteristic of exercise. When exercise stops, excess lactate is rapidly metabolized back to pyruvate, which re-enters the metabolic cycle. This process consumes the extra protons and generates bicarbonate, which spontaneously corrects any acidosis generated. The liver and kidneys have the highest rates of lactate metabolism.

Clinical lactic acidosis is divided into two types, A and B. This division is rather arbitrary, however, because the same mechanism (i.e., an increase in the NADH/NAD ratio) is the root of the metabolic abnormality. Unfortunately, the classification is widely used.

Lactic acidosis associated with tissue hypoxia is labeled type A. Common causes are circulatory shock, extreme hypoxemia, local vascular compromise, carbon monoxide poisoning, or extreme anemia. Shock, the most common cause of lactic acidosis, is the most difficult to treat. Although correction of the acidosis associated with shock is critical, attempts to treat lactic acidosis in this setting with bicarbonate alone are rarely successful. Although pH may be raised somewhat, an increase in intracellular pH enhances phosphofructokinase activity and increases lactate generation by increasing glycolysis. Although some have argued that bicarbonate should not be given to patients with lactic acidosis, it may buy a little time, which may be used to try to reverse the underlying derangement responsible for the lactic acidosis. If this time is not available, all other therapeutic efforts are doomed to failure.

Treatment of type A lactic acidosis consists of improving the circulation and enhancing tissue oxygenation. Correction of fluid deficits, replacement of red cells, and increasing cardiac output are the prime goals. These patients deserve invasive hemodynamic monitoring to allow optimum fluid replacement and use of stimulatory drugs. Local factors that compromise the circulation should be identified and corrected if possible. When acidemia is severe, bicarbonate should be given because acidemia itself decreases cardiac output and impairs organ perfusion. Despite these efforts, however, most of these patients will not survive.

Because conventional treatment of this disorder is so poor, considerable effort has focused on trying to develop new treatments. One of the most interesting possibilities is dichloroacetate. This drug probably works by enhancing the activity of pyruvate kinase, which in turn increases pyruvate utilization by the mitochondria, thus reducing cytosolic pyruvate. All of these effects together prevent lactate generation. The drug clearly lowers lactate levels in both experimental and clinical lactic acidosis, but there is no evidence that it increases survival. At the present time, there is no indication for its clinical use.

Type B lactic acidosis includes a variety of conditions in which organ failure or a drug increases lactate generation or blocks its conversion to bicarbonate. Heavy ethanol intake increases lactate generation, although it is rarely sufficient by itself to cause severe lactic acidosis. The lactate is formed because the metabolism of 1 mole of alcohol generates 2 moles of NADH. When heavy alcohol intake is combined with marked volume contraction and advanced liver disease, lactate levels may rise more than 5 mEq/L. The treatment is volume replacement and glucose administration.

Lactic acidosis may complicate liver failure of any etiology. Serum lactate rises due to the diseased liver's inability to metabolize lactate. Little can be done for these patients unless the liver recovers.

Phenformin, an oral hypoglycemic agent no longer in clinical use, was associated with a high incidence of lactic acidosis. At present, its only use is to induce lactic acidosis in experimental models.

Lactic acidosis may complicate uncontrolled diabetes mellitus. Insulin stimulates pyruvate dehydrogenase and gluconeogenesis; its absence is associated with increased glycolysis and decreased mitochondrial pyruvate utilization. Lactic acidosis may complicate nonketotic hyperosmolar states as well as diabetic ketoacidosis. Therapy should be directed at the diabetes and its associated volume deficits. Lactic acidosis also has been reported in patients with either solid tumors or leukemia. The precise pathophysiology is unknown. Leukemic cells, which may be present in immense numbers, may continue to anerobically metabolize glucose in the test tube and produce spuriously elevated lactate levels. To avoid this problem, blood from these patients should be chilled on ice immediately after it is obtained. This inhibits further metabolism in vitro.

The outcome in type B lactic acidosis may be better than in the hypoxic variety. Insulin, with glucose if needed, will improve lactate metabolism in the diabetic and phenformin-poisoned patient. In alcoholic lactic acidosis, glucose alone may suffice. Patients with liver disease or tumor associated lactic acidosis are not likely to respond to treatment. Bicarbonate should be infused when pH falls to dangerous levels (i.e., below 7.1).

Patients with bacterial overgrowth in blind loops of small bowel and patients with gastrointestinal hypomotility may develop a unique form of lactic acidosis, d-lactic acidosis. The d-lactate, produced by bowel flora, is absorbed and the patient develops mild to moderate acidosis because d-lactate cannot be metabolized. Definitive treatment is reversal of bowel stasis and alteration of the bacterial flora with antibiotics.

Uremic acidosis. Typically, acidosis seen in patients with renal failure is an anion gap acidosis. The increased anion gap is due to the retention of phosphate, sulfate, hippurate, and other solutes. The acidosis is due to the reduction in nephron mass. Although each nephron secretes acid and produces ammonia at an accelerated rate, there are not enough nephrons to excrete the 100 mEq of acid required every day.

Patients with renal insufficiency may also develop hyperchloremic acidosis, which is commonly due to specific tubular defects (see Renal tubular acidosis). Occasionally, however, hyperchloremic acidosis is seen in patients with renal failure who do not have a tubular defect that impairs acidification. These patients are almost invariably volume contracted. Patients with renal failure have, at the single nephron level, maximum sodium bicarbonate reabsorption and maximum distal proton and potassium secretion. Sodium chloride reabsorption, in contrast, is suppressed. When these patients become volume contracted sodium reabsorption is stimulated. Additional sodium can be reabsorbed only as sodium chloride. The resulting reabsorption of sodium at a 1:1 ratio with chloride induces hyperchloremia. Effective treatment of volume contraction corrects the hyperchloremia.

Salicylate intoxication. Salicylate overdose induces respiratory alkalosis, which is commonly followed by anion gap metabolic acidosis. Salicylates directly stimulate the respiratory center to cause respiratory alkalosis. The ensuing metabolic acidosis is mainly the result of increased lactate production induced by increased respiratory effort. Salicylates also inhibit oxidative phosphorylation, which increases the NADH/NAD ratio, which, in turn, increases lactate formation. When salicylate toxicity is suspected, measures appropriate for the treatment of drug overdose should be used. These measures include gastric emptying of retained tablets, either by emesis or lavage, instillation of activated charcoal, and monitoring of drug blood levels. Low level alkaline diuresis should be induced by the judicious administration of bicarbonate to increase renal excretion of the drug. When severe intoxication is present, dialysis should be initiated.

Methanol intoxication. Alcohol dehydrogenase catalyzes the metabolism of methanol to formaldehyde. Formaldehyde is then converted to formic acid. The formaldehyde is responsible for the eye injury associated with methanol ingestion, whereas the formic acid generates the acidosis. Profound metabolic acidosis in an intoxicated patient should implicate methanol as a cause. If methanol levels cannot be promptly obtained, the presence of an osmolar gap is presumptive evidence of methanol intoxication, especially if there are signs of impaired vision or complaints of snowy vision. Funduscopic examination may show retinal hyperemia or edema.

Because ingestion of as little as 30 ml of methanol may

be lethal, treatment should be vigorous and prompt. Because the toxicity is caused by metabolites, rather than the methanol itself, ethanol should be infused to displace methanol from alcohol dehydrogenase; this slows metabolism of the toxin. The poison should then be eliminated by hemodialysis. In the absence of this treatment, mortality is high.

Ethylene glycol. Ethylene glycol (the main component of antifreeze) ingestion produces a profound anion gap acidosis. As is the case for methanol, the toxicity of the compound is caused by its metabolites. The acidosis results from the production of lactate and from the formation of glycolate and oxalate. Central nervous system manifestations are common and range from intoxication and ataxia to coma and convulsions. Cardiopulmonary failure may also be seen. Renal failure, which may be completely or partially irreversible, is an integral feature of the disorder. It is due to renal oxalate deposition, which causes intratubular obstruction. In addition to history, the diagnosis may be facilitated by finding envelope-shaped oxalate crystals in the urine. Treatment is alcohol infusion to deplete alcohol dehydrogenase and prevent metabolism to oxalate and hemodialysis.

Paraldehyde. Though no longer in use, paraldehyde was once popular in the treatment of alcohol withdrawal. Overdose was associated with anion gap acidosis.

Metabolic acidosis with a normal anion gap

Also known as hyperchloremic metabolic acidosis, these disorders can be divided into those of renal and extrarenal origin. By far the most common cause of hyperchloremic metabolic acidosis is diarrhea. Bicarbonate and fluid loss in stool stimulate renal anion conservation, which results in hyperchloremia. Volume expansion with saline allows the kidney to excrete enough acid to correct the disorder. If acidemia is severe, bicarbonate should also be given. Pancreatic fistulas can also cause bicarbonate loss sufficient to induce the syndrome.

Before the invention of the ileal conduit for urinary diversion, ureterosigmoidostomy was often performed. This procedure resulted in colonic exchange of urinary chloride for bicarbonate causing hyperchloremic acidosis.

Hyperalimentation. Depending on the formulation used for total parenteral nutrition, a lowered blood pH with a normal anion gap may develop. This combination occurs more commonly in patients with renal disease. The acidosis is usually not severe and can be corrected by adjusting the amounts of bicarbonate, acetate, chloride, and amino acids in the solution.

Renal tubular acidosis (RTA). Proximal tubular acidification is predominantly concerned with the reabsorption of bicarbonate, whereas distal acidification titrates the nonbicarbonate urinary buffers and lowers the urine pH. Failure of either of these two processes results in hyperchloremic metabolic acidosis of two distinctive types.

Proximal RTA. Proximal RTA is marked by a decrease in the capacity of the proximal tubule to reclaim bicarbonate. The ensuing bicarbonate diuresis causes metabolic acidosis. When the blood bicarbonate concentration falls to the point that filtered load equals the reduced capacity to reabsorb bicarbonate (usually 15 to 18 mEq/L), urinary bicarbonate loss ceases. From this point on, the urinary pH reflects the prevailing acidemia and is less than 5.5. If bicarbonate is administered and the blood bicarbonate concentration is raised to greater than 20 mEq/L, fractional bicarbonate excretion exceeds 15%. The large amount of sodium bicarbonate delivered to the distal nephron and the high levels of aldosterone induced by the bicarbonate diuresis and volume contraction increase urinary potassium losses. Hypokalemia is an integral feature of the disorder.

The disorder is uncommon; it usually occurs as part of the Fanconi syndrome. This syndrome also includes proximal reabsorptive defects for glucose, urate, phosphate, and amino acids, which makes the diagnosis relatively easy. Only a few families have been reported with an isolated defect in proximal bicarbonate reabsorption.

Treatment of proximal RTA with bicarbonate is ineffective because the bicarbonate is excreted as fast as it is given. Bicarbonate administration also increases distal potassium secretion. The best approach to treatment is to induce modest volume contraction with thiazide diuretics. The decrease in volume stimulates residual bicarbonate reabsorptive capacity and results in an increase in the steady state blood bicarbonate.

Distal RTA. The distal forms of RTA occur more commonly than the proximal varieties of RTA, and are all marked by an inability to secrete protons in the collecting duct. It now appears that protons are secreted in these distal nephron segments by two distinct proton ATPase pumps. The first of these pumps is an electrogenic proton ATPase; the second is an electroneutral proton-potassium ATPase, which is related to the gastric acid pump. The combined work of these two pumps allows the collecting duct to generate a 1000:1 proton gradient between urine and blood. Thus the urine pH normally may be as low as 4.5. Because the proton ATPase is electrogenic, its activity is influenced by the electrical environment of the duct. Sodium reabsorption in the cortical collecting duct generates a lumen negative electrical potential, which favors the secretion of positively charged protons into the urine by the proton ATPase. Note that sodium reabsorption thereby influences distal acidification in an indirect manner; no direct sodium-proton exchange occurs.

Aldosterone affects the activity of the proton ATPase in two ways. First, by the stimulation of sodium reabsorption in the cortical collecting duct, which increases the lumen negative potential and subsequently enhances proton secretion, and, second, by direct stimulation of the proton ATPase.

The precise role of the proton-potassium ATPase is not yet fully clarified. The major function of this pump may be potassium reclamation. If so, this pump may be more important in pathologic states than in normal acid-base physiology, but this enzyme may also be an integral part of normal acid excretion. The relative importance of these two pumps to total acidification is not known in either humans or animals. Failure of either might lead to mild distal RTA, failure of both to a more severe variant. Two other aspects of the distal acidification system might lead to acidification defects. First, the maintenance of a three pH unit gradient demands that there is a tight epithelium, which does not allow backleak of secreted acid. A failure here would limit the achievable pH. Second, the effectiveness of distal acidification is greatly affected by the availability of ammonia as a buffer. Acidification will be defective if any of these mechanisms fail.

Traditionally, classic distal RTA is said to be the result of failure of the proton ATPase pump in the absence of any defect in sodium reabsorption or potassium secretion. The potassium losses in the classic syndrome would be due to the passive increase in potassium secretion, which would occur because electrogenic proton secretion no longer shunted out the negative potential generated by sodium reabsorption. The discovery of the proton-potassium exchange pump in the renal collecting duct permits a much simpler hypothesis. If normal proton-potassium ATPase function is required for maintenance of acid-base balance, then a defect of this enzyme might result in both acidosis (from the resulting loss of acid secretion) and hypokalemia (from the loss of distal nephron potassium reabsorption). Indeed, animals given vanadate, an inhibitor of the proton-potassium ATPase in vitro, develop a hypokalemic, hyperchloremic metabolic acidosis, which closely models classic distal RTA. Table 353-2 presents the hypothetical biochemical basis for distal RTA.

Clinically, the disease usually, but not always, begins during childhood. The identification of a large outbreak of distal RTA in northern Thailand has led to the hypothesis that an environmental factor may be inhibiting one or the other distal nephron proton pump.

Becausé of unrelenting acidemia and the exhaustion of blood buffers, the skeleton is titrated to buffer the retained acid. This mobilizes calcium salts from bone and is the cause of both the osteomalacia (or renal rickets) and the nephrocalcinosis and nephrolithiasis typical of this disease.

A similar form of hypokalemic distal RTA is sometimes seen during amphotericin treatment. This disorder results not from failure to secrete protons, but from an inability to maintain pH gradients in the distal nephron. Thus secreted acid back diffuses to the blood.

The key diagnostic feature of the syndrome is hyperchloremic hypokalemic metabolic acidosis associated with a urinary pH persistently above 5.5. If the blood pH is below 7.35, measurement of urine pH with a pH meter is sufficient to make the diagnosis. If the blood pH is higher or there are diagnostic ambiguities, sodium sulfate may be infused or furosemide given orally to test distal nephron function. These agents stimulate distal acidification and normally lower urine pH to below 5.5. They also stimulate urinary potassium excretion and, thus, serve as a test of potassium secretory capacity as well.

Treatment is the daily administration of 60 to 100 mEq of bicarbonate or bicarbonate equivalent such as Shohl's solution. Potassium deficits should also be corrected, although chronic potassium replacement may not be necessary once the initial deficit has been corrected and bicarbonate concentration maintained in the normal range.

Hyperkalemic distal RTA occurs more commonly than the hypokalemic distal RTA. It is most often seen in patients with obstructive uropathy and is also seen in patients with hemoglobin S. Virtually all patients with the disorder have a reduced GFR. The central defect appears to be impaired sodium transport in the cortical collecting duct. Reduced sodium transport at this site decreases the lumen negative potential difference and secondarily slows potassium and proton secretion. These patients also cannot lower urinary pH below 5.5. They are distinguished from the classic form of distal RTA by hyperkalemia and reduced potassium excretion.

Another form of hyperkalemic acidosis is seen in patients with aldosterone deficiency or resistance (Chapter 110). These syndromes differ from the hyperkalemic distal RTA just described in that the urine pH is typically below 5.5 when the patient is acidemic. Aldosterone deficiency or resistance slows the rate of the H-ATPase pump, but does not impair its ability to generate or maintain pH gradients. The acidosis develops because of a failure of ammonia formation and secretion. The decrease in ammoniagenesis is the result of hyperkalemia; aldosterone deficiency itself likely also impairs ammonia formation. The only difference between aldosterone deficiency and resistance is that blood aldosterone levels are low in the former and normal or elevated in the latter. A diagnostic schema for those hyperkalemic syndromes is presented in Table 353-3. These syndromes may be provoked or exacerbated by drugs that in-

Table 353-2. Potential causes of dRTA

Defect	Syndrome
↓ H, K-ATPase activity	Hypokalemic dRTA
↓ H-ATPase activity	Normokalemic dRTA
↓ CCT Na transport	Voltage-dependent (hyperkalemic) dRTA
Aldosterone deficiency	Hyperkalemic metabolic acidosis with low urine pH
↓ Capacity to maintain steep pH gradients	Hyperchloremic metabolic acidosis with normal UpCO*

*The hypokalemia typical of amphotericin induced dRTA is due to increased cell permeability to potassium rather than decreased potassium transport capacity.

Table 353-3. Plasma aldosterone and urine pH in distal renal tubular acidosis

	Urine pH in acidemia	Plasma aldosterone
Aldosterone deficiency	<5.5	Low
Aldosterone resistance	<5.5	Normal or high
Voltage-dependent RTA	>5.5	Normal or high
Combined aldosterone deficiency and voltage-dependent RTA	>5.5	Low

hibit aldosterone release such as heparin or that decrease renal potassium excretion (e.g., potassium-sparing diuretics).

Compensation. Regardless of etiology, metabolic acidosis stimulates ventilation, which results in a fall in PCO_2 averaging about 1.2 times the fall in bicarbonate. The fall in PCO_2 (respiratory compensation) minimizes the fall in pH caused by the decline in bicarbonate. A PCO_2 that is not as low as expected indicates either that the acidosis is of very recent onset or that there is concomitant lung disease. A PCO_2 that is too low for the prevailing bicarbonate suggests that respiratory alkalosis is also present.

Respiratory alkalosis

Respiratory alkalosis is the most common acid-base disorder. It may be due to stimulation of the respiratory center by emotion, central nervous system disease, progesterone excess, or ammonia (see the accompanying box). It is ubiquitous in pregnancy and in liver disease. It is also seen during hypoxia, whether the result of an oxygen-poor environment, heart failure, or lung disease. It is much more common than respiratory acidosis in patients with chronic pulmonary disease. The disorder is treated by confronting the underlying disease, if possible.

Causes of respiratory alkalosis

- Hypoxemia
  - Most pulmonary disease
  - Organic heart disease
    - Congenital heart disease with right to left shunts
    - Congestive heart failure
  - Altitude
- Stimulation of respiratory center
  - Drugs
    - Salicylates
    - Catecholamines
    - Theophylline
    - Nikethemide, ethmivan, doxapram
  - Progesterone excess
    - Pregnancy
    - Cirrhosis
  - CNS disease
    - Subarachnoid hemorrhage
    - Disease of respiratory center
    - Cheyne-Stokes respirations
  - Fever
  - Sepsis
  - Anxiety
- Stimulation of peripheral pulmonary receptors
  - Pneumonia
  - Asthma
  - Embolism
  - Pulmonary edema
  - Pulmonary fibrosis
  - Pleural disease
- Errors of ventilator management

Compensation. Acute respiratory alkalosis is characterized by an increased pH secondary to a fall in Pco_2. The blood bicarbonate is slightly reduced because of buffering but no more than a few milliequivalents per liter. If the respiratory alkalosis persists for 12 to 24 hours, there is a fall in bicarbonate concentration owing to renal bicarbonate excretion and acid retention. Because respiratory alkalosis is the best compensated of the four acid-base disorders, blood pH in chronic respiratory alkalosis is usually normal.

Respiratory acidosis

The acid-base consequences of respiratory acidosis are minor compared to those of hypoxemia produced by ventilatory failure. The presence of respiratory acidosis is prima facie evidence of a severe disorder of pulmonary function, the central nervous system, or the peripheral mechanics of respiration (see the accompanying box). Ensuring adequate oxygenation takes priority over treating the acidosis.

Only a limited number of derangements lead to respiratory failure and acidosis. Central hypoventilation is caused by a number of disorders. It may be iatrogenic; a host of drugs may depress respiration. Neuromuscular disease and

Causes of respiratory acidosis

- Disorders of ventilatory control
  - Central nervous system
    - Depression of respiratory center
      - Anesthetics
      - Drug intoxication
      - Primary central hypoventilation
      - Myxedema
      - Oxygen therapy in chronic hypercapnic patients
      - Sleep
  - Peripheral neuromuscular disease
    - Disorders of peripheral nerves
      - Spinal cord injury
      - Phrenic nerve palsy
      - Guillain-Barré syndrome
      - Myasthenia gravis
      - Paralytic agents
      - Botulism
    - Disorders of muscle
      - Myositis, myopathy, muscular dystrophies
      - Fatigue in hypokalemia, hypophosphatemia
      - Fatigue in obstructive airways disease
- Disorders of pulmonary function
  - Restrictive lung disease
    - Kyphoscoliosis
    - Flail chest
  - Airways obstruction
    - Upper airways obstruction (trachea, larynx, bronchi)
    - Asthma and chronic obstructive pulmonary disease
- Shunts
  - Congenital heart disease with left to right shunt
  - Intrapulmonary shunt
    - Arteriovenous malformation
    - Severe pneumonia, large emboli
- Errors of ventilator management

electrolyte imbalance, particularly hypokalemia, may impair the muscles of breathing. Pulmonary failure may arise because of emphysema, airway obstruction, or vascular shunts. These disorders are best reviewed in the contest of pulmonary disease (Chapter 200).

Compensation. Carbon dioxide retention immediately lowers blood pH and raises blood bicarbonate, the latter because of buffering. Beginning 2 to 3 hours and culminating 2 to 5 days after the start of hypercapnia, the blood bicarbonate rises because of the accelerated renal excretion of acid. The kidney also increases its rate of bicarbonate reabsorption to maintain the high bicarbonate level. The bicarbonate concentration increases 3 to 4 mEq/L for every 10 mm Hg rise in PCO_2. The renal response minimizes the fall in pH but does not completely prevent it.

Because the PCO_2 may change quickly, confusion sometimes arises when a patient with chronic respiratory acidosis has a rapid fall in PCO_2. For example, if a one places a patient with a PCO_2 of 90 mm Hg, a bicarbonate of 40 mEq/L, and a pH of 7.27 on a ventilator and acutely lowers the PCO_2 to 40 mm Hg, buffering will only lower the bicarbonate to 38 and the pH will rise to 7.60. The patient does not have metabolic alkalosis; rather, the patient suffers from overcompensated respiratory acidosis. If the effective volume is normal, the kidney will excrete the extra bicarbonate during the next day and restore the pH to normal. Acetazolamide is often useful to accelerate urinary bicarbonate excretion.

MIXED ACID-BASE DISORDERS

Mixed acid-base disturbances are probably more common than simple disorders and often present a diagnostic challenge. A good history is critical. For example, patients with cirrhosis almost invariably have chronic respiratory alkalosis. Complicated acid-base disturbances in a patient with advanced liver disease may be diagnosed much more easily if the physician assumes that the patient had a preexisting respiratory alkalosis.

Careful analysis of serial blood gas and electrolyte data will often unravel what appears to be a confusing derangement. An patient with asthma who previously had respiratory alkalosis but now is developing respiratory failure as the PCO_2 rises from 20 to 30 mm Hg will have a low bicarbonate and low PCO_2; however, the pH will not be low. The patient does not have metabolic acidosis, which might be the presumptive diagnosis if only one blood gas measurement was available. Serial blood gas determinations will clearly demonstrate that the patient is developing respiratory acidosis on the basis of respiratory alkalosis.

Acid-base nomograms (Fig. 353-1) may be useful if it is remembered that the utility of such devices declines as problems become more complex. When a patient's data are plotted on the nomogram and the point falls within the confidence limits of one of the curves, the implication is that a simple acid-base disorder is present. Careful clinical correlation is essential because mixed disturbances may masquerade as simple ones or may be completely hidden from the graph. For example, consider a patient with vomiting and diarrhea who has a pH of 7.40, and a blood bicarbonate of 24 mEq/L. A good history and awareness of the presence of hypokalemia and hypochloremia result in the correct diagnosis of mixed metabolic acidosis and alkalosis.

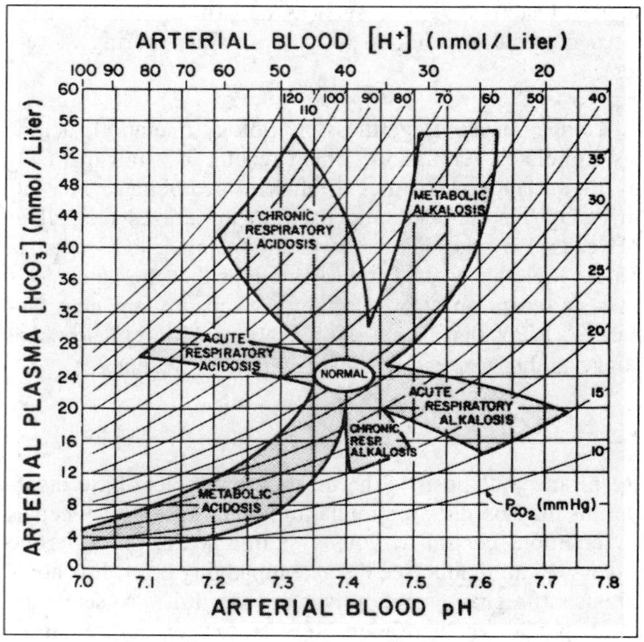

Fig. 353-1. Acid-base nomogram. (Modified from Cogan MG and Rector FC Jr: Acid-base disorders. In Brenner BM and Rector FC Jr, editors: The kidney, Philadelphia, 1986, WB Saunders.)

REFERENCES

Alpern RA et al: Renal acidification mechanisms. In Brenner BM and Rector FC Jr, editors: The kidney, Philadelphia, 1991, WB Saunders.

Cogan MG and Rector FC Jr: Acid-base disorders. In Brenner BM and Rector FC Jr, editors, The kidney, Philadelphia, 1991, WB Saunders.

Emmett M and Seldin DW: Evaluation of acid-base disorders from plasma conjunction. In Seldin DW and Giebisch G, editors: The regulation of acid-base balance, New York, 1989, Raven Press.

Emmett M and Seldin DW: Overproduction acidosis. In Seldin DW and Gebisch G, editors: The regulation of acid-base balance, New York, 1989, Raven Press.

Laski ME, and Kurtzman NA: Use of urinary tests in evaluation of acid-base disorders. In Seldin DW and Giebisch G, editors: The regulation of acid-base balance, New York, 1989, Raven Press.

Laski ME and Kurtzman NA: Acid-base disturbances in pulmonary medicine. In Arieff AI and DeFronzo RA, editors: Fluid, electrolyte, and acid-base disorders, New York, 1985, Churchill Livingstone.

Sabatini S and Kurtzman NA: Pathophysiology of the renal tubular acidosis, Semin Nephrol 11:202, 1991.

Sabatini S and Kurtzman NA: The maintenance of metabolic alkalosis: factors which decrease bicarbonate excretion, Kidney Int 25:357, 1984.

CHAPTER

354 Glomerular Diseases

William G. Couser

Almost half of the 120,000 patients with end-stage renal disease in the United States suffer from some form of glomerular disease. The cost of dialysis and transplant therapy for chronic renal failure now exceeds $4 billion annually. Glomerular diseases may be primary or secondary due to glomerular involvement in a number of systemic illnesses.

The clinical manifestations of glomerular disease can be considered in two broad categories, with overlap between them. Some patients present with acute glomerulonephritis. Signs of glomerular inflammation include proteinuria (usually less than 3.5 g/day and not in the nephrotic range), red cells and red cell casts in the urinary sediment, and often a reduction in renal function that may be associated with sodium and water retention and hypertension. The clinical and pathophysiologic aspects of the acute nephritic syndrome are considered in Chapter 103 (acute nephritic syndrome). Currently recognized glomerular diseases that may cause this syndrome are discussed in detail in this chapter, and a summary of their distinguishing features is presented in Table 354-1. A second group of patients with glomerular disease present with nephrotic range proteinuria (greater than 3.5 g/day in adults) and usually other manifestations of nephrotic syndrome including hypoalbuminemia, edema, hyperlipidemia, and lipiduria. The pathophysiology of proteinuria and the nephrotic syndrome are discussed in Chapters 101 and 104. This chapter describes the clinical and pathologic features of the major glomerular diseases that cause the idiopathic nephrotic syndrome. The features of these diseases are summarized in Table 354-4.

In addition to distinguishing between acute glomerulonephritis and the nephrotic syndrome, it is also useful to separate patients with glomerular disease into those with a primary renal disease and those with some systemic disease associated with major extrarenal manifestations. Glomerular involvement in several systemic diseases is discussed at the end of this chapter.

MECHANISMS AND CONSEQUENCES OF IMMUNE GLOMERULAR INJURY

Most glomerular diseases are mediated by immune mechanisms involving deposition of antibody and/or immune complex formation in glomeruli. Diseases in which immune deposits are not seen, such as minimal change disease (MCD) or idiopathic crescentic glomerulonephritis, are also believed to be immunologically mediated, but the mechanisms are less well understood. Glomerular immune deposits may be continuous, or linear, as in anti-glomerular basement membrane (GBM) disease (see Fig. 354-5, *A*) or discontinuous and granular in various forms of immune complex nephritis (see Fig. 354-2, *B;* 354-3, *B;* 354-5, *B*). Linear deposits represent glomerular deposits of an autoantibody to a GBM antigen. Anti-GBM antibody disposition is relatively uncommon clinically and causes only Goodpasture's syndrome and anti-GBM nephritis without pulmonary hemorrhage.

Granular, or immune complex, deposits are much more common and may be seen at three different sites in the glomerulus: within the glomerular mesangium (IgA nephropathy, lupus nephritis, see Fig. 354-3, *B*), along with the inner, or subendothelial, surface of the capillary wall (lupus, type I membranoproliferative glomerulonephritis, see Fig. 354-10A) and along the outer, or subepithelial, surface of the capillary wall as in membranous nephropathy (see Fig. 354-8, *C*). The locations of these different types of deposits are illustrated schematically in Fig. 354-1. Four factors determine the type of glomerular lesion that results from glomerular immune deposit formation: (1) site of the deposit formation (subepithelial deposits are noninflammatory, subendothelial, and mesangial deposits incite inflammation), (2) mechanism of deposit formations (local immune complex formation is more nephritogenic than preformed complex trapping), (3) biologic properties of the

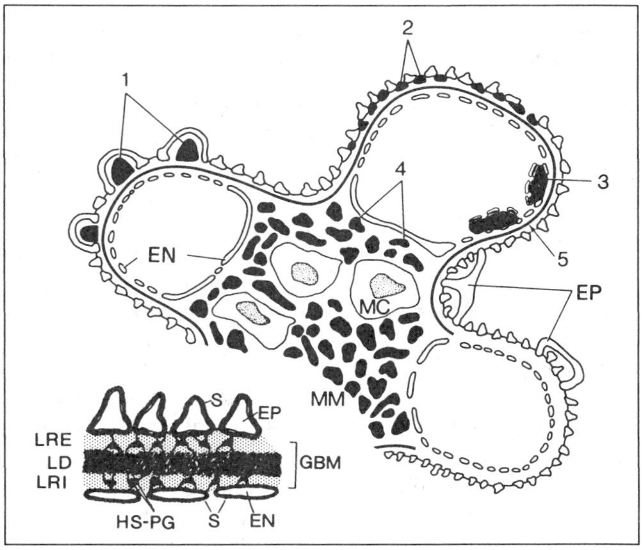

Fig. 354-1. Schematic depiction of intraglomerular sites of immune complex formation. Subepithelial deposits such as those in postinfectious glomerulonephritis *(1)* or membranous nephropathy *(2)* apparently form by local, or in situ, mechanisms. Subendothelial *(3)* and mesangial *(4)* deposits are usually seen together and may form locally or result from the passive trapping of preformed immune complexes from the circulation. Anti-GBM antibody deposits are in a linear pattern within the capillary wall itself *(5)*. The mechanism of formation, composition, quantity, and relative accessibility of each of these deposits to circulating inflammatory cells are the major determinants of the type of lesion produced. The inset illustrates the three layers of the normal glomerular capillary wall, endothelial cells (EN), GBM, and epithelial cells (EP). The negative charge on the capillary wall results from the sialoproteins *(5)* coating the endothelial and epithelial cell surfaces and the heparin-sulfate proteoglycan (HS-PG) anionic sites in the lamina rare interna (LRI) and externa (LRE) of the GBM. (From Alder S and Couser WG: Am J Med Sci 289:55-60, 1985.)

Table 354-1. Summary of primary renal diseases that normally present as acute glomerulonephritis

Diseases	Poststreptococcal glomerulonephritis	IgA nephropathy	Goodpasture's syndrome	Idiopathic crescentic nephritis
Clinical manifestations				
Age and sex	All ages, mean 7, 2:1 male	15-35, 2:1 male	15-30, 6:1 male	Mean 58, 2:1 male
Acute nephritic syndrome	90%	50%	90%	90%
Asymptomatic hematuria	Occasionally	50%	Rare	Rare
Nephrotic syndrome	10-20%	Rare	Rare	10-20%
Hypertension	70%	30-50%	Rare	25%
Acute renal failure*	50% (transient)	Very rare	50%	60%
Other	1-3 week latent period	Follows viral syndromes	Pulmonary hemorrhage Iron-deficiency anemia	None
Recurs in transplants	No	Yes	Only if antibody present	No
Laboratory findings	ASO titers (70%) Positive streptozyme (95%) C3-C9, normal C1, C4	Increased IgA-fibronectin aggregates IgA in dermal capillaries	Positive anti-GBM antibody	Increased anti-neutrophil cytoplasmic antibody (ANCA)
Immunogenetics	HLA D "EN" (9)* ? DR4 (4)	DR4 (4), ? HLA Bw 35	HLA DR2 (16), B7 (5)	None established
Renal pathology				
Light microscopy	Diffuse proliferation	Focal proliferation	Focal diffuse proliferation with crescents	Crescentic GN
Immunofluorescence	Granular IgG, C3	Diffuse mesangial IgA, IgG	Linear IgG, C3	No immune deposits
Electron microscopy	Subepithelial humps	Mesangial deposits	No deposits	No deposits
Treatment	Supportive	None established	Plasma exchange, steroids cyclophosphamide	Steroid pulse therapy, cyclophosphamide
Prognosis	95% resolve spontaneously 5% RPGN or slowly progressive	Slow progression in 25%-50%	75% stabilize or improve if treated early	75% stabilize or improve if treated early

*Relative risk.
RPGN, rapidly progressive glomerulonephritis.

antibodies deposited (complement fixing antibodies produce more injury than noncomplement fixing), and (4) amount of antibody deposited.

The subepithelial immune complex deposits seen in membranous nephropathy are probably all formed locally, or in situ, by one of two mechanisms. An autoantibody response to an antigenic component of normal glomerular epithelial cells results in immune complex formation on the cell surface followed by capping and shedding of the immune complexes from the cell surface into the adjacent lamina rara externa to produce subepithelial deposits. Alternatively, exogenous, nonrenal antigens, particularly if they are positively charged or cationic, may first become localized in the glomerular capillary wall by binding electrically to heparin sulfate-proteoglycan anionic sites in the lamina rara externa (see Fig. 354-1). Antibody binding to these antigens then results in subepithelial immune complex formation and proteinuria.

Regardless of whether subepithelial deposits contain renal or extrarenal antigens, they cause proteinuria by a mechanism that requires assembly of the complement C5b-9 membrane attack complex and does not involve inflammatory cell participation. The lack of inflammatory change is probably because the formation of deposits on the outer surface of the capillary wall renders them inaccessible to circulating neutrophils and macrophages.

Mesangial and subendothelial deposits usually contain exogenous antigens and occur together. Mesangial deposits are present in milder forms of diseases such as class II-III lupus nephritis and IgA nephropathy. Subendothelial deposits appear in addition to the mesangial deposits when the disease is more severe (class IV lupus nephritis, severe IgA nephropathy). Deposits at both sites probably form by similar mechanisms. They may be formed locally or they can result from the passive trapping of preformed immune complexes from the circulation. Glomerular trapping of antigenic macromolecules or of preformed immune complexes is determined by systemic factors such as renal blood flow and mononuclear phagocyte system (MPS) function; properties of the complexes themselves such as size, charge, and avidity; and glomerular properties including charge, permeability, and mesangial uptake and clearing mechanisms.

Because subendothelial and mesangial deposits (and anti-GBM antibody deposits) are accessible to circulating inflammatory cells such as neutrophils and macrophages, such cells localize at the site of deposit formation by immune adherence mechanisms involving Fc or C3b receptors on the cell surfaces and by responding to chemotactic products of complement activation such as C5a. Activated inflammatory cells release proteolytic enzymes and reactive oxygen species believed to cause the capillary wall damage, which results in proteinuria, hematuria, and in some cases leakage of fibrin into Bowman's space to initiate glomerular crescent formation. Crescents represent proliferating parietal epithelial cells of Bowman's capsule and mononuclear cells in a bed of fibrin, which is deposited in part due to tissue factor released by macrophages that migrate through gaps in the capillary wall into Bowman's space. Thus crescents are markers of severe glomerular injury, but not causes of injury. These inflammatory changes are the histologic hallmarks of acute glomerulonephritis.

In addition to these morphologic changes, functional consequences of acute glomerular injury reduce the glomerular filtration rate (GFR). Immune reactions within the glomerulus result in glomerular vasoconstriction with a marked decrease in glomerular plasma flow. In addition to reduced plasma flow, a decrease in the filtering surface area (Kf, LpA) occurs due to the adherence of inflammatory cells to the capillary wall and endothelial cell damage. All of these processes in concert account for the decrease in GFR seen in acute glomerulonephritis. As a compensatory mechanism, there is also increased glomerular synthesis of vasodilatory prostaglandins, primarily PGE_2, which increase glomerular plasma flow and therefore help to maintain the filtration rate.

Finally, immune injury in one portion of the glomerulus may lead to increases in glomerular hydrostatic pressures and plasma flows in other capillary loops and in other glomeruli as a compensatory mechanism to preserve GFR. These increased intraglomerular pressures and flows (hyperfiltration) contribute to maintaining GFR in the short term, but appear to induce glomerular damage and destruction over longer periods of time. The principal morphologic consequence of these adaptive changes is glomerulosclerosis, a lesion characteristic of the chronic stages of most progressive glomerular diseases.

GLOMERULAR DISEASES THAT USUALLY PRESENT AS ACUTE GLOMERULONEPHRITIS (Table 354-1)

Postinfectious glomerulonephritis

Etiology and incidence. The etiology of postinfectious glomerulonephritis is a tissue-invading infection with a nephritogenic organism. Although poststreptococcal glomerulonephritis (PSGN) is the prototype of postinfectious glomerulonephritis, glomerulonephritis may occur after infection with a number of other agents including bacteria, viruses, fungi, protozoa, helminths, and spirochetes. Most of these organisms induce a proliferative glomerulonephritis associated with glomerular immune complex deposits. This section describes only PSGN in detail.

The incidence of streptococcal nephritis varies considerably depending on the source and site of infection, but has diminished markedly in developed countries, due to improved hygiene and health care. PSGN may occur with streptococcal infection at any site, occurs primarily after exposure to a nephritogenic M type, and has a very variable attack rate. Nephritogenic streptococci are usually group A (beta-hemolytic) organisms. M type 12 is the most common source in the United States.

Pathogenesis and pathophysiology. The glomerular injury observed is believed to be consequent to an inflammatory response generated by the formation of immune complex deposits that may contain streptococcal antigens in the mesangium and on the glomerular capillary walls. Several features of this disease including the latent period between the infection and the onset of nephritis, hypocomplementemia, and granular immune complex deposits in glomeruli suggest that the disease is similar to the acute bovine serum albumin (BSA)–serum sickness model in rabbits.

Pathology. The characteristic features of PSGN by light microscopy, immunoflouresence microscopy (IF), and electron microscopy (EM) are illustrated in Fig. 354-2. By light microscopy the lesion is a diffuse proliferative glomerulonephritis (Fig. 354-2, *A*). All glomeruli exhibit a marked hypercellularity with narrowing or occlusion of capillary loops. In about 5% of patients, glomerular crescent formation similar to that in rapidly progressive glomerulonephritis (RPGN) (see later discussion) may be seen.

By IF microscopy coarsely granular deposits of IgG and C3 are seen along the glomerular capillary walls and less conspicuously in the mesangium in the acute phase (Fig. 354-2, *B*). Later C3 may be found without immunoglobulin, and deposits of C3 alone may persist and be detectable for many months.

By EM the immune deposits are seen as discrete, subepithelial, electron-dense nodules, or "humps," (Fig. 354-2, *C*). Humps are usually present at the outset of the disease and persist for about 6 weeks before their gradual resolution makes identification difficult.

Clinical and laboratory features. The onset of clinical signs and symptoms of PSGN occurs after a 1- to 3-week latent period after infection with a nephritogenic strain of group A streptococcus. Nephritis due to a sporadic streptococcal pharyngitis develops in about 5% of infected patients after a latent period of about 10 days. It occurs most commonly in children between 3 and 12 years, usually during the winter and spring. Males are affected twice as commonly as females. Streptococcal pyoderma usually presents in the summer and fall with vesicular lesions on the skin of the extremities, regional adenopathy, and a paucity of systemic symptoms. It may be epidemic. Nephritis occurs in up to 50% of these patients after a latent period of about 3 weeks. Males and females are affected with equal frequency.

PSGN characteristically produces all of the features of the acute nephritic syndrome, which is discussed in Chapter 345. The most common presenting features are the abrupt onset of gross hematuria and a smoky or coffee-colored appearance to the urine accompanied by edema and hypertension. The gross hematuria may last for 1 to 2 weeks, although microscopic hematuria can persist for

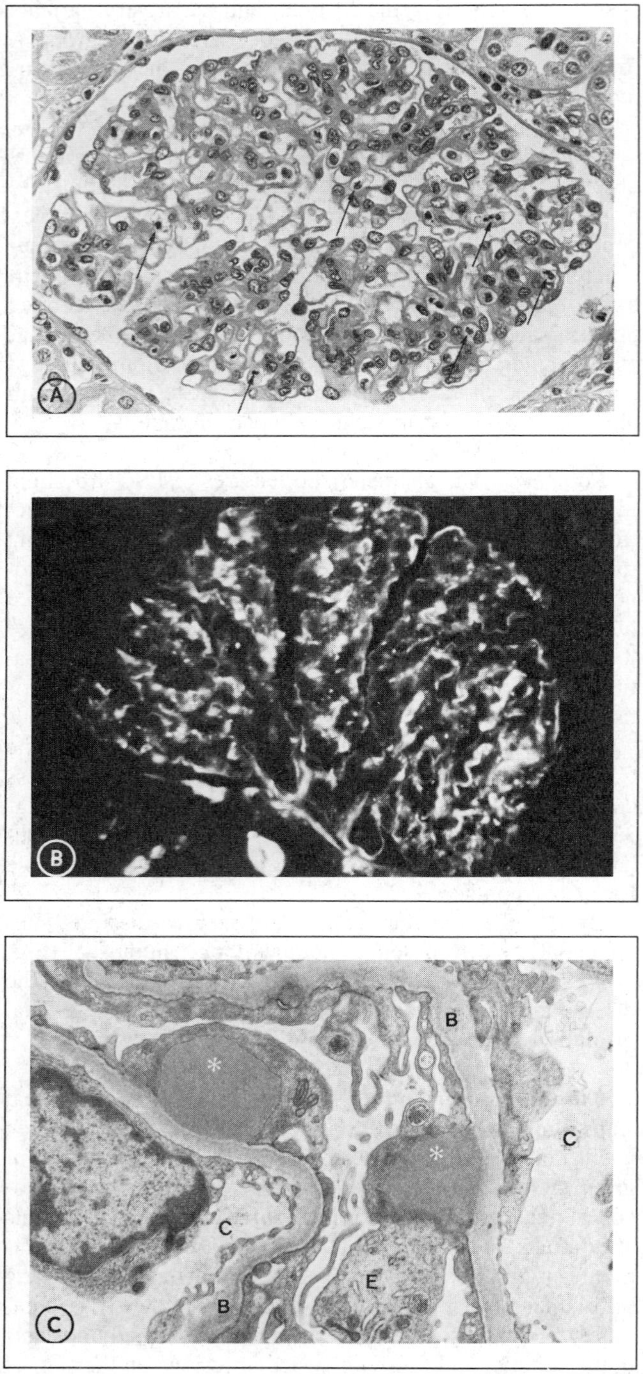

Fig. 354-2. Renal biopsies from a patient with acute poststreptococcal glomerulonephritis. **A,** Light microscopy shows diffuse cellular proliferation with numerous neutrophils *(arrows)* in glomerular capillaries (Hematoxylin-eosin stain; ×375). **B,** Immunofluorescence shows diffuse coarsely granular deposits of IgG on capillary walls and in the mesangium (×400). **C,** Electron microscopy demonstrates two large electron dense "humps" *(asterisks)* on the subepithelial surface of the capillary wall. *B:* basement membrane; *C:* capillary lumen; *E:* epithelial cell (Uranyl and lead stain; ×10,000).

months. Edema is often periorbital initially, but may progress to generalized anasarca with ascites and pleural effusions. Proteinuria is almost invariably present, but daily urine protein excretion is usually less than 3.5 g. However, about 20% of patients will have transient nephrotic range proteinuria at some time during their illness. Hypertension is largely volume-dependent due to renal retention of sodium and water. Both hypertension and edema resolve after the brisk diuresis that heralds recovery. Finally, renal function is decreased to a variable degree ranging from only mild elevations in creatinine and blood urea nitrogen to acute oliguric renal failure requiring dialysis. Renal dysfunction is greater in older patients and patients with nephritis secondary to pharyngitis.

In addition to the classic features of the acute nephritic syndrome mentioned earlier, patients with PSGN may also exhibit other extrarenal signs and symptoms, including congestive heart failure and cerebral symptoms related to hypertension and cerebral edema including headache, nausea and vomiting, and alterations in consciousness, which may progress to convulsions. Abdominal pain, nausea, and vomiting may also be seen.

The diagnosis of acute PSGN is usually supported by laboratory studies. Urinalysis reveals evidence of glomerular inflammation with many red blood cells, red cell casts, occasional white blood cells, and protein. The need to examine a fresh urine specimen to demonstrate red cell casts cannot be overemphasized. The urine is often concentrated with a low urine sodium concentration indicating severe glomerular disease with well-presented tubular function.

Positive cultures for group A beta hemolytic streptococci may be obtained from infected sites in about 25% of patients if treatment has not already been instituted. The most commonly measured serologic parameters are the antistreptolysin O (ASO) titer, which exceeds 200 Todd units within 1 to 3 weeks in about 70% of patients and persists for several months, and the streptozyme test, which is the most sensitive measure of antistreptococcal antibodies available. The ASO titer, however, is often not elevated in patients with nephritis secondary to streptococcal pyoderma.

Levels of C3 are low in over 95% of patients with PSGN during the first 2 weeks of the illness and are usually accompanied by decreased levels of the terminal complement components C5 to C9. The classic pathway components C1, C4, and C2 are often normal, indicating activation predominantly of the alternate complement pathway. Neither the level of antistreptococcal antibody response nor the degree of hypocomplementemia correlates well with the severity or outcome of the renal disease.

With regard to prognosis, about 95% of patients recover normal renal function within 2 months of the onset of the disease, although abnormal proteinuria and hematuria may persist for 1 to 2 years. Spontaneous recovery is the rule even in patients with crescents and disease severe enough to require short periods of dialysis. About 5% of patients with PSGN develop a severe crescentic lesion with prolonged acute renal failure. About half of these patients still recover spontaneously, but the remainder rapidly develop end-stage renal disease. This course is more common in older patients with persistent hypocomplementemia and nephrotic syndrome.

Progression to end-stage renal disease has also occurred in occasional patients after apparent complete recovery from documented episodes of PSGN. In the absence of persistent proteinuria, however, this event appears to be rare. Several prospective studies of large numbers of patients with epidemic forms of acute PSGN have shown no tendency for recovered patients to develop progressive renal disease.

Diagnosis. The differential diagnosis of PSGN includes any of the primary glomerular diseases that cause the acute nephritic syndrome (see Table 354-1), including IgA nephropathy following an upper respiratory tract infection and idiopathic crescentic glomerulonephritis. Both membranoproliferative glomerulonephritis, which may occasionally follow a streptococcal infection, and lupus nephritis are associated with hypocomplementemia and must be ruled out. In classic cases renal biopsy is not required. If atypical features are present, or other findings such as renal failure or persistent hypocomplementemia suggest a crescentic lesion with a poor prognosis, a biopsy should be performed to determine if treatment for RPGN should be considered.

Treatment. The vast majority of patients recover spontaneously regardless of the severity of the initial disease; therefore usually only supportive therapy is indicated. Antibiotic treatment is appropriate if evidence of persistent streptococcal infection is present. Early penicillin therapy may blunt rises in antistreptococcal antibody titers but does not reduce the incidence or severity of poststreptococcal nephritis. Sodium restriction and diuretics are critical in managing or preventing hypertension, edema, and congestive heart failure. Dialysis should be used if necessary. Spontaneous recovery has been reported following up to 31 days of oliguria.

Patients who develop a severe, rapidly progressive course associated with extensive glomerular crescent formation have a form of RPGN and may be considered for treatment as discussed later. In view of the generally good prognosis, however, great caution must be exercised in selecting patients for treatment with any agents that have significant toxicity.

Other postinfectious glomerulonephritides

Subacute bacterial endocarditis (SBE). Some hematuria and proteinuria occur in about 70% of patients with SBE, but renal failure and nephrotic syndrome are uncommon. Renal involvement may be seen with infection of any heart valve and with a wide variety of organisms. Staphylococci and streptococci are most commonly involved. Renal lesions are most severe in patients with prolonged disease or right-sided cardiac involvement in which negative blood cultures may obscure the diagnosis. Associated laboratory abnormalities usually include reduced levels of both classic and alternate pathway complement components. The most common glomerular lesion is a focal proliferative glomerulonephritis often with necrosis and intracapillary thrombi associated with granular immune complex deposits of IgG, IgM, and C3 by IF and mesangial and subendothelial deposits by EM. Both bacterial antigens and specific antibodies to them have been identified in the glomerular deposits of a few patients. Occasional patients with endocarditis develop a crescentic glomerulonephritis with rapid loss of renal function. The disease is usually not progressive, however, and resolves without specific therapy when the cardiac infection is eradicated.

Shunt nephritis. A syndrome quite similar to that in SBE but with more nephrotic than nephritic features has been reported in patients with ventriculoatrial shunts inserted to correct internal hydrocephalus. Infections have usually been with coagulase-negative *Staphylococcus albus*. Proteinuria and glomerular histologic abnormalities, which resemble type I membranoproliferative glomerulonephritis (MPGN), are reversible when the infection is eradicated, a process that requires shunt removal as well as antibiotic therapy.

Nephritis associated with visceral abscesses. An association has been reported between bacterial abscesses at several sites, usually in the lung or abdominal cavity, with or without septicemia, and development of acute nephritis, often with oliguria, crescents, and acute renal failure. In contrast to the previously discussed diseases, patients with this condition commonly have normal serum complement levels, glomerular IF frequently is positive for C3 without immunoglobulins, and no bacterial antigens have been identified in the lesions. The pathogenesis of the glomerular lesion is not clear. The renal lesion is usually reversible if the septic site can be removed.

IgA nephropathy

IgA nephropathy is usually a primary renal disease, but the same renal lesion can be associated with systemic manifestations (usually purpura, arthritis, and gastrointestinal involvement) in the Henoch-Schönlein syndrome, which is discussed later under glomerular involvement in systemic diseases. These two disorders probably present a spectrum of disease manifestations due to a common immunopathogenetic mechanism.

Etiology and incidence. IgA nephropathy is the most common form of acute glomerulonephritis seen in the United States. It is even more common in Asian countries. The etiology of IgA nephropathy is unknown.

Pathogenesis and pathophysiology. The fact that IgA nephropathy frequently follows viral upper respiratory or gastrointestinal tract infections suggests a postinfectious process. The mechanisms leading to glomerular immune deposit formation are unclear, but may involve a mucosal antibody response. IgA containing circulating immune complexes and IgA-fibronectin aggregates are often present, but it is not known if the mesangial deposits result from trapping of these macromolecules or from local immune complex formation in the mesangium. There is also evidence that an IgG autoantibody to a mesangial cell antigen may contribute to the disease. In some patients, extensive capillary wall deposits of IgA may occur and cause heavy proteinuria with a worse prognosis.

Pathology. Fig. 354-3 illustrates the typical light and IF findings in IgA nephropathy. The renal pathology in IgA nephropathy, Henoch-Schönlein purpura, and some cases of focal proliferative lupus nephritis are quite similar; but differentiation between these entities can usually be readily made by clinical criteria. The typical finding by light microscopy is a focal proliferative glomerulonephritis. Small crescents are seen in 100% of patients biopsied at the time of macroscopic hematuria.

In contrast to the focal distribution of changes by light microscopy, IF reveals diffuse deposition of IgA, and often IgG and C3, in the mesangium of all glomeruli (Fig. 354-3, *B*). EM confirms mesangial deposits, and some extension to the subendothelial aspect of the capillary wall in paramesangial areas may be seen, usually in association with more severe glomerular histologic change and proteinuria.

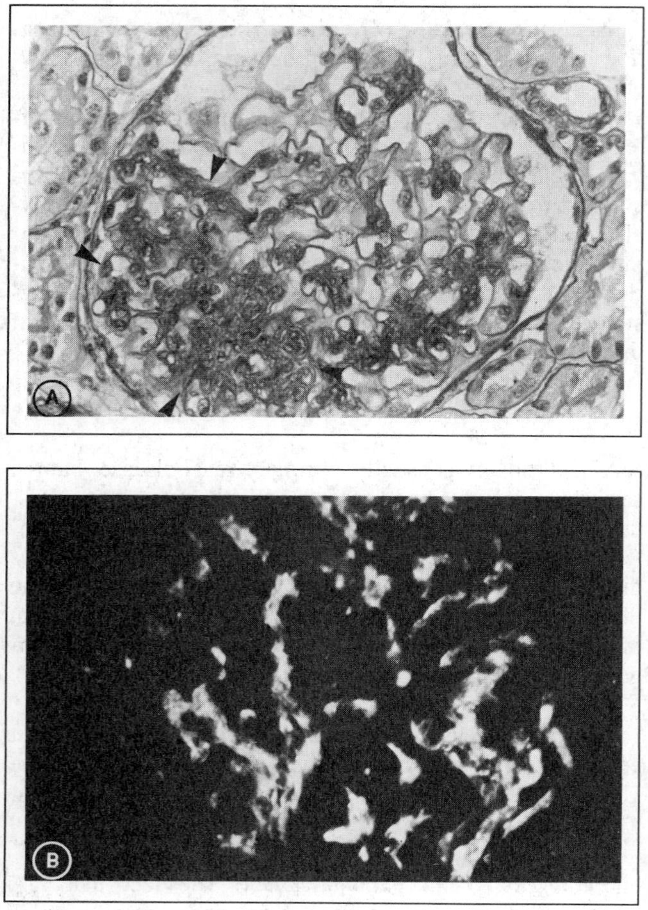

Fig. 354-3. Renal biopsy from a patient with gross hematuria due to IgA nephropathy. Light microscopy **(A)** shows a segmental area of cellular proliferation and mesangial matrix increase *(between arrowheads)* with sparing of adjacent capillary loops (periodic acid-Schiff stain; ×465). Immunofluorescence **(B)** shows nodular deposits of IgA confined to mesangial stalks (×400). Similar biopsy findings are present in the nephritis of Henoch-Schönlein purpura.

Clinical and laboratory features. Half of all patients with IgA nephropathy present with an acute nephritic syndrome usually characterized by gross hematuria that develops coincident with, or 24 to 48 hours after, an upper respiratory tract infection (50%), flulike illness (15%), or episode of gastroenteritis (10%). In contrast to PSGN, there is no significant latent period, and hypertension and edema during acute attacks are uncommon. The disease is one of younger patients, usually 15 to 35 years old, and affects males two to three times more often than females (see Table 354-1). The onset of gross hematuria may be accompanied by dull loin pain and occasionally vague constitutional symptoms. Although some decrease in renal function is common during attacks, acute renal failure is rare. Gross hematuria usually lasts 2 to 6 days. Proteinuria rarely exceeds 1 to 2 g/day; however, about 10% of patients can present with nephrotic syndrome. Some of these patients have extensive capillary wall immune deposits and a poor prognosis. Others have no capillary wall deposits, respond well to steroid therapy, and probably have nephrotic syndrome similar to minimal change disease with superimposed incidental mesangial IgA deposits. Between episodes, persistent proteinuria and microscopic hematuria are common, and these abnormalities bring the remaining patients to medical attention. About half of the patients who experience gross hematuria will have only a single recognized episode. The remainder have recurrent episodes that can continue for decades.

About 50% of patients with IgA nephropathy eventually suffer progressive loss of renal function. This course is more common in adults than children. Although no clinical or laboratory parameters can accurately predict prognosis, the presence of decreased renal function initially, hypertension early in the course, male sex, and proteinuria exceeding 3 g/day are all more common in patients with progressive disease. Occasional patients have extensive crescent formation and may follow a course similar to that described later for RPGN. Mesangial IgA deposits have been shown to recur with high frequency in renal allografts, but they rarely cause acute nephritis or graft loss.

Most patients with IgA nephropathy or Henoch-Schönlein purpura have elevated levels of IgA-fibronectin aggregates, which may be diagnostically useful but are of uncertain pathogenetic significance. Serum complement levels are usually normal. About 50% of patients have elevations in serum levels of IgA. Most patients also have granular deposits of IgA in the dermal capillaries of otherwise normal skin.

Diagnosis. The diagnosis of IgA nephropathy is confirmed by the presence of focal nephritis associated with mesangial IgA deposits in a renal biopsy of a patient with nephritis without clinical or serologic evidence of systemic disease.

Treatment. No specific treatment has been shown to be beneficial in IgA nephropathy. Hypertension may develop early in the course, before significant loss of renal function, and should be treated aggressively. In the rare patient who develops crescentic nephritis with a rapidly progressive course, treatment as discussed later for rapidly progressive glomerulonephritis may be indicated. A subset of patients with nephrotic syndrome and mesangial IgA deposits may respond to oral steroid therapy, similar to patients with minimal change disease (see later discussion).

Loin pain-hematuria syndrome

A cause of recurrent gross hematuria that may be confused with IgA nephropathy is the loin pain-hematuria syndrome. This disorder, which generally affects young women, is characterized by recurrent episodes of gross hematuria associated with dull unilateral or bilateral loin pain and sometimes low-grade fever. Blood pressure and renal function are usually normal. The syndrome has been associated most often with the use of oral contraceptive agents and generally resolves when these agents are discontinued.

Rapidly progressive (crescentic) glomerulonephritis

A third group of patients that may present with an acute nephritic syndrome are those with RPGN. RPGN is not a separate disease entity but rather a clinicopathologic syndrome, which can occur with several systemic and primary renal diseases, and may be initiated by several different pathogenetic mechanisms. Only diseases that produce rapid loss of renal function associated with extensive (usually over 50%) glomerular crescents are referred to as RPGN. Crescents are clusters of proliferating epithelial cells and macrophages found outside of the glomerulus in Bowman's space. Crescents develop after fibrin leakage across the glomerular capillary wall and hence indicate severe capillary wall damage (Fig. 354-4, *A*).

As outlined in the classification system presented in Table 354-2, patients with RPGN can be considered in three broad categories. One group (20%) has crescentic glomerulonephritis mediated by anti-GBM antibody deposition either with pulmonary involvement (Goodpasture's syndrome) or without pulmonary disease (idiopathic anti-GBM nephritis). These two groups of patients are discussed later. Another group (40%) have granular immune complex deposits in glomeruli. These patients may have a crescentic form of a primary renal disease such as PSGN, IgA nephropathy, or type I MPGN or a systemic disease such as lupus nephritis, Henoch-Schönlein purpura, or essential mixed cryoglobulinemia. These diseases can usually be diagnosed by their distinctive clinical and pathologic or serologic features and are discussed in more detail elsewhere in this chapter. A third group of patients with crescentic glomerulonephritis (40%) have disease without glomerular immune deposits. Most of these patients have a form of vasculitis, which may be renal-limited or systemic, and are associated with elevated levels of antineutrophil cytoplasmic antibody (ANCA). Among ANCA positive patients, those

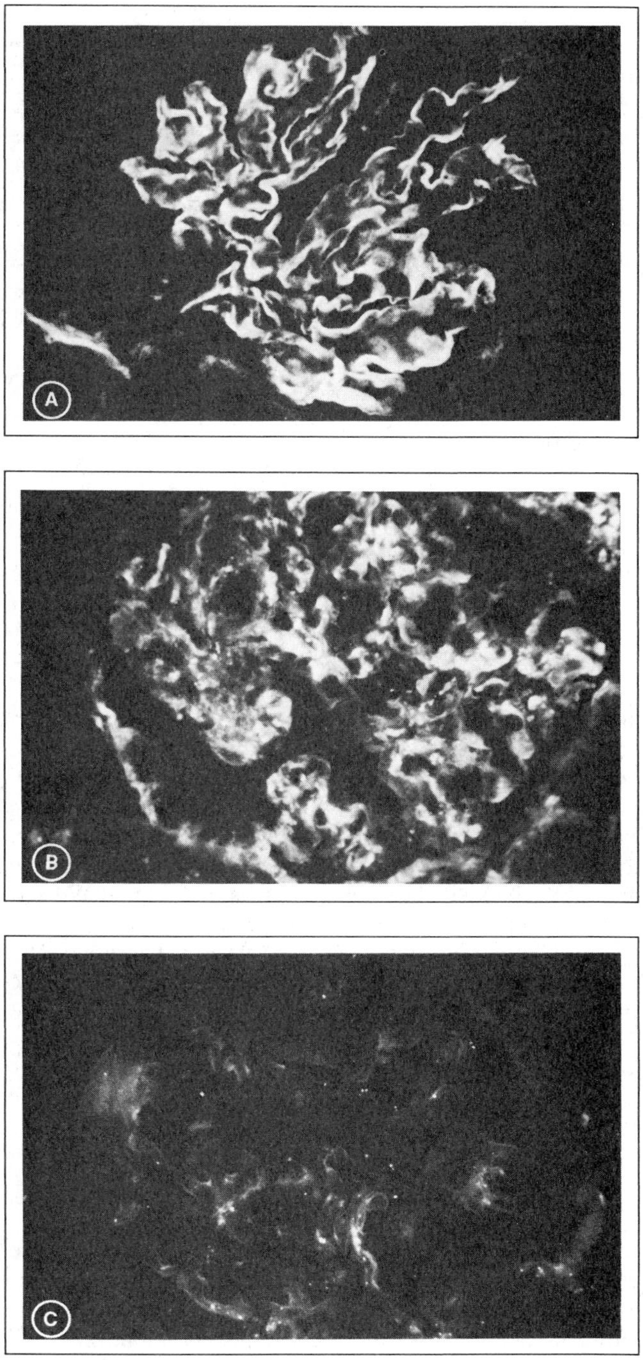

Fig. 354-4. Immunofluorescent staining for IgG in three patients with rapidly progressive glomerulonephritis illustrating the three immunopathogenetic mechanisms that may be present. In **A** IgG is deposited in the continuous, linear pattern along all capillary loops characteristic of anti-GBM antibody deposition. In **B** coarsely granular immune complex deposits are present on capillary walls and in the mesangium in a patient with RPGN due to systemic lupus erythematosus. In **C** there are no significant deposits of IgG in a patient with idiopathic crescentic glomerulonephritis and ANCA (×325).

Table 354-2. Classification of crescentic glomerulonephritis

Category	Primary renal	Systemic
I. Anti-GBM antibody mediated	Idiopathic Complicating membranous	Pulmonary-renal (Goodpasture's)
II. Immune complex mediated	Postinfectious GN IgA nephropathy	Lupus nephritis Henoch-Schönlein purpura
	MPGN type I	Essential mixed cryoglobulinemia
III. No immune deposits		
a. ANCA-positive	Idiopathic crescentic GN	Polyarteritis nodosa Wegener's granulomatosus
b. ANCA-negative	Idiopathic crescentic GN	

with primary renal disease are generally referred to as idiopathic crescentic glomerulonephritis. Other terms sometimes applied to this group of patients include *pauci-immune glomerulonephritis, microscopic polyarteritis nodosa,* or, when the disease follows an initiating allergic event such as a drug reaction, *hypersensitivity vasculitis.* Systemic forms of ANCA-positive vasculitis that involve the kidney include classic polyarteritis nodosa and Wegener's granulomatosis, which are discussed later in the chapter (see Glomerular Involvement in Systemic Diseases). Occasional patients with a lesion similar to that in idiopathic crescentic glomerulonephritis do not have demonstrable ANCA antibodies. Although these patients may have a different disease process, they are clinically similar to ANCA-positive patients and are treated similarly.

RPGN due to antiglomerular basement membrane antibody

Goodpasture's syndrome

Etiology and incidence. Goodpasture's syndrome is a rare disease characterized by a triad of pulmonary hemorrhage, iron deficiency anemia, and glomerulonephritis due to anti-GBM antibody deposition in the lungs and kidneys. It accounts for about 5% of all patients seen with RPGN and less than 1% of all cases of glomerulonephritis. The disease is due to the production and deposition of antibodies to antigens on the alpha-3 chain of type IV collagen. The events that initiate anti-GBM antibody production are not known. Several potential etiologic factors have been implicated, including influenza A viral infection and hydrocarbon solvent exposure. An increased incidence of HLA-DRw2 and B7 antigens has been reported in Goodpasture's syndrome (relative risk 15 to 34 times normal) and is associated with a worse prognosis, suggesting that immunogenetic factors also play a role.

Pathogenesis and pathophysiology. The production of anti-GBM antibody results in the direct binding of IgG in a linear pattern by IF to GBM (see Fig. 354-4, *A*). The immunologic and physiologic consequences of this process have been discussed earlier. In general, anti-GBM disease appears to be self-limited. Renal function can be preserved if glomerular destruction can be minimized until production of pathogenic antibody ceases.

The pulmonary lesions in Goodpasture's syndrome also appear to be mediated by the same anti-GBM antibody that cross-reacts with alveolar basement membrane, but gains access to alveolar basement membrane only if prior lung injury is present. For example, many patients with anti-GBM nephritis and pulmonary hemorrhage are cigarette smokers or have a recent history of exposure to other respiratory toxins or of an influenza-like illness.

Pathology. The histology in Goodpasture's syndrome is that of an initial focal proliferative and necrotizing glomerular lesion that progresses rapidly to diffuse proliferation with crescents as described earlier. The IF findings are diffuse linear deposition of IgG (or rarely, IgA) in a continuous, uninterrupted pattern along the GBM (see Fig. 354-4, *A*) accompanied in most cases by C3 in a similar pattern. Many patients with Goodpasture's syndrome also show linear deposits of IgG along the tubular basement membranes. Anti-GBM antibody deposits cannot be identified by EM.

Clinical and laboratory features. Goodpasture's syndrome is primarily a disease of young white males (male/female ratio, 6:1) with a mean age of 21 who develop hemoptysis, iron deficiency anemia, and RPGN associated with anti-GBM antibody deposits. In most cases the pulmonary manifestations appear first and range from mild hemoptysis with bilateral, fluffy alveolar infiltrates to severe, life-threatening pulmonary hemorrhage with hypoxemia and respiratory failure. About one third of patients with Goodpasture's syndrome die of pulmonary involvement. It must be emphasized that Goodpasture's syndrome is not the only glomerular disease in which both pulmonary and renal manifestations may occur. Other such diseases include systemic lupus erythematosus, Wegener's granulomatosis, Henoch-Schönlein syndrome, mixed cryoglobulinemia, and idiopathic crescentic glomerulonephritis. The term Goodpasture's syndrome is reserved only for those patients with the triad of iron deficiency anemia, pulmonary hemorrhage, and glomerulonephritis mediated by anti-GBM antibody.

Anemia generally parallels the degree of pulmonary involvement and is secondary to blood loss and iron sequestration in the lungs. Although microscopic hematuria and proteinuria usually occur within 2 weeks of the onset of pulmonary disease, some patients may have several exacerbations and remissions of pulmonary disease before nephritis becomes apparent, and occasional patients never develop nephritis.

Renal involvement in Goodpasture's syndrome is initially manifest as microscopic hematuria, which progresses to include proteinuria and decreased renal function. Although rare cases of mild renal disease with spontaneous recovery have been reported, the lesion is usually severe and progressive with rapid development of oliguria and renal failure. The mean time from diagnosis to renal failure is about 3 to 4 weeks. Nephrotic range proteinuria and hypertension are usually not seen, and kidney size is normal.

In addition to the characteristic urinary abnormalities of the acute nephritic syndrome, laboratory abnormalities in Goodpasture's syndrome include iron-deficiency anemia, hemosiderin-laden macrophages in the sputum, and the presence of circulating antibody to human GBM in the serum. Anti-GBM antibodies are detectable by enzyme-linked immunosorbent assay (ELISA) or radioimmunoassay in most patients. Antibody levels roughly parallel activity of the renal disease and usually persist for several months. Serum levels of complement are normal. Infectious complications may increase anti-GBM antibody levels and produce clinical exacerbations of disease.

Diagnosis. The diagnosis of Goodpasture's syndrome is made in patients with pulmonary hemorrhage or alveolar infiltrates and glomerulonephritis associated with positive anti-GBM antibody assays or linear deposits of IgG by IF. The almost uniformly poor prognosis and potential benefit from early treatment in Goodpasture's syndrome make it imperative to establish an accurate diagnosis as quickly as possible. A presumptive diagnosis may be made by demonstrating anti-GBM antibody in the serum in the presence of clinically characteristic pulmonary and renal manifestations.

Treatment. Steroid pulse therapy as described later for idiopathic crescentic glomerulonephritis has been associated with a dramatic improvement in severe pulmonary hemorrhage, but has less effect on the renal lesion. The current treatment of choice for renal involvement in Goodpasture's syndrome is plasma exchange therapy to remove circulating anti-GBM antibody combined with prednisone, 1 mg/kg/day, and cyclophosphamide, 2 to 3 mg/kg/day to inhibit further antibody production. Plasma exchanges of up to 4 L are performed on a daily or alternate day basis until anti-GBM antibody is no longer detectable in the circulation and disease progression has halted. Therapy may require several weeks. Replacement is with albumin, or, when pulmonary hemorrhage is active, with fresh frozen plasma. Overall survival in anti-GBM nephritis appears to be improved by plasma exchange therapy. However, the response rate in patients who are oliguric at the time of presentation or have serum creatinines exceeding 6 mg/dl is very low, again emphasizing the need for early diagnosis. In patients with end-stage renal disease due to anti-GBM nephritis, renal transplantation appears to be a safe and effective form of therapy if it is delayed until anti-GBM antibody is no longer detectable in the serum.

Anti-GBM glomerulonephritis without pulmonary involvement. Over 50% of patients with RPGN mediated by anti-GBM antibodies do not have the pulmonary hemorrhage characteristic of Goodpasture's syndrome and have no other extrarenal manifestations of their disease. In this group of patients the age and sex distribution and the clinical manifestations, course, and prognosis are essentially the same as those described for idiopathic crescentic glomerulonephritis, although patients in their 20s and 30s may be somewhat more commonly affected. Defining the anti-GBM antibody pathogenesis of this disease is essential to select the most appropriate therapy and to avoid recurrent anti-GBM nephritis in transplants. Diagnosis and treatment would be the same as that described for Goodpasture's syndrome.

Idiopathic (pauci-immune) crescentic glomerulonephritis

Etiology and incidence. The most common cause of RPGN is a vasculitic process, which may be confined to the glomerular capillaries (idiopathic or pauci-immune crescentic glomerulonephritis) or part of a systemic disease (microscopic polyarteritis nodosa). In both cases, the disease is associated with elevated levels of antineutrophil cytoplasmic antibody (ANCA) and occurs in the absence of linear or granular immune deposits in the glomeruli. The etiology of idiopathic crescentic glomerulonephritis is not known. In some cases the disease is preceded by a flulike illness with fever, weight loss, and malaise, reflecting a systemic vasculitis. The frequent presence of elevated ANCA suggests that the disorder is autoimmune in nature.

Pathogenesis and pathophysiology. In the idiopathic variety of crescentic glomerulonephritis, capillary wall injury results from some undefined mechanism, which is usually associated with increased levels of ANCA and does not produce glomerular immunoglobulin deposits. The mechanisms of tissue injury in ANCA-positive vasculitis are unclear. They may involve antibody or cell-mediated immune reactions against endothelial surface antigens, some of which may be induced by exposure to inflammatory cytokines, or from neutrophil-induced injury mediated by a reaction of cytokine-activated neutrophils with ANCA, leading to the release of oxidants and proteases. It seems likely that many severe cases of glomerulonephritis are also accompanied by some ischemic acute tubular necrosis. The degree of recovery of renal function depends on whether the underlying disease process resolves spontaneously or whether it can be modified by therapeutic intervention before irreversible glomerular alterations such as thrombosis, necrosis, sclerosis, and scar formation develop.

Pathology. The principal finding by light microscopy in crescentic glomerulonephritis of any cause is the presence of extensive glomerular crescent formation, often with compression of the glomerular tuft (Fig. 354-5, *A*). In most cases over 50% of glomeruli have crescents. Pathology in the glomerular tuft itself is variable. A common finding is a focal segmental necrotizing glomerular lesion. This lesion is generally regarded as indicative of a renal capillary vasculitis, particularly when it occurs in a setting of constitutional symptoms and no immune deposits. Studies have demonstrated that the clinical manifestations and response to therapy of patients with focal necrotizing glomerulonephritis and crescents is much the same, regardless of whether or not histologic evidence of extraglomerular small vessel vasculitis is present. Because many glomerular diseases (see Table 354-2) may be accompanied by glomerular necrosis and crescent formation, these findings alone are not diagnostic of any specific disease entity. Other features in the biopsy, such as diffuse proliferative changes and humps in poststreptococcal glomerulonephritis or granulomata in Wegener's granulomatosis, may assist in the differential diagnosis.

In addition to the glomerular changes, an interstitial infiltrate of mononuclear cells is commonly present and occasionally may assume a periglomerular distribution. Both the severity of the interstitial changes and the percentage

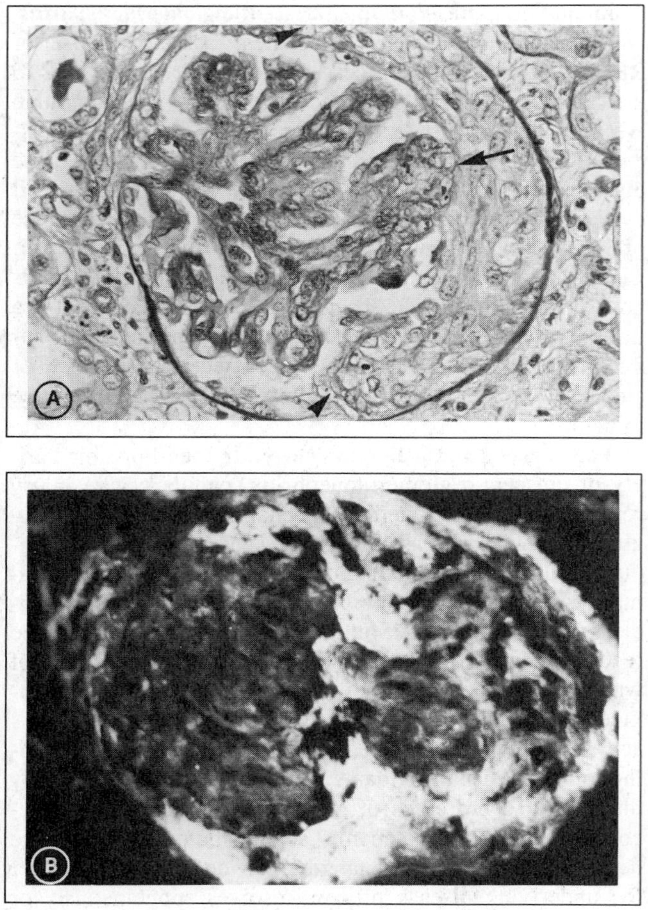

Fig. 354-5. Renal biopsy from a patient with rapidly progressive glomerulonephritis. **A,** Light microscopy demonstrates a large crescent compressing the glomerular tuft, which shows an area of segmental necrosis *(arrow)* (Periodic acid-Schiff stain; ×325). **B,** Immunofluorescent staining shows fibrin deposition in the area of crescent formation (×350).

of glomeruli showing crescent formation correlate roughly with the clinical course and prognosis.

Most patients with idiopathic crescentic glomerulonephritis have no pathogenic glomerular immune deposits by IF (Fig. 354-5, *C*). In all patients, regardless of the underlying disease mechanism, fibrin-related antigens are easily demonstrable in glomerular crescents (Fig. 354-5, *B*).

Findings by EM confirm those by IF. No deposits are seen in anti-GBM disease or crescentic glomerulonephritis with negative IF. Common to all crescentic glomerulonephritides is the presence of discontinuities or gaps in the basement membrane of severely damaged glomeruli through which macrophages and plasma are believed to leak to induce crescent formation.

Clinical and laboratory features. The onset of the disease is usually abrupt but can be insidious, and patients may present either with an acute nephritic syndrome (50%) and rapidly deteriorating renal function or with oliguria, elevated serum creatinines, and the recent onset of signs and symptoms of uremia (50%). The duration of disease from onset to severe renal failure varies from 1 to 2 weeks to a few months. Men are affected twice as often as women, and the median age is 58, although cases have been reported in children and in adults over 80.

Many patients give a history of a recent viral-like syndrome with fever, myalgias, and polyarthralgias. Transient pulmonary infiltrates by radiography or small amounts of hemoptysis are also common, but pulmonary manifestations are rarely of major clinical significance as they are in Goodpasture's syndrome (see earlier discussion). These clinical signs and symptoms are probably consequent to extrarenal vasculitis, which may or may not be demonstrated in a renal biopsy. The presence of focal necrotizing glomerulonephritis in the renal biopsy in such patients is considered diagnostic of a renal vasculitis. In the absence of volume overload, blood pressure is usually normal, edema is absent, and kidney size is normal. Renal failure is the only manifestation of the disease to cause significant morbidity, and the course and prognosis of the renal lesion is the same regardless of whether other systemic manifestations of vasculitis are present.

All patients have proteinuria, hematuria, and usually red blood cell casts. Proteinuria in excess of 3 g/day is unusual, and nephrotic syndrome is rarely seen. A mild anemia is common, and the erythrocyte sedimentation rate is always elevated. Tests for complement anti-GBM antibody and circulating immune complexes are normal or negative. However, levels of ANCA are usually elevated in idiopathic crescentic glomerulonephritis without immune deposits and antibody levels may parallel disease activity.

Diagnosis. The differential diagnosis of crescentic glomerulonephritis includes all of the diseases listed in Table 354-2. When crescentic glomerulonephritis develops as a primary renal disease, patients can generally be divided into ANCA-positive and ANCA-negative groups. ANCA-negative causes of crescentic glomerulonephritis include diseases such as systemic lupus, Henoch-Schönlein purpura, essential mixed cryoglobulinemia, and anti-GBM disease. These entities are discussed elsewhere in this chapter and can generally be readily diagnosed by available serologic tests and biopsy characteristics. ANCA-positive patients include those with Wegener's granulomatosis, polyarteritis nodosa, and the idiopathic or pauci-immune form of crescentic glomerulonephritis. Wegener's granulomatosis is characterized by upper respiratory and pulmonary disease as well as nephritis, and patients with polyarteritis nodosa demonstrate prominent multisystem dysfunction, usually with purpura and necrotizing vasculitis on biopsy. Patients with idiopathic crescentic glomerulonephritis are usually ANCA-positive and have a variant of the syndrome with renal involvement invariably present, extrarenal disease less evident, and usually no extraglomerular vasculitic changes on renal biopsy.

Treatment. The natural history of idiopathic RPGN is difficult to define because virtually all patients have received some form of therapy. Favorable prognostic factors include a young age at the time of onset, a history of a preceding infectious episode, absence of oliguria and hypertension, serum creatinine below 6 mg/dl at presentation and fewer than 50% crescents in the renal biopsy. Response rates approaching 75% have been reported in patients treated with either methylprednisolone pulse therapy or plasma exchange. In pulse therapy, methylprednisolone, 30 mg/kg to a maximum of 3 g, is given intravenously over 20 minutes on a daily or alternate day basis for three doses followed by oral prednisone, 2 mg/kg, which is tapered over several months. About 75% of patients, including some who were oliguric and on dialysis, have shown a dramatic response with a return of renal function to normal or near normal levels. Responses have generally been evident within 5 to 10 days and continued over 4 to 6 weeks. Some patients, however, will progress to renal failure later despite an impressive initial response. Very similar results have been reported in patients treated with intensive plasma exchange (plus prednisone and cyclophosphamide). This treatment is extremely expensive and probably has a higher incidence of complications than pulse therapy, primarily bleeding and infection. Because of the vasculitic nature of idiopathic crescentic glomerulonephritis, most patients are also treated with cytotoxic drugs, usually cyclophosphamide, 1 to 2 mg/kg/day, or pulse intravenous cyclophosphamide, 500 mg/M^2/month. Any patient with signs or symptoms of a systemic vasculitic disease, positive ANCA, or vasculitis or focal necrotizing glomerulonephritis on renal biopsy should receive cytotoxic drug therapy. No data compare the efficacy of daily oral cyclophosphamide versus monthly pulse cyclophosphamide, but the latter appears to be efficacious and associated with fewer side effects in treating lupus nephritis.

The reported experience with renal transplantation in idiopathic crescentic glomerulonephritis is minimal, but the disease appears to recur rarely in allografted kidneys.

GLOMERULAR DISEASES THAT USUALLY PRESENT AS IDIOPATHIC NEPHROTIC SYNDROME

Introduction

The pathophysiology of alterations in the glomerular capillary wall that result in proteinuria, various causes of proteinuria other than glomerular disease, and the clinical consequences of massive urinary protein loss have been discussed in detail in Chapters 343 (Proteinuria) and 346 (Nephrotic Syndrome) and are not reviewed here. However, it is important to be aware that nephrotic syndrome may result from many different diseases. Although the diseases discussed early present most commonly as acute glomerulonephritis and those that follow are usually characterized initially by nephrotic syndrome, this separation is arbitrary. It is also arbitrary to designate a particular value for urine protein excretion, such as the traditional 3.5 g/day, as separating those diseases that usually cause nephrotic syndrome from other glomerular diseases. Thus nephrotic syndrome may be a manifestation of almost any glomerular disease. Moreover, all diseases that can cause nephrotic syndrome are sometimes seen in milder forms or earlier stages with proteinuria, which is not in the nephrotic range. Similarly, the development of the various clinical and biochemical derangements, such as hypoalbuminemia, edema, hyperlipidemia and lipiduria, which are commonly seen in nephrotic syndrome, may be modified by a number of host factors such as GFR, nutritional intake, hepatic disease, and age.

In adults, about one third of patients with nephrotic syndrome have a systemic disease such as diabetes, systemic lupus erythematosus, and amyloid. The remaining two thirds of patients have idiopathic nephrotic syndrome. Most patients with idiopathic nephrotic syndrome have one of three types of glomerular diseases: minimal change (focal sclerosis), membranous nephropathy, or membranoproliferative glomerulonephritis. The most common type is minimal change disease or focal sclerosis in children and membranous nephropathy in adults. The approximate prevalence and clinical features of each of these lesions in large series of children and adults with idiopathic nephrotic syndrome is presented in Table 354-3.

Minimal change disease (MCD, lipoid nephrosis, nil disease)

Etiology and incidence. Despite its relative frequency and association with several clinical events, the etiology of MCD remains unclear. The disease causes idiopathic nephrotic syndrome in about 75% of children and 15% of adults. The incidence varies somewhat in different parts of the world, but it is estimated to affect two to three patients per year per 100,000 population under age 16 in the United States and Europe. Focal glomerular sclerosis (FGS), which is seen in about 10% of children and adults with idiopathic nephrotic syndrome, is treated here as a separate clinical entity (see later discussion). Many authors, however, now regard the histologic lesion of FGS as simply a marker of a more severe form of MCD, which results in structural glomerular damage and is often resistant to steroid therapy.

Pathogenesis and pathophysiology. The pathogenesis of MCD is unknown. Several observations suggest a role for immune factors including the relatively high incidence of atopy and allergic histories in affected children; occasional onset following viral upper respiratory tract infections, immunizations, or hypersensitivity reactions to drugs (particularly NSAIDs) or bee stings; and evidence of cellular hypersensitivity in vitro to some kidney antigens. Recent evidence suggest that T cells from patients with active MCD produce a soluble factor that induces a similar lesion when infused into animals. (See Chapter 346 for a discussion of the pathophysiology of the nephrotic syndrome that characterizes MCD).

Pathology. The biopsy changes in MCD are illustrated in Fig. 354-6. As suggested by the terms *minimal change*, or *nil* disease, glomeruli by light microscopy generally appear entirely normal (Fig. 354-6, *A*). By light microscopy alone the presence of normal glomeruli does not exclude the presence of FGS in unbiopsied glomeruli, nor does it distinguish this disease from early membranous nephropathy. By IF there is no glomerular deposition of immunoglobulins or complement in typical MCD except for occasional traces of IgM or C3 in a nonspecific pattern in the mesangium of some glomeruli (Fig. 354-6, *B*). The only consistent abnormality is seen by EM, which reveals wide-

Table 354-3. Summary of primary renal diseases that present as idiopathic nephrotic syndrome

Diseases	Minimal change disease	Focal glomerular sclerosis	Membranous nephropathy	Membranoproliferative glomerulonephritis	
				Type I	Type II
Frequency*					
Children	75%	10%	<5%	10%	
Adults	15%	15%	50%	10%	
Clinical manifestations					
Age	2-6, some adults	2-6, some adults	40-50%	5%-15%	
Sex	2:1 male	1.3:1 male	2:1 male	2:1 female	
Nephrotic syndrome	100%	90%	80%	60%	
Asymptomatic proteinuria	0	10%	20%	40%	
Hematuria	No	40%	20%	80%	
Hypertension	10%	20% early	Infrequent	35%	
Rate of progression	Does not progress	10 years	50% in 10-20 years	10-20 years	5-15 years
Associated conditions	Allergy to NSAIDs Hodgkin's disease	Heroin nephropathy AIDS	Renal vein thrombosis, cancer, SLE, hepatitis	None	Partial lipodystrophy
Recurs in transplants	Yes	50%	Rarely	30%	90%
Laboratory findings	Manifestations of nephrotic syndrome	Manifestations of nephrotic syndrome	Manifestations of nephrotic syndrome	Low C1, C4, C3-C9	Normal C1, C4; low C3-C9; C3 nephritic factor
Immunogenetics	DR7 (6)†	DR4 (5-6)	DR3 (2-12)	None	DR7 (9)
Renal pathology					
Light microscopy	Normal	Focal sclerotic lesions	Thickened GBM, spikes	Thickened GBM, proliferation, lobulation	Same as type I
Immunofluorescence	Negative	IgM, C3 in sclerotic	Fine granular IgG, C3	Granular IgG, C3	C3 only
Electron microscopy	Foot process fusion	Lesions, foot process fusion	Subepithelial deposits	Mesangial and subendothelial deposits	Dense deposits
Response to steroids	90%	20%-40%, may slow progression	Slows progression	None established	
Other treatment	None	None	Steroids and cytotoxic drugs in high risk patients	None established	

*Approximate frequency as a cause of idiopathic nephrotic syndrome. About 10% of adult nephrotic syndrome is due to various diseases that usually present with acute glomerulonephritis (Table 354-1)

†Relative risk

NSAIDs, nonsteroidal anti-inflammatory drugs; SLE, systemic lupus erythematosus.

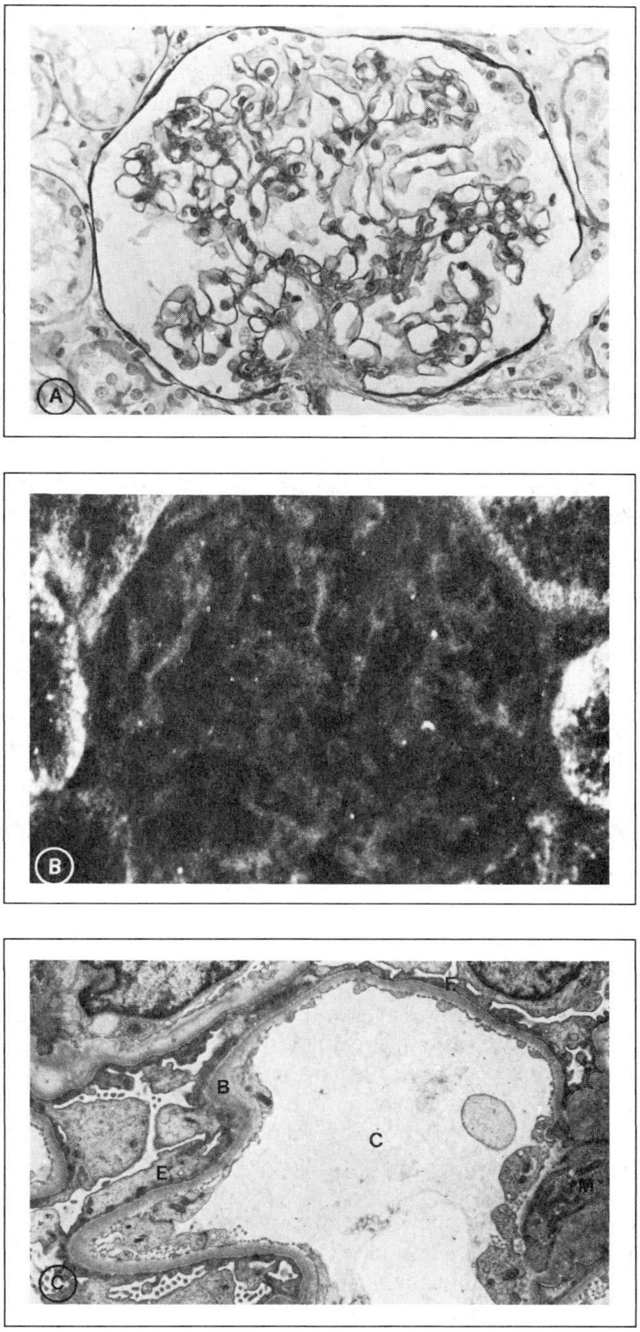

Fig. 354-6. Renal biopsy findings in idiopathic nephrotic syndrome due to minimal change disease. **A,** By light microscopy the glomerulus is normal (periodic acid-Schiff stain; ×600). **B,** Immunofluorescence shows no glomerular immune deposits (×500). **C,** Electron microscopy shows no deposits and diffuse effacement of epithelial cell *(E)* foot processes. *B:* basement membrane; *C:* capillary lumen (Uranyl and lead stain; ×5600).

spread effacement, or "fusion," of epithelial cell foot processes (Fig. 354-6, *C*). Foot process fusion is characteristic of MCD but is not specific. It occurs in all glomerular diseases associated with significant proteinuria.

Clinical and laboratory features. MCD is primarily a disease of childhood, with a peak incidence between 2 and 6 years of age and is the cause of about 75% of childhood nephrotic syndrome (see Table 354-3). It may also occur in adults. Boys are affected twice as often as girls in childhood, but in adults the sex incidence is about equal. The disease virtually always presents as a severe nephrotic syndrome with heavy proteinuria, hypoalbuminemia, edema, hyperlipidemia, and lipiduria. Urine protein excretion exceeding 40 g/day and serum albumin levels of less than 1.0 g% are not unusual. In the absence of significant intravascular volume depletion, blood pressure and renal function are usually normal. However, severe volume contraction may occur and can produce hypotension, prerenal azotemia, and occasional acute oliguric renal failure, which is reversible with volume repletion. Acute renal failure, which may be due to intrarenal edema and may be reversible with diuretic therapy, has also been reported. Edema is common and often progresses to generalized anasarca.

Patients with MCD may suffer a variety of secondary complications of nephrotic syndrome including an increased susceptibility to infection, usually with gram-positive organisms, due to reduced serum levels of IgG; a tendency to form spontaneous thromboses in renal and peripheral veins and pulmonary arteries with thromboembolic phenomena; severe hyperlipidemia; and protein malnutrition due to negative nitrogen balance. In adult patients particular attention must be given to the possibility of an occult lymphoma, because MCD may be associated with Hodgkin's disease. In such patients the nephrotic syndrome often precedes clinical evidence of tumor.

There are no laboratory abnormalities specific for MCD, although most patients have unexpectedly low levels of antibodies to streptococcal antigens (ASO titers). Other abnormalities may occur with severe nephrotic syndrome of any cause. The urinalysis reveals nephrotic changes with proteinuria, free fat, oval fat bodies, and fatty casts. Microscopic hematuria is rare, and gross hematuria and red cell casts are not seen. Proteinuria is generally selective (greater than 90% albumin) in children, but may be nonselective in adults. Occasional patients will exhibit proximal tubular dysfunction with wasting of phosphate, urate, bicarbonate, and amino acids, which results in lowered serum levels of these substances and occasionally leads to rickets or osteomalacia. Tubular dysfunction is presumably related to toxic effects of increased protein and lipid filtration and reabsorption. Serum cholesterol, phospholipids, and triglycerides are elevated. Serum albumin and IgG are low. $Alpha_2$ macroglobulin, IgM, IgE, and clotting factors V, VII, VIII, X, and fibrinogen are often elevated. These elevations, along with the frequent thrombocytosis and hypovolemia, contribute to a hypercoaguable state. T3 resin uptake is often low due to urinary loss of thyroxin-binding globulin, but thyroid function is usually normal.

Diagnosis. In childhood the development of nephrotic syndrome with normal renal function, benign urine sediment, normal blood pressure, and normal complement levels makes the diagnosis of MCD so likely that steroid therapy may be initiated without performing a renal biopsy unless renal function deteriorates or there is no response to therapy. The diagnosis is confirmed if a typical complete remission occurs after steroid therapy. In adults, the diagnosis is made by demonstrating the features of MCD in a renal biopsy.

Course and treatment. The spontaneous remission rate has been variously estimated at 25% to 40%. Despite the relatively high spontaneous remission rate and the fact that MCD probably does not progress to renal failure, the mortality rate from this disease in children was over 50% at 5 years before the use of steroid therapy. Most deaths resulted from bacterial infections or thromboembolic events.

It has never been proved in a controlled study that steroid therapy improves survival in MCD. The response of MCD to steroids, however, is generally dramatic and has led to the widespread belief that such therapy is beneficial. Conventional doses of oral prednisone are 60 mg/M^2/day for children and 1 mg/kg/day for adults, generally given on an alternate-day basis after remission is induced. At least four clinical courses can be identified in treated patients, which appear to be similar in both children and adults.

1. Nonresponders: patients who do not become free of proteinuria after 8 to 12 weeks of therapy generally fail to respond thereafter. In most series this represents about 10% of all patients, and they usually have, or develop, evidence of structural glomerular damage in the form of FGS. The relationship of FGS to MCD is discussed later.
2. Primary responders (90%): most patients (70%) will enter remission and become protein-free within 4 weeks after starting steroid therapy, and more will experience remission within 12 weeks. Of these, about 15% remain protein-free when steroids are tapered after several weeks of remission. The remaining 85% will suffer one or more relapses. Two thirds will have frequent relapses or remain dependent on steroids to maintain remission.
3. Frequent relapsers: relapses occur more than twice a year when steroids are discontinued and persist for many years but are always steroid-responsive. Eventually, spontaneous remission will occur in most of these patients.
4. Steroid-dependent: these patients always relapse when steroids are reduced below a certain level but respond when the dosage is increased.

In the latter two groups of patients (frequent relapsers and steroid-dependent), steroid toxicity may force consideration of alternative approaches to therapy.

Patients who are frequent relapsers or steroid-dependent may suffer long-term consequences of persistent nephrotic syndrome. Such patients can be treated with an alkylating agent, either cyclophosphamide, 2 to 3 mg/kg/day, or chlorambucil, 0.2 to 0.3 mg/kg/day, for 8 to 12 weeks. These agents clearly increase the frequency and duration of subsequent remissions and reduce the need for steroids. Over half of frequently relapsing and steroid-dependent patients treated with a second drug are reported to be in remission 4 years later. The use of such agents should be reserved for patients with severe nephrotic syndrome and steroid toxicity, and must be undertaken with the full knowledge that susceptibility is increased to a host of complications, particularly gonadal failure and an increased incidence of leukemia and probably other malignancies in later life. The management of steroid-resistant nephrotic syndrome with MCD on biopsy is discussed under focal glomerular sclerosis later.

Mesangial proliferative disease

Some patients present with idiopathic nephrotic syndrome and varying degrees of mesangial cell proliferation by light microscopy in the absence of definite focal sclerotic changes. An additional subgroup develops diffuse mesangial deposits of IgM and C3 by IF. Some authors put such patients into separate diagnostic categories such as mesangioproliferative glomerulonephritis or IgM mesangial nephropathy. Mesangial changes tend to be accompanied by more hematuria, a tendency to hypertension, a relatively poor response to steroids, and progressive renal failure due to FGS. Although each of these entities may represent a different disease mechanism, I believe that pure MCD, the various degrees of mesangial pathology seen in some cases of idiopathic nephrotic syndrome, and FGS represent a spectrum of increasingly severe glomerular injury and steroid unresponsiveness probably due to a common underlying mechanism. The approach to the therapy of patients with mesangial proliferation and/or IgM deposits is similar to that in MCD, although treatment is substantially less effective.

Focal glomerular sclerosis

Etiology and incidence. FGS is a histopathologic term that refers to the presence on biopsy of unique sclerosing glomerular lesions in a focal and segmental distribution. It is now clear that similar lesions may occur in a number of chronic glomerular diseases of different etiologies and probably represent a common glomerular response to several types of injury. Focal sclerotic lesions may be present in early biopsies of patients with idiopathic nephrotic syndrome who have changes in most glomeruli consistent with MCD. In this circumstance the lesions are associated with a progressive clinical course and poor response to therapy. A genetic association has been noted with HLA DR4. Patients with the clinical and histologic features of FGS account for about 10% to 15% of all patients with idiopathic nephrotic syndrome in both children and adults (see Table 354-3).

Pathogenesis and pathophysiology. The mechanism that causes the diffuse increase in glomerular permeability in FGS is unknown but may be similar to that in MCD discussed earlier. The focal sclerotic lesions themselves, which ultimately result in glomerular destruction and loss of renal function, may result from injury to the glomerular epithelial cell by this process. These lesions may also occur as a consequence of hemodynamic changes, which produce local increases in glomerular hydrostatic pressure and plasma flow. The development of focal sclerotic glomerular lesions is characteristic of most forms of progressive glomerular disease. Deposits of IgM and C3 are usually seen in sclerotic lesions and probably represent trapping of serum proteins by nonimmune mechanisms in areas of tissue damage.

Pathology. The characteristic lesion of FGS is seen by light microscopy in only some glomeruli (focal). It appears first in juxtamedullary glomeruli and therefore may not be seen in biopsies obtained from the superficial cortex (Fig. 354-7, *A*). Each individual lesion consists of intracapillary deposition of eosinophilic, PAS-positive hyaline material involving portions of one or two lobules in a glomerulus with the other lobules spared (segmental). As in MCD, variable amounts of diffuse mesangial proliferation may be seen and suggest a less favorable prognosis. Loss of renal function develops as sclerotic areas involve more lobules of affected glomeruli, lesions appear in glomeruli near the cortical surface and tubulointerstitial changes become more prominent.

By IF, glomerular deposits of IgM and C3 are present only in the areas of glomerular sclerosis. EM reveals generalized effacement of foot processes in all glomeruli and may show areas of epithelial cell detachment and thickening and folding of the GBM before sclerotic lesions are visible by light microscopy.

Clinical and laboratory features. The clinical features that distinguish FGS from MCD are the more frequent presence of hematuria and hypertension, relative resistance to steroid therapy and progressive loss of renal function; however, there is a wide clinical spectrum in FGS. The mean age is about 20, and the ratio of men/women is about 1.3 : 1. Most patients present with idiopathic nephrotic syndrome, but persistent non-nephrotic proteinuria or hematuria may also be presenting features. Although some microscopic hematuria is seen in 80% of cases, red cell casts are rare. In patients with lesions of FGS on initial biopsies, hypertension and decreased renal function are present in 25% to 50% at the time of diagnosis, and steroid resistance is frequent. Progression to renal failure occurs in an average period of 10 years, although progression over 1 to 2 years ("malignant" focal sclerosis) is not uncommon. The rate of progression is related to the amount of proteinuria. Some patients with documented FGS, however, may retain renal function despite persistent proteinuria, usually without nephrotic syndrome, for over 20 years. In general the prognosis is worse in adults than in children.

About 40% of adult patients are initially steroid-responsive, hypertension and hematuria are not prominent, and renal function is well preserved, although typical lesions of FGS are present on renal biopsies. Despite the presence of histologic lesions of FGS, the prognosis in patients with FGS who respond to steroids is good.

Diagnosis. The differential diagnosis of FGS is that of idiopathic nephrotic syndrome. The diagnosis is made by demonstrating the presence of typical focal sclerotic glomerular lesions on renal biopsy in the absence of other glomerular pathology. In patients with biopsies characteristic of MCD who do not respond to steroid therapy, it is often assumed that lesions of FGS must be present in glomeruli not contained in the biopsy specimen. Several other diseases are associated with idiopathic nephrotic syndrome, progressive renal failure, and a glomerular lesion of FGS, including heroin nephropathy, AIDS, and a nephropathy associated with idiosyncratic reactions to NSAIDs. These lesions are discussed briefly later.

Treatment. An initial trial of steroid therapy as described earlier for MCD is warranted in FGS because up to 40% of patients will respond with a marked reduction in proteinuria as they do in MCD, and these patients have a good prognosis. At the present time the evidence that cytotoxic drugs are of benefit in inducing remission or preserving renal function in steroid-resistant patients with FGS is controversial. Occasional patients who do not respond to conventional oral steroids, however, have entered remission after short-term methylprednisolone pulse therapy or after a course of oral cyclophosphamide, chlorambucil, or cyclosporin. Final conclusions regarding the possible benefit of such therapy must await the outcome of prospective controlled studies. Nonsteroidal anti-inflammatory agents, particularly meclofenamate, have also been reported to reduce protein excretion without lowering GFR in patients with steroid-resistant FGS. Angiotensin-converting enzyme inhibitors may also be useful in managing some patients with steroid resistant nephrotic syndrome, particularly if hypertension is present.

FGS may recur in the transplanted kidney. The likelihood of recurrence is influenced by the rapidity of progression of the original disease to renal failure, the presence of mesangial hypercellularity, and probably the receipt of a relatively well-matched, living, related donor kidney. Patients who progress to renal failure in less than 3 years are at particularly high risk for recurrent disease. In four antigen matches, the recurrence rate may approach 80%, although it is less than 50% for all patients transplanted with FGS. When the disease does recur, it may be manifest as severe proteinuria within hours of transplantation with biopsy evidence of MCD initially and lesions of FGS developing within days leading to graft failure.

Heroin nephropathy

Renal disease in intravenous drug abusers may take several forms including immune complex nephritis related to bacterial endocarditis or visceral abscess, membranous nephropathy or MPGN related to antigen-positive hepatitis, glomerulonephritis as part of a generalized vasculitis, amyloid, AIDS nephropathy, and chronic interstitial nephritis. However, idiopathic nephrotic syndrome occurs with increased frequency in parenteral drug users, and the majority have a lesion similar to FGS. In some centers heroin nephropathy has accounted for over 25% of new cases of FGS seen in adults and over 10% of new cases of end-stage renal disease in young adults. It is most commonly seen in African-American men between 18 and 45 who have been heroin addicts for several years. Most patients have hypertension and impaired renal function in addition to nephrotic syndrome when first seen. The prognosis is poor and progression to renal failure usually occurs within 4 years.

AIDS nephropathy

Proteinuria has been reported in up to 50% of AIDS patients, and 10% may develop nephrotic syndrome. The disorder is more common in African-American patients and patients who have AIDS associated with intravenous drug abuse, but it has been observed in patients without a history of drug abuse and in children, suggesting that an AIDS-specific nephropathy exists. The glomerular lesion in AIDS nephropathy is FGS often accompanied by glomerular viral-like bodies, and the diagnosis of AIDS may be suggested by the renal biopsy. The course is one of progressive loss of renal function.

Adverse reaction to NSAIDs

Occasional patients develop nephrotic syndrome as a consequence of an apparent allergic reaction to NSAIDs. In about half of cases, nephrotic syndrome is accompanied by acute renal failure with lesions of MCD accompanied by interstitial nephritis on biopsy. With persistent proteinuria, glomerular lesions of FGS and loss of renal function may occur.

Membranous nephropathy

Etiology and incidence. Although the inciting event is not known in most cases of membranous nephropathy, in a minority of patients the lesion occurs in association with a variety of identifiable conditions. The best established associations are with persistent hepatitis B antigenemia, autoimmune diseases including lupus, diabetes, thyroiditis, and mixed connective tissue disease, carcinoma, and treatment with several drugs, particularly gold, penicillamine, and captopril. Membranous nephropathy is rare in children, but is the most common cause of idiopathic nephrotic syndrome in adults (see Table 354-3).

Pathogenesis and pathophysiology. Increased glomerular permeability in membranous nephropathy results from the formation of granular immune deposits containing IgG and complement along the subepithelial surface of the glomerular capillary wall and in filtration slit pores. The disease is most likely due to an autoimmune IgG antibody response to an antigen expressed on the surface of the glomerular epithelial cell. Proteinuria is induced by a complement-dependent mechanism that involves assembly of C5b-9 membrane attack complexes. There is also a strong association between idiopathic membranous nephropathy and HLA-DRw3 (relative risk 4), suggesting a genetic susceptibility to this disease, although familial cases are rare. Proteinuria is nonselective. Glomerular destruction occurs slowly due primarily to progressive thickening of the capillary wall, which results from laminin accumulation along the subepithelial surface.

Pathology. The renal pathology in membranous nephropathy is illustrated in Fig. 354-8. By light microscopy, glomeruli in early membranous nephropathy appear normal and cannot be distinguished from MCD (or FGS) unless IF and EM studies are performed. Biopsies later in the course of the disease show an increase in capillary wall thickness but no inflammatory changes or cellular proliferation (Figure 354-8, *A*). When stained with silver methenamine a "spike and dome" pattern may be seen due to projections of excess basement membrane, mostly laminin, between the subepithelial deposits. By IF there is a characteristic, finely granular capillary wall staining for IgG and complement present uniformly throughout all loops in the glomeruli (Fig. 354-8, *B*). Mesangial deposits are usually not seen

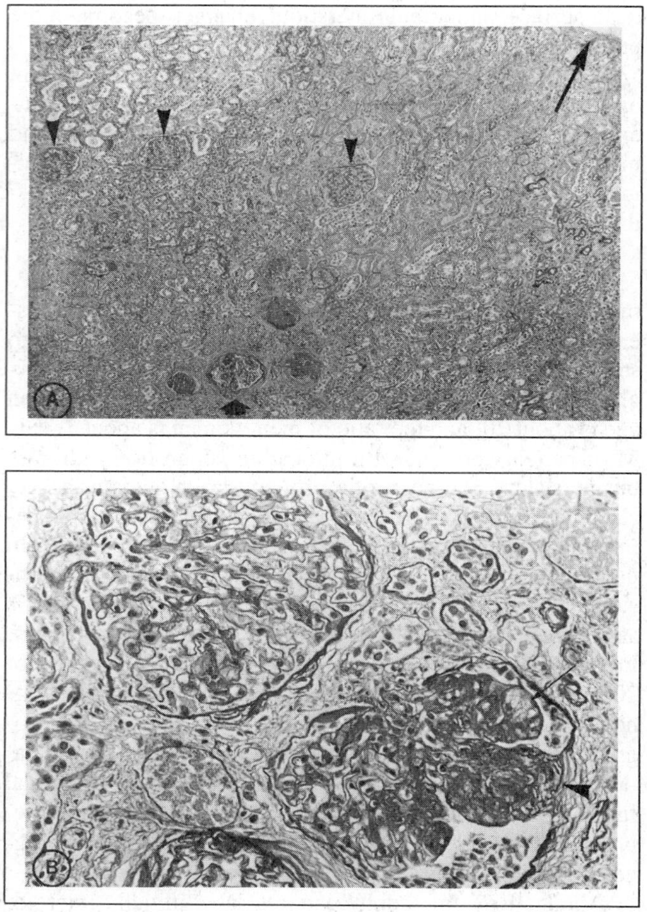

Fig. 354-7. Renal biopsy findings in a patient with steroid-resistant idiopathic nephrotic syndrome and focal glomerular sclerosis. **A,** A low-power light micrograph illustrates the juxtamedullary distribution of sclerotic lesions. Several glomeruli in the deep cortex are totally sclerotic, and one *(short arrow)* has only segmental involvement. Superficial glomeruli *(arrowheads)* near the cortical surface, identified by the *long arrow,* are normal. There is also tubular atrophy and interstitial fibrosis (periodic acid-Schiff stain; ×40). **B,** the glomerulus in the upper left is normal with adhesion to Bowman's capsule *(arrowhead)* and foamy cells *(small arrow)* (Periodic acid-Schiff stain; ×265).

except in the membranous form of lupus nephritis (see later discussion). EM reveals electron-dense deposits in a discontinuous pattern exclusively along the subepithelial surface of the glomerular capillary wall (Fig. 354-8, *C*). As the disease progresses the deposits may gradually become intramembranous and then resolve, leaving areas of lucency in the basement membrane.

Clinical and laboratory features. Membranous nephropathy is a disease of adults with a mean age of 40 to 50 and a male predominance of 2 to 1. Most patients (80%) present with the insidious onset of idiopathic nephrotic syndrome and have normal renal function, although less severe or earlier cases with only asymptomatic proteinuria also occur. Hematuria is relatively uncommon (20%), and the urinalysis usually shows only nephrotic changes. Hypertension is also unusual in the absence of volume overload, and patients may progress to end-stage renal disease without developing increased blood pressure.

The natural history of membranous nephropathy is quite variable. Urine protein excretion may vary widely from day to day and week to week. The spontaneous remission rate is about 25% in adults and 50% in children, but spontaneous remission after the first year of the disease is uncommon. Another 25% of patients have persistent proteinuria but retain stable renal function for decades. About 50% of patients have a slow but progressive loss of renal function over 3 to 10 years. Rarely, previously stable patients may develop rapidly progressive glomerulonephritis with crescents due to a superimposed anti-GBM antibody disease.

Three clinical conditions associated with membranous nephropathy warrant comment. The incidence of secondary renal vein thrombosis in idiopathic membranous nephropathy has been estimated to be up to 40%, but renal vein thrombosis does not appear to alter the severity or course of the renal disease. Renal venography and anticoagulant therapy are undertaken only if thromboembolic complications occur. A second important association is with a variety of carcinomas, especially of the lung, stomach, and colon. Neoplasms have been reported in up to 25% of patients over age 50 with membranous nephropathy. They are often occult when the nephrotic syndrome develops and should be searched for carefully in such patients. Finally, a lesion clinically and pathologically indistinguishable from idiopathic membranous nephropathy is seen in 15% of patients with lupus nephritis (see later discussion). These patients typically have low levels of anti-DNA antibodies and may present with negative antinuclear antibody tests and normal complement levels. This possibility must be kept in mind, particularly in young women presenting with apparently idiopathic membranous nephropathy. There are no laboratory findings specific for membranous nephropathy except as they may occur in association with the conditions listed earlier.

Diagnosis. The diagnosis of membranous nephropathy is made only by demonstrating the characteristic findings described above by light, IF, and EM studies of a renal biopsy specimen.

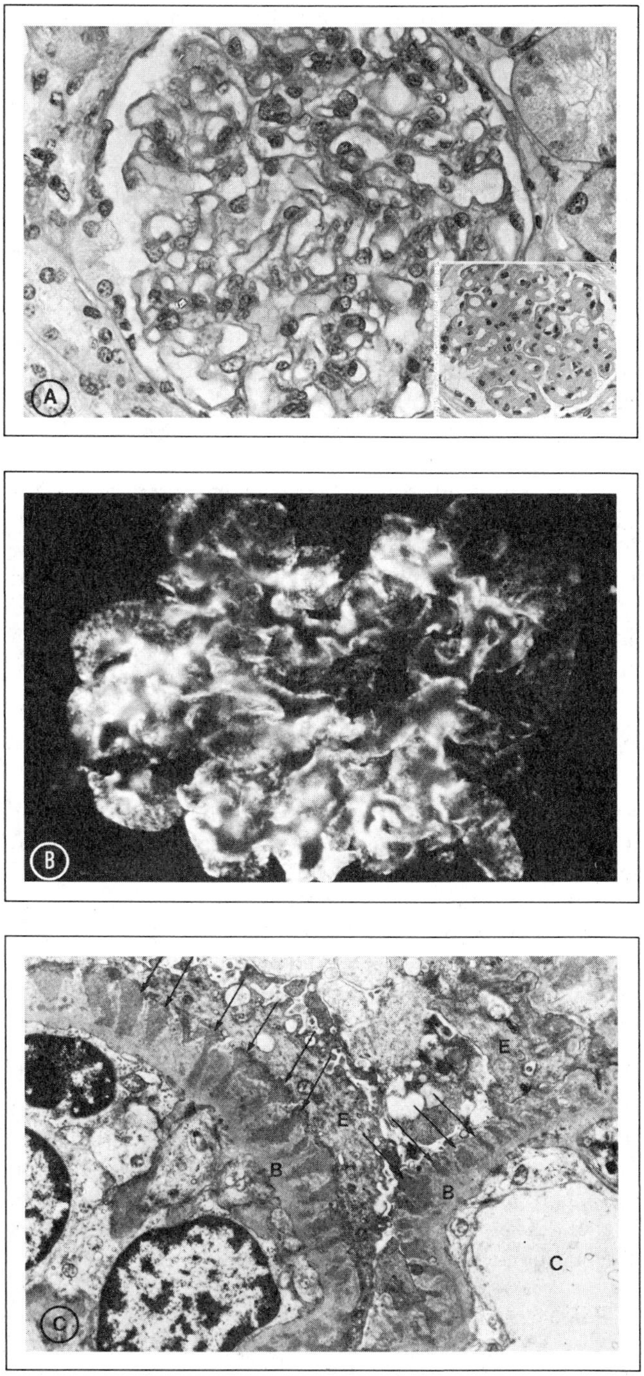

Fig. 354-8. Renal biopsy from a patient with the idiopathic nephrotic syndrome due to membranous nephropathy. **A,** By light microscopy the glomerulus is essentially normal (periodic acid-Schiff stain; ×500). As the disease progresses there is diffuse thickening of the capillary walls without cellular proliferation (*A inset,* Hematoxylin-eosin stain; ×125). **B,** By immunofluorescence finely granular deposits of IgG (and C3) are distributed evenly along all capillary loops (×450). **C,** Electron microscopy shows discontinuous electron dense deposits *(arrows)* along the subepithelial surface of the basement membrane *(B)* and in filtration slit pores with spikelike projections of basement membrane between the deposits. *C:* capillary lumen; *E:* epithelial cells (Uranyl and lead stain; ×500).

Treatment. Treatment of membranous nephropathy remains controversial. Patients who have less than 10 g of proteinuria, normal renal function, and no hypertension tend to do well, particularly if they are female. Poor prognostic signs include proteinuria in excess of 10 g/day, male sex, hypertension, and decreased renal function. A 3-month course of alternate day prednisone therapy, about 2 mg/kg/day, may induce remission in some patients. Better results have been obtained combining steroids, sometimes given with a monthly methylprednisolone pulse, with cytotoxic agents. In patients progressing, or at high risk of progressing, steroid therapy is indicated. Cytotoxic agents should probably be added if any renal functional deterioration occurs. In patients with membranous nephropathy associated with hepatitis B antigenemia, antiviral therapy with alpha-interferon may be useful.

Renal transplantation has been widely used in patients with end-stage renal disease due to membranous nephropathy. Recurrent disease after transplantation has been rare and has occurred only in patients with unusually rapid courses who develop renal failure in 3 years or less after diagnosis. Membranous nephropathy has also been reported to develop de novo in renal transplants and is a common cause of nephrotic syndrome in transplant recipients.

Membranoproliferative glomerulonephritis

At least two major subgroups of MPGN, type I and type II, are recognized. Although their clinical and light microscopic features are similar, differences in other features strongly suggest that different pathogenetic mechanisms are involved. These two subtypes are therefore discussed here as separate entities except in areas where no major distinction is apparent.

Etiology and incidence (types I and II). The etiology of MPGN is not known. The disease causes about 10% of all cases of idiopathic nephrotic syndrome in both children and adults, but is decreasing in frequency. In most series the ratio of type I/type II is about 2:1. In addition to causing the nephrotic syndrome, MPGN is the underlying disease in about 20% of children who present with clinical features of acute glomerulonephritis.

Pathogenesis and pathophysiology

Type I MPGN. Characteristics of type I MPGN include the presence of granular subendothelial and sometimes subepithelial immune complex deposits, low levels of serum complement with classic pathway activation, presence of cryoglobulins and circulating immune complexes, and the development of a very similar lesion in patients with certain chronic infections such as shunt nephritis and chronic hepatitis B and C antigenemia. Although about one third of patients have a history of a recent upper respiratory tract infection, the nature of the stimulus that induces subsequent glomerular immune complex formation has not been defined. The presence of complement deposits, neutrophils, and occasional crescents suggests that glomerular injury in this disease is complement-neutrophil mediated.

Type II MPGN (dense deposit disease). Unlike studies of type I MPGN, IF studies in dense deposit disease generally do not reveal immunoglobulin deposition, and the dense deposits seen by EM are structural lesions in the GBM, and not conventional immune deposits. The process that produces the abnormalities in basement membrane biochemistry and ultrastructure is unclear.

Type II MPGN is now a rare disorder seen primarily in developing countries. In most patients with dense deposit disease, a circulating IgG antibody is present, which is directed against the C3 convertase of the alternate complement pathway (C3Bb) and has been termed C3 nephritic factor, or C3NeF. Most patients also show a persistent reduction in C3, the alternate complement pathway proteins properdin and factor B, and late-reacting complement components, whereas C1, C4, and C2 are normal. C3NeF appears to stabilize the C3Bb C3 convertase resulting in persistent generation of C3b and activation of the alternate complement pathway via the C3b-dependent feedback loop.

Pathology

Type I MPGN. The pathologic findings in type I MPGN are illustrated in Fig. 354-9. Light microscopy reveals diffuse glomerular abnormalities with thickening of the capillary walls and enlargement of glomerular tufts, often in a lobular pattern (Fig. 354-9, *A*). Mesangial cells and matrix are increased, neutrophils are often present, and epithelial crescents may occasionally be seen. The thickened capillary wall is due to interposition of mesangial matrix between GBM and endothelial cells, which gives a characteristic splitting or double contour to the capillary wall ("tram-tracks") when stained with appropriate stains. IF reveals coarsely granular deposits of C3, and often C1q, C4, and properdin, in the mesangium and along the peripheral aspect of the capillary wall (see Fig. 354-9, *B*). These complement components are usually accompanied by IgG and IgM. By EM the typical findings are electron-dense deposits along the subendothelial surface of the peripheral capillary loops and in the mesangium, and the presence of mesangial interposition encircling the capillary loop to varying degrees and separating the lamina densa from endothelial cells with narrowing of the capillary lumen. Occasionally, subepithelial deposits and humps such as those in poststreptococcal nephritis may be seen.

Type II MPGN (dense deposit disease). In dense deposit disease, the findings by light microscopy are similar to those in type I MPGN. IF staining is positive only for C3, which is distributed along the margin of the dense deposits and around dense deposits in the mesangium. Occasional deposits of IgM may be seen, but IgG and early complement components are characteristically absent. EM reveals the presence of a dense, homogeneous osmophilic material replacing the lamina densa of the GBM.

Clinical and laboratory features. The clinical manifestations of MPGN are much more variable than in other glomerular diseases causing the nephrotic syndrome, and there are no consistent differences between types I and II that permit differentiation on clinical grounds. MPGN is a disease

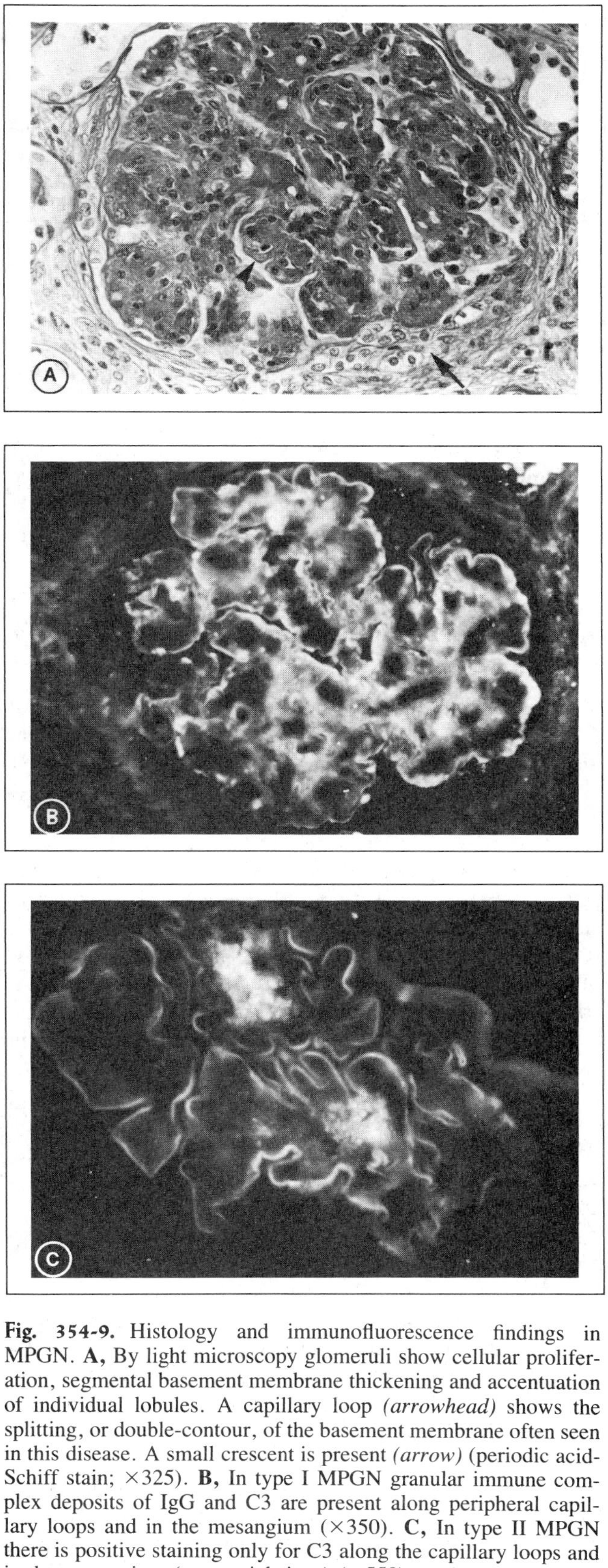

Fig. 354-9. Histology and immunofluorescence findings in MPGN. **A,** By light microscopy glomeruli show cellular proliferation, segmental basement membrane thickening and accentuation of individual lobules. A capillary loop *(arrowhead)* shows the splitting, or double-contour, of the basement membrane often seen in this disease. A small crescent is present *(arrow)* (periodic acid-Schiff stain; ×325). **B,** In type I MPGN granular immune complex deposits of IgG and C3 are present along peripheral capillary loops and in the mesangium (×350). **C,** In type II MPGN there is positive staining only for C3 along the capillary loops and in the mesangium (mesangial rings) (×550).

of children and adolescents usually between the ages of 5 and 15 with only 10% of cases over age 30. MPGN is somewhat more common in females. Onset occurs after an upper respiratory tract infection in many patients. Some cases clearly follow streptococcal infections, and may account for some of the reported cases of chronic poststreptococcal nephritis, but there is no evidence for a streptococcal etiology in most cases. About 20% of all patients present with an acute nephritic syndrome, and about 40% present with nephrotic syndrome, with or without a nephritic component. Nephrotic syndrome develops in over 80% of patients sometime during the course of the disease, and persistent nephrotic syndrome is more common in type II disease. The remaining 40% of patients are detected by finding asymptomatic hematuria or proteinuria on routine examinations. Hypertension is a common early manifestation of MPGN and is present initially in 30% to 50% of patients. Renal function is impaired in about one third of patients at the time of diagnosis.

The course of MPGN, like the clinical presentation, is variable. Within 6 to 10 years about one third of patients progress to chronic renal failure, one third have persistent nephrotic syndrome with relatively stable renal function, and one third have persistent non-nephrotic proteinuria or hematuria. Spontaneous remissions are rare. In the long term (10 to 20 years), at least 50% of patients will progress to end-stage renal disease, and patients with type II MPGN progress more frequently and more rapidly than do patients with type I disease.

The laboratory features of MPGN are not different from other diseases causing nephrotic syndrome except with respect to the complement abnormalities. In type I, serum levels of both classic and alternate pathway complement are reduced at some point during the course of the disease in all patients, but levels tend to fluctuate. Hypocomplementemia is present on a single determination at the time of diagnosis in less than half of patients. There is no correlation between complement levels and disease severity, activity, or prognosis. In type II patients hypocomplementemia is more persistent, but involves only C3 and late-reacting components. C1, C4, and C2 are usually normal. C3NeF is also demonstrable in the serum of most patients with type II MPGN but is rarely present in type I.

Diagnosis. The clinical manifestations of MPGN are indistinguishable from several other glomerular diseases, and the diagnosis can be made only by renal biopsy. The disease should be strongly suspected in adolescent patients with nephrotic syndrome, hematuria, and persistent hypocomplementemia or in patients with partial lipodystrophy.

Treatment. There is no immediate response to oral steroid therapy in MPGN, although alternate day steroid therapy for 2 years has been reported to be beneficial in preserving renal function in children. However, there is no consensus that any form of therapy is beneficial in adults.

Both type I and type II MPGN have been reported to recur morphologically in transplanted kidneys (type I, 30%; type II, 90%). However, less than 25% of such patients develop nephrotic syndrome, and graft loss due to recurrent MPGN is rare.

GLOMERULAR INVOLVEMENT IN SYSTEMIC DISEASES

The various forms of vasculitis are the most common systemic diseases resulting in glomerular involvement. Among the diseases referred to as systemic necrotizing vasculitis, a distinction is made between necrotizing vasculitis involving medium-sized and larger vessels (polyarteritis nodosa), and necrotizing vasculitis involving small vessels and capillaries (microscopic polyarteritis nodosa [PAN] plus several well-defined clinical syndromes including lupus nephritis, Henoch-Schönlein purpura, and mixed essential mixed cryoglobulinemia). The only other common vasculitic syndrome with renal involvement is Wegener's granulomatosis.

Systemic necrotizing vasculitis involving large vessels

Polyarteritis nodosa. PAN is a disease of older patients, which may be associated with drug abuse (particularly amphetamines) and hepatitis B antigenemia. It is usually insidious in onset with arthralgias, weight loss, abdominal and testicular pain, fever, hypertension, and neurologic symptoms as prominent features. PAN is a disease of uncertain pathogenesis, which involves medium-sized blood vessels, and the kidney is affected in over 90% of cases. Pulmonary and skin lesions are rare. Histologically, there are acute inflammatory changes in medium-sized muscular arteries, particularly the arcuate and interlobular vessels with fibrinoid necrosis and subsequent aneurysms (Fig. 354-10). These lesions are generally not seen on renal biopsy and can best be demonstrated by abdominal angiography, which may demonstrate aneurysms in renal, hepatic, and mesenteric vessels.

Renal disease is usually manifest first as hematuria with an active urine sediment and mild proteinuria. The glomerular lesion is primarily an ischemic one in 70% of cases resulting from vasculitic involvement of arcuate and interlobular arteries. In 30% of patients a focal necrotizing glomerulonephritis with crescents similar to the lesions in small vessel vasculitis may be seen, and most of these patients are ANCA-positive. Both types of glomerular involvement can occur in the same patient. Immune deposits are usually not found in the glomerulus, and the pathogenesis of the renal disease is uncertain.

Renal failure is a major cause of death. It may be slowly progressive or develop acutely, often associated with accelerated hypertension. In patients with PAN who develop hypertension and acute renal failure, renal cortical necrosis is common, and there is little reversibility. More commonly, the disease is slowly progressive. Vigorous control of hypertension, use of oral steroids, and the addition of cytotoxic agents such as cyclophosphamide have resulted in 5-year survival rates of over 80% in uncontrolled studies.

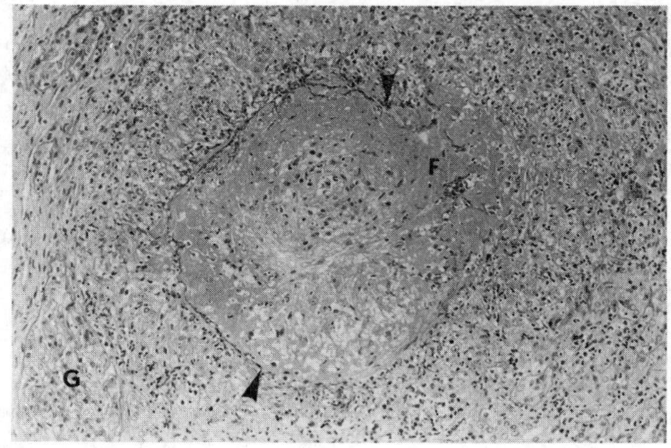

Fig. 354-10. Renal biopsy from a patient with the classic form of polyarteritis nodosa. An arcuate artery shows extensive fibrinoid necrosis *(F)* reduplication of the elastic lamina *(arrows),* occlusion and a perivascular inflammatory cell infiltrate. The glomerulus *(G)* is intact (Periodic acid-Schiff stain; ×375).

Systemic necrotizing vasculitis involving small vessels

Microscopic PAN. Microscopic PAN as a cause of ANCA-positive vasculitis with RPGN is discussed under Idiopathic (pauci-immune) Crescentic Glomerulonephritis.

Systemic lupus erythematosus (SLE). The current diagnostic criteria and clinical manifestations of SLE are considered in more detail in Chapter 177 (Systemic Lupus Erythematosus). This describes only the renal involvement in this common form of systemic necrotizing vasculitis. About 70% of all patients have clinical manifestations of renal disease, which may include microscopic hematuria, proteinuria, acute nephritic syndrome with acute renal failure, and nephrotic syndrome. Renal biopsies reveal abnormalities in most patients regardless of clinical manifestations.

The most common classification system used for renal involvement in SLE is the World Health Organization (WHO) classification, which is based on histopathologic criteria (Table 354-4). In Table 354-4 the WHO classification is presented with the approximate frequency of each lesion, the associated clinical manifestations, and the prognosis.

Class I (normal kidneys, <5%). Only rare patients with diagnostic criteria for SLE have entirely normal kidneys by light microscopy, immunofluorescence, and electron microscopy, as well as an absence of clinical manifestations of glomerular disease.

Class II (minimal or mesangial lupus nephritis, 15%). Class II is the earliest and least severe form of renal involvement in SLE. It is characterized by mesangial deposits of immunoglobulin and C3 with (class IIB) or without (class IIA) focal proliferative changes by light microscopy. These lesions are similar to those illustrated for IgA ne-

Table 354-4. Histologic class, clinical presentation, and prognosis in systemic lupus erythematosus (SLE)

Histologic type	WHO class	Frequency (%)*	Proteinuria	Nephrotic syndrome†	Azotemia‡	Death	Uremic death
Normal	I	<5	0	0	0	0	0
Mesangial	II	15	68	0	12	18	0
Focal proliferative	III	20	100	15	18	30	11
Diffuse proliferative	IV	50	100	87	75	58	36
Membranous	V	15	100	88	20	38	6

*% of patients biopsied with SLE who exhibit this lesion.
†Proteinuria exceeding 3.0 g/24 hr.
‡Serum creatinine > 1.2 mg% or BUN > 25 mg%.

phropathy in Fig. 354-3. Clinical manifestations of proteinuria and hematuria are present in two thirds of patients. Nephrotic syndrome and renal insufficiency, however, are uncommon and do not develop unless there is progression to a more severe lesion, which occurs in about 20% of such patients. Complement levels usually are normal. The 5-year survival rate exceeds 90%, and no specific therapy is indicated for the renal lesion.

Class III (focal proliferative lupus nephritis, 20%). This lesion is a stage in the continuum between mesangial lesions alone and diffuse proliferative lupus nephritis. Focal proliferative changes, as illustrated in Fig. 354-3, are present in less than 50% of glomeruli. Deposits are predominantly mesangial (Fig. 354-3, *B*), but occasional subendothelial deposits may be seen. All patients have proteinuria, but nephrotic syndrome and renal insufficiency occur in less than 20% and often remit after steroid therapy. Serologic abnormalities including hypocomplementemia are more severe than in class II disease. Long-term prognosis with this lesion is also good (90% 5-year survival), but there is a relatively high incidence of transformation to class IV disease resulting in a reduction in 5-year survival to about 70%, with almost half of the deaths occurring from renal failure. The most reliable predictor of progression is probably the presence of subendothelial deposits by EM.

Class IV (diffuse proliferative lupus nephritis, 50%). Class IV is the most severe form of glomerular disease in lupus, with proliferation seen in over 50% of glomeruli, frequently accompanied by crescent formation and necrosis. Extensive mesangial and subendothelial deposits can be seen by IF and EM. Subepithelial deposits may also be present. Proteinuria is seen in all patients, and nephrotic range proteinuria is present in 50% at onset and in 90% at some time during the course of the disease. Renal function is decreased in 75% of patients at the time of presentation, and serologic evidence of disease activity including hypocomplementemia, elevated levels of anti-DNA antibody, and circulating immune complexes are present in most patients. The long-term prognosis of this lesion has improved considerably. Survival rates of over 70% at 5 years are now common. Patients who exhibit a remission of nephrotic syndrome and normalization of serologic parameters within 1 year of starting therapy have the best prognosis.

Class V (membranous lupus nephritis, 15%). About 15% of patients with SLE develop a glomerular lesion that can be indistinguishable from idiopathic membranous nephropathy. Unlike idiopathic membranous nephropathy, the subepithelial deposits usually contain all immunoglobulins ("full house" immunofluorescence) and C3, and some mesangial deposits are usually present. Nephrotic syndrome and slowly progressive renal disease are common. The level and avidity of anti-DNA antibody are often low in such patients who may have undetectable levels of antinuclear antibody at the time of presentation. Some transformation can occur from class V to class IV, and vice versa, but the long-term prognosis for patients with this lesion does not differ significantly from those with class II disease. As in idiopathic membranous nephropathy, there appears to be an increased incidence of renal vein thrombosis. Therapy as discussed under Idiopathic Membranous Nephropathy should probably be given to these patients.

Serologic monitoring. Serologic tests that have been correlated with renal disease activity in SLE include measurements of antibody to double-stranded DNA, particularly if only complement-fixing antibodies are measured, and levels of C3, C4, and CH50, with C4 probably the most sensitive. Although reports of a general correlation between abnormalities in each of these laboratory parameters and disease activity in large numbers of patients have been published, the utility of such measurements in predicting renal disease activity and adjusting therapy in individual patients is minimal. The best parameters for following the activity of renal disease are the serum creatinine level, urine protein excretion, and careful examination of the urine sediment.

Treatment of lupus nephritis. There is general agreement that oral steroids are beneficial in treating lupus nephritis. Usually high dose steroid therapy is given for a period of 4 to 6 weeks and subsequently tapered and adjusted according to response in renal function, serologic parameters, and extrarenal disease. In the two decades since the introduction of steroid therapy, survival rates have increased steadily to over 70% 5-year survival in class IV disease and 90% in other patients.

Benefits from immunosuppressive drug therapy are most apparent in patients with class IV disease. Use of cytotoxic agents should be considered in such patients, particularly when nephrotic syndrome persists, when azotemia does not improve after treatment with oral steroids, when steroid toxicity develops, or when renal function is rapidly deteriorating. Recent studies demonstrate that administration of cyclophosphamide as a monthly IV pulse is as efficacious and less toxic than daily oral administration, and improves renal survival significantly in patients with severe lupus nephritis. In the presence of crescents and rapidly deteriorating renal function, steroid pulse therapy as discussed for idiopathic crescentic glomerulonephritis may be more efficacious than high doses of oral steroids alone. Plasma exchange therapy does not appear useful in the routine management of lupus nephritis.

Henoch-Schönlein purpura. This disease, also referred to as Henoch-Schönlein syndrome or anaphylactoid purpura, is another systemic necrotizing vasculitis of small vessels in which systemic manifestations include palpable purpura (100%) on the extensor surfaces of the legs, arms, and buttocks due to a leukocytoclastic vasculitis of dermal vessels; arthralgias of large joints, usually the knees and ankles (70%); gastrointestinal involvement with colic and bleeding (25%); and renal involvement. About 30% of patients have clinical evidence of renal disease in the form of hematuria or acute nephritic syndrome, and the disease is a common cause of glomerulonephritis before age 15. Except for the systemic manifestations, the disease is similar in its morphologic and clinical characteristics to IgA nephropathy, and the pathogenetic mechanisms are presumably similar. However, Henoch-Schönlein purpura is somewhat more severe, particularly in adults. The typical presentation is with an acute nephritic syndrome, usually without edema or hypertension, developing within 3 months of the onset of other systemic manifestations. In contrast to IgA nephropathy, up to 25% of adults may develop a severe crescentic lesion with RPGN. Nephrotic syndrome has been reported to develop in over 50%, of patients and progressive renal failure occurs in at least 25% of patients. Predictors of progressive disease include presentation with an acute nephritic syndrome, nephrotic syndrome, and crescents. Most patients have self-limited episodes of renal involvement usually lasting 1 week or less; however, recurrences are common.

Laboratory features are not distinctive and do not differ from those described for IgA nephropathy. Elevated levels of IgA-fibronectin aggregates are often present. Renal biopsy may reveal a spectrum of lesions ranging from focal mesangial proliferation to diffuse crescentic glomerulonephritis, but the most characteristic lesion is a focal necrotizing glomerulonephritis in which necrosis and fibrin deposition are more common than in IgA nephropathy. IgA deposits are also present in dermal capillaries of involved or uninvolved skin; and a necrotizing vasculitis may be seen in the arterioles, capillaries, and venules of affected organs including the kidney.

The pathogenesis of Henoch-Schönlein purpura is unknown. The various possible pathogenetic mechanisms are outlined in the discussion of IgA nephropathy. Reports of patients with typical IgA nephropathy who later develop systemic manifestations of this disease, IgA nephropathy and Henoch-Schönlein purpura in identical twins, and similar immunogenetic associations in the two diseases, as well as the clinical, histologic, and immunopathologic similarities, strongly implicates a common underlying disease.

No treatment has been shown to be of benefit in patients with recurrent episodes of acute nephritis or patients with slowly progressive loss of renal function. Short courses of steroids may be useful in controlling systemic manifestations, but usually do not benefit the renal lesion. Patients who develop crescents and a clinical picture of RPGN should be treated as outlined under idiopathic crescentic glomerulonephritis. With focal necrotizing glomerular lesions and deteriorating renal function, the use of cytotoxic agents may be warranted.

Essential mixed cryoglobulinemia. Another systemic necrotizing vasculitis of small vessels that may affect the kidney is essential mixed cryoglobulinemia (EMC). Low concentrations of mixed cryoglobulins, usually type III with polyclonal IgG and IgM with rheumatoid factor activity, are seen in a variety of glomerular diseases, autoimmune disease, vasculidites, and neoplastic syndromes where they rarely produce symptoms. However, type II mixed cryoglobulins, which contain monoclonal rheumatoid factor and polyclonal IgG, are present in EMC associated with vascular purpura, Raynaud's phenomenon, arthralgias, weakness, and glomerulonephritis. The disease begins in middle age and affects women more than men. Fifty percent of patients have renal involvement, which is usually preceded by purpura and arthralgias. The severity of renal disease ranges from microscopic hematuria and mild proteinuria to an acute nephritic syndrome with acute renal failure. Nephrotic syndrome may also be seen and severe hypertension is common. Laboratory findings include a markedly elevated sedimentation rate, cryoglobulins, positive rheumatoid factor, hypocomplementemia, and often hepatitis B antigenemia or evidence of hepatitis C infection. The glomerular lesion is a diffuse proliferative and exudative glomerulonephritis, sometimes accompanied by vasculitis, with large PAS-positive proteinaceous subendothelial deposits present in many capillaries. The deposits are composed predominantly of IgG and IgM, presumably representing the cryoglobulins, with lesser amounts of C3 and fibrin, which exhibit a characteristic fibrillar or crystalloid appearance by EM. Patients with acute nephritic syndrome and renal failure have a poor prognosis. However, over 50% of patients with renal involvement recover with or without therapy, and the survival rate at 10 years is about 75%. No role for steroids or cytotoxic agents alone has been established in this disease, but recent reports suggest that plasma exchange therapy may improve the prognosis in patients with severe renal involvement.

Wegener's granulomatosis. Wegener's granulomatosis is a granulomatous vasculitis, which usually involves the upper and lower respiratory tract and kidneys. The presenting signs are most often respiratory, but renal involvement eventually develops in over 50% of patients and is the cause of death in up to 30%. Hematuria, proteinuria, and mild renal impairment may be seen due to a focal necrotizing and proliferative glomerulonephritis, usually without immune deposits; however, severe necrotizing and crescentic glomerulonephritis may develop rapidly. Necrotizing granulomatous vasculitis may be seen in biopsies of the respiratory tract but is often not evident in renal biopsies. In Wegener's granulomatosis, ANCA are usually positive and titers parallel disease activity. Although the diagnosis can often be made on clinical grounds, a renal biopsy is generally performed early in the disease to identify potentially severe renal involvement, which may be clinically silent, as well as to distinguish Wegener's granulomatosis from other diseases with pulmonary and renal manifestations such as Goodpasture's syndrome, which would be treated differently.

In recent studies, a remission rate of over 90% has been achieved in patients with Wegener's granulomatosis when steroids are used in combination with cyclophosphamide. Many patients have been able to maintain complete remissions and discontinue all drug therapy. Because therapy is more effective in preventing progression than it is in reversing the necrotizing glomerular lesion, early institution of treatment is particularly important with respect to the renal disease.

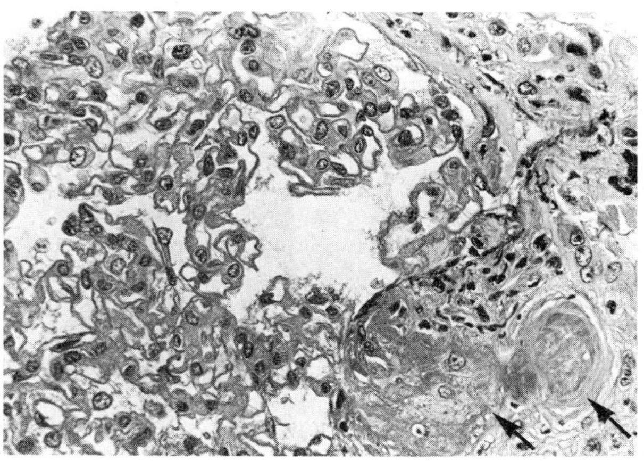

Fig. 354-11. Renal biopsy from a patient with hemolytic-uremic syndrome showing fibrinoid necrosis and occlusion of an afferent arteriole by fibrinoid material *(arrows)*. The glomerulus is normal except for slight mesangial matrix increase (Hematoxylin- eosin stain; ×450).

Thrombotic microangiopathy (hemolytic uremic syndrome and thrombotic thrombocytopenic purpura). Hemolytic uremic syndrome (HUS) and thrombotic thrombocytopenic purpura (TTP) can be referred to collectively as thrombotic microangiopathy, a term that emphasizes that the two diseases can be clinically indistinguishable, probably have a common pathogenesis, and respond to similar therapy.

Hemolytic uremic syndrome. HUS is a syndrome of microangiopathic hemolytic anemia, thrombocytopenia, and renal impairment, which usually occurs abruptly in children 3 to 10 days after episodes of gastroenteritis or viral upper respiratory tract infections. A similar syndrome may occur in adults, often in association with complications of pregnancy or during the postpartum period (postpartum acute renal failure) or associated with oral contraceptives. Up to 60% of children develop acute renal failure, which usually resolves spontaneously with only supportive therapy. Chronic renal failure occurs in only 10% of patients. Laboratory features of the disease include microangiopathic hemolytic anemia, thrombocytopenia, increased reticulocytes, elevated bilirubin levels, reduced haptoglobin levels, and elevations in fibrin split products, usually with only minimal laboratory evidence of disseminated intravascular coagulation. The glomerular lesion is one of the intimal hyperplasia of arterioles and intracapillary fibrin thrombi sometimes with areas of focal necrosis (Fig. 354-11). The anemia and thrombocytopenia presumably result from trapping of platelets and destruction of red cells in areas of capillary thrombosis. The pathogenesis of the syndrome is unknown, but may result from glomerular endothelial cell injury due to an antiendothelial cell antibody with subsequent platelet aggregation, fibrin deposition, and thrombosis. Recent studies have implicated gastroenteritis with verotoxin producing *Escherichia coli* 0157 in many patients.

Children with typical HUS require only supportive therapy, including early dialysis, because the rate of spontaneous recovery is very high. In adults, renal involvement is more severe and development of bilateral cortical necrosis more common. Severe disease is commonly seen in cases associated with pregnancy and oral contraceptives. No treatment has been established to be beneficial in HUS, although aspirin, antiplatelet agents, heparin, fresh frozen plasma infusions, and plasma exchange have all been advocated by some authors. In adults with severe disease treatment with plasma exchange as described later for TTP, the addition of steroids, anti-platelet agents, and aspirin is probably indicated.

Thrombotic thrombocytopenic purpura (TTP). TTP is distinguished from HUS by its more common occurrence in young adults, frequent presence of fever, and neurologic abnormalities, which tend to predominate and cause death and a lesser degree of renal involvement. Acute renal failure occurs in only about 10% of cases. Hematuria is the most common manifestation of renal disease. Mild proteinuria and a serum creatinine in excess of 2 mg/dl occur in only about 50% of cases. Histologically, the renal lesion is the same as that in HUS. The prognosis in TTP is worse than in HUS, with about a 75% mortality rate within 3 months, and spontaneous recovery is rare.

A wide variety of therapeutic regimens have been used in TTP. The most promising results have been obtained with plasma exchange, often using fresh plasma, antiplatelet agents, and steroids. Dramatic clinical remissions have occurred in several patients with apparently severe disease. In refractory cases, splenectomy may confer an additional benefit.

REFERENCES

Balow JE (Moderator): Lupus nephritis, Ann Intern Med 106:79-93, 1987.

Cameron JS et al: Idiopathic mesangial capillary glomerulonephritis. Comparison of types I and II in children and adults and long term prognosis, Am J Med 74:175-185, 1983.

Couser WG: Mediation of immune glomerular injury, J Am Soc Nephrol 1:13-1990.

Couser WG: Rapidly progressive glomerulonephritis. Classification and treatment, Am J Kidney Dis 11:449-464, 1988.

Jennette JC and Falk RJ: Antineutrophil cytoplasmic autoantibodies and associated diseases: a review, Am J Kidney Dis 15:517-529, 1990.

Jindal K et al: Long-term benefits of therapy with cyclophosphamide and prednisone in patients with membranous glomerulonephritis and impaired renal function, Am J Kidney Dis 19:61-67, 1992.

Julian BA et al: IgA nephropathy, the most common glomerulonephrititis world-wide, Am J Med 84:129, 1988.

Meyrier A and Simon P: Treatment of corticol resistant idiopathic nephrotic syndrome in the adult: minimal change disease and focal segmental glomerulosclerosis, Adv Nephrol 17:127, 1988.

Ponticelli C: Prognosis and treatment of membranous nephropathy, Kidney Int 29:927-934, 1986.

Rodriguez-Iturbe B: Epidemic poststreptococcal glomerulonephritis, Kidney Int 25:129-137, 1984.

Savage COS et al: Anti-glomerular basement membrane antibody mediated disease in the British Isles 1980-4, Br Med J 292:301-304, 1986.

CHAPTER

355 Diabetic Nephropathy

Fuad N. Ziyadeh
Stanley Goldfarb

Diabetic nephropathy is currently the major cause of end-stage renal failure in the United States; approximately 30% of all patients entering dialysis programs have lost renal function as a result of diabetes. Although nephropathy is one of the most serious long-term complications of diabetes, only 25% of patients with insulin-dependent diabetes mellitus (IDDM) will ever develop renal failure. Patients with both insulin-dependent (IDDM) and NIDDM develop diabetic nephropathy; the cumulative incidence of this diabetic microvascular complication is uncertain for NIDDM, but it too likely approaches 25% (with a lower incidence in whites and a higher incidence in non-whites such as African-Americans, Native Americans, Mexican-Americans, and Asians). The frequency of diabetic nephropathy among patients with IDDM has probably declined from nearly 50% during the last several decades for uncertain reasons, although the total number of patients afflicted with IDDM and NIDDM appears to be increasing worldwide. The presence of even minor evidence of renal involvement, however, appears to convey a dramatically increased risk of other microvascular and macrovascular complications so that overall mortality is not reduced. The mechanism of this latter association has not been explained as yet but likely reflects a generalized abnormality in small vessels or in organs such as kidney, nerve, or heart.

NATURAL HISTORY

Structural lesions

Kidney structure is dramatically altered in diabetes in virtually all affected patients, even those not destined to develop full-blown diabetic nephropathy (as defined by proteinuria $>$ 500 mg/day and progressive decline in glomerular filtration rate [GFR]). These structural changes include kidney enlargement involving both the tubules and the glomeruli and occurring as early as the first few months after the onset of diabetes. This process involves predominantly hypertrophy (cell enlargement) and, to a lesser extent, hyperplasia (cellular proliferation). The basement membrane of the tubules and the glomeruli also begin to thicken after 2 to 3 years of diabetes. After 3 to 5 years, progressive expansion of the mesangial regions of the glomerulus and of the tubulointerstitial regions of the kidney begin. Renal hypertrophy and basement membrane thickening may play an important role in the pathogenesis of diabetic nephropathy but to this time have been seen in all patients with long-standing diabetes and are not specific signs of overt nephropathy or the potential for progressive nephropathy to develop. Expansion of the mesangial region and tubulointerstitial fibrosis, however, do correlate well with progressive loss of renal function. These latter lesions are specific for the development of nephropathy as detected clinically by the appearance of hypertension, frank proteinuria, and reduced GFR.

The pathologically distinctive lesions of full blown diabetic glomerulopathy require a longer time to appear. The most nearly pathognomonic lesion is nodular diabetic glomerular sclerosis, frequently termed the Kimmelstiel-Wilson lesion. This lesion consists of nodular enlargement of the mesangial compartment of the glomerulus. A roughly similar pattern may be seen in other renal diseases, notably light-chain nephropathy and amyloidosis; however, appropriate immunofluorescent staining, electron microscopy, and historical and laboratory information distinguish these conditions from the nodular glomerular sclerosis of diabetes. More prevalent, and perhaps of greater pathophysiologic significance, is the diffuse rather than nodular enlargement of the mesangium. In addition, sclerotic glomeruli similar to those seen in kidneys with end-stage disease of any cause also accumulate in kidneys of patients with diabetic nephropathy. Another pathognomonic finding is the arteriosclerotic changes in the afferent and efferent arterioles. Although diabetic nephropathy is generally regarded as primarily a glomerular disease because of the presence of proteinuria and clear glomerular structural lesions, abnormalities of the vasculature and tubulointerstitium occur and correlate well with declining functional status. These lesions of the renal tubulointerstitium include chronic interstitial inflammation, fibrosis, and a predisposition to papillary necrosis.

Clinical course

Except for the renal functional abnormalities readily ascribable to the diabetic state, such as polyuria and ketoacidosis, renal function in the first years of IDDM is clinically unremarkable, even though a substantial portion of these patients have abnormally high GFRs. In fact, rarely does a patient with diabetes develop clinically detectable glomerular injury before the diabetes has existed for 10 years. In patients with NIDDM, however, the onset of disease is difficult to date, and hence the interval to renal disease more uncertain. Recent studies of populations that are at high risk for developing NIDDM such as the Pima Indians have suggested that nephropathy occurs in 20% to 30% of patients and that increased GFR is also a common feature of the early stages of NIDDM.

Microalbuminuria (i.e., urinary albumin excretion rates detectable by sensitive assays but below the level detectable by conventional clinical measurement, including dipstick) occurs in patients who go on to develop clinical nephropathy and therefore has been advocated as a useful tool for identifying the patients with diabetes at risk of developing nephropathy. Such microalbuminuric patients have been designated as having *incipient* nephropathy. However, there is a great deal of variation in the rate of microalbuminuria in patients with incipient nephropathy; all patients with diabetes, even those not destined to develop clinical nephropathy, develop intermittent microalbuminuria at times of suboptimal glucose control or strenuous exercise. This variability has reduced the overall utility of the test. Disagreement also exists over the rate of microalbuminuria that represents incipient nephropathy. Normal, nondiabetic individuals excrete <15 μg/min of albumin. It is quite clear that those diabetic patients with >70 μg/min are very likely, within 5 years, to develop gross proteinuria, a highly predictive marker for eventual renal failure. Whether lesser rates of excretion, although above the normal range, are definitely predictive of a high likelihood of clinical nephropathy in the subsequent 5 to 10 years remains controversial. Biopsy studies have shown that glomerular structural lesions are prominent in those patients with >70 μg/min microalbuminuria leading to the hypothesis that microalbuminuria is an **indicator** of rather than a **predictor** of diabetic nephropathy. These questions, however, remain unresolved and the clinical utility of assessing microalbuminuria is not fully established. A patient with diabetes with microalbuminuria should lead physicians to carefully monitor such individuals for even minimal hypertension and to optimize diet and blood glucose control to improve long-term prognosis (vide infra).

Frank proteinuria, detectable by the standard dipstick method, is the usual first indicator of diabetic glomerulopathy and occurs between 10 to 15 years after the diagnosis of IDDM. Over the next 7 to 10 years, those patients developing proteinuria experience a progressive decline in GFR. The rapidity of this decline is quite variable, but on average, patients with overt diabetic glomerulopathy lose 1 ml/min of GFR per month. Most diabetic patients with declining GFRs simultaneously develop obvious arterial hypertension, although many may have had modest elevations in blood pressure before developing proteinuria and declining renal function. During the phase of declining GFR, many patients develop proteinuria of nephrotic proportions with the common features of nephrotic syndrome.

The diagnosis of diabetic nephropathy is generally straightforward in patients with IDDM. The usual criteria are duration of diabetes greater than 10 years, proteinuria, arterial hypertension, and at least some degree of diabetic retinopathy. The urinalysis usually shows no cellular elements and consists merely of bland proteinuria. Rarely, patients with only diabetic nephropathy have hematuria and even red cell casts. Such an active sediment, however, is unusual enough that one should consider the possibility that the patient with hematuria has a renal disease other than diabetic nephropathy. Except in such unusual cases, renal biopsy is usually not required for diagnosis. In patients with NIDDM, however, the diagnosis is more complex. As many as 30% to 40% of patients with NIDDM and obvious renal dysfunction have other forms of renal disease including membranous nephropathy and hypertensive nephrosclerosis if renal biopsy is carried out.

In most respects, the signs and symptoms of renal insufficiency in diabetic nephropathy are similar to those seen in other progressive chronic renal diseases. However, several aspects of diabetes and its nonrenal chronic complications may adversely affect the diabetic patient with progressive renal insufficiency. For example, the propensity to extracellular volume overload that is often associated with renal disease, nephrotic syndrome, and hypertension may be poorly tolerated by a diabetic patient who has concomitant congestive heart failure. The kidney and retina in diabetes may be particularly susceptible to even slight elevations in blood pressure. The anorexia and nausea common to end-stage renal insufficiency are often exacerbated by intestinal autonomic neuropathy and gastroparesis in patients with diabetes. Visual impairment and peripheral vascular disease may further diminish the resiliency of these patients. These lesions may progress or even accelerate in patients. Insulin therapy often must be altered owing to progressive renal disease because the kidney is a major site for catabolism of insulin. Thus many patients with renal insufficiency require reductions in insulin dosage to maintain glucose control without hypoglycemia. Yet another metabolic complication suffered by patients with diabetic nephropathy is the predisposition to hyperkalemia and normal anion gap acidosis out of proportion to their degree of renal insufficiency. Many of these people have low levels of renin and aldosterone secretion that account for these metabolic abnormalities (Chapter 352).

PATHOGENESIS

Hyperglycemia is the central biochemical abnormality of diabetes. The mechanism of tissue and organ dysfunction in diabetes is due to this central feature and is not the result of a discrete mechanism of injury inherited or acquired independently of the hyperglycemic milieu. However, the exact cellular and molecular mediators of structural damage in diabetes continue to be elusive.

Some if not all of the theories of diabetic complications can be implicated in the pathogenesis of nephropathy. First, increased blood flow is a frequent early manifestation of hyperglycemia in a variety of tissues including skin, retina, and heart in early diabetes. Such changes have also been found in the kidney in both clinical and experimental diabetes. Patients with early (during the first 10 years of the disease) IDDM tend to have filtration rates greater than those of nondiabetics—indeed many are above the range of normal subjects. This hyperfiltration of early diabetes is due to increases in plasma flow and, based on data obtained in diabetic animals, a concomitant increase in glomerular capillary hydraulic pressures. Thus the diabetic kidney initially sustains increased renal perfusion and glomerular capillary pressure. The mechanism of this change in tissue blood flow has not been explained, but a number of possible factors include increased vasodilatory prostanoids; nitric oxide; and humoral vasodilators such as glucagon, atrial natriuretic peptide, and insulin-like growth factor-1 (IGF-1), have all been suggested. In addition, the glomerular capillary surface area available for filtration enlarges and contributes to the increase in filtration rate and possibly to the increase in blood flow. The hemodynamic changes of diabetes may contribute to the ultimate occurrence of end-stage renal disease through the injurious effects of high capillary pressures. The mechanistic link between high intraglomerular pressure and vascular injury has not been directly established but could be based on direct pressure injury to endothelium or on increased wall tension leading to altered capillary wall structure and function. The latter could be exacerbated by the increased glomerular size seen in diabetes as discussed later.

Besides alterations in renal hemodynamics, patients with diabetic nephropathy usually develop arterial hypertension. Indeed, those diabetic patients who develop the complication of renal failure may have a co-inherited predisposition to essential hypertension. Recent studies have suggested that this predisposition to arterial hypertension is marked by an increased activity of the sodium-lithium transporter in red blood cells, an abnormality also seen in subsets of nondiabetic essential hypertensives. The combination of arterial hypertension and renal vasodilatation would predictably lead to especially high intrarenal and glomerular capillary pressures.

Several other possible mechanisms could explain renal structural damage in both the tublulointerstitium and glomerulus in diabetes. First, primary vascular injury in diabetes could lead to vascular obstruction and obliteration and could thereby produce a form of ischemic damage to all the parenchymal structures in the kidney.

A series of recent studies has suggested an important role for the *nonenzymatic glycation* of various extracellular proteins in contributing to the altered structure of vascular tissue as well as other renal components including the renal interstitium when exposed to persistent elevation of extracellular glucose levels. *Nonenzymatic glycation* refers to the condensation reaction between a sugar aldehyde or ketone with the ϵ-amino group of lysine or hydroxylysine in proteins; the resultant aldimine (Schiff base) may undergo an Amadori rearrangement. These two compounds comprise the so-called "early glycation products." These products undergo further, slow, and irreversible reactions in vivo to form an array of fluorophors known collectively as advanced Maillard products or "advanced glycation products." Extracellular matrix proteins such as collagens are rich in lysine and hydroxylysine, have a long biologic half-life, and are continuously exposed to ambient levels of glucose in the extracellular fluid. These proteins are good candidates for undergoing substantial glycation in vivo. The advanced glycation end products so produced create extremely abnormal matrix proteins that are capable of trapping albumin within basement membranes, trapping IgG in extracellular matrix, and decreasing the solubility and capacity for degradation of the now abnormally linked collagens. Thus the increased fibrosis and exudative vascular hyalinoses that characterize long-standing diabetes in experimental animals as well as in patients could, in part, be a function of chronic exposure of extracellular matrix proteins to high ambient glucose levels and subsequent nonenzymatic glycation forming long-lived glycation products.

Studies of the alterations of extracellular matrix metabolism in diabetes all suggest that there is an increased production and reduced degradation; both processes may contribute to extracellular matrix accumulation. A number of observations in various tissues suggest that both animals with experimental diabetes and patients have an increased synthesis of a variety of extracellular matrix components including type IV and type I collagens as well as various noncollagenous proteins such as laminin. Vascular hyalinosis and interstitial fibrosis could result from the actions of glucose to stimulate biosynthetic pathways for extracellular matrix synthesis. In vivo and in vitro studies are complementary and strongly suggest that one of the mechanisms of increased interstitial and glomerular collagen formation in diabetes could be the result of the direct actions of glucose to increase collagen gene expression. The cellular mechanism of this action of glucose remains to be determined.

One potential common mechanism for the early tissue dysfunction seen in diabetes is stimulation of activity of the so-called *polyol pathway*. This series of biochemical reactions may be summarized as follows:

(EQ. 1)

$$\text{Glucose} \xrightarrow[\text{NADPH+ H}^+ \;\rightarrow\; \text{NADP}^+]{\text{Aldose Reductase}} \text{Sorbitol} \xrightarrow[\text{NAD}^+ \;\rightarrow\; \text{NADH+ H}^+]{\text{Sorbitol Dehydrogenase}} \text{Fructose}$$

The accumulation of sorbitol was first thought to produce cellular injury because of osmotically induced cell swelling, as the 6-carbon sugar alcohol was poorly diffusible across cell membranes and thus exerted an osmotic pressure. This mechanism may be operative in the lens in diabetes and lead to cataract formation. The cellular content of sorbitol in most tissues, however, does not exceed 200 to 300 μM despite severe hyperglycemia and therefore is a small osmotic burden. Rather, a large body of evidence suggests that increased sorbitol formation produces a fundamental disturbance in cellular *myo*-inositol metabolism and that this disturbance is the proximate cause of the cellular defect induced by polyol pathway activation. In peripheral nerve from rats with acute, streptozotocin-induced diabetes, there is a substantial reduction in energy utilization that is directly related to a reduction in the activity of Na^+, K^+-ATPase. This enzymatic defect is the cause of the delayed motor nerve conduction velocity; this latter functional disturbance is completely reversible by treatment with an aldose reductase inhibitor (ARI), which blocks sorbitol formation. Other biochemical disturbances that have been identified as consequences of polyol pathway activation include increased formation and abnormal cellular localization of protein kinase C, a key component of cell signaling pathways, altered redox potential in the cell as a result of the enhanced rate of reduction of NAD^+, and increased fructosylation of tissues, another form of the nonenzymatic glycation pathway described earlier. Use of ARIs may alter the hemodynamic abnormalities seen in the kidney in early experimental and clinical diabetes and may limit tissue glycation and increased extracellular matrix synthesis in experimental models. Clinical trials of the long-term safety and efficacy of this class of drugs are in progress.

The declining GFR characteristic of diabetic nephropathy most likely results from progressive expansion of the glomerular mesangium causing reduction in the glomerular filtering surface area. The pathway whereby the mesangium expands and glomerular function is thereby lost probably involves the interaction of several abnormalities of the patient's internal environment as described earlier. In addition, global glomerulosclerosis associated with widespread vascular ischemic lesions and tubulointerstitial damage also may contribute to a reduced GFR.

Finally, as mentioned earlier, stimuli to kidney growth in diabetes are uncertain, although recent studies suggest that altered formation of a variety of cytokines including IGF-1 and transforming growth factor beta (TGF-β) may be contributory. Mesangial expansion may be a specific example of how renal and particularly glomerular hypertrophy can be disadvantageous because disproportionate expansion of the mesangial areas appears to be an important contributor to ultimate filtration failure. Besides the possibility of undue mesangial growth with crowding out of the filtering surface area, the increased diameter of the glomerular capillary early in the course of diabetes may confer a mechanical disadvantage through the LaPlace relationship (tension = transmural pressure × vessel radius). Through this relationship, increased capillary diameter would increase wall tension, which may be another injurious component of diabetes-induced renal enlargement.

In summary, the pathogenesis of diabetic nephropathy probably results from several abnormalities of the diabetic milieu. Identified factors are increases in glucose level with arterial and glomerular capillary hypertension, the production of glycated protein products, diabetes-induced extracellular matrix synthesis and accumulation, and excessive renal growth.

PREVENTION AND THERAPY

Most clinical evidence suggests that the more closely glucose is maintained within the normal range, the less likely diabetic nephropathy will occur. Increasing evidence supports a role for strict control to prevent the development of incipient nephropathy and its manifestations including glomerular hyperfiltration, microalbuminuria, and renal hypertrophy. Once definite nephropathy with declining GFR occurs, however, strict control does not alter the rate of deterioration or the nature of the late structural lesions. As discussed in Chapter 168, the strict control of glucose by exogenous insulin is often difficult and may be attended by substantial risks, especially hypoglycemia. Thus at present, the best reasonable control of glucose, usually using more than one insulin injection per day, appears warranted to diminish the risk of long-term renal complications. Once clinical evidence of diabetic nephropathy has appeared, the value of more extreme measures such as continuous subcutaneous insulin infusion or pancreas transplantation to alter the course of established diabetic nephropathy is uncertain.

Control of arterial hypertension with antihypertensive drugs is the most important available measure for retarding the progression of established diabetic nephropathy and retinopathy (Chapter 23). Several clinical trials have demonstrated that reductions of arterial pressure with standard antihypertensive agents can dramatically slow the progressive decline in GFR. The specific antihypertensive regimen must be tailored to the patient's individual needs, but the overriding need to lower elevated arterial pressure with agents cannot be overemphasized. The concomitant appearance of clinically significant autonomic neuropathy with diabetic nephropathy and hypertension can complicate the treatment of hypertension because the patient tends to experience symptomatic hypotension when standing. Nevertheless, continued attempts should be made to use agents less likely to cause orthostatic hypotension, to instruct the patient in standing gradually and to adjust dose schedules to maximize effects of the drug during nighttime because blood pressure control is essential to reduce renal damage. Beta-blocking agents may, in certain patients, mask the symptoms of hypoglycemia, but these agents can be used in many patients with careful instruction and frequent monitoring of glucose levels. Increasingly, calcium channel blockers have been used effectively with minimum side effects. Converting enzyme inhibitors appear to be relatively well tolerated and are effective in controlling proteinuria and reducing progression of renal injury. In particular, they reduce early manifestations such as hyperfiltration and microalbuminuria and may be particularly effective in reducing intraglomerular pressure. These agents may cause hyperkalemia in diabetic patients with nephropathy. In patients with associated renal artery stenosis (more commonly the noninsulin-dependent older patient), these agents may induce reversible acute renal failure. Hence, creatinine and potassium levels should be monitored during treatment with these drugs. Because of the demonstrated importance of hypertension in the progression and perhaps the genesis of diabetic nephropathy, relatively strict criteria for antihypertensive therapy should be applied. Thus careful and repeated follow-up of even minor elevations above average blood pressure levels for age should be standard care of all patients with diabetes. If elevation above average arterial pressure is confirmed, antihypertensive treatment should be promptly initiated.

Dietary protein restriction appears to lessen the progression of a number of progressive renal diseases, including diabetic nephropathy. Available evidence suggests that restriction of dietary protein to the level of 0.8 g of high biologic value protein per kilogram body weight is safe. Careful education and follow-up, usually with the help of a dietitian, are required to effect such a dietary change successfully.

Those patients who develop end-stage renal disease have the same options for renal replacement therapy as do patients with other chronic renal diseases. Patients with diabetic nephropathy, in general, do less well with both hemodialysis and peritoneal dialysis than do patients with nondiabetic uremia and have a generally poorer prognosis after renal transplantation. However, the survival rates for patients with diabetes with all these modes of therapy have improved. Most patients prefer renal transplantation to dialysis because it offers a better quality of life and freedom from the encumbrances of regular dialytic therapy. The relative risks and inconveniences of the major forms of replacement therapy must be considered for each patient, and all forms of therapy should be considered for the diabetic uremic. A major difficulty for patients with diabetes is progressive vascular disease in other organs, notably the central nervous system and peripheral and coronary circulation; substantial mortality due to cardiovascular disease persists even with successful dialysis or transplantation.

REFERENCES

Bjorck S et al: Beneficial effects of angiotensin-converting enzyme inhibition on renal function in patients with diabetic nephropathy, Br Med J 293:471, 1986.

Brenner BM and Anderson S: Glomerular function in diabetes mellitus, Adv Nephrol 19:135-44, 1990.

Brownlee M, Cerami A, and Vlassara H: Advanced glycosylation end products in tissue and the biochemical basis of diabetic complications, N Engl J Med 318:1315, 1988.

Gluck SL and Klahr S: Enlarging our view of the diabetic kidney, N Engl J Med 324:1662, 1991.

Greene DA, Lattimer SA, and Sima AAF: Sorbitol, phosphoinositides, and sodium-potassium ATPase in the pathogenesis of diabetic complication, N Engl J Med 316:1321, 1987.

Kasiske BL et al: Effect of antihypertensive therapy on the kidney in patients with diabetes: a meta-regression analysis, Ann Int Med 118:129, 1993.

Krolewski AS et al: Predisposition to hypertension and susceptibility to renal disease in insulin dependent diabetes mellitus, N Engl J Med 318:140, 1988.

Krolewski AS, et al: Epidemiologic approach to the etiology of type I diabetes and its complications, N Engl J Med 317:1390, 1987.

Mangili R et al: Increased sodium-lithium countertransport activity in red cells of patients with insulin dependent diabetes mellitus, N Engl J Med 318:146, 1988.

Mogensen CE: Prediction of clinical diabetic nephropathy in IDDM patients. Alternatives to microalbuminuria? Diabetes 39:761, 1990.

Myers BD et al: Glomerular function in Pima Indians with noninsulin dependent diabetes mellitus of recent onset, J Clin Invest 88:524, 1991.

Tisher CC and Hostetter TH: Diabetic nephropathy. In Tisher CC and Brenner BM (eds): Renal pathology, Philadelphia, 1989, JB Lippincott.

Zeller K et al: Effect of dietary protein on the progression of renal failure in patients with insulin-dependent diabetes mellitus, N Engl J Med 324:79, 1991.

Ziyadeh FN, Goldfarb S, Kern EFO: Diabetic nephropathy: biochemical and metabolic mechanisms. In Brenner BM and Stein, editors: The kidney in diabetes mellitus. Contemp Issues Nephrol 1989 20, 87-113, 1989.

Ziyadeh FN and Goldfarb S: The renal tubulointerstitium in diabetes mellitus, Kidney Int 39:464, 1991.

CHAPTER

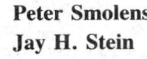

356 Renal Manifestations of Dysproteinemias

Peter Smolens
Jay H. Stein

MULTIPLE MYELOMA

Multiple myeloma, the most common of the dysproteinemias, is frequently complicated by alterations of renal function. These alterations may be manifested by acute or chronic renal failure, proteinuric syndromes, or renal tubular defects. In addition, a number of electrolyte alterations are unique and/or common in patients with multiple myeloma.

Renal failure

Renal insufficiency is commonly seen in patients with multiple myeloma. At presentation, about 50% have a serum creatinine level of greater than 1.5, and 10% to 20% have a serum creatinine concentration above 3.0 mg %. Renal failure requiring renal replacement therapy such as dialysis occurs in 5% to 15%. Of note, renal failure is the presenting manifestation of myeloma in 15% to 25% of patients who have myeloma associated renal failure. Patients who have normal renal function when they first manifest myeloma are unlikely to develop renal failure later. This is due, in large part, to careful appreciation of and response to potential complications of myeloma that may precipitate renal failure as detailed later.

Renal insufficiency is much more common and tends to be more severe in patients with light chain and immunoglobulin D (IgD) type myeloma in contrast to those with the more common IgG or IgA varieties. In most series, patients with more extensive tumor burden are at greater risk of development of renal failure.

Renal pathologic findings in about 50% of patients with myeloma associated renal failure show distinctive, highly eosinophilic light chain–containing casts in the distal nephron, as well as multinucleated giant cells and tubular atrophy (Fig. 356-1). Accordingly, these histologic features have come to be characterized as "myeloma kidney." The remainder of patients are found to have nonspecific interstitial fibrosis and tubular atrophy, acute tubular necrosis, or (less commonly) other lesions such as pyelonephritis, amyloidosis, or "immunoglobulin deposition disease."

A variety of factors (see the box to the right) have been found to contribute to the renal dysfunction that occurs in patients with myeloma.

There is much evidence indicating that the monoclonal immunoglobulin light chains (commonly referred to as Bence Jones proteins [BJPs]) play a critical role in the genesis of the renal failure. As noted, morphologic studies of the kidneys often show a cast nephropathy, and immunofluorescent study of these casts has shown that they are composed (at least in part) of BJPs. Several investigators have shown that the renal failure and distal nephron cast nephropathy can be reproduced by administration of the BJP to experimental animals. Not all patients with Bence Jones proteinuria experience renal failure, however, and experimental studies of BJPs have shown that they are not equally nephrotoxic. Those BJPs that are nephrotoxic may injure the kidney by induction of the formation of obstructing distal nephron casts or by direct tubular cell damage. A recent study has suggested that certain BJPs may alter the tubular reabsorptive capacity of the distal nephron, and the subsequent change in tubular fluid electrolytes may cause normal constituents of the urine in this segment (such as Tamm Horsfall protein) to copreciptate with the BJP, forming the characteristic distal nephron casts. The physicochemical characteristics that determine the nephrotoxicity of BJPs are not known. Factors such as BJP isotype (lambda or kappa), degree of glycosylation or polymerization, and net BJP electric charge have not been found to be predictive of BJP nephrotoxicity. It is possible that certain

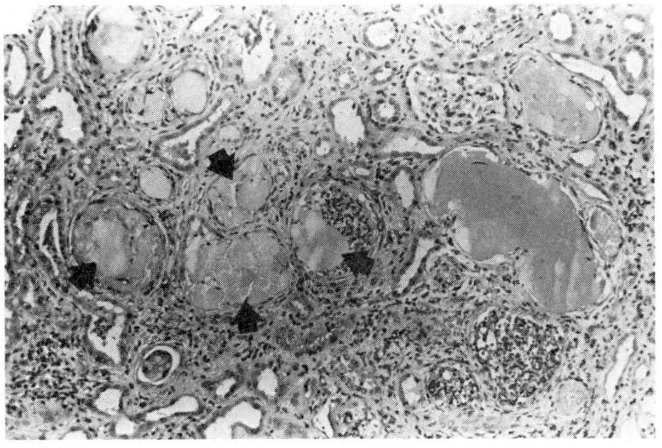

Fig. 356-1. End-stage myeloma kidney, with dense, birefringent intratubular cast formation *(heavy arrows)* and surrounding interstitial reaction. (Photomicrograph courtesy of Michael Kashgarian, Department of Pathology, Yale University School of Medicine.)

Factors that may contribute to myeloma-associated renal failure

Light chain–induced injury (cast nephropathy or direct tubular damage)
Hypercalcemia
Dehydration
Infection
Radiographic contrast media nephropathy
Drug nephropathy (antibiotics, NSAIDs)*
Amyloidosis
Light chain deposition disease
Obstructive nephropathy
Uric acid nephropathy
Hyperviscosity syndrome

*NSAIDs, nonsteroidal anti-inflammatory drugs.

factors may modulate BJP nephrotoxicity. For example, it has been found that modest hypercalcemia can markedly potentiate the nephrotoxicity of certain BJPs in experimental animal models.

Hypercalemia is a very important factor in the renal failure that occurs in these patients. Although it occurs in one third of all patients with multiple myeloma, it is present in up to two third of those with renal failure. Hypercalcemia may contribute to the renal failure in a variety of ways. Urinary concentrating ability may be impaired and polyuria and dehydration may result. Hypercalcemia may also cause vomiting and further exacerbate the volume depleted state. Indeed, up to 50% of patients with myeloma and renal failure are found to be dehydrated on presentation. Hypercalcemia may also suppress glomerular filtration rate (GFR) via its effects on renal hemodynamics, tissue injury from precipitation of calcium salts, and renal outlet obstruction from calcium containing stones.

Drug-induced renal failure is an important and potentially reversible and/or preventable consideration in these patients. They frequently require antibiotics because of their increased risk of infection. Thus they are more likely to experience antibiotic associated acute renal failure (such as aminoglycoside acute renal failure or interstitial nephritis from agents such as methicillin or ciprofloxacin). Bone pain is often considerable in patients with myeloma, and the use of nonsteroidal anti-inflammatory drugs (NSAIDs) for management of the bone pain has also increased the risk of development of acute renal failure.

Prior exposure to intravenous radiographic contrast media has been reported in a number of patients with multiple myeloma who subsequently had acute renal failure. Whether myeloma patients are uniquely predisposed to the nephrotoxic effects of radiocontrast media is currently unclear. The pre-existing renal dysfunction and/or dehydration may have been the factor rather than the myeloma that predisposed these patients to the radiocontrast media nephrotoxicity. Hyperuricemia frequently occurs in myeloma patients, but usually the uric acid concentration does not rise to the levels typically associated with acute uric acid nephropathy. Uric acid stones are a possible but uncommon cause of renal failure. Other potential causes in this population include bladder outlet obstruction by a plasmacytoma, prostatic hypertrophy, or a neurogenic bladder (as may be seen in patients with spinal column complications of myeloma).

Amyloidosis and immunoglobulin deposition disease each occur in approximately 5% to 10% of patients with myeloma and these may be the cause of the renal failure. Rarely, patients with myeloma may experience the hyperviscosity syndrome, and this may lead to renal vascular compromise and subsequent decrement in renal function.

Electrolyte abnormalities associated with multiple myeloma and/or light chain proteinuria

Hypercalcemia
Metabolic acidosis
Low anion gap
Fanconi syndrome (hypophosphatemia, hypouricemia, hypokalemia, acidosis, glucosuria, aminoaciduria)
Hyperuricemia
Spurious elevations in serum calcium and/or phosphate level

Electrolyte abnormalities in myeloma

A variety of electrolyte abnormalities may be observed in patients with multiple myeloma (see the box above). Hypercalcemia, as discussed earlier, is a frequent and major problem in these patients. Rarely, the serum calcium concentration may be spuriously elevated as a result of binding of calcium by the paraprotein. Metabolic acidosis may be a consequence of either a renal tubular acidification defect or the presence of renal failure and diminished capacity to synthesize ammonia. Patients with plasma cell dyscrasias frequently have a low anion gap with values ranging from 5 to 10 mEq/L below normal. The low anion gap appears to be due to the fact that many of the paraproteins are positively charged at a pH of 7.4 and these act as unmeasured cations. The Fanconi syndrome (aminoaciduria, glycosuria, phosphaturia, uricosuria, and proximal renal tubular acidosis) is seen in a small number of myeloma patients. Spurious elevations in serum phosphate level can be seen in 10% of sera containing paraproteins when standard colorimetric techniques are used. This is not a problem when deproteinized serum is examined or enzymatic techniques are used for phosphate level determination.

Renal tubular defects

Patients with multiple myeloma are frequently noted to have defects in urinary concentrating ability and renal acidification. These defects may occur both in patients with renal insufficiency and in those with a relatively well-preserved glomerular filtration rate. Despite the frequency with which these tubular defects may be found in patients with established myeloma, however, they rarely cause specific symptoms or severe alterations in serum electrolyte levels.

In contrast, a relatively small number of patients have been described who do not have the usual manifestations of myeloma but do have clinically significant tubular defects that are believed to be due to the effects of BJPs on the renal tubule. Unlike patients with clear-cut myeloma, these patients come to medical attention because of symptoms related to the tubular disorder such as polyuria generated by nephrogenic diabetes insipidus, or bone and muscle pain caused by the phosphate wasting of the Fanconi syndrome. A variety of tubular defects may be seen in these patients, including renal tubular acidosis, nephrogenic diabetes insipidus, and generalized proximal tubular dysfunction. The BJP excreted by these patients almost invariably is of the kappa type. Renal biopsy results in some, but not all, of these patients have shown distinctive crystalline deposits of the light chain within the tubular cells. Conditions other than plasma cell dyscrasias (such as drug-induced or heavy metal–induced nephropathy) can result in the development of light chain proteinuria and tubular defects similar to those described. These conditions differ from the conditions in plasma cell dyscrasias in that the light chain proteinuria is not monoclonal but polyclonal, and the light chain proteinuria is considered to be the result of the tubular damage and not the cause. Patients with monoclonal Bence Jones proteinuria and tubular disorders usually do not manifest overt myeloma or renal failure even after 10 or more years. Thus therapy should focus on management of the metabolic disorder. Cytotoxic therapy directed against the plasma cell dyscrasia should be withheld until the usual manifestations of myeloma become overt.

Proteinuria and nephrotic syndrome

Bence Jones proteinuria, when searched for with a combination of electrophoresis and immunoelectrophoresis, may be detected in 70% to 80% of patients with multiple myeloma. Many patients are found to excrete 1 to 3 g/day, and some have been reported to excrete 20 g or more daily. In addition, it is not uncommon for these patients to excrete abnormal amounts of albumin in the urine. The amount of albuminuria, however, is usually less than 1 g/day and nephrotic range albuminuria (>3.5 g/day) is found in less than 10% of patients. When nephrotic range proteinuria is observed, it should suggest the presence of renal amyloidosis, immunoglobulin deposition disease (discussed later), or another glomerular lesion. A variety of glomerular lesions, including mesangial proliferation, membranous nephropathy, nil lesion, and crescentic nephropathy, have been reported in patients with plasma cell dyscrasias such as "benign" monoclonal gammopathies and overt myeloma. Whether or not a causal relationship exists between the gammopathy and the glomerulopathy in these patients is not clear. However, significant improvement has been noted in several patients when therapy for the plasma cell dyscrasia was instituted. In view of this, it seems prudent to assume that a causal relationship could exist and to institute treatment to reduce the production of the paraprotein.

Monoclonal immunoglobulin deposition disease

Monoclonal immunoglobulin deposition disease (MIDD) involves the production of abnormal monoclonal immunoglubulins that are prone to tissue deposition. It may be seen in up to 5% to 10% of patients with myeloma and renal impairment. Of patients found to have MIDD, however, 40% to 70% do not meet the criteria for myeloma and do not exhibit overt myeloma in 1 to 5 years of follow-up observation. Patients usually have proteinuria and renal insufficiency. Renal histologic findings are variable, but most patients have thickened tubular and glomerular basement membranes. A most striking lesion, seen in perhaps one third of patients, consists of mesangial expansion and formation of intercapillary nodules similar in appearance to those seen in Kimmelstiel-Wilson (diabetic) glomerulopathy. Immunofluorescence studies reveal that the basement membrane thickening and glomerular nodules are due to deposition of the abnormal monoclonal immunoglubulin. Indeed, if immunofluorescence studies are not made, these patients with glomerular nodules are often incorrectly diagnosed as having diabetic nephropathy. In 90% of cases, the deposited immunoglobulin is a light chain; the light chain is of the kappa isotype in about 80% of these. Why the immunoglubulins in this syndrome are so prone to tissue deposition and to induction of subsequent tissue injury is not certain. Of note, immunoglobulin binding to tissue may be so avid that up to one third of the patients do not have a monoclonal immunoglobulin detectable in the serum or urine, and the diagnosis is only made at immunofluorescence examination of involved tissues. Virtually all of these patients have hypogammaglobulinemia and thus the diagnosis of MIDD should be considered in patients with hypogammaglobulinemia and renal insufficiency. The natural history of this disease is fairly rapid progression to end-stage renal disease. Once the kidney reaches this point, therapy for the plasma cell dyscrasia does not benefit the kidney. If treatment is instituted before that time, however, the deterioration in renal function can usually be halted or partially reversed. Renal transplantation in patients with MIDD and renal failure has frequently been complicated, unfortunately, by loss of transplant kidney function caused by recurrence of the immunoglobulin deposition in the transplanted kidney.

Renal amyloidosis (see Chapter 322)

Diagnosis

The diagnosis of multiple myeloma or isolated Bence Jones proteinuria should be considered in the older patient with acute or chronic renal failure, renal tubular defects, or unexplained proteinuria. A number of laboratory findings should also increase the suspicion that myeloma may be present. Bence Jones proteinuria patients commonly have urine that yields strong positive results for protein when tested with sulfosalicylic acid but only weak positive or nonreactive results in the tests that are specific for albumin (Albustix). Other findings that prompt consideration of multiple myeloma include elevated serum globulin levels, a low or negative anion gap, presence of rouleaux on the peripheral blood smear, and serum calcium level above 9 mg/dl despite renal failure and hyperphosphatemia. The diagnosis of multiple myeloma is confirmed by the finding of monoclonal paraprotein in urine and/or serum, bone marrow plasmacytosis (>15%), and lytic bone lesions or diffuse osteopenia. Ninety-nine percent of these patients are found to have a monoclonal protein in the urine or serum. If serum protein electrophoresis shows hypogammaglobulinemia, one should consider the possibility that light chain or IgD myeloma or monoclonal immunoglobulin deposition disease is present. The reason a serum spike is not seen in these conditions is that light chains are filtered into the urine and serum levels usually do not rise appreciably (unless renal failure is present), and IgD is usually present in very small quantities and 10-fold or greater increases caused by myeloma may still be below the limit of detection with serum protein electrophoresis. Quantitation of serum immunoglobulins in myeloma typically reveals suppression of normal immunoglobulin elements and the high levels of the paraprotein. If nephrotic range albuminuria is present, this should prompt consideration of myeloma associated glomerular diseases such as amyloidosis or immunoglobulin deposition disease or other glomerular processes that may or may not be related to the myeloma. If either condition is suspected, renal biopsy is indicated to confirm the diagnosis. Because the course of patients with myeloma and/or amyloidosis may be complicated by a variety of coagulopathies, one should confirm that clotting and bleeding parameters are normal before proceeding to renal biopsy.

Treatment

The initial approach to the patient with myeloma associated renal failure should include correction of dehydration and forced diuresis if the cardiopulmonary status permits, and correction of hypercalcemia and hyperuricemia. Alkalinization of the urine has been suggested by some clinicians to be beneficial, but because the procedure can promote precipitation of certain BJPs, its use is not recommended unless the effect of pH on the solubility of the particular light chain is known.

Renal ultrasound and/or computed tomography (CT) should be performed to exclude renal outlet obstruction and to estimate the chronicity of the renal failure as suggested by the renal size and structure. Hyperviscosity syndrome should be considered as a cause of the renal failure in patients with myeloma if serum IgA or IgG paraprotein levels are greater than 4 g/dl and in patients with Waldenstrom's macroglobulinemia if the serum IgM level is above 3 g/dl. If hyperviscosity is present, removal of the paraprotein by plasma exchange is indicated.

In view of the important role of BJPs in the genesis of the renal failure, treatment directed at lowering the blood level of BJPs with chemotherapy should be started once the patient is well hydrated. Although the blood BJP level can be lowered much more quickly with plasmapheresis, there is no consensus, as yet, on its efficacy in treatment of myeloma associated renal failure. The sole randomized, prospective study of the effect of addition of plasmapheresis to standard treatment did not show that it conferred any statistically significant advantage in reversing the renal failure. The only patients who were able to discontinue dialysis in that study, however, were those who were treated with plasmapheresis.

Renal biopsy may be useful in patients with renal failure who do not respond to treatment. Several studies have shown that irreversibility of the renal failure is associated with the intensity of cast formation and it has been suggested that aggressive measures such as plasmapheresis might be withheld in patients with this finding. In addition, renal biopsy may reveal the presence of other lesions that were not anticipated.

It should be emphasized that measures taken to prevent renal failure can have a major impact on preserving renal function in patients with myeloma as is attested to by the decreasing rate of renal failure in this population over the past 20 years. Maintaining adequate hydration is extremely important. Diuretics should be used with caution. The serum calcium concentration (corrected for the level of albumin) should be monitored frequently and hypercalcemia should be treated aggressively. Many of these patients have hypoalbuminemia, which may obscure the presence of true hypercalcemia. Patients with myeloma have an increased frequency of infections, which should be treated with the least nephrotoxic antibiotics. Management of bone pain should be attempted with drugs other than NSAIDs if possible. If radiographic imaging is required, one should try to minimize the amount of radiographic contrast agent used and ensure that the patient is well hydrated.

If renal replacement therapy is indicated, either hemodialysis or peritoneal dialysis may be used. Because patients may have lowered levels of normal immunoglobulins and bone marrow suppression, they are at higher risk of hemoaccess device infections if hemodialysis is used, and of peritonitis if peritoneal dialysis is performed. In selected younger patients whose myeloma is in prolonged complete remission, renal transplantation may be performed.

Prognosis

Renal failure in myeloma patients is reversible in about 50% with the use of chemotherapy and the conservative measures outlined. This is in marked contrast to reports in the 1960s and 1970s of improvement in renal function in less than 10%. The likelihood and degree of recovery are inversely related to the rise of serum creatinine level, although recovery can occur even in cases of severe renal failure. About 25% of the patients who require dialysis have sufficient return of function to allow them to discontinue it. Most recovery occurs within the first month, although slow recovery may continue for up to 11 months. If no recovery of function is seen in the first month, subsequent recovery is unlikely. In about 30% of patients with myeloma associated renal failure, renal function deteriorates despite therapy. If renal function worsens in the first month of treatment, progression to end-stage renal failure is to be expected.

Unfortunately, approximately 20% to 30% of patients with myeloma die within 3 months of presentation (generally as a result of progressive myeloma or infection). This risk of early death is increased in those who have renal failure at the time myeloma is diagnosed. In one study of more than 1000 patients the risk was below 10% if serum creatinine level was normal and above 30% if serum creatinine level was greater than 2.2. Median survival of myeloma patients without renal failure treated with Melphalan and prednisone is about 18 to 34 months; that of myeloma patients with end-stage renal failure treated similarly is 10 to 20 months. Whereas the chemotherapy of these patients is more commonly associated with hematologic toxicity caused by the decreased renal clearance of the antimitotic drugs, renal failure does not appear to be the major cause of this shortened survival. The cause of death in these patients is usually unremitting myeloma. Thus the life limiting factor in these patients is usually the progression of the myeloma rather than the presence of the renal failure. Patients who respond to chemotherapy have a higher survival rate. Current more aggressive chemotherapy regimens have been associated with an increased median survival rate in those with renal failure to about 25 months.

Waldenstrom's macroglobulinemia

Renal involvement in Waldenstrom's macroglobulinemia is less common and less severe than that seen in patients with myeloma. Mild to moderate azotemia, often associated with dehydration and/or hyperviscosity, has been reported in about 20% of patients. Severe renal failure is rare. Although proteinuria occurs in about 30% of cases, nephrotic range albuminuria is rare. The most distinctive histologic abnormality seen with renal involvement is IgM deposits (thrombi) in glomerular capillary lumens and subendothelial spaces. Interstitial aggregates of atypical lymphocytes may also be seen. Although light chain proteinuria is seen in about 80% of patients, typical cast nephropathy is unusual. Amyloidosis occurs in 10% to 15% of patients with macroglobulinemia, and amyloid renal involvement is suggested if nephrotic range albuminuria is present. In rare cases, a proliferative glomerulonephritis with renal failure may occur in association with IgM and IgG complexes. A variety of other renal lesions (minimal change nephropathy, membranous nephropathy, crescenteric nephritis) associated with Waldenstrom's macroglobulinemia have been reported, but it is not clear whether the relationship between the Waldenstrom's macroglobulinemia and the nephropathy is causal.

REFERENCES

Alexanian R, Barlogie B, and Dixon D: Renal failure in multiple myeloma: pathogenesis and prognostic implications. Arch Intern Med 150:1693, 1990.

Buxbaum JN et al: Monoclonal immunoglobulin deposition disease: light chain and light and heavy chain deposition diseases and their relation to light chain amyloidosis: clinical features, immunopathology, and molecular analysis. Ann Intern Med 112:455, 1990.

Gallo G: Renal complications of B-cell dyscrasias. N Engl J Med 324:1889, 1991.

Ganeval D et al: Treatment of multiple myeloma with renal involvement. Adv Nephol 21:347, 1992.

Johnson WJ et al: Treatment of renal failure associated with multiple myeloma: plasmapheresis, hemodialysis, and chemotherapy. Arch Intern Med 150:863, 1990.

Kyle RA: Monoclonal gammopathies and the kidney. Annu Rev Med 40:53, 1989.

Pasquali S et al: Long-term survival patients with acute and severe renal failure due to multiple myeloma. Clin Nephrol 34:247, 1990.

Sanders PW et al: Spectrum of glomerular and tubulointerstitial renal lesions associated with monotypical immunoglobulin light chain deposition. Lab Invest 64:527, 1991.

Sanders PW et al: Mechanisms of intranephronal proteinaceous cast formation by low molecular weight proteins. J Clin Invest 85:570, 1990.

Smolens P: The kidney in dysproteinemic states. Am Kidney Fund Newsl 4:27, 1987.

Solomon A: Nephrotoxic potential of Bence Jones proteins. N Engl J Med 324:1845, 1991.

Zucchelli P et al: Controlled plasma exchange trial in acute renal failure due to multiple myeloma. Kidney Int 33:1175, 1988.

CHAPTER

357 Toxic Nephropathy

William F. Finn

It is likely that a significant amount of acute and chronic renal injury results from exposure to various nephrotoxic substances that are found in the environment or encountered as occupational hazards. In addition, the list of diagnostic and therapeutic agents that produce renal injury continues to expand. The susceptibility of the kidney to these toxic agents is in large part a consequence of its intricate anatomic and functional relationships. For example, the blood flow to the kidney per gram of tissue weight is greater than that to any other organ, ensuring that exposure of the kidney to bloodborne toxins is great. Furthermore, the processes of glomerular filtration, tubular reabsorption, and secretion serve to concentrate toxic agents within the kidney itself. As a result of their sophisticated function, renal tubular epithelial cells are particularly vulnerable to the action of metabolic inhibitors. The kidney also possesses various mixed-function oxidases that are useful in the biotransformation of foreign compounds (xenobiotics) into nontoxic metabolites. At times, the process results in the production of more toxic compounds.

Specific agents may produce toxicity directly or as a result of an immune response. Injury may also occur indirectly when the primary damage is elsewhere, causing the liberation of substances that secondarily cause renal injury. The direct toxic effects are determined by the specific chemical properties of the substances, the duration and extent of exposure, and the nature of the host response. They may be manifested as abnormalities in the renal vasculature, dysfunction of the glomerular capillary membranes, or changes in tubular epithelial cell function. Immunologic responses include cytotoxic reactions with complement activation, immune complex reactions, and perhaps a delayed hypersensitivity response.

Host factors may alter renal toxicity by influencing the metabolism of xenobiotics, the renal concentration of toxic agents, the susceptibility to cell injury, or the capacity for repair. It is important to consider that exposure to several agents often produces a synergistic effect. Other important host factors are those related to growth and aging. Not only does renal susceptibility to toxic damage increase with age but at the same time the ability to repair damaged tissue also fades.

Often disregarded is the role of the nutritional status of the individual in determining the susceptibility or tolerance to or the recovery from noxious agents. Finally, certain disease states, particularly those independently involving the kidney, significantly enhance renal toxicity in response to various classes of agents.

The following discussion concentrates on the most important causes of environmental and occupational nephrotoxicity along with the most common causes of nephrotoxicity caused by diagnostic and therapeutic agents.

EFFECT OF ENVIRONMENTAL AND OCCUPATIONAL AGENTS ON THE KIDNEY

Glycols

Glycols are used in solvents in a number of industries. *Ethylene glycol* is the main component in antifreeze and may be ingested as a substitute for alcohol. It is converted to glycoaldehyde with further metabolism to glycolic acid and glyoxylate and eventual irreversible oxidation to oxalate. The initial reaction is dependent on alcohol dehydrogenase, so that simultaneous ingestion of ethyl alcohol and ethylene glycol decreases the oxidation of the latter and modifies its toxicity. The initial manifestations of ethylene glycol poisoning involve the central nervous system and generally coincide with the greatest amount of aldehyde production. Later, pulmonary symptoms predominate and finally, with the deposition of calcium oxalate crystals in the kidney, oxaluria and oliguric acute renal failure supervene. Severe hypocalcemia caused by chelation of calcium ions by oxalate and an overwhelming acidosis aggravated by the production of lactate are hallmarks of this condition. Pyridoxine deficiency markedly increases the amount of ethylene glycol metabolized to oxalate and thus adds to the toxicity. The lethal dose of ethylene glycol is 2 ml/kg, which represents 0.1 g/kg of oxalic acid. The diagnosis should be considered when alcohol-like intoxication without the odor of alcohol, coma with metabolic acidosis and a large anion gap, or massive calcium oxalate crystalluria is observed upon examination of the urine. Crystalluria is demonstrated by needle-shaped crystals of calcium oxalate monohydrate or octahedral "envelopes" of calcium oxalate dihydrate. Treatment is designed to correct the acidosis, prevent the manifestations of hypocalcemia, supply adequate thiamine and pyridoxine, and remove ethylene glycol and its products by means of forced diuresis and/or dialysis. In acute conditions, intravenous treatment with ethyl alcohol, given in a loading dose of 0.6 to 1.0 g/kg over 1 hour, followed by a sustained infusion of 10 to 12 g/hr to maintain the blood level at 100 mg/dl, is effective by virtue of its competition with alcohol dehydrogenase. Other potentially toxic glycols include *ethylene glycol dinitrite, propylene glycol, ethylene dichloride,* and *diethylene glycol*. The latter has been used in the past as a medicinal vehicle in an elixir of sulfanilamide. It is a potent tubular toxin.

Organic solvents

Carbon tetrachloride has been widely used as an industrial solvent and as a household cleaning agent. It is soluble in alcohol, and both hepatic and renal toxicity increase if ethyl alcohol is consumed during the period of exposure. Acute renal failure occurs as a consequence of ingestion or inhalation and exhibits several unusual characteristics. After exposure, a reduction in urine volume may not be apparent for 7 to 10 days. During this time the individual may be symptom free but is more likely to complain of vomiting, abdominal pain, constipation, diarrhea, or fever. The oliguria lasts 1 to 2 weeks. Analysis of the urine reveals more red blood cells and protein than are present in other forms of nephrotoxic acute renal failure. Recovery is expected. *Chloroform* is used chiefly as a refrigerant and as an aerosol propellant and in the synthesis of fluorinated resins. It is also produced during the chlorination of water. Although its primary effect is on the central nervous system and liver, it is also nephrotoxic. Chloroform is thought to be transformed into a toxic product by microsomal metabolism. On this basis, the ingestion of diets high in polybrominated biphenyls, known to be inducers of microsomal enzyme activity, enhances chloroform nephrotoxicity. *Trichloroethylene* is chemically related to both carbon tetrachloride and chloroform and shares with them the propensity for liver and kidney damage. It has a number of industrial applications and has been used as an anesthetic agent for obstetric patients. Acute renal failure has followed inhalation by "solvent sniffers" and in those using cleaning solutions containing this agent. *Toluene* is an aromatic hydrocarbon that has widespread use as an organic solvent. Its potential for renal toxicity has been demonstrated by those who have sniffed toluene-containing substances such as model glues. The maximum allowable concentration of toluene is far exceeded when these compounds are inhaled from paper bags. Although renal damage is generally mild, severe defects in the ability to excrete acid have been noted.

It has been suggested but not proved that prolonged, excessive exposure to various *hydrocarbons,* which interact with as yet unidentified host factors, predispose the kidney to glomerular injury or aggravate injury from other causes. An apparent association with Goodpasture's syndrome with exposure to petroleum products has also been reported. Some have found that previous exposure to hydrocarbon solvents is a common feature among some groups of patients with crescentic glomerulonephritis or proliferative glomerulonephritis. Remissions and exacerbations of the nephrotic syndrome are noted to follow removal from and re-exposure to solvents. A historic relationship between glomerulonephritis and exposure to gasoline vapors has also been described.

Heavy metals

Arsenic is used in insecticides, ant poisons, weed killers, wallpaper, antifouling paint, ceramics, wood preservatives, and glass. The inorganic arsenicals such as arsenic trioxide are more toxic than the organic compounds. Absorption follows inhalation or ingestion. The soluble compounds are readily absorbed via skin and mucous membranes and excreted primarily in the urine. Repeated doses are cumulative. Toxicity results when arsenic combines with sulfhydral enzymes and interferes with cellular oxidative processes. When arsenic is ingested in large amounts, the initial symptoms include a dry, burning sensation in the mouth and throat. This is followed by crampy abdominal pain, severe vomiting, and diarrhea. Vertigo, delirium, and coma are quite obvious manifestations of central nervous system involvement. Death may be caused by circulatory collapse and liver and renal failure. Hemodialysis has been found to be effective treatment for renal failure in some studies. BAL (2, 3,-dimercapto-1-propanol or dimercaprol) is valuable in acute arsenic poisoning. *Arsine* is an extremely toxic gas produced by the action of acid on metal in the presence of arsenic. It is a hazard to workers in metallurgic industries who work with ore contaminated by arsenic. Acute renal failure may accompany arsenic poisoning, which is most likely caused by concomitant cardiovascular collapse and hemolysis. Oliguric acute renal failure is a common complication of arsine (AsH_3) inhalation.

Cadmium is a major by-product of zinc production. It is used in nickel-cadmium batteries; in manufacture of alloys, paints, and glass; in electroplating and soldering; and as a stabilizer in plastics. Cadmium is found in cigarette smoke, seafood, and drinking water. As a result of widespread exposure and a half-life that may exceed 30 years, the body content of cadmium slowly accumulates and may eventually reach about 30 mg. The cadmium content of the food is thought to be the major source of cadmium for the general population. After absorption, cadmium tends to accumulate in the liver and kidney. It is bound to metallothionein, a low-molecular-weight cysteine-rich apoprotein. Accumulation in the kidney continues even as other tissue concentrations fall. It appears that a certain level of cadmium must accumulate within the kidney before overt damage is produced. Urinary excretion increases when defects occur in the tubular reabsorption of metallothionein. Later, as tubular injury progresses to the point of cell death, the renal cortical concentration of cadmium decreases. Thereafter renal cadmium levels may fall despite the fact that liver concentrations continue to rise. Blood values greater than 0.7 μg/dl, urine values above 20 μg/L, and renal cortical concentrations exceeding 200 μg/g wet kidney weight are thought to be associated with toxicity.

Lead has been associated with at least two types of renal impairment. In the more acute form, generalized defects in proximal tubular function result in the Fanconi syndrome with aminoaciduria, glycosuria, and phosphaturia. Serum uric acid levels are generally elevated because of a defect in the tubular secretion of uric acid. Occasionally the urine contains cells with eosinophilic intranuclear inclusions composed of lead and protein. These abnormalities most often occur in children after several months of heavy lead ingestion with blood lead levels usually in excess of 150 mg/dl. Although this impairment is generally rapidly reversible, it is likely that some conditions progress to chronic lead nephropathy, a form of chronic interstitial nephritis. Various factors, such as the amount of calcium in the diet, presence of iron deficiency, and exposure to sunlight and vitamin D, may influence the amount of lead absorbed and the severity of the disease.

Chronic lead nephropathy is qualitatively different from the Fanconi syndrome. It is an indolent disease difficult to separate from other forms of chronic, slowly progressive renal insufficiency. Evidence of excessive lead absorption is supplied by determining urinary lead excretion by the calcium disodium salt of ethylenediaminetetraacetic acid (EDTA) lead mobilization test. The test is performed by measuring the urinary lead excretion after the administration of EDTA. One gram of EDTA is given twice, 8 to 12 hours apart. During this time a 24 hour urine specimen is collected. An excessive body lead burden is indicated by excretion of more than 1000 μg of lead per day. Alternatively, 1 g EDTA in 250 ml of 5% glucose solution may be given intravenously over the course of 1 hour for 3 consecutive days. Excretion of more than 600 μg per 3 days is indicative of excess body lead. Long-term effects of chronic lead exposure have been described in those with occupational exposure, with gout, and with hypertension. Treatment with chelation therapy is effective in cases of acute lead nephropathy and the early renal dysfunction associated with occupational lead exposure, but there is no evidence that such therapy reverses the chronic interstitial disease. Therefore chelation therapy for chronic nephropathy should be instituted with specific guidelines in mind, such as normalization of the EDTA test result and restoration of organ function.

Mercury exists in the form of inorganic salts and gases and organic mercury compounds. In the organic form, mercury is present either as the free metal or in an ionic form such as mercurous or mercuric salt. In the organic form, mercury is bound covalently to at least one carbon atom. Chronic exposure to organic compounds primarily results in central nervous system manifestations, although several distinct renal lesions have been described. Poisoning with inorganic mercury was once a common cause of acute renal failure. Mercury tends to form highly undissociated linkages to sulfhydral groups. The toxic dose of $HgCl_2$ is 0.5 to 2.5 g, with a mean of approximately 1.5 g. After ingestion and before onset of acute renal failure, patients should be treated with intravenous chelation therapy (BAL [British antilewisite], dimercaprol) and induction of diuresis. Chronic exposure to mercury may also be associated with the development of an immune-complex nephropathy manifested as mesangioproliferative glomerulonephritis or as membranous glomerulopathy.

Other heavy metals have been shown to produce clinical acute renal failure, they include *antimony, bismuth, copper,* and *gold*. Bismuth compounds were once prepared as therapeutic agents. Copper ingestion may result from ingestion of fungicide-contaminated feed grains or use of corroded copper-containing hot water heaters. *Gold* has been implicated as a rare cause of acute renal failure, but the nephrotic syndrome is a much more common complication.

Insecticides and herbicides

Nephrotoxicity has been associated with the use of two major catagories of insecticides: the organophosphorus compounds such as *parathion* and the chlorinated hydrocarbons such as *chlordane*. Bipyridinium compounds have been used as herbicides. *Paraquat* reacts with atmospheric oxygen to produce reactive oxygen species. The major toxic effect is on pulmonary tissue although azotemia with evidence of renal tubular damage may be found.

Pigment nephropathy

Myoglobinuria and hemoglobinuria can be produced by exposure to chemical agents. When hemoglobinuria and myoglobinuria accompany acute renal failure it is difficult to define their role in the development of renal damage. Such coexistent factors as abnormalities in blood pressure and the adverse effects of the toxic agents tend to obscure the role of hemoglobinuria and myoglobinuria on renal function.

Radiation

The dose of radiation required to produce renal damage is thought to exceed 2300 R delivered to both kidneys within a 5 week period. A number of variables determine the renal response to radiation, including age, area and technique of irradiation, extent of perirenal fat, and concomitant administration of chemotherapeutic agents. Radiation nephritis has been separated into five clinical categories: acute radiation nephritis, chronic radiation nephritis, asymptomatic proteinuria, benign essential hypertension, and late malignant hypertension.

Carcinogenesis

Exposure to chemical agents has been implicated in the development of neoplasms of the renal parenchyma, renal pelvis and ureter, and urinary bladder. In the late nineteenth century it was first reported that men working in the aniline dye industry had an increased incidence of bladder cancer. Later it was appreciated that bladder cancer was linked to employment in the rubber and electric cable industries and that its development was related to exposure to a number of aromatic amines. Transitional cell carcinoma of the renal pelvis and ureter may be induced by the same exogenous carcinogens that produce bladder tumors. Workers in the aniline dye, rubber, textile, and plastic industries have a higher incidence of these tumors, which account for 7% to 8% of renal neoplasms. Smokers appear to have about twice the bladder cancer rate of nonsmokers. This may reflect increased exposure to such agents as polycyclic aromatic hydrocarbons, dialkylnitrosamines, and aromatic amines, all of which are present in cigarette smoke.

EFFECT OF DIAGNOSTIC AND THERAPEUTIC AGENTS ON THE KIDNEY

Antibacterial agents

Aminoglycoside antibiotics. The aminoglycoside antibiotics include streptomycin, neomycin, tobramycin, kanamycin, gentamicin, and sisomicin, and the semisynthetic compounds netilmicin and amikacin. The aminoglycoside antibiotics are potent tubular toxins. A significant decline in renal function can be expected to occur in 4% to 24% of all patients who receive them and they have been found to be responsible for 7% of all cases of hospital-acquired renal insufficiency. The nephrotoxicity of the aminoglycosides depends in large part on positively charged amino groups that promote binding to anionic, acidic phospholipids on the brush border membranes of proximal renal tubular epithelial cells. Once binding to the membranes of renal tubular epithelial cells occurs, the aminoglycosides undergo pinocytosis, are internalized, and are sequestered in lysosomes. Renal cortical concentrations may be 10 to 100 times that of plasma. Aminoglycoside toxicity is associated with an increase in the number and size of proximal tubular secondary lysosomes. These often contain myeloid bodies, which are lamellar structures consisting of concentrically arranged phospholipid material. Cytoplasmic vacuolization and dilatation of the cisternae of the rough endoplasmic reticulum may occur with eventual mitochondrial swelling and tubular epithelial cell necrosis. An aminoglycoside-induced decline in renal function precedes a decline in the glomerular filtration rate. Early tubular damage may be manifested by increased urinary excretion of tubular enzymes and increased excretion of low-molecular-weight proteins. This may be coupled by renal potassium and magnesium wasting and defects in urine concentrating ability, resulting in decreased urine osmolality and increased urine volume, as seen in nephrogenic diabetes insipidus. Consequently, the acute renal failure associated with aminoglycoside nephrotoxicity tends to be nonoliguric rather than oliguric. Frank tubular necrosis may occur 5 to 10 days after aminoglycoside therapy is begun but is often accelerated if other renal insults are present. The usual course of aminoglycoside nephrotoxicity is eventual resolution, which may be partial or complete. Several risk factors have been associated with aminoglycoside nephrotoxicity, including high doses and/or high serum drug levels (gentamicin or tobramycin peak levels >10 mg/ml and trough levels >2 mg/ml); long duration of therapy; recent aminoglycoside therapy; type of aminoglycoside used; advanced age; liver disease; pre-existing renal insufficiency; serious illness requiring intensive care unit (ICU) admission; shock and/or concurrent nephrotoxic insults; cephalothin, cyclosporine, furosemide, and/or volume depletion; potassium or magnesium depletion; acidosis; and hypoalbuminemia. Surveys suggest that gentamicin is relatively more toxic than tobramycin, followed by amikacin and netilmicin.

Beta-lactam antibiotics. The beta-lactam antibiotics, which include the penicillins, cephalosporins, carbapenems, and monobactams, may produce a variety of hypersensitivity reactions, and it is by this mechanism that renal function is most likely to be impaired. Although the beta lactams are too small to be directly immunogenic, hypersensitivity occurs when their metabolites bind to larger molecules and act as haptens. In the kidney, this may produce an immunologically mediated acute interstitial nephritis that is most commonly encountered with methicillin. The most common clinical manifestations are fever, pyuria, eosinophiluria, eosinophilia, and azotemia. The detection of eosinophiluria may be increased by the use of Hansel's stain. Histopathologically, methicillin-induced acute interstitial nephritis is characterized by a patchy interstitial infiltrate composed mainly of lymphocytes, plasma cells, and eosinophils. Complete recovery occurs in up to 90% of cases. Steroid therapy remains controversial. Acute interstitial nephritis has also been reported with first-generation (cephalothin, cephradine), second-generation (cephalexin), and third-generation (cefotaxime) cephalosporins as well as many of the penicillins. Acute interstitial nephritis may recur at rechallenge with beta lactams other than the original offending agent.

Tetracyclines. Four types of renal dysfunction have been described with the tetracyclines: the Fanconi syndrome, demeclocycline-induced nephrogenic diabetes insipidus, demeclocycline-induced renal failure in cirrhotic patients, and acute interstitial nephritis. In addition, by inhibiting protein synthesis and producing a catabolic state, they may elevate the blood urea nitrogen concentration without changing the glomerular filtration rate, an effect that may worsen azotemia in patients with renal failure.

Polypeptide antibiotics. The polymyxins, polymyxin B and colistin, contain cationic amino groups and may bind to epithelial phospholipids in a manner similar to that of the aminoglycosides. Renal function deteriorates in approximately 20% of patients treated with colistin. The nephrotoxic potential of polymyxin B is similar to that of colistin. Concurrent cephalothin administration increases the risk of colistin-induced nephrotoxicity. Bacitracin is a potent nephrotoxin, producing urinary abnormalities in almost all patients treated and azotemia in 31%.

Macrolide antibiotics. Though not directly nephrotoxic, erythromycin may produce cyclosporine nephrotoxicity by inhibiting hepatic mixed-function oxidases and increasing cyclosporine levels in cyclosporine-treated patients.

Rifampin. Many cases of acute interstitial nephritis have been attributed to rifampin. This complication may be more common in twice- or thrice-weekly therapy or when drug administration resumes after a medication-free interval than it is in continuous daily therapy. Eosinophilia and eosinophiluria may be less common in rifampin-induced acute interstitial nephritis than in methicillin-induced acute interstitial nephritis.

Quinolones. Nephrotoxicity is uncommon in ciprofloxacin and norfloxacin administration, although acute interstitial nephritis with nonoliguric acute renal failure has been reported to be associated with the former.

Sulfonamides. Many of the older sulfonamides were poorly soluble, especially at acid pH, and tended to crystallize in the renal tubules and collecting system, producing intrarenal and extrarenal obstruction with resulting renal colic, hematuria, and acute renal failure. Furthermore their acetylated metabolites tended to be even less soluble and more likely to precipitate than the parent drug. Maintaining a high urine flow rate and alkalinizing the urine lessened this problem. The incidence of renal injury has declined greatly as more soluble sulfonamides have come into use. Sulfadiazine is poorly soluble, as is the acetylated metabolite of sulfamethoxazole. In patients who have preexisting renal insufficiency elevated serum drug levels develop if the dose is not reduced, increasing the risk of sulfonamide-induced nephrotoxicity.

Trimethoprim. Trimethoprim has been reported to block tubular creatinine excretion, increasing the serum creatinine concentration without changing the glomerular filtration rate. It may also interfere with the Jaffe alkaline picrate assay for creatinine, falsely elevating creatinine concentration. Acute interstitial nephritis has been reported to be associated with trimethoprim-sulfamethoxazole. Whether this was caused by the trimethoprim component is unknown.

Antiviral agents

Acyclovir. Acyclovir is active against herpes simplex viruses and against varicella zoster virus. Intracellular conversion to an active form by viral thymidine kinase results in inhibition of herpesvirus deoxyribonucleic acid (DNA) polymerase enzyme. A decline in renal function is more likely to occur in patients with increased serum creatinine concentrations, when given in conjunction with other nephrotoxic agents, or when administered as a rapid intravenous infusion. Consequently, doses need to be adjusted for renal function and given by infusion to prevent intrarenal precipitation.

Foscarnet. Foscarnet is a pyrophosphate analog that inhibits DNA polymerase in herpes viruses and ribonucleic acid (RNA) polymerase in influenza viruses. Its use has been associated with a significant decline in renal function in up to 66% of patients. Examination of renal biopsy specimens has revealed extensive tubular epithelial cell necrosis. The protective effects of hydration with the infusion of 2.5 liters of saline solution per day during the night before the foscarnet therapy and throughout the course of treatment has been demonstrated.

Antifungal agents

The polyene *amphotericin B* is nephrotoxic as a result of a direct toxic effect on renal tubular epithelial cells and renal vasoconstriction. The nephrotoxicity is characterized by potassium wasting, distal renal tubular acidosis, nephrogenic diabetes insipidus, and azotemia. Renal dysfunction occurs in almost all patients treated with this drug and is dose related. The tubular transport abnormalities tend to precede azotemia and are usually reversible. Sodium loading reduces amphotericin B nephrotoxicity by preventing the expected declines in renal blood flow and glomerular filtration rate. Patients receiving amphotericin B should be well hydrated, and the serum electrolyte, blood urea nitrogen (BUN), and creatinine levels should be closely monitored. Saline solution may reverse developing azotemia. In most regimens, amphotericin B is withheld or given only on alternate days if the BUN concentration exceeds 50 g/dl. The imidazole *ketoconazole* is not directly nephrotoxic but may have that effect by increasing cyclosporine blood levels in cyclosporine-treated patients.

Antiprotozal agents

A common side-effect of *pentamidine isethionate* administration is reversible renal and/or hepatic toxicity in approximately 25% of patients. Hypovolemia and diarrheal states in acquired immunodeficiency syndrome patients appear to be important risk factors for increased nephrotoxicity. Pentamidine has also been associated with myoglobinuria and acute renal failure.

Antineoplastic agents

Alkylating agents

Cisplatin. *Cisplatin* is active against a broad range of solid tumors and is particularly useful in the treatment of testicular and ovarian tumors. It is freely filtered at the glomerulus and has great potential for tubular toxicity. Histologic lesions include dilated proximal and distal tubules lined by flattened epithelium and containing intraluminal cast material and sloughing of tubular cells. Necrosis of the epithelial cells lining the collecting ducts may also be seen. Cisplatin nephrotoxicity may result in hypomagnesemia, which stems from impaired tubular conservation of magnesium. It may be accompanied by hypocalcemia, hypokalemia, and sodium wasting. Proteinuria, albuminuria, aminoaciduria, and glucosuria may also occur, but they tend to resolve after withdrawal of the drug. In contrast, the defects of tubular electrolyte handling may persist. The most serious side-effect is an acute dose-related decline in the glomerular filtration rate, which is not completely reversible after cessation of therapy. The toxicity is cumulative, so that each cycle of treatment produces a progressive and often permanent decline in renal function. Proximal tubular cell injury and death may result from inhibition of DNA synthesis, adenosine triphosphate (ATP) synthesis, and/or ATP utilization. Mitochondrial damage may occur and oxygen free radicals may play a role in the evolution of the injury. Volume expansion with intravenous sodium chloride solutions in association with mannitol- or furosemide-stimulated diuresis greatly reduces cisplatin-induced nephrotoxicity. For example, the administration of cisplatin in 250 ml of 3% saline solution over 30 minutes along with an intravenous infusion of normal saline solution with 20 mEg/L of potassium chloride at 250 ml per hour may be effective in reducing nephrotoxicity.

Nitrosoureas. *Streptozocin* is a glycosylated nitrosourea whose primary use is in the treatment of malignant pancreatic islet cell tumors. Unchanged streptozocin is excreted in the urine and concentrated within the kidney. Streptozocin produces renal dysfunction in 28% to 73% of treated patients. The most common abnormality is tubular dysfunction, producing some combination of proteinuria, hypophosphatemia, hypokalemia, renal tubular acidosis, renal glycosuria, and acetonuria. Nephrogenic diabetes insipidus occasionally occurs. In more severe cases, acute tubular necrosis and azotemia develop. Streptozocin is uricosuric and frequently produces hypouricemia. Nephrotoxicity is poorly predictable but may be minimized by reducing the dose by 50% in those patients in whom persistent proteinuria or mild elevations in the serum creatinine concentration develop. *Semustine* is a chloroethyl nitrosourea active against lymphomas, melanoma, and tumors of the brain and gastrointestinal tract. Semustine-induced renal failure is insidious and irreversible; the first indication of renal abnormalities appears at a median of 2 years after the start of therapy. Nephrotoxicity is manifested by a slowly rising serum creatinine concentration and by small kidney size indicated by radiographic or ultrasonographic examination. Glomerular sclerosis, tubular atrophy, and interstitial fibrosis have been reported. *Cyclophosphamide* is a nitrogen mustard that at high doses may impair renal water excretion and produce a dilutional hyponatremia. This represents a self-limiting effect on renal tubular epithelial cells.

Antimetabolites. *Methotrexate* inhibits dihydrofolate reductase, blocking the conversion of dihydrofolate to tetrahydrofolate. Methotrexate is excreted by both glomerular filtration and tubular secretion, and as a result it has a renal clearance exceeding that of inulin. Precipitation of the poorly soluble drug within the distal nephron, producing intrarenal obstructive uropathy, is most widely accepted to be the mechanism of nephrotoxicity. It is a particular problem in high-dose therapy with leukovorin rescue protocols. The incidence of nephrotoxicity can be substantially reduced by hydration and urinary alkalinization although most patients experience a small, reversible decline in glomerular filtration rate (GFR). *Fluoracil* and *floxuridine* are not nephrotoxic but when used in combination with mitomycin C may be associated with the development of the hemolytic-uremic syndrome. *Thioguanine* may be associated with reversible renal failure in approximately 20% of patients receiving individual doses of 700 mg/m^2 or more.

Antitumor antibiotics. *Mitomycin* is used in the palliative treatment of various solid tumors. Nephrotoxicity is a significant dose-related side-effect. The renal failure is characteristic of the hemolytic-uremic syndrome with microangiopathic hemolytic anemia and thrombocytopenia. This occurs in approximately 9% of mitomycin treated patients and is related to total cumulative dose and associated with concurrent fluorouracil treatment. The kidneys demonstrate arteriolar intimal hyperplasia with deposition of fibrin thrombi in the arterioles and glomerular capillaries. Mitomycin C–induced hemolytic-uremic syndrome (HUS) has a high fatality rate, and no treatment has proved effective. *Mithramycin* suppresses osteoclast activity and is most often used to treat tumor-associated hypercalcemia. When it is given on a daily basis, considerable nephrotoxicity occurs with necrosis of proximal and distal tubular cells. Glomeruli are not affected. *Bleomycin*-containing combination regimens may occasionally be associated with the hemolytic-uremic syndrome.

Other agents. *Vincristine* is a vinca alkaloid that promotes antidiuretic hormone (ADH) release and hyponatremia resulting in the syndrome of inappropriate ADH. *Interleukin 2* is an immunotherapeutic agent whose use causes reversible azotemia, accompanied by hypotension, sodium retention, and reduced urine volume in most patients. *Interferon* use is associated with reversible and usually mild proteinuria in 15% to 42% of patients. The enzyme *asparaginase* may produce prerenal azotemia.

Immunosuppressive agents

Cyclosporine is a neutral hydrophobic cyclic polypeptide product of fungal metabolism that is used as a major immunosuppressant in solid organ transplantation. Its hydrophobicity makes it virtually insoluble in water; therefore it must be dissolved in organic solvents such as ethanol and olive oil. Its major limiting feature is its nephrotoxic potential. Several pathogenic mechanisms contribute to the decline in renal function, including physiologic changes in the renal circulation resulting in an increase in renal vascular resistance and a decrease in renal blood flow; anatomic changes in the renal vasculature with or without the presence of microthrombi; and late development of chronic interstitial fibrosis and tubular atrophy. Hypertension, best treated with calcium-channel blocking agents; a tendency to sodium retention; hyperuricemia with an increased incidence of gout; and hyperkalemic, hyperchloremic metabolic acidosis are observed. Cyclosporine nephrotoxicity may be difficult to differentiate from acute renal transplant rejection and may occur despite the use of acceptable dosing schedules, suggesting a role for unidentified patient factors. Cyclosporine nephrotoxicity may be potentiated by urinary tract obstruction, use of nephrotoxic antibiotics or radiocontrast agents, and postoperative acute tubular necrosis. Agents that affect hepatic mixed function oxidases such as erythromycin may markedly elevate blood levels and cause serious renal injury. Vascular lesions may take the form of severe arteriolar hyalinosis or necrosis, which at times is associated with mucoid thickening of the intima. A more severe lesion is associated with thrombocytopenia, which has the features of a thrombotic microangiopathy. This is marked by the development of intimal thickening and an obliterative arteriopathy with fibrin and platelet deposition and occasional thrombus formation. The chronic form of toxicity is characterized by a slow progressive increase in the serum creatinine concentration. Histopathologic examination reveals diffuse interstitial fibrosis, tubular atrophy, and focal glomerulosclerosis.

FK-506 is a new macrolide immunosuppressive agent that has been used alone or in conjunction with cyclosporine in human transplantation. It appears to have side-effects similar to those of cyclosporine.

Nonsteroidal anti-inflammatory drugs

The nonsteroidal anti-inflammatory drugs (NSAIDs) are a group of carboxylic and enolic acid derivatives that are used by an estimated 40 million people in the United States for their antipyretic, anti-inflammatory, and analgesic properties. Nonsteroidal anti-inflammatory drugs exert their major effects through the inhibition of prostaglandin synthesis. In clinical situations involving increased activity of the renin-angiotensin system, acute renal failure may result from enhanced renal vasoconstriction, unopposed by the vasodilatory effect of prostaglandins; this is the most common disorder associated with nonsteroidal anti-inflammatory drugs. Indomethacin accounts for 60% to 70% of the cases reported in the literature. Oliguria and a rise in serum creatinine concentration begin within 24 to 48 hours of drug exposure. The urinalysis finding is usually unremarkable, and the fractional excretion of sodium is less than 1%. Hyperkalemia disproportionate to the degree of renal failure may develop. Dialysis is rarely indicated, and renal function usually returns to baseline after discontinuation of the drug. Predisposing factors include congestive heart failure, cirrhosis, pre-existing renal insufficiency, advanced age, volume depletion, hypertension, and previous diuretic use. Another less common complication of use of nonsteroidal anti-inflammatory drugs is the syndrome of nephrotic range proteinuria and/or acute renal failure associated with acute interstitial nephritis. This syndrome appears to involve an older age group and to have a time course to development of several months. The patients usually have cramps, edema, and oliguria. Recovery is slow and may take weeks to months. The efficacy of steroids is unclear. The renal biopsy result typically shows focal interstitial edema and fibrosis, diffuse or focal monocellular infiltrate, and eosinophils in 30% of specimens. The pathogenesis is still unknown, although current speculation implicates lymphokines and/or leukotrienes. Finally, nonsteroidal anti-inflammatory drugs have been associated with sodium retention in as many as 25% of patients. This problem is usually transient and minor except in patients with severe congestive heart failure or cirrhosis. Nonsteroidal anti-inflammatory drugs may also cause diuretic resistance, impaired urinary diluting ability, and hyperkalemia. Hyperkalemia is more likely in patients with diabetes or renal insufficiency, and in those receiving beta blockers.

Anesthetic agents

Methoxyflurane, which is metabolized in the liver to inorganic fluoride and oxalate, has been associated with nonoliguric acute renal failure and nephrogenic diabetes insipidus. The halogenated anesthetics in current use have dramatically reduced the incidence of this complication.

Radiographic contrast media

Although studies have identified radiocontrast dye as a major cause of acute renal failure in hospitalized patients, the true incidence of this problem is still unknown. The incidence varies from 0.15% to 17%, depending on the type of radiographic procedure and the definition of acute renal failure, which ranges from a rise in serum creatinine concentration of 0.3 mg per deciliter to 2.0 mg per deciliter during the 24 to 48 hours after radiocontrast exposure. The list of purported predisposing risk factors is quite long, but only pre-existing renal insufficiency and diabetes mellitus are consistently recognized. Acute renal failure developed in approximately 50% of diabetic patients with a serum creatinine level greater than 1.5 mg per deciliter and in 76% with a level greater than 5 mg per deciliter. Radiocontrast-induced acute renal failure may be oliguric or nonoliguric. Patients with pre-existing renal insufficiency are more likely to have the oliguric form, which usually lasts for 2 to 5 days with recovery by the seventh day. The urinalysis result may be normal or may reveal multiple tubular epithelial cell and granular casts. The urinary sodium concentration (<10 mEq/L) and fractional excretion of sodium (<0.5%) may be extremely low. A persistent nephrogram for 24 to 48 hours is a characteristic feature. The pathophysiologic mechanisms responsible for the acute renal failure are still unclear. The guidelines for prevention of this disorder are ill defined at present. In patients with pre-existing renal insufficiency and/or diabetes mellitus consideration should be given to an alternative procedure (e.g., sonography, magnetic resonance imaging). Although somewhat controversial, administration of saline solution or mannitol infusions before contrast exposure may be beneficial.

REFERENCES

Bennett WM: Lead nephropathy. Kidney Int 28:212, 1985.

Campese VM et al: Contrast-induced acute renal failure. Adv Exp Med Biol 212:135, 1987.

Consensus statement on the health significance of nephrotoxicity. Toxicol Lett 46:1, 1989.

Dillon JJ and Finn WF: Acute renal failure caused by antibacterial, antifungal, and antineoplastic agents. In Solez K and Racusen LC, editors: Acute renal failure: diagnosis, treatment and prevention. New York, 1991, Marcel Dekker.

Finn WF: Disorders of the kidney and urinary tract. In Tarcher AB, editor: Principles and practice of environmental medicine. Book Company, New York and London, 1992, Plenum Medical.

Gabow PA et al: Organic acids in ethylene glycol intoxication. Ann Intern Med 105:16, 1986.

Garella S and Matarese RA: Renal effects of prostaglandins and clinical adverse effects of nonsteroidal anti-inflammatory agents. Medicine 63:165, 1984.

Hou SH et al: Hospital-acquired renal insufficiency: a prospective study. Am J Med 74:243, 1983.

Myers BD: Cyclosporine nephrotoxicity. Kidney Int 30:964, 1986.

Ozols RF et al: High-dose cisplatin in hypertonic saline. Ann Intern Med 199:19, 1984.

Sensakovic JW et al: Pentamidine treatment of *Pneumocystis carinii* pneumonia in the acquired immunodeficiency syndrome. Arch Intern Med 145:2247, 1985.

CHAPTER

358 Cystic Diseases of the Kidney

Jared J. Grantham

Cysts are the most common structural abnormalities encountered in adult kidneys. By definition, a *cyst* is an epithelium-lined cavity filled with fluid or semisolid material. Nearly all renal cysts are derived from nephrons or collecting duct elements. They begin as tiny hair-sized structures, enlarging in some instances to structures several centimeters in diameter that contain several hundred milliliters of fluid. Generalized cystic diseases are typified by cysts scattered throughout the cortex and the medulla of one or both kidneys. The term *polycystic* is reserved for kidney diseases in which the cysts are diffusely scattered throughout the renal cortex and medulla. In *medullary cystic diseases* the lesions occur principally in the medulla and papilla. The major types of renal cystic disease are outlined in Table 358-1.

SIMPLE OR SOLITARY CYSTS

About 50% of persons above the age of 50 years have one or more renal cysts. These cysts are usually found incidentally in the course of radiographic studies to evaluate hypertension, renal stone disease, hematuria, or urinary tract infection. They are rarely symptomatic. The presence of these cysts does not lead to chronic renal insufficiency. There is no known hereditary connection.

Pathologic features

Simple cysts are usually seen on the outer portion of the kidney cortex, but they can be detected in the medullary and papillary regions. They usually contain a clear fluid that has a composition similar to that of an ultrafiltrate of plasma. Occasionally the cysts may contain blood or pus. They are lined by simple columnar or flat squamous epi-

Table 358-1. Features of renal cystic diseases

	Cortex and medulla				Medulla	
			Polycystic			
	Simple	Acquired	Dominant	Recessive	Sponge kidney	Medullary cystic
Prevalence	Common	>50% of dialysis patients	1:1000	1:16,000	1:5000-1:1000	Rare
Symptoms	Rare	Occasional	Common	Common	Occasional	Common
Inherited	No	No	Yes	Yes	Unknown	Dominant and recessive forms
Kidney size	Normal	Small to large	Large	Large	Normal	Small
Hypertension	Rare	Variable	Common	Common	Rare	Rare
Hematuria	Occasional	Occasional	Common	Occasional	Rare (except with stones)	Rare
Associated conditions						
Azotemia	No	Always	Common	Common	Rare	Common
Liver disease	No	No	40%-60%	100%	No	No
Arterial aneurysm	No	No	10%	No	No	No
Differential diagnosis	Tumor Diverticula of renal pelvis	ADPKD Simple cysts Hippel-Lindau disease	ARPKD Tuberous sclerosis Multiple simple cysts	ADPKD Medullary sponge kidney	Medullary cystic kidney Renal tubular acidosis Idiopathic nephrocalcinosis	End-stage renal disease Medullary sponge kidney

ADPKD, autosomal dominant polycystic kidney disease; ARPKD, autosomal recessive polycystic kidney disease.

thelium. Microdissection studies show that the cysts originate from tubule segments. The mechanism of fluid accumulation in the cysts is unknown. Usually there are only a few simple cysts per kidney, but occasionally they may be so numerous as to be confused with autosomal dominant polycystic kidney disease or with acquired cystic disease. Cysts with diameters of 0.5 to 1.0 cm are common, but a diameter of 3 to 4 cm is not unusual.

Clinical and diagnostic features

Most simple cysts are found on routine urographic examinations. They are more common in adults than in children. Hypertension has been attributed to simple cysts in rare instances. The occasional infected cyst may cause flank pain, pleurisy, fever, and leukocytosis. In most cases, however, the simple cysts are asymptomatic, and the major problem is to differentiate them from malignant masses.

Simple cysts are only rarely associated with renal malignancy. When an asymptomatic renal cyst is discovered incidentally by urography or sonography, further evaluation by computed tomography (CT) may be indicated to rule out the possibility of an associated tumor mass. Sonography with cyst puncture has been used as the cornerstone of screening in the past, but further evaluation with CT has now become more accepted in some centers. Strict criteria for benign cysts by CT scanning are (1) a homogeneous attenuation value near that of water, (2) no enhancement with intravenous contrast material, (3) no measurable thickness of the cyst wall, (4) smooth interface with renal parenchyma. If these criteria are met, the cystic lesion can be followed by periodic sonographic evaluation. If the criteria are not met, the cyst falls into an indeterminant or solid category, and surgical exploration is recommended. Calcification within cystic lesions should raise suspicion of malignancy.

Treatment

There is considerable diversity in the therapeutic approach to the simple cyst. With the use of modern diagnostic tests, most physicians do not advocate surgery if strict CT criteria are met and the mass is asymptomatic. The management of symptomatic renal cysts can take several forms. Most cysts are accessible to percutaneous aspiration for diagnosis. In some cases sclerosing agents can be injected to reduce the reaccumulation of cyst fluid. If the cyst is associated with hypertension and the renal vein renin levels are elevated above normal, drainage of the cysts may be associated with improvement of hypertension. Infected cysts have been drained by percutaneous approaches. Differentiation of infected cysts from renal abscess may be difficult. In this instance an operative approach is usually taken.

AUTOSOMAL DOMINANT POLYCYSTIC KIDNEY DISEASE

Autosomal dominant polycystic kidney disease (ADPKD) is usually recognized in adults between the third and fourth decades of life. The diagnosis is rarely made in infants. In most cases, a family history of renal disease can be elicited on careful questioning. The defective gene is located on the short arm of chromosome 16. The disease exhibits autosomal dominant inheritance with nearly complete penetrance of the gene defect. It is found on all continents and in all races. The prevalence is estimated to be between 1 in 500 and 1 in 1000 with an annual "attack" rate of about 6000 new cases per year in the United States. The disease causes renal insufficiency in 50% of subjects by the age of 70 years, accounts for 6% to 10% of dialysis patients in the United States, and is the third or fourth leading cause of renal failure in adults.

Pathologic features

Polycystic kidneys are impressively enlarged. The cysts are scattered diffusely throughout the kidneys and may vary in size from a few millimeters to several centimeters in diameter. Most of the cysts are filled with straw-yellow colored fluid that resembles urine. Some cysts appear to be filled with blood or thick, putty-like material, which represents old blood. Both kidneys are involved by the process; unilateral polycystic kidney disease has been reported only rarely. Microdissection studies have shown that the cysts originate in all segments of the nephron, including Bowman's capsule, the proximal tubule, the loop of Henle, the distal tubule, the collecting tubule, and the papillary collecting duct. The cysts are lined by a single layer of epithelium that in some instances resembles that seen in the distal nephron. The cells are connected by junctional complexes resembling those seen in proximal and distal tubule segments. Marked hyperplasia of cells and polyp formation have been observed on the interior wall of cysts originating in all the portions of the nephron. Analysis of the cyst fluid reveals cyst fluid to plasma electrolyte concentration gradients for sodium, potassium, chloride, and hydrogen ions. Thus some of the cysts continue to function as nephron segments throughout the life of the patient.

The liver also contains cysts in about 40% to 60% of patients with ADPKD. Females seem to have a greater enlargement of the liver produced by cysts than do males. In some cases the liver cysts are so prominent as to cause portal hypertension or, in rare cases, obstruction of the common bile duct. Liver cysts rarely lead to parenchymal dysfunction.

Arterial aneurysms of the circle of Willis are found in about 10% of patients with polycystic kidney disease. These aneurysms may rupture, causing sudden death. Patients with ADPKD appear to have an increased incidence of aortic aneurysm, abnormalities of the mitral valve and inguinal hernia. Diverticulosis appears to be increased in patients with ADPKD.

Pathophysiology

Although ADPKD is clearly an inherited defect, the primary abnormality causing the cysts is unknown. Renal cysts can be found in utero and in neonates, but renal failure does not develop usually until the fifth or sixth decade of life. As one grows older there appears to be an increase in the size of cystic nephrons in both kidneys. There is associated atrophy and fibrosis of adjacent kidney tissue, which probably underlies the progression to renal insufficiency.

The mechanism by which the cysts enlarge is not known, but several hypotheses have been suggested, all of which incorporate abnormal growth as a central theme. One view holds that abnormal basement membrane material fails to retard the proliferation of the cells. Another suggests that the epithelial cells are more sensitive to normal levels of epithelial growth factors, such as epidermal growth factor; a third suggests that the cells making up the cyst walls are locked in a permanent state of immaturity. In all of these hypotheses, the fluid is thought to derive from glomerular filtrate and transepithelial fluid secretion. Thus the cysts enlarge progressively from the size of a human hair to that of oranges as a result of the proliferation of a thin layer of cells surrounding a large cavity filled with urine-like fluid.

Clinical and diagnostic features

Abdominal pain and hematuria are the most common initial symptoms in patients with ADPKD. Infected renal cysts, secondary to urinary tract infection, are also relatively common. Hypertension occurs in over 50% of patients with ADPKD and often antedates the diagnosis of the disease. Renal insufficiency occurs late in this disorder and is not a presenting feature. There are no distinguishing laboratory features. Patients at various stages of the disease have been found to have mild proteinuria and to excrete lipid bodies in the urine.

The diagnosis of ADPKD can be made by several radiographic tests in patients who are at risk. Sonography is the preferred screening test. When more than five cysts are found in each kidney in a patient with a family history of ADPKD, a secure diagnosis of autosomal dominant polycystic kidney disease can be made. If the sonogram result is equivocal, then computed tomography (CT) is recommended (Fig. 358-1). In advanced cases intravenous nephrotomography can be used to establish the diagnosis, but this is usually not definitive for patients in the early stages of the disease. Because it is important in many instances to exclude the diagnosis of polycystic kidney disease in a patient at risk, I recommend the use of computed tomography when there is any doubt about the diagnosis of ADPKD. Angiography is seldom necessary except when tumor is suspected in a polycystic kidney. Carcinoma has been reported in patients with ADPKD, but this problem is rare. Retrograde pyelography is seldom indicated and should be avoided if at all possible because of the high risk of renal infection.

It is possible to diagnose ADPKD by means of genetic linkage markers on chromosome 16p. For this examination deoxyribonucleic acid (DNA) of at least two relatives (siblings, parent, grandparent, or children) with clinically apparent ADPKD is surveyed together with that of the subject at risk. Genetic markers that flank the ADPKD gene are examined by Southern blotting to determine the extent

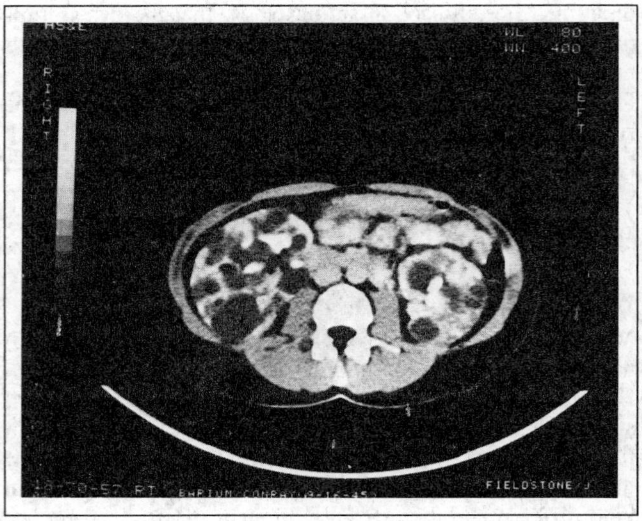

A

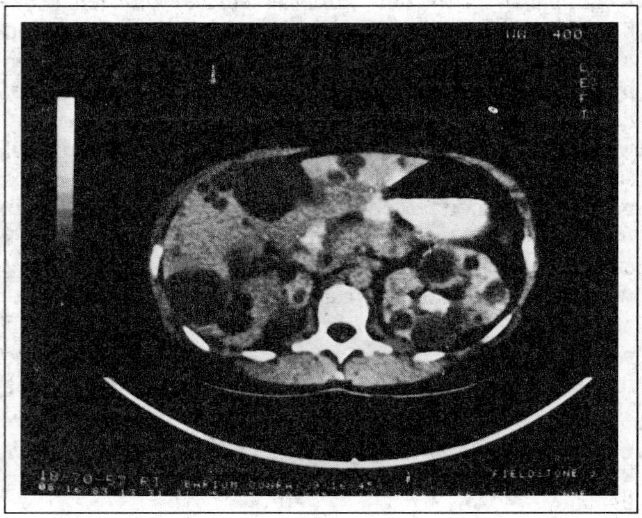

B

Fig. 358-1. Tomogram of autosomal dominant polycystic kidney disease. **A,** Kidney cysts. **B,** Kidney and liver cysts.

to which they are expressed in the individual without clinical ADPKD. In families in which the markers are informative, it is possible to determine an ADPKD genotype in the person at risk with an accuracy exceeding 95%. As a matter of practice, the linkage test has not been widely used because radiologic methods of diagnosis are highly sensitive in adults.

The clinical course of ADPKD is highly variable. Some patients experience minor symptoms throughout life and never progress to end-stage renal disease. More commonly, however, they have bouts of abdominal pain, hematuria, hypertension, or urinary tract infection, and in over half of patients, renal insufficiency develops between the fifth and the sixth decades of life. Gross hematuria in a patient with ADPKD is usually due to rupture of a cyst, but in some cases it may be secondary to infection in the kidney, renal stone, or, in rare cases, a renal tumor. In most patients bed rest, sedation, and hydration result in resolution of the hematuria in a few days. When hematuria persists, more extensive radiologic investigation is indicated.

Urinary tract infection should be treated promptly with bactericidal antibiotics. When a kidney cyst becomes infected, it is important to try to identify the offending organism. When identification is possible, bactericidal therapy should be administered parenterally for at least 2 weeks, followed by long-term oral therapy. Perinephric abscess has been reported in dialysis patients with ADPKD, and this complication requires surgical drainage. Occasionally nephrectomy may be indicated to control renal infection. Renal calculi are found with increased incidence in patients with polycystic kidney disease. Unique pathophysiologic characteristics have not been described for the formation of these calculi.

Most patients with ADPKD require no modification in physical activity or life-style unless they have unusual symptomatic disease. These patients should probably avoid contact sports in which direct blows to the abdomen may be incurred. Pain is managed by specific therapy for the underlying cause, such as stone or infection. Nonsteroidal anti-inflammatory drugs should be avoided because of the risk of papillary injury. In difficult cases surgical unroofing of cysts has proved beneficial in managing renal pain.

Hypertension is usually of the volume-dependent variety. Sodium restriction is effective in the treatment of most patients, but in some it is necessary to add a vasodilator. Diuretics should be used cautiously because of the unknown effect of these drugs on the formation rate of renal cysts. Hemodialysis and peritoneal dialysis are effective means of treating end-stage ADPKD. These patients are also excellent candidates for renal transplantation. In most instances a cadaveric source is chosen because of the hereditary nature of the disease.

Treatment

There is no specific treatment for ADPKD. Recent studies indicate that reducing the protein content of the diet may have a beneficial effect on the rate at which the disease progresses (Chapter 348). Control of blood pressure, urinary tract infection, and renal lithiasis is important to prolong kidney function. Pregnancy does not appear to have an adverse effect when kidney function is normal.

For the time being, only prevention can decrease the incidence of ADPKD. For prevention to be effective, patients with ADPKD must be identified in the early portion of their childbearing years. On the other hand, it is probably not advisable to evaluate all patients at risk for ADPKD to determine whether they have the disorder. One must bear in mind that nothing can be done presently to prevent the progression of the disease, and knowledge of the ailment may affect the patient's employment and insurability.

Patients who have established ADPKD should be advised that it is an autosomal dominant condition and that they can expect each of their children to have a 50-50 chance of inheriting the defective gene. It is also important to emphasize that if the child does not inherit the gene, there is no chance that the same disease will be expressed in his or her progeny. Patients should also be advised of the risk, signs, and symptoms of cerebral aneurysm. Once a patient shows a significant decrease in creatinine clearance, the prognosis for progression of the disease can be judged by the relationship between the reciprocal of the serum creatinine concentration and time.

AUTOSOMAL RECESSIVE POLYCYSTIC KIDNEY DISEASE

Autosomal recessive polycystic kidney disease (ARPKD) is inherited as an autosomal recessive trait. The disease is almost never recognized in the parents. Both parents carry the recessive gene, so each offspring has a one in four chance of having symptomatic disease. ARPKD usually causes the death of the patient within a few hours or days after birth. In milder forms, the renal disease may not be detected until infancy, childhood, or adulthood. The commonly used term "infantile polycystic kidney disease" is technically incorrect; the more correct designation is *autosomal recessive polycystic kidney disease*.

Pathology

Patients with ARPKD who die in infancy usually do not die of renal failure but of underdevelopment of the pulmonary system. The kidneys are enlarged symmetrically and have a spongy character. On microscopic examination the collecting ducts are seen to be widely dilated. In newborns with ARPKD the liver appears relatively normal on gross inspection but almost invariably shows microscopic evidence of diffuse fibrosis. Juvenile patients generally have minimal kidney involvement, with spherical cysts revealed by urography and CT scanning that are very difficult to differentiate from the cysts of ADPKD. However, these individuals have striking liver abnormalities produced by diffuse fibrosis. Portal hypertension is an important complication. Thus there appears to be a spectrum of renal hepatic involvement in ARPKD, with severe kidney disease and mild liver changes at the perinatal end and severe hepatic fibrosis with mild kidney changes in juveniles and young adults.

Clinical and diagnostic features

In children whose kidneys are found to be enlarged at birth, sonography and intravenous nephrotomography are important diagnostic tools. The typical sonogram shows enlarged kidneys with increased echogenicity in the cortex and medulla. In older patients microcystic changes can be observed by CT scanning in those patients who are able to cooperate with the test.

There is no known treatment for ARPKD. Patients who have renal insufficiency can be treated with hemodialysis and peritoneal dialysis. Renal transplantation has been used in selected cases. However, because of the associated fibrosing liver disorder, these patients must be classified as high-risk candidates for renal replacement therapy.

As with other cystic diseases, hypertension, edema, hepatic insufficiency, and urinary tract infection should be treated appropriately.

Parents who give birth to a child with ARPKD should be advised that each of their children will have a one in four chance of having the disease or a one in two chance of being a carrier of the abnormal gene.

ACQUIRED CYSTIC DISEASE

Patients who have been maintained on dialysis regimens, either hemodialysis or peritoneal dialysis, for several years have been observed to have a type of bilateral polycystic kidney disease. Patients with noncystic disorders, such as chronic glomerulonephritis, diabetes mellitus, and interstitial nephritis, who have end-stage renal disease and require dialysis treatment appear to have this peculiar diffuse polycystic kidney disease. In several studies, approximately 50% of patients who had been treated by dialysis longer than 3 years showed signs of acquired polycystic kidney disease. The cysts develop as a consequence of chronic renal insufficiency and may be clinically apparent long before dialysis is instituted.

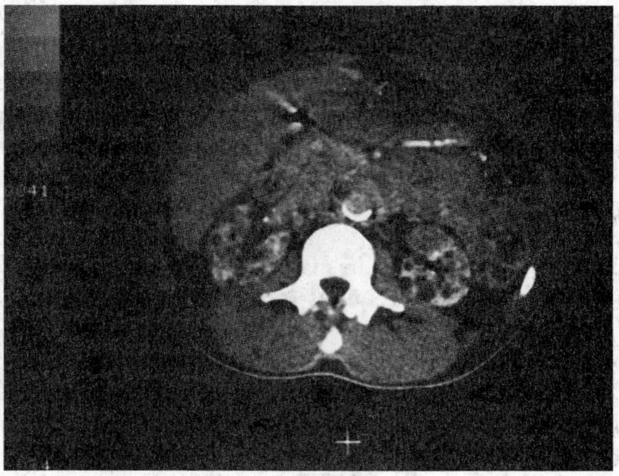

Fig. 358-2. Acquired cystic disease.

Pathologic features

Both kidneys are involved with diffuse cysts, which in some cases may be several centimeters in diameter. The cysts are usually filled with clear fluid, but in some instances they are hemorrhagic. Microscopic examination of the kidneys reveals hyperplasia of the cells lining the inside of many cysts. In some cases microadenomas are found in the cysts' walls, and adenocarcinomas may be found in about 5% of patients with acquired polycystic kidney disease. In several instances, the kidneys have contained adenocarcinoma with metastasis to regional lymph nodes and distant organs.

Clinical and diagnostic features

Recent studies indicate that in patients with long-standing chronic renal insufficiency acquired cystic disease may develop before they enter a dialysis program. In those who do not have acquired cystic disease at the time dialysis is started, the disease will almost certainly develop in a high proportion of patients who have dialysis for long periods. Major clinical manifestations of acquired cystic disease include flank pain and hematuria in association with rupture of hemorrhagic cysts into the urinary tract or into the perinephric region. There are no reported cases of infection in acquired polycystic kidney disease. These patients seem to be unusually susceptible to the development of oxalate stones in the pelvis of the kidney. Erythrocytosis has been associated with acquired cystic disease in a few cases.

The diagnosis is made by sonography in far advanced cases or by CT scan in instances in which the cysts are relatively small (Fig. 358-2). The cysts appear to regress in patients who have successful kidney transplantation and who become nonazotemic.

There is no specific treatment for acquired polycystic kidney disease. When the cystic lesions are associated with solid tumor formation, nephrectomy may be indicated. Kidneys that develop spontaneous bleeding may have to be removed to reduce the risks of severe hemorrhage in the course of hemodialysis and anticoagulation.

JUVENILE NEPHRONOPHTHISIS–MEDULLARY CYSTIC DISEASE

There appear to be at least three diseases in humans that primarily involve the tubular structures of the renal medulla. Medullary cystic disease and juvenile nephronophthisis are familial disorders that appear to be separate and distinct disease entities. By contrast, medullary sponge kidney (discussed separately) occurs only occasionally in members of the same family.

Juvenile nephronophthisis appears to be an autosomal recessive disorder, whereas medullary cystic disease appears to be an autosomal dominant condition. However, these are not rigorous hereditary distinctions but are impressions gained from the study of rather large families with what appear to be two disease processes. The diseases appear to be analogous to the inherited polycystic diseases in that the childhood type, juvenile nephronophthisis, is possibly an autosomal recessive disorder, whereas the type that appears principally in adulthood, medullary cystic disease, appears to be an autosomal dominant process. Some authors are not convinced that the diseases are clearly separable and refer to them collectively as juvenile nephronophthisis–medullary cystic disease complex. Another condition, termed *renal-retinal dysplasia,* encompasses retinal degeneration, familial retinitis pigmentosa, and pigmentary optic atrophy with renal changes similar to those of juvenile nephronophthisis.

Pathology

These various disorders cannot be separated by histologic techniques. In all cases the kidneys are moderately small, and on cut section thinning of the cortex and medulla is revealed. The cortical medullary junction is the site of a variable number of cysts, which range in size from barely perceptible to 2 cm in diameter. The cysts contain clear fluid that resembles normal urine. In some of these cases gross cysts are not visible. As in all cystic diseases, the cysts arise from renal tubules; however, in this instance they originate from medullary nephron structures and collecting ducts.

Clinical and diagnostic features

Within a family structure the disease appears to be inherited in a relatively uniform way. In juvenile nephronophthisis one usually obtains a history of polydipsia, polyuria, pallor, lethargy, and growth retardation. This disease usually progresses to the end-stage before the age of 20 years. In the medullary cystic form seen in adults, the clinical symptoms are similar except for growth retardation. Some cases have been discovered in the sixth and seventh decade of life. These patients may consume extraordinary amounts of water and sodium chloride to accommodate the renal salt and water losses.

The diagnosis is difficult to make by the usual radiographic techniques. Sonography and CT scanning have been useful in patients with clear-cut medullary cysts. But in the last analysis, open renal biopsy that includes medulla is probably the only certain way to make the diagnosis.

The uncertain genetic transmission of these conditions is a problem in genetic counseling. In these individual cases, it is extremely important to obtain a careful family history, so that the dominant or recessive character of the disorder can be ascertained within the family at risk.

MEDULLARY SPONGE KIDNEY

The diagnosis of medullary sponge kidney is usually not made until the fourth or fifth decade of life, when patients have secondary calcifications with passage of urinary stone or infective complications emerge. Progression to end-stage renal failure is uncommon. The incidence of this disease is approximately 1 in 5000 in the general population and perhaps as high as 1 in 1000 in patients studied in urology clinics. Males and females appear to be affected equally. Familial transmission of the disease has been reported on occasion, and there is an occasional association with other congenital problems.

Pathologic features

The external surface of the kidney is normal in this condition, and only on cut section is the abnormality obvious. There is irregular enlargement of the medullary and interpapillary collecting ducts, giving a "Swiss cheese" appearance to the kidney in these regions. The papillary changes are bilateral in most cases. Within an individual kidney one or several papillae may be affected. In some cases the cavity of the cyst may be filled with calculi, but in other instances there is no evidence of calcification in the ectatic collecting ducts.

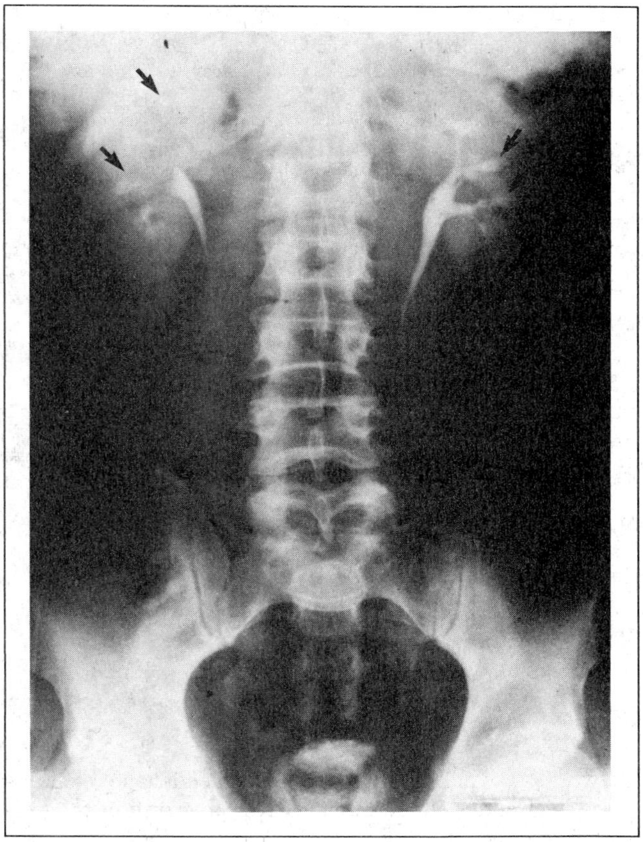

Fig. 358-3. Typical striations in medullary sponge kidney.

Clinical and diagnostic features

The disease is usually noticed in the fourth or fifth decade of life, when it may be associated with gross or microscopic hematuria. Nephrolithiasis with renal colic, loin pain, and secretion of small stones is also a prominent feature. The disease seldom progresses to end-stage renal failure; the most common abnormality is decreased urinary concentrating ability and in rare instances inability to acidify the urine maximally.

The diagnosis is made by intravenous urography, which shows the typical striations in the papillary portions of the kidney produced by the accumulation of contrast material in the dilated collecting ducts (Fig. 358-3). On plain films of the abdomen, calcium precipitates may also be observed in the papillary regions of the kidneys.

There is no known therapy. A causal association of parathyroid adenoma and medullary sponge kidney has been found in several reports. Among all calcium stone formers, women have a greater incidence of medullary sponge kidney than do men. Absorptive hypercalciuria is a common abnormality in sponge kidney that is associated with renal calcification. As a general rule patients should be advised to excrete over 2 liters of urine a day to reduce the opportunity for calcium precipitation in the urine. If a patient has hypercalciuria, thiazide diuretics may decrease urinary calcium excretion.

REFERENCES

Gabow PA, Grantham JJ: Polycystic kidney disease. In Schrier RW and Gottschalk CW, editors: Diseases of the kidney, ed 5. Boston, 1992, Little Brown.

Gabow PA, editor: Polycystic kidney disease. Semin Nephrol 11:595, 1991.

Gardner KD Jr, Bernstein J, editors: The cystic kidney. Boston, 1990, Kluwer.

Grantham JJ: Acquired cystic kidney disease. Kidney Int 40:1443, 1991.

Grantham JJ: Polycystic kidney disease: neoplasia in disguise. Am J Kidney Dis 15:110, 1990.

Reeders ST et al: A highly polymorphic DNA marker linked to adult polycystic kidney disease on chromosome 16. Nature 317:542, 1985.

CHAPTER

359 Glomerular and Interstitial Hereditary Nephropathies

Gerald F. DiBona

Between 10% and 15% of patients with end-stage renal disease have renal failure secondary to some form of progressive hereditary nephropathy. Polycystic kidney disease (Chapter 358) accounts for approximately 70% of these cases. This chapter deals with other hereditary nephropathies that have a documented or highly suggestive genetic pattern.

ALPORT'S SYNDROME

Alport's syndrome is an inherited disorder characterized by the familial occurrence in successive generations of progressive nephritis with evidence of glomerular damage, neural hearing loss, and ocular defects affecting the lens and macula. It is the first hereditary kidney disease as well as the first basement disease for which the gene has been cloned.

Genetics and pathogenesis

Six phenotypic variants are now recognized *(Table 359-1)*. The gene frequency is estimated at 1:5000, resulting in an incidence of 1:10,000 births. By using chromosomal markers the gene for the X-linked form has been located to the middle of the long arm of the X chromosome (Xq21.2-q22.2).

Spear proposed that a genetic defect at a locus governing a structural protein common to the basement membrane of the glomerulus, the anterior lens capsule, and the tectorial membrane of the organ of Corti in the inner ear could explain the association of renal, ocular, and auditory abnormalities. The genetic defect has been localized to the gene for the α_5 chain of type IV collagen (COL4A5), which is located in the q22 region of the X chromosome. Several mutations have been identified, including intragenic deletion, variants, and point mutations. These mutations can be considered to have serious effects on the folding of the globular domain of the α_5 chain of type IV collagen and may explain the pathologic changes observed in the glomerular basement membrane.

Clinical and laboratory findings

The disease usually begins in childhood or adolescence, appearing earlier in males. Initially, there is intermittent or persistent microscopic hematuria. Gross hematuria may occur spontaneously, after exercise, or after a nonspecific upper respiratory infection. Associated with the hematuria are mild intermittent proteinuria, which increases over time, and frequent occurrence of the nephrotic syndrome and hypertension. Renal insufficiency is slowly progressive; end-stage renal failure occurs in the fourth or fifth decade.

Some degree of hearing loss, produced by a bilateral symmetric sensory nerve defect, is an early symptom; deafness occurs in approximately two thirds of affected persons. The incidence, severity, and rate of progression of hearing loss are generally greater in males. Hearing loss can occur as an isolated manifestation or in association with ocular and/or renal abnormalities. Audiometric examinations are required to evaluate affected family members.

Ocular abnormalities include anterior lenticonus, sphe-

Table 359-1. Six phenotypes of dominantly inherited Alport's syndrome

Type	Inheritance	Age at ESRD*	Deafness	Other defects
I	Dominant (X-linked or autosomal)	Juvenile	Yes	Ocular
II	X-linked	Juvenile	Yes	Ocular
III	X-linked	Adult	Yes	None
IV†	X-linked	Adult	No	None
V	Autosomal	?	Yes	Macrothrombocytopenia
VI	Autosomal	Juvenile	Yes	Ocular

*Juvenile type is characterized by intrakindred mean age of onset of ESRD before 31 years in affected males versus after 31 years in the adult type. ESRD, end-stage renal disease.

†Also known as Epstein syndrome (hereditary nephritis, deafness, and macrothrombocytopenia).

rophakia, polar cataracts, perimacular pigmentation, and absence of macular reflex. These macular changes accompany anterior lenticonus. The ocular abnormalities are more frequent and more severe in males. Kindreds with ocular abnormalities have a higher incidence of renal and auditory abnormalities, but any of the three major features (renal, auditory, and ocular abnormalities) may appear in a given patient.

Routine laboratory investigation for immunologic or urologic abnormalities yields consistently negative results. There is no specific biochemical marker of the syndrome in blood or urine.

Pathology

By light microscopy, the findings are nonspecific. In young children, the renal biopsy result may be normal except for an increase in the number of immature glomeruli. Later, there is focal and segmental glomerular hypercellularity consisting of both mesangial and endothelial cells. The mesangial matrix is also increased. There is segmental and diffuse thickening with duplication of the glomerular capillary wall. Progressive glomerular disease is characterized by segmental and global glomerulosclerosis; crescent formation is unusual. The interstitium shows inflammatory cell infiltration, fibrosis, and tubular atrophy. Interstitial lipid-containing foam cells are seen, but their presence is not specific to Alport's syndrome. Immunofluorescence findings are usually normal.

Electron microscopy is the most reliable method of establishing a diagnosis. The earliest changes are focal thinning and thickening of the glomerular basement membrane. There is irregular thickening of the glomerular basement membrane, whose substructure is variously described as splitting, splintering, replication, reticulation, lamination, lamellation, or interweaving ("basket weave") of the lamina densa, and within which there are clear, electron-lucent zones containing small, round electron-dense granulations. There are occasionally similar lesions of the basement membranes of Bowman's capsule and tubular cells. There is fusion of epithelial foot processes, but electron-dense deposits are absent. Diffuse and widespread splitting of the glomerular basement membrane is strongly indicative of Alport's syndrome. In a review of 366 renal biopsies of 310 children with various renal disorders, diffuse and widespread splitting of the glomerular basement membrane was found in 24 of 27 patients with Alport's syndrome and in only 17 of 281 patients with other renal disorders. It has been suggested that Alport's syndrome be redefined as hereditary nephropathy with pathognomonic glomerular basement membrane changes and that the glomerular basement membrane changes be considered one of the criteria for the definition of Alport's syndrome. In rare instances, however, a normal glomerular basement membrane may be observed.

Differential diagnosis

In a patient with persistent hematuria, immunofluorescence and electron microscopy study of a renal biopsy specimen are clearly indicated. In a majority of cases, a definitive diagnosis can be made with these techniques. The finding of characteristic glomerular basement membrane changes should lead the physician to perform further studies to confirm the diagnosis of Alport's syndrome in the patient and in family members.

Berger's disease, or immunoglobulin A (IgA) nephropathy (Chapter 354), a common cause of hematuria in children, adolescents, and young adults, can be differentiated by renal biopsy. In IgA nephropathy, the typical finding by light microscopy is an area of hypercellularity with increased mesangial cells and matrix, often involving only a single lobule in a given glomerulus and with sparing of some adjacent glomeruli. Immunofluorescence reveals diffuse deposition of immunoglobulins in the mesangium of all glomeruli. The principal constituent of these deposits is IgA, which must be demonstrated to establish the diagnosis. Deposition of lesser amounts of IgG is often seen as well. Electron microscopy confirms the immunofluorescence findings by demonstrating small electron-dense deposits predominantly in the mesangium.

Treatment

No form of therapy slows progression to end-stage renal failure. Prompt aggressive treatment of urinary tract and ear infections is advisable. Dialysis and transplantation have been successfully utilized for patients with end-stage renal failure (Chapter 348). Stabilization of progressive hearing loss after successful transplantation and recurrence of the disease in the allograft have been reported. Corneal transplantation and lens extraction may be useful, but there is no treatment for the hearing loss.

FAMILIAL BENIGN ESSENTIAL HEMATURIA

Familial benign essential hematuria appears in childhood as intermittent or persistent hematuria without proteinuria, impairment of renal function, or hearing deficit and is not progressive. Light microscopy reveals normal glomeruli or only minor glomerular abnormalities, and immunofluorescence findings are normal. Electron microscopy shows diffuse and widespread thinning of the glomerular basement membrane, in which attenuation of the lamina densa is particularly prominent. Berger's disease is excluded by negative immunofluorescence findings, and Alport's syndrome may be excluded by absence of diffuse and widespread splitting of the glomerular basement membrane on electron microscopy.

NAIL-PATELLA SYNDROME

Nail-patella syndrome, or hereditary onychoosteodysplasia, is transmitted as an autosomal dominant trait closely linked to the ABO blood group locus. It is characterized by dysplasia of the nails, hypoplasia or absence of the patellae, accessory posterior iliac horns, and elbow deformities with increased carrying angle and limitation of supination and extension. About 50% of affected persons have proteinuria and/or abnormal urinary sediment. Progression to end-stage renal disease occurs in approximately 25% of affected patients. The light microscopy findings are variable and resemble those of Alport's syndrome. The electron microscopy findings in all patients with skeletal abnormalities, regardless of urinalysis or renal function, consist of (1) an irregular nodular thickening of the glomerular basement membrane with intramembranous collagen-like fibrils and (2) localized translucent areas in the glomerular basement membrane and mesangium that have a moth-eaten appearance. The immunofluorescence findings are variable. There is no known specific therapy, but successful dialysis and transplantation have been reported. The disorder does not recur in the transplanted kidney.

FAMILIAL MEDITERRANEAN FEVER

Familial Mediterranean fever is an autosomal recessive disease characterized by recurrent, brief but disabling, self-limited febrile attacks of peritonitis, synovitis, pleuritis, vasculitis, or an erysipelas-like erythema of the lower extremities. It is seen mainly in Sephardic Jews. Increases in serum mono-hydroxy and dihydroxy fatty acids known to cause neutrophil aggregation and decreases in peritoneal fluid C5a-inhibitor, which antagonizes the chemotactic activity of the complement fragment C5a, may participate in the pathogenesis of the acute inflammatory attacks. Systemic amyloidosis (Chapter 254) with renal involvement is a common but insidious complication of familial Mediterranean fever. Renal insufficiency is the major cause of mortality in more than 50% of cases, and renal functional impairment can occasionally precede other features of the disease. Renal involvement, which peaks in the third decade, becomes manifest as proteinuria, at first intermittent, later constant and massive. Renal vein thrombosis is not unusual. The clinical course is progressive, with development of the nephrotic syndrome and eventually end-stage renal failure. Average survival is 7 years after onset of proteinuria and 3 years subsequent to the development of the nephrotic syndrome; survival beyond age 40 is uncommon. Colchicine is effective in relieving the symptoms and frequency of acute extrarenal attacks. Colchicine therapy prevents amyloidosis (taken as proteinuria) and prevents additional deterioration of renal function in patients with amyloidosis who have proteinuria but not the nephrotic syndrome. Renal transplantation is an acceptable alternative to hemodialysis for the treatment of end-stage renal failure, although recurrence of amyloidosis in the renal transplant has been observed.

LIPODYSTROPHY

The syndrome of lipodystrophy is characterized by diminished subcutaneous fat, particularly of the face and upper arms; hirsutism; hyperpigmentation; splenomegaly; hypertension; and diabetes mellitus. Although there is familial aggregation of cases, the mode of transmission is unknown. The most common renal manifestation is asymptomatic proteinuria or the nephrotic syndrome. Renal biopsy reveals membranoproliferative glomerulonephritis, more frequently type II than type I, and there is decreased serum C3 concentration in association with circulating C3 nephritic factor (Chapter 354). The serum complement abnormalities may exist in the absence of clinical evidence of renal disease. The pathogenesis is unknown and there is no known treatment. Renal transplantation has been successfully employed for those patients who progress to end-stage renal failure.

ANDERSON-FABRY DISEASE

Angiokeratoma corporis diffusum, or Anderson-Fabry disease, is an inborn error of glycosphingolipid metabolism resulting from a deficiency of the enzyme alpha-galactosidase A. Inheritance is X-linked recessive, with carrier females displaying no or less marked features of clinical disease. The enzyme deficiency results in widespread tissue accumulation (including in the kidneys) of uncleaved glycososphingolipids, chiefly trihexosyl ceramide. Pain is often the first and usually the most characteristic symptom of the peripheral neuropathy. There are two forms: periodic "crises" of knife-like or burning pain in the limbs, particularly the hands and feet, and chronic acral paresthesias. In the first decade, punctate dark-blue, red, or black nonblanching macules, which evolve into blanching papules, appear in clusters on the skin of the lower trunk, thighs, and scrotum. Corneal opacities, posterior subcapsular cataracts, retinal abnormalities, premature cerebrovascular disease, cardiac involvement, and hypertension are frequently observed. Renal dysfunction is the rule and is evident by the third decade; end-stage renal failure occurs by the fifth decade. Early laboratory findings are hematuria and proteinuria. The urinary sediment may reveal lipid-containing foam cells that have a Maltese cross appearance on polarizing light microscopy. Under electron microscopy the lipid is stored as concentric lamellar inclusions in the lysosomes of the podocytes. These structures have been termed *myelin bodies* because of the resemblance to the myelin that surrounds nerve fibers. These myelin bodies may be noted in several inborn errors of glycosphingolipid metabolism.

Light microscopy reveals lipid deposition in blood vessels, glomerular epithelial cells, Bowman's capsule, and the epithelium of Henle's loop and the distal convoluted tubule. Immunofluorescence findings are normal. Treatment with dialysis and transplantation produces excellent survival rates (83% surviving 33 months). Isolation and characterization of the gene for alpha-galactosidase A have permitted the identification of various molecular defects: partial deletion, duplication, and point mutations.

REFERENCES

Anderson-Fabry Disease: Lancet 336:24, 1990.

Desnick RJ et al: Fabry disease: molecular genetics of the inherited nephropathy. Adv Nephrol 18:113, 1989.

Hostikka SL et al: Identification of a distinct type IV collagen α chain with restricted kidney distribution and assignment of its gene to the locus of X chromosome-linked Alport syndrome. Proc Natl Acad Sci USA 87:1606, 1990.

Kashtan CE et al: Alport syndrome, basement membranes and collagen. Pediatr Nephrol 4:523, 1990.
Nissenson AR and Port FK: Outcome of end-stage renal disease in patients with rare causes of renal failure. I. Inherited and metabolic disorders. Q J Med 73:1055, 1989.
Matzner Y et al: Proposed mechanisms of the inflammatory attacks in familial Mediterranean fever. Arch Intern Med 150:1289, 1990.
Noel LH et al: Inherited defects of renal basement membranes. Adv Nephrol 18:77, 1989.
Shohat M et al: Hypothesis: familial Mediterranean fever—a genetic disorder of the lipocortin family? Am J Med Genet 34:163, 1090.
Tryggvason K: Cloning of Alport syndrome gene. Ann Med 23:237, 1991.

CHAPTER

360 Disorders of Renal Tubular Transport

Sidney Kobrin
Stanley Goldfarb

The production of an ultrafiltration of plasma across the glomerulus causes an enormous load of plasma components to reach the tubular lumen. The tubular cells reabsorb many of these filtered substances from the tubular lumen. Abnormal tubular handling of sodium (Chapter 351), potassium (Chapter 352), and components involved in acid-base homeostasis (Chapter 353) are discussed elsewhere. This chapter focuses on the Fanconi syndrome and selected isolated disorders of renal tubular function.

RENAL GLYCOSURIA

Etiology

Renal glycosuria is defined as the presence of significant amounts of glucose in the urine in the absence of hyperglycemia. This abnormality may occur in a variety of settings. Primary renal glycosuria is an isolated heritable defect that occurs in the absence of other structural or functional abnormalities of the kidney. Congenital glucose-galactose malabsorption is a rare autosomal recessive inherited disorder. It is characterized by intestinal malabsorption of glucose and galactose and renal glycosuria and presents with severe diarrhea at birth. Generalized proximal tubular dysfunction (Fanconi syndrome) may include renal glycosuria. In addition, several more specific tubular defects, such as phosphate wasting and glycinuria, may also be associated with renal glycosuria. Renal glycosuria is commonly seen in pregnancy, the nephrotic syndrome, and, occasionally, advanced renal failure (glomerular filtration rate less than 15 ml/min).

The exact mode of inheritance of the primary form remains to be determined. The early literature on glycosuria suggested that the defect was inherited as an autosomal dominant trait. However, these studies were confounded by investigators' using different definitions and techniques of studying glucose handling, as well as the fact that the expression of the disease shows marked variability in severity even among members of the same family.

Pathophysiology

In normal persons, glucose is almost entirely reabsorbed in the proximal tubule, and less than 100 mg, well below the sensitivity of commonly used dipstick tests, appears in the urine. Glucose transport displays a transport maximum (T_mG): that is, below the saturating filtered load, or T_m, glucose is entirely reabsorbed, whereas the filtered load above T_m is passed into the urine. Theoretically, one might expect glucose to appear in the urine only when filtered load exceeds T_m, but the minimal filtered load, or threshold at which glucose appears in the urine ($F_{min}G$), is usually 70% to 80% of T_m. T_m is normally about 325 mg/min/1.73 m^2, and threshold is about 220 mg/min/1.73 m^2 (equivalent to a blood glucose level of 180 mg/dl). This discrepancy accounts for the so-called splay in the glucose titration curve. Splay could be the consequence of nephronal heterogeneity for glucose reabsorption if filtered load exceeds the reabsorptive capacity of some nephrons before others. Alternatively, splay may be explained by Michaelis-Menten kinetics on the assumption that glucose and its carrier behave as substrate and enzyme, with a finite dissociation constant.

In primary renal glycosuria, glucose titration studies have defined three pathogenetic mechanisms. In type A, T_m is reduced; in terms of the enzyme kinetic model, the number of glucose carriers is reduced, but the affinity of each carrier for glucose is normal. In type B, T_m is normal, but threshold is reduced, and the titration curve has an exaggerated splay. This variant is consistent with a normal number of carrier sites and reduced carrier affinity for glucose. In type O, there is virtual absence of renal tubular glucose reabsorption. Because all types have occurred within one family, they do not appear to be genetically distinct. On histologic examination, the kidney is perfectly normal.

Three patterns of glycosuria have been described in patients with the nephrotic syndrome, including types A and B as described with the primary form as well as a curve characterized by a low point of splay, but an otherwise almost physiologic tracing (type C). The different patterns of glycosuria are displayed graphically in Fig. 360-1.

Diagnosis

The diagnosis of renal glycosuria depends on the following criteria: (1) true glycosuria in the absence of hyperglycemia, (2) a normal glucose tolerance test result, (3) excretion of at least 500 mg glucose/1.73 m^2/day, and (4) exclusion of generalized tubular defects (Fanconi syndrome).

Clinical features

Primary renal glycosuria is generally a benign condition, with only occasional reports of development of hypoglycemia and ketosis during prolonged fasting. The major pur-

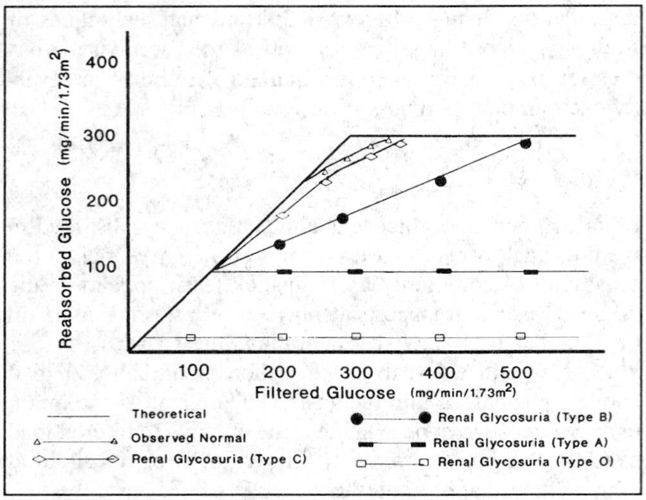

Fig. 360-1. Patterns of glycosuria.

Table 360-1. Aminoacidurias

Amino acid	Clinical disorders	Clinical manifestations
Alpha-amino neutral Tryptophan and others	Hartnup disease	Pellagra-like disorders
Dibasic Cystine Lysine Ornithine Arginine	Cystinuria	Recurrent nephrolithiasis
Dicarboxylic acid Glutamic acid Aspartic acid	Dicarboxylic aminoaciduria	Fasting hypoglycemia and ketoacidosis
Iminoglycines Hydroxyproline Glycine	Iminoglycinuria	No known disease

pose of documenting the primary form of this condition is to exclude diabetes mellitus, the nephrotic syndrome, renal failure, and the Fanconi syndrome from the diagnosis. The early literature suggested that primary glycosuria was a harbinger of diabetes mellitus. However, recent studies suggest that this disorder does not evolve into diabetes mellitus.

AMINOACIDURIA

Amino acids are freely filtered at the glomerulus; more than 95% of these filtered amino acids are then reabsorbed by transport processes located in the proximal tubule. The finding of excessive amounts of amino acids in the urine does not specifically imply a renal disorder. Thus a primary increase in blood levels of amino acids can produce aminoaciduria either as a "spillover" phenomenon or as the result of competition for transport between two structurally similar amino acids. Alternatively, blood levels can be normal, and aminoaciduria can be due to a renal tubular transport defect that is either generalized or specific for a certain type of amino acid. Generalized aminoaciduria is usually part of the Fanconi syndrome. The substrate-specific amino acid transport systems in the kidney and the associated disorders are listed in Table 360-1.

NEUTRAL AMINOACIDURIA: HARTNUP DISEASE

Etiology

Hartnup disease (named for the index family) is inherited as an autosomal recessive trait, and its incidence is 1 in 26,000 live births. The disease represents the apparent failure of synthesis of a transport protein that mediates the intestinal absorption and renal tubular reabsorption of monoaminomonocarboxylic amino acids with neutral or aromatic side chains. These include serine, alanine, threonine, valine, leucine, isoleucine, phenylalanine, tyrosine, glutamine, asparagine, histidine, and tryptophan.

Clinical and laboratory findings

The clinical features of Hartnup disease are similar to those characteristic of pellagra with the exception that the former is intermittent and usually less severe. Nicotinamide deficiency in Hartnup disease results from reduced availability of its precursor, tryptophan, because of both reduced gastrointestinal absorption and increased renal excretion. Patients have a red scaly rash that is exacerbated by exposure to sunlight. Cerebellar ataxia, psychiatric disturbances, and diarrhea are common. Intermittent dystonia without ataxia has been reported. However, these clinical findings are highly variable, and patients in normal physical and mental health have been described. The clinical disorders are subject to exacerbations and remissions, and periods of poor nutrition and excessive sunlight may precipitate clinical attacks. It is also possible that some of the neuropsychiatric manifestations of the disease are due to the absorption of metabolites of the amino acids generated by bacterial action on malabsorbed amino acids within the gut.

Dietary history plus chromatographic analysis of the urine readily distinguishes Hartnup disease from classic pellagra secondary to dietary deficiency. The cornerstone of treatment is the administration of nicotinamide in dosages of 40 to 200 mg per day to prevent pellagra-like disturbances.

DIBASIC AMINOACIDURIA: CYSTINURIA

For a discussion of cystinuria, see Chapter 349.

DICARBOXYLIC AMINOACIDURIAS

Increased renal excretion of glutamic and aspartic acids has been reported in only a few cases but has been detected by genetic screening programs and so may be more prevalent than has been believed. It is an autosomal recessive trait with two forms: Type I is associated with reduced gastrointestinal and renal uptake. In type II, gastrointestinal uptake is normal but renal uptake is impaired. Renal clearance of glutamic and aspartic acids has been found to exceed that of inulin, so an alteration in the bidirectional transport of these compounds is present, with a definite secretory component.

One child described with this disorder was completely normal and the abnormality was detected by screening tests, whereas a second exhibited fasting hypoglycemia, ketoacidosis, and growth retardation. The symptomatic child had a type I defect, and it is postulated that reductions in gastrointestinal uptake combined with renal loss led to a more severe deficiency and consequent impairment of gluconeogenesis. The only available therapy is frequent feeding to prevent hypoglycemia and ketoacidosis.

IMINOGLYCINURIA

Iminoglycinuria is a rare benign disorder characterized by the excretion in urine of excessive amounts of three amino acids, proline, hydroxyproline, and glycine. The underlying defect is believed to be reduced activity of a transport system in the proximal tubule that normally mediates the reabsorption of these amino acids. There are apparently no clinical consequences of this tubular defect.

RENAL PHOSPHATE WASTING SYNDROMES

Hypophosphatemia (Chapter 179) is most commonly seen in acutely ill patients and is usually a consequence of a combination of low dietary intake or malabsorption and a shift of phosphate into cells. Less commonly, hypophosphatemia is due to reduced renal reabsorption of phosphate (i.e., renal phosphate wasting). The causes of renal phosphate wasting are shown in the box below. Primary or secondary hyperparathyroidism may be diagnosed fairly readily by the finding of elevated parathyroid hormone levels and by coexisting disturbances of serum calcium (Chapter 187). Three uncommon causes of renal phosphate wasting, X-linked hypophosphatemic rickets, oncogenic hypophosphatemia, and the Fanconi syndrome, are discussed in the following sections in more detail.

Causes of renal phosphate wasting

Primary hyperparathyroidism

Secondary hyperparathyroidism
Vitamin D deficiency
Dietary
Malabsorption

Lack of 25-(OH)-vitamin D
Liver disease
Phenobarbital, phenytoin

Lack of 1,25-$(OH)_2$-vitamin D_3
Vitamin D–dependent rickets

Primary phosphate transport defect
X-linked hypophosphatemic rickets
Oncogenic hypophosphatemia
Idiopathic hypercalciuria

Fanconi syndrome

X-LINKED HYPOPHOSPHATEMIC RICKETS

Definition and etiology

Various forms of familial hypophosphatemic rickets have been described. The most common form is transmitted via a sex-linked dominant mode of inheritance and is referred to as X-linked hypophosphatemic rickets (XLHR). This syndrome is characterized by hypophosphatemia, inappropriately high urinary phosphate excretion, normocalcemia, normal to lower levels of calcitriol, and the occurrence of rickets in childhood despite normal vitamin D intake. There are also sporadic forms of hypophosphatemic rickets that are probably new X-linked mutations, and rare instances of autosomal dominant inheritance. A variant form, hereditary hypophosphatemic rickets with hypercalciuria, has also been described. This latter syndrome differs from XLHR in that it includes muscle weakness and high serum calcitriol concentrations.

Pathophysiology

The pathogenesis of XLHR has been intensively studied both in affected humans and in a mouse model (Hyp mouse) with very similar clinical, genetic, and biochemical characteristics. Two underlying biochemical abnormalities are present. One is persisting hypophosphatemia, which is explained by reduced capacity of the proximal tubule to transport phosphate; the other is plasma levels of calcitriol that are in the low normal or frankly low range, an inappropriate response because hypophosphatemia normally stimulates the synthesis of this hormone. The abnormality of phosphate reabsorption has been described as one of a reduced tubular maximum for phosphate (reduced T_m). The underlying cause(s) of the reduced phosphate reabsorption and the inappropriately low levels of calcitriol has not been clearly determined in humans. The defect in renal phosphate reabsorption in the mouse model has been localized to the luminal membrane of the proximal tubule. Several studies have indicated the presence of a humoral phosphaturic factor, derived from an extrarenal source, in the mouse model. The inappropriately low plasma calcitriol concentration in the presence of significant hypophosphatemia suggests that the X-linked mutation may also perturb the regulation of renal vitamin D metabolism. The Hyp mouse exhibits a blunted response to activators of calcitriol biosynthesis, as well as increased renal catabolism of this hormone. The increased catabolism is corrected by phosphate supplementation, suggesting that the abnormal vitamin D metabolism is secondary to a disorder in cellular phosphate homeostasis. Interestingly, serum phosphate and calcitriol levels and the T_m for phosphate are very similar in affected males and females.

Bone changes, which include rickets or osteomalacia, stunted growth, and lower limb deformities, define the clinical expression of the disease in XLHR. These skeletal manifestations are caused by a dual abnormality: a renal defect combining phosphate wasting with altered calcitriol metabolism, as described previously, and a bone defect that decreases the ability of the bone-forming cells (osteoblasts and osteocytes) to control mineral deposition in the matrix. As is characteristic of a sex-linked dominant mutation, the bone lesions are fully expressed in male hemizygotes and variably expressed in female heterozygotes. There is no direct correlation between the severity of the bone disease and the degree of hypophosphatemia. Female subjects with hypophosphatemia and no evidence of skeletal involvement have been identified as "carriers" of the trait. These subjects provide evidence that the defect in renal phosphate transport alone cannot explain the abnormal bone phenotype. The reason for this sex dependent difference in expression of the disease in bone and kidney is not clear, but it seems likely that two pathogenetic processes may be acting in parallel in kidney and bone.

Insufficient availability of calcium or phosphate similarly affects cartilage mineralization and induces rachitic changes. However, the effect on osteoid tissue calcification is somewhat different. Calcium deficiency provokes secondary hyperparathyroidism, which stimulates osteoclastic absorption, leading to a progressive decrease in bone mass and osteopenia. By contrast, the phosphate-deficient bone in XLHR is characterized by very little osteoclastic activity because these patients are normocalcemic and secondary hyperparathyroidism does not occur. Therefore despite severe osteomalacia trabecular bone mass is within the normal range in patients with XLHR. This finding may explain the rarity of fractures in these patients. The response to various forms of treatment provides another insight into the bone defect in XLHR. Patients treated with phosphate and vitamin D experience correction of their rickets, but not osteomalacia. When calcitriol is substituted for vitamin D, there is a beneficial effect, including improved and even healed osteomalacia. Some form of osteoblast resistance to vitamin D that can respond only to supraphysiologic levels of calcitriol could explain these findings.

Clinical and laboratory features

The clinical consequence of the reduced serum phosphate level is rickets. Growth retardation to the point of dwarfism and rachitic deformities are primarily seen in the lower extremities. Rickets develops as the infant begins to place weight-bearing stress on the lower extremities. Myopathy, a typical feature of other forms of hypophosphatemia, is rarely seen in XLHR, but adults manifest a variety of rheumatic complaints, including arthralgias and bone pain. The teeth may also be affected by apical abscesses and early decay secondary to abnormal dentine and cementum formation. The dental lesions, analogously to the condition in bone, are more marked in males. Renal phosphate wasting is manifested by a low T_m phosphate/GFR ratio or inappropriately high clearance of phosphate for the reduced serum level. Other abnormalities of tubular or glomerular function are not usually seen, but glycosuria and/or glycinuria has occasionally been reported. The bone biopsy result shows rickets or osteomalacia, depending on the age of the patient. The features of rickets are fairly typical, but as discussed, the osteoclastic activity is less than in osteomalacia associated with hypocalemia and secondary hypoparathyroidism.

Treatment

Adequate treatment requires both oral phosphate and calcitriol administration. Treatment with calcitriol alone does not raise serum phosphate levels, whereas treatment with phosphate alone results in hypocalcemia and secondary hyperparathyroidism. Although the conclusions are still challenged by some authors, most studies have demonstrated that the combination of phosphate and calcitriol administration enhances intestinal absorption of phosphate, heals the lesions of rickets and osteomalacia, and, if given early enough in childhood, significantly improves the growth rate and dramatically decreases the need for corrective osteotomies. Successful phosphate supplementation requires the administration of several daily doses in order to maintain a normal serum phosphate concentration for most of the day and night. The major complication of this therapy is the induction of nephrocalcinosis, which may ultimately result in a decrease in renal function. Frequent renal imaging and assessment of renal function are, therefore, essential. This strategy may allow a timely decrease in the dose or discontinuation of these agents. Whether the treatment should be continued after growth has ceased remains an open question.

ONCOGENIC OSTEOMALACIA

Etiology

Oncogenetic osteomalacia is a rare but fascinating syndrome that bears striking similarity to XLHR, discussed earlier. Patients who have this syndrome develop renal phosphate wasting leading to hypophosphatemia and osteomalacia. Associated with this clinical picture is the presence of unusual mesenchymal tumors of soft tissue or bone, or more generalized disorders of mesenchymal tissue such as fibrous dysplasia of bone and the epidermal nevus syndrome. In each of these settings, surgical resection of diseased tissue has cured the hypophosphatemia and oncogenic osteomalacia.

Pathophysiology

In some patients, no tumor has been identified and the mechanism of the disease is obscure. However, these patients are indistinguishable from those in whom a tumor has been detected. Because these tumors are generally benign, slow growing, and difficult to detect, it is possible that most, if not all, patients considered to have oncogenic osteomalacia may, in fact, have occult neoplasms. It is speculated that these tumors release a humoral factor that inhibits renal phosphate reabsorption and suppresses synthesis of calcitriol. The evidence for this is related to the fact that the biochemical abnormalities have been totally reversed within 24 to 48 hours of surgical removal of some of the tumors.

Clinical and laboratory features

The average age of patients with this syndrome is about 40 years. Men and women are affected equally. The patients show classic clinical and radiologic features of osteomalacia. Presenting symptoms include bone or joint pain, weakness, and difficulty in walking. Serum phosphate levels are uniformly low and alkaline phosphate levels high, whereas values for serum calcium are normal. As in XLHR, levels of parathyroid hormone are normal, but plasma calcitriol levels are inappropriately low for patients with hypophosphatemia. The pathologic features of mesenchymal tumors are generally those of hemangiopericytomas. Occasionally bony tumors resembling osteoblastomas or fibromas have been described. These tumors are usually benign and may be found virtually anywhere in the body. The lesions may be detectable by standard radiologic examination, but the smaller size may make detection difficult. The use of whole-body albumin radionuclide gated blood pool scintigraphy may be useful in demonstrating small peripheral neoplasms.

Treatment

When a tumor cannot be located or completely removed surgically, medical therapy with oral phosphate and calcitriol may heal the bony lesions if serum phosphate levels are normalized. Occasionally, patients have unremitting bone disease refractory to treatment.

FANCONI SYNDROME

Etiology and pathogenesis

Fanconi syndrome is a generalized disorder of proximal tubular transport characterized by excessive urinary excretion of amino acids, glucose, bicarbonate, uric acid, phosphate, potassium, and low-molecular-weight proteins. Incomplete expressions of the syndrome may lack one or more of these abnormalities. The syndrome is usually a secondary consequence of some toxic, immunologic, or metabolic insult. In children, the Fanconi syndrome is usually due to an inborn error of metabolism, whereas in adults the Fanconi syndrome is usually acquired. Fanconi syndrome may rarely arise in a primary idiopathic form. The primary type may occur at any age. It is most commonly sporadic, but familial cases with variable patterns of inheritance also occur. Histologic examination may reveal no specific findings, or tubulointerstitial atrophy and fibrosis. The prognosis is variable: some patients have shown only tubular dysfunction, whereas others have progressed to chronic renal failure over 10 to 30 years.

The various conditions that produce Fanconi syndrome share the feature of deposition in the proximal tubule of a toxic substance, for example, a heavy metal; a normal metabolite that accumulates in excessive amounts; or an abnormal protein (Table 360-2). The precise mechanism by which transport is impaired is uncertain. A leading hypothesis at present is that increased membrane permeability allows enhanced back-leak of solutes from the proximal tubular cell or of peritubular fluid into the tubular lumen.

Table 360-2. Causes of Fanconi syndrome

Inborn	Acquired
Cystinosis (cystine)	Light chain deposition
Wilson's disease (copper)	Multiple myeloma
Galactosemia (galactose-1-phosphate)	Monoclonal gammopathy
	Light chain nephropathy
Hereditary fructose intolerance (fructose-1-phosphate)	Heavy metal poisoning
	Lead, mercury, cadmium, uranium
Tyrosinemia	
Lowe's syndrome	Vitamin D deficiency
Glycogenosis	Renal transplantation
Vitamin D–resistant rickets	Nephrotic syndrome
Cytochrome *c* oxidase deficiency	Amyloidosis
	Sjögren's syndrome
Idiopathic	Drugs
	Anydro-4-epitetracycline
	Methyl-5-chrome
	Maleic acid
	6-Mercaptopurine
	Glue sniffing
	Isofosfamide
	Cis-platinum

Cystinosis is the most common cause of the Fanconi syndrome in children (Chapter 173). It is characterized by deposition of cystine in the conjunctiva, lymph nodes, bone marrow, and kidney. The mechanism of the increased cystine deposition is uncertain but appears to be related to a combination of increased cellular uptake and impaired cystine egress from lysosomes. Inheritance is autosomal recessive. Three forms may be distinguished: The nephropathic form is manifested by tubular dysfunction in infancy and progresses to early renal insufficiency. The adult form is benign, not characterized by renal involvement, and may be detected only by slit lamp examination. An intermediate form appears in adolescence with mild nephropathy and slower progression than in the infantile type. The diagnosis of cystinosis is made by determination of cystine in leukocytes or fibroblasts; by detection of cystine crystals in the conjunctiva, bone marrow, lymph nodes, or rectal mucosa; or by the presence of retinal pigment degeneration. Specific treatment of cystinosis has been unavailing. Renal transplantation has been successful, however, and although cystine crystals have been detected in the transplanted kidney, the Fanconi syndrome has not recurred.

In other hereditary causes of the Fanconi syndrome, the renal functional abnormality can be reversed by halting tissue accumulation of the toxic agent. Wilson's disease is due to copper toxicity, and the Fanconi syndrome, if not far advanced, can be ameliorated by penicillamine. Distal renal tubular acidosis (RTA) may also occur and may cause renal calculi, not otherwise a feature of Fanconi syndrome.

Hereditary fructose intolerance allows the accumulation of fructose-1-phosphate and is fully reversed by dietary fructose restriction. Similarly, galactosemia reflects the accumulation of galactose-1-phosphate, and the Fanconi syndrome is fully reversed by dietary galactose and sucrose restriction. A poorly characterized impaired glycogenolytic response has been associated with Fanconi syndrome, but the specific enzymatic defect has not been defined. Unusually severe glucosuria and hypoglycemia are characteristic. Lowe's syndrome is an X-linked recessive disorder characterized by cataracts and glaucoma, mental retardation, the Fanconi syndrome, and ultimate renal failure. The biochemical basis is unclear.

In adults, the most common cause of the Fanconi syndrome is injury to the proximal tubular cells by light chain deposition. In multiple myeloma or chronic overproduction of monoclonal light chains (Bence Jones protein), filtered light chain is reabsorbed by and accumulates in the proximal tubular cell; it can be identified in renal biopsy specimens by immunofluorescent staining using antisera against the appropriate light chain, and on electron micrographs by the appearance of intracellular crystals, probably representing condensed light chains. Why proximal tubular injury and the Fanconi syndrome develop in only a small proportion of patients with paraproteins and Bence Jones proteinuria is not known. The diagnosis of Fanconi syndrome may precede the recognition of myeloma, sometimes by many years.

Other dysproteinemic states, including amyloidosis and Sjögren's syndrome, are also associated with the Fanconi syndrome, and all these states frequently demonstrate distal tubular defects as well, such as distal RTA and nephrogenic diabetes insipidus (DI). Fanconi syndrome in nephrotic syndrome may also be caused by tubular toxicity produced by filtered and reabsorbed protein, which in this case consists of massive quantities of albumin. However, the Fanconi syndrome is rare in nephrotic syndrome, and a majority of patients have normal amino acid excretion.

Heavy-metal intoxication is caused by lead, cadmium, mercury, and uranium. Acute lead poisoning has produced full-blown Fanconi syndrome, but chronic lead nephropathy is typically associated with decreased uric acid clearance and hyperuricemia. Cadmium toxicity is typically associated with painful osteomalacia, nephrolithiasis, and characteristic hypouricemia in the presence of renal failure. Outdated tetracycline produced the Fanconi syndrome in the 1960s, but the pharmaceutical preparation has been modified so that the responsible degradation product (anhydro-4-epitetracycline) is not formed in currently available preparations. Thus this problem is no longer of clinical significance. Vitamin D deficiency states, including both nutritional deficiency and vitamin D–dependent rickets, have been associated with some features of the Fanconi syndrome, and the mechanism is presumed to be secondary hyperparathyroidism. Aminoaciduria, phosphaturia, and mild bicarbonate wasting (proximal RTA) may occur with both primary and secondary hyperparathyroidism.

Several drugs (Table 360-2) have been associated with the Fanconi syndrome. Recently, the chemotherapeutic agent isofosfamide has been shown to induce the Fanconi syndrome in 4% of a population with underlying normal renal function. The incidence of Fanconi syndrome may be even higher when pre-existent renal function is impaired or other nephrotoxins such as *cis*-platinum have been administered simultaneously.

Clinical features

Glycosuria in the Fanconi syndrome is similar to that seen in hereditary glycosuria and is of no clinical consequence as long as it is recognized as being renal in origin and not indicative of diabetes mellitus. Neither uricosuria nor aminoaciduria has clinical consequences, but the former may cause hypouricemia, which can be readily detected biochemically.

The predominant clinical features of the Fanconi syndrome are acidosis produced by bicarbonate wasting, polyuria caused by osmotic diuresis and hypokalemia, sodium wasting resulting from bicarbonaturia, and rickets or osteomalacia generated by phosphate wasting and probably reduced production of calcitriol. Growth retardation in children is due to acidosis, potassium, and phosphate depletion and possibly to amino acid wasting. Depending on the underlying cause, distal tubular abnormalities, such as distal RTA and nephrogenic DI, and progression to renal insufficiency are frequently associated. Characteristically, tubular abnormalities, such as hypokalemia, hypophosphatemia, and bicarbonate wasting, dominate the early clinical course and are ameliorated or become relatively less important if and as glomerular filtration rate falls.

Proximal bicarbonate wasting produces proximal renal tubular acidosis, characterized by hyperchloremic acidosis and a tendency to hypokalemia; normal urinary acidification when serum bicarbonate is at or below its reduced threshold; normal citrate excretion; and high therapeutic alkali requirements. Distal acidification is usually intact but may be impaired by concomitant potassium depletion or a dysproteinemic state. Hypokalemia is of multifactorial origin and may reflect decreased proximal tubular reabsorption, increased distal delivery of sodium and bicarbonate (particularly after alkali therapy), chronic acidosis, and hyperaldosteronism secondary to volume contraction.

Metabolic bone disease also results from several factors, including phosphate depletion and chronic acidosis. In addition, the conversion of 25(OH)-vitamin D to $1,25(OH)_2$-vitamin D_3 occurs in the proximal tubule and is inhibited in metabolic acidosis and in the maleic acid model of Fanconi syndrome. Thus reduced $1,25(OH)_2$-vitamin D_3 level may be a manifestation of intrinsic proximal tubular dysfunction or a consequence of acidosis and may contribute to metabolic bone disease. Muscle weakness caused by hypophosphatemia has been observed.

Diagnosis

The detection of any of the components of the Fanconi syndrome, including generalized aminoaciduria, proximal

RTA, renal glycosuria, hypophosphatemia with renal phosphate wasting, and hypouricemia with increased fractional excretion of urate, should prompt a search for other components. In its full-blown form the diagnosis should be obvious, but when only two to three components are present, an incomplete Fanconi syndrome must be distinguished from a more specific genetic defect, such as, X-linked hypophosphatemia with glycosuria, and family studies may be helpful. Once Fanconi syndrome is recognized, a specific cause must be sought among the possibilities listed in Table 360-2.

Treatment

Treatment of the underlying cause, when possible, may ameliorate the manifestations of the Fanconi syndrome. When the underlying disease fails to respond to therapy or primary Fanconi syndrome is present, symptomatic therapy focuses on acidosis, hypokalemia, and hypophosphatemic bone disease. Full correction of acidosis, as judged by normalization of serum bicarbonate, is essential to prevent growth retardation in children. Because of bicarbonate wasting, proximal RTA requires alkali supplements far in excess of daily net acid production—up to or more than 2 to 10 mEq/kg/day as sodium bicarbonate or Shohl's solution. The ensuing bicarbonaturia markedly enhances urinary potassium losses, necessitating potassium supplementation, given as phosphate, citrate, or bicarbonate. In adults, there is little evidence that proximal RTA requires treatment with oral alkali.

Similar to those who have X-linked hypophosphatemia (described previously), patients with the Fanconi syndrome and osteomalacia (or rickets) have both hypophosphatemia and reduced plasma levels of calcitriol. Treatment consists of both oral phosphate and calcitriol with the same precautions as when prescribed to patients with X-linked hypophosphatemia.

NEPHROGENIC DIABETES INSIPIDUS

Etiology

The causes of nephrogenic diabetes insipidus are listed in the box above. This chapter focuses on familial nephrogenic diabetes insipidus (FNDI), an X-linked recessive disorder that is fully expressed in males. There is no male to male transmission, and mothers and half of the sisters of affected males are obligate heterozygotes, or carriers. However, as many as two thirds of female carriers manifest a more mild form of the disease and may have a concentrating defect; some have symptomatic polyuria and polydipsia. In addition, female carriers show a blunted response to infusions of desmopressin acetate (DDAVP) with smaller and briefer increases in plasma levels of factor VIIIc and von Willebrand factor. This indicates that the genetic defect has variable penetrance in obligate heterozygotes. An interesting aspect of the disorder is that the ancestry of many apparently unrelated cases has been traced to the ship *Hopewell,* which landed in Nova Scotia in 1761.

Causes of nephrogenic diabetes insipidus

Familial (X-linked recessive)

Electrolyte disorders
Hypercalcemia
Hypokalemia

Tubulointerstitial disease
Obstructive nephropathy
Acute tubular necrosis
Sickle cell anemia
Amyloidosis
Fanconi syndrome
Sjögren's syndrome

Drug-induced
Lithium
Demeclocycline
Amphotericin B
Methoxyflurane
Aminoglycosides
Cisplatin
Rifampin
Foscarnet

Pathophysiology

The pathogenesis of this syndrome is still not entirely clear. Normally vasopressin stimulates adenylate cyclase at the basolateral membrane, and the increased cyclic adenosine monophosphate production enhances water permeability by an incompletely understood mechanism. In FNDI patients, plasma vasopressin levels are appropriate to the serum sodium concentration and osmolality: that is, plasma vasopressin rises linearly as plasma osmolality increases above a threshold level of approximately 280 mOsm/kg. However, urine osmolality remains low despite high endogenous levels of vasopressin and fails to increase in response to administration of either arginine vasopressin or DDAVP, a specific V_2 receptor agonist. (The V_2 receptor mediates the hydro-osmotic effect of vasopressin on the renal tubule via generation of cyclic adenosine monophosphate (AMP), whereas the V_1 receptor mediates the vasoconstriction effect via phosphatidylinositol and intracellular calcium.) Although it is clear that the cause of the polyuria is tubular resistance to the action of vasopressin, the specific nature of the defect leading to resistance is not known. Urinary cyclic AMP levels have been reported to increase in response to vasopressin in some families, whereas in others they do not, so that it is unclear at what step in the sequence of events that leads to increased water permeability the abnormality lies. In patients with familial nephrogenic diabetes insipidus, vascular responses to vasopressin, mediated by the V_1 receptor, are normal, but extrarenal responses to DDAVP, a selective V_2 agonist, are absent. For example, patients with this condition do not show the expected increase in plasma levels of factor VIIIc and von Willebrand factor that normally follow infusion of DDAVP, suggesting that there is a generalized defect in the V_2 receptor in this condition.

Clinical and laboratory findings

Inability to produce concentrated urine leads to increased urine output, hyperosmolality, and thirst. The ability of the patient to avoid dehydration becomes dependent on his or her perception of thirst and access to water. Polyhydramnios may be present at birth, and marked polyuria and polydipsia may appear shortly afterward. In the infant, whose access to water is limited, severe dehydration with fever and circulatory collapse may ensue. Neurologic abnormalities range from lethargy to coma and reflect central nervous system cell shrinkage produced by the hypertonic state. An increased incidence of mental retardation in these patients presumably is due to repeated episodes of hypertonic dehydration in infancy. The main difficulty of those who survive infancy is the inconvenient urge for frequent drinking and voiding, but an intercurrent illness or event that limits access to water can be life-threatening. Laboratory investigation reveals antidiuretic hormone– (ADH)-resistant hyposthenuria in the presence of plasma hypertonicity. The glomerular filtration rate is normal if the patient is not dehydrated, but hyperuricemia is typical even in well-hydrated adults and has been attributed to an increased filtration fraction and enhanced proximal tubular reabsorption. Hydronephrosis, hydroureter, and bladder enlargement may also result from the high urine flow.

Diagnosis

The approach to differentiating the various causes of polyuria is discussed in detail in Chapter 350. The diagnosis of familial nephrogenic DI is usually made in infancy in a child with polyuria and polydipsia who has a family history of the disorder and who fails to respond to exogenous vasopressin administration. This disorder can be differentiated from central DI by absence of response to exogenous vasopressin or by measurement of plasma vasopressin concentrations, which are inappropriately low or absent in central DI.

Other causes of a nephrogenic concentrating defect may be sought from determinations of levels of serum calcium, potassium, and glucose; results of renal function tests; examination of the urinary sediment; and a relevant drug history.

Treatment

In infants with nephrogenic DI, control of solute intake with breast milk or low-solute formulas limits obligatory urine volume. For instance, if the maximum urinary concentration is 100 mOsm per liter, an infant requires 3 liters of urine to excrete a 300 mOsm diet but proportionately less if solute intake is reduced. It is also important that the infant's mother ensure a constant high fluid intake to prevent potentially irreversible neurologic sequelae of dehydration.

Agents that have been used to reduce the degree of polyuria in patients with nephrogenic diabetes insipidus include thiazide diuretics, amiloride, and prostaglandin synthetase inhibitors. Thiazide diuretics probably work by producing mild extracellular fluid volume contraction and thereby enhance proximal tubular fluid reabsorption. As distal delivery of filtrate is reduced, free water excretion is limited. Recently, the combination of a thiazide diuretic and amiloride has been found to have several advantages over a thiazide diuretic alone. The antidiuretic actions of thiazides and amiloride appear to be additive. The combination obviates the need for potassium supplementation, and long-term side-effects are rare. The mechanism of the response to prostaglandin synthesis inhibitors such as indomethacin is unclear, but they probably also act by increasing reabsorption of filtrate at a site proximal to the collecting duct. Although polyuria may not be completely ameliorated by these agents, patient comfort is enhanced.

REFERENCES

Agus ZS: Oncogenic hypophosphatemic osteomalacia. Kidney Int 24:113, 1983.

Burk CD et al: Ifosfamide-induced renal tubular dysfunction and rickets in children with Wilms tumor. J Pediatr 117(2):331, 1990.

Foreman JW and Roth KS. Human renal Fanconi syndrome—then and now. Nephron 51(3):301, 1989.

Foreman JW and Segal S: Aminoaciduria. In HC Gonick and VM Buckalew editors: Renal tubular disorders. New York, 1985, Dekker.

Glorieux FH: Rickets, the continuing challenge. N Engl J Med, 325(26):1875, 1991.

Knoers N and Monnens AH: Amiloride-hydrochlorothiazide versus Indomethacin-hydrochlorothiazide in the treatment of nephrogenic diabetes insipidus. J Pediatr 117(3):499, 1990.

Morris RC, Ives HE. Inherited disorders of the renal tubule. In Brenner BM and Rector FC, editors: The kidney ed 4. Philadelphia, 1991, Saunders.

Scriver CS, Tenenhouse HS, and Glorieux FH. X-linked hypophosphatemia: an appreciation of a classic paper and a survey of progress since 1958. Medicine 70(3):218, 1991.

Verge CF et al: Effects of therapy in X-linked hypophosphatemic rickets. N Engl J Med 325(26):1843, 1991.

CHAPTER

361 Obstructive Uropathy

Saulo Klahr

Obstruction of the urinary tract (obstructive uropathy) affects renal function and structure. *Obstructive uropathy* refers to the structural or functional changes in the urinary tract that impair the flow of urine such that proximal pressure must be raised to transmit the usual flow through the point of anatomic or functional "narrowing." *Hydronephrosis* implies dilatation of the urinary tract. The term *obstructive nephropathy* is used to describe the renal abnormalities that result from urinary tract obstruction. The degree, duration, and location of the obstruction (see the box below) condition the rapidity and extent of functional and pathologic changes in the kidney.

INCIDENCE

Obstructive uropathy is a relatively common disorder. In a large series of autopsies, the prevalence of hydronephrosis was 3.5% to 3.8% and was not different in males and females. Obstructive uropathy occurs at all ages. However, the postmortem incidence of hydronephrosis in children (about 2%), mostly due to congenital anomalies of the urinary tract, is less than that in adults. It was estimated that 166 patients per 100,000 population were hospitalized with a presumptive diagnosis of obstructive uropathy in 1985 in the United States. Obstructive uropathy was the fourth leading diagnosis at discharge (242 patients per 100,000 discharges) among male patients with renal and urologic disorders. In 1985, 387 patient visits per 100,000 population were ascribed to obstructive uropathy in the United States.

PATHOGENESIS AND PATHOPHYSIOLOGY

Urine formation and flow depend on (1) hydrostatic pressure, which decreases progressively from the kidney to the bladder, and (2) ureteral peristalsis. Obstruction to urine flow anywhere in the urinary tract increases the pressure and volume of urine proximal to the obstruction. Significant obstruction impairs renal function, and if the obstruction is severe enough the kidney may be destroyed. Renal injury is probably due to elevated ureteral pressure and decreased renal blood flow, causing ischemia, cellular atrophy, and necrosis. Ureteral peristalsis allows for the generation of the high intraluminal pressures that are necessary for the propulsion of a bolus of urine. Contraction of the circular muscular fibers of the ureter above the bolus of urine prevents the pressure from being transmitted to the kidney. With obstruction, this phenomenon, called *coaptation,* is lost, and high intraluminal pressures can be transmitted upward to the kidney. Hence, a rise in ureteral pressure leads to increased intratubular pressure. The rise in intratubular pressure in turn decreases the net hydrostatic filtration pressure. After 24 hours of obstruction intratubular pressures return to normal in animals with unilateral ureteral obstruction but remain elevated in animals with bilateral ureteral obstruction, although values are less than the peak levels observed at 3 to 6 hours after obstruction. Although there is an increase in renal blood flow initially (2 to 3 hours), this is followed by a progressive decrease such that renal blood flow in the obstructed kidney of dogs is only 20% of control values after 8 weeks of obstruction. The initial rise in renal blood flow is due to increased prostaglandin synthesis. The subsequent decrease in blood flow is mediated by increased release of the vasoconstrictors thromboxane A_2 and angiotensin II. After 24 hours of obstruction the decreases in renal blood flow and hydrostatic glomerular capillary pressure are the main mechanisms responsible for the fall in glomerular filtration rate (GFR). Inhibition of prostaglandin synthesis at this time results in further decreases in renal blood flow and GFR, suggesting that vasodilatory eicosanoids antagonize the vasoconstrictive effects of angiotensin II and thromboxane A_2. Partial obstruction of the urinary tract may lead to similar alterations in renal blood flow and GFR, but in addition tubular defects may be prominent. These include a concentrating defect and decreased excretion of potassium and hydrogen ions. The concentrating defect is due in part to the inability to generate a high osmolar gradient in the renal medulla as a consequence of decreased sodium reabsorption in the thick ascending limb of Henle. There is also a diminished osmotic water reabsorption in the collecting duct in response to vasopressin. The acidifying defect and the decreased potassium excretion are due to impaired proton and potassium secretion in the distal nephron, presumably as a consequence of decreased responsiveness of this segment to aldosterone.

Factors that condition the rapidity and extent of renal abnormalities in obstructive uropathy

Degree of obstruction

Partial or incomplete ("low grade")
Total or complete ("high grade")

Duration of obstruction

Acute (hours or days)
Chronic (months or years)

Location of obstruction

Upper urinary tract

Ureteropelvic junction
Ureter
Ureterovesical junction

Lower urinary tract

Bladder
Urethra

CAUSES OF OBSTRUCTIVE UROPATHY

Obstructive lesions can occur throughout the urinary tract from the renal tubules (uric acid nephropathy) to the urethral meatus (phimosis) (see the box on p. 2762). Obstruction may be due to intrinsic lesions of the urinary tract or to extrinsic causes. *Renal calculi* are the most common cause of *intraluminal obstruction* in the young adult male. Approximately 1 of every 1000 hospital admissions in the United States is related to renal stones, which are three times more frequent in males than in females and have a peak incidence in the second and third decades of life. Calcium oxalate stones are the most common and cause intermittent acute urinary obstruction, which is seldom associated with a significant decrease in renal function. Renal calculi most commonly cause obstruction at the calyx, the ureteropelvic or ureterovesical junction, or the pelvic brim,

Causes of obstructive uropathy

I. Intrinsic causes

- **A. *Intraluminal***
  1. *Intratubular deposition of crystals (uric acid, sulfas)*
  2. *Stones*
  3. *Papillary tissue*
  4. *Blood clots*
- **B. *Intramural***
  1. *Functional*
     - a. Ureter (ureteropelvic or ureterovesical dysfunction)
     - b. Bladder (neurogenic): spinal cord defect or trauma, diabetes, multiple sclerosis, Parkinson's disease, cerebrovascular accidents
     - c. Bladder neck dysfunction
  2. *Anatomic*
     - a. Tumors
     - b. Infection-granuloma
     - c. Strictures

II. Extrinsic causes

- **A. *Originating in the reproductive system***
  1. *Prostate: benign hypertrophy or cancer*
  2. *Uterus: pregnancy, tumors, prolapse, endometriosis*
  3. *Ovary: abscess, tumor, cysts*
- **B. *Originating in the vascular system***
  1. *Aneurysms (aorta, iliac vessels)*
  2. *Aberrant arteries (ureteropelvic junction)*
  3. *Venous (ovarian veins, retrocaval ureter)*
- **C. *Originating in the gastrointestinal tract: Crohn's disease, pancreatitis, appendicitis, tumors***
- **D. *Originating in the retroperitoneal space***
  1. *Inflammations*
  2. *Fibrosis*
  3. *Tumor, hematomas*

Findings that suggest the presence of obstructive uropathy

Flank pain or an enlarged tender kidney
Changes in urine output (anuria, polyuria)
"Bladder symptoms" (decreased stream, hesitancy, incontinence)
Repeated urinary tract infections or infections refractory to "appropriate" treatment
Impaired renal function (elevated BUN* or serum creatinine level)
Gross hematuria
Hypertension
Hyperchloremic metabolic acidosis with hyperkalemia

*BUN, blood urea nitrogen.

where the ureter is crossed anteriorly by the pelvic blood vessels and broad ligament. Most stones are passed spontaneously. If they are not, surgical removal or disintegration of the stones by mechanical means may be necessary. A less common cause of intraluminal obstruction is a sloughed papilla produced by papillary necrosis, which occurs in entities such as sickle cell trait or disease, analgesic abuse, renal amyloidosis, and acute pyelonephritis, particularly when associated with diabetes mellitus. *Intramural causes of obstruction* are either functional or anatomic. The *functional disorders* causing obstruction include ureterovesical reflux, adynamic ureteral segments (usually at the ureteropelvic or ureterovesical junction), and neurogenic dysfunction of the bladder and sphincters. Neurogenic vesical dysfunction (neurogenic bladder) can be caused by upper neuron damage, which may produce involuntary micturition (spastic bladder dysfunction), or by lower spinal tract injury, giving rise to a flaccid atonic bladder. In both settings a significant residual of urine may develop, resulting in ureterovesical reflux, ureteral dilatation, and a significantly increased pressure in the upper urinary tract. The box above lists some of the entities that cause a neurogenic bladder. Certain drugs, such as tranquilizers (diazepam), anticholinergics, antihistaminics, or alpha-adrenergic stimulators, can cause bladder dysfunction and urinary retention. *Anatomic lesions* of the urinary tract resulting in obstruction are less common. *Ureteral strictures* are uncommon and may be due to retroperitoneal surgery or radiation therapy for cervical carcinoma. Rarely, strictures may develop with analgesic abuse or during treatment of genitourinary tuberculosis. *Urethral strictures,* secondary to chronic instrumentation or gonococcal infections are an infrequent cause of obstructive uropathy. *Malignant and benign tumors* of the renal pelvis, ureter, and bladder are uncommon causes of obstructive uropathy.

The *extrinsic causes of urinary tract obstruction* are best classified in terms of the system from which the obstruction originates. Most of the extrinsic lesions that produce obstructive uropathy originate in the reproductive system. Ureteral dilatation is common in pregnant females. The changes are reversible; ureteral dilatation subsides 3 to 4 months after delivery. Pelvic malignancies, particularly carcinoma of the cervix, are a common cause of extrinsic obstruction. In males, prostatic hypertrophy is the most frequent cause of extrinsic obstruction. About 80% of men over 60 years of age have benign prostatic hyperplasia and some evidence of bladder dysfunction. Ten percent of these patients require surgery. In one large series 24% of the patients had the initial complaint of complete urinary retention. Carcinoma of the prostate is another important cause of obstructive uropathy. The combination of benign prostatic hypertrophy and carcinoma of the prostate accounts for the greater occurrence of obstructive uropathy in males than in females after the age of 60. Other lesions that may obstruct the ureter originate in the *vascular system,* the *gastrointestinal tract,* or the *retroperitoneal space* (see the box opposite). Diseases of the retroperitoneum may produce chronic obstruction with few clinical manifestations. Metastasis from tumors of the cervix, prostate, bladder, colon, ovary, and uterus account for 70% of the extrinsic causes of obstruction in the retroperitoneum. Retroperitoneal fibrosis is another cause of ureteral obstruction. A growing number of cases of so-called idiopathic retroperitoneal fibrosis, occurring with equal frequency in both sexes, have been described. The fibrosis usually involves the ureter in the middle third, pulling it toward the midline. In some cases administration of drugs such as methysergide, or other ergot derivatives, may account for the development of retroperitoneal fibrosis.

CLINICAL MANIFESTATIONS AND LABORATORY FINDINGS

Patients with obstructive uropathy may experience acute renal failure, with chronic and slowly progressive symptoms, or with virtually no symptoms or signs. The clinical presentation depends on the duration, severity, and location of the obstruction (see the box on p. 2761) and on the presence or absence of complications. Although the symptoms and signs of obstructive uropathy are often nonspecific, some clinical features are sufficiently distinctive, when present, to suggest the diagnosis of obstruction (see the box on p. 2762).

Flank pain is a common complaint of patients with obstructive uropathy. It is secondary to stretching of the collecting system or renal capsule. Its severity correlates with the rate of distention rather than the degree of dilatation. Pain is more common in acute than in chronic obstruction. Acute ureteral obstruction is characterized by a steady crescendo of flank pain radiating to the groin, testicles, or labia ("classic renal colic"). The acute attack may last less than half an hour or as long as 24 hours. Pain radiating into the flank during micturition is said to be pathognomonic of ureterovesical reflux. On physical examination an *enlarged tender kidney* may be noted. Long-standing obstructive uropathy may increase renal size with readily palpable kidneys. Such patients may have increased abdominal girth or a flank mass. Hydronephrosis is the most common cause of palpable *abdominal mass* in children. *Anuria* occurs with complete bilateral obstruction or with unilateral obstruction in a patient with a solitary kidney. However, with partial obstruction, urine output may be normal or increased (polyuria). A pattern of oligoanuria alternating with polyuria or the presence of anuria should strongly suggest obstructive uropathy. Obstructing lesions of the bladder neck may cause *difficulties in micturition* such as decrease in the force and/or caliber of the urinary stream, intermittency, postvoid dribbling, hesitancy, and nocturia. Urgency, frequency, and urinary incontinence (overflow incontinence) may result from an inability to empty the bladder completely. Infection is a frequent complication in lower urinary tract obstruction. Repeated infections without apparent cause should raise the suspicion of obstruction. Moreover, as long as the obstruction persists, eradication of the infection is exceedingly difficult. Therefore a history of repeated urinary tract infections or persistent infection refractory to antibiotic therapy requires a detailed investigation to exclude obstructive uropathy. A number of patients who have *renal insufficiency* (elevated blood urea nitrogen [BUN] and/or serum creatinine level) may have long-standing, unrecognized obstructive uropathy. Obstructive uropathy may occur in patients with underlying chronic renal disease of another cause and may become manifested by a rapid change in the rate of progression of renal insufficiency. In other patients, however, obstructive uropathy is the sole cause of end-stage renal failure. Occasionally, in patients with retroperitoneal fibrosis, in whom the onset of obstruction is slow and progressive, far-advanced renal failure may be an initial presenting complaint. Urinary tract obstruction should be considered in uremic patients with no previous history of renal disease and a relatively benign urine sediment. *Gross hematuria* may be associated with obstructive uropathy, particularly when the obstruction is due to calculi. Acute or chronic hydronephrosis, either unilateral or bilateral, may be accompanied by a significant elevation in blood pressure. The hypertension could be coincidental or could be due to impaired sodium excretion with expansion of extracellular fluid volume or abnormal release of renin (renin-dependent hypertension). Obstruction may impair the ability of the kidney to excrete acid and potassium, resulting in the development of *hyperchloremic/hyperkalemic metabolic acidosis*. Obstructive uropathy should be considered in elderly individuals without diabetes who have hyperkalemic/hyperchloremic metabolic acidosis.

DIAGNOSIS

The diagnostic approach to a patient with obstructive uropathy depends on the clinical setting and presenting symptoms. The spectrum of the disease encompasses patients who have acute onset of pain to those with acute renal failure and anuria. Thus the approach and the urgency with which the diagnosis must be made are highly variable. When obstructive uropathy is suspected, it is important to inquire about a past history of similar symptoms, presence of urinary tract infection, symptoms of lower urinary tract obstruction, recent surgery, and ingestion of drugs. In hospitalized patients, it is important to characterize the pattern of urine output to determine whether it has changed abruptly, gradually declined, or fluctuates. Physical examination with emphasis on abdominal masses is important. Urinary outlet obstruction should be suspected in elderly patients with an enlarged prostate on palpation. Laboratory procedures provide little help in the diagnosis of urinary tract obstruction. The urine sediment may be normal. The presence of hematuria suggests that the obstructing lesion is a calculus, a sloughed papilla, or a tumor. The presence of bacteriuria, of course, heightens the suspicion of obstructive uropathy. The finding of uric acid crystals in the sediment suggests the diagnosis of acute uric acid nephropathy (Chapter 362). Once this information has been obtained, the diagnostic evaluation will vary depending on the symptom complex and the results obtained during the preliminary assessment of the patient.

In patients who have pain but no decrease in glomerular filtration rate (GFR), the next step is to determine the presence or absence of a renal calculus. This determination can be made by obtaining plain films of the abdomen without injection of contrast media (the kidney, ureter, bladder [KUB] film, see the box on p. 2764). If a calculus is found or if the clinical evidence suggests the passage of a stone,

> **Procedures used to diagnose obstructive uropathy**
>
> Plain abdominal films (KUB)*
> Excretory or intravenous pyelography
> Ultrasonography
> Computed tomography
> Antegrade or retrograde pyelography
> Pressure flow studies (Whitaker test)
>
> *KUB = Kidney, ureter, bladder.

an intravenous pyelogram (IVP) should be performed next. This study helps to determine the degree of obstruction caused by the stone and ascertains whether there is a radiolucent stone. Once a diagnosis of an obstructing calculus has been made, radiologic techniques are essential in the follow-up care. A notable exception to the approach described applies to the pregnant patient with obstructive uropathy. In such a patient radiographic evaluation should be performed only when other diagnostic procedures such as ultrasound or renographic techniques have failed. When renal function is impaired and there is no apparent reason for the decline or when renal insufficiency exists for an apparent reason but abruptly declines, the diagnosis of ureteral obstruction should be considered. Diagnostic ultrasound is the preferred procedure to determine the presence or absence of dilated calices or renal pelvis. Because this procedure is not invasive and is not affected by renal function, it is particularly useful to exclude hydronephrosis in patients with acute or chronic renal failure. Ultrasonography is extremely sensitive in the diagnosis of hydronephrosis, with a reported accuracy greater than 90%. Infrequently, ultrasonography may fail to recognize obstruction in certain conditions. Retroperitoneal fibrosis, for example, may cause significant obstruction with only minimal dilatation. The major drawback of ultrasonography is its extreme sensitivity, resulting in a number of false-positive results. Computed tomography (CT) may be useful as a subsequent study to determine the cause of previously diagnosed obstructive uropathy. This procedure can provide detailed anatomic information but should not be used as an initial procedure because of its high cost, lack of widespread availability, and relatively large radiation dose. Other procedures useful in determining the site of the obstruction are antegrade or retrograde pyelography. Occasionally, pressure flow studies (Whitaker test) may be required to diagnose upper urinary tract obstruction. The test measures pressure differences between the pelvis and the bladder during the infusion at a known rate of fluid into the renal pelvis.

TREATMENT AND MANAGEMENT OF URINARY TRACT OBSTRUCTION

Once the diagnosis of urinary tract obstruction is established, a decision should be made as to whether or not to undertake surgical or instrumental procedures. High-grade or total bilateral obstruction requires intervention as soon as possible. In these patients, the site of obstruction frequently determines the approach. If clinical conditions permit, instrumentation or surgery should be carried out the same day. In some patients dialysis may be necessary before performing any procedure designed to overcome or bypass the obstruction. In some patients with partial unilateral obstruction, especially those with calculi, immediate intervention is not necessary, and attention should be given to the relief of pain, evaluation of renal function, follow-up of urine cultures to detect the presence of urinary infection, and treatment of such infections. Close follow-up observation using intravenous pyelograms may allow evaluation of the progression and location of stones. If infection is present together with obstruction, infections should be treated vigorously, and efforts to correct the obstruction should be made. Prompt relief of partial obstruction is indicated when (1) there are repeated episodes of urinary tract infection, (2) the patient has significant symptoms (flank pain, dysuria, voiding dysfunction), (3) there is urinary retention, and (4) there is evidence of recurrent or progressive renal damage. Patients with lower urinary tract obstruction (urethral and bladder neck obstruction) require surgery if they are ambulatory and have recurrent infections. Obstruction secondary to benign prostatic hyperplasia is not always progressive. Thus a patient with minimal symptoms, no infection, and a normal upper urinary tract may be observed periodically until he or she and the physician agree that surgery is desirable.

A new drug, Proscar (Merck, Sharp & Dohme), an inhibitor of the 5-alpha-reductase (the enzyme responsible for the conversion of testosterone to dihydrotestosterone) is now available for the treatment of benign prostatic hyperplasia. In clinical trials this drug has been shown to ameliorate the symptoms of "prostatism" in about 30% of patients with benign prostatic hyperplasia.

POSTOBSTRUCTIVE DIURESIS

A profound and sometimes prolonged diuresis may follow the relief of obstruction of both kidneys or of a solitary kidney. This diuresis is characterized by marked losses of water, sodium, and other solutes. The mechanisms underlying this syndrome, usually referred to as *postobstructive diuresis,* are not completely clear. Many factors may account for this phenomenon (see the box on p. 2765). One is the volume status of the patient before the relief of obstruction. Individuals who have received large amounts of intravenous or oral fluids before the release of obstruction are often volume expanded. Thus the marked polyuria seen after relief of obstruction may represent a physiologic response to an expanded extracellular fluid volume. Another factor is the accumulation during the period of obstruction of substances such as urea, which are capable of causing an osmotic diuresis. Finally, the inappropriate natriuresis and diuresis observed after release of obstruction may be due in part to increased levels of circulating atrial peptide. This hormone may accumulate during the period of anuria

Potential factors responsible for postobstructive diuresis

Physiologic

Excretion of excess salt and water retained during the period of obstruction

Excessive administration of salt and water after relief of obstruction

Osmotic diuresis resulting from urea retained during the period of obstruction

Pathologic

Excessive urine losses of salt and water unrelated to the volume status of the patient caused by:

- Intrinsic defect in the tubular reabsorption of sodium
- Increased circulating levels of atrial peptide?
- Decreased hydrosmotic response of the distal nephron to antidiuretic hormone

and inhibit sodium and water reabsorption by the renal tubule after relief of the obstruction.

In summary, postobstructive diuresis may be due to the excretion of retained water and electrolytes, to the osmotic effect of retained urea, to the natriuretic effect of atrial peptide, or to a defect in the tubular reabsorption of sodium and water that occasionally results from obstructive uropathy and becomes apparent only after relief of the obstruction.

The management of postobstructive diuresis should include careful and adequate fluid replacement with frequent determination of body weight and plasma and urine electrolytes. These latter measurements provide a rational basis for the amount and composition of fluid to be administered. Urinary losses of fluid and electrolytes should be replaced only to the extent necessary to prevent hypovolemia, hypotension, hypokalemia, hypomagnesemia, and hypohatremia, or hypernatremia.

REFERENCES

Klahr S: New insights into the consequences and the mechanisms of renal impairment in obstructive nephropathy. Am J Kidney Dis 18:689, 1991.

Klahr S: Obstructive nephropathy: pathophysiology and management. In Schrier RW: Renal and electrolyte disorders, ed 4. Boston, 1992, Little, Brown.

Klahr S: Obstructive uropathy. In Glassock RJ, editor: Current therapy in nephrology and hypertension, ed 3. St. Louis, 1992, Mosby-Year Book.

Klahr S and Harris KPG: Obstructive uropathy. In Seldin DW and Giebisch G, editors: The kidney: physiology and pathophysiology, ed 2. New York, 1992, Raven Press.

Stafford SJ: Disorders of Micturition. In Schrier RW and Gottschalk, editors: Diseases of the kidney, ed 4. Boston, 1988, Little, Brown.

Stevens FD and Cook WA: Congenital urologic anomalies. In Schrier RW and Gottschalk CW, editors: Diseases of the kidney, ed 4. Boston, 1988, Little, Brown.

Wilson DR and Klahr S: Urinary tract obstruction. In Schrier RW and Gottschalk CW, editors: Diseases of the kidney, ed 5. Boston, 1993, Little, Brown.

CHAPTER

362 Tubulointerstitial Diseases

Shelley Albert
Eric G. Neilson

Damage to the renal tubulointerstitium is the major and essential contributor to all processes leading to end-stage renal failure. The various causes of tubulointerstitial nephritis as a primary disease account for approximately 15% of lesions leading to acute renal failure and 25% of those leading to chronic renal failure. Furthermore, it has been well documented that changes in glomerular filtration rate (GFR) correlate more strongly with the abnormality of the tubulointerstitium than with glomerular structure. This seeming curiosity results from the combination of interstitial fibrosis, destruction of peritubular capillaries, and reduced performance of the tubular nephron leading to decreased distal solute reabsorption and reduction of filtration via tubuloglomerular feedback. Although this chapter focuses on causes of primary tubulointerstitial nephritis, this correlation should be borne in mind when assessing patients with other progressive glomerular or vascular diseases.

The tubulointerstitial nephropathies can be subdivided into acute and chronic forms, each with distinct causes, abnormalities, and clinical course. Whereas acute interstitial nephritis is often a reversible disease, chronic tubulointerstitial nephritis tends to pursue a relentlessly progressive course, commonly unrecognized until the patient has evidence of end-stage renal failure. In both cases, environmental factors play a major etiologic role and should be carefully sought in the laboratory evaluation of any patient with suspected tubulointerstitial disease.

What, then, in the assessment of a patient with renal disease, should raise suspicion of a primary tubulointerstitial process? In assessing the causes of acute renal failure, a drug history is vital, as is a search for evidence of systemic infection or concurrent disease. On physical examination, findings of fever, a transient maculopapular rash, and flank tenderness, particularly in combination, are suggestive. Eosinophilia is seen in 80% of patients with drug-induced acute interstitial nephritis, and although the classical triad of fever, rash and eosinophilia is found in less than 30% of patients, its presence should strongly suggest the diagnosis. It should be noted, however, that the absence of these symptoms does not exclude a diagnosis of interstitial nephritis, particularly that caused by diuretics or nonsteroidal anti-inflammatory drugs. The urinalysis of acute interstitial nephritis reveals mild to moderate proteinuria (usually less than 1 g/24 hr), gross or microscopic hematuria, white cells, tubular cells and occasionally white cell casts. Eosinophiluria has been suggested as a marker of hypersensitivity-type interstitial nephritis. A recent study confirmed the superiority of Hansel's stain over Wright's stain in examining the urine for eosinophils and noted that a finding of greater than 1% eosinophils in the urine yielded a sensitivity of 63% and specificity of 93% for acute interstitial nephritis. Renal ultrasound reveals normal-sized or enlarged kidneys with increased cortical echogenicity, and gallium scanning may show bilateral increased uptake, although this finding is rather nonspecific. In the absence of a clear-cut clinical picture, renal biopsy is often necessary to direct therapy.

In chronic tubulointerstitial nephritis, these findings are absent. The urinalysis result is typically bland, revealing mild proteinuria, broad granular casts, and few cells. The most suggestive clue to a diagnosis of primary chronic tubulointerstitial disease is evidence of tubular dysfunction (out of proportion to the decrement in GFR), which is often absent in the acute syndrome because of the rapidity of renal functional deterioration. The various causes of chronic tubulointerstitial nephritis tend to damage the renal tubules in a segment-specific manner, although much overlap occurs. Thus the heavy metals and the dysproteinemias often preferentially damage the proximal tubule. This is manifested as a non-anion-gap metabolic acidosis that can be distinguished from a distal acidification defect by the administration of bicarbonate. In proximal renal tubular acidosis (Chapter 353) a bicarbonate load that raises the urine pH to above 7 is accompanied by a low serum bicarbonate and a high (> 70) urine PCO_2 caused by preservation of distal hydrogen ion secretion, which drives the reaction $H^+ + HCO_3^- \rightarrow CO_2 + H_2O$ in the distal lumen. In distal renal tubular acidosis (RTA) the serum bicarbonate level normalizes and the alkaline urine PCO_2 depends on distal hydrogen ion secretion. This proximal acidification defect may or may not be associated with one or more components of the Fanconi syndrome (i.e., glycosuria in the absence of hyperglycemia, phosphaturia, aminoaciduria, uricosuria, and ketonuria). Distal nephron defects include acidification disorders (produced by impaired ammoniagenesis, H^+ ion adenosine triphosphatase [ATPase] impairment, or H^+ ion back leak), hyperkalemia related to aldosterone unresponsiveness, and concentrating defects and can be seen in virtually any of the causes of chronic tubulointerstitial nephritis. Impaired distal sodium reabsorption (salt-wasting nephropathy) resulting in volume depletion is unusual and is generally seen only in medullary cystic disease or obstructive nephropathy. Medullary lesions result in impaired concentrating ability, manifested clinically as polyuria and nocturia, and are common in analgesic nephropathy and sickle cell disease. Other studies that may be helpful in establishing a diagnosis include renal ultrasound, which may reveal hydronephrosis in obstruction, and intravenous pyelography, which can show abnormalities in conditions of reflux nephropathy, papillary necrosis, nephrocalcinosis, and renal tuberculosis. Serum and urine immunoelectrophoresis should be obtained to rule out a plasma cell dyscrasia in the older patient.

PATHOLOGY

The hallmark of acute interstitial nephritis is the infiltration of inflammatory cells into the interstitial compartment with sparing of glomeruli. The infiltrating cell population is composed mainly of T lymphocytes and monocytes, but plasma cells and eosinophils may be seen. Together with interstitial edema, this infiltrate causes the tubules to be pushed away from each other, rather than to lie in close apposition. The tubular basement membrane may be disrupted in more severe cases. Staining of the tubular basement membrane for immunoglobulin G (IgG), IgM, or complement may occasionally be seen by immunofluorescence; both linear and granular patterns have been reported.

In the chronic lesion, the cellular infiltrate is largely replaced by interstitial fibrosis, which accounts for the irregular and contracted gross appearance of the kidney. The tubular epithelial cells are atrophied and the tubular lumina are dilated. It should be noted that *chronic* is a relative term, because fibrotic changes can be seen within 7 to 10 days of initiation of an inflammatory process. Chronic vascular and glomerular changes, consisting of nephrosclerosis and glomerulosclerosis, are often present at later stages of the disease, so that pathologic determination of the primary cause may be impossible.

A third pathologic category, namely, granuloma formation, can be seen in either the acute or the chronic setting. In acute granulomatous interstitial nephritis, the granulomas are sparse and nonnecrotic, giant cells are rare, and an accompanying interstitial infiltrate is common. The granulomas of the chronic lesion contain more giant cells, and if produced by tuberculosis, may be necrotic. Drugs are a common cause of this lesion in acute conditions, and most of the drugs associated with acute interstitial nephritis have been reported to cause granuloma formation. Sarcoidosis or tuberculosis should be considered when granulomas occur in chronic disease. When renal granulomas are found in Wegener's granulomatosis, they are almost always accompanied by glomerular and vascular disorders.

PATHOGENESIS

It is likely that the immune system plays a role in the pathogenesis of a variety of tubulointerstitial diseases, including some that are not traditionally thought of as being immunologic in nature. Tubulointerstitial structures may become the target of immune attack by a number of possible mechanisms. Most of these mechanisms are recognized from work in experimental animals and assumed to occur in human disease. Foreign proteins may bind to renal structures and act as a hapten, initiating an antibody response against the "carrier," as noted in methicillin-induced acute interstitial nephritis with the development of anti–tubular basement membrane antibodies. Drugs or infectious agents that share immunoreactive epitopes with interstitial structures may induce production of cross-reactive antibodies or T cells, which can then attack those structures. Toxins may alter tubulointerstitial proteins or reveal new ones, leading to their recognition as foreign. Finally, self-proteins may become visible to the immune system through increased expression of class II major histocompatibility complex proteins on tubular cells, which are required for antigen recognition by $CD4^+$ T helper cells. Such increased expression has been seen in a variety of human tubulointerstitial nephritides, including some metabolic causes, and indeed tubular cells in vitro are capable of presenting antigen to T helper cells when class II expression is increased. The response against these renal antigens may be modulated by such systems as suppressor T cell populations or idiotypic networks (antibodies and T cells directed against the antigen-binding site of autoantibodies), and only when these protective mechanisms are overcome does the autoimmune response ensue.

The effector limb of the nephritogenic immune response consists of several elements that may function individually or in combination in different human diseases. Humoral mediators, such as antibodies directed against continuous tubular basement membrane components or deposited in the tubulointerstitium as immune complexes, have been identified in isolated instances of human disease, including renal transplant rejection, lupus nephritis, and idiopathic tubulointerstitial nephritis. Cell-mediated immunity appears to predominate in most forms of tubulointerstitial nephritis. When eosinophils are attracted to the tubulointerstitium by chemotactic factors, their activation may lead to the release of various cytotoxic substances, including major basic protein, which has been detected in renal biopsy specimens in acute tubulointerstitial nephritis. T cells may damage tubules through direct cytotoxicity by release of cytolytic agents called perforins, or through delayed hypersensitivity in which lymphokines are released to recruit monocytes and other inflammatory cells.

Numerous insults to the tubulointerstitium are capable of initiating the fibrogenic process. These include inflammatory events located primarily in either the tubulointerstitial or glomerular compartments, obstructing lesions, some drugs, and diabetes mellitus. The two most abundant resident cell types of the tubulointerstitium, the interstitial fibroblasts and, to a lesser extent, the tubular epithelial cells, are both capable of secreting types I and III collagen, the major components of the interstitial matrix. A complex array of mediators can modulate matrix deposition at a number of levels, including fibroblast proliferation and motility, matrix component synthesis, and production of collagenases and other proteases. Most of these mediators are released by circulating cells recruited to the interstitium subsequent to an inciting inflammatory event. Transforming growth factor beta, for example, is released by activated platelets and macrophages, and some T cell subsets. Its actions include stimulation of fibroblast proliferation, increasing the transcription of type I collagen and inhibition of collagenase synthesis. T cells activated in experimental interstitial nephritis can induce fibroblast proliferation, type I collagen secretion, and inhibition of type IV collagen secretion with accompanying tubular atrophy. Other cytokines involved in regulating the fibrogenic response include platelet-derived growth factor, interleukin-1, and gamma interferon. Whether withdrawal of the inciting injury results in degradation of collagen and restoration of the normal interstitial architecture or persistence of an irreversible fibrotic scar depends, in ways that are not well understood, on both the duration of the insult and the balance of the modulatory mediators and cell types present.

ACUTE INTERSTITIAL NEPHRITIS

Acute interstitial nephritis should be considered in the laboratory evaluation of any patient with acute renal failure (see the box below). Although a drug can be established (at least by default) to be the etiologic factor in the majority of cases, it is important to bear in mind the less common possibility of systemic infection as being causative in adults. When a patient is found incidentally to have urinary abnormalities but a primarily nonrenal presentation, the latter diagnosis becomes more likely, particularly in the pediatric age group.

Drugs

Although a multitude of agents have been reported to cause acute interstitial nephritis, far fewer are implicated commonly. The beta-lactam antibiotics (including the cephalosporins) are the best studied group because of the past frequency of methicillin, a drug no longer in common use, as a causative agent. Other frequent offenders include rifampin, generally in association with tuberculosis; sulfonamides; thiazides and furosemide; and cimetidine. It should be noted, however, that acute interstitial nephritis is an uncommon complication of therapy with any of these agents. The onset of renal failure can occur within a few days to several weeks after initiation of therapy with an average delay of about 2 weeks. Renal dysfunction progresses over a

Acute interstitial nephritis

Drugs

Antibiotics

Beta lactams (especially ampicillin, penicillin)
Rifampin
Sulfonamides
Vancomycin
Ciprofloxacin
Cotrimoxazole
Erythromycin
Tetracycline

Nonsteroidal anti-inflammatory drugs

Diuretics

Thiazides
Furosemide
Triamterene
Ethacrynic acid

Miscellaneous

Cimetidine
Phenindione
Phenytoin
Allopurinol
Interferon

Infection

Bacteria

Legionella
Brucella
Diphtheria
Streptococcus

Viruses

Epstein-Barr virus
Cytomegalovirus
Hantavirus

Other

Mycoplasma
Rocky Mountain spotted fever
Toxoplasma

Idiopathic

Anti–tubular basement membrane disease
Tubulointerstitial nephritis and uveitis (TINUsyndrome)
Other

period of days to weeks; rifampin takes a more rapid and severe course and diuretics a more indolent course. The extrarenal manifestations of hypersensitivity in this disease have been discussed.

Acute interstitial nephritis produced by the nonsteroidal anti-inflammatory drugs requires a separate discussion because of several distinct features. Although a typical allergic interstitial nephritis, perhaps accompanied by papillary necrosis, is occasionally seen with these agents, by far the more common picture is one of acute interstitial nephritis associated with nephrotic syndrome. The glomerular lesion is that of minimal change disease, with epithelial foot process fusion on electron microscopy. The hypersensitivity findings of rash, fever, and eosinophilia are typically absent, peripheral edema is common, and the average delay in onset after initiation of therapy is 5.4 months, with a range of 2 weeks to 18 months.

Treatment is aimed first at withdrawal of the offending agent, which results in improvement in renal function within several days in many patients. In the absence of a prompt response, early institution of chemotherapy for patients with biopsy-proven acute interstitial nephritis has been recommended, given the rapidity with which irreversible pathologic changes develop in the tubulointerstitium. This consists, first, of a trial of corticosteroids, in a dose equivalent to 1 mg/kg/day of prednisone. Improvement in renal function should begin within 1 to 2 weeks of initiation of treatment, in which case the course can be discontinued after 4 to 6 weeks. If no improvement is seen within the first 2 weeks, the addition of a second agent such as cyclophosphamide (2 mg/kg/day) may be considered; if it is successful, it should be continued for 1 year with appropriate monitoring of the white blood cell count. Lack of any evidence of improvement after 6 weeks of combined therapy would constitute grounds for discontinuation of both agents. Although this approach has not had a randomized prospective trial, retrospective studies have attested to the beneficial effects of steroids, and anecdotal reports have supported the use of cytotoxic therapy in some patients. Up to one third of patients with drug-induced acute interstitial nephritis (and more in the case of rifampin) require dialytic therapy before resolution of the disease. Attention must also be paid to the effects of tubular dysfunction during the recovery period.

Infection

Although bacteria may invade the renal interstitium directly, renal dysfunction is a rare sequela of *uncomplicated* pyelonephritis in adults. However, a number of systemic infections can be complicated by acute interstitial nephritis (see the box on p. 2767). *Streptococcus* and *Diphtheria* are the most frequent offenders in the pediatric population. In adults the occasional reports of acute interstitial nephritis caused by legionellosis suggests that this infection should be included in the differential diagnosis of the pulmonary-renal syndrome. The human immunodeficiency virus has not been shown to cause isolated interstitial nephritis directly; however, it has been emphasized recently that tubulointerstitial lesions are common in this disease because of a variety of factors. These include opportunistic infections (with cytomegalovirus, cryptococcus, or histoplasmosis), nephrocalcinosis, and acute interstitial nephritis produced by the sulfa derivatives commonly used. Similarly, renal allograft recipients may be susceptible to such causes of infection as Epstein-Barr virus and cytomegalovirus. The various forms of hantavirus infection, including severe hemorrhagic fever in the Far East and self-limited nephropathia epidemica in Northern Europe, have also received attention recently, with isolated reports of infection in Western Europe and North America. Renal failure in infection-related acute interstitial nephritis generally resolves with treatment of the underlying infection, and steroid therapy is usually not needed.

Idiopathic

In a small percentage of cases, no etiologic factor can be identified in a patient with acute interstitial nephritis. In a few of these, circulating anti–tubular basement membrane antibodies have been isolated. Another subcategory includes patients with tubulointerstitial nephritis and uveitis (the so-called TINU syndrome). These patients are usually adolescent females whose biopsy findings show no granulomas and who have no systemic evidence of sarcoidosis. These patients are generally treated with a course of corticosteroids, and many experience a full recovery of renal function over several weeks.

CHRONIC TUBULOINTERSTITIAL NEPHROPATHY

The various causes of chronic tubulointerstitial disease are listed in the box on p. 2769. The etiologic possibilities for a given patient can be narrowed substantially by considering the demographic characteristics of that patient. Thus in the young adult with tubulointerstitial disease, reflux nephropathy or, if the patient is black, sickle disease, should be a major consideration. In the middle-aged woman, analgesic nephropathy should be suspected; in older adults a diagnosis of plasma cell dyscrasia would be the most likely. Obstructive nephropathy is a common diagnosis at any age, and in all cases an occupational history may be helpful.

Toxic/metabolic disorders

Analgesics. Chronic analgesic ingestion has been recognized as a cause of end-stage renal failure for nearly 40 years. The cause and pathogenesis of this complex disease are not fully understood, but certain facts have emerged. The epidemiologic characteristics of analgesic nephropathy vary widely both between and within countries and seems to be largely dependent on the composition and frequency of use of nonprescription analgesics. In Europe in 1986, for instance, the prevalence of analgesic nephropathy among patients with end-stage renal failure varied from 18% in Switzerland to less than 1% in Eastern Europe. It has been noted, however, that there is an inverse relation-

Causes of chronic tubulointerstitial nephropathy

1. **Toxic/metabolic disorders**
   - Analgesics
   - Heavy metals
   - Other toxins
   - Uric acid
   - Oxalic acid
   - Hypercalcemia
   - Hypokalemia
2. **Immunologic conditions**
   - Sjögren's syndrome
   - Transplant rejection
   - Lupus nephritis
3. **Hematopoietic diseases**
   - Sickle cell disease
   - Plasma cell dyscrasias
   - Infiltration
4. **Mechanical disorders**
   - Reflux
   - Chronic obstruction
5. **Vascular diseases**
   - Radiation
   - Arteriolar nephrosclerosis
6. **Hereditary diseases**
   - Medullary cystic disease–familial juvenile nephronophthisis
   - Laurence-Moon-Biedl syndrome
   - Oculocerebrorenal syndrome
7. **Miscellaneous conditions**
   - Granulomatous nephritis
   - Balkan endemic nephropathy

ship between the reported prevalence of analgesic nephropathy and that of nephropathy of unknown cause, suggesting an underestimation of the extent of this problem. In the United States the prevalence varies from 5% to 20% of cases of chronic renal failure.

The main culprit in this disease was previously thought to be phenacetin, the major metabolite of which is acetaminophen. However, despite the legislated removal of phenacetin from analgesic compounds in most countries in the 1970s, the incidence of analgesic nephropathy has not declined. It is now thought that acetaminophen, particularly when taken in combination with aspirin and possibly caffeine, can cause this lesion. A recent case-control study from North Carolina (an area with a high prevalence of analgesic nephropathy) that focused on patients who had chronic renal failure between 1980 and 1982 found an increased risk of renal failure in daily users of both phenacetin and acetaminophen, but not of aspirin in isolation. It is generally believed that at least 1 kg of the analgesic compound must be ingested to produce this lesion (although in this study patients who had ingested as little as 0.4 kg of phenacetin were at risk).

Eighty percent of patients who have analgesic nephropathy are female; commonly they use the product for various chronic pain syndromes and often they exhibit other addictive behavior. The earliest evidence of renal involvement is a defect in urinary concentrating ability, which may be accompanied or followed by acidification defects or salt-wasting. Azotemia occurs late in the disease process and indicates that papillary necrosis, the hallmark of the disease, has already occurred. Intravenous pyelography may be helpful in making the diagnosis by allowing visualization of sloughed papillae (the "ring-shadow" sign); however, this finding is neither sensitive nor specific for analgesic nephropathy. Analgesic abuse is also a risk factor for transitional cell carcinoma of the urinary tract, a disease with a poor prognosis that may be seen more frequently in the coming years as patients with analgesic nephropathy are maintained on dialysis.

The mechanism of analgesic nephropathy most likely involves the concentration of acetominophen in the inner medulla, which is then metabolized by the prostaglandin hydroperoxidase pathway to reactive intermediates that bind covalently to interstitial cell macromolecules, leading to necrosis. Salicylates and nonsteroidal anti-inflammatory drugs may contribute to this process by reducing both glutathione levels (which can prevent covalent binding) and medullary blood flow through prostaglandin inhibition. The process progresses from the inner medulla and eventually involves the tubulointerstitium of the cortex as well.

Treatment of this disease involves withdrawal of the analgesic responsible, which can result in stabilization or improvement in renal function. The physician must be alert, however, to the continued surreptitious use of these agents. Avoidance of volume depletion may also be protective.

Heavy metals. Lead can cause both acute, reversible nephrotoxicity and a chronic irreversible lesion. The acute form, occurring most frequently in children who ingest lead-based paint, results in a Fanconi-like syndrome and is characterized morphologically by the presence of eosinophillic intranuclear inclusion bodies in proximal tubular cells. Chronic exposure over a period of years leads to a nephropathy in which proximal tubular defects are less prominent and the picture is one of progressive azotemia and concentrating defects. This lesion is seen in conditions of either occupational exposure (e.g., among battery or smelter workers) or, in the Southeast United States, among "moonshine" whiskey drinkers who process liquor in automobile radiators. Heavy exposure over a period of many years appears to be required for the development of renal failure. Lead nephropathy, in contrast to other renal diseases, has been associated with the development of saturnine gout, and lead may be a risk factor for hypertension. In the patient with chronic tubulointerstitial nephritis, lead can be diagnosed as an etiologic factor by the ethyldiamine tetraacetic acid (EDTA) chelation test. Urinary excretion of more than 600 μg of lead in the 24 hours following intravenous infusion of 1 g of EDTA is indicative of excess exposure. Treatment (in the patient without evidence of marked interstitial fibrosis) consists of ongoing chelation therapy.

Cadmium exposure, usually occupational (although dietary exposure has been documented in some areas of Japan and Belgium), also leads to a chronic tubulointerstitial nephritis. This is manifested clinically as proximal tubular dysfunction and hypercalciuria with nephrolithiasis. Renal failure is uncommon. No specific therapy (other than avoiding exposure) is available.

Other toxins. Several other agents have been associated with chronic interstitial disease. The nitrosourea compounds carmustine and methyl-CCNU have been demonstrated to cause interstitial fibrosis in cumulative doses of greater than 2000 mg/m^2. *Cis*-platinum produces interstitial fibrosis and renal magnesium wasting, which can be partially prevented by such maneuvers as continuous infusion, vigorous hydration and diuresis, and use of hypertonic chloride content of the vehicle. The immunosuppressive agent cyclosporine, in addition to its well-established role in organ transplantation, is being used with increasing frequency in treatment of a number of autoimmune diseases. It produces, in some cases, both short-term reversible injury and/or chronic damage consisting of glomerular and vascular abnormalities associated with "stripe" fibrosis of the tubulointerstitium. The chronic injury is generally not reversible and may be progressive.

Uric acid. Uric acid can affect the kidney in three ways: Acute urate nephropathy occurs most commonly in the setting of chemotherapy-induced lysis of a lymphoma or leukemia in the patient with a large tumor burden but has also been seen during spontaneous lysis of a solid tumor. The ensuing acute oliguric renal failure, associated with a serum uric acid level greater than 20 mg/dl, results from uric acid crystal deposition in the collecting system. This syndrome is easily prevented in patients undergoing chemotherapy by prophylaxis with allopurinol and hydration, but once established it generally requires temporary dialytic therapy to reduce the uric acid load. Chronic urate nephropathy is now generally thought to be an uncommon clinical entity. Medullary urate crystal deposition is a nonspecific finding at autopsy, and any renal dysfunction found in patients with hyperuricemia can be attributed to concurrent disease, usually hypertension or cardiac disease. Finally, uric acid nephrolithiasis, which can occur in the absence of hyperuricemia, produces renal dysfunction through obstructive mechanisms.

Oxalic acid. Oxalic acid is the metabolic end-product of both endogenous glyoxylic acid and a number of exogenous toxins, so that oxalate nephropathy occurs in several settings. Inherited enzyme deficiencies can produce primary hyperoxaluria, manifested by recurrent calcium oxalate stones and progressive interstitial fibrosis leading to end-stage renal failure and extrarenal oxalate deposition. Prognosis in those patients resistant to pyridoxine (a cofactor for the deficient enzyme) is poor, but combined hepatorenal transplantation has been successfully utilized recently as an enzyme replacement strategy. Ethylene glycol, methoxyflurane, and massive ascorbic acid overdose can all result in acute renal failure generated by oxalate overproduction and deposition in the kidney. In addition, intestinal hyperabsorption of oxalate can occur in ileal disease or bypass, in which luminal calcium, which normally prevents oxalate absorption, is complexed with malabsorbed free fatty acids. Chronic tubulointerstitial nephritis and stone disease can result.

Hypercalcemia. Hypercalcemia has both acute and chronic effects on the kidney. Acutely it produces a vasopressin-resistant concentrating defect associated with hypertension, reduced renal plasma flow, and volume depletion, which can result in acute renal failure. Chronically, calcium deposition along tubular basement membranes, in tubular epithelial cells, and in the interstitium can lead to renal insufficiency and can be visualized radiologically as nephrocalcinosis (Fig. 362-1). Treatment in either case is directed to lowering the serum calcium level and identifying the underlying cause (most commonly, hyperparathyroidism, malignancy, sarcoidosis, or vitamin D intoxication).

Hypokalemia. Prolonged hypokalemia (often caused by laxative or diuretic abuse) occasionally causes proximal tubular vacuolization and possibly interstitial fibrosis morphologically; functionally it is reported to cause reduced glomerular filtration rate and concentrating ability, and increased ammoniagenesis. A recent report found reversible medullary cyst formation in patients with chronic hypokalemia.

Immunologic conditions

Sjögren's syndrome. Sjögren's syndrome is a symptom complex that may occur in isolation (primary) or in association with another autoimmune disease (secondary). It is manifested clinically by dry eyes and dry mouth (sicca syndrome), and by lymphocytic infiltration of other organs. Renal involvement occurs in 40% of patients. A lymphocytic interstitial infiltrate is seen, and clinically a distal tubular

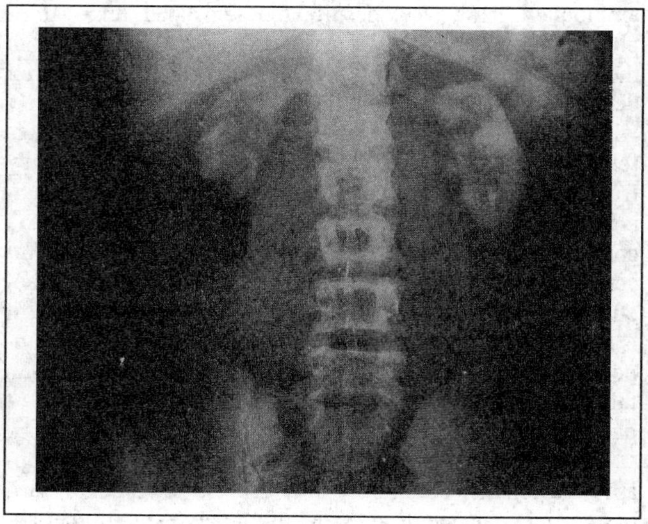

Fig. 362-1. Plain film of a patient with nephrocalcinosis secondary to chronic oxalosis. (Courtesy Dr. Howard Pollack, Radiology Department, University of Pennsylvania.)

acidosis and concentrating defect are common. Azotemia may be seen but renal failure is rare (Chapter 305).

Transplantation. Chronic transplant rejection is a cell-mediated immune process that occurs months to years after transplantation and produces a gradual deterioration in renal function. Pathologically, a typical chronic interstitial nephritis is accompanied by arteriolosclerosis and glomerular basement membrane thickening. Anti–tubular basement membrane antibodies may be detectable. Enhanced immunosuppressive therapy may reverse the process, but progressive graft failure is not uncommon (Chapter 348).

Lupus nephritis. Lupus nephritis commonly involves the tubulointerstitium, often with immune complex deposition along the tubular basement membrane, and the severity of interstitial inflammation correlates with renal function. Tubular functional defects may be prominent in some patients, but by and large, tubulointerstitial involvement in the absence of glomerular disease is uncommon (Chapter 306).

Hematopoetic diseases

Sickle cell disease. The hemoglobinopathy sickle cell disease has several renal effects. Cortical infarcts produced by embolic phenomena, and a glomerulopathy that resembles a normocomplementemic membranoproliferative glomerulonephritis have both been described. Hemoglobin S is particularly susceptible to sickling in the inner medulla because of its relatively hypoxic, hypertonic, and acidic milieu. The consequences of medullary sickling include recurrent episodes of gross hematuria, gradual papillary necrosis that leaves patients more susceptible to infection, and functional defects such as diminished concentrating and acidification abilities. Medullary interstitial fibrosis is a common pathologic finding. A recent study found that 4.2% of patients with sickle cell anemia and 2.4% of those with sickle C disease developed renal failure (which carried a poor prognosis despite dialysis), and that proteinuria, hematuria, hypertension, and severe anemia were all predictors of this outcome.

Plasma cell dyscrasias. Renal involvement in multiple myeloma can take several forms. Although acute renal failure secondary to hypercalcemia, volume depletion, and numerous other factors is common in myeloma, the strongest correlate of progressive chronic renal failure in this disease is urinary light chain excretion (Bence Jones proteinuria). Urinary light chains are not detectable by routine dipstick testing, but the addition of an equal volume of 5% sulfosalicylic acid to the urine produces a precipitate that is proportional to the total protein concentration. Urine immunoelectrophoresis confirms the finding. Urinary light chains in excess of the normal excretion of 6 mg/dl appear to be toxic to tubular cells and in addition may form intratubular casts with Tamm-Horsfall protein in the distal tubule, leading to tubular obstruction. Azotemia caused by urinary light chains generally occurs concurrently with or after the diagnosis of myeloma and is manifested pathologically by "cast" nephropathy: hard, eosinophillic casts surrounded by a giant cell reaction accompanied by tubular atrophy, interstitial fibrosis, and tubular basement membrane staining for light chains by immunofluorescence. Tubular dysfunction in the absence of azotemia, however, may precede a diagnosis of myeloma by years. Various components of the Fanconi syndrome have been noted, almost exclusively in association with kappa light chains, in the absence of any evidence of plasma cell neoplasm. Distal tubular acidosis and nephrogenic diabetes insipidus have been found in myeloma patients, and a number of individuals with both proximal and distal tubular defects, a syndrome that has been termed "combined light chain nephropathy," have been described. The presence of nephrotic-range albuminuria in a patient with urinary light chains should alert the physician to the possibility of glomerular deposition of either lambda or kappa light chains, resulting in amyloidosis or light-chain glomerulopathy, respectively. Management of these patients, in addition to chemotherapy if myeloma is present, includes maintenance of euvolemia and normocalcemia, avoidance of nephrotoxins, and correction of disturbances secondary to tubular defects with the use of sodium bicarbonate administration for distal RTA and thiazide diuretics for nephrogenic diabetes insipidus. Dialysis is appropriate for patients with renal failure, as recovery of renal function may follow chemotherapy.

Infiltration. Leukemic and lymphomatous infiltration of the renal interstitium is a common sequela of these malignancies but only occasionally causes any renal dysfunction and renal failure is rare.

Mechanical disorders

Two clinical entities, reflux and obstruction, can be thought of as producing chronic renal disease through a primary mechanical mechanism, although other factors are clearly involved in the pathogenesis once the disease process has been initiated. Bacterial infection, in particular, may play an important role.

Reflux. Reflux nephropathy is a potentially preventable cause of end-stage renal failure in young adults. Typically an adolescent or young adult exhibits hypertension and renal insufficiency and a history of urinary tract infections or unexplained fevers in childhood. Proteinuria ($>$ 1 g/day) and renal scarring revealed by ultrasound or intravenous pyelography are common, and progression to end-stage disease is the rule.

Intrarenal reflux, that is, the retrograde passage of urine past the papilla and into the nephron, is the pathogenetic hallmark of reflux nephropathy. As this can rarely be visualized directly, the diagnosis of reflux is generally made by the finding of vesicoureteral reflux by voiding cystourethrography. Recent reviews estimate that approximately 40% of children below the age of 5 who have had at least one urinary tract infection have had vesicoureteral reflux without another anatomic abnormality. The incidence of vesicoureteral reflux decreases with age: it is demonstrable in only 5% of adults with urinary tract infection. Whether bacteriuria is required in addition to reflux to cause renal scarring is still a subject of some controversy; new scars have been documented in patients receiving antibiotic prophylaxis. Renal damage produced by sterile reflux is likely an uncommon event, however. In either case, it is thought that under pressure, urine extravasates into the interstitium, and an inflammatory response against either bacterial antigens or normal urinary components such as Tamm-Horsfall protein ensues. The fibrotic healing of inflamed regions results in the radiologic appearance of the reflux kidney, namely, irregular scarring with areas of cortical thinning overlying blunted calices. Once this initial damage has occurred (likely before the age of 5 years), progressive renal functional deterioration can continue in the absence of either further reflux or infection. Focal glomerulosclerosis, most likely on the basis of reduced renal mass, and hypertension, the mechanism of which is unclear, are common sequelae of early renal scarring and are the immediate causes of renal failure.

It is now generally agreed that early intervention is crucial to the prevention of reflux nephropathy. Neither surgical correction of reflux nor medical therapy (i.e., antibiotic prophylaxis) prevents progressive functional deterioration once significant scarring has occurred. For this reason, it has been suggested that all children with a first urinary tract infection should undergo cystographic evaluation once the urine has been sterilized, with the initiation of therapy and close follow-up observation if vesicoureteral reflux is detected. Whether a surgical or medical strategy is chosen depends on the circumstances of the individual case. It should also be noted that the preadolescent, asymptomatic siblings of children with vesicoureteral reflux are themselves at high risk for this disorder and should probably be screened as well.

Obstruction. Prolonged obstruction may be the single most common cause of chronic tubulointerstitial disease. The possible underlying diagnoses are many, but renal calculi, prostatic disease in older men, and carcinoma of the cervix in older women head the list. Other considerations should include papillary necrosis, functional or anatomic abnormalities of the urinary tract, and involvement of the retroperitoneum with tumor or fibrosis. Whatever the cause, the transmission of elevated intratubular pressures to the glomerulus results in a decline in glomerular filtration rate. Renal blood flow, after a transient rise that follows obstruction, declines as well, perhaps as a consequence of thromboxane A_2 production by glomerular epithelial cells. Prolonged obstruction also leads to tubular damage, particularly in the distal nephron, and on pathologic examination interstitial infiltrates may be seen.

Clinically, acute bilateral complete obstruction is marked by anuria and flank pain caused by stretching of the renal capsule and pelvis, as well as pain referable to the underlying cause. In the more insidious forms of obstruction, the disease may be clinically silent. Urine output may be increased in incomplete obstruction as a result of concentrating defects, or there may be alternating polyuria and oliguria if obstruction is intermittent. Evidence of distal tubular dysfunction may include hyperkalemia, metabolic acidosis, vasopressin-resistant concentrating defects, and occasionally salt wasting. Azotemia is present and hypertension is common. The most useful diagnostic screening test is renal ultrasound, which reveals hydronephrosis in the majority of cases. It must be stressed, however, that significant obstruction can coexist with a normal ultrasound examination result, so that further diagnostic studies (such as retrograde or antegrade urography; see Fig. 362-2) should be undertaken when a patient has a normal ultrasound result and a suggestive clinical presentation. Finally, it should be noted that relief of obstruction commonly produces a postobstructive diuresis, a multifactorial condition that often involves a substantial iatrogenic contribution caused by volume loading before relief of obstruction and overly aggressive fluid replacement thereafter. Fluid and electrolyte replacement in these circumstances should be guided by the solute composition of the urine and by clinical assessment of the patient's volume status. Attention to potassium and magnesium losses is also important.

Vascular diseases

Radiation nephritis can occur in an acute, primarily glomerular form within 6 to 12 months after exposure, and in a chronic form thereafter, at which point the tubulointerstitium is the main target. The toxic dose to the kidneys is at least 2300 rad, and currently the disease is usually prevented through the use of shielding. Damage to the vascular endothelium is thought to be the pathogenetic mechanism, and it is therefore not surprising that hypertension is a common finding. In another vascular disease, benign arteriolar nephrosclerosis, chronic vascular and tubulointer-

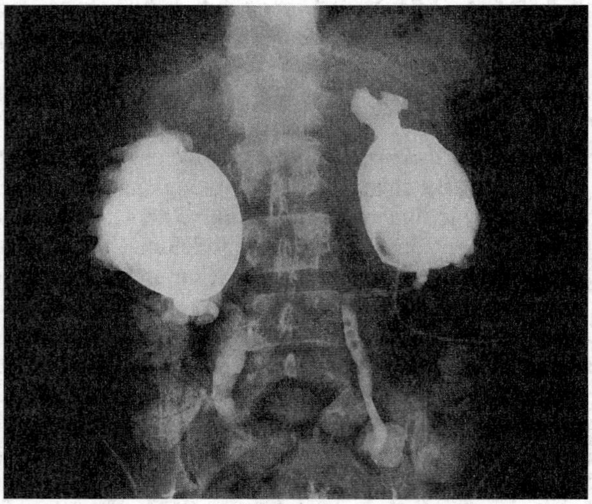

Fig. 362-2. Severe bilateral hydronephrosis secondary to benign prostatic hypertrophy. Antegrade pyelography obtained through percutaneous nephrostomy tubes. (Courtesy Dr. Howard Pollack, Radiology Department, University of Pennsylvania.)

stitial changes may precede the glomerular sclerosis that eventually supervenes. A history of essential hypertension, evidence of other target organ damage, and mild proteinuria suggest the diagnosis.

Hereditary diseases

A number of hereditary diseases can produce tubulointerstitial abnormalities; the most common is juvenile nephronophthisis–medullary cystic disease. The juvenile form of this disease is transmitted in an autosomal recessive manner and results in end-stage renal failure in childhood. An autosomal dominant form in which renal failure is delayed until late middle age also exists. Both diseases are characterized pathologically by cyst formation accompanied by chronic tubulointerstitial changes, with symptoms referable to the latter lesion.

Miscellaneous conditions

Granulomatous nephritis. As noted, granulomatous nephritis represents a distinct pathologic entity that can exist in chronic form. One series identified 14 patients with chronic granulomatous interstitial nephritis. The diagnoses were sarcoidosis in 3 patients and tuberculosis in 3; in the remaining 8 patients no diagnosis could be made and there was no evidence of extrarenal granulomas. Of this latter group, 5 were treated with steroids, to which 4 responded.

Sarcoidosis most commonly affects the kidney through the mechanism of hypercalcemia. Clinically apparent granulomatous involvement of the kidney occurs infrequently but may result in azotemia and tubular dysfunction. Steroid therapy generally leads to improvement in renal function and resolution of granulomas. Tuberculosis can affect the urinary tract at any level, often in the absence of evidence of active systemic disease. Symptoms may include dysuria, hematuria, and flank pain. Abnormalities indicated by examination of the urinary sediment (hematuria, pyuria) and by intravenous pyelography (caliceal deformity, calcifications, and cavitation) are almost universal. Azotemia, however, does not appear to be common in this disease. In one series of 41 patients with urinary tract tuberculosis, only 2 had mild azotemia. Other complications include ureteral stricture, secondary bacterial infection, and stone disease. The diagnosis can be made on the basis of a positive urine culture finding for mycobacterium tuberculosis, which was found in 90% of patients in the cohort mentioned; several specimens should be obtained. Antituberculous chemotherapy is curative in the majority of cases.

Balkan endemic nephropathy. Balkan endemic nephropathy was first described in the late 1940s, and its cause has remained a mystery. The disease primarily affects farm workers living in endemic pockets along the Danube River. At least 20 years' residency in an endemic region appears to be required for this condition to develop. The disease is characterized by proximal tubular dysfunction, tubular proteinuria (especially $beta_2$ microglobinuria), and slow progression to end-stage renal failure; uremia develops by the fifth to sixth decade of life. An increased incidence of transitional cell carcinoma of the renal pelvis and ureters occurs in the same endemic regions and may also strike patients with the nephropathy. At present, prevailing opinion suggests that an environmental factor in combination with a genetic predisposition precipitate Balkan nephropathy. Candidate environmental factors include selenium deficiency, contaminants in drinking water from nearby coal deposits, and ochratoxin (a mycotoxin) contamination of the food chain.

REFERENCES

Arant B: Vesicoureteric reflux and renal injury. Am J Kidney Dis 17:491, 1991.

Beck LH: Requiem for gouty nephropathy. Kidney Int 30:280, 1986.

Cameron JS: Immunologically mediated interstitial nephritis: primary and secondary. Adv Nephrol 18:207, 1989.

Corwin HL, Bray RA, and Haber MH: The detection and interpretation of urinary eosinophils. Arch Pathol Lab Med 113:1256, 1989.

Fang LST: Light-chain nephropathy. Kidney Int 27:582, 1985.

Gregg NJ et al: Epidemiology and mechanistic basis of analgesic-associated nephropathy. Toxicol Lett 46:141, 1989.

Halperin ML and Goldstein MB: Fluid, electrolyte and acid-base emergencies. Philadelphia, 1988, Saunders.

Heeger PS and Neilson EG: Treatment of interstitial nephritis. In Glassock R, editor: Current therapy in nephrology and hypertension, ed 3. Philadelphia, 1992, Decker.

Kuncio GS, Neilson EG, and Haverty T: Mechanisms of tubulointerstitial fibrosis. Kidney Int 39:550, 1991.

Mignon F et al: Granulomatous interstitial nephritis. Adv Nephrol 13:219, 1984.

Morgan SH and Watts RWE: Perspectives in the assessment and management of patients with primary hyperoxaluria type I. Adv Nephrol 18:95, 1989.

Neilson EG: Pathogenesis and therapy of interstitial nephritis. Kidney Int 35:1257, 1989.

Powars DR and et al: Chronic renal failure in sickle cell disease: risk factors, clinical course, and mortality. Ann Intern Med 115:614, 1991.

Sandler DP et al: Analgesic use and chronic renal disease. N Engl J Med 320:1238, 1989.

Seney FD, Burns DK, and Silva FG: Acquired immunodeficiency syndrome and the kidney. Am J Kidney Dis 16:1, 1990.

Simon HB et al: Genitourinary tuberculosis. Am J Med 63:410, 1977.

Ten RM et al: Acute interstitial nephritis: immunologic and clinical aspects. Mayo Clin Proc 63:921, 1988.

Van Ypersele de Strihou C and Méry JP: Hantavirus-related acute interstitial nephritis in Western Europe: expansion of a world-wide zoonosis. QJ Med 73:941, 1989.

CHAPTER

363 Renovascular Diseases

George L. Bakris
Richard M. Slataper

RENOVASCULAR HYPERTENSION

Renovascular hypertension (RVH) is the most common form of curable high blood pressure and is estimated to affect 1% of all hypertensive individuals. It occurs when significant unilateral or bilateral renal artery stenosis causes renal ischemia. The ischemic kidney activates the renin-angiotensin-aldosterone axis, leading to hypertension. Renal artery stenosis is primarily caused by atherosclerosis or fibromuscular dysplasia. The latter condition is rare in blacks. In most cases renal revascularization can preserve renal function and modify or cure the associated hypertension.

PATHOPHYSIOLOGY

The renin-angiotensin system is pivotal in the genesis of RVH (Fig. 363-1). The initial pathogenesis of renovascular hypertension is associated with high renin production. Although plasma renin levels are frequently elevated, renin production is typically suppressed in the unaffected kidney. Significant renal artery stenosis, like hypovolemia or hypotension, induces renin secretion from the juxtaglomerular apparatus. Consequent production of angiotensin II leads to vasoconstriction and aldosterone-mediated sodium retention. Edema, however, usually does not occur in unilateral disease unless renal insufficiency is present. This is related to the normal kidney's ability to "escape" the sodium-retaining effects of aldosterone with a pressure natriuresis. Conversely, in bilateral disease, the resultant increase in intravascular volume and blood pressure ultimately augments renal perfusion and produces mild edema.

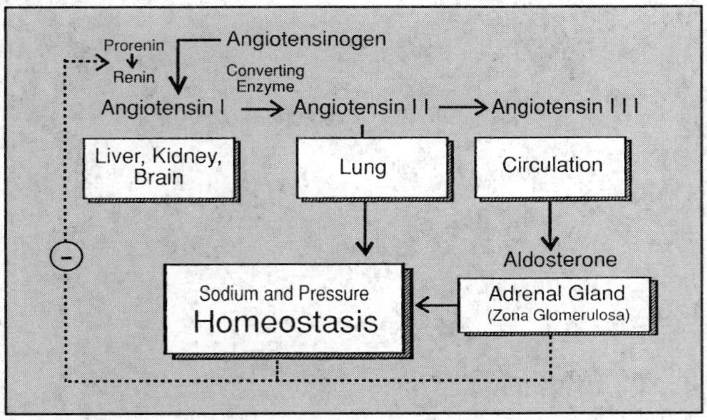

Fig. 363-1. The generation of the Renin-angiotensin-aldosterone (RAA) system and its contribution to salt and blood pressure control. The enclosed boxes represent the areas in the body where the conversions in the RAA system occur.

Renin levels in bilateral disease may eventually normalize as sodium and water retentions become more evident. Thus reduction in renal blood flow ultimately decreases the glomerular filtration rate as well as renal mass and affects both arterial pressure and sodium homeostasis. In individuals who have longstanding disease of either type, hypertension may persist after revascularization as a result of generalized vascular damage, contralateral nephrosclerosis or coexisting essential hypertension.

Renin production is also augmented by prostaglandins in RVH. These prostanoids, however, inhibit conversion of angiotensin I to angiotensin II. Thus most prostaglandins are vasodilatory in spite of their effect on renin release. Recent work suggests that renin production in renovascular hypertension is more prostaglandin-dependent than that of hyperreninemic essential hypertension. This concept serves as the basis for a recently developed test (discussed later) to distinguish RVH from other forms of hypertension.

CLINICAL FEATURES

The likelihood of renovascular hypertension is 10% to 20% in those hypertensive patients with one or more of the following characteristics: severe hypertension as a young adult or after age 50, uncontrollable hypertension at any age, renal insufficiency of unknown cause or after treatment with angiotensin-converting enzyme (ACE) inhibitors, extensive coronary and peripheral vascular disease, and a unilateral small kidney discovered by any previous clinical study. (The most specific physical finding is a continuous epigastric, subcostal, or flank bruit. If a continuous bruit is present, there is a high-correlation with presence of renal artery stenosis.) Individuals with nondiuretic induced hypokalemia (< 2.8 mEq/L) and recent exacerbation of hypertension should also be evaluated for RVH.

Renovascular hypertension develops as a result of significant stenosis (generally $>60\%$) of one main renal artery and occasionally arises from lesions of a distal branch. Two thirds of renal artery stenoses result from atherosclerosis, whereas the various forms of fibromuscular dysplasia are responsible for approximately one third. Atherosclerotic lesions are typically proximal and found more frequently in older males with evidence of extensive vascular involvement. Bilateral disease, azotemia, and recurrent pulmonary edema are also more frequent in this group. Conversely, patients with fibromuscular dysplasia tend to be young white women with no family history of essential hypertension; lesions usually involve the middle and distal segments of the renal artery. Smoking increases the risk of renovascular hypertension in both groups. Extrinsic renal artery compression, by a tumor or retroperitoneal fibrosis, is a rare cause of renovascular hypertension. Other unusual causes include arteritis, embolism, aneurysms, neurofibromatosis, and renal transplantation.

DIAGNOSIS

No ideal screening test exists for detecting renovascular hypertension. The positive predictive value of the currently available tests is considered acceptable only when applied to a population with a high probability of renovascular hypertension. Therefore the goal of patient evaluation for RVH is to assign individuals to low- or high-prevalence groups where the risk-benefit ratio justifies the risk of the next diagnostic or therapeutic intervention. Various tests to help in this evaluation are listed in Table 363-1.

Screening in an office setting has been done by measurement of plasma renin activity (PRA) via routine venapuncture before and 60 minutes after the oral administration of 50 mg of crushed captopril. The *captopril test* result is positive when all of the following criteria are met: (1) a stimulated PRA of 12 ng/ml/hr or more, (2) an increase of at least 10 ng/ml/hr over baseline PRA, (3) a percentage increase in PRA of 150% or more (an increase of 400% or more is required if baseline PRA is less than 3 ng/ml/hr). The patient should be seated during and 30 minutes before the test. A normal sodium diet and discontinuation of ACE inhibitors and diuretics 3 weeks before testing are recommended. Results are often inaccurate in blacks and patients with renal insufficiency or bilateral disease. The high sensitivity and specificity of initial studies have been inconsistently reproduced in recent investigations. *Isotopic renography,* before and after administration of an ACE inhibitor, is a popular noninvasive diagnostic approach with sensitivity and specificity of 85% to 95% that can be easily combined with plasma renin measurement. The angiotensin II–dependent filtration of the stenotic kidney is decreased in the presence of ACE inhibition, resulting in increased retention of isotope on the affected side. Recent modifications have improved accuracy in azotemic patients. *Intravenous digital subtraction angiography* has a similar sensitivity but requires injection of a relatively large amount of contrast material and should be avoided for azotemic patients. Results are inaccurate in patients with decreased cardiac output and in those with distal and branch lesions of the renal arteries. Best results are obtained by injecting contrast material high in the inferior vena cava, where renal vein renins can also be easily collected. Demonstration of increased renin activity in the ischemic kidney and suppressed renin activity in the contralateral kidney has traditionally been used to establish a causal relationship between the stenotic lesion and the resultant hypertension. A *renal vein renin ratio* of 1.5 or greater is believed to predict surgical cure or improvement. Recent prospective trials with and without ACE inhibition have been disappointing, and in some centers the role of renal vein renins has been replaced by ACE inhibitor renography. The *aspirin test* and *exercise renogram* are two recently developed physiologic tests that may eventually be used to distinguish essential from renovascular hypertension. Essential hypertension patients have a presumed exercise-related disturbance of renal hippurate transport not seen in patients with renovascular hypertension. Intravenously administered aspirin decreases the conjectured prostaglandin-mediated renin release in renovascular hypertension, causing blood pressure to fall. Blood pressure is unaffected or rises in individuals who have essential hypertension. Both of these methods are currently being investigated and need further evaluation. *Magnetic resonance imaging* (MRI) and *duplex scanning* are two promising methods for detecting renal artery stenosis (Chapter 341). Neither exposes the patient to the risks of use of contrast medium, radiation, or catheters. Both techniques are best employed when screening for proximal arteriosclerotic stenoses because neither method adequately visualizes distal arterial segments. Duplex scanning has a sensitivity and specificity of roughly 90% and is highly operator-dependent. MRI is slightly more accurate. Neither predicts surgical outcome.

Table 363-1. Tests used in the evaluation of renovascular hypertension

Screening tests	Diagnostic tests	Functional tests (predictive of surgical outcome)
ACE inhibitor renogram*	Arteriogram	ACE inhibit renogram
Captopril test	Intra-arterial digital subtraction angiogram	Renal vein renin ratios/index
Magnetic resonance imaging		Captopril test
Duplex scanning		? Exercise renogram
Intravenous digital subtraction angiogram		? Aspirin test
? Aspirin test		

*ACE inhibitor, angiotensin-converting enzyme inhibitor.

Routine *arteriography* of the renal arteries is considered the gold standard for the diagnosis of renal artery stenosis and in patients with strongly suggestive clinical features is sometimes the first and definitive test (Chapter 341). Functional tests should be performed before arteriography so that angioplasty of suitable lesions may be performed at the time of arteriography. Blood pressure response to correction of the stenosis determines the significance of the lesion. It is important to note that patients who have atherosclerotic disease are at increased risk of development of either catheter-related or radiocontrast-medium-related renal embolic events. The cost and risk of contrast nephropathy in those patients with renal insufficiency (i.e., serum creatinine level 2.5 mg/dl or greater), or increased risk of atheroembolic phenomena (e.g., aneurysms, severe vascular disease), make arteriography an inappropriate screening test. Use of the newer low osmotic radiocontrast agents probably is associated with less renal toxicity and therefore recommended for those at risk. *Intra-arterial digital subtraction angiography* provides very similar images of the renal arteries with less contrast medium and is preferred when patients have renal insufficiency or are otherwise at risk for a contrast reaction.

Hypertension does not improve with correction of the stenotic lesion in approximately one third of older patients. Functional or physiologic tests can help assign a patient to a group likely to improve with revascularization. The predictive value of available functional tests, however, is less than ideal. Clearly, a young patient with a diastolic flank bruit and severe hypertension of recent onset may be referred directly to arteriogram with immediate angioplasty. In an elderly patient with generalized atherosclerotic disease, moderately severe hypertension, and normal renal function a clinician may wish to increase the certainty of the diagnosis with a noninvasive screening test before exposing the patient to catheter-related and contrast-related risks of arteriography. Similarly, once a stenotic lesion is identified one should determine whether it is a consequence or a cause of hypertension. Thus individualized evaluation and therapy are essential.

THERAPY

Optimum management seeks both to control hypertension and to preserve renal function. Angioplasty or revascularization of the affected artery is widely favored as initial therapy for suitable surgical candidates. Unfortunately, medical therapy often provides only brief control of renovascular hypertension, frequently requiring high-dose and multiple-agent treatment. Furthermore, no class of antihypertensive agent has been shown to decrease the progressive nature of most stenoses or prevent reocclusion of atherosclerotic lesions after angioplasty.

Percutaneous transluminal renal angioplasty (PTRA) is a nonsurgical technique that employs balloon catheters to dilate stenotic arterial lesions and can be performed at the time of arteriography. In fibromuscular dysplasia without branch involvement it is the treatment of choice because of a high long-term patency rate. PTRA is considered acceptable therapy for discrete midarterial atheromatous lesions and is associated with a 20% to 30% restenosis rate. Repeat dilation is often successful. Ideally all patients undergoing PTRA should also be surgical candidates because 5% to 6% of patients require emergency surgical repair of the renal artery.

Surgical revascularization is the treatment of choice for branch renal artery lesions and most types of atheromatous lesions. Surgical mortality rate is approximately 2% to 3% for patients with atherosclerotic lesions and negligible for patients with fibromuscular dysplasia. Use of hepatorenal and splenorenal bypass in patients with atherosclerosis has obviated the need for operating on a badly diseased aorta. Nephrectomy is used only when attempts at revascularization are unsuccessful or the ipsilateral kidney is excessively atrophic.

Medical management of blood pressure has markedly improved with the availability of newer antihypertensive agents. ACE inhibitors exhibit effective control of renin-dependent hypertension but may compromise the angiotensin II–dependent blood flow in the ischemic kidney. ACE inhibitors have been associated with acute reversible renal failure in subjects with bilateral renal artery stenosis, stenosis of a solitary kidney, and unilateral stenosis with contralateral renal insufficiency. Calcium channel antagonists are attractive therapeutic alternatives in such cases because they effectively control arterial pressure and tend to preserve renal blood flow. To date, however, there is no convincing evidence that these agents slow the progression of atheromatous lesions in humans. Smoking cessation and hyperlipidemia control slow progression of atherosclerosis and should be pursued. Loss of renal mass is more predictive of worsening perfusion than blood pressure control. Medically treated patients should have periodic assessment of renal size and function. No prospective randomized trials have examined the long-term advantages and risks of medical therapy versus surgery or angioplasty.

RENAL VEIN THROMBOSIS

See Chapter 346.

RENAL ARTERY THROMBOSIS AND EMBOLISM

Thrombosis of the renal artery is nearly always associated with vascular injury. Most commonly arteriosclerosis is the underlying cause. Other predisposing conditions are summarized in the box below. Interestingly, cyclosporin has been shown to suppress the protein C anticoagulant pathway in cultured endothelial cells and may partially explain the increased risk of renal artery thrombosis in renal transplant patients.

The heart is the source of up to 90% of macroemboli. Cardiac conditions leading to macroemboli formation include atrial fibrillation, valvular vegetations, myocardial infarction, cardiomyopathy, and septal defects that can allow right to left passage of a venous thrombosis. Clinical presentations differ with respect to the abruptness of the occlusion, the number of kidneys involved, and the presence or absence of collateral circulation. Slow-developing disease is often insidious, and hypertension may be the only related manifestation (see the discussion of renovascular hypertension). Acute occlusion can be associated with flank or abdominal pain, fever, nausea, vomiting, leukocytosis, and transient gross or microscopic hematuria. Renal function is usually spared in unilateral occlusion, whereas acute oliguric renal failure is typical of bilateral involvement. Renal infarction generally results in sequential elevation of aspartate aminotransferase, lactic dehydrogenase, and alkaline phosphatase levels. Absence of a nephrogram indicated by intravenous pyelography (IVP), contrast computed tomography (CT), or isotopic renogram is highly suggestive

Causes of renal artery thrombosis

Aneurysm
Arteriography
Atherosclerosis
Cyclosporin (rare)
Fibromuscular dysplasia
Heparin-induced thrombocytopenia and thrombosis (rare)
Moyamoya syndrome
Polyarteritis nodosum
Syphilis
Thromboangiitis obliterans

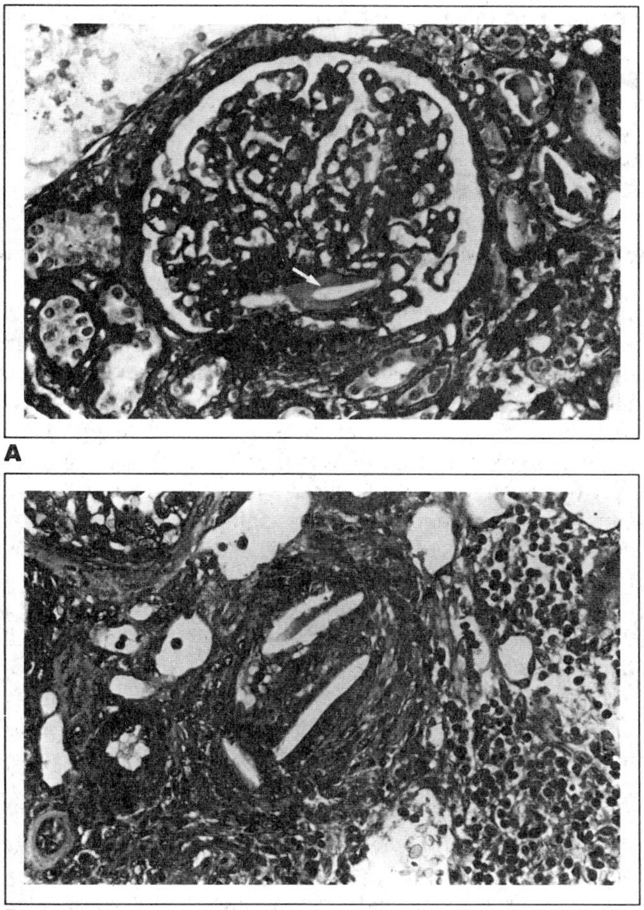

A

B

Fig. 363-2. A, Glomerulus with cholesterol cleft at the hilus (arrow). × 100. **B,** Atheromatous emboli in interlobular artery. × 100. (Photomicrographs courtesy of Melvin Schwartz, M.D.)

of an acute event. Arteriography is diagnostic. Duplex scanning is commonly used to assess renal circulation in transplantation patients. Anticoagulation with or without thrombolytic agents, angioplasty, and revascularization has been employed with success. No therapeutic consensus has emerged to specify which patients are best treated with which methods. Surgical revascularization, especially in young individuals, is generally advocated within 12 hours of occlusion secondary to trauma. Conservative therapy and blood pressure control are the mainstays of management in chronic disease. However, if renal insufficiency is progressive, then revascularization should be considered because successful recovery of renal function 1 to 2 months after occlusion has been described in older individuals with collateral circulation.

RENAL ATHEROEMBOLISM

Small to medium renal artery obstruction by microemboli originating from atheromatous plaques of the aorta characterizes atheroembolic renal disease. Microemboli or cholesterol emboli are composed primarily of cholesterol crystals and their occurrence is usually limited to individuals above the age of 60 with significant atherosclerotic disease. Showers of cholesterol emboli can be released spontaneously or after arteriography, aortic surgery, trauma, and possibly anticoagulation. Protean clinical features make antemortem diagnosis elusive. Periodic renal microinfarction manifests as progressive renal insufficiency and worsening hypertension. A vasculitis-like picture, including pancreatitis, visual disturbances, and painful distal extremities, may be associated with multisystem involvement. Physical features can include livedo reticularis, blue toes, abdominal aneurysm, femoral bruits, and cholesterol emboli of the retinal vasculature. Laboratory findings are transient and nonspecific but can include eosinophiluria (Hansel stain recommended), proteinuria, eosinophilia, azotemia, hypocomplementemia, and elevated sedimentation rate. Diagnosis is made by tissue biopsy of an affected area. On routine preparation the cholesterol crystals are dissolved, leaving the characteristic "cholesterol clefts" in the material occluding a small artery (Fig. 363-2). Renal biopsy has the highest diagnostic yield but skin, muscle, and rectal biopsy may also be diagnostic. There is no recognized effective treatment. Anticoagulation may actually prevent stable plaque formation, thereby liberating cholesterol crystals, and worsen the prognosis.

REFERENCES

Erbsloh-Moller B et al: Furosemide–131 I–hippuran renography after angiotensin-converting enzyme inhibitor for the diagnosis of renovascular hypertension. Am J Med 90:23, 1991.

Garcia-Maldonado M, Kaufman CE, and Comp PC: Decrease in endothelial cell dependent protein C activation induced by thrombomodulin by treatment with cyclosporin. Transplantation 51(3):701, 1991.

Happ T, Clorius JH, and Allenberg JR: Renovascular hypertension: predicting surgical cure with exercise renography. J Vasc Surg 14:200, 1991.

Imanishi M et al: Aspirin test for differentiation of unilateral renovascular hypertension from hyperreninemic essential hypertension. Am J Hypertens 4:761, 1991.

Ives HE and Daniel TO: Vascular disease of the kidney. In Brenner BM, Rector FC Jr, editors: The kidney, ed 4. Philadelphia, 1991, Saunders.

Kalra PA et al: Renovascular disease and renal complications of angiotensin-converting enzyme inhibition therapy. Q J Med 77(282):1013, 1990.

Kent CK et al: Magnetic resonance imaging: a reliable test for the evaluation of proximal atherosclerotic renal artery stenosis. J Vasc Surg 13:311, 1991.

Martinez-Maldonado M: Pathophysiology of renovascular hypertension. Hypertension 17:707, 1991.

Novick AC: Management of renovascular disease: a surgical perspective. Circulation 83(suppl 1):1-167, 1991.

Pickering TG: The role of laboratory testing in the diagnosis of renovascular hypertension. Clin Chem 37:1831, 1991.

Roubidoux MA, Dunnick NR and Klotman PE: Renal vein renins: inability to predict response to revascularization in patients with hypertension. Radiology 178:819, 1991.

Schreiber MJ, Pohl MA, and Novick AC: The natural history of atherosclerotic and fibrous renal artery diseases. Urol Clin North Am 11(3):383, 1984.

Slataper RM and Bakris GL: Secondary hypertension. In Taylor RB, editor: Difficult diagnosis II. Philadelphia, 1992, Saunders.

Sos TA: Angioplasty for the treatment of azotemia and renovascular hypertension in atherosclerotic renal artery disease. Circulation 83(suppl 1):1-162, 1991.

CHAPTER

364 Renal Cell Carcinoma

T. Dwight McKinney

INCIDENCE

Renal cell carcinoma is responsible for about 3% of all malignant neoplasms. It occurs at a rate of 7.5 cases per 100,000 population annually and is the most common renal cancer, accounting for 90% of renal malignancies in adults. Renal cell carcinoma occurs twice as frequently in men as women. Risk factors for the development of renal cell carcinoma include tobacco use, exposure to certain chemicals such as cadmium and nitrosohydrocarbons, acquired cystic disease occurring in end-stage kidneys, and von Hippel-Lindau disease. In the latter autosomal dominant disorder renal cell carcinoma may develop in up to 35% of cases and is frequently bilateral.

PATHOLOGY

Renal cell carcinoma probably arises from proximal tubule cells and may present in three main cell types: clear, granular, and sarcomatoid. Both the cell type and degree of cellular differentiation, in addition to the presence or absence of metastases, are important prognostically; nonmetastatic well-differentiated clear-cell carcinoma has the most favorable prognosis. Thirty percent of patients have metastatic disease at the time of initial diagnosis. The most frequent sites of metastases are the lung, lymph nodes, liver, bone, and adrenal glands. Extension of tumor into the renal veins or inferior vena cava occurs in more than 20% of cases but, unless there is invasion of the vessel wall, does not affect prognosis.

CLINICAL AND LABORATORY MANIFESTATIONS

Renal cell carcinoma may exhibit a variety of clinical and laboratory abnormalities. Isolated microscopic or gross hematuria is the most common presenting symptom and occurs in 40% to 60% of cases. Other manifestations include abdominal or flank pain (20% to 50%), abdominal mass (20% to 45%), weight loss (25% to 35%), fever (10% to 20%), and varicocele (2% to 10%). Hypertension, which may be mediated through the renin-angiotensin system, is present in 15% to 40% of cases. The classic triad of hematuria, abdominal pain, and abdominal mass occurs in less than 10% of cases at initial presentation.

Laboratory manifestations include anemia in 20% to 40% of cases. Rarely (3% to 4%), erythrocytosis, presumably as a result of excessive erythropoietin production, occurs. Hypercalcemia, as a result of bone metastasis or humoral mechanisms, is present in 3% to 6% of cases. Abnormal liver function test results, such as elevation of serum alkaline phosphatase activity, occur in 10% to 40% of patients and may be observed in the absence of hepatic metastases.

DIAGNOSIS

Depending on their availability, a variety of diagnostic procedures may be used to make a presumptive diagnosis and to determine the extent of renal cell carcinoma. Intravenous urography, particularly if combined with nephrotomography, is approximately 95% accurate in differentiating renal cancer from benign processes. Renal ultrasonography is a noninvasive procedure that is approximately 95% accurate and is sensitive in diagnosis if tumors are greater than 3 cm in diameter. Ultrasonography may demonstrate a simple cyst; renal cancer occurring in a simple cyst is rare. If ultrasonography demonstrates a complex cyst, percutaneous cyst puncture can be performed, and cyst fluid can be analyzed for malignant cells, erythrocytes, and fat content, which may suggest the diagnosis of renal cancer. In addition, the cyst wall may be further evaluated after injection of air or radiographic contrast medium. Renal arteriography, particularly if performed with epinephrine infusion, which constricts normal arteries but not tumor vessels, is quite accurate in differentiating benign from malignant renal masses but carries certain risks such as bleeding from the arterial puncture site. Computed tomography with radiographic contrast medium enhancement is currently the most widely available, sensitive, and accurate nonoperative method available for making a presumptive diagnosis of renal cancer and its extent and is the procedure of choice for preoperative staging. If present, involvement of the renal vein, inferior vena cava, regional lymph nodes, and liver by tumor can usually be demonstrated. Nuclear magnetic resonance imaging may be somewhat better than computed tomography in detecting tumor in regional lymph nodes and extension into the renal veins and inferior vena cava. In addition, it is useful in selected patients who have a contraindication to the administration of radiographic contrast medium or if the computed tomography findings are equivocal. Angiography has been largely replaced by computed tomography for diagnosis and staging of renal carcinoma and is used only infrequently nowadays to define the vascular anatomy in planning renal-sparing surgery.

TREATMENT

The prognosis for patients presenting with widespread disease or without metastases but not undergoing operative intervention is dismal, with less than 5% surviving 5 years. For patients without distant metastases the treatment of choice is radical nephrectomy, which includes resection of the regional lymph nodes, ipsilateral adrenal gland, and perinephric fat, and is associated with a higher long-term survival rate than is simple nephrectomy. For patients with bilateral renal cell carcinoma but without tumor elsewhere (approximately 3% of cases), partial bilateral nephrectomies are generally performed. Postoperative survival depends on the stage of the disease. Five-year survival rates range from 50% to 80% for persons with stage I disease (tumor confined to the kidney) to 25% to 50% for those with stage III disease (tumor locally invasive but without distant metastases). The average survival of patients with metastases at the time of nephrectomy is only 6 to 9 months. There appears to be little benefit from postoperative adjuvant radiation, hormonal therapy, or chemotherapy.

Treatment of patients with metastatic renal cell carcinoma is generally unrewarding. A variety of hormonal and chemotherapeutic agents have been evaluated with little success. Recent studies with biologic response modifiers including interleukin-2 combined with lymphokine-activated killer cells or beta interferon have resulted in complete remissions in 6% to 17% and partial remissions in 9% to 61% of patients. These results and ones with other agents such as coumarin and cimetidine suggest that approaches of this type may lead to more successful therapy of metastatic disease. Patients with metastases confined to the lungs have a more favorable prognosis than those with metastases elsewhere. Solitary metastases may be associated with prolonged survival after irradiation or, in exceptional cases, surgical resection. Very rarely, metastatic renal cell carcinoma may undergo regression either spontaneously or after nephrectomy.

TUMORS OF THE UPPER URINARY TRACT

Malignant tumors of the renal pelvis and ureter, usually transitional and less commonly squamous cell carcinomas, account for less than 5% of all adult renal tumors. Malignancies in these locations are much less frequent than those in the urinary bladder. Upper tract tumors are twice as common in men as in women. Predisposing factors include exposure to chemicals such as benzidine and beta naphthylamine, cigarette smoke, chronic analgesic consumption, and Balkan nephropathy.

The most common presenting symptom is painless hematuria, which occurs in 75% of cases. Less frequently, renal colic and urinary urgency and frequency are present. Intravenous urography is generally the first diagnostic procedure performed for the evaluation of hematuria, and its result is almost always abnormal in patients with upper tract tumors. Findings include hydronephrosis, filling defects, decreased or absent excretion of contrast medium by the affected kidney, or a combination of these. Cystoscopy and retrograde pyelograms or ureterorenoscopy is usually performed after intravenous urography. In addition to radiographic or direct visualization of the affected upper urinary tract with these procedures, the bladder and contralateral kidney and ureter can be examined for the presence of simultaneously occurring tumors, and urine and biopsy specimens or brushings can be obtained for cytologic examination. Computed tomography may help to differentiate a radiolucent calculus from a tumor and is useful in determining the extent of tumor. Cytologic examination of voided urine is a useful noninvasive screening procedure that may be employed at any time in the evaluation of patients suspected of having upper tract tumors but is not sufficiently sensitive by itself to exclude the diagnosis.

Treatment of malignant tumors of the renal pelvis and bladder usually consists of radical nephroureterectomy, but local resection of tumor may be appropriate in selected patients, such as those with reduced contralateral renal function. Irradiation and chemotherapy currently appear not to be useful. Close follow-up observation including urinary cytologic evaluation and visualization of the upper tract of the remaining kidney and bladder is mandatory because these tumors are frequently multicentric.

OTHER RENAL TUMORS

Renal *adenomas* are small (less than 2 to 3 cm in diameter) benign tumors that are usually asymptomatic and are discovered incidentally at autopsy or during radiographic examination of the kidneys. Histologically, renal adenomas are quite similar to well-differentiated renal cell carcinoma. Because it may be difficult to exclude renal cell carcinoma, patients with presumed renal adenomas should be followed closely if surgical resection is not performed.

Renal *oncocytoma* is a benign tumor thought to arise from proximal tubular epithelium. In a minority of patients tumors are bilateral. Oncocytoma and renal cell carcinoma can be readily distinguished by histologic examination. However, because these tumors cannot be differentiated by noninvasive means, the diagnosis is usually made at the time of surgery for presumed renal cancer.

Angiomyolipoma of the kidney is a benign tumor (hamartoma) composed of a mixture of blood vessels, smooth muscle, and fatty tissue. The tumor is associated with tuberous sclerosis in 20% to 50% of cases. Angiomyolipomas are generally unilateral and occur more frequently in women except in association with tuberous sclerosis, when they are usually bilateral and present equally in both sexes. Characteristically, angiomyolipomas are asymptomatic and are discovered incidentally. However, they may occur as an abdominal mass or with flank pain and hematuria and, rarely, with massive retroperitoneal bleeding. It is often possible to make a presumptive diagnosis of angiomyolipoma by ultrasonography and computed tomography. However, in some patients surgery may be required to exclude renal cancer.

Sarcomas of the kidney account for 1% to 3% of all malignant renal tumors. A variety of cell types may be seen, including leiomyosarcoma, fibrosarcoma, histiocytoma, rhabdomyosarcoma, angiosarcoma, liposarcoma, chondrosarcoma, and osteogenic sarcoma. The most frequent associated findings are abdominal pain, flank mass, and hematuria. In most patients the disease is metastatic at the time of diagnosis, and the overall prognosis is poor, and most individuals die within 1 year of diagnosis. For patients without metastatic disease, radical nephrectomy is the treatment of choice. A minority of patients respond to currently employed chemotherapeutic regimens. *Wilms' tumor* is the most frequent malignant renal tumor in childhood but is exceedingly rare in adults.

REFERENCES

Buzaid AC and Todd MB: Therapeutic options in renal cell carcinoma. Semin Oncol 16(suppl 1):12, 1989.

Guiliani L et al: Radical extensive surgery for renal cell carcinoma: long-term results and prognostic factors. J Urol 143:468, 1990.

Hartman DS, Aronson S, and Frazer H: Current status of imaging indeterminate renal masses. Radiol Clin North Am 29:475, 1991.

Krigel RL et al: Renal cell carcinoma: treatment with recombinant interleukin-2 plus beta-interferon. J Clin Oncol 8:460, 1990.

Lazzaro B, Gonick P, and Katz SM: Renal cell carcinoma vs. renal oncocytoma: report of a case with overlap features and review of the literature. Urology 37:52, 1991.

Leder RA and Dunnick NR: Transitional cell carcinoma of the pelvicalices and ureter. Am J Roentgenol 155:713, 1990.

Malek RS et al: Renal cell carcinoma in von Hippel-Lindau syndrome. Am J Med 82:236, 1987.

Matson MA and Cohen EP: Acquired cystic kidney disease: occurrence, prevalence, and renal cancers. Medicine 69:217, 1990.

McClennan BL: Oncologic imaging: staging and follow-up of renal and adrenal carcinoma. Cancer 67:1199, 1991.

National Wilms' Tumor Study Committee: Wilms' tumor status report. J Clin Oncol 9:899, 1991.

Parkinson DR et al: Therapy of renal cell carcinoma with interleukin-2 and lymphokine-activated killer cells: phase II experience with a hybrid bolus and continuous infusion interleukin-2 regimen. J Clin Oncol 8:1630, 1990.

Stenzl A and deKernion JB: Pathology, biology and clinical staging of renal cell carcinoma. Semin Oncol 16(suppl 1):3, 1989.

Swanson DA: Systemic treatment for renal cell carcinoma: an overview. Prog Clin Biol Res 350:201, 1990.

Part Ten

Special Topics in Internal Medicine

CHAPTER

365 Occupational and Environmental Health

Leonard J. Gorkun
Waldemar G. Johanson

In 1990, the direct and indirect costs of occupational illness, injuries, and deaths approached $40 billion. The major function of occupational medicine is prevention of illness and injury from stressors in the workplace. This idea was fully appreciated in the eighteenth century by Ramazzini, who introduced the two basic concepts necessary to evaluate the impact of occupation on an individual in his book, *The Diseases of Workers*. First, he taught that physicians should inquire the nature of the patient's trade or occupation; second, it is necessary for the physician to visit the shops, mines, and factories to understand the effects of occupation on the patient. The early development of the field of occupational medicine was a response to the employer's real need to address injury and lost time of employees. Physicians, usually surgeons, were enlisted by employers to reduce effects of injury and consequent disability and lost time. World War II left a diminished male pool of civilians, most of whom had been rejected from military service on the basis of disabilities. To employ this limited group to their physically safe maximum, physicians provided routine pre-employment, periodic, and transfer examinations to determine fitness for assigned tasks. Since the 1950s there has been an abundant, healthy work force and the focus has shifted from sorting out the least disabled to protecting the investment in recruitment and technical training by use of programs to reduce risk by first identifying and controlling work exposure and then modifying lifestyle choices. To date about 1600 physicians have been certified in occupational medicine by the American Board of Preventive Medicine. This is a very small segment of the approximately 500,000 physicians in the United States, which cannot begin to serve all the needs of employees and businesses.

In its report, *The Role of the Primary Care Physician in Occupational and Environmental Medicine,* the Institute of Medicine recognized that most occupationally related problems are seen initially by primary care physicians. Enhanced training in the recognition, treatment, and prevention of occupationally related diseases was recommended as part of training in primary care disciplines. The challenge for the primary care physician is to include consideration of the possible occupational contribution to the medical condition of patients and then use the resultant diagnosis to protect other employees, if possible, from similar consequences.

Disease related to environmental exposures is rarely specific to a particular exposure. Notable exceptions in which a condition is extremely rare in the absence of a specific exposure, or the frequency of a condition is markedly increased in association with a certain exposure have occurred. Mesothelioma is a rare malignant tumor; however, in 80% to 90% of cases occupational exposure to asbestos, especially of the amosite or crocidolite type, is reported. Angiosarcoma of the liver also is a rare tumor. The occurrence of this tumor in two workers at a vinyl chloride plant led to epidemiologic studies that confirmed a relationship between exposure to this agent and the tumor. However, associations such as these are uncommon. The usual circumstance is for patients to seek medical care for a condition that appears to be similar in all respects to illness in unexposed people. The individual physician usually does not have information about other workers with similar exposure so an increased incidence, if present, may not be obvious. In fact, credible evidence of an association between the workplace and a specific disease may require well designed epidemiologic studies.

Three criteria are often used when evaluating a possible association between exposure and the occurrence of a disease: (1) has exposure occurred? (2) is there an effect (adverse health outcome)? and (3) is there a plausible mechanism whereby the effect might be produced by the exposure? The latter has been a stumbling block in the evaluation of several putative exposures. For example, epidemiologic studies have suggested that exposure to electromagnetic fields is associated with adverse health effects although the biologic mechanisms of action remain unknown. A fourth criterion may be added by some: (4) are other factors present that are known to contribute to the effect? The presence of such factors (e.g., smoking in the development of lung cancer) makes the determination of the role of other factors more complicated.

In 1990 there were 6.3 million occupational injuries in the United States; 46% were musculoskeletal, 31.6% lacerations, and 15.8% eye injuries. It was estimated that there were 390,000 disabling occupational illnesses. In addition, NIOSH estimates that there are about 100,000 deaths a year caused by occupational hazards. This is over twice the number of highway deaths in the United States each year. Most workplace fatalities result from motor vehicle accidents, falls, trauma, or electric shocks, which occur in mining, construction, and agriculture.

ORGAN SYSTEM SPECIFICS

Musculoskeletal

Back sprains and strains are among the most common work-related problems. They often result from repetitive handling of heavy objects and materials, and thus people in diverse occupations including truck drivers and nurses are affected. Herniated lumbar disk is a less common condition and is more common in sedentary occupations.

Diagnosis and treatment of back conditions, although extremely important, are the same whether work-related or not. It should be noted, however, that the Worker's Compensation system may affect the patient's history and proper diagnosis, because this system usually requires that a problem be precipitated by a specific event or injury. Although back strains and sprains develop slowly from repeated activity, as opposed to herniated disk or fracture, the worker may focus on a single event to work with the system. History therefore must be diligently explored.

Return to work is sometimes a difficult medical decision for the employee with a resolving back problem. The following general guidelines may be of help:

Very light or sedentary work usually requires infrequent lifting of objects no more than 10 pounds maximum, such as office files and light work objects. Even individuals with 20% permanent partial disability should be able to manage this.

Light work may involve lifting loads up to 20 pounds infrequently and up to 10 pounds more often. Individuals with 10% to 15% permanent partial disability should be able to perform this work.

Medium work should entail lifting up to 50 pounds at a time but up to 25 pounds more often. A person who has 5% permanent partial disability impairment may be able to fulfill this requirement.

Heavy work requires lifting up to 100 pounds at a time and up to 50 pounds more frequently.

Very heavy work requires lifting over 100 pounds and frequent lifting of 50 pounds or more.

NIOSH has produced more detailed guidelines that may be helpful in work assignment taking into account specific employee capabilities. It should be noted that the Americans with Disabilities Act (ADA) requires more specific evaluation of the capability and not the disability of employees and applicants.

Cumulative trauma disorder (CTD), also called repetitive stress injury (RSI), is defined as a disorder of the musculotendinous-osseous-nervous systems that is caused, aggravated, or precipitated by repeated exertions or movements of the body or one of its parts. This category includes carpal tunnel syndrome, various forms of tendinitis, and a variety of less well-defined syndromes. Patients typically experience numbness, tingling, coldness or burning, or chronic pain in the involved part. It is not uncommon for symptoms to persist long after cessation of the activity. CTD occurs in very diverse jobs, such as assembly line work, computer operation, supermarket checkout operation, and even sign language interpretation. It is estimated that CTD now affects 185,000 workers, accounting for nearly one half of all occupational illnesses. It is ironic that devices of workplace automation themselves become the agents of personal injury. Although the causes of CTD remain somewhat controversial, the major precipitating factors are repetition, deviation of joints, force, and absence of rest periods. Systemic illnesses, including rheumatologic conditions, diabetes, and hypothyroidism, may contribute to these problems. Treatment consists of rest, physiotherapy, and perhaps use of nonsteroidal anti-inflammatory drugs. Surgery can be highly effective if an underlying structural problem exists, as is often the case in carpal tunnel syndrome, where release of the carpal ligament may give relief. However, if the ergonomic causes are not addressed, treatment does not produce lasting remission. Prevention of CTD requires redesign of the worksite, including hand tool and keyboard design, so that joints are maintained in a neutral position, as well as inclusion of more frequent rest breaks during repetitive activities. Because CTD now costs employers more than $7 billion in health costs and lost time, it is a problem that demands greater attention.

Hand-arm vibration syndrome may occur in employees who use tools that produce vibrations. It is often called white finger or dead finger for the obvious changes observed. Arterial spasm leads to blanching, loss of sensation, tingling, and clumsiness. Once present, the condition is exacerbated by exposure to cold.

Eye disorders

Eye and visual problems related to occupation usually result from direct exposure to harmful agents and trauma. A more controversial area is the relationship to intense use of video display terminals (VDTs). The visual symptoms in VDT users are now thought to result from improper lighting, ergonomics, and lack of proper corrective lenses when needed, and not to radiation effects.

A good vision conservation program with proper eye protection should almost eliminate that element but may require the use of safety glasses, side shields, goggles, or full face protectors. Treatment for most eye splashes is copious and prolonged lavage. Sterile normal saline solution is preferred, especially in the more severely irritated eye. Persistent irritation, ocular pain, or loss of vision dictates immediate referral. One special radiation effect is that seen in people who view arc welding without filtering protection. Conjunctivitis develops 6 to 24 hours later as a feeling of sand in the eye and may interfere with sleep. It usually resolves within 48 hours.

Cardiovascular disease

Hypertension, smoking, lipid abnormalities, and genetic factors are risk factors underlying 1.5 million myocardial infarctions in the United States each year. These causes are not occupational but point to the economic feasibility of a program for prevention in the workplace. Blood pressure screening and treatment, cholesterol and high-density lipoprotein (HDL) screening, nutritional counseling, smoking cessation, and physical fitness programs can be effectively delivered at the worksite.

In addition to designing and supervising prevention programs, two additional areas should concern the physician in regard to cardiovascular disease and the workplace. One is to match the symptomatic employee with an appropriate level of work and to determine ability to return to work after an event such as myocardial infarction or bypass surgery.

Determining an employee's ability to continue in a job when cardiovascular abnormalities occur or determining his/her ability to return to work after a cardiovascular event requires an evaluation of the physical capacity of the individual and an assessment of the essential aspects of the job. If these are mismatched, another job within or outside the company must be found or disability and/or retirement ensues. Even if the person and the job match in terms of the demands of job and employee ability, employees frequently do not continue or return to the job. Fear, stress, depression, or anxiety may play a role that overrides the reality of the physical capability to do the job. Age is one determinant of this outcome; in one study, 11% of employees below age 55 retired after bypass surgery, compared to 25% of employees above age 55.

Another concern is specific workplace exposure. Carbon monoxide exposure has been associated with an increase in symptoms in workers with cardiovascular disease, presumably caused by lessened oxygen delivery to the myocardium. Garage workers, toll booth collectors, and truckers are some of the workers who may be exposed to high concentrations of carbon monoxide. Nitrates are used to treat cardiovascular disease, but daily exposure in the workplace in the pharmaceutical and especially the explosives industry places workers at risk of angina, myocardial infarction, and even death. Symptoms often occur on Monday morning; they are thought to be due to re-exposure after a period of abstinence. Other agents that have adverse cardiovascular effects are antimony, arsenic, carbon disulfide, cobalt, fluorocarbons, methylene chloride, and heavy metals, especially lead and cadmium.

Hearing

Tone or pitch is measured in hertz (Hz) or cycles per second; intensity of sound is measured in decibels (dB). Instruments used to record the intensity of sound for medical purposes have internal circuitry that allows the measurement to be modified to reflect sounds as heard by the human ear, called the A weighted scale. Results are recorded as "dB(A)." Because the harmonics, overtones, and other variables of human speech are difficult to reproduce consistently, audiograms are conducted with pure tones at frequencies from 500 to 6000 or 8000 Hz although the human ear can hear a range from at least 20 Hz to 20,000 Hz. Results of audiograms are expressed as the number of decibels sound must be increased at a given frequency to be heard by the subject; 0 to 25 dB is usually considered within the range of normal. Up to 40 dB loss may occur before a person realizes he or she has hearing loss. Very low and very high frequencies may be useful to appreciate music, but the range to appreciate speech is 500 through 2000 Hz.

Occupational hearing loss is of two major types. Loss

Factors that impede recognition of hearing loss

Hearing loss develops slowly.
There is no outward visible sign.
Denial by hearing deficient people is common.
Hearing loss is attributed to aging.
Audiograms are not done until loss is severe.

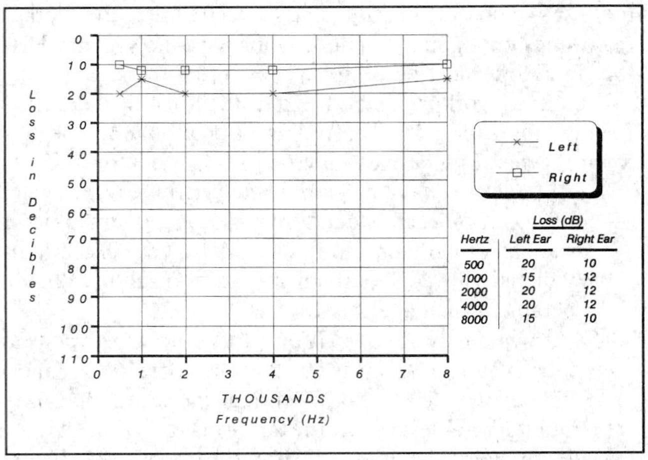

Fig. 365-1. Audiogram of a normal individual.

produced by a single, very loud noise such as in an explosion often affects the ears unequally; the Occupational Safety and Health Administration (OSHA) classifies this type of loss as an injury. The second type is the more common; it results from repeated exposure to loud but not violent noise over long periods, usually years. When exposure occurs only during part of the 24 hour day cycle, as at work, there is often partial or complete recovery before the next exposure. Audiograms can show a temporary decrease in hearing—a temporary threshold shift (TTS)—after exposure to a loud environment. This may not reflect a permanent threshold shift (PTS). Audiograms should be done only after at least 14 hours away from loud noise, including music and other nonworkplace sources. Hearing loss associated with a PTS is referred to by OSHA as an illness and not an injury for reporting purposes.

Hearing loss is often not easily identified for several reasons (see the box below).

No employee should lose hearing if an effective hearing conservation program is established. Such programs begin with a noise survey of the workplace. A walk-through quickly identifies areas that need to be measured. If you

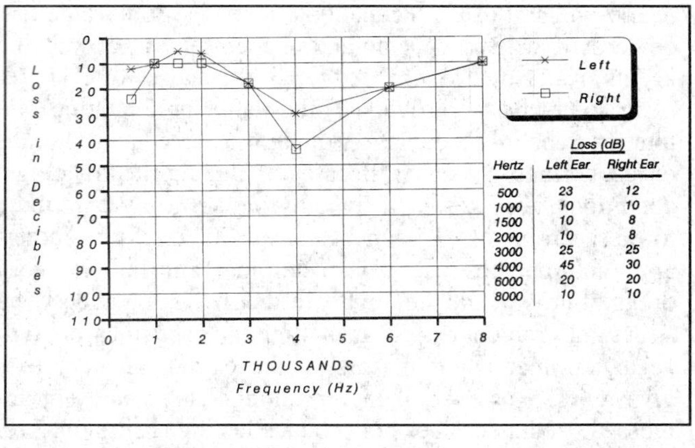

Fig. 365-2. Audiogram demonstrating mild hearing loss at 4000 Hz, characteristic of early noise-induced loss.

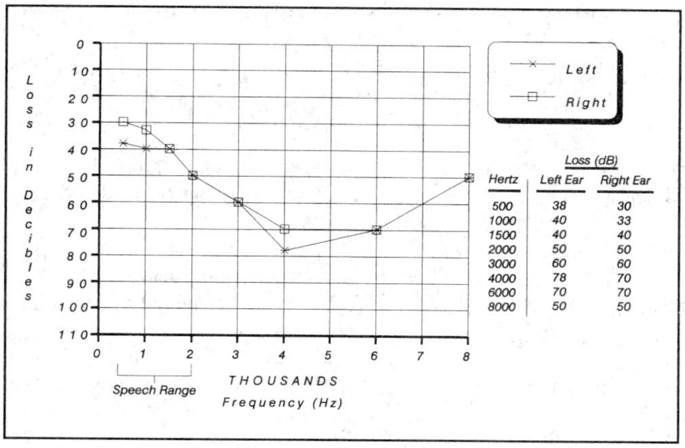

Fig. 365-3. Audiogram showing hearing loss over a wide range of frequencies, characteristic of late noise-induced loss.

must shout to be heard at a 3 foot distance from someone, the noise level is too high to work safely without hearing protection. Employees who must work in an area with a high noise level should have individual exposure monitored by personal dosimetry. A hearing conservation program is required by OSHA standards when ambient noise levels equal or exceed 85 dB(A). Some individuals may suffer hearing loss with steady exposure to no more than 80 dB(A). The amount of time that can be spent in noisy areas and the hearing protection required change as the intensity of noise increases.

Hearing loss associated with normal aging (presbycusis) affects hearing in the 6000 to 8000 Hz range first and then moves to lower frequencies. The loss from noise exposure typically affects hearing at 4000 Hz first and then over the years gradually spreads; eventually it affects the speech range (500 to 2000 Hz) severely enough that the employee notices hearing loss. Fig. 365-1 to 365-3 illustrate these changes. It should be noted that discrimination is the ability to separate sounds in the environment such as speech and background noise. Pure tone audiograms do not determine this, and thus hearing loss may have a much greater social impact than suggested by the audiogram. It is very important to do a baseline audiogram before an employee is assigned to work in a noise monitored area. Because of the many sources of noise, such as previous work assignments, loud music, or other exposure, hearing loss may be present even in young employees before working in a noise monitored area.

Neurologic

The clinical manifestations of neurotoxicity produced by occupational exposure are similar to those that result from other causes. The occupational cause can only be elucidated by a carefully taken occupational history and an inquisitive, perhaps suspicious, attitude. Because hundreds of new materials are introduced yearly into the work environment it is important to catalog all neurotoxic materials and their effects. The problem is that no more than 25% of these materials have been the subject of toxicity studies. Furthermore, the studies that are available usually relate only to acute exposures and in species other than humans. Hence the hypothesized human effects are, at best, extrapolations or educated guesses. Some clinical syndromes have been firmly linked to chemical exposures (Table 365-1).

Table 365-1. Recognized neurologic syndromes associated with chemical exposure

Agent	Area affected	Clinical syndrome
Carbon monoxide, carbon disulfide, manganese	Substantia nigra	Parkinson's syndrome
Toluene, mercury, acrylamide	Cerebellum	Cerebellar degeneration
Triorthocresylphosphate	Posterior column of spinal cord	Similar to neurosyphilis
Leptophos, diethylaminopropriononitrile	Demyelinization of several areas	Spasticity, impotence, urinary retention

Many other agents with adverse effects on the nervous system have been clearly identified: lead, solvents, arsenic, manganese, organophosphates, and insecticides.

Psychiatric

Stress often results from a combination of many demands and little actual or perceived control. There have been various models and testing scales, but life events at and away from work have major impacts. Stress results from changes in the balance between external demands and internal coping abilities. When demands are high but coping skills are high, the results may be viewed as incentive, drive, and motivation. When coping skills are low, even low demands result in overload of the coping skills and mechanisms. The result is stress, which in some individuals is a powerful motivating force that produces a drive to succeed.

Regardless of the actual outcome, perceived heavy demands can be difficult. The appropriate approach is to provide assistance to all employees, on a preventive basis, to improve coping skills. All should be encouraged to participate in the program and use the improved skills whenever they can.

Respiratory

Acute respiratory injury. Many respiratory diseases are caused by exposure to environmental agents, either in the workplace or elsewhere (Table 365-2). Exposure to water-soluble toxic gases such as sulfuric acid, ammonia, or hydrochloric acid causes primary injury in the upper respiratory tract because the gas is scrubbed from the inspired air by mucosal water. This produces inflammation, edema, and even necrosis in the nose, pharynx, larynx, and upper airways. Stridor indicates edema of the larynx and impending severe airway obstruction. Cough and wheezing are due to

Table 365-2. Representative respiratory responses

Site/disorder	Symptoms	Disease	Responsible agents
Acute respiratory injury	Sore throat, hoarseness, stridor, wheezing, cough, dyspnea	Acute nasopharyngitis, laryngitis, bronchitis, pulmonary edema	Sulfuric acid, ammonium, hydrochloric acid, nitrogen dioxide, phosgene
Chronic airway obstruction	Progressive dyspnea, cough, sputum	Chronic bronchitis	Dusts, chlorine, diesel exhaust
		Byssinosis	Cotton dust, flax, hemp
Intermittent airway obstruction	Cough, dyspnea, wheezing	Asthma	TDI, platinum, animal dander, organic dusts
		RADS	Toxic gases
Chronic parenchymal disease	Progressive dyspnea, nonproductive cough	Hypersensitivity pneumonitis	Thermophilic actinomycetes, fungi, bird proteins
		Silicosis	Silica
		Asbestosis	Asbestos

RADS, reactive airway dysfunction syndrome; TDI, toluene diisocyanate.

inflammation of the lower airways, possibly associated with bronchospasm. Chest radiograph findings are usually normal. Diffuse infiltrates, if present, are due to pulmonary edema caused by exposure to a high concentration of soluble gases that exceeds the scrubbing capacity of the upper airways and always indicates a serious injury. Exposure to these soluble agents is always known by the patient because of their irritant properties. Eye irritation, manifested by conjunctival redness, edema, and lid swelling, is usually present, as are redness and itching of exposed skin. Treatment, including irrigation of exposed surfaces, is generally supportive.

Inhalation of water-insoluble gases, such as nitrogen dioxide or phosgene, presents quite a different picture. These gases are often odorless, colorless, and nonirritating to the upper tract. They are not removed in the upper tract and reach the distal airways and alveoli in high concentration. Lung injury is typically delayed for hours and presents as pulmonary edema. Thus the patient may have left the site before the onset of symptoms and examination shortly after exposure may fail to reveal severe, even fatal injury.

Chronic airway disease. Chronic airway obstruction may result from workplace exposures. The best known of these is byssinosis, or "brown lung disease," which occurs in people who work with unprocessed cotton, flax, or hemp. Airborne dusts generated during processing produce both acute and chronic airway responses. Acute symptoms of cough, shortness of breath, and tightness in the chest are often most pronounced after a period away from the mill, hence the name "Monday morning asthma." Pulmonary function declines during the work shift and is lower at the end of the week than at the beginning in susceptible workers. Pulmonary function may be irreversibly lost through continuing exposure. The abnormalities are those of chronic obstructive pulmonary disease (COPD) and are difficult to interpret in individuals who concurrently smoke cigarettes. Once fixed decrements in forced expiratory volume ($FEV_{1.0}$) have developed, avoidance of further exposure does not result in a return to normal.

The mechanism of airway injury is inflammation, apparently caused at least in part by bacterial endotoxin contained in the raw cotton. Prevention requires rigorous dust control and screening of workers so that exposure of individuals with early disease can be reduced before disabling damage occurs.

Chronic airway disease has been reported in survivors of a single acute exposure to corrosive gases. These changes have generally been consistent with chronic airway disease, especially bronchiectasis and bronchiolitis obliterans. Both may produce substantial respiratory impairment and disability. In some patients, persistent wheezing, cough, and dyspnea associated with highly reactive airways appear to have followed a single acute injury. This condition has been termed reactive airway dysfunction syndrome (RADS). Although it is usually impossible to know with certainty that the individual did not have underlying airway disease, this does not appear to be the case for most. The mechanisms leading to these persistent changes are unknown, but chronic bronchial epithelial injury and inflammation have been documented. Management includes prevention of further exposure to inciting agents, including cigarette smoke, and stepped asthmatic care.

Occupational asthma. Many natural substances and synthetic compounds may cause asthma in exposed workers. Workers may become sensitized through immunologic or nonimmunologic mechanisms. Atopic individuals are particularly prone to become sensitized when exposed to natural substances such as animal danders or grain dusts. Synthetic substances appear to sensitize atopic and nonatopic individuals equally well, although there is marked variation among compounds in sensitizing potential. For example, it has been estimated that in 100% of workers exposed to complex platinum salts, but only about 10% of workers exposed to toluene diisocyanate, asthma develops with long-term exposure. Thus there is an important interplay between individual and environmental factors in the development of occupational asthma.

Occupational asthma may be defined as asthma provoked

by exposures in the workplace and is otherwise similar to asthma produced in other settings. Therefore the history of exposure and the development of symptoms in proximity to that exposure are key to the diagnosis. However, asthmatic symptoms and airflow obstruction develop in several differing patterns after exposure, as shown by bronchoprovocation studies in which workers are intentionally exposed in a controlled fashion to substances to which they may be sensitized. One pattern is the acute reaction, in which the subject immediately experiences cough and chest tightness associated with a marked decrease in $FEV_{1.0}$. These reactions are mediated by immunoglobulin E (IgE) and reverse spontaneously or with bronchodilator therapy. Another pattern is the late reaction, in which symptoms develop hours after exposure, also associated with decrements in lung function. These reactions are apparently mediated by more complex factors, including the interplay of various cytokines and other mediators in the airways. Delayed reactions are more protracted, lasting many hours, and are thought to perpetuate a chronic asthmatic state. A third type of reaction is the combination of the early and late responses.

In all patients with asthma, it is important to inquire carefully about possible exposures at work and the timing of symptoms in relation to such exposures. Most patients who have occupational asthma experience significant improvement when removed from exposure. Improvement typically occurs over weekends or holidays, although the lack of improvement in this time frame does not rule out an important occupational component underlying a patient's symptoms.

Pulmonary function tests demonstrate airway obstruction; improvement follows administration of a bronchodilator. In some cases it is desirable to confirm the diagnosis of occupational asthma by demonstrating a significant fall in lung function during the course of a typical work shift. This can be accomplished by simple spirometry or measurement of peak flow performed before going to work, at the end of the shift, and 4 to 6 hours later. Test sensitivity may be increased by taking the measurements after several days away from the workplace. Bronchoprovocation tests performed with known concentrations of specific agents present in the workplace require specialized facilities. Bronchoprovocation tests with a nonspecific agent such as methacholine or histamine have been used to identify the degree of airway reactivity in a given individual. As many as 30% of normal, nonasthmatic young people experience a greater than 20% decrement in $FEV_{1.0}$ after exposure to high concentrations of methacholine; therefore airway responsiveness to these agents should not be interpreted as indicating the presence of asthma. Individuals who demonstrate bronchial reactivity in this way may be at greater risk of development of asthma when exposed to environmental agents, although this is not well established. Conversely, subjects with asthma of whatever cause demonstrate greater bronchial reactivity than nonasthmatics. For these reasons, bronchial provocation with these agents has an uncertain role in the evaluation of subjects suspected of having occupational asthma.

Treatment ideally consists of removal from exposure. In mild cases, preventive treatment with inhaled cromolyn sodium or inhaled corticosteroid may be tried. Avoidance of exposure through workplace controls is usually not effective because the level of exposure required to cause symptoms is low, usually below permissible levels. Treatment is otherwise similar to that of asthma that develops in other settings.

Diffuse pulmonary diseases. Deposition of particulates in the lung elicits widely varying tissue responses. Iron particles cause marked radiographic changes but no inflammatory or fibrotic changes. Pure carbon deposition causes small diffuse lesions indicated radiographically but little or no functional abnormality. Most carbon exposures are also associated with silica or other minerals, as in coal workers' pneumoconiosis, and the cause of the resultant abnormalities is less clear. Some authorities believe that the obstructive lung disease that affects coal miners is due to concurrent cigarette smoking, not to pneumoconiosis.

Fungi and other organic antigenic materials produce marked inflammatory changes in susceptible individuals. Thermophilic actinomycetes are fungi that grow at high temperatures, such as those produced in decomposing organic materials such as hay. Farmers may be occupationally exposed to enormous numbers of the spores of these organisms. Surveys have shown that as many as 70% of midwestern farmers have circulating antibody against thermophilic actinomycetes. Only a small proportion of these individuals have pulmonary abnormalities related to this exposure. The illness produced, called "farmer's lung," takes one of two forms. Some farmers manifest acute symptoms consisting of fever, myalgias, cough, and discomfort in the chest with onset 4 to 8 hours after exposure. These symptoms may be associated with the development of radiographic infiltrates that clear in a few days as symptoms abate if no further exposure occurs. Other individuals do not manifest acute symptoms but instead exhibit chronic and progressive symptoms of nonproductive cough and dyspnea on exertion. Radiographic abnormalities, consisting of diffuse infiltrates of varying intensity, are regularly present but lymphadenopathy and pleural fluid are rare. Abnormal physical findings are limited to the chest and include crackles over involved areas and often wheezing. The latter indicates airway narrowing, and the combination of a diffuse infiltrative process with wheezing on physical examination should suggest the diagnosis of hypersensitivity pneumonitis.

Hypersensitivity pneumonitis occurs in many settings, only some of which are occupational. Pathologically this process is intensely inflammatory and centered on distal bronchioles. Poorly defined granulomas are typical. The causative agent is not demonstrable in lung tissue. With chronic or recurring exposure, diffuse fibrosis with irreversible restrictive abnormalities may result. If pneumonitis is identified early, avoidance of exposure is sufficient therapy as the process is usually self-limiting and reversible. Corticosteroids may be used to hasten recovery but are not needed as a rule.

Crystalline silica causes a form of irreversible and progressive pulmonary fibrosis called silicosis. Exposure to massive concentrations of silica may cause a hyperacute form of silicosis that produces a protein-rich alveolar exudate resembling alveolar proteinosis histologically and pulmonary edema radiographically. This clinical syndrome may develop in as little as 1 year. Such exposures are usually caused by sandblasting in an unprotected environment. Chronic silicosis develops slowly 15 to 20 years after exposure and progresses in the absence of further exposure. The disease predominates in the upper lobes of the lungs for unclear reasons. Because of its effect on lung macrophages, silicosis markedly diminishes host resistance to tuberculosis. Workers with silicosis must be screened for tuberculosis infection by skin testing and, if the finding is positive for tuberculosis, offered preventive therapy.

Asbestosis is a chronic interstitial lung disease caused by deposition of asbestos fibers. It is related to the total dust burden of the lungs and develops 10 to 15 years after exposure. Affected individuals complain of progressive dyspnea on exertion and nonproductive cough. Crackles are present at the lung bases and digital clubbing often occurs. This process is irreversible and unaffected by treatment. Exposure to asbestos also produces pleural plaques, which are calcified areas of pleural thickening, usually over the diaphragm or lateral chest wall. Pleural plaques denote asbestos exposure but do not indicate future development of either asbestosis or mesothelioma.

Mesotheliomas are malignant tumors that arise from the pleura or peritoneum. Patients with mesothelioma have pain in the affected site and fluid accumulation. The fluid is exudative in character and may contain increased amounts of hyaluronic acid. The histologic identification of mesotheliomas is difficult on small biopsy specimens and open biopsies may be required in some cases.

Skin

Work-related skin disorders are common and usually indistinguishable from non-work-related processes of similar nature (Table 365-3). An accurate history of work exposures, preventive measures, and time course is essential to proper diagnosis.

Irritant contact dermatitis. Irritant contact dermatitides are eruptions that appear shortly after exposure to a strong irritating agent; involvement is limited to the areas of exposure. Acid burns tend to appear immediately, whereas burns produced by alkali tend to develop more slowly over several hours so that the initial evaluation may underestimate the extent of injury. Lesions may range from erythema of the skin to vesiculation to necrosis. Sensitive areas such as the finger webs or eyelids may be the only site of involvement. Occlusion, such as that under gloves, tends to promote injury. Healing occurs with varying degrees of scarring, depending on the depth of tissue injury.

Allergic contact dermatitis. Sensitization to a responsible agent and re-exposure cause a different problem. Poison ivy is a well-known example of this process. Metal salts, especially chromium, platinum, and nickel, and certain acrylic monomers may be responsible. Sensitivity to latex gloves or chemicals contained therein has been identified in many health care workers since the advent of universal precautions in the handling of patients and specimens. The diagnosis is based on the history of exposure and lesions at sites of contact. Typical lesions are erythematous scaling patches that may be more pronounced in sensitive areas. Acute responses may be vesicular, and those produced by contact with plants such as poison ivy or sumac are typically linear along the path of contact.

For all forms of contact dermatitis, avoidance of exposure is the best therapy. Wet soaks provide relief for vesicular and weeping eruptions; corticosteroid creams are used for less acute problems.

Contact urticaria. Hives are caused by exposure to agents that release histamine either immunologically through immunoglobulin E (IgE) or nonimmunologically by direct effects on mast cells. Common contacts include shellfish, drugs, and animals. Pruritic, raised plaques develop within moments at the site of contact and persist for several hours. Avoidance of the allergen is advisable as more severe allergic manifestations may result from continuing exposure.

Chloracne. Chloracne is an unusual condition caused by exposure to chlorinated hydrocarbons including dioxins and

Table 365-3. Common occupational skin disorders

Disease	Responsible agents	Mechanisms	Diagnosis
Irritant contact dermatitis	Solvents, acids, alkalis, others	Direct tissue injury	History, compatible eczema
Allergic contact dermatitis	*Rhus,* oleoresin, metals, acrylics	Delayed hypersensitivity	History, compatible eczema, patch tests
Contact urticaria	Animals, drugs	Immunologic (IgE) or nonimmunologic release of histamine	History, controlled exposure
Chloracne	Dioxin, (PCBs) Chlorinated hydrocarbons	Squamous metaplasia of sebaceous glands	History of exposure, appearance

PCBs, chlorobiphenyls; IgE, immunoglobulin E.

polychlorinated biphenyls (PCBs). The clinical presentation may be confused with that of acne vulgaris as the patient has comedones, papules, and cysts. The distribution of lesions in chloracne tends to be more extensive, often including the legs. Hepatic abnormalities or peripheral neuropathy may be present.

Infectious disease

Zoonoses have occurred in the workplace for centuries. In modern times, human immunodeficiency virus (HIV) and hepatitis B infection have replaced anthrax ("wool-sorters' disease"), brucellosis, and other classic illnesses as concerns in the workplace. Health care workers must now abide by OSHA rules issued to prevent exposure to bloodborne pathogens. Tuberculosis has once again become a significant threat to health care workers in some parts of the United States, especially in large cities, where acquired immunodeficiency syndrome (AIDS), drug abuse, and homelessness compound the difficulty of treatment for tuberculosis. The recent emergence of multiple drug resistant tuberculosis (MDRTB) has created real concern over the adequacy of isolation facilities in many hospitals. A number of hospital outbreaks have occurred in which other patients and hospital employees have become infected. In persons with AIDS who become infected with MDRTB pulmonary infiltrates develop within a few weeks and case fatality rates among these patients have been as high as 80%. Hospital workers who become infected with MDRTB present a particular problem because no regimen of prophylaxis is known to be effective against these organisms. Prevention of tuberculosis infection in hospitals and other health care facilities requires major engineering changes. The Center for Disease Control (CDC) has recommended guidelines for hospital facilities for tuberculosis patients that include at least six room exchanges per hour, negative pressure of patient rooms, and exhausting of all air to the outdoors. These measures will be difficult and expensive to achieve for most hospitals.

Ultraviolet lights are effective in reducing the number of viable tubercle bacilli in the air of enclosed places when adequate ventilation cannot be provided. Care must be taken to prevent continuing eye or skin exposure of either patients or employees. However, these lights may reduce the risk of infection when placed in high-risk exposure areas such as emergency rooms or aerosol therapy areas. Personal protective masks are of uncertain benefit, although snugly fitting respirator devices probably do reduce the risk of infection. OSHA currently approves only a dust, mist, and fume (DMF) respirator for this purpose. These devices are uncomfortable when worn for long periods, and compliance is a continuing problem. Prompt recognition of tuberculosis cases and institution of effective antituberculosis therapy are among the best ways to reduce nosocomial infections. AIDS patients may present a particular problem in this regard because of the rapidity with which pulmonary tuberculosis can advance in these patients and the protean manifestations of the infection.

REFERENCES

Demeter SL: The many facts of occupational asthma. Cleve Clin J Med 58(2):137, 1991.

Feuerstein M and Fitgerald T: Biomechanical factors affecting upper extremity cumulative trauma disorders in sign language interpreters. J Occup Med 34(3):257, 1992.

McCunney RJ: Handbook of occupational medicine. Boston/Toronto, 1988, Little Brown.

Merchant JA, editor: Occupational Respiratory Diseases, US DHHS (NIOSH) Publication No 86-102, 1986.

NIOSH Technical Report: Work practices for manual lifting, DHHS (NIOSH), Publication No 81-122, Washington, DC, Government Printing Office, March, 1981.

Pelmear PL and Taylor W: Hand arm vibration syndrome: clinical evaluation and prevention, J Occup Med 33(11):1144, 1991.

Ramazzini B: Demorbis diatriba (Disease of workers), 1713 Revised edition, Chicago, 1940, University of Chicago Press.

Role of the primary care physician in occupational and environmental medicine. Washington, DC, 1988, Institute of Medicine, National Academy Press.

Spengler DM: Back injuries in industry: a retrospective study. I. Overview and cost analysis. Spine 11:241, 1986.

CHAPTER

366 Clinical Toxicology

Richard L. Bauer
William A. Watson

ACUTE POISONING

Acute poisonings are a frequent cause of emergency department visits and intensive care unit hospitalizations of adolescents and adults. Drug abuse and ingestions with suicidal intent are the most common reasons for acute poisonings in adults and have a worse prognosis than accidental poisonings, which predominate in children.

The case fatality rate for poisoning has decreased substantially since 1960, primarily because of added emphasis on prevention, the advent of widespread access to Poison Control Centers, and more effective emergency and in-hospital management. In addition, substitution of benzodiazepines for the barbiturates has resulted in an apparent reduction in severe poisoning episodes and deaths. Physicians should encourage patients to store medicines and household chemicals out of the reach of children, to discard unused prescriptions, and to keep medicines in their original containers.

Emergency therapy

Airway patency, ventilation, and circulatory status should be assessed immediately in poisoning patients (see the box on p. 2790). The airway should be cleared of vomitus and foreign objects, and patients should be positioned on the

Outline of overdose treatment

Airway: Clear of obstruction.
Breathing: Intubate and ventilate as needed.
Circulation: 500 ml IV saline if BP < 90 systolic.
Physical examination: Review major organ systems.
Antidotes and specific therapy if applicable: see Table 366-2.
Decontamination: Rinse eyes, skin as needed. Ipecac syrup–induced emesis or gastric lavage. Activated charcoal and cathartic. Whole bowel irrigation for selected cases.
Consideration of glucose, thiamine, and naloxone for altered mental status.
Enhanced drug elimination in selected cases.
Monitoring of consciousness and vital signs until normal.
Psychiatric consultation before discharge.

side to decrease the risk of aspiration. Intubation with a cuffed endotracheal tube is frequently necessary to prevent aspiration pneumonia. Slow or shallow respirations or blood gas results indicating hypoventilation are indications for assisted ventilation. Symptomatic hypotension that is unresponsive to improved oxygenation and positioning of the patient in the Trendelenburg position should be treated with a fluid challenge of 500 ml normal saline solution given over 30 minutes. A vasopressor such as dopamine or norepinephrine may be required for persistent symptomatic hypotension. Several drugs, such as quinidine, the beta blockers, and the cyclic antidepressants, may cause direct cardiac depression and hypotension. Treatment of these patients should be individualized and may require information from invasive hemodynamic measurements such as the pulmonary artery wedge pressure.

Table 366-1. Complications of drug intoxication

Finding	Common causes*	Finding	Common causes*
Aspiration	Petroleum distillates/hydrocarbons Organophosphates CNS depressants (chloral hydrate) Antidepressants	Hyperthermia	Phenothiazines CNS stimulants Anticholinergics Salicylates Antidepressants
Behavioral disturbances	Anticholinergics Hallucinogens Psychotropic drugs Organic solvents CNS stimulants	Hypothermia	CNS depressants (barbiturates) Alcohols (ethanol) Opiates
Bradycardia	Cardiac glycosides (digoxin) Beta-adrenergic blockers (propranolol) Organophosphates Calcium channel blockers (nifedipine, verapamil)	Ileus	Narcotic analgesics Anticholinergics Antidepressants Meprobamate
		Metabolic acidosis	Salicylates Alcohols (methanol, ethylene glycol)
Cardiac dysrhythmias	CNS stimulants (cocaine) Cardiovascular drugs Antidepressants Theophylline Propoxyphene	Nystagmus	Anticonvulsants CNS depressants Phencyclidine
		Pulmonary edema	Organophosphates Salicylates CNS depressants (ethchlorvynol) Opiates Antidepressants
Coma, hyperreflexia, tachycardia, mydriasis	Antidepressants Anticholinergics/antihistamines Phenothiazines		
Coma, hypotension, flaccidity	CNS depressants (barbiturates, benzodiazepines) Ethanol Opiates	Restlessness, pyrexia, hyperreflexia	Anticholinergics Strychnine Phencyclidine Amphetamines
Hallucinations	Antihistamines/anticholinergics CNS stimulants Organic solvents Hallucinogens (PCP, LSD)	Seizures/hyperreflexia	CNS stimulants (cocaine) Organophosphates Phencyclidine Propoxyphene Antidepressants Theophylline Salicylates Hypoglycemic agents
Hepatic failure	Acetaminophen Carbon tetrachloride *Amanita* mushrooms Isoniazid		
Hyperpnea	CNS stimulants Carbon monoxide Salicylates Alcohols (methanol)	Tachycardia	CNS stimulants Antihistamines/anticholinergics Antidepressants Theophylline

*Substances in parentheses are common examples. CNS, central nervous system; PCP, phencyclidine hydrochloride; LSD, lysergic acid diethylamide.

Diagnosis

The diagnosis of poisoning should be considered in cases of altered consciousness (Chapter 111) or acute psychiatric symptoms. Less commonly, poisoning may be indicated by renal or hepatic failure, a variety of metabolic disorders, hypothermia or hyperthermia, pulmonary edema, or dysrhythmias. Some common physical and laboratory findings associated with specific poisons are listed in Table 366-1.

Efforts should be made to identify and quantitate the substance(s) ingested. Although patients may volunteer this information, the history is often inaccurate. Family and friends, paramedics, and police or fire rescue personnel may supplement the patient's account and should be asked to search for medicine vials or unswallowed tablets that could help identify the drug involved.

Laboratory tests. Quantitative and qualitative laboratory analyses can confirm that poisoning has occurred and help predict prognosis. Quantitative assays are commonly available for salicylates, acetaminophen, iron, lithium, phenobarbital, carbon monoxide, phenytoin, alcohols, and digoxin. Repeat assays obtained after several hours may be used to assess the results of gastric decontamination and initial treatment.

Qualitative tests such as thin-layer chromatography and immunoassays identify specific agents or drug classes but do not quantitate exposure. These tests are useful in confirming that a particular drug has been ingested and are of some value in screening for unknown drugs. Results should be correlated with the history and the clinical picture.

Additional laboratory tests may help identify complications. Arterial blood gases should be assessed in comatose, intubated, or hypotensive patients. Hypoxia and hypercapnia may indicate inadequate ventilation or pulmonary complications such as aspiration or pulmonary edema. Serum electrolyte and blood glucose concentrations should also be determined.

A chest radiograph should be obtained in intubated patients and in patients in whom aspiration or noncardiogenic pulmonary edema are suspected. If dysrhythmias are present or if the poison is known to be cardiotoxic (e.g., antidepressants and quinidine), the electrocardiograph (ECG) should be monitored.

Treatment

The major treatment goals are to decrease the intensity and duration of the poison exposure and to monitor, prevent, or treat potential complications. With the exception of a few specific antidotes and therapies (Table 366-2), treatment is generally limited to careful attention to the airway, breathing, circulation, decontamination, and potential complications (see the box on p. 2790). Frequent measurement of the vital signs is essential to identify those patients in need of intubation and assisted ventilation or circulatory support. Metabolic abnormalities, renal or hepatic failure, and cardiac depression may require invasive monitoring or frequent assessment of electrolytes and cardiopulmonary function.

The aggressiveness of therapy should be based on the clinical status of the patient, the likely complications of the poison, and the quantity of drug ingested. However, be-

Table 366-2. Specific antidotes

Antidote	Poison	Dosages
Naloxone	Opiates (heroin, meperidine, propoxyphene, pentazocine, diphenoxylate)	Loading dose: From 0.4 to 2.0 mg iv; repeat in 2-5 min as necessary Maintenance dose: sufficient to maintain desired level of consciousness
Atropine	Organophosphates	Loading dose: 2 mg iv or im every 2-5 min until hypersalivation is controlled Maintenance dose: sufficient to suppress hypersalivation
Pralidoxime	Organophosphates	Loading dose: 1-2 g iv Maintenance dose: 1-2 g after 2-3 hr
Ethanol	Methanol, ethylene glycol	Loading dose: 0.6-0.7 g/kg Maintenance dose: sufficient EtOH* to maintain serum alcohol level at 100 mg/dl (approximately 125 mg/kg/hr) until methanol, ethylene glycol concentration < 10 mg/dl
Amyl nitrite Sodium nitrite Sodium thiosulfate	Cyanide	Amyl nitrite ampuls inhaled every 2-3 min; monitor blood pressure; then 10 ml 3% sodium nitrite iv over 5 min; then 50 ml 25% sodium thiosulfate over 10 min
Deferoxamine	Iron salts	Hypotensive patients: 10 mg/kg/hr iv for 4 hr; then 5 mg/kg/hr iv for 8 hr, then 2-5 mg/kg/hr iv until serum iron level is less than 100 μ/dl Normotensive patients: 40 mg/kg im every 4-12 hr (total dose should not exceed 6 g/24 hr)
N-Acetylcysteine	Acetaminophen	140 mg/kg po then 70 mg/kg every 4 hr po for 17 doses
Oxygen	Carbon monoxide	100% by face mask or hyperbaric
Flumazenil	Benzodiazepines	Loading dose: 1-5 mg iv Maintenance dose: sufficient to maintain desired level of consciousness

*EtOH, ethylalcohol or ethanol.

cause of frequently inaccurate histories of drug exposure, the indications for therapy with oral charcoal or evacuation of the stomach should be liberal. Patients with a history of drug exposure should be observed for several hours to identify unexpected toxicity, and urine drug screens considered in patients with an atypical clinical course or questionable history of ingestion. Active removal of the drug by hemodialysis, hemoperfusion, or administration of multiple doses of activated charcoal may be considered in these patients, especially if renal or hepatic failure limits normal excretion.

Limiting absorption. Morbidity and mortality from poisoning can be decreased by emptying the stomach of ingested drugs or by binding unabsorbed drug with activated charcoal. These interventions decrease the peak serum concentration and total absorbed dose of drug. In adults who are awake, alert, and cooperative, activated charcoal treatment or ipecac-induced emesis is the usual option. Lavage, after controlling the airway to prevent aspiration, is the preferred therapy in patients who are comatose or uncooperative.

Activated charcoal adsorbs a variety of drugs and prevents their subsequent absorption (Table 366-3). Its effectiveness is increased when given shortly after poison ingestion. The appropriate dose of activated charcoal has not been determined; however, an initial dose of 50 to 100 g mixed with 250 to 500 ml of water to form a slurry appears to be effective and well tolerated. Two or three doses of activated charcoal given at 4 hour intervals may be more effective than a single dose. The activated charcoal–drug compound is eventually excreted in the stool, which may turn black as a result. Although the effectiveness of cathartics in treating overdoses has not been proved, sorbitol (1 to 2 g/kg body weight) or magnesium citrate is often given with the first dose of activated charcoal to facilitate elimination.

Gastric lavage is indicated in patients who are not awake, alert, or oriented. Before lavage in patients exhibiting coma or seizures the risk of aspiration should be minimized by intubation with a cuffed endotracheal tube. A large internal diameter orogastric tube should be used. After the contents of the stomach are aspirated, aliquots (50 to 250 ml) of room-temperature water should be administered and aspirated until no pill fragments or stomach contents are evident. A minimum of 5 L of water is generally required.

Emesis may be used as an alternative to administration of activated charcoal in patients who are awake, alert, and cooperative. It is the preferred therapy when the poison is poorly bound to charcoal. Ipecac syrup is the most appropriate, effective emetic. The recommended dose is 15 to 30 ml in adults and children above age 5, and 15 ml for children between 1 and 5 years old. Ipecac's primary mechanism of action is to stimulate the medullary vomiting center. Ninety percent of patients vomit within 30 minutes. A second dose can be given if vomiting has not occurred in this period; all but 1% of patients respond to two doses.

Protracted vomiting may occur with ipecac. If deterioration in mentation is expected, for example, with cyclic antidepressants, gastric lavage with activated charcoal is preferred. Therapeutic doses of ipecac syrup can produce drowsiness and diarrhea. Ipecac may also induce seizures and is cardiotoxic, although these complications occur almost exclusively in chronic ipecac overdoses.

Table 366-3. Adsorptive capacity of activated charcoal in vitro

Efficiently adsorbed	Poorly adsorbed
Amphetamines	Ferrous sulfate
Chlorpheniramine	Malathion
Diphenylhydantoin	Acids
Aspirin	Alkalis
Propoxyphene	Alcohol
Cyclic antidepressants	Lithium
Chlorpromazine	
Quinine	

Whole bowel irrigation should be considered if there is evidence of continued drug absorption from the gastrointestinal (GI) tract. This situation may occur when sustained release or enteric coated products have been taken, when a large number of tablets (e.g., 100) have been ingested, and when serial serum drug concentrations demonstrate increasing drug concentrations. Whole bowel irrigation is performed by using a balanced electrolyte solution (Golytely). From 500 to 2000 ml per hour is administered orally via a nasogastric tube until the rectal effluent is clear.

Increasing drug excretion. Severe intoxication, deterioration despite therapy, and prolonged coma are potential indications for more aggressive therapies, which include alkalinizing the urine, dialysis, hemoperfusion, and multiple dose activated charcoal (Table 366-4).

Alkaline diuresis. Many drugs are weak acids or bases that exist at least partly in the ionized form in body fluids. Because the renal tubular epithelium is relatively impermeable to charged particles, drugs in the ionized form are trapped in the tubular lumen and excreted in the urine.

The principal indications for alkaline diuresis are severe

Table 366-4. Alternative therapy in severe overdoses*

Alkaline diuresis	Dialysis	Multiple dose activated charcoal
Phenobarbital	Methanol	Theophylline
Salicylate	Isopropyl alcohol	Beta blockers
	Ethylene glycol	Phenytoin
	Lithium	
	Bromides	
	Salicylates	
	Ethanol	

*See text for full description.

phenobarbital and salicylate overdoses. Close monitoring of fluid status, electrolyte concentrations, and urine pH is essential with this treatment. A urinary catheter may be necessary to measure urine output and pH. Sufficient sodium bicarbonate (initially 1 to 2 mEq/kg/hr iv) should be given to maintain the urine pH between 7.5 and 8.5. If the patient is acidotic or is excreting large quantities of fixed acid (i.e., salicylates), a larger initial dose of bicarbonate may be necessary. Urine flow should be adequate, but forced diuresis is not required.

Dialysis and hemoperfusion. Excretion of a few poisons can be increased by hemodialysis or hemoperfusion. Dialysis is most effective with drugs of low molecular weight, a small volume of distribution, low protein binding, and low clearance rates. The clearance of methanol, ethylene glycol, salicylates, and lithium, for example, is increased by dialysis. Hemoperfusion is more effective than dialysis in removing drugs that have high molecular weights, are lipid soluble, and are highly protein bound. Drugs whose elimination rate is increased by hemoperfusion include short- and medium-acting barbiturates, theophylline, methaqualone, and glutethimide. A variety of complications may occur with hemoperfusion, including thrombocytopenia, leukopenia, and a loss of clotting factors.

Indications for dialysis and hemoperfusion include severe intoxication (e.g., coma with depressed respiration, hypotension, and hypothermia), deterioration while receiving adequate treatment, and toxicity associated with high serum concentrations of dialyzable poison.

Multiple dose activated charcoal enhances drug excretion of a limited number of substances with an active enterohepatic circulation. Active and inactive metabolities as well as unchanged drug passively diffuse into the intestinal lumen or are actively secreted in bile. Adsorption onto activated charcoal limits absorbtion of these compounds. Drugs with characteristics similar to those required for hemoperfusion, such as theophylline, are most likely to be effectively removed. The ability of multiple dose activated charcoal to improve the clinical outcome of other overdoses is questionable and has not lived up to earlier expectations.

Treatment of complications

Coma. In patients with a history of drug ingestion, coma should not be assumed to be secondary to drug toxicity. Structural brain lesions, trauma-related injury, and non-drug-associated metabolic encephalopathy need to be considered. Patients with depressed respiration or an absent gag reflex should be intubated.

The case fatality rate of drug overdose patients with a depressed respiratory drive is as high as 5% to 10%, whereas the case fatality rate is less than 1% in patients with lesser degrees of coma. Aspiration pneumonia, which may occur despite intubation, is the most common cause of death in comatose patients. Meticulous respiratory care and maintenance of fluid and electrolyte balance help prevent excess morbidity and mortality.

Cardiopulmonary complications. Hypotension in poisoning patients can be a result of decreased cardiac output, altered capillary permeability, decreased intravascular volume, or decreased vasomotor tone. Hypotension may respond to improved ventilation and oxygenation. If it is persistent, however, 500 ml of normal saline solution should be given intravenously over 30 minutes to treat possible volume depletion or peripheral vasodilatation. If the systolic blood pressure is still less than 90 mm Hg after initial treatment in a symptomatic patient, vasopressors such as dopamine or norepinephrine may be necessary. Hemodynamic monitoring may be required to differentiate volume depletion from heart failure.

Pulmonary edema may occur secondary to direct cardiac toxicity or altered capillary permeability (noncardiogenic pulmonary edema). Patients with noncardiogenic pulmonary edema have normal intracardiac pressures but have interstitial and intra-alveolar infiltrates. Opiates, sedative/hypnotics (especially ethchlorvynol), salicylates, and tricyclic antidepressants are most often implicated. Hypoxia should be treated initially with oxygen by mask, but intubation and ventilation with positive end-expiratory pressure may be required. Overhydration may worsen pulmonary edema and should be prevented.

Dysrhythmias are generally treated with conventional therapy (e.g., lidocaine for ventricular premature contractions). However, interaction of antiarrhythmic therapy with the poison should be prevented. For example, cyclic antidepressants, quinidine, and procainamide have similar effects on the myocardium, and the combination of these drugs should be avoided. Increased cocaine toxicity in animals has been attributed to lidocaine, which should not be used in cocaine overdoses.

Seizures. Seizures may be a direct effect of the poison or of secondary metabolic abnormalities such as hypoglycemia or hypoxia. A prior history of seizures, evidence of electrolyte abnormalities, hypoglycemia, and traumatic or central nervous system structural lesions should be considered in the evaluation. Diazepam or phenobarbital can be used to control seizures. If phenytoin is given, the electrocardiogram should be monitored continuously during administration.

Psychiatric evaluation. Patients who overdose once have an increased risk of subsequent overdoses and death. Many adult patients have a history of previous psychiatric problems such as depression, alcoholism, or schizophrenia. These problems should be identified and therapy initiated before discharge.

COMMON POISONS

Acetaminophen

Acetaminophen is a commonly used analgesic and antipyretic and is frequently a component of nonprescription cold remedies and combination analgesics. Acute doses greater than 150 mg/kg can produce hepatocellular necrosis.

Nausea and vomiting are the earliest symptoms of toxicity. Clinical and biochemical evidence of liver injury is seen 1 to 4 days after ingestion. In severe cases, hepatic failure can lead to encephalopathy, coma, and death. The kidneys and myocardium are less commonly involved.

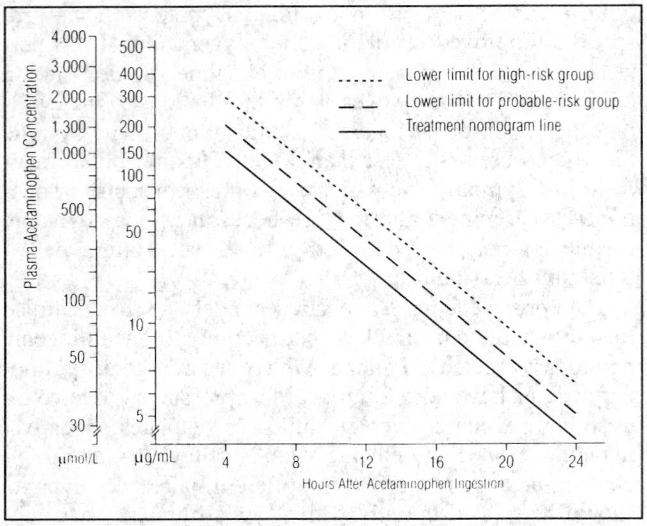

Fig. 366-1. The Rumack Matthews nomogram, relating expected severity of liver toxicity to serum acetaminophen concentrations. (From Smilkstein MJ et al: Ann Emerg Med 10:1058, 1991.)

Hepatocellular injury is the result of metabolism of acetaminophen to a toxic metabolite. This metabolite is normally detoxified by glutathione, but it binds to hepatocytes when glutathione is depleted. Toxicity may occur at relatively lower doses of acetaminophen in patients with decreased glutathione stores, and in the presence of hepatic microsomal enzyme inducers that can increase metabolite formation. *N*-Acetylcysteine is an effective antidote that prevents hepatotoxicity. The loading dose of *N*-acetylcysteine is 140 mg/kg as a 5% solution taken by mouth, followed by 70 mg/kg given every 4 hours for 72 hours. Therapy should be initiated as soon as possible but appears to be effective when started within 16 hours of ingestion. Therapy is indicated if the patient has ingested more than 7.5 g of acetaminophen or has plasma concentrations greater than 150 μ/ml 4 or more hours after ingestion (Fig. 366-1). Nausea and vomiting often occur after *N*-acetylcysteine administration. These symptoms can be minimized by appropriate dilution (i.e., a 5% solution) or if necessary by administration by nasogastric tube. In severely malnourished patients, alcoholics, and those taking enzyme-inducing drugs, the indications for *N*-acetylcysteine therapy probably should be more liberal. Oral activated charcoal should not be used simultaneously with *N*-acetylcysteine; however, activated charcoal followed in 1 hour by lavage may be a useful regimen before starting *N*-acetylcysteine.

Barbiturates

The incidence of barbiturate intoxication has decreased, primarily as a result of the replacement of barbiturates by other hypnotics; however, phenobarbital is still commonly used as an antiseizure medication. Initial symptoms of intoxication include euphoria, ataxia, nystagmus, vertigo, and somnolence. With larger doses, hypothermia, respiratory depression, coma, and cardiovascular collapse appear as cortical and brainstem functions are suppressed.

Phenobarbital concentrations greater than 6 to 8 mg per deciliter are usually associated with coma. Toxicity may be greater than expected at a particular blood concentration because of concurrent ingestion of ethanol or other central nervous system depressants. Chronic barbiturate users may tolerate the drug and display few symptoms despite high serum concentrations.

Support of respiratory and circulatory function is the principal treatment for severe intoxication. Endotracheal intubation, assisted ventilation, and administration of colloids should be instituted as required.

Alkaline diuresis should be considered in severe phenobarbital intoxications but is not effective for other barbiturates. Indications for dialysis or hemoperfusion include deterioration despite supportive therapy and both renal failure and respiratory depression.

Benzodiazepines

The benzodiazepines are widely used to treat anxiety, insomnia, and panic attacks, and clonazepam is used for seizure disorders. Benzodiazepines are generally less toxic than barbiturates. Ingestion of 500 to 1500 mg of diazepam may result in only minor toxicity. Toxic symptoms include drowsiness, ataxia, dizziness, and weakness. The duration of symptoms varies according to the dose and presence of active metabolites. Central nervous system depression may result in stage 1 coma; deeper stages of coma are rare. Other depressants including alcohol are often ingested concurrently. These increase the likelihood of coma, respiratory and cardiovascular depression, and death. Because of the relatively low toxicity of these agents, supportive care and observation are generally sufficient treatment. Activated charcoal, emesis, or gastric lavage should be used to minimize absorption. A benzodiazepine antagonist, flumazenil, in doses of 1 to 5 mg is generally effective in decreasing sedation. Flumazenil should be used cautiously, as seizures have been observed. Benzodiazepine-dependent patients experience withdrawal symptoms after receiving it.

Carbon monoxide

Carbon monoxide is a tasteless, colorless, odorless, nonirritating gas produced by incomplete combustion. Poorly ventilated heating systems, automobile exhaust, and home fires are the most common sources of toxic exposure.

Carbon monoxide has a higher affinity for hemoglobin than does oxygen; it forms carboxyhemoglobin, which decreases oxygen transport. Initial symptoms include headache, irritability, dizziness, nausea, vomiting, and chest pain. Concentrations of carboxyhemoglobin above 30% are considered toxic, although serum concentrations do not always correlate with toxicity. Focal neurologic deficits, coma, seizures, dysrhythmias, myocardial infarction, and cardiovascular collapse occur when carboxyhemoglobin concentrations are above 40% to 50%.

The patient should be removed from the source of exposure and 100% oxygen administered by a nonrebreather mask. Physical activity should be kept to a minimum, and cardiac function should be monitored. One hundred percent oxygen shortens the half-life of carbon monoxide from approximately 250 to 50 minutes. Hyperbaric oxygen further shortens the half-life to approximately 25 minutes and should be considered with severe symptoms or carboxyhemoglobin concentrations greater than 30% to 40%. Oxygen should be continued until symptoms resolve, which generally occurs at carboxyhemoglobin concentrations below 10%. Computed tomographic scanning, which may show focal edematous changes, should be performed if neurologic symptoms persist. These changes usually signify a poor prognosis.

Caustics (acids and alkalis)

Acids and alkalis are common household products found in dishwasher soap and window and drain cleaners. After ingestion, the lips, tongue, and oral cavity are usually affected. The esophagus (especially with alkalis) and stomach (with acids) are often involved, sometimes in the absence of pharyngeal involvement. The extent of damage ranges from mild irritation to acute ulceration and perforation. Acute blood loss may be severe. Late sequelae include esophageal strictures and pyloric stenosis. Inhalation of fumes may produce dyspnea, chest pain, and delayed onset noncardiogenic pulmonary edema.

Immediate therapy after skin exposure should consist of dilution with copious amounts of water. The use of diluents for ingested caustic agents remains controversial. Small quantities (one to two glasses) of water or milk may be useful, but larger volumes may increase toxicity by inducing vomiting, which re-exposes tissues. Emetics should not be given, and gastric lavage should be avoided because of possible oropharyngeal or esophageal perforation. Endoscopy to determine the full extent of esophageal and gastric damage should be performed within 12 to 24 hours of alkali ingestion. When deep or circumferential esophageal lesions are seen, corticosteroids may prevent stricture formation. Severe metabolic acidosis or alkalosis may occur after these ingestions, and acid-base balance should be monitored.

Cocaine

Significant toxicity can be observed after intranasal, oral, pulmonary ("free basing" or "crack"), and intravenous administration of cocaine. Cocaine use is also associated with increased risk of trauma and assault.

The clinical presentation includes restlessness, irritability, hypertension, hyperthermia, tachycardia, and increased respiratory rate. In severe overdoses, tonic-clonic seizures, myocardial infarction, hypotension, and respiratory depression may develop. Cardiac dysrhythmias may cause sudden death. For patients with mild toxicity who manifest tachycardia and mild hypertension, observation and oxygen administration are usually sufficient. Benzodiazepines may be required to treat agitation. Hypertension usually responds to oxygen and benzodiazepines, or labetalol. Seizures should be treated with diazepam. Beta blockers have been associated with hypertension, and studies suggest that antiarrhythmics that prolong myocardial conduction may worsen cocaine cardiac toxicity.

Cyclic antidepressants

Toxicity from cyclic antidepressants includes central nervous system symptoms such as drowsiness, coma, seizures, pulmonary edema, and cardiovascular toxicity. The anticholinergic properties of these drugs produce mydriasis, tachycardia, and decreased gastrointestinal motility. In addition, conduction abnormalities and myocardial depression are common. Prolongation of the QRS interval to more than 100 milliseconds is one sign of severe intoxication. Ingestion of more than 1 g is often associated with severe toxicity, and 2 to 3 g is associated with a mortality rate of approximately 20% with death secondary to myocardial failure and cardiovascular collapse.

Inducing emesis with ipecac syrup is contraindicated because rapid deterioration of the mental status may occur, predisposing the patient to aspiration. Gastric lavage may be useful, particularly if performed soon after ingestion, and activated charcoal inhibits gastrointestinal absorption.

The vital signs and electrocardiogram should be monitored closely. Signs and symptoms indicating toxicity usually develop within 6 to 8 hours of ingestion. Most patients have systemic acidosis, which is both metabolic and respiratory in origin. Careful attention to oxygenation and correction of the acidosis often prevents cardiac toxicity. The serum pH should be maintained at approximately 7.50, using bicarbonate and hyperventilation as needed. Lidocaine and phenytoin may be used to treat ventricular arrhythmias, and diazepam may be used for seizures. Hypotension, most frequently seen with concurrent phenothiazine ingestions, may not respond to intravenous fluids. Norepinephrine or dopamine is required in this situation. Physostigmine, once commonly recommended, is currently indicated only for life-threatening toxicity that does not respond to systemic alkalinization and other conventional measures. Physostigmine can cause seizures, complete heart block, and cholinergic toxicity.

Ethanol and isopropyl alcohol

Of all overdose patients 30% to 50% have consumed significant quantities of ethanol. Ethanol causes central nervous system depression and produces effects ranging from mild ataxia to coma, respiratory depression, cardiovascular collapse, and death. Trauma, hypoglycemia, and other forms of drug ingestion should be considered in the differential diagnosis.

Whole blood ethanol concentrations are related to clinical symptoms. An ethanol concentration greater than 100 mg/dl is usually associated with impairment of psychomotor and cognitive function. Concentrations above 400 mg/dl can result in coma, respiratory depression, and death. Symptoms vary in relation to prior history of drinking, rapidity of ingestion, and individual tolerance.

Comatose patients should have intubation and supportive care. Metabolic abnormalities including thiamine and folate deficiency, hypoglycemia, ketoacidosis, hypokalemia, and lactic acidosis should be identified and treated (Chapter 353).

Isopropyl alcohol is commonly found in rubbing alcohol, aftershave, and window-cleaning solutions. Symptoms are similar to those of ethanol intoxication, although isopropyl alcohol appears to be more potent. Isopropyl alcohol also causes more severe gastrointestinal irritation (often resulting in nausea, vomiting, and abdominal cramps) and more prolonged sedation. The standard enzymatic method of measuring ethanol does not accurately measure isopropyl alcohol concentration. It is metabolized to acetone, which can be detected in the blood, urine, and breath. Treatment is similar to therapy for ethanol intoxication. Hemodialysis should be considered for hypotensive and comatose patients.

Methanol and ethylene glycol

Methanol is commonly found in antifreeze, windshield-washing solutions, and paint thinner. Metabolism to formaldehyde and formic acid results in severe metabolic acidosis, abdominal pain, blindness, seizures, stupor, and coma. Onset of symptoms may be up to 30 hours after ingestion.

Emesis or gastric lavage may be useful if initiated soon after ingestion. Treatment should include correction of the acidosis with bicarbonate and administration of ethanol. Blood ethanol concentrations greater than 100 mg/dl inhibit the metabolism of methanol to formaldehyde and formic acid. Ethanol therapy is indicated when the methanol concentration exceeds 20 mg/dl, when the patient is having significant symptoms, or when there is a history of significant ingestion and blood concentrations are not available. Hemodialysis decreases methanol concentrations and should be combined with ethanol when serum methanol concentrations exceed 50 mg/dl.

Ethylene glycol is metabolized to glycolaldehyde, oxalate, and lactate, which account for its severe toxicity (Chapter 353). In the first 12 hours after ingestion inebriation similar to that caused by ethanol is common. A large anion gap acidosis and presence of urine oxalate crystals suggest the diagnosis. Tachypnea, cyanosis, pulmonary edema, and cardiomegaly develop 12 to 36 hours after ingestion. Renal failure may follow in 2 to 3 days.

Ethanol therapy, which inhibits metabolism to toxic metabolites, is recommended for ethylene glycol concentrations over 20 mg/dl. Hemodialysis is useful with higher serum ethylene glycol concentrations.

Opiates

Morphine, codeine, methadone, hydromorphone, diphenoxylate, and propoxyphene are the most common opiates involved in toxic ingestions. Central nervous system depression produced by these drugs is often profound, and cardiorespiratory failure is the most common cause of death. Acute pulmonary edema is also a potential complication. The narcotic agonist-antagonist pentazocine may produce acute psychiatric symptoms, and fentanyl, propoxyphene, and meperidine have been reported to cause seizures. Patients with cancer using opiates for chronic pain treatment may experience significant toxicity.

Naloxone (Narcan), which is a specific opiate antagonist without agonist properties, is appropriate therapy for all significant opiate overdoses. In adults, from 0.4 to 2.0 mg should be given intravenously. Repeat doses up to a total of 10 mg may be required, especially with propoxyphene or methadone overdoses. Patients using opiates to treat chronic pain should receive lower doses of naloxone initially, so that withdrawal and severe pain are not precipitated. Because the half-life of naloxone is relatively short, a continuous infusion may be required in overdoses of the long-acting opiates, such as methadone. In addition to its central nervous system effects, naloxone may decrease propoxyphene-induced cardiac toxicity and seizures. Patients with significant opiate overdoses merit observation for 24 to 48 hours.

Petroleum distillates

Petroleum distillates may be ingested or inhaled as individual products, or as vehicles for pesticides and other agents. Complications of petroleum ingestion include aspiration pneumonitis and pneumonia, central nervous system stimulation or depression, seizures, and cardiac arrhythmias. Aspiration causes coughing, gagging, and, in severe cases, dyspnea and cyanosis. The pulmonary toxicity of petroleum distillates increases as the surface tension and viscosity decrease and as volatility increases. Fever, increased respiratory rate, decreased breath sounds, rales, wheezes, and leukocytosis may be present. Hepatic and renal damage and sudden death may result from toluene abuse.

In general, emptying the stomach is not recommended for patients who have ingested a small quantity of a petroleum product. Lavage or emesis may be beneficial with ingestions of large quantities or products that contain other toxic chemicals. Pneumonitis is indicated by chest radiograph within 18 hours of exposure.

Treatment of aspiration should include oxygen administration, ventilatory support, and fluids as needed. Epinephrine should be avoided because of the risk of inducing dysrhythmias. Corticosteroids are not beneficial, and antibiotics should not be used for routine prophylaxis.

Phencyclidine

Phencyclidine (PCP, angel dust) can be smoked, ingested, or injected to produce euphoria and hallucinations. Large doses cause disorientation, delusions, sensory anesthesia, analgesia, and behavior that is often violent and self-destructive. Nystagmus, ataxia, bizarre posturing, seizures, hypertension, hyperthermia, and tachycardia are often seen. Very large doses produce apnea and coma.

Mildly intoxicated patients should be placed in a quiet darkened room, as sensory stimulation often increases agi-

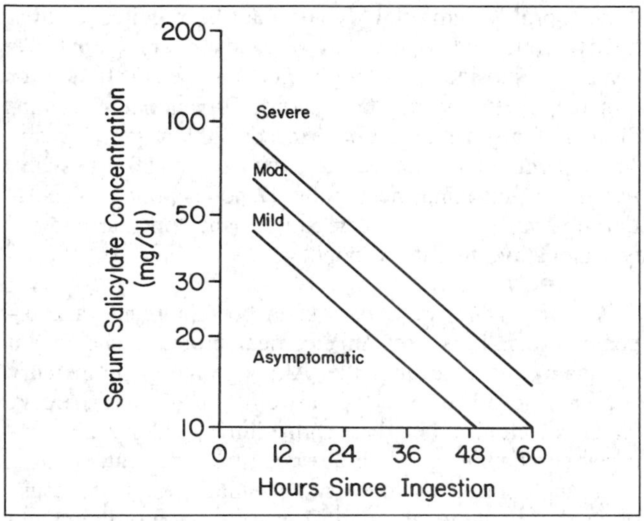

Fig. 366-2. The Done nomogram, relating expected severity of salicylate toxicity with serum salicylate concentration at various intervals after ingestion. (From Done AK: Pediatrics 26:805, 1960.)

tation. Agitation and aggressive behavior generally respond to haloperidol. Nitroprusside may be necessary for severe hypertension.

Salicylates

Symptoms of acute toxicity include nausea, tinnitus, profuse sweating, hyperventilation, seizures, and central nervous system (CNS) depression. Chronic intoxication often causes hyperthermia, confusion, altered consciousness, pulmonary edema, and hypoprothrombinemia.

Salicylates initially produce respiratory alkalosis, followed by metabolic acidosis. The anion gap metabolic acidosis is commonly seen in children and in chronic adult intoxication (Chapter 353). Moderate to severe toxicity generally occurs with single oral doses exceeding 150 mg/kg of body weight. The severity of acute intoxications can be estimated by interpreting serum salicylate concentrations with the Done nomogram (Fig. 366-2). The Done nomogram is not helpful in evaluating chronic intoxication and may underestimate toxicity in the presence of acidosis.

Activated charcoal prevents aspirin absorption. Acid-base, electrolyte, and fluid balance should be monitored closely. Intravenous sodium bicarbonate should be used to correct severe metabolic acidosis. Alkalinization of the urine (discussed earlier) should be performed in patients who are severely toxic as indicated by the Done nomogram. Hemodialysis increases salicylate excretion rates and may be indicated in severely intoxicated patients with pulmonary edema or renal failure.

ENVIRONMENTAL TOXINS

Heavy metals

Lead. In children, ingestion of lead paints found in older residential neighborhoods is a continuing problem. Adults are often exposed to lead in the manufacture of brass, batteries, and glass. Lead bullets, solder, and poorly glazed earthenware are other sources. Lead is stored in the body predominantly in bone but may adversely affect many organ systems, including the central nervous, gastrointestinal, hemopoietic, reproductive, and renal systems. Lead intoxication may present a variety of nonspecific symptoms, including fatigue, weight loss, myalgia, poor ability to concentrate, and paresthesias.

After severe acute exposures, abdominal tenderness with voluntary guarding but no rebound tenderness is the most frequent complaint. Modest elevations of liver enzyme levels and anemia, usually to a mild degree, are frequent. The anemia is usually normocytic, although microcytic anemia (with basophilic stippling) is a more classic but less common presentation. Renal function is usually normal, although a syndrome of hyperuricemia, gout, decreased creatinine clearance, interstitial nephritis, and hypertension occurs. Neuropathy, usually peripheral and often localized to motor nerves, disturbances of memory, seizures, cerebral edema, and encephalopathy, are found. Patients may also experience cardiomyopathy.

The serum lead concentration is the most accurate indicator of recent lead exposure. Concentrations above 80 μ/dl are usually associated with severe toxicity and above 100 μ/dl with encephalopathy. The recommended upper limit for blood lead concentrations is 50 μ/dl in adults (25 μ/dl in children); however, lower concentrations have been found to produce subclinical toxicity, including impairment of renal tubular function, delayed nerve conduction, inhibition of heme biosynthetic enzymes, and hypertension. Urinary lead excretion after a standard dose of calcium ethylenediamine tetraacetic acid (EDTA) can be used to identify lead intoxication in unclear cases.

The source of lead contamination should be determined and patients removed from that exposure. Heavy metal chelators, including intravenously administered dimercaprol (BAL) and calcium EDTA and orally administered penicillamine and succimer, have been used to treat lead poisoning. Toxicity from these agents can be substantial and includes acute tubular necrosis. Therapy should generally be supervised by someone with experience in chelation therapy. Chelation therapy is generally indicated in symptomatic patients with high lead concentrations. Mannitol, dexamethasone, and hyperventilation may be required for cerebral edema. Adequate urinary flow should be ensured when using calcium EDTA because of potential nephrotoxicity caused by the lead-EDTA complex. After an initial course of chelation therapy, serum lead concentrations may again rise. This rebound indicates that the patient has significant body stores of lead and may benefit from several courses of chelation therapy. Long-term treatment with orally administered *D*-penicillamine may be an alternative to repeated courses of calcium EDTA.

Arsenic. Arsenic is used in the manufacture of glass, pesticides, and wood preservatives and has been found to contaminate water, beer, and seafood. Arsenic binds to tissue proteins and is concentrated in the liver, skin, kidney,

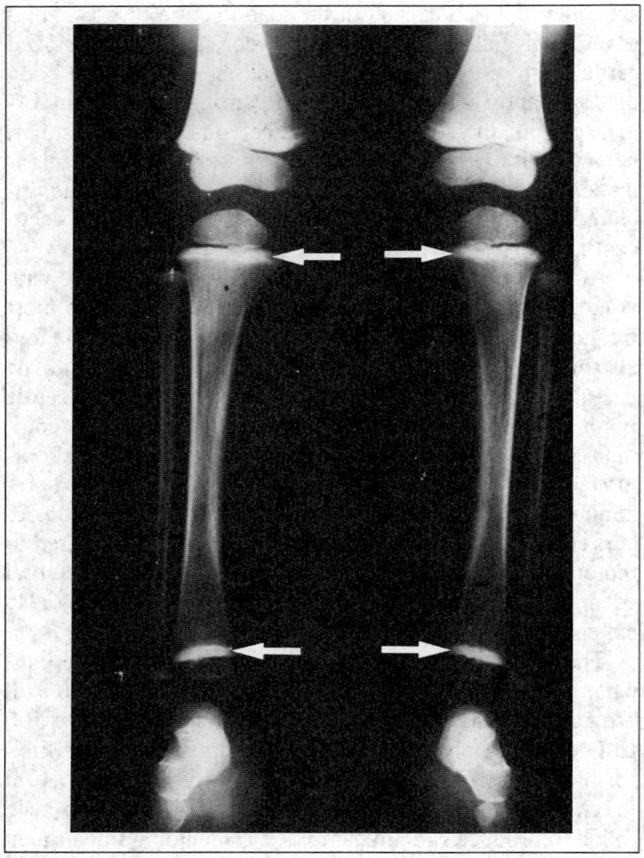

Fig. 366-3. Long bones of a child with chronic lead poisoning showing the lead accumulation in the zones of provisional calcification.

and nervous system. There is also some accumulation of arsenic in bone, but to a lesser extent than of lead.

In humans, the symptoms of acute inorganic arsenic poisoning include severe burning of the mouth and throat, abdominal pain, nausea, vomiting, diarrhea, hypotension, and muscle spasms. Cardiomyopathy, jaundice, renal tubular acidosis, red cell hemolysis, ventricular arrhythmias, coma, seizures, and intestinal hemorrhage may be seen in severe cases.

Chronic arsenic poisoning findings include an irregular, dusky pigmentation and hyperkeratosis of the skin characterized as "rain drops on a dusty road" (Fig. 366-3), painful dysesthesia in the hands and feet, bone marrow depression, transverse white striae of the nails, altered mentation, and occasionally garlic-odor perspiration. Chronic arsenic poisoning is associated with cancer of the skin and lungs.

Diagnostic tests to identify arsenic toxicity are unreliable; however, urinary excretion of arsenic above 100 μ per day does correlate with recent exposure and toxicity. Hair or nail analysis may help to diagnose chronic arsenic poisoning. Concentrations above 1 μ per gram of hair are usually considered diagnostic.

In symptomatic patients, chelation of the arsenic with dimercaprol is indicated. Fluids may be required to treat hypovolemia and to maintain a good urinary output. As symptoms subside, *D*-penicillamine may be substituted for dimercaprol. In asymptotic persons, *D*-penicillamine is indicated if arsenic excretion exceeds 200 μ per day and should continue as long as excretion exceeds 50 μ per day. In chronic poisoning, neuropathy responds poorly to chelation treatment, although dermatitis, pancytopenia, and encephalopathy often do respond.

Mercury. Mercury is present in both inorganic and organic forms. It is used in electrical products and dental amalgams and as a fungicide. Although inorganic mercury is poorly absorbed from the gastrointestinal tract, mercury vapor is well absorbed through the lungs, and organic mercurial compounds are well absorbed from the gut.

In acute inorganic mercury poisonings, the usual cause of death is acute renal failure. Local irritation of the mouth and pharynx may be severe and is accompanied by vomiting, dehydration, and abdominal cramps with bloody diarrhea. Chronic exposure to inorganic mercury may cause gingivitis, speech defects, and tremor. A chronic personalty disorder, termed the Mad Hatter syndrome, characterized by unusual shyness, labile affect, and decline in intellect, may be present.

Organic mercurial compounds have a predilection for the nervous system. Dysarthria, ataxia, paresthesias, and constricted visual fields may develop days to weeks after exposure. Renal involvement is less pronounced than in inorganic mercury poisoning. Organic mercurial compounds cross the placenta and are associated with fetal mental retardation, cerebral palsy, and seizures.

Blood, urine, hair, and nails can be analyzed for mercury. After recent exposures, blood mercury concentrations generally exceed 25 to 50 μ/dl. Urinary excretion of mercury is a good index of total body burden and rarely exceeds 1.5 μ per day in normal individuals.

After acute exposures, toxic patients may be treated with either dimercaprol or penicillamine. These agents are less effective for chronic inorganic mercury poisoning, and *N*-acetyl-dl-penicillamine, which selectively chelates mercury, is probably the most effective treatment.

Pesticides

Cholinesterase inhibitors. Acute poisonings produced by the two types of cholinesterase inhibitors (organophosphates and carbamates) have similar clinical presentations but differ in severity and treatment. Both combine with and inactivate the enzyme acetylcholinesterase, causing the accumulation of acetylcholine, which produces bronchoconstriction, hypersalivation, miosis, abdominal cramping, and hypotension. Muscle fasciculations, weakness, and paralysis can also be seen. Central nervous system effects include restlessness, anxiety, insomnia, convulsions, and coma. Acetylcholinesterase is only transiently inactivated by carbamate insecticides; however, the reaction may be irreversible with the organophosphates. The toxicity associated with carbamate poisoning is usually less severe and has a shorter duration than organophosphate poisoning. In addition to the acute effects of these insecticides, subtle neurologic abnormalities, including problems of abstraction, simple motor skills, and intellectual functioning, may persist long term.

Pesticides are absorbed through the skin or may be ingested and inhaled. Clothes saturated with the poison should be removed and the skin washed with copious quantities of soap and water. Intubation may be necessitated by respiratory paralysis and inadequate control of secretions.

Cholinergic stimulation caused by exposure to these pesticides can be reversed with atropine. Two milligrams of atropine should be given intravenously or intramuscularly every 5 minutes until signs of atropinization occur (red face, dry mouth, mydriasis, tachycardia). Additional doses of atropine may be needed during the first 12 hours after exposure.

Pralidoxime, if given within 36 hours of exposure, partly reactivates cholinesterase after organophosphate poisoning. If muscle weakness and fasciculations persist despite atropine administration, 1 g of pralidoxime in aqueous solution should be given slowly by intravenous infusion. Pralidoxime should not be used in carbamate poisoning, as it may increase the severity of weakness.

Chlorinated hydrocarbons. Chlorinated hydrocarbon insecticides (dieldrin, heptachlor, chlordane, aldrin, endrin) are readily absorbed from the gut and through the skin and lungs. The initial symptoms include behavioral changes, sensory and equilibrium disturbances, seizures, and coma. Respiratory depression, weakness, and involuntary muscle activity may develop in severe cases. The heart may be sensitized to the arrhythmogenic effects of epinephrine, which should be avoided, and hepatocellular necrosis and renal tubular degeneration may develop.

Lavage or emesis, removal of contaminated clothes, and cleansing of the skin are indicated. Seizures can be controlled with diazepam. Stimulants, especially epinephrine, should be avoided, as they may cause ventricular fibrillation. Often these insecticides are dissolved in a petroleum base. Complications of the petroleum solvent should also be considered when choosing therapy.

REFERENCES

Amrein R et al: Flumazenil in benzodiazepine antagonism-actions and clinical use in intoxications and anesthesiology. Med Toxicol 2:411, 1987.

Callaham M and Kassel D: Epidemiology of fatal tricyclic antidepressant ingestion: implications for management. Ann Emerg Med 14:1, 1985.

Ellenhorn MJ and Barceloux DG, eds: Medical toxicology—diagnosis and treatment of human poisonings. New York, 1988, Elsevier.

Gorby MS: Arsenic poisoning. West J Med 149:308, 1988.

Kulig K: Management of poisoning associated with "newer" antidepressant agents. Ann Emerg Med 15:1039, 1986.

Kulling P and Persson H: Role of the intensive care unit in the management of the poisoned patient. Med Toxicol 1:375, 1986.

Litovitz TL et al: 1990 Annual report of the American Association of Poison Control Centers national data collection system. Am J Emerg Med 9:461, 1991.

Paloucek FP and Rodvola KA: Evaluation of theophylline overdoses and toxicities. Ann Emerg Med 17:135, 1988.

Rempel D: The lead exposed worker. JAMA 262:532, 1989.

Smilkstein MJ et al: Efficacy of oral N-acetylcysteine in the treatment of acetaminophen overdose. N Engl J Med 319:1557, 1988.

Watson WA: Factors influencing the clinical efficacy of activated charcoal. Drug Intell Clin Pharm 21:160, 1987.

CHAPTER

367 Substance Abuse

Richard L. Bauer
Abdulhay A. Kadri
Debra K. Hunt

Use of psychotropic substances for recreational or medical purposes has become commonplace in the United States and is in many cases regarded as normal and appropriate. Alcohol is the most commonly used substance; however, surveys suggest that 40% of the population above age 25 years have at some time used marijuana, hallucinogens, cocaine, or heroin. Use of these substances is, in most cases, occasional or experimental; however, excessive and inappropriate use may result in adverse behavioral and health consequences. Alcohol, for example, is involved in 25,000 traffic deaths, and 20,000 persons die of cirrhosis and other alcohol-related diseases annually.

Recognition of substance-induced conditions and diagnosis of pathologic use are essential for successful management. Pathologic use may be substance abuse, a pattern of pathologic use that produces impaired social or occupational functioning, or dependence, the impaired control and continued use of psychoactive substances despite adverse consequences. The symptoms of dependence include the physiologic symptoms of tolerance and withdrawal, drug-seeking behavior, inability to limit intake, and continued use despite social, psychologic, and occupational problems related to the substance abuse. Tolerance is characterized by the need for progressively larger doses of a substance to maintain the desired effect. It is caused by physiologic changes that result from repeated exposure. If the substance is abruptly discontinued, the adaptive changes are unmasked and withdrawal symptoms such as tremor, tachycardia, insomnia, hyperreflexia, and seizures may occur.

The likelihood of withdrawal depends on the quantity and duration of substance use. Minor withdrawal symptoms may be seen after use of as little as 45 mg of morphine daily for 3 days. Moderately severe symptoms are frequent after a regimen of 240 mg of morphine daily for 30 days. Substances with long half-lives (e.g., methadone and phenobarbital) require more prolonged use to cause dependence than substances with short half-lives (e.g., heroin and secobarbital). In addition, withdrawal symptoms associated with long-acting substances are generally milder and appear later than those related to short-acting substances.

Several personality and social factors have been linked to chronic substance abuse. Peer pressure and thrill-seeking behavior are common influences in first-time drug use. Depression, personality disorders, family discord, and a family history of dependence are associated with progression from episodic to chronic substance abuse.

ALCOHOLISM

It is estimated that up to 90% of the adult U.S. population uses alcohol; the amount and frequency used vary from occasional to daily. Most drinkers, especially in the teenage years, experience isolated and brief complications of excessive drinking. However, about 10% of men and 3% to 5% of women are reported by national surveys to meet the Diagnostic and statistical manual of mental disorders, third revised edition (DSMIII-R), criteria for the disease of alcoholism. Genetic and environmental factors contribute to the heterogeneity of drinking behavior. Once established, alcoholism follows a course marked by frequent remissions and relapses. At any one time, more than half of the drinkers who could have met the diagnostic criteria at one time either have become abstainers or drink in a nonalcoholic pattern. The aged drink less frequently and lesser amounts of alcohol and their alcoholism is less identifiable by standard diagnostic criteria.

It is imperative for the physician to manage the patient's overall health with knowledge of the disease of alcoholism, especially if therapy for alcoholism is not initiated. Alcoholics are a heterogeneous population who can best be characterized by their inability to recognize the negative impact of alcohol on their lives. The diagnosis of alcoholism must be contemplated when any patient presents a spectrum of medical complications (see the box) or psychosocial problems, such as marital and family disruption and employment and legal difficulties.

Laboratory testing (e.g., liver function tests or complete blood count) and direct questioning about alcohol use by the physician are of limited sensitivity and specificity, and unreliable as sole diagnostic methods (Table 367-1). The many clinically validated questionnaires, such as the Michigan Alcoholism Screening Test (MAST) and the CAGE, are easily used in the office. The diagnosis of alcoholism is significantly enhanced by interviewing collateral associates of the patient; most alcoholics are diagnosed by family and friends before physician contact or intervention.

Presentation of the diagnosis to the patient must be firm but nonjudgmental. The active alcoholic has major cognitive impairment and does not easily accept alcohol use as the cause of any identified problems. A successful presentation of the diagnosis can be facilitated if the patient has accepting and supportive care givers, preferably family

Table 367-1. Diagnostic tests for alcoholism

		Sensitivity	Specificity
1. CAGE			
C	Have you tried to *cut down* on your drinking?	75	96*
A	Are you *annoyed* by people telling you to stop drinking?		
G	Do you feel *guilty* about your drinking?		
E	Do you drink on first getting up in the morning *(eye opener)* ?		
2. Laboratory studies			
Elevated GGT		54	76
Increased mean corpuscular volume		63	74
Elevated liver function test (OT, PT) results		37	81

*For two or more yes answers in CAGE. GGT, gamma glutamyl transpeptidase; OT, oxaloacetic transaminase; PT, pyruvic transaminase.

Medical complications of alcoholism

Gastrointestinal tract

Esophagitis, gastritis, peptic ulcer
Diarrhea
Pancreatitis
Liver: fatty degeneration, alcoholic hepatitis, cirrhosis
Decreased absorption of folate, vitamin B_{12}, calcium

Cardiovascular system

Exacerbation of angina and congestive heart failure
Hypertension
Cardiomyopathy
Arrhythmias

Metabolic changes

Ketoacidosis, lactic acidosis
Hypomagnesemia, hypocalcemia, hypokalemia
Hyperuricemia
Hypertriglyceridemia

Central nervous system

Acute intoxication
Amnesia
Cerebellar degeneration
Marchiafava-Bignami disease
Central pontine myelinosis
Cerebral atrophy
Myopathy
Withdrawal syndromes: tremulousness, hallucinations, seizures, delirium tremens

Nutritional deficiencies

Wernicke's and Korsakoff's encephalopathies
Folate deficiency
Pellagra

Hematopoietic system

Anemia (direct toxic effect of alcohol, folate deficiency)
Thrombocytopenia

members, in addition to a skilled physician. The effectiveness of physician intervention is well documented.

Complications

The complications of alcoholism encompass the social, psychologic, and physiologic domains. Family disruptions, poor employment history, legal difficulties, physical trauma, mood disorders, serious metabolic imbalances, and pathologic effects on a diversity of organs have been established as sequelae of alcoholism. Life expectancy in alcoholics is 10 to 15 years less than average, partially as a result of increased rates of liver disease, cancers, cardiomyopathy, motor vehicle trauma, and suicide.

Many alcoholics come to the attention of the physician during an illness that precipitates withdrawal symptoms that reveal occult alcoholism. Presenting symptoms include feelings of ill being, restlessness, sleep disorders, and somatic complaints related to the gastrointestinal (GI) tract. However, the irreversible end-organ damage of alcohol (e.g., liver disease, GI bleeding, congestive heart failure, central nervous system disease, and neuropathies) may be the reason the patient enters the health care system. Family members and the spouse may exhibit somatizations or emotional complaints.

Nutritional deficiencies (thiamine and B_{12}) occur despite good dietary intake, as a result of direct toxicity of alcohol, impaired absorption and utilization of nutrients, and toxicity of alcohol metabolites, with resulting neuropathies, bone marrow toxicity, cognitive changes, and intracranial hemorrhages. In the malnourished alcoholic, the resumption of a regular diet during hospitalization can cause severe rhabdomyolysis, hemolysis, and cellular hypoxia caused by acute hypophosphatemia associated with cellular uptake of glucose. The underlying thiamine (vitamin B_1) deficiency is accentuated with the cellular uptake of glucose. B_1 deficiency is a major cause of peripheral neuropathies and Wernicke's disease (ocular disturbances, ataxia, and confusion), which has a 10% to 20% mortality rate if untreated and can become permanent in 80% of these patients. Korsakoff's psychosis (cognitive dysfunction, loss of recent memory, and inability to learn new information) is thought to be a chronic form of Wernicke's disease. Potassium, magnesium, and phosphate deficiencies are common in nutritionally compromised alcoholics.

Fatty liver and alcoholic hepatitis are frequently early manifestations of alcohol use. Of the cases of cirrhosis of the liver in the United States 90% are attributable to alcohol; cirrhosis is the ninth leading cause of mortality in the United States. The amount and duration of alcohol ingestion required to cause cirrhosis vary among individuals and between males and females. Ingestion of more than 1 pint of alcohol (86 proof) daily for 10 years is associated with a 10% risk of cirrhosis and up to 50% risk after 25 years of the same pattern of use. Esophageal varices secondary to portal hypertension may become irreversible, and variceal bleeding is often the immediate cause of death. Gastritis, pancreatitis, and diarrhea are also associated with excessive use of alcohol.

Patients who have cirrhosis may experience hypoglycemia and/or acidosis, the manifestations of which can be easily mistaken for intoxication. The hypoglycemia is due to limited glycogen storage and the high reduced nicotinamide-adenine dinucleotide (NAD)/NAD (NADH/NAD) ratio that depresses gluconeogenesis. The acidosis is due to increased free fatty acid utilization, the de novo synthesis of ketone bodies, and exaggerated lactic acid production with exercise.

Management

Because of the nature of the disease and its impact on the judgment of the patient, involvement of a care giver is essential in treating alcoholics. The initial element of the management plan is the detoxification of the patient, which is followed by a long-term plan to prevent and manage relapse. The prevention of relapse is dependent on the recovery of cognitive function and the medical and social support provided to the patient. When patients are unwilling to enter definitive therapy programs, it is encumbent on the physician to minimize the complications of the disease. There are no data to support the need for hypnotic and sedative agents in the detoxification of every patient.

Withdrawal

Within 4 to 8 hours of the last drink, blood alcohol concentration falls and the symptoms of withdrawal may be manifested. Neither blood alcohol levels nor other serologic markers are helpful in predicting the severity of symptoms or the course of the syndrome. Hyperadrenergism, mood and mental changes, seizures, and delirium tremens form the spectrum of withdrawal symptoms. In some patients, mild autonomic dysfunction, mood disorders, and anxiety that persist up to 6 months after cessation of alcohol therapy increase the risk of relapse.

Tremulousness and irritability mark the onset of the withdrawal syndrome. Within 24 to 48 hours increased tremulousness, diaphoresis, agitation, tachycardia, hypertension, hyperreflexia, and insomnia develop. Patients are generally alert and oriented; however, they may suffer vivid visual and auditory hallucinations they do not recognize as mere hallucinations. Progression to more severe withdrawal complications is seen in 5% to 10% of patients.

A minority of alcoholics may suffer nonfocal multiple or single motor seizures. These seizures are responsive to diazepam, phenobarbital, and carbamazepine, but not to dilantin. The electroencephalogram (EEG) result reverts to normal in the nontraumatic patient. No long-term therapy is indicated but about one third of these patients, especially if benzodiazepine withdrawal is concomitant, progress to delirium tremens (delirium tremors): that is, disorientation, hallucinations (without lucid periods), hyperadrenergism, hypervigilance, and fever. Most cases of delirium tremors are self-limited and resolve within 72 hours, but there is a fatality rate of 10% to 15%.

Detoxification

Most patients can be detoxified as outpatients (see the box below). The essential elements of this strategy are the availability of a home and office support system for the patient and the absence of serious physiologic compromise. An initial evaluation should confirm the absence of major physiologic abnormalities. The patient treated as an outpatient and his or her caregiver are assigned a 24-hour phone contact and seen daily in the office. The treatment plan is indicated in the box below.

Criteria for outpatient detoxification

Patient's willingness to begin treatment

Absence of significant medical problems
- Cardiovascular disease
- Head trauma
- GI bleeding
- Pulmonary compromise
- Hepatic failure
- Nutritional compromise
- Neurologic problems, especially seizures

Absence of significant psychiatric problems
- Depression
- Suicidal potential
- Acute psychosis
- Cognitive impairment

Social setting
- Agreement to long-term follow-up plans
- Alcohol/drug–free place to live
- Home/family support for treatment plans
- Employment modifications

Outpatient detoxification of alcoholics

Nutritional counseling

Education of care giver on potential medical emergencies and professional contact
- Progression of withdrawal symptoms
- Fever
- Mental status changes
- Symptoms of cardiopulmonary compromise
- Nausea or vomiting

Follow-up care
- Daily visits for at least 3 to 5 days
- Thiamine IM daily (100 mg) for at least 3 days
- Monitoring of vital signs
- Reassessment of withdrawal signs and symptoms
- Administration of sedatives and issue daily doses as indicated
- Reassessment of the environment and the care giver

In inpatient detoxifications attention must be given to nutritional problems and comorbidities of the patient. Sedative/hypnotic drugs, if clearly indicated, must be limited to the first 5 to 7 days. Alcoholics are at high risk for addictions, especially with benzodiazepines. Vital signs and fluid status should be monitored particularly closely.

After the detoxification phase most patients require a long-term relapse prevention program. The program is entirely the choice of the patient and the physician. Alcoholics Anonymous is the best known and most accessible program and has no fee.

The use of drugs for maintenance of abstinence is very controversial. Relapse rate is highest in the first 2 to 6 months and often can be predicted by several factors, including persistent depression, anger, memory loss, craving for drugs, and new withdrawal symptoms. Loss of social support also may precipitate relapse. The physician must evaluate all patients for comorbid conditions, such as depression and insomnia, and ensure that adequate medical and social support is available. Visits may need to be more frequent and consultation may be required if relapse appears imminent. Treatment of the commonly associated depressive symptoms with medications is not indicated unless severe psychomotor retardation develops.

OPIOIDS

The opioids are congeners of the naturally occurring alkaloids of opium. Of the opioids, morphine, heroin, codeine, oxycodone, and meperidine are most commonly abused. If dependence develops, drug procurement often dominates the individual's life and often leads to criminal behavior.

Although there are some differences in metabolism and methods of administration, the toxicity and medical complications of these agents are quite similar. Heroin (diacetylmorphine) is more lipid-soluble than morphine, and as such it more readily crosses the blood-brain barrier and causes relatively more intense euphoria and sedation. Heroin is quickly metabolized and is excreted in the urine as free or conjugated morphine. Euphoria, sedation, and analgesia are the desired effects, but overdoses may cause respiratory depression, bradycardia, hypothermia, coma, and death.

Complications

Complications are frequent with both acute overdose (Chapter 366) and chronic opioid abuse. Overdoses may result from variability in the potency of heroin purchased on the street, rapid loss of tolerance after abstinence, and concurrent use of other central nervous system depressants. Nonsterile injection techniques may cause skin abscesses, septic phlebitis, endocarditis, and increased risk of acquired immunodeficiency syndrome. *Staphylococcus aureus* infection is frequent, although gram-negative bacteria, fungi, tetanus, malaria, and other unusual infections also have increased frequency. Other contaminants (talc, quinine, lactose, and cotton fibers) used to dilute the heroin or to prepare the injection may lead to pulmonary hypertension and fibrosis, transverse myelitis, amblyopia, and rhabdomyolysis.

Chronic liver disease, including cirrhosis, chronic persistent hepatitis, chronic active hepatitis, and granulomatous hepatitis, is found in up to 50% of heroin abusers. Concurrent alcohol abuse and hepatitis B infections account for many liver disorders. The nephrotic syndrome with or without progression to renal failure has been described, as has a necrotizing angiitis similar to polyarteritis nodosa.

Withdrawal

In physically dependent opioid users, withdrawal starts within 2 to 48 hours of last use. Abrupt withdrawal of heroin, which has a short half-life, causes prompt and severe withdrawal symptoms. Restlessness, lacrimation, rhinorrhea, and nausea may be followed by mydriasis, muscle aches, diarrhea, piloerection, tachycardia, and hypertension. Symptoms peak at 48 to 72 hours. Higher maintenance doses, greater duration of addiction, and intravenous use of opioids are associated with more intense symptoms. Withdrawal from opioids is rarely fatal, although accompanying illnesses may complicate the clinical course.

Opioids (usually methadone) given to patients in withdrawal quickly relieve symptoms: 10 to 20 mg of methadone, repeated in 2 to 6 hours if needed, may be given orally for moderate and severe withdrawal symptoms. Generally no more than 40 mg of methadone is required in the first 24 hours. Sedation after a single 10 mg dose virtually excludes significant opioid addiction. After 2 days of maintenance therapy designed to produce mild sedation, the methadone can be decreased by 5 to 10 mg daily. Clonidine (0.1 to 0.3 mg) has been used as an alternative therapy because it suppresses many of the autonomic symptoms of withdrawal.

Management

After the initial treatment of withdrawal, referral for maintenance and abstinence treatment should be considered. Outpatient maintenance (generally with methadone) is proscribed by law except in federally regulated treatment centers. Follow-up studies of patients in these programs indicate a 25% to 50% recidivism rate in 1 year. Persons who continue treatment show decreased heroin use, decreased criminal behavior, and increased employment rate. Spontaneous remissions do occur without methadone treatment.

NICOTINE

Currently, 29% of the U.S. adult population are smokers; the rate is declining by 0.5% annually. The Center for Disease Control (CDC) estimates that 434,000 smoking-related deaths occur annually, and over 1.2 million years of life before age 65 are lost each year as a result of smoking.

The addictive potential of nicotine was first reported in the 1940s, but official recognition was delayed for many years. Today the diagnosis of nicotine addiction is well accepted and formally based on DSM III-R criteria. Nicotine dependence scales have been developed for smoking cessation research; however, clinicians can quickly diagnose nicotine dependence with two key questions: "Does the patient smoke within 30 minutes of awakening?" and "Does the patient smoke more than 25 cigarettes per day?" Subjects who seek smoking cessation counseling who respond positively to either question have significantly higher plasma cotinine levels indicating higher nicotine intake. Patients who answer yes to both questions are likely to benefit most from drug therapy.

Withdrawal

The DSM III-R criteria for nicotine withdrawal are daily use of nicotine for at least several weeks and development of at least four signs of withdrawal within 24 hours of abrupt cessation or reduction in use. These signs include craving for nicotine, irritability, frustration or anger, anxiety, restlessness, difficulty in concentrating, decreased heart rate, and increased appetite or weight gain.

Management

Nicotine gum and patches are available to augment quitting attempts. Neither has been effective when used alone; however, when they are used by nicotine-dependent patients, along with physician counseling and follow-up observation, quitting rates can reach 20%. A metaanalysis of smoking cessation techniques found that the strongest predictors of a successful program were (1) number of intervention modalities used (counseling, nicotine replacement, written material, etc.), (2) number of reinforcing visits, and (3) duration of the program. The authors calculated that a cessation program using two modalities in six sessions over a 1-year period would yield a 43% success rate.

One clinical approach to smoking cessation is as follows: (1) identify the smoking habit and assess nicotine dependence, (2) provide a strong, personal message ("Ms. Smith, this is your second episode of bronchitis this year; I think the best thing you could do for your health is to stop smoking"), (3) assess the patient's motivation (willingness to set a quit date), and, if the patient is motivated, (4) set a quitting date, (5) write and jointly sign a contract for the date, (6) prescribe nicotine replacement (especially if the patient is nicotine-dependent) and instruction on its use, and (7) schedule a follow-up visit 2 weeks after the quitting date. When time allows, additional behavioral counseling, such as discussing obstacles to quitting, may further enhance quitting rates. Following this approach can help an additional 4 million people become nonsmokers each year.

COCAINE AND AMPHETAMINES

Recreational use of cocaine has increased in the past decade. Cocaine is usually inhaled nasally; however, it may also be smoked, ingested, or injected. Smoking and injection produce the highest serum concentrations and greatest toxicity, as does use of the free base (produced by heating with diethyl ether). Amphetamines have effects similar to those of cocaine but a substantially longer duration of action.

In low doses, cocaine and amphetamines produce euphoria and a feeling of elation probably as a result of central nervous system release of catecholamines. Larger doses may cause restlessness, tremor, tachycardia, and hypertension (Chapter 366). Cocaine may also cause acute myocardial infarction, cardiac arrhythmias, rupture of the ascending aorta, cerebrovascular accidents, hypertension, hyperpyrexia, and seizures in acute overdoses. Chronic use of cocaine may be associated with rhinitis and nasal mucosal atrophy, and rarely with nasal perforation. Acute and chronic paranoid psychoses have been described with amphetamines and cocaine, and in amphetamine users diffuse vasculitis may develop, leading to renal failure, cerebrovascular accidents, and cor pulmonale.

Withdrawal

Dependence on stimulant drugs is characterized by binge use, the purpose of which is to maintain the euphoria and sense of power that these drugs provide. This is in contrast to dependence on alcohol or opioids, in which avoidance of withdrawal symptoms is the predominant reason for continued use. After bingeing, a period of intense depression, anxiety, and agitation may follow. These symptoms are followed by a period of craving for sleep. Lassitude, sleep disorders, nightmares, depression, and psychomotor retardation may persist for up to 6 to 18 weeks after the period of hypersomnolence. These symptoms are indistinguishable from those of a major depressive episode, and the risk of suicide increases in these individuals. This period of anhedonia may induce a strong craving for the euphoric effects of the drug, and reuse starts another cycle of abuse. Often users of these drugs abuse sedative and anxiolytic drugs to alleviate the unpleasant after-effects of cocaine intoxication.

Management

The first goal of treatment is to stop the cycles of bingeing. Because of the long period of craving for cocaine after withdrawal, many experts believe in patient treatment for up to 5 weeks with a subsequent 5 weeks of evening hospital or extensive group therapy. Practical measures to minimize access to these drugs as well as family and individual therapy and urine drug monitoring are useful components of the intervention. Peer support groups such as Alcoholics Anonymous may be helpful in teaching strategies that prevent relapse. These strategies include avoiding situations in which risk of relapse is high, rehearsing avoidance strategies, and developing drug-free social networks. Antidepressants, such as desipramine, have been shown to ameliorate the withdrawal symptoms and to increase abstinence rates.

REFERENCES

American Psychiatric Association: Diagnostic and statistical manual of mental disorders ed 3. Washington, DC, 1987, American Psychiatric Association.

Bush B et al: Screening for alcohol abuse using the C.A.G.E. questionnaire. Am J Med 82:231, 1987.

Fagerstrom KO: Measuring degree of physical dependence to tobacco smoking with reference to individualization of treatment. Addict Behav 3:235, 1978.

Hays JT and Spickard WA Jr: Alcoholism: early diagnosis and intervention. J Gen Intern Med 2:420, 1987.

Khantzian EJ and McKenna GJ: Acute toxic and withdrawal reactions associated with drug use and abuse. Ann Intern Med 90:361, 1979.

Kottke TE et al: Attributes of successful smoking cessation intervention in medical practice: a meta-analysis of 39 controlled trials. JAMA 259:2882, 1988.

Lam W et al: Meta-analysis of randomized controlled trials of nicotine chewing-gum. Lancet 2:27, 1987.

Schneider NG et al: Nicotine gum in smoking cessation: a placebo-controlled double blind trial. Addict Behav 8:256, 1983.

West LJ et al: Alcoholism. Ann Intern Med 100:405, 1984.

CHAPTER

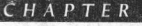

368 Environmental Emergencies, Bites, and Stings

Knox H. Todd

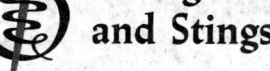

HEAT RELATED DISORDERS

Thermoregulation

Human body temperature varies narrowly around a set point of approximately 37° C despite wide variations in external temperatures. Small interindividual differences in this set point exist, and intraindividual variations occur both diurnally and during the menstrual cycle of ovulating females.

Thermal homeostasis requires a balance between heat gain and loss. At rest, heat is produced primarily in the core of the body by the brain and organs in the abdomen and thorax. With exercise, skeletal muscles become the major generators of body heat. Heat is transferred internally by conduction between adjacent tissues and, more importantly, by forced convection of warmed blood through the cardiovascular system. Two vascular mechanisms regulate heat transfer from the body core to the body surface. First, peripheral blood flow varies directly with environmental temperature. In low environmental temperatures, peripheral vasoconstriction shunts blood flow to the body core. In addition, a countercurrent heat exchange system in the extremities allows the transfer of arterial heat to deep veins in cold environments. With increasing temperatures superficial veins preferentially dilate, facilitating heat transfer to the body surface. The result of these circulatory adjustments is a core to shell temperature gradient that can be increased in cold environments to produce insulation of the body core and decreased in warm environments to facilitate heat loss.

External heat transfer has evaporative and nonevaporative mechanisms. In cold environments, heat is lost primarily by nonevaporative heat transfer through conduction, convection, and radiation. A small amount of heat is lost by insensible evaporation through the skin (transpiration) and respiratory passages. When ambient temperature is greater than skin temperature, all metabolic heat dissipates by evaporation, primarily through sweating.

The center of human thermoregulation is the hypothalamus. Information from warm and cold receptors in the skin, viscera, spinal cord, and hypothalamus itself is integrated in this area, resulting in activation of physiologic and behavioral mechanisms for conserving or dissipating heat. Physiologic responses may include vasoconstriction, vasodilatation, sweating, or shivering. Behavioral responses may include seeking shelter, dressing appropriately, or altering activity levels. These responses are often impaired in victims of thermal stress.

Hyperthermia

Epidemiology. Heat-related deaths often occur in an epidemic fashion in prolonged periods of high temperature and humidity. Typically cases occur after several days of such conditions. Risk factors for heat stroke include advanced age, alcoholism, urban residence, poverty, use of major tranquilizers, and residence on the higher floors of multistory buildings. Factors associated with decreased risk are ability to care for oneself, use of air-conditioning, and decrease in vigorous physical activity during heat waves.

Clinical presentation. Heat illness may present a variety of clinical syndromes. Heat cramps are acute, painful skeletal muscle contractions that usually occur in young adults who are profusely sweating while performing strenuous tasks. The precise mechanism responsible for heat cramps is not clear, but they are believed to result from sodium depletion in acclimatized persons who sweat profusely and replace water losses without salt replacement. The condition responds to rest in a cool environment and oral or intravenous replacement of salts.

Heat exhaustion is a more severe heat syndrome resulting from losses of body water and sodium. Symptoms include weakness, fatigue, headache, nausea, vomiting, diarrhea, and muscle cramps. Patients sweat profusely and body temperature may be mildly elevated. Treatment consists of rest, transfer to a cool environment, and intravenous administration of saline solution.

Heat stroke is a catastrophic condition that occurs when the body's homeostatic mechanisms are unable to prevent marked elevations in core temperature. It occurs in two forms, exertional and classical heat stroke. *Exertional heat stroke* is a disorder of young adults, particularly athletes, soldiers, or laborers who perform strenuous tasks in humid, hot environments. *Classic heat stroke* occurs among elderly, debilitated persons, often in an epidemic fashion during heat waves. Both syndromes are characterized by neurologic disturbances and severe hyperthermia with core temperatures usually greater than 41° C.

Pathophysiology. *Heat stroke* pathophysiology primarily involves the cardiovascular and central nervous systems. Cardiovascular collapse in classic heat stroke is the result of modest fluid depletion and marked decreases in systemic vascular resistance that accompany peripheral vasodilatation. Additionally, cardiac output may be depressed by primary myocardial degeneration caused by direct thermal injury or hypoxia, intramyocardial hemorrhage, or pulmonary vascular hypertension. Pathologic studies of young adult victims of heat stroke have revealed patchy myocardial degeneration, and animal studies have demonstrated decreased myocardial contractility with extreme elevations of core temperature, but the significance of these findings in the typical victim of classic heat stroke is unclear. Cardiac arrhythmias result from primary myocardial damage as well as acid-base and electrolyte disturbances.

Pathologic changes in the central nervous system of heat stroke victims are common; they include cerebral edema, petechiae, and gross hemorrhage; neuronal degeneration; and necrosis, particularly affecting the cerebellum. Brain damage and death are more likely if status epilepticus occurs.

Bleeding disorders, rhabdomyolysis, and acute renal failure are common in exertional heat stroke; however, they are relatively rare in classic heat stroke of the elderly. Proposed mechanisms for bleeding disorders in heat stroke include (1) thermal inactivation of clotting factors, (2) hepatic necrosis with decreased production of clotting factors, (3) thermal destruction of platelets and megakaryocytes, (4) vascular and endothelial damage with increased capillary permeability and release of thromboplastic substances, and (5) primary fibrinolysis. Rhabdomyolysis may occur after prolonged seizures or in the absence of muscular hyperactivity as a result of direct thermal injury or tissue ischemia. Acute renal failure occurs in approximately 25% to 35% of exertional heat stroke cases but in only 5% of classic heat stroke cases. Oliguric acute tubular necrosis is a frequent result of ischemia or myoglobinuric renal failure.

Arterial blood gases often reflect respiratory alkalosis or combined respiratory alkalosis and metabolic acidosis. Hyperventilation is an early response to active or passive heating, and the acidosis is usually due to elevated lactate levels. Common electrolyte abnormalities include hypernatremia or hyponatremia, depending on the relative amount of water and salt loss; hyperkalemia in the setting of renal failure or metabolic acidosis or hypokalemia secondary to potassium loss or respiratory alkalosis. Hypocalcemia, hypophosphatemia, and hypomagnesemia are common. Elevations of amylase, serum glutamic oxaloacetic transaminase (SGOT), bilirubin, uric acid, and creatine phosphokinase (CPK) levels are frequently seen and are of greater magnitude in exertional than classic heat stroke. Venous lactate levels and results of liver function tests may be predictive of outcome.

Differential diagnosis. A number of conditions present in a fashion similar to clinical heat stroke. Systemic infections, particularly meningitis, should be considered and excluded by blood and/or cerebrospinal fluid cultures if necessary. Alcohol or sedative/hypnotic withdrawal may mimic heat stroke with hyperthermia, altered mental status, and seizures. Acute or chronic salicylate intoxication may exhibit the same triad and this diagnosis is often overlooked in the elderly. Other diagnoses that should be entertained include anticholinergic poisoning, thyroid storm, and malignant neuroleptic syndrome.

Prognosis. Factors associated with mortality in heat stroke include advanced age, hypotension on presentation, altered mental status, and initial temperature greater than or equal to 42° C. Prognostic laboratory features include prolonged coagulation times, elevated liver function test results, and increased venous lactate levels.

Treatment. Therapy for heat stroke involves general supportive measures, rapid cooling techniques, and specific treatment of complications. All victims should be transported to a well-equipped emergency center if possible and core temperatures should be continuously monitored. A protected airway should be established, by endotracheal intubation if necessary, and adequate ventilation with 100% oxygen should be given until core temperature is controlled. For altered mental status, intravenous access should be established and glucose, thiamine, and naloxone given. One case series documented a high incidence of hypoglycemia among heat stroke victims.

Rapid cooling of hyperthermic patients is essential; ideally the core temperature should be lowered within 1 hour. Cooling efforts should stop when core temperature reaches 38.5° C to prevent iatrogenic hypothermia. Direct ice application with fanning to promote evaporative heat loss is the most widely used method and results in rapid cooling. Immersion in ice water has been used but is cumbersome and interferes with patient monitoring. An evaporative cooling method using warm air currents and cool mist has been advocated by some and allows for continued vasodilation during cooling. Although this method may allow more effective heat dissipation, it can be argued that peripheral vasoconstriction resulting from ice application is important in managing hypotension. Invasive measures including administration of iced intravenous fluids and iced gastric or peritoneal lavage have been used in cases of malignant hyperthermia but probably have no role in the management of heat stroke. There are no controlled studies comparing different cooling methods. Phenothiazines have been recommended to control shivering resulting from rapid body cooling, but they also lower seizure thresholds, aggravate hypotension, and have anticholinergic effects and should not be used routinely.

Fluid requirements are usually small and replacement should initially consist of 1200 to 1500 ml of crystalloid solution. If hypotension persists, a pulmonary artery catheter should be placed to guide fluid therapy. Dopamine or dobutamine may be required to maintain adequate blood pressure. Acidosis and electrolyte abnormalities should be treated in the standard fashion.

Seizures that complicate heat stroke generate additional body heat, lactate, and myoglobin and should be aggressively treated by anticonvulsants with paralysis if necessary. If elevation of serum CPK level or myoglobinuria indicates rhabdomyolysis, forced diuresis with mannitol and urine alkalinization is indicated to prevent renal failure.

Prevention. Epidemic heat stroke occurs in a predictable fashion during periods of high sustained ambient temperatures, particularly when associated with high humidity and low wind velocity. The military has successfully used indices of climatic heat stress to estimate exertional heat stroke risk and decrease heat-related morbidity among military recruits. Specific temperature/humidity/wind velocity indices indicating heat illness risk for the general public have yet to be widely utilized. Surveillance for heat stroke cases at public hospitals that serve high-risk populations is important to prevention.

Preventive measures during heat waves should include informing the public of risk, spending time in air-conditioned places (commercial malls, public shelters), decreasing strenuous activity, increasing fluid intake, and cautioning those taking major tranquilizers. Salt loading with commercially available salt tablets should be discouraged because of consequent electrolyte abnormalities.

Hypothermia

Epidemiology. Exposure to cold caused 7450 deaths from 1976 through 1985, and most of these were due to hypothermia. Risk factors for hypothermia include extremes of age, alcohol abuse, trauma, and underlying medical conditions.

Pathophysiology. Hypothermia is arbitrarily defined as a core body temperature of less than 35° C. Hypothermia is classified as mild if core temperature is 32° C or above, and profound is less than 32° C.

The earliest physiologic derangement that occurs in mild hypothermia is a rise in central blood volume caused by peripheral vasoconstriction. In subjects with borderline cardiac function, this increase in central blood volume may be sufficient to cause pulmonary edema. Increased central blood volume induces a "cold diuresis," which eventually results in significant intravascular volume depletion. If profound hypothermia develops, this diuresis is exacerbated by depressed renal tubular cell oxidative metabolism and reduced water and sodium reabsorption, causing further volume depletion. In addition, intravascular fluid shifts into the interstitial and intracellular fluid compartments, producing peripheral edema and slight intracellular edema. This intravascular volume depletion results in hemoconcentration and increased blood viscosity. This may account for increases in coronary and cerebral thromboses that occur in low environmental temperatures. Additional reported hematologic effects of hypothermia include thrombocytopenia and disseminated intravascular coagulation.

Cardiac output and heart rate initially increase on exposure to cold, then progressively decrease as core temperature falls. Blood pressure and systemic vascular resistance are maintained by increases in serum catecholamine levels and peripheral vascular tone. At core temperatures below 32° C pulse pressure may be difficult to palpate. Cardiac conduction is delayed and atrial fibrillation with a slow ventricular response is common. Myocardial irritability progressively increases and at temperatures of less than 28° C spontaneous ventricular fibrillation occurs. Osborne or J waves, positive deflections of the R-T segments, are highly suggestive of hypothermia and may be the initial clue to its diagnosis.

Brain metabolism and cerebral blood flow decrease with hypothermia, and increased blood viscosity further impairs cerebral microcirculation. Nerve conduction is slowed, leading to depressed deep tendon reflexes. Pupillary responses are sluggish and eventually disappear. In profound hypothermia, the patient may appear clinically dead. Patients with core temperatures as low as 17° C have been revived, thus resuscitation efforts should not cease until core temperature reaches 30° C.

The pulmonary effects of progressive hypothermia include an early cold-induced increase in bronchial secretions and respiratory depression at extremely low body temperatures. Aspiration pneumonia is common because of this cold-induced bronchorrhea in combination with depressed mental status and decreased cough reflexes.

The oxyhemoglobin dissociation curve is shifted to the left and characterized by increasing affinity for oxygen with decreasing body temperature. This is usually not clinically significant because of concomitantly decreased oxygen requirements in hypothermic tissues. This decrease in metabolic rate and tissue oxygen requirement may account for the survival of some hypothermic patients after prolonged periods of cardiopulmonary arrest. Arterial blood gases usually reveal an acidosis that is multifactorial. A respiratory acidosis secondary to ventilatory failure may be combined with a lactic acidosis secondary to tissue ischemia, muscle shivering, and decreased clearance of lactic acid by the hypothermic liver. During rewarming, lactate levels rise as a result of muscle shivering and mobilization of lactate from reperfused tissues.

Serum electrolyte levels are usually normal. Hyponatremia should suggest a complicating disorder such as hypothyroidism or adrenal insufficiency. Hypophosphatemia has been reported during recovery from hypothermia, and rhabdomyolysis may occasionally occur.

Gastrointestinal motility is decreased and all hepatic functions, including clearance of administered drugs and utilization of glucose, are depressed with hypothermia. Pancreatitis is common; however, amylase values are often elevated in the absence of clinical pancreatitis.

Endocrine responses to hypothermia include decreases in most pituitary hormones, including adrenocorticotropic hormone (ACTH) and antidiuretic hormone (ADH). Thyroid-stimulating hormone (TSH) levels have been reported to rise by some investigators. Serum cortisol and catecholamine levels rise sharply on exposure to cold then progressively fall. Insulin release decreases with body cooling, and peripheral glucose uptake is also depressed, resulting in marked hyperglycemia. These abnormalities are reversed by rewarming. Exogenous insulin given to the hypothermic subject is ineffective until rewarming occurs but may cause iatrogenic hypoglycemia at that time, especially if muscle shivering depletes glycogen stores.

Clinical features. *Chronic* or *urban hypothermia* generally occurs in those with predisposing conditions such as advanced age, alcoholism, or chronic underlying disease. It often exhibits minimal signs and symptoms. The victim may have only mild mental status changes, slurred speech, and incoordination. It is important to remember that extreme environmental conditions are not required to precipitate hypothermia. In subjects with predisposing factors, the diagnosis must be strongly suspected. *Acute* or *immersion hypothermia* occurs in healthy individuals who are exposed to extreme environmental conditions. It has an excellent prognosis if of short duration.

Many medical conditions are associated with hypothermia, and their diagnosis may be obscured in the hypothermic patient. Alcohol is the most common cause of urban hypothermia. Ethanol intoxication impairs behavioral responses and causes cutaneous vasodilatation, anesthesia, and occasionally hypoglycemia. Alcohol is also a risk factor for trauma and environmental exposure. Wernicke's encephalopathy has been reported in association with hypothermia.

Trauma and drug overdose often result in prolonged exposure and hypothermia, and in these settings the precipitating factor may be overlooked. Therapeutic doses of phenothiazines impair shivering thermogenesis and predispose the individual to hypothermia. Patients with skin disorders may lose dermal barriers to heat loss and become hypothermic.

Several metabolic abnormalities predispose to hypothermia, including hypothyroidism, in which low levels of thyroxine and insufficient calorigenesis lead to lower core temperatures. The mortality rate in myxedema is clearly related to the degree of hypothermia. Chronic hypothermia may also mimic myxedema with edema, abdominal distress, ileus, and delayed relaxation phase of deep tendon reflexes. Hypothermia associated with hypoglycemia is common and is found in approximately 50% of cases. Low body temperature may be the only clue to this diagnosis. Diabetic ketoacidosis and, importantly, sepsis are commonly associated with hypothermia.

Hypothalamic disorders including tumors, trauma, or degenerative disease may result in altered thermoregulation. Shapiro's syndrome consists of episodic hypothermia associated with agenesis of the corpus callosum. Idiopathic spontaneous periodic hypothermia without an obvious neurologic lesion has been reported. Spinal cord injury at the first thoracic level interrupts hypothalamic and sympathetic outflow with impaired vasoconstriction and shivering responses to cold exposure.

Treatment. The most common error in evaluating the hypothermic patient is inaccurately measuring core body temperature. Standard thermometers have readings to 34.5° C and are often only shaken down to 34.5° to 36° C. Any patient with an oral temperature of 35° C should have core temperature assessed by a low-reading glass thermometer or thermocouple with a rectal probe. Blood pressures may be difficult to measure because of vasoconstriction and Doppler ultrasound measurements may be necessary.

After establishing the diagnosis of hypothermia, continuous electrocardiographic monitoring is mandatory. The patient is usually markedly volume depleted, and rewarming exacerbates this problem by decreasing peripheral vascular resistance. Early rapid volume expansion with crystalloid solution should be initiated while following blood pressure and urine output. Peripheral veins should be used if accessible; if central venous catheters are necessary, care should be taken to prevent irritation of the myocardium. Military antishock trousers (MASTs) are contraindicated, as the mobilization of cold peripheral blood may precipitate ventricular fibrillation. The patient should be handled gently as the cold, bradycardic heart is extremely irritable and ventricular fibrillation or asystole may be provoked by minor physical trauma during transport, chest compressions, endotracheal intubation, or esophageal probe placement. In profound hypothermia detecting vital signs may be difficult. If spontaneous respirations and a heart beat are detected, chest compressions or pacemaker placement should be avoided even in the absence of a detectable pulse or blood pressure. If electrocardiographic monitoring reveals ventricular fibrillation or asystole, chest compressions and electrical and initial pharmacologic therapy should be attempted; however, the hypothermic heart is relatively resistant to therapy and rapid rewarming measures should be pursued. Defibrillation for persistent ventricular fibrillation should be repeated with every rise in core temperature of 2° to 4° C.

Supplemental oxygen should be provided. Correction of hypoxemia may prevent ventricular fibrillation associated with intubation; thus adequate preoxygenation should precede intubation attempts.

Hypothermia should suggest the diagnosis of hypoglycemia, and this should be ruled out on presentation to the emergency department. Hyperglycemia should be treated only if severe as glucose levels normalize on rewarming.

Empiric antibiotics are controversial, but given that infection is frequently masked by hypothermia, broad-spectrum antibiotics should be considered until culture results are available.

Rewarming techniques include passive external, active external, and active internal methods. For mild hypothermia all techniques work well. Passive external rewarming with an insulating blanket should result in a 0.5° C per hour rise in core temperature. If the rate of rise is slower, a complicating disorder such as hypothyroidism or infection should be suspected.

Active external rewarming techniques such as use of warming blankets or immersion in warm water carry the risk of rewarming shock and core temperature "after drop." With surface rewarming peripheral vascular resistance falls and pre-existing volume depletion may precipitate hypovolemic shock. With active external rewarming a drop in core temperature is often observed before temperature begins to rise. After a drop in temperature this may result from mobilization of peripheral cold blood from the extremities induced by rewarming. Cold blood with high lactate levels returning to the central circulation has been implicated as a cause of ventricular fibrillation during active external rewarming. For these reasons active external rewarming techniques should be avoided, particularly in the elderly.

Active internal rewarming techniques include warm peritoneal, gastric, or colonic lavage; heated inspired oxygen; warm intravenous solutions; partial cardiopulmonary bypass with a heat exchanger; hemodialysis; and thoracotomy with mediastinal lavage. Active core rewarming minimizes rewarming shock and acidosis and avoids core temperature after drop. For the profoundly hypothermic patient with stable cardiac status, a combination of passive external rewarming and heating of oxygen to 42° to 46° C is effective and safe. A portable inhalation rewarming device is presently the only core rewarming mechanism available for use in the field. Intravenous fluids warmed to 40° C may be used; however, add only small amounts of heat to the body. Some authors advise peritoneal dialysis or partial cardiopulmonary bypass with a heat exchanger for stable patients with core temperatures of 28° C or below. In the patient with cardiovascular instability, peritoneal dialysis with rapid 2 L exchanges of potassium-free solution warmed to 40° C is an effective and rapidly instituted method of core rewarming.

There are no randomized, controlled studies of different rewarming techniques. The prognosis of hypothermia is determined principally by the presence or absence of underlying disease rather than by the rewarming method used.

Prevention. Prevention of hypothermia must involve education and efforts directed at members of high-risk populations, particularly chronic alcoholics, the homeless, and the elderly. Provision of shelters for the homeless and fuel assistance programs may have the most pronounced effects.

NEAR-DROWNING

Epidemiology

The term *drowning* refers to death of submersion within 24 hours of the event. *Near-drowning* means that the submersion victim survived for at least 24 hours.

An average of 6503 annual deaths of drowning occurred in the United States from 1978 to 1984. It is a common cause of injury deaths, particularly among young children and young adults. Drowning is second only to motor vehicle accidents as a cause of death in young children.

Drownings occur in recreational areas, pools, and bathtubs, but any collection of water is a potential drowning source. A series of toddler drownings in large-capacity plastic buckets taken home from the workplace was recently reported.

Risk factors for drowning include male sex, home swimming pools, age less than 5 years or 15 to 24 years, and poverty. Among young adults alcohol and other drug use is a common factor. Medical conditions characterized by sudden losses of consciousness such as epilepsy, hypoglycemia, and cardiac arrhythmias may precipitate the submersion event.

Pathophysiology

After submersion, panic ensues, and a period of violent struggling with potential aspiration of fluid occurs. Victims occasionally experience persistent laryngospasm, allowing asphyxiation without aspiration. More commonly, initial breath holding and laryngospasm subside, allowing aspiration with resultant asphyxia and death.

After immersion in cold water, body temperature falls rapidly as the thermal conductivity of cold water is 32 times greater than that of air. If large volumes of cold water are aspirated or swallowed, rapid drops in core body temperature may occur while cardiac activity is still present with resultant central nervous system (CNS) hypothermia. In many cases of cold water immersion, progressive hypothermia results in loss of consciousness and subsequent aspiration and asphyxia. If the victim is supported by a life preserver, aspiration may not occur and deep hypothermia may precede cardiac arrest. Deep core and central nervous system hypothermia may allow for meaningful neurologic recovery after long periods of submersion. In cold water, submersion times of 45 minutes have been reported with full recovery. Given the potential for recovery, particularly in the young after cold water submersion, immediate cardiopulmonary resuscitation and transfer to an emergency department should occur in all cases.

The most pronounced physiologic derangements in near-drowning cases occur in the pulmonary, cardiovascular, and central nervous systems. The cause of death is generally asphyxiation, with resultant cardiac arrest.

With aspiration of water and particulate matter, loss of pulmonary surfactant and alveolar inflammation occurs, with resulting ventilation-perfusion mismatching and decreased pulmonary compliance. Depending on the amount of fluid aspirated, clinical effects may occur immediately or be delayed up to 24 hours.

Myocardial injury and cardiac arrhythmias in near-drowning result from hypoxia and acidosis secondary to asphyxiation. Rarely, ventricular fibrillation may occur secondary to immersion in ice cold water.

Cerebral hypoxia, ischemia, and traumatic spinal cord injury are the major central nervous system insults seen after submersion events. Cerebral injury may continue after resuscitation as a result of increased intracranial pressure and brain edema. Other less common physiologic effects of submersion include electrolyte imbalances, hemolysis, and disseminated intravascular coagulation. Coexisting hypothermia may cause additional derangements.

Clinical presentation and treatment

At the scene, rescue effort must be performed with care to protect the cervical spine from further injury as many near-drownings involve falls or diving with initial cervical spine fracture. All patients should receive supplemental oxygen. Cardiopulmonary resuscitation should begin as soon as is practical during rescue maneuvers. Unless the duration of submersion is known to be long or the patient is known to be normothermic, resuscitation efforts should continue until transfer to an emergency department. The Heimlich maneuver may be used to clear the airway if evidence of upper airway obstruction exists; however, it is not indicated to clear the lower airways of aspirated fluid and increases the risk of aspiration of gastric contents.

After successful cardiopulmonary resuscitation and preferably in the emergency department, neurologic status should be assessed by a standardized classification method (Table 368-1).

Table 368-1. Postsubmersion neurological classification (assessed in emergency room within one hour after rescue)

Category	Description	Glasgow coma scale (10)
A (Awake)	Alert, fully conscious	15
B (Blunted)	Obtunded, stuporous but rousable; purposeful response to pain; normal respirations	10-13
C (Comatose)	Comatose, not rousable; abnormal response to pain; abnormal respirations	
C subcategories (Coma Scale)		
C1 (Decorticate)	Flexion response to pain, Cheyne-Stokes respiration	5
C2 (Decerebrate)	Extensor response to pain, central (?) hyperventilation	4
C3 (Flaccid)	No response to pain, apneustic or "cluster" breathing	3
C4 (Deceased ?)	Flaccid, apneic, no detectable circulation	<3

From Conn AW, Barker GA: Can Anaesth Soc J 31:S38, 1984.

Hospital management involves observation of the minimally symptomatic patient for 12 to 24 hours for evolution of pulmonary injury. Patients with evidence of pulmonary injury on arrival require oxygenation with positive airway pressure by mask or endotracheal intubation, if necessary. Hypothermia should be treated in the usual fashion. Patients with evidence of increased intracranial pressure require cautious diuresis, controlled hyperventilation, and muscular paralysis. Direct measurement of intracranial pressure may be indicated. Although present results are not encouraging, efforts to prevent cerebral injury with barbituates and calcium channel blockers may be useful.

During the evaluation and treatment of near-drowning victims, consideration must be given to other conditions, including cervical spine injury, intracranial mass lesions, and drug intoxication that may have been present on arrival, and complicating conditions, such as pneumonia, that may evolve.

The prognosis of submersion events is related to the age and sex of the victim, time submerged, effectiveness of initial resuscitation efforts, presence and degree of hypothermia, and critical care.

Prevention

In Los Angeles, half of all drownings, and the vast majority of drownings in young children, occur in residential pools. Barrier methods that restrict entry to the pool are required by law in many areas and have been demonstrated to decrease the incidence of this preventable event. Swimming lessons are not advisable until at least age 4 as very early training may actually increase the risk of drowning in children because of increased exposure and increased parental complacency at a time when children are physically unable to coordinate swimming and breathing at the same time.

BITES AND STINGS

Reptiles

Crotalidae. In the United States representatives of the Crotalidae family, or pit vipers, include the rattlesnake, water moccasin or cottonmouth, and copperhead. They may be identified by their characteristic facial pits, between the eye and nostril; elliptical pupils; single row of ventral scales; and triangular head. They account for almost all snake envenomations in the United States, primarily in the southern and southwestern states.

Epidemiology. Victims of snakebite tend to be young adult males. Almost all bites are on the extremities. Bites on the lower extremities are often due to innocent disturbing of snakes, whereas bites on the upper extremities may be more often due to persons' choosing to expose themselves to the risk of snakebites. Alcohol use is often associated with the bite. Snake activity is temperature dependent, with increasing activity in warm weather.

Pathophysiology. Pit viper venom is complex and varies in composition among species. It includes low-molecular-weight enzymatic proteins that cause tissue necrosis, hemolysis, and coagulopathy. Venom is usually deposited subcutaneously, limiting tissue necrosis. If it is deposited within extremity compartments, myonecrosis is more extensive and complicated by increased fascial compartment pressures with resultant ischemia. If venom is injected intravascularly, systemic effects may be rapid and severe. In addition to local tissue necrosis, envenomation can cause disseminated intravascular coagulation, platelet aggregation, and increased vascular permeability, resulting in hypovolemic shock.

Clinical presentation. The severity of envenomation in snakebite is dependent on the amount of venom injected, potency of the venom, and health status of the victim. Many snakebites do not result in sufficient envenomation to cause symptoms. After envenomation occurs, the victim generally feels local pain that is not particularly severe. Local edema occurs rapidly and progresses over hours with purpura and ecchymosis reflecting increased local vascular permeability and tissue necrosis. Significant systemic envenomation is suggested by facial paresthesias, hemodynamic instability, or evidence of coagulopathy.

Treatment. Field treatment of the snakebite victim should consist of immobilization of the extremity and transfer to an emergency department. Local suction devices may be useful. The use of incisions, tourniquets, and cryotherapy is not recommended and may increase morbidity. Recent reports of use of electric shock therapy have not been supported by experimental evidence, and it should not be used. On arrival in the emergency department, severity of envenomation should be assessed by a standardized grading system (see the box above). This will guide therapy, specifically use of antivenin. All moderate or severe envenomations require antivenin. An attempt to identify the species of snake by description or examination of the (preferably dead) animal may be aided by consultation of a herpetologist. Consultation of a regional poison control center is advisable unless the treating physician is experienced in the management of snakebites.

Degrees of crotalid envenomation

No envenomation: fang marks; no local or systemic reactions.

Minimal envenomation: fang marks; local swelling and pain, but no systemic reactions.

Moderate envenomation: fang marks and swelling progress beyond the site of the bite; systemic signs and symptoms, such as nausea, vomiting, paresthesias, and/or laboratory orthostatic changes, hemoconcentration, and mild coagulation parameter changes.

Severe envenomation: fang marks present with marked swelling of the extremity, subcutaneous ecchymosis, severe symptoms, and marked coagulopathy with thrombocytopenia, hypofibrinogenemia, prolonged prothrombin and partial thromboplastin times, increased fibrin split products, increased CPK, proteinuria and hematuria.

From Auerbach PS, Geehr EC: Management of wilderness and environmental emergencies, ed 2, St. Louis, 1989, Mosby-Yearbook.

If the victim has no evidence of envenomation after 6 hours of observation and coagulation profiles are normal, he or she may be released after routine wound care and assessment of tetanus immunity. The snake's mouth harbors gram-negative and anaerobic organisms; thus broad-spectrum antibiotic therapy is indicated in most cases.

Polyvalent Crotalidae antivenin is commercially available from Wyeth Laboratories. It is produced from equine hyperimmune serum by immunizing horses with mixtures of four venoms and an immune system adjuvant. Complications of administration to humans are common and include acute anaphylaxis and anaphylactoid reactions as well as serum sickness.

If it is determined that significant envenomation has occurred and antivenin is indicated, it should be administered as soon as possible. Skin testing before administration of antivenin is recommended but is of limited value because of its poor sensitivity and specificity for predicting anaphylactic reactions. Results of skin testing may guide the physician in assessing need for dilution of antivenin and pretreatment with diphenhydramine.

Antivenin is most effective within 2 hours of the bite. Tissue necrosis after snakebite is related to receiving too little antivenin and receiving it too late. Early use of antivenin controls both extremity intracompartmental pressures and presumably destructive damage of the venom itself.

Routine surgical fasciotomy is of little or no value, and fasciotomy is never a substitute for administration of antivenin. If fasciotomy is considered to be indicated by rising compartmental pressures, prior antivenin administration decreases bleeding complications from the procedure and may altogether obviate the need for fasciotomy.

Prevention. Many snakebites are preventable. One should be alert to the presence of rattlesnakes in warm weather and wear adequate protective clothing when in their territory. Move away from rattlesnakes after recognizing their presence. Do not keep snakes as pets. Children bitten by pet snakes should be evaluated for evidence of abuse.

Elapidae. The Elapidae family includes the eastern and western coral snakes, found in the southeastern United States, and in Arizona and New Mexico, respectively. The elapids have many nonvenomous mimics and may be identified by their round pupils, double row of ventral scales, and distinctive red bordered by yellow band coloration.

Human envenomation by the coral snake is uncommon. The bite produces little pain and envenomation chiefly produces neurologic and cardiologic effects. Limb paresthesias, progressing to ptosis, diplopia, and muscle fasciculation and weakness, occur within hours. Death is rare and results from ventilatory and cardiac failure. The course of envenomation is difficult to predict at the time of presentation. Suspected bites of the eastern coral snake require antivenin treatment. Contact with a regional poison control center is advised, given the infrequent nature of coral snakebites.

Arthropods

Hymenoptera—wasps, bees, and ants

Epidemiology. The order Hymenoptera includes bees, wasps, and ants. An increased risk of exposure to insect stings is found among adult males and those who are occupationally exposed, including beekeepers, house painters, and operators of heavy equipment. Most stings occur in the late summer and early fall. Adults tend to have more serious reactions than children.

The honeybee is widespread and colonies nest in hollow tree trunks or are maintained in commercial hives. Of considerable economic and medical importance is the spread of Africanized bees from Brazil northward. These colonies are more aggressive and easily disturbed than native honeybee colonies and have accounted for many fatal attacks in South America. The first Africanized bee sting in the United States was recently reported in Texas.

Paper wasps and hornets commonly build their nests close to human dwellings, under eaves or in tree branches. Yellow jackets build nests in the ground or in natural cavities in walls or tree trunks.

Ants are widely distributed in the United States, but the species of greatest medical importance is the imported fire ant, which arrived in Alabama early in this century and now infests many of the southern states. These ants have been resistant to control efforts and will likely continue to spread through large sections of the southeastern and western United States.

Pathophysiology. The venom of hymenopteran species consists of a mixture of polypeptide toxins and enzymes. They contain histamine, serotonin, acetylcholine, and a wide variety of allergens. Many of the local reactions to insect stings are due to various vasoactive amines, peptides, and enzymes, but allergic reactions are the more important, resulting in 25 to 40 deaths annually in the United States. Of the general population 1% to 3% report a systemic reaction to insect stings. Some cases of sudden death may represent undiagnosed insect sting anaphylaxis.

Clinical manifestations. Local reactions to insect stings consist of pain, erythema, and edema. Fire ant stings often produce sterile pustules within the first 24 hours, and in a large proportion of victims severe local reactions with extensive edema and erythema develop over the next 2 to 3 days.

Systemic allergic reactions occur within the first few minutes to hours and may include urticaria, nausea, bronchoconstriction, and hypotension. Delayed reactions over the first 1 to 2 weeks after a sting are uncommon; they have included serum sickness as well as immune-mediated nephrotic syndrome, thrombocytopenia, hepatitis, and neurologic disorders.

Treatment. The treatment of an insect sting reaction is straightforward, with cold compresses and antihistamines for local reactions and epinephrine, volume support, pressors, and bronchodilators as needed for the management of anaphylactic reactions.

Prevention. Persons with a history of systemic reactions to hymenoptera stings carry a 35% to 60% risk of anaphylaxis on repeated stings. They should avoid exposure as much as is practical and should not be alone in typical exposure settings. Many hypersensitive persons do not follow advice to change occupation or abandon beekeeping. An epinephrine kit should be prescribed and patients should be instructed in its use.

Venom immunotherapy is extremely effective in preventing systemic reactions in hypersensitive persons. Persons with a history of a systemic sting reaction should be referred to immunotherapy evaluation. Children suffering urticarial reactions only, without airway obstruction or hypotension, are not at increased risk of more severe systemic reactions on repeated stings and should not have immunotherapy.

Lepidoptera

Epidemiology. The Lepidoptera, moths and butterflies, and more specifically their larval forms, the caterpillar, in addition to their potential for economic impact are relatively common but rarely serious causes of human stings. A few species produce poorly characterized venoms contained in spines (setae) found on the surface of the caterpillar. Occupational and recreational exposure to areas of caterpillar infestation results in stings when humans brush against the caterpillar as it clings to vegetation.

The most common species causing human symptoms is the puss caterpillar, *Megalopyge opercularis,* also known as the asp, or perrito ("little dog"), which is approximately 3 cm long and covered with thick brown hairs. It lives in the southeastern United States and causes periodic outbreaks of cutaneous dermatitis in Texas. The incidence of stings is seasonal, usually in the summer and early fall. The gypsy moth caterpillar, *Lymantria dispar,* has been responsible for epidemic dermatitis in the northeastern United States, during late spring and early summer.

Clinical manifestations. Caterpillar dermatitis is characterized by an immediate painful, erythematous, grid-like rash corresponding to points of contract with the venomous setae, or the reaction may be delayed for 24 to 48 hours, with development of papules and vesicles. Systemic symptoms are rare and no deaths directly attributable to lepidoptera have been documented. Stings of *M. opercularis* are particularly painful and symptoms may last for 1 to 2 weeks.

Treatment. Stripping the site of the bite with tape has been reported to be useful in diagnosing the cause of the sting and may remove toxins, thus lessening the severity of the reaction. Microscopic examination may reveal the characteristic setae or spines responsible for introducing the cutaneous toxin. Symptomatic treatment involves analgesics as required for pain; the *M. opercularis* sting often requires parenteral and oral narcotics for relief of severe pain. Topical antipruritic and corticosteroid preparations may provide relief from local pruritus, and systemic corticosteroids have been reported to be effective.

Spiders. There are more than 30,000 known species of spiders, of which only 60 have been implicated in human illness. Most spiders have venom glands, but bites resulting in significant envenomation are rare, likely because venom quantities are small and most bites do not break the skin. In the United States the brown recluse spider *(Loxosceles reclusa)* and the black widow spider *(Latrodectus mactans)* are of importance. They are discussed in the following sections.

Loxosceles species

Epidemiology. The brown recluse spider, *Loxosceles reclusa,* is widely distributed but is concentrated in the central and southwestern United States. It often cohabitates with humans, preferring warm, dry areas such as closets, and woodpiles. The spider has a nondescript appearance, of medium size with varying shades of brown coloration, and a characteristic violin-shaped marking on the dorsal cephalothorax, giving it its common name, "fiddle-back" spider.

Most bites occur during the period from late spring to early fall. The actual incidence of symptomatic bites is difficult to determine. The bite usually results in only minor local symptoms. When bites receive medical attention, the spider is rarely available for identification; thus any necrotic skin lesion suspected to be a spider bite is assumed to be due to the brown recluse, likely causing its incidence to be overestimated. Bites of the brown recluse are much more common than those of the black widow spider (discussed later).

Clinical manifestations. The vast majority of brown recluse spider bites lead to no serious complications and cause only transient skin irritation. *Loxoscelism* is the reaction to bites of the brown recluse; it occurs in two forms: cutaneous, or "necrotic arachnidism," and, rarely, systemic loxoscelism. Symptoms that result from the bite do so within 6 to 12 hours. After an initial transient stinging sensation, local pain and erythema develop; they are followed by a central bleb or pustule. Erythema and edema surrounding the central bleb may display an irregular dependent distribution, corresponding to gravitational spread of venom. As the skin lesion progresses over the first 2 to 3 days, the center becomes violaceous and depressed, with gradual development of a black eschar, which eventually sloughs, leaving a slow healing ulcer of variable size and depth. Necrosis tends to be more extensive and healing slower over areas with more subcutaneous fat. Healing of the ulcer may take weeks or months. The differential diagnosis of this necrotic ulcer is extensive (see the box below). Systemic loxoscelism is rare and occurs more often in children. Findings include fever, rash, hemolysis with resultant renal failure, and disseminated intravascular coagulation. No deaths

Differential diagnosis of *Loxosceles* (brown recluse) bites

Bites of spiders from other genera	Other insects brought in as "spiders"/other lesions
Aphonophena	Solpugids
Steatoda	Ticks (especially Ornithodoros coraceus)
Araneus	Assassin bugs
Argiope	Jerusalem crickets
Heteropoda	Grasshoppers
Misumenoides	Other orthopterans
Chiracanthium	Kissing bug (Triatoma protracta)
Drassodes	Infected flea bites
Lycosa	Imbedded tick mouth parts
Phidippus	Mite
	Bed bug
	Fly bite
	Hymenoptera stings

Admitted misdiagnosis of "brown recluse bite"

Erythema chronicum migrans
Stevens-Johnson syndrome
Lyell's syndrome (toxic epidermal necrolysis)
Erythema nodosum
Erythema multiforme
Periarteritis nodosa
Lymphoid papulosis
Pyoderma gangrenosum
Sporotrichosis
Keratin-mediated response to a fungus
Chronic herpes simplex
Infected herpes simplex
Gonococcal arthritis-dermatitis
Purpura fulminans
Diabetic ulcer
Bed sore
Poison oak
Poison ivy

From Ellenhorn M, Barceloux D: Medical toxicology diagnosis and treatment of human poisoning, New York, 1988, Elsevier.

caused by *L. reclusa* bites have been documented in the United States.

Treatment. Care of a necrotic skin lesion includes the nonspecific care of any wound: frequent cleansing, immobilization, elevation, and tetanus prophylaxis if indicated. Intermittent cool compresses may relieve pain. Antibiotics are indicated only for secondary wound infections, usually caused by the usual streptococcal or staphylococcal pathogens. Dapsone, a leukocyte inhibitor, has been used with largely anecdotal evidence of benefit. Because it may cause massive hemolysis in the presence of G6PD deficiency, levels of this enzyme should be measured. It may also cause methemoglobinemia. Given limited data supporting its efficacy, it should only be given for severe reactions to proven brown recluse spider bites. Surgical excision or skin grafting of any necrotic area should be delayed for 2 to 4 weeks to allow the wound margins to demarcate. The most common error in current management is premature surgical therapy.

Prevention. Prevention of *Loxosceles* bites is difficult. The spider is very resistant to eradication. Avoid habitats if possible. If exposure can be predicted, gloves and a layer of clothing may prevent bites. If a bite does occur and the spider can be retrieved safely, take it to the emergency department for identification.

Latrodectus

Epidemiology. The black widow spider, *Latrodectus mactans,* is found throughout the United States. The spider is shiny black with a red hourglass-shaped marking on the ventral surface. It prefers warm and dry environments and may be found in a wide variety of settings, including woodpiles, barns, and outdoor privies. Most bites occur in the late summer and early fall and are more common in the southwestern United States.

Pathophysiology. The venom of the black widow spider contains no inflammatory substances and causes little local reaction. The important component is alpha latrotoxin, a potent neurotoxin that affects the neuromuscular junction and the sympathetic and parasympathetic nervous systems.

Clinical manifestations. The bite itself is usually painless, and there is little local reaction other than a small area of erythema and edema. Within an hour of the bite, pain develops in muscles near the site and subsequently widespread muscle cramping, with severe pain, abdominal rigidity, and paresthesias may develop.

These systemic symptoms peak at 1 to 6 hours and may last for 24 to 48 hours. The victim may also suffer headaches, nausea, bronchorrhea, and, in severe cases, hypertension, seizures, and altered mental status. Laboratory findings in severe cases include hemoglobinuria, albuminuria, and leukocytosis. Rare deaths have been reported, usually in the very young or old.

Treatment. Most cases of latrodectism are not severe and do not require hospitalization. Muscle cramping and pain may be treated with intravenous calcium gluconate, with sedatives or analgesics as required. Methocarbamol (Robaxin) has also been used but may be inferior to calcium gluconate infusion. Severe presentations may require infusion of standard parenteral antihypertensive agents, such as nitroprusside or labetalol.

An equine antivenin is available but has been used infrequently in the United States. Allergic complications that arise from its use may cause more morbidity than the envenomation itself.

REFERENCES

Auerbach PS and Geehr EC, editors: Management of wilderness and environmental emergencies, ed 2. St Louis, 1989, Mosby.

Conn AW and Barker GA: Fresh water drowning and near-drowning—an update. Can Anaesth Soc J 31:S38, 1984.

Curry SC et al: The legitimacy of rattlesnake bites in central Arizona. Ann Emerg Med 18(6):658, 1989.

Delaney KA et al: Assessment of acid-base disturbances in hypothermia and their physiologic consequences. Ann Emerg Med 18(1):72, 1989.

deShazo RD, Butcher BT and Banks WA: Reactions to and the stings of the imported fire ant. N Engl J Med 323(7):462, 1990.

Elgart GW: Ant, bee, and wasp stings. Dermatol Clin 8(2):229, 1990.

Garfin SR et al: The effect of antivenin on intramuscular pressure elevations induced by rattlesnake venom. Toxicon 23(4):677, 1985.

Gendron BP: Loxosceles reclusa envenomation. Am J Emerg Med 8(1):51, 1990.

Gulaid JA and Sattin RW: Drownings in the United States, 1978-1984. MMWR CDC Surveill Summ 37(1):27, 1988.

Hart GR et al: Epidemic classical heat stroke: clinical characteristics and course of 28 patients. Medicine (Baltimore) 61(3):189, 1982.

Jones TS et al: Morbidity and mortality associated with the July 1980 heat wave in St Louis and Kansas City, Mo. JAMA 247(24):3327, 1982.

Leads from the MMWR: Hypothermia prevention. JAMA 261(4):513, 1989.

Li JT and Yunginger JW: Management of insect sting hypersensitivity. Mayo Clin Proc 67(2):188, 1992.

Moss HS and Binder LS: A retrospective review of black widow spider envenomation. Ann Emerg Med 16(2):188, 1987.

Shama SK et al: Gypsy-moth-caterpillar dermatitis. N Engl J Med 306(21):1300, 1982.

Wilson DC and King LE Jr: Spiders and spider bites. Dermatol Clin 8(2):277, 1990.

CHAPTER

369 Medical Disorders During Pregnancy

Richard S. Abrams
Robert E. Wall

While relatively few medical disorders can prevent pregnancy, virtually the entire spectrum of disease can complicate it. This chapter highlights some of the most frequently encountered medical disorders during pregnancy. Because of the large number of diseases covered, each discussion is brief. In each case, however, the unique interaction of medical disease and pregnancy is emphasized. Recommendations for treatment reflect the understanding that management of serious medical disorders frequently requires the use of medications potentially harmful to the fetus. Yet it is also understood that many untreated medical diseases are potentially just as detrimental to the fetus while jeopardizing the health of the mother as well.

ENDOCRINE DISORDERS

Diabetes mellitus, type I

Beginning in early gestation, glucose and various gluconeogenic amino acids reach the fetus against a concentration gradient by facilitated diffusion. Since maternal loss of glucose and gluconeogenic substrate to the fetus conspires to cause maternal hypoglycemia, it is often necessary to reduce the total daily insulin dosage during the first trimester.

At approximately 24 weeks' gestation, the so-called diabetogenic stress of pregnancy begins. At this time, basal insulin levels are higher than normal nongravid levels, and eating produces a two- to threefold greater outpouring of insulin. Increased plasma insulin is opposed by diminished responsiveness to insulin in the periphery. This insulin resistance is thought to result, at least in part, from the contraregulatory hormones such as human placental lactogen, prolactin, and cortisol produced by the placenta. Thus, in the second half of gestation, insulin requirements predictably increase in women with type I diabetes. In addition, gestational diabetes is most likely to begin at this time.

Major congenital anomalies remain the leading cause of death among infants of diabetic mothers. These anomalies are formed early in gestation, by 8 weeks after the last menstrual period. The teratogenic potential of hyperglycemia has now been confirmed by many animal and human studies. It is therefore mandatory to initiate diabetes education and optimal blood glucose control before conception to prevent major congenital malformations. A useful marker for this treatment goal is the near normalization of maternal glycohemoglobin concentration prior to attempting pregnancy. Similarly, good metabolic control prior to conception reduces the risk of spontaneous abortion to no greater than that of nondiabetic women.

Women with type I diabetes should be evaluated for signs of retinopathy, nephropathy, and hypertension prior to conception. Those with background retinopathy should undergo ophthalmoscopy with the pupils dilated at least monthly. Women in whom active proliferative retinopathy develops during any stage of pregnancy should receive panretinal scatter photocoagulation even if macular edema is aggravated. If severe neovascularization develops during the first trimester that does not respond to appropriate laser therapy, termination of pregnancy should be considered. Pregnancy may be attempted later after successful involution of the neovascularization. In patients with nephropathy, especially those with increased proteinuria, reduced creatinine clearance, or systemic hypertension, daily periods of bed rest, control of blood pressure, and careful glycemic control are essential. Patients should be hospitalized when necessary to meet these goals.

Table 369-1. O'Sullivan criteria for detecting gestational diabetes (100 g oral glucose tolerance test)

Interval	Whole blood* (mg/dl)	Plasma* (mg/dl)
Fasting	90	105
1 h	165	190
2 h	145	165
3 h	125	145

*Values represent two standard deviations above the mean.

Gestational diabetes

Gestational diabetes is defined as carbohydrate intolerance of variable severity with onset during the present pregnancy. The definition applies regardless of whether insulin is used for treatment or the condition persists after pregnancy, but it does not exclude the possibility that glucose intolerance may have antedated the pregnancy.

All pregnant women should be screened for glucose intolerance between the twenty-fourth and twenty-eighth gestational week with a 50 g oral glucose challenge. Screening based on glycosuria or clinical risk factors has been shown to be inadequate. A plasma glucose value of 140 mg per deciliter or greater 1 hour after a 50 g oral glucose dose indicates the need for a full diagnostic glucose tolerance test. It does not, by itself, establish the diagnosis. Diagnosis is based on results of the 100 g oral glucose tolerance test interpreted according to the diagnostic criteria of O'Sullivan and Mahan (Table 369-1).

All patients with gestational diabetes are at significant risk for fetal macrosomia with consequent birth trauma, as well as other neonatal complications, including hypoglycemia, hypocalcemia, and hyperbilirubinemia.

All women with gestational diabetes should receive appropriate nutritional and exercise counseling. If dietary management does not consistently maintain the fasting blood glucose concentration below 105 mg per deciliter or the 2 hour postprandial glucose concentration below 120 mg per deciliter, insulin therapy should be initiated. Oral hypoglycemic agents are contraindicated during pregnancy. If insulin is prescribed, only highly purified nonbeef preparations should be used to minimize antigenicity.

Women who had gestational diabetes should be evaluated at the first postpartum visit by a 2 hour, 75 g glucose tolerance test to detect overt diabetes.

Thyroid disease

Several special considerations of thyroid dysfunction during pregnancy should be kept in mind. First, signs and symptoms of disordered thyroid function may be mimicked by pregnancy itself. Second, increases in thyroid-binding proteins during pregnancy alter standard thyroid function tests. Third, placental transfer of most thyroid hormones is minimal. Finally, most antithyroid drugs freely cross the placenta and are potentially active in the fetal thyroid.

Profound hypothyroidism is often associated with impaired fertility and is uncommon during pregnancy. On the other hand, mild hypothyroidism is a frequent concomitant illness during pregnancy. Therapy consists of full thyroid hormone replacement. When replacement is adequate, thyroid-stimulating hormone levels return to normal, but this may take up to 8 weeks for maximum effect. There is no evidence to suggest that replacement dosages of thyroid medication suppress fetal thyroid function.

Graves' disease is the major cause of thyrotoxicosis in women of childbearing age and thus in pregnancy. The clinical course of Graves' disease is known to vary during gestation. Thyrotoxicosis often improves during pregnancy and worsens postpartum.

Since radioactive iodide therapy is contraindicated during pregnancy, therapeutic options include antithyroid medications and surgery. Two important points require emphasis before specific treatment of hyperthyroidism is considered. First, mild hyperthyroidism appears to be well tolerated during pregnancy. Second, antithyroid drugs freely cross the placenta and are active against the fetal thyroid.

Both propylthiouracil (PTU) and methimazole have been used successfully during pregnancy. PTU crosses the placenta only about one fourth as well as methimazole and is preferred for use during pregnancy. Propranolol has been used during pregnancy to control severe adrenergic symptoms before antithyroid medications have had sufficient time to take effect. Propranolol does not block production of thyroid hormone. Surgery should be reserved for patients with hypersensitivity to antithyroid drugs, for poorly compliant patients, and for the occasional patient in whom reasonable dosages of antithyroid drugs have been ineffective. Patients with Graves' disease who have undergone thyroidectomy may still have high concentrations of thyroid-stimulating immunoglobulin; consequently, their offspring are vulnerable to neonatal thyrotoxicosis.

Hyperparathyroidism

Primary hyperparathyroidism does not appear to impair fertility, but it is known to result in a high rate of fetal complications such as spontaneous abortions, stillbirths, and neonatal tetany. Maternal hyperparathyroidism causes maternal hypercalcemia, which in turn facilitates increased placental calcium transport. High fetal calcium concentrations suppress the fetal parathyroid so that after delivery the neonate is functionally hypoparathyroid. Deprived of its maternal source of calcium, the neonate becomes vulnerable to tetany in the immediate postpartum period.

Medical therapy for hyperparathyroidism during pregnancy is appropriate only for a short period. Surgical exploration of the neck is the recommended treatment for a pregnant patient with rising serum calcium concentration, worsening symptoms, or hyperparathyroid crisis unresponsive to medical therapy. Many authors believe that the high incidence of maternal and neonatal complications associated with hyperparathyroidism makes surgery the treatment of choice even if the disease is mild. Surgery should ideally be performed during the second trimester.

Pituitary adenomas

Prolactin-secreting adenomas account for approximately 30% of all pituitary adenomas. Fewer than 7% of patients with intrasellar microadenomas (size less than 10 mm) manifest clinical evidence of tumor expansion during pregnancy. On the other hand, macroadenomas (size greater than 10 mm) are associated with a 17% incidence of complications during pregnancy. Symptoms of headache, visual disturbance, and nausea are the most common. These symptoms tend to occur most frequently during the first trimester and can be mistaken for symptoms of pregnancy.

For patients with microadenomas treated with bromocriptine to achieve pregnancy, the drug should be discontinued as soon as pregnancy is diagnosed. It is generally accepted that periodic measurement of serum prolactin levels are of minimal benefit during pregnancy, since serum prolactin levels do not always rise with pregnancy-induced tumor enlargement. Because of the low incidence of microadenoma growth during pregnancy, it is not necessary to perform routine visual field testing. Routine clinical evaluation with particular attention to symptoms of headache and visual disturbances constitutes prudent follow-up. For patients with known microadenomas who become symptomatic, immediate computed tomography (CT) scanning or MRI is indicated.

For women with macroadenomas confined to the sella, the risk of enlargement during pregnancy is small. For women with larger macroadenomas that have suprasellar extension, there is a 15% to 35% risk of clinically significant tumor enlargement during pregnancy. Patients with suprasellar extension of their tumors should consider trans-sphenoidal tumor resection prior to conception. Unfortunately, tumor growth during gestation cannot be predicted by prepregnancy tumor size or serum prolactin concentration. Patients at highest risk include those with neurologic or visual symptoms before pregnancy.

All patients with macroadenomas should have monthly neurologic examinations and visual field tests. As with microadenomas, periodic serum prolactin levels are not helpful. CT scanning or MRI should be performed when tumor growth is clinically suspected. Bromocriptine can be used during pregnancy to decrease tumor size rapidly. In previously symptomatic patients with suprasellar extension, continuation of bromocriptine throughout pregnancy is prudent, since sudden reexpansion of the tumor has been reported. Surgery is rarely necessary.

There is no evidence that breast-feeding causes tumor enlargement. Nevertheless, patients with macroadenomas should be followed closely for symptoms or signs of tumor expansion during breast-feeding.

RENAL DISORDERS

Pregnancy is associated with a variety of anatomic and functional changes of the kidneys and lower urinary tract.

calyceal, pelvic, and ureteral dilatation occurs during the first trimester and persists throughout gestation up to 12 weeks postpartum. These changes are most prominent on the right side. Hydronephrosis and hydroureter have direct clinical consequences because urinary stasis contributes to the propensity to develop pyelonephritis in women with asymptomatic bacteriuria.

The most significant alteration in renal function during pregnancy is a progressive increase in the glomerular filtration rate, which begins as early as 2 weeks' gestation. Creatinine and urea production do not increase during pregnancy. Therefore, a serum concentration of creatinine and urea considered normal for a nonpregnant woman may be elevated in the gravida and should be investigated.

Acute renal failure

Acute renal failure during pregnancy most often results from severe preeclampsia or eclampsia. Management of acute renal failure during pregnancy is essentially the same as that for nonpregnant patients (see Chapter 347). Particular attention should be given to fluid and electrolyte balance and adequate nutrition.

Chronic renal failure

Many women with chronic renal disease have diminished fertility. Nevertheless, some patients with moderately severe disease and some who have received renal transplants do conceive. The major determinants of pregnancy outcome in women with chronic renal disease are the presence of hypertension and the severity of pregestational renal insufficiency.

The problem that poses the greatest maternal danger is severe hypertension, with its risk of central nervous system bleeding. Differentiating worsening hypertension and preeclampsia can be difficult.

The severity of renal insufficiency also has a direct effect on the outcome of pregnancy. Pregnancies in women with a pregestational serum creatinine concentration greater than 1.5 mg per deciliter or a creatinine clearance less than 80 ml per minute are associated with an increase in perinatal mortality and the onset or worsening of hypertension.

There is now considerable experience with pregnancy in women who have received renal transplants. These patients are advised to continue the same immunosuppressive therapy that they were receiving prior to conception. The high likelihood of rejection if the drugs are discontinued poses a greater risk to the mother and fetus than does the potential toxicity of the drugs.

HYPERTENSIVE DISORDERS

Hypertension is among the most commonly seen medical disorders of pregnancy. Up to 30% of pregnancies are complicated by hypertension. Chronic essential hypertension accounts for half of all cases. Pre-eclampsia occurs in 7% to 10% of pregnant women. Arterial blood pressure greater than 90 mm Hg diastolic and 140 mm Hg systolic or a rise in blood pressure more than 30 mm Hg diastolic over baseline warrant a diagnosis of hypertension. A useful classification of hypertensive disorders of pregnancy is presented in the box above.

Classification of hypertensive disorders of pregnancy

1. Pre-eclampsia, eclampsia
2. Chronic hypertension ($\geq$ 140/90 mm Hg)
3. Chronic hypertension with superimposed pre-eclampsia/eclampsia
4. Late or transient hypertension

Pre-eclampsia/eclampsia

Diagnosis. Pre-eclampsia is a multiorgan disease unique to pregnancy. The condition is characterized by the development of elevated blood pressure, proteinuria, and generalized edema. Eclampsia is the presence of generalized seizures or coma in a patient with pre-eclampsia. Except in unusual circumstances, pre-eclampsia occurs after 20 weeks gestation and prior to the seventh postpartum day. The vast majority of women who develop pre-eclampsia are nulliparous and frequently at the extremes of their child-bearing years. Chronic hypertension and underlying vascular disease increase the likelihood that superimposed pre-eclampsia will develop. Pregnant women with diastolic blood pressure consistently greater than 75 mm Hg in the second trimester or greater than 85 mm Hg in the third trimester should be observed closely for signs of pre-eclampsia.

It is clinically useful to separate pre-eclampsia into mild and severe disease. In most cases, the development of severe pre-eclampsia requires delivery, regardless of gestational age. The box below lists criteria frequently used to indicate severe disease if any are present. Even in mild

Signs and symptoms of severe pre-eclampsia

1. Blood pressure $\geq$ 160 mm Hg systolic or 110 mm Hg diastolic
2. Proteinuria $>$ 5 g/24 hours or 3+ or 4+ proteinuria as determined by dipstick
3. Oliguria $<$ 400 ml/24 hours
4. Epigastric or right upper quadrant pain
5. Abnormal coagulation tests (thrombocytopenia, prolonged PTT or PT, hypofibrinogenemia)
6. Elevated liver enzymes
7. Pulmonary edema
8. Persistent headache, visual disturbance, lethargy, clonus, or other signs of significant CNS irritability

disease, careful frequent evaluation is necessary because of the possibility of rapid deterioration and the development of eclampsia. Nearly 25% of eclamptics experience their first seizure with "mild" disease.

A subset of severe pre-eclamptic patients develop hemolysis (H), elevated liver enzymes (EL), and low platelets (LP), the so-called "HELLP Syndrome." These patients frequently have little blood pressure change and limited symptoms. The disease is characterized by rapid deterioration and death if prompt delivery and aggressive supportive therapy are not implemented. Unfortunately, this syndrome is frequently misdiagnosed as hepatitis, cholelithiasis, pyelonephritis, or other nonobstetric complications.

Pathophysiology. Diffuse vasospasm and increased sensitivity to vasopressors leading to diffuse endothial injury are present in patients with pre-eclampsia. All organ systems are affected. A decrease in plasma volume and hemoconcentration is typically observed. Most investigators now believe this vasospasm is caused by a relative or absolute deficiency in the production of the vasodilating prostaglandin, PGI_2 (prostacyclin). Some have advocated low-dose aspirin (60-80 mg/day) throughout pregnancy for patients at increased risk for developing pre-eclampsia. This therapy appears to increase the production of prostacyclin, preventing the development of pre-eclampsia. Although low-dose aspirin appears to be safe during pregnancy, this approach to the prevention of pre-eclampsia requires further clinical confirmation.

Management. Although some experts advocate hospital admission for all pre-eclamptic patients, reliable compliant women with mild disease who are remote from term may safely be managed as outpatients with total bed rest and frequent home blood pressure monitoring. Neither sodium nor fluid restriction is indicated. Weekly evaluation of kidney, liver, and coagulation function is mandatory. Weekly or twice-weekly antepartum fetal surveillance is required to ensure adequate placental function. Serial ultrasound evaluation of fetal growth every 2 to 3 weeks is required. Evidence of significant intrauterine growth retardation is an indication for delivery. If maternal and fetal conditions are stable, delivery near term or with biochemical evidence of fetal lung maturity prior to 37 weeks is advisable.

Severe pre-eclampsia or eclampsia requires delivery. Patients should be treated with magnesium sulfate, 4 to 8 grams, given intravenously over 10 to 20 minutes until normal or diminished deep tendon reflexes are achieved. Continuous intravenous administration of magnesium sulfate, 2 to 3 grams per hour, is usually required to maintain diminished reflexes and serum magnesium levels in the therapeutic range of 6 to 8 mEq per L. Respiratory depression can occur rapidly with intravenous infusion and may be reversed by slow intravenous administration of 10 ml of 10% calcium gluconate. Respiratory depression may be aggravated by concurrent use of narcotics or benzodiazepines. Oliguria decreases magnesium excretion, increasing the possibility of respiratory depression.

Arterial blood pressure of 180/110 mm Hg or higher requires treatment. Hydralazine is most often effective when administered in an intravenous bolus of 5 mg to 10 mg. Boluses may be repeated every 15 to 30 minutes if diastolic blood pressure remains at 110 mm Hg. Diastolic blood pressures below 90 mm Hg are undesirable because of the negative impact on uterine and placental blood flow. If blood pressure control is not achieved, labetalol, 50 mg intravenous bolus, may be necessary to lower diastolic blood pressure. Rarely sodium nitroprusside is required to control hypertensive crisis. Because of potential fetal cyanide toxicity, delivery should be prompt once blood pressure is controlled.

Recurrence of seizures in a pre-eclamptic patient requires administration of diazepam 10 mg followed by loading and maintenance infusions of magnesium sulfate as outlined above. Experience with phenytoin in pre-eclamptic seizures has been limited.

Vaginal delivery is usually possible once the patient with severe pre-eclampsia is stabilized. Prostaglandin cervical ripening and oxytocin induction can be used to achieve delivery even in patients with an unfavorable cervix. With rare exceptions, attempts at vaginal delivery should be made in most patients with severe pre-eclampsia or eclampsia. The majority of patients spontaneously begin diuresis within 24 to 36 hours after delivery. Swan-Ganz catheterization and hemodynamic monitoring are rarely required postpartum unless severe oliguria is encountered. Total fluid intake should be maintained at 2000 to 2500 ml per 24 hours.

Prognosis. Most pre-eclamptic primagravidas become normotensive shortly after delivery, although elevated blood pressure can persist in a minority of patients for up to 6 weeks. Hypertension that persists 12 weeks postpartum should be considered chronic and should be appropriately evaluated. The risk of recurrence of HELLP syndrome in subsequent pregnancies appears to be low.

Chronic hypertension

Diagnosis. Without documentation of elevated BP prior to pregnancy, chronic hypertension can only be presumed. The vast majority of patients who present with elevated blood pressure prior to the twentieth week of gestation, however, have chronic hypertension. Signs of long-standing hypertension in the retina or other organ systems strongly suggest the diagnosis. Women with chronic hypertension are at high risk of developing superimposed pre-eclampsia manifest by worsening hypertension, diffuse edema, or proteinuria. In patients with severe labile hypertension, a search for underlying vascular, renal, or endocrine causes should be considered.

Management. Complicating cardiac, renal, neurologic, and retinal disease must be excluded in all women with chronic hypertension, ideally prior to pregnancy. Women with significant hypertension requiring treatment should have their medications reviewed and, if necessary, changed appropriate for pregnancy. Recently use of low-dose aspirin 60-80 mg/day has been advocated to decrease the likelihood of superimposed pre-eclampsia. Patients with mild hypertension *not* on medication are generally treated conservatively during pregnancy with mild sodium restriction, increased bed rest, and daily home blood pressure measurements. Smoking must be eliminated. If blood pressure exceeds 140/100 mm Hg, oral antihypertensive medication is usually administered using the fewest number and safest drugs necessary to maintain diastolic blood pressure near 90 mm Hg. Lowering diastolic blood pressure consistently below 90 mm Hg is not desirable because uterine blood flow may be reduced and fetal growth impaired.

Methyldopa is currently the drug of choice in the United States for treating significant chronic hypertension during pregnancy. Hydralazine has also been used extensively with no evidence of fetal compromise. Use of beta-adrenergic blocking agents during pregnancy was originally condemned, though more recent reports have failed to demonstrate serious fetal or neonatal complications. Infrequent neonatal side effects include mild bradycardia and hypoglycemia. At least two prospective series using labetalol for treatment of chronic hypertension support its safety during pregnancy. The use of diuretics in pregnancy continues to be controversial. As long as maternal electrolytes remain normal, no detrimental effects have been observed in the fetus or neonate when diuretics have been initiated *prior to* pregnancy. Given the other alternatives available for treatment of hypertension during pregnancy, it is inadvisable to initiate diuretics during gestation except in the circumstance of cardiac decompensation. Although oral nifedipine can be an effective agent in the control of acute hypertension during pregnancy, its widespread use to treat chronic hypertension throughout gestation awaits additional study. Angiotensin-converting enzyme (ACE) inhibitors have been associated with impairment of fetal growth, severe oligohydramnios, and anatomic abnormalities in up to 20% of neonates when used in the second and third trimester. Women in their childbearing years treated for chronic hypertension should not be treated with ACE inhibitors unless adequate contraception can be ensured.

Fetal effects. Women with chronic hypertension during pregnancy are at high risk for developing fetal intrauterine growth retardation. Early documentation of fetal age is mandatory with monthly ultrasound evaluation of growth and development in the second half of pregnancy. Weekly antepartum fetal evaluation is mandatory during the last 6 to 8 weeks of pregnancy, or earlier if poor fetal growth is noted. In circumstances of significant fetal growth retardation or suspicious antepartum fetal testing, delivery is indicated regardless of gestational age.

Late or transient hypertension

Hypertension without proteinuria or abnormal edema that develops late in gestation or in the puerperium is referred to as *late* or *transient hypertension*. Blood pressure normalizes by the tenth postpartum day. Often it may be difficult to differentiate transient hypertension from early pre-eclampsia. Almost half of the women with transient hypertension in pregnancy subsequently develop long-standing chronic hypertension.

CARDIOVASCULAR DISORDERS

Normal pregnancy is accompanied by changes in blood volume, heart rate, blood pressure, cardiac output, and ventilation. Cardiac output begins to rise during the first trimester, peaks at an approximate 40% increase by 20 to 24 weeks, then declines during the last 8 weeks of gestation. The increase in cardiac output during early pregnancy is primarily caused by an increase in stroke volume. As pregnancy advances, heart rate increases while stroke volume falls to nonpregnant levels.

Immediately after delivery, with relief of compression on the inferior vena cava, cardiac output may increase as much as 10 to 20 percent. Following this transitory rise in cardiac output, values fall progressively to baseline levels. Nonpregnant levels are reached by the end of the second postpartum week. During the initial postpartum period, relative bradycardia is common.

Most patients with valvular heart disease can successfully complete pregnancy. If necessary, there is ample experience with valvular surgery during pregnancy. Yet, it is extremely important that women with known valvular heart disease be evaluated prior to pregnancy and that, if necessary, corrective surgery be performed before conception.

Mitral stenosis is by far the most common rheumatic valvular lesion encountered in pregnant women. Increased heart rate, blood volume, and transmitral flow are all associated with normal pregnancy and tend to exacerbate the severity of mitral stenosis. Mitral regurgitation generally poses little threat during pregnancy except in severe cases; when volume overload can produce congestive heart failure. Mild aortic stenosis is usually well tolerated. Cardiac catheterization is indicated during pregnancy when aortic stenosis is associated with left ventricular failure, syncope, or angina. Aortic regurgitation is often ameliorated during pregnancy because there is a reduction in total peripheral resistance.

Primary or secondary pulmonary hypertension, Eisenmenger's syndrome, and cardiomyopathy with persistent left ventricular failure all pose an unacceptably high risk of maternal mortality. Women with these conditions should not become pregnant, and those who do conceive should be encouraged to terminate pregnancy in the first trimester.

Marfan's syndrome is associated with aortic dissection and myxomatous degeneration of the aortic and mitral valves. Historically, these patients have been advised to avoid pregnancy. Recent reports, however, suggest a favorable outcome for women with Marfan's syndrome who lack significant cardiovascular involvement.

THROMBOEMBOLIC DISORDERS (see Chapter 217)

Thromboembolic disease is the leading cause of nonobstetric postpartum maternal mortality. In the United States, one half of all thromboembolic events in women younger than 40 years are related to pregnancy. The risk of deep vein thrombophlebitis (DVT) during pregnancy has been reported to be five times higher than in nonpregnant individuals and is probably even higher in the immediate postpartum period. The antenatal risk of DVT is further increased in patients with prior DVT or pulmonary embolism, prolonged bed rest, varicose veins, or obesity, as well as those with a variety of inherited coagulation disorders. Postpartum risks are increased by cesarean delivery (ninefold increase over vaginal delivery).

The diagnosis of deep vein thrombophlebitis or pulmonary embolism may be suspected clinically but usually requires radiographic confirmation.

Initial treatment of pulmonary embolism and iliofemoral thromboembolism includes heparin given intravenously by constant infusion in a dosage sufficient to prolong the partial thromboplastin time (PTT) 1.5 to 2.0 times the control value. Intravenous treatment is usually continued for 7 to 10 days to allow for organization and firm attachment of the thrombus to the vessel wall. In most patients, full-dose intravenous heparin is followed by heparin given subcutaneously, 5000 units every 8 to 12 hours, throughout the remainder of pregnancy and up to 4 to 6 months postpartum. Patients with a single episode of thrombosis confined to a calf vein are less vulnerable to recurrence. In these patients, it is reasonable to treat the acute episode with full-dose intravenous heparin and to follow the patient clinically or with noninvasive techniques throughout the remainder of gestation without the use of prophylactic heparin.

There are insufficient data to conclude which regimen provides the safest maximal protection against recurrent antepartum thrombosis. Participants in the National Institutes of Health Consensus Conference concluded that women with a history of either deep venous thrombosis or pulmonary embolism should be given prophylactic subcutaneous heparin in doses of 5000 units, either two or three times daily, throughout pregnancy and the puerperium.

Unlike heparin, warfarin freely crosses the placenta. Use of warfarin during the first trimester has been associated with a variety of neonatal malformations including nasal hypoplasia, frontal bossing, and short stature with stippled epiphyses. Use during the second and third trimesters has been associated with fetal and placental hemorrhage resulting in fetal death. Warfarin should be avoided throughout pregnancy, and patients already taking warfarin and desiring to conceive should be switched to heparin prior to conception.

Heparin appears to be safe for use during lactation because it does not enter breast milk. Warfarin, on the other hand, minimally enters breast milk, but in at least one study no warfarin levels could be detected in breast-fed infants' plasma.

ASTHMA (see Chapter 300)

Asthma is the most common obstructive pulmonary disease encountered during pregnancy. The effect of pregnancy on asthma is variable, but some generalizations can be made: (1) There is a tendency for asthma to worsen between 28 and 36 weeks of gestation; (2) asthma tends to improve during the last 4 weeks of gestation regardless of the prior course; (3) exacerbations during labor and delivery are rare in women who have been satisfactorily managed throughout gestation; (4) if there has been a change in the clinical course of asthma during gestation, it tends to revert to the pregestational course within the first 3 months postpartum; and (5) the course of asthma is affected similarly from pregnancy to pregnancy.

Management of asthma is altered very little by pregnancy. Medications necessary to control wheezing before conception should not be discontinued merely because of pregnancy. Four classes of drugs form the nucleus of pharmacotherapy: methylxanthines, adrenergic agents, cromolyn sodium, and corticosteroids.

Considerable experience with the use of methylxanthines during pregnancy has been accumulated. There has been no evidence of teratogenicity or fetal injury. The dosage does not usually need to be altered, but it is advisable to measure serum concentrations to ensure a therapeutic response and minimize side effects.

Adrenergic agents are effective bronchodilators used alone or in conjunction with methylxanthines. There has been extensive clinical experience with these drugs during pregnancy with few reports of adverse effects. Administration of adrenergic medication by inhalation provides the most rapid relief of acute asthma with the fewest side effects. Older oral preparations containing phenobarbital should be avoided throughout pregnancy.

Cromolyn sodium prevents release of histamine and is useful for prophylaxis against acute asthma. It has no bronchodilating activity and is not useful for treatment of acute attacks. Cromolyn appears to have no maternal or fetal toxicity.

Acute bronchospasm unresponsive to bronchodilator therapy often improves with the anti-inflammatory effect of corticosteroids. Oral, inhaled, and intravenous corticosteroids are all considered safe for use during pregnancy. Inhaled corticosteroids such as beclomethasone may allow a reduction in the dosage of oral preparations or the frequency of use of beta-sympathomimetic inhalers.

HEPATIC DISORDERS

Acute hepatitis A

Pregnant women with hepatitis A generally do not transmit the infection to their offspring. Presumably, the risk of transmission is limited by the brief viremic period and the lack of fecal contamination during delivery.

Management does not differ from that of nonpregnant patients. In uncomplicated cases, there is no rational basis for restricting protein intake or providing excessive quantities of carbohydrate.

Effective prophylaxis against hepatitis A can be achieved with immune globulin and should be offered to pregnant women with household or sexual contacts who have acute hepatitis A. Staff of child day-care centers where one or more cases of hepatitis A have been recognized are also candidates for immune globulin. Routine administration of immune globulin is not indicated for teachers in elementary or secondary schools in contact with a patient with hepatitis A unless there is evidence of a school- or classroom-centered outbreak. Similarly, routine prophylaxis for hospital personnel, including nurses, is not indicated.

Acute hepatitis B

Infection with the hepatitis B virus (HBV) is a major cause of acute and chronic hepatitis, cirrhosis, and primary hepatocellular carcinoma throughout the world. Fortunately, women who have acute hepatitis B during the first or second trimester rarely transmit the infection to their neonates. On the other hand, women who contract the infection during the third trimester or near the time of delivery have a very high probability of transmitting the virus to their offspring. Mothers positive for both HB_sAg and HB_s Ag infect approximately 70% to 90% of untreated infants. Of these infected infants, up to 90% become HBV carriers; some ultimately develop chronic active hepatitis, cirrhosis, and primary hepatocellular carcinoma. In addition, female carriers may subsequently perpetuate the cycle of perinatal transmission when they become pregnant. Because of the high prevalence of infection with hepatitis B virus, routine screening for Hb_sAg is now recommended for all pregnant women.

Intrahepatic cholestasis of pregnancy

Intrahepatic cholestasis of pregnancy (ICP) results from failure of the liver to excrete bile acids appropriately. Most evidence suggests that this defect is estrogen-related. The disorder tends to recur in subsequent pregnancies or with oral contraceptive use.

Despite the fact that the disease is usually referred to as benign, an increased incidence of preterm labor, stillbirths, fetal distress, and meconium staining has been reported with ICP.

ICP typically occurs during the third trimester and is characterized by generalized pruritus sometimes followed by jaundice. The serum bilirubin concentration usually remains below 5 mg per deciliter. Liver function tests reflect cholestasis without significant evidence of hepatocellular injury.

Relief of pruritus can be achieved with the bile salt-binding resin cholestyramine. Patients should be followed closely for signs of preterm labor and fetal well-being.

Acute cholecystitis

Despite the cholestatic effect of estrogen and impaired gallbladder emptying, there is no proved increased incidence of acute cholecystitis or common duct obstruction during gestation. Cholecystectomy is performed in 1 per 1000 to 3000 pregnancies. Clinical presentation generally does not differ from that in nonpregnant individuals. During late gestation, however, cholecystitis can be confused with the right upper quadrant pain that often accompanies pre-eclampsia. Acute appendicitis during pregnancy may also present with right upper quadrant pain. The presence of gallstones can usually be established with ultrasonography.

Initial management, even when pancreatitis is present, should be conservative. Surgery should be reserved for cases where perforation is suspected, failure to respond to medical therapy within 4 to 5 days, persistent obstructive jaundice, repeated attacks of biliary colic, or patients in whom other acute surgical abdominal diseases (e.g., acute appendicitis) cannot be ruled out.

Acute fatty liver of pregnancy

Acute fatty liver of pregnancy (AFLP) is a relatively uncommon disease of unknown cause. In the past, maternal mortality has been reported to be as high as 80%. A more recent study, however, reported no maternal deaths and a 10% fetal mortality.

The obstetric history of a patient with AFLP parallels pre-eclampsia. The disease presents during the third trimester, with the mean gestational age at onset of 36 weeks. The incidence of AFLP is highest in primiparas and women with multiple gestations.

Initial manifestations are sudden but nonspecific. Nausea, vomiting, and abdominal pain are the most common presenting complaints. The disease can progress to hepatic failure, disseminated intravascular coagulation, renal failure, and/or gastrointestinal bleeding.

Transaminases are typically elevated in the range of 300 to 500 units. Levels above 1000 units suggest fulminant hepatitis. Serum bilirubin may be normal early in the course of AFLP, but it rises if pregnancy is not terminated. Hematologic abnormalities include leukocytosis, microangiopathic hemolytic anemia, and thrombocytopenia. Hypoglycemia is common and may be profound. Liver biopsy is frequently diagnostic but may not be appropriate to perform in the presence of significant coagulopathy.

AFLP is managed by immediate delivery and intensive medical support. Despite appropriate care, the patient's condition may deteriorate further postpartum. In subsequent pregnancies, AFLP does not appear to recur.

DIGESTIVE TRACT DISORDERS

Hyperemesis gravidarum

Hyperemesis gravidarum is a disorder of unknown cause occurring in approximately 3.5 per 1000 pregnancies. The condition is characterized by persistent nausea and vomiting throughout early gestation. As a result of vomiting and poor intake, ketone production, nutritional deficiencies, and fluid and electrolyte disturbances can occur. Thyrotoxicosis, hepatic or gallbladder disease, and hydatidiform mole may present as hyperemesis and should be considered.

In some patients, liquid meal replacement through a pediatric nasogastric tube or total parenteral nutrition may be necessary.

Peptic ulcer disease

It has been suggested that pregnancy ameliorates the severity of peptic ulcer disease. There are few convincing epidemiologic data, however, to support this contention. Moreover, when ulcer symptoms do abate during pregnancy, they often recur within the year after delivery.

Antacids are the treatment of choice for peptic ulcers during pregnancy. The safety of H_2 -receptor antagonists has not been clearly established during pregnancy.

Inflammatory bowel disease

Ulcerative colitis. Ulcerative colitis appears to have little effect on fertility or the course of pregnancy. The incidence of normal live births, congenital anomalies, spontaneous abortions, and stillbirths is similar to that in pregnancies without associated ulcerative colitis. The effect of pregnancy on ulcerative colitis is variable. Of patients whose disease is inactive at the onset of pregnancy, approximately 70% remain free of symptoms throughout gestation. Patients with active disease at the onset of pregnancy do less well. Approximately 70% of these women show no improvement or become worse during pregnancy. Moreover, women who manifest the onset of colitis during pregnancy are more likely to suffer severe, repeated attacks.

Management of ulcerative colitis differs little during pregnancy. Maintenance therapy with sulfasalazine can be continued throughout pregnancy in women with ulcerative colitis who have taken it prior to conception. The drug may also be initiated to treat exacerbations. There is no evidence that the medication should be discontinued near the time of delivery or that use during breast-feeding harms the newborn. If necessary, corticosteroids may be used to manage ulcerative colitis during pregnancy and lactation.

Crohn's disease. Crohn's disease has been associated with decreased fertility and an increased risk of stillbirth. The effects of pregnancy on patients with Crohn's disease are similar to those on patients with ulcerative colitis. If the disease is inactive at the time of conception, it remains so in 80% to 90% of patients. Management is essentially the same as in the nonpregnant patient.

RHEUMATIC DISORDERS

Systemic lupus erythematosus (SLE)

Many reports have suggested that the frequency of exacerbations of SLE is increased during pregnancy and the postpartum period. There are no convincing data, however, to support this concern. The natural history of the disease is variable, and older series were reported before the effective use of corticosteroids or immunosuppressives. The risk of exacerbations does seem to be minimized in patients who are in complete clinical remission at the time of conception.

Pregnancy outcome appears to be related to disease activity. Patients who suffer clinical flares, hypertension, or renal failure have an increased incidence of fetal death, preterm deliveries, and small-for-gestational-age infants. In addition, a subset of women with a high rate of vascular complications and fetal deaths have recently been recognized as having SLE. In some patients, fetal loss may be the sole manifestation of the disease. The presence of antiphospholipid antibodies (lupus anticoagulant and anticardiolipin) are an additional risk factor for fetal loss.

It has been observed that there is a relationship between fetal heart block and maternal SLE. It appears that maternal anti-Ro (SS-A) antibody crosses the placenta and may directly damage fetal cardiac tissue. Only 1% to 5% of the children from mothers with anti-Ro (SS-A) antibody develop transient photosensitive skin rash or permanent congenital heart block. The absence of this antibody in maternal serum suggests that a child is unlikely to be affected.

Many patients with SLE demonstrate spontaneous remission and do not require treatment. However, serious flares involving the kidneys or central nervous system reduce fetal survival and pose a serious threat to maternal well-being. These patients are generally treated with corticosteroids or immunosuppressives. Treatment should not be deferred because of pregnancy.

Rheumatoid arthritis

Most reports indicate that pregnancy has a favorable effect on the clinical course of rheumatoid arthritis. Up to 75% of patients experience a significant remission. Furthermore, remission during one pregnancy often indicates that a similar remission is experienced in a subsequent pregnancy.

Whenever possible, every effort should be made to control arthritic symptoms with adequate rest, physical and occupational therapy, local heat, and if necessary, intraarticular corticosteroid injections. Gold, antimalarials, nonsteroidal anti-inflammatory drugs, and cytotoxic agents should be avoided during pregnancy. Therapeutic dosages of aspirin should be used in preference to these drugs.

All women with rheumatoid arthritis should be evaluated for significant cervical spine disease, especially subluxation, before delivery.

HEMATOLOGIC DISORDERS

Anemia

Because plasma volume increases more than red cell volume, the hematocrit during pregnancy can be expected to fall to as low as 35% by the beginning of the third trimester. Generally, a hemoglobin value of less than 11 g per deciliter defines anemia during pregnancy.

Pure macrocytic anemia in pregnancy with the presence of hypersegmented neutrophils usually represents folate deficiency. Pernicious anemia is extremely rare during pregnancy. Anemia secondary to folate deficiency is frequently combined with iron deficiency and requires oral iron in addition to 1 mg of folic acid daily.

In nonmacrocytic anemia, a low serum ferritin concentration is diagnostic of deficient iron stores. Reticulocytosis can be demonstrated within 2 weeks of oral iron supplementation. Parenteral iron administration is rarely necessary.

Hemoglobinopathy or thalassemia should be suspected in patients who have a previous history of anemia, African or Mediterranean ancestry, and a normal serum ferritin concentration. Hemoglobin electrophoresis is necessary to establish the diagnosis.

The most frequently encountered hemoglobinopathies involve abnormal hemoglobins S and C and beta-thalassemia, either isolated or in combination. Sickle cell trait (Hb AS) is common but comparatively benign. Conversely, sickle cell disease (Hb SS) and hemoglobin SC disease (Hb SC) are frequently complicated by preeclampsia, infection, painful crises, and increased perinatal loss.

Bleeding disorders

Approximately 7% of healthy pregnant women have mild to moderate thrombocytopenia (platelet count 80-150 × 10^9/L). Neither these women nor their offspring manifest abnormal bleeding. This condition has been designated incidental thrombocytopenia of pregnancy and requires no treatment.

Idiopathic thrombocytopenic purpura (ITP). ITP is a common autoimmune disorder in which patients form antiplatelet autoantibodies against platelet-specific antigens. The condition frequently affects young women; consequently, one can anticipate that many patients with ITP will become pregnant while their illness is active. The major concern during pregnancy is whether infants born to mothers with ITP are at risk of serious bleeding during delivery and whether they can be identified before delivery.

Unfortunately, it has been determined that there is no relationship between maternal platelet count and the infant's platelet count. Similarly, measurement of platelet-associated IgG on maternal platelets does not predict neonatal thrombocytopenia. In a prospective series of over 7000 women. Burrows found that severe thrombocytopenia at the time of delivery occurs in less than 5% of infants. Moreover, Burrows found that one of the best predictors of severe neonatal thrombocytopenia is a previously affected infant. He recommends, therefore, that the type of delivery be decided solely on obstetric indications. After delivery a fetal cord platelet count is immediately obtained and the infant's platelet count should be followed carefully over the next week. Maternal indications for treatment of thrombocytopenia should not differ from those for nonpregnant individuals.

Disseminated intravascular coagulation. Disseminated intravascular coagulation (DIC) is associated with a number of complications of pregnancy. Abruptio placentae, amniotic fluid embolus, severe preeclampsia, retained dead fetus, sepsis, and second-trimester abortion can all be associated with DIC. Treatment of the underlying disease including delivery is the mainstay of therapy.

Von Willebrand's disease. Von Willebrand's disease is a group of inherited disorders of platelet function and factor VIII activity. Transfusions of cryoprecipitate or specific clotting factors are necessary if measured factor VIII activity falls below 50% during labor. Patients with type I von Willebrand's disease may also respond favorably to treatment with desmopressin.

INFECTIOUS DISEASES

Sexually transmitted diseases

Gonorrhea. Because the majority of gonorrhea infections are asymptomatic during pregnancy, routine endocervical culture is indicated in high-risk populations. Primary treatment of gonorrhea infections during pregnancy is ceftriaxone 250 mg I.M. once. Diagnostic studies for chlamydia should be performed. Tetracyclines and quinolones are contraindicated.

Syphilis. Because of its detrimental fetal and maternal effects, syphilis must be treated as soon as the diagnosis is confirmed by specific serologic tests. Nonspecific serologic tests (VDRL, RPR) should be performed monthly after treatment. Rising titers indicate inadequate therapy.

Herpes simplex. The incidence of neonatal herpes simplex virus (HSV) appears to be increasing as genital herpes becomes more common. Exposure of the infant to HSV can often be prevented by cesarean delivery if maternal genital herpes lesions are recognized at the onset of labor. Unfortunately, most neonatal HSV infections result from asymptomatic maternal shedding of HSV, as indicated by the fact that only one third of the mothers of infants with neonatal herpes have signs of HSV infections.

Recently, the Infectious Disease Society for Obstetrics-Gynecology has endorsed the following recommendations for women with a history of genital herpes:

A. In women with a history of genital herpes, but without lesions:
   1. Weekly prenatal cultures should be abandoned.
   2. In the absence of genital herpetic lesions, vaginal delivery should be expected (unless other indications for cesarean delivery are present).
   3. To identify potentially exposed neonates, a culture for herpes virus may be obtained from either the mother on the day of delivery or from the neonate.
   4. Isolation is not necessary for the mother.
   5. It is recognized that with such a policy, there is a small risk (approximately 1 per 1000) of neonatal infection.

B. In women with herpetic lesions of the genital tract when either labor or membrane rupture occurs:
   1. Cesarean delivery is a technique that can reduce the risk of neonatal herpes virus infection.
   2. Ideally, cesarean delivery should be performed before or within 4 to 6 hours of membrane rupture, but cesarean delivery may be of benefit in preventing neonatal herpes regardless of duration of membrane rupture.

C. In women with genital herpetic lesions at or near term, but before labor or membrane rupture: cultures collected at 3- to 5-day intervals may be performed to ensure the absence of virus at the time of birth and to increase the likelihood of vaginal delivery.

Viral infections

Cytomegalovirus. Cytomegalovirus (CMV) is the most common congenital viral disease in the United States. From 0.2% to 2.2% of all infants acquire infection during the perinatal period. Infant mortality may be as high as 20% to 30% in primary CMV infections.

Unfortunately, the presence or absence of seroreactivity does not correlate with the presence or absence of the virus on body surfaces or in body secretions. Accurate diagnosis must be established by isolation of the virus from such sites as urine and endocervical secretions. Because there is no satisfactory therapy available for CMV infections in either adults or newborns, it is ideal for women who are pregnant or are contemplating pregnancy and are known to be seronegative to avoid exposure to CMV from such obvious sources as day-care centers and renal dialysis units.

Varicella-zoster. Despite the fact that varicella infections are among the most common communicable diseases in the general population, they are relatively infrequent during pregnancy.

Transmission of the virus to the fetus during the first 20 weeks of gestation has been reported to result in a clinical syndrome of intrauterine growth retardation, hypoplasia of the extremities, cutaneous scars, cortical atrophy, microcephaly, cataracts, chorioretinitis, microphthalmia, and psychomotor retardation. The exact risk of this congenital syndrome is unknown but is probably about 5%.

A more common problem has been maternal varicella in the peripartum period producing neonatal chickenpox. If a mother develops varicella within 4 days before delivery or 2 days after, there is a 25% chance that the newborn will become infected. During this interval, the newborn acquires the virus but is delivered before the mother has produced a varicella-specific antibody response capable of crossing the placenta and protecting the fetus. Such infants may have as high as 30% mortality. When more than 5 days have elapsed between the onset of maternal rash and delivery, sufficient delay has occurred for a maternal antibody response to develop and the fetus is passively immunized, thus ameliorating the severity of the disease. If parturition occurs during the 7-day period of risk for disseminated neonatal infection, newborns should be passively immunized using varicella-zoster immune globulin.

Rubella. Rubella infection during the first trimester can lead to congenital rubella syndrome in up to 80% of fetuses. An estimated 10% to 15% of young adults remain susceptible to rubella, and limited outbreaks continue to be reported, particularly in universities and hospitals. Every effort should be made to vaccinate all nonpregnant young women unless there is proof of immunity or a specific contraindication to the vaccine. Because of the theoretic risk to the fetus, women should be counseled not to become pregnant for 3 months after vaccination.

If a pregnant woman is inadvertently vaccinated or becomes pregnant within 3 months of vaccination, she should be counseled about the theoretic risks of congenital rubella syndrome. She should be reassured, however, that a Center for Disease Control prospective study of susceptible pregnant women who received rubella vaccine within 3 months of conception and who carried their pregnancies to term had a negligible risk of rubella syndrome.

Parvovirus

Infection with parvovirus B_{19} produces a common childhood illness called *erythema infectiosum* or *fifth disease*. This disease is characterized by fever and a lacy macular rash often described as a "slapped cheek" appearance. Because of its affinity to erythroid cells, parvovirus is a common cause of transient aplastic crisis in children and adults. Parvovirus does cross the human placenta and may lead to severe, life-threatening anemia and nonimmune hydrops in the fetus if maternal infection is acquired during pregnancy. The risk of congenital malformation appears negligible. Nonimmune hydrops in the fetus after maternal infection appears to occur in 5% to 10% of cases. Serial ultrasound evaluation of the at-risk fetus is recommended after documented maternal infection. Intrauterine red cell transfusions for the fetus may be necessary to avoid fetal death secondary to anemia.

Acquired immunodeficiency syndrome (AIDS). The human immunodeficiency virus (HIV) may be transmitted from infected women to their offspring by three possible routes: to the fetus in utero through the maternal circulation, to the infant during labor and delivery by inoculation or ingestion of blood and other infected fluids, and to the infant shortly after birth through infected breast milk. Based on currently available information, there is approximately a 25% to 35% rate of perinatal transmission. All women known to be infected with HIV should receive detailed counseling.

Urinary tract infections

Pregnant women are predisposed to infections of the urinary tract because of dilatation of the ureters and collecting systems, smooth muscle relaxation caused by increased progesterone concentrations, and glycosuria.

Between 5% and 10% of pregnant women have asymptomatic bacteriuria. If untreated, up to 25% of these women suffer acute pyelonephritis during pregnancy or the puerperium. Screening urine cultures in all women during early gestation with appropriate treatment and follow-up minimizes the occurrence of significant infection during the third trimester. Patients with treated bacteriuria or a history of frequent urinary tract infections should be screened more frequently. Treatment of asymptomatic bacteriuria can be accomplished with nitrofurantoin or ampicillin. Quinolones are contraindicated. Pyelonephritis should be aggressively managed with hospitalization, rehydration, and intravenous antibiotic therapy based on in-vitro sensitivities. Table 369-2 lists some common antibiotics and special considerations for their use during pregnancy.

Table 369-2. Antibiotic use during pregnancy

Antibiotic	Special considerations during pregnancy
Penicillin G	Safe in nonallergic patients; dosage requirements increased during pregnancy
Ampicillin	Dosage requirements increased during pregnancy; can lower urinary estriols; unconjugated serum estriol unaffected
Amoxicillin	Same as ampicillin
Oxacillin	Dosage requirements increased during pregnancy
Cephalosporins	Dosage requirements increased during pregnancy; some cross-sensitivity in penicillin-allergic patients; may affect urinary estriols; no effect on unconjugated serum estriol
Erythromycin	Generally safe; placental transfer is erratic, but the fetal liver concentrates the drug
Tetracycline	Abnormal fetal teeth and bone development; increased risk of maternal liver and pancreatic disease; contraindicated in pregnancy
Chloramphenicol	May cause "gray baby syndrome"; avoid in pregnancy
Clindamycin	Fetal effects are unknown; may rarely cause pseudomembranous colitis in the mother
Vancomycin	Potential fetal ototoxicity; should be reserved for life-threatening infections in patients allergic to penicillin
Metronidazole	Mutagenic and carcinogenic in animals; may be necessary to use for symptomatic parasitic infections during second and third trimesters
Nitrofurantoin	Generally safe but has been rarely associated with hemolytic anemia in the newborn; few systemic effects
Quinolones	Contraindicated in pregnancy
Sulfonamides	Competes with bilirubin for albumin binding; should not be used in last trimester to avoid neonatal kernicterus
Trimethoprim	Folic acid antagonist; should be avoided during pregnancy unless no alternative available
Aminoglycosides Amikacin Gentamicin Kanamycin Streptomycin Tobramycin	Possible fetal and maternal ototoxicity and renal toxicity; maternal serum levels should be monitored closely but are usually in low range because of rapid renal clearance

NEUROLOGIC DISORDERS

Seizures

Approximately 50% of women with epilepsy have no change in the frequency of their seizures during pregnancy, 40% have more frequent seizures, and 10% have fewer.

All patients treated with anticonvulsants who desire pregnancy should be carefully evaluated regarding the accuracy of the diagnosis of epilepsy and the continuing need for anticonvulsant therapy. Those who require medications should be counseled that there is approximately a 10% risk of congenital malformations in the infants of women treated with phenytoin or phenobarbital during pregnancy. A recent study reported that the risk of congenital anomalies from carbamazepine is even greater. Patients should also be advised that the risk of poor fetal outcome is also high for women who experience grand mal seizures during pregnancy.

To maintain therapeutic concentrations of phenytoin and phenobarbital throughout pregnancy, it is usually necessary to increase the dosage as gestation advances. Patients receiving anticonvulsants should have serum drug concentrations measured at least monthly. Dosages need to be decreased immediately after delivery to avoid toxicity.

Multiple sclerosis

The effect of pregnancy on the course of multiple sclerosis has been variable. Several recent studies have demonstrated that the number and severity of relapses diminish during pregnancy, particularly during the third trimester. In the past, it has been suggested that exacerbations should be anticipated after delivery. Recent reports have not substantiated this concern.

Acute attacks are best managed with bed rest. The use of corticosteroids for severe attacks is advocated by some neurologists, but the efficacy of steroids for multiple sclerosis remains controversial.

REFERENCES

Baker DA: Herpes and pregnancy: new management. Clin Obstet Gynecol 33:2537, 1990.

Briggs GG, Freeman RK, and Yaffe SJ: Drugs in pregnancy and lactation, ed 3. Baltimore, 1990, Williams & Wilkins.

Burrows RF and Kelton JG: Low fetal risks in pregnancies associated with idiopathic thrombocytopenic purpura. Am J Obstet Gynecol 163:1147, 1990.

Centers for Disease Control: Sexually transmitted diseases: treatment guidelines. MMWR 38(suppl 8):1, 1989.

Committee on Technical Bulletins of the American College of Obstetricians and Gynecologists. Human immunodeficiency virus infections. ACOG Tech Bull 165:1, 1992.

Cunningham FG and Lindheimer MD: Hypertension in pregnancy. N Engl J Med 326:927, 1992.

Dalessio DJ: Seizure disorders and pregnancy. N Engl J Med 312:559, 1985.

Dekker GA and Sibai BM: Early detection of preeclampsia. Am J Obstet Gynecol 165:160, 1991.

Donaldson RM: Management of medical problems in pregnancy: inflammatory bowel disease. N Engl J Med 312:1616, 1985.

Hathaway WE and Bonnar J: Hemostatic disorders of the pregnant woman and newborn infant. New York, 1987, Elsevier.

Holmgren U et al: Women with prolactinoma: effect of pregnancy and lactation on serum prolactin and on tumour growth. Acta Endocrinol 111:452, 1986.

Kennedy RL and Darne J: The role of hCG in regulation of the thyroid gland in normal and abnormal pregnancy. Obstet Gynecol 78:298, 1991.

Kitzmiller JL et al: Preconception care of diabetes. Glycemic control prevents congenital anomalies. JAMA 265:731, 1991.

McCune AB, Weston WL, and Lee LA: Maternal and fetal outcome in neonatal lupus erythematosus. Ann Intern Med 106:518, 1987.

Metcalfe J, McAnulty JH, and Ueland K: Heart disease and pregnancy: physiology and management, ed 2. Boston, 1986, Little, Brown.

Metzger BE et al: Proceedings of the third international workshop-conference on gestational diabetes mellitus. Diabetes 40(suppl 2):1, 1991.

Schatz M and Zeigler RS, editors: Asthma and allergy in pregnancy and early infancy. New York, 1992, Marcel Dekker.
Shmoys S and Kaplan C: Parvovirus and pregnancy. Clin Obstet Gynecol 33:268, 1990.
Sibai BM: Diagnosis and management of chronic hypertension in pregnancy. Obstet Gynecol 78:451, 1991.
Sperling RS et al: Treatment options for human immunodeficiency virus-infected pregnant women. Obstet Gynecol 79:443, 1992.
Watson WJ and Seeds JW: Acute fatty liver of pregnancy. Obstet Gynecol Surv 45:585, 1990.

CHAPTER

370 Gerontology and Geriatric Medicine

Michael S. Katz
Meghan B. Gerety
Michael J. Lichtenstein

It is no art to grow old,
It is art to endure it.

Johann Wolfgang von Goethe

Elderly people are subject to deteriorating function, diverse diseases, and environmental challenges that potentiate the development of frailty and the inability to live independently. Geriatric medicine, defined as the medical care of elderly persons, is characterized by the comprehensive assessment and management of the older patient with chronic disability and multiple medical and social problems. The goal of geriatric medicine is generally to optimize function in the elderly patient with debilitating conditions. To accomplish this goal, the physician must combine medical expertise with a knowledge of gerontology (the study of aging) and a recognition that numerous clinical disciplines in addition to internal medicine (e.g., clinical pharmacology, psychiatry, neurology, rehabilitation medicine, nursing) are essential to comprehensive management of the elderly patient.

GERONTOLOGY

Demography and epidemiology of aging

The elderly population of the United States has grown dramatically over the twentieth century and is projected to expand further during the early decades of the next century. The number of persons aged 65 and older increased from 4% of the population in 1900 to 12% in 1987. With the aging of the "baby boom" generation born after World War II, the 65+ age group is anticipated to account for 22% of the population by the year 2030. The growth of the older population reflects improvements in public health, socioeconomic conditions, and medical care that have resulted in decreased mortality rates of all age groups, including elderly persons. Since 1900, life expectancy estimates at birth and at age 65 have increased, respectively, by 25 years and 5 years; currently, life expectancy averages 75 years at birth and 82 years at age 65. The 85 and older age group is the most rapidly growing segment of the U.S. population, and it is expected that more than 100,000 centenarians will be living by the year 2000.

The aging of the population during the twentieth century has heightened the demand for comprehensive health services to increased numbers of older persons susceptible to chronic illness and disability. Although persons 65 and older represent 12% of the population, this group accounts for more than one third of U.S. health care expenditures. Older people undergo more frequent and more prolonged hospitalizations and visit physicians more often than younger individuals. Of people over 65, 85% have at least one chronic illness, and 30% have three or more chronic diseases. One half of community-dwelling persons 65 and older report symptoms of arthritis. Other frequently reported conditions, in order of decreasing prevalence, include hypertension, decreased hearing, heart disease, and visual impairment. Older individuals with chronic illness are subject to functional impairment and eventual loss of the ability to live independently. Most noninstitutionalized persons over 65 maintain adequate basic function, as assessed by personal care activities (basic activities of daily living [basic ADLs], see later discussion). However, one quarter of this population has difficulty performing activities required for independent living (instrumental ADLs). The proportion of older persons institutionalized in nursing homes increases dramatically with age, rising from 1% of those 65 to 74, to 6% of those 75 to 84, and to 22% of the 85+ age group. Current projections indicate that 43% of persons over age 60 will live in nursing homes for some period during their lives.

The three leading causes of mortality in the elderly, accounting for three quarters of all deaths in those 65 and older, are cardiovascular disease (predominantly coronary artery disease), malignant neoplasms (most often of the lung, breast, prostate, and colon), and cerebrovascular disease. Since 1968, mortality rates from coronary artery disease have decreased in all age groups, including those over 65. This decrease is thought to result from risk factor reduction associated with control of hypertension, cessation of cigarette smoking, and decreased cholesterol intake. Over the same period, cancer mortality in elderly persons has increased, probably as a reflection of the decline in mortality from coronary artery disease.

Although disease and disability are common at advanced age, it remains unclear whether the continued growth of the older population into the next century will lead by necessity to increased numbers of debilitated elderly persons requiring extensive medical and social support. Some investigators have argued that disease prevention and health promotion measures might be developed to promote a "compression of morbidity," that is, to delay (or even eliminate) the onset of chronic illness and disability in people surviving to advanced age. The concept of limiting disease morbidity before death has been extended to age-related decrements in function in individuals without disease. It has been observed that physiologic functioning is highly variable among older individuals even though aging populations without discernible disease on the average are characterized by physiologic decline. Thus "normal" aging occurring in the absence of disease has been classified into two categories: *usual,* in which aging is accompanied by typical nonpathologic losses of physiologic function, and *successful,* in which physiologic decline during aging is minimal or even absent. Physiologic losses during usual aging have been attributed to the modifying effects of extrinsic variables (e.g., diet, exercise, psychosocial factors) on basic aging processes. Various extrinsic variables are known to be risk factors for specific diseases common in elderly persons (e.g., coronary artery disease risk factors). Accordingly the gerontologic literature emphasizes the need for future research into strategies by which modifications of lifestyle and environment might reduce morbidity and maintain vitality in increasing numbers of older people.

It is important to note that the aging of the U.S. veteran population has greatly facilitated health services research directed at preventing frailty and maintaining function in elderly persons. The aging of veterans from World War II and the Korean War has led to an especially marked increase in the number of veterans 65 and older. By 1990, more than one half of all males 65 and older were estimated to be veterans. During the 1970s, in early recognition of an enlarging population of older veterans, the U.S. Department of Veterans Affairs (VA, then the Veterans Administration) created a series of regional aging research centers, termed *Geriatric Research, Education and Clinical Centers* (GRECCs), designed to improve the care of elderly veterans. In one prominent example of GRECC-sponsored research, an interdisciplinary approach to comprehensive assessment and management of geriatric inpatients was demonstrated to reduce subsequent hospitalization and also to lower mortality and morbidity. Other VA studies have somewhat surprisingly found that geriatric services provided through established outpatient units such as hospital-based home care and adult day health care have little or no effect on patient outcomes and cost savings. Ongoing studies by the VA continue to evaluate the circumstances under which geriatric assessment and management of both inpatients and outpatients may be optimized.

Biology of aging

Theories of aging. Aging can be defined in biologic terms as those processes occurring during the postmaturational life span that progressively decrease an organism's ability to adapt to environmental change and increase the likelihood of dying. The cellular and organismal mechanisms underlying aging are unknown, although it is generally agreed that aging is likely to result from more than one primary process. Over the years, diverse theories have been proposed in support of a variety of putative aging processes. Many theories of aging have been disproved or otherwise abandoned for lack of supporting evidence; others continue to provide plausible explanations for aging but have yet to be substantiated by conclusive identification of primary aging processes. For descriptive purposes, theories of aging can be classified into two broad categories, according to which aging is attributed to either (1) genetically programmed processes or (2) accumulation of damage to critical cellular or tissue constituents. These two classes of theories, as with many individual theories of aging, are not mutually exclusive.

Genetic theories. Considerable evidence points to a genetic basis for aging. Perhaps the strongest evidence in this regard is the finding that maximum life span is species specific and varies greatly among different species. Compelling evidence for genetic control of life span has also been provided by studies in which selective breeding of *Drosophila melanogaster* and the nematode *Caenorhabditis elegans* has been used to produce populations with increased longevity. The existence in humans of genetic progeroid syndromes (e.g., Werner's syndrome, Hutchinson-Gilford syndrome) characterized by premature occurrence of the aging phenotype further supports a role for genetics in aging. In addition, familial studies of longevity have demonstrated greater similarity between monozygotic twins than between dizygotic twins and nontwin siblings.

Current efforts to delineate the genetic determinants of aging draw on classic evolutionary theory as well as modern molecular biology. It has been suggested that aging evolved as a selected trait conferring advantage to the reproductively fit members of a species by eliminating older individuals in competition for the same resources. Support for this view is limited because animals in the wild do not usually survive to old age. Under these circumstances, aging would not be expected to provide added advantage to younger individuals. Alternative theories postulating genetic control of aging do not presuppose that aging is a selected trait of evolutionary value. For example, aging has been hypothesized to result from the expression of genes that exhibit "antagonistic pleiotropy," that is, have opposite effects on fitness characteristics. In this case, genes selected for early reproductive fitness might also result in decreased fitness and aging later in life. Aging could also be caused by destructive genes expressed only late in the life span, after the period of reproductive fitness; such genes would presumably not be subject to strong negative selection and would thereby be maintained in a species despite their negative effects. Studies to identify specific genes that regulate aging have been conducted in lower organisms such as *C. elegans* and the budding yeast *Saccharomyces cerevisiae*. Mutation of a single gene called *age-1* has been found to lengthen life in *C. elegans,* whereas controlled expression of the viral oncogene v-*Ha-ras* in *S. cerevisiae* prolongs this organism's life span. The relevance of these findings to the genetic control of aging in higher organisms, including humans, is unknown.

Damage theories. Prominent theories advocating the involvement of accumulated damage in aging processes are related conceptually to the longstanding view that metabolic rate is an important determinant of aging. According to this view, the metabolism of fuels necessary to sustain life has deleterious effects on the organism that may cause aging.

Over the past century an inverse relationship between metabolic rate and life span has been observed repeatedly, although not invariably, in mammalian species as well as invertebrates. Other observations, however, have questioned the relationship between metabolic rate and aging. For example, food restriction of rodents is well known to increase life span and retard processes attributable to aging but has no effect on metabolic rate per unit of lean mass. Thus, although not all available data support a metabolic rate hypothesis of aging, several theories suggest possible mechanisms by which essential metabolism of fuels might create damage and thereby hasten aging processes.

Free radical theory. The free radical theory of aging, first proposed in the 1950s and currently under increasing scrutiny, postulates a major role for oxidative metabolism in causing cumulative damage. Highly reactive oxygen species, such as the superoxide and hydroxyl free radicals and also the hydrogen peroxide molecule, are generated in the course of normal oxidative metabolism. These intermediates are thought to cause damage and eventual aging through reactions with nucleic acid, protein, and lipid components of cells. Protective enzymes (e.g., superoxide dismutase, catalase) eliminate toxic oxygen intermediates; and in some instances, transcription of the genes encoding these enzymes declines with age. Therefore to some extent the proposition that free radical damage causes aging is representative of theories invoking a genetic basis for aging.

Glycation theory. Another prominent theory relating fuel utilization to damage and aging holds that toxic effects of glucose may mediate aging processes. Glucose and other reducing sugars undergo nonenzymatic glycation reactions with proteins and nucleic acids to generate glycoadducts termed *advanced glycosylation end-products* (AGEs). It has been proposed that AGEs cause aging by cross-linking or otherwise modifying biologic molecules involved in critical physiologic processes. The glycation theory of aging is especially provocative because recent studies demonstrating prevention of AGE formation by aminoguanidine suggest potential interventions to retard aging processes.

Cellular aging. A distinctive approach to the study of aging has been to use human cells in tissue culture to investigate a cellular basis for aging. This line of research began 30 years ago with the observation that normal human fibroblasts grown in culture exhibit a limited number of population doublings. The doubling capacity of cultured fibroblasts was found to be inversely related to the donor's age and directly related to maximum life span among different species. Findings such as these have led some to contend that aging in vivo is expressed in culture and that aging is an intrinsic characteristic of cells proliferating in vitro. However, others have cautioned against using cultured cells as a model of aging because the relevance of replicative potential in vitro to aging processes in vivo is yet to be established.

Physiologic changes during aging. It is generally agreed that human aging is accompanied by physiologic deterioration. However, studies of the effects of aging on physiologic function are subject to several limitations. First, the physiologic consequences of aging are often difficult to distinguish from the superimposed effects of diseases and lifestyle changes common in elderly persons. Second, physiologic decline is highly variable among elderly persons and also among different organ systems of any given individual. As noted earlier, individual variation may be attributable to factors extrinsic to the primary aging processes. Third, most studies of age differences in physiologic function have been cross-sectional in design. Such studies may fail to identify important cohort effects and secular trends. Despite the limitations of cross-sectional data, longitudinal studies in general confirm a decline in physiologic function with advancing age. Finally, because functional losses during aging reflect diminished homeostatic control mechanisms, age changes in physiologic systems are usually maximal under conditions of stress and may not be demonstrable at rest.

The following sections summarize examples of major physiologic changes observed during human aging.

Body composition and homeostatic regulation. Changes in body composition include a decline in lean body mass (primarily from decreased muscle mass) with a proportionate increase in body fat. These changes are important determinants of physiologic function and therapeutic intervention in elderly persons. For example, reduced muscle mass is thought to account in large part for the decline in maximum oxygen consumption during exercise ($\dot{V}O_{2max}$) demonstrable with increasing age. In addition, increases in body fat may increase the volume of distribution of lipophilic drugs and prolong their pharmacologic actions. Of note, changes in body composition in elderly persons probably result from not only primary aging processes, but also extrinsic factors such as physical inactivity and altered dietary intake. Age changes in homeostatic controls include impaired baroreflex sensitivity, which may predispose older persons to orthostatic hypotension, and diminished thermoregulation, which increases susceptibility to hypothermia and heatstroke.

Cardiovascular function. Numerous studies have been conducted to evaluate functional changes in the cardiovascular system with age. Resting heart rate is unaltered during aging. Cardiac output at rest also does not change with age in healthy subjects carefully screened to exclude coronary artery disease. Systolic blood pressure increases with advancing age as a result of increased arterial stiffness. Although the increase in arterial pressure raises cardiac afterload, resting ventricular function is maintained during aging by a compensatory hypertrophy of the myocardium. During vigorous exercise, heart rate increases to a lesser extent in older persons than in younger individuals. However, in healthy elderly subjects, increases in stroke volume during exercise are greater than in younger persons, and cardiac output is preserved despite the diminished heart rate response to exercise. During exercise the stroke volume in elderly persons is augmented in response to increased end-diastolic volume, according to the Frank Starling mechanism; nonetheless, end-systolic volume in elderly persons is not reduced as much as in younger individuals. It has been emphasized that the cardiovascular responses to exercise in older persons are similar to those in younger individuals exercising in the presence of beta-adrenergic blockade. In this regard, beta-adrenergic responsiveness is known to decline with age in a variety of tissues, including the heart. An age-related increase in plasma catecholamine (norepinephrine) levels has also been documented at rest and during exercise, but the relationship between this finding and decreased adrenergic responses with age has not been clarified.

Pulmonary function. Pulmonary function declines with advancing age. Elastic recoil of the lung decreases during aging, possibly from loss of alveolar attachments to parenchymal elastic fibers. Decreased lung elasticity contributes to age-related increases in functional residual capacity (resting volume of the lungs after a normal expiration) and residual volume (volume remaining after maximum expiration). Loss of elastic recoil, which results in early collapse of peripheral airways during forced expiration, may also account in part for age-associated decreases in forced vital capacity (total volume forcibly exhaled after full inspiration) and the volume forcibly exhaled in 1 second (FEV_1). In addition, decreasing elasticity with age progressively increases the closing volume (lung volume at which peripheral airways collapse) to the extent that in some elderly individuals, airway closure may occur during normal respiration. Arterial oxygen tension (PaO_2) declines with age, largely as a result of a ventilation-perfusion imbalance created by airway collapse in well-perfused areas of the lung. The age-adjusted PaO_2 may be estimated by the equation $PaO_2 = 109 \text{ mm Hg} - 0.43$ (age in years). Diminished ventilatory responses to hypoxia and hypercapnia are demonstrable in elderly persons and are thought to reflect decreased chemoreceptor function.

Renal function. Age-related decrements have been observed in kidney function and the regulation of electrolyte and fluid balance. Anatomic changes of the aging kidney include a gradual decline in mass (especially prominent in the renal cortex), a decrease in the total number of glomeruli, and increased glomerulosclerosis. Glomerular filtration rate, as assessed by creatinine clearance, falls progressively with increasing age. However, the decline in creatinine clearance with age is highly variable, and some individuals evaluated longitudinally over many years exhibit no age-related decrease in creatinine clearance. The kidney's ability to decrease urinary sodium excretion in response to sodium restriction is impaired in older individuals. This defect in sodium conservation may result at least in part from an age-related decline in renin and aldosterone levels documented under basal and stimulated conditions. Several factors contribute to age changes in the regulation of extracellular fluid volume. Vasopressin (antidiuretic hormone) release in response to hypertonic saline infusion is *greater* in older individuals than in younger subjects, reflecting an age-related increase in sensitivity of hypothalamic osmoreceptors. Despite this increase in vasopressin release, kidney responsiveness to vasopressin falls with age, resulting in impaired urinary concentrating ability after water deprivation. In addition, thirst and drinking responses to water deprivation are decreased in elderly individuals. The urinary concentrating defect and reduced thirst in elderly persons increase the risk of dehydration during illness.

Endocrine function. Considerable attention in the endocrine literature has been focused on age changes in glucose metabolism. Glucose tolerance decreases during aging. In healthy aging adults, plasma glucose measured 2 hours after an oral glucose load increases by about 9 mg/dl/decade; fasting plasma glucose increases by 1 mg/dl/decade. The impairment of glucose tolerance at advanced ages is independent of obesity and physical inactivity, which are common accompaniments of aging and can themselves contribute to glucose intolerance. The primary cause of decreased glucose tolerance during aging is insulin resistance in peripheral tissues, especially muscle. Numerous studies have shown that insulin binding to cell receptors does not change with age, and thus a postreceptor abnormality is thought to account for the age-related defect in insulin action. Although insulin secretion may also be impaired with age, circulating insulin levels are not diminished in older individuals, probably because of an age-related decline in insulin clearance. Decreased glucose tolerance during aging does not generally result in glucose levels in the diabetic range. However, as postulated by the glycation theory of aging, moderate elevations in glucose over time could influence the development of physiologic deterioration or age-associated disease. In this regard, fasting plasma glucose and glycosylated hemoglobin are highly correlated in nondiabetic subjects over a wide age range. Epidemiologic data suggest that glucose elevations even within the nondiabetic range increase the risk of cardiovascular disease. It remains to be determined whether the predictive value of glucose is independent of insulin, a known risk factor for cardiovascular disease that may be elevated in elderly individuals with insulin resistance.

Another endocrine variable of potential importance during aging is the growth hormone–insulin-like growth factor 1 (IGF-1) axis. Pituitary secretion of growth hormone declines with increasing age. Many of the anabolic effects of growth hormone are mediated by IGF-1, which is produced by the liver and other tissues in response to growth hormone. As with growth hormone secretion, circulating IGF-1 levels decrease with age. Body composition changes in elderly persons (i.e., reduced lean body mass, increased body fat) resemble those found in nonelderly individuals with growth hormone deficiency. These findings have led to the hypothesis that age-related changes in body composition result at least in part from decreased growth hormone secretion. In support of this hypothesis, a recent study demonstrated that growth hormone administration to healthy elderly men with low IGF-1 levels increased lean body mass and decreased fat mass. Clinical trials of growth hormone administration are currently being extended to frail elderly populations subject to malnutrition and other catabolic conditions.

Immune function. Depressed function of the immune system with aging may predispose elderly persons to infectious diseases and malignancy. An age-related decline in cell-mediated immunity is characterized by decreased proliferation of T lymphocytes in response to mitogenic stimulation. Impaired T cell proliferation with age may be caused by defective intracellular transduction of mitogenic signals. In addition, interleukin 2 (IL-2) synthesis and IL-2 receptor expression, which are required for T cell proliferation, are both decreased with age. Interestingly, only a portion of the T lymphocyte population undergoes functional decline; the mechanisms underlying this heterogeneity of the lymphocyte pool are yet to be identified. Thymic involution and loss of thymic hormones are thought to play a role in decreased T cell function during aging. Age changes in humoral immunity include increased production of autoantibodies, including anti-idiotypic antibodies, and decreased antibody responses to foreign antigens. These changes may reflect age-related alterations in T cell regulation of B cell function.

GERIATRIC MEDICINE

Special considerations in approach to geriatric patients

Atypical presentation of illness. It has been claimed that, in contrast to younger adults, elderly persons have systematically different manifestations of illness. However, many reports describing atypical signs and symptoms of disease are methodologically flawed. Populations studied are often poorly defined and rarely systematically sampled. Study sites, usually teaching hospitals and referral clinics, introduce bias in disease ascertainment and disease severity. Further, the contributions of factors independent of age, such as comorbid disease or disability, are typically not explored. Although it may be inappropriate to conclude that age induces an alteration in host-disease response, there remain many reasons why signs and symptoms of disease in elderly patients may be different than in younger persons. For example, frequent impairments in vision, hearing, and communication can make it difficult to obtain an adequate and accurate history from a frail older person. Acute illness in one system may stress the already reduced reserve capacity of another, producing unrelated signs and symptoms that distract diagnostic efforts away from the correct etiology. In other patients, one chronic illness may be masked by another. An individual with activity limitation from osteoarthritis may not experience angina with severe coronary disease. Finally, treatment for one illness may unmask another previously undiagnosed pathology. Asymptomatic urinary outlet obstruction may become apparent for the first time when a pharmacologic agent with anticholinergic properties provokes urinary retention. Similarly, confusion after administration of a central nervous system (CNS) active drug may be the first sign of underlying cognitive impairment.

Because illness and disability are so often multifactorial in elderly patients, physicians should change their approach to diagnosis and therapy. Even when signs and symptoms appear straightforward, an evaluation to uncover occult contributing disease may be appropriate. Certain nonspecific syndromes are so important that their presentation should be regarded as sentinel events requiring thorough investigation. Failure to thrive, acute change in appetite, decline in self-care capacity, onset of falls, immobility ("taking to bed"), decreased intellectual function, and new incontinence are all such events. The physician who manages only the nonspecific syndrome without further investigation may miss serious acute illness or exacerbation of chronic illness.

Functional status assessment. The effects of age, disease, and environment all interact and express themselves through a common pathway, functional status. *Functional status* is a term used to describe the individual's capacity to function in multiple domains (physical, mental, social, emotional) and at multiple levels (organ function, function of the person as a whole, function of the person in society). Care of the older person should focus on optimizing health and improving or maintaining function. Formal assessment of functional status serves four primary purposes. First, assessment may reveal previously undetected medical or psychiatric problems that warrant evaluation and/or treatment. Second, functional status assessment provides the context within which goals of therapy and intensity of diagnostic evaluation may most appropriately be set. Third, repetition of functional assessment may be used to gauge the impact of therapy. Finally, identification of functional deficits predicts the need for social and environmental interventions. Thus any evaluation of an older or chronically ill patient should be accompanied by an assessment of functional status.

A substantial body of literature has been published over the last decade advocating an interdisciplinary approach to geriatric functional assessment. Interdisciplinary evaluation is comprehensive and includes multiple health professionals evaluating physical, psychologic, social, and environmental function. A screening or case-finding approach is recommended because of the high prevalence of physical disability, depressive symptoms, intellectual impairment, and poor social support among frail elderly persons. The team approach may include primary care physicians, physiatrists, nurses, social workers, psychologists or psychiatrists, pharmacists, and nutritionists in the care of a single patient. However, an interdisciplinary approach may be impractical for physicians in the community. For this reason, a stratified approach to the evaluation of the older patient is preferred, one that progresses in intensity and complexity as illness and functional disability increase (Table 370-1). Three patient categories determine the assessment strategy: (1) apparently healthy elderly persons, (2) frail elderly persons (i.e., functionally impaired or medically ill community-dwelling elderly patients), and (3) institutionalized or severely impaired elderly patients.

Table 370-1 displays supplemental assessments recommended as frailty increases. All are either standardized instruments or semistructured interviews incorporated into the review of systems. Selection of the assessments is designed to aid an individual practitioner perform an appropriate assessment in the context of an office or nursing home practice, where a physician and nurse may be the only members of the interdisciplinary team. Although supplemental assessments increase time required for evaluation, they also

Table 370-1. Geriatric assessment instruments

Domain	Example	Patient category	Assessor	Time required (minutes)
Functional status				
Basic ADLs	Katz ADLs, Lawton PSMS	FE, IE	Questionnaire, MD or assistant	< 5
Instrumental ADLs	Lawton IADLs, OARS ADLs	HE, FE, IE	Questionnaire, MD or assistant	< 5
Cognition	MMSE, SPMSQ	FE, IE	Interviewer administered	10
Gait and balance	Performance-oriented assessment of mobility	FE, IE	MD or other health professional	5-10
Incontinence	Structured history	HE, FE, IE	MD or assistant	< 5
Depression	Geriatric Depression Scale	HE, FE, IE	Questionnaire, MD or assistant	< 5
Social support	OARS Social Support Questionnaire	FE, IE	Questionnaire, MD or assistant	10-15

Modified with permission from Chiodo LK and Gerety MB: Medical evaluation of the geriatric patient. In Katz MS, editor: Geriatric medicine, vol 1. New York, 1991, Churchill Livingstone.

ADLs, Activities of daily living; PSMS, Personal Self-Maintenance Scale; OARS, Older Americans Research and Service Center; MMSE, Mini–Mental State Exam; SPSMQ, Short Portable Mental Status Questionnaire; FE, frail elderly; IE, institutionalized or severely impaired elderly; HE, healthy elderly; MD, physician.

increase diagnostic yield. Self-report questionnaires that can be completed in written form by the patient or caregiver or administered by an office assistant can minimize physician time required for assessment.

Assessment of physical function is essential because dependency predicts institutionalization and mortality independently of disease burden. Physical function can be assessed most simply with basic and instrumental ADLs. Basic ADLs are personal care activities, including bathing, dressing, grooming, toileting, continence, transfers (bed to chair, chair to toilet), and ambulation. Dependence in personal care activities may indicate that the patient requires personal assistance in the home unless the dependency can be relieved. Instrumental ADLs are the skills necessary to survive in a community. They include ability to take medications, manage finances, telephone, shop, keep house, prepare meals, and use transportation. Dependence in these tasks may require social services. A list of instrumental ADL dependencies is much more useful to planning supportive services than a list of traditional medical problems.

Brief instruments are also available to screen for cognitive impairment and depressive symptoms. The Folstein Mini–Mental State Exam or the Pfeiffer Short Portable Mental Status Questionnaire can be administered to the patient by the physician, a nurse, or a trained office assistant. The Geriatric Depression Scale and other self-report instruments that assess depressive symptoms can be completed by the patient as a written questionnaire or administered by the physician or other office personnel. A more extensive discussion regarding assessment and therapy can be found in later sections addressing dementia and depression.

Social function is ideally evaluated by an intake interview that details the patient's financial resources, social supports, and preferences for social intervention. A detailed intake interview is best performed by a trained social worker. A more limited inventory of social and economic supports can be obtained through completion of the OARS (Older Americans Research and Service Center) Social Support Questionnaire or the Medical Outcomes Study Social Support Questionnaire. Both these instruments can be completed by the patient or the caregiver or administered by office personnel. Environmental assessment should ideally be accomplished with a home visit, including a thorough inventory detailing sanitary conditions, safety, and accessibility of the house to the patient. In many team settings, home evaluation is reserved for a physical or occupational therapist. Often, community social workers combine home evaluation with a social intake interview in the same visit. A home access and safety questionnaire completed in the physician's office can substitute for a home evaluation when no professional is available.

Advanced directives. Physicians caring for aged individuals frequently find themselves managing medically futile situations. Identifying futility is difficult, but examples that most individuals would accept as futile include the patient with metastatic progressive cancer or the bedridden, poorly responsive patient with Alzheimer's disease. When caring for these patients, the physician may wish to limit therapy that has a curative intent or unnecessarily prolongs life. However, the act of withholding curative treatment makes it imperative that the physician always provide therapy to improve comfort and care.

When a progressive disease is identified for which no effective therapies exist, it becomes important to know the treatment wishes of the patient and family in advance of a crisis or urgent situation. Ideally the physician has a long-term relationship with the patient and can openly discuss prognosis and treatment options. In 1992, hospitals were mandated to inform patients of their right to obtain advanced directives and choose treatment options. Too often, treatment decisions have to be made without knowledge of the patient's desires or the assistance of surrogate decision makers.

Central to discussing advanced directives with patients is the concept of competence. *Competence* is a legal construct that embodies the individual's ability to make a choice. Competence includes the ability to understand information, appreciate that a choice must be made, comprehend the consequences of each therapeutic option, and express a choice among options. No criterion standards exist for defining and identifying a competent patient; that is, no universally accepted test is available for the diagnosis of incompetence.

The ascertainment of competence is complicated by variability in decision making; some medical decisions are more complex than others. For example, a patient with early dementia may retain the cognitive ability to determine the desirability of nutritional support in the event of severe disability or immobility; persons often do not wish to starve to death or have the sensation of hunger. However, the same patient may not have sufficient cognitive function to make decisions regarding cardiopulmonary resuscitation (CPR). In this case the same patient would be deemed competent to make a decision about nutrition but incompetent to make a decision regarding CPR.

Adults who are fully conscious, are able to communicate, and do not have delirium are assumed to be competent to make decisions on their own behalf unless deemed incompetent in a court of law. Before discussing advanced directives, the physician should assess level of consciousness, cognitive function, and mood and affect to make an assessment of decision-making capabilities. The history and physical examination should focus on problems that may interfere with thought processes. For example, does the patient have a cerebral metastasis, or is the patient taking medications that might induce delirium? Once a determination of the person's decision-making ability is made, the physician may proceed to discussing advanced directives.

Patients may document their wishes and maintain control over care in several ways. Precise requirements for documentation and interpretation of the law vary from state to state. Physicians must be knowledgeable of the requirements and standards of care in the jurisdiction in which they practice. The competent patient may execute a directive to physicians, a durable power of attorney, and documents explicitly outlining treatment preferences.

For the patient who is incompetent and has no directives, the physician must rely on surrogate decision makers. When a family is available, the first-degree next of kin may assist in making treatment decisions. In the absence of a family, the only other option for surrogate decision making is a legal guardian. When family or guardian are unavailable and the patient cannot express treatment preferences, the physician's best medical judgment must be used to guide treatment decisions. In this case the physician must determine the potential risks and benefits of treatment and aim to provide comfort, care, and maximum quality of life.

Directive to physicians. These documents are declarations by competent adults to withhold or withdraw life-sustaining therapy when a medical condition is incurable or irreversible. The directive may be revoked at any time by the patient. When a legally effective directive is executed by a competent individual, it takes precedence over others' wishes and desires. For example, a decision by a terminally ill parent to forego chemotherapy may not be overruled by an adult child or spouse.

Accepted directives vary from state to state but often include the following features. Two physicians must independently document that a condition is terminal and irreversible. The directive must be witnessed by two persons who are not related by blood or marriage to the individual and have no claim on the individual's estate. In addition, the individual's physician may not witness the directive. The directive must be executed in a voluntary manner without any coercion.

A directive to physicians should not be interpreted as an instruction to withhold all treatment. Persons with incurable illnesses often desire care to relieve suffering or treatment for self-limited illnesses such as pneumonia. Too often, physicians who are unfamiliar with the patient see the directive as a reason to withhold all treatment. Patients and their families are often reluctant to execute directives to physicians because they perceive that the quality of medical care and compassion of health care workers decline once a directive is in place. A directive to physicians does not mean "do not care."

Durable power of attorney for health care. Competent patients may wish to have someone make health care decisions on their behalf should they become incapacitated to express their own wishes. Patients may assign "agents" through a durable power of attorney for health care. A power of attorney becomes effective only when patient incompetence is certified in writing by the physician. The requirements for witnessing the power of attorney are similar to those for directives to physicians.

Treatment preferences. Although patients may not wish intensive care to maintain life, they may wish other forms of therapy that provide comfort and maintain quality of life. Accordingly, competent patients may make and document choices regarding a variety of treatment preferences. Examples of such choices include antibiotic therapy for infections, transfusions, and nutritional support.

Surrogate decision makers

Family. When patients are incompetent or cannot otherwise express their desires for medical care, first-degree relatives may consent to or refuse treatment. These relatives include a spouse, parent, adult sibling, or the patient's adult child. Acceptable familial relationships for medical treatment decisions vary among states. The physician must be aware that patients and their surrogate decision makers often disagree in their choices for medical care.

Guardians. Guardianship is put in place when patients are incompetent to manage their own affairs and assign surrogate decision making through a durable power of attorney. An example of a patient for whom guardianship is appropriate is the demented person with no family or social support system. Evidence is brought to a court of law regarding the person's competence. A judge rules on the evidence and may then assign a guardian for the individual. The guardian's responsibilities are to manage the individual's affairs and assist in decision making for health care.

Geriatric clinical pharmacology. Although only 12% of the population are older than 65, this group accounts for 30% of all medication consumption in the United States. Multiple drug use is not only costly but also confers significant clinical risk. Epidemiologic evidence has implicated adverse drug reactions as causal factors in as many as 10% of hospital admissions. Strong associations have been shown between specific drug classes and common disabling conditions in elderly patients. Neuroleptics, long-acting benzodiazepines, and psychoactive drugs have been implicated as risk factors for falls and hip fracture. Cognitive impairment, depression, incontinence, gastrointestinal bleeding, and renal insufficiency have also been linked to drug toxicity in aged persons.

The role of age as a determinant of drug response is controversial. Many studies have convincingly demonstrated that older persons are at greater risk than younger persons for adverse drug events. This association holds across hospital and community settings. Age per se, however, probably confers minimum risk. Indeed, when investigators have controlled for health status and number of medications, the association between age and adverse reactions weakens. It is likely that many interacting factors contribute to variation in drug response and increased susceptibility to adverse drug events. These factors include cumulative burden of chronic and often progressive illness, intermittent acute illnesses, medication number, physician prescribing behavior, and patient compliance. In addition, marked heterogeneity exists among aged individuals in pharmacokinetic and pharmacodynamic responses to drugs.

Table 370-2. Pharmacokinetic and pharmacodynamic changes with aging*

Physiologic change	Pharmacologic effect
Gastrointestinal	
↓ Gastric motility	Negligible
↓ Gastric pH	Negligible
Body composition	
↓ Lean body mass	Water-soluble drugs ↑ Serum concentration, ↓ Vd, ↓ t½
↑ Total body fat	Lipid-soluble drugs ↓ Serum concentration, ↑ Vd, ↑ t½
↓ Albumin	Highly (>90%) protein-bound drugs ↑ Free (active)/bound drug
Metabolism	
↓ Phase I reactions (e.g., oxidation)	Oxidatively metabolized drugs →↓ Metabolism, ↓ clearance, ↑ t½
→ Phase II reactions (e.g., glucuronidation)	No effects
↓ Hepatic blood flow	Drugs with flow-dependent metabolism ↓ Clearance, ↑ t½
Renal function	
↓ Creatinine clearance	Renally excreted drugs ↓ Clearance, ↑ t½
Target organ	
↓ Cellular mass (e.g., brain)	CNS active drugs ↑ Drug effect
↓ Receptor function	
↓ Beta-adrenergic response	Beta-adrenergic drugs ↓ Effect of $beta_1$ active drugs →↓ Effect of $beta_2$ active drugs
↓ Baroreceptor response	Drugs with orthostatic potential ↑ Orthostasis ↓ Heart rate, ↓ blood pressure compensation

From Gerety MB et al: Adverse drug reactions and altered clinical pharmacology in the elderly: a guide for modification of prescribing. In Katz MS, editor: Geriatric medicine, vol 1. New York, 1991, Churchill Livingstone.

* ↑, Increase; ↓, decrease; →, no change; Vd, volume of distribution; t½, half-life.

Age-related changes in pharmacokinetic and pharmcodynamic responses to drugs are outlined in Table 370-2. Changes in renal and hepatic function require adjustment of drug dosage or dosing interval for elderly patients. Creatinine clearance may be estimated using the Cockcroft equation:

$$\text{Creatinine clearance} = \frac{(140 - \text{Age [yr]}) \times \text{Weight (kg)}}{72 \times \text{Serum creatinine (mg/dl)}}$$

(multiply by 0.85 for females)

Patients whose creatinine clearance is less than 50 ml/min should have dosage adjustments for drugs with a narrow therapeutic index and primarily renal clearance. Most clinicians are aware of dosage adjustments required for aminoglycosides, but care must also be taken with other antibiotics, especially ticarcillin, Timentin (ticarcillin and clavulanate), cephalosporins, imipenem, and ciprofloxacin. Other drugs requiring dose adjustment in elderly patients include digoxin, allopurinol, lithium, amantadine, and H_2 blockers. Additional information and dosage adjustment suggestions can be found in other sources.

Hepatic function cannot be easily estimated. Therefore dosage adjustments for drugs handled by the liver are made on the basis of conditions that decrease hepatic function or blood flow. These conditions include congestive heart failure, primary liver diseases, and beta-adrenegic blockade.

Pharmacodynamic properties of specific agents may be altered because of reduced target organ mass or cellular function. This is particularly true of drugs with primary or secondary CNS effects. Such agents should be started at approximately one-half the usual starting adult dose and titrated slowly until the desired therapeutic end-point is achieved.

Physician prescribing behavior should reflect age-associated changes in drug response. To maximize therapeutic benefit and reduce the risk of adverse events, each patient's drug regimen must be carefully tailored, regularly reviewed, and periodically adjusted. New therapy should be initiated only after the need is convincingly demonstrated, goals are clear, an end-point is set, and a strategy for monitoring beneficial and adverse effects is in place.

Following these principles of prescribing is easiest for patients with whom the physician has a long-term relationship. In initial encounters, however, the clinician is often faced with patients with multiple diagnoses and multiple medications. In these patients the certainty of diagnosis and rationale for therapy are often unclear. A mounting body of evidence suggests that it is safe and beneficial to discontinue medications with no apparent indication, even if they have been prescribed for long periods. The best clinical strategy is to discontinue agents one at a time, carefully monitoring for recurrence of the original indication or changes in effectiveness of concomitantly prescribed medications.

Nutrition. Physiologic changes that occur with age often interact with chronic disease and socioeconomic factors to produce poor nutritional status in elderly persons. The U.S. National Health, Examination and Nutrition Survey indicates that older persons often consume as few as 1000 Kcal/day. As many as 60% of hospitalized patients and 50% to 70% of institutionalized persons may have mild to moderate malnutrition. It is often difficult to identify malnutrition with certainty because of coexisting diseases. However, markers of poor nutritional status have clear-cut associations with treatment outcomes. For example, clinical assessments of poor nutritional status are associated with poor surgical outcome. Low serum albumin has a consistent relationship with higher mortality in hospitals, nursing homes, and rehabilitation units.

Numerous factors contribute to inadequate nutrition. Socioeconomic factors include lack of education about appropriate nutrients, inadequate economic resources, and social isolation. Neuropsychologic diseases such as depression and dementia may result in reduced appetite. Functional disability and immobility make it difficult to use transportation, acquire groceries, and prepare food. Age-associated physiologic changes in thirst, taste, and smell may also reduce food consumption. Dental function and periodontal disease, rarely assessed in younger patients, may be important factors in poor nutritional intake in elderly patients.

Assessment of nutritional status in younger persons often involves anthropometric measurements, serum albumin and transferrin levels, total lymphocyte counts, and cell-mediated immune responses to dermal antigen injections. In elderly patients, all these nutritional assessments are less reliable because they are subject to age-associated changes and are also altered by disease.

A simple, clinically oriented evaluation of nutritional status is useful in elderly persons. A nutritionally focused history should elicit changes in weight (significant if >10% weight loss occurs over 6 months or 5% over 1 month) and determine whether weight is stable or still declining. Changes in eating habits or the presence of symptoms that interfere with food intake or digestion should be noted. The physical examination should focus on underlying causes of weight loss as well as signs of malnutrition (cachexia, interosseous wasting, loss of muscle mass) or nutrient deficiency (angular cheilitis or glossitis). Oral examination should include inspection of teeth, gums, fit of dentures, and oropharyngeal lesions that may interfere with mastication or oral intake.

The American Society for Parenteral and Enteral Nutrition has published guidelines suggesting threshold criteria for nutritional intervention. These criteria, however, are not tailored for elderly patients. Supplemental feeding is recommended for persons with obvious malnutrition or borderline nutritional status whenever a prolonged (5 to 7 days) period of hypocaloric intake is anticipated. If nutritional status is uncertain, daily calorie counts should be obtained and supplemental feedings instituted if caloric intake is inadequate. An adequate trial of supplemental oral feeding should be attempted before tube feeding or parenteral nutrition is instituted.

Food delivery systems in hospitals and chronic care institutions do not tailor food to patient preferences and do not appropriately emphasize patient feeding. Restrictive diets ordered in nursing homes and hospitals are often unpalatable, unnecessary, and potentially harmful. Liberalization of food intake to include all foods is preferable for patients with borderline nutritional status, even in those with diabetes or renal, cardiac, or hepatic dysfunction. Between meal snacks, extra meal portions and nutritional supplements are useful but often are unsuccessful because no systematic encouragement is provided to promote intake. If these conservative measures fail, intervention with enteral or parenteral nutrition is imperative.

The risks of enteral and parenteral feeding procedures, although not insubstantial, are outweighed by the morbidity and mortality associated with progressive nutritional decline. Prolonged hypocaloric intake produces anorexia that may be overcome only with up to 10 days of adequate supplementation. Invasive supplementation should be accompanied by formal nutritional consultation. Patients are often reluctant to accept tube feeding but may be persuaded with reassurances that supplementation will be self-limited, may speed recuperation, and will help restore appetite.

Sensory impairment. Hearing and visual impairments are common chronic conditions that limit communication and isolate aged individuals. From a diagnostic perspective, these impairments make it more difficult to obtain a history and evaluate an individual appropriately. Although other specialists may be necessary to rehabilitate sensory impairment, internists must be able to screen for impairment and refer for appropriate management.

Hearing impairment. Clinically significant hearing loss affects one in four persons over 65 years old, although measurable hearing loss affects more than a third of aged individuals. Poor hearing has been associated with increased depressive symptomatology, impaired cognitive functioning, decreased physical activity, and increased social and emotional isolation. These associations persist after adjustment for age, education, and other comorbid conditions, suggesting that hearing loss is an independent etiologic factor in the development of these social disabilities and handicaps.

The frequencies most needed to understand speech include 500, 1000, and 2000 Hz. No universally accepted audiometric definition of hearing loss exists, but an average loss of more than 25 dB at these three frequencies is recognized by most audiologists as evidence for significant hearing impairment. The most common pattern of hearing loss in the elderly is termed *presbycusis* and is characterized by a bilateral high-frequency sensorineural loss. The etiology of presbycusis is undetermined. Other factors that may contribute to hearing loss include prior noise exposure and middle ear disease. Coexisting audiologic conditions, such as tinnitus or central auditory processing disorders (primary problems understanding speech attributable to dysfunction in the brain's auditory centers), may impede successful rehabilitation of hearing loss.

Hearing may be screened quickly, reliably, and inexpensively with self-reports or physical diagnostic tests. The Hearing Handicap Inventory for the Elderly—Screening (HHIE-S) version is the most extensively studied self-report measure. The HHIE-S is a 10-item questionnaire that assesses social and emotional handicaps related to hearing loss. Higher HHIE-S scores are predictive of hearing loss and patient acceptance of audiologic assessment and rehabilitation.

Assessment of hearing should always be preceded by inspection of the ear and removal of any impacted cerumen. A hand-held otoscope with a built-in audiometer provides the only means of producing a standard screening signal at a known distance. All other tests (whispered voice, tuning forks, finger rubs) can help detect hearing impaired individuals but are susceptible to more variability in test administration. When the otoscope/audiometer is used to screen with a 40 dB signal at 1000 and 2000 Hz, sensitivity for detecting hearing loss is 94%. Its specificity is 72% in a physician's office and 90% in an audiologist's office.

To facilitate communication during the clinical interview, the physician should speak clearly and slowly and be positioned in front of the patient so that lip reading may be used to facilitate speech interpretation. Assistive listening devices (ALDs) are useful adjuncts to improve communication. ALDs relieve the difficulty an impaired subject may have in straining to listen, and they also save the interviewer's voice.

Hearing impaired patients with recognized handicap should be referred to an audiologist for full audiometry and the appropriate prescription of a hearing aid. In clinical trials, hearing aids have clearly been demonstrated to cause dramatic improvement in communication function. Improved communication function was also accompanied by improvements in depressive symptomatology and cognitive performance. For patients who cannot afford hearing aids, ALDs provide a less expensive means of general amplification.

Visual impairment. Visual impairment or blindness affects one in six persons aged 75 to 84 and one in four persons aged 85 and older. Total blindness is operationally defined as a visual acuity of 20/200 or worse in the better eye; although only 1% of persons over age 65 meet this definition, they account for most blind persons in the United States. Most impairments, such as loss of accommodation of the lens or corneal abnormalities, are managed with appropriate refraction with glasses or contact lenses. However, a variety of other conditions (macular degeneration, cataracts, diabetic retinopathy, glaucoma) lead to blindness and require ophthalmologic care.

Visual loss leads directly to loss of independence in instrumental ADLs and basic ADLs and decreased physical activity. The greatest threat to a functionally independent aged individual attributable to visual impairment is the loss of driving privileges. Most states require a best corrected visual acuity of 20/40 to operate a car. Visual loss also increases the risk of falls and injury. For example, the 10-year rate for hip fractures is 3% in persons with visual acuity of 20/25 or better, in contrast to a rate of 11% among persons with visual acuity of 20/100 or worse. After adjustment for age, sex, and alcohol and estrogen use, visual loss independently increases the risk of hip fracture twofold to fivefold. In addition to restrictions on activity, vision loss worsens affective symptoms as well. Persons with low vision report increased depressive symptomatology and lower levels of self-esteem and morale.

The internist should screen for visual impairment and, with appropriate referral, take steps to overcome its impact. Near and far vision may be screened effectively using a variety of charts with Snellen letters (or symbols if the patient is illiterate or cognitively impaired). Attention must be paid to fixed distances (14 inches for near vision and 20 feet for far vision) and appropriate illumination of the charts if screening is to be valid. Ophthalmoscopy may identify cataracts or retinal changes of diabetes and macular degeneration. Because the prevalence of vision impairment is so high, age over 65 alone may be used as a criterion for referral to an ophthalmologist if an eye examination has not been performed in the previous 2 years.

A variety of eye impairments may coexist; for example, a patient may have macular degeneration *and* cataracts. The ultimate success of ophthalmologic treatment depends on the severity and combination of impairments. Interventions to improve vision in aged persons with macular degeneration are of limited efficacy. Laser treatment for diabetic retinopathy reduces the risk of progression to blindness over 6 years from 37% to 17%. Diabetic patients should be seen annually by an ophthalmologist. Cataract extraction and intraocular lens implantation improves visual function in selected patients. Persons who are independent, still read the newspaper, drive a car, and take few prescription medications are most likely to benefit from cataract surgery. In patients with glaucoma, reducing the pressure in the eye remains the cornerstone of therapy for preventing blindness.

Hazards of bed rest. Although a time-honored treatment for many illnesses, imposition of bed rest is now understood to pose significant physiologic and psychologic hazards. The physiologic effects of immobility were originally defined in young healthy adult males as part of the space program. Because of marginal reserve in physiologic systems affected by immobilization, elderly persons are particularly prone to adverse effects of bed rest. Understanding the hazards of bed rest is especially important because almost all consequences of immobility are preventable with simple, common-sense maneuvers.

The physiologic consequences of bed rest are global. After less than 2 days of bed rest, blood volume decreases, cardiac output declines, and pulmonary volumes decrease. Urinary concentrating ability decreases, and calcium and nitrogen losses often exceed intake. Appetite decreases and bowel motility slows. Constipation or overflow fecal incontinence may occur. Decreased muscular strength, decreased endurance, and muscle atrophy also occur. Collagen fibers in tendinous and joint capsular structures begin to realign themselves along lines of stress into contractures after only 96 hours. Skin breakdown may begin to occur over bony prominences. Tissue pressure that exceeds capillary pressure for more than 2 hours may produce histologic findings of early tissue necrosis. Addition of shear forces (sliding downward in bed), heat, and humidity may hasten the formation of pressure ulcers. Stasis in the lower extremities and the pelvic venous system increases the risk of deep vein thrombosis. Arterial and venous responses to the upright position are diminished, with resultant postural hypotension. Both peripheral and CNS function are altered. Emotional lability, decreased concentration, poor short-term memory, and diminished intellectual functioning are seen after prolonged immobility.

The effects of bed rest may be prevented or ameliorated using simple precautionary measures and rehabilitation techniques. Assumption of the upright (seated, standing, and/or weight bearing) posture for a few minutes several times a day minimizes fluid, electrolyte, and calcium losses and helps retain vascular tone and baroreflex action. Passive range of motion exercises (i.e., moving joints through full range of motion only once per day) may prevent contractures. A few submaximal contractions of major muscle groups minimize loss of strength. Special attention should be paid to muscle groups important for bed mobility, transfers, and ambulation. These muscle groups include the hip flexors, hip extensors, knee flexors, knee extensors, and trunk musculature. The most effective exercises for these muscle groups in patients who must experience periods of immobility are functional activities, including supine to sit, sit to supine, transfer from bed to chair and chair to bed, sit to stand, and ambulation. Frequent changes of position and time out of bed also prevent pressure ulcer formation. Routine orders for hospitalized elderly patients should include being out of bed for all meals and ambulation at least daily. Nurses and physicians should encourage patients to perform these activities with minimum to no assistance.

The hazards of bed rest are so great that bed rest should be prescribed only when no other alternative exists. Physicians, nurses, and rehabilitation therapists often unwittingly conspire to produce complications of bed rest in the interest of "patient safety," despite the obvious risks of immobility.

Geriatric syndromes

Many of the problems affecting aged individuals should be viewed as syndromes (i.e., collections of signs and symptoms with several potential etiologies). Just as the clinical presentation of heart failure and anemia trigger a differential diagnosis of pathogenetic entities, so should the major geriatric syndromes of dementia, depression, falling, and incontinence. Investigations of established syndromes in other medical subspecialties have led to the understanding of disease mechanisms and effective therapies for the underlying conditions. Currently, the state of the art in studying geriatric syndromes is where the investigation of heart failure was 40 to 50 years ago; only now are we beginning to understand the etiologies of these conditions and what constitutes effective treatment.

Dementia. Dementia (Chapter 118) is a syndrome of global intellectual deterioration. The revised, third edition of the American Psychiatric Association's *Diagnostic and Statistical Manual of Mental Disorders (DSM-III-R)* defines the clinical features that serve as diagnostic criteria for the dementia syndrome. Dementia is characterized by a chronic loss of previously established intellectual ability that interferes with occupational and social function. Memory impairment is essential to the diagnosis and must be accompanied by at least one other deficit in cognitive areas such as language, visuoconstructive function, calculation, abstract thinking, judgment, and executive function. Personality change may also occur, but level of consciousness is maintained. Global cognitive impairment distinguishes the dementia syndrome from the decline in recent memory that often accompanies advanced age ("benign senescent forgetfulness"). Moreover, progressive deterioration with normal attention and alertness differentiate the dementia syndrome from acute confusional states such as delirium.

Dementing illnesses producing intellectual decline occur primarily in later life. The prevalence of dementia increases with age in the general population older than 65. Dementia severe enough to impair the ability to live independently is estimated to occur in 5% of persons older than 65 and 15% to 30% of individuals over 80 to 85. Dementia of lesser severity is thought to occur in more than 10% of the population over 65. Prevalence estimates, together with U.S. census data, suggest that 4 million Americans over age 65 have some degree of dementia. The prevalence of dementia in elderly residents of nursing homes may be as high as 50% to 60%. It is expected that the numbers of older individuals afflicted with dementia will increase as the average age of the older population (especially those over 85) increases.

Alzheimer's disease (Chapter 118) accounts for more than one half of all patients with dementia. The prevalence of Alzheimer's disease may be more common than previously suspected. In a recent community-based study the prevalence rates for probable Alzheimer's disease were 10% of those over the age of 65 and 47% of those older than 85. A widely used set of criteria for the clinical diagnosis of *probable* Alzheimer's disease has been proposed by a work group of the U.S. Department of Health and Human Services Task Force on Alzheimer's disease. The diagnosis requires that dementia be established by clinical examination, formal mental status tests (e.g., Mini–Mental State Examination, Blessed Dementia Scale) and neuropsychologic testing. Deficits must occur in two or more areas of cognition, with progressive worsening of memory and other cognitive function but without disturbance of consciousness. Finally, other disorders (see below) that could account for progressive intellectual decline must be absent. The diagnosis of *definite* Alzheimer's disease requires histopathologic evidence (neuritic plaques, neurofibrillary tangles) rarely obtained premortem.

Dementing disorders other than Alzheimer's disease are discussed in Chapter 118. In autopsy series, 10% to 20% of cases of dementia have been attributed to multiple cerebral infarcts *(multi-infarct dementia),* with an equal number of cases caused by multi-infarct dementia coexisting with Alzheimer's disease. A much lower prevalence (1% to 4%) of multi-infarct dementia has been described in geriatric outpatients with suspected dementia, although this population may exclude patients referred for neurologic rather than geriatric evaluation. Several clinical features distinguishing vascular dementia from Alzheimer's disease have been incorporated into a scoring system (Hachinski Ischemia Score) that is helpful in the diagnosis of multi-infarct dementia. Characteristics suggesting vascular dementia include abrupt onset, history of strokes, focal neurologic findings, stepwise deterioration, emotional incontinence, and history or presence of hypertension.

Much has been written about treatable causes of *reversible* dementia, as contrasted to *irreversible* disorders such as Alzheimer's disease and multi-infarct dementia. Medication toxicity, metabolic disorders such as hypothyroidism, and depression are considered the most common causes of reversible dementia. Cognitive impairment accompanying depression is sometimes called *pseudodementia*. In general, geriatric outpatients with reversible dementia have shorter duration of symptoms, are less demented, and use more prescription drugs than those with irreversible dementia.

Between 10% and 20% of dementias have been classified as "reversible" on the basis of their association with potentially treatable conditions. However, treatment of patients with reversible dementia usually results in only modest, transient improvement of cognitive function. A return to normal mental function is rare, and eventually most treated patients develop progressive deterioration consistent with Alzheimer's disease. Coincidental association of dementia with such disorders as hypothyroidism and depression would not be unexpected given the common occurrence of these different conditions in older persons. It is especially important to recognize that even in patients with "irreversible" dementia, cognitive improvement may follow treatment of coexisting medical disorders. Depression can also occur as a complication of Alzheimer's disease, in which case antidepressant therapy might be expected to improve cognitive dysfunction that is caused by depression. Finally, some treatable conditions such as hearing impairment can produce social isolation and other findings mistakenly attributed to cognitive impairment. These concerns have led some to question the practical significance of reversible dementia and to emphasize instead the treatment of comorbid conditions that contribute to overall loss of function in the demented patient.

A thorough history and physical examination, including neurologic examination and formal mental status testing, usually lead to a suspected diagnosis in the demented patient. Neuropsychologic testing may be required to meet the diagnostic criteria for probable Alzheimer's disease. Initial laboratory evaluation with complete blood cell count, blood chemistries (including electrolytes, glucose, creatinine, calcium), and thyrotropin (preferably a "second-generation" assay to recognize suppressed values associated with hyperthyroidism, as well as high values seen with hypothyroidism) is recommended to identify treatable abnormalities contributing to "reversible" dementia or other dysfunction in the demented patient. Routine screening with other laboratory tests, including neuroimaging by computed tomography (CT) or magnetic resonance imaging (MRI), is controversial. For any given patient the clinical impression derived from the history, physical examination, and initial laboratory evaluation determines whether additional diagnostic procedures are likely to be of benefit. Neuroimaging is probably not applicable to every dementia workup and is recommended especially for patients with recent onset of symptoms, atypical presentation, rapid deterioration, unexplained focal neurologic findings, history of head injury, and manifestations of normal-pressure hydrocephalus (i.e., incontinence or gait disturbance). Neuroimaging may also be useful to reassure patients and caregivers. Positron emission tomography (PET) and single-photon emission computed tomography (SPECT) have demonstrated reduced metabolic activity in the temporal and parietal region of patients with Alzheimer's disease. However, the clinical usefulness of these newer imaging techniques in the diagnostic evaluation of dementia remains to be determined.

Management of the demented patient is directed at treating reversible conditions that exacerbate functional decline and reducing behavioral disturbances through environmental manipulation or pharmacologic therapy (Chapter 118). Education of the patient's caregiver(s) is also an essential aspect of a comprehensive therapeutic plan. Instruction on the nature of the patient's illness and the availability of community respite services can improve patient care as well as reduce caregiver burden and thereby enhance quality of life for the caregiver.

Currently, no effective medical treatments exist for the irreversible dementias. The cholinergic hypothesis of Alzheimer's disease has led to recent clinical trials of the cholinesterase inhibitor tacrine (tetrahydroaminoacridine, THA) as a potential therapeutic agent. Preliminary results suggest that some Alzheimer's disease patients treated with tacrine respond over the short term with clinically meaningful improvement of cognitive function. However, drug toxicity is substantial, and long-term efficacy is unproved. Further studies are required to determine whether tacrine will be recommended in the future as effective treatment for Alzheimer's disease.

Depression. Lifetime risk of experiencing a depressive disorder is 7% to 12% for men and 20% to 25% for women. Depressive symptoms and depressive disorders are seen often in geriatric practices and among frail elderly persons. Prevalence estimates for major depression among elderly persons in the community range from 2% to 4% for men to 4% to 9% for women. Prevalence ranges from 15% to 40% for medically ill elderly patients in clinics, hospitals, and nursing homes. Despite such high estimates, epidemiologic research suggests that depressive disorders do *not* occur more frequently in elderly than in younger persons. Evaluation of birth cohort–specific rates of depression indicates that individuals born in the early twentieth century may be relatively protected from depression. Prevalence estimates are much higher for individuals born after World War II. Thus, although depression is already a major public health problem, it may become even more important in upcoming decades.

Depression is associated with significant functional disability, excess health care utilization, and increased risk of death. The Medical Outcomes Study and other studies have shown that functional disability and health care costs for depressed persons are equivalent to persons with major chronic illnesses, such as chronic lung disease, arthritis, and diabetes. In older individuals, depression is also associated with falls, incontinence, and impaired intellectual function. Although the mood disorder of depression has been shown to be successfully treated with a variety of pharmacologic and psychosocial therapies, it is not known whether improvement of mood is paralleled by improvements in other domains of function.

Despite its prevalence and impact, depression remains an underdiagnosed and undertreated disorder in elderly persons. Primary care physicians, including geriatricians, often do not uncover symptoms in a typical medical encounter. Patients, families, and physicians may mistake low mood, anhedonia, and somatic symptoms of depression as part of aging or chronic illness. Discovery of depression is enhanced by routine use of depression screening questionnaires. Instruments with acceptable sensitivity and specificity in elderly persons include the Geriatric Depression Scale (GDS) and the Brief Carrol Depression Rating Scale (BCDRS). The GDS (15 items) and the BCDRS (12 items) are both brief and have a simple yes/no response format, enhancing feasibility and acceptability. A score above a "depressed" range on a screening instrument, however, is not diagnostic of depression. Only 60% to 70% of individuals with positive scores meet DSM-III-R criteria for the diagnosis of major depression.

Diagnostic criteria for major depression require one of two major symptoms (low mood, anhedonia) to be present. Three or four of the following symptoms must also be present for a total of five symptoms: change in weight, sleep disturbance, psychomotor retardation or agitation, fatigue or low energy, feelings of worthlessness or guilt, difficulty concentrating, and hopelessness or persistent thoughts of death. Symptoms must have persisted for at least 2 weeks and be present most of the day every day. Persons with depressive symptomatology who do not meet criteria for major depression are classified into other categories (e.g., minor depression, dysthymia, nonspecific depression). Less severe depressive disorders have also been shown to be associated with excess disability, morbidity, mortality, and health care utilization. Although clear-cut evidence of treatment benefit exists for major depression, it is unclear to what degree persons with less severe depressive disorders benefit from either psychosocial or pharmacologic therapy.

Drug therapy is effective for major depression. Although most studies demonstrate a high placebo response rate (30% to 40%), drug treatment improves symptoms in up to 60% to 70% of treated individuals. Drugs appear to have no advantage over psychotherapy, and response rates may be somewhat better when both types of therapy are combined. Results of treatment trials in older individuals parallel results in younger populations. Among patients with a first episode of major depression, long-term prognosis may be better for older persons than for younger persons. Benefits of treatment for elderly patients with significant comorbid illnesses are unknown. Most trials of antidepressant therapy have systematically excluded elderly persons and persons with multiple diseases.

Many older individuals do not have access to or desire for psychotherapy. Drug therapy should be instituted for these individuals and for persons in whom symptom severity necessitates a rapid therapeutic response. Antidepressant medications are classified into several pharmacologic categories: tricyclic agents (e.g., desipramine, nortriptyline), heterocyclic agents (e.g., bupropion, trazodone), serotonin reuptake inhibitors (e.g., fluoxetine, sertraline), and monoamine oxidase inhibitors (e.g., phenelzine). No class of agents appears to have any therapeutic advantage over another. Side-effect profiles and cost, however, differ substantially. Selection of a pharmacologic agent therefore may be made on the basis of cost, anticipated side effects, interaction with comorbid disease, and concomitant drug therapy. Table 370-3 compares drugs recommended for use in elderly patients.

Tricyclics, heterocyclics, and monoamine oxidase inhibitors should be started at low doses and increased at the recommended dosing adjustment interval until a therapeutic response is achieved or side effects prohibit further increases. Although published literature suggests that therapeutic response may not be achieved for several weeks or until "full-dose" therapy is reached, many elderly patients achieve remission of symptoms at lower doses. Full doses for elderly persons are one third to one half of full doses for younger persons. Serotonergic reuptake inhibitors are usually started at therapeutic levels and often do not require upward dosage adjustment. In general, use of therapeutic drug levels is not recommended to monitor therapy, since drug response is not reliably related to serum levels. If no response has been achieved after reaching one-half the usual recommended adult dose, it may be prudent to wait several weeks before substituting other therapy. If side effects are intolerable before a therapeutic effect has been achieved, a drug from a different class should be substituted.

After remission, symptomatic breakthrough may occur. A waiting period of several weeks is recommended before therapy is altered, since breakthrough symptoms may often be brief and self-limited. If response is not achieved within this period, a drug from a different class should be substituted. Individuals with depression resistant to two courses of adequate drug therapy should be referred to psychiatric or psychologic professionals for additional evaluation and treatment. Duration of drug therapy is a matter of controversy. Recurrence of major depression typically occurs after brief courses of therapy. Two-year relapse rates for de-

Table 370-3. Frequently used drugs for treatment of depression in elderly patients

Drug Class	Major side effects: Anticholinergic	Sedation	Agitation	Cardiovascular	Drug interaction potential	Dosing interval
Tricyclics						
Desipramine	+	+	−	++	High	Daily (PM)
Nortriptyline	++	++	−	++	High	Daily (PM)
Heterocyclics						
Trazodone	−	+++	−	++	Moderate	Daily (PM)
Bupropion	−	+	+	++	Low	bid-tid
Serotonergics						
Fluoxetine	−	−	++	+	Low	Daily (AM)
Sertraline	−	−	+	+	Low	Daily (AM)
Monoamine oxidase inhibitor						
Phenelzine	++	++	−	+++	High	Daily (PM)

pressed individuals who discontinue drug therapy after 8 to 12 weeks may be as high as 70%. Maintenance drug therapy (full-dose antidepressant drug treatment after remission of symptoms) decreases the likelihood of relapse to 25% to 40%. Minimum recommended duration of therapy is 6 months. Some experts recommend that therapy be continued for as long as 1 year. For individuals with a history of recurrent depression, it may be necessary to continue therapy indefinitely.

Falls. Falling is a major public health problem in the United States. Multiple etiologies contribute to falls. Falls occur when a person's balance is perturbed and the intrinsic mechanisms to correct balance cannot overcome the force of the perturbation. A fall is defined as an event that results in a person coming to rest inadvertently on the ground or other lower level. Exceptions to this definition include falls resulting from loss of consciousness (syncope), sudden paralysis (cerebrovascular accident [CVA] or stroke), or seizure.

One third of community-dwelling persons over 65 years of age fall annually. One half of nursing home residents fall annually. One in six falls results in a soft tissue injury. One in 20 falls results in a fracture, most often of the wrist, ribs, and hip. Injury is the sixth leading cause of death in persons over 65; most of these are fall related. Falls also result in psychologic trauma, leading to reduction in physical activity, anxiety, loss of confidence, and social withdrawal.

In the evaluation of falls, consideration must be given to intrinsic problems (within the patient), extrinsic environmental problems (outside the patient), and their interactions. As persons age, they become less steady, have a stiffer slower gait, and are unable to respond to environmental perturbations as rapidly as younger individuals. Gait and balance evaluation should emphasize structured clinical measures of dynamic balance, that is, performance tasks that require movement and directly assess function. Two such validated clinical tools are available: a structured *performance-oriented assessment of mobility* (POAM) and *functional reach*. These measures identify deficits that increase the risk of falling. The items assessed in the POAM measures of gait and balance are listed in the box below. The POAM is superior to a standard neurologic evaluation in identifying functionally based problems that increase the risk of falling. The POAM identifies balance deficits that may require further evaluation; for example, inability to rise from a chair may indicate proximal muscle weakness or arthritis of the hips or knees.

Functional reach is a simple measure in which patients are asked to reach as far forward as possible without losing balance or shifting base of support. The distance reached with the outstretched arm is measured by a yardstick taped

Items in performance-oriented assessment of mobility

Balance measures

Sitting balance (leaning versus steady)
Ability to rise from chair (number of attempts, assisted versus unassisted)
Immediate standing balance (first 5 seconds)
Standing balance (wide based, narrow based, or assisted)
Sternal nudge (steady, staggers, or falls)
Standing balance, eyes closed (steady versus unsteady)
360-degree turn (continuous versus discontinuous steps)
Sitting down (safe, smooth motion versus unsafe or unsmooth motion)

Gait measures

Gait initiation (hesitation versus no hesitation)
Step length and height (foot clears floor and passes stance foot)
Step symmetry (right and left steps appear equal)
Step continuity
Gait path (straight versus marked deviation)
Trunk (straight versus flexed)
Walk stance (narrow versus broad based)

to the wall. Persons who cannot reach at all have an eightfold increased risk for repeated falls over the ensuing 6 months, in contrast with persons who can reach 10 or more inches.

Other intrinsic factors contributing to falls include neurologic disorders such as cerebellar and vestibular dysfunction. Parkinsonism increases the risk of falling 10-fold. Proprioceptive problems should prompt screening for vitamin B_{12} deficiency and cervical spondylosis. Pre-existing residua from strokes and dementia also increase the risk of falling. Musculoskeletal disorders such as rheumatoid arthritis and osteoarthritis, foot problems (bunions, hammer toes), and primary muscle disorders impair mobility and increase the risk of falling. Postural hypotension from any cause contributes to falls. Among aged individuals, postural hypotension is more likely to occur during the postprandial period.

In contrast to intrinsic factors that increase the risk of falling, extrinsic factors may be readily manageable; correcting these factors may decrease the risk of falling. Poorly fitting shoes providing little support or inadequate traction may lead to tripping and falls. Appropriate footwear should have low heels and firm, nonskid soles. Long, loose garments may also cause tripping.

Most falls occur in and around the home. Structured home safety checks should be done by the family or a case management agency. A fall's location should be reviewed, with special attention to improving safety of the walking surfaces. Slick floors and surfaces (especially in bathrooms), loose rugs, and obstacles (low pieces of furniture, lighting cords) may all predispose to falls and injuries. Poor lighting, especially on stairwells, may lead to a fall. Examples of remedial actions include installation of tub rails, nonslip strips, and tub chairs in bathrooms. Nonslip rugs and removal of obstacles make walking surfaces safer. Providing adequate lighting, handrails, and appropriately sized step rises and keeping steps in good repair make stairways safer.

Specific classes of drugs have been consistently associated with falls and hip fractures. All classes of psychotropic drugs (phenothiazines, butyrophenones, benzodiazepines, antidepressants), especially those with long half-lives and active metabolites, have been shown to increase the risk of hip fracture twofold. A faller's drug regimen should be carefully scrutinized and the use of these agents minimized or eliminated. The evidence that antihypertensives predispose patients to falls and injuries is less compelling, but these agents may increase fall risk by causing postural hypotension. Alcohol is clearly a risk factor for falls and injuries in younger adults, but evidence that alcohol consumption is a contributor to falling in aged individuals is lacking. Persons who use multiple drugs are at increased risk of falling regardless of the class of agents. Medication use should be reviewed frequently to document need, find the lowest effective dose, and reduce the total number of medicines taken.

Appropriate fall management depends on the results of the assessment and the combination of identified risk factors. Some factors (e.g., dim light bulb in a stairwell) are easier to correct than others. Specific disorders contributing to falls should be optimally treated. Sensory impairments, when present, should be appropriately evaluated and rehabilitated. Nonspecific neuromuscular, gait, and balance deficits may often be improved through supervised physical therapy and exercise programs. For example, patients may be taught to transfer safely and to take more time in rising out of a chair. Interventions are now being assessed experimentally to ascertain their effectiveness in fall prevention. Finally, patients and their caregivers should have a means in place to summon help in the event of a disabling fall. For example, call buttons worn around the patient's neck and connected to a central emergency notification system are available.

Urinary incontinence. Urinary incontinence is a common problem, increasing in prevalence with age, functional disability, cognitive impairment, and burden of disease. From 1% to 10% of all community-dwelling elderly persons over age 65 report some degree of incontinence. Approximately 15% to 25% of all hospitalized persons and more than one half of nursing home residents have episodes of incontinence. Cross-sectional surveys of incontinence prevalence may overestimate the burden of incontinence. Only one third to one half of persons who report incontinence have either frequent or troublesome symptoms.

The continence mechanism relies on simultaneous and integrated actions of many physiologic systems. Continence is maintained by a balance between pressure within the bladder *(expulsive forces)* and the bladder outlet *(retentive forces)*. In normal individuals, accumulation of urine in the bladder occurs isotonically, that is, without a rise in bladder pressure. Beta-adrenergic stimulation relaxes detrusor musculature during filling. Alpha-adrenergic stimulation maintains tonic contraction of the bladder neck and the intrinsic urinary sphincter. When a critical volume/pressure threshold is reached, the first desire to void is perceived and may be heightened by an accompanying involuntary detrusor contraction. In response to the urge to void, healthy individuals voluntarily suppress bladder contractions (reducing expulsive pressure) and contract pelvic floor musculature (increasing retentive pressure) until a suitable voiding place is available. Voiding is initiated by cholinergic stimulation of detrusor contraction, together with relaxation of the bladder neck, external sphincter, and pelvic floor musculature.

Cross-sectional studies of older persons have suggested changes in micturition physiology with age and disease. Bladder filling may not be isotonic because detrusor compliance decreases with age. The urge to void and involuntary detrusor contractions may occur at smaller bladder volumes. Older individuals are less able to suppress involuntary detrusor contractions, with a corresponding decrease in ability to postpone voiding. Bladder outlet pressure is probably less affected by age than by disease. Prostatism and urethral stricture may increase bladder outlet pressure. In contrast, postmenopausal or multiparous women may have reduced outlet resistance. Patterns of fluid excretion also change with aging. Although younger individuals excrete most fluid intake during the day, excretion may occur primarily at night in persons of advanced age. Nocturia, a relatively reliable sign of prostatism in younger men, may be less reliable in older men.

Incontinence is usually caused by impairments in more than one element of the continence mechanism. Focal or global neurologic deficits may impair the ability to perceive or respond to urinary urge. Spinal cord disease or autonomic neuropathy may interfere with transmission of efferent and afferent impulses to the bladder. Reduced detrusor contractile function may result from chronic distention secondary to prostatism or urethral stricture. Immobility may prevent timely locomotion to a toilet.

Chronic urinary incontinence is typically classified into one of several syndromes: urge, stress, functional, and overflow incontinence. These syndromes have characteristic symptoms, urodynamic profiles, and potential etiologies but may overlap in as many as one third of incontinent persons *(mixed incontinence)*.

Urge incontinence is involuntary loss of urine associated with a strong desire to void (urinary urgency). Urinary loss is usually of moderate to large volume but varies with the bladder volume required to provoke an involuntary detrusor contraction. Nocturnal episodes of incontinence frequently occur. Although the most common etiologies of urge incontinence are neurologic (e.g., CVA, dementing disorders, upper motor neuron disease), this syndrome often occurs in neurologically normal individuals, especially men with prostatism.

Urodynamic evaluation of the patient with urge incontinence reveals frequent involuntary bladder contractions, many associated with a strong desire to void. However, the amplitude (strength) of bladder contractions varies widely. Indeed, some persons have weak contractions, a condition known as *detrusor hyperactivity with impaired bladder contractility* (DHIC). Instead of complete bladder emptying, individuals with DHIC may void small amounts of urine and have a high postvoid residual. This syndrome has been described in elderly, predominantly female nursing home residents. Its importance and prevalence in a general population is uncertain.

Stress incontinence is the involuntary loss of urine with maneuvers that increase intra-abdominal pressure. Patients describe loss of small to moderate amounts of urine with actions such as coughing, laughing, and sneezing. In women, this condition is typically associated with multiparity, gynecologic surgeries, or menopausal atrophic urethritis. Males usually experience stress incontinence as a result of intrinsic sphincter damage during prostatectomy. Urodynamic studies of persons with pure stress incontinence demonstrate detrusor pressure higher than urethral pressure when the patient voluntarily increases intra-abdominal pressure.

Functional incontinence, which is observed in persons with impaired mobility and/or cognition, is apparently unrelated to neuromuscular disorders of the continence mechanism. Although urodynamic studies may be normal, persons with functional incontinence may be unable to reach the toilet or fail to respond appropriately to the urge to urinate. Although this syndrome is a diagnosis of exclusion, it may be the leading cause of incontinence in hospitalized and institutionalized patients.

Overflow incontinence is characterized by involuntary loss of small to moderate amounts of urine and an overdistended bladder with a high postvoid residual volume. Patients may have almost constant dribbling or intermittent loss of urine. This syndrome is most often secondary to chronic, severe outlet obstruction. Prostatism is the most common cause in men, whereas urinary stricture is the most common cause in women. In individuals with less severe outlet obstruction or relatively weak detrusor contractions, overflow incontinence may be precipitated by drugs that decrease detrusor contractile strength (anticholinergics, smooth muscle relaxants) or increase outlet pressure (alpha-adrenergic agonists). New onset of mechanical obstruction (fecal impaction) or acute changes in mental status may also precipitate urinary retention and overflow incontinence.

Not all individuals with urinary incontinence need evaluation or treatment. Some persons experience relatively little distress or inconvenience with infrequent or small-volume incontinent episodes. Postponement of evaluation may be appropriate until either moderate incontinence occurs or the individual thinks intervention is warranted. A simple severity scale, which focuses on the frequency of incontinent episodes, as well as the attendant social and hygienic consequences, may assist in establishing the threshold for evaluation. The same scheme may also be used to monitor the success of therapy.

The medical evaluation of patients with urinary incontinence should focus on confirming the presence of the disorder, identifying individuals for whom more extensive evaluation may be required, and finding reversible contributing factors or transient causes. The most common transient causes of urinary incontinence are changes in mental status, urinary tract infection, atrophic urethritis, medications, and stool impaction. A history of prior gynecologic and urologic conditions or surgical procedures should be elicited. Associated symptoms such as dysuria, nocturia, hematuria, hesitancy, or change in bowel habits should be determined.

The physical examination should focus on abdominal, pelvic, and rectal findings, including masses, prostatic enlargement, fecal impaction, atrophic urethritis, vaginitis, cystocele, rectocele, or uterine prolapse. Neurologic examination should evaluate general mental status, focal neurologic deficits, autonomic neuropathy, and spinal cord reflexes (bulbocavernosus reflex, perianal wink). Evaluation of the lower urinary tract should include measurement of postvoid residual volume, and may include maneuvers to detect stress incontinence. The Q-tip or pad tests evaluate wetness present after increases in intra-abdominal pressure with a full bladder.

Laboratory evaluation should focus on detection of secondary causes of urinary incontinence, including urinary tract infection, malignancies, and metabolic abnormalities that increase urinary flow. Minimum laboratory evaluation consists of urinalysis, culture and sensitivity, and serum chemistries to determine renal function and presence or absence of hypokalemia, hyperglycemia, or hypercalcemia.

All individuals discovered to have a large postvoid residual volume should undergo evaluation for urinary tract obstruction and detrusor function. If prostatism causing outlet obstruction is thought to be the cause of urinary incontinence and the patient either declines surgery or is a poor surgical candidate, drug therapy may be of benefit. The alpha-adrenergic blocking agents terazocin and prazocin relax prostatic smooth muscle, decrease outlet pressure, and reduce episodes of nocturia in men with prostatism. 5-Alpha-reductase inhibitors (e.g., finasteride) shrink prostate volume and increase urinary flow rates.

Several nonpharmacologic measures used to manage stress, urge, and functional incontinence include scheduled toileting, bladder retraining, pelvic floor exercises, and improved toilet access. Frequent scheduled *toileting* maintains a small volume of urine in the bladder. This small volume reduces the likelihood that an involuntary bladder contraction will occur or that stress leakage will follow changes in intra-abdominal pressure.

Bladder retraining programs are the only therapy known to prolong the interval between perception of the urge to void and onset of incontinence. Retraining is also useful to reduce the frequency of stress incontinent episodes. Bladder retraining should always be accompanied by a scheduled toileting program. Patients should be instructed in the physiology of micturition and the self-limited nature of detrusor contractions. On onset of a contraction, the patient uses relaxation or distraction techniques, together with voluntary contraction of the external sphincter and pelvic floor muscles, until the contraction subsides. The patient should specifically avoid toileting behaviors because such actions increase the strength of involuntary contractions. Combined scheduled toileting and bladder retraining can decrease incontinent episodes by 50% to 75%.

Originally conceived as a treatment for incompetent bladder outlet, *pelvic floor exercises* have been found to be beneficial for urge incontinence. Also known as *Kegel's exercises,* repeated contractions of the pubococcygeus muscle increase bladder outlet resistance. Contractions should be sustained for up to 10 seconds, followed by an equal period of relaxation. Sets of 10 to 30 contractions should be repeated several times a day. Effects may be noted within several weeks, but the exercises must be continued indefinitely because cessation is likely to be followed by recurrence of incontinence.

Incontinent patients may benefit by altering clothing or bathroom facilities to provide more rapid *access* to the toilet. Men or women who wear clothing with many layers (skirts, slips, girdles, garters, hose) or complicated fasteners (hooks, zippers, buttons, belts) may benefit by wearing clothing with elastic waistbands or Velcro closures. A bedside commode can be used for immobile patients or those with nocturnal incontinence.

Drug therapy is a useful adjunct to behavioral modalities in the management of incontinence. Many agents have been tried for urge incontinence, but only a few have been demonstrated to be efficacious. Oxybutynin, a smooth muscle relaxant with anticholinergic properties, and terodiline, a calcium channel blocker with anticholinergic properties, both reduce episodes of incontinence. These agents increase bladder capacity, reduce detrusor pressure, and increase the interval between episodes of urgency. No agent, however, increases the interval between perception of the urge to void and onset of incontinence. Drug therapy is therefore recommended only with a concomitant behavioral program. When behavioral and pharmacologic treatments are used simultaneously in motivated individuals without severe cognitive impairment, incontinent episodes may be reduced by as much as 75%. Individuals who receive no benefit should be considered for further urodynamic evaluation. No treatments have yet been demonstrated to be effective in severely cognitively impaired or institutionalized individuals. Although such persons cannot cooperate with a bladder retraining program, scheduled toileting is recommended. Since pharmacologic agents used for urge incontinence may cause confusion, drugs should be used with great caution in cognitively impaired persons.

Trials evaluating drug therapy for stress incontinence have had mixed results. Alpha-adrenergic agents, such as phenylpropanolamine and tricyclic antidepressants, produce mild increases in bladder outlet pressure. Estrogen replacement therapy (topical or systemic) may be successful in treating postmenopausal urethral atrophy. Trials of estrogen therapy have produced better results when combined with agents known to increase bladder outlet pressure. Drug therapy for stress incontinence is most effective when incontinence is mild to moderate and when accompanied by a program of pelvic floor exercises and scheduled toileting. Persons with intractable stress incontinence may require surgical intervention (artificial sphincter or bladder suspension).

In general, pharmacotherapy is not recommended for individuals with functional incontinence. However, an empiric trial of drug therapy may be warranted if behavioral measures fail and patient/caregiver stress is intolerable. Therapy may be most useful when administered at times of maximum caregiver stress (usually nocturnal incontinent episodes). In the absence of increased postvoid residual volume, small doses of oxybutinin can be tried with careful observation for urinary retention or neurologic side effects. In the patient with increased postvoid residual, empiric therapy with terazocin or prazocin can be tried. Effects should be evident within several weeks of combined drug and behavioral therapy.

REFERENCES

Branch LG, Horowitz A, and Carr C: The implications for everyday life of incident self-reported visual decline among people over age 65 living in the community. Gerontologist 329:359, 1989.

Duncan PW et al: Functional reach: predictive validity in a sample of elderly male veterans. J Gerontol 47:M93, 1992.

Felson DT et al: Impaired vision and hip fracture: the Framingham Study. J Am Geriatr Soc 37:495, 1989.

Finch CE: Longevity, senescence, and the genome. Chicago, 1990, University of Chicago Press.
Gurwitz JH and Avorn J: The ambiguous relation between aging and adverse drug reactions. Ann Intern Med 114:956, 1991.
Harper CM and Lyles YM: Physiology and complications of bedrest. J Am Geriatr Soc 36:1047, 1988.
Hazzard RH et al, editors: Principles of geriatric medicine and gerontology, ed 2. St Louis, 1990, McGraw-Hill.
Katz MS, editor: Geriatric medicine. New York, 1991, Churchill Livingstone.
Katzman R and Jackson EJ: Alzheimer disease: basic and clinical advances. J Am Geriatr Soc 39:516, 1991.
Masoro EJ: Biology of aging: facts, thoughts, and experimental approaches. Lab Invest 65:500, 1991.
Mulrow CD and Lichtenstein MJ: Screening for hearing impairment in the elderly: rationale and strategy. J Gen Intern Med 6:249, 1991.
National Institutes of Health: Geriatric assessment methods for clinical decision making. J Am Geriatr Soc 35:1071, 1987.
National Institutes of Health: Diagnosis and treatment of depression in late life: a consensus statement. Washington, DC, 1991, US Department of Health and Human Services.
Sullivan DH et al: Impact of nutrition status on morbidity and mortality in a select population of geriatric rehabilitation patients. Am J Clin Nutr 51:749, 1990.
Tinnetti ME and Speechley M: Prevention of falls among the elderly. N Engl J Med 320:1055, 1989.
Urinary Incontinence Guideline Panel: Urinary incontinence in adults: clinical practice guidelines. Rockville, Md, 1992, HCPR pub no 92-0038, Agency for Health Care Policy and Research, Public Health Service, US Department of Health and Human Services.

CHAPTER

371 Drug Interactions

Victor A. Yanchick
K. Vincent Speeg, Jr.
Steven Schenker

Most health professionals readily agree that pharmaceutical products can produce dramatic benefits in the diagnosis and treatment of disease and that when properly prescribed and monitored, they can be a major factor in lowering the cost of health care. However, most health professionals are also acutely aware that drugs can be "double-edged swords" and cause patients significant harm and suffering. Each year over 1.5 billion prescriptions are filled in the nation's approximately 55,000 outpatient pharmacies. For a nation of approximately 240 million people this represents an average of about six prescriptions per year per person. The nation's hospitals provide approximately $5 billion worth of drugs and drug products to hospitalized patients annually, representing approximately 15 drug administrations per day for each patient day in the nation's over 7000 hospitals. These figures do not take into account the numbers of drugs administered in nursing homes, mental-health facilities, correctional facilities, health maintenance organizations, and other organized health-care settings, and by physicians who dispense drugs directly to their patients.

This widespread use of medications carries with it a significant set of medical, economic, social, and personal problems. Since 1969 the U.S. Food and Drug Administration has received over 400,000 experience reports. In 1987 the FDA documented 50,000 incident reports that had been filed with this agency. Of these reports, 20,000 involved biologics and 30,000 involved drug products. A total of 12,000 deaths were reported to have been causally linked to adverse drug reactions while 15,000 cases required hospitalization. Most experts feel that these statistics only represent the "tip of the iceberg" and estimate that as many as 90% of all adverse drug reactions go unreported.

DRUG INTERACTIONS

Although adverse drug reactions and drug toxicities can occur when a single drug is administered, the incidence of adverse drug reactions and drug toxicities increases as the number of coadministered drugs increases. Many of these adverse drug reactions and drug toxicities are a result of a *drug interaction,* a situation in which the pharmacodynamic or pharmacokinetic effects of one drug are altered by the concurrent use of another drug (drug-drug interactions), or a situation in which the effects of drugs or nutrients may be affected by the action of the other (drug-nutrient or drug-food interactions). Drug interactions may be either helpful (increased efficacy or diminished toxicity), such as occurs when two drugs with different mechanisms of action are used to treat hypertension, or harmful (decreased efficacy or increased toxicity), such as occurs with the administration of tetracycline derivatives and antacids that contain divalent or trivalent cations or with the concurrent administration of flurazepam and cimetidine.

The prescribing physician usually knows and makes use of the beneficial effects of a specific drug combination. However, undesirable and unwanted consequences often develop unexpectedly when multiple drug therapy is employed, even though many of these interactions involve predictable changes in the pharmacokinetic or pharmacodynamic properties of the drugs. The picture becomes even more complicated when one considers the diversity of the pharmacologic actions that may be present in the agents used in many multiple-drug regimens and the presence of other nondrug factors that may also influence the ultimate outcome of the drug combination. Furthermore, some drugs may interact with other drugs through more than one mechanism of action. For instance, sulfonamides may not only inhibit the metabolism of warfarin but may also displace warfarin from its plasma protein binding sites. In these instances it is often difficult to quantify the ultimate consequences of any given drug combination.

Most drug-drug interactions involve changes in the drug's pharmacokinetics or pharmacodynamics. The same pharmacokinetic and pharmacodynamic principles that determine the behavior of drugs can be applied to predict these drug interactions. Pharmacokinetic interactions involve alteration in the absorption, distribution, metabolism, or excretion of one drug by another agent (see Table 371-1). These interactions are most commonly measured by

Table 371-1. Pharmacokinetic drug interactions

Alterations in absorption

Drugs that may decrease absorption	Drugs that may increase absorption
Antacids	Antacids
Cholestyramine	Metoclopramide
Colestipol	
H_2-receptor antagonists	
Kaolin-pectin	
Metoclopramide	
Mineral oil	
Sulfododecylsulfate	

Examples

Affected drug	Interacting drug	Effect on absorption	Mechanism of action
Tetracycline Derivatives	Di- or trivalent cations	Decreased	Formation of insoluble complex
Digoxin	Aluminum salts	Decreased	Physical adsorption
Cyclosporine	Metoclopramide	Increased	Increased gastric emptying time increases absorption
Digoxin	Metoclopramide	Decreased	Increased gastric emptying time decreases absorption
Warfarin	Cholestyramine	Decreased	Resin binding
Ciprofloxacin	Magnesium-aluminum antacids	Decreased	Complexation
Thyroxine	Colistepol	Decreased	Resin binding
Ketoconazole	Cimetidine	Decreased	Increased pH decreases dissolution

Alterations in cellular uptake or plasma protein binding
Examples

Affected drug	Interacting drug	Consequence
a. Plasma protein binding		
Warfarin	Phenylbutazone Chloral hydrate	Increased free concentration causes increased bleeding risk
Phenytoin	Valproic acid	Increased phenytoin toxicity
Oxazepam	Diflunisal	Increased free concentration causes increased CNS effects
b. Cellular uptake		
Digoxin	Verapamil	Increased digoxin effect

Interactions caused by changes in renal excretion
Examples

Affected drug	Interacting drug	Consequence
Penicillin	Probenecid	Decreased clearance caused by decreased tubular secretion
Methotrexate	Aspirin	Decreased clearance caused by decreased tubular secretion
Oral sulfonylureas	Clofibrate	Decreased clearance caused by decreased tubular secretion
Lithium carbonate	Sodium-depleting diuretics	Increased lithium toxicity caused by decreased lithium clearance
Digoxin	Quinidine	Increased digoxin toxicity caused by decreased digoxin clearance
Digoxin	Amiodarone	Increased digoxin toxicity caused by decreased digoxin clearance
Procainamide	Amiodarone	Increased procainamide toxicity caused by decreased procainamide clearance
Quinidine	Ammonium chloride	Increased clearance caused by decreased tubular reabsorption
Quinidine	Sodium bicarbonate	Decreased clearance caused by increased tubular reabsorption
Aspirin	Sodium bicarbonate	Increased clearance caused by decreased tubular reabsorption

Continued.

Table 371-1. Pharmacokinetic drug interactions—cont'd.

Interactions caused by a change in hepatic metabolism

Inducers of drug oxidation	Inhibitors of drug oxidation
Ethanol (chronic)	Ethanol (acute)
Carbamazepine	Chloramphenicol
Glutethimide	Erythromycin
Barbiturates	Ketoconazole
Phenytoin	Cimetidine
Rifampin	Isoniazid
Primidone	Allopurinol
	Diltiazem
	Ciprofloxacin
	Enoxacin
	Metronidazole
	Omeprazole
	Verapamil
	Amiodarone

Examples

Affected drug	Interacting drug	Consequence
Warfarin	Barbiturates	Increased clearance; decreased activity
Flurazepam	Cimetidine	Decreased clearance; increased activity
Theophylline	Cimetidine	Decreased clearance; increased activity
	Ciprofloxacin	
	Enoxacin	
	Erythromycin	
Digoxin	Rifampin	Increased clearance; decreased activity
Mexiletine	Phenytoin	Increased clearance; decreased activity
Ketoconazole	Rifampin	Increased clearance; decreased activity
Propranolol	Diltiazem	Decreased clearance; increased activity

changes in one or more kinetic parameters such as maximum serum concentration, area under the concentration-time curve, half-life, total amount of drug excreted in the urine, etc. Pharmacodynamic interactions occur when drugs having similar or opposing pharmacological effects are administered concurrently or in situations where the sensitivity or responsiveness of the receptors or tissues to one drug is altered by the actions of another. The pharmacodynamic properties of an agent may be altered independent of changes in its pharmacokinetics. An example of this type of interaction is the increased toxicity of digoxin produced by concurrent administration of potassium-wasting diuretics.

Given the potential for drug interactions, it is surprising that the recognized incidence of this complication is relatively low. In the Boston Collaborative Drug Surveillance Program, which monitored 9900 patients with 83,200 drug exposures, 3600 adverse reactions were found, but only 234 (6.9%) resulted from drug interactions. Of these, 230 were the result of cumulative pharmacologic effects. In another study of 900 hospitalized patients with 114 drug reactions, only 14 (12%) were attributed to drug interactions, and of these, five resulted from cumulative central nervous system depression. Patients on anticoagulant therapy are considered to be at particularly high risk for life-threatening drug interactions. Starr and Petrie reported potential drug interactions in 30% of patients on warfarin and other medications but were able to document such an interaction in only 9%. The importance of drug interactions is most obvious when it is demonstrated in patients receiving interacting drugs who also have other documented risk factors that may influence the severity of drug interactions (see box, p. 2845). These factors can profoundly change the pharmacokinetics and pharmacodynamics of the interacting drugs and contribute to an exaggerated drug response. In presumably normal individuals, plasma half-life can vary several-fold for many drugs (diazepam 9 to 80 hours; dicoumarol, 7 to 74 hours; tolbutamide, 3 to 27 hours), and any interaction between two drugs that results in prolonged plasma half-life of one or the other drug must be considered with this in mind. Disease states may also alter drug pharmacokinetics or pharmacodynamics. For instance, cirrhosis is associated with a decrease in the clearance of many drugs that undergo hepatic oxidation as well as agents that depend on normal hepatic blood flow for elimination. Normal physiologic changes such as declining renal function that occur

Factors that may influence drug-drug interactions

Physiologic factors

Age
Diet
Gender
Genetics
Pregnancy

Pathophysiologic status

Burns
Cardiovascular disease
Cirrhosis
Gastrointestinal disorders (achlorhydria, malabsorption, short bowel syndrome)
Smoking
Alcohol use/abuse
Renal disease
Thyroid disease
Malnutrition

as a normal consequence of aging can have a significant impact on the activity of many drugs that are eliminated primarily by the kidney.

In summary, the ability to predict possible outcomes resulting from the concurrent administration of two or more drugs known or suspected to interact is increased when one understands the basic principles that apply to drug interactions and the nondrug factors that may contribute to altering normal drug response.

PRINCIPLES OF MANAGEMENT

How does one keep track of or anticipate unwanted drug interactions? There is no simple approach to this challenge since a number of factors must be considered when drugs are prescribed. Drug interactions that occur with agents that have a narrow therapeutic index (see below) have a greater potential to create problems than do drugs whose therapeutic index is wide. Similar problems are more likely to occur when the drug interaction involves a compound that demonstrates nonlinear pharmacokinetics (see box above). Physicians should familiarize themselves with these drugs and, if one is prescribed, take extra care to monitor the patient's medication regimen and response to therapy.

Drugs with a narrow therapeutic index*

Aminoglycosides
Aspirin
Digitalis glycosides
Lidocaine
Lithium
Methotrexate
Theophylline
Oral hypoglycemics
Warfarin
Vancomycin
Chloramphenicol
Cyclosporine

*The difference between plasma levels that are subtherapeutic and those that are toxic is small.

Drugs with nonlinear pharmacokinetics*

Aspirin
Bishydroxycoumarin
Ethanol
Naproxen
Phenytoin
Propranolol
Theophylline

*Clearance may decrease as dose increases.

The following are principles that may help physicians approach the problem of drug-drug interactions at the clinical level. They are offered to assist the physician in minimizing the likelihood of prescribing drug combinations that have the potential to precipitate unwanted drug effects.

Identify patient risk factors. In older patients the influence of age on the absorption, distribution, metabolism, and excretion of drugs must be considered a major risk factor. In addition, patients who have impaired renal or hepatic function and disorders such as achlorhydria, diabetes, or cardiovascular disease are at greater risk for undesirable drug interactions. Patients who smoke, use alcohol, or who have dietary deficiencies handle drugs differently and they should be so identified as higher risk patients.

Take a thorough drug history and maintain complete medication records. A complete and up-to-date record of both prescription and nonprescription drugs must be taken, maintained, and utilized. Many avoidable interactions have occurred because the prescribing physician was unaware of prescription medications prescribed by another physician or because the patient used nonprescription medications that were not documented in the patient's records. Studies show that at least 30% of all elderly patients receive drugs from more than one prescriber. Nearly all pharmacies maintain computerized medication profiles for their patients. Recommend that your patients obtain all of their prescription and nonprescription medications from one pharmacy and make sure that this pharmacy maintains and uses these records in filling prescriptions. The pharmacist is often in the best position to detect potential drug-related problems and to inform the prescriber(s) regarding severity of the situation.

Be knowledgeable about the actions of the drugs being prescribed. Physicians should be familiar with the primary and secondary pharmacologic properties of the drugs they prescribe. One must recognize that there is great individual variability in drug metabolism and response of target sites to individual drugs. Thus any changes in these parameters resulting from the addition of other therapeutic agent(s) must be considered in that light. This implies that drug-drug interactions are likely to be clinically significant only if they lead to large changes in drug pharmacokinetics or pharmacodynamics or if they involve a small number of agents that have a narrow therapeutic/toxic ratio. It is helpful to know whether the prescribed drugs are metabolized by the cytochrome P450 oxidase isoenzyme systems in the liver, as happens with warfarin, quinidine, phenytoin, or cyclosporine, or whether the drugs are excreted unchanged primarily by the kidney. It is also very helpful to be familiar with the drugs that have the potential to interfere with the hepatic metabolism of other drugs such as cimetidine and the barbiturates.

Consider therapeutic alternatives. Many documented drug interactions are not absolute contraindications in that they may be allowed to continue if the patient is properly monitored and some dosage adjustment is made to compensate for the altered response. However, in situations in which another agent with similar therapeutic properties and a lesser risk of interacting is available, it should be considered for use.

Avoid complex therapeutic regimens whenever possible. The likelihood of drug interactions increases as the number of drugs taken increases. Whenever a new drug is added to the patient's therapeutic regimen the physician should review the medication profile to determine whether one drug can be discontinued. In addition, the use of medications or dosage regimens that permit less frequent administration may help avoid interactions that result from an alteration of absorption. Dosing schedules should be designed to be as simple as possible to maximize compliance.

Educate the patient. Too often patients know very little about their illnesses, let alone the benefits and problems that may result from their drug therapy. It has been well documented that patients who understand this information are more likely to be compliant with their medications and are more likely to identify drug-induced side effects. Patients should be encouraged to ask questions about their medications and to report any unusual or unexpected responses. Pharmacists should be encouraged to reinforce the directions for the safe and effective use of the prescriptions with the patients and to help the physician monitor the patient's medication regimen and drug response.

Monitor therapy. All patients should be closely monitored not only for the risk of drug-induced problems occurring from drug interactions but also for adverse effects occurring from the use of individual agents and for noncompliance. A low index of suspicion on the part of the prescriber has been cited as one reason why drug interactions are not commonly documented in clinical practice. New symptoms should be suspected as being drug-related until that possibility is excluded. In particular, symptoms in the elderly such as drowsiness, confusion, insomnia, forgetfulness, or irritability are often attributed to the aging process when in fact they may be a result of a drug interaction and can be prevented through dosage adjustment or modification of the therapeutic regimen. The identification of drug-induced illnesses should be a common occurrence in a physician's daily practice.

Individualize therapy. It is well recognized that patients responses to the same drug can vary widely. With many agents, it is difficult to predict drug response when a drug is used alone; the challenge is much greater when drugs are used in combination.

Identify and utilize proper resources for information. It is impossible for the prescribing physician to keep current with the explosion of information dealing with drug interactions. Several useful references list reported drug interactions and many sources summarize the clinical importance of such reports. At least one such reference book should be in the library of all practitioners. It is also highly recommended to utilize the expertise of a pharmacist who is knowledgeable in the area of drug interactions since these individuals can provide excellent consultation and information to the physician and patient alike.

REFERENCES

Benet LZ et al, editors: Pharmacokinetic basis for drug treatment. New York, 1984, Raven.

Geffer ES, editor: Compendium of drug therapy. New York, 1983, Biomedical Information Corporation.

Griffin JP and D'Arcy PF: A manual of adverse interactions. Bristol, England, 1984, Wright.

Hansten PD: Drug interactions: clinical significance of drug-drug interactions. Philadelphia, 1990, Lea & Febiger.

Jick H et al: Comprehensive drug surveillance. JAMA 213:1455, 1970.

Manasse HR Jr: Medication use in an imperfect world: drug misadventuring as an issue of public policy, part 1. Am J Hosp Pharm 46:929, 1989.

May FE, Stewart RB, and Cluff LE: Drug interactions and multiple drug administration. Clin Pharmacol Ther 22:322, 1977.

Perry ZA and Knapp DE: Annual adverse drug reaction report: 1987. Rockville, Md, 1987, U.S. Food and Drug Administration, Office of Epidemiology and Biostatistics, Center for Drug Evaluations and Research.

Shinn AF and Shrewsbury RP: EDI3. Evaluation of drug interactions, ed 3. St. Louis, 1985, Mosby.

Starr KJ and Petrie JC: Drug interactions in patients on long term anticoagulant and antihypertensive adrenergic neuron-blocking drugs. Br Med J 4:133, 1972.

Stewart RB and Cluff LE: Studies on the epidemiology of adverse drug reactions: VI. Utilization and interactions of prescription and nonprescription drugs in outpatients. Johns Hopkins Med J 129:319, 1971.

Tatro DS et al, editors: Drug interactions facts. St. Louis, 1985, Facts and Comparisons.

CHAPTER

372 The Periodic Health Examination

Suzanne W. Fletcher

The periodic health examination is a set of four clinical tasks carried out on asymptomatic persons: taking parts of a history, doing portions of a physical examination, ordering certain laboratory tests, and performing simple preventive maneuvers such as counseling patients or giving them immunizations. These tasks, often called *screening*, are undertaken to promote health and prevent disease or to find disease early in its course so that it can be treated before adverse health outcomes occur.

Over the past several years, the periodic health examination has evolved from the yearly physical examination, a general and untargeted checkup, to a lifetime program of "health protection packages." Certain history items, physical examinations, laboratory tests, immunizations, and counseling procedures are performed based on the age, sex, and risk category of each patient.

When physicians perform periodic health examinations, they usually do so in the context of ongoing care of their patients. Such a practice is called *case finding*, and it implies that the person initiating the examination has assumed the responsibility of following up any abnormality found. If the clinician is not committed to investigation of abnormal results, the examination should not be performed in the first place. Patients undergoing case finding in internal medicine practices frequently are not well and often have many symptoms. Case finding is that part of the examination directed toward medical conditions for which the patient is asymptomatic. For example, a physician practices case finding when he or she performs a periodic clinical breast examination on a patient who is without breast symptoms but who is being seen for diabetes and angina.

Routine physical examinations are among the 20 most frequent reasons for visits to internists' offices in all subspecialties except oncology and nephrology. Internists care for an age group of patients for whom periodic health examinations are recommended with greater frequency than for any other group except pregnant women and very young children.

RECOMMENDATIONS

Several groups have made recommendations for the minimal set of tasks that should be included in periodic health examinations. Figure 372-1 is a summary of recent recommendations for adults made by major groups.

In the history, health behaviors regarding cigarette smoking, alcohol, and seat belt use should be assessed, and appropriate counseling should be given when necessary. Some groups also suggest checking for other health-related behavior such as nutrition, exercise, sexual behavior, substance abuse, and dental care.

Periodic physical examination recommendations are highly targeted and include examinations for hypertension and for breast, cervical, and colorectal cancers. Some groups recommend periodic physical examinations for other cancers as well, including skin, oral, endometrial, testicular, ovarian, thyroidal, and prostatic cancer. Clinical examination for hypothyroidism in postmenopausal women has also been recommended.

Recommended laboratory tests are aimed at breast, cervical, and colorectal cancers as well as hypercholesterolemia. Some groups suggest searching for conditions such as anemia, sexually transmitted diseases, tuberculosis, and low bone mineral content, in high-risk groups. Appropriate immunizations are recommended.

The physician's role in counseling patients about healthful behaviors is growing. Smoking cessation is more likely to be successful with counseling. For control of hypercholesterolemia, the first step is dietary change, and appropriately trained physicians can help patients learn better eating habits. Other healthful behaviors also can be encouraged by physicians.

Examination of Fig. 372-1 shows that recommended procedures and frequencies vary according to patients' ages. For example, carcinoma in situ of the cervix is more common in younger than in older women, and therefore most groups suggest more frequent Papanicolaou smears in young women. Breast cancer, on the other hand, becomes more common as a woman gets older, and recommendations regarding the search for breast cancer reflect this fact. For most women patients, this means that physicians should shift case-finding emphasis from cervical to breast cancer as the woman grows older.

The list of tasks in Fig. 372-1 is short; expert groups currently recommend fewer items than previously. No major group includes routine complete blood counts, urinalyses, chest x-rays, or electrocardiograms. Most of the recommended procedures are also inexpensive, and when possible they should be incorporated into regularly scheduled visits for ongoing care.

Studies have shown that practicing physicians frequently do not perform some examinations that experts recommend with a high degree of consensus, such as tests to detect breast cancer in older women. Meanwhile, they often perform other examinations that are not recommended, such as periodic chest x-rays and electrocardiograms. Periodic health examinations should start with the items listed in Fig. 372-1.

Even when physicians are committed to periodic health examinations, it is not easy to incorporate the performance of indicated examinations into the ongoing care of patients being seen for established diseases. For example, it is difficult to remember that a given patient being seen for hypertension is also due for a breast examination, mammography, and a stool guaiac test. Prompting systems can help. Many practices include in each patient's medical record a flow sheet similar to that in Fig. 372-1; whenever a patient visits the practice, the flow sheet is consulted to see if any

Figure 1. Preventive Care Guidelines for Asymptomatic, Low-Risk Adults: Recommendations from Various North American Health Organizations (1)

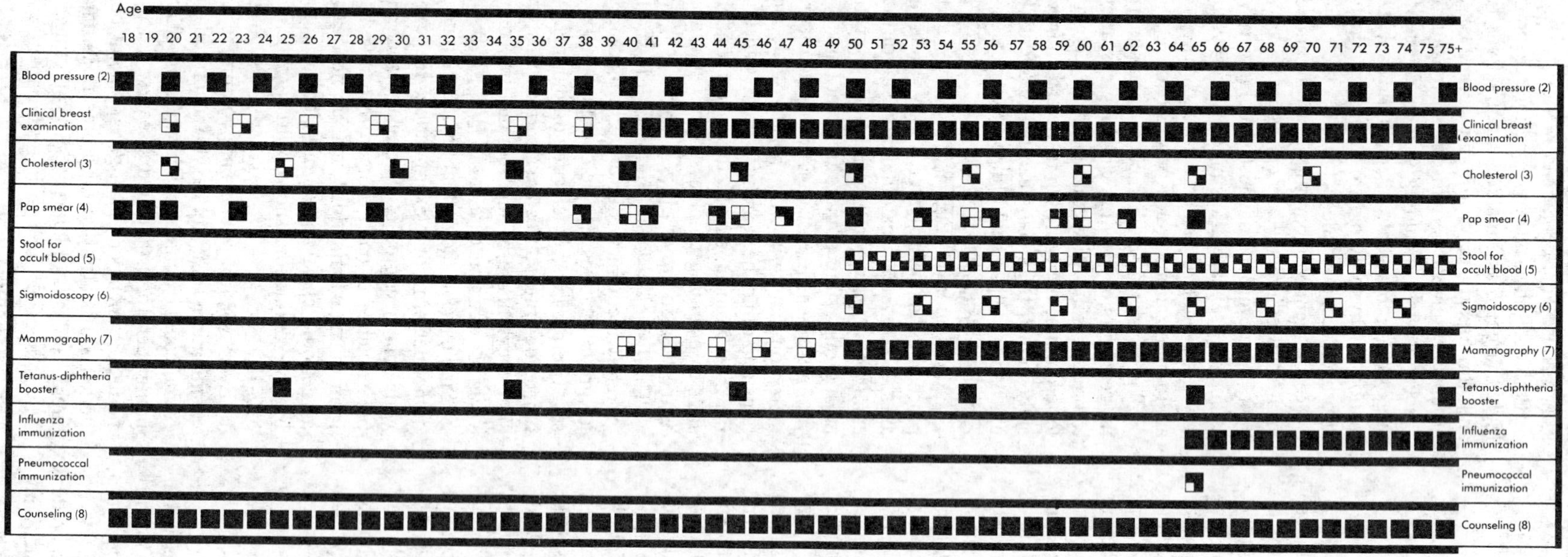

Blackened square indicates that the service is recommended. An empty square indicates that either a recommendation has been made to not provide the service or that no recommendation has been made for or against the service by the particular authority. The placement and spacing of squares indicate a suggested age range and frequency for testing rather than actual ages at which services should be provided.

ACP	USPSTF
CTF	OTHER

ACP American College of Physicians.
USPSTF US Preventive Services Task Force.
CTF Canadian Task Force on the Periodic Health Examination.
Other Immunization Recommendations - CDC Immunization Practices Advisory Committee.
Cholesterol Recommendations - National Cholesterol Education Program Panel on Detection, Evaluation, and Treatment of High Blood Cholesterol in Adults.
Hypertension Recommendations - Joint National Committee on Detection, Evaluation, and Treatment of High Blood Pressure.
Cancer Screening Recommendations - American Cancer Society.

Hayward, Steinberg, Ford, Roizen, Roach

1. This list shows selected, age-specific preventive care services recommended by at least one of the ACP, CTF, or USPSTF, which should be offered to persons who do not have a family history, symptoms, signs, or other diseases that place them at increased risk for preventable target conditions. All authorities stress the importance of determining each person's unique risks for preventable disease in order to individualize preventive care. Strategies for the selective provision of a wider range of services to persons at low and increased risk for particular conditions are found in Tables 2 through 5.
2. The CTF recommends screening at least every 5 years and at every clinical encounter. Others agree or suggest screening every 2 years.
3. The CTF recommends periodic serum cholesterol testing in men between the ages of 35 and 59 years. The USPSTF recommends determinations in middle-aged men and suggests that testing of young men, women, and the elderly may be clinically prudent.
4. ACP and USPSTF do not recommend a Papanicolaou smear for women over 65 years of age who have had consistently normal smears in the previous decade. CTF suggests Papanicolaou smears every 3 years before 35 years of age and every 5 years to 74 years of age, after two normal annual smears folllowing the onset of sexual activity.
5. CTF and USPSTF concluded that there is insufficient evidence to recommend for or against fecal occult blood testing.
6. ACP recommends sigmoidoscopy every 3 to 5 years or air contrast barium enema every 5 years. Neither the CTF nor the USPSTF recommends for or against screening sigmoidoscopy.
7. American Cancer Society recommends annual or biennial mammography for women from 40 to 49 years of age.
8. ACP, USPSTF, and CTF emphasize that all adults should be routinely counseled about tobacco use, nutrition, exercise, sexual behavior, substance abuse, injury prevention, and dental care.

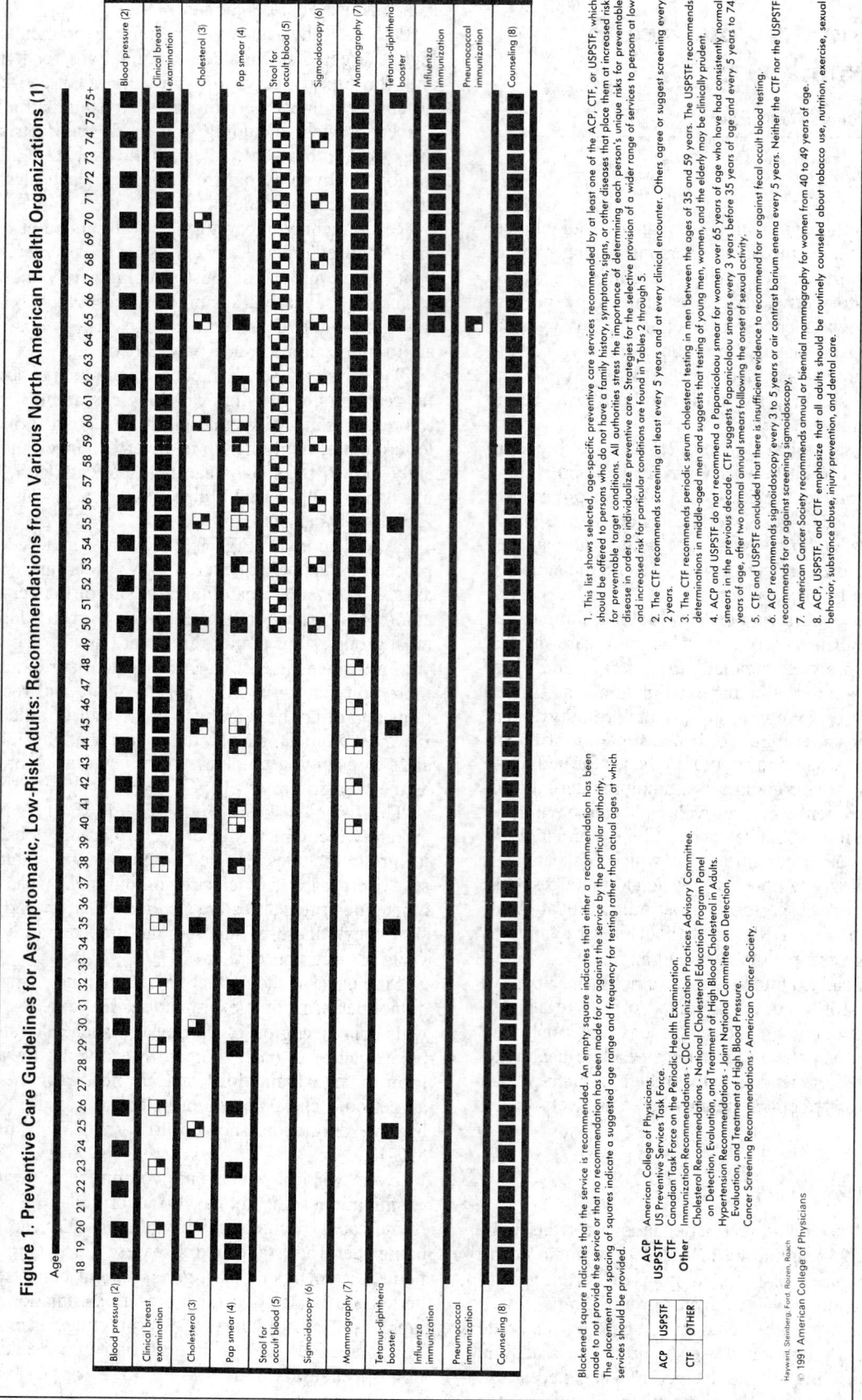

Fig. 372-1. Preventive care guidelines for asymptomatic, low-risk adults: recommendations from various North American health organizations. (From Hayward RS et al: Preventive care guidelines. Ann Intern Med 114:758, 1991. Reprinted with permission.)

procedures are indicated. Computer prompting has also been used to help remind physicians to perform periodic tests.

SCIENTIFIC PRINCIPLES UNDERLYING THE PERIODIC HEALTH EXAMINATION

When physicians undertake periodic health examinations on asymptomatic patients, a decision must be made about which medical problems or diseases should be sought or prevented. This principle sounds straightforward, but often it is not. Thus, a urinalysis, frequently ordered in routine examinations of asymptomatic adults (but not recommended by any of the expert groups represented in Fig. 372-1), might be used to search for any number of medical problems, including diabetes, asymptomatic urinary tract infections, and renal calculi. Before a urinalysis is performed, it is necessary to decide which, if any, of these conditions is worth screening for.

Three criteria have been developed for deciding whether a medical condition should be sought during a periodic health examination. In order of importance, they are (1) the effectiveness of prevention or early treatment for the medical condition, (2) the severity of the condition, and (3) the quality of the proposed screening procedure. A good screening procedure should be sensitive, specific, simple, inexpensive, safe, and acceptable to patients and physicians.

The three criteria are fulfilled better for some conditions than for others, and judgment is involved in reaching decisions. As a result, some recommended procedures listed in Fig. 372-1 are made with much more certainty, scientific evidence, and consensus among various groups than other recommendations. Also, the correct frequency of repeat examinations is undergoing constant modification as more information becomes available.

Physicians who examine their patients for unrecognized disease rarely find the disease. Even "common" diseases are uncommon; for breast cancer, several hundred women must be examined for each case of cancer found. Furthermore, because of low prevalence of disease in asymptomatic individuals, even very accurate tests with good sensitivities and specificities produce many false-positive results. Most abnormalities uncovered during periodic health examinations are not caused by the medical condition being sought. Targeting specific examinations according to a person's age, sex, and risk status helps to increase the prevalence of disease among those examined before the examination is done, thereby cutting down on the number of false-positive test results.

The number of false-positive test results is also related to the number of examinations a physician carries out on a patient. Most physicians do not perform only one or two tests on patients presenting for checkups. Many order several dozen tests, which is easy to do with modern technology and automated blood tests.

A laboratory test result is usually defined as "abnormal" if the result falls outside the range covered by 95% of test results in a large group of people. This means that the more tests a physician orders, the greater the risk of a false-positive test. If the physician orders even five tests, 23% of healthy people will have an abnormal result; with 20 tests, 64%; and with 100 tests, over 99%. The resultant burden of financial, medical, and psychological costs among patients with false-positive test results may be large.

Physicians can guard against this problem by keeping the number of tests they perform to a minimum and by making sure they search only for medical conditions meeting the three criteria outlined above. Such strategies maximize the benefits and minimize the risks and costs of periodic health examinations.

REFERENCES

Eddy DM, editor: Common screening tests. Philadelphia, 1991, American College of Physicians.

Fletcher RH, Fletcher SW, and Wagner EH: Prevention. In Clinical epidemiology: the essentials, ed 2, Baltimore, 1988, Williams & Wilkins.

Hayward RS et al: Preventive care guidelines. Ann Intern Med 114:758, 1991.

U.S. Preventive Services Task Force: The guide to clinical services: an analysis of the effectiveness of 169 interventions. Baltimore, 1989, Williams & Wilkins.

CHAPTER

373 Preoperative Medical Evaluation

Valerie A. Lawrence
Jane Appleby

The goal of preoperative medical evaluation is to decrease operative morbidity and mortality by identifying and treating medical problems that contribute to perioperative risk. Medical complications of surgery are relatively uncommon now, so research in this area is difficult and many clinical issues have not been rigorously studied. However, identifying medical illnesses that increase surgical risk and defining the potential complications will presumably aid in careful management and improve outcome. Also, assessing the additional risk imposed by underlying illnesses can help the physician and patient weigh the potential benefits and risks of a procedure.

Essential to a preoperative medical evaluation is a thorough history and physical examination. Particularly, patients should be asked about past responses to anesthesia and surgery, current medications, smoking habits, and recent acute illness. Also important is a past history of cardiopulmonary disease, bleeding diathesis, and hepatic or renal dysfunction. Physical examination should include an assessment of nutritional status and upper airway abnormalities that may complicate intubation (loose teeth, tracheal deviation), a pulmonary examination, a cardiovascular examination for valvular disease and ventricular dysfunction, plus evaluation for possible coronary artery and peripheral vascular disease.

History, physical findings, and medication should dictate what laboratory data are required. Research has shown that routine screening tests have very low yield for unsuspected abnormal findings and even less yield for abnormalities that affect surgical outcome. The exceptions include a hematocrit when significant operative blood loss is anticipated, a urinalysis before prosthetic, vascular, or neurosurgical procedures or if bladder catheterization is expected, and an electrocardiogram in men older than 40 and women older than 55. If pregnancy cannot be excluded historically, a pregnancy test should be considered. Currently, routine screening for human immunodeficiency virus (HIV) is a very controversial and unresolved issue.

ESTIMATED OPERATIVE RISK

Numerous factors influence operative risk: the site and type of procedure, the method and duration of anesthesia, the condition requiring surgery, and the patient's underlying medical illnesses. Cardiopulmonary complications constitute the great majority of medical complications associated with surgery.

While each surgical procedure has its own inherent risks, the incidence of cardiopulmonary complications is related to the procedure's proximity to the diaphragm. Thoracic and upper abdominal operations cause diaphragm dysfunction and inspiratory pain, thereby reducing postoperative tidal volume and cough effectiveness and increasing the likelihood of significant atelectasis, pneumonia, and ventilatory failure. Procedures lasting over 3 hours increase the likelihood of pulmonary complications and deep venous thrombosis. Vascular procedures, which can be associated with wide swings in blood pressure and heart rate, have a greater risk of perioperative myocardial infarction. Operative risk is generally double for emergent procedures. Nonemergent surgery that does not involve the abdomen, thorax, blood vessels, or brain has a relatively low inherent operative risk.

To a variable degree, all general anesthetic agents depress myocardial contractility. Spinal and epidural anesthesia produce prolonged sympathectomy in the anesthetized area, causing peripheral vasodilation and reduced venous return to the heart. Regional anesthetics have little effect on the cardiovascular system except when absorbed in large quantities. General, spinal, and epidural anesthesia are thought to carry an equal risk of myocardial infarction and cardiac death. Regional anesthesia is usually well tolerated regardless of the patient's clinical status.

The Dripps-American Society of Anesthesiology System (ASA) was developed over 30 years ago for estimating operative mortality resulting from systemic disease. Mortality increases with worse ASA class: class I—healthy; class II—mild systemic disease; class III—severe systemic disease; class IV—incapacitating systemic disease that is a constant threat to life; and class V—moribund and not expected to survive 24 hours with or without operation. Disadvantages of the system are that it is a subjective, relatively gross risk index and that patients with many types of illnesses and different "true" surgical risks are combined, exaggerating the danger in some and minimizing it in others. A further disadvantage is that it does not specifically predict cardiopulmonary complications, which are the major source of surgical risk.

SYSTEMIC RISK FACTORS

Cardiovascular risk factors

Ischemic heart disease. Two large prospective studies are considered classics in identifying risk factors for cardiac complications in mixed populations of patients undergoing a wide variety of noncardiac operations and are the current standards for assessing cardiac risk. (see box below). However, these indices tend to underestimate risk in a significant portion of patients and were derived before current supportive technology. Patients who have had a myocardial infarction (MI) within 6 months of noncardiac surgery are at highest risk of perioperative reinfarction and death. Old studies indicate that the risk of reinfarction is approximately 30% for patients undergoing surgery within 3 months of an MI; it falls to 11% to 16% for surgery within 4 to 6 months and stabilizes at 4% to 6% after 6 months. Short, simple procedures such as cystoscopy, uterine dilation and curettage, and angiography carry a lower risk of infarction than thoracic, vascular, and upper abdominal procedures. Well done prospective trials of invasive hemodynamic monitoring, angioplasty, or coronary artery bypass to reduce the surgical risk of a recent MI have not been done. Therefore, it remains prudent to delay elective procedures until 6 months after an MI. For patients requiring urgent surgery, preoperative coronary angiography, angioplasty, or revascularization and invasive hemodynamic monitoring should be considered. Most perioperative myocardial infarctions occur within 5 days of surgery and the mortality is high. Many perioperative MIs are painless, underscoring the necessity of postoperative surveillance electrocardiograms (ECGs) in patients at risk.

Cardiac risk factors

- Recent myocardial infarction (less than 6 months)
- Angina, unstable or stable class III or IV
- Congestive heart failure
  - Functional class III or IV
  - Elevated jugular venous pressure
  - Third heart sound (S_3)
- Frequent premature ventricular depolarizations
- Moderate to severe valvular aortic stenosis
- Age greater than 70 years
- Poor general medical condition (e.g., hypoxemia, hypokalemia, renal failure, liver disease)
- Intrathoracic, intraperitoneal, vascular, or emergency surgery

Modified from Goldman L et al: N Engl J Med 297:845, 1977; and Detsky AS et al: J Gen Intern Med 1:211, 1986.

Stable angina pectoris slightly increases the risk of perioperative MI and death (1% to 5%). Vigilant anesthesiology, careful intraoperative blood pressure control, continuous ECG monitoring, and appropriate replacement of fluid and blood losses are the best prophylaxis against perioperative arrhythmias, MI, and heart failure. Anti-ischemia and antihypertensive drugs should generally be continued on the day of surgery. Nitrates or beta blockers can be used for empiric prophylaxis against ischemia but short-term perioperative calcium channel blockers may actually increase risk. A stress test may identify patients at increased risk for perioperative myocardial infarction. For patients with ischemic ECG changes at low levels of exercise, coronary angiography before major operations should be considered. For patients who cannot exercise (e.g., because of peripheral vascular disease or degenerative joint disease), dipyridamole-thallium testing may aid in risk assessment.

The risk of perioperative MI and death in patients with unstable angina is probably comparable to that of patients with a recent MI. Elective procedures should be delayed until angina is stable. Coronary angiography and angioplasty or revascularization should be considered. For emergency surgery, patients should have invasive hemodynamic monitoring. Spinal anesthesia may result in a prolonged fall in blood pressure and thus may increase the likelihood of myocardial ischemia.

Because the association between atherosclerotic peripheral vascular disease and coronary artery disease is high, preoperative cardiac assessment for vascular operations poses special problems. History, physical exam, and ECG may underestimate risk and inaccurately predict cardiac outcome. Additional studies may be needed; most commonly used now is thallium stress testing with either exercise or dipyridamole. Several clinical variables appear to categorize risk in combination with thallium stress testing: Q wave on ECG, age greater than 70, history of angina, ventricular ectopy, or diabetes. Those with no clinical markers can often safely go directly to operation without stress testing, while those with three or more clinical markers should often undergo cardiac catheterization to assess the potential risks and benefits of coronary artery bypass surgery first. Of patients with one or two clinical markers, those with no thallium redistribution can usually safely undergo the vascular procedure while those with thallium redistribution should be considered for cardiac catheterization first.

Unfortunately, it is not clear that coronary artery revascularization before vascular surgery improves the short-term operative outcome. Therefore the decision about coronary artery bypass surgery first should rest on the usual criteria (e.g., left main disease, most three-vessel disease) for which there is proven late outcome benefit in survival.

Heart failure. The operative risk associated with congestive heart failure depends on the degree of left ventricular dysfunction. Patients with New York Heart Association (NYHA) functional class I or II failure and no jugular venous pressure elevation are not at significantly high risk of perioperative MI or pulmonary edema. Perioperative management should be conservative, that is, optimization of medical therapy and careful management of fluids, electrolytes, and hematocrit. Patients with NYHA class III or IV heart failure, jugular venous pressure elevation, or a third heart sound (S_3) are at high risk of cardiac complications. Elective surgery should be delayed until heart failure is adequately controlled. Perioperative invasive hemodynamic monitoring has not been carefully evaluated with controlled studies but may be beneficial and is usually recommended.

Arrhythmias. Relevant factors in the incidence and severity of perioperative arrhythmias include underlying ischemic heart disease or left ventricular dysfunction, preoperative history of arrhythmias, depth of anesthesia, presence of aortic stenosis, postoperative infection, hypoxia, hypokalemia, use of digoxin, anemia, and increased levels of circulating catecholamines. Supraventricular tachycardia occurs in about 4% of all surgical patients and should prompt evaluation for congestive heart failure, myocardial infarction, pericarditis, pulmonary embolism, infection, hypoxia, acidosis, hypokalemia, or aggravating drugs such as bronchodilators or epinephrine.

Clinically important ventricular arrhythmias should be controlled prior to operation. If surgery cannot be delayed, lidocaine may be used. Patients on chronic antiarrhythmic therapy should receive their usual oral dose the morning of surgery and as soon as possible after the operation. Patients taking quinidine may have prolonged neuromuscular blockade after exposure to neuromuscular blockers, and their respiratory status should be followed closely.

Heart block. Left or right bundle branch block or right bundle branch block plus left anterior hemiblock does not confer a significant risk of perioperative second- or third-degree heart block. Asymptomatic patients with bifascicular block should have continuous intraoperative ECG monitoring but usually do not require a prophylactic temporary pacemaker. Symptoms of high-grade atrioventricular block, sinus node failure, and noncongenital second- or third-degree heart block should be evaluated and treated before elective procedures.

The presence of a permanent pacemaker does not increase surgical mortality. Discharge of pacing impulses from demand pacemakers, however, may be inhibited by electrocautery. Ground connections for cautery should be placed as far from the chest as possible. If pacemaker inhibition still occurs, the pacemaker should be set in a fixed-rate mode.

Valvular heart disease. Valvular heart disease reduces the patient's ability to meet perioperative demands for increased cardiac output, increases the risk of bacterial endocarditis, and in patients with prosthetic valves, may require modification of chronic anticoagulation. In general, mildly symptomatic patients (NYHA class I or II) tolerate surgery well, except those with aortic stenosis. For noncardiac surgery, hemodynamically important aortic stenosis increases perioperative mortality to about 13%, primarily from arrhythmias and pulmonary edema, compared to about 2% for other valvular disease. Patients with severe aortic stenosis should undergo valve replacement before elective, noncardiac operations with general or spinal anesthesia.

Mitral stenosis increases the risk of perioperative atrial fibrillation. Preoperative administration of digoxin or beta receptor antagonists may slow the ventricular rate if atrial fibrillation occurs. For mitral and aortic regurgitation, risk of noncardiac surgery depends on the degree of left ventricular volume overload and decompensation. Well-compensated lesions pose little increased risk. Patients with moderate to severe regurgitation should have invasive hemodynamic monitoring and cautious afterload reduction if surgery cannot be delayed. Patients with moderate to severe aortic regurgitation are extremely sensitive to bradycardia and vasodilation. Valve replacement should be considered in patients with functional class III or IV valvular disease.

Patients with valvular heart disease undergoing procedures that produce transient bacteremia are at risk for bacterial endocarditis. Clean operations, such as orthopedic, ophthalmologic, and plastic surgical procedures, do not require prophylaxis. Antibiotic prophylaxis should be given to patients with disease of their native valves, hypertrophic cardiomyopathy, atrial septal defect (primum only), most congenital cardiac malformations, prosthetic valves, and vascular grafts and patches. For patients with mitral valve prolapse, prophylaxis is not recommended without documented regurgitant flow.

Perioperative management of patients on chronic anticoagulant therapy depends on its indication. Patients who should have minimal interruption of anticoagulation include those with mechanical prosthetic valves in the mitral position, dialysis patients whose shunts have previously clotted, and patients with demonstrated risk of embolization. While warfarin is discontinued, full-dose heparin therapy can be used preoperatively, stopped 6 to 12 hours before surgery, and then restarted postoperatively when risk of surgical rebleeding is acceptably low. For other patients, including those with prosthetic aortic valves, discontinuation of warfarin (3 or 4 days preoperatively to several days postoperatively) without heparinization is reasonable.

Hypertension. While it is preferable that patients be normotensive, diastolic blood pressures less than 110 mm Hg may not be associated with greater operative risk. Further, rapid manipulation of blood pressure preoperatively, especially with diuretic-induced changes in volume status, may increase the likelihood of intraoperative lability in blood pressure. Exceptions are patients with ischemic heart disease or congestive heart failure, in whom the increased afterload combined with anesthetic-induced myocardial depression may increase the risk of ischemia or left ventricular dysfunction. Patients with diastolic blood pressures greater than 120 mm Hg are at increased risk and should have better control before surgery.

In hypertensive patients, intraoperative blood pressure is labile regardless of the degree of control preoperatively. Most antihypertensive drugs should be continued up to the time of operation. Options for patients who are NPO include parenteral methyldopa, hydralazine, propranolol, labetalol, enalapril, nitroprusside, and sublingual nifedipine or transdermal clonidine. A patient taking diuretics should have a serum potassium level measured preoperatively; if it is less than 3 mEq per liter (3.5 mEq/liter for patients on digoxin), elective procedures should be delayed for potassium repletion.

Pulmonary risk factors

Anesthesia and surgical site. Incidence of complications is greatest with thoracic and upper abdominal operations, less with lower abdominal procedures, and least with peripheral procedures. Prolonged anesthesia (more than 2 to 3 hours) is also associated with pulmonary complications. General anesthesia decreases tidal volume, expiratory reserve volume (ERV), and sigh frequency. As ERV approaches closing volume, small airway collapse produces diffuse atelectasis in all patients undergoing general anesthesia. Patients with elevated closing volumes (from bronchitis, emphysema, cigarette smoking) or pre-existing depression of ERV (from obesity, neuromuscular disease, skeletal abnormalities) are particularly susceptible to these changes. Consequently, the likelihood of significant atelectasis and hypoxemia is increased.

General anesthesia also impairs lung defense mechanisms by increasing airway secretions and depressing lower airway ciliary clearance and cough reflex, thus promoting tracheobronchial bacterial colonization. Patients with pre-existing lower airway colonization or defects in airway clearance are especially likely to convert airway closure to pneumonia.

Aspiration of gastric contents occurs in 7% to 16% of patients undergoing general anesthesia. Nasogastric tubes, autonomic dysfunction (e.g., diabetes), drugs that relax the lower esophageal sphincter, and emergency operations increase the risk of aspiration. Neutralization of gastric acid with H_2-receptor blocking agents or antacids reduces the morbidity of aspiration.

Spinal anesthesia itself has little effect on pulmonary function, but prolonged immobilization may lead to gravity-dependent atelectasis. Paralysis of lower thoracic nerve roots may decrease tidal volume and cough effectiveness. For lower abdominal and lower extremity surgery, spinal and general anesthesia probably have equal risk of pulmonary complications.

Nearly one half of patients undergoing abdominal procedures develop small pleural effusions within 3 days of operation. The effusion usually occurs on the side of surgery and resolves within 3 to 4 days.

Infection. Acute upper and lower respiratory tract infections increase the risk of aspirating infected secretions, atelectasis, pneumonia, and possibly laryngospasm on intubation. Elective procedures should be delayed until acute infections have resolved. Patients with chronic bronchitis have excessive tracheobronchial secretions, a propensity for bronchospasm, and bacterial colonization of their lower airways. These patients should have aggressive postoperative pulmonary toilet. Preoperative antibiotics should be considered but there is not good evidence regarding their use.

Asthma. Patients with asthma may have exacerbations in the perioperative period, partly related to the irritant effect of dehumidified, highly oxygenated inspired air, increased airway secretions, aspiration, or administration of mast cell degranulating drugs. Preoperative preparation includes bronchodilator therapy and treatment of bronchitis, if present. Patients with severe asthma may benefit from high-dose oral steroids beginning 1 week before surgery. In general, patients should be without wheezes at the time of induction.

Chronic obstructive pulmonary disease. Operative risk depends on the extent of underlying functional pulmonary impairment and the type of procedure. Unfortunately, pulmonary function tests and arterial blood gas analysis only roughly correlate with the likelihood of pulmonary complications. Maximum voluntary ventilation, FEV_1, and $PaCO_2$ are the more reliable predictors of outcome. Roughly, risk of pulmonary complications is low when FEV_1 is greater than 2.0 liters, moderate for FEV_1 of 1.0 to 2.0 liters, and high with FEV_1 less than 1.0 liter. Hypercarbia, more than hypoxemia, identifies patients who may be difficult to wean from mechanical ventilation.

No single spirometric test accurately predicts complications. Further, critical appraisal of the evidence about spirometry's predictive value indicates it is a poor screening test. Rather than being obtained routinely, preoperative spirometry should be used to define clinically apparent lung disease that has not been previously characterized, to determine if there is a bronchodilator response, when hypercarbia is suspected, or to assess other factors important to clinical decisions. Patients should not be denied potentially high-benefit surgery on the basis of marginal pulmonary function alone. With very careful management, many such patients can do well. In addition to pre-existing lung disease, other factors such as type of procedure, smoking history, volume of airway secretions, obesity, age, duration of anesthesia, and presence of other medical illnesses should be considered. Restrictive lung disease increases operative risk, but less so than chronic obstructive disease. However, cor pulmonale markedly increases risk. Lung resection is a special situation, and risk assessment requires more sophisticated tests and the guidance of pulmonary specialists.

Prophylaxis of pulmonary complications. Ceasing cigarette smoking is recommended, but airway secretion may actually increase in the first few days after cessation. The necessary period of abstinence to reduce complications is not clear, but appears to be about 2 months. For reversible airways disease, aerosolized bronchodilators and corticosteroids should be the primary therapy. If the patient has a purulent cough, antibiotics in the week before surgery may be helpful. Postoperatively, incentive spirometry and early mobilization appear to be the most powerful prophylactic measures. Chest percussion has not been shown to be better than incentive spirometry and should be used in a case-specific basis only.

Prevention of thromboembolism (see Chapter 217). Risk factors for postoperative deep venous thrombosis (DVT) include venous stasis (venous insufficiency, history of DVT, congestive heart failure), obstruction to venous return (obesity, pregnancy), age greater than 40, prolonged immobilization, hypercoagulable states (malignancy, oral contraceptive use, pregnancy, nephrotic syndrome), lower-extremity orthopedic procedures, and prostatectomy. For those undergoing thoracic or abdominal surgery, low-dose subcutaneous heparin (5000 units 2 hours before surgery and 5000 units every 8 to 12 hours postoperatively until the patient ambulates normally) significantly reduces the likelihood of DVT and pulmonary embolism. Operative complications are not significantly increased, although wound hematomas are slightly more frequent.

Heparin prophylaxis is also effective but less so for hip and knee surgery, open prostatectomies, and gynecologic cancer operations. Alternative regimens include two-step warfarin (begin 10 days before surgery, with prothrombin time [PT] at 2 to 3 seconds prolonged, then postoperatively give approximately twice the dose to increase PT to 1.5 times control), adjusted-dose heparin (3500 units s.c. t.i.d. begun 2 days before surgery; check partial thromboplastin time [PTT] 6 hours after morning dose, and adjust heparin dose by 500 to 1000 units to keep PTT at 30 to 40 seconds), and pneumatic compression. Although further studies are needed, low-molecular-weight heparin appears to be as effective as standard subcutaneous heparin in preventing postoperative DVT in high-risk patients and may produce fewer bleeding complications.

When anticoagulation is contraindicated, external pneumatic compression of the lower extremities is effective. Leg elevation and elastic stockings are only marginally effective in preventing clot formation. For neurosurgical procedures, low-dose heparin is recommended for extracranial operations and pneumatic compression for intracranial procedures.

Hematologic risk factors

Most patients with mild to moderate anemia (hematocrit 20% to 30%) do not require preoperative transfusion before major surgery unless significant blood loss is expected. In general, it is wise to delay elective surgery until the cause of anemia is determined because some hematologic diseases require special perioperative management and occult disease may affect risk/benefit considerations for a procedure.

A platelet count of 80,000 to 100,000/μl is adequate in patients undergoing major surgical procedures. Minor surgery not involving the airway or blood vessels is usually safe with 30,000 platelets/μl. Patients with dysfunctional platelets, regardless of the total count, may have a higher incidence of perioperative hemostatic complications. Aspirin should be avoided for 1 to 2 weeks before noncardiac surgery. Other nonsteroidal anti-inflammatory drugs that inhibit platelet function can be stopped 1 to 2 days before surgery.

Endocrine risk factors

The stress of anesthesia and surgery increases insulin and corticosteroid requirements. Diabetic patients have a higher incidence of postoperative wound and genitourinary infections, which may increase insulin requirements. Conversely, surgical resolution of infection, sepsis, and shock reduces postoperative insulin requirements.

Perioperative insulin requirements depend on the degree of glucose control and type of therapy before surgery. Oral hypoglycemic agents should be discontinued the day of surgery. In patients whose fasting serum glucose values are below 200 mg per deciliter, perioperative insulin is generally not required. Insulin-dependent diabetics and those with poor control need perioperative insulin. Several regimens are effective: (1) half the usual morning dose of insulin before surgery; (2) one third the usual daily dose of insulin before surgery and one third after; or (3) continuous infusion of 8 to 10 units of regular insulin in 5% glucose solution. Patients receiving supplemental insulin should have intravenous glucose until oral intake is adequate. Postoperatively, serum glucose should be checked regularly to guide insulin dosage.

Inability to meet perioperative requirements for corticosteroids may lead to adrenal crisis. Patients receiving adrenal-suppressing doses of steroids for a period of 1 week or more during the previous year, those currently taking corticosteroids, or those with a suspect pituitary-adrenal axis should receive supplemental corticosteroids perioperatively. In cases of maximum stress, adequate replacement is hydrocortisone 100 mg intravenously or intramuscularly at midnight before surgery, the morning of surgery, and then every 6 to 8 hours for 24 hours or until postoperative complications resolve. Replacement should then be tapered over several days.

Hypothyroidism increases sensitivity to sedative and anesthetic agents and impairs ventricular function, ability to excrete a free water load, and ventilatory response to $PaCO_2$. However, available evidence suggests that mild to moderate hypothyroidism usually does not significantly increase surgical risk. When feasible, it is probably prudent to delay elective operations until replacement therapy is adequate. An important exception may be patients with angina undergoing coronary artery bypass surgery; risk of ischemia may increase with full thyroid replacement. Close attention should be paid to postoperative respiratory and volume status and serum sodium concentration.

Hyperthyroid patients undergoing surgery are at increased risk of thyroid storm. Elective operations should be delayed until the patient is euthyroid. For emergent or urgent operations, propranolol usually controls cardiovascular manifestations of hyperthyroidism and prevents thyroid storm.

Gastrointestinal and hepatic risk factors

Anesthetic agents generally reduce blood flow to the liver and enhance the risk of surgery in patients with liver disease. Morbidity usually results from postoperative gastrointestinal bleeding, hepatic encephalopathy, acute renal failure, and infection. The operative mortality associated with acute liver disease is difficult to separate from the prognosis of the disease itself. Acute viral hepatitis, for example, has a 9% overall operative mortality, while 85% of patients with acute fulminant hepatic failure die after surgery. Alcoholic hepatitis also increases operative risk. Acute hepatitis is a relative contraindication to surgery, but the degree of risk is not well quantitated. The usual recommendation is to delay elective procedures until liver function tests have remained normal for 1 month.

Most data about operative risk of chronic liver disease come from patients undergoing portosystemic shunting procedures. Serum bilirubin greater than 10 mg per deciliter, albumin less than 3 g per deciliter, prothrombin time greater than 4 seconds above control, poorly controlled ascites, encephalopathy, and poor nutritional status are associated with increased risk of operative complications and death.

Perioperative management of patients with liver disease includes meticulous attention to fluids, electrolytes, and the dosage of hepatically metabolized drugs, plus preoperative lactulose or neomycin to decrease risk of encephalopathy in those with poor prognostic indicators or history of encephalopathy. Hypoglycemia and hypokalemia are more likely with nasogastric sectioning and decreased oral intake.

Peptic ulcer disease, gastritis, and reflux esophagitis can be exacerbated by stress of surgery and nasogastric tubes. The incidence of upper gastrointestinal bleeding can be reduced with H_2-receptor antagonists or hourly administration of antacids. Preoperative parenteral hyperalimentation should be considered for patients with malnutrition (e.g., inflammatory bowel disease, malabsorption syndrome) to improve wound healing and reduce postoperative infection, but the large Veterans Affairs Cooperative Trial did not find it to be effective in reducing complications in all patients.

Renal risk factors

Whether renal insufficiency is glomerular, interstitial, or obstructive, impaired creatinine clearance and azotemia affect surgical risk. Mild to moderate impairment does not significantly alter operative morbidity if volume depletion and nephrotoxic drugs are avoided or if dosage is appropriately modified and potassium administration is monitored. As the glomerular filtration rate approaches 25 ml per minute, complication rates increase. Elderly patients are at risk of obstructive uropathy from prostatic hypertrophy or anticholinergic drugs. Patients with nephrotic syndrome are more susceptible to intravascular volume depletion, infection, and vascular thrombosis.

Patients with severe renal failure on chronic dialysis have only a 2% to 4% mortality for major elective surgery, but operative morbidity approaches 60%. Incidence of hyperkalemia, shunt or fistula thrombosis, pneumonia, wound infection, postoperative hypoventilation, pulmonary edema, and bleeding complications are increased. Maintaining serum potassium below 5 mEq per deciliter, replenishing bicarbonate stores, and controlling hypertension appear to reduce surgical risk. Dialysis within 24 hours of surgery is generally safe and may reduce the postoperative rise in serum potassium. A hematocrit of 20% to 30% is usually well tolerated. If transfusion is required, washed cells should be considered because of reduced potassium load.

REFERENCES

Collins R et al: Reduction in fatal pulmonary embolism and venous thrombosis by perioperative administration of subcutaneous heparin. Overview of results of randomized trials in general, orthopedic, and urologic surgery. New Engl J Med 318:1162, 1988.

Detsky AS et al: Predicting cardiac complications in patients undergoing noncardiac surgery. J Gen Intern Med 1:211, 1986.

Eagle KA et al: Combining clinical and thallium data optimizes preoperative assessment of cardiac risk before major vascular surgery. Ann Intern Med 110:859, 1989.

Gersh BJ et al: Evaluation and management of patients with both peripheral vascular and coronary artery disease. J Am Coll Cardiol 18:203, 1991.

Goldman L et al: Multifactorial index of cardiac risk in noncardiac surgical procedures. N Engl J Med 297:845, 1977.

Guidelines for electrocardiography: A report of the American College of Cardiology/American Heart Association Task Force on Assessment of Diagnostic and Therapeutic Cardiac Procedures (Committee on Electrocardiography). J Am Coll Cardiol 19:473, 1992.

Kroenke K: Preoperative evaluation: the assessment and management of surgical risk. J Gen Intern Med 2:257, 1987.

Lawrence VA, Page CP, and Harris GD: Preoperative spirometry before abdominal operations: a critical appraisal of its predictive value. Arch Intern Med 149:280, 1989.

Levine MN et al: Prevention of deep vein thrombosis after elective hip surgery: a randomized trial comparing low molecular weight heparin with standard unfractionated heparin. Ann Intern Med 114:545, 1991.

Lubin MF, Walker HD, and Smith RB, editors: Medical management of the surgical patient. Boston, 1988, Butterworth.

Merli GJ and Weitz HH, editors: Medical management of the surgical patient. Philadelphia, 1992, W.B. Saunders.

National Institutes of Health Consensus Conference: Prevention of venous thrombosis and pulmonary embolism. JAMA 256:744, 1986.

Roizen MF: Routine preoperative evaluation. In Miller RD, editor: Anesthesia, ed 2. New York, 1986, Churchill Livingstone.

Veterans Affairs Total Parenteral Nutrition Cooperative Study Group: Perioperative total parenteral nutrition in surgical patients. N Engl J Med 325:525, 1991.

CHAPTER

374 The Fiduciary Concept: A Basis for an Ethics of Patient Care

Henry S. Perkins

Effective patient care requires more than technical knowledge of diagnosis and therapy; it also requires an understanding of the physician-patient relationship. This chapter describes the fiduciary concept and its usefulness as an ethical basis for a physician's decisions within the physician-patient relationship. The term *fiduciary concept* refers to the physician's commitment to promote the patient's interests as the patient defines them.

THE FIDUCIARY CONCEPT

Originating in Roman law, the fiduciary concept has usually applied to relationships in which one person entrusts the management of his or her property to a second person. That second person is expected to make decisions that benefit the first person and not to profit from him or her unfairly.

Because patient care resembles managing a valuable trust, the fiduciary concept has recently been applied to the physician-patient relationship. The patient's request for help and the physician's offer to give it initiate the physician-patient relationship. The physician thereby becomes a fiduciary, or trustee, for the patient. The patient entrusts his or her body and its medical management to the physician to serve the patient's vital medical interests. These interests often include prolonging life, relieving symptoms, and restoring function. Yet some patients may define other medical interests as vital to them. The fiduciary concept, as applied to the physician-patient relationship, emphasizes the importance of treating each patient as an individual, respecting the patient's definition of his or her vital medical interests, and encouraging the patient to participate in decisions about care to the extent he or she wishes.

Three factors form the basis for the physician's fiduciary commitment to promote the patient's interests as the patient defines them. First, disease makes patients less able than healthy people to protect their own interests and thus leaves them more vulnerable to harm. Revelation of highly personal information during diagnostic work-up and therapy increases patients' vulnerability. Second, the physician's technical knowledge, familiarity with medical culture, and usually better health gives the physician considerably greater ability to influence clinical care than the patient has. Third, society gives physicians many privileges and expects physicians to reciprocate by helping the vulnerable sick.

Nonetheless, important constraints limit the physician's

duty to help: established professional practices, legality, personal conscience, availability of medical expertise and material resources, and commitments to other patients and to family. For example, established professional practice, legality, and perhaps personal conscience should prevent the internist from "mercifully" hastening the death of an end-stage cancer patient with an intentional overdose of morphine. (Instead, the internist should help relieve the patient's suffering by maximizing physical comfort and addressing the patient's emotional and spiritual needs.) Similarly, the internist's family commitments justify referring an acutely ill asthmatic to another qualified doctor when the patient calls the internist at home during the internist's vacation. Patient noncompliance, however, does *not* eliminate the physician's duty to help. That duty ends only when all medical problems are resolved, the patient dismisses the physician, or the physician gives the patient sufficient notice to find another physician. A seizure patient, for instance, takes her phenytoin erratically. When she does not take it, her seizures recur. The patient's noncompliance does not justify the internist's discharging the patient from the clinic without giving her sufficient notice to find another physician.

These examples illustrate the fallacy of two popular conceptions of the physician-patient relationship. First, though fiduciary in character, the physician-patient relationship does not require physician altruism. The physician need not completely abandon personal interests to promote the patient's. Such selflessness is probably impossible. The physician, of course, must sometimes sacrifice his or her immediate interests to deliver good, timely patient care. In return, the physician can expect proper payment, courtesy from patients, and opportunities for intellectual growth. Second, the physician-patient relationship is not a contract in the usual sense. Physician and patient do not initiate the relationship by negotiating their respective duties in detail. Instead, the physician pledges loyalty to the patient without a reciprocal pledge from the patient. The physician can hope the patient communicates honestly and cooperates with therapy, but the physician cannot demand such behavior as a contractual duty.

DECISION MAKING USING THE FIDUCIARY CONCEPT

A popular framework for analyzing ethical issues in patient care—and a sensible approach to many physicians—helps identify four kinds of values underlying any particular case. The first kind of value, *patient preferences,* refers to the competent patient's wishes to accept or reject the diagnostic tests and therapies recommended by the physician. The second kind of value, *medical considerations,* refers to the physician's opinion about diagnosis, prognosis, and management; the consultants' advice about diagnostic work-up and management; and information from relevant empirical studies. (Note that medical facts and established practices, which underlie medical considerations, by themselves do not determine how the physician should resolve ethical issues in a particular patient's care.) The third kind of value, *quality-of-life judgments,* refers to judgments by others about the value to the patient of his or her life circumstances. And the fourth kind of value, *contextual factors,* refers to the benefits and burdens to others that result from decisions about the patient's care. Common contextual factors include the wishes of the family or physician concerning the patient's care, the value of that care for teaching or research, the legal liability of the hospital, and the costs of that care to society. Nearly all ethical issues in patient care arise because of conflicts between two or more of these kinds of values.

The physician can use this analytical framework to gather information pertinent to a particular ethical issue in patient care, but the framework does not guide the physician to a particular decision. The fiduciary concept does that by helping determine the importance of each kind of value. The fiduciary concept suggests a hierarchy appropriate for most cases. Specifically, patient preferences should usually carry the greatest weight in the decision because they reflect the patient's interests most accurately. Medical considerations should carry the next greatest weight because they structure the ethical issue in the context of the case and help define the range of solutions that might benefit the patient. Quality-of-life judgments and contextual factors should carry the least weight in decisions about ethical issues. Rooted in the opinions and interests of people other than the patient, these two kinds of values run the greatest risk of compromising the patient's interests and thereby undermining the fiduciary concept. Nonetheless, quality-of-life judgments and contextual factors may justifiably predominate whenever patient preferences are unknown and medical considerations indicate short survival or extremely poor physical or mental outcome.

The fiduciary concept also encourages the physician to seek wide consultation when facing any ethical issue in patient care. Through consultation with other health professionals, a medical ethicist, or a hospital ethics committee, the physician can check for biases that may undermine patient interests, can obtain constructive criticism of solutions being considered, and can identify alternative solutions. A shared understanding of the fiduciary concept and a shared analytic framework such as the one described above provide the common ground necessary for physician and consultant to discuss ethical issues fruitfully.

A case illustrates decision-making using the fiduciary concept and the analytic framework above. A demented, elderly Jehovah's Witness develops generalized lymphadenopathy and severe anemia with a hematocrit of 15%. Her internist suspects lymphoma but cannot rule out treatable tuberculosis without a lymph node biopsy. The internist knows that the patient, comfortable despite her dementia, has enjoyed her life at the nursing home. Before she became too demented to make decisions for herself, the patient always accepted fully aggressive treatment—excluding blood transfusions—for her illnesses. However, the family doubts that the biopsy and any subsequent treatment are justified. Remembering her as a vibrant, intelligent woman, the family believes the patient would not find her demented existence worthwhile and, thus, would not want it prolonged. In addition, worried about potential legal liability, the consulting surgeon balks at performing the biopsy without the authority to transfuse.

The internist structures the ethical issue in this case by using certain important medical considerations: the severity of the anemia, the differential diagnosis of generalized lymphadenopathy, and the usual indications for lymph node biopsy. These considerations define the ethical issue as follows: despite the risk of bleeding, should the surgeon perform a lymph node biopsy in this severely anemic patient to rule out tuberculosis? The internist also uses medical considerations to define possible solutions: not to biopsy, to biopsy and to transfuse if necessary, or to biopsy but not to transfuse under any circumstances.

Having defined the ethical issue and its possible solutions, the internist uses the fiduciary concept to weigh the available information and to make a patient-care decision. Guided by his knowledge of the patient's prior wishes and decisions, the internist concludes that she would accept the biopsy as promoting her interests but would refuse transfusions. Furthermore, unlike the family who rarely visits the patient in the nursing home, the internist believes the patient enjoys her blissful though demented life there. When the internist wins the family over to that viewpoint, they consent to the biopsy. The surgeon agrees to perform the biopsy without transfusion as long as the hospital's ethics committee approves the plan beforehand. The committee approves it, and the surgeon performs the biopsy.

In this case the internist follows the usual hierarchy implicit in the fiduciary concept. In making the decision to pursue the biopsy, the internist gives more weight to patient preferences (as inferred from the patient's prior wishes and decisions) than to medical considerations (such as the usual practice to transfuse a patient with such a low hematocrit), quality-of-life judgments (such as the family's initial opinion that the patient would not find her demented life worthwhile), and contextual factors (such as the surgeon's anxiety over legal liability).

MANAGING COMMON ETHICAL ISSUES IN PATIENT CARE

The fiduciary concept can help the physician manage common ethical issues such as withholding or withdrawing life-support therapy, assessing patient decision-making capacity, performing informed consent properly, and avoiding the pitfalls of cost containment.

Withholding or withdrawing life-support therapy

The fiduciary concept defines two justifications for withholding or withdrawing life support: patient refusal and futility of the therapy. Either justification provides sufficient grounds for withholding or withdrawing therapy.

Patient refusal means that an informed, rational patient believes life-support therapy is contrary to his or her interests and therefore refuses it. For example, an alert middle-aged man, admitted for an acute myocardial infarction, refuses medication, laboratory tests, and continued hospitalization. He understands that refusing treatment may hasten his death, but he insists on going home "to be left alone." When attempts to dissuade the man fail, the physician discharges him and plans follow-up by telephone.

Futility of therapy means therapy cannot achieve any functional goals the patient would choose. The physician typically considers only complex functional goals for the patient (such as resuming gainful employment or living independently), but the patient may have much simpler goals (such as watching television or seeing his or her grandchildren). Because therapy can almost always achieve some simple goals the patient might have, futility can be used only rarely as a justification for withholding therapy.

Nonetheless, many medical ethicists consider therapy that maintains mere biologic existence without hope for cognitive function as futile and thus recommend discontinuation of such therapy. For example, a woman remains persistently vegetative 4 months after cardiac arrest. She has already contracted a pneumonia and two urinary tract infections. The consulting neurologist believes the patient cannot recover any physical or mental function. Because the patient has previously expressed no wishes about life support, the decision about providing antibiotics in the future depends on whether they will help achieve any of the patient's presumed functional goals for therapy. When questioned, the family and friends say that before the cardiac arrest the patient enjoyed keeping house and visiting her friends, and she would probably set those activities as minimum therapeutic goals now. However, antibiotics cannot achieve these goals or even the goal of returning the patient to a cognitive state, but can merely maintain her vegetative state. The internist attending the patient concludes that further antibiotic therapy is futile for helping achieve her presumed functional goals. After explaining this viewpoint to the family, the internist writes an order to withhold antibiotics but to continue aggressive comfort and hygiene measures. Although consultation with the family is desirable, their concurrence with a decision based on futility is not required.

Controversy exists over whether the fiduciary concept ever permits withholding nutrition and fluids. Most scholars in law and medical ethics, however, appear to favor the view that withholding nutrition and fluids is permissible if the patient explicitly refuses them or if they would cause burdens to the patient disproportionate to their benefits. Imminently dying patients probably present the clearest case of feedings with burdens disproportionate to their benefits.

Assessing patient decision-making capacity

The fiduciary concept implies that patients who have sufficient decision-making capacity should be encouraged to participate in medical decisions about themselves and to promote their own interests. However, the concept also implies that patients who lack sufficient decision-making capacity have their interests protected and promoted by others. Decision-making capacity means the ability to understand information relevant to a decision, to deliberate logically about options and their probable consequences, to make a choice consistent with one's own values, and to communicate that choice.

The physician should consider that a patient has sufficient decision-making capacity until proven otherwise. An elderly woman has a chronic dementia with intermittent lucidity and confusion. Considering a no-resuscitation order, the internist asks the patient about her wishes when she is lucid. She says she wants no cardiopulmonary resuscitation, and the internist honors that wish. Minors with sufficient decision-making capacity should ordinarily be allowed to make medical decisions for themselves. A 16-year-old girl requests birth control pills from her family's internist. After discussing the social and medical implications with the patient and being satisfied that her decision is informed, the internist may ethically prescribe the pills.

The vegetative, the severely demented, and the comatose lack all four conditions for decision-making capacity. Physicians should ensure that these patients have appropriate proxy decision-makers. Family members often serve adequately as informal proxies. But when patient and family interests conflict or when family members disagree about what to do, physicians should request that a court declare the patient incompetent and appoint an official guardian. As fiduciaries for patients lacking decision-making capacity, physicians should determine whether the decisions of either informal family proxies or official guardians reflect patients' presumed wishes. If these decisions do not, physicians should challenge them and, if necessary, arrange for review by a court. For example, a comatose elderly man is admitted to the hospital after an auto accident. Computerized tomography shows a large subdural hematoma, and the consulting neurosurgeon recommends immediate surgery to drill burr holes. The patient's only relative prefers medical treatments and refuses to consent to the surgery. Assuming the patient would want every chance to live, the internist on the case questions the relative's decision and applies to a court for guidance. The judge authorizes the emergency surgery to save the patient's life.

A recent influential law promotes advance directives, documents by which patients can request or refuse therapy for a future time when they cannot make or express medical decisions for themselves. The most familiar advance directives are durable powers of attorney for health matters and directives under state natural death acts. Physicians should encourage patients to sign such directives and should honor the wishes they express.

Informed consent

The fiduciary concept clarifies the purpose of informed consent: to facilitate the informed, rational patient's decision-making about his or her care, not to protect the physician or the hospital from lawsuits. Before any major medical decision, the physician should disclose to the patient the risks and benefits of all medically acceptable options and should make a recommendation based on the physician's perception of the patient's values. The physician should then allow the patient to express a preference.

A good ethical standard of disclosure (and the legal standard in some states) is what a reasonable patient would want to know under the circumstances. Withholding from the patient important information about diagnosis, prognosis, or therapy is usually not justified. Patients want this information, and it almost never harms them. For example, a patient with metastatic lung cancer has already received maximal radiotherapy. The oncologist counsels him about options for future care: hospice care or an experimental drug trial. Though realizing some risk to subject recruitment, the oncologist correctly warns the patient not to expect the trial to benefit him directly. The oncologist explains the trial is intended to determine toxicity and will probably benefit only future patients. Nonetheless, the patient chooses the drug trial over hospice care to "make a contribution to science."

Cost containment

The fiduciary concept also reinforces the physician's duty to serve patient interests despite recent pressures to reduce costs and conserve resources. Cost containment measures are ethically permissible so long as they do not significantly compromise patients' interests. Only patient refusal or lack of benefit—not cost containment—justifies withholding therapy. Thus, the physician may discontinue mechanical ventilation for the irreversibly comatose patient to comply with the patient's wishes but not to save money for the hospital.

CONCLUDING REMARK

The fiduciary concept provides solid grounds for making decisions about ethical issues in patient care. For some issues the fiduciary concept suggests to the physician a particular solution. For other issues the concept helps the physician narrow choices to several ethically acceptable options. The final choice among these options may justifiably depend on institutional policy, physician preference, or other nonfiduciary considerations. Yet the physician must always act as trustee for the patient and ensure that the patient's interests guide medical management.

REFERENCES

Council on Ethical and Judicial Affairs, American Medical Association: Decisions near the end of life. JAMA 267:2229, 1992.

The Hastings Center: Guidelines on the termination of life-sustaining treatment and the care of the dying. Briarcliff Manor, NY, 1987, The Hastings Center.

Holder AR: Minors' rights to consent to medical care. JAMA 257:3400, 1987.

Jonsen AR, Siegler M, and Winslade WJ: Clinical ethics: a practical approach to ethical issues in clinical medicine. New York, 1992, McGraw-Hill.

Perkins HS: Another ethics consultant looks at Mr. B.'s case. J Clin Ethics 1:126, 1990.

President's Commission for the Study of Ethical Problems in Medicine and Biomedical and Behavioral Research: Deciding to forego life-sustaining treatment. Washington, DC, 1983, U.S. Government Printing Office.

President's Commission for the Study of Ethical Problems in Medicine and Biomedical and Behavioral Research: Making health care decisions. Washington, DC, 1982, U.S. Government Printing Office.

Siegler M: Decision-making strategy for clinical-ethical problems in medicine. Arch Intern Med 142:2178, 1982.

Steinbrook R and Lo B: Artificial feedings: solid ground, not slippery slope. N Engl J Med 318:286, 1988.

Appendix

Immunization Schedule for Adults

Adult immunization in the United States

Age group (years)	Vaccine/toxoid					
	Td*	Measles	Mumps	Rubella	Influenza	Pneumococcal
18-24	x	x	x	x		
25-64	x	x†	x	x		
≥ 65	x				x	x

From Update on adult immunization. MMWR 40:RR-12, Nov 15, 1991.
*Td, tetanus + diphtheria toxoids, adsorbed for adult use (contains 5 Fl units tetanus + 2 Fl units diphtheria vs childhood vaccine, which contains 5 Fl units tetanus + 12.5 Fl units diphtheria).
†Indicated for persons born in 1957 or later.

ADMINISTRATION SCHEDULE

Td (toxoids, not live): Primary: two doses IM at least 4 weeks apart, third dose 6 to 12 months after second. Booster: every 10 years.

Measles (Attenuvax) (live virus vaccine): Unless contraindicated,* one dose (0.5 ml) sc preferably in outer aspect upper arm. Booster not required.

Measles + rubella (M-R Vax) (live virus): Unless contraindicated* (do not give to pregnant women), one dose (0.5 ml) sc as with measles. Booster not required.

Measles + rubella + mumps (MMR) (live virus): Unless contraindicated* (do not give to pregnant women), one dose (0.5 ml) sc as with measles. Booster not required.

Rubella (Meruvax) (live virus): As with measles + rubella (contraindicated in pregnant women).

Mumps (Mumpsvax) (live virus): As with measles (not contraindicated in pregnant women).

Rubella + mumps (Biavax) (live virus): As with measles + rubella (contraindicated in pregnant women).

Influenza (killed virus): One dose (0.5 ml) IM. Annual reimmunization with current vaccine recommended.

Pneumococcal (Pneumovax 23, Pnu-Immune 23) (pure antigens, 23): One dose (0.5 ml) sc. Revaccination contraindicated except possibly individuals at high risk (nephrotic syndromes, renal failure, transplant recipients HIV who received vaccine > 6 years before).

From Sanford JP, editor: Guide to antimicrobial therapy 1992. Dallas, 1992, Antimicrobial Therapy. Reprinted with permission from the publisher.
*Review package insert for specific product being administered.

Index

B

C

D

E

F

G

H

I

J

K

L

M

N

O

P

S

T

U